The Clinical Practice of Emergency Medicine

The Clinical Practice of Emergency Medicine

Third Edition

Editor-in-Chief

Ann Harwood-Nuss, MD, FACEP

Professor of Emergency Medicine
Associate Dean of Educational Affairs
University of Florida Health Science Center
Jacksonville, Florida

Senior Editor

Allan B. Wolfson, MD, FACEP, FACP

Professor of Emergency Medicine
Program Director, Affiliated Residency in Emergency Medicine
University of Pittsburgh
Pittsburgh, Pennsylvania

Associate Editors

Christopher H. Linden, MD, FACEP
Associate Professor and Director
Regional Poisoning Treatment Center
Department of Emergency Medicine
University of Massachusetts
Worcester, Massachusetts

Suzanne Moore Shepherd, MD, FACEP
Associate Professor
Department of Emergency Medicine
Hospital of the University of Pennsylvania
Philadelphia, Pennsylvania

Phyllis Hendry Stenklyft, MD, FACEP
Associate Professor and Division Chief
Pediatric Emergency Medicine
University of Florida Health Science Center
Jacksonville, Florida

LIPPINCOTT WILLIAMS & WILKINS
A **Wolters Kluwer** Company
Philadelphia • Baltimore • New York • London
Buenos Aires • Hong Kong • Sydney • Tokyo

Acquisitions Editor: Anne M. Sydor
Developmental Editor: Sarah Fitz-Hugh
Supervising Editor: Mary Ann McLaughlin
Production Service: Colophon
Manufacturing Manager: Colin Warnock
Cover Designer: Karen Quigley
Compositor: Maryland Composition
Printer: Québecor-World Color

530 Walnut Street
Philadelphia, PA 19106 USA
LWW.com

Printed in the USA

Library of Congress Cataloging-in-Publication Data

The clinical practice of emergency medicine / Ann L. Harwood-Nuss.— 3rd ed.
p. ; cm.
Includes bibliographical references and index.
ISBN 0-7817-1680-2
1. Emergency medicine. I. Title: Emergency medicine. II. Harwood-Nuss, Ann.
[DNLM: 1. Emergencies. 2. Emergency Medicine. WB 105 C6406 2000]
RC86.7 .C534 2000
616.02'5—dc21

00-042410

Care has been taken to confirm the accuracy of the information presented and to describe generally accepted practices. However, the authors, editors, and publisher are not responsible for errors or omissions or for any consequences from application of the information in this book and make no warranty, expressed or implied, with respect to the currency, completeness, or accuracy of the contents of the publication. Application of this information in a particular situation remains the professional responsibility of the practitioner.

The authors, editors, and publisher have exerted every effort to ensure that drug selection and dosage set forth in this text are in accordance with current recommendations and practice at the time of publication. However, in view of ongoing research, changes in government regulations, and the constant flow of information relating to drug therapy and drug reactions, the reader is urged to check the package insert for each drug for any change in indications and dosage and for added warnings and precautions. This is particularly important when the recommended agent is a new or infrequently employed drug.

Some drugs and medical devices presented in this publication have Food and Drug Administration (FDA) clearance for limited use in restricted research settings. It is the responsibility of health care providers to ascertain the FDA status of each drug or device planned for use in their clinical practice.

10 9 8 7 6 5 4 3 2 1

Dedication

To my parents, with love—Dr. Arthur Harwood and Nyta Harwood
Ann Harwood-Nuss

To my family; to my mentors; and to the emergency medicine residents
at the University of Pittsburgh,
who continue to teach me something new every day.
Allan B. Wolfson

To my family; friends; mentors; colleagues; and students, past,
present, and future.
And especially to my loving wife, Jeanne, an ED nurse and source of joy
and inspiration, without whose support I would not be able to do this.
Christopher H. Linden

To John, whose patience, humor, and love I treasure, and to the many colleagues,
students, and residents who have contributed to my education and practice
happiness far more than I can ever repay. Enjoy!
Suzanne Moore Shepherd

To Jerry, Gerald, and Erin for their unconditional love, support, and patience; to
my parents and neighbors; and to the staff
and patients of the Shands Jacksonville Pediatric Emergency Department.
Phyllis Hendry Stenklyft

Preface

The Clinical Practice of Emergency Medicine (CPEM) was written to serve as a comprehensive reference with a rapidly accessible collection of clinically relevant material. We have made every effort to ensure that the third edition is current, thorough, and readable, with little waste of words, features crucial in the setting of a busy emergency department. This uniquely formatted book was designed to include not only succinct discussions of basic disease processes and differential diagnosis, but also key information on the role of the consultant, patient disposition, indications for admission, acceptable alternatives to admission (i.e., outpatient treatment), guidelines for transfer, medico-legal issues, and clinical pitfalls. The Pitfalls section is particularly valuable in that it delineates the most common errors in the care of the emergency patient, as well as those points most critical for the reader to recall. It "gently reminds the busy clinician to be careful and rethink the issues in patient management one more time before discharge . . ."

As the editors planned the third edition, we made a conscious effort to respond to our readers' suggestions and observations about the first two editions. We also felt an obligation to respond to the changing environment of medicine.

As in the first two editions, the editors agreed that the text should be written by academic and practicing emergency physicians, those most capable of orienting the discussion toward the undifferentiated emergency patient. On occasion, however, we called upon our colleagues in other medical specialties to contribute certain areas of expertise. We are deeply appreciative of their efforts.

The preface would be incomplete without acknowledging the enormous time, talent, energy, and effort expended by the editors and contributing authors. There is a daunting sense of responsibility when one undertakes a task such as this. To produce a readable, accurate, concise work demands literally thousands of hours. When we see the text used in our busy Emergency Departments, whether to review therapy, disposition options, or pathophysiology, the rewards are obvious.

Ann Harwood-Nuss

Contributing Authors

Cynthia K. Aaron, MD
Department of Emergency Medicine
UMass Memorial Healthcare
Worcester, Massachusetts

Stephanie B. Abbuhl, MD
Associate Professor
Department of Emergency Medicine
University of Pennsylvania School of Medicine
Medical Director
Emergency Department
Hospital of the University of Pennsylvania
Philadelphia, Pennsylvania

Talaat A. Abdelmoneim, MD
Department of Pediatrics
Long Island College Hospital
Brooklyn, New York

Lina Abujamra, MD
Pediatric Emergency Medicine Fellow
Department of Emergency Medicine
University of Florida Health Science Center
Jacksonville, Florida

Norberto Adame, Jr., MD, FACEP
Assistant Professor
Department of Emergency Medicine
Maricopa Medical Center
Phoenix, Arizona

Mark C. Adams, MD
Methodist Hospital Institute for Kidney Stone Disease
Indianapolis, Indiana

Stephen L. Adams, MD, FACP, FACEP
Emergency Department
Northwestern Memorial Hospital
Chicago, Illinois

Richard V. Aghababian, MD
Professor and Chair
Department of Emergency Medicine
University of Massachusetts Medical Center
UMass Memorial Healthcare
Worcestor, Massachusetts

John Alcock, MD
Department of Emergency Medicine
University of New Mexico Health Sciences Center
School of Medicine
Albuquerque, New Mexico

E. Jackson Allison, Jr., MD, MPH, FACEP
Associate Dean and Professor
Department of Emergency Medicine
State University of New York Upstate Medical Center
Physician Executive and Director of Emergency Medicine
Department of Veterans Affairs Medical Center
Syracuse, New York

Janet G. Alteveer, MD
Assistant Professor
Department of Emergency Medicine
UMDNJ–Robert Wood Johnson Medical School
Assistant Director
Department of Emergency Services
Cooper Hospital/University Medical Center
Camden, New Jersey

James T. Amsterdam, DMD, MD
Professor of Clinical Emergency Medicine
Department of Emergency Medicine
University of Minnesota
Minneapolis, Minnesota
Head
Emergency Medicine Department
Regions Hospital
St. Paul, Minnesota

Eric Anderson, MD
Department of Emergency Medicine
MetroHealth Medical Center
Cleveland, Ohio

Mark J. Ault, MD
Professor of Clinical Medicine
Department of Medicine
University of California Los Angeles
Director
Division of General Internal Medicine
Cedars–Sinai Medical Center
Los Angeles, California

Agoritsa Baka, MD
Fellow, Pediatric Emergency Medicine
Department of Pediatrics
Emory University School of Medicine
Children's Healthcare of Atlanta
Atlanta, Georgia

Katherine Bakes, MD
Department of Emergency Medicine
Harbor–UCLA Medical Center
Torrance, California

Robert A. Barish, MD
Associate Professor and Chief
Director of Emergency Medical Services
Division of Emergency Medicine
University of Maryland School of Medicine
Baltimore, Maryland

William G. Barsan, MD
Professor
Department of Surgery
University of Michigan Health System
Chief
Emergency Department
University of Michigan Hospitals and Health Center
Ann Arbor, Michigan

Brigitte M. Baumann, MD
Chief Resident
Department of Emergency Medicine
Hospital of the University of Pennsylvania
Philadelphia, Pennsylvania

Edward J. Bayne, MD
Clinical Assistant Professor
Department of Pediatrics
University of Florida Health Science Center
Jacksonville, Florida

Bruce M. Becker, MD, MPH
Assistant Professor
Brown University School of Medicine
Attending Physician
Department of Emergency Medicine
Rhode Island and Miriam Hospitals
Providence, Rhode Island

Ronald S. Benenson, MD
Assistant Professor
Department of Emergency Medicine
Pennsylvania State University
Hershey, Pennsylvania
Associate Residency Director
Department of Emergency Medicine
York Hospital
York, Pennsylvania

Guy I. Benrubi, MD
Professor and Associate Chair
Department of Obstetrics and Gynecology
University of Florida Health Science Center
Jacksonville, Florida

Nicolas H. Benson, MD
Professor
Department of Emergency Medicine
East Carolina University School of Medicine
Pitt County Memorial Hospital
Greenville, North Carolina

Theodore I. Benzer, MD, PhD
Instructor
Division of Emergency Medicine
Department of Emergency Medicine
Harvard Medical School
Attending Physician
Department of Emergency Medicine
Massachusetts General Hospital
Boston, Masschusetts

Anthony R. Berner, MD
Instructor
Department of Emergency Medicine
University of Massachusetts Medical School
Worcester, Massachusetts
Associate Chairman
Department of Emergency Medicine
Newton-Wellesley Hospital
Newton, Massachusetts

Joseph Bernstein, MD
Assistant Professor
Department of Orthopaedic Surgery
Hospital of the University of Pennsylvania
Philadelphia, Pennsylvania

Howard A. Bessen, MD, FACEP
Clinical Profesor
Department of Medicine
University of California Los Angeles
Los Angeles, California
Director
Emergency Medicine Residency Program
Department of Emergency Medicine
Torrance Memorial Medical Center
Torrance, California

Phillip I. Bialecki, MD, MHE
Assistant Professor
Department of Emergency Medicine
Ohio University College of Medicine
Athens, Ohio
Associate Director of Research
Department of Emergency Medicine
Doctors' Hospital
Columbus, Ohio

C. J. Biddle, PhD, CRNA
Professor
Graduate Program in Anesthesia
Virginia Commonwealth University
Richmond, Virginia

Elisabeth F. Bilden, MD
Instructor of Clinical Surgery
Toxicology Fellow
Department of Surgery (Emergency Medicine)
University of Arizona College of Medicine
Attending Physician
Department of Emergency Medicine
University Medical Center
Tucson, Arizona

Louis S. Binder, MD
Professor
Department of Emergency Medicine
University of Illlinois at Chicago College of Medicine
Attending Physician
Department of Emergency Medicine
University of Illinois Medical Center
Chicago, Illinois

Dale S. Birenbaum, MD
Assistant Professor
Department of Emergency Medicine
University of Florida Health Science Center
Gainesville, Florida

Frank Birinyi, MD, FACEP
Department of Emergency Medicine
The Ohio State University Medical Center
Columbus, Ohio

Adrienne J. Birnbaum, MD
Assistant Professor
Department of Emergency Medicine
Albert Einstein College of Medicine
Residency Program Director
Department of Emergency Medicine
Jacobi and Montefiore Medical Center
Bronx, New York

Diane M. Birnbaumer, MD, FACEP
Assistant Professor of Medicine
University of California Los Angeles
Los Angeles, California
Associate Residency Director
Department of Emergency Medicine
Harbor–UCLA Medical Center
Torrance, California

Paul Blackburn, MD
Department of Emergency Medicine
Maricopa Medical Center
Phoenix, Arizona

Eric T. Boie, MD
Clinical Instructor
Department of Emergency Medicine
Mayo Medical School
Staff Physician
Department of Emergency Medicine
Saint Mary's Hospital
Rochester, Minnesota

Edward B. Bolgiano, MD
Assistant Professor of Surgery
University of Maryland School of Medicine
Director of Emergency Medicine
Bon Secours Hospital
Baltimore, Maryland

G. Randall Bond, MD
Professor
Departments of Emergency Medicine and Pediatrics
Medical Director
Poison and Drug Information Center
University of Cincinnati
Cincinnati, Ohio

Laura J. Bontempo, MD
Instructor
Division of Emergency Medicine
Northwestern University Medical School
Attending Physician
Emergency Department
Northwestern Memorial Hospital
Chicago, Illinois

Pierre Borczuk, MD
Instructor
Department of Medicine
Harvard Medical School
Attending Physician
Department of Emergency Medicine
Massachusetts General Hospital
Boston, Massachusetts

Marc Borenstein, MD, FACEP, FACP
Associate Professor of Clinical Medicine
Department of Medicine
Columbia College of Physicians and Surgeons
Vice-Chair and Residency Program Director
Department of Emergency Medicine
St. Luke's–Roosevelt Hospital Center
New York, New York

William Bozeman, MD
Assistant Professor
Department of Emergency Medicine
University of Florida Health Science Center
Jacksonville, Florida

Jefferson D. Bracey, DO, FACEP
Assistant Professor
Department of Surgery
University of Nevada School of Medicine
Las Vegas, Nevada
Assistant Director
Department of Emergency Medicine
St. Rose Dominican Hospital
Henderson, Nevada

G. Richard Braen, MD
Professor and Chairman
Department of Emergency Medicine
School of Medicine and Biomedical Sciences
State University of New York at Buffalo
Buffalo General Hospital
Buffalo, New York

John A. Brennan, MD
Clinical Assistant Professor
Department of Emergency Medicine
UMDNJ–Robert Wood Johnson Medical School
New Brunswick, New Jersey
Director of Pediatric Emergency Medicine
Department of Emergency Medicine
St. Barnabus Health Care Services
Livingston, New Jersey

Jeffrey Brent, MD, PhD
Associate Clinical Professor
Departments of Medicine, Surgery, and Pediatrics
University of Colorado Health Sciences Center
Denver, Colorado

Stephen W. Bretz, MD
Instructor of Clinical Medicine
Attending Physician
Division of Emergency Medicine
University of California Davis Medical Center
Sacramento, California

Judith C. Brillman, MD
Associate Professor/Residency Director
Department of Emergency Medicine
University of New Mexico Hospital
Albuquerque, New Mexico

Geoffrey Broocker, MD, FACS
Walthour–DeLaPerreire Professor of Ophthalmology
Residency Program Director
Department of Ophthalmology
Emory University School of Medicine
Chief of Service, Ophthalmology
Grady Memorial Hospital
Atlanta, Georgia

Daniel Brookoff, MD
Associate Director of Internal Medicine and Transitional Residency Programs
Methodist Hospital
Memphis, Tennessee

David F. M. Brown, MD
Instructor
Harvard Medical School
Assistant Chief
Department of Emergency Medicine
Massachusetts General Hospital
Boston, Masschusetts

Thomas A. Brunell, MD, MA
Resident
Department of Emergency Medicine
UMass Memorial Healthcare
Worcester, Massachusetts

James H. Bryan, MD, PhD, FACEP
Assistant Professor
Department of Medicine
Oregon Health Sciences University
Staff Physician
Emergency Medicine Service
Veterans Affairs Medical Center
Portland, Oregon

Randall M. Bryant, MD
Assistant Professor
Department of Pediatrics
University of Florida Health Science Center
Director of Interventional Electrophysiology and Pacing
Nemours Children's Clinic
Wolfson Children's Hospital
Jacksonville, Florida

Sharona Bryant, MD
Division of Toxicology
Hahnemann Medical College of Pennsylvania
Department of Emergency Medicine
Division of Toxicology
Mercy Health Systems
Philadelphia, Pennsylvania

Joseph A. Buckwalter, MS, MD
Professor and Chair
Department of Orthopaedic Surgery
University of Iowa
Iowa City, Iowa

Mary C. Burke, MD
Assistant Professor
Department of Emergency Medicine
UMass Memorial Healthcare
Worcester, Massachusetts
Chief
Department of Emergency Medicine
Milford–Whitinsville Regional Hospital
Milford, Massachusetts

Keith K. Burkhart, MD, FACMT, FACEP
Professor
Departments of Emergency Medicine and Pharmacology
The Pennsylvania State University
Medical Director
Central Pennsylvania Poison Center
The Milton S. Hershey Medical Center
Hershey, Pennsylvania

Michael J. Burns, MD
Instructor
Department of Medicine
Harvard Medical School
Director
Division of Toxicology
Beth Israel Deaconess Medical Center
Boston, Massachusetts

Laurie Jeanne Burton, MD
Assistant Professor
Department of Pediatrics
Emory University
Attending Physician
Division of Pediatric Emergency Medicine
Children's Healthcare of Atlanta
Hughes Spalding Children's Hospital
Atlanta, Georgia

Clifton Callaway, MD
Assistant Professor
Department of Emergency Medicine
University of Pittsburgh Medical Center
Pittsburgh, Pennsylvania

Karen Camasso–Richardson, MD
Assistant Professor
Department of Pediatrics
Case Western Reserve University
Staff, Pediatric Emergency Medicine
Rainbow Babies and Children's Hospital
Cleveland, Ohio

Maureen Campbell, DO, FACEP
Clinical Faculty
College of Osteopathic Medicine
Nova Southeastern University
Associate Staff
Emergency Department
Cleveland Clinic, Florida
Ft. Lauderdale, Florida

Donna A. Caniano, MD
Professor of Surgery and Pediatrics
The Ohio State University College of Medicine and Public Health
Surgeon-in-Chief
Children's Hospital
Columbus, Ohio

Thomas R. Caraccio, PharmD, ABAT
Assistant Professor
Department of Emergency Medicine
State University of New York at Stony Brook
Stony Brook, New York
Assistant Professor of Pharmacology and Toxicology
New York College of Osteopathic Medicine
Old Westbury, New York
Clinical Manager
Long Island Regional Poison and Drug Information Center
Winthrop University Hosptial
Mineola, New York

Leslie S. Carroll, MD
Instructor
Department of Emergency Medicine
Thomas Jefferson University Hospital
Philadelphia, Pennsylvania

David D. Cassidy, MD
Attending Physician
Emergency Medicine Residency Program
Orlando Regional Medical Center
Orlando, Florida

William K. Chiang, MD
Assistant Professor
Department of Surgery/ Emergency Medicine
New York University
Assistant Director
Emergency Department
Bellevue Hospital Center
New York, New York

Theodore A. Christopher, MD
Associate Professor
Department of Surgery (Emergency Medicine)
Jefferson Medical College
Chief
Department of Emergency Medicine
Thomas Jefferson University Hospital
Philadelphia, Pennsylvania

Carl R. Chudnofsky, MD
Assistant Professor
Department of Emergency Medicine
University of Michigan
Ann Arbor, Michigan
Chairman
Department of Emergency Medicine
Hurley Medical Center
Flint, Michigan

James E. Cisek, MD, FACEP
Associate Professor
Department of Emergency Medicine
Virginia Commonwealth University
Medical Director
Virginia Poison Center
Medical College of Virginia Hospitals
Richmond, Virginia

David M. Cline, MD
Assistant Residency Director
Clinical Associate Professor
Department of Emergency Medicine
University of North Carolina
Chapel Hill, North Carolina
Education Director
Department of Emergency Medicine
Wake Medical Center
Raleigh, North Carolina

Joseph E. Clinton, MD, FACEP
Chief of Service
Department of Emergency Medicine
Hennepin County Medical Center
Minneapolis, Minnesota

Thomas E. Collins, MD
Senior Clinical Instructor
Department of Surgery
Case Western Reserve University
EMS Director
Department of Emergency Medicine
Metro Health Medical Center
Cleveland, Ohio

Stephen A. Colucciello, MD
Clinical Associate Professor
Department of Emergency Medicine
University of North Carolina at Chapel Hill
Assistant Chairman
Department of Emergency Medicine
Carolinas Medical Center
Charlotte, North Carolina

William F. Coombs, MD
Attending Physician
Emergency Department
Miami Children's Hospital
Miami, Florida

David M. Cosentino, MD
Clinical Instructor
Department of Emergency Medicine
University of Florida Health Science Center
Jacksonville, Florida

Carol C. Coulson, MD
Assistant Professor
Departments of Obstetrics, Gynecology and Radiology
The Penn State Geisinger Health System
Director
Inpatient and Obstetric Services
The Milton S. Hershey Medical Center
Hershey, Pennsylvania

Gerard R. Cox, MD, MHA, FACEP
Clinical Assistant Professor
Military and Emergency Medicine
Uniformed Services University of the Health Sciences
Bethesda, Maryland
White House Physician
White House Medical Unit
Washington, DC

Sandra A. Craig, MD
Clinical Instructor
Department of Surgery
University of North Carolina
Chapel Hill, North Carolina
Associate Residency Director
Department of Emergency Medicine
Carolinas Medical Center
Charlotte, North Carolina

R. Kemp Crockett, MD
Director of Emergency Medicine
Department of Pediatrics
Miami Children's Hospital
Miami, Florida

Barbara Insley Crouch, PharmD, MSPH
Associate Professor (Clinical)
Department of Pharmacy Practice
College of Pharmacy, University of Utah
Director
Utah Poison Control Center
Salt Lake City, Utah

Joseph J. Currier, MD
Department of Emergency Medicine
UMass Memorial Healthcare
Worcester, Massachusetts

Steven C. Curry, MD
Associate Professor of Clinical Medicine
University of Arizona College of Medicine
Director
Department of Medical Toxicology
Good Samaritan Medical Center
Phoenix, Arizona

Kevin M. Curtis, MD
Department of Emergency Medicine
Hospital of the University of Pennsylvania
Philadelphia, Pennsylvania

Rita K. Cydulka, MD
Associate Professor and Residency Director
Departments of Surgery and Emergency Medicine
Case Western Reserve University–MetroHealth Medical Center
Cleveland, Ohio

Richard C. Dart, MD, PhD
Associate Professor
Department of Emergency Medicine
University of Colorado
Director
Rocky Mountain Poison and Drug Center
Denver Health Medical Center
Denver, Colorado

Mohamud R. Daya, MD
Associate Professor and Attending Physician
Department of Emergency Medicine
Oregon Health Sciences University Hospital
Portland, Oregon

Peter M. C. DeBlieux, MD
Associate Clinical Professor
Departments of Emergency Medicine, and Pulmonary and Critical Care
Louisiana State University
Program Director
Department of Emergency Medicine
Charity Hospital
New Orleans, Louisiana

Karen DeFazio, MD
Instructor
Department of Emergency Medicine
UMass Memorial Healthcare
Worcester, Massachusetts
Attending Physician
Department of Emergency Medicine
Milford–Whitinsville Regional Hospital
Milford, Massachusetts

Beth Anne DeGennaro, MD
Department of Emergency Medicine
Mount Sinai–NYU Medical Center/Health Systems
New York, New York

Christopher J. Degnen, MD
Clinical Instructor
Department of Medicine
Harvard Medical School
Boston, Massachusetts
Attending Physician
Emergency Department
Lahey Clinic
Burlington, Massachusetts

David Della-Giustina, MD
Clinical Assistant Professor
Department of Military and Emergency Medicine
Uniformed Services University of the Health Sciences
Bethesda, Maryland
Residency Director
Department of Emergency Medicine
Madigan Army Medical Center
Fort Lewis, Washington

Romano DeMarco, MD
Junior Resident
Department of Urology
Indiana University Hospital
Indianapolis, Indiana

Lucian K. DeNicola, MD
Professor
Department of Pediatrics
University of Florida Health Science Center
Wolfson Children's Hospital
Jacksonville, Florida

James W. Dennis, MD
Department of Surgery
Division of Vascular Surgery
University of Florida Health Science Center
Jacksonville, Florida

Heeten J. Desai, MD
Department of Emergency Medicine
Vanderbilt University School of Medicine
Nashville, Tennessee

Jeffrey Desmond, MD
Lecturer
Division of Emergency Medicine
Department of Surgery
University of Michigan Medical School
Ann Arbor, Michigan

James P. d'Etienne, MD
Chief Resident
Department of Emergency Medicine
University of Florida Health Science Center
Jacksonville, Florida

Edward T. Dickinson, MD, FACEP
Assistant Professor
Director of EMS Field Operations
Department of Emergency Medicine
Hospital of the University of Pennsylvania
Philadelphia, Pennsylvania

Lynnette Doan-Wiggins, MD, JD
Assistant Professor
Department of Surgery
Loyola University Stritch School of Medicine
Department of Emergency Medicine
Loyola University Medical Center
Maywood, Illinois

J. Ward Donovan, MD
Associate Professor of Medicine
Pennsylvania State University College of Medicine
Director
Central Pennsylvania Poison Center
The Milton S. Hershey Medical Center
Hershey, Pennsylvania

Daniel R. Douglas, MD
Adjunct Assistant Professor
Department of Emergency Medicine
Oregon Health Sciences University
Staff Physician
Department of Emergency Medicine
Providence St. Vincent Medical Center
Portland, Oregon

Marc Downing, MD
Clinical Instructor
The Ohio State University College of Medicine
Assistant Chief Resident
Children's Hospital
Columbus, Ohio

Robert P. Dowsett, BM, BS
Medical Director
Department of Emergency Medicine
Westmead Hospital
Sydney, Australia

William H. Dribben, MD
Assistant Professor
Department of Emergency Medicine
Washington University
Division of Emergency Medicine
Barnes-Jewish Hospital
St. Louis, Missouri

Jeffrey Dubin, MD
Department of Emergency Medicine
Washington Hospital Center
Washington, DC

William R. Dubin, MD
Professor
Department of Psychiatry
Temple University School of Medicine
Belmont Center for Comprehensive Treatment
Philadelphia, Pennsylvania

Ellen M. Dugan, MD, FACEP
Associate Professor and Assistant Chairman
Department of Emergency Medicine
Georgetown University Medical Center
Washington, DC

Susan M. Dunmire, MD, FACEP
Associate Professor
Department of Emergency Medicine
University of Pittsburgh Medical Center
Pittsburgh, Pennsylvania

Sophia Dyer, MD
Fellow in Medical Toxicology
Department of Pediatrics
Harvard Medical School
Children's Hospital
Massachusetts Poison Control System
Boston, Massachusetts

Philip A. Edelman, MD
Associate Professor of Medicine
Director of Toxicology and Clinical Services
Division of Occupational Medicine and Toxicology
School of Medicine and Health Sciences
George Washington University Medical Center
Washington, DC

Joanne Edney, MD
Staff Physician
Denver General Hospital
Denver, Colorado

Charles L. Emerman, MD
Associate Professor and Chair
Department of Emergency Medicine
Case Western Reserve University School of Medicine
Metrohealth Medical Center
Cleveland, Ohio

Javier I. Escobar, II, MD
Pediatric Emergency Medicine Fellow
Department of Emergency Medicine
University of Florida Health Science Center
Jacksonville, Florida

Phillip G. Fairweather, MD
Clinical Assistant Professor
Department of Emergency Medicine
Mount Sinai School of Medicine
New York, New York
Associate Attending
Emergency Medical Department
Elmhurst Hospital Center
Elmhurst, New York

Samir M. Fakhry, MD, FACS
Assistant Professor
Department of Surgery
University of North Carolina at Chapel Hill
Chapel Hill, North Carolina

Jay L. Falk, MD, FACEP
Clinical Professor
Department of Medicine
University of Florida
Gainesville, Florida
Academic Chairman
Department of Emergency Medicine
Orlando Regional Medical Center
Orlando, Florida

James A. Feldman, MD
Associate Professor
Department of Emergency Medicine
Boston University School of Medicine
Vice Chair–Clinical Performance
Department of Emergency Medicine
Boston Medical Center
Boston, Massachusetts

Ronald M. Ferdman, MD
Assistant Professor of Clinical Pediatrics
Keck School of Medicine
University of Southern California
Attending Physician
Division of Clinical Immunology and Allergy
Children's Hospital Los Angeles
Los Angeles, California

Robert P. Ferm, MD, FAAP, FACEP, FACMT
Assistant Professor
Department of Emergency Medicine
University of Massachusetts Medical School
Attending Physician
Department of Emergency Medicine
UMass Memorial Healthcare
Worcester, Massachusetts

Francis M. Fesmire, MD, FACEP
Assistant Professor of Medicine
University of Tennessee College of Medicine
Director
Heart/Stroke Center
Erlanger Medical Center
Chattanooga, Tennessee

Susan S. Fish, PharmD, MPH
Associate Professor
Department of Emergency Medicine
Boston University School of Medicine and School of Public Health
Vice Chair for Research
Department of Emergency Medicine
Boston Medical Center
Boston, Massachusetts

Timothy C. Flynn, MD, FACS
Professor of Surgery
University of Florida College of Medicine
Chief of Surgery
Veterans Affairs Medical Center
Gainesville, Florida

Michael J. Foley, MD
Department of Emergency Medicine
Indiana University School of Medicine
Department of Emergency Medicine
Methodist Hospital–Clarian Health Partners
Indianapolis, Indiana

Phil Fontanarosa, MD
Adjunct Associate Professor of Medicine
Division of Emergency Medicine
Northwestern University Medical School
Chicago, Illinois

Alan T. Forstater, MD
Clinical Assistant Professor of Surgery (Emergency Medicine)
Jefferson Medical College
Attending Physician
Department of Emergency Medicine
Thomas Jefferson University Hospital
Philadelphia, Pennsylvania

Brent Furbee, MD, FACMT
Assistant Clinical Professor
Department of Emergency Medicine
Indiana University School of Medicine
Medical Director
Indiana Poison Center
Emergency Medicine Trauma Center
Methodist Hospital
Indianapolis, Indiana

Brendan R. Furlong, MD, FACEP
Associate Medical Director
MedStar Transport
Department of Emergency Medicine
Washington Hospital Center
Washington, DC

Gregory G. Gaar, MD, FAAP, FACEP, FAACT
Clinical Associate Professor
Department of Pediatrics
University of South Florida College of Medicine
Director
Saunders Pediatric Emergency Care Center
Tampa General Hospital
Tampa, Florida

Daniel S. Gabbay, MD
Department of Emergency Medicine
Hospital of the University of Pennsylvania
Philadelphia, Pennsylvania

David F. Gaieski, MD
Instructor
Department of Emergency Medicine
Hospital of the University of Pennsylvania
Philadelphia, Pennsylvania

E. John Gallagher, MD
Professor of Medicine
Albert Einstein College of Medicine
Director
Department of Emergency Medicine
Bronx Municipal Hospital
Bronx, New York

Lucille Gans, MD, FACEP
Clinical Instructor
University of Massachusetts Medical School
UMass Memorial Healthcare
Worcester, Massachusetts

Pierre Gaudreault, MD, FRCP(C)
Clinical Associate Professor
Department of Pediatrics
University of Montreal
Chief
Clinical Pharmacology/Toxicology Unit
Hopital Sainte–Justine
Montreal, Quebec, Canada

Michael O. Gayle, MD, FRCPC, FAAP, FCCM
Associate Professor
Department of Pediatrics
University of Florida Health Science Center
Nemours Children's Clinic
Pediatric Intensivist
Department of Pediatrics and Anesthesia
Wolfson Children's Hospital
Jacksonville, Florida

Joel M. Geiderman, MD, FACEP
Department of Medicine
Division of Emergency Medicine
University of California Los Angeles Hospital and Clinics
Director and Co-Chair
Department of Emergency Medicine
Cedars–Sinai Medical Center
Los Angeles, California

Richard D. Gerkin, Jr., MD
Medical Director
Phoenix Fire Department Health Center
Medical Toxicologist
Samaritan Regional Poison Center
Good Samaritan Medical Center
Phoenix, Arizona

Michael A. Gibbs, MD, FACEP
Associate Professor of Emergency Medicine
University of North Carolina at Chapel Hill
Residency Program Director
Department of Emergency Medicine
Carolinas Medical Center
Medical Director, MedCenter Air
Chapel Hill, North Carolina

Brian P. Gilligan, MD
Fellow, Pediatric Emergency Medicine
Department of Emergency Medicine
Unversity of Florida Health Science Center
Jacksonville, Florida

Yevgeniy Gincherman, MD
Emergency Physician
Department of Emergency Medicine
Suburban Hospital
Bethesda, Maryland

Timothy G. Givens, MD
Assistant Professor
Department of Pediatrics
University of Louisville
Associate Medical Director
Emergency Department
Kosair Children's Hospital
Louisville, Kentucky

Jonathan Glauser, MD, FACEP
Assistant Clinical Professor
Case Western Reserve University
Attending Staff
Department of Emergency Medicine
Cleveland Clinic Foundation
Cleveland, Ohio

George W. Go, MD
Staff Physician
St. John's Medical Center
Longview, Washington

Steven A. Godwin, MD
Assistant Professor and Assistant Residency Director
Department of Emergency Medicine
University of Florida Health Science Center
Jacksonville, Florida

Jay M. Goldman, MD, FACEP
Senior Physician
The Permanente Medical Group
Department of Emergency Medicine
Kaiser Foundation Hospital (Hayward)
Hayward, California

Federico Gonzalez, MD, FACS
Clinical Associate Professor
Section of Plastic Surgery
Kansas University Medical Center
Kansas City, Kansas

John E. Gough, MD, FACEP
Associate Professor
Department of Emergency Medicine
East Carolina University School of Medicine
Attending Physician
Emergency Department
Pitt County Memorial Hospital
Greenville, North Carolina

Deepi G. Goyal, MD
Department of Emergency Medicine
Saint Mary's Hospital–Mayo Clinic
Rochester, Minnesota

Vicente H. Gracias, MD
Assistant Professor of Surgery
Division of Traumatology and Surgical Critical Care
Hospital of the University of Pennsylvania
Philadelphia, Pennsylvania

Louis G. Graff, IV, MD, FACP, FACEP
Associate Professor
Department of Traumatology and Emergency Medicine
University of Connecticut Medical School
Farmington, Connecticut
Associate Director
Department of Emergency Medicine
New Britain General Hospital
New Britain, Connecticut

Thomas P. Graham, MD, FACEP
Assistant Clinical Professor
Department of Medicine/Emergency Medicine
University of California Los Angeles School of Medicine
Attending Physician
Department of Emergency Medicine
UCLA Medical Center
Los Angeles, California

Andis Graudins, MB
Clinical Lecturer
Department of Medicine
Sydney University
Sydney, Australia
Consultant Toxicologist
Departments of Emergency Medicine and Clinical Pharmacology
Westmead Hospital
Westmead, New South Wales, Australia

Michael I. Greenberg, MD
Department of Emergency Medicine
Hahnemann–Medical College of Pennsylvania
Philadelphia, Pennsylvania

Constance S. Greene, MD
Program Director
Department of Emergency Medicine
Cook County Hospital
Chicago, Illinois

Neena Gupta, MD
Department of Emergency Medicine
St. Barnabus Medical Center
Livingston, New Jersey

Alan H. Hall, MD, FACEP
Clinical Assistant Professor
Department of Preventive Medicine and Biometrics
University of Colorado School of Medicine
Denver, Colorado

Christine Haller, MD
Department of Medicine and Pharmacology
University of Minnesota
Division of Clinical Pharmacology and Toxicology
Hennepin County Medical Center
Minneapolis, Minnesota

Thomas J. Haronian, MD
Section of Emergency Medicine
Brown University School of Medicine
Department of Emergency Medicine
Rhode Island and Miriam Hospitals
Providence, Rhode Island

James L. Harper, MD
Assistant Professor
Department of Pediatrics
University of Nebraska Medical Center
Omaha, Nebraska

Richard S. Hartoch, MD
Assistant Professor
Department of Emergency Medicine
Oregon Health Sciences University
Portand, Oregon

Stephen C. Hartsell, MD, FACEP
Associate Professor
Department of Surgery
Division of Emergency Medicine
University of Utah School of Medicine
Salt Lake City, Utah

Ann Harwood-Nuss, MD, FACEP
Professor of Emergency Medicine
Associate Dean of Educational Affairs
University of Florida Health Science Center
Jacksonville, Florida

Elizabeth A. Hatfield, MD
Attending Physician
Department of Emergency Medicine
St. Lukes Hospital
Milwaukee, Wisconsin

Alan C. Heffner, MD
Department of Emergency Medicine
Carolinas Medical Center
Charlotte, North Carolina

Mary A. Hegenbarth, MD
Associate Professor
Department of Pediatrics
University of Missouri–Kansas City School of Medicine
Attending Physician
Division of Emergency Medicine
Children's Mercy Hospital
Kansas City, Missouri

Irvin N. Heifetz, MD
Assistant Professor
Department of Emergency Medicine
UMass Memorial Healthcare
Worcester, Massachusetts

Michael B. Heller, MD
Clinical Professor of Medicine
Temple University School of Medicine
Philadelphia, Pennsylvania
Department of Emergency Medicine
St. Luke's Hospital
Bethlehem, Pennsylvania

Sean O. Henderson, MD
Assistant Professor
Department of Emergency Medicine
University of Southern California
Medical Director–Main Emergency Admitting
Department of Emergency Medicine
LAC+USC Medical Center
Los Angeles, California

Gregory W. Hendey, MD, FACEP
Assistant Clinical Professor
Department of Medicine
University of California
San Francisco, California
Residency Director
Department of Emergency Medicine
University Medical Center
Fresno, California

Barry H. Hendler, DDS, MD
Associate Professor
School of Dental Medicine
Director of Continuing Medical Education
Co-ordinator of Laser and Cosmetic Surgery
Department of Oral and Maxillofacial Surgery
Hospital of the University of Pennsylvania
Philadelphia, Pennsylvania

Philip L. Henneman, MD, FACEP
Clinical Professor and Chair
Department of Emergency Medicine
Tufts University School of Medicine
Boston, Massachusetts
Baystate Health System
Springfield, Massachusetts

Fred M. Henretig, MD
Professor
Departments of Pediatrics and Emergency Medicine
University of Pennsylvania School of Medicine
Director
Section of Clinical Toxicology
Division of Emergency Medicine
Children's Hospital of Pennsylvania
Philadelphia, Pennsylvania

Gregory L. Henry, MD
Clinical Professor
Department of Surgery
Section of Emergency Medicine
The University of Michigan Medical School
Vice President
Emergency Physician Medical Group
Ann Arbor, Michigan

Mel Herbert, MD
Department of Emergency Medicine
University of California Los Angeles School of Medicine
UCLA Medical Center
Los Angeles, California

Robert D. Herr, MD, FACEP, FACP
Associate Professor and Attending Physician
Emergency Department
University of Arkansas Hospital
Little Rock, Arkansas

Thomas J. Higgins, Jr., MD
Department of Medical Toxicology
Good Samaritan Regional Poison Center
Good Samaritan Medical Center
Phoenix, Arizona

Kendall Ho, MD, FRCPC
Associate Dean and Director
Division of Continuing Medical Education
University of British Columbia
Assistant Professor
Division of Emergency Medicine
Vancouver Hospital and Health Sciences Center
Vancouver, British Columbia, Canada

Robert S. Hockberger, MD
Professor of Medicine
Division of Emergency Medicine
University of California Los Angeles School of Medicine
Los Angeles, California
Chair
Department of Emergency Medicine
Harbor–UCLA Medical Center
Torrance, California

Alan Hodgdon, MD, FACEP
Emergency Medical Director
Mercy Providence Hospital
Pittsburgh, Pennsylvania

Dee Hodge III, MD
Associate Professor
Department of Pediatrics
Washington University School of Medicine
Associate Director
Clinical Affairs for Emergency Services
St. Louis Children's Hospital
St. Louis, Missouri

Gwendolyn L. Hoffman, MD, FACEP
Associate Professor
Department of Emergency Medicine
Michigan State University College of Human Medicine
East Lansing, Michigan
Residency Director
Department of Emergency Medicine
Spectrum Health/MSU Program in Emergency Medicine
Spectrum Health-Downtown
Grand Rapids, Michigan

Jerome R. Hoffman, MD
Professor of Clinical Medicine
Division of Emergency Medicine
University of California Los Angeles School of Medicine
Los Angeles, California

Robert S. Hoffman, MD
Assistant Professor of Clinical Surgery and Emergency Medicine
New York University School of Medicine
Director
Fellowship in Medical Toxicology
Director
New York City Poison Center
Attending Physician
Department of Emergency Services
Bellevue Hospital Center
New York, New York

Judd E. Hollander, MD
Associate Professor and Director of Clinical Research
Department of Emergency Medicine
Hospital of the University of Pennsylvania
Philadelphia, Pennsylvania

Lisa Horton, MD
Affiliate Assistant Professor
Department of Pediatric Emergency Medicine
University of Maryland School of Medicine
Baltimore, Maryland

John M. Howell, MD, FACEP
Associate Professor and Chair
Department of Emergency Medicine
Georgetown University Medical Center
Washington, DC

David S. Howes, MD, FACEP
Associate Professor of Clinical Medicine
Emergency Medicine Residency Program Director
Department of Emergency Medicine
University of Chicago Hospital
Chicago, Illinois

Kathleen C. Hubbell, MD
Clinical Associate Professor
Department of Medicine–Emergency Medicine
Louisiana State University School of Medicine
Director, Accident Room
Department of Emergency Medicine
Medical Center of Louisiana–Charity Hospital
New Orleans, Louisiana

John F. Huddleston, MD
Professor
Department of Obstetrics and Gynecology
University of Florida Health Science Center
Jacksonville, Florida

Kaveh Ilkhanipour, MD
Physician Quality Manager
Mercy Providence Hospital
Pittsburgh, Pennsylvania

John Isaacs Jr., MD
Associate Chairman and Associate Professor
Department of Otolaryngology
University of Florida Health Science Center
Jacksonville, Florida

Alexander P. Isakov, MD
Department of Emergency Medicine
UMass Memorial Healthcare
Worcester, Massachusetts

Richard J. Iseke, MD
Assistant Professor
Department of Emergency Medicine
UMass Memorial Healthcare
Worcestor, Massachusetts
Director, Emergency Services
Lawrence General Hospital
Lawrence, Massachusetts

Eugene Izsak, MD
Department of Emergency Medicine
Children's Hospital of Virginia
Norfolk, Virginia

Geoffrey Jackman, MD
Pediatric Emergency Medicine Fellow
Department of Pediatrics
Emory University School of Medicine
Children's Healthcare of Atlanta
Atlanta, Georgia

Dag Jacobsen, MD, PhD
Professor and Director
Medical Intensive Care Unit
Ullevaal University Hospital
Oslo University
Oslo, Norway

Sheldon Jacobson, MD, FACP, FACEP
Professor
Department of Emergency Medicine
Mount Sinai School of Medicine
Chairman
Department of Emergency Medicine
Mount Sinai–NYU Medical Center/Health Systems
New York, New York

Andy Jagoda, MD, FACEP
Associate Professor and Residency Site Director
Department of Emergency Medicine
Mount Sinai Medical Center
New York, New York

Paul A. Janson, MD
Instructor
Department of Family Medicine
Tufts University
Boston, Massachusetts
Staff Physician
Department of Emergency Medicine
Lawrence General Hospital
Lawrence, Massachusetts

David Anthony Jerrard, MD
Associate Professor of Surgery
Department of Medicine
University of Maryland
Clinical Director
Emergency Department
Veterans Affairs Hospital
Baltimore, Maryland

Lindsey Alan Johnson, MD
Clinical Assistant Professor
Department of Pediatrics
Pediatric Inpatient Medical Director
University of Florida Health Science Center
Jacksonville, Florida

B. Tilman Jolly, MD
Associate Professor of Emergency Medicine and Environmental and Occupational Health
The George Washington University Medical Center
Washington, DC

James L. Jones, MD
Associate Clinical Professor
Department of Obstetrics and Gynecology
University of Florida Health Science Center
Jacksonville, Florida

Robert C. Jorden, MD
Clinical Professor of Emergency Medicine
University of Arizona College of Medicine
Chairman
Department of Emergency Medicine
Maricopa Medical Center
Phoenix, Arizona

Madeline Matar Joseph, MD
Assistant Professor
Department of Emergency Medicine
University of Jacksonville Health Science Center
Jacksonville, Florida

Steven M. Joyce, MD, FACEP
Professor
Department of Surgery
Division of Emergency Medicine
University of Utah Hospital & Clinics
Salt Lake City, Utah

Hanif Kamal, MD
Pediatric Infectious Disease Fellow
Department of Pediatrics
The Nemours Children's Clinic
Jacksonville, Florida

Richard M. Kaplan, MD, MS
Clinical Assistant Professor
Department of Emergency Medicine
University of Pittsburgh
Staff Physician
Emergency Department
West Penn Hospital
Pittsburgh, Pennsylvania

Michael A. Kaufman, MD
Resident
Department of Emergency Medicine
Case Western Reserve University
Metro Health Medical Center
Cleveland, Ohio

Andrew M. Kaunitz, MD
Professor and Assistant Chairman
Department of Obstetrics & Gynecology
University of Florida Health Science Center
Director
Menopause and Gynecologic Services
University of Florida Medicus Women's Center
Jacksonville, Florida

Thomas E. Kearney, PharmD, ABAT
Clinical Professor
University of California San Francisco School of Pharmacy
Managing Director
San Francisco Division California Poison Control System
San Francisco, California

Gabor D. Kelen, MD, FRCP(C), FACEP
Professor and Director
Department of Emergency Medicine
Johns Hopkins University School of Medicine
Emergency Physician-in-Chief
Johns Hopkins Hospital
Baltimore, Maryland

John J. Kelly, DO, FACEP
Associate Professor
Department of Medicine
Temple University School of Medicine
Adjunct Associate Professor of Emergency Medicine
Medical College of Pennsylvania
Hahnemann University
Interim Chairman
Department of Emergency Medicine
Albert Einstein Medical Center
Philadelphia, Pennsylvania

Christopher S. Kennedy, MD
Assistant Professor
University of Missouri-Kansas City School of Medicine
Attending Physician
Department of Pediatrics
Children's Mercy Hospital
Kansas City, Missouri

Taryn Kennedy, FRCSI, FRCS(ed)
Instructor
Department of Emergency Medicine
UMass Memorial Healthcare
Worcester, Massachusettes
Director of Emergency Services
Department of Emergency Medicine
Marlborough Hospital
University of Massachusetts Health System
Marlborough, Massachusetts

Blaine A. Kent, MD
Departments of Emergency Medicine and Anaesthesiology
Dalhousie University
Queen Elizabeth II Health Sciences Centre
Halifax, Nova Scotia, Canada

Stuart G. Kessler, MD
Clinical Associate Professor
Vice Chair
Department of Emergency Medicine
Mount Sinai School of Medicine
New York, New York
Director
Department of Emergency Medicine
Elmhurst Hospital Center
Elmhurst, New York

Naghma S. Khan, MD
Division Director
Pediatric Emergency Medicine
Department of Pediatrics
Emory University
Medical Director
Department of Emergency Medicine
Children's Healthcare of Atlanta at Egleston
Hughes Spalding Children's Hospital
Atlanta, Georgia

Joseph D. Kim, MD
Department of Emergency Medicine
Thomas Jefferson University Hospital
Philadelphia, Pennsylvania

Donna Kinser, MD
Associate Professor
Department of Emergency Medicine
University of California, Davis
Sacramento, California

J. Douglas Kirk, MD, FACEP
Associate Professor and Assistant Chief
Department of Emergency Medicine
University of California Davis Medical Center
Sacramento, California

Niranjan Kissoon, MD
Department of Pediatrics and Anesthesia
Wolfson Children's Hospital
Jacksonville, Florida

Kenneth W. Kizer, MD, MPH, FACEP, FACMT, FAACT
Distinguished Professor
Department of Emergency and Military Medicine
Uniformed Services University of the Health Sciences
Bethesda, Maryland
President and Chief Executive Officer
The National Quality Forum
Washington, DC

Jane F. Knapp, MD
Professor
Department of Pediatrics
University of Missouri–Kansas City School of Medicine
Director
Division of Emergency Medicine
Children's Mercy Hospital
Kansas City, Missouri

Michael O. Koch, MD
Professor and Chairman
Department of Urology
Indiana University Hospital
Indianapolis, Indiana

Katalin I. Koranyi, MD
Professor of Clinical Pediatrics
Department of Pediatrics
The Ohio State University College of Medicine
Attending Physician
Department of Pediatrics
Children's Hospital
Columbus, Ohio

Carissa J. Kostecki, MD
Fellow, Pediatric Emergency Medicine
University of Louisville
Kosair Children's Hospital
Louisville, Kentucky

Ron Forrest Koury, DO
Resident Physician
Department of Emergency Medicine
University of Kentucky–Chandler Medical Center
Lexington, Kentucky

Kevin R. Kowaleski, MD
Department of Emergency Medicine
Children's Hospital of Virginia
Norfolk, Virginia

David A. Kramer, MD
Residency Director
Department of Emergency Medicine
York Hospital
York, Pennsylvania

Richard S. Krause, MD
Assistant Clinical Professor
Department of Emergency Medicine
School of Medicine and Biomedical Sciences
State University of New York at Buffalo
Buffalo General Hospital
Buffalo, New York

Edward P. Krenzelok, PharmD
Professor
Departments of Pharmacy and Pediatrics
University of Pittsburgh
Director
Pittsburgh Poison Center
Children's Hospital of Pittsburgh
Pittsburgh, Pennsylvania

Kenneth W. Kulig, MD
Clinical Associate Professor
Department of Surgery
Division of Emergency Medicine and Trauma
University of Colorado
Chief
Department of Medicine
Porter Adventist Hospital
Denver, Colorado

Donald B. Kunkel, MD
Medical Director,
Samaritan Regional Poison Center
Good Samaritan Medical Center
Phoenix, Arizona

Steven C. Larson, MD
Assistant Professor
Department of Emergency Medicine
Hospital of the University of Pennsylvania
Philadelphia, Pennsylvania

Kenneth Leong, MD
Burn Fellow
Department of Plastic Surgery
Kansas University Medical Center
Kansas City, Kansas

William Levin, MD
Assistant Professor of Emergency Medicine
New York Medical College
Emergency Department
Metropolitan Hospital Center
New York, New York

M. Andrew Levitt, DO, FACEP
Associate Professor
Department of Medicine
University of California San Francisco
San Francisco, California
Director of Research
Department of Emergency Medicine
Alameda County Medical Center
Oakland, California

William J. Lewander, MD
Associate Professor
Department of Pediatrics and Emergency Medicine
Brown University
Director
Pediatric Emergency Medicine
Hasbro Children's Hospital
Providence, Rhode Island

Marc Linares, MD
Attending Physician
Emergency Department
Miami Children's Hospital
Miami, Florida

Christopher H. Linden, MD, FACEP
Associate Professor
Department of Emergency Medicine
University of Massachusetts Medical School
Worcester, Massachusetts
Staff Physician
Department of Emergency Medicine
Milford–Whitinsville Regional Hospital
Milford, Massachusetts

Louis J. Ling, MD
Professor
Department of Emergency Medicine
University of Minnesota
Medical Director
Hennepin Regional Poison Center
Hennepin County Medical Center
Minneapolis, Minnesota

James E. Lingeman, MD
Director of Research
Methodist Hospital Institute for Kidney Stone Disease
Indianapolis, Indiana

Jeffrey F. Linzer, MD
Assistant Professor of Pediatrics
Division of Emergency Mecine
Emory University School of Medicine
Vice Section Chief Emergency Services
Children's Healthcare of Atlanta
Attending Physician
Hughes Spalding Children's Hospital
Atlanta, Georgia

Toby L. Litovitz, MD
Professor
Department of Emergency Medicine
Georgetown University
Director
National Capital Poison Center
Washington, DC

Robert C. Luten, MD
Professor
Department of Emergency Medicine
University of Florida Health Science Center
Jacksonville, Florida

Sharon Elizabeth Mace, MD
Associate Professor
Department of Emergency Medicine
Ohio State University
Columbus, Ohio
Clinical Director, Observation Unit
Director
Pediatric Education/Quality Improvement
Cleveland Clinic Foundation
Cleveland, Ohio

Darryl J. Macias, MD
Assistant Professor
Department of Emergency Medicine
University of New Mexico Health Sciences Center
School of Medicine
Albuquerque, New Mexico

Ronald B. Mack, MD
Associate Professor of Pediatrics
Bowman Gray School of Medicine at Wake Forest University
Attending Physician
Brenner Children's Hospital
Winston–Salem, North Carolina

H. Trent MacKay, MD, MPH
Special Assistant for Obstetrics and Gynecology
Contraception and Reproductive Health Branch
CPR/NICHD/NIH
Bethesda, Maryland

Brian D. Mahoney, MD, FACEP
Associate Professor
Program in Emergency Medicine
University of Minnesota
Medical Director
Emergency Medical Services
Hennepin County Medical Center
Minneapolis, Minnesota

William K. Mallon, MD
Associate Professor
Department of Emergency Medicine
University of Southern California School of Medicine
Residency Director
Department of Emergency Medicine
LAC + USC Medical Center
Los Angeles, California

James Manning, MD
Associate Professor
Department of Emergency Medicine
University of North Carolina at Chapel Hill
Chapel Hill, North Carolina

Anthony S. Manoguerra, PharmD, ABAT
Professor of Clinical Pharmacy
Department of Clinical Pharmacy
University of California San Francisco
San Francisco, California
Director, San Diego Division
California Poison Control System
University of California San Diego
San Diego, California

Nizar F. Maraqa, MD
Fellow
Division of Infectious Disease
University of Florida Health Science Center
Jacksonville, Florida

Juan A. March, MD, FACEP
Associate Professor and Chief
Division of Emergency Medical Services
Department of Emergency Medicine
East Carolina University School of Medicine
Attending Physician
Emergency Department
Pitt County Memorial Hospital
Greenville, North Carolina

Catherine A. Marco, MD
Assistant Professor
Department of Surgery
Medical College of Ohio
Attending Physician
Department of Emergency Medicine
St. Vincent Mercy Medical Center
Toledo, Ohio

Steven M. Marcus, MD
Associate Professor
Department of Pediatrics
University of Medicine and Dentistry–New Jersey Medical School
Executive Director
New Jersey Poison Information and Education System
Newark Beth Israel Medical Center
Newark, New Jersey

Vincent J. Markovchick, MD
Professor
Department of Surgery
University of Colorado
Medical Director
Denver 911 Paramedics
Medical Director
Denver Fire Department EMTs
Denver, Colorado

Daniel R. Martin, MD
Associate Professor
Department of Emergency Medicine
The Ohio State University Medical Center
Columbus, Ohio

Marcus L. Martin, MD
Chairman and Professor
Department of Emergency Medicine
University of Virginia Hospital
Charlottesville, Virginia

Thomas P. Martin, MD
Department of Emergency Medicine
Western Pennsylvania Hospital
Pittsburgh, Pennsylvania

John A. Marx, MD
Clinical Professor
Department of Emergency Medicine
University of North Carolina at Chapel Hill
Chapel Hill, North Carolina
Chair
Department of Emergency Medicine
Carolinas Medical Center
Charlotte, North Carolina

James J. Mathews, MD
Professor of Medicine
Northwestern University Medical School
Chief
Division of Emergency Medicine
Northwestern Memorial Hospital
Chicago, Illinois

Thom A. Mayer, MD, FACEP, FAAP
Clinical Professor
Department of Emergency Medicine and Pediatrics
Georgetown University and George Washington University
Washington, DC
Director of Flight Services
Chairman
Department of Emergency Medicine
Inova Fairfax Hospital
Falls Church, Virginia

Kathryn McCans, MD
Assistant Professor
Department of Emergency Medicine
UMDNJ-Robert Wood Johnson Medical School
Camden, New Jersey

Margaret M. McCarron, MD
Professor
Departments of Medicine and Emergency Medicine
University of Southern California
Chief Physician
Drug Information Center
LAC+USC Medical Center
Los Angeles, California

Mary A. McCormick, PharmD
Assistant Clinical Professor
Department of Traumatology and Emergency Medicine
Administrative Director
Connecticut Poison Control Center
University of Connecticut Health Center
Farmington, Connecticut

James H. McCrory, MD
The Children's Hospital
Macon, Georgia

Maureen D. McCollough, MD, MPH
Assistant Professor
Department of Medicine
University of California Los Angeles School of Medicine
Los Angeles, California
Director of Pediatric Emergency Medicine
Department of Emergency Medicine
Olive View–UCLA Medical Center
Sylmar, California

Alison J. McDonald, MD, FACEP
Clinical Adjunct Assistant Professor
Departments of Surgery and Emergency Medicine
Thomas Jefferson University
Philadelphia, Pennsylvania
Director of Emergency Medicine
Kennedy Memorial Hospital
Turnersville, New Jersey

Robin McFee, DO, MPH
Assistant Professor
Department of Preventive Medicine
State University of New York–Stony Brook
Medical Director
Seabury Barn Adolescent Health Program
Stony Brook, New York

Douglas McGee, DO
Associate Professor and Associate Residency Director
Department of Emergency Medicine
Thomas Jefferson University
Albert Einstein Medical Center
Philadelphia, Pennsylvania

Samuel A. McLean, MD, MPH
Resident
Department of Emergency Medicine
Boston Medical Center
Boston, Massachusetts

Thomas G. McLoughlin, Jr., MD
Department of Emergency Medicine
University of Florida Health Science Center
Jacksonville, Florida

Ted A. McMurry, MD
Medical Director
Emergency Trauma Center
St. John's Regional Health Center
Springfield, Missouri

Robert M. McNamara, MD
Professor and Chief
Division of Emergency Medicine
Temple University Hospital
Philadelphia, Pennsylvania

Don Mebust, MD
Senior Resident
Emergency Medicine Residency Program
University of California Los Angeles
Los Angeles, California

C. Crawford Mechem, MD, FACEP
Assistant Professor
Department of Emergency Medicine
Hospital of the University of Pennsylvania
EMS Medical Director
Philadelphia Fire Department
Philadelphia, Pennsylvania

Moss H. Mendelson, MD
Assistant Professor
Department of Emergency Medicine
Eastern Virginia Medical School
Norfolk, Virginia

Jeffrey G. Michael, DO
Instructor of Pediatrics
Department of Pediatrics
University of Missouri–Kansas City School of Medicine
Pediatric Emergency Medicine Fellow
Department of Emergency Medicine
The Children's Mercy Hospital
Kansas City, Missouri

Samir Midani, MD
Division of Infectious Diseases and Immunology
Department of Pediatrics
The Nemours Children's Clinic
Jacksonville, Florida

Daniel Mines, MD
Fellow
Division of General Internal Medicine
Center for Clinical Epidemiology and Biostatistics
University of Pennsylvania Medical Center
Philadelphia, Pennsylvania

Joyce M. Mitchell-Savinsky, MD
Clinical Instructor
Department of Internal Medicine
Case Western Reserve University School of Medicine
Residency Program Director
Department of Emergency Medicine Services
PHS–Mt. Sinai Medical Center
Cleveland, Ohio

Howard C. Mofenson, MD, FAAP, FAACT, FACMT
Professor of Pediatrics and Emergency Medicine
State University of New York–Stony Brook
Stony Brook, New York
Medical Director
Long Island Regional Poison Control Center at Winthrop
University Hospital
Mineola, New York

Brian Mongillo, MD
Instructor
Department of Emergency Medicine
UMass Memorial Healthcare
Worcester, Massachusetts
Attending Physician
Department of Emergency Medicine
Milford–Whitinsville Hospital
Milford, Massachusetts

Jeffrey A. Moody, MD
Methodist Hospital Institute for Kidney Stone Disease
Indianapolis, Indiana

Gregory P. Moore, MD
Associate Clinical Professor
Department of Emergency Medicine
Clarian Health Partners
Indiana University
Attending Physician
Department of Emergency Medicine
Methodist Hospital
Indianapolis, Indiana

Gregory J. Moran, MD, FACEP
Associate Professor of Medicine
Department of Emergency Medicine
University of California Los Angeles School of Medicine
Los Angeles, California
Director of Research
Department of Emergency Medicine
Olive View–UCLA Medical Center
Sylmar, California

Lawrence Mottley, MD, MHSA, FACEP
Clinical Associate Professor
Department of Emergency Medicine
Boston University School of Medicine
Boston, Massachusetts

Michael F. Murphy, MD, FRCP
Associate Professor
Departments of Emergency Medicine and Anaesthesiology
Dalhousie University
Queen Elizabeth II Health Sciences Centre
Halifax, Nova Scotia, Canada

Deborah Mulligan-Smith, MD, FAAP, FACEP
Associate Clinical Professor
Community Health and Family Medicine
University of Florida
Medical Director
Pediatric Services and Emergency Medical Services for Children
North Broward Hospital District
Ft. Lauderdale, Florida

Daniel A. Muse, MD
Staff Physician
Department of Emergency Medicine
Faulkner Hospital
Boston, Massachusetts

Khaled Mutabagani, MD
Department of Pediatric Surgery
Children's Hospital
Columbus, Ohio

Vinay M. Nadkarni, MD
Assistant Professor
Thomas Jefferson University
Philadelphia, Pennsylvania
Attending Physician
duPont Hospital for Children
Wilmington, Delaware

Jeffrey B. Nemhauser, MD
EIS Officer
Medical Section
Hazard Evaluations and Technical Assistance Branch
Division of Surveillance, Hazard Evaluations, and Field Studies
National Institute for Occupational Safety and Health
Cincinnati, Ohio

Kenneth J. Neuberger, MD
Clinical Assistant Professor of Surgery (Emergency Medicine)
Jefferson Medical College of Thomas Jefferson University
Attending Physician
Department of Emergency Medicine
Thomas Jefferson University Hospital
Philadelphia, Pennsylvania

Edward Newton, MD
Associate Professor
Department of Emergency Medicine
University of Southern California
Vice-Chairman
Department of Emergency Medicine
LAC+USC Medical Center
Los Angeles, California

Valerie Dobiesz Neylan, MD
Assistant Professor
Department of Emergency Medicine
University of Illinois
Associate Residency Director
Department of Emergency Medicine
University of Illinois Hospital
Chicago, Illinois

Constance G. Nichols, MD
Assistant Professor
Department of Emergency Medicine
UMass Memorial Healthcare
Worcester, Massachusetts

James T. Nieman, MD
Professor
Department of Medicine
University of California Los Angeles School of Medicine
Department of Emergency Medicine
Harbor–UCLA Medical Center
Torrance, California

Valerie C. Norton, MD
Assistant Professor
Department of Emergency Medicine
Vanderbilt University
Nashville, Tennessee

Robert C. Nuss, MD
Professor
Department of Obstetrics and Gynecology
University of Florida Health Science Center
Jacksonville, Florida

Martin O'Bryan, MD
Department of Emergency Medicine
Swedish Medical Center
Denver, Colorado

Jonathan S. Olshaker, MD
Professor
Departments of Surgery and Medicine
University of Maryland Medical Center
Chief
Emergency Care Services
Veterans Affairs Medical Center
Baltimore, Maryland

Kent R. Olson, MD, FACEP
Clinical Professor of Medicine and Pharmacy
University of California San Francisco
Medical Director, San Francisco Division
California Poison Control System
San Francisco, California

Hisham A. Omran, MD
Clinical Instructor
Department of Pediatrics
University of Missouri Kansas City
Pediatric Emergency Medicine Fellow
Division of Emergency Medicine
Children's Mercy Hospital
Kansas City, Kansas

Joseph P. Ornato, MD, FACC, FACEP
Professor and Chairman
Department of Emergency Medicine
Virginia Commonwealth University's Medical College of Virginia
Richmond, Virginia

David Overton, MD, MBA, FACEP, FACP
Professor
Department of Emergency Medicine
Michigan State University College of Human Medicine
East Lansing, Michigan
Director
Emergency Medicine Program
Michigan State University Kalamazoo Center for Medical Studies
Kalamazoo, Michigan

Julide Ayse Ozan, BHS
Physician Assistant–Certified
Department of Emergency Medicine
University of Florida Health Science Center
Jacksonville, Florida

Edward A. Panacek, MD
Professor
Department of Medicine
Residency Program Director
Division of Emergency Medicine and Medical Toxicology
University of California Davis
Davis, California

Paul M. Paris, MD, FACEP, LLD (HON)
Professor and Chairman
Department of Emergency Medicine
University of Pittsburgh School of Medicine
Pittsburgh, Pennsylvania

Katerina T. Parmele, MD
Department of Emergency Medicine
Mercy Hospital
Pittsburgh, Pennsylvania

Steven J. Parrillo, DO, FACEP
Associate Professor
Department of Emergency Medicine
Philadelphia College of Osteopathic Medicine
Attending Physician and Faculty
Department of Emergency Medicine
Albert Einstein Medical Center
Philadelphia, Pennsylvania

Ian D. Paul, MD
Department of Emergency Medicine
Boston Medical Center
Boston, Massachusetts

Paul R. Pentel, MD
Professor
Department of Medicine and Pharmacology
University of Minnesota
Director
Division of Clinical Pharmacology and Toxicology
Hennepin County Medical Center
Minneapolis, Minnesota

Paul E. Pepe, MD, MPH, FACEP, FCCM, FCCP
Professor and Chairman
Department of Emergency Medicine
University of Texas Southwestern Medical Center
Dallas, Texas

Jeanmarie Perrone, MD
Assistant Professor
Co-Director
Division of Toxicology
Department of Emergency Medicine
University of Pennsylvania
Attending Physician
Emergency Department
Hospital of the University of Pennsylvania
Philadelphia, Pennsylvania

Shawna J. Perry, MD
Director Clinical Operations
Assistant Professor and Assistant Chair
Department of Emergency Medicine
University of Florida Health Science Center
Jacksonville, Florida

David J. Peter, MD, FACEP
Assistant Professor
Department of Emergency Medicine
Northeastern Ohio Universities College of Medicine
Rootstown, Ohio
Attending Physician
Department of Emergency Medicine
Akron General Medical Center
Akron, Ohio

Anne L. Peters, MD
Associate Professor of Medicine
Division of Endocrinology
University of California Los Angeles School of Medicine
Director
Clinical Diabetes Program
UCLA Medical Center
Los Angeles, California

Norman E. Peterson, MD
Professor
Division of Urology
Denver Health Medical Center
Denver, Colorado

James A. Pfaff , MD
San Antonio Uniformed Health Education Consortium Chief
Department of Emergency Medicine
Brooke Army Medical Center
San Antonio, Texas

Paul A. Pitel, MD
Chair
Department of Pediatrics
Nemours Children's Clinic
University of Florida Health Science Center
Jacksonville, Florida

Stephen J. Playe, MD
Assistant Professor
Department of Emergency Medicine
Tufts University School of Medicine
Boston, Masschusetts
Residency Program Director
Department of Emergency Medicine
Baystate Medical Center
Springfield, Massachusetts

Anthony P. Pohlgeers, MD
Assistant Director
Department of Pediatric Emergency Medicine
Wolfson Children's Hospital
Jacksonville, Florida

Charles V. Pollack, Jr., MA, MD, FACEP
Clinical Associate Professor of Surgery (Emergency Medicine)
University of Arizona College of Medicine
Tucson, Arizona
Chairman
Department of Emergency Medicine
Maricopa Medical Center
Phoenix, Arizona

Peter T. Pons, MD
Associate Professor
Division of Emergency Medicine
Department of Surgery
University of Colorado Health Sciences Center
Attending Physician
Department of Emergency Medicine
Denver Health Medical Center
Denver, Colorado

Dana Pope, MD
Staff Physician
Department of Emergency Medicine
St. Francis Hospital
Federal Way, Washington

Robert S. Porter, MD
Clinical Assistant Professor
Department of Surgery
Thomas Jefferson University
Staff Physician
Department of Emergency Medicine
Albert Einstein Medical Center
Philadelphia, Pennsylvania

Louis G. Poulos, DO
Assistant Professor and Assistant Director of Clinical Operations
Department of Emergency Medicine
University of Illinois Hospital
Chicago, Illinois

Franklin D. Pratt, MD
Assistant Clinical Professor of Emergency Medicine
Department of Medicine
University of California Los Angeles
Los Angeles, California
Medical Co-Director
Department of Emergency Medicine
Torrance Memorial Medical Center
Torrance, California

Michael T. Pulley, MD, PhD
Assistant Professor
Department of Neurology
University of Florida Health Science Center
Jacksonville, Florida

Kimberly S. Quayle, MD
Assistant Professor of Pediatrics
Department of Pediatrics
Washington University School of Medicine
Medical Director
Transport Service
St. Louis Children's Hospital
St. Louis, Missouri

Bruce Quinn, MD
Clinical Assistant Professor
Department of Medicine
University of Miami School of Medicine
Attending Physician
Pediatric Emergency Department
Jackson Memorial Hospital
Miami, Florida

T. Eugene Ragland, MD, FACEP
Clinical Assistant Professor
Department of Surgery–Emergency Services
University of Michigan
Associate Director
Department of Emergency Services
St. Joseph Mercy Hospital
Ann Arbor, Michigan

Mobeen H. Rathore, MD
Professor and Chief
Pediatric Infectious Diseases/Immunology
Assistant Chairman
Research and Academic Affairs
Department of Pediatrics
University of Florida Health Science Center
Jacksonville, Florida

Eileen M. Raynor, MD
Assistant Professor
Department of Otolaryngology
University of Florida Health Science Center
Jacksonville, Florida

Kevin M. Reilly, MD
Associate Professor and Director
Department of Emergency Medicine
Albany Medical Center
Albany, New York

Patrick M. Reilly, MD
Assistant Professor
Division of Traumatology and Surgical Critical Care
Department of Surgery
University of the Hospital of Pennsylvania
Philadelphia, Pennsylvania

Erica E. Remer, MD, FACEP
Staff Physician
Section of Emergency Medicine
The Cleveland Clinic Foundation
Cleveland, Ohio

Francis P. Renzi, MD
Associate Professor
Department of Emergency Medicine
Associate Chair
Director Residency Program
UMass Memorial Healthcare
Worcester, Massachusetts

Marc C. Restuccia, MD
Assistant Professor
Department of Emergency Medicine
University of Massachusetts Medical School
Medical Director
Emergency Medicine System
UMass Memorial Healthcare
Worcester, Massachusetts

Iris M. Reyes, MD
Assistant Professor
Director of Quality Assurance
Department of Emergency Medicine
Hospital of the University of Pennsylvania
Philadelphia, Pennsylvania

David M. Richardson, MD
Clinical Assistant Professor
Department of Medicine
Pennsylvania State University College of Medicine
Hershey, Pennsylvania
Attending Physician
Department of Emergency Medicine
Lehigh Valley Hospital
Allentown, Pennsylvania

Silvana Riggio, MD
Clinical Associate Professor
Department of Psychiatry
Mount Sinai School of Medicine
New York, New York

Elizabeth Rincon, MD
Pediatric Emergency Medicine Fellow
Department of Emergency Medicine
Miami Children's Hospital
Miami, Florida

Patrice M. Ringo, MD
Emergency Physician
Department of Emergency Medicine
Southern Regional Medical Center
Riverdale, Georgia

Ralph J. Riviello, MD, FAAEM
Assistant Professor and Attending Physician
Department of Emergency Medicine
University of Virginia Medical Center
Charlottesville, Virgina

Raymond J. Roberge, MD, MPH, FAAEM, FACMT
Clinical Associate Professor
Department of Emergency Medicine
University of Pittsburgh School of Medicine
Vice-Chairman
Department of Emergency Medicine
Western Pennsylvania Hospital
Pittsburgh, Pennsylvania

James R. Roberts, MD, FAAEM, FACMT
Professor and Chair
Department of Emergency Medicine
Director
Division of Toxicology
Medical College of Pennsylvania/Hahnemann University
Drexel University School of Medicine
Mercy Health Systems
Philadelphia, Pennsylvania

Rebecca R. Roberts, MD
Co-Director
Division of Research
Department of Emergency Medicine
Cook County Hospital
Chicago, Illinois

Robert M. Rodriguez, MD
Department of Emergency Medicine
Highland General Hospital
Oakland, California

Christopher C. Rose (deceased)

S. Rutherfoord Rose, PharmD, FAACT
Associate Professor
Department of Emergency Medicine
Virginia Commonwealth University
Director
Virginia Poison Center
Medical College of Virginia Hospitals
Richmond, Virginia

Peter Rosen, MD, FACEP
Professor
Residency Director
Department of Emergency Medicine
University of California San Diego
San Diego, California

Steven Rosenzweig, MD
Clinical Associate Professor
Division of Emergency Medicine
Jefferson Medical College
Attending Physician
Thomas Jefferson University Hospital
Philadelphia, Pennsylvania

Todd C. Rothenhaus, MD
Assistant Residency Director
Department of Emergency Medicine
Boston University School of Medicine
Attending Physician
Department of Emergency Medicine
Boston Medical Center
Boston, Massachusetts

Richard E. Rothman, MD
Department of Surgery
Medical College of Ohio
Toledo, Ohio

Douglas A. Rund, MD, FACEP
Professor and Chairman
Department of Emergency Medicine
The Ohio State University Medical Center
Columbus, Ohio

Micheal D. Rush, MD
Assistant Residency Director and Assistant Professor
Department of Emergency Medicine
University of Missouri–Kansas City School of Medicine
Attending Physician
Department of Emergency Medicine
Truman Medical Center
Kansas City, Missouri

Dawn Ruskosky-Sollee, PharmD
Clinical Assistant Professor
College of Pharmacy
Department of Emergency Medicine
University of Florida Health Science Center
Assistant Director
Florida Poison Information Center
Clinical Toxicology Service
Shands Jacksonville
Jacksonville, Florida

Richard J. Ryan, MD, FACEP
Assistant Professor
Department of Emergency Medicine
University of Cincinnati
Medical Director
Department of Emergency Medicine
The Jewish Hospital
Cincinnati, Ohio

Alfred Sacchetti, MD
Assistant Clinical Professor
Department of Emergency Medicine
Thomas Jefferson University
Philadelphia, Pennsylvania
Research Director
Department of Emergency Medicine
Our Lady of Lourdes Medical Center
Camden, New Jersey

Annie T. Sadosty, MD
Chief Resident
Department of Surgery
Division of Emergency Medicine
University of Maryland
Baltimore, Maryland

Philip N. Salen, MD
Attending Physician
Emergency Medicine Residency of the Lehigh Valley
St. Luke's Hospital
Bethlehem, Pennsylvania

Leonard Samuels, MD
Narberth, Pennsylvania

Darrell C. Sandel, MD
Medical Intensive Care Unit
Ullevaal University Hospital
Oslo University
Oslo, Norway

Arthur B. Sanders, MD, MHA
Professor
Section of Emergency Medicine
Department of Surgery
University of Arizona
Attending Physician
Department of Emergency Medicine
University Medical Center
Tucson, Arizona

John P. Santamaria, MD, FAAP, FACEP
Clinical Associate Professor
Department of Pediatrics
University of South Florida School of Medicine
Co-Medical Director
After Hours Pediatrics
Tampa, Florida

Lisa Santer, MD
Department of Emergency Medicine
University of Florida Health Science Center
Jacksonville, Florida

Eric Savitsky, MD
Assistant Professor
Department of Medicine
University of California Los Angeles School of Medicine
Emergency Medicine Residency Program
Los Angeles, California

Alok Saxena, MD, FACEP
Attending Physician
Departments of Emergency Medicine and Trauma
University Medical Center
Las Vegas, Nevada

Anne Schaefer, MD
Fellow, Pediatric Hematology
Washington University School of Medicine
St. Louis Children's Hospital
St. Louis, Missouri

David A. Schaeffer, MD, FAAP, FATS
Assistant Professor
Mayo Medical School Jacksonville
Division Chief of Pulmonology, Allergy, and Immunology
Department of Pediatrics
Nemours Children's Clinic
Medical Director of Respiratory Care
Wolfson Children's Hospital
Jacksonville, Florida

Jeffrey Schaider, MD
Assistant Professor
Department of Emergency Medicine
Rush Medical College
Associate Chairman
Department of Emergency Medicine
Cook County Hospital
Chicago, Illinois

Jay L. Schauben, PharmD, ABAT
Clinical Professor
University of Florida Health Science Center
Director
Florida Poison Information Center
Jacksonville, Florida

Raquel M. Schears, MD
Assistant Professor
Department of Emergency Medicine
Hospital of the University of Pennsylvania
Philadephia, Pennsylvania

Daniel T. Schelble, MD
Chairman
Department of Emergency Medicine
Akron General Medical Center
Akron, Ohio

Frederick M. Schiavone, MD
Associate Professor
Department of Emergency Medicine
University Medical Center School of Medicine
Residency Program Director
Department of Emergency Medicine
University Hospital
Stony Brook, New York

Eric W. Schmidt, MD
Assistant Professor
Department of Emergency Medicine
UMass Memorial Healthcare
Worcester, Massachusetts

Marc B. Schnapper, MD
Resident
Department of Emergency Medicine
Ohio State University
Columbus, Ohio

Robert E. Schneider, MD
Academic Faculty
Department of Emergency Medicine
Carolinas Medical Center
Charlotte, North Carolina

Sandra M. Schneider, MD, FACEP
Professor and Chair
Department of Emergency Medicine
University of Rochester
Chief
Department of Emergency Medicine
Strong Memorial Hospital
Rochester, New York

Robert D. Schremmer, MD
Instructor
Department of Pediatrics
University of Missouri–Kansas City School of Medicine
Pediatric Emergency Medicine Fellow
Department of Pediatrics
The Children's Mercy Hospital
Kansas City, Missouri

Robert A. Schwab, MD
Vice Chair and Associate Professor
Department of Emergency Medicine
University of Missouri–Kansas City School of Medicine
Clinical Director
Department of Emergency Medicine
Truman Medical Center
Kansas City, Missouri

Byron C. Scott, MD, FACEP
Medical Director
Emergency Department
Baylor/Richardson Medical Center
Richardson, Texas

Phillip A. Scott, MD
Lecturer
Director, Emergency Stroke Team
Section of Emergency Medicine
University of Michigan
Ann Arbor, Michigan

David C. Seaberg,
Department of Emergency Medicine
University of Florida Health Science Center
Jacksonville, Florida

Charles M. Seamens, MD, FACEP
Assistant Professor
Department of Emergency Medicine
Vanderbilt University Medical Center
Nashville, Tennessee

Timothy Seay, MD
Regional Medical Director
Department of Emergency Medicine
Greater Houston Emergency Services
Conroe, Texas

Donna L. Seger, MD
Assistant Professor
Department of Emergency Medicine
Vanderbilt University School of Medicine
Medical Director
Middle Tennessee Poison Center
Nashville, Tennessee

Rebecca A. Seip, MD
Senior Attending Physician
Department of Emergency Medicine
Allegheny General Hospital
Pittsburgh, Pennsylvania

Clare T. Sercombe, MD
Program in Emergency Medicine
University of Minnesota
Hennepin County Medical Center
Minneapolis, Minnesota

Linda L. Settle, MD
Department of Emergency Medicine
Children's Healthcare of Atlanta
Atlanta, Georgia

Harry W. Severance, MD, FACEP
Assistant Professor
Division of Emergency Medicine
Department of Surgery
Duke University School of Medicine
Attending Physician
Duke University Medical Center
Durham, North Carolina

Michael W. Shannon, MD, MPH
Assistant Professor of Pediatrics
Harvard Medical School
Associate in Medicine
Children's Hospital
Staff Toxicologist
Massachusetts Poison Control System
Boston, Massachusetts

Ghazala Q. Sharieff, MD
Assistant Clinical Professor
Departments of Medicine and Pediatrics
University of California San Diego
Attending Physician
Department of Pediatric Emergency Medicine
Children's Hospital and Health Center
San Diego, California

Kathy N. Shaw, MD, MSCE
Associate Professor of Pediatrics
University of Pennsylvania School of Medicine
Chief
Division of Emergency Medicine
Children's Hospital of Philadelphia
Philadelphia, Pennsylvania

Suzanne Moore Shepherd, MD, DTMH, FACEP
Associate Professor
Director of Education and Research
PENN Travel Medicine
Department of Emergency Medicine
Hospital of the University of Pennsylvania
Philadelphia, Pennsylvania

Robert Shesser, MD, MPH
Professor
Department of Emergency Medicine
George Washington University School of Medicine
Washington, DC

Richard D. Shih, MD
Residency Director
Department of Emergency Medicine
Morristown Memorial Hospital
Morristown, New Jersey

Lee W. Shockley, MD
Assistant Professor
Department of Surgery
Division of Emergency Medicine
University of Colorado
Residency Program Director
Department of Emergency Medicine
Denver Health Medical Center
Denver, Colorado

William H. Shoff, MD
Assistant Professor
Director
PENN Travel Medicine
Department of Emergency Medicine
Hospital of the University of Pennsylvania
Philadephia, Pennsylvania

Robert Sigillito, MD
Departments of Emergency Medicine, Pulmonary and Critical Care
Louisiana State University
Charity Hospital
New Orleans, Louisiana

Harold K. Simon, MD
Associate Professor
Department of Pediatrics
Emory University School of Medicine
Section Chief of Emergency Medicine
Children's Healthcare of Atlanta
Attending Physician
Hughes Spalding Children's Hospital
Atlanta, Georgia

Robert Simon, MD
Professor
Department of Emergency Medicine
Rush Medical College
Chairman
Department of Emergency Medicine
Cook County Hospital
Chicago, Illinois

Adam Singer, MD
Department of Emergency Medicine
State University of New York at Stony Brook
Stony Brook, New York

Jonathan I. Singer, MD, FAAP, FACEP
Professor
Departments of Emergency Medicine and Pediatrics
Wright State University School of Medicine
Staff Physician
Department of Emergency Medicine
Children's Medical Center
Dayton, Ohio

Madhumita Sinha, MD
Pediatric Emergency Medicine Fellow
Department of Emergency Medicine
Children's Hospital Medical Center of Akron
Akron, Ohio

Marco L. A. Sivilotti , MD, MSc
Assistant Professor
Department of Emergency Medicine
University of Massachusetts Medical School
Attending Physician
Emergency Department
UMass Memorial Healthcare
Worcester, Massachusetts

Corey M. Slovis, MD, FACP, FACEP
Professor and Chairman
Department of Emergency Medicine
Vanderbilt University Medical Center
Nashville, Tennessee

Alan Jon Smally, MD, FACEP
Associate Professor
Department of Traumatology and Emergency Medicine
University of Connecticut School of Medicine
Farmington, Connecticut
Senior Attending Physician
Department of Emergency Medicine
Hartford Hospital
Hartford, Connecticut

Martin J. Smilkstein, MD
Assistant Professor
Department of Emergency Medicine
Oregon Health Sciences University
Medical Director
Oregon Poison Center
Portland, Oregon

Mark Smith, MD
Clinical Professor
Department of Emergency Medicine
The George Washington University School of Medicine and Health Sciences
Chair
Department of Emergency Medicine
Washington Hospital Center
Washington, DC

Rodney Smith, MD
Emergency Medicine and Trauma Center
Methodist Hospital of Indiana
Indianapolis, Indiana

Brian K. Snyder, MD
Assistant Clinical Professor
Department of Emergency Medicine
University of California San Diego
San Diego, California

Peter L. Sosnow, MD, FACEP
Adjunct Assistant Professor
Department of Emergency Medicine
Albany Medical College
Chief
Emergency Medicine
Albany Memorial Hospital
Albany, New York

Peter E. Sokolove, MD
Assistant Professor of Clinical Medicine
Division of Emergency Medicine
University of California Davis
Davis, California
Associate Residency Director
Division of Emergency Medicine
University of California Davis Medical Center
Sacramento, California

Amy S. Spangler, RN, MS, PNP
Department of Emergency Medicine
Children's Hospital of Virginia
Norfolk, Virginia

William H. Spivey (deceased)

David G. Spoerke, MD
Phytotoxicology Consultant
Bristlecone Enterprises
Lakewood, Colorado

Sarah A. Stahmer, MD, FACEP
Associate Professor
Residency Program Director
Department of Emergency Medicine
UMDNJ-Robert Wood Johnson Medical School
Cooper Hospital/University Medical Center
Camden, New Jersey

J. Stephan Stapczynski, MD
Chair
Department of Emergency Medicine
University of Kentucky College of Medicine
Medical Director
Emergency Department
University of Kentucky Hospital
Lexington, Kentucky

Mary B. Staten-McCormick, MD, FACEP
Assistant Clinical Professor
Michigan State University College of Human Medicine
East Lansing, Michigan
Clinical Staff
Department of Emergency Medicine
Bronson Methodist Hospital
Kalamazoo, Michigan

Mark T. Steele, MD
Associate Professor
Department of Emergency Medicine
University of Missouri–Kansas City School of Medicine
Chairman
Department of Emergency Medicine
Truman Medical Center
Kansas City, Missouri

Christopher P. Steidle, MD
Northeast Indiana Urology
Fort Wayne, Indiana

Barry Steinberg, MD, DDS, PhD, FACS
Chief
Department of Maxillofacial Surgery
University of Florida Health Science Center
Jacksonville, Florida

Phyllis Hendry Stenkylft, MD, FAAP, FACEP
Associate Professor and Division Chief
Pediatric Emergency Medicine
University of Florida Health Science Center
Jacksonville, Florida

Mary H. Stewart, MD
Senior Instructor
Department of Emergency Medicine
Case Western Reserve University School of Medicine
Attending Physician
Emergency Department
MetroHealth Medical Center
Cleveland, Ohio
Director, Emergency Department
Allen Memorial Hospital
Oberlin, Ohio

C. Keith Stone, MD
Associate Professor
Department of Emergency Medicine
University of Kentucky
Lexington, Kentucky

Jeffrey R. Suchard, MD
Medical Toxicology Fellow
Department of Medical Toxicology
Good Samaritan Regional Medical Center
Phoenix, Arizona

John B. Sullivan, Jr., MD
Associate Dean for Clinical Affairs
Associate Professor of Emergency Medicine
University of Arizona Health Sciences Center
Medical Director, Arizona Poison Center
Tucson, Arizona

Stuart P. Swadron, MD
Clinical Instructor
Department of Emergency Medicine
University of Southern California School of Medicine
Chief Resident
Department of Emergency Medicine
LAC + USC Medical Center
Los Angeles, California

David A. Talan, MD, FACEP, FIDSA
Professor
University of California Los Angeles School of Medicine
Chair
Department of Emergency Medicine
Olive View-UCLA Medical Center
Sylmar, California

Janet Talbot-Stern, MD
Clinical Senior Lecturer
Department of Surgery
University of Sydney
Director
Emergency Department
Royal Prince Alfred Hospital
Sydney, Australia

Ellen H. Taliaferro, MD
Associate Professor
Division of Emergency Medicine
Department of Surgery
University of Texas Southwestern Medical School
Medical Director
Violence Intervention and Prevention Center
Parksand Health and Hospital Systems
Dallas, Texas

David A. Tanen, MD
Department of Medical Toxicology
Good Samaritan Regional Medical Center
Phoenix, Arizona

Milton Tennenbein, MD, FRCPC, FAAP, FAACT, FACMT
Professor
Departments of Pediatrics, Medicine, and Pharmacology
University of Manitoba
Director
Emergency Services
Children's Hospital
Winnipeg, Manitoba, Canada

Harold A. Thomas, Jr., MD
Associate Professor
Department of Emergency Medicine
Oregon Health Sciences University
Portand, Oregon

Laura B. Thomas, MD, DMD
Resident
Department of Emergency Medicine
Hospital of the University of Pennsylvania
Philadelphia, Pennsylvania

Stephen H. Thomas, MD
Instructor
Department of Medicine
Harvard Medical School
Attending Physician
Department of Emergency Medicine
Massachusetts General Hospital
Boston, Massachusetts

Brian R. Tiffany, MD, PhD
Co-Director of Research
Department of Emergency Medicine
Maricopa Medical Center
Phoenix, Arizona

Wenzel Tirheimer, MD
Department of Emergency Medicine
Ohio State University
Columbus, Ohio

Asad Tolaymat, MD
Professor
Department of Pediatrics
University of Florida Health Science Center
Chief
Department of Nephrology
Nemours Children's Clinic
Jacksonville, Florida

Andrew R. Topliff, MD
Toxicology Fellow
Hennepin Regional Poison Center
Minneapolis, Minnesota

Alexander T. Trott, MD
Professor
Department of Emergency Medicine
University of Cincinnati College of Medicine
Associate Chief of Staff
University Hospital
Cincinnati, Ohio

Jeffrey Tucker
Assistant Professor of Pediatrics and Emergency Medicine
University of Connecticut School of Medicine
Department of Emergency Medicine
Connecticut Children's Medical Center
Hartford, Connecticut

Michael A. Turturro, MD, FACEP
Clinical Associate Professor
University of Pittsburgh School of Medicine
Department of Emergency Medicine
Vice Chair and Director of Academic Affairs
Department of Emergency Medicine
Mercy Hospital of Pittsburgh
Pittsburgh, Pennsylvania

Robert C. Urbanic, MD
Department of Emergency Services
St. Joseph Mercy Hospital
Ann Arbor, Michigan

Phyllis A. Vallee, MD
Assistant Professor
Department of Internal Medicine
Case Western Reserve University
Cleveland, Ohio
Associate Residency Director
Department of Emergency Medicine
Henry Ford Hospital
Detroit, Michigan

Verena T. Valley, MD, RDMS
Associate Professor
Ultrasound Director
Department of Emergency Medicine
University of Mississippi Medical Center
Jackson, Mississippi

Laurie Vande Krol, MD
Assistant Professor
University of Colorado Health Sciences Center
Staff Emergency Physician
Denver General Hospital
Denver, Colorado

Henry C. Veldenz, MD, FACS
Assistant Professor
Department of Surgery/Vascular
University of Florida Health Science Center
Jacksonville, Florida

Gregory A. Volturo, MD, FACEP
Vice-Chair
Department of Emergency Medicine
University of Massachusetts Medical School
UMass Memorial Healthcare
Worcester, Massachusetts

Scott R. Votey, MD
Associate Professor
Department of Emergency Medicine
University of California Los Angeles School of Medicine
Co-Director
UCLA Emergency Medicine Residency Program
UCLA Medical Center
Los Angeles, California

David J. Vukich, MD
Professor and Chair
Department of Emergency Medicine
University of Florida Health Science Center
Jacksonville, Florida

Paula S. Wadbrook, MD
Resident
Department of Emergency Medicine
Maricopa Medical Center
Phoenix, Arizona

Ron M. Walls, MD, FRCPC, FACEP
Associate Professor of Medicine
Division of Emergency Medicine
Harvard Medical School
Chairman
Department of Emergency Medicine
Brigham and Women's Hospital
Boston, Massachusetts

Frank G. Walter, MD, FACEP, FACMT
Associate Professor
Department of Surgery (Emergency Medicine)
University of Arizona College of Medicine
Director of Clinical Toxicology
Department of Emergency Medicine
University Medical Center
Tucson, Arizona

James J. Walter, MD
Professor of Clinical Medicine
Chief
Section of Emergency Medicine
University of Chicago
Chicago, Illinois

Richard Y. Wang, DO
Assistant Professor
Department of Medicine
Brown University
Director
Division of Medical Toxicology
Department of Emergency Medicine
Rhode Island Hospital
Providence, Rhode Island

Kevin R. Ward, MD
Assistant Professor and Director of Research
Department of Emergency Medicine
Virginia Commonwealth University Medical College of Virginia
Richmond, Virginia

Gary S. Wasserman, DO, FAAP, FACMT
Professor of Medicine
Department of Pediatrics
University of Missouri–Kansas City School of Medicine
Chief
Section of Medical Toxicology
The Children's Mercy Hospital
Kansas City, Missouri

D. Shannon Waters, MD
Resident
Department of Emergency Medicine
University of Kentucky Medical Center
Lexington, Kentucky

William A. Watson, Pharm. D.
Professor
Department of Surgery
University of Texas Health Sciences Center
Managing Director
South Texas Poison Center
San Antonio, Texas

Paul M. Wax, MD
Associate Professor and Attending Physician
Department of Emergency Medicine
University of Rochester School of Medicine
Strong Memorial Hospital
Rochester, New York

Robert L. Wears, MD, MS, FACEP
Professor
Department of Emergency Medicine
University of Florida Health Science Center
Jacksonville, Florida

Elizabeth A. Wedemeyer, MD
Associate Clinical Professor
Department of Pediatrics
Columbia University School of Medicine
Assistant Attending Pediatrician
Presbyterian Hospital
New York, New York

Scott D. Weir, MD
Attending Physician
Department of Emergency Medicine
Hospital of Saint Raphael
New Haven, Connecticut

Larry D. Weiss, MD, JD, FACEPO
Clinical Associate Professor
Assistant Chief of Academic Affairs
Section of Emergency Medicine
Louisiana State Tulane University School of Medicine
New Orleans, Louisiana

Howard A. Werman, MD
Associate Professor
Department of Emergency Medicine
Ohio State University College of Medicine and Public Health
Medical Director, MedFlight
Columbus, Ohio

J. M. Whitworth, MD
Professor
Department of Pediatrics
University of Florida Health Science Center
Jacksonville, Florida

James A. Wilde, MD, FAAP
Assistant Professor
Departments of Emergency Medicine and Pediatrics
Medical College of Georgia
Augusta, Georgia

Abigail R. Williams, RN, JD, MPH
Managing Partner
Abigail Williams and Associates, PC
Worcester, Massachusetts

Kenneth A. Williams, MD, FACEP
Associate Professor
Department of Emergency Medicine
University of Massachusetts
Worcester, Massachusetts
Attending Physician
Department of Emergency Medicine
Rhode Island Hospital
Providence, Rhode Island

Donald C. Willis, MD
South Florida Perinatal Medicine
Miami, Florida

Gabriel R. Wilson, MD
Chief Resident
Department of Emergency Medicine
New York Medical College Affiliated Hospitals
New York, New York

Lance D. Wilson, MD
Clinical Instructor
Department of Emergency Medicine
Case Western Reserve University
Research Director
Department of Emergency Medicine
PHS–Mt. Sinai Medical Center
Cleveland, Ohio

Michael D. Witting, MD
Assistant Professor
Department of Surgery
Division of Emergency Medicine
University of Maryland
Attending Physician
Department of Emergency Medicine
Mercy Hospital
Baltimore, Maryland

Richard Wolfe, MD
Assistant Professor of Medicine
Division of Emergency Medicine
Harvard Medical School
Chairman
Department of Emergency Medicine
Beth Israel Deaconess Medical Center
Boston, Massachusetts

R. Wayne Wolfram, MD
Department of Emergency Medicine
Children's Hospital of Virginia
Norfolk, Virginia

Allan B. Wolfson, MD, FACEP, FACP
Professor of Emergency Medicine
Department of Emergency Medicine
University of Pittsburgh
Program Director
University of Pittsburgh Affiliated Residency in Emergency Medicine
Pittsburgh, Pennsylvania

Robert H. Woolard, MD, FACEP
Chairman
Section of Emergency Medicine
Brown University School of Medicine
Physician-in-Chief
Department of Emergency Medicine
Rhode Island and Miriam Hospitals
Providence, Rhode Island

Alan D. Woolf, MD, MPH
Associate Professor
Department of Pediatrics
Harvard Medical School
Director
Program in Clinical Toxicology
Department of Medicine
Children's Hospital
Boston, Masschusetts

Martha S. Wright, MD
Assistant Professor
Department of Pediatrics
Case Western Reserve University
Associate Director
Pediatric Emergency Medicine Services
Rainbow Babies and Children's Hospital
Cleveland, Ohio

Todd Wylie, MD
Department of Emergency Medicine
University of Florida Health Science Center
Jacksonville, Florida

Collette Ditz Wyte, MD
Assistant Clinical Professor
Department of Emergency Medicine
Wayne State University
Detroit, Michigan
Associate Research Director
Department of Emergency Medicine
Beaumont Hospital
Royal Oak, Michigan

Roger Yang, MD
Department of Emergency Medicine
Harbor–UCLA Medical Center
Torrance, CA

Donald M. Yealy, MD
Professor and Vice Chairman
Department of Emergency Medicine
University of Pittsburgh Medical Center
Pittsburgh, Pennsylvania

Robert Zalenski, MD
Associate Professor
Director of Clinical Research
Departments of Emergency Medicine and Cardiology
Wayne State University School of Medicine
Attending Physician
John D. Dingell Veterans Administration Hospital and Detroit Receiving Hospital
Detroit, Michigan

Elisa Alter Zenni, MD
Clinical Assistant Professor
Department of Pediatrics
University of Florida Health Science Center
Jacksonville, Florida

David N. Zull, MD
Associate Professor of Medicine
Northwestern University School of Medicine
Chicago, Illinois

Leslie S. Zun, MD
Associate Professor
Department of Emergency Medicine
Finch University
Chicago Medical School
Chairman
Department of Emergency Medicine
Mt. Sinai Medical Center
Chicago, Illinois

Contents

SECTION III TRAUMA
Suzanne Moore Shepherd

PART I. *General Considerations*

PART II. *System Considerations*

PART III. *Orthopedic Considerations*

PART IV. *Special Considerations*

PART V. *Special Procedures*

SECTION IV GENERAL MEDICAL EMERGENCIES
Allan B. Wolfson

PART I. *Cardiovascular Disease*

SECTION V PEDIATRICS
Phyllis Hendry Stenklyft

PART I. *Resuscitation*

PART II. *Signs and Symptoms*

PART III. *Specific Diseases*

PART IV. *Pediatric Trauma*

PART V. *Administrative and Clinical Issues*

SECTION VI TOXICOLOGY
Christopher H. Linden

The Clinical Practice of Emergency Medicine

INTRODUCTION

The Approach to the Emergency Department Patient

Robert L. Wears

. . . in the physician or surgeon, no quality takes rank with imperturbability. . . . Imperturbability means coolness and presence of mind under all circumstances, calmness amid storm, clearness of judgment in moments of grave peril, immobility, impassiveness, or, to use an old and expressive word, *phlegm*. It is the quality which is most appreciated by the laity though often misunderstood by them; and the physician who has the misfortune to be without it, who betrays indecision and worry, and who shows that he is flustered and hurried in ordinary emergencies, loses rapidly the confidence of his patients.

Sir William Osler, *Æquanimitas*

INTRODUCTION

It is one thing to practice medicine in an emergency department (ED); it is quite another to practice emergency medicine. The effective practice of emergency medicine requires an approach, a way of thinking, and personality characteristics different from all other medical specialties.

Its physical limitation to the ED is perhaps the least important of emergency medicine's characteristics. Five factors have led emergency physicians to develop a unique approach to the patient: the pressure of time and volume, the variety of conditions faced, the paucity of information, the limitation of therapeutic options, and the constraint of disposition.

Time and Volume Pressure

More than any other specialty, emergency physicians deal with patients as turbulent flow in a constricted channel. In a true emergency, seconds to minutes may make the difference between life and death or serious disability. In these situations, emergency physicians, contrary to much of their previous training, must be prepared to "treat first and ask questions later."

Also, the time available for an emergency physician to evaluate and think about any given patient is severely limited by the demands of other patients being managed concurrently. In most practices, during the busiest part of the day, an emergency physician has on average only 10 to 15 minutes per patient for evaluation, testing, treatment, disposition, and documentation. Whether this is adequate or not is immaterial; the reality is that no more time is available.

The combination of time and volume pressures forces emergency physicians to be much more aware of priorities among patients. While trauma surgeons occasionally face triage conditions, emergency physicians are the only practitioners who routinely make (at least mental) triage decisions every day.

Variety of Conditions

As a specialty in breadth rather than depth, emergency physicians must manage a wider variety of conditions than any other specialists, save perhaps family practitioners. In addition, unlike other specialists, emergency physicians must shift domains rapidly. Practicing emergency medicine is like carefully lining up a putt, then dropping the putter, picking up a tennis racket to return a volley or two, quickly side-stepping an onrushing tackler, and then returning to sink the putt.

Paucity of Information

Emergency physicians frequently deal with episodes of real or perceived crises in illnesses of whose past course they are unaware. Old records are often unavailable and patients' recall is limited in scope and reliability. The information-gathering options available in the ED are similarly limited. Only a small subset of the vast diagnostic armamentarium is available to the emergency physician promptly.

Limited Therapeutic Options

Options for treatment are limited as well. Often, emergency physicians can provide only temporizing or symptomatic treatment, while definitive management must be deferred to another specialist. In addition, in emergency situations, the tolerance for therapeutic errors, whether of omission or commission, is more limited than in nonemergencies.

Although one may not realize it when viewing the chaotic, turbulent frothing of a busy ED, emergency medicine possesses a certain elegance enforced by these constraints. There is an attractive intellectual simplicity in meeting the challenge of providing timely, accurate care using primarily one's own hands and brain, supplemented by a few limited laboratory and imaging tests.

Constraint of Disposition

Every patient interaction an emergency physician has must soon be ended. This forces emergency physicians to focus on the "bottom line." No matter how uncertain the diagnosis, no matter how much extended observation or testing might help, every patient encounter in the ED ultimately reduces to three binary decisions: Is the patient sick or not sick? If sick, should I treat or not treat? If I should treat, should I admit or discharge? These questions must be answered despite the lack of definitive information, the lack of time to collect or consider additional information, or the lack of availability of advice from colleagues and consultants.

A FRAMEWORK FOR APPROACHING THE EMERGENCY DEPARTMENT PATIENT

Because there are many sources outlining the mechanics of history taking and physical examination, this section will not cover those areas in detail, but will instead concentrate on how they are different in emergency medicine.

The first question to be asked on initial approach to a patient in the ED is, "Do I need to resuscitate this patient?" Corollaries to this question are, "How great is the threat?" and "How soon must I act?" The first question is usually answered in the first few seconds at the bedside and is as often based on an overall *gestalt* of the chief complaint and patient's general appearance as on specific complaints or vital-sign abnormalities.

In true emergencies, the usual sequence of history, physical examination, laboratory testing, and treatment is altered by the need to take rapid action. In the most extreme cases, the sequence becomes treatment, physical examination, laboratory testing, and history.

When action is urgently required, the emergency physician

must commit to it unhesitatingly. This requires mental preparedness; there will not be time to ponder the benefits and risks of the various options for managing acute upper airway obstruction. The thinking required must be invested ahead of time, and a plan of action internalized by the physician before the situation requiring it arises.

Often, if action is to be effective it must be initiated before all the information bearing on the decision is available. This requires a "bias toward action" in the emergency physician's mind. While this is occasionally a source of criticism from other specialists who fail to understand emergency medicine, in the proper circumstances it can save lives. A simplistic example of bias toward action would be putting a patient with chest pain on a cardiac monitor on arrival to the ED; clearly the diagnosis of heart disease has not yet been made, so it is not certain that the monitor is truly "needed," but the physician anticipates a potential need and acts without waiting for confirmation. A more dramatic example is sudden upper airway obstruction, where the decision to perform a cricothyroidotomy must be made promptly; to wait until the need is clear may be to wait too long.

Part of the art of emergency medicine is the ability to reliably discriminate between cases requiring urgent action and those allowing a more measured approach. The bias toward action should not be used as an excuse for an indiscriminate, "shoot-from-the-hip" approach to the patient; it is a tool that the emergency physician can learn to use effectively.

Bedside Evaluation

If resuscitation or other urgent interventions are not required, then the usual framework for patient evaluation (history, physical, laboratory, treatment, disposition) can be used. In the ED, certain factors will require more or less emphasis, or alteration, however.

Patients and physicians in EDs are generally complete strangers, and thus patients have legitimate questions about the emergency physicians they have just met: Are they capable? Can they be trusted? Therefore, the first task faced by the emergency physician, even before the task of information gathering begins, is to build a working relationship with the patient right away.[7]

The initial contact the physician makes should be social—an introduction. This should include everyone in the room, and should be accompanied by physical contact—a handshake or touch. This establishes a tone of personal respect for the patient and helps enlist the family, if present, in an alliance with the physician. As early as possible the physician should show empathy with the patient by acknowledging recognition of an apparent need. Most commonly and most easily this can be done by an offer to relieve apparent pain, if appropriate.

The body language of the physician–patient encounter is important. Often in the ED, the standing physician presides over the supine, frequently disrobed patient, presenting an authoritarian image that can be threatening to patients. As often as possible, therefore, the physician should sit down while conducting the initial interview, ideally bringing her head to the same level as the patient's. This is especially important in dealing with children, but should not be neglected in adult patients.

The information-gathering phase of the encounter should begin with a general, open-ended question, such as, "How can I help you?" It is important to remember that both parties, not just the physician, are interested in gathering information at this time. Patients' desires for information, explanation, and reassurance are great, and are seldom met by physicians.[1,8] One way emergency physicians can meet this almost insatiable need for information early in the encounter is by commenting about findings during the physical examination: "Your heart sounds normal," or "Your throat looks red."[7]

Given the time pressures of emergency medicine, physicians typically fear losing control of the interview and attempt to keep the patient focused and on target. Observations of physician–patient interactions have shown that patients are interrupted by the physician on average about 18 seconds after they begin to relate their history, but that if uninterrupted, 80% can get their story out within 1 minute.[2] Physicians' time concerns are real, but if the physician dominates the interview, the patient will become passive and volunteer little[4]; the physician will then have to spend additional time extracting information later. In addition, the chief complaint may not always be mentioned first; failure to wait for the true chief complaint to emerge can lead to false trails and lost time.[7] Considering the gain in rapport with the patient and the potential for mischief with early interruption, it seems wise for emergency physicians to discipline themselves to be quiet for the first 60 seconds of the interview (Table 1).

Disposition

Once the initial assessment is completed, the physician should outline the plan to the patient, and should give an honest estimate of about how long it will take. It is also useful to provide some anticipatory guidance about the probable outcome, particularly in complex, chronic problems that are unlikely to be resolved in an ED evaluation. During the wait for laboratory results, consultations, or observation, the patient and family should be updated periodically on progress and asked if there is anything they need.

Finally, once a disposition is reached, the plan should be carefully and clearly communicated to the patient and family. Particularly if the patient is to be discharged, specific instructions about follow-up and reasons to return to the ED should be covered. Because patients are likely to have difficulty retaining a series of detailed explanations or instructions, it is most helpful if they are given in written form. Having a printed instruction sheet does not relieve the physician of the obligation to instruct the patient, but it does help to reinforce those instructions once the patient has left the ED.

A FRAMEWORK FOR DECISION MAKING IN EMERGENCY MEDICINE

Medicine is essentially about making decisions; in emergency medicine, this general property of medicine is intensified. Because a great deal of medical decision making occurs at a subconscious level, it is surprising to many to learn that there is a formalism for making and assessing the quality of medical decisions. Although it seems unrealistic to expect that clinicians will adopt a formal decision-making model in their practices, some useful insights into the nature of decision making in the ED can be gained by such models.

TABLE 1. Rules to Guide the Bedside Evaluation of the Emergency Department Patient

Introduce yourself to everyone.
Shake hands.
Sit down.
Relieve pain early.
Don't interrupt.
Provide information.
Explain what will happen.
Provide updates.
Be helpful.

Management, Not Diagnosis

Traditionally, medicine has focused on diagnosis as the central important task of the clinician. Emergency medicine makes it clear that this is erroneous: In medicine in general and especially in emergency medicine, the central task is not diagnosis; it is management. Often a diagnosis cannot be made under the constraints of an ED evaluation; the great insight that emergency physicians have contributed to their colleagues in other specialties is the notion that there need not always be a diagnosis. If one can be made, it is extremely helpful, but if not, decisions must still be made and actions must still be taken.

In addition, patients want more than simply a diagnosis. They want explanation and reassurance. For example, parents will not be satisfied to know that their child's abdominal pain is due to gastroenteritis; they want to know that it is not appendicitis. Simply providing the diagnosis, however correct, dismisses the parents' concerns and will leave them unsatisfied. By empathizing with their fears, the physician can strengthen rapport with the family and take a position as their friend and ally, rather than a remote authority. Thus, the intellectual task is to come up with a reasonable plan of management, which may include, but not be limited to, making a diagnosis.

Decision Thresholds

The concept of decision threshold[6] clarifies many decisions emergency physicians make, and adds specificity to the often used but more vague concept of "index of suspicion." Consider the following hypothetical scenario of the simplest possible decision problem in emergency medicine: There is only one disease under consideration, and there are only two possible actions—to treat or not treat—based on the emergency physician's assessment of the patient. In this scenario, there are four possible outcomes: The patient either has the disease, and may be treated or not treated, or does not have the disease, and is treated or not treated. The correct management decision will depend on the values of these outcomes, and on the probability that a particular patient (or group of patients) actually has the disease in question.

If the patient is almost certainly nondiseased (i.e., the probability of disease is near 0), then the correct decision is obviously to not treat, since treatment entails costs and risks of its own. Conversely, if the patient surely has the disease (probability near 1), then the correct decision is just as obviously to treat, since the costs and risks of treatment are outweighed by the negative consequences of failing to treat. Therefore, there must be some *threshold* probability between 0 and 1 at which the decision is a toss-up; either choice will produce about the same outcome. This treatment threshold need not (and frequently does not) coincide with the diagnostic thresholds that clinicians have traditionally been taught. Thus, the clinician's task is not necessarily to make a diagnosis, but to discover whether the probability of disease is clearly over or clearly under the treatment threshold, and to act accordingly.

The threshold approach can be extended to more complex problems. For example, a more realistic scenario would allow use of a diagnostic test to improve the physician's initial assessment. Now there are two decision thresholds. At very low probabilities of disease, it is better not to test and to treat no one, because the outcome of large numbers of false positives erroneously treated outweighs that of the occasional diseased patient detected. Similarly, at very high probabilities, it is better not to test, but to treat everyone, because the consequences of large numbers of false negatives erroneously denied treatment outweigh the occasional nondiseased patient spared unnecessary treatment. At intermediate probabilities, testing and treating only those patients with a positive test will produce the best overall outcome. Thus, the clinician's task is to decide whether a given patient's probability of disease lies either below the no treat–test threshold, or above the test–treat threshold. Testing is useful only in changing the management decision in the area between the two thresholds. While there may be other benefits to testing besides producing a change in management (e.g., reducing uncertainty, or clarifying prognosis), the threshold approach provides a rationale for understanding physicians' differing choices when faced with what superficially seem to be similar clinical scenarios.

In framing decision making in this way, it is important to note that a very broad idea of "test" is used. Anything that helps physicians revise their probability assessments is considered a test in this sense, so a therapeutic trial, or a period of observation, or a clinical scoring system, or a practice guideline can all be considered "tests" because they help physicians sort out probabilities of diseases. McNutt et al.[5] have provided interesting evidence that physicians' diagnostic and management performance improves when they receive the nonverbal cues that accompany face-to-face communication, even though this "test" occurs largely at a subconscious level.

The way in which emergency physicians determine whether they have crossed an action threshold seems to be by the use of naturalistic or "event-driven" decision making.[4] This contrasts strongly with the algorithmic or analytical decision-making process taught in medical school. Naturalistic decision making is effective in settings characterized by ill-defined problems; dynamic, uncertain environments; shifting, unclear, or competing goals; tight but nonlinear or hidden coupling between actions and their effects; time pressure; high stakes; and scant opportunity for learning by trial and error.

The decision-making process can be broken into several phases. First, the physician classifies the current situation as typical or atypical, based on matching critical cues to stored patterns or schemata. If the situation is typical, then the stored patterns will evoke a customary set of responses. If not, variations of customary responses are considered first, and then novel, "one-of-a-kind" responses. Clearly, experience is critical in developing a sufficiently rich set of stored schemata such that the vast majority of clinical problems can be recognized and dealt with by a preplanned response.

Next, the physician engages in serial evaluation of the available courses of action, beginning with the most typical response, and evaluating each by mentally simulating the expected outcomes. Once a sufficiently satisfying action is discovered, it is implemented. In other words, there is generally not a search for the best of all possible responses, but for a sufficiently good response. The payoff for accepting a good but not necessarily best response is that decisions can be quick and almost effortless. In fact, a great deal of physicians' expertise seems to lie in their ability to constructively perceive the problem, which seems to lead automatically to a solution without much conscious effort. This contrasts sharply to the slow and laborious analytic approach of exhaustively considering all the possibilities and eliminating them one by one until the best option is identified.

Learning this method of decision making is not easy. It can be gained with experience, and is generally communicated by narratives of meaningful cases.[3] It does not appear to be attainable through application of a formal (such as decision) analysis. Such methods have their place, but they have not proven useful in helping medical students or residents to become physicians.

COMMON PITFALLS

There are three common pitfalls in the approach to the patient in the ED.

- The first is tunnel vision. Here the physician, in single-minded pursuit of the disposition, fastens onto a single complaint (typically the first offered) without waiting to be sure that the patient's *chief* complaint has been elicited. A related error is the premature closure of hypothesis generation (e.g., assuming that chest pain is due to myocardial ischemia without first mentally ruling out the possibilities of aortic dissection, esophageal rupture, or pericarditis).
- The second pitfall is just the opposite: an inability to see the forest for the trees. Here the physician fails to rank findings in any order of importance, is reluctant to close off hypothesis generation, or is unable to integrate the findings into a small number of explanations. This is frequently manifested by procrastination in decision making, perhaps hidden behind a cascade of laboratory testing. The ability to simultaneously entertain a modest number of possible explanations for the patient's problem without prematurely settling on one, or letting the number in contention grow too large, is the "golden mean" between these two problems.
- The final pitfall is failure to attend to the patient. Time "gained" by failing to attend to the social interaction with patient and family is likely to be lost later, as missing information may not be extracted except by persistent questioning, leaving the physician at risk of pursuing many false passages before happening across the true trail.

References

1. Adamson TE, Tschann JM, Gullin DS, et al. Physician communication skills and malpractice claims: a complex relationship. *West J Med* 1989;150:356–360.
2. Beckman HB, Frankel RM. Effect of physician behavior on the collection of data. *Ann Intern Med* 1984;101:692–696.
3. Klein GA. *Sources of power: how people make decisions.* Cambridge, MA: MIT Press, 1998.
4. Klein GA, Orasanu J, Calderwood R, et al., eds. *Decision making in action: models and methods.* Norwood, NJ: Ablex Publishing Co, 1993.
5. McNutt RA, Evans AT, Wallsten TS, et al. The effect of visual information on physicians' estimates of acute ischemic heart disease and their decisions to admit. *Med Decis Making* 1993;13:393(abst).
6. Pauker SG, Kassirer JP. The threshold approach to clinical decision making. *N Engl J Med* 1980;302:1109–1117.
7. Rosenzweig S. Emergency rapport. *J Emerg Med* 1993;11:775–778.
8. Waitzkin H. Doctor-patient communication: clinical implications of social science research. *JAMA* 1984;252:2441–2446.

SECTION I

Section Editor: Suzanne Moore Shepherd

Chief Complaint

CHAPTER 1
Chest Pain

Robert Zalenski and Rebecca R. Roberts

The challenge in accurately diagnosing chest pain arises from some important neuroanatomic facts. First, neither the quality nor the intensity of pain produced by the nerves coming from the thoracic viscera is specific for any single organ system. Spasm of the esophagus, ischemia of the heart, or distention of the great vessels can produce feelings of pressure, aching, or burning. Pain can be severe, minimal, or even absent during the course of life-threatening conditions such as an acute myocardial infarction.

Second, the location and radiation of the pain do not reliably identify the specific organ system involved. Thoracic organ pathology can produce pain that is referred outside the thorax to the epigastrium, neck, or jaw. Conversely, cervical pathology from a ruptured cervical disk can produce pain in the shoulder and around the clavicle. Abdominal pathology, such as a ruptured ectopic pregnancy, can produce chest and scapular pain due to diaphragmatic irritation.

The anatomic explanation for referred pain is simple: Somatic afferent nerves from the skin and muscle of the arms enter the same dorsal root nerve pools as the visceral afferent nerves from the heart, esophagus, and other thoracic organs. Activation of this nerve pool by visceral afferents can stimulate the somatic afferent nerves. The brain interprets the pain as coming from the arm, muscle, or joint innervated by the pooled somatic afferents. Pain from the heart can be perceived as pain in the upper inner arm, forearm, or axilla, because both areas synapse in the dorsal roots T1–T5.[7] Also, because dorsal nerve segments overlap three segments above and below a particular level, thoracic pain can be referred to the neck or abdomen. Therefore, to identify the organ system and the disease process, the physician must rely on the duration and frequency of the pain, the setting in which it occurs, the aggravating and relieving factors, and associated symptoms.

ORGAN SYSTEMS

The five major thoracic organ systems are listed in Table 1.1. The most common etiologies that affect these organs can be categorized as structural disruption, infarction or ischemia, infection, and inflammation.

DIFFERENTIAL DIAGNOSIS

The historical features of chest pain are useful in establishing the "pretest" probability for each disease in the differential. Such probabilities guide the choice and interpretation of further diagnostic tests.

Acute myocardial infarction (AMI) produces a nonlocalized pressure, ache, or burning, the intensity of which ranges from severe pain to minimal discomfort. The pain is usually substernal and in the left chest, but can occur between the umbilicus and the neck. It frequently radiates to the shoulder or left arm and lasts several hours.

TABLE 1.1. Common Causes of Chest Pain

Organ System/Etiology	Chest Pain	Associated Symptoms
CARDIOVASCULAR		
Acute myocardial infarction	Pressure, aching, burning	Dyspnea, palpitations, nausea, diaphoresis, radiation
Aortic dissection	Sudden, severe, tearing	Back pain, neurovascular deficits
Unstable angina	Same as AMI except episodic	Same as AMI
Pericarditis	Sharp, pleuritic	Fever, dyspnea
Myocarditis	Same as AMI or pericarditis	Dyspnea, palpitations, CHF
RESPIRATORY		
Pulmonary embolus	Sharp pleuritic or central ache	Dyspnea, cough, hemoptysis, leg swelling, risk factor
Pneumothorax	Sudden, sharp, pleuritic	Dyspnea, cough
Pneumomediastinum	Variable	Risks: cocaine, COPD, iatrogenic procedures
Pneumonia	Sharp, pleuritic	Cough, fever, dyspnea
Pleuritis	Sharp, pleuritic	Cough, fever
Mediastinitis	Variable	Fever, dyspnea, sepsis
Tumor	Chronic, variable	Weight loss
ESOPHAGEAL		
Rupture: Boerhaave's	Sudden, severe	Vomiting, hematemesis
Esophageal spasm	Similar to AMI	Reflux, nausea
Reflux esophagitis	Burning, worse supine	Reflux, nausea, sore throat
ABDOMINAL DISORDERS		
Gastrointestinal	Constant, related to food	Vomiting, abdominal pain, GI bleeding
Cholecystitis	Constant or colicky	Vomiting, abdominal pain, jaundice, fever
Ruptured ectopic pregnancy	Sharp, pleuritic	Abdominal pain, vaginal bleeding, shoulder pain
MUSCULOSKELETAL		
Ruptured cervical disc	Pain on neck movement	Neurologic signs, pain referred in root distribution
Costochondritis	Sharp, pleuritic	Localized tenderness and inflammation
Herpes zoster	Burning, lancinating	Dermatomal distribution of pain, rash, paresthesias
Postherpetic neuralgia	Burning, lancinating	History of zoster

Stuttering presentations may last 12 to 24 hours. Determining the onset of constant pain is essential in deciding whether the patient is eligible for thrombolytic therapy. Dyspnea, diaphoresis, nausea, and weakness are frequently associated symptoms. Occasionally, pain is felt only in a referred area, such as the arm, or via the vagus nerve, in the ear. Elderly and diabetic patients often present without pain, and this diagnosis must be suspected with the presentation of syncope or confusion.[1]

Pain features not suggestive of AMI include stabbing, knifelike sensations or radiation to areas outside of cervicothoracic nerve segments, such as the legs or flanks.[5] Very brief pain (lasting less than 5 seconds) or pain that is clearly pleuritic or exactly reproduced by bending or palpation is not likely to be of cardiac origin.[12]

The pain of angina is similar to that of AMI but is of shorter duration. A clear exertional pattern is helpful to the diagnosis; pain can also be provoked by effort, emotion, or exposure to cold. Prompt relief within 5 minutes from sublingual nitroglycerin is suggestive of angina but can also occur with esophageal spasm or placebo. Pain that is relieved with exertion and brought on by rest is not anginal. Angina is unstable when it increases in severity (duration, intensity, frequency), occurs with reduced activity or at rest, or has been present for less than 4 weeks. This diagnosis requires hospital admission.

Aortic dissection classically produces a severe tearing pain in the anterior chest radiating to the back, flank, or arm. The patient sometimes feels pain traveling down the back as the dissection extends distally. Its onset is sudden, but it may be intermittent or wax and wane. Uncommonly, it presents as a myocardial infarction or as a chronic pain that has become worse. The pain has no relieving factors, and writhing, diaphoresis, dyspnea, nausea, and vomiting are commonly associated. Associated symptoms, such as weakness, paralysis, syncope, and numbness or pain in an extremity, are also common and more specific for dissection.

Pericarditis produces a sharp or aching pain in the precordium that may radiate to the scapula, neck, or shoulder. Unlike AMI, it has a long duration (days), and can be continuous and severe. It is usually made worse by lying down or breathing (thus the associated "shortness of breath"). Patients may insist on leaning forward to make themselves more comfortable.

Myocarditis can present with associated pericarditis. It also uncommonly masquerades as a myocardial infarction.[13] Antecedent viral illness and younger age are diagnostic clues, but an in-hospital evaluation is necessary for definitive diagnosis of this uncommon cause of chest pain.

The most common presentation of pulmonary embolism (PE) is dyspnea, pleuritic pain, or hemoptysis.[20] About 85% of cases of PE present with one or more of these nonspecific symptoms. Tachypnea is common, but tachycardia is found in only a minority of proven cases of PE. Large pulmonary emboli can produce circulatory collapse with syncope due to acute pulmonary hypertension and right heart failure. PE is mistaken for AMI about 7% of the time.[19] Chest pain that is strictly reproducible is not consistent with PE.

Pneumothorax may produce a severe, sudden stabbing pain in the affected side, or it may be asymptomatic. It has no characteristic pain radiation. It is made worse by breathing, is relieved by splinting, and is associated with shortness of breath and nonproductive cough. Pleurisy, an inflammation of the parietal pleura, is similar but does not have the associated symptoms or radiographic findings. Pneumonia can also cause pleuritic pain, but its association with productive cough, shortness of breath (at rest or exertion), and fever is a helpful differentiating feature.

Pain may be due to an esophageal source. Pain from esophageal spasm is often indistinguishable from angina in quality, intensity, location, and radiation. Spasm has been described as a perfect mimic of acute ischemia. Esophageal reflux is a midline epigastric discomfort usually described as indigestion or burning. It lasts minutes to hours, and is worse after eating and lying down. It is associated with belching but not shortness of breath, and tends to be chronic.

Relief with antacids does not reliably rule out pain from cardiac ischemia. Esophageal rupture produces pain in the anterior chest, back, or epigastrium. Rupture occurs in the setting of increased barotrauma from retching or prolonged vomiting or coughing. Vomiting that occurs before the pain suggests esophageal rupture, not AMI.[14] Dysphagia and occasionally hemoptysis are the initial symptoms. Life-threatening mediastinitis and sepsis develop if esophageal rupture goes untreated.

MAJOR EMERGENCY ENTITIES

The following immediately or potentially life threatening diseases of the thoracic organ systems must be considered in every patient who presents to the emergency department with chest pain.

Acute Myocardial Infarction and Ischemia

Occlusion of a coronary vessel resulting in death of heart muscle can present as a catastrophic condition, with malignant dysrhythmias, pump failure, or myocardial rupture, or as a completely compensated minimally painful state. It is by far the most common chest pain emergency, accounting for 40 of 1000 hospital admissions.[2] Although the Framingham study risk factors of smoking, hypertension, diabetes, family history, and elevated cholesterol further increase the likelihood of developing AMI or angina over a period of years, they are not helpful in making the diagnosis in the acute care setting. Nevertheless, the physician should document, for medicolegal purposes, the presence of risk factors in all patients with chest pain. The symptoms of coronary vasospasm may be very similar to those of AMI or angina due to occlusive disease.

Emergency physicians frequently evaluate pain associated with recent cocaine use. Such patients commonly have vasospasm, and indeed have a lower confirmed rate of myocardial infarction than non–cocaine-related admissions.[3] Vasospastic ischemic pain is more common than AMI.

Electrocardiographically, even in patients without ischemia, ST segment elevation is present nearly 40% of the time due to repolarization abnormalities. Unless the presentation of AMI is classic, these abnormal baseline findings make it helpful to have an old ECG without ST elevation, or serial ECGs showing evolving ST elevation in the emergency department, before deciding to give thrombolytic therapy.

Thrombolytic therapy, percutaneous coronary interventions, adjunctive treatment with antithrombotic and antiplatelet agents, and treatment in the coronary care unit have significantly lowered case fatality and reinfarction rates, making it imperative to diagnose AMI in the emergency department. Unstable angina is just as important to recognize, because 10% to 20% of confirmed cases proceed to infarction. Heparin, glycoprotein IIB/IIIA and ACE inhibitors, and vasodilators, or more invasive procedures such as coronary revascularization and intraaortic balloon pumping, may be required to treat recurrent pain or associated heart failure or shock.

Dissection of the Thoracic Aorta

This disruption in the intimal layer of the aorta allows blood to track between the media and adventitia. Aortic rupture is an ever-present threat. Untreated dissection has a mortality rate of 90%; fortunately, it is responsible for fewer than 1 in 1000 hospital admissions.[2] Progression of the dissection can cause severe organ damage to the spine, brain, kidneys, bowel, and heart, including AMI and cardiac tamponade. The patient must be carefully examined for evidence of these complications. Hypertension is the most common risk factor, although younger patients with Marfan or Ehlers-Danlos syndromes may have dissection due to cystic medial necrosis.

Pulmonary Embolism

Pulmonary embolism (PE) is an obstruction of the pulmonary arterial system due to clot, which usually embolizes from deep femoral or pelvic veins. In addition to dyspnea, pleuritic pain, and hemoptysis, it can produce acute respiratory failure or right-sided heart failure, as evidenced by cyanosis, hypotension, increased jugular venous pressure, and a loud S2 or right heart gallop. The hospitalization rate is 2 in 1000.[2] Mortality from PE itself is uncommon and is usually due to recurrent emboli. Recognition of such predisposing conditions as immobilization, recent surgery, hypercoagulability, and low-flow circulatory states is critical to raising the clinician's diagnostic suspicion. A high degree of suspicion is especially important, because PE often presents with subtle, nonspecific findings.[22]

Tension Pneumothorax and Esophageal Rupture

Tension pneumothorax occurs when air escapes from the lung into the thoracic cavity, shifting the mediastinum to one side and compromising right-sided heart filling. Dyspnea, diaphoresis, tachycardia, tachypnea, and hypotension commonly result. Jugular vein distention, tracheal deviation, decreased breath sounds, and percussion tympany are noted on physical examination. Pneumothorax may be spontaneous or secondary to trauma, infection (such as tuberculosis and AIDS), or the rupture of emphysematous blebs. Patients with tension pneumothorax require immediate needle thoracostomy and subsequent placement of a chest tube.

Esophageal rupture can occur in the cervical esophagus, but it usually occurs in the distal esophagus. Conditions associated with retching, vomiting, and coughing, such as ethanol abuse, hyperemesis gravidarum, and status asthmaticus, predispose patients to this rare but important disease.[21]

DIAGNOSTIC APPROACH

After verifying or establishing initial patient stability, the diagnostic approach proceeds from a consideration of age, sex, specific clinical presentation, and preexisting conditions or risk factors for the specific emergency entities. The history and physical examination are essential for differentiating these entities and detecting their complications.

The chest x-ray is key to the detection of pneumothorax, heart failure, pneumonia, and a widened mediastinum, as seen in aortic dissection. Mediastinal or subcutaneous air can be a clue to devastating conditions such as mediastinitis or esophageal rupture. Diagnosis of certain entities may require more advanced imaging modalities, such as CT scanning, MRI, angiography, or cardiography. Transesophageal echocardiography is sensitive, specific, and practical for the emergency department diagnosis of aortic dissection.[9]

Diagnosing PE continues to be clinically challenging.[22] Arterial blood gas studies are useful to assess the severity of hypoxemia and response to therapy. A normal PO_2 is present about 10% of the time in the patient with PE. The Prospective Investigation of Pulmonary Embolism Diagnosis (PIOPED) study provided insights into the limitation of the ventilation/perfusion scan.[18] If the clinical presentation and scan results are both high or low probability, the diagnosis can be confirmed or excluded with a high degree of confidence.

If the clinical probability is intermediate or high, then a low-probability or even a normal scan does not rule out PE, and angiography is suggested. More recently, new algorithms for the evaluation of suspected PE include testing for the predisposing deep venous thrombosis using ultrasound.[8,11,15,22] Newer tests that appear promising for patients with nondiagnostic ventilation/perfusion scans include thin-slice spiral CT scans of the chest and quantitative D-dimer assays.[6,10]

A 12-lead ECG may be of significant diagnostic value in many of the clinical entities under consideration when determining the cause of chest pain. In the patient with AMI, it may also help to guide therapy. On ECG, regional ST elevation of 1 mm (0.1 mV) in two leads is a requirement for the administration of thrombolytic therapy. ST segment depression in leads opposite (i.e., reciprocal) to the ST segment elevation is helpful in confirming subtle ST elevation. Diffuse ST elevation with associated PR depression (most frequent in lead II) suggests pericarditis; low-voltage or electrical alternans suggests an effusion. In PE, the ECG most commonly shows T-wave inversions in the anterior leads.[19] Serial ECGs may be useful with recurrent pain or to detect AMI evolution or reperfusion.

The emergency department ECG is a simple prognostic indicator for in-hospital complications. In stable, pain-free patients who are being admitted to rule out AMI, an ECG without ST segment changes, Q waves, T-wave inversion, or left bundle branch block is associated with a very low (less than 1%) incidence of life-threatening complications. When an ST segment elevation of 0.1 mV is present in the right ventricular lead V4R in the setting of inferior AMI, suggesting coincident right ventricular infarction, complication rates are higher than when it is absent.[23]

Diagnostic decision tools, such as an algorithm for risk assessment in AMI[5] or a single numerical probability for acute ischemia,[16] have been developed and validated. More recently, Goldman and associates have developed and tested a new algorithm for predicting short-term complication rates using ECG findings, presence of heart failure, low blood pressure, and worsening angina.[4]

New approaches to the potentially ischemic patient in the emergency department are being implemented, such as the use of serial cardiac markers, continuous 12-lead ECGs, and early provocative testing (e.g., stress-testing the patient on an exercise treadmill).[17,24] These are well suited for an "emergency chest pain center," a program of the emergency department organized specifically for treating and ruling out coronary syndromes.

The diagnostic value of the cardiac troponins is well established, but myoglobin has yet to find its diagnostic niche. Resting sestamibi scanning is an excellent modality for risk stratification, but emergency echocardiography to assess regional wall motion abnormalities has yet to find its role. These technologies were comprehensively reviewed in a recent NIH report.[25] It is hoped that these techniques will advance our ability to diagnose and exclude AMI and acute ischemia in the emergency department.

References

1. Bayer AJ, Chadha IS, Farag RR, et al. Changing presentation of myocardial infarction with increasing old age. *J Am Geriatr Soc* 1986;34:263.
2. Ehxhauser A, Andrews RM, Fox SF. Clinical classifications for health policy research: discharge statistics by principal diagnosis and procedure. *Agency Health Care Policy Res* 1993;93:43.

3. Gitter MJ, Goldsmith SR, Dunbar DN, et al. Cocaine and chest pain: clinical features and outcome of patients hospitalized to rule out myocardial infarction. *Ann Intern Med* 1991;115:277.
4. Goldman L, Cook EF, Johnson PA, et al. Prediction of the need for intensive care in patients who come to emergency departments with acute chest pain. *N Engl J Med* 1996;334:1498–1504.
5. Goldman L, Cook EF, Brand DA, et al. A computer protocol to predict myocardial infarction in emergency department patients with chest pain. *N Engl J Med* 1988;318:797.
6. Holbert JM, Costello P, Federle MP. Role of spiral computed tomography in the diagnosis of pulmonary embolism in the emergency department. *Ann Emerg Med* 1999;33:520–528.
7. Horwitz L, Groves B. *Signs and symptoms in cardiology*. Philadelphia: JB Lippincott Co, 1985:5.
8. Hull RD, Feldstein W, Pineo GF, et al. Cost effectiveness of diagnosis of deep vein thrombosis in symptomatic patients. *Thromb Haemost* 1995;74:189–196.
9. Hwang JJ, Shyu KG, Chen JJ, et al. Usefulness of transesophageal echocardiography in the treatment of critically ill patients. *Chest* 1993;104:861.
10. Janssen MCH, Heebels AE, deMetz M, et al. Reliability of five rapid D-dimer assays compared to ELISA in the exclusion of deep venous thrombosis. *Thromb Haemost* 1997;77:262–266.
11. Kearon C, Ginsberg JS, Hirsh J. The role of venous ultrasonography in the diagnosis of suspected deep venous thrombosis and pulmonary embolism. *Ann Intern Med* 1998;129:1044–1049.
12. Lee TH, Cook EF, Weisberg M, et al. Acute chest pain in the emergency room. *Arch Intern Med* 1985;65:60.
13. Narula-Jagat AU, Khaw-Ban AN, William DEC Jr, et al. Recognition of acute myocarditis masquerading as acute myocardial infarction. *N Engl J Med* 1993;328:100.
14. Nehra D, Beynon J, Pye JK. Spontaneous rupture of the oesophagus (Boerhaave's syndrome). *Postgrad Med J* 1933;59:214.
15. Perrier A, Desmarais S, Miron M, et al. Non-invasive diagnosis of venous thromboembolism in outpatients. *Lancet* 1999;353:190–195.
16. Selker HP, Beshansky JR, Griffit JL, et al. Use of the acute cardiac ischemia time-insensitive predictive instrument to assist with triage of patients with chest pain or other symptoms suggestive of acute cardiac ischemia. A multicenter, controlled trial. *Ann Intern Med* 1998;129:845–855.
17. Roberts RR, Zalenski RJ, Mensah EK, et al. Costs of an emergency department-based accelerated diagnostic protocol vs hospitalization in patients with chest pain. *JAMA* 1997;278:1670–1676.
18. Saltzman HA, Abass A, Greenspan RH, et al. Value of the ventilation/perfusion scan in acute pulmonary embolism. *JAMA* 1990;263:2754.
19. Sashara AA, Hyers TM, Cole CM, et al. The urokinase pulmonary embolism trial: a national cooperative study. *Circulation* 1990;47:11–86.
20. Stein PD, Terrin ML, Hales CA, et al. Clinical, laboratory, roentgenographic, and electrocardiographic findings in patients with acute pulmonary embolism and no pre-existing cardiac or pulmonary disease. *Chest* 1991;199:598.
21. Taylor MB. *Gastrointestinal emergencies*. Baltimore: Williams & Wilkins, 1992:24.
22. Wells PS, Ginsberg JS, Anderson DR, et al. Use of a clinical model for safe management of patients with suspected pulmonary embolism. *Ann Intern Med* 1998;129:997–1005.
23. Zalenski RJ, Rydman RJ, Sloan EP, et al. The emergency department electrocardiogram and hospital complications in myocardial infarction patients. *Acad Emerg Med* 1996;3:318–325.
24. Zalenski RJ, McCarren M, Roberts F, et al. An evaluation of a chest pain diagnostic protocol to exclude acute cardiac ischemia in the emergency department. *Arch Intern Med* 1997;157:1085–1091.

CHAPTER 2
Abdominal Pain

Beth Anne DeGennaro and Sheldon Jacobson

Evaluation of the patient with abdominal pain is one of the frequent problems encountered in emergency medicine, and one of the most challenging. The difficulties related to evaluation stem from several factors. Diverse processes involving intraabdominal as well as extraabdominal diseases may give rise to pain patterns that are similar because of the manner in which abdominal pain is perceived. Most conditions that produce abdominal pain usually evolve over time: Localizing signs or other significant acute intraabdominal symptoms acquire a characteristic pattern that will permit specific diagnosis.

PATHOPHYSIOLOGY

Pain produced by disease of the intraabdominal organs is either visceral or deep somatic. The afferent visceral neurons are mainly of the small C-fiber unmyelinated type that ascend in the sympathetic chain. The fibers enter the spinal cord by way of the dorsal root ganglia and travel with the somatic sensory fibers to the cerebral cortex.

Stimulation of the visceral afferent fibers, usually by chemical irritants or distention, is perceived as a poorly localized, aching pain. In general, visceral pain is referred to the abdominal wall in relation to the embryonic origin of the diseased organ. Diseases of organ systems derived from the embryonic foregut (the stomach, duodenum, liver, and pancreas) cause upper abdominal or epigastric pain. Midgut processes (the small bowel and right colon) present with periumbilical pain. Diseases of the hindgut-derived structure (the distal colon and urogenital system) cause lower abdominal pain.

Deep somatic pain results from irritation of the parietal peritoneum and mesenteric root. These structures are innervated by myelinated sensory afferent fibers distributed by way of the segmental peripheral nerves. Deep somatic pain is intense and well localized. The early periumbilical pain of appendicitis is typical of visceral pain, whereas the right lower quadrant pain caused by local peritoneal irritation is a deep somatic pain.

ORGAN SYSTEMS

The intraabdominal structures that give rise to abdominal discomfort are complex and varied. Pain may arise from perturbation of the intestinal tract, the biliary tree, the pancreas, the genitourinary system, the vascular system, the abdominal wall and its apertures, the vertebral bodies, and segmental nerves.

Abdominal pain can also be referred from contiguous body cavities or from distant sites. Thus, a patient with basilar pneumonia may present with abdominal pain, or a patient with an inferior myocardial infarction may present with epigastric distress.

Toxic-metabolic and systemic diseases can cause abdominal pain. Some of these are diabetic ketoacidosis, lead intoxication, porphyria, vasculitis, neurosyphilis, and familial Mediterranean fever.

DIFFERENTIAL DIAGNOSIS

In taking the history, note the nature of the onset of pain. Patients who have a rapid onset of severe pain with minimal time for pain buildup should be assumed to have a ruptured viscus until proven otherwise. It may represent a perforated peptic ulcer, a ruptured ectopic pregnancy, or a ruptured colonic diverticulum. In women the menstrual history must be documented, and menstruating patients with acute abdominal pain must be evaluated as if they have an ectopic pregnancy until proven otherwise.

Associated signs and symptoms may be as important as the pain pattern itself. Thus, the presence of vomiting and the type of vomitus and the presence of diarrhea, blood in the stool, obstipation, fever, dysuria, vaginal discharge, and vaginal bleeding must be determined.

Often, a logical sequence of events and associated signs and symptoms are fairly consistent among patients who undergo the same abdominal process. Patients with small bowel obstruction develop abdominal distention, nausea, and bloating, followed by vomiting, periumbilical colicky pain, and only late loss of bowel sounds and obstipation. The initial signs and symptoms are nonspecific and may be confused with those of gastritis or other nonspecific gastrointestinal infections. The evolution of the process, however, is fairly typical when taken in context.

The history should also detail the type, location, pattern, and referral of the pain; relieving and exacerbating factors; and prior occurrences. Note underlying significant medical problems and prior surgical problems and procedures. Therapeutic and recreational drug and alcohol use should be carefully defined. Finally, as with all emergency department patients, document avocational and vocational exposures.

The physical examination should include a rectal temperature, full vital signs including orthostatic vital signs, a cardiopulmonary evaluation, a genitourinary examination, an examination for hernias, and a complete abdominal and rectal examination.

The abdominal examination is much less precise than the cardiac and pulmonary evaluation because of the diffuse nature of visceral pain and in no small part because of the variability of pain thresholds. The patient presenting with a rigid abdomen, absent bowel sounds, and classic "peritoneal" signs offers little difficulty, but this classic presentation of the acute surgical abdomen is relatively uncommon.

The abdominal examination begins with the observation of the patient's position and breathing. This often neglected aspect of the clinical examination can yield vital information. One should be able to answer the following questions: Is the patient in respiratory distress? Is the abdomen distended? Does the abdomen move with respiration? Is there voluntary or involuntary guarding? Is there visible peristalsis? Is there evidence of an abnormal vascular pattern? Are the legs kept flexed? Is the patient icteric?

Auscultation of the abdomen for the presence or absence of bowel sounds is useful for diagnosing obstruction and perforation, but localization of bowel sounds to a specific quadrant of the abdomen is not. The presence of systolic rushes temporally associated with the patient's colicky pain can help in the diagnosis of early intestinal obstruction. The physician must listen for several minutes before truly saying that the bowel sounds are absent. In general, the statement that the patient has diminished or hyperactive bowel sounds has no intrinsic meaning except as an indication that bowel sounds are present.

In a patient with a distended abdomen and absent bowel sounds, "peritoneal irritation" becomes the major diagnostic entity; next, carry out light percussion of the abdomen to define areas of tenderness. Also, in a patient suspected of having ruptured a viscus, it is helpful to percuss the right upper quadrant for liver dullness, because liver dullness may be absent with free intraabdominal air. A false-positive sign can be seen, however, when a distended hepatic flexure overlies the liver. If peritoneal irritation is not suspected, percussion can be limited to the evaluation for hepatomegaly and splenomegaly, and for tympany in the case of bowel obstruction and distention.

Then proceed directly with light palpation for organomegaly, tenderness, and masses. If the patient has minimal discomfort with light palpation, the pressure should be gradually increased until the pressure itself becomes slightly uncomfortable. The examiner should attempt to localize the discomfort further by having the patient grade each sector of the abdomen. The presence of referred tenderness is an important sign of localized peritoneal irritation. In appendicitis, deep palpation in the left lower quadrant can cause discomfort referred to McBurney's point (Rovsing's sign).

Next, examine the patient for inguinal, umbilical, femoral, and ventral hernias. The umbilical, inguinal, and femoral rings should be defined and explored. In all older patients, a bimanual examination of the epigastrium for an aortic aneurysm is mandatory. The pelvic and rectal examinations, including heme testing of stool, are then performed.

An intraabdominal source of discomfort must be differentiated from pain originating in the abdominal wall from such diverse conditions as a rectus muscle hematoma, a segmental neuropathy, or an internal hernia within the abdominal wall. This differentiation is facilitated by having a patient perform either a sit-up or a leg lift (Carnett's test). Deep palpation of the abdomen is performed while the patient is maintaining the maneuver. If the process is in the abdominal wall, the discomfort of palpation is increased, but with pain originating within the abdomen the discomfort is decreased. Once a full examination is performed, it is essential to remember that serial examinations of the abdomen are often the most helpful adjunct to the diagnosis and treatment of abdominal pain.

MAJOR EMERGENCY ENTITIES

Several abdominal conditions require immediate or urgent surgical intervention. Perforated viscus, ruptured abdominal aortic aneurysm, acute appendicitis, ischemic bowel, and strangulated hernia are included in this group. Identification of entities that mandate such emergent surgical care is imperative, and delays in diagnosis may prove costly. In addition, some conditions (e.g., small bowel obstruction and acute pancreatitis), although they may not necessarily require surgery, must be identified expeditiously so that hospitalization and appropriate supportive care can prevent morbidity and allow treatment of comorbid conditions.

About 50% of patients who present to an emergency department with abdominal pain cannot be diagnosed on the initial visit. Most of these patients have a minor, self-limiting illness for which a specific diagnosis is not possible or even necessary. Some patients, however, have a subacute presentation of a serious surgical or medical illness, and these patients must not be lost to follow-up. Having the same physician who established the initial baseline data follow the patient ensures that subtle changes will be readily detected.

If the patient is to be followed by a consultant, this person must see the patient in the emergency department before discharge or immediately after discharge. Follow-up should be as often as every 12 hours if the patient is not improving. If follow-up cannot be arranged or if patient compliance is an issue, the patient should be admitted to the hospital.

Because of the difficulty in evaluating these patients and the large number of possible diagnostic entities and pitfalls to diagnosis, an approach has evolved that casts a wide safety net and, it is hoped, minimizes the potential for serious errors or delays in diagnosis. In several situations, however, there is a high potential for serious errors in diagnosis and management. Patients in the "coronary-prone years" with upper abdominal pain must have an immediate electrocardiogram and cardiopulmonary examination in a manner completely analogous to the approach to patients who present with chest pain (see Chapter 1). The patient who presents with a leaking abdominal aortic aneurysm is often misdiagnosed on initial evaluation. To prevent this serious lapse in diagnosis, all older patients should have a bimanual examination for an upper abdominal expansile mass. In addition, all older patients presenting with an initial episode of "renal colic," usually with left flank as well as upper abdominal pain, should have an immediate emergency study to rule out a leaking aortic aneurysm.

The relative frequency of ectopic pregnancy requires that all premenopausal patients have a thorough evaluation for this condition. Patients with ruptured ectopic pregnancies can present with shock, shoulder pain, diffuse abdominal pain, and right upper quadrant pain, as well as with the typically localized lower quadrant pain.

DIAGNOSTIC APPROACH

Initial evaluation of any patient with abdominal pain must include a thorough history, a physical, and baseline laboratory studies. The most important issues in the history are the pain pattern and associated signs and symptoms. The diagnosis is evident in approximately one half of patients after this part of the evaluation is complete.

Most of the diagnostic tests available to the emergency physician that help to support acute evaluations are neither sensitive nor specific enough to play a significant role in the evaluation process. However, exceptions to this rule (such as the finding of free intraperitoneal air on the abdominal film) do exist. All diagnostic studies must be used judiciously in conjunction with a full history and physical exam. An initial evaluation plan should include a complete blood count, keeping in mind that a normal white blood cell count should not dissuade you from ordering a further workup; an increased white count will increase your suspicion for serious pathology.

All patients need a urinalysis, and all premenopausal women with abdominal pain should have a pregnancy test. Most patients require measurement of glucose, electrolyte, blood urea nitrogen, and creatinine levels to help guide fluid and electrolyte repletion, to provide a baseline for those who will receive intravenous medications or contrast media, and to assist in the diagnosis of metabolic disturbances that can present with abdominal pain. Determination of the serum lipase level is useful when pancreatitis is considered in the differential diagnosis. A lipase level is a more sensitive and specific test to obtain for suspicion of pancreatitis than an amylase level, as amylase can be produced by several organs and may be elevated in alcoholic patients without pancreatitis.

Serum transaminases, bilirubin, alkaline phosphatase, and a prothrombin time are helpful laboratory tests in patients with a tender right upper quadrant when the differential includes hepatitis as well as cholecystitis. Other specialized testing and imaging techniques of the abdomen, such as ultrasonography, CT scanning, and radionuclide scanning of the biliary tree, may be extraordinarily helpful in selected cases.

Plain films of the abdomen are useful in cases in which one is looking for free air in the abdomen and in patients in whom intestinal obstruction is a major consideration. The finding of appendicolithiasis, said to be diagnostic of appendicitis, is uncommon in adults, and its absence should not influence the decision-making process.

More than 90% of renal calculi are radiopaque; therefore, an abdominal film, in combination with ultrasonography, is helpful when considering the diagnosis of renal colic. An intravenous pyelogram or helical noncontrast CT should be obtained to confirm the diagnosis. Helical CT offers the added benefit of viewing other organ systems and is very helpful in evaluating the presence of an abdominal aortic aneurysm (AAA) and appendicitis.

Ultrasound has emerged as a useful bedside adjunct in the emergency department. Right upper quadrant scans will help in the diagnosis of gallstones and acute cholecystitis. Abdominal aortic aneurysms may be identifiable by ultrasound. Ultrasound remains the invaluable test of choice for rapid identification of ectopic pregnancies. Used in conjunction with KUB plain films, ultrasound can also be helpful in the evaluation of renal colic.

Helical CT scans are useful in the diagnosis of renal colic, appendicitis, diverticulitis, abdominal abscesses, and AAA. These exams may be performed with or without contrast, depending on the diagnosis in question and the patient's renal function. While the helical CT is a very useful tool, the emergency physician must remember not to send an unstable patient out of the department for this evaluation unless appropriate monitoring can be maintained.

Approximately 50% of patients will not have a definitive diagnosis made on their first visit. Patients in this group are usually not sick enough to require hospitalization and are followed as outpatients. After discharge, the problem remits spontaneously in most patients; a few (8% to 10%) continue to have pain and require further evaluation. In this group, a diagnosis is made on the basis of findings on diagnostic studies and reexamination. The choice of which imaging techniques to use is made on an individual basis: They include CT scanning, biliary imaging, intravenous urography, and upper and lower gastrointestinal series. At this point, peptic ulcer disease may be definitely diagnosed, and unsuspected pancreatic or biliary tract disease uncovered. Here, too, an occasional patient with inflammatory bowel disease has this diagnosis made based on radiographic or endoscopic findings. For persistent abdominal pain of unknown origin, diagnostic laparoscopy may prove to be useful.

The elderly patient who presents with abdominal complaints can become a diagnostic dilemma. Such patients may have intraabdominal free air or free pus within the abdomen, with few objective findings until late in their course. A "sluggish" leukocyte and febrile response to infection in the elderly may compound this diagnostic challenge. Elderly patients with ill-defined abdominal pain should also be evaluated for an ischemic bowel syndrome. The initial presentation of ischemic bowel is often that of midabdominal pain associated with nausea and vomiting and minimal objective findings. Metabolic acidosis is a characteristic early concomitant. If there is evidence of metabolic acidosis, an ileus pattern is present on the abdominal film, and no other diagnosis is probable, then immediate surgical consultation is mandatory. Early angiographic and surgical intervention should reduce the very high mortality of this condition.

Some patients initially diagnosed as having gastroenteritis return with the classic findings of acute appendicitis or small bowel obstruction. A patient with gastroenteritis must have gastritis, manifested by vomiting, and enteritis, manifested by diarrhea. If the diagnosis of gastroenteritis is made without evidence of both upper and lower gastrointestinal involvement, the diagnostic accuracy is questionable, and major surgical conditions can be overlooked.

Once a definitive diagnosis has been made, few would argue against administering a potent analgesic agent to the patient with severe abdominal pain. The dogma that the "premature" administration of an analgesic agent may alter the abdominal examination and delay the diagnostic process is clearly incorrect. Several studies have shown that analgesia actually may help evaluation and diagnosis by decreasing patient anxiety, thus allowing a more accurate physical examination. Of course, if one is following a patient sequentially, the administration of analgesics requires that a new baseline be established for purposes of comparison. Exercise caution when discharging any patient with undiagnosed abdominal pain who has received narcotics for pain control.

COMMON PITFALLS

- Formulating a definitive diagnosis can be extremely difficult, for the aforementioned reasons. In addition, the difficulty in diagnosing more occult processes often results in a delay in diagnosis. Indeed, it is far better to follow these patients without a diagnostic label while workup is being pursued than to mislabel them initially. Once a patient is given a diagnostic label, extraordinary efforts and circumstances may be required before the erroneous label is reconsidered.

Bibliography

Aach RD. Abdominal pain. In: MacBryde CM, Blacklow RS, eds. *Signs and symptoms*, 6th ed. Philadelphia: JB Lippincott Co, 1983.

Bughosim TF, Milloy TD, Vukor LE. Acute abdominal pain in the elderly. *Ann Emerg Med* 1990;19:1383.

Chase CW, Barker DE, Russell WL, et al. Serum amylase and lipase in the evaluation of acute abdominal pain. *Am Surg* 1996;62(12):1028–1033.

Colucciello SA, Lukens TW, Morgan DL. Assessing abdominal pain in adults: a rational, cost-effective, and evidence-based strategy. *Emerg Med Pract* 1999;1(1).

Easter DW, Cuschieri A, Nathanson LK. The utility of diagnostic laparoscopy for abdominal disorder of 120 patients. *Arch Surg* 1992;127:379.

Graam A, Henby C, Mobley J. Laparoscopic evaluation of acute abdominal pain. *J Laparosc Surg* 1991;1:165.

LoVecchio F, Oster N, Sturmann K, et al. The use of analgesics in patients with acute abdominal pain. *J Emerg Med* 1997;15(6):775–779.

Pace S, Burke TF. Intravenous morphine for early pain relief in patients with acute abdominal pain. *Acad Emerg Med* 1996;3(12):1086–1092.

Rao PM, Rhea JT, Novelline RA, et al. Helical CT technique for the diagnosis of appendicitis: prospective evaluation of a focused CT appendix examination. *Radiology* 1997;202:139–144.

Reynolds SL, Jaffee DM. Diagnosing abdominal pain in a pediatric emergency department. *Pediatr Emerg Care* 1992;8(3):126.

Simmen HP, Secrutins M, Ratzer A. Emergency room patients with abdominal pain unrelated to trauma: prospective analysis in a surgical university service. *Hepatogastroenterology* 1991;38:279.

Spiro HM. An internist's approach to acute abdominal pain. *Med Clin North Am* 1993;77:963.

Walters DT et al. Abdominal pain. *Prim Care* 1986:13:3.

CHAPTER 3
Cough

Frank Birinyi and Douglas A. Rund

Cough is a common symptom faced by emergency department physicians. Often, the history and physical examination provide a diagnosis, effective treatment is recommended, and the patient is discharged home. In other situations, cough may herald a serious underlying condition, and hospital admission is required.

Cough is a protective mechanism. Along with the mucociliary elevator, cough acts to clear secretions and foreign material from the respiratory tree. Physiologically, the act of coughing is a reflex, initiated by stimulation of cough receptors. Receptors lie predominantly within the proximal portions of the pulmonary tree: the larynx, trachea, and larger bronchi. Smaller populations reside within the terminal bronchioles, as well as in the pharynx, sinuses, pleura, pericardium, and diaphragm. Receptors are activated by various factors: excess mucus production, environmental irritants (cigarette smoke, noxious gases, dust, allergens), aspiration, inflammation (secondary to microbial invasion), or thermal factors (hot or cold air). Cough receptors can also be mechanically stimulated by pressure or extrinsic tension exerted by tumor, adenopathy, or aortic aneurysm. Stimulation of cough receptors gives rise to afferents that are conveyed centrally by the vagus, glossopharyngeal, trigeminal, and phrenic nerves. A discrete central cough center has not been demonstrated.

The typical cough consists of an initial deep inspiratory phase. This is followed by glottic closure, contraction of the thoracic and abdominal expiratory muscles, and an increase in the intrapulmonary pressures. The sudden opening of the glottis provides for the explosive expiration of air at high velocities, with subsequent clearance of secretions and foreign particles. These high velocities vibrate the vocal cords, secretions, tracheobronchial walls, and adjacent lung parenchyma, creating the characteristic sound of a cough.[3]

CLINICAL PRESENTATION

A cough productive of purulent sputum is generally a reliable indication of infection within the respiratory tract. Infections involving the most proximal portion include sinusitis, pharyngitis, rhinitis, and the common cold. Although these infections are usually associated with a productive cough, initially the cough may be nonproductive. More distal infections include bronchitis, pneumonia, and abscess. With viral etiologies, the sputum is usually clear or mucoid; purulent sputum suggests bacterial involvement.

A predominantly nonproductive cough is usually seen with the inhalation of environmental irritants and nonrespiratory sources of cough. These include masses that exert extrinsic pressure on the trachea and bronchi, such as an aneurysm, tumor, foreign body, and adenopathy. Less common etiologies of cough include irritation of the diaphragm, pleura, or pericardium.

DIFFERENTIAL DIAGNOSIS

Cough and its character are not diagnostic. It is the association of cough with other signs and symptoms that is usually suggestive of the underlying pathology.

Urgent Causes

Chest pain (not associated with the cough itself) or dyspnea generally accompanies cough when urgent conditions are present. Congestive heart failure, usually of a mild degree, can present with cough as a predominant symptom. A careful history regarding cardiac risk factors, orthopnea, dyspnea, and dyspnea on exertion, along with a careful examination of the lungs and chest x-ray usually clarifies this situation. Pulmonary embolism can also present as cough, but the primary symptoms usually include chest pain (frequently pleuritic) and dyspnea. Another urgent consideration in the patient with cough is foreign body. Choking and stridor are typically present with large foreign bodies in the proximal airway, but cough may be the predominant symptom with a smaller or more distal foreign body.

Acute Causes

Upper Respiratory Tract

The most common etiology for cough in a normal person is a viral upper respiratory tract infection, the common cold. Common symptoms include rhinorrhea and sore throat; fever, chills, sweats, headache, hoarseness, sneezing, postnasal discharge, and constitutional malaise and myalgias may also be seen. Patients in whom severe headache and systemic complaints (myalgias, malaise) predominate are more likely to have influenza. Rhinitis should be considered in patients with significant nasal symptoms. A history of atopy, seasonal exacerbations, itchy and watery eyes, and a profuse thin rhinorrhea suggests an allergic rhinitis. Patients with conjunctival injection along with their cough, pharyngitis, fever, headache, myalgia, and malaise may have pharyngoconjunctival fever, typically caused by adenovirus.

Patients with sinusitis complain of head congestion, fullness, toothache, headache, or facial pain. They may or may not have rhinorrhea or postnasal drainage. Patients with laryngitis typically develop hoarseness and frequently have associated infection, either above or below the vocal cords. Cough secondary to tracheitis or tracheobronchitis is typically associated with substernal burning. Patients who have had a tonsillectomy occasionally develop lingual tonsillitis and complain of dysphagia, odynophagia, and a foreign-body sensation.

Lower Respiratory Tract

Acute bronchitis is a common cause of cough (or change in chronic cough) in emergency department patients. Sputum production is a hallmark of bronchitis. Hemoptysis can be caused by vigorous coughing in bronchitis, but it also raises the suspicion of pneumonia, pulmonary embolism, tumor, bronchiectasis, or tuberculosis. Productive sputum is also suggestive of pneumonia. Pain is not an unusual symptom in pneumonia, and not uncommonly precipitates the emergency department visit. In patients with pneumonia, the clinical appearance varies widely. Pneumococcal pneumonia, classically characterized by rust-colored sputum, presents with fever and shaking chills; the patient appears ill. Mycoplasmal pneumonia, on the other hand, is typically associated with low-grade fever, scanty mucus production, hacking cough, headache, and minimal systemic symptoms; affected patients may wait a week before seeking a medical evaluation. Aspiration pneumonia should be suspected in elderly or obtunded patients. Purulent and putrid sputum suggests an anaerobic infection such as a lung abscess. Sputum that is thick, tenacious, excessive, and difficult to expectorate is seen in bronchiectasis. These patients have a history of poorly treated and recurrent infections, resulting in impaired bronchial clearance and chronic colonization of the airways by microorganisms.

Cough is a symptom that all asthmatics experience as a consequence of their disease. Other symptoms of asthma, which can occur singly or in combination, are chest tightness, wheezing, and dyspnea. Patients with asthmatic bronchitis lack a history of asthma, but present with cough and bronchospasm. These patients, because they are unfamiliar with wheezing, frequently describe their chest as having "congestion." *Cardiac asthma* refers to those patients whose congestive heart failure precipitates bronchospasm.

A wide variety of parenchymal pulmonary infections may manifest cough symptoms. Symptoms of tuberculosis include hemoptysis, weight loss, weakness, and fever. Specific fungal infections are associated with specific geographic regions. Coccidioidomycosis is common in the Southwest, and histoplasmosis in the Ohio and Mississippi River valleys. *Pneumocystis carinii, Mycobacterium tuberculosis,* and *Mycobacterium avium* complex are associated with decreased host resistance from chemotherapy and other forms of immunosuppression, and with underlying HIV infection.

Chronic Causes

Acute illnesses such as the common cold seldom last longer than 3 weeks. Patients who present with symptoms of longer duration should be considered to have chronic cough. Chronic bronchitis is the most common cause of chronic cough. By definition, chronic bronchitis requires a chronic productive cough for 3 months in each of 2 consecutive years.[2] The cough is typically worse on arising in the morning. Superimposed acute infection changes sputum color and quantity. Although tumor can produce a cough, bronchogenic carcinoma is not a common cause of chronic cough. Primary bronchogenic cancer should be suspected in smokers with a change in their cough, persistent hoarseness, clubbing, weight loss, evidence of metastatic disease, or the triad of chest pain, cough, and hemoptysis.

In patients who do not smoke and who have a normal chest x-ray, postnasal drainage is the most frequent cause of chronic cough. This postnasal drainage is usually secondary to sinusitis and rhinitis. The cough is short, frequent, and worse at night or when the patient is supine. Allergic etiologies are associated with seasonal exacerbations. Asthma, in addition to causing acute cough, is another common cause of chronic cough. Cough and wheezing occurs in all asthmatics; however, dry cough without wheezing is the sole symptom of cough-variant asthma. Patients with cough-variant asthma, like classic asthmatics, demonstrate airway hyperresponsiveness with pulmonary function testing.[7] Gastroesophageal reflux disease is also capable of causing a chronic cough as an isolated symptom. Less common etiologies of cough include mediastinal masses such as tumor (thymoma, thyroid cancer, teratoma, neurofibroma, Hodgkin disease, metastatic malignancy) and granulomatous disease (tuberculosis, sarcoid).

Some patients complain of a persistent cough following a respiratory tract infection. This has been described as postinfectious cough, and is attributed to airway inflammation with or without transient airway hyperresponsiveness.[5] The diagnosis is one of exclusion. Pertussis patients initially develop a nonspecific upper respiratory tract infection; as the upper respiratory tract symptoms wane, severe coughing paroxysms develop. Adult pertussis patients, unlike children, lack the characteristic inspiratory whoop at the end of a coughing paroxysm. Cough is an adverse side effect of all angiotensin converting enzyme inhibitors, including captopril (Capoten), lisinopril (Zestril, Prinivil), enalapril (Vasotec), fosinopril (Monopril), quinapril (Accupril), ramipril (Altace), moexipril (Univasc), trandolapril (Mavik), and benazepril (Lotensin).[6]

EMERGENCY DEPARTMENT EVALUATION

History

The most common cause of cough is a viral upper respiratory tract infection, the common cold. The cough is secondary to secretions from the nasopharynx stimulating cough receptors in the hypopharynx and larynx. Therefore, patients should be carefully questioned if the cough represents a throat-clearing maneuver, if they note a sensation of a throat tickle or secretions draining from the back of the nose into the throat, and if there is nasal congestion or discharge. The cough may last 2 to 3 weeks. A cough lasting longer than 3 weeks is unlikely to be an acute viral upper respiratory tract infection, except with back-to-back infections.

Patients with a cough lasting longer than 3 weeks have chronic cough. Chronic bronchitis is the most common etiology. Chronic bronchitis patients invariably have a long history of smoking and usually note a productive cough on awakening. Postnasal drainage, in addition to being the most common cause of an acute cough, is also the most common etiology of chronic cough in patients without chronic bronchitis. Bronchospasm should be suspected in those patients whose cough follows exposure to cold air, strong odors, smoke, or exercise. Gastroesophageal reflux disease is suggested in patients with heartburn, a sour taste in the mouth, and persistent regurgitation. Pertussis should be suspected in patients who present with severe paroxysms of cough following an upper respiratory tract infection.

Sputum production is indicative of a microbial infection

within the respiratory tract. A predominantly nonproductive cough should lead the emergency physician to consider etiologies other than infection. Angiotensin converting enzyme inhibitors are capable of causing a troublesome cough in 6% to 14% of patients taking any of the antihypertensives from this class.[6] Patients with malignancy may have pulmonary metastasis, because the lung is the most common metastatic site.

Physical Examination

A general body habitus demonstrating cachexia and weight loss suggests chronic and potentially life threatening conditions. Abnormal vital signs, such as elevated temperature, tachypnea, abnormal pulse oximetry, and tachycardia, should heighten the suspicion for significant underlying pathology.

With upper respiratory tract infection, the nasopharynx may be swollen and erythematous, with secretions. The oropharynx may have a cobblestone appearance, and drainage or mucus may be seen adherent to the posterior pharyngeal wall. Tonsillar exudates may be seen in pharyngitis. In patients at risk for immunocompromise, the oropharynx should be inspected for candidiasis. Sinusitis presents with sinus tenderness; rhinorrhea may or may not be present. One should palpate the neck for adenopathy secondary to metastasis or infection.

Inspection of the lungs can ascertain an expanded anteroposterior diameter in patients with chronic bronchitis. With an acute exacerbation of chronic bronchitis, retractions (subcostal, intercostal, suprasternal, and supraclavicular) may be noted. Auscultation determines the presence of bronchospasm from any cause, such as asthma, acute or chronic bronchitis, congestive heart failure, pneumonia, or pulmonary embolism. Patients with localized rales may have early consolidation and inflammation from pneumonia; alternatively, the rales may be secondary to proximal obstruction by foreign body, tumor, or adenopathy. Pleural rub is associated with pulmonary embolism, lobar pneumonia, pulmonary infarction, and pleuritis. Breath sounds diminish when any process obstructs sound transmission from the patient's airways to the listener's ears. This finding is due most commonly to pneumonia and pleural effusion. Dullness to percussion clinically confirms this diagnosis. The patient should be examined for adenopathy if there is suspected malignancy, immunocompromise, or HIV infection.

Laboratory and Radiographic Evaluation

The laboratory and radiographic evaluation is dependent on the suspected underlying pathology as well as host factors. A chest x-ray is indicated for those patients with chronic cough, risk factors, significant underlying morbidity, and an abnormal physical examination, and for those with abnormal pulse oximetry. Comparison of current x-ray films with old films may help to make a new diagnosis or measure progression of disease. Pneumonias present not only with frank infiltrates, but also with interstitial patterns and pleural effusions. In the immunocompromised, *Pneumocystis carinii* pneumonia should be suspected in the setting of hypoxia and a normal or near-normal chest x-ray.

Cardiac asthma should be considered in patients with cardiomegaly and increased vascular markings. Aspiration pneumonia is usually seen in the dependent areas of the lung, reflecting the patient's position at the time of the aspiration. Tumor and abscess can also be found. A primary tumor may be subtle, with metastatic disease in the mediastinum more prominent radiographically. Other findings in patients with tumor include atelectasis and pleural effusions. Metastases to the lung parenchyma tend to be multiple and bilateral.

In patients with a change in a chronic cough, a chest x-ray should be obtained in order to eliminate the possibility of a mediastinal tumor or adenopathy. Bronchogenic carcinoma is very unlikely when the chest x-ray is normal. Adenopathy may compress or deviate the trachea and mainstem bronchi. Bilateral hilar adenopathy, frequently out of proportion to a patient's symptoms, may be seen in sarcoidosis. Cavities, with air–fluid levels can be secondary to bacteria, fungi, and tuberculosis. The lung apex is the usual site of tuberculosis. Rib fractures (particularly at the lateral portion of the rib), pneumothorax, and pneumomediastinum are occasionally seen with severe paroxysms of coughing.

Patients without significant underlying illness who present with cough and involvement limited to the upper respiratory tract generally do not require further evaluation beyond the history and physical examination, provided that their vital signs (including pulse oximetry) are normal. On occasion sinus films or soft-tissue neck films are obtained. Sinus films may demonstrate air–fluid levels, and mucosal thickening of the maxillary sinuses may be appreciated in patients with chronic sinusitis. Sinus films may be normal, however, in patients with sinusitis.

Neck films using a soft-tissue technique are helpful when evaluating patients for lingual tonsillitis and epiglottitis. Soft-tissue air on neck films can be seen with pneumomediastinum; these patients complain of neck pain after forceful coughing. The effect of the associated Valsalva maneuver may be rupture of a pulmonary bleb, with dissection of air along the bronchial tree to the mediastinum and subsequently into the neck.

The sputum Gram stain and culture and sensitivity studies are essential for appropriate antibiotic selection and management of infectious pneumonias. If the patient is unable to produce sputum spontaneously, a specimen may be induced by the respiratory therapist. Sputum staining for acid-fast bacilli can be diagnostic, and sputum cytology is a low-risk diagnostic test when neoplasm is suspected. Cultures for pertussis should be obtained from the posterior nasopharynx, using nasopharyngeal swabs.

Blood work may be obtained for emergency department patients felt to be potential admissions. Bacterial infections may result in elevation of the white blood cell count with a left shift, but lack of an elevated count does not exclude bacterial infection. The elderly, particularly in the face of an overwhelming infection, may fail to generate a leukocytosis. A viral infection, on the other hand, manifests lymphocytosis with a normal or depressed white blood cell count. A marked leukocytosis with an increase in lymphocytes characterizes pertussis. An elevated eosinophil count may be seen with parasitic infiltration, eosinophilic pneumonia, or allergies. An arterial blood gas is indicated when pulse oximetry is abnormal. If *Legionella* is suspected, a urine for *Legionella* antigen may be collected.

Immunocompromised adults, especially those with AIDS or at risk for AIDS, should receive a chest x-ray and pulse oximetry. A CD4 count should be drawn if none has been done recently; a CD4 lymphocyte count greater than 200/μL makes clinically significant opportunistic lung infection unlikely.

EMERGENCY DEPARTMENT MANAGEMENT

The emergency department physician should attempt a reasoned approach to determine the underlying cause, because specific therapy of cough has a high likelihood of success. When urgent conditions are present, cough is usually associated with significant dyspnea and chest pain, and the patient appears ill. In these situations, a brief history can be obtained from the paramedics, family, or patient regarding cardiac and pulmonary disease, medications, and similar events in the past. A physical examination can be carried out quickly regarding the body habitus, neck veins, auscultation of the lungs and heart, and peripheral edema. An i.v., supplemental oxygen, and cardiac monitoring, if not already begun by the paramedics, are established immediately.

In nonurgent situations, the basis for management begins with the history and physical examination. An older patient with productive cough, tachypnea, fever, and mental obtundation deserves a prompt portable chest x-ray. An i.v. is established, supplemental oxygen is begun, and labwork, old charts, and old chest-rays are ordered. For patients found to have pneumonia, antibiotics may be started in the emergency department once sputum has been obtained. If a specimen cannot be obtained or induced within 1 hour, antibiotics are nevertheless started. In the elderly with acute cough, it is especially important to have a high index of suspicion for serious disorders such as congestive heart failure, pulmonary embolism, and aspiration, because the classic signs and symptoms may be absent or minimal.

The management of the older patient who does not appear quite so ill can proceed with the labwork, chest x-ray, and old charts and old chest x-rays being ordered in the routine fashion. Usually, this scenario involves an older patient with a cough and underlying chronic disease, such as lung or heart disease.

For the previously healthy patient who does not appear ill, and whose vital signs (including pulse oximetry) are unremarkable, evaluation is frequently limited to the history and physical examination. Asthmatics are treated in the usual fashion, with inhaled beta-2-agonists and steroids. Patients felt to have asthmatic bronchitis or cough-variant asthma should have a chest x-ray and usually benefit from inhaled beta-2-agonists. Pre- and posttreatment peak expiratory flows are helpful to monitor their response to treatment.

DISPOSITION

Hospital admission to a general medical bed is usually warranted in those patients with hypoxemia and lower tract diseases such as pneumonia, asthma, chronic bronchitis, abscess, and tumor. A cardiac monitor may or may not be required if the patient has heart disease. Hospital admission is also indicated if i.v. medications such as antibiotics are necessary. The final criterion for hospital (or observation unit) admission is the appearance of critical illness. These are generally older patients who are vulnerable to bacteremia, sepsis, complications from their medications, and worsening of their clinical condition. Their chest x-rays may appear normal initially, but after i.v. hydration, pneumonia becomes apparent on subsequent films.

Consultation with a specialist is indicated for those patients with serious and significant exacerbations of their underlying disease, such as chronic bronchitis. Consultants also may be utilized for patients with less common etiologies of cough, such as lung abscess and tuberculosis, so that appropriate antibiotics, antituberculous agents, and isolation procedures can be promptly initiated. Patients without hypoxemia suspected of having *Pneumocystis carinii* pneumonia may be discharged, provided that arrangements have been made for outpatient continued diagnostic workup and provided that the patient can be followed closely for progression of disease and toxicity.

If transfer to another hospital is necessary, patients may be transferred, provided their conditions have been evaluated and they are stable. Ground transport should have oxygen, i.v., and cardiac monitoring capabilities when appropriate. For patients transferred with conditions such as pneumonia, the first dose of antibiotics should be started in the emergency department prior to transport.

Patients with acute cough felt to have a cold and viral upper respiratory tract infection may be reassured and discharged. Antitussives shown to be effective toward postnasal drainage include the antihistamine–decongestant combinations, dexbrompheniramine maleate/pseudoephedrine sulfate (Drixoral Cold & Allergy) 6 mg/120 mg b.i.d. and azatadine maleate/pseudoephedrine sulfate (Trinalin Repetabs) 1 mg/120 mg b.i.d.[5] Sedation is the primary side effect. Initiating therapy once a day at bedtime for several days prior to b.i.d. therapy may be helpful. Some improvement in cough is usually seen in several days to 2 weeks after the initiation of therapy.

Acute sinusitis patients with postnasal drainage also benefit from these same antihistamine–decongestant combinations, along with antibiotics and nasal decongestants such as 0.05% oxymetazoline hydrochloride (Afrin, Dristan) b.i.d. for 2 to 3 days. Safe and effective treatment of allergic rhinitis includes intranasal corticosteroids such as Flonase (fluticasone), 50-mg spray b.i.d., and second-generation nonsedating antihistamines such as fexofenadine (Allegra), 60 mg b.i.d., or loratadine (Claritin), 10 mg q.d. Optionally, a nasal spray such as 0.05% oxymetazoline hydrochloride may be used b.i.d., but for no more than 3 to 5 days. Its continued use for more than 5 to 7 days may result in rhinitis medicamentosa.[8] Outpatient allergy testing may be useful in patients who have allergic rhinitis, a seasonal component to a cough, or a cough associated with specific allergens, such as pollen or animal dander.

Patients with bronchitis or pneumonia (and normal pulse oximetry) may be discharged with appropriate prescriptions and instructions regarding follow-up with their personal physician. Older patients with the potential for worsening of their clinical condition should see their physicians in 2 to 3 days. Ipratropium bromide (Atrovent), administered q.i.d. via a metered-dose inhaler and spacer device or via nebulization, and smoking cessation are effective antitussives in chronic bronchitis. Cough-variant asthma patients may be discharged after instruction on the use of an albuterol metered-dose inhaler administered via a spacer device, two puffs q.i.d. Daily inhaled antiinflammatories, such as cromolyn (Intal) q.i.d. or corticosteroids (Vanceril) b.i.d. are usually beneficial. A short course of oral corticosteroids may be necessary for refractory cases.[7]

For cough induced by angiotensin converting enzyme inhibitor, switching to another angiotensin converting enzyme inhibitor or decreasing the dose is usually not beneficial. Angiotensin II receptor antagonists such as losartan (Cozaar) or valsartan (Diovan) may be used as an alternative, or a different class of hypertensive agent can be prescribed.[1,6] Resolution of angiotensin converting enzyme inhibitor cough usually occurs within 4 weeks after discontinuing the drug.[6] Patients felt to have postinfectious cough do not require specific treatment; the cough is self-limited and resolves spontaneously.

In patients without a history of chronic bronchitis, whose chest x-rays are normal, and who do not take angiotensin converting enzyme inhibitors, chronic cough is almost always secondary to postnasal drainage, asthma, or gastroesophageal reflux disease.[4] Effective treatment of postnasal drainage includes dexbrompheniramine maleate/pseudoephedrine sulfate, 6 mg/120 mg b.i.d., or azatadine maleate/pseudoephedrine sulfate, 1 mg/120 mg b.i.d. If the postnasal drainage is secondary to a chronic sinusitis, then antibiotics and a nasal decongestant such as 0.05% oxymetazoline hydrochloride are given in addition to the antihistamine–decongestant combination. The nasal decongestant is recommended b.i.d. for 5 days, the antihistamine–decongestant b.i.d. for a minimum of 3 weeks. Asthmatics are treated in the usual fashion, with beta-2-agonist aerosols delivered by hand-held metered-dose inhalers and a spacer device, or administered by a nebulizer. Steroids, either inhaled or oral, are also indicated. For patients felt to have chronic cough secondary to gastroesophageal reflux disease, antireflux measures and acid suppression with H_2 antagonists, proton pump inhibitors, or prokinetic drugs are indicated.

Nonspecific antitussives may be prescribed when the underlying etiology of cough is unknown, or when the definitive therapy has not had a chance to work. Antitussives shown to be effective include codeine, 30 to 60 mg PO q.d. or 20 mg PO b.i.d.; dextromethorphan, 10 to 20 mg q.i.d. for 10 days or 20 mg b.i.d. for 3 days; and the combination dexbrompheniramine maleate/pseudoephedrine sulfate, 6 mg/120 mg b.i.d.[5]

COMMON PITFALLS

- The most common etiology of cough in emergency department patients is a viral upper respiratory tract infection, the common cold.
- In patients with cough secondary to postnasal drainage, the combination of a first-generation antihistamine and a decongestant is more effective than the newer nonsedating antihistamines, probably because the newer agents lack the anticholinergic properties of the older first-generation antihistamines.
- Patients who complain of chest congestion should be examined carefully for wheezing.
- Chronic cough (i.e., lasting longer than 3 weeks) is seen most frequently in chronic bronchitis.
- All angiotensin converting enzyme inhibitors are capable of causing a chronic cough.
- In patients without chronic bronchitis and a normal chest x-ray (and who do not take angiotensin converting enzyme inhibitors), the three most common causes of chronic cough are postnasal drainage, asthma, and gastroesophageal reflux disease.

References

1. Abramowicz M, ed. Valsartan for hypertension. *Med Lett* 1997;39:43.
2. American Thoracic Society. Standards for the diagnosis and care of patients with chronic obstructive pulmonary disease. *Am J Respir Crit Care Med* 1995;152:S77.
3. Bouros D, Siafakas N, Green M. Cough. In: Roussos C, ed. *The thorax.* New York: Marcel Dekker Inc, 1995:1335.
4. Irwin RS. Cough. In: Irwin RS, Curley FJ, Grossman RF, eds. *Diagnosis and treatment of symptoms of the respiratory tract.* Armonk, NY: Futura Publishing, 1997:1.
5. Irwin RS, Boulet LP, Cloutier MM, et al. Managing cough as a defense mechanism and as a symptom—a consensus panel report of the American College of Chest Physicians. *Chest* 1998;114:133S.
6. Lacourcière Y, Brunner H, Irwin R, et al., and the Losartan Cough Study Group. Effects of modulators of the renin-angiotensin-aldosterone system on cough. *J Hypertens* 1994;12:1387.
7. Patrick H, Patrick F. Chronic cough. *Med Clin North Am* 1995;79:361.
8. Rachelefsky GS. Pharmacologic management of allergic rhinitis. *J Allergy Clin Immunol* 1998;101:S367.

CHAPTER 4
Dyspnea

C. Keith Stone and D. Shannon Waters

Dyspnea refers to difficult, labored, or uncomfortable breathing. Dyspnea is a symptom of many disorders that involve alterations or abnormalities in gas exchange, pulmonary circulation, respiratory mechanics, O_2-carrying capacity of the blood, or cardiovascular function. Dyspnea results when ventilatory demand exceeds respiratory function. A mismatch between supply and demand of oxygen and failure of CO_2 elimination is at the basis of dyspnea.

A person with normal breathing capacity may require a large increase in ventilatory demand before dyspnea is produced. On the other hand, in a person with a preexisting diminished respiratory capacity, a small increase in ventilatory demand may produce significant shortness of breath (SOB). Because the perception of dyspnea is also mediated by psychological and cultural factors,[2] it may be helpful to assess breathing difficulty in terms of diminished ability to perform specific daily functions, such as housework or climbing stairs.

The pathophysiology of dyspnea is complex. However, an understanding of the basic principles behind respiration is necessary to understand the cause and treatment of dyspnea in a given disorder. Chemoreceptors in the blood and brain, as well as mechanoreceptors in the airways, lungs, and chest wall, are involved in the automatic regulation of the level and pattern of breathing.[2] The carotid and aortic bodies and central chemoreceptors in the medulla sense changes in the partial pressure of oxygen (PO_2), partial pressure of carbon dioxide (PCO_2), and pH of the blood and transmit signals back to brainstem respiratory centers that adjust breathing. These receptors cause changes in the rate of ventilation[12] to maintain blood–gas and acid–base homeostasis.[2] In most individuals, the most profound stimulus to the central nervous system respiratory control center is normally the arterial carbon dioxide tension (PCO_2). An increase in PCO_2 of 1.5 mm Hg from the normal level of 40 mm Hg may produce a doubling of ventilation. Arterial oxygen tension and pH are other factors that significantly influence ventilation. In the patient with chronic obstructive pulmonary disease (COPD) and hypercarbia, the arterial oxygen tension may be the most influential factor affecting respiratory drive.

Afferent impulses from vagal receptors in the airways and lungs also exert important influences on the level and pattern of breathing. Feedback of afferent information from lung and chest wall mechanoreceptors provides respiratory motor and premotor neurons with important information regarding the mechanical status of the ventilatory pump, as well as changes in length and force of contraction of the respiratory muscles.[2] Elastic resistance of the lung to stretch, airway flow resistance, and tissue friction must be overcome for breathing to proceed. Elastic resistance is the most significant of these factors at normal respiratory rates. At rates faster than 15 breaths per minute, airway resistance becomes more important.

Listed in Table 4.1 are the most frequently encountered causes and the most common etiologies of acute dyspnea seen in the emergency department (ED). Dyspnea may result from respiratory, cardiovascular, hematologic, neuromuscular, metabolic, or psychogenic derangement. Most commonly, cardiovascular and respiratory disorders are the cause, with the degree of derangement proportional to the resultant dyspnea.

CLINICAL PRESENTATION

Patients presenting to the ED with dyspnea often complain of SOB. Depending on their level of distress and any preexisting respiratory problems, they may appear comfortable or may exhibit varying degrees of distress. Once the initial examination assures that the airway is patent and oxygenation adequate, a thorough history must be obtained.

Pertinent questions in the history can provide valuable infor-

TABLE 4.1. Causes of Acute Dyspnea

UPPER AIRWAY OBSTRUCTION	NEUROMUSCULAR
Angioedema	Guillain-Barrè syndrome
Epiglottitis	Myasthenia gravis
Foreign body	**METABOLIC/SYSTEMIC**
CARDIOVASCULAR	Anaphylaxis
Congestive heart failure	Anemia
Pulmonary edema	Hyperthyroidism
Cardiac tamponade	Sepsis
Acute coronary ischemia	Acidosis
Cardiac dysrhythmias	Salicylate intoxication
Pulmonary embolus	Obesity
PULMONARY	**PSYCHOGENIC**
Aspiration	Hyperventilation syndrome
Asthma	
COPD exacerbation	
Pneumonia	
Pneumothorax	
Pleural effusion	
Adult respiratory distress syndrome	
Toxic inhalation	

mation and diagnostic clues to the cause of dyspnea. The duration of dyspnea; associated chest pain or palpitations; precipitating factors such as exertion, exercise, or anxiety; associated paresthesias of the mouth and fingers; the number of pillows the patient uses to sleep; concomitant coughing or sputum production; exercise tolerance; tobacco use; recreational drug use; and occupational history are several important factors that can help narrow the differential diagnosis.[12] Trepopnea, the presence of dyspnea in one lateral position but not the other, may be the result of unilateral lung disease, unilateral pleural effusion, or, occasionally, chronic obstructive pulmonary disease (COPD). Paroxysmal nocturnal dyspnea, breathlessness that occurs while sleeping, is usually associated with left ventricular failure. Orthopnea, or the presence of dyspnea in the recumbent position, is also associated with left ventricular failure, but can be associated with COPD.

Although, in most patients, dyspnea may be readily apparent to the examiner, certain populations are not able to relay a history of shortness of breath. The very young, the very old, and those with diminished mental capacity may present only with tachypnea[11] or an altered level of consciousness. In these patients, it is important to keep respiratory difficulty in the differential diagnosis. On physical examination, the patient's vital signs, mental status, assumed position, use of accessory muscles, conjunctival and mucous membrane color, skin and nailbed color, upper airway examination, neurologic examination, and cardiovascular and pulmonary examinations may give valuable clues to the etiology. Problems with oxygenation may be easily revealed by pulse oximetry, and difficulty with CO_2 elimination may be revealed by arterial blood gas determination in the patient who is unable to relay an adequate history.

DIFFERENTIAL DIAGNOSIS

Upper Airway Obstruction

Obstruction of the upper airway may be the consequence of a diverse group of entities, including foreign-body aspiration, epiglottitis, croup, angioedema, peritonsillar or retropharyngeal abscess, or neuromuscular dysfunction. The nature of the presenting picture depends on the site and degree of the obstruction, as well as the underlying cause. Cough, stridor, dyspnea, aphonia, or hoarseness may be present. Although many of these conditions do not usually cause complete airway obstruction, rapid deterioration is possible in these patients, and the emergency physician must be ready to provide immediate airway intervention.

Epiglottitis is an important cause of respiratory distress due to upper airway obstruction, although it is seen significantly less frequently with the use of HiB vaccine. The incidence is greatest in children 2 to 4 years old. The onset is characteristically abrupt, with a mild upper respiratory infection progressing within hours to high fever, lethargy, and difficulty in swallowing oral secretions. Respiratory distress and stridor are the most consistent signs. Restlessness, anxiety, and tachycardia are also often present.

In adults, the presentation of epiglottitis is typically less dramatic, and dyspnea may be minimal or absent. Fever and sore throat are the most common complaints. Consequently, the diagnosis is often delayed in adults.

Congestive Heart Failure

Congestive heart failure (CHF) is a clinical condition that develops when cardiac output becomes insufficient to meet systemic metabolic demands.[1] Acute failure of the left ventricle to eject a normal quantity of blood may cause fluid to accumulate in the pulmonary interstitium, alveoli, and bronchioles, thereby producing pulmonary edema. In addition to interfering with gas exchange, transudation of fluid into the perialveolar spaces reduces pulmonary compliance. Acute precipitating factors of CHF include increased Na intake, noncompliance with CHF medications, acute myocardial infarction (MI), arrhythmia, or anemia. The most common causes of CHF are coronary artery disease and hypertension,[1] although valvular heart disease, cardiomyopathy, and renal failure are other common entities.

The patient with dyspnea of cardiac origin generally presents to the ED with complaints of dyspnea on exertion that is relieved by rest. Other pertinent information obtained on history includes the presence of orthopnea, paroxysmal nocturnal dyspnea (PND) relieved by standing or walking, peripheral edema, and fatigue.

The physical examination may reveal jugular venous distention (JVD), rales, diminished breath sounds, cardiac gallop, cardiac arrhythmias, peripheral edema, hepatomegaly, and ascites.[1] Pulmonary edema may also lead to bronchospasm and cardiac wheezing, so-called cardiac asthma. Chest radiography may reveal cardiomegaly, pulmonary vascular redistribution, Kerley B lines, pleural effusion, and peribronchial cuffing. An uncommon but quickly fatal cardiac cause of dyspnea is ventricular septal rupture post-MI. Although rare, prompt diagnosis is crucial if potential life-saving measures, such as surgery, are to be employed.[17]

Chronic Obstructive Pulmonary Disease

The American Thoracic Society defines *COPD* as a disease state characterized by the presence of airflow obstruction due to chronic bronchitis or emphysema.[3] The airflow obstruction is often continuous and progressive and, in contrast to asthma, dyspnea is usually always present. *Chronic bronchitis* is defined as the presence of a chronic, productive cough for 3 months in each of 2 successive years in which other causes of chronic cough have been eliminated.[3] *Emphysema* is defined as abnormal permanent enlargement of the air spaces distal to the terminal bronchioles, accompanied by destruction of bronchiolar walls but without obvious fibrosis.[3] Although COPD is a chronic disorder, exacerbations of diminished respiratory function often bring patients to the ED.

COPD exacerbations are usually caused by a worsening of airflow obstruction due to increased bronchospasm, increased sputum production from superimposed respiratory infection, environmental irritants (such as tobacco smoke), or cardiovascular deterioration. The patient may present with progressive dyspnea, increased sputum production, and audible wheezing. Hypoxemia, tachypnea, cyanosis, and agitation may be seen. Signs of hypercarbia, such as confusion, stupor, inadequate respiratory effort, or apnea, may be seen and indicate severe compromise with impaired gas exchange.[3] These patients attempt to improve ventilation by sitting forward, using pursed-lip exhalation, and using accessory muscles of respiration in order to overcome the increase in airflow resistance that accompanies bronchoconstriction and dynamic airway collapse.[10] Auscultation may reveal a combination of diminished breath sounds, a prolonged expiratory phase, wheezes, or rales. The chest radiograph may reveal an increased anterior–posterior diameter, flattened diaphragms, hyperinflated lungs, attenuation of the peripheral lung markings, and, in cases of superimposed infection, an infiltrate.

Asthma

Asthma is a chronic inflammatory disease, clinically characterized by recurrent episodes of wheezing, chest tightness and discomfort, dyspnea, and cough. Exacerbation is characterized by an early phase, which chiefly consists of bronchospasm, edema, and obstruction; and a late phase, which is caused primarily by the inflammatory response. Numerous triggers may cause an exacerbation. Among them are respiratory infections, allergens, cold air, exercise, cigarette smoke, emotional stress, outdoor pollutants, and other factors associated with seasonal changes.[15] Viral upper respiratory infections may be the most common cause of acute asthma exacerbations.[15] Duration of symptoms for greater than 24 hours suggests a greater component of inflammation in the absence of any evidence of infection.

Patients with an asthma exacerbation present to the ED with the complaints of SOB, wheezing, cough, and chest tightness.[15] The physical examination may reveal an increased AP diameter of the chest due to air trapping, tachypnea, wheezing, and mild-to-severe respiratory distress. Auscultation may be misleading in the case of severe obstruction; wheezing may be absent, as bronchial airflow is diminished to such an extent that no sound is audible. Chest radiographs may be normal, reveal signs of airway obstruction (such as in COPD), demonstrate a pneumothorax or pneumomediastinum, or, in the case of a precipitating infection, reveal an infiltrate.

It is important to remember that the preeminent contributing factor to death in acute asthma remains the failure to administer appropriate treatment, typically because the patient or physician underestimates the severity of the attack.[15] Therefore, it is important to treat not only based on the patient's symptoms, but also based on clinical parameters and ancillary studies.

Pneumonia

Pneumonia classically presents as an acute febrile illness with cough and purulent sputum production. Dyspnea results from alveolar obstruction secondary to sputum production, bronchiole obstruction due to mucous plugging, increased work of breathing, and hypoxia.

Pneumonia should be suspected in patients with newly acquired lower respiratory symptoms (cough, sputum production, and/or dyspnea), especially if these symptoms are accompanied by fever, altered breath sounds, and rales.[4] *Streptococcus pneumoniae* remains the most common etiology of community-acquired pneumonia, even in the immunocompromised host.[4] Patients with atypical pneumonia caused by *Mycoplasma pneumoniae, Legionella pneumophila,* and *Chlamydia psittaci* may present with an insidious or subacute onset, moderate fever, and less purulent sputum. Headache, nonproductive cough, myalgias, arthralgias, and malaise may predominate.[4] Immunosuppressed patients may present with staphylococcal pneumonia or pneumonia caused by opportunists such as *Pneumocystis carinii*, mycobacteria, or fungal organisms.

The physical examination in pneumonia may reveal rales, egophony or vocal resonance, increased vocal fremitus, or bronchial breath sounds. A chest radiograph may demonstrate lobar consolidation, as in bacterial pneumonia; patchy infiltrates, suggesting staphylococcal pneumonia, *Haemophilus influenzae,* or gram-negative pneumonia; interstitial infiltrates, suggesting *Mycoplasma, Legionella,* or *Pneumocystis*; or cavitary lesions, as in tuberculosis;[6] or, as seen in up to 30% of *Pneumocystis carinii* pneumonia (PCP), it may be entirely normal.[4] A sputum Gram stain performed in the ED may also provide valuable clues to the cause of the pneumonia. Early recognition is important, so that appropriate antibiotic treatment may be rendered promptly.

Pneumothorax

Pneumothorax, or air in the pleural cavity, can occur spontaneously or as the result of trauma. Normally, the visceral and parietal pleura are in close apposition, but when the potential space between the two is occupied by gas, the lung can no longer fully expand. Depending on the amount of air within the pleural space, respiratory compromise results. Spontaneous pneumothorax typically occurs in tall, thin, young males. The cause of the pneumothorax is the rupture of a subpleural bleb, which is usually apical in location. Spontaneous pneumothorax also may be seen in patients with asthma, COPD, and tuberculosis, and in AIDS patients with PCP. Traumatic pneumothorax results from blunt or penetrating injury to the chest. Hemothorax, pulmonary contusion, and bronchial rupture[9] may accompany the pneumothorax.

Patients may present to the ED in obvious respiratory distress or may complain of dyspnea and chest pain. Auscultation may reveal unilateral diminution of the breath sounds associated with increased tympany on percussion. Signs of imminent cardiovascular collapse, such as hypotension, mediastinal shift, and the aforementioned findings, may herald a tension pneumothorax, which should be promptly relieved prior to any further examination or diagnostic studies. Subcutaneous emphysema also may be present. Chest radiography may reveal an obvious pneumothorax or may be more subtle. In the supine patient, the only sign of a pneumothorax may be an abnormally prominent costophrenic angle on the AP or PA view. A spontaneous pneumomediastinum also may present as dyspnea or chest pain. Although uncommon, this entity should be suspected in the setting of cocaine freebasing or inhalational drug use.[13]

Pulmonary Embolism

Pulmonary embolism (PE) is an obstruction of the pulmonary artery or one of its branches by an embolus, usually a blood clot derived from the leg or pelvic veins. The diagnosis of PE is often subtle and may be difficult. Despite attempts to identify a reliable, cost-effective, and readily available test to use in the noninvasive diagnosis of PE, significant inadequacies of both sensitivity and specificity have hindered all such efforts to date.[8]

The most common symptom in a patient with PE is dyspnea. Chest pain and cough are also not infrequent complaints.[16] Frequent signs of PE include tachypnea and tachycardia. Although embolism may present as pulmonary infarction, with the acute onset of pleuritic pain, hemoptysis, and an audible pleural friction rub, such a presentation is uncommon. PE may also mimic other entities. Associated fever and cough may suggest pneumonia, while associated rib tenderness or pleuritic chest pain may suggest a musculoskeletal etiology.

Clinical suspicion plays a key role in the decision to pursue an evaluation for acute PE.[16] Patients at high risk include those who have had a previous PE or DVT, a recent surgery, or a recent immobilization; those with a malignancy or cardiopulmonary disease; those with lower extremity or pelvic trauma; and women during pregnancy or in the postpartum period.[16] Laboratory analysis should include an arterial blood gas, which may reflect hypoxemia and/or hypocarbia. The arterial–alveolar oxygen gradient is classically increased and, in combination with blood–gas analysis, may contribute to the formulation of a higher clinical suspicion.[8] A ventilation–perfusion scan, spiral computed tomography scan, and pulmonary angiogram, used in conjunction with the clinical pretest probability and duplex Doppler evaluation of the lower extremities, will help the physician determine the likelihood of the presence of PE and the necessity of anticoagulation and admission.

Psychogenic Hyperventilation

Dyspnea can also occur as a somatic manifestation of psychiatric disorders, such as anxiety disorder, with resultant hyperventilation.[12] Patients with hyperventilation syndrome are often seen in the ED. Tachypnea and anxiety are the predominant findings. The patient may complain of paresthesias around the mouth and the fingers. Carpopedal spasm also may be present. The patient may give a history of obtaining relief of dyspnea with exertion, which is not a typical feature of organic disorders producing difficulty breathing. The presence of respiratory alkalosis without hypoxemia on arterial blood–gas analysis is characteristic, as is a normal arterial–alveolar oxygen gradient. Given that a number of important processes produce respiratory alkalosis (e.g., salicylate, intoxication, PE, and anemia), psychogenic hyperventilation should be a diagnosis of exclusion.

EMERGENCY DEPARTMENT EVALUATION

The most important initial treatment in the evaluation of dyspnea is to secure the airway and assure oxygenation and circulation. In cases of obvious severe distress, this may mean endotracheal intubation and mechanical ventilation, whereas mild-to-moderate distress may warrant only the use of oxygen initially. Once the ABCs have been addressed, the physician should perform a rapid, complete history and physical examination, as the cause of the dyspnea may be readily identified.[12]

It is important to remember that many of the common diseases that produce dyspnea share many physical findings. Intermittent adventitious sounds (crackles or rales) are heard in a variety of illness, such as COPD, CHF, and pulmonary fibrosis, and are not specific for any one disease entity. Continuous adventitious sounds (wheezes) may also be produced by a variety of illnesses (Table 4.2), and are almost always a sign of airflow obstruction. Stridor (a loud and harsh-sounding wheeze with a crowing or musical sound of fixed pitch) can be heard, predominantly during inspiration, when the trachea, bronchus, or larynx is obstructed. The presence of other signs and symptoms, such as fever and purulent sputum production in pneumonia, or JVD and gallop rhythm in CHF, significantly supplement the auscultatory findings in establishing the diagnosis in a dyspneic patient.

TABLE 4.2. Causes of Wheezing

UPPER RESPIRATORY TRACT
Angioedema
Foreign body
Tumor
Infection
LOWER RESPIRATORY TRACT
Anaphylaxis
Asthma
Aspiration
Bronchiolitis
COPD
Foreign body
VASCULAR
Adult respiratory distress syndrome
Congestive heart failure
Pulmonary embolus
EXTRATHORACIC
Carcinoid
Factitious

Pulse oximetry is an easy, noninvasive monitoring technique that allows continuous, reliable measurements of oxygen saturation while avoiding repeated arterial punctures.[14] Every person that presents to the ED complaining of dyspnea should have his or her oxygen saturation recorded. Use of the pulse oximeter does have several limitations, however. First, because of the shape of the oxyhemoglobin dissociation curve, measurement of oxygen saturation is relatively insensitive in detecting changes in PaO_2 at high levels of oxygenation. In patients receiving supplemental oxygen, for example, a substantial drop in PaO_2 may be unaccompanied by any change in saturation. In addition, the curve has a steep downward slope normally commencing at a saturation of 91% corresponding to a PaO_2 of 60 mm Hg, and even relatively modest desaturation below this level represents a significant decline in PaO_2.[14] The curve may also shift due to changes in body temperature and pH. Pulse oximetry may be inaccurate in reflecting oxygen saturation in the presence of high carboxyhemoglobin levels, methemoglobinemia, severe anemia, and low-perfusion states. Finally, pulse oximetry does not relay any information regarding PCO_2.

Measurement of arterial blood gases may be necessary in evaluating patients who present with dyspnea. Blood gases demonstrate the severity of gas exchange impairment and are useful as diagnostic tools, as well as for establishing a baseline for monitoring therapy. In disease states such as COPD and asthma, measurement of the carbon dioxide level and degree of acidosis can provide valuable information about the severity of the exacerbation and may be more helpful than oxygen saturation at guiding treatment. The physician should use discretion, however, when obtaining blood gases. In cases of mild dyspnea due to asthma or COPD exacerbation, a normal oxygen saturation on room air pulse oximetry, and other noninvasive diagnostic studies, such as spirometry (FEV1 or FVC), may be adequate.

If a blood gas is obtained, the A-a oxygen gradient may be

calculated. The most common formula used for calculation is as follows:

$$A\text{-}a = [150 - (1.2 \times PCO_2)] - \text{arterial } PO_2$$

This formula is accurate at sea level, where the alveolar partial pressure of oxygen is 150 mm Hg. The normal gradient should be around 10 in a young person and may increase to no more than 20 as a person ages. A quick way to calculate a patient's normal A-a gradient is to add one-tenth of the patient's age plus 10. Patients in whom hypoxemia is caused by alveolar hypoventilation alone, such as those with drug overdose or neuromuscular disease, have a normal A-a gradient. On the other hand, in hypoxemia produced by ventilation–perfusion mismatch, right-to-left shunting, and diffusion barrier, such as typically occur in COPD, parenchymal lung disease, PE, and pneumonia, the A-a gradient is increased.

The chest radiograph is a valuable diagnostic tool in elucidating the cause of dyspnea and should be obtained in most cases. Diagnostic radiographic findings can be expected in certain entities, such as pneumonia, PE, and pneumothorax. However, the chest radiograph may be entirely normal, even when significant illness is manifested by dyspnea, such as with PE.

Chest radiographic findings may also be minimal in certain conditions, such as aspiration or toxic inhalation, when the study is obtained as part of the initial evaluation. Also, the presence of radiographic abnormalities does not necessarily imply that a given illness is producing the current episode of dyspnea. For example, the radiograph of the patient with COPD manifests various abnormalities, but a given episode of dyspnea may be unrelated to the chronic findings displayed on the radiograph. In addition, the presence of chronic radiographic changes in such instances may render the appearance of acute disease processes, such as CHF or pneumonia, less apparent.

Special views of the chest may be in order in certain circumstances. An expiratory view may accentuate the presence of a small pneumothorax, because the constant volume of the intrapleural air is accentuated by the reduced size of the hemithorax on expiration. The lateral decubitus view may confirm the presence of a pleural effusion. Inspiratory–expiratory, or positional, films may indicate a bronchial foreign body. Other radiographic studies, such as a lateral view of the neck in suspected epiglottitis, also may be in order.

Measurement of the pulsus paradoxus may prove helpful to the physician in detecting certain causes of dyspnea, such as pericardial tamponade or pediatric asthma.[5] The paradoxical pulse is obtained by inflating a blood pressure cuff above the systolic pressure, then slowly deflating it until the first systolic sound is heard during expiration. After noting this pressure, the cuff is further deflated until systolic sounds are heard throughout the respiratory cycle. The difference of pressure is normally 4 to 5 mm Hg, and pulsus paradoxus is present when the value is greater than 10. This test is accurate in identifying patients with moderate-to-severe asthma.

Peak flow meters are inexpensive instruments that provide a rapid bedside measure of airway function,[15] and may provide additional useful information during the management of asthmatic patients. With proper instruction on use and good patient cooperation, the physician can make a rapid and objective assessment of the patient's condition and can also use sequential peak flow measurements as an additional measure of the effectiveness of therapy. Knowledge of the patient's baseline peak flow is the best guide to therapy.[15]

Other diagnostic studies may be helpful when evaluating a patient with dyspnea. An ECG can show abnormalities of heart rate and rhythm, or evidence of ischemia, injury, or infarction.[12] An ECG also may be helpful in evaluating patients with a suspected pulmonary embolus, although suggestive changes are present in only a minority of patients. Anemia is an important cause of dyspnea,[7] and a check of the patient's hemoglobin or hematocrit may be useful as part of the workup. Rarely, bedside laryngoscopy or bronchoscopy may provide a definitive diagnosis, especially in the case of upper airway obstruction or suspected foreign body.

EMERGENCY DEPARTMENT MANAGEMENT

Management of the dyspneic patient in the ED depends on the patient's baseline respiratory status, the cause of the current respiratory decline, and the degree of respiratory distress. The goal of the treatment of dyspnea is to correct the underlying disorder causing the symptoms. Unfortunately, in many patients, treatment of the underlying cause is ineffective or only partly effective, and dyspnea persists.[10] (Specific therapies can be found in the chapters devoted to each of the differential diagnoses.)

Every patient who complains of SOB should have pulse oximetry performed and, at least initially, be provided with supplemental oxygen. If the clinical condition warrants mechanical ventilation, the physician must be prepared to intubate promptly and should have all necessary material at the patient's bedside. The history and physical examination will suggest the choice of other appropriate diagnostic studies; that is, suspected pneumonia will require the performance of a chest radiograph and sputum Gram stain and culture, or a patient with a history of chest pain will need to have an ECG performed to help evaluate the likelihood of significant ischemic heart disease. Once a preliminary diagnosis is made, treatment should be appropriately tailored to alleviate the patient's SOB. A patient with COPD or asthma exacerbation may benefit from inhaled beta-adrenergic agents and intravenous or oral steroids.[3,15] A patient in CHF may benefit from nitrates and diuretics.[1] Many of the disorders producing dyspnea share similar ED interventions, although the underlying pathologies may be different.

DISPOSITION

The disposition of the dyspneic patient depends on the cause of the respiratory difficulty, the severity of the respiratory compromise, and the success of the ED treatment. Any patient with continuing dyspnea, despite treatment, should be admitted for further evaluation. Depending on the clinical condition and diagnosis, the patient may need observation in the general ward, on telemetry, or in the intensive care unit. The patient may be safely discharged home if he or she has improvement in or resolution of SOB and an appropriate diagnosis, such as mild asthma exacerbation, has been made. When considering discharge in dyspneic patients, it is important to assure that they are back to their baseline respiratory status, will be able to obtain the medications prescribed, are capable of caring for themselves at home, and will have adequate, prompt follow-up care.

COMMON PITFALLS

- Do not rely on pulse oximetry alone to gauge a patient's respiratory status; it gives no information about pCO_2.
- If a tension pneumothorax is suspected, do not wait for radiographic confirmation before decompressing the pleural space.
- The chest radiograph may be totally normal in PE.
- Do not withhold oxygen for fear of blunting the hypoxic respiratory drive in a patient with COPD; correct the hypoxia first.

- Absence of wheezing in a patient with asthma or COPD in respiratory distress indicate severely obstructed airways.

ACKNOWLEDGMENT

The authors gratefully acknowledge the contribution of George Sternbach, who wrote the previous version of this chapter.

References

1. Albrich, JM. Congestive heart failure: a state-of-the-art review of clinical pitfall, evaluation, and recent advances in drug therapy (Part I). *Emerg Med Rep* 1997;18:159.
2. American Thoracic Society. Dyspnea. Mechanisms, assessment, and management: a consensus statement. *Am J Respir Crit Care Med* 1999;159:321.
3. American Thoracic Society. Standards for the diagnosis and care of patients with chronic obstructive pulmonary disease. *Am J Respir Crit Care Med* 1995;152:S78–S106.
4. Bartlett JG, Breiman RF, et al. Community-acquired pneumonia in adults: guidelines for management. *Clin Infect Dis* 1998;26:811–838.
5. Bulloch B, Ruddy RM. Asthma update: managing asthma in the pediatric emergency department. *Pediatr Emerg Med Rep* 1998;3:39–50.
6. Cunha BA. TB pneumonia. *Emerg Med* 1998;30:102–111.
7. Hetzel TM, Losek JD. Unrecognized severe anemia in children presenting with respiratory distress. *Am J Emerg Med* 1998;16:386–389.
8. Jones JS, Neff TL, et al. Use of the alveolar-arterial oxygen gradient in the assessment of acute pulmonary embolism. *Am J Emerg Med* 1998;16:333–337.
9. Lin MY, Wu MH, et al. Bronchial rupture caused by blunt chest injury. *Ann Emerg Med* 1995;25:412–415.
10. Manning HL, Schwartzstein RM. Pathophysiology of dyspnea. *N Engl J Med* 1995;333:1547–1553.
11. Margolis P, Gadomski A. Does this infant have pneumonia? *JAMA* 1998;279:308–313.
12. Morgan WC, Hodge HL. Diagnostic evaluation of dyspnea. *Am Fam Physician* 1998;57:711–716.
13. Panacek EA, Singer AJ, et al. Spontaneous pneumomediastinum: clinical and natural history. *Ann Emerg Med* 1992;21:1222–1227.
14. Schnapp LM, Cohen NH. Pulse oximetry uses and abuses. *Chest* 1990;98:1244–1249.
15. Silverman R. Acute asthma in adults. *Emerg Med* 1999;3:79–91.
16. Susec O, Boudrow D, et al. The clinical features of acute pulmonary embolism in ambulatory patients. *Acad Emerg Med* 1997;4:891–897.
17. Yahia S, Brodyn NE, et al. Emergency use of echocardiography in a post-myocardial infarction patient with acute dyspnea. *Am J Emerg Med* 1996;14:33–36

CHAPTER 5
Fever and Night Sweats

Harold A. Thomas Jr. and James H. Bryan

> Humanity has but three great enemies: fever, famine, and war; of these, by far the greatest, by far the most terrible, is fever.
>
> Sir William Osler

Fever is one of the oldest and most widely recognized signs of disease and accounts for approximately 6% of adult and 20% to 30% of pediatric visits to the emergency department. While the exact temperature that constitutes a fever is debatable, most consider a rectal temperature of 38°C in children and a temperature of 38.3°C in adults to represent a fever. Although fever has been recognized as a pathologic sign for at least 2500 years, and despite Sir William Osler's acclamation, it is still unclear whether fever represents the physician's ally or foe.

Regulation of body temperature is under the control of the preoptic area of the anterior hypothalamus. This area acts like a thermostat, continuously balancing heat production and heat loss. It constantly receives input from central receptors, which monitor the temperature of blood perfusing the brain, and peripheral receptors, which monitor skin temperature.

Heat production is controlled in several ways. The basal metabolic rate is under the direct control of the hypothalamus and can be varied, depending on the demand for heat production. The basal metabolic rate may be altered by varying the level of circulating thyroxine, which increases cellular metabolism. In addition, the fastest and most sensitive way in which the body increases heat production is by increasing muscle activity (shivering when cold, or the shaking chill of a fever).

The principal method of body heat loss is to vary the volume of blood flowing to the skin's surface. Blood flow to the fingertips can vary more than 100-fold over different environmental temperatures. The exocrine sweat glands can also contribute to heat loss. Sweating cools the body by vaporization (conversion of a liquid to a vapor). After acclimatization to a hot environment, up to 4 L of sweat can be produced each hour.

The hypothalamic thermostat has an inherent set-point of about 37°C. The normal circadian rhythm exhibits daily variations of up to 2°C. Temperatures are lowest around 4 a.m. and then gradually increase until they peak between 6 and 10 p.m. The reason for this circadian rhythm is unclear, but, unlike other circadian rhythms, such as cortisol secretion, it is not reversed in shift workers who are awake at night and sleep during the day. Most fevers follow this pattern, being higher in the evening and lower in the morning.

Elevation of the hypothalamic set-point appears to be mediated by cytokines. Exogenous pyrogens such as microorganisms, as well as toxins and metabolic byproducts of these organisms, act to stimulate the release of cytokines from lymphocytes, monocytes, and macrophages. While the detailed mechanism by which cytokines produce fever is not clear, it is believed that they travel via the bloodstream to the hypothalamus, where they act to increase prostaglandin synthesis, primarily prostaglandin E2 (PGE2). The resulting increase in prostaglandins causes an elevated cyclic adenosine monophosphate (cAMP) level, resulting in an elevated hypothalamic set-point. This elevated set-point increases body temperature by affecting peripheral vasoconstriction and internal heat production. Fever is maintained until pyrogen levels fall or until prostaglandin production is inhibited. Aspirin, ibuprofen, and acetaminophen exert their antipyretic effects by blocking central hypothalamic prostaglandin synthesis, without any effect on circulating endogenous pyrogen. Corticosteroids can block the release of endogenous pyrogen as well as inhibit prostaglandins, but are nevertheless relatively weak antipyretics.

Cytokines produced in response to pyrogens include interleukins (ILs), tumor necrosis factor (TNF), and interferons (IFNs). Because of the complex interaction between cytokines, the exact role each plays in the production of fever is difficult to establish. Different pyrogens appear to induce different cytokines. It is generally believed that bacteria and their products of metabolism typically provoke release of IL-1. However, an intravenous injection of lipopolysaccharide (a compound used to model systemic bacterial infections) induces a large rise in IL-6 while minimally increasing IL-1 and TNF.[3] In contrast, viral proteins appear to stimulate IFN. In addition to elevating temperature, IL-1 induces the liver to produce acute phase reactants, including C-reactive protein (CRP), which are responsible for the elevated erythrocyte sedimentation rate (ESR) associated with some fevers. IFN, although a potent pyrogen, does not enhance production of acute-phase reactants. Although not supported by data, this is the rationale behind the expectation of an elevated ESR and CRP level with a bacterial fever but not with one of viral etiology.

Other physiologic parameters that affect body temperature are exercise, the menstrual cycle, and the environmental temperature. Strenuous exercise can significantly elevate temperature. During a race, marathon runners may have temperatures as high as 41°C. There is a rapid fall to normal, usually over 30 minutes, after cessation of activity. At ovulation, there is a 0.5°C increase in temperature that persists until just before the next menses. In a group of normal volunteers, elevation of the room temperature from 20°C to 30°C resulted in an increase in rectal temperature from 36.7°C to 37.3°C.

Not all elevations of body temperature necessarily constitute a fever. A true fever is an elevation of body temperature caused by a change in the hypothalamic set-point. This new elevated set-point causes the body to engage its normal heat-generating mechanisms to elevate the temperature until the new set-point is reached. In contrast, in hyperthermia a true fever does not exist; rather, the body attempts to maintain a normal temperature, but its homeostatic mechanisms are overwhelmed. Some causes of hyperthermia include heat exhaustion or heat stroke, vigorous exercise, hyperthyroidism, hypothalamic stroke or tumor, burns, malignant hyperthermia, and the use of amphetamines, phenothiazines, or anticholinergic drugs. In adults, temperatures greater than 41.5°C almost always represent hyperthermia and not a true fever. Additionally, in middle-aged to elderly patients who present with what appears to be a septic syndrome, chronic salicylate intoxication should be considered. Fever above 38°C, an elevated white blood cell count with an associated bandemia, decreased systemic vascular resistance, and evidence of multisystem organ failure all have been documented in cases of chronic salicylate intoxication. A careful inquiry into a history of a chronic inflammatory condition or chronic use of one of the myriad salicylate-based antiinflammatory agents (e.g., aspirin, Pepto-Bismol, salsalate, oil of wintergreen) is important in avoiding the significant morbidity and mortality associated with this condition.

The phenomenon of night sweats represents a nocturnal fluctuation in the hypothalamic set-point, causing a slight rise in body temperature that leads to reactive perspiration. Night sweats are most commonly related to tuberculosis or lymphoma, but are also seen in elderly patients with disorders of catecholamine excess and in solid malignancies. Gobbi and colleagues evaluated temperature fluctuations in patients with Hodgkin disease who complained of night sweats and found that their body temperature rose 0.5°C to 1.5°C within 30 minutes before sweating began. The temperature fluctuations were not enough to awaken the patients, but the discomfort related to the sweating was.[7]

Many metabolic abnormalities are associated with the febrile state. There is a 7% increase in the basal metabolic rate for each 0.55°C increase in temperature. Fever alone can cause significant proteinuria as well as achlorhydria, both of which resolve when the fever resolves. Fever increases both the oxygen tension (PO_2) and the carbon dioxide tension (PCO_2), and shifts the oxyhemoglobin dissociation curve to the right, resulting in lower oxygen saturation. Fever also seems to lower the seizure threshold, causing febrile seizures in children without a predisposition to epilepsy. Fever also can cause reactivation of latent herpes simplex infections (fever blisters).

The value of fever to the host remains a subject of debate, but evidence suggests that fever may have a significant protective effect. Neutrophils and lymphocytes are most active at elevated temperatures. In addition, higher temperatures decrease the level of serum iron, a substrate that many bacteria need in order to replicate. When iron levels are experimentally kept in the normal range, increased mortality is noted for a given inoculum of bacteria. Fever also seems to inhibit certain viruses, such as coxsackievirus and poliovirus. Experimental evidence on poikilotherms also suggests the benefit of fever. Lizards and goldfish exhibit a higher mortality when kept in a cooler environment and infected with bacteria. Both seek a warmer environment after infection, and those allowed to do so demonstrate significantly greater survival. The only two human infections in which elevation of temperature is of proven value are neurosyphilis and disseminated gonorrhea. Interestingly, neither of these diseases is associated with a significant natural fever.

There is, however, some evidence that argues against a protective effect of fever. Mice infected with tetanus spores or streptococci had decreased survival with an elevation of temperature. Mice and possibly humans are more susceptible to pneumococcal infections when febrile.

CLINICAL PRESENTATION

Most febrile patients present to the emergency department with a chief complaint of fever. However, some patients may present with more generalized complaints. Elderly patients may complain of general malaise or not feeling well; parents may bring in infants who are eating poorly or appear lethargic. In these patients, fever may be an incidental finding.

In children, fevers documented at home should be treated as real, even in the absence of a documented fever in the emergency department. Additionally, in children with subjective fevers, one study showed that mothers have an overall accuracy of 79%, with positive and negative predictive values of 68% and 88%, respectively.[8] Further, bundling of infants has been shown to have no effect on the rectal temperature of healthy infants, so elevated rectal temperatures should not be attributed to bundling.[9]

DIFFERENTIAL DIAGNOSIS

Infection

Infection is the most common cause of fever. Infection may originate in any portion of the body and lead to a febrile response. Much of the emergency physician's time is spent ascertaining the source of the fever and attempting to differentiate a viral from a bacterial etiology.

Drug Fever

While any drug can cause a febrile reaction, penicillin and penicillin analogues are the most frequent causative agents. The fever typically begins 7 to 10 days after the patient starts taking the drug, and there is an associated rash in 18% of cases and eosinophilia in 22% of cases. Drugs that are commonly associated with a drug fever are listed in Table 5.1. Drug fever is always a diagnosis of exclusion.

Neoplastic Diseases

While many different malignancies and tumors may produce fever, leukemia, Hodgkin disease and non-Hodgkin lymphoma, hepatoma, and atrial myxoma are the most common. Because the underlying disease or its treatment often leaves the patient immunosuppressed, however, it is important to eliminate occult infection as the etiology of the fever.

Central Nervous System Lesions

Structural lesions, head trauma, and strokes can cause elevated temperature either by direct destruction of the hypothalamic

TABLE 5.1. Drugs Commonly Associated with Drug Fevers

ANTIBIOTICS	
Cephalosporins	
Isoniazid	
Nitrofurantoin	
Penicillins	
Rifampin	
Sulfonamides	
ANTICANCER DRUGS	
Bleomycin	
Streptozotocin	
ANTICONVULSANTS	
Carbamazepine	
Phenytoin	
Barbiturates	
CARDIAC DRUGS	
Hydralazine	
Methyldopa	
Nifedipine	
Procainamide	
Quinidine	
NSAIDS	
Ibuprofen	
Salicylates	
OTHERS	
Cimetidine	
Iodides	

thermoregulatory center (hypothermia is more likely) or, more commonly, by blood irritating of the central receptors in the preoptic area.

Rheumatologic and Connective Tissue Disorders

Fever may be the only initial manifestation of many connective tissue and rheumatologic disorders. In systemic lupus erythematosus (SLE), fever is the initial symptom in 5% of the cases. In older patients, temporal arteritis may present as recurrent fevers with no identifiable source.

Drug Ingestion

Drugs associated with elevated temperature include cocaine, amphetamines, belladonna alkaloids, tricyclic antidepressants, and monoamine oxidase inhibitors. As discussed previously, older patients with chronic salicylate poisoning are also prone to fever.

Pulmonary Embolus

Approximately two-thirds of patients with a pulmonary embolus will exhibit a fever. While the majority of these fevers are low grade, temperatures may exceed 39.5°C in up to 10% of the cases.

Factitious Fever

Factitious or self-induced fever should be suspected if the history is suspicious, if other vital signs do not correlate with the degree of fever, or if the patient does not appear ill. Patients may have an underlying psychiatric disorder, such as a personality disorder or psychosis, or there may be an issue of secondary gain (e.g., work avoidance). Factitious fever is most common in females. Many are health care professionals or have a medical background. The easiest way to detect a factitious fever is to simultaneously measure temperatures at two or more body sites (e.g., oral and rectal), or measure the temperature of a freshly voided urine sample, which should reflect the true core temperature.

EMERGENCY DEPARTMENT EVALUATION

At presentation, it is important to obtain an accurate temperature measurement. Unfortunately, this measurement is commonly overlooked for the sake of convenience. Recorded temperatures may vary widely depending on the method used to obtain them. Rectal temperatures have long been the gold standard, but because of the invasiveness and relative difficulty of obtaining them, easier methods, such as oral, axillary, and tympanic temperatures, are often employed. Multiple studies have shown that none of these alternative methods consistently provides a temperature comparable to the rectal temperature. In addition, there appears to be no standard correction factor that may be used to improve their accuracy.

The rectal temperature, which most accurately reflects the core temperature, tends to be, on average, 0.7°C higher than a simultaneously obtained oral temperature. Oral temperatures can, in fact, vary more than 1.6°C, depending on where the probe is positioned in the mouth. In addition, the respiratory rate also influences oral temperatures. Tandberg and Sklar[17] found that the oral temperature decreased by almost 0.5°C for each increase of 10 in the respiratory rate. Kresovich-Wendler and associates[15] evaluated several characteristics in patients who were found to be afebrile on oral temperature measurement (mean temperature, 37.4°C) but febrile on rectal temperature measurement (mean temperature, 39.2°C). The two variables that most accurately predicted a wide disparity between the two measurements were a heart rate above 115 beats per minute and the presence of mouth breathing.[15]

While axillary temperatures are generally felt to be approximately 1°C lower than rectal temperatures, they have repeatedly been shown to be unreliable and miss many patients with significant fevers. In a large study[2] of over 1100 pediatric patients, there was a greater discrepancy between axillary and rectal temperatures shortly after the onset of fever (1.04°C) than 2 hours after a temperature elevation (0.53°C). In addition, this study showed there was no reliable correction factor that would allow conversion of axillary to rectal temperatures.[2]

The latest innovation for obtaining temperatures is the tympanic thermometer. Although this method is frequently employed because it is noninvasive and rapid, numerous studies in both adults and children have shown that temperatures obtained tympanically are a poor reflection of the rectal temperature. In one study of pediatric patients less than 6 years old, the correlation between rectal and tympanic temperatures was best (r = 0.83) in afebrile patients (T less than 100.5°F) and significantly worse (r = 0.61) in febrile patients.[13] Like oral and axillary temperatures, no single correction factor will allow conversion of tympanic to rectal temperatures. The discrepancy in this study was present despite the use of the rectal equivalency setting on the tympanic thermometer.

A patient with a low-grade fever may suffer from an acute, life-threatening condition, while another with a much higher temperature may have a benign viral infection. The source of the fever may be readily apparent, or it may remain undiagnosed after weeks of sophisticated evaluation. While pediatric patients often require a more extensive evaluation, history and physical alone can identify the etiology of a fever in the majority of adults.

History

Important points in the history include

1. Associated symptoms (e.g., vomiting, dysuria, cough, shortness of breath, joint pain, rashes)
2. Duration and magnitude of fever
3. Close contacts with similar illness
4. Occupational, travel, or recreational exposure
5. History of diseases associated with immunocompromise (e.g., HIV), diabetes, chronic renal failure, blood dyscrasia, alcohol or drug abuse, chronic lung disease, or cardiac valve disease
6. Presence of medical hardware (e.g., prosthetic valves)
7. History of recent hospitalizations, which might suggest nosocomial infections
8. Current medications, particularly antibiotics and antipyretics, and duration of use
9. Allergies

Physical Examination

The most important observation on the physical examination is the general overall appearance and mental status of the patient. Specifically, does the patient look well or toxic? Does the patient have an altered mental status, which might indicate infection or sepsis, especially in the elderly? Vital signs should be obtained, including pulse oximetry in selected patients with respiratory signs or symptoms. In the presence of a fever, the pulse can be expected to increase by 10 beats per minute for each 0.55°C increase in temperature. Some diseases are associated with a relative bradycardia for the degree of fever (pulse–temperature dissociation). This association is classically seen with typhoid fever, but it can be seen in legionnaire disease, mycoplasmal infections, drug fever, factitious fever, and some viral syndromes. In addition, patients taking beta-blockers may have no change in their pulse in response to a fever. The earliest sign of septic shock is an inappropriately elevated pulse. Tachypnea and dyspnea are suggestive of pulmonary disease, while tachypnea without dyspnea may indicate sepsis or metabolic acidosis of any cause. The history will frequently direct the physician to the most likely source of the infection. In the absence of localizing symptoms, a thorough examination should be undertaken. The entire body should be examined for rashes, skin breakdown or decubiti, cellulitis, "track marks," or lymphadenopathy. Rashes may suggest a viral exanthem, vasculitis, meningococcemia, Rocky Mountain spotted fever, Lyme disease, or toxic shock syndrome (staphylococcal or streptococcal). Lymphadenopathy associated with fever may suggest malignancy, autoimmune disorders, or infection. Tender, localized adenopathy is usually associated with an infection in the region drained by the involved nodes. The most common cause of acute generalized adenopathy is infectious mononucleosis. Nodes secondary to malignancy are usually painless, rubbery, and firm.

The head and neck should be examined for scleral icterus, which might indicate hepatitis or cholecystitis. Examination in and around the ears may reveal otitis externa or media, or suggest mastoiditis. The oropharynx may show evidence of pharyngitis, peritonsillar or retropharyngeal abscess, or periodontal infection. Sore throat, drooling, and fever may suggest epiglottitis in children or adults. While children should be examined in the operating room, the adult epiglottis may be visualized by direct or indirect laryngoscopy in the ED.

The chest should be examined for indications of a pulmonary or cardiac cause of fever. Localized rales or rhonchi suggest pneumonia. As x-ray findings frequently lag behind physical findings, an early pneumonia may not be visible on x-ray. A pericardial rub is indicative of pericarditis, and a new heart murmur should suggest endocarditis, especially in intravenous (i.v.) drug users. However, functional murmurs may increase due to fever-induced tachycardia.

The abdomen should be examined for signs of peritoneal irritation or ascites. Localized pain may suggest cholecystitis, appendicitis, pancreatitis, or diverticulitis. Suprapubic pain suggests a urinary tract infection. A rectal examination may demonstrate evidence of a perirectal abscess or prostatitis. In patients with a urethral discharge, a detailed sexual history should be obtained. A swollen or painful testicle suggests epididymoorchitis or torsion. In women, a pelvic examination should be performed to evaluate for sexually transmitted diseases, cervical motion or upper tract tenderness suggestive of pelvic inflammatory disease, or tuboovarian abscesses.

Examination of the musculoskeletal system is often overlooked in febrile patients, but examination of the spine may reveal tenderness suggestive of osteomyelitis, discitis, or epidural abscess (especially in i.v. drug users). A detailed examination of the extremities may demonstrate a septic or inflamed joint, or it may suggest osteomyelitis, myositis, or deep venous thrombosis. In i.v. drug users, skin-popping and track-mark sites should be examined for evidence of cutaneous abscesses, crepitance suggestive of soft-tissue infection, and infected pseudoaneurysms.

Laboratory Evaluation

While no test exists that easily identifies patients with serious infections, a thorough understanding of certain basic laboratory tests can greatly enhance patient evaluation. The white blood cell (WBC) count is the oldest and best-known screening test used to differentiate serious bacterial infections from other disorders. In adults, however, its discriminatory value is not as great as most expect. In a study of febrile adults with unexplained fever after careful physical examination, only 56% of those subsequently shown to have a bacterial source had a WBC count over 15,000/μL. In addition, an elevated WBC count is nonspecific. Neutrophilia can occur secondary to emotional or physical stress, acute or chronic inflammation, benign or malignant tumors, myeloproliferative disorders, asthma, seizures, or medications such as steroids, lithium, or epinephrine. Neutrophil counts over 30,000/μL have been reported secondary to strenuous exercise, seizures, and lithium use.[19] In addition, patients with low WBC counts (less than 1,000/μL) are at significant risk for occult bacterial infections.

A "left shift" is only slightly more useful. A total neutrophil band count greater than 1500/μL was found in approximately one-third of patients with unexplained fever, of which only half proved to have bacterial infections. Table 5.2 lists the effect of several noninfectious processes on the WBC count. From these data, it is apparent that the WBC count is neither sensitive nor specific for bacterial infection.

Certain changes in neutrophil morphology are associated with bacterial infections. Toxic granulations are small, dark cytoplasmic inclusions found in 75% of bacteremic patients. They can also be seen in patients with vasculitis and in those who are on chemotherapy. Döhle bodies are round or oval cytoplasmic inclusions seen in 29% of bacteremic patients, as well as in patients with burns, trauma, or neoplasms, or during pregnancy. Cytoplasmic vacuolization has the best correlation with significant bacterial disease. In one study, 91% of patients with more than 10% vacuolization had bacteremia. Cytoplasmic vacuolization has not proved useful in pediatric studies.

TABLE 5.2. Noninfectious Processes That May Alter WBC Counts

Cause	WBC Count	Comment
Burns, fractures, epinephrine injection	Leukocytosis with neutrophilia but no "left shift"	WBC increase immediate; lasts 2–3 h
Corticosteroids, Cushing syndrome	Leukocytosis with neutrophilia, "left shift," eosinopenia	Onset 18 h after oral dose; duration 24 h after last dose
Diabetic ketoacidosis	Leukocytosis with "left shift"	Up to 25,000/μL
Addison disease	Lymphocytosis, neutropenia, eosinophilia	

Measurement of acute-phase reactants, ESR and CRP, is often used to help recognize patients with serious occult infections. The results can be misleading, as these tests are neither sensitive nor specific. The ESR is often used as a screening test for temporal arteritis, bacterial endocarditis, tuberculosis, osteomyelitis, and occult bacteremia in children.[11]

A major disadvantage of the ESR is the 1-hour time to complete the test (ESR is the distance, in millimeters, that red blood cells in citrated blood fall in 1 hour). In a recent study of 192 patients,[11] no patients with elevated sedimentation rates (greater than 20 mm in males, greater than 30 mm in females) had an ESR less than 5 mm at 30 minutes. Therefore, values less than 5 mm at 30 minutes should allow the physician to conclude that the ESR is normal while waiting only half the normal time of the test.[11] When the ESR is elevated, no conclusion can be made prior to the 1-hour time frame.

Several newer tests have been developed to measure the ESR more rapidly (e.g., the zeta sedimentation rate, which determines the ESR in 4 minutes). Unfortunately, these tests require more expensive equipment, and they are not accurate at high ESR values.

CRP, an acute-phase reactant in serum, is more sensitive and specific and rises faster than the ESR, but again it is not particularly useful in the emergency department. While many small studies have indicated that an elevated CRP may be useful in detecting acute intraabdominal infections, a recent metaanalysis of 22 studies using CRP to aid in the diagnosis of appendicitis found a combined sensitivity and specificity of only 62% and 66%, respectively.[10] The individual studies showed a wide range of sensitivities (40% to 99%) and specificities (27% to 90%), believed to be due in part to the wide variation of cut-off values used. With the few exceptions noted previously, both the ESR and CRP are probably best used for following the resolution of a known disease.

There is no consensus on the value of screening for streptococcal pharyngitis in febrile patients with a sore throat. Throat cultures may be falsely positive (in the case of a carrier state) or falsely negative. The sensitivity of commercial rapid streptococcal screens varies between 55% and 96%, with specificities between 50% and 98%. In addition, the rapid screens test only for streptococcal disease and not for other causes of pharyngitis, such as gonococcus, *Chlamydia*, or *Mycoplasma*. Consequently, it is debatable whether cultures or rapid screens should be obtained or whether treatment should be based solely on clinical suspicion (sore throat, fever, lymphadenopathy, lack of other upper respiratory tract symptoms, or recent exposure to group A streptococcus).

An appropriately performed urinalysis demonstrating pyuria and bacteriuria in patients with suprapubic pain, dysuria, frequency, or hesitancy supports a diagnosis of urinary tract infection (UTI). In young adult women, urine cultures are probably not necessary at the time of initial diagnosis. In older women, men, children, and patients with comorbid diseases, and in cases resistant to therapy, urine cultures are recommended. In one study of febrile children less than 1 year old,[12] the frequency of a UTI was approximately 5%, whether or not a UTI was suspected. In this study, the sensitivity of pyuria (greater than 5 WBC/hpf) and bacteriuria on urinalysis for detecting a UTI was 54% and 86%, respectively.[12] In addition, in adults in whom there is a high clinical suspicion but a negative urinalysis, urine cultures should be obtained and initial treatment based on the degree of suspicion. The formation of significant levels of nitrites or leukocytes in the urine occurs over time (up to 6 hours), and individuals with urinary frequency may thus have a falsely negative urinalysis.

Because acute diarrhea is usually self-limited, stool evaluation is rarely helpful or necessary. In the evaluation of chronic diarrhea, traveler's diarrhea, or antibiotic-associated diarrhea, or in cases in which there are a cluster of causes, evaluation for fecal leukocytes is the most useful test. The presence of fecal leukocytes is 82% sensitive and 83% specific for detecting bacterial diarrhea.[6] Stool should be tested for *Clostridium difficile* toxin if there is a history of recent antibiotic use. The presence of ova or parasites is indicative of a parasitic etiology for diarrhea. In patients with presumed viral or benign disease, stool cultures are probably not necessary in the absence of fecal leukocytes. Cultures are indicated in any patient who appears toxic, has been exposed to other patients with enteritis, or is at risk for unusual pathogens or parasitic diseases. In travelers from malarious areas, malaria should also be considered, as it may present with fever, gastrointestinal (GI) symptoms, and anemia, but without cells in the stool.

Like many laboratory tests, there is no consensus on the value of routine blood cultures in febrile patients. The incidence of bacteremia in the emergency department has been reported to vary from 2.6% to as high as 10.7% of febrile patients. The higher figures generally come from tertiary referral centers, the lower figures from community hospitals. Most community hospitals report approximately equal numbers of gram-positive and gram-negative bacteremia, whereas university centers report a much higher incidence of gram-negative bacteremia. Mortality from bacteremia ranges from 20% to 40%; there are no data, however, on mortality for clinically unsuspected bacteremia.

Several studies have shown that blood culture results rarely alter the treatment of patients with either community-acquired pneumonia (CAP) or nosocomial pneumonias. In one study of 517 patients admitted for CAP, cultures were positive in only 6.6% (34) of patients, and of those the culture results altered therapy in only seven patients (1.4% of the total). Of these seven, six were already on drugs to which the organism was sensitive, and the change was made to a cheaper, narrow-spectrum drug.[5]

Sklar and Rusnak[16] examined the value of outpatient blood cultures in febrile adults discharged from the emergency department. In this study, 5 of 86 patients subsequently proved to have positive blood cultures. All were contacted, and four were subsequently admitted. No long-term morbidity was noted.[16] Of these patients, three were diagnosed with endocarditis and one with pyelonephritis. The fifth patient, who refused to return for admission, had presumed pneumococcal endocarditis. Each of the patients with endocarditis had identifiable risk factors (two with murmur and a history of rheumatic fever, one on dialysis and with a murmur, and one i.v. drug abuser). Other studies have shown that patients with underlying illnesses, most commonly diabetes, are at greater risk for bacteremia, and this study seems to support those findings. Therefore, it might prove prudent to limit outpatient blood cultures to febrile patients who have underlying diseases or risk factors

For inpatients, the current recommendations are to obtain cultures in patients with fever and signs of sepsis (hypotension, tachycardia, fevers, chills), in those with altered mental status, in ill-appearing patients with unexplained leukocytosis, and in immunocompromised patients. In addition, some recommend blood cultures to identify the causative organism in pneumonia, osteomyelitis, meningitis, or septic arthritis, but in general, it is preferable to obtain cultures directly from the infected site. Cultures are rarely helpful adjuncts in the management of immunocompetent patients with simple infections such as cellulitis, orchitis, dental infections, and most CAPs.

Lumbar puncture to obtain cerebrospinal fluid (CSF) for analysis is recommended in patients with fever, headache, photophobia, and signs of meningeal irritation such as nuchal rigidity or Kernig's or Brudzinski's sign. However, signs of meningeal irritation are frequently absent, especially in the very young or old; one must have a low threshold to perform a lumbar puncture in these patients. The CSF should be routinely analyzed for protein, glucose, Gram stain, and cell count with differential. In selected cases, a VDRL/RPR for syphilis, viral cultures, or tests for bacterial antigens should be added.

Various antigenic tests are available; they have the advantage of identifying a specific organism when positive. Latex agglutination is rapid, economical, and noninvasive. Better results are obtained with urine than with serum or CSF, presumably because the antigens are more concentrated in urine. Unfortunately, these tests historically have had a high specificity (greater than 99%) but a low sensitivity. The sensitivity is best for *Haemophilus influenzae* and group B streptococci (61% and 67%, respectively) and much worse (7%) for *Streptococcus pneumoniae*.[1] Fortunately, children have much less morbidity with pneumococci than with *H. influenzae*. In addition, the importance of detecting *H. influenzae* has diminished with the decline in documented cases as a result of the introduction of the *H. influenzae* vaccine. While there may be a theoretical advantage in identifying the causative organism, one study[1] has shown that, in clinical practice, treatment and disposition decisions are made without utilizing the latex agglutination results. Latex agglutination is less useful in adults because they are at risk for many more pathogens. Commercial reagents are available only for *Streptococcus pneumoniae, Neisseria meningitidis, H. influenzae,* and group B streptococci.

Enzyme-linked immunosorbent assay (ELISA), an immunologic test, is much more sensitive in detecting pneumococci than is latex agglutination. The ELISA is positive in 76% of cases. Quicker means of identifying organisms grown in blood cultures is also available. DNA probes have been developed that, when mixed with the growth from positive blood culture bottles, directly and rapidly identify *Staphylococcus aureus, S. pneumoniae, Escherichia coli, H. influenzae, Enterococcus* sp., and *Streptococcus agalactiae*. This method uses a chemiluminescent probe that detects the rRNA of the target organism.

Radiologic Studies

Routine chest radiographs are commonly obtained in patients who present with fever without an obvious source. This practice is largely based on studies that show lack of auscultatory findings in up to 25% of patients with infiltrates on chest radiographs. Better sensitivity should be obtained, however, when auscultatory findings are correlated with respiratory symptoms such as tachypnea, shortness of breath, or cough. In infants and children, chest radiographs are currently recommended only in patients with fever and signs or symptoms of a lower respiratory tract infection (e.g., rales, rhonchi, wheezing, retractions, tachypnea, stridor, cough). In one study[4] of 197 febrile infants less than 3 months old, 40 had no respiratory signs or symptoms. Radiographs in these 40 were normal in all but four, and the only abnormality present in these four was hyperinflation.

Signs or symptoms should guide the need for other radiologic studies. Plain films may reveal osteomyelitis in patients with fever and bone pain, but bone scans are more sensitive. Abdominal radiographs may identify free air (bowel perforation), appendicoliths or focal ileus (appendicitis), thumbprinting or gas in the bowel wall (mesenteric ischemia), or pneumobilia or gallstones (cholecystitis). Patients with fever and abdominal pain may benefit from an ultrasound to evaluate for the presence of cholecystitis, pelvic inflammatory disease, or a tuboovarian abscess. Computed tomography scans should be used in selected patients to evaluate for appendicitis, abdominal abscess, or diverticulitis. Magnetic resonance imaging should be considered in i.v. drug abusers with back pain and fever to rule out epidural abscess.

EMERGENCY DEPARTMENT MANAGEMENT

While antipyretics are frequently used in febrile patients who are significantly uncomfortable or tachycardic, their use should always be weighed against any potential benefit of the fever, as well as the inherit toxicity of the medication. In spite of popular belief, the response to antipyretics does not allow the differentiation between serious (e.g., bacterial) and nonserious (e.g., viral) infections. In addition, some practitioners believe there is an unwarranted phobia of fever in children, resulting in knee-jerk administration of antipyretics without first judging the overall appearance of the child (i.e., when febrile, does the child look toxic, or is he or she active and playful?). When a decision is made to use antipyretics and there are no contraindications, adults should receive oral doses of 650 to 1000 mg acetaminophen or 800 mg ibuprofen. Children should receive 15 to 20 mg per kilogram acetaminophen orally or 30 to 40 mg per kilogram rectally. Ibuprofen dosed at 10 mg per kilogram orally may be used in children over 6 months of age. Because of the potential for dehydration in febrile infants less than 6 months old, ibuprofen is not recommended because it may increase the risk of kidney damage.

The choice of antibiotics should, when possible, be based on the type and site of infection. Septic patients should be started on broad-spectrum antibiotics after appropriate specimens for culture are obtained. Suggested antibiotic regimens for the initial treatment of sepsis are listed in Table 5.3. It is probably best not to initiate antibiotics in a febrile patient with an unknown source who appears nontoxic or is not thought to be septic.

DISPOSITION

When considering the disposition of the febrile patient, the single most important consideration is his or her general health. A young person with no medical problems has a very slight chance of developing a serious infection (with the exception of i.v. drug abusers). As the age and presence of underlying medical problems increase, the chance of serious occult infection in-

Table 5.3. Suggested Antibiotic Regimens for the Initial Treatment of Septic Patients

Patient	Antibiotic
Neonate (<1 wk old)	Cefotaxime (50 mg/kg i.v. q12h) *plus* ampicillin (25 mg/kg i.v. q8h)
Neonate (1 wk–2 mo)	Cefotaxime (50 mg/kg i.v. q8h) *plus* ampicillin (25 mg/kg i.v. q6h)
Infant/child	Cefotaxime (50 mg/kg i.v. q8h) *or* ceftriaxone (100 mg/kg i.v. q24h)
Adult	Ticarcillin/clavulanic acid (3.1 g i.v. q6h) *or* piperacillin/tazobactam (3.375 g i.v. q6h) or imipenem (500–1,000 mg i.v. q8h) *or* meropenem (1 g i.v. q8h)

creases and makes admission advisable. Keating and associates[14] found that 95% of patients who were older than 60 years and had a temperature above 101°F (38.3°C) on admission to the emergency department had a serious infection, with 92.5% requiring admission. Wasserman and colleagues[18] reported that the sensitivity and specificity of fever (37.5°C or greater) as an indicator of bacterial infection in an elderly patient were 50% and 86%, respectively. The sensitivity and specificity of a WBC count above 14,000/μL were 44% and 88%, respectively, and the sensitivity and specificity of a band percentage on the differential of 6% or higher were 32% and 93%, respectively. All patients with fever, elevated WBC, and bandemia meeting the previously described criteria were diagnosed with bacterial infections. Only 6% of the patients with none of the criteria described were diagnosed with bacterial infection.[18]

Any patient with unexplained fever and neutropenia or malignancy should be admitted for a full "septic" workup. Patients with diabetes are at special risk, as discussed, as are patients who are taking corticosteroids. Alcoholics are also considered to be immunosuppressed and at increased risk. They have many alterations in their host defenses and may require admission for infections that are often treated on an outpatient basis among other populations.

The postsplenectomy patient is at special risk for developing clinically inapparent bacteremia, usually from *S. pneumoniae*. Such patients often have fever and a flulike syndrome as their only complaints. Even when these patients are promptly diagnosed and started on antibiotics, there is a 50% to 75% mortality; they should all be encouraged to be immunized against *S. pneumoniae*.

If good follow-up can be arranged, specimens for cultures can be obtained in the emergency department, and the nontoxic, low-risk patient can be discharged and rechecked in 24 hours, when initial culture results become available. Continued follow-up or contact is necessary until cultures are confirmed negative.

COMMON PITFALLS

- When a fever is important to the evaluation and management of a patient, the temperature should be obtained rectally.
- Do not ignore parental reports of fever in infants who are afebrile on arrival to the emergency department.
- Do not attribute fever in infants to overbundling.
- In adults and the elderly, the WBC count should be interpreted cautiously when used to judge the seriousness of an infection.
- The response to antipyretics does not help differentiate serious from nonserious infections.

References

1. Adcock PM, Paul RI, Marshall GS. Effect of urine latex agglutination tests on the treatment of children at risk for invasive bacterial infection. *Pediatrics* 1995;96:951.
2. Anagnostakis D, et al. Rectal-axillary temperature difference in febrile and afebrile infants and children. *Clin Pediatr* 1993;32:268.
3. Blatteis CM, Sehic E. Cytokines and fever. *Ann N Y Acad Sci* 1998;840:608.
4. Bramson RT, et al. The futility of the chest radiograph in the febrile infant without respiratory symptoms. *Pediatrics* 1993;92:524.
5. Chalasani NP, et al. Clinical utility of blood cultures in adult patients with community-acquired pneumonia without defined underlying risks. *Chest* 1995;108:932.
6. DuBois D, Binder L, Nelson B. Usefulness of the stool Wright's stain in the emergency department. *J Emerg Med* 1988;6:483.
7. Gobbi PG, et al. Night sweats in Hodgkin's disease: a manifestation of preceding minor febrile pulses. *Cancer* 1990;65:2074.
8. Graneto JW, Soglin DF. Maternal screening of childhood fever by palpation. *Pediatr Emerg Care* 1996;12:183.
9. Grover G, et al. The effects of bundling on infant temperature. *Pediatrics* 1994;94:669.
10. Hallan S, Asberg A. The accuracy of C-reactive protein in diagnosing acute appendicitis—a meta-analysis. *Scand J Clin Lab Invest* 1997;57:373.
11. Harrow C, Singer AJ, Thode HC. Facilitating the use of the erythrocyte sedimentation rate in the emergency department. *Acad Emerg Med* 1999;6:658.
12. Hoberman A, et al. Prevalence of urinary tract infection in febrile infants. *J Pediatr* 1993:123:17.
13. Hooker EA. Use of tympanic thermometers to screen for fever in patients in a pediatric emergency department. *South Med J* 1993;86:855.
14. Keating HJ, et al. Effect of aging on the clinical significance of fever in ambulatory adult patients. *J Am Geriatr Soc* 1984;32:282.
15. Kresovich-Wendler K, Levitt MA, Yearly L. An evaluation of clinical predictors to determine need for rectal temperature measurement in the emergency department. *Am J Emerg Med* 1989;7:391.
16. Sklar DP, Rusnak R. The value of outpatient blood cultures in the emergency department. *Am J Emerg Med* 1987;5:95.
17. Tandberg D, Sklar D. Effect of tachypnea on the estimation of body temperature by an oral thermometer. *N Engl J Med* 1983;308:945.
18. Wasserman M, et al. Utility of fever, white blood cells, and differential count in predicting bacterial infections in the elderly. *J Am Geriatr Soc* 1989;37:537.
19. Young GP. CBC or not CBC? That is the question. *Ann Emerg Med* 1986;15:367.

CHAPTER 6
Edema

J. Stephan Stapczynski

Edema is the presence of increased interstitial (extravascular) fluid that becomes clinically detectable. Edema may be localized to one portion of the body or generalized throughout many areas of the body. Severe generalized edema is termed *anasarca*. An increased amount of interstitial fluid may also accumulate in potential body cavities, such as the pleural space or peritoneal cavity, producing the conditions of hydrothorax or ascites, respectively. The amount of fluid necessary to produce detectable edema depends on its distribution. Localized edema of the lips (like that seen with acute allergic angioedema) is evident with the accumulation of only a few milliliters, whereas the generalized edema of congestive heart failure (CHF) requires an increase of several liters of body water to be detected.

The pathogenesis of edema is intimately connected with the concept of total body water and its division into various components. Total body water is responsible for approximately 70% of body weight; roughly two-thirds is intracellular, and one-third is extracellular. Extracellular water is approximately one-fourth intravascular and three-fourths interstitial. Because water is freely diffusible across most cell membranes, there is a constant exchange between these compartments. Under steady-state conditions, the relative amounts found in each compartment are determined by the interplay between hydrostatic and oncotic forces as represented by the Starling equation.

$$\text{Fluid accumulation} = K[(P_c - P_{if}) - \sigma(\pi_p - \pi_{if})] - Q_{lymph}$$

with

K = hydraulic conductance
P_c = mean intracapillary hydrostatic pressure
P_{if} = mean interstitial hydrostatic pressure
σ = reflection coefficient of oncotically active macromolecules
π_p = plasma oncotic pressure
π_{if} = interstitial fluid oncotic pressure
Q_{lymph} = lymphatic flow

Intravascular hydrostatic pressure tends to force fluid out of vessels into the interstitium, and plasma oncotic pressure tends to draw it back. The usual intensity of these forces *in vivo* is such that there is bulk flow of fluid out of the capillaries into the interstitial space. Overexpansion of the interstitial volume and clinical edema are prevented by the lymphatics, which return excess interstitial fluid to the vascular space. The edematous disorders can be classified according to which component of the Starling equation is deranged.

Increased capillary permeability can be due to mechanical, toxic, chemical, thermal, immunologic, or radiation damage to vascular endothelium.[1] Edema associated with focal inflammation or infection is produced by increased capillary permeability caused by the chemical or immunologic mediators of inflammation. As capillaries become more permeable, plasma protein leaks into the interstitial space and interstitial oncotic pressure rises, drawing more fluid out of the vessels. A new steady state is reached when increased interstitial pressure balances the other forces. Edema fluid resulting from capillary leak has a relatively high protein content and tends not to "pit" under the examiner's fingertip pressure.[1]

Vasomotor tone provided by the autonomic nerves is an important factor in maintaining the integrity of the venous and lymphatic microcirculation. Neurologic illness or injuries that affect the autonomic nervous system can promote the development of edema. Patients with hemiplegic cerebrovascular accidents (CVAs) tend to develop unilateral edema on the paralyzed side, especially if the involved side is dependent. Likewise, vasodilation—either local or systemic—can lead to the development of edema. Nonsteroidal antiinflammatory agents, monamine oxidase inhibitors, beta-adrenergic blockers, and other vasodilators may produce edema as a side effect.

Increased capillary hydrostatic pressure can be generalized due to an elevated systemic venous pressure, which unbalances the Starling equation throughout the systemic circulation. Edema usually becomes manifest where the hydrostatic forces are greatest—in the legs during upright posture. Many systemic causes of edema lead to renal retention of sodium and an increase in total body water, further exaggerating the formation of edema. Increased capillary hydrostatic pressure can be localized to a portion of the vascular system due to venous outflow obstruction, venous valvular incompetence, or prolonged upright posture. Patients with venous hypertension have increased skin blood flow and a defective vasoconstrictive response to upright posture; both are associated with a marked increase in capillary filtration. Prolonged dependency of the legs without muscle activity will cause edema in healthy people.

Reduced plasma oncotic pressure is usually due to decreased levels of plasma albumin, the most oncotically active plasma protein. Conditions such as starvation, malabsorption, protein-losing enteropathies, cirrhosis, nephrotic syndrome, and severe catabolic states may cause hypoalbuminemia. Edema from hypoalbuminemia tends to pit slowly but easily and to accumulate in the soft tissues about the eyelids, especially when the patient is supine.

In most capillary beds, the interplay between hydrostatic and oncotic forces is such that there is a consistent flow of fluid out of the vascular system into the interstitial space. The accumulation of excess interstitial fluid is prevented by lymphatic flow, but if the regional lymphatics are blocked, then edema can develop.[8] Because of the high protein content that develops in the interstitial space, lymphedema tends to be brawny, nonpitting, and resistant to treatment. Lymphedema tends to accumulate in the interstitial tissues, whereas edema from venous disease collects in the subfascial areas. In primary lymphedema, the problem appears to be an abnormality in the cutaneous and subcutaneous lymphatic channels. Secondary lymphedema is caused by obstruction of lymph flow in the regional lymph nodes or lymphatic channels. In Western countries, the most common causes of lymphedema are neoplastic infiltration, surgical resection, and irradiation of regional lymph nodes.[8]

In some conditions, edema develops without clear-cut imbalances in the Starling equation. These include hyperthyroidism, hypothyroidism, and idiopathic (cyclic) edema. Idiopathic edema is a syndrome with several manifestations, the most characteristic being edema formation during orthostasis, with resolution during recumbency. Weight gains of more than 4 lb during the day are common. The syndrome is found almost exclusively in women of childbearing age. Edema formation is aggravated by several factors, including the menstrual cycle, obesity, increased salt ingestion, heat, prolonged standing, and drugs (Table 6.1). The most consistent observation in attempting to unravel the pathogenesis of idiopathic edema has been that of an increase in capillary permeability with loss of effective arterial volume when the patient is in an upright position. As discussed later, this leads to expansion of body water and greater edema. Some patients initially thought to have idiopathic edema may have subclinical hypothyroidism. Others may have subtle CHF or edema caused by wearing tight clothes.

In understanding the production of edema, it is important to distinguish between primary events (such as diminished cardiac output or decreased serum albumin levels) and secondary responses. Many, if not most, of the primary processes lead to a decrease in effective arterial volume by reducing blood volume or cardiac output. This diminished arterial volume leads to renal underperfusion and increased retention of sodium. To preserve normotonicity, water excretion also decreases. The resultant overexpansion of body water tends to restore effective arterial volume, albeit at the expense of overexpansion of the other fluid compartments, especially the interstitial space. For example, edema caused by cirrhosis tends to be initially localized in the abdomen because the portal venous system is obstructed. However, as ascites volume increases, effective arterial volume decreases, and secondary renal retention of sodium leads to expansion of total body water. Therefore, a disorder that may initially be localized can become generalized. Although edema can be distinguished as that which is usually generalized or usually localized, exceptions are common.

TABLE 6.1. Classification of Edema According to Cause (Example)

EDEMA CAUSED BY INCREASED CAPILLARY PERMEABILITY
Mechanical damage (contusions)
Toxic and chemical damage (infiltration of antineoplastic agents into the subcutaneous tissues)
Infection (cellulitis)
Thermal damage (burns)
Immunologic damage (allergic angioedema)
Radiation damage (radiation therapy)
Loss of autonomic tone (CVA)
Loss of local metabolic responsiveness (sometimes edema seen with nonsteroidal antiinflammatories)
Inhibition of kinase II by ACE inhibitors
Drug-induced vasodilation (beta-blockers, calcium channel blockers, direct vasodilators)
EDEMA CAUSED BY INCREASED CAPILLARY HYDROSTATIC PRESSURE
Generalized Increase in Venous Pressure
Congestive heart failure
Constrictive pericardial disease
Renal (acute glomerulonephritis, acute renal failure)
Pulmonary artery hypertension (cor pulmonale)
Drugs that promote renal retention of sodium (steroids, estrogens, vasodilators)
Focal Increase in Venous Pressure
Venous obstruction of isolated vein (deep venous thrombosis, superior vena cava syndrome, tight-fitting garments)
Incompetent venous valves (chronic venous insufficiency)
Prolonged orthostasis (dependent edema)
EDEMA CAUSED BY DECREASED PLASMA ONCOTIC PRESSURE
Starvation
Malabsorption
Hepatic failure
Nephrotic syndrome
Extensive protein loss through skin (burns)
Inflammatory bowel disease
Cushing syndrome
Preeclampsia
EDEMA CAUSED BY LYMPHATIC OBSTRUCTION
Primary
Congenital
Acquired (lymphedema praecox)
Secondary (Obstructive)
Toxic or chemical damage
Neoplastic infiltration
Traumatic or surgical damage
Radiation damage
EDEMA CAUSED BY ENDOCRINE DISTURBANCES
Hypothyroidism
Hyperthyroidism
Hormone replacement (corticosteroids, estrogen, progesterone, testosterone)
IDIOPATHIC EDEMA

CLINICAL PRESENTATION

Edema is clinically important because it motivates patients to seek medical attention. Occasionally, localized or generalized edema can produce serious or life-threatening effects when vital organs are obstructed. For example, laryngeal edema can cause asphyxia. In some patients with chronic obstructive pulmonary disease (COPD), peripheral edema may be a marker of pulmonary decompensation with right-sided heart failure.[14] Other complications directly attributable to edema include local skin breakdown, respiratory compromise, and cardiovascular impairment.

Because hydrostatic forces are important in producing or exacerbating edema, generalized edema due to a number of causes (particularly CHF) is usually first noted in dependent body parts, such as the feet and pretibial areas when the patient is sitting or standing and the presacral areas if the patient is bedridden. Edema caused by hypoalbuminemia tends to accumulate in the periorbital loose tissues, and patients first notice puffiness about the eyes on arising in the morning. Some patients may notice tightness in the hands when edema of the fingers makes it difficult to slip rings on and off. Edema caused by increased hydrostatic pressure or hypoalbuminemia is usually soft and pitting. Lymphedema, edema caused by increased vascular permeability, and edema seen with thyroid disease tend to be firm and nonpitting. Primary lymphedema, or edema of systemic etiology, may be uncomfortable but is usually not frankly painful.

Another cause of lower extremity swelling is lipedema, a

lipodystrophy that can be confused with lymphedema.[11] Lipedema produces symmetric swelling with soft fatty tissue, extending from the proximal thighs to the ankles, exhibiting prominent malleolar fat pads, but sparing the feet. Lipedema is more common in women, and produces soft, minimally pitting swelling that is often tender. Other family members may be affected. Lipedema does not produce the skin changes common in lymphedema. Lipedema also does not appear to predispose the limb to infection, whereas lymphedema may be complicated by episodes of cellulitis.

Edema confined to a single limb is usually due to obstruction of the draining veins or lymphatics.[7] Patients with hemiplegic CVAs may develop unilateral edema due to loss of autonomic innervation to the paralyzed side of the body, and the edema is more prominent when the affected side is dependent. Asymmetric leg edema, usually on the left side, may also be seen in elderly bedridden patients due to iliac vein obstruction.[12] Unilateral extremity edema can been seen in limbs with arteriovenous fistulas (placed for hemodialysis) or arterial bypass grafts (performed for ischemic disease).[13] In both cases, edema appears to result from arterial pressure reaching the venous and capillary beds, promoting fluid extravasation due to increased intravascular pressure. Lymphatic disruption during arterial exposure may also play a role. Edema of the neck, face, and shoulders is common in superior vena caval obstruction. Isolated facial edema can be seen with angioedema and other allergic reactions.

Sustained edema produces changes in the overlying skin, causing it to thicken and eventually become scarred. Occasionally, edema may produce local vasodilation and a slight erythematous appearance of the skin, but marked redness or warmth usually indicates local inflammation or infection. Prolonged venous stasis leads to a change in skin pigmentation and, occasionally, skin breakdown and chronic ulceration (usually just above the medial malleolus).

DIFFERENTIAL DIAGNOSIS

Edema is one of the classic signs of inflammation. A major differential diagnostic consideration, therefore, in patients with edema is whether focal inflammation or infection is present. The problem is complicated by the observation that patients with one cause of edema (such as CHF or cirrhosis) may be susceptible to other causes of edema (such as deep vein thrombosis or cellulitis). Clues to inflammation or infection include marked redness, warmth, significant pain, and lymphangitis.

Several disorders may present with leg pain and swelling, mimicking some of the edematous disorders. Erythema nodosum, an inflammatory disease involving the cutaneous and subcutaneous blood vessels, may present with acute (less than 72-hour) unilateral or bilateral lower extremity edema. A leaking or ruptured popliteal (Baker's) cyst of the knee may produce calf swelling and pain. An acute tear of the medial head of the gastrocnemius muscle presents as pain in the medial mid-calf area and may mimic deep venous thrombosis. Reflex sympathetic dystrophy often presents with swelling as an early sign, in addition to the other symptoms of burning pain, hyperesthesia, and skin changes. Malignancies of bone, cartilage, and soft tissues may produce unilateral limb swelling.

An important suspicion is the possibility of the development of an acute venous obstruction in a patient with chronic leg edema caused by CHF or venous insufficiency. Helpful clues include a sudden increase in edema over a short time (less than 72 hours), erythema and/or warmth, and increased edema confined to one leg.

EMERGENCY DEPARTMENT EVALUATION

The initial assessment of edema should focus on the following issues: (1) the distribution, (2) the presence of pitting versus nonpitting, (3) the time course of its onset, (4) the pattern of progression, (5) any variability throughout the day, and (6) the presence of associated erythema, warmth, or pain.[3,5,7,9]

The first distinction to make is whether edema is generalized or focal. Focal edema is usually caused by local venous obstruction, lymphatic obstruction, or inflammation.[7] Marked warmth, redness, and pain indicate inflammation. The sudden onset of edema in the face or lips is typical of allergic angioedema or angioedema associated with angiotensin converting enzyme (ACE) inhibitors or other drugs.[6] The incidence of ACE-inhibitor angioedema has been estimated to be one to 12 cases per 1000 patients treated.[10] Most cases present within 1 week after onset of therapy. Unilateral leg edema is most commonly caused by chronic venous insufficiency.[7] Other clues that support this diagnosis are chronic skin changes, hyperpigmentation, and ulcerations.

Generalized edema is common in a number of systemic diseases and functional abnormalities. In CHF, other signs of left or right heart failure will usually be evident, such as cardiomegaly, elevated jugular venous pressure, hepatojugular reflux, third and fourth heart sounds, and pulmonary rales. Patients with cirrhosis who develop edema usually have other stigmata of liver disease and ascites. In patients with generalized edema, the urine should be checked for the presence of protein and cells. Moderate-to-large proteinuria detected with a standard urine dipstick strongly suggests renal disease. Patients with acute glomerulonephritis or acute renal failure occasionally present with edema. Chronic renal failure is a rare cause of edema, because most patients can balance their fluid status despite markedly low urine output. Measurement of serum albumin levels is necessary to detect patients in whom hypoalbuminemia (less than 2.5 g/dL) is a causative factor.

The production of pitting requires firm pressure over a bony area for at least several seconds. Slow pitting and recovery are common in hypoalbuminemia-related edema. Nonpitting edema is characteristic of lymphedema, increased vascular permeability, and thyroid disease, and is sometimes seen in longstanding cases of edema due to other causes.

Edema that develops over 24 to 48 hours is most consistent with acute inflammation or venous obstruction.[7,9] Lower extremity edema, often asymmetric, is common in elderly patients who live in chronic care facilities. A predisposition to left-sided edema has been noted.[12] Compression of the left common iliac vein and the accompanying lymphatics by the right iliac artery were proposed to explain this observation. If no obstructive cause can be found on physical examination (inguinal or supraclavicular lymphadenopathy, abdominal or pelvic mass, or signs of deep venous thrombosis), further investigation of elderly patients with asymmetric or unilateral left-sided edema is not felt to be warranted.

Recurrent edema is characteristic of idiopathic edema. Variability of edema throughout the day is often seen because of the influence of hydrostatic forces in edema formation, but it is most marked in idiopathic edema. The diagnosis of idiopathic edema requires the exclusion of other causes and is supported by an abnormal water-loading test. Normally more than 65% of a standard oral water load (20 mL/kg) is excreted within 4 hours, regardless of body position. Patients with idiopathic edema excrete a normal amount when recumbent but excrete less than 65% when they remain upright during the 4 hours.

Pain is unusual in primary lymphedema. It is also unusual in other systemic causes of edema.

The inguinal lymph nodes should be checked for enlargement. Venous valvular incompetence can be checked with the Brodie-Trendelenburg test.

EMERGENCY DEPARTMENT MANAGEMENT

Treatment is directed toward the underlying cause, as identified by the clinical evaluation. There is little benefit, and potential harm, to the empiric treatment of edema with diuretics. Drug-induced iatrogenic edema is common and, when possible, the responsible drugs should be changed or stopped. Angioedema is treated with beta-adrenergic agonists, antihistamines, and steroids.[6] Angioedema secondary to ACE inhibitors is generally refractory to epinephrine, antihistamines, and steroids.[4,10] The only treatment that has been shown to be clearly beneficial is discontinuation of the agent. Those patients with venous and arterial disease who present with peripheral edema and chronic skin ulcers benefit from layered compression bandage therapy and should be referred to a wound treatment specialist for evaluation.[2,5]

DISPOSITION

Patients with edema may require admission for evaluation and treatment of the underlying cause, such as CHF, COPD, or cirrhosis. Patients with angioedema affecting the upper airway should be observed closely; such swelling may suddenly worsen. ACE-inhibitor–induced angioedema is usually refractory to treatment, may persist, and may relapse after improvement.[4] It is prudent that patients with angioedema of the face and neck be observed carefully; overnight observation or hospitalization is common practice. Patients with angioedema affecting solely the face, without evidence of airway involvement, and who improve dramatically while in the emergency department, can be discharged after a period of observation.

COMMON PITFALLS

Edema is a sign, not a diagnosis. The common pitfalls associated with the assessment of edema are

- Failing to distinguish between focal and generalized distributions of edema
- Ignoring the local complications of edema
- Failing to detect the presence of cellulitis in patients with chronic edema
- Failing to elevate a swollen body part to promote resolution of edema
- Using diuretics overzealously to treat edema
- Failing to educate the patient about the causes of edema and the value of simple measures, including bed rest and dietary salt restriction

References

1. Agostini A, Cicardi M, Porreca W. Peripheral edema due to increased vascular permeability: a clinical appraisal. *Int J Clin Lab Res* 1992;21:241.
2. Bowering CK. Use of layered compression bandages in diabetic patients. Experience in patients with lower leg ulceration, peripheral edema, and features of venous and arterial disease. *Adv Wound Care* 1998;11:129.
3. Ciocon JO, Fernandez BB, Ciocon DG. Leg edema: clinical clues to the differential diagnosis. *Geriatrics* 1993;48(5):34, 45.
4. Finley C, Silverman MA, Nunez AE. Angiotensin-converting enzyme inhibitor-induced angioedema: still unrecognized. *Am J Emerg Med* 1992;10:550.
5. Hofman D. Oedema and its treatment. *J Wound Care* 1998;7[Suppl]:S10.
6. Kwong KY, Maalouf N, Jones CA. Urticaria and angioedema: pathophysiology, diagnosis, and treatment. *Pediatr Ann* 1998;27:719.
7. Merli GJ, Spandorfer J. The outpatient with unilateral leg swelling. *Med Clin North Am* 1995;79:435.
8. Mortimer PS. The pathophysiology of lymphedema. *Cancer* 1998;83:2798.
9. Powell AA, Armstrong MA. Peripheral edema. *Am Fam Physician* 1997;55:1721.
10. Pylypchuk GB. ACE-inhibitor versus angiotensin II blocker-induced cough and angioedema. *Ann Pharmacother* 1998;32:1060.
11. Rudkin GH, Miller TA. Lipedema: a clinical entity distinct from lymphedema. *Plast Reconstruct Surg* 1994;94:841.
12. Sloane PD, Baldwin R, Montgomery R, Hargett F, Hartzena A. Left-sided leg edema of the elderly: a common variant of true iliac compression syndrome. *J Am Board Fam Pract* 1993;6:1.
13. Soong CV, Barros Aab. Lower limb oedema following distal arterial bypass grafting. *Eur J Vasc Endovasc Surg* 1998;16:465.
14. Weitzenblum E, Apprill M, Oswald M, et al. Pulmonary hemodynamics in patients with chronic obstructive pulmonary disease before and during an episode of peripheral edema. *Chest* 1994;105:1377.

CHAPTER 7
Approach to Coma and Transient Loss of Consciousness

Rebecca A. Seip and Marcus L. Martin

PATHOPHYSIOLOGY

Consciousness is the result of the interaction between the reticular activating system and the cerebral cortex. The general state of alertness and wakefulness occurs in the reticular activating system, a group of neurons in the brain stem. The cognitive functions, or an awareness of the environment, are a cerebral cortical function. For a human to be fully conscious, both of these systems must be functioning.

An altered level of consciousness may be clinically characterized as a progression through various stages. Drowsiness or lethargy may be the first change seen: There is slightly decreased wakefulness and decreased interaction with the environment. The patient may be aroused by verbal stimuli. A worsening in the severity of these changes leads to obtundation, which may progress to stupor, in which the patient may be awakened only briefly by vigorous stimulation. Coma is the state in which the patient cannot be awakened by any environmental stimuli.

ORGAN SYSTEMS

Central nervous system (CNS) function can be impaired at a cellular or structural level. If impaired at a structural level, there is focal destruction of the CNS anatomy. This may result from increased intracranial pressure, with mechanical compression of CNS structures, or from direct destruction due to tumors, trauma, or intracerebral hemorrhage. A malfunction in almost any of the other organ systems may impair CNS function at a cellular level. This dysfunction may occur with hypothyroidism or adrenal insufficiency; with disturbances of electrolyte regulation, which produce hypo- or hypernatremia or hypercalcemia; or with other metabolic disturbances, such as hypoglycemia or hyperosmolar states. Illnesses resulting in renal or hepatic damage may cause uremia and hepatic encephalopathy. Hypoxia from a pulmonary or cardiac etiology may also affect CNS function. Hypotension with decreased intracranial perfusion may result from a cardiac etiology, sepsis, or volume loss from gastrointestinal (GI) bleeding or organ trauma.

Due to the interrelationships between various organ systems, CNS dysfunction may result from a combination of organ system failures, such as hepatorenal syndrome or a large myocardial infarction causing hypotension and heart failure, with resulting pulmonary compromise and hypoxia. External environmental or toxic insults may also cause CNS depression at the cellular level through a direct toxic effect or secondarily through damage to other organ systems.

In general, when the CNS is impaired at a cellular level, diffuse CNS depression ensues, producing no focal findings on the clinical examination. Two exceptions are hypoglycemia and hepatic failure, in which focal findings may be seen. Pupillary light reflexes remain intact, except when the CNS depression is caused by toxins that affect pupillary size, such as anticholinergics or opiates.

There may be focal findings on examination when a destructive process causes structural damage to a specific area of the CNS. However, a localized problem may also cause a secondary diffuse process. This may be seen with the postictal state following a seizure, in cerebral edema secondary to a tumor, or in a subarachnoid hemorrhage secondary to a ruptured aneurysm.

DIFFERENTIAL DIAGNOSIS

The differential diagnosis of coma is extensive. In the emergency department, a thorough history and physical examination will help narrow the possibilities. The list of etiologies may be divided into several groups (Table 7.1).

TABLE 7.1. Differential Diagnosis of Transient Loss of Consciousness and Coma

METABOLIC CAUSES
Electrolyte Disorders
Hypernatremia
Hyponatremia
Hypercalcemia
Hypoglycemia
Hypermagnesemia (coma due to respiratory depression, hypoxia, hypotension)
Diabetic ketoacidosis
Hyperosmolar states
Hypothyroidism
Thyrotoxicosis
Adrenal insufficiency
Hepatic encephalopathy
Uremia
Thiamine deficiency (Wernicke encephalopathy)
VASCULAR CAUSES
Hypertension
Hypotension
Vasculitis
CVA (thrombotic or hemorrhagic)
Subarachnoid hemorrhage (aneurysm or AVM)
NEUROLOGIC ETIOLOGIES
Tumor
Hydrocephalus
Status epilepticus
TRAUMA
Subdural hematoma
Epidural hematoma
Cerebral contusion
Diffuse cerebral edema
INFECTIOUS ETIOLOGIES
Meningitis
Encephalitis
Intracranial abscess
Sepsis
TOXICOLOGIC ETIOLOGIES
Carbon monoxide
Ethanol, methanol, isopropyl alcohol, ethylene glycol
Drug abuse and overdose
ENVIRONMENTAL ETIOLOGIES
Heatstroke
Hypothermia
High-altitude cerebral edema (HACE)
Near-drowning
Dysbarism

MAJOR EMERGENCY ENTITIES

In the evaluation of any patient with mental status changes or frank coma, an hypoxic etiology must always be considered and ruled out. After evaluating and treating for hypoxia, other major emergency entities must be considered.

Hypoglycemia

A common cause of altered mental status is hypoglycemia. This is most common in patients on insulin therapy. It may be due to dosage errors, missed meals, a change in exercise pattern, or erratic absorption from injection sites. Interaction with other drugs, such as alcohol, beta-blockers, or salicylates, may also lead to hypoglycemia. The oral hypoglycemic agents, including the first- and second-generation sulfonylureas and newer agents such as troglitazone, may also produce hypoglycemia. The half-life of these agents is long, so the patient should be admitted for appropriate glucose supplementation and careful monitoring.

The following drugs can potentiate the action of the oral hypoglycemics: clonidine, ethanol, beta-blockers, monoamine oxidase inhibitors, sulfonamides, coumarin anticoagulants, and salicylates. Ethanol and salicylates are two common substances that may, by themselves, induce hypoglycemia. The predominant cause of hypoglycemia until age 2 is salicylate ingestion; alcohol predominates in the succeeding 8 years. Insulin and the oral hypoglycemics, alone or with alcohol, predominate until age 50. Over age 60, the oral hypoglycemics are the most important cause.

Renal or hepatic disease with impairment of function increases the risk that a patient will develop hypoglycemia. Beta-blockers may inhibit the warning signs for hypoglycemia, although sweating is minimally affected. Hypoglycemia may also be seen in other medical conditions, such as sepsis.

When blood glucose levels begin to fall (50 to 70 mg/dL), symptoms of CNS excitation appear; these may include anxiety, tremor, sweating, and occasionally hallucinations. With a fall to the range of 20 to 50 mg/dL, further symptoms appear, including clonic convulsions, loss of consciousness, hyperreflexia, pupillary dilation, and tachycardia. As the glucose level continues to fall, progressive CNS depression and coma may occur. Brain stem reflexes are preserved until late. Primitive movements such as sucking and pouting movements of the lips, forced grasping, or extensor plantar responses may be seen as cortical control is removed. Loss of consciousness is usually preceded by a period of confusion, but it may occur suddenly. Focal neurologic signs may be present during a hypoglycemic episode due to the effect on cells that are especially sensitive or lack an adequate arterial blood supply.

Hyperglycemia

At the other end of the spectrum is diabetic ketoacidosis (DKA). This may be seen in the emergency department as the initial presentation of new-onset juvenile diabetes, in a known diabetic with poor compliance, or in a diabetic with a precipitating stressful event, such as infection. Acute myocardial infarction or treatment with steroids may also be a factor. A history of polyuria, polydipsia, nausea, vomiting, or abdominal pain may be obtained. Weight loss may be a complaint in new-onset diabetes. The patient is commonly dehydrated. Acetone breath or Kussmaul respirations may be present. Mental status changes, including coma, may be seen.

Hyperosmolar hyperglycemic nonketotic coma is more typically seen in an older patient with an undiagnosed or mild type II diabetes who experiences a precipitating severe illness. Gram-negative pneumonia, uremia with vomiting, and acute viral illness are the most commonly reported predisposing conditions. The patient typically has a longer history of symptoms before admission than in DKA and commonly presents in a coma. Mortality figures vary from 40% to 70%, in contrast to 1% to 10% in DKA.

Adrenal and Thyroid Emergencies

Adrenal and thyroid emergencies are not commonly seen in the emergency department, but it is important to keep them in mind in the differential diagnosis of coma, as life-saving treatments are available. In a patient with suspected myxedema coma, a history may reveal prior symptoms of hypothyroidism. The patient may have a history of thyroid problems, such as Graves disease, which may result in hypothyroidism. The treatment of Graves disease with radioactive iodine is associated with a relatively high incidence of eventual hypothyroidism. A surgical scar on the neck should alert the physician to the possibility of thyroid or parathyroid dysfunction. A history of noncompliance with thyroid medications may be obtained from the family.

Clinically, hypothermia to 36°C or less may be seen, blood pressure may be normal or hypotension may occur, and the pulse is generally bradycardic. Periorbital and pretibial nonpitting edema and macroglossia may be present. The patient's hair may be dry, with loss of the lateral eyebrows. The cardiac examination may be consistent with a pericardial effusion. On neurologic examination, the muscle relaxation phase of the deep tendon reflexes is classically delayed. Laboratory studies may reveal hyponatremia, hypoosmolarity, and an elevated creatine phosphokinase.

Thyroid storm rarely presents as coma. Confusion, agitation, or occasionally hallucinations may occur. Hyperthermia above 38°C and tachycardia, with or without cardiac failure, are noted. A precipitating event such as trauma or infection must be sought.

Acute adrenal crisis may occur due to an acute exacerbation of chronic adrenal insufficiency, rapid cessation of chronic steroids, or adrenal hemorrhage, which is usually secondary to sepsis. Stressors such as infection, trauma, or surgery may precipitate an adrenal crisis. Nausea, vomiting, abdominal pain, and fever may be noted. Hypovolemic shock may develop, and the mental status may deteriorate into lethargy and coma. An Addison disease patient maintained on chronic glucocorticoid replacement may not develop dehydration and hypotension until late in the course of adrenal crisis, as mineralocorticoid secretion is usually preserved.

Hypertension

In a patient with severe hypertension who presents with mental status changes, the cause may be primary hypertensive encephalopathy or an intracranial bleed. A subarachnoid hemorrhage due to a ruptured aneurysm or an arteriovenous malformation usually presents with diffuse findings. The patient may have only mild preceding mental status changes but may present comatose. The classic history is the sudden onset of a severe headache associated with nausea and vomiting. A patient may give a history of prodromal headaches in the preceding weeks. Sudden transient loss of consciousness is seen in 45% of patients. If a subarachnoid hemorrhage is suspected and the computed tomography (CT) scan is negative, a lumbar puncture must be performed. In a small percentage of patients with subarachnoid hemorrhage, the CT scan is normal.

Toxic Causes

Overdose of a wide variety of medications or illicit substances may produce a variety of mental status changes that may progress to coma. Appropriate diagnosis requires an adequate history and familiarity with the constellation of signs and symptoms that may appear in specific toxicologic emergencies.

High doses of benzodiazepines may produce sedative–hypnotic effects. Cardiac depression is usually minor, as is respiratory depression; however, respiratory depression may become a problem if benzodiazepines are combined with other CNS depressants, in the elderly, or in patients with underlying respiratory disease. Opiates and barbiturates produce more severe respiratory depression. Hypotension is commonly seen with barbiturate overdoses and may also be seen with opiates. Miosis is usually present with opiates (an exception is meperidine, in which mydriasis may be seen). Glutethimide, formerly used as a sedative–hypnotic, has properties similar to those of the barbiturates; patients generally present with dilated pupils, and the drug tends to produce a fluctuating level of consciousness. The coma may be prolonged, lasting up to several days. Pulmonary edema is most commonly seen with intravenous heroin overdose, but may be present in other opiate or barbiturate intoxications. Cutaneous bullae and hypothermia may occur with barbiturate overdoses.

Alcohol intoxication, depending on the degree of tolerance, may produce a somnolent, difficult-to-arouse patient with varying degrees of respiratory depression. Ingestion of substitute substances such as methanol, ethylene glycol, or isopropyl alcohol may also occur. Ingestion of isopropyl alcohol can present as stupor in a known alcoholic or as an encephalopathy of unknown cause in persons with hidden addictions. Along with CNS depression, GI effects (abdominal pain, gastritis, nausea, or vomiting) and cardiac toxicity can occur. The major metabolite of isopropyl alcohol is acetone; as such, the severe anion-gap metabolic acidosis seen in methanol and ethylene glycol poisoning is not seen with isopropyl poisoning. In methanol intoxication, the patient may present with visual changes ranging from blurred vision to blindness. Calcium oxalate crystals may be present in the urine of patients who have ingested ethylene glycol. The osmolal gap should be calculated; any discrepancy that cannot be attributed to ethanol ingestion must be explained.

Ingestion of tricyclic antidepressants may produce rapid mental status changes, seizures, and cardiovascular effects. Sinus tachycardia is most commonly noted. The QRS complex may become widened. Atrial and ventricular dysrhythmias may occur. Anticholinergic effects such as delayed gastric emptying, decreased bowel sounds, and mydriasis may be present.

Acetaminophen and salicylate levels should always be obtained. A history of prior tinnitus and vomiting may lead the clinician to suspect salicylate intoxication. Chronic salicylism in the elderly is often subtle. Respiratory alkalosis in adults or metabolic acidosis in children may be seen.

Carbon monoxide or cyanide inhalation should be suspected

if the patient has been involved in a fire. Carbon monoxide poisoning should also be suspected in colder weather, particularly if the patient or others in the household have experienced flulike symptoms. Arterial blood gas levels may show a normal PO_2, but the measured hemoglobin saturation will be low. Cyanide interferes with the cellular use of oxygen; therefore, mixed venous PO_2 will be high, as cells cannot use the available oxygen. Cyanide also causes a severe metabolic lactic acidosis.

DIAGNOSTIC APPROACH

The initial assessment of a patient presenting with coma or transient loss of consciousness should be performed in a relatively short time and should be focused on stabilization. The state of consciousness is determined by both the cerebral cortical and midbrain ascending reticular activating systems. Key observations will help confirm whether the disease is of the brain stem or hemispheres.

Before the patient arrives in the emergency department, field personnel should assist with airway support and administer oxygen. The spine is immobilized and stabilized. Intravenous access is obtained, and cardiac monitoring is ongoing. Bedside evaluation of blood sugar is performed, and the patient should receive glucose if hypoglycemic. Any of the support mechanisms not performed by field personnel are initiated immediately in the emergency department.

The history, physical examination, and serial neurologic examinations are of utmost importance. Often, however, little information is available before intervention is required to protect the brain against irreversible damage. Life-threatening and reversible processes causing coma or altered level of consciousness should be addressed; these include hypoxia, hypoglycemia, poisoning, infections, increased intracranial pressure secondary to trauma, and other mechanisms, such as alteration in body temperature. Evaluation of the cardiorespiratory status and blood glucose takes precedence over investigation of other potential etiologies. Avoid giving a large glucose load to a patient who may not be hypoglycemic, because it may worsen any brain injury.

The history is obtained while stabilizing the patient. Information should include the abruptness of change in mental status, preceding events, medical history, current medications, and use of toxic agents. The clothing should be checked for suicide notes and drug bottles, and any medical alert tags should be noted. After the ABCs have been addressed, the patient is evaluated for signs of head trauma, including pupillary asymmetry and reactivity, hemotympanum, and Battle's sign. The level of consciousness is documented, and the Glasgow Coma Scale used to quantify the patient's condition. Vital signs, including a core body temperature, are assessed.

Examination of the patient's eyes may be the single most important assessment in the evaluation of coma. An unresponsive patient who has open eyes may appear awake but may actually be in a state of akinetic mutism. These patients may be abulic (with long delays in response to stimulation) secondary to hydrocephalus, frontal meningioma, metastatic or primary tumor, hemorrhage, or contusion. Other causes of akinetic mutism include psychiatric disorders such as catatonia and dissociative states, and the "locked-in syndrome," which refers to patients who are paralyzed but in fact awake. This syndrome may be due to pontine infarct, but high cervical spinal cord injuries and severe drug-related dystonias can be causative. The fundi are examined for lack of venous pulsation or other evidence of papilledema, which would suggest increased intracranial pressure.

Eye movements are generated by the brain stem. The shape and size of pupils and their reactions are recorded. Reactive asymmetric pupils differing in size by 1 to 2 mm can be seen in 10% of normal people. Pupils are more likely to remain equal and reactive in cases of metabolic and drug etiology; a fixed, unilaterally dilated pupil suggests transtentorial herniation. Local trauma or topical mydriatics can also cause unilateral dilation. The patient with a possible head or neck injury presents a problem with the performance of the doll's-eye maneuver (oculocephalic reflex).

Ice water caloric testing (oculovestibular reflex) can be performed to induce nystagmus, in which the slow phase is driven by the brain stem and the fast phase is driven by the cortex. This test, done correctly in a comatose patient, helps differentiate a brain stem lesion from a hemispheric lesion. If the brain stem is normal, the eyes will turn conjugately toward the side where ice water is flushed into the ear. This is the slow phase of the eye movement. If the hemispheres are intact, the slow phase of eye movement will be followed by a fast phase, in which the eyes move away from the side of the water infusion. This fast phase is a jerking movement. Stimulation of the cornea will cause an eye blink if the fifth and seventh cranial nerves are intact, another method to evaluate brain stem function.

Respirations are observed. Apneustic breathing, characterized by deep inspiration followed by a long apneic phase and only a few breaths per minute, suggests brain stem failure. Ataxic breathing is an ominous sign of brain stem failure. Normal or Cheyne-Stokes respiration indicates good brain stem function. However, Cheyne-Stokes respiration may be due to bilateral dysfunction of structures deep in the cerebral hemispheres or diencephalon, bilateral cerebral infarctions, or hypertensive encephalopathy. When Cheyne-Stokes respiration is noted, metabolic diseases as well as incipient transtentorial herniation should be considered.

The neck is flexed to check for nuchal rigidity if there is no contraindication. Rigidity of the neck suggests meningeal inflammation due to meningitis or subarachnoid hemorrhage. Empiric antibiotic coverage is immediately initiated in cases highly suspicious of meningitis. Antibiotic coverage should not be delayed by the diagnostic workup (i.e., inability to perform lumbar puncture due to delay in obtaining a head CT).

The patient's posture is noted. Decorticate and decerebrate posturings are abnormal postures that may be recognized in the comatose patient. Decorticate posturing, characterized by flexor positioning of the upper extremities and extension, internal rotation, and plantar flexion in the lower extremities, suggests injury to the brain above the level of the midbrain. Decerebrate posturing is characterized by arms that are extended, adducted, and hyperpronated; legs that are extended with feet plantar flexed; clenched teeth; and opisthotonus. Decerebrate posturing occurs in patients with infarcts of the brain stem rostral to the midpons and also in patients with large cerebral hemorrhages that destroy or compress the lower thalamus and midbrain. This motor pattern typically emerges in the wake of lesions of the internal capsule or cerebral hemisphere that interrupt the corticospinal pathways. Clinical disease patterns often cloud the demarcation between decerebrate and decorticate posturing, and motor responses can shift back and forth depending on the location of the lesion and pressure effects on the upper brain stem.

Suggested steps in the management of the comatose patient are as follows:

1. Establish and maintain airway patency and protect the patient from aspiration.
2. Administer oxygen.
3. Provide adequate ventilation.
4. Support circulation.
5. Establish intravenous access and draw blood for rapid glucose determination; evaluation of electrolytes, calcium, and renal and liver function; drug screen; blood gas determina-

tion; complete blood count; magnesium; thyroid function studies; platelet count; prothrombin time; and partial thromboplastin time.

If indicated by the rapid glucose determination, administer glucose as 25 to 50 mL of 50% dextrose solution to adults and 2 mL per kilogram of 25% dextrose solution to children. To avoid precipitating acute Wernicke-Korsakoff syndrome in a thiamine-deficient patient, give 100 mg thiamine in conjunction with the glucose. Patients should receive multivitamins in the initial bag of intravenous solution. Give 2 to 4 mg of naloxone intravenously in adults, and 0.01 to 0.1 mg per kilogram in children. Measures to decrease intracranial pressure include hyperventilation to reduce PCO_2 to about 26 to 30 mm Hg and administration of intravenous mannitol (0.5 to 1.0 g per kilogram). Fluid restriction may be necessary, and ultimately cerebrospinal fluid may need to be drained by intraventricular catheter. Seizures are treated and seizure precautions taken. Normalize body temperature. An electrocardiogram is obtained, pulse oximetry applied, and a Foley catheter placed.

After the initial treatment of reversible causes and stabilization, definitive workup and therapy are instituted to prevent further CNS damage. In addition to diagnostic laboratory studies, plain radiographs (cervical spine series, chest x-ray), head CT scan and magnetic resonance imaging, carotid duplex studies, Doppler studies, and a lumbar puncture may prove helpful.

There are three primary pathologic processes that produce coma: expanding mass lesions that secondarily destroy the reticular activating system, brain stem lesions that directly damage the reticular activating system, and metabolic disorders that disrupt brain stem function.

The mnemonic AEIOU-TIPPS (Table 7.2) helps organize the approach for specific treatment and antidote administration. In carbon monoxide poisoning, patients immediately receive high-flow oxygen. Hyperbaric treatment may also be indicated. Patients suspected of meningitis receive intravenous antibiotics without delay. Patients intoxicated with ethanol receive supportive care and careful observation, and determination that methanol, ethylene glycol, or isopropyl alcohol is not responsible for their presentation. All metabolic causes, such as hypothyroidism, adrenal insufficiency, and electrolyte abnormalities, receive specific treatment.

Operable lesions are definitively treated by a neurosurgeon and may include clipping of aneurysms, resection of arteriovenous malformations, and evacuation of hematomas, abscesses, and tumors. Nimodipine may help prevent brain injury and improve outcome after subarachnoid hemorrhage. In subarachnoid hemorrhage patients who exhibit sustained systolic blood pressure greater than 180 mm Hg, antihypertensive treatment may be beneficial. Elevated blood pressure should be managed in ischemic stroke, but caution must be used, because the response to therapy may be exaggerated. In ischemic stroke patients, various neuroprotective agents are currently being evaluated. The use of tissue plasminogen activator within 3 hours of stroke onset should be appropriately considered.

The approach to coma and transient loss of consciousness must be systematic. Orderly evaluation, with simultaneous stabilization, is of the utmost importance. Early recognition and correction of reversible causes and prevention of further brain damage by definitive intervention are the basic principles of treatment in patients with altered consciousness.

TABLE 7.2. Mnemonic for Coma and Transient Loss of Consciousness

A	—	alcohol
E	—	epilepsy, electrolytes, encephalopathy
I	—	insulin
O	—	opium
U	—	urea (metabolic)
T	—	trauma
I	—	infection
P	—	psychiatric
P	—	poison
S	—	shock

T for tumor, and **E** for environmental causes such as heatstroke, hypothermia, and high-altitude injuries should also be considered.

COMMON PITFALLS

- Not approaching the patient with transient loss of consciousness in a systematic fashion
- Not intervening in a timely fashion to prevent reversible causes of brain damage
- Not observing hypoglycemic patients who take oral hypoglycemic agents for an appropriate amount of time or providing adequate glucose supplementation

Bibliography

Alberts MJ. tPA in acute ischemic stroke. *Neurology* 1998;51[3 Suppl 3]:S53–S55.
Alguire PC. Rapid evaluation of comatose patients. *Postgrad Med* 1990;87(6):223.
Arieff AL, Carrol H. Nonketotic hyperosmolar coma with hyperglycemia: clinical features, pathophysiology, renal function, acid-base balance, plasma-cerebrospinal fluid equilibria, and the effects of therapy in 37 cases. *Medicine* 1972;51:73.
Ashton CH, Teoh R, Davies DM. Drug-induced stupor and coma: some physical signs and their pharmacological basis. *Adverse Drug React Acute Poison Rev* 1989;8(1):1.
Burger AG, Philippe J. Thyroid emergencies. *Baillieres Clin Endocrinol Metab* 1992;6(1):77.
Chan JCN, Cockram CS. Drug-induced disturbances of carbohydrate metabolism. *Adverse Drug React Toxicol Rev* 1991;10(1):1.
Guidelines for CPR and emergency cardiac care: special resuscitation situations. American Heart Association. *JAMA* 1992;268:2242.
Howton JC. Thyroid storm presenting as coma. *Ann Emerg Med* 1988;17:343.
Kitabchi AE, Murphy MB. Diabetic ketoacidosis and hyperosmolar hyperglycemic nonketotic coma. *Med Clin North Am* 1988;72:1545.
Kleeman CR. Metabolic coma. *Kidney Int* 1989;36:1142.
LeRoux PD, Winn HR. Management of the ruptured aneurysm. *Neurosurg Clin North Am* 1998;9(3): 525–540.
Myers L, Hays J. Myxedema coma. *Crit Care Clin* 1991;7(1):43.
Peterson J. Coma. In: Rosen P, ed. *Emergency medicine: concepts and clinical practice,* 3rd ed. St. Louis: Mosby–Year Book, 1992.
Plum F, Posner J, eds. *Diagnosis of stupor and coma,* 2nd ed. Philadelphia: FA Davis Co, 1972.
Rich J, Scheife RT, Katz N, et al. Isopropyl alcohol intoxication. *Arch Neurol* 1990;47:322.
Samuels MA. A practical approach to coma diagnosis in the unresponsive patient. *Cleve Clin J Med* 1992;59:257.
Seltzer HS. Drug-induced hypoglycemia: a review of 1418 cases. *Endocrinol Metab Clin North Am* 1989;18:163.
Starkman S. Altered mental status. In: Hamilton GC, Sanders AB, Strange GR, et al., eds. *Emergency medicine: an approach to clinical problem-solving.* Philadelphia: WB Saunders, 1991.
Williams GH, Dluhy RG, Thorn GW. Diseases of the adrenal cortex. In: Isselbacker KJ, Adams RD, Braunwald EB, et al., eds. *Harrison's principles of internal medicine,* 9th ed. New York: McGraw-Hill, 1980.

CHAPTER 8
The Weak Patient

Phillip G. Fairweather and Andy Jagoda

Patients presenting to the emergency department with a complaint of weakness pose a great diagnostic challenge for the physician. This nonspecific complaint has myriad causes, and a systemic evaluation is critical. Specific attention to potentially life-threatening etiologies is the principal focus, and diligence in data gathering is essential to the establishment of a diagnosis. A detailed history and physical examination guide the selection of diagnostic studies in these challenging cases. Though rarely encountered, when approaching the patient with a complaint of weakness, consideration is given to disorders such a botulism, myasthenia gravis, and Guillain-Barré syndrome because of their associated high morbidity and mortality. The emergency physician should have a high clinical suspicion for these and all other disorders that can precipitously compromise the respiratory and functional status of their patients. Accepting the challenge and proceeding in an organized fashion can offer great reward for the patient and physician.

The complaint of "dizziness" may accompany that of "weakness," and, at times, patients use these terms interchangeably. There is considerable overlap in their etiologies. In the ambulatory care setting, dizziness is the most common presenting complaint in patients over the age of 75.[1] *Weakness* is defined as a decrease in muscle strength or power. It may be a focal symptom, involving a single muscle group, or it may be generalized. Dizziness is imprecisely interpreted by patients and may be used to describe lightheadedness, disequilibrium, disorientation, confusion, or vertigo. The emergency physician must appreciate the distinction between these symptoms and endeavor to understand the patients' intended meaning. This chapter specifically addresses those patients who present with a complaint of "weakness."

EMERGENCY DEPARTMENT EVALUATION

An exhaustive history and physical examination must often be performed to uncover the subtle details essential in establishing the cause of a patient's complaint of weakness. The patient's definition of *weakness* must first be clarified. Whether the weakness is focal muscle weakness or generalized fatigue must be determined early in the evaluation. If muscular weakness is meant, then the clinician must determine whether it is focal or generalized, proximal or distal. The history of present illness should focus specifically on the acuity of onset and duration of symptoms, exacerbating and mitigating factors, and presence of associated symptoms.[4] Sudden onset of weakness may suggest botulism, while a slower progression may suggest the Guillain-Barré syndrome or myasthenia gravis, although these illnesses may also have accelerated courses. The weakness of myasthenia gravis may fluctuate, and a careful history is needed to elicit a progression of symptoms throughout the day or an association with exercise or repeated activity, such as chewing or combing one's hair. Recent illness, other medical problems, recent vaccination, occupational history, travel history, history of tick bites, use of medication, and use of recreational drugs are important in assessing the patient complaining of weakness. A thorough review of systems should include inquiry about recent weight loss, fever or sweats, visual changes (including diplopia), difficulty swallowing, joint or muscle pain, palpitations, change in bowel habits, and skin rashes.

The patient's age is an important consideration in developing the differential diagnosis in a patient with weakness. The elderly have a higher incidence of comorbid medical conditions than do their younger counterparts and are at higher risk of acute central nervous system and cardiovascular events. They are more likely to present with occult infections and metabolic disorders that are symptomatically manifested as weakness.[4] In the pediatric age group, infantile botulism and intussusception are two rare but important considerations. Infantile botulism may be seen in children days old to over 1 year of age. This variant of botulism is much more common than food-borne or wound botulism, and it presents with weakness, poor tone, poor suck, or constipation.

On the physical examination, orthostatic monitoring and oxygen saturation should be included in the vital signs. Supplemental oxygen is indicated if hypoxemia is present; the airway must be secured if there is a potential for imminent compromise. Tachycardia, with or without hypotension, suggests volume depletion or toxic drug ingestion. Rectal temperature measurement is particularly important, because infection frequently presents with nonspecific complaints, such as weakness. A blood glucose level should be obtained early during the evaluation, as hypoglycemia may present with an array of symptoms, including weakness. The ears, sinuses, thyroid, and cardiac status should be assessed, and there should be a careful evaluation for signs of trauma, which may suggest physical abuse. A rectal examination, including a guaiac test for occult blood, is recommended.

The neurologic examination begins early in the course of the patient's evaluation with the assessment of the mental status. Altered mental status, including confusion, slowness, or agitation, may represent underlying disease or toxic exposure; suspicion of cognitive defects should prompt a formal mental status evaluation. Cranial nerve testing in the patient with a complaint of weakness focuses on the motor examination. Ptosis, usually symmetric but sometimes unilateral, can be an early sign of myasthenia. When myasthenia is a consideration, having the patient hold an upward gaze for several minutes is helpful in assessing for fatigue. Difficulty with accommodation can be the earliest sign of weakness due to botulism and does not occur with myasthenia. Diplopia due to weak oculomotor muscles must be assessed, with an emphasis on the evaluation of the sixth cranial nerve. The abducens is the longest cranial nerve and the most sensitive to toxins such as botulism or to increased pressure from intracranial mass lesions.

The remainder of the neurologic examination in the patient complaining of weakness concentrates on motor strength, deep tendon reflexes, and assessment for muscle atrophy and fasciculations. Upper and lower motor neuron diseases present with the important distinguishing characteristics listed in Table 8.1. Upper motor neurons arise in the cerebral cortex and their axons extend through the subcortical white matter, internal capsule, brainstem, and spinal cord, where they synapse directly with lower motor neurons or interneurons, fine-tuning motor activity. Lower motor neuron cell bodies lie in the brainstem motor nuclei and anterior horn of the spinal cord. Their axons extend to the skeletal muscles they innervate. The weakness of upper motor neuron disease is generally unilateral, the Babinski sign is present, muscle tone is increased, deep tendon reflexes are increased, and no fasciculations are visible or palpable. In general, distal muscle groups are more severely affected than are proximal groups.

Lower motor neuron disease affects single muscle groups. Flexors and extensors are equally compromised in an extremity.

TABLE 8.1. Upper Versus Lower Motor Neuron Weakness

Clinical	Upper Motor Neuron	Lower Motor Neuron
Weakness	Weakness greater in the arm extensors and leg flexors; weakness often on only one side	Weakness often in one muscle group; extensor same as flexor
Deep tendon reflexes	Increased	Decreased
Muscle tone	Increased	Decreased
Fasciculation	None	Present
Muscle atrophy	None	Severe
Babinski sign	Present	Absent

TABLE 8.2. Medical Research Council Grading of Strength

Grade	Definition
5	Normal strength
4	Active movement against gravity and resistance
3	Active movement against gravity (no resistance from physician)
2	Active movement with gravity eliminated (no resistance from physician)
1	Flicker or trace contraction
0	No visible or palpable contraction

Deep tendon reflexes and muscle tone are decreased with lower motor neuron disease. Absent reflexes may also indicate Guillain-Barré syndrome or other systemic processes such as hypothyroidism or hypokalemia. Muscle atrophy and fasciculation are long-term results of lower motor neuron lesions. The presence of fasciculations with upper motor neuron signs, such as hyperreflexia, is suggestive of amyotrophic lateral sclerosis. Fasciculations in the setting of a toxic exposure point to organophosphate poisoning. Table 8.2 lists the Medical Research Council's strength grading from 0 to 5, which permits standardization of documentation between examiners.

Lower motor neuron diseases can arise from a muscle-based disorder, a neuropathic-based disorder, or a myoneural junction source. Table 8.3 illustrates several symptoms, physical signs, and laboratory findings that distinguish the etiologies of lower motor neuron weakness. Weakness due to a myopathy tends to involve proximal muscle groups, while neuropathic disease (Guillain-Barré syndrome) affects distal muscle groups. Myoneural junction diseases have a more distal distribution and are particularly inclined to affect respiratory and bulbar muscle groups (myasthenia gravis and botulism).

When psychogenic weakness is considered in the differential diagnosis, several maneuvers may be helpful. Weak muscles give way to pressure in a smooth fashion, but psychogenic weakness usually results in a jerking or sudden release. In a patient with upper extremity weakness from organic disease, making a fist should not result in wrist extension (unless there is an isolated lesion of the flexor tendons); in functional states, the wrist extends as the patient tries to make a fist. In patients with psychogenic bilateral lower extremity weakness, attempts to lift one leg against resistance result in the other leg firmly thrusting downward, while in patients with organic disease, the downward thrust is diminished or absent.

DIFFERENTIAL DIAGNOSIS

The differential diagnosis of the weak patient is extensive, and no single list can cover every possible cause. Division of the etiologies into broad categories, such as infectious, toxic, metabolic, endocrinologic, structural, mechanical, and rheumatologic, permits a more organized approach to this extensive list. A complete history and physical examination should direct the physician to one of these categories. Other diagnostic testing may then be used to further hone the diagnosis.

All infections can potentially cause weakness, either through nonspecific mechanisms, such as those seen with mononucleosis or hepatitis, or from specific toxins affecting neuromuscular function, such as those in poliomyelitis, botulism, Guillain-Barré syndrome, or tick paralysis. Sinus and ear infections can affect the labyrinthine system and produce lightheadedness or vertigo. The human immunodeficiency virus can directly or indirectly cause the full spectrum of weakness, from nonspecific fatigue to neuropathies and myelopathies. Chronic fatigue syndrome, thought to be viral in origin, requires an extensive workup to exclude all other processes before the diagnosis can be established, and it is not a diagnosis that should be made in the emergency department.[6]

Toxins, including prescription drugs, can produce generalized weakness: There are usually no focal findings on examination (Table 8.4). In one study of 106 patients with a chief complaint of weakness or dizziness, 9% of all patients and 20% of those over age 60 had symptoms attributed to prescription medications.[7] Drugs associated with vasodilation, bradycardia, or diuresis can produce orthostatic blood pressure changes, and patients who are taking them may present with the complaint of weakness. Other drugs can cause myopathies or neuropathies. Carbon monoxide poisoning commonly presents with weakness, emphasizing the importance of a complete occupational and social history in evaluating the patient. Toxins that act at the neuromuscular junction, such as the organophosphates and the carbamates, can cause weakness, fasciculations, or paralysis. Heavy metal poisoning presents with diffuse weakness that is slowly progressive and often associated with CNS findings.

All metabolic derangements can present with weakness, including hypoxia and alterations in serum glucose, potassium, sodium, and calcium.[5] Hypokalemia may be induced by drugs or gastrointestinal losses, or it can be secondary to familial periodic paralysis. Familial periodic paralysis, which may also be due to hyperkalemia, is characterized by profound weakness that often spares the respiratory muscles.[3] Anemia often presents with a complaint of weakness and lightheadedness due to the associated decreased oxygen delivery and hypotension.

Hypothyroidism is the most common endocrine cause of weakness and is often initially misdiagnosed. Thyrotoxic periodic paralysis can present with weakness as a primary complaint, probably mediated through hypokalemia.[2] Adrenal insufficiency, perhaps the most life-threatening endocrine etiology of weakness, may present with hypotension, hyperkalemia, and hyponatremia. It is a diagnosis that must be considered in weak patients on chronic steroid therapy. Diabetics often complain of weakness. Weakness in these individuals may

TABLE 8.3. Myopathy Versus Neuropathy Versus Myoneural Junction Disease

Clinical	Myopathy	Neuropathy	Myoneural Junction
Distribution	Proximal > distal	Distal > proximal	Diffuse, especially bulbar and respiratory muscles
Reflexes	Decreased	Decreased	Normal
Sensory involvement	–	+	–
Atrophy	±	±	–
Fatigue	±	±	+
Serum CPK	Normal to elevated	Normal	Normal

CPK, creatine phosphokinase.

TABLE 8.4. Commonly Used Drugs and Other Substances Associated with Weakness
MYOPATHIES
Steroids
Alcohol
Heroin
Clofibrate
Epsilon-aminocaproic acid
Diuretics
Laxatives
Amphotericin
D-penicillamine
Cimetidine
Procainamide
NEUROPATHIES
Carbon monoxide
Heavy metals
Polychlorinated biphenyls
Isoniazid
Nitrofurantoin
Gold
NEUROMUSCULAR JUNCTION DISEASE
Organophosphates
Carbamates

be due to either hypo- or hyperglycemia or to a neuropathy. Neuropathies predispose to silent myocardial infarction and to vasomotor instability.

Weakness is a prominent complaint of most rheumatologic diseases and occasionally is the primary presenting symptom. Systemic lupus erythematosus, polymyositis, dermatomyositis, polymyalgia rheumatica, and particularly myasthenia gravis must all be considered in patients presenting with symmetric weakness.

Structural lesions often cause focal weakness. Lesions in the spinal canal can result in weakness that is symmetric and distal to the site of compromise. Lesions in the frontal lobes, basal ganglia, and cerebellum can cause disequilibrium. Brainstem infarcts can present with difficulty with swallowing, talking, or respiration, in addition to weakness.

Mechanical causes of weakness are associated with lightheadedness or presyncope and include postural hypotension, carotid and vertebral artery insufficiency, cardiac dysrhythmias, vasovagal events, and states of decreased cardiac output.

Radiographic and Laboratory Examination

Clinical suspicion gathered from the history and physical examination guides further testing. In general, a complete blood count, serum chemistry, and urinalysis are obtained. A sedimentation rate is helpful if rheumatologic disease is suspected. A Monospot test, liver function tests, and thyroid function tests are sometimes indicated. Heavy metal screening and red blood cell acetylcholinesterase level are required in selected cases, but these are rarely available to the emergency physician while the patient is in the department. Carboxyhemoglobin is indicated in suspected cases of carbon monoxide poisoning. A serum creatine phosphokinase and aldolase are helpful in cases of suspected myopathy.

Pulse oximetry and arterial blood gas analysis are indicated in cases of suspected pulmonary dysfunction. Pulmonary function testing, including vital capacity and maximum inspiratory force, is recommended when respiratory muscle compromise is suspected. An electrocardiogram and cardiac monitoring have a low diagnostic yield in patients with generalized weakness, though they may be helpful when dysrhythmias or electrolyte abnormalities are suspected. Rarely, more specialized laboratory testing is indicated in the evaluation of the weak patient in the emergency department. Patients with suspected Guillain-Barré syndrome require cerebrospinal fluid analysis. This characteristically exhibits fewer than 50 lymphocytes per milliliter, a normal sugar, and an elevated protein. A Tensilon test should be considered in patients with suspected myasthenia gravis. Computed axial tomography or magnetic resonance imaging with intravenous contrast best evaluates structural lesions in the brain or spinal canal.

EMERGENCY DEPARTMENT MANAGEMENT

The focus of the emergency physician's approach to the patient complaining of weakness is to rule out the life-threatening diagnoses, specifically those diagnoses that can progress to cardiopulmonary compromise (Table 8.5). After airway patency is established, patients are assessed for adequacy of respiration. Certain patients, based on the history and physical examination, must be assessed for hypoxemia, hypercapnia, or carboxyhe-

TABLE 8.5. Acute Life-Threatening Causes of Weakness

Cause	History	Physical	Laboratory	Treatment
Myasthenia gravis	Chronic weakness, improves with rest	Double vision, muscle fatigue, improves with rest	Positive Tensilon test	Thymectomy, AChE inhibitors
Guillain-Barré	Recent infection, progressive weakness distal to proximal	Distal sensory loss, lost reflexes, no visual deficits	CSF with elevated protein, < 50 WBCs	Supportive care, plasma exchange, gamma globulin
Botulism	Acute onset; canned, pickled, smoked food	Blurred or double vision	None	Supportive care, equine antitoxin
Adrenal insufficiency	Acute weakness associated with stress	Hypotension, hyperpigmentation	Hyperkalemia, hyponatremia	Hydrocortisone
Organophosphate poisoning	Occupational exposure, progressive weakening	Miosis, fasciculations, muscarinic dysfunction	Decreased RBC AChE	Atropine, pralidoxime
Carbon monoxide poisoning	Occupational or social exposure	Nausea, vomiting, coma, headache, dizziness	Elevated carboxyhemoglobin	100% oxygen, hyperbaric oxygen
Hypokalemia	Familial, GI, or renal loss	Diffuse weakness	Low serum potassium	Potassium

AChE, acetylcholinesterase; CSF, cerebrospinal fluid; WBCs, white blood cells; RBC, red blood cell; GI, gastrointestinal.

moglobinemia. Assessment of pulmonary function with measurements of tidal volume and vital capacity may be valuable, especially in patients with suspected myasthenia gravis; patients with a vital capacity less than 1.5 L are possible candidates for intubation.

Potentially unstable patients require intravenous access, pulse oximetry, and cardiac monitoring. Regular reassessment throughout the emergency department stay is necessary to avoid missing deterioration in the patient's status. Specific interventions depend on the diagnosis. Sedating drugs should be avoided in anxious patients who are hypoxemic. Drugs that interfere with myoneural junction function, such as the aminoglycosides, should be avoided in patients with suspected myasthenia gravis. Hypoglycemia is treated with dextrose, and hypokalemia with potassium. Hydrocortisone, 100 mg intravenously, should be given to patients with suspected adrenal insufficiency. Patients with periodic paralysis do not have a total body deficit of potassium, but instead have an alteration in intra- and extracellular potassium levels; therefore, the potassium must be carefully corrected to avoid inducing hyperkalemia. Patients who are weak due to toxins require specific antidotes when available. Significant carbon monoxide poisoning is an indication for hyperbaric oxygen treatment; organophosphate poisoning requires the use of atropine and pralidoxime. Heavy metal poisoning is treated with chelation therapy.

DISPOSITION

Patients with progressive symptoms or those with suspected or confirmed disease with a known progressive course, such as myasthenia gravis, Guillain-Barré, or botulism, must be admitted to an intensive care setting regardless of their initial appearance. Early consultation with appropriate specialists is recommended, and a comprehensive management plan should be determined. No laboratory tests should be ordered unless results will be available before emergency department discharge or careful follow-up has been arranged.

COMMON PITFALLS

- Not taking the complaint seriously, and thus not performing a detailed history and physical examination
- Failing to obtain a drug and toxin exposure history and missing an occupational exposure, drug-induced myopathy, or drug-induced adrenal insufficiency
- Diagnosing a psychogenic etiology or the chronic fatigue syndrome in the emergency department
- Not recognizing absent reflexes as an early manifestation of the Guillain-Barré syndrome
- Failing to distinguish periodic paralysis from hypokalemia induced by drugs, gastrointestinal loss, or other etiologies

References

1. Baloh R. Dizziness in older people. *J Am Geriatr Soc* 1992;40:713.
2. Bergeron L, Sternbach G. Thyrotoxic periodic paralysis. *Ann Emerg Med* 1988;17:843.
3. Cannon L, Bradford J, Jones J. Hypokalemic periodic paralysis. *J Emerg Med* 1986;4:287.
4. Chew W, Birnbaumer D. Evaluation of the elderly patient with weakness: an evidence based approach. *Emerg Med Clin North Am* 1999;17:265.
5. Knochel J. Neuromuscular manifestations of electrolyte disorders. *Am J Med* 1982;72:521.
6. Schluederberg A, Straus S, Peterson P, et al. Chronic fatigue syndrome research: definition and medical outcome assessment. *Ann Intern Med* 1992;117:325.
7. Skiendzielewski J, Martyak G. The weak and dizzy patient. *Ann Emerg Med* 1980;9:353.

SECTION II

Section Editor: Ann Harwood-Nuss

Surgical Emergencies

PART I

Emergency Aspects of Ophthalmology

CHAPTER 9

The Ophthalmic Examination

Geoffrey Broocker

Ocular emergencies usually create an atmosphere of mystery, intrigue, and fear for the nonophthalmic physician. One should approach the eye and the visual system with the same basic thought processes as for other body systems (Fig. 9.1).

HISTORY

Often, the history provides enough information to establish a reasonable differential diagnosis, allowing the physician to focus on the appropriate segment of the visual system. Key historical points include age, trauma, family history, systemic illnesses, occupation, allergies, and ocular history. It is essential to know whether the patient had any previous visual problems or wears glasses.

Common Complaints

Pain and Discomfort

It is often difficult to identify the source of pain because of the sensory overflow from various segments of the fifth cranial nerve (e.g., acute angle-closure glaucoma may present with pain in the frontal sinus region). Discomfort may be localized according to specific symptoms. Discomfort related to the anterior ocular surface or lids usually involves burning, itching, tearing, and foreign-body sensation. Orbital or periorbital discomfort may involve eye muscle fatigue, sinus congestion, and vascular headaches, all of which are nonocular causes. These, along with ocular and intracranial pathology, are best described as dull aches or pressure. Ocular inflammatory disorders (including episcleritis, scleritis, and acute glaucoma) are common, but in-

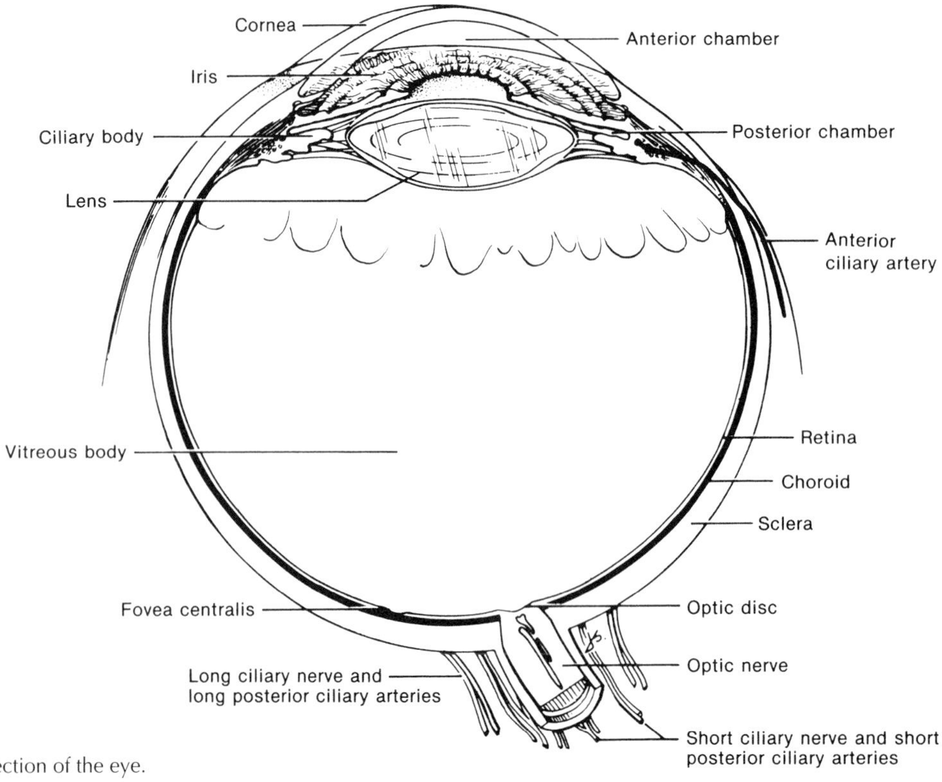

Figure 9.1. Cross section of the eye.

tracranial pathology (arteritis, aneurysm, pituitary apoplexy, and tumors) is not.

Photophobia

Photophobia is a common type of discomfort particular to ophthalmic disease. It is the hallmark of uveal inflammation (e.g., iritis or uveitis of any cause). It may also occur in corneal, retrobulbar, and meningeal inflammatory conditions.

Discharge

Discharge is due primarily to anterior surface disorders and is addressed in Chapter 10.

Tearing

Tearing, most often reflex in origin, indicates abnormal surface irritation from dysfunctional lubrication (chemical and infectious sources) and injured epithelium (corneal foreign body or abrasion). The dry-eye syndrome is therefore a common cause of tearing.

Redness and Swelling

Redness and swelling are signs of congestion; they may be due to the release of inflammatory mediators. Allergens and infectious agents contribute to anterior surface signs. The orbital outflow disorders (congestive) are of concern; they include trauma, thyroid ophthalmopathy, orbital cellulitis, orbital inflammatory syndromes, cavernous sinus thrombosis, and fistulas. Intraocular inflammation tends to cause circumlimbal redness (ciliary flush) or generalized redness, but usually does not cause swelling. Exceptions to this are endophthalmitis and some cases of scleritis.

Changes in Appearance

A sense of urgency arises most often when there is an acute change in appearance. A common example is the subconjunctival hemorrhage. Although usually benign, it may be more ominous in the setting of possible penetrating trauma. Swelling and mass effect are noted with chalazia and dacryocystitis (over the lacrimal crest region). Proptosis may be due to a retrobulbar mass effect (thyroid ophthalmopathy, mucocele, tumor, and fistula).

Visual Disturbances

Visual disturbances are a frequent complaint and are often related to a nonocular cause. Blurred vision may originate from refractive errors all the way through the visual system to occipital cortex disorders. A good clinician should use the history as a starting point in the evaluation. *Glare* or *halos* are common disturbances. They are usually the result of light-scatter phenomena from unclear ocular media (mucinous tear film, corneal edema of any cause, corneal epithelial abnormalities, cataract, or vitreous haze). *Spots* or *floaters* are commonly degenerative opacities within the vitreous; they may, however, indicate red or white blood cells in the aqueous or vitreous. The sudden appearance of floaters may be clinically important.

Transient visual loss is a potentially serious problem. If uniocular, consider the anterior circulation and pathways. If binocular, consider generalized hypoperfusion, posterior circulation, or pathways from the chiasm back to the occipital cortex.

Diplopia

Diplopia may be due to serious underlying disease. A major point is whether it is uniocular or binocular (Does it disappear when one eye is covered?). Uniocular diplopia is generally due to pathology within the eye, binocular diplopia to ocular motility disturbances (cranial nerve palsies or muscle disorders). Whether the diplopia is horizontal or vertical may be key information. Horizontal diplopia is significant and may imply possible intracranial pathology (third- or sixth-nerve palsies caused by increased intracranial pressure, tumor, or aneurysm). Painful ophthalmoplegias are important and suggest intracranial disease. Pupil-sparing third-nerve palsies are usually vascular in origin (diabetes).

Dizziness

Dizziness can be categorized as lightheadedness, which may be a manifestation of hypoperfusion, and vertigo, in which objects appear to be spinning. Vertigo is usually associated with nystagmus.

THE OCULAR EXAMINATION

Visual acuity is the key vital sign in ophthalmology. A Snellen chart (or equivalent), near card, or description of visual ability from any source (e.g., finger counting or newsprint) is necessary before proceeding with further examination. It is critical to evaluate each eye separately. Most physicians tend to focus only on the symptomatic eye. *The physician must be certain that the nonexamined eye is completely covered while checking the vision in the other eye.* Patients often look around hands and occluders and through fingers in an attempt to perform well. Carefully document the visual acuity, and note whether it was checked with or without glasses. If the vision is subnormal, consider rechecking the vision through pinholes, which optically correct most refractive errors. If the vision improves significantly, one must consider a refractive abnormality.

A "step back and look" approach to the inspection of the eye and adnexa is critical. By going right to the slit lamp or direct ophthalmoscope, one may miss key findings such as small puncture wounds in the eyelid. Evert the upper lids to look for retained foreign bodies. An applicator stick can be used to provide a fulcrum for the lid. The lid margins are often a source for anterior surface disorders of the eye and should be carefully inspected for erythema, crusting, lash loss, and irregularity. A marginal laceration, especially near the nasal canthus, should be referred for proper repair.

The pupillary examination, often labeled PERRLA (pupils equal, round, reactive to light, and accommodation), is one of the most important tests of the integrity of the anterior visual pathway. Iris color and pupil size and shape are important. Drugs and trauma (blunt or sharp) affect these circumstances. Iritis tends to cause miosis as well as adhesions to the lens (posterior synechiae). Systemic and topical medications may dilate or constrict the pupil, depending on parasympathetic or sympathetic effects. Narcotics, barbiturates, psychotropics, and psychedelic drugs affect the pupil size, depending on their toxicity and whether the patient is in withdrawal. Essential anisocoria (inequality in diameter of pupils) occurs in a significant percentage of the normal population. Horner syndrome and tonic pupil (Adie's pupil) cause anisocoria. The anisocoria of Horner syndrome may be accentuated in dim illumination and diagnosed pharmacologically. Adie's pupil has a light-near dissociation (minimal light reaction, greater for accommodation) and is generally larger than the Argyll Robertson pupil. Dorsal midbrain syndromes also create this finding but are associated with paresis of upward gaze and retraction nystagmus. Trauma may cause pupillary dilation through sphincter injury or miosis from traumatic iritis. Ruptures can be seen on slit-lamp examination. *Corneoscleral lacerations are often plugged with a segment of iris, creating a peaked pupil toward the laceration.*

The deafferented, or Marcus Gunn, pupil has ocular and neurologic significance. Using a bright light, the physician should check the pupils individually for size, shape, and direct reaction.

The physician can view the consensual response in the other eye. By swinging the light directly from one eye to the other and back again, the midbrain can sample the intensity of input from each eye. For example, in retrobulbar neuritis, if the light swings from the normal eye to the eye with the problem, the midbrain quickly interprets a relative reduction in input and the efferent response is subsequently less. The examiner will see the pupil dilate instead of constrict. One must be careful not to confuse this with hippus (rhythmic wavering pupil). A bright light and a notable initial constriction differentiate these two. If both optic nerves are equally damaged, the examiner cannot demonstrate the Marcus Gunn pupil because there is no *relative* difference.

Ocular position and motility are part of the "step back and look" approach. Exophthalmos and enophthalmos are usually obvious. Enophthalmos is commonly seen in severe orbital floor fractures. A tethered inferior rectus causing marked upgaze restriction may also be seen. The extraocular movements involve a complex coordination of frontomesencephalic and cerebellomesencephalic interactions through the third, fourth, and sixth cranial nerves. Any disturbance in intracranial processing or in midbrain or cranial nerve function, or an intraorbital or cranial nerve or muscle abnormality may result in an imbalance in ocular position response. This includes abnormalities in primary gaze (straight ahead) or congruity of gaze in the six cardinal positions (left, right, up and right, up and left, down and right, down and left). Esotropia (cross-eye) can be seen by observing the light reflex off the cornea to be temporal to the central cornea; exotropia (walleye) can be seen by observing the light reflex nasal to the central cornea. This can be documented by the cover–uncover test. Ask the patient to fixate on a distant object or target; cover and then uncover each eye. The deviated eye straightens when the normal eye is covered (opposite to the direction of the original deviation). An esotropic eye moves temporally when the normal eye is covered. Vertical deviations can be noted by the higher eye, which is labeled a hypertropia. The light reflex is lower on the cornea in the hypertropic eye than in the other eye. During cover testing, that eye moves downward when the normal eye is covered. It is a challenge to determine whether the origin of the motility disturbance is inherited, acquired, neural, muscular, or some combination.

The eyes are just the anteriormost extension of the visual system. Probably the single most important test of the "total" system is the visual field. Defects in the visual field may indicate injury anywhere from the retina to the occipital cortex (Fig. 9.2). Abnormalities in visual field testing may occur before the patient has actual visual complaints. Performing formal visual field assessment by perimetry is difficult in the emergency setting, but simple confrontation fields (Fig. 9.3) may produce the information required for localization. The examiner is the "control" and faces the patient. Targets (e.g., fingers) in 45-degree intervals are used to test the peripheral field, one eye at a time. Gross hemianopic defects (homonymous or bitemporal), as well as isolated defects, can be easily described. The Amsler grid (Fig. 9.4) is an ancillary test that assesses the visual field of the central 10 degrees of vision. Because this is the macular projection of the retina, it provides useful information on central retinal disorders (hemorrhage, edema, and degeneration). The Amsler grid is essentially a "tile floor" pattern with a central dot. Using one eye at a time, the patient fixates on this dot and is asked to describe wavy lines or missing areas. Principal findings are metamorphopsia (wavy distortion) and scotomas (blind spots) of macular lesions or optic nerve disorders (e.g., toxic amblyopia and optic neuritis).

Because the central retina and optic nerve are essentially a

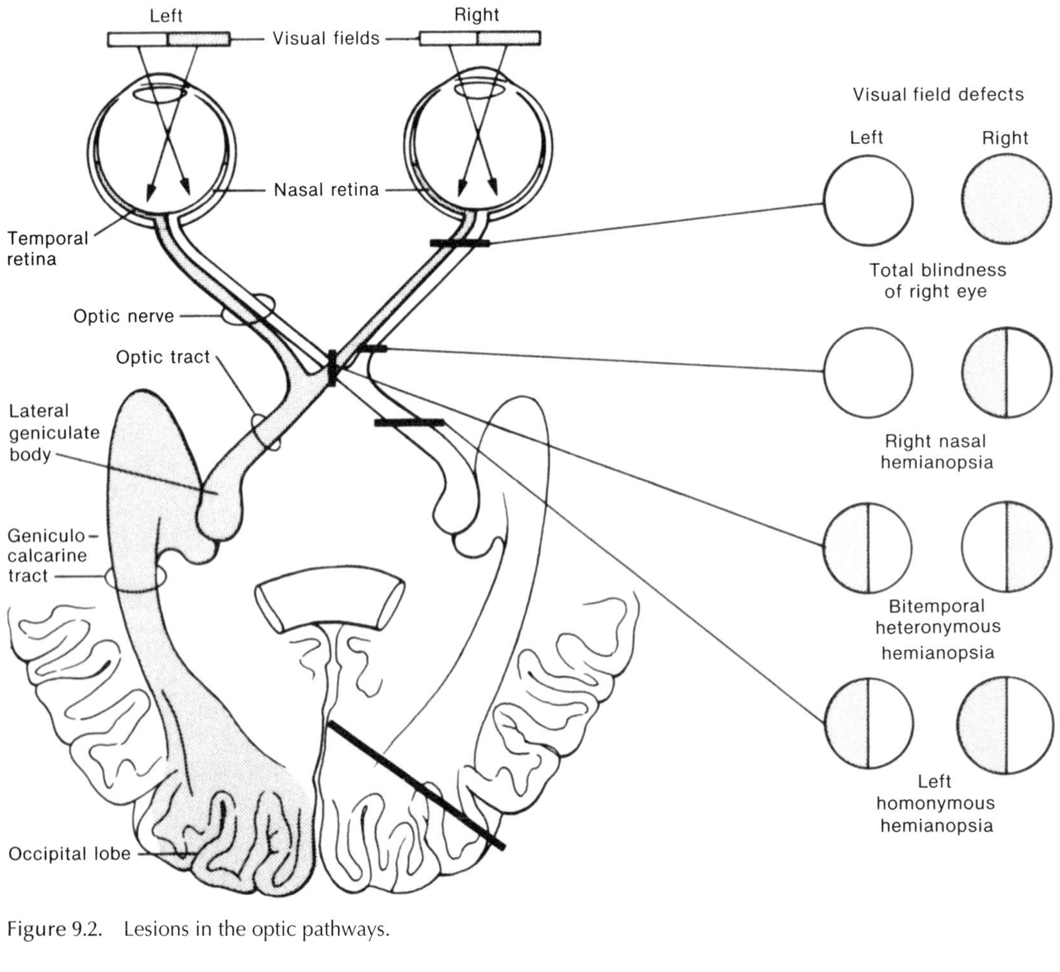

Figure 9.2. Lesions in the optic pathways.

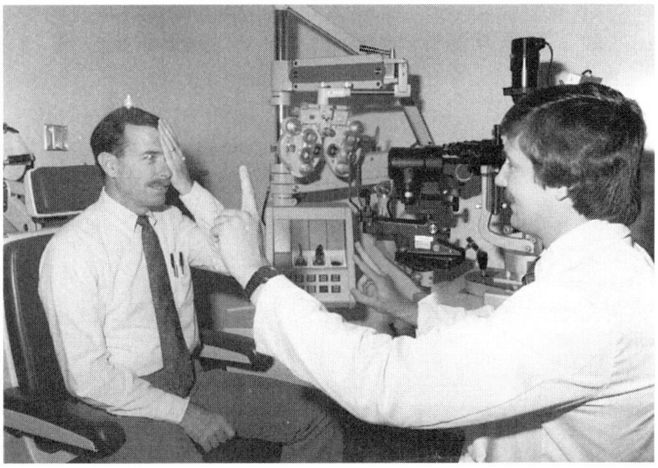

Figure 9.3. Performing confrontation fields.

color projection system, even simple analysis of color perception may help isolate the problem. Color vision testing can be performed using many techniques, but in the emergency setting, the testing of the central red saturation is a good way to localize the problem to the central retina or optic nerve. Using the red bottle top of a dilating or cycloplegic agent (e.g., tropicamide [Mydriacyl] or phenylephrine hydrochloride [Mydfrin]), the examiner can ask the patient to quantitate the "degree" of red seen in each eye ("If this is a dollar's worth of red in the good eye, how much is it worth in the other?"). If the response reveals desaturation, macular or optic nerve disease may be present.

THE PHYSICAL EXAMINATION

Every physician should develop proficiency using the penlight. A bright penlight is helpful for pupil evaluation and is also useful in assessing the lids and anterior surface of the eye. Loupe magnifiers should be used if available. Many penlights are equipped with a cobalt blue filter that can be used with fluorescein application. The light should be moved across the eye to

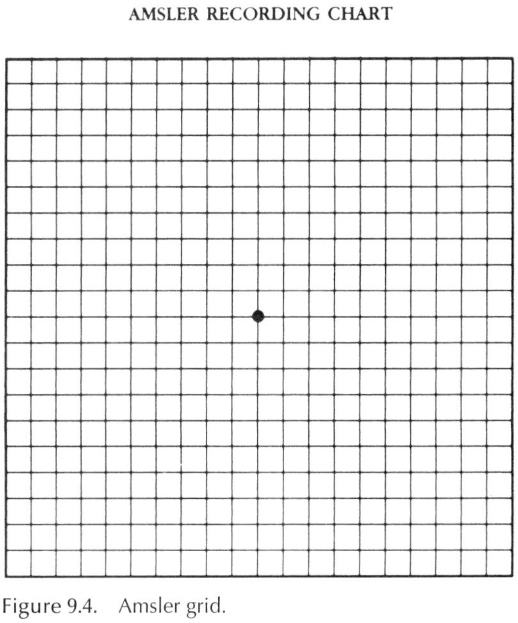

Figure 9.4. Amsler grid.

perceive the glassy reflective surface of the cornea. Epithelial abrasions and edema can be identified from the discontinuity in the reflections. It is useful to compare the findings with those of the other eye. The patient should be asked to look up while the lower lid is pulled down to evaluate the lower cornea and globe. *Foreign bodies commonly are located under the upper lid.* The examiner should look for discharge and areas of inflammation.

Fluorescein is a stain picked up by severely damaged or absent epithelial cells (corneal abrasion). It changes color in the presence of abnormal pH. A dark flow in a green-yellow background is seen if aqueous humor is present from a corneal laceration.

Slit-Lamp Examination

The anterior segment of the eye is best examined with the slit-lamp biomicroscope. The view of the anterior segment anatomy is astounding under high magnification. In the presence of injury or infection, the slit-lamp examination is mandatory. The patient's head is positioned in the chin rest, with the forehead against the bar. The black line on the right vertical pole next to the patient's face is aligned with the level of the eyes. The examiner sets the oculars (usually to 0) and then adjusts the interpupillary distance, as with binoculars. The light source is moved to 45 degrees from the examiner–patient axis, and the chassis is adjusted forward or backward to bring the eye into focus. The examination is started on low magnification (10×). Once the eye is in focus, the magnification may be increased. Fine adjustments are made with the joystick. On some models, the up–down control is on the joystick. The beam is adjusted to a slit rather than a full circle. The three-dimensional box seen on the cornea shows the 0.5-mm thickness. With the slit lamp, the extent and level of corneal injuries can be assessed. The lids, conjunctiva, cornea, anterior chamber, and irises of both eyes should be examined systematically.

The *lid margins* may demonstrate information related to "the red eye." Lacerations may be appreciated, especially in the nasal canthal region, where the identification of a canalicular laceration is critical.

The *conjunctiva* has epibulbar and tarsal components. The examiner should look for discharge, follicles (lymphoid aggregates characteristic of certain viral, toxic, or allergic conditions), chemosis (subconjunctival fluid swelling), and hyperemia. Small foreign bodies can be swept from under the upper lid during the slit-lamp examination.

The examination of the *cornea* involves the following:

1. Epithelium: to detect abrasions, edema, ulcers, and foreign bodies
2. Stroma: to detect primarily edema, but also deep ulcers, deep scars, and penetration
3. Endothelium: to detect keratitic precipitates (white cells on the endothelium). These precipitates are a hallmark of iritis. Penetration through this layer is called a *laceration.*

The size and shape of the findings are noted. A drawing of front and side views is helpful.

The *anterior chamber* is bounded by the cornea and iris and is filled with aqueous. Its depth can be assessed by adjusting the slit beam. By narrowing the beam into a small column of light, the examiner may see a cellular reaction (iritis) as well as flare (light scatter caused by inflammatory proteins in the aqueous). Red or white blood cells may be present in the anterior chamber. Red blood cells usually result from trauma; the layering of these cells in the anterior chamber is called a *hyphema.* Sometimes, pigment dispersion (granules of pigment) is difficult to differentiate from mild diffuse red blood cells. White blood cells are present in iritis; the layering of these cells in the anterior chamber is called a *hypopyon.*

The *iris–lens* examination involves noting pupil dysfunction, which may include traumatic tears in the sphincter or adhesions to the anterior lens capsule (posterior synechiae). The iris may plug corneoscleral lacerations (thereby peaking the pupil) or be torn at its root (iridodialysis). Opacities of the lens are defined as cataract opacities and may be due to many causes. Injury to the anterior capsule of the lens in penetrating trauma has diagnostic and surgical significance, because these lenses generally become rapidly opaque and incite tremendous inflammation.

The Ocular Fundus Evaluation

The ophthalmoscope can be used to magnify the anterior surface of the eye, using the higher, black-numbered lenses. Impaired view may be due to cloudy media (e.g., corneal and lens opacities, and vitreous blood), but it can also be due to unusual refractive errors. One tip for better viewing is to have the patient wear his or her corrective lenses while undergoing this test. It is expected that the refractive correction has made the patient "normal-sighted." If the examiner and patient are "normal-sighted," generally a –2 or –3 lens (the red 2 or 3) allows a comfortable view of the fundus.

The *optic nerve head* should be evaluated for margins, shape, and cup. The examiner should be aware of anomalies, such as small disks with little or no cup and central vessels with multiple early bifurcations. Spontaneous venous pulsations should be noted. Hemorrhages and blurred margins can be critical findings, and should be compared with findings in the other eye. The *macula* should be examined with attention to the presence of hemorrhages, exudates, and edema. It is important to note if these findings are generalized (diabetic or hypertensive retinopathy) or localized (any vascular retinopathy, especially occlusive disease). It is difficult to determine the layer of retinal bleeding, especially when the bleeding is subretinal. Deep hemorrhages tend to be small and irregular. Superficial hemorrhages are flame-shaped. Edema makes the retina look gray-white. In central retinal artery occlusion and other causes of a thickened nerve fiber layer of the retina (e.g., Tay-Sachs disease), one will see a distinctive, central red area called the *cherry-red spot*. This represents the visualization of the normal choroidal circulation through the one area of the retina where the nerve fiber layer is absent (fovea centralis).

Recognition of vascular retinopathies has important implications. The *retinal vessels* are a mirror of the body's microcirculation in a host of systemic processes.

Finally, *intraocular pressure* should be evaluated. The intraocular pressure is to the eye what the blood pressure is to the cardiovascular system. Normal values range from 10 to 21 mm Hg, and are measured in various ways:

Indentation tonometry. The Schiøtz tonometer is cumbersome, can spread infection, and may create its own trauma, but it is relatively easy to use.

Applanation tonometry. The applanation tonometer is accurate, easy to use, and mounted on most slit lamps. Figure 9.5 shows the hand-held model.

Tonometer pens are electronic devices that are easy to use and relatively accurate, but very expensive (see Fig. 9.5).

Noncontact tonometers are for screening only; they may be inaccurate.

Pneumotonometers are effective and relatively easy to use, but somewhat expensive to maintain; they must be calibrated.

Manual assessment of the tensions may be crude and inaccurate. The eyeball is palpated through closed lids in a gentle balloting motion. Each eye is compared with the other. The examiner's eye may be used as a control. By measuring the intraocular pressure with a tonometer and then doing finger tensions, the examiner may become more proficient. *This method should be avoided in recently operated globes or if lacerations are suspected.*

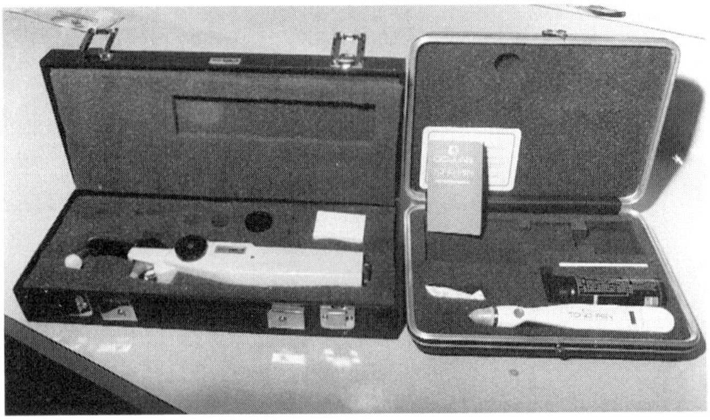

Figure 9.5. Hand-held applanation tonometer (**left**) and tonometer pen (**right**).

DISPOSITION

Role of the Consultant

The urgency of referral depends on multiple factors. Through a careful history and physical examination, the emergency physician should be able to arrive at a diagnosis. Medicolegally, one can never be faulted with a phone consult with the ophthalmologist, documenting the details. Providing the necessary information to the ophthalmologist is the key to an effective consultation. The minimum information the consultant needs includes the patient's age, chief complaint, ocular history (and any pertinent medical history), and visual acuity in both eyes, as well as any other pertinent findings.

COMMON PITFALLS

- In the setting of trauma, epibulbar (subconjunctival) hemorrhage associated with a history of high-velocity or potentially lacerating objects (e.g., glass, metal) suggests the possibility of ocular penetration, especially if the vision is diminished (vitreous hemorrhage).
- A key piece of information often missing on the emergency department evaluation is the patient's visual acuity. Each eye must be assessed while occluding the other. The use of a pinhole is extremely useful when vision is reduced. Improved vision through the pinhole suggests routine referral for refraction and glasses, thus avoiding an unnecessary urgent consultation or expensive diagnostic testing.
- "Red-top" ocular medication bottles are mydriatic–cycloplegic agents. The vast majority of dilated pupils presenting in the emergency setting are pharmacologic in origin. Other findings, such as horizontal diplopia, motility disturbance, and ptosis of the lid, suggest more serious neuroophthalmic etiologies.
- Headache is a common complaint, and may have an ocular origin. Be aware that shared sensory influx from a host of anterior cranial and facial structures (e.g., the paranasal sinuses) can refer pain to the orbit and periorbital regions.
- Anterior visual pathway and carotid circulation problems tend to be associated with uniocular visual loss; posterior pathways and vertebrobasilar circulation problems often present with binocular complaints (check for hemianopia).

- Penlight diagnoses are difficult. Use the slit-lamp biomicroscope, if available, to examine the eye. Turn the light intensity rheostat down low when turning on the slit lamp to avoid blowing out expensive bulbs and also to reduce patient discomfort from high-intensity light.
- Excess fluorescein should be avoided when evaluating ocular surface problems or checking intraocular pressure.
- Avoid the indiscriminate use of topical antibiotics in serious ocular infections without first obtaining adequate samples for culture and sensitivities.
- The emergency physician should not be afraid to use topical anesthetics to aid in the evaluation of the eye, especially in the setting of trauma (to reduce lid spasm). However, these agents retard corneal epithelial wound healing; hence, discharging a patient with a topical anesthetic is a medicolegal risk and should always be avoided.
- Pupillary dilation may be essential to visualize the posterior segment of the eye (optic disk and retina) for proper diagnosis. A weak mydriatic should be used and *documented in the record*. Tropicamide 0.5% or 1.0% should be used because it is short-acting (4 to 6 hours) and relatively easy to reverse with miotics. The incidence of precipitating angle-closure glaucoma in the general population is extraordinarily low (about 2:10,000). If there is concern with regard to this problem or compromising the pupillary examination neurologically, the appropriate specialist should be called to assist in the decision.
- Topical corticosteroids, used alone or in combination with other topical medications, should be used only after proper consultation by phone.
- Even though ocular medications are most often delivered topically, there are significant systemic side effects seen with certain agents, especially those that treat glaucoma (e.g., beta-blockers). Punctal compression, to avoid drainage down the nasolacrimal system into the posterior nasopharynx (subsequently swallowed), will reduce this problem.

Bibliography

Bartlett J, et al. *Ophthalmic drug facts*. St. Louis: Facts & Comparisons, 1999.

Colenbrander A. Principles of ophthalmology. In: Tasman W, Jaeger EA, eds. *Duane's clinical ophthalmology*, vol. 1, chapter 63. Philadelphia: Lippincott Williams & Wilkins, 1998.

Glaser J. Neuro-ophthalmic examination: general consideration and special techniques. In: Tasman W, Jaeger EA, eds. *Duane's clinical ophthalmology*, vol. 2, chapter 3. Philadelphia: Lippincott Williams & Wilkins, 1998.

Mannis MJ, Plotnick R. Bacterial conjunctivitis. In: Tasman W, Jaeger EA, eds. *Duane's clinical ophthalmology*, vol. 2, chapter 5. Philadelphia: Lippincott Williams & Wilkins, 1998.

Patel KH, Javitt JC, et al. Incidence of acute angle closure glaucoma after pharmacologic mydriasis. *Am J Ophthalmol* 1995;120(6):709–717.

Pavan-Langston D. *Manual of ocular diagnosis and therapy*, 4th ed. New York: Lippincott-Raven, 1995.

Physician's desk reference for ophthalmology, 26th ed. Montvale, NJ: Medical Economics Data Production Co, 1998.

Tate GW Jr, Safir A. The slit lamp: history, principles, and practice. In: Tasman W, Jaeger EA, eds. *Duane's clinical ophthalmology*, vol. 1, chapter 59. Philadelphia: Lippincott Williams & Wilkins, 1998.

Vaughan D. *General ophthalmology*, 15th ed. Stamford, CT: Appleton & Lange, 1998.

CHAPTER 10
Acute Eye Infections

Robert S. Porter

The red eye poses a diagnostic challenge to everyone, including the ophthalmologist. Infection is only one cause, and a diligent search must be made for other etiologies. This chapter addresses ocular infections of the anterior surface (conjunctiva and cornea). Intraocular infections also occur, but are much rarer and are not discussed in detail.

Conjunctivitis is the inflammation of the mucous membrane that covers the anterior sclera and inner eyelids. Infection of the conjunctiva is one of the most common causes of red eye treated in the emergency department, and usually is viral or bacterial. Most cases are self-limited, but serious complications can occur. The conjunctiva contributes to the formation of the tear film, and severe conjunctivitis may result in scarring and an abnormal tear film. Because the precorneal tear film is an important optical surface determining clarity of vision, treatment must be accurate and the patient followed carefully.

Keratitis is an inflammation of the cornea. The corneal epithelium may be involved in a superficial manner (with punctate erosions or ulceration), or there may be deeper involvement with infiltration. Quite often there is simultaneous involvement of the conjunctiva as well. Keratitis is usually quite painful and can be associated with either viral or bacterial disease. The intact corneal epithelium is normally an effective barrier against bacterial organisms, with several exceptions, including *Neisseria gonorrhoeae, Corynebacterium diphtheriae, Listeria monocytogenes,* and *Haemophilus aegyptius*. However, any damage to the corneal epithelium can permit access by a wide variety of other organisms. Because corneal scarring is one of the leading causes of blindness worldwide, aggressive, appropriate treatment is essential.

Endophthalmitis is infection or inflammation of the intraocular tissues. This can result from direct inoculation or hematogenous spread of organisms. *Panophthalmitis* is the term used when infection also involves the orbital soft tissues. These conditions typically require subconjunctival or intravitreal as well as systemic antibiotics and must be managed by an ophthalmologist.

VIRAL PATHOGENS

There are three viral pathogens of particular note: the adenoviruses, herpes simplex, and herpes zoster viruses.

Adenovirus infection is very common and highly transmissible. Infection starts in one eye and several days later becomes bilateral, with significant watery discharge and follicles (Fig. 10.1). Preauricular adenopathy is common, and there is marked discomfort, which may persist for weeks. It is quite common to see serious progression as the immunologic response increases. Development of pseudomembranes may indicate corneal injury not present on the initial examination. Epidemic keratoconjunctivitis is caused by adenovirus types 8 and 19 and is highly contagious. This is the classic "pinkeye."

Occultly contaminated equipment in ophthalmology offices is a leading cause of outbreaks. Contact with infected persons in physicians' offices, emergency departments, and schools is also a source. The period of contagion is roughly 2 weeks after onset

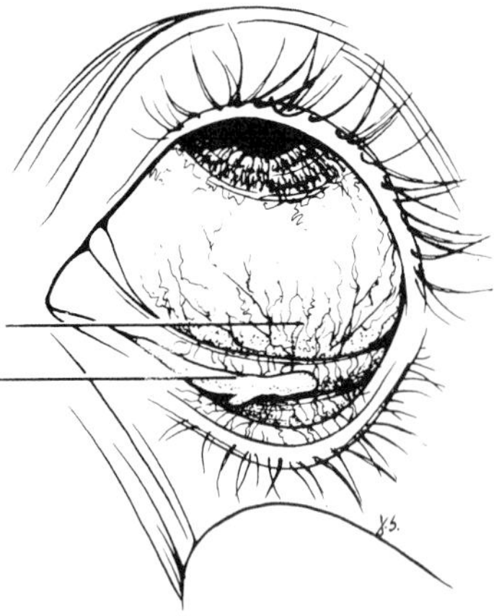

Figure 10.1. Viral infection.

of symptoms. Adenoviral keratoconjunctivitis does not respond to topical antiviral agents. Supportive care includes isolation, cool compresses, ocular decongestants, lubricants, and a broad-spectrum antibiotic to prevent secondary overinfection. Evaluation of therapeutic response is not always easy. Knowledge of the course of this condition will ease patient expectations as to the therapeutic response. Progressive visual loss, increasing discomfort, and pseudomembrane formation are indications for urgent referral. Reduced discharge, swelling, and hyperemia indicate therapeutic success.

Herpes simplex conjunctivitis may present with unilateral conjunctival hyperemia associated with a clear discharge. Other findings may include lid vesicles or ulcerations in early or primary cases. Corneal spread can occur rapidly, resulting in a dendritic ulcer (Fig. 10.2). Ophthalmologic consultation is indicated once the diagnosis is made. In simple, early epithelial herpes, mechanical debridement is an important aspect of treatment and should be done by an ophthalmologist. Topical vidarabine 3%, trifluorothymidine 1%, or idoxuridine 0.5% may be used in consultation with the ophthalmologist.

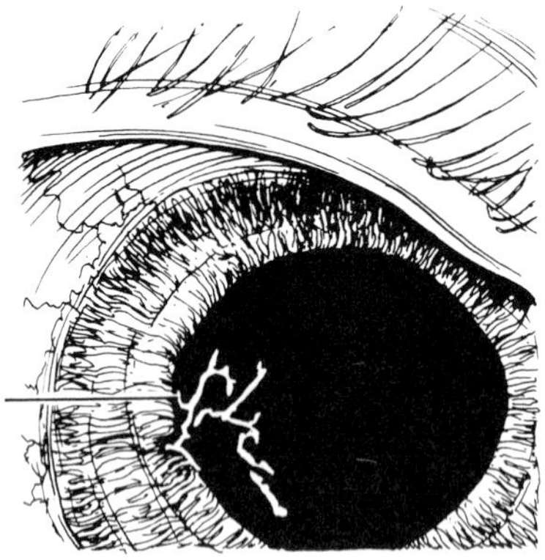

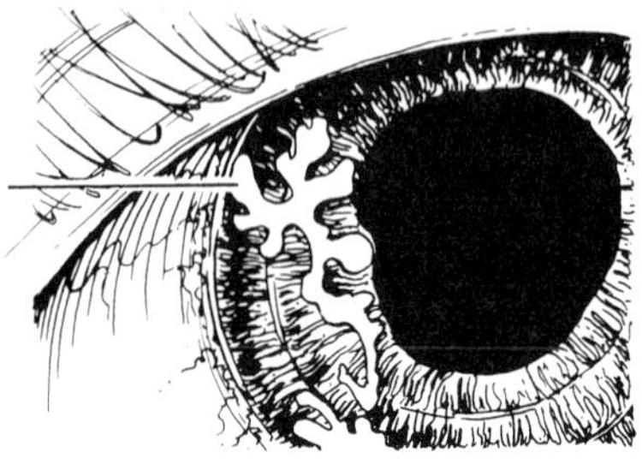

Figure 10.2. Herpes simplex keratitis. **(A)** Early epithelial dendritic ulcer. **(B)** More advanced or geographic ulcer.

Herpes zoster ophthalmicus, ocular involvement, should be suspected, especially if the nasociliary branch of the fifth cranial nerve is involved. Punctate keratopathy, lid vesicles, or dendritic infiltrates may be present. In fact, herpes zoster may mimic herpes simplex. Early ophthalmologic consultation may be indicated. Systemic steroids to avoid postherpetic neuralgia should not be administered by an emergency physician. Topical cycloplegics and steroids are beneficial. There is evidence that systemically administered acyclovir may diminish the severity of the process and postherpetic neuralgia when administered early in the course of the disease. When iritis is present, intraocular pressure may be elevated.

Bacterial Pathogens

The pathogens of greatest clinical importance and frequency include *Staphylococcus, Haemophilus,* pneumococci (and other streptococci), *Neisseria gonorrhoeae,* diphtheroids, coliforms, *Pseudomonas, Proteus,* and *Moraxella.* Of lesser frequency, but still important, are Parinaud's oculoglandular syndrome (cat-scratch fever) and luetic and tuberculous disease. Mucopurulent conjunctivitis is most commonly caused by *Staphylococcus aureus,* followed by *Streptococcus pneumoniae* and *Haemophilus influenzae.* The onset is often acute and unilateral but may rapidly become bilateral. Crusting of the lids is common. *Epidemic forms* can be caused by pneumococci and *Haemophilus. Gram stain and culture are usually unnecessary unless the case is quite severe, is unresponsive to therapy, or occurs in a compromised host.*

Treatment consists of warm compresses, lubricants, and broad-spectrum antibiotics (drops during the day and ointments at bedtime). Commonly used antibiotics include sulfacetamide 10%, gentamicin 0.3%, Polytrim, and Neosporin. The sulfa drugs are less sensitizing than neomycin. Chloramphenicol is least sensitizing. Bacterial conjunctivitis should be notably improved in 48 hours.

Gonococcal conjunctivitis usually causes unilateral conjunctival hyperemia, a severe purulent discharge with associated edema, and erythema of the lids. The population at risk includes neonates, sexually active adults, and health-care workers. The incubation period is from 1 to 3 days. Culture and Gram stain should be done and will reveal gram-negative intracellular diplococci. The patient should be seen by an ophthalmologist immediately and may require admission for systemic therapy and frequent irrigation of the eye, because the gonococcus can penetrate the intact cornea. Topical antibiotics, irrigation, and parenteral penicillin or cephalosporins are used. Single-dose ceftriaxone may allow for selected outpatient therapy.

Pseudomonas aeruginosa is a very aggressive ocular pathogen, producing an adherent mucopurulent, yellow-green exudate and a "ground glass" appearance of the cornea adjacent to the ulcer. Perforation and extension of the infection to the sclera are major concerns.

Fungal Pathogens

The common fungal pathogens include *Actinomyces, Aspergillus, Blastomyces, Candida, Coccidioides, Mucor* (in diabetics), and *Sporothrix.* Fungal infection is generally not fulminant. Patients taking corticosteroids and those with suppressed immune systems are at risk. *A history of trauma involving vegetable matter is important.* Beneath the corneal infiltrate, an endothelial plaque may be seen. The hypopyon associated with this type of corneal infection may contain fungal elements. Gram and Giemsa stains and cultures are essential. Fungal blepharoconjunctivitis can be controlled with lid hygiene and compresses. If the physician identifies fungal elements on corneal ulcer smears, natamycin 5% suspension (Natacyn) should be given every hour after appropriate consultation.

Rickettsial Disease

It is difficult to diagnose rickettsial disease of the eye. Rocky Mountain spotted fever and scrub typhus can cause anterior surface ocular problems. History, other lesions, clinical suspicion, and complement fixation may aid in the diagnosis. Treatment may be curative with systemic tetracycline or chloramphenicol.

Chlamydia

Mucopurulent inclusion conjunctivitis is extremely common, especially in sexually active young adults (Fig. 10.3). The diagnosis is made by the lack of organisms on Gram stain and a positive immunofluorescent antibody screen. The presence or history of a urethral discharge may suggest concomitant gonococcal disease. Conjunctival scrapings may be helpful acutely. Systemic therapy is necessary and includes erythromycin or tetracycline, 1 g daily (250 mg every 6 hours) for 3 to 4 weeks (doxycycline 100 mg b.i.d. is preferred). Ocular therapy (topical sulfa or erythromycin) is supportive only and not curative. Partners should be referred for treatment. Neonatal inclusion conjunctivitis occurs several days to 2 weeks after birth. The treatment is similar, but topical therapy with sulfacetamide 10%, q.i.d. for 3 weeks, is more effective. Systemic therapy with erythromycin is necessary in the neonate due to concomitant pneumonitis. Trachoma continues to be a major cause of inflammatory blindness worldwide, although it is not prevalent in the United States.

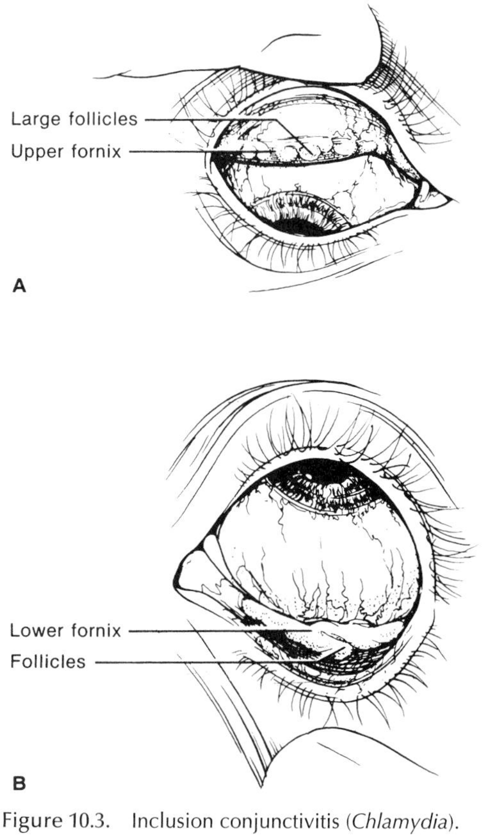

Figure 10.3. Inclusion conjunctivitis (*Chlamydia*).

Parasitic Disease

Acanthamoeba is a growing concern, especially in contact lens wearers. Pediculosis (*Phthirus pubis*) affects the lids, brows, and ocular surface. Toxocariasis (*Toxocara*) and toxoplasmosis (*Toxoplasma*) are principally diseases that affect the retina and uvea.

Clinical Presentation

The hallmark of anterior surface infection is the red eye. In addition, discomfort, discharge, lid crusting, sticking, photophobia, and visual loss are often seen. Unfortunately, there are many noninfectious causes of these symptoms as well (Table 10.1), and there is much overlap of findings. A careful history can be helpful in sorting them out. Inquire about known eye conditions, contact lens use, previous trauma, use of eye medications, and contact with infected people. Symptoms of systemic illness or infection are particularly important, especially any that might increase suspicion of an immunocompromised state.

Eye infections can be bilateral or unilateral. Herpetic disease is usually unilateral. Adenoviral infections generally start in one eye and "ping-pong" to the other after several days. Posttraumatic iritis is limited to the injured eye, but be alert for secondary infection of a traumatic corneal lesion. Allergens tend to involve both eyes.

Most of the inflammatory and infectious eye conditions cause a discharge, but purulent discharge should increase suspicion of bacterial infection. History of trauma involving vegetable matter (e.g., tree branch) may implicate fungal disease as the cause of infection. Contact lens wearers are especially prone to all types of infectious disease, as well as to ischemic injury from overwear syndrome and toxic infiltrates from old or contaminated lenses.

DIFFERENTIAL DIAGNOSIS

Although infection is a common cause of the red eye, many processes mimic infectious disease of the anterior ocular surface (see Table 10.1):

Allergic reactions
Airborne irritants
Foreign bodies
Chemical or thermal burns
Medicamentosus (common)
Trauma
Vascular conditions (carotid–cavernous sinus fistulas, blood dyscrasias)
Orbital inflammatory or congestive diseases (e.g., thyroid ophthalmopathy)
Glaucoma (acute and neovascular)
Uveitis (includes episcleritis or scleritis)
Neoplasia (squamous and meibomian cell carcinoma)
Mucocutaneous syndromes (ocular pemphigoid, Stevens-Johnson syndrome)
Dry eye syndromes

This is a sizable list because many conditions cause a release of vasoactive substances (e.g., histamine and prostaglandins), resulting in redness, discharge, or both. To complicate matters, however, these noninfectious conditions may create a milieu conducive to secondary bacterial infection. For example, any irritation may cause the patient to rub the eye and either transfer agents from the hand or create mild trauma, serving as a nidus for infection. Conversely, certain bacteria (most often staphylococcal lid infections) are occasionally associated with hypersensitivity reactions.

TABLE 10.1. Differential Diagnosis of Red Eye

Factor	Infectious Keratitis Conjunctivitis	Iritis	Angle-Closure Glaucoma	Allergic/Toxic	Traumatic
Type of Injection	Diffuse epibulbar and tarsal conjunctiva	Diffuse, ciliary flush	Diffuse	Diffuse epibulbar and tarsal conjunctiva	Diffuse (hemorrhagic)
Discharge	Viral: watery, occasional, pseudomembranes Bacterial: purulent, occasional pseudo-membranes Fungal: mucopurulent	Watery	Watery	Watery (± mucoid)	Watery
Itching	Minimal	None	None	Moderate to severe	None
Preauricular Node	Viral: fairly common Bacterial: occasional Fungal: occasional	None	None	None	None
Vision	Usually normal, may become markedly decreased if corneal involvement	Usually blurred	Usually markedly blurred (corneal edema)	Usually normal, unless corneal involvement	Usually markedly blurred (corneal, intraocular blood, retinal injury, etc.)
Pain	Usually mild but can be severe (especially adenovirus); more irritation than photophobia	Photophobia	Usually severe, but significant number have little dis-comfort	Usually very little, mostly irritation	Usually severe
Cornea	Usually clear unless epithelium involved; loses glassy appearance; infiltrates appear white	Usually clear	Generalized haze	Usually clear	If corneal injury, may be hazy
Intraocular Pressure	Usually normal (elevated in zoster uveitis)	Usually down or normal; occa-sionally up	Elevated	Normal	May be normal, up or down (even with perforation)
Pupils	Usually normal	Usually smaller; poorly reactive	Middilated (little or no reaction)	Normal	May be large, normal, small, or irregular
Scrapings/ Stains	Viral: monocytic Bacterial: PMNs + stain inclusions Fungal: PMNs + stain			Eosinophils may be present (e.g., vernal)	

PMNs, polymorphonuclear leukocytes.
Modified from Vaughan D, Asbury T. *General ophthalmology*, 11th ed. Los Altos, Calif.: Lange Medical Publications, 1986.

EMERGENCY DEPARTMENT EVALUATION

After taking a careful history, as described, visual acuity testing of both eyes is the first step in the physical examination of the eye. This should be performed prior to instillation of any medication. After this, direct inspection of the eye, followed by slit-lamp examination, should be done with attention to the following anatomic structures.

Lids

Crusting of the lids is common in bacterial overgrowth, infection, and dermatologic conditions (seborrhea). Ulcerations are common in herpetic and staphylococcal infections. Lice (*Phthirus*) may also be seen. Lid eversion should be performed if indicated (foreign body, pseudomembranes).

Conjunctiva

Note the presence of chemosis or discharge (serous, mucoid, or mucopurulent). Follicles represent lymphoid aggregates, which are a hallmark of acute adenoviral disease, but are, on occasion, seen in other cases of infectious, toxic, and allergic conjunctivitis. Membranes, or fibrinous pseudomembranes, are seen in severe conjunctivitis associated with adenovirus, occasionally in other conditions (such as *S. pneumoniae* and diphtheria), and rarely in herpetic disease. Hemorrhage is usually petechial but may be more extensive, as in adenovirus, hemorrhagic conjunctivitis virus, *Haemophilus*, and *S. pneumoniae*. An acute, markedly purulent conjunctivitis should be thoroughly and rapidly evaluated before treatment. Corneal perforation is possible, especially in conditions such as gonococcal disease.

Cornea

The hallmark of epithelial injury, especially in viral disorders, is punctate areas of cell loss. These appear as stained specks with fluorescein and are diagnostic of adenovirus (superficial punctate keratopathy). However, many other conditions may mimic this, including herpetic disease, so consider additional clues. Ulceration implies a larger epithelial defect and is important to identify. Immediate referral is indicated in this setting because of the potential for permanent scarring or perforation. The ulceration description should include size, shape, and anterior stromal involvement. Herpetic ulcers are usually dendritic or geographic. Bacterial and fungal ulcers tend to be round with fluffy white borders and extend into the anterior stroma (Fig. 10.4). They are usually associated with a purulent discharge and lid-sticking. Infiltrates are epithelial, subepithelial, or stromal collections of inflammatory cellular debris that are nonspecific but common in viral (adenoviral, herpetic), chlamydial (inclusion), bacterial (in association with the ulcerative defect), and hypersensitivity reactions (small and near limbus).

Anterior Chamber

The presence of white blood cells in the aqueous is the hallmark of iritis (uveitis), which occurs with severe anterior surface infections (herpetic disease, adenovirus). The grading of the reaction (1+ to 4+) of these cells correlates with the severity of the iritis. Layering of the cells in the anterior chamber is called a *hypopyon* and is a hallmark of severe ulceration of the cornea and endophthalmitis. Usually seen with bacterial and fungal infection, *a hypopyon warrants immediate consultation and referral*. In the presence of a small corneal ulcer without hypopyon, *consult first*. After stains and cultures have been performed, cover with "heavy" topicals (e.g., topical ciprofloxacin [Ciloxan 0.3%] every 30 to 60 minutes). Fortified drops are most often used and are prepared by the pharmacy. If a hypopyon is present, or the ulcer is large or multiple, this is an ocular emergency, and the ophthalmologist should be called. Infectious ulcers of the cornea tend to be more central, whereas hypersensitivity immune ulcers (e.g., rheumatoid and staphylococcal) tend to be peripheral.

Other Physical Findings

Preauricular lymphadenopathy is an important sign of adenoviral conjunctivitis, but it may be seen in severe bacterial infection (streptococcal and neisserial). It is classically seen in Parinaud's oculoglandular syndrome, in which the nodes are very large and tender and occasionally draining. Distant skin ulcerations or vesicles, including the lids, suggest herpetic disease (simplex or zoster), as well as impetigo. *Moraxella* and *Staphylococcus* tend to cause ulceration and maceration in the lateral canthal regions.

Diagnostic Aids

Fluorescein

The ocular surface is stained with a moistened, sterile fluorescein strip and viewed with a slit lamp. A small quantity is used. The examiner should look for areas of epithelial loss on the conjunctiva and cornea. The noninfected eye is stained first.

Rose Bengal

Rose bengal is not used as frequently, but it does indicate devitalized epithelium. A small amount should be used; a slit lamp is generally required. It is occasionally helpful in the diagnosis of herpetic ulcers. The dendritic pattern of a herpetic ulcer may appear similar to that of a healing corneal abrasion. The margins of a healing abrasion are healthy, with proliferating epithelial cells, and do not stain with rose bengal. The margins of a herpetic dendritic ulcer contain actively infected epithelial cells that are devitalized and pick up the red stain.

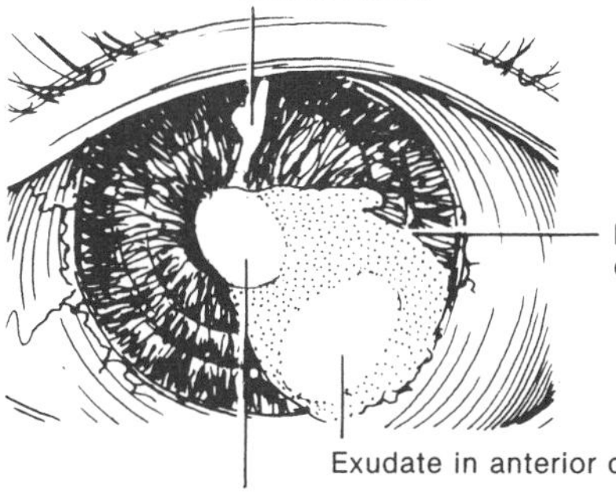

Figure 10.4. Bacterial or fungal corneal ulcer.

Laboratory Studies

Routine conjunctival infections are not cultured, but it is appropriate, in the setting of a severe or unusual purulent conjunctivitis, to perform Gram and Giemsa stains of the material. After cultures, conjunctival scrapings should be taken. A flamed platinum spatula that has cooled is gently scraped across the anesthetized tarsal conjunctiva. The material is spread thinly on a glass slide. Corneal scraping of ulcers must be performed at the slit-lamp biomicroscope, preferably by an ophthalmologist; it is essential before initiation of antibiotics. Conjunctival cytology of cell types and the identification of intracytoplasmic inclusions are also helpful. In culturing organisms, blood, chocolate, and Sabouraud dextrose agar, and thioglycollate broth are basic media for corneal ulcers. *At a minimum, culturettes of conjunctival exudates should be placed into liquid culture media.* Viral and chlamydial studies are available at large medical centers but are generally not performed in the emergency setting. Deeper ocular infections (endophthalmitis) typically require culture of the anterior chamber and/or vitreous prior to treatment. This should be performed by an ophthalmologist. Evaluation of other body fluids is occasionally necessary. For example, a urethral discharge may help determine a possible gonococcal or Reiter's conjunctivitis.

EMERGENCY DEPARTMENT MANAGEMENT

It is important to avoid contagion. In the setting of ocular infection, it is essential to maintain clean equipment and to avoid checking the intraocular pressure, unless absolutely necessary, because of the risk of spreading contamination with the tonometer. The emergency physician is at risk to contract or spread these highly contagious diseases and should be fastidious about hand-washing. Appropriate medical excuses need to be offered to school-age children and health-care workers.

Table 10.2 lists antibiotics for topical use. It is important to avoid mixing bacteriostatic antibiotics (e.g., erythromycin) with bactericidal antibiotics (e.g., bacitracin). Certain bacteriostatic antibiotics (e.g., sulfa) can be bactericidal at the high levels delivered in topical preparations; therefore, hospital sensitivity profiles may not be reliable.

Be aware of antibiotics with increased sensitizing ability. Neomycin, a major component of Neosporin, is highly sensitizing and should be avoided. It may mask evaluation of response as well as create reactions that look worse than the original condition. Sulfa agents, bacitracin, and aminoglycosides can create a similar picture, but much less frequently. There have been cases of Stevens-Johnson–like reactions to topical sulfa. By prescribing only a small amount at a time and no multiple refills, patient retention of old medications that may be contaminated can be avoided.

Severe anterior surface disorders can result in iritis, with the potential to cause subsequent scarring of the pupil to the lens (posterior synechiae), as well as iris to cornea (peripheral anterior synechiae). Cycloplegics are essential and improve patient comfort. Longer acting cycloplegics (scopolamine, homatropine, and atropine) may be necessary. Although corticosteroids play an important role in the management of iritis and may reduce corneal scarring, their use in the emergency setting is controversial, and they should be used only in consultation with the ophthalmologist.

It is important to understand the immunologic inflammatory consequences after proper antibiotic coverage (usually corneal

TABLE 10.2. Antibiotics for Topical Use

GENERAL PRINCIPLES OF ADMINISTRATION

Topical antibiotics are given four times daily for simple infection, more frequently or fortified for serious infection (ulcers, gonorrhea). The most common infectious pathogens are *Staphylococcus aureus, Haemophilus* species, pneumococci, and *Staphylococcus epidermidis.* Even when sensitivity testing shows resistance to many of these antibiotics, they may still be effective because of their high concentration (e.g., sulfa).

ANTIBACTERIAL AGENTS

Bacitracin: Effective against most gram-positive organisms as well as diphtheroids, *Haemophilus,* and *Actinomyces.* Ointment form and in mixture with polymixin B (Polysporin). Fortified drops for ulcers prepared fresh only by pharmacy.

Chloramphenicol: Effective against many gram-positive and gram-negative organisms, especially *Haemophilus, Moraxella, S. aureus,* group B streptococci, and diphtheroids. Solution (0.5%) and ointment (1%) (Chloroptic, Econochlor, others). Low allergy index.

Ciprofloxacin: A fluoroquinolone currently used for corneal ulcers caused by many staphylococcal and streptococcal species, and *Pseudomonas aeruginosa.* This commercially available preparation (Ciloxan, 0.3%) permits outpatient management of simple corneal ulcers. Low allergy index.

Erythromycin: Effective against gram-positive organisms, diphtheroids, *Haemophilus, Actinomyces,* and *Neisseria.* Only in ointment form (0.5%) (Ilotycin). Very effective for staph or rosacea blepharitis.

Gentamicin: Effective against most gram-negative organisms, especially *Pseudomonas,* as well as gram-positive organisms, including *Staphylococcus* species. Highly effective broad-spectrum agent, but has fairly high sensitizing as well as potential toxic effects. Available in solution and ointment form (Genoptic, Garamycin, Gentacidin).

Neomycin: Wide range of effectiveness (like gentamicin) but even more sensitizing and potentially toxic to corneal epithelium. Usually in mixtures in solution or ointment (Neosporin, Ocutricin).

Norfloxacin: A fluoroquinolone similar to ciprofloxacin, but approved as a 0.3% solution (Chibroxin) for conjunctivitis caused by a wide variety of gram-positive and gram-negative organisms.

Polymyxin B: Fairly effective against most gram-negative organisms (not effective against *Proteus* or *Neisseria*). Available only in mixtures (Neosporin, Polysporin, Polytrim, and others).

Sulfacetamide: Effective against a wide range of gram-positive and gram-negative organisms; some *Staphylococcus* species, pneumococci, *Haemophilus, Moraxella,* and *Chlamydia.* Available in solution (10%, 15%, and 30%) and ointment form (10%) (Bleph-10, Sulamyd, others). Potential for allergy is fairly high.

Tetracycline: Effective against many *Staphylococcus, Streptococcus* species, also gonococci, *Actinomyces, Haemophilus,* a few gram-negative organisms, and *Chlamydia.* Available in solution and ointment (1%) (Achromycin). Allergy index is not bad, but irritating.

Tobramycin: Similar in activity to gentamicin, as a 0.3% solution (Tobrex).

Trimethoprim: Effective against many staphylococcal and streptococcal species and *Haemophilus.* In combination with polymyxin B (Polytrim), it has a wide range of efficacy. It is not recommended for children under 2 years of age. Very low allergy index.

ANTIFUNGAL AGENTS

Natamycin: Effective against many filamentary and yeast forms. Drug of choice for most mycotic corneal injuries. Available as Natacyn, 5% suspension.

Flucytosine: Effective against candida and cryptococcus. Solution 1% (Ancobon).

Miconazole: Approved for candida, cryptococcus, and aspergillus. Available as 1% solution (Monistat):

ANTIVIRALS

Idoxuridine: First antiherpetic drug available. Does not penetrate corneal epithelium well, but has been on market longest and fairly safe. Available as 0.1% solution and 0.5% ointment (Stoxil, Herplex). Resistance well known.

Vidarabine: Fairly effective by today's standards. Penetrates cornea only fairly well and is somewhat toxic to the epithelium (as is idoxuridine). Needs to be applied only five times daily (but ointment is annoying), rather than every 2 hours, as with most antiviral drops. Available as a 3% ointment (ARA-A, Vira-A).

Trifluorothymidine: Most popular antiviral for herpetic disease. Penetrates cornea fairly well. Toxic to epithelium. Available in 1% solution (Viroptic) and must be initiated at an every-2-hour dosage until ulcer is healing.

Acycloguanosine: Available for just about every other part of the body *except* the eye. In investigational studies, it is highly effective in the treatment of ocular herpetic disease. It has a low toxicity. Acyclovir is available topically for genital use. It has a systemic preparation that has been helpful in reducing morbidity in herpes zoster (shingles), as well as for systemic zoster or simplex involvement.

infiltrates). Ophthalmologic referral is indicated because of the possible indication for corticosteroid therapy.

The goal should be to do a thorough examination and treat ocular infection in a way that will least harm the patient. Sulfacetamide 10% or Polytrim solutions given four to six times daily for several days will clear most simple surface infections. Gentamicin, tobramycin, and several quinolone solutions are currently available and are extremely helpful, but they may be more beneficial when reserved for special situations. Chronic use will cause eye toxicity and permit resistant organisms and fungal overgrowth. Drops are aesthetically superior and provide high levels quickly; however, they are cleared by tear drainage too quickly. Ointments reduce this clearing effect as well as the irritation, but cause blurred vision. Use of ointments (polymyxin–bacitracin combinations) may be particularly helpful at bedtime. For the previously stated reasons, drops are better used in adults, but ointments may be more efficacious in children.

DISPOSITION

Role of the Consultant

Immediate consultation is indicated in the following circumstances:

Purulent conjunctivitis associated with a corneal infiltrate, ulcer, or hypopyon. Risk factors include trauma and contact lens history.

A hyperacute conjunctivitis with a history or Gram stain suggesting gonococcal disease

Membranous conjunctivitis. Secondary injury to the cornea or severe corneal epithelial injury may occur.

Consultation within 24 to 48 hours:

Relatively severe conjunctivitis or keratitis that suggests possible herpetic disease, especially if it is near the visual axis

Consultation within 3 to 7 days:

Bacterial conjunctivitis that does not improve within 48 hours
Viral disease that is nonmembranous with intact vision. Adenoviral disease (e.g., epidemic keratoconjunctivitis) may show persistent signs of involvement for weeks!

Indications for Admission

Emergency admissions are rare, but are required for endophthalmitis; occasionally, severe or recalcitrant corneal ulcers, and *Neisseria* conjunctivitis with corneal infiltrates may also require hospital admission. It is uncommon to admit a patient with herpes simplex or zoster. The principal goal for admission is systemic therapy, frequent topical antibiotic administration, and subconjunctival or intravitreal injections. Topical therapy may need to be administered every 30 to 60 minutes (and prepared fortified).

Special Considerations

Outpatient care may be possible, but many patients are incapable of intensive care at home. Most patients with corneal ulcers should be rechecked in 24 hours. Moderately severe cases of bacterial conjunctivitis should be seen in 48 to 72 hours. Referral should be based on progression of the disease, lack of response, increased pain, and decreased vision.

COMMON PITFALLS

- *The red eye is not always infected!*
- High-risk situations for purulent conjunctivitis should be sought and include conjunctival pseudomembranes, posttraumatic reaction, and contact lens wear.
- Multiple antibiotics are often used when progression of the infection is really due to hypersensitivity (Neosporin) or toxicity to the drug. Prolonged therapy creates the same risk as overtreating systemic infection with regard to the emergence of resistant organisms or fungal growth.
- Initiating antibiotic therapy before diagnostic studies are performed may force the ophthalmologist into "shotgun" therapy.
- *The indiscriminate use and distribution of topical anesthetics and corticosteroids are to be condemned.*

Bibliography

Colenbrander A. Principles of ophthalmology. In: Tasman W, Jaeger EA, eds. *Duane's clinical ophthalmology*, vol. 1. Philadelphia: JB Lippincott Co, 1992.

Glaser J. Neuro-ophthalmic examination: general consideration and special techniques. In: Tasman W, Jaeger EA, eds. *Duane's clinical ophthalmology*, vol. 2. Philadelphia: JB Lippincott Co, 1992.

Mannis MJ. Bacterial conjunctivitis. In: Tasman W, Jaeger EA, eds. *Duane's clinical ophthalmology*, vol. 1. Philadelphia: JB Lippincott Co, 1992.

Pavan-Langston D. *Manual of ocular diagnosis and therapy*, 2nd ed. Boston: Little, Brown and Company, 1986.

Physician's desk reference for ophthalmology, 22nd ed. Montvale, NJ: Medical Economics, 1994.

Tate GW Jr, Safir A. The slit lamp: history, principles, and practice. In: Tasman W, Jaeger EA, eds. *Duane's clinical ophthalmology*, vol. 1. Philadelphia: JB Lippincott Co, 1992.

Vaughan D, Asbury T. *General ophthalmology*, 11th ed. Los Altos, CA: Lange Medical, 1986.

CHAPTER 11
Common Ophthalmic Medications

Geoffrey Broocker

The information provided here describes representative therapeutic preparations for many ocular conditions. Please refer to compendiums such as the *Physician's Desk Reference for Ophthalmology* for a thorough listing with pharmaceutical manufacturers' specifications. Frequency of medication applications depends on the agent used and the severity of the condition being managed.

DIAGNOSTIC MEDICATIONS

These agents facilitate the ability to examine the eye.

Stains

These are topical solutions that highlight epithelial abnormalities of the cornea and conjunctiva.

Fluorescein: Sterile paper strips are preferred to the 2% solutions, owing to ease of contamination of the latter.

Rose bengal: This 1% solution stains devitalized corneal–conjunctival epithelium; it is helpful in differentiating a herpetic corneal ulcer from a healing abrasion.

Anesthetics

These are topical solutions that promote patient cooperation for the examination; they are also used in conjunction with the aforementioned stains. Anesthetics are usually required for determining intraocular pressure.

Tetracaine hydrochloride (Pontocaine): 0.5% to 1.0% solution, lasts for 15 minutes; may sting

Proparacaine hydrochloride (Ophthetic, Ophthaine): 0.5% solution, less irritating

Cocaine (0.25% to 0.5%): Effective but highly toxic to the corneal epithelium

Mydriatics and Cycloplegics

These are used diagnostically or therapeutically to dilate the pupil (mydriasis) and/or paralyze the ciliary body (cycloplegia). This permits evaluation of the internal ocular structures and gauges the baseline refractive error of the eye by blocking accommodation. In addition, these agents prevent synechiae formation (adhesions of the iris to lens and cornea) by reducing intraocular inflammation through stabilization of the blood–aqueous barrier. These agents are capped in *red*.

Phenylephrine hydrochloride (Neo-Synephrine, Mydfrin): Vasoconstricts the surface vessels and dilates the pupil without cycloplegia; 2.5% solution is the strength recommended because of a higher incidence of cardiovascular side effects with 10%. Dilation capability varies, used alone, and may last up to 4 hours, depending on the amount of pigmentation of the iris.

Tropicamide (Mydriacyl 0.5% and 1.0%): Provides an excellent short-term dilation of the pupil, plus cycloplegia (4 to 6 hours). Relatively easy to reverse (if concerned about potential angle-closure glaucoma); used most often by ophthalmologists

Cyclopentolate hydrochloride (Cyclogyl 0.5%, 1.0%, and 2.0%): Best short-term cycloplegic for determining refractive error, may last for 6 hours up to a day!

Homatropine hydrobromide (1%, 2%, and 5%): Lasts for a few days and is useful for short-term on low-level inflammation (iritis) caused by trauma or abrasions

Scopolamine hydrobromide (Hyoscine 0.25%): Lasts for 3 to 5 days and is more effective for long-term inflammation seen postoperatively or in severe uveitis

Atropine sulfate (0.25% to 2.0% solution, 0.5% and 1.0% ointment): Lasts for 10 to 14 days; most commonly used postoperatively and in severe uveitis. Corneal epithelial and systemic toxicities are important to note.

THERAPEUTIC AGENTS

Lubricants

The precorneal tear film is the most important layer of the eye with regard to comfort and vision. Abnormalities of this complex multilayered film are responsible for a large percentage of surface complaints (burning, itching, foreign-body sensation, epiphora, and blurred vision that vacillates with blinking). Artificial lubricants are an effective but temporary treatment for any condition that causes this "dry-eye syndrome."

Artificial tears: These agents (Table 11.1) usually contain various methylcellulose compounds, but synthetics are available. Trends toward successful use involve the "thickness" of the solution and single-use, nonpreserved packets. Frequency of use, especially when preserved, multiuse bottles are selected, can have limited return on symptoms. Overall, these agents not only are benign, but also relieve most anterior surface irritation from any cause. *Be liberal in dispensing these agents!*

Bland lubricating ointments (Hypotears, Lacri-Lube): Especially helpful for lubrication during sleep or conditions with incomplete lid closure (e.g., general anesthesia, seventh-nerve palsies). Nonpreserved varieties without lanolin are preferable.

Antibiotics

Refer to Table 11.2.

Antiinflammatories

These agents are used most often to suppress allergic (i.e., immunologic) reactions of the eye of all types, both externally and internally. It may be necessary to suppress severe external inflammation to avoid corneal scarring or permanent tear-film abnormalities. Within the eye, these agents help to prevent scarring (synechiae) and subsequent development of glaucoma. Topical application often allows excellent penetration into the anterior chamber. This category is divided into steroid and nonsteroid (NSAID) varieties.

Steroid Antiinflammatory Agents

These are very effective in blocking pathways of inflammation. A significant portion of the population will raise their intraocular pressure in response to prolonged use of these agents (generally 2 weeks or more). Because of this and infectious concerns, ophthalmic initiation and follow-up may be necessary.

Medrysone 1% (HMS): Mild steroid, few side effects. Used for surface allergy problems

Fluorometholone 0.1% (FML): Slightly more potent, with fewer side effects than prednisolone and dexamethasone. As fluorometholone acetate 0.1% (Flarex), potency comparable to prednisolone acetate 1% due to better penetration

Rimexolone 1% (Vexol): Similar profile to that of fluorometholone, but with a lower propensity to raise intraocular pressure

TABLE 11.1 Artificial Tear Preparations

Agent in Solution	Trade Name Concentration	Preservative
Carboxymethylcellulose	*Refresh Tears* (0.5%)	Boric acid
	Refresh Plus (0.5%)	Preservative-free
	Celluvisc (1%)	Preservative-free
Hydroxyethylcellulose	*Comfort Tears* (0.005%)	Benzalkonium chloride
	Adsorbotear (0.4%)	Thimerosal
	Tear Gard	Preservative-free
Hydroxypropylmethylcellulose	*Isopto Plain/Isopto Tears* (0.5%)	Benzalkonium chloride
	Tearisol (0.5%)	Benzalkonium chloride
	Ultratears	Benzalkonium chloride
	Bion Tears (0.3%)	Preservative-free
	Tears Naturale (0.3%)	Benzalkonium chloride
	Tears Naturale II	Sodium borate
	Tears Naturale Free	Preservative-free
	Nature's Tears (0.4%)	Benzalkonium chloride
	OcuCoat (0.8%)	Benzalkonium chloride
	OcuCoat PF (0.8%)	Preservative-free
Polyvinyl alcohol	*Liquifilm* (1.4%)	Chlorbutanol
	HypoTears (1%)	Benzalkonium chloride
	HypoTears PF (1%)	Preservative-free
	Akwa Tears (1.4%)	Benzalkonium chloride
	Dry Eyes (1.4%)	Benzalkonium chloride
	Murine (0.5%)	Benzalkonium chloride
	Tears Plus (1.4%)	Chlorbutanol
Glycerin	*Dry Eye Therapy* (0.3%)	Preservative-free
Polycarbophil	*AquaSite*	Preservative-free

TABLE 11.2. Antibiotics for Topical Use

GENERAL PRINCIPLES OF ADMINISTRATION

Topical antibiotics are given four to six times daily for simple infections, more frequently or fortified for serious infection (corneal ulcers, gonorrhea). The most common infectious pathogens are *Staphylococcus aureus, Haemophilus* species, *Pneumococcus,* and *Staphylococcus epidermidis.* Even though sensitivities show resistance to many of these antibiotics, they may still be bacteriocidal because of their high concentration (e.g., sulfa).

ANTIBACTERIAL AGENTS

Bacitracin: Effective against most gram-positive organisms, also diphtheroids, *Haemophilus,* and *Actinomyces.* Commercially in ointment form and in popular mixture with polymyxin B (Polysporin). Fortified drops for ulcers prepared fresh only.

Chloramphenicol: Effective against many gram-positive and gram-negative organisms, especially *Haemophilus, Moraxella, S. aureus,* group B streptococci, and diphtheroids. Solution (0.5%) and ointment (1%) (Chloroptic, Econochlor, others). Low allergy index. Usage has diminished due to concern for aplastic anemia and large group of alternative choices.

Ciprofloxacin: Topical formulation of the systemic medication; a fluoroquinolone, with broad-spectrum activity. It is currently indicated for ulcers and conjunctivitis caused by various staphylococcal and streptococcal strains, and *Pseudomonas aeruginosa.* Its overall effectiveness in the general clinical setting is currently beneficial because it allows for ambulatory care of most corneal ulcers. It has a very low allergy index. Solution is 0.3% (Ciloxan).

Erythromycin: Effective against gram-positive organisms, diphtheroids, *Haemophilus, Actinomyces,* and *Neisseria.* Only in ointment form (0.5%) (Ilotycin). Very effective for staph or rosacea blepharitis.

Gentamicin: Effective against most gram-negative organisms, especially *Pseudomonas,* as well as gram-positive organisms, including *Staphylococcus* species. Highly effective broad-spectrum agent, but has fairly high sensitizing as well as potential toxic corneal epithelial effects. Available in solution and ointment form. (Genoptic, Garamycin, Gentacidin).

Neomycin: Wide range of effectiveness (like gentamicin), but even more sensitizing and potentially toxic to corneal epithelium. Usually in mixtures in solution or ointment (Neosporin, Ocutricin).

Norfloxacin: Approved for treatment of bacterial conjunctivitis with efficacy that parallels ciprofloxacin. (Chibroxin 0.3%).

Olfloxacin: Similar indications and coverage as ciprofloxacin. (Ocuflox).

Polymyxin B sulfate: Fairly effective against most gram-negative organisms (except *Proteus* or *Neisseria*). Available mostly in ointment form and only in mixtures (Neosporin, Polysporin, others). Available also in solution with trimethoprim (Polytrim).

Sulfacetamide sodium: Effective against a wide range of gram-positive and gram-negative organisms, some *Staphylococcus* species, pneumococci, *Haemophilus, Moraxella,* and *Chlamydia.* Available in solution (10%, 15%, and 30%) and ointment form (10%) (Bleph-10, Sulamyd, others). Potential for allergy is fairly high.

Sulfisoxazole diolamine: Similar in coverage and effect as sulfacetamide (Gantrisin).

Tetracycline (oxytetracycline): Effective against *Streptococcus* species, *Haemophilus ducreyi,* a few gram-negatives, and *Chlamydia.* Allergy index is not bad, but irritating. Available primarily in combination with polymyxin B in Terramycin ointment.

Trimethoprim sulfate: Effective against some staphylococcal and streptococcal strains, as well as *Haemophilus* species. In combination with polymyxin B (Polytrim), it has a wide range of effectiveness. Its safety and effectiveness has not been determined under 2 months of age. Very low allergy index.

ANTIFUNGAL AGENT

Natamycin: Effective against many filamentary and yeast forms. Drug of choice for most mycotic corneal injuries (and only ocular formulation commercially available). Available as Natacyn, 5% suspension.

ANTIVIRALS

Idoxuridine: First antiherpetic drug available. Does not penetrate corneal epithelium well, but has been on market longest and fairly safe. Available as 0.1% solution and 0.5% ointment (Stoxil, Herplex). Resistance occurs. Can be toxic to corneal epithelium.

Vidarabine monohydrate: Available as a 3% ointment (ARA-A, Vira-A) only and is fairly effective. It penetrates the cornea only fairly well, and is somewhat toxic to the epithelium. Needs to be applied only five times daily (but ointment is annoying), rather than every 2 hours, as with most antiviral drops.

Trifluridine (trifluorothymidine): Most popular antiviral for corneal herpetic disease, and penetrates cornea fairly well. Toxic to epithelium, like others. Available in 1% solution (Viroptic) and must be initiated at an every-2-hour dosage until ulcer is healing.

Acyclovir sodium (acycloguanosine): Available topically for just about every other part of the body *except* the eye. It is highly effective in the treatment of ocular herpetic disease (deep corneal and intraocular involvement) given systemically. It has a low toxicity. Acyclovir is available topically for genital use. The systemic preparation has been helpful in reducing morbidity (especially postherpetic neuralgia) in herpes zoster (shingles), as well as for ocular zoster or simplex involvement. Must be given intravenously for retinal involvement (retinal necrosis syndromes) and in immunocompromised patients (HIV).

Therapy for CMV retinitis: Even though these agents are not used topically, their frequency of use in AIDS patients with CMV retinitis, and occasionally other viral retinopathies, deserves mention.

Cidofovir: Used systemically for CMV retinitis (Vistide).

Foscarnet sodium: Used systemically for CMV retinitis (Foscavir).

Ganciclovir sodium: Most common agent used for systemic therapy, but often injected intravitreally to enhance effectiveness in setting of advanced disease. Transscleral intraocular implant better tolerated and efficacious (but must be replaced over time).

Loteprednol etabonate 0.5% (Lotemax): Relatively new preparation with high potency and lower propensity to raise intraocular pressure.

Prednisolone acetate and phosphate 0.125% and 1.0% (Pred Mild, Pred Forte, Inflamase Forte): Potent and highly effective for anterior segment inflammation. High risk for side effects (intraocular pressure and infection, especially herpes simplex facilitation)

Dexamethasone 0.1% (Decadron): Potent and highly effective. Very high risk for side effects

Nonsteroidal Antiinflammatory Agents

Recent emphasis on these therapies used topically have paralleled systemic usefulness. Although there is therapeutic overlap, the Food and Drug Administration has recommended indications for each of these agents.

Flurbiprofen 0.03% (Ocufen): Used to keep the pupil dilated during cataract surgery

Diclofenac 0.1% (Voltaren): Used for postoperative inflammation after cataract surgery

Ketorolac 0.5% (Acular): A product developed for allergic conjunctivitis
Suprofen 1% (Profenal): Used to keep the pupil dilated during cataract surgery

Antibiotic–Steroid Combinations

A number of products are available with broad-spectrum antibiotics combined with varying concentrations of potent topical corticosteroids (e.g., TobraDex tobramycin/dexamethasone) both in drop and ointment forms. These formulations may be helpful in postoperative circumstances, but they should be reserved for other conditions, with ophthalmic consultation.

Antiglaucoma Agents

These either suppress aqueous production or increase outflow facility, or both. Because the ciliary body and muscle are critical determinants of the intraocular pressure (with regard to aqueous production and outflow), autonomic agents and their blockers may affect the intraocular pressure. Carbonic anhydrase inhibitors block aqueous production because this enzyme is essential in the active production of aqueous humor. The most recent addition to the management regimen includes topical prostaglandins, which act in a different manner by reducing outflow through a uveoscleral route.

Miotics (cholinergic agonists): *Pilocarpine* 0.5% to 10%; *carbachol* 0.75%, 1.5%, and 3.0%; *echothiophate iodide* (phospholine iodide) 0.06% to 0.25%: Rarely cause systemic problems, but use of depolarizing agents in general anesthesia (succinylcholine) is contraindicated in patients taking phospholine. Miotics make the pupils small; usually capped in *green* (pilocarpine and carbachol).
Adrenergic agents: *Epinephrine* compounds 0.5% to 2.0%, *dipivalyl epinephrine* 0.1% (Propine): Tolerance develops commonly, and the eyes turn red! These products have *white* caps.
Alpha-2 agonists: *Apraclonidine* 0.5% and 1.0% (Iopidine), *brimonide tartrate* 0.2% (Alphagan): Reduce aqueous production and may increase uveoscleral outflow. Alphagan has fewer side effects. As with most adrenergic agents, ensure that the patient does not have a problem with cardiovascular sensitivity. Beware of use with MAO inhibitors.
Beta-blockers: *Timolol* 0.25% and 0.5% (Timoptic), *betaxolol* 0.25% (Betoptic-S), *levobunolol* 0.5% (Betagan), *metipranolol* 0.3% (OptiPranolol), and *carteolol* 1% (Ocupress): Most have *yellow* caps and may cause beta-blocker side effects (heart and lung). Betoptic is cardioselective (beta-1) and has fewer side effects, but also has less ocular efficacy. Cardiac sensitivity and adverse effects on libido and serum cholesterol are reasons to swing toward use of newer agents.
Carbonic anhydrase inhibitors: *Oral Agents: Acetazolamide* (Diamox 250-mg tablets, 500-mg capsules) and *methazolamide* (Neptazane 50 mg) are the principal agents used. These are mild diuretics and may facilitate potassium depletion when given chronically. If glaucoma therapy is given systemically, the incidence of side effects goes up dramatically. These agents are sulfa-related compounds; therefore, allergic reactions can occur. They may also precipitate renal stones in susceptible patients. *Topical Agents: Dorzolamide hydrochloride* 2% (Trusopt), and *brinzolamide* 1% (Azopt) offer fewer side effects, but they are not as efficacious in reducing the intraocular pressure as are the oral agents. Dorzolamide also comes in a combination form, with the beta-blocker timolol, as Cosopt.
Osmotic agents: *Oral glycerin* (Osmoglyn) 50% to 75% (1.0 to 1.5 g/kg) over ice, frequently produces nausea and vomiting; *isosorbide* 45% (Ismotic), 1.5 g/kg, will lower the pressure adequately over 1 to 2 hours, a preferred agent in diabetic patients. A rapid response is most often accomplished with a 20% solution of mannitol, 1 to 2 g/kg i.v. over 30 to 45 minutes. These agents are used emergently to shrink the vitreous and rapidly lower the intraocular pressure. It is essential to know the patient's fluid, renal, and cardiovascular status before using these compounds.

OCULAR ALLERGIC CONDITIONS

Surface reactions to a host of airborne agents (e.g., pollen, dust) and irritants can cause conjunctival swelling (chemosis), redness, itching, and tearing. Management of these reactions should start conservatively with cool compresses and decongestant–antihistamine combinations. More aggressive therapy can involve more potent topical antihistamines, mast-cell inhibitors, topical NSAIDs (see previous discussion), and corticosteroids.

Ocular Decongestants

These agents, many of which are available over the counter, are topical solutions used to whiten the eye. Although overtly effective, the utilization of these agents often hinders timely diagnosis and treatment of the condition that presents as "the red eye." Chronic use of these agents causes tolerance and eventual worsening of the vascular dilatation. A few of these agents may also include a mild topical antihistamine, which may be a useful way to initiate therapy for mild allergic phenomena. When an antihistamine is present, the decongestant product will usually include the suffix "-A" to indicate such.

Naphazoline hydrochloride (Naphcon, Vasocon, others): Contain preservatives that may be sensitizing
Phenylephrine hydrochloride (Prefrin, Relief, others): These compounds are not as stable, and are also preserved (except for Relief).
Tetrahydrozoline hydrochloride (Murine, Visine, others): Available over the counter, also preserved
Oxymetazoline hydrochloride (OcuClear, Visine L.R.): Similar to tetrahydrozoline but more potent

Antihistamines

Along with the combination antihistamines used with the previously noted decongestants, these agents have been marketed specifically for ocular allergy management.

Levocabastine hydrochloride 0.05% (Livostin): Very effective, but does sting on administration
Emedastine difumarate 0.05% (Emadine): Has effects similar to those of previous agent

Mast-cell Stabilizers

Seasonal allergy disorders usually revolve around IgE-mediated (Type I) hypersensitivity reactions. This involves the release of histamine and many vasoactive substances that create the signs and symptoms of allergy. By blocking the mast-cell release of these vasoactive substances, symptomatology is relieved. Because this affects only unsensitized mast cells, the effects of these agents take days to weeks to work properly.

Cromolyn sodium 4% (Crolom, Opticrom): Used extensively in Europe, became popular in the United States in 1980s, especially in the management of vernal conjunctivitis
Lodoxamide tromethamine 0.1% (Alomide): May have somewhat

different mechanism of action (calcium influx on mast cell), but almost as effective

Olopatadine hydrochloride 0.1% (Patanol): Has inherent antihistaminic effects and also appears to have mast-cell–stabilizing capability

COMMON PITFALLS

- Avoid the indiscriminate use of topical antibiotics in serious ocular infections without first obtaining adequate samples for culture and sensitivities.
- Topical corticosteroids, used alone or in combination with other topical medications, should be used only after proper consultation by phone.
- Even though ocular medications are most often delivered topically, there are significant systemic side effects seen with certain agents, especially those that treat glaucoma (e.g., beta-blockers). Punctal compression, to avoid drainage down the nasolacrimal system into the posterior nasopharynx (subsequently swallowed), will reduce this problem.

Bibliography

Bartlett J, et al. *Ophthalmic drug facts.* St. Louis: Facts & Comparisons, 1999.

Colenbrander A. Principles of ophthalmology. In: Tasman W, Jaeger EA, eds. *Duane's clinical ophthalmology,* vol. 1, chapter 63. Philadelphia: Lippincott Williams & Wilkins, 1998.

Glaser J. Neuro-ophthalmic examination: general consideration and special tecniques. In: Tasman W, Jaeger EA, eds. *Duane's clinical ophthalmology,* vol. 2, chapter 3. Philadelphia: Lippincott Williams & Wilkins, 1998.

Mannis MJ, Plotnick R. Bacterial conjunctivitis. In: Tasman W, Jaeger EA, eds. *Duane's clinical ophthalmology,* vol. 2, chapter 5. Philadelphia: Lippincott Williams & Wilkins, 1998.

Patel KH, Javitt JC, et al. Incidence of acute angle closure glaucoma after pharmacologic mydriasis. *Am J Ophthalmol* 1995;120(6):709–717.

Pavan-Langston D. *Manual of ocular diagnosis and therapy,* 4th ed. Boston: Lippincott-Raven, 1995.

Physician's desk reference for ophthalmology, 26th ed. Montvale, NJ: Medical Economics Data Production Company, 1998.

Tate GW Jr, Safir A. The slit lamp: history, principles, and practice. In: Tasman W, Jaeger EA, eds. *Duane's clinical ophthalmology,* vol. 1, chapter 59. Philadelphia: Lippincott Williams & Wilkins, 1998.

Vaughan D. *General ophthalmology,* 15th ed. Stamford, CT: Appleton & Lange, 1998.

CHAPTER 12

Acute Visual Disturbances

Catherine A. Marco

Loss of vision, whether unilateral or bilateral, partial or complete, is an emergent ophthalmologic complaint, and requires rapid and thorough evaluation and management. Emergent evaluation includes taking the relevant ocular history, examination of the eyes and other relevant systems, pertinent laboratory evaluation, determination of the differential diagnosis, and rapid institution of appropriate therapy. Consultation with an ophthalmologist and/or other appropriate specialists is often indicated.

CLINICAL PRESENTATION

Patients with visual loss or visual disturbance may present with a variety of symptoms. Typically, any degree of visual loss is disturbing to the patient and may lead to early evaluation; however, some patients may procrastinate and not seek medical evaluation. A thorough history can be crucial and the most efficient approach to the wide differential diagnosis of visual disturbances.

Several historic points may be particularly useful in determining the etiology of symptoms. The onset of symptoms, whether gradual or abrupt, transient or persistent, constant or waxing and waning, may be of importance. The unilateral or bilateral nature of the disturbance, and association of pain, may be valuable in the differentiation of certain disorders. Associated symptoms, including systemic symptoms (fever, weakness, rash, etc.), previous history of similar symptoms, history of trauma, and other ocular symptoms, including eye pain, redness, discharge, and so forth, should be sought when obtaining historical information from the patient.

DIFFERENTIAL DIAGNOSIS

Visual disturbance or visual loss may represent any of myriad clinical disorders. Some of the more common entities are summarized in Table 12.1. In general, any abnormality of the cornea, lens, vitreous, retina, optic nerve, optic tract, optic radiations, or occipital cortex should be considered.

EMERGENCY DEPARTMENT EVALUATION

Complete details of the ophthalmologic examination are included in Chapter 9. Specifically, when evaluating the patient with loss of vision or visual disturbance, of primary importance are visual acuity and visual field testing.

Visual acuity can be measured with a Snellen eye chart. The acuity of each eye should be tested independently, with the patient's usual visual correction, if available. For patients who normally wear corrective lenses, but which are unavailable for testing, pinhole testing can be easily performed by creating a device with paper and "pinholes" created with an 18-gauge needle. For patients unable to adequately read from the eye chart, their ability to count fingers, detect movement, and perceive light and dark should be evaluated.

Visual field testing can be useful in determining the extent of visual loss and in developing the appropriate differential diagnosis. Eyes should be tested independently. The confrontation technique may be employed, in which the examiner presents variable numbers of fingers in various visual fields, and asks the patient to count the fingers, while maintaining a forward gaze. Each quadrant should be tested for both eyes. More advanced visual field testing can be performed by an ophthalmologist.

Additionally, the examination should evaluate the external and slit-lamp appearance of the cornea and conjunctiva, and trauma, foreign bodies, hyphema, infection, corneal opacities, and other abnormalities should be ruled out. Intraocular pressure (IOP) should be measured, using a hand-held tonometer, applanation tonometry, or Schiøtz tonometer. Glaucoma is discussed in greater detail in Chapter 13.

Pupils should be evaluated, utilizing the swinging flashlight test. Pupillary response can be valuable in differentiating afferent from efferent defects. The normal response is bilateral pupillary constriction in response to bright light in either pupil.

Funduscopic examination should be performed using a

TABLE 12.1. Differential Diagnosis of Selected Causes of Visual Disturbance

Disease Process	Symptoms	Clinical Findings	Ancillary Tests	Management
Giant-cell arteritis	Painless visual loss, sudden or gradual, headache, myalgias	Optic nerve edema, temporal artery tenderness	Elevated ESR	Steroids, ophthalmic consultation
Optic neuritis	Painful visual loss, pain with EOM	APD, elevation of optic disc		Consider steroids in patients with MS; ophthalmic consultation
Uveitis	Eye pain, blurred vision, photophobia	Cells in anterior or posterior chamber, flare in aqueous humor		Topical steroids, cycloplegics, ophthalmic consultation
Central retinal artery occlusion	Sudden, painless, profound visual loss	APD, pallor of retina, cherry red fovea		Globe massage, paracentesis, acetazolamide, inhaled carbogen, ophthalmic consultation
Central retinal vein occlusion	Sudden, painless visual loss	Retinal hemorrhages, venous dilation, optic disc edema		Ophthalmic consultation
Amaurosis fugax	Monocular visual loss (transient)		Carotid and cardiac studies	ASA, neurologic consultation
Vitreous hemorrhage	Visual floaters, cobwebs, or severe visual loss	Diminished or absent red reflex ("eight ball" hemorrhage)		Treatment of underlying condition; ophthalmic consultation
Retinal detachment	Acute, painless visual disturbance; filmy, cloudy vision; peripheral monocular visual loss ("veil")	Gray/translucent detached area with folds, bulging appearance		Ophthalmic consultation
Macular degeneration	Gradual, painless disturbances; spots in visual field; distortion of straight lines	Drusen, macular pigment clumps		Ophthalmic consultation
Diabetic retinopathy	Gradual visual disturbances, scotomas	Multiple retinal hemorrhages, macular edema		Ophthalmic consultation
Ischemic optic neuropathy	Painless, diminished visual acuity	APD, pale, elevated optic disc		Ophthalmic consultation
TIA	Transient binocular visual loss	Normal	Carotid, cardiac studies	Neurologic consultation, ASA
Cortical blindness	Sudden or gradual, complete visual loss or homonymous hemianopia, HA	Papilledema, other neurologic findings	CT, MRI, LP	Neurologic consultation, therapy of underlying disorder
Migraine HA	Transient visual loss	Normal		Neurologic consultation; see Chapter 203
Glaucoma	Sudden, painful visual disturbance, ABD pain, N/V	Optic nerve pallor and cupping	Elevated IOP	Topical beta-blocker; miotic, carbonic anhydrase inhibitor; ophthalmic consultation; see Chapter 13
CMV retinitis	Sudden or gradual visual disturbance	Retinal hemorrhages, areas of pale retinal necrosis ("tomato and cheese pizza" appearance)	Consider CT/MRI	Foscarnet or ganciclovir, ophthalmic consultation
Methanol	Transient visual disturbance, N/V, HA	Hyperemic, swollen optic discs, cherry red spot		ETOH, see Chapter 351
Functional visual loss	Variable symptoms	Normal	Optokinetic nystagmus	Psychiatric consultation

This table represents only a summary of certain disorders, and is not an exhaustive information source for the above disease states.
ESR, erythrocyte sedimentation rate; EOM, external otitis media; APD, afferent pupillary defect; MS, multiple sclerosis; TIA, transient ischemic attack; CT, computed tomography; MRI, magnetic resonance imaging; LP, lumbar puncture; IOP, intraocular pressure; CMV, cytomegalovirus.

hand-held ophthalmoscope. Pupillary dilation may be required to perform an adequate examination of the retina. In particular, the optic disc, macula, and retina should be evaluated for any abnormalities.

Radiographic evaluation (including magnetic resonance imaging [MRI] or computed tomography [CT]) may be indicated in cases in which intracranial pathology or mass lesions involving the optic nerve or globe are suspected. Patients presenting with complaints related to loss of vision require a complete ophthalmologic examination, which should include measurement of visual acuity, visual field testing, tonometry, and slit-lamp examination.

EMERGENCY DEPARTMENT MANAGEMENT

Numerous disease processes can produce visual disturbance or visual loss. The most commonly encountered are discussed next. This discussion is not an exhaustive review of ophthalmologic disorders, but a summary of salient points relevant to the emergency physician.

Inflammatory Processes

Giant-cell Arteritis

Giant-cell arteritis (GCA), an inflammatory disease of medium and large arteries, typically affects patients over the age of 60, with a female predominance of 3:1. Peak incidence occurs between the ages of 70 and 80. Patients may present with malaise, headache, fever, anorexia, jaw claudication, pain over the temporal or occipital arteries, and painless visual loss secondary to ischemic optic neuropathy, or cranial nerve palsies. Diagnostic tests include an elevated erythrocyte sedimentation rate (ESR) (typically 80 to 100 mm within the first hour; elevated in 98% of documented cases) and an abnormal temporal artery biopsy. Findings and symptoms may be atypical (ESR may be normal, there may be no visual involvement, etc.) Early administration of corticosteroids (80 to 120 mg of prednisone per day, or intravenous methylprednisolone, 1 g per day) may prevent blindness and other long-term visual defects, as well as contralateral eye involvement (common within 10 days without treatment), and may provide dramatic pain relief. Patients may have a 34% chance of improvement in visual function after steroid therapy.[8] A biopsy should be performed within 7 to 10 days of steroid initiation, although a negative biopsy does not exclude GCA.[14,16]

Optic Neuritis

Optic neuritis is an inflammatory disorder from varying etiologies, including multiple sclerosis, sarcoidosis, systemic lupus erythematosus, leukemia, syphilis, collagen vascular diseases, alcohol abuse,[13] idiopathic, or other causes.[5] Most patients (65%) have pain with eye movement. Typically, there is an afferent pupillary defect, and elevation of the optic disc may be seen on funduscopic examination. Visual field defects may be noted. Although treatment with oral steroids has not been shown to be beneficial (and may even be harmful), treatment with intravenous methylprednisolone may be indicated for patients with suspected multiple sclerosis. Although steroids do not affect recovery, they have been shown to delay the onset of symptoms of multiple sclerosis. Consultation with an ophthalmologist is indicated for patients with suspected optic neuritis.[5]

Uveitis

Uveitis, inflammation of the iris, ciliary body, or choroid, may cause visual impairment. Uveitis may be caused by Reiter syndrome, ankylosing spondylitis, sarcoidosis, tuberculosis, collagen vascular disorders, and other diseases. Treatment with topical corticosteroids and cycloplegic agents is often effective. Systemic steroids may be indicated in severe cases. Therapy of the underlying disorder should be undertaken.[5,6]

Vascular Events

Central Retinal Artery Occlusion

Central retinal artery occlusion (CRAO) often presents with sudden, painless visual loss (Fig. 12.1). There may be a history of transient visual loss prior to this event. The cause is often due to emboli from carotid plaques, cardiac valves, fat emboli, arteriosclerosis, or a host of other underlying disorders, including such entities as collagen vascular disease, hypotension, sickle cell disease, and GCA. Elderly patients are more commonly affected, and men are more commonly affected than are women. Visual loss is typically profound, with 90% of patients sustaining losses that range from counting fingers to light perception. An afferent pupillary defect may be present. Physical findings include pallor of the involved retina, "cherry-red spot" of the fovea, "boxcars" of the arterioles, and opacification of the superficial retina. Branch RAO may occur and may present with sudden loss of visual field and reduction in visual acuity. The long-term prognosis is related to the duration of symptoms prior to resolution. Full vision may be restored if resolved within 1 to 2 hours.[12] Treatment is often unsatisfactory, but should be offered, and it may include intermittent globe massage in an attempt to dislodge an embolus (moderate pressure for 5 seconds and release for 5 seconds), anterior chamber paracentesis (to decrease IOP and increase retinal perfusion), intravenous acetazolamide (to decrease IOP), inhaled carbogen (oxygen–carbon dioxide mixture of 95%/5%) to induce retinal vasodilation and increase retinal pO_2.[15] Hyperbaric oxygen and nifedipine have also been reported as successful therapies.[1] Other treatment offered by an ophthalmologist may include ophthalmic artery infusion of urokinase or tissue plasminogen activator.[10]

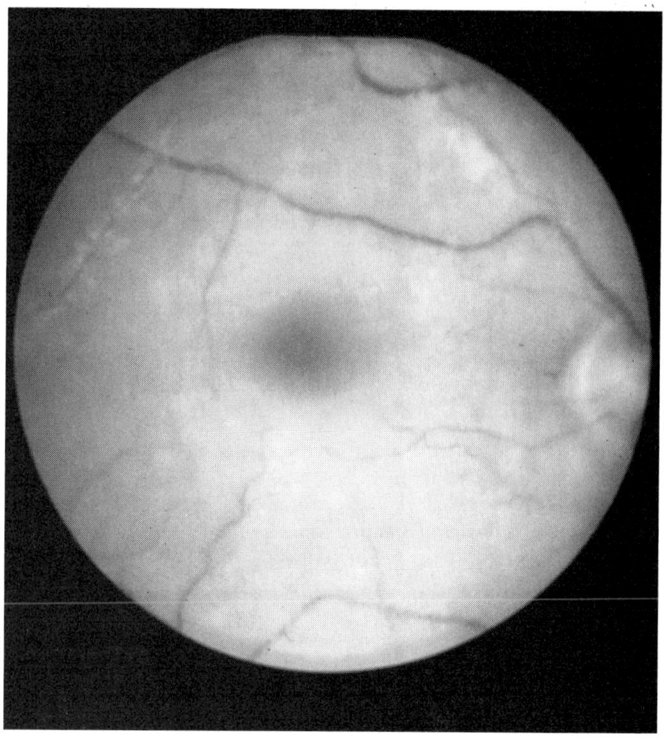

Figure 12.1. Central retinal artery occlusion.

Central Retinal Vein Occlusion

Patients with central retinal vein occlusion (CRVO) typically present with painless, sudden loss of vision. (Fig. 12.2). Most patients are over the age of 50, and many also have significant cardiovascular disease. Other associated disorders include hypertension, glaucoma, venous stasis, diabetes mellitus, and collagen vascular disorders. Physical findings may include retinal hemorrhage, which may be pronounced and diffuse, venous dilatation, cotton-wool spots, and optic disc edema. Treatment

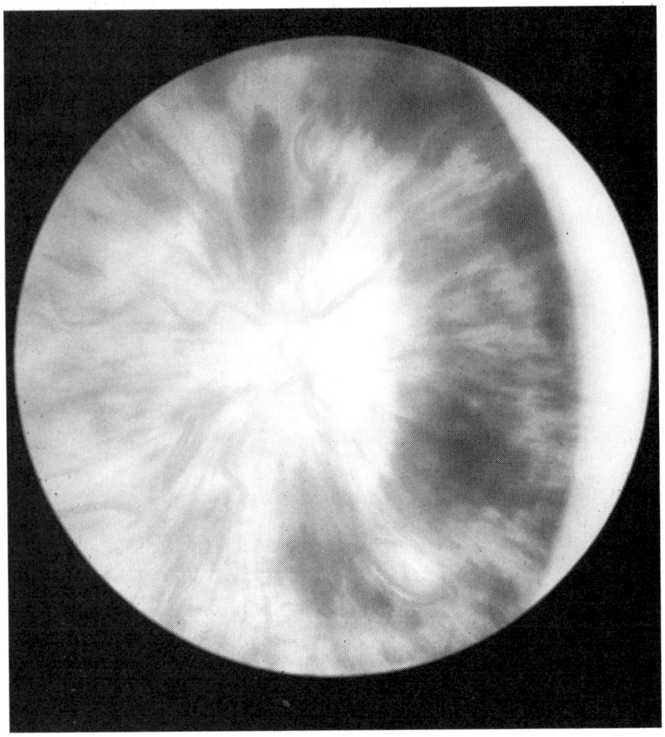

Figure 12.2. Central retinal vein occlusion.

is often unsuccessful, but should include a careful evaluation of the probable etiology in order to prevent contralateral eye involvement. Spontaneous resolution may occur in some cases. Treatment offered by an ophthalmologist may include panretinal laser photocoagulation.

Branch RVO may occur, and may have segments of intraretinal hemorrhage. Complications may include macular edema, ischemia, and neovascularization with associated vitreous hemorrhage. Laser photocoagulation has an important role in the treatment of branch RVO, which has a better prognosis.[4]

Amaurosis Fugax

Amaurosis fugax, a unilateral transient obstruction of a retinal artery, may cause temporary loss of vision (up to 15 minutes). The visual loss is often described by the patient as a curtain being drawn across the visual field. Amaurosis fugax is usually caused by cholesterol emboli or fibrin–platelet emboli, and may be associated with carotid artery disease, cardiac arrhythmias, anemia, sickle cell disease, hypertension, or episodic hypotension. Carotid and cardiac studies may be indicated to determine the source of the emboli. Treatment with aspirin should be initiated, and ophthalmologic consultation obtained.

Ischemic Optic Neuropathy

Ischemic optic neuropathy is typically found in patients over the age of 50, and often presents with painless decreased visual acuity. This disorder may result from an infarction of the optic nerve (90% of cases) or from GCA (10% of cases). An afferent pupillary defect may be found, as well as a pale, elevated optic disc.

Vitreous and Retinal Disorders

Vitreous Hemorrhage

Vitreous hemorrhage typically presents with acute unilateral painless loss of vision, and may be accompanied by symptoms of "floaters" or "cobwebs." Associated visual disturbances may be mild or severe, depending on the extent of the hemorrhage. The normal red reflex of the fundus is absent. Diffuse, dark, particulate opacities may be seen, or if severe, a black uniform reflex ("eight ball hemorrhage") will be seen instead of the normal retinal red reflex. Vitreous hemorrhage may be associated with numerous disorders, including diabetes, trauma, malignancy, CRVO, leukemia, anemia, and thrombocytopenia. Management includes ophthalmologic consultation and treatment of any underlying condition.

Diabetic Retinopathy

Diabetic retinopathy may be divided into proliferative and nonproliferative. It may occur in Type I or Type II diabetes mellitus. Nonproliferative diabetic retinopathy is a progressive microangiopathy. Symptoms may be mild or nonexistent, and may include hue discrimination abnormalities, scotomas, contrast sensitivity, or a variety of other visual complaints. Physical findings include multiple hemorrhages throughout the retina and macular edema. Proliferative retinopathy refers to ischemia as a result of microvascular occlusions, and may present with cotton-wool spots, retinal vein beading, and irregular dilation of the retinal capillary bed. Sudden visual loss may occur with massive vitreous hemorrhage from fragile neovascularization or from retinal detachment. Treatment by an ophthalmologist is indicated, and may include laser photocoagulation.

Retinal Detachment

Retinal detachment refers to a separation of the two layers of the retina: the pigment epithelium and neurosensory retina (Fig. 12.3). The most common type, rhegmatogenous, occurs as a result of tears, holes, or breaks in the sensory layer of the retina. It may be associated with advancing age, male gender, significant myopia, diabetes mellitus, sickle cell disease, or ocular contusion or penetrating injury, or it may be idiopathic. Additionally, exudative or traction types of retinal detachment may be seen. Symptoms include photopsia (light flashes), floaters, or a shower of black dots in the periphery secondary to hemorrhage

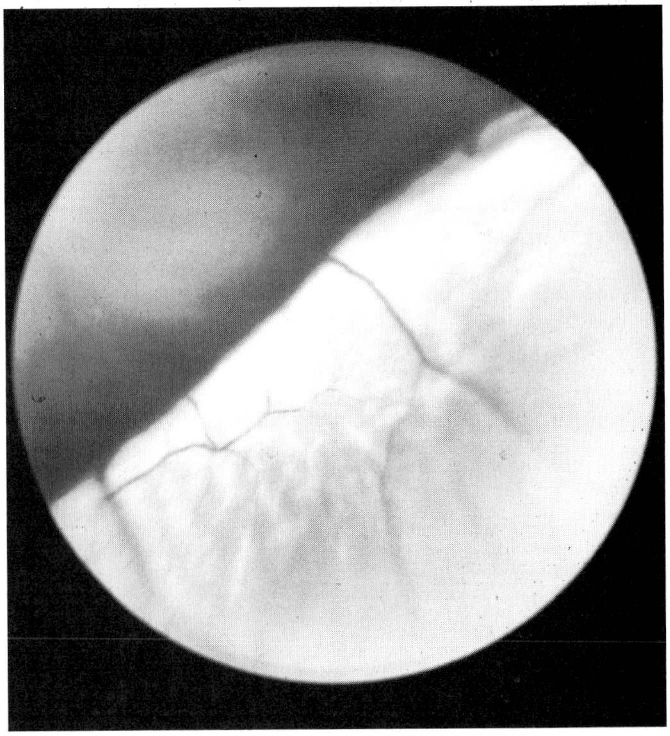

Figure 12.3. Retinal detachment.

into vitreous humor, or a sensation of a shadow or curtain obscuring the visual field. Visual acuity may be normal if the macula is unaffected, or severely impaired if involved. On examination, the detached area may appear gray, opaque, or translucent. Folds may be seen. Vessels may appear dark red. Ophthalmologic consultation is indicated, and therapy may include diathermy, laser photocoagulation, or other intraocular surgical therapies. Symptoms often resolve within 1 week.

Macular Degeneration

Macular degeneration is the most common cause of permanent blindness among older patients. The incidence is associated with advanced age, family history, tobacco history, race (Caucasian), and gender (slight female predominance). The etiology is unknown. Symptoms include blurred vision, visual distortion, scotoma, or central visual loss. Physical findings include drusen (yellow-white deposits beneath the pigment epithelium) and clumps of pigment throughout the macula. Treatment includes laser photocoagulation and the use of low-vision aids, under the care of an ophthalmologist.[2,12]

Neurologic and Structural Disorders

Cerebrovascular Accident

Cerebrovascular accidents (CVAs) and transient ischemic attacks may be associated with visual loss. A bilateral homonymous hemianopsia may result from involvement of the optic tract or occipital lobes. Involvement of both occipital lobes may produce complete blindness (cortical blindness). Treatment should be initiated in consultation with a neurologist.

Other Etiologies of Cortical Blindness

Cortical blindness may be caused by such entities as ischemia, mass lesions, hydrocephalus, anoxia, encephalitis, meningitis, edema, or hemorrhage into the occipital lobe(s).[3,11] Evaluation should be conducted promptly, and may include CT, MRI, and lumbar puncture.

Compression of the Optic Chiasm

The optic chiasm may be compressed by mass lesions such as pituitary adenomas, meningiomas, craniopharyngiomas, or aneurysms. These patients may present with bitemporal hemianopia. Treatment of the underlying disorder should be undertaken by the appropriate consultant.

Infectious Processes

Although some infectious processes cause symptoms of visual disturbance (such as blurring), most are not associated with reduction of visual acuity or loss of peripheral visual fields.

Cytomegalovirus Retinitis

Cytomegalovirus (CMV) retinitis may present with sudden or gradual visual loss when the infection invades the macula. It is seen primarily in immunocompromised patients, such as those with AIDS, or those on chemotherapy, or after organ transplantation. Findings include retinal hemorrhagic areas combined with zones of white retinal necrosis ("tomato and cheese pizza" appearance). Early treatment with intravenous antiviral therapy (foscarnet or ganciclovir) is indicated, in consultation with an ophthalmologist.[17]

Glaucoma

Patients with glaucoma may present with acute or chronic visual loss. Visual field testing may indicate a diminished perception in the nasal region. Optic nerve pallor and cupping is seen on examination. Elevated IOP (often 50 to 70 mm Hg) is typically found. Early initiation of therapy is indicated and includes a miotic (e.g., pilocarpine), topical beta-blocker (e.g., timolol), a carbonic anhydrase inhibitor (e.g., acetazolamide), mannitol or glycerin, and topical steroids. A more detailed discussion of glaucoma is found in Chapter 13.

Malignancies of the Eye

Although space does not permit a detailed study of ophthalmologic malignancies, it is prudent for the emergency physician to have an awareness of the spectrum of malignancies that may affect vision. Benign intraocular tumors may include retinal angiomas or astrocytic hamartomas. Malignant intraocular tumors include retinoblastoma (tumor of childhood, usually under age 1, presenting with leukocoria or strabismus) and malignant melanoma. Metastatic tumors may involve the eye, most often with choroidal metastasis. Patients with cancer of the breast, lung, gastrointestinal tract, melanoma, kidneys, prostate, and thyroid may have choroidal metastases.[9] Complications of intraocular malignancies that affect vision include hemorrhage from tumor vascularization, retinal detachment, retinal degeneration, and retinopathy. Abnormal physical findings should alert the physician to the importance of timely ophthalmologic follow-up.

Toxicologic Effects

Methanol Toxicity

Methanol toxicity is associated with transient visual disturbances. Symptoms and signs usually occur within 18 to 48 hours of the ingestion. Associated symptoms include nausea, vomiting, headache, or abdominal pain. Findings include hyperemic, swollen optic discs, with retinal edema. A cherry-red spot may be observed.[7] Treatment of methanol toxicity is discussed in Chapter 351.

Other Toxins

Numerous other toxins that may be associated with visual disturbances include carbon monoxide, lead, salicylates, sulfonamides, ergots, tin, quinine, barbiturates, chemotherapy, and nitroglycerin. Visual loss is usually bilateral, and therapy consists of the appropriate treatment of the underlying condition.[14]

Eye Disorders Associated with Systemic Disease

Patients with vascular disease may develop hemorrhages of various types, including preretinal, linear, punctate, subretinal, and white central hemorrhages (Roth's spots). Additionally, there may be acute ocular ischemia due to infarction of the optic disc (ischemic optic neuropathy), which presents with sudden visual loss, and a pale, swollen optic disc. It may be caused by GCA, hypertension, or arteriosclerotic disease. Other causes of ocular ischemia may include choroidal infarction, retinal infarction, and transient retinal ischemia (amaurosis fugax). Patients with AIDS may present with toxoplasmosis, candidal endophthalmitis, herpes zoster ophthalmicus, or optic neuropathy.

Many other systemic disorders are associated with abnormal ocular complaints, and include metabolic, infectious,[4] endocrine, autoimmune, granulomatous, hematologic, vascular, malignancies, connective tissue, and other disorders. Generally, the primary disorder should be treated, and ophthalmologic consultation should be obtained in a timely fashion.

Functional Visual Loss

The diagnosis of functional visual loss should always be a diagnosis of exclusion. There may be a variety of complaints, but no abnormalities are seen on examination. The swinging flashlight test, IOP, and external and funduscopic examinations are normal. Optokinetic responses may be tested in a cursory fashion in the emergency department by passing a tape measure, or sheet of paper with prominent vertical lines, rapidly before the affected eye(s). Another simple test involves placing a mirror before the patient's face and rocking the mirror from side to side. The presence of optokinetic nystagmus (following movements with rapid returns to the primary position of the eye) indicates that vision is present. Additionally, patients feigning blindness may demonstrate an inability to oppose outstretched forefingers while bringing outstretched arms together; this ability would not ordinarily be affected by blindness. Additional tests to differentiate organic from functional visual loss should be conducted by an ophthalmologist.

DISPOSITION

For the majority of patients with acute visual loss, consultation with an ophthalmologist is indicated. The severity and nature of the disease process will dictate whether emergent or urgent consultation is necessary. Patients considered for hospital admission should be those who require intravenous medications, surgery, or other invasive procedures, or for whom serious worsening of vision is imminent.

COMMON PITFALLS

- Failure to consider the diagnosis of glaucoma in atypical presentations
- Failure to measure intraocular pressure
- Failure to test visual fields adequately
- Failure to administer steroids rapidly to patients with giant cell arteritis
- Delay in treatment of central retinal artery occlusion

References

1. Alexander LJ. Age-related macular degeneration: the current understanding of the status of clinicopathology, diagnosis and management. *J Am Optom Assoc* 1993;64:822–837.
2. Beiran I, Reissman P, Scharf J, et al. Hyperbaric oxygenation combined with nifedipine treatment for recent-onset retinal artery occlusion. *Eur J Ophthalmol* 1993;3:89–94.
3. Forrester JV. Uveitis: pathogenesis. *Lancet* 1991;338:1498–1501.
4. Hoover BW, Stack LB. Acute bilateral blindness. *Acad Emerg Med* 1996;3:1056–1059.
5. Janda AM. Sudden nontraumatic visual loss. *Postgrad Med* 1992;91:111–125.
6. Keltner JL, Johnson CA, Spurr JO, et al. Visual field profile of optic neuritis. *Arch Ophthalmol* 1994;112:946–953.
7. La Vene D, Halpern J, Jagoda A. Loss of vision. *Emerg Med Clin North Am* 1995;13:539–561.
8. Liu GT, Glaser JS, Schatz NJ, et al. Visual morbidity in giant cell arteritis. *Ophthalmology* 1994;101:1779–1785.
9. McKellar MJ, Hidajat RR, Elder MJ. Acute ocular methanol toxicity: clinical and electrophysiological features. *Aust N Z J Ophthalmol* 1997;25:225–230.
10. Makino A, Soga T, Obayashi M, et al. Cortical blindness caused by acute general cerebral swelling. *Surg Neurol* 1988;29:393–400.
11. Newell FW. *Ophthalmology: principles and concepts,* 8th ed. St. Louis: Mosby–Year Book, 1996:305–308.
12. Schumacher M, Schmidt D, Wakhloo AK. Intra-arterial fibrinolytic therapy in central retinal artery occlusion. *Neuroradiology* 1993;35:600–605.
13. Shimozono M, Townsend JC, Ilsen PF, et al. Acute vision loss resulting from complications of ethanol abuse. *J Am Optom Assoc* 1998;69:293–303.
14. Varma R. *Essentials of eye care: the Johns Hopkins Wilmer handbook.* Philadelphia: Lippincott-Raven Publishers, 1997:357–380.
15. Vaughan DG, Asbury T, Riordan-Eva P. *General ophthalmology.* East Norwalk, CT: Appleton & Lange, 1995:187–188.
16. Weinberg DA, Savino PJ, Sergott RC, et al. Giant cell arteritis: corticosteroids, temporal artery biopsy, and blindness. *Arch Fam Med* 1994;3:623–627.
17. Zun LS. Acute visual loss. *Emerg Med Clin North Am* 1988;6:57–72.

CHAPTER 13
Acute Angle-Closure Glaucoma

William Bozeman

Glaucoma is a group of disorders characterized by an intraocular pressure (IOP) elevated to a degree sufficient to result in loss of vision. The clinical presentations and underlying pathologic mechanisms within this group of disorders are diverse. The two common classifications of primary glaucoma—open-angle glaucoma and angle-closure glaucoma—occur in about one of 50 Americans over age 35, and represent overall the second leading cause of blindness in the United States.[22]

Primary angle-closure glaucoma accounts for 6% of all patients with glaucoma, and occurs in 0.6% of the general population. Primary acute angle-closure glaucoma is less common among Blacks than among Whites; however, the chronic form is more common in Blacks, Eskimos, and Southeast Asians. Women are affected three times more often than are men.

There are three clinical types of primary angle-closure glaucoma. The chronic form is often subtle and difficult to diagnose, with a gradual visual loss over a prolonged period. The subacute, or intermittent, form is characterized by periodic episodes of mild pain, blurred vision, and halos. In contrast, manifestations of the acute form of angle-closure glaucoma are dramatic, with the sudden onset of unilateral ocular pain and decreased visual acuity. Without appropriate therapy, acute angle-closure glaucoma is devastating and can result in blindness within a few days. A high index of suspicion by the astute emergency physician will lead to prompt diagnosis and treatment of acute angle-closure glaucoma.

AQUEOUS HUMOR DYNAMICS AND THE ANTERIOR CHAMBER ANGLE

Aqueous humor is produced by the ciliary body. In the normal eye, the aqueous humor first fills the posterior chamber and then passes between the posterior surface of the iris and the lens to enter the anterior chamber (Fig. 13.1). The iris touches the lens only at the pupillary margin.[2] Once the aqueous humor circulates within the anterior chamber, it leaves through the trabecular meshwork of the anterior chamber angle and enters Schlemm's canal (Fig. 13.2). The aqueous then passes from Schlemm's canal to episcleral vessels by way of collector channels in the sclera (Fig. 13.3). The level of IOP at any time represents a balance between the rate of formation of aqueous humor

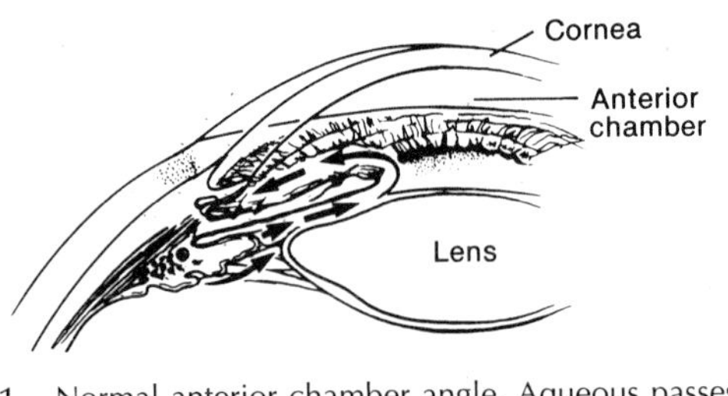

Figure 13.1. Normal anterior chamber angle. Aqueous passes from the posterior chamber through the pupil into the anterior chamber and out through the trabecular meshwork.

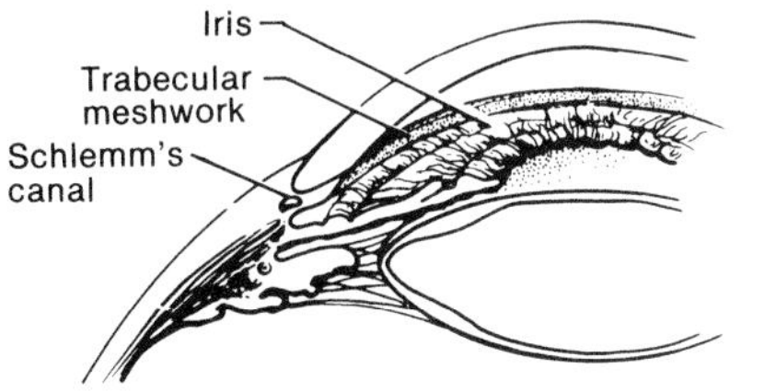

Figure 13.2. Normal appearance of anterior chamber angle.

and the resistance to outflow from the anterior chamber. In glaucoma, the elevated IOP is due to an obstruction to outflow from the anterior chamber, rather than to higher-than-normal rates of aqueous production.

Obstruction to outflow from the anterior chamber occurs in both open-angle and angle-closure glaucoma. The location and mechanism of the resistance to outflow distinguish these two conditions. In open-angle glaucoma, the angle is open, and the aqueous has access to the trabecular meshwork to exit the anterior chamber. Although the exact nature of the resistance to outflow is not completely understood, the obstruction to outflow is located in the tissue between the trabecular meshwork and Schlemm's canal. In angle-closure glaucoma, the peripheral iris touches the trabecular meshwork and blocks the flow of aqueous to the trabecular meshwork. This apposition between the iris and the trabecular meshwork may be temporary or may become permanent if pathologic adhesions develop. These adhesions, known as peripheral anterior synechiae, can occur in eyes with narrow angles, inflammation, fibrovascular proliferation, and previous surgical intervention (Fig. 13.4).

Predisposition and Pathophysiology

Several anatomic features predispose an eye to angle-closure glaucoma. A shallow anterior chamber, which results in excessive narrowing of the entrance to the angle, can be occluded more easily than an anterior chamber of normal depth. In a shallow anterior chamber, the area of lens–iris contact is greater than normal. This lens-to-iris apposition impedes the flow of aqueous from the posterior chamber to the anterior chamber through the pupil. A pressure differential results between the posterior and anterior chambers, with a slightly higher pressure in the posterior chamber. This condition, known as relative pupillary block, produces a forward bowing of the peripheral iris and results in contact between the iris and the trabecular meshwork, thereby closing the angle (Fig. 13.5).

Eyes prone to develop greater-than-usual degrees of pupillary block are at risk to develop angle-closure glaucoma. Hyperopic (farsighted) eyes are smaller than average (shorter anterior-to-posterior length). These eyes have greater iris-to-lens contact and an increased risk for angle-closure glaucoma. In

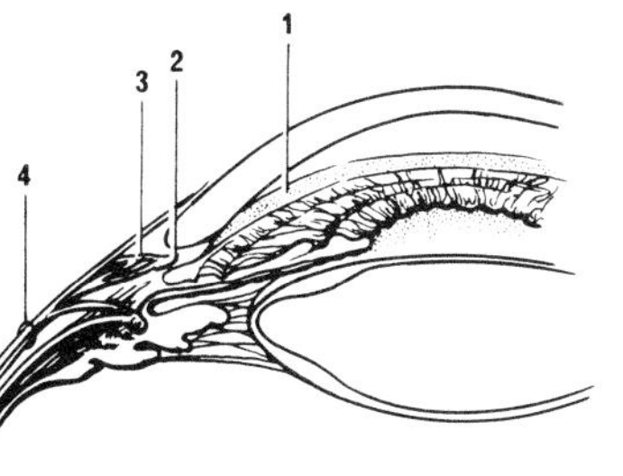

Figure 13.3. Pathway of aqueous out of the anterior chamber is through *(1)* the trabecular meshwork, *(2)* Schlemm's canal, and by way of *(3)* collector channels to *(4)* the episcleral vessels.

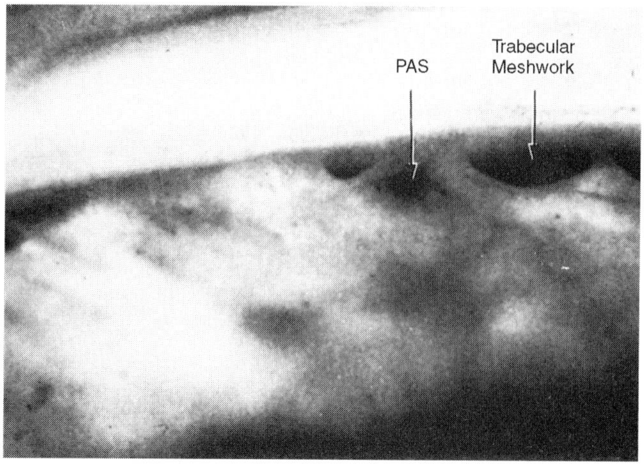

Figure 13.4. Peripheral anterior synechiae *(PAS)*. These abnormal adhesions of the iris to the trabecular meshwork are seen in angle-closure glaucoma.

addition, the lens size and position are major factors in the degree of relative pupillary block. For example, the development of a cataract may thicken the lens and increase the contact of the posterior surface of the iris to the lens, resulting in an increase in pupillary block. These anatomic relations—the size of the eye and the position of the lens—predispose to angle closure. The actual event that triggers an attack of acute angle closure is often identified as a pharmacologic or physiologic event that alters the balance between the aqueous humor dynamics and the pathologic anatomic relations.

In predisposed eyes, pupillary dilatation is the most significant event that can precipitate an acute angle-closure attack. During dilatation, the peripheral iris becomes more flaccid and may be pushed against the trabecular meshwork, closing the angle. There is usually sudden and complete blockage to aqueous outflow. When the pupil is middilated, 5 to 7 mm, both relative pupillary block and peripheral laxness of the iris are greatest.[15] If the pupil continues to dilate beyond the midposition, the peripheral chamber angle deepens as pupillary block is reduced. Such a widely dilated pupil may be at risk to develop angle closure if it assumes the precarious middilated position during constriction.

Pupillary dilatation may occur in response to pharmacologic agents or physiologic situations, such as low illumination, stress, and fatigue.[9,20] Two general classifications of topical and systemic medications most often implicated in precipitating acute angle-closure glaucoma are the parasympatholytics and the sympathomimetics. Parasympatholytics, such as atropine, and sympathomimetics, such as 10% phenylephrine, as well as many over-the-counter medications with anticholinergic or sympathomimetic activity, can produce pupillary dilatation and precipitate angle closure (Table 13.1).[5,11,18] Although uncommon, a third class of medications that can induce angle closure comprises the topical parasympathomimetics, such as pilocarpine. Often used to treat angle closure, topical parasympath-

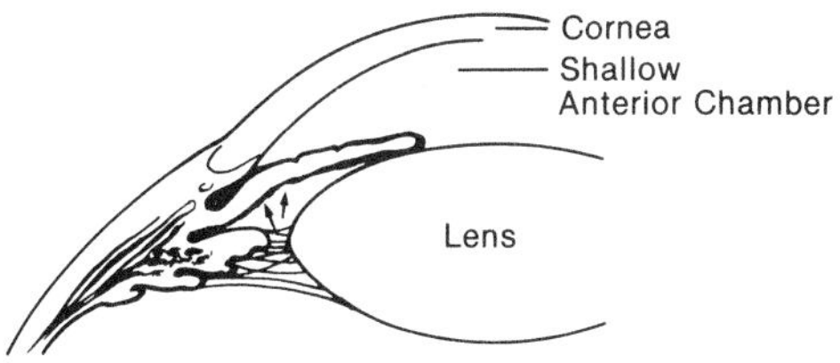

Figure 13.5. Angle closure with pupillary block. The angle is closed as the iris is pushed up against the trabecular meshwork.

TABLE 13.1. Commonly Used Pharmacologic Preparations That Can Precipitate Angle Closure

Nonproprietary Name	Trade Name
DIRECT OR INDIRECT SYMPATHOMIMETIC ACTIVITY	
Prescription Sympathomimetics	
Epinephrine compounds	
Epinephrine bitartrate	Primatene Mist, Bronkaid
Epinephrine hydrochloride	Epifrin (ophthalmic solution
Epinephrine borate	Epinal (ophthalmic solution)
Norepinephrine	
Levarterenol	
Norepinephrine bitartrate	Levophed-bitartrate
Terbutaline	Brethaire, Brethine
Amphetamine compounds	
Dextroamphetamine sulfate	Dexedrine, Obetrol
Hydroxyamphetamine	Paredrine (ophthalmic solution)
Nonprescription Sympathomimetics	
Propylhexedrine	Benzedrex (nasal inhaler)
Naphazoline hydrochloride	Privine (nasal inhaler)
Tetrahydrozoline hydrochloride	Visine (ophthalmic solution)
	Tyzine (nasal inhaler)
Oxymetazoline hydrochloride	Afrin
Pseudoephedrine hydrochloride	Actifed, Sudafed, Afrinol
Monoamine Oxidase Inhibitors	
Tranylcypromine sulfate	Parnate
Phenelzine sulfate	Nardil
Isocarboxazid	Marplan
DIRECT OR INDIRECT ANTICHOLINERGIC ACTIVITY	
Mydriatic and Cycloplegic Agents	
Atropine sulfate	
Scopolamine hydrobromide	
Homatropine hydrobromide	
Cyclopentolate hydrochloride	
Tropicamide	
Antispasmodics	
Dicyclomine hydrochloride	Bentyl
Oxyphencyclimine hydrochloride	Daricon
DIRECT OR INDIRECT ANTICHOLINERGIC ACTIVITY *(contd.)*	
Antipsychotics	
Chlorpromazine hydrochloride	Thorazine
Thioridazine hydrochloride	Mellaril
Trifluoperazine hydrochloride	Stelazine
Haloperidol	Haldol
Phenothiazines Used in the Treatment of Nausea and Vomiting	
Chlorpromazine	Thorazine
Perphenazine	Trilafon
Prochlorperazine	Compazine
Promethazine	Phenergan
Antihistamines Used in Hypersensitivity Reactions and Motion Sickness	
Ethanolamines	
Diphenhydramine hydrochloride	Benadryl
Dimenhydrinate	Dramamine
Alkylamines	
Chlorpheniramine maleate	Chlor-Trimeton, Dristan, Sine-Off
Brompheniramine maleate	Dimetane
Piperazines	
Hydroxyzine hydrochloride	Atarax
Hydroxyzine pamoate	Vistaril
Meclizine hydrochloride	Antivert
Tricyclic Antidepressants	
Tertiary amines	
Imipramine	Tofranil
Amitriptyline	Elavil, Limbatrol, Triavil
Doxepin	Adapin, Sinequan
Secondary amines	
Nortriptyline	Pamelor
Protriptyline	Vivactil
Desipramine	Norpramin, Pertofrane
Miscellaneous Drugs for Parkinsonism	
Trihexyphenidyl hydrochloride	Artane
Benztropine mesylate	Cogentin
Ethopropazine hydrochloride	Parsidol

omimetics that produce miosis can, in some eyes, aggravate relative pupillary block by increasing the area of surface contact between the iris and the lens. However, in general, miotics tend to make the peripheral iris more taut and decrease the forward bowing into the peripheral angle.

CLINICAL PRESENTATION

Symptoms

In acute angle-closure glaucoma, outflow of aqueous is suddenly and completely halted. This cessation is associated with a marked elevation of IOP, which can occur within 30 to 60 minutes.[17] This acute pressure rise with distention of the ocular coats causes a sudden onset of severe pain that may be either localized to the eye, orbit, or brow, or generalized, as a severe headache. Vagal stimulation with the onset of sudden, severe pain often results in nausea and vomiting. On occasion, the gastrointestinal distress dominates the presenting clinical picture, leading to an erroneous diagnosis of a gastrointestinal illness or an acute surgical abdomen. Blurring vision or the onset of rainbow-colored halos may occur simultaneously or shortly after the onset of pain (Table 13.2).

TABLE 13.2. Diagnosis of Acute Angle-Closure Glaucoma

HISTORY
Acute onset of pain
Exposure to dim illumination (i.e., movie theater)
Emotional upset or fatigue
Precipitating medications (anticholinergics, sympathomimetics)
SYMPTOMS
Pain
Blurred vision/halos around lights
Loss of vision
Nausea
Vomiting
SIGNS
Conjunctival injection
Corneal edema (light reflex irregular or steamy appearance)
Middilated, nonreactive pupil
Evidence of a narrow angle (fellow eye should also appear narrow)
Anterior chamber cells—no keratic precipitates

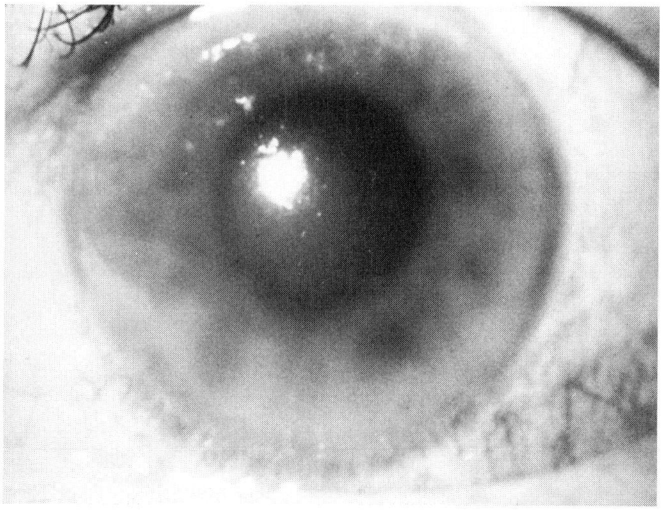

Figure 13.6. This eye demonstrates the hallmarks of acute angle-closure glaucoma: perilimbal injection, corneal edema, and a middilated nonreactive pupil.

Clinical Signs and Clinical Course

On presentation, the patient with acute angle-closure glaucoma has a unilateral red eye with congested episcleral and conjunctival blood vessels, nonreactive middilated pupil, corneal edema, shallow anterior chamber, and high IOP (Fig. 13.6). Although mild anterior chamber inflammation is common, keratic precipitates (aggregates of white blood cells) on the corneal endothelium are not a typical finding.

The IOP is usually high, 60 to 90 mm Hg (less than 21 mm Hg is considered normal). However, if the attack has been prolonged, and the ciliary body becomes ischemic and aqueous production is reduced, the IOP may be low. The anterior chamber appearance is shallow. Corneal involvement varies with the duration of the attack. The cornea is usually hazy or steamy-appearing with epithelial edema. Diffuse stromal edema ensues after prolonged exposure to elevated IOP.

The untreated course of acute angle-closure glaucoma is varied. An attack damages the corneal endothelium, the lens, the retinal ganglion cell layer, and the optic nerve. The amount of damage depends more on the duration of an attack than on the degree of pressure elevation.[3] The lens may develop *glaukomflecken* (tiny, white focal opacities beneath the lens capsule) as a result of lenticular ischemia. A generalized cataract may occur months to years after the attack. Optic nerve damage is often generalized.[10] In some patients, the attack will continue and, if untreated, will result in pain and permanent blindness within 2 to 3 days. Visual prognosis improves with the initiation of prompt, effective treatment.[6]

DIFFERENTIAL DIAGNOSIS

The differential diagnosis of the acutely painful red eye includes corneal disease such as keratitis, ulcer, erosion, foreign body, and keratoconjunctivitis (Table 13.3). Causes not related to the corneal surface include acute iritis or anterior uveitis, acute angle-closure glaucoma, episcleritis, scleritis, orbital cellulitis, periorbital cellulitis, and septic cavernous sinus thrombosis. Most conditions are readily distinguished by a careful history and examination. Other ophthalmic disorders that more closely mimic acute angle-closure glaucoma are glaucomatocyclitic crisis, neovascular glaucoma, glaucoma secondary to iritis or uveitis, and the lens-induced glaucomas (Fig. 13.7).

Glaucomatocyclitic Crisis

The chief complaint in glaucomatocyclitic crisis is recurrent attacks of visual blurring and halos. IOP is elevated and the conjunctiva moderately injected. In contrast to acute angle-closure glaucoma, pain is an occasional complaint but not a prominent feature. Additionally, the anterior chamber is deep, few cells are present in the anterior chamber, and keratic precipitates are on the corneal endothelium.

TABLE 13.3. Differential Diagnosis of Acute Angle-Closure Glaucoma

	Conjunctivitis	Keratitis	Iritis	Acute Angle-Closure
Vision	Normal	Normal/blurred	Normal/blurred	Marked decrease in vision
Pain	None or minor; "irritated"	Moderate to severe; "sharp, irritated"	Moderate to severe; "ache, worse in light"	Severe/associated with nausea and vomiting
Discharge	Tearing	Tearing Purulent if infected	None	None to tearing
Conjunctiva	Diffuse injection	Perilimbal to diffuse injection	Diffuse injection	Prominent perilimbal vessel dilation associated with diffuse injection
Pupil	Size: normal Reaction to light: normal	Normal Normal	Constricted Minimal reaction	Middilated Minimal or no reaction
Cornea	Clear or fine punctate erosions; slight haze	Minimal to moderate punctate erosions; hazy to opacification	Minimal to severe hazy to steamy	Minimal to severe hazy to steamy
Intraocular Pressure	Normal	Normal	Low to elevated	Elevated If prolonged attack, may be low
Anterior Chamber	Normal depth No cells	Normal depth Minimal cells	Normal depth (can be shallow) Moderate-to-severe cell/KP present	Shallow (both eyes are shallow) Minimal-to-moderate cell No KP present

KP, keratic precipitates.

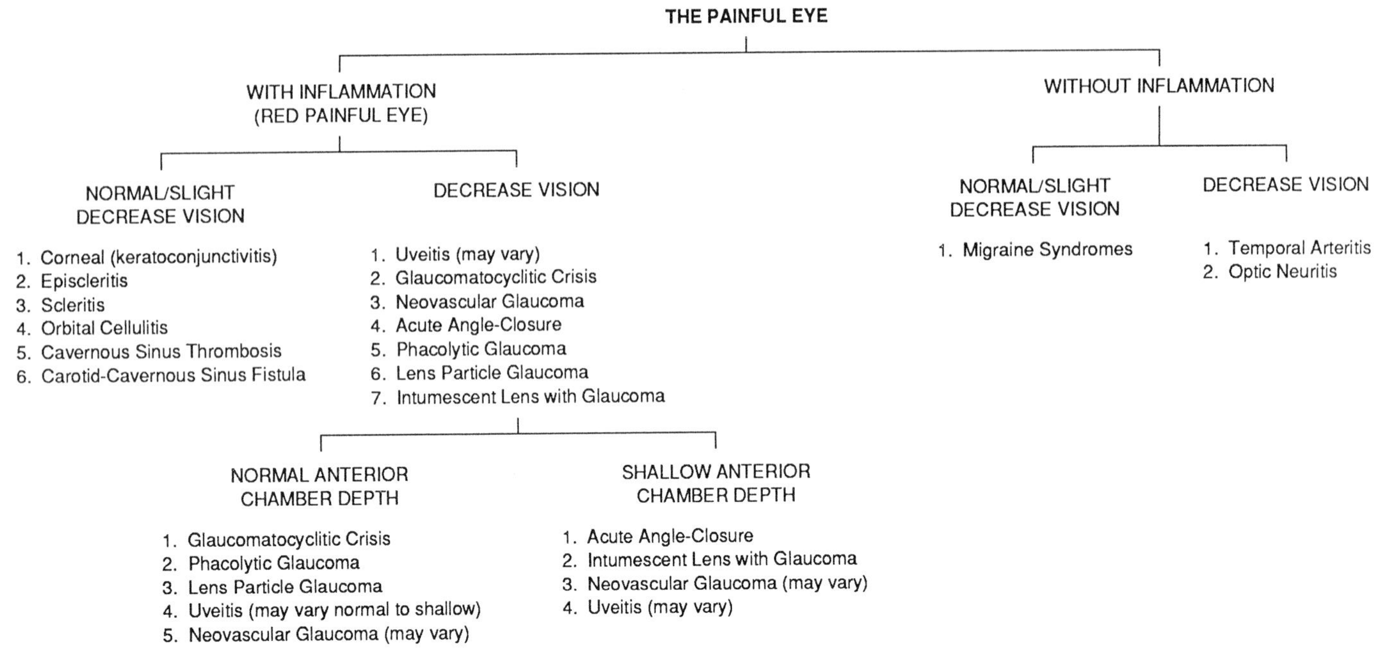

Figure 13.7. Differential diagnosis of the painful eye.

Neovascular Glaucoma

Patients with neovascular glaucoma often present with a chief complaint of a painful red eye that has had severe loss of vision months before inflammation of the eye occurred. Clinical findings include high IOP, corneal edema, anterior chamber inflammation, and usually a normal-depth anterior chamber.

Neovascular glaucoma is usually secondary to one of several retinal disorders, and occasionally is associated with other ocular or extraocular conditions. The two most common associations are proliferative retinopathy of diabetes mellitus and retinal vascular occlusion. The underlying stimulus for neovascularization is hypoxia. The neovascularization of the iris, known as rubeosis iridis, can be seen on slit-lamp biomicroscopy as randomly oriented vessels on the surface of the iris.[23] These vessels typically progress to the anterior chamber angle, where a fibrovascular membrane covers the trabecular meshwork, preventing outflow of aqueous.[21] In the early stage of neovascularization, the anterior chamber depth is normal. Only actual examination of the angle structures by gonioscopy, a technique using the slit lamp and a mirror to view the angle, would reveal the vascular membrane. If the neovascularization is progressive, a secondary form of angle closure develops as the fibrovascular membrane contracts, pulling the iris to the trabecular meshwork, which leads to the development of peripheral anterior synechiae. Anterior chamber depth is often normal, but it can be shallow in the periphery.

To distinguish neovascular glaucoma from acute angle-closure glaucoma, a history of diabetes mellitus or previous severe loss of vision before the acute attack is helpful. Also, the pupil is often miotic, and tufts of neovascular vessels may be evident.

Acute Iritis

The clinical presentation of acute iritis with secondary glaucoma is typically mild-to-moderate pain, photophobia, and blurred vision. The onset is gradual, in contrast to acute angle-closure glaucoma. Clinical findings may mimic angle closure, with conjunctival perilimbal injection (the conjunctiva adjacent to the cornea) and corneal edema. Distinguishing characteristics include miotic pupil, keratic precipitates, and a normal anterior chamber depth (Fig. 13.8).

Phacolytic Glaucoma

The typical patient with phacolytic glaucoma presents with the acute onset of a unilateral painful red eye. Similar to angle-closure glaucoma, the examination reveals a high IOP and conjunctival injection. The cornea may be either edematous or clear at the time of presentation. In contrast to acute angle-closure glaucoma, the anterior chamber depth appears normal, there is moderate-to-marked anterior chamber cell reaction, keratic precipitates are present, and a mature or hypermature (liquid cortex) cataract can be seen (Fig. 13.9). The cause of phacolytic glaucoma is the release of soluble lens protein into the aqueous, which leads to elevated IOP. With the availability of modern

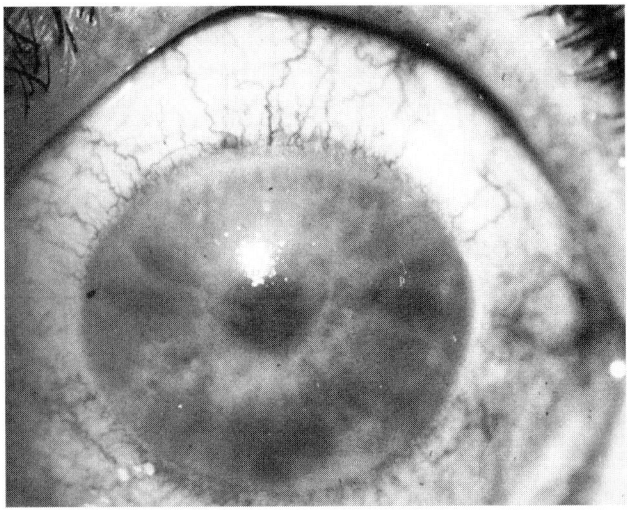

Figure 13.8. Acute iritis. This eye demonstrates the perilimbal injection and corneal edema that is common to both acute iritis and acute angle-closure glaucoma. The constricted miotic pupil seen here is characteristic of acute iritis.

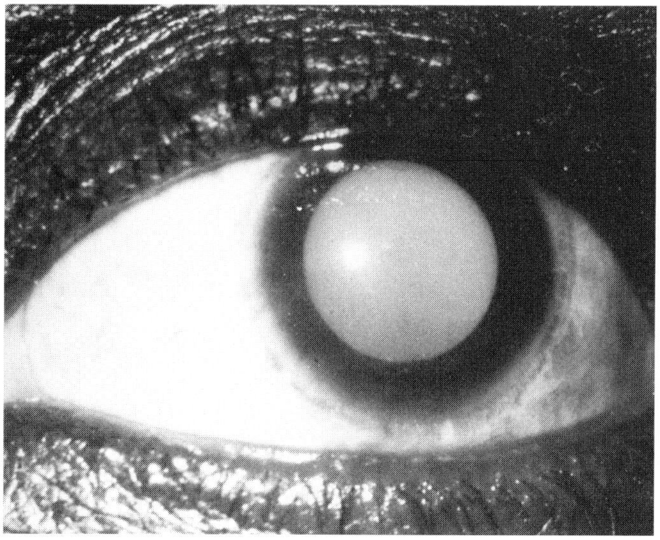

Figure 13.9. Phacolytic glaucoma. This eye demonstrates the milky-white lens of a hypermature cataract.

cataract surgery, phacolytic glaucoma is a rare cause of acutely elevated IOP.

Lens Particle Glaucoma

Lens particle glaucoma is associated with either spontaneous or traumatic disruption of the lens capsule. The presentation in the setting of spontaneous disruption is the acute onset of a unilateral painful red eye. In the case of trauma, either surgical or accidental, the onset is soon after the inciting event. The IOP is elevated, the conjunctiva injected. In contrast to angle-closure glaucoma, the anterior chamber is of normal depth, the pupil is often miotic, and lens cortical material is present in the anterior chamber (Fig. 13.10). The particulate lens material reduces outflow in the trabecular meshwork, with resultant increased IOP.[4]

Intumescent Lens

Characterized by a gradual, painless loss of vision in the involved eye over many years, intumescent lens is associated with the development of an advanced cataract. The patient presents to an emergency department when secondary angle closure occurs as the cataract changes configuration by absorbing water and swelling. Similar to acute angle-closure glaucoma, the anterior chamber depth is shallow, the IOP is elevated, and the eye is painful. In contrast to acute angle-closure glaucoma, the intumescent (swollen, mature) lens is readily evident (Fig. 13.11).[16] This is a rare cause of secondary angle closure.

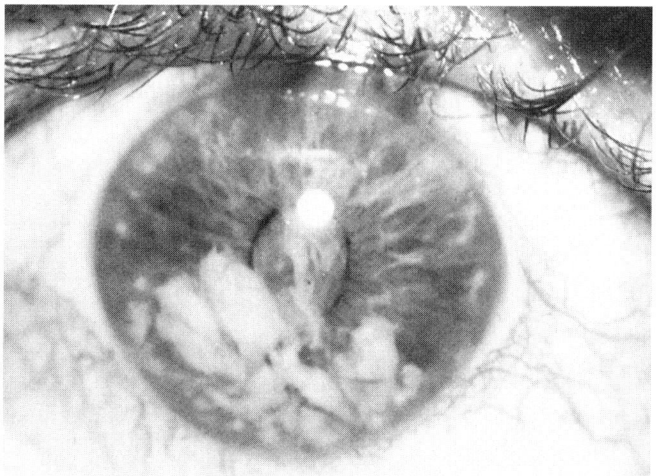

Figure 13.10. Lens particle glaucoma. The fluffy white material seen here in the anterior chamber is lens cortex. This eye had a spontaneous rupture of the lens capsule in a mature cataract.

EMERGENCY DEPARTMENT EVALUATION

History

A careful history is an essential part of the emergency department evaluation of acute angle-closure glaucoma, to establish the diagnosis and plan appropriate therapy. Question the patient about the following factors:

Onset of symptoms (sudden, gradual, subsequent to accidental or surgical trauma)
Previous symptoms similar to those of the current complaint (brief episodes of pain, blurred vision, and halos around lights)
Visual acuity in the affected eye as well as in the fellow eye
Pain in or about the eye
Discharge or secretions from the eye (tearing is common with ocular pain; however, a purulent discharge may indicate an infectious cause)
Medical history of asthma or congestive heart failure and history of drug allergies (particularly sulfa drugs).

Physical Examination

Visual Acuity

Visual acuity is probably one of the most important evaluations done during the ocular examination. If a distance or near visual acuity cannot be recorded due to inability to read the chart, the following should be recorded, including the distance at which each is tested: finger counting, hand motions, light perception, or no light perception. As is often the case in evaluating an acutely painful red eye, severe lacrimation or blepharospasm may prevent the examiner from testing visual acuity. These problems can be temporarily relieved in some cases with a topical anesthetic such as proparacaine hydrochloride or tetracaine hydrochloride.

Lids and Adnexa

The lids and adnexa are first observed. Edema and erythema of the lids are common to most of the conditions that present with

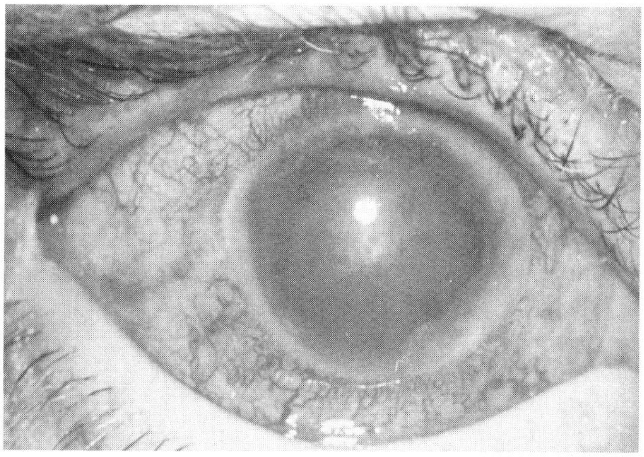

Figure 13.11. Intumescent lens. The large opaque cataract is associated with an acute-onset glaucoma.

a painful red eye. Some clues to diagnosis may include the following:

1. An enlarged preauricular node in the setting of viral conjunctivitis
2. Localized swelling in the lid that is painful, as in a hordeolum (stye)
3. Lid edema and erythema in association with fever, indicating periorbital or orbital cellulitis (history of paranasal sinus infection or previous trauma)
4. Proptosis associated with lid edema and erythema, indicating orbital cellulitis (check for fever) or cavernous sinus thrombosis (check for cranial nerve involvement)
5. Decreased visual acuity associated with lid edema and erythema (consider acute angle-closure glaucoma, neovascular glaucoma, and lens-induced glaucoma).

Conjunctiva

The conjunctiva is often nonspecifically injected; however, observation of the pattern of injection may be of some assistance. Perilimbal injection may indicate acute iritis or angle closure. Segmental injection characterizes episcleritis, and diffuse injection more commonly typifies keratoconjunctivitis. The presence of purulent discharge should alert the physician to a possible infectious cause (Fig. 13.12).

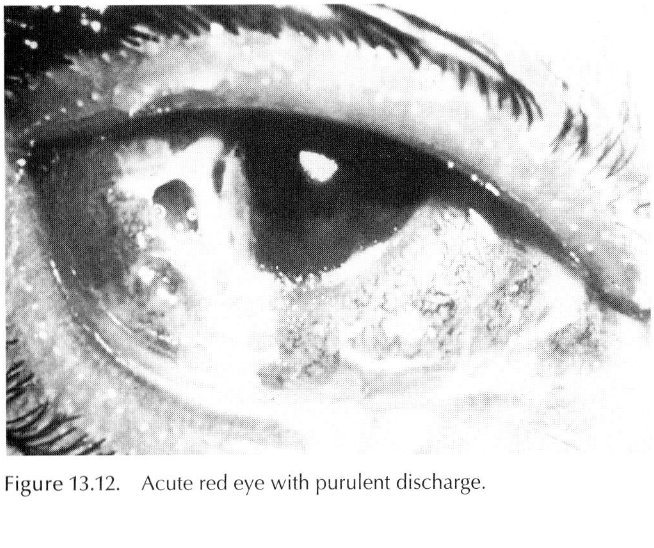

Figure 13.12. Acute red eye with purulent discharge.

Cornea

A slit-lamp examination, using a small quantity of fluorescein, helps identify corneal disease such as keratitis, ulcer, erosion, or foreign body as a possible cause of the painful red eye. Corneal edema, either epithelial (hazy) or diffuse stromal (steamy), should be noted. The rapid elevation of IOP is often associated with corneal decompensation.

Anterior Chamber

Assessment of the anterior chamber depth is essential in the evaluation of the painful red eye and the diagnosis of acute angle-closure glaucoma. An accurate determination can be done with gonioscopy, a technique performed by an ophthalmologist. In the emergency department, an adequate estimation of the anterior chamber depth can be accomplished with an oblique flashlight and a slit-lamp examination.

Oblique Flashlight Test. To perform the oblique flashlight test (Fig. 13.13), a penlight is directed to the temporal side of each eye, perpendicular to the corneal limbus. The examiner shines the light across the eye from the temporal side. In an eye with a normal-depth anterior chamber, the entire iris is illuminated. In an eye with a narrow angle or shallow anterior chamber depth, a shadow is cast on the nasal side of the iris.[22]

A

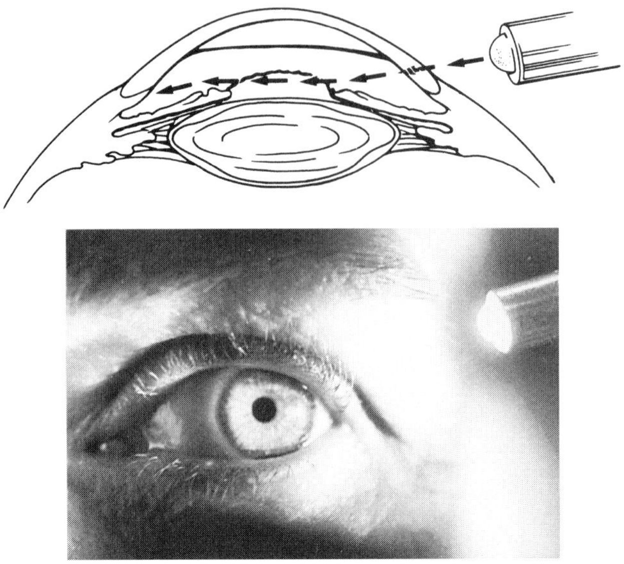

B

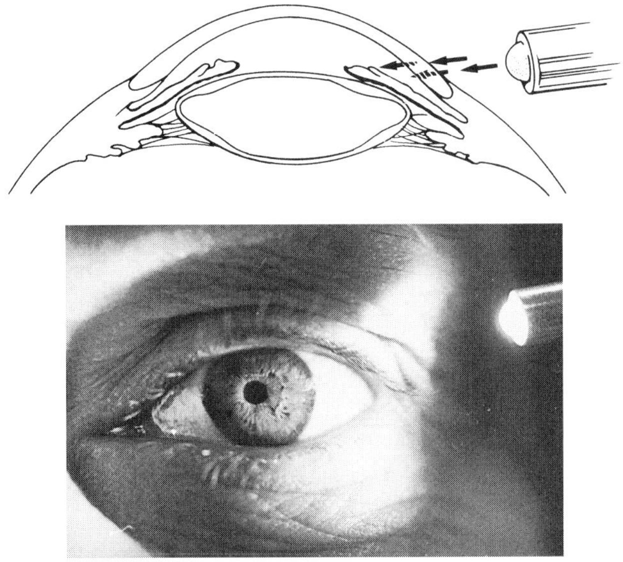

Figure 13.13. Flashlight test for wide and narrow angles. **(A)** Wide angle: Entire iris is illuminated. **(B)** Narrow angle: Only temporal half of iris is illuminated. (Photo courtesy of D.R. Anderson, M.D.)

Slit-Lamp Examination. The central and peripheral anterior chamber depth can be estimated during the slit-lamp examination. Van Herick and associates developed a technique for making this estimate. A narrow slit beam of light is directed obliquely to allow an estimate of corneal thickness and of the distance between the corneal beam to the beam on the surface of the iris. The anterior chamber depth is measured and expressed in terms of corneal thickness (Fig. 13.14). When the depth is less than one-fourth of the corneal thickness, the anterior chamber angle is extremely narrow. If the angle is closed, the iris will be seen in contact with the cornea. Both the affected and the nonaffected eye are evaluated. The fellow eye in acute angle-closure glaucoma may vary slightly but will have similar anatomic relations and appear narrow. If a unilateral shallow chamber is detected, the diagnosis of acute angle-closure glaucoma is doubtful.

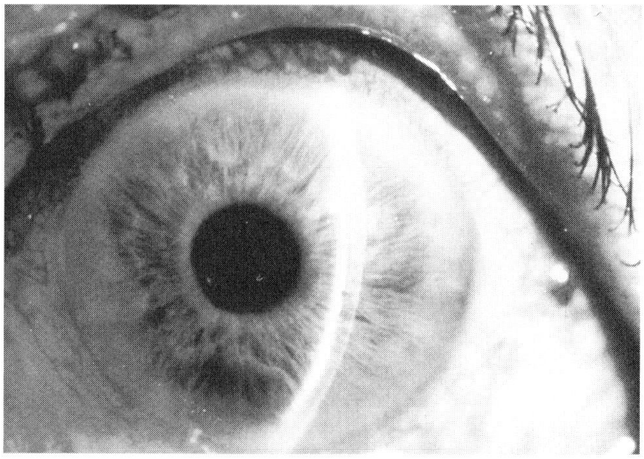

Figure 13.14. Shallow anterior chamber estimation using narrow slit beam on slit-lamp examination.

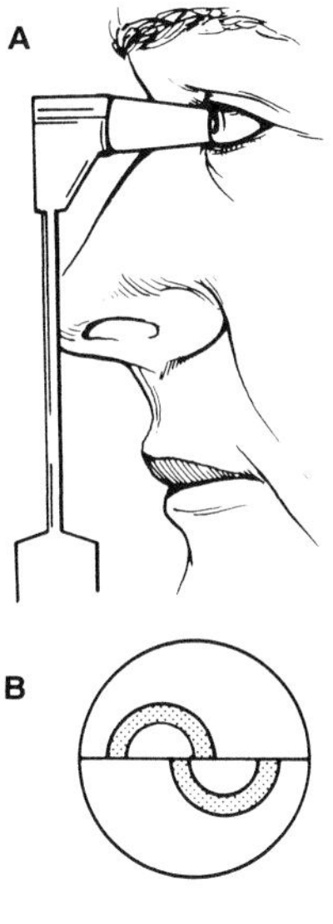

Figure 13.15. Applanation tonometry. (A) The tonometer tip should just contact the patient's cornea. (B) Viewed through the slit lamp are two fluorescent semicircles aligned edge to edge.

Pupils

The size and shape of the pupil and its reaction to light are recorded for each eye. Unequal pupil size (anisocoria) is noted, specifically with respect to the involved, red, painful eye (see Table 13.2). A middilated nonreactive pupil is characteristic of acute angle-closure glaucoma. In contrast, the pupil in acute iritis is miotic (constricted) and poorly reactive (see Fig. 13.8).

Lens

A mature (opaque) or hypermature (liquid cortex) lens may be associated with lens-induced glaucoma (see Figs. 13.9–13.11). Phacodonesis, movement of the lens, indicates a dislocated or subluxed lens. This may occur secondary to trauma,[7] or it may be part of a systemic syndrome, most notably Marfan syndrome. The dislocated lens may increase pupillary block and result in a secondary angle-closure glaucoma.

Intraocular Pressure

The range of IOP considered normal is from about 10 to 21 mm Hg (mean, 16 ± 2.5 mm Hg).[20] Three commonly used tonometers available in the emergency department are the air-puff noncontact tonometer, the Schiøtz tonometer, and the applanation tonometer.

Air-Puff Noncontact Tonometer. The air-puff tonometer measures the IOP without the application of topical anesthesia and without contact between the instrument and the eye. A 3-millisecond puff of air is blown against the cornea. The pressure is calculated by the amount of corneal flattening. This tonometer is not as accurate as the Schiøtz or applanation tonometer, but it has the advantage of use without contact with the eye.

Schiøtz Tonometry. Schiøtz, or indentation, tonometry determines IOP by measuring the indentation of the cornea produced by a known weight. Each instrument is accompanied by a graph that expresses the scale readings in millimeters of mercury. To perform Schiøtz tonometry, the patient is placed in a supine position and a drop of a local anesthetic, such as proparacaine hydrochloride or tetracaine hydrochloride, is instilled. The patient is asked to look upward and fix on some object in the distance. While separating the lids, the instrument is gently placed in a vertical position directly over the cornea, and the plunger is allowed to rest completely on the eye. With the instrument held steady, the pointer will stay fixed at a value on the scale. Readings between 3 and 6 with a 5.5-g weight will be accurate. Readings below 3 are inaccurate, and a 7.5-g weight should be added. Falsely elevated IOPs are associated with excessive lid squeezing or inadvertent pressure on the globe. Falsely low IOPs are associated with high myopia (nearsightedness), thyroid disease, and previous ocular surgery.

Applanation Tonometry. The applanation tonometer is usually mounted on a slit-lamp biomicroscope, but it can be hand-held. In applanation tonometry, the cornea is flattened, and the IOP determined by measuring the applanating force and the area flattened. To perform applanation tonometry, a local anesthetic and fluorescein are instilled into the lower cul-de-sac. Correctly positioned at the slit lamp, with the chin in the chin rest and the forehead firmly against the headband, the patient is asked to look straight ahead. Using the cobalt blue light, the examiner gently contacts the anterior corneal surface with the tonometer tip (Fig. 13.15). On contact, two fluorescein semicircles are seen. The semicircles should be aligned by turning the calibrated dial until the inner border of each semicircle just touches. This reading is multiplied by 10 and is the measurement of the IOP in millimeters of mercury.

Laboratory Studies

Due to vagal stimulation with the sudden increase in IOP, patients with acute angle-closure glaucoma frequently present with nausea and vomiting. The duration and severity of these symptoms may necessitate obtaining appropriate studies to assess metabolic imbalance and dehydration. In elderly patients on multiple medications, including diuretics, serum electrolyte levels should be measured before initiating medical treatment with carbonic anhydrase inhibitors or hyperosmotics.

EMERGENCY DEPARTMENT MANAGEMENT

Acute angle-closure glaucoma is an ophthalmic emergency. Once the diagnosis has been established in the emergency department, the immediate goal is twofold: to obtain appropriate consultation with an ophthalmologist and to decrease the elevated IOP. If examination by a ophthalmologist is imminent, therapy should be delayed. However, if prompt consultation is unavailable, therapy to decrease IOP should be initiated.

Therapy to reduce IOP is directed at decreasing aqueous production, increasing aqueous outflow, and reducing vitreous volume by dehydrating agents. A combination of topical agents and systemic medications directed toward these three goals is often effective in reducing IOP. The therapeutic options used in the medical management of acute angle-closure glaucoma are discussed next. The exact therapy used should be tailored to each patient's medical status.

Corneal Indentation

When IOP is 50 mm Hg or greater, topical miotics are ineffective due to ischemia of the iris constrictors. In this situation, a quick maneuver to lower IOP is corneal indentation.[1] As the cornea is indented, the aqueous is displaced and forced into the peripheral anterior chamber, which temporarily opens the angle. This results in an immediate decrease in IOP and, on occasion, can abort an attack. If, however, the attack is long-standing, it is unlikely that the aqueous can be forced through regions of iris to the trabecular meshwork adhesions (peripheral anterior synechiae). The advantages of corneal indentation are that it is rapid and may break an attack without additional medical intervention. The disadvantage is that corneal epithelium may be disrupted, which can complicate further therapy.

Corneal indentation is performed with topical anesthetics, and the patient is seated or in a reclining position. Any smooth instrument or a cotton-tipped applicator can be used, but the Goldmann applanation prism is readily available and easily held. The prism is held with the fingers to the patient's cornea and firm pressure applied for about 30 seconds (Fig. 13.16).

Topical Therapy

Timolol Maleate

Timolol maleate (Timoptic solution, 0.25% and 0.5%) is a nonselective beta-blocker. Lowering of IOP occurs by decreasing aqueous humor formation. Timoptic solution should be used with caution in patients with known conditions that are contraindications for the use of systemic beta-blockers, such as asthma, heart block, and heart failure. Side effects include decreased pulse rate, bronchial spasm, and altered mental state. *The recommended dosage for treating acute angle-closure glaucoma* is Timolol 0.5% solution, one or two drops at 10- to 15-minute intervals initially for three doses, and then one drop every 12 hours.

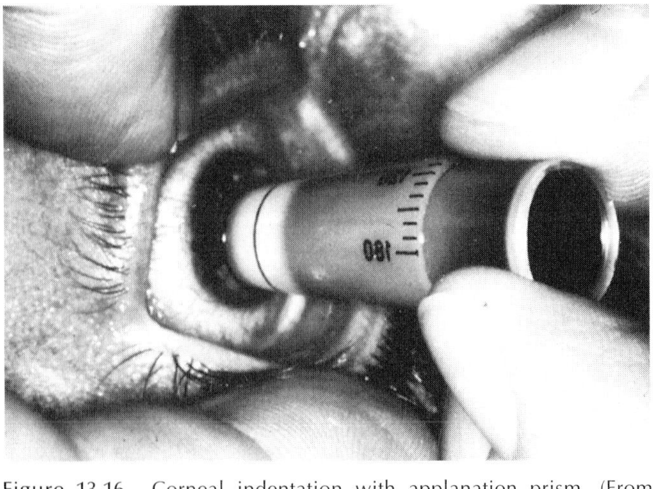

Figure 13.16. Corneal indentation with applanation prism. (From Anderson DR. Corneal indentation to relieve acute angle-closure glaucoma. *Am J Ophthalmol* 1979;88:1091, with permission.)

Pilocarpine Hydrochloride 1% and 2%

Pilocarpine is a direct-acting parasympathomimetic miotic agent. The mechanism of action in acute angle-closure glaucoma is mechanical. With miosis, the peripheral iris is pulled taut and away from the trabecular meshwork. Ocular side effects include a brow ache and diminished night vision. Systemic side effects, such as sweating, tremors, bradycardia, and hypotension, are uncommon in routine use of pilocarpine. However, these complications have been observed as a result of too frequent administration in the treatment of acute angle-closure glaucoma. *The recommended dosage for treating acute angle-closure glaucoma* is pilocarpine 2%, one drop every 30 minutes until the pupil constricts, and then one drop every 6 hours. *Note:* Miotics cause congestion of the iris stroma and aggravate inflammation; for this reason, concentrations higher than 2% are seldom used in an acute attack. Pilocarpine is not recommended if the diagnosis of acute angle-closure is unclear, or if the patient presents with a unilateral shallow anterior chamber.

Prednisolone Acetate

Topical corticosteroids reduce inflammation. The complications of long-term steroid use are not seen in the acute situation. *The recommended dosage for treating acute angle-closure glaucoma* is prednisolone acetate 1% (PredForte), one drop every 30 minutes to 1 hour until surgical treatment is completed.

Apraclonidine

Apraclonidine is a topical alpha-2 agonist used in chronic glaucoma. IOP is lowered by reduction of aqueous humor production, and effects are additive to those of topical beta-blockers.[9] Success in acute angle-closure glaucoma treatment has also been reported, and its use should be considered.[8] *The recommended dosage for treating acute angle-closure glaucoma* is Apraclonidine 0.5% solution, two drops (single administration).

Systemic Therapy

Acetazolamide

Acetazolamide is a carbonic anhydrase inhibitor that inhibits aqueous humor formation. Similar to sulfonamides, it must be given with caution in patients who have a history of allergy to sulfa drugs. Metabolic and, possibly, respiratory acidosis can occur with the use of carbonic anhydrase inhibitors; this medication should be avoided in patients with significant respiratory disease. Hypokalemia can be seen with acute therapy. *The recommended dosage for treating acute angle-closure glaucoma* is acetazolamide (Diamox), 500 mg i.v. every 12 hours; or if a patient can tolerate oral administration, acetazolamide (250-mg tablets), 500 mg PO every 6 hours.

Mannitol

Mannitol is a hyperosmotic that can be administered parenterally. It can aggravate or precipitate congestive heart failure and should be used cautiously in patients at risk for this problem. Mannitol lowers IOP by increasing the blood osmolality. This creates a gradient between the blood and the vitreous and draws water from the vitreous cavity. Side effects include headache, mental confusion, congestive heart failure, and dehydration. *The recommended dosage for treating acute angle-closure glaucoma* is mannitol 20%, 1 to 2 g/kg i.v. over 30 to 60 minutes.

Glycerin and Isosorbide

These hyperosmotic agents can be administered by mouth in patients able to tolerate oral medications. Glycerin should be avoided in diabetic patients because it can produce hyperglycemia and ketosis. Isosorbide is not metabolized to sugar and is a useful oral hyperosmotic in diabetics. *The recommended dosage for treating acute angle-closure glaucoma* is glycerin 75% (Glyrol), 1.0 to 1.5 g/kg PO (on ice with juice), or isosorbide 45% (Ismotic), 1.5 g/kg PO. *Note:* The hyperosmotic agents (mannitol, glycerin, and isosorbide) should not be used simultaneously.

Surgical Therapy

The definitive treatment of angle-closure glaucoma is release of pupillary block by an iridectomy. Laser iridectomies have replaced incisional iridectomies.[13] Laser surgery is usually completed after the resolution of acute angle-closure glaucoma. At times it is necessary to perform an iridectomy emergently in an eye that is medically unresponsive.[12] These cases generally involve patients who have delayed medical attention longer than 24 hours.

DISPOSITION

Role of the Consultant

Acute angle-closure glaucoma is an ophthalmic emergency. Consultation with an ophthalmologist should occur immediately.

Indications for Admission

Intractable Pain, Nausea, and Vomiting

Due to vagal stimulation as a consequence of the rapid and severe elevation of IOP, patients who present with acute angle-closure glaucoma are systemically ill and usually require admission. Analgesic and antiemetic agents may be given if the patient is having severe pain, nausea, or vomiting.

Intensive Medical Therapy and Monitoring

Parenteral administration of medications should be done in the hospital so that the patient can be closely observed for possible untoward reactions. IOP should be monitored every 2 to 3 hours to reevaluate whether the eye is responding to medical therapy. If the eye is responding and IOP is decreasing, then therapy should be continued. If the eye is not responding well to medical maneuvers and the IOP remains elevated, laser surgery (either iridectomy or iridoplasty) should be done within 2 to 4 hours.[17]

Transfer Considerations

If the initial receiving hospital cannot obtain an ophthalmology consult, therapy should be initiated and the patient transferred. This should be conducted expeditiously, because delay in treatment is detrimental to the visual prognosis.[6]

COMMON PITFALLS

- The diagnosis of acute angle-closure glaucoma is often difficult and delayed because the systemic complaints of pain, nausea, and vomiting are given primary attention. The overzealous treatment of these complaints (i.e., administration of analgesics and anticholinergics) may hinder a careful ophthalmologic examination and can exacerbate an angle-closure attack.
- Any patient with a painful red eye and decreased vision is considered an ophthalmic emergency and requires prompt consultation with an ophthalmologist.

ACKNOWLEDGMENT

The authors gratefully acknowledge the contribution of Alana L. Grajewski and Richard K. Parrish II who wrote the previous version of this chapter.

References

1. Anderson DR. Corneal indentation to relieve acute angle-closure glaucoma. *Am J Ophthalmol* 1979;88:1091.
2. Chandler PA, Grant WM. *Glaucoma,* 2nd ed. Philadelphia: Lea & Febiger, 1979:132.
3. David R, Tessler Z, Yassar T. Long-term outcome of primary acute angle-closure glaucoma. *Br J Ophthalmol* 1985;69:261.
4. Epstein DL, Jedziniak JA, Grant WM. Obstruction of aqueous outflow by lens particles and by heavy-molecular-weight soluble lens proteins. *Invest Ophthalmol Vis Sci* 1978;17:272.
5. Hall SK. Acute angle-closure glaucoma as a complication of combined beta-agonist and ipratropium bromide therapy in the emergency department. *Ann Emerg Med* 1994;23:884.
6. Hillman JS. Acute closed-angle glaucoma: an investigation into the effect of delay in treatment. *Br J Ophthalmol* 1979;63:817.
7. Jarrett WH. Dislocation of the lens: a study of 166 hospitalized cases. *Arch Ophthalmol* 1967;78:289.
8. Krawitz PL, Podis SM. Use of apraclonidine in the treatment of acute angle closure glaucoma. *Arch Ophthalmol* 1990;108:1208.
9. Morrison JC, Robin AL. Adjunctive glaucoma therapy: a comparison of apraclonidine to dipivefrin when added to timolol maleate. *Ophthalmology* 1989;96:3.
10. Murphy MB, Spaeth GL. Iridectomy and primary angle-closure glaucoma. *Arch Ophthalmol Vis Sci* 1974;91:114.
11. Reuser T, Flanagan DW, Borland C, Bannerjee DK. Acute angle-closure glaucoma occurring after nebulized bronchodilator treatment with ipratropium bromide and salbutamol. *J R Soc Med* 1992;85:499.
12. Rich R. Argon laser treatment for medically unresponsive attacks of angle-closure glaucoma. *Am J Ophthalmol* 1982;94:197.
13. Rivera AH, Brown RH, Anderson DR. Laser iridotomy vs. surgical iridectomy: have the indications changed? *Arch Ophthalmol Vis Sci* 1985;103:1350.
14. Roden DR. The prevalence and cost of glaucoma. In: *Glaucoma detection and treatment: proceedings of the First National Glaucoma Conference.* Sponsored by the National Society to Prevent Blindness, Tarpon Springs, FL, 1980:20.
15. Rutkowski PC, Thompson HS. Mydriasis and increased intraocular pressure. *Arch Ophthalmol* 1972;87:21.
16. Shields MB. Disorders of the lens. In: *A study guide to glaucoma.* Baltimore: Williams & Wilkins, 1982:271.
17. Simmons JR, Belcher CD III, Dallow RL. Primary angle-closure glaucoma. In: Duane TD, Jaeger EA, eds. *Clinical ophthalmology,* vol. 3, rev. ed. New York: Harper & Row, 1987:1.
18. Singh J, O'Brien C, Wright M. Nebulized bronchodilator therapy causes acute angle-closure glaucoma in predisposed individuals [Letter]. *Respir Med* 1993;87:559.
19. Spaeth GL. The normal development of the human anterior chamber angle: a new system of descriptive grading. *Trans Ophthalmol Soc UK* 1971;91:709.
20. Stamper RL, Bellows AR. Angle-closure glaucoma. In: Stamper RL, Bellows AR, eds. *Basic and clinical science course of the American Academy of Ophthalmology.* Section 8:72. San Francisco: American Academy of Ophthalmology, 1986–1987.
21. Tasman W, Margargal LE, Augsburger JJ. Effects of argon laser photocoagulation on rubeosis iridis and angle neovascularization. *Ophthalmology* 1980;87:400.
22. Vargas E, Drance SM. Anterior chamber depth in angle-closure glaucoma. Clinical methods of depth determination in people with and without the disease. *Arch Ophthalmol Vis Sci* 1973;90:438.
23. Wand M, Dueker DK, Avello LM, et al. Effects of panretinal photocoagulation on rubeosis iridis, angle neovascularization, and neovascular glaucoma. *Am J Ophthalmol* 1978;86:332.

CHAPTER 14

Orbital and Periorbital Infections in Children and Adults

David A. Kramer and Ronald S. Benenson

Orbital and periorbital infections are relatively rare and affect children more frequently than adults. When they do occur, they can be life-threatening. The terms *orbital cellulitis* and *periorbital cellulitis* are often used interchangeably, although the single

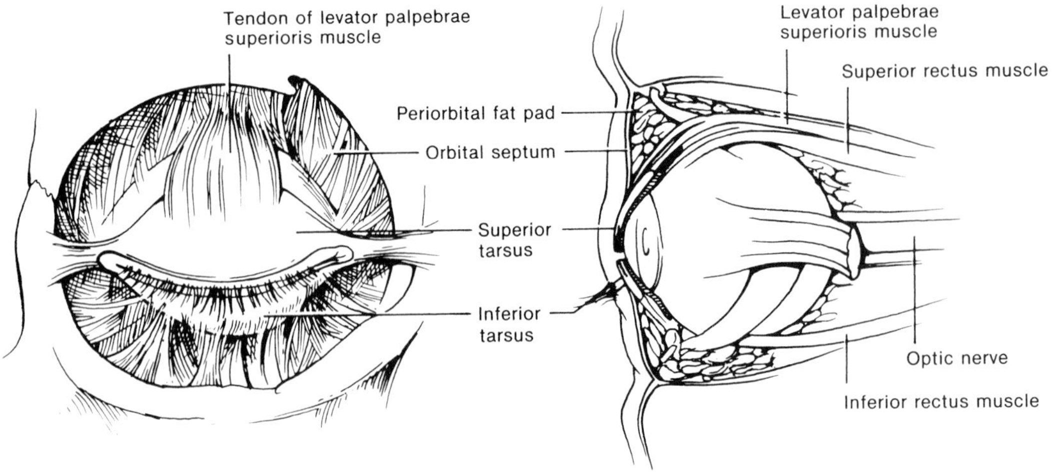

Figure 14.1. View of orbit–orbital septum.

most important step in managing these diseases is to differentiate the two. *Orbital (postseptal) infection* is anatomically defined as inflammation of any of the tissues within the orbit posterior to the orbital septum. A more anatomically correct term than periorbital cellulitis is *preseptal cellulitis*. This term includes any inflammation anterior to the orbital septum, a sheetlike layer of fascia that separates the orbit from the eyelids (Fig. 14.1). Preseptal cellulitis is invariably present in orbital infection, as are chemosis and proptosis.

ETIOLOGY

Seventy-five percent of all cellulitides (periorbital and orbital) have an identifiable predisposing factor, and 50% are directly attributable to sinusitis, upper respiratory tract infection, and otitis media with effusion.

The orbit is a cone-shaped cavity, and the inferior, medial, and superior walls are immediately adjacent to the paranasal sinuses. It is easy to see why infections can lead to cellulitis (Fig. 14.2).

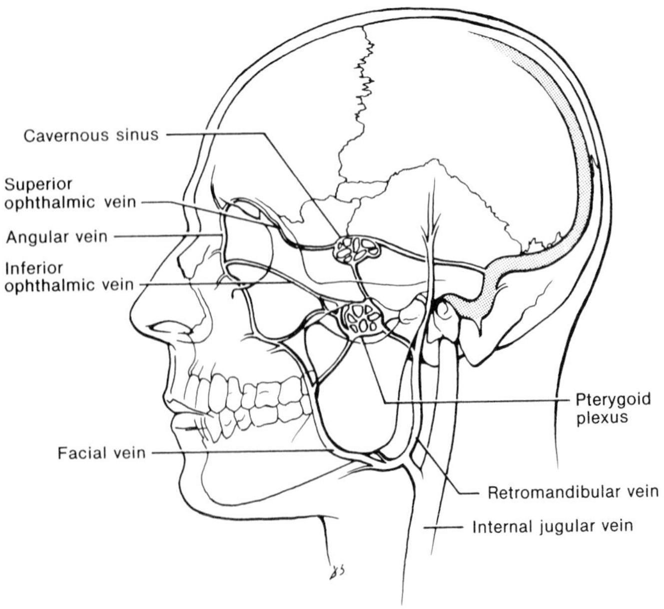

Figure 14.2. Perinasal veins (valveless) and cavernous sinus.

The bacterial pathogens involved in orbital and periorbital cellulitis are presumed to be the same pathogens causing the predisposing condition: chronic or acute sinusitis; upper respiratory tract infection; localized skin infection or inflammation, including chalazion, hordeolum, dacryocystitis, and impetigo; trauma; otogenous and dental infections; postsurgical infections; and many other rarer causes. In the minority of patients from whom bacterial pathogens are isolated, *Staphylococcus aureus, Staphylococcus epidermidis, Streptococcus pneumoniae,* and streptococcal species including microaerophilic *Streptococcus milleri* are most commonly cultured. Other occasionally reported pathogens include *Moraxella catarrhalis,* nontypable *Haemophilus influenzae, Bacteroides* spp., *Peptostreptococcus* spp., *Eikenella corrodens,* and *Pseudomonas aeruginosa,* as well as mixed bacterial cultures. Even when there is strong evidence of hematogenous spread, blood cultures are positive only 11% to 34% of the time.

The advent of *H. influenzae* type B (HiB) vaccine has changed the age-related etiologies of orbital and periorbital cellulitis. In two series of children with orbital or periorbital cellulitis, the only positive cultures for HiB were recorded prior to 1988 and in patients who did not receive the HiB vaccine. Streptococcal species are now the most commonly isolated pathogens in children. In the setting of local infection or trauma, regardless of age, *S. aureus* or beta-hemolytic streptococci are likely to be causative. Older patients tend to have staphylococcal and streptococcal infections. In the setting of sinusitis, the causative organisms are those usually involved in either chronic or acute sinusitis. Anaerobes tend to predominate in chronic sinusitis (Fig. 14.3).

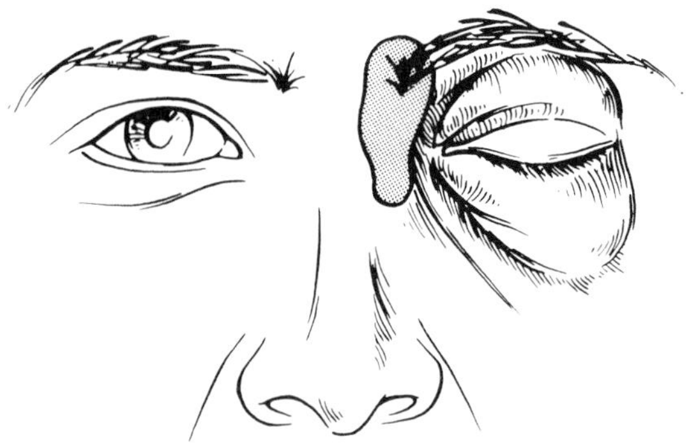

Figure 14.3. Orbital cellulitis (from sinusitis).

CLINICAL PRESENTATION

Patients experiencing orbital infection have ocular pain and to varying degrees exhibit internal and external ophthalmoplegia, pupillary paralysis, and decreased visual acuity, even to the point of blindness. They may also develop increased intraocular pressure and loss of sensation along the trigeminal nerve (V1 and V2). Preseptal cellulitis, chemosis, and proptosis are present. Diffuse impairment of extraocular movements occurs when the globe is displaced by abscess.

Patients with preseptal cellulitis present with erythema, edema, warmth, and closure of the palpebral fissures; one or both eyes may be involved. Fever is more common than in orbital infection. In contrast to orbital infection, there should be no complaints of ocular pain, pain with movement of the globe, or ocular tenderness, or any limitation of globe mobility. If present, these symptoms suggest postseptal (i.e., true orbital) infection.

Immunocompromised Patients

Mycotic infections can present as an orbital infection in diabetic or other immunocompromised patients, as well as in patients with physical conditions causing metabolic acidosis, such as renal failure, cirrhosis, leukemia, and lymphoma. The patient usually presents with complaints of sinus congestion, rhinitis, and facial and orbital pain, and on examination may have proptosis, ophthalmoplegia, and visual loss. These infections are important because, although uncommon, orbital phycomycosis can cause thrombotic vasculitis, necrosis, and rapid orbitocerebral extension and can be fatal in 75% of patients. *P. aeruginosa* infections in immunocompromised patients reportedly can cause a necrotizing infection similar to the mycotic infections, with equally poor prognosis.

Pediatric Versus Adult Presentations

The literature does not allow for detailed differentiation between these two groups. In general, patients with periorbital cellulitis tend to be younger than those with orbital cellulitis, although orbital cellulitis has been described in neonates. Both infections are more common in childhood, both present acutely, and both may appear in a subacute form due to inadequate antibiotic therapy.

DIFFERENTIAL DIAGNOSIS

The patient who presents with apparent periorbital cellulitis should be presumed to have orbital cellulitis until the latter can be ruled out. Nearly 75% of all patients with an "acute orbit" have periorbital cellulitis. The other 25% have orbital cellulitis, subperiosteal abscess, orbital abscess, or cavernous sinus thrombosis. Differentiating among these serious infections is difficult because they share many features.

A *subperiosteal abscess* presents much like orbital cellulitis. There may be significant tenderness between the orbital margin and the globe itself. Extraocular movement impairments may be limited to a particular muscle group, with the eye "looking away" from the intraorbital location of the abscess. The globe may be displaced by the abscess.

An *orbital abscess* resembles orbital cellulitis. It is located in the postseptal tissues. Ophthalmologic findings of venous congestion and disk edema may be more prominent than in orbital cellulitis. Pus may spread into the lid and conjunctiva. There is pronounced exophthalmos, ophthalmoplegia, and visual impairment. The globe may be displaced due to mass effect.

Cavernous sinus thrombosis frequently presents unilaterally, followed by bilateral axial proptosis with paralysis of cranial nerves III, IV, and VI. It is extremely difficult to distinguish from orbital cellulitis until infection spreads across the anterior and posterior intercavernous sinus and bilateral involvement occurs. Dilatation of the episcleral veins is a classic feature and the first sign of worsening beyond orbital involvement. Venous engorgement of the fundus and pupillary fixation and dilatation also suggest cavernous sinus thrombosis.

Periorbital cellulitis may be confused with *allergic periorbital swelling*. If there is uncertainty about the diagnosis, the swelling and erythema should be marked with a pen, epinephrine or diphenhydramine administered, and the patient reexamined in 2 hours. Cellulitis frequently spreads across the pen lines, whereas the swelling in the allergic patient who receives epinephrine or diphenhydramine should regress.

EMERGENCY DEPARTMENT EVALUATION

Diagnosing the cause and extent of inflammation is problematic. While performing the physical examination, remember the following:

1. Pure preseptal (periorbital) cellulitis may present with sufficient swelling to inhibit visual acuity and ocular motility.
2. Fever is absent in as many as 24% of all patients with preseptal and postseptal infections.
3. Unilateral involvement is the rule rather than the exception for both periorbital and orbital cellulitis.

Blood cultures should be taken for children, but are of little value for adults. For orbital cellulitis, blood cultures are negative in two-thirds of children and in 90% to 95% of adults. Cultures of eyelid aspirates and eye secretions also correlate poorly with blood culture results and are *not* useful unless there is a clear source of cutaneous infection. Cultures of cerebrospinal fluid are recommended only for infants in whom meningeal signs are clearly present.

Sinus films do not differentiate between orbital cellulitis and orbital abscess and have been replaced by computed tomography (CT) scan. CT scanning of the orbit is advocated in all children with periorbital swelling in whom postseptal infection cannot be ruled out by examination. Most authors advocate obtaining coronal as well as axial CT views to locate superomedial subperiosteal or orbital abscesses that might be missed on axial views alone. There is no advantage to using contrast rather than noncontrast CT scanning. CT scans identify a subperiosteal abscess or orbital abscess in only 80% of cases. Diagnosis of orbital infection remains a clinical one. CT scanning does contribute to the selection of a surgical approach for abscess drainage once the patient has been admitted, or if the patient has failed to improve on parenteral antibiotics. Ultrasound has been advocated because of its lack of ionizing radiation and its ability to discriminate between fluid and soft-tissue density. A magnetic resonance scan offers another alternative for identification of patients requiring surgical treatment.

EMERGENCY DEPARTMENT MANAGEMENT

Treatment should not be delayed in favor of extended diagnostic workup. In adults, if the infection appears to be localized to the preseptal tissues only and is not severe, antibiotics can be given orally on an outpatient basis. Antibiotics should cover *S. aureus*, group A *Streptococcus*, and Enterobacteriaceae. First-generation cephalosporins or penicillinase-resistant synthetic penicillins should be given. For the adult with signs of serious infection, first-generation cephalosporins, penicillinase-resistant synthetic penicillins, or second- or third-generation parenteral cephalosporins and vancomycin or ticarcillin/clavulanate or ampicillin/sulbactam are appropriate alternatives.

In children, only the mildest cellulitis should be treated on an outpatient basis. Even this is controversial; some authorities recommend admission and parenteral antibiotics for all children with periorbital cellulitis. Either cefuroxime 20 to 30 mg/kg/d every 12 hours or amoxicillin/clavulanate potassium (Augmentin) 40 mg/kg/d every 8 hours may be used with equal efficacy. In cases of trauma or infection in which the suspicion of staphylococcal infection is high, dicloxacillin 25 to 40 mg/kg/d every 6 hours or, in the penicillin-allergic patient, erythromycin 40 mg/kg/d every 6 hours may be given. The condition should be treated for at least 7 to 10 days. If the infection appears to be secondary to sinusitis, treatment should last at least 2 to 3 weeks and antibiotic coverage should be aimed at organisms that cause sinusitis (anaerobic bacteria). If outpatient treatment has been selected, the patient should be reexamined the next day, preferably by a specialist.

If there is any question about the extent of the infection, intravenous antibiotics should be initiated without delay. In the child under age 5 in whom sinusitis is believed to be the source or in whom no clear cause can be found, antibiotic coverage for gram-positive cocci, including resistant *S. pneumoniae,* should be initiated until culture results are available.

Most authors also advocate coverage for anaerobes, including *Bacteroides* spp. and microaerophilic *S. milleri.* The most frequently recommended combination is a beta-lactamase–resistant penicillin, such as nafcillin 150 mg/kg/d every 6 hours, and chloramphenicol 50 to 100 mg/kg/d every 6 hours (this dose is halved for neonates). Alternatively, a high-dose second-generation cephalosporin active against gram-positive organisms, such as cefuroxime 75 to 100 mg/kg/d every 8 hours or cefotaxime, may be used along with metronidazole for anaerobic coverage. *Ampicillin is no longer recommended.* The dose of cefuroxime should be increased to 240 mg/kg/d in cases of associated meningitis.

In the penicillin-allergic patient, either vancomycin 40 mg/kg/d every 6 hours or clindamycin, combined with chloramphenicol, is a reasonable choice. For patients with infection clearly related to a skin lesion, nafcillin is recommended. For the penicillin-allergic patient, vancomycin is recommended.

DISPOSITION

Role of the Consultant

Any sign of true orbital (postseptal) infection in patients of any age mandates hospital admission for intravenous antibiotic treatment. It should prompt an urgent otolaryngologic and ophthalmologic consultation as well. The infected orbit may need emergency surgical exploration and drainage if there is no improvement within 24 to 48 hours, or if visual acuity worsens.

Indications for Admission

Mild preseptal cellulitis in the adult may be treated on an outpatient basis, but only if the patient can be reexamined by an ophthalmologist the next day. If a trial of outpatient treatment is chosen, the first dose of the selected oral antibiotic should be given before discharge from the emergency department. If the periorbital swelling is considerable or involvement deep to the preseptal tissues is evident, intravenous antibiotics should be started in the emergency department before admission to the hospital, in consultation with the admitting physician. Children with periorbital cellulitis should be assessed with caution; only the mildest of infections may be managed on an outpatient basis.

Transfer Considerations

Transfer is required if orbital cellulitis is suspected and an ophthalmologic surgeon is unavailable. The emergency physician should arrange immediate transfer while antibiotics are being given. An advanced life-support unit is necessary only in severe cases, such as a patient with signs of cavernous sinus thrombosis.

COMMON PITFALLS

- The most important action is to differentiate periorbital (preseptal) from orbital (postseptal) infection. All but the mildest cases of periorbital cellulitis warrant admission.
- Periorbital cellulitis may be easily confused with allergic periorbital swelling.
- Tests that are of *little value* in differentiating periorbital from orbital cellulitis include white blood cell counts and sinus films, cultures of eyelid aspirates or eye secretions, routine cerebrospinal fluid cultures (in the absence of meningeal signs), and blood cultures in adults.
- CT scanning is the diagnostic test of choice. Contrast-enhanced CT appears to be no more useful than noncontrast CT in differentiating the type and extent of infection.
- Ultrasound may be less useful in children under age 4 because of redundant mucosa in the young child.
- Antibiotic coverage should be directed at the underlying etiology, most commonly sinusitis. Consider coverage for resistant *S. pneumoniae.*

Bibliography

Andrews TM, Myer CM. The role of CT in the diagnosis of subperiosteal abscesses of the orbit. *Clin Pediatr* 1992;31:1.

Barone SR, Aiuto LT. Periorbital and orbital cellulitis in the *Hemophilus influenzae* era. *J Pediatr Ophthalmol Strabismus* 1997;34:293.

Dudin A, Othman A. Acute periorbital swelling: evaluation of management protocol. *Pediatr Emerg Care* 1996;12:16.

Handler LC, et al. The acute orbit: differentiation of orbital cellulitis from subperiosteal abscess by CT. *Neuroradiology* 1991;33:1.

Lahgam-Brown JJ, Rhys-Williams S. CT of acute orbital infection: the importance of coronal sections. *Clin Radiol* 1989;40:5.

Lessner A, Stern GA. Preseptal and orbital cellulitis. *Infect Dis Clin North Am* 1992;6:4.

Moloney JR, et al. The acute orbit: preseptal (periorbital) cellulitis, subperiosteal abscess, and orbital cellulitis due to sinusitis. *J Laryngol Otol* 1987;12[Suppl]:1.

Paerregaard A, Lund I. Periorbital and orbital cellulitis in children. *Ugeskr Laeger* 1995;157:6576.

Sadow KB, Chamberlain JM. Blood cultures in the evaluation of children with cellulitis. *Pediatrics* 1998;101:E4.

Schwartz GR, Wright SW. Changing bacteriology of periorbital cellulitis. *Ann Emerg Med* 1996;28:617.

Skedros, DG, et al. Subperiosteal orbital abscess in children: diagnosis, microbiology, and management. *Laryngoscope* 1993;103(Pt 1):1.

Slavin ML, Glaser JS. Acute severe irreversible visual loss with sphenoethmoiditis—"posterior" orbital cellulitis. *Arch Ophthalmol* 1987;105:345.

Williams SR, Carruth JAS. Orbital infection secondary to sinusitis in children: diagnosis and management. *Clin Otolaryngol* 1992;17:6.

PART II

Emergency Aspects of Dental and Oral Surgery

CHAPTER 15

Toothache and Common Periodontal Problems

Alan Hodgdon

Pain in the jaw and other facial structures is a common presenting complaint in most emergency departments. It is the job of the emergency physician to determine which of these complaints demands immediate therapy and which can be ameliorated until a dentist or oral-maxillofacial surgeon is available. The majority of dental-related problems can be treated with simple therapy.

A thorough medical history and review of systems should be obtained before oral examination and treatment begin. Many chronic diseases, from clotting disorders to cancers, can be manifested by oral problems. In addition, fatal anaphylaxis can occur from antibiotics prescribed for oral infections, just as in cases of severe systemic diseases. Because manipulation of the oral cavity causes transient bacteremia, certain patients should be identified to receive antibiotics before invasive procedures.

The information presented here is restricted to those patients whose main pathology is confined to the oral cavity. If obvious facial cellulitis, fever, or Ludwig's angina is present, the reader is referred to Chapter 18, "Dental, Oral, and Salivary Gland Infections."

TOOTH ANATOMY

To understand how an apical abscess develops and how other common tooth pathologies cause pain, it is important to briefly review some points about tooth anatomy. First, the enamel is the hard outer surface of the teeth. When the enamel is intact, it is white and shiny.

Under this surface lies the dentin. It is off-yellow and sensitive to both pain and infection. It is composed of dentin tubules, which connect this structure directly to the pulp cavity, where the nerve and blood supply of the tooth live. The dentin, then, is a very important structure. When it is exposed by either caries or trauma, it should be covered. This reduces pain and lessens the chance for infection, which can track along the tubules to the dental pulp.

The periodontal ligament is an important structure for holding the tooth in position. This structure is very cellular and fragile. This is why when a tooth is knocked out of the mouth, the tooth may be held under running water to remove gross contamination but should not be scrubbed. The scrubbing process removes the periodontal ligament, and the tooth will then not "take" when reinserted.

Teeth are numbered, usually by the method of Fig. 15.1. In other words, numbering starts with the third molar at the posterior of the right upper jaw, proceeds forward and around to the third molar of the left upper jaw, then drops down and proceeds forward from the left third molar of the lower jaw, ending with the no. 32 tooth, the posterior third molar of the lower right jaw. The more practical method is just to name the tooth involved, keeping in mind the dental formula. The dental formula states that the mouth can be divided into four quadrants, each having the following teeth: a central incisor, a lateral incisor, a canine tooth, two premolars, and three molars (the last, or third, molar is the wisdom tooth). Using this simple formula, all of the teeth can be properly identified.

ORAL EXAMINATION

Emergency department management is based on a thorough history, as described, and an adequate physical examination of the mouth. First, the patient's general appearance should be noted, concentrating on facial symmetry. Evaluate for facial edema, localized external areas of tenderness, erythema, and obvious lesions. The lymph nodes in the neck, including the submandibular and preauricular regions, are palpated.

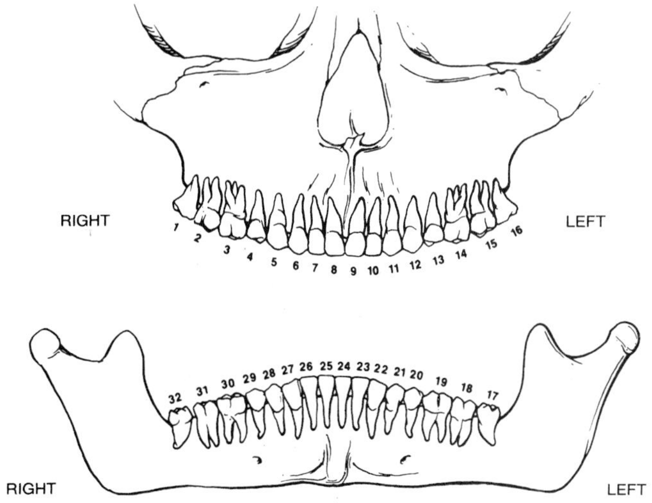

Figure 15.1. Identification of teeth (dental arches widely spread).

With a tongue blade in each hand, with good lighting from either a headlamp or a good overhead light, both hands should be free to feel in the mouth and hold the tongue blades. After you have gloved and are holding a tongue blade in each hand, ask the patient to open his or her mouth. Evaluate first for trismus. This is noted almost immediately by the inability to fully open the mouth. The distance can be objectively measured by the distance between the central incisors, usually greater than 35 mm, but it is acceptable to estimate the ability of the patient to open the mouth. When mouth opening is limited by pain, it usually indicates infection in the muscles of the face and is an indication for further examination.

Proceeding from the outside in, and from the anterior of the mouth toward the back, evaluate the soft-tissue structures for pathology. Do this first before looking at the teeth, because most tooth pathologies cause problems with the surrounding gingiva. Begin at the inferior lip, looking for erosions, state of dentition, erythema, abscess, and areas of inflammation. Then proceed to the posterior mucosa, and evaluate the posterior oropharynx, then the tongue. Evaluate the actual teeth, focusing on areas noted in the initial visual inspection or by evaluating areas of pain described by the patient. There are ways to use heat or cold to stress the nerves of the teeth, but the percussion test works the best and is relatively sensitive. Simply percuss the occlusal surface of the tooth, and if the nerve is inflamed, this will usually elicit pain. When you elicit tenderness on examination in an area, be specific. This helps in determining whether tooth pathology is old or new and helps guide therapy. It is helpful to keep in mind that old, dead teeth are usually not painful, because the root of the tooth is already dead. The acutely infected and dying teeth are painful.

After the gingiva and tooth structures are evaluated with the tongue blades, focus on the area of pathology, carefully identifying the pathology noted. Look closely at the tooth surfaces and the gingiva associated with the suspected tooth, and attempt to move the tooth. Loose teeth and recession of the gingival structures indicate advanced periodontal disease. Palpate the tongue and floor of the mouth and examine the mucosa for lesions. If the mouth is unusually dry, make note of this as well.

With the history and physical examination conducted in an organized manner, the following diseases can be diagnosed and appropriate management begun. Pathologies described are divided into those of the actual teeth versus those of the supporting structures of the teeth.

DISEASES OF THE TEETH

Dental Caries

Dental caries, or tooth decay, are the most common cause of toothache seen in the emergency department and the most common cause of tooth loss worldwide. This is obviously not an acute process, but eventually the pain increases until often the patient "can't take it any longer." Pain is associated with exposure of the dentin and, in advanced cases, with irritation of the pulp. Associated periodontal disease may contribute to the pain. The whole process is caused by a complex interaction of susceptible teeth, with bacteria, mostly *Streptococcus mutans,* in the proper acidic media. As such, caries of the teeth, as well as periodontal diseases in general, are bacterial in nature. Plaque is associated with this process; build-up of plaque and lack of proper dental care are largely responsible for this preventable disease.

The patient usually complains of dull pain, often exacerbated by hot or cold foods. Percussion of the involved tooth and evaluation of the associated mucosa will help determine appropriate pain medication prior to referral. Unless pulpitis or other pathology is evident on examination, antibiotics are not indicated. Definitive therapy involves excavation and filling (by a general dentist) of the dental areas involved.

Pulpitis

Pulpitis is inflammation of the confined structures of the pulp cavity. The most common cause is extension of infection from dental caries. The most common symptom is pain, as the vascular and nerve bundles lie herein. The patient complains of severe pain, often throbbing and shooting in character. The pain is exacerbated by thermal changes. Pulpitis is usually acute, but chronic pulpitis also can occur. Here the pain is less intense and less temperature sensitive. Emergency department treatment includes adequate analgesia and arranging for follow-up care by a dental practitioner. In cases of severe pain, urgent dental consultation may be advisable. Definitive treatment involves excavation and filling of the underlying dental caries, and usually a root canal. Root canal therapy removes the structures of the root (the nerve and vascular bundle) and thereby may avoid tooth extraction. Endodontic therapy is expensive and requires patient compliance.

Periapical Abscess

When dental caries are left unchecked for prolonged periods, the infection tracks to the pulp cavity, causing pulpitis. Over time, this is followed by extension of the infection to the cancellous bone of the dentoalveolar ridge. Here the infection usually spreads to the buccal, lingual, or palatal cortical bone and can usually be seen and palpated. Clinically, the tooth is usually nonvital and is sensitive to both percussion and thermal testing. It is important to identify a periapical abscess, as it is readily treated with incision and drainage (I and D) by experienced emergency physicians or by a dental consultant.

The area is identified by erythema, tenderness, and distension. Apical block anesthesia is done by injecting a small volume of lidocaine in the soft gingival sulcus near the root of the tooth, and incision and drainage can be carried out easily under this simple local anesthesia. Drainage of this infection can prevent the further tracking of the infection to other areas of the face and neck. As with any abscess, I and D is the treatment of choice, as antibiotics do not penetrate well into the area of abscess. After I and D, and after any oral procedure, the patient should swish and spit with warm salt solution until the spit is clear and a quick reexamination of the mouth can be performed.

After drainage of an abscess, the antibiotic of choice is penicillin (penicillin V potassium 500 mg q.i.d. or 1 g b.i.d.) or clindamycin 350 mg q.i.d. Erythromycin or another macrolide is also an acceptable choice. The patient should be given instructions for a follow-up visit with a dental consultant within 1 to 2 days.

Definitive treatment involves either extraction of the tooth or excavation and filling of the underlying dental caries, followed by root canal. The procedure chosen depends on the health of the involved teeth and supporting structures, and how compliant the patient is expected to be. Root canal therapy requires a patient who can comply with more than one office visit and follow instructions.

A common pitfall of periapical abscess occurs when the emergency physician attempts to avoid an I and D of the abscess by treating the patient with antibiotics. This is often related to a certain lack of experience or knowledge and puts the patient at risk for extension of the infection.

PERIODONTAL DISEASES

Periodontal disease is often thought of as gum disease. Actually, the periodontium consists of the supporting structures of the gingiva, periodontal ligament, and alveolar bone. Periodontal disease is actually a group of diseases. The two most important in terms of frequency are gingivitis and periodontitis.The most common cause of periodontal disease is poor dental hygiene, with the subsequent build-up of plaque, resulting in both dental caries and subsequent periodontal disease. As with dental caries, bacterial interplay with susceptible structures precipitates the inflammation and degeneration of the structures affected. Many systemic diseases also are associated with periodontal diseases, the most common being insulin- and noninsulin-dependent diabetes, human immunodeficiency virus (HIV) infection, and cardiovascular diseases. Additionally, hormonal factors and drug reactions can cause specific types of periodontal disease.

Neither gingivitis nor periodontitis is by itself an emergency, but the complications of these diseases result in many emergency department visits each year, so a basic understanding of these processes is important.

Gingivitis

Gingivitis is an inflammatory process of the gingiva, characterized by a change in the normal contour of the gingiva, with erythema, edema, and, often, discharge. Despite changes in the gingiva, the junctional epithelium that covers the inferior portion of the tooth is maintained intact and the tooth is not loosened. Treatment of gingivitis is local containment of the plaque (which is a causative factor), or treatment of the systemic disease, when it is a factor.

Periodontitis

Periodontitis is also an inflammatory condition of the gingival tissues, but is characterized by loss of attachment of the periodontal ligament and the bony support of the tooth. It is thought to represent an extension of gingivitis, although only a few gingivitis sites make this transition. The destruction of these supporting structures of the tooth does not proceed in a steady manner, but seems to progress in bursts related to unknown factors. In the elderly, periodontitis continues to be a significant cause of tooth loss. Evidence of periodontitis should be noted on examination and the patient referred to a dentist for evaluation and treatment.

Periodontal Abscess

When periodontitis is advanced, the associated bone loss can result in localized pockets forming around the tooth. These pockets can become infected, resulting in pain, erythema, and frank abscess. This type of abscess differs from the periapical abscess, because the tooth may still be healthy and no caries need be present.

Initial treatment consists of local anesthesia, usually an apical block, followed by I and D by either the emergency physician or dental consultant. Antibiotics are usually not indicated unless the abscess is extensive. The patient should be referred to a dentist for further management, which usually involves physical removal of the periodontal pocket by excision or curette.

Pericoronitis

Pericoronitis is inflammation, usually followed by infection, of the gingival tissue overlying the crown of an impacted tooth. As the tooth attempts to erupt through this gingiva (operculum), the area becomes inflamed and secondarily infected. This usually involves the wisdom teeth (third molars), and the severity can range from mild inflammation to a significant, spreading facial infection.

Emergency treatment is based on severity, but usually involves oral antibiotic administration of penicillin (penicillin V potassium 500 mg q.i.d. or 1 g b.i.d.), or clindamycin 350 mg q.i.d. Erythromycin or another macrolide is also an acceptable choice. Adequate pain medications should be given and urgent referral to an oral surgeon should be made. Definitive treatment usually involves excision of the impacted tooth.

Acute Necrotizing Ulcerative Gingivitis

Acute necrotizing ulcerative gingivitis (ANUG), also called trench mouth, is an intraoral infection characterized by erythema and hyperemia of the gingiva, fetid breath, bleeding gums, and friability of the mucosa. White plaques and areas of ulceration are usually evident and a pseudomembrane that bleeds with manipulation may be present. Systemic symptoms are often present, such as fever, malaise, or dehydration. The disease occurs mostly in teen-agers and is associated with factors such as malnutrition, smoking, stress, or poor personal hygiene. Such factors favor the proliferation of fusiform and spirochete bacteria as responsible for the infection.

ANUG is treated by local mouth care, such as gentle debridement of lesions with a cotton-tipped swab soaked with hydrogen peroxide. Antibiotics are usually indicated (penicillin, clindamycin, or erythromycin), especially if fever or adenopathy is present. Pain medications should be administered and referral to a dental consultant arranged. Bony destruction can occur as a consequence of ANUG, so follow-up is important.

MOUTH LESIONS

There are a multitude of causes of lesions of the mouth, including ulcers. Some of the more common etiologies of ulcerations are described next. It should be noted, however, that many systemic diseases have dermatologic manifestations that can first make their appearance as lesions in the mouth. These diseases include pemphigus, erythema multiforme, lichen planus, Stevens-Johnson, Behçet, various hemorrhagic disorders, and neoplasms. If a lesion looks suspicious, the patient should be referred to a dental consultant for further evaluation and potential biopsy.

Aphthous Ulcers

These lesions are common, with about one-third of people manifesting one in their lifetime. Often, they are recurrent and characterized by a round, symmetrical, shallow lesion with a yellowish exudate. These ulcers are usually 0.5 to 1.0 cm in diameter and are painful. A burning sensation is often noted in the area just before eruption. The etiology is unknown. Treatment consists of general mouth care instructions and dyclonine hydrochloride topically for pain.

Acute Herpetic Gingivostomatitis

This is an acute infection, usually noted in children less than 6 months of age. It represents the first infection with herpes, and as such, presents with a classic prodrome of illness, followed by lymphadenopathy and fever. The oral lesions are usually multiple, shallow, round, and discrete ulcers with a red halo of inflammation. The gingiva are usually inflamed and painful as well. Acute treatment is symptomatic, ensuring control of fever and adequate hydration. A "swizzle" of equal parts viscous lidocaine, Maalox, and Benadryl can be given for symptomatic relief of oral pain.

Allergic Stomatitis

This condition causes localized or generalized swelling and inflammation of the gingiva, usually with no systemic symptoms. Burning is a predominant symptom. Diagnosis is by history, and treatment is avoidance, once the inciting allergen is identified.

Traumatic Ulcers

These can be caused by thermal injury, chemicals, or even bites, such as sustained during seizures. Aspirin is a common chemical burn, when applied topically on painful teeth or gums. As the burn resolves and the mucosa sloughs, a painful, red, bleeding surface often remains. Treatment for these ulcers is good general mouth cleansing and avoidance of the chemical or trauma.

COMMON PITFALLS

- A good general history, including susceptibility to allergies, is important. Failure to obtain a history potentially exposes patients to antibiotics and analgesics to which they may be allergic. In addition, procedures are often performed on those who should have antibiotic prophylaxis, and this may be neglected inadvertently.
- Failing to refer patients for routine dental care after noting poor oral hygiene and dental caries. Tooth loss is often preventable when follow-up dental care is made available and utilized.
- Failing to drain an abscess cavity when one is noted. Administration of antibiotics alone does not constitute adequate treatment in the presence of an abscess.

Bibliography

Burt BA, Eklund SA. *Dentistry, dental practice and the community.* Philadelphia: WB Saunders, 1999.

Dewhurst SN, et al. Emergency treatment of orodental injuries: a review. *Br J Oral Maxillofac Surg* 1998;36:165–175. Heasman P, et al. *Periodontology.* New York: Churchill Livingstone, 1997.

Kidd EA. The operative management of caries. *Dental Update* 1998;25:104–108, 110.

Kidd EA, Joyston-Bechal S. *Essentials of dental caries: the disease and its management.* Oxford: Oxford University Press, 1997.

Killoy WJ. Chemical treatment of periodontitis: local delivery of antimicrobials. *Int Dent J* 1998;48:305–315.

Oliver RC, Brown LJ. Periodontal diseases and tooth loss *Periodontology 2000* 1993;2:117–127.

Orstavik D, Pitt Ford T. *Essential endodontology.* Blackwell Science, 1998.

Pihlstrom BL, Ammons WF. Treatment of gingivitis and periodontitis. Research Science and Therapy Committee of the American Academy of Periodontology. *J Periodontol* 1997;68:1246–1253.

Stock C, et al. *Color atlas and text of endodontics.* Mosby-Wolfe, 1995.

Wade DN, Derns DG. Acute necrotizing ulcerative gingivitis-periodontitis: a literature review. *Milit Med* 1998;163:337–342.

CHAPTER 16

Postoperative Complications from Oral and Maxillofacial Surgery

James T. Amsterdam

This chapter outlines postoperative complications from oral and maxillofacial surgery (OMFS) that may present to the emergency physician. OMFS procedures involve major facial surgery done in the hospital (e.g., osteotomies of facial bones) and minor procedures done in the office (e.g., removal of teeth). Patients may be referred to the emergency department directly from the surgeon's office after an intraoperative complication, or may have developed a problem several hours or days after hospital discharge or completion of office surgery.

OMFS postoperative complications are unique for two reasons: First, the airway may be compromised, and second, the patient may be in intermaxillary fixation (teeth wired together or secured with elastics). OMFS postoperative complications fall into the following general categories:[5]

Intermaxillary fixation (teeth/jaws "wired" closed or secured with elastics):
- Airway concerns
- Emergency release of intermaxillary fixation for vomiting

Bleeding:
- After tooth extraction and alveolar bone surgery
  - After periodontal surgery
  - Postoperative midface osteotomy procedure

Swelling:
- Postextraction infection
  - Surgical edema and hematoma
  - Salivary gland obstruction
- Fracture of mandible during tooth extraction
- Sudden change in occlusion (bite)
- Office anesthesia complication
- Aspiration versus swallowed instrument, packing, or tooth

The three steps for initial evaluation are the following:

1. Ensure an adequate airway.
2. Control bleeding.
3. Obtain a history of the surgical procedure (what, when, and by whom).

After initial evaluation and stabilization, contact the treating OMF surgeon or the ear, nose, and throat (ENT) consultant.

INTERMAXILLARY FIXATION

Intermaxillary fixation (IMF) consists of tying the upper and lower teeth together with stainless steel wires or elastics. This is a common method of stabilizing the upper and lower jaws to allow for healing of jaw osteotomy procedures, jaw fractures, and jaw reconstruction procedures. Complications are rare, and the need to release the IMF on an emergency basis is infrequent. The critical reason to cut the fixation is vomiting. If release of IMF during the first 4 weeks after surgery is necessary, reoperation may be necessary or the surgical result will be compromised. The typical duration of this method of fixation is 4 to 8 weeks, during which time the patient must consume only liquids. Speech is usually difficult to understand, and most patients lose 10% to 20% of their weight while the jaws are wired together. If an acrylic surgical bite splint is interposed between the teeth, the oral airway can be greatly restricted. Edema can further restrict the oral airway. If, in addition to a restricted oral airway, the patient has a restricted nasal airway, then breathing becomes difficult. During the first 2 weeks after surgery when IMF is used and some surgical edema remains, some patients become anxious about breathing and adequate nutrition, and may present to the emergency department. Usually, reassurance and possibly a nasopharyngeal airway are all that are needed for treatment. Vomiting while in IMF is frightening to the patient but should not require release of IMF, unless the emesis cannot be cleared.

Release of IMF can be done on an emergency basis when access to the airway is mandatory. Examples of such situations are trauma, significant airway restriction due to acute infection or surgical edema, and a severe medical emergency, such as status epilepticus, septic shock, or cardiac arrest.

Release of IMF is accomplished by using small wire cutters to cut all the wires that cross from one dental arch to the other (all wires traversing from the upper teeth to the lower teeth). There may be three to eight wire loops (six to 16 wires) to cut. Occasionally, rubber bands are used to hold the teeth together, and these can be cut with a scalpel or scissors. Release of IMF with wires may be time consuming to those untrained in placing IMF. Consider emergency blind nasotracheal intubation or cricothyroidostomy in extremely acute situations. If wires are cut and not removed, small loose wires will remain in the mouth. All patients with IMF should have wire cutters or scissors with them.

MANAGEMENT

Evaluation and treatment involve the following:

1. Analyze blood gas levels or capnometry.
2. Monitor with a pulse oximeter.
3. Assess the work of breathing and the possibility of fatigue.
4. Consider a nasopharyngeal airway.
5. Release IMF in extreme cases by cutting the vertical wires between dental arches with wire cutters or by cutting the elastic bands with a scalpel or scissors.
6. Consider cricothyroidostomy or nasotracheal intubation when immediate airway access is necessary and no experienced person is available to release the wire IMF.

DISPOSITION

If the IMF needs to be cut, the OMFS or ENT consultant should be called immediately. Otherwise, discharge or admission of the patient is totally dependent on the presenting complaint.

COMMON PITFALLS

- Failure to recognize that the IMF can result in aspiration if the patient is unable to clear the airway by expelling vomitus between the teeth
- Being too quick to cut the IMF when doing so may not be necessary
- Hesitancy to cut the IMF when doing so is necessary
- Discharging the patient or sending the patient to the floor without a wire cutter or scissors and instructions as to when to cut the IMF

BLEEDING

Bleeding (from the mouth or nose, or both) is one of the more common postoperative complications. Normally, a small amount of bleeding mixes with saliva during the first 12 hours after many intraoral procedures. Significant hemorrhage must be differentiated from this type of bleeding. Problematic hemorrhage is usually apparent during an office procedure or within the first 12 hours. It is important to obtain a history of aspirin or nonsteroidal antiinflammatory drug (NSAID) use.

Prolonged bleeding from a simple tooth extraction in the absence of a coagulopathy is usually minor and can be controlled with oral gauze packs. For removal of lower wisdom teeth, the incidence of problem bleeding is 0.5% to 1.1% intraoperatively and 0.5% to 0.8% postoperatively.[6] Possible sources of bleeding include the extraction socket, inferior alveolar artery, posterior superior alveolar artery, long buccal artery, facial artery, palatine artery, lingual artery, and maxillary artery.

Bleeding after Tooth Extraction or Alveolar Bone Surgery

The most significant hemorrhage related to alveolar bone surgery in the mandible is from damage to the inferior alveolar neurovascular bundle that runs in a bony canal below the roots of the posterior teeth. Damage to this structure can occur during[4] surgical removal of teeth, odontogenic tumors, and cysts and the placement of endosseous dental implants.[4]

MANAGEMENT

1. Reassure the patient.
2. Keep the patient's head elevated 45 degrees.
3. In the case of postextraction bleeding, simply biting on gauze may not be sufficient to stop the bleeding. The gingiva around the extraction site should be infiltrated with 1% or 2% lidocaine with 1:50,000 or 1:100,000 epinephrine. The anesthesia helps the patient to bite with more force. The vasoconstrictor helps to decrease capillary oozing. If bleeding persists, the socket should be packed with Gelfoam, Surgicel, or Avitene. The packing usually must be secured with a black silk suture. If bleeding persists, see the following item (item 4).
4. Decide whether the bleeding is caused by an anatomic problem or by a coagulopathy, including excessive aspirin use.
5. Consider a hematocrit and coagulation screen, type and crossmatch, and intravenous fluids.
6. Consider OMFS or ENT consultation for persistent or severe hemorrhage for possible suturing, electrocautery, or extraoral cutdown on facial, lingual, or external carotid arteries. Emergency ligation of the external carotid artery is seldom necessary; local control is preferred.

Persistent Bleeding from Palate Secondary to Palatine Artery Injury

MANAGEMENT

1. Apply pressure to the bleeding site with 4×4-in. gauze packs. An assistant or the patient holds the packing by hand. Administration of a local anesthetic with a vasoconstrictor is again useful (see previous management section).
2. If bleeding continues after 30 to 60 minutes of pressure, the OMFS or ENT consultant will need to ligate or cauterize the artery.

Delayed Bleeding after Midface Osteotomy

Delayed bleeding after midface osteotomy involves bleeding from the nose and nasopharynx, or acute swelling of the upper cheeks (unilaterally or bilaterally) within 2 weeks after surgery. Many patients have a small amount of bleeding from the nose after midface osteotomy procedures (e.g., segmental osteotomy and Le Fort I, II, III) due to disruption of the nasal mucosa and pooling of blood in the maxillary sinuses. This minor nasal bleeding must be differentiated from significant hemorrhage. The incidence of severe postoperative bleeding after Le Fort I osteotomy is 0.75%.[1,3]

MANAGEMENT

1. Consider a balloon nasal pack as the first option in significant bleeding, because it simultaneously occludes the posterior, middle, and anterior nasal cavities.
2. Consider arteriography for significant bleeding to rule out an arteriovenous fistula or a pseudoaneurysm.
3. Hospital admission is probably necessary for observation, reoperation, or embolization.
4. Notify the OMFS or ENT surgeon immediately.

DISPOSITION

If bleeding can be controlled by the aforementioned measures, the patient can be safely discharged. In the case of postextraction bleeding, the patient needs to be instructed not to smoke, use straws, or spit. These actions all create a negative pressure in the mouth, which leads to clot dislodgment and rebleeding. Of course, the patient should be asked to refrain from aspirin- and NSAID-containing products. Persistent bleeding requires OMFS or ENT consultation.

COMMON PITFALLS

- Failure to follow a sequential approach to postoperative oral hemorrhage
- Failure to use local anesthesia and a vasoconstrictor for pain and hemorrhage control
- Ordering a coagulopathy workup before trying simple measures
- Failure to order a coagulopathy workup when simple measures fail
- Failure to obtain OMFS or ENT consultation when revision of the surgical area may be required for hemorrhage control

SWELLING

Patients may present with acute swelling after OMFS procedures because of concern over the airway or swallowing, or for an explanation. The swelling may be from a hematoma, surgical edema, acute cellulitis, or abscess.

Hematoma and Surgical Edema

Office procedures that may result in hematoma or surgical edema significant enough to warrant an emergency department visit are procedures in the floor of the mouth (e.g., excision of mandibular tori, excision of the sublingual gland, and removal of a stone from the salivary gland duct).

MANAGEMENT

1. The airway is the primary concern.
2. Have the patient sit up and lean forward.
3. Perform appropriate monitoring (e.g., pulse oximetry). Consider admission for observation.
4. With obvious airway compromise, consider the following interventions, in order of preference: insertion of a nasopharyngeal airway, oral or nasal endotracheal intubation, cricothyroidostomy, or tracheostomy.
5. Consider prophylactic antibiotics with both hematoma and surgical edema in the floor of the mouth to avoid development of a Ludwig's angina type of infection.

Postextraction Infection

A common reason for an emergency department visit is the rapid progression of an infection after removal of an impacted mandibular third molar (wisdom tooth). This can involve several tissue spaces, including the parapharyngeal space. Edema and infection in the masticator space cause trismus (limited mouth opening due to muscle spasm), making examination of the oropharynx difficult. The incidence of infection is 0.6% to 2.5%.[2]

MANAGEMENT

1. Obtain the patient's history: when and by whom the surgery was done, immunocompromise, preoperative infection and antibiotic use, current antibiotics.
2. Determine if there is significant limitation of mouth opening; examine the oropharynx for parapharyngeal swelling.
3. Check temperature and extent of swelling (e.g., whether it involves submandibular or submental spaces and extends across the midline). (See Chapter 18.)
4. If the airway is compromised, consider inserting a nasopharyngeal airway. Cricothyroidostomy or tracheostomy is seldom necessary but must be considered for severe cases. If a definitive airway is necessary, a nasoendotracheal intubation is attempted first if trismus is present.
5. Consider admission for intravenous antibiotics and surgical incision and drainage in the operating room. Consult the OMF or ENT surgeon.
6. If trismus and swelling are minimal, oral antibiotics and daily outpatient follow-up for 3 or 4 days are essential.

DISPOSITION

Disposition in the case of postoperative swelling or infection is based on the severity of the condition. Mild postoperative swelling that is not compromising the airway, and should not compromise the airway, can be managed on an outpatient basis. If there is any doubt, the OMFS or ENT consultant should see the patient. Some with postoperative infections can be managed as outpatients. However, because fascial planes of the head and neck can be violated during surgery, a very high index of suspicion is necessary for the potential for infection to spread.

COMMON PITFALLS

- Failure to recognize the potential for airway compromise from swelling or postoperative infection
- Failure to recognize the potential for the spread of infection through the fascial planes of the head and neck

Swelling of Salivary Glands Due to Obstruction of Ducts

Acute swelling of the submandibular gland(s) and, occasionally, the parotid can occur. Surgical edema or a suture obstructing the opening can result from intraoral surgery or placement of intraoral acrylic surgical stents. Swelling typically is mildly tender, without signs of infection. The patient may present hours to 3 days postoperatively.

MANAGEMENT

1. Examine the salivary ducts for any obstruction that can be eliminated (e.g., sutures or acrylic stents) and consult the OMF surgeon. If edema is the only cause of the obstruction, the swelling will resolve in 3 to 4 days.
2. Antibiotics may be important, especially if the surgery was for removal of a salivary duct stone that was causing chronic partial obstruction.

DISPOSITION

Patients with swelling secondary to a salivary gland or salivary duct obstruction can generally be discharged for follow-up the next day. Analgesia and antibiotics are important. The patient should refrain from eating sour foods.

COMMON PITFALLS

- Failure to recognize mechanical obstruction of a duct that should be relieved.
- Failure to treat for infection due to the stasis of saliva.

Fracture of the Mandible from Extraction of Teeth

Fracture of the mandible typically results from removal of impacted lower wisdom teeth.

MANAGEMENT

1. Evaluation and treatment are the same as for any jaw fracture.
2. Application of a Barton's bandage to immobilize the jaw (Fig. 16.1) is seldom necessary, as prompt OMFS or ENT consultation is required.

Sudden Change in Occlusion

A sudden change in occlusion (bite) during the postoperative period (after jaw osteotomy, fracture repair, or mandibular reconstruction in which rigid internal fixation was used without IMF) can occur due to failure of the internal fixation. Failure of external fixation devices (transcutaneous pins and bars) is readily apparent. The patient will present with a malocclusion (shifting of the bite) that occurred suddenly. There may be mild-to-moderate pain aggravated by jaw movement.

MANAGEMENT

1. Evaluation is the same as for fractures of the mandible. Treatment is usually reoperation, although emergency admission is typically unnecessary.

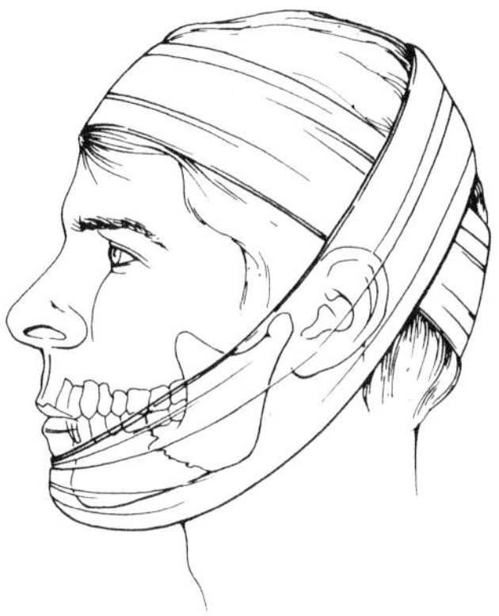

Figure 16.1. Barton's bandage.

2. Notify the OMF surgeon: It may be desirable to stabilize the mandible immediately by IMF.

DISPOSITION

A fracture of the jaw secondary to an extraction or the disruption of occlusion is a major problem. The OMFS or ENT consultant should be notified immediately. Nondisplaced jaw fractures can be treated with antibiotics, analgesia, soft diet, and referral to the office the next day. Such fractures are normally treated with IMF that is placed in the office. Displaced fractures require immediate consultation and admission. Disruption of IMF and the occlusion may require reoperation.

COMMON PITFALLS

- Failure to consider jaw fracture as an etiology of postextraction pain
- Failure to place a patient with a jaw fracture on antibiotics
- Failure to recognize the clinical significance of a displaced occlusion
- Failure to consult the OMFS or ENT

Complications from Outpatient Sedation and Anesthesia

Drugs used for office sedation are narcotics, benzodiazepines, barbiturates, and occasionally ketamine. A patient may be transported to the emergency department from a doctor's office because of complications related to such sedation. The most frequent event is loss of an adequate airway, or prolonged hypoventilation, which leads to cardiovascular complications.

MANAGEMENT

Complications from outpatient office sedation are treated according to the patient's condition.

Aspiration or Swallowed Foreign Bodies

Teeth, dental restorations, bone, drill bit, packing, or dental instruments may all be swallowed or aspirated. Usually, the situation is not life-threatening. Evaluation includes the probable location of the object and whether arrangements need to be made to remove it. Packing aspiration is the most serious, as it can drape over the carina.

MANAGEMENT

1. Obtain a description of the object and the events surrounding the aspiration or swallowing.
2. Order a chest x-ray or abdominal radiograph to determine whether the object is in the lungs, stomach, or bowel.
3. Consider a pulmonary or gastrointestinal consult to remove the object by flexible fiberoptic endoscopy. Small, blunt objects may be allowed to pass, without intervention, through the gastrointestinal tract. Sharp or pointed objects in the gastrointestinal tract and objects in the lungs should be removed as quickly as possible.
4. Deeply aspirated packing at the level of the carina is devastating, because both bronchi may be obstructed.

DISPOSITION

Aspirated foreign bodies that appear to be in the gastrointestinal tract can generally be managed on an outpatient basis if there is no potential for perforation. If the potential for perforation exists, the gastrointestinal endoscopist should be called. Tracheobronchial aspiration requires immediate pulmonary consultation.

COMMON PITFALLS

- Failure to recognize tracheobronchial aspiration
- Failure to summon immediate assistance if deep aspiration of a pack below the cords and above the carina is suspected

ACKNOWLEDGMENT

The author gratefully acknowledges the contribution of R. Gregory Smith who wrote the previous version of this chapter.

References

1. Lanigan DT, West RA. Management of postoperative hemorrhage following the Le Fort I maxillary osteotomy. *J Oral Maxillofac Surg* 1984;42:367.
2. Lanigan DT, Hey JH, West RA. Aseptic necrosis following maxillary osteotomies: report of 36 cases. *J Oral Maxillofac Surg* 1990;48:142.
3. Lanigan DT, Hey JH, West RA. Major vascular complications of orthognathic surgery: hemorrhage associated with LeFort I osteotomies. *J Oral Maxillofac Surg* 1990;48:561.
4. Lanigan DT, Hey JH, West RA. Hemorrhage following mandibular osteotomies: a report of 21 cases. *J Oral Maxillofac Surg* 1991;49:713.
5. Peterson LJ. Prevention and management of surgical complications. In: Peterson LJ, Ellis E, Hupp JR, et al., eds. *Contemporary oral and maxillofacial surgery*. St. Louis: Mosby, 1988.
6. Sisk AL, Hammer WB, Shelton DW, et al. Complications after removal of impacted third molars. *J Oral Maxillofac Surg* 1986;44:855.

CHAPTER 17
Temporomandibular Joint Disease

Barry H. Hendler

TEMPOROMANDIBULAR SYNDROME

The temporomandibular joint (TMJ) consists of the mandibular condyle (the posterior extension of the mandible covered by the meniscus or articular disk) that articulates in the temporal fossa. The temporal fossa is bordered anteriorly by the articular eminence. When the mandible closes, the condyle moves posteriorly and superiorly in the temporal fossa. Therefore, on opening, the condyle moves anteriorly and inferiorly, guided by the articular eminence.

Temporomandibular myofascial pain dysfunction syndrome, or simply TMJ syndrome, is a complex neuromuscular disturbance, possibly resulting from and definitely aggravated by occlusal disturbances and the anatomy of the TMJ. Other entities, such as trauma, psychological tension, and neuromuscular habits (e.g., bruxism and clenching), contribute to the problem. Patients who present to the emergency department frequently complain of nonspecific unilateral facial pain generalized to the region of the TMJ. The pain is dull, and increases throughout the day with continued jaw motion. Clinical examination frequently reveals spasm of the masseter muscle externally and the internal pterygoid intraorally. There is usually limitation of opening, with deviation toward the affected side. TMJ x-rays are usually normal unless there is associated temporomandibular degenerative joint disease (osteoarthritis).

CLINICAL PRESENTATION

The term *internal derangement* of the TMJ alludes to any disturbance between the articular components within the joint. It implies a localized structural derangement that interferes with the smooth function of the joint. It has recently been applied primarily to changes in the disk–condyle relation, with the disk most commonly displaced in an anteromedial direction. Internal derangement also produces pain or functional disturbance in the masticatory system and is often a result of TMJ neuromuscular dysfunction. The patient should be questioned about the presence or history of joint noises. Patients with internal derangement almost always have or have had joint noises. The noise is usually described as either clicking or crepitus. Crepitus is considered to represent advanced disease and occurs as a result of movement across irregular surfaces. This may also indicate a perforation of the disk or its attachments. This is especially true when degenerative changes are observed on radiographs.

Typically, the patient with internal derangement reports a clicking TMJ followed by a period of no joint noise. When the disk is anteriorly displaced and does not reduce to a normal position during opening, the patient will have limited opening, or a "closed-lock" condition. This condition may be either intermittent or persistent. The emergency physician should measure the interincisal maximum opening, which is usually limited to 20 mm (normal, 35 to 50 mm).

Arthritic TMJ may present with pain and crepitation. There may be periods of pain exacerbation and remission. As in other arthritides, there is often morning stiffness that wears off with function during the day, as opposed to the TMJ syndrome, which worsens as the day progresses.

RADIOGRAPHIC STUDIES

Routine radiographic evaluation of the TMJ should include a panoramic view, which is the easiest to read and requires the least sophisticated technique. The emergency physician can also order a TMJ series or tomograms of the joints, taken in both open and closed positions. Tomograms avoid superimposition of other anatomic structures that make a regular TMJ series difficult to read. The panoramic survey and tomograms are necessary to distinguish arthritis, TMJ pain dysfunction syndrome, or internal derangement. Degenerative joint disease (osteoarthritis) may involve one or both of the TMJs. Films may demonstrate flattening of the condylar head, erosions, or osteophyte formation. Rheumatoid arthritis should also be considered, but a good history should clarify the diagnosis. When any type of internal derangement is suspected, a computed tomography scan of the joints should be ordered to assess bony architecture (i.e., arthritis). Magnetic resonance imaging is essential to assess disk position; arthrography can be used to assess disk perforation.

DIFFERENTIAL DIAGNOSIS

When the diagnosis of TMJ dysfunction is considered, the emergency physician should rule out pain of odontogenic origin. Tooth pain or sore teeth, in the absence of odontogenic pathology, may indicate bruxism. Headaches are a common complaint of patients with a TMJ disorder. Patients with an internal derangement frequently complain of headaches on the affected side, but no specific diagnostic pattern has been documented. Because headaches are such a common complaint, one should not assume that an internal derangement is the cause unless more specific diagnostic evidence is present. Headaches associated with internal derangement frequently emanate from the TMJ and radiate to temporal-orbital-occipital areas. This frequently follows jaw function and may be relieved with an occlusal splint or other therapies directed toward internal derangement.

Earache is a common complaint. Tinnitus and occasional dizziness may also be noted. Ear pathology should be considered and ruled out before assuming that an earache is due to TMJ disease.

Neck ache and shoulder pain are often reported by patients with TMJ disorders. These complaints are not specifically diagnostic, but may reflect a more generalized muscle disorder. In general, all pain is exacerbated by chewing.

MANAGEMENT AND DISPOSITION

TMJ pain or dysfunction, regardless of cause, is treated initially by a combination of physiotherapy (moist heat for 15 minutes four times a day) and a soft diet for 2 weeks. Analgesics such as nonsteroidal antiinflammatory agents or aspirin–codeine combinations are effective in addition to muscle relaxants and tranquilizers such as diazepam. Bite plates (occlusal splints) are used to reposition the mandible to relieve spasm, correct oral habits, and "recapture" a displaced disk.

A documented internal derangement is usually referred to an oral and maxillofacial surgeon, who may perform arthroscopy or arthroplasty to correct disk position permanently or to reconstruct arthritic joints.

COMMON PITFALLS

- TMJ dysfunction is often called the "great impostor" because it mimics so many other facial pain syndromes.
- The physician who fails to understand disk displacement may confuse it with muscle spasm. A history of joint noise is critical in this regard.

TEMPOROMANDIBULAR JOINT DISLOCATION

In acute dislocation of the mandible, the condyle moves too far anteriorly in relation to the eminence and becomes locked. The

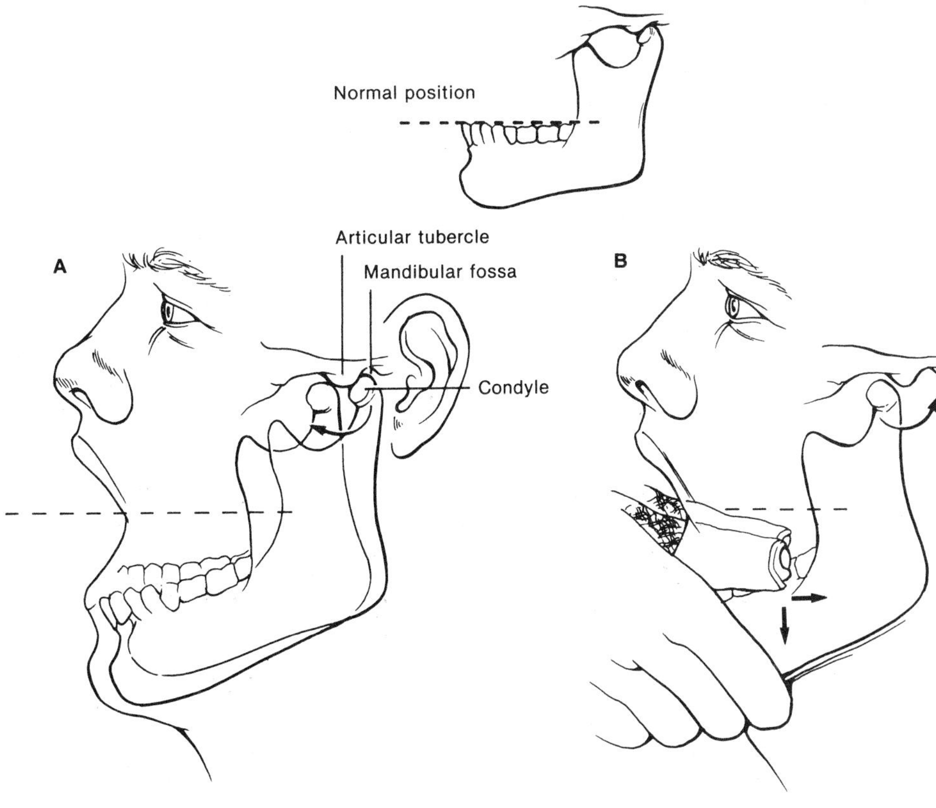

Figure 17.1. **(A)** Temporomandibular joint dislocation and **(B)** reduction.

mouth is in open position as opposed to "closed-lock" position (Fig. 17.1). Subsequent muscular trismus prevents the condyles from moving back into the temporal fossa. The spasm of the external pterygoid, masseter, and internal pterygoid muscles, and associated edema, result in extreme discomfort and anxiety. Predisposing factors include anatomic disharmony between the fossa and the anterior articular eminence, weakness of the capsule forming the TMJ ligaments, and torn ligaments. Dislocation is likely to occur during maximum opening (yawning or laughing). Although the TMJ is a double joint, the dislocation may be bilateral or unilateral. Palpation of the TMJs may reveal them to be anterior to the articular eminence. Radiographs should be taken to rule out a fracture, as the clinical picture and occlusal disturbances of both fracture and dislocation are similar.

An understanding of TMJ anatomy is important for proper manual reduction. It may be helpful to relieve the patient's anxiety and intense muscle spasm with intravenous diazepam, 5 to 10 mg, titrated by slow injection. When the patient is sufficiently relaxed, the physician should face the patient and grasp the mandible with both hands, one hand on each side, with the thumbs (wrapped with gauze) placed on the occlusal surfaces of the posterior teeth (see Fig. 17.1). The fingertips are placed around the inferior border of the mandible in the region of the angle. Downward pressure is applied to free the condyles from their position anterior to the eminence. The chin is then pressed backward after the jaw has been forced downward. The mouth closes and the condyle returns to its position in the fossa. Because of severe muscle spasm, the jaw may snap back quickly, so the physician must be aware.

Postreduction instructions include a soft diet for 1 to 2 weeks, avoidance of wide opening of the mandible, and the use of analgesics and muscle relaxants. Patients who chronically dislocate the TMJ and those who suffer acute recurrences may be helped by a Barton bandage (see Chapter 16) or elastic and Velcro jaw "bra" applied around the head to prevent maximum opening for 2 weeks, but this is seldom done. Severe cases may require intermaxillary wiring and fixation for added control. Patients who have suffered dislocation of the TMJ should be referred to an oral and maxillofacial surgeon for follow-up because surgical alteration of the eminence may be necessary.

Bibliography

Bronstein SL, Tomasetti BJ, Ryan DE. Internal derangements of the TMJ: correlation of arthrography with surgical findings. *J Oral Surg* 1981;39:572.

Chase DC, Dolwick MF, Hendler BH, et al. TMJ disorders—diagnosis. *Patient Care* 1983;17:21.

Chase DC, Dolwick MF, Hendler BH, et al. TMJ disorders—treatment. *Patient Care* 1984;18:1.

Kaplan A. *Temporomandibular disorders.* Philadelphia: WB Saunders, 1991.

Laskin D. Medical management of TMJ disorders. *Oral Maxillofac Surg Clin North Am* 1995;7:?.

Swartz JD, Hendler BH. High-resolution CT in evaluation of TMJ disease. *Head Neck Surg* 1985;7:409.

Taro A. *TMJ arthroscopy: a diagnostic and surgical atlas.* Philadelphia: JB Lippincott Co, 1993.

CHAPTER 18
Dental, Oral, and Salivary Gland Infections

James T. Amsterdam

The presentation of dental, oral, and salivary gland infections in the emergency department can vary from a patient with a simple complaint of pain or gingival swelling to a toxic patient with massive facial swelling and a compromised airway. Variable factors include the origin and location of the infection and the degree to which the infection has been contained or has spread to the deep spaces of the head and neck. The most common focus of infection is odontogenic, in addition to exposure to trauma or surgery that may violate the natural anatomic barriers of the fascial planes of the head and neck, resulting in deep-space infection.[2,3,10,11]

The key to diagnosis and management of dental infections and space infections of the head and neck is an understanding of the fascial planes of the head and neck (Fig. 18.1). Cellulitis of odontogenic origin usually involves the middle and lower part of the face and neck. Although such infections are generally well contained, in a debilitated host or in the case of a virulent organism, rapid spread of infection may be fatal.[1,3–5,7–9]

The fascial spaces of the head and neck are potential spaces filled with loose areolar tissue that can rapidly break down when subjected to infection. In the case of oral infection, the deep cervical fascia is the most important. The deep cervical fascia consists of several layers that surround the neck, including the superficial and investing layer that attaches to the inferior border of the mandible and splits to form the masticator space. Other important spaces include the lateral pharyngeal space (lateral to the pharynx and medial to the masticator space), the retropharyngeal space (between the deep cervical and prevertebral fascia), and the pharyngomaxillary space (from the base of the skull to the hyoid bone), which communicates with all deep spaces (see Fig. 18.1).[1,3,13–15]

The mylohyoid muscle of the mandible divides the sublingual (superior) and submaxillary (inferior) spaces. The submental space is anterior to the sublingual space. Infection involving the submaxillary, sublingual, and submental spaces with elevation of the tongue is called *Ludwig's angina*, a serious infection with a potential for airway obstruction (Fig. 18.2).[1,3,10,12]

Infections that affect the midface involve the canine space, which is commonly infected by abscessed anterior maxillary teeth, and the buccal space, which is superficial to the buccinator and frequently infected by the molar teeth. Infections in these areas are especially important because of the possibility of cavernous sinus thrombosis due to the fascial venous system.[6]

DIFFERENTIAL DIAGNOSIS

Before attributing any swelling of the face or the head and neck to dental infection, other entities should be considered. Tumors may present as nonspecific swellings and may be hard to distinguish from advanced primary infections if secondary infection is present. Viral infections, especially those that involve the salivary glands (e.g., mumps), can present as swellings. Less com-

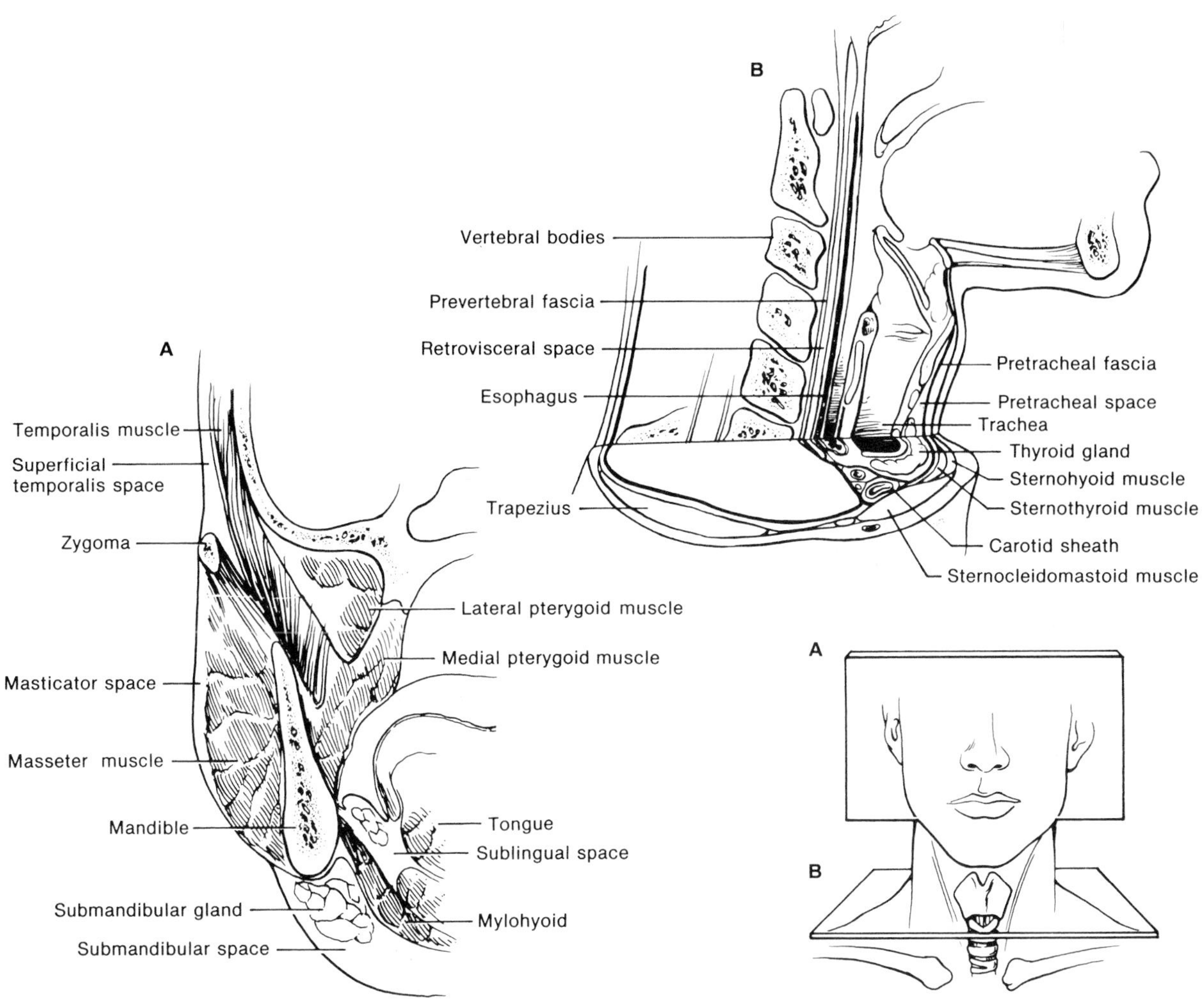

Figure 18.1. Fascial planes of the head and neck. **(A)** Coronal section of the head. **(B)** Cross section of the fascial planes of the neck.

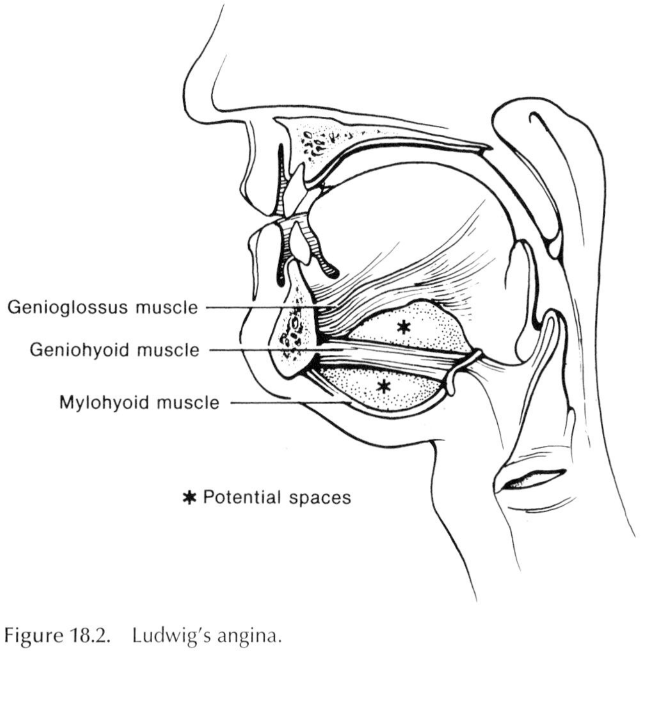

Figure 18.2. Ludwig's angina.

mon infections are scrofula (tuberculous cervical lymphadenitis) and actinomycosis. Failure to respond to conventional therapy should lead the clinician to suspect some complication (tumor or uncommon infection). Certain fungal infections, although rare, are more common in the head and neck regions, such as mucormycosis. Fungal infections should be considered in immunocompromised patients, such as those with diabetes or the human immunodeficiency virus (HIV).[3]

Submaxillary and parotid gland disease is not uncommon. These patients have a history of increasing pain when eating, and they are especially affected by sour foods. Submandibular gland infection is generally caused by *Streptococcus* secondary to stasis of saliva from obstruction caused by a stone. *Staphylococcus* is more commonly involved in parotid gland infections. Infectious parotitis is seen in the elderly and especially in diabetics. This entity is usually bilateral and associated with fever and toxicity. Autoimmune diseases, such as Sjögren syndrome and Mikulicz disease, can also cause facial swelling due to enlargement of the salivary glands (Figs. 18.3 and 18.4).[3]

EMERGENCY DEPARTMENT MANAGEMENT

Initial management of oral, dental, and salivary gland infections begins with localization of the infection. Most infections are of odontogenic origin and localized to a specific tooth. Patients with dental pain should be examined for the presence of infec-

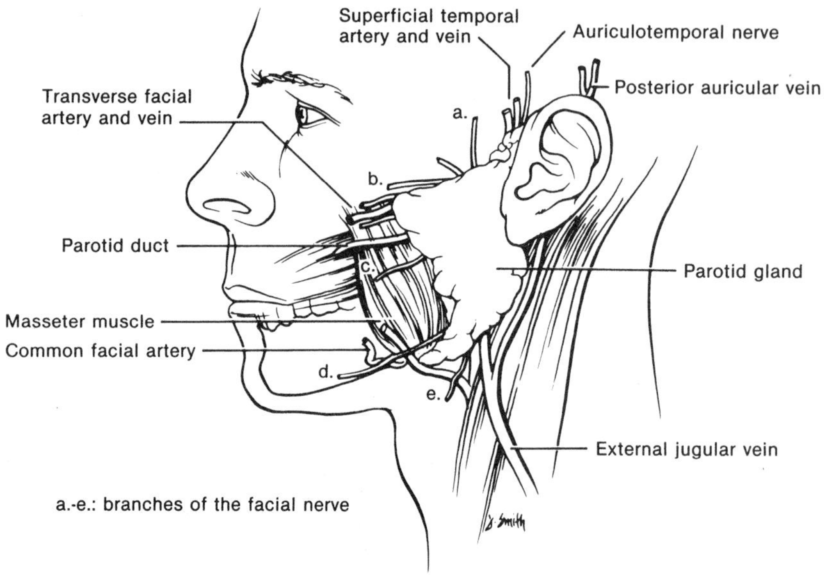

Figure 18.3. Normal anatomy of the parotid gland.

tion. Pain to percussion with a tongue blade indicates involvement at the apex of the tooth (periapical abscess). Tender swelling over the gingiva adjacent to a tooth may indicate either a periodontal abscess or extension of a periapical abscess through the cortex of bone into the subperiosteal space. Differentiating these entities without a dental radiograph can be difficult. Management in either case would consist of a conservative incision, drainage, and antibiotic therapy (phenoxymethyl penicillin or erythromycin 250 mg four times a day).[1,5]

A fluctuant abscess requires drainage, because antibiotics are no cure for pus. The gingiva should be anesthetized superficially with 2% lidocaine/1:100,000 epinephrine. A stab incision is made toward the alveolar bone and must extend through the periosteum if no pus is initially encountered; blunt dissection is performed with a mosquito hemostat. The area is irrigated, and, if there is room, a Penrose or iodoform drain can be placed. The drain should be secured with a black silk suture. In the case of these localized infections, there is no need to open the abscess beyond a stab incision. The drain will allow for continued drainage and the source of the infection will be eliminated with extraction of the tooth, root canal (endodontic) therapy, or periodontal therapy.[4]

The presence of cellulitis indicates that there has been spread of infection. The emergency physician must then determine the following: (1) the extent of involvement of contiguous spaces, (2) the potential for spread of infection to the fascial planes of the head and neck, and (3) potential for airway compromise. Once extensive involvement is recognized, it is the role of the oral and maxillofacial surgeon to compartmentalize the spread of infection and determine the site of the initial focus, so that pus can be evacuated under controlled conditions in the operating room.[1]

Table 18.1 summarizes the essential features of odontogenic and parapharyngeal space infections.

The presence of more serious infections is determined by common physical signs and symptoms. After 3 to 5 days, clinical signs are usually apparent. Fever is present. Any involvement of the internal pterygoid or the masseter muscle will result in trismus (muscle spasm causing inability to open the mandible). The presence of trismus limits visibility of the oropharynx and makes the clinical diagnosis of retropharyngeal involvement difficult. If a toxic patient with trismus should vomit, the danger of aspiration is high because the emesis cannot be quickly evacuated. Therefore, patients with severe trismus need an aggressive workup (including a computed tomography scan of the retropharyngeal space) and admission for hydration and parenteral antibiotics. The oral cavity may be visualized under general anesthesia at the time of incision and drainage. The presence of Ludwig's angina requires aggressive attention to the airway. This may include nasoendotracheal intubation, tracheostomy, or observation in an intensive care environment where such procedures can be rapidly undertaken.[1,3]

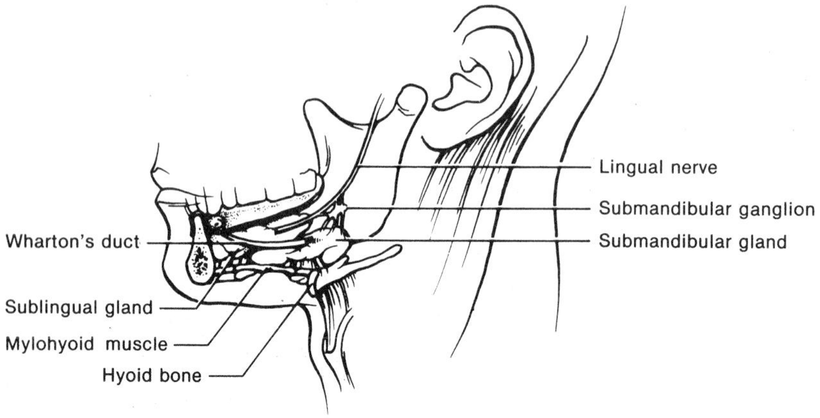

Figure 18.4. Normal anatomy of the submandibular gland.

TABLE 18.1. Essential Features of Odontogenic and Parapharyngeal Space Infections

Fascial Space Anatomic Area	Pathophysiology	Clinical Presentation	Diagnosis/ Treatment	Disposition	Pitfalls
Periapical abscess	Local confinement may occur, or extension through cortex	Acute or chronic odontalgia Pain with percussion No visible swelling	Periapical lucency on Panorex; analgesics/ABX	Dental referral	Consider extension to deeper space
Subperiosteal	Contained by periosteum of local alveolar bone	Vestibular, palatal, or sublingual swelling/ fluctuance	Stab incision to alveolar bone, irrigation ± drain, analgesics/ABX	Dental/oral surgery f/u 24–48 h	Failure to penetrate periosteum with incision; failure to avoid palatine vessels; failure to provide SBE prophylaxis, if indicated
Canine space	Anterior maxillary teeth origin with perforation above levator oris m.	Obliteration of nasolabial groove; may spontaneously drain near medial canthus	Analgesics/ABX; needle aspiration if unsure of abscess (intraoral approach)	OMFS consult if fluctuant/extensive; 24 h f/u for local cellulitis	May produce periorbital cellulitis if untreated; patient must return if eye closes
Buccal space	Premolar/molar teeth origin with perforation beyond buccinator m.	Massive cheek swelling	Analgesics/ABX; fluctuance usually easy to palpate	OMFS consult for abscess drainage; 24 h f/u for cellulitis	May be confused with erysipelas; in child, consider buccal cellulitis *(H. influenzae)*
Masticator spaces: Submasseteric Pterygomandib-ular Temporal	Mandibular molar origin. These 3 spaces freely communicate and are bound by fascia around the muscles of mastication.	Trismus is the clinical hallmark. Extraoral swelling may be absent with deep temporal or pterygomandibular space infection.	Patients often dehydrated → may require fluid resuscitation; CT scan may confirm diagnosis.	OMFS consult; hospitalize for trismus, toxicity, or severe dehydration	Failure to document trismus (<1 cm intercanine opening); pterygomandib-ular space swelling may mimic a peritonsillar abscess
Sublingual space	Anterior mandibular teeth with perforation above the mylohyoid line; communicates posteriorly with submandibular space	Sublingual edema, ± tongue elevation; minimal extraoral swelling; often crosses midline with bilateral swelling	Airway assessment; i.v. antibiotics; fluid resuscitation if dehydrated	OMFS consult; strongly consider hospitalization unless well localized with close f/u	Failure to recognize threat to airway; failure to involve consultant early
Submandibular space	Mandibular molar origin with perforation below the mylohyoid line; communicates anteriorly with submental and posteriorly with sublingual spaces	Prominent extraoral swelling beneath the mandible	Airway assessment; i.v. antibiotics	OMFS consult; see "sublingual"	Often the precursor of Ludwig's angina
Submental space	Anterior mandibular teeth with perforation below the mentalis m.	Prominent chin swelling extending back to the hyoid bone	Airway, i.v. antibiotics	OMFS consult; see "sublingual"	Communication with submandibular space may lead to Ludwig's angina.
Ludwig's angina	Bilateral sublingual, submandibular, and submental space involvement	"Brawny edema" of the neck; upper airway obstruction with stridor	Airway stabilization; broad-spectrum antibiotics	Immediate OMFS or ENT consult; prepare for OR	Failure to be prepared for a surgical airway; almost 100% mortality if untreated (most from airway compromise)

(continued)

TABLE 18.1. *(Continued)*

Fascial Space Anatomic Area	Pathophysiology	Clinical Presentation	Diagnosis/ Treatment	Disposition	Pitfalls
Parapharyngeal infections: Lateral space and retropharyngeal space	Multiple etiologies: Odontogenic, tonsillitis, pharyngitis, foreign body	Pharyngeal bulging, dysphagia, trismus; posterior compartment of lateral space may not produce intraoral swelling; nuchal rigidity with prevertebral involvement	CT scan defines location and extent of abscess; lateral neck x-ray may show retropharyngeal abscess	OMFS consult (if felt odontogenic); ENT consult for peritonsillar or pharyngeal origin	Differentiating from peritonsillar abscess may be quite difficult
Mediastinitis	Two routes of spread: deep cervical planes, carotid sheath	Chest pain, severe dyspnea, systemic toxicity	Mainly clinical Dx; widened mediastinum on CXR possible	Intravenous antibiotics; hospitalize	Failure to consider Dx, even when odontogenic source may have cleared
Cavernous sinus thrombosis	Thrombophlebitis or septic emboli spread via facial veins	Ocular pain, orbital edema, retinal hemorrhages early; CN III, IV, V, VI deficits; commonly spreads to contralateral side	Usually dramatic findings; CT scan or MRI may confirm Dx	Hospitalize	Failure to consider Dx

ABX, antibiotics; DX, diagnosis; f/u, follow-up; m., muscle; OMFS, oral/maxillofacial surgeon; CT, computed tomography; i.v., intravenous; ENT, ear, nose, and throat; OR, operating room; CN, cranial nerve; MRI, magnetic resonance imaging.

Odontogenic infections are caused by oral flora; in the absence of deeper spread, appropriate antibiotic coverage includes penicillin or clindamycin. Penicillin is the antibiotic of choice for the treatment of most orofacial infections, with the exception of some *Bacteroides* species. High-dose penicillin G (12 million U/d) is required for Ludwig's angina. Second- or third-generation cephalosporins are useful in cases that involve *Bacteroides* or penicillin allergy, although cross-over sensitivity must be considered. Ampicillin/sulbactam (Unasyn) also provides excellent anaerobic coverage. Clindamycin is a useful alternative, but potential side effects should be monitored, especially when oral therapy is initiated. Erythromycin is also a useful alternative to penicillin, but it is more difficult to administer intravenously. Chloramphenicol is reserved for extreme situations in which there is no alternative therapy.[1,3,7]

Failure of an oral infection to respond within 24 hours of penicillin therapy suggests infection with an anaerobic bacteria (*Bacteroides fragilis*).

Parapharyngeal space infections (sublingual, submandibular, submaxillary, lateral pharyngeal, retropharyngeal, and pretracheal) are polymicrobial. Appropriate antibiotic therapy includes penicillin G (high-dose) and metronidazole or cefoxitin. Alternative therapy may include clindamycin or ticarcillin/clavulanate (Timentin).

DISPOSITION

Role of the Consultant

Patients with a simple periapical abscess can be managed with the institution of intraoral saline rinses, analgesia, and oral antibiotics. As discussed, a simple incision and drainage may be indicated. Follow-up should be arranged the next day with the oral and maxillofacial surgeon or the family dentist.[1,4]

Indications for Admission

All patients with suspicion of extension of infection to the fascial spaces of the head and neck should be admitted. Facial cellulitis with closure of the eye indicates potential spread of infection to the periorbital spaces and increased potential for cavernous sinus thrombosis. Patients with extensive trismus cannot be adequately evaluated by clinical examination. Patients with Ludwig's angina or impending Ludwig's angina (i.e., involvement of the three spaces without elevation of the tongue) are at risk for immediate airway obstruction and should be admitted. Such airway obstruction can occur precipitously and without warning, so anticipation is necessary. In most cases, the patient is admitted to the oral and maxillofacial surgeon. When the cause of the infection is unclear, the patient may be managed by an otorhinolaryngologist. Many cases are managed jointly by both services.

Transfer Considerations

If the initial receiving hospital has no surgical backup in the area of the head and neck, the patient should be transferred expeditiously to an appropriate facility. Blood cultures should be obtained and antibiotics instituted after consultation with the receiving physician. Special attention should be given to the airway. Advanced life-support personnel should be used. In the case of Ludwig's angina, it may be necessary to establish a definite airway before transfer in order to adequately stabilize the patient.

COMMON PITFALLS

- All patients with complaints of orofacial pain or swelling must be carefully examined for the presence of infection and extension of infection from the initial focus.
- The emergency physician should aggressively manage a patient in whom infection may be extending or has a high probability of extending. This is especially important if the infection has the potential to spread to the mediastinum or involve the airway, both of which can be fatal.
- Many patients fear dentists and, when sent home, return only when the situation is far advanced. Follow-up should always be recommended within 12 to 24 hours, and the patient should always be encouraged to return to the emer-

gency department in the case of high fever, increasing swelling, inability to open the mouth, difficulty swallowing, or inability to open the eye.

ACKNOWLEDGMENT

The author gratefully acknowledges the contribution of Byron Thompson who wrote the previous version of this chapter.

References

1. Amsterdam JT. Dental emergencies. In: Rosen P, et al., eds. *Emergency medicine: concepts and clinical practice,* 4th ed. St. Louis: CV Mosby, 1998.
2. Amsterdam JT. Dental caries. In: Honigman B, ed. *Emergindex.* Denver: Emergency Information Center, 1993.
3. Amsterdam JT, Hendler BH. Deep space infections of the head and neck. In: Callaham ML, ed. *Current practice of emergency medicine,* 2nd ed. Philadelphia: BC Decker, 1991.
4. Amsterdam JT. Emergency dental procedures. In: Roberts J, Hedges J, eds. *Clinical procedures in emergency medicine,* 3rd ed. Philadelphia: WB Saunders, 1998.
5. Amsterdam JT, Hendler BH, Rose LF. Dental emergencies. In: Schwartz G, et al., eds. *Principles and practice of emergency medicine,* 2nd ed. Philadelphia: WB Saunders, 1986.
6. Dice WH, Pryor GJ, Kilpatrick WR. Facial cellulitis following dental injury in a child. *Ann Emerg Med* 1985;11:541.
7. Hendler BH. Maxillofacial fractures. In: Tintinalli JE, Ruiz E, Krome R, et al., eds. *Emergency medicine—a comprehensive study guide,* 4th ed, chapter 204. New York: McGraw-Hill, 1996.
8. Hendler BH, Amsterdam JT. Infection of dental origin. *Curr Top Emerg Med* 1981;2:1.
9. Hendler BH, Quinn PD. Fatal mediastinitis secondary to odontogenic infection. *J Oral Surg* 1978;36:308.
10. Kruger GO. *Textbook of oral and maxillofacial surgery,* 5th ed. St. Louis: CV Mosby, 1979.
11. Osbon DB. Facial trauma. In: Irby WB, ed. *Current advances in oral surgery.* St. Louis: CV Mosby, 1965.
12. Rose LF, Hendler BH, Amsterdam JT. Temporomandibular disorders and odontic infections. *Consultant* 1982;22:110.
13. Sicher H. *The propagation of dental infections in oral anatomy.* St. Louis: CV Mosby, 1965.
14. Solinitsky U. The fascial compartments of the head and neck in relation to dental infections. *Bull Georgetown U Med Center* 1954;7:86.
15. Thoma KH. *Oral surgery,* 5th ed. St. Louis: CV Mosby, 1969.

PART III

Emergency Aspects of Otolaryngology

CHAPTER 19

Adult Epiglottitis

Michael F. Murphy and Blaine A. Kent

The evaluation and management of epiglottitis requires clinical acumen, preplanning, teamwork, and therapeutic expertise to avert tragedy.

Scrutiny of the events surrounding the death of George Washington in 1799 suggests the diagnosis of epiglottitis, although, at the time, his death was attributed to quinsy. Clinical descriptions of epiglottitis appeared in the eighteenth century,[13] and the condition was more accurately defined in the early part of the twentieth century.[13,24] In the late 1930s and early 1940s, a precise clinicopathologic and bacteriologic definition was achieved, although subsequent clinical data implicated epiglottitis as a disease of childhood only. However, ample evidence currently supports an adult form of epiglottitis.[13,16]

Available demographic data demonstrate that epiglottitis occurs in adults of all ages.[3,15,16] It does not appear to have a predilection for season or race, but there is a preponderance of male patients.[6,11,21] The true incidence of epiglottitis is difficult to ascertain because the index of suspicion for the diagnosis varies among clinicians.[2] The incidence is estimated to be in the vicinity of 1 to 4 per 100,000 adults per year.[3,11,21] The causes of epiglottitis include infection, trauma, burns, and some medical disorders.

PATHOPHYSIOLOGY

Inflammatory disorders of the laryngeal region may affect either supraglottic structures (supraglottitis, epiglottitis) or infraglottic structures (laryngotracheitis). Strictly speaking, the term *supraglottitis* more appropriately defines the condition[2] because the pathologic changes involve not only the epiglottis, but also the aryepiglottic folds and false cords. However, tradition persists with the terminology of *epiglottitis*.

The larynx serves several purposes: It connects the hypopharynx with the trachea, maintaining airway patency; it serves as a valve to protect the airway during swallowing; and it allows for vocalization (Fig. 19.1). The supraglottic area is set obliquely down and back and is bounded anteriorly by the epiglottis, laterally by the aryepiglottic folds and posteriorly by the interarytenoid fold. The mucosa of the supraglottic area is continuous with that of the hypopharynx above and the larynx and trachea below (Fig. 19.2). The glossopharyngeal nerve provides sensory innervation on pharyngeal surfaces of the larynx. The laryngeal surface is supplied by the superior laryngeal branch of the vagus, which is also the major motor nerve to the intrinsic laryngeal musculature. Some authors believe that this functional relation explains laryngospasm and the exuberant autonomic activity associated with stimulation of the laryngeal surface of the epiglottis during laryngoscopy.

The pathologic picture varies according to the causative agent and the extent of the process. The gross findings vary from slight erythema and edema of an isolated portion of the supraglottis to global involvement with intense inflammation, edema, and airway obliteration.[21] Microscopic examination reveals superficial and deep ulceration of the epithelium. Polymorphonuclear leukocyte infiltration is intense, and microabscess formation may be noted. Necrosis of vascular walls, smooth muscle, and apocrine glands is present. Edema on the lingual surface of the epiglottis may be minimal because the mucosa adheres to the cartilage. Elsewhere, no such limiting feature exists, and the mucosa is free to swell. Inferiorly, the limit of edema is the vocal cords, where the mucosa is tightly adherent.

The precise pathophysiology of total airway obstruction is not well defined, but numerous factors are involved: mucosal edema; aspiration of secretions, leading to laryngospasm of the inflamed, hyperesthetic larynx; inspissation of secretions; and

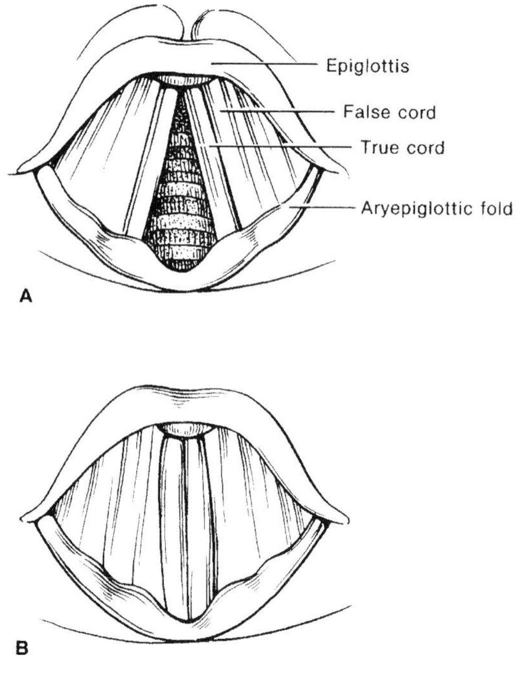

Figure 19.1. **(A)** Larynx in respiration. **(B)** Larynx during phonation.

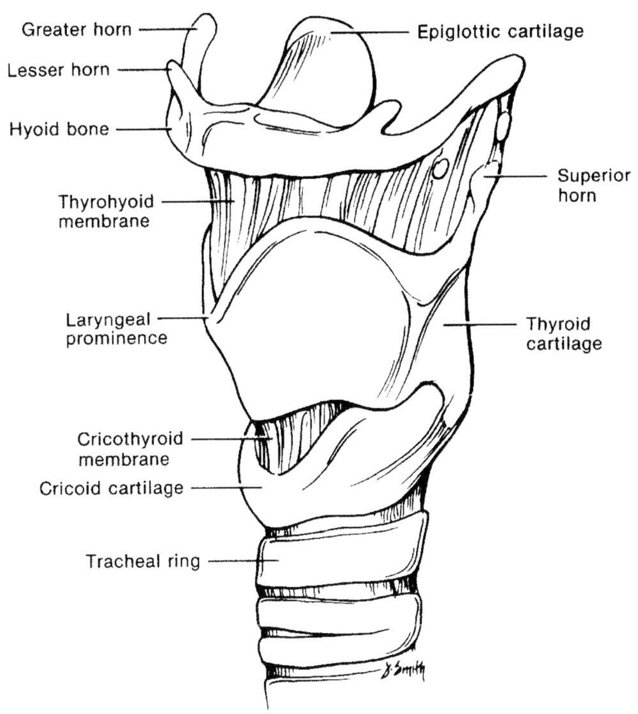

Figure 19.2. Normal anatomy of the larynx.

fatigue. The patient's reluctance to lie flat suggests that mechanical factors related to the size of the swollen epiglottis are probably significant. It is highly unlikely, however, that an edematous, rigid epiglottis will fall or be aspirated into the glottis and cause obstruction. Abscess formation may occur, contributing to airway compromise. Respiratory distress correlates with the degree of narrowing of the airway and indicates increased resistance to airflow. Resistance is proportional to $1/r^4$ (r = radius). Thus, a 2-mm change in radius produces a 16-fold change in resistance.

BACTERIOLOGY

The identification of a responsible infectious agent in adult epiglottitis has proven difficult. In adults, the yield from blood cultures ranges from 10% to 30%.[6,11] Surface cultures of the epiglottis and pharynx have proven useful in some instances[2,3]; however, in numerous cases, there is no growth or they are positive for commensals only.

This has led some investigators[5] to suggest that epiglottitis exists in two forms: (1) as part of a bacteremic illness, or (2) as a local infection. Of the bacteremic illnesses, *Haemophilus influenzae* type B is the most common bacterium found in the blood cultures of adults. Cases with proven bacteremia run a more fulminant course. *Streptococcus pneumoniae* bacteremia is associated with the immunocompromised host (malignancy, steroid dependency, AIDS).[19] The local infection may have a bacterial, viral, or fungal etiology; this form of the disease tends to run a more benign course. *H. influenzae* and beta-hemolytic streptococci are the most common causes of the local form. Herpes simplex is the only virus isolated in adults to date.[10] However, influenza and parainfluenza viruses have been isolated in children. Fungi implicated are *Aspergillus* and *Candida*.[4]

Other bacteria isolated include *S. pneumoniae*, beta-hemolytic streptococci, staphylococci, *Haemophilus parainfluenzae*, *Streptococcus viridans*, and *Fusobacterium necrophorum*, *Klebsiella pneumoniae*,[21] *E. coli*,[23] and *Neisseria* spp.[8] Aspiration of gasoline, thermal and chemical burns, and trauma have all been cited as causes of noninfectious epiglottitis.[12,14] Sarcoidosis has been reported to lead to chronic epiglottitis.

CLINICAL PRESENTATION

Any patient presenting with a possible diagnosis of epiglottitis or airway obstruction should be evaluated for urgent and rapid nonsurgical or surgical airway control in an acute care area with a high ratio of nursing support and equipment to patients. Personnel with expertise in airway intervention should be summoned if they are not available on site.

The presentation of epiglottitis in an adult is often less dramatic than in a child. Most children present in respiratory distress with impending airway obstruction. The clinical course of epiglottitis in the adult is variable. It can be mild and pose little threat to the patient, or it can be severe, resulting in total airway obstruction and death.[6,11,15,16,21] Typically, adult epiglottitis presents as a sore throat out of proportion to physical findings, dysphagia, a muffled "hot potato" voice, and respiratory distress or dyspnea. Some authors include hoarseness, but others say that hoarseness is atypical.[20]

For purposes of discussion, the clinical presentation may be categorized into a spectrum that varies from a fulminating course developing over hours to a subacute form smoldering for days to weeks:

Category 1: Severe respiratory distress, imminent or actual respiratory arrest. Patients in category 1 typically report a history of a brief but rapidly progressive illness. Blood culture often reveals *H. influenzae* type B.

Category 2: Intermediate condition with moderate-to-severe symptoms and signs of potential airway compromise. Patients in category 2 are at considerable risk. Their symptoms (inability to swallow or lie supine, dyspnea, and severe sore throat) and signs (muffled voice, stridor, and the use of accessory muscles) should alert the clinician to this risk. The emergency physician should prepare to intervene if the airway should suddenly deteriorate, and then undertake further evaluation of the airway.

Category 3: Mild-to-moderate illness without indications of potential airway compromise. Patients in category 3 may report a 3- to 14-day history of a sore throat and pain on swallowing, with minimal physical findings on examination. A patient can rapidly progress from category 3 to 2 or 1 with little warning.

DIFFERENTIAL DIAGNOSIS

Coexisting conditions can always complicate diagnosis and treatment, and extra care is required in potentially life-threatening situations. If epiglottitis is suspected, even if an associated condition has been diagnosed, definitive diagnostic maneuvers should be undertaken. Possible associated conditions include peritonsillar or retropharyngeal abscess, foreign body, angioedema, pharyngitis, inhalation or ingestion of a toxic substance, acute thyroiditis, epiglottic hematoma, and thermal injury.

EMERGENCY DEPARTMENT EVALUATION

Because the potential exists for rare sudden airway obstruction and death despite a "benign" presentation,[11,15,16] the patient with possible epiglottitis should be evaluated in an acute resuscitation area with high-density nursing and should not be left alone, due to the risk of sudden airway obstruction without warning.

The diagnosis of epiglottitis depends first on its being considered. *Symptoms in excess of physical findings are the hallmark.* The patient may be tachypneic and tachycardic and have pharyngitis. Some patients describe exquisite tenderness on palpation of the thyroid cartilage.[1] Twenty percent to 30% of patients become moderately to severely ill, with signs of airway compromise, drooling, stridor, and cyanosis.

There is no typical time course for epiglottitis. The period from onset to presentation may be hours to days. Sore throat and odynophagia, with or without dysphagia, are consistent findings.[15,21] Fever may or may not be present. There may be voice changes, chills, dyspnea, and pain on tongue protrusion.

A recent study found that dyspnea was the only intubation risk factor (n = 51) that predicted the need for aggressive airway management. Dyspnea had a positive predicted value of 62% and a negative predicted value of 100% as a symptom suggesting the need for intubation.[11]

Patients in whom epiglottitis is suspected must undergo indirect (mirror) or direct (fiberoptic) laryngoscopy.[17] In the past, there was controversy as to whether manipulation of the oropharynx could lead to airway compromise. This concern persists in children, but there is little evidence to support the concern in adults.[1,13] Fiberoptic laryngoscopy is the diagnostic evaluation of choice. It is well tolerated and allows an excellent view of the supraglottis.[7,16]

Soft-tissue lateral neck x-rays can also be helpful. Several abnormalities may be evident, including enlargement of the epiglottis (thumb sign) and aryepiglottic folds, and ballooning of the hypopharynx. One study[20] suggested that epiglottic and aryepiglottic widths greater than 8 mm and 7 mm, respectively, indicated acute epiglottitis. However, a 10% to 20% false-negative rate exists. Another study[18] indexed both epiglottic and aryepiglottic width to third cervical vertebral body width and epiglottic width to epiglottic height and found that ratios greater than 0.5, 0.35, and 0.6, respectively, were 100% sensitive for epiglottitis. These results were derived from 33 patients, of which only six were adults. A more recent article described the qualitative evaluation of the presence or absence of a deep, well-defined vallecular air space running parallel to the pharyngotracheal air column that approaches the level of the hyoid bone in lateral soft-tissue neck radiographs. This well-defined space was absent in all 26 consecutive confirmed cases of adult epiglottitis in this study. Additionally, the investigators found a 98.2% sensitivity and 99.5% specificity in correctly identifying adult epiglottitis when random case controlled radiographs were examined by blinded participants. The authors suggest that this may be a useful diagnostic screen in patients who do not require immediate airway intervention.[9]

EMERGENCY DEPARTMENT MANAGEMENT

Emergency departments must be committed to preplanned, cooperative teamwork to prevent disaster for the patient with epiglottitis. The cooperative effort must involve the departments of emergency medicine, anesthesiology, and surgery (ear, nose, and throat in some centers), similar to a trauma team. Protocols for in-hospital management should draw on intensive care and infectious disease expertise. In community hospitals, preplanning must address optimal use of available resources, transfer agreements, and the exigencies of transport.

All emergency departments must be equipped to intervene in acute upper airway emergencies with endotracheal intubation or cricothyroidostomy. Additional emergency airway management equipment includes bag and mask devices with deflatable positive-pressure relief ("pop-off") valves and jet ventilators. Transcricoid jet ventilation via small-caliber catheters, while associated with barotrauma hazards, provides adequate ventilation and oxygenation until more definitive airway management can be achieved.

The issue of airway management is controversial and depends on available resources and personal skill. Sudden airway obstruction is rare, but always a possibility in epiglottitis.[11,15] Most adult patients (greater than 70%) present with no respiratory symptoms or signs (category 3) and can be safely observed for progression in an intensive care unit.[14]

Patients presenting in categories 1 and 2 must be judged individually. Patients in extremis or with totally obstructed airways must receive definitive airway management in the emergency department (Fig 19.3). Patients with mild dyspnea or respiratory complaints could be observed and monitored in the intensive care setting. The remainder should undergo definitive airway management in the controlled setting of the operating room, and subsequently be admitted to the intensive care unit.

Patients taken to the operating room should be accompanied by a physician skilled in airway management. Once in the operating room, a surgeon skilled in surgical airway management and rigid bronchoscopy should be scrubbed and ready in case orotracheal intubation is impossible or fails. An inhalation induction aided by the judicious use of intravenous sedation is the recommended anesthetic technique.[6,16,23] The antibiotic of choice on empiric grounds is cefuroxime, cefotaxime (up to 2 g i.v. every 4 hours), or ceftriaxone (1 to 2 g per day i.v., given every 12 hours); alternative therapy includes ampicillin–sulbactam (Unasyn) 1.5 to 3.0 g every 6 hours i.v., or trimethoprim–sulfamethoxazole. These provide coverage for group A *S. pneumoniae, Staphylococcus pyogenes,* and *H. influenzae.*[6,22]

Some authors have advocated the use of corticosteroids, but scientific evidence supporting their efficacy is lacking.[11] In the case of angioedema, however, steroids may be lifesaving. Aerosolized epinephrine and racemic epinephrine are not thought to be useful.

Helium–oxygen mixtures may buy time while preparing for definitive management. The density of helium is less than that of nitrogen and produces reduced airway resistance, improved gas flow, and decreased work of breathing. The emergency physician must be aware of the relative concentrations of helium and oxygen in the mixture, as various standard preparations exist.

DISPOSITION

All patients with epiglottitis, whether or not they are intubated, should be admitted to an intensive care unit.[11,15] If they are to be observed, personnel and equipment necessary for emergency airway intervention must be immediately available.[16] Resolution of the disease is monitored by fiberoptic laryngoscopy.[1] The ability of a patient to breathe around an occluded endotracheal tube with its cuff deflated is a good test for the suitability for extubation.[1,11] This usually can occur 48 to 72 hours after intubation or admission to the hospital. Oral antibiotics may replace intravenous antibiotics at that time and should be continued for 14 days.

If *H. influenzae* type B is isolated, case contacts should receive rifampin. If there are children under age 4 in the household, all household contacts should be treated.

Transfer Considerations

Transfer may be necessary if the appropriate specialists and intensive care setting are unavailable. However, no patient in category 1 or 2 should be transferred unless airway control has

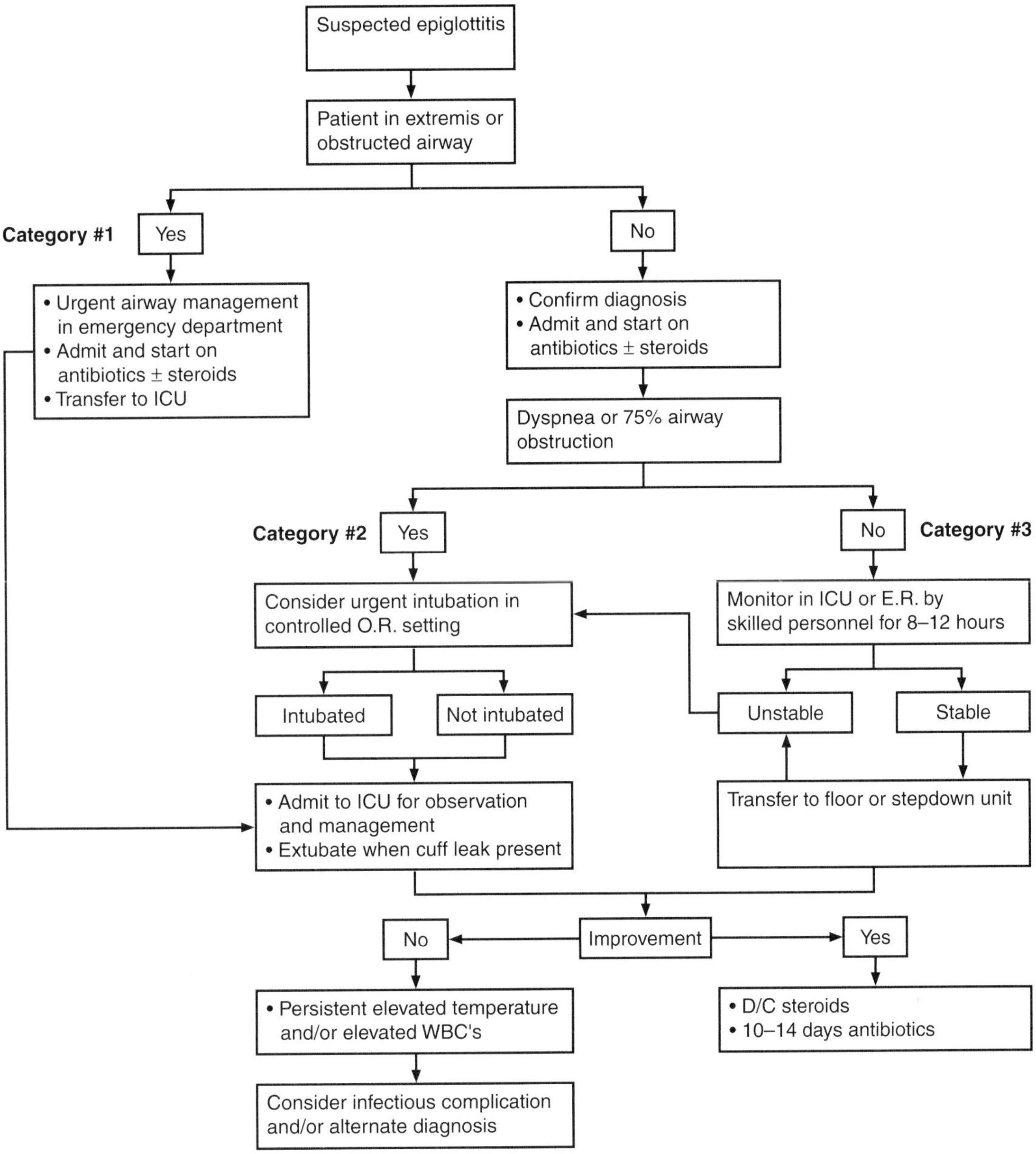

Figure 19.3. Treatment algorithm for acute epiglottitis. (Modified from Hébert PC, Ducic Y, Boisvert D, et al. Adult epiglottitis in a Canadian setting. *Laryngoscope* 1998;108:64, with permission.)

been achieved. If patients in category 3 require transfer, they should be accompanied by personnel and equipment necessary to establish an airway.

COMMON PITFALLS

- The literature is replete with case histories documenting delays in the diagnosis of epiglottitis. Physicians are generally unaware of the adult form of the disease; thus, the most common pitfall is the failure to consider the diagnosis.
- Airway management for the patient with epiglottitis should be undertaken by an experienced physician.
- Elective blind nasal intubation is contraindicated.[25]
- The possibility of sudden airway obstruction should always be considered.
- All patients with even mild dyspnea require close monitoring in an appropriate setting.

References

1. Andreassen UK, Baer S, Nielsen TG, et al. Acute epiglottitis: 25 years' experience with nasotracheal intubation, current management policy and future trends. *J Otolaryngol* 1992;106:1072.
2. Baker AS, Eavey RD. Adult supraglottitis (epiglottitis) [Editorial]. *N Engl J Med* 1986;314:1185.
3. Berg AS, Trollfors B, Nylén O, et al. Incidence, aetiology, and prognosis of acute epiglottitis in children and adults in Sweden. *Scand J Infect Dis* 1996;28:261.
4. Bolivar R, Gomez LG, Luna M, et al. *Aspergillus* epiglottitis. *Cancer* 1983;51:367.
5. Carenfelt C. Etiology of acute infectious epiglottitis in adults: septic vs. local infection. *Scand J Infect Dis* 1989;21:53.
6. Carey MJ. Epiglottitis in adults [Review]. *Am J Emerg Med* 1996;14:421.
7. Dixon J, Black JJ. Adult epiglottitis: an important cause of airway obstruction. *J Accid Emerg Med* 1998;15:114.
8. Donnelly TJ, Crausman RS. Acute supraglottitis: when a sore throat becomes severe. *Geriatrics* 1997;52:65.
9. Ducic Y, Hébert PC, MacLachlan L, et al. Description and evaluation of the vallecula sign: a new radiological sign in the diagnosis of adult epiglottitis. *Ann Emerg Med* 1997;30:1.
10. Giani G, Quirino T, Sacrini F, et al. Supraglottitis due to herpes simplex virus type I in an adult. *Clin Infect Dis* 1996;22:382.

11. Hébert PC, Ducic Y, Boisvert D, et al. Adult epiglottitis in a Canadian setting. *Laryngoscope* 1998;108:64.
12. Kornak JM, Freije JE, Campbell BH. Caustic and thermal epiglottitis in the adult. *Otolaryngol Head Neck Surg* 1996;114:310.
13. Mayo-Smith MF, Hirsch PJ, Wodzinski SF, et al. Acute epiglottitis in adults. *N Engl J Med* 1986;314:1133.
14. Mayo-Smith MF, Spinale J. Thermal epiglottitis in adults: a new complication of illicit drug use. *J Emerg Med* 1997;15:483.
15. Mayo-Smith MF, Spinale JW, Donskey CJ, et al. Acute epiglottitis. An 18 year experience in Rhode Island. *Chest* 1995;108:1640.
16. Park KW, Darvish A, Lowenstein E. Airway management for adult patients with acute epiglottitis: a 12-year experience at an academic medical center (1984–1995). *Anesthesiology* 1998;88:254.
17. Phelan DM, Love JB. Adult epiglottitis: is there a role for the fibreoptic bronchoscope? *Chest* 1984;86:783.
18. Rothrock SG, Pignatello GA, Howard RM. Radiologic diagnosis of epiglottitis: objective criteria for all ages. *Ann Emerg Med* 1990;19:978.
19. Rothstein SG, Persky MS, Edelman BA, et al. Epiglottitis in AIDS patients. *Laryngoscope* 1989;99:389.
20. Schumaker HM, Doris PE, Birnbaum G. Radiologic parameters in adult epiglottitis. *Ann Emerg Med* 1984;13:588.
21. Solomon P, Weisbrod M, Irish JC, et al. Adult epiglottitis: the Toronto hospital experience. *J Otolaryngol* 1998;27:332.
22. Spalding M, Ala-Kokko TI. The use of inhaled sevoflurane for endotracheal intubation in epiglottitis. *Anesthesiology* 1998;89:1025.
23. Trollfors B, Nylén O, Carenfelt C, et al. Aetiology of acute epiglottitis in adults. *Scand J Infect Dis* 1998;30:49.
24. Warshawski J, Havas TE, McShane DP, et al. Adult epiglottitis. *J Otolaryngol* 1986;15:362.
25. Wurtule P. Nasotracheal intubation: a modality in the management of acute epiglottitis in adults. *J Otolaryngol* 1984;13:118.

CHAPTER 20

Acute Infections of the Adult Pharynx and Laryngitis

William Levin and Gabriel R. Wilson

PHARYNGOTONSILLITIS

Sore throat affects patients of all ages and is one of the most common complaints in the outpatient setting. The term *sore throat* has become synonymous with acute pharyngotonsillitis because it is the most common cause of pain in the oropharynx. Tonsillitis and pharyngitis are somewhat difficult to separate because of the overlap of the infectious process. Many experienced physicians will arbitrarily label the recent onset of enlarged, erythematous painful tonsils *acute tonsillitis,* whereas a diffusely erythematous pharynx without obvious tonsillar enlargement or in a patient without tonsils is considered a pharyngitis. When both areas are involved, the term *pharyngotonsillitis* is used.

Transmission of most causes of pharyngitis is by person-to-person contact through droplets of saliva. The causes include multiple bacteria, viruses, and fungi. Acute streptococcal pharyngitis caused by group A beta-hemolytic streptococci (GABHS) has received the most attention, because it was demonstrated in the 1950s that rheumatic fever could be prevented by treating the preceding pharyngitis. Less than 1% of patients with untreated group A beta-hemolytic streptococcal throat infections will develop rheumatic fever; and of those, 1.8% will develop fourth-degree rheumatic heart disease.[1] Furthermore, whether treated or not, patients with group A beta-hemolytic streptococcal infections may develop poststreptococcal glomerulonephritis.

GABHS account for 10% to 15% of sore throats in adults.[2] Other groupable streptococci (C and G), as well as *Neisseria gonorrhoeae, Staphylococcus aureus, H. influenzae,* and *Corynebacterium diphtheriae,* also cause pharyngitis. Viral agents are probably the most common etiology, including enteroviruses, adenoviruses, rhinoviruses, apoinfluenza virus, and Epstein-Barr virus, the causative pathogen of infectious mononucleosis (IM). Candidiasis may be seen in the pharynx of the immunocompromised patient, or in the patient taking antibiotics or inhaled steroids. A sore throat does not always represent a pharyngotonsillitis, and thus the history and physical examination are necessary to exclude peritonsillar abscess, retropharyngeal abscess, and other potentially life-threatening processes.

CLINICAL PRESENTATION AND DIFFERENTIAL DIAGNOSIS

Despite a multitude of studies and despite many clinicians' seemingly clear-cut algorithms, it remains an impossible task to differentiate bacterial from nonbacterial infections of the pharynx. Many primary care physicians with reliable patients tend to use throat cultures to determine which pharyngitides are due to GABHS. A classic study in children from 1971, however, showed that over 50% of children with sore throats and positive throat cultures had no significant rise in ASO or anti-DNAase B titers—meaning GABHS were not likely the source of the infection.[3] Furthermore, a negative throat culture does not always mean that GABHS are not present in the pharynx.[4]

Other clinicians use the physical examination findings to help guide the diagnosis; however, the error rate among experienced physicians in differentiating GABHS from viral pharyngitis is 20% to 40%.[3,4] There is a slight trend toward bacterial pharyngitis if the patient has fever, pharyngeal erythema, pharyngeal exudate, tender cervical adenopathy, headache, and absence of cough and rhinorrhea. Viral infections are typically accompanied by conjunctivitis, nasal congestion, hoarseness, cough, aphthous ulcers on the soft palate, and myalgias. It must be recognized, though, that these are trends that have poor statistical correlation with positive throat cultures and rises in ASO titers.

The pharyngitis that accompanies IM is exudative with grossly enlarged tonsils, especially in younger patients. Petechiae may be present on the soft palate. A concurrent lymphadenopathy may be present, with hepatomegaly and splenomegaly also possible. Fever is usually present.

Diphtheria is no longer a common cause of pharyngitis, but its presentation should still be recognized and considered, especially in the patient who has recently come from another country and has not received a full set of vaccinations. Usually anorexia, malaise, and a low-grade fever will be followed 1 to 2 days later by a gray or white membrane that adheres to the tonsils.

Patients with pharyngitis who present with severe pain on swallowing (odynophagia) may be dehydrated from lack of oral intake; they will also have increased insensible fluid loss from fever. Other complications from pharyngitis involve progression to peritonsillar cellulitis, abscess, or retropharyngeal abscess, and are addressed later.

EMERGENCY DEPARTMENT EVALUATION

Examination should begin with assessing the patency of the airway and surveying the presence and severity of tonsillar hypertrophy. If the patient does not have severely enlarged tonsils, and yet appears to have trouble breathing or swallowing, other etiologies, such as epiglottitis, must immediately be considered. In this circumstance, a soft-tissue lateral x-ray of the neck should be accomplished rapidly, with airway management equipment easily accessible.

Typically, erythema of the tonsils or pharyngeal mucosa is seen. Exudate or adherent membrane may be present on the tonsils. The neck and jaw angle should be palpated for the presence of enlarged nodes. A throat culture may be considered (see below).

Patients appearing dehydrated, with dry oral mucosa, may have an intravenous line placed and electrolytes drawn. A complete blood count will usually not add relevant information, but may be drawn. A Monospot heterophile agglutination test may be performed if IM is a diagnostic consideration.

EMERGENCY DEPARTMENT MANAGEMENT

Admission should be considered whenever a complication of pharyngotonsillitis is identified. The two most common reasons for admission are dehydration and the presence of peritonsillar cellulitis or abscess. A patient who cannot swallow cannot maintain adequate oral intake or take medication, and may deteriorate if managed as an outpatient. Intravenous hydration, antibiotic administration, and observation may be accomplished in the emergency department (ED); those patients who measurably improve may be discharged with 24-hour follow-up. Admission should always be considered for patients with unreliable follow-up or poor social circumstances.

When deciding to treat a pharyngitis in the ED, the clinician must weigh the benefits of decreasing the chance of the patient developing acute rheumatic fever and communicating the infection to others, against the chance of the patient developing an adverse reaction to the antibiotic prescribed. Treating a GABHS pharyngitis may decrease the severity of the symptoms 12 to 24 hours earlier, but this is of questionable significance. In addition, consistently overtreating patients theoretically may prompt GABHS resistance to penicillin.

There is no good strategy at this time to avoid all of the aforementioned complications. There are a few helpful algorithms that, with patient discussion and input, will allow the emergency physician to choose a logical course of action. One approach is to treat all patients and not culture. This approach recognizes the lack of reliable follow-up in the emergency setting, as well as the inaccuracy of throat culture results. It exposes many patients unnecessarily to penicillin, but will not miss a case of GABHS pharyngitis. It is probably the strategy that is most cost-effective, will relieve symptoms the soonest, and provide greatest patient satisfaction by expediting their disposition.[4]

Strategy 2 is to culture all patients and treat none (unless the culture returns positive). This strategy seeks to avoid overtreating patients with viral pharyngitis, as only around 10% to 15% of pharyngitis is due to GABHS. It can only be implemented in an ED with the resources in place for following up culture results and recontacting patients. Patients in an inner-city hospital setting may not have home telephones or may give inaccurate contact information, so this may not be a viable alternative. A variation in this strategy is to begin treatment in the ED and have the patient call back for culture results in 2 days. If the results are negative, the antibiotics are stopped.

DISPOSITION

Patients who appear toxic or have severe odynophagia who do not measurably improve after hydration and observation should be admitted.

Nontoxic-appearing patients who can tolerate oral fluids and medications may be discharged. If the patients are being treated for a presumed GABHS pharyngitis, a 10-day course of penicillin can be prescribed. While the traditional regimen has been 250 mg to 500 mg every 6 hours, 1000 mg every 12 hours has been shown to be just as effective.[5,6] In addition, compliance with a b.i.d. regimen is significantly higher than a q.i.d. course.

Patients who are definitely not allergic to penicillin may be given the choice of a single injection of 1.2 million U of Benzathine penicillin. As the intramuscular may be painful, this should be done only after discussing the options with the patient. Alternatives include cephalexin 1 g b.i.d., or cefadroxil 500 mg b.i.d.

Patients with allergies to penicillin may be given erythromycin base 250 mg to 333 mg t.i.d. Azithromycin and clarithromycin have not been as well studied, but may be alternatives.

Patients diagnosed with infectious mononucleosis should be instructed to follow up with their primary physician in 7 days. They should be advised to avoid contact sports if there is the possibility of splenomegaly.

All discharged patients should have clear instructions to return for worsening odynophagia, worsening unilateral odynophagia, inability to tolerate oral fluid intake, or lack of improvement after 48 hours.

COMMON PITFALLS

- Consider acute epiglottitis or supraglottitis, especially in a patient who presents with sudden, severe pharyngitis, drooling (because it hurts to swallow), and respiratory distress. Adults usually have a more gradual onset over several days, and are less likely to develop sudden airway compromise unless they present later in the progression of the swelling.
- Do not give ampicillin to a patient with suspected mononucleosis. The resulting rash helps make the diagnosis and does not imply ampicillin allergy, but can be uncomfortable.
- Do not miss abscesses, which usually require hospitalization, intravenous penicillin, and drainage. Peritonsillar abscesses and cellulitis make the tonsillar pillar bulge toward the midline. Retropharyngeal abscesses and epiglottitis may require soft-tissue lateral neck films to visualize.
- Consider gonococcal pharyngitis in patients with a suggestive history. Patients will have a mild clinical syndrome and require special cultures on Thayer-Martin medium.

RETROPHARYNGEAL ABSCESS

The retropharyngeal space lies between the fascia, which is densely adherent to the paraspinal muscles, and the posterior pharyngeal mucosa, which can be seen directly through the open mouth. There are three fascial layers with intervening potential spaces, but the important point is that these potential spaces extend to the mediastinum and offer a direct, unimpeded path for the spread of infection.

Retropharyngeal abscess is primarily a disease of young children and occurs when lymph nodes in the retropharyngeal space become infected. These lymph nodes involute by puberty. In adults, retropharyngeal abscess is predominantly caused by ingested foreign bodies, such as fishbones that penetrate the posterior pharyngeal wall.[5,7] Other causes include blunt and penetrating neck wounds, which have the potential to develop the delayed complication of an abscess, and iatrogenic injuries secondary to intubation or endoscopy. Uncommon causes include Pott disease (cervical tuberculosis), sinusitis, and otitis media. Retropharyngeal abscesses tend to be polymicrobial, with streptococcus, staphylococcus, and anaerobes most commonly recovered when cultured.

CLINICAL PRESENTATION

The patient presents with fever, neck pain, and sore throat out of proportion to the oropharyngeal findings. Other possible findings include odynophagia, neck swelling, drooling, torticollis, meningismus, cervical adenopathy, and stridor. If the abscess is high in the neck, nasal obstruction and a hyponasal voice result. The voice may sound muffled if the swelling is above the level of the larynx, or sound normal if the abscess is lower in the neck. As the swelling increases, difficult or noisy breathing may occur. Chest pain associated with these symptoms strongly suggests mediastinal extension.

On examination, patients appear toxic, dehydrated, and febrile. The head is held stiff; and passive or active motion of the head is painful. Inspection of the neck does not reveal any redness or swelling, although anterior displacement of the larynx may be appreciated. Palpation of the neck reveals deep tenderness only. Fluctuance is not always palpated because of the thickness of the intervening tissue. Unlike the presentation of a peritonsillar abscess, there is no trismus with uncomplicated retropharyngeal abscess, and direct visualization of the posterior wall should be possible. The area of the abscess may appear erythematous, boggy, and displaced forward toward the uvula if the abscess is located at this level (Fig. 20.1). A process more caudal in the neck may show no abnormalities on oral examination. Palpation of the posterior wall may confirm the diagnosis, but because of the risk of rupturing the abscess into an already compromised airway, *this maneuver is not recommended.*[8]

Possible complications of a ruptured abscess are many and grave. The airway is at risk, either from obstruction of the airway by a growing abscess, or from sudden rupture of the abscess with subsequent aspiration or asphyxia. Direct extension inferiorly through the fascial planes can lead to mediastinitis. Extension laterally into the parapharyngeal space and carotid sheath can lead to jugular vein thrombosis (Lemierre disease), hemorrhage from the carotid artery or jugular vein, cranial nerve (IX, X, XII) deficits, or Horner syndrome. Overwhelming sepsis may occur, especially in immunocompromised patients.

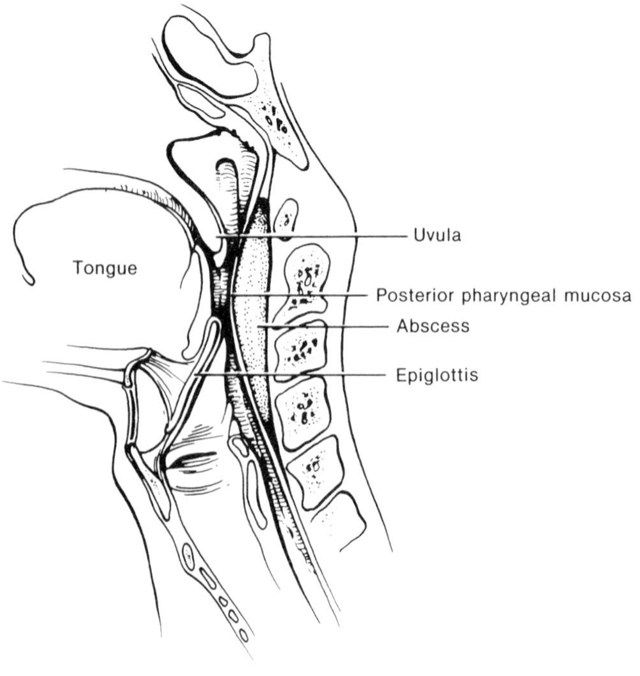

Figure 20.1. Retropharyngeal abscess.

DIFFERENTIAL DIAGNOSIS

Meningitis and other deep neck infections may present similarly, though examination and radiography will clarify the diagnosis. Bulges on the posterior wall are not necessarily of inflammatory etiology, and may occur from hematoma (e.g., in the anticoagulated patient), osteophyte of the cervical spine, neoplasm, or persistent lymph node. History will aid in differentiating these from an abscess.

EMERGENCY DEPARTMENT EVALUATION

Retropharyngeal abscess is a true medical emergency. Airway impingement or obstruction and abscess rupture can occur at any time; therefore, careful monitoring of the patient, as well as expedient evaluation and management, are essential in averting a potentially disastrous outcome. Equipment for emergency management of the airway, including a tracheostomy set, must be available, and the patient must be carefully monitored for respiratory distress. An intravenous line should be established and fluids started. A complete blood count, electrolytes, and blood cultures may be drawn, though these tests usually have little role in the patient's initial management. The lateral neck soft-tissue view is the most important initial diagnostic test in evaluating the retropharyngeal space and, along with a chest x-ray, should be undertaken immediately. Positive findings include air in the retropharyngeal space, an air–fluid level posterior to the pharynx or esophagus, and widening of the retropharyngeal soft tissues. Abnormal swelling of the retropharyngeal space is suggested when the posterior border of the air column is greater than 7 mm from the anterior border of the body of C2, or 20 mm from C6. Soft tissue wider than one-third the width of the body of C2, or the full width of the body of C6, also suggests abnormality. A normal lateral neck film effectively eliminates this diagnosis. A chest x-ray should be reviewed for mediastinitis.

A contrast-enhanced computed tomography (CT) scan of the neck and chest should be obtained in short order in patients suspected of having retropharyngeal abscess; in addition to establishing the diagnosis with certainty, it will define the extent of the lesion in the spectrum of cellulitis to abscess.

EMERGENCY DEPARTMENT MANAGEMENT

Advanced airway management equipment, including a tracheostomy set, should be stationed at the bedside. The patient should be monitored carefully. Intravenous fluids and intravenous antibiotics—high-dose penicillin (6 million U every 6 hours) and metronidazole (500 mg every 6 hours after a 1-g loading dose), or cefoxitin (2 g every 8 hours)—should be started immediately. An otolaryngology consult should be obtained early. Patients will likely be admitted to the intensive care unit or directly to the operating room. Definitive management includes incision and drainage under carefully controlled circumstances. The presence of mediastinitis mandates a significantly more extensive debridement by a thoracic surgeon.[9] Incision and debridement for retropharyngeal cellulitis is at the discretion of the otolaryngologist.

While there are no case reports of patients exhibiting respiratory decompensation during CT scan, the physician is well advised to watch the patient closely and have advanced airway management equipment and personnel readily available.

COMMON PITFALLS

- Be prepared for airway obstruction and rupture of abscess.
- Palpation of the posterior pharyngeal wall risks rupture of the abscess.
- The lateral neck film is the most useful initial test for retropharyngeal disease.

- A contrast-enhanced CT of the neck is the preferred diagnostic test.

PERITONSILLAR CELLULITIS AND ABSCESS

Peritonsillar abscess is a complication of tonsillitis, whether from group A streptococcus or infectious mononucleosis.[10] It occurs more frequently in teen-agers and younger adults, but it can present at any age, especially in immunocompromised or diabetic patients. The abscess forms in the potential space between the lateral aspect of the tonsillar capsule and the superior constrictor muscle of the pharynx. When tonsillitis spreads beyond the tonsil capsule, inflammation in this space results in cellulitis and then abscess if left untreated. Abscess cultures tend to be polymicrobial, with the frequent presence of group A beta-hemolytic streptococci and anaerobes such as *Bacteroides*.

CLINICAL PRESENTATION

Typically, a younger patient (though rarely under 10 years old) will present with worsening sore throat pain and fever of 2 days' duration or more. As the pain increases, it localizes to one side and radiates to the ipsilateral ear. It is accompanied by odynophagia and dysphagia, which eventually result in drooling and dehydration. The patient may tilt the head toward the painful side. Trismus may result, though, if severe, it suggests parapharyngeal abscess. The key in differentiating severe tonsillitis from peritonsillar abscess is the localization of the pain.

There is a continuum of illness from tonsillitis to peritonsillar abscess. The patient may present at any point, and symptoms and treatment vary accordingly. The early stage is inflammation without fluid collection, or peritonsillar cellulitis; there is absent or mild trismus, fullness on the side of the affected tonsil, and unilateral erythema extending onto the soft palate. The palate is not bulging, nor is the uvula displaced.

At the other extreme is abscess with trismus that makes examination of the oral cavity difficult. The ipsilateral soft palate is markedly erythematous and swollen. The tonsil is displaced downward and medially, and the uvula is pushed contralateral (Fig. 20.2). The breath is foul-smelling.

Local complications include extension into the contiguous deep neck spaces (e.g., parapharyngeal abscess), with the possible catastrophic consequences of erosion into the carotid artery, or thrombosis of the internal jugular vein (Lemierre disease). Airway obstruction, mediastinitis, sepsis, and descending necrotizing fasciitis are other infrequent complications. Most complications occur in diabetic or immunocompromised patients, or in patients who were neglected or noncompliant with an initial antibiotic regimen.

DIFFERENTIAL DIAGNOSIS

Unilateral enlargement of a tonsil may occur from squamous cell carcinoma, lymphoma, leukemia, vascular lesions, or neoplasms of the lateral pharyngeal space. Such an enlargement can usually be distinguished from abscess by history and presentation. Lateral neck abscess of dental origin may be confused with peritonsillar abscess, but a history of toothache should serve to differentiate the two.

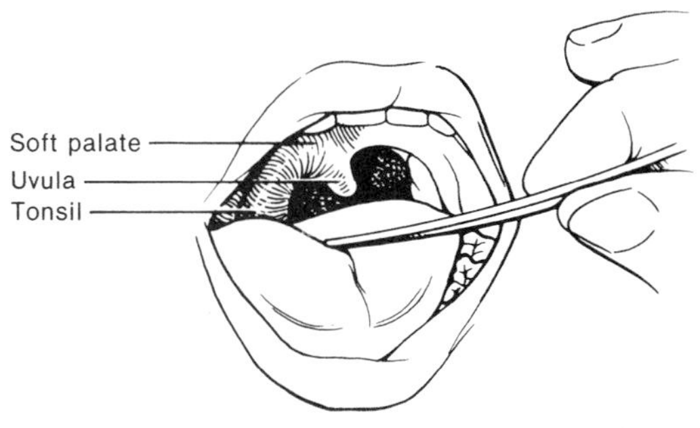

Figure 20.2. Peritonsillar abscess.

EMERGENCY DEPARTMENT EVALUATION AND MANAGEMENT

After examination, a complete blood count, serum electrolytes, Monospot, and throat culture should be obtained. Intravenous fluids should be started to correct the dehydration that is usually present, and intravenous antibiotics initiated. Penicillin (1 to 2 million U every 4 hours) or clindamycin (600 mg every 8 hours) are good choices.[11] Early cellulitis may be treated with hydration and antibiotics alone, though to differentiate abscess from inflammation may require needle aspiration. For abscesses, needle aspiration will provide significant relief.

The emergency physician may consult an otolaryngologist or, if experienced, can undertake diagnostic and therapeutic needle aspiration.[12] Great care must be taken regarding direction and depth of approach to avoid puncturing the carotid artery. A useful depth guide can be created by removing the plastic needle cap (or sheath) from an 18-gauge needle and cutting off the distal 2 cm with scissors. One then carefully replaces the modified needle cap over the needle. With patients in the sitting position, hunched slightly forward, apply topical anesthetic to the posterior pharynx. Instruct patients that although they will feel an initial puncture, the procedure will likely reduce their pain significantly. Aiming posterolaterally toward the medial aspect of the enlarged tonsil, insert the 18-gauge needle with 2-cm depth guide into the abscess and withdraw the plunger, aspirating any available fluid. Send the aspirate for culture and Gram stain.

Depending on the outcome of the aforementioned procedure or consultation with an otolaryngologist, disposition may vary. Uncomplicated, nonimmunocompromised patients who are able to tolerate oral antibiotics and fluids may be discharged with otolaryngology follow-up in 24 hours. Patients with more complex cases should be admitted to the hospital for intravenous hydration and antibiotics. If the previously described procedure does not relieve severe symptoms, or if there is any suspicion of spread of infection beyond the peritonsillar area, a contrast-enhanced CT should be ordered immediately. A small percentage of peritonsillar abscesses will not respond to needle aspiration, and will require incision and drainage.

COMMON PITFALLS

- Failure to recognize an impending abscess. This usually results in a repeat visit within a day or two when the patient fails to improve.
- Needle aspiration may be done by the emergency physician, but only with great care by those experienced in the procedure.
- Asymmetric swelling of the pharynx is always abnormal, even if asymptomatic; further evaluation is warranted.

LARYNGITIS

Laryngitis is manifested by hoarseness. When acute, the change in voice is secondary to vocal cord edema from inflammation or vocal cord trauma. Viral upper respiratory tract infection (URI) is the most common cause of acute laryngitis, and is usually accompanied by cough, sore throat, or rhinorrhea.

Hoarseness may be exacerbated by thick secretions adhering to the vocal cords, or by the vigorous coughing that occurs with a URI. Acute hoarseness also may occur after prolonged shouting, or in opera singers or other vocalists with frequent or lengthy performances.

Typical agents causing URI with laryngeal involvement include parainfluenza viruses 1 and 2, adenoviruses, rhinoviruses, and coronaviruses. Bacterial superinfection may cause a more virulent illness. *Staphylococcus aureus* and *H. influenzae* have been implicated.

Hoarseness lasting longer than 4 weeks suggests a different and potentially more serious group of etiologies.

CLINICAL PRESENTATION

Hoarseness with other associated symptoms may be the presentation of life-threatening illness and should prompt immediate evaluation of the airway. A patient with impending airway obstruction complains of shortness of breath and may present with stridor, air hunger, drooling, and voice change. This is an emergency and not simple laryngitis.

Most commonly, acute laryngitis results from viral URI and is easily recognized when the patient presents with cough, sore throat, low-grade fever, and rhinitis. Hoarseness is due to inflammation of the vocal cords, edema from coughing, or tenacious secretions.

If the laryngitis is not from an obvious URI, the patient should be questioned about prolonged shouting, singing, or injury to the anterior neck. Sudden voice changes from overuse will be self-limited. Voice changes due to injury require further evaluation, as edema or hematoma can be progressive and impinge on the airway.

A change of voice that persists more than 3 weeks should be considered chronic; possible etiologies include vocal cord nodules, cysts, or granulomas; malignant laryngeal tumors; neurologic disorders; and gastroesophageal reflux.

EMERGENCY DEPARTMENT EVALUATION

Patients with a change of voice should be questioned about whether the change is acute or chronic, and if acute, rapid assessment of the airway should be accomplished. After patients relate the onset and duration of the laryngitis, they should be questioned about associated symptoms, underlying medical problems, and injuries to the anterior neck. Patients with a URI-associated laryngitis usually present a few days into their illness. Patients with sudden onset or rapid progression of symptoms are most vulnerable to airway obstruction and require careful, prompt evaluation. Patients should be examined for signs of impending airway obstruction, such as shortness of breath or stridor. They also should be checked for findings suggestive of URI, such as mild fever, pharyngeal erythema or edema, rhinitis, and cough. In viral URI, laboratory tests are not helpful.

A soft-tissue lateral x-ray of the neck should be obtained to exclude epiglottitis or to help evaluate neck trauma. If the patient appears toxic or if more than a URI is suspected, a complete blood count may be helpful. Arterial blood gas determination is not helpful, because relatively normal values are maintained until there is clinically obvious deterioration. Intravenous fluid may be considered if the patient is dehydrated and has more than a simple URI.

Flexible fiberoptic laryngoscopes can be used by experienced emergency physicians to evaluate cases of neck trauma with voice change. Laryngoscopy can also be used to evaluate causes of airway impingement.

EMERGENCY DEPARTMENT MANAGEMENT

Acute viral laryngitis requires simple symptomatic management. Mucolytics and expectorants such as guanefisin and iodinated glycerol are useful and well tolerated. Decongestants also can be used. Antihistamines have no role in this setting. Antibiotics are reserved for patients with known immunocompromised states, or in patients with a course prolonged more than a week, in which bacterial superinfection is possible. Increased fluid intake as well as room air humidification are also helpful. Patients with signs of airway obstruction or a history of neck trauma require otolaryngology consultation.

Patients whose acute laryngitis is secondary to vocal cord overuse should be advised to rest their voice, which includes abstaining from whispering. For the special circumstance of vocalists with acute laryngitis who will need to sing within 48 hours, voice rest should be prescribed and an intramuscular injection of dexamethasone given if they have objective evidence of vocal cord edema. Singers should drink a lot of water, use a humidifier, and rest their voices, but they should do warm-up exercises prior to the performance. Severe laryngitis mandates canceling the concert.[2,13]

DISPOSITION

Patients with simple URI may be discharged and instructed to follow up with their primary physician as needed. A 10- to 14-day duration of symptoms may be expected. Patients who are hoarse from voice overuse should be instructed to completely rest their voices; these patients should be advised to follow up with an otolaryngologist if their voices have not normalized in 2 weeks. All patients with chronic laryngitis require otolaryngology referral for complete evaluation.

COMMON PITFALLS

- In the setting of acute hoarseness, a missed diagnosis of epiglottitis can be fatal. The physician must remain alert to the clinical picture that suggests more than simple laryngitis.
- All patients with chronic laryngitis must be referred to an otolaryngologist to rule out malignancy, neurologic disorders, and other etiologies. The importance of this follow-up must be stressed to the patient.

References

1. Arkkila E, et al. Peritonsillar abscess associated with infectious mononucleosis. *ORL J Otorhinolaryngol Relat Spec* 1998;60:159.
2. Brown DE. *Infections of the deep fascial spaces of the head and neck: a manual.* American Academy of Ophthalmology and Otolaryngology, 1978.
3. Dubois D, et al. Rapid diagnosis of group A strep pharyngitis in the emergency department. *Ann Emerg Med* 1986;15:157.
4. Fyllingen G, et al. Phenoxymethylpenicillin two or three times daily for tonsillitis with beta-hemolytic streptococci group A: a blinded, randomized, and controlled clinical study. *Scand J Infect Dis* 1991;23:553.
5. Gilbert DN, et al. *Sanford guide to antimicrobial therapy.* Antimicrobial Therapy Inc, 1999.
6. Green SM. Acute pharyngitis: the case for empiric antimicrobial therapy. *Ann Emerg Med* 1995;25:404.
7. Helleman K, et al. Curr Ther Respir Clin 1988:43:374.
8. Herzon FS. Peritonsillar abscess: incidence, current management practices, and a proposal for treatment guidelines. *Laryngoscope* 1995;105:1.
9. Kieff DA, et al. Selection of antibiotics after incision and drainage. *Otolaryngol Head Neck Surg* 1999;120:57.
10. Kline JA, et al. Streptococcal pharyngitis: a review of pathophysiology, diagnosis, and management. *J Emerg Med* 1994;12:665.
11. Pichichero ME. Group A streptococcal tonsillopharyngitis: cost-effective diagnosis and treatment. *Ann Emerg Med* 1995;25:390.
12. Postma GN, et al. The professional voice. *Otolaryngol Head Neck Surg* 1998;000:00.
13. Putto A. Febrile exudative tonsillitis: viral or streptococcal. *Pediatrics* 1987;80:6.
14. Roberts JR. Streptococcal pharyngitis. In: Roberts JR, ed. *Robert's practical guide to common medical emergencies.* 1996:177.
15. Sharma HS. Retropharyngeal abscess: recent trends. *Auris Nasus Larynx* 1998;25:403.

CHAPTER 21
Sinusitis

Eric T. Boie

Upper respiratory complaints including sinusitis are among the most common disorders encountered by the emergency physician. It is estimated that 14% of the U.S. population, approximately 30 million people, are treated annually for diseases of the paranasal sinuses.[11] Billions of dollars are spent on physician visits, prescription and over-the-counter medications, and workdays lost secondary to sinus disease. Sinus disease is usually a harmless inconvenience; however, it occasionally presents as a fulminant, life-threatening entity in the emergency department (ED).

Sinusitis is an inflammatory disease of the paranasal sinuses resulting from infectious, allergic, or autoimmune processes.[16] *Rhinosinusitis* has been proposed as a more precise definition, as inflammation frequently involves the nasal passages, and sinusitis without rhinitis is rare.[10] Sinusitis can be further classified as acute, subacute, or chronic based on duration of symptoms. *Acute sinusitis* lasts 3 to 4 weeks, with complete resolution of symptoms either spontaneously or with treatment. *Chronic sinusitis* is defined by persistent symptoms for more than 3 months despite maximum therapy. In *subacute sinusitis,* symptoms last from 3 weeks to 3 months.[1]

The exact incidence and prevalence of sinusitis is difficult to determine due to lack of rigid criteria defining sinus disease. Occurrence among men equals that among women. Children are more often affected than are adults; from 0.5% to 2.0% of upper respiratory infections (URIs) in adults and 5% to 10% of URIs in children are complicated by acute bacterial sinusitis.[7,8] Sinus disease in the United States is more prevalent in the Midwest and South compared with the Northeast and West.[10] Chronic sinusitis affects 5% to 15% of urban dwellers, and the prevalence of chronic sinusitis is increasing.[1]

The human sinuses are composed of four paired, sterile cavities lined with ciliated epithelium. Maxillary and ethmoid sinuses are present at birth. Frontal and sphenoid sinuses develop in the seventh and tenth year of life, respectively.[9] Individual sinus anatomy is highly variable, with frontal sinuses absent in 2% to 5% of the population.[12] The posterior ethmoid and sphenoid sinuses empty into the superior meatus. The frontal, anterior ethmoid, and maxillary sinuses empty into the ostiomeatal complex within the middle meatus. Obstruction of the ostiomeatal complex (OMC) due to inflammation, anatomic abnormality, or other pathology is the critical event in the development of acute sinusitis.[9] Maxillary sinusitis is most common, followed by ethmoid, frontal, and sphenoid, in descending order of frequency.[11]

Most cases of sinusitis follow a viral URI. Viruses injure the sinus epithelium, resulting in ciliary dysfunction and a massive inflammatory cascade. Ciliary dysfunction results in mucostasis, and the damaged epithelium is highly susceptible to secondary bacterial invasion from the contiguous nasal passages. Inflammation results in occlusion of the OMC, obstructing sinus drainage and creating a hypoxic, hypercarbic, acidic environment that is ideal for bacterial growth.[7] Multiple factors contribute to the development of sinusitis that does not follow a URI, including dental infection, ciliary dysfunction, occlusion of the OMC, and immunodeficiency. Five percent to 10% of acute maxillary sinusitis occurs due to contiguous spread of dental infection.[1] Ciliary motility disorders, both congenital (Kartagener syndrome) and acquired, predispose to sinusitis. Inflammatory changes of allergic or infectious origin can result in OMC occlusion. Anatomic abnormalities such as polyps, enlarged adenoids, or malignancies can do likewise. Nasal foreign bodies also result in OMC obstruction and can lead to sinusitis: 95% of nasally intubated patients develop sinusitis.[1] Immunocompromised patients, including those with steroid dependence, cystic fibrosis, the human immunodeficiency virus (HIV), diabetes, neutropenia, cancer, chronic renal disease, and organ transplants, are all more susceptible to the development of sinusitis and are more likely to have severe disease.[1]

Infectious sinusitis can be of viral, bacterial, or fungal origin. Viral rhinosinusitis is 20 to 200 times more common than bacterial sinusitis.[2] Over 200 viruses have been implicated in acute sinusitis, with subtypes of *rhinovirus, parainfluenza,* and *influenza* virus being the most common.[5] *Streptococcus pneumoniae* (30%), nontypeable *Haemophilus influenzae* (20%), *Moraxella catarrhalis, Staphylococcus aureus,* other streptococcal species, and anaerobes of dental origin compose the primary pathogens in acute bacterial sinusitis.[7] Antibiotic resistance is a growing concern. One-third of *Haemophilus* isolates and nearly all of *Moraxella* strains are beta-lactamase producing, and up to half of pneumococcal strains display penicillin resistance.[11] *Pseudomonas* is an important pathogen in patients with cystic fibrosis and HIV. The bacteriology of chronic sinusitis is not as well defined; however, anaerobes, gram negatives, and staphylococcal species are most frequently implicated.[9] Fungal sinusitis presents either as an acute fulminant or a chronic indolent process. The former occurs in those who are significantly immunocompromised. Mucoraceae species, including *Rhizopus, Mucor,* and *Absidia,* cause necrotizing invasive disease most often in patients with diabetic ketoacidosis.[4] *Aspergillus* species are becoming a more common pathogen, manifesting in one of three chronic forms in immunocompetent adults: indolent invasive, mycetoma ("fungus ball"), and allergic fungal sinusitis. The last is the most recently described and frequent form of fungal sinusitis in the United States.[13]

CLINICAL PRESENTATION

The clinical presentation of acute sinusitis is highly variable. Most of the presenting chief complaints are nonspecific and may include purulent nasal discharge, nasal congestion, facial pressure, dental pain, ear pain, fever, headache, cough, fatigue, halitosis, or diminished sense of smell. Such symptoms are almost indistinguishable from those of a viral URI, thus *duration* of symptoms becomes critical in diagnosis. A patient with cold symptoms that do not resolve after 7 to 10 days has a high likelihood of having acute bacterial sinusitis.[2] Criteria have been established to aid in the diagnosis of acute bacterial sinusitis, as outlined in Table 21.1. In patients with more than 7 days of symptoms, acute bacterial sinusitis is probable if two major factors or one major and two minor factors are present.[11] The presentation of acute sinusitis in children differs from that of adults. Children with sinusitis most commonly present with rhinorrhea and cough, and there is often coexistent otitis.[7] Children under

TABLE 21.1. Major and Minor Factors for Diagnosis of Acute Sinusitis

Major[a]	Minor
Facial pain or pressure	Headache
Purulent nasal discharge	Cough
Fever	Fatigue
Nasal congestion	Halitosis
Nasal obstruction	Dental pain
Hyposmia or anosmia	Ear pain/pressure

[a]Diagnosis requires two major *or* one major and two minor factors in a patient with symptoms for more than 7 days (from the Task Force on Rhinosinusitis).[2]

the age of 5 are less likely to complain of facial pain, dental pain, and headache.[8] Periorbital edema occasionally is the presenting sign in a child with ethmoid sinusitis.[7] Unilateral sinus drainage in a child should alert the astute emergency physician to the possibility of a nasal foreign body.[8] Chronic sinusitis in adults and children may present similarly to acute sinusitis, but symptoms tend to be more vague and less severe.[9]

Systemic toxicity, mental status changes, severe headache, and fever are signs and symptoms indicative of more serious sinus disease or its complications.[12] The emergency physician needs to maintain a heightened awareness for these ominous markers, as early identification and treatment is critical in decreasing associated morbidity and mortality. Both acute and chronic sinusitis can present initially with complications. Complications occur most frequently in teen-age males.[12] The most worrisome complications involve the orbit or intracranial cavity. Periorbital cellulitis is the most common complication of sinusitis, usually originating from the ethmoid sinuses.[17] Periorbital cellulitis must be differentiated from orbital cellulitis, where rates of visual loss approach 10%.[5] Intracranial complications of sinusitis include meningitis, osteomyelitis, cavernous sinus thrombosis, and intracranial abscesses (epidural, subdural, and intracerebral). Meningitis is the most common intracranial complication of sinusitis, as it is estimated that 15% of cases may be of paranasal sinus origin.[12] Extension of acute frontal sinusitis with suppurative inflammation of cortical bone results in the famed "Pott's puffy tumor," a condition requiring aggressive surgical and antimicrobial therapy.[17] Cavernous sinus thrombosis classically presents with periorbital edema, exophthalmos, papilledema, and cranial nerve III, IV, and VI palsies. Intracranial abscesses will usually present with fever and acute neurologic signs. Fortunately, such severe complications of sinusitis are rare. However, long-term morbidity approaches 33%, with blindness, hemiparesis, seizure disorders, and cognitive impairment as some of the more common postmorbid states.[12] A much less severe complication of sinus disease is asthma instability. Although no cause-and-effect relationship has been definitively established, it is widely believed that sinusitis exacerbates asthma.[14]

Special consideration must be given to the immunocompromised host with sinus complaints, as invasive fungal sinusitis is much more common in this population. Patients are typically toxic and may present with moldy-smelling, thick, brown or black nasal discharge. Nasal crusting is prominent, and perforation of the palate, nasal septum, or cribriform plate may be apparent.[13] The invasive organisms cause ischemic necrosis of the bone and mucosa, with hematogenous invasion of the orbit, skin, and brain. Progression to coma and death can occur within hours. Interestingly, acute fungal sinusitis is relatively rare in acquired immune deficiency syndrome (AIDS) patients, presenting as a late-stage phenomenon when CD4+ counts drop below 50/μL.[13] *Aspergillus* is the most common fungal pathogen in this group.

DIFFERENTIAL DIAGNOSIS

The differential diagnosis for sinusitis is broad, as the signs and symptoms of sinus disease are neither sensitive nor specific. Viral URI, nasal polyps, cocaine abuse, allergic rhinitis, vasomotor rhinitis, and rhinitis medicamentosa all may present with symptoms of nasal discharge and congestion. Cerebral spinal fluid rhinorrhea should be considered in a patient with a history of head trauma. Persistent unilateral nasal discharge with epistaxis is concerning for neoplasm or nasal foreign body.[11] Tension, cluster, and migraine headaches, as well as dental disease, are alternative diagnoses in the patient whose sinus disease manifests as cephalgia or facial pain. Patients with fever deserve particular attention, as pyrexia may be a manifestation of simple sinusitis or severe central nervous system (CNS) infection, such as meningitis or intracranial abscess.

EMERGENCY DEPARTMENT EVALUATION

Acute sinusitis is a diagnosis based primarily on clinical history and physical findings (see Table 21.1). Unfortunately, physical examination findings may not prove helpful, as none are specific for acute sinusitis.[5] Findings in a patient with sinusitis may include mucosal hyperemia, purulent rhinorrhea, nasal airway congestion, crusting of the anterior nares, and facial pain. However, palpable facial tenderness is a poor indicator of underlying sinus infection, and "purulent" discharge is not a reliable indicator of bacterial sinusitis.[7] Transillumination has been used as a diagnostic aid, as opacification to transillumination of frontal or maxillary sinuses was a marker of a fluid-filled, infected sinus. Transillumination actually has poor correlation with the presence of fluid, poor intraobserver consistency, and poor specificity. Thus, it is of little use in the diagnosis of acute sinus disease.[5,7]

Radiographic imaging has little role in the diagnosis of acute sinus disease in the ED. The clinical significance of abnormal findings on imaging studies is debatable. Plain radiographs both underestimate and overestimate disease and have poor correlation with computed tomography (CT) findings.[5,7] Abnormal findings are common in a large proportion of asymptomatic individuals, and findings of air–fluid levels, sinus opacification, or mucosal thickening rarely lead to a change in management.[5] CT scan has become the modality of choice for sinus imaging, but also may be oversensitive in detecting "disease."[6] Eighty-seven percent of patients with viral URIs have abnormalities consistent with sinusitis on CT.[1] In a study of healthy, asymptomatic children aged 1 to 2, 69% had abnormal sinus CT scans.[7] It is neither medically necessary nor economically feasible to CT scan every patient with symptoms of sinusitis. CT scans are most helpful after maximum medical therapy in patients undergoing consideration for surgical treatment, and thus should be reserved for the consulting specialist.[5] Use of CT in the ED should be limited to those patients in which serious complications of sinusitis are suspected.[6]

Nasal cultures are not helpful in the diagnosis of acute sinusitis, as growth correlates poorly with cultures from sinus aspirates.[1] Sinus aspiration is neither practical nor routinely performed in the ED. Blood tests are necessary only in patients who show signs of systemic toxicity, show signs of CNS involvement, or have significant comorbid disease or immunosuppression.

The lack of a simple diagnostic test makes the diagnosis of sinusitis challenging, but also creates a tendency to label many common colds as sinusitis.[11] Duration and severity of symptoms may provide clues in the diagnosis. In acute bacterial sinusitis, symptoms generally worsen after 5 days, persist for at least 10 days, and are much more severe than those associated with a viral URI.[2]

EMERGENCY DEPARTMENT MANAGEMENT

The goal of therapeutic intervention in acute sinusitis is threefold: to relieve obstruction of the OMC, to restore mucociliary clearance, and to reestablish sinus sterility through eradication of infection.[9] As acute sinusitis is not purely an infectious process, antimicrobial therapy alone will likely fail.[11] Combination treatment with antibiotics, topical steroids, nasal decongestants, mucoevacuants, anticholinergics, antihistamines, and nonpharmacologic measures may provide the best symptomatic and therapeutic outcome.

Antibiotics have been the mainstay of treatment for acute sinusitis, but great controversy exists regarding indications for use, choice of antimicrobial agent, and duration of therapy. Mild cases of rhinosinusitis with symptoms lasting less than 7 days are most likely viral in etiology, and the temptation to prescribe antibiotics for these patients should be resisted.[2,20] The natural course of untreated acute sinusitis is unknown, but it is estimated that 40% to 50% of cases would resolve spontaneously.[7,16] Antimicrobial therapy is often cited as necessary to avoid development of complications of acute sinus disease; however, there is no prospective evidence to support this conclusion.

In patients meeting the diagnostic criteria for sinusitis with progressive or nonresolving symptoms for more than 7 days, use of a first-line antimicrobial agent is appropriate.[2] Table 21.2 lists the commonly used first- and second-line antimicrobials for acute sinusitis. Amoxicillin is still highly effective and is the first-line agent of choice in acute sinusitis.[7,20] Newer, more expensive antibiotics do not appear to be more effective than amoxicillin or trimethoprim plus sulfamethoxazole (TMP-SMX) in patients with uncomplicated sinusitis.[3,20] Most studies suggest that almost any antibiotic results in clinical improvement greater than 85% of the time.[16] Although no prospective study has established the optimum duration of therapy, a 10- to 14-day course is generally accepted as adequate.[8,11] A small number of studies have shown 3 days of therapy as equally effective, but this is not yet an accepted practice.[15] Second-line agents should be initiated if there is progression of symptoms after 2 to 3 days of initial therapy.[2,7]

The use of topical steroids in acute sinusitis is attractive, as they are potent antiinflammatories with few side effects. Studies have demonstrated improved symptom relief, but the clinical efficacy of topical steroids is uncertain.[1,5] Steroids are generally well tolerated, with local irritation and bleeding as the most common side effects.[5]

Topical alpha-adrenergic agonists, such as oxymetolazone, have been used to decrease mucosal edema, promoting sinus drainage and ventilation. These agents should not be used for more than 3 days, as this may elicit rhinitis medicamentosa due to rebound vasodilation. Oral systemic decongestants (ephedrine, pseudoephedrine, phenylephrine, phenylpropanolamine, etc.) also can be taken, but side effects, including nervousness, insomnia, hypertension, and tachycardia, may limit their use. Despite the extensive use of these agents, their efficacy remains unclear.[10]

The mucoevacuant guaifenesin can be used to increase mucous flow and decrease mucous viscosity.[1] Side effects are minimal but may include abdominal discomfort and emesis.[5]

Topical anticholinergics such as ipratropium bromide may reduce rhinorrhea, and thus can also be used as adjunctive therapy.[1] Antihistamine use in acute sinusitis remains controversial. While antihistamines may decrease rhinorrhea, some argue that their use is contraindicated, as they increase mucous viscosity, leading to inspissation and outflow obstruction.[8] Nonpharmacologic therapy such as steam inhalation and saline douching provide symptomatic relief by softening crusts and moisturizing dry mucosa.

All of these adjunctive therapies are based largely on anecdote and personal preference, as there is little evidence that these additions make a great impact on clinical outcome.[8,10] It is likely that the longer acute sinusitis is treated, the more the natural course of infection is seen; that is, spontaneous resolution occurs regardless of what is done.[11]

Special consideration is needed for managing sinusitis in children, the elderly, and immunocompromised patients. Although debated, because children experience more URIs than do adults, the incidence of acute sinusitis in children may be higher. Sinusitis should be considered in any child with respiratory symptoms not improving after 10 days.[8] Any child with recurrent acute sinusitis, or chronic sinusitis despite aggressive therapy, should be referred for evaluation for cystic fibrosis or underlying immune dysfunction.[9,14] In elderly patients, the threshold to treat acute sinusitis should be lower, as aggressive medical intervention may be important in reducing morbidity in this group.[5] In immunocompromised patients, increased alertness for fulminant sinusitis and its complications is necessary. Sinusitis is one of the most common problems affecting HIV-positive patients.[18] The treatment of acute sinusitis is essentially the same regardless of HIV status, except for duration of antimicrobial therapy (21 days is standard).[19] When CD4+ counts fall below 200, opportunistic sinus infections become more common and more resistant to standard therapy.[18]

TABLE 21.2. Antibiotic Therapy Alternatives in Acute Sinusitis[16]

FIRST-LINE THERAPY
Amoxicillin
Trimethoprim and sulfamethoxazole (TMP/SMX)
Erythromycin–sulfamethoxazole
SECOND-LINE THERAPY
Amoxicillin–clavulanate
Cefixime
Cefpodoxime proxetil
Cefprozil
Cefuroxime axetil
Levofloxacin
Trovafloxacin
FIRST- OR SECOND-LINE THERAPY
Azithromycin
Clarithromycin

Second-line therapy is indicated when symptoms progress during the first 48 to 72 hours of first-line therapy.

DISPOSITION

Most patients with acute, uncomplicated sinusitis can be safely discharged with instructions to return to the ED or to follow up with their regular doctor if symptoms are worsening or not improving within 2 to 3 days. Patients should be educated on the signs of potential intracranial extension (severe headache, vomiting, confusion) and advised to return to the ED immediately for the same. Patients with sinus symptoms lasting longer than 1 month despite a complete course of therapy should be referred to an otolaryngologist for CT imaging and further evaluation.[11]

Any patient with severe headache, altered mental status, systemic toxicity, meningeal signs, or visual complaints suggestive of intraorbital or intracranial extension requires aggressive management to prevent the significant morbidity and mortality associated with complicated sinus disease. Administration of broad-spectrum antibiotic therapy, most appropriately a third-generation cephalosporin plus vancomycin, should not be delayed by diagnostic procedures.[16] Early antibiotics, followed by CT, lumbar puncture, and consultation of ear, nose, and throat; neurosurgery; and ophthalmology where appropriate, is critical.[11] The majority these patients will require admission to the intensive care unit.

Transfer to a referral center is necessary if specialist consultation is not readily available for patients with serious complications of sinus disease. Appropriate stabilization efforts and intravenous antibiotic therapy should be initiated prior to transfer. Advanced cardiac life support–capable transport by ground or air is necessary for patients with intracranial complications.

COMMON PITFALLS

- Obtaining radiographic imaging in the setting of acute, uncomplicated sinusitis adds little to the work-up except cost.

There is rarely a role for imaging in acute sinusitis, unless complications are present.[6]

- Using antibiotics in patients with symptoms consistent with sinusitis of less than 7 days' duration should be avoided. Antibiotics are often inappropriately dispensed for viral rhinosinusitis, which is 20 to 200 times more common than acute bacterial sinusitis.[2]
- Patients with symptoms of sinusitis with marked headache and fever must be carefully evaluated to avoid missing early indicators of intracranial extension of acute sinus disease.
- Elderly, diabetic, HIV-positive, and other immune suppressed patients demand a keen awareness, as they are at greater risk for more severe sinusitis and its complications.
- Remember that despite its prevalence, the classifications, diagnostic criteria, clinical management, and ideal treatment options of acute sinusitis are largely anecdotal and without a prospective, evidence-based foundation.

References

1. Anonymous. Infectious rhinosinusitis in adults: classification, etiology and management. International Rhinosinusitis Advisory Board. *Ear Nose Throat* 1997;76(12):1–22.
2. Ahuja GS, Thompson J. What role for antibiotics in otitis media and sinusitis? *Postgrad Med* 1998;104(3):93–99, 103–104.
3. de Ferranti SD, et al. Are amoxicillin and folate inhibitors as effective as other antibiotics for acute sinusitis? A meta-analysis. *BMJ* 1998;317(7159):632.
4. Eloy P, Bertrand B, et al. Mycotic sinusitis. *Acta Otorhinolaryngol Belg* 1997;51(4):339–352.
5. Evans KL. Recognition and management of sinusitis. *Drugs* 1998;56(1):59–71.
6. Hudgins PA, Mukundan S. Screening sinus CT: a good idea gone bad? *Am J Neuroradiol* 1997;18(10):1850–1854.
7. Incaudo GA, Wooding LG. Diagnosis and treatment of acute and subacute sinusitis in children and adults. *Clin Rev Allergy Immunol* 1998;16(1-2):157–204.
8. Isaacson G. Sinusitis in childhood. *Pediatr Clin North Am* 1996;43(6):1297–1318.
9. Josephson GD, Gross CW. Diagnosis and management of acute and chronic sinusitis. *Compr Ther* 1997;23(11):708–714.
10. Kaliner MA, Osguthorpe JD, et al. Sinusitis: bench to bedside. Current findings, future directions. *J Allergy Clin Immunol* 1997;99:S829–S848.
11. Maltinski G. Nasal disorders and sinusitis. *Prim Care* 1998;25(3):663–683.
12. Mansfield EL, Gianola GJ. Intracranial complications of sinusitis. *J La State Med Soc* 1994;146(7):287–290.
13. Morpeth JF, Rupp NT, et al. Fungal sinusitis: an update. *Ann Allergy Asthma Immunol* 1996;76(2):128–140.
14. Nishioka GJ, Cook PR. Paranasal sinus disease in patients with cystic fibrosis. *Otolaryngol Clin North Am* 1996; 29(1):193-205.
15. Pichichero ME, Cohen R. Shortened course of antibiotic therapy for acute otitis media, sinusitis and tonsillopharyngitis. *Pediatr Infect Dis J* 1997;16(7):680–695.
16. Poole MD. Antimicrobial therapy for sinusitis. *Otolaryngol Clin North Am* 1997;30(3):331–339.
17. Rao VM, el-Noueam KI. Sinonasal imaging. Anatomy and pathology. *Radiol Clin North Am* 1998;36(5):921–939.
18. Rombaux P, Bertrand B, et al. Sinusitis in the immunocompromised host. *Acta Otorhinolaryngol Belg* 1997;51(4):305–313.
19. Tami TA. The management of sinusitis in patients infected with the human immunodeficiency virus (HIV). *Ear Nose Throat* 1995;74(5):360–363.
20. Werk LN, Bauchner H. Practical considerations when treating children with antimicrobials in the outpatient setting. *Drugs* 1998;55(6):779–790.

CHAPTER 22
Rhinitis

Michael J. Foley and Gregory P. Moore

Rhinitis and other nasal disorders are generally not life-threatening conditions, but they are responsible for frequent emergency department (ED) visits, restricted activities, loss of productivity, discomfort, and decreased quality of life. It is established that 40 million Americans will have a nasal disorder annually, resulting in millions of visits and significant health-care dollars spent on diagnosis and treatment.[5] Allergic rhinitis alone affects approximately 20% of the U.S. population,[12] and the cost of medication for nasal obstruction is approximately 5 billion dollars annually.[17]

Rhinitis is the most frequent of the upper respiratory infections and can be broadly categorized into noninfectious and infectious types. Acute rhinitis is the usual manifestation of a common cold and, by definition, lasts less than 3 weeks. Chronic rhinitis lasts longer than 3 weeks and can occur in conditions characterized by granuloma formation (e.g., tuberculosis, syphilis, histoplasmosis). Simple viral infections (e.g., adenovirus) of the nasopharynx are the most common cause of rhinitis. Other infectious causes are bacterial or fungal. Allergic (seasonal or perennial) rhinitis is the largest cause of noninfectious rhinitis. Other noninfectious causes include vasomotor, atrophic, gustatory, hormonal, granulomatous, drug-induced, and idiopathic rhinitis.

Anatomic abnormalities associated with rhinitis may include septal deformities, nasal valvular collapse, septal hematomas, abscess, neoplasms, foreign bodies, and choanal atresia in children. These should be considered when evaluating this chief complaint. It is important to investigate patients presenting with clear, watery rhinorrhea for a possible cerebrospinal fluid (CSF) leak. CSF rhinorrhea is often unilateral and associated with surgery or trauma, but cases of spontaneous leaking have been described. There is no reliable method for distinguishing CSF from nasal mucus in the ED, despite the continued use of glucose indicator sticks and the formation of a halo effect on filter paper.

Allergic rhinitis is an immunologically based inflammatory condition triggered by exposure to an allergen. Antibodies (immunoglobulin M [IgM]) specific for the allergen are produced, and they subsequently attach to mast cells in the nasal mucosa. Later, when reexposure occurs, the allergen attaches to IgE on mast cells, causing the release of inflammatory mediators (the most important being histamine). *Seasonal allergic rhinitis,* by definition, has a seasonal variation in symptoms, with the common allergens being pollens (tree, grass, ragweed) and molds. *Perennial allergic rhinitis* can be more difficult to diagnose and occurs on the majority of days throughout the year. The most common allergen responsible for perennial allergic symptoms is the house dust mite.[8] Animal dander (cats, dogs, horses) is another common nonseasonal allergen. A thorough history will help distinguish these two forms of rhinitis.

Nonspecific environmental triggers such as irritants (smoke, strong odors, fumes), temperature changes, humidity, and air conditioning are responsible for a condition known as *vasomotor rhinitis.* Rhinorrhea and nasal obstruction are the predominant symptoms, rather than sneezing or pruritis. Due to the rare nature of this entity, vasomotor rhinitis should be a diagnosis of exclusion.

Atrophic rhinitis occurs with atrophy of the nasal mucosa and commonly causes loss of smell and taste. Nasal and sinus surgery may result in cases of secondary atrophic rhinitis.

Certain medications affecting peripheral vascular tone have been associated with *drug-induced rhinitis.* Beta-blockers (systemic and topical ophthalmic), angiotensin converting enzyme inhibitors, birth control pills, chlorpromazine, aspirin, and other nonsteroidal antiinflammatory drugs have all been implicated. Prolonged use (greater than 5 days) of topical nasal vasoconstricting agents in the form of drops, sprays, or inhalers may result in a condition called *rhinitis medicamentosa.* Tachyphylaxis and rebound nasal congestion lead to a cycle of shorter duration of relief and, thus, more frequent use.

Gustatory rhinitis is a self-limiting form of rhinitis that occurs while eating spicy or hot foods and is a common condition of the elderly. *Hormonal rhinitis* may develop during puberty, pregnancy, thyroid conditions, or changes with age (e.g., in postmenopausal women).

Many drugs, such as cocaine, amphetamines, and amyl nitrate, are abused via the intranasal route. These patients have chronic rhinitis and inflammation of the nasal mucosa, and may develop bloody nasal drainage, mucosal ulcerations, or frank septal perforation.

CLINICAL PRESENTATION

Most patients with nasal disorders have symptoms of nasal obstruction and/or rhinorrhea. Other symptoms include postnasal drip, hyposmia (diminished sense of smell) or anosmia (absence of the sense of smell), congestion, and sneezing. A good question to initially ask of all rhinitis patients is, "What is your primary symptom?" This may identify the specific etiology and thus aid therapy (Table 22.1).

Patients with infectious rhinitis have symptoms consistent with the common cold, with the exception of fungal infections, which have more chronic manifestations. Patients with allergic rhinitis describe profuse rhinorrhea, conjunctivitis, sneezing, and continuous or seasonal exacerbations. Eliciting a history of chronic nasal vasoconstricting agent use leads to the diagnosis of rhinitis medicamentosa. These patients usually have continuous nasal congestion and clear rhinorrhea.

It is essential to obtain a thorough medication history when evaluating a patient for drug-induced rhinitis. Hormonally induced rhinitis of pregnancy begins during the second month of gestation and terminates with delivery. Asking about a recent history of trauma helps in screening a patient for CSF rhinorrhea or septal hematoma. Investigate concomitant pulmonary symptoms, as rhinitis may be associated with asthma or other pulmonary disorders.

Compared with allergic rhinitis, patients with vasomotor rhinitis generally have less sneezing and pruritis. Patients with atrophic rhinitis commonly lose taste or smell and have recurrent epistaxis and a foul odor to the nasal discharge. Any bloody nasal discharge should alert the physician to a possible diagnosis of intranasal drug abuse, intranasal foreign body, neoplasms, or angiofibroma (i.e., young males).

DIFFERENTIAL DIAGNOSIS

Specific clues in the history help narrow the differential diagnosis. Unilateral symptoms are associated with structural abnormalities. Allergic rhinitis should be suspected after a careful history of known exposure to allergens. The ED physician should suspect an intranasal foreign body in children with chronic, unilateral, purulent nasal drainage.

Nasal neoplasms are rare, but the emergency physician should consider the diagnosis in any patient with unilateral nasal obstruction, bleeding, or pain. Cystic fibrosis may present as rhinorrhea with nasal polyps in children. Rare disorders that cause rhinitis include Wegener's granulomatosis, sarcoidosis, CSF rhinorrhea, and nasal polyposis.

EMERGENCY DEPARTMENT EVALUATION

Following a thorough but directed history, the physical examination should focus on the head and neck. It is optimal to gather all the necessary equipment before examination of the nasal structures (similar to the approach to epistaxis). Palpate the nose for masses and tenderness. The nose and nasal mucosa should be examined with a head mirror or headlight. Rhinoscopy with a nasal speculum allows evaluation of only the anterior one-third to one-half of the nasal cavity. The remainder of the nasal cavity can be examined with a fiberoptic nasopharyngoscope, if available. Determining whether there is unilateral obstruction helps in the differential diagnosis. Evaluate the mucosal surface and look for foreign bodies or tumors. Caution must be exercised not to confuse large swollen turbinates with nasal polyps. Polyps are pale gray, lack sensation, and are mobile. Turbinates have a pink mucosal surface, are tender to palpation, and are relatively firm to palpation. Define the character of the nasal drainage as primarily clear and watery or thick and purulent. Palpate the maxillary and frontal sinuses and examine the oropharynx, ears, eyes, neck, and lungs to rule out conditions presenting with symptoms similar to those of rhinitis.

Ancillary laboratory tests are generally not helpful in the ED setting. To raise the suspicion for fungal rhinitis, cancer, or other rare nasal conditions, the ED physician should consider whether the patient may be immunocompromised in any way. These patients also need to be evaluated for sepsis syndromes with a complete blood count, blood culture, and chest x-ray. If sinusitis is suspected, plain films of the sinuses have been found to have low yield. Limited (5-mm slices) coronal computed tomography (CT) of the sinuses has become the standard radiographic study to evaluate the sinuses.

Non-ED testing, such as nasal mucociliary clearance, peak nasal inspiratory flow, olfactory nerve testing, swabs, smears, biopsies, allergy skin testing, IgE serologic testing, endoscopy, and nasal cytology, may be done in conjunction with an allergist or otolaryngologist in the outpatient setting. Outcomes of patients with rhinitis are much improved when the etiology is specifically identified.

EMERGENCY DEPARTMENT MANAGEMENT

Prevention of attacks by avoidance of precipitating factors should be recommended. Perennial allergic rhinitis may be controlled by reducing exposure to house dust mites and animal dander. This effort may completely relieve the symptoms of rhinitis without

TABLE 22.1. Common Causes of Rhinitis

Symptoms	Etiology	Discharge	Distinguishing Factors	Treatment
Unilateral or bilateral	Sinusitis	Mucopurulent	Facial pain, fever	Antibiotic, decongestant
Unilateral	Foreign body	Mucopurulent	Foul odor	Removal
Unilateral	CSF leak	Clear	Surgery, trauma	Neurosurgical consult
Bilateral	Allergic	Clear	Pruritis	Antihistamines, corticosteroids, decongestants
Bilateral	Vasomotor	Clear, bloody	Lose taste, smell	Supportive
Bilateral	Intranasal drug abuse	Bloody	Other signs of drug abuse	Cessation of drug abuse
Bilateral	Rhinitis medicamentosa	Clear	Use of nasal vasoconstrictors	Stop medication
Bilateral	Hormonal	Clear	During puberty or pregnancy	None
Bilateral	Gustatory	Clear	Associated with eating	Self-limited

the need for medical management. Following avoidance, the next line of therapy is medical treatment to provide symptomatic relief. The three main medical therapies for symptomatic relief are antihistamines, decongestants, and corticosteroids.

Oral antihistamines are the cornerstone of medical therapy and are highly effective in controlling watery rhinorrhea, itching, and sneezing. Their main mechanism of action is via blocking of the H1 histamine receptors. First-generation antihistamines such as diphenhydramine (Benadryl) and chlorpheniramine (Chlor-Trimeton) easily penetrate the blood–brain barrier due to their high lipophilicity. They frequently cause sedation and altered motor skills and are therefore not recommended in school-aged children or in adults who will be driving or operating heavy machinery. Patients may also have urinary retention, constipation, dry eyes, and tachycardia due to the anticholinergic side effects. This side-effect profile led to the development of second-generation antihistamines such as astemizole (Hismanal), cetirizine (Zyrtec), fexofenadine (Allegra), loratadine (Claritin), and terfenadine (Seldane). The second-generation antihistamines are relatively nonsedating due to less lipophilicity and have improved patient tolerance but are considerably more expensive. The ED physician should be aware of potential drug interactions with all of the first-generation and most of the second-generation agents, as they are metabolized by the cytochrome P-450 system. Topical antihistamines such as azelastine (Astelin) also may be effective, but they are still under investigation for use in patients with rhinitis.

Decongestants reduce nasal congestion by decreasing vasodilation, resulting in less edema and blood flow to the nasal mucosa. Their mechanism of action is via stimulation of alpha-receptors. Topical agents include phenylephrine (Neo-Synephrine) HCl 0.5% and oxymetazoline (Afrin) HCl 0.05%. They should be used for only 3 to 5 days, as extended use may result in rebound vasodilation and increased nasal congestion. Systemic agents (alpha-adrenergic agonists) include pseudoephedrine (Sudafed) and phenylpropanolamine. These agents have been studied extensively and seem to be safe for use in patients with controlled hypertension.[13,15] The use of decongestants in patients with uncontrolled hypertension may lead to stroke or severe hypertension. There are also a variety of medications with decongestant–antihistamine combinations.

Corticosteroids are the primary pharmacologic treatment for allergic rhinitis. Nasal steroids act on both the immediate- and the late-phase reactions. Examples include beclomethasone (Vancenase, Beconase), budesonide (Rhinocort), flunisolide (Nasalide, Nasarel), fluticasone (Flonase), and triamcinolone (Nasacort). These agents generally have a delayed clinical response, and patients should be advised to expect that nasal steroids will take at least 1 week to become efficacious. Minimal adverse effects include nasal irritation and epistaxis. Systemic steroid therapy is rarely indicated in cases of allergic rhinitis.

The primary advantage of cromolyn sodium is prophylactic use before allergen exposure, with the greatest benefit in patients with high IgE levels and considerable exposure to the offending allergen.[4] Anticholinergics such as ipratropium (Atrovent) 0.3% nasal spray effectively control rhinorrhea by reducing the volume of nasal secretions by blocking parasympathetic nerve transmission.

Special considerations are the use of decongestants in patients with uncontrolled hypertension[13,15] and the use of sedating medications in the elderly and school-aged children. The use of terfenadine or astemizole in conjunction with macrolide antibiotics (e.g., erythromycin or clarithromycin) or antifungal agents (e.g., ketoconazole) may result in life-threatening cardiac toxicity (QT interval prolongation and ventricular tachycardia).

Other treatment options that are unavailable in the ED include desensitization to allergens (e.g., pollens) and surgery. Surgical treatment may be necessary after failed medical management, especially for a deviated nasal septum or nasal polyps. By correcting these two conditions, topical medications may have better access to the nasal mucosa.

DISPOSITION

Almost all patients seen in the ED for rhinitis can be discharged home. All of the medications discussed are relatively simple to administer and are commonly used in the outpatient setting. Referral to a specialist (allergist or otolaryngologist) may be considered with progression of symptoms, complications, or the need for nasal endoscopy, CT scans, or allergy skin testing. This specialized evaluation allows a much clearer understanding of the pathophysiology in specific nasal disorders.

COMMON PITFALLS

- Failure to focus on the history and physical examination
- Not considering comorbid diseases in patients with rhinitis (e.g., hypertension, immunocompromised states, current use of macrolide antibiotics)
- Failure to obtain a good medication history (including over-the-counter medications)
- Failure to consider intranasal drug use as a cause of nasal congestion and rhinitis
- Missing an intranasal foreign body in young children with chronic nasal discharge
- Misidentification of turbinates as nasal polyps
- Avoid the use of terfenadine or astemizole in conjunction with macrolide antibiotics (e.g., erythromycin or clarithromycin) or antifungal agents (e.g., ketoconazole). This combination may result in life-threatening cardiac toxicity.
- Be aware that the use of decongestants in patients with uncontrolled hypertension may lead to stroke or severe hypertension.

References

1. Bascom R. Environmental factors and respiratory hypersensitivity: the Americans. *Toxicol Lett* 1996;86(2–3):115–130.
2. Casiano RR, Lasko DS. Diagnosis and management of rhinosinusitis. *Hosp Physician* 1999;January:25–39, 64.
3. Ferguson BJ. Allergic rhinitis. Recognizing signs, symptoms, and triggering allergens. *Postgrad Med* 1997;101:110–116.
4. Guarderas JC. Rhinitis and sinusitis: office management. *Mayo Clinic Proc* 1996;71(9):882–888.
5. Kopke RD, Jackson RL. Rhinitis. In: Bailey BJ, ed. *Head and neck surgery—otolaryngology*, vol. 1. Philadelphia: JB Lippincott Co, 1993:269–289.
6. Lund V, Aaronson D, Bousquet J, et al. International consensus report on the diagnosis and management of rhinitis. *Allergy* 1994;49[Suppl 19].
7. Lynn M, Snoey E, Bosker G. Allergic disease update—sneezing, wheezing, and getting the red out: clinical classification and outcome: effective pharmacotherapy. *Emerg Med Rep* 1997;18(25):245–256.
8. Mackay IS, Durham SR. ABC of allergies: perennial rhinitis. *BMJ* 1998;316(7135):917–920.
9. McCue JD. Safety of antihistamines in the treatment of allergic rhinitis in elderly patients. *Arch Fam Med* 1996;5(8):464–468.
10. Meltzer EO, Schatz M, Zeiger RS. Allergic and nonallergic rhinitis. In: Middleton, E Jr, Reed CE, Ellis EF, eds. *Allergy: principles and practice*, vol. 2, 3rd ed. St. Louis: Mosby, 1988:1253–1289.
11. Naclerio RM, Solomon W. Rhinitis and inhalant allergens. *JAMA* 1997;278(22):1842–1848.
12. Naclerio RM. Allergic rhinitis. *N Engl J Med* 1991;325:860–869.
13. Petrulis AS, et al. The acute effect of phenylpropanolamine and brompheniramine on blood pressure in controlled hypertension: a randomized double-blinded crossover trial. *J Gen Intern Med* 1991;6(6):503–506.
14. Rachelefsky G. Childhood asthma and allergic rhinitis: the role of leukotrienes. *J Pediatr* 1997;131(3):348–355.
15. Sands CD, et al. Effect of phenylpropanolamine hydrochloride on blood pressure in Korean patients with hypertension controlled by hydrochlorothiazide. *Clin Pharmacol* 1992;11(2):168–173.
16. Sibbald B, Rink E. Epidemiology of seasonal and perennial rhinitis. Clinical presentation and medical history. *Thorax* 1991;46:859–901.
17. Wood RP III, Jafek BW, Eberhard R. Nasal obstruction. In: Bailey BJ, ed. *Head and neck surgery—otolaryngology*, vol. 1. Philadelphia: JB Lippincott Co, 1993:302–328.

CHAPTER 23
Mastoiditis

James A. Pfaff

Before the advent of antibiotics, there was a 20% incidence of complications of otitis media, with mastoiditis being the most predominant. Since then, mastoiditis has become relatively rare, with a reported incidence as low as 0.004% of all patients who have had otitis media.[17] While uncommon, mastoiditis can result in significant and even life-threatening complications. There have been reports of a recent increased resurgence of this disease.[9]

Mastoiditis is best defined as an inflammatory process of the pneumatic spaces of the temporal bone caused by middle ear suppuration; it is really a continuum of disease processes. It is classified into both acute and chronic forms. The mastoid air cells communicate with the middle ear cavity by way of the aditus ad antrum. These cells are lined with epithelium that is continuous with the epithelium lining the tympanic cavity and are inflamed during an episode of acute otitis media. When the aditus ad antrum is blocked, a closed space develops, causing stasis of secretions and the resultant inflammatory cascade. The inflammation may be confined to the periosteum or extend through it, with ultimate decalcification and resorption of the bony septum of the mastoid bone,[4] a condition generally known as coalescent mastoiditis. According to Bluestone and Klerrie,[1] there are a number of directions to which the resulting inflammation can then spread: (1) back through the aditus ad antrum, with spontaneous resolution; (2) lateral to the surface of the mastoid process, resulting in a subperiosteal abscess (at present, the most common complication of mastoiditis); (3) anteriorly, forming an abscess below the auricle or behind the sternocleidomastoid, resulting in an abscess (known as Bezold's abscess); (4) medially to the petrous portion of the temporal bone (a rare condition known as petrositis); or (5) posteriorly to the occipital bone, resulting in osteomyelitis of the calvarium (a condition known as Citelli abscess).

The incidence of subperiosteal abscess has increased; nearly 50% of patients diagnosed with coalescent mastoiditis also have a subperiosteal abscess.[20] In addition to the aforementioned abscesses, additional complications of mastoiditis include lateral sinus thrombosis, brain abscess, epidural and subdural abscesses, meningitis, otic hydrocephalus, leptomeningitis, suppurative labyrinthitis, sigmoid sinus thrombosis, and facial nerve paralysis.[6]

Chronic mastoiditis is a complication of chronic otitis media, resulting in fibrosis of the mucoperiosteum, mucosal edema, granulation tissue, and bone abnormalities. It is usually characterized by chronic otorrhea through a patent ventilating tube or a perforation of the tympanic membrane (TM) that has been present for more than 2 months.[14] Patients may or may not have an associated cholesteatoma, which is a cystlike mass formed by the ingrowth of squamous epithelium into the middle ear, either through the perforated TM or by retraction of the TM. Its presence will determine the type of therapy given in chronic disease. This disease should be considered in patients with long-standing ear disease, persistent aural discharge, pain, granulation tissue, or cholesteatoma that is refractive to medical therapy.[8]

There is an additional, well-described entity known as latent or masked mastoiditis. This usually results from resolution of overt middle ear disease without resolution of disease within the temporal bone. The patient often appears to have clinical resolution of symptoms when, in fact, there is subsequent subclinical disease that can result in bony destruction, until serious complications such as intracranial involvement occur.

Because acute mastoiditis is often a complication of acute otitis media, it has been reported that the organisms causing it are similar, yet this is not always the case.[15] While *Streptococcus pneumoniae* is the most common organism isolated, *Streptococcus pyogenes, Staphylococcus aureus,* gram-negative organisms such as *Pseudomonas aeruginosa* and *Proteus,* and anaerobes have all been isolated in acute disease. This prevalence may be related to improved culture techniques for the organisms and not necessarily to a change in virulence.[12] *S. aureus, Pseudomonas,* and *Proteus* are the most common organisms involved in chronic disease, although there may be a high incidence of associated anaerobes.[12] Up to 20% to 30% of all cases may fail to yield an isolated organism.[13] In immunocompromised patients, *Aspergillus, Mycobacterium tuberculosis,* other atypical *Mycobacterium* sp., and *Pneumocystis carinii* have all been described, with the latter infection unique to acquired immunodeficiency disease (AIDS) patients.[10] These infections have a slower and more indolent course than do acute diseases. Given the increasing prevalence of disease caused by *M. tuberculosis,* this pathogen should be considered in both the immunocompromised and the immunocompetent host in the presence of mastoiditis and otitis media that are not responding to traditional therapy.

Mastoiditis in children less than 1 year old was thought to be uncommon, given the lack of mastoid pneumatization, but there may be a relative increased incidence from the preantibiotic era. This may be related to the use of antibiotics and the difficulty in detecting the disease in younger age groups.[7] As is the case in otitis media, there appears to be a predilection for the male gender. Mastoiditis has also been described as a complication of leukemia, mononucleosis, sarcoma of the temporal bone and Kawasaki disease.[16]

CLINICAL PRESENTATION

There is usually, but not always, a preceding otitis media, but in one series, 55% of patients with the diagnosis of acute mastoiditis did not have otitis media.[6] The percentage of patients who have previously been on antibiotics ranges from 36% to 71%; their use does not have a protective effect.[11] Postauricular pain is the most common symptom (98%); headache and otalgia also are seen. The patient may have a toxic or lethargic appearance, with a history of decreased appetite or irritability. On examination, fever is present in 83% of patients; up to 76% of patients have postauricular tenderness, swelling, and erythema.[20] The auricle may be displaced forward and laterally, although in children less than 1 year old, the displacement may be downward and lateral due to the mastoid not being fully developed.[5] There may be swelling of the posterior aspect of the external auditory canal, especially in the presence of a subperiosteal abscess.[4] On otoscopic examination, the TM is abnormal in 88% of patients; it may be thickened, opaque, and bulging, with decreased mobility; the TM may be normal in 10%.[18] The disease should be considered in the case of otitis media that is not resolving.

Increasing headache, otalgia, fever, postauricular pain, swelling, or change in the consistency of the otorrhea in patients with chronic otitis media should alert the emergency physician to the possibility of mastoiditis. Patients with chronic mastoiditis will have a perforated TM and otorrhea, and they may have a cholesteatoma. The cholesteatoma may appear to have white or yellow debris on the TM or an abnormality of the TM contour if it is confined to the middle ear.

Patients with masked or latent disease have a smoldering course, with recurrent or prolonged symptoms, little or no fever, and a variable pain picture preceded by a latent period after the apparent resolution of an acute otitis media.[8] Patients may not have retroauricular swelling, and their TM may be intact or perforated. The first sign of this subclinical disease may manifest as serious complications, such as meningitis or an intracranial abscess.

DIFFERENTIAL DIAGNOSIS

Localized scalp infections, such as furuncles or due to trauma, will often present with postauricular swelling. Reactive lymphadenopathy from systemic infections of the head and neck region can also be easily mistaken for mastoiditis. Systemic lymph node disorders from viral infections or neoplastic disease can present with postauricular swelling. If there is swelling of this area in an adult with a history of tobacco use, a neoplastic source should be considered. Rhabdomyosarcoma, eosinophilic granuloma, and brachial cleft abnormalities mimic the findings of mastoiditis in infants.[19]

EMERGENCY DEPARTMENT EVALUATION

Mastoiditis should be considered in any patient with posterior auricular pain and swelling and in patients with a history of otitis media that is not resolving, particularly in the presence of fever and otalgia. Any patient with a history of chronic otitis media with posterior auricular swelling and pain should also have mastoiditis ruled out. Be particularly wary in the immunocompromised host or very young patient with persistent otitis media. The diagnosis of masked or latent mastoiditis should be considered in any patient presenting with an intracranial infection without an obvious source.

Laboratory testing of the disease is not useful. While leukocytosis and an increased erythrocyte sedimentation rate are often present, they are neither sensitive nor specific for the disease. Blood cultures are generally not positive. Of course, a lumbar puncture should be performed in all patients manifesting signs and symptoms of meningitis.

In the past, radiographs were the main modality used in evaluation of the mastoid. Often, radiographs reveal clouding of the mastoid space and bony abnormalities, but they are generally unhelpful and at other times misleading.[2] Computed tomography (CT) is more useful in defining the extent of the disease, as well as intratemporal and intracranial complications. Contrast-enhanced CT may further define complications such as lateral sinus thrombosis. The usefulness of magnetic resonance imaging for this disease has not been extensively studied.

EMERGENCY DEPARTMENT MANAGEMENT AND DISPOSITION

Treatment of mastoiditis depends on the probable etiology and the extent of the disease. All patients with the diagnosis of mastoiditis require otolaryngologic consultation and intravenous antibiotic therapy in the emergency department. Toxic-appearing patients or those with intracranial complications may require intensive care admission and probable neurosurgical referral. For the patient who requires admission, parenteral antibiotics are indicated for acute mastoiditis with only periosteal involvement. In general, decisions about admission, myringotomy, tympanostomy tubes, and mastoidectomy are made by the consulting physician.

The need for surgical treatment, such as myringotomy, tympanostomy tubes, and mastoidectomy may be required if acute disease does not resolve, or progresses. Risk factors for possible early surgical intervention include the presence of fever, leukocytosis, and proptosis of the auricle. A therapeutic mastoidectomy may be required.[6]

The antibiotics selected should be effective for *S. pneumoniae,* the most commonly isolated pathogen. They also should be able to penetrate the blood–brain barrier. Initial selections may include third-generation cephalosporins, such as ceftriaxone (1 g every 12 hours) or cefotaxime (1 g every 4 hours), or a combination of a semisynthetic penicillin and chloramphenicol.[16] Concern for anaerobic bacteria may result in the addition of Flagyl.[12] Immunocompromised patients may require antifungal or antituberculous agents; the use of these should be made in conjunction with otolaryngologic and infectious disease specialists.

The use of daily parenteral antibiotics for ambulatory patients has been advocated if there is close follow-up by an otolaryngologist and an infectious disease specialist.[3] Alternatively, for less severe disease, outpatient treatment includes the traditional regimens used for otitis media: amoxicillin, Bactrim, Augmentin, or the cephalosporins.

Patients who fail to improve within 24 to 72 hours and have evidence of coalescent disease, a subperiosteal abscess, or intracranial disease are candidates for mastoidectomy. The treatment of chronic mastoid disease is controversial, with some authors feeling that mastoiditis without cholesteatoma is a reversible process that can benefit from medical therapy and aural drainage.[4] Mastoid surgery is required for those patients with chronic disease and a cholesteatoma. Antibiotic coverage should include agents specific against *Pseudomonas,* such as ticarcillin-clavulanate. The otolaryngologist is responsible for the decision regarding surgical intervention. Transfer arrangements should be made if no specialty consultation is available.

COMMON PITFALLS

- Failure to consider mastoiditis in a patient with otitis media that has not resolved in a timely manner
- Failure to consider the presence of latent or masked mastoid disease in toxic-appearing infants or immunosuppressed patients without other apparent sources of infection
- Failure to recognize the significant intracranial or intratemporal complications that can still occur in patients with middle ear disease
- Failure to consider a complication of middle ear disease as the cause of ear drainage

References

1. Bluestone CD, Klerrie JO. Intratemporal complications and sequelae of otitis media. In: Bluestone CD, Stool SE, eds. *Pediatric otolaryngology.* Philadelphia: WB Saunders, 1990:521.
2. Bitar CN, Luka EA, Steele RW. Mastoiditis in children. *Clin Pediatr* 1996;35:391.
3. Eihorn M, Fliss DM, Leiberman A, et al. Otolaryngology and infectious disease team approach for outpatient management of serious pediatric infections requiring parenteral antibiotic therapy. *Int Pediatr Otorhinolaryngol* 1992;24:245.
4. Fliss DM, Leiberman A, Dagan R. Acute and chronic mastoiditis in children. *Adv Pediatr Infect Dis* 1997;13:165.
5. Ginsberg CM, Rudey R, Nelson JD. Acute mastoiditis in infants and children. *Clin Pediatr* 1980;19:549.
6. Gliklich RE, Eavers RD, Iannuzi RA, et al. A contemporary analysis of acute mastoiditis. *Arch Otolaryngol Head Neck Surg* 1996;122:135.
7. Harley EG, Sdralis T, Berkowitz RG. Acute mastoiditis in children: a 12 year retrospective study. *Otolaryngol Head Neck Surg* 1997;116:26.
8. Holt GR, Gates GA. Masked mastoiditis. *Laryngoscope* 1983;93:1034.
9. Hoppe JE, Koster S, Bootz F, et al. Acute mastoiditis relevant once again. *Infection* 1994;22:178.
10. Lalwani AK, Sooy CD. Otologic and neurotologic manifestations of acquired immunodeficiency syndrome. *Otolaryngol Clin North Am* 1992;25:1183.
11. Luntz M, Keren G, Nusen S, et al. Acute mastoiditis revised. *Ear Nose Throat J* 1994;73:648–654.
12. Maharj D, Jadvat A, Fernandes CM, et al. Bacteriology in acute mastoiditis. *Arch Otolaryngol Head Neck Surg* 1987;113:514.

13. Moloy PJ. Anaerobic mastoiditis: a report of two cases with complications. *Laryngoscope* 1982;92:1311.
14. Myer CM. Diagnosis and management of mastoiditis in children. *Pediatr Ann* 1991;20:622.
15. Nadal D, Herman P, Bauman A, et al. Acute mastoiditis: clinical, microbiological and therapeutic aspects. *Emerg J Pediatr* 1990;145:560.
16. Nadol JB, Eavery RD. Acute and chronic mastoiditis: clinical presentation, diagnosis and management. *Curr Clin Top Infect Dis* 1995;15:204.
17. Palva T, Virtanen H, Maknenein J. Acute and latent mastoiditis in children. *J Laryngol Otol* 1985;99:127.
18. Pfaltz CR, Griesmer C. Complications of acute middle ear infections. *Ann Otol Rhinol Laryngol* 1984;112:133.
19. Scott TA, Jackler RK. Acute mastoiditis in infancy: a sequela of unrecognized acute otitis media. *Otolaryngol Head Neck Surg* 1989;101:683.
20. Speigel JH, Lustig LR, Lee DC, et al. Contemporary presentation and management of a spectrum of mastoid abscesses. *Laryngoscope* 1998;108:82

CHAPTER 24
Nasal Hemorrhage

Todd C. Rothenhaus and Ian D. Paul

Epistaxis is a frequent problem seen by the emergency physician. It is estimated that up to a seventh of the population will have at least one episode of epistaxis in their lifetime. The incidence is bimodal, with a peak from the ages of 2 to 10, and a broader peak between the ages of 50 and 80.[7] Nasal hemorrhage occurs most commonly in the dry,[22] and colder,[8,16] months. Most cases are minor; of patients presenting to the emergency department (ED), more than 90% can be definitively managed by the emergency physician. While most patients require follow-up with an otolaryngologist, only 5% to 10% of cases will require an ED consultation for management or admission.

CLINICAL PRESENTATION

Blood is supplied to the nasal mucosa from terminal branches of both the internal and external carotid arteries.[1] The anterior and posterior ethmoidal arteries, branches of the internal carotid system, supply both the septum and lateral aspect of the nose superiorly. The sphenopalatine artery, also part of the internal carotid system, supplies the turbinates and meati posteriorly and the inferoposterior portion of the nasal septum. The superior labial artery, a branch of the external carotid artery, and the greater palatine artery, a branch of the internal carotid artery, supply the anterior portions of the septum and floor of the nasal cavity.

Nasal hemorrhage may present in a number of ways. Frequently, bleeding is minor and arrests in triage with properly performed compression of the nose. Although patients may attempt a number of unusual and unfounded techniques to arrest epistaxis, while in the ED, they should be instructed to firmly grasp and pinch the entire, soft, anterior portion of the nose and hold pressure for 10 to 15 minutes. If bleeding is not easily controlled, or there is any suspicion of airway compromise or hemodynamic instability, the patient should be brought directly to the treatment area.

Approximately 90% of nosebleeds are considered anterior, which means the bleeding can be visualized in the anterior portion of the nasopharynx. Anterior hemorrhage most frequently arises from Kiesselbach's plexus (also known as Little's area), an anastomotic network of vessels on the anterior portion of the

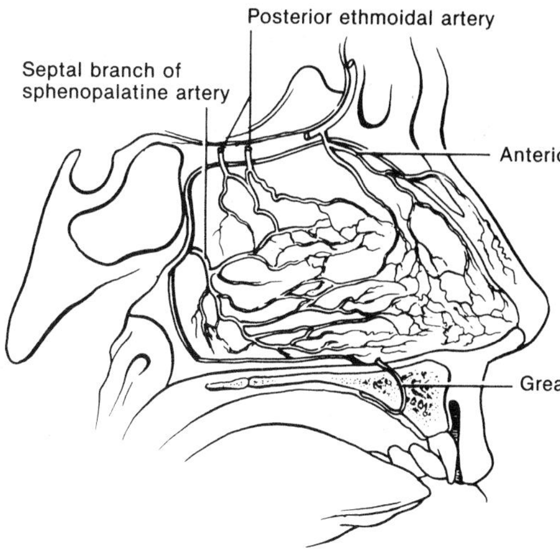

Figure 24.1. Blood supply to Kiesselbach's plexus.

nasal septum (Fig. 24.1). Posterior hemorrhage cannot be visualized directly, tends to be more severe, and is not amenable to simple outpatient therapy. Except in cases of trauma, epistaxis is typically localized to one side of the nose, and the source is frequently a single bleeding point.

Occasionally, patients present with massive epistaxis that is initially confused with hemoptysis or hematemesis. If fresh blood is not clearly dripping out of the nose, examine the oropharynx under suitable light; blood dripping from the posterior nasopharynx confirms nasal hemorrhage.

DIFFERENTIAL DIAGNOSIS

Most cases of nasal hemorrhage are spontaneous and idiopathic. Other causes include facial trauma,[3] nose-picking (epistaxis digitorum), foreign bodies (especially in children,[7] the mentally retarded, and elderly institutionalized patients), and nasal or sinus infections. Iatrogenic causes include nasogastric and nasotracheal intubation, surgical complications, and overzealous treatment of self-limited hemorrhage. Hypertension has long been thought to be associated with epistaxis. However, whether hypertension predisposes to epistaxis remains unclear.[13] A deviated septum is a risk factor for recurrent epistaxis, as drying and cracking of the superficial nasal mucosa occurs at sites of turbulent airflow. Use of topical nasal steroid sprays may produce epistaxis through irritation of the nasal mucosa by the propellant.

Children nearly always present with anterior epistaxis associated with local irritation or recent respiratory infection.[7] Allergic rhinitis has been implicated as a common cause of recurrent epistaxis in children.[15]

Posterior hemorrhage should raise suspicion for juvenile nasopharyngeal angiofibroma in young males, or squamous cell carcinoma in the Asian population. Osler-Weber-Rendu syndrome is characterized by a lack of contractile elements in the muscular wall of vessels, leading to arteriovenous malformations. Patients with acquired immunodeficiency syndrome (AIDS) may have thrombocytopenia from idiopathic thrombocytopenic purpura (ITP), splenomegaly, or drug use, or may present with a qualitative platelet disorder that may predispose to bleeding.[20] Table 24.1 lists some of the many causes of epistaxis.

EMERGENCY DEPARTMENT EVALUATION

A thorough, directed history and physical examination allows the physician to determine the etiology and site of the bleeding,

TABLE 24.1. Causes of Epistaxis

Spontaneous or idiopathic
Trauma
Digital trauma
Facial fractures
Foreign body
Infection
Bacterial rhinitis or sinusitis
Nasal diphtheria
Tumors
Juvenile angiofibroma
Paranasal sinus tumors
Surgery
Chemical irritants
Systemic toxins
Medications
Aspirin
NSAIDs
Warfarin
Heparin
Dipyridamole
Coagulopathy
Thrombocytopenia
Chemotherapy
ITP
DIC
Hemophilia
Von Willebrand disease
Hepatic failure
Leukemias
Venous congestion
CHF
Mitral stenosis
Forceful coughing or nose-blowing
Other
Osler-Weber-Rendu syndrome
Barotrauma
Endometriosis
Allergic rhinitis

NSAIDs, nonsteroidal antiidnflammatory drugs; ITP, idiopathic thrombocytopenic purpura; DIC, disseminated intravascular coagulation; CHF, congestive heart failure.

effect control, and make the appropriate disposition. However, if the patient is bleeding profusely, is hemodynamically unstable, or is extremely apprehensive, an initial attempt should be made to control or slow the bleeding before a lengthy history is obtained. The patient's vital signs, as well as extent, duration, and initial side of hemorrhage, should be noted.

Question patients about past episodes of epistaxis, hypertension, or hepatic or other systemic disease. Easy bruising or prolonged bleeding after minor surgical procedures suggests the possibility of coagulopathy, and recurrent episodes of epistaxis, even if self limited, should raise suspicion for nasal pathology. Use of alcohol and medications, especially aspirin, nonsteroidal antiinflammatory agents, and warfarin (Coumadin), as well as subcutaneous heparin and dipyridamole, should also be sought, as these not only predispose to epistaxis, but also make treatment more difficult.[8,12]

EMERGENCY DEPARTMENT MANAGEMENT

As with all patients presenting to the ED, attention should first be directed toward the ABCs. Massive hemorrhage may require endotracheal intubation. Rapid control of epistaxis associated with multiple trauma or significant facial injuries is best secured with epistaxis balloons,[10] with consideration given to immediate otolaryngology consultation and angiography to rule out internal carotid artery injury.[6] Nontrauma patients with massive epistaxis should be spared lengthy attempts at locating a bleeding source and also be managed with nasal balloons or Foley catheter balloon and anterior packing (discussion follows). Patients with severe hemorrhage should receive intravenous crystalloid infusion, as well as continuous cardiac monitoring and pulse oximetry.

If bleeding is severe, blood should be sent for hematocrit and type and cross-match. If the patient relays a history of easy bruising, recurrent frequent epistaxis, a history of platelet disorders, neoplasia, or recent administration of chemotherapy,[8] a complete blood count is warranted. While a international normalized ratio (INR) and partial thromboplastin time (PTT) are generally not indicated unless warfarin use or liver disease is suspected,[8] a bleeding time is an excellent screen for bleeding disorders. Excessively high blood pressure contributes to hemorrhage and makes bleeding difficult to control, but should be managed carefully. Control of bleeding reduces patients' anxiety, and is frequently all that is necessary to reduce blood pressure.

Treatments at the disposal of the emergency physician include topical vasoconstrictors, chemical or electrical cautery, nasal packing using prefabricated nasal tampons or epistaxis balloons, or traditional nasal packing. Every ED should have a prepackaged epistaxis tray or have key materials readily available (Table 24.2).

Preparation is the key to successful management of epistaxis. Both the patient and physician should be adequately gowned. Droplet spread of blood occurs with sneezing and coughing, so gloves and protective eyewear should be worn.[1,20] Adequate light should be provided by a headlamp with an adjustable, narrow beam.

Position the patient upright or leaning slightly forward. Adjust the chair so that the patient is just below eye level. The patient's head should be comfortably positioned against the headrest to prevent sudden movements during treatment. Have

TABLE 24.2. Equipment Used for Management of Nasal Hemorrhage

ENT chair
Headlamp
Nasal speculum (short and long)
Bayonet forceps
Frazier suction tips (no. 7 and 9)
Yankauer suction tip
Emesis or kidney basin
Gowns
Rubber gloves
Silver nitrate sticks
Electrocautery (optional)
Cotton balls
Dental roll
4×4s
Facial tissue
0.5×72.0-in. petrolatum gauze
Antibacterial ointment (Neosporin, Polysporin, or Bacitracin)
0-silk sutures (straight needle)
Silk tape
Tongue depressors
Small plastic cups
Foley catheters (16F or 18F with 30-mL balloon)
Red rubber catheters (two 8F)
Cocaine 4% topical
Pontocaine 2%–4% or lidocaine 2%–4% topical
Phenylephrine 0.25% solution
Epinephrine 1:1,000 for topical use
Prepackaged nasal balloons
Merocel nasal sponges
Avitene, Surgicel, Oxycel, or Gelfoam
Porcine fat

the patient hold a kidney or emesis basin under the chin to catch blood running from the nose or mouth.

Have the patient blow the nose to clear the nasopharynx, even if bleeding has ceased, as local fibrinolytic activity can result in recurrence of epistaxis or persistent oozing. An initial attempt to locate the bleeding site should then be undertaken. The nasal speculum is used to spread the nares vertically, with the instrument held in such a manner that the index finger rests on the bridge of the nose for stabilization. Begin the examination at Kiesselbach's plexus, moving superiorly and posteriorly along the nasal septum, and conclude with the turbinates and lateral wall. Particular attention should be directed to Kiesselbach's plexus, the posterior floor of the nasal cavity, the junction of the anterior third and posterior two-thirds of the nasal septum,[8] and the high anterior septum. With a well-illuminated and thorough examination, a bleeding point can almost always be identified.

If the point of bleeding is identified and is not bleeding too briskly, application of oxymetazoline (Afrin) alone, or in combination with chemical cautery, has been shown to be effective in the management of anterior epistaxis.[11] Electrical cautery has little advantage over silver nitrate.[21] Cautery should be performed properly to avoid complications. The tip of the applicator should be rolled gently over the mucosa until a grey eschar forms. If bleeding is very light or has stopped and the mucosa is dry, wetting the tip of the applicator may be necessary. Brisk bleeding may be slowed by cauterizing the four quadrants around the bleeding site or any identifiable vessel just proximal to the area. Diffuse or extensive cautery should be avoided, and only one side of the septum should be cauterized at one time, to avoid septal necrosis or perforation.

If bleeding is brisk, pledgets soaked with an anesthetic–vasoconstrictor solution should be inserted into the nose on the side of the bleeding to effect hemostasis and provide anesthesia. Dental roll is particularly unsuited for this purpose, as it does not conform to the contours of the nasal cavity, and once impregnated, tends to hold solutions tenaciously. An acceptable pledget can be fashioned by unwinding a cotton ball, placing the strip between the jaws of bayonet forceps, and winding the fibers around the end of the forceps to form a tight circular band. This then is pulled off the forceps and soaked in 4% cocaine or a 1:1 solution of 4% topical lidocaine and epinephrine (1:1,000). Multiple pledgets may be placed, one above the other, onto the floor of the nasal cavity, and allowed to remain in place for 10 to 15 minutes. Alternatively, if accessible, the point of bleeding can be injected with 0.5 to 1.0 mL of 1% lidocaine with epinephrine 1:100,000 using a 27-gauge needle. If application of vasoconstriction alone fails to stop the bleeding, then cautery may be tried over the now well anesthetized area.

If a bleeding point cannot be localized, yet bleeding continues, the approximate depth of the bleeding site can be localized using a small Frazier suction catheter. Place the catheter at the nares and tilt the patient's head slightly forward so that the suction captures all bleeding. Gently advance the catheter forward along the floor of the nose until blood returns from the nares. Once the approximate depth of the bleeding site is localized, another attempt at slowing or arresting the bleeding, using soaked pledgets, may then be made.

If this fails to arrest the hemorrhage, anterior nasal packing should be performed. At this point, it may be a good idea to reconsider whether bleeding is posterior, because placing a posterior pack will necessitate removing any anterior packing. In addition, if the site of bleeding is from one of the meati, or from the medial surface of a turbinate, packing may prove to be of little value, and attempts to arrest the bleeding with other methods will be needed.

Traditional anterior nasal packing has been supplanted by preformed nasal tampons or epistaxis balloons. Merocel nasal packing is an effective and quick method to control epistaxis.[1,18] After sufficient anesthesia is obtained, hold the Merocel at a 45-degree angle and insert it into the nasal cavity for a distance of 1 to 2 cm. Rotate the Merocel into the horizontal plane and, with firm pressure, push the Merocel straight backward into the nasal cavity. Merocel is supplied for both anterior or anterior–posterior hemorrhage. If an anterior–posterior sponge is employed, it should be inserted until it touches the back wall of the posterior nasal space. If the pack does not fully rehydrate with blood, then saline should be applied. Secure the drawstring to the cheek. Traditional anterior nasal packing should be used if a septal deformity precludes the use of Merocel.[18]

Epistaxis balloons (intranasal balloon catheters) are particularly useful in cases of intractable or posterior hemorrhage. Radiographic evidence has shown that these catheters work through multiple mechanisms, including direct tamponade of the bleeding vessel, tamponade of supplying vessels, occlusion of the posterior choana, and pressure on the inferior and middle turbinate arteries. Balloons are available in either anterior (single-balloon) or anterior–posterior (double-balloon) models. A valve affords access to each balloon. After checking the integrity of the balloons, the catheter is copiously covered with water-based lubricant or viscous lidocaine (petroleum-based materials may cause delayed rupture of the balloon[17]) and the catheter is inserted along the floor of the nose. The balloon should be inflated slowly to minimize pain. Air may be used initially, but saline or sterile water should be used in patients in whom the balloon will remain for more than a few hours.

Traditional anterior nasal packing is difficult for the novice, and should not be attempted until sufficient anesthesia is obtained. The nose should be packed with sterile petrolatum ribbon (0.5 to 1.0 in. wide) gauze, to which is added an antibacterial ointment to prevent the possibility of toxic shock syndrome. Soaking material used for prolonged packing in topical vasoconstrictors may lead to prolonged absorption and is contraindicated.[19] Packing begins by grasping the ribbon about 6 in. from its end with the bayonet forceps. The ribbon is then placed in the nasal cavity as far back as possible, ensuring that the free end still protrudes from the nose. This first pass is then pressed onto the floor of the nasopharynx with the closed bayonets. The ribbon is then grasped about 4 to 5 in. from the nasal alae, the nasal speculum is repositioned so that the lower blade holds the ribbon against the lower border of the nasal alae, and a second strip is brought into the nose and pressed downward. This process is continued superiorly in a stair-step fashion until there is no room left in the nose. Both ends of the ribbon must protrude from the anterior end of the nose, and the ipsilateral nostril is covered with a piece of gauze and secured with tape.

Other alternatives to the traditional anterior nasal pack include calcium sodium alginate (Kaltostat), Oxycel, Avitene, and balloon tamponade. Topical thrombogenic agents such as gelatin sponge (Gelfoam) and microfibrillar collagen powder (Avitene) are useful in cases of epistaxis associated with coagulopathy when applied directly to the bleeding area. Packing with porcine fatty tissue is especially helpful in patients with thrombocytopenia or qualitative platelet disorders.

In the absence of either a suitable epistaxis balloon or a patient able to tolerate lengthy nasal packing, suitable nasal tampons can be constructed by cutting off the fingers of a sterile latex glove, packing them with rolled gauze or cotton balls, and securing the open ends with a silk suture. Two or three of these are then slathered in antibacterial ointment and placed in the nasal cavity, one above the other, until acceptable tamponade is achieved. If the ends of the silk sutures are left long, a dental roll may be secured outside the nasal alae to prevent the tampons from slipping into the nasal pharynx and causing obstruction.

Control of Posterior Epistaxis

Bleeding that begins with the sensation of blood in the posterior pharynx, bleeding that cannot be localized anteriorly, or bleeding that fails to arrest with anterior packing is considered posterior and will need to be managed in consultation with an otolaryngologist. However, bleeding should be controlled by the emergency physician using one of a number of available techniques.

The traditional method of posterior packing is cumbersome and should be replaced with the use of an epistaxis balloon or inflatable Foley catheter. Balloon catheters are easier to install, and equally efficacious, when compared with traditional posterior nasal packs.[2] Regardless of technique, posterior packing occludes the posterior choanae only, and requires some form of anterior pack. Once both the posterior choana and the anterior nares are occluded, the entire nasopharynx fills with blood. Hence, if the posterior pack dislodges, a large amount of blood can be aspirated.[4] Posterior packs are uncomfortable and fraught with complications, including hypoxia, hypercarbia, exacerbation of obstructive sleep apnea, aspiration, hypertension, bradycardia, arrhythmias, myocardial infarction, and death.[5,23] Inflatable balloon catheters designed with a central airway may limit or reduce hypoxia.

If an epistaxis balloon is used, the catheter is first placed as far into the nose as is possible. Next, the posterior balloon is inflated slowly with 4 to 5 mL of water or saline and the catheter is pulled gently forward to fit snugly in the posterior choana. Finally, the anterior balloon is filled with saline until the bleeding stops, the pain is too great, or bowing of the septum is noted. Pressure necrosis and adhesions may result from overinflation, and the amount of fluid placed in each balloon should be recorded.

If a Foley catheter is to be used, a 12F to 16F catheter with 30-cc balloon is placed into the nose along the floor of the nasopharynx until the tip is visible through the mouth in the posterior pharynx. It is then slowly inflated with 15 mL of saline, pulled anteriorly until it is firmly set against the posterior choanae, and secured into place with an umbilical clamp wrapped around dental roll or matted 4×4s to avoid direct pressure necrosis of the ala or columnella.

A traditional posterior pack is fashioned from 4×4-in. gauze rolled into a 1-in. roll and secured with three silk sutures or umbilical tapes. This pack is brought into position in the posterior choana by passing two small, red rubber catheters through each nostril and back out of the mouth, securing each of the two outer sutures to the catheters and pulling the catheters out of the nose again, drawing the pack through the mouth and into position. Each of the sutures is tied together over a gauze buttress to prevent pressure necrosis of the columnella. The third suture is brought out through the mouth and taped to the cheek to facilitate removal.

DISPOSITION

Because of the number of serious causes of epistaxis, including tumors in the elderly and foreign bodies in children, all patients who present to the ED with epistaxis should receive follow-up for a complete nasal examination. Patients should be instructed to avoid blowing the nose, straining, bending over, and participating in sports or other strenuous activity, and to sneeze with their mouth open. Home humidifiers and saline nasal sprays may be helpful in drier, colder months, and patients should avoid any manipulation of the nose. Discontinuation of offending drugs should be individualized and based on the particular indications for each. Patients with a grossly excoriated anterior mucosa should be instructed to gently apply topical antibiotic ointment to the site. Children with recurrent epistaxis and no known bleeding disorder should be referred for coagulation studies.

All patients with anterior packing should receive follow-up with an otolaryngologist in 48 to 72 hours. Anterior nasal packing prevents normal surgical drainage of the sinuses (and frequently the eustachian tubes), and patients should be placed on a penicillin or first-generation cephalosporin. Oral pain medications also should be provided.

All patients with posterior packing need to be admitted, and consideration should be made toward obtaining an arterial blood gas analysis. Clinicians should also strongly consider admitting frail, elderly, cardiac, or chronic obstructive pulmonary disease patients who require anterior packing. Many consulting otolaryngologists are opting for early management of posterior bleeds with endoscopic cautery under direct visualization in the operating suite, early surgical control using arterial ligation, or referral to invasive radiology for selective arterial embolization.[9,14] If time permits and bleeding is not severe, early consultation may spare patients with posterior nasal hemorrhage the discomfort of posterior packing altogether.

COMMON PITFALLS

- Failure to prepare the necessary equipment for control of epistaxis leads to unnecessary inconvenience and delays.
- Epistaxis in young children is rare and should prompt a search for a foreign body.
- Failure to identify the source of bleeding or to place an anterior pack properly leads to rebleeding and necessitates a return to the ED for repacking.
- Failure to identify posterior epistaxis until after an anterior pack has been placed necessitates completely unpacking the nose so a posterior pack can be placed.

References

1. Alvi A, Joyner-Triplett N. Acute epistaxis. *Postgrad Med* 1996;99(5):83–96.
2. Cook PR, Renner G, Williams F. A comparison of nasal balloons and posterior gauze packs for posterior epistaxis. *Ear Nose Throat J* 1985;64:446–449.
3. Chen D, Cheung SW. Epistaxis originating from traumatic pseudoaneurysm of the internal carotid artery: diagnosis and endovascular therapy. *Laryngoscope* 1998;108.
4. Davis JP. Respiratory obstruction associated with use of the Brighton epistaxis balloon. *J Laryngol Otol* 1993;107(2):140–141.
5. Fairbanks DN. Complications of nasal packing. *Otolaryngol Head Neck Surg* 1986;94:412–415.
6. Ghorayeb BY, Kopaniky DR, Yeakley JW. Massive posterior epistaxis. *Arch Otolaryngol Head Neck Surg* 1988;114:1033–1037.
7. Guarisco JL, Graham HD. Epistaxis in children: causes, diagnosis, and treatment. *Ear Nose Throat J* 1989;68:522–538.
8. Jackson KR, Jackson RT. Factors associated with active, refractory epistaxis. *Arch Otolaryngol Head Neck Surg* 1988;114(8):862–865.
9. Jassar P, Sissons G. A case of intractable epistaxis. *J Laryngol Otol* 1997;11:1192–1194.
10. Keen MS, Moran WJ. Control of epistaxis in the multiple trauma patient. *Laryngoscope* 1985;95:874–875.
11. Krempl GA, Noorily AD. Use of oxymetazoline in the management of epistaxis. *Ann Otol Rhinol Laryngol* 1995;104(9 Pt 1):704–706.
12. Lavy J. Epistaxis in anticoagulated patients: educating an at-risk population. *Br J Haematol* 1996;95:195.
13. Lubianca-Neto JF, Fuchs FD. A study of the association between epistaxis and the severity of hypertension. *Am J Rhinol* 1998;12:269.
14. Moreau S, Valdazo A. Supraselective embolization in intractable epistaxis: review of 45 cases. *Laryngoscope* 1998;108:887.
15. Murray B, Milner R. Allergic rhinitis and epistaxis in children. *Ann Allergy Asthma Immunol* 1995;74(1):30–33.
16. Nunez DA, McClymont LG, Evans RA. Epistaxis: a study of the relationship with weather. *Clin Otolaryngol* 1990;15:49–51.
17. Ong CC, Odutoye T. An observation of the effects of paraffin paste on nasal epistaxis balloons. *Acta Otorhinolarygol Belg* 1996;50(3):171–175.
18. Pringle MB, Brightwell AP. The use of Merocel nasal packs in the treatment of epistaxis. *J Laryngol Otol* 1996;110:543.
19. Ross GS, Bell J. Myocardial infarction associated with inappropriate use of topical cocaine as treatment for epistaxis. *Am J Emerg Med* 1992;10:219–222.
20. Rothstein SG, Schneider KL, Kohan D, et al. Emergencies in AIDS patients: the otolaryngologic perspective. *Otolaryngol Head Neck Surg* 1991;104(4):545–548.
21. Toner JG, Walby AP. Comparison of electro and chemical cautery in the treatment of anterior epistaxis. *J Laryngol Otol* 1990;104(8):617–618.
22. Viducich R, Gerson L. Posterior epistaxis: clinical features and acute complications. *Ann Emerg Med* 1995;25(5):592–596.
23. Wetmore SJ, Scrima L, Hiller FC. Sleep apnea in epistaxis patients treated with nasal packs. *Otolaryngol Head Neck Surg* 1988;98:596–599.

CHAPTER 25
Foreign Bodies in the Ear, Nose, and Throat in Children and Adults

Raquel M. Schears

FOREIGN BODIES IN THE EAR

Complaints of aural foreign bodies occur routinely in the emergency department (ED), especially in children.[4,21] A recent 5-year study of 191 patients presenting to an ED or referred to an ear, nose, and throat (ENT) clinic, identified 27 different objects inserted in the ears of patients ranging in age from 10 months to 17 years, with 74% of patients less than 8 years of age.[2] Heading the list of objects were beads, followed by plastic toys, pebbles, insects, and popcorn kernels.

Despite this documented frequency, there is a paucity of information regarding the treatment of aural foreign bodies. Perhaps this explains the high ENT referral rate following unsuccessful attempts at removal in the ED.[6] Additionally, in pediatric-aged patients, the smaller size of the anatomic structures, coupled with their exquisite sensitivity, and the variable degree of patient cooperation impede object retrieval. Retained foreign bodies or trauma caused by repeated attempts at removal of objects from the external auditory canal (EAC) can lead to significant morbidity.

CLINICAL PRESENTATION

The presentation of a foreign body in the EAC differs depending on the patient's age. Adults typically complain that something is in the ear. Usually, this occurs after the patient has inserted an object into the EAC, which then becomes lodged, or when an insect crawls into the ear while the patient is asleep. What motivates children to stick stuff in their ears has not been well studied. It seems more associated to the presence of preexisting irritation than to etiologies of cognitive impairment, imitation of adult behavior, or playing make-believe.[9] Diagnosing EAC foreign bodies in infants, preverbal children, or cognitively impaired adults can be much more difficult. The inability to communicate or fears of punishment often obscures the history. In this situation, common presenting signs and symptoms include otalgia, tugging at the ear, bleeding, otorrhea, tinnitus, or hearing deficits. Unusual symptoms, such as persistent coughing and hiccups, also have been reported.[2,18]

DIFFERENTIAL DIAGNOSIS

The differential diagnosis includes otitis media, otitis externa, cerumen impaction, tympanic membrane perforation, cholesteatoma, and EAC trauma, including lacerations or hematomas.

EMERGENCY DEPARTMENT EVALUATION

A pertinent history regarding previous ear infection, disease, or trauma (including tympanic membrane perforation) is obtained prior to any instrumentation. The size and shape of the foreign body, along with the dynamics and duration of placement in the EAC, are ascertained. Associated symptoms, such as perception of foreign body movement, hearing loss, vertigo, or gait disturbances, are elicited. If a patient complains of severe ear pain due to object movement or sound within the ear, the presence of a live insect should be suspected. In this instance, most patients will be incapable of completing the usual history and physical examination prior to intervention. Various solutions have been instilled to kill or paralyze insects before removal. Microscope immersion oil has been shown *in vitro* to suffocate and still cockroaches most quickly.[17] Anecdotally, mineral oil or 2% lidocaine has also been used successfully. Personal and home hygiene concerns should be discussed later in the patient encounter.

Most of the EAC has a very thin layer of epithelium that is exquisitely sensitive and highly vascular. Its cylindrical shape with two points of anatomic narrowing (Fig. 25.1) helps explain why objects easily inserted may not exit spontaneously. Removal becomes more difficult when the objects are located within the medial two-thirds of the EAC. Patients must be positioned comfortably and examined gently. Forewarning patient of the anticipated discomfort, and advising them to remain still during the examination, minimizes pain and prevents further advancement of the foreign body. Retracting the pinnae in a posterosuperior direction to straighten the canal, and using a hand-held halogen otoscope with a large-sized speculum, will optimize views of the EAC and tympanic membrane. Children usually require restraint, and possibly sedation, to receive a proper examination. It is best to have the child seated on the parent's lap, with the child's arms and torso held securely by the parent. Another adult should assist by holding the child's head immobile for the examination. Nitrous oxide has been suggested as a useful adjunct to the examination in children and adults.[6]

EMERGENCY DEPARTMENT MANAGEMENT

There are several different tools and described techniques for foreign body removal. EDs should keep a prepared tray containing the instruments and equipment needed (Table 25.1). As

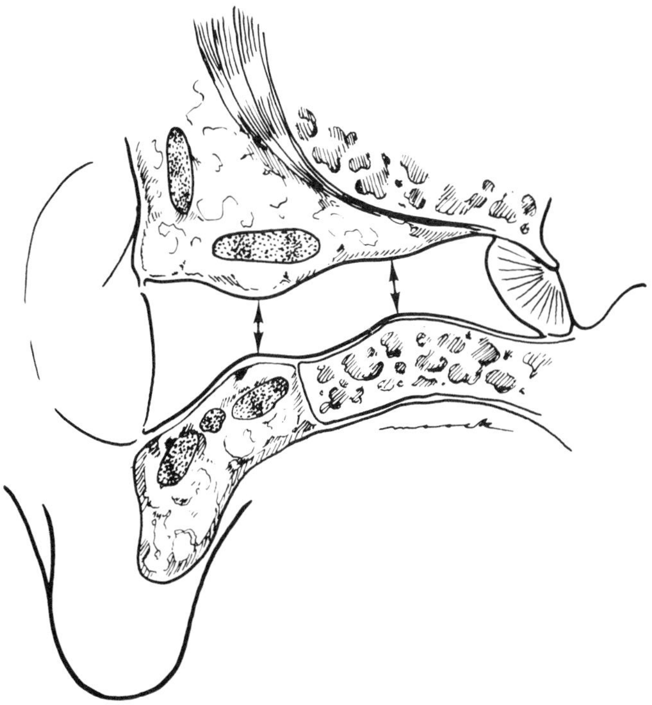

Figure 25.1. The anatomic narrowing of the external auditory canal.

TABLE 25.1. Equipment Tray for Foreign Body Removal

Foreign-body forceps **(A)**	Barnes tip suction **(I)**
Bayonet forceps **(B)**	Schuknecht foreign-body remover **(J)**
Alligator forceps **(C)**	Fogarty biliary catheter
Hartman forceps **(D)**	Cyanoacrylate glue
Nasal speculum **(E)**	Topical Lidocaine (4%)
Right-angle hook **(F)**	Topical vasoconstrictor
Ear curette **(G)**	Auralgan
Frazier suction tube **(H)**	

Letters in parentheses refer to Figure 25.2.

in the examination, adequate patient cooperation is essential for successful removal and to reduce the risk of complications. Analgesia and sedation, with agents such as ketamine, are often required to achieve this cooperation and are preferred over physical restraint.

Irrigation often removes aural foreign bodies expediently and is minimally invasive. As a prerequisite, tympanic membrane integrity must be confirmed by pneumatoscopy. Tap water or saline solutions are suitable irrigants and should be warmed to body temperature to prevent patient discomfort and dizziness during the procedure.[10] Commercial irrigator systems used for cerumen removal are available for this purpose. Alternatively, a 14- or 16-gauge angiocatheter attached to a 60-mL syringe works effectively. Irrigation should be avoided in the treatment of hygroscopic substances, such as vegetables, beans, or rice. Given the potential for swelling worsening the impaction, direct instrumentation for removal is advised.

Irrigation is absolutely contraindicated in the removal of disk batteries. Moisture promotes the breakdown of the battery casing, which allows the concentrated alkali electrolyte contents to leak into the EAC. Tissue damage secondary to liquefaction necrosis and electrolysis can be severe.[2] Disk batteries need prompt removal under direct visualization. Repeated attempts at removal in the ED are also strongly discouraged, as bleeding will lead to similar complications.

Suction can also be used to remove impacted foreign bodies, especially those with smooth contours. The flange tip of flexible intravenous tubing can be inserted adjacent to smooth foreign bodies under direct visualization, and suction then applied.[9,21] This technique is minimally invasive and presents little risk should an uncooperative patient move during the procedure. Alternatively, various suction tips, such as the Frazier or Barnes tip, and the Schuknecht foreign body remover are advocated for use in these situations[2] (Fig. 25.2). Unfortunately, the potential for complications is higher when rigid instruments are used within the EAC.

Certain irregularly shaped objects, including insects, lend themselves to direct manipulation with alligator forceps under direct visualization via an otoscope. Microscopic inspection of the retrieved insect is advised to confirm that it has been removed completely. Organic material may be carefully crushed and brought out in sections if object dimensions prevent intact removal.

Alligator forceps should not be used with round, smooth objects or those with polished convex surfaces, such as disk batteries, due to the risk of medially advancing the object deeper into the EAC. In this instance, the right-angle hook can be used to reach beyond the object to coax it out.[2,6] Cyanoacrylate glue can be used to adhere the object to an applicator (e.g., the end of a straightened paper clip, a swab stick, or bristles of a fine paint brush).[25]

Once the object has been removed, the EAC and tympanic membrane are carefully reexamined for the presence of aural trauma, including abrasions, lacerations, or inflammation. Clinicians should complete a bilateral examination for detection of multiple or previously missed foreign bodies. Given the sensitive nature of the EAC, a topical anesthetic such as antipyrine–benzocaine (Auralgan) is recommended for a few days following a foreign body removal. Patients with an inflamed EAC can be treated with antibiotic otic drops and follow up with their doctor.

DISPOSITION

If the emergency physician cannot remove the aural foreign body easily or if more than minor canal trauma is sustained during the attempted removal, the patient is referred to an ENT clinic within 12 to 24 hours. Putty impaction is a problematic foreign body and also falls into this semiurgent follow-up category. Putty had been recommended to plug or waterproof the EAC in children with tympanostomy tubes. These products are difficult to extract, with piecemeal removal the norm.[20] Large impacted pieces usually require otomicroscopic removal to avoid EAC trauma.

Immediate ENT consultation in the ED is necessary for retained disk batteries, or sharp objects wedged against the EAC or tympanic membrane, when standard removal attempts have failed.

Indications for operative extraction usually involve sharp or wedged objects, especially in patients with existent injury to the

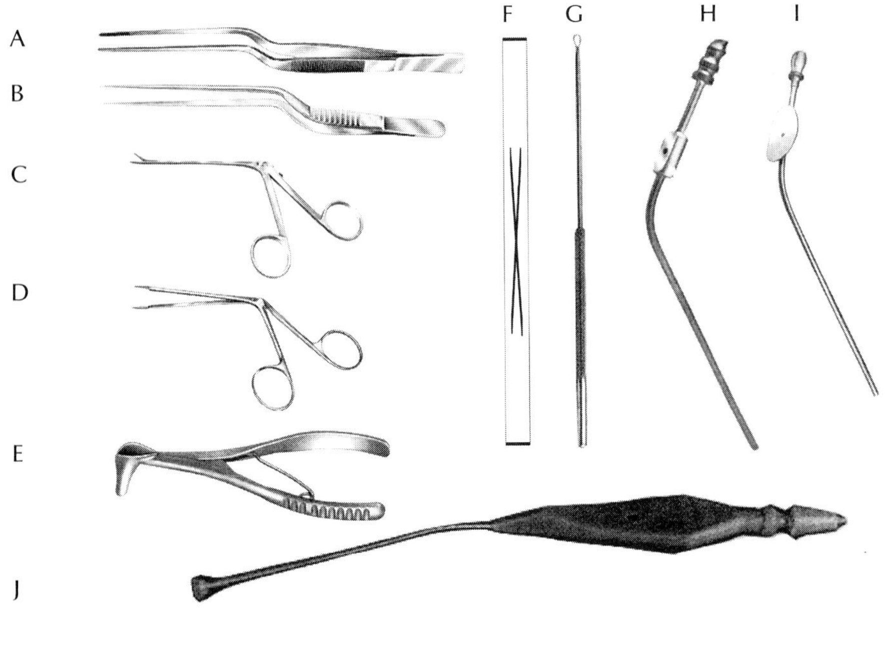

Figure 25.2. Selected instruments used for foreign-body removal. **(A)** Foreign body forceps. **(B)** Bayonet forceps. **(C)** Alligator forceps. **(D)** Hartman forceps. **(E)** Nasal speculum. **(F)** Right-angle hook. **(G)** Ear curette. **(H)** Frazier suction tube. **(I)** Barnes suction tube. **(J)** Schuknecht foreign-body remover.

EAC or tympanic membrane. Age at presentation has also been shown to be the most significant factor associated with the need for general anesthesia. In one study,[2] fully 88% of patients needing operative removal were children under 7 years of age at the time of presentation. These children would not tolerate repeat attempts at object removal.

COMMON PITFALLS

- The diagnosis of an aural foreign body is frequently missed because it is not suspected or is misdiagnosed in the setting of draining ear infections. All children under age 8 presenting to the ED should have both ears examined.
- Failure to recognize special circumstances involved in the management of foreign bodies such as disk batteries, putty, and insects, especially in young children
- Failure to consult ENT early for unsuccessful object removal in the ED. Persistence in removal attempts should be discouraged, as they cause decreased patient cooperation, increased risk of trauma, and increased likelihood of operative extraction.
- Failure to recheck the EAC after foreign body removal leads to missed or retained foreign bodies

FOREIGN BODIES IN THE NOSE

Nasal foreign bodies seem limited only by the dimensions of the patients' nares, and they occur predominantly in preschoolers. Food, followed by beads, paper, and parts of toys, are the common picks for insertion in the worst offenders, children aged 2 to 3 years old.[4,7] Disk batteries remain the foreign bodies with the greatest potential for significant permanent morbidity.[1] Myiasis, or parasitic involvement, of the nose has been reported in the tropical regions of the United States, particularly among compromised hosts: diabetics, the elderly, and the chronically ventilator dependent. Fly maggots, ascarids, and worms are among the most commonly reported animate foreign bodies.[26]

The nasal cavity has three turbinates along the lateral wall, which impair visualization and facilitate foreign-body entrapment. Differentiating between the child with a simple upper respiratory infection and the one with a purulent discharge due to a stashed gumball continues to challenge clinicians.

CLINICAL PRESENTATION

Patients presenting to the ED for this problem usually come in two varieties: the obvious patient, observed to have placed an object into the nose; and the obscure patient, classically presenting with foul pus copiously pouring out of a single nostril. Other presenting complaints include unilateral nasal obstruction, epistaxis, intermittent sneezing, or nasal pain with fever. Occasionally, nasal or facial cellulitis can be the only clue to a long-standing foreign body. Another rarely reported presentation is that of bad body odor, or bromhidrosis, without any nasal symptoms.[23] Harbored objects can go undetected in asymptomatic patients for extended periods, with incidental discovery on routine radiographs. Patients with parasitic involvement frequently report bilateral symptoms and elevated temperature.

DIFFERENTIAL DIAGNOSIS

The differential diagnosis of this entity includes simple sinusitis, tumor, and epistaxis unrelated to a foreign body. Nasal polyps also may mimic a foreign body.

EMERGENCY DEPARTMENT EVALUATION

A thorough, yet gentle physical examination is performed to minimize patient anxiety. Position the patient's head upright, for tilting the head backward (neck extended) limits the view obtained of the roof of the nasal cavity. Unlike for aural foreign bodies, sedation to aid examination or removal of nasal foreign bodies is rarely necessary, given the greater dimensions of the nasal vestibule and reduced mucosal sensitivity. Nasal obstruction can be confirmed visually by placing a mirror under the patient's nose and noting an absence of condensation moisture at the opening of the affected nostril during breathing. The sinuses are transilluminated for air–fluid levels or opacification and are percussed to assess for tenderness reflective of concurrent sinusitis.

To perform an adequate examination of the nasal cavity interior, a strong light source, preferably on a headlamp, and the largest nasal speculum the nostril can accommodate are best. For greatest visualization, insert the speculum until it is flush with the opening of the nostril and perpendicular to the nose. If a foreign body is not located on the initial direct examination, the nasal mucosa is prepared for further exploration by inserting cotton-tipped swabs soaked with either a 4% cocaine solution or a 1:1 mixture of a topical vasoconstrictor and anesthetic. Such nasal cavity preparation reduces mucosal inflammation, potential for bleeding, and patient discomfort.

Most foreign bodies are located immediately anterior to the middle turbinate or on the floor of the nasal cavity just below the inferior turbinate. Nasal radiographs may be helpful if a foreign body is strongly suspected but not seen on examination. Glass objects larger than 2 mm and gravel larger than 1 mm are radiopaque. Organic materials such as wood are best seen by computed tomography (CT) scan.[13]

EMERGENCY DEPARTMENT MANAGEMENT

Many techniques have evolved for noninvasive removal of nasal foreign bodies,[7] and the emergency physician should be familiar with several options. Perhaps the simplest technique is to encourage the cooperative patient to blow his or her nose with the unaffected nostril occluded. For this maneuver to be successful, the nasal cavity must be adequately prepared with topical vasoconstrictors. For children too young to cooperate, a useful variation on this technique, the positive pressure method,[3] may be all that is necessary for object expulsion. The key elements are to keep the patient's unaffected nostril occluded, while the parent blows a puff of air into the child's mouth. Alternatively, an Ambu bag and a tight-fitting mask can be used instead of the mouth-to-mouth technique. No studies have been undertaken to document the safety or efficacy of this method.

Long alligator forceps are the best instrument for removing irregularly shaped or compressible objects. The flange-tipped suction catheter connected to wall suction can be used to remove round or smooth-surfaced objects.[7,9] Alternatively, a Fogarty biliary catheter can be passed beyond such round objects, inflated with 1 or 2 mL of fluid, and then pulled backward to bring the object within easy grasp.[21]

Other rigid devices, including the right-angle hook, can be positioned behind objects to retrieve them by withdrawing the instrument and object together. Removal of disk batteries is particularly amenable to this method.[1,7] Recall, that disk battery retrieval is a considerably more delicate endeavor than removal of most other foreign bodies. Because these batteries are capable of producing rapid tissue destruction on contact with moisture present in the nasal cavity, care must be taken to avoid bleeding or crushing the battery casing. In the case of vegetable matter, minimal manipulation is advised, to reduce the potential for disintegration and possible retention.

When using these techniques, care must be taken to avoid aspiration of the foreign body. This complication occurs when the object is pushed further into the posterior nasopharynx during the removal attempt. If the foreign body is precariously perched, such that aspiration seems a significant risk, removal should occur in the operating room after the airway has been protected.

Removal of parasitic infestations is best left to ENT. Usually by the time the infestation is detected, serious tissue destruction has already occurred. Extensive irrigation and debridement, in combination with antiparasitic medications, are used to eradicate the infestation.[26]

Once successful foreign body removal is achieved, the nasal cavity must be carefully reinspected. Evidence of multiple foreign bodies, trauma, pressure necrosis, or secondary infection is noted. If significant epistaxis has been induced during the removal procedure, 3 days of nasal packing is prudent. Patients leaving the ED with either nasal packs in place or evidence of sinusitis secondary to foreign-body impaction need oral antibiotics and close follow-up. Therapy should cover skin and upper respiratory flora. In the case of sinusitis, 14 days of therapy is recommended. Patients with nasal packs should receive prophylaxis until the packs are removed. Antibiotics prevent the increased likelihood of sinusitis and toxic shock observed with packing.

DISPOSITION

Urgent referral within 12 to 24 hours to an ENT clinic should be made when a nasal foreign body is strongly suspected but cannot be confirmed in the ED. Referral is also appropriate to follow up focal sinusitis or limited facial cellulitis treated with oral antibiotics and discharged from the ED.

Immediate ENT consultation is obtained in cases of (1) a disk battery that cannot be removed, (2) animate infestation with significant tissue destruction, (3) any case in which attempts at removal place the patient at risk for aspiration, and (4) extensive infection (e.g., spreading cellulitis).

COMMON PITFALLS

- Missed foreign body because the diagnosis was not considered or the examination was inadequate
- Aspiration of the foreign body because the object was pushed further into the nasopharynx during the removal attempt
- Missed or retained foreign body because reexamination was not performed after initial object removal
- Increased patient morbidity due to failure to consult ENT early for unsuccessful removal attempts or special circumstances such as disk batteries and parasitic infestations
- Failure to diagnose and treat sinusitis caused by foreign body impaction

FOREIGN BODIES IN THE THROAT

A foreign body in the throat is a common complaint in the ED, and it tends to occur at the extremes of age. Children often present with symptoms consistent with partial or complete airway obstruction due to foreign body aspiration. Tragically, aspiration is the cause of death in at least 300 children each year in the United States, with those under 2 years of age being the most commonly affected.[24] Overall, up to 80% of foreign bodies accidentally aspirated or ingested occur in the pediatric population. The foreign bodies children choose tend to be small objects such as peanuts, or objects not usually thought of as ingestible (e.g., coins, toys, screws, safety pins).

In adults with an intact swallowing mechanism, the upper airway is protected and throat foreign bodies tend to lodge in the posterior oropharynx. Elderly patients who wear dentures are at increased risk for throat foreign bodies because of the associated decrease in the palatal sensation and secondary impairment of swallowing. Other sources of functional, neuromuscular, and anatomic impairments of swallowing also increase in incidence with age. Likewise, the presence of structural cerebral dysfunction or altered sensorium, or desire for secondary gain may predispose patients to having a throat foreign body. In one prospective study of adults presenting to or referred to an ENT service for foreign body sensation, only 31% actually had a true foreign body, though most could associate the onset of symptoms to eating fish or chicken.[14]

CLINICAL PRESENTATION

Aspiration of a foreign body is the most common cause of acute airway obstruction. Symptoms of partial airway compromise include cough, choking, and dyspnea. Stridor places the foreign body in the laryngotracheal area, while wheezing and retractions indicate a bronchial location. Likewise, gastrointestinal impaction can occur at several levels. Odynophagia favors a pharyngeal foreign body, while dysphagia, drooling, and inability to eat suggest lower esophageal obstruction.

Children often present late, with vague histories and nonspecific symptoms, or may be asymptomatic following foreign body ingestion. Another pediatric presentation is that of partial airway compromise because of extrinsic compression from an intraesophageal foreign body pressing on the posterior aspect of the immature trachea.

Acute esophageal impactions in adults typically present within 12 hours of symptoms that began while eating either fish or chicken.[12,14] Adults can reliably localize the position of the object. Patients who sense an object in the area under the mandibular angle often have impaction in the pharynx, including the base of the tongue, tonsils, vallecula, and pyriform recesses. Overall, these areas are the most common sites where sharp objects impale. If patients point lateral to the trachea and superior to the clavicle, the object is usually lodged in the cervical esophagus just below the cricopharyngeus muscle. Finally, patients with substernal chest pain often harbor an esophageal object at the level of the aortic arch or gastroesophageal junction. Symptoms that help predict an actual retained foreign body include severe pain at rest, inability to swallow secretions, otalgia, cough, dysphagia, hoarseness, and lateralizing pain that may progress.[12,14]

DIFFERENTIAL DIAGNOSIS

In children, the differential diagnosis includes croup, epiglottitis, reactive airway disease, pneumonitis, neoplasm, and a foreign body in the lower esophagus.

In adults, the most common diagnosis after a true foreign body is residual oropharyngeal trauma, after a spontaneously relieved obstruction. Infection, abscess, neoplasm, and distal esophageal impaction also are possible etiologies.

EMERGENCY DEPARTMENT EVALUATION

Regardless of patient age, the foremost goal of the emergency physician is to differentiate the patient presenting with airway involvement from the one with pharyngoesophageal signs and symptoms. A foreign body causing partial obstruction of an airway can suddenly result in a complete obstruction. Total airway obstruction causes the patient to spiral rapidly through three stages: alert, awake, and apneic; then unconscious with a pulse; followed by cardiopulmonary arrest.

Children with partial airway compromise and symptoms of a throat foreign body require vigilant observation and readiness to intervene immediately to manage the airway. If possible, the emergency physician should examine the cooperative child's oropharynx to diagnose the foreign body. However, if the child is uncooperative, examination of the oropharynx and use of restraint or sedation should be avoided pending radiographic studies.

Radiographic investigation can be vital to diagnosing the presence of a foreign body. Anterior–posterior (AP) and lateral soft-tissue neck radiographs should be obtained to make the diagnosis of radiopaque laryngeal or esophageal foreign body and to exclude epiglottitis from the differential. Similarly, standard two-view chest radiographs are indicated to assess the substernal esophagus and airways for radiopaque objects. If these radiographs are obtained off-site, experienced personnel must accompany the patient to assess airway status constantly and be prepared to intubate immediately.

In general, an AP film will show an *esophageal* coin face-on, while the lateral film will depict a *tracheal* coin edge-on.[12,21] Comparison radiographs, such as inspiratory and expiratory phase films and decubitus films, can aid in the diagnosis of aspirated foreign body. An expiratory view should demonstrate air-trapping and mediastinal shift in the setting of an endobronchial obstruction. Dependent positioning in a normal lung will force air out on expiration, allowing the hemidiaphragm to rise. However, with an endobronchial foreign body acting like a ball-valve, air-trapping occurs on expiration. This results in abnormal hyperaeration and failure of the hemidiaphragm to rise in dependency. Confirmed aspirated foreign bodies or suspicion of radiolucent objects in the lungs mandate immediate pulmonary consultation. Direct bronchoscopy, CT, and occasionally magnetic resonance imaging (MRI) can be useful adjunctive studies for certain radiolucent objects.[16]

In adults and cooperative children, there are several physical examination findings that suggest foreign-body presence. Specifically, pooling of oral secretions, presence of stridor or inspiratory wheeze, and subcutaneous emphysema of the neck due to esophageal perforation are found. A careful examination of the posterior oropharynx should be made, with special attention to the tonsillar fossae and posterior tongue, where objects are often missed.[14,27] Dentition is assessed for missing teeth or dentures. If the initial examination is unrevealing, the lower portion of the pharynx is examined. A dental mirror and laryngoscope with a # 3 MacIntosh blade can be used to depress the tongue for better visualization. Obvious foreign bodies noted on the initial examination may be removed using bayonet or Magill forceps. A more extensive examination can be performed using fiberoptic nasolaryngoscopy. The area of the vallecula and the piriform recesses should be scrutinized carefully. Any oropharyngeal lacerations or abrasions are noted, and can fully mimic the presence of a true foreign body.

Soft-tissue films of the adult neck are less valuable in the diagnosis of oropharyngeal foreign body due to their low sensitivity and specificity.[14] Similarly, more than 30% of radiolucent masses are undetected on initial radiographs.[12] ENT consultation should be obtained promptly if the diagnosis of foreign body is confirmed in the ED or if a falsely negative initial examination is suspected. Often, an endoscopic evaluation, esophagram, or CT will be modalities for further patient assessment.

EMERGENCY DEPARTMENT MANAGEMENT

Apnea in the ED must trigger immediate action by the emergency physician. First, perform a jaw thrust maneuver to open the airway. Examine the pharynx for the presence of a foreign body. If present, remove it with a finger sweep, suction, or forceps. Proceed to direct laryngoscopy and one attempt to remove any deeper obstruction, if visualized. Persistent apnea strongly suggests a subglottic foreign body, requiring an open cricothyrotomy in patients over 12 years old, or needle cricothyrotomy in underaged children.[8] Once an emergency airway is established, provide oxygen and ventilate.

The type of foreign body and its dimensional characteristics influence the likelihood of airway obstruction or esophageal impaction, which directly affect management. For example, children ingest mostly inorganic foreign bodies (coins, pins, and toys) but tend to aspirate particulate organic material (peanuts, food, and seeds). Adults usually present with large food bolus obstructions within the esophagus and less commonly, the airway. Overall, when a foreign body is ingested, 80% to 90% will enter the gastrointestinal tract, with the remainder landing in the tracheobronchial tree.[27]

Ingested foreign bodies that are smooth, round, and smaller than a penny will pass uneventfully in most children and adults.[11,12,14,15] Disk batteries in the esophagus are an exception and constitute a true emergency. They should be promptly removed endoscopically to avoid well-described fatalities due to esophageal corrosion, necrosis, and perforation.[19,27] For other such impacted objects (coins, toys, etc.), extraction can occur using nonendoscopic methods (Foley catheter, magnetic tube) or endoscopic techniques. The interventional removal strategy chosen should take cost into consideration. The success rate for removal is 95% to 100%, and the complication rate is 0% to 2%, regardless of technique used.[19,22]

The standard Foley catheter method[22,27] is to insert a 12F to 16F Foley nasally or orally to below the level of the foreign body, with the patient in the Trendelenburg position on a fluoroscopy table. The balloon is inflated with barium contrast and the catheter is slowly withdrawn, backing the object out of the esophagus. Magnetic foreign bodies are extracted by magnetic tube also under fluoroscopy.[11] After successful removal, an esophagram is performed to confirm the integrity of the esophagus.

Sharp objects are likely to perforate immediately; therefore, open safety pins, razor blades, toothpicks, and so forth, require immediate endoscopic retrieval, and that failing, surgical intervention.[5,15]

Another "time bomb" is the cocaine-packed condom, intentionally ingested by drug traffickers. Fatalities have been reported when these condoms rupture in the gastrointestinal tract. Large packets that become impacted in the esophagus can be confirmed on plain film. With this ingestion, endoscopic removal is contraindicated because of the associated risk of condom rupture. Emergency surgical intervention is considered as first-line therapy.[15,22,27]

Completely obstructing esophageal food (or meat) impactions are almost exclusively seen in adults, and should be urgently removed endoscopically.[22,27] However, a variety of chemical means had been reported in the literature previous to the advent of endoscopy for esophageal disimpaction. *Papain* was recommended to enzymatically dissolve a meat bolus. Unfortunately, its nonspecific action was also shown to weaken the esophageal wall and lead to perforation.[15,22] The use of *gas-forming* agents fell to similar complications. *Glucagon* may help with lower obstructions by decreasing tone at the gastroesophageal junction alone, to allow an object to pass. It has several unpleasant side effects, however, and is contraindicated in patients with pheochromocytoma, insulinoma, or hyperglycemia, or in those suspected of having a sharp foreign body. Anecdotal success with *atropine, benzodiazepines, calcium channel blockers,* and *nitroglycerin* has not been significantly better than with glucagon.[15] Basically, the risks associated with most of these agents—depressing the gag reflex and promoting aspiration or esophageal perforation due to vomiting—continue to prevent their widespread application.

DISPOSITION

ENT consultation should be obtained in all cases of retained laryngeal foreign body or when the possibility cannot be excluded. Flexible bronchoscopy with channel biopsy forceps may be used to remove objects not accessible with bayonet forceps. Patients found to have minor pharyngeal trauma as the basis of their symptoms may be safely discharged. The possibility of subsequent infection must always be discussed with the patient.

COMMON PITFALLS

- Significant morbidity and mortality have occurred in cases in which the airway was not aggressively managed in children with a laryngeal foreign body. Partial obstruction may become complete obstruction at any time.
- Laryngeal foreign body must be considered in children who present with croup, particularly those who do not respond well to conventional therapy.
- Deep-tissue abscess and mediastinitis are potential complications of missed laryngeal or pharyngeal foreign bodies.
- There is a high incidence of underlying esophageal pathology in cases of esophageal food bolus impaction. These patients should have a follow-up swallowing study to evaluate for this possibility once the acute problem is relieved.

References

1. Alvi A, Bereliani A, Zahtz, GD. Miniature disc batteries in the nose: a dangerous foreign body. *Clin Pediatr* 1997;427.
2. Ansley JF, Cunningham MJ. Treatment of aural foreign bodies in children. *Pediatrics* 1998;101:638.
3. Backlin SA. Positive-pressure technique for nasal foreign body removal in children. *Ann Emerg Med* 1995;25:554.
4. Baker MD. Foreign bodies of the ear and nose in childhood. *Pediatr Emerg Care* 1987;3:67.
5. Blaho KE, Merigian KS, Winbery SL, et al. Foreign body ingestions in the emergency department: case reports and review of treatment. *J Emerg Med* 1998;16:21.
6. Bressler K, Shelton C. Ear foreign body removal: a review of 98 consecutive cases. *Laryngoscope* 1993;103:367.
7. Brownstein DR, Hodge D. Foreign bodies of the eye, ear and nose. *Pediatr Emerg Care* 1988;4:215.
8. Craig RM. Esophageal disorders: inflammatory disease, foreign bodies and esophageal obstruction, and caustic injury. *Hosp Physician Gastroenterol Board Rev Manual* 1998;4:1.
9. Das SK. Aetiological evaluation of foreign bodies in the ear and nose. *J Laryngol Otol* 1984;98:989.
10. Ernst AA, Takakuwa KM, Letner C, et al. Warmed versus room temperature saline solution for ear irrigation: a randomized clinical trial. *Ann Emerg Med* 1999;34:347.
11. Hachimi-Idrissi S, Corne L, Vandenplas Y. Management of ingested foreign bodies in childhood: our experience and review of the literature. *Eur J Emerg Med* 1998;5:319.
12. Hess GP. An approach to throat complaints: foreign body sensation, difficulty swallowing, and hoarseness. *Emerg Med Clin North Am* 1987;5:313.
13. Howell JM, Chisholm CD. Wound care. *Emerg Med Clin North Am* 1997;15:417.
14. Jones NS, Lannigan FJ, Salama NY. Foreign bodies in the throat: a prospective study of 388 cases. *J Laryngol Otol* 1991;105:104.
15. Karjoo M. Caustic ingestion and foreign bodies in the gastrointestinal system. *Curr Opin Pediatr* 1998;10:516.
16. Kavanagh PV, Mason AC, Muller NL. Thoracic foreign bodies in adults. *Clin Radiol* 1999;54:353.
17. Leffler S, Cheney P, Tandberg D. Chemical immobilization and killing of intra-aural roaches: an in vitro comparative study. *Ann Emerg Med* 1993;22:1795.
18. Lossos I, Breuer R. A rare case of hiccups. *N Engl J Med* 1988;318:711.
19. McGahren ED. Esophageal foreign bodies. *Pediatr Rev* 1999;20:129.
20. Muntz H. The use of Silly Putty as an ear plug. *Arch Otolaryngol Head Neck Surg* 1995;121:354.
21. Pons P. Foreign bodies. In: Rosen P, ed. *Emergency medicine,* 3rd ed. St. Louis: Mosby, 1992.
22. Stack LB, Munter DW. Foreign bodies in the gastrointestinal tract. *Emerg Med Clin North Am* 1996;14:493.
23. Stegman JC. Unusual presentation of nasal foreign bodies. *Am J Dis Child* 1987;141:239.
24. Tariq M, Beg M. A foreign body in the bronchus still presents problems. *Int J Clin Pract* 1999;53:81.
25. Thompson MP. Removing objects from the external auditory canal. *N Engl J Med* 1984;311:1365.
26. Werman HA. Removal of foreign bodies of the nose. *Emerg Med Clin North Am* 1987;5:253.
27. Webb WA. Management of foreign bodies of the upper gastrointestinal tract: update. *Gastrointest Endosc* 1995;41:39.

CHAPTER 26
Acute Hearing Loss

John H. Isaacs, Jr.

Acute hearing loss has not been well defined. For the purposes of this chapter, however, it is defined as a loss of hearing that causes the patient to come to the emergency department.

The overall incidence of acute hearing loss is unknown because of the diversity of diseases involved. Sudden neurosensory hearing loss (NSHL) is estimated to occur in 5 to 20 patients per 100,000.[1,5] It most commonly occurs in patients in their sixth decade.[1]

There are two major groups of patients presenting with acute hearing loss. The first includes those whose hearing loss is due to conductive problems. Occasionally, a patient suffers acute hearing loss from both conductive and neurosensory problems. For example, a temporal bone fracture may damage the eighth nerve or the cochlea, as well as the tympanic membrane and the ossicles; it may also block conduction through the presence of a blood clot in the middle ear or external auditory canal. The second group includes those who suffer sudden NSHL (i.e., loss due to pathology in, or medial to, the cochlea). Sudden NSHL is defined as any hearing loss, ranging from instantaneous loss to that which occurs over a period of time (up to several days). Varying degrees of NSHL must be documented on an audiogram.[1,6,11,17] Because audiometric testing equipment is unavailable in the emergency department, such definitions are of little use to the emergency physician.

PATHOPHYSIOLOGY

The pathophysiology depends on the underlying disease process. Sound is conducted through the external auditory canal and vibrates the eardrum, which in turn vibrates the ossicles and the fluids of the inner ear. Any disruption of the ossicles, the middle ear, or conduction of noise to the eardrum can cause a conductive hearing loss.[12] NSHL is caused by problems in the cochlea and central auditory pathway, which are generally problems with hair cell function or the acoustic nerve or brain stem.

ETIOLOGY

The etiology also depends on the disease process that has caused the hearing loss. In many cases of conductive loss, the cause can be determined and sometimes treated in the emergency department. Some causes of NSHL are well known and understood (ototoxic drugs, noise exposure, perilymph fistula, temporal bone trauma).[1,2] In these cases, the cause frequently can be determined through the history, and the appropriate treatment begun. Idiopathic sudden NSHL is thought to have various causes, including viral infection,[18,20] vascular problems, and autoimmune disease.[1,3,4,6,9,20] The cause in an individual case, however, is often unknown.

OUTCOME

Most conductive hearing losses respond well to treatment or improve without treatment (e.g., cerumen impaction, acute otitis media). Ossicular problems and tympanic membrane perforations can usually be repaired with surgery. Recovery of acute NSHL depends on the underlying cause; most known causes, such as trauma or ototoxic drugs, have a fairly poor prognosis. In cases of sudden idiopathic hearing loss, patients with the least hearing loss tend to do better; those with more severe hearing loss generally do not do as well, even with treatment. Children and those over 40 years of age have a poorer prognosis.[1] Patients with vertigo have a poorer prognosis.[1,6,13] If the patient truly has NSHL, particularly if it is profound, the physician should remember the poor prognosis and not be overly optimistic with the patient.

CLINICAL PRESENTATION

The typical presentation of a patient with sudden hearing loss is an ambulatory patient complaining of unilateral hearing loss, sometimes noted because of an inability to use the phone with that ear. There may be other complaints, such as vertigo, pain, aural drainage, facial nerve paralysis, or trauma. These associated problems may be so severe as to override the hearing problem; in some cases, the patient may not even complain of the hearing loss immediately. Occasionally, the patient will not know how long the hearing loss has been present; in such instances, it can usually be assumed to have been only a few days. Sudden hearing loss is usually not life-threatening; however, diabetic patients develop malignant external otitis, which, if untreated, has a mortality rate of 70% to 80%. Additional signs and symptoms depend on the underlying cause of the acute hearing loss.

DIFFERENTIAL DIAGNOSIS

Because acute hearing loss is a presenting complaint or a finding with multiple causes, it is more appropriate to consider possible causes rather than a differential diagnosis. Causes of conductive hearing loss, such as foreign body, acute infection, or cerumen impaction, can usually be determined and treated. In some cases, the cause of NSHL can be defined (e.g., ototoxic drugs), but in many cases it is idiopathic. Tables 26.1 and 26.2 list common causes of acute hearing loss.

EMERGENCY DEPARTMENT EVALUATION

History

The history is the most important element when evaluating acute hearing loss, particularly in the emergency department where auditory testing is unavailable. The physician should inquire about

1. Pain or drainage from the ear, which may indicate infection
2. A precipitating event, such as airplane travel or scuba diving (barotrauma)

TABLE 26.1. Differential Diagnosis of Conductive Hearing Loss

Causes		Signs/Symptoms
Otitis media and externa	Acute otitis media	Red TM Pain on pushing in tragus Pain better after drainage
	Acute serous otitis	Fluid/air bubbles No erythema
	External otitis	Pain on pulling pinna Pain *not* better with drainage
Tumors	Osteoma	Smooth Nonpainful History of past discomfort in cold water
	Squamous cell carcinoma	Bleeding Irregular ulcer that will not heal
	Glomus tumor	Red mass behind TM that blanches No pain
	Cholesteatoma	Check attic area Often squamous debris
Trauma	Barotrauma	Plane flight Scuba
	Temporal bone fracture	Loss of consciousness Ossicular chain disruption Blood in middle ear TM damage
	Trauma to external auditory canal or traumatic ossicular dislocation	TM or ossicular dislocation History of slap; Q-tip injury; physical exam
Impaction/Obstruction	Blood clot in ear	Could be from head wound
	Foreign body	History and physical exam will confirm
	Cerumen	Physical exam will confirm

TM, tympanic membrane

TABLE 26.2. Differential Diagnosis of Neurosensory Hearing Loss

Causes		Symptoms/Signs
External agents or injury	Temporal bone fracture	Damage to cochlea or auditory nerve
		History
		X-rays
	Barotrauma	Scuba or airplane
	Ototoxic drugs[21]	History; usually bilateral
		Erythromycin
		Vancomycin
		Aminoglycosides
		Loop diuretics
		Salicylates
		Antineoplastic drugs (cistplatin, DFMO)
	Noise exposure	History; usually bilateral
	Inner ear hemorrhage	Anticoagulants
	Acoustic trauma	History
	Toxic agents[22]	History
		Carbon monoxide
		Lead
		Mercury
		Arsenic
		Gold
		Aniline dyes
Disease-induced	Ménière disease	Episodic vertigo
		Fluctuating hearing
		Tinnitus
	Acoustic neuroma	Difficult diagnosis; some vertigo or unsteadiness, special tests required, CT, MRI
	Autoimmune disorder[9]	History as indicated
		Sed rate/labs as indicated
	Multiple sclerosis	Difficult diagnosis
		History of other neurologic signs
	Vascular accidents, including small cerebellar strokes	Vascular disease history, CT
	Perilymph fistula/internal rupture of inner ear membranes	History of trauma, straining, lifting
	Metastatic disease to temporal bone	History
		X-ray
	Meningitis	Fever, headache, nuchal rigidity
	AIDS[14,23]	HIV testing
		History
		Viral or *Cryptoccocus neoformans*
	Migraine	History
	Buerger disease	History
	Viral[18]	CMV, rubella, varicella zoster, measles, mumps, etc.
	Bacterial infection	
	Syphilis	FTA
	Malingering	Difficult; will often respond to voice when not being "tested"
	Sarcoidosis[1]	History[1], chest x-ray and neuro

3. Placement of a foreign body, which is usually, but not always, known
4. Exposure to ototoxic drugs or toxins[2]

The social history, including workplace, may indicate exposure to noise or toxic substances. The use of a cotton-tipped applicator can cause cerumen impaction or trauma to the tympanic membrane or middle ear, resulting in a blood clot in the ear canal, tympanic membrane damage, or ossicular disruption. Temporal bone fractures are associated with trauma and, usually, loss of consciousness. The history may reveal that hearing gradually worsened and was then completely lost (as with noise exposure). True episodic loss of hearing suggests Ménière disease, but the classic triad of episodic vertigo, fluctuating hearing loss, and tinnitus is necessary to make the diagnosis of Ménière disease. If this is the initial episode, Ménière disease may be suspected but not diagnosed.

Vertigo is an important complaint and is important prognostically in patients with NSHL. Its presence is associated with a worse prognosis. Vertigo is also a common complaint in patients with acoustic neuromas. Associated neurologic signs and symptoms may suggest multiple sclerosis. A history of vascular disease, such as stroke or myocardial infarction, may implicate vascular disease as the etiology of acute hearing loss. A history of human immunodeficiency virus (HIV) or HIV risk factors can help define the cause of hearing loss.[1,14] Systemic illness, such as mumps, can cause hearing loss and should be explored. Tertiary syphilis can cause hearing loss; an FTA-ABS or equivalent testing must be done. Autoimmune disease (lupus, etc.) may precipitate an event of NSHL.

Possible reasons for secondary gain should be sought, which would lead to the diagnosis of pseudohypacusis (malingering).

Finally, the physician should ensure that any problems with hearing are not caused by language or mental status problems.

Physical Examination

The history should guide the physical examination. Vital signs may hint at a possible cause of the hearing loss. For example, fever may indicate meningitis or viral illnesses; an elevated blood pressure may suggest vascular disease.

The cranial nerves should be tested, with special emphasis on the facial nerve. When testing for facial nerve function, the physician should ensure that the movement is truly due to the seventh cranial nerve. For example, the eye can close by simply relaxing the third cranial nerve; eye closure must be forceful. The mouth can be moved by the masseter muscle, which is innervated by the fifth cranial nerve. Also, movement of the forehead on one side can cause apparent slight movement on the opposite side.

The ears should be examined with an otoscope. If temporal bone fracture or communication with the central nervous system (CNS) is suspected, sterile instruments should be used. Wax is not naturally present in the medial aspect of the ear canal (near the eardrum). If wax is present, it has been pushed in (by means of a cotton-tipped applicator or a shower), or it is not wax. A cholesteatoma should be suspected if there is a crusting on the eardrum, particularly on the superior aspect, over the pars flaccida.

Cerumen impactions may be removed by irrigation; however, the physician should ensure the eardrum is intact before irrigating the ear canal. Manipulation of the ear canal may stimulate the vagus nerve, especially in the elderly, causing mild cough or even cardiac arrest. In some cases, the wax may be too dry and impacted for removal by irrigation or under direct vision. Mineral oil drops, which are less toxic and less likely to cause a reaction than commercially available wax removal preparations, are an alternative (four drops four times a day for a week or two). Frequently, this will soften the wax, allowing it to drain on its own. If the wax does not drain on its own, suctioning under direct vision by an otolaryngologist or a primary care physician can remove the impaction.

Palpation of a tender mastoid tip may indicate mastoiditis. The temporomandibular joint should also be palpated.

Special Tests

Perilymph Fistulas

The physician instructs the patient to close his or her eyes and walk straight ahead; the physician then taps the patient on the shoulder and has him or her turn 180 degrees in the direction tapped. Turning in the direction of the fistula will cause unsteadiness.[16]

Tuning Fork Testing

The best frequency to use is 512 Hz; lower frequencies may cause the patient to *feel* the vibrations rather than actually *hear* the tuning fork.

The two tests most commonly performed are the Weber and the Rinne. The Weber test is traditionally performed by placing the base of the fork in the midline of the forehead. However, this test can also be done, and with better results, by testing the middle of the upper teeth, provided the patient does not have dentures. When doing the Weber test, the fork should be pressed firmly against the skull or teeth. A good contact between the base of the tuning fork and the skull is necessary to make the skull vibrate. If the sound is localized to one ear, there is either a conductive hearing loss in that ear or NSHL in the opposite ear.

The Rinne test should be done on each ear. It is "positive" if it is normal. Place the base of the tuning fork over the mastoid tip and press firmly; then, immediately take the tuning fork off and hold it next to the external ear canal. Ask the patient which is louder. Normally, air conduction is heard better (and therefore louder) than bone conduction. Louder bone conduction indicates a conductive hearing loss. Unfortunately, the Rinne test detects only large conductive losses (about 40 decibels). Thus, a lesser but significant conductive hearing loss yields a positive (i.e., normal) Rinne test.

Audiometry

Although it is best to test hearing with an audiometer operated by a qualified audiologist, it is usually possible in the emergency department to get some idea of the patient's ability to hear. Start speaking in a whisper and continue to speak louder and louder until the patient can hear. Note the distance and the approximate level of volume at which the patient can hear (i.e., whisper, soft conversation, normal conversation, loud voice, yelling). A noisemaker can be used to mask hearing in the normal ear. Malingerers and pseudohypacusis patients frequently respond to off-hand comments or requests spoken in a normal or soft voice when they believe they are not being tested.

Audiometric testing should be obtained if possible. However, if the patient has a readily identifiable cause of hearing loss, such as acute otitis media, serous otitis media, hemotympanum, external otitis, cerumen impaction, or foreign body, audiometric testing should probably be delayed until the underlying problem is treated.

Laboratory Evaluation and Special Studies

Laboratory evaluation in the emergency department depends on the suspected underlying cause. A patient with a cerumen impaction does not need a diagnostic work-up. If no clear cause for the sudden hearing loss is noted, the following tests may be indicated: HIV, antinuclear antibodies, sedimentation rate, complete blood count, renal profile, rheumatoid factor, immunoglobulin-E, thyroid function test (thyroid-stimulating hormone, T3, T4), prothrombin time, partial thromboplastin time, platelet count, serum electrolytes, glucose, VDRL, and FTA-ABS. Other tests may be indicated by history[15] (e.g., lipid studies, rheumatoid factor, antinuclear antibody). Tests that may be ordered in consultation with a specialist include an audiogram, auditory brain stem response, electronystagmogram, magnetic resonance imaging and CT scanning of the temporal bones.[8] A CT scan on a patient with simple acute otitis media may show fluid in the mastoid, and the radiologist will diagnose mastoiditis. This should not be treated any differently than acute otitis media unless there are clinical signs of mastoiditis, such as erythema, tenderness, protrusion of pinna, and, occasionally, fluctuance.

EMERGENCY DEPARTMENT MANAGEMENT

Simple causes of hearing loss, such as acute otitis media, external otitis, or cerumen impaction, can be treated in the emergency department. Foreign bodies can sometimes be removed, particularly in an older patient. Some problems, such as barotrauma and serous otitis media, require minimal treatment or close observation only. Ototoxic medications should be discontinued. Suspected malingering may require psychiatric evaluation; audiologic testing confirms malingering.

Generally accepted, recommended treatments for sudden hearing loss include observation, bed rest, and a low-salt diet. Treatment for a possible perilymph fistula includes these as well as sedation and absolute bed rest with the patient's head elevated. In some cases, if NSHL is confirmed, steroids may be given, particularly if HIV infection is not present.[11,14,19] External otitis is frequently treated with ear drops containing neomycin and polymyxin B sulfates and hydrocortisone (Cortisporin). If an eardrum perforation is suspected, the suspension, not the solution, should be used; the suspension is less irritating and painful to the middle ear mucosa. Allergic reaction to neomycin is common. If the patient seems to be getting worse or not responding to Cortisporin drops, it may be due to an allergic reaction, necessitating a different medication.

Even in simple cases, it is probably wise to obtain an audiogram at some point in the patient's treatment. In all other cases, it is best to refer the patient to an otolaryngologist for treatment and further care.

DISPOSITION

Except for straightforward problems, consultation with an otolaryngologist should be obtained in most cases of sudden hearing loss. Ideally, the patient should be seen within 2 to 3 days; some studies have shown benefit if treatment is started within 7 days,[10] 10 days,[11] or 16 days.[7] The case can probably be discussed immediately with an otolaryngologist on the phone, and the timing of further consultation can be determined at that point.

Generally, patients with sudden hearing loss do not require admission to the hospital. The major exception is perilymph fistula. These patients require sedation and absolute bed rest. Depending on the social and home situation, it may be necessary to admit the patient to administer this treatment. For patients not admitted, close follow-up is indicated. After cleaning a cerumen impaction in an elderly patient, the patient may need evaluation for an underlying presbycusis, which may need further study and treatment. All follow-up can be accomplished by either a primary care physician or an otolaryngologist, depending on the severity and underlying problem.

If the patient must travel to consult a specialist, air travel is contraindicated in perilymph fistulas and in barotrauma cases, unless a specially pressurized plane is used.

COMMON PITFALLS

- Because acute hearing loss is a symptom or sign of multiple medical conditions, the disease that causes it may be either diagnosed and treated with relative simplicity, or of a nature that is undefinable and untreatable in the emergency department.
- History is frequently the key to diagnosis, and must include specific inquiry regarding recent infection; prior hearing or neurologic problems; occupational or recreational noise exposure; recent flying, diving, or high-altitude travel; and any self-instrumentation of the ear. Failure to elicit history in these areas may lead the emergency physician in the wrong direction.
- The emergency physician must methodically examine the ear and related structures (e.g., temporomandibular joint), perform a complete neurologic examination, remove cerumen from the external auditory canal to visualize the tympanic membrane, and, when appropriate, perform bedside hearing tests along with a fistula test. This will help avoid the error of diagnosing an "ear infection" with no objective findings to support the diagnosis.
- The emergency physician should take special care with respect to treatment in two situations. First, foreign body removal requires special techniques and should be performed with a clear strategy (see Chapter 25). Second, otitis externa should be treated with a drug in suspension in the case of tympanic membrane perforation or when the physician cannot visualize the tympanic membrane because of debris.
- A major pitfall is to offer a prognosis that is too optimistic. It may create or reinforce unreasonable expectations on the part of the patient, leading to dissatisfaction with the medical care received.

References

1. Arts H. Differential diagnosis of sensorineural hearing loss: In: Cummings C, Fredrickson J, Harker L, et al., eds. *Otolaryngology—head and neck surgery.* Chicago: Mosby–Year Book, 1998:148.
2. Brookhouser PE, GrundFast KM. General sensorineural hearing loss. In: Cummings C, Fredrickson J., Harker L, et al., eds. *Otolaryngology—head and neck surgery.* Pediatrics Volume. Chicago: Mosby–Year Book, 1998:32.
3. Byl FM. Sudden hearing loss: 8 years' experience and suggested prognostic table. *Laryngoscope* 1984; 94:647 (referencing VanCaneghem D. LaSurdité subite. *Acta Otorhinolaryngol Belg* 1958;12:5–17).
4. Cole RR, Jahrsdoerfer RA. Sudden hearing loss: an update. *Am J Otolaryngol* 1988;9:211.
5. Fetterman BL, Saunders JE, Luxford WM. Prognosis and treatment of sudden sensorineural hearing loss. *Am J Otolaryngol* 1996; 17:529.
6. Guyla AJ. Sudden sensorineural hearing loss: an otologic emergency. *Compr Ther* 1996;22:217.
7. Kubo T, Tohru M, Asai H, et al. Efficacy of defibrinogenation and steroid therapies on sudden deafness. *Arch Otolaryngol Head Neck Surg* 1988;9:211.
8. Mark AS, Seltzer S, Nelson-Drake J, et al. Labyrinthine enhancement on gadolinium enhanced MRI in sudden deafness and vertigo: correlation with audiologic and electronystagmographic studies. *Ann Otol Rhinol Laryngol* 1992;101:459.
9. McCabe B. Autoimmune sensorineural hearing loss. *Ann Otol Rhinol Laryngol* 1979;88:585.
10. Megighian D, Bolzan M, Barion Nicholai P. Epidemiological considerations in sudden hearing loss: a study of 183 cases. *Arch Otorhinolaryngol* 1986;243:250.
11. Miyake H, Yanagita N. Therapy of sudden deafness. *Acta Otolaryngol (Stockh)* 1988;Suppl 452:27.
12. Nadol JB. Hearing loss. *N Engl J Med* 1993;329:1092.
13. Nakashima T, Yanagita N. Outcome of sudden deafness with and without vertigo. *Laryngoscope* 1993;103:1145.
14. Real R, Thomas M, Gerwin J. Sudden hearing loss and AIDS. *Otolaryngol Head Neck Surg* 1987;97:409.
15. Schweinfurth JM, Parnes S, Very M. Current concepts in the diagnosis and treatment of sudden sensorineural hearing loss. *Eur Arch Otorhinolaryngol* 1996;253:117.
16. Singleton G. Evaluation of the dizzy patient. In: Bailey BJ, ed. *Head and Neck Surgery—Otolaryngology.* Philadelphia: JB Lippincott Co, 1993.
17. Terayama Y, Ishibe Y, Matsushima J. Rapidly progressive sensorineural hearing loss (rapid deafness). *Acta Otolaryngol (Stockh)* 1988;Suppl 456:43.
18. Wilson W. The relationship of the herpes virus family to sudden hearing loss: a prospective clinical study and literature review. *Laryngoscope* 1986;96:870.
19. Wilson WR, Byl FM, Laird N. The efficacy of steroids in the treatment of idiopathic sudden hearing loss. *Arch Otolaryngol* 1980;106:772.
20. Wilson W, Veltri R, Laird N, et al. Viral and epidemiologic studies of idiopathic sudden hearing loss: a prospective clinical study and literature review. *Otolaryngol Head Neck Surg* 1983;91:653.
21. Rybak S, Matz G. Effects of toxic agents. In: Cummings CW, Fredrickson JM, Harker LA, et al., eds. *Otolaryngology—head and neck surgery,* 2nd ed. St. Louis: Mosby–Year Book, 1992.
22. Brookhouser PE. Sensorineural hearing loss in children. In: Cummings CW, Fredrickson JM, Harker LA, et al., eds. *Otolaryngology—head and neck surgery,* 2nd ed, chapter 176. St. Louis: Mosby–Year Book, 1992.
23. Kwartler JA, Linthicum FH, Jahn AF, et al. Sudden hearing loss due to AIDS-related cryptococcal meningitis—a temporal bone study. *Otolaryngol Head Neck Surg* 1991;104:265.

CHAPTER 27
Vertigo and Labyrinthine Disorders

Eileen M. Raynor and Robert D. Herr

Just as dizziness is the complaint of abnormal orientation in space, vertigo is the abnormal feeling of motion, either of the person or of his or her environment.[17] Although the prevalence of dizziness in unselected emergency patients is unknown, data from the National Ambulatory Medical Care Survey show

TABLE 27.1. Etiology of Dizziness in 125 ED Patients

Etiology	Percentage
Peripheral vestibular disorder	43
Cardiovascular	21
Unknown	10
Medication-induced	7
Posttraumatic	6
Other	6
Psychogenic	6
Hyperventilation	5
Endocrine	4
Infectious	3
Seizure	2
Anemia	2
Ménière syndrome	1
Multiple sensory deficit	1

Adapted from Herr R, Zun L, Mathews J. A directed approach to the dizzy patient. *Ann Emerg Med* 1989;18:664–672.

dizziness as a chief complaint in 2.6% of all patients, increasing to nearly 7% in patients by age 85 (Table 27.1).[14,15] Distinguishing vertigo from lightheadedness, loss of balance, or nonspecific dizziness is important, because the patient with true vertigo is significantly more likely to have a labyrinthine disorder.[3,4,16] Labyrinthine disorders are not life-threatening, and specific treatment is unavailable. The challenge is to identify patients with serious causes of vertigo and dizziness. Regardless of cause, vertigo can be disabling, recurrent, and refractory to treatment.[3,16,17]

True vertigo is described as an illusion of movement. It is often accompanied by nystagmus and is due to a vestibular system lesion in the brain stem, eighth cranial nerve, or labyrinth. The most important step for the emergency physician is to determine whether the vertigo is due to a peripheral or central cause.

About 85% of patients with vertigo have *peripheral vertigo*, with dysfunction of the vestibular organs. The term *peripheral vestibular disorder* is applied to patients with rotational vertigo, nausea, or vomiting, with no sign of brain stem deficit. In addition to these labyrinthine symptoms, cochlear symptoms may be present as aural fullness, tinnitus, or hearing loss. Tinnitus can be described as a hissing sound, high-pitched ringing, bells, or machinery-like roaring. Peripheral vertigo has multiple etiologies, including infection (labyrinthitis), ototoxicity from chemotherapy, autoimmune/allergic (Ménière) or traumatic (benign paroxysmal positional vertigo [BPPV], temporal bone fracture). Episodes may recur and even be debilitating, or they may gradually decrease over time. In most cases, cure is unavailable, and treatment is targeted at rehabilitation. Causes of peripheral vertigo are listed in Table 27.2.

Central vertigo has a more insidious onset and is frequently accompanied by neurologic symptoms, since the cause is a central nervous system (CNS) lesion. It may be due to ischemic changes from a cerebrovascular accident (CVA), multiple sclerosis, or intracranial tumor. Often the patient will describe a feeling of disorientation; however, true vertigo may also be present. This "lesion," when induced by drugs or metabolic abnormalities, is considered "systemic" or "global" by some authors.[1,12] Common causes of central vertigo are listed in Table 27.3.

Table 27.4 summarizes the characteristics of peripheral and central vertigo. Miscellaneous causes of vertigo are listed in Table 27.5.

TABLE 27.2. Causes of Peripheral Vertigo

Benign paroxysmal positional vertigo: Vertigo occurs mainly with change of head position, such as tilting the head backward or lying down, usually lasting only minutes. Episodes of vertigo may persist for days to months. Examination shows normal hearing and position-elicited nystagmus.

Acute labyrinthitis: Sudden onset of vertigo, increasing over 1 to 3 hours, then abating over days, in a patient who lacks other neurologic signs. Transitory episodes recur for up to 6 weeks. Most often seen in healthy adults; may follow an upper respiratory infection.

Vestibular neuronitis: Acute onset of vertigo, nausea, and vomiting without cochlear symptoms, with recurrent or concurrent upper respiratory infection.[1] Symptoms last 2 days to 6 weeks. Mild transitory episodes may recur over 12 to 18 months. Examination shows normal hearing. The exact cause is obscure, but it is believed to result from unilateral vestibular paralysis from a viral infection of the nerve.[1]

Ménière disease: Classically described as a triad of hearing loss, tinnitus, and vertigo. The vertigo is of abrupt onset, lasts for minutes to hours, and is accompanied by tinnitus, sensorineural hearing loss that fluctuates over long periods, and feeling of unilateral ear fullness. Attacks range from several per week to every few years. All forms have the common mechanism of endolymphatic absorption defect leading to endolymphatic hydrops and, often, rupture.

Labyrinthine concussion: Vertigo caused by head trauma that dislodges otoconia, leading to unequal loads on the macular beds and imbalance between the two otoliths.[1]

Cholesteatoma: Middle ear neoplasm with any of the following symptoms: facial twitching, various degrees of deafness (conductive or sensorineural) with loss of labyrinthine function. A positive insufflation test can indicate a cholesteatoma that has eroded the bone over the lateral semicircular canal.

Ototoxic drugs: Those in most common use are furosemide, the antimalarials (chloroquine, quinine), aminoglycosides, and cisplatin.

Labyrinthine infarction/ischemia: Symptoms are identical to those of vertebrobasilar insufficiency: Patients present with isolated episodes of vertigo of abrupt onset, lasting a few minutes, and associated with no other neurologic signs. They have nystagmus and a Nylen-Barany test that indicates peripheral vertigo. Progression to other signs of vertebrobasilar insufficiency or infarction is common. Patients with history of atherosclerosis should be seen by an otolaryngologist if attacks continue.[18]

Perilymphatic fistula: A history of vertigo after sneezing, nose-blowing, or barotrauma suggests perilymphatic fistula. Perilymphatic fistula most commonly results from head trauma. By insufflating the ear, the onset of vertigo and nystagmus is considered a positive test. Symptomatic treatment is usually sufficient, but surgical repair may be necessary.

Rupture of the round window: Overpressure leads to intractable vertigo. The ear canal should be examined. Granulation tissue in a patient with diabetes suggests malignant otitis externa. This commonly follows instrumentation of the ear canal, can cause lesions of cranial nerves VII and VIII, and requires assessment for basilar skull osteomyelitis.

Cerumen impaction: This may lead to hearing loss in one or both ears and is found in 25% of adults; the incidence increases with age.[19] Cerumen removal may resolve the vertigo. The tympanic membrane should be examined. A cholesteatoma appears as a built-up layer of epidermoid cells.

Tympanic membrane rupture, otitis media, and serous otitis with effusion: Rupture suggests barotrauma; all can cause peripheral vertigo that can become serious if it is untreated, is associated with mastoiditis, or occurs in an immunocompromised patient.

TABLE 27.3. Causes of Central Vertigo

Cerebral concussion: History of recent head trauma with a nonfocal neurologic examination. The dizziness is usually more lightheadedness than true vertigo and does not worsen with positional changes unless accompanied by a component of labyrinthine concussion. The patient complains of other sequelae of head injury—a prominent headache made worse by mental or physical effort, feeling dazed and unsteady, nausea, hyperacusis, and poor concentration.[20]

Cerebellar pontine angle tumor: Presents as loss of CN VIII function with hearing loss, vertigo, and nystagmus. Dizziness may vary from mild unsteadiness to true vertigo. There may also be lesions of CN V, VII, IX, XII. Cerebellar examination may show gait abnormality or unilateral ataxia. Unlike Ménière disease, vertigo does not completely abate between attacks.

Acoustic neuroma: Tumor of CN VIII, usually beginning on the vestibular branch; incidence highest in the fifth decade. It manifests early as cochlear symptoms with high-frequency deafness, followed months to years later by chronic vertigo. In advanced stages headache, ipsilateral ataxia, and palsy of CN V, VII, or X may develop.

Cerebellar infarction: May result from occlusion of the vertebral or posterior inferior cerebellar artery, from atherosclerosis or, in younger patients, from a twisting injury of the neck causing stretching, then dissection of the vertebral artery. This causes sudden onset of severe vertigo with nausea, vomiting, and sometimes severe retroauricular pain. Examination shows ipsilateral ataxia with severe nystagmus. Cranial nerve deficits may coexist (commonly CN V, IX, X, or XI) and indicate infarction of the adjacent brain stem.

Cerebellar hemorrhage: Vertigo occurs with occipital headache, repeated vomiting, and inability to stand or walk. Examination shows ipsilateral facial nerve weakness and diminished corneal reflex, dysarthria, and dysphagia. Gaze is conjugately affected and the patient cannot look toward the side of the hemorrhage from ipsilateral sixth nerve weakness. Vertical eye movements are maintained. Progression of cerebellar bleeding causes stupor, then coma from brain stem compression. Death follows rapidly without surgical decompression.

Vertebrobasilar insufficiency: In addition to vertigo, the patient may complain of posterior lobe symptoms of bilateral visual blurring, dimness, or blindness, and brain stem symptoms such as nausea, dysarthria, dysphagia, perioral numbness, or weakness or paresthesias of all four limbs. Symptoms are transient and follow abrupt change in posture or compression of the vertebral artery by movement of the neck, particularly hyperextension, or by osteoarthritis of the cervical spine. Examination may reveal a bruit over the subclavian artery.

Complex partial (temporal lobe) seizure: Focal seizure of the superior temporal cortex causes a prodrome of vertigo and auditory hallucinations followed by automatic behaviors such as lip-smacking, chewing, or walking in a daze and not responding to external stimuli. It is most prevalent in young adults and teenagers. Two-thirds of the patients have had generalized seizures at some time.

Orthostatic dizziness: A momentary interruption in cerebral circulation found in patients with orthostatic hypotension or the bedridden.[1] The onset is after arising abruptly. Lightheadedness may be accompanied by visual dimming or spots. Syncope may follow.

Hypertensive dizziness: Ill-defined; may be an adjustment of cerebral blood flow. Dizziness resolves when blood pressure normalizes.

Basilar artery migraine: Usually affects young women with family history of migraine. Vertigo is accompanied by unilateral, suboccipital headache, vomiting, and dysarthria. Visual prodrome is usually absent.[1]

Ethanol intoxication: This syndrome is well known. Eye movements can be in all directions with dysconjugate gaze; however, pupils should always react to light.

Other drugs: Commonly prescribed medications include phenytoin, salicylates, and phenothiazines. Over 800 over-the-counter medications list dizziness as a side effect in handbooks of adverse drug effects.

TABLE 27.4. Characteristics of Peripheral and Central Vertigo

	Peripheral	Central
Intensity	Moderate to intense	Mild to moderate
Temporal pattern	Brief, episodic	Chronic, continuous
Onset	Abrupt	Gradual
Nystagmus	Rotatory/ horizontal	Any kind, including bizarre vertical
Nausea/vomiting	Common	Uncommon
Hearing loss	Possible	Unlikely
Neurologic deficits	Otherwise none	Often present

From Edwards FJ. Overcoming the diagnostic challenges of dizziness, vertigo, and syncope. *Emergency Medicine Reports*. Atlanta: American Health Consultants, Jan. 10, 1994.

TABLE 27.5. Miscellaneous Causes of Vertigo or Dizziness

Hyperventilation syndrome: A noncentral and nonperipheral cause of vertigo reported in up to 23% of patients with dizziness.[21,22] Vertigo follows hyperventilation, sometimes during a panic attack. Typically, the patient has perioral and extremity numbness and dizziness. While usually associated with lightheadedness, hyperventilation has been shown to precede true vertigo in some patients.[21] An evaluation may be indicated based on clinical judgment, especially for the patient with true vertigo.

Motion sickness: A perceptual disorientation in healthy people due to rapid changes in position. A sensation of lightheadedness or impending faint without vertigo (often with dimming of vision) suggests a transient decrease of blood to the brain.

Impending faint: Caused by conditions that cause true syncope—vasovagal near-syncope, orthostatic hypotension, blood hyperviscosity syndromes, cardiac dysrhythmia, or cardiac valvular abnormality.

Nonvertiginous "dizziness": May be due to stumbling or falling that is without any head sensation.[21] The workup should be directed toward evaluating sensory neuropathy, or poor vision that causes falls.

CLINICAL PRESENTATION AND EMERGENCY DEPARTMENT EVALUATION

History

The history is critical to determination of the differential diagnosis. Identifying the length of duration, associations with head movement, inciting events, associated symptoms, and underlying medical conditions will guide the examiner in the appropriate direction.[3,6] Most young patients with vertigo have some type of peripheral vestibular disorder.[16] Serious causes of dizziness, although more common in older patients, do occur in the young and must be considered in all patients with vertigo. No single test is completely sensitive at detecting serious causes of dizziness, so the approach is a mixture of clinical judgment and ancillary testing. Underlying conditions that may be contributing to the problem include diabetes, certain medications (particularly antidepressants, beta-adrenergic blockers, and calcium channel blockers), migraine headaches, cardiovascular disease, or significant psychiatric history.

If the symptoms suggest central vertigo, consider a new or increased dose of medication, diabetes or hypoglycemia, hypo-

or hyperthyroidism, anemia or polycythemia, atherosclerosis, neck injury or arthritis, CVAs of the brain stem, cerebellar infarction or hemorrhage, or vertebrobasilar insufficiency.[8] A history of epilepsy suggests that partial complex (temporal lobe) seizure may be the cause of vertigo. A history of cancer or lymphoma might implicate a metastatic brain tumor. Fever and headache suggest that meningitis, encephalitis, or brain abscess should be evaluated. Peripheral vertigo may be present in coexistence with central vertigo, and any patient with neurologic signs should undergo further evaluation.[4,12]

The duration of the vertiginous episodes greatly assists in the diagnosis. Vertigo lasting seconds and associated with head movement is often benign paroxysmal positional vertigo (BPPV) or vertebrobasilar insufficiency.[8] Vertigo lasting minutes to hours may be Ménière disease, otosyphilis, Cogan syndrome, or recurrent vestibulopathy. Vertigo lasting days and associated with severe nausea and occasional hearing changes is most likely labyrinthitis (vestibular neuritis), although migraine vestibulopathy is also a possibility.[3,6]

Physical Examination

Orthostatic hypotension, carotid sinus hypersensitivity, and dysrhythmia can cause vertigo.[3,11] Lying and standing vital signs are desirable, but many patients either refuse to move or are too unsteady to stand. A directed physical examination should focus on the cranial nerves (especially hearing), cerebellar function, nystagmus, and positional testing. Vesicles on the auricle suggest Ramsay Hunt disease as a central cause of vertigo. The external auditory canal and tympanic membrane should be examined for any abnormality, as cholesteatoma, acute otitis media, and even cerumen impactions may cause vertigo.

Any cranial nerve abnormality strongly suggests a central process. Most commonly, a lesion of the seventh cranial nerve results in facial nerve paresis; a central seventh lesion is suggested by unilaterally decreased eye closing and smiling with intact forehead wrinkling due to crossover innervation.[1,16] Loss of cranial nerves III, IV, and VI is revealed by a dysconjugate gaze in a particular direction; all directions should be tested (see Chapter 60).

Lesions of the eighth nerve may result in decreased hearing. Sensorineural hearing loss should be ruled out by testing hearing to whispered voice or to rubbing fingers, or with a portable hearing screener. Decreased hearing in one ear requires further evaluation, as it may be sensorineural and signify asymmetry of function of the eighth cranial nerve.[9,10] Because most sensorineural loss reduces high-frequency tones, with tinnitus frequently present, a portable hearing screener that tests different frequencies is useful.[2]

Tuning fork tests may be helpful in identifying a unilateral sensorineural hearing loss or a conductive hearing loss. If the patient has bilateral sensorineural hearing losses, the tuning fork test will be equivocal. The base of a vibrating tuning fork placed on the midline of the forehead (the *Weber test*) relies on bone conduction; it is normally heard equally in both ears. Decreased sound in one ear implies either a sensorineural loss in that ear or a conductive hearing loss in the other ear. A vibrating tuning fork should be heard longer in air than through bone. In the *Rinne test*, the base of a vibrating tuning fork is applied on the mastoid bone. When the patient no longer feels it vibrating, it is quickly moved in front of the ear. Patients with normal conductive and sensorineural systems will still hear it vibrating. Sensorineural hearing loss is suspected if the hearing is equally reduced by both routes, but air conduction is still better than bone conduction.[14] In contrast, in conductive hearing loss, the sound is felt longer by bone than through air.

Cerebellar function is tested by finger-to-nose testing, rapidly alternating hand movements, and the heel-to-shin test. Past pointing or poor coordination suggest multiple sclerosis, cerebellar hemorrhage, or infarction. Station and gait are usually abnormal during acute vertigo and have little discriminatory value. The Fakuda test involves marching in place with the eyes closed and is considered positive for a peripheral lesion when the patient leans or falls to the affected side.

The most helpful physical findings are nystagmus and positional testing. Nystagmus can be characterized as peripheral or central by observing it in a darkened room. Peripheral nystagmus is suppressed with fixation of gaze (opened eyes in a lit room) and is enhanced when the patient looks in the direction of the fast component. Peripheral nystagmus is typically horizontal or rotatory and is worsened with head movement.[4,6] Central nystagmus may be of any type; however, nystagmus that is vertical, dysconjugate, direction-changing, or not suppressed by visual fixation is *always* central[4,6] (Table 27.6).

If nystagmus is subtle or absent, the patient should undergo the Dix-Hallpike maneuver (Table 27.7). The patient is asked to sit near the top of the gurney in a room with the lights dimmed, with enough room to hang the head off the end of the gurney. He or she is brought rapidly from sitting to lying, with the head tilted backward 45 degrees below the horizontal and to the left 45 degrees from midline, with eyes open. A positive test is defined as either the onset of nystagmus, reproduction of the vertigo, or both. After 30 seconds, the patient is brought to the upright position and the test repeated with the patient's head turned to the right. Any positive test should be repeated after a few minutes to see if either the nystagmus or vertigo is less pronounced or "fatigable."

Laboratory Testing

Significant electrolyte abnormalities are confined largely to patients taking diuretic medications or those who have a history of electrolyte abnormalities.[3,4] Occult metabolic causes of central vertigo are unlikely, but routine glucose measurement should be done to screen for hypoglycemia. Unsuspected significant

TABLE 27.6. Nystagmus from Central and Peripheral Lesions

	Central	Peripheral
Direction	Any direction	Usually rotatory or horizontal
Laterality	May be one eye	Both eyes
Visual fixation	Enhances nystagmus	Suppresses nystagmus
Effect of gaze toward side of fast component	Does not enhance nystagmus	Enhances nystagmus

TABLE 27.7. Dix-Hallpike Maneuver—Central vs. Peripheral Vertigo

	Central	Peripheral
Negative test	Does not help localize the lesion	5–30 s
Latency	None	
Fatiguability	None	Yes
Duration	Sustained	Transient

hypoglycemia is found in about 3% of patients. A complete blood count will identify patients with anemia or polycythemia and an elevated SED rate may point to rheumatoid arthritis or systemic lupus erythematosus. Otosyphilis will be identified with a positive FTA-ABS or MHA-TP.

Radiologic Imaging

If central vertigo is suspected, further evaluation is needed. Structural CNS lesions should be sought by either emergent head computed tomography (CT) or magnetic resonance imaging (MRI) with gadolinium scanning. These should be selected with regard to whether suspicion tilts toward intracranial tumor, cerebellar infarction or hemorrhage, acoustic neuroma, or multiple sclerosis.[12]

Other Studies

Electronystagmography (ENG) is a noninvasive means of detecting eye movements by recording corneoretinal potentials on a moving strip recorder; it may be useful acutely. ENG can often distinguish central from peripheral vertigo as well as identify which ear is the affected side.[10,13] This test is usually performed by an audiologist. An audiogram should also be done to evaluate whether there is a hearing loss related to the disorder.

Routine electrocardiograms are abnormal in 20% of dizzy patients age 45 and older.[8] Significant findings occur in 3%; these are mostly predicted by a history of cardiac disease.[11] The vestibular labyrinth is particularly vulnerable to ischemia and infarction in patients with a history of atherosclerosis (see Table 27.2).[12]

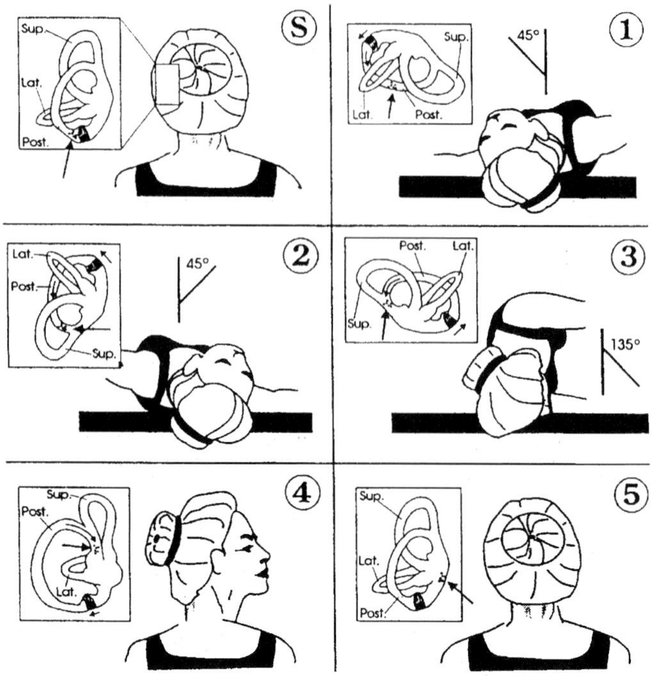

Figure 27.1. Epley Maneuver. Positioning sequence for left posterior semicircular canal as viewed by operator (behind patient). *(Box)* Exposed view of labyrinth, showing migration of particles (*large arrow*). *(S)* Start—patient seated (oscillator applied). *(1)* Place head over end of table, 45 degrees to left. *(2)* Keeping head tilted downward, rotate to 45 degrees right. *(3)* Rotate head and body until facing downward 135 degrees from supine. *(4)* Keeping head turned right, bring patient to sitting position. *(5)* Turn head forward, chin down 20 degrees. Pause at each position until induced nystagmus approaches termination, or for T (latency + duration) seconds if no nystagmus. Keep repeating entire series (1–5) until no nystagmus in any position.

EMERGENCY DEPARTMENT MANAGEMENT

After the ABCs have been addressed, the patient older than age 45 should have an intravenous line, oxygen, and heart monitor until a cardiovascular cause of vertigo can be reasonably excluded. Symptomatic treatment should begin immediately. Intravenous boluses of isotonic crystalloid should be given to the orthostatic patient, unless a history of congestive heart failure requires a more judicious hydration regimen. Because many dehydrated patients do not manifest orthostatic changes, fluid should also be given to the patient who is vomiting or having prolonged nausea.

Drug overdose or drug toxicity should be managed according to the ingestant, time since ingestion, and overall condition of the patient.

Central vertigo should be managed as a priority. Acute onset of a structural CNS abnormality, manifested by an abnormal neurologic examination, requires that neurology or neurosurgery consultation be obtained. Head CT scanning is usually done, but its inability to see the posterior fossa often requires either clinical diagnosis or referral for MRI. The decision to obtain an MRI is best discussed with the specialist.

The patient with labyrinthitis will probably feel better with hydration and time. All unnecessary movement should be avoided. The patient who is vomiting might benefit from intravenous droperidol (2.5 to 5.0 mg). There is no evidence as to the superiority of any one antivertigo medication, but antihistaminic and anticholinergic medications seem to help. Choices include meclizine (Antivert, 25 mg orally three times a day), diazepam (Valium, 5 mg once per day orally), diphenhydramine (Benadryl, 25 mg orally four times a day), and transdermal scopolamine (0.5-mg disc every 3 days). Because the elderly are prone to become confused after using scopolamine, it should be avoided in these patients.[3,15]

BPV or BPPV is easily managed with the Epley maneuver. This maneuver is similar to the Dix-Hallpike and begins with the patient sitting up, then laying him or her back, with the affected ear held at a 45-degree angle and the head extended until the vertigo resolves. The head is then turned to the opposite side and held at a 45-degree angle with extension. The patient is then rotated up on that side, with the head looking down at about 135 degrees; once the vertigo is resolved, the patient is seated upright, with the head sideways. The head is then turned forward. This procedure is repeated until there is no nystagmus or vertigo in any of the positions. The patient is then told to stay in an upright position for 24 to 48 hours. A soft cervical collar may be beneficial as well[5,7](Fig. 27.1). This procedure should not be performed in patients with cervical spine injuries or degenerated joint disease.

An acute attack of Ménière disease may be managed as a labyrinthitis, but the patient should be referred to an otolaryngologist for follow-up.

Perhaps as valuable as medication is performing Cawthorne's head exercises each morning and afternoon (Table 27.8). They worsen the vertigo while they are being performed, but they habituate the vestibular system, thereby allowing the vertigo to improve over time, often long enough to perform a required task.

DISPOSITION

The patient with vertigo should be given time off from work or school. Patients should be cautioned, in writing, to avoid driving, working at heights, or operating heavy equipment until episodes have resolved completely.

TABLE 27.8. Cawthorne's Balance Exercises

1. Eye Exercises	Looking up, then down—at first slowly, then quickly. 20 times. Looking from one side to the other—at first slowly, then quickly. 20 times. Focus on finger at arm's length, moving it 1 ft in each direction and back again. 20 times.
2. Head Exercises	Bend head forward, then backward with eyes open—slowly, later quickly. 20 times. Turn head from side to other side—slowly, then quickly. 20 times. As dizziness improves, head exercises should be done with eyes closed.
3. Sitting	While sitting, shrug shoulders. 20 times. Turn shoulders to right, then to left. 20 times. Bend forward and pick up objects from ground and sit up. 20 times.
4. Standing	Change from sitting to standing and back again. 20 times with eyes open. Repeat with eyes closed. Throw a small rubber ball from hand to hand above eye level. 20 times. Throw ball from hand to hand under one knee. 20 times.
5. Moving About	Walk across room with eyes open, then closed. 10 times. Walk up and down a slope with eyes open, then closed. 10 times. Walk up and down steps with eyes open, then closed. 10 times. Any game involving stooping or turning is good.

Exercises are to be done for 15 to 30 minutes twice a day.

These exercises help your central nervous system adjust to the current function of your inner ear balance mechanism and will lead to a decrease in your symptoms of positional dizziness. You may omit any exercises that do not cause dizziness.

Patients discharged with peripheral vertigo should be told that recurrence is likely, and that they should return for any symptoms of central dizziness. The symptoms appearing on the head injury checklist are useful, except that "dizziness or staggering while walking" is crossed off. Outpatient referral is indicated either to the primary provider for follow-up or to an otolaryngologist for further evaluation and management.

In the elderly, falls are especially dangerous, due to decreased strength and bone mass. Such patients should be discharged only if they are steady on their feet. Order a walker and encourage its use to prevent a fall if and when the dizziness recurs.[15]

Immediate consultation with a neurologist is indicated for the patient with signs of a new CNS abnormality. Immediate consultation with an otolaryngologist is indicated for the following: signs of otitis media in an immunocompromised patient, malignant external otitis, signs of perilymphatic fistula or cholesteatoma, or sudden sensorineural hearing loss with or without vertigo. Consultation with either a specialist or a neurologist should be considered in patients with vertigo of unknown etiology, in those with a history of cardiovascular disease, or those whose vertigo does not improve in the emergency department. Patients with a history of atherosclerosis and suspected labyrinthine ischemia should be seen by an otolaryngologist if attacks continue.[6,8]

Admission is indicated for signs of central vertigo, vertigo caused by dysrhythmia, and vertigo that is disabling or associated with persistent vomiting, and for patients who cannot be safely discharged because they lack household help. Admission to a bed with continuous cardiac monitoring is indicated for patients with suspected vertigo from dysrhythmia.

Transfer is indicated for emergent neurologic or neurosurgical consultation or monitoring that is unavailable locally. In most cases, advanced cardiac life-support transport is indicated, owing to possible progression of a CNS lesion or need to treat a symptomatic dysrhythmia.

COMMON PITFALLS

- Most, but not all, young patients have a peripheral vestibular disorder.
- Medication-induced vertigo is common.
- A common error is to delay intravenous hydration in hopes that the nauseated patient will be able to drink or that the nonorthostatic patient is well hydrated.
- Orthostatic vital signs are often hard to define and interpret in vertiginous patients.
- Failure to recognize neurologic signs and symptoms in association with the vertigo
- Do not discharge a vertiginous patient who lives alone.
- Falls in the elderly may cause hip fractures. Consider admission for all elderly patients who are unsteady. Those discharged should be encouraged to use a walker.
- Provide return instructions and a referral to all discharged patients.

References

1. Adams RD, Victor M. *Principles of neurology*. New York: McGraw-Hill, 1993.
2. Alvord LS. Handheld screening audiometers: reliability factors of a new screening tool. *Hear Instr* 1991;42(10):49.
3. Baloh RW. Vertigo. *Lancet* 1998;352:1841–1846.
4. Baloh RW. Differentiating between peripheral and central causes of vertigo. *Otolaryngol Head Neck Surg* 1998;119:55–59.
5. Bernard ME, Bachenberg TC, Brey RH. Benign paroxysmal positional vertigo: the canalith repositioning procedure. *Am Fam Physician* 1996;53(8):2613–2616.
6. Buttner U, Helmchen C, Brandt T. Diagnostic criteria for central versus peripheral positioning nystagmus and vertigo: a review. *Acta Otolaryngol* 1999;119:1–5.
7. Epley JM. Particle repositioning for benign paroxysmal positional vertigo. *Otolaryngol Clin North Am* 1996;29(2):323–1.
8. Gomez CR, Cruz-Flores S, Malkoff MD, et al. Isolated vertigo as a manifestation of vertebrobasilar ischemia. *Neurology* 1996;47:94–97.
9. LaRouere MJ, Seidman MD, Kartush JM. Medical and surgical treatment of vertigo. In: Jacobson GP, Newman CW, Kartush JM, eds. *Handbook of balance function testing*. St. Louis: Mosby, 1993:338.
10. Kentala E. Characteristics of six otologic diseases involving vertigo. *Am J Otolaryngol* 1996;17:883–892.
11. Kinney EL, Wright RJ. Should echocardiography be used to screen dizzy patients? *Angiology* 1988;October:902.
12. Kim GW, Heo JH. Vertigo of cerebrovascular origin proven by CT scan or MRI: pitfalls in clinical differentiation from vertigo of aural origin. *Yonsei Med J* 1996;37:47–51.
13. Shi M, Yu X, Niu H, et al. The value of electronystagmography in differential diagnosis of vertigo. Hunan I Ko Ta Hsueh Hsueh Pao 1997;22:156–158.
14. Sloane PD. Dizziness in primary care: results from the National Ambulatory Medical Care Survey. *J Fam Pract* 1989;1:33.
15. Sloane PD. Evaluation and management of dizziness in the older patient. *Clin Geriatr Med* 1996;12(4):785–801.
16. Turbiak TW, Reich JJ. Ear emergencies. In: Stair TO, ed. *Practical management of eye, ear, nose, mouth, and throat emergencies*. Rockville, MD: Aspen Systems, 1986:68.
17. Turbiak TW, Miller G. Vertigo and labyrinthine disorders. In: Harwood-Nuss A, ed. *Emergency medicine*. Philadelphia: JB Lippincott Co, 1991:91.
18. Grad A, Baloh RW. Vertigo of vascular origin: clinical and nystagmographic features in 84 cases. *Arch Neurol* 1989;46:281.
19. Gleitman RM, Ballachanda BB, Goldstein DP. Incidence of cerumen impaction in the general adult population. *Hear J* 1992;45:28.
20. Evans RW. Postconcussive syndrome: an overview. *Tex Med* 1987;83:49.
21. Drachman DA, Hart CW. An approach to the dizzy patient. *Neurology* 1972;22:323.
22. Herr RD, Zun L, Mathews JJ. A directed approach to the dizzy patient. *Ann Emerg Med* 1989;18:664.

CHAPTER 28
Acute Otitis Media in Adults

Harry W. Severance

Acute otitis media (AOM) is a well-recognized disease, but there is disagreement over its definition and classification. International symposia have attempted to develop a uniform system of classification, but unanimity has not yet been achieved.[1,11,15]

Figures 28.1 and 28.2 present the anatomy of the middle ear. AOM has a rapid, short course of signs and symptoms of inflammation of the middle ear without reference to etiology or pathogenesis. An effusion is almost always present in the middle ear space. Acutely appearing effusions are usually assumed to be suppurative (generated by bacterial pathogens)—hence the use of terms such as *suppurative, purulent,* or *bacterial* otitis media. Terms such as *nonsuppurative, serous,* or *secretory* are used for effusions that do not appear to be suppurative. These effusions also can present acutely. Classically, nonsuppurative effusions are thought to be nonbacterial; however, bacteria and other pathogens have been isolated from these effusions. There is also frequent difficulty in differentiating suppurative from nonsuppurative effusions without invasive techniques.[1] Therefore, classification and nomenclature in this area remain perplexing.

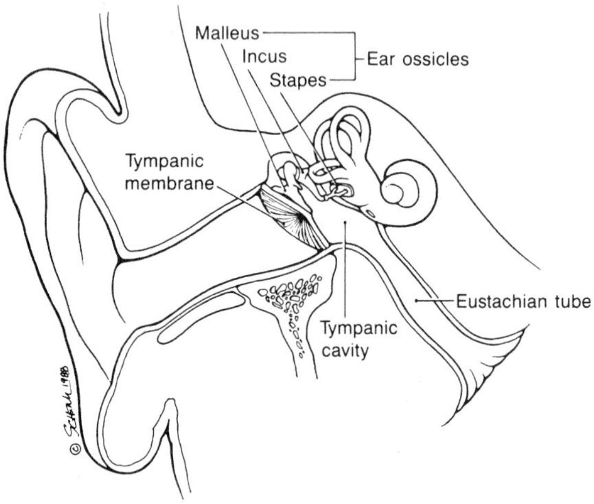

Figure 28.1. Anatomy of the middle ear.

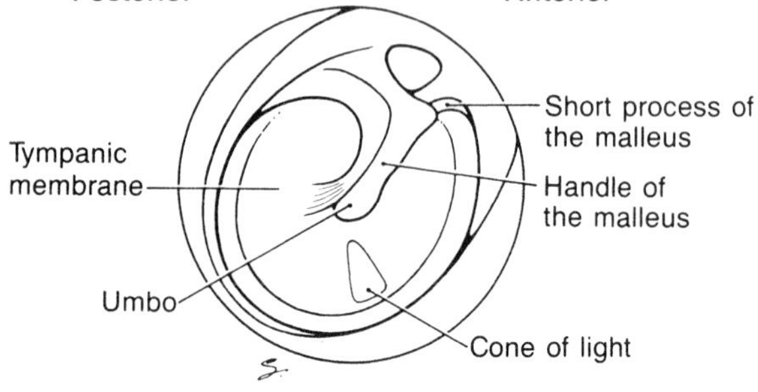

Figure 28.2. Anatomy of the tympanic membrane.

The term *acute* implies a rapid onset and brief presence of signs and symptoms, present for a period usually consisting of hours or days, and for all presentations of AOM, including nonsuppurative forms, no more than about 3 weeks.[1]

EPIDEMIOLOGY

Although AOM is one of the most common and well-reported diseases of children,[5,13,14,16,17,19] it is infrequently reported in adults.[2,4,18] Textbooks usually mention adult disease in anecdotal or associative terms only. Surveys by government and private agencies often lump adult cases with pediatric cases or use a wide age range for grouping, which makes evaluation difficult. Various agencies, institutions, and governments have differing age divisions for pediatric and adult populations, which complicates statistical comparisons of available data. Often, no great effort is made to separate acute and chronic forms of otitis in adults. Therefore, quantifying AOM in adults is difficult at best with existing data.

However, in a 1980 survey by the U.S. National Center for Health Statistics, with 1869 primary care physicians sampled, 20% (2.4 million) of the 11.7 million reported visits for otitis media were in patients older than 15 years. Seventy-two percent (1.85 million) of these visits were associated with the acute form. A 1987 National Disease and Therapeutic Index survey of 2130 office-based physicians recorded 465,000 visits for AOM among patients age 10 or older, with 304,000 visits for those age 20 or older. The same study noted almost 3.9 million visits by patients 20 years or older for unspecified otitis media. A similar study in 1970 also noted about 4 million cases.

There is little other epidemiologic information on adults in the current literature. However, the epidemiology of pediatric disease has been studied intensively, and adult disease has been assumed to follow similar patterns.

ETIOLOGY

The etiology of AOM has been studied in large pediatric populations over many years. Adult etiologies have been assumed to be similar, although no such broad-based studies have been reported. The most frequent organism is *Streptococcus pneumoniae,* which is found in 30% to 39% of cases. The relative incidence of pneumococcal infection is thought to rise with increasing age into adulthood. The second most common organism is *Haemophilus influenzae,* which occurs in about 20% to 30% of pediatric cases.[4] *H. influenzae* is more common in, but not limited to, younger age groups. Some more recent studies of older children and one study of a small number of adults have identified *H. influenzae* in equally high proportions.[4] *Moraxella* (formerly *Branhamella*) *catarrhalis* accounts for 3% to 15% of cases, and may be increasing in incidence.[4,7,12,14]

Chlamydia and *Mycoplasma* species have been reported.[10] Respiratory viruses are frequently associated with AOM.[7,10] Viruses are being studied intensively in association with pediatric presentations of AOM, and these studies have suggested a greater role for viruses in the etiology of AOM.[6–8] They predispose patients to subsequent bacterial infections, or may be the primary causative agent. Viruses in the middle ear may hinder the clinical response to antimicrobial therapy. Investigators report viral isolates either alone or in conjunction with bacteria in up to 30% of middle ear samples from pediatric AOM populations.[7,8] The most common species are influenza virus, rhinovirus, respiratory syncytial virus, adenovirus, and parainfluenza virus.[7,8] The relationship of viruses to adult cases of AOM is currently unknown, but is thought to be significant.

Adult microbiologic information is almost nonexistent compared with the wealth of pediatric information. Two prospective studies of adults cultured purulent middle ear effusions. In one study, involving 88 patients, the predominant organism was *S. pneumoniae* (62.5%), followed by *Staphylococcus aureus* (11.5%), *H. influenzae* (10.5%), *Streptococcus pyogenes* (7.3%), and other bacterial pathogens (8.8%). Some patients had multiple pathogens. The other study involved 34 patients; 26% grew *H. influenzae* and 21% grew *S. pneumoniae* from middle ear cultures.[4] Only 9% of the cultured organisms were beta-lactamase producing. In 26% of patients there was no growth on the cultures.[4]

PATHOPHYSIOLOGY

The pathogenesis of AOM in adults is thought to be similar to that in children. The onset of symptoms nearly always follows an upper respiratory infection. Rarely, barotrauma is the inciting event. The major acute predisposing factor is obstruction or dysfunction of the eustachian tube.[10] Hyperemia and edema of the mucosa at the pharyngeal portion of the eustachian tube is the typical obstructing event. This prevents normal ear ventilation and thus allows exudative and transudative fluid collections in the middle ear. Bacteria, viruses, and other pathogens are thought to be transferred to this fluid media by way of the eustachian tube. Some believe that isolation of fluid media in the closed space of the middle ear allows colonization by existing microbes, producing causative agents different from those that caused the primary infection. However, one recent adult study that simultaneously cultured purulent middle ear effusions and nasopharyngeal exudates demonstrated the same pathogens 97% of the time.

Colonizing microbes may proliferate within the middle ear space, thus activating the host's inflammatory defense system. Cytokines such as interleukin-1 and tumor necrosis factor are activated. Secondary mediators are, in turn, produced, including histamine, interferons, and leukotrienes. Circulating leukocytes then migrate to the site of infection and release proteolytic enzymes and free radicals, which, while attacking the targeted microbes, may also inadvertently damage host tissues. The local host damage may result in viscous effusions and chronic histologic changes, resulting in hearing impairment.[8]

Other predisposing factors include previous otitis infection; congenital, traumatic, or infectious damage to the eustachian tube; and damage to the tympanic membrane (TM). Other obstructive processes, such as nasopharyngeal tumors, can give rise to AOM. Researchers are exploring a possible link between exposure to cigarette smoke and AOM in children and adults.[8]

If no microbial pathogens can be identified in middle ear fluid collections, the pathophysiology is thought to result entirely from eustachian tube dysfunction or obstruction.

Barotrauma or aerotitis is a subset of eustachian tube dysfunction induced chiefly by technologic advances. Barotrauma is most common after air travel, although other causes include rapid elevator descents or descents into deep water such as with scuba diving, although it can occur even in a deep swimming pool. Cases can occur during travel over hills or mountains, especially if descent is rapid, such as in motor vehicles. Barotrauma is most commonly induced by a rapid descent, which produces a rapid increase in ambient atmospheric pressure that is significantly greater than middle ear pressure. Such rapid changes necessitate an active opening of the eustachian tube through contraction of the levator and tensor veli palatini muscles, allowing ambient air to be drawn into the middle ear space, thereby equalizing pressure. If the pressure change is too rapid for active middle ear air exchange, or dysfunction of the eustachian tube prevents this exchange, barotrauma results. Uncorrected negative pressure in the middle ear space causes retraction of the TM, immobility of the TM and ossicles, conductive hearing loss, and, if middle ear pressure is not equalized, transudation of serum and bleeding. If the ambient pressure change is rapid or great enough, TM rupture can also occur.

NATURAL HISTORY

Most cases of adult AOM resolve without sequelae. A few adults develop complications, but exact percentages are not known. The most common acute complication in adults is TM perforation and drainage of the effusion. Less common complications are secondary to local spread of infection and include mastoiditis, facial paralysis, subdural empyema, brain abscess, and meningitis. Adults with normal immunologic function seldom develop these complications. Pneumonic or meningeal spread occurs most often in children; the incidence in adults is unknown. Chronic, untreated otitis media can lead to such local complications as nonhealing TM perforations, cholesteatomas, and chronic hearing loss. The effects of vaccines against various infective microbes implicated in AOM are being studied in pediatric populations. The potential impact of these interventions on the natural history of adult presentations of AOM is unclear.

CLINICAL PRESENTATION

In adults, the usual presenting complaint is ear pain or discomfort.[4] Often, only one ear is affected, and the ear may have been the site of previous infection. There is usually a history of concurrent or recent upper respiratory tract infection.[4] Other presenting complaints may include hearing difficulty, tinnitus, and vertigo. Fever is variable. In one prospective study, a symptomatic triad of otalgia, impaired hearing, and upper respiratory tract infection was present in almost 100% of patients, with elevated temperature in only 9%.[4]

Adults present more commonly than children with spontaneous TM rupture and serosanguineous or purulent discharge from the affected ear. Although the incidence of systemic spread from adult AOM is unknown, high fever and signs of systemic toxicity in the adult with ear pain should cause the examiner to consider a diffuse process and compromised immune system.

In one study in which adults delayed seeking initial evaluation, significant complications were present at the initial presentation. Therefore, the initial examination should include a search for potential complications.

There are two major categories of complications resulting from otitis media: otologic and intracranial.[6] Otologic complications include TM perforation, mastoiditis, petrositis, facial nerve paralysis, and labyrinthitis. Intracranial complications include extradural abscess, subdural abscess, brain abscess, meningitis, lateral sinus thrombosis, and otic hydrocephalus. Many of these complications used to occur in untreated suppurative otitis media and have been significantly reduced in the era of antibiotic therapy, especially local otologic complications. Systemic complications from otitis media, such as bacteremia, pneumonia, and meningitis, are infrequent in adults.

Adults who present with symptoms of otitis media and high fever or signs of systemic toxicity or localized spread should receive a thorough examination. A white blood cell count, blood cultures, chest radiograph, and cerebral spinal fluid studies should be done, as indicated.

DIFFERENTIAL DIAGNOSIS

Almost any disease process of the head and neck can refer pain to the ear. Dental caries or abscesses commonly refer pain to the ear, as does sialoadenitis or temporomandibular joint syndrome. Sinusitis and pharyngitis can present as ear pain. Acute glaucoma and other optic diseases are occasionally referred to the ear. Otitis externa and soft-tissue infection in proximity to the auricle must be differentiated from otitis media. In most cases, a careful evaluation should produce the correct diagnosis.

EMERGENCY DEPARTMENT EVALUATION

Head and Neck

The evaluation of ear pain should include a thorough examination of the head and neck to rule out other causes. Teeth and gums are examined and percussed. The oral cavity and nasopharynx are inspected for inflammation, sinusitis, and other diseases. Parotid, submandibular, and submaxillary glands are palpated and the temporomandibular joints examined. The soft tissue around the auricle is inspected and palpated. The auricle and tragus are manipulated. The neck is inspected and palpated, and the carotids are auscultated for bruits. The eyes are briefly examined to rule out signs of glaucoma or other ocular pathology.

Middle Ear

The hallmark of the middle ear examination is otoscopic visualization of the TM: An examination for ear pain or other otitis media–related symptoms is incomplete without it. Wax, debris, and discharge that obstruct visualization must be removed. The TM is noted for appearance, landmarks, and light reflex. Signs suggestive of otitis media are loss of normal concavity of the membrane, bulging or retraction of the membrane, visual loss of the bony landmarks, and erythema or an opaque or bluish appearance of the membrane. A fluid level or bubbles behind the TM also may be seen. Findings from barotrauma-induced otitis media are usually the same as for other types of nonsuppurative AOM, although hemotympanum or membrane rupture can be seen.

Pneumatic otoscopy has classically been the most sensitive and simple bedside test for the presence of effusion behind the TM and should be part of the routine examination. Pneumatic otoscopy does not define whether the effusion is suppurative or nonsuppurative.

The hand-held acoustic otoscope reportedly is a reliable test for the presence of middle ear effusions.[9] In one study, the acoustic otoscope was shown to detect effusions with equal facility in adults and children.[9]

Tympanocentesis and myringotomy of the middle ear are the most accurate invasive tests to evaluate middle ear effusions. These procedures not only detect the presence and nature of effusions (purulent vs. serous), but also provide material for culture and Gram stain. These procedures are normally reserved for the otolaryngologist.

EMERGENCY DEPARTMENT MANAGEMENT

Antimicrobial Therapy

Uncomplicated otitis media, presenting acutely with an effusion present, is usually assumed to be suppurative (bacterial). *S. pneumoniae, H. influenzae,* and, more recently, *M. catarrhalis* are the usual pathogens, with *S. pneumoniae* and *H. influenzae* thought to be the two most common organisms in adults.[2] The presence of beta-lactamase–producing strains has been increasing significantly in pediatric populations over the past decade, and is suspected to be likewise increasing in adults.[2,8] Amoxicillin (500 mg orally three times a day for 10 days) and, more recently, trimethoprim-sulfamethoxazole (TMP-SMX) (double strength twice a day for 10 days) remain the first-line drugs of choice for adult populations, though resistance to these drugs is increasing.

Patients whose signs and symptoms continue after initial antibiotic therapy or those who are allergic to penicillins or TMP-SMX should receive alternative antibiotics. Alternative selections include one of the new macrolides (azithromycin or clarithromycin); one of the newer cephalosporins; the second-generation agents cefaclor, loracarbef, cefuroxime axetil, or cefprozil; and third-generation drugs such as cefpodoxime proxetil or cefixime; or alternative penicillins such as amoxicillin-potassium clavulanate.[2,8] Fluoroquinolones, such as ciprofloxacin, are currently being studied as possible second-line antimicrobials for AOM, as is intramuscular injection of the third-generation cephalosporin ceftriaxone.[8] Second-line, broader spectrum antibiotics should also be considered in patients at high risk for complications, such as those with diabetes or other types of relative or total immunocompromise. Choices in alternative antibiotic therapy must also take into account any allergic history, as well as the spectrum of activity of the chosen agent.

All presentations of AOM complicated by TM perforation should be treated with an antibiotic regimen.

Supportive Therapy

Supportive therapy includes fever control, relief of otalgia, and treatment of associated upper respiratory symptoms. Acetaminophen or ibuprofen is thought to be adequate to treat pyrexia and otalgia in most adults. Short-term narcotic analgesia may be appropriate for adults with severe otalgia. However, severe otalgia without significant TM bulging should prompt a search for other causes of the pain. Otalgia and other symptoms should improve significantly over the first 24 to 48 hours after appropriate antibiotic therapy begins; failure to respond is a cause for concern. Therefore, when prescribing outpatient narcotic analgesia, such prescriptions should cover only this initial period. Patients who experience continued otalgia or other symptoms should be instructed to return for further evaluation.

Myringotomy has been recommended for adults with severe otalgia and a bulging TM. This technique allows almost instantaneous pain relief and provides material for culture, and should be considered for adults with these symptoms.

Decongestants and antihistamines are effective in reducing the symptoms of an upper respiratory infection, and should be considered in adults. This is especially valuable for barotrauma-induced AOM.

TM perforations associated with AOM usually resolve spontaneously without sequelae. Purulent discharge through the perforation may result in an eczematoid external otitis. Topical ear drops consisting of a steroid–antibiotic mixture are often prescribed. However, if such drops enter the middle ear space through the perforation, they may cause a chemical ototoxicity.[3] Therefore, there is no consensus concerning this therapy.

DISPOSITION

Role of the Consultant

Adults with uncomplicated AOM can be safely discharged on antibiotics and symptomatic therapy. Patients should be instructed to seek follow-up for worsening symptoms or for symptoms of systemic illness. Follow-up examination of the ear after completion of therapy has not been evaluated in adults. All patients with TM perforation secondary to AOM should receive a follow-up evaluation to confirm healing of the membrane.

Patients who return with continued symptoms despite therapy should be reevaluated for other causes. In their absence, a trial of an alternative antibiotic should be instituted. These patients should be told to return immediately for any worsening of symptoms. Follow-up at the completion of antibiotic therapy is mandatory.

Patients with persistent otorrhea secondary to TM rupture that continues after initial antibiotic therapy should be referred to an otolaryngologist.[3] Patients whose symptoms persist after the second course of antibiotics also should be referred to an otolaryngologist.

Patients who return during or after therapy with any worsening of symptoms should receive consultation by an otolaryngologist. Myringotomy should be considered in patients with worsening symptoms, especially if the diagnosis is in question, severe pain is present, or infectious complications occur.

Patients with known immunocompromise or other disabling illness should have early referral. An otolaryngologist or primary physician must assess the results of therapy. Tympanocentesis or myringotomy may be necessary to determine the etiology.

Patients with signs of systemic toxicity or localized or intracranial infectious complications deserve an immediate and thorough examination. Immediate consultation is indicated. Hospital admission and parenteral antibiotics may be indicated.

Indications for Admission

Symptoms or signs of chronic or acute sequelae of AOM should be evaluated by an otolaryngologist. Subsequent treatment or hospitalization is based on the nature and severity of the symptoms. Most adults are successfully treated as outpatients, but the rare adult with systemic toxicity or severe localized spread should be admitted.

Transfer Considerations

Special consideration is necessary for patients who requires air transport. These patients must be transported at low altitudes, usually under 1000 feet, or in pressurized aircraft. Inability to equilibrate middle ear pressure and high altitudes can lead to TM rupture or localized spread of pathogens to adjacent tissues.

COMMON PITFALLS

- Failure to visualize the TM
- Failure to test the mobility of the TM
- Confusing a ruptured TM with drainage with otitis externa

References

1. Bluestone CD. State of the art: definitions and classifications. In: Lim DJ, et al., eds. *Proceedings of the third international symposium: recent advances in otitis media with effusion*. Philadelphia: BC Decker, 1984:1.
2. Bluestone CD. Otitis media. In: Johnson JT, Yu VL, eds. *Infectious diseases and antimicrobial therapy of the ears, nose and throat*. Philadelphia: WB Saunders, 1997:273.
3. Cahill L, Jehle D. Otitis. In: Reisdorff EJ, Roberts MR, Wiegenstein JG, eds. *Pediatric emergency medicine*. Philadelphia: WB Saunders, 1993:617.
4. Celin SE, Bluestone CD, Stephenson J, et al. Bacteriology of acute otitis media in adults. *JAMA* 1991;266:2249.
5. Giebink GS. Epidemiology and natural history of otitis media. In: Lim DJ, et al., eds. *Proceedings of the third international symposium: Recent advances in otitis media with effusion*. Philadelphia: BC Decker, 1984:5.
6. Giebink GS. Infection of the middle and inner ear. In: Schlossberg D, ed. *Infections of the head and neck*. New York: Springer-Verlag New York, 1987:64.
7. Giebink GS. Otitis media update: pathogenesis and treatment. *Ann Otol Rhinol Laryngol* 1992;101:21.
8. Hoppe HL, Johnson CE. Otitis media: focus on antimicrobial resistance and new treatment options. *Am J Health Syst Pharm* 1998;55:1881.
9. Jehle D, Cottington E. Acoustic otoscopy in the diagnosis of otitis media. *Ann Emerg Med* 1989;18:396.
10. Klein JO. Otitis externa, otitis media, mastoiditis. In: Mandell GL, et al., eds. *Principles and practice of infectious disease*, 4th ed. New York: Churchill Livingstone, 1995:579.
11. Klein JO, Tos M, Hussel B, et al. Definitions and classifications. *Ann Otol Rhinol Laryngol* 1989;98(Pt 2, Suppl 139):10.
12. Kovatch AL, Wald ER, Michaels RH. Beta-lactamase-producing *Branhamella catarrhalis* causing otitis media in children. *J Pediatr* 1983;102:261.
13. McFadden DM, Berwick DM, et al. Age-specific patterns of diagnosis of acute otitis media. *Clin Pediatr* 1985;24:571.
14. Odio CM, Kusmiesz H, et al. Comparative treatment trial of Augmentin versus cefaclor for acute otitis media with effusion. *Pediatrics* 1985;75:819.
15. Paparella MM, Bluestone CD, et al. Definition and classification. *Ann Otol Rhinol Laryngol* 1985;94:8.
16. Pukander J, Sipila M, et al. Occurrence of and risk factors in acute otitis media. In: Lim DJ, et al., eds. *Proceedings of the third international symposium: recent advances in otitis media with effusion*. Philadelphia: BC Decker, 1984:9.
17. Schnore SK, Sangster JF, et al. Are antihistamine decongestants of value in the treatment of acute otitis media in children? *J Fam Pract* 1986;22:39.
18. Shambaugh GE, Girgis TF. Acute otitis media and mastoiditis. In: *Otolaryngology*, vol II: *Otology and neuro-otology*, 3rd ed. Philadelphia: WB Saunders, 1991:1343.
19. Shurin PA, Giebink GS, et al. Epidemiology and natural history. *Ann Otol Rhinol Laryngol* 1985;94:10.

CHAPTER 29
Acute Otitis Externa

Harry W. Severance

Otitis externa (OE) is a general term encompassing all of the irritative and infective processes that involve the skin of the external auditory canal.[3,15,19] There are several systems for dividing the types of OE. One generally accepted system divides it into three major groups: *inflammatory OE,* in which the pathogenesis involves infectious pathogens, *eczematoid (allergic) OE,* and *seborrheic OE.*[3] Inflammatory OE can be further subdivided into acute forms, in which the predominant pathogens are bacterial, and chronic forms, in which fungal organisms predominate.

Acute inflammatory otitis is by far the most common type of OE presenting to emergency physicians. It is defined as an inflammatory condition of the auricle, ear canal, or the outer surface of the tympanic membrane (TM).[15,19] Acute inflammatory OE can be further subdivided into diffuse and localized forms.[3,12,15] Acute diffuse OE ("swimmer's ear") is the most common of all external ear infections.[3,12,15,19] Acute localized OE is commonly an infection involving a hair follicle in the area of the ear canal.[3,12] The initial presentations of these two processes are similar.

ACUTE DIFFUSE OTITIS EXTERNA

EPIDEMIOLOGY

Acute diffuse OE is found in all age groups, in all climates, and in all seasons. However, the incidence is greatly increased during the summer, especially among swimmers (hence the term *swimmer's ear*).[3,19,22,26] The spectrum of disease produced by this entity ranges from mild itching and irritation of the ear to excruciating pain, swelling, purulent discharge, and systemic illness.[19,24]

ETIOLOGY

Excessive wetness or dryness of the canal, trauma, or a change in the canal environment makes the ear canal epithelium vulnerable to infection by endogenous bacteria, virulent exogenous bacteria, or other microbial pathogens.[2] Normal flora of the external canal include *Staphylococcus epidermidis, Corynebacterium* (diphtheroids), *Micrococcus* sp., and occasionally *Staphylococcus aureus, Streptococcus viridans,* and anaerobic bacteria such as *Propionibacterium acnes.*[2,11,12,15,19] Common pathogenic exogenous bacterial organisms are *Pseudomonas aeruginosa, Enterobacter aerogenes, Proteus vulgaris, Klebsiella pneumoniae, S. aureus,* and non–group-A streptococci.[2,7,10,12,16,19,20,26] *P. aeruginosa* is the most commonly isolated bacterium.[2,8] Fungal organisms are rarely seen as the sole infecting organism in acute disease, but are most often found in hot, moist environments, or among those with immune compromise.[3,5,15,19] Commonly cultured fungal organisms are *Aspergillus niger, Candida* sp., *Actinomyces,* or yeasts.[3,5,8,19] Herpesvirus hominis and varicella-zoster also may cause external otitis.[2,8]

ANATOMY

Figure 29.1 shows the anatomy of the external ear. The adult external auditory canal is about 24 to 35 mm long and ends medially at the TM.[11,12,15,16] In the adult, the distal third of the canal is supported by the cartilaginous base of the auricle; the proximal two-thirds of the canal passes through the temporal bone. This ratio is reversed in infants and small children.[2] A constriction, the isthmus, is present at the juncture of the cartilaginous and osseous portions of the canal and limits the entry of wax and foreign bodies to the area near the TM.[12,15] The canal forms an S shape with a slight upward and backward orientation; this likewise discourages foreign-body entry.[15] The epithelium of the canal originates on the outer surface of the three-layered TM and migrates outward at 1.5 to 2.0 mm a month.[1,15,16] The skin of the canal is thicker in the cartilaginous portion and includes a well-developed dermis and subcutaneous layer. The skin lining the osseous portion is thinner and firmly attached to the periosteum, lacking dermal papilla and subcutaneous tissue.[11] Hair follicles are numerous in the outer third and sparse in the inner two-thirds of the canal.[12]

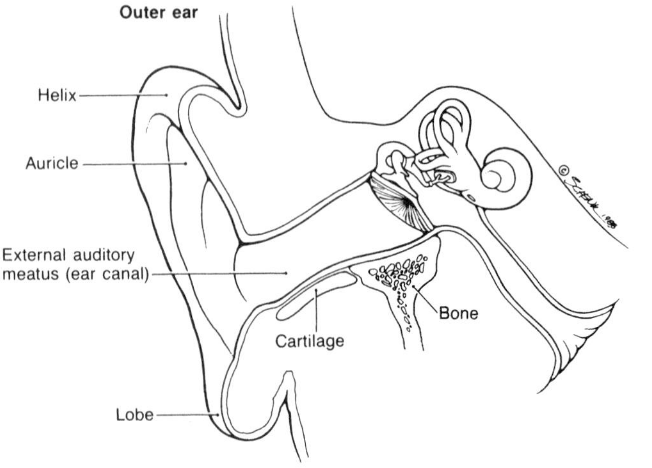

Figure 29.1. Anatomy of the external ear.

The external canal is equipped with barriers to prevent contamination of the canal and injury to the TM.[16,17] The outward movement of keratinized epithelium, along with the normal mandibular chewing motion, propels keratinized debris and cerumen outward.[5,15,16,24] The concentration of hair follicles and secretions of the numerous sebaceous and cerumen (apocrine-type) glands in the outer third of the canal, along with the S shape and isthmus of the canal, further prevent entry of foreign objects.[11,14–16] The waxy, water-repellent cerumen is a mixture of secretions from the sebaceous and apocrine glands in this area and the desquamated keratin layer from the stratum corneum. It protects by several mechanisms, including mechanical obstruction, stickiness, the water-repellent action of the lipids and waxes, bacteriostatic and bactericidal effects, and the presence of lysozyme and immunoglobulins.[11,14–16,23] Acidic pH plays a protective role, and possibly so does the presence of trace metals.[15,16,23]

PATHOPHYSIOLOGY

The usual precipitating factor in acute OE is the introduction of infectious organisms into the epithelium of a previously traumatized ear canal in which protective defenses have been disrupted.[2,16] Usual traumatic mechanisms are foreign bodies (cotton-tipped applicators, pencils), prolonged wetness (water sports, bathing, increased environmental humidity), or excessive dryness (previous infection, dermatoses, insufficient cerumen).[2] Various sequences of events have been proposed to explain the evolution of acute OE.[5,16] In general, disruption of or interference with any of the protective mechanisms of the external canal can lead to OE. Predisposing factors include previous ear surgery or TM rupture,[5,20] a narrow or abnormally angled canal,[5,18] and excessive or decreased cerumen production.[5] Even in the presence of predisposing factors, trauma and introduction of infectious agents into the canal are the immediate precipitating factors. In the most common scenario of infection, swimming pool water with an alkaline pH and commonly containing *Pseudomonas* organisms is introduced into a previously traumatized ear canal, often producing an episode of acute, diffuse OE.

NATURAL HISTORY

After the inciting event, symptoms develop over several hours or days. The spectrum of disease can range from mild to severe. Left untreated, the infection can resolve, persist as a chronic infection, or, with some organisms (usually *Pseudomonas*), progress over weeks or months to malignant (necrotizing, invasive) OE.[9,17] This entity is seen almost exclusively in diabetics and other immunocompromised patients, although there are reports that it occasionally progresses from initially uncomplicated diffuse OE in nonimmunocompromised swimmers.[9] Malignant OE can result in a high incidence of neurologic sequelae or death.[4,6,7,9,18,25]

CLINICAL PRESENTATION

Patients presenting with mild-to-moderate acute OE may complain only of itching or irritation in the affected ear, often heightened by manipulation of the auricle or tragus.[2,3,15,16,19] In more severe presentations, the severity of pain and tenderness may seem disproportionate to the degree of inflammation, probably due to compression of nerve fibers. Edema and erythema are present and the canal may be closed. There is usually a discharge described as yellowish, greenish, or watery. Fungal infections produce a dark or cheesy discharge. Frequently, the canal is so tender and swollen that the entire ear canal and TM cannot be adequately visualized. In such cases, complete otoscopic examination should be delayed until the acute swelling subsides.[2] If the canal is visualized, it often appears pale, soggy, and edematous, occluded by cerumen and desquamated epithelium.[19] The TM, if visualized, may appear normal, opaque, or erythematous. It may have normal mobility or, if the drum is thickened, reduced response to insufflation.[2]

In more severe infections, there can be periauricular inflammation, cellulitis, lymphadenitis, and erythema.[2,16,19] Fever is variably present[2,19] and pain can be intensified by any manipulation of the jaw or the affected side of the face.[19] Such presentations often result from combined infections with *Pseudomonas* sp. and *Streptococcus pyogenes* or from *S. aureus*.[2]

DIFFERENTIAL DIAGNOSIS

Many different diseases can produce ear pain. Locating the source of pain helps narrow the differential. The examiner usually can rule out otitis media by findings specific to the outer ear and canal. Pain on manipulation of the auricle and tragus is usually evidence against otitis media.[19] If the TM can be visualized and mobility is normal, otitis media is not present. A serosanguineous discharge from the affected ear may represent a ruptured TM secondary to acute otitis media or penetrating trauma to the ear canal. Signs and symptoms of toxicity, facial nerve palsy, or meningeal signs are present in malignant OE.[6,7]

Other diagnoses in the differential include adjacent disease processes with pain referred to the area of the ear canal: parotitis, periauricular adenitis, mastoiditis, dental abscess, temporomandibular joint pain, sinusitis, tonsillitis, or pharyngitis.[2,15,16,19]

In cases of ear canal occlusion when severe pain and edema prevent adequate cleaning and visualization, excluding middle ear infection on the initial examination may be difficult.[15]

EMERGENCY DEPARTMENT EVALUATION

Emergency department evaluation includes manipulation of the auricle and tragus. The periauricular area is inspected for inflammation, cellulitis, folliculitis, or eczematous conditions. The canal is inspected and its condition noted. The TM is visualized, on initial examination if possible, and its mobility tested to rule out otitis media. Any exudate is cultured.[19] Fungal cultures are included if the history is suggestive, the exudate is cheesy or black, or a candidal rash is present.

In elderly patients with diabetes and other immunocompromised patients with otorrhea and intense ear pain, the possibility of malignant OE must be considered. A white blood cell count (WBC) and erythrocyte sedimentation rate (ESR) are obtained in these patients.[17] Signs of systemic toxicity, local extension of infection to periauricular areas, nuchal rigidity, or facial nerve palsy are sought.

If the WBC or ESR is more than mildly elevated, or any of the aforementioned signs are present, evaluation for malignant OE proceeds. This is especially true in patients who have had symptoms for weeks or months or in those who return with worsening or unresolved symptoms after previous evaluation and therapy.

Evaluation consists of proving spread of infection to the mastoid or base of the skull. Numerous radiologic techniques are used in this assessment. Plain films, including tomographic views, and computed tomography (CT) scanning can detect the bony erosions of advanced disease but are often of little help in early presentations.[9] Technetium and gallium scanning are reported to be much more sensitive (than even CT scanning) in detecting early disease, and are preferred by many otolaryngologists.[9,13,17] However, low specificity and decreased availability in emergency departments limit their usefulness. CT scanning is the current modality of choice for defining the anatomic extent of disease.[13,17] However, significant destruction of trabecular bone is often necessary to define osteomyelitis by CT scanning.[13,17] CT scans are generally more available to emergency physicians. The value of magnetic resonance imaging (MRI) is currently under investigation, but in small numbers of patients it has detected the presence of disease at least as well as CT scanning.[9,17]

EMERGENCY DEPARTMENT MANAGEMENT

Basic management of acute OE includes aural hygiene, elimination of microbes, and analgesics. Hygiene involves cleansing of the ear canal and is considered by many to be the single most important part of therapy.[3,15,16] For mild infections, dry-mopping with a small tuft of cotton attached to a wire applicator may be sufficient; sometimes it is even curative.[15] In more severe infections, with an inflamed, edematous canal with cheesy secretions and debris, removal by suctioning is recommended.[5,15,16] If appropriate suctioning devices are unavailable, one author suggests using a trimmed infant feeding tube attached to a De Lee suction device.[15] Others suggest that in severe cases, suctioning should be done using the operating microscope. After all major debris and exudate are removed, careful irrigation with warm, sterile saline or a 2% acetic acid solution is recommended to complete the cleansing. Forceful irrigation is contraindicated, as it could traumatize further the macerated epithelium of the canal and actually promote suprainfection. After irrigation is complete, the canal must be dried. Several techniques have been used, including suction or instillation of a drying solution of dilute alcohol.[2] Some authors suggest using a hair dryer.[15,16] In severe cases, this regimen must be repeated at regular intervals until inflammation has subsided.

Topical otic solutions are recommended by many for eliminating microbes and acidifying the canal in most cases of acute inflammatory OE. There is no consensus, however, on a solution of choice. Many are recommended and available, ranging from acetic acid preparation (2%) and half-strength Burow's solution (aluminum acetate, 1:20) to topical antibiotic preparations containing neomycin (active against gram-positive organisms and also against some gram-negative organisms, notably *Proteus* sp.) with either colistin or polymyxin (active against gram-negative bacilli, notably *Pseudomonas* sp.). Some of these commercially available solutions contain other ingredients, such as corticosteroids, to reduce inflammation.[12,21,26] Most solutions seem to be effective if used in conjunction with the other recommended treatment measures. There are anecdotal reports that neomycin-containing solutions produce a contact dermatitis, but the actual incidence in one trial was found to be 0.1%.[9] Otic solutions are preferable to suspensions, except in TM perforation or the presence of a ventilation tube.

In canals that are severely inflamed and edematous, an ear wick may be necessary for the application of otic solutions.[19] Expandable ear wicks of hydroxycellulose or similar materials are available and are reported by some to be preferable to cotton or gauze, although the latter are still recommended.[15,24] The wick is placed about 10 to 12 mm into the outer third of the canal, and otic drops are placed directly on the wick.[2,15] If wicks are required, steroid-containing solutions may have an advantage in hastening the reduction of inflammation. Ear wicks are usually used for 24 to 48 hours and then removed. Often they spontaneously fall out as inflammation subsides.

Otic solutions are applied to the affected canal three or four times daily, two to four drops per application. Seven to 10 days of therapy with resolution of symptoms is reasonable.[5,11]

Pain from OE can be intense, and some patients may require narcotic analgesia during the initial evaluation, cleaning, and wick insertion and during the first 24 to 48 hours of treatment.[2,3,11,15] Oral codeine or hydrocodone is effective.[2,3] Continued severe pain after therapy begins should prompt reevaluation. Mild, locally applied dry heat often helps in pain management.[2,3]

During treatment, introduction of water into the ear canal must be avoided. Swimming is prohibited. Showers should be brief and hair-washing infrequent and followed by instillation of otic drops.[16] When bathing, shower caps, ear plugs, or other devices to prevent entry of water into the ear canal can be considered.[24]

Oral antibiotics are generally unnecessary for mild-to-moderate cases of acute diffuse OE. In the vast majority of uncomplicated cases, these local measures should bring about resolution of symptoms. Oral antibiotics have been recommended in patients with more severe presentations, such as intense pain, fever, or lymphadenitis, or in patients who require ear wick insertion.[2,5,12] Cultures of ear aspirates should be obtained in all such patients. Oral antibiotics are also recommended for patients with occluded ear canals who have symptoms, signs, or history suggestive of otitis media, such as upper respiratory infections, fever, or sore throat.[24]

There are no firm guidelines for empiric oral antibiotic therapy for cases of acute OE presenting without complications. Penicillinase-resistant penicillins, trimethoprim–sulfamethoxazole, erythromycin, tetracycline, cephalosporins, and ciprofloxacin have all been advocated for initial empiric therapy.[5,12,19] Culture results and evolution of the patient's condition should guide modifications to therapy. In the patient begun on an oral antibiotic who is improving, with cultures that indicate good sensitivity, continuation for a 10-day course with resolution of symptoms is reasonable. Almost all cases resolve with the aforementioned measures.

Parenteral antibiotics are occasionally required in the rare patient with symptoms of systemic toxicity,[2] or in the patient with a progressive or unresponsive infection. Cultures of ear aspirate should be done on all such patients and the possibility of malignant OE considered, especially in predisposed patients.

A combination of an aminoglycoside and an antipseudomonal penicillin should be started.[12,15] If *S. aureus* infection is suspected, a cephalosporin or penicillinase-resistant penicillin is the initial therapy. Treatment is adjusted as culture results indicate. For patients with proven or suspected malignant OE, the infectious agent is almost invariably *P. aeruginosa,* and admission with parenteral antibiotic therapy is mandatory.[3] Currently recommended initial parenteral treatment consists of an aminoglycoside in combination with an antipseudomonal penicillin, or an appropriate third-generation cephalosporin. Newer studies have reported good results with single agents such as ceftazidime or cefoperazone.[9,11] The usual parenteral treatment period has been 4 to 6 weeks,[3,11,12] with oral ciprofloxacin after about 1 week in responding cases.[9,11]

DISPOSITION

Most patients with acute diffuse OE may be discharged home with instructions for good aural hygiene, topical antibiotic drops, and symptomatic therapy, including analgesia.[26] Discharge instructions should include avoiding water sports during therapy and for up to 2 to 4 weeks after resolution of symptoms. A 10-day follow-up is encouraged.

Elderly patients with diabetes or other immunocompromising diseases who are seen for OE should receive close follow-up and monitoring to prevent the rapid onset of malignant OE.[24]

Patients with obstructed canals, with ear wicks inserted, or with severe pain (especially those whose initial otoscopic examination was limited due to pain and swelling), and patients on oral antibiotics or narcotic analgesics should be reevaluated in 12 to 24 hours to ensure that symptoms are resolving and to allow completion of a thorough otoscopic examination. As swelling subsides, polyps, neoplasms, foreign bodies, or otitis media not visible on the initial examination may be revealed.[24]

Patients with severe edema, exudative discharge, and pain may require periodic, aggressive hygiene with irrigation, suctioning, and drying of the ear canal daily until symptoms regress. Otolaryngologic consultation should be considered in patients who require multiple daily visits for hygiene.

All patients with worsening of symptoms or failure to respond to initial management should be evaluated by an otolaryngologist. For patients with worsening symptoms, consultation should be immediate to consider possible hospitalization and parenteral antibiotic therapy.

Admission and parenteral antibiotic therapy are required for patients with systemic toxicity, meningeal signs, or facial palsy. A workup to rule out malignant OE is indicated, including lumbar puncture, CT scanning (possibly MRI), and bone scans.

ACUTE LOCALIZED OTITIS EXTERNA

Acute localized OE is usually caused by an infected hair follicle in the cartilaginous ear canal (aural furunculosis), which, in adults, consists of the outer third of the canal.[2,3,12,16] More rarely, eczema, seborrhea, impetigo, warts, or herpetic eruptions can produce localized OE.[15]

The epidemiology and etiology are similar to those of acute diffuse OE, but in most cases the infecting organism is *S. aureus*.[2,3] The pathophysiology is similar to that of acute diffuse otitis media: Most cases are caused by direct trauma to the ear canal, although occasionally they are secondary to a blocked sebaceous gland.[3] The natural history of untreated acute OE is that of acute diffuse OE.

CLINICAL PRESENTATION

Itching and pain of the affected ear are the usual presenting symptoms. Physical findings are similar to those of diffuse otitis, except that a localized swelling or pustule (abscess) may be identified in the cartilaginous ear canal.[1] Local adenopathy is common. Often, the canal is swollen shut, impairing the differentiation of localized from diffuse OE. A discharge is not often present in localized otitis media until the abscess ruptures.[3]

DIFFERENTIAL DIAGNOSIS AND EMERGENCY DEPARTMENT EVALUATION

The differential diagnosis and evaluation of acute localized OE are the same as for acute diffuse OE.

EMERGENCY DEPARTMENT MANAGEMENT

Management of a localized otitis follows the same guidelines as for diffuse otitis. The vast majority of cases respond to good aural hygiene as described previously, topical otic solutions, and analgesia. If a discrete, painful lesion is identified, incision and drainage may be necessary, especially if pain is significant. If localized cellulitis is present, an oral systemic antibiotic active against *S. aureus* (dicloxacillin or a cephalosporin) should be instituted for 10 days.

DISPOSITION

Symptoms of acute localized OE should resolve within a few days after initiation of treatment, especially with continued good hygiene. Cases that worsen or fail to respond should be referred to an otolaryngologist; worsening cases should receive immediate evaluation. Patients who have undergone incision and drainage and those receiving antibiotics for associated cellulitis should receive a mandatory follow-up in 12 to 24 hours.

COMMON PITFALLS

- Confusing OE with otitis media
- Misdiagnosis of a ruptured TM with purulent drainage as OE
- Underdiagnosing OE when symptoms of toxicity or malignant OE are present

References

1. Alberti PWRM. Epithelial migration on the TM. *J Laryngol Otol* 1964;78:808.
2. Arnold JE. The ear. In: Nelson WE, ed. *Nelson's textbook of pediatrics,* 15th ed. Philadelphia: WB Saunders, 1996:1804–1826.
3. Austin DF. Diseases of the external ear. In: Ballenger JJ, Snow JB, eds. *Diseases of the nose, throat, ear, head and neck,* 15th ed. Baltimore: Williams & Wilkins, 1996:974–988.
4. Babiatzki A, Sade J. Malignant external otitis. *J Laryngol Otol* 1987;101:205.
5. Bell DN. Otitis externa. *Postgrad Med* 1985;78:101.
6. Cohen D, Friedman P. The diagnostic criteria of malignant external otitis. *J Laryngol Otol* 1987;101:216.
7. Cohen D, Friedman P, Eilmon A. Malignant external otitis versus acute external otitis. *J Laryngol Otol* 1987;101:211.
8. Fairbanks D. Otic topical agents. *Otolaryngol Head Neck Surg* 1980;88:327.
9. Giamarellou H. Malignant OE. The therapeutic evolution of a lethal infection. *J Antimicrob Chemother* 1992;30:745.
10. Havelaar AH, Bosman M, Borst J. OE by *Pseudomonas aeruginosa* associated with whirlpools. *J Hyg (Lond)* 1983;90:489.
11. Hirsch BE. Infections of the external ear. *Am J Otolaryngol* 1992;13:145.
12. Klein JO. Otitis Externa, otitis media, mastoiditis. In: Mandell GL, Bennett JE, Dolin R, eds. *Principles and practice of infectious diseases,* 4th ed. New York: Churchill Livingstone, 1995:579–585.
13. Kraus DH, Rehm SJ, Kinney SE. The evolving treatment of necrotizing external otitis. *Laryngoscope* 1988;98:934.
14. Main T, Lim D. The human external auditory canal secretory system—an ultrastructural study. *Laryngoscope* 1976;86:1164.
15. March SM. Infections of the external ear. *Pediatr Infect Dis* 1985;4:192.
16. Marcy SM. External otitis due to infection. *Pediatr Infect Dis* 1985;4(Suppl 3):S27.
17. Rubin J, Yu VL. Malignant external otitis: insights into pathogenesis, clinical manifestations, diagnosis, and therapy. *Am J Med* 1988;85:391.
18. Salit IE, McNeely DJ, Chait G. Invasive external otitis: review of 12 cases. *Can Med Assoc J* 1985;132:381.
19. Schuller DE, Schleuning AJ. Infection and inflammation of the ear. In: Schullers DE, Schleuning AJ, eds. *DeWeese and Saunders' textbook of otolaryngology,* 8th ed. St. Louis: Mosby, 1994:403–433.
20. Seyfried PL, Cook RJ. OE infections related to *Pseudomonas aeruginosa* levels in five Ontario lakes. *Can J Public Health* 1984;75:83.
21. Slack R. A study of three preparations in the treatment of OE. *J Laryngol Otol* 1987;101:533.
22. Springer GL. Freshwater swimming as a risk factor for OE: a case-control study. *Arch Environ Health* 1985;40:202.
23. Stone M, Fulghum RS. Bactericidal activity of wet cerumen. *Ann Otol Rhinol Laryngol* 1984;93:183.
24. Turbiak TW, Reich JJ. Ear emergencies. In: Stair TO, ed. *Practical management of eye, ear, nose, mouth, and throat emergencies.* Rockville, MD: Aspen Systems, 1986:35.
25. Uri N, Kites R, Meyer W, et al. Necrotizing eternal otitis. *J Laryngol Otol* 1984;98:1083.
26. Wadsten C, Bertilsson CA, Sieradzki H, et al. A randomized clinical trial of two topical preparations in the treatment of external otitis. *Arch Otorhinolaryngol* 1985;242:135.

CHAPTER 30
Nontraumatic Upper Airway Obstruction

Joseph E. Clinton

The physician who faces an awake patient who is experiencing rapidly progressive airway obstruction knows the meaning of apprehension. Evaluation, differential diagnosis, and emergency intervention all must occur simultaneously. The window of time for effective intervention before irreversible injury occurs is so small that little margin for error exists. Progressive airway compromise exemplifies the need for anticipation, preparation, and practice to deal with the responsibility of emergency airway management.

Effective emergency management requires early recognition of a high-risk clinical situation and anticipation of further deterioration in the airway status. This approach allows intervention to occur at the proper time, before the situation becomes desperate. The necessary therapy is likely to be less traumatic to the patient if practiced early in a controlled manner. Preparation of equipment, drills of the emergency team, and practice of technique all contribute to lessen the margin for error and improve patient outcome.

This chapter presents an overview of nontraumatic conditions that affect upper airway patency. The focus here is on the development of the airway obstruction, its recognition, and early management.

CLINICAL PRESENTATION

Nontraumatic airway obstruction is often insidious in onset. Once begun, the process may further deteriorate gradually or decompensate suddenly without warning. Neither the person eating a large piece of steak nor the adult with epiglottitis expects that he or she will soon be suffocating when the event is in its early stages. Obstruction occurs abruptly in the first case; hours may pass during the obstructive process in the second. The emergency physician must understand the disease processes at work and be prepared to intervene quickly when necessary.

Several factors may affect the type of presentation manifest by a given patient. The site of the obstruction, the size of the obstructing agent, and associated spasm and edema are important determinants of the presentation.[16] Historical factors may simplify the diagnosis. Physical findings may be nonspecific, or simply serve to separate patients into a category of obstruction.

Spectrum of Respiratory Distress

Airway obstruction proceeds from no clinical findings to obvious distress with a patient in an agonal state. The pattern of increasing obstruction is first manifest by some subjective findings of respiratory distress by the patient. The initial subjective finding may appear as "wheezing" with both an inspiratory and an expiratory component. Further obstruction alters the finding to stridor. Next, the airway obstructs completely and the patient struggles, loses consciousness, and will die without effective intervention to restore airway patency.

Apprehension, agitation, and struggling develop as obstruction increases. The fear in the eyes of a conscious patient experiencing airway obstruction is apparent. The patient's discomfort is transmitted to all who are present at the time. A nonproductive atmosphere of near hysteria can develop in the absence of an organized approach to relieve the obstruction. One of the benefits of public education on the choking victim has been to provide instruction that channels energies from useless activity into airway-clearing maneuvers. Deaths from choking numbered 3300 in the United States in 1997. Sixty-eight percent of those deaths occurred in individuals over age 65, and 54% in those over age 75. A smaller incidence peak occurs in the newborn to age 4 group.[12]

Although airway obstruction by a foreign body, such as food, occurs suddenly, obstruction by an expanding mass effect within the upper airway is more insidious. Abscesses may obstruct the airway by their location. Expanding hematomas behave similarly. Edema and soft-tissue swelling owing to infection or allergy behave slightly differently because of a more diffuse mass effect.

Signs to anticipate in the patient suspected of developing airway obstruction vary slightly, depending on the cause, but some generalization can be made. The habitus of the patient is important to note. An upright posture with the neck extended in the sniffing position is characteristic in the patient with supraglottic obstruction, such as epiglottitis. Forcing a supine position in such a patient for the convenience of the medical team is disastrous. Pursing of the lips is commonly noted in patients who are struggling for air. An asymmetrical mass may increase in size during the observation period.

DIFFERENTIAL DIAGNOSIS

The differential diagnosis of upper airway obstruction includes several causes for the obstruction. Foreign-body obstruction, infection, hypersensitivity, hemorrhagic disorders, extrinsic mass, and neoplasia all may result in the syndrome of upper airway obstruction. The patient's presentation may quickly narrow the diagnosis, or the diagnosis may remain a mystery until late in the patient's course.

Foreign-Body Obstruction

The classic example of upper airway obstruction by a foreign body is the "cafe coronary." Food that causes an obstruction has often been poorly masticated. The victim may have painful or poorly fitting dentures or otherwise poor dentition that hampers chewing. Alcohol consumption is often implicated in the condition. This type of obstruction usually occurs in the supraglottic area and responds to the airway maneuvers prescribed by the American Heart Association.[3]

Aspirated toys or smaller pieces of food may pass the vocal cords and produce obstruction in the subglottic area. These obstructions may be intermittent and aggravated by the head-down position, which allows gravitational movement of the object to an obstructive position. Back blows and the head-down position may actually worsen these obstructions.[12,16] The clinical presentation of a subglottic foreign body may be one of localized wheezing and atelectasis of obstructed pulmonary segments as the foreign body becomes lodged in a bronchus.

Any object that can fit in the mouth may produce airway obstruction given proper circumstances. The broad range of possibilities is best approached by attempts to differentiate supraglottic and subglottic obstructions. The site of the obstruction affects management decisions. A supraglottic obstruction that is not removable may be bypassed by tracheal intubation or surgical airway placement. A subglottic obstruction may require a more difficult airway decision, depending on its location. Magill forceps may allow removal of foreign bodies under direct vision.[20] A recently described aspiration technique using a blunted endotracheal tube, wall suction, and a meconium aspirator or "Y" connector to the tube can greatly facilitate removal of subglottic foreign bodies such as balloons and steak.[15]

Infection

Cellulitis of oropharyngeal structures produces a treacherous setting in which airway compromise develops with little notice in a patient who has dysphonia and limited communication capacity. Ludwig's angina (cellulitis of the sublingual space) can quickly obstruct the airway. The condition is a true otolaryngologic emergency that requires airway maintenance and antibiotic therapy. Retropharyngeal or laryngeal abscess can cause gradual obstruction owing to expansion and catastrophic deterioration through sudden rupture into the airway.[8,14] The natural history of these conditions needs to be kept clearly in mind when evaluating the emergency patient.

Hypersensitivity

Anaphylaxis can present suddenly after exposure to a known or unrecognized antigenic stimulus. When its representation is in the form of laryngeal edema, prompt intervention is needed to interrupt the obstructing process. A delay in the initiation of medical therapy may force surgical intervention in order to save the patient's life. Food, drug, and insect sting allergies are commonly encountered causes of anaphylactic airway emergencies. A history of exposure may depend on the patient's ability to communicate, which is directly related to the degree of airway compromise that is present.

Hereditary angioneurotic edema (HANE) is an autosomal dominant condition that is manifested by sudden edema of the face, hands, abdominal viscera, and airway.[11] Episodes may be triggered by minor trauma, emotional distress, and surgery. No race or sex predilection exists, and family history may be negative. HANE is most commonly characterized by a complement deficiency of C_1 esterase inhibitor (C_1 INH). The postulation is that the excess of a C_2 kinin develops because of the inhibitor deficiency, and the C_2 kinin is responsible for the increased capillary permeability seen in HANE.[8] Management of the condition is discussed in a later section.

Angiotensin converting enzyme (ACE) inhibitor agents for control of hypertension have become a new cause of angioedema in patients previously free of the condition.[9,13] Moderate-to-complete airway obstruction may occur. The drugs must be discontinued in patients experiencing this adverse reaction to prevent recurrence.

Hemorrhagic Disorders

The widespread use of anticoagulants for the treatment of cardiac and cerebrovascular disease has increased the population at risk for spontaneous hematoma formation. Spontaneous hematomas may develop throughout the body without any special predilection to one area. When the pharynx, the airway, or soft tissues surrounding these structures are involved, airway compromise is a predictable consequence.

Warfarin-predisposed patients have been reported with airway compromise owing to hematoma of the sublingual space, retropharynx, and hypopharynx.[1] The syndrome is marked by rapid, unexpected deterioration of a person who, in most cases, was previously healthy. Pain is often noted early, frequently preceding other symptoms. Signs of airway obstruction may develop before the examiner's eyes. Physical examination often reveals an area of swelling, frequently without ecchymosis. Soft-tissue radiography of the neck, computerized tomography, and indirect laryngoscopy are often useful. Close observation during the evaluation period is essential to avoid unrecognized abrupt deterioration with adverse outcome.

Extrinsic Mass

Unusual causes of airway obstruction owing to an extrinsic mass are occasionally seen. An example is the development of an obstruction in the esophagus caused by achalasia.[18] The distended esophagus impinges on the airway in the neck and produces recurrent airway obstruction that disappears when the esophageal obstruction is cleared. Cystic lesions of various types may produce a similar syndrome that may require temporary airway support until the lesion is removed.[6]

Neoplasia

Direct or indirect airway obstruction may result from neoplastic disorders. Laryngeal carcinoma and intrinsic airway tumors produce a gradually developing obstruction that may be mistaken for bronchospastic disease. Bypass of the laryngeal lesion by intubation or cricothyrotomy reveals an abrupt decrease in airway resistance. The abrupt resistance change localizes the disease to a site above the distal end of the tracheal tube. Tumor masses extrinsic to the airway may impinge on its lumen in a manner similar to that described for cystic lesions.[7] Bronchogenic carcinoma or lymphomas may produce a superior vena caval syndrome leading to airway obstruction.[9]

Congenital tumors of the oropharynx or neck may present immediate and unexpected airway emergencies at birth. Such a condition requires immediate availability of neonatal resuscitation capabilities and surgical readiness.[17]

Kaposi's sarcoma of the trachea has presented with airway obstruction. Death followed hemorrhage of the tumor when it was incised in an attempt to provide surgical airway support during obstruction.

EMERGENCY DEPARTMENT EVALUATION

Regardless of the cause of the obstruction, the emergency physician must first gauge its severity by quickly placing the patient in one of four categories: (1) stable, deterioration risk low; (2) stable, deterioration risk high; (3) compromised respiration; or (4) agonal state. Once this immediate classification has been made, the evaluation and therapy process can proceed with the appropriate degree of fervor.

A patient in the first category has been determined to be stable and at low risk of deterioration. This categorization is the most hazardous for the emergency physician to make. It implies that the patient can be evaluated at a leisurely pace with a minimal degree of observation. Such a patient will prove the physician wrong most often because the opportunity exists to do so. Airway-obstructing lesions notoriously deteriorate unexpectedly in patients who looked well minutes before the decompensation. Classification of a patient in the first category implies a certainty of diagnosis that is usually absent during initial evaluation. Although the patient may be placed in this category after an observation and data-collection period, it is seldom appropriate to place a patient with suspected airway compromise in this category early in the evaluation period.

The second category reflects the appropriate degree of concern during initial evaluation of any patient in whom airway obstruction is suspected. The risk of deterioration calls for constant observation, with equipment in readiness to intervene if necessary. Measures intended to arrest the underlying obstructive process should be instituted as soon as possible.

The third category, with established airway compromise, calls for immediate decision on airway implementation. The emergency physician must quickly assess the likelihood of success with a medical approach before airway establishment by intubation or surgical approach is required. The judgment must be made using clinical experience. An arterial blood gas analysis may help with the decision when it can be obtained immediately, but often such testing only delays needed therapy.

The last category, with the patient in an agonal state, represents the most straightforward, immediate evaluation and therapy situation. The airway must be established immediately. No other consideration takes precedence.

EMERGENCY DEPARTMENT MANAGEMENT

Airway management is the second part of the evaluation and therapeutic tightrope that must be walked when dealing with upper airway obstruction. The differential diagnosis coupled with the severity assessment will guide the therapeutic approach.

Modifying Factors

The patient who has been classified as stable and at high risk of deterioration is a candidate for attempts to improve status without physical airway intervention. Medical interventions are most effective when directed at a specific cause, but a few nonspecific interventions may be of benefit early. Oxygen supplementation should be initiated in all cases. Consideration needs to be given to nebulization therapy with racemic epinephrine or beta-2 agents and steroids to decrease edema in hypersensitivity or croup syndromes. If infection is a possibility, then appropriate antibiotic therapy should be considered. Bleeding disorders need supplementation of coagulation factors to arrest the process.

A mixture of 80% helium and 20% oxygen has been suggested as a temporizing measure in patients with airway obstruction caused by tumors.[10] The density of the mixture is one-third that of air. The increased flow of gas allowed by the decreased density may improve oxygenation in selected patients with narrowed upper airways. Application of the gas mixture in other types of airway obstruction has been limited. Concern over use of the technique in patients with progressive obstructive disease centers around the possibility that the mixture will delay definitive management of the condition. Temporary cessation of the helium mixture might abruptly lead to complete obstruction while breathing room air in this scenario.

Treatment Directed at Cause

The likelihood that foreign-body obstruction exists should prompt airway-clearing maneuvers to be implemented according to widely accepted protocols described by the American Heart Association.[3] Failure to clear the airway should lead to more aggressive airway-establishment maneuvers.

Mortality in children with epiglottitis seems to be reduced when a controlled, aggressive approach to airway intervention occurs. Those who undergo controlled airway establishment seem to have a lower mortality than those whose management is characterized by close observation with airway intervention as needed.[5] Similar statistics are not available in the adult patient, but experience has shown that they, too, may deteriorate unexpectedly and need to be monitored constantly until the infection recedes. Preparation for surgical airway placement must be constant.

The patient with a hemorrhagic disorder with associated warfarin therapy requires some medical therapy to reverse the coagulopathy. Vitamin K enhances clotting factor synthesis in the liver. Levels of dependent factors II, VII, IX, and X begin to increase 2 hours after vitamin K administration, with significant elevation in 6 to 8 hours, and are frequently normal in 24 hours.[17] The most rapid correction of the clotting abnormality is by administration of fresh-frozen plasma or prothrombin complex concentrates. Airway obstruction is an indication for rapid reversal, which means fresh-frozen plasma administration in most cases. Fewer side effects are seen with plasma than with the concentrates.[17] Plasma is, therefore, the preferred emergency management.

Airway-Opening Maneuvers

Airway-opening maneuvers such as chin lift, head tilt, and oral and nasal airways are most useful in patients with a decreased level of consciousness.[3] The situation is quite different if the comatose state is a result of hypoxia owing to airway obstruction. Patients who are suffering from an airway obstructive process need more than these devices provide. Specific medical therapy and more aggressive airway intervention therapy are usually indicated.

Nonsurgical Management

A patient with significant airway compromise who does not improve with medical intervention will often require tracheal intubation. Blind nasotracheal or orotracheal intubation will suffice in many cases in which the decision is made before the airway is completely obstructed. Rapid-sequence orotracheal intubation will facilitate intubation.[19] Whether it will facilitate removal of the airway obstruction depends on its etiology and location. The physician must weigh the risks of paralysis against its potential benefit in each case. Inability to remove an obstructive agent or to secure the airway with tracheal intubation is an indication to pursue surgical approaches to the airway.[2]

Surgical Management

Transtracheal needle ventilation using a high-pressure oxygen source to supply intermittent ventilation provides adequate ventilation in cases in which exhalation can still occur through the upper airway. The presence of a ball-valve mechanism of the obstruction will allow exhalation to occur. The technique is a temporizing measure that allows time to secure the airway by other, more definitive means.

Cricothyrotomy is the emergency surgical airway of choice for most airway-obstructing lesions.[14] If the offending lesion is subglottic, such as a laryngeal abscess, hematoma, or tumor, then tracheostomy is preferred over cricothyrotomy.

Providing details of the procedural approach to airway management is beyond the scope of this chapter. A more lengthy discussion of the procedures and the logic behind their use can be found elsewhere.[3,8]

DISPOSITION

Role of the Consultant

The development of protocols for treatment of the wide variety of obstructive conditions needs to be begun by the emergency physician. A cooperative team effort needs to be organized by personnel from the emergency, anesthesia, otolaryngology, pediatric, and medicine departments who will be dealing with the patients, depending on the cause. Treatment of pediatric epiglottitis is an excellent example of the type of cooperative efforts that can optimize results. Communication and agreement on management should occur in advance for common, recurrent clinical problems, such as epiglottitis. The cooperative approach developed with these cases will carry over to optimize management of the more unusual causes of airway obstruction.

Indications for Admission

The patient with airway obstruction needs to be under constant observation in an intensive care unit until the risk of airway obstruction has passed. A good example of an attempt to separate high-risk from low-risk croup patients has been developed by Davis. A scoring system to assist with decision making in children with croup is based on clinical findings. A score of 0 to 15 is given based on the presence of stridor, retraction, air entry, skin color, and mental status. The patient is given a score of 0 to 3 for each of the five findings. The total score is then determined. Patients with a score of less than 5 may be treated at home with mist therapy. Those with a score higher than 5 should be admitted for at least a trial of racemic epinephrine, and possibly steroids, and close monitoring for deterioration that necessitates intubation. Similar scoring mechanisms might apply to other reversible causes of airway obstruction. Whenever doubt exists as to the immediate future course of a patient with airway obstruction, intensive care unit admission is mandatory.

COMMON PITFALLS

- The emergency physician should be aware of untoward events that might occur after relief of the obstruction. These include local trauma, infection, and other hazards of airway intubation. A prominent concern when dealing with airway obstruction is the sudden pulmonary edema after the obstruction has been relieved; the mechanism development is unclear but is presumably related to the sudden decrease in hydrostatic pressure. Treatment is supportive and may include diuresis.[4]
- The most common mistake when dealing with airway obstructive disease is to underestimate the potential for deterioration. A complacent attitude fosters poor preparation, surprise deterioration, mismanagement, and tragic outcome. Upper airway obstruction is an emergency condition that requires maximal preparation.
- The second most common mistake is to relax monitoring to the point where deterioration goes unnoticed. All the time invested in preparation, drills, and skill maintenance is wasted if the disease process is not treated with the respect it deserves.

References

1. Boster SR, Bergin JJ. Upper airway obstruction complicating warfarin therapy with a note on reversal of warfarin toxicity. *Ann Emerg Med* 1983;12:711.
2. Clinton JE, McGill JW. Basic airway management and decision-making. In: Roberts JR, Hedges JR, eds. *Clinical procedures in emergency medicine,* 3rd ed. Philadelphia: WB Saunders, 1998:115.
3. Emergency Cardiac Care Committee and Subcommittees A. Guidelines for cardiopulmonary resuscitation and emergency cardiac care. *JAMA* 1992;268:2171–2299.
4. Galvis AG. Pulmonary edema complicating relief of upper airway obstruction. *Am J Emerg Med* 1987;5:294.
5. Glover DM, Wilson CB. Pediatric infections. *Emerg Med Clin North Am* 1985;3:25.
6. Henderson LT, Dennehy JCI, Teichgraeber J. Airway obstructing epiglottic cyst. *Ann Otol Rhinol Laryngol* 1985;94:473.
7. Holinger LD, Birholz JC. Management of infants with prenatal ultrasound diagnosis of airway obstruction by teratoma. *Ann Otol Rhinol Laryngol* 1987;96:61.
8. Jackson C. The larynx in typhoid fever. *J Med Sci* 1905;130:845.
9. Kalia S, Tintinalli JE. Emergency evaluation of the cancer patient. *Ann Emerg Med* 1984;13:723.

10. McGee DL. Helium-oxygen therapy in the emergency department. *J Emerg Med* 1997;15:291–296.
11. Moore GP, Hurley WT, Pace SA. Hereditary angioedema. *Ann Emerg Med* 1988;17:1082–1086.
12. National Safety Council. *Accident facts, 1998 edition.* Itasca, IL: National Safety Council, 1998:9.
13. Pigman EC, Scott JL. Angioedema in the emergency department: the impact of angiotensin-converting enzyme inhibitors. *Am J Emerg Med* 1993;11:350–354.
14. Ramsey PG, Weymuller EA. Complications of bacterial infection of the ears, paranasal sinuses, and oropharynx in adults. *Emerg Med Clin North Am* 1985;3:143.
15. Ruiz E, Stolzenberg BT, Bowker DB, et al. Total obstruction of the trachea by foreign bodies: a practical solution to a rapidly fatal problem. *J Emerg Med* 1998;16[Suppl 2]:81S(abst).
16. Salcedo L. The difficult pediatric airway, foreign body aspiration. *Anesth Clin North Am* 1998;16:885–892.
17. Tepas JJ, Deen HG, McArtor R. Giant cystic choristoma of the head and neck in a neonate: successful management of a life-threatening respiratory emergency. *J Pediatr Surg* 1982;17:184.
18. Turkot S, Golzman B, Kogan J, et al. Acute upper-airway obstruction in a patient with achalasia. *Ann Emerg Med* 1997;29:687–689.
19. Walls RM. Rapid-sequence intubation in head trauma. *Ann Emerg Med* 1993;22:1008–1013.
20. Westfal R. Foreign body airway obstruction: when the Heimlich maneuver fails [Letter]. *Am J Emerg Med* 1997;1:103.

CHAPTER 31

The Neck Mass in Adults and Children

Ted A. McMurry

The neck mass is a complaint or finding that may accompany many disorders. It may be congenital or acquired, infectious or neoplastic, benign or malignant.[4] In children, most neck masses are relatively common and minor, whereas the incidence of neoplastic lesions is high in adults. In neither group does the neck mass commonly present as an acutely emergent or life-threatening problem.

CLINICAL PRESENTATION

An accurate history and careful physical examination are critical in the evaluation of the neck mass. The primary goal is to determine the most likely site and cause. The history should address the seven cardinal symptoms of head and neck disease: dysphagia, odynophagia, referred pain with swallowing, hoarseness, stridor, speech disorder, and globus phenomenon.[15] Dysphagia and odynophagia need not be present concomitantly but may allow the patient to localize the lesion to the upper aerodigestive tract. Referred pain is typically to the ear and has the same significance as odynophagia. A major concern suggested by neck pain is the presence of an infection or disease process extending to the deep spaces of the neck. Masses or space-occupying lesions can present as problems with speech or as airway obstruction, the latter the most likely emergency the physician may encounter with the neck mass. The globus phenomenon is the sensation of a lump in the throat that is present between meals and may be described as excessive postnasal drip, "worms" in the throat, trouble swallowing saliva, or excessive mucus. The globus phenomenon is not associated with difficulty swallowing food.[15]

Other important historical features include the use of tobacco in any form, the excessive use of alcohol,[1] previous radiation exposure of the neck, current or recent illnesses, current or recent injuries, infection of the head and neck, travel history, animal exposure, and other associated local or systemic symptoms. Specific questions about the mass include duration, changes or fluctuations in size, associated pain or inflammation, and sites of any drainage.

A good physical examination is critical and includes a thorough evaluation of the scalp, face, skin, nose, ears, oral cavity, dental structures, pharynx, nasopharynx, and the mass itself. Also included in this examination are indirect visualization of the nasopharynx and larynx with a mirror and headlight, and digital palpation of the nasopharynx and base of the tongue. The neck mass is examined and palpated for size, shape, consistency, mobility, and tenderness. When attempting to determine whether a neck mass may be a lymph node, it is important to recognize the location of the normal chain of cervical lymph nodes (Fig. 31.1). Figure 31.2 shows the anterior and posterior cervical triangles in the neck formed by the sternocleidomastoid muscle medially and the midline of the neck anteriorly and posteriorly. The importance of these triangles and normal lymph node distribution will become apparent as one reviews the differential diagnosis of the neck mass.

DIFFERENTIAL DIAGNOSIS

The differential diagnosis of a neck mass is extensive and depends on the patient's age. The "80% rule" states that 80% of isolated neck masses in children are benign[15]; in adults, 80% of nonthyroid neck masses are neoplastic and 80% of neoplastic masses are malignant. Furthermore, 80% of these malignant masses are metastatic and 80% of the primary tumors are located above the clavicle.[4,12]

Infectious Neck Mass

The most common cause of a benign neck mass in children is cervical adenopathy secondary to an upper respiratory tract infection, usually of viral origin. Acute cervical lymphadenitis is most often caused by bacteria, with beta-hemolytic streptococci and *Staphylococcus aureus* the most common isolated organisms. Anaerobic bacterial infection should be considered if a dental infection is present. The child with acute cervical lymphadenitis is often febrile and tends to appear toxic. The inflamed cervical mass is warm, erythematous, and tender.[5] Cat-scratch disease is generally a self-limiting, benign, ipsilateral, lateral adenopathy[5] that typically follows a scratch from a cat or, rarely, a dog or monkey bite. The etiologic organisms are *Bartonella quintana* and *Bartonella henselae,* fastidious gram-negative bacteria.[11] Although the adenopathy typically resolves in about 3 months,[17,20] the clinical course may be shortened with antibiotic therapy (e.g., azithromycin for 5 days), and incision and drainage of the nodes is discouraged.

The most common viral cause of acute cervical lymphadenitis is mononucleosis. It is typically associated with fever, anorexia, malaise, pharyngitis, or an exudative tonsillitis. However, the very young child may demonstrate only cervical adenopathy and a mild upper respiratory tract infection.[10,20]

Other potential but uncommon sources of infectious neck masses include *Haemophilus influenzae,* anaerobic bacteria, psittacosis, histiocytosis, toxoplasmosis, tuberculous adenitis (scrofula), actinomycosis, brucellosis, typhoid, and syphilis. Deep neck infection is a serious but uncommon problem that may

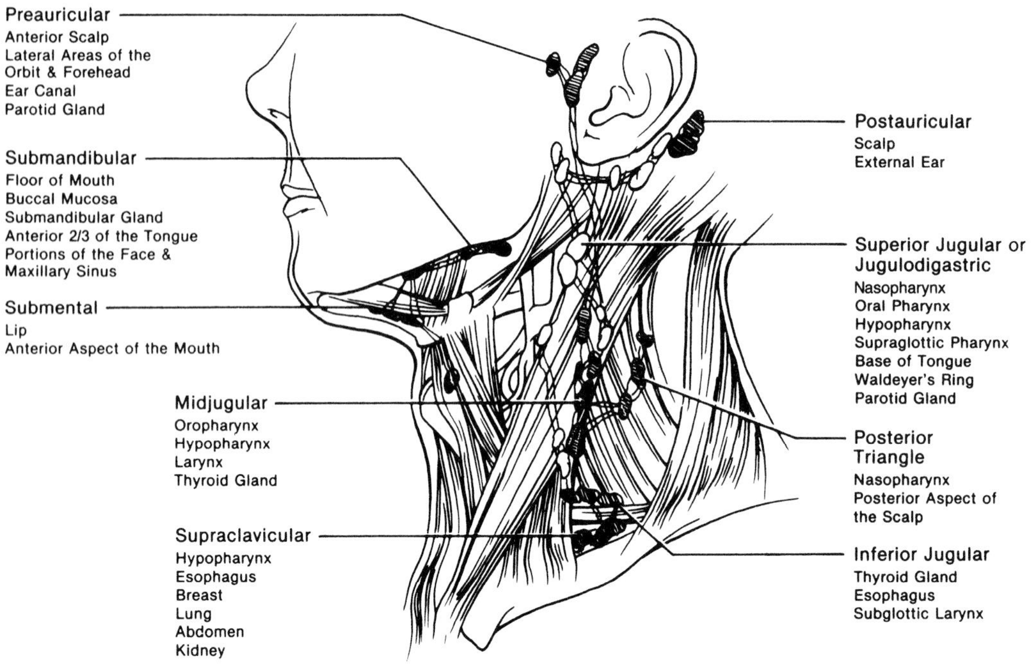

Figure 31.1. Major cervical nodes and drainage patterns.

lead to life-threatening complications such as airway obstruction, septicemia, erosion into the carotid artery, and extension into the mediastinum. Ninety percent of deep neck space abscesses occur in either the retropharyngeal, the lateral pharyngeal, or the submandibular space.[4,13] *S. aureus* and hemolytic streptococci are the pathogens most frequently found in children. Anaerobic streptococci and *Bacteroides* may occur in adults, especially when dental infection is the primary underlying problem.[19]

With increasing numbers of geriatric patients, especially those from nursing homes and those who are victims of self-neglect, infections of the salivary glands and submandibular space are seen. These infections are associated with poor oral hygiene, dental disease, dehydration, and general debilitation. Parotid gland infection, cellulitis, and abscess of the floor of the mouth or submandibular space (Ludwig's angina) are common examples (Fig. 31.3).

As AIDS becomes more prevalent, it will probably assume greater importance in the differential diagnosis of the neck mass in both children and adults.

Congenital Neck Mass

About 6% of neck masses are congenital.[3] The most common of these are thyroglossal duct cysts, dermoid cysts, branchial cleft

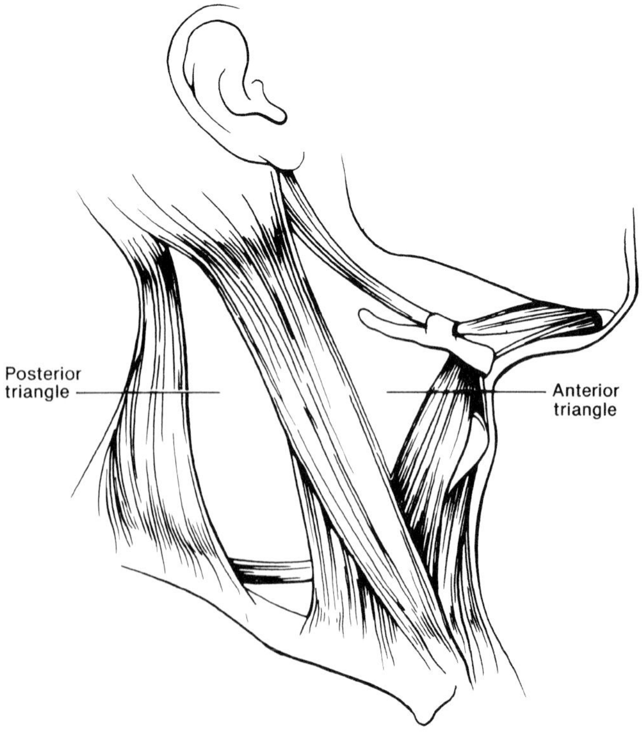

Figure 31.2. Anterior and posterior triangles of the neck.

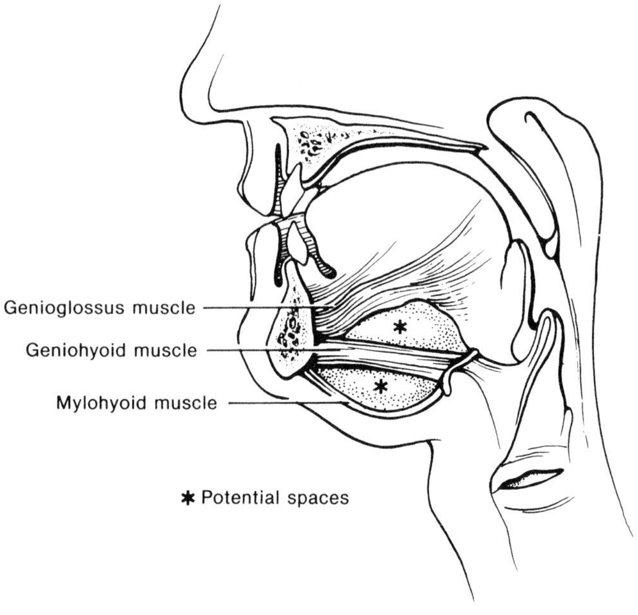

Figure 31.3. Ludwig's angina.

cysts, and cystic hygromas (lymphangiomas). The first two present as midline neck masses; the latter two, typically as lateral neck masses.

Thyroglossal duct cyst is the most common benign congenital neck mass (Fig. 31.4).[6] The thyroglossal duct is a microscopic thread of undifferentiated epithelial cells, a remnant of the embryogenic development of what becomes the pyramidal lobe of the thyroid gland. It descends from a position at the base of the tongue, through the hyoid bone to the inferior portion of the neck, where it fuses with the lateral aspects of the thyroid gland.[16,18] For unknown reasons, the remnant of undifferentiated cells may become activated and differentiate into one of the epithelial cell forms or into glandular tissue (including thyroid tissue). It can be located anywhere from the base of the tongue to the thyroid gland, but it is commonly adjacent and inferior to the hyoid bone.[9] The cyst tends to be fluctuant, smooth, rounded, well defined, and nontender. Although the size is usually 1 to 2 cm, it may fluctuate in size. It can also become infected. There is no significant sex prevalence, and although it may present at any age, the vast majority occur between 1 and 9 years of age, with a peak incidence between 3 and 5 years. The mass is typically discovered by a parent, who reports its intermittent presence. The mass becomes more visible with hyperextension of the neck. One study of midline cervical masses found that movement of the mass with swallowing or tongue protrusion was common but not pathognomonic of a thyroglossal duct cyst. However, an infrahyoid position and a history of inflammation and fluctuating size were helpful in differentiating between a thyroglossal duct cyst, an epidermoid cyst, and a midline enlarged lymph node.[9] Serious complications or emergencies associated with thyroglossal cysts are rare, even though up to 30% develop an associated sinus that drains and serves as the route of recurrent infection.[16] Surgical excision of the cyst and tract is necessary to prevent recurrent infection.

An epidermoid cyst is the most common of the dermoid cysts that occur in the head and neck.[4] An estimated 27% of midline cervical masses are dermoid or epidermoid cysts.[4,9] Typically, an epidermoid cyst is a nontender midline cervical mass that moves with the overlying skin and tends not to fluctuate in size or become inflamed. The submental and infrahyoid areas are the most common locations. Dermoid cysts are more common in children under 5 years of age, but may be acquired at any age as a result of a prior puncture wound. Again, serious complications or emergencies associated with dermoid cysts are rare, and the treatment is surgical excision.

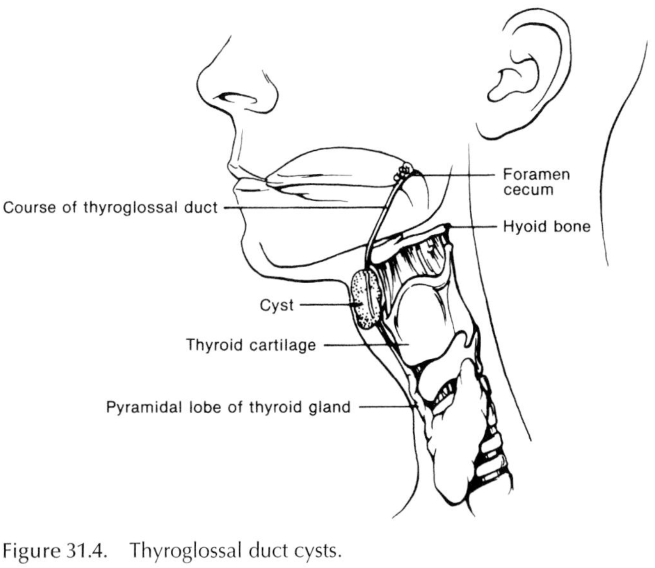

Figure 31.4. Thyroglossal duct cysts.

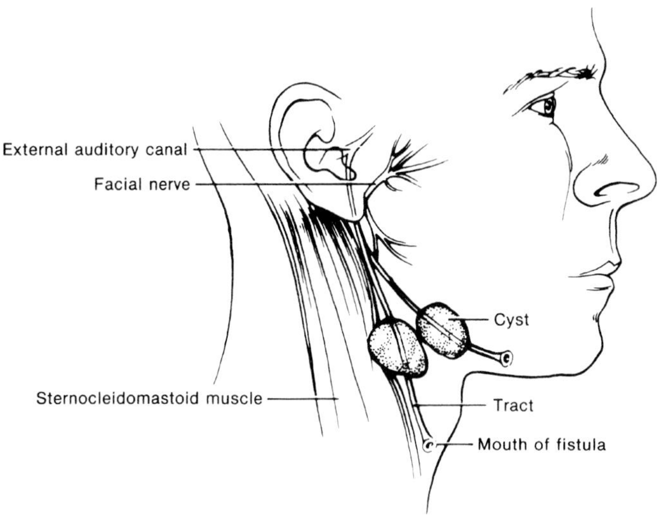

Figure 31.5. Branchial cleft cyst.

Branchial anomalies may present as cysts, sinuses, or fistulas. The second branchial cleft is responsible for most anomalies, of which cysts are the most common (Fig. 31.5). The cysts are usually lined with squamous epithelium, less commonly with a columnar epithelium. They lie anterior to and in the middle third of the sternocleidomastoid muscle. There is no sex prevalence. They occur with equal frequency on either side of the neck. The cyst may develop at any age, although it may be more common in adults. When the cyst does develop in childhood, it occurs more often in the early school years.[15] The cyst typically is rounded, nontender, slightly mobile, and of variable firmness. It may gradually increase in size, and may appear to enlarge with upper respiratory tract infections. Infections of the cyst are uncommon.

Branchial sinuses are relatively uncommon. They may open internally or externally. Almost all that open externally on the side of the neck result from the second branchial cleft or groove.[16] Branchial sinuses are usually noted at birth, with the external sinus opening anterior to the lower third of the sternocleidomastoid muscle. The rare internal sinus opens into the tonsillar fossa. A fistula occurs when the tract has both an internal and an external opening. First branchial cleft anomalies with the external sinus opening in the external auditory canal require special precautions because of the proximity to the facial nerve and parotid gland. Acute, serious complications or emergencies arising from branchial cleft anomalies are uncommon. The treatment is elective surgical excision of the cyst, sinus, or fistula.

Cystic hygromas and lymphangiomas are congenital masses of lymphatic tissue thought to arise from lymphatic sacs. The cysts are thin-walled and lined with endothelial cells, and may be isolated or clustered. Eighty percent to 90% are located in the posterior triangle of the neck.[8,18] Sixty-five percent present at birth, 80% are noted in the first year of life, and 90% are found before the end of the second year. There is no sex prevalence, and the masses occur with equal frequency on either side of the neck.[4,7,18] The masses can be smooth, rounded or lobulated, soft, and compressible, and they can be transilluminated. An increase in size may occur with an upper respiratory tract infection. Although they tend to be asymptomatic, they may become large enough to cause difficulty with swallowing or breathing due to compression of the trachea. Emergencies are uncommon. The accepted treatment is surgical excision, although some surgeons prefer expectant observation in the asymptomatic mass in anticipation of a spontaneous regression.

Another congenital lateral neck mass is the hemangioma, a vascular anomaly present at birth that usually regresses spontaneously. The hemangioma is a bluish, nonpulsatile mass with a "bag of worms" texture located in the area of the parotid gland.[15] Airway compromise can occur if the mass reaches sufficient size to encroach on the upper airway.

Other uncommon congenital neck masses include thyroid cysts, parotid gland cysts, and thymus remnants.

Neoplasms in Children

Benign neoplasms in children that present as neck masses include hemangiomas, lymphangiomas, fibromas, neurofibromas, and lipomas. Only 20% of neck masses in children are malignant. Of these, more than 50% are lymphomas in the Hodgkin disease and histiocytic lymphoma (lymphosarcoma) groups.

Malignant neck neoplasms in children tend to be single, nontender, and fast-growing, and are located in the posterior triangle of the neck. Age is a key element in the occurrence of the various malignant neck neoplasms. From ages 1 to 5, neuroblastoma, rhabdomyosarcoma, histiocytic lymphoma, and Hodgkin disease are more common. In the older child, histiocytic lymphoma and Hodgkin disease occur equally often. The adolescent most commonly acquires Hodgkin disease. Even though histiocytic lymphomas occur twice as often as the Hodgkin lymphomas in children, they present with nearly equal frequency in the head and neck. Eighty percent of Hodgkin disease and only 40% of histiocytic lymphomas present with a neck mass.[14,20] Histiocytic lymphomas occur at any age, whereas Hodgkin disease is very uncommon before age 5, peaking between ages 5 and 9.[4,19] Rhabdomyosarcoma is the most common solid tumor of the head and neck in childhood and is one of the most common tumors in children under age 6. It is less common in non-Whites. Rhabdomyosarcoma presents with rapid growth in the orbit, nasopharynx, ear, mastoid, face, or tongue. The neuroblastoma is the most common solid tumor in children overall, but it presents as a neck mass only about 5% of the time.[19] Five percent of malignant neck neoplasms are thyroid cancer (medullary, papillary, mixed papillary, or follicular). There is a 2:1 female predominance. Roughly three-fourths of preadolescent children with a single thyroid nodule have a thyroid cancer.[14] About 25% of neurofibromas and neurofibrosarcomas present in the neck and head, but they represent only 5% of malignant head and neck neoplasms. Unlike in the adult, metastatic squamous cell cancer that presents as a neck mass occurs in less than 1% of the total neck masses in children.

Adult Neoplasms

Benign neck neoplasms in the adult are of the same origin as those found in children but are significantly less common. Only 20% of adult neck masses are benign. Neck neoplasms account for 5% of all cancers. It is estimated that up to 90% of malignant neck masses in patients over age 50 are metastatic.[5,15] Most often, squamous cell carcinoma from a primary site in the upper aerodigestive tract metastasizes to the lymph nodes of the upper, middle, and lower aspects of the neck. When a neoplasm below the clavicle metastasizes to the neck, it tends to involve the supraclavicular nodes. Figure 31.1 shows the lymph node groups and the anatomic areas from which metastasis occurs.

In nine out of ten cases, the primary site for a metastatic node can be found with a careful history and physical examination. Of those with an occult primary lesion, roughly three-fourths have a primary lesion in the head and neck; the remainder have a primary lesion below the clavicle. Lymph node spread is an ominous development, reducing the chance of control of most head and neck cancers by at least 50%.[2]

Benign and malignant thyroid disease should always be in the differential diagnosis. This includes simple goiter, primary thyroid cancer, and metastatic thyroid cancer. Difficulty swallowing and voice change are especially suggestive of thyroid cancer in the presence of a thyroid mass or enlargement. Papillary and follicular carcinomas are the more common forms of thyroid cancer in the adult. Graves disease and autoimmune thyroiditis should also be considered when there is an enlarged or painful thyroid with associated weight loss, tachycardia, and tremors.

Three-fourths of salivary gland tumors are in the parotid gland, and one-sixth of these parotid tumors are malignant.[4] A painful mass in the parotid gland that is adherent to the skin or deep tissues suggests a malignant neoplasm (see Fig. 18.3 in Chapter 18).

Carotid body tumors are typically small, nontender, horizontally mobile masses that overlie the bifurcation of the common carotid artery. Their size increases slowly over years, and they may produce symptoms secondary to their size. Although surgical excision is the recommended therapy for small tumors in healthy patients, significant morbidity and mortality are associated with their removal.

EMERGENCY DEPARTMENT MANAGEMENT

A thorough history and examination of the head and neck are essential. The nasopharynx, base of the tongue, and larynx are examined both by digital palpation and by indirect mirror visualization. Critical complications or emergencies associated with neck masses are very uncommon, but when they occur they are almost always caused by airway compromise from tracheal displacement and compression or from upper airway obstruction by a mass. Infectious complications such as sepsis, deep neck space infection, and extension into the mediastinum are other life-threatening problems. A rare complication is erosion into the carotid sheath and subsequent rupture of the carotid artery. Appropriate blood tests include a complete blood count, Monospot, and thyroid function studies. Radiographic studies may include posteroanterior and lateral views of the chest, a sinus series, and a lateral view of the neck. Needle aspiration of a neck mass in the emergency department is not recommended. A neck mass of presumed inflammatory or infectious origin, including infected congenital cysts, can be treated with observation and antistaphylococcal antibiotics for up to 2 weeks. However, prolonged or repetitive courses of antibiotics are to be avoided. Endoscopic examination, sialography, ultrasound, computed tomography scan, magnetic resonance imaging, angiography, an upper gastrointestinal series, barium enema, and biopsies are usually unnecessary in the emergency department, but may be completed by the consultant(s).

DISPOSITION

Role of the Consultant

Consultation in the emergency department with a surgeon skilled in head and neck surgery is required for any patient with signs or symptoms of airway compromise or if there is suspicion of a deep neck space infection. Any adult, especially one over age 40, with a history of tobacco or heavy alcohol use who presents with a neck mass of any size requires referral within a reasonably short time to a surgeon skilled in head and neck surgery. Children should be treated according to the most likely cause of the mass and referred to their primary physician within 2 weeks if the mass has not resolved or is changing shape. Children with a lymph node greater than 3 cm should be referred for evaluation regardless of their age. Children with an asymptomatic mass of presumed congenital origin should be referred for follow-up with their primary physician or a surgeon skilled in head and neck surgery.

Indications for Admission

The patient with a compromised airway or suspected deep neck space or mediastinal infection must be admitted. The toxic-appearing child or adult who cannot swallow or tolerate oral fluids adequately should also be admitted for intravenous antibiotic therapy and hydration.

Transfer Considerations

If the receiving hospital has no surgical backup, an emergent transfer to an appropriate hospital willing to accept the patient should be accomplished, because a tracheostomy or surgical exploration may be required in the presence of a compromised airway or deep neck space infection.

COMMON PITFALLS

- An incomplete or inadequate history and physical examination will result in the failure to find an apparent primary lesion in an adult. Do not focus on the neck mass or the lesion only. Ninety percent of the primary lesions can be determined from the history and physical examination.
- Failure to recognize the significant incidence of malignancy of neck masses in the adult results in delays in evaluation and definitive treatment.
- Failure to educate parents on the need for follow-up if their child has a suspicious cervical lymph node or mass also results in delays in definitive evaluation.

References

1. Andiman WA. The Epstein-Barr virus and EB virus infections in childhood. *Pediatrics* 1979;95:171.
2. Baker HW. Principles of management of cancers of the head and neck. In: McKenna RJ, Murphy GP, eds. *Fundamentals of surgical oncology,* 1st ed. New York: Macmillan, 1986.
3. Cramer LM, Chase RA. Plastic and reconstructive surgery. In: Schwartz SI, Lellehei RC, Shires GI, et al., eds. *Principles of surgery,* 2nd ed. New York: McGraw-Hill, 1974.
4. Damion J, Hybels RL. The neck mass. *Postgrad Med* 1987;6:75.
5. Everts EC, Echevarria J. Disease of the pharynx and deep neck infections. In: Paparella MM, Shumrick DA, eds. *Otolaryngology,* 2nd ed. Philadelphia: WB Saunders, 1980.
6. Gray SW, Skandalakis JE. *Embryology for surgeons.* Philadelphia: WB Saunders, 1972.
7. Haller JA Jr. Pediatric surgery. In: Schwartz SI, Lellehei RC, Shires GI, et al., eds. *Principles of surgery,* 6th ed. New York: McGraw-Hill, 1994.
8. Holt GR, Daily WW. Mass in the neck—a diagnostic challenge. *Mo Med* 1976;73:230.
9. Knight PJ, Hamoudi AB, Vassy LE. The diagnosis and treatment of midline neck masses in children. *Surgery* 1983;5:603.
10. Lake AM, Oski F. Peripheral lymphadenopathy in childhood. *Am J Dis Child* 1978;132:357.
11. La Scola B, Raoult D. Cultures of *Bartonella quintana* and *Bartonella henselae* from human samples: a 5-year experience. *J Clin Microbiol* 1999;37(6):1899.
12. Maisel RH. When your patient complains of a neck mass. *Geriatrics* 1980;35:409.
13. Maran AG. Neck masses. In: Maran AG, Stell PM, eds. *Clinical otolaryngology.* St. Louis: CV Mosby, 1979.
14. May M. Neck masses in children: diagnosis and treatment. *Ear Nose Throat J* 1978;57:136.
15. Moloy P. How to (and how not to) manage the patient with a lump in the neck. *Prim Care* 1982;9:269.
16. Moore KL. *The developing human—clinically oriented embryology.* Philadelphia: WB Saunders, 1973.
17. Ortiz JA, Hudkins C, Komblut A. Adenitis, adenopathy, and abscesses of the head and neck. *Emerg Med Clin North Am* 1987;5:359.
18. Pounds LA. Neck masses of congenital origin. *Pediatr Clin North Am* 1981;28:841.
19. Snow JB. Masses of the neck. *Introduction to otorhinolaryngology.* Chicago: Year Book, 1979.
20. Zitelli BJ. Neck masses in children: adenopathy and malignant disease. *Pediatr Clin North Am* 1981;28:813.

CHAPTER 32
Emergency Aspects of Head and Neck Neoplasms

Eileen M. Raynor

The stereotype of patients with head and neck neoplasms as 50- to 60-year-old men who smoke and drink to excess must not mislead the emergency physician. Neoplasms of the upper aerodigestive tract often occur in persons of all ages and both sexes who may neither smoke nor drink. Oral cancer is not uncommon in men and women who have used smokeless tobacco for more than 15 years. Major salivary gland tumors affect both sexes, are not related to smoking or drinking, and usually occur in people aged 40 to 60. The oral and pharyngeal mucosae are frequent sites of Kaposi's sarcoma in people with acquired immunodeficiency syndrome (AIDS).[6]

People who present to the emergency department with a neoplasm of the head and neck may be divided into two groups: (1) those whose tumors are symptomatic but who are unaware that they harbor a neoplasm and (2) those who know of their tumor. People in the first group are primarily diagnostic problems, whereas those in the second group are management problems.

UNDIAGNOSED NEOPLASMS

A neoplasm of the head or neck is normally symptomatic early in its course,[2] and symptoms are similar to or identical with symptoms of infection of the upper aerodigestive tract. Emergency physicians must not overlook neoplasm as a cause of these complaints:

1. A sore throat of more than 3 weeks' duration in a person over age 40 is cancer until proved otherwise.
2. Hoarseness or voice change that persists longer than 4 weeks in an adult over 40 is cancer until proved otherwise.
3. An otherwise unexplained unilateral serous effusion of the middle ear in an adult over 40 suggests cancer of the nasopharynx.
4. A nonhealing ulcer involving the mucous membrane of the upper aerodigestive tract for more than 2 weeks in an adult over 40 suggests cancer.
5. A solitary lump in the neck in an adult should be regarded as a neoplasm until proved otherwise.

Differentiating between infection and a tumor begins with a thorough history and a complete physical examination, with special attention to the upper aerodigestive tract (Fig. 32.1). With the aid of the fiberoptic endoscope, emergency physicians should be able to visualize the entire upper aerodigestive tract. Descriptions of standard techniques of the head and neck examination, including the use of fiberoptic endoscopes and rigid scopes, can be found in current otolaryngology textbooks.

Head and neck squamous cell carcinomas are usually ulcerative, locally expansive, and invasive. Carcinomas of the nasopharynx and of the base of the tongue are exceptions to this generalization, as these tumors may initially be entirely submucosal.

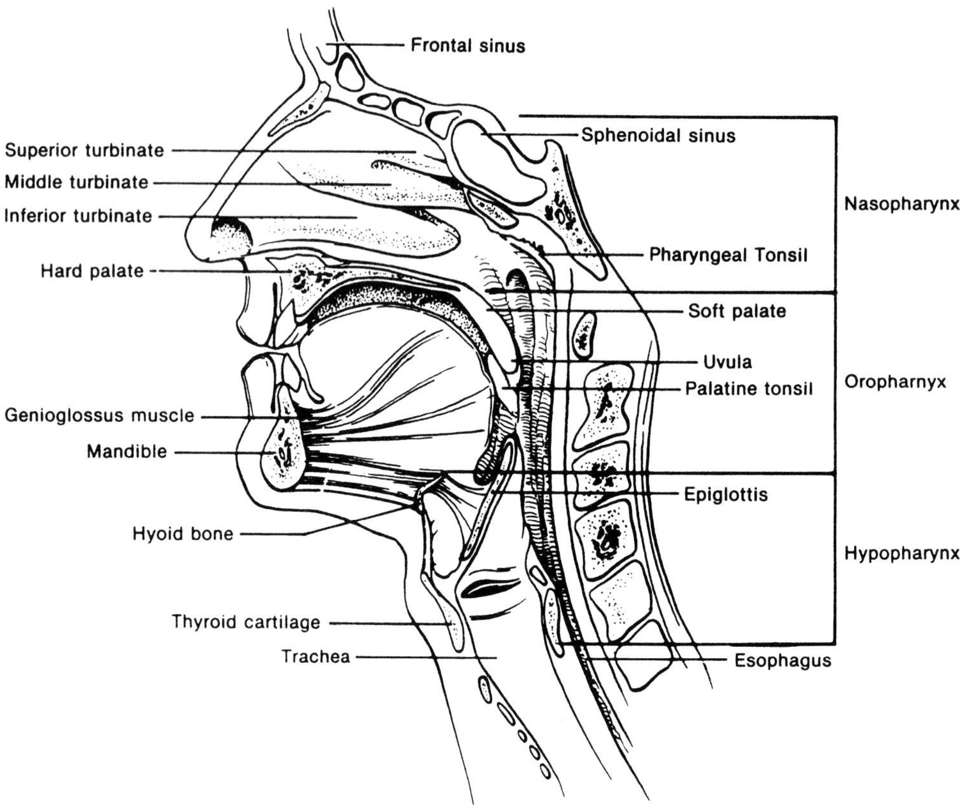

Figure 32.1. Sagittal view of head and neck.

Carcinoma of the Nasopharynx

Carcinoma of the nasopharynx most often makes its presence known by a unilateral enlargement of an upper jugular lymph node.[10] Significant symptoms are epistaxis, nasal obstruction, congestion, and bloody sputum. Carcinoma of the nasopharynx also presents as a unilateral obstruction of the eustachian tube. This causes a sense of fullness or pressure and hearing loss in the affected ear. Otoscopic examination reveals either a retracted eardrum or fluid in the middle ear. Visualization of the nasopharynx shows a tumor mass in the vicinity of the affected ear's eustachian tube cushion.

The differential diagnosis includes nasopharyngitis (viral or bacterial), lymphoma, and human immunodeficiency virus (HIV)-associated adenoid hypertrophy. Viral or bacterial nasopharyngitis is associated with diffuse inflammation of the entire nasopharynx and frequently a purulent exudate. Nasopharyngitis is often accompanied by pharyngitis. Lymphoma and HIV adenoidal hypertrophy both demonstrate a mass of lymphoid tissue which may obstruct the choana.

Emergency treatment includes control of any epistaxis, pain relief, and treatment of infection, if present. When a nasopharyngeal tumor is suspected, referral is indicated. No biopsy should be done in the emergency department. The patient should be referred to an otolaryngologist for follow-up, usually within 3 to 5 days.

COMMON PITFALLS

- Failure to associate an otherwise unexplained unilateral upper jugular cervical lymph node with carcinoma of the nasopharynx
- Failure to associate an otherwise unexplained unilateral middle ear effusion in an older adult with carcinoma of the nasopharynx
- Failure to visualize the nasopharynx

Neoplasms of the Nose and Paranasal Sinuses

Squamous cell carcinomas of the nose and maxillary sinus constitute the majority of tumors found in this area. These tumors often occur in older persons, predominantly male, with a median age of 60 years. Patients with squamous cell carcinoma of this area come to the emergency department because of epistaxis, nasal airway obstruction, and persistent nasal discharge. They may also present complaining of facial swelling or a palate mass. Good lighting and a nasal speculum are essential for adequate visualization of the nasal cavity. Fiberoptic endoscopes may be used if they are available. Examination reveals an ulcerative, exophytic tumor mass of varying size involving the lateral wall or the floor of the nose. Epistaxis associated with these tumors is rarely profuse.

The differential diagnosis includes mucosal melanoma, extramedullary plasmacytoma, juvenile nasopharyngeal angiofibroma, nasal foreign body, and septal hematoma. Melanomas may occur in the nose, particularly on the septum, as well as in the nasopharynx and oropharynx.[8] They typically have a similar presentation as squamous cell carcinoma in the same location. Extramedullary plasmacytoma occurs in 40% of patients with a history of multiple myeloma and presents as an erythematous, friable nasal mass with frequent epistaxis. Juvenile nasopharyngeal angiofibromas occur in pubescent males and present with epistaxis (often unilateral) and nasal obstruction. Foreign bodies are usually accompanied by unilateral rhinorrhea that is often purulent. Septal hematomas may be due to trauma and demonstrate a widened septum, and associated ecchymosis.

If the emergency physician detects or strongly suspects an intranasal tumor, treatment should be directed toward achieving hemostasis by local tamponade using absorbable packing. Biopsies of the tumor should not be done, due to the risk of significant bleeding. The patient should be referred to an ear, nose, and throat (ENT) consultant for further evaluation.

COMMON PITFALLS

- Failure to visualize the site and cause of epistaxis
- Failure to consider cancer as the cause of the problem
- Inability to visualize the nasal cavity adequately

Carcinoma of the Mouth (Including Lips and Anterior Two-Thirds of the Tongue)

The person with carcinoma of the mouth usually comes to the emergency department because of a sore, nonhealing ulcer or oral bleeding. If the ulcer is on the anterior tongue, the person will also complain of exacerbation of the pain with tongue motion. Physical examination reveals a discrete mucous membrane ulceration and varying amounts of local induration.

The differential diagnosis includes herpetic ulcer, aphthous ulcer, lichen planus, pemphigus vulgaris, pemphigoid, and traumatic ulceration secondary to dentures.[7] It is usually impossible to differentiate between these diseases by history and physical examination, except in an obvious case of carcinoma. If the ulcer has not healed in 2 weeks with application of various topical or systemic agents, or if it is associated with a neck mass, the emergency physician should arrange for the person to be seen by a consultant within 3 to 5 days. The emergency physician should not biopsy the ulcer, but should provide adequate analgesics, either systemic or topical, to relieve pain until the patient can be seen by the consultant. Diagnosis is usually made by biopsy of the lesion and the surrounding mucous membrane.

COMMON PITFALLS

Failure to consider cancer as the cause of the ulcer

Carcinoma of the Posterior Third of the Tongue

A patient with carcinoma of the posterior third of the tongue characteristically complains of a sore throat that persists longer than 2 weeks and some degree of dysphagia. The patient often notes that the sore throat did not improve with antibiotics, but worsened. Direct visualization may show an ulcerating lesion, but frequently there is no mucosal aberration. The base of the tongue and neck should be digitally palpated; this will reveal an area of induration or a discrete mass.

The differential diagnosis includes a lingual thyroid gland, lingual tonsillitis, and lymphoma. A lingual thyroid gland is usually situated in the midline directly beneath the cecal foramen, whereas an early carcinoma of the posterior tongue is usually a unilateral lesion. Lingual tonsillitis ordinarily occurs in an adult who has previously undergone palatine tonsillectomy, and is recognized by the presence of diffuse inflammation, fever, and an elevated white blood cell (WBC) count. Lingual tonsillitis improves with antibiotic therapy.

When carcinoma of the base of the tongue is diagnosed or strongly suspected, the emergency physician should evaluate the patient's airway, hydration, and ability to swallow. The results of that evaluation dictate the disposition. If the tumor is sufficiently large, the patient may have dyspnea, especially in the supine position. In this case, an otolaryngologist should be consulted for airway management. If the person cannot maintain hydration or swallow sufficiently to obtain pain relief with oral medication, the emergency physician must arrange admission, preferably to a head and neck surgical oncologist. If no specialist is available, arrangements should be made for transfer to a hospital that has appropriate personnel. If the person can swallow adequately to maintain hydration and obtain pain relief with oral medication, the emergency physician must arrange for the patient to be seen within 3 to 5 days by the oncologic surgeon.

COMMON PITFALLS

- Failure to visualize the base of the tongue
- Failure to palpate the base of the tongue digitally
- Failure to adequately assess the airway

Carcinoma of the Oropharynx

Carcinomas that arise in the oropharynx usually involve either the palatine tonsil or the soft palate. Often, the patient complains of a persistent sore throat, some degree of dysphagia, and fetid breath. Physical examination shows an ulcerative lesion that may contain impacted food debris.

The differential diagnosis for tonsillar lesions includes lymphoma and granulomatous infections. When the soft palate is the tumor's primary site, neoplasms of minor salivary gland origin must also be considered. The diagnosis is made through a biopsy of the lesion and the surrounding mucous membrane. The biopsy should be performed by an otolaryngologist.

Visualization of the tumor may be difficult due to trismus from invasion of the pterygoid muscles. This presentation may be similar to that of a retropharyngeal or parapharyngeal abscess. An elevated WBC and fever will be present in patients with an abscess; however, a computed tomography (CT) scan with contrast will clearly differentiate between tumor and abscess.

When carcinoma of the oropharynx is diagnosed or strongly suspected, hydration and ability to swallow should be assessed. If the patient can maintain hydration and obtain pain relief from oral medication, the emergency physician should arrange for follow-up care within 3 to 5 days with a head and neck oncologic surgeon. If the patient's swallowing function is compromised, the emergency physician must arrange admission to a head and neck surgical oncologist.

COMMON PITFALLS

Failure to consider cancer as the cause of the ulcerative lesion

Carcinoma of the Larynx

A patient with carcinoma of the larynx may present to the emergency department with a constellation of symptoms, ranging from persistent hoarseness to chronic sore throat, cough, and shortness of breath. Laryngeal neoplasms are readily visible to direct and indirect laryngoscopy. When visualizing the larynx, the examiner must note the location and size of the tumor, vocal cord function, and airway adequacy.

The differential diagnosis includes vocal cord nodule (singer's nodes), vocal cord polyp, Reinke's edema of the vocal cord, hemorrhage into the cord, granulomas of the cords, leukoplakia of the cords, juvenile papillomatosis, tuberculosis, sarcoid, syphilis, acute epiglottitis, and acute laryngitis.

When carcinoma of the larynx is diagnosed or strongly suspected, the emergency physician must evaluate the laryngeal competence (adequacy of the airway for respiration and the ability of the larynx to prevent tracheal aspiration). Suspected epiglottitis is not a contraindication to fiberoptic laryngoscopy. If laryngeal function is impaired, supportive measures, such as supplemental oxygen, endotracheal intubation, or emergency tracheostomy, are indicated. The greater the airway obstruction, the more cautious one should be in administering narcotics or relaxants to avoid precipitating respiratory obstruction. An otolaryngologist should be contacted for emergency consultation for probable hospitalization. If the larynx is competent, the emergency physician must arrange for follow-up care with an otolaryngologist. The urgency of this follow-up visit depends on the patient's status.

COMMON PITFALLS

- Failure to visualize the larynx
- Underestimating the degree of laryngeal obstruction

Major Salivary Gland Neoplasms

Tumors of the parotid gland are about four times more common than tumors of the submandibular gland. These neoplasms grow slowly and are essentially symptom-free; indeed, most are benign.[9] Often, another person discovers the growth and points it out to the affected person. The sudden awareness of the tumor may prompt a visit to the emergency department. Other patients relate their tumor to a sore throat or some minor trauma. These patients usually do not seek attention until the tumor size alarms them.

The differential diagnosis includes acute parotitis, sialolithiasis with obstruction of the duct, Sjögren syndrome, and the benign lymphoepithelial lesion seen in HIV patients.

Physical examination may reveal a discrete tumor mass in a major salivary gland. The mass is usually firm, but a Warthin's tumor (benign cystadenoma) often feels cystic. If "stripped," the gland produces clear saliva. Acute parotitis usually has an abrupt onset. The gland is diffusely enlarged and very tender. "Stripping" the gland produces purulent saliva. Stones that obstruct the duct also become abruptly symptomatic; eating greatly exacerbates the pain and swelling, and stripping produces no saliva. Frequently, stones can be palpated along the course of the duct. The vast majority of stones are found in Wharton's duct (of the submandibular gland). Sjögren syndrome usually produces diffuse bilateral parotid enlargement. "Stripping" the gland produces thick mucoid saliva or none at all. Benign lymphoepithelial lesions are often multiple, bilateral cystic masses involving the parotid glands. Clear saliva is produced upon stripping the gland.

When a major salivary gland neoplasm is diagnosed, the emergency physician should arrange for follow-up care with an otolaryngologist. Because these tumors are slow-growing and most are benign, there is no urgency for the referral. No attempt should be made to incise and drain cystic salivary gland masses or to perform excisional or incisional biopsies in the emergency department. A CT scan or sialography may be useful in identifying duct occlusion from stones. A CT scan will also help in differentiating the type of tumor as well as its extent.

COMMON PITFALLS

Misdiagnosing intrinsic salivary gland tumors as inflamed lymph nodes

Unknown Primaries

Carcinoma of unknown primary will present with an enlarging neck mass, often accompanied by multiple enlarged lymph nodes.[2] The patient may complain of pain but often is brought in to the emergency department because of the mass' appearance. The patient may have systemic symptoms of fever, nightsweats, and weight loss, and if the mass is sufficiently large, they may exhibit torticollis.

The differential diagnosis of a unilateral neck mass includes branchial cleft cyst, lymphadenitis, lymphoma, tuberculosis, sarcoid, cat-scratch fever, actinomycosis, carotid body tumor, metastatic cancer, and squamous cell carcinoma. Diagnosis is made by fine-needle aspiration (FNA), preferably by an otolaryngologist. Branchial cleft cysts are anterior to the sternocleidomastoid and feel cystic to palpation. Lymphadenitis is usually accompanied by fever and leukocytosis, whereas lymphoma often presents with multiple lymph nodes and systemic symptoms, including nightsweats, fever, and weight loss. Sarcoid, acute mononucleosis and cat-scratch fever often involve multiple lymph nodes bilaterally. Tuberculosis and actinomycosis may present as a draining neck mass; actinomycosis is often associated with recent dental work or oral surgery. Carotid body tumors are pulsatile and occur in the upper third of the neck.

A contrasted CT scan of the neck is helpful for determining cystic from solid masses, and the presence of heterogeneity is more consistent with a malignant neoplasm. Open biopsy is to be discouraged; however, FNA is often extremely helpful. Unless the mass is compromising vital structures, arrangement can be made for follow-up with an otolaryngologist within 3 to 5 days. If there is a concern for airway compression, the head and neck surgeon should be contacted immediately.

COMMON PITFALLS

- Failure to evaluate the upper aerodigestive tract for evidence of the primary
- Failure to consider metastatic cancer
- Inadequate evaluation of vital structures

PREVIOUSLY DIAGNOSED NEOPLASMS

Patients with known head and neck neoplasms often seek emergency care because of complications associated with therapy or complications secondary to the neoplasm. Complications of therapy include dislodged feeding tubes, mucositis, dehydration, nausea, vomiting, a dislodged voice prosthesis, an obstructed tracheostomy tube, dysphagia, airway obstruction, and severe pain. Complications secondary to the neoplasm are hemorrhage, wound infection, salivary fistula, esophageal obstruction, and airway obstruction.

COMPLICATIONS ASSOCIATED WITH THERAPY

Feeding Tubes

Feeding tubes (nasogastric [NG], gastrostomy, or feeding jejunostomy) are used to secure entry to the gastrointestinal tract for nutrition and hydration. Most often, this follows extensive primary resection, salvage surgery, and radiation therapy.

NG tubes are difficult to secure for long periods, so accidental removal is seen. It is usually possible to replace the NG tube, but the head and neck surgeon should be contacted for specific instructions, because he or she may prefer that no attempt be made to reintroduce the NG tube.

Gastrostomy tubes are less prone to accidental removal because they are anchored by a balloon-tipped catheter or via a mushroom-tipped tube. However, balloons may rupture and deflate, resulting in accidental removal. The stomach is often sutured in the vicinity of the gastrostomy ostia to the anterior abdominal wall to minimize the possibility of a gastric leak even if the tube comes out. This maneuver makes it easier to change the gastrostomy tube.[3] When confronted with a dislodged gastrostomy tube, the emergency physician should contact the surgeon for instructions about which type and size tube to reinsert, if the patient has not brought the tube along. A gastrostomy fistula will contract quickly if the tube is left out for more than a few hours. If this has occurred, the fistula can be dilated to its original size by *gently* passing a series of catheters of increasing diameter. Excessive force can lead to a ruptured viscus, false passage into the peritoneal cavity, and hemorrhage. Once the tube has been replaced, its intragastric position should be checked by instilling and removing a small amount of sterile water or saline solution, or by aspiration of gastric contents.

Jejunostomy feeding tubes are seldom dislodged because they are sutured to the abdominal wall. If one comes out, the emergency physician should contact the attending surgeon.

Voice Prosthesis

After total laryngectomy, patients may elect to have a small tracheoesophageal (TE) fistula established so they can use a vocal prosthesis for speech. This prosthesis frequently dislodges. Although patients who use the prosthesis are taught how to insert the device, their attempts at insertion are not always successful. Occasionally, the prosthesis is lost. A TE fistula will close rapidly if patency is not maintained. If the emergency physician does not have experience in inserting a vocal prosthesis, the procedure should not be attempted. Patency of the TE fistula can be ensured by passing a 16F Foley or red rubber catheter through the tracheal puncture into the distal esophagus. The catheter can be secured to the neck or chest wall. Once patency of the TE fistula is ensured, the prosthesis may be reinserted by the surgeon or speech pathologist at a convenient time. A vocal prosthesis is small and can be aspirated into the distal tracheobronchial tree. The irritation of the prosthesis usually causes a chronic cough. If the prosthesis cannot be accounted for, a chest radiograph is indicated to rule out aspiration.

Radiation Therapy and Chemotherapy

Radiation therapy and chemotherapy are frequently associated with nausea, vomiting, mucositis, and dysphagia. The patient may seek emergency care for dehydration and inability to obtain pain relief from oral medications. Radiation therapy may produce significant laryngeal edema that causes airway obstruction. Emergency treatment for such patients depends on the severity of dehydration, dysphagia, and airway compromise.

Tracheostomy Tube

A tracheostomy tube obstructs for one of three reasons: (1) the tube is occluded by secretions, (2) the tube is lying outside the tracheal lumen, or (3) the tube is blocked by an overinflated cuff. The quickest solution is to remove the entire tracheostomy tube; this should result in immediate improvement in the airway. An obturator should always be used when reinstating the tracheostomy tube. Once the tube has been replaced, a sterile catheter should be passed into the trachea to confirm the intraluminal position of the tube. A tracheocutaneous (TC) fistula more than 72 hours old will not close immediately on removal of a tracheostomy tube. However, if the tracheostomy tube has been out for a number of hours before the person gets to the emergency department, it may not be possible to reinsert the tube until the TC fistula has been gently dilated using the graduated tube technique. The caveats for this technique are the same as those listed under the section for the gastrostomy tube.

Patients who have undergone total laryngectomy have a permanent stoma, which is the termination of the upper airway. The stoma may become occluded with thick secretions and crusts producing dyspnea. Removal of the crusts will immediately improve the airway. The patient may also present with bleeding from the stoma site. This is usually due to granulation tissue around the stoma. The bleeding is easily controlled by cauterization of the granulation with silver nitrate. Stomal stenosis may occur after radiation therapy and can produce dyspnea. In this case, the stoma can be gently dilated and a tracheostomy or laryngectomy tube inserted to ensure patency.

COMMON PITFALLS

- Using excessive force when replacing feeding tubes
- Failure to preserve the TE fistula after a vocal prosthesis becomes dislodged
- Failure to rule out aspiration of a voice prosthesis
- Failure to check the intraluminal position of a tracheostomy tube by passing a sterile catheter into the distal trachea
- Failure to recognize a laryngeal stoma obstruction

COMPLICATIONS SECONDARY TO NEOPLASM

HEMORRHAGE

Hemorrhage from a ruptured vessel is associated with an active enlarging tumor, prior irradiation, wound infection, or a salivary fistula.[1,5] Of head and neck vessels, rupture of the carotid artery is most frequent, but rupture of the lingual artery is also seen. Catastrophic hemorrhage is often heralded by a "sentinel" bleeding episode, which may be manifested by coughing up a moderate amount of blood or bleeding from the neck. Often, the sentinel bleeding has ceased by the time the patient arrives in the emergency department. The emergency physician should be aware that a life-threatening situation may exist. If examination reveals a blood clot over the area of the carotid artery or the surface of the tongue, no attempt should be made to remove the clot. The quiet interval should be used to begin an intravenous infusion of saline solution and to draw a blood specimen for hemoglobin, hematocrit, and type and crossmatch. The patient needs constant observation, because bleeding may recur.

Catastrophic hemorrhage from the carotid artery may be external through the neck or internal into the hypopharynx. Internal hemorrhage is uniformly and rapidly fatal due to aspiration of large quantities of blood. External hemorrhage can be controlled by directly occluding the carotid artery. Definitive treatment of carotid artery rupture usually involves ligation of the artery, although, in selected cases, angiography and embolization of the carotid artery is successful.[1] Definitive surgery is best done in the operating room.

Massive bleeding from rupture of the lingual artery at the base of the tongue requires the emergency physician to simultaneously maintain the airway and occlude the ruptured vessel. The patient should be in an upright position. The blood should be removed with suction and then pressure applied to the base of the tongue with a tonsil sponge or 4×4-in. gauze pad on a curved hemostat. If the airway cannot be maintained while achieving hemostasis, an emergency cricothyrotomy may be required. The patient must be taken to the operating room for definitive surgical treatment as rapidly as possible.

Airway Obstruction

Airway obstruction secondary to an enlarging neoplasm will result in a visit to the emergency department. Obstruction can be mild or severe. Supplemental oxygen should be given before and during laryngoscopy. Visualization of the larynx is critical in planning immediate treatment and allows the emergency physician to quantify the degree of obstruction and its location, and the feasibility of intubation directly or with the aid of a fiberoptic endoscope. Occasionally, the airway obstruction is severe enough that the patient must immediately be intubated, or else undergo a tracheostomy or cricothyrotomy. Rapid intubation with the guidance of a fiberoptic bronchoscope can often prevent the need for a tracheostomy. Tracheostomies are best performed in the operating room, but the emergency physician may need to perform a cricothyrotomy if the airway cannot be maintained.

Salivary Fistulas

Salivary fistulas may develop weeks or months postoperatively. They are more common in patients who received preoperative radiation therapy.[5] The appearance of a salivary fistula is often frightening to the patient. Patients who have undergone a laryngectomy and develop a fistula may present with aspiration pneumonia. The emergency physician should suction and divert the salivary stream away from the trachea by opening and packing the wound lateral to the trachea. The surgeon should be consulted at this stage. The emergency physician may be asked to pass an NG tube. Once the saliva has been diverted or absorbed and an NG tube has provided a feeding bypass, the patient will require instruction on use of the NG tube for alimentation. The patient needs to follow-up with his or her otolaryngologist as soon as possible for management of the fistula.

Pain

Constant pain is a hallmark of the later stages of uncontrolled head and neck neoplasms. Although oral medication can often control such pain, the cancer patient may present to the emergency department because of inability to obtain pain relief. The attending surgeon should be made aware; the emergency physician should instruct the patient in alterations in the analgesic dosage, timing, or both, to achieve adequate pain control.

COMMON PITFALLS

- Failure to recognize a sentinel hemorrhage
- Underestimating the degree of airway obstruction
- Inability to establish an airway or perform a cricothyrotomy

References

1. Morrissey DD, Anderson PE, Nesbit GM, et al. Endovascular management of hemorrhage in patients with head and neck cancer. *Arch Otolaryngol Head Neck Surg* 1997;123:15–19.
2. Nguyen C, Shenouda G, Black M, et al. Metastatic squamous cell carcinoma to cervical lymph nodes from unknown primary mucosal sites. *Head Neck* 1994; 58–63.
3. Raynor EM, Williams MF, Martindale RG, et al. Timing of percutaneous endoscopic gastrostomy tube placement in head and neck cancer patients. *Otolaryngol Head Neck Surg* 1999;120:479–482.
4. Richtsmeier WJ, Scher RL. Telescopic laryngeal and pharyngeal surgery. *Ann Otol Rhinol Laryngol* 1997;106:995–1001.
5. Righi PD, Weisberger EC, Krakovits PR. Wound complications associated with brachytherapy for primary or salvage treatment of head and neck cancer. *Laryngoscope* 1998;107:1464–1468.
6. Schiff NF, Annino DJ, Woo P, et al. Kaposi's sarcoma of the larynx. *Ann Otol Rhinol Laryngol* 1997;106:563–567.
7. Shklar G, McCarthy PL. *The oral manifestations of systemic disease.* Boston: Butterworths, 1976.
8. Stern SJ, Guillamondegui OM. Mucosal melanoma of the head and neck. *Head Neck* 1991;1:22–27.
9. Sur RK, Donde B, Levin V, et al. Adenoid cystic carcinoma of the salivary glands: a review of 10 years. *Laryngoscope* 1997;107:1276–1279.
10. Vasef M, Ferlito A, Weiss L. Nasopharyngeal carcinoma, with emphasis on its relationship to Epstein-Barr virus. *Ann Otol Rhinol Laryngol* 1997;106:348–356.

PART IV

Emergency Aspects of General Surgery

CHAPTER 33

Emergencies of Artificial Conduits

Karen DeFazio and Brian Mongillo

Patients presenting to the emergency department with artificial conduits are commonplace. Complications of these devices range from minor inconveniences for the patient to life-threatening emergencies. Emergency physicians must be aware of the purpose, structure, and proper maintenance of these devices so they will be prepared for complications. In addition, physicians must recognize systemic pathology independent of the devices.

RESPIRATORY DEVICES

The tracheostomy tube is an airway appliance seen frequently in the emergency department. Patients receive tracheostomies because of underlying respiratory or neurologic conditions that require airway management. Complications include local infection, bleeding, obstruction, air leaks, and accidental or intentional removal.

Infection and Hemorrhage

Local wound infection is managed with regular cleaning and antibiotics as indicated. Hemorrhage early after placement of a tracheostomy is often local and superficial and can be managed conservatively. If hemorrhage persists, evaluation of the coagulation status is suggested. Acute, profuse bleeding around a well-established tracheostomy is most likely due to erosion into an artery, such as occurs in tracheoinnominate artery fistula. A sentinel bleed of small amounts may be the only warning sign prior to life-threatening hemorrhage. Fluid resuscitation and blood transfusion may be necessary if the patient is hypotensive. Bleeding may be controlled with hyperinflation of the tracheostomy tube cuff or by endotracheal intubation of the patient after removal of the tracheostomy tube to allow placing a finger in the stoma to compress the innominate artery against the sternum. All arterial bleeding requires surgical consultation.[9]

Obstruction of a Tracheostomy

Obstruction from mucus may be life-threatening. Suctioning can be attempted with an endotracheal suction catheter, but this may not be successful. Saline injected through the catheter loosens dried mucus. If suctioning does not improve ventilation, or if there is a mechanical problem with the tracheostomy tube (e.g., cuff air leak), the tube should be removed and replaced.

Replacement of Tracheostomy Cannula

Tracheostomy tubes may be cuffed or uncuffed and may come with an inner cannula that can be removed for cleaning. The patient's head should be extended to facilitate placement. A replacement tube should be the same type as the original. In an emergency, however, replacement with a smaller size is preferred if maintaining a patent airway depends on it. Removal and replacement of tracheostomy tubes should follow the curved path of the tube itself. When inserting a new tube, the obturator should be in place to facilitate insertion, then removed when completed. A well-positioned tube can be advanced gently with little resistance. If force is necessary to place the tube, efforts should cease because of the possibility of creating false passages, bleeding, and edema. The safest way to ensure proper placement of a tracheostomy tube is to use a thin red rubber catheter as a guide. The catheter can be placed through the existing tracheostomy before removal. If the tracheostomy tube has accidentally fallen out, the catheter may be placed directly through the stoma. Once the old tracheostomy tube is removed, the new tube without the obturator can be passed over the catheter into place. The red rubber catheter can then be removed.

If the tracheostomy tube cannot be replaced and the airway is in jeopardy, the physician should consider oral endotracheal intubation. The original indication for the tracheostomy, however, may hamper attempts at endotracheal intubation (e.g., laryngeal malignancy). If respiratory distress persists after adequate tube replacement, the physician must not overlook other causes (pneumothorax, pulmonary embolus, or cardiac pathology).

VASCULAR CONDUITS

Indwelling central venous access is essential in patients who require chronic therapy, such as chemotherapy, hyperalimentation, lengthy antimicrobial therapy, hemodialysis, and ambulatory heparin therapy. Most outpatients requiring these devices are immunocompromised. The most serious complications are line sepsis and central venous thrombosis. Artificial conduits of the vascular system include catheters for short-term use, catheters for long-term use, subcutaneous devices, large-bore catheters used for hemodialysis, and arteriovenous fistulas.

Short-term catheters are single- and triple-lumen catheters inserted percutaneously into the central circulation. They allow

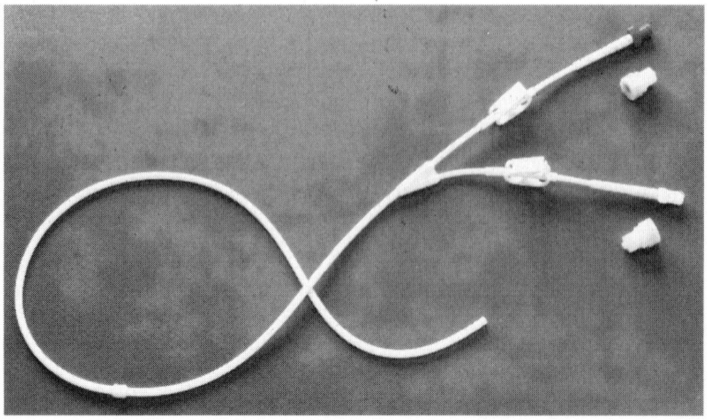

Figure 33.1. Hickman catheters are available with one, two, or three lumens. (Courtesy of Bard Access Systems, Inc.)

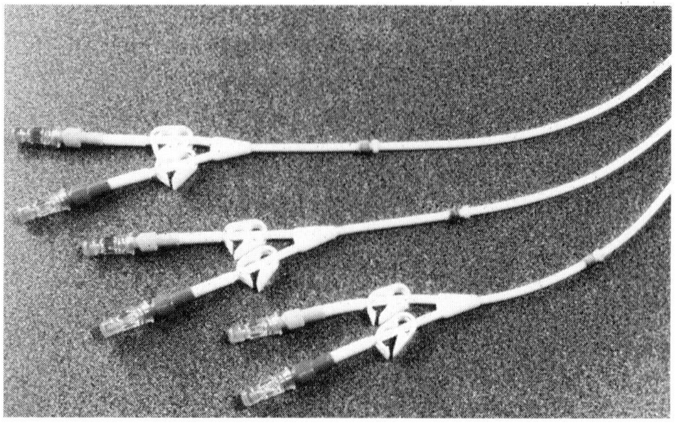

Figure 33.3. Large-bore catheters for hemodialysis. (Courtesy of Bard Access Systems, Inc.)

for phlebotomy and delivery of medications and blood products for up to 3 weeks. If a central line is used for phlebotomy, the port should be prepared with povidone–iodine. In a triple-lumen catheter, the longest port is prepared (the proximal lumen port). The catheter is flushed with normal saline and brisk blood return is ensured. Before phlebotomy, fluids or medications infusing through the other ports are held for 15 minutes. Five milliliters of blood are aspirated and discarded. Then the blood needed for phlebotomy is drawn. If giving medications, normal saline should be used to flush the catheter between medications. The final step after access is to flush with 5 mL heparin (100 U/mL).[2] To prevent air embolism, whenever the protective cap is removed from a port, the catheter arm should be clamped off until intravenous tubing or a syringe is attached.

Common *long-term catheters* include the Broviac and Hickman (Fig. 33.1).[8] Access to the double-lumen Hickman catheter is gained in much the same way as with triple-lumen catheters. The catheters have a clamp that should be kept locked except during phlebotomy and administration of fluids and medications.

Subcutaneous devices (Port-A-Cath, Infus-A-Port) are surgically implanted and have subcutaneous infusion ports in continuity with a central Silastic catheter. The port chamber is visible and palpable on the chest wall (Fig. 33.2). Access to these devices is gained using aseptic technique, by inserting a 20- or 22-gauge, Huber-point, right-angled needle into the infusion port chamber. The relatively small gauge needle limits the speed of administration of fluid, blood, or medication. Heparin should be instilled after each use, but these catheters rarely undergo thrombosis.[8]

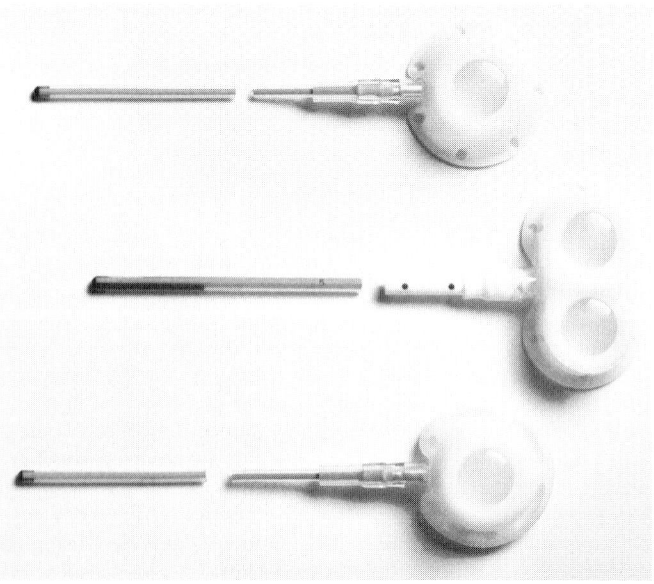

Figure 33.2. Infusion ports are subcutaneously placed and attached to a catheter placed in a central vein. (Courtesy of Bard Access Systems, Inc.)

Large-bore catheters used for hemodialysis (Fig. 33.3) are most often temporizing measures until permanent arteriovenous access sites mature. These Silastic, double-lumen, high-flow catheters are placed in a central vein and provide temporary access for hemodialysis for up to 8 weeks. After dialysis, each lumen is flushed with 2500 U of heparin. These catheters are used *solely* for dialysis; phlebotomy and medication and fluid administration should *not* be done—except in an emergency, when all other means of standard venous access have failed. Strict aseptic technique must be used. Blood must be aspirated before giving medications or fluids because of the heparin within the lumens.

Arteriovenous fistula (Cimino-Brescia fistula) is the preferred vascular access for long-term hemodialysis. A normal patent fistula should have a palpable thrill and an auscultatory bruit. The arteriovenous fistula should not be accessed in the emergency department except under urgent circumstances when attempts at standard methods of intravenous access have failed. To gain access to the fistula, the area is prepared with povidone–iodine and an intravenous catheter is placed in the usual fashion. When complete, the catheter is removed and gentle local pressure is applied to avoid hemorrhage.

Complications of Vascular Conduits

Thrombosis

Thrombosis is one of the most common complications of indwelling venous catheters. The risk increases with greater diameter, length, and rigidity of the catheter. The incidence of thrombotic complications can be reduced by changing the catheter frequently. Catheters must also be routinely flushed with 5 mL of heparin (100 U/mL) after use. Patients with a history of, or increased risk for, thrombosis can also be placed on low-dose warfarin therapy. In general, the implantable Port-A-Cath rarely develops thrombotic complications.[8]

Thrombosis is related to the formation of a fibrinous sheath around the catheter that begins almost immediately after placement. Thrombosis must be suspected if blood cannot be aspirated from the catheter. Urokinase 5000 IU (1 mL) is indicated, and the solution is injected slowly into each port of the catheter. After waiting 5 minutes, the syringe is removed aseptically, a 5-mL syringe is connected to the catheter, and aspiration is attempted.

Aspiration attempts are repeated every 5 minutes. If the catheter is not open within 30 minutes, it is capped and the urokinase is allowed to remain in the catheter for 60 minutes before another attempt is made. A second injection may be necessary in resistant cases. When patency is restored, 5 mL of blood is aspirated to ensure removal of all drug and residual clot. If thrombolysis does not restore patency, the catheter must be replaced.

The complications of thrombus formation include extravasation and embolism. Thrombus formation around a venous catheter can lead to fixation of the catheter against the vessel wall, with subsequent perforation of the vessel. This can cause extravasation of the material being infused. Superior vena cava syndrome due to extravasation of 5-fluorouracil (5-FU) has been reported. Acute-onset vena cava syndrome produced by thrombosis of the superior vena cava in a patient receiving adjuvant chemotherapy through a Hickman catheter has been reported. After angiographic diagnosis, fibrinolytic therapy with streptokinase brought about complete resolution of the superior vena cava syndrome.[19] Vessel wall perforation has occurred with infusion of 5-FU into the pericardium and into the lung parenchyma, causing chemical pericarditis and a necrotizing chemical pneumonitis. Thrombosis associated with false aneurysm formation and hemorrhage into the mediastinum, as well as perforation of the heart with cardiac tamponade, also has been reported.[3,8,15]

Because of clot formation on the tips of venous catheters, there is the potential for pulmonary embolism during flushing, manipulation, and changing over a guidewire. However, the actual occurrence of a clinically significant pulmonary embolus is rare.[6] An air embolism is possible if air is allowed to enter the venous circulation. If this is suspected, the patient is positioned in the left lateral decubitus position in Trendelenburg and stabilized with 100% oxygen and intravenous access. Supportive measures are instituted.

Care should be taken while manipulating catheters because of the risk of displacement, cardiac dysrhythmias, and perforation or rupture of the external catheter. A Hickman catheter repair kit is available that includes silicone adhesive, injection caps, and an external catheter segment with clamps.

Thrombosis is the most common complication of the arteriovenous fistula. If a patient states that the palpable thrill in the access is lost, a vascular surgeon should be consulted immediately for possible thrombectomy. The chance of successfully reopening a thrombosed access appears to be related to the time elapsed since thrombosis occurred.

Hemorrhage

Hemorrhage from an arteriovenous fistula, a life-threatening complication, can be from the dialysis puncture site, accidental trauma, infection, aneurysm, or pseudoaneurysm. Gentle pressure is applied to the area and the extremity is elevated. Care must be taken not to occlude and possibly thrombose the vessel by compressing too firmly. An auscultatory bruit should be present during compression to ensure the fistula is not occluded. Gelfoam soaked in topical thrombin can be applied to the wound to assist in hemostasis. If indicated, a complete blood count (CBC), platelet count, prothrombin time (PT), and partial thromboplastin time (PTT) are ordered. These patients must be observed in the emergency department or admitted for observation. Recurrent or prolonged bleeding requires surgical consultation because of its association with aneurysms, pseudoaneurysms, or infection.

Other complications of arteriovenous fistulas include carpal tunnel syndrome, distal venous stasis, and vascular insufficiency or "steal" syndrome.

Infections

Infections are common with indwelling catheters and arteriovenous fistulas. Local infections are usually manifested by fever, erythema, tenderness, and purulent drainage. Not all patients with local infections require catheter removal or admission; reliable patients with localized infection who are not febrile, toxic, or immunocompromised may be treated as outpatients. The decision to discharge a patient or to remove a catheter, and the choice of antibiotic, are made in conjunction with the patient's primary care physician, nephrologist, hematologist, or oncologist. Cultures from the catheter, blood cultures from a distant site, and cultures from the local wound site are obtained and the patient is treated with an oral semisynthetic penicillin or first-generation cephalosporin to cover both staphylococci and streptococci. If treated as an outpatient, a follow-up evaluation is needed in 24 hours.

Any febrile patient with a fistula or indwelling catheter without an obvious source of infection must be treated presumptively for an access infection. Patients with leukocytosis or neutropenia, tachycardia, and hypotension are admitted. These patients are treated with intravenous antibiotics effective against gram-positive and gram-negative organisms. Triple broad-spectrum antibiotics are needed for the neutropenic patient.

The decision to remove the indwelling catheter should be made in conjunction with the primary care physician. Most available data indicate that catheter removal does *not* usually influence the outcome of sepsis or local infection.[12] Septic shock, however, warrants catheter removal. Blood cultures should be drawn from the line before its removal, and the catheter tip should also be cultured.

Dialysis patients are at high risk for infectious complications involving the access device. Infections involving arteriovenous fistulas usually result from contamination at the time of puncture for dialysis and are usually caused by staphylococci. Superficial soft-tissue infections overlying arteriovenous fistulas can usually be treated on an outpatient basis with a single dose of intravenous vancomycin, because this medication is not dialyzable. If the patient is discharged, outpatient follow-up in 24 hours must be arranged with the nephrologist. An infection that involves the fistula itself can be serious, leading to thrombosis and hemorrhage. If this is suspected, or if the patient is febrile with signs of sepsis, admission is indicated. Special consideration can be made for the reliable hemodialysis patient who has a fever but otherwise feels well and has no tachycardia, leukocytosis, neutropenia, or signs of sepsis. This patient may be treated as an outpatient after a thorough search for infection is made, blood cultures are obtained, intravenous vancomycin is given, and the nephrologist is consulted. Some nephrologists, however, prefer to admit all febrile dialysis patients.

GASTROINTESTINAL CONDUITS

Artificial conduits of the gastrointestinal (GI) tract fall into two categories: (1) catheters to feed and administer liquids in the proximal GI tract and (2) ostomies of the distal GI tract for expulsion of stool and decompression. Both have similar complications secondary to involvement with the GI tract, but they also present with problems unique to the mechanics of the device.

The use of enteral feeding tubes has increased in recent years for patients who cannot feed themselves but have functional GI tracts. The emergency physician is most likely to encounter this in the institutionalized patient with a neurologic deficit. Gastrostomy, gastrojejunostomy, and jejunostomy tubes are the most common. Complications due to feeding, extraluminal migration, accidental removal of the tube, and tube blockage are encountered.

The physician must first rule out life-threatening conditions. Patients who are overfed or who have decreased gastric motility may easily aspirate stomach contents, resulting in pneumonia. Decreased gastric motility and large feeding residuals may be secondary to small bowel obstruction, systemic infection, or ischemic bowel.[17] GI hemorrhage may occur from erosions of the device into the gastric mucosa.

If the physician suspects that a feeding tube is not in the lumen of the stomach or intestine, a radiologic study with contrast is obtained to confirm placement. Tubes must not be used for feeding if the location is in doubt, because of possible intraperitoneal contamination. Accidental injury to the device tract may cause contamination of the peritoneum by GI contents, resulting in peritonitis. Tubes that have migrated within the gut lumen may result in bowel obstruction caused by the internal anchor or balloon of a Foley catheter.

Patients with blocked feeding tubes are usually brought to the emergency department after standard attempts at irrigation have failed. Once there is obstructing material within the lumen of the tube, further irrigation is unlikely to relieve the obstruction. The practice of using wires or stylets to unblock tubes may be dangerous, because once beyond the visualized exterior portion of the tube there is always the chance of causing a tube puncture. A safe, effective method of unclogging jejunostomy tubes involves the use of a Fogarty arterial embolectomy catheter.[4] The catheter is advanced into the feeding tube, monitoring the length of catheter advanced so as not to penetrate further than the length of the feeding tube itself. (This length can be measured by comparing it with stock feeding tubes of the same type as the indwelling tube.) If the catheter cannot pass easily, the distal balloon can be inflated, which helps dislodge the obstruction. With the balloon deflated, the catheter can be advanced further. Once the catheter has been passed almost to the end of the feeding tube, it is withdrawn while the balloon is intermittently inflated. The Fogarty catheter should *not* be withdrawn from the tube while the balloon is continually inflated: This may dislodge the feeding tube. This procedure can be repeated as many times as needed. A tube study with water-soluble contrast should be performed to confirm patency and position.[4]

A tube that cannot be unblocked, or a tube that has accidentally come out, must be replaced. In the rare instance of a jejunostomy tube that cannot be unclogged, attempts to change the tube with a guidewire should be referred to a surgeon. If a feeding tube is removed or has fallen out, the tract may begin to close unless it has been established for a long time. Even though clogged, the tube can act as a stent until adequate replacement can be arranged. A tube should not be electively removed unless it can be replaced in a timely manner.

A gastrostomy tube can easily be replaced with passage of a Foley catheter through the tract. Gentle, constant pressure with the tip lubricated is usually successful. Placement can be confirmed by auscultation over the stomach with air insufflation, as well as aspiration of stomach contents. If placement is in question, it can be confirmed with a radiologic study. Before inserting the gastrostomy tube, an anchor should be placed over the tube to prevent it from advancing further than desired. The anchor can be made from a latex catheter segment 3 cm long; holes are cut on either side and the feeding tube is placed through them, creating a crossbar-shaped apparatus. A clamp is inserted through the openings, and the feeding tube pulled through the anchor. Placement of the anchor can be adjusted to the proper depth before the catheter is inserted in the stoma. About 1 cm of feeding tube should show between the abdominal skin and the crosspiece.[7]

If a feeding tube must be removed, the physician must know what type of tube was placed. A Foley catheter replacement tube is the easiest to remove by deflating the balloon. Other types of tubes stabilized by small "mushroom" anchors may be removed with traction through the stoma. Other types may be sutured in place or have a large anchoring apparatus that cannot be pulled through. The external portion of the tube does not always indicate the type of anchoring apparatus. Cutting the tube at the skin and pushing the remaining stump of the tube back into the stomach should be avoided unless endoscopic removal is planned. Intestinal obstruction is possible, especially in children. Removal of certain catheter designs can be facilitated by passing a stylet through the tube; this distends and elongates the internal "mushroom," allowing easier removal.

Colostomies and ileostomies are conduits between the intestinal lumen and the abdominal wall. A colostomy from the distal colon expels relatively dry feces. Right-sided colostomies and ileostomies produce more liquid material, and the increased liquid output makes care more difficult and skin irritation more likely. Daily output of an ileostomy should be between 500 and 1000 mL, discharging frequently throughout the day. Ileostomies are usually covered by an open-ended pouch that can be emptied easily, because frequent removal of a close-ended pouch would promote skin breakdown. Colostomies usually have a closed pouch because of the decreased frequency of emptying. All pouches should have no more than 1/16- to 1/8-in. clearance around the stoma, or skin breakdown will occur. Continent ileostomies consist of a pouch with a nipple that can be cannulated to remove intestinal products.

During the immediate postoperative period, the most dangerous complication of an ostomy is gangrene of the stoma. This is caused by a decreased blood supply to the artificially formed "anus." The visible mucosa should be pink and moist; dark or black mucosa suggests gangrene. It is impossible to tell how far the gangrene extends from an external examination; it may involve the intraperitoneal area and lead to peritonitis. These patients must be taken to the operating room and the wound opened to determine the extent of involvement and to resect the gangrenous segment.

Strictures and prolapse of the stoma are also seen; the latter is more common in ileostomies. A prolapsed stoma can be manually reduced but often recurs. Stoma retraction may occur and is usually secondary to increased tension on the bowel. Clinically, the stoma will appear to be level with the skin or below it.[5] Skin breakdown is more common around ileostomies due to the more erosive material. Abscess formation can occur around colostomies or ileostomies. Peristomal fistula is seen in the setting of ileostomy performed for Crohn disease. Patients with ileostomies may also be prone to diarrhea and severe electrolyte disturbances. Food blockage of an ileostomy may result in complaints of abdominal pain, decreased output, or increased watery output. The patient may also provide a history of eating foods that are poorly digested.

Life-threatening complications and threatened integrity of the ostomy require surgical evaluation. Improved maintenance of appliances and prevention of skin breakdown are facilitated by skilled ostomy care nurses.

URINARY CONDUITS

Artificial conduits of the urologic system facilitate urine drainage. Indwelling urethral and suprapubic catheters are used for bladder management. Infection is the most common complication. The urinary tract of patients with indwelling catheters is usually colonized by organisms (bacteriuria). Urinary tract infection occurs when there is microbial invasion of the tissues of the urinary tract. Infection results from either bacteria ascending from the perineum along the catheter, or with blockage of prostatic and ejaculatory ducts. Patients with catheters in place longer than 10 days almost always develop an infection. Infection from the urethra and bladder may cause pyelonephritis and sepsis.

Bladder and renal calculi are important complications of urinary stasis and infection. Urethral strictures and, less commonly, urethral diverticula also occur. Both can lead to recurrent infection, hematuria, urinary extravasation, abscess formation, and urethrocutaneous fistulas.[21] Fournier's gangrene is a life-threatening complication. Ischemic necrosis of the glans penis in a diabetic with an indwelling catheter has been reported, as has penile necrosis.[20] Other complications of urethral catheters include laceration, erosion, and hypospadias of the penile urethra.[16,18]

A distinct disadvantage of urethral catheters, when compared with suprapubic catheters, is the potential trauma to the urethra if the catheters are pulled out without deflating the balloon. This usually occurs in demented or mentally ill patients. In most cases, a new catheter can be replaced easily without resistance. If this is not possible, a urologist must be consulted.

Occasionally, the balloon will not deflate for removal of the catheter. One technique for balloon deflation is to pierce the balloon with a sharp instrument. Although this can be done blindly, fluoroscopic or ultrasonographic guidance can be used. With gentle traction, the balloon is drawn against the bladder neck and is punctured with a 25-gauge spinal needle. In men, this can be done suprapubically. In women, it can be done through the anterior vaginal wall,[13] or the needle can be introduced along the catheter transurethrally. These methods can lead to fragmentation of the balloon in the bladder; cystoscopy is necessary to remove the fragments and prevent a stone from forming around the foreign body.

The safest method is to cut off the adapter for the balloon channel. This alone may deflate the balloon if the problem is in the adapter. A well-lubricated, flexible angiographic guidewire or no. 26 orthopedic wire suture is inserted into the balloon channel and rotated. This should relieve the obstruction and allow the water to drain from the balloon.[10]

Regardless of which method is used, the balloon should always be inspected carefully after removal. If pieces are missing, a cystoscopy must be arranged to retrieve the balloon fragments from the bladder.

The external urine-collecting device, or condom catheter, can also cause complications: urinary tract infections, skin breakdown, and decubitus ulcers. Allergic reactions to the catheter material may also occur. Tight placement of the external catheter on the penis may cause pressure sores, erosion, and even partial gangrene or amputation of the penis.[21] Severe edema and maceration of the penile skin can develop. Urethral constriction by the external catheter can cause proximal urethral dilatation, diverticulum formation, and, potentially, urinary extravasation, abscesses, and fistula formation.[21]

Patients who do not have a functional bladder may have a urinary diversion and wear a bag appliance to collect urine.[11] A cutaneous ureterostomy is a cutaneous stoma made from the ureter. Common complications include infection, necrosis of the stoma, and stomal stenosis. Infection can be treated with local wound care and oral antibiotics if the patient is not febrile, immunocompromised, or septic. If infection of the urinary tract is suspected, the patient may require admission and intravenous antibiotics. Stenosis and necrosis of the stoma require urologic consultation.

Urinary diversion by a bowel conduit consists of diverting the urine to a short bowel segment, usually the ileum, that is directed to the anterior abdominal wall. Complications include infection; intestinal obstruction; stoma necrosis, stenosis, and hemorrhage; parastomal hernia; and upper urinary tract deterioration secondary to infection or ureterointestinal obstruction. Infections can be local or involve the upper urinary tract. Upper tract infections are common secondary to chronic bacteriuria in association with a refluxing conduit. These patients may require hospitalization and intravenous antibiotics.

To obtain a clean urine specimen from a bowel conduit, a double-catheter specimen is taken. The tip of a 20F red rubber catheter is cut off. A smaller 12F or 14F red rubber catheter is inserted and held retracted inside the larger one. Both are inserted into the stoma so that a clean urine specimen can be obtained from the smaller catheter; the larger catheter is used to protect the smaller one from bacterial contamination.

Bowel conduits may have complications related to intestinal surgery (ileus or intestinal obstruction due to adhesions); consultation is necessary. Ureterointestinal obstruction can also occur, often secondary to malignancy. Gradual contraction of the stoma site occurs in most patients; if significant, this requires stomal revision. Bleeding can occur if there is superficial separation of the bowel mucosa from the stoma. The treatment is good stoma care. Stomal necrosis requires urgent consultation. Parastomal hernia formation is treated as any abdominal wall hernia.

Ureteral stents (Fig. 33.4) are used to ensure urine flow from the kidney. Common complications are obstruction, migration, and infection. All stents result in some morbidity (irritative voiding symptoms, hematuria, and flank pain during micturition). To some degree, all stents undergo encrustation by mineral deposition. This can be minimized by maintaining a dilute urine and preventing infection. In addition, acidification of the urine may help prevent encrustation.[1] If obstruction is suspected, an ultrasound, renal scan, or intravenous pyelogram is useful. Urologic consultation is necessary. Migration of the stent must also be ruled out in patients with persistent pain or significant bleeding. A kidney–ureter–bladder view is obtained, and the stent's position is checked. The proximal curl should be overlying the kidney, the distal curl overlying the bladder. There is an increased incidence of vesicoureteral reflux after stent placement, so urinary tract infections are common.

The Tenckhoff catheter (Fig. 33.5) is the most widely used catheter in patients on chronic ambulatory peritoneal dialysis. It is made of silicone rubber and has one or two cuffs made of Dacron velour. The cuff permits collagen tissue ingrowth between the fibers, which anchors the catheter. Complications occurring during long-term use of peritoneal catheters include local infections, peritonitis, catheter malfunction, cuff extrusion, and pericatheter hernias. Local infections are common at the skin exit site and are usually secondary to staphylococci. A culture should be taken, and antistaphylococcal antibiotic therapy started. Close follow-up and meticulous exit-site care are necessary. These superficial infections can progress to subcutaneous tunnel infections. The skin should be cleansed daily, and the

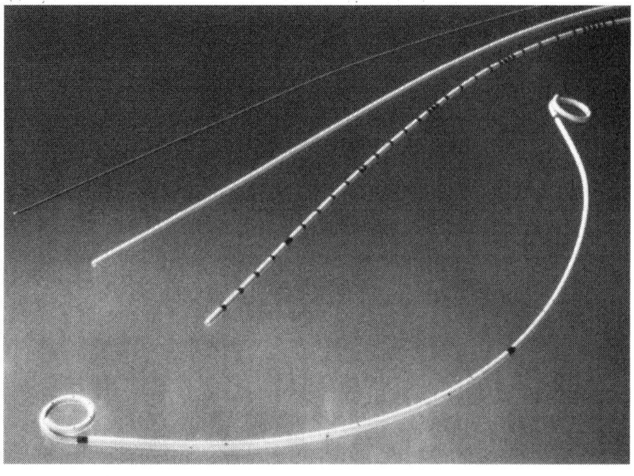

Figure 33.4. Ureteral indwelling, double-pigtail stent set. The coiled ends of the double-pigtail stent prevent migration. (Courtesy of Cook Urological Inc.)

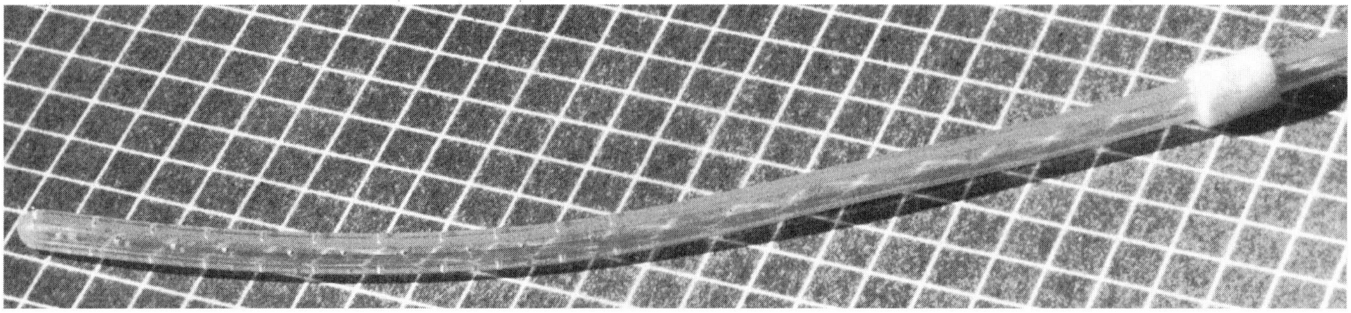

Figure 33.5. Tenckhoff peritoneal catheter. This catheter is surgically implanted through the lower abdominal wall. (Courtesy of Bard Access Systems, Inc.)

catheter immobilized to prevent trauma and tension. If infection is suspected to involve the subcutaneous cuff or the catheter tunnel, or if the patient shows signs of peritonitis, the patient is admitted for intravenous antibiotics with surgical consultation. Cuff extrusion can occur following infection or can result from pressure necrosis of the skin at the catheter exit site. Catheter replacement is necessary.

Tenckhoff catheter malfunction usually involves obstruction of the catheter. Two-way obstruction is usually secondary to intraluminal occlusion by fibrin clots. These can be dislodged by forceful irrigation with a syringe or dissolved by fibrinolytic agents. One-way or outflow obstruction presents as reduction in drainage flow, complete failure to drain, or abdominal pain during drainage or infusion. This is caused by displacement of the catheter in the upper abdomen, encasement of the catheter by adhesions or omentum, or catheter obstruction by incarceration of tissue within the side holes. Catheter revision or replacement is usually necessary. Slow drainage from the catheter may be secondary to constipation and responds well to bowel stimulation by enema. This should be ruled out first before looking for a mechanical cause of catheter failure. Surgical consultation is necessary before catheter manipulation. Pericatheter hernias are managed as any abdominal wall hernia. The physician must be suspicious of peritonitis whenever there is leakage around the catheter.

NEUROSURGICAL CONDUITS

The ventriculoperitoneal (VP) shunt diverts cerebrospinal fluid (CSF) to the peritoneal cavity in hydrocephalus. Shunt malfunction and infection may be neurosurgical emergencies.

VP shunts comprise three parts: an intracranial ventricular catheter, a shunt device, and a distal catheter. The intracranial catheter is usually positioned with the distal tip in the front horn of a lateral ventricle. Most shunts have some type of one-way valve to prevent reflux. Shunts can have one or two chambers and can be dome-shaped or cylindrical. They can be tested by digital pressure on the pumping chamber to demonstrate shunt patency both distally and proximally. The emergency physician must know the type of shunt the patient has in order to test it properly. If it cannot be pumped easily, a distal obstruction is likely; if the chamber does not refill easily, there is probably a proximal obstruction. Shunts are labeled with radiopaque material to make radiologic study possible when evaluating for obstruction.

Mechanical obstruction of VP shunts is the most common complication. Obstruction can be caused by disconnection, kinking of tubing, valve and reservoir leakage, and blockage by CSF cellular elements. Clinically, the signs of obstruction are those of increased intracranial pressure. Patients have headache, decreased level of consciousness, nausea, and vomiting. Sudden obstruction may progress rapidly to herniation and death if untreated. By evaluating the function of the pumping chamber, it may be possible to tell whether the obstruction is distal or proximal, but leakage or disconnection cannot be ruled out. Plain radiographs of skull, chest, and abdomen will help determine what type of shunt is present and may demonstrate kinking or disconnection. Cranial computed tomography scanning determines the intracranial position and other pathology, such as hematoma. Puncture and drainage of the reservoir may relieve increased intracranial pressure if there is a distal obstruction, but most obstructions are proximal and this will not help. Ventricular puncture by the neurosurgeon may be life-saving.

Infection can be a serious complication; most infections are caused by *Staphylococcus epidermidis*. Ninety percent of infections occur within the first 4 months after insertion.[14] The patient may have nonspecific symptoms such as nausea and vomiting, fever, and erythema over the device. All patients with suspected shunt infections are admitted for intravenous antibiotics. In addition to CSF infection, patients may have peritonitis from the distal tube eroding into abdominal organs or from contamination from a primary shunt infection. In the patient with a VP shunt and an acute abdomen, aspiration of the shunt may rule out shunt infection as the source of peritonitis.

COMMON PITFALLS

- Sepsis must be ruled out in febrile patients with an indwelling central venous catheter or an arteriovenous fistula.
- A central venous dialysis catheter or arteriovenous fistula should not be used for access in the emergency department unless standard attempts at intravenous access have failed and access is important.
- The patient with a stoma and fever or signs of sepsis should be examined for necrosis or gangrene of the stomal mucosa.
- The intracranial pressure should be assessed in patients with obstructed VP shunts; the intracranial pressure may rise rapidly, requiring immediate neurosurgical consultation.

References

1. Adams J. Renal stents. *Emerg Med Clin North Am* 1994;12(3):749.
2. Anderson AJ, Krasnow SH, Boyer MW, et al. Hickman catheter clots: a common occurrence despite daily heparin flushing. *Cancer Treat Rep* 1987;71:651.
3. Barton B, Hermann G, Weil R. Cardiothoracic emergencies associated with subclavian hemodialysis catheters. *JAMA* 1983;250:2660.
4. Bentz ML, Tollett CA, Dempsey DT. Obstructed feeding jejunostomy tube: a new method of salvage. *J Parenter Enter Nutr* 1988;12:417.
5. Borkowski S. Pediatric stomas, tubes and appliances. *Pediatr Clin North Am* 1998;45(6):1419.
6. Cervia J, Caputo T, Davis S, et al. Septic pulmonary embolism complicating a central venous catheter. *Chest* 1990;98:1526.
7. Collure D. A technique of anchoring a catheter in a feeding gastrostomy. *Am J Surg* 1982;144:370.

8. Ferrara B. Thrombotic complications of the Hickman catheter. *J Fla Med Assoc* 1987;74:255.
9. Hackeling T, Triana R, Ma J, et al. Emergency care of patients with tracheostomies: a 7 year review. *Am J Emerg Med* 1998;16(7):681.
10. Hessl JM. Removal of Foley catheter when balloon does not deflate. *Urology* 1983;22:219.
11. Hollander JB, Diokno AC. Urinary diversion and reconstruction in the patient with spinal cord injury. *Urol Clin North Am* 1993;20:465.
12. Jacobs MB, Yeager M. Thrombotic and infectious complications of Hickman-Broviac catheters. *Arch Intern Med* 1984;144:1597.
13. Kleeman FJ. Techniques for removal of Foley catheter when balloon does not deflate. *Urology* 1983;21:416.
14. Madsen MA. Emergency department management of ventriculoperitoneal CSF shunts. *Ann Emerg Med* 1986;15:1330.
15. Manheimer F, Aranda C, Smith RL. Necrotizing pneumonitis caused by 5-fluorouracil infusion: a complication of a Hickman catheter. *Cancer* 1992;70:554.
16. McDowell G, Hayden L, Wise H. Penile necrosis secondary to an indwelling Foley catheter. *J Urol* 1987;138:1243.
17. McGovern R, Borkin JS, Goldberg RI, et al. Duodenal obstruction: a complication of percutaneous endoscopic gastrostomy tube migration. *Am J Gastroenterol* 1990;85:1037.
18. Merguerian PA, Erturk E, Hulbert WC, et al. Peritonitis and abdominal free air due to intraperitoneal bladder perforation associated with indwelling urethral catheter drainage. *J Urol* 1985;134:747.
19. Morales M, et al. Superior vena cava thrombosis secondary to Hickman catheter and complete resolution after fibrinolytic therapy. *Support Care Cancer* 1997;5(1):67.
20. Nacey JN, Delahunt B, Neale TJ, et al. Ischemic necrosis of the glans penis: a complication of urethral catheterization in a diabetic man. *Aust N Z J Surg* 1990;60:819.
21. Selzman A, Hampel N. Urologic complications of spinal cord injury. *Urol Clin North Am* 1993;20:453.

Bibliography

Massry SG, Glossack RJ, eds. *Textbook of nephrology.* Baltimore: Williams & Wilkins, 1989.

Roberts JR, Hedges J, eds. *Clinical procedures in emergency medicine,* 2nd ed. Philadelphia: WB Saunders, 1991.

Schrier RW, Gottschalk CW, eds. *Diseases of the kidney,* vol. 3, 5th ed. Boston: Little, Brown and Company, 1993.

Shackelford RT, Zuidema GD, eds. *Surgery of the alimentary tract,* 2nd ed. Philadelphia: WB Saunders, 1982.

Walsh P, Retik A, Stamey T, et al., eds. *Campbell's urology,* 6th ed. Philadelphia: WB Saunders, 1992.

CHAPTER 34

Surgical Causes of Abdominal Pain

Robert M. McNamara

Acute abdominal pain accounts for approximately 5% to 10% of all presenting complaints in the emergency department (ED).[5] The cause is nonspecific or unknown in most cases; in 14% to 40% of cases, the cause is surgical.[5,6] The challenge for the emergency physician is significant because roughly one-third have an atypical presentation.[19] In the ED, the disease is often in its least advanced stage, and the signs and symptoms are poorly defined. Efforts to reach a correct initial diagnosis are often vital. In the elderly patient, an ED misdiagnosis results in a mortality rate nearly 2.5 times higher than if the correct diagnosis is made and the patient is admitted.[7]

A complete and accurate history and physical examination are the keys to determining whether abdominal pain is surgical in nature. Diagnostic testing is often misleading or causes undue delay; it should never be a substitute for a complete history and physical examination.[18] An understanding of the physiology and mechanisms of the three types of abdominal pain (visceral, somatic or parietal, and referred) is valuable to the clinician.

Visceral Pain

Visceral nerve fibers are found within the muscular walls of hollow organs and the capsules of solid organs. They are stimulated primarily by stretching, distention, and excessive contractions. Visceral pain is characteristically deep, dull, aching or cramping, and poorly localized. The afferent impulses reach the spinal cord through several midline nerve trunks. As a result, visceral pain is usually felt in the midline.[8,9] Several viscera can share a common pathway and cause pain in the same area. For example, afferents of the stomach, gallbladder, and pancreas combine in the celiac plexus, and visceral pain from all three organs can be felt in the epigastrium. The visceral peritoneum and viscera are insensitive to touch, so pure visceral pain may be unaccompanied by tenderness, although the patient may typically move about or be restless.[9,14]

Parietal (Somatic) Pain

The parietal peritoneum is sensitive to noxious stimuli because of somatic sensory innervation. Afferent fibers travel to a specific level of the spinal cord from T6 to L1, making this pain more localized.[8,9] It is characteristically sharper and aggravated by stimulation of the parietal peritoneum with movement, coughing, or walking.[22] The patient with parietal pain will generally lie still.[5] Parietal pain in the surgical abdomen may develop acutely (ulcer perforation) or can follow visceral pain (appendicitis), in which visceral distention progresses to inflammation. The presence of true parietal pain usually indicates a surgical cause of abdominal pain.

Referred Pain

Pain felt at a site other than that of the primary noxious stimulus is called referred pain. Most visceral pain is of this type, but use of this term usually implies pain felt at a distant or extraabdominal location from the diseased organ. Referred pain occurs in an area supplied by the same neurosegment as the involved organ.[8] The stimulus is usually intense and most often secondary to an inflammatory lesion.

CLINICAL PRESENTATION

Only through careful performance of the history and physical examination can the emergency physician avoid missing a subtle presentation of early surgical disease or ascribing a surgical cause to a nonabdominal or medical cause of abdominal pain.

History

Pain is a subjective experience, largely affected by psychological traits, ethnic and cultural background, and events surrounding its occurrence. Full patient cooperation should be sought and, if possible, sufficient time allowed for the patient to adequately describe what he or she is feeling. An ordered approach is helpful and should cover the following areas.

Time of Onset

Pain that awakens the patient from sleep is almost always significant.[18] The length of time a pain has been present should be correlated with the expected findings for the diagnosis under consideration. For example, a high temperature would not be expected early in the course of an appendicitis. Some suggest that abdominal pain that has been present for 6 or more hours usually requires surgical intervention.[18]

Mode of Onset

A sudden, severe onset of pain, especially if coupled with weakness or fainting, implies a surgical condition of a serious nature. An abdominal vascular accident, perforation, or torsion of a viscus must be considered with this history. A ruptured or dissecting aneurysm, ulcer perforation, volvulus, or ruptured ectopic pregnancy may have such a presentation.[1,18] Such a precipitous onset with relatively unimpressive findings on examination is characteristic of an abdominal vascular accident. The absence of a sudden onset does not rule out the aforementioned conditions, especially in the elderly. For example, less than half of the patients over the age of 70 with a perforated ulcer report the sudden onset of abdominal pain.[7]

A less acute but still abrupt onset is suspicious for surgical disease, often with visceral obstruction (cholecystitis and small bowel obstruction), but also includes nonsurgical entities (renal colic and pancreatitis). Pain that begins gradually and maximizes slowly is characteristic of an inflammatory process that may be surgical (appendicitis) or medical (salpingitis).[22]

Progression Since Onset

Sustained improvement of an untreated pain is generally reassuring that the condition is nonsurgical. Progression can be diagnostic, as with appendicitis, in which a poorly described midline visceral pain becomes a localized parietal pain.[22] It may also guide the rate of intervention, such as when the intermittent pain of a bowel obstruction becomes constant, raising the possibility of vascular compromise.

Location

When pain is parietal, basic anatomy usually indicates the involved organs. Visceral pain is poorly localized but can be expected to occur in a constant midline location. Upper tract lesions down to the duodenum will cause epigastric pain. Disease of the small intestine and proximal colon, including appendicitis, localizes periumbilically, whereas colonic and pelvic diseases are noted in the hypogastrium.[9]

Character

The severity of pain usually parallels the magnitude of the condition. Excruciating pain is typical of a perforated ulcer, mesenteric ischemia,[15] or a dissecting or ruptured aneurysm. Compromise of visceral circulation by gastric or colonic volvulus also causes severe pain. However, severe pain is not always surgical (pancreatitis), and the individual pain threshold should be evaluated as well.

True colicky pain is intermittent, rhythmic, and the hallmark of small bowel obstruction, but it can also be seen with simple gastroenteritis. Biliary colic, although related to an obstructive process, is usually steady. In the elderly patient, altered pain perception or underreporting of pain severity can create significant diagnostic problems.[3] Therefore, any abdominal pain in the elderly must be evaluated carefully.

Radiation and Referral

Referred pain patterns may be virtually diagnostic. Biliary tract disease typically causes upper abdominal pain that radiates to the ipsilateral shoulder or scapula. Pain of renal origin often radiates to the groin or testes[18]; diaphragmatic irritation may cause shoulder pain.

Influencing Factors

Pain aggravated by coughing, walking, or movement is typical of pain of parietal origin and usually indicates a surgical lesion.[9] It is useful to ascertain the effects of transport to the ED. A patient with peritoneal irritation may indicate increased abdominal pain due to jarring of the vehicle on an uneven road surface. Pleuritic pain can indicate diaphragmatic irritation[18] or be a clue to a nonabdominal cause.[14] Relieving factors, particularly medication, should also be ascertained.

Previous Episodes

Recurrent episodes of a similar pain usually indicate a medical condition.[14] Serious pathology, however, such as mesenteric ischemia, can present as recurrent pain. Efforts should be made to uncover the results of any previous investigation of the abdominal pain.

Associated Symptoms

Gastrointestinal symptoms are common with both surgical and nonsurgical conditions. In surgical diseases, however, the abdominal pain nearly always precedes vomiting, whereas the converse is true in 75% of cases of gastroenteritis or nonspecific causes.[5] An important exception to this is Boerhaave syndrome, in which severe pain from esophageal rupture follows vomiting or retching. In other surgical conditions, vomiting ranges from nearly universal (small bowel obstruction) to uncommon (ulcer perforation).

The character and quality of the vomiting should be investigated. Violent retching with little vomitus and severe epigastric pain is characteristic of gastric volvulus. Vomiting that progresses from gastric contents to bilious to feculent is virtually diagnostic of small bowel obstruction.[18]

Anorexia is an important symptom; it is felt that the presence of hunger should raise doubts about the diagnosis of appendicitis.[18] However, a pooled analysis of several studies on appendicitis indicated a sensitivity of only 68% for anorexia.[22] Diarrhea does not rule out a surgical condition. For example, diarrhea is often reported by patients with appendicitis,[22] mesenteric infarction,[21] and even bowel obstruction.[8]

Associated weakness or fainting should raise suspicion for a serious condition. In one series, syncope was part of the presenting picture in 23% of patients with a ruptured abdominal aortic aneurysm.[1]

Further History

A pertinent review of systems, medical history, and social history must not be forgotten. Genitourinary and cardiopulmonary symptoms may indicate a nonsurgical cause of pain. Gynecologic history is important in detecting ectopic pregnancy or distinguishing salpingitis from appendicitis. The presence of pregnancy may alter certain diagnostic tests. Pregnancy also may obscure the presentation, especially in appendicitis.[22] A list of current medications should be obtained, paying particular attention to drugs that can cause pancreatitis and peptic ulcer disease. The social history, particularly in regard to alcohol use, must not be neglected.

Physical Examination

Patient cooperation should be established through reassurance and a careful explanation of what is to be done and why. The patient's clinical condition often limits the extent of the examination before intervention, but efforts for completeness are essential. The primary focus is on the vital signs, the abdominal examination, and the adjacent organs.

General Appearance and Attitude

Pallor and diaphoresis are strong indicators of a serious condition. Many patients may appear deceivingly well.[18] The patient with peritoneal irritation will lie immobile, reluctant to move, and may lie curled up to ease tension on the irritated peritoneum. Those with visceral pain tend to be restless in bed.[9,18]

Vital Signs

A rectal temperature should be obtained. A high fever early in the course of a surgical cause of abdominal pain is uncommon, except in cholangitis. A normal temperature is often seen in appendicitis[22] and in most patients with mesenteric infarction[21]; it should not lead the clinician astray. Tachycardia and hypotension associated with pain of recent onset suggest hemorrhage from a ruptured abdominal aneurysm or an ectopic pregnancy. Tachypnea may indicate a nonabdominal cause of the pain or metabolic acidosis.[14]

Abdominal Inspection and Auscultation

Distention is common with large bowel obstruction, including cecal and sigmoid volvulus. Auscultation is one of the least valuable and potentially misleading steps in the examination.[18] Total silence is uncommon, and other, more reliable signs are usually present with peritonitis.

Palpation

Palpation is the most critical step. The goal is to define an anatomic area of maximal tenderness. This allows a narrowing of the diagnostic possibilities. Warm hands, verbal preparation, and a gentle manner yield the best results. Relaxing the abdominal muscles by thigh flexion also permits a better examination.[18] Palpation should begin in the area farthest from the expected site of maximal tenderness.[18] Gentle palpation usually suffices, and the use of one finger may aid localization. Pure visceral pain may be unaccompanied by tenderness.[9,14] The presence of masses and organomegaly is determined and the size of the abdominal aorta ascertained in older patients.

Rebound tenderness is significant pain elicited by sudden release of a deeply palpating hand. This is distressing to the patient and, while sensitive for the presence of peritonitis, this test has an unacceptable false-positive rate (specificity of 50%).[10] It is recommended that more reliable information may be obtained with light percussion or gentle rocking of the pelvis.[9] Rigidity is a significant sign of peritonitis. Voluntary guarding should be assessed with the thighs flexed and the patient taking a deep breath.

In the older patient, guarding or muscular rigidity may be absent despite serious intraabdominal pathology and peritoneal irritation.[3] This may be partially attributed to the relatively thin musculature of the abdominal wall in older patients. For example, only 21% of those over the age of 70 with a perforated ulcer present with epigastric rigidity.[7] Palpation of the elderly abdomen must be done carefully to detect subtle increases in muscle tone, as this may indicate a serious underlying condition.

Other Signs

Inflammation over the psoas muscle can be detected by passive thigh extension and may indicate appendicitis. Hypogastric pain on internal rotation of the flexed thigh may be due to an abscess overlying the obturator internus.[22] Having the patient raise up on the toes and then drop on the heels, or striking of the heels, may indicate peritonitis. This is reportedly more accurate than rebound for appendicitis.[10,11] The cough test, which involves having the patient cough and observing for flinching, grimacing, or moving of the hands toward the abdomen, has been reported to have a sensitivity of 78% and a specificity of 79% for peritonitis.[4]

Further Examination

All hernial orifices should be inspected, with care taken not to overlook the femoral canal. The pelvic examination yields information regarding salpingitis, ectopic pregnancy, and ovarian problems. The rectal examination is recommended for appendicitis but is not specific for appendicitis.[22] In males, a testicular examination should be done to assess for epididymitis or torsion.

Femoral pulses are usually normal in a ruptured aneurysm, but a dissecting aneurysm may cause an inequity.[18] Special attention to the lung, heart, and flanks and to skin lesions should assist in detecting nonsurgical causes of pain.

DIFFERENTIAL DIAGNOSIS

It is inevitable that a certain percentage of laparotomies reveal no surgical lesions. The emergency physician can decrease this percentage by ensuring that the initial history and physical examination are performed accurately and by being aware of the variety of conditions that can cause abdominal pain (Table 34.1, Fig. 34.1).

In the patient with upper abdominal pain, myocardial infarction, pulmonary embolism, spontaneous pneumothorax, and pulmonary infections must be considered.[14] Genitourinary disease, including testicular torsion, pyelonephritis, renal colic, and ovarian cysts, can cause significant abdominal pain.[14] Salpingitis is one condition commonly mistaken for appendicitis.[22]

Pancreatitis is an important medical cause of pain that leads to unnecessary surgery. Diabetic ketoacidosis, adrenal crisis, hypercalcemia, sickle cell anemia, black widow spider bites, and plumbism may cause an acute abdomen. Joint symptoms combined with a rash may indicate systemic lupus erythematosus or Henoch-Schönlein purpura, whereas a rash alone may establish the diagnosis of herpes zoster. Uncommon familial causes include acute intermittent porphyria, familial Mediterranean fever, and hereditary angioneurotic edema. The spinal nerves may be the source of pain with spinal tuberculosis, discitis, vertebral osteomyelitis, Paget disease, or malignancy.[14]

TABLE 34.1. Causes of Acute Abdominal Pain in the Emergency Department

Cause	Percentage of Cases
Nonspecific abdominal pain	41–46
Appendicitis	4–24
Cholecystitis	2.5–9
Gastroenteritis	7
Salpingitis	2–7
Urinary tract infection	3–5
Small bowel obstruction	2.5–4.0
Renal colic	1.5–4.0
Constipation	2
Pancreatitis	1–2
Diverticulitis	1–2
Dyamenorrhea	1–2
Ectopic pregnancy	<1
Ovarian cyst	<1
Incomplete abortion	<1
Abdominal aneurysm	<1

Compiled from Brewar RJ, Golden GT, Hitch DC, et al. Abdominal pain: an analysis of 1000 consecutive cases in a university hospital emergency room. *Am J Surg* 1976:131;219; deDombal FT. Acute abdominal pain—an OMGE survey. *Scand J Gastroenterol* 1979;14[Suppl]:29; and Wilson DH. *Practitioner* 1979;222:480.

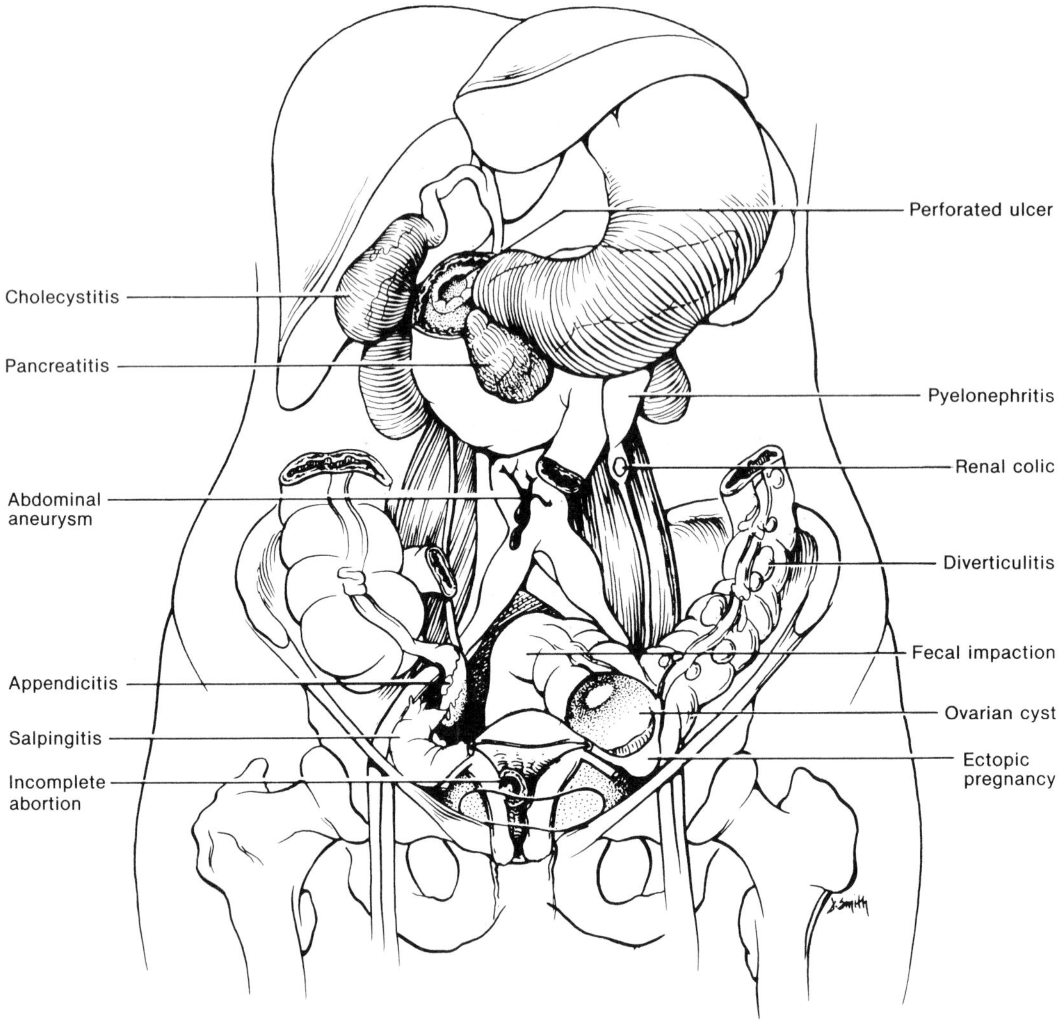

Figure 34.1. Surgical causes of abdominal pain.

EMERGENCY DEPARTMENT EVALUATION

When the presentation is undifferentiated, the most important points to remember are to avoid overreliance on diagnostic tests and to perform sequential examinations until the disease process is clarified.[18]

Sensitive, rapid pregnancy tests are available and are routinely indicated in women of childbearing age. A urinalysis may indicate pyelonephritis or a kidney stone. A complete blood count is routinely ordered. However, one study found that only 71% of patients under age 65 and 37% of those age 65 or older who required surgery for acute abdominal pain had a white blood cell (WBC) count greater than 10,000.[5] Ten percent of those with appendicitis have a normal WBC count.[17] In elderly patients, 21% with appendicitis have a normal WBC count.[16] A serum lipase or amylase may be useful if pancreatitis is a consideration. An elevated serum lactate may be seen in mesenteric ischemia.

The utility of plain abdominal radiographs is controversial. They are extremely helpful in small bowel obstruction. In ulcer perforation, up to 40% of patients may have no free air demonstrated on plain radiographs.[12] Computed tomography (CT) scanning can detect small amounts of free air and may be useful in suspected perforated ulcer when the plain radiographs are normal or equivocal. Ultrasound and CT scanning are valuable in the diagnosis of aneurysm, cholelithiasis, ectopic pregnancy, and ureterolithiasis.[20] The intravenous pyelogram, if normal on the 5-minute film, provides strong evidence against renal colic as the diagnosis. Other causes, particularly a ruptured aneurysm, should be considered.

The value of repeated examinations in nondifferentiated, acute abdominal pain cannot be overemphasized. Sustained improvement points to a nonsurgical cause; a worsening condition suggests surgical disease. An unexpected worsening may indicate the urgent need for laparotomy. The use of intensive observation and sequential examinations has successfully increased diagnostic accuracy in appendicitis.[23]

EMERGENCY DEPARTMENT MANAGEMENT

The specific therapy for each surgical cause of abdominal pain is covered in other chapters. Initial therapy includes intravenous volume replacement with isotonic fluid and gastrointestinal decompression by nasogastric suction.

The timing of narcotic analgesia is controversial. The surgeon's arrival may be delayed. The relief of severe pain is humane and may enable a more accurate history and physical examination.[2,13] Judicious doses of intravenous narcotics (titrated morphine sulfate, 2 to 5 mg i.v.) should be considered after the initial examination for patients in severe pain. If the surgeon is hostile to this approach, one must be immediately available for consultation. Naloxone, if deemed necessary, may be given to reverse the analgesic.

DISPOSITION

Urgent consultation with the appropriate surgical or gynecologic specialist is required in cases of hemodynamic compromise or suspicion of an acute vascular event. Peritonitis or the probable diagnosis of a surgical cause of pain should be quickly followed by consultation. Many cases, however, will be unclear initially, and consultation may be appropriately delayed.

A definitive or high-probability surgical cause of abdominal pain mandates admission to the hospital. If, after initial evaluation, the diagnosis is unclear, consultation may be obtained or a period of observation undertaken. If repeated evaluations over 4 hours have not clarified the situation, consultation or admission may be advisable. Elderly patients merit special consideration, as up to one-third with acute abdominal pain require surgery.[7]

It may be impossible to rule out appendicitis within the first 12 hours of abdominal pain. The surgical conditions most likely to be discharged are appendicitis and small bowel obstruction.[5] A patient who is discharged after an evaluation of abdominal pain should be instructed to return if his or her condition worsens or if the pain or vomiting persists beyond 6 to 8 hours. Benign causes of vomiting are usually self-limited. Antiemetics or narcotic analgesics are seldom indicated on discharge.

Most surgical causes of abdominal pain are adequately handled by the general surgeon. Guidelines for transfer may be found for individual entities in the corresponding chapter.

COMMON PITFALLS

- Inadequate history and physical examination are the most common sources of error in diagnosing a surgical cause of abdominal pain.
- The rebound tenderness test lacks specificity and should be replaced by gentle percussion or indirect tests, such as the cough test.
- Pain perception and the muscular response to peritoneal irritation may be altered in the older patient.
- For most findings there is a definite percentage of exceptions. This is especially true with (1) the WBC count, anorexia, and appendicitis; (2) free air and perforated ulcers; and (3) bowel obstruction and diarrhea. Overreliance on diagnostic testing should be replaced by dependence on sequential evaluation.
- The patient should not be discharged on antiemetics or narcotic analgesics.

References

1. Akkerssdijk GJ, van Bockel JH, Ruptured abdominal aortic aneurysm: initial misdiagnosis and the effect on treatment. *Eur J Surg* 1998;164:29.
2. Attard AR, Corlett MJ, Kidner NJ, et al. Safety of early pain relief for acute abdominal pain. *BMJ* 1992;305:554.
3. Bender JS. Approach to the acute abdomen. *Med Clin North Am* 1989;73:1413.
4. Bennett DH, Tambeur LJ, Campbell WB. Use of the coughing test to diagnose peritonitis. *BMJ* 1994;308:1336.
5. Brewer RJ, Golden GT, Hitch DC, et al. Abdominal pain: an analysis of 1000 consecutive cases in a university hospital emergency room. *Am J Surg* 1976;131:219.
6. deDombal FT. Acute abdominal pain—an OMGE survey. *Scand J Gastroenterol* 1979;14[Suppl]:29.
7. Fenyo G. Acute abdominal disease in the elderly. Experience from two series in Stockholm. *Am J Surg* 1982;143:751.
8. Hickey MS, Kiernan GJ, Weaver KE. Evaluation of abdominal pain. *Emerg Med Clin North Am* 1989;7:437.
9. Jung PJ, Merrell RC. Acute abdomen. *Gastroenterol Clin North Am* 1988;17:227.
10. Liddington MI, Thomson WH. Rebound tenderness test. *Br J Surg* 1991;78:795.
11. Markle GB. Heel-drop jarring test for appendicitis [Letter]. *Arch Surg* 1985;120:243.
12. Maull KL, Reath DB. Pneumogastrography in the diagnosis of perforated peptic ulcer. *Am J Surg* 1984;148:340.
13. Pace S, Burke TF. Intravenous morphine for early pain relief in patients with acute abdominal pain. *Acad Emerg Med* 1996;3:1086.
14. Purcell TB. Nonsurgical and extraperitoneal causes of abdominal pain. *Emerg Med Clin North Am* 1989;7:721.
15. Ottinger LW, Austen WG. A study of 136 patients with mesenteric infarction. *Surg Gynecol Obstet* 1967;124:251.
16. Owens BJ, Hamit HF. Appendicitis in the elderly. *Ann Surg* 1978;187:392.
17. Sasso RD, Hanna EA, Moore DL. Leukocytic and neutrophilic counts in acute appendicitis. *Am J Surg* 1970;120:563.
18. Silen W, ed. *Cope's early diagnosis of the acute abdomen,* 19th ed. New York: Oxford University Press, 1996.
19. Staniland JR, Ditchburn J, deDombal FT. Clinical presentation of acute abdomen: study of 600 patients. *BMJ* 1972;3:393.
20. Sternbach G. Abdominal ultrasound. *Ann Emerg Med* 1986;15:295.
21. Uruyama H, Ohtake H, Kawakami Y, et al. Acute mesenteric vascular occlusion: analysis of 39 patients. *Eur J Surg* 1998;164:195.
22. Wagner JM, McKinney WP, Carpenter JL. Does this patient have appendicitis? *JAMA* 276:1589.
23. White JJ, Santillara M, Haller JA. Intensive in-hospital observation: a safe way to decrease unnecessary appendectomy. *Am Surg* 1975;41:793.

CHAPTER 35

Abdominal Mass

David D. Cassidy

Patients with an abdominal mass present to the emergency department with various characteristics and consequences. An abdominal mass noticed initially by the patient may have been present for days, months, or years, or it may be discovered by the emergency physician as a new finding. The consequences of the process involved may have no influence on the patient's health, or they may cause significant disease or death. The extent of the emergency department evaluation may vary from a few minutes of discussion and physical examination to extensive laboratory and radiologic procedures leading to emergent surgery.

The incidence of patients presenting to emergency departments with abdominal masses is unknown. Often, abdominal masses as such are not coded in medical records departments; rather, they are coded as definitive diagnoses. Additionally, when discussed in medical records and literature reviews, it is not always clear whether the masses were palpable or discovered radiologically.

For the purposes of this chapter, an *abdominal mass* is defined as a palpable mass anterior to the paraspinous muscles, lying between the symphysis pubis and the costal margin. Masses palpable only on pelvic examination are discussed briefly here but are discussed in more detail in Chapter 87.

The final diagnosis of an abdominal mass may include a normal abdominal organ, as palpated in a thin patient, or abnormal shapes of physiologically normal abdominal organs. Also included are organs affected by a pathologic process and abnormal fluid collections. Occasionally, organs not usually present in the abdomen may present as palpable masses in this location.[16] Diffuse collections of air from a perforated viscus or bowel obstruction, ascitic fluid, and normal abdominal adipose tissue are not discussed in this chapter.

Normal organs often palpated in thin patients include the inferior margin of the liver, Riedel's lobe, kidney, cecum, sigmoid

TABLE 35.1. Differential Diagnosis of Abdominal Mass

INFECTION	METABOLIC AND CONGENITAL
Liver	Pancreas
Hepatitis	Pancreatitis
Hepatic abscess	Pancreatic pseudocyst
Cholecystitis	Liver and spleen
Paraintestinal abscess	Cirrhosis
Appendicitis	Amyloidosis
Diverticulitis	Storage diseases
Crohn disease	Cysts
Ulcerative colitis	Renal
Pararenal abscess	Hepatic
Spleen	Splenic
Mononucleosis	Pancreatic
Splenic abscess	
Mesenteric adenitis	**MECHANICAL AND TRAUMATIC**
NEOPLASM	
Liver	Vascular
Hepatoma	Aneurysm
Adenoma	Fistula
Metastatic disease	Hepatic vein occlusion (liver)
Gastric carcinoma	Congestive heart failure (liver)
Lymphoma	Portal hypertension (spleen)
Spleen	Bowel obstruction
Bowel	Intussusception
Lymph nodes	Volvulus
Primary bowel neoplasms	Urinary obstruction (bladder)
Renal and adrenal neoplasms	Biliary obstruction (gallbladder)
Gynecologic neoplasms	Constipation
Peritoneal and omental metastatic disease	Hernias
Abdominal wall neoplasms	Hematomas
Lipomas	Splenic
Sarcomas	Duodenal
Neuromas	Abdominal wall
Metastatic disease	

colon, aorta, and gravid uterus. Abnormal organs may be affected by various processes, including infection, neoplasm, metabolic disorders, mechanical factors, and external trauma (Table 35.1). Abnormal fluid collections, in addition to abscesses of the aforementioned organs, may include congenital cysts of the kidney, liver, spleen, and urachus. Infectious fluid collections may include any of these cysts secondarily infected, as well as loculated peritonitis, peritoneal abscess, and hydatid cysts.

CLINICAL PRESENTATION

The acuteness or chronicity of the development of signs or symptoms associated with an abdominal mass often determines the need for emergent therapy versus care delivered on an outpatient basis with appropriate follow-up. The development of sudden abdominal pain with a rapidly expanding abdomen suggests the presence of an abdominal aortic aneurysm, which requires emergent surgical therapy. Likewise, a child with progressive abdominal pain and development of an enlarging mass over a short period of time may exhibit findings suggestive of intussusception.[28] The intermittent presence of an abdominal mass may be due to a spigelian hernia.[11] Stable, nonemergent, chronic problems include palpable stool due to constipation or the large cirrhotic liver that, if accompanied by portal hypertension, may also include a palpable spleen.

The onset of new symptoms associated with chronic problems may require emergency therapy. The onset of pain and fever in a patient with palpable kidneys secondary to polycystic kidney disease may indicate the presence of either pyelonephritis or bleeding into the kidney. Similarly, nausea, vomiting, fever, and leukocytosis in a patient with a history of biliary colic may indicate cholecystitis complicating cholelithiasis.

Often, new symptoms associated with an abdominal mass may provide important clues to the diagnosis. Pain is probably the most common symptom associated with an abdominal mass (see Chapter 34). The presence of an abdominal mass in a patient with pain suggestive of pancreatitis may indicate a pancreatic pseudocyst.[6] As always, the duration, severity, location, quality, and radiation of pain are important factors to consider in patients with pain and an abdominal mass.

Gastrointestinal symptoms are often useful in determining the cause. Nausea and vomiting suggest the presence of either hepatitis or obstruction of a hollow viscus. Constipation may be due to bowel obstruction secondary to tumor or localized inflammation, such as appendicitis or diverticulitis. Anorexia is often present in appendicitis, hepatitis, and malignancy. The presence of an abdominal mass and diarrhea suggests chronic pancreatitis with pseudocyst formation, an abscess associated with chronic colitis, or a secretive process associated with villous adenoma. Although upper gastrointestinal bleeding and a left upper quadrant mass may be due to bleeding esophageal varices (with associated portal hypertension and splenomegaly), such bleeding with a pulsatile abdominal mass and back pain suggests an aortoenteric fistula.[14] Lower gastrointestinal bleeding and abdominal mass may be secondary to malignancy or to an inflammatory process with abscess formation, such as diverticular disease or colitis. Constipation, diarrhea, or a decrease in stool caliber is observed in colon cancer and tuberculous enteritis.

Genitourinary signs and symptoms may also help to determine the cause of an abdominal mass. Urinary hesitancy or urgency in the presence of a lower abdominal mass may suggest bladder distention secondary to urethral obstruction or urine retention caused by an anticholinergic medication such as a phenothiazine. The presence of hematuria suggests polycystic kidney disease, renal cell tumor, or, in the setting of an abdominal aortic aneurysm, aortocaval fistula.[25]

Signs and symptoms of upper respiratory tract infection, such as sore throat and cough, along with a left upper quadrant mass could indicate splenomegaly secondary to mononucleosis.

Constitutional signs and symptoms such as fever, chills, and weight loss help to narrow the diagnostic probabilities in patients with abdominal masses. Those with hepatomegaly, fever, and anorexia may have hepatitis. If such patients also have nightsweats and weight loss, the possibility of hepatic tuberculosis increases.[10] Those with clinical pancreatitis who also have abdominal masses and fever are more likely to have pancreatic phlegmon.[27] Fever, in addition to an abdominal aortic aneurysm, greatly increases the likelihood of a mycotic aneurysm, with a much higher mortality rate.[22] Fever may also be present in any abdominal abscess and is often present with lymphoma.

The importance of a complete history and physical examination cannot be overemphasized. This is well illustrated in a case report by McAuley and associates.[21] A patient with precipitous high-output cardiac failure, a pulsatile abdominal mass, and unilateral lower extremity venous engorgement was found to have an abdominal arteriovenous fistula. The axiom of unifying all findings under one diagnosis is clearly useful in patients with abdominal masses.

DIFFERENTIAL DIAGNOSIS

The most important characteristic of an abdominal mass is its location. Size is also important, as illustrated by the fact that very

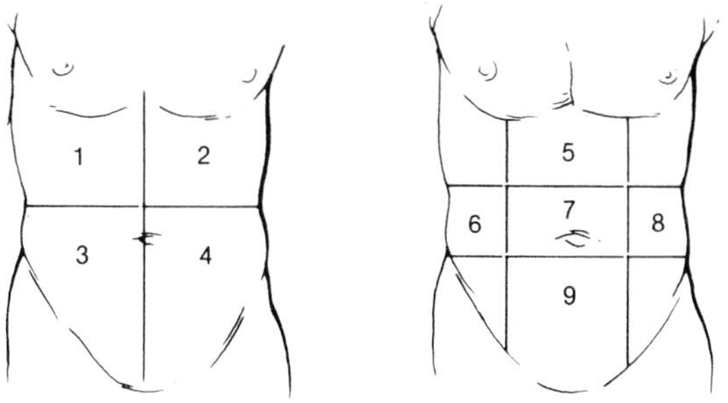

Figure 35.1. Regions of the abdomen. *(1)* Right upper quadrant. *(2)* Left upper quadrant. *(3)* Right lower quadrant. *(4)* Left lower quadrant. *(5)* Epigastric. *(6)* Right flank. *(7)* Umbilical. *(8)* Left flank. *(9)* Suprapubic.

large right upper quadrant masses are more likely to be neoplastic hepatic disease.[5] Similarly, the consistency of a mass can lead to a diagnosis. A rock-hard or nodular mass suggests a neoplasm; tenderness, an acute inflammatory process. For example, a nontender, palpable gallbladder is likely to be neither acute nor inflamed, and may be due to obstruction caused by a neoplasm. Mobility of a mass indicates that it is not attached to the abdominal wall or retroperitoneal tissue. Pulsation of the mass indicates that it is vascular in origin and may be due to an aortic aneurysm.

In Fig. 35.1, the abdomen is divided into nine overlapping areas: two upper and lower quadrants, three midline areas, and the bilateral flank regions. Table 35.2 lists the normal contents of each region. With very large masses and organomegaly, displacement of organs and masses is common. The location of various abdominal masses is shown in Fig. 35.2.

Right Upper Quadrant

Masses in the right upper quadrant usually represent either the liver or the gallbladder. A rock-hard liver suggests malignancy or cirrhosis. Tender hepatomegaly in a patient who has jaundice, anorexia, nausea, and vomiting, but is otherwise hemodynamically stable, most likely indicates hepatitis. If the patient appears toxic with fever, leukocytosis, or left shift, the possibility exists of an intrahepatic abscess. A detailed history and thorough physical examination may delineate unusual causes of hepatomegaly. A travel history may suggest a possible amebic abscess or parasitic cyst. A patient with signs of right heart failure may have congestive hepatomegaly. Enlargement of one lobe of the liver may result from tumor, high bile duct obstruction,[15] or hepatic vein occlusion.[4]

The gallbladder may be palpable in acute obstructive biliary colic without infection. Such a patient has intermittent pain without fever or leukocytosis. When accompanied by fever and leukocytosis, however, a tender right upper quadrant mass without a firm edge, suggesting a hepatic origin, should raise the possibility of cholecystitis. A nontender, palpable gallbladder with jaundice suggests a possible malignancy in the head of the pancreas or the ampulla of Vater.

TABLE 35.2. Normal Contents of the Abdomen

Right upper quadrant	Umbilical
Liver	Stomach
Gallbladder	Duodenum
Colon	Other small bowel
Right kidney	Colon
Right adrenal gland	Aorta, vena cava
Epigastric	Lymph nodes
Gallbladder	Omentum
Stomach	Left flank
Colon	Colon
Pancreas	Small bowel
Aorta	Kidney
Lymph nodes	Right lower quadrant
Left upper quadrant	Cecum
Spleen	Appendix
Stomach	Lymph nodes
Pancreas	Ovary
Left kidney	Suprapubic
Left adrenal gland	Distended bladder
Right flank	Small bowel
Liver	Sigmoid colon
Colon	Enlarged uterus
Small bowel	Left lower quadrant
Right kidney	Sigmoid colon
	Lymph nodes
	Ovary

Left Upper Quadrant

Left upper quadrant masses are generally due to splenic enlargement, and may involve pathology of gastric or pancreatic origin. Sudden, painful splenic enlargement may be due to a traumatic subcapsular hematoma. This can occur with minimal or no trauma when pathologic splenomegaly preexists, such as in patients with mononucleosis. Infections such as endocarditis and malaria may cause splenomegaly. Extremely large spleens in American adults are most often due to chronic myelocytic leukemia, portal hypertension, or myelofibrosis. A normal spleen may be displaced by a subphrenic process such as an abscess.[26] A left upper quadrant mass found in a patient presenting with abdominal distention, nausea, vomiting, and a succussion splash suggests a possible gastric malignancy or ulcer causing gastric outlet obstruction. Rarely, a left upper quadrant mass results from a foreign body in the stomach.

Epigastrium

A pulsatile mass in the epigastrium strongly suggests an abdominal aortic aneurysm. If such a mass is associated with pain, shock, or pulse disparity in the lower extremities, rupture or dissection of the aneurysm must be considered. Although pancreatic pseudocysts may be located anywhere in the abdomen, they are frequently found in the epigastrium. Such masses may be associated with shock if hemorrhage in the pseudocyst cavity occurs. Pancreatic cancer may result in a palpable mass, which is associated with aching pain, often in conjunction with wasting, anemia, and, occasionally, painless jaundice.

Periumbilical Region

Periumbilical masses may extend into other quadrants of the abdomen, epigastrium, or suprapubic region. Well-localized masses in the periumbilical region often include an umbilical hernia sac. This may be congenital, a result of surgery, or associated with blunt trauma to the abdomen.[9] The contents of such a hernia can include stomach, omentum, bowel, or adipose tissue, and should be distinguished from abdominal wall masses such as lipoma or hematoma.[24] Lymph node masses in the paraaortic region of the retroperitoneum and mesentery are palpable as a deep mass. These lymph nodes, when enlarged because of malignancy or chronic infection, are often relatively nontender. A Sister Mary Joseph's nodule is a palpable lymph node in the abdominal wall suggestive of metastatic disease from a primary gastrointestinal malignancy.

Suprapubic Region

Masses in the suprapubic region are often pelvic organs, confirmed on pelvic examination (see Chapter 87). Occasionally, a

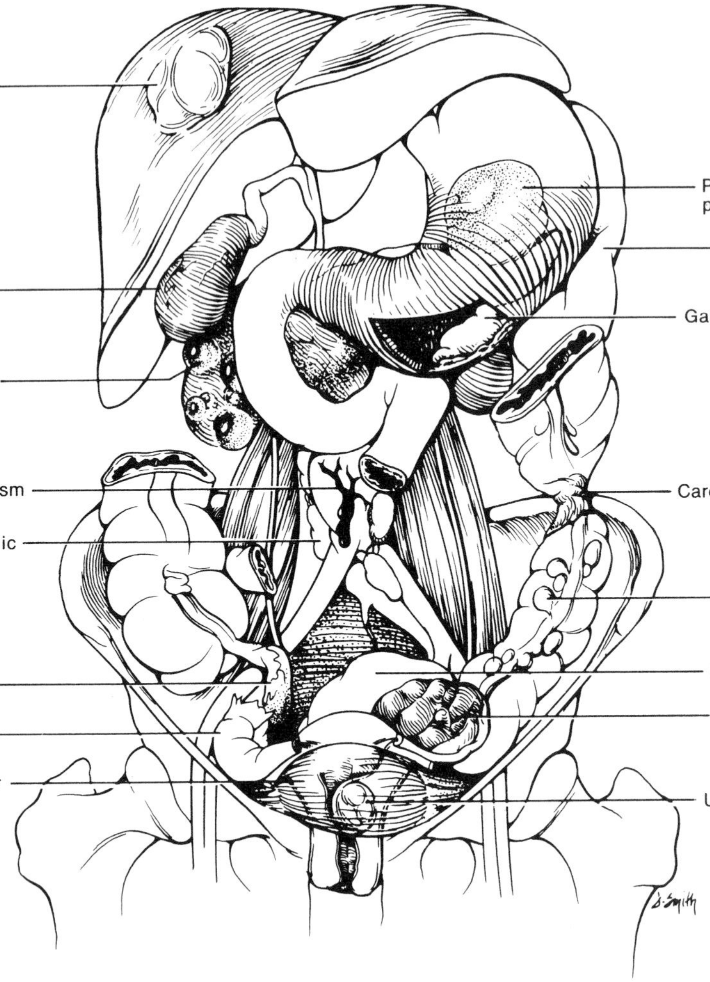

Figure 35.2. Abdominal mass.

distended bladder, which is normally midline, smooth, and moderately tender, is mistaken for a mass of other origin, such as the uterus. The distinction is often made after urinary catheterization.

Right Lower Quadrant

A mass palpated in the right lower quadrant in a healthy, thin adult is often a normal cecum. However, if it is associated with weight loss, occult blood in the stool, or a change in bowel habits, a malignancy or gastrointestinal tuberculosis should be considered. The patient with a mass and a classic history of appendicitis, but with symptoms present for more than 24 hours, possibly has an appendiceal abscess.

Left Lower Quadrant

Most left lower quadrant masses are related to the sigmoid colon. In a person who is otherwise healthy, a mass that changes shape or size may be normal stool in the sigmoid colon. A patient with diverticular disease, colitis, or malignancy may present with left lower quadrant mass and fever, suggesting a paracolic abscess.

Flank Region

Flank masses caused by kidney enlargement are often mistaken for other organs. If a mass is palpated in one flank, the other flank should also be examined for possible bilateral palpable kidneys, suggesting cystic disease. The presence of a varicocele and renal mass indicates a possible renal malignancy with renal vein thrombosis. In the right flank, a Riedel's lobe may be palpated and may occasionally be mistaken for the gallbladder or right kidney. However, close examination reveals that this mass is continuous with the liver. The sausage-shaped mass associated with intussusception is often felt in the right flank between the right upper and lower quadrants. This mass may move with time in a direction consistent with that of the colon. The additional findings of paroxysmal pain and currant-jelly stool provide further evidence for intussusception.

Finally, masses that involve abdominal organs need not be localized to the region in which the organ is usually found. Tumors of the small intestine and colon may be located in any of the abdominal regions rather than in the epigastrium.[19] The spleen, when greatly enlarged, may be palpable in the right upper quadrant.[3] When congenital failure or acquired laxity of splenic attachments occurs, the spleen may be found anywhere in the abdomen or pelvis.[7] The variants of situs inversus viscerum, although rare, must be mentioned. This disorder is suggested in the patient with heart tones on the right side or a grossly abnormal electrocardiogram.

EMERGENCY DEPARTMENT EVALUATION

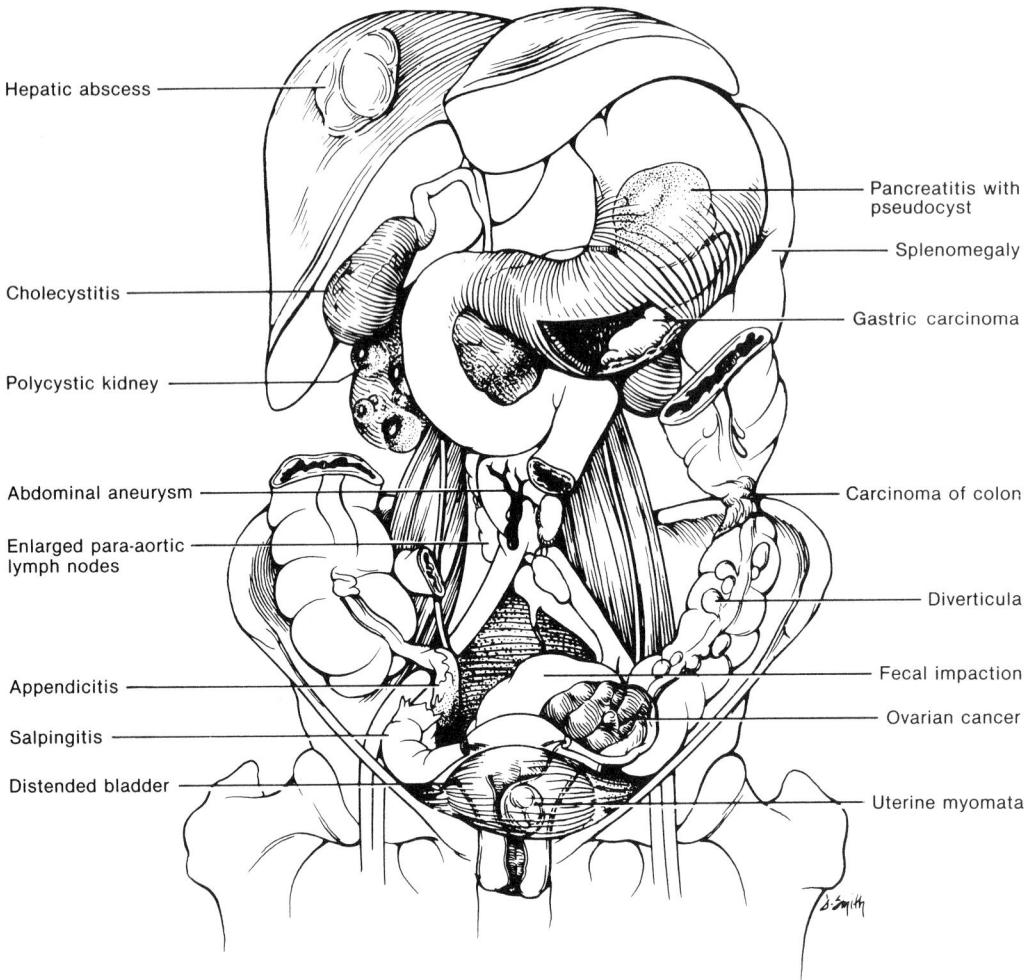

A patient who presents to the emergency department with an abdominal mass that has not been previously evaluated should undergo thoughtful evaluation. If the cause of the mass can be determined without question and found to be of a benign nature, laboratory evaluation may be unnecessary. If the cause is unknown, the patient should undergo testing for occult blood in the stool, electrolytes, a complete blood count with differential, and blood urea nitrogen and creatinine. If hepatocellular dysfunction or malnutrition is suspected, prothrombin time and liver function tests should be performed. If vomiting or diarrhea has been present, electrolytes should be measured. When metastatic disease is suspected, the blood count may reveal the presence of anemia or thrombocytopenia, and an SMA-23 may show hypercalcemia, hypomagnesemia, or elevated alkaline phosphatase (bone or liver). An unexpected abnormal laboratory value may be the only finding that steers the physician toward a correct diagnosis. For example, an elevated serum amylase level may lead to the diagnosis of pancreatic pseudocyst.[6] Although many laboratory tests do not have high predictive values for any given pathologic process, they may become abnormal in the course of a disease process. An unexpected rise in the values of liver function tests, especially the alkaline phosphatase, may suggest that a neoplastic mass distant from the liver has metastasized to the liver.

Other aspects of the emergency department evaluation must also be individualized. For patients who cannot void or who have an undiagnosed lower abdominal mass, catheterization of the urinary bladder often helps rule out urinary retention. A nasogastric tube should be placed in patients with occult blood in the stool or persistent vomiting. Patients in shock, with signs of peritoneal inflammation, or those who appear toxic should have an arterial blood gas determination in addition to the laboratory evaluation, urinary catheterization, and nasogastric tube placement.

Radiologic studies provide the greatest diagnostic assistance in determining the cause of an abdominal mass. Although plain films of the abdomen seldom lead to a specific diagnosis, they are useful in determining the presence and, occasionally, the origin of abdominal masses. Both flat and upright films of the abdomen should be obtained in most cases. Occasionally, a nonpalpable mass is seen on plain films due to displacement of other organs, such as an abdominal aortic aneurysm displacing bowel on a cross-table lateral view of the abdomen. Plain abdominal films indicate the presence of an abdominal aortic aneurysm in 55% to 85% of cases, but a negative examination does not rule out the diagnosis. Accordingly, additional imaging with computed tomography (CT) scanning or ultrasound must be performed.[13,20] A gas pattern in a mass displacing the bowel may suggest an abscess. Eighty-five percent of kidney stones and 15% of gallstones are visualized on plain abdominal films. An appendolith is thought by some to be diagnostic of appendicitis and may, after perforation, indicate an appendiceal abscess. Ingested foreign bodies can be seen on plain films and are most common in children and psychiatric patients. The presence of bowel gas outside the peritoneal cavity seen in inguinal and spigelian hernias is also useful.[11]

Ultrasonography can be used to determine the nature of abdominal masses. Often, the presence of cholelithiasis and biliary obstruction is determined by ultrasonography, as are subcapsular splenic hematomas, hydronephrosis, and aneurysms. Ultrasonography can also help in differentiating abdominal wall hematomas from incisional hernias postoperatively,[24] in detecting intussusception,[1] and in determining the cause of colonic masses, such as stool.[8] Ultrasound has been suggested as the best initial investigative tool to use in the emergency department evaluation of abdominal masses. It has positive and negative predictive values of 99% and 97%, respectively.[2] Advantages to using ultrasound include its noninvasive and portable nature, its accuracy in detecting the size of abdominal aortic aneurysms, and its usefulness in determining both intraperitoneal and intracapsular fluid accumulations. Unfortunately, ultrasound is operator-dependent and limited by obesity and gaseous distention of the bowel.[17] Emergency physicians can become proficient in goal-directed ultrasound examinations.[23]

CT scanning provides cross-sectional imaging of the entire abdominal, pelvic, and retroperitoneal structures with a high diagnostic accuracy. With the addition of intravenous contrast, vascular structures are clearly delineated and the parenchyma of many organs are enhanced.[18] Oral contrast allows for enhanced visualization of the bowel and the bowel wall. Although CT scanning and ultrasound sensitivities are both close to 100% in detecting abdominal aortic aneurysms, CT scanning has greater accuracy in determining size, detecting thrombus, defining cranial–caudal extent, demonstrating involvement with other vascular structures, and detecting a leak.[12] CT scanning is not limited by obesity and bowel gas but does require the patient to leave the department, thus creating management problems in the case of hemodynamic instability. Newer spiral CT scanners shorten scanning times considerably.

EMERGENCY DEPARTMENT MANAGEMENT

As always, life-saving measures should be instituted before evaluation. The ABCs should be attended to, and the treatment of shock should be initiated before other forms of evaluation and treatment are undertaken.

Certain emergencies require immediate recognition by the emergency physician. An abdominal aortic aneurysm (see Chapter 52), during rupture or dissection, often presents with severe pain and shock. Patients in shock are frequently "shotgunned" with rapid volume expansion. However, the pulsatile, expanding abdominal mass is often overlooked because of guarding or obesity. Careful physical examination of the abdomen and a search for other physical findings must be performed in the initial stages of resuscitation. Early blood transfusion and immediate consultation with a vascular surgeon are key factors in determining the outcome in a ruptured aortic aneurysm.

A splenic subcapsular hematoma may also present as an abdominal mass. This possibility should be considered in all patients with tender, palpable spleens, even if a history of trauma is not present. Often the initial, normal hematocrit markedly decreases after volume resuscitation with crystalloid. Ultrasonography or CT scanning can often confirm the diagnosis.

Some abdominal masses may lead to bowel obstruction (see Chapter 42). The patient with severe vomiting should be considered to have a possible bowel obstruction and should be treated accordingly, with nasogastric suction and intravenous fluids.

Patients with rupture of, or hemorrhage into, a pancreatic pseudocyst may deteriorate rapidly due to third-space losses from peritonitis or hypovolemia from hemorrhage. In addition to a possible history of pancreatitis, such patients may have an elevated serum amylase or lipase level.

Gallbladder disease (see Chapter 39) may cause problems ranging from simple biliary colic to cholecystitis with severe toxicity. Patients in the latter group with palpable gallbladders may have an empyema of the gallbladder, which necessitates immediate surgical consultation and treatment.

DISPOSITION

All the problems noted in the preceding section necessitate consultation with either a general or a vascular surgeon as soon as the diagnosis is considered. The precise diagnosis of these problems need not be made before the initial consultation. Patients who present with fever, peritoneal signs, or intractable pain also require surgical consultation after completion of the initial evaluation. Admission to the hospital is the usual disposition of these patients.

Many patients with abdominal masses may be evaluated as outpatients. Determining the best method of evaluation depends somewhat on the preferences of the patient, physician, and institution, as well as consideration of relative costs. The availability and reliability of the patient also must be considered. Referral should be to a primary care provider who can assume responsibility for coordinating further studies.

COMMON PITFALLS

- The physician may initially fail to include a vital diagnosis in the early differential. Patients in shock require early evaluation for possible abdominal aortic aneurysm or pancreatic pseudocyst. Conversely, patients with huge lower abdominal masses often undergo extensive evaluation because urinary retention was not considered.
- Failure to do an adequate initial physical examination may result in a delayed or missed diagnosis.
- Inadequate documentation of findings may result in the failure of subsequent caregivers to recognize progression of disease.
- Inadequate resuscitation and failure to obtain timely surgical consultation may adversely affect the outcome.
- Failure to arrange for realistic, accomplishable follow-up plans for outpatient evaluation may result in patients being lost to follow-up. Many patients who are referred are not recognized as being unable to follow through with referrals because of alcoholism, transportation problems, language barriers, or financial concerns. These factors may dictate the need for admission.

References

1. Alessi V, Salerno G. The "hay-fork" sign in the ultrasonographic diagnosis of intussusception. *Gastrointest Radiol* 1985;10:177.
2. Baker CS, Lindsell DRM. Ultrasound of the palpable abdominal mass. *Clin Radiol* 1990;41:98.
3. Barloon TJ, Lu C. Lymphoma presenting as an abdominal mass involving an ectopic spleen. *Am J Gastroenterol* 1984;79:684.
4. Becker CD, Scheidegger J, Marincek B. Hepatic vein occlusion—morphologic features on computed tomography and ultrasonography. *Gastrointest Radiol* 1986;11:305.
5. Berezin A, Seltzer SE. Differential diagnosis of huge abdominal masses visualized on CT scans. *Comput Radiol* 1984;8:95.
6. Bodurtha AJ, Dajee H, You CK. Analysis of 29 cases of pancreatic pseudocyst treated surgically. *Can J Surg* 1980;23:432.
7. Collins JC, Cheek RC. Chronic torsion of the spleen. *Am Surg* 1976;42:427.
8. Derchi LE, Musante F, Biggi E, et al. Sonographic appearance of fecal masses. *J Ultrasound Med* 1985;4:573.
9. Fullerton JC, Saltzstein ED, Peacock JB. Traumatic hernia of the anterior abdominal wall. *J Emerg Med* 1984;1:213.
10. Gallinger S, Strasberg SM, Marcus HI, et al. Local hepatic tuberculosis, the cause of a painful hepatic mass—case report and review of the literature. *Can J Surg* 1986;29:451.
11. Ginaldi S. Spigelian hernia. *Ann Emerg Med* 1987;16:455.
12. Gnomes MN, Choyke PL. Pre-operative evaluation of abdominal aortic aneurysms: ultrasound or computed tomography? *J Cardiovasc Surg* 1987;28:159.
13. Gnomes MN, Schellinger D, Hufnagel C. Abdominal aortic aneurysm—diagnostic review and new techniques. *Ann Thorac Surg* 1979;27:479.
14. Grigsby WS, Eitzen EM, Boyle DJ II. Aortoenteric fistula: a catastrophe waiting to happen. *Ann Emerg Med* 1986;15:731.
15. Hadjis NS, Hemingway A, Carr D, et al. Liver lobe disparity consequent upon atrophy—diagnostic, operative and therapeutic considerations. *J Hepatol* 1986;3:285.
16. Hansen GR, Laing FC. Sonographic evaluation of a left ventricular aneurysm presenting as an upper abdominal mass. *J Clin Ultrasound* 1980;8:151.
17. Harris JH. *The radiology of emergency medicine*, 3rd ed. Baltimore: Williams & Wilkins, 1993:623.
18. Kapoor R, Hemmer K, Herbert O, et al. Abdominal computed tomography. *Arch Intern Med* 1983;143:249.
19. Khaw H, Sottiurai VS, Craighead CC, et al. Ruptured abdominal aortic aneurysm presenting as symptomatic inguinal mass—report of six cases. *J Vasc Surg* 1986;4:384.
20. Loughran CF. A review of the plain abdominal radiograph in acute rupture of abdominal aortic aneurysms. *Clin Radiol* 1986;37:383.
21. McAuley CE, Peitzman AB, DeVries EJ, et al. The syndrome of spontaneous iliac arteriovenous fistula: a distinct clinical and pathophysiologic entity. *Surgery* 1986;99:373.
22. McNamara MF, Roberts AB, Bakshi KR. Gram-negative bacterial infection of aortic aneurysms. *J Cardiovasc Surg* 1987;28:453.
23. Plummer D. Principles of emergency ultrasound and echocardiography. *Ann Emerg Med* 1989;18:1291.
24. Rankin RN, Hutton L, Grace DM. Postoperative abdominal wall hematomas have a distinctive appearance on ultrasonography. *Can J Surg* 1985;28:84.
25. Salo JA, Verkkala K, Ketonen P, et al. Diagnosis and treatment of spontaneous aortocaval fistula. *J Cardiovasc Surg* 1987;28:180.
26. Snape J, Baker AR, Rees Y. Pseudosplenomegaly as a result of subphrenic abscess. *Postgrad Med* 1986;62:29.
27. Sostre CF, Flournoy JG, Bova JG, et al. Pancreatic phlegmon: clinical features and course. *Dig Dis Sci* 1985;30:918.
28. Trenkner SW, Wilson JAP, Coon WW, et al. Enteric intussusception presenting as a rapidly enlarging mass. *Am J Gastroenterol* 1986;81:480.

CHAPTER 36

Abdominal Pain in the Elderly

Diane M. Birnbaumer and Katherine Bakes

People over the age of 65 are the fastest-growing segment of the population and currently account for 13% of the United States census.[19] The impact of the elderly on the practice of emergency medicine is undeniable. The elderly make up 19% of emergency department visits; two-thirds of these patients are admitted, a clear indicator of the acuity of their presentation. The elderly account for 43% of all hospital emergency department admissions and 47% of admissions to critical care units. By the year 2030, 20% to 21% of the population will be over the age of 65, and the fastest growing subset of the population is people over the age of 85.

Conditions that cause abdominal pain in the elderly are usually more serious and more urgent than in younger patients (Table 36.1). Seventy-five percent of elderly patients who present to the emergency department with abdominal pain have a diagnosis made in the emergency department, and in contrast to younger patients, most will have a surgical disease. Even those who have no obvious cause found after evaluation in the emergency department may still have significant disease; 10% of these patients with "abdominal pain of unclear etiology" are diagnosed with cancer within 6 months of presentation.

Among patients hospitalized with abdominal pain, the diagnosis of a disease that requires surgical intervention occurs twice as often in the 65-and-older group, and mortality is increased tenfold (Table 36.2). The fact that 50% to 63% of elderly patients with abdominal pain are admitted to the hospital, 20% go directly from the emergency department to the operating room, and 13% die postoperatively[14] shows that abdominal pain in the elderly is a potentially serious and potentially life-threatening problem.

TABLE 36.1. Acute Abdominal Pain in Patients Under and Over Age 50

Under 50 (6,317 cases)	%	Over 50 (2,406 cases)	%
Nonspecific abd. pain	39.5	Nonspecific abd. pain	20.9
Appendicitis	32.0	Cholecystitis	15.7
Cholecystitis	6.3	Appendicitis	15.2
Obstruction	2.5	Obstruction	12.3
Pancreatitis	1.6	Pancreatitis	7.3
Diverticular disease	<0.1	Diverticular disease	5.5
Cancer	<0.1	Cancer	4.1
Hernia	<0.1	Hernia	3.1
Vascular	<0.1	Vascular	2.3

From Telfer S, Fenyo G, Holt PR, et al. Acute abdominal pain in patients over 50 years of age. *Scand J Gastroenterol* 1988;144[Suppl]:47.

TABLE 36.2. Abdominal Emergencies in the Elderly: Diagnosis and Mortality in Patients Above Age 70

	Cases		*Mortality*	
Diagnostic Category	*n*	%	*n*	%
Acute biliary	66	33	2	3
Intestinal obstruction	51	25		
Incarcerated hernia	16		0	0
Adhesions	11		0	0
Miscellaneous benign	8		2	25
Malignant	16		10	62
Appendix	27	14	0	0
Perforated viscus	20	10	3	15
Gastrointestinal bleeding	19	9	1	5
Trauma	6	3	2	33
Miscellaneous	11	6	4	36
Total	200	100	24	12

From Reiss RR, Deutsch A. Emergency abdominal procedures in patients above 70. *J Gerontol* 1985;40:154.

Emergency physicians must be familiar with the differences in evaluating and treating elderly patients as compared with their younger counterparts.

Social Differences

The elderly differ from younger patients both socially and medically, making evaluation a challenge. The vast majority of the elderly live independently, often alone. Due to a fear of loss of independence, they may delay presentation to medical care when they develop symptoms and thus present much sicker than if they had been evaluated promptly. The elderly patient may have a complicated medical and surgical history and may be taking multiple medications. The elderly may have more than one process occurring, further compounding the difficulty of evaluation.

Physiologic Changes

The physiologic changes of the renal, immune, cardiac, pulmonary, and homeostatic systems decline with age. Changes that occur with aging alter the presentation of abdominal pain, as well as the evaluation and natural history of the process. The elderly patient may have a delayed febrile response or delayed elevation in white blood cell count compared with a younger patient with the same medical condition. The omentum shrinks with age and is therefore less able to wall off intraabdominal processes, so the elderly patient may develop peritonitis earlier than a younger patient. Muscle mass, including abdominal musculature, decreases with age, and patients with significant intraabdominal processes may not manifest the guarding or rebound expected with peritoneal irritation.

Expanded Diagnoses

The number and type of diagnostic possibilities increase with age. In addition to the usual causes of abdominal pain seen in all age groups, vascular disease is more common in the elderly, with increased risk for vascular events such as myocardial infarction, mesenteric ischemia, and intraabdominal aneurysms. Cancer is more common in the elderly. The elderly are more likely to develop complications from other intraabdominal processes, such as appendicitis or cholecystitis.

DIFFERENTIAL DIAGNOSIS

The differential diagnosis of abdominal pain in the elderly is extensive. The vast majority of the diagnosable causes of abdominal pain in the elderly patient are surgical problems requiring admission and possibly urgent or emergent surgery (see Table 36.2). In order of decreasing frequency, the diagnosable causes of abdominal pain in the elderly are as follows:

1. Biliary colic or cholecystitis (12% to 33%)
2. Nonspecific abdominal pain (15%)
3. Intestinal obstruction (hernias, adhesions, malignancies; 12% to 25%)
4. Appendicitis (5% to 14%)
5. Perforated viscus (7% to 10%)
6. Gastrointestinal bleeding (9%)
7. Pancreatitis (7%)
8. Diverticular disease (6%)
9. Vascular (mesenteric ischemia, aortic aneurysm; 2%)

Other important causes of abdominal pain include peptic ulcer disease (PUD) and nephrolithiasis. In addition, nonabdominal diseases can cause acute abdominal pain, including pneumonia, acute myocardial infarction, diabetic ketoacidosis, and drug toxicity. As mentioned, although 15% to 25% of elderly patients will have no discernible cause of their abdominal pain identified in the emergency department, up to 10% will be diagnosed with cancer within 6 months; the most common site is the colon.

Each of the following diseases is discussed in depth in a separate chapter in this text. The focus of the discussion here is to isolate features applicable to the elderly.

Biliary Tract Disease

Biliary tract disease is the most common diagnosable cause of abdominal pain in the elderly, accounting for 12% to 33% of all cases of abdominal pain. The incidence of gall bladder disease increases with age; almost 50% of those over age 70 have gallstones. The stereotype of female preponderance is eliminated once both sexes reach age 65; the ratio of females to males with stones decreases to 1:1 at this point. Most elderly patients present with typical symptoms, but up to 25% have no history of biliary tract disease. Up to 10% of the elderly have acalculous cholecystitis. On examination, up to 25% have no abdominal pain, and only 50% with cholecystitis will have peritoneal signs. Fever and leukocytosis are seen in 30% and 40%, respectively.[5] Liver function tests may be nonspecific but typically show the usual pattern consistent with gallstone disease. Because elderly patients may lack fever, peritoneal signs, or elevation in the white count, it is prudent to obtain an imaging study of the biliary tree. HIDA scan and ultrasound are excellent tests to rule out cholecystitis and its complications.

Emergency department management includes intravenous hydration if indicated. Nasogastric suctioning is unnecessary unless the patient has severe nausea, vomiting, or ileus. Intravenous antibiotics to cover enteric gram-negative aerobes and anaerobes should be given. Ampicillin, gentamicin, and metronidazole provide effective initial coverage. Pain medication and urgent surgical consultation are also indicated.

Almost 80% of patients present with complications of biliary tract disease (cholecystitis, cholangitis, or pancreatitis); jaundice, high fever, and generalized peritonitis suggest severe complications from gallstones, and up to 43% of the elderly will present with jaundice.[5] There is also a significantly higher incidence of emphysematous cholecystitis, gangrene, gallstone ileus, and perforation (8% to 10%). Perforation of the gallbladder has a mortality rate of 15% to 25%. Cholangitis may present with mental status changes and septic shock in up to 43% of patients.[20] Emphysematous cholecystitis is seen almost exclusively in the elderly. The diagnosis is suggested on plain films by gas in the gallbladder or biliary tree. The overall mortality of the elderly patient with cholecystitis is nearly 10%,[5] and one study showed mortality rates were twice as high in men.[17]

Intestinal Obstruction

Bowel obstruction is the second most common cause of abdominal pain in the elderly that required surgery. The sites may be viewed as occurring in thirds: one-third of obstructions occur in the large bowel, and one-third in the small bowel, and one-third are due to hernias. The most common causes of small bowel obstruction are postsurgical adhesions and hernias. The most common cause of large bowel obstruction is malignancy; sigmoid volvulus and fecal impaction cause the remainder of large bowel obstructions. The elderly are predisposed to volvulus due to a sedentary lifestyle, chronic constipation, and medications that alter bowel motility. Sigmoid volvulus accounts for 70% of cases of volvulus in the elderly (− old). Cecal volvulus and other, rarer forms of volvulus, such as transverse colon or gastric volvulus, may occasionally be seen.

Most patients present with the acute or subacute onset of paroxysms of colicky abdominal pain in the umbilical or hypogastric region. Nausea, vomiting, and constipation are extremely common. Prior surgical procedures and changes in bowel habits are critical issues to determine.

On examination, the presence of fever may indicate peritonitis. Although the abdomen is frequently tender, tenderness may be minimal. Peritoneal signs suggest strangulation or perforation. A careful search for scars and hernias (particularly in the inguinal and femoral regions) is indicated. An examination of the genitalia and rectum may reveal cancer or impaction.

Laboratory studies are not usually helpful. Plain abdominal films are useful in making the diagnosis. If the obstruction is early, a nonspecific ileus pattern may be seen. Multiple air–fluid levels and distended loops of bowel on plain films are characteristic. In some cases, the films may demonstrate a volvulus, gallstone ileus, or bezoar. Sigmoid volvulus can be diagnosed by plain film most of the time. A "bird's beak" in the left lower quadrant and a single, dilated loop of large bowel suggest volvulus. Cecal volvulus may demonstrate a single, large, round, distended loop of bowel, usually in the lower quadrants.

Emergency department treatment includes nasogastric suctioning and intravenous fluids. Patients may "third space" large amounts of fluid into the bowel, so monitoring fluid status is critical. Close observation of the cardiopulmonary status is critical. A Foley catheter allows monitoring of urine output.

Urgent surgical consultation is indicated. Volvulus is a surgical emergency. Sigmoid volvulus may be initially treated with colonoscopy, barium enema, or a rectal tube. However, many patients ultimately require surgery, as there is a significant incidence of recurrence.

Pancreatitis

Pancreatitis is the most common nonsurgical cause of acute abdominal pain in the elderly. Its incidence increases with age, and it is usually secondary to biliary tract disease, peptic ulcer disease, or complications from therapeutic agents. The presentation is characterized by the gradual onset of severe and continuous epigastric pain accompanied by nausea and vomiting. Fever is uncommon unless the disease is secondary to another process. Although most patients complain of pain, severe tenderness on examination is uncommon. An elevated serum amylase and lipase level and leukocytosis are characteristic. Plain films of the abdomen may reveal localized ileus (sentinel loop) or a more generalized pattern of ileus.

Appendicitis

Appendicitis accounts for 5% to 7% of all acute abdominal emergencies in the elderly. Whereas 20% of younger patients are perforated at the time of surgery, 44% of elderly patients with appendicitis are perforated with gangrene or abscess at the time of laparotomy.[10] This high rate of perforation is multifactorial and includes the more tenuous circulation to the appendix, other host factors, and delays in presentation, diagnosis, and treatment. In one study, only 15% of patients presented within 24 hours of the onset of pain. Up to 50% of elderly patients are misdiagnosed preoperatively.

Virtually all elderly patients with appendicitis present with abdominal pain, but only 35% will demonstrate the typical pattern of epigastric pain that moves to the periumbilical region and then to the right lower quadrant. Up to 17% of patients will have no right lower quadrant pain at all,[2] and, more often, elderly patients present with vague, poorly defined abdominal pain.

Fever is a poor indicator of appendicitis, although there may be some temperature elevation in up to 60% of patients. An important clue to diagnosis is right lower quadrant tenderness, present in 86% of the elderly patients with appendicitis. Approximately half of patients will have peritoneal signs in the emergency department.[2]

Emergency department evaluation includes a thorough history and physical examination. White blood cell counts are elevated in up to 80% of patients.[2] Plain abdominal radiographs are not helpful except to exclude other processes. The most suggestive finding on plain films is an appendicolith in the right lower quadrant. A persistent, abnormal gas collection suggests abscess formation. Abdominal ultrasound may be useful, but it has not been studied in the elderly.

Treatment includes keeping the patient NPO, administering antibiotics that cover abdominal flora, and obtaining surgical consultation. Complications include perforation, gangrenous appendicitis, and abscess formation. Mortality approaches 25% in patients over age 75.

Peptic Ulcer Disease

The incidence of PUD and its complications are increased in the elderly.[6] This increase in incidence is multifactorial: an increase in the incidence of *Helicobacter pylori,* use of nonsteroidal antiinflammatory drugs (NSAIDs), an increase in the number of parietal cells, alterations in acid secretion and the gastric mucosal barrier, increased tobacco use, and decreased compliance with treatment.[6,9,11] The proportion of duodenal to gastric ulcers decreases with age, dropping from 66% in those younger than 65 to 42% in those older than 65.[9] Signs and symptoms depend on the stage of the disease and possible complications. Up to 94% of the elderly with bleeding secondary to PUD have been found to have no epigastric pain at all.[9] Less severe symptomatic presentations include gnawing or burning pain localized to the epigastrium, substernal, or periumbilical area. Other initial manifestations include gastrointestinal bleeding, perforation, anemia, poor appetite, or weight loss. In people older than 65, one study reported that 65% of patients presented with atypical pain characterized by nausea, vomiting, loss of appetite or weight, melena, or no symptoms at all.[9] Ten percent of patients present with an acute abdominal process.

The risk of gastrointestinal bleeding from PUD increases with age, as 50% of elderly patients are found to be bleeding at presentation.[9]

Examination of the elderly patient with PUD should focus on signs of perforation or bleeding. Abnormal vital signs may indicate acute bleeding. The skin, nail beds, and conjunctiva may be pale if the patient is anemic. The abdomen should be examined, particularly for tenderness. The elderly patient may not demonstrate peritoneal signs, even with a perforation. A rectal examination should be done to check for occult blood, melena, and masses.

Laboratory evaluation includes a complete blood count and electrolytes, as well as type and crossmatch for blood in patients in whom bleeding is suspected. Anemia may be noted.

All patients with epigastric pain should have an electrocardiogram to rule out an acute myocardial infarction.

An upright chest radiograph or left lateral decubitus film should be ordered if perforation is suspected. These films show free air in 50% to 90% of those who have perforated; instilling 500 mL of air through a nasogastric tube can increase the yield.

Initial treatment includes intravenous fluids and blood resuscitation in hypotensive patients in whom bleeding is suspected. Early endoscopy should be considered and has been shown to decrease mortality in one study.[1] Pharmacologic treatment of PUD in the elderly is controversial. Histamine H2 receptor antagonists have not been found to affect risk of rebleeding, number of transfusions needed, or the need for surgery, but may decrease the mortality rate. The use of proton pump inhibitors is even more controversial, as one study found a decrease in the complication of PUD yet an increase in mortality in the elderly.[7] Misoprostol, a prostaglandin inhibitor, is the most promising drug to prevent the development of 40% of ulcers in patients using NSAIDs.[6] Patients with perforation should have a nasogastric tube placed and be kept NPO; urgent surgical consultation is required. Age and bleeding are independent risk factors for mortality from PUD, with a 13% mortality rate from bleeding in patients over age 74.[9] Although perforation rates are not higher in the elderly, the mortality rate is higher because the elderly often present with minimal or atypical signs and symptoms, with consequent delays in diagnosis and treatment.

Diverticular Disease

Diverticular disease is common in the elderly, accounting for 9% of acute surgical admissions.[3] Prevalence increases with increasing age, with at least 50% of patients over age 60 having the disease. The sigmoid colon is involved in up to 90% of cases. Diverticulitis represents an inflammatory response to a diverticulum that has ruptured into surrounding tissue. It is a common cause of abdominal pain in the elderly.

The most common complications of diverticular disease are lower gastrointestinal bleeding (15% will have at least one bleeding episode) and diverticulitis (30%). Diverticular bleeding is usually painless but can be massive. Patients with diverticulitis may have microperforations that cause mild symptoms or may develop macroperforations that cause the patient to become significantly ill.

The elderly patient with diverticular disease may present with bloating and constipation; diverticulitis may cause abdominal pain, more often on the left side and often worsened during bowel movements.

On examination, patients with significant macroperforation are often febrile. The abdomen is tender to palpation in the left lower quadrant, although suprapubic or generalized tenderness is also seen. Diffuse abdominal tenderness suggests frank perforation and peritonitis. Twenty percent have a palpable left lower quadrant mass. Evaluation should include a rectal examination.

Laboratory studies and radiographs are seldom useful, because the diagnosis is clinical. Abdominal films may demonstrate free air in the peritoneum if perforation of the diverticula has occurred. Computed tomography (CT) scanning can be useful, especially when an abscess is present. The white blood count may or may not be elevated in diverticulitis; patients may be anemic from diverticular bleeding.

Emergency department treatment of diverticulitis includes intravenous hydration and intravenous antibiotics to cover colonic flora. Diverticular bleeding should be treated with intravenous access and fluid and blood resuscitation as necessary. Surgical consultation is indicated in patients with symptomatic diverticular disease. Gastrointestinal bleeding in the elderly generally requires urgent localization of the site of hemorrhage and hospitalization.

Mesenteric Ischemia

Acute mesenteric ischemia or infarction (AMI) is a rare but grave cause of abdominal pain in the elderly, with a mortality rate of 85%. Predisposing factors include vascular disease, the use of vasoconstricting drugs as well as digitalis and diuretics, advanced age, prior thromboembolic events, hypotension or hypovolemia, and heart disease (particularly left ventricular aneurysms, atrial fibrillation, or valvular disease).

There are several variants of AMI, and the presentation varies depending on the location, degree of collateral circulation, and underlying disease. Thrombosis may be manifested by an insidious onset of pain, anorexia, and diarrhea with or without blood loss in the stool. An acute mesenteric occlusion from an embolus or thrombus usually presents with catastrophic pain, minimal or no tenderness, and bloody diarrhea or Hemoccult-positive stool. If the process is advanced, cardiovascular collapse may be a prominent feature.

Mesenteric artery embolism accounts for 30% of cases; the source of emboli is most often the heart. These patients often present with the abrupt onset of severe abdominal pain. Mesenteric artery thrombosis tends to have a more gradual onset of abdominal pain; there may be a history of intestinal "angina." *The cardinal feature of AMI is pain out of proportion to the examination.* Patients with abdominal tenderness may have infarcted bowel causing peritoneal irritation. Bowel sounds are variable. Gastrointestinal bleeding is common and ranges from Hemoccult-positive stool to frank hematochezia.

The emergency department evaluation must be done quickly, for time is of the essence in AMI. Tests in patients with suspected AMI include electrolyte levels, blood urea nitrogen, creatinine, a complete blood count, an arterial blood gas, urinalysis, and type and screen for blood. The white count is elevated in up to 90% of patients; it often exceeds 15,000/μL, with a left shift of the differential. Prothrombin time (PT), partial thromboplastic time (PTT), liver function tests, and a serum phosphate may also be indicated. Abdominal films may show an ileus, "thumb-printing" of the bowel wall, air in the portal system, or air in the bowel wall. Nasogastric suctioning, intravenous fluids, and monitoring of the patient's cardiovascular status are critical. Vasopressors should be avoided or stopped. Antibiotics that cover bowel flora should be given. Emergent surgical and radiographic consultation should be obtained as soon as the diagnosis is suspected. Both ultrasound and CT scanning can be useful if the diagnosis is uncertain, but angiography is the diagnostic test of choice; it may also offer therapeutic options in some patients.

Constipation/Impaction

Slowing of gut motility, sedentary lifestyles, and medications may combine to produce constipation or fecal impaction. This is a common complaint, particularly among nursing home patients. Constipation that is of recent onset, however, should trigger an investigation, because it may be a symptom that indicates intestinal cancer. Paradoxic diarrhea is seen with the passage of loose, watery stools past an incompletely obstructing fecal mass.

The abdomen should be thoroughly observed for scars, hernias, and masses. The rectal examination may demonstrate a fecal mass; this should be digitally removed.

Miscellaneous Causes

Other causes of abdominal pain in the elderly include inflammatory bowel disease, intraabdominal abscess, prostatitis, aortic aneurysm, nephrolithiasis, pyelonephritis, and urinary retention. Acute myocardial infarction, congestive heart failure, pneumonia, thyroid disease, diabetic ketoacidosis, and drug toxicity can also cause abdominal pain.

EMERGENCY DEPARTMENT EVALUATION

History

An accurate history may be difficult to obtain; it may require patience and diligence. Elderly patients may be unable to give a cogent history due to dementia or residua of a stroke. They may not be able to hear the physician's questions. In addition to talking to the patient, consulting primary care physicians and family members and reviewing the patient's medical record may be necessary to evaluate the elderly patient fully. Information about the patient's medical and surgical history and a list of the patient's medications is of great value. Nonabdominal processes may also present as abdominal pain, so obtain a history of cardiac or pulmonary complaints (cough, shortness of breath, fever, or chest pain). Pneumonia, pulmonary embolism, and myocardial infarction may cause pain in the epigastrium and confuse the patient and the physician. A history of hypertension or heart disease may be a clue to the patient with mesenteric ischemia or abdominal aortic aneurysm.

Avoid making a premature diagnosis. The classic stereotype is the elderly patient with a history of nephrolithiasis who insists he is having a kidney stone; in fact, the pain may be due to a ruptured abdominal aneurysm.

The localization and progression of the pain can give clues as to the diagnosis. Although "typical" pain patterns are seen in elderly patients, the older patient may complain only of vague or poorly defined symptoms despite having a condition that may be life-threatening. The timing of the onset of the pain is important; pain of abrupt onset often signals a catastrophic event, such as rupture of an abdominal aortic aneurysm, perforation of a viscus, obstruction of a viscus, or mesenteric ischemia; nephrolithiasis may also present in this manner. Pain of rapid but not abrupt onset may also be caused by catastrophic events but is more characteristic of obstruction, infection, or inflammation. Pain that worsens over several hours to days is usually inflammatory or infectious. Pain out of proportion to physical findings suggests mesenteric ischemia or renal stone disease.

Physical Examination

In no group is it more important to examine the entire patient than it is in the elderly. The patient's general appearance often provides clues; his or her mental status and state of hydration and the color and moisture of the skin should be noted. Vital signs must be evaluated, but elderly patients may have normal vital signs despite significant disease. Elderly patients with infections may not develop fever; in fact, they may present afebrile or hypothermic. Tachycardia and tachypnea may be due to pain, early sepsis, intravascular volume depletion, hypoxia, acidosis, or hemorrhage. A normal or slightly decreased blood pressure in a normally hypertensive elderly patient may be a sign of sepsis, volume depletion, or hemorrhage.

A thorough cardiovascular and pulmonary examination is mandatory. It may reveal nonabdominal causes of the abdominal pain.

The abdomen should be observed for surgical scars, distension, and masses. Auscultation for bruits and bowel sounds should be done. Palpation of the abdomen for masses, tenderness, guarding, and rebound may be revealing, but the elderly patient may not guard or have rebound and may have only vague abdominal tenderness, even in the presence of significant intraabdominal disease. Special care should be made to evaluate the patient for ventral, incisional, inguinal, and femoral hernias. Femoral pulses should be assessed. The back should be inspected for deformity and assessed for bony or flank tenderness or masses.

All elderly patients should have a rectal examination, looking for tenderness, blood, and masses. A male patient with lower abdominal discomfort should have his prostate evaluated for tenderness or masses. A female patient should have a pelvic examination performed unless the pain is localized to the upper quadrants or she has had a hysterectomy and bilateral oophorectomy. Studies have shown that rectal and pelvic examinations are infrequently performed and often yield abnormal findings.[13] In the latter situation, a visual inspection of the vulva is prudent.

Laboratory Studies

All elderly patients with upper abdominal pain, nausea, or vomiting should have an electrocardiogram to rule out myocardial infarction.

Once a differential diagnosis is formulated, appropriate laboratory examinations should be ordered. Although testing patterns should be adjusted to accommodate the higher return among elderly patients, normal laboratory values do not rule out surgical disease in the elderly.[15] A urinalysis provides useful information regarding possible kidney stones or urinary tract infection. A complete blood count may be helpful if the patient is anemic (indicating acute or chronic bleeding) or if the patient's white blood count is elevated; however, *the white count is commonly normal in an elderly patient with significant infection and should not be used as a criterion of infection.*[15] The white blood count differential should be checked, as elderly patients may have only a left shift to indicate infection, and a bandemia may be associated with a higher risk of mortality.[13] Electrolytes may be helpful in patients taking diuretics, and an anion gap may indicate early sepsis or diabetic ketoacidosis. A digoxin level should be ordered in patients taking this drug. Liver function tests, amylase, and lipase are indicated in patients with suspected biliary tract or pancreatic disease. A blood gas should be obtained in patients with suspected mesenteric ischemia.

Radiographic Studies

Studies on the cost effectiveness of radiographs have greater application to younger patients with abdominal pain. It is important to have a low threshold for ordering tests on the elderly, particularly those for whom the diagnosis is unclear. A chest radiograph will provide information about intrathoracic processes that may be causing abdominal pain. Taken upright, it may reveal intraperitoneal air. In patients unable to tolerate an upright film, a left lateral decubitus film can be used to evaluate for the presence of free air, paying attention to the area above the liver as well as the region near the right iliac crest. Abdominal films should be inspected for dilated loops of bowel, air–fluid levels, free air, ascites, calcifications, stones (less than 10% of gallstones are present on plain radiographs), air in the bowel wall or bowel wall thickening ("thumb-printing") consistent with mesenteric ischemia, or air in the biliary tree or gallbladder.

Ultrasound evaluation may be helpful in a few selected abdominal conditions. In cholecystitis, both ultrasound and nuclear scintigraphy reach sensitivities and specificities of 95%. Ultrasound is the test of choice for detecting gallstones, while HIDA scan is slightly more sensitive in diagnosing cholecystitis.[18] When arteriography is not readily available, intestinal ischemia secondary to arterial occlusions may be diagnosed by ultrasound. An absent Doppler signal from a visualized superior mesenteric artery or celiac artery (only feasible in about 60% of patients due to body habitus) has been found to be pathognomonic for total vessel occlusion. In appendicitis, ultrasound can be diagnostic, although it should never be ruled out by a negative study.

CT is the test of choice for many conditions. CT is especially useful if an intraabdominal abscess is suspected, as in diverticulitis (seen in one-third) or chronic appendicitis. In diverticulitis without abscess formation, CT may show bowel wall thickening, mesenteric inflammation, or air in the bladder or vagina secondary to fistula formation.[8] One study found CT to be comparable to colonoscopy at picking up diverticular disease in patients over 70 years of age.[12] In appendicitis, CT may show circumferential appendiceal wall thickening (greater than 2 mm), and 25% will demonstrate an appendicolith. Mesenteric stranding, an inflammatory mass, or a "target sign" may also be seen.[8] In mesenteric ischemia, CT can be helpful if the diagnosis is in question and the patient is stable. Findings may include gas in the bowel wall, nonenhancing bowel wall, or thrombotic mesenteric vessels. Depending on the diagnostic criteria, sensitivity has been found to range from 60% to 100% and specificity from 60% to 90%.[4,8,21] Angiography and nuclear medicine studies also may be helpful when indicated.

EMERGENCY DEPARTMENT MANAGEMENT

Initial stabilization of the elderly patient is no different from that of any other patient. Attention to life-threatening problems must occur (ABCs). Fluid challenges should be given cautiously and their effect observed with frequent, if not continuous, monitoring of vital signs (including pulse, blood pressure, and pulse oximetry). Patients should receive no food or liquids by mouth until a diagnosis has been made. Vascular access should be established in most patients. Hydration with normal saline or blood products will depend on the volume status. Coexisting heart or lung disease must be considered. Nasogastric suctioning should be done in patients with suspected gastrointestinal bleeding, perforated viscus, mesenteric ischemia, or bowel obstruction. Antibiotics are indicated if infection is suspected. A Foley catheter is indicated in the ill patient.

DISPOSITION

Many elderly patients with abdominal pain have an underlying cause that requires hospitalization and possibly emergent surgery. *Surgical consultation and admission should be considered in most elderly patients with abdominal pain, particularly if the pain has persisted for more than 6 hours.* In patients with an unclear diagnosis, at a minimum emergency department observation is prudent for several hours, with frequent examinations. If the patient is to be discharged, a follow-up appointment within 12 to 24 hours must be arranged. The patient and family members should be instructed to return immediately for any worsening of pain or change in status. Family members and the patient's private physician should be involved in discharge arrangements.

COMMON PITFALLS

- The elderly underreport symptoms, delay seeking care, have comorbid diseases, and have altered immune and physiologic responses. The result is significantly greater morbidity and mortality for any given abdominal process in the elderly patient.
- The elderly are at least twice as likely to require surgery as their younger counterparts with abdominal pain.
- In general, the classic descriptions do not always apply to the elderly and should not be relied on for diagnosis.
- The elderly patient with abdominal pain may have a potentially lethal process despite a nonspecific or even relatively benign examination and normal laboratory studies.
- Information from family members, medical records, and treating physicians should be sought to obtain a complete medical history.
- Elderly patients with abdominal pain may benefit from emergency department observation, serial examinations, and radiographic testing.
- Exercise extreme caution when considering discharging elderly patients with abdominal pain. These patients should be reevaluated within 12 to 24 hours after discharge.
- Nonabdominal processes (myocardial infarction or pneumonia) may present as abdominal pain in the elderly.

References

1. Chow LW, Gertsch P, Poon RTP, et al. Risk factors for rebleeding and death from peptic ulcer in the very elderly. *Br J Surg* 1998;85:121.
2. Elangoran S. Clinical and laboratory findings in acute appendicitis in the elderly. *J Am Board Fam Pract* 1996;9:75.
3. Elliott TB, Yego S, Irvin TT. Five-year audit of the acute complications of diverticular disease. *Br J Surg* 1997;84:535.
4. Frager D, Baer JW, Medwid SW, et al. Detection of intestinal ischemia in patients with acute small-bowel obstruction due to adhesions or hernia: efficacy of CT. *AJR* 1996;166:67.
5. Gonzalez JJ, Sanz L, Grana JL, et al. Biliary lithiasis in the elderly patient: morbidity and mortality due to biliary surgery. *Hepatogastroenterology* 1997;44:1565.
6. Griffin MR. Epidemiology of nonsteroidal anti-inflammatory drug–associated gastrointestinal injury. *Am J Med* 1998;104(3A):23S.
7. Hasselgren G, Blomqvist A, Eridsson S, et al. Short and long term course of elderly patients with peptic ulcer bleeding—analysis of factors influencing fatal outcome. *Eur J Surg* 1998;164:685.

8. Johnson GL, Johnson PT, Fishman EK. CT evaluation of the acute abdomen: bowel pathology spectrum of disease. *Crit Rev Diagn Imaging* 1996;37(3):163.
9. Kemppainen H, Raiha I, Sourander L. Clinical presentation of peptic ulcer in the elderly. *Gerontology* 1997;43:283.
10. Korner H, Sondenaa K, Soreida JA, et al. Incidence of acute nonperforated and perforated appendicitis: age-specific and sex-specific analysis. *World J Surg* 1997;21:313.
11. Lazzaroni M, Porro GB. Treatment of peptic ulcer in the elderly. *Drugs Aging* 1996;9(4):251.
12. Liscomb G, Loughrey G, Thakker M, et al. A prospective study of abdominal computerized tomography and colonoscopy in an elderly population. *Eur J Gastroenterol Hepatol* 1996;8:887.
13. Marco CA, Schoenfeld CN, Keyl PM, et al. Abdominal pain in geriatric emergency patients: variables associated with adverse outcomes. *Acad Emerg Med* 1998;5(12):1163.
14. Miettinen P, Salonen A, Lahtinen J, et al. The outcome of elderly patients after operation for acute abdomen. *Ann Chir Gynaecol* 1996;85:11.
15. Parker JS, Vukov LF, Wollan PC. Abdominal pain in the elderly: use of temperature and laboratory testing to screen for surgical disease. *Fam Med* 1996;28:193.
16. Perko MJ, Just S, Schroeder TV. Importance of diastolic velocities in the detection of celiac and mesenteric artery disease by duplex ultrasound. *J Vasc Surg* 1997;26:228.
17. Russell JC, Walsh SJ, Reed-Fourquet LR, et al. Symptomatic cholelithiasis: a different disease in men? *Ann Surg* 1998;227(2):195.
18. Sanson TG, O'Keefe KP. Evaluation of abdominal pain in the elderly. *Gastrointest Emerg* 1996;14(3):615.
19. Strange GR, Chen EH. Use of emergency departments by elder patients: a five-year follow-up study. *Acad Emerg Med* 1998;5(12):1157.
20. Sugiyama M, Atomi Y. Treatment of acute cholangitis due to choledocholithiasis in elderly and younger patients. *Arch Surg* 1997;132:1129.
21. Taourel PG, Deneuville M, Pradel JA, et al. Acute mesenteric ischemia: diagnosis with contrast-enhanced CT. *Radiology* 1996;199:632.

CHAPTER 37

Breast Masses and Breast Infection

John M. Howell and Ellen M. Dugan

Effective emergency department evaluation of a breast mass depends on recognition of two major processes: cancer and infection. A breast abscess usually occurs in lactating women, but it may also represent inflammatory carcinoma in the elderly.[8,11,14,16,17] Cancer, on the other hand, may present in a manner similar to fulminant mastitis.[11,17] Experienced physicians can diagnose only 70% of breast cancers by examination alone.[17] The initial evaluation of a breast mass may be difficult, challenging, and highly relevant to ultimate patient outcome.

DIFFERENTIAL DIAGNOSIS

The differential diagnosis for breast mass includes cancer, mastitis, Paget disease, benign neoplasms, lipoma, fat necrosis, Mondor disease, and abscess.

CLINICAL PRESENTATIONS

Cancer

One out of nine women in the United States develops breast cancer. This disease is diagnosed in 180,000 patients annually.[1] Risk factors for breast cancer are listed in Table 37.1. In women under 25 years of age, fewer than 5% of breast masses are malignant. The incidence of breast cancer rises significantly during child-bearing years, and by the age of 70 more than 75% of breast masses are malignant.[2,10] Discussions of breast cancer histopathology and staging are beyond the scope of this chapter and are contained elsewhere.[14]

Masses that are smooth, movable, and firm with distinct margins are usually benign (Table 37.2).[17] Seventy-five percent to 80% of cancerous lesions are hard and cartilaginous, with distinct edges that are serrated and irregular.[14] However, 20% to 25% of cancerous nodules are less hard and less fibrotic in consistency, making accurate clinical diagnosis more difficult.[14]

Cancerous nodules are usually located in the upper outer quadrant.[14,17] Associated skin changes range from none to local edema or frank ulceration.[14,17] Fibrosis may shorten Cooper's ligament and cause skin dimpling, a process also seen in fat necrosis.[14,17] Bloody nipple discharge suggests ductal carcinoma, or it may reflect the presence of an intraductal papilloma.[17]

Lymph nodes involved in the spread of breast cancer are initially rubbery and shotty, but eventually they become hard and matted with progressive infiltration.[14] Axillary glands are most commonly involved, although spread to the parasternal and supraclavicular regions may also occur.[14,17]

Once in the lymphatic system, breast cancer cells disseminate to the lung, liver, and bony skeleton.[14] Patients suspected of metastatic breast cancer should have a complete blood count, measurement of serum levels of calcium, electrolytes, and liver enzymes, and chest radiography.

Erythema, edema, tenderness, and induration are late skin changes in the setting of breast cancer, but they also may be seen in acute mastitis.[5,16] Most breast infections occur 1 to 3 months postpartum,[8,14,16,17] so mastitis or abscess in a nonlactating woman, as well as delayed resolution of a puerperal infection, is a warning sign of inflammatory cancer.[12]

Benign Neoplasms

Fibroadenomas are the most common benign neoplasms of the breast.[14] They usually present during the third to fourth decade of life and are spherical, firm, mobile, and well defined.[14] Fibroadenomas should be removed to rule out cancer and preclude continued enlargement.[14] Fibrocystic disease causes cyclic pain and swelling of one or both breasts just before menses.[11] The nodules or cysts range from 2 or 3 mm to several centimeters in diameter.[14] They are firm, round, distinct, and rubbery, and they transilluminate.[14] Women with fibrocystic disease should be followed longitudinally because their risk of breast cancer is three to five times that of the general population.[17] Conservative treatment includes a well-fitting brassiere, heat, and analgesics.[11] Danazol, an androgen derivative, may be effective if hormonal treatment is indicated.[16]

Fat Necrosis

Fat necrosis may present as a tender lump in the breast. This follows trauma in 50% of cases.[11,14,17] The mass usually does not enlarge,[8,10] but nipple retraction may be seen. Excision for definitive diagnosis is indicated.[11]

Lipomas

Lipomas are superficial and occur in any quadrant of the breast. Mammography is usually diagnostic.

Mondor Disease

Mondor disease is thrombosis of the lateral thoracic or thoracoepigastric veins as they traverse the breast.[11] The inflamed

TABLE 37.1. Established and Probable Risk Factors for Breast Cancer

Risk Factor	Comparison Category	Risk Category	Typical Relative Risk
Family history of breast cancer	No 1st-degree relatives affected	Mother affected before the age of 60	2.0
		Mother affected after the age of 60	1.4
		Two Ist-degree relatives affected	4.6
Age at menarche	16 yr	11 yr	1.3
		12 yr	1.3
		13 yr	1.3
		14 yr	1.3
		15 yr	1.1
Age at birth of 1st child	Before 20 yr	20–24 yr	1.3
		25–29 yr	1.6
		≥30 yr	1.9
		Nulliparous	1.9
Age at menopause	45–54 yr	After 55 yr	1.5
		Before 45 yr	0.7
		Oophorectomy before 35 yr	0.4
Benign breast disease	No biopsy or aspiration	Any benign disease	1.5
		Proliferation only	2.0
		Atypical hyperplasia	4.0
Radiation	No special exposure	Atomic bomb (100 rad)	3.0
		Repeated fluoroscopy	1.5–2.0
Obesity	10th percentile	90th percentile:	
		Age, 30–49 yr	0.8
		Age, ≥50 yr	1.2
Height	10th percentile	90th percentile:	
		Age, 30–49 yr	1.3
		Age, ≥50 yr	1.4
Oral contraceptive use	Never used	Current use[a]	1.5
		Past use[a]	1.0
Postmenopausal estrogen-replacement therapy	Never used	Current use all ages	1.4
		Age, <55 yr	1.2
		Age, 50–59 yr	1.5
		Age, ≥60 yr	2.1
		Past use	1.0
Alcohol use	Nondrinker	1 drink/day	1.4
		2 drinks/day	1.7
		3 drinks/day	2.0

[a]Relative risks may be higher for women given a diagnosis of breast cancer before age 40.
Adapted from Harris JR, Lippman ME, Veronesi U, et al. Breast cancer. *N Engl J Med* 1992;327:319.

vein is characteristically tubular and may cause retraction of the skin. Mondor disease is self-limited and usually diagnosed with ease.[11]

Idiopathic Granulomatous Mastitis

Idiopathic granulomatous mastitis (IGM) is a rare *inflammatory* breast disease of unknown etiology. The clinical presentation is similar to that of mammary carcinoma, and IGM can be misdiagnosed as carcinoma. IGM is associated with women who have experienced childbirth and oral contraceptive use. Treatment consists of resection or corticosteroids. There is a 38% recurrence rate following treatment.[7]

TABLE 37.2. Physical Findings Suggestive of Benign and Malignant Breast Masses

Benign	Malignant
Soft or firm on palpation	Firm or hard on palpation
Discrete, regular margins	Indistinct margins
No attachments	Attached to skin or deep fascia
More likely to be tender	Less likely to be tender
No discharge	Bloody discharge
No skin changes	Dimpling of overlying skin or nipple retraction
Mobile	Less likely to be mobile

Mastitis and Abscess

Most breast abscesses occur 1 to 3 months postpartum, but postmenopausal women may also develop mastitis.[8,14,16,17] A postpartum breast abscess is caused by normal skin pathogens that invade through cracks in the nipple.[15] Breast milk is an ideal culture medium. Unrecognized infection coalesces into abscesses, usually located away from the areola.[17] Staphylococci are the most common causative agents[5,14,15]; streptococci are cultured less often.[8] Preventive measures include nipple hygiene (cleaning), hand washing, cleansing the infant's skin, and early recognition.[5,14,17]

Postmenopausal breast abscesses are distinct from puerperal forms in cause and presentation. Causative bacteria include *Escherichia coli*,[12] group D streptococci,[6] staphylococci,[12] and anaerobes, including *Bacteroides* sp.[15] These abscesses are often found in the subareolar region in association with ductal ectasia, a chronic inflammation of major ducts below the nipple and areola. Recurrence rates after simple incision and drainage exceed 39%.[3] Mamillary fistulas occasionally form between the areola and infected lactating glands.[8,9]

Although most breast abscesses occur postpartum, cancer may mimic mastitis.[17] Mastitis or abscess in a nonlactating woman and delayed resolution of a puerperal infection are warning signs of inflammatory cancer.

Tuberculosis remains the most common cause of persistent breast abscess.[14,17]

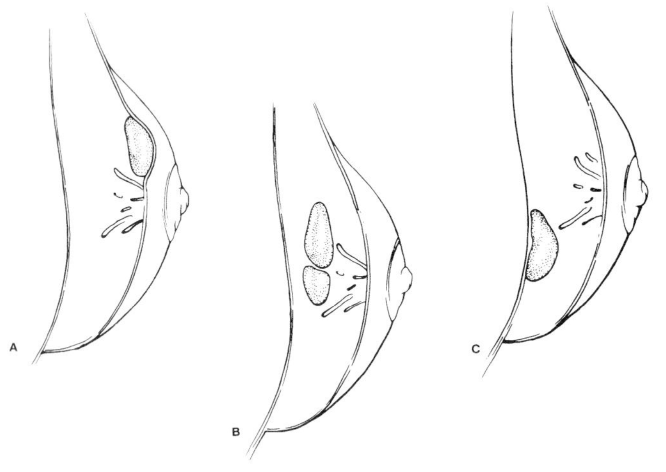

Figure 37.1. Breast abscesses. **(A)** Superficial abscess. **(B)** Intramammary abscess. **(C)** Retromammary abscess.

Chronic infection also occurs after inadequate drainage of partitioned areas within an abscess.[17] Untreated chronic infection may result in substantial morbidity and cosmetic deformity.[17]

Mastitis in the lactating breast causes pain, fever, erythema, edema, tenderness, and induration. Fluctuance in a centrifugal location is the hallmark of a superficial abscess. Intramammary and retromammary loculations occur deep in breast tissue and near the pectoralis musculature, respectively (Fig. 37.1).[16] For this reason, fluctuance may not be readily apparent.[16] The breast appears indurated, and the patient withdraws to palpation.[14] Paradoxically, decreasing induration and diminished pain may reflect the need for wide incision and drainage.[17]

Postmenopausal breast abscesses are commonly subareolar. A mamillary fistula is identified by expressing pus from the nipple or areola.[15] Nipple retraction and inversion are also observed.[12]

Chronic abscess presents as an indolent mass in a woman with history of tuberculosis or breast incision and drainage.[14,17]

Paget disease of the nipple reflects carcinoma of the mammary ducts underlying the areola.[14,17] The nipple initially appears dry, scaling, cracked, and eczematoid.[14,17] The condition may progress to chronic skin inflammation and a surface crust. Subareolar fullness may or may not be palpable.[14]

EMERGENCY DEPARTMENT MANAGEMENT

Simple mastitis in the lactating woman, without abscess formation, is treated with antimicrobials that are effective against staphylococci and streptococci.[5,8] Dicloxacillin (250 to 500 mg four times a day), or erythromycin (250 to 500 mg four times a day) in penicillin-allergic patients, is appropriate. Breast milk should be cultured for aerobes and anaerobes.[5] Feedings may be discontinued for up to 48 hours if there is concern about infant diarrhea; however, drainage must be accomplished by continued feeding or pump.[5,8,16] Local heat should be applied.[17]

Superficial abscesses may be drained and treated in the emergency department if there is no fever or toxicity. Incision and drainage may be performed by an emergency physician or a surgeon who is qualified to perform this procedure. Incision is performed in a curvilinear manner along skin lines[14] or in a radial manner.[16] A circumareolar approach may also be used.[8,17] Care should be taken to ensure that there are no loculations that might result in a chronic abscess. In superficial abscesses, needle aspiration has been successful in a few patients (C.M. Magnant, *personal communication*, 1994). Culture (anaerobic and aerobic) and Gram stain of the drainage should be performed.[8] The patient should be given antimicrobials and instructed in the same local measures as for simple mastitis. Patients should be educated about causal factors, symptoms, and how to avoid recurrent episodes of mastitis.[4]

DISPOSITION

Mastitis

Role of the Consultant

Patients with nontoxic mastitis or superficial abscess should be reevaluated in 24 hours. Mamillary fistulas should be referred to a surgeon for excision and definitive closure.[8,9,12] Postmenopausal intramammary abscesses necessitate surgical consultation because of the high recurrence rate after simple drainage.[11,15] Incision and drainage of superficial abscesses may be referred to a surgeon for cosmetic reasons if the emergency physician is not skilled in the procedure.

Indications for Admission

Women with marked temperature elevation or toxic appearance should be admitted and placed on intravenous antibiotics that are effective against staphylococci and streptococci. Women with simple infections that do not improve or that worsen after 24 hours should also be admitted. Patients with deep intramammary and retromammary abscesses are hospitalized for operative drainage.[16]

Transfer Considerations

Women transferred for operative care should be stable, without evidence of septic shock. Antimicrobials should be initiated by the referring hospital and pain controlled before transfer.

Suspected Breast Cancer

Role of the Consultant

Women suspected of having breast cancer should be referred immediately to a consultant who is experienced in the diagnosis and management of breast disorders. Mammography may be used to evaluate suspicious breast masses in women who are not pregnant and are at least age 20. Arrangements may be made for mammography to be performed on an outpatient basis. If mammography is performed, a subsequent visit to a specialist is important. About 18% of mammograms show a false-negative result for breast cancer,[3] so patients should be counseled that a negative study does not necessarily mean the absence of disease.[13]

Indications for Admission

Patients with suspicious breast masses need not be admitted unless either breast cancer is advanced on presentation, with intractable pain or serious secondary infection, or family or socioeconomic factors place admission in the patient's best interest. In general, the initial evaluation of suspicious breast masses is done on an outpatient basis.

Transfer Considerations

Consider transfer or referral when no physician experienced in the management of breast disorders is available.

COMMON PITFALLS

- Inflammatory cancer may present with erythema, edema, and tenderness. Infection in a nonlactating breast and failure of a postpartum infection to abate in a timely manner should suggest the possibility of cancer.

- Inadequate drainage of a breast abscess may lead to chronic infection with substantial morbidity and cosmetic deformity.
- Subareolar abscesses in postmenopausal women are usually associated with ductal ectasia (chronic subareolar inflammation) and may recur, requiring removal of the involved duct system. These patients require surgical consultation.
- Subareolar abscesses may also present with mamillary fistula, demonstrated clinically by expressing pus from the nipple area. Surgical removal of the tract and definitive closure are indicated.

References

1. Boring CC, Squires TS, Tong T. Cancer statistics. *CA Cancer J Clin* 1992;42:19.
2. Brinton LA, DeVesa SS. Etiology and pathogenesis of breast cancer. In: Harris JR, Lippman ME, Morrow M, et al., eds. *Diseases of the breast.* Philadelphia, Lippincott–Raven Publishers, 1996.
3. Donegan WL. Evaluation of a palpable breast mass. *N Engl J Med* 1992;327:937.
4. Fetherston C. Management of lactation mastitis in a western Australian cohort. *Breastfeed Rev* 1997;5(2):12–19.
5. Fiorica JV. The breast. In: Danforth DN, Scott JR, Di Saia PJ, et al., eds. *Danforth's obstetrics and gynecology,* 8th ed. Philadelphia: Lippincott Williams & Wilkins, 1999.
6. Harris JR, Lippman ME, Veronesi U, et al. Breast cancer. *N Engl J Med* 1992;327:319.
7. Imoto S, Kitaya T, Kotama T, et al. Idiopathic granulomatous mastitis: case report and review of the literature. *Jpn J Clin Oncol* 1997;27(4):274–277.
8. Iglehart JD. The breast. In: Sabiston DC, ed. *Textbook of surgery: the biological basis of modern surgical practice,* 15th ed. Philadelphia: WB Saunders, 1997.
9. Lambert ME, Bates CD, Sellwood RA. Mamillary fistula. *Br J Surg* 1986;73:367.
10. Ligon RE, Stevenson DR, Diner W, et al. Breast masses in young women. *Am J Surg* 1980;140:779.
11. Magnant CM. Fat necrosis, hematoma and trauma. In: Harris JR, Lippman ME, Morrow M, et al., eds. *Diseases of the breast.* Philadelphia: Lippincott–Raven, 1996.
12. Maier WP, Berger A, Derrick BM. Periareolar abscess in the nonlactating breast. *Am J Surg* 1982;144:359.
13. *Physician Insurers Association of America Cancer Study—March 1990.* Pennington, NJ: Physician Insurers Association of America, 1990.
14. Rush BF. Breast. In: Schwartz SI, ed. *Principles of surgery,* 5th ed. New York: McGraw-Hill, 1989.
15. Scholefield JH, Duncan JL, Rogers K. Review of a hospital experience of breast abscesses. *Br J Surg* 1987;74:469.
16. Warden TM, Fourre MW. Incision and drainage of cutaneous abscesses and soft tissue infections. In: Roberts JR, Hedges JR, eds. *Clinical procedures in emergency medicine,* 2nd ed. Philadelphia: WB Saunders, 1991.
17. Wilson RE. The breast. In: Sabiston DC, ed. *Textbook of surgery,* 13th ed. Philadelphia: WB Saunders, 1986.

CHAPTER 38
Esophageal and Gastric Neoplasms

Jonathan Glauser

ESOPHAGEAL NEOPLASMS

The prognosis for esophageal cancer is grim and has remained unchanged in recent years. Long-term survivors are rare. Only 30% of patients present with nonmetastatic disease. Five-year survival rates range from 7% to 20% in reports of operable, small squamous cell carcinomas treated with surgery. Survival after diagnosis averages from 2 to 4 months if demonstrable metastases are present, to 8 to 14 months if "curative" surgery has been performed with chemotherapy added. Overall, 80% to 90% die within 2 years of diagnosis.

Prognosis depends on lymph node spread, metastases, and the depth of extension of the tumor (Table 38.1). When all of these are favorable (stages I or II), the 5-year survival rate is 50%. Unfortunately, one-third of patients have inoperable advanced cancer when first seen.

Squamous cell carcinomas and adenocarcinoma of the esophagus constitute the fifth most common cancer in men in the United States (Fig. 38.1). They account for an estimated 9,800 deaths per year in the United States, with an incidence of 2 to 5 per 100,000 in White men and a somewhat higher incidence in Blacks (17/100,000). The overall age-adjusted incidence in the United States in 1987 was 3.9 persons per 100,000, with an overall age-adjusted mortality of 3.4 per 100,000, reflecting the high mortality rate for this malignancy. There were 12,100 new cases diagnosed in the United States in 1995, with 12,500 new cases expected in 1997.

Epidemiologic studies identify certain risk factors for the development of esophageal cancer. Heavy use of alcohol and tobacco, including tobacco swallowing, and nutritional deficiencies in vitamins A and C, riboflavin, zinc, and molybdenum have been implicated. Diets rich in fresh fruit and vegetables seem to be protective. Salicylate and nonsteroidal antiinflammatory medication use may also decrease risk of esophageal cancer. A disproportionate number of patients are of low socioeconomic status. Carcinoma of the esophagus has been associated with chronic iron deficiency and the Plummer-Vinson syndrome. It has been also associated with achalasia, reflux esophagitis, hiatal hernia, corrosive esophagitis and strictures from lye, and scleroderma. Occupational exposure to tetrachloroethylene, as for dry cleaners, and to toluene, as for shoemakers, paint mixers, and rubber cement mixers, appear to also

TABLE 38.1. TNM Staging for Esophageal Cancer

PRIMARY TUMOR (T)			
TX	Minimum requirements to assess the primary tumor cannot be seen		
T0	No evidence of primary tumor		
Tis	Preinvasive carcinoma (carcinoma *in situ*)		
T1	Tumor invades into but not beyond the submucosa		
T2	Tumor invades into but not beyond the muscularis propria		
T3	Tumor invades into the adventitia		
T4	Tumor invades contiguous structures		
REGIONAL LYMPH NODES (N)			
Cervical esophagus (cervical and supraclavicular lymph nodes)			
NX	Lymph nodes cannot be assessed		
N0	No demonstrable metastasis to regional lymph nodes		
N1	Regional lymph nodes contain metastatic tumor		
Thoracic esophagus (nodes in the thorax, not those of the cervical, supraclavicular, or abdominal areas)			
N0	No nodal involvement		
N1	Nodal involvement		
DISTANT METASTASIS (M)			
MX	Distant metastasis cannot be assessed		
M0	No evidence of distant metastasis		
M1	Distant metastasis present		
Stage I	Stage II	Stage III	Stage IV
T1N0M0	T2N0M0	T3N0M0	Any T, Any NM_1
	T1N1M0	T3N1M0	
	T2N1M0	T4N1M0	

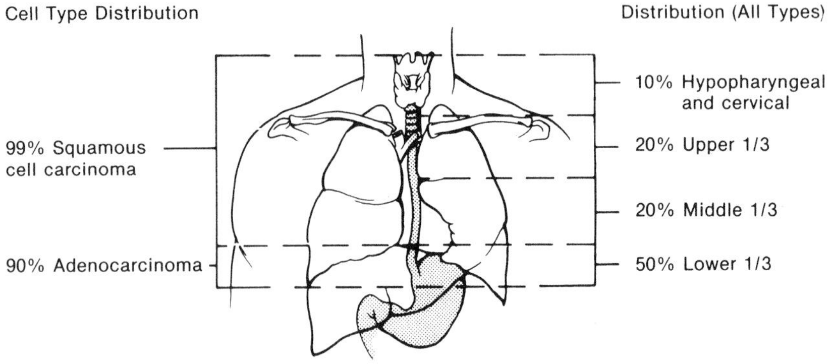

Figure 38.1. Locations of cancer of the esophagus. (From Schwartz SI, et al. *Principles of surgery,* 5th ed. New York: McGraw-Hill, 1989, with permission.)

be risks for the disease. A disproportionate number of patients with squamous cell carcinoma have had a partial gastrectomy.

Adenocarcinoma arising from Barrett's esophagus is thought by some to be gastric cancer. It accounts for as many as 60% of tumors confined to the lower esophagus and almost half of all esophageal cancers. Barrett's esophagus, or columnar cell-lined esophagus, is considered to be a premalignant lesion. It may present as adenocarcinoma in childhood, and attempts at control of Barrett's esophagus with agents such as omeprazole or with antireflux operations have met with mixed success.

Chronic ingestion of nitrosamines found in some salted foods, tannins in hot tea and other beverages, certain fungi that are contaminants of corn and produce fumonisins, betel nut chewing, opium, and thermal mucosal irritants have been cited as risk factors for esophageal cancer. Familial factors, such as tylosis, are rare.

Esophageal carcinomas may develop in association with other tumors of the upper aerodigestive tract, for example, cancers of the tonsil and palate, which may also arise after exposure to a carcinogen such as tobacco smoke.

Gastrointestinal involvement with Kaposi's sarcoma occurs in 50% to 70% of patients with Kaposi's sarcoma and the acquired immunodeficiency syndrome (AIDS). Lesions may appear as violaceous nodules on endoscopy or as dark red macules and may bleed, although they are generally asymptomatic. Primary lymphoma of the esophagus associated with AIDS has been reported. Malignant melanoma, mesenchymal tumors and small cell carcinomas are unusual primary malignancies of the esophagus; breast cancer is the most common tumor that metastasizes to the esophagus.

CLINICAL PRESENTATION

More than 90% of all esophageal neoplasms are malignant. Patients with benign tumors may present with bleeding or dysphagia but usually experience no symptoms. Benign tumors may be distinguishable from carcinoma only after surgical removal.

The earliest and most constant presenting symptom of esophageal cancer is dysphagia—initially of solids, later of liquids. One-half to two-thirds of the esophageal circumference must be involved with gross tumor to produce dysphagia, or when the diameter has been narrowed to approximately 13 mm. Total dysphagia occurs when the lumen is constricted to 4 mm in diameter. A vague retrosternal discomfort or a sensation of slow food passage may be perceived.

Weight loss, often of 9 to 10 kg over 2 or 3 months, may be due to dysphagia or to anorexia from widespread disease.

Pain may occur only on eating (odynophagia), reflecting mediastinal involvement, or it may be persistent. It is an ominous sign. Pain may be located in the epigastrium, substernally, or in the midback.

Excessive salivation may lead to aspiration, cough, and pulmonary infection. Patients may present with lung abscesses or pneumonia. Tracheoesophageal fistulas are quite common and may be due to the disease or to radiation therapy. Cough or hemoptysis may be a presenting sign. Regurgitation of undigested food may occur.

Other presenting signs depend on the extent of involvement of the tumor. Hoarseness, paralysis of the diaphragm, and gastric retention occur with invasion of the recurrent laryngeal, phrenic, and vagus nerves, respectively. Lymphadenopathy may be noted in the neck. Erosion into a bronchus may cause mediastinitis; erosion into the aorta may result in massive bleeding. Malignant pleural effusion or malignant ascites indicates unresectable disease.

Rarely, these tumors present with hormonal abnormalities. Hypercalcemia has been reported, sometimes with ectopic parathyroid hormone production from bony metastases. The syndrome of inappropriate secretion of antidiuretic hormone may result from pneumonia or from narcotic administration.

The emergency physician may see acute problems at any stage of this disease, as complications of both therapy and the disease itself.

The most common complication from radiation is esophageal stricture. Occasionally, patients may develop pericarditis, radiation pneumonitis, myocarditis, or spinal cord damage from radiation. Pneumonitis may not be due to aspiration, but to prior radiation therapy. Brain radionecrosis may result in increased intracranial pressure and herniation syndrome. Pneumopericardium with pericardial tamponade has occurred after surgical resection of esophageal cancer.

EMERGENCY DEPARTMENT EVALUATION AND MANAGEMENT

In the emergency department, a chest film may show a pleural effusion, pneumonia, lung metastases, or an air–fluid level from total esophageal obstruction. Liver function studies, determination of serum electrolyte and calcium levels, and a complete blood cell count should be performed. Fecal occult blood testing over 3 consecutive days may be positive in as few as 20% of cases, and is an insensitive screen.

If esophageal neoplasm is suspected, it may be appropriate to obtain a barium swallow. The results of a barium swallow test are nearly always abnormal in symptomatic patients. In 90% of cases, the presence of stenosis, mass effect, or esophageal narrowing with a ragged mucosal pattern is diagnostic. Double-contrast esophagography obtained by coating the esophageal mucosa with barium and distending the lumen with air is especially useful in demonstrating early cancers or fistulas.

Esophagoscopy can define the site of the lesion, the extent of the circumferential involvement, and the length of involvement. Fiberoptic endoscopy also permits biopsy and cell scraping. Brushings combined with multiple biopsies can confirm a diagnosis of malignancy in over 95% of cases. Lugol's iodine or toluidine blue staining may differentiate normal tissue from neoplastic tissue or Barrett's epithelium.

Computed tomography (CT) is the best noninvasive method for assessing local spread of disease, but it is not accurate for detecting lymphatic spread. More invasive, but useful, studies for staging include bronchoscopy (to detect tracheal invasion) and mediastinoscopy. A bone scan should be obtained in patients with bone pain, as well as plain films of the area. Endoscopic ultrasonography (EUS) has been used to assess the extent of the circumferential involvement of tumor with the surrounding structures and may be the most accurate method for clinical staging. EUS is more accurate than CT for detecting involvement of regional lymph nodes. Magnetic resonance imaging (MRI) may be useful in assessing the relation of esophageal cancer to mediastinal structures, such as the aorta or trachea, as well as in detecting liver metastases.

Staging may also involve laparoscopy, thoracotomy, or thoracoscopy.

TREATMENT AND PROGNOSIS

Irradiation, surgical resection, or both, are the preferred modes of treatment. Surgical resection and irradiation provide a 2-year survival rate of 28% versus 11% for irradiation alone. Overall 5-year survival after surgery is cited at under 10%. Operative mortality from esophagectomy is approximately 8%. The surgical procedure may entail lymphadenectomy of varying degree or colon replacement of the esophagus. Often, treatment is palliative to relieve dysphagia and to allow enteral nutrition. Endoscopic mucosectomy for early esophageal cancer is an alternative, if the cancer is limited to the mucosa. Patients may undergo cervical esophagostomy, feeding gastrostomy, tracheostomy, or esophageal bypass. Bougie dilatation has been performed to facilitate passage of food. Laser opening of the occluded esophagus has a lower mortality rate and fewer complications than tube insertion and may be effective 80% of the time in palliating obstruction. Other methods for relieving tumor obstruction endoscopically include photodynamic therapy (PDT) utilizing light sensitizing agents and bipolar electrocoagulation (BTP or BICAP) to deliver thermal energy to the surface of the tumor. The emergency physician will need to be able to recognize various prosthetic devices, such as the Proctor-Livingstone or Celestin tube placed through the esophageal obstruction to facilitate passage of liquid or pureed diets. A Celestin tube has its own antimigration device detectable on film. A variety of self-expanding metal stents (SEMS) are commercially available.

Chemotherapy has an insignificant role in therapy for esophageal cancer. There are reports of remissions of 2 to 5 months in 5% to 50% of patients using a variety of agents, chiefly cisplatin, 5-fluorouracil, mitomycin-C, bleomycin, Taxol, vindesine, and vinblastine. Radiation therapy has been used alone or in combination with chemotherapy or surgery. Complications of radiation, such as esophagitis, stricture formation, transverse myelitis, the Brown-Sequard syndrome, pericardial effusion, or constrictive pericarditis, may cause presentation to the hospital.

COMMON PITFALLS

- The importance of early detection of esophageal carcinoma cannot be overstated. About 33% of patients have inoperable, advanced cancer when first seen.
- The earliest and most constant presenting symptom of esophageal cancer is dysphagia, initially with solids and later with liquids.
- Epigastric pain is an ominous symptom.
- The most common complication of radiation therapy is stricture of the esophagus.
- Pneumonitis may occur as the result of aspiration or from prior radiation therapy.
- In the emergency department, if esophageal cancer is suspected, it may be appropriate to obtain a barium swallow. In symptomatic patients, the barium swallow is nearly always abnormal.

GASTRIC NEOPLASMS

The incidence of gastric carcinoma has declined in the United States in the past 65 years, from approximately 50 per 100,000 in 1930 to 6 per 100,000 today—7.4 and 3.4 per 100,000 in males and females, respectively. However, it is still the sixth highest cause of cancer death in men in the United States, with 14,000 deaths annually and 22,400 new cases per year anticipated in 1997.

There is an increased incidence of the disease after age 50; it is unusual in persons younger than the age of 30. The mean age of diagnosis in the United States is 63. Neoplasm after partial gastric resection has been reported. The average delay in diagnosis is more than 10 months, due in part to patient denial and self-treatment with over-the-counter medications for "heartburn" and "gas" and to medical reluctance to work up common presenting complaints. The 5-year survival remains approximately 15% to 20%. The best hope for improving this figure lies in early diagnosis and possibly in screening asymptomatic patients, since 5-year survival for stage 0 gastric cancer may be over 95%, while it is 2% for stage IV disease. The latter has been effective in Japan, where gastric carcinoma is quite common (88 per 100,000) and surgical cure rates approach 50%. In the United States, approximately two-thirds of patients are at stage III or IV at the time of diagnosis.

Men are affected more frequently than are women. A genetic component may be involved, especially if first-degree relatives have had gastric carcinoma. Familial adenomatous polyposis and hereditary nonpolyposis colorectal cancer may be risk factors for gastric carcinoma. Diet has been implicated, especially a high intake of salted, pickled, or smoked foods, and, possibly, nitrates as precursors to carcinogenic nitrosamines. Mucosal changes associated with pernicious anemia may be premalignant, as are adenomatous gastric polyps. Smoking confers a slightly increased risk, as may the presence of type A blood. A role for *Helicobacter pylori* in causing atrophic gastritis that might be a precursor to gastric cancer has been suggested. This organism has been linked to mucosa-associated lymphoid tissue (MALT) lymphoma of the stomach as well. Pernicious anemia and the human immunodeficiency (HIV) virus have been linked to atrophic gastritis and to gastric lymphoma, respectively. Fresh vegetables, vitamin C, refrigeration of foods, wheat bran, and citrus fruits have all been proposed to be protective.

CLINICAL PRESENTATION

The patient may appear pale or cachectic with a low-grade fever. The most common symptom of gastric carcinoma is epigastric pain. This may be a mild ulcer-type pain, occurring after meals, or it may be continuous. Although the characteristics of the pain are nonspecific, the patient tends not to be symptom-free for more than 1 month at a time. There may be a vague postprandial fullness or burning. Dysphagia may be present, especially with tumors of the cardia. The average duration of symptoms before diagnosis is 6 to 10 months.

Weight loss of more than 3 kg is present in at least 40% of patients and suggests more advanced disease. Nausea and vomiting may be present, especially with pyloric tumors.

Unexplained anemia, melena, weakness, and hematemesis may also be presenting signs. Malaise, bloating, and anorexia are nonspecific symptoms of gastric cancer. There is some evidence of gastrointestinal bleeding in one-third of patients, but it is usually not severe.

Gastric obstruction with anorexia, upper abdominal fullness, and occasional vomiting of undigested food are less frequent presentations of a variety of gastric tumors. Rarely, a tumor may perforate and present with peritonitis, sepsis, or gastrocolic fistula.

Gastric cancer may spread through four separate mechanisms: (1) venous spread to the liver or more distant sites, such as the adrenals, bone, kidneys or lungs; (2) transperitoneal spread to the liver surface or ovary; (3) direct extension to the pancreas, mesocolon, or esophagus; and (4) lymphatic spread to the esophageal, paraaortic, and neck nodes.

Manifestations of advanced disease include a palpable abdominal mass, ascites, liver metastases, and palpable lymph nodes, especially a left supraclavicular node (Virchow), or left axillary (Irish's).

Jaundice may be due to either hepatic metastases or biliary obstruction at the hepatic portal. In women, metastases to the ovary may cause pelvic pain or mass, and an enlarged ovary (Krukenberg tumor) may be palpable on pelvic examination. Lung metastases with or without pleural effusion may cause shortness of breath. Cutaneous manifestations of gastric cancer include dermatomyositis, acanthosis nigricans, and multiple seborrheic keratoses. Infiltration of the umbilicus is called Sister Mary Joseph's nodule. Metastases to the prerectal pouch may be palpable as Blumer's shelf or present as mechanical bowel obstruction. There may be pain from bone involvement or neurologic symptoms from brain or meningeal metastases. Nephrotic syndrome, thrombophlebitis, and myopathy may occur.

If the tumor is detectable on physical examination, it is usually not curable. In fact, fewer than 10% of patients with symptoms have early gastric cancer (EGC) (cancer confined to the mucosa and submucosa).

Although 95% of gastric cancers are adenocarcinomas, approximately 5% of gastric malignancies are lymphomas. These will present as an abdominal mass, anemia, hematemesis, or perforation. Leiomyosarcomas are uncommon. Five-year survival with these rare types approaches 50% with surgical excision and radiation therapy.

Gastric carcinoids are rare and usually asymptomatic. If symptomatic, they present with bleeding, dyspepsia, or pain. Amine precursor uptake and decarboxylation (APUD) cells are diffused throughout the gastrointestinal tract. The carcinoid syndrome of flushing, diarrhea, asthma, cyanosis, and right-sided valvular heart disease is more frequently produced by intestinal tumors.

EMERGENCY DEPARTMENT EVALUATION

Diagnostic workup may be started in the emergency department and includes chest film, liver function studies, complete blood cell count, and abdominal ultrasonography or computed tomography (CT). The chest x-ray may demonstrate thickened and infiltrated gastric folds, or abnormal mass lesions. Liver scan or biopsy, endoscopy, lymph node biopsy, or evaluation of pleural or peritoneal effusions may reveal metastases.

Immunochemical fecal occult blood testing for 3 consecutive days will be positive in only 24% of gastric cancers, and is an insensitive test. Low pepsinogen I levels of a low pepsinogen I/II ratio may herald atrophic gastritis, but is of little screening value in the emergency department.

A routine upper gastrointestinal series is insensitive and without value in the diagnosis of EGC. Double-contrast upper gastrointestinal studies are more sensitive and the only type of barium meal examination that is capable of diagnosing EGC. Fiberoptic gastroscopy with biopsy and brush cytology is the *gold standard* for diagnosis. It can differentiate cancer from lymphoma and confirm the presence of carcinoma suspected by radiography. In combination with radiography it is 90% accurate in diagnosing gastric cancer. Endoscopic ultrasonography may be more accurate than CT in staging the depth of primary gastric tumors. CT scanning is useful in identifying liver metastases and in providing information about nodal involvement and extragastric tumor involvement, including peritoneal seeding and spread to the ovaries and rectal shelf. CT of the chest may reveal pulmonary metastases.

Serum carcinoembryonic antigen (CEA) is not sensitive or specific enough to have a role in the diagnosis of gastric cancer. Other tumor markers proposed, such as tumor necrosis factor-alpha and interleukin-6, seem not to be well correlated with tumor stage. Gene alterations may be detectable as mutation/deletion of *p53,* or mutations of APC, MCC, or DCC, but they do not have clinical significance as yet to the practice of emergency medicine.

EGC is curable in 90% of cases, regardless of lymph node involvement. The key is early diagnosis. History, physical examination, and radiographic studies cannot diagnose EGC.

The role of esophagogastroduodenoscopy (EGD) in the United States remains to be defined. Advocates of EGD note that complication rates are low (0.1%) and that it is often better tolerated than an upper gastrointestinal series. EGD is advisable if dyspepsia persists for more than 7 to 10 days or if improvement occurs but symptoms persist for 6 to 8 weeks. Some believe that gastroscopy is mandatory for all gastric ulcers; others believe that if radiographic findings are typically benign, with complete and sustained healing at 6 weeks, EGD is unnecessary.

TREATMENT AND PROGNOSIS

In the United States, the prognosis for patients with gastric carcinoma is bleak, with overall 5-year survival at 10% to 15%. Survival rates of EGC are 90% to 100%; unfortunately, only 6% with gastric cancer have EGC. The best predictor of survival after curative surgical resection is the presence or absence of serosal involvement. Table 38.2 lists staging and TNM classification, with survival rates by stage.

Surgical resection provides the only opportunity for cure, but 10% to 20% of patients are not explored; approximately half of those who undergo surgery have nonresectable tumors. Of the remainder who are operated on with curative intent (50%), the 5-year survival is 26% to 33%. *Curative resection* is defined as removal of all gross disease with negative surgical margins. The median survival of "surgically cured" patients ranges from 33 to 47 months. Operative mortality averages 8%. Over 50 different reconstructive procedures have been described, and laser/electrocautery ablation may need to be repeated to provide temporary relief. Indications for surgery include diagnosis suggested on an upper gastrointestinal series or confirmed on biopsy, obstruction, perforation, and bleeding.

Some patients undergo palliative procedures only, such a gastrojejunostomy, yttrium-aluminum-garnet (YAG) laser to control bleeding or restore patency, or plication of the tumor to control perforation.

TABLE 38.2. TNM Classification of Gastric Cancer

PRIMARY TUMOR (T)		
T1	Tumor is limited to mucosa and submucosa regardless of its extent or location.	
T2	Tumor involves the mucosa and the submucosa (including the muscularis propria), and extends to or into the serosa, but does not penetrate through the serosa.	
T3	Tumor penetrates through the serosa without invading contiguous structures.	
T4	Tumor penetrates through the serosa and invades the contiguous structures.	
NODAL INVOLVEMENT (N)		
N0	No metastases to regional lymph nodes	
N1	Involvement of perigastric lymph nodes within 3 cm of the primary tumor along the lesser or greater curvature	
N2	Involvement of the regional lymph nodes, more than 3 cm from the primary tumor, which are removable at operation, including splenic, celiac, and common hepatic nodes	
N3	Involvement of other intraabdominal lymph nodes that are not removable at operation, such as the paraaortic, hepatoduodenal, retropancreatic, and mesenteric nodes	
DISTANT METASTASIS (M)		
M0	No (known) distant metastasis	
M1	Distant metastasis present	
		5-year Survival
Stage 1	Nodes negative Mucosal or submucosal involvement only	90%–100%
Stage 2	Invasion of muscularis or serosa, negative nodes	50%
Stage 3	Positive nodes, no residual tumor	10%
Stage 4	Any distant metastases Any positive lymph nodes with macroscopic or microscopic residual tumor	0%–3%

Chemotherapy produces no significant difference in survival rates but produces tumor regression in 10% to 25% of cases. Median survival for recurrent or inoperable gastric carcinoma can be improved from 3 to 6 months untreated to 9 to 11 months with chemotherapy. The most frequently used agents are 5-fluorouracil, mitomycin-C, cisplatin, etoposide, epirubicin, leucovorin, doxorubicin, and methotrexate. Taxotere, CPT-11, Taxol, and S-1 are newer agents. The emergency physician should watch for neutropenia, thrombocytopenia, anemia, nausea/vomiting, diarrhea, infection, phlebitis/thrombosis, nephrotoxicity, neurotoxicity, and hepatotoxicity in patients on chemotherapy.

COMMON PITFALLS

Pathophysiology

- The average delay in diagnosis is more than 10 months and is due to patient denial and self-treatment with over-the-counter medications for "heartburn."
- The most common symptom of gastric cancer is epigastric pain; most patients will not be symptom-free for more than a month at a time.
- Weight loss and dysphagia may be present, with the former suggestive of advanced disease.
- Diagnostic evaluation may begin in the emergency department if gastric cancer is suspected. A routine upper gastrointestinal tract series is without value. Double-contrast upper gastrointestinal study is the only type of barium study capable of diagnosing EGC.
- Fiberoptic gastroscopy is the gold standard for diagnosis.

Bibliography

Alexander HR, Kelsen DG, Tepper JC. Cancer of the stomach. In: Devita VT Jr, Hellman S, Rosenberg SA, eds. *Cancer: principles and practice of oncology.* Philadelphia: Lippincott, 1997:1021–1054.

American Joint Committee on Cancer. Beahrs OH, Henson DE, Hutter RVP, et al., eds. *Manual for staging of cancer,* 3rd ed. Philadelphia: JB Lippincott Co, 1998:63–67.

El-Bayoumy K, Chung JR, Reddy BS, et al. Dietary control of cancer. *Exp Biol Med* 1997;216:211–223.

Forman D. *Helicobacter pylori* infection and cancer. *Br Med Bull* 1998;54(1):71–78.

Hill ME, Cunningham D. Medical management of advanced gastric cancer. *Cancer Treat Rev* 1998;24:113–118.

Huang JQ, Sridhar S, Chen Y, et al. Meta-analysis of the relationship between *Helicobacter pylori* seropositivity and gastric cancer. *Gastroenterology* 1998;114:1169–1179.

Kono S, Hirohata T. A review on the epidemiology of stomach cancer. *J Epidemiol* 1994;4:1–11. Kuipers EJ. Review article: relationships between *Helicobacter pylori,* atrophic gastritis and gastric cancer. *Aliment Pharmacol Ther* 1998;12[Suppl 1]:25–36.

Lambert R. An overview of the management of cancer of the esophagus. *Gastrointest Endosc Clin North Am* 1998;8(2):415–435.

Murikami A, Otani T, Nakaniski K, et al. Diagnostic validity of fecal occult blood test for detecting gastroenterological cancers. *Jpn J Cancer Res* 1992;83:141–145.

Poulin EC, Schlachta CM, Mamazza J. Operative treatment of malignancy: management of esophageal stenosis. *Gastrointest Endosc Clin North Am* 1998;8(2):435–450.

Sasako M, Mann GB, Cornelis JH, et al. Report of the Eleventh International Symposium of the Foundation for Promotion of Cancer Research: basic and clinical research in gastric cancer. *Jpn J Clin Oncol* 1998;28(7)443–449.

Sleisenger MH, Fordtran JS. *Gastrointestinal disease, pathophysiology/diagnosis/management,* 6th ed. Philadelphia: WB Saunders, 1998.

CHAPTER 39

Acute Diseases of the Gallbladder

Lance D. Wilson

Gallbladder disease is a common problem presenting to emergency departments, primarily because of the high prevalence of gallstones. About 25% of women and 15% of men over age 50 have gallstones. In the United States, over 600,000 cholecystectomies are performed yearly, contributing to the $5 billion annual cost of gallbladder disease.[2] Emergency physicians are confronted with a wide range of gallbladder pathology and should be familiar with the natural history of gallbladder disease to better understand the variable presentations of acute gallbladder disease and acute complications of chronic disease.

PATHOPHYSIOLOGY

The gallbladder acts as a reservoir off the common bile duct (CBD) that receives, concentrates, and secretes bile to assist in intestinal absorption of fat and fat-soluble vitamins. Gallstones form when cholesterol is supersaturated in the bile, leaves solution, and crystallizes on a matrix of calcium and other bile constituents. In the United States, about 90% of gallstones are cholesterol or mixed cholesterol stones. Once formed, gallstones may dissolve, remain unchanged, or grow larger.[12]

Risk factors for gallstone formation are those that predispose to increased concentrations of cholesterol in the bile and include increased age, obesity, female sex, family history, ethnicity, and hyperlipidemia. Crohn disease, ileal resection, and rapid weight loss are associated with decreased bile salts and are also risk factors for gallstone formation. About 10% of gallstones are formed of calcium bilirubinate (pigment stones); these are associated with hemolytic anemias, cirrhosis, biliary tract anomalies, and infections.[2]

Most gallbladder pathology is secondary to gallstones. However, about 10% of cases of acute cholecystitis are acalculous. Acalculous cholecystitis classically occurs in inpatients after major surgery, burns, trauma, or sepsis. After a major insult, bile stasis and low arterial inflow probably lead to gallbladder inflammation, infection, and, eventually, necrosis of the gallbladder wall. However, patients do present to the emergency department with acalculous cholecystitis. Over 70% of cases occur in outpatients, typically elderly men with significant atherosclerotic disease.[11] Acalculous cholecystitis must be considered in patients with acquired immunodeficiency syndrome (AIDS), who may present with cholecystitis and cholangitis secondary to cytomegalovirus and *Cryptosporidium* infection. Acute acalculous cholecystitis has a mortality rate that may be as high as 67%.[6]

CLINICAL PRESENTATION

It is helpful to view cholelithiasis (the presence of gallstones) in three stages: asymptomatic, symptomatic, and complicated. Complicated cholelithiasis includes such conditions as acute cholecystitis and its complications, choledocholithiasis (stones in the CBD), and the acute complications of chronic gallstones.[12]

Asymptomatic Cholelithiasis

Most people with asymptomatic gallstones remain asymptomatic. About 10% to 20% of people with asymptomatic gallstones develop complications over 20 years, or about 1% each year.[7] When patients with previously asymptomatic gallstones become symptomatic, nearly all develop pain, rather than cholecystitis or other acute complications, so they can be managed expectantly. With some exceptions, prophylactic cholecystectomy is not indicated.[7,12]

Symptomatic Cholelithiasis

Many people present to the emergency department with mildly symptomatic gallstones. Pain is caused by distention of the gallbladder as it contracts against stones obstructing the gallbladder neck or cystic duct. Typically, mild biliary pain is a vague midline discomfort, usually associated with nausea. The term *biliary colic* is a misnomer, as biliary pain is constant and lasts more than 1 hour and usually less than 5 hours. Pain typically occurs in the evening and is rarely postprandial. The vague nature and nonspecific location of the discomfort makes it often mistaken for gastritis, gastroenteritis, or other benign abdominal pathology. If the process continues, pain may become more severe, may become localized to the epigastrium or the right upper quadrant (RUQ), may radiate to the back or scapula, and may be associated with vomiting.[4]

Complicated Cholelithiasis

Complications of gallstones include acute cholecystitis and its complications, CBD stones, cholangitis, and complications of chronic gallstones. All are potentially life-threatening and require prompt recognition and treatment.

Acute Cholecystitis

In acute cholecystitis, the gallbladder neck or cystic duct is obstructed; the persistently increased intraluminal pressure, along with irritation from bile and stones, leads to mucosal damage, inflammation of the gallbladder wall, and, eventually, ischemia. In about 65% of cases, bacteria (usually enteric gram-negative bacteria and occasionally anaerobes) are cultured from bile. Bacterial suprainfection plays a role in some cases.[12] In acute cholecystitis, pain is typically sharp and more localized to the RUQ, with variable radiation to the epigastrium or back. Nausea and vomiting are common. Low-grade fever and tachycardia are usually present. Murphy's sign (respiratory arrest during deep inspiration while palpating the RUQ) or localized peritonitis may be elicited. In up to a third of cases, a swollen, tender gallbladder is palpated. Typically, a leukocytosis with left shift is present, and mild increases in liver function tests, alkaline phosphatase, and bilirubin are seen in 30% to 40% of patients.[9] Laboratory tests can be normal and fever can be absent, especially in the diabetic or chronically debilitated patient, and must not be relied on to make the diagnosis.[12] Patients are rarely septic; if sepsis is present, consider more complicated conditions, especially ascending cholangitis.

Complications of Acute Cholecystitis

Gallbladder perforation usually occurs in the setting of an acute or chronic cholecystitis, typically in the elderly, debilitated, or diabetic patient. The gallbladder usually becomes gangrenous and then perforates. The perforation normally walls off to form an empyema, but occasionally a bile leak occurs and leads to bile peritonitis.[9] Rarely, acute cholecystitis is complicated by infection with a gas-forming organism, leading to emphysematous cholecystitis. This typically occurs in diabetics and elderly men with vascular disease. Emphysematous cholecystitis is a serious condition with an overall mortality of 15%; mortality in uncomplicated acute cholecystitis is 4%.[5]

Common Duct Stones

Gallstones in the CBD are termed *choledocholithiasis*. Stones usually form in the gallbladder and migrate from the cystic duct, but they can form primarily in the biliary tree. Presentation is usually similar to that of acute cholecystitis but can be variable and sometimes more subtle. Patients may have jaundice if symptoms last more than 24 hours.[7] Choledocholithiasis usually causes an elevation in alkaline phosphatase and conjugated bilirubin, consistent with extrahepatic obstruction. Increases in amylase and lipase are variable. Four percent to 8% of patients with gallstones develop acute pancreatitis, which can vary from mild pain to severe pancreatitis, with massive fluid shifts and cardiovascular collapse.[8] Biliary tract and pancreatic tumors can present with abdominal pain, pancreatitis, and jaundice, but the presentation is typically more indolent, and 50% of patients do not have pain.

Ascending Cholangitis

Ascending cholangitis must be considered in any septic patient who presents with signs and symptoms of acute biliary tract disease, especially if the patient is diabetic, elderly, or debilitated. Ascending cholangitis is a bacterial infection of the biliary system, most frequently associated with CBD stones and obstruction. Classically, it presents with Charcot's triad of RUQ pain, jaundice, and fever and chills; if mental status changes and shock occur, this is considered Reynold's pentad. Ascending cholangitis seldom presents classically, so it must be considered in any septic patient without a source. Mortality approaches 40%.[3]

Complications of Chronic Cholelithiasis

In chronic and occasionally in acute cholecystitis, gallbladder–enteric fistulas may form, causing pain, aerobilia, or infection. Rarely, a gallstone may pass through a fistula into the small bowel and lodge in the ileocecal valve, causing a small bowel obstruction (gallstone ileus). Fistulas have been described between the gallbladder and the duodenum, stomach, colon, pleura, and other organs. Chronically inflamed gallbladders can become calcified, leading to the radiographic finding of a "porcelain gallbladder." These patients have a 25% risk of developing gallbladder cancer, which normally occurs in less than 1% of patients with chronic cholelithiasis.[4,12]

DIFFERENTIAL DIAGNOSIS

When patients present with complaints attributable to gallbladder disease, a wide range of both intraabdominal and extraabdominal processes must be considered (Table 39.1). Elderly or debilitated patients are often difficult to assess and require ancillary studies to rule out life-threatening disease.

EMERGENCY DEPARTMENT EVALUATION

Despite the diversity in acute gallbladder pathology, evaluation should follow a relatively straightforward sequence based on the patient's clinical status (Table 39.2). The goal of the emergency physician is to rule out life-threatening problems and, if gallbladder pathology is suspected, to rule out acute cholecystitis and other complicated acute gallbladder disease. If the patient presents with pain or other symptoms attributable to gallstones and is well and not dehydrated or vomiting, referral for outpatient ultrasound and follow-up is appropriate. No further emergency department workup is necessary. In the sicker patient with severe pain or dehydration and possibly fever, further workup is indicated, including a complete blood count, electrolytes, liver function tests, bilirubin, amylase, lipase, and urinalysis.

Radiographic Studies

The diagnosis of acute cholecystitis and its complications is primarily radiographic. Plain radiographs are most helpful for ruling out bowel obstruction or other causes of abdominal pain, although gallstones are visible on plain radiographs in about 10% of cases.

TABLE 39.1. Differential Diagnosis of Acute Diseases of the Gallbladder

Complications of gallstones
Acute cholecystitis
Hepatitis
Pancreatitis
Peptic ulcer disease
Esophageal disease, with or without perforation
Appendicitis
Bowel obstruction
Colonic pathology
Pelvic inflammatory disease
Fitz-Hugh–Curtis syndrome/perihepatitis
Renal colic
Pyelonephritis
Pneumonia
Pulmonary embolism
Acute myocardial infarction
Aortic dissection
HELLP syndrome

Because of its availability and low risk, ultrasound is the first-line method of evaluating the gallbladder and biliary tree. Gallstones alone do not make the diagnosis of acute cholecystitis. Other signs, such as a thickened gallbladder wall, sludge in the gallbladder, gallbladder distention, pericholecystic fluid, and focal tenderness are suggestive, with a sensitivity of more than 95% for acute cholecystitis.[10] Ultrasound is also helpful in making the diagnosis of complications of acute cholecystitis. A dilated CBD or intraluminal stone is diagnostic of choledocholithiasis. Free fluid suggests gallbladder perforation. Ultrasound can also assess other extrabiliary causes of RUQ pain in the liver, kidney, or pancreas.[10,12]

Cholescintigraphy with 99m-iminodiacetic compounds tests the patency of the cystic duct. Failure to visualize the gallbladder is highly sensitive for acute cholecystitis.

Hepatobiliary scanning is usually used when there is a high suspicion for acute cholecystitis, with an equivocal or negative ultrasound scan. However, some recommend it as the initial study for acute cholecystitis.[12]

Computed tomography (CT) scanning is reserved for patients with atypical presentations or possible concomitant intraabdominal pathology or complications.

EMERGENCY DEPARTMENT MANAGEMENT AND DISPOSITION

Emergency department management of symptomatic cholelithiasis includes hydration, antiemetics, and analgesia. These patients can usually be sent home with appropriate follow-up. If acute cholecystitis or another complicated presentation of gallbladder disease is considered, prompt consultation with a general surgeon is mandatory. Attention to the patient's volume and electrolyte status, antiemetics, and nasogastric tube placement is recommended. Analgesia, typically with intramuscular nonsteroidals or meperidine, is appropriate after surgical consultation.[1]

If the patient is febrile and acute cholecystitis is suspected, antibiotics are probably indicated, but this should be discussed with the consultant. The patient who is septic or is suspected of having ascending cholangitis, perforation, or emphysematous cholecystitis should be given antibiotics promptly after blood cultures. Typical biliary pathogens include enteric gram-negative bacteria or gram-positive species such as enterococcus or streptococci. Anaerobic species, particularly *Clostridium* and *Bacteroides fragilis,* occur in approximately 10% to 15% of cases, usually in the elderly or with obstructive disease. Appropriate coverage would include an intravenous antipseudomonal penicillin such as ticarcillin/clavulanate 3.1 g q6h or piperacillin/tazobactam 3.75 g q6h. Alternative regimens, especially if anaerobes are suspected, include a cephalosporin or an aminoglycoside plus clindamycin or metronidazole.[3]

Definitive treatment for symptomatic gallstones is usually surgical, with laparoscopic cholecystectomy standard treatment versus open cholecystectomy.[12] Oral dissolution therapy is used to dissolve gallstones, occasionally in conjunction with extracorporeal shock-wave lithotripsy in patients who are substantial surgical risks or do not want surgery.[4]

In patients who present with pain, fever, or jaundice after laparoscopic cholecystectomy, one must consider the increasingly recognized complications of the procedure, including biliary injury and fistulas, wound infections, and intraabdominal abscesses, which may present weeks to months after surgery.[12]

Definitive treatment for acute cholecystitis and complicated gallstone disease is almost always surgical. Most surgeons prefer urgent cholecystectomy (open or laparoscopic) rather than delayed surgery. In patients with CBD duct stones, endoscopic sphincterotomy or dilatation to relieve obstruction followed by

TABLE 39.2. Features That Differentiate Diseases of the Gallbladder

Cholelithiasis	Acute Cholecystitis	Gallstone Ileus	Choledocholithiasis	Cholangitis
PRESENTATION				
Usually asymptomatic, biliary colic in RUQ or epigastric pain (severe, persistent), nausea, vomiting	Pain in RUQ, severe usually associated with meal; nausea, vomiting	Abdominal distention, pain, vomiting; usually elderly patient, 65–77 years; associated medical disorders frequent (diabetes, cardiovascular disease, h/o gallbladder disease)	May be asymptomatic; pain in RUQ	Usually elderly patient; h/o biliary tract disease; colicky RUQ pain, fever, chills
PHYSICAL				
Asymptomatic—normal exam, biliary colic—tenderness (RUQ, epigastrium)	Temperature elevation classically; tachycardia, peritoneal irritation in RUQ (+ Murphy's sign); palpable mass in RUQ + 1/3 of patients; clinical jaundice, unusual	Appears acutely ill, dehydrated, abdominal distention, abdominal pain on palpation, clinical jaundice unusual	Normal exam, or common duct obstruction; clinical jaundice, RUQ tenderness	RUQ tenderness, clinical jaundice (mild); temperature 104°F–105°F; Charcol's triad/Reynold's pentad not always present: hypothermia not uncommon
LABORATORY				
WBC count normal, hepatic enzymes normal, bilirubin normal	Leukocytosis (may be absent); liver chemistries—slight elevation; bilirubin may reach 4.0 mg/dL	Leukocytosis (mild); electrolyte imbalance and dehydration —↓ Na^+, ↓ Cl^-, ↓ K^+, ↑ BUN; bilirubin not elevated	Asymptomatic—normal common bile duct obstruction; ↑ bilirubin, ↑ alkaline phosphatase, ↑ transaminase (minimal)	Leukocytosis >20,000 or <10,000 with left shift; bilirubin ↑ slight, alkaline phosphatase ↑
RADIOGRAPHS				
Ultrasonography → stones	Abdominal films not diagnostic; help to rule out other conditions. Ultrasonography—high sensitivity; specificity and accuracy for cholecystitis. Tc-HIDA scans useful in equivocal cases or acalculous cholecystitis.	Abdominal films—pneumobilia, evidence of mechanical bowel obstruction; stone in GI tract	Abdominal films rule out other diseases; ultrasonography—stones in CBD, dilation of CBD, if obstruction	Abdominal film—pneumobilia may be present
DIFFERENTIAL DIAGNOSIS				
When biliary colic present—gastric/duodenal ulcer, pancreatitis, hepatitis, renal colic, gastroesophageal reflux, angina, hiatal hernia	Appendicitis, perforated ulcer, acute pancreatitis, hepatitis, RLL pneumonia	Other causes of intestinal obstruction (hernia, adhesions, tumor)	Causes of obstructive jaundice: tumor in CBD, hepatic duct, head of pancreas, ampullar, duodenal	Nonsuppurative cholangitis; amebic/pyogenic hepatic abscess

cholecystectomy, or open cholecystectomy with CBD exploration, is performed.[8] Most patients with ascending cholangitis need some type of urgent biliary decompression. All patients with gallbladder perforation, emphysematous cholecystitis, or gallbladder empyema need emergent surgery.[9]

COMMON PITFALLS

- Acute complications of gallstone disease must be considered and recognized, particularly in the elderly and debilitated.
- Remember to consider cholecystitis or cholangitis in the elderly, diabetic, or debilitated patient who presents with fever of unknown origin, change in mental status, or other nonspecific complaints.
- Symptomatic gallstones should be considered in patients with mild or atypical presentations, such as nausea, dyspepsia, or vague abdominal pain.
- Always consider acute gallbladder disease in the pregnant woman with abdominal pain.
- Always obtain timely surgical consultation when complications of gallstone disease are considered.

References

1. Akriviadis EA, Hazigavriel M, Kapnias D, et al. Treatment of biliary colic with Diclofenac: A randomized, double-blind, placebo-controlled study. *Gastroenterology* 1997;113:225.
2. Diehl A. Epidemiology and natural history of gallstone disease. *Gastroenterol Clin North Am* 1991;20:1.
3. Elsakr R, Johnson DA, Younes Z, et al. Antimicrobial treatment of intra-abdominal infections. *Dig Dis* 1998;16:46.
4. Kalser S. National Institutes of Health Consensus Development Conference statement on gallstones and laparoscopic cholecystectomy. *Am J Surg* 1993;165:390.
5. Lee BY, Morilla C. Acute emphysematous cholecystitis: a case report and review of the literature. *N Y State J Med* 1992;92:406.
6. Leiva JI, Etter El, Gathe J, et al. Surgical therapy for 101 patients with acquired immunodeficiency syndrome and symptomatic cholecystitis. *Am J Surg* 1997;174:414.
7. Patino JF, Quintero GA. Asymptomatic cholelithiasis revisited. *World J Surg* 1998;22:1119.
8. Pellegrini C. Surgery for gallstone pancreatitis. *Am J Surg* 1993;165:515.
9. Reiss R, Deutsch AA. State of the art in diagnosis and management of acute cholecystitis. *Dig Dis* 1993;11:55.
10. Saini S. Imaging of the hepatobiliary tract. *N Engl J Med* 1997;336:1889.
11. Savoca P. The increasing prevalence of acalculous cholecystitis in outpatients. *Ann Surg* 1990;211:433.
12. Strasberg S. Cholelithiasis and acute cholecystitis. *Baillieres Clin Gastroenterol* 1997;11:643.

CHAPTER 40

Surgical Causes of Jaundice

Byron C. Scott and Jay L. Falk

Jaundice is a yellow discoloration of the skin, body fluids, and other viscera resulting from elevated levels of bilirubin in the serum. The numerous etiologies of jaundice are broadly categorized as either medical or surgical. Surgical jaundice is synonymous with extrahepatic biliary obstruction; medical jaundice encompasses all entities responsible for bilirubin overproduction, defective bilirubin metabolism, and impaired intrahepatic bilirubin excretion. This differentiation has practical importance in guiding patients to the appropriate specialist.

Extrahepatic obstruction can be distinguished from other causes of jaundice on the basis of the history, physical examination, and clinical laboratory findings in up to 90% of cases.[2,7,10] Invasive and noninvasive testing is used selectively to confirm clinical suspicions and to further delineate the nature and extent of the pathologic process.

CLINICAL PRESENTATION

Patients presenting with extrahepatic obstruction often report that the jaundice was first noticed by a family member or friends. Typically, the patient is an older person who denies constitutional symptoms. Cholestasis, a term that describes impairment of either intrahepatic or extrahepatic bile flow, is characterized by pruritus, pale stools, and dark urine. Abdominal pain suggests the presence of gallstones or pancreatitis; weight loss implies a malignant process. The patient must be questioned about previous biliary surgery, exposure to infectious hepatitis, alcohol intake, travel history, the use of drugs such as chlorpromazine and oral contraceptives, and chronic medical conditions.

The general appearance of a patient presenting with extrahepatic obstruction is typically that of someone who is "more yellow than sick."[5] Evidence of sepsis, including fever and toxic appearance, is evident when the obstruction is complicated by bacterial cholangitis. Abdominal findings vary according to the cause of obstruction. Epigastric tenderness suggests a pancreatic process; right upper quadrant tenderness is more suggestive of choledocholithiasis. Hepatomegaly can be seen in both medical and surgical jaundice. A palpable, nontender gallbladder represents malignant common duct obstruction (Courvoisier's law), especially if jaundice is painless.

DIFFERENTIAL DIAGNOSIS

The differential diagnosis of the patient who presents to the emergency department with jaundice is listed in Table 40.1. Despite the large number of potential etiologies, a careful history and physical examination can often narrow the differential diagnosis considerably. The selected use of laboratory tests guided by the clinical evaluation can rapidly pinpoint a definitive diagnosis.

EMERGENCY DEPARTMENT EVALUATION

Simple laboratory tests can be helpful in diagnosing surgical jaundice. In cases of extrahepatic obstruction, icterus typically results from elevated levels of conjugated bilirubin. Icterus resulting from hepatocellular disease may also be due primarily to conjugated bilirubin. Bilirubin fractionation is most useful in separating out diseases in which serum bilirubin levels are primarily unconjugated, such as hemolysis or ineffective erythropoiesis.[6] The

TABLE 40.1. Differential Diagnosis of Jaundice

PREHEPATIC	**EXTRAHEPATIC OBSTRUCTION**
Hemolysis	Common duct stone
Sickle cell disease	Biliary stricture
Other hemoglobinopathies	Bacterial cholangitis
Ineffective erythropoiesis	Ampullary carcinoma
Crigler-Najjar syndrome	Cholangiosarcoma
Gilbert syndrome	Gallbladder carcinoma
Prolonged fasting	Pancreatitis
Neonatal jaundice	Pancreatic carcinoma
Drugs	Pancreatic pseudocyst
HEPATOCELLULAR	Sclerosing cholangitis
Hepatitis	Hemobilia
Infectious	Duodenal diverticula
Alcoholic	Ascariasis
Autoimmune	Congenital choledochal cyst
Toxin	Caroli disease
Drug-induced	Recurrent pyogenic cholangitis
Cirrhosis	Postlaparoscopic cholecystectomy complications
Postischemia	Congenital biliary atresia
Hemochromatosis	Diaphragmatic defects
INTRAHEPATIC CHOLESTASIS	
Cholestatic jaundice of pregnancy	
Dubin-Johnson syndrome	
Drugs	
Rotor syndrome	
Benign recurrent cholestasia	
Familial syndromes	

severity of hyperbilirubinemia may suggest the cause of obstruction. Malignancy causes the highest average levels, often in the range of 10 to 30 mg/dL. Choledocholithiasis typically results in a transient rise in the bilirubin level, rarely exceeding 15 mg/dL.[11] Hepatic parenchymal disease is characterized by elevation of both conjugated and unconjugated bilirubin levels.

Alkaline phosphatase is synthesized in the epithelial cells of hepatic cholangioles as well as in bone and intestine. In the presence of biliary tract obstruction, alkaline phosphatase of hepatic origin results in elevated serum levels. High serum alkaline phosphatase levels are not pathognomonic of extrahepatic biliary obstruction, but when accompanied by conjugated hyperbilirubinemia, this possibility should be strongly suspected.[6]

Liver function tests along with an amylase or lipase can differentiate hepatocellular from cholestatic or obstructive pictures.[7,10] Transaminase levels are typically very high in hepatocellular disease but tend to be only moderately elevated in surgical jaundice.

Surgical jaundice may be accompanied by prolonged prothrombin times because of the inability of bile salts to reach the gut and assist in the absorption of vitamin K. This abnormality responds to parenteral injections of vitamin K over a 3-day period. Failure to respond implies the presence of hepatic parenchymal disease.[6]

Plain films of the abdomen are of limited value in the evaluation of jaundice. Only 20% of gallstones are radiopaque. Intrabiliary air may be visible, or an emphysematous gallbladder.[6]

The history of possible hepatitis exposure coupled with markedly elevated transaminase levels points to infectious hepatitis. Alcoholic liver disease is suggested by a history of alcohol abuse in combination with the physical stigmata of alcoholic liver disease. Exposure to hepatotoxins such as Amanita or carbon tetrachloride may suggest the diagnosis. Specific parenchymal disease may be diagnosed by liver biopsy in selected cases.[1]

Perhaps the most difficult distinction to make is between intrahepatic cholestasis and extrahepatic obstruction, because both cause an elevation in conjugated bilirubin levels. Currently, ultrasonography or computed tomography (CT) scanning can be used to demonstrate the dilated biliary ducts seen with obstruction. Both have similar sensitivities and positive predictive values, but ultrasonography is the diagnostic study of choice because of its lower cost and easier availability. CT scanning provides information about the level and nature of an obstruction and may be especially useful in identifying pancreatic masses.[8,9]

Once obstruction has been confirmed by one of these imaging techniques, prompt referral to a general surgeon is indicated. Management may include involvement by both a surgeon and a gastroenterologist.[4] The invasive techniques of transhepatic cholangiography (THC) or endoscopic retrograde cholangiopancreatography (ERCP) are reserved for equivocal cases or those in which corrective surgery is planned. These techniques may be used to bypass obstructions in a palliative or curative manner. THC is superior when a proximal lesion is suspected; ERCP is superior for distal lesions.[9]

EMERGENCY DEPARTMENT MANAGEMENT

Patients presenting to the emergency department with obstructive jaundice are generally not toxic or in need of resuscitation. Rather, thorough evaluation to identify coexistent conditions that might delay or even preclude surgical decompression is required. In patients who have been vomiting or not eating, assessment of hydration status, electrolytes, and nutritional status is indicated.

One entity that requires prompt intervention is bacterial cholangitis.[12] The potential for deterioration from sepsis is significant, and blood cultures must be obtained and parenteral antibiotics initiated. Bacteriologic organisms include *Enterobacter* sp. (68%), enterococci (14%), *Bacteroides* (10%), and *Clostridium* sp. (7%). Appropriate regimens include any of the following: antipseudomonal penicillin; ampicillin, gentamicin, and metronidazole; imipenem/cilastatin; ticarcillin/clavulanate; piperacillin/tazobactam; ampicillin/sulbactam; cefoxitin plus an antipseudomonal aminoglycoside; a third-generation cephalosporin and metronidazole or clindamycin; and aztreonam and clindamycin.[3,7,12] Ceftriaxone should probably be avoided, because it has been associated with biliary sludging.[7] Patients who display signs of significant toxicity may require aggressive intervention with intravenous fluids, supplemental oxygen, cardiac monitoring, nasogastric suction, and bladder catheterization before expeditious disposition to a critical care unit or surgery.

DISPOSITION

Role of the Consultant

Because little can be done in the emergency department in the way of definitive therapy for patients with extrahepatic obstruction, surgical consultation should be obtained once the diagnosis is suspected. The surgeon should decide whether further evaluation is necessary or whether sufficient information is available to proceed to laparotomy.

Indications for Admission

Patients with bacterial cholangitis should be hospitalized for parenteral antimicrobial therapy. If there is no evidence of infection, most cases of obstruction can be further evaluated and treated in an outpatient setting. Intractable pain, intractable emesis, or evidence of associated pancreatitis should result in immediate consultation rather than a referral. Most such cases are appropriately managed in the hospital.[11]

Transfer Considerations

Most patients can be successfully evaluated at the local institution. Critically ill patients with obstruction and cholangitis should receive resuscitative fluids, intravenous antibiotics, and possibly cholecystectomy before transfer to a center with sophisticated imaging and critical care services.

COMMON PITFALLS

- Patients with simple biliary colic must be differentiated from those cases complicated by cholangitis or pancreatitis. Patients with cholangitis can deteriorate rapidly and develop septic shock and the multiple organ dysfunction syndrome. Likewise, patients with pancreatitis can develop the systemic inflammatory response syndrome. Accordingly, the clinical assessment should be accompanied by the appropriate laboratory assessment to avoid misdiagnosis.
- Critically ill patients with cholangitis require emergent drainage of the biliary tree. Those with pancreatitis require urgent surgical consultation to orchestrate the timing and type of decompressive intervention.

References

1. Bouchier IAD. Diagnosis of jaundice. *BMJ* 1981;283:1282.
2. Frank BB, et al. Clinical evaluation of jaundice: guidelines of the patient care committee of the American Gastroenterological Association. *JAMA* 1989;262:3031.

3. Gilbert DN, Moellering RC, Sande MA. *The Sanford guide to antimicrobial therapy.* Hyde Park, NY: Antimicrobial Therapy, Inc., 1999.
4. Huang J, Christian W, Bebb J, et al. Decision making in surgery: the management of obstructive jaundice. *Br J Hosp Med* 1997;57:40.
5. Marin GA. Differential diagnosis of jaundice—hepatocellular vs. obstructive disease. *Postgrad Med* 1987;81:178.
6. Nakeeb A, Pitt HA. The jaundiced patient. In: Miller TA, ed. *Modern surgical care: physiologic foundations and clinical applications,* 2nd ed. St. Louis: Quality Medical Publishers, 1998.
7. O'Connor KW, Snodgrass PJ, Swonder JE, et al. A blinded prospective study comparing four noninvasive approaches in the differential diagnosis of medical vs. surgical jaundice. *Gastroenterology* 1983;84:1498.
8. Rossi RL, Traverso LW, Pimentel F. Malignant obstructive jaundice. *Surg Clin North Am* 1996;76:63.
9. Scharschmidt BF, Goldberg HI, Schmid R. Approach to the patient with cholestatic jaundice. *N Engl J Med* 1983;308:1515.
10. Schenker S, Blaint J, Schiff L. Differential diagnosis of jaundice: report of a prospective study of 61 proved cases. *Am J Dig Dis* 1962;7:449.
11. Way LW. Biliary tract. In: Way LW, ed. *Current surgical diagnosis and treatment,* 10th ed. Los Altos, CA: Lange Medical Publications, 1994.
12. Westphal JF, Brogard JM. Biliary tract infections. *Drugs* 1999;57:81.

CHAPTER 41
Acute Appendicitis

Brian K. Snyder

Acute appendicitis can mimic virtually any intraabdominal process; therefore, to know acute appendicitis is to know well the diagnosis of acute abdominal pain.[10]

Appendicitis is an acute inflammatory process of the appendix resulting from obstruction of the lumen with subsequent bacterial invasion, distention, ischemia, and ultimate rupture. As traditionally taught, appendicitis presents with initial periumbilical pain, which later migrates to the right lower quadrant (RLQ). Anorexia, nausea, and vomiting are associated symptoms. Physical examination reveals a low-grade fever and RLQ tenderness, with guarding and rebound as the process progresses. Laboratory evaluation reveals a leukocytosis with neutrophilia. Unfortunately, this classic presentation occurs in only a minority of cases and the diagnosis may be difficult to make. In one large series, diagnostic accuracy averaged only 85%, with a 19% perforation rate. A percentage of the perforation rate is surely from delayed diagnosis. Incidence of perforation increases with the extremes of age, and perforation is associated with greater morbidity and mortality.[1]

The lifetime risk of appendicitis is 8.6% for males and 6.7% for females, with an annual incidence of 1.1:1,000. The male-to-female ratio for appendicitis is 1.4:1, although females have a higher rate of negative appendectomies. The peak incidence for males is between 10 and 14 years, and for females, between 14 and 19 years. Appendicitis rates are 1.5 times higher for Whites than for non-Whites, and are higher in summer.[1] The etiology of these differences is unknown, but temporospatial clustering and outbreaks of appendicitis point to an infectious agent as a cause of some cases of appendicitis.[3]

The normal, uninflamed appendix is a hollow visceral structure with a closed distal end arising from the cecum; on average, it is 9.5 to 10.0 cm in length. Although the density of immune cells in lymphoid follicles in the appendix suggests an immunologic role, the function of the appendix is unknown.[6] Its anatomic position can be anterior (postilial, preilial, and pelvic) or posterior (retrocecal and subcecal), and many appendices are mobile (Fig. 41.1).[9] The traditional surface landmark for the location of the appendix is McBurney's point, which is located 1.5 to 2.0 in. from the inferior aspect of a line drawn from the anterior superior iliac spine point to the umbilicus. However, barium studies reveal that most appendices lie inferior to this point; therefore, making clinical decisions based on the presence or absence of pain or tenderness at exactly McBurney's point is unjustified.[20]

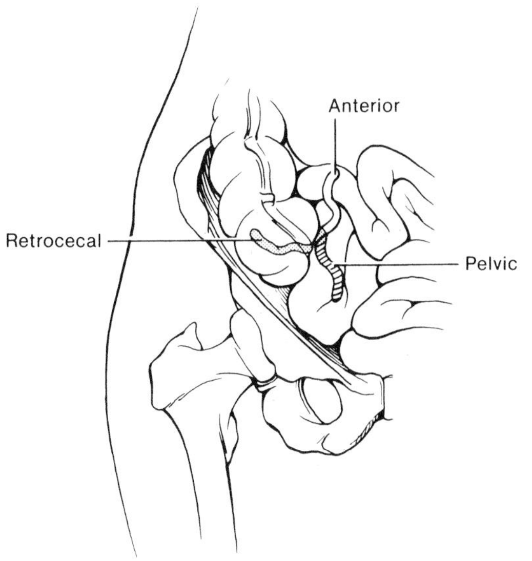

Figure 41.1. Anatomic position of the appendix.

PATHOPHYSIOLOGY

The common pathophysiologic event in appendicitis is obstruction of the lumen. Obstruction can be from lymphoid hyperplasia, intraluminal objects (fecaliths, foreign bodies, or parasites) or tumors (carcinoid, adenocarcinoma, or metastatic tumors). A variety of inflammatory conditions can result in hyperplasia of appendiceal lymphoid follicles that progresses until the appendiceal wall itself obstructs the lumen. Conditions noted for this process include respiratory infections, mumps, mononucleosis, amebiasis, and bacterial gastroenteritis.

Crohn disease can affect the appendix.[35] Patients with the acquired immunodeficiency syndrome can have other processes of the appendix, including Kaposi's sarcoma, lymphoma, or opportunistic infections (e.g., cytomegalovirus).[33]

Once the appendiceal lumen is obstructed, mucus secretion within the appendix raises intraluminal pressures until lymphatic and venous return is impaired. Ischemic injury to the mucosa results, followed by bacterial invasion of the appendiceal mucosa and submucosa. Continued inflammation and bacterial proliferation result in perforation of the appendix and spillage of inflammatory cells and bacteria into the peritoneum, resulting in peritonitis. At times, the peritoneal infection is contained by the omentum and a periappendiceal abscess forms.[35]

CLINICAL PRESENTATION

History

The characteristic clinical presentation of acute appendicitis is abdominal pain in association with anorexia, nausea, and vom-

TABLE 41.1. Signs and Symptoms of Acute Appendicitis

	Nonperforated (%)	Perforated (%)	All Cases (%)
SYMPTOMS			
Abdominal pain	99.6	99.3	99.6
Epigastric at onset	74.4	70.1	73.5
Constant RLQ	25.5	29.1	26.0
Anorexia			92
Nausea	78.0	79.8	78.3
Vomiting	51.8	64.2	54.2
Migration of pain	52.3	38.0	49.6
Fever	16.3	39.6	20.8
Diarrhea	15.0	22.4	16.4
Constipation	8.3	14.2	9.4
Lucid interval[a]	3.2	11.2	4.8
SIGNS			
Abdominal tenderness			
Direct RLQ	99.6	99.3	99.6
Referred RLQ	26.3	18.6	24.9
Lower abdominal	7.8	21.6	10.6
Generalized	9.6	21.6	11.9
Right-sided rectal tenderness	48.7	41.8	47.4
Local rigidity over RLQ	26.3	45.5	30.1
Generalized rectal tenderness	11.4	19.4	12.9
Rebound tenderness	4.8	4.5	4.8
Positive psoas test	4.8	3.7	4.7
Generalized rigidity	0.7	12.7	3.1
Palpable mass in RLQ	0.5	3.7	1.2

[a]*Lucid interval* refers to a period of time after perforation in which pain is temporarily lessened; some authorities do not consider this a legitimate phenomenon.

Data from Lewis FH, Holcroft JW, Boey J, et al. Appendicitis: a critical review of diagnosis and treatment in 1000 cases. *Arch Surg* 1975;110:677; and Pieper R, Kager L, Näsman P. Acute appendicitis: a clinical study of 1018 cases of emergency appendectomy. *Acta Chir Scand* 1982;148:51.

iting[23,27] (Table 41.1). About 50% of patients present within 24 hours of the onset of symptoms, 33% between 24 and 48 hours and the rest thereafter. Abdominal pain occurs in nearly 100% of patients, is epigastric in onset in 74%, and migrates to the RLQ in 50%. Anorexia is present in 92% of patients, accompanied by nausea and vomiting in 78% and 54% of patients, respectively.

Physical Examination

Although often regarded as a reliable clinical feature of appendicitis, fever is reported in only 21% of all cases and in only 16% of cases of appendicitis uncomplicated by perforation.

The most reliable sign of acute appendicitis is RLQ tenderness, present in nearly 100% of patients. Twenty-five percent of patients demonstrate referred RLQ tenderness under remote palpation (Rovsing's sign); rigidity in the RLQ is present in 30% of patients. Nearly 50% of patients demonstrate right-sided rectal tenderness.

The most significant complication of acute appendicitis is perforation, which either leads to generalized peritonitis and sepsis or is contained as an intraabdominal abscess. The mortality rate of perforated appendicitis is 1.66%, seven times greater than that of patients undergoing appendectomy for simple, acute appendicitis (0.24%) and 12 times greater than that of appendectomy of a normal appendix (0.14%).[40] Clearly, the clinician must try to diagnose cases of simple acute appendicitis before perforation occurs.

There are few reliable clinical features that distinguish nonperforated from perforated appendicitis (see Table 41.1). The duration of symptoms tends to be longer in patients with perforation (greater than 48 hours). Signs that suggest perforation include lower or generalized abdominal tenderness, local or generalized rigidity over the RLQ, the presence of a palpable RLQ mass, and generalized rectal tenderness.[27]

Pediatric, geriatric, and pregnant patients deserve special mention. Because diagnosis often is more difficult in these groups, their morbidity and mortality is greater.

Pediatric Patients

Children's appendices have a much thinner wall than that in the adult, allowing more rapid mucosal penetration and subsequent perforation. Perforation rates average 37% to 59% in children under age 13. In children under age 3, the perforation rate increases to 67% to 79%. The inability of the very young to verbalize their symptoms contributes to the difficulty in diagnosis.[11,15,29] Diarrhea is a presenting complaint in about a third of appendicitis patients under the age of 3[11,19] (see Chapter 260).

Geriatric Patients

Only 20% of patients over age 60 who are diagnosed with appendicitis present with the classic nausea, vomiting, RLQ tenderness, and an elevated white count or shift. Consequently, the perforation rate is 67% to 90%. The mortality rate is 4.6%, 23 times greater than that of patients younger than age 60[1,18] (see Chapter 36).

Pregnant Patients

The physiologic changes of pregnancy, especially during the second and third trimesters, impede the diagnosis and create a physiologic environment that suppresses the normal host response to inflammation. As the uterus enlarges, the appendix

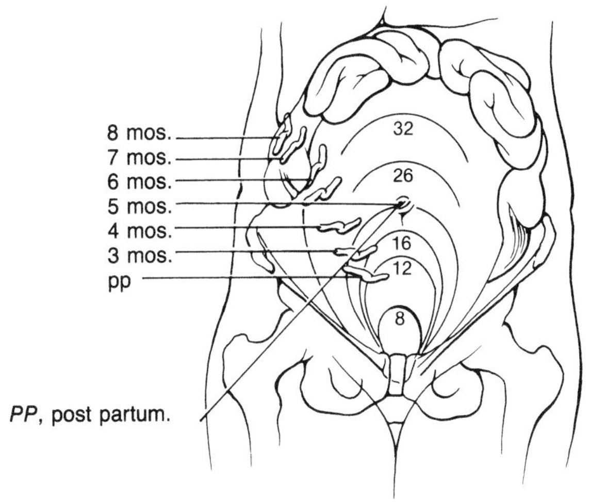

Figure 41.2. Changes in appendiceal position during pregnancy.

rotates in a counterclockwise direction out of the pelvis (Fig. 41.2). In addition, as the expanding uterus lifts the abdominal wall away from the appendix, the omentum is less available to wall off the infectious process following perforation. Diffuse peritonitis develops preferentially over a periappendiceal abscess. The increase in serum steroids during pregnancy diminishes the inflammatory response and facilitates a more rapid and overwhelming peritonitis.[26] These physiologic and anatomic processes result in a perforation rate of 43%.[37] The maternal mortality rate remains low at 0.7%, but fetal mortality may approach 8.5%.[26]

DIFFERENTIAL DIAGNOSIS

A variety of conditions mimic appendiceal inflammation[1] (Table 41.2); the diagnostic accuracy of appendectomy for suspected acute appendicitis is only 85%. Disorders most commonly associated with removal of a normal appendix despite clinical suspicion of acute appendicitis include mesenteric lymphadenitis, other diseases of the appendix, and gynecologic ailments. The greatest diagnostic difficulties are encountered in women of childbearing age. The overall diagnostic accuracy for females is 77%; in contrast, males have a diagnostic accuracy of 91%.[1]

TABLE 41.2. Differential Diagnosis of Acute Appendicitis

Discharge Diagnoses Most Commonly Recorded After Negative Appendectomy	Percentage
Other diseases of the appendix (colic, concretion, Meckel's diverticulum, fecalith, fistula, intussusception, mucocele)	19.4
Other appendicitis (chronic, recurrent, relapsing, or subacute)	16.5
Mesenteric lymphadenitis	22.0
Abdominal pain	12.2
Gastroenteritis, noninfectious	6.4
Cholelithiasis	4.1
Ovarian cyst	5.5
Uterine leiomyoma	4.3
Endometriosis	4.0
Lymphoid hyperplasia of the appendix	3.1
Cervicitis, endocervicitis	2.7

Other considerations in the differential diagnosis include regional enteritis, perforated peptic ulcer, diverticulitis, carcinoma of the bowel, ureteral calculi, pelvic inflammatory disease, mittelschmerz.

Data from Addis DG, Shaffer N, Fowler S, et al. The epidemiology of appendicitis and appendectomy in the United States. *Am J Epidemiol* 1990;132:910.

EMERGENCY DEPARTMENT EVALUATION

Appendicitis should be suspected based on the history and physical examination. The emergency clinician should be particularly aggressive in evaluating the very young, the elderly, and the pregnant patient, as the morbidity and mortality rates of acute appendicitis in these subpopulations far exceed those of others. No laboratory or radiographic study is completely sensitive for acute appendicitis, but several are commonly relied on for their supportive value.

Laboratory Studies

Acute appendicitis is classically associated with leukocytosis with a left shift. In one large study, 88% of adult patients with acute appendicitis had a white count of over 10,000 cells/μL, and 94% had a leukocytosis *or* a neutrophilia above 75%. Specificity was only 76% and 62%, respectively. Approximately 10% of patients with acute appendicitis have normal leukocyte and neutrophil counts.[22] Unfortunately, the leukocyte count is nonspecific, being reported as low as 38%.[2] Further complicating matters, the normal range for the leukocyte count changes with age. By calculating likelihood ratios, one finds that the leukocyte count has minimal effect on the probability of disease, except for the extremes of the leukocyte count. However, only a small minority of patients will have such leukocyte values.[36] Some authors advocate serial leukocyte counts and progressive leukocytosis as suggestive of acute appendicitis. Studies regarding the clinical utility of sequential leukocyte counts are inconclusive, and it appears that utility, if any, is limited to a small percentage of the total patient population.[13,25,38]

Urinalysis, often obtained in the evaluation of abdominal pain, cannot be relied on to distinguish disease of the urinary tract from that of the appendix. In one study of patients with histologically confirmed acute appendicitis, 30% had an abnormal urinalysis, regardless of the position of the appendix. In those with either a ruptured or inflamed appendix in the retrocecal or pelvic position, abnormal urinalysis was detected in 50%. Diagnostic decisions should *not* be based on the presence of pyuria or bacteriuria.[34]

Imaging Studies

Radiologic studies should be reserved for those with equivocal symptoms and physical findings. In cases of strongly suspected appendicitis, time-consuming diagnostic procedures should not be used. One study demonstrated that patients who had a barium enema as part of their workup had significantly longer delays from presentation to surgery. Because the incidence of perforation is directly related to the interval between symptom onset and surgery, tests that may delay definitive therapy should be used with caution.[28]

Plain radiographs are often obtained in suspected appendicitis; a variety of radiographic findings may be seen, including a fecalith, localized ileus, or obscuration of fat–tissue interfaces.[17] These findings are nonspecific and the diagnostic yield is low.[7] Plain radiographs should be obtained only when other diagnoses are high in the differential (e.g., bowel obstruction).

A barium enema can used to evaluate potential appendicitis on the premise that a normal appendix can be filled with barium but an obstructed appendix will not allow the passage of barium. Generally, a barium enema is highly accurate in the diagnosis of appendicitis, although false-positive examinations occur and there is a relatively high incidence of technical failure.[17]

Labeled white blood cell scanning provides good sensitivity (90% to 97%) and specificity (89% to 97%). A major disadvantage of such nuclear medicine studies is that although early positive studies are possible, the procedure can take up to 4 hours to complete.[5,32]

Abdominal ultrasonography is often used in the evaluation of appendicitis. When obstructed, the appendix appears as a blind-ended, immobile, noncompressible structure that cannot be displaced under direct pressure from the ultrasound probe. An appendix that is visualized on ultrasound examination is considered diagnostic of appendicitis. If the appendix cannot be seen, appendicitis is excluded. Unfortunately, ultrasonography is nondiagnostic in 3% to 11% of cases due to pain, guarding, obesity, or overlying gas. Sensitivity ranges from 75% to 89% and specificity from 86% to 100%. Poorer results are obtained in early appendicitis, perforation, and retrocecal appendicitis.[17] Ultrasound is the preferred modality in pregnant patients and is highly sensitive in this population.[24]

Helical computed tomography (CT) scanning of the abdomen is fast and highly accurate in the evaluation of acute appendicitis. The sensitivity of unenhanced helical CT is approximately 90%; with the addition of rectal or intravenous contrast, the sensitivity increases up to 97% to 98%.[14,21,30] Specificity is equally high at 94% to 97%. Findings include a fecalith, an inflamed appendix, stranding in the surrounding fat or periappendicular fluid, phlegmon, or abscess[6] (Fig. 41.3). Helical CT in the evaluation of appendicitis appears to be cost effective, and its use may decrease the negative laparotomy and perforation rates.[30,31] Furthermore, CT often provides an alternative diagnosis. In addition, it is useful in the assessment of cases of suspected perforated appendicitis with periappendiceal abscess formation, which may be treated conservatively or with percutaneous drainage and interval appendectomy.[41]

Diagnostic laparoscopy, especially for women of childbearing age, has advocates. It is highly accurate and safe.[8]

EMERGENCY DEPARTMENT MANAGEMENT AND DISPOSITION

The patient suspected of having acute appendicitis should be given nothing by mouth. Intravenous access is indicated to ensure hydration. Surgical consultation should be obtained promptly, as timely appendectomy of an inflamed but nonperforated appendix is of paramount importance. If acute appendicitis is suspected but in doubt, radiologic study, emergency department observation, or admission for inpatient observation with sequential examination is an alternative. Observation is a safe and effective way to distinguish patients with appendicitis from those without.[12,16]

Although traditional edict warns that analgesia will obscure the diagnosis in acute abdominal pain, the use of narcotics has not been shown to increase the number of delayed or missed diagnoses.[4] The judicious use of short-acting narcotics is reasonable in patients with acute abdominal pain while evaluation is in progress, especially those in which a radiologic procedure is to be performed or surgical consultation is delayed.

COMMON PITFALLS

- Abdominal pain and tenderness are present in nearly 100% of patients with appendicitis; other clinical features are less reliable.
- Fever occurs in only 16% of patients with acute appendicitis; its presence is more suggestive of appendiceal perforation.
- Reliance on the leukocyte count is unwarranted and usually leads to false reassurance.
- Helical CT appears to be highly accurate in diagnosing appendicitis, although no test is fail-proof.
- Caution is advised in evaluating the young, the elderly, pregnant women, and women of childbearing age. The diagnosis is often elusive, and many patients proceed to perforation.
- When in doubt, admit the patient for observation to an emergency department observation area or surgical service for sequential physical examinations.
- The missed diagnosis of appendicitis remains one of the most frequent malpractice claims against emergency physicians.

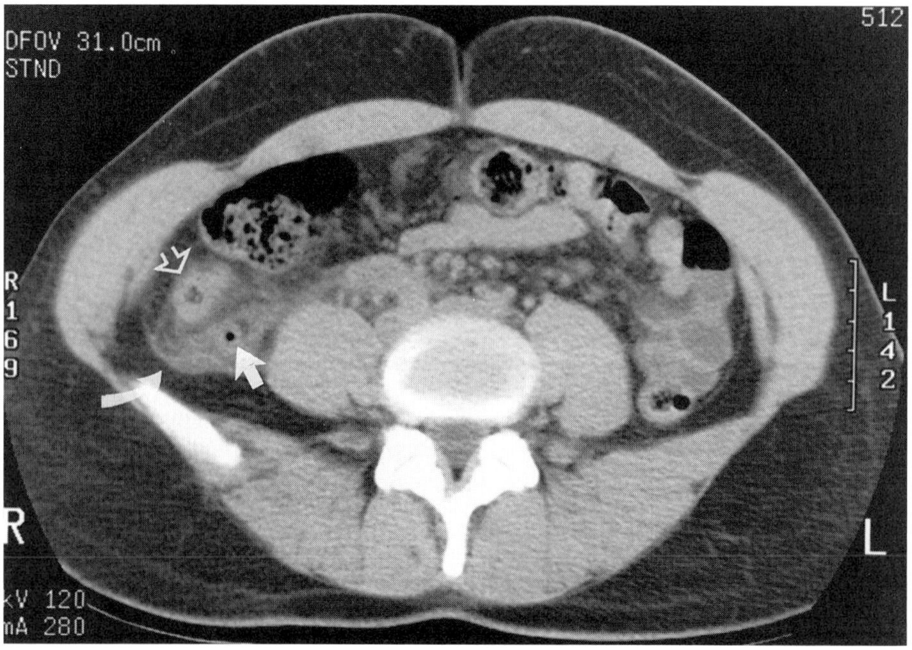

Figure 41.3. CT appearance of appendicitis.

Document all examinations, laboratory results and their interpretations, and conversations with consultants, including their opinion, advice, and therapeutic plan.[39]

- For patients being discharged with indefinite diagnoses, provide clear, legible instructions explicitly detailing conditions meriting a return visit for further evaluation.

References

1. Addis DG, Shaffer N, Fowler S, et al. The epidemiology of appendicitis and appendectomy in the United States. *Am J Epidemiol* 1990;132:910.
2. Alvarado A. A practical score for the early diagnosis of acute appendicitis. *Ann Emerg Med* 1986;15:557.
3. Andersson R, Hugander A, Thulin A, et al. Clusters of acute appendicitis: further evidence for an infectious aetiology. *Int J Epidemiol* 1995;24:829.
4. Attard AR, Corlett MJ, Kidner NJ, et al. Safety of early pain relief for acute abdominal pain. *BMJ* 1992;305:554.
5. Barron B, Hanna C, Passalaqua AM. Rapid diagnostic imaging of acute nonclassic appendicitis by leukoscintigraphy with sulesomab, a technetium 99m-labelled antigranulocyte antibody Fab′ fragment. *Surgery* 1999;125:288.
6. Bjerke K, Brandtzaeg P, Rognum TO. Distribution of immunoglobulin-producing cells is different in normal human appendix and colon mucosa. *Gut* 1986;27:667.
7. Boleslawksi E, Pannis Y, Benoist S. Plain abdominal radiography as a routine procedure for acute abdominal pain of the right lower quadrant: prospective evaluation. *World J Surg* 1999;23:262.
8. Borgstein PJ, Gordijn RV, Eijsbouts QAJ, et al. Acute appendicitis—a clear-cut case in men, a guessing game in women: a prospective study on the role of laparoscopy. *Surg Endosc* 1997;11:923.
9. Buschard K, Kjaeldgaard A. Investigation and analysis of the position, fixation, length and embryology of the vermiform appendix. *Acta Chir Scand* 1973;139:293.
10. Cope Z. The differential diagnosis of appendicitis. In: Silen W, ed. *The early diagnosis of the acute abdomen,* 19th ed. New York: Oxford University Press, 1996:88.
11. Daehlin L. Acute appendicitis during the first three years of life. *Acta Chir Scand* 1982;148:291.
12. Dolgin SE, Beck RA, Tartter PI. The risk of perforation when children with possible appendicitis are observed in the hospital. *Surg Gynecol Obstet* 1992;175:320.
13. Errikson S, Granstrom L, Carlstrom A. The diagnostic value of repetitive preoperative analyses of C-reactive protein and total leukocyte count in patients with suspected acute appendicitis. *Scand J Gastroenterol* 1994;29:1145.
14. Funaki B, Grosskreutz SR, Funaki CN. Using unenhanced helical CT with enteric contrast material for suspected appendicitis in patients treated at a community hospital. *AJR* 1998;171:997.
15. Gamal R, Moore TC. Appendicitis in children aged 13 years and younger. *Am J Surg* 1990;159:589.
16. Graff L, Radford MJ, Werne C. Probability of appendicitis before and after observation. *Ann Emerg Med* 1991;20:503.
17. Hoffmann J, Rasmussen O. Aids in the diagnosis of acute appendicitis. *Br J Surg* 1989;76:774.
18. Horattas MC, Guyton DP, Wu D. A reappraisal of appendicitis in the elderly. *Am J Surg* 1990;160:291.
19. Horwitz JR, Gursoy M, Jaksic T, et al. Importance of diarrhea as a presenting symptom of appendicitis in very young children. *Am J Surg* 1997;173:80.
20. Karim OM, Boothroyd AE, Wyllie JH. McBurney's point—fact or fiction? *Ann R Coll Surg Engl* 1990;72:304.
21. Lane MJ, Katz DS, Ross BA, et al. Unenhanced helical CT for suspected acute appendicitis. *AJR* 1997;168:405.
22. Lau WY, Ho YC, Chu KW, et al. Leukocyte count and neutrophil percentage in appendectomy for suspected appendicitis. *Aust N Z J Surg* 1989;59:395.
23. Lewis FH, Holcroft JW, Boey J, et al. Appendicitis: a critical review of diagnosis and treatment in 1000 cases. *Arch Surg* 1975;110:677.
24. Lim HK, Bae SH, Geo GS. Diagnosis of acute appendicitis in pregnant women: value of sonography. *AJR* 1992;159:539.
25. Lyons D, Waldron R, Ryan T, et al. An evaluation of the clinical value of the leucocyte count and sequential counts in suspected appendicitis. *Br J Clin Pract* 1987;41:794.
26. Mahmoodian S. Appendicitis complicating pregnancy. *South Med J* 1992;85:19.
27. Pieper R, Kager L, Näsman P. Acute appendicitis: a clinical study of 1018 cases of emergency appendectomy. *Acta Chir Scand* 1982;148:51.
28. Preston CA, Karach SB. The influence of gender and use of barium on morbidity and mortality in acute appendicitis. *Am J Emerg Med* 1989;7:253.
29. Putnam TC, Gagliano N, Emmens RW. Appendicitis in children. *Surg Gynecol Obstet* 1990;170:527.
30. Rao PM, Rhea JT, Novelline RA, et al. Effect of computed tomography of the appendix on treatment of patients and use of hospital resources. *N Engl J Med* 1998;338:141.
31. Rao PM, Rhea JT, Rattner DW, et al. Introduction of appendiceal CT; impact on negative appendectomy and appendiceal perforation rates. *Ann Surg* 1999;229:344.
32. Rypins EB, Kipper SL. 99mTc-hexamethylpropyleneamine oxime (Tc-WBC) scan for diagnosing acute appendicitis in children. *Am Surg* 1997;63:878.
33. Savioz D, Lirionia A, Zurbuchen P, et al. Acute right iliac fossa pain in acquired immunodeficiency: a comparison between patients with and without acquired immunodeficiency syndrome. *Br J Surg* 1996;83:644.
34. Scott JH, Amin M, Harty JI. Abnormal urinalysis in appendicitis. *J Urol* 1983;129:1015.
35. Silen ML, Tracy TF. The right lower quadrant "revisited." *Pediatr Clin North Am* 1993;40:1201.
36. Snyder BK, Hayden SR. Accuracy if the leukocyte count in the diagnosis of acute appendicitis. *Ann Emerg Med* 1999;33:565.
37. Tamir HL, Bongard FS, Klein SR. Acute appendicitis in the pregnant patient. *Am J Surg* 1990;160:571.
38. Thompson MM, Underwood MJ, Dookeran KA. Role of sequential leucocyte counts and C-reactive protein measurements in acute appendicitis. *Br J Surg* 1992;79:822.
39. Trautlein JJ, Lambert R, Miller J. Malpractice in the emergency room: a critical review of undiagnosed appendicitis cases and legal actions. *Qual Assur Util Rev* 1987;2:54.
40. Velanovich V, Satava R. Balancing the normal appendectomy rate with the perforated appendicitis rate: implications for quality assurance. *Am Surg* 1992;58:264.
41. Yamini D, Vargas H, Bongard F, et al. Perforated appendicitis: is it truly a surgical urgency? *Am Surg* 1999;64:970.

CHAPTER 42
Bowel Obstruction

Philip L. Henneman

Intestinal obstruction is a common disorder that has been recognized by physicians for centuries. It accounts for approximately 4% of patients presenting to an emergency department with nontraumatic abdominal pain of less than 7 days' duration. The challenge to the emergency physician is to promptly identify the patients with bowel obstruction from the many patients presenting to an emergency department with abdominal pain and vomiting, without doing multiple tests and without delaying treatment, admission, and surgical consultation.

Intestinal obstruction was associated with a 60% mortality in 1900. This has decreased to approximately 5% due to early recognition, aggressive stabilization with fluid resuscitation, simple nasogastric decompression, and, in most cases, surgical intervention. Mortality can still result from strangulation, bowel infarction, and resulting sepsis. Early recognition and initiation of treatment are the only way for the emergency physician to minimize major morbidity or mortality.

Intestinal obstruction accounts for about 20% of all acute surgical admissions. The obstruction most commonly affects the small intestine but involves the colon in up to 20% of patients. The vast majority of bowel obstructions are due to postoperative adhesions, accounting for 50% of small bowel obstructions. Other common causes include hernias and neoplasm in adults and intussusception, hernias, and congenital abnormalities in children. Feces, foreign bodies, strictures, abscesses, trauma, and volvulus are other less common causes.

The stomach, small bowel, biliary tract, and pancreas collectively secrete 8 to 10 L of fluid daily. Almost all of this volume is reabsorbed in the large bowel. Obstruction prevents the flow of fluid and other intraluminal contents to the colon, resulting in accumulation in the more proximal sections of the bowel. This causes a gradual distention of the bowel proximal to the obstruction, and increasing intraluminal pressure. As pressure increases within the bowel, hypersecretion of fluid into the bowel develops, and absorption from the bowel is retarded. Volume losses into the intraluminal space are variable but can be up to 9 L in 24 hours, causing significant depletion of intravascular volume. Further increases in intraluminal pressure result in capillary and lymphatic obstruction with resulting edema of the bowel wall. Retrograde peristalsis eventually develops, resulting in vomiting by the patient. If allowed to progress, venous and finally arterial obstruction will occur. Bacterial overgrowth occurs in the stagnant bowel contents. Hemorrhagic necrosis, gangrene of the bowel, and leakage of contaminated contents finally develop, resulting in bacterial peritonitis and sepsis. It is the goal of therapy to prevent these life-threatening complications.

CLINICAL PRESENTATION

Bowel obstruction should be considered in all patients with abdominal pain and vomiting, especially if they have a history of previous abdominal surgery or colorectal cancer. Pain is the initial and primary complaint, although it may be poorly appreciated or communicated in patients with altered or impaired mental status. The pain is usually intermittent and colicky, with cramps occurring every 3 to 10 minutes, depending on the location of obstruction. Vomiting generally follows the development of abdominal pain. The more proximal the obstruction, the earlier vomiting develops; in obstruction of the colon, vomiting may not develop for 24 to 48 hours. Although obstipation (i.e., no passage of feces or flatus) is the rule once obstruction is complete, the passage of stool and flatus may continue until the distal bowel is evacuated. Diarrhea may even occur when there is partial obstruction. Late in the course, abdominal distention may develop. This may be subtle to the physician, but the patient is often aware of this change.

The patient's vital signs usually reflect the degree of volume depletion and in general are only modestly altered until late in the disease process. Hypotension and tachycardia imply advanced disease. Gangrenous bowel, however, may be present without fever or tachycardia.

A helpful sign in diagnosing early small bowel obstruction is the auscultatory finding of crescendo–decrescendo rushes of high-pitched peristalsis sounds coincident with the patient's colic. Bowel sounds eventually decrease and disappear with overdistention and infarction of the bowel.

Abdominal tenderness is variable but usually present in most patients. The determination of rebound tenderness is often complicated by the presence of distended bowel, which may give a false-positive result of increased pain with rapid decompression of the abdominal wall. The absence of percussion tenderness (tapping on the abdomen) or pain with jostling of the patient's gurney or bed implies that peritoneal signs are not present. It is important to realize that the absence of local tenderness or rebound does not exclude the possibility of vascular compromise or infarction.

It is important to ask about and examine for the presence of an external hernia. An incarcerated hernia may be easily reducible with immediate relief of the intestinal obstruction.

In a recent, prospective study of 48 patients with bowel obstruction, the clinical variables most useful in diagnosing bowel obstruction were history of previous surgery, history of constipation, age over 50, vomiting, distended abdomen, and increased bowel sounds. Variables not classified as helpful in this study included sex, progress of complaint in relation to the onset of pain, nausea, history of similar complaints, guarding, and the severity of pain.

DIFFERENTIAL DIAGNOSIS

There are multiple reasons a patient may have abdominal pain and vomiting, including cholecystitis, hepatitis, pancreatitis, peptic ulcer disease, appendicitis, myocardial infarction, nonspecific abdominal pain, and pregnancy, to name a few. The presence of right upper quadrant tenderness should help to differentiate hepatobiliary disease. Elevated lipase or amylase will identify pancreatitis. Patients with peptic ulcer disease may have heme-positive stool. Appendicitis usually presents with right lower quadrant tenderness. The absence of abdominal tenderness may imply cardiac etiology in an elderly patient with risk factors. Patients with kidney stones may complain of abdominal pain but do not usually have abdominal tenderness. An electrocardiogram (ECG) may help diagnose myocardial ischemia, and patients with kidney stones usually have hematuria. A pelvic examination and pregnancy test will identify the pregnant patient. Colicky pain can be associated with appendicitis, cholelithiasis, kidney stones, or gastroenteritis. Diarrhea occurs in all patients with gastroenteritis but is an uncommon complaint in patients with bowel obstruction. Uremia and hepatitis can be associated with abdominal distention (ascites) and vomiting. Ascites and peripheral edema do not occur with bowel obstruction. The presence of jaundice should direct the emergency physician to the diagnosis of liver disease. Finally, air–fluid levels on abdominal x-rays are a common finding in patients with gastroenteritis, but frequent diarrhea, lack of distended loops of bowel, and fecal leukocytes or heme-positive stool will help in making the correct diagnosis.

EMERGENCY DEPARTMENT EVALUATION

The general appearance of the patient will help determine the overall status of the patient (i.e., sick or not sick). A complete history and physical examination are critical in making the diagnosis of bowel obstruction. Ill-appearing patients require supportive treatment (e.g., monitor, intravenous fluid, etc.) before a complete history can be obtained. Inspection of the patient's vital signs is critical to determine the patient's volume status and risk of infection. Tachycardia and hypotension should prompt the emergency physician to provide immediate fluid resuscitation. The presence of fever indicates an infectious etiology to the patient's symptoms and implies bowel infarction if bowel obstruction is diagnosed. Evaluation of the skin will help to identify jaundice in the patient with hepatobiliary disease or poor capillary refill in a patient in shock. Auscultation of the lungs may reveal a pulmonary cause of the patient's symptoms. Inspection of the abdomen may reveal distention or surgical scars. Auscultation of the abdomen may reveal crescendo–decrescendo, decreased, or absent bowel sounds. Gentle palpation of the abdomen demonstrates areas of tenderness, the presence of ascites or a mass, and the presence of guarding or rebound tenderness. Gentle tapping of the patient's costovertebral angle should be undertaken to determine the presence or absence of tenderness, which would imply renal disease. Pelvic examination is appropriate in all women with abdominal pain, looking for discharge, cervical motion or adnexal tenderness, or masses—none of which are usually present in patients with bowel obstruction. Rectal examination and testing of stool for occult blood, although critical to the evaluation of all patients with abdominal pain, should be delayed until an upright abdominal x-ray is obtained in patients with a high clinical suspicion of bowel obstruction. Digital examination may introduce air into the rectum, confusing the determination of complete bowel obstruction. Inspection and examination for an external hernia may identify the cause of a patient's complaints and lead to early reduction and relief of an obstruction.

The most important diagnostic test for bowel obstruction is the upright abdominal x-ray. Patients who are too ill to stand can undergo a left lateral decubitus abdominal x-ray, which will

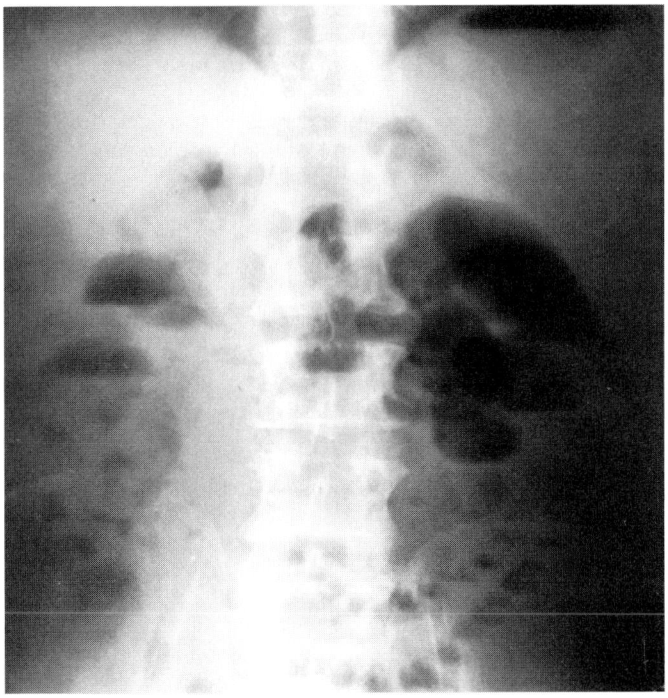

Figure 42.1. "Stepladder" pattern of air–fluid levels on upright view in patient with small bowel obstruction.

reveal the same findings. X-ray findings in bowel obstruction include dilated loops of bowel, air–fluid levels, and strings of air pockets called the "string of beads" sign (Figs. 42.1 and 42.2). In approximately 5% of patients with bowel obstruction, the abdominal x-ray is normal; if the bowel lumen is completely full of fluid, it will not show the characteristic interface of air and fluid. Absence of air in the rectum may be a sign of obstruction unless the rectal examination was performed before the abdominal x-ray. Air within the distal portions of the bowel may occur if the obstruction is only partial.

Patients with bowel obstruction may have metabolic abnormalities from profuse vomiting, third spacing of fluid into the

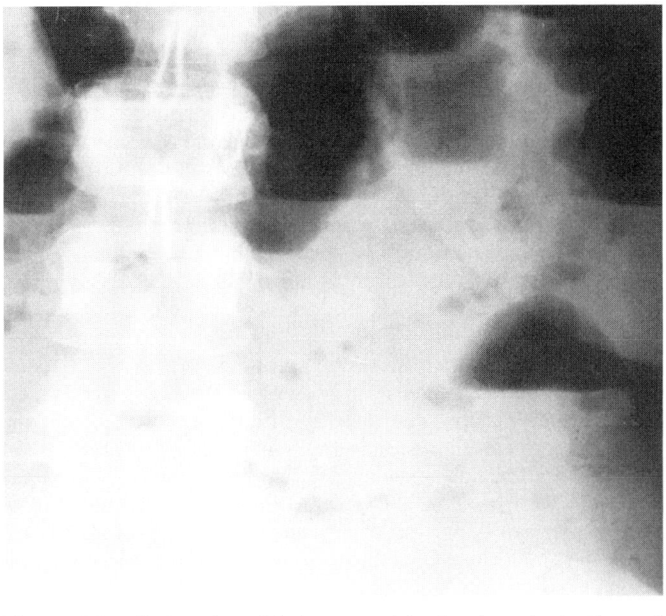

Figure 42.2. "String of pearls" sign on upright view in patient with small bowel obstruction.

lumen of the bowel, and resulting dehydration. Once the diagnosis of bowel obstruction is made, electrolytes, blood urea nitrogen, and creatinine results should be obtained and abnormalities corrected. A complete blood count may reveal an elevated white blood cell count in an elderly patient without other signs of early sepsis, but this finding is nonspecific. A hemoglobin or hematocrit may be elevated from hemoconcentration or decreased from hemorrhagic complications of bowel necrosis or chronic blood loss from a malignancy.

EMERGENCY DEPARTMENT EVALUATION

Patients with abdominal pain and vomiting should be brought promptly into the emergency department and evaluated. If appropriate because of abnormal vital signs or significant history, the patient should be placed on a cardiac monitor. The patient should be undressed and placed in a gown. An intravenous line should be started, and signs of hypovolemia should initiate prompt fluid resuscitation with normal saline. Blood samples can be drawn at the time of intravenous line placement and held until appropriate laboratory work is ordered. Patients who are vomiting or nauseated should be treated with an antiemetic (e.g., chlorpromazine) to make them more comfortable. After initial stabilization and treatment, a complete history and physical examination should be taken. Laboratory tests should be ordered based on the physician's differential diagnosis. If cardiac disease remains in the differential, an ECG should be performed. The patient should then undergo an upright or left lateral decubitus abdominal x-ray, depending on the patient's condition.

In general, the diagnosis of bowel obstruction is made with an abdominal x-ray. If plain radiographic findings are negative and clinical suspicion is high, abdominal computed tomography (CT) should be utilized, as it is superior to ultrasound and plain films in determining the level and cause of obstruction. In the vast majority of cases, abdominal CT is not necessary from the emergency physician's perspective, although it may help the surgeon decide the cause of the obstruction.

On confirmation of the diagnosis and after discussing the planned clinical course with the patient, a nasogastric tube should be inserted, after anesthetizing the nasal passage and posterior pharynx, and attached to intermittent suction. The gastric contents should be visualized to determine the presence or absence of blood. The patient should be given intravenous narcotic analgesics for relief of abdominal discomfort. Surgical consultation should be obtained and the patient admitted to the hospital. Febrile patients or those with evidence of peritonitis should also be given antibiotics as soon as possible to cover bowel flora.

DISPOSITION

Patients with bowel obstruction should be admitted to the hospital. Determining the appropriate hospital bed depends on the patient's condition and comorbid illnesses. Surgical consultation should be obtained promptly, with direct communication by the emergency physician. The challenge for the surgeon is to determine whether strangulation has occurred and whether the patient requires acute operative management or whether a trial of observation (12 to 24 hours) and bowel rest can be attempted.

Stable patients may be transferred if the patient requests it or consents to transfer. Unstable patients should not be transferred.

COMMON PITFALLS

- Delay in promptly and adequately treating a patient's hypovolemia

- Delay or failure to treat a patient's symptoms with antiemetics and narcotic analgesics
- Extensive laboratory and radiographic testing that delays the diagnosis and early consultation with a surgeon
- Delay or failure to place a nasogastric tube after making the diagnosis of obstruction
- Misinterpretation of abdominal x-rays in a patient with air–fluid levels due to gastroenteritis

Bibliography

Bass KN, Jones B, Bulkley GB. Current management of small-bowel obstruction. *Adv Surg* 1997;31:1.

Bohner H, Yang Q, Franke C, et al. Simple data from history and physical examination help to exclude bowel obstruction and to avoid radiographic studies in patients with acute abdominal pain. *Eur J Surg* 1998;164:777.

Greenfield RH, Henneman PL. Disorders of the small intestine. In: Rosen P, Barkin R, Braen R, et al., eds. *Emergency medicine: concepts and clinical practice,* 4th ed. St. Louis: CV Mosby, 1998:2005.

Lopez-Kostner F, Hool GR, Lavery IC. Management and causes of acute large-bowel obstruction. *Surg Clin North Am* 1997;77:1265.

Suri S, Gupta S, Sudhakar PJ, et al. Comparative evaluation of plain films, ultrasound and CT in the diagnosis of intestinal obstruction. *Acta Radiol* 1999; 40:422.

CHAPTER 43
Hernias

Sharon Elizabeth Mace

A hernia is the protrusion of a part or structure or organ through the tissues that normally contain it. This all-inclusive definition would include abdominal wall hernias as well as other hernias, such as diaphragmatic hernias and internal hernias. Hernias of the abdomen are, by far, the most common type of hernia and are the focus of this chapter. Hernias are commonly encountered in clinical practice. It is estimated that 5% of the population has a hernia. Herniorrhaphy accounts for 10% to 15% of all the procedures in a general surgical practice, with about 500,000 such operations performed in the United States each year. Herniorrhaphy is the most common operation in general surgical practice.

CLASSIFICATION

Hernias can be classified as an external, internal, or interparietal hernia. An external hernia protrudes completely through the abdominal wall to the outside and, thus, can be seen and palpated. Examples of external hernias include incisional, umbilical, inguinal, and femoral hernias. An interparietal hernia is a rare hernia in which the hernial sac is contained within the abdominal wall. An internal hernia is a hernia in which the herniated part or organ occurs within the confines of a body cavity. Internal hernias include diaphragmatic hernias, hernias through a tear in the mesentery or omentum, and hernias through the foramen of Winslow into the lesser sac. Internal hernias are much less common than external hernias and can be very difficult to diagnose.

Hernias of the abdominal wall involve protrusion of part of the abdominal contents beyond the normal confines of the abdominal wall. Hernias can occur wherever there is a weakness in the abdominal wall. The weakness or defect allows protrusion of peritoneum and abdominal contents. The abdominal wall contains various fascial and muscular layers, which are designed to contain the contents of the abdomen. Hernias represent a failure of the abdominal wall (and its component parts) to contain the enclosed peritoneum and other abdominal structures or viscera. The intestines are the most common structure that undergoes herniation, but all intraperitoneal structures can herniate, from a tiny piece of omentum to part of or an entire organ, such as the bowel, bladder, kidney, or liver.

DEFINITIONS

A *reducible hernia* is a hernia in which the protruding or herniated structures can be returned through the abdominal wall defect back into the abdominal cavity. An irreducible hernia is one in which the protruding or herniated structures cannot be returned through the abdominal wall defect back into the abdominal cavity. Another term for irreducible hernia is *incarcerated hernia,* which is sometimes mistakenly used to imply that an irreducible hernia is about to become strangulated.

A *strangulated hernia* is one in which the blood supply to the herniated structures or viscus is compromised. Gangrene will occur in the strangulated viscus if the vascular compromise is not relieved. Strangulation of a hernia is a life-threatening situation with significant associated morbidity and mortality. Strangulation requires emergency treatment and surgical intervention. Hernias that have a small neck or opening and a fairly large sac have a tendency to strangulate. As the size of the hernial orifice increases, the likelihood of strangulation decreases. All strangulated hernias are irreducible or incarcerated, but not all irreducible or incarcerated hernias are strangulated.

Groin hernias, which include inguinal hernias (both direct and indirect; Figs. 43.1 and 43.2) and femoral hernias (Fig. 43.3), are the most common, accounting for 85% of all hernias (80% groin, 5% femoral). If umbilical and incisional hernias were added to the category of groin hernias, they would comprise 95% to 98% of all hernias.

Other, much rarer abdominal wall hernias include epigastric, pelvic, lumbar, and spigelian hernias. Epigastric hernias are ones that occur in the midline of the abdominal wall between the umbilicus and the xiphoid. Pelvic hernias are rare and involve the protrusion of abdominal contents through areas in the floor of the abdominal cavity. The obturator hernia, which is the most common of the pelvic hernias, involves herniation through the obturator foramen and generally occurs in elderly women. Lumbar hernias occur in the superior and inferior lumbar triangles, which are two naturally weak regions of the posterior abdominal wall. Spigelian hernias are protrusions of abdominal contents lateral to the rectus abdominis muscle through the external oblique fascia.

Ventral hernias include umbilical, epigastric, and spigelian hernias. Incisional hernias can be another type of ventral (anterior) hernia. Incisional hernias constitute about 10% of all hernias and result from postincisional weakness of the anterior abdominal wall.

Umbilical hernias are common in infants, occurring in up to 65% of African American infants versus 10% of Caucasian infants. The majority of umbilical hernias in infants close spontaneously, usually by age 2, and rarely incarcerate or strangulate. Conversely, umbilical hernias in adults often incarcerate, with strangulation occurring in 20% to 30%. Ulceration and perfora-

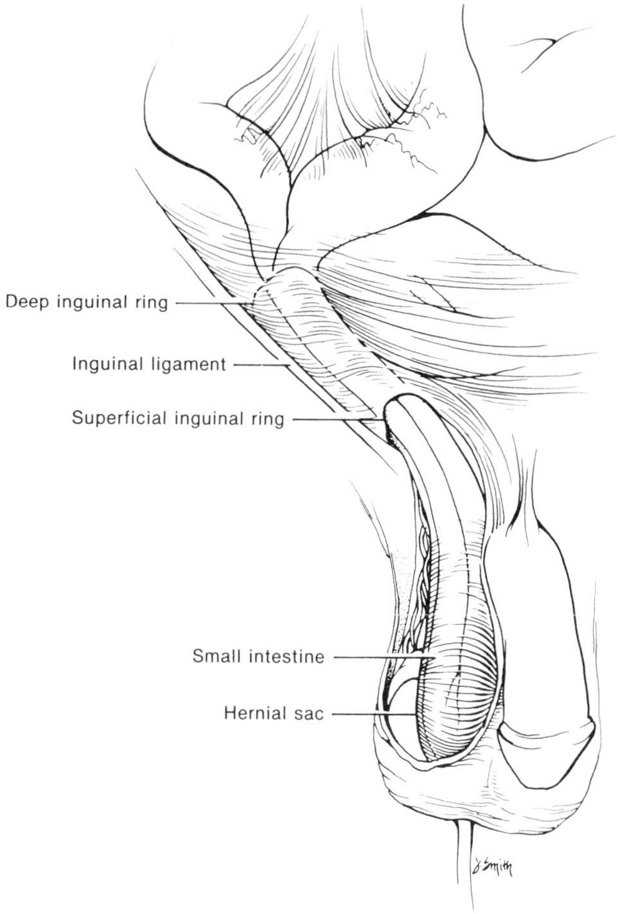

Figure 43.1. Indirect inguinal hernia.

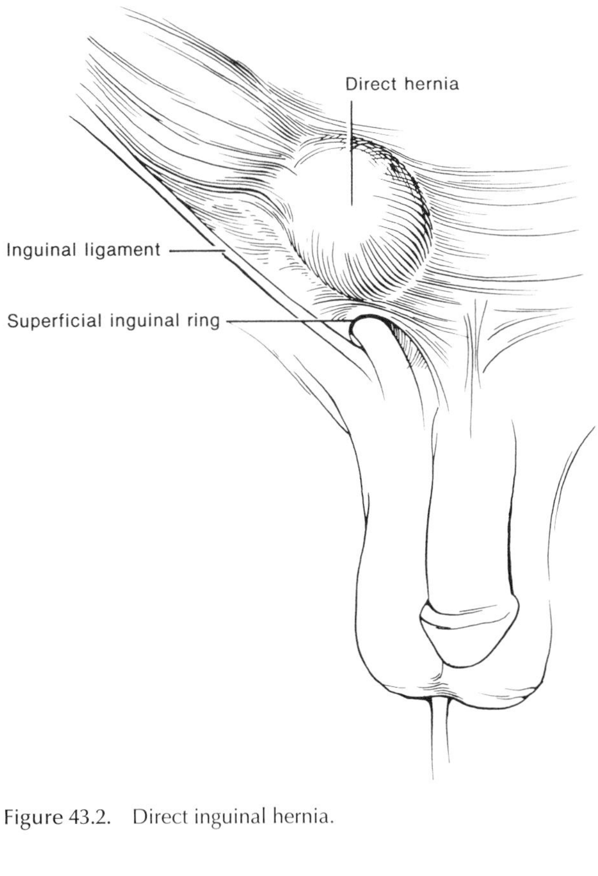

Figure 43.2. Direct inguinal hernia.

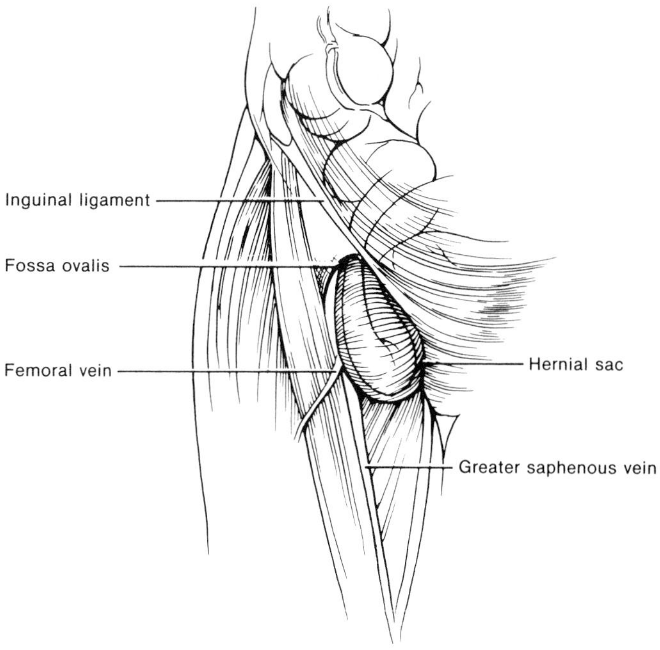

Figure 43.3. Femoral hernia.

tion can also occur in adults with umbilical hernias, complications that are associated with high morbidity and mortality, especially in cirrhotic patients. Patients with increased intraabdominal pressure (such as ascites, pregnancy, or obesity) have a higher incidence of umbilical hernias, which occur in 20% of patients with cirrhosis and ascites.

Groin Hernias

The inguinal hernias (direct and indirect) and the femoral hernia are the three types of groin hernias. Anatomic location distinguishes the inguinal hernias from the femoral hernia. The inguinal hernias are above, or superior to, the inguinal ligament, while the femoral hernia is below, or inferior to, the inguinal ligament. The two types of inguinal hernias—direct and indirect—are also differentiated based on anatomy. With an indirect hernia, the protruding abdominal contents pass through the internal (or deep) inguinal ring and into the inguinal canal and lie lateral to the inferior epigastric vessels. With a direct hernia, the protruding abdominal contents lie medial to the inferior epigastric vessels and protrude through a weak area in the aponeurosis of the transversus abdominal muscle in Hesselbach's triangle (or the inguinal triangle). Hesselbach's triangle is an area bounded by the inferior epigastric artery (on the lateral aspect), the lateral border of the rectus abdominis muscle (on the medial aspect), and the inguinal ligament (on the inferior border). Of all inguinal hernias, about two-thirds are indirect inguinal hernias and one-third are direct inguinal hernias.

An indirect inguinal hernia transverses the deep inguinal ring into the inguinal canal and follows the path of a patent processus vaginalis. The processus vaginalis is formed during male fetal development to allow the descent of the testes from their original retroperitoneal site into the scrotum. If the processus vaginalis fails to close off after birth, an indirect hernia may occur that could allow abdominal contents to progress down the inguinal canal, even into the scrotum. In girls, the processus vaginalis follows the round ligament, while, in boys, the processus vaginalis follows the spermatic cord.

Inguinal hernias are much more frequent in boys than in girls because there is a much smaller aperture for the round ligament compared with the spermatic cord. Because of this embryology, childhood hernias are usually indirect hernias. Indirect inguinal hernias commonly incarcerate, while direct inguinal hernias almost never incarcerate.

A femoral hernia is the protrusion of abdominal contents between the femoral vessels (artery and vein) and the lacunar ligament in the femoral canal. Because of the narrow neck or opening, femoral hernias frequently incarcerate. Because of differences in the structure of the pelvis, femoral hernias occur almost exclusively in women. However, because of the rarity of femoral hernias, the most common hernia in a woman is an indirect inguinal hernia, not a femoral hernia.

CLINICAL PRESENTATION AND EVALUATION

Most hernias are asymptomatic and are usually found by chance, either by the patient or by the physician on a routine physical examination. The most common presenting complaints of a hernia are swelling and/or pain and discomfort.

If there is an acute incarceration, there may be the sudden onset of severe pain with nausea and vomiting. The pain occurring with an acute incarcerated hernia is caused by edema and inflammation of the herniated structures and the surrounding tissues. Incarcerated hernias are the second most common cause of bowel obstruction in the United States, with postoperative adhesions being the most common cause of bowel obstruction. If strangulation is present, the patient may present with signs and symptoms of bowel obstruction and/or perforation.

Occasionally, the initial symptoms may be somewhat misleading. In some patients, the pain from an incarcerated groin hernia may be located in the epigastrium because of traction on the abdominal contents from the hernia. In other patients, strangulation can occur without any symptoms and signs of bowel obstruction when only part of the bowel wall is herniated. This occurs with a Richter's hernia, one in which only one side of the intestinal wall is within the hernia sac.

Pain and/or hypesthesia located along the medial aspect of the thigh, radiating to the knee, due to irritation of the obturator nerve (Howship-Romberg sign) occurs in 50% of patients with an obturator hernia.

Physical examination should include inspection and gentle palpation for any bulges or masses. Cooperative patients may be asked to cough or strain, which increases intraabdominal pressure, in an attempt to demonstrate the hernia. Palpation of the external inguinal ring in a male patient may also be helpful in detecting an inguinal hernia.

In patients with an incarcerated hernia, the swelling is tender, and they may have a low-grade fever and tachycardia.

In patients with a strangulated hernia, signs and symptoms of bowel obstruction, peritonitis, perforation, abscess, and even septic shock may be present. Leukocytosis with a left shift is usually present, although this finding may not occur in geriatric patients. Dehydration with electrolyte abnormalities and an elevated blood urea nitrogen often occur. Acute abdominal series radiographs are indicated. The upright chest roentgenogram is necessary to rule out free air under the diaphragm resulting from perforation or dead bowel. The flat plate and upright abdominal films may demonstrate bowel obstruction and occasionally a hernia sac.

DIFFERENTIAL DIAGNOSIS

The most common diagnoses to consider in a patient presenting with a groin mass are inguinal hernia, enlarged inguinal lymph node(s), and hydrocele of the spermatic cord. Other less common etiologies include lipoma, saphenous vein varix, psoas abscess, and incarcerated ovary.

EMERGENCY DEPARTMENT MANAGEMENT

Patients with hernias can be grouped into three categories: (1) asymptomatic or minimal symptoms (swelling or mild discomfort), with a spontaneously reducible hernia; (2) irreducible but not strangulated hernia; and (3) strangulated hernia.

Patients in category 1 should be given discharge instructions, which include the warning signs of incarceration and strangulation, and told to avoid exercise and straining. They need referral to general surgery for evaluation for elective herniorrhaphy.

If the irreducible hernia is acute (and there is no evidence for strangulation), nonsurgical reduction should be done. Cool compresses may be placed over the hernia site to diminish local blood flow and decrease intraluminal gas pressure. Appropriate sedation is given. If the patient has a groin hernia, the patient is placed in approximately a 20-degree Trendelenburg position. The hernia may spontaneously reduce. If not, gentle manipulation may be attempted. Slow, steady compression ("gentle-taxis") is used, not forceful attempts.

Once reduction is achieved, herniorrhaphy within a few days is ideal. This allows local edema to resolve. Because the incidence of recurrence is high, urgent surgery is recommended. If the hernia cannot be reduced, emergency surgery is done as soon as fluid and electrolyte abnormalities are corrected. Complications of nonsurgical or manual hernia reduction include partial reduction and hernia reduction in masse. Hernia reduction en masse is a rare complication in which the hernia sac is manipulated into the preperitoneal space. This gives the false impression that the hernia has been reduced, although it is still incarcerated and at risk for strangulation.

Surgical management is mandatory for all incarcerated hernias that cannot be reduced and for all strangulated hernias. Supportive care prior to surgery usually includes fluid resuscitation and antibiotics.

COMMON PITFALLS

- Failure to diagnose a small hernia
- Misdiagnosis of a hernia for other causes of a groin mass
- Failure to identify an incarcerated or strangulated hernia
- Failure to make an appropriate referral to a surgeon
- Failure to make a timely diagnosis and aggressively resuscitate a patient with a strangulated hernia

Bibliography

McArthur KE. Hernias and volvulus of the gastrointestinal tract. In: Feldman M, Scharschmidt BF, Sleisenger MH, eds. *Sleisenger and Fordtran's gastrointestinal and liver disease—pathophysiology/diagnosis/management,* vol. 1, 6th ed. Philadelphia: WB Saunders, 1998:317.

Moody FG, Calabuig R. Abdominal cavity: anatomy, structural anomalies, and hernias. In: Yamada T, Alpers DH, Powell DW, et al., eds. *Textbook of gastroenterology,* vol. 2, 2nd ed. Philadelphia: JB Lippincott Co, 1995:2278.

Wantz G. Abdominal wall hernias. In: Schwartz SI, Shires GT, Spencer FC, et al., eds. *Principles of surgery,* vol. 2, 7th ed. New York: McGraw-Hill, 1999:1585.

CHAPTER 44
Colonic Neoplasms

Jonathan M. Glauser

Colorectal cancer is the second most common cancer in the United States and in other developed countries, excluding skin cancer; it is exceeded in incidence and mortality only by lung cancer. Colorectal cancer accounts for 20% of all deaths from malignant disease in the United States and 14% of newly diagnosed cancer cases in both men and women. Most cancer cases occur in patients older than 40 years, with 90% of cases diagnosed after the age of 50. The peak incidence is in the seventh decade; the median age of colorectal cancer death is 68. However, 4% to 6% of cases occur in young adults aged 20 to 40 years. The mortality rate in the United States is 26 per 100,000 per year. The number of new cases in the United States is rising, with 145,000 new cases in 1987 and 152,000 new cases in 1993. Approximately 6% of the U.S. population develops cancer of the colon and rectum, and 6 million Americans alive today will die of the disease. The cure rate is 40% to 44%; the mortality for men is unchanged since 1960 and only slightly improved for women.

The American Cancer Society estimates that 75% of the 61,000 deaths in 1991 from colorectal cancer could have been prevented by early diagnosis and treatment. Other groups believe that modification of diet by decreasing animal fat intake, increasing fiber intake in the form of whole-grain cereals, fruit, and vegetables, and avoidance of specific chemicals such as cellulose, uronic acid, and carotene may lower the incidence of colorectal cancer. The role of the emergency physician in the detection and prevention of colorectal cancer may be significant. The process of change from normal mucosa to premalignant adenoma to frank invasion of surrounding tissues by carcinoma takes about 5 to 10 years. The natural history of the disease affords the physician a large window of opportunity for screening and detection. Predisposing factors may be elicited by history (Table 44.1).

TABLE 44.1. Predisposing Conditions for Colorectal Cancer

- Familial polyposis—nearly 100% chance of developing cancer by age 40 years
- Gardner, Turcot, and Peutz-Jeghers syndromes (rare and inherited) correlate with development of adenomas in colon and subsequent cancer.
- Patient history of colon cancer, adenomatous polyps, or breast, ovarian, or uterine cancer
- Inflammatory bowel disease—up to one-third of ulcerative colitis deaths due to colon cancer. Crohn disease may be premalignant, especially when age at onset is younger than 21 years.
- Male homosexuality—risk factor for anorectal cancer, primary rectal lymphomas, Burkitt's-like lymphoma, and Hodgkin disease of rectum
- Hereditary nonpolyposis colorectal carcinoma—biomarkers are being sought for this familial aggregation of colorectal cancer exhibiting mendelian segregation.
- Diet—an inverse correlation exists between dietary fiber intake and colorectal carcinoma; other implicated dietary factors may include red or processed meat, fat, and alcohol (high beer intake possibly due to nitrosamines). Fruits, vegetables, and refined grains may be protective.
- Chronic constipation
- Job-related exposure to toluene, xylene (printers), other carcinogens (workers in insulation, chemical plants, synthetic rubber manufacturing, oil refineries)
- Sedentary lifestyle
- High body mass index (BMI), overweight
- *Streptococcus bovis* bacteremia/endocarditis

CLINICAL PRESENTATION

The most common presentations for colonic neoplasms include bleeding, weight loss, pain, obstruction, and change in bowel habits.

Bleeding

Bleeding from cancer is frequently self-limited and seldom presents as massive hemorrhage. Rectal bleeding may be occult or intermittent and is the most common sign of rectal cancer, particularly among patients older than age 40 years. Rectal bleeding should never be attributed to hemorrhoids without proper evaluation. Colorectal malignancy is present in 10% of patients older than age 40 years with new onset of rectal bleeding. Blood that coats the exterior of a formed stool is likely to have originated from the anal canal or rectum; if blood is admixed with feces, the bleeding source is usually higher in the colon.

Anemia

Although uncommon, severe anemia in colorectal cancer is usually caused by iron deficiency from chronic blood loss. However, liver dysfunction from metastatic disease or drug toxicity may cause a functional folate deficiency that results in anemia. In addition, microangiopathic hemolytic anemia has been reported with colonic malignancies. Fatigue, shortness of breath, and angina may all be secondary to anemia.

Obstruction

Rectal cancer often presents with tenesmus, but obstruction is uncommon. Left-sided colon tumors produce obstructive symptoms and changes in bowel habits. Right-sided colon tumors generally remain clinically silent because of the large-caliber and fluid stool, but a mass in the right side of the abdomen is the first sign of cancer in 10% of patients. Obstruction tends to occur at the sigmoid where stool is driest. The tumor may result in intussusception, or it may cause a volvulus due to fixation of the bowel wall by the tumor. In most patients, the ileocecal valve is incompetent, and both large and small bowel obstruction may occur simultaneously. For the 15% of patients in whom the ileocecal valve is competent, the vascular supply to the cecal wall is cut off, resulting in necrosis and perforation. Bowel obstruction and perforation have been associated with poor prognosis.

Constipation has been listed both as a frequent complaint and as a predisposing factor along with laxative abuse. Narrow-caliber stools, stool consistency changes, and a feeling of incomplete bowel emptying are all suggestive symptoms.

Perforation and Abscesses

Intestinal perforation may be localized and present with a tender mass or with generalized peritonitis. A psoas or a thigh abscess may occur. Thigh emphysema and right hip pain, as well as Fournier's gangrene of the scrotum with perineal erythema, induration, and blistering, have been described after a perforated cecal carcinoma. Fistulas between the colon and pelvic organs are possible sequelae of perforation.

Metabolic Disturbances

Metabolic disturbances may develop from either the primary neoplasm or metastatic cancer. Hypokalemia and diarrhea are well-recognized features of villous adenomas, which have high potential for malignant change. Hypercalcemia may be caused by either bone metastases or, rarely, elaboration of a parathyroid hormone–like substance by the tumor. Adrenal insufficiency caused by metastases has been reported.

Hormonal Abnormalities

There are unusual cases of colon tumors that elaborate hormones. These arise from cells with the capacity for amine precursor uptake and decarboxylation (APUD) cell tumors. Carcinoid tumors, the best-known type, secrete serotonin, kallikrein, and certain tachykinins. Patients may present with flushing, diarrhea, abdominal pain, asthma, and right-sided valvular heart disease. Treatment consists of surgical removal of the tumor, administration of serotonin antagonists such as cyproheptadine for the diarrhea, and chemotherapy. Metastatic disease, especially to the liver, is usually widespread at the time of diagnosis. Colon cancer has also been found to elaborate adrenocorticotropic hormone as well as an insulin-like hormone. Flushing attacks simulating the carcinoid syndrome may also occur with Verner-Morrison syndrome of hypersecretion of vasoactive intestinal peptide (VIPoma), although these tumors most often arise from the pancreas.

Metastatic Disease

Metastatic disease can have widely varying manifestations. Liver, lungs, bone, ovaries, adrenals, and the peritoneal cavity are most commonly involved. If the liver is invaded, coagulation defects may ensue. Thromboembolic events resulting from mucin-producing adenocarcinomas of the colon have been reported. Metastatic tumor to the lumbosacral spine may cause back pain and spinal cord compression. Approximately one-fourth of patients with colorectal cancer exhibit evidence of hematogenous spread on initial evaluation.

DIFFERENTIAL DIAGNOSIS

In the differential diagnosis, include any entity that may present with strictures, rectal bleeding, mass lesions, abdominal pain, or change in bowel habits. Diverticular disease, benign tumors, inflammatory bowel disease, ischemic bowel disease, tubercular and fungal infections, irritable bowel disease, infectious diarrhea, and medication-induced diarrhea all must be considered. Hemorrhoidal bleeding is generally benign and is a diagnosis of exclusion in the elderly.

EMERGENCY DEPARTMENT EVALUATION

Gastrointestinal complaints must be aggressively pursued; the average duration of symptoms of colonic neoplasms is 6.5 months before diagnosis. Only by shortening this period can mortality and morbidity be reduced. More aggressive screening may be warranted for high-risk groups such as first-degree relatives of individuals with familial adenomatous polyposis, members of hereditary colorectal cancer families, patients with colorectal adenomas or with previous colorectal cancer, and patients with inflammatory bowel disease.

The American Cancer Society recommendations for screenings are as follows:

- Men and women older than age 50 years should have a fecal Hemoccult test every year.
- Men and women older than age 50 years with none of the high-risk factors for colorectal cancer should have sigmoidoscopic examinations annually until two consecutive examinations are normal; thereafter, examinations should be every 3 to 5 years.
- Men and women older than age 40 years should have a digital rectal examination every year.

Several means of screening are available to the emergency physician, although many of them are not well tailored to emergency settings.

Digital Rectal Examination

Digital rectal examinations may detect 10% of colorectal cancers. This change from the 30% detection rate cited two decades ago reflects a proximal redistribution of colonic neoplasms. A shelflike deformity located anteriorly above the prostate (Blumer's shelf) may indicate metastatic tumor.

Occult Blood Testing

Stool should be tested for occult blood. The test can detect as little as 2 to 3 mL of blood in stool. A person may normally lose 0.62 mL of blood daily into the gastrointestinal tract. If two fecal occult blood smears are tested daily for 3 days, the clinical sensitivity for colon cancer approaches 80% to 93%. Emergency physicians do not have the opportunity to test multiple specimens, however; nor do they test patients who are on low-peroxidase diets. (Broccoli, turnips, cantaloupe, and radishes, among other foods, contain peroxidase.) The pseudoperoxidase activity of hemoglobin produces a blue color when hydrogen peroxide is applied to filter paper impregnated with guaiac. False-positive reactions may be produced by animal hemoglobin in meat or by nonhemoglobin peroxidases in stool from food and bacteria. Aspirin or other nonsteroidal antiinflammatory drug use may cause positive occult blood test result, while ingestion of ascorbic acid or other antioxidants may cause a false-negative test result. It has been estimated that annual fecal occult blood testing has the potential to cause a 15% to 33% reduction in colorectal cancer mortality.

Proctosigmoidoscopy

Proctosigmoidoscopy has been proposed as a diagnostic tool in the emergency department to evaluate colitis, sigmoid masses, or rectal bleeding. The rigid proctoscope is 25 cm long and, in theory, can detect 25% to 35% of colorectal cancers. Before undergoing this procedure, which is uncomfortable to the patient, the patient must use one or two Fleet enemas. Furthermore, most physicians do not routinely pass the scope beyond 17 cm of colon. The flexible fiberoptic 60-cm sigmoidoscope permits trained operators to reach those 50% to 64% of colorectal cancers that are in the lower half of the descending colon. Although the flexible sigmoidoscope is better tolerated by patients and can be advanced to 50 cm 75% of the time, its use in the emergency department may be impractical because patients are usually not adequately prepared and because most emergency physicians are unaccustomed to the procedure and to the biopsy technique. Patient flow and acuity often preclude performance of this procedure, which may have to be repeated by the gastroenterologist or surgeon.

Barium Enema and Colonoscopy

Barium enema and colonoscopy are excellent screening and diagnostic tests and should be undergone by high-risk patients in alternate years. Total colonoscopy detects synchronous cancers in 2% to 5% of cases and concurrent adenomas in 40% to 50% of colon cancers; it also enables biopsy and polypectomy of lesions. The major limitation of colonoscopy is that the cecum cannot be visualized in 10% to 36% of cases. Advanced or multiple distal polyps found on flexible sigmoidoscopy heralds the presence of an advanced proximal polyp—villous, malignant, or larger than 10 mm in diameter—in more than 5% of cases, making colonoscopy a valuable diagnostic tool, even after sigmoidoscopy.

Double-contrast barium study may detect 92% to 94% of cancers subsequently found within a 3-year period, but it is of little value in screening if only symptoms of benign disease are present. It is more sensitive than the single-contrast technique for detection of polyps, early inflammatory bowel disease, and lesions of the rectum.

Serum Carcinoembryonic Antigen

Serum carcinoembryonic antigen is seldom available in the emergency department and has low sensitivity and specificity for colorectal cancer, although it is of preoperative value as a prognostic factor. It is most useful for early detection of metastatic cancer after curative resection of colorectal cancer. Positivity approaches 100% as dissemination occurs, and it suggests investigation for residual or metastatic disease. Healthy patients, patients with other malignancies, and patients with inflammatory bowel disease may test falsely positive. Its sensitivity for Dukes stage 1 and B tumors is 36%; for stage C, 74%; and for stage D colon cancers, 83%. It is the most cost-effective means of detecting potentially curable recurrent disease; a "low" cut-off of 3.0 ng/mL, or 2.5 ng/mL on two consecutive tests, has been suggested as the screening level for metastatic disease.

Magnetic Resonance Imaging, Computed Tomography, Ultrasonography, and Molecular Genetics

The role of magnetic resonance imaging (MRI), computed tomography (CT), and ultrasonography in the emergency setting is not well defined, although they have occasionally been useful in the diagnosis of colorectal cancer. MRI may be useful in preoperative staging of colorectal cancer, but it is no more sensitive than CT in diagnosing pericolonic tumor extension and regional lymph node metastases. Angiographic CT and the use of T1-weighted spin echo images are the state-of-the-art imaging modalities for metastatic deposits in the liver. Endocavitary ultrasound is of some value in staging rectal cancer, being somewhat more sensitive than CT for detecting local tumor extension.

Tumor cells in the colon are characterized by phenotypic changes that are the result of qualitative alterations in gene expression. Genes altered in sporadic colorectal cancer include *ras* genes, APC, DCC, and *p53* tumor-suppressor genes, among others. Molecular genetics may have clinical uses in the future.

Monoclonal Antibody Imaging

Monoclonal antibody imaging is used for improved lesion detection. The monospecific antibody to a tumor-associated antigen is tagged with a radioactive moiety and administered either intraperitoneally or intravenously to detect tumor spread.

Surveillance and Recurrence

More than 500,000 people in the United States have surveillance to identify metastases, local recurrence, or a second primary cancer. A typical follow-up schedule may entail examinations every 3 months during the first postoperative year, every 4 months in year 2, and every 6 months thereafter through year 5. Monitoring of carcinoembryonic antigen and liver function tests are typical. Liver ultrasound is sensitive for detection of metastases greater than 1 to 2 cm in diameter; chest radiography has been suggested every 6 months to detect pulmonary spread. The yield of positron-emitted tomography and MRI for tumor surveillance is not better than less expensive studies.

TREATMENT AND SURVIVAL

Treatment of colorectal cancer is surgical. Once distant metastases have occurred, there is evidence that survival may be prolonged by surgery. Resection in appropriately selected patients with liver metastases can improve survival. As many as 25% to 32% of patients have been reported to be disease-free 5 years after resection of hepatic, pulmonary, or locally recurrent metastases. Sites for spread of tumor are typically liver, local recurrence, abdomen, lungs, retroperitoneum, ovary, and abdominal wall.

The mean 5-year survival of all patients with colorectal cancer is 40% to 45% (Tables 44.2 and 44.3). The cure rate has not changed substantially in three decades. Median survival is 3.5 years; this ranges from more than 10 years for *in situ* disease to a mean of 0.8 years for distant disease at the time of diagnosis. Five-year survival rate for localized colorectal cancer is 85% versus 55% for regional disease and 5% to 6% for distant disease.

For rectal cancer alone, 5-year survival rates approximate 88% to 93% for Dukes A node-negative rectal cancer, 71% to 85% for Dukes B cancer, and 29% to 41% for node-positive Dukes C cancer.

TABLE 44.2. Colorectal Cancer Staging[a]

STAGE I
Carcinoma in situ: Tis NO MO
Tumor invades submucosa: T1 NO MO
Tumor invades muscularis propria: T2 NO MO
STAGE II
Tumor invades through muscularis propria into subserosa or into nonperitonealized pericolic or perirectal tissues: T3 NO MO
Tumor perforates the visceral peritoneum or directly invades other organs or structures: T4 NO MO
STAGE III
Any degree of bowel wall perforation with regional lymph node metastasis
N1: 1 to 3 pericolic or perirectal lymph nodes involved
N2: 4 or more pericolic or perirectal lymph nodes involved
N3: Metastasis in any lymph node along a named vascular trunk
Any T N1 MO
Any T N2, N3 MO
STAGE IV
Any invasion of bowel wall with or without lymph node metastasis, but with evidence of distant metastasis
Any T Any N M1

[a]Dukes B (corresponds to stage II) is a composite of better (T3, NO, MO) and worse (T4, NO, MO) prognostic groups, as is Dukes C (corresponds to stage III) (Any T, N1, MO) and (Any T, N2, N3, MO).

T, primary tumor; N, regional node; M, metastasis; 0–4, progressive increase in size or involvement.

Data from American Joint Committee on Cancer. *Manual for staging of cancer*, 4th ed. Philadelphia: JB Lippincott Co, 1992.

TABLE 44.3. Survival Rates of Patients with Colorectal Cancer

Astier-Collier Classification[a]	5-Year Survival
A: Limited to mucosa	90%–100%
B_1: Extension into but not through muscularis propria. Negative nodes.	85%
B_2: Extension through muscularis propria. Negative nodes.	65%–85%
C_1: Extension into but not through muscularis propria. Positive regional nodes.	50%–60%
C_2: Extension through muscularis propria. Positive regional nodes.	25%–45%
D: Distant metastasis (liver, lung, bone, or adjacent organ invasion)	5%

[a]Modified Dukes classification.

Patients with disseminated colon cancer merit limited palliative resection to abort bleeding and to manage obstruction.

Chemotherapy, although it cannot effect a cure or improve the survival rate, may cause temporary improvement in 15% to 25% of patients. Levamisole and 5-fluorouracil (5-FU) are used most frequently for Dukes C (Astier-Collier C1 and C2, TNM stage III), often with leukovorin (folinic acid). Fluorouracil has been given via direct intrahepatic arterial infusion or, investigationally, via portal vein infusion, as well as via conventional systemic means. Fluorouracil may cause nausea, vomiting, diarrhea, oral ulcers, gastrointestinal ulceration, abnormal liver function studies, and bone marrow depression. Thrombocytopenia and mild leukopenia are the most common hematologic effects. Levamisole has caused arthralgias, nausea, fatigue, dermatitis, taste changes, and mild hematologic depression. Folinic acid has been used to enhance the inhibition of DNA synthesis; alfa-2a recombinant interferon may act synergistically with 5-FU. Dacarbazine (DTIC) has been used for malignant APUD tumors. The emergency physician may be called on to manage side effects or complications of these drugs. Hepatic artery catheter infusion of fluorouracil has been associated with local complications, including biliary sclerosis, cholecystitis, chemical hepatitis, and gastric ulceration. New, promising chemotherapeutic options not in common use include folate-based thymidylate synthase inhibitors such as raltitrexed, oral fluorinated pyrimidines such as capecitabine, topoisomerase I inhibitors such as topotecan and irinotecan, and platinum compounds such as oxaliplatin.

Radiation in colonic cancer is more problematic than in rectal cancer because of the natural tissue constraints in the abdomen. Adjuvant radiation therapy reduces the risk of pelvic recurrence in patients with rectal cancer; the role of radiation in the adjuvant treatment of colon cancer is investigational. Possible advantages of radiation therapy must be balanced against the risks of radiation proctitis and small bowel damage.

Immunotherapy using monoclonal antibodies has shown promise in isolated cases and is investigational at this time. Radiolabeled monoclonal antibodies that can be used in the detection of metastatic lesions from colorectal cancer may be linked to cytotoxic agents for immunotargeted therapy.

Bibliography

American Cancer Society. *Cancer facts and figures.* Atlanta: American Cancer Society, 1996, pub. no. 5008.96.

American Joint Committee on Cancer. *Manual for staging of cancer,* 4th ed. Philadelphia: JB Lippincott Co, 1992.

Centers for Disease Control and Prevention (CDC). Screening for colorectal cancer—United States, 1992–1993, and new guidelines. *MMWR* 1993;45(5):107–110.

Fletcher RH. Carcinoembryonic antigen. *Ann Intern Med* 1986;104:66.

Goldberg RM, Fleming TR, Tangen CM, et al. Surgery for recurrent colon cancer: strategies for identifying resectable recurrence and success rates after resection. *Ann Intern Med* 1998;129:27–35.

Graham RA, Wang S, Catalano PJ, et al. Postsurgical surveillance of colon cancer: preliminary cost analysis of physician examination, carcinoembryonic antigen testing, chest x-ray, and colonoscopy. *Ann Surg* 1998;228(1):59–63.

Hill MJ. Diet and cancer: a critical review of scientific evidence. *Eur J Cancer* 1995;Prev 4[Suppl]:3.

Hsing AW, McLaughlin JK, Chow WH, et al. Risk factors for colorectal cancer in a prospective study among U.S. white men. *Int J Cancer* 1998;77:549–553.

Mandel JS, Bond JH, Church TR, et al. Reducing mortality from colorectal cancer by screening for fecal occult blood. *N Engl J Med* 1993;328:1365–1371.

Potter JD, Slattery M, Bostick R, et al. Colon cancer: a review of the epidemiology. *Epidemiol Rev* 1994;15:499–545.

Potter SL, Tong T, Bolden S, et al. Cancer statistics, 1997. *CA Cancer J Clin* 1997;47:5–27.

Schottenfeld D, Winawer SJ. Cancers of the large intestine. In: Schottenfeld D, Fraumeni JF Jr, eds. *Cancer epidemiology and prevention,* 2nd ed. New York: Oxford University Press, 1996.

Steele GD. The National Cancer Data Base report on colorectal cancer. 1994;74:1979–1989.

Screening guidelines for colorectal cancer. *Scand J Gastroenterol Suppl* 1992;192:123.

Sleisenger MH, Fordtran JS. *Gastrointestinal and liver disease,* 6th ed. Philadelphia: WB Saunders, 1998.

Winawer SJ, Fletcher RH, Miller L, et al. Colorectal screening: clinical guidelines and rationale. *Gastroenterology* 1997;112:594–642.

CHAPTER 45

Colonic Diverticular Disease

Michael D. Witting and Annie T. Sadosty

In the Western world, the increasing prevalence of diverticular disease parallels the advancing age of the population.[1] The prevalence of diverticular disease rises from 5% in persons younger than age 40, to 30% in those older than age 50, to 50% in those older than age 70, and to 66% in those older than age 85.[3] Diverticulosis is equally common among men and women. The disease has widely differing prevalence rates in various geographic areas and ethnic groups. The lower rates of diverticular disease seen in people of Eastern ethnicity increase with Western migration. This is believed to be secondary to the adoption of a Western diet, which is typically lower in fiber than the traditional Eastern diet.[1]

The common causative agent for the development of diverticulosis appears to be a reduction in dietary fiber content. The pathophysiology is related to a pressure gradient between the colonic lumen and the serosa and areas of relative weakness in the bowel wall. Very high intraluminal pressure can develop within short segments of the colon. According to Laplace's law of pressures within a cylinder, pressure equals tension divided by radius. Accordingly, the descending and sigmoid colons, which have narrow lumens, have the greatest intraluminal pressures. This pressure causes herniation of diverticula at the points where the intramural vessels penetrate the circular muscle layer, usually between the mesenteric and antimesenteric taenia. Increased fiber enlarges the lumen size, thereby decreasing the intraluminal pressure.

The sigmoid colon is involved in more than 90% of patients with the disease, and in approximately half of the patients it is the only segment of the bowel involved. The cecum is involved in 2%, the ascending colon and rectum in 4% each, and the transverse colon in 10% (Fig. 45.1).

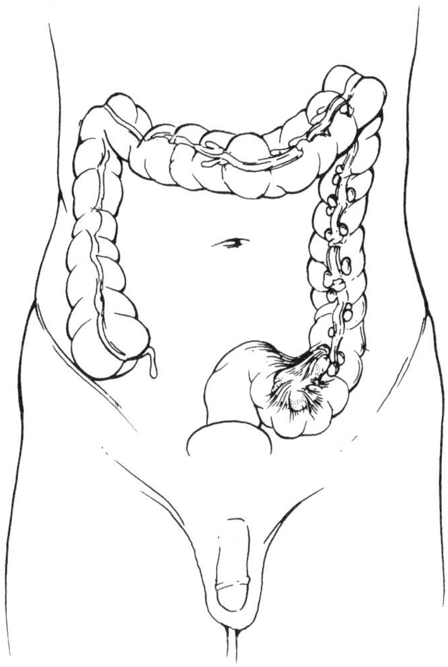

Figure 45.1. Diverticulitis with abscess.

Most persons with diverticulosis remain asymptomatic throughout their lives.[1] In a large series of ambulatory patients with diverticulosis, followed for an average of 5.6 years, 17% eventually showed signs of diverticulitis.[1] The longer a patient has diverticulosis, the greater is the probability of complications, primarily diverticulitis and bleeding. There is no relationship, however, between the number and size of diverticula and the incidence of complications or probability of recurrent disease. The use of nonsteroidal antiinflammatory drugs is an etiologic factor in the development of diverticulitis.[3]

Diverticulitis results from inflammation of diverticula, resulting in microperforation or macroperforation (abscess, fistula, peritonitis, or obstruction). Diverticular bleeding results from an arterial lesion in the vasa recta, characterized by eccentric intimal thickening, altered internal elastic lamina, and focal medial thinning.[6] A disproportionately high tendency exists for diverticula on the right side of the colon to hemorrhage. One theory holds that the wider necks and domes of right-sided diverticula cause greater exposure to injurious factors than for left-sided diverticula.[6] Bleeding from diverticulosis is massive in about one-fourth of patients in whom it occurs and mandates transfusion in approximately one-third.[12] Fortunately, the vast majority of diverticular bleeding ceases spontaneously.

CLINICAL PRESENTATION

Patients with diverticulosis present to the emergency physician with three common patterns: (1) mild left lower quadrant pain; (2) acute left lower quadrant pain, tenderness, and fever; and (3) massive lower gastrointestinal (GI) bleeding.

Mild Left Lower Quadrant Pain (Painful Diverticular Disease)

Diverticulosis most frequently presents as left lower abdominal pain. The pain is usually dull, crampy, and intermittent and is often alleviated by the passage of flatus or stool. Signs of infection are absent.

Acute Left Lower Quadrant Pain, Tenderness, and Signs of Infection (Acute Diverticulitis)

Patients with acute diverticulitis classically present with abrupt-onset, severe, constant left lower quadrant pain; localized tenderness; and fever, leukocytosis, or other signs of systemic toxicity.

Occasionally, the pain and tenderness occur in the left upper quadrant. Patients may present with a picture of a ruptured viscus with diffuse tenderness, rebound, guarding, and diminished or absent bowel sounds. Rarely, diverticulitis may present with signs of fistulization, such as pneumaturia and draining infections of the lower abdomen or medial aspect of the upper thigh. Diverticulitis often presents atypically in immunocompromised patients, such as those with acquired immunodeficiency syndrome (AIDS), renal failure, or diabetes, and those receiving immunosuppressive therapy. In these patients, fever, abdominal pain, or abdominal tenderness may be absent.[8] Additionally, the incidence of free perforation, a rare complication in the immunocompetent, is much higher in immunocompromised patients.[4,8,10]

Massive Lower Gastrointestinal Bleeding (Diverticulosis)

Patients may present with painless, massive rectal bleeding. Such bleeding is characteristically sudden, often profuse from the onset, and more frequent in older persons. The blood is usually bright or dark red, and although the patient may feel faint, initial hypotension is not common.

DIFFERENTIAL DIAGNOSIS

Diverticulosis

When diverticulosis presents as mild, sometimes colicky left lower quadrant pain, it must be differentiated from irritable bowel syndrome, Crohn disease, and colon cancer.

Acute Diverticulitis

Acute diverticulitis must be distinguished from more severe presentations of Crohn disease, ulcerative colitis, and ischemic colitis, although diverticulitis and inflammatory bowel disease may coexist. Vascular catastrophe, such as aortic rupture or dissection or mesenteric ischemia, is generally distinguished by pain out of proportion to physical findings. In women, diverticulitis that presents as a left lower quadrant mass has been misdiagnosed as a gynecologic mass.[8] High fever, leukocytosis, and left lower quadrant mass should suggest a perforation and abscess. This may be due to inflammatory bowel disease, colon cancer, sigmoid volvulus, iatrogenic perforation of the rectosigmoid, or a tuboovarian abscess.[7] Right-sided diverticulitis, a rare disease seen primarily in Asian populations, may mimic acute appendicitis.[13]

Diverticular Bleeding

Diverticular bleeding must be distinguished from other causes of profuse lower GI bleeding, such as angiodysplasia, ischemic colitis, and, occasionally, ulcerative colitis and colonic or rectal cancer. Upper GI hemorrhage occasionally presents as rectal bleeding and hemodynamic instability.

EMERGENCY DEPARTMENT EVALUATION

Left Lower Quadrant Pain

Historical information should focus on GI symptoms, previous similar attacks, prior diagnostic studies, and change in bowel habits. The duration of the attack, characteristics of the pain, and history of fever should also be elicited. With diverticulitis, the pain may be intermittent, crampy, and associated with nausea and vomiting. The attack may be associated with either constipation or diarrhea.

The physical examination should take careful note of the patient's temperature, pulse rate, and blood pressure. Complete abdominal, pelvic, and rectal examinations are essential. In rare cases, tenderness may be found only on rectal examination. Palpation may reveal the outline of the sigmoid colon as a rope-like mass. Minimal tenderness and mobility point to an irritable colon; a large, sausage-like, markedly tender fixed mass points to diverticulitis. Signs of peritonitis and the presence of a mass on pelvic and rectal examinations are important to note. Abdominal x-ray films (flat and upright) should be obtained to look for a mass in the left lower quadrant as well as for free air. A complete blood cell count should be requested with a differential white blood cell count. Leukocytosis with a left shift is compatible with the diagnosis of diverticulitis.

Lower Gastrointestinal Bleeding

The history should focus on the onset, color, amount, and frequency of bloody bowel movements. A history of previous attacks, bleeding tendencies, and bowel habits is important.

Hemodynamic instability should be assessed (blood pressure, pulse, and orthostatic changes). Abdominal and rectal examinations are particularly critical. The abdominal examination should focus on areas of tenderness and the presence or absence of a mass. The rectum should be palpated for masses, and the color of the blood in the rectal vault examined. If rectal bleeding is significant, nasogastric intubation can exclude active upper GI bleeding. If there is brisk, bright red bleeding, anoscopy can exclude anorectal causes such as internal hemorrhoids.

EMERGENCY DEPARTMENT MANAGEMENT

Painful Diverticular Disease

For the patient with left lower quadrant pain with no mass or signs of infection, institution of a high-fiber diet is effective in relieving pain. Anticholinergic agents have long been used, but their efficacy remains unproved. A follow-up flexible sigmoidoscopy should be done to rule out rectal cancer.

Diverticulitis

For the patient in whom the diagnosis of severe diverticulitis is highly probable, an intravenous line should be started, nasogastric tube inserted, specimens for blood and urine cultures collected and sent to the laboratory, and intravenous antibiotics begun. Acute diverticulitis can be diagnosed solely on clinical grounds. In cases in which the diagnosis is unclear, computed tomography, contrast enema, or ultrasonography can be performed. Controversy abounds as to which is the ideal initial study of choice. Such factors as patient stability, the diagnoses considered, body habitus, and the individual institution's relative expertise may influence a clinician's choice of diagnostic test.

Computed tomography offers the advantages of evaluating vascular structures, correctly estimating the extent of diverticulitis, and allowing possible percutaneous abscess drainage, and it is less invasive than contrast enema evaluation.[5] Contrast enema is less expensive and has comparable or greater accuracy in diagnosing diverticulitis[10,11] and is superior to computed tomography in diagnosing cancer.[10] Though it has been stated that barium enema evaluation is contraindicated in patients with acute diverticulitis, several modern studies have confirmed the safety of water-soluble contrast enema.[10,12] A few centers have reported high accuracy in diagnosing diverticulitis with ultrasonography.[9,10,12] Sigmoidoscopy should be avoided in patients with acute diverticulitis.

For both complicated and uncomplicated diverticulitis, antibiotics should target gram-negative rods and anaerobic bacteria. Cefoxitin, a combination antibiotic such as ampicillin–sulbactam, and the combination of clindamycin and an aminoglycoside are good choices. Outpatient management for mild cases may include a combination of metronidazole and either trimethoprim–sulfamethoxazole or ciprofloxacin or monotherapy with amoxicillin/clavulanate.

Diverticular Bleeding

For the patient with massive lower GI bleeding, two large-bore intravenous lines (16-gauge or larger) should be inserted. A specimen should be drawn and sent for type and crossmatch for 4 to 6 U of blood. A Foley catheter should be placed. Lactated Ringer's solution should then be infused at a rate depending on the patient's vital signs and cardiac status. If the patient is not stabilized after 2 L of crystalloid infusion, a central venous line should be inserted and blood given. Fluid resuscitation should be aimed at restoring urine output to a rate of approximately 1 mL/kg/h.

DISPOSITION

A surgical consultation should be requested for patients in whom the diagnosis of acute diverticulitis is suspected and in all patients with rapid lower GI bleeding. Clearly, the patient with lower GI bleeding who is hemodynamically unstable should have an immediate surgical consultation.

Indications for Admission

Patients with diverticulitis complicated by abscess or fistula formation, obstruction, or free perforation should be admitted to a surgical service. Patients suspected of having severe acute diverticulitis and those with gross lower GI bleeding must be admitted. Obviously septic patients, those with severe concomitant diseases, and those with massive GI bleeding should be admitted to an intensive care unit.

Outpatient management should be limited to immunocompetent patients with mild uncomplicated diverticulitis. Severely immunocompromised patients with diverticulitis should be admitted, even those with benign-appearing presentations.

COMMON PITFALLS

- Although less frequently encountered in patients younger than age 40, diverticulosis is relatively more likely to be complicated and require surgery in younger patients than in older patients.[2]
- The classic signs and symptoms of diverticulitis are often absent in immunocompromised patients. These patients have a higher incidence of free perforation, failure of medical therapy, and postoperative morbidity and mortality.[8,10]

References

1. Almy TP, Howell DA. Diverticular disease of the colon. *N Engl J Med* 1980;302:324.
2. Cunningham MA, Davis JW, Kaups KL. Medical versus surgical management of diverticulitis in patients under age 40. *Am J Surg* 1997;174:733.
3. Deckmann RC, Cheskin LJ. Diverticular disease in the elderly. *J Am Geriatr Soc* 1993;40:986.

4. Ferzoco LB, Raptopoulos V, Silen W. Acute diverticulitis. *N Engl J Med* 1998;338:1521.
5. Hulnick DH, Megibow AJ, Balthazar EJ, et al. Computed tomography in the evaluation of diverticulitis. *Radiology* 1984;152:491.
6. Meyers MD, Alonso DR, Gray GF, et al. Pathogenesis of bleeding colonic diverticulosis. *Gastroenterology* 1976;71:577.
7. Naliboff JA, Jongmire-Cook SJ. Diverticulitis mimicking a tuboovarian abscess. *J Reprod Med* 1996;41:921.
8. Perkins JK, Shield CF, Chang FC, et al. Acute diverticulitis. *Am J Surg* 1984;148:745.
9. Pradel JA, Adell J, Taourel P. Acute colonic diverticulitis: prospective comparative evaluation with US and CT. *Radiology* 1997;205:503.
10. Roberts P, Abel M, Rosen L, et al. Practice parameters for sigmoid diverticulitis—supporting documentation. *Dis Colon Rectum* 1995;38:125.
11. Smith TR, Kyunghee CC, Morehouse HT, et al. Comparison of computed tomography and contrast enema evaluation of diverticulitis. *Dis Colon Rectum* 1990;33:1.
12. Vernava AM, Moore BA, Longo WE, et al. Lower gastrointestinal bleeding. *Dis Colon Rectum* 1997;40:846.
13. Wong SK, Ho YH, Leong AP, et al. Clinical behavior of complicated right-sided and left-sided diverticulosis. *Dis Colon Rectum* 1997;40:344.

ACKNOWLEDGMENT

The authors acknowledge the substantial contribution of Dr. C. Gene Cayton, the author of the chapter in the first edition of this book.

CHAPTER 46
Perianal, Rectal, and Anal Diseases

Leonard Samuels

The anorectal area is the site of few true emergencies but many uncomfortable conditions. The posterior quarters are so often a source of irritation that the idioms most frequently used to describe "irritations" refer to it. Hemorrhoids, abscesses, perirectal infection, functional disorders, and cancer are discussed in this chapter. The reader is referred elsewhere in this text for a discussion of proctitis.

ANATOMY

The anus is variously defined, but an accepted definition is the terminal large bowel from the dentate line distally to where the external margins of the anal canal meet. The anal opening is an elliptical orifice. The anatomy of the perianal soft tissue is easier to understand if one considers the region as made up of concentric layers. The central core is the anal canal; the first ring, the mucosa; the second, the internal sphincter; and the third, the levator and external sphincter. The inner visceral tube is composed of smooth muscle with autonomic innervation. The outer muscular group is funnel shaped, of skeletal muscle, with somatic innervation. Beyond this outer muscular layer, the fatty tissue of the buttocks extends to the dermis and epidermis of the skin surfaces.

The rectum is approximately 20 cm long and the most distal portion of the large bowel. It has no peritoneal covering; this distinguishes it from the sigmoid, which is completely invested with peritoneum. The primary purpose of the rectum is as a storage cavity for stool.

THE FUNCTION OF CONTINENCE

The rectum could not serve as a storage cavity for stool if there were no mechanism to keep the stool within it until the proper time for passage. The angulation of the anorectal system (60 degrees between the axis of the rectum and the anal canal) aids continence through the creation of a flap valve effect.[10] The angle is present except during defecation or when the hips are flexed more than 90 degrees. The anal canal generally has higher pressures than the rectum, a gradient vital to the preservation of continence. The gradient exists because the anorectal ring, comprising the internal and external sphincters and the puborectalis muscle, creates pressure through contraction. If the layers of the ring are cut completely, incontinence inevitably results.

ANORECTAL ABSCESSES

Anorectal abscesses are serious because they may spread rapidly, dissecting into deep-tissue spaces. Perianal abscesses are located immediately adjacent to the anus; there is no induration noted on rectal examination. Ischiorectal abscesses are deeper, with diffuse and lateral perianal swelling; induration is present on rectal examination. Intersphincteric, intermuscular, and supralevator abscesses generally do not have external signs, but swelling and tenderness at various depths are noted during rectal examination (Fig. 46.1).

CLINICAL PRESENTATION

Ischiorectal and perianal abscesses normally present as severe perianal pain and a "boil." Patients with deeper perirectal abscesses often present with fever, systemic toxicity, and a sensation of rectal fullness or heaviness. Although simple ischiorectal and perianal abscesses are the most common, an abscess may

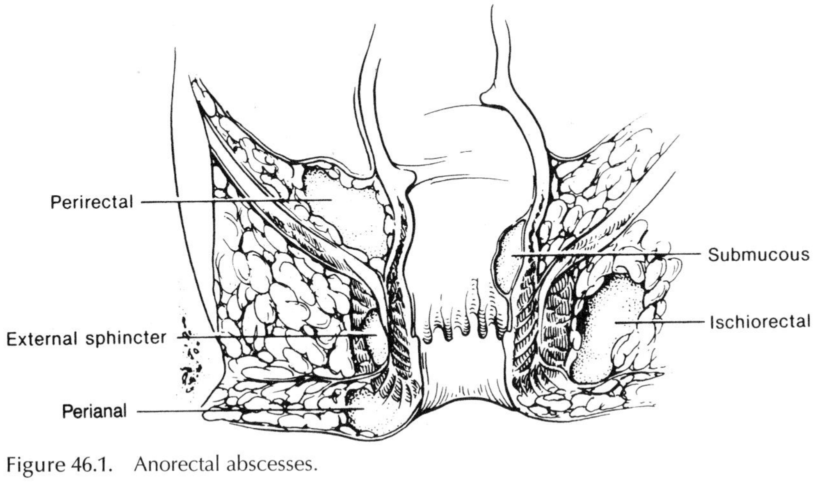

Figure 46.1. Anorectal abscesses.

track into several tissue planes and have deep components in addition to superficial ones. On occasion, a perirectal abscess may extend intraabdominally and cause systemic toxicity, peritonitis, and an abdominal or a pelvic mass.

Anorectal sepsis in severely neutropenic patients is common and deadly. Pyrexia and pain develop early, but because of the neutropenia, swelling and fluctuance develop late if at all. Therapy should include anaerobic coverage and a third-generation cephalosporin or broad-spectrum penicillin, possibly combined with an aminoglycoside. When fluctuance is present, or if cellulitis progresses despite antibiotics, surgery may be lifesaving.[3]

DIFFERENTIAL DIAGNOSIS

Swelling and pus can be present owing to a local abscess or a sinus tract from a distant source. Pilonidal abscess, Bartholin gland abscess, deep perirectal abscess, and, rarely, intraabdominal abscess fistula (Crohn disease) can generate sinus tracts that may initially resemble a superficial buttocks abscess. Careful palpation is the most useful technique to differentiate a sinus tract from an abscess.

Coexisting and predisposing illnesses should also be sought. They include inflammatory bowel disease, tuberculosis, various blood dyscrasias, sepsis, diabetes, and corticosteroid therapy. Local trauma and local infectious processes (such as hidradenitis suppurativa, infected hair follicles, or a poorly healing episiotomy) also predispose toward abscess development.

An aneurysm in the rectal region may simulate an abscess. Abscess aspiration results in accurate diagnosis and prevents catastrophe.

EMERGENCY DEPARTMENT EVALUATION AND MANAGEMENT

The extent of a perirectal abscess and its anatomic location are usually determined with a careful digital examination. The emergency physician should drain only relatively superficial abscesses that can be drained through perianal skin (ischiorectal and perianal abscesses). Adequate drainage is important.

Some authors recommend culture of the abscess by needle aspiration before drainage. Although *Escherichia coli, Staphylococcus aureus,* and fecal anaerobes are the most common organisms in perirectal abscesses, other organisms also cause abscesses. Antibiotic prophylaxis at least 1 hour but less than 2 hours prior to incision and drainage should be given to patients with clinically (as opposed to only echocardiographically) detectable valvular disease, with prosthetic valves, or with a history of endocarditis, rheumatic fever, or congenital heart disease.[1] Antibiotic prophylaxis is reasonable in patients who are immunocompromised, but no standard guidelines exist. Amoxicillin-clavulanic acid or ampicillin-sulbactam is a good choice, and clindamycin is a good choice in penicillin-allergic patients.[1] For penicillin-allergic patients unable to take oral antibiotics or patients who are known to carry methicillin-resistant *S. aureus,* vancomycin is the preferred drug.

Incision and drainage should be performed with the patient prone or in the jackknife position with the buttocks taped apart. Local anesthesia may be adequate, but many patients suffer less if given meperidine or morphine. The incision should be radial; removal of an ellipse of skin may be helpful in facilitating drainage. Loculations should be broken up with a hemostat, and the wound should be copiously irrigated. Loose packing with a single piece of gauze should be removed in 48 hours. Sitz baths encourage drainage. Routine abscesses usually heal without the patient needing antibiotics. Indications for antibiotic therapy include systemic toxicity, a large area of cellulitis, lymphangitis, and immunocompromise. Patients with these symptoms should be considered for admission.

Drainage of multiple abscesses may result in a residual fistula that will require further attention. The patient should be warned of this possibility and referred for follow-up surgery.

DISPOSITION

Deep abscesses with systemic symptoms necessitate urgent surgical consultation for drainage and admission to the hospital. Prompt therapy is important to prevent spread of the infection and septic shock. Poor outcomes have been associated with delay in therapy, inadequate treatment, and significant concomitant disease.

COMMON PITFALLS

- Failure to identify a deep abscess
- Failure to identify an abscess as complex or of pilonidal origin
- Treatment in the emergency department of an abscess that requires extensive surgical management
- Failure to identify conditions that warrant preincisional antibiotics

ANAL FISSURES

PATHOPHYSIOLOGY

Anal fissures begin as abrasions that cause anal sphincter spasm; this leads to a vicious cycle of spasm, inadequate drainage, and repeated injury to the anal opening during stool passage. The chronically inflamed tissue of the chronic fissure becomes resistant to healing.

CLINICAL PRESENTATION

The patient complains of pain and mild bleeding on stooling. The acute fissure appears as a slitlike radial cut on examination. The chronic fissure has the appearance of a midline ulcer with a skin tag and enlarged papilla. In both lesions, the skin surrounding the fissure appears normal. "Type A" patients seem to be more prone to develop fissures.

DIFFERENTIAL DIAGNOSIS

The appearance of an acute anal fissure is usually so clear that it is seldom misdiagnosed. A chancre may be mistaken for a fissure, but chancres are nontender. Tuberculosis, Crohn disease, ulcerative colitis, human immunodeficiency virus (HIV), leukemia, and syphilis predispose to anal fissures, and these fissures may be unusually severe, multiple, or not in the usual midline posterior anal location.[9] A careful examination of the perianal region is required to detect the ulceration of a chronic fissure behind the concealing skin tag.

EMERGENCY DEPARTMENT EVALUATION AND MANAGEMENT

Anal abrasions and acute and subacute fissures require good anal hygiene and a high-residue diet. A shower or brief sitz bath directly after stooling cleanses the area and reduces irritation.

The goal is to permit early healing before the tissue is permanently altered by the irritation process. Traditional treatment for chronic fissures is surgery. Recently, medical treatments such as topical glyceril trinitrate or local injection of botulinum toxin have been demonstrated to be fairly effective in promoting healing. Any treatment plan requires referral.[4,6,8]

COMMON PITFALLS

- Failure to recognize an atypical fissure as a sign of more serious disease
- Failure to recognize and refer patients with chronic fissure

ANORECTAL FISTULAS

CLINICAL PRESENTATION AND EMERGENCY DEPARTMENT EVALUATION

An anorectal fistula is an abnormal communication between the anorectum (primary opening) and another site, usually after drainage of an anorectal abscess. The tract is usually single. A fistula or sinuses in the perianal area can also originate from nonanorectal sites, such as diverticulitis of the sigmoid colon, appendicitis, inflammatory bowel disease, periurethral infection, and presacral tumors.

EMERGENCY DEPARTMENT MANAGEMENT

Anorectal fistula is treated by uncapping the fistula and allowing it to heal outward from its base. The procedure should be performed by a surgeon and not in the emergency department.[6] Treatment that necessitates incision through the anorectal ring can result in incontinence.

HEMORRHOIDS

CLINICAL PRESENTATION AND EMERGENCY DEPARTMENT EVALUATION

Hemorrhoids are varicose veins at the rectal outlet and are the most frequent cause of rectal bleeding. Increased pressure in the hemorrhoidal veins is thought to be the major predisposing factor. Conditions believed to cause rectal venous outflow obstruction include pregnancy and bearing down when stooling (increased abdominal pressure), repeated storage of firm stool in the rectal ampulla (local obstruction of venous return), and hepatic fibrosis (shunting of venous return).

Internal hemorrhoids occur above the anorectal line. They are covered by mucosa and are insensitive to painful stimuli. These features differentiate them from external hemorrhoids. When thrombosis is present, hemorrhoids may be painful and a hard clot is palpable in the hemorrhoidal vessels. Hemorrhoids may itch but are usually not painful unless thrombosis is present. When pain is the chief complaint and hemorrhoidal disease is not extreme, another source for the pain should be carefully sought.

EMERGENCY DEPARTMENT MANAGEMENT

Acute exacerbations of hemorrhoidal disease characterized by prolapse of part of the anal canal and thrombophlebitis of the hemorrhoidal plexus require conservative treatment with stool softeners, sitz baths, pain-relieving ointment or suppository, and analgesics. Topical hydrocortisone is of value only if there is itching. With the exception of chronic or constantly prolapsed internal hemorrhoids, most episodes of hemorrhoidal disease are self-limited. A thrombosed external hemorrhoid can be treated conservatively or surgically. After local anesthesia, the clot can be evacuated through a short incision made over the clot. Sitz baths and a pad to absorb the oozing are helpful after treatment. If bleeding is heavy, packing with Surgicel for a few hours or overnight reliably produces hemostasis. A thrombosed internal hemorrhoid should be managed by a surgeon.

RECTAL PROLAPSE

Rectal prolapse is a full-thickness protrusion of a portion of the distal rectum through the anal opening. The protrusion has a tubular appearance with concentric folds on the end. Mucosal prolapse occurs when the rectal mucosa loses its connection to the underlying muscle and protrudes out the anal opening; it differs from rectal prolapse in that there is no protrusion of muscle and the protruding tissue forms a circle with radial grooves. Internal rectal prolapse occurs when the upper rectum and sigmoid prolapse into the rectal ampulla but not through the anal orifice. Internal rectal prolapse is found primarily in women.[3] They may complain of incontinence of flatus or feces, tenesmus, rectal pressure, pelvic fullness or pain, lower back pain, or a sensation of incomplete evacuation.

EMERGENCY DEPARTMENT EVALUATION AND DIFFERENTIAL DIAGNOSIS

A patulous anus is commonly found when repeated rectal prolapse is the presenting complaint. If the lesion has reduced at the time of examination, the most effective way to provoke prolapse is to have the patient strain. Rectal pain from rectal prolapse is uncommon and should suggest a secondary lesion or incarceration. Occasionally, a polyp or rectal tumor may protrude through the anus and simulate prolapse. Examination after reduction helps to differentiate the conditions. Mental illness, multiple sclerosis, tabes dorsalis, and cauda equina syndrome are associated with rectal prolapse, although they are responsible for only a small percentage of cases.

EMERGENCY DEPARTMENT MANAGEMENT

Reduction of most prolapses can easily be accomplished in the emergency department, but such reduction is usually short-lived. Incarceration of a rectal prolapse necessitates emergency operative therapy. It can progress to strangulation, bleeding secondary to ulceration, and rupture. Adults eventually require surgery for recurrent rectal prolapse. Most authorities recommend early surgery, because once incontinence develops from weakening of the sphincter, surgery to correct the prolapse may not restore continence.[6]

IMPACTION

Impaction is generally the result of inadequate regulation of stool consistency, although anatomic factors, such as denervation and stricture, also may play an important role in selected cases. The maintenance of a lumen of normal caliber for the rectal outlet depends on the regular passage of a formed stool and explains why chronic diarrhea predisposes to impaction.

Constipation, the most common cause of impaction, can itself be caused by many conditions. Diabetes, lead poisoning, uremia, opiates, sedatives, iron supplements, and immobilization all can cause constipation. Insufficient fluid intake prevents bulk from exerting a softening effect and can even cause bulk to be the impacting agent. Pain or partial obstruction can delay the passage of stool, as can poor bowel habits or psychological factors, leading to a more inspissated stool.

Most fecal impactions occur in the rectum.[10] If impaction is located in the rectum on digital examination, it is still important to assess for other masses on abdominal examination. Impaction may result in diarrhea, with only liquid stool able to make its way past the impaction. The impaction often weakens sphincter tone, resulting in chronic passage of watery stool.

Most impactions necessitate urgent treatment. Mineral oil enemas may be effective, if used several times a day, in softening and lubricating the impaction. When digital disimpaction is required, the disruption of the impaction should be gentle to avoid trauma to the rectal wall. Injury may cause a subsequent abscess. Nonrectal impactions, obstructive symptoms, fever, and dehydration warrant consultation and admission.

MISCELLANEOUS CONDITIONS

ANAL PRURITUS

Pruritus ani results from mucus secretion from internal rectal prolapse, pinworm eggs, pubic lice, or scabies. Idiopathic anal pruritus usually presents as a nocturnal itch in a tense person. Thickened, lichenified perianal skin is characteristic. Ice alleviates the itch, as may sitz baths and good anal hygiene. A shower directly after stooling may be helpful.

VENEREAL DISEASE AND WARTS

Condylomata acuminata is caused by the human papillomavirus. The warts may be pedunculated or sessile. Patients with even modestly compromised cellular immunity are more vulnerable to wart infection, but the warts are also very contagious among nonimmunocompromised persons. Most human papillomavirus infections, including most that predispose toward malignant transformation, do not result in visible warts.[11] Condylomata acuminata are four to 13 times more prevalent in the population of patients seen in sexually transmitted disease clinics than in the general population.[7] No therapy totally eradicates the human papillomavirus, but various locally destructive therapies can temporarily destroy visible warts.[5]

Condylomata lata are wartlike lesions caused by syphilis. They are smoother than anogenital warts and are nearly always moist. Syphilis should be recognized and treated by the emergency physician. Treatment includes benzathine penicillin G, 2.4 million U i.m., or a 10-day course of tetracycline or erythromycin. Venereal diseases such as herpes simplex, lymphogranuloma venereum, and gonorrhea can also manifest as rectal diseases.

RECTAL ULCERS

Rectal ulcers, which occur particularly in acquired immunodeficiency syndrome (AIDS) patients, are very painful and often hard to treat. Many are idiopathic, probably of viral origin. The differential diagnosis includes syphilis, chancroid, tuberculosis, herpes, lymphoma, sarcoma, carcinoma, mycobacterium avium, intracellulare, *Cryptococcus neoformans,* and chlamydia.[3]

CARCINOMA

The symptoms of anal cancer are often indistinguishable from those of benign lesions. The most common symptoms are pain and bleeding. A palpable mass is present in 25% of cases; pruritus is present in about 15% of cases. In about 25% of cases, patients are asymptomatic and cancer is detected by routine rectal examination. The predictive value in older persons of a positive guaiac test result for colorectal carcinoma is 5% to 10%. In addition, adenomas are found in 30% to 40% of patients with positive guaiac test results. Squamous cell tumors account for 80% to 95% of anal tumors.[5] Adenocarcinomas are common in the rectum. Risk factors for colorectal carcinoma include prior adenoma, family history of large bowel cancer, personal history of breast or uterine carcinoma, exposure of pelvis to radiation, and presence of ureterosigmoidostomy. Familial polyposis, ulcerative colitis, and Crohn disease of the colon are more severe risk factors. Leukemic infiltration into the anal area can result in severe anal pain but in minimal physical findings, except for superficial induration. The patient may appear quite ill. The white blood cell count is usually diagnostic. Persistent coccygeal pain suggests a tumor of neural origin in the coccyx and lower back. Spasmodic pain is more characteristic of benign conditions such as coccygodynia, a syndrome (secondary to trauma) of sharp pains precipitated by movement of the coccyx.

PILONIDAL DISEASE AND HIDRADENITIS SUPPURATIVA

Pilonidal disease is a syndrome of infection in the presacral midline that causes sinus tracts, abscesses, and pits. Hidradenitis suppurativa is a chronic inflammatory disease that originates in areas of apocrine sweat glands and results in superficial, often multiple, and interconnected abscesses. Treatment of both conditions involves incision and drainage of abscess cavities, moist heat or soaks, and antibiotics. Both conditions necessitate more extensive surgical procedures by a surgeon for definitive treatment; otherwise, recurrence is inevitable.

References

1. Dajani AS, Taubert KA, Wilson S, et al. Prevention of bacterial endocarditis. Recommendations by the American Heart Association. *JAMA* 1997;227(22):1794.
2. Eu KW, Seow-Choen F. Functional problems in adult rectal prolapse and controversies in surgical treatment. *Br J Surg* 1997;84(7):904.
3. Gilliland R, Wexner SD. Complicated anorectal sepsis. *Surg Clin North Am* 1997;77(1):115.
4. Giorgio M, Cassetta E, Gui D, et al. A comparison of botulinum toxin and saline for the treatment of chronic anal fissure. *N Engl J Med* 1998;338(4):217.
5. Janicke DM, Pundt MR. Anorectal disorders. *Emerg Med Clin North Am* 1996;14(4):757.
6. Kamm MA. Fortnightly review: faecal incontinence. *BMJ* 1998;316(7230):528.
7. Koutsky L. Epidemiology of genital human papilloma virus infection. *Am J Med* 1997;102(5A):3.
8. Loder PB, Kamm MA, Nichols RJ. "Reversible chemical sphincterotomy" by local application of glyceril trinitrate. *Br J Surg* 1994;81:1386.
9. Lund JN, Scholefield JH. Aetiology and treatment of anal fissure. *Br J Surg* 1996;83:1335.
10. Rasmussen OO, Christiansen J. Physiology and pathophysiology of anal function. *Scand J Gastroenterol* 1996;31[Suppl 216]:169.
11. Rhea WG, Bourgeois BM, Sewell DR. Condyloma acuminata: a fatal disease? *Am Surg* 1998;64(11):1082.

PART V

Emergency Aspects of Vascular Surgery

CHAPTER 47
Nontraumatic Carotid Artery Emergencies

James W. Dennis

There are essentially two major conditions relating to the carotid artery that demand urgent evaluation and treatment if a patient is to achieve maximal recovery: (1) acute cervical thromboembolic disease and (2) spontaneous carotid dissection. Although less common than some peripheral vascular problems, these two entities are widely prevalent etiologies to stroke, the third leading cause of death in the United States, occurring in over one-half million people annually. Historic data indicate that approximately 35% to 40% of strokes are lethal and over 70% of those recovering will have some permanent neurologic deficit.[10] This morbidity extracts a high socioeconomic cost as productive, contributing individuals are often transformed into assistance-dependent members of society. Rapid diagnosis and initiation of treatment help to minimize the potential devastating loss of neurologic function and maximize the chances of returning a patient to an independent lifestyle.

ACUTE THROMBOEMBOLIC DISEASE OF THE CAROTID ARTERY

Over the years, several manifestations of acute thromboembolic events involving the cervical carotid artery have been identified and given various descriptive terms. These include transient ischemic attack (TIA), crescendo TIAs, reversible ischemic neurologic deficit (RIND), fluctuating stroke (stuttering hemiplegia), progressing stroke (stroke in evolution), and established stroke. TIA and RIND are addressed in this chapter.

TRANSIENT ISCHEMIC ATTACK

A TIA is defined as any focal neurologic deficit lasting less than 24 hours (usually less than 1 hour) with complete resolution. Crescendo TIAs represent a succession of TIAs in which each succeeding event is more severe than the previous TIA or the time interval is shortening between attacks. Amaurosis fugax is a unique type of TIA that is defined as temporary, monocular loss of vision, often appearing as a curtain coming down or across the visual field. The natural history of a TIA resulting from carotid artery occlusive disease has been documented in a review of several nonoperative series.[20] Untreated patients have a permanent stroke risk of approximately 7% annually for the first 5 years (or about one-third overall), which can be reduced to about one-half of that with antiplatelet agents.[13] Crescendo TIAs represent a more ominous picture, although the exact risk in these patients is poorly defined because most are treated surgically on an urgent basis.[11]

Of utmost importance, any patient presenting with these symptoms mandates immediate evaluation to determine the cause of the TIAs. Etiologies other than carotid artery disease include cardiac emboli, migraine headaches, intracerebral aneurysms or space-occupying lesions, nerve palsies, inflammatory arteriopathies (Takayasu disease) and intraocular abnormalities, usually of the retina. A good physical examination often reveals evidence of the source. Along with a meticulous neurologic examination, particular attention should be paid to the presenting blood pressure, the heart auscultation, the cervical auscultation, and the funduscopic examination.

In most instances, a carotid duplex ultrasound (US) is the best means by which to rule in or out the presence of significant vascular disease. The accuracy of these noninvasive examinations approach 95% in experienced hands and is the deciding factor if further intervention, either arteriogram or surgery, is warranted.[5] If the US clearly shows a high-grade stenosis (75% to 80%), many surgeons will perform a carotid endarterectomy on that basis alone[16] (Fig. 47.1). Less severe lesions or those examinations demonstrating ulcerative plaques usually require arteriography, which more clearly shows the anatomy, to determine whether this represents the probable etiology of the TIA. The value of a computed tomography (CT) scan in these circumstances is debatable. Although it does rule out intracranial lesions, studies have shown CT findings to be both predictive and unpredictive of the outcome following surgery.[15] Those with a normal US should undergo a CT scan and echocardiogram on an urgent basis. Anticoagulation with intravenous heparin is not usually needed unless there appears to be a delay in the evaluation and treatment.

REVERSIBLE ISCHEMIC NEUROLOGIC DEFICITS AND STROKES

RINDs are defined as acute focal neurologic deficits that last longer than 24 hours but completely resolve. Fluctuating strokes demonstrate a waxing and waning of the severity of the neurologic deficit, progressing strokes show a continual gradual worsening over several days, and established strokes have stable, fixed deficits. Although it is impossible to determine if and when a fixed neurologic deficit will resolve, these patients should all be treated in a similar manner. A prompt, yet thorough physical ex-

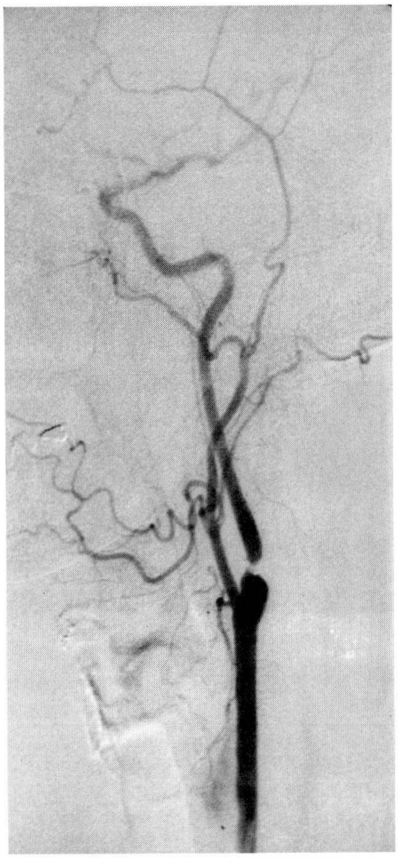

Figure 47.1. Arteriogram of an internal carotid artery high-grade stenosis at the typical location just past the carotid bifurcation. Atherosclerotic lesions similar to this are often the etiology of TIAs and strokes.

amination should be done and a CT scan obtained to rule out intracranial hemorrhage. Until recently, little more than supportive care could be given to individuals presenting with acute strokes. Studies have now demonstrated a better long-term clinical outcome if the deficit is less than a few hours old and the patient can be started on thrombolytic agents. Several protocols are being used. A large multicenter, prospective, randomized study utilizing intravenous tissue plasminogen activator (TPA) within 3 hours of a stroke resulted in a 30% increase in the number of patients having little or no disability at 3 months.[12] This improvement comes with a price, however, as the risk of symptomatic intracranial hemorrhage increased from 0.6% to 6.4% with this treatment. A more recent study showed a similar benefit in patients up to 7 hours following the onset of their stroke.[18] Another technique uses urokinase through an intraarterial catheter placed in the carotid artery within 4 to 6 hours of a stroke.[8] If the internal carotid artery can be recanalized, the prognosis is significantly better than that for permanent occlusions. The latter arteriographic technique also allows good visualization of the carotid anatomy and avoids the need for US. These more aggressive approaches require that a dedicated team of neurologists, interventional radiologists, and vascular surgeons be available at all times. These factors limit the applicability of these approaches in smaller, nonteaching hospitals. Low-molecular-weight heparin has also been used acutely, with significant improvement in neurologic recovery at 6 months over placebo.[9]

Patients presenting more than 6 to 7 hours after a stroke began should generally undergo a CT scan of the head and US of the carotid arteries unless another obvious source of the stroke is identified. Very high grade stenoses or intraluminal thrombus will usually require anticoagulation with intravenous heparin and earlier than normal surgical intervention.[7] If these tests are negative, the patient should be admitted for monitoring, further workup as to the etiology of the stroke and hypertension control as needed.

ACUTE CAROTID ARTERY DISSECTION

Dissection of the carotid artery is a less common but equally devastating cause of acute cerebrovascular insufficiency. Although well described in the trauma literature, carotid dissections can occur spontaneously with common, everyday neck movements, or with no inciting event at all. Similar to TIAs, the early, accurate diagnosis and initiation of treatment of dissections can often determine the severity of the long-term neurologic deficit resulting from these lesions.

PATHOGENESIS

Underlying etiologies of spontaneous carotid dissection are varied. They include congenital anomalies, infections of the pharynx, syphilis, and arterial wall defects such as Marfan syndrome, cystic medial necrosis, fibromuscular dysplasia, arteritis, and atherosclerosis.[1,6] The initiating event appears to be a tear in the intima of the internal carotid artery or intramural hemorrhage, which may result from any of the aforementioned factors. Also, it is thought that stretching of the vessel over the lateral articular processes of the first two cervical vertebrae may play a role in some instances.[19] This hyperextension of the neck may go unrecognized or may result from everyday movements such as coughing or even washing hair.

In most instances, the dissection begins 2 to 3 cm beyond the carotid bifurcation or, less commonly, slightly more distal in the midcervical internal carotid artery. It usually extends up to the point where the internal carotid artery enters the petrous canal. As blood progresses up the false channel within the medial layer of the arterial wall, the true lumen becomes compressed and either narrowed or occluded. At other times, microemboli may travel to the distal cerebral circulation, the false lumen may reenter into the true lumen, or, rarely, pseudoaneurysms may develop in the thinned-out arterial wall.

CLINICAL PRESENTATION

Carotid dissection can occur in all ages, from very young children to the elderly, with the majority occurring in middle age. In a large series of 30 patients at one institution, the most common symptoms were TIAs (56%), completed stroke (30%), amaurosis fugax (17%), severe headache (20%), neck pain (13%), tinnitus (7%), and incomplete Horner syndrome (3%).[14] There is often a delay between the inciting event and the development of the clinical symptoms; this delay may range from hours to days. A thorough history and physical examination, along with a high index of suspicion, are needed to identify these problems early in their course. A carotid duplex US represents the quickest means by which to detect an abnormality in the internal carotid artery and should be done as soon as possible.[17] This will often indicate a severe stenosis or occlusion, which should lead to an urgent arteriogram.

ARTERIOGRAPHIC FINDINGS

Two types of arteriographic pictures of carotid dissections are seen. The most common type is that of a very narrowed segment of the internal carotid artery a few centimeters from the bifurcation to the base of the skull (Fig. 47.2). This is known as the "carotid string sign" and is quite characteristic of a dissection. This type of narrowing may also be seen in the more distal internal carotid artery, depending on where the intimal tear or

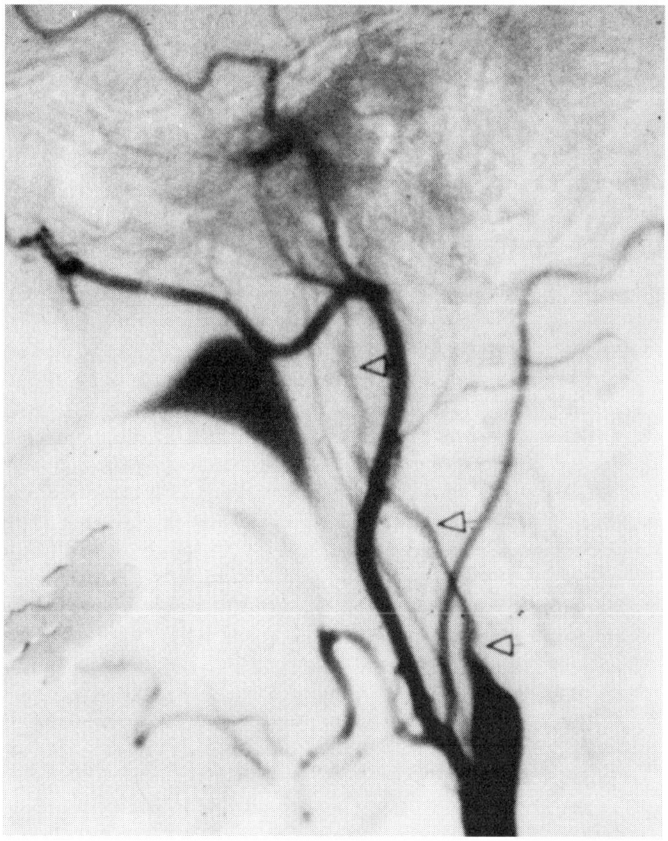

Figure 47.2. Arteriogram showing the most common finding seen in acute carotid dissection. The long, irregular, narrowed segment of the internal carotid artery is known as the "carotid string sign." (Reprinted with permission from Okuhn SP, Stoney RJ. In: Bergan JJ, Yao JST, eds. Vascular surgical emergencies. Orlando: Grune & Stratton, 1987:125–137.)

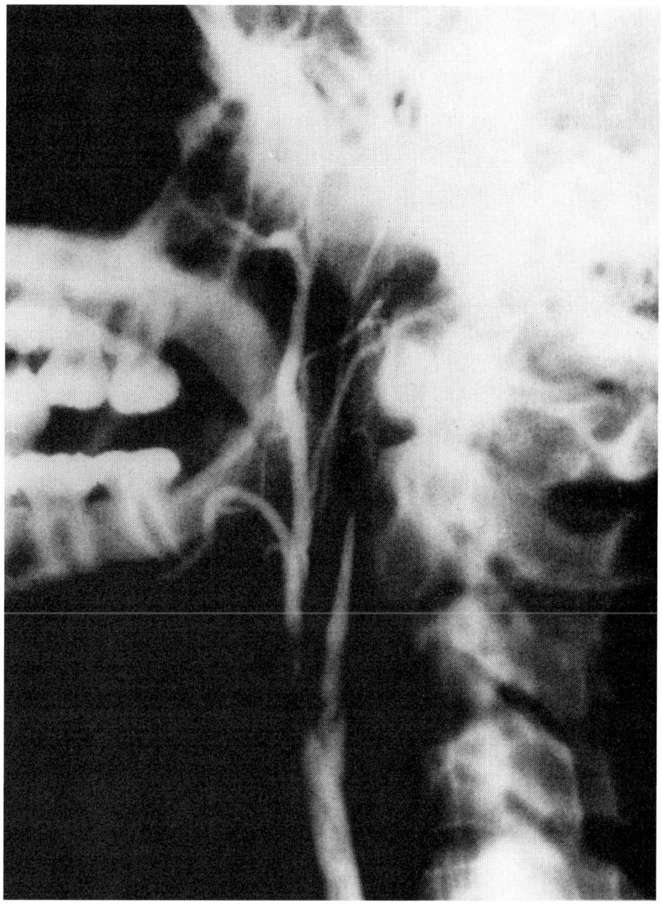

Figure 47.3. Arteriogram demonstrating the "dunce's cap," which represents an acute occlusion of the internal carotid artery following dissection. This may later disappear as the thrombus propagates proximally to the bifurcation. (Reprinted with permission from Okuhn SP, Stoney RJ. In: Bergan JJ, Yao JST, eds. Vascular surgical emergencies. Orlando: Grune & Stratton, 1987:125–137.)

medial hemorrhage begins. The second commonly seen pattern is that of a tapered occlusion of the internal carotid artery several centimeters after the bifurcation (Fig. 47.3). This is called a "dunce's cap." If some time has passed since the occlusion occurred, the internal carotid may be thrombosed back to the bifurcation, making it difficult to distinguish from atherosclerotic occlusive disease that had progressed to thrombosis. Other findings often seen on an arteriogram include delay in the column of contrast reaching the brain; a small filling defect at the base of the dissection, representing an intimal flap (with or without thrombus); and distal middle cerebral artery emboli.

TREATMENT

Once the diagnosis of carotid dissection has been established, the best results are generally obtained by anticoagulation with intravenous heparin, followed by oral anticoagulants for up to a year.[14,17] Care must first be taken to ensure that no intracerebral hemorrhage exists or that no carotid pseudoaneurysm has developed. Anticoagulation helps maintain patency of the narrowed lumen and prevents emboli from occurring. In most cases, the true lumen will normalize within a few months, with recurrence a very rare event. This medical management has been shown to be superior to the direct surgical intervention that was initially attempted in the 1960 and 1970s.[4]

In some instances, surgery may be beneficial if the diseased segment of artery is surgically accessible. This would include patients with recurrent emboli despite anticoagulation, those with pseudoaneurysms, and those with documented progressive stenoses. In these cases, resection of the diseased artery and interposition grafting is most commonly done. If the distal end of the dissection cannot be approached and the back pressure is measured at 70 mm Hg or more, the carotid can be ligated with little risk of stroke.[3] More recently, placement of internal carotid stents have been reported to be moderately successful in some acute carotid dissections.[2] The long-term durability and safety of these endovascular techniques is yet to be determined.

References

1. Anderson CA, Collins CG Jr, Rich NM, et al. Spontaneous dissection of the internal carotid artery associated with fibromuscular dysplasia. *Am Surg* 1980;46:263–271.
2. Dejjani GK, Monsein LH, Laird JR, et al. Treatment of symptomatic cervical carotid artery dissections with endovascular stents. *Neurosurgery* 1999;44(4):755–761.
3. Ehrenfeld WK, Stoney RJ, Wylie EJ. Relation of carotid stump pressure to safety of carotid artery ligation. *Surgery* 1983;313:1191–1195.
4. Ehrenfeld WK, Wylie EJ. Spontaneous dissection of the internal carotid artery. *Arch Surg* 1976;111:1294–1298.
5. Eikenboom BC, Ackerstaff RGA, Ludwig JW, et al. Digital video subtraction angiography and duplex scanning in assessment of carotid disease: comparison with conventional angiography. *Surgery* 1983;94:821–829.
6. Friedman WA, Day AL, Quisling RG, et al. Cervical carotid dissecting aneurysms. *Neurosurgery* 1980;7:207–212.
7. Gasecki AP, Ferguson GG, Eliasziw M, et al. Early endarterectomy for severe carotid artery stenosis after a nondisabling stroke: results from the North American Symptomatic Carotid Endarterectomy Trial. *J Vasc Surg* 1994;20(2):288–295.
8. Gonner R, Remonda L, Mattle H, et al. Local intra-arterial thrombolysis in acute ischemic stroke. *Stroke* 1998;29(9):1894–1900.
9. Kay R, Wong KS, Yu YL, et al. Low-molecular-weight heparin for the treatment of acute ischemic stroke. *N Engl J Med* 1995;333(24):1588–1593.
10. Matsumoto N, Whisnant JP, Kurland LT, et al. Natural history of stroke in Rochester, Minnesota, 1955 through 1969: an extension of a previous study, 1945 through 1954. *Stroke* 1973;4:20–25.

11. Mentzer RM, Finkelmeier BA, Crosby IK, et al. Emergency carotid endarterectomy for fluctuating neurological deficits. *Surgery* 1981;89(1):60–64.
12. National Institute of Neurological Disorders and Stroke rt-PA Stroke Study Group, The. Tissue plasminogen activator for acute ischemic stroke. *N Engl J Med* 1995;333(24):1581–1587.
13. North American Symptomatic Carotid Endarterectomy Trial Collaborators. Beneficial effects of carotid endarterectomy in symptomatic patients with high-grade carotid stenosis. *N Engl J Med* 1991;325:445–453.
14. Okuhn SP, Stoney RJ. Carotid Artery Dissection. In: Bergan JJ, Yao JST, eds. *Vascular surgical emergencies*. Orlando: Grune & Stratton, 1987:125–137.
15. Pritz MB. Timing of carotid endarterectomy after stroke. *Stroke* 1997;28:2563–2567.
16. Thomas GI, Jones TW, Stavney LS, et al. Carotid endarterectomy after Doppler ultrasonographic examination without angiography. *Am J Surg* 1986;151:616–620.
17. Treiman GS, Treiman RL, Foran RF, et al. Spontaneous dissection of the internal carotid artery. A nineteen year clinical experience. *J Vasc Surg* 1996;24(4):597–607.
18. Trouillas P, Nighoghossian N, Laurent D, et al. Thrombolysis with intravenous rtPA in a series of 100 cases of acute carotid territory stroke. *Stroke* 1998;29(12):2529–2540.
19. Welling RE, Saul TG, Tew JM Jr, et al. Management of blunt injury to the internal carotid artery. *J Trauma* 1987;27:1221–1226.
20. Wiebers DO, Whisnant JP. Epidemiology. In: Warlow C, Morris PJ, eds. *Transient ischemic attacks*. New York: Marcel Dekker Inc, 1982:8–20.

CHAPTER 48

Emergency Aspects of Peripheral Vascular Insufficiency

Henry C. Veldenz

The presentation of a patient with an ischemic limb to the emergency department represents both a challenge and an opportunity in assessment and management. Guided by history and physical examination skills, this encounter can be readily directed to the appropriate outcome for the patient. Once the acuity and severity of the ischemic limb has been elucidated, disposition, ranging from outpatient follow-up to emergency surgery, can be selected.

Lower extremity peripheral vascular occlusive disease (LEPVOD) occurs in the patient population at risk for cardiovascular disease.[1,3,5] It is merely a regional manifestation of the underlying systemic disease of atherosclerosis. Thus, hypertension, hypercholesterolemia, tobacco abuse, diabetes mellitus, end-stage renal disease, and inactivity are prevalent among these patients.

The incidence of LEPVOD has been stable over the past decade. Hypercoagulable states, however, are recognized with an increasing frequency.[4] When LEPVOD becomes clinically apparent, the *levels* of occlusive disease that may affect a patient also have a corresponding *collateral bed* that carries circulation in times of need. However, unlike the named arterial level involved in the occlusive process, the collateral circulation is a high-resistance vascular system, explaining diminished flow in states of increased flow demand. This state plays a role in both occlusive and embolic situations.

Important to the management of the ischemic limb are the *timing* and the *severity* of the ischemia. Presentations that represent chronic disease of minimal severity, such as intermittent claudication, are handled differently from the acute, profound ischemia of an acute aortic embolic occlusion. The timing and severity of presentation *are* related to the patient's underlying anatomy and pathophysiology.

CLINICAL PRESENTATION

The presentation of vascular insufficiency is heavily dependent on the underlying pathology. A person with a macrovascular embolus will potentially manifest all six of the P's of acute ischemia: pain, pallor, pulselessness, poikilothermia, paresthesias, and paralysis. The most important symptom will be pain, with the sensory and motor changes occurring early in the course.

The patient with chronic occlusive disease will also complain of pain, but unlike that of a patient with an acute embolic occlusion, the pain will have been present for a period of days to weeks. The acute sensory and motor deficits are absent; instead, patients exhibit a spectrum of chronic changes. Typical chronic trophic changes are also seen in chronic occlusive disease; if the LEPVOD is severe enough for long enough, the patient may also have frank tissue loss demonstrated by ischemic ulceration or actual gangrene.

The patient with intermittent claudication will give a history of pain in a leg or legs with walking a set, short distance. This distance is almost always reproducible. The leg is symptomatic *distal* to the level of occlusive involvement. The degree of disability is related to the presence of collateral development. An anatomic level of LEPVOD is usually present, such as a superficial femoral artery occlusion producing *calf* claudication or an external iliac artery occlusion producing *calf and thigh* claudication.

Ischemic rest pain occurs in the forefoot or the toes. It can also be described by the term *metatarsalgia*. In the very elderly, pain may not be the chief complaint; instead, the patient may complain of symptoms of sleep deprivation from untreated pain. It takes two anatomic levels of occlusion, requiring flow through two high-resistance collateral beds in series, to produce ischemic rest pain. Ischemic rest pain does not occur in the calves, nor is it cramping of the calves at rest. The patient with ischemic ulceration or gangrene also has two or more levels of occlusion. Rest pain is present if the neural changes have not progressed too far. Also, a history of a prior trivial trauma may have incited the tissue loss.

To illustrate these concepts, consider the following scenarios: the presence of one-block right calf claudication combined with normal pulses, except absent right popliteal and tibial pulses, indicates a right superficial femoral artery occlusion. The profunda femoris collaterals provide limb viability. However, the presence of rest pain in the right foot, perhaps with a beginning ischemic toe ulcer, would also have calf and thigh claudication with minimal ambulation and absent pedal, popliteal, and femoral pulses. In this scenario, the collateral beds of the hypogastric and profunda arteries cannot provide enough nutritive flow at rest. Symptoms and findings are distal to the right iliac and femoral artery occlusions in this situation.

DIFFERENTIAL DIAGNOSIS

Knowledge of common syndromes with similar presenting complaints is essential. Claudication can be confused with other musculoskeletal or neurologic conditions, such as fibromyalgia, osteoarthritis, sciatica, lumbar back syndromes, or spinal stenosis. However, vascular claudication is consistently reproducible by the same degree of exertion and is relieved by the same degree of rest. The other conditions can produce discomfort at rest, have different inciting factors, and are inconsistently related to variable exertion.

Ischemic rest pain also can be mimicked by other neurogenic, muscular, or skeletal conditions. Diabetic neuropathy is the most common condition; it can also coexist with rest pain. The presence in the contralateral foot of the "stocking and glove" distribution and associated numbness may aid in the distinction. In addition, "burning" attributed to diabetic neuropathy is different from the usual gnawing, aching, "pins and needles," or "on fire" descriptions of the foot in ischemic rest pain. In both claudication and rest pain, the diagnosis of LEPVOD can be strongly suggested by physical examination. The patient with signs of actual tissue loss *may* have a similar differential diagnosis. (Trauma and infection are also considered, but are usually apparent from the history or physical.)

EMERGENCY DEPARTMENT EVALUATION

The timing of the pain helps determine acuity. The degree of secondary skin, sensory, and motor changes suggests the severity. Location of the pain helps determine the location of the process. Additional history of comorbid diseases is important to obtain.

The examination is the most cost-effective tool for the assessment of LEPVOD. While physician extenders, students, and junior residents can and should participate in patient care and evaluation, the accuracy of the vascular examination is an experience-dependent process.[2]

Initial inspection of all extremities provides the traditional starting point, with uninvolved limbs providing key "normal" references for changes. Skin quality, color, and tissue loss are inspected. The stethoscope can detect bruits (signifying noise from turbulent flow) in the carotid, femoral, and, possibly, the popliteal systems. The carotid, brachial, radial, ulnar, femoral, popliteal, dorsal pedal, and posterior tibial pulses should be palpated bilaterally. Each should be charted in a manner that another examiner can tell whether the initial pulses were normal, diminished, or absent. A given pulse will be *diminished* below a stenosis, while a given pulse is *absent* distal to an occlusion. Excellent collateral development can transmit enough flow to create a diminished pulse, but this event is unusual.

Additional maneuvers can be noninvasive yet provocative for ischemic changes that confirm a diagnostic impression. Elevation pallor is induced when an affected extremity is raised 2 to 3 ft above the heart. A normal or mildly ischemic leg will still have capillary refill against the gradient created. An extremity with two or more levels of occlusive disease will pale with this maneuver. This pallor should be evident even in dim fluorescent lights. A follow-up maneuver is to try to induce dependent rubor. The pale foot is dangled over the edge of a bed or chair, rendered dependent to gravity. It will become a plethoric red or purple over 60 to 90 seconds, demonstrating the pooling of blood into chronically vasodilated distal circulatory beds.

Diagnostic studies before consultation or disposition are probably rare if vascular surgical support is available. Laboratory profiles of renal function and coagulation help facilitate possible arteriography. Correction of other concomitant cardiovascular, pulmonary, or metabolic abnormalities is appropriate. Plain radiography of an affected foot with gangrene or signs of infection can be helpful. Foreign bodies, soft-tissue gas, and osteomyelitis can change aspects of management.

Noninvasive vascular laboratory examination, such as the continuous-wave Doppler instrument or duplex ultrasound, serves only to confirm impressions to which a solid history and physical should give rise. A common troublesome situation is that of a patient with a limb threatened by ischemia, but with good "Dopplerable" pulses.

The Doppler units have exquisite sensitivity for any moving column of blood. The presence of a strong signal can lull the emergency physician into a false sense of security. *In sum, the absence of a pulse is better evidence of ischemia than the Doppler signal is evidence of adequate perfusion.*

EMERGENCY DEPARTMENT MANAGEMENT

Initial management is based on the severity of the ischemic process. Claudication does not require urgent management. Ischemic rest pain is serious and may result in major limb loss if untreated.

Intravenous hydration is appropriate if either angiographic or operative treatment is indicated. Anticoagulation with heparin should be coordinated in consultation with a vascular specialist. The presence of tissue loss requires the additional assessment for the possibility of infection. Erythema secondary to cellulitis, and not dependent rubor, may require institution of antibiotics. Antibiotics should cover for the diabetic foot, with its typical gram-negative and anaerobic organisms. Moreover, if wet gangrene or soft-tissue air is identified, urgent intervention is necessary.

DISPOSITION

In most if not all presentations for LEPVOD, the patient can benefit from a vascular consultation. The patient with claudication can usually be referred for outpatient care. It is a chronic condition that can be electively managed outside of the emergency department. A patient with an acute embolus needs urgent vascular consultation. Frequently, this presentation will result in emergency thromboembolectomy. However, the surgeon involved with this decision needs to see the patient as soon as possible in order that the correct operative or percutaneous approach for revascularization can be instituted.

The presence of rest pain implies two levels of occlusive disease and significant potential for limb loss. While the need and timing for revascularization are typically urgent, the eventual treating vascular consultant should make this decision. Emergency department consultation is appropriate for this patient. Signs of limb loss, such as ischemic ulcers, dry or wet gangrene, or infections, are also appropriate reasons for emergency vascular consultation. Many times, the consultant will request an arteriogram, but this decision should be made by the vascular surgeon, because the arteriogram might delay the time to operative revascularization. In the more severe and urgent situations, the consulting surgeon will decide on admission or direct transfer to the operating room.

In smaller facilities, the availability of vascular surgery consultation may have bearing on some decisions. The absence of surgeons or arteriographic capability may mandate patient transfer. Patients with the urgent situation of rest pain can transfer via ground services. Acute embolic ischemia, profound rest pain with neurologic deterioration, or ascending infections may require rapid transfer to a receiving hospital with vascular surgery services. Aeromedical transport is appropriate if available.

COMMON PITFALLS

- A common troublesome situation is one in which the patient with a threatened limb from ischemia "has good Dopplerable pulses." The Doppler units have exquisite sensitivity for any moving column of blood, and the presence of a strong signal can lull the emergency physician into a false sense of security. *Remember, the absence of a pulse is better evidence of ischemia than the Doppler signal is evidence of adequate perfusion.*
- Many times, the consultant will request an arteriogram, but this decision should be made by the vascular surgeon, because the arteriogram might delay the time to operative revascularization
- The presence of rest pain implies two levels of occlusive disease and significant potential for limb loss. While the need

and timing for revascularization are typically urgent, the eventual treating vascular consultant should make this decision in the emergency department.

- The examination is the most cost-effective tool for the assessment of LEPVOD. While physician extenders, students, and junior residents can and should participate in patient care and evaluation, the accuracy of the vascular examination is an experience-dependent process.

References

1. Dossa CD, Shepard AD, Amos AM, et al. Results of lower extremity amputations in patients with end stage renal disease. *J Vasc Surg* 1994;20:14–19.
2. Endean ED, Sloan DA, Veldenz HC, et al, Performance of the vascular physical examination by residents and medical students. *J Vasc Surg* 1994;19:149–154.
3. Levy PJ, Gonzalez MF, Hornung CA, et al. A prospective evaluation of atherosclerotic risk factors in young adults with premature lower extremity atherosclerosis. *J Vasc Surg* 1996;23:36–45.
4. Levy PJ, Hornung CA, Haynes JL, et al. Lower extremity ischemia in adults younger than forty years of age: a community-wide survey of premature atherosclerotic arterial disease. *J Vasc Surg* 1994;19:873–881.
5. Valentine JR, Grayburn PA, Eichorn EJ, et al. Coronary artery disease is highly prevalent among patients with premature peripheral vascular disease. *J Vasc Surg* 1994;19:668–676.

CHAPTER 49
Septic Thrombophlebitis

Timothy C. Flynn

Although venous thrombosis is an entity commonly seen in the emergency department, septic thrombophlebitis is relatively rare. The most common cause of septic thrombophlebitis is the introduction of an intravenous catheter used for therapeutic infusions. Up to 30% of catheters cause thrombosis of the veins into which they are inserted, but fewer than 1% to 2% cause bacteremia.[2] Immunocompromised patients and burn patients are at highest risk for developing this potentially lethal complication.[8,9]

Insertion of a catheter into a vein provides ready access and a favorable environment for the multiplication of microorganisms. A catheter in the lumen of a vein destroys the vascular endothelium. The resultant exposure of the media then promotes fibrin deposition and thrombosis. If a sufficient volume of clot develops, local defense mechanisms may be overwhelmed, because there is no chance for macrophages and other cells of bacterial defense to be deposited in the clot itself. Even if meticulous care is taken in the insertion of the catheter and maintenance of the catheter site, blood-borne microorganisms may be introduced into the thrombus from remote septic sources, especially in the burn patient, whose wound is a repository for bacteria.

Intravenous drug abuse is an increasingly important cause of septic thrombophlebitis and probably the most common cause seen by the emergency physician.[1] Substances injected by addicts are extremely toxic to the endothelium and are likely to promote thrombosis. This toxicity, combined with the usual lack of sterility of the injectate, injection site, and injection apparatus, predisposes this group of patients to a septic thrombus. A drug abuser may present with any accessible vein affected, including veins in the head and neck, deep veins (femoral or subclavian), and even the penile veins.

Local inflammatory processes may also lead to septic thrombophlebitis, and patients with this condition may be encountered in the emergency department. Although less frequently seen in this era of aggressive antibiotic therapy, in the past this was a common and almost universally fatal problem, particularly in the postpartum or postabortal patient.[3,4] Septic sites in the pelvis or neck region provide a ready source of bacteria that invade the local venous drainage system.[10] Thrombosis is induced as a result of the inflammatory process, and the clots become a culture medium for the growth of microorganisms, thereby further promoting clot in the local region and then dissemination into the bloodstream, resulting in sepsis.

Once established, a septic vein can give rise to septic emboli.[5] Clot contaminated with microorganisms dispersed into the pulmonary vasculature can result in multiple areas of infarction and abscess formation. Bacteremia from septic veins also can result in endocarditis or infections of previously placed prosthetic material, such as heart valves and arterial prostheses.

CLINICAL PRESENTATION

Superficial septic thrombophlebitis usually presents as an erythematous, tender cord proximal to the site of a previous venous cannulation or injection site.[2] Although the patient is usually febrile, there may be minimal physical findings in peripheral veins, especially in infected deep veins. The patient may appear septic, with all the classic signs of pulmonary and cardiovascular collapse, or there may be few signs of sepsis, except persistent fever.[4]

DIFFERENTIAL DIAGNOSIS

A diagnosis of septic thrombophlebitis should be considered in any patient with a peripheral or central venous line who has a fever that persists after removal of the catheter. One must also consider this entity in patients who have pelvic inflammatory disease and fail to respond to usual treatment. In the burn patient, the fever workup should include a careful inspection of all current and previous cannulation sites, because this process is so common in this patient population. The same careful inspection of venous sites should be done for the immunocompromised patient and the intravenous drug user. The diagnosis is frequently one of exclusion and is often overlooked in patients with multiple problems or other sources of sepsis.

EMERGENCY DEPARTMENT EVALUATION

Examination of all catheter or injection sites is critical and may be especially challenging in the drug addict. Once a peripheral vein has been identified as a potential site of sepsis, every effort should be made to obtain a culture, either of the clot or of pus expressed from the vein. It may be necessary to make a small incision over the vein to express the clot, although removing the catheter and milking the clot back through the catheter site is usually enough. Aspiration of the clot or instillation of sterile nonbacteriostatic saline solution into the region, followed by aspiration, can be attempted, but these maneuvers seldom yield positive results. Cutdown sites should be opened, the tie on the vein removed, and the vein milked. All clot and suppurative material should be cultured for both aerobic and anaerobic organisms.[11] A Gram stain may be helpful in directing initial therapy.

Deep veins and central veins are not amenable to direct physical examination, but B-mode ultrasonography and computed tomography are useful in establishing whether there is clot present in these veins. The presence of clot does not necessarily indicate invasion by microorganisms; however, suspicion must be raised if there is clot identified in the septic patient.

Septic thrombophlebitis in the pelvic or cervical region is almost invariably associated with other inflammatory processes in the region. It is an uncommon but serious postpartum complication, occurring in roughly one in 2,000 deliveries.[7] Examination of the pelvis may show tenderness or induration in the pelvic side wall, and there may be a cervical discharge. However, particularly in postpartum patients, physical signs may be lacking and only certain clinical features will suggest infected pelvic veins. These patients often have high-spiking fevers and mild ileus and respond poorly to broad-spectrum antibiotics. They may or may not have positive blood cultures. A positive blood culture without frank abscess suggests septic thrombophlebitis. In the cervical region, suppurative thrombophlebitis is often associated with undrained abscesses in the peritonsillar and deep cervical tissue. Computed tomography may be useful in identifying undrained abscesses as a source of bacteria that can invade clots. Any therapeutic modality directed toward the vein needs to be done after adequate treatment of the local abscess.

EMERGENCY DEPARTMENT MANAGEMENT

Clearly the most difficult task is to identify a vein as the possible source of sepsis in patients who have a variety of other possible septic foci. In the patient with a classic presentation (fever, a cord extending proximally from an intravenous site, erythema, and pain), the first line of therapy is usually removal of the catheter, elevation of the extremity, and local application of heat. These patients should receive broad-spectrum antibiotics (vancomycin). The most common offending organisms are gram positive, especially *Staphylococcus aureus.* In hospitalized patients or immunocompromised patients, a variety of gram-positive or gram-negative organisms may be the cause of sepsis. If the patient fails to defervesce within 24 to 36 hours, complete surgical excision of the vein is necessary. Although this procedure can be done under local anesthesia at bedside, it is preferable to take the patient to the operating room for complete removal of the vein and tributaries that have clot in them.

In patients who have central or deep vein clot or suspected pelvic or cervical septic thrombophlebitis, attempts at resection are fraught with hazard. Therapy includes administration of broad-spectrum antibiotics and systemic anticoagulation. The addition of anticoagulation to the regimen has improved patient outcome.[2,6] Anticoagulation prevents further accumulation of thrombus and allows the body's thrombolytic processes to clear the thrombus as the source of bacterial infection. Fibrinolytic therapy may be considered, although there is no literature regarding its use, and one must be concerned about the creation of septic emboli as the clot breaks up.

DISPOSITION

Role of the Consultant

Patients with suspected septic thrombophlebitis from an indwelling central catheter should be followed by their primary physicians. In some patients, this catheter may be the only site of venous access; removal of the catheter may present a major problem. The catheter should not be removed until it is demonstrated that clot is present and infected; catheter-related sepsis may be treated solely by changing the catheter over a wire, allowing continued access to the venous system. Patients with suspected pelvic or cervical abscesses and suppurative thrombophlebitis should be seen by a gynecologic and an ear, nose, and throat surgeon, respectively. Many of these patients may have areas of undrained pus that require further surgical procedures. Infectious disease consultants are quite helpful in antibiotic therapy selection pertinent to the microflora prevalent in the community. General surgery consultation may be necessary for those patients who require peripheral vein excision.

Indications for Admission

All patients suspected of having a septic vein should be admitted for intravenous antibiotic therapy. The degree of systemic toxicity dictates whether the patient requires monitoring in the intensive care setting. Outpatient management is not appropriate.

Transfer Considerations

Few of these patients require transfer emergently. Patients with either central lines or peripheral lines should be returned to their primary physicians for follow-up.

COMMON PITFALLS

- The most common pitfall is the failure to consider this entity in patients who present with fever. This is especially true in the addict population or in the patient with pelvic septic thrombophlebitis. A delay in diagnosis may result in septic pulmonary emboli, endocarditis, or seeding of a previously uninfected prosthesis.
- Primary prevention by the emergency physician relies on recognition that any intravenous line is a portal of entry for bacteria and a potential site of thrombosis.
- Many patients require emergency intravenous access; breaks in sterile technique are common. This may be unavoidable in the emergency department, but the intravenous lines or cutdowns should be removed as soon as possible once a stable situation is achieved. Most hospitals have policies that require rotation of intravenous sites every 72 hours to prevent contamination and subsequent suppuration. Careful attention to catheter insertion technique and the proper care of catheter sites by a dedicated team of nurses are the first line of defense against this potentially lethal complication.

References

1. Ang AK, Brown OW. Septic deep vein thrombosis. *J Vasc Surg* 1986;4:563.
2. Baker CC, Peterson RSR, Sheldon GF. Septic phlebitis: a neglected disease. *Am J Surg* 1979;138:97.
3. Collins CG. Suppurative pelvic thrombophlebitis. *Am J Obstet Gynecol* 1970;108:681.
4. Dunn LJ, Van Voorhis LW. Enigmatic fever and pelvic thrombophlebitis. *N Engl J Med* 1967;276:265.
5. Griffith GL, Maull KI, Sachatello CR. Septic pulmonary embolization. *Surg Gynecol Obstet* 1977;144:105.
6. Josey WE, Staggers SR. Heparin therapy in septic pelvic thrombophlebitis: a study of 46 cases. *Am J Obstet Gynecol* 1974;120:228.
7. Keogh J, MacDonald D, Kelehan P. Septic pelvic thrombophlebitis: an unusual treatable postpartum complication. *Aust N Z J Obstet Gynaecol* 1993;33:204.
8. Missavage AE, McManus WF, Pruitt BA. Suppurative thrombophlebitis. In: Earnst CB, Stanley JC, eds. *Current therapy in vascular surgery.* Toronto: BC Deckker, 1987.
9. O'Neill JA, Pruitt BA, Foley FD, et al. Suppurative thrombophlebitis—a lethal complication of intravenous therapy. *J Trauma* 1968;8:256.
10. Yau PC, Norante JD. Thrombophlebitis of the internal jugular vein secondary to pharyngitis. *Arch Otolaryngol* 1980;106:507.
11. Zinner MJ, Zuidema GD, Lowery BD. Septic nonsuppurative thrombophlebitis. *Arch Surg* 1976;111:122.

CHAPTER 50

Complications of Vascular Grafts

Timothy C. Flynn

Because vascular surgeons operate on patients with progressive, multisystem disease, complications are common and tend to be either life- or limb-threatening. The diagnosis and management of these complications are difficult, and the outcome is often not good. Because patients with vascular disease are frequent users of the health-care system, clinicians seeing the patient should be aware of the common procedures performed and the possible complications likely to occur.

In general, vascular procedures are done for either aneurysmal or occlusive disease. The most commonly performed *carotid* procedure is an endarterectomy, which involves opening the artery, scraping out the diseased intima and media, and then closing the arteriotomy either primarily or with a patch. *Aortic* procedures for either occlusive or aneurysmal disease almost always involve the implantation of a synthetic graft in the abdomen or chest. *Infrainguinal* procedures call for the implantation of a graft to bypass occluded segments of the femoral, popliteal, or tibial vessels that cause limb-threatening ischemia. Autogenous vein is the preferred conduit for these procedures, although some surgeons still use synthetic grafts for bypasses to the above-knee popliteal segment. For a variety of reasons, surgeons may perform *extraanatomic* procedures, most commonly axillobifemoral or femoral–femoral bypasses. These are usually reserved for high-risk patients or when infection is present in the usual site of graft insertion. Although autogenous materials have been tried in these positions, synthetic grafts seem to have a better patency and are preferred. *Vascular access* procedures for patients on dialysis are either arteriovenous fistulas or synthetic arterial-to-venous grafts.

The ideal graft material has yet to be developed. All currently available arterial substitutes have some major drawback. *Synthetic* grafts are all either Dacron or polytetrafluoroethylene (PTFE). Neither material allows for the development of an endothelial-lined intima in the human, and thus grafts are prone to thrombosis, anastomotic stenosis, and infection. Due to modern manufacturing techniques, structural failure in the graft itself is rare and grafts of these materials are successfully used with acceptable rates of complication, especially in vascular reconstructions of the aorta and its major branches. *Autogenous* grafts are those in which the patient's own tissue is used. Saphenous vein is the most readily accessible and easiest to use autogenous conduit. It can be harvested and reversed or used *in situ* after valve disruption. When saphenous vein is not available, arm veins may be used with a very reasonable patency. Autogenous grafts maintain some degree of thrombosis resistance and are less likely to become infected. Because of the exposure of these venous structures to arterial pressures, intimal hyperplasia and fibrosis can occur, resulting in graft failure. *Homografts* are conduits made from veins from other humans. The most common of these is the human umbilical vein graft. These grafts were thought to be superior to synthetic grafts in the infrapopliteal position but were found to be prone to the development of pseudoaneurysms over time and are rarely used today. Cryopreserved saphenous veins have also been tried but have an unacceptable patency.

Vascular grafts are subject to a variety of significant complications. The most common problems likely to be encountered in the emergency department are

1. Progressive stenosis and occlusion
2. Infection
3. Erosion into contiguous structures
4. Disruption of the suture line, resulting in false aneurysm

PROGRESSIVE STENOSIS AND OCCLUSION

Depending on the size of graft insertion, as many as 15% to 80% of grafts will fail within 5 years. The combination of thrombogenicity and progress of atherosclerotic disease in the inflow and outflow tracts can lead to graft thrombosis. In addition, intimal proliferation in the sites of both proximal and distal anastomosis contribute to graft stenosis and occlusion. Thrombosis can also occur in response to graft infection, and any patient with graft thrombosis should be evaluated for this as well. Grafts that fail within the first 30 days of insertion usually do so as a result of a technical problem. Autogenous grafts that fail within the first year frequently do so because of a problem in the vein graft itself, usually sclerosis at a site of previous recannulized thrombosis or a fibrotic stricture developing at a valve site. Grafts that fail after this period of time frequently do so as a result of disease progression or anastomotic stricture.[4]

CLINICAL PRESENTATION

More often than not, graft stenosis is asymptomatic until the sudden occlusion of the graft results in the return of symptoms. These include an increase in claudication, rest pain, or the development of gangrene. Loss of a previously palpable pulse in the distal vessels after a bypass graft even in an asymptomatic patient is a grave finding, and these patients should be considered to have developed a thrombosis and be referred for possible angiography. This should be done even if Doppler signals are present. Acutely ischemic extremities with loss of sensation and motor function are a true emergency and have a relatively short time-window to have the ischemia relieved. The return of a previously healed ulcer may be the first sign of graft failure, and the patency of the graft should be investigated if this occurs. Conversely, because grafts are often placed for long-standing atherosclerosis, thrombosis may not lead to critical ischemia, due the presence of well-established collateral circulation. In such situations, the patient may relate a sudden decrease in the distance that can be walked without pain. Such cases should be approached with the same intensity as the ischemic patient, because once the graft has occluded, thrombosis of the distal arterial tree can occur and threaten the limb.

DIFFERENTIAL DIAGNOSIS

Most clinicians should be familiar with the classic signs of acute ischemia and not mistake these for other entities that can cause limb weakness, including stroke or nerve compression. The history of a previous graft or the finding of the typical groin or leg scars should prompt graft failure to be in the differential diagnosis of any lower extremity limb complaint.

EMERGENCY DEPARTMENT EVALUATION

In evaluating graft stenosis or acute thrombosis, one of the most important adjuncts to decision making is the patient's previous medical records, especially the reports of previous clinical examinations, angiograms, operative reports, and noninvasive laboratory studies. The patient should be queried about the onset of symptoms and their progression and compare findings with a time when the graft was functioning well. Accurate pulse examination is a skill that takes time and considerable effort to develop. Objective quantification of limb ischemia can be obtained by doing an ankle–brachial index. This is performed by placing a blood pressure cuff above the ankle and listening for return to flow at the best pedal artery and comparing this with the higher of the two arm pressures. A change of 0.15 from previous measurements is considered significant and should prompt further investigation, either a duplex scan or angiogram. Physical examination of the extremity should also include motor and sensory examination. Light touch is lost early with ischemia, although it may be difficult to test because many of the patients already have a neuropathy. Motor loss usually begins in the anterior compartment with loss of dorsiflexion at the ankle and great toe. This should be tested by holding up the leg at the calf and asking the patient to move the ankle and great toe. The foot should be isolated to avoid being misled by gross movement of the limb by the thigh muscles. History, physical examination, pulse check, and ankle–brachial index should be adequate to make the diagnosis of a failing or thrombosed graft.

EMERGENCY DEPARTMENT MANAGEMENT

Management consists of early vascular surgery consultation and heparinization, if the consultant agrees. Heparinization can prevent thrombosis of major inflow and outflow vessels and especially the smaller arteries distal to the graft thrombosis. Timing of heparinization must be considered with the need for possible angiography and the use of thrombolytic agents. Because patients with peripheral vascular disease have a high incidence of coronary disease, changes in the central circulatory status may lead to thrombosis. Graft thrombosis may be precipitated by myocardial infarction, atrial fibrillation, congestive heart failure, or volume depletion. It is important for the emergency physician to evaluate the cardiac and fluid status of the patient as rapidly as possible. Normalizing the patient's cardiac and fluid parameters may well correct an ischemic state even if the graft is occluded. If it appears that the patient will need surgical intervention or angiography, a complete blood cell count should be obtained, levels of electrolytes and creatinine should be determined, and prothrombin time and partial thromboplastin time should be measured.

DISPOSITION

The patient with an acutely threatened extremity will require urgent operative intervention, with the success for limb salvage determined by the anatomic situation and the time since the onset of the ischemic state. Delays of more than 4 to 6 hours decrease the likelihood of success. With a less urgent state, angiography and thrombolysis may be considered after consultation with the vascular surgeon. If transfer is required, heparinization before transport is mandatory in most instances and should not be delayed while transportation arrangements are made. An experienced vascular surgeon should be consulted and all pertinent information, including history, previous operations, and previous noninvasive studies, should be transmitted. Optimization of cardiac and fluid states should be attempted in the timeframe of the transfer, but delays for such therapy should be avoided, especially in patients who have a severely ischemic extremity. Patients thought to have a failing graft, as evidenced by progression of symptoms or a fall in the ankle–brachial index, should be seen by the vascular surgeon as soon as possible.

COMMON PITFALLS

- Failure to recognize the change in the patient's extremity status as graft thrombosis
- Failure to consult the old chart for previously recorded examinations and to recognize that loss of a palpable pulse or a decline of 0.15 in the ankle–brachial index is significant
- Failure to evaluate the central circulatory status and overall cardiovascular status of the patient, with special emphasis on the identification of possible embolic sources and the presence of a low-flow state
- Failure to heparinize, with subsequent extension of thrombosis into the microvasculature that may result in limb loss
- Failure to refer the acutely ischemic extremity to an appropriate surgeon to address the ischemia

GRAFT INFECTION

Infections can be relatively acute after graft placement or can occur years later. They can present as sepsis or be indolent, producing gradual dissolution of a vascular anastomosis. Acute infections are usually caused by *Staphylococcus aureus* or gram-negative rods, appearing 5 to 7 days postoperatively. Occasionally, wounds that appear to be intact at the time of discharge may be seen within the first 30 days manifesting signs of infection. Graft infections may also appear at a much later time, up to years after implantation. These infections are frequently caused by *Staphylococcus epidermidis*.[2]

CLINICAL PRESENTATION

Acute graft infections frequently produce erythema, warmth, or fluctuance over the graft itself or, more commonly, over the anastomosis. The groin is the most common place to become infected, due to its proximity to the perineum, the disruption of lymphatic channels, and the difficulty of keeping the area clean, especially in the obese patient. In addition to gross infections, lymphatic leaks are not uncommon after groin incisions. These frequently result in copious drainage of clear lymph fluid from the incision. Occasionally, there is no leakage and the patient will present, in the early postoperative period, with a mass in the groin that is nontender and without erythema. This is most commonly a lymphatic fluid collection in the subcutaneous tissue or around the graft. In any event, any drainage from a wound that is over a vascular graft has potential for serious graft infection and limb loss.

Infections in grafts that have been implanted for long periods of time present special diagnostic problems. Transient bacteremia is probably the cause of such infections. Urinary tract infections, pneumonia, and dental procedures or other surgical manipulation can result in blood-borne bacteria. Normal vascular endothelium probably protects against bacterial adhesion, and because most prosthetic grafts never become completely endothelialized, the patient with a prosthetic implant is always susceptible to bacterial invasion. Common physical signs of a chronic infection are swelling, erythema, and fluctuance under a vascular incision. In more indolent infections, patients can present with a fever of unknown origin or with septic thrombi that present as painful abscesses distal to the graft. Unexplained fever in the patient with a vascular implant is another presentation of vascular infection.

EMERGENCY DEPARTMENT MANAGEMENT

Any swelling or drainage of any sort (whether purulent or clear), should prompt a consultation with the vascular surgeon. Treatment of a possible graft infection with oral antibiotics without consultation should not be attempted. Virtually all the prosthetic grafts that become infected will require removal, because the ultimate outcome of vascular infection is an anastomotic disruption and hemorrhage. Adjuncts to diagnosis, such as plain films and ultrasonography, are usually not helpful. A computed tomographic scan is useful to identify perigraft fluid collections. Although it may be difficult at times to make a diagnosis of graft infection, the presence of air bubbles in the fluid or fluid surrounding the graft should be considered a sign of graft infection. All patients with a prosthetic graft infection should be admitted and initially treated with intravenously administered antibiotics while the arrangements are made to excise the infected material. Wound infections involving purely autogenous material can sometimes be managed without excision. However, even these grafts are at risk for an anastomotic disruption and hemorrhage. Fluctuance over a vascular incision should *never* be drained in the emergency department because uncontrolled hemorrhage may ensue.

DISPOSITION

All suspected graft infections should be seen by the vascular surgeon, preferably the individual who implanted the graft. If a vascular surgeon is not available, then the patient should be transferred to a vascular surgeon. The patient should be started on antibiotics to cover *Staphylococcus* and gram-negative rods before transfer.

COMMON PITFALLS

- Outpatient antibiotics are not appropriate therapy for cellulitis, drainage, or fluctuance over a prosthetic or autogenous graft.
- One should never drain a fluctuant area over the graft site.
- It is important to recognize graft thrombosis as possibly being due to graft infection.
- Lymphatic leaks are a serious condition that can lead to graft infection unless appropriately treated.

EROSION INTO CONTIGUOUS STRUCTURES

Probably the most life-threatening complication is the erosion of a graft into adjacent structures. This most commonly involves the erosion of the abdominal aortic graft into the gastrointestinal tract. If this occurs at the proximal aortic suture line and involves both the native aorta and graft, exsanguinating hemorrhage can ensue (aortoduodenal fistula). However, graft erosion can occur in any part of the bowel and any part of the graft. If this does *not* occur at a suture line, it is called a perigraft fistula and most often presents as a more chronic bleeding state.[3]

CLINICAL PRESENTATION

Physical examination usually produces no findings, although the palpation of a false aneurysm of the aorta or iliac is possible. In patients with erosions at the proximal graft anastomosis, the patient may present with cardinal or sentinel bleeding. This occurs when there is massive bleeding into the gastrointestinal tract, resulting in vomiting or acute rectal evacuation of blood. The patient rapidly becomes hypotensive. The area of the aortoenteric fistula clots, and, for a period of time, stability is reached. Unless promptly treated, the patient will then die of a second massive hemorrhage. Patients with perigraft fistulas bleed through the interstices of the graft and from the eroded bowel wall edges. These patients frequently present with more chronic bleeding, with guaiac-positive stools and anemia. This may be difficult to diagnose.

EMERGENCY DEPARTMENT MANAGEMENT

Patients who have an aortic graft and present with massive gastrointestinal hemorrhage, with either hematemesis or hematochezia, should have aortoenteric fistula strongly considered. Although other sources of bleeding are possible, prompt consultation with a vascular surgeon is indicated. In the unstable patient, emergency laparotomy with endoscopy prior to the incision is usually performed. A delay in operative intervention will result in death.

In the patient with a graft in place and a guaiac-positive stool and anemia who is hemodynamically stable, a further workup for other sources of bleeding should be undertaken. This would include upper and lower endoscopy, bleeding scans, and contrast gastrointestinal studies. Computed tomography may also be helpful. If this workup is negative for a site of bleeding and the patient persists with gastrointestinal bleeding, an exploratory operation should be undertaken to rule out a graft enteric fistula. No other tests can definitively rule out this entity, other than celiotomy. Aortography in these patients may be undertaken to plan the possible reconstruction should the graft have to be removed, but it is not diagnostic for a graft-enteric fistula.

Graft erosion is seldom a problem in other areas, except for an erosion through the skin, exposing the graft itself. Such exposed grafts should be considered infected, usually in their entire length, because either the erosion was caused by an infection or infection occurred after the erosion. After exposure and infection, disruption of the suture line can be expected, producing massive hemorrhage. Exposed grafts warrant immediate vascular consultation and rapid operative intervention.

DISPOSITION

The treatment of aortoduodenal fistula requires the highest level of care and expertise. Mortality is high. Patients should be transferred immediately to a vascular surgeon because bleeding may occur at any time. Patients should have blood samples drawn for typing and crossmatch and undergo correction of the blood loss. Hypertension should be avoided because this may result in loss of the blood clot that is preventing exsanguination. It is of utmost importance that operative intervention not be delayed for an extensive workup.

COMMON PITFALLS

- An aortoenteric fistula should be suspected in a patient with an implanted graft who presents with upper or lower gastrointestinal hemorrhage or anemia.
- Routine or extensive workup (i.e., barium enema, upper gastrointestinal series, arteriography, and computed tomography) on patients with implanted grafts with occult or overt gastrointestinal bleeding may delay timely operative intervention.
- Emergent vascular consultation should be obtained for patients with massive bleeding and intraabdominal grafts.

- An exposed graft should be considered an infected graft that requires operative intervention.

ANASTOMOTIC DISRUPTION OR FALSE ANEURYSMS

A true aneurysm is a localized dilatation of the vessel usually caused by weakening of the media. A false aneurysm is the result of a disruption of the graft arterial suture line with the walls of the aneurysm formed by the collagenous scar around the anastomosis. A false aneurysm usually presents as a pulsatile mass or bulge at a previous anastomosis. As many as 10% to 15% of femoral anastomoses will ultimately result in a false aneurysm. It is thought that most are the result of an underlying low-grade infection that is subclinical and without signs of cellulitis, erythema, or sepsis. Seldom is a false aneurysm due to failure of the suture material or the graft itself. False aneurysms need to be repaired because of their tendency to occlude or produce distal emboli, resulting in limb ischemia.[1]

CLINICAL PRESENTATION

False aneurysms that appear in the abdominal cavity can be either at the proximal aortic suture line or at the iliac suture line. Sometimes, they can be palpated more easily in the area of the umbilicus (aortic) or low in the right or left lower quadrant. Usually, they produce no symptoms until rupture occurs, at which time symptoms typical of any other aneurysm rupture may occur. These include back pain, pain radiating to the testis or thigh (especially with iliac ruptures), anemia, or hemorrhagic shock. Occasionally, ureteral obstruction due to false aneurysms at the iliac anastomosis can occur. The most common site for false aneurysms is in the groin, where they usually present as a slowly enlarging pulsatile mass.

In the absence of overt infection, the wound is usually well healed. However, if the false aneurysm gets large enough, it may result in skin erosion. Patients who present with distal emboli after a previous aortobifemoral bypass should be examined for the presence of a false aneurysm in the groin, because this is one source for the embolic material. Likewise, acute occlusions of one limb of the graft may be secondary to the development of a false aneurysm. Venous obstruction with leg swelling can also occur, and occasionally, neurologic symptoms with nerve compression of the femoral nerve can be seen. False aneurysms are more common with the use of prosthetic material. However, they can occur with autogenous grafts either in the groin or distally. Many of these will be accompanied by signs of infection.

EMERGENCY DEPARTMENT EVALUATION AND MANAGEMENT

The emergency physician should consider the presence of a false aneurysm whenever physical examination of the groin anastomosis reveals an abnormally prominent pulsation or the patient reports a change in the appearance of the groin. Ultrasonography with color flow duplex can be helpful in making the diagnosis. Computed tomography is often required to evaluate the proximal anastomoses, as well to be sure that a low-grade infection involving the graft is not present. In addition, the contralateral limb of the graft should be investigated. Occasionally, an anastomotic false aneurysm in the groin may rupture, with acute expansion and hemorrhage. These are seldom life-threatening, but they may result in considerable blood loss and represent a vascular emergency. Vascular surgeons should be consulted whenever the emergency physician believes the anastomosis in the groin is not perfectly normal or if he or she feels abnormal pulsations in the abdomen with a graft in place.

DISPOSITION

Complications of graft insertion should be handled by a vascular surgeon. An anastomotic false aneurysm should be seen by a vascular surgeon in the emergency department.

COMMON PITFALLS

- A false aneurysm should not be mistaken for an abscess or cyst. Do *not* attempt drainage either percutaneously or with an incision.
- In the presence of an abdominal graft, lower abdominal pain or pain radiating to the testis or thigh should suggest rupture of an anastomotic false aneurysm.
- A proximal anastomotic false aneurysm should always be considered as a source of distal emboli or as a cause of acute graft occlusion.
- The other sites of anastomosis should be investigated in patients who have a false aneurysm at one anastomosis.
- The patient's complaint of a change in the pulsatile nature of the groin is significant and should be investigated.

References

1. Downs AR. Anastomotic aneurysms. In: Ernst CB, Stanley JC, eds. *Current therapy in vascular surgery*. Toronto: BC Deckker, 1991:447.
2. Moore WS, Deaton DH. Infections in prosthetic vascular grafts. In: Moore WS, ed. *Vascular surgery*. Philadelphia: WB Saunders, 1993:694.
3. Peck JJ, Eidemiller LR. Aortoenteric fistulas. *Arch Surg* 1992;127:1191.
4. Quinones-Baldrich WJ. Acute arterial and graft occlusion. In: Moore WS, ed. *Vascular surgery*. Philadelphia: WB Saunders, 1993:648.

CHAPTER 51
Aortic Dissection and Thoracic Aortic Aneurysms

Shawna J. Perry

AORTIC DISSECTION

Aortic dissection is the most frequent catastrophic event involving the aorta. First recognized postmortem by Morgagni in 1761, aortic dissection remains a diagnostic challenge to the emergency physician because of its nonspecific presentation, variable population at risk, and time pressure for diagnosis. Delays or errors in diagnosis can have devastating consequences.

Dissection of the aorta begins with an intimal tear, usually proximal (60%) in the ascending portion of the thoracic aorta.[12]

The site of the initial intimal tear is usually at the aortic root or between the origin of the left subclavian artery and the ligamentum arteriosum. These two areas of the aorta are relatively fixed, and it is believed that maximum stress is applied to these areas during systole. The intimal tear allows blood to penetrate down to the media separating intima from adventitia. The length of time required to dissect the entire aorta can be seconds, with the dissection proceeding either distally or proximally. *Reentry tears* occur distal to the initial site, creating an alternate path for aortic blood flow through a *false lumen*. An intramural hematoma can develop within this false lumen, minimizing flow and occasionally causing dilation. A small number of patients develop an intramural hematoma with no evidence of a communicating tear.[13] The dissection may dilate as the flow of blood through the false lumen increases or an intramural hematoma organizes. The term *dissecting aneurysm* is frequently used because of this pathologic finding, but it is done so incorrectly, as this is not a true aneurysm (see later discussion of thoracic aortic aneurysms). Spontaneous rupture is common and is most often into the pericardium. Dissections with an open false lumen and tear beginning high in the aorta have a poor prognosis.[12]

The cause of the intimal tear is unknown and the role of a structural defect of the aortic wall remains unclear. Histologic changes of recurrent injury and repair of the aorta in patients with Marfan syndrome and within the wall of a dissection may contribute to the process. Hypertension is the most common predisposing factor to dissection and is seen in up to 78% of descending aortic dissections.[24,25] It is not yet known why one hypertensive person will undergo dissection and another will not. Marfan syndrome is a widely recognized risk factor that carries a mortality rate of greater than 90% in the event of dissection or aneurysm rupture. Other risk factors for aortic dissection are congenital abnormalities of the aorta, such as bicuspid valve and coarctation. Dissection has also been reported in pregnancy, with half having evidence of systemic hypertension.[18] Connective tissue diseases such as Turner syndrome and systemic lupus erythematous, as well as cocaine use and trauma (iatrogenic and blunt), have all been associated with aortic dissection.[2,14,21,22] Aortic dissection is *not* due to atherosclerotic disease. Dissection is most likely a multifactorial disease, with hypertension the principal risk factor.

CLASSIFICATION

DeBakey originally classified aortic dissections into three categories according to the origin of the dissection: type I, involving the entire length of the aorta; type II, beginning in the ascending aorta (the aortic root to the left subclavian); and type III, originating from the area distal to the left subclavian.[7] The Stanford classification is a simpler scheme that divides dissections into type A, involving the ascending aorta, and type B, confined to the descending aorta and beginning after the left subclavian[6] (Fig. 51.1). This more widely used nomenclature aids in determining treatment options and prognosis.

Type A dissections are more common (80%) and are considered surgical emergencies. Possible complications at presentation of type A dissections may include aortic rupture, cardiac tamponade, and aortic valve insufficiency. Heparinization is used in the operative repair, and restoration of flow may result in intracerebral hemorrhage. Type B dissections are managed medically unless they are complicated by rupture, vascular occlusion, acute expansion, or impending rupture. Up to one-fourth of patients with type B dissection require urgent operation for hemorrhage, limb or organ ischemia, intractable pain, or progression of dissection. Paraplegia is a significant complication of surgical intervention for type B dissections.

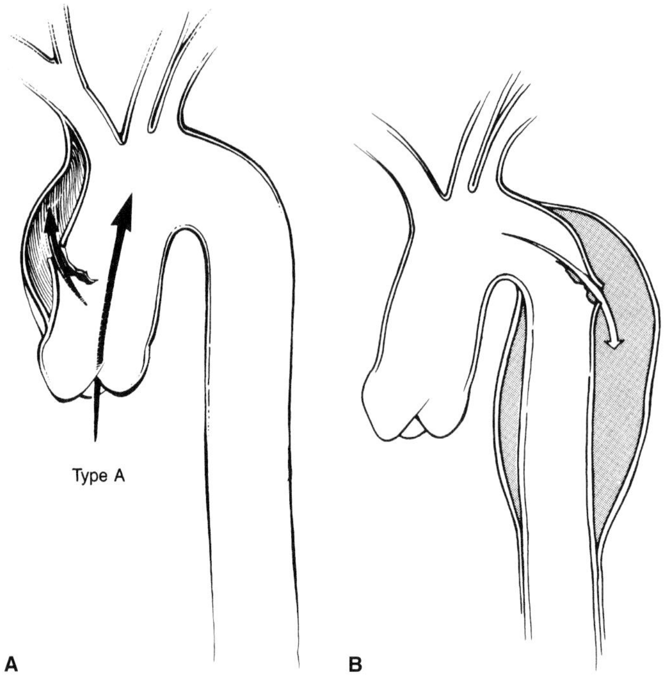

Figure 51.1. Classification of aortic dissections. **(A)** Dissection of ascending aorta. **(B)** Dissection of descending aorta.

MORTALITY

The most common cause of death for untreated dissections is rupture of the aortic wall into the pericardial sac at the level of the right lateral wall of the aorta, where the adventitia is thinnest. Rupture is most often into the pericardial sac, the pleural space, or the mediastinum. Death may also occur due to congestive heart failure or myocardial infarction.

The mortality rate of patients with untreated type A dissection is 75%, and the rate for surgically treated type A dissection is 15% to 20%.[8] Risk factors for death are (1) older age, (2) hypertension, (3) preoperative cardiopulmonary resuscitation, (4) hemodynamic instability, and (5) lack of retrograde cerebral perfusion.[12,13] Mortality postoperatively ranges from 16% to 35%, with a 5-year survival of 55% to 80%.[6,11,20] Reoperation after initial surgery is a very poor prognostic sign.

The medical therapy and surgical mortality rates for uncomplicated type B dissections are the same (32% to 36%); therefore, medical therapy is used first line in uncomplicated patients.[17] The use of beta-blockers and afterload-reducing medication appears to decrease the risk of extension or dilation of the dissection. It does not stop the progression of the disease indefinitely, and aortic replacement will eventually be needed.[26] Five-year survival for uncomplicated type B dissection is 48% to 60%.[11,15] Type B dissections complicated by rupture, vascular occlusion, acute expansion, or impending rupture have a surgical mortality ranging from 26% to 75%.[9] Controversy exists over whether medically managed type B dissections would be better served by earlier surgical intervention.[7,11,15]

CLINICAL PRESENTATION

To make the diagnosis of aortic dissection, the emergency physician must include it in the differential diagnosis at presentation. Sudden onset of pain in the chest or in conjunction with back pain is the most prevalent symptom.[1,23,24] The pain is severe and is frequently described as dull and pressure-like. With this presentation, history should focus on identifying risk factors for aortic dissection, especially hypertension and Marfan syndrome. The pain of aortic dissection is classically described as "ripping" or "tearing"; however, studies have more frequently demonstrated this with nondissecting pathology.[1] In addition to pain in the chest and back, accompanying locations for discomfort include the neck, throat, mandible, abdomen, and leg. Patients may also complain of pain in the lower back, pelvis, and a lower extremity.[24] No pain at all accompanies 15% to 20% of dissections.[25]

On examination, the patient may clinically appear to be in shock, exhibiting cool and diaphoretic skin, yet paradoxically have a normal or elevated blood pressure. The majority of patients present this way, but nearly one-fourth will present hypotensive due to leaking at the dissection site or rupture. A variety of signs and symptoms can result due to vascular compromise from the dissection or proximity to the dissection site. The majority are neurologic (33%), with syncope, altered mental status, cerebrovascular accident, paraplegia, or visual disturbances.[1] Syncope is the initial complaint in less than 10% of patients, but decreased level of consciousness occurs more frequently. Syncope may be a sign of the development of hemopericardium or cardiac tamponade.[24] Other associated findings with dissection are cardiac tamponade and congestive heart failure. Cardiovascular collapse is seen most often with type A dissection. Proximity to the dissection site or developing hematoma can cause hoarseness (laryngeal nerve compression), dyspnea, or stridor with wheezing (tracheal compression) and dysphagia (esophageal compression). On examination, initial hypertension is very common (systolic greater than 150 mmHg), but the patient may still appear clinically in shock. The presence of hypotension strongly suggests a type A dissection, a rupture of either type of dissection, or a dissection into the brachiocephalic artery. Gastrointestinal symptoms include midepigastric pain, hemorrhage, or melena secondary to splanchnic vessel infarctions and are frequently misdiagnosed as a primary abdominal pathology. Renal artery involvement may lead to hematuria, flank pain, oliguria, or uncontrollable hypertension due to excess renin release.

Head and neck examination may reveal the presence of jugular venous distension secondary to congestive heart failure, cardiac tamponade, or an expanding hematoma around the aorta causing outflow obstruction. Aortic insufficiency murmur occurs in 16% to 20% of patients, resulting from proximal dissection causing dilation of the aortic valve ring and loss of commissural support of the aortic valve.[1]

Poor prognostic factors include pleural effusion, cardiac tamponade, and pericardial friction rub. The presence of these signs implies leakage of the dissection into the pericardial space. The abdominal examination may reveal tenderness to palpation or rigidity. Rarely, a pulsatile mass is palpable.[13] Examination of the limbs may reveal unequal, decreased, or absent peripheral pulses in 50% of cases. A complete deficit of pulse is found in 8% to 10% of patients.[24,25] Differential blood flow to the extremities is often manifested by a marked discrepancy in blood pressure between arms and between the arms and legs, should dissection extend the entire length of the aorta. Rare but reported initial presentations of dissection have included hemoptysis, superior vena cava syndrome, right atrium or ventricular rupture, and deep vein thrombosis.[13,24] Cranial nerve deficits secondary to dissection into the carotid arteries, or motor deficits secondary to distal dissection of spinal arteries, may also be present.[13]

DIFFERENTIAL DIAGNOSIS

Chest pain with associated back pain is the most prevalent symptom of aortic dissection; therefore, the differential diagnosis is broad and contains numerous other life-threatening conditions. Myocardial infarction is the principal diagnosis of exclusion, as well as cerebrovascular accident in patients with neurologic symptoms. Misdiagnosis of either could result in the use of thrombolytic therapy and increased risk of death from exsanguination. Other diagnoses to exclude are pulmonary embolism, thoracic aneurysm, pneumothorax, multilobar pneumonia, mediastinal cyst or tumor, pericarditis, pancreatitis, cholelithiasis, cholecystitis, perforated viscus, and peripheral vascular disease.

The diagnosis of aortic dissection should be considered in the presence of the following:

- History of hypertension
- History of connective tissue disease or congenital aortic abnormalities
- Aortic insufficiency with chest and/or back pain
- Atypical chest or back pain
- Presence of acute neurologic symptoms (rare with myocardial infarction)
- Diminished or absent peripheral pulses (especially if reappear)
- Syncope
- Chest pain in pregnancy (third trimester)
- Trauma
- Acute unexplained left ventricular failure
- Flank pain and hematuria without an obvious source
- Presence of multiple sites of ischemia

EMERGENCY DEPARTMENT EVALUATION

Patients suspected of aortic dissection should be managed aggressively in anticipation of impending leak or rupture. The patient should be placed on a cardiac monitor and intravascular access established with at least two large-bore catheters (16-gauge or larger). A blood specimen should be drawn and sent for type and crossmatch. Initial laboratory studies should include a complete blood cell count; determination of serum levels of electrolytes, amylase, and cardiac enzymes; urinalysis; and a 12-lead electrocardiogram (ECG). Although routine laboratory studies are not usually helpful in the diagnosis of aortic dissection, they may rule out other causes. The complete blood cell count often reveals leukocytosis. If a sufficient amount of blood has accumulated in the false lumen, the hematocrit may be low. Renal artery involvement may result in increased blood urea nitrogen and creatinine levels, as well as hematuria, indicating ischemia or infarction of the kidney. A normal creatinine phosphokinase level is useful in distinguishing dissection from myocardial infarction. A small number of patients, however, dissect proximally into the right coronary artery and suffer a myocardial infarction. ECG changes compatible with myocardial infarction and pericarditis can be seen in approximately 25% of patients with dissection.

The most available radiologic study for the emergency physician is the chest radiograph, to assist in the diagnosis of aortic dissection. In 65% to 85% of cases, the chest radiograph demonstrates some abnormality.[1,24] A widened mediastinum is the most common finding, but a left-sided pleural effusion or an indistinct aortic knob may also be seen (Fig. 51.2). The deviation of a calcified aortic intima by greater than 6 mm from the outer wall of the aorta is considered pathognomonic of dissection. Other findings suggestive of dissection are the double density sign (a false lumen that is less radiopaque than the true lumen), tracheal deviation, and an irregular aortic contour. Unfortunately, a normal chest radiograph does not exclude the diagnosis. If the diagnosis of dissection is considered, radiographic confirmation is required by either aortography, computed tomography (CT) or transesophageal echocardiography (TEE).[16]

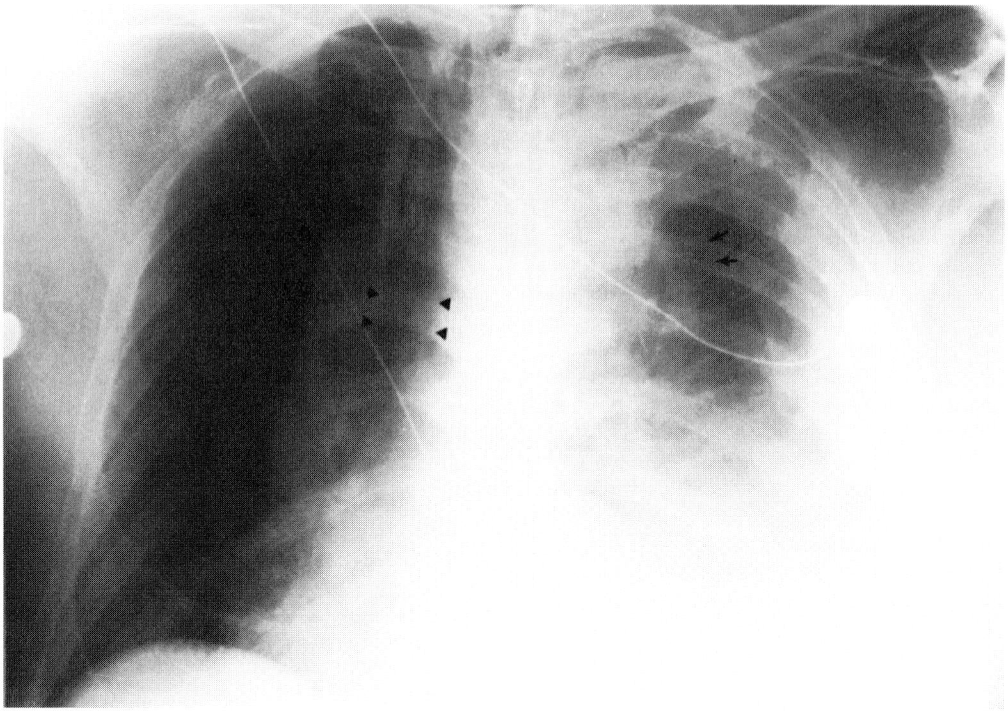

Figure 51.2. Chest x-ray film of a 65-year-old woman with type A dissection. Note the widened mediastinum, indistinct aortic knob *(arrows)*, tracheal deviation *(triangles)*, and left pleural effusion.

The aortogram is still considered the "gold standard" for diagnosis of aortic dissection (sensitivity and specificity greater than 90%), but it has the disadvantages of a large contrast dye load, of being a time-consuming procedure, and of having a significant false-negative rate if the false lumen is thrombosed. In addition to confirming the diagnosis, the aortogram reveals the extent of dissection, the condition and patency of the distal vessels, and the pattern of blood flow in the true and false lumens. False-positive results are seen in any process that causes thickening of the aortic wall, such as a clotted aneurysm, mediastinal hematoma, neoplasms, or periaortic fat.

CT is used as a supplement to aortography and in some institutions has replaced it for making the diagnosis of dissection. The advantages of CT are (1) superior visualization of fluid collection in the pericardium, pleura, and mediastinum; (2) demonstration of distal vessel patency; (3) noninvasiveness; and (4) sensitivity and specificity equal to aortography. Its main disadvantages are the necessary exposure to contrast dye for the examination and its inability to localize the site of the intimal tear. Spiral CT, with its three-dimensional reconstruction feature, is more expedient and has demonstrated improved delineation of the intimal tear and assessment of the great vessels.[19] Spiral CT does not show greater sensitivity or specificity than TEE or magnetic resonance imaging (MRI).[23]

TEE is frequently used as the first diagnostic study in suspected dissection, if it is available. It has a sensitivity and specificity of 99% and 98%, respectively. The goals of TEE in aortic dissection are (1) to confirm the diagnosis, (2) differentiate true and false lumens, (3) localize the intimal tear, (4) evaluate left ventricular wall motion, (5) determine the presence of fluid collections, and (6) detect aortic insufficiency. It demonstrates a diagnostic accuracy of 100% for aortic insufficiency and cardiac tamponade. TEE provides limited ability to evaluate the great vessels and coronary vessels. Complications of transient atrioventricular (AV) block, bradycardia, and asthma can occur during introduction of the probe.[10] Images may be limited in obese or emphysematous patients. TEE is often combined with CT.

MRI has a sensitivity and specificity no better than those of TEE or CT, and it is seldom used in the emergent setting because of cost, length of time needed for the study, and relative unavailability. MRI and TEE combined have the same sensitivity and specificity as TEE and CT.[23]

EMERGENCY DEPARTMENT MANAGEMENT

The most important aspects of emergency department management are the reduction of arterial blood pressure and the forceful contractility of the left ventricle. These measures should be initiated before confirmatory tests are performed if clinical suspicion for dissection is high. Reductions in these aspects of the cardiovascular system have developed empirically in an attempt to limit the propagation of a dissection.[26] Systolic blood pressure control is important because the rate of dissection is directly proportional to the blood pressure, especially to the rate of rise of arterial blood pressure. The systolic blood pressure should be maintained at 100 to 110 mm Hg or the lowest level compatible with adequate renal and cerebral perfusion. The drug of choice to control blood pressure is intravenous nitroprusside at the initial rate of 0.5 to 1.0 μg/kg/min. Oral agents should never be used.

Once a systolic blood pressure of 100 mm Hg is achieved, intravenous beta-antagonist therapy should also be used to suppress the reflex tachycardia from the initiation of nitroprusside and concomitant rise in arterial pressure. The target heart rate is between 60 and 80 beats per minute. Appropriate beta-antagonists include intravenous esmolol (0.5 mg/kg loading dose over 1 minute, infusion rate of 0.05 mg/kg/min) or intravenous propranolol (0.5 to 1.0 mg increments at 5 minute intervals). Intravenous labetalol is an alternative to the nitroprusside and beta-antagonist therapy for patients with mild hypertension and no contraindications of chronic obstructive pulmonary disease or asthma. Congestive heart failure, heart block, and bradycardia are contraindications for propranolol use. Oral agents should never be used in the acute setting of aortic dissection.

DISPOSITION

Management of the patient with aortic dissection requires urgent multispecialty involvement. The radiologist should be consulted emergently to obtain the appropriate diagnostic procedures. The cardiothoracic surgeon should also be notified. Once the diagnosis of dissection has been made, an internist may need to be consulted for medical management. All patients suspected of having acute aortic dissection should be admitted to an intensive care unit. Indications for transfer include inadequate facilities or personnel to definitively make the diagnosis or treat the condition. If transfer is indicated, air transport should be used to minimize the time required. If only ground transport is available, an ACLS unit should be used.

COMMON PITFALLS

- The most common mistake is failure to consider the diagnosis of aortic dissection.
- Unexplained, severe, and sustained chest pain (especially with associated back pain) must be evaluated with aortography, CT, or TEE to rule out dissection.
- A radiologist and a cardiothoracic surgeon should be consulted early.
- The most important aspect of emergency department management is control of the blood pressure and heart rate.
- Arrange immediate transport to the nearest appropriate hospital if your facility has inadequate resources for diagnosis and management of dissection.

THORACIC AORTIC ANEURYSMS

Thoracic aortic aneurysm is very insidious in onset and presentation. It is defined as a localized or diffuse dilation of the aorta to a diameter of greater than 5 to 6 cm. Dilation is the result of an undermining of the overall strength of the aortic wall by direct loss of supportive proteins such as elastin and collagen. Once the wall of the aorta is weakened, there is progressive alteration in anatomy, with the growing diameter and thinning wall that lead to dilation and rupture. Turbulent flow can lead to thrombus formation. Causes for the undermining of the aortic wall are listed in Table 51.1.

The prevalence is 5.9 new aneurysms per 100,000 person-years based on retrospective studies. Its incidence is equal between men and women, with an increasing prevalence with advancing age. Risk factors are hypertension, advanced atherosclerotic disease, and smoking.[3] The natural history of thoracic aneurysms is progressive dilation and rupture, with a 76% mortality rate at 2 years in untreated patients and a 30% mortality rate after surgical repair.[5]

TABLE 51.1. Diseases Contributing to Thoracic Aortic Aneurysms

Atherosclerosis
Coarction of the aorta
Cystic medial necrosis
Giant cell arteritis
Marfan syndrome
Mycotic aneurysms
Seronegative spondyloarthropathies
Syphilis
Tuberculosis
Takayasu's arteritis

Aneurysm diameter is a significant risk factor for rupture. The median size at time of rupture is 6.0 cm for ascending aneurysms and 7.2 cm for descending aneurysms. The risk of rupture increases 25.2% for ascending diameters greater than 6.0 cm, with a 38% increase in risk for descending diameters greater than 7.2 cm.[4] The estimated increase in diameter is 0.2 to 0.32 cm per year.[3] In patients with Marfan syndrome, rupture occurs at smaller diameters. Surgical intervention is therefore planned according to the patient's stability at time of diagnosis and diameter of the aneurysm as monitored over time. Surgical mortality ranges between 15% and 20%.

The most common scenario for diagnosis of thoracic aneurysm is as an incidental finding on chest x-ray. Occasionally, patients will present with aortic regurgitation murmurs or with symptoms directly related to impingement of thoracic structures by the aneurysm. Aortography, CT, and TEE can be used to evaluate suspected aneurysms. If the diagnosis has not been made previously, aneurysms suspected in the emergency department should be evaluated at the time of presentation, even if asymptomatic. Consultation with a thoracic surgeon is recommended in this setting to determine treatment plan. Those patients not needing immediate surgical repair should have periodic outpatient diagnostic tests to monitor the aneurysm diameter.

In cases of rupture or impending rupture, the patient will present with deep, aching or throbbing chest or back pain. A sudden escalation of pain and hypotension are signs of aneurysm rupture. Rupture may also present as cardiopulmonary arrest secondary to intrathoracic or intraabdominal hemorrhage, should the aneurysm extend beyond the diaphragm. Bedside transthoracic and transabdominal echo can be of assistance in locating large collections of fluid. Disposition is determined by consultants based on the aneurysm diameter, risk of rupture, and surgical risk to the patient.

References

1. Armstrong WF, Bach DS. Clinical and echocardiographic findings in patients with suspected acute aortic dissection. *Am Heart J* 1998;136:1051.
2. Bordeleau L, Cwinn A. Aortic dissection and Turner's syndrome: case report and review of the literature. *J Emerg Med* 1998;16:593.
3. Cambria RA, Gloviczki P. Outcome and expansion rate of 57 thoracoabdominal aortic aneurysms managed nonoperatively. *Am J Surg* 1995;170:213.
4. Coady MA, Risso JA. Surgical intervention criteria for thoracic aortic aneurysms: study of growth rates and complications. *Ann Thorac Surg* 1999;67:1922.
5. Crawford ES, DeNatale MD. Thoracoabdominal aortic aneurysm: observations regarding the natural course of the disease. *J Vasc Surg* 1986;3:578.
6. Dailey PO, Trueblood HW. Management of acute aortic dissections. *Ann Thorac Surg* 1970;10:237.
7. DeBakey ME, Henley WS. Surgical management of dissecting aneurysms of the aorta. *J Thorac Cardiovasc Surg* 1965;49:130.
8. Erlich M, Fang C. Perioperative risk factors for mortality inpatients with acute type A dissection. *Circulation* 1998;98[Suppl II]:II-294.
9. Elefteriades JA, Lovoulos CJ. Management of descending aortic dissection. *Ann Thorac Surg* 1999;67:2002.
10. Erbel R, Hellmut O. Effect of medical and surgical therapy on aortic dissection evaluated by transesophageal echocardiography: implications for prognosis and therapy. *Circulation* 1993;87:1604.
11. Fann JI, Smith JA. Surgical management of aortic dissection during a 30-year period. *Circulation* 1995;92[Suppl II]:II-113.
12. Fuster V, Halperin JL. Aortic dissection: a medical perspective. *J Cardiovasc Surg* 1994;9:71313.
13. Hirst AE, Varner JJ. Dissecting aneurysm of the aorta: a review of 505 cases. *Medicine* 1958;37:217.
14. Hussain KM, Chandna V. Aortic dissection in a young corticosteroid-treated patient with systemic lupus erythematosus. *Angiology* 1998;49:649.
15. Juvonen T, Ergin MC. Risk factors for rupture of chronic type B dissections. *J Thorac Cardiovasc Surg* 1999;117:776.
16. Keren A, Kim CB. Accuracy of biplane and multiplane transesophageal echocardiography in diagnosis of typical acute aortic dissection and intramural hematoma. *J Am Coll Cardiol* 1996;28:627.
17. Miller DC. The continuing dilemma concerning medical versus surgical management of patients with acute type B dissections. *Semin Thorac Cardiovasc Surg*

1993;5:33.
18. Nolte JE, Rutherford RB. Arterial dissections associated with pregnancy. *J Vasc Surg* 1995;21:515.
19. Oliver TB, Murchison JT. Spiral CT in acute non-cardiac chest pain. *Clin Radiol* 1999;54:38.
20. Pansini S, Gagliardotta PV. Early and late risk factors in surgical treatment of acute type A dissection. *Ann Thorac Surg* 1998;66:779.
21. Perron AD, Gibbs M. Thoracic aortic dissection secondary to crack cocaine ingestion. *Am J Emerg Med* 1997;15:507.
22. Rogers FB, Osler TM. Aortic dissection after trauma: case report and review of the literature. *J Trauma* 1996;41:906.
23. Sommer T, Fehske W. Aortic dissection: a comparative study of diagnosis with spiral CT, multiplanar transesophageal echocardiography, and MR imaging. *Radiology* 1996;199:347.
24. Spitell PC, Spittell JA. Clinical features and differential diagnosis of aortic dissection: experience with 236 cases (1980 through 1990). *Mayo Clin Proc* 1993;68:642.
25. Torossov M, Singh A. Clinical presentation, diagnosis, and hospital outcome of patients with documented aortic dissection: The Albany Medical Center experience, 1986–1996. *Am Heart J* 1999;137:154.
26. Wheat MW, Palmer RF. Treatment of dissecting aneurysms of the aorta without surgery. *J Thorac Cardiovasc Surg* 1965;50:364.

CHAPTER 52
Abdominal Aortic Aneurysm

Robert L. Wears

The timely recognition of an abdominal aortic aneurysm (AAA) is a major challenge to the emergency physician. The presentation may be confusing, accurate diagnosis difficult, and the cost of delay or misdiagnosis devastating. AAA is the most common cause of unexpected death following discharge from the emergency department (ED),[16] and is one of the eight high-risk areas for medical malpractice litigation in emergency medicine.[14]

AAAs (defined as a 50% or greater increase in aortic diameter[12]) are present in nearly 2% of the elderly.[7] The prevalence is increasing,[3,24] even after adjusting for improved methods of detection. As the proportion of the population older than 60 years of age grows, emergency physicians can expect to encounter patients suffering from AAAs more frequently.

The etiology of AAA remains obscure. A variety of evidence suggests that atherosclerosis alone is not the principal cause; smoking is the single most important risk factor,[19] but familial, biochemical, and hemodynamic factors have all been implicated.[7,12,15] Most patients are male, but the prevalence of AAA increases with increasing age in both sexes[31]; it is roughly as common (approximately 5%) in 90-year-old women as it is in 80-year-old men.[7]

The natural history of the AAA is one of gradual expansion (although sudden changes in size may occur), followed by rupture, exsanguination, and death,[32] although occasional cases of chronic contained rupture have been reported, with survival following rupture of weeks to months.[13] Most AAAs are symptomless until rapid expansion or leakage occurs; indeed, the onset of symptoms referable to the aneurysm is a bad prognostic sign. Eighty percent of patients with untreated, symptomatic AAAs will be dead within 1 year of the onset of symptoms (33% in 1 month, and 74% in 6 months).[30]

The risk of rupture and death depends on the size of the aneurysm. Aneurysms less than 4.0 cm in diameter are at low risk for rupture.[6] For diameters between 4.0 and 5.0 cm, the 5-year risk is between 3% and 12%, and for diameters greater than 5.0 cm, between 25% and 41%.[7] However, there is considerable difference of opinion among vascular surgeons about the risk of rupture, and better data are needed.[18]

Early detection and elective repair of AAAs leads to increased life expectancy, even in elderly patients.[8,32] Operative mortality for elective surgery is roughly 2% to 7% in all age groups,[27] compared with the very high mortality of rupture (90% overall; 50% to 75% in patients who present to the ED in shock,[7] 20% if not in shock[30]). Because rupture of an AAA is inevitable given enough time, elective resection is generally recommended for aneurysms of 5.0 cm or more.[7] Although some have extended this indication to AAAs as small as 4.0 cm,[11,15] a randomized, controlled trial of active ultrasonic surveillance versus immediate repair of small aneurysms has shown no evidence favoring early operation.[26]

CLINICAL PRESENTATION

AAAs typically present in three ways: asymptomatic, symptomatic, and ruptured. Physical examination is the key to recognition, because about half of asymptomatic AAAs are palpable.[29] The sensitivity of physical examination depends on the size of the aneurysm, ranging from about 50% for aneurysms between 4 and 5 cm to 76% for those between 5 and 6 cm.[20] Unfortunately, this sensitivity is not high enough to confidently rule out an aneurysm based on a negative physical examination. Most palpable aneurysms are found in the epigastrium, extending to the paraumbilical areas on both sides of the midline. False-positive physical findings are common, illustrating the difficulty of the diagnosis.[1]

Asymptomatic Aneurysm

Occasionally, an AAA is discovered on routine examination for another, clearly unrelated problem. Frequently, the aneurysm is noted on abdominal plain films.[22] The emergency physician's task in this setting is to confirm that the aneurysm is truly asymptomatic.

Symptomatic Aneurysm

Patients who are hemodynamically stable but who have symptoms referable to an AAA can present in a variety of ways, and so are easily misdiagnosed. In fact, almost half of all AAAs are misdiagnosed on their initial presentation.[2,23] Abdominal, low-back, or flank pain is the cardinal symptom of AAA, but it is nonspecific. The pain may be associated with syncope at the time of onset. The discomfort occasionally radiates to the testis or leg, causing the symptoms to be attributed to renal colic, inguinal hernia, or lumbar spine disease. The pain is usually not much affected by movement and can vary considerably in location.[25] Radicular findings[21] or hematuria[28] may occasionally be present, further misleading the physician.

Less common presentations of symptomatic AAA include hydronephrosis or leg swelling (usually left) from compression, new onset or worsening of hypertension (secondary to renal artery compression), testicular swelling, or evidence of peripheral embolization. Aortovenous or aortocaval fistulas are uncommon, and usually present as high-output failure with marked distention of the lower abdominal and leg veins, accompanied by more typical evidence of AAA, such as abdominal mass and back pain.[4]

About 10% of symptomatic AAAs present with severe pain and marked abdominal tenderness.[30] Because these patients have the appearance of an acute abdomen, identifying them as "emergent" cases is not as much of a problem as in other symptomatic patients, even though the presumptive diagnosis may be erroneous (e.g., perforated viscus).

An uncommon, acute presentation of a symptomatic AAA is gastrointestinal bleeding secondary to an aortoenteric fistula.[9] Such bleeding may be massive and can distract the emergency physician from suspecting vascular disease. In particular, aortoenteric fistula should be assumed whenever a patient who has had a previous repair of an AAA presents with gastrointestinal bleeding.

Finally, symptomatic AAA may present acutely as complete aortic occlusion with a clinical picture similar to that of a saddle embolus or acute Leriche syndrome. This complication requires prompt operation and still carries an approximate 50% mortality.[30]

Ruptured Aneurysm

The classic triad of findings in ruptured AAA is back pain, hypotension, and a pulsatile abdominal mass, but all three findings are present in only about half the patients who survive to reach the ED.[17] Therefore, the presence of any one of these findings in a patient with a known AAA is sufficient to make the diagnosis of rupture without confirmatory testing.[7] Unfortunately, most patients presenting with ruptured AAAs have no prior knowledge of their aneurysm.[29] Rupture of an AAA is correctly diagnosed preoperatively about in 70% of patients[23]; mortality increases dramatically with misdiagnosis.[10]

DIFFERENTIAL DIAGNOSIS

The differential diagnosis of AAA includes the differentials of shock and the acute abdomen. If shock is present, the differential typically includes acute myocardial infarction, hemorrhagic pancreatitis, perforated viscus, and mesenteric infarction. In patients whose presentation is less severe, renal or biliary colic, diverticulitis, and lumbosacral disc disease also need to be considered. Because these conditions are more common than AAA, it is useful to consider the differential diagnosis in reverse; for example, when entertaining a diagnosis of renal colic in a patient over age 60, AAA should be considered.

EMERGENCY DEPARTMENT MANAGEMENT

The ED management of a patient with a suspected AAA must be tailored to the patient's presentation.

Asymptomatic Aneurysm

If the AAA is clearly and unequivocally unrelated to the patient's symptoms, the patient should be referred promptly to a vascular surgeon for further evaluation and possible elective repair. An abdominal ultrasound examination may be useful in establishing the presence or absence of AAA, but it cannot provide evidence that the AAA is not ruptured, leaking, or expanding.

Symptomatic Aneurysm

An aneurysm producing symptoms should be assumed to be ruptured, rapidly expanding, or otherwise complicated (infected, dissecting). Therefore, although these patients may appear hemodynamically stable, prompt surgical consultation should be obtained, and preparations for fluid resuscitation and operative repair should be made by placing several large-bore intravenous lines and sending blood for type and crossmatch, hemoglobin, renal function, and coagulation studies. Vigorous fluid resuscitation should not be started unless there is evidence of peripheral hypoperfusion,[7] and hypertension should be controlled if present.[29] Patients presenting as an acute abdomen or patients with known AAA and any one of the findings in the classic triad require immediate surgery without the usual preoperative evaluation and preparation, as rupture is either imminent or has already occurred but has been temporarily confined to the retroperitoneum.[7] In less acute presentations, radiologic imaging may be helpful in selected cases but should not be ordered indiscriminately.

Ruptured Aneurysm

Patients in shock from a ruptured AAA need rapid resuscitation and prompt operation. Except in unusual circumstances, these patients should be transported to the operating room as quickly as possible without waiting for diagnostic testing or stabilization. A policy of immediate operation in such circumstances maximizes the patients' chances of survival. Even if it is discovered that a ruptured AAA is not present, many of these patients will have another surgical condition requiring operation, so the risk of unnecessary laparotomy is not great.[33]

Radiologic Imaging

Plain films of the abdomen are occasionally helpful in the diagnosis of AAA, in that calcified walls are visible in about one-half of cases.[22] Fusiform calcifications show the presence of an aneurysm, but not whether it is enlarging or leaking. Absent or "normal" aortic calcifications are of no value in ruling out the diagnosis. Therefore, plain films should not be ordered to evaluate the presence of an AAA or its complications.

Abdominal ultrasonography is useful in quickly and accurately establishing the presence of an aneurysm with almost 100% sensitivity.[7] However, it is not reliable in determining whether rupture has occurred or in estimating the proximal and distal extent of the aneurysm. Its role in the ED lies in rapidly establishing the presence of AAA at the bedside when there is doubt.

Computed tomography provides greater detail than ultrasound and a more accurate measure of size. It is particularly useful in identifying leakage, rupture, or complications of AAA.[34] Because computed tomography takes more time and requires intravenous contrast and removal of the patient from the ED, it should be limited to stable patients in whom precise information is required. Magnetic resonance imaging also provides detailed images but is expensive, not widely available, and contraindicated in patients with pacemakers or metallic implants or clips; therefore, it currently offers no substantive advantage over ultrasound or computed tomography.[7]

Aortography is useful in selected cases in planning the operative repair of AAAs, but should not be used for diagnosis or to establish size. The decision to use angiography should be left to the surgical consultant, who may need information about renal or iliofemoral involvement, mesenteric artery stenosis, or suspected visceral lesions (e.g., horseshoe kidney).[5]

DISPOSITION

Patients who are truly asymptomatic should be referred promptly to a vascular surgeon for further evaluation for elective resection. Patients with a symptomatic AAA should be admitted for close observation. These patients will require prompt surgery if it becomes clear that the aneurysm is the source of their symptoms. Patients who present with rupture of their AAA obviously should go straight to the operating room.

Role of the Consultant

All patients with suspected symptomatic or ruptured AAAs should have a prompt surgical consultation, preferably with a vascular surgeon. Patients in whom the AAA is truly an incidental finding may be referred for later consultation if otherwise appropriate.

Indications for Admission

All patients with symptomatic AAAs should be admitted to the hospital for close observation and further investigation. One should assume that abdominal or back pain in the presence of AAA is due to sudden expansion or rupture.

Transfer Considerations

If the initial receiving hospital does not have sufficient surgical capability to treat an AAA, transfer to a more appropriate institution may be indicated. The decision to transfer may be a difficult one for patients who present with cardiovascular instability. The current hospital's capabilities, the length of time in transit, and the likelihood of survival to the second hospital must be considered.

COMMON PITFALLS

- AAAs are frequently misdiagnosed, especially in the obese; therefore, any palpable abdominal pulsation in an obese patient should be suspected of being an AAA, even if a mass cannot be clearly discerned. Back pain is a common symptom, and because peritoneal signs may not be present unless free rupture into the abdominal cavity has occurred, the emergency physician may be misled to one of the common misdiagnoses of AAA, such as renal colic or lumbosacral disease. Because early recognition of AAA is most important to ensure maximum survival, it is a sound practice to perform a physical examination specifically aimed at ruling out an aneurysm in all patients over 50 who present with abdominal or back pain.
- A second pitfall is assuming that an aneurysm discovered on physical examination is incidental and not the source of the patient's symptoms. Any back or abdominal pain in the presence of a pulsatile abdominal mass should be considered to be due to an expanding or leaking aneurysm unless there is overwhelming evidence to the contrary.
- A third pitfall includes abbreviating an ED evaluation due to "gatekeeping" or managed care concerns. AAAs are not immediately obvious, and patients and physicians may have difficulty negotiating the preauthorization requirements of medical plans. These factors should not be allowed to prevent a thorough assessment of the older patient with back or abdominal pain.[35]

References

1. Beede SD, Ballard DJ, James EM, et al. Positive predictive value of clinical suspicion of abdominal aortic aneurysm: implications for efficient use of abdominal ultrasonography. *Arch Intern Med* 1990;150:549–551.
2. Bengtsson H, Bergqvist D. Ruptured abdominal aortic aneurysm: a population-based study. *J Vasc Surg* 1993;18:74–80.
3. Bickerstaff LK, Hollier LJ, Van Peenen HJ, et al. Abdominal aortic aneurysms: the changing natural history. *J Vasc Surg* 1984;1:6–12.
4. Calligaro KD, Savarese RP, DeLaurentis DA. Unusual aspects of aortovenous fistulas associated with ruptured abdominal aortic aneurysms. *J Vasc Surg* 1990;12:586–590.
5. Campbell JJ, Bell DD, Gaspar MR. Selective use of arteriography in the assessment of aortic aneurysm repair. *Ann Vasc Surg* 1990;4:419–423.
6. Cronenwett JL, Murphy TF, Zelenock GB, et al. Actuarial analysis of variables associated with rupture of small abdominal aortic aneurysms. *Surgery* 1985;98:472–483.
7. Ernst CB. Abdominal aortic aneurysm. *N Engl J Med* 1993;328:1167–1172.
8. Goldstone J. Aneurysms of the aorta and iliac arteries. In: Moore WE. ed. *Vascular surgery: a comprehensive review.* Philadelphia: WB Saunders, 1993:401–421.
9. Grigsby WS, Eitzen EM, Boyle DJ II. Aortoenteric fistula: a catastrophe waiting to happen. *Ann Emerg Med* 1986;15:731.
10. Hoffman M, Avellone JC, Plecha FR, et al. Operation for ruptured abdominal aortic aneurysms: a community-wide experience. *Surgery* 1982;91:597.
11. Hollier LH, Taylor LM, Ochsner J. Recommended indication for operative treatment of abdominal aortic aneurysms. *J Vasc Surg* 1992;15:1046–1056.
12. Johnston KW, Rutherford RB, Tilson MD, et al. Suggested standards for reporting on arterial aneurysms. *J Vasc Surg* 1991;13:452–458.
13. Jones CS, Reilly MK, Dalsing MC, et al. Chronic contained rupture of abdominal aortic aneurysms. *Arch Surg* 1986;121:542–546.
14. Karcz A, Holbrook J, Burke MC, et al. Massachusetts emergency medicine closed malpractice claims: 1988–1990. *Ann Emerg Med* 1993;22:553–559.
15. Katz DA, Littenberg B, Cronenwett JL. Management of small abdominal aortic aneurysms: early surgery vs watchful waiting. *JAMA* 1992;268:2678–2686.
16. Kefer MP, Hargarten SW, Jentzen J. Death after discharge from the emergency department. *Ann Emerg Med* 1994;24:1102–1107.
17. Kiel CS, Ernst CB. Advances in management of abdominal aortic aneurysm. *Adv Surg* 1993;26:73–98.
18. Lederle FA. Risk of rupture of large abdominal aortic aneurysms. Disagreement among vascular surgeons. *Arch Intern Med* 1996;156(9): 1007–1009.
19. Lederle FA, Johnson GR, Wilson SE, et al. Prevalence and associations of abdominal aortic aneurysm detected through screening. Aneurysm Detection and Management (ADAM) Veterans Affairs Cooperative Study Group. *Ann Intern Med* 1997;126(6):441–449.
20. Lederle FA, Simel DL. Does this patient have abdominal aortic aneurysm? *JAMA* 1999;281(1):77–82.
21. Lodder J, Cheriex E, Oostenbroek R, et al. Ruptured abdominal aortic aneurysms presenting as radicular compression syndromes. *J Neurol* 1982;227:121–124.
22. Loughran CF. A review of the plain abdominal radiograph in acute rupture of abdominal aortic aneurysms. *Clin Radiol* 1986;37:383–387.
23. Marston WA, Ahlquist R, Johnson G, et al. Misdiagnosis of ruptured abdominal aneurysms. *J Vasc Surg* 1992;16:17–22.
24. Melton LJ III, Bickerstaff LK, Hollier LH, et al. Changing incidence of abdominal aortic aneurysm. *Am J Epidemiol* 1984;120:379–386.
25. Merchant RF Jr, Cafferata HT, DePalma RG. Pitfalls in the diagnosis of abdominal aortic aneurysm. *Am J Surg* 1981;142:756–758.
26. Participants in the UKSAT. Mortality results for randomised controlled trial of early elective surgery or ultrasonographic surveillance for small abdominal aortic aneurysms. *Lancet* 1998;352:1649–1655.
27. Paty PS, Lloyd WE, Chang BB, et al. Aortic replacement for abdominal aortic aneurysm in elderly patients. *Am J Surg* 1993;166:191–193.
28. Phillips SM, King D. The role of ultrasound to detect aortic aneurysms in "urological" patients. *Eur J Vasc Surg* 1993;7:298–300.
29. Rothrock SG, Green SM. Abdominal aortic aneurysms: current clinical strategies for avoiding disaster. *Emerg Med Rep* 1994;15:125–136.
30. Scobie TK. Abdominal aortic aneurysms: how can we improve their treatment? *Can Med Assoc J* 1980;123:725–729.
31. Scott RA, Ashton HA, Kay DN. Abdominal aortic aneurysm in 4237 screened patients: prevalence, development and management over 6 years. *Br J Surg* 1991;78:1122–1125.
32. Szilagyi DE, Smith RF, DeRusso FJ, et al. Contribution of abdominal aortic aneurysmectomy to prolongation of life. *Ann Surg* 1966;164:678–699.
33. Valentine RJ, Barth MJ, Myers SI, et al. Nonvascular emergencies presenting as ruptured abdominal aortic aneurysms. *Surgery* 1993;113:286–289.
34. Weinbaum FI, Dubner S, Turner JW, et al. The accuracy of computed tomography in the diagnosis of retroperitoneal blood in the presence of abdominal aortic aneurysm. *J Vasc Surg* 1987;6:11–16.
35. Young GP, Lowe RA. Adverse outcomes of managed care gatekeeping. *Acad Emerg Med* 1997;4:1129–1136.

CHAPTER 53

Mesenteric Ischemia and Infarction

Kendall Ho and Ron M. Walls

Mesenteric ischemia is the failure of normal oxygenation of the small or large intestine due to interruption of vascular flow (Fig. 53.1). The consequences of this failure of oxygenation occupy a spectrum that ranges from intermittent, nonspecific intestinal symptoms to frank gut infarction with death of the patient.[1,3,4,7,9,13,14,17,18,20,21,23,24,26] Unfortunately, despite increasing literature and medical familiarity with the lethal nature of the condition, mortality remains well over 50%, primarily attributable to delay in diagnosis.[9,20,21] Mortality rates of less than 50% have been achieved with aggressive diagnostic and therapeutic approaches.[13,14,26]

Acute mesenteric ischemia (AMI) is much more common than chronic mesenteric insufficiency. The vascular interruption in AMI can be divided into three categories: arterial occlusion, venous occlusion, and nonocclusive mesenteric ischemia (NOMI). Of the 70% to 80% of all AMI due to vascular occlusion,[3] embolus to the superior mesenteric artery (SMA) accounts for nearly half the cases, while SMA thrombosis accounts for a further 10%.[14] Strangulated small or large bowel due to herniation, adhesions, or volvulus is another major cause of acute vascular occlusion.[20] An estimated 5% to 15% of AMI are due to venous thrombosis.[4,23] While historically thought to be rare, NOMI is increasingly being recognized, especially in systemically and critically ill patients, with periods of markedly reduced blood flow.[21] A chronic syndrome of inadequate mesenteric blood flow without complete vascular occlusion or bowel infraction, also termed *intestinal angina,* may uncommonly occur.[14,20]

Once ischemia is established, the pathologic sequence is identical, regardless of the causative mechanism. Four major factors contribute to the extent and severity of ischemia: hypoxic injury, reperfusion injury, toxic luminal factors, and bacteria and toxins.[20] Hypoxia initially causes epithelial and submucosal damage, followed by full-thickness involvement and eventual loss of bowel integrity with continuing oxygenation failure. Should perfusion be restored in ischemic regions, generation of superoxides and free radicals could add further insult to already damaged tissues. Toxic luminal substances, such as hydrochloric acid and digestive enzymes, penetrate the edematous and porous intestinal mucosal barrier to cause further cellular damage. Bacterial invasion and toxin excretion lead to systemic sepsis.[20] Hypotension, due to blood and fluid losses and exacerbated by sepsis, leads to further compromise of vascular flow to the gut, and the process becomes self-propagating. In the most severe cases, AMI can lead to the development of multiorgan dysfunction syndrome (MODS).[17,20]

All attempts to establish reliable diagnostic criteria for the condition have failed because the symptoms are nonspecific and the presentation is often unremarkable until the compromised gut (and often the patient) is not salvageable. In one series, over half of the patients who underwent laparotomy were immediately closed when the surgeon discovered the advanced state of the intraabdominal infarction.[18]

This disorder has a distinct epidemiologic preference for the elderly.[1,17,18,20,21,24,26] Many patients have evidence of significant preexisting cardiac diseases, especially congestive heart failure.[1,7,18,20,24,26] Postoperative and critically ill patients, and those exposed to vasospastic substances such as norepinephrine, cocaine, or digoxin, are at an increased risk of developing NOMI.[13,17,20,21]

CLINICAL PRESENTATION

History

Presentation to the emergency department is highly variable. Unfortunately, the only symptom that is virtually universally

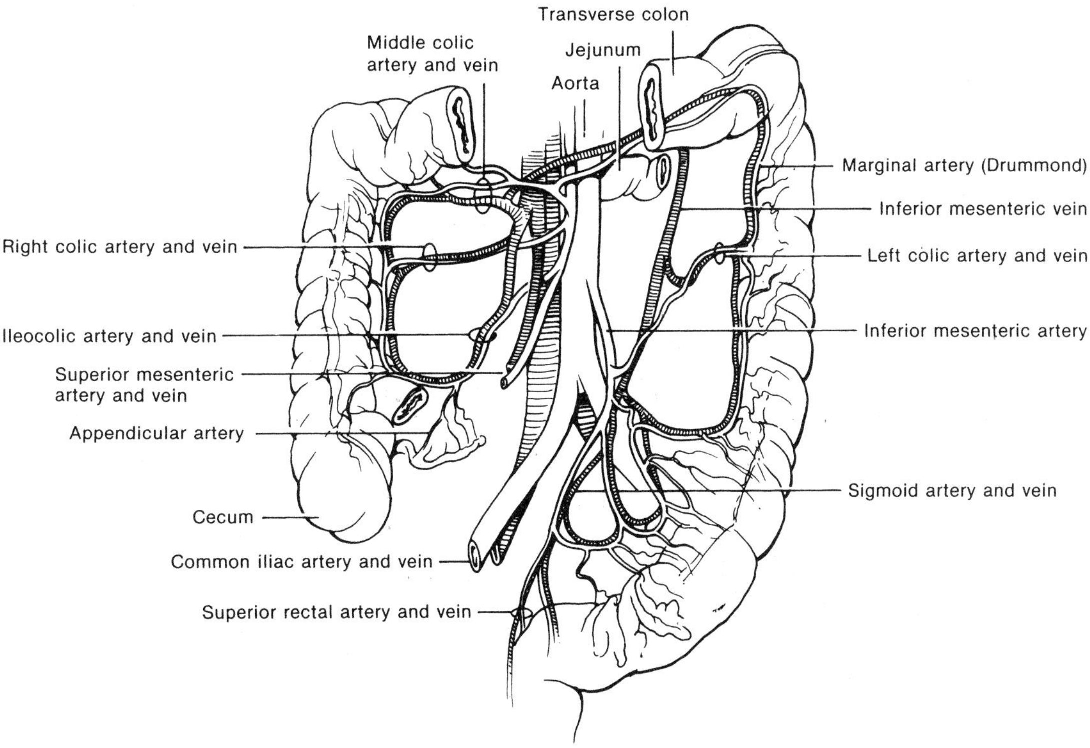

Figure 53.1. Vascular supply to the colon.

present is abdominal pain, which may be localized or diffuse and may have either a colicky or constant character.[1,3,7,13,18,20,26] Patients with NOMI may be free of pain in up to 25% of cases, but these patients will have recently experienced episodes of shock, cardiac arrest, cardiac dysrhythmia, or other hypotensive crises and so will usually present in an inpatient setting.[14] Suddenness of onset is a useful, but not completely reliable symptom, because pain may develop over seconds, minutes, hours, or even days or weeks, depending on the underlying process.[1,9,20] However, sudden onset of severe abdominal pain with minimal physical findings mandates consideration of AMI.[9,14,20] Vomiting, diarrhea, or both will be reported or observed frequently, and sometimes vomitus or stool may be obviously bloody.[3,13,14,20,26] Weight loss is invariably present in chronic mesenteric ischemia.[20] Nausea and anorexia, often long standing, will be reported in some cases.[11] A small number of patients will complain of abdominal fullness or distention.[1]

Historically, the patient will usually have a combination of the following: advanced age, a history of significant cardiovascular disease, a history of thromboembolic events, and concurrent medication with digitalis and a diuretic.[1,7,18,20,26] The patient may report episodes of vague abdominal fullness or discomfort after meals, and unexplained weight loss is often present, if sought.[18] However, most patients will present with AMI without a preceding history of intermittent or chronic symptoms.

Physical Examination

The physical examination may be remarkably normal, especially in retrospect after the diagnosis is ultimately made. The patient may appear completely well apart from the presenting pain. Twenty percent to 40% will appear dehydrated, some to the point of frank circulatory shock.[1,18] Fever and modest tachycardia are often, but not invariably, present.[1,7] Hematemesis or melena may occur. Abdominal examination is fully normal in only a very few cases. However, abnormalities, when noted, are often mild and belie the catastrophic nature of the disease. Signs of peritoneal irritation will be present to some degree in 30% to 50% of cases.[1,7,18] Less urgent abdominal findings, such as increased or decreased bowel sounds, localized or diffuse tenderness, distention, bruit, or mass, will be present to some degree in virtually all cases. Most patients will have occult blood in the stool, especially later on in the course of the process.[20] In fact, occult blood loss in the stool may precede abdominal symptoms.[14]

Approximately 10% of patients will present in crisis, with catastrophic hemodynamic collapse, signs of severe systemic toxicity, altered mental status, and signs of frank peritonitis.[1] Although the need for operative intervention is immediately obvious in this type of presentation, the outcome is universally fatal.

DIFFERENTIAL DIAGNOSIS

The differential diagnosis of abdominal pain in the elderly is notoriously difficult (see Chapter 36). Symptoms are often vague or poorly represented. The patient may have other serious medical illness or dementia, which interferes with the history and examination. Physical examination is unreliable in the elderly and may be falsely reassuring.

Nevertheless, abdominal pain in a patient older than 50 years of age must be considered representative of an ominous process until thorough medical evaluation proves this not to be the case. The differential diagnosis is myriad and mirrors that of abdominal pain in any other age group with one exception: As the patient ages, the likelihood of vascular disease increases. This introduces the entire spectrum of vascular disorders to the differential diagnostic list: aneurysm, dissection, renal vascular disease, mesenteric vascular disease, myocardial infarction, and systemic embolization. Other considerations, such as diverticulitis, appendicitis, volvulus, obstruction, perforation, peptic ulcer disease, gallbladder disease, pancreatitis, splenic infarction, inflammatory disease, malignancy, gastrointestinal hemorrhage, and functional bowel disease, are discussed elsewhere in this text.

The principal diagnostic approach is the determination of whether a surgical condition is present and, if so, whether the situation is urgent. In mesenteric ischemia, although both of these criteria are universally present, they are rarely appreciated.

EMERGENCY DEPARTMENT EVALUATION AND MANAGEMENT

Patients older than 50 years of age presenting with abdominal pain undergo an appropriate and timely diagnostic workup to ensure that serious conditions, especially mesenteric ischemia, are not missed. Over 80% of patients presenting to emergency departments with mesenteric ischemia will be misdiagnosed or will undergo extensive and time-consuming evaluations, thus ensuring their mortality.[4,11,22] Even when the condition is suspected, the patient may have a bad outcome. In one series, four patients diagnosed with intestinal angina at the time of admission were admitted to the hospital without aggressive diagnostic or therapeutic intervention.[18] The value of an aggressive approach to the diagnosis and management of AMI is stressed in the literature.[9,10,13,14,20]

Emergency department evaluation is dictated by the patient's condition. When the patient presents in hemodynamic or septic crisis, immediate therapeutic measures must precede definitive diagnosis. Patency of the upper airway must be ensured, and the ability of the patient to maintain the airway and to ventilate and oxygenate adequately must be assessed. High-flow oxygen, preferably by mask, should be administered. Examination of the airway and chest, supplemented by determination of arterial blood gases, will determine the need for immediate intubation. Two intravenous lines should be established and crystalloid solution administered to replenish intravascular volume. The degree of volume depletion should be determined and, although patients are elderly, crystalloid should be rapidly administered, because the hypovolemia is known to aggravate the mesenteric hypoperfusion. Rapid bedside determination of serum glucose level should be performed, with intravenous glucose administered as indicated. Blood samples should be obtained, and laboratory blood tests, including complete blood cell count, electrolytes, amylase, urea, creatinine, glucose, coagulation parameters, and crossmatch, should be ordered.

Additional studies may be indicated. Continuous electrocardiographic monitoring should be instituted and a 12-lead surface electrocardiogram obtained. The ultimate diagnosis in these cases may be obscured by the systemic nature of the presentation, and the prognosis is grim.

In patients with no hemodynamic compromise, the presentation most suggestive of ischemia is abdominal pain that is disproportionate to physical findings. Aggressive, early investigation of ischemia should be undertaken in these patients, especially if they are elderly and have risk factors for AMI and if there is not another satisfactory explanation for the pain. Delaying investigation of suspected AMI until more prominent abdominal findings are present will substantially increase mortality.[9,20] In all cases, it is advisable to establish intravenous access, because the patient's condition may deteriorate rapidly, especially if the presenting problem is vascular. After a thorough history and physical examination, laboratory specimens should be obtained, as indicated earlier.

Laboratory Studies

Unfortunately, laboratory studies are so nonspecific they are of little help. Although it has been said that the principal use of the laboratory in mesenteric ischemia is to exclude other entities,[20] this is often not possible. In fact, misdiagnosis often follows erroneous interpretation of the laboratory results, such as when a modest elevation of the serum amylase value leads to an incorrect attribution of the patient's condition to acute pancreatitis. Nevertheless, laboratory studies should be performed and carefully interpreted.

The hemoglobin value is almost universally elevated due to hemoconcentration late in the course of the disease, but it may be normal earlier.[1] Leukocytosis is present in almost all cases and is often marked. Approximately 25% of patients will have white blood cell (WBC) counts of 10,000 to 15,000/μL, 50% will have WBC counts of 15,000 to 30,000/μL, and 25% will exceed 30,000/μL.[1,7,20] Serum amylase determination will show a modest elevation, somewhere in the range from the upper limit of normal to twice normal, about half the time.[1,7,20] Occasionally, profound elevations are seen. Metabolic acidosis is widely thought to be a universal companion of gut ischemia, presumably on the basis of the anaerobic metabolism initiated by the ischemic process. This belief is not supported by the literature, and one large series noted normal serum bicarbonate levels in all 60 patients in the study.[1] However, acidosis, if present, is a significant finding. Other laboratory findings, such as azotemia, hyperbilirubinemia, elevated enzyme and inorganic phosphate levels, and other, more exotic determinations are of no diagnostic value.[9,20,24,26] In the end, none of these laboratory tests have been shown to be sensitive or specific in discriminating mesenteric ischemia from other intraabdominal pathologic processes.[17,20,21]

Imaging

Plain radiography is likewise nonspecific. Abdominal gas may be absent, sparse, or normal or may demonstrate an ileus pattern.[1,9,10,16,20] In the majority of cases, the films will be normal or not suggestive of any particular pathologic process.[14,16,20] The finding of gas in the intestine wall or in the portal venous system invariably occurs only late in the process.[20] Thumbprinting of the intestinal mucosa, shown in relief against air or barium, is strongly suggestive but not specific.[20] The definitive test in the evaluation of a patient with suspected mesenteric ischemia is aortic and mesenteric biplanar angiography.[1,2,9,10,20] In cases of vascular occlusion, this modality can accurately identify the location of vascular occlusion and scrutinize atherosclerotic changes in all vessels. Demonstration of characteristic mesenteric vasoconstriction in the absence of pancreatitis, shock, or vasopressor therapy is diagnostic of NOMI.[14] Angiography also allows the selective infusion of vasodilating or thrombolytic agents directly into the affected vessels as a therapeutic maneuver.[5]

Computed tomography (CT) scanning is emerging as a reasonable and noninvasive alternative if clinical suspicion of mesenteric ischemia is low to moderate. Intraperitoneal free fluid, visualization of thrombus in splanchnic arteries or veins, and abnormal bowel wall characteristics such as wall thickening, pneumatosis, or streaky mesentery are highly suggestive findings.[9,23] One series of 54 cases suggested that CT might be as sensitive as angiography in detecting mesenteric infarction.[16] In addition, CT has some advantages over angiography in evaluating other possible causes of the abdominal process. CT with intravenous contrast can increase diagnostic accuracy in demonstrating venous thrombosis, nonenhancement of arteries, or signs of intestinal necrosis, including pneumatosis or portal vein gas.[9,15,22] However, if mesenteric ischemia is strongly suspected, angiography should still be the first-line diagnostic procedure over CT with intravenous contrast.

Early experience with duplex ultrasound with Doppler signal analysis shows that it has promise as a screening tool for mesenteric ischemia.[8,10,12,17,22] This modality demonstrates low-flow states by estimating splanchnic arterial and venous flow.[8,12,17] However, its utility is limited, as there is a great variation in vascular flow between normal and affected subjects. Furthermore, duplex ultrasound cannot demonstrate anatomy to assist in surgical planning, and its image quality can be easily affected by patient movement and bowel gases.[9,16]

Magnetic resonance (MR)[6,10] and MR angiography[11,19] are potential imaging techniques for noninvasive screening of mesenteric ischemia. However, limited experience with this modality and its infrequency of emergent availability in most institutions limit the consideration of MR in the diagnosis and management of AMI at this time.

The advantages of using laparoscopy to diagnose mesenteric ischemia include bedside performance in unstable patients, direct visualization of bowel appearance, and serial performances or a second look in following patients' progress.[27] Its disadvantages include visualization of the serosal surface only and inability to detect mucosal ischemia, the induction of pneumoperitoneum that may further impair splanchnic blood flow, and inability to detect pulses of the bowel vasculature.[27] The concomitant use of pulse oximetry, measurement of intraluminal PCO_2, together with laparoscopy, may enhance diagnostic accuracy, as there is a strong association between gastrointestinal ischemia and an increased intraluminal PCO_2 in animal and human models.[17,25]

Ultimately, only extreme vigilance will lead to the diagnosis. *Elderly patients who present with abdominal pain, especially those with risk factors for mesenteric ischemia, must undergo a rapid diagnostic sequence leading to a sound provisional diagnosis. The additional features of pain out of proportion to the physical examination, significant leukocytosis, clinical signs of dehydration or hemoconcentration, unexplained acidosis, or the other clinical features of mesenteric ischemia outlined earlier, mandate consideration of early angiography to confirm or exclude the diagnosis.* Proponents of aggressive therapy advocate angiographic studies with selective papaverine infusion for patients older than 50 years of age with risk factors for AMI who experience a sudden onset of abdominal pain that persists for more than 2 hours without establishment of an alternate diagnosis.[9,14,20]

Early surgical consultation must be sought in cases of suspected mesenteric ischemia because delay may prove fatal. Many patients will have harbored their symptoms at home for a protracted period before presentation to a hospital, and time may be short. Waiting for "confirmation" of the diagnosis by development of significant metabolic acidosis, circulatory collapse, frank peritoneal signs, definitive findings on plain radiography, or other unambiguous events places the patient in profound jeopardy. If any reasonable doubt exists as to the diagnosis, and the patient is not in obvious need of immediate laparotomy, angiography should be obtained. Admission to hospital with a diagnosis of "rule out mesenteric ischemia" is not acceptable, and many of these patients have their diagnoses made only at autopsy, or at laparotomy when the disease has progressed to frank infarction.

DISPOSITION

Role of the Consultant

Mesenteric ischemia is a surgical disease. Temporizing measures, such as selective papaverine infusion during angiography, do not obviate the need for revascularization or resection,[1–3,7,9,10,13,14,18,20,21,24,26] except in a small number of cases.[5,9,14,20] Surgical and radiographic consultation should be sought early.

Indications for Admission

The decision to admit an elderly patient with undiagnosed abdominal pain should not be difficult. The list of serious causes of abdominal pain in the undiagnosed elderly patient significantly outweighs the list of trivial or benign conditions. In addition, elderly patients with "benign" conditions, such as biliary colic, often fare poorly and deteriorate precipitously. In patients with a clear diagnosis that is not believed to require hospitalization, close consultation with the patient's primary physician and early follow-up examination are mandatory. When the diagnosis is in doubt, or when the patient carries an established prior diagnosis such as "diverticulosis" but appears to be developing another acute process, admission and early surgical consultation are indicated.

Transfer Considerations

If facilities for vascular surgery or invasive radiography are not present in the institution of presentation, immediate general surgical consultation should be sought. The advisability of transfer of the patient versus laparotomy without preceding angiography depends on local circumstances and the patient's condition.

COMMON PITFALLS

- The most common pitfall in mesenteric ischemia is, ironically, failure to make the diagnosis while the patient is still living or salvageable. Extreme vigilance, appropriate interpretation of the diagnostic aids outlined previously, and institution of an aggressive diagnostic and therapeutic approach improve diagnostic accuracy and decrease morbidity. Admission of a patient with suspicion of mesenteric ischemia to a hospital mandates immediate surgical consultation and angiography. Without angiography, the condition will only become apparent when it is too late to save the patient.
- Perhaps the greatest pitfall is the reluctance to obtain angiography. Angiography carries a low risk of morbidity, which is even more appealing when balanced against a universally fatal condition. Early radiographic consultation and refusal to "wait until morning" are essential to a good outcome.
- From the medicolegal standpoint, it is of paramount importance to establish a sound diagnosis in all patients presenting with abdominal pain. Young patients without physical or laboratory suggestion of an acute surgical process can often be discharged with close and meticulous follow-up. This practice becomes less prudent in the elderly, and consultation and admission should be considered in any uncertain circumstances.

References

1. Andersson R, Parsson H, Isaksson B, et al. Acute intestinal ischemia. *Acta Chir Scand* 1984;150:217.
2. Batellier J, Kieny R. Superior mesenteric artery embolism: eighty-two cases. *Ann Vasc Surg* 1990;4:112.
3. Boley SJ, Brandt LJ, Veith FJ. Ischemic disorders of the intestine. *Curr Probl Surg* 1978;15:1.
4. Boley SJ, Kaleya RN, Brandt LJ. Mesenteric venous thrombosis. *Surg Clin North Am* 1992;72:183.
5. Bull PG, Hagmuller GW, Kreuzer W. New aspects in the diagnosis and management of acute mesenteric infarction. *Int J Angiol* 1993;2:51.
6. Burkart DJ, Johnson CD, Reading CC, et al. MR measurements of mesenteric venous flow: prospective evaluation in healthy volunteers and patients with suspected chronic mesenteric ischemia. *Radiology* 1995;194:801.
7. Clavien P-A, Muller C, Harder F. Treatment of mesenteric infarction. *Br J Surg* 1987;74:500.
8. Danse EM, Laterre PF, Van Beers BE, et al. Early diagnosis of acute intestinal ischaemia: contribution of colour Doppler sonography. *Acta Chir Belg* 1997;97:173.
9. Eldrup-Jorgensen J, Hawkins RE, Bredenberg CE. Abdominal vascular catastrophes. *Surg Clin North Am* 1997;77:1305.
10. Geelkerken RH, van Bockel JH. Mesenteric vascular disease: a review of diagnostic methods and therapies. *Cardiovasc Surg* 1995;3:247.
11. Gehl HB, Bohndorf K, Klose KC, et al. Two-dimensional MR angiography in the evaluation of abdominal veins with gradient refocused sequences. *J Comput Assist Tomogr* 1990;14:619.
12. Gentile AT, Moneta GL, Lee RW, et al. Usefulness of fasting and postprandial duplex ultrasound examinations for predicting high-grade superior mesenteric artery stenosis. *Am J Surg* 1995;169:476.
13. Kaleya RN, Boley SJ. Acute mesenteric ischemia. *Crit Care Clin* 1995;11:479.
14. Kayela RN, Sammartano RJ, Boley SJ. Aggressive approach to acute mesenteric ischemia. *Surg Clin North Am* 1992;72:157.
15. Kim JY, Ha HK, Byun JY, et al. Intestinal infarction secondary to mesenteric venous thrombosis: CT-pathologic correlation. *J Comput Assist Tomogr* 1993;17:382.
16. Klein HM, Lensing R, Klosterhalfen B, et al. Diagnostic imaging of mesenteric infarction. *Radiology* 1995;197:79.
17. Kolkman JJ, Groeneveld ABJ. Occlusive and non-occlusive gastrointestinal ischaemia: a clinical review with special emphasis on the diagnostic value of tonometry. *Scand J Gastroenterol* 1998;33[Suppl 225]:3.
18. Kwaan JHM, Connolly JE. Prevention of intestinal infarction resulting from mesenteric arterial occlusive disease. *Surg Gynecol Obstet* 1983;157:321.
19. Li, King. Mesenteric occlusive disease. *MRI Clin North Am* 1998;6:331.
20. Montgomery RA, Venbrux AB, Bulkley GB. Mesenteric vascular insufficiency. *Curr Probl Surg* 1997;34:943.
21. Newman TS, Magnuson TH, Ahrendt SA, et al. The changing face of mesenteric infarction. *Am Surg* 1998;64:611.
22. Rahmouni A, Mathieu D, Golli M, et al. Value of CT and sonography in the conservative management of acute splenoportal and superior mesenteric venous thrombosis. *Gastrointest Radiol* 1992;17:135.
23. Rhee RY, Gloviczki MD. Mesenteric venous thrombosis. *Surg Clin North Am* 1997;77:327.
24. Sitges-Serra A, Mas X, Roqueta F, et al. Mesenteric infarction: an analysis of 83 patients with prognostic studies in 44 cases undergoing a massive small-bowel resection. *Br J Surg* 1988;75:544.
25. Tollefson DFJ, Wright DJ, Reddy DJ, et al. Intraoperative determination of intestinal viability by pulse oximetry. *Ann Vasc Surg* 1995;9:357.
26. Urayama H, Ohtake H, Kawakami T, et al. Acute mesenteric vascular occlusion: analysis of 39 patients. *Eur J Surg* 1998;164:195.
27. Zamir G, Reissman P. Diagnostic laparoscopy in mesenteric ischemia. *Surg Endosc* 1998;12:309.

PART VI

Emergency Aspects of Orthopedic Surgery

CHAPTER 54

Painful Syndromes of the Hand and Wrist

Jeffrey B. Nemhauser and Michael I. Greenberg

This chapter addresses specific disorders that constitute the larger group of problems known as *repetitive motion disorders*. Repetitive motion disorders are a group of musculo-tendinous maladies that are generally associated with workplace or occupational etiologies. Injuries due to repetitive motions are quite common and appear to be increasing in incidence. In 1980, these injuries were noted to comprise about 18% of all reported work-related injuries. In 1990, they were reported to make up approximately 48% of all work injuries. United States Bureau of Labor Statistics data in 1994 reported over 92,500 repetitive stress injury cases involving the upper extremity. These injuries were reported to be associated with over 37,000 days of work lost. The economic impact of these injuries is enormous and represents one of the most pressing problems in occupational health and safety today.

CARPAL TUNNEL SYNDROME

Carpal tunnel syndrome (CTS) is a commonly occurring entrapment neuropathy involving the median nerve at the wrist and represents the most common of all peripheral compression neuropathies.[10]

At the level of the wrist, the median nerve exists in an anatomic tunnel or canal that is formed dorsally by the carpal bones and volarly by the fibrous, but rigid, transverse carpal ligament (Fig. 54-1). The flexor tendons and their accompanying sheaths also lie within this anatomic tunnel. The tunnel begins approximately at the level of the volar wrist crease and extends distally approximately three centimeters. Despite the fact that the carpal tunnel is open at both of its ends, the canal maintains the essential physiologic properties of a closed compartment. When intracanal interstitial pressure becomes elevated above a critical threshold, capillary blood flow rates are reduced below that which is essential for the maintenance of median nerve viability and function. Any condition that tends to decrease the internal area of the canal or increase the volume of the anatomical contents of the canal could theoretically induce carpal tunnel syndrome by resulting in impingement of the median nerve.

Numerous specific clinical conditions have been causally associated with the development of the carpal tunnel syndrome. However, it is important to remember that the idiopathic variety is probably the most common. Some authors have suggested that persons who happen to have an anatomically small canal (on a genetic basis) are more likely to develop this syndrome.[7] In addition, rheumatoid arthritis, diabetes, myxedema, and pregnancy are noted to be frequent causes of carpal tunnel syndrome. Acute fracture of the distal radius as well as fracture and dislocation of the carpus can result in carpal tunnel syndrome by either direct trauma to or compression of the median nerve secondary to bleeding. Infections involving bacterial, viral, or fungal etiologies can cause synovitis, which may result in local nerve compression with the ultimate development of CTS. Any space-occupying lesion such as tumors, as well as osteophytes resulting from malunited fractures or degenerative joint disease, can result in the development of median nerve compression with CTS symptoms.

The 1994 Bureau of Labor Statistics data indicate that about 9% of cases are associated with typing and key entry jobs, 6% with repetitive use of tools, and 12% with repetitive grasping motions. Carpal tunnel syndrome occurs more frequently in women in a ratio of greater than 2:1. Females account for over 78% of all cases. CTS is noted to be a condition of middle age and is typically seen most often in the age range of 40 to 60 with the mean age at diagnosis reported to be 50 for men and 51 for women.

CLINICAL PRESENTATION

The classically recognized clinical presentation of CTS involves paresthesias and pain at the radial aspect of the palm of the hand, frequently increased at night. The modern view of the etiology of this syndrome involves forceful, repeated hand motion associated with work. CTS is often a bilateral condition with the patient typically complaining of numbness, tingling, burning, or paresthesias in the hand along the distribution of the median nerve (the thumb, index, middle, and radial aspect of the ring fingers). These symptoms characteristically awaken the patient from sleep and may be relieved by shaking the hand and wrist. A nocturnal pain pattern is often the hallmark of CTS and as the syndrome progresses, the occurrence of symptoms may be seen to increase. The symptoms are often exacerbated by activities that maintain the wrist flexed, such as driving, holding a book, and by use of the hand such as with knitting, sewing, and hammering. Patients may also complain of weakness or clumsiness in the hand manifested by difficulty with fine motor functions such as picking up objects, holding things, and buttoning clothing.

Physical examination may reveal decreased sensation to light

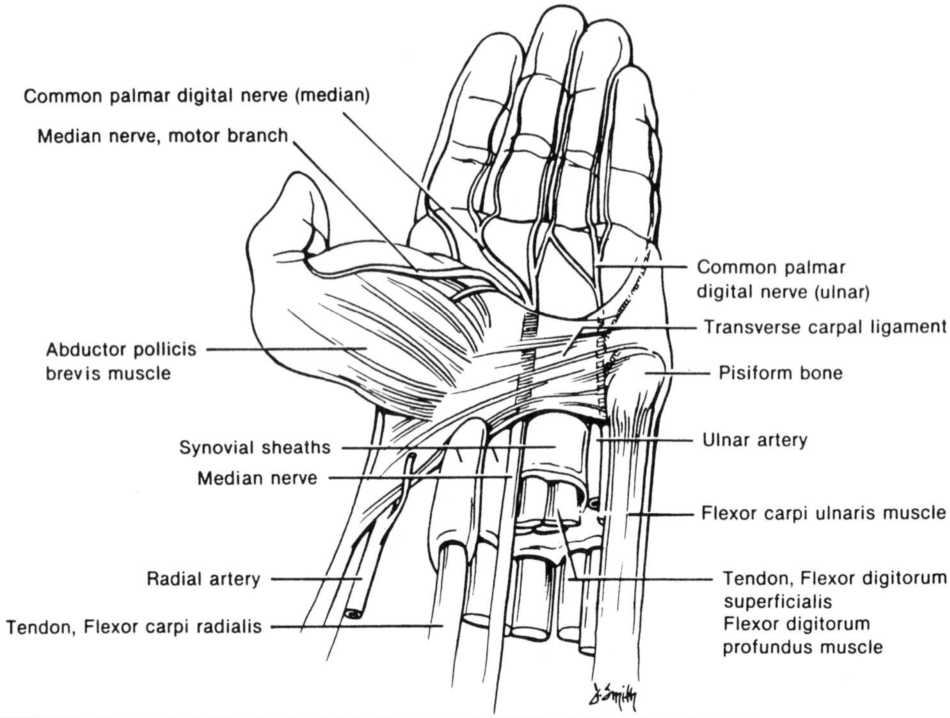

Figure 54.1. View of the carpal tunnel. The median nerve and flexor tendons, which are in the tunnel, lie below the transverse carpal ligament that forms the roof of the tunnel.

touch or decreased two-point discrimination in the median nerve distribution. Phalen's wrist-flexion test and Tinel's sign are frequently noted to be positive with carpal tunnel syndrome.[6,11] Phalen's test is considered to be positive if holding the wrist in complete, but unforced, flexion for 30 to 60 seconds reproduces or exaggerates the numbness and paresthesias in the median nerve distribution. Tinel's sign is positive if light tapping over the median nerve at the wrist causes a tingling sensation distally along the median nerve.

Phalen's test is believed to be more useful in the diagnosis of carpal tunnel syndrome.[11] In more advanced cases there may be weakness of the median-innervated thenar muscles, the abductor pollicis brevis, and the opponens. Thenar atrophy is best seen as a guttering appearance along the radial aspect of the thenar eminence that exposes the first metacarpal. In cases of carpal tunnel syndrome caused by an inflammatory synovitis (rheumatoid arthritis), there may be swelling along the volar aspect of the wrist.

Recent attempts to develop consensus criteria for the diagnosis and classification of CTS have been described. The first principle elucidated by these attempts is that no "gold standard" currently exists for the diagnosis of CTS. Rather, a combination of electrodiagnostic study results in conjunction with symptomatology will be expected to provide the most accurate diagnostic information. The use of electrodiagnostics alone is not considered sufficient to make the definitive diagnosis of CTS.

DIFFERENTIAL DIAGNOSIS

The clinical manifestations of carpal tunnel syndrome are most often characteristic and consequently there is seldom confusion with other entities. Occasionally, the clinical presentation may be unusual and consideration may need to be given to other entities that share characteristics with carpal tunnel syndrome.

Cervical root irritation, especially at the C6 and C7 levels, secondary to either a herniated cervical disc or osteoarthritis with encroachment on the neural foramina, may produce numbness in the median-innervated fingers, with pain radiating to the shoulder. However, cervical root pathology usually causes radicular symptoms that are seldom bilateral and that are worse at night.

Compression of the median nerve in the proximal forearm (pronator syndrome) may also present with numbness in the radial three and one-half digits and weak thenar muscles. However, in this case, Phalen's test would be expected to be negative and Tinel's sign would be positive in the forearm rather than at the wrist. In this case, nocturnal awakening is unlikely, and there would be pain in the volar forearm both subjectively and with palpation.

EMERGENCY DEPARTMENT EVALUATION

The diagnosis of carpal tunnel syndrome is usually made by a careful history and physical examination. Radiographs of the wrist, including a carpal tunnel view, may show structural abnormalities such as callus, osteophytes, and calcific deposits. Cervical spine films may be useful if clinical symptoms suggest the presence of a cervical radiculopathy. Thyroid function tests, fasting blood sugar, erythrocyte sedimentation rate, rheumatoid factor, antinuclear antibodies, determination of serum calcium and uric acid levels, and a white blood cell count with differential may all be useful when clinically indicated.

EMERGENCY DEPARTMENT MANAGEMENT

The initial treatment for the majority of patients involves conservative care. Wrist splints in neutral or slight extension can be worn when symptoms arise, especially at night. The patient should be told to avoid any upper extremity activities that obviously aggravate the symptoms. When underlying medical conditions are suspected (e.g., hypothyroidism, rheumatoid arthritis, gout) appropriate referral to either orthopedic or plastic surgeons with special expertise in treating CTS is required. Diuretics may be useful if carpal tunnel syndrome is associated with pregnancy but should be given only in consultation with the patient's obstetrician.

EMERGENCY DEPARTMENT DISPOSITION

All patients presenting in the emergency department with symptoms of carpal tunnel syndrome should be referred to appropriate specialists for further evaluation and treatment. Outpatient electromyographic and nerve conduction studies are useful when trying to differentiate carpal tunnel syndrome from other causes of similar symptoms or when objective signs of carpal tunnel syndrome are absent but the history and subjective symptoms are compatible with carpal tunnel syndrome. These studies are not generally ordered from the emergency department but would be reserved for the consultant.

The injection of corticosteroids into the carpal canal can result in substantial symptomatic improvement, sometimes even complete relief. However, following steroid injection, the symptoms will often recur.[8] Surgical decompression of the carpal canal is the treatment of choice for those patients who fail conservative care. Indications for operation include muscle weakness, thenar atrophy, and no response to or recurrence after conservative treatment. Surgery involves what is known as carpal tunnel release (CTR), consisting of the division of the transverse carpal ligament. This surgery generally affords good results. However, recurrence of symptoms is seen in up to 20% of patients with as many as 12% requiring reoperation. More recently, endoscopic surgical release procedures have been successful.

References

1. Green DP. Diagnostic and therapeutic value of carpal tunnel injection. *J Hand Surg* 1984;9A:850.
2. Katz RT. Carpal tunnel syndrome: A practical review. Saint Louis University School of Medicine, Missouri. *Am Fam Physician* 1994;49:1371, 1385.
3. Kuschner SH, Ebramzadeh E, Johnson D, Brien WW, Sherman R. Tinel's sign and Phalen's test in carpal tunnel syndrome. *Orthopedics* 1992;15:1297.
4. Mackinnon SE, Novak CB: Repetitive strain in the workplace. *J Hand Surg* 1997;2–18.
5. Mascola JR, Rickman LS. Infectious causes of carpal tunnel syndrome: Case report and review. *Rev Infect Dis* 1991;13:911.
6. Okutsu I, Ninomiya S, Takatori Y, Hamanaka I, et al. Results of endoscopic management of carpal tunnel syndrome. *Orthop Rev* 1993;22:81.
7. Phalen GS. The carpal tunnel syndrome: Seventeen years' experience in diagnosis and treatment of six hundred and fifty-four hands. *J Bone Joint Surg [Am]* 1966;48:211.
8. Rempel D, Evanoff B, Amadio PC, et al. Consensus criteria for the classification of carpal tunnel syndrome in epidemiologic studies. *Am J Pub Health* 1998;88;1447.
9. Szabo RM. Acute carpal tunnel syndrome. *Hand Clinics* 1998;14;419.
10. Slater RR, Jr, Bynum DK. Diagnosis and treatment of carpal tunnel syndrome. *Orthop Rev* 1993;22:1095.
11. Skandalakis JE, Colborn GL, Skandalakis PN, McCollam SM, Skandalakis LJ. The carpal tunnel syndrome: I and II. *Am Surg* 1992;58:72.

GUYON'S CANAL (ULNAR TUNNEL) SYNDROME

The ulnar nerve, originating from both C8 and T1 nerve roots, is formed from the medial cord of the brachial plexus. Following an anatomically tortuous course through the upper extremity, the nerve is susceptible to compressive forces at multiple locations along its course. At the elbow, the ulnar nerve travels through the cubital tunnel, which is the most common site for ulnar nerve compression. Neuropathy secondary to cubital tunnel pathology must be ruled out before a diagnosis is made of ulnar nerve compression at the wrist.

The ulnar nerve, primarily a motor and sensory nerve for the hand, does not give off important branches in the proximal upper extremity. On its entrance into the hand, the ulnar nerve provides the primary motor innervation to the intrinsic muscles therein.

The ulnar nerve innervates the abductor and opponens digiti minimi and flexor digiti minimi brevis (the hypothenar muscles); the lumbrical muscles of the fourth and fifth fingers, all of the interossei, the adductor pollicis, the medial head, and, occasionally, the lateral head of the flexor pollicis brevis are also innervated by the ulnar nerve. The ulnar nerve also supplies sensation for a significant part of the hand, which includes the palmaris brevis and the skin over the hypothenar eminence. The superficial branch of the nerve continues and divides into the common palmar digital nerves, which divide distally to form the proper digital nerves to the ulnar side of the fifth finger and the adjacent sides of the fifth and fourth fingers.

Together with the ulnar artery, the ulnar nerve passes into the wrist on the radial side of the pisiform bone via an anatomic space first described in 1861.[6] This space, the loge or canal of Guyon, is a 4-cm-long channel located between the pisiform carpal bone and the hook of the hamate.[7] The anatomy of this small space is complex.

Within the loge of Guyon, the ulnar nerve bifurcates into deep (motor) and superficial (sensory) branches. In 1969, Shea and McClain divided the canal of Guyon into three anatomic zones based on the landmarks of bifurcation.[3] Zone I represents that part of the canal that contains the ulnar nerve prior to its division into its component motor and sensory branches. Zone II is that part of the tunnel encompassing the deep motor branch distal to the bifurcation of the nerve. The sensory branch of the ulnar nerve travels through zone III of the loge of Guyon.[6] These anatomic divisions allow a more precise localization of lesions within the wrist. Lesions at the wrist, whether mass lesions, anatomic abnormalities, traumatic injuries, or ulnar artery disorders, may produce a predictable set of complaints and physical findings, depending on the level of impingement within Guyon's canal.

CLINICAL PRESENTATION

Patients exhibiting ulnar nerve compression at the level of the wrist typically present complaining of wrist pain that radiates into the ulnar two digits.[6] Patients should be asked about a history of previous falls onto an outstretched hand, which may have resulted in an occult hamate fracture. A fracture here may impinge on the nerve as it passes through zone I or zone II (or both) of Guyon's canal. Fractures of the hook of the hamate have been reported to account for 14% of all cases of ulnar nerve compression in the wrist.[3]

Patients should also be asked about repetitive trauma in both vocational and avocational settings. Repeated blows to the ulnar side of the hand and use of pneumatic tools have been implicated as potential causes of ulnar neuropathy at the wrist. Holding the wrist in forced hyperextension during such activities as bicycling may also predispose to this condition.[3] Interestingly, each of these activities has been mentioned as a cause for other painful wrist syndromes, which are discussed elsewhere in this chapter.

Physical examination of a patient complaining of a painful wrist and hand begins at the neck.[5,6] Painful or limited range of motion may suggest the presence of cervical disc disease. This should be followed by axial compression of the cervical spine, which may elicit radiculopathic pain from a compressed nerve root.

The elbow must be examined for evidence of swelling or deformity, inflammation, or masses. The ulnar nerve should be carefully palpated and percussed to assess for the presence of increased irritability. Identification of a focal site of irritation must then be compared with the opposite extremity; nearly one-fourth of normal subjects exhibited a positive Tinel's sign on percussion of the ulnar nerve.[5]

A careful assessment of the wrist and hand can help identify the level and, possibly, the exact location of an ulnar neuropathy.[6] Examination of the wrist and hands has five main components: localization of point tenderness, examination of the vascular supply, provocative testing of the nerve supply, and sensory and motor testing.[3]

Fractures of the hook of the hamate are a frequent cause of ulnar neuropathy at the loge of Guyon. They are the most common reason for symptoms from zones I and II when there is a history of trauma. Eliciting tenderness with careful palpation may indicate an occult new fracture or a poorly healed old fracture.

A determination of the patency of the ulnar artery is the second part of a focused examination of the wrist and hand. An Allen test performed on both hands will help the clinician to ascertain ulnar artery contribution to hand perfusion. The artery should also be palpated for the presence of tenderness, aneurysmal dilatation, and thrills. Arterial thrombosis or aneurysms can cause localized pressure on the ulnar nerve within Guyon's canal. Ulnar artery thrombosis has been reported as the most common cause of isolated sensory symptoms from ulnar nerve compression.[3]

Provocative testing of the ulnar nerve supply to the hand is accomplished by performing both the Tinel and Phalen tests. Percussion of the ulnar nerve at the level of Guyon's canal may elicit paresthesias to the fifth digit and the ulnar half of the fourth digit. Similarly, paresthesias in the distribution just described may result from having the patient allow his or her wrists to fall into complete volar flexion. This is considered a positive Phalen's sign.[1]

The sensory and motor examination of the hand should focus on identification, where possible, of the level of the ulnar nerve lesion. For example, impaired sensation to the ulnar dorsum of the hand (both light touch and two-point discrimination) is suggestive of an ulnar nerve lesion proximal to the wrist. Weakness to the FDP muscles of the fourth and fifth digits is similarly suggestive of more proximal compression.

Nerve compression within zone I of Guyon's canal will usually present with mixed motor and sensory findings.[3,6] Patients will exhibit weakness of the ulnar-innervated muscles in the hand, and will manifest sensory deficits to the palmar surface of the hypothenar eminence and to the ulnar two digits of the hand.

Zone II compression of the ulnar nerve results in motor branch paresis of the ulnar nerve. Wasting of the intrinsic muscles of the hand in the first dorsal interosseous space is evidence of chronic motor branch neuropathy. Further evidence of motor branch weakness can be elicited by asking the patient to extend his or her fingers. A distal ulnar neuropathy will result in a severe claw hand deformity.[6] The long flexor muscles flex the distal interphalangeal and proximal interphalangeal joints of the fourth and fifth digits. The long extensor muscles hyperextend the metacarpophalangeal joints of the same digits. The loss of intrinsic muscle function to the hand, however, results in an inability to maintain extension of the digits at the distal interphalangeal and proximal interphalangeal joints.[1]

Wartenberg's sign, an inability to abduct the fifth finger while holding the digits of the hand in extension, may be present with ulnar motor weakness. This is less likely to be present, however, with an isolated zone II injury, because the motor branch to the abductor digiti minimi exits prior to this portion of the canal. Interosseous muscle function can be evaluated by asking the patient to cross the index and middle fingers. This test is known as the Scott Earle test. Froment's sign is present when the adductor pollicis muscle, innervated by the ulnar nerve, is weak. This sign is elicited by having the patient tightly hold a piece of paper between the thumb and the radial side of the index finger. The examiner then attempts to pull the paper from the patient. Flexion at the thumb interphalangeal joint (indicating weakness of the adductor pollicis muscle) results in a positive Froment sign. Comparison with the patient's other hand should be performed.[1,5]

Injuries or compression of the ulnar nerve in zone III of Guyon's canal involves the superficial sensory branch of the nerve. Of the three zones of the canal, this is the least likely to exhibit pathology.[6]

DIFFERENTIAL DIAGNOSIS

Lesions at any location along the length of the ulnar nerve or the nerve roots from which it arises may be responsible for symptoms of wrist or hand pain. More proximal lesions, such as cervical disc disease affecting the C8 or T1 nerve roots, must be considered. (Evaluation of the cervical spine has already been described). Identification of painful and/or limited cervical motion merits further study to rule in or rule out a lesion at this level as the cause for a patient's symptoms.

Brachial plexus pathology may also be responsible for symptoms in the distribution of the ulnar nerve. Pancoast's tumor, an apical tumor of the lung, can exert pressure on or grow into the brachial plexus, resulting in symptoms distant from the primary site.[5] A careful examination would, therefore, include palpation of the supraclavicular region of the affected extremity for mass lesions. And, if clinical suspicion warrants, a posteroanterior (PA) and lateral radiograph of the chest should be ordered.

Thoracic outlet syndrome may also result in a brachial plexopathy. The diagnosis of this entity may be made by provocative testing. One such maneuver is the so-called hands-up test, in which the patient is asked to make a fist and then abduct the shoulder to 90 degrees and externally rotate the upper extremity. In the presence of thoracic outlet syndrome, this activity can trigger and reproduce the patient's symptoms.[7]

Distal median nerve function and the presence of an associated carpal tunnel syndrome must be excluded when examining a patient with complaints in the distribution of the ulnar nerve.

Whereas the most common cause for ulnar nerve compression lies at the cubital tunnel of the elbow, within the wrist itself it is the presence of a ganglion that accounts for the majority of atraumatic ulnar neuropathy.[4,6] Bednar[3] reported that, in the absence of trauma, 86% of patients presenting with a combined motor and sensory finding had a ganglion compressing the nerve. Anomalous muscle bellies and other anatomic variants, including lipomas, giant cell tumors, schwannomas, thickened ligaments, bipartite hamuli, and pisiform-hamate coalitions constitute another large class of entities responsible for ulnar nerve compression at the wrist.[3] It is unlikely, however, that a precise diagnosis of one of the aforementioned causes would be made in the emergency department.

Hamate fractures, ulnar artery thrombosis, repetitive trauma neuropathies (hypothenar hammer syndrome), and rheumatoid tenosynovitis are other potential causes of ulnar nerve compression. The presence of other joints affected by rheumatoid arthritis may help identify this disease as a potential cause of ulnar nerve compression at the wrist.[3]

EMERGENCY DEPARTMENT EVALUATION

The diagnosis of ulnar nerve compression at the wrist is usually made with a history and physical examination. Radiographs of the wrist may prove valuable for identifying the presence of a hamate fracture or malunion. A history of trauma, recent or remote, coupled with bony point tenderness should raise the clinician's index of suspicion. Special views of the wrist or tomograms may provide additional confirmatory evidence if initial plain films do not reveal a fracture.

Complaints referable to the elbow or to the cervical spine also merit obtaining radiographs of each of these structures. Similarly a PA and lateral chest radiograph should be obtained if one is at all concerned about the possibility of an intrathoracic mass lesion causing a brachial plexus neuropathy. It is unlikely that additional laboratory studies, in the absence of supporting clinical signs or symptoms, will provide useful information in the diagnosis of this entity.

EMERGENCY DEPARTMENT MANAGEMENT

The treatment of ulnar nerve compression at the wrist may be initiated in the emergency department. As with other compressive neuropathy syndromes, in the absence of an identifiable cause, a trial period of 1 to 3 months of nonoperative intervention is recommended.[3] The application of a wrist splint, avoidance of activities that aggravate symptoms, and use of nonsteroidal anti-inflammatories have been advocated.[6] Depending on the underlying cause of the neuropathy, symptoms may or may not resolve during this time. Referral for an outpatient workup by a hand surgeon is also the responsibility of the emergency department physician, and should be arranged prior to the patient's departure. For those patients who present with an identifiable cause for their symptoms, a more urgent follow-up is indicated.

DISPOSITION

Outpatient workup of ulnar nerve compression falls under the purview of the hand surgeon, who may obtain electromyographic and nerve conduction studies.[6] These studies are valuable in establishing a diagnosis. Inasmuch as the majority of causes of ulnar nerve compression neuropathy at the wrist are due to anatomic pathology, treatment for this condition is usually surgical.[2]

COMMON PITFALLS

- Perform a thorough physical examination on both upper extremities, as some abnormal findings may be physiologic and not pathologic. Comparing one side to the other is also a good technique to identify subtle pathology.
- Examine the entire course of the ulnar nerve from its origin at the nerve roots of the cervical spine to its distal end point in the digits of the hand. Ulnar neuropathy may be due to compressive forces at one or more locations along the length of the nerve.
- Consider anomalous innervations of the hand and perform a thorough evaluation of both ulnar and median nerve function to identify potential pathology.
- Remember that the most common cause of compressive ulnar neuropathy at the wrist is atraumatic anatomic pathology, which is probably most amenable to surgical repair. The most common traumatic cause of ulnar nerve compression at the wrist is fractures of the hook of the hamate.
- Examination of the painful wrist and hand involves five main components: localization of point tenderness, examination of the vascular supply, provocative testing of the nerve supply, and sensory and motor testing.

References

1. American Society for Surgery of the Hand. *The hand: Examination and diagnosis*, 3rd ed. New York, Churchill Livingstone, 1990.
2. American Society for Surgery of the Hand. *The hand: Primary care of common problems*, 2nd ed. New York, Churchill Livingstone, 1990.
3. Bednar MS. Ulnar tunnel syndrome. *Hand Clin* 1996;12(4):657–664.
4. Bozentka DJ. Cubital tunnel syndrome pathophysiology. *Clin Orthop Rel Res* 1998;351:90–94.
5. Idler RS. General principles of patient evaluation and nonoperative management of cubital tunnel syndrome. *Hand Clin* 1996;12(2):397–403.
6. Khoo D, Carmichael SW, Spinner RJ. Ulnar nerve anatomy and compression. *Orthop Clin North Am* 1996;27(2):317–338.
7. Tetro AM, Pichora DR. Cubital tunnel syndrome and the painful upper extremity. *Hand Clin* 1996;12(4):665–677.

THE HYPOTHENAR HAMMER SYNDROME

In 1934, a classic report provided the basis for the definition of the hypothenar hammer syndrome (HHS): evidence of distal ulnar artery injury following a history of trauma to the palm.[3] The distal ulnar artery lies most exposed to potential trauma at the base of the hypothenar eminence, just distal to the volar carpal ligament. At this location, the artery is no longer protected within Guyon's canal and is covered only by skin, subcutaneous fat, and (in 85% of the population) the palmaris brevis muscle.[3] Given its susceptible position, the ulnar artery is easily compressed between hard objects and the hook of the hamate.[4,5] This can occur any time that the hypothenar aspect of the base of the palm is subjected to trauma.

HHS is most commonly seen in those individuals who use the palms of their hands to push, pound, or hammer as part of their daily work activities.[4,6] Metal workers, automobile mechanics, lathe operators, and machinists are all at risk. The prevalence of HHS among carpenters has been reported to be as high as 14%.[5] This syndrome has also been found in workers who regularly use high-speed hand-held vibratory tools,[4] such as air hammers, drills, chain saws, sanders, and impact wrenches. HHS is not, however, limited specifically to this population.

Injuries to the distal ulnar artery, not unlike those caused by industrial occupational trauma, have also been seen in athletes. Baseball catchers, racquet handlers (tennis, badminton, etc.), and martial artists have all been reported as having an increased risk for developing HHS.[3] The increasing popularity of mountain biking has led to the discovery that these athletes are also prone to developing injuries of the ulnar artery. Table 54.1 lists a variety of sports that have also been implicated as potential causes HHS.

Repetitive ulnar artery injury, whether from work or sport, can result in traumatic vasospasm, thrombosis, or aneurysm formation.[4–6] Various combinations of these lesions are also possible and can complicate both diagnosis and management. Prolonged distal ulnar or digital arterial vasospasm can occlude affected blood vessels. If the source of irritation is eliminated, however, vasospasm and occlusion are reversible phenomena and a normal arterial supply may be restored.[4]

More severe trauma to the ulnar artery can damage the internal elastic lamella, leading to formation of intraarterial thrombi.[3] Embolization of traumatized intima and thrombus cause digital ischemia by occluding the end arterial supply to the fingers.[4,6] Ischemia may also occur as a result of reflex vasospasm. Thrombosis involving the adventitia may affect periarterial sympathetic fibers, resulting in vasospasm that limits surrounding collateral circulation.[6]

TABLE 54.1. Sports Reported to Cause HHS[6]

Baseball	Softball
Badminton	Karate
Handball	Weight lifting
Football	Hockey
Frisbee	Mountain biking

True palmar aneurysms may develop if the media of the arterial wall is damaged primarily.[4]

CLINICAL PRESENTATION

HHS is a treatable cause of digital ischemia that should be considered in the differential diagnosis of patients presenting with complaints of symptomatic digital ischemia.[5] As described earlier, the patient is classically a male laborer with a history of blunt trauma to his dominant hand.[4,5] Clinical findings in HHS include a male predominance, unilateral hand involvement, and acute onset of pain, followed by the more gradual development of a severe Raynaud's phenomenon (i.e., increased sensitivity of the digits to exposure to cold).[3] In a patient exhibiting Raynaud's phenomenon, coldness in the fingers of the dominant hand without a history of triphasic color changes and a lack of thumb involvement is highly suggestive of a diagnosis of HHS.[5]

The most typical occupational history of a patient with HHS includes frequent, repetitive, but comparatively minor hypothenar trauma. The daily trauma may be so much a part of the patient's regular activities that it goes unrecognized or is otherwise ignored. Careful inquiry about work and recreation is mandatory.[5]

At presentation, a patient may complain of one or more episodes of acute, lancinating pain over the hypothenar eminence that occur after striking a blow with the palm of the hand.[4] This pain typically radiates into the fourth and fifth fingers, and a dull, aching hypothenar pain may then ensue. Other patients describe an immediate pain episode that resolves completely over time. Then, days to weeks to months afterward, ischemic finger symptoms develop as a consequence of a slowly progressing thrombosis of the ulnar artery.[6]

Physical findings in HHS are largely localized to the hypothenar eminence and the digits of the affected hand. Prominent calluses over the hypothenar eminence provide a clue about recurrent trauma to this area.[5] Moreover, tenderness to palpation over the hypothenar area may indicate the presence of an ulnar artery aneurysm. Further examination may reveal the fingers or fingertips to be cold, pale, mottled, atrophic, or ulcerated.[4,5] The Allen test should be performed as part of the physical examination. A positive test suggests that either the superficial volar arch is incompletely developed or, as in the case of HHS, that the distal ulnar artery is occluded or stenotic.[4]

DIFFERENTIAL DIAGNOSIS

Many conditions are known to cause ischemia of the upper extremity. Collagen vascular diseases and various vasculitides and coagulopathies may each result in poor perfusion of the hand and fingers.[4] These disorders, however, tend to be systemic and have more generalized findings than does HHS.

Buerger disease (thromboangiitis obliterans), like HHS, affects primarily young males. Raynaud's phenomenon and hand or digital pain are historic features shared by these two conditions. The upper extremity examination of a patient with Buerger disease may be indistinguishable from someone with HHS, including an absent or diminished ulnar pulse.

Two elements may be helpful in differentiating one condition from the other. Buerger disease is found almost exclusively in cigarette smokers. Conversely, tobacco use is not a prerequisite for the development of HHS. Buerger disease is often a systemic condition involving not only the upper extremities, but also the lower ones. HHS is confined to the upper extremity only and is most often unilateral in its presentation. In the absence of clarifying historic or physical features, referral for arteriography or, potentially, arterial biopsy may be required to confirm or rule out the diagnosis of Buerger disease.

High-speed hand-held vibratory tools are known to cause both HHS and the hand–arm vibration syndrome (HAVS). Whereas both of these conditions can result in Raynaud's phenomenon of the digits of the dominant hand, the underlying pathology is different. HHS is caused by ulnar artery injury and may be differentiated from HAVS by a careful history and vascular examination at the patient's wrist.[5]

EMERGENCY DEPARTMENT EVALUATION

The emergency physician must not forget to obtain both a vocational and an avocational history from a patient presenting with complaints of hand and wrist pain. While the history will often lead the clinician to the proper diagnosis, a thoughtful and deliberate physical examination is also necessary. Performing and documenting the results of the Allen test is an important part of the physical examination. The modified Allen test is performed with the patient in a seated position. The hands, palms facing up, should be resting on the knees. The clinician then compresses the radial artery with one thumb and the ulnar artery with the other thumb, thereby externally occluding the arterial supply to the hand. The patient next rapidly clenches and opens the first several times to exsanguinate the palm. If there is pathology in the ulnar artery, the palm will remain pallid after the clinician releases his or her thumb from that vessel. Blood supply will return to the palm only after the pressure on the radial artery is removed. A pencil Doppler instrument may be used in conjunction with the Allen test to confirm the patency of the arterial blood supply to the hand.[1,5] This examination should be performed at both wrists.

EMERGENCY DEPARTMENT MANAGEMENT

Most patients with HHS will respond to proper therapy when promptly initiated. The emergency physician should therefore begin treatment after making the diagnosis of this condition. At a minimum, local wound care of necrotic or ulcerated digits can take place in the emergency department. Additional conservative measures that may be offered include counseling on the avoidance of cold environments and cessation of smoking,[5] because both will exacerbate HHS. Patients should be encouraged to wear mittens or gloves to help keep their hands and fingers warm and protected.

Aspirin and a calcium channel blocker (diltiazem or nifedipine) may be prescribed and are considered appropriate initial therapeutic agents.[3] With proper therapeutic intervention, the prognosis for HHS is good, and surgery is generally not indicated. Patients need to understand, however, that response to therapy is predicated on the elimination of the underlying trauma source. In some instances, this may require a change of occupation.[5]

DISPOSITION

Referral to a hand surgeon for angiographic studies and ongoing management is proper and necessary. Arteriography can reveal ulnar artery irregularity or aneurysms. Occlusion of the ulnar artery segment overlying the hook of the hamate is considered pathognomonic of HHS.[5] Multiple digital artery occlusions, secondary to embolization, may also be seen.

Conservative, nonsurgical modalities are favored for the treatment of HHS, except in the case of ulnar artery aneurysm. In this instance, resection of the aneurysm is performed in order to avoid or prevent further digital embolization.[3] Surgical repair is still the preferred method of treatment for this condition.[7]

COMMON PITFALLS

- Manual laborers presenting with pain to the dominant hand need a careful historic review of their daily occupational activities in order to establish a history of regular hypothenar trauma. Identification of calluses over the hypothenar eminence can provide a clue to this history.
- Recall that some athletes and even people who use canes or walkers are susceptible to ulnar artery trauma.
- Buerger disease is an important part of the differential diagnosis of HHS and must be ruled out. Angiography or arterial biopsy may be required to make the diagnosis. An important clinical clue is that Buerger disease tends to be a systemic condition and will involve both upper extremities.
- An occluded ulnar arterial supply to the hand (given the proper clinical history) is very highly suggestive of the diagnosis of HHS.
- HHS is a treatable condition, provided that the source of trauma is eliminated. The emergency department physician must introduce and then reinforce this concept once the diagnosis of HHS is made.

References

1. American Society for Surgery of the Hand. *The hand: Examination and diagnosis*, 3rd ed. New York, Churchill Livingstone, 1990.
2. American Society for Surgery of the Hand. *The hand: Primary care of common problems*, 2nd ed. New York, Churchill Livingstone, 1990.
3. Applegate KE, Spiegel PK. Ulnar artery occlusion in mountain bikers. *J Sports Med Phys Fitness* 1995;35:232–234.
4. Conn J, Bergan JJ, Bell JL. Hypothenar hammer syndrome: posttraumatic digital ischemia. *Surgery* 1970;68(6):1122–1128.
5. Duncan WC. Hypothenar hammer syndrome: an uncommon cause of digital ischemia. *J Am Acad Dermatol* 1996;34(5):880–883.
6. Müller LP, Rudig L, Kreitner K-F, et al. Hypothenar hammer syndrome in sports. *Knee Surg Sports Traumatol Arthrosc* 1996;4:167–170.
7. Wheatley MJ, Marx MV. The use of intra-arterial urokinase in the management of hand ischemia secondary to palmar and digital arterial occlusion. *Ann Plast Surg* 1996;37(4):356–363.

DE QUERVAIN'S TENOSYNOVITIS/ DE QUERVAIN SYNDROME

De Quervain's tenosynovitis, a not infrequent cause of wrist pain, is the most common tendinitis of the extensor tendons of the hand and wrist.[2] De Quervain syndrome is a nonsuppurative tenosynovitis of the first dorsal compartment of the wrist.[6–9] The first dorsal compartment, like the other dorsal compartments of the wrist, is a "tunnel" through which the tendons of the hand's extrinsic extensor muscles pass.

The first dorsal compartment of the wrist overlies the styloid process of the radius. This compartment contains the tendons of the abductor pollicis longus (APL) and the extensor pollicis brevis (EPB).[7] The APL tendon inserts at the base of the dorsum of the thumb's metacarpal, and the EPB tendon inserts at the base of the thumb's proximal phalanx. At the level of the wrist, these tendons and their synovial sheaths lie sandwiched between the carpal bones and a fibrous band called the dorsal (extensor) retinaculum.

Typically the extrinsic tendons of the wrist glide easily through the fibroosseous canals defined by the carpal bones on one side and the extensor retinaculum on the other. The APL and EPB work in tandem to hold the thumb in abduction.[7] De Quervain syndrome represents a derangement in the normal gliding of the APL and/or the EPB tendons and, therefore, an impairment in thumb abduction.

Several hypotheses exist as to the underlying cause of de Quervain's tenosynovitis. Authors suggest that de Quervain syndrome is due to a myxoid degeneration of the tendon sheaths of the first dorsal compartment.[3]

TABLE 54.2. Vocational and Avocational Causes of de Quervain's Tenosynovitis[7]

Working at a typewriter or adding machine
Excessive writing
Washing or wringing clothes
Chopping wood
Cutting cloth with heavy scissors
Sewing, knitting, weaving
Working on a grinder or buffing machine
Fitting rubber rings over a pipe
Operating machine keyboards, sewing machines, lathes, drills, presses, grinders, and switchboards
Prolonged piano playing
Playing a reed instrument and supporting its weight on the right thumb

Chronic inflammation resulting from overuse is another postulated cause of this syndrome. According to this theory, overuse of sheathed tendons leads to a failure of inherent lubrication mechanisms.[4] Over time, friction between tendons and their synovial sheaths causes inflammatory changes in these structures. The tendon hypertrophies and the intrinsic diameter of the sheath narrows in response to inflammation. This further impedes the smooth gliding of the tendon through its synovial sheath.

A third theory explaining the pathophysiology of de Quervain's tenosynovitis identifies the condition to be the result of thickening of the extensor retinaculum overlying the first dorsal compartment.[7]

Despite various pathophysiologic theories, nearly all authors agree as to the etiology of de Quervain syndrome. Persistent repetition of specific tasks beyond the point of fatigue is commonly implicated.[7] These tasks frequently involve repeated pronation and supination of the forearm combined with forceful exertion of the thumb.

Other reported activities that can lead to a tenosynovitis of the first dorsal compartment include performing tasks that may be new or unfamiliar to the patient. Many patients begin to have symptoms within days of starting a new job or resuming an old one after a holiday.[5,7] Table 54.2 lists jobs and activities previously reported to result in de Quervain's syndrome. Minor blunt trauma and rheumatoid arthritis have also been identified as possible causes of de Quervain syndrome.

CLINICAL PRESENTATION

Pain at the radial styloid is a classic and defining symptom of de Quervain's tenosynovitis. Although the pain is more or less constant, it is exacerbated by thumb abduction, ulnar deviation of the wrist, and simple grasping. Holding the thumb at rest, in contrast, may offer only minimal relief. Previous trials of nonsteroidal antiinflammatory drugs or acetaminophen use tend to provide little, if any, symptomatic relief.

The pain, usually described by patients as severe in quality, has also been reported as a "stiffness."[7] In more advanced cases, patients may also note swelling and crepitus at the site of maximal pain. Pain can radiate proximally into the forearm or distally to the thumb. Occasionally, the pain may be so intense that sleep is disturbed. Other patients may complain of weakness or an inability to use the affected hand due to debilitating pain.

Another hallmark of de Quervain syndrome is a history of gradual onset of pain in the absence of fracture or acute trauma.[7] De Quervain syndrome typically affects women more than men (approximately 10 to 1) between the ages of 35 and 55.

Examination of the patient with de Quervain's tenosynovitis begins with a careful inspection of the forearm and wrist. Mild

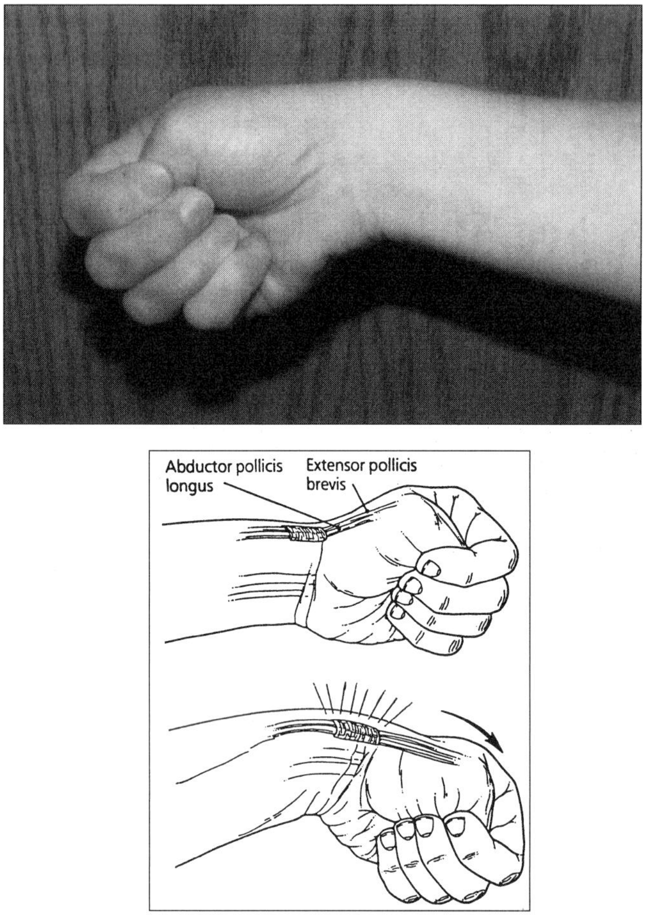

Figure 54.2. Finkelstein's test.

cases may exhibit only subtle, localized swelling at the radial styloid.[6,7] A more extensive fusiform swelling and, possibly, erythema can characterize more severe cases.

Palpation of the first dorsal compartment should be approached gently. Tenderness or crepitus at the radial styloid is highly suggestive of de Quervain syndrome.[8] A positive Finkelstein test, however, is diagnostic of this condition.[7] The Finkelstein test requires that the patient flex the thumb into the palm and then grasp it with the other fingers of the hand. The patient then actively ulnarly deviates the wrist[1] (Fig. 54.2). Severe, sharp pain (a positive test) is pathognomonic of tenosynovitis of the first dorsal compartment.[2,6] It is important to distinguish the sharp pain of de Quervain syndrome from a "pulling sensation" in the same anatomic distribution.[4] The latter is more indicative of a diagnosis of radial nerve entrapment, not tenosynovitis.

DIFFERENTIAL DIAGNOSIS

The superficial branch of the radial nerve crosses the APL and the EPB muscles in the distal forearm and then divides into terminal branches before entering the hand. The anterior terminal branch of the radial nerve, which provides sensation to the dorsum of the thumb, passes into the hand almost directly over the extensor retinaculum of the first dorsal compartment.[7] Radial nerve entrapment, therefore, should be ruled out of the differential diagnosis using the previously described technique.

Arthritis at the carpal–metacarpal (CMC) joint of the thumb is another differential diagnosis that may be excluded by the emergency department physician.[6] The pain in CMC arthritis is more accurately localized to the basal joint of the thumb, not to the first dorsal compartment. Moreover, the clinician can elicit or aggravate CMC arthritis pain by grinding the first metacarpal on the trapezium.[2] This procedure does not stretch the APL or EPB tendons and will therefore not cause pain in a patient with de Quervain syndrome. The clinician must also be alert to rule out fractures of the radial styloid, scaphoid, or trapezium.[6] A clinical history of trauma and plain film radiographs should suffice to include or exclude fractures from the diagnosis.

Intersection syndrome, another tenosynovitis of the radial extensor tendons, may be confused with de Quervain syndrome. Like de Quervain's tenosynovitis, intersection syndrome is a nonsuppurative process that develops after repeatedly performing a novel activity.[6] Patients will present complaining of radial wrist pain.

Examination of patients with intersection syndrome generally reveals swelling, pain, and crepitus in a more proximal and ulnar distribution than is seen in de Quervain syndrome.[6,9] Tenderness is localized not to the area of the radial styloid, but to the region where the radial wrist extensors of the second dorsal compartment and the tendons of the first dorsal compartment intersect.[5]

EMERGENCY DEPARTMENT EVALUATION

Diagnosis of de Quervain syndrome rests on obtaining a history of overuse of the thumb and eliciting a positive Finkelstein test. The medical literature reports no objective confirmatory electrodiagnostic tests or studies. Plain film radiographs in the absence of fracture or arthritis are usually nondiagnostic.[7]

EMERGENCY DEPARTMENT MANAGEMENT

Several methods exist for treating de Quervain's tenosynovitis. The least invasive techniques (rest, application of heat, and immobilization with a thumb spica splint) are, by themselves, ineffective for treating this condition.[6] They may be used, however, as adjunctive therapies to the mainstays of treatment: steroid injection and, when necessary, surgical release. Steroid injection into the tendon sheaths of the first dorsal compartment is an effective treatment for de Quervain syndrome that may be employed by the emergency department physician.

Between 70% and 80% of patients with de Quervain syndrome will respond to steroid injection.[5,9] One recent article cited a success rate of 84% after either one or two steroid injections into the first dorsal compartment.[8] Steroids may even be used alone without subsequent splinting or immobilization. Several studies have shown no advantage to using immobilization as a therapeutic modality after (or in the absence of) steroid injection.[7]

A corticosteroid preparation such as methylprednisolone acetate is a good choice for injection into the tendon sheath, as it tends to provide long-lasting relief. Approximately 2 cc of steroid should be drawn up and mixed in a syringe with 0.5 cc of lidocaine.[2] Using a 25- or 27-gauge needle helps minimize the pain of injection. Although techniques vary according to author, most agree that the needle should be passed through the skin at the distal end of the first dorsal compartment. One source suggests inserting the needle through the tendon sheath and tendon until it touches the radius.[6] As the needle is slowly withdrawn and as it exits the tendon, resistance will fall and the steroid–lidocaine mixture will easily be injected into the tendon sheath (Fig. 54.3). Forced injection of steroids into a tendon is not desirable.

A successful injection of the steroid–lidocaine mixture can be identified by the clinician feeling the medication track distally along the tendons. Immediate relief of pain (due to the presence of the lidocaine in the injected mixture) is also a good marker for accuracy of placement.[8] Patients need to be advised that it may take several days for the steroid to begin relieving their pain and

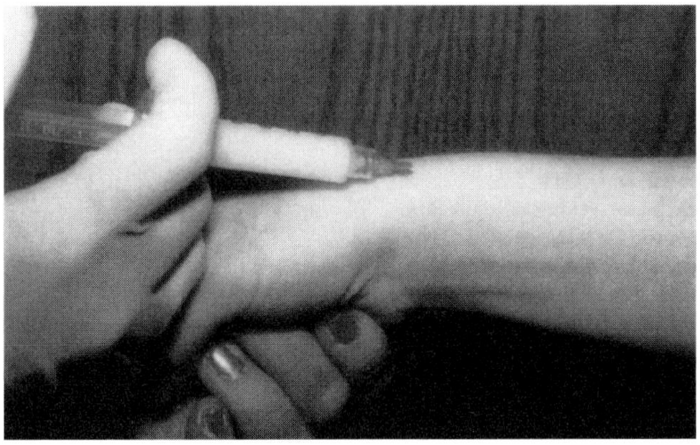

Figure 54.3. Corticosteroid injection into the tendon sheath.

References

1. American Society for Surgery of the Hand. *The hand: examination and diagnosis*, 3rd ed. New York, Churchill Livingstone, 1990.
2. American Society for Surgery of the Hand. *The hand: primary care of common problems*. 2nd ed. New York, Churchill Livingstone, 1990.
3. Clarke MT, Lyall HA, Grant JW, et al. The histopathology of de Quervain's disease. *J Hand Surg [Br]* 1998;23(6):732–734.
4. Goldman RH. Cumulative trauma syndrome: an occupational hazard. *Emerg Med* 1991;23(2):25–45.
5. Higgs PE, Mackinnon SE. Repetitive motion injuries. *Annu Rev Med* 1995;46:1–16.
6. Higgs PE, Young VL. Cumulative trauma disorders. *Clin Plast Surg* 1996;23(3):421–433.
7. Moore JS. De Quervain's tenosynovitis. *Occup Environ Med* 1997;39(10): 990–1002.
8. Rankin ME, Rankin EA. Injection therapy for management of stenosing tenosynovitis (de Quervain's disease) of the wrist. *Nat Med* 1998;90(8):474–476.
9. Zingas C, Failla JM, Van Holsbeck M. Injection accuracy and relief of de Quervain's tendinitis. *Hand Surg* 1998;23(1):89–96.

that, in the meantime, there is the possibility of a postinjection flare reaction. This painful phenomenon, sometimes seen after injection of steroids, is generally self-limited and usually resolves after a couple of days.

Failure of steroid injection to achieve a cure does occur in a small but significant percentage of those with de Quervain syndrome. These failures are believed to be due to the presence of a separate EPB compartment that is smaller and deeper than the APL compartment. If a patient has multiple sheaths within the first dorsal compartment but only one of them is injected, steroids are not likely to be effective in treating de Quervain syndrome.[6] Patients must be counseled about this possibility and advised to seek appropriate follow-up care with a hand surgeon if adequate relief is not achieved after one or two steroid injections. As a curative modality, surgery can also fail if the tendon sheath of the EPB compartment is not identified and released.

DISPOSITION

A referral to a hand surgeon is entirely appropriate when one considers that 20% to 30% of steroid injection attempts will not alleviate the pain of this condition.[6] Failure to achieve a cure after two or three injections over a 3- to 5-week period indicates the necessity for surgically releasing the stenotic tendon sheath or sheaths.[2] In general, surgically dividing the sheath(s) within the first dorsal compartment is a curative procedure.

Because multiple sheaths may lie within the compartment, the surgeon must carefully inspect this area to be certain that all sheaths have been released.

COMMON PITFALLS

- A positive Finkelstein test is virtually diagnostic for de Quervain's tenosynovitis.
- Fractures of the radial styloid and arthritis at the CMC joint of the thumb are two important differential diagnoses to be excluded. Radiographs and careful physical examination can help to rule out these possibilities.
- Radiographs in de Quervain syndrome are most likely to be normal or possibly reveal some soft-tissue swelling.
- Long-acting steroid combined with lidocaine is often curative and can be used in the emergency department to treat this condition. Patients should be warned about the possibility of postinjection flare reaction and the possibility of failure of this treatment.

CHAPTER 55
Hand Infections

Carl R. Chudnofsky

ESSENTIAL ANATOMY

The nail plate inserts into a depression on the dorsum of the finger called the proximal nail fold, which divides the proximal nail fold into superficial and deep epithelial surfaces called the dorsal roof and ventral floor, respectively. The eponychium, commonly called the cuticle, is a horny layer extension of the proximal nail fold that extends a short distance onto the dorsum of the nail. It seals the potential space between the nail plate and the proximal nail fold. Laterally, the proximal nail fold is continuous on either side with the lateral nail folds or paronychium. The soft tissue under the distal free edge of the nail is called the hyponychium (Fig. 55.1).[1]

The distal pulp space of a finger or thumb is composed of fat globules that are divided into small fascial compartments by 15 to 20 vertical fibrous septa (see Fig. 55.1). The presence of these compartments has a substantial impact on the pathophysiology and management of pulp space infections.

The flexor tendons are surrounded by a tendon sheath that is composed of an outer fibrous sheath and an inner synovial sheath. The inner synovial sheath has a visceral and parietal layer with a potential space between them. The tendon sheaths of the index, middle, and ring fingers extend from the midpalmar crease to just beyond the distal interphalangeal joints. The tendon sheath of the flexor pollicis longus tendon begins at the base of the distal phalanx of the thumb and extends to the pronator quadratus muscle in the wrist. Between the base of the thumb metacarpal and the wrist, the tendon sheath of the flexor pollicis longus tendon is called the radial bursa. The tendon sheath surrounding the flexor tendons of the little finger begins just distal to the distal interphalangeal joint and, like the tendon sheath of the flexor pollicis longus tendon, ends at the pronator quadratus muscle in the wrist. The ulnar bursa is that part of the tendon sheath between the fifth metacarpal and the pronator quadratus muscle (see Fig. 55.1). The radial and ulnar bursas communicate with each other in 50% to 80% of patients.[7,19]

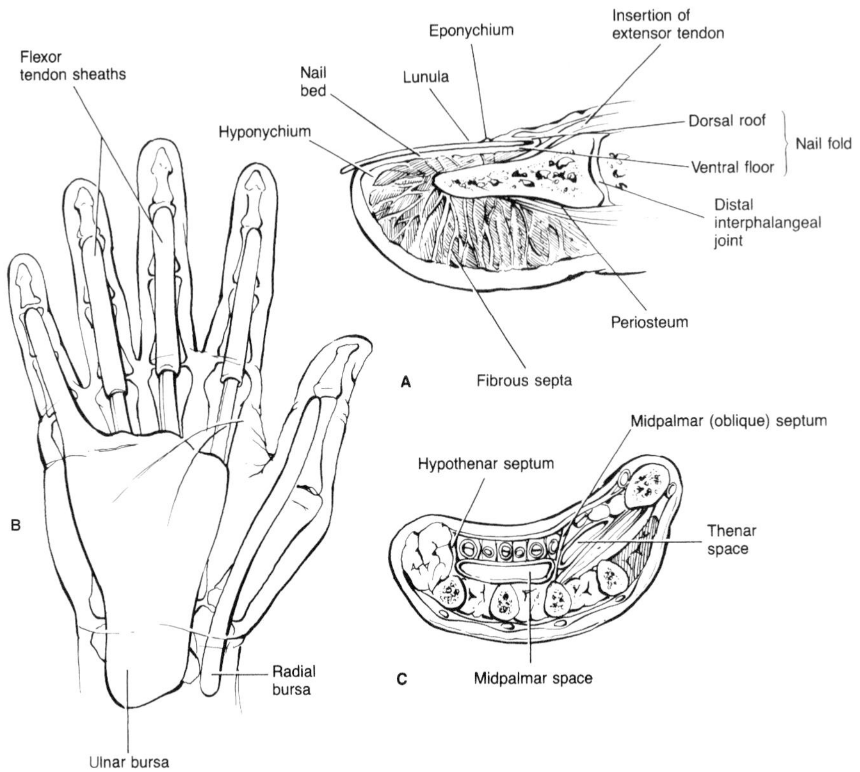

Figure 55.1. Anatomy. (**A**) Fingertip and nail bed. (**B**) Flexor tendon sheaths. (**C**) Deep palmar spaces.

The hand contains several fascial spaces that are potential sites of infection. The most frequently infected spaces are the deep palmar spaces, which include the thenar space, the midpalmar space, and the hypothenar space, and the web spaces (see Fig. 55.1). The thenar space is bounded on its ulnar side by the vertical septum between the third metacarpal and the long finger profundus and radially by the lateral edge of the adductor pollicis. The adductor pollicis also forms the dorsal roof of the compartment. The midpalmar space lies deep to the flexor tendons. Radially it is bordered by the vertical septum between the third metacarpal and the long finger profundus and ulnarly by the hypothenar muscles. The dorsal roof is formed by the fascia over the second and the third palmar interossei and the third and fourth metacarpals.[7] The hypothenar space contains the hypothenar muscles. It is bordered radially by a fibrous septum from the fifth metacarpal to the palmar fascia.[17]

MICROBIOLOGY

The majority of hand infections are caused by *Staphylococcus aureus* and *Streptococcus* species. Anaerobes, alone or in combination with aerobic bacteria, are seen in approximately 30% of all hand infections and in 40% of infections secondary to human bite or clenched-fist injury and intravenous drug abuse.[20] Gram-negative organisms are rare in normal hosts but are common in patients with diabetes mellitus or a depressed immune system.[15] Methicillin-resistant *S. aureus* is a frequent pathogen in intravenous drug abusers.[7] Polymicrobial infections are relatively common, particularly with infections caused by bite wounds and intravenous drug abuse.[20] Chronic hand infections may be caused by atypical mycobacteria, particularly *Mycobacterium marinum,* a common cause of hand infections occurring in aquatic environments.[8] Immunocompromised patients may be infected with a variety of fungi, including *Candida albicans,*[21] *Coccidioides immitis,*[10] and *Aspergillus flavus.*[11]

HISTORY AND PHYSICAL EXAMINATION

A careful and detailed history and physical examination are essential in the diagnosis and management of hand infections. Important historical information is listed in Table 55.1.

A history of trauma, especially penetrating trauma, is frequently obtained from patients with a hand infection. The type of trauma and the setting in which it occurred can provide valuable clues to the causative organism. For example, infections from injuries occurring at home or in industry are caused predominantly by gram-positive organisms.[7] Cat bites are commonly infected with *Pasteurella multocida,* while infected human bite wounds or clenched-fist injuries are frequently caused by *Eikenella corrodens* and other oral flora.[6,20] The progression of symptoms may also be helpful in determining the type of bacteria present. Streptococcal infections evolve over 24 to 48 hours and are more often associated with cellulitis and lymphangitis. In contrast, *S. aureus* is more likely to cause a suppurative infection that develops over 3 to 6 days. Chronic infections are more often due to fungi or atypical mycobacteria.[7] The nature and location of pain and swelling may be helpful in determining the location and severity of infection, while the duration of symptoms can be an important determinant of the need for surgical inter-

TABLE 55.1. Important Historical Information in Patients with a Hand Infection

Nature and setting of any preceding trauma
Progression of symptoms
Nature and location of local symptoms
Duration of symptoms before arrival
Associated extraextremity symptoms
Underlying medical problems
History of intravenous drug abuse
Current medications

vention. Associated symptoms may aid in gauging the severity of infection and the choice of initial antimicrobial therapy. For example, a urethral or endocervical discharge in a patient with a suspected flexor tenosynovitis suggests the possibility of disseminated gonorrhea.[18] Finally, the presence of underlying medical problems (e.g., diabetes mellitus, cancer, and acquired immunodeficiency syndrome [AIDS]), intravenous drug abuse, and the use of certain medications, particularly immunosuppressive agents, frequently have a significant impact on the diagnosis, treatment, and microbiology of hand infections.

On physical examination, the position of the hand and fingers at rest and the presence of any wounds or breaks in the continuity of the skin should be noted. The location and nature of any swelling, fluctuance, erythema, warmth, or tenderness should be carefully documented. The hand and individual digits should be put through a full range of motion. Any limitation or pain with movement should be clearly described. A thorough and well-documented neurovascular assessment is mandatory.

PARONYCHIA

Paronychia is an infection involving the lateral nail fold (paronychium). It is the most common infection of the hand.[17,22] It results from mechanical separation of the eponychium from the nail plate with subsequent invasion of bacteria or fungi.[15] Common causes of a paronychia include hangnails, manicuring, and nail biting.[7,19] Individuals whose hands are repeatedly submerged in water (e.g., dishwashers) seem to be particularly susceptible.[15] Extension of the infection to involve the adjacent eponychium and proximal nail fold is called an eponychia.[2,17]

CLINICAL PRESENTATION

Pain, swelling, and redness usually begin in the proximal portion of the lateral nail fold in the area adjacent to the eponychium. If ignored or untreated, it may extend to involve the onychium and proximal nail fold (i.e., eponychia) or, rarely, to the lateral nail fold on the opposite side (i.e., run-around infection).[2,17,19] The involved tissue is usually very tender. Fluctuance is generally present but may be absent early in the course of the infection. In severe infections, pus may extend beneath the nail. Large amounts of subungual pus may result in a floating nail. Systemic signs and symptoms such as fever or tachycardia are unusual.

DIFFERENTIAL DIAGNOSIS

The differential diagnosis of an acute paronychia includes herpetic whitlow, a chronic paronychia, and a felon. Herpetic whitlow is a viral infection caused by the herpes simplex virus. It can usually be differentiated from a paronychia by careful history and physical examination (see the section on herpetic whitlow). A chronic paronychia is a smoldering infection frequently caused by *C. albicans*. It is most common in diabetics and in middle-aged women whose hands are frequently exposed to water containing irritants or alkali.[17] Patients usually complain of a waxing and waning infection. Pain and tenderness are less severe in comparison to an acute paronychia.[16] A severe infection may be confused with a felon. However, rather than subungual pus or fluctuance of the nail folds, patients with a felon have tense swelling of the distal pulp space.

EMERGENCY DEPARTMENT EVALUATION

The diagnosis of a paronychia is made by history and physical examination. Radiographs may be useful in selected situations (e.g., trauma, suspicion of a foreign body) but are generally not helpful. Laboratory testing is unnecessary in the majority of patients.

EMERGENCY DEPARTMENT MANAGEMENT

If the diagnosis is made before the accumulation of pus, management is nonsurgical and includes an oral antimicrobial agent effective against *Staphylococcus* and *Streptococcus* species (Table 55.2) and warm soaks. Rest and elevation of the affected part are helpful adjuncts. Once fluctuance has been identified, however, surgical drainage must be performed. The method of drainage depends on the severity of the infection.

A digital block provides anesthesia for drainage. Local preparation includes cleansing the digit with povidone–iodine or a similar agent. Hemostasis is obtained by placing a 1-in. Penrose drain securely around the proximal portion of the affected digit.

Superficial infections are drained by inserting a no. 11 blade between the nail and eponychium. The eponychium is lifted away from the nail to drain the pus (Fig. 55.2). If necessary, the blade can then be swept around to incise the lateral nail fold. The incision should be made tangential to the dorsolateral curve of the nail, with the blade directed away from the nail bed and nail matrix to avoid injury to these structures. After drainage, a small gauze wick should be inserted between the eponychium and nail to facilitate continued drainage.

If pus is present under the adjacent portion of the nail, one-fourth of the nail on that side should be removed for adequate drainage to occur (see Fig. 55.2).[7,19,22] The portion of nail to be removed is first separated from the underlying nail bed by inserting a small hemostat or iris scissors beneath the distal free edge of the nail and gently opening and closing the instrument as it is worked proximally toward the eponychium. Once separated, an iris scissors is used to cut longitudinally along the nail from the distal edge to the eponychium. The nail is then gently removed with the aid of a Kelly clamp. If this does not allow complete drainage of pus, an incision can be made into the lateral nail fold as previously described. A gauze wick is inserted to promote drainage.

If pus is discovered under the dorsal roof of the proximal nail fold or beneath the nail in the nail fold, or if the patient presents with a floating nail, drainage requires removal of the proximal one-third of the nail.[7,17,19,22] However, controversy exists as to whether incision of the eponychial tissue is necessary for adequate drainage.

If the infection involves the eponychium and one lateral nail fold (in addition to pus under the dorsal roof or nail root), some authors recommend making a single incision starting at the midpoint of the lateral nail fold and extending it proximally to the base of the nail.[16,17] The eponychial tissue and lateral nail fold are bluntly elevated from the nail, and the proximal one-third of the nail is removed (Fig. 55.3) If a run-around infection is present, Neviaser[24] and Siegel and Gelberman[26] recommend making an incision in each lateral nail fold as just described. The entire eponychium is gently elevated as a flap to expose the underlying nail root, and the proximal one-third of the nail is excised using iris scissors (see Fig. 55.3).[17,19] In contrast, Zook[29] maintains that it is not necessary to make incisions in the eponychium. He agrees that the proximal portion of the nail must be removed, but argues that an incision in the eponychium will frequently not heal primarily in the face of infection and may result in a notch or square corner in the

TABLE 55.2. Recommendations for Initial Antimicrobial Therapy of Hand Infections[a]

Infection	Initial Antimicrobial Therapy[b]	Comments
Felon/paronychia	Cephalexin 500 mg PO q.i.d. for 7 days	Cefazolin should be used for admitted patients.
Severe infections[c]	Cefazolin 1 g i.v., and penicillin G 2 million units i.v.	Ceftriaxone 1 g i.v. is given for flexor tenosynovitis due to disseminated gonorrhea.
Diabetic/immuno-compromised patients	Cefazolin 1 g i.v., and penicillin G 2 million units i.v., and gentamicin 1.0 mg/kg i.v., or aztreonam 12 g i.v.	High incidence of gram-negative organisms
Intravenous drug abuser	Cefazolin 1 g i.v., and vancomycin 1 g i.v.	High incidence of methicillin-resistant *Staphylococcus aureus*
Herpetic whitlow	None	Consider acyclovir for suppression of recurrent attacks and for severe infection in immunocompromised patients.

[a]Agents or a combination of agents with similar coverage may be substituted. Alternatives for penicillin- and/or cephalosporin-allergic patients are discussed in the text.
[b]Initial antimicrobial therapy should be adjusted as the results of culture and sensitivity tests become available.
[c]Flexor tenosynovitis, web space abscess, and palmar space infection.

eponychium. Unfortunately, there are few scientific data regarding the optimal approach. If a floating nail is present, incision of the eponychia tissue is probably unnecessary because removal of the nail can be easily performed by pushing back the lateral nail fold and excising the loose nail (see Fig. 55.3). However, if the nail is partially adherent it may be difficult to remove the proximal portion without incising one or both sides of the eponychium. Regardless of which technique is used, after removal of the proximal portion of the nail, a gauze wick should be placed between the eponychium and exposed nail to prevent adhesion of the eponychium to the nail bed and to facilitate continued drainage.

DISPOSITION

The majority of patients with a paronychia may be discharged from the emergency department. The affected digit should be

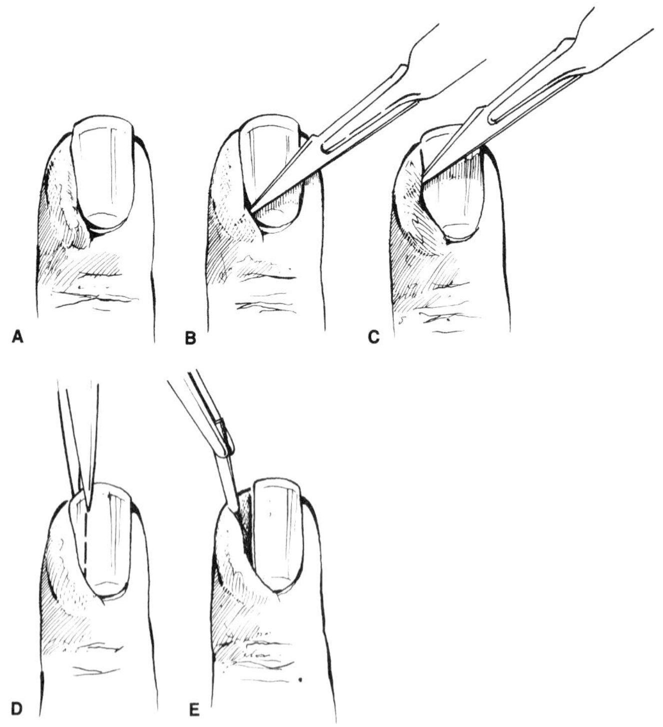

Figure 55.2. Drainage of a paronychia. **(A)** Superficial paronychia. **(B)** Elevation of the eponychia using a no. 11 blade. **(C)** If necessary, the lateral nail fold may be incised to achieve adequate drainage. **(D)** A more extensive paronychia with pus extending under the adjacent portion of the nail. **(E)** Removal of the adjacent one-fourth of the nail to drain the subungual pus. If removal of the nail does not allow complete drainage, the lateral nail fold may be incised as in **(C)**.

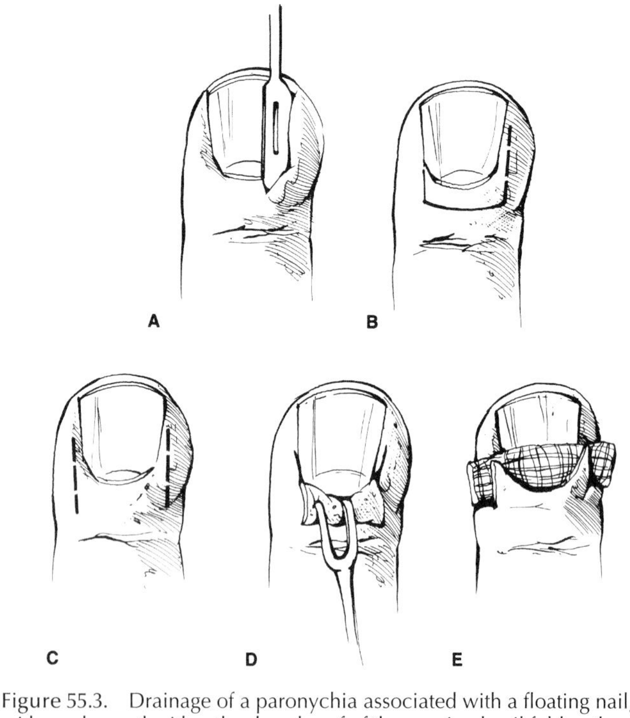

Figure 55.3. Drainage of a paronychia associated with a floating nail, or with pus beneath either the dorsal roof of the proximal nail fold or the nail within the proximal nail fold. **(A)** Elevation of the eponychial fold with a flat probe to expose the base of the nail for excision of a floating nail. **(B)** Placement of an incision to drain the eponychium and lateral nail fold and to elevate the eponychial fold for excision of the proximal one-third of the nail. **(C–E)** Incisions and procedure for elevating the entire eponychial fold for excision of the proximal one-third of the nail. A gauze pack prevents premature closure of the cavity. (Redrawn from Neviaser RJ. Infections. In: Green DP, ed. *Operative hand surgery,* 3rd ed. New York: Churchill Livingstone, 1993:1023.)

kept clean and dry. Elevation should be stressed to help diminish pain and swelling. Patients with a small superficial paronychia should be rechecked at 24 hours. At this time, the gauze wick is removed and the patient is started on warm soaks. For larger, more extensive infections, the drain should remain in place for 48 to 72 hours before beginning warm soaks.[17] An oral antimicrobial agent effective against *S. aureus* and *Streptococcus* species is indicated if there is surrounding cellulitis (see Table 55.2). The need for admission is rare, but it should be considered for those patients who have an extensive surrounding cellulitis or lymphangitis, particularly in high-risk individuals such as diabetics, those on immunosuppressive agents, and patients with AIDS. Consultation with a hand surgeon is recommended for all high-risk patients presenting with a severe infection.

COMMON PITFALLS

- Failure to recognize the need for surgical drainage. If the presence of pus is suspected, drainage should be performed.
- Failure to remove the adjacent portion of the nail when subungual pus is present. If this is not done, adequate drainage may not occur.
- Failure to place a wick between the eponychium and nail plate after drainage. This may result in reaccumulation of pus and, if the proximal portion of the nail was removed, adhesions between the aponychium and underlying nail bed.

FELON

A felon is an infection of the distal pulp space of a finger or thumb. It occurs more commonly in the right hand, with the thumb and index finger most frequently affected.[15] The infection frequently results from a puncture wound to the tip of the digit. A subcutaneous abscess rapidly forms in the pulp space, breaking down the fibrous septa as it expands. If left untreated, the infection may extend to the distal phalanx, causing osteomyelitis, or to the skin, resulting in necrosis and a draining sinus on the volar surface of the fingertip.[17] Moreover, because the fibrous septa create a closed space within the fingertip, pressure from the expanding abscess and associated edema can lead to ischemia of the pulp space and, ultimately, slough of the tactile portion of the finger pad.

CLINICAL PRESENTATION

The patient with a felon typically presents with a red, swollen, and painful fingertip. There is a history of penetrating trauma in approximately two-thirds of cases, but this is not necessary to make the diagnosis.[16] Early in the course of the infection, the patient usually complains of an aching pain that increases when pressure is applied to the fingertip. The pain rapidly becomes severe and throbbing. Systemic signs and symptoms are rare. On examination, the fingertip is extremely tender and there is erythema and swelling of the distal pulp space. As a rule, the swelling does not extend proximal to the distal interphalangeal joint.[7] Fluctuance is generally present within 48 hours.[17] In some cases, the abscess will point, while in others there will be a more diffuse collection of pus. If the infection has spread toward the skin, a draining sinus may be visible on the volar surface of the fingertip. In advanced cases, there may be necrosis of the tactile portion of the finger pad. Other complications of an untreated felon include necrosis of the distal phalanx secondary to osteomyelitis, pyogenic arthritis of the distal interphalangeal joint, and, rarely, a flexor tenosynovitis from proximal extension. [2,7,17]

DIFFERENTIAL DIAGNOSIS

The differential diagnosis of a felon includes herpetic whitlow, cellulitis of the fingertip, and a severe run-around infection. (Herpetic whitlow is discussed later in this chapter.) In cellulitis of the fingertip, fluctuance is usually absent, and pain, tenderness, and swelling are less severe. In addition, unlike a felon, cellulitis will often spread proximal to the distal interphalangeal joint. Patients with a severe run-around infection have fluctuance of the eponychium and both lateral nail folds. In contrast, the fluctuance associated with a felon is much greater in the distal pulp space.

EMERGENCY DEPARTMENT EVALUATION

The diagnosis of a felon is made by history and physical examination. Radiographs of the affected digit are recommended to assess for osteomyelitis. Gram stain and culture and sensitivity testing of spontaneous or surgically obtained drainage will aid in making a bacteriologic diagnosis and help guide the choice of antimicrobial agent. Other laboratory tests (e.g., complete blood cell count, electrolytes, glucose) may be helpful in certain patients, such as those with a complication of an untreated felon (e.g., pyogenic arthritis, flexor tenosynovitis, osteomyelitis) or those with significant underlying medical disorders (e.g., diabetes mellitus, AIDS, cancer). In general, however, laboratory testing is unnecessary.

EMERGENCY DEPARTMENT MANAGEMENT

If the patient presents in the early stages of the infection (i.e., before the onset of fluctuance), management includes an oral antimicrobial agent and supportive care. The antimicrobial chosen should be effective against *Staphylococcus* and *Streptococcus* species (see Table 55.2). Supportive measures include rest, immobilization, and elevation of the affected extremity. Surgical drainage is indicated when there is fluctuance present or if associated swelling threatens to interrupt blood flow to the distal pulp space. Although the presence of pus may be difficult to assess in some patients, it is usually present if the process has been going on for more than 48 hours.[17]

The basic goal of surgical intervention is to provide adequate drainage without creating a disabling scar or unstable fat pad, injuring the digital artery and nerve, or violating the flexor tendon sheath, causing an iatrogenic flexor tenosynovitis.[17] In the past, several surgical approaches have been recommended (Fig. 55.4). Many of them however, are associated with a high incidence of unacceptable complications and are therefore no longer recommended (Table 55.3) At the present time, the unilateral longitudinal approach is the technique most often employed.[7,17,19]

Before drainage, a tourniquet (sterile Penrose drain) should be placed around the proximal portion of the digit, as described previously. The unilateral longitudinal incision is made dorsal to the neurovascular bundle on the ulnar side of the index, long, and ring fingers or on the radial side of the thumb and little finger. The incision starts approximately 0.5 cm distal to the distal flexion crease and extends in a straight line to a point in line with the beginning of the hyponychium (see Fig. 55.4). The blade is carefully inserted deeper and deeper until the abscess is entered. The opening of the cavity is enlarged using a small Kelly clamp

TABLE 55.3. Surgical Approaches for Draining a Felon

Surgical Approach	Indications	Complications	Comments
Unilateral longitudinal incision	All felons	Injury to the neurovascular bundle	Technique of choice for most felons; incision should be made dorsal to the neurovascular bundle.
Longitudinal volar incision	Presence of a draining sinus or pointing on the volar fat pad	Sensitive scar on the tactile surface of the digit	Incision should not cross the distal flexion crease; if a sinus is present, necrotic skin edges should be debrided.
Transverse volar incision	Pointing in the center of the volar fat pad	Sensitive scar on the tactile surface of the digit; injury to the neurovascular bundle	Offers no advantage over the longitudinal volar incision
Through-and-through incision	All felons	Injury to the neurovascular bundle; potential for an unstable fat pad	Rarely, if ever, necessary for adequate drainage
Hockey stick or J incision	Severe infections	Unsightly, tender scar; unstable fat pad; rare skin slough	Not recommended for routine use
Fish-mouth incision	Severe infections	Unsightly, tender scar; unstable fat pad; skin slough	No longer recommended

until complete evacuation is achieved. Blunt rupture of all the fibrous septa should be avoided because it frequently results in an unstable fat pad. The cavity is irrigated with saline, and the wound is packed with 0.25-inch gauze packing. The hand is splinted and elevated, and the patient is started on an oral antimicrobial agent effective against *Staphylococcus* and *Streptococcus* species (see Table 55.2). The gauze pack is removed in 48 hours, at which time the patient is started on warm soaks.

For patients with a draining sinus or pointing abscess on the volar surface of the fingertip a midline longitudinal incision is recommended.[13,17] Because the abscess cavity lies directly under the draining sinus or area of pointing, a midline longitudinal incision made directly through this area produces excellent drainage with few complications. The incision is made through the sinus (or over the area of pointing), starting 0.5 cm distal to the distal flexion crease, and extends to the beginning of the hyponychium (see Fig. 55.4). Care should be taken not to cross the distal flexion crease because this may result in a disabling scar. The incision is deepened until the abscess cavity is entered. A small Kelly clamp is used to gently widen the opening and ensure complete drainage. After drainage, the cavity is irrigated with saline; but in contrast to the unilateral longitudinal approach, no packing is necessary. Instead, the application of a thick coat of zinc oxide (or similar agent) will keep the exudate from drying up and closing the wound, and it will enhance sequestration of the necrotic core.[13] A bulky dressing is applied, and the distal extremity is immobilized and elevated.

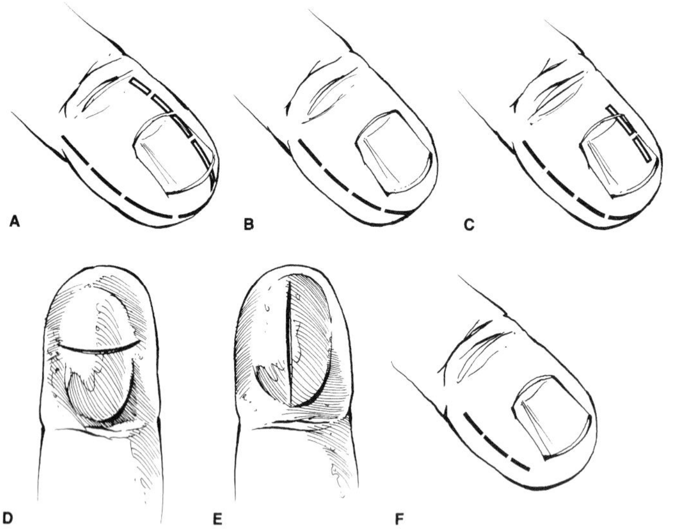

Figure 55.4. Incisions for drainage of felons. **(A)** Fish-mouth incision. This approach has significant complications and should be avoided. **(B)** Hockey stick or J incision. This should be reserved for an extensive or severe abscess or felon. Its routine use is no longer recommended. The incision should be more dorsal at the tip than shown (i.e., at the junction of the skin and nail bed). **(C)** Incision for through-and-through drainage of a felon is rarely, if ever, necessary. Again, the distal incision should be at the junction of the skin and the nail bed. **(D)** Volar drainage. Useful if the abscess points volarward, but this incision risks injury to digital nerves. **(E)** Alternative volar approach. Less risk to digital nerves but should not touch or cross the distal interphalangeal flexion crease. **(F)** Unilateral longitudinal approach. (Redrawn from Neviaser RJ. Infections. In: Green DP, ed. *Operative hand surgery,* 3rd ed. New York: Churchill Livingstone, 1993: 1025.)

DISPOSITION

Most patients with a felon may be discharged from the emergency department. Patients should be encouraged to keep the affected digit clean and dry. Elevation of the involved extremity will help decrease pain and swelling and facilitate healing. The patient should be reevaluated in 48 hours, at which time the gauze wick is removed and warm soaks initiated. If a zinc oxide dressing is used, it should be changed every 2 days. An oral antimicrobial agent effective against *Staphylococcus* and *Streptococcus* species is also recommended (see Table 55.2). In addition, a few days of an oral narcotic analgesic (e.g., oxycodone or hydrocodone with acetaminophen) will be appreciated by most patients. The need for admission is rare but should be considered for a severe infection in high-risk individuals such as immunocompromised patients and diabetics. Consultation is recommended for these patients before making a final disposition. Moreover, patients who develop a pyogenic arthritis, flexor tenosynovitis, osteomyelitis, or an ischemic digit will require immediate consultation and admission.

COMMON PITFALLS

- Failure to recognize the need for surgical drainage. If the patient has been symptomatic for 48 hours or more, the presence of pus is highly likely and the pulp space should be surgically drained. Moreover, if swelling is so severe that it could compromise distal blood flow, the finger should be opened regardless of whether pus is present.

- Improperly placed incisions. For example, a volar incision that crosses the distal flexion crease may cause a disabling scar, while a lateral incision not made dorsal to the neurovascular bundle may result in permanent sensory loss or ischemia of the distal fat pad.
- Blunt rupture of all the fibrous septa. This is no longer recommended because it frequently results in an unstable fat pad.
- Failure to diagnose osteomyelitis. Therefore, all patients with a suspected felon, particularly those with long-standing symptoms, should undergo radiologic evaluation. For patients with suspected osteomyelitis, but in whom plain films are normal or equivocal, a bone scan should be arranged.

HERPETIC WHITLOW

Herpetic whitlow is a viral infection of the fingertip caused by type 1 or type 2 herpes simplex virus. In the past, the disease was thought to be most common in medical and health-care professionals. However, researchers in one study found that individuals most often affected are adults with genital herpes and patients of all ages with herpetic gingivostomatitis.[4] The infection most often affects the distal pulp space and, occasionally, the proximal and lateral nail folds.[4] The fingers are affected more often than the thumb. Herpetic whitlow is self-limited and usually resolves in 3 to 4 weeks. About 20% of patients experience recurrent infections that tend to be less severe than the original.[3]

CLINICAL PRESENTATION

Patients initially have pain and dysesthesia or burning of the distal phalanx. This is usually followed by swelling and erythema. Despite associated swelling, however, the distal pulp space usually remains soft.[16] This helps to differentiate herpetic whitlow from a felon, in which there is tense swelling of the distal pulp space. One or more small vesicles then appear and often coalesce to form bullae. On examination, tenderness is present, but usually much less severe than that seen with bacterial infections.[17] Some patients may have associated fever, lymphadenopathy, lymphangitis, and constitutional symptoms.[3] The vesicles may contain fluid that is clear, turbid, or occasionally hemorrhagic but not purulent. If purulence is present, it suggests a secondary bacterial infection[9] After 10 days, the vesicles or bullae will begin to crust over. Shortly after this, the area peels to reveal normal skin.

DIFFERENTIAL DIAGNOSIS

The differential diagnosis of herpetic whitlow includes a felon and a paronychia. The features differentiating these conditions have been described previously in this chapter.

EMERGENCY DEPARTMENT EVALUATION

The diagnosis of herpetic whitlow is usually clinical. It can often be confirmed in the emergency department by a Tzanck smear. This is performed by first unroofing a vesicle and scraping the base with a wooden applicator. The scrapings are spread on a slide and allowed to air dry or are fixed with ethyl alcohol. The slide is stained with Giemsa or Wright stain or with methylene blue and examined for the presence of multinucleated giant cells.[3] If the Tzanck smear is negative or unable to be performed, a culture can be obtained. This is more sensitive than a Tzanck smear, but results take up to 48 hours. Electron microscopy and the fluorescent antibody test are complicated by both false-positive and false-negative results, and serologic tests often require more than a week to become positive.[3]

EMERGENCY DEPARTMENT MANAGEMENT

Management of herpetic whitlow is symptomatic. The digit is covered with a dry dressing to reduce the spread of infection. An oral analgesic and aspiration of tense vesicles may be helpful in relieving pain. The use of acyclovir has not been evaluated in a large, prospective, controlled trial, but several anecdotal reports have documented suppression of recurrent attacks with oral acyclovir.[5,14] Topical acyclovir has not been shown to be effective in the treatment of herpetic whitlow. Incision and drainage is contraindicated because it can result in secondary bacterial infection.

DISPOSITION

Patients with herpetic whitlow may be discharged from the emergency department. A follow-up visit is arranged in 7 to 10 days with the primary care physician or a hand specialist. Discharge instructions should include signs of secondary bacterial infection. If there is a suspicion of an associated bacterial infection (i.e., a paronychia or felon), consultation with a hand surgeon is highly recommended.

COMMON PITFALLS

Misdiagnosing herpetic whitlow as a felon or paronychia requiring incision and drainage. Surgical intervention causes unnecessary discomfort and may lead to secondary bacterial infection.

FLEXOR TENOSYNOVITIS

Infection of a flexor tendon sheath can be one of the most devastating hand infections encountered in clinical practice. It is most commonly caused by a penetrating injury, particularly at the distal and proximal flexion creases where the tendon sheaths are more superficial. It may also result from direct extension of a neighboring infection and, rarely, by hematogenous or lymphatic spread. The thumb, index finger, and middle fingers are the digits most commonly involved, and the right hand is affected about twice as often as the left hand.[16] If not recognized and treated early, purulence within the tendon sheath can destroy the delicate gliding mechanism. Persistent infection leads to the formation of adhesions, resulting in severe limitation of movement. If allowed to continue, the infection will eventually destroy the blood supply to the tendon, producing tendon necrosis.

CLINICAL PRESENTATION

Patients with flexor tenosynovitis complain of severe pain, swelling, and limited motion of the affected digit. There is a history of penetrating trauma in approximately 90% of cases.[16] Kanavel[16] described four cardinal signs of flexor tenosynovitis: (1) excessive tenderness over the course of the sheath but limited to the sheath, (2) symmetric enlargement (edema) of the whole finger, (3) a flexed position of the finger at rest, and (4) excruciating pain on passive extension the finger, most marked at the proximal end. The latter is the most valuable of these signs and may be the only one present very early in the disease process.[17] In established infections, swelling frequently involves the dorsum of the hand. This is most commonly due to lymphatic drainage from the affected digit, rather than from extension of infection. Dorsal swelling is usually less than that seen with a thenar or midpalmar space infection. If the patient does not seek medical treatment early, the infection may spread to one of the deep palmar spaces, especially the thenar space and midpalmar space, or to adjacent bone or joints, causing an associated osteomyelitis or septic arthritis, respectively.

Infection of the tendon sheath of the little finger or thumb may extend to involve the ulnar bursa and radial bursa, respectively. Patients with involvement of the ulnar bursa will develop severe pain and tenderness in the palm and wrist. There is usually swelling of the entire hand, and dorsal edema becomes more pronounced. The other fingers become sensitive to touch and assume a semiflexed position. Any attempt at passive extension of the fingers is resisted because of severe pain. Similarly, patients with involvement of the radial bursa will develop severe pain and tenderness over the thenar eminence and radial aspect of the wrist. The thenar eminence becomes swollen, but usually not to the degree of a thenar space infection. Swelling over the dorsum of the hand also becomes more prominent. The hand is usually held in moderate flexion and radial deviation. In contrast to patients with infection of the ulnar bursa, patients with infection of the radial bursa do not have pain or limitation of movement of the other fingers. If this occurs, it usually means the infection has spread from the radial bursa to the ulnar bursa, causing a "horseshoe abscess."

DIFFERENTIAL DIAGNOSIS

The differential diagnosis of flexor tenosynovitis includes a palmar space infection, cellulitis, osteomyelitis, and septic arthritis. However, the diagnosis of flexor tenosynovitis can usually be made if a detailed physical examination is performed, with emphasis on the four cardinal signs described by Kanavel.[16] The finding of excruciating pain on passive extension of the digit is particularly helpful because it is often present early in patients with flexor tenosynovitis and is generally not seen with other hand infections. (Palmar space infections are discussed later in this chapter.) Patients with a cellulitis of the digit have symptoms and physical findings that are usually less severe than those associated with flexor tenosynovitis. In particular, tenderness is localized to the area affected with cellulitis, the digit is not held flexed, and severe pain with passive extension of the digit is generally lacking. Likewise, patients with osteomyelitis and septic arthritis tend to have findings that are more localized to the infected bone or joint, respectively.

EMERGENCY DEPARTMENT EVALUATION

The diagnosis of flexor tenosynovitis is made by history and physical examination. Radiographs of the affected digit are recommended to look for a foreign body and osteomyelitis. A complete blood cell count may be helpful in identifying those individuals with systemic involvement. Blood cultures are indicated in patients with evidence of systemic infection. Urethral or endocervical cultures for *Neisseria gonorrhoeae* may be useful in the appropriate clinical setting. Other tests should be based on the patient's presenting complaints, underlying medical problems, and the need for operative drainage.

EMERGENCY DEPARTMENT MANAGEMENT

Emergency department management of suspected flexor tenosynovitis includes elevation and immobilization of the affected hand, intravenous antimicrobial therapy, and relief of pain. Antimicrobial therapy should be broad spectrum, aimed at both gram-positive aerobic bacteria as well as anaerobic organisms (see Table 55.2). Intravenous cefazolin and penicillin G are recommended initially.[20] Gentamicin or aztreonam should be added for suspected gram-negative infection (i.e., infection in a diabetic or immunocompromised patient). Nafcillin can be used in place of cefazolin for gram-positive coverage, but, unlike cefazolin, it does not have activity against gram-negative organisms. It also has poor anaerobic coverage. In patients with a nonanaphylactic allergy to penicillin (i.e., patients who can safely be given a cephalosporin), cefoxitin provides coverage for common gram-negative and gram-positive bacteria, as well as many anaerobic organisms.[20] Vancomycin and clindamycin may be used in patients with a cephalosporin or severe penicillin allergy. Patients with evidence of disseminated gonorrhea should receive intravenous ceftriaxone. Finally, patients with severe pain will benefit from a parenteral narcotic while awaiting surgical consultation.

DISPOSITION

All patients with suspected flexor tenosynovitis require immediate consultation with a hand surgeon and admission to the hospital. Patients presenting greater than 48 hours after the onset of symptoms require drainage in the operating suite. If the patient presents within the first 24 to 48 hours, conservative therapy with continued elevation and immobilization, intravenous antimicrobial agents, and close observation may be attempted. If the patient's condition is not markedly improved within 24 hours or if physical findings are not resolved within 2 days, surgical drainage is indicated.[7,17] The choice of conservative versus operative management is best left to the consulting surgeon.

COMMON PITFALLS

- Failure to make the diagnosis on initial presentation. A careful history and physical examination, with close attention to the cardinal signs of flexor tenosynovitis and a low threshold for consultation and admission, will help avoid a late diagnosis.
- Sending the patient with equivocal findings home without having been seen by the consulting surgeon. The emergency physician should stand firm on admitting all patients with suspected cases of flexor tenosynovitis and should be adamant that the consulting hand surgeon see the patient in the emergency department or shortly after admission. This request should be clearly documented in the emergency department record.

WEB SPACE (COLLAR BUTTON) ABSCESS

An infection of a web space usually results from a break in the skin surrounding an infected palmar blister. Consequently, it is seen most often in individuals who do manual labor. If left untreated, the infection spreads dorsally to the dorsal subcutaneous space and deep into the palmar web space. This creates an hourglass configuration to the abscess, hence the term *collar button abscess*. Rarely, an untreated infection in the web space between the index and middle fingers will spread medially to involve the other two web spaces.[2]

CLINICAL PRESENTATION

Patients usually complain of pain and swelling of the involved web space and surrounding palm. Systemic signs and symptoms are unusual in uncomplicated infections. Examination reveals tenderness and swelling of the affected web space. Anteroposterior pressure over the web space elicits severe discomfort.[2] Swelling may be more prominent on either the palmar or the dorsal aspect, depending on the nature of the infection.[17] Because of pus and swelling, the fingers adjacent to the affected web space are held abducted at rest. Patients with a neglected web space abscess may present with signs of tendon sheath or palmar space involvement. Untreated infections may also dissect distally along the course of the lumbricals, leading to tissue slough.[2] Rarely, the infection will spread to involve the dorsal subaponeurotic space.[2] If this occurs, patients will have pain, tenderness, and fluctuance involving the dorsum of the hand.

DIFFERENTIAL DIAGNOSIS

The differential diagnosis of a web space abscess includes a dorsal subcutaneous space infection, an infected palmar blister, and a deep palmar space infection. As with other infections of the hand, a careful history and physical examination will lead to the appropriate diagnosis. In a dorsal subcutaneous space infection, the fingers are not held abducted at rest and palmar tenderness is minimal or absent. Although infection of a palmar blister usually precedes a web space abscess, pain and tenderness are mild in comparison and are localized over the blister, not the web space. Furthermore, swelling is usually minimal and, when present, does not involve the dorsum of the hand. The findings associated with a deep palmar space infection vary with the involved space. (Palmar space infections are discussed later in this chapter.)

EMERGENCY DEPARTMENT EVALUATION

The diagnosis of a web space infection is made by history and physical examination. Radiographs of the affected hand are recommended if a foreign body or osteomyelitis is suspected. Gram stain and culture and sensitivity testing of spontaneous drainage will aid in making a bacteriologic diagnosis and help guide the choice of antimicrobial agent. A complete blood cell count may be helpful in identifying those individuals with a more diffuse infection. Blood cultures are indicated in patients with evidence of systemic infection. Additional tests should be based on the patients' presenting complaints, their underlying medical problems, and institutional requirements for drainage in the operating suite.

EMERGENCY DEPARTMENT MANAGEMENT

Emergency department management includes elevation of the affected hand, antimicrobial therapy, and pain control. Initial antimicrobial therapy is the same as described for flexor tenosynovitis (see Table 55.2). Pain should be treated with a parental analgesic.

DISPOSITION

All patients with a suspected web space infection require immediate consultation with a hand surgeon and admission to the hospital. Definitive management requires drainage in the operating suite.

COMMON PITFALLS

- Diagnosing a primary dorsal space infection because of the presence of dorsal edema
- Failure to recognize palmar involvement when dorsal edema is more prominent
- Failure to obtain consultation early in the evaluation process

PALMAR SPACE INFECTIONS

The palm of the hand contains three fascial spaces that are important sites of infection: the thenar space, the midpalmar space, and the hypothenar space. The compartments may become infected from direct penetrating trauma; from contiguous infection, such as a tenosynovitis or osteomyelitis; or, rarely, from hematogenous seeding. Deep space infections may be associated with significant morbidity and permanent loss of function; thus, prompt diagnosis and treatment are essential.

CLINICAL PRESENTATION

The clinical presentation of patients with a palmar space infection depends on which space is involved. However, any patient may present with fever, chills, and other manifestations of a serious infection. A thenar space infection causes severe pain and tenderness and tense swelling of the thenar eminence. Because lymphatic drainage from the palm is directed dorsally, there is usually marked dorsal edema as well. However, there is little, if any, tenderness over the dorsum of the hand. Fluctuance is often present in the web space between the thumb and index finger. The thumb is held abducted and flexed; passive adduction produces severe pain. In contrast, patients with a midpalmar space infection have pain and tenderness over the central palm. There is marked fluctuance and swelling of the midpalmar space, resulting in a loss of normal palm concavity. In severe infections, there is frequently a bulge or convexity of the palm, a finding considered by Mann[23] to be almost pathognomonic of a midpalmar space infection. As with other serious hand infections, there is also edema over the dorsum of the hand, but no tenderness, erythema, or fluctuance. Motion of the middle and ring fingers is painful and limited.[17] Infection of the hypothenar space is rare. There is pain and fullness over the hypothenar eminence, with a noticeable lack of swelling in the palm and fingers.

DIFFERENTIAL DIAGNOSIS

The differential diagnosis of a palmar space infection includes a cellulitis or superficial abscess of the palm, a web space infection, and flexor tenosynovitis. Once again, the history and physical examination are the keys to the correct diagnosis. Both a cellulitis and a superficial (subcutaneous) abscess of the palm produce pain and tenderness that may not be localized to a particular space. In addition, they cause far less palmar swelling, and dorsal edema is minimal or absent. Moreover, unless there is digital involvement, movement of the fingers or thumb causes little, if any, discomfort. The findings associated with a web space abscess and flexor tenosynovitis have already been described.

EMERGENCY DEPARTMENT EVALUATION

The diagnosis of a palmar space infection is made by history and physical examination. Radiographs of the affected hand are recommended to look for a suspected foreign body, osteomyelitis, or gas in the tissues. A complete blood cell count may be helpful in identifying those individuals with a severe infection. Blood cultures are indicated in patients with evidence of systemic infection. Additional tests should be based on the patients' presenting complaints and underlying medical problems and on institutional requirements for admission and drainage in the operating suite.

EMERGENCY DEPARTMENT MANAGEMENT

Emergency department management of a palmar space infection includes elevation and immobilization of the affected hand, broad-spectrum intravenous antimicrobial therapy, and pain control. Once again, antimicrobial therapy is the same as for other serious hand infections (see Table 55.2). A parenteral analgesic such as morphine or meperidine is indicated for patients with severe discomfort.

DISPOSITION

All patients with a suspected palmar space infection require immediate consultation with a hand surgeon and admission to the hospital. Definitive management requires drainage in the operating suite.

COMMON PITFALLS

- Failure to appreciate the presence of a palmar space infection, particularly early in the disease process. Therefore, it is essential to maintain a high index of suspicion and consider the possibility of a palmar space infection in any patient who presents with erythema, swelling, and tenderness of the palm.
- Misinterpreting the presence of dorsal edema as a dorsal hand infection
- Sending home patients who have an equivocal examination, without their having been examined by the consulting surgeon. Thus, evaluation in the emergency department by the consulting hand surgeon is mandatory before releasing any patient with a suspected palmar space infection.

References

1. Boles SD, Schmidt CC. Pyogenic flexor tenosynovitis. *Hand Clin* 1998;14:567.
2. Chudnofsky CR, Sebastian S. Special wounds: nail bed, plantar puncture, and cartilage. *Emerg Med Clin North Am* 1992;10:801.
3. Crandon JH. Common infections of the hand. In: Grayson TH, ed. *Flynn's hand surgery*, 4th ed. Baltimore: Williams & Wilkins, 1991:762.
4. Feder HM, Long SS. Herpetic whitlow: epidemiology, clinical characteristics, diagnosis, and treatment. *Am J Dis Child* 1983;137:861.
5. Gill MJ, Arlette J, Buchan K. Herpes simplex virus infection of the hand: a profile of 79 cases. *Am J Med* 1988;84:89.
6. Gill M, Buchan K, Arlette J, et al. Acyclovir therapy for herpetic whitlow [Letter]. *Ann Intern Med* 1986;105:631.
7. Goldstein EJC, Barones MF, Miller TA. *Eikenella corrodens* in hand infections. *J Hand Surg* 1983;8:563.
8. Gunther SF, Gunther SB. Diabetic hand infections. *Hand Clin* 1998;14:647.
9. Hausman MR, Lisser SP. Hand infections. *Orthop Clin North Am* 1992;23:171.
10. Hoyen HA, Lacey SH, Graham TJ. Atypical hand infections. *Hand Clin* 1998;14:613.
11. Hurst LC, Amadio PC, Badalamente MA, et al. *Myobacterium marinum* infection of the hand. *J Hand Surg* 1987;12:428.
12. Hurst LC, Gluck R, Sampson ST, et al. Herpetic whitlow with bacterial abscess. *J Hand Surg* 1991;16:311.
13. Iverson RE, Vistnes LM. Coccidioidomycosis tenosynovitis in the hand. *J Bone Joint Surg* 1973;55:413.
14. Jebson PJL. Infections of the fingertip—paronychias and felons. *Hand Clin* 1998;14:547.
15. Jones NF, Conklin WT, Albo VC. Primary invasive aspergillosis of the hand. *J Hand Surg* 1986;11:425.
16. Kanavel AB. *Infections of the hand*. Philadelphia: Lea & Febiger, 1939:17.
17. Kilgore ES, Brown LG, Newmeyer WL, et al. Treatment of felons. *Am J Surg* 1975;130:194.
18. Kono M, Stern PJ. The history of hand infections. *Hand Clin* 1998;14:511.
19. Kour AK, Looi KP, Pho RWH. Hand infections in patients with diabetes. *Clin Orthop Rel Res* 1996;331:238.
20. Laskin OL. Acyclovir and suppression of frequently recurring herpetic whitlow. *Ann Intern Med* 1985;102:494.
21. Louis DS, Jebson PJL. Mimickers of hand infections. *Hand Clin* 1998;14:519.
22. Mann RJ, Peacock JM. Hand infections in patients with diabetes mellitus. *J Trauma* 1977;17:376.
23. Mann RJ. *Infections of the hand*. Philadelphia: Lea & Febiger, 1988.
24. Neviaser RJ. Infections. In: Green DP, ed. *Operative hand surgery*, 3rd ed. New York: Churchill Livingstone, 1993:1021.
25. Rosenfeld N, Kurzer A. Acute flexor tenosynovitis caused by gonococcal infection: a case report. *Hand* 1978;10:213.
26. Siegel DB, Gelberman RH. Infections of the hand. *Orthop Clin North Am* 1988;19:779.
27. Spiegel JD, Szabo RM. A protocol for the treatment of severe infections of the hand. *J Hand Surg* 1988;13:254.
28. Yuan RTW, Cohen MJ. *Candida albicans* tenosynovitis of the hand. *J Hand Surg* 1985;10:719.
29. Zook EG. The perionychium. In: Green DP, ed. *Operative hand surgery*, 3rd ed. New York: Churchill Livingstone, 1993:1303.

CHAPTER 56
Low Back Pain

David Della-Giustina

Back pain is a complaint that is commonly seen in the emergency department (ED), affecting up to 90% of the population at some point in their lives. With an annual incidence of 5%,[9] back pain is second only to upper respiratory illness as a reason for physician visits.[12] Up to 85% of patients with low back pain will have no definite etiology determined for their symptoms.[15] Fortunately, despite the lack of a definite etiology, almost 90% of patients will have resolution of their symptoms within 1 month.[1] In the approach to the patient with back pain, patients may be categorized into three groups: (1) back pain in adults, (2) back pain with sciatica, and (3) back pain in children. By far, the majority of patients with back pain seen in the ED fall into the first category.

Sciatica is defined as a radicular pain into the leg in the distribution of a lumbar nerve root; it is often accompanied by a neurosensory or motor deficit.[9] Sciatica is less common than back pain without sciatica, afflicting only 1% of patients with low back pain.[9] There are many etiologies for sciatica, but most commonly it is due to a herniated disc. Generally, patients with sciatica have a more protracted course than routine back pain patients, with only 50% of patients with sciatica recovering within 1 month. However, of all patients with sciatica, only 5% to 10% will require surgery.[9]

Children are a separate category, because back pain is a rare complaint in children and more likely to be due to a serious etiology. The differential diagnosis for the child with back pain is different from that of the adult, and it varies further based on the age of the child. Due to the higher potential for serious disease, the approach to the child with back pain must be more aggressive than for the adult.

CLINICAL PRESENTATION

The clinical presentation of the patient with back pain ranges from the patient with mild pain who requires a work excuse to the patient with the severe, unrelenting pain of an epidural abscess. More important than recognizing a particular "classic" presentation for the various diseases is the thorough evaluation of each patient, with a focus on the *red flags* found in the history and physical examination that should raise suspicion for serious disease (Table 56.1).

History

Back pain is differentiated into three categories based on the duration of the symptoms: acute (less than 6 weeks), subacute (between 6 and 12 weeks), and chronic (greater than 12 weeks). Pain that is subacute or chronic raises a red flag because 90% of back pain episodes resolve within 4 to 6 weeks. Patients who have had back pain for 6 weeks or more require further diagnostic evaluation.

Patients older than 50 or younger than 18 years also raise a red flag due to the higher probability of pathology, such as tumor or infection. Patients under age 18 have a higher likelihood of congenital and bony abnormalities, such as spondylolysis and spondylolisthesis. In those over age 50, causes such as fracture, vascular disease, tumor, pancreatitis, and other intraabdominal or retroperitoneal processes are more common.

A history of trauma suggests fracture and is usually a readily available historical clue. In an otherwise healthy patient, a major mechanism (motor vehicle crash or a fall from a significant height) is required to cause vertebral fracture. However, one must realize that in the patient with osteoporosis, even minor trauma may result in fracture.

A history of radicular pain (sciatica) suggests nerve root or spinal cord compression or inflammation. Patients with sciatica commonly complain more of the leg symptoms than the back pain. In addition to the radicular symptoms, one must inquire about neurologic deficits such as weakness, paresthesias, anesthesia, gait disturbances, and bowel and bladder incontinence. Any neurologic deficit raises a red flag for compression of at least a single spinal nerve root, but may signal compression of the cauda equina or spinal cord. Bilateral or rapidly progressive symptoms, or urinary or fecal incontinence, are very worrisome and suggest cauda equina syndrome or spinal cord compression.

TABLE 56.1. Red Flags in the History and Physical Exam

HISTORY
Pain greater than six weeks
Age less than eighteen or over fifty
History of trauma
Sciatica
Neurological complaints (paresthesias, anesthesia, weakness)
Incontinence of bowel or bladder
Night pain
Unrelenting pain despite rest and analgesics
Fever, chills, and night sweats
History of injection drug use
History of cancer
PHYSICAL EXAM
Fever
Patient writhing in pain
Point vertebral tenderness
Neurological deficits
Positive straight leg raise

The typical description for a benign etiology of back pain is that of a dull, aching pain that usually worsens with movement but improves with rest and lying still. Atypical pain features, such as night pain and unrelenting pain despite rest and appropriate or even supernormal analgesic use, raise red flags for infection or tumor. Other atypical features associated with a herniated disk include pain that is worsened with prolonged sitting, coughing, or the Valsalva maneuver, and relieved by lying supine.[7] Finally, bilateral sciatica pain that worsens with activities such as prolonged standing, walking, and back extension, and is relieved by rest and forward flexion is consistent with spinal stenosis.

Constitutional symptoms, such as fever, chills, nightsweats, malaise, and an undesired weight loss, are all red flags that suggest infection or malignancy. The significance of these symptoms is increased if the patient has additional infectious risk factors, such as injection drug use, immunocompromise, recent bacterial infection, or recent genitourinary or gastrointestinal procedure.

A history of cancer or a history suggestive of undiagnosed cancer raises the suspicion for spinal metastases. Back pain is the initial symptom in 96% of these cases.[13] The malignancies at high risk to metastasize to the spine include breast, lung, thyroid, kidney, prostate, myeloma, lymphoma, and sarcoma.

Physical Examination

The physical examination is directed toward verifying neurologic complaints, identifying neurologic deficits, and uncovering red flags (see Table 56.1). The presence of fever raises a concern for infection with a specificity of 98% for bacterial infection. However, it is insensitive, ranging from 27% for tuberculosis osteomyelitis to 50% for pyogenic osteomyelitis and 83% for spinal epidural abscess.[8]

The patient who is writhing in pain should suggest a serious etiology, because, most often, patients with a benign etiology for back pain find more relief lying still. In the patient who is writhing in pain, one should consider etiologies such as a rupturing abdominal aortic aneurysm, nephrolithiasis, vertebral osteomyelitis, and epidural abscess. All patients with back pain require an abdominal examination. Specifically, one is evaluating for bruits, masses, tenderness, and an enlarged, pulsatile aorta consistent with an aortic aneurysm.

Examination of the back should include a search for evidence of underlying infection or trauma. Inspect the back, looking for contusion or swelling consistent with trauma, and erythema, warmth, or drainage consistent with infection. Point tenderness to percussion of the vertebral bodies is found with bacterial infection with a sensitivity of 86% and a specificity of 60%.[8] Straight-leg testing is performed to evaluate for evidence of herniated disc. A positive test is a reproducible radicular pain that radiates below the knee. This pain is usually relieved by decreasing the elevation, and is worsened by ankle dorsiflexion. Reproduction of the patient's back, buttock, or thigh pain is not a positive test. A positive straight-leg raise test is 80% sensitive for a L4-5 or L5-S1 herniated disc (Fig. 56.1). Radicular pain in the affected leg when elevating the asymptomatic leg (positive crossed straight-leg raise test) is highly specific, yet insensitive, for nerve root compression by a herniated disc.[8]

The neurologic examination is the most important part of the physical examination. The examination should evaluate lower extremity strength, sensation, and reflexes. Rectal examination does not need to be performed on all patients with back pain; however, it should be performed in those patients with red flags and neurologic signs or symptoms; in men in whom prostatic disease is probable; and in those with severe pain. On rectal examination, one is evaluating for sensation, tone, masses, and evidence of perirectal abscess.

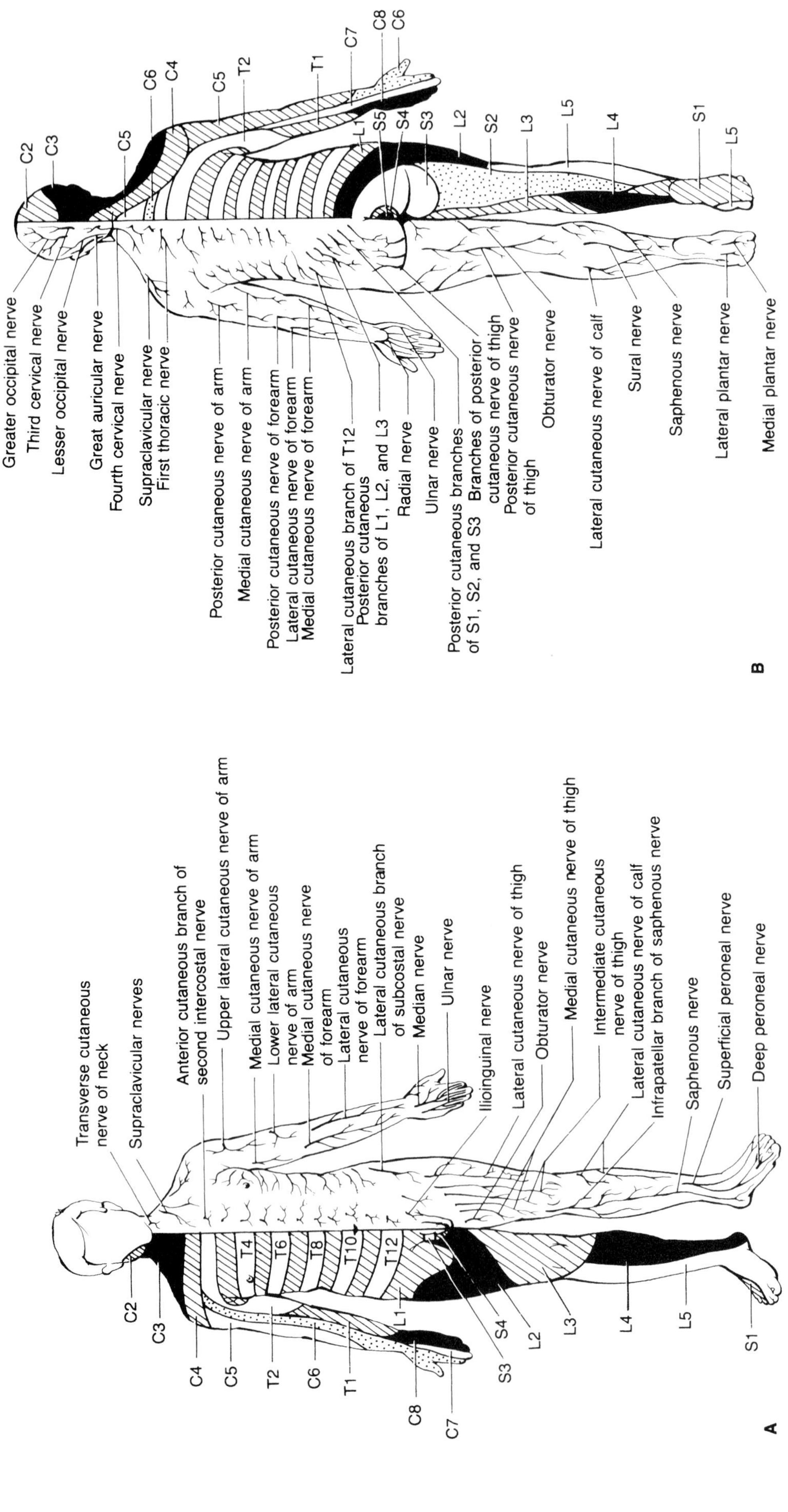

Figure 56.1. Sensory dermatomal segments. **(A)** Anterior view. **(B)** Posterior view.

DIFFERENTIAL DIAGNOSIS

Back Pain in Adults

Acute Lumbosacral Strain

The majority of patients seen in the ED for acute low back pain have symptoms that fall into the category of acute lumbosacral strain (Fig. 56.2). This syndrome is known by many other names, such as mechanical back pain, back sprain/strain, and lumbago, but it is essentially an episode of acute low back pain without sciatica or any neurologic deficits.

The patient typically complains of mild-to-moderate pain in the lumbar area that may radiate to the buttocks or thigh, and is worsened by activity and relieved with rest. The inciting incident is usually unremarkable, varying from an unusual posture for a period of time to lifting a heavy object. Physical examination typically reveals mild paraspinal tenderness, negative straight-leg raise testing, normal neurologic examination, and no other significant findings. The investigation of red flags, if any, from the history and physical examination is negative. Because 90% patients will see spontaneous resolution of their symptoms within 4 weeks, there is no need to perform diagnostic testing unless red flags are uncovered. This saves the patient unnecessary pain, expense, and radiation exposure.

The treatment for these patients should focus on the areas of activity modification, analgesia, manipulation, and other modalities. In terms of activity modification, patients should continue their routine daily activities as they can tolerate, using pain as the limiting factor. Routine activity has been demonstrated to allow more rapid recovery than either bed rest or back mobilizing exercise.[10] Appropriate analgesia is paramount in treating the patient with acute lumbosacral strain. The primary treatment regimen should involve acetaminophen alone or in combination with a nonsteroidal antiinflammatory drug (NSAID). When employing NSAIDs, one must consider that no single NSAID has been shown as being most effective.[5] Thus, one should initiate therapy with a less expensive agent such as ibuprofen, naproxen, or indomethacin. Additionally, NSAIDs should be used with caution in patients at risk of adverse effects, such as the elderly and those with peptic ulcer disease or renal disease. Opiate analgesics should also be prescribed for patients with moderate-to-severe back pain. The prescriptions for these medications are best limited to 1 to 2 weeks' duration due to the risk of sedation, addiction, and constipation. Manipulation is a controversial area of treatment. Although safe and recommended as effective by the 1995 AHCPR guidelines, more recent literature shows it is no more effective than exercises and only minimally more effective than giving the patient an instructional booklet.[3] The use of other physical modalities, such as traction, TENS units, diathermy, and ultrasound, is ineffective.[1]

Spinal Infections

Vertebral osteomyelitis and spinal epidural abscess are uncommon etiologies for back pain. However, due to the potential morbidity and mortality that result from missed infection, one needs to remain vigilant concerning these possibilities. These infections occur more commonly in injection drug users, the immunocompromised, diabetics, and the elderly, most often due to hematogenous spread with *Staphylococcal aureus*. Patients usually present with moderate-to-severe back pain accompanied by fever, chills, unrelenting pain, nightsweats, and weight loss. With epidural abscess, the patient may have concomitant sciatica and neurologic symptoms. Additionally, some patients with epidural abscess may present in sepsis. The peripheral white blood cell (WBC) count may be elevated or normal, but the erythrocyte sedimentation rate (ESR) is universally elevated.[11] One should always consider back pain in an injection drug abuser as a spinal infection until proven otherwise.

Back Pain with Sciatica

The differential diagnosis for sciatica includes all etiologies that cause compression or inflammation of the spinal nerve roots, cauda equina, and spinal cord (Table 56.2). The major cause of sciatica is herniated disc. However, in the ED one should consider other etiologies, including spinal stenosis and compression of the cauda equina or spinal cord by tumor, infection, or hematoma.

Herniated Disc

Although sciatica affects only 1% of patients with low back pain, it is present in almost all patients with a symptomatic herniated disc. Ninety-eight percent of herniated disks involve either the L4-5 or L5-S1 intervertebral disks.[9] Herniated disc most commonly occurs in patients during the fourth or fifth decades of life. Often, patients complain of weeks of nonradicular low back pain preceding the onset of the radicular symptoms. The radicular symptoms are the hallmark of the nerve root compression and usually become the prominent symptom, with a diminution of the back pain. Clinically, the diagnosis of herniated disc is made by localizing the pain to an isolated nerve root and

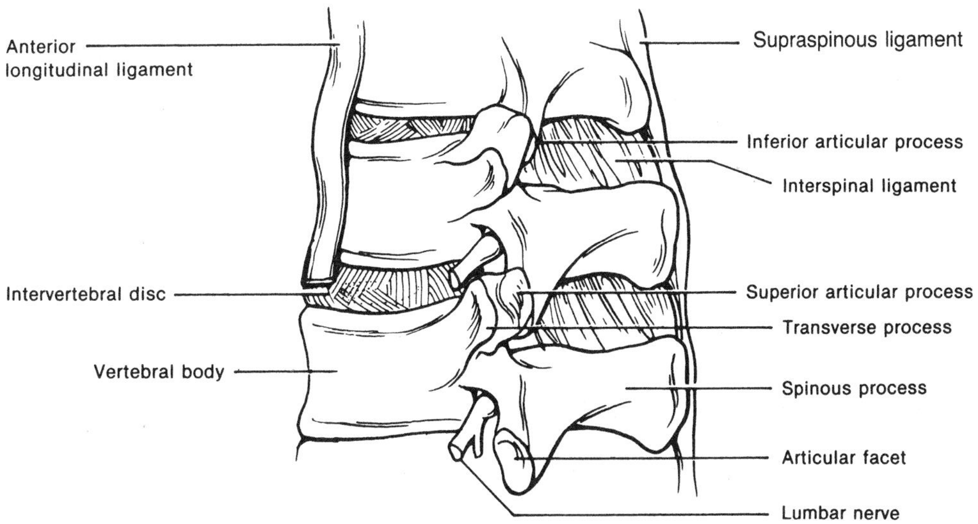

Figure 56.2. Normal anatomy of the lumbar spine.

TABLE 56.2. Differential Diagnosis of Sciatica

LUMBOSACRAL NERVE ROOT LESION
Disc herniation
Neoplasm
Infection (bone, disc, epidural space, nerve)
Spondylosis
Spondylolisthesis
Spinal stenosis
Subarachnoid hemorrhage
Arachnoiditis
Arachnoid cyst
Paget's disease
LUMBOSACRAL PLEXUS LESION
Hematoma
Pregnancy
Pelvic tumors (uterine, bladder, prostate)
Endometriosis
Aneurym of common iliac or hypogastric artery
Endometriosis
SCIATIC NERVE LESION
Trauma
Entrapment
Ischemia
Tumor
REFERRED LEG PAIN
Degenerative disc
Facet joint disease
Bone tumor
Osteoarthritis of the hip
Sacroiliac joint disease
Spinothalamic tract lesion

Modified from Bay JW. Other causes of low back pain and sciatica. In: Hardy RW, ed. *Lumbar disc disease*, 2nd ed. New York: Raven Press, 1993, with permission.

demonstrating neurologic dysfunction in the distribution of that nerve root. Finally, positive straight-leg raise testing increases the probability of herniated disc, especially if the crossed straight-leg raise test is positive. If a diagnosis of herniated disc is entertained, one should ensure that there are no multiple nerve roots involved. The treatment regimen for herniated disk mirrors that for acute lumbosacral strain, including the use of routine activity as opposed to bed rest,[14] with the exception that manipulation should be used with extreme caution.

Cauda Equina Syndrome

Cauda equina syndrome and spinal cord compression present in a similar fashion to acute lumbosacral strain with one major difference: the presence of neurologic involvement. These syndromes are due to compression of the cauda equina or spinal cord by tumor, herniated disc, infection, or hematoma. The patient usually presents with minimal to moderate back pain and sciatica in association with bilateral neurologic deficits and incontinence. The physical examination will demonstrate evidence of bilateral nerve root involvement. The most common sensory deficit found in cauda equina syndrome occurs over the buttocks, perineum, and posterior–superior thighs in the "saddle" distribution.[8] Urinary retention is the most consistent finding in cauda equina syndrome (sensitivity 90%).[8] This proves useful in the patient with a benign history and physical examination but who complains of urinary incontinence. By evaluating a postvoid residual, a negative test (no urinary retention) makes it extremely unlikely that the patient has incontinence due to cauda equina syndrome.[8] All patients with suspected cauda equina syndrome or spinal cord compression require emergency neurosurgery consultation, high-dose steroid therapy, and emergent magnetic resonance imaging (MRI) to determine the etiology.

Spinal Stenosis

Spinal stenosis is a narrowing of the lumbar spinal canal that may occur at single or multiple spinal levels. It is a cause of chronic back pain (usually chronic) that may have associated sciatica. The symptoms, which usually begin in the sixth decade, include low back pain aggravated by prolonged standing and spinal extension, and relieved by rest and forward flexion. The classic symptom for spinal stenosis is pseudoclaudication, although this is seen in only 60% of patients. Pseudoclaudication is pain of the lateral legs that occurs with walking, and is relieved with rest. It is termed *pseudoclaudication* because it is caused by neurologic compression, not arterial insufficiency.[6]

Back Pain in Children

Children rarely present to the ED with complaints of back pain. When they do, however, one must perform a more thorough diagnostic evaluation, as there is a much higher probability of a serious treatable etiology. The history should be directed toward those questions asked of the adult. Additionally, one must ask about a recent increase in physical activity or involvement in sports such as football, dance, and gymnastics. These activities increase the likelihood of spondylolysis or spondylolisthesis. The physical examination should specifically note the absence of birthmarks, such as café au lait spots, indicative of neurofibromatosis, as well as midline skin abnormalities of the back that may indicate underlying developmental spinal abnormalities. Etiologies to consider in the child under age 10 are discitis, tumor, and osteomyelitis. Etiologies for those age 10 and older include spondylolysis, spondylolisthesis, Scheuermann disease, tumor, vertebral osteomyelitis, herniated disc, and ankylosing spondylitis. All children without an obvious etiology for their back pain should be evaluated with a complete blood count (CBC), ESR, urinalysis (UA), and plain spinal radiography.

EMERGENCY DEPARTMENT EVALUATION

The ED evaluation must concentrate on the identification of red flags in the history and physical examination (see Table 56.1). The presence of red flags will direct the diagnostic evaluation and treatment regimens. The absence of red flags means that it is unlikely that the patient has significant disease, and, thus, no diagnostic tests are required.

Laboratory Testing

If the patient has red flags raised for infection or tumor, one should obtain a CBC, a UA, and an ESR. With infection, the WBC count may be normal or elevated, but the ESR is universally elevated. The UA can be positive in infection if it is the source of hematogenous spread, but it is otherwise normal. The CBC, UA, and ESR are usually normal with tumor unless there is specific involvement of the hematologic or urinary system.

Radiography

Plain Radiography

Plain spinal radiographs should always be obtained in children or in adults when there is concern of fracture, spinal infection, or tumor, or if neurologic dysfunction is present. In adults, only anteroposterior (AP) and lateral views of the lumbar spine are necessary. Oblique views and a cone-down view of L5-S1 add minimal information and more than double the radiation exposure.[9] In children, the oblique views should be obtained after reviewing the AP and lateral views because these additional views may demonstrate spondylolysis or spondylolisthesis, common problems in children. It is not necessary to obtain initial plain radiographs in suspected disc herniation. However, they may be obtained to rule out other etiologies for the radicular symptoms, such as fracture, tumor, or infection.

Magnetic Resonance Imaging

The imaging examination of choice for most emergent back symptoms is MRI. It is the gold standard test for cauda equina syndrome, spinal cord compression, spinal infection, herniated disc, and spinal hematoma. MRI provides the best resolution of the spinal cord and spinal canal as well as disc disease. In cases of suspected cauda equina syndrome, obtain an MRI of the lumbosacral spine only, especially if a midline herniated disc is suspected as the etiology. In cases of suspected spinal cord compression, one should obtain an MRI of the entire spine for two reasons. First, there is a risk of false localization to a spinal level on physical examination. Second, in metastatic spinal cord compression there is a 10% risk of asymptomatic metastases distant from the affected site that may alter the treatment regimen. Although it is the gold standard for disk herniation, MRI should rarely be ordered from the ED to evaluate for a herniated disc. For suspected herniated disc, a spinal MRI is ordered on a routine basis after the patient fails to respond to 4 to 6 weeks of conservative management.

Computed Tomography Scan

Computed tomography (CT) scanning is superior to MRI in evaluating the bony architecture of the spine, especially in the assessment of a vertebral fracture. However, it provides less resolution of the spinal cord and spinal canal than does MRI. When used in conjunction with myelography (CT-myelogram), CT scanning approaches MRI and should be considered the imaging method of choice in the patient who is unable to undergo an MRI.[4]

EMERGENCY DEPARTMENT MANAGEMENT

For the majority of patients with low back pain, with or without sciatica, the primary issue is appropriate pain management. A good approach for adults is to utilize acetaminophen 1000 mg orally in combination with an NSAID, such as ibuprofen 800 mg orally, in the ED. The use of the injectable NSAID ketorolac should be reserved for the patient who is unable to tolerate an oral NSAID. If the pain is more severe, administer intravenous opiates such as morphine sulfate 0.1 mg/kg or meperidine 0.5 to 1.0 mg/kg initially, followed by titration until the patient is comfortable.

The patient with a suspected cauda equina syndrome or spinal cord compression requires treatment with high-dose dexamethasone, followed by emergent spinal imaging with plain films and MRI. The exact dexamethasone dose is controversial and ranges from 10 mg to 100 mg intravenously. A rational approach is to administer 10 mg to the patient with equivocal signs of compression and 100 mg to the patient who has more significant findings, such as partial or complete paraplegia, saddle anesthesia, or incontinence with poor rectal tone.[2] Regardless of the exact dose given, these patients require the steroid administration before obtaining the imaging studies. Plain spinal radiographs are taken of the area of suspected spinal involvement. If possible, the MRI should be obtained emergently and not delayed until the next day.

In the patient with suspected spinal infection, obtain at least two sets of blood cultures, as these are frequently positive. Additionally, one should discuss the need for antibiotics in the ED with the consultant prior to their administration. Patients with paralysis or sepsis due to infection require antibiotics. These patients may require open biopsy with culture of the site, and the administration of antibiotics may cause the biopsy culture to be falsely negative. If given empirically, the choice of antibiotic should be directed against *S. aureus,* such as cefazolin 2 g intravenously. If a source for the infection is found, such as the urinary tract, antibiotics should be appropriate for that source.

DISPOSITION

Patients with acute lumbosacral strain and sciatica can be discharged home with primary care physician follow-up in 2 to 4 weeks. They should be treated with acetaminophen and NSAIDs, such as ibuprofen 800 mg three times daily, unless contraindicated. Most patients may benefit from a short course (1 to 2 weeks) of opiate analgesia, such as hydrocodone or oxycodone. If patients have a deficit in a single nerve root consistent with a herniated disc, the primary care physician should see the patient within 7 to 10 days. All patients suspected of having a cauda equina or spinal cord compression syndrome require emergent MRI and consultation in the ED by a spine surgeon. If known or suspected metastatic disease is present, an oncologist should also be consulted. All patients with suspected spinal infection require hospital admission and spinal MRI within 24 hours or earlier if there is any neurologic involvement.

Transfer

Transfer to another facility is necessary in the patient with suspected spinal infection, cauda equina syndrome, or spinal cord compression if the facility evaluating the patient is unable to obtain an appropriate imaging study (MRI or CT-myelogram) or has no spine surgeon on staff. These patients are safe to transport utilizing a BLS ground transport unit, unless they have unstable vital signs. In patients with suspected cauda equina syndrome or spinal cord compression, steroids should be administered before the transfer.

COMMON PITFALLS

- Always consider a rupturing abdominal aortic aneurysm in the patient over age 55 with acute low back pain.
- There is no need to obtain diagnostic tests in the patient with low back pain and no "red flags."
- Children with back pain have a much higher incidence of serious diagnosable etiologies and should be evaluated with a CBC, ESR, UA, and plain spinal radiography, unless a definite benign etiology is determined.
- Always consider spinal infection in the immunocompromised patient or the injection drug user with back pain, especially if a fever is present.
- The treatment regimen for patients with lumbosacral strain and back pain with sciatica comprises routine activity as tolerated, acetaminophen, NSAIDs, and short-term opiate analgesics.
- Patients with suspected herniated disc do not require imaging with MRI unless they fail to improve within 4 to 6 weeks.
- In patients with suspected cauda equina syndrome or spinal cord compression, high-dose dexamethasone should be initiated prior to imaging studies.

References

1. Bigos S, Bowyer O, Braen G, et al. Acute low back problems in adults. Clinical practice guideline. *Quick reference guide number 14.* Rockville, MD: U.S. Department of Health and Human Services, Public Health Service, Agency for Health Care Policy and Research, AHCPR Pub. No. 95-0643, December 1994.

2. Byrne T. Spinal cord compression from epidural metastases. *N Engl J Med* 1992;327(9):614.
3. Cherkin D, Deyo R, Battie M, et al. A comparison of physical therapy, chiropractic manipulation, and provision of an educational booklet for the treatment of patients with low back pain. *N Engl J Med* 1998;339(15):1021.
4. Deen HG. Diagnosis and management of lumbar disk disease. *Mayo Clin Proc* 1996;71(3):283.
5. Deyo R. Drug therapy for back pain: which drugs help which patients. *Spine* 1996;21:2840.
6. Deyo R. Rethinking strategies for acute low back pain. *Emerg Med* 1995;28(11):38.
7. Deyo R, Loeser J, Bigos S. Herniated lumbar intervertebral disc. *Ann Intern Med* 1990;112:598.
8. Deyo R, Rainville J, Kent D. What can the history and physical examination tell us about low back pain. *JAMA* 1992;286:760.
9. Frymoyer J. Back pain and sciatica. *N Engl J Med* 1988;318:291.
10. Malmivaara A, Hakkinen U, Aro T, et al. The treatment of acute low back pain—bed rest, exercise, or ordinary activity. *N Engl J Med* 1995;332:321.
11. Martin R, Yuan H. Neurosurgical care of spinal epidural, subdural and intramedullary abscesses and arachnoiditis. *Orthop Clin North Am* 1996;27(1):125.
12. Mazanec D. Back pain: medical evaluation and therapy. *Cleve Clin J Med* 1995;62:163–168.
13. Schmidt R, Markovchick V. Nontraumatic spinal cord compression. *J Emerg Med* 1992;10:189.
14. Vroomen P, de Krom M, Wilmink J, et al. Lack of effectiveness of bed rest for sciatica. *N Engl J Med* 1999;340:418.
15. White A, Gordon S. Synopsis: Workshop on idiopathic low-back pain. *Spine* 1982;7(2):141.

CHAPTER 57
Common Foot Disorders

Valerie Dobiesz Neylan and Louis G. Poulos

Foot pain is a common complaint in the emergency department; foot disorders can be extremely debilitating. Nontraumatic causes of foot pain are usually chronic or subacute in nature. In the vast majority of cases, such pain is caused by overuse conditions or improperly fitting shoes.

Foot injuries rank second only to knee injuries as the most common injuries associated with sports. The emergency physician can often provide symptomatic relief as well as definitive care. Special attention needs to be given to diabetic patients with foot disorders, as they are at high risk for serious complications.

FOREFOOT PAIN

The forefoot includes the metatarsals and the phalanges. Abnormalities in this region involve the skin, toenails, and joints.

SUBUNGUAL HEMORRHAGE (BLUE OR BLACK TOENAIL SYNDROME)

Painful and black toenails are often a result of improper footwear, resulting from the toenails' rubbing on the undersurface of the shoe or the foot sliding forward to jam the toes. If the symptoms are acute, the treatment is to drain the hematoma with nail trephination, which can be done using a heated paper clip or an electrocautery. To prevent recurrence, the patient can be instructed to use a metatarsal pad under the metatarsal heads or a tongue pad underneath the tongue of the shoe.

ONYCHOCRYPTOSIS (INGROWN TOENAIL)

Ingrown toenails are often the result of poorly fitting shoes, abnormal nail growth, or poor nail-cutting. A sharp edge of the nail pierces the epidermis of the sulcus and penetrates the dermal tissues. The hallux of male adolescents is most often involved. Symptoms include pain, swelling, erythema, and purulent drainage of the affected toe. Treatment is directed at the severity of the wound.

Warm soaks are helpful in mild-to-moderate cases. If a paronychia is present, partial nail ablation is indicated. Utilizing a digital nerve block and local anesthetic, an oblique wedge of nail should be dissected free of the sulcus and inflamed tissue with a scalpel. Phenol or a cotton pledget can be applied to the nail edge. If pus is present, oral or topical antibiotics are indicated. A nonsteroidal antiinflammatory agent is appropriate for pain. Definitive treatment should be with a podiatrist or orthopedic surgeon.[6]

MORTON'S INTERDIGITAL NEUROMA

Morton's neuroma is caused by repetitive trauma compressing the interdigital nerve between the third and fourth metatarsal heads. It is seen in patients who are runners, dancers, and basketball players, and in those who have to stand for long periods of time. Symptoms are sharp, stabbing pain and paresthesia between the toes.

Diagnosis is made clinically by pinching between the metatarsal heads and simultaneously using the other hand to compress the forefoot with pressure on the first and fifth metatarsal heads. This maneuver will elicit pain and possibly a palpable mass or an audible click, known as Mulder's click. Treatment includes ice in acute cases, orthotics, rest, steroid injections, and possible surgical excision.[7]

METATARSAL STRESS FRACTURES

Stress fractures are the result of repetitive loading forces, causing the bone to fatigue, rather than of an acute event. Metatarsal bones are a common site of stress fractures. The most common metatarsal stress fracture occurs at the neck of the second metatarsal. This injury is more common in patients with Morton syndrome (the first ray shorter than the second).[1]

Symptoms include localized pain that is worsened by activity or weight bearing and is relieved with rest. Plain x-rays typically do not reveal stress fractures until 10 to 14 days after they occur. Bone scans are helpful but not practical in the emergency department setting. The condition is treated by having the patient avoid weight bearing on the site for 4 to 6 weeks, applying ice, and administering nonsteroidal antiinflammatory drugs.

BUNIONS (HALLUX VALGUS)

Bunion deformity occurs most commonly at the first metatarsophalangeal (MTP) joint. The deformity consists of lateral deviation of the hallux and medial deviation of the first metatarsal. The etiology is unclear but may be hereditary biomechanical abnormalities and improperly fitting shoes. Symptoms are pain and erythema at the MTP joint. Treatment in the emergency department is focused on analgesia with nonsteroidal antiinflammatory drugs and patient education on proper shoes. In severe cases, surgical correction in indicated.[7]

BLISTERS, CALLUSES, AND CORNS

Excessive localized pressure or friction between the foot and improperly fitted shoes or from constant sliding of the foot inside a shoe can result in blisters, calluses, and corns. Blisters result from shearing forces, causing fluid to accumulate within the layers of the skin. There is some controversy regarding the treatment of blisters. Several options exist in management, including leaving the blister intact, debridement, and aspiration.

Calluses develop from excessive pressure, causing hypertrophy of the squamous cell layer of the epidermis on skin that is normally thick, such as the sole. A callus is painless and may be diffuse or localized. Treatment includes regular debridement with a callus file, pumice stone, or scalpel.

A corn is a painful conical thickening of skin with recurrent pressure; the apex of the cone points inward and causes pain. Corns usually occur over bony prominences such as the fourth or fifth toe. When they occur in moist areas, such as between the toes, they are called soft corns. Treatment is aimed at prevention with appropriate footwear and padding proximal to the lesions to relieve pressure. These lesions should be aggressively pursued and treated in diabetic patients because of the risk of infection and long-term sequelae.

PLANTAR WARTS (VERRUCA VULGARIS)

Plantar warts are caused by the human papillomavirus and are painful when the patient puts weight on them. Callus formation over the wart is common. Distinguishing warts from calluses may be difficult. Warts occur at any site, whereas calluses appear only on pressure areas. Pinching around the lesion, producing pain, supports an underlying wart. If the hyperkeratotic area is scraped, the underlying wart typically bleeds and has a spotted appearance, representing thrombosed vessels.

Treatment in the emergency department consists of application of pressure-relief dressing and administration of analgesics and topical solutions containing salicylic acid. Refractory warts may require laser or surgical excision.[2,4]

HINDFOOT PAIN

PLANTAR FASCIITIS

The plantar fascia is a band of connective tissue on the plantar surface of the foot that extends from the calcaneal tuberosity to the metatarsal heads. Irritation and microtears due to overuse and repetitive heel strikes cause inflammation of the fascia, resulting in heel pain, often in the morning. This entity accounts for 10% of running injuries and primarily afflicts the middle-aged, the elderly, and athletes. Physical examination findings are of point tenderness over the medial calcaneal tuberosity, reproduction of pain with passive dorsiflexion of the ankle or toes, or heel pain with standing on the toes. Treatment is focused on relaxing the tension on the fascia and includes rest, ice, stretching the gastrocnemius muscle, arch taping, use of orthotics, administration of nonsteroidal antiinflammatory drugs, and advising the patient to wear proper shoes.[4,5]

CALCANEAL STRESS FRACTURES

The cause of calcaneal stress fractures is repetitive stresses. Patients typically present with insidious onset of heel pain aggravated by weight-bearing activities. On examination, there is localized tenderness over the medial or lateral aspects of the calcaneus, and pain is elicited by squeezing the calcaneus from both sides, the heel "squeeze" test. Radiographs are typically normal initially or show a typical sclerotic appearance on the lateral view parallel with the posterior margin of the calcaneus. Treatment is conservative rest, administration of nonsteroidal antiinflammatory drugs, and advising the patient not to put weight on the site.

ACHILLES TENDINITIS

Achilles tendinitis is caused by overuse and is seen most commonly in middle-aged or older adult distance runners. Inflammation of the tendon results in pain 3 to 6 cm above the tendon insertion. Tenderness anterior to the tendon is more consistent with retrocalcaneal bursitis. Treatment includes rest, ice, heel lifts, nonsteroidal antiinflammatory drugs, ultrasound, stretching of the gastrocnemius and soleus muscles, and, rarely, surgery.[3]

RETROCALCANEAL BURSITIS

Retrocalcaneal bursitis is an inflammation of the bursa that lies between the Achilles tendon and the posterior border of the calcaneus. Symptoms begin early in activity and are exacerbated by dorsiflexion of the foot. Tenderness is just anterior to the Achilles tendon (deep) and posterior to the calcaneus. Hindfoot swelling is often present. The treatment is rest and administration of nonsteroidal antiinflammatory medications. The patient is instructed on stretching exercises and use of a heel lift. This condition also may be treated with steroid and local anesthetic injections.

GENERALIZED FOOT CONDITIONS

BROMHIDROSIS

Malodor of the feet is caused by keratin decomposition in the presence of hyperhidrosis or excessive production of sweat. A corynebacterial overgrowth or fungal colonization may occur, worsening the condition. Treatment includes measures to reduce sweat production and to control secondary infection. Use of talcum powder, spray deodorants, and absorbent insoles may be helpful.

TINEA PEDIS

The most common fungal infections of the skin are on the feet. Footwear, because it causes moisture and warmth between the toes, predisposes to this condition; communal activity promotes its spread.

There are three types of tinea pedis. One involves maceration and desquamation in the lateral toe spaces, the second manifests as episodes of unilateral acute vesiculation on the soles, and the third includes dry redness and diffuse scaling over the soles. Symptoms are extreme itching, burning, and irritation on the soles of the foot and between the toes. Treatment includes a variety of agents, such as tolnaftate, clotrimazole, and miconazole. These agents should be used twice daily. Widespread infections and cases involving the nails are treated with systemic griseofulvin, terbinafine, or the imidazoles.

DISPOSITION

Foot problems are a frequent presenting complaint in the emergency department. The vast majority can be diagnosed easily and treated symptomatically. Patients should be referred to a primary care physician, a podiatrist, or an orthopedic surgeon for definitive care.

COMMON PITFALLS

- Failure to aggressively manage diabetic patients with foot disorders; the risk of complications is high if such patients are inadequately treated.
- Failure to recognize metatarsal stress fractures, which are common and may not be visualized radiographically. If a stress fracture is suspected, treat it conservatively with avoidance of weight bearing.
- Failure to distinguish between plantar warts and calluses. It is important to diagnose accurately, because management and treatment are different for the two conditions.

References

1. Caillet R. *Foot and ankle pain,* 3rd ed. New York: F.A. Davis, 1997.
2. Dunagin WG. Verruca vulgaris. In: Rakel RE, ed. *Conn's current therapy.* Philadelphia: WB Saunders, 1988.
3. Galloway MT, Jokl P, Dayton OW. Achilles tendon overuse injuries. *Clin Sports Med* 1992;11:771.
4. Lorimer DL, French G, West S. *Neale's common foot disorders: diagnosis and management,* 5th ed. London: Churchill Livingstone, 1997.
5. Quaschnick MS. The diagnosis and management of plantar fasciitis. *Nurse Pract* 1996;21:50.
6. Roberts JR, Hedges JR. *Clinical procedures in emergency medicine,* 3rd ed. Philadelphia: Saunders, 1998.
7. Van Wyngarden TM. The painful foot, part I: common forefoot deformities. *Am Fam Physician* 1997;55(6):2207.

CHAPTER 58
Bone and Soft-Tissue Neoplasms

Joseph A. Buckwalter

Emergency physicians cannot be expected to definitively diagnose, stage, and treat musculoskeletal neoplasms. However, they should recognize the clinical manifestations of these neoplasms and initiate appropriate management. Failure to do so can delay diagnosis, compromise the results of treatment, and lead to unnecessary complications. Unfortunately, early diagnosis of bone and soft-tissue neoplasms may be difficult, because they do not have a uniform clinical presentation. They may appear in any part of the musculoskeletal system in patients of any age. They may cause severe pain, massive swelling, and pathologic fracture, or they may be asymptomatic. The wide variety of benign and malignant musculoskeletal neoplasms and their rarity make categorization of these lesions difficult. Furthermore, the presentation of some common benign disorders of the skeleton and soft tissues closely resembles neoplasm. Table 58.1 lists some of the disorders that resemble neoplasms, benign neoplasms, malignant primary neoplasms, and neoplasms that commonly metastasize to bone.

CLINICAL PRESENTATION

Bone and soft-tissue neoplasms usually come to the attention of the patient or physician because of pain, swelling, or loss of musculoskeletal function. Less frequently, *they are discovered incidentally* when an examination or imaging study is performed for other reasons.

Pain

Not all musculoskeletal neoplasms cause pain. When they do, patients often describe the pain as a progressive, deep aching that may interfere with normal activities, awaken them at night, or prevent sleeping. It is usually not relieved by rest and may be referred to another location. For example, a tumor about the hip may cause aching pain extending down the thigh to the knee or pain limited to the knee. A tumor of the cervical spine may cause pain radiating down the arm. Pain associated with neoplasms of the lumbar spine or pelvis may be felt in the buttock, thigh, or leg.

Swelling

Although many neoplasms present as firm, easily palpable, well-defined masses or as diffuse swelling of an extremity, others are not so easily identified by physical examination. Tumors confined within bone cannot be palpated. Deep soft-tissue tumors may produce only a slight increase in limb circumference rather than a discrete mass or easily detected diffuse swelling. This is particularly characteristic of deep soft-tissue tumors of the thigh, hip, and shoulder. These lesions may reach a large size without causing pain or producing a discrete mass, particularly in obese or muscular patients. Intrapelvic, intraabdominal, and intrathoracic musculoskeletal neoplasms may also grow quite large before they cause physical signs that indicate their presence.

Loss of Function

The loss of function associated with musculoskeletal tumors is commonly due to pain, a neurologic deficit, or a pathologic fracture. The neurologic deficit may be slowly progressive, such as that caused by a soft-tissue sarcoma of the posterior thigh that gradually compresses the sciatic nerve. Alternatively, the neurologic deficit may be acute, as in the sudden compression of the spinal cord from rapid enlargement of a primary or metastatic spinal tumor. The presence of a neoplasm should be suspected in any patient who fractures a bone after minor trauma. In these patients, the plain radiographs usually show some irregularity of the bone near the fracture site. Even in patients with a history of significant trauma, an irregularity of the bone should lead the physician to suspect the possibility of a pathologic fracture secondary to a bone neoplasm.

Incidental Discovery

An unsuspected neoplasm may be revealed by an evaluation performed for other reasons. Physical examination may reveal the presence of a soft-tissue or bone mass that the patient has not noticed. Radiographs or other imaging studies ordered to evaluate an acute injury may demonstrate a bone or soft-tissue neoplasm. For this reason, the physician should carefully review all parts of radiographs and other imaging studies, not just the area of an acute injury.

DIFFERENTIAL DIAGNOSIS

Table 58.1 lists many of the lesions to be considered in the differential diagnosis of bone and soft-tissue neoplasms. The references indicated in the table provide detailed descriptions that will aid in distinguishing these lesions.

TABLE 58.1. Differential Diagnosis of Bone and Soft-Tissue Neoplasms

Disorders That Resemble Neoplasms	Benign Lesions	Malignant Neoplasms	Metastatic Neoplasms
BONE			
Fracture			
Metabolic bone diseases	Eosinophilic granuloma	Myeloma	Lung
Hyperparathyroidism	Aneurysmal bone cyst	Osteosarcoma	Breast
Paget disease	Bone-forming lesions	Parosteal osteosarcoma	Kidney
Osteomalacia	Osteoid osteoma	Chondrosarcoma	Thyroid
Osteoporosis	Osteoblastoma	Ewing sarcoma	Prostate
Infection	Osteoma	Fibrosarcoma	Gastrointestinal tract
Bone infarct	Cartilage-forming lesions	Malignant fibrous histiocytoma	
Simple cyst	Osteochondroma	Angiosarcoma	
	Enchondroma	Adamantinoma	
	Chondromyxoid fibroma	Chordoma	
	Chondroblastoma	Lymphoma	
	Fibrous lesions	Malignant vascular tumor	
	Fibrous cortical defect		
	Fibrous dysplasia		
	Giant cell tumor		
SOFT TISSUE			
Hematomas			
Myositis ossificans	Lipoma	Liposarcoma	Rare
Thrombophlebitis	Angiolipoma	Fibrosarcoma	
Infection	Lymphangioma	Malignant fibrous histiocytoma	
Ganglion	Neuroma	Leiomyosarcoma	
Pseudoaneurysms	Neurofibroma	Rhabdomyosarcoma	
Arteriovenous malformation	Fibromatoses	Synovial sarcoma	
Keloid	Superficial	Malignant schwannoma	
Nodular fascilitis	Deep	Malignant vascular tumor	
Fat necrosis	Giant cell tumor of tendon sheath		
	Elastofibroma		

Data from references 1 through 6.

Many injuries, infections, developmental disorders, and diseases of unknown cause that affect the musculoskeletal system may closely resemble neoplasms. For example, stress fractures can mimic bone-forming neoplasms, including osteosarcomas. Osteomyelitis and Ewing sarcoma may be difficult to distinguish based on the history, physical findings, and plain radiographs. Fibrous dysplasia can cause pathologic fractures and resemble a malignant neoplasm. In some patients, the radiographic and clinical presentation of Paget disease appears almost identical to that of metastatic carcinoma of the prostate.

A malignant bone neoplasm should be suspected in any patient whose radiographs show evidence of bone destruction. Radiographic evidence of bone destruction, particularly irregular loss of bone, suggests the presence of a neoplasm (Figs. 58.1 and 58.2). Figures 58.3 and 58.4 show a typical appearance of a metastatic carcinoma of the breast. This is by far the most common cause of an impending pathologic fracture that would be seen in the emergency department. With the exception of infection, most benign bone lesions do not produce irregular permeative destruction of bone. A soft-tissue sarcoma should be suspected in any patient with an enlarging soft-tissue mass. A history of progressive deep, aching pain that is not relieved by rest and interferes with normal activities and sleep should also suggest the possibility of a musculoskeletal neoplasm. Not all musculoskeletal neoplasms, even malignant lesions, cause pain.

EMERGENCY DEPARTMENT EVALUATION

The initial evaluation of a patient with a suspected musculoskeletal neoplasm should include a careful history, physical examination, and plain radiographic studies. The physician should determine the duration of symptoms and signs, with particular attention to the pattern of pain and any possible loss of musculoskeletal function.

The presence of other illnesses should be determined. Specific risk factors for metastatic tumors (i.e., lung, breast, prostate, thyroid, kidney) should be addressed. Physical examination should include the following:

Size of any lesions
Tenderness
Bruits
Skin color
Temperature changes
Neurologic function
Joint effusions and range of motion
Pulses
Changes in limb circumference
Muscle strength
Presence or absence of enlarged lymph nodes
Whether lesions are fixed to the skin, tendons, muscles, or bones

Radiographs in two planes should be taken. Depending on the results of this initial evaluation, it may be appropriate to order laboratory studies and more extensive imaging studies. Computed tomography, magnetic resonance imaging, arteriography, technetium bone scanning, and ultrasonography may be used to assess the relation of the lesion to other structures and to determine the extent and stage of the lesion. A comprehensive physical examination, chest radiograph, chest and abdominal computed tomography, renal ultrasound studies, and mammography may be appropriate to determine the source of an apparent metastatic lesion.

Although failure to order sophisticated imaging studies occasionally delays the diagnosis of bone and soft-tissue neoplasms, more common errors include failure to perform a

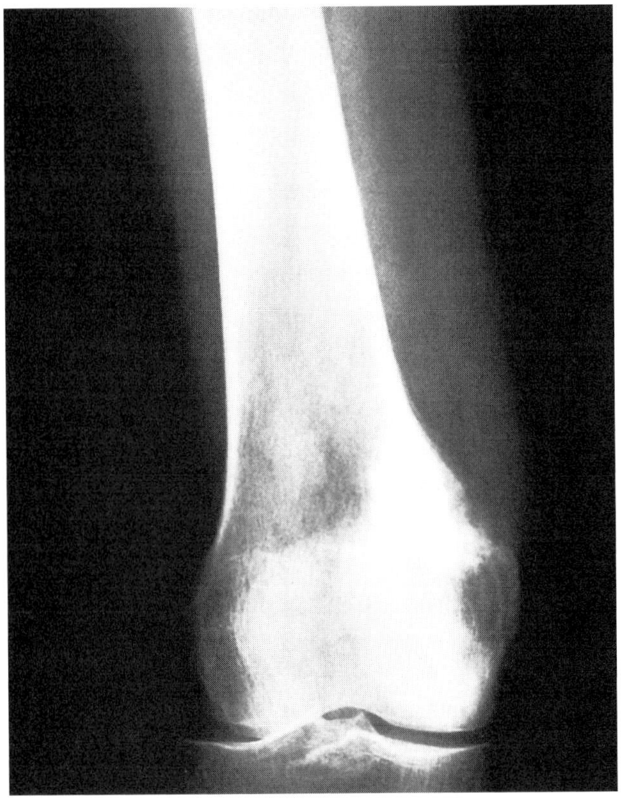

Figure 58.1. A destructive bone-forming lesion of the distal femoral metaphysis. Notice the destruction of the medial femoral condyle, the new bone formation in the region of bone destruction, and the elevation of the periosteum. These features are characteristic of osteosarcomas.

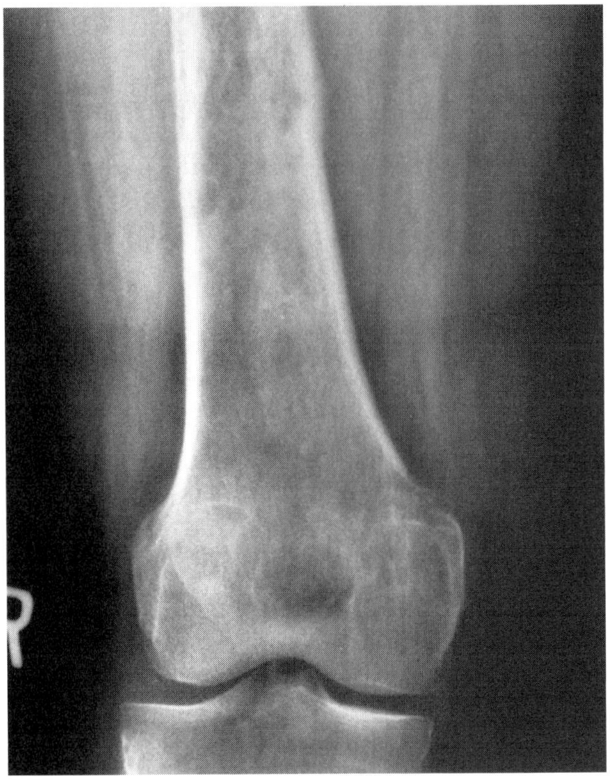

Figure 58.3. A destructive, primarily lytic metastatic lesion from a carcinoma of the breast. Notice the irregular destruction of the distal femoral shaft extending into the femoral metaphysis.

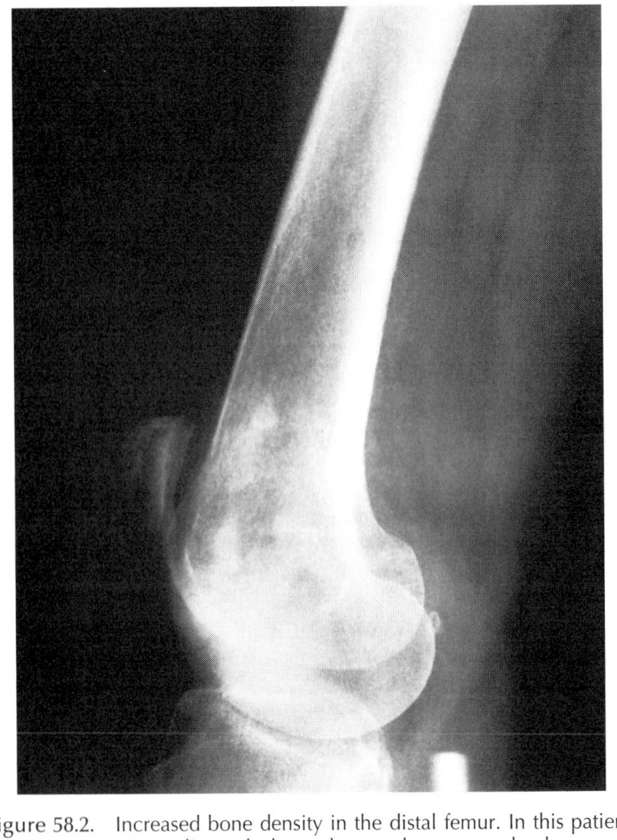

Figure 58.2. Increased bone density in the distal femur. In this patient, the anteroposterior radiograph shows the neoplasm more clearly.

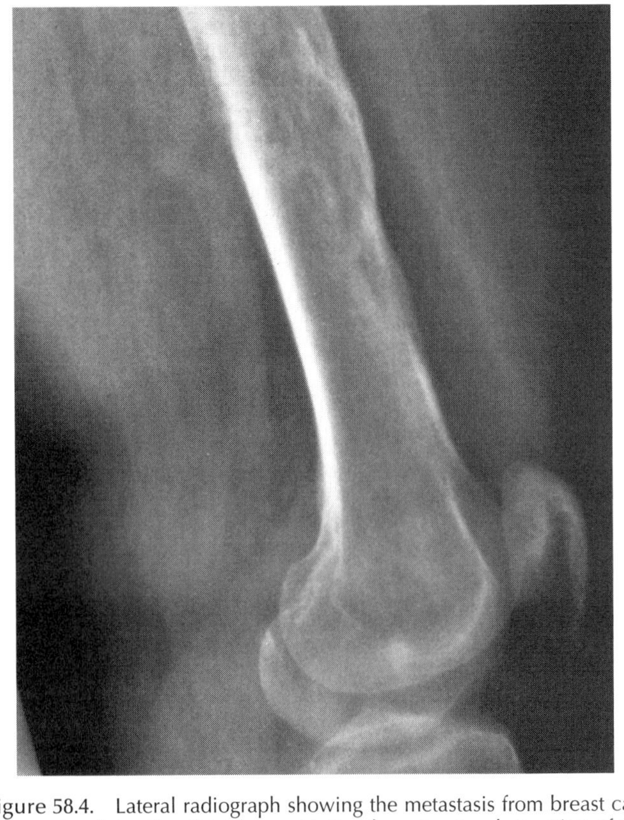

Figure 58.4. Lateral radiograph showing the metastasis from breast carcinoma involving the distal femur. Notice the extensive destruction of the anterior femoral cortex as well as the region of the posterior femoral cortex. This extensive lesion has significantly weakened the femoral shaft and is highly likely to result in a pathologic fracture. This patient should be immediately protected and referred for prophylactic internal fixation of this lesion as well as for comprehensive evaluation.

thorough physical evaluation, including a neurologic and orthopedic examination, failure to note abnormalities on plain radiographs, failure to recognize a pathologic fracture, and failure to obtain consultation for evaluation of suspicious lesions.

EMERGENCY DEPARTMENT MANAGEMENT

Most patients with suspected neoplasms of bone and soft tissue do not require emergency treatment. However, patients with severe pain, compromise of neurologic or vascular function, pathologic fracture, or an impending pathologic fracture may require urgent treatment. Severe pain associated with a musculoskeletal neoplasm may indicate bleeding into the lesion, pressure on nerves, an increase in compartment pressure, a pathologic fracture, or an impending pathologic fracture. Patients with pathologic fractures should be splinted appropriately, and consultation should be sought. Patients with impending fractures should be protected to avoid a fracture that may compromise definitive treatment. The presence of a neurologic deficit, particularly a deficit caused by spinal cord compression, requires emergency consultation and definitive treatment. Biopsy of a musculoskeletal lesion is seldom appropriate as an emergency procedure. Biopsies should be planned carefully and almost always preceded by appropriate staging studies. Inappropriate biopsies may fail to obtain satisfactory tissue for diagnosis, cause unnecessary contamination of tissue compartments and other complications, including infection and excessive bleeding, and spread the tumor beyond its original location.

DISPOSITION

Role of the Consultant

Patients with a suspected bone or soft-tissue neoplasm should be referred to an orthopedic surgeon with experience in the treatment of musculoskeletal neoplasms. If possible, consultation should be obtained before ordering staging studies (computed tomography, magnetic resonance imaging, and bone scans). In the patient with severe intractable pain, a neurologic deficit or an impending neurologic deficit, or a pathologic or impending pathologic fracture, consultation should be sought immediately.

Indications for Admission

Patients with suspected musculoskeletal neoplasms generally do not need to be admitted unless there is uncontrollable pain, evidence of neurovascular compromise, impending neurovascular compromise, pathologic fracture, or impending fracture. Patients with these conditions should be admitted for definitive evaluation, staging, possibly biopsy, and definitive treatment. Patients who do not require admission should be referred to an orthopedic surgeon before discharge from the emergency department. The patient should be instructed that urgent evaluation by a consultant is essential.

Transfer Considerations

The management of patients with musculoskeletal neoplasms frequently requires consultants in musculoskeletal oncology, medical oncology, radiation therapy, musculoskeletal pathology, and musculoskeletal radiology. A neurosurgeon, thoracic surgeon, or general surgeon and radiologist may also be helpful in the management of complex problems. For this reason, patients with bone and soft-tissue neoplasms should be cared for at centers with these specialists and should be transferred to these centers expeditiously. Patients with pathologic fractures or impending fractures of the long bones should have their limbs stabilized before transfer.

COMMON PITFALLS

- Failure to detect a musculoskeletal neoplasm. In part because neoplasms of bone and soft tissue occur infrequently, physicians may not consider neoplasm when confronted with complaints of pain, swelling, and loss of musculoskeletal function, and with incidental, unexplained physical findings or abnormalities on imaging studies. If the emergency physician suspects a musculoskeletal neoplasm, the patient should be referred for more extensive evaluation.
- Failure to refer to a consultant. Occasionally, a lesion may be identified, but the patient is not referred for definitive evaluation. This may occur when a patient has other medical problems or an acute traumatic injury. The possible neoplasm may be noted, but because attention is focused on other problems, the patient is not referred for evaluation of the possible tumor.
- Failure to recognize a neurologic deficit or a potential neurologic deficit. Patients with possible bone and soft-tissue neoplasms should have a thorough neurologic examination. Tumors of the limbs may compress peripheral nerves. Even more serious problems are compression of the spinal cord owing to tumors in or about the spine and destruction of the vertebrae, leading to spinal cord compression.
- Failure to recognize a pathologic fracture. A fracture that occurs after minimal trauma should alert the physician to the possibility of a pathologic fracture. The radiographs of the fractured bone should be inspected carefully for any abnormalities that might indicate the presence of an underlying neoplasm. If it is difficult to determine whether an underlying neoplasm is present, but the fracture occurred after minimal trauma, the patient should undergo more extensive evaluation. If this does not reveal evidence of a neoplasm, the patient should be either referred for consultation or followed carefully.
- Failure to recognize an impending pathologic fracture. This problem is most frequently seen in patients with metastatic disease (see Figs. 58.3 and 58.4). In these patients, it is essential to evaluate the skeleton for the presence of metastatic tumor. Areas of particular concern include the spine, the femur, and the tibia.
- Inappropriate biopsy. Patients with suspected musculoskeletal neoplasms usually should not have a biopsy until appropriate staging studies have been performed and the patient has been evaluated by an orthopedic surgeon with experience in the management of these problems. Inappropriate aspiration or incisional or excisional biopsies can disseminate tumor, cause bleeding and infection, and fail to provide diagnostic tissue. Needle aspiration of a soft-tissue mass in the emergency department may seem like a simple, quick, safe way to make a diagnosis, but it can cause bleeding and infection and may fail to provide diagnostic tissue.

References

1. Enneking WF. *Musculoskeletal tumor surgery.* New York: Churchill Livingstone, 1983.
2. Enzinger FM, Weiss SW. *Soft tissue tumors,* 2nd ed. St. Louis: CV Mosby, 1988.
3. Mirra JM. *Bone tumors: clinical radiologic and pathologic correlations.* Philadelphia: Lea & Febiger, 1989.
4. Resnick D, Niwayama G. *Diagnosis of bone and joint disorders.* Philadelphia: WB Saunders, 1981.
5. Schajowicz F. *Tumors and tumorlike conditions of bones and joints.* New York: Springer-Verlag, 1981.
6. Sim FH. *Diagnosis and management of metastatic disease.* New York: Raven Press, 1988.

PART VII
Emergency Aspects of Neurosurgery

CHAPTER 59
Intracranial Neoplasms

Collette Ditz Wyte and Elizabeth A. Hatfield

Intracranial neoplasms (INs) are benign or malignant tumors located within the cranial cavity. They include masses that arise from or are metastatic to the pituitary or pineal glands, meninges, intracranial portion of the cranial nerves, intracranial blood vessels, or the brain tissue itself.[14]

About 75% of central nervous system (CNS) tumors in children are infratentorial, whereas 75% of such tumors in adults are supratentorial. The most common brain tumors in adults are metastatic tumors, malignant gliomas, meningiomas, and pituitary adenomas. Cerebellar astrocytomas, medulloblastomas, and fourth ventricle ependymomas predominate in children.

Gliomas are neoplasms of glial lineage and constitute 50% of primary INs.[14] They include multiple types, from the highly malignant glioblastoma multiforme to the relatively benign astrocytoma. These tumors have a predilection for the cerebral hemispheres in adults. Increasing age of the patient correlates with poor prognosis.

Meningiomas are the second most common adult brain tumor, constituting 20% of primary INs.[14] They are histologically benign, slow-growing tumors of arachnoid tissue and are usually very vascular. Of all INs, meningiomas have the highest association with extraneural tumors. Meningiomas usually compress but do not invade brain tissue. Changes in the underlying skull are frequent and may be seen on plain radiograph. They also contain a high concentration of progesterone receptors, rendering them hormone sensitive.

Pituitary adenomas represent 15% of all primary INs.[14] Only one-third of the patients reveal the characteristic sign of bitemporal hemianopia from compression of the optic chiasm by superior extension of the tumor. Some patients present with only endocrine symptomatology, such as secondary amenorrhea, galactorrhea, impotence, and Cushing syndrome. Diagnosis is aided by an enlarged sella turcica on lateral skull films, a pituitary mass on computed tomography (CT), or an abnormal signal on magnetic resonance imaging (MRI). An elevated serum prolactin level is present in two-thirds of these patients.

Acoustic neuroma is a benign schwannoma of the eighth cranial nerve that is usually located within the internal auditory meatus. It constitutes 7% of all primary INs.[6] More than 95% of patients with this tumor present with unilateral neurosensory hearing loss.[6] Other symptoms include tinnitus, vertigo, dysequilibrium, facial paresthesias, dysphagia, and hoarseness.

Metastatic tumors are the most common IN in late middle life and account for 20% to 30% of all adult INs. Lung and breast cancers are the number one primary tumors in men and women, respectively. Malignant melanoma, hypernephromas, and colon carcinomas complete the five most frequent primary lesions.

Cerebral metastases, like emboli, tend to be found along the middle cerebral artery distribution in the parietal lobe. They are usually multiple. Thus, a neurologic examination and enhanced CT or MRI findings of several lesions should suggest the possibility of metastatic disease.

Meningeal carcinomatosis is a diffuse infiltration of the meninges by tumor cells that can occur with systemic cancer. Clinical suspicion is warranted in the presence of multifocal neurologic signs and symptoms, and suspicion is verified by an abnormal cerebrospinal fluid (CSF) analysis, typically revealing increased intracranial pressure (ICP), increased protein concentration, decreased glucose, pleocytosis, and, occasionally, malignant cells.

EPIDEMIOLOGY

Overall, the incidence of brain tumors is 5 to 9 per 100,000 population and may be increasing.[14] Nine thousand to 12,000 persons die of brain tumors yearly, which is just slightly more than the annual number of deaths caused by drowning. Brain cancer is the second leading cause of cancer-related deaths in children and the fourth leading cause of cancer-related deaths in middle-aged men.

The incidence, type, location, and prognosis of brain tumors are all age related. The incidence of primary INs increases steadily with advancing age, with the first peak occurring in early childhood and the second and highest peak occurring between the fifth and sixth decades.

Metastatic cancer has only a 1:100,000 incidence in persons younger than age 35, but the incidence increases rapidly thereafter, reaching more than 30:100,000 by age 60.[14] Eighteen percent of all patients with systemic cancer have evidence of metastatic brain tumors. Half of this group show neurologic symptoms. Ten percent of cerebral metastases are diagnosed before the discovery of the primary tumor.[14]

Whereas females have an increased incidence of meningiomas, pituitary adenomas, and schwannomas, males have an increased incidence of gliomas, brain metastases, and brain tumors in general.[14]

ETIOLOGY

There is a well-known role of heredity in the neurophakomatoses, most notably von Recklinghausen neurofibromatosis, von Hippel-Lindau hemangioblastoma, and tuberous sclerosis. Most brain tumors, however, do not reflect a genetic pattern. Embryologic factors are responsible for the rare congenital tumors, such as pineoblastomas, teratomas, and germinomas.

Oncogenic virus injections and chemical carcinogens have been shown to produce CNS tumors in animals, but their role in humans is speculative. Trauma has been implicated by some to be the cause of brain tumors, for example, development of meningiomas along cranial fracture lines. This is highly controversial. The role of radiation and irradiation also remains controversial. In the vast majority of cases, the cause remains idiopathic.

PATHOPHYSIOLOGY

There are two major mechanisms for symptoms produced in INs. First, increased intracerebral pressure produces nonspecific symptoms such as headache, vomiting, mental status changes, and disturbances in consciousness. These symptoms may be more noticeable in the early awakening hours, since cerebral vasodilation accompanies sleep, therefore producing a paroxysmal increase in ICP. This rise in ICP may be caused directly by the tumor mass or by associated cerebral edema, which is a localized area of tissue swelling secondary to altered capillary permeability. The rise in ICP is normally a combination of the two. Occasionally, ICP is raised secondary to obstruction of CSF flow, venous system drainage, or meningeal absorption. Chronically elevated ICP can itself decrease CSF absorption, therefore causing a cyclical worsening of ICP.

The second mechanism is tissue destruction or irritation. This may be due to infiltration or compression of normal brain tissue adjacent to the tumor. It may also be caused by displacement of brain matter and compression of neural tissue at sites distant from the tumor, with the most significant example being uncal herniation.

NATURAL HISTORY

The symptomatology and prognosis depend on the growth characteristics of the tumor and its location in the cranial cavity. A slow-growing tumor in a relatively silent brain region can reach enormous size without producing neurologic symptoms. Elevated ICP syndrome may actually be the first clinical presentation in these patients. Alternatively, small tumors in proximity to vital CNS structures may produce early profound focal neurologic symptoms. Accordingly, the terms *benign* and *malignant* have less importance with INs than with other masses, because a histologically benign tumor may be lethal by virtue of its location in the brain.

CLINICAL PRESENTATION

A slow onset and gradual worsening of symptoms are typical for INs.

Signs and Symptoms

Headache

A recent onset or change in the character of a headache may signal the presence of an IN. Although most patients with headache do not have tumors, 60% to 90% of patients with brain tumors complain of headache at some point in their illness, and 20% have headache as the initial symptom.

Headaches caused by INs are described as steady, nonthrobbing, dull, aching pain relieved by analgesics. They may be so mild and intermittent at first that the patient mentions them only as a response to direct questioning. With tumor growth, the headaches become more severe, more frequent, and persistent. In addition to a progressive nature, other characteristics of tumor-induced headaches include early-morning occurrence, aggravation by Valsalva maneuvers, and association with vomiting, particularly in the absence of preceding nausea. Any headache—no matter the character—associated with seizure activity, abnormal mental status, focal neurologic signs, or papilledema is due to IN until proven otherwise.

Tumor-induced headache is secondary to either increased ICP or traction on pain-sensitive structures. The structures in the cranial cavity that are sensitive to pain include major arteries, veins, dura mater, and cranial nerves. Therefore, headache is a poor localizing sign. However, supratentorial expanding lesions typically produce pain in the frontal or vertex regions, because these structures are most commonly innervated by the trigeminal nerve. Posterior fossa structures, on the other hand, are innervated by the ninth and tenth cranial nerves and the first three cervical nerves; therefore, infratentorial masses usually cause pain in the occipital and upper posterior cervical spinal regions.

Seizures

New onset of seizure activity is another common presentation of patients with IN. Thirty-five percent of cerebral tumors are associated with seizure activity, and seizures are the initial symptom in 15%. Although seldom seen with infratentorial tumors (less than 3%), seizures occur in approximately half the patients with supratentorial masses. Aside from being supratentorial, the other tumor features predisposing to epileptogenicity are slow-growing neoplasms, such as benign astrocytomas, and tumors that involve the cortex, such as meningiomas.

In patients younger than age 20, the incidence of cerebral tumors causing epilepsy is almost negligible at 0.02%. In patients with new onset of seizure activity and focal neurologic deficits, the incidence of tumor increases to 50%. Half of the patients without history of prior seizure who present with status epilepticus also have IN. Besides initial status or focal neurologic findings, clinical suspicion of IN should also be aroused in any patient older than age 20 with a first episode of seizure, particularly if the seizure is followed by a prolonged postictal period or Todd paralysis. The risk of IN is also increased if the seizure has focal motor, sensory, or psychomotor features.

Particular subsets of seizure are seen, depending on the tumor location. Generalized or focal motor seizures are produced by frontal lobe neoplasms. Complex partial seizures are often manifested by temporal lobe lesions. Absence seizures are usually not a complication of INs.

Mental Status

Mental status or behavioral changes are commonly seen with IN, particularly with frontal and temporal lobe lesions. Because of their often subtle nature, such changes may be overlooked until focal neurologic signs develop. Often patients are unaware of changes in their behavior, but alterations of mental status may be disclosed by questioning their families and friends. Case reports exist that describe patients who presented with emotional lability or other inappropriate behavior who were later diagnosed with a brain tumor. Symptoms can mimic a depressive disorder or Alzheimer disease, with a predominance of apathy, irritability, restlessness, depression, loss of spontaneity, or memory loss. Bilateral frontal lobe tumors (i.e., "butterfly" glioblastoma) that result in inappropriate and antisocial behavior may be confused with affective or schizophrenic disorders. These various changes in mental status seem to occur most often with rapidly growing tumors, such as glioblastomas.

Focal Neurologic Deficits

Progressive focal neurologic defects may also be produced by intracranial masses. Common findings include aphasia, hemiparesis, sensory or visual deficits, and cranial nerve palsies. The sixth cranial nerve is involved most commonly because it has the longest intracranial course. These findings must be differentiated from a number of other intracranial lesions, such as cerebrovascular accident (CVA), transient ischemic attacks (TIAs), and intracerebral hemorrhagic disorders. The characteristic unique to IN-induced focal neurologic deficits is that these deficits tend to be slow in onset, with only gradual increase in severity. Rarely, the onset of symptoms is sudden, and intraneoplastic hemorrhage must then be a consideration.

Miscellaneous

Vomiting occurs in 70% of patients with IN, but it is the presenting symptom in only 10%. It is characteristically projectile, unrelated to food, more frequent in the early waking hours (as is headache), and usually not preceded by nausea. Like headache and papilledema, it is one of the cardinal signs of chronically increased ICP. Other rare initial presentations of IN include vertigo or dysequilibrium, irreversible coma, and acute blindness.[3] Remote symptoms include neurogenic pulmonary edema and cardiopulmonary collapse.[5]

Presentation by Location

Clinical presentation depends on the presence or absence of elevated ICP and the location of the tumor. Mixed clinical pictures are often present, because tumors usually spread to involve more than one brain region. Frontal lobe tumors may produce personality change, particularly in respect to acquired social behavior. Uninhibited behavior may be prominent, and reflected in the use of inappropriate language or actions without regard for their effect on others. Apathy and poor hygiene are common. A severe decline in intellect and memory may also ensue. These changes develop slowly over months to years, until an obvious dementia occurs. Patients may also experience loss of bladder control. Generalized tonic–clonic seizures and jacksonian or partial motor seizures are also characteristic of frontal lobe tumors.

The occipital lobe is very small and seldom affected by tumors. When present, they are manifested by visual agnosia or alexia, highly congruent hemianopia, and, rarely, seizures. When seizures do occur, they are often preceded by visual hallucinations consisting of unformed flashes of light and color.

Parietal lobe neoplasms present as dysphasia if the dominant lobe is affected and as dyspraxia if the nondominant lobe is involved. Sensory loss, inattention, homonymous hemianopia, and loss of opticokinetic nystagmus also occur.

Temporal lobe masses can also present with personality changes, but these tend to be subtler than those associated with frontal lobe tumors. They are characterized by alterations in affect, imitating psychotic disorders rather than the demented picture of frontal lobe tumors. Other symptoms include complex partial seizures with prodromal gustatory, olfactory, auditory, or formed visual hallucinations and upper quadrantic homonymous hemianopia.

Cerebellar tumors, although rare in adults, cause dysmetria, hypotonia, ataxia, nystagmus, and "cerebellar fits," which are episodes of intermittent decerebrate rigidity.

Emergent Problems

Although the *sine qua non* of IN is slow, progressive deterioration in clinical status, occasionally a rapid decline occurs. This is often caused by an acute increase in ICP that develops in minutes to hours and is characterized by a sudden and marked increase in headache, with stiff neck, opisthotonus, facial flushing or pallor, and drowsiness that may progress to coma. Characteristically, the patient develops bradycardia with an elevation of blood pressure. This is termed *the Cushing response* and is the physiologic rise in systemic blood pressure as a consequence of increased ICP. This is compensatory to maintain adequate cerebral perfusion pressure (CPP = MAP − ICP). Reflex bradycardia secondary to elevated mean arterial pressure (MAP) is another component of this response. The respiratory rate slows and deepens and may progress to a Cheyne-Stokes pattern. This acute alteration in ICP is usually caused by an intracranial hemorrhage; however, it can be seen with hemorrhage into an IN. Such hemorrhages occur with glioblastoma multiforme and metastatic brain tumors.[10]

Acute hydrocephalus is rare but can occur with tumors blocking the fourth ventricle in children or the foramen of Monroe in adults. It is a life-threatening emergency in which ventricular decompression is urgently needed. Intraventricular tumors can also cause intermittent obstruction, owing to a ball–valve mechanism. When this occurs, there is a clinical pattern of severe headache followed by altered levels of consciousness and even coma that may resolve spontaneously only to recur.

Sudden death is a rare but devastating complication of IN and is most often secondary to uncal herniation.[5] A pressure rise within one hemisphere, rather than a general increase in pressure, can displace the uncus and hippocampal gyrus of the temporal lobe between the free edge of the tentorium and the midbrain. In the early stages of uncal herniation, the patient classically presents with an ipsilateral dilated pupil with contralateral hemiparesis, Babinski's sign, and spastic hypertonicity. This phase progresses to a stage at which both pupils become fixed and dilated, with oculomotor paresis, nonresponsiveness to caloric testing, bilateral Babinski's signs, and decerebrate response to pain. Terminally, the patient develops hyperventilation, which slows near death. The pulse rate rises and the blood pressure falls, producing the clinical syndrome of neurogenic shock.

Cerebellar herniation is more common in posterior fossa tumors. Another cause of sudden death, this is protrusion of the cerebellar tonsil through the foramen magnum, causing acute hydrocephalus and cardiorespiratory and vagal disturbances with pyramidal tract abnormalities. An upward herniation of the cerebellum through the incisura is also possible, but this is rare.

DIFFERENTIAL DIAGNOSIS

Depending on which of the multiple presentations occurs, IN can be mimicked by a multitude of neurologic and psychiatric disorders.

Headache

Migraine headaches share similar characteristics with IN-induced headaches. They are intermittent but not worse in the early waking hours, as are IN headaches. They are often associated with vomiting that is preceded by nausea, whereas nausea may be lacking in tumors. Classic migraine aura consisting of scintillating scotomas, visual field defects, hemiplegia, or hemiparesis may be mistaken for neurologic deficits associated with a tumor. Whereas in tumors these deficits are progressive, in migraine headaches they are fleeting. Although the migraine headache is typically unilateral, it is a throbbing, severe pain, unlike the characteristic dull aching of a tumor. Also, the duration of a migraine headache is hours to days, which is usually longer than the duration of a tumor-induced headache.

Muscular or tension headaches also resemble IN-induced headaches because of their occipital location and dull, aching nature. However, they are not associated with vomiting, neurologic deficits, seizures, or changes in mental status. They are also not progressive. CT or MRI would distinguish an IN from a migraine or tension headache.

Cerebrovascular Accident

Tumors occasionally present in an apoplectic manner and mimic stroke, particularly if there is hemorrhage into the tumor. Such hemorrhage occurs in glioblastomas and metastatic bronchogenic carcinoma, melanoma, renal carcinoma, and choriocarcinoma.[10] Normally CVA presents as a sudden onset of nonprogressive focal signs that may improve over time. IN characteristically has an insidious onset with progressive worsening of symptoms over time. Patients with nonhemorrhagic CVA seldom complain of headache and often have a history of hypertension or other evidence of arteriosclerosis. The distinction between tumor and CVA may be made with CT.

TIAs are characterized by fluctuant neurologic findings that do not progress, unlike those caused by brain tumors. CT or MRI in TIAs is unremarkable, and carotid Doppler studies are indicated for follow-up.

Brain Abscess

Brain abscesses are characterized by headache, papilledema, pyramidal signs, and seizures. Often the patient will present with tachycardia, fever, leukocytosis, and other signs of infectious etiology. The patient may give a history of head injury, previous meningeal symptoms, or rheumatic or cyanotic heart disease. However, in chronic brain abscess, these latter signs and symptoms may not be present. It may be difficult to distinguish an abscess from a neoplasm, even with enhanced CT or cerebral angiography. A brain biopsy may then be necessary for definitive diagnosis.

Acute infection of the meninges may simulate symptoms of brain tumors. The diagnosis may be made on examination of the CSF after a negative CT scan.

Subdural Hematoma

Chronic subdural hematoma may also present as headache, papilledema, and seizure disorder. The initial injury may have been so mild as to be forgotten, or it may have occurred in a patient too inebriated or demented to remember the incident. CT or MRI can readily differentiate between a chronic subdural hematoma and a tumor. Acute subdural hematoma is readily distinguished from IN because there is usually a clear history of head trauma.

Pseudotumor Cerebri

Pseudotumor cerebri is a syndrome consisting of nonspecific intermittent headache, papilledema, constricted visual fields, and an enlarged blind spot. It is often seen in obese young women with menstrual irregularities. Conditions associated with pseudotumor cerebri include ovarian dysfunction, Addison disease, Cushing disease, adrenocorticosteroid therapy or withdrawal, hypoparathyroidism, pregnancy, menarche, use of oral contraceptives, vitamin A abuse, tetracycline usage in infancy, and intracranial venous sinus thrombosis. Pain in this case is secondary to cerebral swelling causing traction on pain-sensitive structures. Diagnosis can be aided by a negative CT scan combined with a lumbar puncture that reveals increased opening pressure.

Dementia

Mental slowness or memory loss may be the only presenting symptom in frontal lobe neoplasms, as well as in Alzheimer or Pick disease. Precedent changes in personality or alterations in micturition are more indicative of frontal lobe tumors, and therefore should be sought. CT or MRI is useful in ruling out IN.

Delirium

Delirium may be a presenting symptom in IN. Drug abuse, metabolic abnormality, hypoxia, hypoglycemia, vitamin deficiency, and endocrinopathy are generally included in the differential diagnosis. Here again, CT or MRI would be helpful to exclude IN.

Psychoses

Psychiatric disorders such as depression may be mimicked by frontal lobe masses, whereas affective and schizophrenic-like disorders may be noted with temporal lobe masses. These symptoms may be ameliorated by psychotropic medication, even when the cause is IN. CT or MRI is helpful in excluding IN.

Demyelination

Multiple sclerosis and other demyelinating disorders can be distinguished clinically by their multiplicity of signs and symptoms and remitting course. MRI has proved superior to CT in making the distinction between such disorders and IN. A combination of clinical findings, CSF analysis, and evoked potential responses is diagnostic.

Seizure Disorder

IN should be considered in any adult with new onset of seizure, especially when the seizure is associated with focal neurologic signs or prolonged postictal stage. Electroencephalographic focal findings confirmed by a mass on a CT or MRI scan are diagnostic.

Intracranial Aneurysm

Giant aneurysms may present as mass lesions and can seldom be differentiated from tumor by CT or MRI. Angiography is usually necessary.

Hydrocephalus

Hydrocephalus may be caused by an obstructing neoplasm or by multiple other disorders. CT or MRI is warranted.

Intracerebral Hemorrhage

Hypertensive intracerebral hematoma and vascular malformations are mimicked by spontaneous hemorrhage in certain vascular tumors. They may all present as sudden headache, coma, stupor, hemiparesis, and bloody CSF. Although a hemorrhagic lesion can be seen on CT scan with all of these, intravenous contrast medium enhancement may show a margin of tumor surrounding a central clot in a bleeding tumor.

EMERGENCY DEPARTMENT EVALUATION

Emergency department evaluation of a suspected IN should begin with a careful history. Direct questioning regarding change in behavior or affect, visual disturbances, weakness, changes in sensation or speech, history of headache or vomiting, and new onset of seizures should be elicited.

Physical Examination

The physical examination should include a detailed neurologic and mental status examination. The most frequent finding in IN is papilledema. It is seen in 50% to 90% of these patients, depending on the stage of the tumor. Therefore, a funduscopic examination is imperative. These patients do not necessarily complain of visual disturbance, because papilledema does not interfere with visual acuity, but causes an enlargement of the physiologic blind spot. Consequently, visual field confrontation testing must also be performed. Papilledema is a nonspecific, nonlocalizing consequence of increased ICP. Therefore, small tumors such as pituitary adenomas, slow-growing astrocytomas, and brainstem gliomas may be present in the absence of papilledema. Even with an increase in ICP, papilledema may be absent if the patient has a high degree of myopia or if there is a preexistent or resultant optic neuritis from chronic papilledema itself. Venous pulsations, although not always visible, rule out increased ICP when seen. In addition to papilledema and optic atrophy, visual disturbances in brain tumors may include diplopia or visual field defects.

In addition to these various ophthalmic findings, focal neurologic deficits may be identified on neurologic examination, including hemiparesis, positive Babinski sign, cranial nerve palsies, dysarthria, ataxia, dysphasia, and abnormalities in sensation. These signs may have localizing potential, but this is usually lost in the presence of increased ICP. Serial neurologic examinations are essential in any patient suspected of having an IN. Patients who present with acutely elevated ICP may manifest headache, meningismus, bradycardia and hypertension, and altered levels of consciousness. The classic ipsilateral fixed and dilated pupil with contralateral hemiparesis or terminal findings of bilateral fixed and dilated pupils, decerebrate posturing, hypoventilation, tachycardia, and hypotension signify an impending herniation and demand immediate treatment.

In patients suspected of having brain malignancies, a thorough breast, pulmonary, abdominal, and skin examination should be performed to identify possible primary malignancies.

Laboratory Studies

Laboratory workup of patients with suspected IN or of patients who present with altered mental status, new-onset seizures, focal neurologic deficits, or evidence of elevated ICP include complete blood cell count, drug screen, and determination of serum levels of electrolytes (including calcium and magnesium), glucose, and blood urea nitrogen. These are ordered to rule out metabolic or infectious abnormalities. Baseline and serial serum osmolalities should be obtained if mannitol therapy is to be initiated. Liver function tests and measurement of serum ammonia levels may be helpful if hepatic encephalopathy is in the differential diagnosis. Coagulation studies and type and crossmatch should be ordered if urgent neurosurgical intervention is a consideration.

Radiologic Studies

The major diagnostic tool available for the emergency department evaluation of IN is CT. It defines the anatomic location of a neoplasm and, in many instances, predicts pathologic features. For example, smoothly marginated, homogeneous tumors favor benign disease, whereas irregular, inhomogeneous tumors favor malignancy. More important, CT may be used to rule out IN in suspected patients, because the accuracy of CT for diagnosing brain tumors is approximately 85% in nonenhanced studies and rises to 95% when intravenous contrast agents are used conjunctively. INs appear as abnormal lesions that may displace surrounding structures. Adjacent cerebral edema is often visualized as a low-density halo surrounding the mass. The lesion is further circumscribed with intravenous contrast medium, which outlines the more vascular periphery of the tumor. Multiplicity of tumor suggests metastatic disease.[1] Most metastatic tumors that are 1 cm or greater are visualized with CT.

Due to greater sensitivity, lack of ionizing radiation, and multiplanar imaging capability, MRI has replaced CT as the first-line imaging study for most patients with subacute or chronic neurologic disease.[1] For the emergency department patient, however, because of implanted or attached metal devices and ferromagnetic life-support systems that cannot be brought into the scanning arena, CT remains the imaging modality of choice.

In addition, MRI remains more costly and less readily available. The long scanning time for MRI (45 to 60 minutes, compared with 5 to 10 minutes for CT) requires a cooperative, immobile patient. A faster (10- to 15-minute) dual-plane MRI protocol is currently being studied, however.[8]

Cerebral angiography, although invasive and no longer routinely used, may still be necessary after a CT or MRI study, at the neurosurgeon's discretion. The main indication for IN is to eliminate the possibility of a giant aneurysm or vascular malformation as a cause of the CT abnormality. It is also used as a vascular road map to aid in either stereotactic needle biopsy or preoperative planning.

Miscellaneous Studies

Lumbar puncture is relatively contraindicated in the presence of an IN, but it may be warranted after a negative CT scan if meningeal carcinomatosis, meningitis, or subarachnoid hemorrhage is suspected. Ultrasound waves cannot penetrate bone; therefore, ultrasonography is used only intraoperatively to aid in tumor localization.[7] Monoclonal antibodies and gene therapy are being studied for use in both the diagnosis and treatment of IN, but much more work needs to be done in this field before these antibodies can be clinically useful.[4,9,13]

EMERGENCY DEPARTMENT MANAGEMENT

Prehospital Care

Management of patients with IN is directed at associated symptoms and complications. Field management should follow the ABCs of emergency medicine: providing airway control, ventilation, and stabilization of circulation with cervical spine immobilization, as necessary. An intravenous line should be established at a keep-vein-open (KVO) rate unless hypotension is present.

Acute Intervention

Once the patient's cardiopulmonary system is stabilized, acute intervention depends on the presentation of the patient. When a confused or comatose patient presents to an emergency department, one should consider administering 50% dextrose, naloxone (Narcan), and thiamine (vitamin B_1) to address the more common or easily treatable causes of coma, such as hypoglycemia, narcosis, and Wernicke encephalopathy.

The patient should be placed on a cardiac monitor and vital signs should be closely followed.

Seizures

Prevention of further seizures or treatment of a patient actively experiencing seizures should be done without further depressing mental status when possible. Phenytoin loading (10 to 15 mg/kg injected i.v. piggyback over 20 minutes) is the therapy of choice. Diazepam or lorazepam should be given to actively seizing patients to control status, in addition to phenytoin. Phenobarbital is reserved as a last-line drug because of CNS depression, but when necessary it may be given 2 to 3 mg/kg initially to a total of 15 to 18 mg/kg.

Increased Intracranial Pressure

For patients suspected of elevated ICP, the head of the bed should be raised 20% to 30% to aid cerebral venous outflow and thus potentiate ICP lowering. Fluids should be given at KVO rate unless the patient is simultaneously hypotensive. In this situation, shock management supersedes and isotonic fluid resuscitation is warranted. In the absence of hypotension, 0.9% normal saline administered at KVO rate is preferred over dextrose 5% in water or other hypotonic solutions, because the latter may precipitate or aggravate cerebral edema.

Hyperventilation

Patients with IN seldom present with acute elevation of ICP, but when they do, emergent treatment is necessary. There is concern that hyperventilation may further insult brain tissue, by inducing secondary ischemia.[2,17] However, intubation with hyperventilation is the fastest method to decrease ICP and should be initiated in the patient with radiographic or clinical evidence of herniation. The goal is to keep P_{CO_2} between 25 and 30 mm Hg. This can be titrated and monitored with serial arterial blood gas measurements. As the partial pressure of carbon dioxide is lowered in the circulation, the cerebrovascular bed constricts, reducing cerebral blood flow (CBF). A rule of thumb is that CBF is reduced by 2% per millimeter of mercury decrease in P_{CO_2}. This in turn reduces the ICP. Excessive hyperventilation with a resultant P_{CO_2} below 20 mm Hg restricts cerebral perfusion and may result in ischemic sequela. Oxygen supplementation is used to ensure adequate tissue oxygenation and to prevent hypoxia, which itself is a stimulus for ICP elevation.

Controlled rapid-sequence orotracheal intubation protects against the transient rise in ICP associated with laryngoscopy and endotracheal tube insertion.[15] Preoxygenation and a reduced or priming dose of a neuromuscular blocking agent are administered initially to prevent hypoxia and fasciculations, respectively. The patient is then given a sedative–hypnotic (i.e., 3 to 5 mg/kg of sodium thiopental) and a short-acting neuromuscular blocking agent (i.e., 1.0 to 1.5 mg/kg succinylcholine). Pulse oximetry, continuous monitoring, and CO_2 monitoring are recommended.

Most investigators conclude that 100 mg lidocaine given intravenously 1 to 5 minutes before intubation lowers the risk of transient ICP elevation. The mechanism of action includes cough reflex suppression, increased cerebrovascular resistance, and decreased cerebral blood volume during a period of profound sympathetic stimulation.

Osmotic Agents

Osmotic agents include urea, glycerol, and mannitol, of which mannitol is the agent of choice. These drugs are used in patients with ICP elevation in an attempt to stabilize them until surgical decompression is available.

Osmotic agents are effective in decreasing cerebral edema only in regions of the brain where the blood–brain barrier is intact. The current recommended dose of mannitol is 1 g/kg (range, 0.25 to 2.0 g/kg) of a 20% solution by intravenous infusion over 20 to 30 minutes. Because of potential rebound phenomenon (a secondary rise in ICP as mannitol is taken up by the CNS cells), the smallest effective dose of mannitol should be used. Lower doses are less likely to cause electrolyte and osmotic disturbances. No matter what dose is used, electrolytes, serum osmolality, blood pressure, urine output, and ICP (when possible) should be monitored. Serum osmolality should be maintained under 310 mOsmol. If the cause of ICP elevation is thought to be an intracranial hemorrhage, mannitol should be used with caution, because it can result in extension of the bleed. Glycerol may be given orally or intravenously, but it is seldom used, because the major complications of hemolysis, acute renal failure, and hyperosmolar coma may occur. Its effectiveness also rapidly decreases after the first day of usage.

Loop Diuretics

Furosemide (Lasix) therapy is recommended in adjunct with mannitol to lower ICP with less elevation of serum osmolality or electrolyte disturbance. For this reason, it has been recommended by some authors to be used alone in the very young or elderly. Furosemide is effective even in the absence of an intact blood–brain barrier, and thus reduces cerebral edema in the pathologic regions of the brain, where osmotic diuretics are ineffective. It also decreases CSF production and sodium influx into the CNS. The recommended dose is 0.5 to 1.0 mg/kg given by i.v. push, and the onset of action is 15 to 20 minutes.

Corticosteroids

Cerebral edema secondary to IN continues to be one of the most widely accepted indications for dexamethasone therapy. Initial dosage is 10 mg given by i.v. push, followed by 4 mg every 6 hours for 48 hours, with tapering over the next 5 to 7 days. Dexamethasone has a delayed effect in decreasing cerebral edema.[11]

Miscellaneous

Barbiturate coma, using pentobarbital or thiopental, to control elevated ICP is typically done as a last resort by the neurosurgical–anesthesiology team in the intensive care unit and is not recommended in the emergency department setting. ICP monitoring, in an attempt to keep ICP less than 20 mm Hg, is also postponed until the patient is in the intensive care setting.

Although hypertension is primarily a problem associated with intracranial hemorrhage and not with IN, bleeding into an IN may occur. In this setting, hypertension is usually transient and secondary to ICP elevation. In these cases, hyperventilation, mannitol, and furosemide will all produce a reduction in the blood pressure by lowering the ICP. In a patient whose blood pressure is not adequately controlled with ICP reduction, the key to management is to lower the blood pressure slowly so as to avoid cerebral ischemia.

Nitroprusside (50 μg in 500 mL dextrose 5% in water, at 0.51 μg/kg/min and increased every 5 minutes as necessary to a maximum of 8 μg/kg/min) acts as an arterial and venous dilator. There is concern that the vasodilatory effects of nitroprusside may elevate the ICP by increasing cerebral blood flow. Labetalol, on the other hand, acts as an α_1- and β-adrenergic blocker and has no effect on CBF and no reflex tachycardia. To retain the minute-to-minute control one has with nitroprusside, a labetalol drip should be initiated at 2 mg/min and titrated up to 6 mg/min. Recalling the formula CPP = MAP − ICP, in the absence of malignant hypertension associated with intracranial bleeding or cardiac ischemia, one should err on the side of hypertension to avoid cerebral ischemia.

Therapeutic response of acute intervention is assessed by continuous ICP monitoring when appropriate. In the emergency department, serial neurologic examinations and continuous cardiac and vital sign monitoring suffice.

DISPOSITION

Definitive long-term therapy for IN combines surgical removal or debulking of the tumor, if it can be performed without compromising brain function, with adjunctive irradiation and chemotherapy.[12,17]

Role of the Consultant

Neurosurgical consultation is mandatory in all patients with IN. A stat consult is warranted with status epilepticus or suspected ICP elevation. Likewise, all patients with IN are admitted to the neurosurgical unit. Those without significant ICP elevation and with stable vital signs may be admitted to a nonmonitored bed, while those who require hyperventilation or osmotic agents require intensive care monitoring.

Transfer Considerations

In rural or community-based facilities, it may be necessary to transfer patients to a hospital where neurosurgical consultants are readily available. In the absence of clinical or CT evidence of significant cerebral edema, this may be done by a basic life-support unit. If impending herniation or elevated ICP is a concern, either based on clinical examination or by evidence of a midline shift on CT, an advanced cardiac life-support unit or helicopter transport team is warranted. Intubation with hyperventilation and supplemental oxygen, corticosteroids, mannitol, and seizure control should all be initiated before transfer.

COMMON PITFALLS

- Unenhanced CT alone cannot completely exclude IN.
- Because of the nonspecific quality of an IN headache, the diagnosis of brain tumor is often missed initially. Neurologic follow-up is essential in all patients in whom the cause of headache is not reasonably certain.
- An appropriate history and physical examination must be done on all patients, even those with primarily psychiatric symptoms.
- A careful neurologic examination must be done, no matter how trivial the chief complaint seems.
- There are no consistently reliable indicators of elevated ICP.
- Not everyone with elevated ICP has papilledema.
- Withholding mannitol and diuretics in a patient who displays signs of impending herniation while awaiting CT confirmation or neurosurgical consultation is unwise.

References

1. Campbell BG, Zimmerman RD. Emergency magnetic resonance of the brain. *Top Magn Reson Imaging* 1998;9:208.
2. Chestnut RM. Medical management of severe head injury: present and future. *New Horiz* 1995;3:581.
3. Dunniway HM, Welling DB. Intracranial tumors mimicking benign paroxysmal positional vertigo. *Otolaryngol Head Neck Surg* 1998;118:429.
4. Fueyo J, Gomez-Manzano C, Yung WK, et al. The functional role of tumor suppressor genes in gliomas: clues for future therapeutic strategies. *Neurology* 1998;51:1250.
5. Gleckman AM, Smith TW. Sudden unexpected death from primary posterior fossa tumors. *Am J Forensic Med Pathol* 1998;19:303.
6. Harner SG, Laws ER Jr. Clinical findings in patients with acoustic neurinoma. *Mayo Clin Proc* 1983;58:721.
7. Jodicke A, Deinsberger W, Erbe H, et al. Intraoperative three-dimensional ultrasonography: an approach to register brain shift using multidimensional image processing. *Minim Invasive Neurosurg* 1998;41:13.
8. Medina LS, Zurakowski D, Strife KE, et al. Efficacy of fast screening MR in children and adolescents with suspected intracranial tumors. *Am J Neuroradiol* 1998;19:529.
9. Miettinen M, Chatten J, Paetau A, et al. Monoclonal antibody NB84 in the differential diagnosis of neuroblastoma and other small round cell tumors. *Am J Surg Pathol* 1998;22:327.
10. Nutt SH, Patchell RA. Intracranial hemorrhage associated with primary and secondary tumors. *Neurosurg Clin North Am* 1992;3:591.
11. Poungvarin N. Effects of dexamethasone in primary supratentorial intracerebral hemorrhage. *N Engl J Med* 1987;136:1229.
12. Saran FH, Driever PH, Thilmann C, et al. Survival of very young children with medulloblastoma (primitive neuroectodermal tumor of the posterior fossa) treated with craniospinal irradiation. *Int J Radiat Oncol Biol Phys* 1998;42:959.
13. Sasaki M, Plate KH. Gene therapy of malignant glioma: recent advances in experimental and clinical studies. *Ann Oncol* 1998;9:1155.
14. Walker AE, Robins M, Weinfeld FD. Epidemiology of brain tumors: the national survey of neoplasms. *Neurology* 1985;35:219.
15. Walls RM. Airway management. *Emerg Clin North Am* 1993;11:53.
16. Young RF. Radiosurgery for the treatment of brain metastases. *Semin Surg Oncol* 1998;14:70.
17. Yundt KD, Diringer MN. The use of hyperventilation and its impact on cerebral ischemia in the treatment of traumatic brain injury. *Crit Care Clin* 1997;13:163.

CHAPTER 60
Cranial Nerve Emergencies

Michael T. Pulley

The evaluation of cranial nerve function in the emergency department is a critical part of the neurologic examination. A detailed cranial nerve examination can be performed rapidly and is very helpful in establishing localization of lesions, especially when consciousness is impaired and assessment of sensory and motor function is difficult. Dysfunction of the individual cranial nerves may occur but, often, there is involvement of other cranial nerves or "long tracts," which helps to pinpoint the lesion.

CRANIAL NERVE I (OLFACTORY)

CLINICAL PRESENTATION

The olfactory nerve subserves the sense of smell but is also important in the perception of taste. Difficulty perceiving odors is most often due to intranasal conditions such as the common cold. The olfactory epithelium is connected to the olfactory bulb by sensory axons projecting through the cribriform plate of the ethmoid bone. Fracture of the ethmoid bone with trauma may cause loss of smell and leakage of cerebrospinal fluid (CSF rhinorrhea). Rapid deceleration of the head can cause shearing forces that tear the olfactory axons and produce loss of smell. The location of the olfactory bulbs on the floor of the frontal fossa makes them susceptible to compression from space-occupying lesions in the frontal lobes, but this effect usually develops gradually. Associated findings may include disinhibition or personality change.

DIFFERENTIAL DIAGNOSIS

As stated, the most common causes for altered smell are intranasal, including the common cold. Traumatic disruption of olfactory fibers needs to be considered. Frontal lobe mass lesions include tumors (meningioma, glioma) and abscesses.

EMERGENCY DEPARTMENT EVALUATION

The sense of smell is tested using common odors such as coffee or fruit. Each nostril should be tested individually, and precise identification is not important. Irritating stimuli such as ammonia should be avoided, as they result in stimulation of the trigeminal nerve. If CSF rhinorrhea is suspected, the fluid can be analyzed to determine whether it has the characteristics of CSF. A computed tomography (CT) scan of the head should be performed to rule out fractures, contusions of the frontal lobes from coup/contrecoup injuries, or pneumocephalus. Associated findings in the setting of a mass lesion may include papilledema.

EMERGENCY DEPARTMENT MANAGEMENT

Management of these patients is typically directed to the associated injuries, as trauma is the most common cause.

DISPOSITION

Role of the Consultant

Neurosurgical consultation may be required to assess the need for urgent surgery if there is evidence of increased intracranial pressure (ICP) or CSF rhinorrhea.

Indications for Admission

Patients with CSF leaks should be monitored for evidence of possible infection, as the barrier to pathogens entering the brain has been breached.

Transfer Considerations

If a mass lesion or significant traumatic brain injury is detected, transfer to a facility with neurosurgical capability is required.

COMMON PITFALLS

As patients with frontal lobe tumors may behave strangely, they may be felt to have a psychiatric basis of their complaint of loss of smell or taste. Unusual odors may indicate temporal lobe seizures.

CRANIAL NERVE II (OPTIC)

CLINICAL PRESENTATION

Dysfunction of the optic nerve leads to complaints of blurred vision or loss of vision. The correct characterization of the pattern of visual loss is key to establishing the localization and possible etiologies. Monocular dysfunction implies an abnormality of the retina or optic nerve. Bitemporal hemianopsia (loss of the temporal half of the visual field of both eyes) localizes to the optic chiasm. Retrochiasmal lesions produce homonymous (the same in both eyes) visual field defects (Fig. 60.1).

DIFFERENTIAL DIAGNOSIS

Acute monocular visual loss is typically due to vascular causes. The classic history of "a shade being pulled down" that is described for amaurosis fugax need not be present. The source of the emboli that cause the visual loss in most cases is atheroscle-

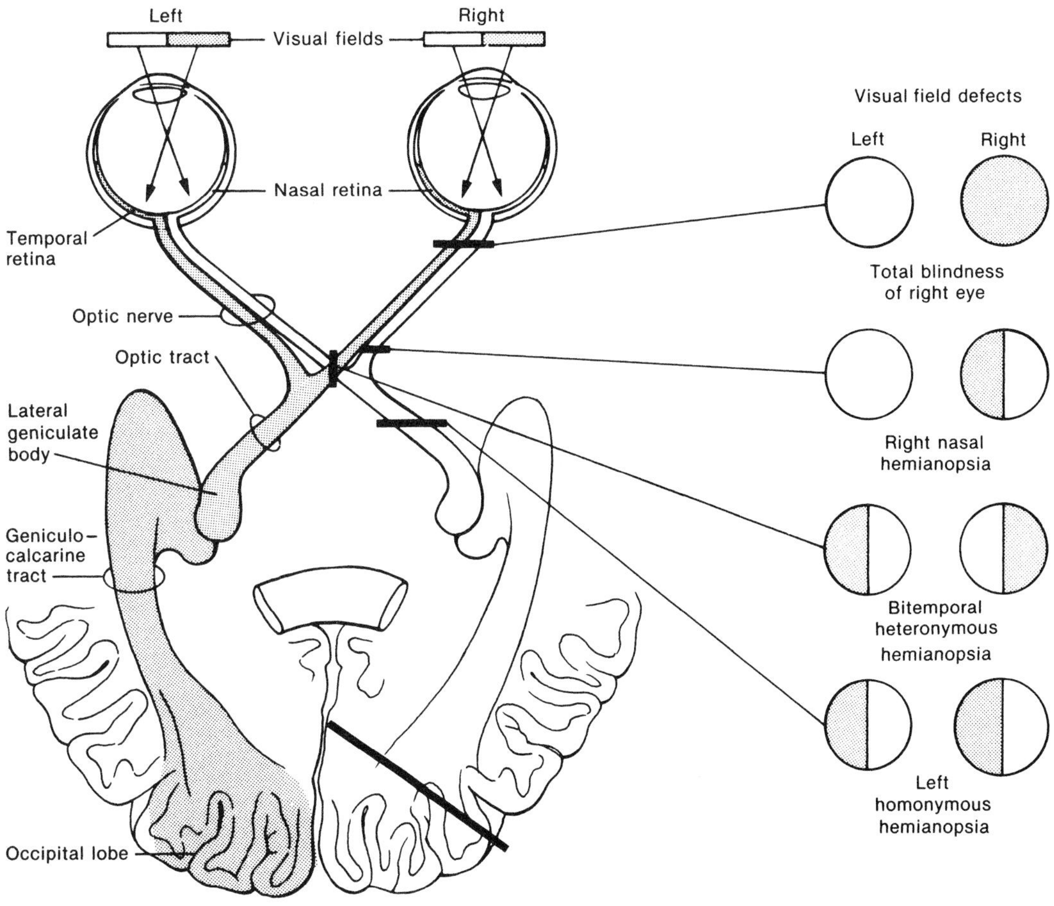

Figure 60.1. Lesions in the optic pathways.

rotic disease of the carotid artery. This may lead to other transient ischemic attacks (TIAs) in the ipsilateral hemisphere. However, temporal arteritis, which is often associated with headache and/or jaw claudication in patients over age 60, needs to be considered. Other pathology of the retina or globe, such as hemorrhage or central retinal vein occlusion, should be kept in mind. Symptoms of optic neuritis[3] usually include blurriness rather than loss of vision, and possibly eye pain (especially with eye movement). Slowly developing papilledema due to an intracranial mass in "noneloquent" parts of the brain or pseudotumor cerebri may also cause blurring or loss of vision, often accompanied by headache. Acute angle-closure glaucoma can lead to rapid loss of vision associated with eye or head pain.

EMERGENCY DEPARTMENT EVALUATION

Testing of optic nerve function involves assessment of visual acuity, visual fields, pupillary light reflex, and the funduscopic examination. Acuity should be assessed with glasses or by using a pinhole to compensate for refractive errors. Visual field testing at the bedside is performed on each eye, using the confrontation method to compare with one's own visual fields. The funduscopic examination is frequently difficult in patients with poor cooperation, cataracts, or periorbital edema. The goal is to exclude papilledema, retinal hemorrhage, or markedly increased intraocular pressure (increased optic cup-to-disc ratio). Absence of papilledema does not exclude acutely increased ICP, because it takes time to develop. An afferent pupillary defect is typically found with optic neuritis.

Papilledema and visual field defects require evaluation with a CT scan. If this is normal, a lumbar puncture to measure opening pressure and to exclude an indolent infectious etiology such as cryptococcus should be performed in the setting of papilledema. A sedimentation rate and C-reactive protein should be ordered if temporal arteritis is suspected. Measurement of intraocular pressure should be performed if glaucoma is considered.

EMERGENCY DEPARTMENT MANAGEMENT

Management is dependent on the etiology of visual loss. Recurrent episodes of monocular visual loss with resolution or in association with other TIAs may be an indication to start the patient on intravenous (i.v.) heparin (with no bolus on initiation) until the vasculature can be evaluated by ultrasonography or arteriography. Optic neuritis is somewhat less likely to lead to future development of multiple sclerosis if treated with i.v. steroids, and this can be initiated as soon as the diagnosis is established. Temporal arteritis should be treated with a high dose of oral steroids (60 to 80 mg of prednisone per day) to prevent visual loss. This should *not* be postponed until temporal artery biopsy can be performed, as it does not reduce the yield and the risk of visual loss is high. Although papilledema is usually caused by increased ICP, this does not need to be treated acutely with mannitol or hyperventilation unless there is decreased level of consciousness or deterioration of neurologic status.

DISPOSITION

Role of the Consultant

Consultation with a neurologist should be obtained in cases of amaurosis fugax, visual field defects, and suspected optic neuritis. If retinal or other intraocular pathology is suspected, it may be necessary to consult an ophthalmologist. If papilledema is due to an intracranial mass, a neurosurgical opinion should be obtained.

Indications for Admission

Amaurosis fugax or visual field defects require admission for workup. Optic neuritis should be treated with high-dose i.v. steroids as an inpatient. If papilledema is due to a mass, admission for possible surgery is usually required. Temporal arteritis can be managed on an outpatient basis with close follow-up and arrangement for a temporal artery biopsy.

Transfer Considerations

Mass lesions require the availability of neurosurgical evaluation and management. The patient should be transferred to an alternative facility if this is not available.

COMMON PITFALLS

- Patients are notoriously poor at characterizing the pattern of visual loss. They often state that they have lost vision in an eye when a field defect is present. Also, patients are often unaware of visual field loss, particularly when associated with parietal lobe dysfunction. As such, omission of visual field testing leads to misdiagnosis or improper localization of the lesion.
- Difficulty visualizing the fundi leads to the temptation to use dilating eye drops, but they should be avoided unless intracranial pathology has been definitely excluded. Patients who have papilledema are sometimes treated for increased ICP unnecessarily, which may make the treatment ineffective when it is really needed.

CRANIAL NERVES III, IV, AND VI (OCULOMOTOR, TROCHLEAR, AND ABDUCENS)

CLINICAL PRESENTATION

The cranial nerves that control eye movements are discussed together, as dysfunction of any produces diplopia or dysconjugate gaze. The third nerve supplies all of the extraocular muscles except the lateral rectus (sixth; abduction of the eye) and the superior oblique (fourth; inferior nasal movement and intorsion of the eye). The levator palpebrae superioris (elevation of the lid) and pupillary constrictor muscles are also supplied by cranial nerve three. A complete third nerve lesion results in marked ptosis, diplopia and a "blown" (dilated) pupil. The eye is deviated laterally due to unopposed action of the lateral rectus, and the superior oblique cannot be tested well.

Partial third nerve palsy due to extrinsic compression causes dysfunction of the more superficial parasympathetic fibers, resulting in pupillary dilatation. Ischemia of the nerve (often painful at onset) spares the pupillary fibers while the remaining functions are affected. Diplopia is most prominent when moving the eyes in the direction of function of the paretic muscle. Thus, with sixth nerve palsy, diplopia is maximal on lateral gaze ipsilaterally. Patients with fourth nerve lesions unconsciously compensate for diplopia by developing a head tilt toward the unaffected side and complain of diplopia when walking down steps (looking down and in).

DIFFERENTIAL DIAGNOSIS

Isolated third cranial neuropathies are most often due to ischemia and present with pain at onset. The most common underlying cause is diabetes, and a similar presentation can be seen with fourth and sixth cranial nerve palsies. Isolated fourth nerve palsy is most often due to trauma that may be relatively minor. The sixth nerve has the longest intracranial course of the cranial nerves and travels along the base of the skull, bending over the ridge of the petrous portion of the temporal bone. It is susceptible to stretch as a nonspecific effect of increased ICP (the false localizing sign). Infection in the mastoid or middle ear may spread to involve the petrous bone and cause a sixth nerve palsy that may be associated with facial pain (Gradenigo syndrome).[1]

Combined dysfunction of the nerves supplying the extraocular muscles may result from lesions in areas where they are in close proximity to one another. This includes the cavernous sinus and the superior orbital fissure,[1] where associated findings help to localize the lesions. Cavernous sinus lesions may cause dysfunction of the trigeminal nerve (first and second divisions) or the sympathetic fibers as they travel with the carotid artery. In the superior orbital fissure, associated involvement of the frontal, lacrimal, or nasociliary branches of the first division of the trigeminal nerve may occur. Cavernous sinus thrombosis or carotid–cavernous fistula is associated with proptosis of the eye and dilation of the scleral vessels ipsilaterally.

Conditions that affect the extraocular muscles but not the nerves need to be considered. Myasthenia gravis causes fluctuating and fatigable diplopia and ptosis that may be associated with limb weakness, dysarthria, dysphagia, or shortness of breath. Thyroid ophthalmopathy and orbital pseudotumor are other etiologies of abnormal extraocular movement.

Finally, multiple sclerosis or ischemic disease of the brainstem can cause an intranuclear ophthalmoplegia (INO). This is due to a lesion in the medial longitudinal fasciculus, which functionally connects the third and sixth nuclei to allow conjugate lateral gaze. When attempting to look in the affected direction, the ipsilateral eye abducts, but the contralateral eye cannot adduct, and there is nystagmus of the abducting eye with diplopia.

EMERGENCY DEPARTMENT EVALUATION

The key is determining which eye movements are abnormal and whether there are associated findings. The most dangerous scenario is the development of a dilated pupil in a patient who has reduced responsiveness. This is an indication of herniation, and the patient should be intubated, hyperventilated, and given mannitol i.v. to attempt to decrease ICP. If a brainstem lesion is suspected based on associated findings, a CT scan should be performed to exclude a hemorrhagic etiology. Detection of proptosis, Horner syndrome, or facial numbness indicates the need to evaluate the cavernous sinus. This can be achieved with contrasted magnetic resonance imaging (MRI), if available, or conventional angiography.

EMERGENCY DEPARTMENT MANAGEMENT

A "blown" pupil should be treated as an extreme emergency with impending death. As such, the usual measurers to lower ICP should be instituted, as mentioned earlier. Cavernous sinus thrombosis may be related to infections that require institution of antibiotics.

DISPOSITION

Role of the Consultant

Neurosurgical consultation is required for patients who have herniation syndromes, if they survive the initial insult. A neurologist's opinion should be sought in cases involving long tract findings or facial numbness in association with eye movement abnormalities, as this implies the possibility of brainstem lesions.

Indications for Admission

A brainstem lesion, herniation, or cavernous sinus involvement requires admission for further workup.

Transfer Considerations

Transfer to a facility with neurosurgical backup is required after stabilization of patients who have evidence for herniation. The remaining problems can typically be worked up without need for transfer, as long as CT scanning is available.

COMMON PITFALLS

- Rarely, patients will unwittingly put drugs (e.g., cocaine) in their eyes; the presence of a "blown" pupil in an otherwise awake and alert patient without any other evidence of neurologic dysfunction raises that possibility.
- Myasthenia gravis can present with eye movement abnormalities mimicking lesions of cranial nerves three, four, and six.
- If patients have any associated shortness of breath or dysphagia, they require admission for close monitoring and immunomodulatory therapy.

CRANIAL NERVE V (TRIGEMINAL)

CLINICAL PRESENTATION

Isolated dysfunction of the fifth cranial nerve is rare. The most common presentation is the excruciating facial pain seen in trigeminal neuralgia (tic douloureux[2]). This pain is lancinating and brief; aggravated by cold, chewing, yawning, touching the face, or shaving; may be referred to the teeth or mouth; most commonly involves the distribution of the second division of the trigeminal nerve (V_2); and may be seen in patients with multiple sclerosis. Pain in the distribution of the trigeminal nerve may herald the onset of herpes zoster (shingles). This is most troubling when the first division of the trigeminal nerve (V_1) is involved, as the cornea may be affected.

Facial numbness is not unusual with ischemic lesions of the brain or brainstem, but the presence of other symptoms or signs indicates this is not of peripheral origin. A lesion in the lower medulla or upper brainstem may affect the spinal nucleus of the trigeminal nerve. This can cause an unusual pattern of sensory loss known as an "onion skin." This describes concentric circles beginning at the mouth and extending farther out on the face. Cavernous sinus syndromes may involve V_1 and/or V_2, with resulting numbness in those distributions.

Weakness of the muscles of mastication due to a lesion of the trigeminal nerve is exceedingly rare.

DIFFERENTIAL DIAGNOSIS

Facial pain can also result from migraine headache, cluster headache, dental problems such as abscesses, and temporomandibular joint (TMJ) syndrome. Jaw claudication (pain with chewing) occurs in temporal arteritis, and there may be fatigue of the jaw muscles with chewing tough foods in myasthenia gravis.

Perioral numbness may be due to panic attack if the other characteristic features are present (feeling of impending doom, heart racing, feeling of air hunger, dizziness). Facial numbness or pain may also be psychogenic, but this is a diagnosis of exclusion.

EMERGENCY DEPARTMENT EVALUATION

Facial pain evaluation should include a careful inspection and palpation of the oral cavity to rule out dental problems. With herpes zoster, special attention should be given to the cornea.

The evaluation of trigeminal nerve function should involve testing light touch, pinprick, and the corneal reflexes. Involvement of other cranial nerves might suggest a brainstem or cavernous sinus lesion. Rule out any long-tract signs, which might indicate a cortical or subcortical localization.

EMERGENCY DEPARTMENT MANAGEMENT

Trigeminal neuralgia responds best to treatment with carbamazepine, gabapentin, or phenytoin. Herpes zoster should be treated with acyclovir. Trigeminal distribution herpes zoster in an immunocompromised host is an indication for i.v. acyclovir.

DISPOSITION

Role of the Consultant

If there is suspicion that the patient may have an ischemic etiology of facial numbness, a neurologic consultation should be obtained. Involvement of the cornea in herpes zoster warrants evaluation by an ophthalmologist.

Indications for Admission

Trigeminal distribution herpes zoster in an immunocompromised host is an indication for admission and i.v. therapy. Ischemic etiologies of facial numbness require admission for further workup.

Transfer Considerations

Patients with facial pain or numbness rarely require transfer unless CT scanning is not available.

COMMON PITFALLS

- Perioral numbness due to the "onion skin" arrangement of trigeminal representation in low medullary or very high cervical spine lesions may mistakenly be passed off as a panic attack or hyperventilation.
- Patients with trigeminal neuralgia may be convinced that they have dental problems even after this diagnosis has been excluded by a dentist.
- Isolated sensory loss involving the chin due to involvement of the mental branch of the trigeminal nerve has been said to be a sign of underlying malignancy until proven otherwise.
- A reduced corneal reflex is not necessarily indicative of brainstem or trigeminal nerve dysfunction as it may be seen in cortical or subcortical lesions.

CRANIAL NERVE VII (FACIAL)

CLINICAL PRESENTATION

The most common isolated cranial neuropathy is facial nerve or Bell's palsy. The presentation usually involves pain behind the ear, followed by decreased ability to move the ipsilateral side of the face. It can progress to inability to close the eye, with drying and irritation. There may be difficulty maintaining saliva in the mouth and pocketing of food in the lax jaw. Patients rarely complain of difficulty with taste, although taste may be absent from the anterior two-thirds of the tongue, if tested. Sounds may seem louder in the affected ear (hyperacusis).

Although the patients often complain that the face feels numb, there is no loss of sensation when tested (although it may feel "different" on that side). Rarely, there is in the external auditory canal an associated herpes zoster lesion, which receives sensory innervation from the facial nerve (Ramsay-Hunt syndrome). Bilateral facial weakness (facial diplegia) can occur in isolation. There are also involuntary movements involving half of the face, termed *hemifacial spasm*.

DIFFERENTIAL DIAGNOSIS

The primary distinction to be made is whether there is an upper motor neuron or lower motor neuron pattern of the facial weak-

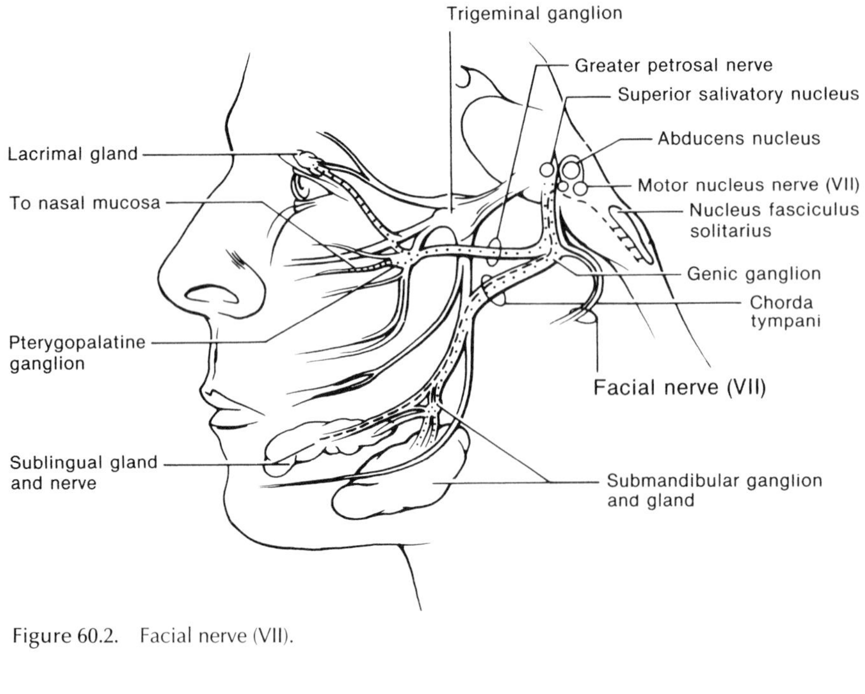

Figure 60.2. Facial nerve (VII).

ness. Because the corticobulbar pathway supplies input to both sides of the forehead, this is spared in the case of an upper motor neuron lesion. Possible etiologies of facial nerve palsy include herpes zoster, Lyme disease, sarcoidosis, and Guillain-Barré syndrome, although Bell's palsy is the most common. Myasthenia gravis may also cause acute facial weakness that is usually bilateral (Fig. 60.2).

EMERGENCY DEPARTMENT EVALUATION

Determination of the absence or presence of forehead involvement is the first objective. Next, exclude active herpes zoster lesions. Then, decide on the severity of the facial weakness—can the patient close the eye? If there is bilateral facial weakness, is there more widespread weakness or loss of reflexes, which might suggest myasthenia gravis or Guillain-Barré syndrome?

EMERGENCY DEPARTMENT MANAGEMENT

If the facial weakness is prominent, the cornea will require protective treatment. This usually involves the patient using artificial tears while awake and placing an eye lubricant in the eye, with the eye covered by a patch, at night. There is controversy about the routine use of steroids and, more recently, the use of acyclovir to treat Bell's palsy; these issues have not been resolved.[4]

DISPOSITION

Role of the Consultant

- If there is any question regarding the differentiation of an upper motor neuron versus lower motor neuron pattern of facial weakness, a neurologist should be consulted. Associated findings of weakness or areflexia, which might suggest Guillain-Barré syndrome, warrants neurologic evaluation as well.

Indications for Admission

If the facial weakness is due to an ischemic etiology, the patient will require admission for further workup. Facial weakness associated with Guillain-Barré also justifies admission for close observation.

Transfer Considerations

Facial weakness can usually be evaluated without the need for transfer to another facility.

COMMON PITFALLS

- Do not forget to protect the cornea and caution the patient regarding the possibility of worsening weakness, which can lead to inability to close the eye.

CRANIAL NERVE VIII (VESTIBULOCOCHLEAR)

CLINICAL PRESENTATION

Dysfunction of the vestibular portion of the eighth nerve manifests as vertigo. Patients frequently complain of feeling "dizzy," but when questioned describe a sense of movement or spinning. Nausea and vomiting are frequently associated symptoms. Hearing loss or tinnitus indicates dysfunction of the cochlear portion of the nerve.

DIFFERENTIAL DIAGNOSIS

Benign paroxysmal positional vertigo (BPPV) is the most common etiology, particularly in the older population. The patient notices that turning the head in a particular direction causes intense vertigo (usually with a brief delay after moving), associated with nausea and vomiting, that quickly subsides. "Central" vertigo due to brainstem or cerebellar dysfunction tends to occur without delay and does not usually have a positional predilection. Labyrinthitis is also associated with severe feelings of vertigo, but it is usually more persistent than that seen with BPPV. Ménière disease involves recurrent attacks of vertigo, associated with roaring tinnitus and progressive loss of hearing. Migraine headaches are also associated with vertigo. Drugs, including alcohol, cause vertigo and need to be considered in any patient with this complaint. Acute unilateral hearing loss can be seen with ischemia involving the cochlear artery, a branch of the anterior inferior cerebellar artery. Patients may become suddenly aware of hearing loss that develops insidiously, such as that caused by an acoustic neuroma. Other cerebellopontine angle tumors, such as meningioma, need to be considered in the differential diagnosis of hearing loss, especially if there is associated facial weakness or numbness.

EMERGENCY DEPARTMENT EVALUATION

The eyes should be observed for spontaneous nystagmus, and then in all directions of gaze. Vertical nystagmus suggests central dysfunction or a toxic etiology. A provocative test known as the Dix-Hall-Pike maneuver (or Nylen-Barany maneuver) should be performed. The patient is asked to position himself or herself on the stretcher such that, when supine, the neck will just meet the end. The patient is rapidly moved from a seated to a supine position with the neck extended approximately 30 degrees and the head turned such that one ear faces the ground. The patient is questioned regarding the appearance of vertigo, and the eyes are observed for nystagmus. If positive, the patient tends to forcibly close the eyes, so they cannot be observed. The keys are to determine whether there is a clear asymmetry of the vertigo response, whether there is a delay between moving the patient and onset of symptoms, and whether there is fatigue of the response. If there is any question regarding the possibility of alcohol or drug ingestion, appropriate laboratory studies should be obtained. Hearing should be tested in each ear by using a finger rub or watch. A tuning fork can be used to look for evidence of lateralization of hearing (to the good ear with sensorineural hearing loss) or reduced air conduction (on the side with conductive hearing loss).

EMERGENCY DEPARTMENT MANAGEMENT

If patients have significant associated vomiting, they may become dehydrated and require fluid or electrolyte replacement. Medications to treat vertigo include the benzodiazepines and meclizine.

DISPOSITION

Role of the Consultant

If there is uncertainty regarding the differentiation of central versus peripheral vertigo, consultation with a neurologist or an ear, nose, and throat (ENT) specialist should be sought.

Indications for Admission

Central nystagmus that is not induced by drugs or alcohol suggests a brainstem lesion, which is an indication for admission.

Transfer Considerations

Transfer may be necessary if neurologic consultation is not available.

COMMON PITFALLS

BPPV causes severe vertigo, and the pattern on provocative testing (Dix-Hall-Pike) of delayed vertigo and fatigue of the response are characteristic. A few beats of nystagmus on far lateral gaze are frequently seen in normal individuals as they break visual fusion of the image. This can be evaluated by simply moving the test finger back a few degrees or not moving to the extremes of gaze.

CRANIAL NERVES IX AND X (GLOSSOPHARYNGEAL AND VAGUS)

CLINICAL PRESENTATION

Isolated dysfunction of cranial nerve nine or ten is quite rare. The primary manifestation of the dysfunction is difficulty swallowing. Occasionally, dysarthria due to decreased palatal movement may be the presenting symptom. A rare presentation of ninth cranial nerve dysfunction is glossopharyngeal neuralgia. This is similar in characteristics to trigeminal neuralgia but involves the throat and is precipitated by swallowing or tongue movement.

DIFFERENTIAL DIAGNOSIS

The majority of patients who have dysphagia on a neurologic basis have ischemic lesions in the cortex, subcortical areas, or brainstem. The dysphagia is much more prominent and is a presenting complaint in the case of brainstem lesions, particularly in the lateral medulla. Oral or nasal tumors need to be considered, especially in those with a history of smoking. Myasthenia gravis can cause palatal dysfunction, with a resulting nasal speech as well as nasal regurgitation of liquids on attempted swallowing. Involvement of these nerves at the base of the skull as they exit through the jugular foramen (by metastases to the bone or skull fracture) is often accompanied by involvement of the spinal accessory nerve.[5]

EMERGENCY DEPARTMENT EVALUATION

The function of the palate should be assessed by having the patient say "ah" while watching for clear deviation of the uvula to one side, and also testing the gag reflex bilaterally. Because most cases of difficulty swallowing are not due to isolated dysfunction of cranial nerves nine or ten, associated findings to suggest ischemic lesions (hemiparesis, Horner syndrome, etc.) or neuromuscular disease should be carefully sought.

EMERGENCY DEPARTMENT MANAGEMENT

If patients' swallowing dysfunction is severe enough to impair the ability to safely swallow their own saliva, they may require intubation to prevent aspiration. This is usually required only when there is associated depressed level of consciousness. If the dysfunction is less prominent, simply keeping the patient NPO until they can be thoroughly evaluated by a speech pathologist may be all that is required.

DISPOSITION

Role of the Consultant

If there is a question of ischemic neurologic dysfunction of the brain or brainstem, a neurologist should be consulted. In the event of pain involving the throat that does not seem to involve a simple strep infection, an ENT evaluation may be indicated.

Indications for Admission

If patients have severe swallowing dysfunction, they will need admission for i.v. fluids, and perhaps nasogastric tube feeding if it is not resolving rapidly. Palatal dysfunction due to a stroke necessitates admission for determination of the underlying etiology.

Transfer Considerations

Patients with dysphagia can usually be evaluated and treated without need for transfer.

COMMON PITFALLS

If there is concern regarding patients' ability to swallow, do not allow them to take anything by mouth until they can have a formal swallowing evaluation. Missing a few meals will not do any long-term harm, but a case of aspiration pneumonia can be deadly.

CRANIAL NERVE XI (SPINAL ACCESSORY)

CLINICAL PRESENTATION

Dysfunction of the spinal accessory nerve is almost never seen in the emergency setting. The function of this nerve is purely motor, supplying the sternocleidomastoid (SCM) and trapezius muscles. It is very superficial in location and can be injured with penetrating trauma of the neck. This results in a drooping shoulder or winging of the scapula that is maximum on abduction of the arm and weakness of the SCM. Shoulder pain may be a prominent complaint with trapezius weakness. SCM weakness results in difficulty rotating the head in the opposite direction.

DIFFERENTIAL DIAGNOSIS

Winging of the scapula can be produced by weakness of the trapezius, serratus anterior, or rhomboid muscles. The portion of the scapula protruding and the position producing maximal winging allow differentiation. With serratus anterior weakness, the medial and inferior borders protrude, and this is accentuated with the arms outstretched in front of the body, especially with pushing against a wall. With rhomboid weakness, the superior and medial borders protrude, and this is accentuated by elevating the arm over the head. With trapezius weakness, the inferior angle is rotated medially, and this is accentuated by abducting the arms. Pain and drooping of the shoulder are much more likely to be caused by dislocation or rotator cuff injuries. The spinal accessory nerve may be involved in cases of idiopathic inflammatory brachial plexopathy (Parsonage-Turner syndrome), which usually involves the upper trunk of the brachial plexus. The accessory nerve may be damaged in the jugular foramen along with the glossopharyngeal and vagus nerves.[5]

EMERGENCY DEPARTMENT EVALUATION

Other potential causes for shoulder drooping or pain are evaluated by palpating the shoulder, performing range of motion, and testing for weakness. Shoulder x-rays may be necessary. Testing for winging of the scapula with the arm in various positions, as outlined earlier, should be performed. Associated dysfunction of cranial nerves nine and ten needs to be excluded, and, if there is evidence of involvement of all three, a CT scan of the head with bone windows to examine the jugular foramen is indicated.

EMERGENCY DEPARTMENT MANAGEMENT

Providing analgesia for pain and, possibly, a sling due to drooping of the shoulder as a result of trapezius weakness are the primary concerns in managing patients with accessory nerve dysfunction.

DISPOSITION

Role of the Consultant

Referral to a neurologist to evaluate the cause of scapular winging and to perform electromyography, if deemed necessary, can be accomplished in the outpatient setting.

Indications for Admission

A skull base lesion causing a jugular foramen syndrome is an indication for admission.

Transfer Considerations

Dysfunction of cranial nerve eleven can be evaluated and treated without transfer.

COMMON PITFALLS

- Weakness of the SCM causes difficulty rotating the chin away from the affected side (recall the origin and insertion of the muscle to understand its action).

CRANIAL NERVE XII (HYPOGLOSSAL)

CLINICAL PRESENTATION

The function of the hypoglossal nerve is purely motor; it supplies the ipsilateral tongue. Dysfunction results in weakness that manifests as deviation toward the side of the weakness with protrusion. Abnormal movements of the tongue may be seen with drug-induced movement disorders such as tardive dyskinesia.

DIFFERENTIAL DIAGNOSIS

Isolated weakness of the tongue is rare. Often, there is associated facial weakness, reduced gag, or extremity weakness with an upper motor neuron lesion. Skull fractures may involve the hypoglossal nerve, but they tend to be associated with other severe injuries. Brainstem strokes causing tongue weakness are unusual. Myasthenia gravis may cause weakness of the tongue that is asymmetric and usually associated with some facial weakness, diplopia, or palatal dysfunction.

EMERGENCY DEPARTMENT EVALUATION

Ensuring that the patient does not have associated dysfunction of cranial nerves nine or ten, which may make it difficult to protect the airway, is paramount.

EMERGENCY DEPARTMENT MANAGEMENT

Ensuring the ability to maintain a patent airway is the primary goal. If there is severe tongue weakness, insertion of an oral biteguard may be required to prevent the tongue from moving posteriorly and blocking the airway.

DISPOSITION

Role of the Consultant

Because the most common cause for tongue weakness or deviation is brain ischemia, neurologic consultation is usually indicated.

Indications for Admission

Tongue weakness is most often due to stroke, and this should be evaluated on an inpatient basis.

Transfer Considerations

Transfer is needed only if the patient requires neurologic evaluation that is not available.

COMMON PITFALLS

Patients who have conversion disorder will occasionally deviate the tongue to the "wrong" side (away from the hemiparesis), believing that if it is weak, it will not move toward the side of weakness.

BRAINSTEM ISCHEMIA

CLINICAL PRESENTATION

Vascular disease affecting the brainstem (vertebrobasilar stroke or TIA) is common. There are characteristic symptoms that increase the likelihood of brainstem localization, especially when seen in combination. These include diplopia, vertigo, dysphagia, dysarthria, facial sensory loss, ataxia, abnormal breathing patterns, or altered level of consciousness. The presence of "crossed" findings (sensory or motor disturbances that involve one side of the face and the contralateral body) or Horner syndrome also suggests a brainstem lesion. The appearance of multiple symptoms localizing to the brainstem in a stepwise fashion can indicate basilar artery thrombosis, which carries a high risk for death or severe disability.

DIFFERENTIAL DIAGNOSIS

Nonischemic etiologies of brainstem dysfunction, such as hemorrhage, demyelinating disease, and brainstem tumors, need to be considered. The CT scan helps to exclude hemorrhage, and the evolution and associated findings usually allow differentiation of stroke from tumor or demyelination.

EMERGENCY DEPARTMENT EVALUATION

The emergence of tissue plasminogen activator (TPA) as an option for acute stroke intervention has led to the need for very rapid evaluation of patients who may benefit. Thus, neurologic examination, routine laboratory studies, and establishment of an i.v. should be performed early. Also, rapid CT scanning is critical to decision making. Involvement of a "stroke team" or neurologist experienced in administration of TPA is desirable. Assuring that the patient can protect the airway is of great importance with dysphagia or depressed level of consciousness.

EMERGENCY DEPARTMENT MANAGEMENT

TPA should be considered in patients that present and are evaluated within 3 hours. If there is concern for basilar artery thrombosis, institution of i.v. heparin may be appropriate.

DISPOSITION

Role of the Consultant

If there is any question regarding brainstem ischemia, a neurologist should be consulted.

Indications for Admission

Brainstem strokes and TIAs are indications for admission to establish the etiology. Failure to treat the underlying cause can lead to severe morbidity or death.

Transfer Considerations

If the emergency department initially evaluating the patient does not administer TPA for acute stroke and the patient presents early enough that he or she may be a candidate, then transfer to an alternative facility is indicated.

COMMON PITFALLS

- Cortical and subcortical lesions may cause dysfunction that suggests a brainstem location. This is most likely due to interruption of the corticobulbar pathways or central projections of sensory pathways.
- The most common abnormalities that lead to erroneous assignment of the problem to the brainstem are facial weakness, facial numbness, tongue deviation, decreased gag reflex, reduced corneal reflex, and dysarthria.

References

1. Brazis PW, Masdeu JC, Biller J. *Localization in clinical neurology*. Boston: Little, Brown and Company, 1996.
2. Fromm GH. Trigeminal neuralgia and related disorders. *Neurol Clin* 1989;7:305–319.
3. Hutchinson WM. Acute optic neuritis and the prognosis for multiple sclerosis. *J Neurol Neurosurg Psychiatry* 1976;39:283–289.
4. Roob G, Fazekas F, Hartung HP. Peripheral facial palsy: etiology, diagnosis and treatment. *Eur Neurol* 1999;41(1):3–9.
5. Wilson-Pauwels L, Akesson EJ, Stewart PA. *Cranial nerves: anatomy and clinical comments*. Philadelphia: BC Decker, 1988.

PART VIII

Emergency Aspects of Urology

CHAPTER 61

Male Urologic Infections

David S. Howes and Erica E. Remer

It is important to separate infectious diseases of the male reproductive organs from diseases of the male urinary tract. Complaints of dysuria, urgency, frequency, and hesitancy may indicate urethritis, lower urinary tract infection (cystitis), pyelonephritis, or disease of any of the organs connected or adjacent to the urethra, bladder, ureters, or kidney. Consideration must also be given to disease of the prostate, vas deferens, seminal vesicles, epididymides, and testes, because these organs are contiguous with the male urinary tract and patients with these disorders may present with similar symptoms.

Despite the classic teaching that women have more frequent urinary tract infections (UTIs), if all forms of male-specific infections, such as urethritis and epididymitis, are included in the incidence of UTI, occurrence rates are probably equal in both sexes during the adult years. If prostatitis is added to the incidence of cystitis, men probably have more UTIs after the fifth decade.[8]

CLINICAL PRESENTATION

History

The hallmark of UTI is dysuria. Other symptoms include urgency and increased frequency of urination in small amounts, cloudy or foul-smelling urine, and hematuria. In the older man, difficulty in initiation of voiding, dribbling, or a less forceful urinary stream suggests the presence of prostatism. The emergency physician should inquire about fever, chills, and back, suprapubic, or perineal pain. A history of prior UTI and diagnostic or operative procedures of the urinary tract is important. Information concerning the patient's sexual preferences and recent sexual contacts, prior sexually transmitted diseases (STDs), and significant complicating medical conditions, such as diabetes, kidney transplant, or other potential immunosuppressive conditions, should be sought.[7,13,16,19]

Physical Examination

As with all emergency department (ED) patients, general condition, vital signs, and fever should be noted. Toxic patients should have intravenous lines started immediately. The abdomen should be examined for masses, bladder fullness, bruits, and tenderness or guarding. The back must be checked for masses, bruits, and costovertebral angle tenderness; the scrotum should be examined for tenderness and masses; the urethra should be inspected for discharge or sores; the prepuce should be retracted and inspected; perianal sores, rectal tenderness, perineal tenderness, and prostatic tenderness should be sought. Specific attention should be given to the presence of groin sores or lymphadenopathy and the presence of penile lesions.

Laboratory Studies

The hallmark of UTI is the presence of leukocytes and bacteria in otherwise uncontaminated urine. Diagnosis of a UTI in males does not require obtaining urine by the "clean-catch midstream voided urine" or catheterization.[18] In males, there appears to be no significant difference in numbers of contaminating organisms obtained with clean-catch versus routine voiding samples. In the male, 10^3 colony-forming units (CFUs) per milliliter of a single organism is sufficient to diagnose true infection. In the ED, a positive leukocyte esterase dip test is sufficient to establish the presence of pyuria. A white blood cell count of 2 to 5 per high-power field or greater on microscopic examination corresponds to significant bacteriuria as well.[8]

Although a simple urinalysis does not reliably localize infection within the male genitourinary tract, the clinical picture and epidemiologic features of the patient's presentation will usually separate cystitis and pyelonephritis from disorders of the prostate or urethra and genitalia. If the history is suspicious for urethritis and laboratory confirmation is desired, smears for Gram stain, immunofluorescence assay, or culture for *Chlamydia* and urethral culture for gonorrhea may be done. These are most accurate when the patient has not voided for several hours. A contrary and pragmatic view is that, in the man with clinical urethritis, the presence of leukocytes on dipstick leukocyte esterase test or microscopic examination of urine is more sensitive as a screening tool than a positive microscopic examination of a urethral smear for leukocytes.[20]

If a UTI is suspected on clinical grounds, the presence of leukocytes in the urine should be sought and a urine culture should be obtained; blood cultures are indicated in the patient with presumed pyelonephritis. Although cultures are not useful in initial ED management, this information will help to guide future antibiotic choice in the event of failure to respond to initial therapy.

URETHRITIS

Urethritis is the most common urologic infection in men. It is important to appreciate that in the young male who is sexually active, dysuria with or without discharge is almost always due to urethritis. Isolated infection of the bladder or the kidney (the "classic" UTI) is rare in young, otherwise healthy males.

Urethritis has traditionally been classified as either gonococcal or nongonococcal. With easy and accurate *Chlamydia* identification techniques, it is now apparent that this is an artificial separation because both chlamydial and gonorrheal infections are commonly present in the same patient and are often contracted from the same contact.

The Centers for Disease Control and Prevention estimates that there are between 800,000 and 1 million cases of gonorrhea per year, the incidence being strongly influenced by prevalent sexual attitudes and preferences. Because nongonococcal and chlamydial urethritis are not reportable diseases, an estimate of the number of affected patients is more difficult to determine. The reported incidence of nongonococcal urethritis in Great Britain exceeds the incidence of gonorrhea by a ratio of almost 2:1, and similar findings are reported for Sweden.[2]

Gonococcal Urethritis

CLINICAL PRESENTATION

A purulent urethral exudate noted a few days after a sexual encounter, associated with dysuria, is the most common presentation in symptomatic heterosexual men. The usual incubation period is between 3 and 5 days, but it may extend to 14 days or more.

EMERGENCY DEPARTMENT EVALUATION

A Gram stain of the urethral exudate obtained by swabbing the urethra (in symptomatic men) is a reliable method for the diagnosis of gonorrhea. The specificity is 95% to 98%, and the sensitivity is 83% to 95% when typical gram-negative intracellular diplococci are found. To obtain a specimen from a male without exudate, a calcium alginate–tipped swab (Calgiswab) should be gently inserted 2 to 3 cm into the anterior urethra. Cultures on Thayer-Martin or similar culture media should be obtained.

EMERGENCY DEPARTMENT MANAGEMENT

Treatment has been well studied and is frequently updated by the Centers for Disease Control and Prevention (Table 61.1).[2] The increasing incidence of penicillinase-producing *Neisseria gonorrhoeae* worldwide has led to the use of third-generation cephalosporins or the fluoroquinolones. Patients should also be started on antichlamydial therapy (doxycycline or azithromycin).

TABLE 61.1. Treatment of Gonococcal Urethritis

CURRENT TREATMENT OF CHOICE	
Ceftriaxone	125 mg i.m. single dose
All treatment for gonorrhea should be followed by doxycycline, 100 mg two times a day for 7 days, or azithromycin, 1.0 g PO single dose, due to the high percentage of patients who are also infected with *Chlamydia*.	
ALTERNATIVE TREATMENTS	
Ofloxacin	400 mg PO single dose
or	
Ciprofloxacin	500 mg PO single dose
or	
Norfloxacin	800 mg PO single dose
or	
Cefixime	400 mg PO single dose

Adapted from Gilbert DN, Moellering RC; Sande MA. *The Sen ford guide to antimicrobial therapy*. Dallas: Antimicrobial Therapy, Inc., 1999.

DISPOSITION

All patients with gonococcal urethritis should be rechecked after therapy to ensure a cure. Referral to an STD clinic is appropriate. Emphatic counseling should be given to ensure that the medication is taken and that the patient's sexual partners are also examined and treated. Single-dose therapy with ceftriaxone or one of the fluoroquinolones and azithromycin ensures compliance.

COMPLICATIONS

From 1% to 3% of patients with gonococcal infections develop hematogenous spread of the organism that may involve joints, meninges, heart, and skin. Strains that disseminate are usually nonvirulent in their primary site, and the original infection is often minimally symptomatic. In addition to the complications of bacteremia, local spread may involve the vas deferens, prostate, paraurethral glands, epididymis, and adjacent soft tissues (Table 61.2). Severe urethral inflammation may result in a urethral stricture.[2]

Chlamydial Urethritis

There is little question that *Chlamydia trachomatis* causes the majority of sexually transmitted diseases in the United States.[2,15] The prevalence is high in heterosexuals and adolescents. Gonorrheal coinfection is common.

CLINICAL PRESENTATION

The clinical features of chlamydial urethritis resemble those of gonorrhea but are generally less severe; the discharge is often thinner and less purulent, but there is sufficient overlap in signs and symptoms to make clinical distinction unreliable. *Chlamydia* has an incubation period of 1 to 3 weeks, but it may extend as long as 45 days.[1,2]

EMERGENCY DEPARTMENT EVALUATION

The laboratory diagnosis of chlamydial urethritis has been based on a urethral smear of epithelial cells utilizing immunofluorescence techniques. Most hospital laboratories do not have the capacity to accurately identify *Chlamydia* with tissue culture. A technique using an enzyme-linked immunosorbent assay on urine samples has been developed and looks promising. Its sensitivity is equivalent to, if not better than, urethral sampling techniques, and specimen collection is better tolerated. Improvement in this technology will allow inexpensive, ef-

TABLE 61.2. Infectious Sequelae of Gonorrhea

Epididymitis	Conjunctivitis
Prostatitis	Dermatitis
Endocarditis	Vasculitis
Meningitis	Tenosynovitis
Arthritis (both septic and reactive)	

fective widespread screening of populations at risk, such as military personnel, sexually active adolescents, and individuals who seek advice for contraception or STD testing.[5,20]

EMERGENCY DEPARTMENT MANAGEMENT

Doxycycline, 100 mg twice a day for 6 days, is associated with excellent cure rates, good compliance, and few side effects. To date, there are no known tetracycline-resistant strains of *Chlamydia*. From a public health viewpoint, azithromycin in a single 1-g oral dose is as effective as doxycycline, and compliance is ensured by dispensing it in the ED.[14] Other antibiotics that have been effective include erythromycin and trimethoprim–sulfamethoxazole (cotrimoxazole). Both of these agents have cure rates between 85% and 95% when given for at least 7 days. For those patients who cannot tolerate the tetracyclines, either erythromycin base, 500 mg, or erythromycin ethyl succinate, 800 mg, should be taken four times a day; or cotrimoxazole double-strength (e.g., Bactrim DS) twice a day; all regimens are to be continued for at least 7 days. The fluoroquinolones have antichlamydial activity as well: ofloxacin, 300 mg twice a day or levofloxacin, 500 mg a day, either for a 7-day course.[1,6]

COMPLICATIONS

Complications of chlamydial infections include epididymitis and possibly prostatitis. In contrast to females who may become infertile because of chronic chlamydial infection, exposure to *Chlamydia* in the male does not appear to lead to infertility.[2,8]

Nongonococcal, Nonchlamydial Urethritis

Nongonococcal, nonchlamydial urethritis is a "wastebasket" diagnosis for all cases in which the infection is neither gonorrheal nor chlamydial. As greater facility with identification and isolation of pathogenic commensal organisms is gained, more specific causes of nongonococcal, nonchlamydial urethritis may be found. Up to 25% of nongonococcal urethritis may be caused by *Ureaplasma (Mycoplasma)* species. There is good evidence that implicates *U. genitalium* as a cause of urethritis.

Reports show a high incidence of urethral *Trichomonas vaginalis* in men with symptoms of urethritis whose female partners had symptomatic *Trichomonas* vaginitis.[9] In other studies of the cause of nongonococcal urethritis, *Candida, Gardnerella,* and *Bacteroides* species; *Staphylococcus saprophyticus; Corynebacterium genitalium;* and various viruses, including herpes, are isolated on occasion.[2] After *Chlamydia, Ureaplasma,* and gonorrhea have been eliminated as the cause of urethritis, about 30% of cases remain without apparent cause.

TREATMENT

Doxycycline (100 mg given twice daily for 7 days) is effective against most *Ureaplasma* species. If doxycycline fails, azithromycin, 1 g in a single oral dose, should be given. These organisms respond poorly to sulfonamides.

Although all types of nongonococcal urethritis respond initially to antibiotic therapy, recurrence of symptoms is found in up to 50% of cases. In this instance, more prolonged therapy with doxycycline for 14 to 28 days is advised. Erythromycin may be used as an alternative for those patients who cannot tolerate doxycycline. Ofloxacin, 300 mg orally every 12 hours for 7 days, is another alternative.[1,2]

Recurrent Urethritis

If a patient presents to the ED with a recurrent urethritis despite adequate therapy for both *Chlamydia* and gonorrhea, the patient may either have been reinfected by his partner(s) or represent treatment failure. The partner(s) of the patient with recurrent infection should be examined, and treatment ensured. If the patient presents with recurrent nongonococcal, nonchlamydial urethritis and both he and his partner(s) have had appropriate therapy, *Trichomonas, Candida,* and herpes simplex virus should be sought as possible pathogens.[9]

PROSTATITIS

Prostatitis is a poorly defined but common syndrome of prostatic inflammation. Its manifestations include a wide range of pelvic, urinary, or ejaculatory symptoms with or without a tender prostate or evidence of bacterial infection. It is estimated that up to 50% of men experience some form of prostatitis. Symptomatic prostatitis syndromes can be classified into four subcategories (Table 61.3) on the basis of the bacterial findings on culture and on the microscopic examination of the expressed prostatic secretion or the presence of pyuria[10]: (1) acute bacterial prostatitis, (2) chronic bacterial prostatitis, and (3) chronic prostatitis/chronic pelvic pain syndrome (CP/CPPS) of either the inflammatory or (4) noninflammatory subtypes. Both acute and chronic bacterial prostatitis are characterized by bacteriuria that can be localized to the prostate. Urine, prostatic secretions, and semen usually show evidence of leukocytes, and frequently the offending organism is cultured from these secretions.

Acute bacterial prostatitis is most often seen in younger men, whereas chronic infection is seen in older men. The latter may not complain of symptoms of prostatitis. In younger men, the role of *Chlamydia* is uncertain. In men with acquired immunodeficiency syndrome, the prostate may harbor *Cryptococcus neoformans*.[11]

TABLE 61.3. Classification of Symptomatic Prostatitis

	Acute Bacterial[a]	Chronic Bacterial	*Chronic Prostatitis/Chronic Pelvic Pain Syndrome*	
			Inflammatory	Noninflammatory
Evidence of inflammation[b]	+	+	+	0
Culture positive (EPS)	+	+	0	0
Culture positive (bladder)	+	+	0	0
Etiology	Coliforms	Coliforms	???	???
Rectal examination	Very abnormal	Usually normal	Usually normal	Normal

[a]Prostatic massage should be avoided.
[b]Expressed prostatic secretion (EPS) positive for leukocytes; pyuria often present.

About 90% of symptomatic men have CP/CPPS of either inflammatory or noninflammatory subtypes. Inflammatory CP/CPPS is a nonbacterial prostatitis in which inflammation is present but no cause can be found. Noninflammatory CP/CPPS, formerly referred to as *prostatodynia,* shares many of the symptoms of bacterial or nonbacterial prostatitis but lacks signs of inflammation and is not associated with UTI.[10,12]

Acute Bacterial Prostatitis

EMERGENCY DEPARTMENT EVALUATION

Acute bacterial prostatitis is easy to diagnose and treat. It usually presents as an acute illness with fever, chills, and pain in the lower back, the rectal area, or the perineal area. The patient often complains of painful sitting (e.g., the sensation of "sitting on a hot coal"). Systemic symptoms of malaise, arthralgia, and myalgia may also be present. These may appear several days before the local prostatic inflammation produces symptoms of dysuria, frequency, and urgency. The patient frequently is toxic at the time of the ED visit. The diagnosis is suggested once perirectal pathology has been eliminated. Occasional patients present with acute urinary retention; this combination of obstruction and infection may progress to sepsis.[11,12]

Examination of the prostate may be difficult because it is exquisitely painful. The prostate is swollen, tender, warm, and firm to touch. In the patient with classic signs and symptoms of acute bacterial prostatitis, a finding of exquisite external perineal tenderness is probably sufficient to make the diagnosis and a digital rectal examination of the prostate may be deferred. Massage of the prostate is *contraindicated* because of possible hematogenous spead of bacteria. Because the prostate surrounds the urethra, cystitis often accompanies acute prostatitis and a urine culture will usually reveal the infecting organism. The swelling of the acutely inflamed prostate may cause complete urinary retention; this combination of obstruction and infection may progress to sepsis.[11,12]

EMERGENCY DEPARTMENT MANAGEMENT

Acute prostatitis is responsive to antibiotics. For the less toxic patient, appropriate antibiotics include trimethoprim–sulfamethoxazole, ofloxacin, ciprofloxacin, or other fluoroquinolones. Antibiotic therapy should be continued for a minimum of 4 weeks in all patients. Referral is important, as complete resolution of symptoms may take weeks to months and most men will require ongoing consultation (mostly reassurance) during convalescence.[1,2,11,12]

Toxicity, fever, urinary retention, concurrent underlying disease, and altered immune response are indications for hospitalization and the administration of intravenous antibiotics. Parenteral ampicillin and an aminoglycoside such as tobramycin are an appropriate empiric therapy. The subsequent choice of antibiotics is ideally made from sensitivity testing of bacteria grown from urine cultures.

Instrumentation of the urinary tract should be avoided. If the patient has acute urinary retention from prostatitis, catheterization may be painful and could potentially result in hematogenous release of bacteria. Until antibiotics and rest allow the inflammation to subside, a suprapubic catheter may be necessary. Urologic consultation is indicated.

Fluid replacement, antipyretics, narcotic analgesics, and stool softeners should be given. Nonsteroidal antiinflammatory drugs and spasmolytics are useful for milder pain. Bedrest frequently makes the patient more comfortable. Hospitalization of the toxic patient ensures that appropriate supportive care is maintained.

The patient may experience irritative voiding symptoms for several months after completion of therapy; nonsteroidal antiinflammatory agents, such as ibuprofen, have been anecdotally useful. A firm, hard prostate may also be noted for the same duration, but if this condition persists, the possibility of an underlying malignancy must be considered.

CHRONIC BACTERIAL PROSTATITIS

Chronic bacterial prostatitis encompasses only 10% of all cases of prostatitis, but it is probably the most common cause of recurrent UTI in men. In most, the pathogen is *Escherichia coli,* but *Pseudomonas, Proteus* species, *Enterobacter, Klebsiella,* and enterococci are also found. The usual picture of chronic prostatitis is of relapsing dysuria, occasionally associated with perineal discomfort and associated epididymitis. A prolonged course of an oral fluoroquinolone is indicated. Many urologists recommend a trial of an alpha-adrenergic blocking agent such as finasteride in addition to antibiotic therapy in cases of recent or frequent relapse.[3]

Prostatic calculi are common and may be visible on pelvic films. In most instances, stones cause no apparent harm and require no therapy. However, these stones can serve as the nidus for recurrent infection from bacteria, and surgical removal of infected calculi may be indicated in follow-up consultation with a urologist.

NONINFLAMMATORY CHRONIC PROSTATITIS/CHRONIC PELVIC PAIN SYNDROME (FORMERLY PROSTATODYNIA)

When the patient has symptoms referable to the prostate, with no inflammatory cells in the expressed prostatic secretion and no bacteria cultured from the prostatic fluid, the syndrome is designated noninflammatory CP/CPPS, an entity formerly referred to as *prostatodynia*. There are likely multiple etiologies for this symptom complex. This new terminology recognizes the limited understanding of the causes of this syndrome in most patients and the possibility that organs other than the prostate gland may be important in the pathogenesis of chronic pelvic pain in males.[10] Clearly, the treatment of this entity is in the urologist's domain.

In the older patient with symptoms of prostatism and no evidence of inflammation (i.e., no pyuria or leukocytes in expressed prostatic secretions), it is reasonable to offer an alpha-adrenergic agent such as finasteride or a natural product such as saw palmetto extract. The patient should seek urologic consultation in follow-up.[23]

PROSTATIC ABSCESS

Prostatic abscess is now rare, except in immunosuppressed patients. A fever despite antimicrobial treatment, increasing rectal symptoms, and persistent leukocytes should suggest a prostatic abscess. Rectal examination usually reveals a fluctuant mass, the hallmark of the prostatic abscess. Occasionally, only a firm, tender prostate is found because of the anterior location of the abscess. Urologic consultation is indicated. Hospitalization and intravenous antibiotics are necessary for these seriously ill patients.

SEMINAL VESICULITIS

Seminal vesiculitis is difficult to separate clinically from prostatitis, and probably includes elements of prostatitis because of the con-

TABLE 61.4. Treatment of Epididymitis

ALL CASES	
Gram stain of urethral swab or urine sediment	
Culture of gonorrhea, immunofluorescence for Chlamydia	
Examination for concurrent STD	
PRESUMED STD ETIOLOGY	
Ceftriaxone	250 mg i.m.
or	
Ciprofloxacin	500 mg PO
and	
Doxycycline	100 mg PO two times per day for 10 days
ALTERNATIVE REGIMEN	
Ofloxacin	300 mg PO two times per day for 10 days
PRESUMED BACTERIAL (COLIFORM) ETIOLOGY	
Ofloxacin	200 mg PO two times per day for 14 days
or	
Ciprofloxacin	500 mg PO two times per day for 14 days
or	
Trovafloxacin	200 mg PO daily for 14 days
Urine culture	
Look for predisposing genitourinary pathology	
OPTIONAL THERAPY (ALL CASES)	
Scrotal support	
Nonsteroidal antiinflammatory drugs	

tiguous spread of the infection or inflammatory condition. If the patient presents with hematospermia, evaluation and treatment should be the same as for prostatitis. Urologic referral is appropriate.

EPIDIDYMITIS

Acute epididymitis is an inflammatory process of the epididymis, with scrotal pain, swelling, and tenderness, usually resulting from infection.[4,21,22] Epididymitis is covered in detail in Chapter 67.

Once the diagnosis of acute epididymitis has been established, a presumptive etiology is made on the basis of age.[2,5] For men younger than age 35, or if an STD is believed to be the causative agent, coverage for gonorrhea and chlamydial infection is indicated (Table 61.4). For men who are older than age 35, or are the insertive partners in anal intercourse, coliforms must be covered (see Table 61.4).

If the patient appears toxic, admission and intravenous antibiotics are indicated. An aminoglycoside or third-generation cephalosporin is an appropriate choice for the patient with presumed coliform etiology.

CYSTITIS AND PYELONEPHRITIS

Cystitis

PREDISPOSING CAUSES

In males, the long anatomic distance of the urethra discourages retrograde travel of organisms from the penile meatus to the bladder. Factors associated with an increased risk for infection include congenital anomalies, such as hypospadias, and instrumentation of the urethra. After 3 days of indwelling urinary catheter drainage, virtually 100% of patients have a UTI. Autoerogenous intraurethral insertion of foreign objects may precipitate cystitis. Trauma to the urethra or bladder may allow dissemination of organisms.

Cystitis without trauma or instrumentation is rare in young men and is usually a secondary manifestation of upper urinary tract disease, diabetes, chronic prostatitis, nephrolithiasis, tumor, congenital malformation, or mechanical obstruction.[16] Of these, chronic prostatitis, prostatism in older men, and prior instrumentation are the most common predisposing causes. Abnormalities are found in up to 80% of males who present with a UTI without antecedent trauma or instrumentation. It is particularly important to ensure that urinary obstruction is not present, because the combination of infection and obstruction is an important, preventable cause of sepsis.

EMERGENCY DEPARTMENT EVALUATION AND MANAGEMENT

A thorough history and physical examination should be done. The genitalia, rectum, and abdomen are examined, and urinalysis and culture of urine are performed. Postvoiding urethral catheterization may be indicated to assess residual urine volume in patients who relate symptoms of prostatism such as hesitancy, dribbling, and incomplete bladder-emptying sensation. Intravenous pyelography or ultrasonography may be indicated. If the patient is younger than age 35, urethritis must be considered because it can masquerade as cystitis. In this case, antimicrobial therapy should cover the STDs discussed earlier. For patients with clinically apparent cystitis and patients older than age 35, therapy for coliforms should be instituted while awaiting culture results: cotrimoxazole double-strength (Bactrim DS) two times per day for 10 days, or a fluoroquinolone such as ofloxacin 400 mg orally twice daily for 10 days, or ciprofloxacin 500 mg orally twice daily for 10 days. In view of the high percentage of abnormalities associated with male UTI, frequency of other related genitourinary infections, and the difficulty in determining the precise site of infection by clinical criteria, short courses of antimicrobial agents are ill advised in men.[8]

DISPOSITION

Cystitis is commonly associated with other urinary tract pathology. Therefore, the evaluation must be continued beyond the ED, and referral is always appropriate. Patients with a known history of instrumentation, congenital malformation, and symptomatic prostatic hypertrophy should be referred to a urologist, with consultation before discharge.

Pyelonephritis

Pyelonephritis presents in a similar manner in both males and females. Predisposition to infection from underlying urinary tract disease or abnormality is more common in males, and a thorough search for these problems in males with suspected pyelonephritis is indicated. It should be appreciated that pyelonephritis is a common presenting condition in the older man with prostatism.

PREDISPOSING CAUSES

Abnormal anatomy, such as ureteral ectopia, bifid ureter, or renal scarring from prior renal infections, predisposes to infection of the kidney. Other common predisposing causes include abnormal physiology from neurologic trauma, urinary retention from prostatism, acute prostatitis or other cause, underlying renal disease, and the presence of a foreign body, such as a stone or an indwelling catheter.

ETIOLOGY

E. coli is the most common causative organism, accounting for more than 90% of infections. It is followed in frequency by *Enterobacter, Klebsiella, Proteus, Pseudomonas,* and enterococcal species. *Staphylococcus aureus* infections are usually associated with blood-borne spread, and a primary source should be diligently sought. Gram-positive organisms are unusual causative agents and are associated with diabetes, an immunocompromised host, or tumor of the urinary tract.[7,13,19]

EMERGENCY DEPARTMENT MANAGEMENT

Men with symptoms of pyelonephritis should be strongly considered for admission and parenteral antibiotic therapy. Urine should be obtained for culture and sensitivity testing before therapy is initiated. If patients have had rigors, chills, hypotension, or a temperature greater than 102° (39°C), blood cultures are indicated as well. Patients who appear toxic, are nauseated or vomiting, or have a temperature greater than 102° (39°C) should be hospitalized and treated with parenteral antibiotics directed against *E. coli* and other common enteric coliforms.

Parenteral therapy for pyelonephritis includes the following:

Ampicillin, 1 g every 6 hours, and gentamicin, 1 mg/kg every 8 hours
Ciprofloxacin, 200 to 400 mg every 12 hours
Ofloxacin, 200 to 400 mg every 12 hours
Ceftriaxone, 1 to 2 g daily

Oral therapy may be begun after defervescence of fever. The fluoroquinolones (e.g., ofloxacin, norfloxacin, ciprofloxacin, or others) are the drugs of choice, and therapy should be given for 14 days.[15]

Nursing home patients and patients who have recently been hospitalized or instrumented should be presumed to have a nosocomial infection, and antibiotic therapy should be chosen that includes pseudomonal coverage, for example, an aminoglycoside, ceftazidime, an extended-spectrum penicillin such as piperacillin/tazobactam, or imipenam.[1,19]

The patient with ureteral colic and fever and chills should be suspected of having a ureteral obstruction and an infection. Pyelonephritis in the presence of an obstruction can rapidly progress to a renal abscess, with subsequent loss of renal tissue and sepsis. In addition to immediate urologic consultation, blood and urine cultures should be obtained, followed by intravenous pyelography or renal ultrasonography and intravenous administration of antibiotics.[17]

COMMON PITFALLS

- "Cystitis" in a young, sexually active male with dysuria is most likely to be urethritis.
- A careful search should be done for associated STDs in the young male who presents with symptoms of urethritis.
- Instructions should be provided regarding the need for the patient's sexual partner(s) to obtain evaluation and treatment.
- Prostatic massage in a patient with acute bacterial prostatitis may lead to bacteremia or sepsis.
- One should not assume that all perineal discomfort is prostatitis.
- The postvoid residual urinary volume should be checked in the older man who presents with symptoms of prostatism and acute UTI.
- Strong consideration should be given for parenteral administration of antibiotics in the male with pyelonephritis and toxicity.

References

1. Abramowicz M. The choice of antibacterial drugs. *Med Lett Drugs Ther* 1998;40:33.
2. Anonymous. 1998 guidelines for treatment of sexually transmitted diseases. Centers for Disease Control and Prevention. *MMWR* 1997;46:1.
3. Barbalias GA, Nikiforidis G, Liatsikos EN. Alpha-blockers for the treatment of chronic prostatitis in combination with antibiotics. *J Urol* 1998;159:883.
4. Bennett RT, Gill B, Kogan SJ. Epididymitis in children: the circumcision factor? *J Urol* 1998;160:1842.
5. David LM, Natin D, Walzman M, et al. Urinary symptoms, sexual intercourse and significant bacteriuria in male patients attending STD clinics. *Genitourin Med* 1996;72:266.
6. Gilbert DN, Moellering RC, Sande MA. *The Sanford guide to antimicrobial therapy*. Dallas: Antimicrobial Therapy, Inc., 1999.
7. Goossens H, Sprenger MJW. Community acquired infections and bacterial resistance. *BMJ* 1998;317:654.
8. Hooten TM, Stamm WE. Diagnosis and treatment of uncomplicated urinary tract infection. *Infect Dis Clin North Am* 1997;11:647.
9. Krieger JN, Jenny C, Verdin M, et al. Clinical manifestations of trichomoniasis in men. *Ann Intern Med* 1993;118:844.
10. Krieger JN, Nyberg L, Nickel JC. NIH consensus definition and classification of prostatitis. *JAMA* 1999;282:236.
11. Leigh DA. Prostatis—an increasing clinical problem for diagnosis and management. *J Antimicrob Chemother* 1993;32[Suppl A]:1.
12. Lipsky BA. Prostatitis and urinary tract infection in males: what's new, what's true? *Am J Med* 1999;106:327.
13. Lloyed S, Zervos M, Mahayni R, et al. Risk factors for enterococcal urinary tract infection and colonization in a rehabilitation facility. *Am J Infect Control* 1998;26:35.
14. Martin DH, Mroczkowski TF, Dalu ZA. A controlled trial of a single dose of azithromycin for the treatment of chlamydial urethritis and cervicitis. *N Engl J Med* 1992;326:921.
15. Mombelli G, Pezzoli R, Pinoja-Lutz G, et al. Oral vs intravenous ciprofloxacin in the initial empiric management of severe pyelonephritis or complicated urinary tract infections: a prospective randomized clinical trial. *Arch Intern Med* 1999;159:53.
16. Patterson JE, Andriole VT. Bacterial urinary tract infections in diabetes. *Infect Dis Clin North Am* 1997;11:735.
17. Pearle MS, Pierce HL, Miller GL, et al. Optimal method of urgent decompression of the collecting system for obstruction and infection due to ureteral calculi. *J Urol* 1998;160:1260.
18. Prandoni D, Boone MH, Larson E, et al. Assessment of urine collection technique for microbial culture. *Am J Infect Control* 1996;24:219.
19. Rosser CJ, Bare RL, Meredith JW. Urinary tract infections in the critically ill patient with a urinary catheter. *Am J Surg* 1999;177:287.
20. Sadof MD, Woods ER, Emas SJ. Dipstick leukocyte esterase activity in first-catch urine specimens: a useful screening test for detection of sexually transmitted diseases in the adolescent male. *JAMA* 1987;258:1932.
21. Sawyer EK, Anderson JR. Acute epididymitis: a work-related injury? *N J Nat Med Assoc* 1996;88:385.
22. Suzer O, Oscan H, Kupeli S, et al. Color Doppler imaging in the diagnosis of the acute scrotum. *Eur Urol* 1996;32:457.
23. Wilt TJ, Ishani A, Stark G, et al. Saw palmetto extracts for treatment of benign prostatic hyperplasia. *JAMA* 1999;280:1604.

CHAPTER 62
Urinary Tract Infections in Women

Eric T. Boie, Deepi G. Goyal, and Annie T. Sadosty

Urinary tract infections (UTIs) in women are among the most common problems encountered by the emergency physician. Twenty percent to 40% of women will have a UTI sometime in their lifetime,[2,25] and estimates place annual incidence of infection between 3% and 10%. Women are 30 times more likely than men to suffer a UTI, and of those women affected, 20% have more than three UTIs per year.[10] It is not surprising, then, that complaints related to the urinary tract account for 7 million annual outpatient visits (1.6 million emergency department [ED] visits), 1 million hospitalizations, and billions of dollars in health-care costs annually.[12,25]

UTIs comprise a collection of diseases that can be classified based on both the anatomy and the complexity of the disease. Anatomically, upper UTIs involve the kidney, resulting in pyelonephritis. Pyelonephritis may be chronic, subclinical, or acute, with this chapter focusing on management of the latter. Lower UTIs involve the urethra and bladder, resulting in acute urethritis and acute cystitis, respectively.

UTIs can be further classified as complicated or uncomplicated. A complicated UTI is associated with a condition that increases risk for acquiring infection, failing therapy, or suffering increased morbidity.[13,28] These associated conditions may be structural (obstruction, catheterization, renal calculi), metabolic (diabetes, pregnancy, chronic renal failure), or functional (impaired host [AIDS, neutropenia] or unusual pathogen). Table 62.1 lists many of these factors that place a patient at risk for a complicated UTI. Complicated UTIs can range in severity from simple cystitis to urosepsis with shock; thus, it is the associated conditions, not severity of disease, that make a UTI complicated. Some authors argue that true uncomplicated UTIs only occur in nonpregnant, healthy adult women with no neurologic or structural dysfunction.[2] Eighty percent of UTIs fall into this group.[25]

The urinary tract is normally an enclosed, protected, and sterile mucosal surface. Washout of bacteria by urine flow is the primary host defense against infection.[33] This process is nearly continuous in the upper tract but only intermittent in the lower. Uropathogens are generally not virulent, but instead are highly adapted to ascend, colonize, and grow in the urinary tract, subsequently causing cell damage and infection.[33] The colon is the primary reservoir for most uropathogens. Over 95% of infections result from enteric bacteria ascending the urinary tract.[2] Although the exact process of ascent is unknown, enteric bacteria colonize the vagina and periurethral area, ascend the urethra into the bladder, multiply in the urine, reflux into the ureters, and ultimately colonize and invade the renal parenchyma.[33] Factors that alter urine washout, change the characteristics of the urine, or facilitate entry of bacteria into the urinary tract increase risk for development of a UTI. The primary risk factors in young healthy women for development of an uncomplicated UTI are sexual intercourse and diaphragm use with spermicide.[12] Less than 5% of UTIs result from hematogenous spread during septicemia. These organisms tend to be more virulent, causing severe pyelonephritis or even microabscesses within the kidney.[2]

TABLE 62.1. Risk Factors for Development of Complicated Urinary Tract Infection

1. Hospitalization
2. Catheterization/urinary tract instrumentation
3. Pregnancy
4. Anatomic/functional abnormalities
5. Childhood UTI (prior to age 12)
6. Symptoms > 7 days prior to treatment
7. Diabetes Mellitus
8. Immunosuppression (cancer, chronic renal failure, AIDS, drug or alcohol abuse)
9. Elderly
10. Recent antibiotic use
11. Urinary retention
12. Sickle cell trait and anemia
13. Incompetent vesicourethral valve

Developed from articles by Ronald/Harding[28] and Bacheller/Bernstein[2]

The most common uropathogens responsible for development of a UTI are enteric gram-negative bacilli of the class Enterobacteriaceae. *Escherichia coli* is responsible for over 80% of UTIs in reproductive-aged females.[10] *Staphylococcus saprophyticus* causes 5% to 20% of UTIs in this group, with other enterics such as *Klebsiella, Enterobacter,* enterococcus, *Proteus, Pseudomonas,* and Group B *Streptococcus* causing the balance of infections. Hospitalized, catheterized, and immunosuppressed patients tend to suffer UTIs from more virulent bacteria as well as *Candida.*[2] *E. coli* infections are much less common in this group, causing less than 40% of infections.[25]

CLINICAL PRESENTATION

Asymptomatic Bacteriuria

Asymptomatic bacteriuria is simply the presence of bacteriuria in a patient with no symptoms of cystitis or pyelonephritis. This condition is most common in elderly and pregnant women. The incidence of asymptomatic bacteriuria increases with age to as high as 40% in women over 60. Thirty percent of individuals become symptomatic within 1 year.[10] Identification of asymptomatic bacteriuria in elderly women is of questionable benefit, as no association with excess morbidity and mortality has been demonstrated. In contrast, it is critical that the emergency physician identify asymptomatic bacteriuria in a pregnant woman. While only 4% to 7% of pregnant women will have asymptomatic bacteriuria, 30% of these will subsequently develop pyelonephritis if untreated.[10] Asymptomatic bacteriuria has also been implicated in stillbirth and preterm labor, but this remains controversial.

Acute Cystitis

Acute cystitis is most commonly seen in reproductive-aged women. The most typical symptoms include dysuria, frequency, urgency, and suprapubic or abdominal discomfort. Hematuria occurs in up to 40% of women with acute cystitis.[13] More general complaints may also be described, such as fatigue, malaise, irritability, and diaphoresis.[18] Fever (greater than 38°C) and severe abdominal pain are rare, and should make the emergency physician consider upper tract disease or alternative diagnoses. Microscopic urinalysis reveals pyuria, bacteriuria, and, frequently, hematuria.

Acute Recurrent Cystitis

Acute recurrent cystitis is defined as three or more episodes of acute cystitis within a year. It occurs in 20% of individuals with acute cystitis, usually as the result of separate episodic uncomplicated infections.[2] Individuals with recurrent cystitis should be identified for consideration of UTI prophylaxis.[25]

Acute Urethritis

Acute urethritis presents with symptoms nearly identical to those of cystitis. There may be a coexistent cervicitis and vaginal discharge. Pyuria without evidence of bacteriuria is common on urinalysis (UA), with subsequent cultures growing minimal uropathogens. *Chlamydia trachomatis, Neisseria gonorrhoeae,* and the herpes simplex virus are the usual causative organisms.

Acute Pyelonephritis

Acute pyelonephritis can present with variable severity, from a mild cystitis-like illness with flank pain to a more severe illness with fever, chills, nausea, vomiting, sweats, and flank and/or abdominal pain. Absence of cystitis symptoms is not uncommon.[25] Costovertebral angle tenderness is a common physical finding. UA reveals pyuria, bacteriuria, hematuria, and white blood cell casts; the latter are highly specific for acute pyelonephritis.

Urosepsis

Urosepsis is most likely to manifest in women with indwelling catheters, immunosuppressive disorders, urinary obstruction, complicated UTIs, or serious underlying medical problems. Elderly women from extended care facilities are at greatest risk. Typically, such patients present with nonspecific signs and symptoms, including fever, confusion, weakness, tachycardia, tachypnea, and dehydration. Family members or nursing home staff may provide valuable history, as the patient often cannot provide one herself. If alert, the patient may complain of incontinence, abdominal pain, thirst, dyspnea, or even cough.[9] Fever is often present, but hypothermia is not unusual. Examination will usually reveal dehydration or compensated shock, but delayed presentation may result in severe hypotension and septic shock.

Symptomatic Catheterized Patients

Urinary catheterization is responsible for the vast majority of nosocomial UTIs. Incidence of infection for indwelling catheters is 5% per catheter-day.[2] Such UTIs are, by definition, complicated, with manifestations ranging from mild suprapubic pain, bladder spasms, and incontinence around the catheter to fulminant sepsis. All symptomatic catheterized patients should be treated with broad-spectrum antibiotic therapy.[25]

DIFFERENTIAL DIAGNOSIS

The emergency physician should be aware that ED patients differ from those of other outpatient settings. Patients presenting with urinary symptoms to an inner-city ED are more likely to have gynecologic disease (vaginitis, pelvic inflammatory disease, and sexually transmitted disease), upper tract disease, and social circumstances that complicate access to care and follow-up when compared with other outpatient settings.

The differential diagnosis of acute dysuria includes the following: acute urethritis, acute cystitis, and vaginitis. Generally, urethritis is characterized by a more gradual onset and occurs in patients who have concomitant vaginal symptoms. Urgency, frequency, and urinary incontinence commonly accompany the dysuria of acute cystitis. The bladder, when infected or inflamed, contracts spasmodically to create these symptoms. Vaginitis is common and presents with external dysuria and vaginal discharge. Frequency and urgency are lacking because the bladder is not involved.

Flank pain typical of pyelonephritis is common in other diseases as well. Patients with unilateral costovertebral angle tenderness may have renal calculi, perinephric abscesses, renal infarcts, and neoplastic or traumatic processes.

The emergency physician must base the differential diagnosis on the presenting complaint, then narrow it with additional history, physical examination, and laboratory examination.

EMERGENCY DEPARTMENT EVALUATION

History

Historical information of importance includes the nature of the dysuria (external or internal), the duration of symptoms, and accompanying symptoms of urgency, frequency, incontinence, abnormal vaginal discharge, external genital lesions, fever, back pain, hematuria, or foul-smelling urine. A detailed sexual history, including the possibility of pregnancy, the number of partners, and the type of birth control method used, is also prudent. The medical history should be explored in an effort to identify any factors that would make an otherwise uncomplicated UTI complicated (see Table 62.1).

Physical Examination

The examination begins with an assessment of vital signs and hydration status. Examination of the genitourinary tract includes assessment of costovertebral angle tenderness, suprapubic mass, or tenderness, and examination of the external genitalia and urethra. A pelvic examination should be performed in women in whom the diagnosis is unclear and in women whose history suggests a diagnosis of either urethritis or vaginitis. It is important to note the presence or absence of indwelling catheters, as they place the patient at risk for a complicated UTI.

When combined with a good history, a careful physical examination should enable the physician to identify patients with urosepsis, acute cystitis, and acute pyelonephritis, and should allow the physician to predict whether the patient has a complicated or uncomplicated infection.

Urinalysis Collection

A urine specimen should be collected by the method most appropriate for the patient's clinical status and capacity to cooperate with cleansing guidelines. In the presence of obesity, menstrual blood, copious vaginal discharge, or an anatomic abnormality, the preferred method for obtaining a urine specimen is an in-and-out urethral catheterization of the bladder. The main risk is induction of UTI, but this occurs less than 1% of the time in a normal host.[29] For nonmenstruating, thin patients lacking vaginal discharge, a clean-catch UA can be utilized. The sample should be a midstream specimen obtained after perineal cleansing with gauze moistened by either saline or tap water. No benefit has been proven from soap cleansers.[13] Some experts suggest that urine from a freshly wet diaper can be collected for accurate analysis.[3] Regardless of the means by which the urine is obtained, the specimen should be processed promptly after collection, as stagnation increases colony counts.

Dipstick Chemical Tests/Urine Microscopy

The nitrite test depends on bacterial reduction of nitrate to nitrite. The test is more likely to be positive with gram-negative bacteria. It may be falsely negative in the presence of low-count UTIs, dilution, antimicrobial therapy, and infections caused by non–nitrate-reducing bacteria such as *S. saprophyticus, Acinetobacter,* and enterococcus.[10,25] While the negative predictive value of a nitrite test ranges from 0.27 to 0.70, the positive predictive value is 0.96.[25] Thus, a positive nitrite test strongly suggests the presence of bacteriuria, while a negative test does not exclude it. The leukocyte esterase test detects the presence of neutrophil granules and connotes pyuria greater than or equal to 8 to 10 white blood cells per high-power field.[2] The sensitivity for the leukocyte esterase test ranges from 0.75 to 0.90, while the specificity is more precisely defined as being 0.95.[25] False-positive results have been reported with *Trichomonas,* and false-negative results have been seen in UAs with dipsticks positive for glucose and ketones.[4]

The ease of use and availability of these tests can assist the emergency physician in identifying UTIs. Generally, a completely negative dipstick analysis corresponds to a negative microscopy evaluation, although 5% of UAs with negative dipstick results are found to have abnormal urine microscopy.[4] Urinary microscopy has been shown to change patient management in only 5% of patients,[16] and, therefore, consideration must be paid to both the turn-around time and the cost of each test. A urine dipstick costs approximately 30 cents and takes a few minutes to perform, whereas a microscopic UA costs approximately $12 and takes nearly an hour to complete.[16] For cases in which the diagnosis is clear, a dipstick should suffice. Full microscopic evaluation may be of assistance in the more complicated cases and in cases in which false-negative or false-positive results are expected. Understanding the limitations of the nitrite and leukocyte esterase tests better enables the clinician to decide when to employ microscopic analysis.

Gram Stain

Few institutions employ urine Gram stain, but in places where it is available, it can be very helpful. A Gram stain of unspun urine that reveals 1 to 2 bacteria per high-power field or a Gram stain of spun urine that reveals 20 bacteria per high-power field corresponds to greater than 10^5 colony-forming units (CFU) per milliliter of urine.[21]

Urine Culture

Isolation and quantification of uropathogens in culture may help differentiate the various UTIs. Asymptomatic bacteriuria requires 10^5 CFU per milliliter of uropathogen cultured from an asymptomatic patient. Counts of 10^5 CFU per milliliter have historically been used in diagnosing acute cystitis and acute pyelonephritis. However, it was found that 30% to 50% of patients with UTIs had less than 10^5 CFU per milliliter of uropathogen on culture.[10] Early or subsiding infections, partially treated infections, diuretic use, recent voiding, and obstruction can explain low colony counts ("low-count UTIs").[10] New standards have been set at 10^3 and 10^4 CFU per milliliter for cystitis and pyelonephritis, respectively. Any symptomatic catheterized patient with greater than 10^2 CFU per milliliter of uropathogen on culture is considered infected. Patients with acute urethritis typically have less than 10^2 CFU per milliliter despite pyuria and typical cystitis symptoms.[25]

The vast majority of young, otherwise healthy women with probable UTI do not need cultures or sensitivity tests. Urine cultures should be obtained in any woman with potential for a complicated UTI; acute bacterial pyelonephritis; fever without focus; relapsing UTI; recently treated, documented UTI; fever and neutropenia; indwelling bladder catheterization; or sepsis.[35]

Other Laboratory Studies

Patients with urosepsis, acute bacterial pyelonephritis, or complicated UTI should have creatinine assessed, as renal dysfunction may occur with upper tract infections. Old literature speaks of the necessity of blood cultures in the setting of acute pyelonephritis. New literature suggests that blood cultures are unnecessary because they rarely assist with clinical decision making. Blood cultures are positive in 18% to 29% of patients with pyelonephritis, but several studies have shown that the results of the blood cultures never or rarely (less than 2%) affected a change in antimicrobial therapy.[17,20,34] Similarly, several studies have shown little to no discrepancy between the organism cultured from the urine and that cultured from the blood.[20] Because blood cultures are costly and often do not add to the clinical evaluation, careful thought should be given as to whether they are necessary. In the adult patient with a UTI, blood cultures are recommended when the diagnosis is unclear, when urine culture cannot be obtained (catheterization impossible), or when bacteremic seeding of the kidneys is possible (endocarditis).[20] They need not be performed for routine pyelonephritis. Vaginal cultures can be helpful when vaginitis and urethritis are likely, though their results are not available for initial management decisions. A pregnancy test is indicated if pregnancy is possible.

Imaging Studies

Radiologic imaging of the woman with uncomplicated UTI is seldom indicated. Routine imaging of women with pyelonephritis is also not recommended, as 75% of adults with pyelonephritis have normal anatomy.[13] Indications for emergent or urgent imaging are not clearly defined, but in general, patients who are severely ill, patients who fail to respond to appropriate antimicrobial therapy, and patients with recurrence within 3 days of finishing treatment may deserve radiographic evaluation in the form of either ultrasonography or computed tomography.

EMERGENCY DEPARTMENT MANAGEMENT

Urosepsis

Prehospital management and immediate resuscitative efforts are necessary for women with urosepsis. Airway management and the provision of supplemental oxygen, intravenous crystalloids, and antibiotics are the mainstays of care. Administration of appropriate antimicrobial agents should begin in the ED as soon as possible. Although urine and blood cultures should ideally be obtained prior to the administration of antibiotics, culture acquisition should not delay the administration of appropriate therapy. Examples of suitable antibiotic choices include a third-generation cephalosporin, imipenem–cilastatin, ticarcillin–clavulanate, or ampicillin in combination with an aminoglycoside. See Table 62.2 for intravenous therapy.

Uncomplicated Cystitis

Patients with cystitis can be treated with oral antimicrobial agents as outpatients. Due to growing concerns about antimicrobial resistance, increasing attention has been placed on the choice of antimicrobial therapy and its duration. *In vitro* studies have found increasing resistance of common urinary pathogens to commonly used agents.[7,11,15] As with all antimicrobial therapy, the choice of agent must be tailored to regional susceptibility patterns. Despite the increasing resistance of many urinary pathogens to trimethoprim–sulfamethoxazole (TMP/SMX), this agent remains an extremely well tolerated and effective agent in most of the United States.[6,11,14,19,27] Furthermore, there are increasing data to suggest that overuse of fluoroquinolones is leading to increasing uropathogen resistance.[5,6,15,23] Overall, TMP/SMX remains an excellent first-line agent for most cases of uncomplicated UTIs. For patients with a contraindication to TMP/SMX or those in an area where resistance is a significant concern, fluoroquinolones or nitrofurantoin remain viable alternatives. Several experts feel that if treating with nitrofurantoin, a 7-day regimen is more effective than a 3-day one.[10,13] Beta-lactam antibiotics cannot be advocated as first-line agents in patients without contraindications to the aforementioned agents due to the high incidence of resistance to these drugs.[11,27] Three-day regimens of treatment seem to confer an advantage over single-dose therapy in terms of the incidence of symptom recurrence. This is thought to be due to the inability of the single-dose regimens to eradicate uropathogens from the vagina, urethra,

TABLE 62.2. Treatment Regimen for Urinary Tract Infections

Condition	Characteristic Pathogens	Recommended Treatment	Recommended Duration of Treatment
Acute uncomplicated cystitis	*E. coli, S. saprophyticus, P. mirabilis, K. pneumonia*	Trimethoprim/Sulfamethoxazole (TMP/SMX) 160 mg/800 twice daily	3 days
		Fluoroquinolones (Ciprofloxacin 500 mg twice daily, Ofloxacin 200 mg twice daily, Levofloxacin 250 mg once daily, lomefloxacin 400 mg once daily, Enoxacin 200 mg twice daily)	3 days
		Cefixime 500 mg once daily	3 days
		Nitrofurantoin monohydrate/macrocrystals (Macrobid) 100 mg twice per day	7 days[3,5]
Asymptomatic bacteriuria in pregnancy	*E. coli, S. Saprophyticus, P. mirabilis, K. pneumonia*	Nitrofurantoin monohydrate/macrocrystals (Macrobid) 100 mg twice per day	3 days
		Sulfisoxazole 500 mg four times per day	3 days
		Cephalexin 250–500 mg four times per day	3 days
		TMP/SMX (160 mg/800 mg) twice daily (relatively contraindicated in 1st and 3rd trimesters)	3 days
Recurrent cystitis	*E. coli, S. saprophyticus, P. mirabilis, K. pneumonia*	Consider prophylaxis with: TMP/SMX 40/200 mg, Nitrofurantoin 50 mg, Norfloxacin 200 mg, Cephalexin 250 mg, Trimethoprim 100 mg daily OR Consider postcoital prophylaxis with TMP/SMX 40/200 mg	6 months
Acute uncomplicated pyelonephritis (outpatient treatment)	*E. coli, S. saprophyticus, P. mirabilis, K. pneumonia*	Consider parenteral loading with Gentamicin 3–5 mg/kg or Ceftriaxone 1 g IV followed by: TMP/SMX (160 mg/800 mg) twice daily	10–14 days
		Fluoroquinolones (Ciprofloxacin 500 mg twice daily, Ofloxacin 200 mg twice daily, Levofloxacin 250 mg once daily, lomefloxacin 400 mg once daily, Enoxacin 200 mg twice daily)	10–14 days
Acute uncomplicated pyelonephritis (severe illness requiring hospitalization)	Same as above	Gentamicin 5 mg/kg IV once daily	Daily until clinically improved, followed by 10–14 days of oral therapy above
		Ceftriaxone 1 g IV once daily	Daily until clinically improved, followed by 10–14 days of oral therapy above
		Fluoroquinolones (Ciprofloxacin 500 mg IV twice daily, Ofloxacin 200–400 mg IV twice daily, Levofloxacin 500 mg IV once daily)	Daily until clinically improved, followed by 10–14 days of oral therapy above
Complicated urinary tract infection (outpatient therapy)	E. coli, *Proteus* species, *Klebsiella* species, *Pseudomonas* species, *Serratia* species, enterococci, Staphylococci	Fluoroquinolones (Ciprofloxacin 500 mg twice daily, Ofloxacin 200 mg twice daily, Levofloxacin 250 mg once daily, lomefloxacin 400 mg once daily, Enoxacin 200 mg twice daily)	10–14 days
Complicated urinary tract infection (severe illness requiring hospitalization)		Gentamicin 5 mg/kg IV once daily with ampicillin 1 g IV every 6 hours	Daily until clinically improved, followed by 10–14 days of oral therapy above
		Ceftriaxone 1 g IV once daily	Daily until clinically improved, followed by 10–14 days of oral therapy above
		Ticarcillin-Clavulanate 3.2 g IV every 8 hours	Daily until clinically improved, followed by 10–14 days of oral therapy above
		Aztreonam 1 g IV every 8–12 hours	Daily until clinically improved, followed by 10–14 days of oral therapy above
		Imipenem-cilastatin 250–500 mg IV every 6–8 hours	Daily until clinically improved, followed by 10–14 days of oral therapy above
		Fluoroquinolones (Ciprofloxacin 500 mg IV twice daily, Ofloxacin 200–400 mg IV twice daily, Levofloxacin 500 mg IV once daily)	Daily until clinically improved, followed by 10–14 days of oral therapy above

and rectum.[13,14] For patients with severe dysuria, a 1- to 2-day course of a urinary analgesic, such as phenazopyridine 200 mg three times per day, is also advisable. See Table 62.2 for alternative antimicrobial regimens.

Uncomplicated Pyelonephritis

Patients with pyelonephritis who are febrile and vomiting should be treated with antipyretics, antiemetics, and intravenous fluids. Antimicrobial therapy is similar to that for patients with uncomplicated cystitis. Many authors advocate the use of single-dose parenteral therapy followed by oral therapy for a duration of 10 to 14 days.[26,32] Acceptable parenteral agents include gentamicin or third-generation cephalosporins. Because some patients develop worsening symptoms within 24 to 36 hours of ED discharge, early follow-up is recommended.[26] Other acceptable regimens for the management of pyelonephritis are listed in Table 62.2.

Complicated Urinary Tract Infections

In general, agents used for the treatment of complicated UTIs are similar to those used for uncomplicated infections,[24] with the specific agent chosen on the basis of known or presumed susceptibilities of the infecting organism. Due to the structural abnormalities inherently associated with complicated infections, a longer course of therapy is warranted to effectively sterilize the urinary tract. In addition, close follow-up is mandatory to ascertain effective cure. Acceptable agents for the treatment of complicated UTIs are listed in Table 62.2.

Urinary Tract Infections Complicating Pregnancy

Antibiotics commonly used to treat UTIs are contraindicated in pregnancy. TMP/SMX is relatively contraindicated in the first trimester due to its inhibition of folate metabolism, and is contraindicated in the third trimester due to its potential to cause kernicterus in the newborn. Fluoroquinolones may damage growing cartilage and epiphyses of long bones, contraindicating their use in pregnancy. Other viable alternatives for treating the parturient with cystitis include nitrofurantoin, sulfisoxazole, and cephalexin.[21] Due to the high incidence of complications affecting both the mother and the fetus, pyelonephritis in pregnancy has historically been an infection treated as an inpatient.[21] Recent studies, however, have shown that patients may be managed as outpatients with close follow-up.[1,22] If outpatient management is elected, 10 to 14 days' treatment is recommended, as is consultation with the patient's obstetrician to assure close follow-up.

Asymptomatic Bacteriuria

Treatment of asymptomatic bacteriuria is not advocated except during pregnancy.[30] Pregnant women with bacteriuria have a markedly increased risk of acute pyelonephritis and the accompanying risks of prematurity and low-birth-weight infants.[30] Treatment is again directed at the etiologic organism. Recommended regimens include 3-day courses of amoxicillin, an oral cephalosporin, or nitrofurantoin.[30]

Recurrent Cystitis

Women with more than three UTIs within 1 year may benefit from longer term prophylactic therapy. Postcoital prophylaxis with one-half of a TMP/SMX tablet (40/200 mg) may benefit those whose recurrences have clearly been related to intercourse.[8,25] Continuous daily prophylaxis for 6 months with TMP/SMX, nitrofurantoin, norfloxacin, cephalexin, or trimethoprim has also been shown to decrease the morbidity of recurrent UTIs.[25] Unfortunately, approximately 40% to 60% of these women will reestablish their pattern of frequency of infections within 6 months of discontinuing prophylactic therapy.[31]

DISPOSITION

Role of the Consultant

Consultants are seldom required for uncomplicated UTI in women. Patients with cystitis do not require follow-up unless symptoms worsen or recur. Uncomplicated acute pyelonephritis may be referred to primary care physicians for subsequent management. As noted, pregnant women with pyelonephritis require close follow-up, and consultation with their obstetricians is advised. Some women with complicated UTI may require urologic and medical consultation.

Indications for Admission

Patients with urosepsis and serious underlying medical problems may require critical care admission if they are hemodynamically unstable, require mechanical ventilation, or have complicating medical conditions. Patients with complicated pyelonephritis or uncomplicated pyelonephritis associated with toxicity are candidates for hospital admission (serious medical conditions, dehydration with inability to maintain a normovolemic state, and inability to take oral medication). The young, nonparous, otherwise healthy woman with acute, uncomplicated, and nontoxic pyelonephritis may respond within hours of initiating appropriate therapy and may be subsequently managed as an outpatient.

COMMON PITFALLS

- Failure to consider the diagnosis of UTI in the septic patient
- Failure to consider the diagnosis in the elderly patient with altered mentation
- Failure to collect a clean urine specimen and failure to recognize a contaminated UA. The lower the ratio of leukocytes to squamous cells in the urine specimen, the more likely it is that the leukocytes are simply vaginal contaminants; if a predominance of squamous cells is seen, a second urine specimen must be collected.
- Failure to properly interpret the urine microscopic examination or chemical dipsticks
- Failure to perform a pelvic examination when indicated
- Failure to recognize complicated UTI
- Failure to ensure appropriate, timely follow-up
- Unnecessarily treating asymptomatic, nonparous bacteriurics

References

1. Angel J, O'Brien W, Finan M, et al. Acute pyelonephritis in pregnancy: a prospective study of oral versus intravenous antibiotic therapy. *Obstet Gynecol* 1990;76:28–32.
2. Bacheller C, Bernstein J. Urinary tract infections. *Med Clin North Am* 1997;81:719–730.
3. Belmin J, Hervias Y, Avellano E, et al. Reliability of sampling urine from disposable diapers in elderly incontinent women. *J Am Geriatr* 1993;41:1182–1186.
4. Bonnardeaux A, Somerville P, Kaye M. A study on the reliability of dipstick urinalysis. *Clin Nephrol* 1994;41:167–172.
5. Cormican M, Morris D, Corbett-Feeney G, et al. Extended spectrum beta-lactamase production and fluoroquinolone resistance in pathogens associated with community acquired urinary tract infection. *Diagn Microbiol Infect Dis* 1998;32:317–319.
6. Ditmanson L, Apgar D. Uncomplicate the treatment of uncomplicated urinary tract infections. *Arch Intern Med* 1996;156:111–113.
7. Dyer I, Sankary T, Dawson J. Antibiotic resistance in bacterial urinary tract infections, 1991 to 1997. *West J Med* 1998;169:265–268.

8. Engel J, Schaeffer A. Evaluation of and antimicrobial therapy for recurrent urinary tract infections in women. *Urol Clin North Am* 1998;25:685–701.
9. Eykyn S. Urinary tract infections in the elderly. *Br J Urol* 1998;82[Suppl 1]:79–84.
10. Faro S, Fenner D. Urinary tract infections. *Clin Obstet Gynecol* 1998;41:744–754.
11. Gupta K, Scholes D, Stamm W. Increasing prevalence of antimicrobial resistance among uropathogens causing acute uncomplicated cystitis in women. *JAMA* 1999;281:736–738.
12. Hooton T, Scholes D, Hughes J, et al. A prospective study of risk factors for symptomatic urinary tract infection in young women. *N Engl J Med* 1996;335:468–474.
13. Hooton T, Stamm W. Diagnosis and treatment of uncomplicated urinary tract infection. *Infect Dis Clin North Am* 1997;11:551–581.
14. Hooton T, Winter C, Tiu F, et al. Randomized comparative trial and cost analysis of 3-day antimicrobial regimens for the treatment of acute cystitis in women. *JAMA* 1995;273:41–45.
15. Iqbal J, Rahman M, Kabir M, et al. Increasing ciprofloxacin resistance among prevalent urinary tract bacterial isolates in Bangladesh. *Jpn J Med Sci Biol* 1997;50:241–246.
16. Jou W, Powers R. Utility of dipstick urinalysis as a guide to management of adults with suspected infection or hematuria. *South J Med* 1998;91:266–269.
17. MacMillan M, Grimes D. The limited usefulness of urine and blood cultures in treating pyelonephritis in pregnancy. *Obstet Gynecol* 1991;78:745–748.
18. Malterud K, Baerheim A. Peeing barbed wire: symptom experiences in women with lower urinary tract infection. *Scand J Prim Health Care* 1999;17:49–53.
19. McCarty J, Richard G, Huck W, et al. A randomized trial of short-course ciprofloxacin, ofloxacin, or trimethoprim/sulfamethoxazole for the treatment of acute urinary tract infection in women. *Am J Med* 1999;106:292–299.
20. McMurray B, Wrenn K, Wright S. Usefulness of blood cultures in pyelonephritis. *Am J Emerg Med* 1997;15:137–140.
21. Millar L, Cox S. Urinary tract infections complicating pregnancy. *Infect Dis Clin North Am* 1997;11:13–26.
22. Millar L, Wing D, Paul R, et al. Outpatient treatment of pyelonephritis in pregnancy: a randomized controlled trial. *Obstet Gynecol* 1995;86:560–564.
23. Naber K. Fluoroquinolones in urinary tract infections: proper and improper use. *Drugs* 1996;52[Suppl 2]:27–33.
24. Nicolle L. A practical guide to the management of complicated urinary tract infection. *Drugs* 1997;53:583–592.
25. Orenstein R, Wong E. Urinary tract infections in adults. *Am Fam Physician* 1999;59:1225–1234.
26. Pinson A, Philbrick J, Lindbeck G, et al. ED management of pyelonephritis in women: a cohort study. *Am J Emerg Med* 1994;12:271–278.
27. Preston S, Abdel-Rahman S, Nahata M. Empiric treatment of uncomplicated urinary tract infections. *Ann Pharmacother* 1998;32:1231–1233.
28. Ronald A, Harding G. Complicated urinary tract infections. *Infect Dis Clin North Am* 1997;11:583–592.
29. Sobel J, Reinhart H. Antibacterial host factors in the urinary tract. *Adv Intern Med* 1991;36:131–150.
30. Stamm W, Hooton T. Management of urinary tract infections in adults. *N Engl J Med* 1993;329:1328–1334.
31. Stapleton A, Stamm W. Prevention of urinary tract infection. *Infect Dis Clin North Am* 1997;11:719–733.
32. Sundman K, Arneborn P, Blad L, et al. One bolus dose of gentamicin and early oral therapy versus cefotaxime and subsequent oral therapy in the treatment of febrile urinary tract infection. *Eur J Microbiol Infect Dis* 1997;16:455–458.
33. Sussman M, Gally D. The biology of cystitis: host and bacterial factors. *Annu Rev Med* 1999;50:149–158.
34. Thanassi M. Utility of urine and blood cultures in pyelonephritis. *Acad Emerg Med* 1997;4:797–800.
35. Werman H, Brown C. Utility of urine cultures in the emergency department. *Ann Emerg Med* 1986;15:302–307.

CHAPTER 63
Calculous Disease of the Kidney and Bladder

James E. Lingeman, Jeffrey A. Moody, Christopher P. Steidle, and Mark C. Adams

Urinary tract stone disease, or urolithiasis, affects persons of all ages. From 2% to 5% of the general population may be expected to develop a urinary calculus during their lifetime. This incidence is variable according to the geographic location (climate) and season. The concept of "stone belt," or geographic areas with unusually high incidences of urinary calculi, is well accepted.[3] The highest incidence of stone disease is in the southeastern United States during the summer. The incidence of stone disease in Whites is reported to be approximately twice that in Blacks and Asians. The male-to-female ratio is approximately 2:1. The disease is relatively uncommon in patients younger than the age of 15, with the highest incidence during the third and fourth decades of life. The economic impact of urolithiasis is enormous. The estimated cost to society in the United States exceeds $1 billion annually.[24]

Urinary calculi consist of four basic crystalline types: calcium salts, struvite, uric acid, and cystine. The underlying pathophysiology of stone formation in the urinary tract requires that urine be supersaturated with the involved salt. The presence of a stone in the urinary tract implies that, in addition to supersaturation, there may be a lack of urinary inhibitors of crystallization or an increase in urinary particle (crystal) retention. Stones that contain calcium salts are by far the most common type of stone encountered (Table 63.1). Struvite (ammoniomagnesium phosphate) is the second most common type and is inextricably associated with infection with urea-splitting organisms. The most common urea-splitting organism is *Proteus*, but urea may also be split by *Klebsiella*, *Staphylococcus* species, and *Providencia*. Uric acid stones in their pure form are less common, occurring with an estimated frequency of 10%. Cystine stones are rare, representing less than 1% of all stone disease. Patients who form cystine stones do so due to an autosomal recessive genetic disorder. The primary defect in cystinuria involves an abnormality in the transport of the dibasic amino acids, resulting in excessive concentrations of the relatively insoluble amino acid cystine in the urine.

The natural history of urinary calculi is variable, but recurrence is common. Up to 75% of patients develop a recurrent calculus after either spontaneous passage or operative removal of a stone.[15] Stone recurrence is often delayed, with long periods between stone episodes. The most obvious consequences of an undiagnosed stone are loss of renal function and hypertension secondary to hydronephrosis.

CLINICAL PRESENTATION AND EVALUATION

The clinical presentation of urinary stone disease is often characteristic. Although pain is usually the reason for an emergency department visit, hematuria and symptoms of urinary tract infection are also common complaints. The history should include history of prior stone disease, family history of stone disease, history of urinary tract infections, and the character of the pain. Stone disease is rare in children and, when encountered, may indicate a genetic disorder or an overt metabolic disorder. A family history of stone disease is commonly present. A history of prior urinary tract infections, especially with urea-splitting organisms, may be an important diagnostic clue and a harbinger of a true urologic emergency—an obstructing stone associated with infection.

TABLE 63.1. Distribution of Various Stone Types (by Predominant Compound)[a]

Calcium oxalate	72%
Infection stones (struvite and carbonate apatite)	16%
Uric acid	6%
Cystine	1%
Other	5%

[a]Crystallographic analyses of 49,000 stones from Beck Analytical Services, Indianapolis, IN.

The pain of renal colic is an acute clinical event secondary to the acute distention of the renal pelvis and upper ureter. Renal colic is visceral in nature, with waxing and waning of symptoms. Typically, the pain associated with an upper urinary tract calculus is localized to the flank. Because of the similar embryologic origin of the gonads and renal unit, pain may be referred to the ipsilateral testis or labia. As the stone moves down the ureter, the pain may move anteriorly from the flank to the ipsilateral lower quadrant. The pain may be referred to the testis when the stone is near the ureterovesical junction. Additionally, as the stone nears the bladder, symptoms of frequency and urgency may be manifested. Gastrointestinal symptomatology, such as nausea and vomiting, is frequently present, with the nausea being the most marked at the peak of the colic episode. Using the constellation of acute pain onset, flank pain, hematuria, and positive kidney–ureter–bladder (KUB), a 90% predictive diagnostic accuracy has been reported.[7]

The physical examination of the patient with urolithiasis is an essential part of the initial evaluation. Patients with renal colic are usually writhing in pain, unable to find a comfortable position, in contradistinction to patients with peritonitis, who typically lie quietly, because any movement aggravates their pain. Tachycardia and tachypnea are common. Hypertension may be present secondary to sympathetic stimulation from the pain. A temperature above 38°C (100.4°F) usually implies a concomitant urinary tract infection and the possibility of urosepsis. The abdominal examination may disclose costovertebral angle tenderness secondary to an acutely hydronephrotic kidney. Auscultation may disclose diminished bowel sounds, because ileus commonly accompanies renal colic. Peritoneal signs can occur if pyelonephritis is present, but they usually signify surgical causes of abdominal pain, such as appendicitis, pelvic inflammatory disease, diverticulitis, or a perforated viscus. The testes should be examined to rule out other causes of testicular pain.

It is vitally important to be certain that an obstructive calculus does not coexist with urinary infection, because such patients are at significant risk for the development of urosepsis.

The most important initial laboratory examination is the urinalysis. The patient with urolithiasis almost always has hematuria. In rare instances, a patient with a completely obstructed ureter may not have hematuria. The urinalysis may reveal the presence of crystalluria. Crystals of calcium oxalate, the coffin lids of struvite, and the hexagonal crystals of cystine are easily recognized. A pH greater than 7.5 in a fresh urine specimen indicates infection with urea-splitting organisms. Culture of the urine should always be performed. Serum electrolyte levels are usually normal; however, prolonged vomiting may lead to metabolic alkalosis. Hyperchloremic metabolic acidosis occurs with renal insufficiency or distal renal tubular acidosis. Serum creatinine levels are usually normal but can be slightly elevated in cases of complete obstruction. Hypercalcemia (calcium level higher than 10.2 mg/dL) in a patient with nephrolithiasis almost invariably signals the presence of primary hyperparathyroidism. Leukocytosis is common due to demargination of white blood cells caused by the stress of renal colic.

DIFFERENTIAL DIAGNOSIS

The differential diagnosis of a patient with suspected urinary calculus is protean (Table 63.2). Urologic diseases that simulate urolithiasis may be divided by anatomic site. Upper tract diseases include renal infarct, which results in sudden pain, hematuria, and leukocytosis, and produces a characteristic rise in serum transaminase levels, especially serum lactic dehydrogenase. Renal tumors may present as acute hemorrhage into the tumor, producing symptoms that are similar to those of a renal stone. The upper ureter may be obstructed by urothelial tumors, blood clots (especially in anticoagulated patients), and sloughed renal papillae. Sloughed renal papillae are seen in patients with sickle cell disease, analgesic abuse, and diabetes mellitus. Ureteral obstruction may be secondary to prior urologic instrumentation, tuberculosis, ureteral strictures, surgery, intrinsic urothelial tumors, or metastasis from tumors such as breast cancer. Nonurologic causes of diseases that stimulate urolithiasis are commonly due to intraabdominal or retroperitoneal conditions such as peritonitis, abdominal aortic aneurysm, retroperitoneal lymphadenopathy from tumors (the most common of which is lymphoma), and retroperitoneal fibrosis.

TABLE 63.2. Diseases That Simulate Urolithiasis

Urologic Disease	Nonurologic Disease
Upper urinary tract	Intraabdominal
Renal infarct	Peritonitis (esp. appendicitis)
Renal parenchymal tumors	Biliary colic
Urothelial tumors	Intestinal obstruction
Papillary necrosis	Vascular
Pyelonephritis	Abdominal aortic aneurysm
Hemorrhage (blood clot)	Superior mesenteric artery occlusion
Ureter	Retroperitoneal
Urothelial tumors	Retroperitoneal lymphadenopathy or
Hemorrhage (blood clot)	Retroperitoneal fibrosis
Prior surgery (e.g. stricture)	Tumor
Metastatic tumors	Gynecologic
Lower urinary tract	Cervical cancer
Urothelial tumors	Endometriosis
Urinary retention	Ovarian vein syndrome
	Musculoskeletal

A Münchausen-like syndrome is seen uncommonly in the emergency department evaluation of suspected urolithiasis (Table 63.3).[9] These patients are typically itinerant and quite knowledgeable about urolithiasis. They usually give a history of uric acid urolithiasis and a contrast medium allergy, usually of an anaphylactic nature. The hematuria that is always present initially resolves when the urine is collected in the presence of a nurse or physician. These patients usually require large dosages of intravenous or intramuscular narcotics to alleviate pain. This group of patients poses a significant management problem for the physician, because, by the time drug-seeking behavior is recognized, the patient has already been medicated. The evaluation of suspected malingering includes urinalysis (to be certain that no coexistent urinary tract infection exists) and computed tomography (CT). Virtually all stones are readily visible on non–contrast-enhanced abdominal CT scans, and, additionally, hydronephrosis and pyonephrosis may be ruled out. The burden of proof is on the physician to rule out a *bona fide* pathologic process.

TABLE 63.3. Münchausen-like Syndrome/Narcotic-seeking Patients

History of multiple narcotic allergies
History of uric acid lithiasis
History of contrast allergy
Multiple prior stone events
Itinerant
Factitious hematuria
Noncooperative

EMERGENCY DEPARTMENT EVALUATION

Radiologic studies are essential in establishing the diagnosis of urolithiasis. Approximately 90% of urinary calculi are radiopaque, and most are visible on the KUB radiograph. Radiolucent stones include uric acid, xanthine, triamterene, matrix stones, and, most commonly, small calcium oxalate stones. Calcium-containing calculi must be at least 2 mm in diameter to be visible on plain radiographs (Fig. 63.1). Other calcifications that may be visible on the KUB view include costochondral calcification, gallstones, undigested pills, splenic artery calcifications, renal artery aneurysms, abdominal aortic aneurysms, calcified mesenteric lymph nodes, stool, and phleboliths (Table 63.4). Phleboliths are common in North America and usually appear in middle age. They are a consequence of Western diet and represent thrombosed pelvic veins that become calcified. They usually appear well rounded and normally reside below a line drawn between the ischial spines. It should be established before contrast administration whether calcifications are truly intrarenal. This may be established by oblique films, nephrotomograms, or CT. Additionally, ileus of the small bowel may be observed usually secondary to sympathetic stimulation produced by renal irritation. Intravenous pyelography (IVP or excretory urography) or CT is necessary for the initial diagnosis of urolithiasis, regardless of whether a calcification is evident on a plain KUB film (Table 63.5). If an obstructed nephrogram is visualized, it is wise to obtain delayed films (Fig. 63.2). Extravasation occasionally occurs with complete obstruction and subsequent rupture of a calyceal fornix (Fig. 63.3). Extravasation is usually self-limited and benign if the duration of obstruction is short and infection is absent. It is important to identify patients with prior contrast medium reactions and preexisting renal insufficiency before IVP. Good alternatives to excretory urography in patients with renal insufficiency and serum creatinine levels greater than 2 mg/dL or a history of severe contrast reactions, such as laryngospasm and cardiovascular collapse, include ultrasonography and CT. Ultrasonography detects both lucent and opaque renal stones as well as hydronephrosis. However, most ureteral stones cannot be identified using ultrasonography. CT provides excellent demonstration of renal and ureteral calculi, including radiolucent calculi, and gives information regarding the presence or absence of hydronephrosis. In addition, CT may provide useful information about other retroperitoneal and intraabdominal conditions.

Spiral or helical CT has emerged as the diagnostic procedure of choice in many emergency departments for the evaluation of patients with suspected urolithiasis. With sensitivity and specificity of 98%,[26] no other noninvasive diagnostic procedure can

TABLE 63.4. Calcifications Seen on a Radiograph That Simulate Urolithiasis

Vascular	Phleboliths
Abdominal aortic aneurysm	Prostatic calculi (in enlarged gland)
Renal artery aneurysm	Calcified costochondral junction
Splenic calcification	Splenic granulomas
Aortic calcification	Adrenal calcification
Hypogastric calcification	Chronic pancreatitis
Nephrocalcinosis	Sacral bone islands
Calcified lymph node	Undigested pills
Gallstones	

TABLE 63.5. IVP Signs of an Obstructing Ureteral Calculus

Obstructive (intense) nephrogram
Extravasation (pyelosinus backflow)
Columnization
Ureteropyelocaliectasis (dilatation)

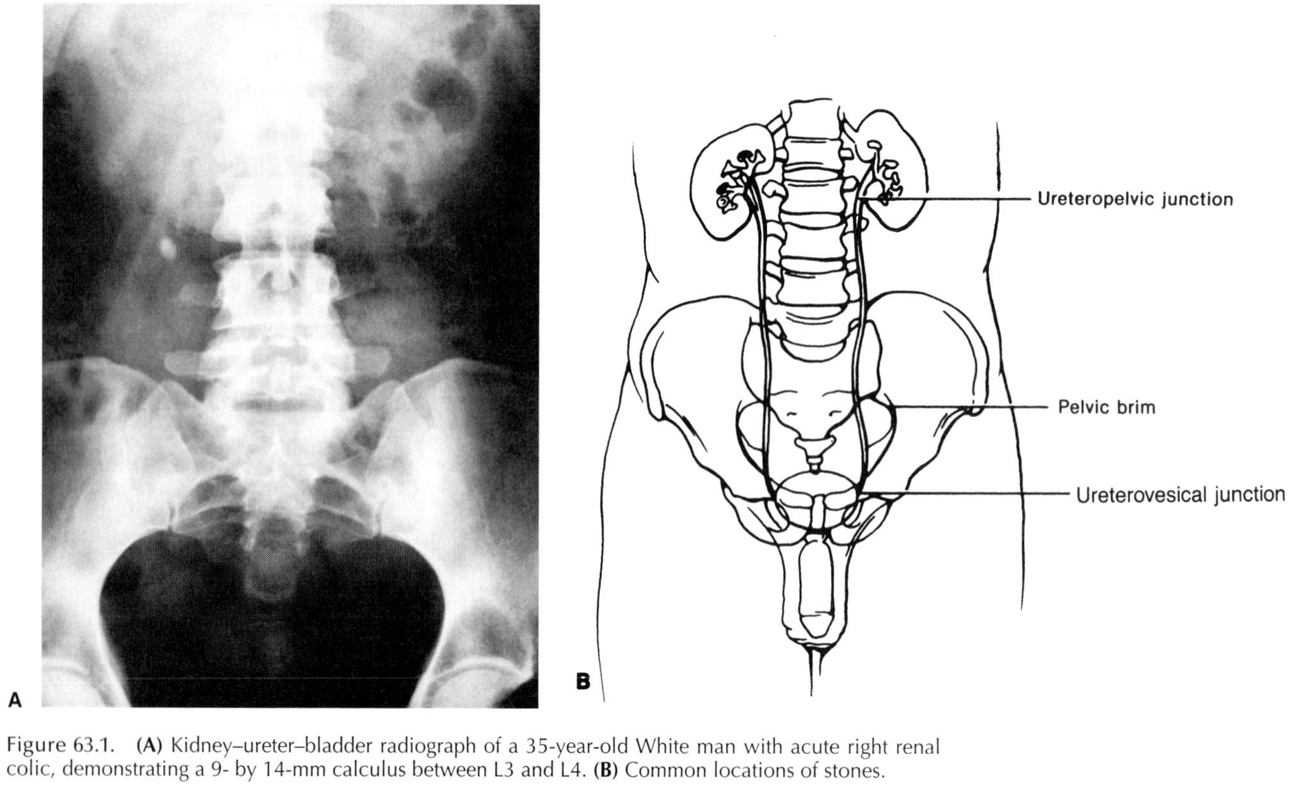

Figure 63.1. **(A)** Kidney–ureter–bladder radiograph of a 35-year-old White man with acute right renal colic, demonstrating a 9- by 14-mm calculus between L3 and L4. **(B)** Common locations of stones.

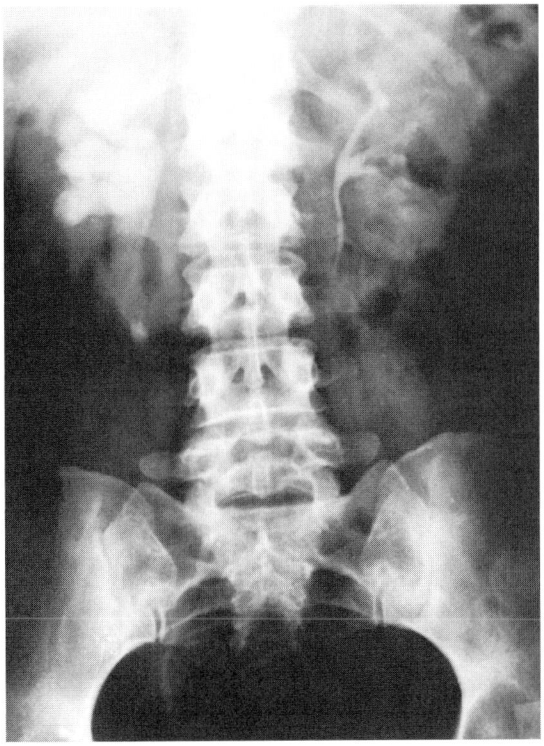

Figure 63.2. Intravenous pyelogram of the patient in Fig. 63.1A, demonstrating marked dilation of the renal collecting system and ureter proximal to the calculus. A stone of this size has a less than 10% chance of spontaneous passage, and, therefore, immediate urologic intervention is appropriate.

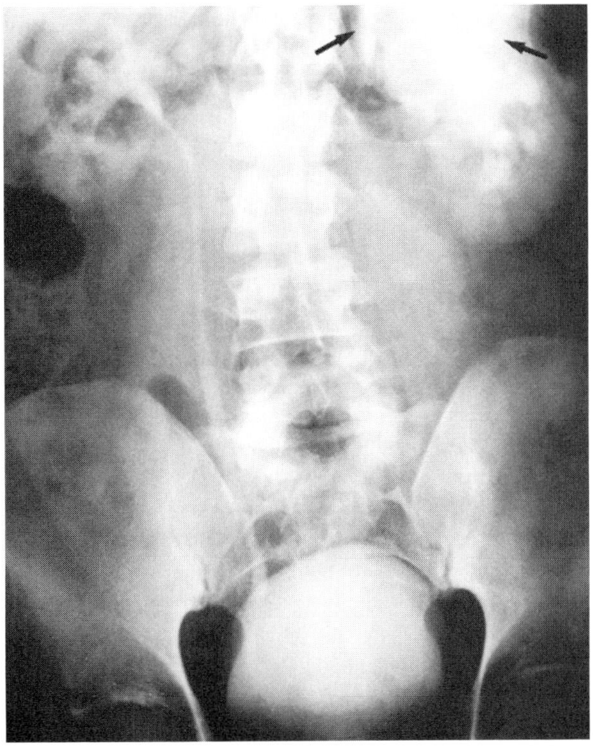

Figure 63.3. Intravenous pyelography of a 45-year-old White man with acute left renal colic, demonstrating extravasation in the region of the left renal pelvis (*arrows*). Extravasation characteristically occurs with small distal ureteral calculi. The calculus is not visible in this instance.

equal non–contrast-enhanced spiral CT. Further, non–contrast-enhanced spiral CT is a more rapid test than IVP and avoids the risks associated with intravenous contrast administration. Spiral CT scanning is also useful for the accurate prediction of ureteral obstruction, aiding in the decision of whether and how to treat symptomatic patients.[8] Spiral CT scanning has even been used experimentally to predict stone composition *in vitro*, but has yet to be proven in human studies.[17,21] The main disadvantage of CT is its greater expense compared with IVP. Also, unless a KUB is obtained, radiolucent stones (mainly uric acid) cannot be distinguished from radiopaque stones.

EMERGENCY DEPARTMENT MANAGEMENT

Most patients with stones present to the emergency department with pain as their predominant symptom. The goals of the emergency physician are to make the proper diagnosis and provide relief of the pain. If the pain is typical colic, or if the patient has had similar pain with previous stones, then pain medication should be administered immediately without waiting for the results of IVP or CT. If the pain is atypical and an intraabdominal process is suspected, pain medication is usually withheld until the correct diagnosis is established. Once significant delay in function is noted on the initial films of an IVP, the patient should be medicated appropriately, because it may take hours to obtain delayed films. Morphine and meperidine (Demerol) are the usual parenteral narcotics used in treating colic, and large and repeat doses of either may be necessary to relieve the initial pain. Once the initial ureteral spasm is relieved, however, the patient's pain often will be quite mild, if it returns at all. Anticholinergic, spasmolytic, or antiinflammatory medications, commonly used in Europe, have not been found to be useful in the United States.

Pain management for patients with renal colic was traditionally confined to parenteral narcotics with the side-effect profile of nausea, pruritus, sedation, and potential respiratory depression. The mechanism of action of narcotics only controls the pain response without acting on the mechanism that initiates the painful stimuli in renal colic. The introduction of ketorolac tromethamine (Toradol), a parenteral nonsteroidal antiinflammatory drug that can be given both intravenously and intramuscularly, has been a major advance for the control of renal colic.

The pain of ureteral colic is mediated by prostaglandins released by the ureter in response to obstruction. Prostaglandins act to increase peristaltic action of the ureter to aid in passage of the stone,[23] but they also sensitize nociceptors to stimuli such as bradykinin, inducing pain and visceral responses to prostaglandins (nausea, vomiting). Ketorolac acts via inhibition of the prostaglandin synthesis pathways, and, when given parenterally, is very effective in relieving the pain and nausea of ureteral obstruction, with equal or more efficacy than parenteral narcotics.[5] Ketorolac, used for a variety of painful emergency department diagnoses, decreased visual analog pain (VAP) scores by 37 mm (0 to 100 mm VAP scale) and was most effective for colic.[2]

Ketorolac should be used with caution in patients with a history of gastrointestinal bleeding, renal insufficiency, or cardiovascular disease. Acute decreases in renal blood flow (35% decrease) were noted after acute infusion of Toradol in a unilateral ureteral obstruction dog model.[20] Acute, transient renal failure occurred in six patients with cardiovascular disease when given ketorolac.[6]

Nausea and vomiting are common with ureteral colic and can be exacerbated by narcotics. In such patients, administration of an antiemetic agent is appropriate, as is vigorous fluid replacement if dehydration has occurred.

DISPOSITION

Once the diagnosis of a stone has been made and the patient has been made comfortable, proper disposition of the case should be made in conjunction with the consulting urologist who will be responsible for the patient's ultimate care (Table 63.6). The most common factor that necessitates patient admission is pain that is refractory to oral pain medications. Once the patient has been made comfortable with intramuscular or intravenous narcotics, an oral agent (codeine, oxycodone [Percodan], meperidine, hydromorphone [Dilaudid], or ketorolac) should be prescribed for any recurrence of pain. If pain relief is inadequate, admission will be necessary for pain control. Persistent nausea and vomiting and urinary extravasation are other indications for admission.

Infection in the presence of an obstructing stone is a urologic emergency that necessitates not only admission, but also immediate urologic intervention. This situation essentially represents an abscess with ready vascular access by way of the renal circulation. The appropriate therapy for this, as with an abscess, is drainage. The obstructed renal unit can be drained either by cystoscopy and passage of a ureteral catheter or by placement of a percutaneous nephrostomy tube. Both procedures can readily be accomplished under local anesthesia. Antibiotics alone are not adequate therapy in these circumstances, because the patient can suffer from continued bacteremic showering, progression to frank urosepsis, and rapid destruction of function of the involved kidney until drainage is achieved. Stabilization of ongoing sepsis and vascular instability should not take precedence over drainage in these patients, because improvement may not occur until the septic source is removed. Effective drainage can be achieved rapidly, and delay in drainage can lead to significant mortality.

Other factors deserve consideration in determining the disposition of the patient. Patients with high-grade obstruction by IVP are more likely to require intervention and admission. Patients with a solitary kidney or underlying intrinsic renal disease are more likely to suffer from a significant decrease in overall renal function with any degree of obstruction; therefore, the threshold for admission of such patients is lower. In addition, the likelihood that the patient will be able to pass the calculus without intervention should be considered. Factors to weigh in this regard include the duration of symptoms and size of the obstructing stone. Ureteral calculi less than 5 mm in size usually pass spontaneously, whereas those over 8 mm rarely do.[25]

TABLE 63.6. Indications for Admission

Obstruction with infection[a]
Pain not controlled by oral analgesics
Persistent nausea and vomiting
Urinary extravasation
Hypercalcemic crisis
RELATIVE INDICATIONS FOR ADMISSION
High-grade obstruction
Solitary kidney
Intrinsic renal disease
Size of obstructing stone
Duration of symptoms
Social situation

[a]Potential urologic emergency.

TABLE 63.7. Current Options for Urolithiasis Management (in Order of Decreasing Invasiveness)

1. Open surgery
2. Percutaneous nephrostolithotomy
3. Ureteroscopy
4. Extracorporeal shock wave lithotripsy
5. Observation

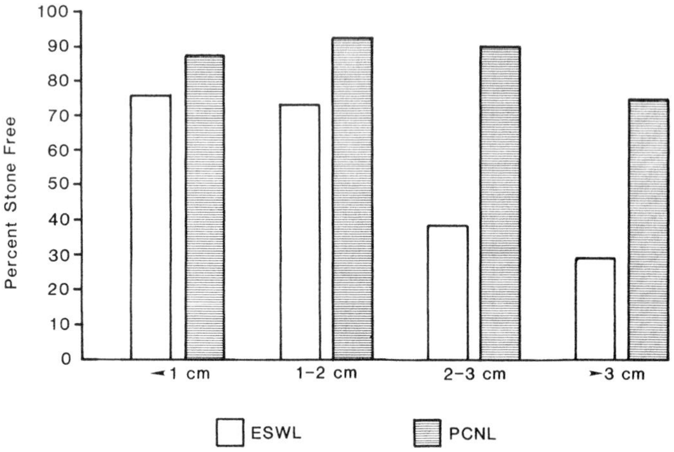

Figure 63.4. Percentage of patients who are stone-free after extracorporeal shock wave lithotripsy (ESWL) and percutaneous nephrostolithotomy (PCNL), stratified by initial stone size. Most ureteral calculi are less than 2 cm in diameter.

Most patients who present to an emergency department with calculi, after evaluation and relief of their pain, will not meet any of these criteria for emergent admission and may be discharged. Sufficient oral narcotic agents and an oral antiemetic agent should be prescribed, as necessary. Prophylactic antibiotics are not used. Patients should be instructed to strain their urine and save any solid material for analysis. They should be told to return or seek attention for recurrent severe pain, persistent vomiting, or the onset of fever. Outpatient urologic follow-up should be arranged within 2 weeks.

CURRENT TREATMENT

Several technologic advancements have revolutionized the treatment of symptomatic urolithiasis in the last two decades (Table 63.7). The most important of these advancements has been the development of extracorporeal shock wave lithotripsy (ESWL*). This technology, pioneered by the Dornier HM3 lithotriptor, has proved effective in the management of 85% to 90% of urolithiasis cases.[4,10,13,14] Various new lithotriptors that use a variety of energy sources and stone localization systems and have lower anesthesia requirements have been introduced.[16] Patients with large stones (i.e., more than 2 cm in diameter) and staghorn calculi, particularly when associated with hydronephrosis, are much less likely to become stone-free with ESWL monotherapy (Fig. 63.4). In addition, cystine stones fragment poorly with ESWL.

Another important technologic advance is percutaneous nephrostolithotomy, which involves the establishment of a tract from the skin into the renal collecting system through which stones can be fragmented with ultrasonic, laser, electrohy-

* ESWL is a registered trademark of Dornier Medical Systems, Inc., Marietta, Georgia.

draulic, or pneumatic devices and removed using various endoscopes, grasping forceps, and stone baskets. This technique is complementary to ESWL in that it is appropriate for larger and harder renal calculi that cannot be treated successfully with ESWL (Fig. 63.5).[10–13]

Ureteral calculi can be managed effectively with either ESWL or another new technique, ureteroscopy. Previously, ureteral calculi that necessitated intervention were managed with either blind basketing by way of the cystoscope or ureterolithotomy. The development of rigid and flexible ureterorenoscopes now allows visualization of the entire ureter from the bladder to renal pelvis and removal of ureteral calculi under direct vision. Again, various energy sources (ultrasound, laser, electrohydraulic, pneumatic) can be used through the ureteroscope to fragment stones if necessary. Ureterorenoscopy is most successful when applied to stones in the distal ureter. However, success rates decrease and complication rates increase when proximal ureteral calculi are approached with this technique. In general, upper ureteral calculi tend to be managed with ESWL, while ureteroscopy is still commonly used for distal ureteral stones.[14,22] The American Urological Association has released a peer-reviewed, literature-based set of guidelines for the treatment of ureteral stones.[22] These guidelines are designed to give both the urologist and the general practitioner an outline for the management of ureteral stones, based on size and location in the ureter. Most (98%) of ureteral stones less than 5 mm will pass spontaneously, if the associated symptoms can be controlled and no concomitant infection exists. Proximal ureteral stones less than 1 cm can be treated with ESWL. Distal ureteral stones less than 1 cm can be treated with either ESWL or ureteroscopy. Nearly all upper urinary tract calculi can now be treated without open surgery, and the only indication for open intervention is the need for a coincident reconstructive operation.[1]

In addition to the treatment of existing symptomatic stones, an important goal for the urologist is to prevent further stone formation. Medical therapy based on a careful metabolic stone

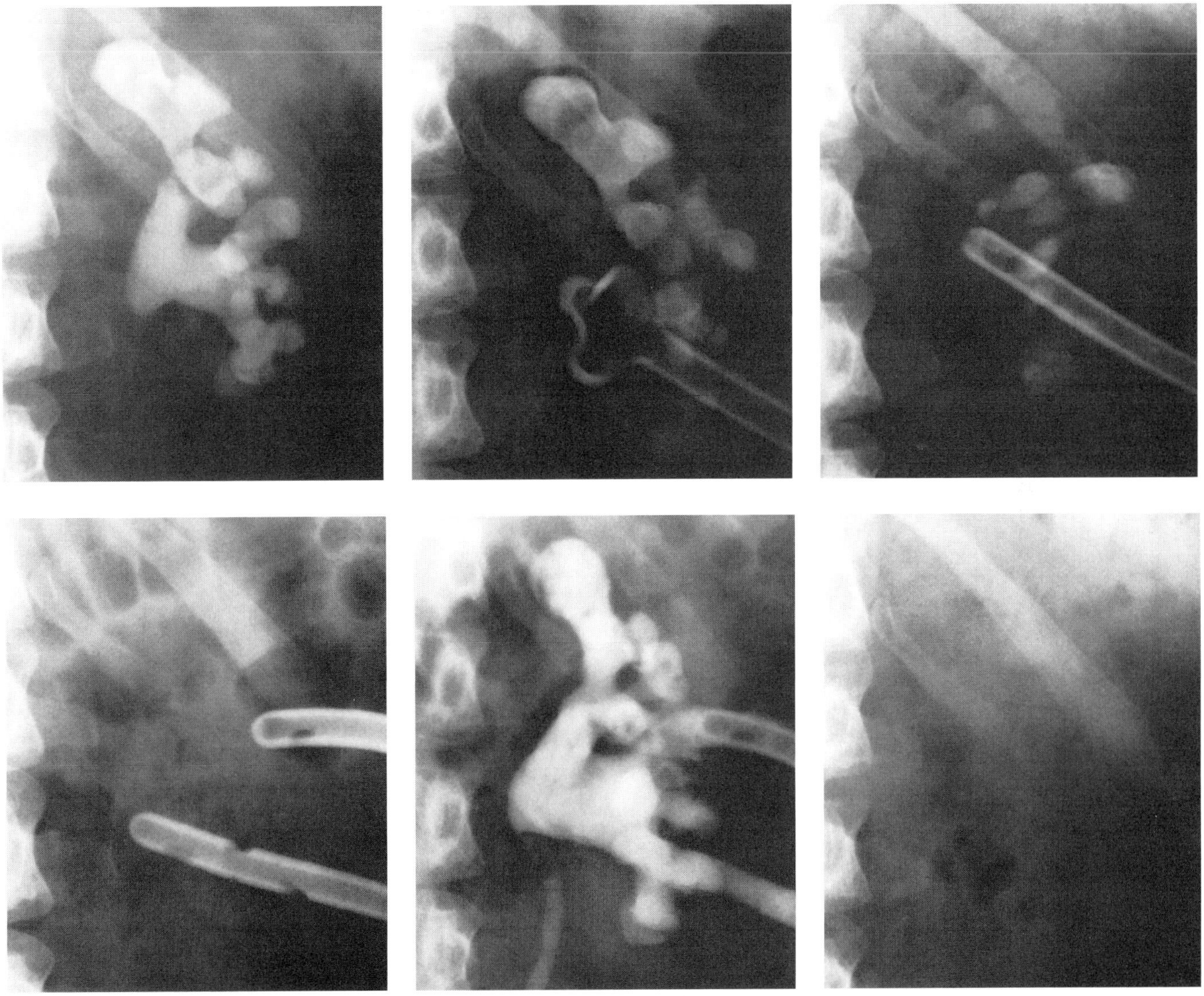

Figure 63.5. **(A)** Combined percutaneous nephrostolithotomy (PCNL) and extracorporeal shock wave lithotripsy (ESWL) for staghorn calculi. This 35-year-old White woman presented with a *Proteus* urinary tract infection and was found to have a large complete left staghorn calculus. **(B)** The stone was approached initially with PCNL, but numerous stone fragments remained scattered throughout the rather complex renal collecting system. **(C)** These fragments were then treated with two sessions of ESWL, greatly reducing the remaining stone material. **(D, E)** A second PCNL was then performed, requiring a second nephrostomy tube to effect complete stone removal. **(F)** The patient remains free of stone and infection 2 years after therapy.

evaluation can dramatically reduce the incidence of recurrent stone formation.[18,19] Such evaluation should begin in the emergency department by checking serum electrolyte levels (looking for distal or type I renal tubular acidosis) and serum calcium level (hypercalcemia usually indicates primary hyperparathyroidism). More detailed studies (i.e., 24-hour urine collections) should be delayed for 2 to 4 weeks after resolution of an acute stone event.

VESICAL CALCULI

Vesical calculi occur predominantly in males. Endemic urate calculi, once prevalent in young males, have virtually disappeared from industrialized societies. Most bladder calculi now present during adult life and are secondary to bladder outlet obstruction or foreign bodies in the bladder, such as an indwelling catheter. Calcium oxalate is the most common constituent of bladder calculi in the United States, although the incidence of struvite and hydroxyapatite calculi is higher than in the kidneys.

Typical symptoms of vesical calculi are pain on voiding and hematuria. The pain may be dull or sharp and is often severe at the end of micturition or with exercise or sudden movement. Hematuria often occurs at the end of voiding. Interruption of the urinary stream from impaction of the stone at the bladder neck may occur. Frequency, urgency, and dysuria are present in up to 50% of patients. Urinary tract infection is common, especially if an indwelling catheter is present. Some patients, especially those with prostatic enlargement, have no symptoms directly referable to the calculi but present only with symptoms of outflow obstruction.

The diagnosis of vesical calculi can be suspected from the history, and they rarely may be palpable on physical examination. Feeling a stone "clink" with a urethral sound is an age-old technique of detecting bladder calculi. Such stones are often apparent on plain radiographs, and cystoscopy is both diagnostic and therapeutic.

Once the diagnosis of a vesical stone has been made in the emergency department, it may be appropriate to anchor an indwelling Foley catheter if the patient has significant bladder outflow obstruction or cystitis. The patient should then be referred to a urologist, because successful treatment requires not only removal of the stone, but also relief of outflow obstruction, correction of bladder stasis, and removal of foreign bodies whenever possible.

References

1. Assimos DG, Boyce WH, Harrison LH, et al. The role of open stone surgery since extracorporeal shock wave lithotripsy. *J Urol* 1989;142:263–267.
2. Bartfield JM, Kern AM, Raccio-Robak N, et al. Ketorolac tromethamine use in a university-based emergency department. *Acad Emerg Med* 1994;1:532–538.
3. Boyce WH, Garvey FK, Strawcutter HE. Incidence of urinary calculi among patients in general hospitals: 1948–1952. *JAMA* 1956;161:1427.
4. Chaussy C, Fuchs G. Erfahrungren mit der Extrakorporalen Stosswellenlithotripsie nach funf Jahren klinischer Andwendung. *Urologe A* 1985;24:305–309.
5. Cordell WH, Wright SW, Wolfson AB, et al. Comparison of intravenous ketorolac, meperidine, and both (balanced analgesia) for renal colic. *Ann Emerg Med* 1996;28:151–158.
6. Corelli RL, Gericke KR. Renal insufficiency associated with intramuscular administration of ketorolac tromethamine. *Ann Pharmacother* 1993;27:1055–1057.
7. Elton TJ, Roth CS, Berquist TH, et al. A clinical prediction rule for the diagnosis of ureteral calculi in emergency departments. *J Gen Intern Med* 1993;8:57–62.
8. Fielding JR, Fox LA, Heller H, et al. Spiral CT in the evaluation of flank pain: overall accuracy and feature analysis. *J Comput Assist Tomogr* 1997;21:635–638.
9. Jones WA, Cooper TP, Kiviat MD. Munchausen syndrome presenting as urolithiasis. *West J Med* 1978;128:185–188.
10. Kahnoski RJ, Lingeman JE, Coury TA, et al. Combined percutaneous and extracorporeal shock wave lithotripsy for staghorn calculi: an alternative to anatrophic nephrolithotomy. *J Urol* 1986;135:679–681.
11. Lam HS, Lingeman JE, Barron M, et al. Staghorn calculi: analysis of treatment results between initial percutaneous nephrostolithotomy and extracorporeal shock wave lithotripsy monotherapy with reference to surface area. *J Urol* 1992;147:1219–1225.
12. Lam HS, Lingeman JE, Mosbaugh PG, et al. Evolution of the technique of combination therapy for staghorn calculi: a decreasing role for extracorporeal shock wave lithotripsy. *J Urol* 1992;148:1058–1062.
13. Lingeman JE, Coury TA, Newman DM, et al. Comparison of results and morbidity of percutaneous nephrostolithotomy and extracorporeal shock wave lithotripsy. *J Urol* 1987;138:485–490.
14. Lingeman JE, Newman D, Mertz JH, et al. Extracorporeal shock wave lithotripsy: the Methodist Hospital of Indiana experience. *J Urol* 1986;135:1134–1137.
15. Marshall V, White RH, De Saintonge MC, et al. The natural history of renal and ureteric calculi. *Br J Urol* 1975;47:117–124.
16. Moody JA, Evan AP, Lingeman JE. Extracorporeal shock wave lithotripsy. In: Weiss R, O'Reilly P, George N, eds. *Principles of urology*, vol. 1. London: Harcourt Mosby, 1999 *(in press)*.
17. Mostafavi MR, Ernst RD, Saltzman B. Accurate determination of chemical composition of urinary calculi by spiral computerized tomography. *J Urol* 1998;159:673–675.
18. Pak CY. Medical management of nephrolithiasis. *J Urol* 1982;128:1157–1164.
19. Pak CY, Britton F, Peterson R, et al. Ambulatory evaluation of nephrolithiasis. Classification, clinical presentation and diagnostic criteria. *Am J Med* 1980;69:19–30.
20. Perlmutter A, Miller L, Trimble LA, et al. Toradol, an NSAID used for renal colic, decreases renal perfusion and ureteral pressure in a canine model of unilateral ureteral obstruction. *J Urol* 1993;149:926–930.
21. Saw KC, Lingeman JE, McAteer JA, et al. Spiral CT scan for predicting stone composition: the effect of CT collimation and stone size. In: *American Urological Association national meeting*, vol. 1. Dallas: AUA Press, 1999.
22. Segura JW, Preminger GM, Assimos DG, et al. Ureteral Stones Clinical Guidelines Panel summary report on the management of ureteral calculi. *J Urol* 1997;158:1915–1921.
23. Selmy GI, Hassouna MM, Khalaf IM, et al. Effects of verapamil, prostaglandin F2 alpha, phenylephrine, and noradrenaline on upper respiratory tract dynamics. *Urology* 1994;43:31–35.
24. Shuster J, Schaeffer RL. Economic impact of kidney stones in white male adults. *Urology* 1984;24:327–331.
25. Ueno A, Kawamura T, Ogawa A, et al. Relation of spontaneous passage of ureteral calculi to size. *Urology* 1977;10:544–546.
26. Vieweg J, Teh C, Freed K, et al. Unenhanced helical computerized tomography for the evaluation of patients with acute flank pain. *J Urol* 1998;160:679–684.

CHAPTER 64
Genitourinary Neoplasms

Romano DeMarco and Michael O. Koch

RENAL NEOPLASMS

Renal cell carcinoma (RCC) is the most common primary tumor of the kidney. It accounts for 85% of all primary renal neoplasms[12] and 90% to 95% of renal malignancies. Primary carcinomas of the renal pelvis or ureter account for approximately 8% of all renal neoplasms.[12] A number of rare sarcomas account for the remainder of renal neoplasms.

Approximately 5% of solid renal parenchymal masses are benign in nature. The most common neoplasm is an oncocytoma. Oncocytomas do not appear to have any malignant potential. Other benign lesions are the fat-containing tumor; angiomyolipoma, which is seen in patients with tuberous sclerosis; and renal adenomas, which are probably just small, low-grade renal malignancies.

Nephroblastoma (Wilms' tumor) occurs primarily in children and contributes around 5% of cases, with approximately 600 new cases each year.[20]

Approximately 30,000 new cases of RCC are diagnosed annually in the United States, with 18,000 yearly mortalities.[17] Most cases of RCC occur sporadically, however a small percentage have a hereditary association, including Von Hippel-Lindau, tuberous sclerosis, and adult polycystic kidney disease.[24] RCC is more common in Scandinavians and North Americans, with a lower incidence in people of Asian and African descent. It is most common in adult males, with a male-to-female ratio of 2:1. Its onset in patients is typically in their fifth to sixth decade of life. Moderate cigarette consumption is a proven risk factor for RCC.

CLINICAL PRESENTATION

RCC has been coined "the internist's tumor" because of its baffling presenting signs and symptoms. The classically described triad of flank pain, abdominal mass, and hematuria for RCC is seen in only about 10% of patients at presentation and usually represents advanced disease. An increasing number of incidental RCCs are being diagnosed secondary to the prevalent use of radiographic imaging, done most frequently for nonurologic indications. As many as 25% to 40% of patients are diagnosed with RCC after incidental detection of a mass by ultrasound or computed tomography (CT) scan.[16] Incidentally discovered tumors tend to be smaller than those that cause symptomatic presentation and are more amenable to surgical resection.

Hematuria is the most common presenting symptom, followed by abdominal mass, pain, and weight loss. Hematuria, gross or microscopic, is usually observed only if the tumor has invaded the collecting system, and is most commonly seen with large tumors. This is in contrast to tumors of the renal pelvis or ureter, in which hematuria is usually gross and painless, occurring earlier.

Palpation of an abdominal or flank mass is more commonly found in thin patients or the pediatric population, with tumors of the lower pole more easily palpable. The mass is generally firm and nontender and moves with diaphragmatic excursion.

Flank pain is noted as a presenting sign in less than 20% of cases. As the tumor enlarges, it may encroach on the psoas and quadratus lumborum muscle, causing severe back pain. Occasionally, an acute varicocele is found as the presenting sign. Classically, this varicocele does not decompress with recumbency. A right-sided varicocele, in particular, should raise concerns of an underlying renal malignancy.

Up to 35% to 40% of patients with RCC have metastatic disease at the time of presentation.[3] The most common sites are the lungs, bone, and liver. Bony metastases are generally lytic and painful. Patients may present with pathologic fractures.

RCC is associated with a wide variety of paraneoplastic syndromes. One well-known clinical manifestation of RCC is Stauffer syndrome, which was first described in 1961 as a reversible cause of hepatic dysfunction in a patient with RCC.[11] This syndrome occurs in 15% of patients with typical laboratory findings of elevated alkaline phosphatase, prothrombin time, and total bilirubin. These abnormalities should return to baseline after nephrectomy, and, if not, suggest the presence of metastatic disease. RCC is the malignancy most commonly associated with fever of unknown origin. This fever is probably due to a pyrogen or other growth factor. Hypercalcemia occurs in 10% to 15% of patients with RCC. This may occur secondary to bony metastases, a tumor-released parathyroid hormone–related peptide, or elevated prostaglandin levels. Anemia is the most common systemic manifestation of RCC, with 20% to 30% of patients being anemic at time of presentation. This anemia usually resembles normochromic or normocytic indices; however, hematuria or bleeding into the tumor can occasionally be the cause. Erythrocytosis, defined as hematocrit greater than 55 or hemoglobin greater than 15, occurs in almost 4% of patients. This is secondary to elevated levels of erythropoietin. It does not affect white blood cells or platelets and resolves after nephrectomy.

DIFFERENTIAL DIAGNOSIS

As noted earlier, the presentation of renal tumors can be quite varied. The differential diagnosis of hematuria and flank pain includes renal calculi and pyelonephritis. Retroperitoneal masses may arise from any neoplastic process of the kidneys, perinephric organs, and retroperitoneal space. Neoplastic processes involving the colon, stomach, esophagus, pancreas, spleen, liver, small intestine, and retroperitoneal primary tumors and metastases must enter the differential diagnosis.

The most common renal mass seen on radiologic imaging is a simple renal cyst. One autopsy series identified a 50% incidence of simple cysts after the age of 50.[13] One can usually make a diagnosis of a classic benign simple cyst by following strict CT and sonographic criteria. Cysts are typically round, thin walled, and homogenous, and have no internal echoes or densities. Other clinical entities to consider when evaluating a renal mass include hematoma, abscess, infarct, vascular malformation, renal pseudotumor, angiomyolipoma, oncocytoma, and metastatic carcinoma.

The finding of a renal pelvic or calyceal filling defect is usually secondary to a radiolucent stone. These stones account for approximately 10% of all calculi and are usually uric acid. However, filling defects in the renal pelvis and ureter may represent a neoplastic process, papillary necrosis, or blood clot.

EMERGENCY DEPARTMENT EVALUATION

A patient with hematuria and flank pain should have a urinalysis, complete blood count (CBC), and creatinine sent. If the urinalysis demonstrates pyuria or bacteriuria, a urine culture should be obtained. The initial imaging study for the evaluation of flank pain and hematuria is traditionally an intravenous pyelogram (IVP), because a renal calculus is foremost in the differential. However, noncontrast spiral CT scans of the abdomen and pelvis are equivalent in sensitivity for stones and allow for the avoidance of contrast.

Once a renal parenchymal mass is identified, it is up to the urologist to determine whether it is consistent with a benign renal cyst or solid malignancy. Renal sonography is the best study in determining whether a renal mass seen on IVP or noncontrasted CT scan is cystic or solid, while a contrasted CT scan of the abdomen and pelvis is the most sensitive study for the diagnosis of RCC. For tumors less than 3 cm, the sensitivities of IVP, ultrasound, and CT scan are 67%, 79%, and 94%, respectively.[1] An IVP filling defect requires a retrograde pyelogram for definitive diagnosis. If an RCC is discovered, a general metabolic panel should be obtained to rule out a significant metabolic disturbance requiring immediate management.

EMERGENCY DEPARTMENT MANAGEMENT

Patients should have their pain alleviated. Intravenous fluid resuscitation and serial hematocrits are rarely needed but may be required for hypotension, tachycardia, or severe nausea and vomiting.

DISPOSITION

Role of the Consultant

Outpatient workup by the urologist is usually standard for any suspicious renal mass, and an appointment should be made. Emergency physicians should explain to the patient the necessity of follow-up, so that the urgency of the referral is not ignored.

Indications for Admission

Patients with severe pain or significant metabolic abnormalities from metastatic disease may need admission for pain control and management. Severe hematuria with urinary clot retention or hemodynamic instability may necessitate hospitalization.

Transfer Considerations

Transfer is usually not needed; however, there should be a referral to a urologist experienced in surgical management of RCC.

COMMON PITFALLS

- A renal tumor might not be considered in the forefront of diagnoses because the symptoms usually resemble more common urinary diseases.
- Intravenous pyelograms are easily misread. The more common diagnoses of renal calculi and pyelonephritis are often made on the basis of clinical suspicion and from radiographs of less than perfect quality. The emergency department IVP is not performed with a bowel preparation, and the detail is often inadequate to reveal renal parenchymal or epithelial tumors.
- The final diagnosis of a renal tumor can be difficult; the emergency physician should ensure appropriate and timely referral to a urologist.
- Emergency personnel should remember that relatively minor renal trauma can cause unexpectedly severe bleeding if a renal tumor is present, particularly in children.

TREATMENT COMPLICATIONS

Nephrectomy

Radical nephrectomy is the treatment of choice for RCC. This can be performed through a transabdominal, flank, or thoracoabdominal approach. The most common postoperative complication after radical nephrectomy is an ileus, which is particularly common after a transabdominal approach. The most immediate life-threatening complication after nephrectomy is hemorrhage, most often from the ligated renal vessels. This complication is rare. Other sources include splenic or hepatic injury, liver tear, or lumbar vessels. Bleeding may be insidious, becoming apparent some days after surgery. It should be suspected in the emergency patient with tachycardia, orthostatic hypotension, anemia, or abdominal pain.

Pneumothorax is an uncommon event during a transabdominal nephrectomy, but it is much more likely after a flank nephrectomy. It is usually evident at the time of surgery but should be considered in the postoperative patient who is short of breath.

Postoperative abdominal pain may be due to problems more serious than ileus or incisional pain. Dissection in the retroperitoneum can result in injury to the duodenum or pancreas, with resultant pancreatitis. Traction on or injury to the superior mesenteric artery can cause bowel ischemia.

A subtle, but serious postoperative problem after radical nephrectomy is adrenal insufficiency, characterized by weakness, malaise, and hyponatremia and hyperkalemia. This will occur in the patient with previous removal of the contralateral kidney and adrenal, but it also may occur in the elderly patient with borderline adrenal function preoperatively.

Chemotherapy

Metastatic renal cell cancer is resistant to standard chemotherapy, and these agents are very infrequently used for this disease. Immunotherapy with interferon and/or interleukin-2 (IL-2) has shown some antitumor effect but significant toxicity. Patients receive interferon subcutaneously one to five times weekly. Most experience a flulike syndrome of fever, malaise, chills, and myalgias. Confusion and lethargy can be seen when high doses are used. IL-2, administered intravenously or subcutaneously in low doses, has considerably more toxicity and results in a "capillary leak" syndrome that is characterized by fever, hypotension, oliguria with fluid retention, renal failure, pulmonary edema, and hepatic dysfunction. These dose-related side effects usually resolve within 24 to 72 hours after administration. Although the patient is usually hospitalized for therapy, delayed manifestations may present after discharge. Many patients receive modified doses as outpatients.

BLADDER CARCINOMA

Bladder cancer is the fourth most common malignancy in men after prostate, lung, and colorectal cancer, accounting for 5.5% of all cancer cases.[4] In women, it is the eighth most common cancer, accounting for 2.3% of all cancers. Approximately 50,500 new cases are diagnosed annually, with 10,000 deaths occurring yearly. Bladder cancer usually strikes patients in their sixth and seventh decades. Multiple risk factors include smoking and exposure to aromatic amines, phenacetin, and acrolein, a metabolite of cyclophosphamide. Transitional cell cancers account for 90% of the histologic tumors, while the remainder are squamous cell carcinoma or adenocarcinoma.

CLINICAL PRESENTATION

More than 70% of patients present initially with intermittent, painless, gross hematuria.[14] Clot retention may be seen in approximately 20% of patients. Irritable voiding symptoms such as frequency, urgency, and dysuria often are associated with tumors involving the bladder trigone and ureteral orifices, particularly carcinoma *in situ* (CIS). Patients may present with flank pain from ureteral obstruction. Rarely, patients present with symptoms of advanced disease, such as weight loss or abdominal or bone pain. Up to 20% of patients have no specific symptoms, with the tumor being discovered during evaluation of microscopic hematuria.

DIFFERENTIAL DIAGNOSIS

The differential diagnosis of painless, gross hematuria includes infectious cystitis, hemorrhagic cystitis, glomerulonephritis, urinary calculi, and other tumors of the genitourinary system. Irritative voiding symptoms may be present with prostatitis, cystitis, and lower urinary tract calculi.

EMERGENCY DEPARTMENT EVALUATION

The patient with gross hematuria and clot formation should have a serum creatinine and CBC drawn. A large urethral catheter (22F) may be necessary if there is suspected bladder outlet obstruction due to clot formation. Intravenous access for fluid administration and possible IVP may be needed. An IVP should be obtained in all patients with gross, painless hematuria unless contraindicated. A renal ultrasound examination should be obtained in place of an IVP in a pregnant patient, while an ultrasound or noncontrast CT scan is needed for a patient with contrast allergy or significant renal insufficiency.

EMERGENCY DEPARTMENT MANAGEMENT

If blood clots are present, the bladder is irrigated until the return is clear. Normal saline irrigation may be needed to irrigate a bladder cleared of clots. A three-way catheter for constant irrigation may be used, but this is not as important as placement of a catheter large enough to remove clots (22F or larger). A catheter is not necessary if urinary retention from clot retention is not suspected. Urologic consultation should be obtained. All of these patients eventually require cystoscopy, although this can be done in the urologist's office at follow-up.

DISPOSITION

Role of the Consultant

Outpatient workup by the urologist is standard, although management of clot retention may require admission.

Indications for Admission

Patients with significant hematuria or clot retention should be admitted. If ureteral obstruction or pyelonephritis is suspected, admission is advisable.

Transfer Considerations

The availability of a urologist may necessitate transfer if admission for management of gross hematuria or ureteral obstruction is necessary.

COMMON PITFALLS

- Bladder tumors are often misdiagnosed as urinary tract infections. Most physicians do not obtain a urine culture when treating cystitis. Unfortunately, the urinalysis can show white blood cells in patients with both tumor and infectious cystitis.
- In the older patient with hematuria or irritative voiding symptoms, a urine culture should be obtained.

Treatment Complications

The diagnosis of bladder cancer is usually accomplished by cystoscopy with transurethral biopsy. Tumors are completely removed transurethrally if possible. Bleeding into the bladder is the most common complication, but bladder perforation, bowel perforation, and obstruction of the ureteral orifice may occur.

Bladder tumors that are limited to the mucosa are generally treated transurethrally, while tumors that grow deeper into the muscle generally necessitate complete eradication.

INTRAVESICAL THERAPY

Intravesical chemotherapy is used for the treatment of superficial bladder cancer, and for patients at high risk for tumor recurrence, multiple tumors, and CIS. Bacillus Calmette-Guérin (BCG) is an attenuated strain of *Mycobacterium bovis* that has stimulatory effects on the immune system and is used in therapy for superficial bladder carcinoma. It commonly causes cystitis in up to 90% of patients. Patients that present with high fever, shaking chills, and hypotension should be suspected of having BCG sepsis. This occurs in less than 0.4% of patients, and these patients should be hospitalized immediately, started on broad-spectrum antibiotics, and given isoniazid and rifampin.[15] BCG sepsis is very uncommon if the bladder is allowed to heal prior to instillation.

Intravesical chemotherapeutic agents such as mitomycin-C and Thiotepa may cause chemical cystitis. Suprapubic pain and pyuria are sometimes observed in addition to irritative voiding symptoms. Skin rash, usually in a palmar and facial distribution, and palmar desquamation are observed often with the use of mitomycin-C. Thiotepa is generally more well tolerated than mitomycin-C, with mild cystitis and irritative voiding symptoms occurring in 15% to 30% of patients. The major adverse side effects of Thiotepa are leukopenia and thrombocytopenia due to systemic absorption, which can be increased due to recent tumor resection, extensive tumor, or concurrent cystitis.

Multiagent systemic chemotherapy is the standard treatment for patients with nonresectable or metastatic disease. The usual agents include cisplatin, methotrexate, vinblastine, doxorubicin, or carboplatin with inherent toxicities.

RADICAL CYSTECTOMY

The most common complications found in patients after radical cystectomy are wound infections, postoperative intestinal obstruction, which is usually transient, and atelectasis/respiratory complications. Less common complications include myocardial infarction, pneumonia, and pyelonephritis. Incidence of urinary leakage at ureteroenteric anastomosis has been reduced secondary to the use of indwelling ureteral stents. A pelvic abscess may occur after a missed rectal injury during surgery or urinary leak. Hence, patients presenting with fever, pelvic or perineal pain, and fluctuance on rectal examination should be assessed appropriately with CBC, CT scan, and drainage, if an abscess is found.

URINARY DIVERSION

The standard form of urinary diversion after cystectomy for the past 40 years has been an ileal conduit. In this procedure, a 12- to 16-cm segment of ureter carries the urine from the ureters to a cutaneous stoma. It has no reservoir function. From many patients' standpoints, it has an unacceptable impact on body image. The most commonly associated, long-term complications of ileal conduits are parastomal hernias and either ureteral strictures or upper tract stone disease, leading to renal damage.

Continent urinary diversions, either a cutaneous continent urinary reservoir (CUR) or a bladder substitute (neobladder), are being used at many institutions with almost equal frequency to conduit diversions. All continent urinary diversions are made from a segment of either small or large bowel. A CUR has an entry stoma on the abdomen wall that the patient is required to catheterize every 4 to 6 hours to drain the reservoir. These stomas are easy to conceal and offer an appliance-free lifestyle. The most commonly performed CUR diversions are the "Indiana pouch" and the "Kock pouch."

For selected patients with a bladder substitute following cystectomy, a neobladder can be created in which an intestinal reservoir made from either small intestine or a combination of small and large intestine is constructed and then anastomosed to the ureters and urethra. Many different configurations have been described, with the "Studer bladder" and the "hemi-Kock" probably being the most common. Most patients are able to void spontaneously, and only a few require intermittent catheterization for adequate drainage. Daytime urinary control is usually excellent, while a significant portion of patients require protective incontinence pads at night.

The unique, acute complications of urinary diversion are primarily related to the intestinal and urinary anastomoses. Urinary extravasation can occur at the anastomosis between the bowel and ureter or at the enteroenterostomy. These most commonly occur during the initial hospitalization, but can occur after discharge. Urinary extravasation presents as oliguria or anuria, elevated blood urea nitrogen and serum creatinine levels, ileus, and abdominal or flank pain. The most sensitive test for detecting a leak from the ureterointestinal anastomoses is a contrasted CT scan. Leaks can occur along the suture lines of a CUR or neobladder. These are best detected by filling the pouch with contrast under fluoroscopy. In a continent urinary reservoir or bladder substitute, the balloon should never be inflated in the neourethra or the catheterizing tract. Under intermittent fluoroscopic observation, water-soluble contrast is infused in the loop until adequate distension of the bowel segment is seen.

Distal obstruction of the ileal loop can lead to urinary leak or hydronephrosis when the obstruction is chronic. Catheterizing the stoma and draining more than 20 cc of urine implies inadequate emptying. Gentle exploration with a gloved finger may reveal a fold or fascial edge.

A continent diversion may develop an obstruction of the catheterizing tract, and the patient may not be able to get a catheter into the reservoir. This may be due to a fold in the catheterizing tract, a false passage secondary to previous catheterizations, or angulation of the stomal tract. The emergency physician should try gentle catheterization with the patient in several positions (e.g., standing, supine, or lying on the side). Manipulation of a catheter into the conduit or reservoir or the insertion of a percutaneous drainage tube under fluoroscopy or ultrasound guidance by an interventional radiologist or urologist may have to be arranged. Pouch rupture because of retention is a rare but potentially fatal complication and is more common in the neurologically impaired patient who fails to empty, in part owing to impaired sensation. Stricture of the anastomosis between the urethra and bladder substitute may present as severe urinary hesitancy, decreased stream, fever, and flank pain. A catheter placed in the urethra will meet obstruction at the neobladder–urethral anastomosis. This requires immediate urologic consultation.

Leakage at the site of the bowel anastomosis can occur in the first month postoperatively and usually presents with peritonitis. These patients usually present with abdominal pain, nausea, vomiting, and signs of a surgical abdomen. These patients need emergent surgical exploration.

A more common presentation to the emergency department is nausea and vomiting due to a paralytic ileus. This is transient and resolves with nasogastric suction and bowel rest. A mechanical bowel obstruction can occur at any time. This usually occurs secondary to adhesions, but anastomotic strictures and internal hernias are also causes. A patient suspected of having a bowel complication should be made NPO, resuscitated with intravenous fluids, and admitted. When there is severe nausea or vomiting, a nasogastric tube should be placed.

Flatplate and upright abdomen radiographs may demonstrate free air under the diaphragm or dilated bowel.

The incidence of pyelonephritis in patients with a urinary diversion is approximately 10% to 20% and can be a major source of morbidity and mortality, particularly in the patient with coexisting renal dysfunction.[23] The chronic bacteria of the bowel segment serves as a persistent source of ascending infection. When drainage is impaired, pyelonephritis can occur. Positive urine cultures do not correlate with the occurrence of pyelonephritis. Most patients with ileal conduits and CUR diversions are chronically colonized with bacteriuria. In contrast, many patients with neobladders have sterile urine. Treatment is not indicated in the absence of symptoms after any form of urinary diversion. Clinical signs, including flank pain and fever, should direct antibiotic therapy. The presence of mucus in the urine is not a specific sign of infection. Although mucus production increases in the presence of an infection, it is a normal finding in patients with bowel exposed to urine.

Metabolic complications can result from absorption of solutes through the permeable bowel wall and can be minimized by avoiding prolonged contact of urine and bowel. Ileum and colon both are associated with the potential for hyperchloremic metabolic acidosis, producing a non–anion gap acidosis. However, this acidosis is rarely significant in a patient with normal renal function.

Ureteral obstruction usually occurs at the ureteroenteric anastomosis, but may occur more proximally. The incidence is approximately 15%, and the risk is present throughout the life of the anastomosis, emphasizing the need for long-term monitoring. A patient may present with flank pain and be found to have hydronephrosis on IVP or ultrasound. Stomal stenosis occurs in 5% of adults. It is more common in the pediatric population and is preventable through construction of a well-vascularized, everted stoma.

Calculus disease results from persistent infection, hypercalciuria associated with chronic acidosis, enteric hyperoxaluria associated with the use of large amounts of ileum, and infection. Infection stones are associated with urea-splitting organisms, such as *Proteus, Klebsiella,* and *Pseudomonas.* Treatment includes stone removal, elimination of factors that cause residual urine, adequate oral intake, adequate bladder irrigation, and aggressive treatment of infection.

DIFFERENTIAL DIAGNOSIS

After transurethral resection or biopsy, a bladder perforation should be suspected in someone with abdominal pain, anuria, oliguria, and fever. After a cystectomy, ileal conduit or continent diversion, urinary leakage, ureteral obstruction, bowel anastomosis leakage, and bowel obstruction or ileus should be considered in a patient with similar symptoms.

EMERGENCY DEPARTMENT EVALUATION

A careful history is important to direct the examination. All patients are examined for signs of peritonitis. A white blood cell, serum creatinine, and flatplate and upright abdominal radiographs should be obtained. Urine should be sent for analysis and culture. If flank pain is present, an IVP or ultrasound should be obtained.

EMERGENCY DEPARTMENT MANAGEMENT

The postoperative patient's surgeon should be notified. If a consultant is not available, a patient with abdominal pain after a resection or biopsy of the bladder should have a large-bore catheter placed. If bladder perforation is suspected, a low-pressure cystogram should be obtained.

The patient with a ureteral obstruction needs admission for percutaneous nephrostomy. Intravenous antibiotics are given to any patient at risk for sepsis, including those with suggested urinary obstruction and peritonitis. Patients with intestinal anastomotic leaks or urinary leaks from urinary reservoirs generally require surgical repair.

DISPOSITION

Role of the Consultant

The role of the consultant is to facilitate management of all postoperative complications. Urologic consultation should be obtained for the instrumentation of any urinary diversion.

Indications for Admission

Any patient suspected of having bowel obstruction, peritonitis, ureteral obstruction, or bladder perforation should be admitted.

Transfer Considerations

The availability of a urology consultant may necessitate transfer. If the procedure was performed at the same institution as the emergency department, transfer should not be needed unless the radiology or intensive care facilities are inadequate.

COMMON PITFALLS

- Dismissal of "usual and expected postoperative pain" may overlook a potentially serious problem.
- Ureteral obstruction with infection can cause urosepsis.
- Bowel obstruction, peritonitis, or bladder perforation with intraperitoneal extravasation can be fatal.

CARCINOMA OF THE PROSTATE

Carcinoma of the prostate is the most common malignancy in American men as well as the second leading cause of cancer deaths in men.[18] In 1996 there were an estimated 317,000 new cases of prostate cancer diagnosed and 41,4000 deaths from the disease. Carcinoma of the prostate has been associated with age, race, dietary factors, and other environmental factors. This malignancy is found almost two times more often in African-American men than in Caucasians.

CLINICAL PRESENTATION

Prostate cancer may be diagnosed incidentally on screening of men with the digital rectal examination, elevated prostate-specific antigen (PSA) level, or as a result of specific symptoms. However, most men who require treatment for prostate cancer seek medical attention through the emergency department only after experiencing symptoms of their disease, with bladder outlet obstruction or vesical irritability being the most common presentation. In the pre-PSA era, regional symptoms consisting of back, leg, and perineal pain were present in 20% to 40% of patients at diagnosis. Hematuria and constitutional symptoms (weight loss, fatigue, and generalized weakness) were found in 10% to 15%. [18] Several studies suggest that 20% to 25% of patients with urinary retention harbor an identifiable prostate cancer. In one series, 19% patients had spinal cord compression as the first indication of carcinoma.[22] The ischium, lumbosacral spine, and thoracic spine are the three most common sites for bony involvement.

The treatment of prostate cancer is determined by the extent of the disease. Radical prostatectomy, external beam radiation therapy, or brachytherapy are the options for locally controlled disease without evidence of metastatic disease. For patients with metastatic disease, androgen ablation, either medical or surgical, is indicated. Chemotherapy is utilized in patients with hormone refractory disease.

DIFFERENTIAL DIAGNOSIS

The main differential diagnoses for local voiding symptoms include benign prostatic hyperplasia (BPH) and prostatitis. The acute onset of symptoms in prostatitis contrasts to the insidious onset of prostate cancer. The symptoms of bladder outlet obstruction are similar regardless of the cause of the enlargement. These entities can also coexist, however. The differential diagnosis of a prostate nodule includes a benign prostatic nodule, induration secondary to focal prostatitis, and prostatic calculi. Approximately 50% of suspicious lesions on digital rectal examination actually represent cancer on prostate biopsy.

EMERGENCY DEPARTMENT EVALUATION

The patient presenting with symptoms of prostatism and bladder outlet obstruction should have a thorough abdominal examination to palpate for a distended bladder and a digital rectal examination to evaluate the prostate. A urinalysis and urine culture should be sent to rule out infection. Electrolytes and serum creatinine should also be checked. A PSA level may be drawn, with specific instructions given for the patient to follow up the results with a local urologist. Any patient with severe bone pain should have appropriate radiographs taken to rule out a pathologic fracture. A careful neurologic evaluation is indicated with a presumed diagnosis of prostate cancer with complaints of significant back pain or lower extremity weakness to rule out spinal cord compression. Any patient with severe back pain and/or an abnormal neurologic examination should undergo an emergency spinal magnetic resonance imaging or CT scan to exclude cord compression. A bone scan is usually not indicated during an emergency department evaluation.

EMERGENCY DEPARTMENT MANAGEMENT

Any patient suspected of having urinary retention should be catheterized. Marked polyuria may ensue after relief of the bladder outlet obstruction. This postobstructive diuresis may produce electrolyte abnormalities.

Patients with bone metastases can present with severe pain and associated neurologic dysfunction secondary to spinal cord compression. Palliation with aggressive administration of narcotic analgesics should be employed. Patients with persistent back pain and known skeletal involvement on bone scans with or without neurologic findings are at high risk for cord compression. This medical emergency should first be treated with high doses of intravenous glucocorticoids. These patients should be monitored closely for changes in neurologic status. They are generally treated with emergent external beam radiotherapy. Occasionally, surgical decompression may be necessary if there is spinal instability. All of these patients should receive immediate androgen ablation, either by surgical castration or the administration of high-dose ketoconazole, which blocks steroid synthesis.

Patients with metastatic disease are treated with androgen-deprivation therapy. This is accomplished by bilateral orchiectomies or, pharmacologically, with luteinizing hormone–releasing hormone (LH-RH) agonists and/or antiandrogens. A patient beginning LH-RH therapy has a transient stimulation of LH secretion, with subsequent increase in testosterone during the first 2 to 3 weeks of treatment. Thus, a patient may present to the emergency department with symptoms exacerbated by his hormonal therapy. Frequently, patients will be treated with both LH-RH agonists and an antiandrogen to block this flare phenomenon.

DISPOSITION

Role of the Consultant

In the absence of complicating factors such as urinary retention, severe pain, or spinal cord compression, the urology evaluation can be arranged on an outpatient basis. The consultant may be needed to relieve urinary obstruction or evaluate a patient with an impending spinal cord compression.

Indications for Admission

Any patient with urinary retention, intractable pain from bony metastases, or signs of neurologic impairment should be admitted.

Transfer Considerations

A patient in urinary retention who cannot be catheterized or undergo diversion with a suprapubic tube may need transfer if urologic consultation cannot be obtained. An oncologist, family practitioner, or internist can admit a patient with painful bony metastases for pain control. If a neurosurgeon is unavailable for evaluation and management of spinal cord compression, transfer may be required.

COMMON PITFALLS

Cord compression should be considered in any man with prostate cancer and back pain.

TREATMENT COMPLICATIONS

Radical Prostatectomy

After radical prostatectomy, patients may have an indwelling catheter for up to 3 weeks. Should a patient present to the emergency department in the immediate postoperative period with a catheter dislodged or removed, the emergency department physician can attempt to replace the catheter. If there is any resistance, the attempt should be terminated. If necessary, a catheter may have to be reinserted under direct cystoscopic guidance.

Patients may also present in urinary retention following the removal of their urethral catheter. Vesicourethral strictures occur in less than 10% patients.[6] These patients may need placement of a suprapubic catheter if urethral catheterization is unsuccessful.

Pulmonary embolism and deep venous thrombosis occur in 4% and 3% of patients, respectively. Wound infection, rectal injury, and pelvic lymphoceles all occur in less 5% of patients. However, a patient with a rectal injury not recognized at the time of surgery may present with signs of sepsis and abdominal and pelvic pain. The rectal examination may reveal a fluctuant mass.

Impotence, which occurs approximately 50% of the time, and urinary incontinence with a less than 3% occurrence rate, should be referred to a local urologist for treatment.

External Beam Radiation Therapy

The complications and morbidity associated with external beam radiation therapy most commonly involve the lower gastrointestinal and urinary tracts. Sixty percent of patients develop mild urinary symptoms, most commonly increased frequency, nocturia, urgency, or mild rectal morbidity, including rectal discomfort, tenesmus, or diarrhea.[18] These symptoms usually appear during the third week of treatment and resolve within days to weeks after completion. Less than 5% of patients require hospitalization for complications secondary to radiation therapy.

Patients presenting with severe urinary symptoms or tenesmus should be managed supportively. Daily intake of psyllium (Metamucil) may help to curb frequent bowel movements, while sitz baths may decrease the local irritation and help relieve pain. Hydrocortisone (Anusol-HC) suppositories may be helpful for rectal irritation or bleeding. Diarrhea may be treated appropriate agents, while phenazopyridine (Pyridium) and oxybutynin (Ditropan) and alpha blocking agents can be used for irritable voiding symptoms.

Hormonal Therapy

Patients suffering from prostate cancer usually benefit symptomatically from medical or surgical castration. Patients usually have pain relief and improved performance status following castration. Wound infections and scrotal hematomas are the most common complications following bilateral orchiectomies. Men sometimes suffer from hot flashes and sweating following surgical castration. Megestrol acetate (Megace) may provide symptomatic relief for these symptoms.

Luteinizing hormone-releasing hormone (LH-RH) agonists have become the standard non-surgical therapy for metastatic prostate cancer. These agents are injected as a depot intramuscularly or subcutaneously and maintain constant release for a 30-180 day period of castration levels. Side effects include impotence, hot flashes in up to 60% and sweating in about 10% of patients.[21] Under treatment with LH-RH agonists, a stimulation of testosterone secretion occurs during the first two to three weeks. This may stimulate tumor growth and may increase such clinical symptoms as bone pain.

TESTICULAR CARCINOMA

Testicular carcinoma is a rare form of malignancy, but it is the most common malignancy in men between the ages of 15 and 35 years.[9] In 1995 the incidence of testicular cancer in White males in the United States had increased to 4.5 cases per year per 100,000 population, up from 2.88 cases per year per 100,000 in the U.S. Army between 1940 and 1947.[7,10] However, there has not been an increase in cases in African American males during this same period.

CLINICAL PRESENTATION

The most common presentation of testicular carcinoma is painless swelling of one testis. Patients may also complain of fullness, dull ache, pain, or infertility. Any solid, hard mass in the scrotum should be considered a germ cell tumor until proven otherwise. Testicular tumors may be confused with epididymitis, orchitis, torsion, hydrocele, spermatocele, varicocele, or trauma.

Approximately 40% to 50% of patients have metastatic disease at the time of initial presentation, with 10% presenting with manifestations of metastatic disease.[5,19] Symptoms may include hemoptysis or shortness of breath from lung metastases, back pain from retroperitoneal adenopathy, gastrointestinal symptoms from direct gastrointestinal involvement or mass effect, gynecomastia from elevated serum beta human chorionic gonadotropin (bhCG) level, or a neck mass from suprahilar adenopathy. Up to 90% of patients with testis cancer have elevated alpha-fetoprotein (AFP) or bhCG levels. Ten percent of patients with testicular cancer have a history of cryptorchidism. Patients also have a 5% chance of developing a contralateral tumor, most often metachronously.

Inguinal orchiectomy is used for both diagnosis and treatment of testicular cancer. The primary lymphatic drainage from the testis follows the gonadal vessels into the retroperitoneum. Retroperitoneal lymph node dissection thus may be necessary for accurate staging of early lesions or removal of advanced metastatic disease.

DIFFERENTIAL DIAGNOSIS

The differential diagnosis of testicular masses includes epididymitis, hydrocele, torsion, spermatocele, hematocele, hematoma, and orchitis. Transillumination can help define a hydrocele and spermatocele. Testicular ultrasound should always be performed in any patient with a testicular mass.

EMERGENCY DEPARTMENT EVALUATION

The patient should have a thorough genital examination in the standing position. Scrotal ultrasonography should be obtained in any patient in whom a mass does not readily transilluminate. bhCG and AFP serum markers should be drawn for anyone with a suspicious testicular mass and are helpful in staging and follow-up.

EMERGENCY DEPARTMENT MANAGEMENT

If the diagnosis of a testicular tumor is suspected, a urologic consultation is needed.

DISPOSITION

Most patients are taken to the operating room expeditiously. If not taken the day of the evaluation, the patient should be discharged only after appropriate arrangements are made.

Role of the Consultant

The ultimate diagnosis and welfare of the patient are the responsibility of the consultant.

Indications for Admission

The patient with signs and symptoms referable to metastases should be admitted.

Transfer Considerations

A patient may be transferred to facilitate urologic consultation.

COMMON PITFALLS

Delay in diagnosis occurs in nearly half of patients presenting with testicular tumors. The average time elapsed from the time the patient noticed the mass to surgical diagnosis is nearly 6 months. Misdiagnosis of testicular tumors as inflammatory or infectious conditions and underemphasizing the urgency of the diagnosis are common causes of delay. These patients need immediate urologic evaluation.

TREATMENT COMPLICATIONS

Inguinal Orchiectomy

The initial step in the diagnosis and treatment of testicular cancer is the inguinal orchiectomy. Wound infection and scrotal hematoma are the most common complications. Complications are infrequent, but a spermatic vessel that is not securely ligated may cause significant inguinal and retroperitoneal blood loss. Orchiectomy for testis cancer is done through an inguinal approach to avoid contamination of scrotal lymphatics.

Retroperitoneal Lymph Node Dissection

Retroperitoneal lymph node dissection (RPLND) is frequently part of the staging and treatment for testicular cancer. The patients who undergo this surgery for *low-stage* disease are mostly young, vigorous, and fit, without extensive disease and debilitating chemotherapy. Hence, the occurrence of early or late complications is minimal. Damage to the postganglionic sympathetic nerve fibers may cause loss of seminal emission and, therefore, a dry ejaculate. With proper surgical techniques, this complication can be avoided in almost all patients. The most common complication of primary RPLND (no previous chemotherapy) is wound infection in 4.8%, with small bowel obstruction occurring in less than 2.5% of patients.[8]

The patients who have RPLND after chemotherapy for residual tumor mass are at a higher risk for serious, life-threatening complications. The most common serious complication in these patients is adult respiratory distress syndrome.[2] Bleomycin, a chemotherapeutic agent used to treat testes germ cell tumors, can produce an acute interstitial pneumonia and permanent fibrotic lung changes. Avoiding high concentrations of oxygen in these patients and overzealous fluid resuscitation with crystalloids helps prevent respiratory insufficiency. Hence, the emergency department physician should be cognizant of this to prevent exacerbating bleomycin lung toxicity.

Tumor adherence to the great vessels and retroperitoneal structures may result in subadventitial dissection of the aorta. If unnoticed at the time of surgery, delayed aortic rupture is possible. Occasionally, the weakened wall is replaced with an artificial tube graft. A delayed aortic–duodenal fistula may occur if there is an injury to the duodenum and if there is a weakened aortic wall. This is a devastating complication and is almost always fatal.

Patients may develop thromboses of the vena cava or iliac or pelvic veins following extensive dissection. Symptoms of pulmonary embolus, lower extremity edema, or pain should prompt the diagnosis and treatment.

Chylous ascites, due to leakage from large, uncontrolled retroperitoneal lymphatic channels, may become evident well after discharge from the hospital. Patients will have abdominal distention and, occasionally, respiratory distress if the ascites is advanced. Drainage is usually not indicated. Treatment consists of bedrest and a strict medium-chain triglyceride diet. Prolonged ileus, delayed small bowel obstruction, and pancreatitis are other gastrointestinal complications that must be considered after RPLND.

Patients may also present with flank pain following RPLND. The ureters that delineate the lateral margins of dissection may be injured from transection or devascularization. The patients thus can have a urinoma, hydronephrosis, or a urinary fistula through the incision.

References

1. Amendola MA, Bree BL, Pallack HM, et al. Renal cell carcinoma—resolving a diagnostic dilemma. *Radiology* 19XX;88:166.
2. Baniel J, Foser RS, Rowland RG, et al. Complications of post chemotherapy retroperitoneal lymph node AV, dissection. *J Urol* 1995;153:976.
3. Bono Lovisolo JA. Renal cell carcinoma: diagnosis and treatment. State of the of art. *Eur Urol* 1997;1:47.
4. Boring CC, Squires TS, Tong T, et al. Cancer statistics—1995. *Cancer J Clin* 1995;45:2.
5. Borl GJ, Vogelzang NJ, Goldman A, et al. Impact of delay in diagnosis on clinical stage of testicular cancer. *Lancet* 1981;2:970.
6. Catalona WJ. Nerve sparing radical retropubic prostatectomy. In: Glenn JF, ed. *Urologic surgery*. Philadelphia: JB Lippincott Co, 1991:56.
7. Dixon FJ, Moore RA. Tumors of the male sex organs. *Atlas of tumor pathology, section VIII, fascicles 31b and 32.* Washington, DC: Armed Forces Institutes of Pathology, 1952.
8. Donohue JP. Radical orchiectomy and retroperitoneal lymph node dissection. In: Oesterling JE, Richie JP, eds. *Urologic oncology*. Philadelphia: WB Saunders, 1997:36.
9. Einhorn LH, Richie JP, Shipley WU. Cancer of the testis. In: DeVita VT, Hellman S, Rosenberg SA, eds. *Cancer: principles and practice of oncology*, 4th ed. Philadelphia: JB Lippincott Co, 1993:37.
10. Feuer EJ, Brown LM, Kaplan RS. Testis. In: Miller BA, Gloechler LA, Harvery BF, et al., eds. *SEER cancer statistics review 1973–1990*. Bethesda, MD: National Institutes of Health, 1993.
11. Fletcher MS, Parkham DA, Pryor JP, et al. Hepatic dysfunction in renal cell carcinoma. *Br J Urol* 1981;53:533.
12. Garnick MB, Richie JP. Renal neoplasia. In: Brenner BM, Rector FC Jr, eds. *The kidney*, 4th ed. Philadelphia: WB Saunders, 1991:37.
13. Glassberg KI. Renal dysplasia and cystic disease of the kidney. In: Walsh PC, Retik AB, Vaughan ED, Wein AJ, eds. *Campbell's urology*. Philadelphia: WB Saunders, 1998:59.
14. Green LF, Hanash KA, Farrow GM. Benign papilloma or papillary cancer of the bladder? *J Urol* 1973;110.
15. Lamm DL, van der Meijden APM, Morales A, et al. Incidence and treatment of complication of bacillus Calmette-Guerin intravesical therapy in superficial bladder cancer. *J Urol* 1992;147.
16. Motzer RJ, Russo P, Nanus DM, et al. Renal cell carcinoma. *Curr Probl Cancer* 1997;21:4.
17. Parker SL, Tang T, Bolden S, et al. Cancer statistics, 1996. *Cancer J Clin* 1996;65:5.
18. Prenta KJ. Epidemiology and etiology of prostate cancer. In: Raghavan D, Scher HI, Leiber SA, et al., eds. *Principles and practice of genitourinary oncology*. Philadelphia: Lippincott–Raven Publishers, 1997:36.
19. Presti JL. Testicular cancer: an overview. In: Crawford ED, Das S, eds. *Current genito-urinary cancer surgery*. Philadelphia: Lea & Febiger, 1990:34.
20. Prouse OA, Reddy PP, et al. Pediatric genitourinary tumors. *Curr Opin Oncol* 1998;10.
21. Schroder FH. Endocrine treatment of prostate cancer. In: Walsh PC, Retik AB, Vaughan ED, Wein AJ, eds. *Campbell's urology*. Philadelphia: WB Sanders, 1998:89.
22. Smith EM, Hampel N, Ruff RL, et al. Spinal cord compression secondary to prostate carcinoma: treatment and prognosis. *J Urol* 1993:149.
23. Sullivan JW, Grabstald H, Whitmore WF. Complications of ureteroileal conduit with radical cystectomy: review of 366 cases. *J Urol* 1980;124.
24. True LD, Grignon D. Pathology of renal cancers. In: Raghavan D, Scher HI, Leiber SA, et al., eds. *Principles and practice of genitourinary oncology*. Philadelphia: Lippincott–Raven Publishers, 1997:77.

CHAPTER 65
Urinary Incontinence and Retention

Norman E. Peterson

URINARY INCONTINENCE

Urinary incontinence is not an emergency condition. It may be tolerated for lengthy periods before attention is sought. Proper management depends on accurate distinctions between stress, urge, and true incontinence and recognition of potential contributions from infection, drugs or medication, sustained bladder overdistention, neuropathologic deficits, obstruction, anatomic factors, and so forth. Emergency management is limited to assessment for contributory pathology (bladder distension, neurologic deficit), and urologic referral.

Stress Urinary Incontinence

Stress urinary incontinence (SUI) refers to involuntary urine spillage during abrupt increases in intraabdominal pressure (cough, sneeze, straining, laughing, sudden activity). SUI is often associated with multiparity and obesity, which are incriminated in reducing anatomic support for normal vesical urethral positioning, resulting in transfer of intraabdominal pressure from a bladder-closing to a bladder-opening mode. Neither obesity nor multiparity is a prerequisite, however. Other risk factors include diabetes, corticosteroid therapy, radiation therapy, and previous relapsing or unsuccessful antiincontinence surgery. Chronic vesical overdistension may accrue from blunted appreciation of symptoms, as with senility, diabetes, mental retardation, or depressed states of consciousness. The sensory neurogenic bladder characteristic of diabetes can produce chronic vesical overdistension and ultimate detrusor dysfunction; this complication may be interdicted by timed voiding, intended to prevent bladder overdistension.

Although SUI is primarily an adult female complaint, men and children are not exempted and require equally comprehensive assessment for potential etiologies, emphasizing obstructed voiding, operative history (prostatic resection), and neurologic factors. Important diagnostic data are frequently provided by voiding cystourethrography.

EMERGENCY DEPARTMENT EVALUATION

The diagnosis of SUI begins with confirmation of involuntary expulsion of urine. Severity may be quantified by documenting use and frequency of incontinence pads, and by whether the patient will consider a surgical remedy.

History alone is frequently diagnostic; support is provided by demonstrating urine loss with coughing and correction by digital urethral support (Marshall test). Other diagnostic adjuncts include cystoscopic disclosure of bladder neck opening by coughing and by radiographically delineating reduction or loss of the normal posterior urethrovesical angle, reflecting anatomic nonsupport. In addition, videourodynamic imaging may verify anatomic descent of the urethrovesical complex, thereby distinguishing SUI from incontinence resulting from unstable bladder contractions. Sophisticated urodynamic evaluation, including leak-pressure management, is particularly important after standard remedies have failed.

When predisposing or contributing factors are identified, diagnosis of SUI may require sophisticated urodynamic evaluation of vesical and urethral status and activity. Accurate diagnosis is crucial to avoidance of postoperative voiding dysfunction, usually manifested by chronic catheter differentiation that is required to avoid inappropriate surgery for vesical hyperactivity, which is managed by nonsurgical methods.

MANAGEMENT

Management of SUI is usually surgical, involving restoration of normal vesicourethral positioning by fixation of the paraurethral connective tissue to the symphyseal periosteum or to Cooper's ligament. Several methods are available for this purpose, including open suprapubic or vaginal needle suspension techniques. In selected patients, periurethral injection of bovine cross-linked collagen may be applicable. Although suprapubic methods are traditionally more reliable and more durable, anterior vaginal suspension procedures are convenient in patients undergoing vaginal surgery for other purposes.

SUI may be exaggerated by chronic bladder distension or incomplete emptying, and symptoms may be reduced to manageable levels if bladder emptying is improved. Patients with mild symptoms of SUI occasionally improve with Kegel exercises, weight reduction, estrogen replacement, or electrostimulation methods, involving operative positioning of electrodes within selected spinal foramina and a generator in a subcutaneous pocket.

Vaginal pessary may be attempted in poor operative candidates. SUI may also respond to pharmacologic manipulation, involving either vesical relaxation with anticholinergic drugs, increasing outlet resistance with alpha-agonist agents, or both.

Urgency Incontinence

Urgency incontinence describes a sudden, compelling urge to void that cannot be suppressed, and it affects both sexes and all age groups. Less severe cases involve the urgency syndrome without incontinence. Voiding volumes are typically small, often coexisting with urinary frequency. Dysuria is not a consistent feature in the absence of urinary tract infection, and a normal urinary sediment without inflammatory components or bacteria suggests emotional, functional, or neurologic contributions. Nonpathologic urgency and incontinence is not uncommon in the first several years of life, even after apparent bladder control has been achieved. Absence of coexisting neurologic or obstructive symptoms makes spontaneous recovery likely, and awareness of this phenomenon may help to avoid unnecessary sophisticated urodynamic and radiographic testing. Simple observation and anticholinergic therapy are usually adequate.

Patients with obstructed voiding may display uninhibited bladder contractions or hypercontractility, leading to urgency with or without incontinence; these symptoms often subside after relief of obstruction. Examples of obstruction range from detrusor–sphincter dyssynergy and posterior urethral valves in boys to benign prostatic hypertrophy (BPH) in men. Symptoms that may coexist with urgency incontinence include enuresis, infection, and prostatism (frequency, nocturia, tenesmus, incomplete emptying, and reduced voiding dynamics).

DIFFERENTIAL DIAGNOSIS

Inflammatory irritation usually reflects urinary infection. Other potential etiologies of urgency incontinence include urethral syndrome, interstitial cystitis, radiation cystitis, some medications (bacillus Calmette-Guérin [BCG], cyclophosphamide), and carcinoma *in situ*. Essential to diagnosis is examination of the urinary sediment, urine culture (when bacterium is present), cystoscopy, urine cytology, and bladder biopsy. Many of the potentially responsible disorders share the common feature of reduced bladder capacity owing to painful bladder filling. Diurnal frequency, often with urgency, is dominant. In contrast, a functional or nonpathologic etiology is more likely in the patient who describes daytime frequency without nocturia, a conclusion supported by noninflammatory urinary sediment.

The urethral syndrome is a common disorder in women who manifest recurrent episodes of urgency, frequency, and dysuria with noninflammatory urinary sediment and negative urine culture. This disorder is commonly interpreted as infection, and standard or extended courses of antibiotics are frequent. Patients may describe improvement during treatment, with prompt relapse thereafter. Urinary sediment often reveals squamous epithelial cells regardless of age or estrogen status. Episodes are typically cyclic, occasionally induced by intercourse. Treatment should be symptomatic, avoiding antibiotics when bacteriuria is not present. Urethral dilatation often benefits recalcitrant cases.

Interstitial cystitis usually affects women and typically commences in the third decade. This disorder involves an idiopathic, noninfectious, inflammatory cystitis extending into the muscularis and causing varying degrees of frequency, urgency, and dysuria, which may become disabling. Subsequent vesical fibrosis progressively reduces bladder capacity to degrees that may become intolerable. Clinical benefit is variably claimed for numerous remedies, including amitriptyline, antihistamines, calcium channel blockers, bladder hydrodilation, bladder instillations (silver nitrate, oxychlorosene, dimethyl sulfoxide, BCG, steroids), and many others. Clinical responses are often partial, incomplete, or transitory, sometimes culminating in bladder augmentation or cystectomy/urinary diversion. Oral sodium pentosan polysulfate has been introduced as specific therapy for interstitial cystitis, with encouraging early clinical results. Diagnosis of interstitial cystitis, particularly in men, requires biopsy exclusion of potential competing diagnoses, including inflammatory carcinoma *in situ*.

True Incontinence

True incontinence occurs without urgency or increased abdominal pressure and is usually the consequence of urinary fistula or disruption of the continence apparatus. Urinary fistula may result from trauma, prolonged third stage of parturition, malignant erosion, or defects associated with ischemia(operative, chemical, radiation).

Traumatic, malignant, or surgical damage to the male external urethral (e.g., radical prostatectomy and traumatic avulsion of the membranous urethra sphincter) may result in continuous urinary incontinence. True incontinence in women may result from destruction of normal urethral elasticity by radiation or urethral surgery (usually multiple), producing the "drain-spout urethra," or by uterine procidentia that effaces normal posterior urethrovesical angulation.

True incontinence resulting from developmental anomalies is occasionally encountered, particularly in younger age groups. Examples include ectopic ureteral drainage (distal to the bladder outlet in females; distal to the external sphincter in males) or urethral duplication in males involving channels originating in the bladder and bypassing the external sphincter.

Excretory urography, retrograde ureterography, voiding cystourethrography, retrograde urethrography, panendoscopy, and bladder instillations (chromocystography) may establish the diagnosis of urinary fistula.

Damage to the external urethral sphincter or loss of urethral elasticity is verifiable by radiographic studies or urodynamic evaluation. Conventional bladder-neck suspension often fails in such patients, as opposed to success rates as high as 94% with fascial sling or periurethral injection procedures. Artificial urinary sphincter implantation is a final option for patients with sphincteric incompetence who fail conservative remedies.

URINARY RETENTION

Urinary retention describes an inability to void or to expel the bladder contents, resulting in bladder distension and its sequelae. Retention must, therefore, be distinguished from anuria, which represents either interruption of urine production by the kidney from vascular or parenchymal disorders or obstruction to urine delivery to the bladder.

CLINICAL PRESENTATION

Acute urinary retention is typically manifested by a palpable and severely uncomfortable bladder, with discomfort exaggerated by pressure applied suprapubically (Credé). Chronic urinary retention is often encountered in senile, diabetic, or neurologically compromised patients manifesting frequent small-volume expulsions of urine characteristic of overflow incontinence. A chronic uriniferous odor is characteristic, as well as an apparent indifference to the discomfort of vesical overdistention. Patients with intermediate cases may suffer only urinary frequency or SUI.

Causes of urinary retention are usually obstructive, exemplified by BPH in senior men. Other etiologies may be inflammatory, neurogenic, or pharmacologic. Retention in women is rare and classically ascribed to emotional or psychogenic disturbances, but urodynamic investigations have identified organic etiologies in most cases studied. Pediatric obstructions are predominantly congenital and may severely damage immature nephrons; these manifestations may be obvious in prenatal ultrasound screening and functionally critical in the neonatal period.

DIFFERENTIAL DIAGNOSIS AND EMERGENCY DEPARTMENT EVALUATION

Differential Diagnosis in the Male

Adult male urinary retention is statistically most common with BPH, which is characterized by insidious progressive obstruction, usually in the sixth decade or later. Symptoms (prostatism) include hesitancy, frequency, urgency, a sense of incomplete bladder emptying, and diminution in size and force of the voided stream. Digital rectal examination discloses smooth, symmetric, homogeneous prostatic enlargement devoid of nodular induration. Similar symptoms in a younger patient with an unenlarged prostate are usually attributable to fibromuscular contracture of the vesical outlet (median bar). A history of enuresis, epididymitis, or nocturia is not unusual.

Prostatic cancer rarely obstructs voiding. Indurated nodularity is the classic clinical manifestation. Serum prostate-specific antigen (PSA) correlates with the likelihood, extent (stage), and aggressiveness of prostate cancer. Additional diagnostic information may accrue from serum prostatic acid phosphatase, osteoblastic metastasis, ureteral obstruction, and the ratio of serum protein-bound to protein-unbound levels of PSA. Final diagnosis relies on tissue sampling of biopsy or operative specimen. The advised response to abnormal digital rectal examination or elevated PSA is transrectal needle biopsy after antibiotic pretreatment, with transrectal ultrasonographic guidance as indicated.

Voiding may also be obstructed by infectious or inflammatory processes such as urethritis and prostatitis, with restoration of normal voiding after temporary catheter drainage and antibiotic therapy. Obstruction from tuberculosis, bilharziasis, and echinococcosis has also been documented, although presently relegated to virtual historic interest. Gonococcal urethral stricture has also become a clinical rarity owing to avoidance of chronic, untreated infection. Contemporary stricture disorder more often follows violent or iatrogenic trauma. Urinary retention is not a feature of nongonococcal (chlamydial) urethritis. Miscellaneous causes of urinary retention in men have been cataloged (Table 65.1).

Differential Diagnosis in Children

Pediatric urinary retention often results from developmental anomalies. Nonurologic disorders frequently coexist and usually predominate in significance. Obstructive and developmental insults to the immature kidney are variable and may be manifested neonatally or variably thereafter by sepsis, azotemia, failure to thrive, urinary infection, and voiding disorders. Prompt and comprehensive diagnosis is imperative, and urinary drainage is paramount. Pediatric urinary obstruction and retention are exemplified by posterior urethral valves in boys, hydrocolpos resulting from vaginal stenosis or imperforate hymen in girls, and prolapsing or dissecting ureterocele in either sex, particularly with duplicate renal pelves and ureters. Pediatric urinary retention produces a palpably distended blad-

TABLE 65.1. Miscellaneous Causes of Urinary Retention in Men

Documented Connections	Anecdotal Connections
Prostatic metastases from kidney and penis	Hypogastric artery aneurysms
Leukemic infiltration of prostate	Urethral calculi
Malignant retroperitoneal fibrosis (fibrous histiocytoma)	Sickle cell syndrome
	Prostatic infarction
Bladder and urethra malignancies	Bladder clots
Pelvic nerve plexus injury during surgical intervention for testis and rectal tumors	Inappropriate antidiuretic hormone secretion
	Cysts of prostate, seminal vesical, muellerian duct, ejaculatory duct, or Cowper's gland
Vincristine-infusion neuropathy	
Infectious perivesical fat necrosis	Inflammatory rectal or perirectal processes
Idiopathic perivesical fibromatosis	Various functional disorders

From Peterson NE. Urinary retention. In: Wolfson AB, Harwood-Nuss A, eds. Renal and urologic emergencies. New York: Churchill Livingstone, 1986.

der, overflow incontinence, a vulnerability to infection, and complications including ureteral obstruction or reflux with hydroureteronephrosis, respiratory distress, renal functional depression with azotemia, and extravasated urinary ascites.

Pediatric urinary retention may also derive from congenital neuropathology, exemplified by lumbosacral myelomeningocele or sacral agenesis. Retention syndromes in older children are more commonly functional, including the primary megacystis syndrome (girls) and transitory external sphincter hyperspasticity (boys), both of which are considered to be learned phenomena and amenable to relearning and biofeedback-type management. Megacystis is attributed to infrequent voiding, culminating in chronic vesical overdistention and potentially permanent detrusor damage. External sphincter spasm may result from deliberate avoidance of painful voiding during infection or from efforts to prevent incontinence during uninhibited detrusor contradiction. Urodynamic evaluation is diagnostic. Less severe cases tend to resolve spontaneously. Miscellaneous causes of urinary retention in children are given in Table 65.2.

Neuropathologic Causes

Normal urinary storage and voiding dynamics require complex coordination between autonomic and somatic innervation, smooth and skeletal muscle, and spinal reflex circuits subject to brain and brainstem modification. Voiding disturbances contribute to 20% of all urologic complaints, of which 25% have a neurogenic basis.

Urinary retention is characteristically a dominant feature of disorders such as *spinal cord trauma or myelodysplasia* at or below the level of the motor nuclei governing detrusor and sphincteric activity (spinal segments S-2 to S-4, vertebral level L-2). Such lesions interrupt the spinal reflex arc and produce areflexic (flaccid) bladder dysfunction. Traumatic lesions may be transitory (spinal shock), with full recovery of bladder dysfunction after variable intervals of intermittent self-catheterization. More severe injuries produce increasing levels of voiding dysfunction, maximizing at complete irreversibility. Neurologic insult above the level of the spinal micturition center produces reflex (spastic or hypertonic) voiding, with varying degrees of detrusor–sphincter dyssynergy (external sphincter spasm during bladder contraction). High-pressure voiding dynamics are then established, with potential complications including urgency incontinence, infected residual urine, ureteral reflux, pyelonephritis, stone formation, detrusor collapse, and chronic renal failure. Therapeutic options include pharmacologic relaxation of the bladder and external sphincter, intermittent self-catheterization, and biofeedback relearning methods. More severe and recalcitrant cases may require external sphincter ablation or bladder augmentation procedures. Resistance to standard therapeutic measures may require diagnostic refinements provided only by urodynamic or electromyographic investigation.

Miscellaneous spinal neurologic disorders capable of producing voiding dysfunction include spinal lipomeningocele, sacral dysgenesis, sacrococcygeal teratoma, presacral or spinal neuroblastoma, operative neurologic injury, encephalitis, meningitis, epidural abscess, and spinal osteomyelitis.

Back pain, gait disturbance, and bladder dysfunction that lack overt explanation arouse suspicion of a *spinal cord tumor.* Back pain in children may be associated with cerebral palsy, vertebral epiphysitis, disk herniation, or spinal cord tumor. Ninety percent of patients with *multiple sclerosis* eventually develop lower urinary tract symptoms: 50% experience incomplete bladder emptying, 25% have detrusor instability with urgency and incontinence, and 25% display bladder atony and urinary retention. Deteriorating voiding patterns often parallel advancing neuropathology. Management is symptomatic, including intermittent self-catheterization, anticholinergic suppression, alpha-adrenergic antagonism, and so on.

Landry-Guillain-Barré syndrome is an idiopathic polyradiculopathy that may be induced by viral infection, vaccination, surgery, or other infections. Anterior root and anterior horn cell involvement results in predominantly areflexic motor neuropathy with minimal sensory loss. Urologic symptoms affect 30% of patients, dominated by motor paralysis and urinary retention. Voiding symptoms are often of secondary importance to progressive afebrile symmetrical motor weakness or paralysis. Symptoms peak at 4 weeks in 90% of patients. Functional recovery is variable and usually stable at 6 months. Urologic management is limited to temporary intermittent self-catheterization.

Isolated bladder atony and urinary retention that develop in an otherwise healthy patient is often the result of viral infection, most frequently herpes simplex or herpes zoster. Incubation periods of 7 to 21 days are characterized by fever, malaise, and 2 to 4 days of dermatomal pain evolving into erythema, then papular and vesical eruption. Infection can traverse both visceral and somatic nerves and therefore produce skin eruption and bladder atony. Neuropathy may be bilateral despite unilateral cutaneous involvement. Isolated visceral nerve involvement may produce urinary retention without cutaneous or other manifestations. Reversibility is prompt and complete, and interval therapy requires only intermittent self-catheterization.

The Shy-Drager syndrome is an uncommon adult-onset multisystemic degenerative process that affects the cerebellum and brainstem. It produces autonomic deficits with parkinsonian features, orthostatic hypotension, impotence, anorectal dysfunction, and urgency incontinence or urinary retention. Urologic symptoms often provoke the initial presentation. Therapy for the urinary retention component involves intermittent self-catheterization.

Additional disorders potentially accountable for neuropathologic urinary retention syndromes include diabetes mellitus, tabes dorsalis, pernicious anemia, poliomyelitis, syringomyelia, and inflammatory polyradioculopathies.

Pharmacologic Agents Causing Voiding Dysfunction

Bladder smooth muscle (detrusor) is innervated by beta-adrenergic receptors under chronic stimulation to produce muscle relaxation, and therefore compliant filling. In contrast, the smooth

TABLE 65.2. Miscellaneous Causes of Urinary Retention in Children

Imperforate hymen
Vaginal atresia
Bladder diverticulum
Benign hyperplasia of the posterior urethra, similar to adult prostate
Cystic enlargement of prostatic utricle (the fused caudal remnant of otherwise repressed muellerian ducts, located at prostatic apex)
Anterior urethral valve
Obstructed congenital duplications of bladder and urethra
Fungal bezoars
Malignancies of bladder, prostate, and urethra
Urethral meatal stenosis, ulceration, and concretions
Inflammatory lesions of the prostate and urethra
Vesical and urethral calculi
Foreign bodies
Constipation

From Peterson NE. Urinary retention. In: Wolfson AB, Harwood-Nuss A, eds. Renal and urologic emergencies. New York: Churchill Livingstone, 1986.

muscle vesical outlet and proximal urethra are innervated predominantly by alpha-adrenergic receptors under chronic stimulation to produce contraction and increased outlet resistance (urinary continence). The external urethral sphincter is predominantly skeletal muscle under chronic stimulation to produce contraction and continence. The act of voiding involves coordinated reversal of these three functions. Table 65.3 summarizes agents that may inadvertently lead to voiding dysfunction. Table 65.4 lists preferred drug therapy for alleviating dysfunctional voiding.

TABLE 65.3. Drugs That Contribute to Urinary Incontinence

BETA-ADRENERGIC STIMULATION (DETRUSOR RELAXATION)
Isoproterenol (Isuprel)
Progesterone
Atropine
ALPHA-ADRENERGIC STIMULATION (VESICAL OUTLET CONTRACTION)
Ephedrine sulfate
Pseudoephedrine (Sudafed)
Phenylephrine (Neo-Synephrine)
Phenylpropanolamine (Ornade, appetite suppressants)
Imipramine (Tofranil)
Estrogen, estradiol
Levodopa, dopamine, epinephrine
Antihistamine
Bromocriptine (Parlodel)
Mercurial diuretics
Nortriptyline (Aventyl, Nortylin)
Phenothiazines
Testosterone
Amphetamines
Amitriptyline (Elavil, Triavil)
Benztropine mesylate (Cogentin)
Hydralazine (Apresoline)
Isoniazid
Morphine sulfate
MUSCULOTROPIC DETRUSOR RELAXATION
Propantheline (Pro-Banthine)
Methantheline (Branthine)
Belladonna
Oxybutynin (Ditropan)
Flavoxate (Urispas)
Dicyclomine (Bentyl)
Hyoscyamine (Cystospaz)
Imipramine (Tofranil)
Estrogen
Emepronium bromide
Diazepam (Valium)
Terbutaline
Indomethacin
Nifedipine

TABLE 65.4. Pharmacotherapy for Voiding Dysfunction

Storage	Emptying
DETRUSOR	
Urecholine	Pro-Banthine Flavoxate (Urispas) Oxybutynin (Ditropan)
VESICAL OUTLET	
Dibenzyline Prazosin (Minipress) Terazosin (Hytrin) Doxazosin (Cardura) Tamsulosin (Flomax)	Ephedrine Pseudoephedrine
EXTERNAL SPHINCTER	
Diazepam (Valium) Dantrium Baclofen	

EMERGENCY DEPARTMENT MANAGEMENT

Urinary Drainage

Bladder drainage provides both symptomatic relief from urinary retention and clinical stabilization during evaluation. Most episodes of urinary retention are amenable to well-lubricated 13F to 16F urethral catheterization by straight (Robinson) catheter for simple decompression or by balloon (Foley) catheter for sustained drainage. Mechanical obstructions that can inhibit bladder access include urethral stricture (from prior trauma, instrumentation, or infection), urethral false passage (from prior or concurrent instrumentation), vesical outlet contracture, benign or malignant prostatic urethral obstruction, and extrinsic local compression. Alternate methods to achieve bladder access may be necessary, and urologic consultation is advisable. Obstruction at the level of the vesical outlet or prostatic urethra that impedes passage of a straight catheter may yield to an angulated (coude) catheter. Alternatively, a malleable, semirigid mandrin may be inserted within the catheter and bent into a suitable curvature for manipulation, as with a metal urethral sound. This procedure is best restricted to performance by *experienced personnel*.

Urethral stricture and false passage often coexist and may inhibit routine catheterization. False passages may be bypassed by the mandrin catheter technique. Alternatively, a combination of flexible filiform guides may be maneuvered across obstruction and false passages into the bladder; progressively larger follower catheters are then attached for sequential dilatation and drainage. Filiform follower attempts are also best restricted to performance by experienced personnel. Failure of these maneuvers usually requires escalation to endoscopic or operative methods.

When urologic consultation is not readily available, temporary relief may be provided by suprapubic trocar cystostomy (commercial) or insertion of a small drainage tube into the bladder through a large-bore needle. Requirements include a palpable bladder and the absence of prior suprapubic surgery. If there is doubt about bladder distention (as in the obese patient), ultrasound confirmation is advisable. These procedures require a simple midline puncture one fingerbreadth about the symphysis pubis, with the trocar or needle directed slightly caudally and then advanced until urine is returned. The catheter or tubing is then advanced, the needle is withdrawn, and drainage secured in position.

A noteworthy exception to indication for prompt urethral catheterization pertains to the patient with pelvic fracture, prostate displacement on rectal examination, or blood at the urethral meatus. Suspected urethral trauma should be investigated initially by retrograde ureterography. Confirmation of urethral injury mandates urologic consultation and management. Catheterization should be deferred and drainage established otherwise.

Patients with chronic obstructive uropathy usually require continuous urinary drainage. The patient in otherwise good health with no ancillary requirements for hospital care may be discharged from the emergency department with Foley catheter drainage collected into a leg bag. Follow-up should be arranged before discharge and include a thorough discussion and understanding of events that recommend a prompt medical response.

Urinary retention related to drugs or medication requires referral to the prescribing physician for recommended adjustment or substitution therapy.

Patients in whom a neurogenic cause of retention is suspected mandate appropriate neurologic referral.

Bibliography

Awad SA, Gajewski JB, Sogbein SK, et al. Relationship between neurological and urological status in patients with multiple sclerosis. *J Urol* 1984;132:499.

Caplan LR, Kleeman FJ, Berg S. Urinary retention probably secondary to herpes genitalis. *N Engl J Med* 1977;297:920.

Crooks KK. The protean aspects of posterior urethral valves. *J Urol* 1981;126:763.

Crooks KK. Urethral strictures following transurethral resection of posterior urethral valves. *J Urol* 1982;127:1153.

Field PL, Stephens FD. Congenital urethral membranes causing urethral obstruction. *J Urol* 1974;111:250.

Fontanarosa PD, Roush WR. Acute urinary retention. *Emerg Med Clin North Am* 1988;6:419.

Guttman L, Frankel H. The value of intermittent self-catheterization in the early management of traumatic paraplegia and tetraplegia. *Paraplegia* 1966;4:653.

Hastie KJ, Dickinson AJ, Ahmad R, et al. Acute retention of urine; is trial without catheter justified? *J R Coll Surg Edinb* 1990;35:225.

Higgins PM, et al. Management of acute retention of urine; a reappraisal. *Br J Urol* 1991;67:365.

Jacobs SC, Herbert LA, Piering WF, et al. Acute motor paralytic bladder in renal transplant patients and anogenital herpes infection. *J Urol* 1980;123:426.

Jellinek EH, Tulloch WS. Herpes zoster with dysfunction of bladder and anus. *Lancet* 1976;2:1919.

Koch MO. Fluid and electrolyte abnormalities in urologic practice. *AUA update series,* lesson 12, vol. XI. Houston: AUA Off Ed, 1992:90–95.

Kogan BA, Solomon MH, Diokno AC. Urinary retention secondary to Landry-Guillain-Barré syndrome. *J Urol* 1984;131;197.

Lockhart JL, Webster GD, Sheremata W, et al. Neurogenic bladder dysfunction in the Shy-Drager syndrome. *J Urol* 1981;126:119–121.

McGuire EJ, Savastano JA. Urodynamic findings and long-term outcome management of patients with multiple sclerosis. *J Urol* 1984;132:173.

O'Reilly PH, Brooman PJC, Farah NB, et al. High-pressure chronic retention: incidence, etiology and sinister implication. *Br J Urol* 1986;58:644.

Pavlakis AL, Siroky MB, Kran RJ. Neurogenic detrusor areflexia. *J Urol* 1983;129:1182.

Peterson NE. Urinary retention. In: Wolfson AB, Harwood-Nuss A, eds. *Renal and urologic emergencies.* New York: Churchill Livingstone, 1986.

Purkerson ML, Blaine ED, Stokes TJ, et al. Role of atrial peptide in the natriuresis and diuresis that follows relief of obstruction in rats. *Am J Physiol* 1989;256(4 Pt 2):F583.

Stine RJ, Avila JA, Lemons MF, et al. Diagnostic and therapeutic urologic procedure. *Emerg Med Clin North Am* 1988;6:547.

CHAPTER 66
Cutaneous Lesions of the Male Genitalia

Stephen W. Bretz

Despite increased public awareness regarding sexually transmitted diseases (STDs), emergency physicians are not uncommonly confronted with patients complaining of genital lesions. As many individuals do not have other care providers, emergency physicians are in a unique position not only to diagnose and treat these diseases, but also to counsel patients on prevention.

Effective emergency department screening and treatment is especially important given the clear association and increased risk of human immunodeficiency virus (HIV) transmission in the setting of ulcerative and nonulcerative STDs.[7] In general, agents cause either local primary genital lesions or a syndrome of genital ulcers and regional lymphadenopathy (ulcer-node syndrome).

Primary genital lesions are caused by trauma, Behçet disease, drug eruptions, scabies, pediculosis, molluscum contagiosum (MC), or human papillomavirus (HPV). The prevalence of primary genital lesions is uncertain, but trauma or HPV (genital warts) is probably the most common cause.

The syndrome of genital ulceration(s) and regional lymphadenopathy (ulcer-node syndrome) may be caused by lymphogranuloma venereum (LGV), granuloma inguinale, chancroid, herpes simplex virus (HSV), and syphilis. Of the six classic venereal diseases (gonorrhea, syphilis, genital herpes, chancroid, LGV, and donovanosis), only gonorrhea is *not* characterized by cutaneous lesions; *all* are commonly associated with regional lymphadenopathy. The Centers for Disease Control and Prevention reports that there are 500,000 new cases of genital herpes per year in the United States, 29,000 cases of early syphilis, 665 cases of chancroid, and 170 new cases of LGV.

It is important to note that the relative incidence of these disorders varies significantly by geographic area, especially outside of the United States. For instance, chancroid is about as common as gonorrhea in the Far East, while in the United States, chancroid is about a thousand times less common than gonorrhea. Despite rigorous testing, up to 25% of patients who present with genital ulcers will have no laboratory-confirmed diagnosis.

CLINICAL PRESENTATION/DIFFERENTIAL DIAGNOSIS

Primary Genital Lesions

The causes of genital ulceration, cellulitis, maculopapular eruption, abscess, eschar, and vesicular lesions are legion. HPV, pediculosis, MC, and scabies all cause primary genital lesions (Table 66.1). A history of trauma or exposure to an infected partner may or may not be present.

Pediculosis Pubis

The agent of pediculosis pubis, *Phthirus pubis,* causes lesions that are frequently erythematous and pruritic. The occurrence in a communal living situation is well described. Symptoms usually start about 3 days after exposure. Although the lesions are generally erythematous papules, they may appear hemorrhagic, possibly because of an anticoagulant material that is deposited at the time of feeding. Intense itching often results in excoriations that predispose to secondary bacterial infection. Although largely confined to the pubic region, the parasite may migrate to other hairy parts of the body, particularly the eyebrows and eyelids (blepharitis).

TABLE 66.1. Characteristics of Primary Genital Lesions

Disorder	Feature
HPV	Multiple verrucous papules/varying size sessile or "fine reticulate" pattern
Phthirus pubis pediculosis	Severely pruritic and erythematous papular lesions especially around hair follicles/excoriations Secondary infection is common May be associated with blepharitis with eyebrow involvement
Scabies	Intensely pruritic lesions with linear furrowing More commonly in the perineal region
MC	Umbilicated, non-pruritic papules Can be erythematous with superinfection

Treatment is accomplished with application of Lindane 1% shampoo to the affected area for 4 minutes, and then rinsing or permethrin 1% to affected areas for 10 minutes. Lindane should not be used on children under 2 years old or on pregnant or lactating females. Retreatment in 7 to 10 days (to kill newly hatched lice) may be required.

Genital Warts

Genital warts are verrucous-like eruptions caused by HPV, with approximately 90% of cases due to types 6 and 11. Many subtypes of HPV have been linked to the development of dysplasia and squamous cell (penile and anal) cancer, although types 6 and 11 have lower neoplastic potential then other subtypes. Patients with genital warts frequently have other STDs.

Condyloma acuminatum is a hyperplastic papilloma and the most common manifestation of genital HPV infection. The lesion of condyloma acuminatum typically appears as raised or flat, wartlike papules, usually multiple. A large wart may show "satelliting," a phenomenon in which the large wart is surrounded by smaller lesions.

Lesions of condyloma acuminatum are usually painless and nonpruritic. Some subclinical lesions may be appreciated with gauze application of 5% acetic acid to the penile shaft, and then examining the skin for white patches with a 10× lens. Although podophyllin is widely used in the treatment of genital warts, many authorities believe that cryotherapy is preferable. Laser therapy as well as surgical excision may be preferred for extensive or recurrent warts. Patients must be informed of neoplastic potential and have appropriate follow-up and possible biopsy for atypical or persistent warts.

Molluscum Contagiosum

A DNA virus in the poxvirus family that is usually transmitted by direct contact causes MC. While this disorder is transmitted by casual contact, especially in the pediatric population, adults with genital lesions usually acquire it through sexual contact. The incubation period is variable, but is usually between 2 and 8 weeks. The lesions are usually nonpruritic, nonerythematous papules with central umbilication.

The infection is usually self-limited, with the lesions lasting weeks to years, although the lesions can be more disseminated in immunocompromised states. Lesions normally resolve without scarring. Removal of the lesions is possible with cryotherapy with liquid nitrogen or by topical application of podophyllin, trichloroacetic acid, or bichloroacetic acid. No emergent therapy is needed.

Scabies

The mite *Sarcoptes scabiei* causes scabies. The incidence of scabies has increased in the United States since 1974. Conditions of poverty, poor hygiene, overcrowding, malnutrition, and sexual promiscuity are contributory factors. The infection produces intense itching and areas of excoriation in a characteristic pattern on the penis, scrotum, axillae, buttocks, elbows, and interdigital web spaces. Sensitization to the burrowing mites and eggs that are laid occurs over 1 to 4 months and causes a characteristic pruritic skin eruption. Skin lesions, however, can be vesicular, pustular, or papular in nature.

Sensitization may take weeks to develop when an individual is first infected. Reinfection is possible, and, if left untreated, scabies may persist for decades. A nodular variant of scabies occurs in a small percentage of patients with pruritic, reddish brown nodules on the scrotum, penis, and axillae. Lymphadenopathy is rarely seen. Scabies can be difficult to differentiate from pediculosis pubis, although the presence of lesions on the scrotum and penis would be more consistent with scabies.

Treatment consists of applying Permethrin cream 5% to the entire body below the neck, and rinsing off after 8 hours. Lindane 1% can alternatively be used in a similar fashion. There is some evidence to support the use of ivermectin (200 μg/kg or 0.8% cream), especially in immunocompromised patients with disseminated lesions or in patients with repeated infestations.[12]

Ulcer-Node Syndrome

The ulcer-node syndrome may be caused by genital herpes, LGV, chancroid, granuloma inguinale, or syphilis. Any genital ulcer may be accompanied by regional lymphadenopathy. The morphology of the ulcer(s) and lymphadenopathy may be of some diagnostic help, but none of the clinical characteristics is specific. In STD clinics, the clinical impression of a genital ulcer may be incorrect in almost half of all cases.

Unfortunately, genital herpes, syphilis, LGV, and chancroid may appear identical. The papule is the initial lesion of syphilis; chancroid may begin as a papule or pustule; the initial lesion of LGV may be papular or vesicular. Genital herpes begins with multiple vesicular lesions that tend to occur in clusters. Rapid erosion can lead to ulceration that is similar to and indistinguishable from the other causes of ulcer-node syndrome. The lesions are usually painless in syphilis but painful in chancroid and primary herpes.

Lymphadenopathy is similarly of minimal diagnostic help. The appearance of inguinal or femoral adenopathy without a genital ulcer is common in LGV, but can also occur in chancroid. Lymph nodes frequently become fluctuant with chancroid and LGV. Lymphadenopathy is often bilateral in syphilis and genital herpes, but usually unilateral in chancroid and LGV. The adenopathy of syphilis and LGV is usually less painful than that caused by genital herpes. The adenopathy of chancroid is usually unilateral and suppurative.

Table 66.2 provides a summary of the recommended treatments for each of the specific diseases associated with the ulcer-node syndrome.[2]

Genital Herpes (Herpesvirus Hominis)

It is estimated that more than 45 million Americans, or one in every four to five, has a genital herpes infection. A half-million new cases are reported per year, making it the most common cause of genital ulcers.[2,10] Approximately 80% of these cases are caused by HSV-2, while HSV-1 accounts for the remaining 20%. In the general adult population, antibodies to HSV-1 are noted in 70% to 90%, while approximately 22% have antibodies to HSV-2. Infection rates after exposure vary, but an individual who regularly has sexual intercourse with an infected partner has a 10% chance of acquiring the disease each year.[8]

There are five stages of the infection: primary, latent, shedding, recurrent, and disseminated. An incubation period of 2 to 12 days for primary infection and 1 to 7 days for recurrent herpes has been well described. Systemic symptoms such as fever, myalgias, and headache coincide with the onset of genital lesions that usually occur on the shaft or glans of the penis.

The initial lesions are painful vesicles with surrounding erythema that go on to form shallow, tender ulcers. The ulcers may coalesce to form lesions akin to chancroid or syphilis. The lesions tend to resolve in 5 to 10 days, but may persist for weeks. Two to 3 weeks after the onset of symptoms, tender, nonfluctuant inguinal lymphadenopathy can be appreciated bilaterally. Complications include aseptic meningitis, sacral radiculopathy, extragenital lesions, transverse myelitis, and encephalitis.

Urethral involvement can cause dysuria and urinary retention, although these symptoms are rare in males. Herpetic sacral radiculomyelitis may also develop, causing urinary retention, neuralgias, and obstipation. In the latent phase, the virus remains dormant in nerve root ganglia. During the shedding phase, patients are asymptomatic. Though the actual rate is unknown, shedding is estimated to occur during 1% of the asymptomatic days. Recurrence is common and is seen in up to 90% of

TABLE 66.2. Recommended Treatment for Ulcer-Node Syndromes

Syndrome/Causative Agent	Therapy	Alternative Therapy
Syphilis		
Primary/secondary and early latent	Benzathine Penicillin G 50,000 units/kg IM up to 2.4 million units as a single dose	Doxycycline 100 mg po bid × 2 wks; Tetracycline 500 mg po qid × 2 wks
Late latent/tertiary	Benzathine Penicillin G 50,000 units/kg IM up to 2.4 million units each week × 3 wks	Doxycycline 100 mg po bid × 4 wks; Tetracycline 500 mg po qid × 4 wks
Neurosyphilis	Penicillin G 3–4 million units IV q 4 hours × 10–14 days; Procaine Penicillin 2.4 million IM q day and probenecid 500 mg po qid × 10–14 days	
Granuloma inguinale	TMP/SMZ 1 tab po bid × 3 wks; Doxycycline 100 mg po bid × 3 wks	Cipro 750 mg po bid × 3 wks; E-mycin 500 mg po qid × 3 wks
LGV	Doxycycline 100 mg po bid × 3 wks	E-mycin 500 mg po qid × 3 wks
Chancroid	Ceftriaxone 250 mg IM single dose; Azithromycin 1 g po single dose	Cipro 500 mg po bid × 3 days; E-mycin 500 mg qid × 7 days
HSV (first episode)	Acyclovir 400 mg po tid × 7–10 days; Famciclovir 250 mg po tid × 7–10 days	
HSV (recurrent)	Acyclovir 800 mg po bid × 5 days; Famciclovir 125 mg po bid × 5 days	

Based on recommendations in 1998 Guidelines for Treatment of Sexually Transmitted Diseases, U.S. Department of Health and Human Services, Centers for Disease Control and Prevention. Cipro, ciprofloacin; E-mycin, Erythromysin

patients during the first year.[1] Subsequently, patients average between five and eight episodes per year. Viral shedding from lesions is shortened from an average of 11 days to 3 to 4 days.

Daily suppressive therapy may have a role in several instances: in patients with more than six recurrences per year, in immunocompromised patients, and for the purpose of decreasing subclinical shedding (which may prevent transmission).[2,11] Daily suppressive therapy consists of acyclovir 400 mg twice a day or famciclovir 250 mg twice a day.[2,5]

Though the diagnosis is often made clinically, diagnostic tests for HSV infection are especially important when the diagnosis is unclear. Viral isolation by culture is the "gold standard" diagnostic test, but does not help with management within the emergency department, as results can take up to 10 days. Sensitivity is approximately 90% for primary lesions, 40% for recurrent lesions, and 25% for crusted lesions.

Viral antigen detection is an alternative, using direct fluorescent assay or enzyme-linked immunosorbent assay (ELISA). ELISA tests are available but may only be positive after a lengthy lag period following the initial infection. Polymerase chain reaction (PCR) testing is not as readily available, but it is probably the most sensitive test available. The Tzanck test, looking for multinucleated giant cells and intranuclear inclusions, has a limited application, given its lower sensitivity.

Patient education is very important, especially given the commonness of this disease and its social ramifications. Many individuals who are infected with HSV-2 do not carry the diagnosis of genital herpes; rather, they have a mild or unrecognized infection and shed virus intermittently. Thus, an individual may transmit the disease unknowingly. Likewise, the current sexual partner may not be the source.

Lymphogranuloma Venereum

LGV, a systemic infection that affects the genital lymphatic tissue, is caused by *Chlamydia trachomatis.* This entity is rare in the United States, with most cases being associated with travel and sexual contact in tropical and subtropical countries. Outbreaks in the United States have been observed in the Midwest and Southeast. The incubation period is 3 to 30 days.

Because of its evanescent and rapidly healing nature, the genital ulcer is seen in only 5% to 15% of patients. Unlike all other causes of ulcer-node disease, LGV is distinguished not by prominent ulcers, but by lymphadenopathy without cutaneous ulcers. The second stage follows in 3 to 4 weeks and is characterized by the formation of inguinal buboes, along with systemic symptoms such as malaise, fatigue, and headache.

The buboes, which are usually unilateral, become progressively larger until they spontaneously drain. A draining sinus tract is often the initial finding. LGV may progress, if untreated, to a third stage with anorectal fissures and strictures. In homosexual males, this entity may present as proctitis.

Given the transient nature of the ulcers that are seen in the first stage of LGV, patients who have the disease usually present with tender lymphadenopathy with overlying violaceous skin. The "groove sign," which results from lymphadenopathy on opposing sides of Poupart's ligament, is characteristic of LGV, but it is noted in only about 20% of cases.

The LGV serotype of *Chlamydia trachomatis* is difficult to culture, but one can attempt to culture the organism from genital specimens or aspiration of a bubo. For the diagnosis, there is greater reliance on an LGV complement fixation test, which is generally available. A titer of greater than 1:64 suggests LGV, while a titer of less than 1:16 reliably excludes LGV. Microimmunofluorescence antibody testing is not commonly available but is more sensitive and specific. The buboes may be aspirated, but incision and drainage should be avoided.

Chancroid

Haemophilus ducreyi is the causative agent of chancroid. The incidence of chancroid is much greater in developing countries (20/100,000 compared with 0.5/100,000 in the United States). The peak incidence in the United States was 5035 cases in 1987. Just 773 cases were reported in 1994, with an overwhelming male predominance (ranging from 3:1 to 25:1). Most cases are associated with localized outbreaks in urban centers. There is some evidence to support the assertion that circumcision may reduce the risk of this disorder.

This organism has an incubation period of approximately 3 to 5 days, after which small papules form. Within 1 to 2 days the papules ulcerate to form painful lesions with irregular, nonindurated borders that are clearly demarcated. Sixty percent of patients have tender lymphadenitis, usually unilateral. The lymph nodes rapidly become fluctuant with erythematous, overlying skin. Spontaneous rupture of the formed bubo is common. Aspiration of painful nodes may be necessary, but incision and drainage should be avoided.

Chancroidal ulcers may be difficult to distinguish from syphilis. The ulcers of chancroid tend to be deeper and more painful, with ragged margins and tender unilateral adenopathy. Indeed, chancroid and syphilis may coexist and are often indistinguishable. Genital herpes may also mimic chancroid; most "apparent" chancroid is due to HSV. The current CDC clinical definition for a probable case of chancroid requires (1) one or more painful genital ulcers, (2) a negative dark-field examination or serologic test for syphilis performed at least a week following the appearance of the ulcer, and (3) a clinical presentation atypical for herpes or a negative herpes culture.[2] Laboratory diagnosis is difficult. The utility of a Gram stain is limited because of a wide-ranging sensitivity (10% to 90%), and culture of *H. ducreyi* requires selective media, yielding a sensitivity of less than 80%.[2] Newer techniques, such as PCR, will likely yield more sensitive and specific tests.

Syphilis

Of all the diseases that present as a genital ulcer, syphilis, caused by *Treponema pallidum,* is the most important when one considers the potential morbidity for untreated infection. The number of new cases reported has varied in the United States, with a peak of 45,000 cases in 1990. Subsequently, this number fell to 8,551 in 1997, of which approximately two-thirds were male. In 1997, the overall incidence was 3.2 per 100,000 in the United States.[3] The rate of syphilis in urban areas is five times higher than overall rates. As well, there seems to be a correlation between drug activity and syphilis rates in counties that border some interstate highways.[4]

The incubation period is about 1 to 3 weeks. The singular ulcer, typical of primary syphilis, usually presents at the site of inoculation 1 to 3 weeks after exposure. Thus, it is important to examine the perianal and oral cavities, as well as the genitalia, especially among the homosexual population.

Characteristically, the ulcer (chancre) is painless, indurated, and nonexudative, with a smooth base and raised, firm borders. Inguinal lymphadenopathy consists of moderately enlarged bilateral (70%) or unilateral painless lymph nodes. The rash of secondary syphilis, characterized by local or diffuse mucocutaneous lesions, may appear before the chancre is healed (6 to 8 weeks). These lesions can be macular, papular, or even pustular.

Tertiary syphilis is the term applied to gummas and cardiovascular syphilis, most commonly aortitis associated with medial necrosis and aneurysm. Neurosyphilis (syphilitic meningitis, parenchymatous syphilis, or meningovascular syphilis) can occur from months to many years after the onset of disease. Tabes dorsalis, often seen with optic atrophy, reflects demyelination of the posterior columns and dorsal roots, but it is usually seen only after 25 to 30 years of infection. For the purposes of treatment, the term *latent* applies to currently asymptomatic patients who have positive serologic studies, with a negative cerebrospinal fluid examination. Furthermore, the disease is termed *early latent* if it is within the first year of infection, and *late latent* if more than a year has passed and the patient has not been treated.

Dark-field microscopy with immunofluorescent staining is the only widely available means by which to make an absolute diagnosis of syphilis. A negative microscopic examination, however, does not rule out the diagnosis. Every patient with genital ulceration should be tested for syphilis with the nontreponemal tests and rapid plasma reagin (RPR) and Venereal Disease Research Laboratory (VDRL) tests. There is some evidence to support screening serologic studies in the emergency department in areas where the incidence is high, such as urban areas.[6] The sensitivity of these two tests approaches 80% in primary syphilis and essentially 100% in secondary syphilis. Positive tests should be confirmed with a fluorescent treponemal antibody absorption (FTA-ABS) or microhemagglutination assay for *T. pallidum* (MHA-TP). After treatment, repeat VDRL titers should be taken at 3, 6, 8, and 12 months. If treatment was successful, one should expect a fourfold decrease at 3 months and an eightfold decrease at 6 months.[2]

Presumptive treatment must be provided to every individual who has had sexual contact within the 90 days prior to his or her partner's diagnosis of primary, secondary, or early latent syphilis. If the exposure occurred more than 90 days before the sex partner's diagnosis of primary, secondary, or early latent syphilis, the patient should have serologic testing, but if follow-up is questionable, treatment should be provided.[2] Despite the fact that *T. pallidum* remains sensitive to penicillin, it is important to note that procaine penicillin, which has a shorter half-life, is not a satisfactory substitute for benzathine penicillin.

Granuloma Inguinale

Granuloma inguinale is a rare cause of genital lesions, especially in the United States, where fewer than 30 cases are identified each year. It is sometimes referred to as donovanosis and the causative agent is *Calymmatobacterium granulomatis*. The incubation period varies from weeks to months, after which painless, progressively enlarging ulcers develop. Due to their increased vascularity, the lesions have a "beefy red" appearance and bleed with minimal contact. Initially, there is no significant lymphadenopathy, but painless, granulating lymph nodes may be noted due to direct spread of infection to the lymph nodes, which may progress to pseudobuboes. Diagnosis of granuloma inguinale is established by the presence of Donovan bodies on microscopy of a biopsy specimen, because this organism is exceedingly difficult to culture.

Other Diagnostic Considerations for Genital Ulcers

Although uncommon, genital ulcers may be due to granuloma inguinale, candidiasis, tularemia, Behçet syndrome, neoplasia, amebiasis, psoriasis, lichen planus, fixed drug eruption, and mycobacteria.

DISPOSITION

Distinguishing primary genital lesions (genital warts, scabies, and pediculosis pubis) from genital ulcers has important therapeutic implications. Unfortunately, the emergency physician often does not have bacteriologic or virologic tests available for definitive diagnosis. All patients with ulcers or inguinofemoral lymphadenopathy, however, should have serologic testing for syphilis.

Given the poor follow-up that is common among many emergency department patients, presumptive treatment is often appropriate. For instance, if both chancroid and syphilis are suggested, empiric treatment with erythromycin plus penicillin G benzathine (2.4 million units given i.m.) may be indicated. The rationale for this regimen is that although erythromycin is effective for chancroid and most cases of syphilis, 10% of cases of early syphilis will persist with erythromycin, similarly, short courses of ceftriaxone also mask early syphilis.

Specialists in infectious diseases or dermatology may need to be consulted, but rarely on an emergent basis. It is essential that patients be discharged with the appropriate follow-up and encouraged to refer sexual contacts for screening. Patients should also be referred for HIV testing, as strong evidence suggests that both ulcerative and nonulcerative STDs promote the transmission of HIV.[7] Although admission is rarely indicated, patients with fever and signs of systemic illness should be carefully evaluated prior to discharge. As well, immunocompromised patients, especially those with disseminated disease, often require admission.

COMMON PITFALLS

- Failure to consider and test for other, concurrent STDs in the patient with an identified STD
- Failure to distinguish LGV or chancroid from syphilis and genital herpes
- Failure to recognize the need to aspirate (rather than incise and drain) large inguinal buboes that are extremely painful or unresponsive to antibiotics
- Failure to treat a patient for syphilis in addition to the primary treatment, when one is uncertain whether the patient has syphilis
- Failure to adequately educate the patient, attain appropriate follow-up, and stress the importance of treatment for sexual partners

References

1. Benedetti J, Corey L, Ashley R. Recurrence rates in genital herpes after symptomatic first-episode infection. *Ann Intern Med* 1994;121:847–854.
2. Centers for Disease Control and Prevention. 1998 Guidelines for treatment of sexually transmitted diseases. *MMWR* 1998;47(no. RR-1)
3. Centers for Disease Control and Prevention. Primary and secondary syphilis—United States, 1997. *MMWR* 1998;47:493–497.
4. Cook RL, Royce RA, Thomas JC, et al. What's driving an epidemic? The spread of syphilis along an interstate highway in rural North Carolina. *Am J Public Health* 1999;89(3):369–373.
5. Diaz-Mitoma et al. Oral famciclovir for the suppression of recurrent genital herpes. *JAMA* 1998;280:887–892.
6. Ernst AA, Farley TA, Martin DH. Screening and empiric treatment for syphilis in an inner-city emergency department. *Acad Emerg Med* 1995;2(9):765–772.
7. Fleming DT, Wasserheit JN. From epidemiological synergy to public health policy and practice: the contribution of other sexually transmitted diseases to sexual transmission of HIV infection. *Sex Transm Dis* 1999;75(1):3–17.
8. Marr L. *Sexually transmitted diseases*. Baltimore: The Johns Hopkins University Press, 1998.
9. Martin DH, Mroczkowski TF. Dermatologic manifestations of sexually transmitted diseases other than HIV. *Infect Dis Clin North Am* 1994;8(3):533–582.
10. Oliver L, Wald A, Kim M, et al. Seroprevalence of herpes simplex virus infections in a family medicine clinic. *Arch Fam Med* 1995;4(3):228–232.
11. Wald A, Zeh J, Barnum G, et al. Suppression of subclinical shedding of herpes simplex virus-2 with acyclovir. *Ann Intern Med* 1996;87:69–73.
12. Walton SF, McBroom J, Mathews JD, et al. Crusted scabies: a molecular analysis of *Sarcoptes scabiei* variety hominis populations from patients with repeated infestations. *Clin Infect Dis* 1999;29(5):1226–1230.

CHAPTER 67
Acute Scrotal Mass

Robert E. Schneider

The acute scrotal mass can be a challenging differential diagnosis. The three most common diagnoses are torsion of the testis/spermatic cord, acute epididymitis, and torsion of the appendix testis or epididymis. Less frequent diagnoses include orchitis, acute hydrocele, spermatocele, varicocele, spermatic granuloma, and inguinal hernia. The ischemic insult from testicular torsion makes acute scrotal pain a true surgical emergency. The evaluation most often is difficult, even though a careful history and physical examination narrow the possibilities.

The male external genitalia must be examined systematically in both the supine and standing positions. The former prevents the patient from retreating during the examination, while the latter provides optimum positioning to evaluate the lie of each testis, the presence or absence of both a varicocele or an inguinal hernia. After quickly assessing the penis and retracting the foreskin to expose the glans, both testes are compared for size and consistency. A testis is best examined with two hands, one palpating and assessing the testicular consistency while the other evaluates the epididymis. The normal testis should be examined first to provide a baseline. The testes normally are oriented vertically with a slight and variable forward tilt. The rubbery consistency should be homogeneous and similar to the thenar eminence of the thumb. The surface is smooth. A normal testicle is 6.0 cm long by 4.0 cm wide by 2.5 cm thick. The testes should be freely mobile within the scrotum (Fig. 67.1). Any palpable mass is described in relationship to the testis, epididymis, spermatic cord, or as a separate entity. All masses should be transilluminated with a penlight or flashlight placed in contact with the posterior scrotal wall and the findings described as positive (does transilluminate) or negative (does not transilluminate).

The epididymis is a discrete, sausage-shaped structure 1 cm thick, usually located on and firmly attached to the posterior

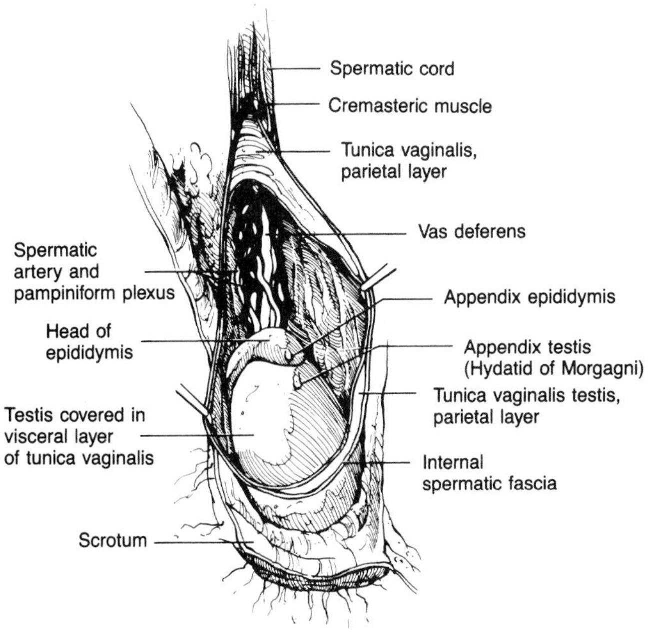

Figure 67.1. Normal anatomy of the scrotum.

wall of the testicle. In 7% of patients, it is anteriorly oriented. The epididymal head, or globus major, is the thickest portion and lies on the top of the testis. The body of the epididymis is a continuation of the head and tapers to the tail, or globus minor, which is contiguous with the vas deferens. The 1×3-mm testicular and epididymal appendages are not normally palpable, but are most commonly located anteriorly, near the upper pole of the testis and the head of the epididymis.

From the testis, the spermatic cord can be palpated ascending into the fascial cleft of the subcutaneous external inguinal ring. The vas deferens is a firm tubular structure lying within the 1.5- to 2.0-cm-diameter cord. The spermatic arteries are not palpable and the veins are palpable only when enlarged (varicocele). In the standing position, a cough or Valsalva maneuver while palpating the external inguinal ring may elicit an overt hernia or, most often, an impulse consistent with an early tear in the fascial ring. This maneuver also may elicit or accentuate a varicocele.

TESTICULAR TORSION

Torsion of the testis has an incidence of one in 4000 males. It can occur at any age but is most common between the ages of 12 and 18 years.[21] Testes predisposed to torsion lack posterior fixation to the scrotal wall and have an abnormally high attachment of a voluminous tunica vaginalis (Fig. 67.2). The tunica vaginalis normally fixes the testis and epididymis to the posterolateral surface of the scrotum (see Fig. 67.1). However, complete envelopment of the testis by the tunica vaginalis permits rotation of the testis (clapper) within the tunica (bell), resulting in the classic "bellclapper" deformity.[16]

The resultant ischemic event is an emergency. Initially, the testis and cord twist within the tunica vaginalis, causing occlusion of the venous sytem. Arterial flow is subsequently decreased by both the twisting mechanism and the secondary edema consequent to venous occlusion. The degree of testicular damage is related to the duration and extent of vascular occlusion. There are no serum markers to identify the ischemic process. Partial arterial flow may persist with less than 540 degrees to 720 degrees of rotation until edema results in complete occlusion. The variable degree of testicular ischemia makes the absolute window for testicular viability unknown. Testicular salvage times emanate from animal data and show that damage occurs after 2 hours of complete cessation of blood flow. A history of continuous pain for 24 hours is usually associated with an infarcting testis. A salvage rate of 100% following manual or surgical detorsion within 6 hours of ischemic onset is often quoted.[4] However, following acute detorsion, nearly half of the involved testes atrophy by more than 20%.[1] An atrophic testicle may have impaired fertility. Significant preexisting testicular histologic abnormalities have been shown to antedate the acute ischemic event.[12] Therefore, consequent fertility damage to a contralateral testicle from ipsilateral torsion is unlikely.[11]

CLINICAL PRESENTATION

Sudden onset of testicular pain and swelling is the classic presentation for testicular torsion. Unfortunately, in the majority of cases, the history is nonspecific and misleading and should not be used alone to diagnose the acute scrotal mass.[14] Pain is most often present or is a significant part of the event.[21] Pain can be acute or insidious in onset and mild to excruciating in intensity.

Often, the pain is abdominal and may mimic acute gastroenteritis. In one study, scrotal pain with radiation to the abdomen or inguinal region occurred in 50% of patients with testicular torsion, whereas abdominal or inguinal pain without scrotal pain occurred in 12.5%.[10]

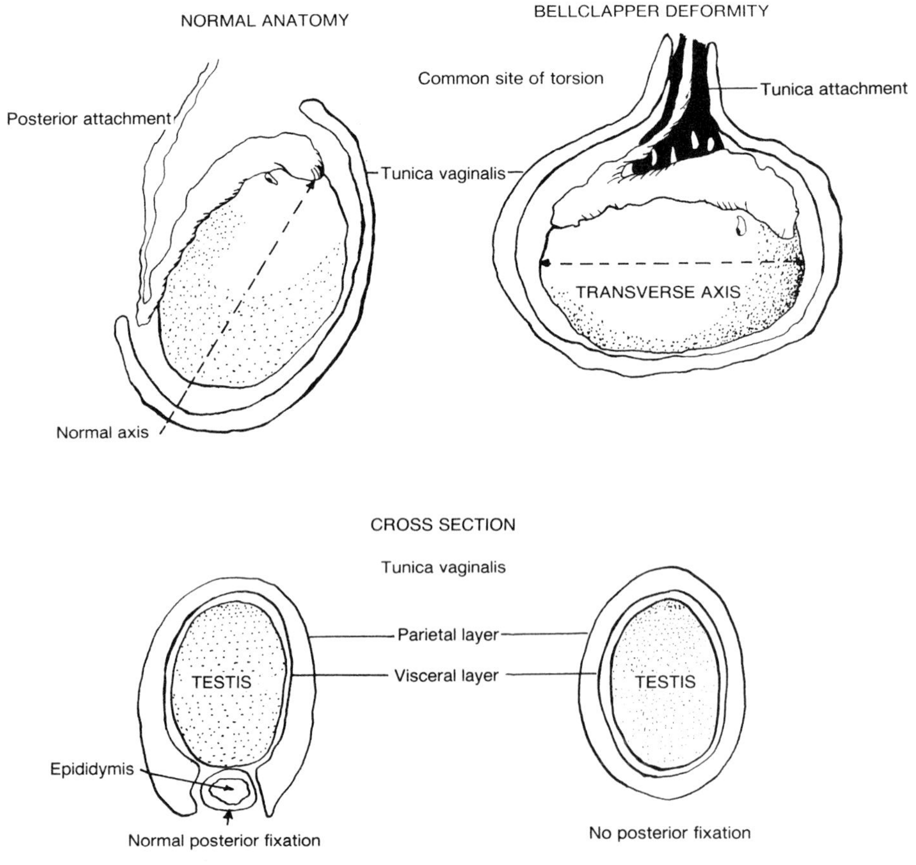

Figure 67.2. Bellclapper deformity.

A history of a similar event can be elicited in half of the patients and results from previous episodes of torsion followed by spontaneous detorsion. Approximately half of patients report the onset of pain during sleep. Cold weather, sexual arousal, and scrotal trauma are often important inciting events. Nausea, vomiting, and low-grade fever are common clinical findings. Voiding symptoms such as dysuria, urgency, and hesitancy are rarely described.

Physical examination reveals either a painful or often nonpalpable testis that has elevated cephalad in the hemiscrotum due to the twisting and foreshortening of the spermatic cord. Engorgement of the testicle and secondary swelling of the scrotum are usually present. Instead of lying in the usual vertical orientation, the affected testis is often found lying horizontally in the scrotum due to its abnormal mobility within the tunica vaginalis.

The epididymis may be malrotated anteriorly but is usually nontender when palpated. Chronicity of the event usually results in the epididymis becoming globally enlarged and sausage-shaped anatomically. The spermatic cord tends to become thickened in the area of torsion. Elevation of the testis does not relieve the discomfort (Prehn's sign) as it does in epididymitis, because torsion is primarily an ischemic event, not an inflammatory process. With the passage of time, however, testicular torsion evolves into a secondary inflammatory process. Laboratory data are nonspecific and not helpful. One-third of patients have a nonspecific leukocytosis of more than 10,000 white blood cells per cubic millimeter, and almost all patients have a normal urinalysis.[10,15]

When these classic findings are absent, the entire hemiscrotum is usually swollen, tender, and firm. A reactive hydrocele may have developed.[13] The overlying scrotal skin rapidly develops redness and edema, and within a few hours, the testis and epididymis are no longer anatomically separable. In a series of 206 patients with torsion, 42% presented with swelling and precluded palpation of the intrascrotal contents.[15] Finally, the hemiscrotum becomes an amorphous, painful scrotal mass referred to as "missed torsion."

The ipsilateral loss of the cremasteric reflex with testicular torsion and its preservation in most cases of epididymitis is a soft finding and certainly not diagnostic of one event or the other.[20] The cremasteric reflex is a superficial skin reflex mediated by spinal nerves T-12 to L-2, elicited by stroking the skin of the inner aspect of the ipsilateral thigh in an upward motion, resulting in contraction of the cremasteric muscle and elevation of the testis by at least 0.5 cm. This is best demonstrated with the patient in the supine, frogleg position and requires the absence of any inflammatory process in the overlying scrotal skin. Occasionally, the cremasteric findings are equivocal and unreliable in severe epididymitis associated with marked overlying scrotal skin inflammation.

DIFFERENTIAL DIAGNOSIS

In an adolescent, acute scrotal swelling is torsion until proven otherwise. The differential diagnosis includes acute epididymitis, torsion of the testicular or epididymal appendices, orchitis, testicular tumor, inguinal hernia, and traumatic hydrocele or hematocele. Age does not preclude the diagnosis of testicular torsion. A series of 243 patients with testicular torsion revealed that 31% were prepubertal, 60% were 12 to 18 years old, 5% were older than 30 years, and isolated case reports in the elderly continue to be reported.[8]

Acute epididymitis, the most common entity mistaken for testicular torsion, is rare before puberty. Sixty percent of patients with epididymitis are older than 30 years. Epididymitis classically has a more gradual onset than testicular torsion. The diagnosis of epididymitis is in the history and must be pursued compulsively. Usually, a history of urinary tract infection, painful voiding, urethral discharge, or an indwelling urethral catheter suggests the diagnosis of epididymitis. A work or exercise history consistent with a lot of lifting, straining, or events that increase intrapelvic pressure favors epididymitis (roofer, construction worker, weight lifter). A history of previous episodes of testicular pain suggests testicular torsion. Nausea with vomiting is more common in testicular torsion. The physical examination may not be helpful, and often times is confusing.

A thorough understanding of the pathophysiology of epididymitis is imperative when examining the scrotal contents. The retrograde development of epididymitis dictates that the pain often originates in either abdominal lower quadrant, then migrates down into the scrotum. Initially, the testicular pain is felt in the globus minor or the tail of the epididymis. This is usually disclosed as a firm, hard mass at the inferior portion of the normally smooth testis. If the diagnosis is missed or delayed, the inflammatory process will ascend into the body, then to the head, or globus major, of the epididymis, producing the large sausage-shaped mass often found on the posterior surface of the testis. In the late stages of either disease process, the tenderness and diffuse swelling that often accompany torsion and epididymitis can obscure any discernible physical findings.

Primary orchitis is very rare. In fact, if this is your diagnosis, consultation with a colleague is recommended for confirmation. A history of mumps orchitis and manifestations of a systemic illness should be present. Otherwise, orchitis seldom occurs unless it represents contiguous spread of infection from the epididymis to the testis (epididymoorchitis). In primary orchitis, the onset of testicular pain and swelling is more gradual and global. The epididymis is normal. The spermatic cord may be tender but is not indurated or thickened.

Torsion of a testicular or epididymal appendage can cause venous engorgement with subsequent arterial occlusion and infarction. The appendix testis is the most common appendage to twist.[10] It is usually located anteriorly, near the upper pole of the testis. Appendiceal testicular torsion occurs in the same age group as testicular torsion. Sudden onset of scrotal pain without radiation is the most common presentation. The onset of pain may not be as rapid as that of testicular torsion and may occur intermittently and then progress over 3 to 5 days. The symptoms are usually less severe than in testicular torsion. Nausea and vomiting occur more often in testicular torsion than in appendiceal torsion. Diagnostically, early in the process, the testicular appendage may be palpated separately as a tender mass at the head of the testis. The often-referenced "blue dot" sign refers to a small, tender, infarcted (blue), pealike structure seen through the hormonally unstimulated, prepubertal scrotal skin held taught over the head of the testis.[10] Localized tenderness in the head of the testis without comparable mass or erythema of the scrotal skin, however, is more commonly found in appendiceal torsion.[14] Excision of the twisted appendage is the standard treatment, although nonsurgical observation has been successful because autoinfarction is the consequence. Surgical exploration is often required in delayed cases to confirm the diagnosis of appendiceal torsion and exclude testicular torsion.

Carcinoma of the testis is the most common cancer in males age 15 to 35 years, a similar age range for the occurrence of testicular torsion.[22] The initial diagnosis is incorrect 25% of the time; the most common misdiagnosis is epididymitis. Symptoms from testicular tumors normally have a more gradual onset. Pain is not generally a major complaint for testicular tumor, although 10% of patients with intratesticular tumor hemorrhage can experience the sudden onset of pain. On examination, the affected testicle is characteristically not tender. The testis may be generally enlarged and feel heavy to the patient, but, more often, a distinct, firm, intratesticular mass is palpated by the examiner. The scrotum usually has less erythema and edema than in testicular torsion, and, on palpation, the affected testicle can be separated from the other normal intrascrotal structures. In a delayed presentation, a testicular tumor can appear similar to missed testicular torsion. Ten percent of testicular tumors have a reactive hydrocele, which can obscure palpation. Signs of metastatic disease, such as an abdominal mass, lower extremity edema, neurologic abnormalities, lumbar back pain, or weight loss, may be present in up to 10% of patients with testicular tumors. The urinalysis is usually normal.

Incarcerated scrotal hernias account for less than 2% of acute scrotal masses, but may present with a history similar to that of testicular torsion. The young age of the patient and the associated unrelenting nausea and vomiting tend to support this diagnosis. Abdominal pain and groin pain are usually present. The scrotal hernia can usually be palpated extending into the groin, and the testis may be displaced lower in the scrotum.

A traumatic hydrocele and hematocele are included in the differential diagnosis because a trauma history also accompanies 5% to 10% of cases of testicular torsion. The testis is usually not as painful as in testicular torsion, and the epididymis and spermatic cord, if palpable, are in their normal positions. Swelling often obscures the examination, and ancillary tests are recommended to confirm the diagnosis.

EMERGENCY DEPARTMENT EVALUATION

A rapid presumptive diagnosis of testicular torsion should be suspected on the basis of the history and physical findings. Because the presentation most often is variable and the scrotum develops erythema from many causes, testicular torsion must be the primary consideration for any scrotal complaint in the young and the adolescent.

Diagnostic tests, such as color Doppler ultrasound or radionuclide testicular scintigraphy, are always adjunctive and should never delay urologic consultation, attempted manual detorsion, and scrotal exploration.[25] These adjunctive tests are not required to make the diagnosis.

Imaging

Radionuclide imaging assesses testicular perfusion with a sensitivity that approaches that of color Doppler ultrasound.[5,25] Despite a 90% to 100% accuracy rate in defining testicular blood flow, testicular scintigraphy provides little anatomic information, is labor intensive, and is often unavailable in the middle of the night. It is radiologist-reader–dependent. In early testicular torsion, the scan demonstrates relatively decreased or absent testicular blood flow to the affected testis, and a "cold spot" on delayed images corresponds to the nonperfused testis. After 7 hours of relatively continuous ischemia, the nonperfused testis develops a reactive edema and hyperemia. The scan may display a halo of increased tracer activity (i.e., the rim sign) around the cold testis, often confused with and appearing quite similar to acute epididymitis. In acute epididymitis, relatively increased global perfusion to the affected hemiscrotum is seen. A nuclear scan cannot reliably differentiate torsion of a testicular or epididymal appendage from epididymitis, but it is helpful in confirming testicular blood flow and eliminating testicular torsion as the cause of the patient's pain.

A normally perfused testis with a surrounding lucency from accumulated fluid is seen with a hydrocele. A testicular tumor usually demonstrates increased radioisotope uptake in comparison with its contralateral mate. A color Doppler ultrasound is the preferred diagnostic modality for suspected testicular tumor.

Color Doppler ultrasound yields the most information in evaluation of the acute scrotum because it provides information about both anatomy and arterial perfusion. It can determine whether a mass is intratesticular or extratesticular and is particularly applicable when swelling or a reactive hydrocele has made physical examination difficult or impossible. The normal testis has characteristic echoes that are homogeneous and finely granular, whereas the epididymis is distinguished by its coarser texture. A typical testicular tumor is detected as a hypoechoic, inhomogeneous mass within the testis. Epididymitis displays a thickened and enlarged epididymis. Abscess cavities may be apparent within both the testes and epididymis.

Recommendations for Imaging

Although color Doppler ultrasound and radionuclide scans are helpful, an aggregate clinical impression derived from a thorough history and physical examination is more important. The imaging test used often depends on the consultant, the availability of the examination, the quality of the equipment, and the experience of the technician and radiologist-reader. Adjunctive tests should never delay operative exploration. Imaging may be obtained while waiting for an operating suite, but it is imperative that the examining physician remember that testicular torsion is diagnosed at surgical exploration. Once the diagnosis of testicular torsion is suspected, immediate urologic consultation is initiated. Meticulous charting and documentation of the history and physical examination, the suspected diagnosis and need for scrotal exploration, as well as the time course for all of these events, are imperative.[4]

If the urologist requests adjunctive testing, this must be documented in the emergency department record. The urologist should be informed that an attempt at manual detorsion will be made while awaiting the patient's transfer to the operating room or the radiology suite, and documentation carried out should the urologist discourage or request that detorsion not be attempted.

EMERGENCY DEPARTMENT MANAGEMENT

Manual detorsion is successful in 30% to 70% of patients.[6] Spontaneous or successful manipulative preoperative testicular detorsion results in a 100% testicular salvage rate.[4] Manual detorsion can be attempted with the patient standing or supine, but most often is done with the patient supine, in bed, or on a stretcher, with the physician standing on the patient's right side.[23] Classically, the patient is placed in the frogleg lithotomy position to allow total access to his scrotum and testis. The patient must be informed that manual detorsion is a painful maneuver. Light sedation or spermatic cord block may be done to lessen the patient's discomfort. A spermatic cord block allows multiple detorsion attempts and experimentation with direction, but it eliminates pain relief as an end point to judge successful detorsion. Most testes twist in a lateral to medial direction, so manual detorsion is initially attempted from medial to lateral, similar to opening a book; that is, the patient's right testis is detorsed in a counterclockwise direction, and the left testis in a clockwise direction. The testis is rotated 180 degrees in one direction and maintained in position. Further rotation is continued as necessary.

If the initial detorsion increases the pain, the detorsion should be attempted in the opposite direction. One to three turns is usually sufficient. The detorsion is stopped when either the anatomy is restored or the testicular pain is relieved. Both should occur promptly. Significant swelling makes the initial detorsion maneuver more difficult and there is much less chance of success.

Ideally, manual detorsion should be followed by surgical exploration to confirm success and pex both testes, because torsion is an anatomic abnormality and tends to be bilateral. There have not been any reported cases of recurrent ischemia in the interval between successful manual detorsion and orchiopexy.

The technique of spermatic cord block is simple.[25] The spermatic cord is palpated and encircled with the nondominant hand at the scrotal inguinal junction. Three to four injections with 1% plain lidocaine are made at different angled approaches with a 25-gauge, 1.5-in. needle.

An alternative method can be instituted if the cord cannot be palpated because of severe pain or pronounced swelling. After palpating the pubic tubercle, a needle is inserted vertically downward 1 cm below and medial to the pubic tubercle onto the anterior aspect of the pubic bone. Repeated slow injections should be made at different angles, attempting to infiltrate the area around the ilioinguinal nerve and genital branch of the genitofemoral nerve. The duration of a successful lidocaine spermatic cord block is about 1 to 3 hours.

DISPOSITION

Role of the Consultant

The urologist or general surgeon is obligated to establish a final diagnosis and perform definitive orchiopexy or orchiectomy, depending on the operative findings. Selected ancillary tests must not delay surgical exploration. When securing operative consent, the consultant should explain the need for bilateral orchiopexy, the possibility of orchiectomy, and the option for placement of a testicular prosthesis. An unequivocally infarcted testis is usually removed at exploration to lessen the chance for persistent pain and promote resolution of the inflammatory process. Bilateral orchiopexy is always required, because the anatomic defect is present bilaterally.

Indications for Admission

All patients suspected of having testicular torsion should be admitted and taken to the operating suite. Observation and serial examinations are not useful in the management of suspected testicular torsion. Preoperative emergency department laboratory studies should be completed quickly to expedite surgery. If preoperative manual detorsion successfully reestablishes testicular blood flow, arrangements for delayed orchiopexy can be made by the consultant. The urologist or general surgeon is ultimately responsible for any planned or self-directed delay in scrotal exploration and orchiopexy.

Transfer Considerations

The unavailability of a urologist, general surgeon, or immediate operating room facilities, warrants prompt transfer. The lack of radionuclide scanning or color Doppler ultrasonography does not effect the treatment; that is, the patient needs to undergo attempted manual detorsion and surgical exploration.

COMMON PITFALLS

- Misdiagnosis and delays in attempted testicular detorsion are common pitfalls in the evaluation of acute scrotal pain.
- Fifty percent of testes lost because of testicular torsion are associated with initial misdiagnosis. The quintessential history and physical examination are often misleading. An antecedent history of trauma most often misleads the examiner.
- Relying on a single "classic" differentiating parameter, such as age, characteristic onset of pain patterns, or physical examination findings, can erroneously convince the examiner that testicular torsion is not present.
- Referred pain to the abdomen can suggest gastroenteritis, a common misdiagnosis.
- Scrotal erythema and swelling tend to promote a diagnosis of infection, rather than initial ischemia with subsequent inflammatory sequelae.
- Delayed presentation precludes a meaningful examination, and the ability to work through a limited differential diagnosis.
- Many authorities maintain that diagnosis based on history, physical findings, and laboratory results is impossible and that prompt exploration should be carried out in every case. Ideally, careful physical examination should promote selective scrotal exploration, but, most often, the examiner finishes indecisive, which necessitates urologic consultation and scrotal exploration.
- Unnecessary delays in consulting with a urologist or general surgeon may result while awaiting ancillary tests. The examiner should not delay consultation to obtain adjunctive tests. The emergency physician must initiate prompt consultation and timely preoperative laboratory testing to minimize these delays.
- If testicular torsion is a consideration, the emergency physician cannot accept or be talked into an alternative diagnosis by the consultant over the telephone. Absolute documentation of telephone consultations is imperative, as occasionally the consultant will attempt to shift the responsibility for diagnosis back to the emergency physician.
- Manual detorsion by the emergency physician is the most rapid means of reestablishing blood flow to an ischemic testis. However, the ultimate responsibility for confirming detorsion, testicular viability, and definitive fixation to the scrotal wall rests with the urologist or general surgeon.

ACUTE EPIDIDYMITIS

Inflammation or infection that is limited to the epididymis and causes acute pain and swelling of gradual onset is termed *acute epididymitis*. Epididymoorchitis implies extension of the inflammation or infection onto the adjacent testis. Epididymitis occurs in less than one in 1,000 men per year and is the most common cause of acute scrotal pain.[18] It is primarily a disease of adults and seldom occurs before puberty unless there is an associated anatomic abnormality of the lower urinary tract that promotes urinary tract infection. Epididymitis most often results from retrograde spread of infected urine down the vas deferens into the globus minor, or tail, of the epididymis. Occasionally, reflux of sterile urine causes the same inflammatory process (i.e., chemical epididymitis).[3]

In men younger than age 35 years, the organisms most often responsible are those that cause urethritis: *Chlamydia trachomatis* and *Neisseria gonorrhoeae*.[18,24] In men older than age 35 years, bacteriuria caused by obstructive urinary disease is more common, and *Escherichia coli*, enterococci, *Pseudomonas*, and *Proteus* predominate. Tuberculous epididymitis is rare. Any organism may invade the epididymis in association with a systemic infection, such as blastomycosis and meningococcus. *Candida* and *E.*

coli epididymitis have been seen in patients with acquired immune deficiency syndrome. Amiodarone (Cordarone) has been associated with drug-induced epididymitis confined to the globus major, or head, of the epididymis.

In the prepubertal patient, coliform bacteria predominate. Nongonococcal bacterial epididymitis in a boy younger than age 10 years should prompt a thorough diagnostic evaluation for genitourinary anomalies or neurogenic bladder disease, as underlying urogenital abnormalities exist in 47% of prepubertal patients with bacterial epididymitis.[2,3] A negative urine culture is evidence against an anatomic anomaly.

Initially, gradual development of scrotal pain, swelling, and inflammation occurs when only a small portion of the epididymis or vas deferens is involved. With progression, the globus minor of the epididymis becomes involved and extends superiorly into the body, then into the globus major, or head, of the epididymis if not diagnosed and treated appropriately. The eventual large, red, hot, swollen scrotal mass of epididymoorchitis may indirectly compress the terminal branches of the spermatic artery and vein, causing testicular ischemia—hence, the importance of early diagnosis and aggressive management. Bacteria can also invade an ischemic testis, leading to testicular and epididymal abscesses.

CLINICAL PRESENTATION

The gradual onset of scrotal pain and swelling peaks over a period of 3 to 24 hours. The pain can be sharp and often radiates to the groin and either lower abdominal quadrant, simulating appendicitis or diverticulitis, but, commonly, the only complaint is a dull ache in the scrotum.

Irritative voiding symptoms, such as frequency, dysuria, and urgency, occur in 10% to 20% of patients.[14,24] A history of fever is not common. On occasion, a debilitated or immunocompromised patient may present with bacteremia. A history of recent cystoscopy, an indwelling urethral catheter, urinary tract infection, or genitourinary surgery should be sought, especially in older men. Similarly, a thorough history of sexual relationships, previous exposures to sexually transmitted disease, work-out routines, and job-related duties (any activity that promotes a Valsalva maneuver or increases intrapelvic pressure and promotes retrograde flow of sterile or infected urine) must be evaluated. Body builders who lift a lot of weight, and roofers and construction workers who climb and do a lot of heavy lifting, are prototypes for the development of epididymitis.

Nausea occurs in 15% of patients.[13] Bilateral epididymal involvement occurs in 10% of cases. Rarely, abdominal pain attributed to infection involving the vas deferens and spermatic cord is the sole initial and presenting symptom. This has been mistaken for appendicitis or diverticulitis.[24]

On examination, a localized, indurated, tender portion of the epididymis may be palpated inferiorly and separate from a less painful testis. Eventually, the entire epididymis becomes involved, and the distinction between the testis and epididymis is less evident. The involved testis hangs low in an erythematous and edematous scrotum. Most often, testicular discomfort can be relieved by scrotal elevation and support (a positive Prehn's sign), as epididymitis is an inflammatory process. A urethral discharge is present in 10% of patients.[24]

Progression of the infection can result in scrotal wall fixation to the underlying testis and epididymis and epididymal abscess formation. More commonly, an erythematous, edematous scrotum overlies an amorphous, tender mass.

DIFFERENTIAL DIAGNOSIS

The differential diagnosis of epididymitis includes torsion of the testis or its appendages, torsion of an epididymal appendage, testicular tumor, orchitis, and inguinal hernia. (These were discussed in the section on testicular torsion.) A reactive hydrocele may be the lone physical finding, prompting a search for its primary (very young infant) or secondary cause. Any inflammatory or traumatic event that prevents the parietal tunica vaginalis from absorbing viscerally secreted fluid will promote the development of a hydrocele. Most often, the posteriorly located epididymis is palpable even though the anterolateral surface of the testis is obscured by a hydrocele. Ultrasonography is the test of choice to evaluate the intrascrotal contents if definitive palpation is obscured by a secondary hydrocele. Tumors of the epididymis and spermatic cord are rare.

EMERGENCY DEPARTMENT EVALUATION

After the history and physical examination, a urinalysis and urine culture should be obtained. A properly collected urinalysis shows pyuria or bacteriuria in 50% of patients.[15] A small number of patients have a urethral discharge that can be Gram-stained. The white blood cell count is commonly elevated, nonspecific, and not helpful in the differential diagnosis. Color Doppler ultrasound can confirm testicular blood flow and help differentiate epididymitis from testicular torsion. It can also aid in the evaluation of the epididymis for enlargement and abscess formation. If gram-negative bacteremia is suspected, blood cultures should be obtained and intravenous fluids and broad-spectrum antibiotic therapy initiated as quickly as possible.

EMERGENCY DEPARTMENT MANAGEMENT

Aggressive initial management of acute epididymitis is crucial to reduce the potential morbidity associated with this disease process. Complete bedrest, scrotal elevation with ice applied to the affected epididymis for 10 minutes three times per day, organism-specific antibiotic therapy, nonsteroidal antiinflammatory drugs, narcotic pain medication, and stool softeners are the initial treatment modalities recommended for acute epididymitis. Patients are instructed to observe strict bedrest, getting up only to eat or go to the bathroom. Once pain-free in bed, they are encouraged to be ambulatory with a scrotal supporter and are instructed emphatically not to lift or strain, especially when having a bowel movement, as this will promote a recurrence of the pathophysiologic inflammatory process.

Antibiotics are prescribed in all cases. Despite an infectious cause, cultures of the urine and urethral discharge may be negative. If there is a history of sexually transmitted disease or if the causative organism is not known, a single 125-mg intramuscular dose of ceftriaxone (Rocephin) is administered in the emergency department. This is followed by a 7-day course of doxycycline 100 mg orally every 12 hours, ofloxacin (Floxin) 400 mg orally every 12 hours for 7 days, or, alternatively, azithromycin (Zithromax) 1 g orally as a single dose in the emergency department prior to discharge.[7] Men older than 35 years who are suspected of having a urinary tract infection caused by enteric gram-negative bacilli or *Pseudomonas* should be initially treated based on the suspected organism, with their treatment altered, if necessary, based on the results of the emergency department urine culture. Empiric treatment for gram-negative rods and gram-positive cocci should be initiated with ciprofloxacin 500 mg orally every 12 hours for 7 to 10 days. Therapy with trimethoprim–sulfamethoxazole (TMP-SMX) (Septra or Bactrim) 1 tablet every 12 hours or ofloxacin (Floxin) 400 mg every 12 hours is an excellent alternative. Urology follow-up is encouraged within 5 to 7 days.

DISPOSITION

Role of the Consultant

Immediate urologic consultation should be obtained if testicular torsion is considered. Outpatient management of epididymitis is appropriate in most cases. Urologic follow-up should be arranged for 5 to 7 days, unless worsening of the patient's condition necessitates an earlier visit. All pediatric cases of epididymitis require urologic consultation to evaluate the potential for lower urinary tract anomalies and urinary obstruction as the cause of the epididymitis.

Indications for Admission

Adult patients with suspected bacteremia or severe constitutional symptoms, including intractable pain or nausea and vomiting, require hospitalization and parenteral antibiotics. Patients in whom the physical examination and ultrasonography are equivocal for abscess formation should also be admitted for antibiotic therapy and serial ultrasound examinations.

Hospitalization is required for severe cases of epididymitis or when an epididymal or testicular abscess is suspected. Selected epididymotomy or epididymectomy may prevent testicular damage when an abscess is diagnosed. Occasionally, orchiectomy may be the most time-efficient and definitive treatment option.

Transfer Considerations

The unavailability of a urologist may necessitate transfer if operative intervention is necessary. Most cases of epididymitis can be treated initially by emergency physicians.

COMMON PITFALLS

- Delayed presentation can make initial assessment quite difficult. Scrotal swelling associated with both epididymitis and testicular torsion can be identical after a few days.
- Testicular torsion and testicular tumors can be overlooked unless there is a high index of suspicion.
- Epididymitis is the most common misdiagnosis in cases of testicular tumor and testicular torsion.
- Bladder outlet obstruction and urinary retention must be considered in the older patient with epididymitis.
- An incomplete history and a poor understanding of scrotal anatomy are commonly the reasons why epididymitis is misdiagnosed on initial evaluation.

ORCHITIS

Acute orchitis, by definition, is a primary infection of the testis and, as such, is rare. Most often, orchitis is seen as a secondary infection related to an initial epididymal infection. Orchitis may occur during a systemic illness in which systemic seeding of the testis occurs with *E. coli, Klebsiella, Pseudomonas, Staphylococcus,* and *Streptococcus*. Most commonly, influenza, infectious mononucleosis, tuberculosis, syphilis, and amebiasis cause orchitis. The latter pathogens occur most often in immunocompromised patients.

Mumps orchitis occurs in males systemically infected with the virus, but seldom before puberty. About 15% to 20% of postpubertal males with mumps develop orchitis. The onset of the testicular swelling normally occurs 3 to 7 days after the development of parotitis. One-third of men with mumps orchitis, however, do not have parotitis. One-third of cases may be bilateral. Atrophy results in about 50% of involved testes.

CLINICAL PRESENTATION

The usual presentation of orchitis is high fever, nausea, vomiting, and gradual onset of testicular pain radiating to the groin. There are usually no urinary or urethral symptoms. The testis is uniformly enlarged and tense and tender to palpation, while the epididymis is normal. A reactive hydrocele, cutaneous erythema, and scrotal enlargement are common and may make palpation of the testis difficult.

DIFFERENTIAL DIAGNOSIS

When there is systemic infection, the differential diagnosis is not difficult. In the absence of systemic features, epididymoorchitis and testicular torsion must be considered. The onset of epididymoorchitis is slower than that of orchitis, which is slower than the onset of testicular torsion. In orchitis, palpation of the cord and epididymis reveals the spermatic cord to be much less thickened and the epididymis to be in its normal posterior position.

EMERGENCY DEPARTMENT EVALUATION

Because orchitis is, most often, part of a systemic process, attention should be directed at the primary disease. In the minority of patients with orchitis as the main manifestation, an examination should be accompanied by a urinalysis. Pyuria may imply a primary epididymal process with extension to the testis (epididymoorchitis). Orchitis is such a rare diagnosis that a color Doppler ultrasound should be done to confirm normal testicular blood flow, thus eliminating testicular torsion from the differential diagnosis.

EMERGENCY DEPARTMENT MANAGEMENT

Treatment for mumps orchitis is generally supportive with bedrest, scrotal elevation, and analgesics. Resolution requires 1 to 3 weeks. Steroid therapy is probably not helpful. Making incisions in the testicular tunica albuginea early in the course of the disease has been tried as a means of reducing intratubular pressure but has shown no appreciable benefit. Atrophy occurs in about 50% of affected testes, regardless of treatment.

HYDROCELE AND OTHER DISORDERS OF THE SPERMATIC CORD

A hydrocele is the most common cause of nonacute intrascrotal swelling. It is an accumulation of serous fluid in the potential space between the visceral and parietal layers of the tunica vaginalis that normally envelopes and fixes the anterolateral aspect of the testis and epididymis to the posterior scrotal wall, preventing testicular torsion. Most hydroceles are found in older patients, and an underlying cause is not identified. A sudden onset of a symptomatic hydrocele can occur secondary to epididymitis, trauma, or tumor.

Approximately 10% of testicular tumors have a reactive hydrocele as the presenting complaint.[10] In pediatric hydroceles, congenital failure of the tunica vaginalis to obliterate after birth allows communication between the scrotum and the peritoneum, creating a hydrocele or hernia. These "communicating hydroceles" acutely enlarge and shrink depending on patient activity, as peritoneal fluid and occasionally a loop of intestine fill the scrotum when the patient is in the upright position and spontaneously decompress when the patient is supine. This is the classic history of scrotal swelling that vanishes when the child sleeps.

CLINICAL PRESENTATION

Most hydroceles in adults develop gradually and are asymptomatic. A chronically enlarging hydrocele may present as scrotal enlargement associated with a heavy sensation, occasionally radiating to the groin. An acute hydrocele may present with pain, depending on the inciting event.

The classic hydrocele is a cystic, pear-shaped mass located anterior to the testis and epididymis. It often obscures definitive palpation of the testis. Transillumination most often reveals a translucent mass surrounding an opaque testicular shadow. A hydrocele should be confined to the scrotum, with a normal spermatic cord above it. Rarely, a hydrocele of the spermatic cord can be palpated in the region of the external inguinal canal.

DIFFERENTIAL DIAGNOSIS

The most common disorders to consider in the differential diagnosis include spermatocele, varicocele, traumatic hematocele, and inguinal hernia.

A hematocele is blood or a blood clot within the potential space between the two leaves of the tunica vaginalis. It occurs most often after needle aspiration of a hydrocele, but it can accompany testicular torsion or trauma. A cystlike mass, similar to a hydrocele, can be felt on examination. However, the mass does not transilluminate. Following trauma, this type of swelling may become quite large. Ultrasonography can differentiate blood from less echogenic hydrocele fluid and reveal a ruptured testis or testicular tumor. In the absence of a reasonable history or diagnostic ultrasonography, a hematocele should be explored.

A spermatocele is a common cystic mass lying above and posterior to the testis. Spermatoceles are retention cysts arising from the epididymis and contain spermatozoa.[10] Usually painless, these masses may alarm the patient about a possible testicular tumor. A spermatocele is usually soft, freely mobile, and lucent on transillumination, but may become firm in a chronic state. Most spermatoceles are less than 1 cm in size, but can become as large as 10 cm. It is not possible to differentiate a spermatocele from a lipoma or other adnexal mass by palpation alone. Combining the examination with ultrasonography can usually confirm the diagnosis. Excision is required only when the size of the spermatocele causes pain or there is a question regarding the diagnosis.

A varicocele is a dilatation of the testicular pampiniform venous plexus.[2] A varicocele is usually a chronic condition, but the acute appearance of a varicocele, especially on the right side, can herald a retroperitoneal tumor, tumor adenopathy, renal cell carcinoma, or renal vein thrombosis. Varicoceles are more common on the left than on the right and usually present as a mass above the testis, often referred to as a "bag of worms" because of the multiple torturous vessels imprinting the scrotal skin. Nearly 20% of men have a left varicocele of some degree.[23] The left side predominates because the left testicular vein drains perpendicularly into the left renal vein without valves to reduce hydrostatic pressure, as compared with the right testicular vein, which drains obliquely into the inferior vena cava. Right-sided varicoceles are only seldom seen without a concomitant left varicocele.

Most varicoceles are asymptomatic, but if symptoms occur, they are usually limited to the upright position (increased gravity) and include heaviness on the affected side that is usually relieved by assuming a supine position. Most often, reassurance suffices.

An inguinal hernia may present as an acute swelling in the scrotum. The clinical history is variable and not helpful. The exception is an incarcerated hernia that occurs most commonly during the first year of life and is accompanied by signs of peritoneal irritation or obstruction (i.e., nausea and/or vomiting). Most hernias may be palpated in the superior scrotal and inguinal regions.[10] Transillumination is usually not helpful. The auscultation of bowel sounds in the hemiscrotum may help to identify a hernia. Uncomplicated reduction of bowel through the inguinal defect into the abdominal cavity confirms the diagnosis.

A sperm granuloma is an inflammatory response to sperm that have entered the interstitium; it can occur in the epididymis, vas deferens, or testis. A sperm granuloma is most commonly found at the site of a previous vasectomy or in the epididymis following an epididymotomy. A sperm granuloma is generally small and asymptomatic, but, at times, presents as a palpable, painful intrascrotal mass. This creates a problem only in differentiating the granuloma from a testicular tumor. The physical and ultrasound examinations demonstrate an extratesticular mass that is usually confluent with the epididymis or vas deferens. Rarely, testicular granulomas require diagnostic exploration. Emergency department treatment consists of antiinflammatory agents and pain medication.

EMERGENCY DEPARTMENT EVALUATION

Many hydroceles preclude palpation of the testis. Transillumination is insensitive in eliminating tumor as the inciting cause. Often, the history suggests epididymitis as the cause, but the epididymis is hidden by the hydrocele. Epididymitis should be suspected if the urinalysis discloses pyuria. Scrotal ultrasonography is the diagnostic test of choice for detecting masses within the testis; it is the best modality to image the epididymis through a hydrocele.

EMERGENCY DEPARTMENT MANAGEMENT

The priority in emergency department evaluation of hydroceles is disclosing the etiology. Underlying reversible causes should be treated. Very infrequently, aspiration of the hydrocele is required to permit adequate examination and provide relief from painful swelling. The technique involves anterior aspiration through an 18-gauge, pliable venous catheter inserted over a needle cannula.

The indwelling, flexible, atraumatic tip prevents damage to the opposing testicle during collapse of the hydrocele and can be positioned in the most dependent area of the scrotum to ensure adequate drainage. The maneuver is not definitive because recurrence is guaranteed. Surgical exploration is necessary if a palpable mass remains poorly defined. Otherwise, the treatment of hydroceles is elective, being indicated when the size of the scrotum is unacceptable cosmetically or interferes with physical activity.

DISPOSITION

The acute development of a hydrocele requires referral based on the suspected underlying cause.

COMMON PITFALLS

Dismissal of a newly developed hydrocele as a benign process may delay diagnosis of an underlying testicular malignancy.

OTHER DISORDERS PRESENTING AS A SCROTAL MASS

Infectious disorders of the scrotal skin and urethra can present as an acute scrotal mass. Primary abscesses of the scrotal skin occur from infections of the hair follicles or sweat glands. These are common and similar to abscesses anywhere else on the body. These types of abscess are limited to the superficial layers of the scrotal skin.

Deep scrotal infection usually arises from infection of the lower urinary tract or perirectal disease. Commonly, such infections originate from extravasation of infected urine as a result of urethral instrumentation or urethral stricture disease and periurethral abscess formation. Infection also may originate from perirectal and ischiorectal abscesses. Often, the etiology is not clear. These abscesses are rooted deep in the perineum and may spread extensively by the time they cause obvious cutaneous lesions. Spread of infection to the urethral corpus spongiosum may result in bacteremia. Eventually, the tunica albuginea is penetrated, with spread to Buck's fascia. Once Buck's fascia is invaded, the next barrier is Colles' fascia. Infection may spread anteriorly along Colles' fascia to involve the scrotum, resulting in an acute scrotal mass.

Fournier's gangrene, or idiopathic synergistic necrotizing fasciitis, is a rapidly spreading subcutaneous infection that presents as massive scrotal swelling, with progression to necrosis of the scrotal wall within 24 hours if not recognized or treated. The average age of the patient is 55 years, and immunocompromised patients have a higher incidence of occurrence.[17] Diabetics, steroid users, chronic alcohol abusers, or patients with the human immunodeficiency virus are at risk. The typical organisms include hemolytic streptococci, *Bacteroides fragilis, E. coli,* and *Clostridium* species.

CLINICAL PRESENTATION

Superficial scrotal skin abscesses seldom cause difficulty in diagnosis. A localized area of erythema with a smaller area of suppuration is found on examination. Most patients are afebrile and without constitutional symptoms. No laboratory work is required. Superficial abscesses may be incised and drained under local anesthesia in the emergency department.

Deep scrotal abscesses and early Fournier's gangrene can present as generalized scrotal swelling. The onset may occur several days after instrumentation of a urethral stricture or in an inadequately treated diabetic with an initial superficial skin abscess. The patient may have a history of perirectal disease. Pain is usually intense, but initial physical examination of the affected area can be devastatingly subtle. Fever and other constitutional symptoms are often present. A diabetic patient may present with ketoacidosis. The scrotal contents often cannot be palpated because the entire scrotum is edematous, red, tense, and warm. Frequently, no localized area of fluctuation is detected.

DIFFERENTIAL DIAGNOSIS

Scrotal edema from congestive heart failure or lymphatic obstruction can occasionally appear similar to scrotal infection. Concomitant anasarca or edema of the lower extremities shifts the differential diagnosis away from an infectious cause. Occasionally, edema of the scrotum occurs as a result of an allergic reaction. The scrotum should not be tender to palpation and the erythema is considerably less. Constitutional symptoms, including fever, are absent. Cellulitis of the scrotum may present with significant edema. This is rare without an underlying cause, but it can occur. Less tenderness should be found in an otherwise healthy patient, but the distinction from a deep abscess may be difficult to ascertain. Epididymoorchitis that has progressed to suppuration and overlying skin fixation can present with scrotal swelling similar to that seen with a deep scrotal abscess. Often indistinguishable on examination, both require surgical drainage.

EMERGENCY DEPARTMENT EVALUATION

Rapid diagnosis and treatment of bacteremia are the principles of initial management. If the diagnosis remains in question, ultrasonography has the ability to detect abscess cavities within fascial planes and is helpful in differentiating cellulitis from a deep abscess. A plain pelvic radiograph (KUB) occasionally demonstrates subcutaneous air. If urethral obstruction is suspected as the inciting cause, a urethral catheter should be placed into the bladder. If obstruction is encountered, an immediate urethrogram may be diagnostic. The rectum and perineum should be examined carefully for induration and fluctuance.

EMERGENCY DEPARTMENT MANAGEMENT

Fournier's gangrene requires aggressive medical and surgical resuscitation, intravenous fluids, broad-spectrum antibiotics (Unasyn, Timentin, or piperacillin). These modalities should be instituted as soon as possible, and urologic consultation obtained while alerting the operating room for aggressive surgical debridement. If perirectal disease is suspected, a general surgeon must also be consulted, as a temporizing colostomy will most likely be required.

DISPOSITION

Role of the Consultant

Surgical drainage with wide debridement and antibiotic therapy must be instituted rapidly because of the extremely aggressive nature of Fournier's gangrene. Postoperative hyperbaric oxygen therapy is recommended and will promote wound healing.[17]

Indications for Admission

Patients with complex scrotal abscesses should be admitted through the operating room. Cellulitis of the scrotum can be difficult to distinguish from a secondary skin reaction associated with a deeper infection. Cellulitis requires intravenous antibiotics, serial examinations, and close follow-up.

Transfer Considerations

Patients should be transferred if surgical consultation or intensive care beds are not available.

COMMON PITFALLS

- The most common mistake involves underestimating the severity of an infection. With Fournier's gangrene, a delay of 4 to 8 hours can make a significant difference in morbidity.
- In the very early stages, most severe scrotal infections mimic cellulitis, and the clinician may mistakenly be tempted to treat the problem on an outpatient basis with oral antibiotics without aggressive follow-up.

Acknowledgment

The author gratefully acknowledges the contribution of Douglas Swartz, who wrote the previous version of this chapter.

References

1. Anderson JB, Williamson RLN. The fate of the human testes following unilateral torsion of the spermatic cord. *Br J Urol* 1986;58:698.
2. Bar-Charma N, Palmer LS, Cohen S, et al. The adolescent varicocele: when to treat. *Emerg Med* June 3, 1993:73.
3. Bennett RT, Bhagwant G, Kogan SJ. Epididymitis in children: the circumcision factor? *J Urol* 1998;160:1842.
4. Boyarsky S, Steinhardt GF, Onder R. Medical aspects of testicular torsion. *Mo Med* 1990;87:359.
5. Burks DD, Markey BJ, Burkland TK, et al. Suspected testicular torsion and ischemia: evaluation with color Doppler sonography. *Radiology* 1990;175:815.
6. Cattolica EV. Preoperative manual detorsion of the torsed spermatic cord. *J Urol* 1985;133:803.
7. Centers for Disease Control and Prevention. 1998 Guidelines for treatment of sexually transmitted diseases. *MMWR* 1998;47(RR-1):1.
8. Dixon AR, Sayers RD. Testicular torsion in older men [Letter]. *BMJ* 1987;295:269.
9. Friedman SC, Sheynkin YR. Acute scrotal symptoms due to perforated appendix in children: case report and review of literature. *Pediatr Emerg Care* 1995;181.
10. Gilchrist BF, Lobe TE. The acute groin in pediatrics. *Clin Pediatr* 1992;31:488.
11. Gold SJ. *Physicians medical law letter* [monograph] New York: Prof Liability Pub, 1987.
12. Hagen P, Buchholz MM, Eigenmann J, et al. Testicular dysplasia causing disturbance of spermiogenesis in patient with unilateral torsion of the testis. *Urol Int* 1992;49:154.
13. Harwood-Nuss AL. Genitourinary disease. In: Rosen P, ed. *Emergency medicine,* 4th ed. St. Louis: CV Mosby, 1996:1539.
14. Knight PJ, Vassy LE. The diagnosis and treatment of the acute scrotum in children and adolescents. *Ann Surg* 1984;200:664.
15. Lee LM, Wright JE, McLaughlin MG. Testicular torsion in the adult. *J Urol* 1983;130:93.
16. Muschat M. The pathological anatomy of testicular torsion, an explanation of its mechanism. *Surg Gynecol Obstet* 1932;54:758.
17. Paty R, Smith AD. Gangrene and Fournier's gangrene. *Urol Clin North Am* 1992;19:149.
18. Prater JM, Overdorf BS. Testicular torsion: a surgical emergency. *Am Fam Physician* January 15, 1991;44:834.
19. Procedures for your practice—testicular detorsion. *Patient Care* 1991:143.
20. Rabinowitz R. The importance of the cremasteric reflex in acute scrotal swelling in children. *J Urol* 1984;131:89.
21. Rabinowitz R, Hulbert WC. Acute scrotal swelling. *Urol Clin North Am* 1995;22:101.
22. Rowland G, Donohue JP. Scrotum and testis. In: Gillenwater JY, Grayhack JT, Howards SS, Duckett JW, eds. *Adult and pediatric urology,* 2nd ed. Chicago: Year Book, 1991:1565.
23. Schneider RE. Urologic procedures. In: Roberts JR, Hedges JR, eds. *Clinical procedures in emergency medicine,* 3rd ed. Philadelphia: WB Saunders, 1998:957.
24. Schwab R. Acute scrotal pain requires quick thinking and plan of action. *Emerg Med Rep* 1992;13:11.
25. Wilbert DM, Schaerfe CW, Stern WD, et al. Evaluation of the acute scrotum by color-coded doppler ultrasonography. *Urology* 1993;149:1475.

CHAPTER 68
Miscellaneous Urologic Conditions

Douglas McGee

Emergency physicians are required to evaluate and treat afflictions of the male and female genital tracts. This chapter defines these clinical entities and provides treatment recommendations. Disorders of the penis, including balanoposthitis, phimosis, paraphimosis, and priapism, and disorders of the female genitourinary tract, including Bartholin gland abscess, vaginal foreign bodies, and imperforate hymen are discussed. Infectious disorders of the genital tract, nephrolithiasis, cutaneous genitourinary disease, and acute scrotal pain are covered elsewhere in this text.

DISORDERS OF THE FORESKIN AND GLANS PENIS

Balanoposthitis[14,20]

Balanitis refers to inflammation of the glans penis. *Posthitis* refers to inflammation of the prepuce of the penis. Because balanitis and posthitis usually occur together, *balanoposthitis* correctly describes a male with inflammation of the glans and prepuce. Balanitis is more common in uncircumcised men who exercise poor hygiene, but it may affect young boys. Patients with balanoposthitis present with a prepuce and glans that is edematous, erythematous, fissured, and painful. Various skin changes are possible based on the etiology. The differential diagnosis of balanoposthitis is divided into infectious and noninfectious causes. Fungal infections with *Candida albicans* cause itching and burning of the penis, accompanied by white discharge, discrete ulcerated papules, and white, cheesy plaques. Group B streptococci, *Gardnerella vaginalis,* and mixed anaerobes have been isolated from men with balanoposthitis. Secondary syphilis and condyloma lata may infect the glans. Protozoal infections with *Trichomonas vaginalis* and amoebiasis have been reported. Genital herpes may cause necrotizing balanoposthitis, and human papillomavirus (HPV) can induce genital warts on the glans or foreskin. Noninfectious causes of balanoposthitis include trauma, latex allergy, and various dermatoses. Dermatologic lesions include psoriasis, lichen planus, erythema multiforme, and a variety of premalignant and malignant lesions. When balanoposthitis is severe, phimosis may occur and precipitate urinary retention.

The emergency department (ED) evaluation is usually limited to the history and physical examination. Test the patient for diabetes mellitus when infection with *C. albicans* is suspected. Perform serologic testing for syphilis when this organism is suspected. Acetic acid whitens the superficial epithelial skin layer when applied to lesions infected with HPV. Meticulous hygiene, including retraction of the foreskin and cleansing of the glans penis and prepuce, is the mainstay of treatment. Direct the treatment of infectious balanoposthitis toward the offending organism. Treat fungal infections of the glans with topical antifungal agents. Use metronidazole to treat *Gardnerella,* anaerobic infection, and *Trichomonas* infections. Treat secondary syphilis according to established guidelines.

Treat patients who have balanoposthitis as outpatients except when they have associated medical diseases, such as diabetes. This group requires hospital treatment. When phimosis is present and causes urinary retention, consultation in the ED with a urologist may be required to relieve the phimosis to allow for free drainage of urine. All patients with balanoposthitis require follow-up with their primary physician and may benefit from urologic evaluation for circumcision. Refer patients with skin lesions suspicious for precancerous changes or malignancy to a dermatologist for evaluation.

Phimosis

When the foreskin is not retractable behind the glans penis, the condition is termed *phimosis.* Physiologic phimosis is present until normal adhesions between the foreskin and glans have separated. Although most young boys are able to retract the foreskin by puberty, retraction is usually possible at an earlier age.[5,7] As normal secretions accumulate and epithelial sloughing occurs, smegma is formed. Smegma assists in the separation of the foreskin from the glans and is normal. Parents may confuse smegma with infectious penile discharge if expressed from the penis. Pathologic phimosis, or simply phimosis, occurs when retraction of the foreskin is not possible after puberty or when the foreskin was previously retractable.[5]

Asymptomatic phimosis does not require emergent treatment. Reassure concerned parents when physiologic phimosis is present. Do not encourage them to attempt forceful retraction. When severe phimosis causes urinary retention or interferes with placement of a urinary catheter, a slit made in the dorsal aspect of the foreskin facilitates access to the urethral meatus.[14,18] After achieving adequate local anesthesia of the penis with a dorsal nerve block or ring block placed at the base of the penis, gently separate adhesions between the foreskin and glans with a hemostat. Place one jaw of the hemostat inside the dorsal foreskin, taking care not to include the urethral meatus or glans. Close the hemostat on the foreskin, crushing it for 3 to 5 minutes. Incise the crushed foreskin with straight scissors. The crushed edges rarely bleed but may require absorbable suture for hemostasis if they separate. Although some patients are satisfied with the cosmetic appearance of the foreskin after the dorsal slit procedure, the urologist may perform definitive circumcision.

Paraphimosis

Paraphimosis occurs when the retracted foreskin is not replaced, usually after cleansing or catheter insertion. Paraphimosis requires definitive treatment in the ED. After foreskin retraction, the constricting phimotic ring causes progressive edema, impairs venous return, and threatens the viability of the glans. Although most patients complain of pain and usually provide a history of foreskin retraction, debilitated, uncircumcised patients may not provide this history. Do not confuse paraphimosis with balanitis in these patients.

After adequate sedation or penile anesthesia, attempt manual reduction. Place fingers of both hands behind the phimotic ring and foreskin while applying gentle, steady pressure on the glans with the thumbs.[5,14,18] Gauze placed under the fingers may improve traction on the foreskin while bringing it over the glans, but lubricants are rarely helpful. Several other techniques are described to treat paraphimosis; application of these techniques should be guided by the physician's skill and training in the maneuvers. A 21-gauge needle can be used to puncture the edematous foreskin; manual compression after puncture allows the escape of enough edema fluid to facilitate reduction.[2,14] Blood aspirated from the glans after a tourniquet is placed at the base of the penis may allow reduction.[17] Subdermal hyaluronidase injected into the edematous foreskin facilitates dispersion of edema fluid and may make reduction possible.[6] Granulated sugar has been applied to the edematous glans and foreskin to extract tissue water and ease reduction.[13] When less aggressive methods fail, the phimotic ring is incised with a scalpel to facilitate foreskin reduction.[18] Prevention is key; ED personnel must replace the foreskin after urinary catheter placement.

Priapism

Priapism is characterized by a prolonged, painful, unwanted penile erection, usually in the absence of sexual stimulation. The physiologic balance achieved between venous outflow and arterial dilatation of the corpora cavernosa controls erectile function. Priapism occurs when normal physiologic blood flow is altered. Today, medications used to treat erectile dysfunction in men (papaverine, prostaglandin E1, etc.) cause most cases of priapism.[4,9] It is uncommon in boys, unless sickle cell disease is present, and it is rare in neonates.[19] Patients with priapism present to the ED complaining of penile pain and persistent erection, even after ejaculation. The mean time to presentation in one series of 34 patients was 30 hours.[9] The penis is erect and painful to palpation. The corpora cavernosa is engorged, but, in contrast to normal erections, the corpus spongiosum and glans penis are flaccid.

The differential diagnosis is divided into "low-flow" and "high-flow" priapism.[9] Simply stated, low-flow priapism results from impaired venous outflow. High-flow priapism results from abnormally increased arterial flow.

Low-flow priapism is far more common than high-flow priapism and is often caused by vasoactive drugs that cause engorgement of the corpora cavernosa. Impaired venous outflow causes sludging, thrombosis, acidosis, and decreased oxygen tension within the corporal bodies. This pathophysiologic cascade causes the irreversible cellular damage and corporal fibrosis responsible for the long-term complications of low-flow priapism. Intracavernosal agents used for erectile dysfunction, antihypertensive agents, psychotropic drugs, cocaine, and ethanol are among the drugs that have been implicated. Leukemia, sickle cell anemia, and a variety of neoplastic etiologies are also responsible for priapism.[9,16]

High-flow priapism is uncommon and usually results from trauma to the penis or perineum.[12] Arterial fistula formation between the cavernosal artery and the corporal bodies increases arterial flow into the penis that exceeds venous outflow.

The history usually suggests the etiology of the patient's priapism. Careful attention to prescription or illicit drug use may help determine whether these agents are responsible. Suspect sickle cell disease among patients at risk when the history of sickle cell disease is unknown. Elicit the history of prior episodes of priapism and record the onset of erection. On examination, the penis is painful to palpation and the corporal bodies are engorged, but the glans and the corpus spongiosum are soft. Some authors recommend blood gas analysis of blood aspirated from the corporal bodies to assist in identifying the etiology.[9,18] Low pH, low oxygen tension, and high carbon dioxide levels suggest low-flow, venous obstruction. Blood gas parameters similar to arterial blood suggest high-flow priapism, a condition usually seen after trauma.

Emergency physicians must treat priapism when the urologist is not immediately available for consultation. Most cases of priapism encountered in the ED treatment will be low-flow priapism. There is conflicting literature describing terbutaline's efficacy in priapism. Some small clinical trials have demonstrated that oral terbutaline is more effective than placebo in achieving detumescence[15]; others have found no benefit.[8] Because of its relative safety in patients without hypertension or coronary artery disease, a trial of subcutaneous terbutaline (0.25 to 0.5 mL injected subcutaneously, repeated in 20 minutes if needed), or 5 mg of oral terbutaline, repeated in 15 minutes, may be attempted.[18] When sedation, analgesia, and/or terbutaline do not result in detumescence, corporal aspiration and irrigation is indicated.[9,18] Anesthetize the penis and aspirate 30 to 60 mL of blood from a single corporal body at the 10 o'clock or 2 o'clock position. Do not puncture the glans. Anastomoses between the corporal bodies obviate the need for bilateral aspiration. When the erection persists after aspiration, a careful injection of phenylephrine into the punctured corpus cavernosum may be done (Fig. 68.1). One milligram of phenylephrine is diluted in 9 mL of sterile saline to achieve a concentration of 1000 μg per milliliter. Inject 200-μg aliquots of phenylephrine up to three times to achieve detumescence. Monitor the blood pressure and rhythm when repeated injections are required. If this treatment fails to relieve the erection, urologic evaluation for corporal body shunting is required. If the urologist is unavailable, transfer the patient to definitive care. Sickle cell patients with priapism require analgesia, hydration, supplemental oxygen, and, when traditional antisickling measures fail, red blood cell exchange transfusion.[16]

Emergent therapy in the ED is not required for high-flow priapism because it does not cause the ischemic injury seen in low-flow priapism. Order Doppler flow ultrasonography of the penis and perineum to document arteriovenous fistulas when suspecting high-flow priapism.[12]

BARTHOLIN GLAND ABSCESS, VAGINAL FOREIGN BODIES, IMPERFORATE HYMEN

The Bartholin glands are located in the labia minora and drain by a duct that exits between the hymen and the labium. These glands are not normally palpable but can form asymptomatic cysts or become infected and abscessed. Patients between 20 and 30 years of age present complaining of a painful, indurated mass located lateral to the vaginal introitus.[1,11] The infection is polymicrobial and may contain *Neisseria gonorrhoeae* and *Chlamydia trachomatis*. The differential diagnosis of Bartholin gland swelling includes sebaceous cysts, mucoid cysts, and various benign and malignant vulvar masses. Other cystic lesions (e.g., inclusion cysts, Gartner duct cysts, and endometriosis) can occur but are rarely confused with a Bartholin gland abscess.[11]

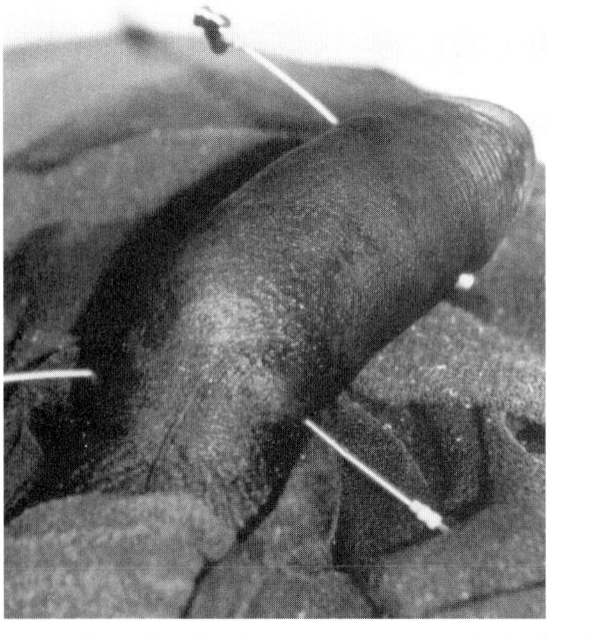

Figure 68.1. The penis undergoing corpus cavernosum injection for priapism.

Prescribe sitz baths, analgesics, and gynecologic follow-up when the abscess has pointed and ruptured spontaneously. As is true for most abscesses, antibiotics after drainage are not routinely given. If the abscess has not drained spontaneously, it is appropriate in the ED to perform incision and drainage and the placement of a Word catheter.[3,11] Insert the catheter through a 1.0- to 1.5-cm stab incision made in the abscess just inside the hymenal ring. Tuck the free end of the catheter into the vagina; it should remain in place for at least 4 weeks to allow fistula formation. The patient should be referred to a gynecologist for follow-up within 5 to 7 days. If a Word catheter is not available, perform a traditional incision, drainage, and packing. Patients with Bartholin gland abscesses are usually treated as outpatients but should be referred to a gynecologist for reevaluation. Recurrent abscesses or abscesses treated with simple incision and drainage may require marsupialization by a gynecologist.

Vaginal bleeding or spotting, discharge, and odor suggest a vaginal foreign body, particularly in the prepubertal female.[10] Adult female patients usually provide a history of foreign-body insertion, but young girls usually do not. Although curious children may inadvertently place some objects in the vagina, vaginal foreign bodies are often placed as part of sexual abuse. Recurrent pelvic pain, recurrent urinary tract infection, and retroperitoneal perforation have been reported in association with vaginal foreign bodies. When vaginal foreign bodies are found in young girls, sexual abuse must be suspected. Patients require the multidisciplinary approach, diligence, respect, and attention to evidence collection that is afforded any victim of suspected sexual abuse. Small children may require intravenous sedation or anesthesia and the expertise of a pediatric gynecologist to remove the foreign body. Thorough speculum examination and removal with forceps are usually sufficient for vaginal foreign bodies that cannot be recovered by the patient.

When primary amenorrhea is present, the differential diagnosis in the adolescent female with abdominal pain includes imperforate hymen, demonstrated by a bulging hymen that is dark in color due to retained menstrual blood.[5] Refer patients with suspected imperforate hymen to a gynecologist.

COMMON PITFALLS

- Phimosis is normal in young boys and does not require treatment in asymptomatic adults.
- Paraphimosis can look like balanitis unless the emergency physician recognizes that the foreskin is retracted.
- ED personnel should take great care to always return the foreskin to its anatomic location after retraction.
- Priapism is a urologic emergency that requires ED treatment in coordination with the consulting urologist. Red cell exchange therapy may be necessary when priapism occurs in a patient with sickle cell disease.
- Vaginal foreign bodies in girls should always raise the possibility of sexual abuse.

References

1. Aghajanian A, Bernstein L, Grimes DA. Bartholin's duct abscess and cyst: a case control study. *South Med J* 1994;87:26–29.
2. Barone JG, Fleisher MH. Treatment of paraphimosis using the "puncture" technique. *Pediatr Emerg Care* 1993;9:298–299.
3. Blumstein H. Incision and drainage. In: Roberts JR, Hedges JR, eds. *Clinical procedures in emergency medicine*. Philadelphia: WB Saunders, 1998:643.

4. Broderick GA. Intracavernous pharmacotherapy. *Urol Clin North Am* 1996;23:111–126.
5. Brown MR, Cartwright PC, Snow BW. Common office problems in pediatric urology and gynecology. *Pediatr Clin North Am* 1997;44:1091–1115.
6. DeVries CR, Miller AK, Packer MG. Reduction of paraphimosis with hyaluronidase. *Urology* 1996;48:464–465.
7. Golubovic Z, Milanovic D, Vukadinovic V, et al. The conservative treatment of phimosis in boys. *Br J Urol* 1996;78:786–788.
8. Govier FE, Jonsson E, Kramer-Levien D. Oral terbutaline for the treatment of priapism. *J Urol* 1994;151:878–879.
9. Harmon WJ, Nehra A. Priapism: diagnosis and management. *Mayo Clin Proc* 1997;72:350–355.
10. Herman-Giddens ME. Vaginal foreign bodies and child sexual abuse. *Arch Pediatr Adolesc Med* 1994;148:195–200.
11. Hill DA, Lense JJ. Office management of Bartholin gland cysts and abscesses. *Am Fam Physician* 1998;57:1611–1616.
12. Ilkay AK, Levine LA. Conservative management of high flow priapism. *Urology* 1995;46:419–424.
13. Kerwat AS, Stephenson B. Reduction of paraphimosis using granulated sugar. *Br J Urol* 1998;82:755.
14. Langer JC, Coplen DE. Circumcision and pediatric disorders of the penis. *Pediatr Clin North Am* 1998;45:801–812.
15. Low FC, Jarow JP. Placebo-controlled study of oral terbutaline and pseudoepinephrine in management of prostaglandin E1-induced prolonged erections. *Urology* 1993;42:51–53.
16. Powars DR, Johnson CS. Priapism. *Hematol Oncol Clin North Am* 1996;10:1363–1372.
17. Raveenthiran V. Reduction of paraphimosis: a technique based on pathophysiology. *Br J Surg* 1996;83:1247.
18. Scheinder RE. Urologic procedures. In: Roberts JR, Hedges JR, eds. *Clinical procedures in emergency medicine*. Philadelphia: WB Saunders, 1998:947.
19. Walker JR, Casale AJ. Prolonged penile erection in the newborn. *Urology* 1997;50:796–799.
20. Waugh MA. Balanitis. *Dermatol Clin* 1998;16:757–762.

PART IX

Emergency Aspects of Obstetrics

CHAPTER 69

Complications of Fertility Regulation Methods

Andrew M. Kaunitz

Although modern methods of contraception are extremely safe, use of each method is associated with a certain incidence of complications. In this chapter, complications associated with hormonal contraceptives, intrauterine devices (IUDs), and barrier and spermicidal contraceptives are addressed. Evaluation and management of several of the more serious complications (e.g., thromboembolic disease and pelvic infections) are covered elsewhere. Fortunately, complications of contraception are infrequent and usually minor.

HORMONAL CONTRACEPTIVES

Oral contraceptives (OCs) were introduced in 1960. Since that time, the dose of estrogen and progestin in each tablet has declined dramatically. The use of low-dose OCs (less than 50 mg ethinyl estradiol) and more sophisticated prescribing practices have resulted in a marked reduction in the risk of complications.[6] The incidence of deep venous thrombosis and pulmonary embolism in women currently using low-dose OCs is two to four times higher than in nonusers.[10] Because thromboembolism is rare in reproductive-age women (four to ten cases annually per 100,000 women), the attributable risk of thromboembolism associated with OC use is approximately six to 30 annual cases per 100,000 users.[13] The two- to fourfold increased risk of thrombosis associated with OC use contrasts with a six- to 15-fold increased risk associated with pregnancy.[13] Use of low-dose OCs does not increase the risk of coronary artery or cerebrovascular disease.[15,18] Healthy, nonsmoking women who are older than age 35 can safely use OCs until menopause.

Hypertension and migraine headaches have traditionally been thought to be increased by the use of OCs. However, it is unclear that a causal relationship between OC use and these two entities exists.[12,24] Provided careful follow-up is maintained, otherwise healthy, nonsmoking, well-controlled hypertensive women younger than age 35 can use combined OCs. Otherwise, hypertensive women should use progestin-only or nonhormonal contraceptives. Continuous administration of low-dose combined OCs can prevent menstrual migraines.[22] However, if OC use is accompanied by worsening migraine intensity or frequency, OCs should be discontinued in favor of progestin-only or nonhormonal methods. A recent randomized, double-blind, placebo-controlled trial found that use of a specific OC formulation (triphasic norgestimate) did not cause headaches.[11]

Many laypersons believe that OCs cause cancer. Published studies have demonstrated that OC use does not increase the risk of breast cancer and that the risks of endometrial and ovarian cancer are substantially reduced by OCs.[6]

Although the low-dose OC has improved safety, it has also produced two bothersome side effects: breakthrough bleeding and absence of withdrawal bleeding. Breakthrough bleeding tends to occur early in the use of OCs, often resolving with time. A vaginal speculum examination should be performed to exclude such pathologic conditions as vaginitis, cervicitis,[9] a cervical polyp, or carcinoma. If the patient has not taken her OCs appropriately, or if pregnancy is suspected, a pregnancy test should be performed.

When breakthrough bleeding persists in a woman using a low-dose estrogen OC, adding extra estrogen (e.g., 1.25 mg conjugated equine estrogen or its equivalent) in the first 7 days of the OC pack for several months may resolve this problem.[7] The emergency physician may initiate these pharmacologic changes after consultation with a clinician, who will provide follow-up.

In the early 1990s, two highly effective, long-acting, progestin-only contraceptives became available in the United States: levonorgestrel subdermal implants (Norplant) and injectable depot medroxyprogesterone acetate (Depo-Provera).[8] Implants can provide up to 5 years of contraception. Depo-Provera is administered by deep intramuscular injection every 3 months.

Menstrual changes are the most common side effect among women using continuous progestin-only methods. Most women using Norplant experience an irregular bleeding pattern during the first year following implant insertion; this declines to one-third of users by the fifth year. Approximately one-third of women experience regular cycles during their first year, increasing to two-thirds by the fifth year of implant use. Pregnancy testing should be performed in Norplant users when amenorrhea abruptly occurs in women who had experienced regular cycles.[17] Although pregnancies occur only rarely in implant users, should a pregnancy be diagnosed, the likelihood of an ectopic implantation is higher than in women using no contraceptive method. Although women using Depo-Provera may also experience irregular bleeding initially, over three-fourths of long-term users experience amenorrhea. As with women taking OCs, women experiencing irregular bleeding during use of Norplant or Depo-Provera can be treated with oral estrogen (conjugated estrogen 1.25 mg or its equivalent daily) after vaginal examination to rule out infectious or neoplastic causes of bleeding.

Occasionally, wound infection occurs after implant placement. Some of these infections are the result of the ends of the implant being placed too close to the incision, thus preventing wound healing. Women with infection resulting from Norplant insertion should be treated with antibiotics effective against *Staphylococcus aureus* and referred to a physician knowledgeable about contraceptive implants. In most cases, the implants will be removed.

Headache is commonly reported by women using Norplant.[20] Most headaches do not have features of migraines and may resolve over time. However, because cases of idiopathic intracranial hypertension have been reported, retinal examination should be performed in implant users with headaches.

Some women develop ovarian cysts[16] that may cause lower abdominal discomfort. More often, they are asymptomatic and noted incidentally during pelvic examination. Ovarian cysts in Norplant users should be managed expectantly. Surgical intervention is rarely necessary and should be reserved for cases in which a cyst fails to resolve or when torsion or rupture is suspected.

INTRAUTERINE DEVICES

Two intrauterine devices (IUDs) are currently marketed in the United States. The most widely used IUD, the Copper T 380A, is currently approved for 10 years of use. The progesterone-releasing IUD must be replaced annually. After decades of controversy, the association between pelvic inflammatory disease (PID) and IUD use is now better understood. When IUD insertion is performed in women at low risk for sexually transmitted diseases, the risk of PID appears no higher than in nonusers.[23] Emergency physicians may be confronted by a number of IUD-associated problems: coexistent PID, pregnancy, expulsion, and perforation.

When women wearing an IUD present with PID, antibiotic therapy should be initiated. In this setting, most clinicians recommend IUD removal once antibiotic therapy has been initiated. Antibiotics should cover both gonococci and *Chlamydia*. Guidelines for admission are essentially the same as for those patients without an IUD (see Chapter 82, "Pelvic Inflammatory Disease"). If outpatient therapy is appropriate, close follow-up should be arranged (48 to 72 hours post–emergency department visit). If PID occurs in a woman who has been wearing an IUD for 5 years or longer, a tuboovarian abscess caused by *Actinomyces israelii* may be present. High-dose intravenous penicillin (or clindamycin in penicillin-allergic patients) is the drug of choice.[1]

Pregnancy occurs in less than one woman per 100 users of Copper T 380A IUDs annually. The risk of miscarriage, preterm labor, and sepsis is increased, however, and the incidence of spontaneous abortion may be a high as 50%. The risk of losing the pregnancy is reduced by removing the IUD. If the tail of the IUD is visible on vaginal speculum examination, gentle traction should be used to remove the IUD. This should be performed by a clinician experienced with IUDs. If the tail is not visible, no effort should be made to probe for it. In this setting, if the woman does not want to have an abortion, she should be advised to seek medical attention if signs of infection (fever, abdominal pain, bleeding, or cramping) occur. Some clinicians have reported successful sonographically assisted IUD removal when the string is not visible.[21]

Because the Copper T 380A is an extremely effective contraceptive, few intrauterine or ectopic pregnancies occur. However, when an accidental pregnancy does occur in an IUD user, an ectopic pregnancy will be present in approximately 5% (Copper T 380A) or 15% (progesterone-releasing IUD) of cases.[19] Complaints of vaginal bleeding, abdominal pain, or amenorrhea in IUD users should be carefully evaluated for the possibility of an ectopic pregnancy.

Between 3% and 10% of patients have spontaneous expulsion of an IUD within a year of insertion.[3] Although a patient's inability to feel her IUD may represent expulsion or perforation, most often a correctly positioned device is found. On examination, the IUD tail may be obscured by cervical mucus. If a tail is not seen, plain films can be used to determine the presence or absence of the IUD. In this setting, however, vaginal ultrasonography may be necessary to accurately localize the device. Partial expulsion may be associated with intermenstrual bleeding or cramping. The IUD tail often lengthens and the tip of the IUD may be felt in the vagina by the woman or her sexual partner. A partially expelled IUD is usually visible or palpable during vaginal examination and should be removed.

Most IUD perforations through the uterine wall occur at the time of insertion. With modern IUDs, the incidence of perforation is substantially less than 1%. An uncomplicated perforation may be managed by laparoscopy or laparotomy. Although not an emergency, early removal of intraabdominal copper-bearing IUDs minimizes adhesion formation. Some IUD perforations are not noted until intraabdominal bleeding or infection results. Immediate gynecologic consultation is appropriate.

BARRIER AND SPERMICIDAL CONTRACEPTIVES

Barrier methods and spermicides prevent sexually transmitted diseases, including human immunodeficiency virus infection. Few complications result from the use of condoms, diaphragms, and vaginal spermicides containing nonoxynol 9. Allergies to the latex in condoms and diaphragms, the spermicide nonoxynol 9, or the lubricants or vehicles may result in local reaction on the vaginal mucosa or penis. Nonlatex condoms and diaphragms are commercially available. Use of diaphragms with spermicidal jelly or condoms with spermicidal foam may increase the risk of urinary tract infection.[4]

Toxic shock syndrome has been reported in users of the diaphragm.[2] Risk can be minimized by not leaving diaphragms in place longer than 24 hours and by avoiding their use during menses. Displacement or breakage of a barrier contraceptive increases the risk of pregnancy. Postcoital (emergency) contraception (see Chapter 88, "Sexual Assault") is most effective if used within 72 hours of intercourse. The availability of a prescription emergency contraceptive kit (Preven, Gynétics, Somerville, NJ) should facilitate use of this underutilized approach to fertility regulation.

RISK OF ECTOPIC PREGNANCY IN THE SETTING OF CONTRACEPTIVE OR STERILIZATION FAILURE

In general, women who use contraception experience a lower risk of ectopic pregnancy than sexually active women using no birth control. Oral, injectable, and copper intrauterine contraceptives markedly reduce users' absolute risk of experiencing an intrauterine or ectopic pregnancy. The only two contraceptive methods that do not reduce users' overall ectopic risk are progestin-only OCs (minipills) and the progesterone IUD (Progestasert, Alza, Palo Alto, CA).

When pregnancy occurs in a contraceptive user or sterilized woman, the likelihood that the pregnancy is ectopic is 33% in sterilized women, 6% in copper IUD users, 17% in Norplant users, and 23% in women using the progesterone IUD.[5,14] Therefore, when emergency physicians diagnose pregnancy in sterilized women or those using intrauterine or implantable contraception, prompt vaginal sonography and prompt follow-up measures to monitor for possible ectopic pregnancy are mandated.

References

1. Case records of the Massachusetts General Hospital: case 10-1992. *N Engl J Med* 1992;326:692.
2. Centers for Disease Control. Toxic shock syndrome and the vaginal contraceptive sponge. *MMWR* 1984;33:43.
3. Chi I-C. The TCU380A (AG), MLCU375, and NOVA-TIUDs and the IUD daily releasing 20 mcgm levonorgestrel—four pillars of IUD contraception for the nineties and beyond? *Contraception* 1993;47:325.
4. Hooton TM, Hillier S, Johnson C, et al. *Escherichia coli* bacteriuria and contraceptive method. *JAMA* 1991;265:64.
5. Kaunitz AM. Revisiting progestin-only OCs. *Contemp OB/GYN* 1997; December:91.
6. Kaunitz AM. Oral contraceptive estrogen dose considerations. *Contraception* 1998;58[Suppl 3]:15S.
7. Kaunitz AM. Oral contraceptives. In: Stovall TG, Ling FW, eds. *Gynecology for the primary care physician*. Philadelphia: Current Medicine Group, 1999;83.
8. Kaunitz AM. Contraceptive choices. In: Nobel J, ed. *Textbook of primary care medicine*, 3rd ed. St. Louis: Mosby, *(in press)*.
9. Krettek JE, Arkin SI, Chaisilwattana P, et al. *Chlamydia trachomatis* in patients who used oral contraceptives and had intermenstrual spotting. *Obstet Gynecol* 1993;81:728.
10. Lidegaard Ø, Edström B, Kreiner S. Oral contraceptives and venous thromboembolism: a case-control study. *Contraception* 1998;57:291.
11. Lippman JS, Godwin A, Olson W. The tolerability of a triphasic norgestimate/EE containing OC: results from a double-blind, placebo-controlled trial. Abstract presented at the 46th Annual Meeting of the American College of Obstetricians and Gynecologists, New Orleans, 1998; Redmond G, Godwin AJ, Olson W, Lippman JS. Use of placebo controls in an oral contraceptive trial: Methodological issues and adverse event incidence. *Contraception* 1999;60:81.
12. Mattson RH, Rebar RW. Contraception methods for women with neurologic disorders. *Am J Obstet Gynecol* 1993;168:2027.
13. Ory H. Cardiovascular safety of oral contraceptives—what has changed in the last decade? *Contraception* 1998;58[Suppl 3]:9S.
14. Peterson HB, Xia Z, Hughes JM, et al. The risk of ectopic pregnancy after tubal sterilization. *N Engl J Med* 1997;336:762.
15. Pettiti DB, Sidney S, Bernstein A, et al. Stroke in users of low-dose oral contraceptives. *N Engl J Med* 1996;335:8.
16. Shoupe D, Horenstein J, Mishell DR, et al. Characteristics of ovarian follicular development in Norplant users. *Fertil Steril* 1991;55:766.
17. Shoupe D, Mishell DR, Bopp BL, et al. The significance of bleeding patterns in 30 Norplant implant users. *Obstet Gynecol* 1991;77:256.
18. Sidney S, Siscovick D, Petitti D, et al. Myocardial infarction and use of low-dose oral contraceptives: a pooled analysis of 2 US studies. *Circulation* 1998;98:1058.
19. Sivin I. Dose and age-dependent ectopic pregnancy risks with intrauterine contraception. *Obstet Gynecol* 1991;78:291.
20. Sivin I, Mishell DR Jr, Darney P, et al. Levonorgestrel capsule implants in the United States: a 5-year study. *Obstet Gynecol* 1998;92:337.
21. Stubblefield P, Fuller A, Foster S. Ultrasound-guided intrauterine removal of intrauterine contraceptive devices in pregnancy. *Obstet Gynecol* 1998;72:961.
22. Sulak PJ, et al. Extending the duration of active oral contraceptive pills to manage hormone withdrawal symptoms. *Obstet Gynecol* 1997;89:179.
23. Walsh T, Grimes D, Frezieres R, et al. Randomised controlled trial of prophylactic antibiotics before insertion of intrauterine devices. *Lancet* 1998;351:1005.
24. Woods J. Oral contraceptives and hypertension. *Hypertension* 1988;11[Suppl II]:II-11.

CHAPTER 70
Pregnancy Testing

Howard A. Werman

Pregnancy testing is seldom performed in the emergency department to detect the presence of a normal pregnancy. Rather, it is used for a specific subset of clinical circumstances that mandate the need for a rapidly performed and extremely sensitive test to exclude the possibility of pregnancy. Among the currently accepted emergency department uses of pregnancy testing are the following:

- To exclude an ectopic pregnancy
- To determine whether a pregnancy existed before the assault in cases of rape
- To exclude pregnancy in women who are to be treated with medications that may be contraindicated in pregnancy
- To exclude pregnancy in women who must undergo extensive radiographic procedures
- To evaluate blunt and penetrating abdominal trauma in women
- To exclude pregnancy in women with certain suspected medical conditions that may be harmful to the fetus (i.e., rubella, herpes cervicitis, alcoholism)
- To detect a possible underlying cause in cases of intentional overdose or toxic ingestion and to provide advice regarding the effect of the ingested substance(s) on the pregnancy

The diagnosis of pregnancy is established by detecting the presence of human chorionic gonadotropin (hCG).[3] The detection of hCG in the serum or urine does not guarantee a normally located or properly developing fetus. hCG is a glycoprotein hormone that is produced by trophoblastic cells of the placenta. The major biologic effect of hCG is maintenance of the corpus luteum. The hormone is composed of two subunits: α and β.

There are three other glycoprotein hormones that share an almost identical α subunit: luteinizing hormone (LH), follicle-stimulating hormone, and thyroid-stimulating hormone. The β subunit, however, is specific to hCG and is therefore a highly specific indicator of pregnancy.

After implantation of the ovum in the endometrium, trophoblastic cells initiate placental development with rapidly rising levels of hCG (Fig. 70.1). hCG can be detected by qualitative urine or serum pregnancy tests as early as 6 to 9 days after implantation. Levels of 50 IU/L may be reported as early as 1 week after implantation, although individual variation exists. This represents the lowest level of hCG to which most newer urine pregnancy tests are sensitive. One day after a missed menses, the levels are generally in excess of 100 IU/L. Serum hCG levels double every 1.4 to 2.1 days, until they peak at approximately 60 days after implantation. Thereafter, hCG levels plateau and remain detectable up to 3 weeks after delivery. Quantitative serum measurements should be interpreted with great caution, however, because there is marked biologic variation in the levels for each patient at a given point in the pregnancy. Urine hCG levels closely parallel serum values.[11]

hCG levels also remain elevated after elective or spontaneous termination of pregnancy and after removal of an ectopic pregnancy.[5,7] The half-life of hCG after termination of pregnancy is approximately 1.5 days, and clearance depends on the stage at which the pregnancy was terminated as well as the underlying reason for loss of the pregnancy. Patients with induced abortions have a detectable level of hCG up to 60 days (median, 30 days) after termination of pregnancy, whereas patients with

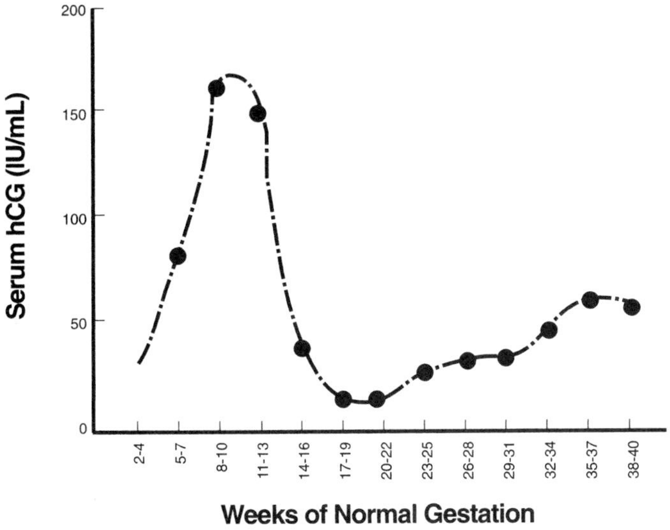

Figure 70.1. Fluctuation of serum human chorionic gonadotropin (hCG) during normal intrauterine gestation. (Adapted from Varma K, Larraga L, Selenkow HA. Radioimmunoassay of serum human chorionic gonadotropin during normal pregnancy. *Obstet Gynecol* 1971;37:10.)

spontaneous abortions and those with ectopic pregnancy may have positive pregnancy tests for up to 35 days (median, 19 days) and 31 days (median, 8.5 days), respectively (Fig. 70.2).

CLINICAL PRESENTATION

Pregnancy should be considered in any woman of childbearing age who presents to the emergency department. A careful gynecologic and sexual history should be taken for all potentially childbearing women, particularly when one of the conditions listed earlier may exist. Pregnancy can often be inferred from certain subjective observations made by the patient and from objective physical findings, but it should always be confirmed by laboratory testing and, when appropriate, imaging modalities. This is particularly true for certain populations, such as adolescents or poisoned patients, in whom establishing the diagnosis of pregnancy can be difficult based on the history and physical examination.[16,17]

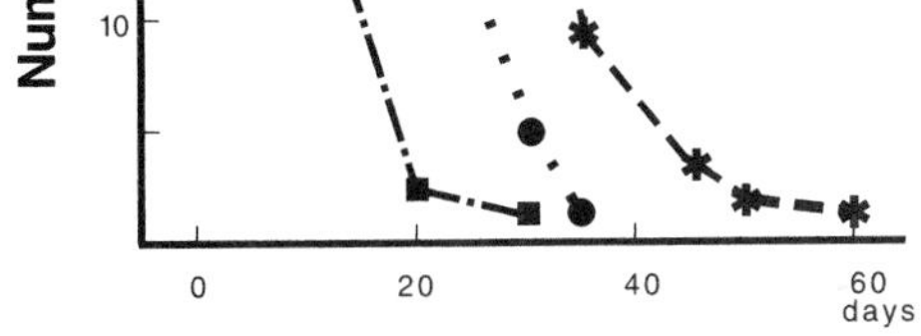

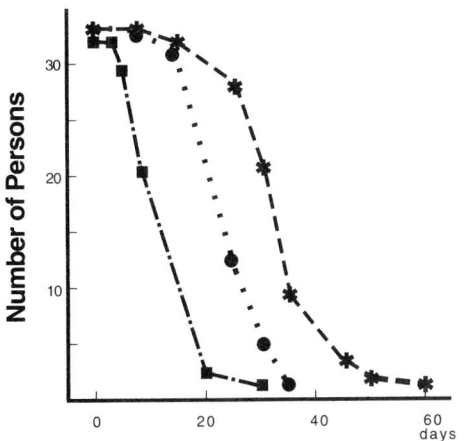

Figure 70.2. Number of patients with detectable levels of hCG β subunit (less than 10 IU/L) in serum after induced abortion, spontaneous abortion, and ectopic pregnancy, by time. *Right curve* indicates women with induced abortion. *Middle curve* indicates women with spontaneous abortion. *Left curve* indicates women with ectopic pregnancy. (Redrawn after Steier JA, Bergsjo P, Myking OL. Human chorionic gonadotropin in maternal plasma after induced abortion, spontaneous abortion, and removed ectopic pregnancy. *Obstet Gynecol* 1984;64:391.)

Cessation of menses is the first symptom of pregnancy in most patients. This is reliable only if the patient had previously experienced regular menstruation. Additionally, some women experience bleeding after implantation of the fertilized ovum, and this may be misinterpreted as a normal menstruation. Ten percent of women seen in the emergency department who reported a previous normal menstrual cycle and denied that there was any chance of pregnancy were later found to be pregnant.[10] Other symptoms that are often described include sensitivity of the nipples, fullness and tingling of the breasts, nausea, vomiting, bladder irritability, urinary frequency, and fatigue. Quickening, or the sensation of fetal movement, is usually noted after the sixteenth week of pregnancy.

Among the early physical findings in pregnancy is Hegar's sign, which is softening of the lower uterine segment. This sign may be present as early as 1 to 2 weeks after a missed menses. It may be accompanied by a blue discoloration of the cervix (Chadwick's sign) or softening of the cervix (Goodell's sign). A darkening of the breast areola is noted. The pregnancy is accompanied by enlargement of the uterus. The uterine fundus can be appreciated above the pelvic brim at approximately 12 weeks. Finally, the appearance of fetal heart tones after 10 weeks of pregnancy can be used to establish the diagnosis.

Positive or negative results from recently performed home pregnancy tests should be interpreted with great caution in patients presenting to the emergency department. These tests are often performed incorrectly, and the results may be inaccurate.[13]

EMERGENCY DEPARTMENT EVALUATION

There have been many technologic advances in the area of pregnancy testing over the past few years, making older diagnostic techniques, such as bioassay and agglutination inhibition tests, obsolete.

Because of the emergency physician's need for a sensitive test that can be performed rapidly, only two types of pregnancy tests should be considered for use in the emergency department. These are the β-specific hCG radioimmunoassays (RIAs) for serum and the β-specific enzyme-linked immunosorbent assay (ELISA). RIAs require 1 to 2 hours to perform and are able to detect from 5 to 40 IU/mL. They have a reported specificity of 99%. The primary use of these tests is in quantitative testing, discussed later in this chapter.

In the ELISA test, a substrate is added to the patient's urine specimen, which has been previously labeled with an enzyme-linked antibody. In the presence of hCG, the enzyme acts on the added substrate to produce a characteristic color change. Urine ELISA tests may require as little as 3.5 minutes to perform and can detect levels as low as 10 to 75 IU/L (many newer tests claim a sensitivity of 20 IU/L). They have a reported specificity of 99%. Serum ELISA tests require a longer period of time to process but are sensitive to a lower level of hCG.

Several quantitative measures of hCG are available. These tests may be particularly useful in detecting abnormal pregnancies (such as ectopic pregnancies) if the levels are followed every 48 hours. A rise in the serum hCG level of less than 20% or a fall in the levels has a 100% predictive value for fetal demise (or ectopic pregnancy).[4] Additionally, a quantitative value of more than 50,000 IU/L makes the diagnosis of ectopic pregnancy unlikely.[14]

The measurement of serum progesterone levels using a direct RIA has shown promise in discriminating normal and abnormal gestations.[8] Levels of progesterone below 25 ng/mL are strongly suggestive of an abnormal gestation, including ectopic pregnancy.[15] Levels less than 5 ng/mL identify nonviable pregnancies with a high degree of accuracy. Unfortunately, the test is not widely available for emergency department evaluation.

Transvaginal ultrasonography can be used in the emergency department to determine the presence of an intrauterine pregnancy. A gestational sac should be detectable at approximately 4 weeks when the serum hCG is above 400 to 800 IU/mL. In the skilled hands of an observer who frequently performs ultrasonography, the technique is invaluable. Unfortunately, this is not always the case in hospital emergency departments at all hours.

COMMON PITFALLS

- There are several situations in which the use of serum or urine pregnancy tests may lead to incorrect results. False-negative urine pregnancy tests can result from dilute urine specimens. This is why a morning first-void urine is used to test for pregnancy under normal circumstances. This approach, however, is not practical for emergency department patients. Cartwright[2] found that all of the women with false-negative pregnancy results in his study were patients with a urine specific gravity below 1.015. This problem was alleviated by using 20 drops of urine instead of the recommended 5 drops.
- False-negative urine pregnancy tests have also been noted in patients with ectopic pregnancy when hCG levels are generally less than expected for dates. False-negative rates of greater than 10% have been demonstrated, even with the newer urine pregnancy tests.[1,6,9]
- False-positive results have also been a problem with both urine and serum pregnancy tests. It must be remembered that pregnancy tests detect hCG and do not *per se* test specifically for pregnancy.
- False-positive tests occur in less than 1% and are most commonly seen in postmenopausal women. Trophoblastic tumors (hydatidiform mole, choriocarcinoma) secrete hCG and will yield false-positive pregnancy results. Trophoblastic cells are not the only cells that are capable of secreting hCG. hCG has been secreted by a variety of tumors, including gastrointestinal neoplasms, lymphoma, leukemia, myeloma, sarcoma, breast carcinoma, bronchogenic carcinoma, adrenocortical carcinoma, renal cell carcinoma, and melanoma. More important, normal tissues such as ovary, pituitary gland, lung, liver, kidney, spleen, and stomach contain biologically inactive hCG. As lower levels of hCG are detected by both urine and serum tests, more false-positive results are expected.
- Older pregnancy tests that do not utilize specific hCG β-subunit antibodies will give false-positive results in the presence of LH. This may occur in patients with LH-secreting conditions (e.g., menopausal women, ovariectomy, hypothyroidism), in patients on phenothiazines or methadone, or in patients with immunologic disease. Proteinuria can produce false-positive results when agglutination inhibition tests are used.

References

1. Barnes RB, Roy S, Yee B, et al. Reliability of urinary pregnancy tests in the diagnosis of ectopic pregnancy. *J Reprod Med* 1985;30:827.
2. Cartwright PS. Performance of a new enzyme-lined immunoassay urine pregnancy test for the detection of ectopic pregnancy. *Ann Emerg Med* 1986;15:1198.
3. Chard T. Pregnancy tests: a review. *Hum Reprod* 1992;7:701.
4. Collins WP. Early pregnancy tests. *Br J Obstet Gynecol* 1990;97:204.
5. Pittaway DE. hCG dynamics in ectopic pregnancy. *Clin Obstet Gynecol* 1987;30:129.
6. Romero R. Human chorionic gonadotropin assay sensitivity on screening for ectopic pregnancy [Letter]. *Am J Obstet Gynecol* 1986;155:681.
7. Saver MN. New methods for diagnosis and management of ectopic pregnancy. *Resid Staff Phys* 1987;33:39.
8. Steier JA, Bergsjo P, Myking OL. Human chorionic gonadotropin in maternal plasma after induced abortion, spontaneous abortion, and removed ectopic pregnancy. *Obstet Gynecol* 1984;64:391.
9. Tsokos N, Masters AM, Boyne P. Emergency serum and urine hCG analyses with the "Tandem ICON" procedure. *Aust N Z J Obstet Gynaecol* 1986;26:284.
10. Ramoska EA, Saccheti AD, Neppo M. Reliability of patient history in determining the possibility of pregnancy. *Ann Emerg Med* 1989;18:48–50.
11. Naryshkin S, Aw TC, Filstein M, et al. Comparison of the performance of serum and urine hCG immunoassays in the evaluation of gynecologic patients. *Ann Emerg Med* 1985;14:1074–1076.
12. O'Connor RE, Bibro CM, Pegg PG, et al. The comparative sensitivity and specificity of serum and urine hCG determinations in the ED. *Am J Emerg Med* 1993;11:431–436.
13. Daviaud J, Fournet D, Ballongie C, et al. Reliability and feasibility of pregnancy home-tests: laboratory validation and diagnostic evaluation by 638 volunteers. *Clin Chem* 1993;39:53–59.
14. Stovall TG, Ling FW. Ectopic pregnancy diagnostic and therapeutic algorithms minimizing surgical interventions. *J Reprod Med* 1993;38:807–812.
15. Stovall TG, Kellerman AL, Ling FW, et al. Emergency department diagnosis of ectopic pregnancy. *Ann Emerg Med* 1990;19:1098–1103.
16. Causey AL, Seago K, Wahl NG, et al. Pregnant adolescents in the emergency department: diagnosed and not diagnosed. *Am J Emerg Med* 1997;15:125–130.
17. Jones JS, Dickson K, Carlson S. Unrecognized pregnancy in the overdosed or poisoned patient. *Am J Emerg Med* 1997;15:538–541.

CHAPTER 71

Drugs in Pregnancy

Mary H. Stewart

Pregnant women are frequently evaluated and treated by emergency physicians. As a result, emergency physicians prescribe medications for gravid women more often than any other group of physicians, with the exception of obstetricians. It is therefore necessary that they have an understanding of the effect of a variety of medications on the pregnant patient as well as her fetus.

Between one- and two-thirds of all pregnant women will take at least one medication during pregnancy.[18] The most commonly used drugs are antimicrobial agents, antiemetics, tranquilizers, and analgesics.[18] It is estimated that half of the pregnancies in North America are unplanned, thereby exposing thousands of fetuses to drugs before the women are aware they are pregnant.[14] The actual risks of most drugs during pregnancy are unknown. No medication can be considered as proven "safe" during pregnancy.[29] The use of any medication during pregnancy requires that the need to treat the mother be balanced against the potential adverse effects to the fetus. Additionally, the risk of drug use during pregnancy must be balanced against the risk of uncontrolled disease.[29] Major malformations occur in 2% to 4% of all newborns; 1% of these can be attributed to medication in general.[29] Although the absolute numbers of abnormalities due to medications are relatively low, these are thought to be potentially the most preventable birth defects.[29] This chapter has a twofold focus: (1) medications commonly used in the emergency department for the treatment of urgent or emergent conditions and (2) medications frequently prescribed on an outpatient basis.

MATERNAL AND FETAL DRUG RESPONSES

Maternal and fetal drug responses are influenced by two factors during pregnancy. First, pregnancy-induced changes in maternal physiology can cause alterations in the absorption, distribution, and elimination of drugs in the mother. Second, the placental–fetal unit affects the amount of drug entering the fetal circulation, the fraction of drug metabolized by the placenta, and the distribution and elimination of the drug by the fetus.[18]

TERATOLOGY

Birth defects are generally considered to be structural defects of the newborn. These may be divided into three categories: (1) malformations that are structural defects caused by intrinsic problems in embryologic differentiation or development; (2) disruptions that occur when normal fetal development has been disrupted, such as a limb amputation as a result of amniotic bands; and (3) deformations of a normally differentiated part, such as Potter's facies.[31] During the time between conception and implantation, the embryo is relatively insensitive to teratogenic effects. This time is associated with an "all or none" response in which the embryo either survives unharmed or dies.[31] The conceptus is most susceptible to major organ malformations during the period of embryogenesis, from 4 to 12 weeks after the onset of the last menstrual period.[29] After organogenesis, a teratogen can affect the growth of organs, the size of the organs, or their function. Toward the end of pregnancy, drugs may directly affect the fetus and newborn, causing complications at the time of delivery or with postnatal care.

FOOD AND DRUG ADMINISTRATION CLASSIFICATION

In 1979, the Food and Drug Administration (FDA) developed five categories for use in drug labeling to provide a better assessment of fetal risk. These categories are not perfect and have resulted in some ambiguous statements. This may create difficulty in counseling and may produce anxiety in women. These categories have not been consistently upgraded with the acquisition of new data.[14] The Teratology Society advocates development of a new system utilizing an evidence-based, narrative approach.[14] Countries such as Sweden, Australia, Switzerland, and Denmark have different classification systems; however, all are based on stratification of fetal risk.

Class A. Controlled human studies have shown no risk to the fetus.

Class B. Either (1) animal studies have shown no risk and no human studies have been done, or (2) animal studies have shown an adverse effect, but this has not been confirmed in humans.

Class C. Either (1) animal studies have shown an adverse effect and there are no controlled human studies, or (2) there are no studies in animals or humans.

Class D. There is a demonstrated human fetal risk, but the benefit of use may outweigh the risk.

Class X. Studies have demonstrated human risk and the risk outweighs any possible benefit. These agents are contraindicated in women who are or may become pregnant.

Many agents have dual categories, which reflect safe use during one portion of pregnancy and unsafe use in another. Examples include ibuprofen (B/D) and sulfonamides (B/D).[14]

Physicians can consult several teratogen information services to receive current, evidence-based information on the safety of drugs during pregnancy. In Canada, The Motherisk Program in Toronto is accessible by phone or World Wide Web as are the Organization of Teratology Information Services in the United States and several state organizations.

Motherisk Program: (416)813-6780; http://www.motherisk.org
Organization of Teratology Information Services: (801)328-2229; http://orpheus.ucsd.edu/ctis/

DRUG THERAPY DURING PREGNANCY

Safety

Fetal safety is a major concern in guiding the selection of drugs prescribed during pregnancy. Effective drugs that have been in use for a long time are thus preferred over newer preparations. Exposure should be decreased by using the smallest effective dose for the shortest duration possible. No drug should be prescribed during pregnancy without a clear need.

Analgesics

Acetaminophen

Acetaminophen is the analgesic and antipyretic drug of choice at any time during pregnancy. Large population-based studies have shown no increase in congenital malformation with the use of acetaminophen or paracetamol.[19,27]

Aspirin

Aspirin is the drug most frequently taken during pregnancy. It readily crosses the placenta. Some case-controlled studies have reported associations between aspirin use in pregnancy and congenital malformations. The Collaborative Perinatal Project in the United States studied more than 50,000 pregnancies and failed to show low-dose aspirin as a cause of stillbirth, reduced birth weight, teratology, or an increase in perinatal deaths.[30] The Michigan Medicaid Surveillance Study, which investigated 1709 pregnancies in which exposure to aspirin occurred during the first trimester, also failed to demonstrate an increase in congenital malformations.[24]

The use of high-dose aspirin in the second half of pregnancy is more controversial. Pregnant women treated with more than 3 g per day for rheumatoid arthritis during the second half of pregnancy were found to have prolonged gestation and labor. High-dose aspirin given near to delivery has been demonstrated to cause bleeding tendencies and central nervous system (CNS) hemorrhage in the newborn, particularly in premature infants.[24] The near-term use of aspirin may cause constriction or closure of the fetal ductus arteriosus due to the inhibition of prostaglandin synthetase.[26]

Nonsteroidal Antiinflammatory Drugs

Nonsteroidal antiinflammatory drugs (NSAIDs) (e.g., ibuprofen, indomethacin, naproxen, sulindac, diclofenac) have been predominantly studied in their role as tocolytic agents. These drugs are reversible inhibitors of prostaglandin synthetase and inhibit premature uterine contractions. Fetal exposure to NSAIDs has been associated with premature closure of the ductus, resulting in pulmonary hypertension.[26] A reduction in amniotic fluid is also associated with the use of these drugs.[24] The Michigan Medicaid Surveillance Study collected data from 3178 first-trimester exposures to ibuprofen and found no teratogenicity of the drug. In addition, when ibuprofen was used as a tocolytic (115 cases), the effects noted on the ductus and amniotic fluid volume were reversed with the discontinuation of the drug.[24] Experience with most NSAIDs in humans is limited, and it must be suspected that all agents that inhibit prostaglandin synthesis can cause adverse effects during pregnancy. Therefore, the potential toxicity of NSAIDs is the basis for the recommendation that they be used judiciously and not in the third trimester.[24,26]

Opiates

Morphine, meperidine, and oxycodone are safe analgesic agents during pregnancy and have not demonstrated any teratogenic effects.[3] The use of codeine appears to be safe. Codeine has been associated with certain congenital defects; the significance of which is unknown.[3] The use of any opiate can produce respiratory and CNS depression in the newborn. This may be safely reversed in the infant with administration of naloxone. Chronic use of opiates during pregnancy may result in neonatal addiction and withdrawal.[3]

Antiasthmatics

Asthma complicates approximately 1% of pregnancies and may be associated with increased risk of prematurity and low birth weight.[29] The risks of drug use during pregnancy must be weighed against the risks of uncontrolled asthma. No asthma medication to date meets the criteria for FDA Class A.[29]

Beta-Mimetics

Albuterol, metaproterenol, and terbutaline have been used safely in pregnancy. There is no increased risk of congenital malformation associated with these agents.[8,29] Limited data are available on the use of oral beta-agonists in early pregnancy. All beta-agonists have been used in the third trimester to prevent premature labor; however, in therapeutic doses, they do not appear to prolong term labor.[3,8,29] Hyperglycemia may be present transiently, and neonatal hyperglycemia can also occur.[3]

Epinephrine

Epinephrine has been theorized to reduce uterine blood flow, and some studies have shown an increase in congenital malformations with its use.[3,8] Other studies have not demonstrated this increase.[29] Generally, the severity of disease in women requiring epinephrine is worse than in those who do not receive this drug, and epinephrine may indeed be the causative factor in this association. Epinephrine is, therefore, only relatively contraindicated in pregnancy and may be used when other agents fail.

Theophylline

Theophylline compounds are considered safe during pregnancy. There is no increase demonstrated in congenital malformations.[29] Theophylline may accumulate during the third trimester as a result of decreased clearance. Thus, maternal drug levels should be followed closely. There are reports of neonatal transient theophylline toxicity as well.[3,8,29] Current asthma practice suggests that theophylline should be used for pregnant patients whose asthma is otherwise not controlled.[29]

Sodium Cromoglycate

No fetal compromise or congenital malformations have been reported with the use of cromolyn.[8,29] Cromolyn is the recommended drug for prophylaxis in pregnant women.[29]

Corticosteroids

Aerosolized corticosteroids are the preparation of choice for pregnant patients. Beclomethasone dipropionate has been studied the most, but all are considered safe.[8,29] A spacer device should be used to enhance respiratory tract penetration and minimize oral deposition and systemic effects. Corticosteroids are indicated for the treatment of severe asthma in pregnancy.[29] The current literature neither confirms nor excludes adverse effects of systemic steroids on the incidence of low birth weight or preeclampsia.[29] Some steroids are used to enhance pulmonary lung maturity.[8] The use of steroids when necessary to control asthma is considered significantly more beneficial than the risk of uncontrolled disease in the pregnant patient.[8,29]

Anticoagulants

Heparin

Heparin does not cross the placenta and is of no direct risk to the fetus. It is the anticoagulant of choice in the pregnant patient.[3] There may be a significantly increased risk of antepartum hemorrhage.

Warfarin

The coumarin derivatives are contraindicated in pregnancy due to their high association with congenital malformations (approximately 30% of cases).[3] The greatest risk occurs between the sixth and ninth weeks of gestation; however, CNS malformations may occur with exposure at any time during pregnancy.

Thrombolytics

There is limited information on the use of thrombolytics in pregnancy. Though there have been successful case reports, the complications of these agents are well known and the risk of antepartum hemorrhage is significant.

Anticonvulsants

The risk of birth defects in healthy, pregnant women is 2% to 4% and rises to 4% to 6% in pregnant women taking one antiepileptic drug.[6] Exposure to these agents presents the greatest risk to the fetus from the third to eighth week after conception.[6] The teratogenic effects are worsened with the use of combination therapy.[6] Women who require medication should be maintained on the most effective agent with the lowest teratogenic potential.[8] Generalized seizures during pregnancy may cause increased risk of spontaneous abortion or hypoxic injury. There are case reports of intrauterine death after one isolated seizure.[32] The Antiepileptic Drug Pregnancy Registry is the first North American registry for pregnant women taking any antiepileptic drug. Contact may be made by

Phone: (800)233-2334
World Wide Web: http://neuro-www2.mgh.harvard.edu/aed/registry.nclk

Phenytoin (Class D)

Phenytoin is considered a human teratogen. It is estimated that 7% to 10% of children exposed will develop intrauterine growth retardation, motor and developmental delays, facial dysmorphia, and limb abnormalities.[8] As many as 3% may have major malformations, including cleft lip or palate and microcephaly.[8] Neonatal coagulopathy as a result of deficiency of the vitamin K–dependent coagulation factors is another complication of phenytoin therapy. It may be prevented by administration of vitamin K to the mother during the last trimester or to the infant art birth.[6,8] Phenytoin also decreases serum folic acid levels, which is reported to cause megaloblastic anemia and neural cord defects.[6,8] This responds well to folic acid supplementation.[8]

Carbamazepine (Class C)

There have been reports of craniofacial defects, hypoplastic fingernails, and developmental delays in infants exposed to carbamazepine.[6,8] As with phenytoin, folic acid deficiency may lead to neural tube defects; folate should be supplemented and antenatal alpha-fetoprotein testing considered.[8]

Phenobarbital (Class D)

Phenobarbital may contribute to folic acid deficiency and coagulation defects, as does phenytoin.[8] Neonatal depression and withdrawal syndromes may also be seen. The literature implicating phenobarbital as a teratogen is inconclusive, with one large study showing no evidence of teratogenic risk.[8] Therefore, phenobarbital is probably considered safe in pregnant epileptics.

Valproic Acid (Class D)

Valproic acid is teratogenic in animals and humans.[3,6,8] It readily crosses the placenta and concentrates in the fetus. Neural tube defects occur in approximately 2.5% of exposed pregnancies.[8] The teratogenic effects of phenytoin, phenobarbital, or carbamazepine are worsened by the addition of valproic acid.[6] Valproic acid should not be considered for women of childbearing age.[6]

Trimethadione (Class X)

Trimethadione is the most potent teratogenic anticonvulsant. It is associated with an 80% rate of malformation and frequent spontaneous abortions. It should not be used in pregnancy.[8]

Benzodiazepines (Class D)

Benzodiazepines readily cross the placenta and accumulate in the circulation of the embryo.[23] The literature remains divided as to whether benzodiazepines cause an increase in congenital malformations. A recent study demonstrated no difference in the prevalence of congenital abnormalities between women taking benzodiazepines and controls.[32] Third-trimester treatment of women with diazepam has been shown to cause apnea, hypotonia, and hypothermia in the newborn.[32] In chronically treated patients, tremor, irritability, and hypertonia as a result of withdrawal may be seen in some infants.[32]

New Antiepileptic Drugs

Felbamate, gabapentin, lamotrigine, and topiramate are newer agents available for the treatment of epilepsy. There is little clinical information regarding their use and safety in pregnant women.[6,8]

Antimicrobials

Penicillins

Beta-lactam antibacterials are the oldest class of antibacterials used in the treatment of infections during pregnancy.[18] They are water-soluble, cross the placenta by diffusion, circulate in the fetus, are excreted into the amniotic fluid, and recycle in the fetus by gastrointestinal absorption. Penicillins and their derivatives have not been shown to be associated with congenital malformations and are considered safe in pregnancy.[3,6,8,18] They are all listed as FDA category B.[9]

Erythromycin

Erythromycin is considered safe for use in pregnancy.[3,9] The estolate form of erythromycin is associated with hepatotoxicity in the mother and should be avoided in pregnancy. It is listed as FDA category B.[9]

Azithromycin

Azithromycin is a relatively new macrolide with a prolonged half-life. No studies for safety in pregnancy have been done in humans. It is listed as FDA category B.[9]

Clarithromycin

Clarithromycin has been used in pregnancy to treat or prevent *Mycobacterium avium* complex (MAC) in human immunodeficiency virus (HIV)-positive women. No studies of its safety in pregnancy have been done in humans. It is listed as FDA category C.[9]

Cephalosporins

Cephalosporins are considered safe during pregnancy. Though controlled studies are lacking, there are no reported cases of congenital malformation. All of these are listed as FDA category B.[3,9] First- and second-generation cephalosporins have been shown to have lower plasma concentrations in pregnant women than those in nonpregnant women. This is felt to occur because of increased volume of distribution and faster clearance.[18] However, a study of ceftriaxone (third-generation) in pregnant women demonstrated the pharmacologic behavior to be similar to that in nonpregnant women.[18]

Imipenem

Imipenem is the first in a new class of antibiotics, the carbapenems. It is administered with cilastin, a dipeptidase inhibitor that prevents nephrotoxicity.[9] There is limited experience with this drug during pregnancy, and it is rarely indicated. It is FDA category C; no teratogenicity has been reported.[2,9]

Sulfonamides

The sulfonamides readily cross the placenta. Their use in the third trimester should be avoided because they compete with bilirubin for albumin-binding sites and may cause kernicterus.[3,9] Sulfonamides are FDA category B. Trimethoprim is a folate agonist and is therefore not recommended in pregnancy; it is FDA category C.[9]

Tetracyclines

Tetracycline use during pregnancy may result in genitourinary and limb abnormalities. It chelates calcium and results in staining of the teeth and bones.[3,9] Tetracyclines are associated with hepatotoxicity in the mother and should be avoided in pregnancy.[3,9] They are FDA category D.

Chloramphenicol

There is no reported association between chloramphenicol use and the development of congenital malformations. It is considered safe through much of pregnancy but should be avoided near term because of case reports of cardiovascular collapse or "gray baby."[3]

Aminoglycosides

Aminoglycosides should be used in pregnancy to treat gram-negative bacteria resistant to less toxic alternatives. Gentamicin is the aminoglycoside of choice in pregnancy. It is listed as FDA category C.[9] Kanamycin and streptomycin may cause hearing loss from damage to cranial nerve VII.[2,3]

Clindamycin

Clindamycin may be used in pregnant women who are allergic to penicillin or erythromycin. No human studies have been done; there is no evidence of teratogenicity in animal models.[2] It is FDA category B.[9]

Metronidazole

Metronidazole should be avoided in the first trimester. Human studies are conflicting, but animal models demonstrate carcinogenesis.[3] Some practitioners use it during the latter half of pregnancy because no human teratogenesis has been found.[3,9] It is FDA category B.[9]

Nitrofurantoin

Nitrofurantoin is safe during pregnancy. It should be avoided in the third trimester because it can cause hemolysis in infants who are glucose-6-phosphate dehydrogenase deficient.[3,9] It is FDA category C.

Fluoroquinolones

Fluoroquinolones should be avoided in pregnancy because they have been associated with irreversible arthropathy secondary to cartilage damage. They are potentially mutagenic and teratogenic in humans.[2,3]

Antituberculous Agents

Isoniazid (INH) is considered part of the optimal treatment of tuberculosis in pregnant women. It is considered significantly more beneficial than the risk of untreated tuberculosis in the mother or fetus. It is FDA category C.[3,9] Rifampin crosses the placenta and has been implicated in congenital abnormalities in case reports. The benefit of rifampin also outweighs the risk of untreated disease in pregnancy and should be used along with ethambutol when indicated. It is FDA category C.[3,9] Ethambutol also crosses the placenta but has not been associated with any congenital defects. It is considered safe in pregnancy (FDA category B).[3,9]

Antifungal Agents

Nystatin is poorly absorbed from skin, mucous membranes, and the gastrointestinal tract. It is considered safe for use in pregnancy. Clotrimazole and miconazole use in pregnancy has not been shown to be associated with fetal abnormality and is considered safe.[3] Oral terbinafine is category B and is the likely oral agent of choice.[10] Griseofulvin is embryotoxic and teratogenic in animals. There are two reports of conjoined twins in human pregnancies.[10] Ketoconazole is category C and has caused syndactyly, oligodactyly, and cataracts in animals. It can also block androgens and may interfere with genital development of male fetuses.[10] Itraconazole is also category C and has caused skeletal defects, encephalocele, and macroglossia in animals.[10]

Pyrethroids

Pyrethroids are the treatment of choice for scabies and lice during pregnancy. Lindane has been used safely, but its neurotoxicity makes it a second-line agent.[10] In animals, lindane is not teratogenic, but the Michigan Medicaid Surveillance Study suggested an increased risk of hypospadias with first-trimester exposure.[3]

Antivirals

Acyclovir has been used during all stages of pregnancy and has not been associated with adverse effects on the fetus or newborn.[2,10] The experience with valacyclovir and famciclovir is more limited, and their safety has not been assessed.[2,10] The Centers for Disease Control and Prevention (CDC) recommends that the first clinical episode of genital herpes simplex virus (HSV) infection in a pregnant woman be treated with oral acyclovir.[2] Intravenous acyclovir is indicated for life-threatening maternal viral infections such as disseminated HSV or herpes zoster.[2,10]

Zidovudine is effective for reducing the maternal–fetal transmission of HIV without causing significant toxicity in the fetus or newborn.[2,24] Most women exposed to or diagnosed with HIV in pregnancy should be treated as nonpregnant patients.[24] The combination of zidovudine with other retroviral drugs should be discussed with the patient and recommended when appropriate.[5,24] The use of any of the protease inhibitors can be associated with hyperglycemia or the development of diabetes. This may be exacerbated in pregnancy, and patients should be instructed on recognition of symptoms of hyperglycemia. Such women should be closely followed for the development of hyperglycemia.[24]

Physicians may report cases of prenatal exposure to antiretroviral drugs to the Antiretroviral Pregnancy Registry, PO Box 13398, Research Triangle Park, NC 27709-3398; phone: (919)483-9437 or (800)722-9292, ext. 38465; fax: (919)315-8981.

Topical Preparations

The topical agents polysporin, erythromycin, bacitracin, neomycin, and gramicidin have not been shown to be teratogenic and are safe during pregnancy.[3,10] There are insufficient data on mupirocin and fusidic acid, but they appear to be safe.[10]

Cardiovascular Drugs

Antidysrhythmic Agents

All antidysrhythmic agents cross the placenta to some extent.[7] The doses of agents that are renally excreted may need to be increased during pregnancy to compensate for increased renal clearance.[7]

Digoxin

Digoxin has a long history of safe use during pregnancy. It is not teratogenic and not associated with adverse fetal effects when given in appropriate doses.[7] Digitalis toxicity during pregnancy has been associated with fetal death and miscarriage, presumably due to hypoperfusion.[7]

Adenosine

Adenosine is an endogenous purine nucleoside with a very short half-life. It has no demonstrated teratogenicity or adverse fetal effects and is as effective in terminating AV node–dependent tachycardias in pregnancy as it is in nonpregnant patients.[7]

Class IA Agents

Teratogenicity has not been associated with quinidine, procainamide, or disopyramide.[7] Of these, quinidine has the longest history of use in pregnancy. Quinidine and procainamide are considered safe during pregnancy.[7] Disopyramide has a more limited history and has been shown to cause contractions in pregnancy; thus, cautious use is indicated.[7]

Class IB Agents

Lidocaine is not known to be teratogenic. The risk of lidocaine is minor when appropriate doses are utilized. In large doses, it has been associated with low Apgar scores and neonatal lidocaine toxicity.[7] Mexiletine is structurally related to lidocaine and freely crosses the placenta. Data in pregnant women are limited, but mexiletine has not been associated with teratogenicity.[7]

Class IC Agents

Flecainide and propafenone cross the placenta, but neither has been shown to cause fetal adverse effects or teratogenicity.[7] These agents should be used cautiously, as they have not been extensively studied in humans.[7]

Class II Agents

Beta-blockers, particularly propranolol, have been used with considerable experience in pregnancy. No teratogenicity is demonstrated with these agents, and they are considered safe for use.[7] Some adverse effects have been noted, including intrauterine growth retardation (IUGR), fetal bradycardia, premature labor, neonatal hypoglycemia, respiratory depression, and bilirubinemia.[7] If necessary, glucagon may be given during labor to counteract the bradycardic and hypoglycemic effects of beta-blockade.[7]

Class III Agents

Amiodarone and its metabolite, desethylamiodarone, have limited ability to cross the placenta. Amiodarone has a high iodine content and has been associated with fetal goiter, neonatal hypothyroidism (approximately 9% of exposures), and growth retardation. Other reported adverse effects include fetal bradycardia, prolonged QT, prematurity, and possibly death. Given these effects and the prolonged half-life of amiodarone, it should be used in pregnancy only when absolutely necessary.[7]

Limited data are available on the use of sotalol during pregnancy. It has not been shown to be teratogenic, but transient neonatal bradycardia has been reported. It should be used cautiously and infants monitored for bradycardias.[7]

Ibutilide has not been studied in pregnant women. In high doses, it has been demonstrated to be teratogenic in animal studies. Due to limited data and potential teratogenicity, ibutilide is not recommended in pregnancy.[7]

Class IV Agents

The greatest experience with calcium channel blockers in pregnancy has been with verapamil. It has not been shown to be teratogenic and is generally considered safe in pregnancy, as are the other calcium antagonists.[7] Intravenous use carries an increased risk of maternal hypotension and subsequent fetal hypoperfusion. Animal studies have suggested a relationship between diltiazem and skeletal deformities and even fetal death. Because of this, verapamil is the drug of choice among calcium antagonists.[7] It should be noted, however, that adenosine and beta-blockers are preferred over calcium antagonists in the management of supraventricular tachycardia in pregnancy.[7]

Antihypertensive Agents

Fetal wastage in untreated patients with mild chronic hypertension is up to 16%. In those with severe hypertension (greater than 160/100), it is as high as 40%. Therapy must be monitored carefully to prevent maternal hypotension and resultant placental hypoperfusion.[2,8]

Angiotensin Converting Enzyme Inhibitors

The three most common angiotensin converting enzyme inhibitors are captopril, enalapril, and lisinopril. These agents are avoided in pregnancy because during the last half of pregnancy they are associated with severe fetal renal toxicity that can lead to *in utero* anuria and oligohydramnios, structural defects of the cranium and kidneys, and hypotension and anuria in the newborn.[2]

Diuretics

The thiazide diuretics and furosemide are not teratogenic but should be used cautiously. An increase in perinatal mortality and congenital defects has been associated with these agents, probably related to decreased maternal plasma volume, resulting in placental hypoperfusion.[2,8]

Methyldopa

The most commonly used antihypertensive agent is methyldopa. It has been the drug of choice for more than 30 years; it is effective and lacks fetal or neonatal adverse effects.[8]

Beta-Blockers

Propranolol is the most commonly used beta-blocker for hypertension in pregnancy. Atenolol is cardioselective but may have a higher risk of IUGR than propranolol, especially when started in the first trimester.[8] Labetalol is a combined alpha- and beta-blocker and appears to be without risk of teratogenicity.[8] Labetalol has been shown to increase pulmonary surfactant and may be advantageous, especially in premature infants.[2,8] As with beta-blockers, neonates should be monitored for bradycardias for 24 to 48 hours.[8]

Hydralazine

Hydralazine is a vasodilator with a direct effect on arterioles. It is the drug of choice to control acute exacerbations of hypertension.[2,8] Hydralazine has been found to be safe and without risk of teratogenicity.[8] Changes in fetal heart rate occur when the drug is given, but they are apparently without significant sequelae.[8]

Calcium Channel Blockers

Nifedipine should be reserved for cases in which other agents have failed to control hypertension in pregnancy. It has been shown to be teratogenic in animal models at high doses. No excess teratogenicity has been found in human models. IUGR and fetal death have been reported.[8]

Cough and Cold Preparations

Antihistamines

Diphenhydramine in pregnancy has been associated with a number of minor anomalies. It is not recommended in pregnancy.[3] The antihistamines chlorpheniramine, pheniramine, and tripelennamine have not demonstrated teratogenicity and are probably safe.[3] Brompheniramine has been shown to cause birth defects and should not be used.[11] Astemizole was studied prospectively in a group of 114 women in which the incidence of major malformation was found to be within the expected rate for the general population. Astemizole was not associated with perinatal complication or IUGR.[20] Although the power of this study was limited, the results are encouraging. Further study is necessary to determine fetal risk.

Decongestants

Sympathomimetic drugs such as ephedrine, phenylephrine, phenylpropanolamine, and pseudoephedrine are commonly used decongestants and are combined with other agents to alleviate symptoms of allergy and upper respiratory tract infection. Pseudoephedrine is known to be teratogenic in animals; no human teratogenicity has been reported.[3] Phenylpropanolamine has been implicated in the causation of gastroschisis when used during the first trimester.[22] Although otherwise considered not to be teratogenic, sympathomimetics have been shown to be associated with minor malformations such as inguinal hernia and clubfoot.[22] Some of these agents have been shown to cause significant tachycardias and hypertensive episodes with even a single therapeutic dose.[22] These effects may be particularly damaging in pregnancy; thus, decongestant medications should be used cautiously.

Expectorants

Guaifenesin is safe for use during pregnancy. Iodinated compounds should be avoided to prevent fetal goiter as a result of iodine crossing the placenta.

Antitussives

Dextromethorphan is safe for use in pregnancy.

Gastrointestinal Medications

Antacids

Antacids are used by 30% to 50% of women for the relief of heartburn during pregnancy; most are well tolerated.[4] There are limited data concerning the effect of antacids on the fetus. No teratogenicity is observed in animal studies. Currently, the use of most aluminium-, magnesium-, and calcium-containing antacids are acceptable for use in pregnancy at therapeutic doses.[4] Sodium bicarbonate should not be used, as it can cause metabolic alkalosis and fluid overload in both the mother and the fetus.[4] Compounds containing magnesium trisilicate, when used in high doses, can cause nephrolithiasis, hypotonia, respiratory distress, and cardiovascular compromise in the fetus.[4]

Mucosal Protectants

Sucralfate is not systemically absorbed and is therefore commonly used during pregnancy.[4] In one study, sucralfate was demonstrated to completely relieve symptoms of heartburn and reflux more effectively than lifestyle changes in controls.[4]

Histamine H_2 Receptor Antagonists

Few published safety reports on the use of cimetidine in pregnant women exist. The Michigan Medicaid Surveillance Study reported 460 newborns exposed to cimetidine. No association between cimetidine and congenital defects could be demonstrated.[4] Ranitidine is the only H_2 receptor antagonist whose efficacy has been studied in pregnancy. Twice-daily doses reduced symptoms and antacid use compared with the baseline. Little literature is available on the use of famotidine in human pregnancy. Animal studies show no evidence of teratogenicity or fetotoxic effects.[4] Safety data are limited in the use of nizatidine during pregnancy. Data from animal studies are conflicting, but there have been reports of abortions, low fetal weights, and malformations with high doses.[4]

H_2 receptor antagonists thus appear to be well tolerated during pregnancy, with the possible exception of nizatidine, and are efficacious in the treatment of heartburn in pregnancy. The use of these drugs should be limited to those patients not responding to lifestyle changes, antacids, and sucralfate.[4]

Promotility Agents

Metoclopramide has not been associated with teratogenicity in animals. In the Michigan Medicaid Surveillance Study, 192 newborns were exposed to metoclopramide; 10 major birth defects were reported and eight were expected based on the general population rate of malformation, which was not statistically significant.[4] Further study is needed to assess fetal safety. Metoclopramide has been found to increase milk production and has been used as a lactation stimulant.[8] Cisapride was recently evaluated for safety during pregnancy in a Canadian cohort study. One hundred twenty-nine women were exposed to cisapride during pregnancy. The investigators found no difference in rate of minor or major congenital malformation between this cohort and the control group. Although the power of this study was limited, the investigators feel that cisapride can be used safely in pregnant women when nonsystemic drugs and H_2 receptor antagonists fail to control symptoms.[4]

Proton Pump Inhibitors

Omeprazole crosses the placenta, but animal studies fail to show evidence of teratogenicity.[17] A recent Swedish cohort study failed to demonstrate an effect on the rate of congenital malformation when omeprazole was used during pregnancy. The investigators concluded that the present data indicate no evidence of teratogenicity with omeprazole use and that the individual risk of an exposed pregnancy is negligible.[13] No reports are available to date on the safety of lansoprazole during pregnancy.[4]

Antiemetics

The use of antiemetics should be considered after conservative measures to alleviate nausea and vomiting have failed. Pyridoxine has been found to be useful for nausea and vomiting during pregnancy for a few days, but the effect decreases over time. Pyridoxine is not known to be teratogenic.[8]

Trimethobenzamide, prochlorperazine, and promethazine are commonly prescribed antiemetics. These agents have been studied and have not been shown to be teratogenic.[3,8] The use of phenothiazines is associated with a small risk of hypotension, and they should be reserved for patients with hyperemesis gravidarum.

Laxatives

Agents acting locally in the gastrointestinal tract are safe for use during pregnancy. These include castor oil, senna, bisacodyl, milk of magnesia, magnesium citrate, Epsom salts, and the phosphate salts of sodium and potassium. Stool softeners such as the docusates are safe for use in pregnancy.[3]

Hypoglycemics

Insulin is safe in pregnancy. Oral hypoglycemics are contraindicated because they cross the placenta and may cause fetal hypoglycemia.[3]

Local Anesthetics

Most local anesthetics have not been shown to be teratogenic and are safe for use in pregnancy.[21] Bupivacaine and mepivacaine should be used cautiously and may be associated with fetal bradycardia. It is recommended that all local anesthetics be used in the minimum dose required for effective pain control.[21]

Combination tetracaine, epinephrine, and cocaine (TAC) is contraindicated in pregnancy because epinephrine and cocaine are suspected teratogens.

Immunizations

Few vaccines have been officially tested in pregnant women. Because of the theoretical risk to the fetus, live vaccines should not be administered during pregnancy or to those likely to become pregnant in the ensuing 3 months.[28] It is also best to avoid any form of immunization during the first trimester, if possible.[28] High fevers during the first trimester have been associated with neural tube defects, and this may occur as a result of immunization. Commonly used immunizations that are safe for use in pregnancy include tetanus toxoid, tetanus–diphtheria toxoid, tetanus immune globulin, rabies human diploid cell vaccine, rabies immune globulin, hepatitis B vaccine, hepatitis B immune globulin, varicella zoster immune globulin, and pooled immune globulins. Hepatitis A vaccine should be used only if clearly indicated; it is FDA category C mainly because of the risk of febrile response.[28] The influenza vaccine may be given in the second or third trimesters.[28]

Psychotropics

Antidepressants

Tricyclic antidepressants (TCAs) are widely prescribed in reproductive-age women. There is no significant association between first-trimester use of TCAs and congenital malformation.[15] One study demonstrated antidepressant withdrawal symptoms in newborns of women who took TCAs.[15]

Selective serotonin reuptake inhibitors (SSRIs), such as sertraline and fluoxetine, are popular agents for the treatment of depression. Studies show no increase in rates of major malformations, miscarriage, stillbirth, or prematurity in groups taking SSRIs compared with controls.[1,15,16] There is little information available on the safe use of newer agents such as moclobemide, venlafaxine, and nefazodone during pregnancy.[1]

Amphetamines can cause clinically significant maternal hypertension and have potential teratogenic effects. The use of stimulants during pregnancy should be avoided because they have not been shown to be safe.[1]

Mood Stabilizers

Lithium is associated with an increased risk of cardiovascular abnormalities.[1,15] The "floppy-baby" syndrome, in which the infant is hypotonic, cyanotic, and sucks poorly is felt to be the result of lithium toxicity. Lithium has also been reported to effect neonatal thyroid function.[1]

Carbamazepine and Valproic Acid

See the section on anticonvulsants.

Antipsychotics

The best studied neuroleptic agents in pregnancy are the phenothiazines and haloperidol. Several large, prospective studies have failed to demonstrate significant teratogenic risk.[15] Some authorities recommend discontinuation of antipsychotics 5 to 10 days prior to delivery to decrease the chances of neonatal extrapyramidal symptoms.[15] Information on the safety of the newer antipsychotics, such as clozapine, risperidone, olanzapine, and zuclopenthixol, is predominantly in the form of case reports. Thus far, no evidence of teratogenicity has been reported.[1]

HYPERBARIC OXYGENATION

Hyperbaric oxygenation is the treatment of choice in the pregnant patient experiencing decompression sickness, arterial gas embolism, severe carbon monoxide poisoning, or gas gangrene. The use of hyperbaric oxygenation may be life-saving for the mother and prevent fetal abnormality or demise in these circumstances.[12]

COMMON PITFALLS

- Consider every female of reproductive age (ages 10 to 50?) a potential antenatal patient.
- There should be a clear medical indication every time a drug is used in pregnancy.
- Use the lowest effective dose.
- Discourage self-medication.
- Use agents that have been widely used in pregnancy (over newer agents).
- Explain how to take all prescribed drugs.
- Drugs that are absolutely contraindicated include brompheniramine, warfarin, the quinolones, and the tetracyclines.
- Denying pharmacologic therapy to a patient for a *bona fide* medical condition because she is also pregnant does not help her and may place the mother and fetus at risk for adverse outcome.

References

1. Austin MP, Mitchell PB. Psychotropic medications in pregnant women: treatment dilemmas. *Med J Aust* 1998;169(8):428–431.
2. Briggs GG. Medication use during the perinatal period. *J Am Pharm Assoc* 1998;38(6):717–726, 726–727.
3. Briggs GG, Freeman RK, Yaffee SJ. *Drugs in pregnancy and lactation,* 5th ed. Baltimore: Williams & Wilkins, 1998.
4. Broussard CN, Richter JE. Treating gastro-oesophageal reflux disease during pregnancy and lactation; what are the safest options? *Drug Saf* 1998;19(4):325–337.
5. Carpenter CC, Fischl MA, Hammer SM. Antiretroviral therapy for HIV infection in 1998. *JAMA* 1998;280(1):78–86.
6. Chang SI, McAuley JW. Pharmacotherapeutic issues for women of childbearing age with epilepsy. *Ann Pharmacother* 1998;32(7-8):794–801.
7. Chow T, Galvin J, McGovern B. Antiarrhythmic drug therapy in pregnancy and lactation. *Am J Cardiol* 1998;82(4A):581–621.
8. Colie CF. Medications in pregnancy. *Curr Opin Obstet Gynecol* 1996;8(6):398–402.
9. Dashe JS, Gilstrap LC. Antibiotic use in pregnancy. *Obstet Gynecol Clin* 1997;24(3):617–629.
10. Guenther L. Skin drugs in pregnancy—which ones to use. *Derm Nsg* 1997;9(4):233–236, 265.
11. Ives TJ, Tepper RS. Drug use in pregnancy and lactation. *Pharmacother Prim Care Physician* 1990;17:623.
12. Jennings RT. Women and the hazardous environment: when the pregnant patient requires hyperbaric oxygen therapy. *Aviat Space Environ Med* 1987;58:370.
13. Kallen B. Delivery outcome after the use of acid-suppressing drugs in early pregnancy with special reference to omeprazole. *Br J Obstet Gynaecol* 1998;105(8):877–881.
14. Koren G, Pastuszak A, Ito S. Drugs in pregnancy. *N Engl J Med* 1998;338(16):1128–1136.
15. Kuller JA, Katz VL, McMahon MJ, et al. Pharmacologic treatment of psychiatric disease in pregnancy and lactation: fetal and neonatal effects. *Obstet Gynecol* 1996;87(5 Pt 1):789–794.
16. Kulin NA, Pastuszak A, Koren G. Are the new SSRIs safe for pregnant women? *Can Fam Physician* 1998;44:2081–2083.
17. Lalkin A, Magee L, Addis A, et al. Acid-suppressing drugs in pregnancy. *Can Fam Physician* 1997;43:1923–1924.
18. Loebstein R, Lalkin A, Koren G. Pharmacokinetic changes during pregnancy and their clinical relevance. *Clin Pharmacokinet* 1997;33(5):328–343.
19. McElhatton PR, Sullivan FM, Volans GN, et al. Paracetamol poisoning in pregnancy: an analysis of outcomes of cases referred to the teratology information service of the National Poison Information Service. *Hum Exp Toxicol* 1990;9:147.
20. Mazzotta P, Koren G. Nonsedating antihistamines in pregnancy considering astemizole. *Can Fam Physician* 1997;43:1509–1511.
21. Moore PA. Selecting drugs for the pregnant dental patient. *J Am Dent Assoc* 1998;129(9):1281–1286.
22. Onuigbo M, Alikhan M. Over-the-counter sympathomimetics: a risk factor for cardiac arrhythmias during pregnancy. *South Med J* 1998;91(12):1153–1155.
23. Ornoy A, Arnon J, Shechtman S. Is benzodiazepine use in pregnancy really teratogenic? *Reprod Toxicol* 1998;12(5):511–515.
24. Ostensen M, Ramsey-Goldman R. Treatment of inflammatory rheumatic disorders in pregnancy: what are the safest treatment options? *Drug Saf* 1998;19(5):389–410.
25. Public Health Service Task Force recommendations for the use of antiretroviral drugs in pregnant women infected with HIV-1 for maternal health and for reducing perinatal HIV-1 transmission in the United States. *MMWR* 1998;47(RR-2):1–30.
26. Rayburn WF. Connective tissue disorders and pregnancy. Recommendations for prescribing. *J Repro Med* 1998;43(4):341–349.
27. Rudolf AM. Effects of aspirin and acetaminophen in pregnancy and in the newborn. *Arch Intern Med* 1981;141:358.
28. Samuel BU, Barry M. The pregnant traveler. *Infect Dis Clin North Am* 1998;12(2):325–354.
29. Schatz M. Asthma treatment during pregnancy. What can be safely taken? *Drug Saf* 1997;16(5):342–350.
30. Slone D, Heinonen OP, Kaufman DW, et al. Aspirin and congenital malformations. *Lancet* 1976;1:1373–1375.
31. Wilson JG, Fraser FC. *Handbook of teratology*. New York: Plenum Publishing, 1977.
32. Zahn CA, Morrell MJ, Collins SD, et al. Management issues for women with epilepsy: a review of the literature. *Neurology* 1998;51(4):949–956.

CHAPTER 72
Complications of Induced Abortions

James L. Jones and Andrew M. Kaunitz

Approximately 1.6 million abortions are performed in the United States annually, making abortions among the most frequently performed surgical procedures in the United States.[12,13] Each year, approximately 3% of all reproductive-age American women have abortions.[11] These women tend to be young and unmarried.

Since abortions became legal in the early 1970s, the average gestational age among women having them has declined. Currently, approximately one-half of all abortions are performed before the eighth week of pregnancy, and more than

85% are done in the first 12 weeks of pregnancy.[6] Nearly 99% of induced abortions are accomplished by curettage, and almost 90% are performed in outpatient settings.

After legalization of abortions, deaths from induced abortion plummeted in the United States.[3,19,20] The risk of death associated with induced abortion in the first 8 weeks of pregnancy is one per 200,000 abortions,[1] a death rate 20 times lower than that associated with childbirth.[15]

Serious complications of legal abortion are infrequent.[7] In one study based on 170,000 first-trimester procedures, a major complication rate of less than one per 1000 abortions was noted.[10] Nevertheless, because so many abortions are performed, it is not unusual for physicians working in emergency settings to encounter problems related to legal termination of pregnancy.

Abortion complications likely to be encountered by emergency physicians reflect the techniques employed during the abortion, the gestational age of the pregnancy, the underlying medical status, and the age of the patient. Common complications of induced abortion include hemorrhage, intrauterine infection and sepsis, intrauterine blood clots, retained products of conception, continuing pregnancy, and ectopic pregnancy. Gynecologic referral or consultation is appropriate for patients presenting with these clinical problems.

EMERGENCY DEPARTMENT EVALUATION

The workup of patients with potential complications of induced abortion should include a history emphasizing gestational age at termination, method used for the abortion, and the nature of the current complaint. If possible, the physician who performed the procedure should be contacted to ensure that the history is accurate.

Physical examination of the patient should include the patient's vital signs, with a tilt test for orthostasis. A general physical examination is performed, with attention to the abdominal and pelvic examination. A bimanual examination is performed after a vaginal speculum examination. A pelvic ultrasound may be helpful if the examination is inadequate or if the patient is obese. An ultrasound may also be helpful in identifying a hemoperitoneum and in ruling out incomplete evacuation of the uterus or an ectopic pregnancy. Emergency department physicians should remember that an enlarged corpus luteum may be mistaken in this clinical setting for an ectopic pregnancy.

Initial laboratory studies should include a complete blood cell count. A type and screen may also be ordered if the patient gives a history of heavy vaginal bleeding or if an operative procedure is anticipated. A urine pregnancy test performed soon after an abortion should be positive and provides little information to the clinician. A single quantitative human chorionic gonadotropin (hCG) drawn after a termination of pregnancy also provides little information. Serial quantitative hCGs, drawn 48 hours apart, may be helpful if there is any question of a continuing or an ectopic pregnancy. If a serial quantitative hCG level rises or plateaus, this would be suspicious for an ectopic or failed attempted abortion.

DIFFERENTIAL DIAGNOSIS AND EMERGENCY DEPARTMENT MANAGEMENT

Postabortion complications include postabortion bleeding, acute hematometra, hemorrhage, postabortion infection, continuing pregnancy, incomplete evacuation, and ectopic pregnancy.

Postabortion Bleeding

Excessive postabortion vaginal bleeding is usually of uterine or cervical origin. A vaginal speculum examination allows determination of the source of the bleeding. Even minor cervical lacerations from the use of a tenaculum for cervical manipulation can present as delayed vaginal bleeding. Minor cervical bleeding can be controlled with topical application of silver nitrate or Monsel's solution during a vaginal speculum examination. More recalcitrant bleeding may require placement of a suture or the use of electrocautery.

If evaluation of the vagina and cervix is negative and blood is coming from the cervical os, the uterus is the source of bleeding. Uterine bleeding in this setting is usually due to retained products of conception or acute hematometra. The history and a bimanual pelvic examination to determine the size of the uterus may help differentiate an acute hematometra from retained products of conception. The risk of hemorrhage is greater with medical approaches to abortion, such as methotrexate.[9]

Acute Hematometra

Acute hematometra occurs in 0.2% to 1.0% of abortions.[14] Typically, severe and progressive lower abdominal cramping occurs within several hours of the abortion. Vaginal bleeding may be minimal, because the hematoma is obstructing the outflow tract. The pelvic examination reveals a markedly distended and tender uterus. Hypotension, anemia, and fever are not present. Prompt suction evacuation of the uterus can be performed without anesthesia or cervical dilation. Symptomatic relief occurs on evacuation of the blood. Unless the patient is hypertensive, ergonovine maleate or methylergonovine (0.2 mg i.m.) should be administered to induce contraction of the uterus. Alternatively a 10-mg prostaglandin E2 suppository can be given rectally.

Retained Products of Conception

Retained products of conception after an induced abortion may result in bleeding, infection, or both. Occurring in approximately 1% of suction curettage patients, this complication is found more often after the use of local, rather than general anesthesia.[7] Typically, within 1 week of the abortion the patient complains of cramping and heavy bleeding, which may be accompanied by fever. It may be difficult to distinguish between conditions caused by retained products of conception and infection.

Reaspiration of the uterus will confirm the diagnosis. If the pelvic examination reveals an enlarged uterus, significant amounts of fetal or placental tissue may be present. In this setting, it would be wise to perform the uterine evacuation in an operating room. If the patient is febrile, the possibility of intrauterine infection should be strongly considered, and antibiotics should be initiated before the patient undergoes uterine evacuation.

Other Causes of Postabortion Bleeding

Rarely, bleeding continues despite appropriate medical therapy. Persistent, unexplained uterine bleeding should alert the clinician to the possibility of a bleeding diathesis. The most common bleeding diathesis among women of reproductive age is von Willebrand disease.

Uterine perforation may also present as heavy vaginal bleeding. Perforation of the uterine fundus with a blunt probe or cervical dilator usually does not cause significant complications and often can be managed with close observation alone. Perforation with a curette or suction cannula risks injury to abdominal contents and requires laparoscopy or laparotomy to rule out bowel injury.[17] Heavy vaginal bleeding from a uterine perforation associated with injury to the pelvic vasculature may result in a broad-ligament hematoma. In this setting, prompt, exploratory laparotomy may be appropriate.[2] Finally, uterine bleeding may be a presenting sign of an underlying postabortion infection.

Postabortion Infection

The legalization of abortion has greatly reduced morbidity and mortality from septic abortion.[3] Risk factors for postabortion infection include retained products of conception, gonococcal or chlamydial endocervical infections, and procedures not performed in aseptic conditions. Uterine tenderness, fever, and excessive bleeding occurring 3 to 7 days postoperatively are the hallmarks of postabortion infection. Sepsis and shock are uncommon. The organisms responsible for postabortion infections are similar to those that cause pelvic infections in nonpregnant women. Antibiotic guidelines for treating pelvic inflammatory disease are applicable to postabortion infections and include ceftriaxone (250 mg in a single i.m. dose) with doxycycline (0.1 g PO twice daily for 14 days), or amoxicillin/clavulanate (Augmentin) and doxycycline (see Chapter 82, "Pelvic Inflammatory Disease"). Coverage against anaerobic pathogens should be included in any antibiotic regimen.

The primary treatment for postabortion infection is suction curettage. Antibiotics should be administered in advance of the procedure. Because of an increased risk of hemorrhage, reaspiration of an infected uterus should be performed in an operating room and the patient admitted for intravenous antibiotic therapy.

Infection after Illegal Abortion

Few young physicians practicing in the United States have cared for women experiencing complications of criminal abortion. If the movement to outlaw abortion succeeds, however, emergency physicians will need to learn lessons first taught in the days of illegal abortion. In that era, deaths from illegal abortion often outnumbered maternal deaths associated with childbirth. Self-induced abortions were often attempted using catheters, knitting needles, or open wire coat hangers. When catheters were used, soap, Lysol, and detergents were the agents most commonly introduced into the uterus. After infusion of these noxious substances into the pregnant uterus, necrosis of the intrauterine contents, thrombosis of uterine and pelvic vasculature, hemolysis, and disseminated intravascular coagulation commonly occurred. Abortions also were attempted by physicians with inadequate training, or instrumentation was done by nonmedical personnel. Uterine perforation was common.

Women experiencing complications of illegal abortion tend to present later than women with complications of legal abortion.[8] In addition, such women often deny uterine instrumentation.[4] Both of these factors can combine to make evaluation and treatment of complications of illegal abortion particularly challenging.

Ledger's recommendations regarding the evaluation and management of patients with suspected septic abortion remain useful.[18] High-spiking fevers are characteristic of women with septic abortions. Hypotension and leukopenia strongly support the diagnosis of sepsis. Blood cultures and frequent monitoring of the urinary output are appropriate. During vaginal speculum examination, a Gram stain of any cervical leukorrhea present should be obtained, because it may suggest a gonococcal or clostridial infection. Swabs for *Chlamydia* and *Neisseria gonorrhoeae,* as well as conventional aerobic culture, should also be performed. A bimanual pelvic examination not only assesses uterine size, but also determines whether there is evidence of extrauterine infection. Both advanced gestation (greater than 12 weeks) and extrauterine extension are associated with the most serious infections and may therefore require therapy more extensive than intravenous antibiotics and uterine curettage.

In patients at risk for serious infection, supine and upright radiography should be obtained, searching for intraperitoneal or myometrial gas. The presence of such gas mandates intraabdominal surgical evaluation so the possibility of bowel and uterine damage can be assessed. Rarely, radiographs of women with sepsis after illegal abortion demonstrate layered myometrial gas in an "onion skin" pattern. This finding indicates myometrial necrosis caused by clostridial infection and mandates laparotomy with hysterectomy.

Women with infections after illegal abortion but without the previously described signs or symptoms should be managed with antibiotic therapy and uterine curettage (see section on infections after legal abortion).

Continuing Pregnancy

Continuation of pregnancy after abortion is the result either of failure to abort an intrauterine pregnancy or of ectopic pregnancy.[16] Performing the abortion at or before 6 weeks' gestational age or the presence of a uterine anomaly increases the risk of failure. The absence of chorionic villi in the abortion specimen, continuing symptoms of pregnancy, progressive lower abdominal pain, and a plateau or increase in serial quantitative serum hCG levels suggest a continuing pregnancy. It is important to remember, however, that sensitive urine pregnancy tests may remain positive for weeks after termination of a first-trimester pregnancy (see Chapter 70, "Pregnancy Testing").

Physical examination may suggest an ongoing intrauterine pregnancy. This diagnosis should be confirmed with pelvic ultrasonography, using a vaginal probe if possible. If ultrasonography fails to reveal an intrauterine pregnancy, an ectopic pregnancy should be assumed (see Chapter 74, "Ectopic Pregnancy").

Medical Termination of Pregnancy

Medical methods of abortion were originally developed for nonsurgical management of ectopic pregnancy and are gaining wide acceptance as primary methods of abortion, especially before 8 weeks' gestation.[9] The currently available methods include methotrexate, which is used with or without misoprostol, an oral prostaglandin. RU-486, or mifepristone, is not approved for use in the United States. Side effects are minimal and include mild nausea and stomatitis. There is an increased risk of incomplete evacuation of the uterus with medical abortion, and the time to resolution of the pregnancy is prolonged compared with dilation and evacuation. In a series of 300 patients, approximately 9% of women undergoing medical termination of pregnancy subsequently required dilation and evacuation.[5]

References

1. Atrash HK, Mackay T, Binkin NJ, et al. Legal abortion mortality in the United States: 1972 to 1982. *Am J Obstet Gynecol* 1987;156:605.
2. Berek JS, Stubblefield PG. Anatomic and clinical correlates of uterine perforation. *J Obstet Gynecol* 1978;135:181.
3. Cates WC Jr, Rochat RW, Grimes DA, et al. Legalized abortion: effect on national trends of maternal and abortion-related mortality (1940 through 1976). *Am J Obstet Gynecol* 1978;132:211.
4. Creinin MD, Burke AE. Methotrexate and misoprostol for early abortion: a multicenter trial. *Contraception* 1996;54(1):19–22.
5. Creinin MD, Vittinghoff E, Schall E, et al. Medical abortion with oral methotrexate and vaginal misoprostol. *Obstet Gynecol* 1997;90(4 Pt 1):611–616.
6. Centers for Disease Control. Abortion surveillance, United States, 1988. In: CDC surveillance summaries, June 1991. *MMWR* 1991;40(SS-2):15.
7. Grimes DA, Cates WC Jr. Complications of legally induced abortion: a review. *Obstet Gynecol Surv* 1979;34:177.
8. Grimes DA, Cates WC Jr, Selik RM. Fatal septic abortion in the United States, 1975–1977. *Obstet Gynecol* 1981;57:739.
9. Grimes DA. Medical abortion in early pregnancy: a review of the evidence. *Obstet Gynecol* 1997;89(5 Pt 1):790–796.

10. Hakim-Elahi E, Tovell HM, Burnhill MS. Complications of first trimester abortion: a report of 170,000 cases. *Obstet Gynecol* 1990;76:129.
11. Henshaw SK, Forest JD, Van Vort JV. Abortion services in the United States, 1984 and 1985. *Fam Plann Perspect* 1987;19:63.
12. Henshaw SK, Koonin LM, Smith JC. Characteristics of U.S. women having abortions, 1987. *Fam Plann Perspect* 1991;23:75.
13. Kaunitz A. Complications of legal and illegal abortion. In: Benrubi G, ed. *Obstetric and gynecologic emergencies.* Philadelphia: JB Lippincott Co, 1993.
14. Kaunitz AM, Grimes DA. First trimester abortion technology. In: Corson SL, Derman RJ, Tyrer LB, eds. *Fertility control.* Boston: Little, Brown and Company, 1985:63.
15. Kaunitz Am, Hughes J, Grimes DA, et al. Causes of maternal mortality in the United States. *Obstet Gynecol* 1985;65:605.
16. Kaunitz AM, Rovira EZ, Grimes DA, et al. Abortions that fail. *Obstet Gynecol* 1985;66:533.
17. Lauersen NH, Birnbaum S. Laparoscopy as a diagnostic and therapeutic technique in uterine perforations during first-trimester abortions. *J Obstet Gynecol* 1973;117:522.
18. Ledger WJ. *Infection in the female,* 2nd ed. Philadelphia: Lea & Febiger, 1986.
19. Santamarina BA, Smith SA. Septic abortion and septic shock. *Clin Obstet Gynecol* 1970;13:291.
20. Studdiford WE, Douglas GW. Placental bacteremia: a significant finding in septic abortion accompanied by vascular collapse. *Am J Obstet Gynecol* 1956;71:842.

CHAPTER 73

Vaginal Bleeding in Early Pregnancy

Edward Newton and Sean O. Henderson

Emergency physicians are frequently called upon to evaluate patients with vaginal bleeding. This entity ranks among the top ten reasons for a visit to the emergency department (ED).[27] After menarche, vaginal bleeding is most often an integral part of the normal reproductive cycle. However, it may also signal the presence of serious illness, particularly if the patient is pregnant. Assessment of patients with vaginal bleeding is complex because of the broad range of diagnostic possibilities, from completely benign (e.g., normal menses) to life-threatening (e.g., ectopic pregnancy).

With the increased availability of certain bedside diagnostic techniques, including ultrasensitive, rapid tests for beta human chorionic gonadotropin (βhCG) and ultrasound (US), the role of the emergency physician in diagnosing and treating the various causes of pathologic vaginal bleeding has become more prominent in recent years. There has also been an increasing trend toward outpatient management of clinically stable patients with threatened or completed abortion, and even unruptured ectopic pregnancy. For these patients, the bulk of their medical care occurs in the ED. As a result, the level of medical sophistication required to manage these cases in the ED has increased as well.

DIFFERENTIAL DIAGNOSIS

Vaginal bleeding in the pregnant patient evokes a unique differential diagnosis compared with the nonpregnant state. In addition, the stage of pregnancy is important to determine, as the differential diagnosis of vaginal bleeding changes significantly over the course of the gestation. This chapter focuses on vaginal bleeding in the early stage of pregnancy (i.e., less than 20 weeks' gestation). Ectopic pregnancy is dealt with in Chapter 74. The causes of vaginal bleeding in early pregnancy are shown in Table 73.1.

TABLE 73.1. Differential Diagnosis of Vaginal Bleeding in Early Pregnancy

Implantation bleeding
Ectopic pregnancy
Heterotopic pregnancy
Spontaneous Abortion
Threatened abortion
Missed abortion
Complete abortion
Incomplete abortion
Septic abortion
Criminal or self-induced abortion
Complications of therapeutic abortion
Molar pregnancy
Bleeding from vaginal or cervical lesions

There is a complex interaction between fetal and maternal hormones that is required for successful fertilization, migration, and implantation of the embryo, and development of the embryo and fetus to a viable stage. Disruption of the normal hormonal environment, maternal illness, abnormal physical characteristics of the fallopian tubes or uterus, and fetal chromosomal abnormalities can all result in fetal loss.

CLINICAL PRESENTATION

Patients frequently present to the ED with a complaint of abnormal vaginal bleeding that may be accompanied by lower abdominal or lower back pain. One of the essential early components of the initial evaluation, and a major branch point in the diagnostic process, is to determine whether the patient is pregnant. Often, the patient is unaware of the pregnancy, particularly if her usual menstrual cycles are irregular.

Pregnancy is frequently complicated by vaginal bleeding. Approximately 20% to 25% of all pregnancies manifest vaginal bleeding at some point, yet more than half of these pregnancies continue to term.[11,18] First-trimester bleeding accounts for over 80% of bleeding during pregnancy.

The exact clinical presentation depends on the underlying cause. However, patients present with variable amounts of vaginal bleeding, ranging from slight "spotting" to massive hemorrhage. The severity of bleeding is not helpful in diagnosing a specific condition, although it has important implications for the hemodynamic stability of the patient. The location and nature of the patient's pain occasionally suggest one diagnosis over another. Pain from ectopic pregnancy progressively increases until the point of rupture. The resulting hemoperitoneum may cause left shoulder pain (Kehr's sign) due to irritation of the diaphragm by free intraperitoneal blood. On pelvic examination, adnexal tenderness and an adnexal mass can often be palpated. Patients with threatened abortion have crampy pelvic pain, with radiation to the lower back as the uterus contracts and the cervix dilates. The uterus may be slightly tender and irritable, but the adnexa are nontender. Completed abortion usually results in progressive diminution of pain and bleeding as the cervix closes and the uterus contracts. Incomplete abortion is associated with more severe pain and bleeding because retained products of conception (POCs) prevent uterine contraction and hemostasis. Septic abortion is associated with fever, pelvic pain, and uterine tenderness. Depending on the stage of infection, the patient may manifest all of the typical findings of gram-negative septic shock.

The normal physiologic adjustments of pregnancy include expansion of plasma volume, dilutional anemia, increased cardiac output, resting tachycardia, mild hypotension, and respiratory alkalosis. These physiologic changes alter the clinical presentation of a pregnant patient with significant hemorrhage. Because of the expanded plasma volume, up to 40% of blood volume can be lost before the typical signs of shock occur. Conversely, uterine blood flow is at increased risk when maternal hemorrhage occurs as blood is shunted preferentially from the placental to the maternal circulation.[16] Serious fetal distress can occur while the mother remains relatively asymptomatic.

Psychological Effects of Spontaneous Abortion

Most patients with spontaneous abortion experience a normal sense of grief for the loss of an anticipated child. However, a significant number of patients who experience spontaneous abortion are at risk for developing a major depressive episode within the following 6 months. Spontaneous abortion often evokes guilt regarding minor trauma or other actions that most likely bear no relation to the miscarriage. In addition, the abrupt change in the patient's hormonal milieu resembles the postpartum state, during which depression is relatively common. Risk factors for developing major depression include nulliparity and a history of infertility. Maternal age, trimester in which the miscarriage occurs, and socioeconomic status are not predictive of depression following spontaneous abortion.[20]

Implantation Bleeding

It is traditionally taught that after the fertilized ovum completes its migration through the fallopian tube toward the uterus, the process of embedding the morula in the uterine lining produces a small amount of vaginal bleeding. This is expected to occur within the first 4 weeks of pregnancy and may be misconstrued as an abnormally light and late menstrual period. Although there is little clinical or experimental evidence that implantation bleeding actually occurs, it would account for the relatively common occurrence of vaginal bleeding in very early pregnancy, at a time before other causes typically present.

Ectopic Pregnancy

Ectopic pregnancy must be considered in all cases of vaginal bleeding in early pregnancy, as it is by far the most lethal condition to be considered. The incidence of ectopic pregnancy has increased significantly over the past 20 years and is particularly high in patients who have undergone treatment for infertility and in patients with a history of a previous ectopic pregnancy, tubal infections or surgery, and intrauterine device (IUD) use.[1]

The clinical presentation of ectopic pregnancy ranges from dramatic to subtle, depending on whether the ectopic has ruptured, as well as its location and size. Patients with a ruptured ectopic pregnancy may present in hemorrhagic shock, with massive hemoperitoneum and variable amounts of vaginal bleeding. At the other extreme, the ectopic pregnancy may be relatively asymptomatic and be discovered during elective US examination. It may be particularly difficult to distinguish between an ectopic pregnancy and a complete abortion, because, in both cases, the uterus is empty on US examination and the βhCG levels may be lower than expected by dates. The reader is also referred to Chapter 74, "Ectopic Pregnancy."

Spontaneous Abortion

Abortion is defined as the death and subsequent passage of a fetus weighing less than 500 g or a fetus of less than 20 weeks' gestational age. The true incidence of spontaneous abortion is unknown, as many occur prior to a missed menstrual period and before the diagnosis of pregnancy can be made clinically. Estimates of the overall rate of spontaneous abortion range from 31% to 78%.[17] Of those pregnancies that become clinically apparent, approximately 20% will threaten to abort and 10% will spontaneously abort. There is a biphasic distribution of spontaneous abortion. During the first 10 weeks, fetal demise, with subsequent miscarriage, is most commonly due to fetal chromosomal abnormalities. Analysis of aborted material reveals that almost 70% have trisomies at various locations, representing new mutations. A second peak occurs from weeks 14 to 18, during which maternal illness, uterine abnormalities, placental factors, and incompetence of the cervix are primarily responsible. Spontaneous abortion in the second half of pregnancy is almost exclusively attributable to incompetence of the cervix and premature labor.[17] Several additional risk factors have been identified, including a history of pelvic inflammatory disease (PID), infertility, previous spontaneous abortion, and lower level of education.[23]

The pathophysiology of spontaneous abortion is incompletely understood. Immunologic factors account for 30% of cases. Antiphospholipid antibodies have been implicated as a cause of recurrent abortion that may be amenable to treatment with low-dose salicylate and corticosteroids.[7] If both parents share many human leukocyte antigens, the trophoblast may not induce the production of blocking maternal antibodies that prevent immunologic rejection of the fetus. Thus, consanguinity also results in a higher rate of spontaneous abortion. Uterine abnormalities that may preclude normal gestation include large leiomyomas, or septate uterus. Cervical incompetence occurs when the cervix progressively thins and dilates due to gravitational forces, previous trauma, or premature labor. It is a more important factor in the mid- and third trimesters and may result in recurrent abortion. Chronic maternal illnesses, such as renal failure, diabetes (diabetic ketoacidosis), drug abuse, and malnutrition, are associated with increased fetal loss. All of these conditions tend to produce recurrent spontaneous abortion. Fetal chromosomal abnormalities are common and are not usually recurrent, so that subsequent pregnancies may be normal. Episodic maternal illnesses, such as abdominal trauma, use of certain drugs and medications, and infections are commonly associated with fetal loss. Of particular importance among infections are pyelonephritis, listeriosis, toxoplasmosis, rubella, cytomegalovirus, and herpes simplex I and II (TORCH syndrome).[6]

The underlying cause of the spontaneous abortion usually cannot be determined in the ED, and parents should be reassured that their actions did not cause the miscarriage. They should be referred for genetic counseling to determine the prospects for future normal pregnancies. Patients with recurrent abortion should be referred to an infertility specialist if they wish to conceive successfully.

Spontaneous abortion can be categorized into four distinct entities:

1. Threatened abortion
2. Complete abortion
3. Incomplete abortion
4. Missed abortion

In addition, patients may present to the ED with complications following therapeutic abortion, self-induced abortion, and criminal abortion. Septic abortion may complicate any of these entities but is more common with incomplete abortion or criminal abortion.

Threatened Abortion

Threatened abortion is marked by the onset of vaginal bleeding or lower abdominal pain, without cervical dilation, during the first half of pregnancy. Patients present with vaginal bleeding that ranges from spotting to profuse, and they may have gradual onset of lower abdominal contractions and pain. Approximately 20% of pregnancies present with some degree of vaginal bleeding during pregnancy. Of these, half will spontaneously abort and half will continue past 20 weeks' gestation. The threatened abortion may be considered inevitable when the cervix is dilated and membranes are ruptured or visible in the cervical os.

There have been numerous attempts to identify a simple test that can distinguish between those threatened abortions that have a chance of continuing and those that are destined to abort. The advantages of such a test are that a patient can be counseled immediately regarding the likely outcome of the pregnancy, unnecessary prolonged bedrest can be avoided, and arrangement for elective D and C can be made.

Norms for several serum markers of pregnancy have been established, including hCG, human placental lactogen (hPL),[24] progesterone,[8,9] CA-125,[21,22] and early pregnancy factor (EPF).[26] Levels of these markers vary significantly when the fetus or placenta fails to develop normally. CA-125 is released by exposed decidua and is undetectable in normal pregnancies but elevated when there is decidual damage. One study found that all patients with vaginal bleeding for more than 3 days and elevated levels of CA-125 proceeded to spontaneous abortion.[21] Conversely, EPF has been found to be reduced in abnormal pregnancies and may be useful in predicting viability of the pregnancy. Unfortunately, there is sufficient overlap between the results seen in normal pregnancies and those seen in abnormal pregnancies that these tests cannot be relied on completely. The most promising marker is serum progesterone. A serum progesterone level less than 14.2 ng/mL in asymptomatic and 10.5 ng/mL in symptomatic patients suggests failure of the pregnancy,[8] whereas another study found that levels greater than 11 ng/mL indicate a good prognosis for viability when no definite intrauterine pregnancy was seen on US.[30] However, serum progesterone levels are not routinely available in the ED, and the clinical utility of these tests remains to be established.

Probably the most useful prognostic factor is the presence or absence of a detectable fetal heartbeat on US in a grossly normal-appearing fetus after 9 weeks' gestation. If the heartbeat is absent, all of the pregnancies will eventually abort. If a heartbeat is present, approximately 95% of the pregnancies will continue until at least 20 weeks.[18]

Another finding on US that may be highly accurate in later pregnancy complicated by threatened abortion is the measurement of cervical length. In one study,[19] cervical length less than 20 mm predicted spontaneous abortion with 100% accuracy.

Pregnancies that survive an episode of threatened abortion are at higher risk for congenital malformations, low birth weight, prematurity, low APGAR scores, and postpartum hemorrhage in the mother.[33]

Complete Abortion

Complete abortion occurs when all fetal and placental components are expelled from the uterus. Typically, this occurs after a period of threatened abortion, although it may be mistaken as a menstrual period if it occurs during the first month of pregnancy. Occasionally, a patient brings the aborted material to the ED. This material should be examined by a pathologist to determine whether fetal tissue and chorionic villi are present or whether abnormalities such as partial molar pregnancy exist.

The distinction between complete abortion and ectopic pregnancy is often difficult. In both cases, serum hCG will be elevated to a level somewhat lower than expected for dates and the uterus may be firm and smaller than expected for dates. Depending on the size of the abortus and the amount of time since the abortion was completed, the cervical os will be open to varying degrees in a complete abortion, in contrast to an ectopic pregnancy. Clinically completed abortion patients often experience a diminution of abdominal pain and vaginal bleeding once the POCs have been expelled. In contrast, patients with ectopic pregnancy most often experience progressive symptoms, including worsening pain and evidence of continued blood loss and hemoperitoneum. However, the clinical distinction may require a period of observation to establish whether the symptoms are increasing or abating. Obviously, presence of expelled POCs is important in making this distinction, and all POCs should be examined by a pathologist. Occasionally, a decidual cast is passed during an ectopic pregnancy, and this may be mistaken for POCs. The presence of fetal tissue or chorionic villi should be confirmed by pathologic examination to avoid this error. In ectopic pregnancy, ultrasonic examination may reveal a complex adnexal mass, but often ectopic pregnancy must be inferred by the absence of an intrauterine pregnancy. In both cases, a small amount of blood may be seen but no POCs are visualized within the uterine cavity. It is important to identify the uterine endometrial stripe on US that is present in complete abortion but absent in ectopic pregnancy.

Rarely, in heterotopic pregnancy, an ectopic pregnancy can coexist with a complete abortion. Consequently, pelvic US is essential in all cases of clinically diagnosed complete abortion to examine the adnexa and to determine whether any residual material remains in the uterus.

Incomplete Abortion

Incomplete abortion occurs when some, but not all, of the POCs are expelled vaginally. This occurs more commonly after the tenth week of gestation, whereas complete abortion is more common prior to the tenth week. Because the placental surface is larger and the uterus is unable to completely contract, this condition often is associated with more active bleeding and pain than is completed abortion. Examination of passed tissue is indicated to verify that it is actually of placental or fetal origin rather than just clotted blood or a decidual cast. In most cases, fetal demise has occurred up to 2 weeks previously, and US examination reveals no identifiable fetal structures, but rather, an amorphous collection of tissue and blood.

Missed Abortion

Missed abortion occurs when there is fetal demise but uterine contractions do not occur and the fetus is retained for 4 weeks or more. There may be scant vaginal bleeding at the onset, but this resolves and the patient is often asymptomatic. Most missed abortions terminate spontaneously within 2 weeks of diagnosis. The uterus stops enlarging and may decrease in size. Secondary symptoms of pregnancy, such as breast enlargement, regress and βhCG levels fall progressively. No fetal heartbeat is seen on US, and variable degrees of abnormality are seen, depending on the duration of fetal demise and subsequent degeneration. Often, the placenta is visualized but there is no fetal tissue within the gestational sac.

Prolonged retention of a missed abortion can result in disseminated intravascular coagulation (DIC). This complication is seen more often when the fetal demise occurs during the second trimester, but it can occur at any time during pregnancy and mandates a more aggressive approach in management

Septic Abortion

Serious infection can occur whenever the cervix opens and the uterus is exposed to vaginal flora. All forms of spontaneous and therapeutic abortions may be complicated by infection, but the risk is greatest when tissue remains in the uterus (missed abortion or incomplete abortion) or when the uterus has undergone instrumentation (amniocentesis, D and C, criminal abortion). The most common infecting agents are *Escherichia coli, Streptococcus fecalis,* and, occasionally, *Clostridia perfringens*.[2] Patients present with a septic appearance, including fever, chills, abdominal pain, and weakness. Although the white blood cell count is often elevated in normal pregnancy, elevation beyond 16,000/mL is abnormal and reinforces the diagnosis of septic abortion. On pelvic examination, there is often a purulent vaginal discharge, cervical motion tenderness, and an exquisitely tender uterus. Extension of the infection to produce peritonitis can occur.

Therapeutic Abortion

In recent years, therapeutic abortion is produced pharmacologically rather than surgically. For pregnancies between 4 and 8 weeks, administration of various combinations of misoprostol and mifepristone result in abortion in 92% to 97% of early pregnancies (less than 50 days). Many of these therapeutic abortions are managed on an outpatient basis because of the inherent delay in producing a pharmacologic abortion. Some of these patients subsequently present to the ED with a completed abortion or with complications of abortion. Complications include incomplete abortion (1.8%) and prolonged bleeding (0.4%).[28] Management is identical to that of complete or incomplete abortion, depending on the success of the procedure. The reader is also referred to Chapter 72.

Molar Pregnancy

Hydatidiform mole, invasive mole, and choriocarcinoma are three forms of trophoblastic disease that may present with vaginal bleeding. The incidence of molar pregnancy is one in 1,800 to one in 5,000 pregnancies and is higher in elderly primiparas and Asians. Both malignant and benign forms of trophoblastic disease are characterized by high levels of βhCG, which is a reliable serum marker for following the progression of the disease.

Patients with a molar pregnancy present with a variety of symptoms, but almost all experience vaginal bleeding at some point during the pregnancy. Other clinical findings suggestive of complete molar pregnancy include uterine size that is large for gestational age (50%), more frequent occurrence of hyperemesis gravidarum (26%) due to excessive βhCG production, occurrence of preeclampsia or eclampsia in the first or second trimesters (12% to 27%), and, rarely, vaginal passage of grape-like clusters of hydropic vesicles.[25] In addition, patients with molar pregnancy may present with pulmonary insufficiency, hyperthyroidism, ascites, and multiple, large theca lutein cysts.

The incidence of these findings is much lower in cases of partial molar pregnancy, and many of these cases go undetected. Diagnosis of this condition is essential because of its malignant potential and relative curability by chemotherapy. Approximately 5% of partial molar pregnancies undergo malignant transformation. There are rare case reports of a molar pregnancy coexisting with a twin fetus that can develop normally to term. Management of these cases is clearly difficult and should be in the hands of high-risk obstetrics specialists.

Diagnosis of molar pregnancy is made by an US that shows a characteristic "snowstorm" or "soap bubble" pattern of uterine contents, by the presence of very high (greater than 100,000-U) serum levels of βhCG, or by pathologic examination of curetted material.

Metastases from systemic embolization of trophoblastic material occur in 15% to 20% of cases. Consequently, the level of serum hCG is monitored until it normalizes. If the hCG level fails to normalize within 6 weeks, chemotherapy is initiated, with good cure rates.

Bleeding from Vaginal Lesions

Occasionally, vaginal bleeding may occur during pregnancy from nonobstetric causes such as vaginal or cervical erosions, trauma, infection, adenomas, and carcinomas. Bleeding from these causes is usually of the spotting type, and careful examination of the vaginal walls and cervix usually reveals the cause. Carcinoma of the cervix can certainly occur during childbearing years, and PAP smear or formal biopsy is indicated for suspicious lesions. Endocervical polyps can grow under the hormonal stimulation of pregnancy. They may bleed spontaneously or as a result of relatively minor trauma. Vaginal candidiasis may be associated with a small amount of bleeding as the vaginal mucosa becomes friable. A standard wet mount helps distinguish between the normal increase in vaginal secretions during pregnancy and candidiasis.

EMERGENCY DEPARTMENT EVALUATION AND MANAGEMENT

Unstable Patients with Vaginal Bleeding

All patients presenting with vaginal bleeding require at least urgent medical evaluation, and occasional patients require immediate resuscitation. As in all emergency presentations, patients with massive blood loss from any source require stabilization and resuscitation prior to eliciting historic details or performing laboratory investigations. Patients with evidence of massive blood loss, as reflected by significant hypotension, tachycardia, diminished alertness, syncope, or pallor, or obvious massive vaginal blood loss require the immediate infusion of crystalloid (up to 2 L) and should have two large-bore intravenous lines placed for this purpose. Blood should be obtained for immediate determination of hemoglobin level and coagulation profile, and to type and crossmatch for possible transfusion. If crystalloid infusion is insufficient in restoring normal vital signs and mental status, infusion of type O-negative blood is indicated pending the availability of crossmatched blood. Coagulation defects are corrected by infusion of whole blood or fresh-frozen plasma and platelets as required. Frequent reassessment of vital signs, monitoring of cardiac rhythm and pulse oximetry, supplemental oxygen, and placement of a Foley catheter are indicated to gauge the patient's response to resuscitation.

As resuscitation continues, evaluation of the source of blood loss can be made. Pelvic examination often reveals a large amount of clotted blood, which should be removed with ring forceps. Occasionally, POCs are evident, protruding from the cervical os, and, if possible, these should be removed with ring forceps as well to allow the uterus to contract. Vaginal or cervical lacerations can be sutured. If blood loss continues to be brisk, the vaginal vault can be tightly packed with gauze as a temporizing measure to tamponade bleeding. Infusion of oxytocin will cause uterine contraction and may reduce blood loss but will also trap any POCs that remain in the uterus. Urgent consultation with an obstetrician is indicated to provide definitive care and admission. Performing a D and C can control most vaginal hemorrhage. Rarely, the only means of controlling hemorrhage entails invasive procedures such as emergency hysterectomy or embolization or ligation of the internal iliac arteries.[29,32]

Stable Patients with Vaginal Bleeding

The vast majority of patients presenting with vaginal bleeding have no, or only minor, evidence of the hemodynamic effects of blood loss. Bleeding is often associated with crampy lower abdominal or lower back pain due to uterine contractions. A systematic approach combining history, physical findings, and appropriate laboratory and imaging techniques will reveal an accurate diagnosis in a high percentage of these cases.

It is essential to determine whether the patient is pregnant, and this is readily and rapidly accomplished by measuring serum or urine βhCG. Bedside qualitative testing for hCG is indicated in all reproductive-age females presenting with vaginal bleeding, abdominal or back pain, syncope, or menstrual irregularity. The only appropriate reasons for omitting qualitative hCG testing are the presence of an obvious pregnancy, a previously positive pregnancy test, and a previous hysterectomy.[18] All forms of birth control, including tubal ligation, have a measurable failure rate, especially if patient compliance is less than optimal. Consequently, hCG testing should be conducted regardless of a history of birth control. hCG testing is highly accurate (serum 100%, urine hCG 99%) in diagnosing pregnancy by the time of the first missed menstrual period (hCG 50 to 250 IU/L). Currently used tests for hCG are sensitive to a level of 25 IU/L. The use of quantitative hCG is essential in interpreting US results in early pregnancy and should be obtained routinely if the qualitative test is positive.

History

Once the presence of pregnancy is established, essential historic information includes the time of the last normal menstrual period, previous pregnancies and parity, complications of previous pregnancies, amount and duration of bleeding, whether any fetal tissue has been passed, and symptoms referable to blood or volume loss, such as syncope, weakness, fatigue, dizziness, difficulty breathing, or chest pain.

It is also important to elicit information regarding medications, allergies, and medical and surgical histories, particularly treatment for infertility that predisposes to heterotopic pregnancy.

Physical Examination

After a general physical examination, abdominal and pelvic examinations are indicated in all cases of vaginal bleeding occurring during the first 20 weeks of pregnancy. A pelvic examination should be deferred during the second half of pregnancy because of the risk of precipitating massive bleeding from a placenta previa.

An abdominal examination may reveal evidence of peritoneal irritation, including diminished bowel sounds, involuntary guarding, and rebound tenderness due to hemoperitoneum. After the twelfth week, the uterus may be palpable. Fetal heart tones are audible with a fetoscope by the twelfth week and should be recorded as a routine component of the vital signs.

A pelvic examination reveals variable amounts of blood in the vaginal vault. The character of the blood should be noted, because bright red blood indicates continuing hemorrhage, whereas a brownish discharge suggests that bleeding has stopped spontaneously. The presence of blood clots indicates more significant bleeding than does an unclotted bloody discharge. After evacuating the blood by swabbing or suction, the vault is inspected for bleeding lesions. The cervix is examined for lesions, tenderness on movement (Chandelier's sign), softening and bluish discoloration (Chadwick's sign); for patency of the external and internal ostia to ring forceps; and for active bleeding. POCs that are visible in the os are removed, if possible, with ring forceps. Bimanual examination of the uterus gives an estimate of gestational age and reveals tenderness or masses. Adnexal masses such as corpus luteum cysts are common in pregnancy, but a tender adnexal mass suggests ectopic pregnancy. Exquisite uterine tenderness to palpation suggests endometritis and possible septic abortion.

Pelvic Ultrasound

One of the most important changes in the management of vaginal bleeding in early pregnancy is the use of portable bedside US performed by emergency physicians. Numerous studies validate the accuracy and efficiency of the use of US in this setting.[4,10] Transabdominal US can detect intrauterine pregnancy by the fifth to sixth week, and transvaginal US can detect it by weeks 4.5 to 5.0. It is essential to determine whether the uterus contains a normal fetus. The typical findings in early pregnancy include visualization of an endometrial stripe, the yolk sac by the fifth week, and the fetal pole and fetal heartbeat by weeks 5.5 to 7.0.[3]

TREATMENT OF SPECIFIC CONDITIONS

Fetomaternal Hemorrhage during Spontaneous Abortion

Theoretically, fetomaternal hemorrhage (FMH) can occur by the end of the fourth week of pregnancy. Studies to determine the incidence of FMH during spontaneous abortion reveal conflicting results. One study found an incidence of 0%,[15] and another found an 11% incidence of positive Kleihauer-Betke tests in patients with threatened abortion.[31]

Most authors now recommend that RhoGAM be administered to Rh-negative mothers who present with threatened or other forms of abortion. During the first trimester, "mini RhoGAM" is given at a dose of 50 μg i.m.; later in pregnancy, a regular dose of 300 μg is used.

Threatened Abortion

Management in this case includes admission to the hospital for spontaneous abortion to occur or for D and C. Treatment for threatened abortion is largely supportive. The standard recommendations to avoid sexual intercourse and vaginal douching and to remain at bedrest for 48 hours are unproved in terms of efficacy in preventing spontaneous abortions but are somewhat intuitive. Administration of exogenous hCG has been shown experimentally to be more effective than bedrest in preventing threatened abortion and may prove useful clinically in the future.[13] Treatment with exogenous progesterone has been found ineffective.

Complete Abortion

Management of complete abortion is controversial. In the past, virtually all of these patients underwent D and C to remove all potentially retained tissue and blood. Recently, many of these patients have been successfully managed expectantly with analgesia and other supportive measures. Although D and C results in fewer days of bleeding, it requires admission and a surgical procedure with some attendant risks, particularly uterine perforation, as well as greater cost. This decision can be guided by US. Patients with fluid only in the uterine cavity can be managed expectantly; those with fluid and solid POCs should undergo D and C.[5]

Incomplete Abortion

Bleeding and pain generally are more severe with incomplete abortion than with other forms of abortion. Consequently, parenteral analgesia is often indicated, and the extent of bleeding and need for transfusion should be determined. Pelvic examination often reveals retained POCs in the cervical os, and these should be removed by ring forceps, if possible. This often allows the uterus to contract more completely, producing hemostasis. Visualization of retained placenta by US generally mandates removal by D and C or suction curettage, as these patients are at risk for profuse, prolonged bleeding and infection. Some patients with incomplete abortion can be managed conservatively. One study found that if no POCs were seen on US, neither D and C nor expectant management resulted in any complications. However, if POCs were visualized on US, conservative management resulted in a much higher complication rate (40% vs. 2.5%) compared with D and C.[14]

Septic Abortion

Treatment depends on the degree of sepsis but should always include culture and sensitivity of the discharge, parenteral antibiotics, and admission for evacuation of the uterine contents after the patient has been resuscitated and therapeutic serum levels of antibiotics are obtained. Occasionally, patients with septic abortion may require vigorous resuscitation with fluid infusion, central venous pressure monitoring, pressors, and high-dose antibiotics for septic shock and rapidly progressive infection. Emergency hysterectomy may be required, so emergent obstetric consultation is indicated. Antibiotic treatment should include broad-spectrum anaerobic and gram-negative coverage.

DISPOSITION

Pregnant patients who present with significant anemia or massive vaginal bleeding requiring infusion of more than 1 L of crystalloid or blood to restore normal vital signs, and those with ongoing significant blood loss or vaginal packing, require immediate consultation with an obstetrician and admission to the hospital. Patients with vaginal bleeding beyond the twentieth week are often admitted directly to the obstetric service for monitoring and investigation.

Patients with suspected ruptured ectopic pregnancy require admission and operative treatment. However, hemodynamically stable patients with an unruptured ectopic pregnancy may be managed as outpatients in consultation with the obstetrician, with administration of cytotoxic agents and the provision of early obstetric follow-up.

Patients in whom no clear diagnosis can be made may require admission to the hospital for further investigation, such as laparoscopy or hysteroscopy, to determine the cause of bleeding.

Abortion

Spontaneous complete abortion patients with minimal bleeding and pain can be discharged home after a brief period of observation and instructions to return to the ED if bleeding or pain increases or if fever occurs. They can be followed by an obstetrician within 24 hours in an outpatient setting. Psychological counseling should be offered for patients demonstrating a severe grief reaction to the fetal loss. Patients with recurrent abortion should be referred for genetic counseling as well.

The vast majority of patients with threatened abortion are currently managed as outpatients. Although the efficacy is unproved, standard discharge instructions recommend 24 to 48 hours of bedrest and avoidance of sexual intercourse or vaginal douching. Patients are instructed to return to the ED if bleeding or pain worsens, or if fever occurs, and to bring any passed fetal or placental tissue with them if abortion occurs. Follow-up within 24 to 48 hours is arranged with an obstetric specialist.

Patients with inevitable abortion are admitted to the labor and delivery service, under the care of an obstetrician, for completion of the abortion. All patients with septic abortion are admitted to the hospital for administration of parenteral antibiotics and, ultimately, removal of the fetus and placenta. Patients in septic shock are managed in an intensive care setting and may require large volumes of fluids, invasive monitoring, and pressor agents to reverse shock.

Disposition of patients with incomplete abortion is more controversial. Traditionally, these patients were admitted for D and C. Recently, studies have shown that expectant management may be as safe and effective as D and C in managing these cases. This decision should be made in consultation with the obstetric specialist who will follow the patient. Adequate pain management must be ensured if the patient is to be managed as an outpatient.

COMMON PITFALLS

- The emergency physician should be aware that a significant number of patients who experience spontaneous abortion are at risk for developing a major depressive episode within the following 6 months.
- One of the most common pitfalls is the failure to suspect pregnancy as the etiology of abdominal pain or vaginal bleeding in reproductive-age females. Often, patients provide inaccurate information regarding sexual activity, compliance with birth control, and the timing of the last menstrual period. It is essential to determine whether the patient is pregnant, and the best means of accomplishing this is by routinely measuring βhCG in all reproductive-age females with abdominal pain or vaginal bleeding.
- In mothers with uncertain dates, a US done at 5 weeks' gestation may visualize a yolk sac that is mistaken for an empty gestational sac. Subsequent therapeutic evacuation of the uterus may terminate a viable pregnancy.
- Failure to administer appropriate doses of RhoGAM to block maternal isosensitization may result in erythroblastosis fetalis in subsequent pregnancies after FMH during spontaneous abortion. Although studies show conflicting results on the incidence of FMH, it is prudent to administer RhoGAM to Rh-negative mothers with vaginal bleeding beyond the fourth week of pregnancy.
- Ectopic pregnancy: Passage of a decidual cast that is present with ectopic pregnancy may mimic passage of fetal and placental tissue. Similarly, patients who have undergone D and C may still harbor an ectopic pregnancy if only the uterine decidual cast is removed at D and C. Consequently, it is essential to verify the pathologic examination of tissue obtained through spontaneous abortion or D and C. The absence of chorionic villi and fetal tissue on pathologic examination should prompt further investigation for possible ectopic pregnancy.
- A pseudogestational sac may be seen in 10% to 20% of ectopic pregnancies. This may be misinterpreted as the "double-ring sign" of an intrauterine pregnancy, causing the diagnosis of ectopic pregnancy to be inappropriately dismissed.
- Diagnosis of heterotopic pregnancy is difficult. The presence of a viable intrauterine fetus on US may cause the clinician to incorrectly exclude the possibility of concurrent ectopic pregnancy. This is particularly true in patients undergoing ovarian stimulation treatment for infertility, because, in this group, the incidence of heterotopic pregnancy may be as high as one in 100.

- *Molar pregnancy:* Failure to submit aborted material for pathologic examination may result in failure to diagnose a partial molar pregnancy. Consequently, the opportunity to intervene with chemotherapy may be lost or long-delayed.

References

1. Aboud E. A five year review of ectopic pregnancy. *Clin Exp Obstet Gynecol* 1997;24:127–129.
2. Allan A. Vaginal bleeding in early pregnancy. *Practitioner* 1994;238:310–315.
3. Brennan DF. Ectopic pregnancy—Part II: diagnostic procedures and imaging. *Acad Emerg Med* 1995;2:1090–1097.
4. Burgher SW, Tandy TS, Dawdy MR. Transvaginal ultrasound by emergency physicians decreases patient time in the emergency department. *Acad Emerg Med* 1998;5:802–807.
5. Cetin A, Cetin M. Diagnostic and therapeutic decision-making with transvaginal sonography for first trimester spontaneous abortion, clinically thought to be complete or incomplete. *Contraception* 1998;57:393–597.
6. Chamberlain G. Vaginal bleeding in early pregnancy. *BMJ* 1991;302:1141–1143.
7. Coulam CB, Clark DA, Kutteh WH. Current clinical options for diagnosis and treatment of recurrent spontaneous abortion. *Am J Reprod Immunol* 1997;38:57–74.
8. Cunningham DS, Brodnik RM, Rayl DL, et al. Suboptimal progesterone production in pathologic pregnancies. *J Reprod Med* 1993;38:301–305.
9. Dart R, Dart L, Segal M, et al. The ability of a single serum progesterone value to identify abnormal pregnancies in a patients with beta-human chorionic gonadotropin values less than 1000 mIU/mL. *Acad Emerg Med* 1998;5:304–309.
10. Durham B, Lane B, Burbridge L, et al. Pelvic ultrasound performed by emergency physicians for the detection of ectopic pregnancy in complicated first trimester pregnancies. *Ann Emerg Med* 1996;29:338–347.
11. Everett C. Incidence and outcome of bleeding before the 20th week of pregnancy: prospective study from general practice. *BMJ* 1997;315:32–34.
12. Everett CB, Preece E. Women with bleeding in the first 20 weeks of pregnancy: value of a general practice ultrasound in detecting fetal heart movement. *Br J Gen Pract* 1996;46:7–9.
13. Harrison RF. A comparative study of human chorionic gonadotropin, placebo, and bed rest for women with early threatened abortion. *Int J Fertil Menopausal Stud* 1993;38:160–165.
14. Hurd WW, Whitfield RR, Randolph JF, et al. Expectant management versus elective curettage or the treatment of spontaneous abortion. *Fertil Steril* 1997;68:601–606.
15. Kuller JA, Laifer SA, Portney DL, et al. The frequency of transplacental hemorrhage in patients with threatened abortion. *Gynecol Obstet Invest* 1994;37:229–231.
16. Mason E, Rosene-Montella K, Powrie R. Medical problems during pregnancy. *Med Clin North Am* 1998;82:249–269.
17. McBride WZ. Spontaneous abortion. *Am Fam Physician* 1991;43:175–182.
18. McKennett M, Fullerton JT. Vaginal bleeding in pregnancy. *Am Fam Physician* 1995;51:639–646.
19. Murakawa H, Utumi T, Hasegawa I, et al. Evaluation of threatened preterm delivery by transvaginal ultrasonographic measurement of cervical length. *Obstet Gynecol* 1993;82:829–832.
20. Neugebauer R, Kline J, Shrout P, et al. Major depressive disorder in the six months after miscarriage. *JAMA* 1997;277:3838.
21. Noci I, Biagiotti R, Periti E, et al. Maternal CA 125 levels in first trimester abortion. *Eur J Obstet Gynecol Reprod* 1995;60:35–36.
22. Ocer S, Bese T, Saridogan E, et al. The prognostic significance of maternal serum CA 125 measurement in threatened abortion. *Eur J Obstet Gynecol Reprod Biol* 1992;46:137–142.
23. Parazzini F, Chatenoud L, Tozzi L, et al. Determinants of risk of spontaneous abortions in first trimester pregnancy. *Epidemiology* 1997;8:681–683.
24. Pedersen JF, Ruge S, Sorensen S. Depressed levels of human placental lactogen in first trimester vaginal bleeding. *Acta Obstet Gynecol Scand* 1995;74:27–29.
25. Rose PG. Hydatidiform mole: diagnosis and management. *Semin Oncol* 1995;22:149–156.
26. Shahani SK, Moniz CL, Brdekar AD, et al. Early pregnancy factor as a marker for assessing embryonic viability in threatened and missed abortion. *Gynecol Obstet Invest* 1994;37:73–76.
27. Smith EE, Cantrill SV, Campbell M, et al. Clinical policy for the initial approach to patients presenting with a chief complaint of vaginal bleeding. ACEP clinical policy. *Ann Emerg Med* 1997;29:435–458.
28. Spitz IM, Bardin CW, Benton L, et al. Early pregnancy termination with mifepristone and misoprostol in the United States. *N Engl J Med* 1998;338:1241–1247.
29. Thavarasah AS, Sivalingam N, Almohdzar SA. Internal iliac and ovarian artery ligation in the control of pelvic haemorrhage. *Aust N Z J Obstet Gynaecol* 1989;29:22–25.
30. Valley VT, Mateer JR, Aiman EJ, et al. Serum progesterone and endovaginal sonography by emergency physicians in the evaluation of ectopic pregnancy. *Acad Emerg Med* 1998;5:309–313.
31. Von Stein GA, Munsick RA, Stiver K, et al. Fetomaternal hemorrhage in threatened abortion. *Obstet Gynecol* 1992;79:383–386.
32. Yamashita Y, Harada, M, Yamamoto H, et al. Transcatheter arterial embolization of obstetric and gynaecological bleeding: efficacy and clinical outcome. *Br J Radiol* 1994;67:530–534.
33. Zhang J, Olshan A, Cai WW. Birth defects in relation to threatened abortion. *Epidemiology* 1994;5:341–344.

CHAPTER 74

Ectopic Pregnancy

G. Richard Braen and Richard S. Krause

One of the leading causes of maternal morbidity and mortality in the United States is ectopic pregnancy. It is also a major factor in decreasing the future fertility of the affected woman and is aptly called an unqualified disaster in human reproduction.[9] Fetal wastage is virtually 100%. Unfortunately, the frequency of ectopic pregnancies in the United States has increased by fivefold since 1970.[3] Pooled data indicate that the current incidence of ectopic pregnancy is 16.8 per 1000 pregnancies (1.7% of all pregnancies in women in the United States will be ectopic).[33] Furthermore, it is estimated that of 100 women with a history of ectopic pregnancy, approximately 50% will be infertile, 35% to 40% will subsequently have a successful pregnancy, and 10% to 15% will experience a second ectopic pregnancy.[20]

Ectopic pregnancy is the result of implantation of a fertilized ovum at a site other than the endometrium of the uterine cavity. The most frequent site of implantation is the lateral two-thirds of the fallopian tube (80%) (Fig. 74.1). About 15% implant in the medial one-third. Interstitial or cornual implantation occurs in approximately 3% of ectopic gestations. Interstitial and abdominal implantations carry the greatest risk of mortality because of their hemorrhagic tendencies.[10] Extratubal ectopic gestations occur in about 5% of cases: in the ovary (3%), within the abdominal cavity (2%), or in the cervix (rare). Combined intrauterine and extrauterine gestations (heterotopic pregnancy) were formerly very rare, with an estimated incidence of one in 30,000 pregnancies.[34] Combined pregnancies are now estimated to occur in up to one in 3000 normal patients and 1 in 100 patients being treated with assisted reproductive technologies.[12]

The most common predisposing factors include intrinsic or extrinsic abnormalities of the fallopian tube and abnormal development of the embryo itself. Abnormalities of the fallopian tube have been extensively studied and are believed to be the most important cause of ectopic pregnancies. The most common source of tubal pathology is pelvic inflammatory disease (PID).[31] The risk of ectopic pregnancy is known to be several times more likely among women with a history of salpingitis.[32] All pathogens, including *Chlamydia* and gonococci, are believed to cause tubal distortion and scarring, which adversely affect tubal patency and motility. Subacute infection with less virulent organisms may actually increase the amount of residual tubal pathology because diagnosis and treatment may be delayed.[13] Up to 64% of fetuses associated with ectopic pregnancy are abnormal.[22] However, it is not known whether these abnormalities cause altered transit through the fallopian tube or whether they result from the poor growth environment of the ectopic implantation site.[27]

There are multiple risk factors for developing an ectopic pregnancy. Table 74.1 lists several important population characteristics. The numerical risk assigned to each population characteristic applies to a pregnant woman with that particular characteristic. Table 74.1 is most useful in assessing the relative risk a woman has of harboring an ectopic gestation if she is known to be pregnant. However, up to 42% of women with ectopic pregnancy have no historic risks factors.[33]

Age at the time of conception is a relative risk factor for developing an ectopic pregnancy. The percentage of pregnancies that are ectopic increases with maternal age and is threefold greater in the older age group than in the younger.[25]

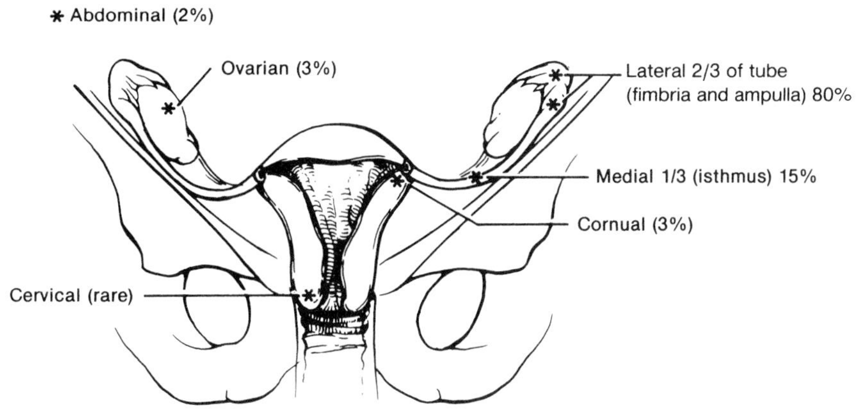

Figure 74.1. Sites of implantation in ectopic pregnancy.

Fourteen percent of all pregnancies in women with an intrauterine device (IUD) are ectopic. The IUD does not prevent ovulation, as does the oral contraceptive, but interferes with intrauterine implantation of the ovum. Therefore, a woman wearing an IUD is potentially at risk for tubal implantation if her ovum becomes fertilized. Additionally, IUD wearers are frequently subjected to delayed diagnosis of ectopic pregnancy.[27] Health-care providers may confuse the symptoms caused by an ectopic pregnancy with those related to the mechanical or inflammatory response of an IUD (which indeed may be identical) and fail to consider the possibility of an ectopic gestation in an IUD wearer.[14]

PID is almost universally accepted as the major causative factor for ectopic pregnancies. An epidemic of PID is occurring in the United States.[7] Major risk factors for PID are age in the 20s, divorce, and marital separation.[29] Rates for non-White women are 1.4 to 2.5 times higher than those for White women.

Ectopic pregnancy must be considered after tubal sterilization procedures. Sixteen percent of women who become pregnant after tubal sterilization have an ectopic gestation. In most cases, this probably represents partial recanalization with access of the sperm to the ovum but impaired passage of the fertilized ovum to the uterine cavity. Like IUD wearers, patients who have had prior tubal sterilization are frequently subjected to a delay in diagnosis of ectopic gestation. Physicians often neglect to consider this diagnosis early in the presentation.

Women who have had an elective abortion within the preceding 2 weeks and present with symptoms referable to the genital tract are at risk of having an undiagnosed ectopic pregnancy. Confirmation of the products of uterine extraction is necessary to exclude the diagnosis of ectopic pregnancy. This is a frequent problem in large urban clinics with a high incidence of therapeutic abortions performed with unreliable follow-up.[28]

The major life-threatening condition associated with an ectopic pregnancy is intraabdominal hemorrhage with shock. Refractory hemorrhagic shock is the cause of death in approximately 85% of fatalities from ectopic pregnancy.[10] Misdiagnosis by physicians contributes to one-half of the fatalities.[10] It is common for an emergency physician to evaluate a patient with a ruptured ectopic pregnancy with a history of several prior visits for abdominal pain or vaginal bleeding.

TABLE 74.1. Rates of Ectopic Pregnancy for Various Population Subgroups

Population Characteristic	Ectopic Pregnancies As a Percentage of Total Pregnancies in Each Population Group
Overall	0.94
Age	
15–19 yr	0.45
20–29 yr	0.82
30–39 yr	1.42
Contraception	
Oral contraceptives	0
Barrier	0.002
IUD	14.0
One or more episodes of salpingitis (by laparoscopy)	6.9
Prior tubal sterilization	16.0
Prior ectopic pregnancy	11.2

Adopted from Westrom L, Bengtsson L, March PA. Incidence, trends and risks of ectopic pregnancy in a population of women. BMJ 1981;282:15.

CLINICAL PRESENTATION

Any patient with lower abdominal pain or vaginal bleeding with a positive pregnancy test in the first trimester should be suspected of having an ectopic pregnancy. The "classic" triad of amenorrhea, vaginal bleeding, and abdominal pain is neither sensitive nor specific for ectopic pregnancy. Only 15% of patients with ectopic pregnancies present with this classic picture. Only 14% of patients with the classic constellation of signs and symptoms actually have an ectopic gestation.[26]

Abdominal pain is the most common symptom and is reported in more than 97% of patients. Abnormal vaginal bleeding is present in 55% to 86% of cases.[1,15,21,28,30] A "normal" menstrual history is obtained in 15% to 30% of patients. Abdominal pain occurs *without* bleeding in up to one-third of patients. It should be emphasized that consideration of an ectopic pregnancy is based on a history of abdominal pain and a positive pregnancy test in the first trimester. The quality, character, and location of the pain are highly variable.[15] It may be cramping, colicky, steady, or dull. Flank or lower back pain may be noted, or tenesmus may occur from rectal irritation caused by blood in the cul-de-sac.[6] The pain may be localized to either lower quadrant or may be generalized, suggesting hemoperitoneum.[1,15] Profuse vaginal hemorrhage occurs in the minority of cases and suggests rupture of a cornual implantation.[7]

Vital signs are often normal, except in those patients with significant blood loss. This will be manifested by orthostatic hypotension, tachycardia, or frank shock. Paradoxic bradycardia may be seen. Any woman of childbearing age who presents with signs of hemorrhagic shock without historic or physical evidence of trauma has a ruptured ectopic pregnancy until proved otherwise. Fever is seldom present.

Tenderness on pelvic examination is the most common sign and is present in 83% to 97% of cases.[1,15,21,28] The physical findings depend on whether intraperitoneal irritation has occurred from leakage or rupture of the ectopic gestation.

A palpable mass may represent the ectopic gestation or be felt on the side opposite the ectopic gestation, possibly representing a corpus luteum cyst rather than the ectopic pregnancy.[21] Transmigration of the fertilized ovum to the opposite tube is presumed to have occurred in these cases.[17]

A recent study utilized sophisticated statistical methods to identify findings on history and physical that are predictive of ectopic pregnancy. Patients with ectopic pregnancy were more likely to have moderate-to-severe sharp abdominal pain with abdominal or pelvic tenderness and a small uterus on physical examination. Peritoneal signs were uncommon but highly predictive of ectopic pregnancy. Risk factors strongly predictive of ectopic pregnancy included infertility, use of an IUD, tubal ligation, or other pelvic surgery. Patients with these characteristics are at especially high risk for ectopic pregnancy. However, no combination of factors confirmed or excluded the diagnosis of ectopic pregnancy with a high degree of certainty.[8]

DIFFERENTIAL DIAGNOSIS

Given the broad spectrum of patient complaints and physical findings, the differential diagnosis of ectopic pregnancy is proportionally broad. The most common pelvic conditions that share clinical aspects of ectopic pregnancy include PID, threatened or incomplete abortion, corpus luteum or follicular cyst, ovarian cyst with a twisted pedicle, endometriosis, gastrointestinal disorders, dysfunctional uterine bleeding, mittelschmerz, and intrauterine pregnancy.

PID is the diagnosis most commonly confused with ectopic pregnancy.[13] The signs and symptoms may be identical and the same population is at risk. A significant percentage of normal intrauterine pregnancies are associated with pelvic pain and vaginal bleeding in the first trimester, as are almost all cases of nonviable intrauterine pregnancies. Rupture of a corpus luteum cyst of pregnancy is associated with a positive pregnancy test, pain, and a tender pelvic mass—identical symptoms of an ectopic pregnancy. Serous cul-de-sac fluid may help to differentiate the two.

Gastrointestinal disorders to be differentiated include appendicitis, diverticulitis, irritable bowel syndrome, and gastroenteritis. Nephrolithiasis should also be considered.

Patients who merit special consideration are those with a history of tubal ligation or other pelvic surgery, an IUD in place or recently removed, or a recent history of an elective or spontaneous abortion. An especially high risk group is those undergoing treatment of infertility with embryo transfer procedures or ovulation-inducing agents. These patients are at increased risk of mortality because of the *failure to consider ectopic pregnancy.*

EMERGENCY DEPARTMENT EVALUATION

The evaluation of suspected ectopic pregnancy may be organized into three general categories based on hemodynamic stability (Table 74.2).

The history should emphasize the patient's reproductive past, menstrual history, and risk factors, and a chronologic review of the nature and intensity of the symptoms.

The physical examination should focus on changes associated with normal pregnancy and signs of peritoneal inflammation or significant blood loss. Uterine size, adnexal masses, appearance of cervix and os, and rectal examination should be noted. Serial abdominal examinations may aid in the assessment. A pelvic examination should be repeated only as necessary because of the concern that overly aggressive palpation may precipitate rupture.

TABLE 74.2. Categories for Evaluating Suspected Ectopic Pregnancy Based on Hemodynamic Stability

CATEGORY A
Patients presenting in hypovolemic shock
CATEGORY B
Patients of reproductive age presenting with complaints and physical findings indicative of an acute abdoman but who are hemodynamically stable
CATEGORY C
Patients presenting with abdominopelvic complaints suggestive of an ectopic pregnancy but who are clinically judged to be at low risk of immediates deterioration.

Laboratory studies should include a urinalysis and a pregnancy test. For patients in categories A and B (see Table 74.2), a hematocrit and a blood bank specimen are necessary. Other laboratory tests are nonspecific and seldom useful in establishing the diagnosis of ectopic pregnancy.

Sensitive urine pregnancy tests with a human chorionic gonadotropin (hCG) threshold of 20 IU/L should be used as a screening test for possible ectopic gestation. The current generation of urine hCG assays using monoclonally derived, enzyme-tagged antibodies meets this sensitivity requirement. These assays allow detection of pregnancy at 1 week postconception (3 weeks' gestation). Almost all patients with an ectopic pregnancy will have a positive pregnancy test if the threshold for hCG is 20 IU/L.[4] The chance for a false-negative result exists when the serum hCG level is low and the urine is dilute (specific gravity less than 1.010).[2] A patient highly suspected of harboring an ectopic gestation with a dilute urine and a negative urine pregnancy test should have a serum β-hCG radioimmunoassay.

Patients in category C (see Table 74.2) may benefit from quantitative serum hCG level determinations. Serum β-hCG levels rise exponentially during the first 6 weeks of gestation and peak at approximately 100,000 mIU/mL. A single quantitative serum β-hCG value serves as an objective substitute for a menstrual history (i.e., it dates the pregnancy). This becomes important because one-third of patients with an ectopic pregnancy cannot recall the date of their last menstrual period. The irregular bleeding associated with ectopic gestation clouds certainty about the duration of amenorrhea in others. Serial quantitative serum β-hCG levels double every 2 days in early *intrauterine* pregnancies. Abnormal gestations, both intrauterine and extrauterine, have prolonged doubling times.[18] Patients in whom serum β-hCG levels do not increase by more than 66% (1.66-fold increase) in 48 hours are likely to harbor an abnormal pregnancy and should have further evaluation.[23] Serial serum quantitative β-hCG determinations can be used in stable patients to more accurately detect a nonviable intrauterine or ectopic gestation.

The gestational sac of a normal intrauterine pregnancy becomes visible with transabdominal ultrasonography at 5 to 6 weeks' gestation, corresponding to a quantitative β-hCG of 6000 to 6500 mIU/mL.[16] With transvaginal sonography, a gestational sac is commonly visualized when the β-hCG level exceeds 1000 mIU/mL.

This level of β-hCG is often referred to as the discriminatory zone.[18,19] Intrauterine pregnancy or findings suggestive of an ectopic gestation may be seen with very low β-hCG levels. β-hCG levels should therefore not be used as a basis for delaying ultrasonography when ectopic pregnancy is suspected.

Ultrasonography is operator dependent and has a high incidence of nonspecific findings with gestational ages earlier than 5 to 6 weeks. With transvaginal ultrasonography, a gestational sac is identified and localized outside the uterus in about 62% of ectopic pregnancies.[33] False-negative and false-positive results occur in up to 25% of patients.[5] Although a positive diagnosis of ectopic pregnancy can be made by identifying an extrauterine gestation, this is a rare finding. In practice, ultrasonography is more helpful in excluding the diagnosis when it demonstrates an intrauterine pregnancy, because the combined gestation is so rare.

The correlation of ultrasonographic findings with quantitative serum β-hCG levels increases the accuracy of diagnosis in ectopic pregnancy. This is especially true if the quantitative β-hCG level is above the discriminatory zone.[18,19] The absence of a gestational sac with a serum β-hCG titer above the discriminatory zone has a sensitivity of 100%, a specificity of 96%, a positive predictive value of 86%, and a negative predictive value of 100% for the diagnosis of ectopic pregnancy.[24] The ultrasonographic absence of an intrauterine sac, with hCG levels below the discriminatory zone, does not allow the definitive diagnosis of an ectopic pregnancy.

In summary, urine hCG testing screens for pregnancy and ultrasonography locates it. A single quantitative serum β-hCG assay is used to date the pregnancy and increase the accuracy of ultrasonographic results, while serial quantitative levels merely tell the clinician whether the pregnancy is behaving in a normal biochemical manner.

Because pregnancy can be biochemically detected at approximately 1 week of gestation but may not be located reliably with ultrasonography until 5 to 6 weeks of gestation, a 4- to 5-week period of uncertainty exists. During this period, a pregnancy can be detected but often cannot be located by noninvasive means. Laparoscopy performed on all patients in the period of uncertainty results in a high incidence of unnecessary diagnostic laparoscopies for normal intrauterine pregnancies.[26] Therefore, patients in category C (see Table 74.2) during the period of uncertainty, who are stable and reliable, are best evaluated by se-

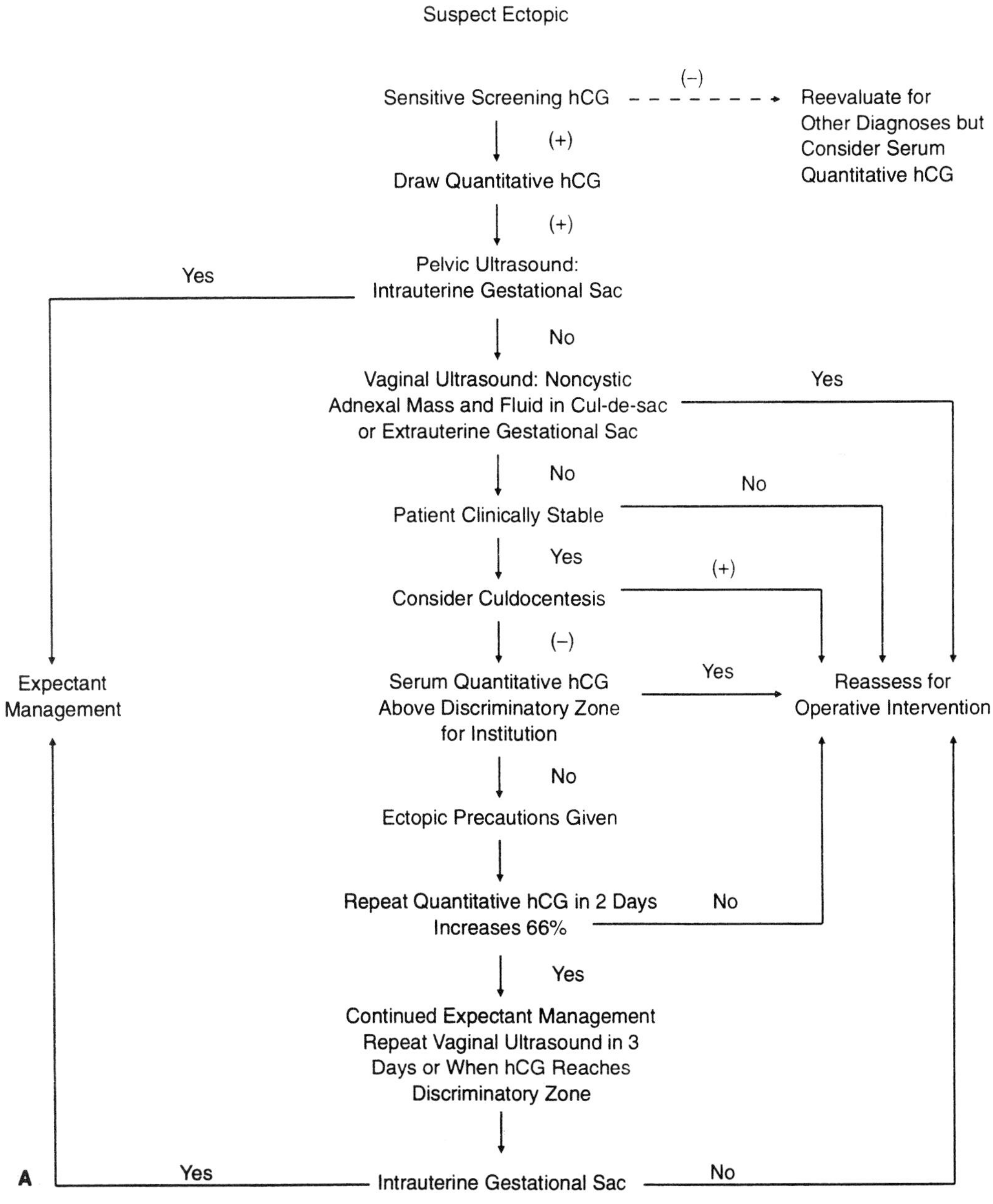

Figure 74.2. Algorithm for evaluation and management of suspected ectopic pregnancy. **(A)** When ultrasonography is not readily available. *(figure continues)*

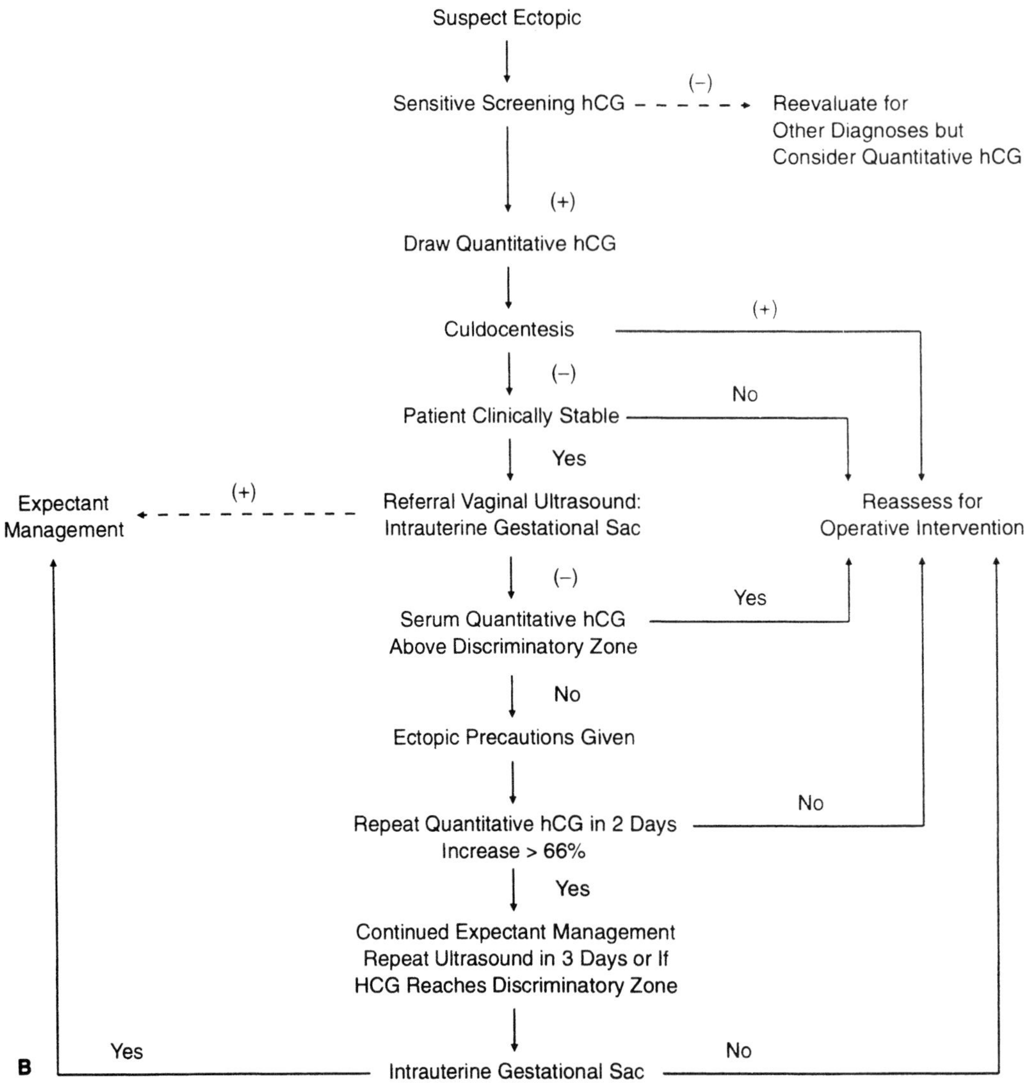

Figure 74.2. *(continued)* **(B)** When ultrasonography is available. (From Wolcott HD, Stock RJ, Kaunitz AM. Ectopic pregnancy. In: Benrubi G, ed. *Obstetric and gynecologic emergencies*. Philadelphia: JB Lippincott Co, 1994, with permission.)

rial serum quantitative β-hCG level, provided that an initial sonogram is nondiagnostic. Failure of β-hCG levels to increase normally places a patient at higher risk for an ectopic or other abnormal pregnancy.

Culdocentesis is a simple, rapid, and accurate method of detecting intraperitoneal blood. It may be used when ultrasonography is not immediately available or when ultrasonography results are equivocal. A positive test is one in which nonclotting blood is aspirated from the cul-de-sac with a hematocrit higher than 15%. A "dry tap" is nondiagnostic. A negative tap occurs when clear fluid is obtained. When positive, the test will identify a ruptured or leaking ectopic pregnancy with high sensitivity and moderate specificity.[11] Patients in categories B and C are likely to benefit from both ultrasonography and culdocentesis. However, if either modality delays operative intervention in category A patients, it should not be used, because findings will not alter management, but delay treatment.

EMERGENCY DEPARTMENT MANAGEMENT

Management is guided by the patient's hemodynamic status, reliability for follow-up, and the availability of ultrasonography (Fig. 74.2).[33] *Patients in category A* should be treated for hemorrhagic shock: The patient should be placed in the Trendelenburg position and administered high-flow oxygen by nonrebreather mask. Two large-bore peripheral intravenous lines should be established and crystalloid infusion begun. Baseline blood samples should be obtained in addition to a clot tube for the blood bank. Transfusion with O-negative, type-specific, or fully crossmatched blood should be considered after crystalloid infusion, depending on the infusion urgency and response of the patient to initial therapy. Immediate gynecologic consultation for laparotomy should be obtained.

Patients in category B are stable but have potential for rapid progression to category A. Anticipation of fluid resuscitation and rapid confirmation of the diagnosis dictate the course of evaluation and management. One or two large-bore intravenous lines should be established. Baseline blood studies include complete blood cell count, Rh typing, and typing and screening for potential blood replacement. A sensitive urine pregnancy test must also be performed. Ultrasonography should be used if immediately available. Culdocentesis is used if ultrasonography results are nondiagnostic or if ultrasonography is not available. Patients in category B, by definition, have an acute abdomen. Therefore, they warrant urgent consultation.

Patients in categories A and B present few problems in evaluation and management. *Patients in category C,* who are stable and ambulatory, pose the greatest diagnostic and management problems. Figure 74.2 provides a useful management scheme. The evaluation of a possible ectopic pregnancy starts with a urine pregnancy test on *all* women of childbearing age who present with abdominopelvic pain. The *only exception* is the woman who has had a hysterectomy. The presence of an IUD, tubal ligation, a partner with a vasectomy, or incidental trauma should not deter consideration of an ectopic pregnancy. The diagnosis should be pursued until reasonably ruled out.

DISPOSITION

Role of the Consultant

Given the broad spectrum of presentations and the lack of pathognomonic findings in suspected ectopic pregnancy, there should be a low threshold for requesting consultation from the gynecology, radiology, and surgery services.

Consultation should be obtained for patients in category A or B. Early notification of consulting services may allow early mobilization of operating room personnel. The timing for consultation in category C patients is more flexible and dependent on local resources, consultant availability, and whether the patient has a previously established relationship with a gynecologist. Category C patients with a positive culdocentesis should *not* be discharged from the emergency department before specialty consultation. Category C patients with a negative or diagnostic culdocentesis fall into a gray zone, and the timing of consultation depends on the patient's symptoms and potential for clinical deterioration. Other category C patients in whom culdocentesis was omitted because of minimal symptoms may be discharged with careful instructions and outpatient follow-up.

Indications for Admission

All patients in categories A and B require admission. Category C patients may be discharged with gynecologic follow-up in 48 hours, except in the following instances:

- Positive culdocentesis
- Progressive symptomatology or physical findings
- When no intrauterine pregnancy can be visualized on ultrasonography in a symptomatic patient with a reliable menstrual history that dates the pregnancy at 5 to 6 weeks' gestation or in a patient with a quantitative serum β-hCG level above the discriminatory zone
- Patients unreliable for follow-up

The usual timing of follow-up is 48 hours, the standard sampling interval for quantitative serum β-hCG levels. Most outpatients will be evaluated by this method. All patients discharged from the emergency department with ectopic pregnancy in the differential diagnosis should be placed in an Expectant Management Register to ensure follow-up, track serial hCG levels, or call-back for an emergency department recheck, should that be necessary. A management system should also be in place to follow up on the products of uterine extraction in women who undergo uterine evacuation procedures in the emergency department for suspected incomplete abortion. If the pathology report shows "no chorionic villi," ectopic pregnancy is the likely diagnosis and the patient should return for further evaluation.

Alternative Therapy for Unruptured Ectopic Pregnancies

Patients with unruptured ectopic pregnancies may be treated using alternative therapeutic options. Methotrexate may be used for these cases when given orally, intramuscularly, or intravenously, along with leucovorin rescue to prevent toxicity to bone marrow. Regimens exist that include single-dose methotrexate/leucovorin with minimal toxicity to the patient.

Patients treated medically for ectopic pregnancy may experience abdominal pain 3 to 7 days after treatment. This is thought to be secondary to methotrexate-induced tubal abortion. It may be difficult to differentiate expected pain from pain due to rupture of a persistent EP. Patients presenting with abdominal pain in this timeframe following methotrexate administration should have a complete blood count and ultrasound to rule out significant free fluid in the cul-de-sac, and should be evaluated for other causes of abdominal pain. The patient may need consultation and/or admission to the hospital for observation. Hemodynamic instability and/or falling hematocrit would require surgical intervention.

Stable patients with an ectopic pregnancy and no cardiac activity on ultrasound may be followed with serial examination and repeat quantitative β-hCG levels. If the levels continue to fall, no invasive interventions may be necessary. In addition to the repeat β-hCG levels, repeat transvaginal ultrasonic scanning should be considered to ensure reabsorption of the embryo.[1]

Transfer Considerations

In general, patients should be transferred only if there is no operating facility and an ectopic pregnancy has been diagnosed or if an ectopic pregnancy is strongly suspected but diagnostic resources are unavailable. Stable patients and patients in hypovolemic shock who undergo successful volume resuscitation may be transferred with appropriate personnel. Intravenous access is necessary.

It is important that the receiving physician be provided with all available information so that he or she may contribute to the management and transfer plan.

COMMON PITFALLS

- The most common pitfall is failure to consider the diagnosis of ectopic pregnancy, especially in women with few symptoms.
- Ultrasonography, culdocentesis, and serum β-hCG level determinations are of limited sensitivity and specificity.
- In making a diagnostic decision, clinical findings consistent with ectopic pregnancy should outweigh any single negative test result.
- Delays have been documented in cases that involve women who have undergone tubal sterilization, women with an IUD in place or recently removed, and women who have undergone a recent spontaneous or therapeutic abortion. Ectopic pregnancy does occur in these groups and must be ruled out.

References

1. Carson SA, Buster JE. Ectopic pregnancy. *N Engl J Med* 1993;329:1174.
2. Cartwright PS. Performance of a new enzyme linked immunoassay for the detection of ectopic gestation. *Ann Emerg Med* 1986;15:1198.
3. Centers for Disease Control. Ectopic pregnancy surveillance, United States, 1970–1987. *MMWR* 1988;39(554):9.
4. Christensen H, Thyssen H, Schebye O, et al. Three highly sensitive "bedside" serum and urine tests for pregnancy compared. *Clin Chem* 1990;36:1686.
5. Chinn DH, Callen PW. Ultrasound of the acutely ill obstetrics and gynecology patient. *Radiol Clin North Am* 1983;21:585.
6. Cohen AW, ed. *Emergencies in obstetrics and gynecology.* New York: Churchill Livingstone, 1981.
7. Curran JW. Economic consequences of pelvic inflammatory disease in the United States. *Am J Obstet Gynecol* 1980;138:848.
8. Dart R, Kaplan B, Varaklis K. Predictive value of history and physical examination in patients with suspected ectopic pregnancy. *Ann Emerg Med* 1999;283–290.

9. DeCherney AH. Ectopic pregnancy. In: Kase NG, Weingold AB, eds. *Principles and practice of clinical gynecology*. New York: John Wiley and Sons, 1983:483.
10. Dorfman SF, Grimes DA, Cates W, et al. Ectopic pregnancy mortality, United States, 1979 to 1980: clinical aspects. *Obstet Gynecol* 1984;64:386.
11. Eisinger SH. Culdocentesis. *J Fam Pract* 1981;13:95.
12. Gamberoella FR, Marrs RP. Heterotopic pregnancy associated with assisted reproductive technology. *Am J Obstet Gynecol* 1999;160:1520–1523.
13. Gonzalez FA, Waxman M. Ectopic pregnancy: a prospective study on differential diagnosis. *Diagn Gynecol Obstet* 1981;3:101.
14. Gump DW, Gibson M, Ashikaya T. Evidence of prior pelvic inflammatory disease and its relationship to *Chlamydia trachomatis* antibody and intrauterine contraceptive device use in infertile women. *Am J Obstet Gynecol* 1983;146:153.
15. Helvancioglu A, Long EM, Yang SL. Ectopic pregnancy, an eight-year review. *J Reprod Med* 1979;22:87.
16. Hill LM, Breckle R, Wolfgram KR. An ultrasonic view of the developing fetus. *Obstet Gynecol Surv* 1983;38:375.
17. Iffy L, Gasser RF. Tubal pregnancy. *Obstet Gynecol* 1976;47:380.
18. Kadar N, Caldwell B, Romero R. A method of screening for ectopic pregnancy and its indications. *Obstet Gynecol* 1980;58:162.
19. Kadar N, Devore G, Romero R. Discriminatory HCG zone: its use in the sonographic evaluation for ectopic pregnancy. *Obstet Gynecol* 1981;58:156.
20. Metha L, Young ID. Recurrence risk for common complications of pregnancy—a review. *Obstet Gynecol Surv* 1987;42:218.
21. Pagano R. Ectopic pregnancy: a seven year survey. *Med J Aust* 1981;2:586.
22. Poland BJ, Dill FJ, Stylbo C. Embryonic development in ectopic human pregnancy. *Teratology* 1976;14:315.
23. Romero R. Understanding and treating first trimester vaginal bleeding. *Contemp Obstet Gynecol* 1983;21:6.
24. Romero R, Kadar N, Jeanty P, et al. The value of the discriminatory HCG zone in the diagnosis of ectopic pregnancy. *Obstet Gynecol* 1985;66:357.
25. Rubin GL, Peterson HB, Dorfman SF, et al. Ectopic pregnancy in the United States, 1970 through 1978. *JAMA* 1983;249:1725.
26. Schwartz RO, DiPietro DL. Beta HCG as a diagnostic aid for suspected ectopic pregnancy. *Obstet Gynecol* 1980;56:197.
27. Scott J, DiSaia PJ, Hammond C, et al., eds. *Danforth's obstetrics and gynecology*, 7th ed. Philadelphia: JB Lippincott Co, 1994.
28. Tancer ML, Delke I, Veridiano NP. A fifteen year experience with ectopic pregnancy. *Surg Gynecol Obstet* 1981;152:179.
29. Washington AE, Cates W, Zaidi AA. Hospitalizations for pelvic inflammatory disease: epidemiology and trends in the United States, 1975 to 1981. *JAMA* 1984;251:2529.
30. Weinstein L, Morris MB, Dotters D, et al. Ectopic pregnancy—a new surgical epidemic. *Obstet Gynecol* 1983;61:698.
31. Westrom L. Effect of acute pelvic inflammatory disease on fertility. *Am J Obstet Gynecol* 1975;121:707.
32. Westrom L, Bengtsson L, Mardh PA. Incidence, trends and risks of ectopic pregnancy in a population of women. *BMJ* 1981;282:15.
33. Wolcott HD, Stock RJ, Kaunitz AM. Ectopic pregnancy. In: Benrubi G, ed. *Obstetric and gynecologic emergencies*. Philadelphia: JB Lippincott Co, 1994.
34. Yaghoobian J, Pinck RL, Ramanathan K, et al. Sonographic demonstration of simultaneous intrauterine and extrauterine gestation. *J Ultrasound Med* 1986;5:309.

CHAPTER 75
Common Medical Diseases in Pregnancy

John F. Huddleston and Donald C. Willis

Asthma in Pregnancy

Asthma complicates 0.4% to 1.3% of pregnancies,[13] and there is evidence that the percentage is increasing.[1] The effect of pregnancy on the asthma is variable, and the course in one pregnancy may not be predictive of that in subsequent pregnancies. In a survey of retrospective studies that included more than 1000 patients, asthma was unchanged in half, improved in 29%, and worsened in 21%.[25] The severity of asthma before pregnancy appears to correlate with the response to pregnancy. If the asthma is mild before pregnancy, its severity is usually unchanged; in patients with severe asthma before pregnancy, the asthma may become even worse.[10] When the disease is sufficiently controlled to obviate hospitalization, the tendency for poor fetal growth among similarly complicated pregnancies requiring hospitalization was not observed.[21]

Fetal mortality has been associated with severe asthma (uncontrolled episodes of wheezing).[11] Older studies showed that poor control of asthma was associated with increased fetal mortality. However, in more recent studies that included severe asthmatics and the use of β_2 agonists, theophylline, and corticosteroids to maintain adequate control of asthma, maternal deaths were eliminated and fetal loss was reduced to that of the general population. It has become apparent that the control of asthma is essential to improve maternal and fetal outcome, even if corticosteroids are required.[13,21] Congenital malformation rates are not increased among infants of asthmatic mothers.

The National Institutes of Health published its report of the Working Group on Asthma and Pregnancy in 1992. This provides an excellent review of the management of asthma in pregnancy.[16]

Pulmonary Physiology During Pregnancy

Mechanical and hormonal changes that occur during pregnancy affect the respiratory system. Respiratory rate is relatively unchanged, but tidal volume is increased, resulting in hypocapnia and a tendency toward chronic respiratory alkalosis. Arterial pCO_2 values of 27 to 32 mm Hg are normal for pregnancy, compared with 38 to 45 mm Hg for nonpregnant women. The importance of this fact is that a pregnant woman with respiratory symptoms and an arterial pCO_2 of 40 mm Hg or higher has at least mild pulmonary failure. A compensatory renal bicarbonate loss occurs, with a reduction of serum levels to 18 to 21 mEq/L during pregnancy (normal, 24 to 30 mEq/L). This partially compensates for the respiratory alkalosis, but a slightly alkaline pH of 7.40 to 7.47 is normal during pregnancy. The bicarbonate loss results in a lower buffering capacity, which assumes importance in clinical conditions such as diabetic ketoacidosis, in which the need for buffering of metabolic acids is strong (see the later section, "Diabetes in Pregnancy").

Lung compliance is unchanged in pregnancy, but airway conductance is increased and total pulmonary resistance is reduced. Total breathing capacity, forced vital capacity, peak expiratory flow rate (PEFR), and forced expiratory volume in 1 second (FEV_1) are not affected by pregnancy. Because of elevation of the diaphragm, functional residual capacity and residual volumes are somewhat reduced.

DIFFERENTIAL DIAGNOSIS

The differential diagnosis of asthma in the pregnant patient is essentially the same as in the nonpregnant patient (see Chapter 146). Specific to pregnancy, the differential diagnosis of severe respiratory distress includes recurrent pulmonary emboli, acute left ventricular heart failure with pulmonary edema due to peripartum cardiomyopathy, and amniotic fluid embolism.

Peripartum cardiomyopathy is associated with the onset of congestive heart failure among women with no prior history of heart disease. Although it can occur during the last month of pregnancy or within the first 5 months after delivery, most cases are found in the first 3 months postpartum.[26] It is more common among older, Black multiparas, frequently those who have experienced preeclampsia. The presence of mural thrombi with resulting pulmonary embolism is not uncommon. The cause is unknown.

Amniotic fluid embolism typically presents with severe respiratory distress, cyanosis, shock, and disseminated intravascular coagulation. The onset of symptoms is sudden and catastrophic. Patients are frequently not resuscitable. An important feature in the diagnosis is that bronchospasm is rare with this entity.

EMERGENCY DEPARTMENT EVALUATION

Clinical evaluation of a pregnant patient with acute asthma is very similar to that of a nonpregnant woman. The physical examination should include evaluation of the level of consciousness and of the use of accessory respiratory muscles, measuring the pulse and respiratory rates, looking for pulsus paradoxus (more than a 10-mm Hg drop in systolic blood pressure during inspiration), auscultation of the lungs, and measurement of FEV_1 or PEFR. The following physical findings may indicate severe airway obstruction and the need for hospitalization:

Altered sensorium
Tachycardia greater than or equal to 120 to 130 beats per minute
Respiratory rate of greater than 30 breaths per minute
Pulsus paradoxus of more than 18 mm Hg
FEV_1 less than 1 L
An arterial pCO_2 level exceeding 40 mEq/L

Although these findings often correlate with severity of disease, their presence can be seen with less severe asthmatic attacks, or they may even be absent when severe airway obstruction is present.[9] The amount of wheezing does not always correlate with the severity of functional derangement. Caution is appropriate when trying to judge the severity of an asthmatic attack based on physical findings. However, an FEV_1 of less than 1 L is a fairly reliable indicator of severe airway obstruction, and an arterial pCO_2 exceeding 40 mEq/L reliably predicts respiratory failure after the first trimester of pregnancy.

Laboratory Evaluation

Laboratory evaluation for an acute asthmatic attack may include a complete blood cell count with differential, sputum analysis, arterial blood gas (ABG) analysis, and pulmonary function testing.

A routine ABG analysis for all asthmatic patients is controversial. Some authors recommend routine ABG determination, while others base the need on clinical findings or response to initial therapy. However, among pregnant women, it is probably safest to obtain an ABG analysis, unless the attack is obviously mild or response to therapy is rapid. Severe hypoxia or hypercapnia, both potentially detrimental to the fetus, should be rapidly detected and treated. There should be no adverse risk to the fetus when the oxygen saturation is greater than or equal to 95%. Mild asthma reflects a normal or slightly reduced pCO_2, whereas more severe airway obstruction results in normal or elevated pCO_2 with arterial hypoxemia. In normal pregnancy, ABGs reflect a compensated respiratory alkalosis resulting from hyperventilation.[13] The pH generally ranges from 7.40 to 7.47 and the $PaCO_2$ from 25 to 32 mm Hg. Arterial PO_2 is normally 100 mm Hg, or slightly higher.

Probably the most reliable indicator of severity of airway obstruction and response to treatment is the FEV_1 or PEFR. An FEV_1 of less than 1 L can be an indication of severe airway obstruction and need for hospitalization. Repeat ABG analysis is often of little value when the FEV_1 is greater than 1 L.

Chest Radiography

Although routine chest films are not recommended in the evaluation of asthma during pregnancy, they should be done if pneumonia or pneumothorax is suspected and for patients who do not respond to standard therapy. Proper shielding of the abdomen is important.

Exposure of the developing fetus to radiation can potentially lead to birth defects (first trimester only), fetal growth retardation, microcephaly, and mental retardation when such exposure is excessive.[3] An exposure of 5 rad or less is thought to be safe for the developing fetus; a routine posterolateral chest film exposes the fetus to less than 0.04 rad.[3] When the abdomen is shielded with a lead apron, radiation exposure to the fetus is negligible.

Chest radiographs are altered by pregnancy. The diaphragm elevates progressively during pregnancy. This elevation causes the heart to rotate on its axis and shift to the left. As a result, cardiac size appears increased, making the identification of moderate cardiomegaly difficult. As a result of increased pulmonary blood flow, lung markings may also be increased, erroneously suggesting the diagnosis of mild congestive heart failure.

EMERGENCY DEPARTMENT MANAGEMENT

The management of asthma in the pregnant patient is essentially the same as in nonpregnant patients. Treatment with theophylline, β_2 agonists, or corticosteroids should not be withheld because of pregnancy. It has become apparent that the control of asthma, even if corticosteroids are required, is essential to improve maternal and fetal outcomes.[13] A suggested management outline is shown in Figure 75.1. The Centers for Disease Control and Prevention has recommended that patients with chronic asthma, including pregnant women, receive yearly influenza immunization, but that, in pregnant patients, this be limited to the second and third trimesters.[6]

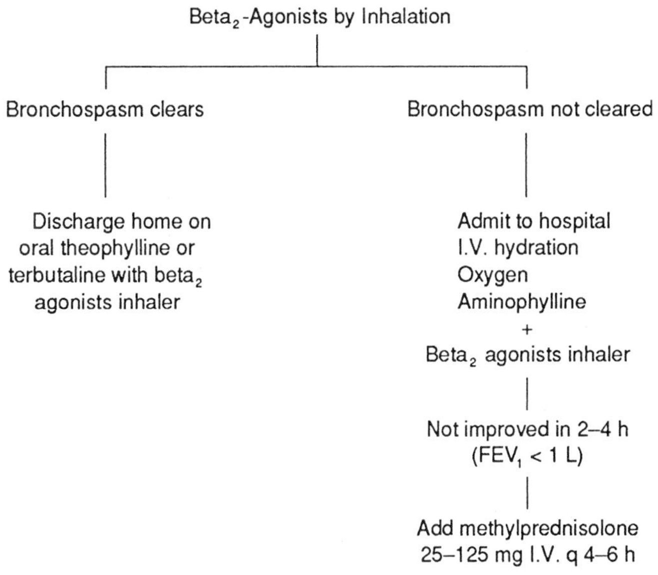

Figure 75.1. Suggested management of asthma in pregnancy.

TABLE 75.1. Medications Used to Treat Asthma during Pregnancy

CONSIDERED SAFE
Aminophylline
Theophylline
β-Adrenergic agonists
Terbutaline
Isoetharine
Albuterol
Metaproterenol
Corticosteroids
Prednisone
Prednisolone
Methylprednisolone
Beclomethasone dipropionate (by inhalation)
Cromolyn sodium
CONTROVERSIAL
Epinephrine
CONTRAINDICATED
Iodine expectorants

Drugs Used to Treat Asthma in Pregnancy

Drugs used to treat asthma in pregnancy are listed in Tables 75.1 and 75.2.

β-Adrenergic Agonists

Selective β_2 agonists are potent bronchodilators and the initial treatment of choice in acute asthma during pregnancy. Although β_2 agonists can be given by subcutaneous injection, intravenous (i.v.) infusion, or aerosol inhalation, the aerosolized method is preferred. Inhalation by nebulizer or metered dose produces a more rapid onset of action, minimizes adverse systemic effects, and is as effective as i.v. therapy.[20] Although isoetharine has been used with success, more selective β_2 agonists, such as metaproterenol and albuterol, are recommended. For maximal benefit, the aerosol should be slowly inhaled over 5 to 6 seconds, followed by a short period of breath holding, and then slowly exhaled. Even patients who take β_2 agonists on an outpatient basis may respond to this inhalation therapy.

There are no reports linking the use of β_2 agonists with congenital birth defects. These agents do cross the placenta and can result in fetal tachycardia, usually less than 175 beats per minute. Long-term use during pregnancy has not been associated with adverse perinatal outcome. Infants followed up to 12 months of age have shown no harmful effects.[4]

Certain β_2-adrenergic agents (e.g., terbutaline) are used to inhibit uterine contractions as therapy for preterm labor. These agents can precipitate pulmonary edema in otherwise healthy women. Fortunately, pulmonary edema has not been reported with treatment of asthma. Diabetic ketoacidosis has also been associated with β-adrenergic therapy for preterm labor. These agents are best avoided among pregnant diabetic women with asthma. Patients with migraine headaches should probably not be given parenteral terbutaline.

Epinephrine

The use of epinephrine in pregnancy is controversial. Greenberger and Patterson[13] favor subcutaneous epinephrine as the treatment of choice during pregnancy. Chung and Barnes[7] advise that epinephrine is best avoided during pregnancy because of its ability to decrease uterine blood flow and, possibly, to cause congenital malformations. Epinephrine has been associated with an increased incidence of fetal malformations when used in the first 4 months of pregnancy.[15] In monkeys treated with intraarterial epinephrine, uterine artery vasoconstriction and reduced uterine profusion were demonstrated.[17] However, intraarterial injection of epinephrine in monkeys may have little or no application to the subcutaneous use of epinephrine among pregnant women. Selective β_2 agonists, on the other hand, cause either no change or an increase in uterine blood flow.[1,5] There are no advantages, and there are possible disadvantages, to the use of epinephrine over the more selective β_2 agonists. Although controversial, epinephrine use in pregnancy should be replaced by the more selective β_2 agonists.

TABLE 75.2. Drugs Used to Treat Acute Asthma in Pregnancy

Drug	Dose	Comment
β AGONISTS		
Terbutaline (subcutaneous)	0.25 mg	After 15–30 min a second dose of 0.25 mg may be given. Patients not responding to a second dose should be admitted to the hospital for intravenous aminophylline and corticosteroid therapy.
Albuterol	1–2 puffs (90 μg/puff)	Repeat every 4–6 h.
Metoproterenol	2–3 puffs (0.65 mg/puff)	Repeat every 3–4 h.
Metoproterenol sulfate	0.3 mL 5% solution in 2.5 mL saline	Repeat every 4 h.
Isoetharine	0.5 mL 1% solution in 1.5 mL saline	Initial use every 1–2 h as needed, and then every 3–4 h.
AMINOPHYLLINE		
Loading dose[a]	5.6 mg/kg (not to exceed 400 mg)	Give over 20–30 min.
Maintenance dose	0.5 mg/kg/h	
CORTICOSTEROIDS		
Methylprednisolone	25–125 mg I.V.	Repeat every 4–6 h. High-dose therapy with 125 mg every 6 h may be preferred, because it will result in a more rapid improvement. Taper after improvement and start an oral corticosteroid such as prednisone 40–60 mg/d. Taper prednisone over next 1–2 wk.

[a]Patients not currently taking theophylline.

Theophylline

Theophylline is less effective as a bronchodilator than the β_2 agonists, but when it is used in combination with them, there is an additive effect, because they have different modes of action. During pregnancy, patients who do not respond to β_2 agonist therapy should be considered for hospital admission and intravenous therapy with aminophylline. Aminophylline is the water-soluble salt of theophylline, which readily crosses the placenta and induces fetal levels similar to or higher than maternal levels.[2] No teratogenic effect has been demonstrated in human studies. In the newborn, metabolism and excretion of theophylline are limited, resulting in a half-life two to three times that in an adult. After delivery, newborns can maintain adult therapeutic levels (1020 μg/mL) for up to 18 hours.[2] Neonatal toxicity can occur in the absence of maternal toxicity, owing to increased neonatal sensitivity and slower elimination of the drug.[2] To avoid such toxicity, the dose of aminophylline should be reduced in pregnancy. Patients who are not currently taking theophylline should receive a loading dose of 5 to 6 mg/kg, not to exceed 400 mg intravenously over 20 to 30 minutes. In patients who have taken the drug sporadically, half the loading dose should be used; it is best to eliminate it completely if the patient has adhered to an adequate oral regimen. One must remember that the loading dose is based on *actual* body weight and the maintenance infusion is based on *ideal* body weight, rather than current pregnancy weight.

A continuous infusion dose should not exceed 0.5 mg/kg/h to avoid fetal toxicity. Smokers and adolescents (younger than age 20) rapidly metabolize aminophylline and may require a higher dose (0.7 mg/kg/h). Higher doses can be used during pregnancy if serum levels are followed. The serum theophylline level should be measured about 10 hours after therapy is initiated and daily thereafter. Therapeutic levels for theophylline are 10 to 20 μg/mL. However, during pregnancy, levels higher than 12 μg/mL should be avoided to prevent toxicity to the baby. Hyperactive fetal movement and fetal tachycardia may be seen when theophylline levels exceed these limits. Toxicity in the newborn, including tachycardia, jitteriness, and irritability, is only occasionally observed, but can occur even with neonatal blood levels that are therapeutic in the adult. Thus, the recommendations regarding dosage reduction are even more important in late pregnancy, or whenever delivery is likely.

Corticosteroids

Most patients respond to a β agonist alone or in combination with i.v. aminophylline. If improvement (FEV_1 remains less than 1 L) is not apparent, corticosteroid therapy is recommended. During pregnancy, there should be no hesitation to add corticosteroids in the management of asthma. The early administration of corticosteroids is an important part of therapy when asthma is severe or resistant. Patients who are already taking oral corticosteroids for asthma should receive i.v. corticosteroids as part of the initial therapy. Although methylprednisolone (25 mg i.v. every 4 to 6 hours) is effective, high-dose corticosteroid therapy (e.g., 125 mg methylprednisolone every 6 hours) may be preferred, because it results in a more rapid improvement.[14] Improvement should occur within 1 hour after corticosteroid treatment is started, with maximal effect in 6 to 8 hours.

Cortisol and other corticosteroids freely cross the placenta, but they are rapidly converted by the fetoplacental unit into a less active form, cortisone.[19] After maternal ingestion, prednisone is rapidly converted to its active form, prednisolone. However, prednisolone is poorly transferred across the placenta, and fetal levels are considerably lower than maternal levels.

Corticosteroids have been shown to induce fetal malformations in certain animal species (cortisone acetate has been demonstrated to induce cleft palate in rabbits).[8] Corticosteroids, including prednisone, have been used extensively during pregnancy and have little, if any, effect on the developing fetus.[4] They are not considered teratogenic in humans. For patients with severe asthma, corticosteroid therapy is preferable and causes less fetal or maternal risk than poorly controlled asthma during pregnancy.

An inhaled corticosteroid, beclomethasone dipropionate, has permitted significant reduction or discontinuation of prednisone in corticosteroid-dependent asthmatic patients. The use of a topically active corticosteroid with minimal systemic effects appears logical for use in pregnancy. Inhaled beclomethasone and its metabolites that appear in the systemic circulation are highly protein bound, accounting for the lack of systemic effects. Little systemic absorption occurs after the use of two puffs (100 mg) four times daily. However, when used in dosages exceeding those recommended, beclomethasone has been shown to cause adrenal suppression.[23,24] The use of a spacer should be considered to reduce oropharyngeal candidiasis, improve respiratory tract penetration, and reduce potential systemic effects.

Available information suggests that beclomethasone dipropionate is safe during pregnancy when administered in recommended doses. Greenberger and Patterson[12] reported the safe use of beclomethasone during 45 pregnancies.

Disodium Cromoglycate (Cromolyn Sodium)

Cromolyn sodium inhibits release of histamine from mast cells and is useful as a prophylactic agent in some patients with asthma. It is not effective for treatment of acute asthmatic attacks. It is poorly absorbed after inhalation, so the amount available for transfer across the placenta is insignificant. Studies in both animals and humans have failed to show any teratogenic or other adverse effects when cromolyn sodium is used throughout pregnancy.[7]

Newer Drugs for the Treatment of Asthma

Several drugs, marketed over the past 5 years but with limited data concerning safety in pregnancy, may have roles under specific situations.[22] Nebulized ipratropium might be used for acute asthmatic symptoms not responding to β_2-agonist therapy. Nedocromil probably can be continued in a patient with persistent asthma who was well-controlled on it prepregnancy. Inhaled salmeterol could definitely be considered for the gravida inadequately controlled on moderate doses of inhaled steroids.

Antibiotics

Bacterial pneumonia and bronchitis can initiate an acute asthmatic attack. If sputum analysis demonstrates polymorphonuclear leukocytes and few or no eosinophils, infection must be suspected. Treatment with ampicillin or erythromycin (500 mg PO every 6 hours) or with a cephalosporin such as cefaclor (250 mg PO every 8 hours for 10 days) is recommended. Erythromycin may slow aminophylline metabolism and necessitate a lower continuous infusion dose. Antibiotic therapy should not be used unless there is evidence of infection. Patients with pneumonia or a febrile respiratory tract infection may benefit from i.v. antibiotic treatment.

Supportive Therapy

Because most patients with acute asthma are dehydrated, i.v. hydration with 5% dextrose in 0.5 normal saline at 100 to 125 mL/h is beneficial. Oxygen by nasal cannula at 2 to 3 L/min should be administered after an initial ABG analysis is obtained. Patients with carbon dioxide retention may benefit from humidified oxygen at 3 to 7 L/min by Venturi mask to deliver optimal oxygen without causing further carbon dioxide retention. A pO_2 of greater than 70 mm Hg or an oxygen saturation greater than or equal to 95% should be achieved. Oxygen administration to reduce hyperventilation, even with mild asthma in pregnancy, may be beneficial. Human studies suggest that maternal hyperventilation resulting in reduced pCO_2 and maternal alkalosis may decrease fetal oxygen tension by inducing uterine artery vasoconstriction and causing a shift of the oxyhemoglobin dissociation curve to the left.[26]

DISPOSITION

During pregnancy, patients who develop pneumonia or require i.v. therapy for an acute asthmatic attack should be considered for hospital admission. The same patients could benefit from consultation with specialist(s) in maternal–fetal, pulmonary, or internal medicine. The attending obstetrician or obstetric service should be notified. Although procedures vary among institutions, many obstetric services prefer to have all pregnant patients admitted to their service, with specialists in internal medicine or pulmonary medicine acting in a consultative role.

COMMON PITFALLS

- Judging the severity of an asthmatic attack based on physical findings may be misleading.
- Appropriate treatment with theophylline, β agonists, and corticosteroids should not be withheld because of pregnancy. It is apparent that the control of asthma, even if corticosteroids are required, is essential to improve maternal and fetal outcomes.
- Although controversial, epinephrine use in pregnancy should be replaced by the more selective β_2 agonists.
- Perinatal toxicity to theophylline can occur in the absence of maternal toxicity, owing to the baby's increased sensitivity and slower elimination of the drug. To avoid such toxicity, the i.v. dose of aminophylline should be reduced in pregnancy.
- Oxygen administration, even with mild asthma in pregnancy, should be used to reduce hyperventilation. This may be beneficial, because human studies suggest that maternal hyperventilation and alkalosis can reduce the amount of oxygen released to the fetus.[18]

References

1. Alexander S, Dodds L, Armson BA. Perinatal outcomes in women with asthma during pregnancy. *Obstet Gynecol* 1998;92:435.
2. Arwood LL, Dasta JF, Friedman C. Placental transfer of theophylline: two case reports. *Pediatrics* 1979;63:844.
3. Brent RL. The effects of embryonic and fetal exposure to x-ray, microwaves, and ultrasound. *Clin Obstet Gynecol* 1983;26:484.
4. Briggs GG, Freeman RK, Yaffe SJ. *Drugs in pregnancy and lactation,* 2nd ed. Baltimore, Williams & Wilkins, 1986;366, 422.
5. Caritis SN, Mueller-Heubach E, Morishima HO, et al. Effect of terbutaline on cardiovascular state and uterine blood flow in pregnant ewes. *Obstet Gynecol* 1977;50:603.
6. Centers for Disease Control. Prevention and control of influenza during pregnancy. *MMWR* 1984;33:253.
7. Chung KF, Barnes PJ. Prescribing in pregnancy: treatment of asthma. *BMJ* 1987;294:103.
8. Fainstat T. Cortisone-induced congenital cleft palate in rabbits. *Endocrinology* 194;55:502.
9. Fischl MA, Pitchenik A, Gardner LB. An index predicting relapse and need for hospitalization in patients with acute bronchial asthma. *N Engl J Med* 1981;305:783.
10. Gluck JC, Gluck PA. The effects of pregnancy on asthma: a prospective study. *Ann Allergy* 1976;37:164.
11. Gordon M, Niswander KR, Berendes H, et al. Fetal morbidity following potentially anoxigenic obstetric conditions: VII. Bronchial asthma. *Am J Obstet Gynecol* 1970;106:421.
12. Greenberger PA, Patterson R. Beclomethasone dipropionate for severe asthma during pregnancy. *Ann Intern Med* 1983;98:478.
13. Greenberger PA, Patterson R. Management of asthma during pregnancy. *N Engl J Med* 1985;312:897.
14. Haskell RJ, Wong BM, Hansen JE. A double-blind randomized clinical trial of methylprednisolone if status asthmaticus. *Arch Intern Med* 1983;143:1324.
15. Heinonen OP, Slone D, Shapiro S. *Birth defects and drugs in pregnancy*. Littleton, MA: Publishing Sciences Group, 1977;345.
16. Luskin AT, Clark S, Frederiksen M. *Executive summary: management of asthma during pregnancy*. NIH publication No. 933279A. Bethesda, MD: National Institutes of Health, 1992.
17. Misenhimer HR, Margulies SI, Panigel M, et al. Effects of vasoconstrictive drugs on the placental circulation of the rhesus monkey. *Invest Radiol* 1972;7:496.
18. Moya F, Morishima HO, Shnider SM, et al. Influence of maternal hyperventilation on the newborn infant. *Am J Obstet Gynecol* 1965;91:76.
19. Murphy BEP, Clark SJ, Donald IR, et al. Conversion of maternal cortisol to cortisone during placental transfer to the human fetus. *Am J Obstet Gynecol* 1974;118:538.
20. Pierce RJ, Payne CR, Williams SJ. Comparison of intravenous and inhaled terbutaline in the treatment of asthma. *Chest* 1981;79:506.
21. Schatz M. Interrelationships between asthma and pregnancy. *J Allergy Clin Immunol* 1999;103:S330.
22. Shatz M. Asthma and pregnancy. *Lancet* 1999;353:1202.
23. Toogood JH, Lefcoe NM, Haines DSM, et al. A graded dose assessment of the efficacy of beclomethasone dipropionate aerosol for severe asthma. *J Allergy Clin Immunol* 1977;59:298.
24. Toogood JH, Lefcoe NM, Haines DSM, et al. Minimum dose requirements of steroid-dependent asthmatic patients for aerosol beclomethasone and oral prednisone. *J Allergy Clin Immunol* 1978;61:355.
25. Turner ES, Greenberger PA, Patterson R. Management of the pregnant asthmatic patient. *Ann Intern Med* 1980;6:905.
26. Walsh JJ, Burch GE. Postpartal heart disease. *Arch Intern Med* 1961;108:817.

Sickle Cell Disease in Pregnancy

Compared with normal pregnancies, those complicated by sickle cell anemia (SS disease) are associated with significantly higher rates of maternal and perinatal morbidity and mortality.[9,10,12,13] With improved prenatal care, maternal mortality has declined from a rate as high as 30% to the current rate of about 2%.[11] It must be appreciated, however, that this 2% rate is more than 200 times the general maternal mortality rate in this country. Maternal morbidity is primarily due to vasoocclusive "crises," which result from abnormal, sickled transformation of erythrocytes (frequently the result of infection, hypoxemia, acidosis, or dehydration), sludging and obstruction of blood flow to the microcirculation, and resultant ischemia (causing pain) and infarction. The etiology of maternal mortality among these women is related to the same pathophysiology and includes congestive heart failure (2% to 20%), pulmonary embolism (including embolism from infarcted bone marrow, 20% to 40%), and preeclampsia, which is a common complication of this disorder.

The overall fetal wastage is approximately 30%, owing to an increased risk of spontaneous abortion, stillbirth, prematurity, and intrauterine growth retardation. This increase in pregnancy wastage is probably related to thrombotic events in the placenta, as well as to maternal morbidity. Pathologic features in the umbilical vein have been found with maternal SS disease.[3]

The frequency and severity of vasoocclusive crises vary greatly among parturients. Although controversial, many authors believe that pregnancy worsens the disease, with an increase in frequency of such crises, especially during labor and the postpartum period.[8] Prompt recognition and intervention are vital for optimal maternal and fetal outcomes.

Sickle cell–thalassemia (SThal) disease and sickle cell–hemoglobin C (SC) disease are treated similarly to sickle cell disease in pregnancy, although the obstetric courses with these hemoglobinopathies are typically not as severe as with SS disease.

CLINICAL PRESENTATION

During pregnancy, most crises are vasoocclusive and occur most often in the latter half of pregnancy. They follow a typical pattern of recurring attacks of sudden pain, most often affecting the extremities, abdomen, chest, and vertebrae.

Although infrequent in pregnancy, hemolytic crisis is characterized by the sudden onset of severe anemia and a low reticulocyte count. Aplastic crisis is usually self-limited and associated with infection, especially with parvovirus B-19. This has proved fatal in pregnancy when sensitization from prior blood products prohibits transfusion.

DIFFERENTIAL DIAGNOSIS

When a known SS disease patient presents to the emergency department with pain, the physician must determine whether it is due to the usual vasoocclusive pathophysiology. If so, is it associated with an infection? If not, is the pain caused by a surgical or obstetric disorder (Table 75.3)? The diagnosis of vasoocclusive crisis is one of exclusion, and other causes of pain may become clear only after failed response to management. Consultation with a perinatologist or hematologist is prudent.

A reason for the pain crisis should always be sought. First on the list is infection. This will be discovered in about 25% of SS gravidas and is associated with one-third of all maternal deaths in SS patients. In pregnancy, the most common infections are pneumonia, cystitis or pyelonephritis, and osteomyelitis. After delivery, endometritis should always be considered. *Escherichia coli* and *Salmonella* replace pneumococci as the major offending organisms in bacterial sepsis. *Mycoplasma* should also be considered in cases of pneumonia.

EMERGENCY DEPARTMENT EVALUATION

Diagnostic laboratory tests include complete blood cell count with reticulocyte count, clean-catch urinalysis with culture, and hemoglobin electrophoresis for percentage of hemoglobin A. Crisis is unlikely if the hemoglobin A percentage is higher than 40% to 50% (which in SS and SC patients always represents red cells persisting from a prior transfusion). Other laboratory tests should be based on potential organ complications, with recommendations by the appropriate specialist.

Hemodilution of pregnancy normally causes a relative lowering of the hematocrit. Also, the white blood cell (WBC) count may increase to 10,000 to 16,000/μL in the absence of infection. Both total and segmental leukocytes increase during pregnancy, as well as with infection and vasoocclusive crisis. However, a substantial rise in the WBC count with an increase in band (nonsegmented) leukocyte level above 1000/μL is often seen with significant bacterial infection. Nucleated red blood cells, common with the intense hemolysis that is part of SS disease, may be counted as WBCs in certain automated systems; this fact must be considered in evaluating high "WBC" results.

TABLE 75.3. Differential Diagnosis for Vasoocclusive Sickle Cell Crisis

PREGNANCY-RELATED	MEDICAL
Threatened abortion	Pneumonia
Ectopic pregnancy	Pyelonephritis or cystitis
Ovarian cyst with or without torsion	Drug addiction
Degenerating leiomyoma	Thrombophlebitis
Abruptio placentae	Pulmonary embolism
Severe preeclampsia	**SURGICAL**
	Appendicitis
	Cholelithiasis
	Pancreatitis

A complete physical examination is mandatory. Ultrasonography is recommended if the differential diagnosis includes any of the pregnancy-related problems listed in Table 75.3. After initial emergency department evaluation, continuous electronic fetal monitoring is indicated after the pregnancy has reached a gestational age of about 24 weeks.

EMERGENCY DEPARTMENT MANAGEMENT

All pregnant women with SS disease should be admitted to the hospital if there is any suspicion of crisis or infection. Care should be in a medical center with a specialist and subspecialist who are knowledgeable in the management of the gravida with SS disease. If these facilities are not readily available, the patient should be stabilized and transferred to the nearest perinatal center where maternal–fetal medicine and hematology subspecialists are available.

Management of SS disease in a pregnant patient is similar to that in a nonpregnant patient and involves rest, adequate nutrition, hydration, oxygen, and analgesia:

1. The patient should be admitted to the hospital or transferred to the appropriate center, when indicated.
2. Hydration, in the absence of congestive heart failure, should be provided (D_5LR 1000 mL over 2 hours and then 125 to 150 mL/h).
3. Acetaminophen is the preferred analgesic for milder pain. If narcotics are required, satisfactory results usually can be achieved with a combination of meperidine (50 to 100 mg) or butorphanol (1 to 2 mg) in combination with promethazine (25 mg) given intravenously or intramuscularly. Although the potential for narcotic addiction is high with SS disease, adequate analgesia should not be withheld if the likelihood for actual pain is high.
4. Prophylactic antibiotics are not indicated, but appropriate antibiotics should be initiated immediately if infection is suspected or diagnosed by physical examination or laboratory testing.
5. Oxygen should be delivered by nasal cannula at 2 to 4 L/min.
6. Unless the patient has severe preeclampsia or congestive heart failure, invasive central monitoring and Foley catheterization are to be avoided, to minimize the risk of iatrogenic infection.
7. Partial exchange transfusion has been considered the cornerstone of management for the prevention as well as treatment of crisis during pregnancy.[5,6] Initially performed as a cumbersome, manual technique, most such procedures are now done by continuous-flow erythrocytapheresis.[7] With the added risk of acquired immunodeficiency syndrome transmission through blood products (with current blood-banking practices, only about one in a half-million transfusions), the risks versus benefits of this therapy must be carefully explained to the patient. Some specialists are now restricting partial exchange transfusions to patients with severe or recurrent crises. Most vasoocclusive crises are now managed without the use of simple blood transfusion(s). The transfusion of two to four units may still be required when the initial hematocrit is less than 15% or for women in active labor with crisis.[4] With the multiple-unit transfusions, there are also risks of alloimmunization complicating future cross-matching or causing a delayed transfusion reaction.[2]

DISPOSITION

As with other medical complications in pregnancy, it is most appropriate to consult the patient's obstetrician or the obstetric service in teaching hospitals. Consultation with maternal–fetal medicine or hematology is then at the obstetrician's discretion. Maternal–fetal medicine physicians can play an important role in the management of SS disease and other medical problems in pregnancy, because of their obstetric background and expanded training in the field of high-risk pregnancy. Genetic counseling is extremely valuable, because prenatal diagnosis is possible[1] and has recently been expanded to preimplantation diagnosis in at-risk women undergoing *in vitro* fertilization.[14]

Indications for Admission

Any pregnant woman with SS disease who is suspected of having a crisis or infection should be admitted to the hospital.

Transfer Considerations

Care of the SS parturient is best done at a center with appropriate subspecialists experienced in the management of SS disease. If such subspecialists are not readily available, strong consideration for transfer is indicated. Hydration, oxygen, and appropriate analgesics should be initiated before transfer. Because of the decrease in oxygen tension with altitude, ground transportation is ideally suited for most transports. Helicopters fly at about 2000 feet above ground level for flights less than 100 miles and 3000 to 5000 feet for flights over 100 miles. Fixed-wing aircraft are theoretically pressurized to ground level.

Sickle Cell Trait in Pregnancy

One in 12 Black Americans carries the sickle cell trait (SA hemoglobin). This condition is asymptomatic, with normal hemoglobin concentrations. Sickling occurs only with severe hypoxia (pO_2 less than 15 mm Hg). General anesthesia is well tolerated.

During pregnancy there is no increase in maternal mortality or fetal loss. Although still asymptomatic, these SA patients may become more anemic than expected during pregnancy. As with SS disease, prenatal diagnosis is available when both partners are hemoglobin S (or C or thalassemia) carriers.

The only increased risk during pregnancy is a doubling in the expected risk of asymptomatic and clinical urinary tract infections in SA gravidas, so appropriate surveillance with urine cultures should be performed.[12] This risk is due to reduced oxygen tension in the renal medulla, causing local sickling with ischemia. The result is renal disease manifest by hematuria and an inability to concentrate urine.

References

1. Adinolfi M, Sherlock J. First trimester prenatal diagnosis using transcervical cells: an evaluation. *Hum Reprod Update* 1997;3:383.
2. Brumfield CG, Huddleston JF, DuBois LB, et al. A delayed hemolytic transfusion after partial exchange transfusion for sickle cell disease in pregnancy. *Obstet Gynecol* 1984;63:13S.
3. Decastel M, Leborgne-Samuel Y, Alexandre L, et al. Morphological features of the human umbilical vein in normal, sickle cell trait, and sickle cell disease pregnancies. *Hum Pathol* 1999;30:13.
4. Koshy M. Sickle cell disease and pregnancy. *Blood Rev* 1995;9:157.
5. Martin JN, Martin RW, Morrison JC. Acute management of sickle cell crisis in pregnancy. *Clin Perinatol* 1986;13:853.
6. Morrison JC, Blake PG, Reed CD. Therapy for the pregnant patient with sickle hemoglobinopathies: a national focus. *Am J Obstet Gynecol* 1982;144:268.
7. Morrison JC, Morrison FS, Floyd RC, et al. Use of continuous flow erythrocytapheresis in pregnant patients with sickle cell disease. *J Clin Apheresis* 1991;6:224.
8. Morrison JC, Propst MG, Blake PG. Sickle hemoglobin and the gravid patient: a management controversy. *Clin Perinatol* 1980;7:273.
9. Morrison JC, Ruvinsky ED, Nicholls ET. Sickling and pregnancy: a worrisome combination. *Contemp Obstet Gynecol* 1981;18:125.
10. Pollack CV Jr. Emergencies in sickle cell disease. Department of Emergency Medicine, Maricopa Medical Center, Phoenix, Arizona. *Emerg Med Clin North Am* 1993;11:365.
11. Powars DR, Sandhu M, Niland-Weiss J, et al. Pregnancy in sickle cell disease. *Obstet Gynecol* 1986;67:217.
12. Pritchard A, Scott DE, Whalley PJ, et al. The effects of maternal sickle cell hemoglobinopathies and sickle trait on reproductive performance. *Am J Obstet Gynecol* 1972;117:662.
13. Ranney HM. The spectrum of sickle cell disease. University of California, San Diego. *Hosp Pract* 1992;27:133, 141, 149.
14. Xu K, Shi ZM, Veeck LL, et al. First unaffected pregnancy using preimplantation genetic diagnosis for sickle cell anemia. *JAMA* 1999;281:1701.

Diabetes in Pregnancy

Prior to the discovery and beginning availability of insulin in 1921, pregnancy was uncommon among diabetic women and was associated with high maternal and fetal mortality rates. With modern prenatal care and improved glycemic control, maternal mortality now is nearly as low as that of the general population and perinatal mortality has decreased to 3% to 5%. Although much improved, this perinatal mortality rate is still above the 1% to 2% seen in the general population.[1]

The incidence of major malformations, now the major cause of perinatal death, is three to four times higher among offspring of diabetic women and accounts for almost half of all their perinatal losses. It is believed that these anomalies are caused by hyperglycemia during embryogenesis. Using rat and mouse embryo cultures, hyperglycemia (but not hypoglycemia) has been demonstrated to cause birth defects in rodents.[4] Maternal glucose readily crosses the placenta, so that maternal (and thus fetal) hyperglycemia during human organogenesis may also explain the increased risks of fetal malformations. Insulin is a large molecule that does not cross the placenta. The fetus does not begin its own insulin production until 9 to 11 weeks' gestation. However, fetal hyperinsulinemia, produced in response to fetal hyperglycemia, acts as a major fetal growth factor, leading to the excessive fetal growth that is so often an undesirable finding in poorly controlled diabetic pregnancies.[9]

Improvement in pregnancy outcome among diabetic women now depends on achieving a euglycemic state before the time of conception and for the subsequent 6 to 8 weeks, during which the majority of organogenesis occurs. Diabetic embryopathy thus evolves early in gestation, probably by the seventh week of pregnancy. Because women often do not see their obstetricians until after this critical time, it is the role of family physicians, internists, and emergency physicians to inform and advise women of childbearing age of the importance of achieving optimal glycemic control before pregnancy. Ideally, this degree of metabolic stability should be in place before contraceptive efforts are dropped in anticipation of the planned pregnancy. Maintaining excellent control during early pregnancy, when gestational nausea frequently upsets the gravida's ability to follow a consistent meal plan, is especially challenging. Only through patient education and physician awareness can the perinatal mortality and morbidity rates among diabetic women be minimized.[4,5,9,11]

PATHOPHYSIOLOGY

Accelerated Fasting Ketosis

The developing fetus depends primarily on glucose for energy requirements and on amino acids for protein synthesis. Glucose is transferred across the placenta by facilitated diffusion. Fetal glucose levels are only 10 to 20 mg/dL below maternal levels. In part, owing to the siphoning of glucose by the fetus, maternal glucose levels after a 12- to 14-hour fast are 15 to 20 mg/dL lower during pregnancy. This results in a decreased insulin release with an elevated blood level of ketoacids. Ketoacid levels are up to four times higher in normal pregnancy after an overnight fast. The term *accelerated starvation ketosis* describes the fasting hypoglycemia, decreased insulin concentration, and ketonemia. The lower glucose concentration after an overnight fast explains the frequent occurrence of hypoglycemic symptoms when breakfast is skipped. For this reason, it is important that pregnant women have some caloric intake in the mornings. Quickly evolving ketosis represents the ease by which the dreaded diabetic ketoacidosis (DKA) may appear.

Insulin Requirements during Pregnancy

During the first half of pregnancy, insulin requirements are typically stable or may decrease due to (1) the transplacental siphoning of glucose by the fetus, (2) the decreased oral intake resulting from gestational nausea and vomiting, and (3) the early-pregnancy estrogen and progesterone elevations, which cause (except in the type 1 diabetic woman) beta-cell hyperplasia and increased insulin secretion.

Over the second half of pregnancy, insulin requirements can increase by 100% or more over prepregnancy levels. Human placental lactogen, produced in large quantities by the placenta and a major cause of gestational diabetes, is structurally related to growth hormone and is the most important cause of insulin resistance during pregnancy.

Classification

In 1949 White described a classification to help determine the likely outcome and aid in the management of diabetic women during pregnancy. The classification is based on (1) duration of disease, (2) age at onset, and (3) underlying vascular involvement (Table 75.4).

The emergency physician may be called on to treat pregnant diabetic women for complications relating to normal pregnancy as well as for special problems associated with diabetes.

Diabetic Ketoacidosis

DKA during pregnancy is associated with a 50% (per episode) fetal loss rate. Early recognition and treatment improve both maternal and fetal outcomes. During pregnancy, DKA may develop rapidly, with relatively low serum glucose levels of only 200 to 300 mg/dL. The readily available free fatty acids (ketogenic substrates) and the accelerated renal loss of bicarbonate related to hypocarbia, both normal pregnancy findings, are factors favoring this rapidity of development.[2]

DIFFERENTIAL DIAGNOSIS

Hypoglycemic Coma

Onset is usually rapid, without other symptoms that are associated with DKA. The serum concentration of glucose is low. Urine ketones are negative.

Nonketotic Hyperosmolar Coma

Dehydration is the major problem, with a blood urea nitrogen level greater than or equal to 70 mg/dL commonly found. Hyperglycemia is marked, with levels as high as 1000 mg/dL.

Alcoholic Ketoacidosis

These patients are usually not diabetic but are often alcoholics with poor nutrition. Ketosis is present, but the serum glucose level is normal.

Uremic Acidosis

Ketosis is mild or not present.

Starvation Ketosis

The differential diagnosis between starvation ketosis and DKA is made difficult because of the accelerated starvation ketosis seen during pregnancy (see previous discussion of pathophysiology). The accelerated metabolic response to starvation in pregnancy results in serum ketone levels that are up to four times higher than in the nonpregnant state. The presence of ketonemia or ketonuria (usually mild) with low or normal serum glucose levels suggests starvation ketosis, and excludes DKA. Treatment consists of increasing dietary or intravenous (i.v.) carbohydrates.

EMERGENCY DEPARTMENT EVALUATION

It is important to identify an infectious site that could precipitate DKA. Most patients have an altered sensorium, ranging from drowsiness to coma. Other physical findings include evidence of dehydration and rapid, shallow respiration, often with a fruity breath odor due to acetone.

Because home glucose monitoring by capillary blood is standard care for the diabetic woman during pregnancy, a careful review of recent glucose values, if available, is often beneficial.

TABLE 75.4. Classification of Diabetes in Pregnancy

Class	Age at Onset (y)	Duration (y)	Vascular Disease	Treatment
A	Any	Any	O	Diet and insulin
B	>20	<10	O	Insulin
C	10–19	10–19	O	Insulin
D	≤10	≥20	Benign retinopathy	Insulin
F	Any	Any	Nephropathy	Insulin
R	Any	Any	Retinopathy	Insulin
H	Any	Any	Heart disease	Insulin

GESTATIONAL DIABETES

Class	Fasting Glucose Level		Postprandial Glucose Level
A-1	<105 mg/dL	and	<120 mg/dL
A-2	≥105 mg/dL	or	≥120 mg/dL

From American College of Obstetricians and Gynecologists. *Management of diabetes mellitus in pregnancy.* ACOG technical bulletin no. 92. Washington, DC: ACOG, 1986.

Laboratory Tests

Initial blood studies should include complete blood cell count; serum determinations of glucose, electrolytes, bicarbonate, urea nitrogen, creatinine, and ketones; and arterial blood gas analysis. A Foley catheter should be placed and left to monitor urine output and urine ketone concentration; urinalysis with culture should be ordered. Other laboratory tests and cultures should be obtained as indicated by history and physical examination. The serum tests and arterial gases should be repeated every 2 hours during the initial phase of treatment.

EMERGENCY DEPARTMENT MANAGEMENT[2]

Regular insulin (6 to 10 U) should be administered by i.v. push, and then a continuous infusion of insulin in normal saline (50 U regular insulin in 500 mL saline [1 U/10 mL]) is begun at 6 to 10 U/h. If the serum glucose value does not fall by 30% in 2 hours, the insulin dose rate should be doubled. Because the gravida with DKA generally presents with a fluid deficiency of 3 to 6 L, 1,000 mL sodium chloride 0.45% should be given over the first hour, and then 300 to 500 mL/h. When serum glucose reaches 250 to 200 mg/dL, the insulin infusion rate should be halved and the i.v. fluid type should be changed to dextrose 5% in sodium chloride 0.45%. When the serum glucose value falls to less than 150 mg/dL and the serum ketone level is decreasing, insulin should be given at a basal rate of 1 to 2 U/h.

If the pH remains less than 7.30 and is not rising, the insulin dose should be increased, despite a falling blood glucose value. Dextrose 5% in water should be infused at 200 mL/h in order to avoid hypoglycemia and possibly even cerebral edema, a usually irreversible and fatal condition that may be precipitated if severe hyperglycemia is reversed too rapidly.

Rapid correction of acidosis in the pregnant woman is important because of the tremendous fetal risk. *In utero* fetal resuscitation may occur with correction of maternal hyperglycemia and acidosis. For mild acidosis (pH greater than 7.10), bicarbonate is generally not given. If pH is less than 7.10, 88 mEq sodium bicarbonate in 1,000 mL sodium chloride 0.45% should be administered.

DKA is accompanied by a shift in the potassium from the intracellular to the extracellular compartment. A normal or even elevated serum potassium level before initiation of treatment may mask total body potassium depletion. Once the acidosis is becoming corrected, hypokalemia may become obvious. To avoid hypokalemia, potassium chloride (40 mEq/L) should be added to the i.v. fluids when the serum potassium level, measured every 2 hours, falls into the mid-normal range.

The effects of maternal acidosis on the fetus are not fully understood. However, DKA is frequently associated with sudden fetal death. Postulated mechanisms include the following:

- Acidosis may have a direct effect on the fetus. Although no large studies are available, it appears that fetal distress may result from maternal acidosis. The likely explanation is that an unfavorable tenacity for oxygen to fetal hemoglobin develops in the presence of acidosis (Bohr effect). Case presentations have demonstrated decreased fetal heart rate variability and late decelerations (both signs of fetal distress) among monitored fetuses during the course of maternal DKA. With correction of maternal hyperglycemia and acidosis, fetal monitoring returned to normal.
- Dehydration resulting in hypovolemia with decreased placental perfusion can lead to fetal hypoxia and lactic acidosis.
- High lactic acid levels may predispose the fetal brain to hypoxic injury.
- Fetal hyperglycemia increases the fetal oxygen demand.

When the fetus has reached a viable gestational age (24 weeks), continuous electronic fetal monitoring is generally used. If the fetus appears compromised, cesarean delivery should be delayed until the mother is metabolically stable. Fortunately, correction of the maternal acidosis and hyperglycemia may also correct the fetal compromise and allow pregnancy to continue.

DISPOSITION

Role of the Consultant

Under optimal conditions, consultation with one physician qualified to manage both the pregnancy and the DKA would provide the most efficient care for patient management. Such management is possible in centers where maternal–fetal medicine physicians are available. However, in many hospitals, care must be divided between internists or endocrinologists for management of the DKA and an obstetrician to oversee the fetal condition.

Transfer Considerations

Patients with DKA should not be transferred until therapy has begun and the condition is stable or improving. Continuing care should be at a facility that has an obstetrician or maternal–fetal medicine physician available to assess fetal status.

OTHER PROBLEMS ASSOCIATED WITH DIABETES IN PREGNANCY

Urinary Tract Infection or Pyelonephritis

Urinary tract infections are more common during pregnancy among diabetic women. Early diagnosis and treatment of bacteriuria and cystitis can prevent the development of pyelonephritis. Pyelonephritis, a common antecedent of DKA during pregnancy, requires hospital admission for administration of i.v. antibiotics and metabolic surveillance (see later section, "Urinary Tract Infection in Pregnancy," for treatment recommendations).

Preeclampsia

The frequency of preeclampsia is greatly increased among women with diabetes. Compared with a 5% to 8% incidence in the normal population, as many as 25% of pregnancies among diabetic women become complicated by preeclampsia.[14] Patients may present with asymptomatic hypertension or with complaints such as headache, epigastric or right upper quadrant pain, visual disturbances, and eclamptic seizures. The combination of preeclampsia and diabetes significantly increases the risk of perinatal loss. Immediate consultation with the obstetric service is advised if blood pressure elevation (greater than or equal to 140/90) is detected.

Yeast Vulvovaginitis

Vaginal pruritus caused by yeast infection is frequently seen among diabetic women during pregnancy. Presenting complaints include vaginal itching, dysuria, and dyspareunia. The diagnosis is confirmed by culture or microscopic identification of mycelia or pseudohyphae on direct microscopy in a potassium hydroxide 10% preparation. During pregnancy, miconazole nitrate 2% cream (Monistat) applied daily for 7 days or clotrimazole 100-mg vaginal tablets at bedtime for 7 days provides prompt resolution in most patients.

Significant Decrease in Fetal Movement

Pregnancy among diabetic women is associated with an increased risk of stillbirth. Decreased fetal movement may be an early warning sign of impending fetal demise. Any pregnant woman who perceives a significant decrease in fetal movement after the twenty-fourth week of pregnancy should be evaluated. Immediate consultation with the obstetric service for antepartum fetal heart rate testing is prudent.

Myocardial Ischemia

Any diabetic woman with complaints suggesting myocardial ischemia should be thoroughly examined. Ischemic heart disease is unusual among diabetic women during pregnancy, it but carries a grave prognosis. Most such patients have been at least 30 years of age. The outcome in one study of 12 women with myocardial infarctions occurring either before or during pregnancy reported a 66% maternal mortality rate.[12] Because of the poor prognosis, termination of pregnancy with permanent sterilization is recommended for any diabetic woman with ischemic heart disease.

Childbirth Complicated by Macrosomia with Possible Shoulder Dystocia

The delivering physician should be able to perform appropriate maneuvers for safe delivery if shoulder dystocia occurs. The possibility of this complication, often associated with poor control of glucose levels, should always be considered prior to attempted vaginal delivery of a diabetic woman.

Visual Loss Due to Diabetic Retinopathy

The pregnant woman with preexisting diabetes should have an ophthalmic examination for early detection of diabetic retinopathy. Although once thought to be hastened by pregnancy, background diabetic retinopathy may not adversely be affected by it.[7] Some women with long-standing, poorly controlled diabetes also have proliferative retinopathy, which (unless prepregnancy laser therapy has been performed) has the potential for vitreous hemorrhage and permanent loss of vision. Delivery is indicated in such women if progressive visual loss occurs. Macular edema has been recognized among pregnant diabetic women and is usually associated with hypertension and proteinuria.[13]

Preterm Labor

β-Sympathomimetic drugs, such as terbutaline, used to treat preterm labor can cause extreme elevations in glucose levels and even DKA in diabetic women. If treatment of preterm labor is necessary, i.v. magnesium sulfate has no effect on blood glucose and is the drug of choice.

Maternal Glucose Control

The ability to make frequent capillary blood glucose measurements at home has reduced both maternal and perinatal mortality and morbidity.[9] Home glucose monitoring has become an important part of prenatal care for diabetic women, especially those requiring insulin.[6,16] Such glucose determinations are made one to four times daily, depending on recent glucose control. When a diabetic gravida presents to the emergency department, the physician should inquire about the availability of recent data from home glucose monitoring.

Capillary blood glucose determinations have shown a good correlation with plasma samples, especially in the fasting state. However, after carbohydrate ingestion, values differ from plasma levels by as much as 15%, with capillary values being higher.[15]

Urine testing for glucose has no role in the management of diabetes during pregnancy. Even during normal pregnancy, glucose can occasionally be detected in the urine. The cardiac output increases by 40% during pregnancy, accompanied by a similar increase in renal perfusion and glomerular filtration rate. These increases lead to more filtered substrate, in this case, glucose. If tubular reabsorption is not equally increased, glucosuria may be present, even at low blood glucose levels. It is necessary for the pregnant diabetic to rely on capillary glucose monitoring to determine optimal insulin dosage. Thus, urine testing for glucose has been virtually abandoned during pregnancy. However, there remains a place for the home measurement of urine ketones, especially when hyperglycemia is persistent.

Insulin Management during Pregnancy

Most diabetic women require split-dose or multiple injections of regular and NPH insulin to achieve adequate control. Traditionally, the total dose of insulin is given as two-thirds in the morning and one-third at night. The starting morning dose consists of two-thirds NPH and one-third regular; the evening dose is one-half NPH and one-half regular. This "ideal" insulin regimen will vary, depending on capillary glucose surveillance. During pregnancy, perinatal morbidity and mortality are related to the degree of glycemic control; therefore, the goal of insulin therapy during pregnancy is blood glucose levels that are essentially in the euglycemic range (fasting, 60 to 90 mg/dL; 2 hours after each meal, 90 to 120 mg/dL).

Oral Hypoglycemic Agents

The level of glycemic control achieved with oral agents is not satisfactory during pregnancy. These agents readily cross the placenta and may lead to stimulation of fetal insulin secretion. High fetal insulin concentration is associated with fetal macrosomia and resultant myocardial hyperplasia, stillbirth, and delayed fetal lung maturation. For these two reasons, oral hypoglycemic agents have no use in pregnancy. On the other hand, oral agents have not been associated with birth defects among humans.

DISPOSITION

Role of the Consultant

Diabetes in pregnancy is a high-risk situation for mother and fetus. Optimal prenatal care requires either a maternal–fetal medicine physician or an obstetrician experienced in the management of diabetes in pregnancy. Maternal–fetal medicine physicians are specially trained in the management of such pregnancies. If such a subspecialist is not available, the combined efforts of an obstetrician to oversee management of the pregnancy and an internist to assist in insulin adjustments are advised.

Indications for Admission

Admission is indicated when poor glucose control remains uncorrected after 3 to 4 days of home glucose monitoring and insulin adjustment, as well as when complications are present, including hyperemesis gravidarum, DKA, preeclampsia, pyelonephritis, dehydration, and febrile illness (viral or bacterial).

COMMON PITFALLS

- The main cause of fetal loss among diabetic women is birth defects. This risk can be reduced only by achieving euglycemic control at the time of conception and throughout the first 7 to 10 weeks of pregnancy.

- Because perinatal outcome is related to glycemic control, acceptable blood glucose levels during pregnancy are significantly lower than for the nonpregnant woman.
- Urine glucose testing during pregnancy is altered by the increased glomerular filtration rate and has been abandoned.
- During pregnancy, DKA can occur with blood glucose levels as low as 200 to 300 mg/dL.
- As a result of accelerated starvation ketosis, ketones in the urine and even in the blood can occur with normal blood glucose levels.

GESTATIONAL DIABETES

Approximately 3% of pregnant women will develop gestational diabetes. Because of the insulin resistance caused by the placental hormone, human placental lactogen, the maternal response at meals is characterized by hyperinsulinemia and higher glucose concentrations than in the nonpregnant state. Some women cannot increase their insulin secretions to meet this demand and will develop hyperglycemia after meals. These women have gestational diabetes. Only about 15% of gestational diabetics will eventually develop fasting hyperglycemia and require insulin therapy. Human placental lactogen production is a reflection of placental mass, so carbohydrate intolerance in gestational diabetes is generally not present until after 26 to 28 weeks of pregnancy. Because these women are euglycemic during early pregnancy, there is no increased risk for fetal malformations.

DIAGNOSIS

Most experts recommend gestational diabetes screening for all women during pregnancy, a practice currently followed by practically all obstetricians in the United States.[3] A 50-g oral glucose load is given without regard to the last meal, and a serum glucose determination is made 1 hour later. A value higher than 140 mg/dL is considered abnormal, and a 100-g oral 3-hour glucose tolerance test (OGTT), following 3 days of unrestricted activity and carbohydrate intake, is performed.

The currently accepted upper limits of normal serum glucose values for this OGTT are 105, 190, 165, and 145 mg/dL fasting and 1, 2, and 3 hours after ingestion, respectively. If two or more values are elevated, the diagnosis of gestational diabetes is made, the woman is prescribed a diabetic diet, and glucose surveillance is begun. Selective screening, a lower 1-hour glucose screening threshold, and somewhat lower acceptable values for the 3-hour OGTT have recently been proposed and challenged.[10]

EMERGENCY DEPARTMENT MANAGEMENT

The diet typically prescribed is a 30- to 35-cal/kg (ideal body weight) American Diabetic Association diet. The woman is then followed with fasting and 2-hour postprandial serum glucose determinations every 1 to 2 weeks, although the necessity of measuring the postpartum value has been questioned if the fasting values remain normal.[8] Gestational diabetes is associated with two major risks. Fifteen percent of women will develop fasting hyperglycemia (greater than or equal to 105 mg/dL) and require insulin. Fetal macrosomia with resulting birth trauma is a major risk. When delivering a patient with gestational diabetes, the physician should be able to perform appropriate maneuvers if shoulder dystocia occurs. Hypoglycemia may develop in the newborn soon after delivery. Approximately 60% of gestational diabetics develop overt diabetes later in life.

References

1. American College of Obstetricians and Gynecologists. *Diabetes and pregnancy.* ACOG technical bulletin no. 200. Washington, DC: ACOG, 1994.
2. Brumfield CG, Huddleston JF. The management of diabetic ketoacidosis in pregnancy. *Clin Obstet Gynecol* 1984;27:50.
3. Gabbe S, Hill L, Schmidt L, et al. Management of diabetes by obstetrician-gynecologists. *Obstet Gynecol* 1998;91:643.
4. Hagay Z, Reece EA. Diabetes mellitus in pregnancy and periconceptional genetic counseling. *Am J Perinatol* 1992;9:87.
5. Hare JW. Gestational diabetes mellitus: levels of glycemia as management goals. *Diabetes* 1991;40[Suppl 2]:193.
6. Homko CJ, Sivan E, Reece EA. Is self-monitoring of blood glucose necessary in the management of gestational diabetes? *Diabetes Care* 1998;21[Suppl]:B118.
7. Horvat M, MacLean H, Goldberg L, et al. Diabetic retinopathy in pregnancy: a 12-year prospective study. *Br J Ophthalmol* 1980;64:389.
8. Huddleston JF, Cramer MK, Vroon DH. A rationale for omitting two-hour postprandial glucose determinations in gestational diabetes. *Am J Obstet Gynecol* 1993;169:257.
9. Landon MB, Gabbe SG. Fetal surveillance in the pregnancy complicated by diabetes mellitus. *Clin Perinatol* 1993;20:549.
10. Metzgar BE, Coustan DR. Summary and recommendations of the Fourth International Workshop-Conference on Gestational Diabetes. *Diabetes Care* 1998;21[Suppl]:B161.
11. Ratner RE. Clinical review 47: gestational diabetes mellitus: after three international workshops do we know how to diagnose and manage it yet? *J Clin Endocrinol Metab* 1993;77:1.
12. Silfen SL, Wapner RL, Gabbe SG. Maternal outcome in class H diabetes mellitus. *Obstet Gynecol* 1980;6:749.
13. Sinclair SH, Nesler C, Foxman B, et al. Macular edema and pregnancy in insulin dependent diabetes. *Am J Ophthalmol* 1984;97:154.
14. Taylor R, Vanderpump M. New concepts in diabetes mellitus: I. Treatment, pregnancy and aetiology. Human Metabolism Research Centre, Newcastle upon Tyne, UK. *Postgrad Med J* 1994;70:418.
15. Varner MW. Efficacy of home glucose monitoring in diabetic pregnancy. *Am J Med* 1983;75:592.
16. Weiner CP, Faustich MW, Burns J, et al. Diagnosis of gestational diabetes by capillary blood samples and/or portable reflectance meter: derivation of threshold values and prospective validation. *Am J Obstet Gynecol* 1987;156:1085.

Urinary Tract Infection in Pregnancy

Urinary tract infection (UTI) is one of the most common medical complications in pregnancy and is a frequent cause of emergency department visits.[1,9] Females have a higher rate of UTIs than males, presumably because of the shorter urethra, the easy entry of bacteria into the bladder during sexual intercourse, and incomplete bladder emptying. The physiologic changes of pregnancy worsen the risk for UTI and render the upper tract more susceptible to infection.

In pregnancy, the bladder has decreased tone and increased capacity. These changes increase stasis and the risk for vesicoureteral reflux, especially in women who had urologic procedures as children to correct such reflux.[2] The ureters are physiologically dilated, due to a decrease in ureteral muscle tone and peristalsis, secondary to progesterone increases during pregnancy. In addition, there is ureteral compression by the enlarged pregnant uterus and the enlarged ovarian veins, and the urine is made nutritionally rich from nutrients filtered by the glomeruli in excess of the tubular capacity for their resorption.

The typical microbiologic isolates in UTI are similar in pregnant and nonpregnant patients.[11] *Escherichia coli* accounts for over 75% of all isolates. Other gram-negative aerobes, such as *Klebsiella* and *Proteus,* are also commonly isolated. Both enterococci and group B streptococci have been implicated in UTI. *Staphylococcus saprophyticus* is also an occasional uropathogen.

CLINICAL PRESENTATION

In pregnancy, UTI may be divided into asymptomatic bacteriuria (ASB), cystitis, and pyelonephritis. Both untreated ASB and cystitis may progress to upper tract (renal) infection, especially pyelonephritis.

By definition, the pregnant patient with ASB has no urinary tract symptoms. Four percent to 7% of all pregnant women have bacteria in their bladders without symptoms. The importance of this fact is that if the ASB is left untreated, about 25% of pregnant patients will develop pyelonephritis during pregnancy, labor, or the immediate puerperium. This percentage represents most of the 1% to 2% of all gravidas who will suffer from pyelonephritis.[4] Therefore, all pregnant patients ideally should be screened for ASB at the time of the first prenatal visit. Many women, however, do not seek prenatal care, early or ever, and many of these same women use the emergency department for various complaints.

Although there are no studies clearly showing a favorable cost-to-benefit ratio, a urinalysis or urine culture performed on such women during an emergency department visit for any complaint would probably be prudent. The usual definition of ASB requires that a single pathogen be isolated at a concentration greater than 100,000 colony-forming units (CFUs) per milliliter; however, the pregnant patient in the emergency department who has an uncontaminated urinalysis with bacteria and leukocytes should be treated. Eradication of ASB will largely prevent progression to pyelonephritis.

Cystitis commonly presents as urinary frequency, urgency, and dysuria. Suprapubic discomfort and tenderness are variably noted. However, UTI confined to the bladder does *not* result in fever or costovertebral angle tenderness. A urine culture with a single pathogen at greater than 100,000 CFU/mL is considered pathognomonic for infection. However, it has been clearly shown that, in symptomatic patients, a concentration of greater than 100 CFU/mL in the *bladder* urine is sufficient to confirm the diagnosis and justify treatment. The caveat here is that care must be taken to exclude vulvovaginal contamination, lest the diagnosis of cystitis be overcalled. The spun (and occasionally unspun) urine sediment reveals numerous leukocytes and rod-shaped bacteria, which may or may not be motile. Appropriately and promptly treated patients with cystitis typically respond quickly and have a good prognosis. Inadequate or delayed therapy may result in progression to pyelonephritis and its possible complications.

Classically, the gravida with pyelonephritis presents with chills, fever, flank pain, nausea, vomiting, urinary frequency and urgency, and dysuria.[9] The presence of fever with costovertebral angle tenderness in a patient with a positive, uncontaminated urinalysis or urine culture is diagnostic. As noted, the prevalence rate of pyelonephritis in pregnancy is 1% to 2%. This infection is always serious, but it can be more so in the pregnant patient. Gravid women may develop preterm labor, which may result in preterm delivery. Although the direct mechanism linking pyelonephritis and preterm labor has not been elucidated, it is postulated that bacterial endotoxin may result in cytokine or prostaglandin release from the decidua or membranes,[8] or that some bacteria release precursors of prostaglandins that are important in the initiation and maintenance of labor. Pyelonephritis, therefore, may lead to perinatal wastage.

Pyelonephritis may have other serious consequences in pregnancy.[10] Approximately 20% of gravidas with this infection have transient renal dysfunction with decreased creatinine clearance.[4] About 15% of these gravidas have bacteremia, so blood cultures are prudent. Uncommonly, septic shock may develop, even after treatment has begun.[7] Prolonged fetal bradycardia, not representing fetal distress but due to maternal hypothermia, also may be seen.[5] Adult respiratory distress syndrome has been reported as a consequence of urosepsis in such patients.[3] Very rarely, acute renal failure may result from pyelonephritis during pregnancy.[13]

EMERGENCY DEPARTMENT MANAGEMENT

Because ASB may progress to cystitis and pyelonephritis during pregnancy, gravid women who have not received prior prenatal care or undergone prior urinary screening tests should have a urinalysis to exclude ASB. Initially, a clean-catch urine specimen can be obtained; however, vulvovaginal contamination is common in pregnant women, and graphic instructions should be given to promote proper collection technique. Catheterization should be avoided if possible. In an uncontaminated urine specimen (no or few epithelial cells), the presence of rod-shaped bacteria indicates ASB. Such a urine specimen should be sent for culture. More than 100,000 CFU/mL of a single urinary pathogen is considered diagnostic. Treatment, however, should begin with the urinalysis findings and not await the culture results.

Treatment for ASB in the pregnant patient consists of 7 to 10 days of amoxicillin (500 mg PO every 6 hours), nitrofurantoin (100 mg PO three to four times per day), or a short-acting sulfonamide (with or without sulbactam). Because both nitrofurantoin and sulfonamides can displace bilirubin from its albumin-binding sites, with resultant neonatal hyperbilirubinemia, these two drugs should be avoided in the third trimester. Amoxicillin is the drug of choice in the third trimester. In areas where a high percentage of gram-negative aerobes (such as *E. coli*) show ampicillin resistance, cephalexin (250 mg every 6 hours) is an acceptable alternative.[6]

Patients with symptoms of cystitis should likewise provide a clean-catch urine specimen for urinalysis and culture. The presence, in an uncontaminated specimen, of leukocytes and rod-shaped bacteria confirms the diagnosis of cystitis. A urine culture should also be done; in symptomatic patients, only greater than 100 CFU/mL are required to demonstrate an infection. Although catheterization should be avoided, it may be necessary in symptomatic patients from whom an uncontaminated specimen cannot be obtained. Treatment of cystitis is the same as that of ASB.[6]

Pyelonephritis requires prompt and appropriate attention. The diagnosis of pyelonephritis is most commonly made with the finding of a positive urinalysis, fever, and costovertebral angle tenderness. Because of the possible complications of renal infection, pregnant patients with pyelonephritis should, with rare exception, be hospitalized. Many of these patients are dehydrated. Clinical management includes intravenous (i.v.) hydration, i.v. antibiotics, antipyretics, and close observation for septic shock and renal dysfunction.

Because the predominant pathogens are gram-negative aerobes, ampicillin (2 g i.v. every 6 hours) or ceftriaxone (1 to 2 g/d) is a good initial drug. Again, however, if a high percentage of the gram-negative aerobes (especially *E. coli*) shows resistance to ampicillin, then cefazolin (1 g i.v. every 6 hours) is the drug of choice. With the exception of patients who appear septic, are allergic to the initial therapy, or are not responding to the initial therapy, aminoglycosides should be avoided because of the high prevalence of transient renal dysfunction.[15] If the patient appears septic, therapy with ampicillin or cefazolin plus an aminoglycoside (1.0 mg to 1.5 mg/kg every 8 hours) should be initiated. All pregnant patients who receive aminoglycosides should have a serum creatinine level determined to exclude renal dysfunction, and then serum monitoring of aminoglycoside levels.[16] Ciprofloxacin is not recommended for use in pregnancy, because adequate human studies are not available.

If the patient does not respond within 48 hours, the clinician should consider the possibility of a resistant organism or urinary tract obstruction. Antibiotic changes appropriate to now-available culture and sensitivity data, intravenous pyelography, or ultrasonography may be appropriate.

DISPOSITION

Patients with cystitis or pyelonephritis are at risk for preterm labor and delivery.[8] Therefore, any pregnant patient with these infections should be evaluated for contractions and have her cervix examined. After midpregnancy, the presence of frequent contractions (more than 3 per hour) should be ruled out with an external fetal monitor. The preterm presence of frequent contractions or of an effaced or dilated cervix should prompt an evaluation by the obstetric consultant. Like pyelonephritis, preterm labor is an indication for admission and treatment with both antibiotics and tocolytic agents, such as terbutaline or magnesium sulfate. In the presence of urosepsis and overzealous hydration, pulmonary edema may be precipitated by the use of i.v. catecholamines, such as terbutaline.

An important consideration for pregnant patients with any UTI is follow-up. Pregnant patients with a prior UTI have a high rate of recurrence. In a retrospective analysis of pyelonephritis, 60% of patients required rehospitalization for a UTI.[12] Close follow-up with repetitive urine cultures to identify ASB for the remainder of pregnancy is important to prevent reinfection. If ASB is subsequently found, it should be treated as outlined previously. Another option to prevent reinfection in patients with a prior UTI is antibiotic suppression, usually accomplished with nitrofurantoin (100 mg PO every night), for the remainder of the pregnancy; such a regimen has been shown to reduce recurrence of bacteriuria to 8%.[14] Because close monitoring or suppression is commonly necessary, the patient's obstetrician should be notified of the infection or arrangements made to ensure prenatal care and appropriate follow-up.

References

1. Andriole VT, Patterson TF. Epidemiology, natural history, and management of urinary tract infections in pregnancy. *Med Clin North Am* 1991;75:359.
2. Bukowski TP, Betrus GG, Aquilina JW, et al. Urinary tract infections and pregnancy in women who underwent antireflex surgery in childhood. *J Urol* 1997;11:551.
3. Cunningham FG, Lucas MJ, Hankins GV. Pulmonary injury complicating antepartum pyelonephritis. *Am J Obstet Gynecol* 1987;156:797.
4. Gilstrap LC, Cunningham FG, Whalley PJ. Acute pyelonephritis in pregnancy: an anterospective study. *Obstet Gynecol* 1981;57:409.
5. Hankins GD, Leicht T, Van Hook JW. Prolonged fetal bradycardia secondary to maternal hypothermia in response to urosepsis. *Am J Perinatol* 1997;14:217.
6. Hooten TM, Stamm WE. Diagnosis and treatment of uncomplicated urinary tract infection. *Infect Dis Clin North Am* 1997;11:551.
7. Mabie WC, Barton JR, Sibai B. Septic shock in pregnancy. *Obstet Gynecol* 1997;90:553.
8. Mazor M, Furman B, Bashiri A. Cytokines in preterm parturition. *Gynecol Endocrinol* 1998;12:421.
9. Nathan L, Huddleston JF. Acute abdominal pain in pregnancy. *Obstet Gynecol Clin North Am* 1995;22:55.
10. Schieve LA, Handler A, Hershow R, et al. Urinary tract infection during pregnancy: its association with maternal morbidity and perinatal outcome. *Am J Public Health* 1994;84:405.
11. Stamm WE, Counts GW, Running KR, et al. Diagnosis of coliform infection in acutely dysuric women. *N Engl J Med* 1982;307:463.
12. Stamm WE, Hooton TM. Management of urinary tract infections in adults. *N Engl J Med* 1993;329:1328.
13. Ventura JE, Villa M, Mizraji R, et al. Acute renal failure in pregnancy. *Ren Fail* 1997;19:217.
14. Van Dorsten JP, Lenke RR, Schifrin BS. Pyelonephritis in pregnancy: The role of in-hospital management and nitrofurantoin suppression. *J Reprod Med* 1987;32:897.
15. Vercaigne LM, Zhanel GG. Recommended treatment for urinary tract infection in pregnancy. *Ann Pharmacother* 1994;28:248.
16. Wing DA, Hendershott CM, Debuque L, et al. A randomized trial of three antibiotic regimens for the treatment of pyelonephritis in pregnancy. *Obstet Gynecol* 1998;92:249.

CHAPTER 76
Infections in Pregnancy

Carol C. Coulson

Infections in pregnancy affect not only the infected patient, but also the fetus and the course of the pregnancy. The stage of pregnancy influences the physician's choice of therapy. Those who care for pregnant women must modify both their approach and their treatment of infections in this population. Physicians often need to choose more aggressive management, because infections are tolerated less well in pregnancy. An example is the pregnant patient with pyelonephritis who requires hospitalization for antibiotic treatment, whereas most nonpregnant patients with this disorder can be managed as outpatients. The choice of drug therapy is also guided by information regarding teratogenicity and toxicity to the fetus. The way drugs are prescribed in pregnancy may differ from therapy for nonpregnant patients. The presenting signs and symptoms of infection of various organ systems in the pregnant patient are usually identical to those in the nonpregnant patient. However, special considerations regarding diagnostic procedures and management are key to resolving infections with the least morbidity to the pregnant patient and fetus.

RESPIRATORY TRACT INFECTIONS

Pneumonia

In the preantibiotic era, maternal mortality from antepartum pneumonia was high. More recently, antibiotic therapy has contributed to an overall downward trend in both maternal and fetal morbidity and mortality, although pneumonia remains a potentially serious complication of pregnancy. There is no evidence that pregnancy places the mother at increased risk for acquiring a respiratory tract infection. Therefore, pregnant patients presumably encounter the same risks as nonpregnant patients in comparable health. Underlying chronic diseases, especially asthma, and maternal smoking may influence the incidence of pneumonia in pregnancy as in the nonpregnant patient.[15]

Cough, sputum production, and fever are the hallmarks of pneumonia. Physical examination often reveals a mildly ill patient with fever. Auscultation and percussion confirm the presence of infiltrates or lobar consolidation. Evaluation should consist of obtaining a sputum sample to check for white blood cells and perform a Gram stain and culture. Blood cultures should be performed, along with a complete blood cell count and differential. The diagnosis is supported by a chest radiograph with abdominal shielding to evaluate the extent of infiltrates. For the fetus, there is minimal radiation (usually less than 1 rad) with an anteroposterior, lateral, and occasional oblique chest film. Lobar consolidation is more consistent with bacterial infection, while patchy infiltrates are seen with a viral infection. The two most common organisms that cause pneumonia in this population are *Streptococcus pneumoniae* and *Mycoplasma pneumoniae*.

Treatment usually includes admission and intravenous antibiotics. Although pneumonia can be treated in the outpatient setting in the nonpregnant patient, normal physiologic changes of pregnancy decrease functional residual lung capacity in the gravid patient. Because of less reserve, hospitalization for most pregnant patients with pneumonia is prudent. Although there are no studies indicating that pregnant patients with pneumonia are sicker than nonpregnant patients, there remains a risk for the development of fulminant illness, including septic shock and acute respiratory distress syndrome. Optimal therapy for pneumococcal pneumonia (penicillin V potassium [Pen Vee-K], 500 mg PO four times daily for 7 to 14 days) differs from therapy for mycoplasmal infection (erythromycin, 250 to 500 mg PO four times daily for 14 days). An effort should be made to distinguish the two, using history, physical examination, and serologic and laboratory information.

Viral Infections (Respiratory)

Viral infection in general, but particularly influenza, predisposes to bacterial superinfection. Patients should be watched closely for worsening symptoms. Influenza vaccination is not contraindicated in pregnancy and is, in fact, recommended for women with underlying medical conditions.[1] Other upper respiratory tract infections such as laryngitis and bronchitis in previously healthy patients without chronic asthma are caused by various viral agents. These usually do not require antibiotic therapy. Symptomatic and supportive care with particular attention to hydration is often sufficient. Some infections may create enough inflammatory response in the respiratory tract to constitute reactive airway disease. Appropriate symptomatic treatment is indicated. Upper respiratory tract viral infections are also the most common precursors of acute bacterial sinusitis via a variety of mechanisms. The symptoms, evaluation, and treatment of sinusitis do not differ based on pregnancy status, with the exception of abdominal shielding for radiographs when needed.

Tuberculosis

Tuberculosis is another respiratory tract infection that may be detected in pregnancy. It is often asymptomatic, but it should be suspected in a patient with lethargy, respiratory complaints, and recent immigration from an endemic area. A chest radiograph demonstrates patchy parenchymal infiltrates with adenopathy and pleural effusion. Although tuberculin skin testing is valuable in pregnancy, definitive diagnosis relies on demonstration of *Mycobacterium tuberculosis* in sputum culture. Multidrug therapy with isoniazid (300 mg PO daily) plus rifampin (600 mg PO daily) for a minimum of 9 months is the regimen of choice for active disease.[14] Ethambutol (2.5 g PO daily) should be added if drug resistance is suspected. Pyridoxine (vitamin B_6, 50 mg PO daily) should be administered concomitantly with isoniazid to prevent potential neurotoxicity. Rifampin has been reported to cause hemorrhagic disease of the newborn. To prevent this complication, prophylactic administration of vitamin K in the third trimester is recommended. Streptomycin should not be used, due to the risk of fetal ototoxicity. The patient should be referred to her obstetrician or the local health department for follow-up of drug toxicity, congenital disease in the newborn, and chemoprophylaxis of the infant.[9]

Pneumocystis carinii Infection

In the pregnant woman with respiratory compromise who is positive for human immunodeficiency virus (HIV) infection, the differential diagnosis must include *Pneumocystis carinii* pneumonia (PCP). Although there are no pathognomonic clinical features, the fever, dyspnea, and hypoxemia seen in patients with PCP are usually quite profound. Rales are frequently absent. The chest radiograph shows diffuse interstitial pneumonitis and air bronchograms. Definitive diagnosis relies on demonstration of the organism in lung tissue by means of percutaneous or open lung biopsy or bronchoalveolar lavage. Hospitalization is warranted for oxygen therapy, supportive care, and antibiotic treatment with trimethoprim–sulfamethoxazole or pentamidine. If left untreated, PCP is universally fatal.

Summary

The most important consideration in the pregnant patient with an upper respiratory tract infection, regardless of theoretical expectations of the clinical course of the infection, is the concern that adequate oxygenation be maintained. Maternal hypoxia affects fetal oxygenation. Although some recommend that all pregnant patients with pneumonia undergo PO_2 assessment, clinical judgment must be used in deciding which patient does *not* need an arterial blood gas analysis. Overall, if there is a question regarding adequate oxygenation, an arterial blood gas analysis should be performed.

VIRAL INFECTIONS

Viral syndromes in pregnancy pose variable risks to the unborn fetus. Maternal morbidity and mortality are rare. Therefore, emergency department management involves supportive care and prevention of communication to other potentially pregnant women (including personnel and other patients).

Torch

TORCH (*t*oxoplasmosis, *o*ther [hepatitis B virus, varicella zoster], *r*ubella, *c*ytomegalovirus, and *h*erpesvirus) is discussed below.

Varicella (chickenpox) is associated with a pathognomonic vesicular outbreak. *Rubella (German measles)* is rare but may cause malaise and generalized fatigue. Viremia and transmission by respiratory droplets can occur before a rash develops for varicella (10 to 21 days) and after exposure in rubella infections (10 to 21 days). The diagnosis of varicella is most often made clinically on the basis of the pathognomonic skin eruption, although serologic confirmation is available. The diagnosis of rubella is made by a fourfold rise in immunoglobulin-G (IgG) serum titers or IgM-specific tests. Serum for IgG determination should be drawn initially and then 2 to 3 weeks later, with both specimens run simultaneously to assess increasing IgG titer over time.[6] Infection in early pregnancy (first trimester) causes the most fetal harm and can result in congenital abnormalities of the cardiac, neurologic, musculoskeletal, and ophthalmic systems. These patients should be referred to an obstetrician for counseling and follow-up. It is critical that the patient call her obstetrician before entering the office to avoid exposing other patients to the virus. Rubella vaccine for nonimmune patients should not be administered in pregnancy or within 3 months prior to conception.

Infection in late pregnancy by either virus seldom affects pregnancy outcome. In the immunosuppressed state of pregnancy, however, evolution of *varicella pneumonia* should always be considered. Varicella pneumonia in pregnancy increases the risk of maternal complication and death, with mortality as high as 40%. The patient suspected of having varicella pneumonia should be admitted to the hospital because acute respiratory distress syndrome may develop rapidly.

Peripartum varicella infection (from 5 days before delivery through 2 days after delivery) places the fetus at high risk for morbidity and mortality. Passive transmission of protective maternal antibodies to the disease has not yet occurred in this window. In addition, premature labor is always a concern, particularly in the presence of infection. Attempts should be made to determine whether the patient is in labor by asking about contractions (abdominal tightening and back pain). Patients who are suspected of being in labor should be sent to the labor and delivery room for evaluation.

Varicella zoster immune globulin (VZIG) should be administered to susceptible pregnant women within 96 hours of exposure to the disease in hopes of tempering the severity of the illness. There is *no* evidence that administration of VZIG to this population will prevent maternal viremia, fetal infection, or congenital varicella syndrome. VZIG can be obtained from the American Red Cross.

Most adults infected with *cytomegalovirus* (CMV) are essentially asymptomatic. Unfortunately, CMV is the most common cause of intrauterine infection. Documented in 0.5% to 2.5% of all deliveries, CMV infection has a wide range of effects, ranging from rare but significant neurologic damage in the fetus to simply producing an asymptomatic carrier state accompanied by viral shedding. In light of the difficulty of diagnosis due to its asymptomatic presentation and low incidence of fetal morbidity, clinicians are limited to obtaining laboratory data and confirming seroconversion.

Toxoplasmosis, a protozoan infection, is usually asymptomatic. Rarely, the patient may present with a mononucleosis-like picture. Most infections are self-limited without significant complications. Many newborns are asymptomatic. No increase in fetal death is observed. For the rare affected newborn, a constellation of central nervous system and ophthalmic problems may be noted. If toxoplasmosis or CMV infection is suspected in pregnancy, the patient should be referred for counseling and serologic testing.

Mumps virus, a paramyxovirus, is transmitted by respiratory secretions. Typically, the patient presents with fever, malaise, myalgia, and anorexia, followed by parotitis in 24 hours. Treatment of mumps is supportive, and there is no observed increase in maternal morbidity or mortality. Mumps infection in the first and second trimesters may be associated with increased fetal loss. However, there is no fetal congenital disorder clearly associated with maternal mumps infection.

Human parvovirus B19 is the etiologic agent of erythema infectiosum (fifth disease). Presentation in adults is frequently that of a flulike illness with fever, adenopathy, arthralgias, and arthritis, particularly of the hands. Rash is usually absent. Up to 20% of those infected may remain asymptomatic. Serologic testing for IgG- and IgM-specific antibodies to human parvovirus B19 is available and should be used if exposure is suspected. Parvovirus infection is associated with an increased risk of fetal hydrops and stillbirth.[12] It has been described, as well, in conjunction with a variety of fetal anomalies (causation is unclear) and congenital anemia. The patient should be referred to an obstetrician for counseling, follow-up serologies, and ultrasonography. Infection appears to confer lifelong immunity

Herpesvirus infection in pregnancy raises concern for neonatal transmission associated with vaginal delivery. From 4% to 8% of infants delivered through the infected birth canal of a mother with recurrent herpes will acquire the infection. The neonatal infection rate approaches 50% with vaginal delivery if the maternal herpes outbreak is primary. Approximately 25% of infants infected during delivery will die of disseminated disease. Patients often complain of pain from acute lesions of the perineum. Accurate emergency department diagnosis is critical for management in later stages of pregnancy by the patient's obstetrician. A herpes culture should be obtained from the base of suspicious lesions with a cotton-tipped swab. (Calcium alginate swabs have been found to inactivate the herpesvirus.) Accurate documentation of the status of the membranes is paramount. If uterine contractions and rupture of the membranes have occurred, the patient should be transferred immediately to the labor suite. The emergency physician should provide supportive care, including analgesics and suggestions about hygiene (e.g., Burow's solution soaks to the perineum). The use of acyclovir in pregnancy has been reported in over 300 cases.[2] Although there is no indication of fetal toxicity, use of acyclovir continues to be dictated by the severity of maternal illness. Acyclovir therapy may be indicated for disseminated herpes simplex virus (HSV) or varicella pneumonia. Routine use to ameliorate severity or duration of recurrent outbreaks has not been studied in pregnant subjects, although suppressive doses are used frequently in HIV-positive gravidas with severe or frequent herpes outbreaks.

Viral hepatitis in pregnancy in the United States follows the same disease course as in nonpregnant patients. Fetal morbidity and mortality are not increased.[11] Diagnosis is made by serologic identification of specific viral antigens and antibodies. Symptoms include malaise, nausea, vomiting, fatigue, and nonspecific gastrointestinal symptoms. The symptoms of hepatitis are similar to those of morning sickness.

Jaundice, icteric sclera, and dark urine may be seen. However, spider angiomas and palmar erythema are normal findings in pregnancy. Serum transaminase levels are not altered in pregnancy, so elevated values may indicate hepatitis. A threefold to fourfold elevation of alkaline phosphatase levels is usual in pregnancy due to placental production. Acute hepatitis A virus (HAV) may be diagnosed by detecting IgM anti-HAV serologically, whereas hepatitis B virus (HBV) is seen with hepatitis B surface antigen. Hepatitis B e antigen should also be determined if the surface antigen for hepatitis B is positive, because "e" positivity correlates with infectivity and indicates an increased risk for fetal transmission.

Therapy for pregnant patients is similar to that for nonpregnant patients. Hospitalization is recommended for the patient who is unable to maintain fluids or who is severely debilitated. All patients with elevated coagulation studies (prothrombin time, partial thromboplastin time) require hospitalization.

For pregnant women at high risk for hepatitis B, immune-specific vaccine and globulin can be given safely during pregnancy for preventive purposes. The usual dose for hepatitis B vaccine is 1 mL intramuscularly, followed by repeat doses 1 and 6 months later. Because the vaccine is made of purified proteins, placental transmission is not a risk. Prophylaxis given at the same time as the vaccine can be administered as an intramuscular injection of hepatitis B–specific immunoglobulin (0.06 mL/kg as soon as possible after exposure). Pregnant women exposed to hepatitis A should be given gamma globulin prophylactically (0.62 mL/kg within 2 weeks of exposure).

Hepatitis C (blood-borne non-A, non-B hepatitis) is diagnosed by the detection of either hepatitis C–specific antibody or hepatitis C–specific RNA. Seventy-five percent of patients are asymptomatic and anicteric.[10] The distinction between hepatitis C and other viral liver infections is important because up to 50% of patients with hepatitis C maintain abnormal chemical markers for liver disease more than 1 year after diagnosis. This is presumptive of chronic active hepatitis and predisposes the patient to cirrhosis. Pregnancy does not appear to alter the course of disease. Vertical transmission to the fetus has not been reported in the absence of detectable hepatitis C–specific RNA. Interferon treatment is contraindicated in pregnancy.[10]

Hepatitis D (delta hepatitis) can infect only in the presence of hepatitis B. Acute coinfection is not usually more virulent than hepatitis B alone and presents with a similar clinical picture. However, superinfection, which occurs when delta hepatitis develops in a chronic carrier of hepatitis B, generally leads to more severe disease, including cirrhosis and portal hypertension.

Serologic detection of hepatitis D is limited because the anti-delta antibody is transient unless chronic infection develops. Management strategy for delta hepatitis involves the prevention of hepatitis B infection through vaccination.

Clinically, hepatitis E (enteric non-A, non-B hepatitis) presents with gastroenteritis and hepatitis similar to HAV. Routine serologic testing is unavailable at this time. Hepatitis E should be suspected in any gravida with appropriate history in whom tests for HAV, HBV, and HCV are negative. The course of the disease in pregnancy is not well documented. Treatment is generally supportive.

Hepatitis G, also known as GBV-C, has been described. It frequently coexists with hepatitis C and, similarly, is transmitted parenterally. Vertical transmission to the fetus, however, is much more common with hepatitis G. Its clinical role in acute and chronic liver disease is unclear.[17]

GASTROINTESTINAL INFECTIONS

Nausea and vomiting can occur at any time in pregnancy, although morning sickness typically occurs in the first trimester. If accompanied by diarrhea or malaise, the differential diagnosis includes viral gastroenteritis (rotavirus, Norwalk virus) and bacterial food poisoning. Nausea, vomiting, and chronic fatigue may also suggest the possibility of hepatitis.

Gastroenteritis in pregnant patients is similar to gastroenteritis in nonpregnant patients. Viral gastroenteritis has a variable incubation period and is brief and self-limited. Symptoms include nausea and vomiting with or without a low-grade temperature. Therapy is usually supportive, with fluids and rest. Of major concern in pregnancy, however, is dehydration and the ability to maintain oral intake. In the patient with a large amount of ketonuria, hospitalization may be recommended for intravenous supplementation and correction of electrolyte imbalance.

Bacterial gastroenteritis (caused by *Salmonella, Shigella, Campylobacter, Staphylococcus, Bacillus cereus, Clostridium,* or *Vibrio* species) may occur in pregnancy. Symptoms begin abruptly with nausea and crampy abdominal pain, often followed by diarrhea. High fever (greater than 38.5°C [101.3°F]) and chills are often present. The volume of diarrhea may be large. Mucus and blood may be present. Diagnosis is made from fresh stool cultures. Dehydration may be significant, and hospitalization is often necessary. Antibiotics for *Salmonella* and *Shigella* infections are not standard in the healthy adult nonpregnant population but should probably be initiated in pregnant patients who are moderately to severely affected, because therapy may decrease the duration of symptoms. Ampicillin (500 mg PO four times daily for 5 days) is recommended. Although not often seen in residents of the United States, parasitic infections in pregnant women can be found in recent immigrants from Southeast Asia and Latin America and in travelers. Parasitic infections may be less well tolerated by pregnant women because of altered immune function. Seemingly benign intestinal infections in the nonpregnant patient may cause increased morbidity during pregnancy. Fatal peritonitis with invasive parasitic disease has been described.[5] Additionally, some parasites cross the placenta to infect the fetus. Parasites are most often spread by the fecal–oral route. Symptoms range from mild gastrointestinal complaints of constipation and flatulence to severe illness with massive bloody diarrhea and fever. History and physical examination may also reveal a variety of constitutional signs and symptoms, especially anorexia, weight loss, hepatomegaly, jaundice, and skin lesions. Besides supportive care, treatment of specific infections depends on the expected course. Unfortunately, many agents used to treat parasitic infections are also teratogenic. Table 76.1 lists parasitic infections that require treatment and drug regimens considered safe in pregnancy.[5]

BREAST INFECTION

Breast symptoms of infectious cause (mastitis and breast abscess) must be differentiated from engorgement in the postpartum period (see Chapter 37). Engorgement (breast congestion with milk) usually occurs within the first week after delivery. Breasts become firm and warm, and patients complain of diffuse tenderness. Low-grade fever may accompany engorgement. In contrast to bilateral breast engorgement, mastitis is unilateral, painful, and often accompanied by a high fever. Caused by coagulase-positive *Staphylococcus aureus* transmitted from the newborn's oropharynx, treatment includes cephalexin (Keflex, 500 mg) or dicloxacillin (500 mg PO) four times daily for 1 week. *Toxic shock syndrome* caused by *S. aureus* associated with puerperal mastitis has been reported.[7] Because the organism is shared between mother and child, continued breastfeeding is allowed. Decompression of the breast through breast pumping or breastfeeding may accelerate resolution of mastitis. Symptomatic relief of pain can be achieved by warm showers, expression of milk, use of a supportive bra, and analgesics. Nipples may be lubricated with lanolin agents to prevent fissure formation.

Abscess formation should be suspected when focal fluctuance and increased tenderness are found or when clinical signs and symptoms of suspected mastitis do not subside after several days of oral antibiotic therapy. Incision and drainage along with continued antibiotic therapy are needed. Incision and drainage of these lesions should *not* be attempted in the emergency department, because such lesions often dissect deeply and widely in tissue planes. Breastfeeding on the affected side should be deferred until the abscess is cleared.

URINARY TRACT INFECTIONS

Asymptomatic bacteriuria, defined as greater than 10^5 colony-forming units (CFU) per milliliter obtained on culture, is present in 2% to 10% of all pregnant women. Patients with diabetes or sickle cell disease are at high risk for developing urinary infection in pregnancy. Twenty percent to 40% of pregnant women with untreated bacteriuria develop acute pyelonephritis (see Chapter 75).[13]

Treatment with antibiotics includes sulfisoxazole (500 mg four times daily; not to be used late in pregnancy), cephalexin (500 mg four times daily), or nitrofurantoin (100 mg four times daily) for 1 week. Ampicillin (500 mg four times daily for 7 days) may be used. However, up to 30% of *Escherichia coli* urinary tract infections may be resistant. Single-dose therapy is *not* recommended in the pregnant patient, although 3-day regimens are effective in most otherwise healthy pregnant women.[16] Quinolone therapy must be avoided, because these drugs are teratogenic in animal models. Follow-up is important.

When pyelonephritis is suspected by the presence of fever and flank pain, complications such as septic shock and preterm labor may occur. All pregnant patients with pyelonephritis should be admitted for intravenous hydration and antibiotic therapy with a cephalosporin or an aminoglycoside.

Urethritis should be considered in patients with dysuria, white blood cells in the urinalysis, and *negative* urine cultures. A urethral culture for *Chlamydia trachomatis* should be done. Erythromycin is appropriate therapy.

TABLE 76.1. Important Intestinal Parasites During Pregnancy

Parasite	Gastrointestinal Site	Clinical Problems	Epidemiology and Life Cycle	Drugs to Use in Pregnancy if Indicated
Protozoa				
Giardia lamblia	Duodenum, upper jejunum	Diarrhea, flatulence, malabsorption	Multiplies in gut, cyst Worldwide; animal reservoir Food and water borne	Paromomycin Metronidazole
Entamoeba histolytica	Colon	Dysentery, extraintestinal invasion	Multiplies in gut, cyst Worldwide; human reservoir Food and water borne	Paromomycin Metronidazole for hepatic abscess
Helminths				
Enterobius vermicularis (pinworm)	Colon	Pruritus ani Pruritus vulvae	Eggs mature extraintestinally Feces-finger-food borne Worldwide	Pyrantel pamoate
Trichuris trichiurae (whipworm)	Colon	Rectal prolapse	Eggs mature extraintestinally Feces-finger-food borne Worldwide	Mebendazole
Ascaris lumbricoides	Small and large intestine	Migration, obstruction	Eggs mature extraintestinally Feces-finger-food borne Worldwide	Pyrantel pamoate
Hookworm				
Necator americanus: *Ancylostoma braziliense*	Small intestine	Anemia, hypoproteinemia, larval dermatitis	Geographically limited Eggs must hatch and larvae mature in soil	Pyrantel pamoate
Strongyloides stercoralis	Jejunum	Anemia, hypoproteinemia, hyperinfection syndrome	Autoinfective Worldwide	Thiabendazole
Hymenolepis nana (dwarf tapeworm)	Jejunum	Hyperinfection syndrome	Autoinfective Worldwide	Paromomycin Niclosamide
Tapeworms	Small intestine	Megaloblastic anemia	Intermediate hosts limit range	Niclosamide
Taerig solium *T. saginata* *Diphyllobothrium latum*		Malnutrion (*D. latum*), cysticercosis (*T. solium*)	*T. solium*, pigs *T. saginate*, cattle *D. latum*, freshwater fish	
Flukes Schistosomes	Mesenteric veins Liver and biliary tract	Egg- or worm-induced granulomas (schistosomes)	Intermediate hosts limit range	Praziquantel
Liver flukes (*Clonorchis, Opisthorchis*)		Cholangitis, obstructive jaundice (liver flukes)	Schistosomes, snail Liver fluke, snail, and fish	

From D Alauro F, Lee RV, Pao-In K, et al. Intestinal parasites and pregnancy. *Obstet Gynecol* 1985;66:639.

SKIN INFECTIONS

Pthirus pubis (crab louse) and *Sarcoptes scabiei* (scabies) may present a problem in pregnant patients. Crab lice can be found in pubic hair, usually attached at the base of a hair or adjacent skin, and are transmitted through close physical contact. These nits can be found in other areas of the body as well, such as axillary and perianal hairs and eyelashes. The scabies mite causes pruritus from focal skin burrowing and intradermal deposition of eggs. Irritation is most often found on the back of the arms and legs and between the fingers. Excoriations may be the most obvious sign. Diagnosis is made by inspection, using a hand lens, of the high-yield areas. Because these infections are spread by intimate contact, family members need to be examined as well.

Other recommendations for improving hygienic situations should be given, such as washing all infected clothing, including bed sheets, and treating appropriate contacts. Both skin infections can be transmitted from mother to child through intimate contact. The finding of the crab louse should alert caretakers to the possibility of the presence of other venereal diseases, such as gonorrhea and chlamydial infection. Pyrethrins (RID), applied at night and washed off in the morning, are acceptable in pregnancy. Lindane (Kwell) has caused concern because of its suspected neurotoxic effect. If pyrethrins are not effective, referral to an obstetrician should be made for supervised lindane use in symptomatic patients.

VAGINAL, CERVICAL, AND OTHER LOWER GENITAL TRACT INFECTIONS

Vaginitis and Cervicitis

Lower genital tract discharge is most often vaginal but may be due to cervicitis. Evaluation of the vagina and cervix should include a speculum examination, testing the pH of vaginal secretions with phenaphthazine paper (Nitrazine), wet mount, and cultures of the cervix for *Neisseria gonorrhoeae* and *Chlamydia*. The differential diagnosis for a vaginal discharge in a pregnant patient should also include rupture of the membranes. This should be suspected in all pregnant patients, and a careful history obtained. Was a gush of fluid present? Is clear fluid present? Are contractions present? If there is suspicion of ruptured membranes, an assessment should be performed.

Pregnancy may be accompanied by a vaginal discharge that is physiologic or abnormal. Many women note an increase in asymptomatic vaginal secretions. A physiologic vaginal discharge occurs in pregnancy due to increased hormonal status; it is normally white and nonirritating and may drain onto the undergarments. Wet mount evaluation is remarkable for an acidic pH (less than 4.5) and numerous epithelial cells.

Pathologic vaginal irritations are caused by *Trichomonas vaginalis, Candida,* and bacterial vaginosis (previously called nonspecific vaginitis or *Gardnerella vaginalis* infection) (see Chapter 85).

It has been suggested that *T. vaginalis* may play a role in the pathogenesis of preterm labor and premature rupture of the membranes.[8] At this point, however, no consistent recommendations exist. Treatment for *T. vaginalis* infection may be initiated for patients who are symptomatic with annoying malodorous and copious discharge. Motile organisms can be seen on microscopic analysis of secretions, and the pH is higher than 4.5. Single-dose therapy with metronidazole (2 g PO) is recommended, although multidose therapy (250 mg PO three times daily) should be used for recurrent cases. Sexual partners should be treated to prevent reinfection. The treatment of pregnant women with metronidazole (when used after 12 weeks of pregnancy) results in no increased risk of complications. *T. vaginalis* or bacterial vaginosis may suggest that the patient has a concomitant sexually transmitted disease (caused by *N. gonorrhoeae* or *Chlamydia*). The emergency physician may want to culture for these at the same visit.

Candida albicans is normally present in 10% to 20% of patients. In physiologic quantities, its presence causes no symptoms. With overgrowth of *Candida,* a patient's chief complaint is often pruritus with or without notable discharge. The vulva may also be irritated and result in extreme itching. The classic "cottage cheese" discharge is seen in only 10% to 20%. Hyphae and buds on the wet mount potassium hydroxide slide confirm the diagnosis. The vaginal pH is less than 4.5. Antifungal vaginal cream (clotrimazole [Gyne-Lotrimin] or miconazole nitrate 2% [Monistat], one applicator per vagina at bedtime for 5 to 7 nights), is recommended. Nystatin is not recommended. However, if no other agent is available, nystatin is not contraindicated but must be used twice daily for 14 days. Candidal vaginal infections are not associated with obstetric complications. Only symptomatic patients need to be offered treatment.

More than half of all patients with bacterial vaginosis are symptomatic. Symptomatic patients present with a chief complaint of a fishy, foul odor instead of vulvar or vaginal pruritus or discharge. Examination is remarkable for the lack of inflammation of vulva or vagina, hence the name *vaginosis*. Diagnosis is confirmed by (1) a positive amine test when potassium hydroxide is added to a slide with vaginal secretions, (2) a wet mount showing "clue" cells (epithelial cells studded with bacteria), (3) *Lactobacillus* morphotypes less than background bacteria, and (4) pH higher than 4.5. All patients should be offered treatment with metronidazole (500 mg PO twice daily for 5 to 7 days after first trimester) or clindamycin (300 mg PO three times daily for 7 days). Alternative therapy with intravaginal clindamycin cream or metronidazole gel may be considered, although systemic oral therapy may reduce the risk of pregnancy complications, while intravaginal treatment may not. Evidence suggests that patients with bacterial vaginosis are at increased risk for preterm premature rupture of the membranes, preterm labor, intraamniotic infection, and postpartum endometritis.[8]

Cervical infection (cervicitis) is characterized by cervical friability, erythema, ulcers, and discharge that is cloudy or purulent. *N. gonorrhoeae* and *Chlamydia* cause both symptomatic and asymptomatic cervicitis, and either may present as a yellow-green cervical discharge. However, both gonococcal and chlamydial infections may produce *no* mucopurulent discharge. A finding of excessive white blood cells on the wet mount examination in the presence of no visible pathogens should alert the clinician to the possibility of a sexually transmitted disease.

Gonorrhea and Chlamydial Infection

Although 75% to 90% of women with gonorrhea are asymptomatic, aggressive diagnosis and treatment are important. Obstetric complications from gonorrheal infections include premature rupture of membranes, preterm delivery, and chorioamnionitis (infection of the uterine cavity with a fetus *in utero*). Specimens from women with other venereal diseases (trichomoniasis, bacterial vaginosis, and chlamydial infection) and from patients with mucopus or complaints of a vaginal discharge should be cultured. All partners of culture-positive women need to be identified and treated. Patients with known exposure to *N. gonorrhoeae* or *Chlamydia* should be offered antibiotic therapy. Pregnant women with sexually transmitted diseases are also at risk for acquiring HIV infection.

The emergency department evaluation may include a Gram stain of endocervical material for gram-negative diplococci, but culture is the only means by which definitive diagnosis can be made. Cervical cultures are positive in 80% of patients with gonorrhea. Simultaneous chlamydial cultures should be performed, because 20% to 50% of all patients with gonorrhea have concomitant chlamydial infection. Although culture on select media was the standard for detection of *N. gonorrhoeae* and *Chlamydia* in the past, amplification techniques with ligase chain reaction (LGR) or polymerase chain reaction (PCR) are more reliable, widely available, and, often, less costly. Rapid antigen detection methods have not proved to have high yields.

Treatment of gonorrhea in pregnancy consists of ceftriaxone (125 mg i.m. in a single dose), cefixime (400 mg PO in a single dose), or spectinomycin (2 g i.m. in a single dose) for those who cannot tolerate cephalosporin, and concomitant macrolide therapy for chlamydial infection (erythromycin [500 mg PO four times daily for 7 days] or azithromycin [1 g PO in a single dose]. Alternative therapy with amoxicillin (500 mg PO three times daily for 7 days) is acceptable if erythromycin cannot be tolerated. Tetracyclines and the quinolones are contraindicated in pregnancy because of possible adverse fetal effects. The effect of *Chlamydia* on obstetric outcome is less clear; with cervical chlamydial infection, the goal is to prevent neonatal transmission. This occurs in 60% of newborns born to infected mothers and is manifested as conjunctivitis (50%) or late neonatal pneumonia (10%). It is most important to eradicate chlamydial infections in patients who are close to delivery. If a patient far from term demonstrates a chlamydial infection, treatment may also be offered at this time.

Other Sexually Transmitted Diseases and Lower Genital Tract Infections

Other lower genital tract infections, such as lymphogranuloma venereum, granuloma inguinale, and chancroid, are rare in the United States.

Human Papillomavirus Infection

The incidence of human papillomavirus (HPV) infection, a lower genital tract infection, has risen dramatically in the past decade. HPV may be isolated by DNA identification in a number of tissues, including cervix, vagina, and vulva. It manifests itself most often as genital warts. Of the more than 60 serotypes, three are associated with cervical dysplasia and carcinoma (the so-called high oncogenic risk serotypes 16, 18, 33). There are no current recommendations to treat HPV infections in pregnancy. Cytotoxic agents such as podophyllin or 5-fluorouracil are contraindicated in pregnancy. Cesarean delivery is not indicated to prevent neonatal exposure to lower genital tract HPV. For patients with condylomata of sufficient size that vaginal delivery may be obstructed, referral should be made to an obstetrician who is capable of performing electrocautery, cryotherapy, or laser ablation of the lesions.

Syphilis

Syphilis in pregnancy is diagnosed either from a positive screening nontreponemal antibody test (Venereal Disease Research Laboratory [VDRL] test or rapid plasma reagin [RPR] test), followed by a positive fluorescent treponemal antibody absorption test (FTA-ABS), or when serologic tests are ordered because of clinical suspicion (painless lower genital tract lesions). The Centers for Disease Control and Prevention recommends penicillin G benzathine (2.4 million units i.m.). Subsequent treatment depends on the duration and stage at diagnosis. Pregnant patients allergic to penicillin should be desensitized before treatment. Transmission to the fetus is possible at any gestational age. Fetal complications include intrauterine death, preterm labor, and development of early congenital syphilis. Treatment should be initiated as early as possible, and all pregnant patients should have a screening test for syphilis.

Human Immunodeficiency Virus Infection

The majority of women infected with HIV are of reproductive age. The presence of other sexually transmitted diseases, particularly those characterized by genital ulcers or inflammation, increases the risk of HIV acquisition and transmission. Pregnant women with HIV are susceptible to the same spectrum of opportunistic infections as nonpregnant patients. Particular awareness for persistent HSV, PCP, central nervous system toxoplasmosis, esophageal candidiasis, and CMV retinitis with vision loss is paramount. The detection of acquired immunodeficiency syndrome (AIDS)–related neoplasms and infections may be obscured by the normal findings of pregnancy. HIV positivity does not appear to affect the course of pregnancy, nor does pregnancy appear to influence the early progression of HIV.[3] The 1994 report of the AIDS Clinical Trial Group protocol number 076 (ACTG-076) clearly demonstrates the safety and benefits of zidovudine use during pregnancy complicated by HIV infection, primarily a substantial reduction in the perinatal transmission of HIV.[4] The benefits of combination therapy with antiretroviral agents and viral protease inhibitors are well established in the nonpregnant population. Thus, multidrug regimens in pregnancy are also recommended.[3]

INFECTIONS RELATED TO PREGNANCY

Chorioamnionitis

All fevers in pregnancy need to be explained. It is crucial to exclude chorioamnionitis, an infection of the amniotic cavity with the fetus *in utero*. If the diagnosis is *not* made, complications occur, including premature rupture of membranes, preterm labor, maternal sepsis, fetal sepsis, and maternal or fetal death. The diagnosis is suggested by fever and uterine tenderness without contractions. Fetal tachycardia may also be present due to maternal fever. Leukocytosis is often present; and if the membranes are ruptured, the fluid may be foul smelling. If chorioamnionitis is suspected, an obstetrician should be consulted to admit the patient to the hospital for antibiotic therapy, amniocentesis, or delivery. Appropriate laboratory studies include complete blood cell count, urinalysis and urine culture, blood cultures, and cervical cultures for *N. gonorrhoeae* and *Chlamydia*.

Wound Infection

Various other infections may occur after vaginal or cesarean delivery. Wound infection after cesarean delivery may occur early (12 to 48 hours after delivery) or later (4 to 8 days after delivery). In either case, the presentation involves fever and wounds that appear infected. Early infections are more virulent. Cellulitis of the skin margins may be present and tender. Group A or group B streptococci or clostridia are seen in early infection. Infected wounds should be opened entirely, drained, and packed. Dressings should be changed during delayed healing. Patients with large wound infections should be admitted so they can receive antibiotics (ampicillin or cephalosporins) and wound care.

Late wound infections are also accompanied by fever and frequently drain infected material. They are most often caused by mixed organisms. Opening and packing the wound should suffice. The fascia should be examined to assess its integrity. Admission is indicated; patients with wounds that do not improve within 24 hours of debridement should receive broad-spectrum antibiotics.

Episiotomies may become superficially infected, or the fascia may become involved in more extensive infection. For superficial infection with local erythema and tenderness, the perineal incision should be opened to allow drainage and spontaneous healing. No attempt should be made to repair the infected wound. Sitz baths in warm water with or without salt are helpful for cleaning and symptomatic relief. If an abscess is suspected, the patient should be referred for incision and drainage.

Necrotizing fasciitis, a deep infection involving the fascia, is a serious process. Spread along fascial planes occurs quickly and results in sepsis and sometimes death. The key to diagnosis is the appearance of cool, necrotic skin, often with a serosanguineous exudate. If this condition is suspected, an obstetrician or surgeon should by notified and plans made for admission, antibiotic therapy, fluid and electrolyte support, and immediate debridement in the operating room.

Postpartum endometritis is associated with fever, uterine tenderness, and foul lochia. It may occur after vaginal or cesarean delivery. Urinary tract infection with suprapubic tenderness needs to be excluded. Complete blood cell count, urinalysis, and blood cultures may be helpful. An obstetrician should be consulted.

References

1. American College of Obstetricians and Gynecologists. *Immunization during pregnancy.* ACOG technical bulletin no. 160. Washington, DC: American College of Obstetricians and Gynecologists, 1990.
2. Andrews EB, Yankaskas BC, Cordero JF, et al. Acyclovir in pregnancy registry: six years' experience. *Obstet Gynecol* 1992;79:7.
3. Centers for Disease Control and Prevention. Public Health Service task force recommendations for the use of anteretroviral drugs in pregnant women infected with HIV-1 for maternal health and for reducing perinatal HIV-1 transmission in the United States. *MMWR* 1998;47(RR-2):1–30
4. Connor EM, Sperling RS, Gelber R, et al. Reduction of maternal-infant transmission of human immunodeficiency virus type I with Zidovudine treatment. Pediatric AIDS Clinical Trial Group Protocol 076 Study Group. *N Engl J Med* 1994;331(18):1173.
5. D'Alauro F, Lee RV, Pao-In K, et al. Intestinal parasites and pregnancy. *Obstet Gynecol* 1985;66:639.
6. Dascal A, Libman MD, Mendelson J, et al. Laboratory tests for the diagnosis of viral disease in pregnancy. *Clin Obstet Gynecol* 1990;33:218.
7. Davis D, Gash-Kim TZ, Heflernan EJ. Toxic shock syndrome: case report of a postpartum female and a literature review. *J Emerg Med* 1998;16(4):607–614.
8. Gibbs RS, Romero R, Hillier SL, et al. A review of premature birth and subclinical infection. *Am J Obstet Gynecol* 1992;166:1515.
9. Hamadeh MA, Glassroth J. Tuberculosis and pregnancy. *Chest* 1992;101:114.
10. Hunt CM, Carson KL, Sharara AI. Hepatitis C in pregnancy. *Obstet Gynecol* 1997;89(5 Pt 2):883–890.
11. Hunt CM, Sharara AI. Liver disease in pregnancy. *Am Fam Physician* 1999;59(4):829–836.
12. Levy R, Weissman A, Blomberg G, et al. Infection by parvovirus B19 during pregnancy: a review. *Obstet Gynecol Surv* 1997;52(4):254.
13. Lucas MJ, Cunningham FB. Urinary infection in pregnancy. *Clin Obstet Gynecol* 1993;36:821.
14. Miller KS, Miller JM Jr. Tuberculosis in pregnancy: interactions, diagnosis, and management. *Clin Obstet Gynecol* 1993;39(1):120–142.
15. Richey SD, Roberte SW, Ramin KD, et al. Pneumonia complicating pregnancy. *Obstet Gynecol* 1994;84:525.
16. Stamm WE, Hooton TM. Management of urinary tract infections in adults. *N Engl J Med* 1993;329:1328–1334.

17. Zanetti AR, Tanzi E, Romano L, et al. Multicenter trial on mother-to-infant transmission of GBV-C virus. The Lombardy Study Group on Vertical/Perinatal Hepatitis Viruses Transmission. *J Med Virol* 1998; 54(2):107–112.

Bibliography

American College of Obstetricians and Gynecologists. *Antimicrobial therapy for obstetric patients*. ACOG technical bulletin no. 245. Washington, DC: American College of Obstetricians and Gynecologists, 1998.

American College of Obstetricians and Gynecologists. *Perinatal viral and parasitic infections*. ACOG technical bulletin no. 177. Washington DC: American College of Obstetricians and Gynecologists, 1998.

American College of Obstetricians and Gynecologists. *Pulmonary disease in pregnancy*. ACOG technical bulletin no. 224. Washington, DC: American College of Obstetricians and Gynecologists, 1996.

American College of Obstetricians and Gynecologists. *Viral hepatitis in pregnancy*. ACOG technical bulletin no. 248. Washington, DC: American College of Obstetricians and Gynecologists, 1998.

Gilstrap LC III, Faro S, eds. *Infections in pregnancy*, 2nd ed. New York: Wiley-Liss, 1997.

Pastorek JG II. The ABCs of hepatitis in pregnancy. *Clin Obstet Gynecol* 1993;36:843

Sweet RL, Gibbs RS, eds. *Infectious diseases of the female genital tract*, 3rd ed. Baltimore: Lippincott Williams & Wilkins, 1995.

CHAPTER 77

Hypertensive Disorders of Pregnancy

Sean O. Henderson and Edward Newton

High blood pressure (BP) complicates 8% to 10% of all pregnancies, 20% of pregnancies in young nulliparas, and 40% to 50% of the pregnancies of women carrying twins.[17] Preeclampsia, a hypertensive disorder characterized by vasospasm and coagulation abnormalities, is a leading cause of fetal and maternal morbidity and death. Eclampsia occurs in approximately one of 2000 (0.05% to 0.2%) deliveries, and the incidence of it is higher in women who do not have appropriate prenatal care.[3,16]

Historically, maternal mortality from eclampsia, the most severe form of hypertension in pregnancy, ranges from 1% to 20% of all deliveries, although most current reports place mortality at approximately 5%.[21] In such severe forms of preeclampsia–eclampsia, intracerebral hemorrhage has been identified as the final event in over 50% of the patients who die. The mother is also at risk from the repeated seizure activity, which may lead to aspiration pneumonia, pulmonary edema, acute renal failure, or hypoxemia and acidemia.[21] Abruptio placentae and subsequent maternal disseminated intravascular coagulopathy (DIC) may also be present. Finally, cardiovascular collapse may occur from overaggressive treatment or massive intracerebral hemorrhage.

The effects on the fetus are similarly dramatic. Combined with the compromised uteroplacental perfusion caused by the characteristic vasospasm, the effects of multiple convulsions result in 10% to 28% fetal mortality.[3]

Causes of hypertension in pregnancy are multiple. The American College of Obstetrics and Gynecology in 1972 attempted to unify these entities by identifying four categories of hypertension associated with pregnancy:

1. Preeclampsia–eclampsia
2. Chronic hypertension
3. Preeclampsia superimposed on chronic hypertension
4. Transient hypertension

Hypertension in this definition is a level of 140/90 mm Hg or an increase of 30/15 mm Hg from baseline. In 1988, the World Health Organization (WHO) defined preeclampsia as BP exceeding 140/90 mm Hg after the twentieth week and proteinuria exceeding 0.3 g/24 h. The presence of edema is not a factor in the WHO definition.

PATHOPHYSIOLOGY

The pathophysiology of preeclampsia–eclampsia is unclear. Several theories have been proposed, most of which involve the uteroplacental circulation. Normal pregnancy is characterized by an increase in prostaglandin I2 (prostacyclin). In patients with preeclampsia–eclampsia, vasospasm peripherally may be stimulated by an increase in the vasoactive prostaglandin, thromboxane, with a simultaneous lower-than-normal production of prostacyclin.[17] The severe vasospasm that occurs exceeds the ability of the cerebral autoregulatory system, and seizure activity results.

Another suggested theory is based on the supposed presence of a single recessive or dominant gene with subsequent inadequate placentation.[9] The hypoxia and hypoperfusion that result disturb the functioning of the placental endothelial cells, with changes in circulating vasoactive substances and the sensitivity of the vascular bed to same.[9]

It does appear that both mother and fetus contribute to the risk of preeclampsia. When a woman becomes pregnant by a man who has been the father of a preeclamptic pregnancy in a different woman, the risk of preeclampsia is 1.8 times that of normal.[14]

CLINICAL PRESENTATION

Preeclampsia–Eclampsia

Preeclampsia is a condition of pregnancy that occurs most often after the twentieth week of gestation. In nulliparous patients it occurs most commonly near term. By definition, it is characterized by hypertension, proteinuria, generalized edema, and any of the following: hemoconcentration, hypoalbuminemia, hepatic dysfunction, coagulation abnormalities, and increased urate levels. Preeclampsia may progress rapidly to the convulsive phase of the disease, eclampsia.[17]

This life-threatening complication is usually preceded by warning signs and symptoms, such as headaches, epigastric pain, hyperreflexia, visual disturbances, and rising blood pressure (BP). Seizures may appear, however, without any warning signs or symptoms in a patient without previously recognized preeclampsia.[3] Factors predisposing to preeclampsia–eclampsia include nulliparity, diabetes mellitus, multiple gestations, extremes of age, hydatidiform mole, fetal hydrops, and genetic inheritance.[17] Preeclampsia regresses rapidly after delivery, and its signs and symptoms usually abate within 48 hours postpartum. The risk of eclampsia does continue postpartum, however, as 13% to 37% of cases have been reported in the postpartum period. The differential diagnosis of altered mental status in a postpartum patient should include eclampsia. Although there have been reported cases of postpartum seizures attributed to eclampsia up to 23 days postpartum, the vast majority occurs within the first 24 hours after delivery.

The HELLP syndrome, a variant of preeclampsia, is characterized by hemolytic anemia (H), elevated liver enzymes (EL), and low platelets/thrombocytopenia (LP), as well as by the classic hypertension, edema, and proteinuria.[3]

It is possible for patients to suffer from seizures even in the mild form of preeclampsia. A division of preeclampsia into mild and severe forms is useful for both disposition and prognosis. Severe preeclampsia exists when any of the following are present in a patient with a BP of 140/90 mm Hg and proteinuria greater than 0.3 g/24 h:

1. BP greater than or equal to 160/110 mm Hg on two occasions 6 hours apart with patient at rest
2. Proteinuria greater than 5 g/24 h
3. Urinary output less than or equal to 400 mL/24 h
4. Cerebral or visual disturbances
5. Epigastric or hepatic pain
6. Pulmonary edema or cyanosis
7. Platelet count lower than $100 \times 10^3/\mu L$.

Chronic Hypertension

BP greater than or equal to 140/90 in the period before pregnancy or before the twentieth week of gestation is considered chronic hypertension. Hypertension diagnosed for the first time during pregnancy and persisting beyond the forty-second postpartum day is also classified as chronic hypertension.[17] Differentiation of chronic hypertension from preeclampsia is important, as the latter necessitates inpatient management, while the former may be treated on an outpatient basis. Chronic hypertension typically occurs in the older, multiparous woman, often with a history of hypertension in a previous pregnancy. The presence of chronic hypertension increases the risk of developing superimposed preeclampsia, abruptio placenta, intrauterine death, and accelerated or malignant hypertension.

Preeclampsia Superimposed on Chronic Hypertension

Any existing hypertensive disease predisposes the gravid woman to the development of preeclampsia–eclampsia. Rather than being defined by a specific value, this diagnosis is usually made if the BP increases by 30 mm Hg (systolic) or 15 mm Hg (diastolic) in the presence of proteinuria or generalized edema.

Transient Hypertension

Transient hypertension is defined as the development of hypertension during pregnancy or within the first 24 postpartum hours without other signs of preeclampsia or preexisting hypertension. The BP usually returns to normal within 10 days after delivery, but elevated BP has a high rate of recurrence in later pregnancies. It may also be predictive of eventual hypertension.[17]

DIFFERENTIAL DIAGNOSIS

The diagnostic dilemma in a gravid patient with hypertension revolves primarily around distinguishing between chronic hypertension, transient hypertension, and preeclampsia. Transient hypertension is characterized by the presence of increased systolic or diastolic pressures in the absence of any other of the classic signs of preeclampsia (i.e., generalized edema or proteinuria). The patient with chronic hypertension will have a history of hypertension that antedates the twentieth week of pregnancy. Causes of hypertension in this group of patients are similar to those in the nongravid patient population.

Although eclampsia may exist simultaneously with chronic hypertension, seizures prior to the twentieth week of gestation or after 48 hours postpartum are generally not considered attributable to eclampsia and should be worked up and treated as in the general population. Some causes to consider include idiopathic epilepsy, trauma, systemic lupus erythematosus, chronic alcohol use, dialysis, electrolyte or metabolic disturbances, ischemic encephalopathy, drug withdrawal, infection, toxin exposure, primary brain or metastatic tumor,[7] stroke, intracranial hemorrhage, psychogenic (pseudoseizure), or status postepidural anesthesia.[3,8]

EMERGENCY DEPARTMENT EVALUATION

Preeclampsia–eclampsia should be suspected in the presence of headache, blurred vision, scotomata, epigastric pain, diastolic BP greater than 100 mm Hg, increasing serum creatinine, consumptive coagulopathy, or abnormal transaminases.

Postpartum eclampsia may occur in up to 30% of patients with preeclampsia, usually within the first 12 to 24 hours and rarely beyond the forty-eighth hour. Anecdotal reports of seizures occurring 3 to 23 days postpartum have been attributed to eclampsia, but they are controversial.[8] Patients with late postpartum eclampsia frequently present with complaint of headache, visual disturbances of several days' duration, or epigastric discomfort followed by convulsions. Hypertension is present, as are the characteristic proteinuria and edema.

Computerized tomography of eclamptic encephalopathy shows low attenuation areas in the cortex, with consistent involvement of the posterior areas and occasionally the basal ganglia. In more severe cases, intracerebral hemorrhage may be present.[8,15]

Laboratory testing should include an evaluation of electrolytes, including sodium and bicarbonate, as well as liver function tests, to rule out the presence of the HELLP syndrome. A complete blood count with platelets and DIC screen may be indicated. The urine should be screened for protein; an electrocardiogram and a chest radiograph are indicated to search for hypertensive complications, such as ischemia or congestive heart failure. The fetus should be monitored continuously for signs of distress.

EMERGENCY DEPARTMENT MANAGEMENT

Chronic Hypertension and Transient Hypertension

In the vast majority of cases (90%), mild-to-moderate (preexisting) essential hypertension is associated with good outcome for both mother and child.[4] Conditions that may prompt pharmacologic management include advanced maternal age (over 40 years of age), evidence of end organ damage, intrauterine growth retardation, history of previous perinatal death, or hypertension of greater than 15 years' duration. The presence of any one of these factors should prompt consideration of pharmacologic intervention, regardless of the BP.

Treatment of the hypertensive disorders of pregnancy varies according to the BP and the presence of other signs and symptoms of preeclampsia–eclampsia. The only definitive care for preeclampsia–eclampsia is delivery of the fetus. Pharmacologic therapy serves as a temporizing measure only.

For the emergency physician who is not an expert in the treatment of preeclampsia–eclampsia, hydralazine is the first-line drug of choice for BP control (where the diastolic BP is less than 110 mm Hg). Magnesium sulfate is the drug of choice for the control of seizures.[16] The final step in the treatment of preeclampsia–eclampsia involves termination of the pregnancy with the least harm to the infant and mother. In cases in which there is evidence of advanced disease or of impending eclampsia, delivery is indicated, regardless of the age of the fetus. In these cases, evacuation of the uterus is the only measure that will halt the advance of the disease.[17] Delivery should also occur if there is evidence of fetal distress.

For milder cases of the disease, or in cases in which it is unclear whether preeclampsia is present, temporizing measures, such as bedrest or prophylactic $MgSO_4$ therapy, may be indicated.

While the course of preeclampsia is usually gradual, 16% of cases of eclampsia occur without warning. It is advisable that all eclamptic patients (especially those with less than 36 weeks' gestation) be managed at a tertiary care center with the capability of managing high-risk obstetric and neonatal cases.[12]

Initial Treatment for Eclampsia

- Maintain oxygen delivery to both mother and fetus.
- Minimize the aspiration risk by placing the mother in the left lateral decubitus position.
- Invasive hemodynamic monitoring is indicated only for patients with complications such as pulmonary edema or continued oliguria.[17]
- In most cases, volume replacement therapy is not indicated except as needed to maintain urine output of 1 to 2 cc/kg/h. Because of the capillary leaks that accompany preeclampsia, aggressive fluid therapy may actually precipitate pulmonary or cerebral edema.[4]
- Monitor urine output using a Foley catheter.
- Treat the seizure with one of the following established protocols.

Seizure Therapy

Magnesium Sulfate. Magnesium sulfate is the drug of choice for eclampsia in the United States.[20] Several regimens have been proposed, the most common being Pritchard's (intramuscular) and Zuspan's (intravenous).[19] A comparison of these protocols favors the use of Pritchard's protocol in an effort to raise and maintain maternal magnesium levels sufficiently high to be of benefit.[10] The goal of therapy is to raise the maternal magnesium plasma level to 5 to 8 mg/dL. A commonly used loading dose of 4 g will achieve such a therapeutic maternal plasma level; the effect, however, is transient, and the level will fall within 60 minutes. Thus, a more recent recommendation is a loading dose of 6 g initially, followed by 2 to 3 g intravenously (i.v.) per hour.[17] The specific regimens are detailed in Table 77.1.

Continue the magnesium sulfate administration until 24 hours after delivery. Signs of improvement will include a decrease in BP, improvement in sensorium, and an increase in urine output. Magnesium is excreted by the kidney, so in those cases in which urinary output is decreased or in the presence of renal failure, magnesium doses should be adjusted to avoid toxicity. When magnesium toxicity is suspected (Table 77.2), calcium gluconate 1 g may be administered slowly. The effect of the calcium is transient; therefore, continuous monitoring of the patient is warranted. Although there may be an initial decrease in BP for the first 30 to 45 minutes after the initiation of $MgSO_4$ therapy, the drug itself is not an antihypertensive agent. As such, one of the medications detailed below should be added to the treatment regimen to control the BP and minimize further end organ damage.

Postdelivery, fetal magnesium may have equilibrated with the mother's, causing hypotonia, respiratory depression, or hypotension. Calcium gluconate may be administered to the infant in those cases.[21]

TABLE 77.1. Drug Therapy for Eclampsia

Magnesium Sulfate Dosing Regimen	
PRITCHARD (INTRAMUSCULAR)	
Loading dose:	4 g i.v. over 3–5 min plus 10 g i.m.
Maintenance dose:	5 g i.m. every 4 h
ZUSPAN	
Loading dose:	4 g i.v. over 5–10 min
Maintenance dose:	1–2 g i.v. every hour

TABLE 77.2. Effects of Magnesium Sulfate on the Mother

Serum Level (mg/dL)	Clinical Effects
1.5–2.5	Normal
4–8	Therapeutic for seizure prophylaxis
8–12	Loss of patellar reflexes, double vision, flushing, somnolence, slurred speech
15–17	Muscle paralysis
30–35	Cardiac arrest

Dilantin. Phenytoin has historically been the drug of choice in Europe for the control of eclamptic seizures. It provides prolonged seizure protection and has an antihypoxic effect.[11] Recently, however, phenytoin does not appear to be as effective in controlling eclamptic seizures as magnesium sulfate. When compared with $MgSO_4$, phenytoin has no effect on labor outcome.[13]

In cases in which status epilepticus due to eclampsia occurs, intubation and muscular paralysis are indicated. Other options include the administration of a short-acting barbiturate such as sodium amobarbital (250 mg) or a benzodiazepine.

Antihypertensive Therapy

The goal of antihypertensive therapy is to reduce BP without adverse effects on the fetus. Acute antihypertensive treatment is indicated when the diastolic BP is greater than 105 mm Hg; the goal is to reduce it to 90 to 100 mm Hg. Placental hypoperfusion must be avoided.[17] Targets for BP control include a systolic BP of 140 to 150 mm Hg and a diastolic pressure between 90 and 100 mm Hg. Specific medications to be used in the treatment of this disorder include the following.

Hydralazine. Hydralazine is a vasodilator and the most commonly used agent. It is recommended as the first-line agent. Although it may be used as continuous intravenous medication, intermittent bolus injections appear to be more sensible. The initial bolus is 5 mg over 1 to 2 minutes, with repeated doses of 5 to 10 mg every 20 to 30 minutes as indicated by initial response. Once the desired effect is obtained, additional doses are repeated as necessary.

If a total dose of 20 mg is administered without therapeutic response, other hypertensive agents should be considered. Side effects of hydralazine include hypotension (reported more often in preeclamptics than in gravidas with chronic hypertension), headache, tremulousness, nausea, vomiting, and tachycardia. Neonatal thrombocytopenia has also been reported.

Diazoxide. A potent arteriolar vasodilator, diazoxide is recommended for the occasional patient who is refractory to hydralazine. The use of 30 mg "miniboluses" is recommended; they may be administered every 5 minutes as needed. Diazoxide may cause arrest of labor, which can be overcome by oxytocin. Other effects include maternal and neonatal hyperglycemia due to suppression of insulin release and displacement of highly protein bound drugs (like Dilantin), resulting in increased toxicity.

Labetalol. Labetalol is both an alpha and beta blocker and appears to have a faster onset of action and an absence of reflex tachycardia when compared with hydralazine. Follow the initial dose of 10 mg i.v. with a doubled dose every 10 minutes until the desired BP is achieved or until 300 mg is injected. Continuous infusion may be started at 1 to 2 mg/min (no more than 1 mg/kg) to control BP and run at 0.5 mg/min for maintenance.

Nifedipine. The oral calcium channel blocker nifedipine is no longer recommended for the emergency control of hypertension. It has potent uterine muscle relaxant properties that can increase the risk of uterine atony and postpartum hemorrhage.

Nitroprusside. A potent vasodilator, nitroprusside is reserved for patients who are unresponsive to more conventional therapy. Nitroprusside has a rapid onset of action and is reversible with discontinuation of therapy. The drug is metabolized to cyanide and thiocyanate, which may cross the placenta. Low doses of nitroprusside have not been associated with clinically evident fetal toxicity.

Captopril. The angiotensin converting enzyme inhibitor captopril is reserved for postpartum use, as it has been demonstrated to have adverse effects on the renal perfusion of the fetus.

Nimodipine. An intravenous calcium channel blocker, nimodipine has been suggested as both an antihypertensive and an antiseizure medication in the setting of eclampsia.[1] It causes a decreased vascular resistance, and, therefore, a decreased mean arterial pressure, without affecting peripheral oxygen delivery. Initial reported studies on the use of nimodipine as single-agent therapy for eclampsia are promising but small.

Diuretics. Overall, diuretics are not used as first-line therapy. They cause little harm to the fetus. Most patients experiencing the sequelae of preeclampsia–eclampsia, however, are hemoconcentrated and not in need of further volume contraction. Because the uteroplacental circulation may already be compromised, diuretics should be reserved for those patients with documented congestive heart failure or fluid overload.[17]

Prevention

A number of randomized trials have demonstrated the benefit of low-dose aspirin therapy in reducing the incidence of gestational hypertension in pregnant women at risk for this condition.[18] Although more recent trials in larger patient populations show less of a protective effect, the benefit in a high-risk group of patients (previous preeclampsia, chronic hypertension, multiple gestation, and diabetes mellitus) appears to outweigh the small increase in bleeding complications and abruptio placentae associated with salicylate use.[4,5]

Magnesium sulfate is well established as prophylaxis for eclampsia.[6,19] Concerns over the delay of spontaneous or induced labor have not been validated.[13] In patients who are preeclamptic and receiving $MgSO_4$, the incidence of eclampsia falls from 1.2% to 0.3%.

Another suggested prophylactic measure is the use of calcium supplementation during pregnancy. Although the mechanism of action is unclear, the rates of hypertensive disorders among nulliparous women receiving such supplementation (e.g., 2 g daily) during pregnancy were shown to be lower than in the control group.[2]

DISPOSITION

Hypertension (Chronic and Transient)

Nonmedical management should be considered for individuals not at high risk for preeclampsia–eclampsia. In certain cases—in which the patient has a history of hypertension preceding the pregnancy, and the systolic BP is 140 mmHg or the diastolic BP is 90 to 99 mmHg in the appropriate clinical setting (after 20 weeks' gestation)—patients may serve a short stay in the hospital to rule out preeclampsia and be discharged home with close follow-up.

Role of the Consultant

Because the definitive therapy for eclampsia is delivery of the fetus, an obstetrician should be consulted as soon as the diagnosis is entertained. In cases in which preeclampsia is suspected or newly diagnosed, the need for admission should be determined after discussion with the obstetrician. Discharge should occur only if close follow-up is feasible.

Indications for Admission

Patients with severe preeclampsia and eclampsia must be admitted to monitored settings after appropriate consultation with the obstetrician. Some cases of early preeclampsia and hypertension in pregnancy may be managed on an outpatient basis if follow-up is available and the patient is compliant. Such decisions should follow appropriate emergency department interventions, including discussion with the obstetrician.

Transfer

Except in those cases in which a higher level of care is needed, patients experiencing symptomatic preeclampsia or those with eclamptic seizures are not candidates for transfer. The dynamic nature of the disease, the need for continuous monitoring during therapy, and the high fetal and maternal mortality make this disease inappropriate for interfacility transfer.

COMMON PITFALLS

- Making the diagnosis of preeclampsia may be difficult for the emergency physician, because the three classic clinical signs—hypertension, proteinuria, and edema—may not occur simultaneously, may be present as part of another disease process, or may be present as part of a normal pregnancy.[17]
- The emergency physician must be aware of and monitor the patient's serum magnesium levels during treatment for eclampsia to prevent overtreatment as well as undertreatment.
- When BP is measured by different observers at different times, the values may vary. Characteristically, the BPs reflect the altering vasospasticity and cardiovascular reactivity of the patient. Higher pressures should not be disregarded in the face of subsequent lower observed pressures.[23]

- Seizure activity in the third trimester of pregnancy or immediately after delivery that is not responsive to magnesium sulfate mandates immediate computed tomography scan and lumbar puncture to exclude other etiologies of seizures.[22]

References

1. Anthony J, Mantel G, Johanson R, et al. The haemodynamic and respiratory effects of intravenous nimodipine used in the treatment of eclampsia. *Br J Obstet Gynaecol* 1996;103:518.
2. Belizam JM, Villar J, Gonzalez L, et al. Calcium supplementation to prevent hypertensive disorders of pregnancy. *N Engl J Med* 1991:325:1399.
3. Brady WJ, Dehnke DJ, Carter CT. Postpartum toxemia: hypertension, edema, proteinuria and unresponsiveness in an unknown female. *J Emerg Med* 1995;13:643.
4. Burrows R, et al. Report of the Canadian Hypertension Society Consensus Conference-2. Nonpharmacologic management and prevention of hypertension disorders in pregnancy. *Can Med Assoc J* 1997;157:907.
5. CLASP. CLASP: a randomized trial of low-dose aspirin for the prevention and treatment of preeclampsia among 9364 pregnant women. *Lancet* 1994;343:619.
6. Coetzee EJ, Dommisse J, Anthony J. A randomized controlled trial of intravenous magnesium sulfate versus placebo in the management of women with severe preeclampsia. *Br J Obstet Gynaecol* 1998;105:300.
7. Delanty N, Vaughn CJ, French JA. Medical causes of seizures. *Lancet* 1998;352:383.
8. Druelinger L. Postpartum emergencies. *Emerg Med Clin North Am* 1994;12:219.
9. Erkkola R. Can preeclampsia be predicted and prevented? *Acta Obstet Gynecol Scand* 1997;76:598.
10. Graham KM. Magnesium sulfate in eclampsia. *Lancet* 1998;351:1061.
11. Gulmezoglu AM, Duley L. Use of anticonvulsants in eclampsia and preeclampsia: survey of obstetricians in the United Kingdom and Republic of Ireland. *BMJ* 1998;316:975.
12. Jagoda A, Riggis S. Emergency department approach to managing seizures in pregnancy. *Ann Emerg Med* 1991;20:80.
13. Leveno KJ, Alexander JM, McIntire DD, et al. Does magnesium sulfate given for prevention of eclampsia affect the outcome of labor? *Am J Obstet Gynecol* 1998;178:707.
14. Lie RT, Rasmussen S, Brunborg H, et al. Fetal and maternal contributions to risk of preeclampsia: population based study. *BMJ* 1998;316:1343.
15. Manfredi M, Beltramello A, Bongiovanni LG, et al. Eclamptic encephalopathy: imaging and pathogenetic considerations. *Acta Neurol Scand* 1997;96:277.
16. Murphy C. Hypertensive emergencies. *Emerg Med Clin North Am* 1995;13:973.
17. Probst BD. Hypertensive disorders of pregnancy. *Emerg Med Clin North Am* 1994;12:73.
18. Sibai BM, Cartis SN, Thom E, et al. Prevention of preeclampsia with low dose aspirin in healthy, nulliparous pregnant women. *N Engl J Med* 1993;329:1213.
19. Sibai BM, Graham JM, McCubbin JH. A comparison of intravenous and intramuscular magnesium sulfate regimens in preeclampsia. *Am J Obstet Gynecol* 1984;150:728.
20. The Eclampsia Trial Collaborative Group. Which anticonvulsant for women with eclampsia? Evidence from the Collaborative Eclampsia Trial. *Lancet* 1995;345:1455.
21. Usta IM, Sibai BM. Emergent management of puerperal eclampsia. *Obstet Gynecol Clin North Am* 1995;22:315.
22. Witlin AG, Friedman SA, Egerman RS, et al. Cerebrovascular disorders complicating pregnancy—beyond eclampsia. *Am J Obstet Gynecol* 1997;176:1139.
23. Zuspan FP. Problems encountered in the treatment of pregnancy-induced hypertension. *Am J Obstet Gynecol* 1978;131:591.

CHAPTER 78
Emergencies of Late Pregnancy

Moss H. Mendelson

Although women in the second half of pregnancy (greater than 20 weeks' gestation) commonly have their own physician, some emergent problems require intervention and stabilization by the emergency physician and rapid consultation with an obstetrician. Because a potentially viable second "patient" exists after 23 to 24 weeks, the approach must consider alterations in physiology, differential diagnosis, medications and doses, as well as the potential need to rescue the fetus to prevent its demise. The most common problems of late pregnancy encountered in the emergency department (ED) are vaginal bleeding, shortness of breath, and coma or seizure.

VAGINAL HEMORRHAGE IN LATE PREGNANCY

Vaginal bleeding after 20 weeks of gestation is not uncommon, occurring in about 4% of pregnancies.[10] It can, however, be frightening to the patient as well as the physician. Definitive treatment, if required, should be performed by an obstetrician. The emergency physician must stabilize the patient hemodynamically and should be aware of the differential diagnosis, the studies necessary to define the problem, as well as the indications for transfer if limited facilities exist for management of the premature or distressed newborn.

Abruptio placentae, separation of part of the placenta from the uterine wall, accounts for about 30% of bleeding in the second half of pregnancy. Risk factors include hypertension, increased maternal age, and a history of smoking. In addition, abdominal trauma with transmission of forces to the uterus may cause shearing of the placenta from its attachments. Cocaine use has also been implicated as a cause of placental abruption.[3] *Placenta previa*, which accounts for about 20% of third-trimester bleeding, is a placenta that overlaps the cervix to varying degrees. Placenta previa is more common with a uterus scarred from previous cesarean section and with advanced maternal age. Of placentas that overlie the cervix at 20 weeks' gestation (up to 20% of pregnancies), less than 10% of these remain so at delivery.[7] The other 50% of patients who experience late bleeding often have no definite cause identified. It is believed that most episodes of bleeding represent small marginal separations of the placenta, but this cannot usually be proven. Other causes include vaginal or cervical trauma, lower genital tract infections, polyps, or hemorrhoids.

The pregnant patient undergoes several changes in cardiovascular physiology that are crucial to remember. Maternal blood volume expands by about 1.5 L during a normal pregnancy, resulting in a dilutional anemia that is physiologic (hematocrit 32% to 34%). Pregnant patients also manifest a baseline increase in heart rate (90 to 100 beats per minute) and stroke volume, resulting in a cardiac output 30% to 40% higher at term than seen in the nonpregnant state. Systematic vascular resistance is decreased, however, and the net hemodynamic result of these changes is a blood pressure lower than the nonpregnant state. Finally, the uteroplacental bed does not have any autoregulatory function; placental blood flow is determined strictly by maternal blood pressure and cardiac output. Because of the expanded intravascular volume, signs of extensive blood loss can occur late, and significant fetal hypoperfusion may exist before maternal signs of shock are apparent. Pregnancy is also associated with a rise in concentration of many clotting factors (especially fibrinogen), resulting in an hypercoagulable state.

CLINICAL PRESENTATION AND DIFFERENTIAL DIAGNOSIS

The patient with bleeding after 20 weeks' gestation may present with a spectrum from painless spotting or bloody mucoid discharge to dark or exsanguinating bleeding and severe uterine pain. Placenta previa is most often seen as bright red, painless vaginal spotting. The bleeding is rarely severe (except during labor or after pelvic examination with probing of the cervical os). The patient may be aware of an abnormal placental location. The patient with abruptio placentae more often has dark, variable bleeding, accompanied by uterine tenderness and irritability, manifested by intermittent or steady cramping. Bleeding between the placenta and uterine wall may result in significant occult blood loss, with maternal tachycardia or even hypotension, but without evidence of significant external bleeding. Fetal distress (heart rate out of the normal range of 120 to 160 beats per minute) may also occur if a significant degree of separation has occurred. Abruptio placentae may also trigger maternal coagulation, resulting in evidence of consumptive coagulopathy, with bleeding from needlesticks, urine, and other sites.

EMERGENCY DEPARTMENT EVALUATION

The patient with vaginal bleeding should first be assessed hemodynamically. With significant maternal blood loss, fluid resuscitation is begun. Blood should be sent for complete blood cell count, prothrombin time, partial thromboplastin time, and fibrinogen levels. The patient's blood should be typed and crossmatched, and fresh-frozen plasma or fresh whole blood may be needed. The mother's Rh type should be determined and a Kleihauer-Betke test sent to determine whether significant fetomaternal transfusion has occurred.[1] The fetus should be evaluated for signs of distress: bradycardia less than 120 beats per minute, tachycardia more than 160 beats per minute, decelerations after uterine irritability, or loss of beat-to-beat variability during continuous fetal monitoring.

History should include known obstetric problems or ultrasonographic diagnoses. Other historical information includes amount of bleeding, passage of clots, character of blood (bright red or dark, older blood), presence of uterine cramping or pain, prior cervical or vaginal lesions or infection, drug use, and history or evidence of abdominal trauma (including domestic violence). The abdominal examination should confirm uterine size as well as the presence of contractions or tenderness to palpation. Vaginal examination *should not be performed* in the ED if adequate obstetric backup is available, and should be preceded by ultrasonography whenever possible to diagnose or exclude placenta previa.

Ultrasonography remains the diagnostic modality of choice for late-pregnancy bleeding.[12] The major purpose of ultrasonography is to locate the placenta and its relationship to the cervix. Additionally, information regarding gestational age and general fetal well-being may be obtained. Transabdominal ultrasound (TAS) is usually performed first, but is noted to have a false positive rate of 2% to 6% for placenta previa. False positives can be caused by obesity, a posterior placenta, a full bladder, or a focal myometrial contraction. Endovaginal sonography (EVS) eliminates many of these false positives and has been proven safe in many studies. While TAS is easily performed in the ED, the role of EVS in the ED assessment of vaginal bleeding in late pregnancy is less well defined.[11]

On the other hand, the ultrasonography findings in abruption are variable and are affected by the type of abruption (retroplacental, subchorionic) and the timing of the study in relationship to the onset of bleeding. Retroplacental bleeding may have a sonographic appearance very similar to that of a normal placenta, creating an area of thickened placenta or an area mistaken for a fibroid or contraction. Marginal bleeding may be recognized sonographically as a hematoma, though the amount of apparent blood collection seen may significantly underestimate true losses. Evidence of abruption by ultrasound is helpful to the obstetrician in developing a care plan for the patient, and can be followed with serial examinations. A negative study does not eliminate abruption from the differential, and, in fact, a patient with late pregnancy bleeding and an ultrasound negative for placenta previa is often assumed to have abruption. With abruption, fetal monitoring becomes the primary tool for management decisions.[11]

A vaginal examination is ideally performed after ultrasonography in an operating suite capable of converting to an emergent surgical delivery with fetal resuscitation in the event that severe bleeding is triggered. If immediate obstetric consultation is not available, patients with significant bleeding should be prepared for transport to a facility that is able to provide a wide range of resuscitative services. If the bleeding is not severe, a cautious vaginal examination in the ED is rational, preferably after placenta previa has been excluded with ultrasonography. The purpose of the examination is to exclude hemorrhoidal bleeding or vaginal or cervical lesions that cause bleeding. Neither fingers nor instruments should be placed in the cervical os, because uncontrolled bleeding from a placenta previa can be triggered by such manipulation.

EMERGENCY DEPARTMENT MANAGEMENT AND DISPOSITION

Prehospital triage of the woman with bleeding after 24 weeks' gestation (a uterus above the umbilicus provides a rough measure) should be to a facility that can manage a potentially high-risk or premature delivery. Management consists of assessment of the amount of bleeding from evidence at the scene and degree of bleeding at the perineum (if a private evaluation of this can be made), administration of maternal supplemental oxygen, positioning of the patient on her left side, and intravenous administration of fluids en route.

The ED should ideally be a place of cardiovascular stabilization and triage only. If the mother has hemodynamic compromise secondary to hemorrhage, fluid resuscitation should be initiated rapidly with crystalloid. Appropriate bloodwork is initiated, including coagulation tests, as noted earlier. In the mother with rapid exsanguination, O-negative blood transfusion may be required. Fresh whole blood or packed cells with fresh-frozen plasma may be needed if abruptio placentae is suspected, because this can cause consumption of clotting factors. Fetal heart rate should be quickly measured, with initiation of continuous monitoring if possible. Rapid transport to the obstetric suite is the goal.

In the patient with less emergent bleeding, referral to the obstetric unit is preferred for definitive diagnosis. The standard method of evaluation is ultrasonography followed by vaginal examination in a delivery suite, where the discovery of a fetus-threatening placenta previa can be treated with rapid delivery. In the patient with a presumed or visible abruptio placentae, admission to a high-risk prepartum unit for continuous monitoring after labor deck diagnosis is appropriate. A cautious vaginal examination in the ED may be appropriate, particularly in a hospital where transfer will be needed if no simple bleeding source is found. Continued fetal well-being should always be documented if the patient spends any significant time in the ED, because hypovolemia is frequently detected by signs of fetal distress before maternal vital sign changes. If the mother is Rh-negative (with an unknown or Rh-positive father) or if a positive Kleihauer-Betke test is positive for fetomaternal hemorrhage, RhoGAM should be administered in a dose determined by the number of milliliters of fetal cells calculated to be in the maternal circulation (300 μg/15 mL fetal red blood cells).[14]

Interfacility transfer to a high-risk unit should be accomplished after initial diagnosis or assessment by an obstetrician and is usually performed by specialized obstetric or high-risk neonatal transport units. In general, predelivery transport is safest and is associated with the best outcome, but it must be accomplished in a controlled fashion, with personnel capable of supporting the mother and managing fetal distress or a premature delivery en route.

COMMON PITFALLS

- Vaginal examinations should be limited to visual inspection of the perineum and vaginal vault to look for obvious noncervical bleeding sources. Fingers or instruments should *never* be placed in or near the cervix, because uncontrolled bleeding from a placenta previa can result.
- Coagulopathy should be considered in patients with severe hemorrhage, because clotting factors are consumed when significant bleeding occurs with abruptio placentae, and coagulopathy can seriously compromise the mother's ability to limit uterine bleeding.

SHORTNESS OF BREATH IN LATE PREGNANCY

Breathlessness is a common symptom in pregnancy. A respiratory alkalosis is common, with normal P_{CO_2} levels in pregnancy of 27 to 32 mm Hg. "Dyspnea," the sensation of increased breathing effort, is likewise common, particularly in the first two trimesters. It usually improves after about 28 weeks and is thought to be related in some women to progesterone-induced stimulation of the respiratory center. The alveolar–arterial P_{CO_2} gradient increases to a mean of about 14 mm Hg near term in the sitting position and may be as high as 20 mm Hg in the supine position. Arteriolar–alveolar gradients greater than 20 mm Hg are clearly abnormal, but those between 10 and 20 mm Hg are difficult to interpret.[13]

Respiratory physiology in pregnancy shows important changes in response to the stress of illness or injury. Oxygen consumption normally increases by 25%, and residual volume is impaired, particularly in late pregnancy, resulting in poor reserve when a pulmonary insult occurs. The fetus is more sensitive than the mother to a hypoxic insult, because fetal hemoglobin is "left shifted." Tachypnea causes an alkalosis that leads to constriction of the uteroplacental vascular bed and decreased fetal blood flow.[13]

CLINICAL PRESENTATION AND DIFFERENTIAL DIAGNOSIS

Respiratory distress presents in pregnancy much as it does in the nonpregnant patient. Predominant signs include increased rate or depth of breathing, use of accessory muscles or other evidence of increased work of breathing, and cyanosis if oxygenation is significantly impaired. Increased respiratory effort may be combined with other clinical evidence of infection in the patient with sepsis or another infectious cause. Wheezing may be caused by asthma, but amniotic fluid embolus, pulmonary embolus (PE), or simple pneumonia must also be considered.

Differentiating normal pulmonary changes of pregnancy from respiratory distress caused by illnesses requiring treatment may be difficult. PE occurs with increased frequency in pregnancy due to the hypercoagulability and stasis induced by pregnancy, as well as the vessel trauma that occurs at delivery. Amniotic fluid embolus is a rare but frequently fatal cause of respiratory distress and cardiovascular collapse due to amniotic fluid (with antigenic foreign debris) entering the maternal circulation and being filtered in the pulmonary vascular bed. Other potential causes of respiratory distress include asthma,[6] respiratory insufficiency from systemic infection or sepsis, pneumonia, or other nonpregnant etiologies.

EMERGENCY DEPARTMENT EVALUATION

Assessment of the pregnant patient with respiratory distress is similar to that of nonpregnant patients. A pertinent history includes prior respiratory risk factors such as asthma, smoking, or hypercoagulability independent of pregnancy itself. Proximate symptoms should be sought, such as fever, sputum production, and the nature and location of associated chest pain. Physical examination focuses on the lungs and clues to bronchospasm, local or diffuse consolidation, or fluid overload. Vital signs include an accurate respiratory rate, temperature, and pulse oximetry as an initial screen. In any patient with increased work of breathing, arterial blood gases (ABGs) are necessary to accurately assess oxygenation (P_{O_2}) and ventilation (P_{CO_2}). Chest radiography is safe and usually necessary in the pregnant patient with respiratory symptoms of significance. X-ray beams with a margin greater than 10 cm from the fetus give a negligible radiation exposure, and shielding can be done in late pregnancy to minimize exposure and reassure the patient.

PE remains a significant cause of maternal morbidity and mortality in pregnancy. The period of highest risk for thromboembolism remains unsettled in the literature. Recent studies suggest that most deep venous thromboses associated with pregnancy occur in the antepartum period, though two-thirds of PEs are noted in the postpartum period. Increased venous stasis, in combination with increases in coagulation factor levels, and interactions are the most important risk factors. Other factors, such as prolonged bedrest, prior thrombotic disease, and intercurrent illness, also contribute. The clinical presentation can be confusing, as many normal, near-term patients give a history of dyspnea and leg discomfort and have tachypnea and lower extremity swelling on examination. Because of the immediate morbidity and mortality associated with PE and the longer term implications of having the disease (prolonged heparin therapy, prophylaxis during subsequent pregnancies, future use of contraceptives), the emergency physician treating pregnant patients with significant respiratory complaints should be aggressive in pursuing the diagnosis.

The workup for PE in pregnancy proceeds in a stepwise fashion, and does not deviate much from the workup in nonpregnant patients. Chest radiography is indicated, and ABGs are usually assessed, though results of the latter can be difficult to interpret, as outlined earlier. Ventilation–perfusion (V/Q) scanning is often the initial study of choice, followed by angiography if the V/Q scan neither confirms nor rules out PE. The total amount of radiation exposure during workup for PE is small if shielding is used and should never be a barrier to making a diagnosis. A patient undergoing chest x-ray, V/Q scanning, and angiography (brachial approach) has an average fetal exposure of 0.5 rad, a level not considered to pose any fetal risk.[4,8] Some authors favor lower extremity studies (ultrasonography or impedance plethysmography) prior to angiography in patients with low- or intermediate-probability V/Q scan results. A positive noninvasive study ends the workup, and the patient is treated for PE. However, a normal lower extremity study is inconclusive and requires subsequent angiography. About half of patients with equivocal V/Q scan results and negative lower extremity studies have angiographically proven PE.

EMERGENCY DEPARTMENT MANAGEMENT AND DISPOSITION

The pregnant patient with respiratory distress requires pulse oximetry, supplemental oxygen, adequate fluids, and positioning on her left side to maximize uterine perfusion. This can be initiated in the prehospital phase, although little else can or should be done (as with other patients with respiratory distress) until a definitive diagnosis is made. Respiratory support and control of ventilation should be prompt if it is indicated, because the fetus is disproportionately affected by respiratory acidosis or hypoxia. Conservative and prompt therapy for hypoxia and increased work of breathing is recommended, because pregnancy impairs normal maternal compensatory mechanisms and reserve. The threshold for admission or intubation of pregnant patients with respiratory distress is *much lower* than in nonpregnancy.

Treatment of asthma in pregnancy is similar to that in nonpregnancy (see Chapter 75). Inhaled β-agonists are the mainstay of acute therapy. Epinephrine can be used if these fail, but it has the theoretic disadvantage of α-stimulation (which causes uterine contraction). Both inhaled prophylactic corticosteroids and oral prednisone are safe, and their use should be encouraged.

Treatment of PE is problematic because warfarin is contraindicated in pregnancy. In the ED, intravenous heparin should be started when the diagnosis of PE is made, with an intravenous load of 70 to 100 U/kg (5,000 to 10,000 U). The subsequent infusion dose is 1000 U/h, aiming for an activated partial thromboplastin time 1.5 to 2.5 times control.[8] Because warfarin (Coumadin) causes a multitude of fetal abnormalities, heparin, which is too large to cross the placenta, is given subcutaneously, usually twice daily, to maintain anticoagulation until 2 to 6 weeks postpartum. Patients who have received thrombolytic treatment for massive pulmonary embolism without adverse fetal outcome have been reported.[2] The role of low-molecular-weight heparin is evolving, and there are limited data that it is safe in pregnancy. However, no clear consensus recommendations regarding its use in pregnant patients have emerged.[8]

Patients with significant respiratory impairment should usually be managed jointly by an obstetrician and an internist. Fetal well-being is optimized by maintaining maternal oxygenation and acid–base balance aggressively and by minimizing the work of breathing.

COMMON PITFALLS

- Failure to appreciate the lack of respiratory reserve in late pregnancy
- Failure to aggressively treat asthma due to fear of harming the fetus
- Reluctance to pursue all ancillary studies that are appropriate in the pregnant woman with possible PEs due to concerns about fetal radiation exposure

SEIZURES AND ALTERED LEVEL OF CONSCIOUSNESS

Clinical Presentation and Differential Diagnosis

Central nervous system problems such as seizure and coma have a wide differential diagnosis in pregnancy. The most common cause of seizures in pregnancy is epilepsy. In about 40% of women with epilepsy, seizure frequency increases in pregnancy; this is particularly common in patients with poor prior control.[5] "Noncompliance" is believed to be a common cause, although several factors may be at work, including decreased medication intake due to nausea and maternal concerns about teratogenicity of antiseizure medicines. Indeed, the risk of congenital defects is increased two- to threefold in patients with epilepsy. The relative contribution of drugs needed to manage seizures, epilepsy itself, or prolonged acidosis from maternal seizures is unknown.

The differential diagnosis of seizures in a nonepileptic patient should include eclampsia; other primary central nervous system events, including thrombotic or hemorrhagic stroke; and drug toxicity (cocaine, cyclic antidepressants, and isoniazid most commonly cause seizures). Rarely, an amniotic fluid embolus or a PE can present as seizure.

Coma has a similar differential diagnosis, with a postictal state due to seizure from epilepsy or eclampsia as the most common consideration. Stroke must be considered in the patient whose condition does not reverse rapidly or who has a focal deficit. Pregnant diabetics have increased metabolic demands as well as peripheral insulin resistance, and they may be more prone to either hyperglycemia or hypoglycemia. Overdose is not uncommon in pregnancy and should be considered in the patient with a decreased level of consciousness or a picture consistent with a toxic syndrome.

EMERGENCY DEPARTMENT EVALUATION

Assessment of the seizing patient usually consists of emergent interventions to ensure an adequate airway and oxygenation and to stop the seizure. Focal signs should be noted. Once the seizure is terminated, clues to eclampsia (hyperreflexia, proteinuria, persistent hypertension, and marked edema) should be sought. Obstetric history (including symptoms of preeclampsia), history of epilepsy or diabetes, compliance with current medications, use of other current medications, including alcohol and antidepressants, and risk factors for thrombosis are all determined. The physical examination should include a detailed neurologic examination for focal findings and trauma. Evaluation of the comatose patient also includes all of the aforementioned, in addition to a determination of the depth of coma.

When appropriate, laboratory studies should include rapid glucose determination and measurement of antiseizure medication levels. A toxicology screen may be useful in the patient with suspected overdose, as may be an electrocardiogram (to detect cardiac effects of cyclic toxicity).

Computed tomography is rarely useful in the known epileptic or in the eclamptic whose neurologic examination normalizes with standard therapy. It may be useful to detect intracranial hemorrhage, however, in the patient with focal or persistent deficits or continued coma. In all other patients, it is a standard part of the evaluation of the patient with an otherwise unexplained, sudden central nervous system event.

EMERGENCY DEPARTMENT MANAGEMENT AND DISPOSITION

Airway protection is paramount in the comatose patient and in the patient with seizures. Intubation should be considered early, because the fetus suffers disproportionate injury from hypoxia, hypercarbia, and acidosis. Treatment of seizures of unknown etiology can be accomplished safely in pregnancy with either benzodiazepines or phenytoin. Both of these have been reported to be effective in eclamptic seizures, but if the clinical diagnosis is eclampsia, magnesium sulfate is still the medication of choice (and discussed more fully in Chapter 77).

Benzodiazepines, while contraindicated as Food and Drug Administration category D drugs, are safe for acute use and preferable to hypoxia and acidosis of persistent seizure activity. If respiratory depression occurs in the mother, intubation should be performed. Due to the changes in phenytoin pharmacokinetics, a regimen has been proposed of a 10 mg/kg initial intravenous load (not to exceed 50 mg/min), followed by 5 mg/kg given intravenously 2 hours later. If seizure activity is sustained, completion of the total 15 mg/kg load should be performed more promptly.[9]

In general, while the differential considerations may be altered by pregnancy, emergent treatment of the comatose patient or patient with seizures is unchanged. Indeed, it is even more important to minimize the hypoxic, hypercarbic, and acidotic insults of seizure or coma in pregnancy, due to the increased susceptibility of the fetus to these metabolic derangements. Admission is required for control of persistent seizures and for management of the comatose patient. Both a neurologist and an obstetrician may need to be involved, unless the patient has clear evidence of eclampsia.

COMMON PITFALLS

- Eclampsia should be considered in any comatose patient or patient with seizures in the third trimester, and clues to this systemic disease should be sought.
- Hypertension and coma may be seen in hemorrhagic central nervous system events, and a computed tomographic scan should be considered if the patient with presumed eclampsia does not respond promptly to magnesium sulfate.

References

1. Cardwell MS. Ultrasound diagnosis of abruptio placentae with fetomaternal hemorrhage. *Am J Obstet Gynecol* 1987;157:358.
2. De Swiet M. Thromboembolism. *Clin Haematol* 1985;14:643.
3. Fleming AD. Abruptio placentae. *Crit Care Clin* 1991;7:865.
4. Ginsberg JS, Rainbow AJ, Coats G. Risks to the fetus of radiologic procedures used in the diagnosis of maternal venous thromboembolic disease. *Thromb Haemost* 1989;61:189.
5. Jagado A, Riggio S. Emergency department approach to managing seizures in pregnancy. *Ann Emerg Med* 1991;20:80.
6. *Management of asthma during pregnancy.* NIH publication No. 93-3279A. Bethesda, MD: National Institutes of Health, 1993.
7. Newton ER, Barss V, Cetrulo CL. The epidemiology and clinical history of asymptomatic midtrimester placenta previa. *Am J Obstet Gynecol* 1984;148:743.
8. Toglia MR, Weg JG. Venous thromboembolism during pregnancy. *N Engl J Med* 1996;335:108.
9. Ryan G, Lange IR, Naugler MA. Clinical experience with phenytoin prophylaxis in severe preeclampsia. *Am J Obstet Gynecol* 1989;161:1297.
10. Sholl JS. Abruptio placentae: clinical management in nonacute cases. *Am J Obstet Gynecol* 1987;156:40.
11. Phelan MB, Valley VT, Mateer JR. Pelvic ultrasonography. *Emerg Med Clin North Am* 1997;15:789.
12. Treacy M, Smith C, Rayburn W. Ultrasound in labor and delivery. *Obstet Gynecol Surv* 1990;45:213.
13. Weinberger SE, Weiss ST, Cohen WR, et al. Pregnancy and the lung. *Am Rev Respir Dis* 1980;121:559.
14. Wible-Kant J, Beer AE. Antepartum Rh immune globulin. *Clin Perinatol* 1983;10:343.

CHAPTER 79

Emergency Delivery and Related Topics

Lynnette Doan-Wiggins

The past century witnessed a marked improvement in prenatal and obstetric care. During the past 60 years, maternal mortality has decreased markedly from 582 per 100,000 live births in 1935 to 7.5 per 100,000 live births in 1982, with this number remaining relatively constant through 1996.[4,6] From the viewpoint of safer care during labor, the outstanding advance during the twentieth century has been the great increase in the proportion of inhospital deliveries.[6]

The degree to which the emergency physician interacts in the process of labor and delivery varies among institutions, depending on the availability and readiness of inpatient obstetric services. The role of the emergency physician may be only to determine the patient is in active labor and to order transport directly to the labor and delivery area. Alternatively, in a hospital with little or no obstetric services, the emergency physician may be called on to manage a complicated delivery and neonatal resuscitation until transfer to a more comprehensive facility is possible.[7]

Labor is defined as the coordinated effective sequence of involuntary uterine contractions resulting in progressive effacement and dilatation of the cervix. This, coupled with the voluntary bearing-down efforts of the mother, results in *delivery*, the actual expulsion of the products of conception.

Labor is normally divided into three stages. The first stage begins when uterine contractions reach sufficient force to cause dilatation and effacement of the cervix and ends when the cervix is completely dilated. Although the average duration of the first stage of labor averages 8 hours in the nulliparous patient and 5 hours in the parous woman, there is marked individual variation.[6] The second stage of labor begins when the cervix is completely dilated and ends with delivery of the infant. The duration of this stage is highly variable, with a median of 50 minutes in nulliparas and 20 minutes in multiparas.[6,7] In general, if the second stage lasts greater than 2 hours, abnormal labor has developed.[6] The third stage of labor begins after delivery of the infant and ends with delivery of the placenta, with the placenta usually delivering spontaneously within 20 to 30 minutes.[7,9]

The cardinal movements of labor describe the positional changes the fetus undergoes that allow the fetal head to pass through the pelvis. A normal delivery involves fetal engagement, descent, flexion, internal rotation, extension, external rotation, and expulsion[6,7,9] (Fig. 79.1).

CLINICAL PRESENTATION

Peripartum events that require emergent attention include fetal distress, preterm labor, and imminent delivery. Timely recognition and intervention are essential for good maternal and fetal outcomes.

Fetal Distress

During the third trimester, normal baseline fetal heart rate is 120 to 160 beats/min, with heart rate varying considerably from beat to beat.[2,6,7] Rates above or below this range may indicate fe-

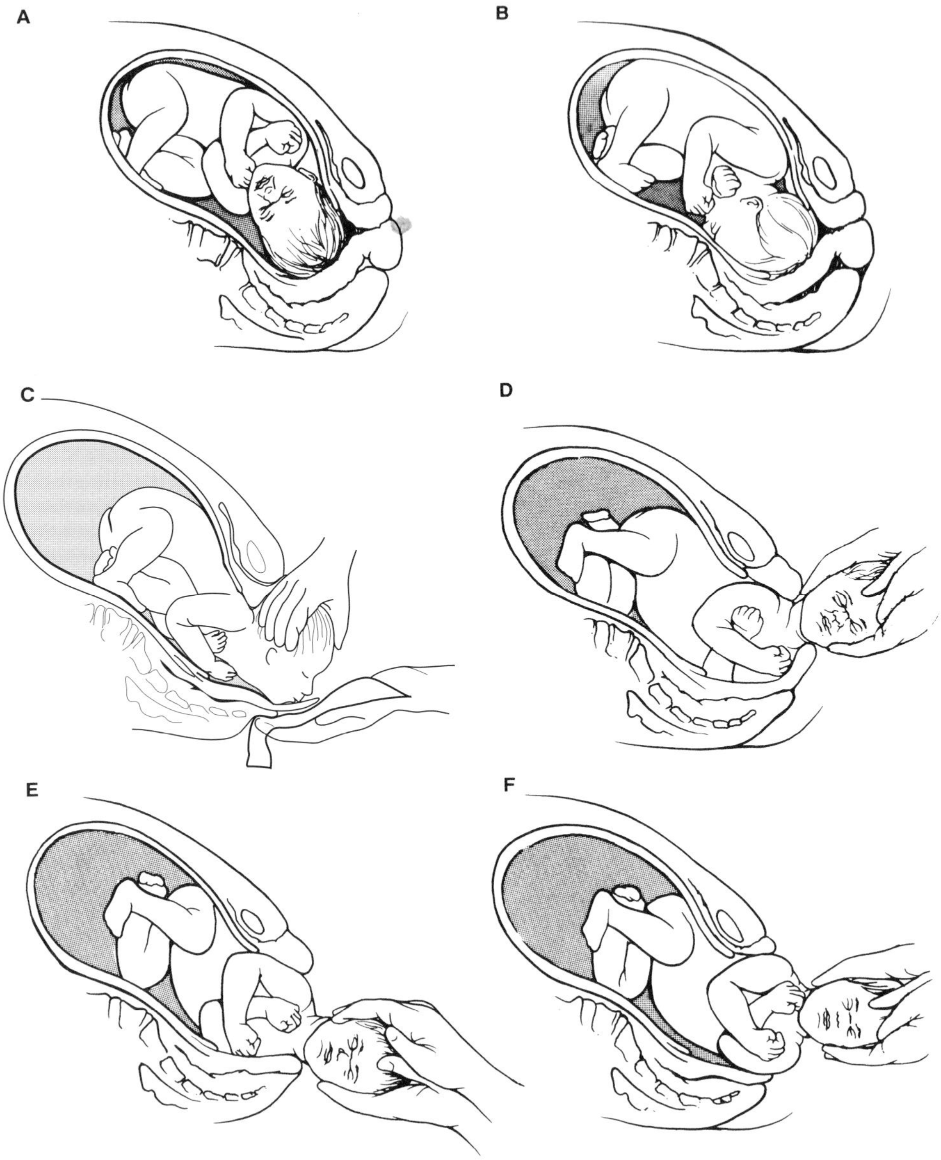

Figure 79.1. Mechanism of labor and delivery for vertex presentations. **(A)** Engagement, flexion, and descent. **(B)** Internal rotation. **(C)** Extension and delivery of the head, using the modified Ritgen maneuver. After delivery of the head, the infant's nose and mouth should be suctioned and the neck checked for encirclement of the umbilical cord. **(D)** External rotation, bringing the thorax into the anteroposterior diameter of the pelvis. **(E)** Delivery of the anterior shoulder. **(F)** Delivery of the posterior shoulder. Note that after delivery, the head is supported and used to gently guide delivery of the shoulder. Traction should be minimized.

tal distress. Fetal tachycardia occurs when fetal heart rate is greater than 160 beats/min.[6,7] Brief accelerations in fetal heart rate (i.e., those lasting less than 20 seconds) occur commonly during labor and are probably a physiologic response to fetal movement.[2,6] In contrast, persistent fetal tachycardia commonly occurs in response to maternal fever or medications but may also indicate early fetal distress.[2,6]

Fetal bradycardia occurs when fetal heart rate falls below 120 beats/min.[6,7] Like brief accelerations in fetal heart rate, decreases in fetal heart rate that reach their nadir with the peak of the contraction and end with or slightly after the end of a contraction (early decelerations) are physiologic and are probably the result of vagal nerve stimulation due to compression of the fetal head.[2,6] In contrast, decelerations that persist significantly after a contraction (late decelerations) and those that occur independently of uterine contractions (variable decelerations) are ominous and may represent uteroplacental insufficiency and cord compression, respectively.[2,6] If prolonged fetal monitoring during labor is necessary in the emergency department (ED), fetal heart rate should be assessed at the end of and for 60 seconds after a contraction at 15-minute intervals during the first stage of labor and at 5-minute intervals during the second stage.[2,6]

Preterm Labor

Preterm labor, that is, labor occurring prior to the completion of 37 weeks of gestation, is a major cause of preterm delivery, a complication that affects approximately 5% to 10% of all births.[1,13] Early identification of preterm labor allows timely intervention aimed at stopping or at least slowing the process. *Preterm labor,* as in term labor, is defined as uterine contractions with sufficient intensity, duration, and frequency to produce progressive effacement and dilatation of the cervix. Uterine contractions alone, therefore, do not indicate labor is occurring.[6,9]

Imminent Delivery

Imminent delivery occurs late in the second stage of labor and is heralded by an uncontrollable urge to push by the laboring woman and, with descent of the fetus, the urge to defecate. Signs on examination include rectal or perineal bulging and crowning of the fetal head.[6]

DIFFERENTIAL DIAGNOSIS

Abdominal cramping in women at or near term should prompt the consideration of labor. *True labor* is characterized by a regular sequence of uterine contractions that results in dilatation and effacement of the cervix and descent of the fetus. More common in late pregnancy and parous women, *false labor*, or Braxton-Hicks contractions, are characterized by brief, irregular contractions not accompanied by descent of the fetus or changes in the cervix (Table 79.1). Although false labor may stop spontaneously, it may rapidly convert to the effective contractions of true labor. A period of observation is, therefore, frequently necessary.[6] The passage of blood-tinged cervical mucus, or *"bloody show,"* is a rather common and dependable sign of the approach of labor. Bloody show must be distinguished from more active vaginal bleeding during labor, which suggests placenta previa or abruption and in which vaginal examination is contraindicated.[6,7]

Spontaneous rupture of the membranes (SROM) usually occurs during the course of active labor but occurs before labor in approximately 8% of cases.[6] SROM is indicated by the passage of a variable amount of normally clear or slightly turbid fluid from the vagina and may be verified if amniotic fluid is seen extruding from the cervical os or is found in the vaginal fornix on sterile speculum examination.[6,7] Amniotic fluid may be differentiated from vaginal fluid by placing a drop of fluid on Nitrazine paper. The pH of amniotic fluid is 7.0 to 7.5; that of vaginal fluid is between 4.5 and 5.5. A pH above 6.5 is consistent with ruptured membranes.[6] Detection of ruptured membranes is important for three reasons: Labor may be imminent; if the presenting fetal part is not already fixed in the pelvis, cord prolapse and compression are likely; and the risk of intrauterine infection is increased if delivery is delayed for 24 hours or more.[6,7,9] Rupture of the membranes before the onset of labor at any stage of gestation is referred to as *premature rupture of the membranes* (PROM).[6] When PROM occurs prior to 37 weeks' gestation, it is termed *preterm premature rupture of the membranes*.[6,9]

EMERGENCY DEPARTMENT EVALUATION

The evaluation of a patient over 20 weeks' gestation who presents to the ED complaining of contractions, SROM, or bloody show includes a history, physical examination, and ancillary studies as indicated. The pace of the evaluation is determined by the stage of labor, maternal and fetal well-being, and the probable disposition of the patient. The patient interview covers prior obstetric and gynecologic history, as well as general medical and surgical history, including any intercurrent illness. The current pregnancy is reviewed for prenatal care and complications. The quality, frequency, and severity of contractions are elicited. The occurrence of bloody show (as distinguished from vaginal bleeding) or SROM is detailed.[7]

TABLE 79.1. True Versus False Labor

Consideration	True Labor	False Labor
Contractions	Regular, ↑ severity and frequency	Irregular, no change in severity, frequency
Discomfort	Abdominal, lower back	Lower abdominal
Sedation	No effect	Relieves discomfort
Cervix	Progressive change over time	No change over time

Adapted from Cunningham FG, et al., *Williams' Obstetrics*, 19th ed. Norwalk, CT: Appleton & Lange, 1993.

The physical examination focuses on both maternal and fetal health. Maternal vital signs are assessed and a general physical examination performed. Elevated blood pressure, particularly when accompanied by headache or visual disturbances, proteinuria, or epigastric or right upper quadrant pain, suggests preeclampsia.[6] Fever may indicate amnionitis, pyelonephritis, or other infectious complications.

The abdominal examination focuses on estimating fetal age and location. Between 20 and 34 weeks' gestation, measurement of fundal height (i.e., the distance from the pubic symphysis to the fundus) in centimeters approximates the gestational age in weeks.[6] The maneuvers of Leopold, found in any standard obstetric text, are performed during the latter months of pregnancy to assess fetal lie, position, and presentation. *Lie* refers to the relation of the long axis of the fetus to that of the mother and is either longitudinal (greater than 99% of term pregnancies) or transverse. *Presentation*, or presenting part, refers to that portion of the fetus that is foremost in the birth canal and is the part felt through the cervix on sterile vaginal examination. In longitudinal lies, the presenting part is usually either the fetal head (vertex or cephalic presentation) or the feet or buttocks (breech presentation). *Position* refers to the relation of the presenting part to the birth canal and may be either left or right.[6,7] At or near term, vertex presentation occurs in about 96% of all pregnancies, but is more variable before term. At 29 to 32 weeks, 14% of all pregnancies have sonographically been determined to be breech; at 33 to 36 weeks, the number falls to approximately 9%.[6]

Unless there has been bleeding in excess of a bloody show or PROM is suspected, a sterile digital (not speculum) vaginal examination is performed to assess the progress of labor and confirm fetal presentation and position. Palpation of the cervix is used to assess effacement, dilatation, and fetal station.[6,7] *Cervical effacement*, or thinning, is estimated by comparing the palpated length of the cervical canal with that of the nongravid or uneffaced cervix (about 2 cm) and is expressed as a percentage from 0% to 100%. The completely effaced cervix is usually less than 0.25 cm thick.[6,7] *Cervical dilatation* is the average diameter of the cervical os on palpation, with 10 cm representing full dilatation.[6,7] *Fetal station* refers to the level of the presenting fetal part in the birth canal in relation to the ischial spines (which define "0" station). The birth canal above and below the spines is divided into fifths: +5/5 station indicates that the presenting part has reached the perineum. If the vertex is at 0 station or below, engagement of the fetal head has usually occurred; that is, the biparietal plane of the fetal head has passed through the pelvic inlet.[6]

If there is a question of PROM, a sterile speculum examination is done prior to digital examination to determine the presence of amniotic fluid in the vagina, as previously noted. Because the incidence of chorioamnionitis, the most common complication of PROM, is directly proportional to the number of digital vaginal examinations performed following membrane rupture, if amniotic fluid is identified, digital examination is deferred.[6,9] If bleeding in excess of a bloody show has occurred, vaginal examination is contraindicated in the ED.[7]

In addition to the tests associated with SROM, blood should be sent for hemoglobin or hematocrit, and maternal blood type, if not on record. Urine should be examined for glucose and protein, if indicated.[6]

Fetal evaluation primarily involves Doppler assessment of the fetal heart rate, as discussed previously. Ultrasound may augment the process. The region of the abdomen in which fetal heart sounds are heard most clearly varies with fetal presentation and the degree to which the presenting part has descended. After engagement, fetal heart sounds are loudest below the umbilicus in vertex presentations and above in breech presentations. To avoid confusion of maternal and fetal heart sounds, the maternal pulse should be palpated as the fetal heart rate is auscultated.[7]

MANAGEMENT OF DELIVERY

Although transfer to the labor and delivery suite is always preferable to delivery in the ED, occasionally there will be inadequate time to safely effect transfer.[9] Imminent delivery occurs late in the second stage of labor and is characterized by uncontrollable bearing-down movements of the mother; pressure on the rectal tissue, resulting in the urge to defecate; and perineal bulging, with eventual crowning of the fetal head.[6,7]

When delivery is imminent in the ED, a large-bore intravenous line of crystalloid solution should be started and the patient placed on a stretcher with her hips and knees partially flexed, the thighs abducted, and the soles of the feet placed firmly on the stretcher. An inverted bedpan placed beneath the patient's buttocks will provide additional space for delivery.[7] Although complete sterility is not a priority, when time permits, the perineum should be cleansed, the perineal area draped, and the physician gowned and sterilely gloved.[6,7] Eye protection and a mask should also be worn by the physician.

The mechanism of labor consists of engagement of the presenting part, flexion, descent, internal rotation, extension, external rotation or restitution, and expulsion (see Fig. 79.1). Maternal expulsive efforts are usually spontaneous and effective, and delivery of the infant occurs spontaneously. Occasionally, maternal coaching is necessary to help coordinate bearing-down efforts. In this case, the mother is instructed to take a deep breath at the beginning of each contraction, hold it, and push throughout the duration of the contraction. Pushing should not extend beyond the completion of the contraction.[6]

Normal Spontaneous Vertex Delivery

Spontaneous vertex delivery includes three phases: delivery of the head, delivery of the shoulders, and delivery of the body and legs. Gentle, gradual, controlled delivery is desirable to avoid maternal and fetal injury. As the fetal head delivers via the process of extension, the physician places one hand over the occiput, providing gentle pressure for control. When the fetal head distends the vaginal introitus to a diameter of 5 cm or more, the other hand, preferably draped with a sterile towel, may exert forward pressure on the chin of the fetus through the perineum just in front of the coccyx in a modified Ritgen maneuver (see Fig. 79.1C). This maneuver extends the neck at the proper time, protecting the maternal perineal muscles. The head is gently supported during subsequent delivery of the forehead, face, chin, and neck.

After the head has been delivered, the infant's face is quickly wiped and the mouth and nose suctioned with a bulb syringe to minimize the chance of aspiration during delivery of the thorax. A finger is then passed around the fetal neck to assess for nuchal cord, found in 25% of deliveries. If found, the cord is gently loosened and slipped over the infant's head. If this cannot be done easily, the cord is doubly clamped and cut and the infant delivered *promptly*.[6,7]

In most cases, the infant's shoulders are born spontaneously. Delivery may be aided by grasping the sides of the head and exerting gentle downward traction until the anterior shoulder appears beneath the symphysis pubis. The head is then gently lifted upward to aid delivery of the posterior shoulder (see Fig. 79.1). The remainder of the body usually follows without difficulty. After the shoulders have been freed, delivery may be assisted by *gentle* traction on the head, if necessary. Injury to the neck or brachial plexus can occur from direct pressure on the axilla or oblique traction on the neck during delivery.[6,7]

After delivery, the neonate is held with the head slightly lower than the body to facilitate drainage of accumulated mucous and bronchial secretions while the nose and mouth are thoroughly suctioned.[9] The neonate is kept at or slightly below the level of the perineum until clamps are applied to the umbilical cord 4 to 5 cm and 2 to 3 cm away from the fetal abdomen. The cord is then cut, usually 30 to 60 seconds after delivery.[6,7] The newborn is quickly dried and bundled to prevent cooling.[7,9]

The placenta is delivered during the third stage of labor, usually spontaneously and within 5 to 30 minutes of delivery.[6,9] Signs of placental separation include a globular, firmer uterus that rises in the abdomen as it contracts, a sudden gush of blood, and lengthening of the umbilical cord. Intraabdominal pressure produced by the mother's bearing-down efforts may be enough to effect complete expulsion of the placenta. If maternal force alone is insufficient, delivery may be aided by applying gentle pressure through the abdominal wall to lift the uterine fundus cephalad while keeping the umbilical cord slightly taut. This maneuver is repeated until the placenta appears at the introitus, when it is gently lifted out of the vagina. Trailing membranes are gently removed with traction. Excessive traction on the placenta should never be used and can result in inversion of the uterus. Following delivery, the placenta is examined for completeness.[6,7,9]

After delivery of the placenta, gentle uterine massage and an oxytocic agent are used to stimulate uterine contractions. Oxytocin is the most commonly used oxytocic. Typically, 20 U of oxytocin is added to 1000 mL of normal saline and given intravenously at a rate of 10 mL/min for several minutes until the uterus is firmly contracted and bleeding is controlled. The infusion rate is then reduced to 1 to 2 mL/min. Oxytocics should not be used before delivery of the placenta, because resultant uterine contractions may entrap the placenta or an undiagnosed second twin.[6,7,9]

Episiotomy

Prior to the early 1990s, greater than 60% of women in the United States received an episiotomy during childbirth, most as a routine procedure.[16] Its use was justified by the prevention of severe perineal tears, better future sexual function, and a reduced incidence of urine and fecal incontinence.[10,16] More recent studies, however, have determined that the routine use of episiotomy results in an equal or greater incidence of third- and fourth-degree perineal lacerations, postpartum perineal pain, urinary incontinence, and dyspareunia.[10,14,16] Therefore, the routine use of episiotomy has been abandoned for a more selective approach.[6,7,10] Indications for selective episiotomy include breech delivery, shoulder dystocia, occiput posterior presentations, and imminent perineal tear.[6,7]

Generally, the midline episiotomy is preferred over the mediolateral in the ED because of ease of performance and repair, less blood loss, and more rapid and comfortable healing.[6,7] The episiotomy should be timed so that it precedes trauma to the maternal tissues and fetus but avoids excessive blood loss before delivery. With vertex presentations, the episiotomy should be performed when the fetal head begins to distend the perineum and the fetal head becomes visible to a diameter of 3 to 4 cm during a contraction.[6,7] The incision may be made with a scalpel or scissors and extends through the skin, subcutaneous tissue, vaginal mucosa, urogenital septum, and the superior fascia of the pelvic diaphragm. If a scalpel is used, a tongue blade should be placed between the infant's head and maternal perineum while the perineum is incised.[7]

Repair of the episiotomy is deferred until after the placenta is delivered and after inspection and repair of the cervix and upper vaginal canal. Absorbable suture is used, with the goals of restoring anatomy and achieving hemostasis with a minimum of suture material. A variety of techniques are used and can be found in several standard textbooks.[6,7]

COMPLICATED DELIVERIES

Preterm Labor

If preterm labor exists and delivery is not imminent, consultation is advised, with immediate transfer to the labor and delivery area for monitoring and assessment of fetal maturity. When appropriate obstetric facilities are not available, attempts to arrest labor should be initiated in the ED.[7]

Although a number of drugs and other interventions have been used to inhibit preterm labor, unfortunately, none has been found to be completely effective.[1,6,13] Initial management includes supplemental oxygen, placing the mother in the left lateral decubitus position, and intravenous hydration with 500 mL of crystalloid solution.[1,7,9] If contractions persist and cervical changes are documented despite these basic interventions, pharmacologic tocolytic therapy is indicated (Table 79.2).[1,6,7,9,13] Although tocolytic therapy has not been shown to inhibit preterm labor for greater than 48 hours, this brief delay may allow maternal transfer to a tertiary care center or delay delivery sufficiently to improve fetal maturation with glucocorticoids.[1,6,13] In addition to the first-line tocolytics noted in Table 79.2, nifedipine has been demonstrated to be a potentially effective tocolytic with few adverse fetal effects.[1,6,13] Because fetal viability is rare prior to 24 weeks' gestation and fetal outcome at 34 to 37 weeks is similar to that at term, tocolytic therapy is generally not recommended outside of this age range.[1,13]

Preterm PROM may herald the onset of preterm labor and is a risk factor for the development of intrauterine infection. All women with preterm PROM, therefore, should be admitted for assessment of labor and consideration for antibiotic, tocolytic, and fetal maturation therapy.[6,9]

Fetal Distress

If fetal distress is suspected on the basis of changes in fetal heart rate, changing maternal position, typically into the lateral recumbent position, and administration of maternal oxygen may be beneficial.[2,7] In the absence of bleeding, a vaginal examination should be performed to rule out cord prolapse.[2,7] If immediate obstetric services are not available, tocolytic therapy to decrease uterine contractions and improve fetoplacental blood flow until delivery can be accomplished should be considered.[2,7] The definitive therapy for persistent fetal distress is delivery of the infant, either vaginally or by cesarean section.[2,6,7]

Cord prolapse usually occurs at the same time as rupture of the membranes and is diagnosed by palpation of the umbilical cord on vaginal examination or by visualization of the cord protruding through the introitus. Cord prolapse occurs during labor in approximately 0.2% of pregnancies and is more frequently seen with abnormal fetal presentation, multiple gestations, low birth weight, and prematurity.[6,17] The management of cord prolapse is directed at sustaining fetal life until delivery is accomplished, usually by cesarean section. If immediate obstetric services are not available, tocolytic therapy may be instituted.[7,12] Compression on the umbilical cord is minimized by placing the patient in the knee–chest or deep Trendelenburg position and exerting manual pressure through the vagina to lift and maintain the presenting part away from the prolapsed cord.[7,9] Some physicians recommend instilling 500 to 700 mL of saline into the bladder to maintain cord decompression.[7,12]

Shoulder Dystocia

Complicating less than 2% of all vaginal deliveries, *shoulder dystocia* refers to impaction of the fetal shoulders in the pelvic outlet after delivery of the head in vertex presentations.[3,8,18] Although more common in infants weighing greater than 4000 g, shoulder dystocia cannot be reliably predicted from any antepartum risk factors.[6,8,18] Impaction of the fetal shoulders and thorax in the maternal pelvis prohibits adequate respiration, and compression of the umbilical cord frequently compromises fetal oxygenation, making shoulder dystocia a serious and, at times, fatal complication of delivery.[9,18]

The goal of management is to minimize the time between delivery of the head and delivery of the body. Assistance, including that of an obstetrician and pediatrician, should be sought.[7,18] Excessive traction on the fetal head and fundal pressure should be avoided, because these maneuvers can worsen shoulder impaction and increase the incidence of permanent brachial plexus injury in the infant.[6,9,18]

Several techniques to manage shoulder dystocia have been described that result in successful delivery in a significant number of cases. Use of the McRoberts' maneuver has been well documented and consists of hyperflexion of the maternal thighs onto the maternal abdomen.[6–8,18] Alternatively, moderate suprapubic pressure may be applied to the maternal abdomen by an assistant while gentle traction is exerted on the fetal head.[6,7,18] Recently the "all-fours" maneuver has been described and consists of placing the mother on her hands and knees to effect delivery without the aid of additional maneuvers.[3] If none of these techniques is successful, rotational manipulation of the

Table 79.2. Tocolytic Agents[7]

Agent	Initial Dose	Subsequent Dose[a]
Terbutaline[b]	0.25 mg subcutaneously, or 2.5–5.0 μg/min i.v. infusion	May repeat every 20 to 60 min, or ↑2.5–5.0 μg/min every 20 min
Ritodrine	50–100 μg/min i.v. infusion	↑50 μg/min every 10 to 20 min to maximum dose of 350 μg/min
Magnesium sulfate	4–6 g i.v. over 20 min	2–4 g/h i.v. infusion

[a]Except as noted, endpoint is cessation of uterine contractions or signs of drug toxicity.
[b]Although commonly used as a first-line tocolytic, terbutaline is not approved by the Food and Drug Administration for this use.

fetal shoulders, aided by a wide midline episiotomy, may effect delivery. These maneuvers are described elsewhere.[6,7,9,18]

Breech Presentation

When compared with cephalic presentations, breech delivery is associated with an increased incidence of preterm delivery, low birth weight, umbilical cord prolapse, uterine and congenital abnormalities, and perinatal morbidity and mortality.[6,7,20] Breech delivery should be suspected in preterm deliveries and is confirmed by demonstrating the firm ballotable head in the uterine fundus. Sonography can also be used to confirm breech presentation.[6]

Breech delivery is difficult because successively larger and less compressible parts of the fetus are born, culminating in delivery of the fetal head, which may be trapped by an incompletely dilated cervix. In addition, umbilical cord prolapse is more common. In general, delivery is easier and perinatal morbidity and mortality reduced when the breech infant is born spontaneously at least to the level of the umbilicus. Techniques for assisting and extracting the breech infant differ with the type of breech presentation and are detailed in several textbooks.[6,7]

Meconium-stained Amniotic Fluid

Meconium-stained amniotic fluid occurs in approximately 8% to 15% of all deliveries and results in meconium aspiration syndrome in 2% to 6% of these neonates.[5,19] When meconium-stained fluid is identified during delivery, it is generally agreed that thorough suctioning of the infant's nares and mouth with a bulb syringe or DeLee suction trap should be performed prior to delivery of the shoulders.[5,6,19] Subsequent suctioning of the hypopharynx under direct visualization, followed by intubation with suctioning of the lower airway, is indicated in depressed neonates, those who have passed thick or particulate meconium, and those in which inadequate oropharyngeal suctioning was performed during delivery.[5,6] Whether vigorous infants with thinly meconium-stained fluid require intratracheal suctioning is controversial.[5,6,19]

Perimortem Salvage

Perimortem cesarean section should be performed in any woman who suffers a cardiac arrest after 24 weeks' gestation and is unresponsive to brief resuscitation.[11,15] Fetal survival is related to fetal maturity, time from maternal death to delivery, the effectiveness of cardiopulmonary resuscitation on the mother, and, in certain circumstances, the availability of neonatal intensive care facilities.[7,11] The chances of fetal survival are greatest if delivery is completed within 5 minutes of maternal arrest.[11] Following cesarean delivery, maternal resuscitation may be improved through increased maternal venous return.[11]

Prior to cesarean section, maternal resuscitation should be aided by placing the mother in the left lateral decubitus position at 15 degrees or by manually displacing the uterus off the inferior vena cava. Maternal oxygen via an endotracheal tube, cardiac compressions, and fluid resuscitation, if indicated, are initiated and continued throughout the procedure.[11,15] Delays to assess fetal heart tones or gestational age should be avoided.[15] Emergent obstetric and pediatric consultation should be requested concurrent with initiation of the procedure.[15] Because cesarean delivery may improve maternal hemodynamics, maternal resuscitation should be continued after delivery.

DISPOSITION

The best place for delivery is in the labor and delivery suite. In hospitals with full obstetric services, unless the patient is crowning, there is usually time to transport the mother to the in-house obstetric unit.[9]

Patients in preterm labor and those in whom other complications of pregnancy have been identified should be delivered in a tertiary care center whenever possible. Generally, antepartum maternal transport is more desirable than postpartum, especially with fetal prematurity.[1,9,13] The issue of transfer to an appropriate facility is best decided in consultation with the attending obstetrician. Parity, progress of labor, fetal and maternal condition, time involved in transport, the sophistication of in-house services, and response to initial therapy are factors to consider in deciding the appropriateness of transfer. Indications for transfer include preterm labor, PROM, preeclampsia–eclampsia, third-trimester bleeding, multiple gestations, and known fetal abnormalities. Ultimately, the transfer decision is made on a case-by-case basis, preferably in consultation with an obstetrician. When the decision is made to transfer the patient, minimally an ACLS unit should be used. Aeromedical transport or the presence of a qualified nurse or physician may also be indicated.

COMMON PITFALLS

- Failure to recognize imminent delivery may lead to a transfer that places mother and infant at increased risk for poor outcome.
- Failure to recognize meconium-stained amniotic fluid and to perform meticulous airway care during and immediately after delivery may lead to subsequent fetal aspiration, morbidity, and mortality.
- Manipulation of the fetus during delivery should be gentle and smooth. Excessive traction, particularly to accomplish shoulder delivery, may lead to significant fetal injury, often with long-term disability.
- Excessive traction to the umbilical cord during delivery of the placenta can cause uterine inversion or tearing of the placenta.

References

1. American College of Obstetricians and Gynecologists. Preterm labor. ACOG technical bulletin no. 206. *Int J Gynecol Obstet* 1995;50:303–313.
2. American College of Obstetricians and Gynecologists. Fetal heart rate patterns: monitoring, interpretation, and management. ACOG technical bulletin no. 207. *Int J Gynecol Obstet* 1995;51:65–74.
3. Bruner JP, Drummond SB, Meenan AL, et al. All-fours maneuver for reducing shoulder dystocia during labor. *J Reprod Med* 1998;43:439–443.
4. Centers for Disease Control and Prevention. Maternal mortality—United States, 1982–1996. *JAMA* 1998;280:1042–1043.
5. Cleary GM, Wiswell TE. Meconium-stained amniotic fluid and the meconium aspiration syndrome. An update. *Pediatr Clin North Am* 1998;45:511–529.
6. Cunningham FG, MacDonald PC, Gant NF, et al., eds. *Williams' obstetrics,* 20th ed. Stamford, CT: Appleton & Lange, 1997.
7. Doan-Wiggins L. Emergency childbirth. In: Roberts JR, Hedges JR, eds. *Clinical procedures in emergency medicine,* 3rd ed. Philadelphia: WB Saunders, 1998:988–1015.
8. Gherman RB, Goodwin T, Murphy T, et al. The McRoberts' maneuver for the alleviation of shoulder dystocia: how successful is it? *Am J Obstet Gynecol* 1997;176:656–661.
9. Gianopoulos JG. Emergency complications of labor and delivery. *Emerg Med Clin North Am* 1994;12:201–217.
10. Helewa ME. Episiotomy and severe perineal trauma: of science and fiction. *Can Med Assoc J* 1997;156:811–813.
11. Katz VL, Dotters DJ, Droegemueller W. Perimortem cesarean delivery. *Obstet Gynecol* 1986;68:571–576.
12. Katz Z, Shoham Z, Lancet M, et al. Management of labor with umbilical cord prolapse: a 5-year study. *Obstet Gynecol* 1988;72:278–281.
13. Keirse MJ. New perspectives for the effective treatment of preterm labor. *Am J Obstet Gynecol* 1995;173:618–628.
14. Klein MC, Gauthier RJ, Robbins JM, et al. Relationship of episiotomy to perineal trauma and morbidity, sexual dysfunction, and pelvic floor relaxation. *Am J Obstet Gynecol* 1994;171:591–598.
15. Lanoix R, Akkapeddi V, Goldfeder B. Perimortem cesarean section: case reports and recommendations. *Acad Emerg Med* 1995;2:1063–1067.

16. Lede RL, Belizan JM, Carroli G. Is routine use of episiotomy justified? *Am J Obstet Gynecol* 1996;174:1399–1402.
17. Murphy DJ, MacKenzie IZ. The morbidity and mortality associated with umbilical cord prolapse. *Br J Obstet Gynaecol* 1995;102:826–830.
18. Naef RW, Morrison JC. Guidelines for management of shoulder dystocia. *J Perinatol* 1994;14:435–441.
19. Peng TC, Gutcher GR, Van Dorsten JP. A selective aggressive approach to the neonate exposed to meconium-stained amniotic fluid. *Am J Obstet Gynecol* 1996;175:296–301.
20. Rayl J, Gibson PJ, Hickok DE. Fetus-placenta-newborn: a population-based case-control study of risk factors for breech presentation. *Am J Obstet Gynecol* 1996;174:28–32.

CHAPTER 80

Postpartum Emergencies

Moss H. Mendelson

The postpartum patient presenting to the emergency department may be suffering from any of a diverse number of diseases exclusive to or more prevalent in the postpartum period. Many of these problems are life-threatening.

In the third trimester, maternal blood volume is 35% to 50% above normal, the plasma volume is increased by 1,200 mL, and the red blood cell volume by 250 mL. Cardiac output is increased by about 1.5 L/min; 600 mL/min of blood flows through the placental site at term. Consequently, uterine and ovarian veins handle a 60-fold increase in volume during pregnancy. In addition, the hypercoagulable state of pregnancy and the trauma from delivery predispose to body-wide thrombosis in the puerperium, experienced as deep venous thrombosis (DVT) or cerebrovascular accident.[9]

The postpartum uterus returns to its nonpregnant anatomic shape and position by loss of cellular fluid and protein and consequent reduction in cell size. This involution is ongoing during the weeks after delivery. Most involution (about 40%) occurs in the first week postpartum. The uterus resumes its intrapelvic position by 2 weeks and normal size by palpation at 6 weeks postpartum. Vaginal bleeding generally diminishes several hours after delivery to a red-brown discharge, which may last through day 3 or 4 postpartum. A mucopurulent discharge may wax and wane over 4 to 6 weeks.[9]

The mean time to ovulation is 70 to 75 days in nonlactating mothers and 190 days in those who lactate; elevated prolactin levels are responsible for the delay in women who nurse. Menstruation resumes by about 12 weeks in most nonlactating women (mean, 7 to 9 weeks) but may be delayed in breastfeeding mothers up to 36 months.[9]

POSTPARTUM HEMORRHAGE

CLINICAL PRESENTATION

The causes of postpartum hemorrhage may be divided into early (less than 24 hours) and late (greater than 24 hours, less than 6 weeks) presentations (Table 80.1). Early postpartum hemorrhage is most often due to uterine atony. Bleeding can be brisk, and shock can develop rapidly. Maternal vital signs are often falsely reassuring, and blood loss can be hidden within the uterus and/or pelvis, making recognition of significant bleeding difficult in some cases.[18] Late causes of hemorrhage include infection, delay in placental site involution, and retained placental parts. There may also be a normal, transient increase in bleeding in the second postpartum week due to sloughing of the eschar that covers the placental attachment site.[7,13]

TABLE 80.1. Causes of Postpartum Hemorrhage

EARLY HEMORRHAGE (<24 H)
Uterine atony
Genital tract laceration
Retained placental parts
Placenta accreta
Hematoma
Uterine inversion
Uterine rupture
Coagulopathy
LATE HEMORRHAGE (UP TO 6 WK)
Infection (endometritis)
Retained placental parts
Delayed placental site involution
Sloughing of placental site eschar

DIFFERENTIAL DIAGNOSIS

Early Postpartum Hemorrhage

Uterine atony is responsible for most cases of early postpartum hemorrhage. Failure of the uterine corpus to contract properly allows continued blood loss from the placental site. Myometrial dysfunction occurs more frequently if the uterus has been overdistended (multiple gestations, hydramnios, multiparity, macrosomia); if there has been precipitous or prolonged labor, general anesthesia, or previous postpartum hemorrhage; if leiomyomas or amnionitis is present; or if fetal demise or amniotic fluid embolus occurs. Adherent fragments of placenta can also interfere with myometrial contractile function.

Minor pelvic trauma occurs in almost all deliveries. However, some vaginal and cervical lacerations may lead to severe hemorrhage. Pelvic vessels can be injured in the process of delivery, causing a pelvic hematoma. Vulvar hematomas are the most common; because the bleeding is bounded by superficial fascial planes, the hematoma usually dissects to the skin and is visible. Deeper vaginal hematomas can be occult and accumulate a significant amount of blood, distending into the pelvic space under the peritoneum. Patients may present with complaints of rectal pressure. Retroperitoneal hematomas are the least common but most dangerous type of hemorrhage. They are associated with significant blood loss, usually the result of trauma to a branch of the hypogastric artery, and can present with shock.

Retained placenta is a common cause of both immediate and late postpartum hemorrhage. Premature, assisted delivery of the placenta increases the risk for retained fragments, with resultant impairment of full uterine contraction and development of hemostasis. *Placenta accreta,* an abnormally deep attachment of the placenta to the myometrium, is suspected if placental delivery is difficult and no cleavage plane between placenta and uterus is found at manual exploration.[9]

Uterine inversion is uncommon.[15] Inversion is usually recognized soon after delivery of the placenta, and is more likely if traction is exerted on the umbilical cord. If the uterine corpus passes through the cervix, the inversion is complete; if not, it is incomplete, and may be occult. The patient presents with acute onset of abdominal pain, hemorrhage (average loss, 2 L), and shock. Often, hypotension occurs before significant visible blood loss.[31]

Uterine rupture is catastrophic and often results in fetal and even maternal demise, although the clinical spectrum of morbidity is broad. Factors associated with a rupture include previous curettage, cesarean section (especially with a high uterine incision) or rupture, hydramnios, multiple fetuses, and placenta accreta. Although more common in a previously scarred uterus, rupture of the nonscarred uterus does occur.

Coagulopathy can complicate postpartum hemorrhage that occurs from any source. Additionally, abruption, amniotic fluid embolus, and pregnancy-induced hypertensive disease can cause consumptive coagulopathies that then cause postpartum hemorrhage.

Late Postpartum Hemorrhage

The differential diagnosis of late postpartum hemorrhage includes endometritis, retained placental parts, placental site subinvolution or eschar sloughing, and resumption of menses.

EMERGENCY DEPARTMENT EVALUATION AND TREATMENT

The evaluation of the patient with postpartum bleeding should begin with an assessment of the extent of blood loss and the presence of hypovolemia and shock. If present, shock is treated as the rest of the evaluation proceeds. In all cases of significant immediate postpartum bleeding, laboratory studies should include a complete blood count and coagulation studies. Early establishment of vascular access is critical. The patient is typed and crossmatched, and fresh-frozen plasma should be available.[18]

Abdominal and bimanual examinations are necessary to identify the size, position, shape, and tone of the uterus, and the placenta (if available) should be inspected for completeness. If the uterus feels boggy and uterine atony is suspected, manual massage is performed: One hand massages in a circular fashion on the abdomen, with intravaginal fingers massaging the uterus upward. Massage may cause temporary uterine contraction, with recurrent bleeding after relaxation.[7] Pharmacologic treatment (Table 80.2), started concomitantly, includes drugs that cause increased uterine muscular tone (oxytocin, prostaglandins, and ergot alkaloids). Intravenous infusion of oxytocin is first-line treatment.

If bleeding continues, the birth canal should be inspected for trauma. Vaginal or cervical lacerations longer than 2 cm or those that are bleeding are repaired. Adequate exposure is needed, which can require general anesthesia.[27] With persistent bleeding or a placenta that appears incomplete, digital exploration of the uterine cavity may be indicated to look for retained placental fragments or uterine rupture. If placental elements remain, an obstetrician is consulted for uterine cavity curettage with a gauze sponge over the fingers.[7]

Management of uterine inversion includes manual restoration of uterine anatomy, followed by removal of the placenta if it remains attached. Manual replacement through the vagina is usually successful. The uterus is compressed between both hands intravaginally and gradually replaced. General anesthesia or tocolytics may be required to allow adequate uterine relaxation. Only after replacement of the uterus is oxytocin started.[31]

Refractory bleeding from any source may require emergent surgical intervention or arterial catheterization and embolization. Uterine rupture, once diagnosed, almost always requires surgery. Retroperitoneal hematomas frequently require surgery or embolization. Increasingly, angiographic embolization is being utilized in refractory cases of bleeding. Very high success rates for embolization have been cited, even cases that have failed traditional surgical intervention. Availability (time to catheter placement) and comfort and skill levels of the personnel involved can influence its use.

Imaging

Ultrasonography may aid in narrowing the differential in stable patients with both early and late postpartum hemorrhage. Ultrasound of the uterine cavity can be used to help rule out retained placental tissue by demonstrating a normal uterine stripe. Ultrasound may also be able to distinguish between retained tissue (echogenic mass) and a large intrauterine clot (sonolucent). Occult hematomas can be identified and those patients rapidly triaged to angiography and subsequent embolization. Computed tomography (CT) scanning, although more time consuming, may also show hematomas that would be amenable to percutaneous drainage.[23] It is unclear whether the advent of rapid spiral CT scanning will change imaging algorithms for patients with postpartum hemorrhage.

Curettage

Traditional therapy of late postpartum hemorrhage has been curettage. However, placental tissue is often not retrieved, and bleeding may worsen after the procedure. With the ability of uterine ultrasound to rule out retained placental parts, initial therapy now relies on pharmacologic management, using the drugs in Table 80.2. If bleeding stops, the patient is observed. Curettage may be indicated if bleeding persists or if retained placenta is seen by ultrasound.[7] Endometritis should be considered if late bleeding is accompanied by fever or abdominal tenderness (discussion follows).

DISPOSITION

Many causes of early postpartum hemorrhage are best treated in the labor and delivery suite, where obstetric surgical facilities, including general anesthesia and skilled personnel, are avail-

TABLE 80.2. Medical Management of Uterine Atony

Drug	I.M. Dose	I.V. Administration	Side Effects
Oxytocin	10 U	20–30 U in 1 L NS at 200 mL/h	Hypotension if given as bolus; cramping
Ergonovine maleate	0.2 mg		Cramping
Methyl-ergonovine	0.2 mg		Cramping
15-methyl-prostaglandin	0.25 mg		Nausea and vomiting

NS, normal saline.

able. In the emergency department, treatment of the unstable patient begins with vascular access, aggressive fluid therapy, oxytocin, and mobilization of appropriate resources. The disposition of a patient with late postpartum hemorrhage depends on the amount of bleeding, the response to initial therapy, and the probable cause of the bleeding. Decisions are best made in consultation with the patient's obstetrician.

COMMON PITFALLS

- Visually estimating blood loss is not an accurate method. Young women may have significant blood loss without developing typical signs of hypovolemia, making recognition of significant bleeding difficult in some cases.
- Be aware that intravenous boluses of oxytocin can cause hypotension.
- Uterine atony is the most common cause of postpartum hemorrhage. If it responds rapidly to manual massage, oxytocin should be given as well to prevent subsequent relaxation.
- Genital tract lacerations are the second most common cause of postpartum hemorrhage. Blood loss may be excessive if these are not considered and ruled out by visual inspection early on.

PUERPERAL FEVER

CLINICAL PRESENTATION

Fever above 100.4°F (38°C) on any 2 of the first 10 days postpartum (not including the first 24 hours) is considered significant. This definition may cause delay in the diagnosis of potentially life-threatening infections in patients who either do not mount a fever to 38°C, or who develop serious bacteremia and sepsis in the first 24 hours postpartum. Persistent fever after the first 24 hours of the postpartum period warrants investigation.

Fever may be classified as early (less than 48 hours) or late (greater than 48 hours, less than 6 weeks). Patients may present with symptoms and signs that make the diagnosis obvious, such as findings associated with respiratory or urinary tract infection. Many causes of puerperal fever, however, have nonspecific presentations. Lower abdominal pain may be due to persistent contractions or inflammation. Vaginal discharge can be scant or profuse in the face of metritis or normal involution. Abdominal tenderness and foul-smelling lochia are nonspecific signs, as are tachycardia and decreased bowel sounds. Wound sites should always be examined for tenderness, dehiscence, induration, edema, erythema, and discoloration.[25] Mastitis presents initially with fever, flulike symptoms, and, usually, a localized, painful site in the affected breast, with erythema and induration. There have also been reports of toxic shock syndrome from *Staphylococcus aureus* mastitis.[11] Septic thrombophlebitis may present with refractory fever or symptoms of pulmonary embolism (PE).

DIFFERENTIAL DIAGNOSIS

Early infections (within 48 hours) most often occur in the uterus and peritoneum following cesarean section (often polymicrobial) or are related to the urinary or respiratory tracts. Late infections (after more than 48 hours) include uterine infection following vaginal delivery (usually the result of ascending endogenous organisms), abdominal and episiotomy wound infections, breast infections, and complications of uterine infection (such as abscess or thrombophlebitis). Anaerobic bacteria, *Chlamydia, Mycoplasma,* and *Ureaplasma urealyticum* are often responsible for late infections.[28] Table 80.3 outlines common causes of puerperal fever.

Endometritis is infection of the endometrium (the decidua and adjacent myometrium), but often the process extends beyond the uterus into the parametrial tissue, causing a diffuse pelvic cellulitis. The incidence of postpartum uterine infection is 1% to 6% in vaginally delivered women.[7] Cesarean section increases both the frequency and the severity of infection: Endometritis occurs in up to 10% to 20% of patients undergoing cesarean section, despite prophylactic antibiotics.[29] Other risk factors include premature rupture of membranes, prolonged time from rupture of membranes to delivery, the number of cervical examinations performed, intrauterine manipulation, preterm labor, and low socioeconomic status. Endometritis can lead to sepsis, peritonitis (rare), adnexal infections (most often perisalpingitis), pelvic abscess, septic pelvic thrombophlebitis, parametrial phlegmon, and toxic shock syndrome. Salpingitis is uncommon.[7]

Most endometritis is the result of ascending (polymicrobial) infection of normal cervicovaginal flora or preexisting genital tract infection. The placental attachment site and the tissue

TABLE 80.3. Causes of Puerperal Fever

Site	Examples	Comment
Pelvic	Endometritis	Single most common cause of puerperal fever; suspect especially after cesarean section
	Wound infection	Requires local exploration and opening
	Fasciitis	
	Pelvic abscess	Diagnosed by ultrasound
	Septic thrombophlebitis	Suspect with failure to respond to antibiotics for endometritis
Urinary	Pyelonephritis	Catheterized U/A for diagnosis
Pulmonary	Atelectasis	Consider aspiration if general anesthesia
	Pneumonia	
Breast	Engorgement	Within 24–28 hours; diffuse, bilateral erythema and distention
	Milk stasis	
	Mastitis	Fever, flulike symptoms; focal erythema and tenderness
	Breast abscess	
Other	Bacteremia	
	Sepsis	
	Endocarditis	
	I.V. site	
	Viral syndrome	

U/A, urinalysis.

trauma associated with delivery provide good growth media for bacteria. The role of *Chlamydia* in postpartum endometritis is unsettled.[20]

Wound infections complicate 1.5% to 13.0% of deliveries. Most infections are caused by skin or genital tract flora. Common pathogens include *S. aureus,* groups A and B streptococci, *Escherichia coli, Proteus* spp., and anaerobes (especially *Clostridium* and *Bacteroides*). If cesarean section is performed emergently or amnionitis is present, a higher rate of wound infection is noted. Many patients initially are diagnosed with endometritis, but despite antibiotic therapy continue to spike temperatures because they require debridement and drainage. Complications of wound infection include synergistic bacterial gangrene (especially with clostridial species), necrotizing fasciitis (most commonly a group A beta-hemolytic streptococcal infection), wound dehiscence, and toxic shock syndrome.[4,7]

Episiotomy and pelvic floor infections complicate less than 1% of deliveries. The fascial anatomy dictates the depth and spread of the infection and may obscure the findings. Causative bacteria include streptococci and staphylococci, gram-negative enterics, and *Bacteroides* spp. Most infections are superficial and mild, limited to the skin and superficial fascia in the area adjacent to the episiotomy. More extensive disease can involve Scarpa's fascia, causing a potentially life-threatening necrotizing fasciitis.[9]

Septic pelvic thrombophlebitis develops from an infection of the placental site and associated thrombosed myometrial veins. Once established, the process can proceed beyond the local venous system to include the vena cava. Most often the process is unilateral, usually right-sided. Septic pelvic thrombophlebitis is most common following cesarean section.[7]

One percent to 2% of postpartum women develop mastitis, which is usually seen between weeks 2 and 6 after delivery. *S. aureus* is the most common causative agent.

Engorgement of the breasts consists of distended, firm, nodular breasts in the first 24 to 48 hours postpartum, while lacteal secretion is developing. The condition is painful and often associated with mild transient fever. Milk stasis is the result of incomplete emptying of the milk glands. This noninfectious process can complicate the evaluation of the febrile postpartum patient and can progress to sporadic infectious mastitis.

EMERGENCY DEPARTMENT EVALUATION

After a detailed obstetric history is taken, the examination focuses on the genital tract, wounds, the breasts, and the urinary and respiratory systems. Examination may reveal tenderness of the lower abdomen and a purulent or foul-smelling lochia. The uterus is tender and possibly boggy, with parametrial thickening and pain. If an adnexal mass is palpable, it might represent an abscess or an infected hematoma. The entire perineum and genital tract are inspected for signs of infection from a laceration or episiotomy. A rectovaginal examination should help identify parametritis or other abscesses or hematomas. Although unusual, a retropsoas abscess is suggested if there is diffuse hip or pelvic pain, fever, a tender rectal area, and painful ambulation.

Laboratory evaluation should include blood cultures, a complete blood count, and a urinalysis. Endometrial culture should be considered but may be difficult to interpret because of cervical contamination. Chest x-ray may be indicated; plain films of the pelvis may reveal soft-tissue gas if fasciitis is present.

Imaging studies may be helpful in puerperal fever, particularly when the source is unclear or there is no clinical response to 48 to 72 hours of appropriate antibiotic therapy. CT scanning in endometritis shows intrauterine debris, fluid, and gas in some patients. Ultrasound may reveal endometrial gas, which is sometimes associated with infection but is also seen in clinically well women. Ultrasound, CT scanning, and magnetic resonance imaging can be helpful in the diagnosis of several occult, intrapelvic, infectious sources, such as abscess, infected hematoma, and septic thrombus. Generally, ultrasound is the first-line test of choice; a CT scan can be performed if initial ultrasound is negative. Pelvic venography may be required to diagnose septic thromboses.[3,17]

EMERGENCY DEPARTMENT MANAGEMENT

Endometritis is treated empirically, without endometrial cultures, and the patient is followed closely. If the patient is toxic or has underlying medical problems (e.g., diabetes) or the clinician suspects anaerobic infection, clindamycin and gentamicin or clindamycin and a second-generation cephalosporin (cefoxitin) are given. Single-agent parenteral therapy has also been suggested: Cefoxitin, cefotaxime, mezlocillin, and piperacillin successfully treat the most common aerobic pathogens and some anaerobic pathogens. Ampicillin–sulbactam (Unasyn), ticarcillin–clavulanate (Timentin), and imipenem are also effective single, broad-spectrum antibiotics.[8,19]

Although most require admission, in patients with mild endometritis, oral agents are appropriate: The quinolones have the broadest range of activity against the pathogens likely to be involved in infection.[19] Patients with endometritis who do not respond to treatment within 48 to 72 hours require further workup to detect resistant organisms, wound infection, abscess formation, infected hematomas, and septic thrombophlebitis. Treatment of wound infection may include opening and debriding the area under adequate anesthesia. If more than local cellulitis is suspected, exploration under general anesthesia should be considered.[25] Fascial necrosis is a surgical emergency requiring immediate consultation: Mortality approaches 100% in patients treated with antibiotics alone and drops to 50% with combined surgical and pharmacologic treatment. Abscesses and some superficial hematomas can be incised and drained.

If septic thrombophlebitis is suspected, heparin and antibiotics for 7 to 10 days are usually necessary. The incidence of heparin-related bleeding in the postpartum state is low (1% to 2%).[9]

Mastitis is usually sufficiently treated with a penicillinase-resistant antibiotic.[1] With prompt treatment, mastitis usually resolves within 48 hours. If an abscess has formed, incision and drainage is necessary.[12] If breast infection is not present but milk stasis develops, more efficient emptying of the breast is needed. Nursing should continue, and treatment includes breast support, ice, and analgesia. If the patient is not breastfeeding, and conservative methods are insufficient to relieve pain, suppression of lactation may be helpful. Bromocriptine has been withdrawn for lactation suppression, but other agents are available. Consultation with the obstetric service is indicated.

DISPOSITION

The disposition varies with the type and severity of illness. If the patient is toxic (from any source), inpatient parenteral antibiotic therapy is indicated. Patients with abscesses, septic thrombophlebitis, or complicated wound infections also require inpatient therapy.

COMMON PITFALLS

- Necrotizing fasciitis is life-threatening; it requires emergent surgical consultation, aggressive debridement, and antibiotic therapy. Despite prompt, appropriate treatment, mortality is significant.

- Failing to consider nongynecologic sources of postoperative infections, such as urinary tract infection, may lead to a delay in diagnosis and inappropriate initial therapy.
- Do not assume that breast pain and fever in the first 2 to 4 days postpartum are caused by mastitis. Engorgement often causes these symptoms and does not require antimicrobials.

MEDICAL DISEASES

The postpartum patient may suffer exacerbations of a medical condition. Also, the onset of many diseases occurs during the weeks after delivery, including previously subclinical thyroid disease and autoimmune disorders. Postpartum ischemic necrosis of the anterior pituitary (Sheehan syndrome) may develop if severe postpartum hemorrhage with shock has occurred.[9]

HYPERTENSIVE DISEASE

Pregnancy-related hypertension is classified as preeclampsia and eclampsia, chronic hypertension, preeclampsia superimposed on chronic hypertension, and transient hypertension.[6] The occurrence of these diseases antepartum is discussed in Chapter 77.

NEUROLOGIC DISEASE

Half of all thromboembolic events in women under age 40 in the United States occur in relation to pregnancy and the puerperium. The risk of both hemorrhagic and ischemic *stroke* is at its maximum in the 6 weeks postpartum, and stroke remains responsible for a significant number of maternal deaths. The increased risk of ischemic stroke seems to be due to spontaneous thrombosis, possibly related to heightened coagulability. The relative risk of maternal cerebral artery occlusion is 8.7 (95% confidence interval, 4.6 to 16.7) in the postpartum period. The middle cerebral artery is the most common site of occlusion. Predisposing factors such as preeclampsia, chronic hypertension, diabetes, and hypotensive episodes are found in about one-third of patients. Stroke can present as new-onset seizure, and if so, must be differentiated from eclampsia. Embolic sources should be considered in pregnant patients suffering an acute ischemic stroke.[14] CT scanning, performed acutely and followed by lumbar puncture if needed, is used to exclude hemorrhage.[21] *Cortical venous thrombosis* is also reported, particularly 1 to 4 weeks postpartum. Initial symptoms are variable and may include headache, lethargy, and vomiting. Seizures are common (up to 30%), and hemiplegia may occur (gradual onset). Care is supportive, although prophylactic anticonvulsant therapy is usually given. Most authors do not recommend anticoagulation, as bleeding frequently follows clot resolution. Mortality may be as high as 20%, despite aggressive supportive treatment.[21,24]

Postpartum women also have an increased incidence of idiopathic *Bell's palsy*. The course and expression of the disease are unaltered by pregnancy. In a distinct syndrome known as *postpartum cerebral angiopathy*, the patient presents with headache, vomiting, seizures, and focal neurologic signs. Angiography shows multiple areas of segmental narrowing in the cerebral arteries; these usually clear spontaneously.

THROMBOEMBOLIC DISEASE

The risk of thromboembolic disease in pregnancy is roughly five times higher than in the nonpregnant population. Though most thromboses develop in the antepartum period, recent data indicate that two-thirds of pulmonary embolisms occur in the postpartum period. PE remains a significant cause of maternal death. Virchow's triad—stasis, changes in maternal coagulation, and vessel damage from delivery (especially cesarean section)—predisposes to thrombosis development.[26]

Diagnosing DVT and PE can be difficult in the puerperium. Leg edema and calf soreness are common postpartum. Arterial blood gas analysis shows a normal respiratory alkalosis secondary to hormone stimulation. Pelvic thrombosis is often clinically silent until PE occurs. A protocol of ventilation–perfusion scanning, noninvasive lower extremity studies, and pulmonary angiography may be needed to make or exclude the diagnosis (see discussion in Chapter 78). Treatment includes intravenous heparin and is similar to treatment in nonpregnant patients. Postpartum patients with DVT or PE usually require a total daily dose of 25,000 to 40,000 U of heparin.[4,21]

PERIPARTUM CARDIOMYOPATHY

Peripartum cardiomyopathy is the development of cardiac failure in the last month of pregnancy or in the first 5 postpartum months, in the absence of an identifiable cause for the cardiac failure or of prior demonstrable heart disease. The incidence is reported to be between one in 1,300 and one in 15,000 deliveries. Ninety-seven percent present in the first 2 postpartum months. The disease is more common in older multiparous women and in patients with twin gestations. Patients often have superimposed preeclampsia, obesity, or coexisting obstetric infection or anemia. Clinically, patients present with left ventricular failure. Renal insufficiency can also be seen. Most patients have nonspecific but abnormal electrocardiograms, demonstrating ST-T wave changes, left ventricular hypertrophy or bundle-branch block, atrial fibrillation, and atrial and ventricular premature contractions. An echocardiogram shows four-chamber enlargement and abnormalities of left ventricular contractility. The workup is directed at excluding other causes of heart failure. Primary therapy is bedrest, sodium restriction, digoxin, and diuretics. Anticoagulation is considered if cardiac dilatation is pronounced. Patients can become refractory to medical management, and overall maternal mortality ranges from 25% to 50% in the long term. Ten percent to 20% of patients die during their first hospitalization. If the heart size returns to normal, the prognosis is good; cardiomyopathy that persists after 6 months is a poor prognostic sign. PE is a common complication.[10,16]

POSTPARTUM PSYCHIATRIC DISEASE

A woman's risk of psychiatric admission peaks in the first postpartum year. Fifty percent to 70% of postpartum patients experience "maternity blues." Typically starting on postpartum day 3 or 4, this is a mild depression most prevalent in the first 2 weeks. It is probably a normal reaction to the stresses of childbirth. Common symptoms include tearfulness, irritability, and lability.[9]

Clinically diagnosable depression occurs in about 7% to 10% of women; in half of these patients, the symptoms were not present during or before the pregnancy. Risk factors include maternal personality traits such as anxiety, neuroticism, and cognitive style; poor marital adjustment; poor social support systems; and an excess of life events. Stresses during the pregnancy and labor may also contribute.[5,22,30]

Postpartum psychosis is rare (0.25% incidence). Usually, the disease has a rapid onset in the first few days postpartum; mania is a common presentation. Postpartum psychosis is thought

TABLE 80.4. Drug Therapy in Lactating Mothers[a]

Compatible	Caution or Temporary Cessation Required	Contraindicated
Phenytoin	Metronidazole (12°–24°)	Cytotoxic agents
Acetaminophen	Radiopharmaceuticals	Bromocriptine
Aminophylline	Salicylates	Ergotamine
ACE inhibitors	Antihistamines	Lithium
Propranolol	Phenobarbital	Gold salts
Coumadin	Benzodiazepines	Methimazole
Prednisone	Ephedrine	
Digoxin	Pseudoephedrine	
Antibiotics	Haloperidol	
Oral contraceptives	Cimetidine	
Alcohol		
Caffeine		

[a]Applies to standard, normal dosages; high dosages of some agents may be potentially harmful for the infant.
ACE, angiotensin converting enzyme.

to represent exacerbation of preexisting disease. The duration of illness is usually 2 to 3 months.[9]

THERAPEUTIC DRUGS IN LACTATION

Most drugs ingested by the mother are secreted in breast milk in levels that are not thought to be pharmacologically significant to the infant. Two rules prevail: The infant will receive 1% to 2% of the maternal dose of most drugs, and the higher the maternal blood drug level, the higher the breast milk concentration of the agent. Antibiotics are among the most commonly prescribed agents and may alter the infant's bowel flora, interfere with culture results from an infant's infectious workup, and cause allergic reactions and drug sensitization. Scheduling maternal dosages just after nursing or just before the infant goes to sleep may minimize fetal exposure.[2] Table 80.4 summarizes the relative risks of therapy with some common drugs.

References

1. Albert JR, Morrison JC. Neurologic diseases in pregnancy. *Obstet Gynecol Clin North Am* 1992;19:765.
2. Briggs GG, Freeman RK, Yaffe SJ. *Drugs in pregnancy and lactation*, 3rd ed. Baltimore: Williams & Wilkins, 1990.
3. Brown CEL, Dunn DH, Harrell R, et al. Computed tomography for evaluation of puerperal infections. *Surg Gynecol Obstet* 1991;172:285.
4. Chatelain SM, Quirk JG. Amniotic and thromboembolism. *Clin Obstet Gynecol* 1990;33:473.
5. Cox JL, Murray D, Chapman G. A controlled study of the onset, duration and prevalence of postnatal depression. *Br J Psychol* 1993;163:27.
6. Cunningham FG, Lindheimer MD. Hypertension in pregnancy. *N Engl J Med* 1992;326:927.
7. Cunningham FG, MacDonald PC, Gant NF, et al., eds. *Williams' obstetrics*, 19th ed. Norwalk, CT: Appleton & Lange, 1993.
8. Faro S, Hammill HA, Maccato M, et al. Ticarcillin/clavulanate for treatment of postpartum endometritis. *Rev Infect Dis* 1991;13[Suppl 9]:S758.
9. Gabbe SG, Nielbyl JR, Simpson JL, eds. *Obstetrics: normal and problem pregnancies.* New York: Churchill-Livingstone, 1986.
10. Homans DC. Peripartum cardiomyopathy. *N Engl J Med* 1985;312:1432.
11. Kalstone C. Methicillin-resistant staphylococcal mastitis. *Am J Obstet Gynecol* 1989;161(1):120.
12. Karstrup S, Solvig J, Nolsoe CP, et al. Acute puerperal breast abscesses: US-guided drainage. *Radiology* 1993;188:807.
13. Khong TY, Khong TK. Delayed postpartum hemorrhage: a morphological study of causes and their relation to other pregnancy disorders. *Obstet Gynecol* 1993;82(1):17.
14. Kittner SJ, Stern BJ, Feeser BR, et al. Pregnancy and the risk of stroke. *N Engl J Med* 1996;335:768.
15. Lago J. Presentation of acute uterine inversion in the emergency department. *Am J Emerg Med* 1991;9:239.
16. Lee W. Clinical management of gravid women with peripartum cardiomyopathy. *Obstet Gynecol Clin North Am* 1991;18:257.
17. Lev-Toaff AS, Baka JJ, Toaff ME, et al. Diagnostic imaging in puerperal febrile morbidity. *Obstet Gynecol* 1991;78(1):50.
18. Lowe TW. Hypovolemia due to hemorrhage. *Clin Obstet Gynecol* 1990;33:454.
19. Martens MG, Faro S, Maccato M, et al. Susceptibility of female pelvic pathogens to oral antibiotic agents in patients who develop postpartum endometritis. *Am J Obstet Gynecol* 1991;164:1383.
20. McGregor JA, French JI. *Chlamydia trachomatis* infection during pregnancy. *Am J Obstet Gynecol* 1991;164:1782.
21. Milliez J, Dahoun A, Boudraa M. Computed tomography of the brain in eclampsia. *Obstet Gynecol* 1990;75:975.
22. Phillips LHC, O'Hara MW. Prospective study of postpartum depression: 4.5 year follow-up of women and children. *J Abnorm Psychol* 1991;100:151.
23. Sherer DM, Abulafia O, Anyaegbunam AM. Intra- and early postpartum ultrasonography: a review. Part II. *Obstet Gynecol Surv* 1998;53:181
24. Smolke GA, Cox SM, Cunningham FG. Cerebrovascular accidents complicating pregnancy and the puerperium. *Obstet Gynecol* 1991;78:37.
25. Soper DE, Brockwell NJ, Dalton HP. The importance of wound infection in antibiotic failures in the therapy of postpartum endometritis. *Surg Gynecol Obstet* 1992;174:265.
26. Toglia MR, Weg JG. Venous thromboembolism during pregnancy. *N Engl J Med* 1996;335:108.
27. Varner M. Postpartum hemorrhage. *Crit Care Clin* 1991;7:883.
28. Watts DH, Eschenbach DA, Kenny GE. Early postpartum endometritis: the role of bacteria, genital *Mycoplasmas* and *Chlamydia trachomatis*. *Obstet Gynecol* 1989;73(1):52.
29. Watts DH, Krohn MA, Hillier SL, et al. Bacterial vaginosis as a risk factor for post-cesarean endometritis. *Obstet Gynecol* 1990;75:52.
30. Wolman WL, Chalmers B, Hofmeyr GJ, et al. Postpartum depression and companionship in the clinical birth environment: a randomized, controlled study. *Am J Obstet Gynecol* 1993;168:1388.
31. Zahn CM, Yeomans ER. Postpartum hemorrhage: placenta accreta, uterine inversion and puerperal hematomas. *Clin Obstet Gynecol* 1990;33:422.

PART X

Emergency Aspects of Gynecology

CHAPTER 81

Gynecologic Causes of Abdominal Pain

Patrice M. Ringo

The spectrum of gynecologic diseases that can present with abdominal pain is substantial. The emergency department (ED) physician must differentiate gynecologic from nongynecologic, acute from chronic, and benign from catastrophic causes in a timely, accurate, and efficient manner.

TABLE 81.1. Causes of Pelvic Pain in Women

Gynecologic	Nongynecologic
MILD VISCERAL	

PID (mild)
Ovarian cyst (stretch)
Menstrual disorders
  Myomata
  Dysfunctional uterine bleeding
Ectopic pregnancy (unruptured)
Endometriosis
	Appendicitis (early)
	Cystitis/pyelonephritis
	Hepatitis
	Gastroenteritis
	Diverticulitis (early)
	Proctitis
	Hemorrhoids

SEVERE VISCERAL	
Ovarian torsion Ectopic pregnancy PID (severe)	Infection/inflammation (severe) Incarcerated hernia Ischemic bowel Bowel obstruction Gallbladder colic Renal colic
SUDDEN PERITONEAL	
Ectopic pregnancy Ovarian cyst rupture Hydrosalpinx rupture Pyosalpinx rupture Mittelschmerz	Ruptured spleen Ruptured abdominal aneurysm Perforated viscus Other ruptured viscus (hollow or blood filled)
PROGRESSIVE PERITONEAL	
PID	Appendicitis Inflammatory bowel disease Cholecystitis/diverticulitis

CLINICAL PRESENTATION AND DIFFERENTIAL DIAGNOSIS

The approach to the woman with pelvic pain should be systematic and address three important questions:

1. What type of pain does the patient have?
2. Is the patient pregnant?
3. What nongynecologic etiologies need to be considered?

The presentations of various gynecologic causes of pelvic pain can be grouped by the different clinical syndromes commonly seen (Table 81.1). The skill of diagnosis resides in the ability to recognize patterns.[22] Visceral nerves innervating the abdominal and pelvic organs, as well as the visceral peritoneum, cause dull, aching, poorly localized pain. The somatic nerves innervate the parietal peritoneum (as well as the overlying muscle and skin). Stimulation of these nerves causes the more classic sharp "peritoneal pain," with well-localized peritoneal irritation exacerbated by movement.[1] The type of pain also governs the appropriate ancillary studies to obtain.

Mild Visceral Pain

Mild visceral pain is dull, aching pain with tenderness localized to the visceral organ involved. The purpose of the physical examination is to localize the most likely source involved. The differential consists of various causes of infection or inflammation, such as uncomplicated pelvic inflammatory disease (PID), ovarian cyst distension, menstrual cramping, uterine myomata, and endometriosis, as well as infections of the gastrointestinal and urinary systems (discussion follows).

Pelvic Inflammatory Disease

PID is discussed more fully in Chapter 82. Uncomplicated PID pain is most often bilateral. The pathogenesis of PID remains unclear. It appears to result from the ascension of bacteria to the upper female genital tract. The ensuing signs and symptoms are a result of the inflammatory reaction.[23] Onset is more frequent within 1 week of menses (possibly because ascendance of infection occurs more readily when the cervical os is open during menstruation), but the pain may be subacute and develop over several days. Uncomplicated PID is characterized by a dull lower abdominal pain. If infection extends beyond the endometrium and tubes, pain can become more severe and peritoneal irritation is seen. Clinical signs and laboratory parameters tend to be nonspecific, a fact that makes diagnosis difficult.[25] They can include fever, vaginal discharge, cervical motion tenderness, uterine or adnexal tenderness, and, rarely, a mass. Risk factors include multiple sex partners, prior PID, young age, and either no contraception or the use of an intrauterine device.[12,13] More recently, there has also been reported an increased risk of

PID with vaginal douching.[27] Mild symptoms of low abdominal pain and uterine tenderness may be the only signs of PID, although pathologic changes may still be significant with clinically mild disease. PID may be difficult to differentiate from surgical diseases, such as appendicitis.

Two complications of PID alter the clinical presentation. *Fitz-Hugh-Curtis syndrome* (*perihepatitis*) occurs when inflammation of the liver capsule causes adhesions to develop between the liver and surrounding abdominal wall. It occurs in about 4% to 14% of all cases of salpingitis, and may precede PID signs and symptoms in up to 20% of cases. Fitz-Hugh-Curtis can also occur after an acute episode of perihepatitis as a result of a recent PID infection, although in many cases there may be no history of PID or sexually transmitted disease (STD).[3] The pain associated with Fitz-Hugh-Curtis is in the right upper quadrant, and is pleuritic and often severe. The pain may also radiate to the right shoulder. Neither anorexia nor a significant increase in hepatocellular enzymes is usually seen. The differential includes acute cholecystitis, pulmonary embolus, and pneumonia, as well as pyelonephritis and urinary calculus.[19]

Tuboovarian abscess (TOA) may occur with severe PID, particularly when caused by or associated with anaerobic organisms. TOA is the most common intraabdominal abscess in premenopausal women. TOAs represent the most serious and dangerous complication of adnexitis. The mortality of PID has been reported to be as high as 8.6% when associated with rupture.[14] Some TOAs are detected when PID fails to resolve with appropriate antibiotic treatment. In a recent study, *Neisseria gonorrhoeae* and *Chlamydia trachomatis* were evident in 28% of women with TOA.[17] In other cases, sterile hydrocele or pyosalpinx results from a remote acute infection. Risk factors for TOA include PID risk factors as well as recent surgery or instrumentation.[26] The most common signs and symptoms include abdominal pain, fever, and a palpable pelvic mass.[17] Patients usually have continued, severe pain after treatment for PID (often unilateral), but a pelvic mass is palpated only if the patient is not too tender. Rupture of an abscess causes sudden, frank pain due to peritoneal contamination, and it is a gynecologic emergency.

Dysmenorrhea

Primary dysmenorrhea occurs in adolescents, usually within 1 to 2 years of menarche. Pain due to myometrial contractions occurs just before or coincident with menstruation, and it is described as severe, crampy, and suprapubic. It tends to occur with every menstrual period and may be incapacitating, particularly for the first 1 to 2 days of menses. Physical examination shows midline tenderness over the uterus with otherwise normal findings. Secondary dysmenorrhea can occur at any age in a menstruating woman and is most often associated with endometriosis. The rate of dysmenorrhea decreases with increasing age. In a study of 165 university students aged 17 to 19, dysmenorrhea caused absenteeism or loss of activity at least once for 42% of the women studied. The most significant associated risk factors were early age at menarche, long menstrual periods, smoking, alcohol intake, and weight (greater than the 90th percentile).[10]

Sexual abuse has also been strongly associated with dysmenorrhea and chronic pelvic pain. In a study of 581 nonpregnant women ages 18 to 45 with complaints of dysmenorrhea and chronic pelvic pain, there was a childhood incidence of sexual abuse of 26% and an adult incidence of 28%.[11]

Uterine Myomata

Fibroid tumors of the uterus are common, particularly during later reproductive years. Myomata often cause heavy, irregular, and crampy menses. These tumors may undergo ischemia, necrosis, hemorrhage, or torsion. Torsion causes a sharp increase in severity of visceral pain. Physical examination in a patient with fibroids reveals a tender, enlarged, and often irregular uterus. Myomata may also interfere with fertility and increase the risk of spontaneous abortions.[9]

Endometriosis

Endometriosis is the implantation of hormonally responsive endometrial tissue outside of the uterine cavity. Implants can occur anywhere in the abdomen or pelvis as well as other areas of the body. More extensive lesions tend to correlate with severity of reported pelvic pain.[6,20] The cyclical nature of the associated symptoms can sometimes be of assistance in the history. Approximately 50% will flare with menses. Symptoms are those of secondary dysmenorrhea in older women, with dyspareunia and abdominal, pelvic, or back pain due to stretch of contiguous organs or masses of endometrial tissue. Complications such as rupture of an endometrioma can lead to sudden pain from free peritoneal bleeding.

Severe Visceral Pain

Clinically severe visceral pain is characterized by poorly localized, nonperitoneal pain with disproportionately severe signs and symptoms, such as vomiting, pallor, restlessness, and diaphoresis. Several potential surgical diseases may cause this clinical picture, but the lack of peritoneal signs may give the clinician false reassurance that the disease process is less urgent.

Adnexal Torsion

Torsion of the ovary or other adnexal structures is a gynecologic emergency. Common predisposing factors include pregnancy, ovarian hyperstimulation syndrome, and ovarian or paraovarian cyst disease. Almost always, the ovary is enlarged; malignancy is rare. Follicular cysts are the most common type of cyst found on laparoscopic examination.[5] The pain associated with torsion is generally intense, severe, and unilateral, with frequent radiation to the back or thigh. The pain may be associated with nausea and vomiting, and an adnexal mass is often palpable. Because the ovary and the kidney have the same innervation (T_{10-11}), the clinical picture is very similar to that of renal colic. Other nongynecologic causes of severe visceral pain include bowel ischemia and bowel obstruction.

Sudden Somatic Pain

Ectopic Pregnancy

Ectopic pregnancy (EP) is discussed in Chapter 74; it is the most common concern in the woman with sudden somatic pain. It is important to remember that while catastrophic pain in association with missed menses and vaginal bleeding is the classic presentation for EP, other clinical features are seen in EP. As skills at early diagnosis improve, diagnosis of EP without frank intraperitoneal rupture is becoming more common. Early stretch and growth of the ectopic gestation in the fallopian tube can result in mild pain caused by tubal distension and contraction. Intermittent leakage of blood, which often precedes rupture by several days, will cause mild, focal, and intermittent peritoneal irritation, which is often poorly characterized by the patient.

In a recent study of 441 patients, in which 13% were diagnosed with an EP, the signs and symptoms that were most predictive of EP were pain reported as moderate to severe, lateral or sharp, peritoneal signs, cervical motion tenderness, or lateral or bilateral abdominal or pelvic tenderness. Risk factors predictive of EP included a history of infertility or use of an intrauterine device, prior tubal ligation, or other pelvic surgery.[7]

Because of the diversity of presentations, almost half of ectopic pregnancies are still missed on initial physician contact.[2]

Mittelschmerz

Mittelschmerz is unilateral adnexal pain at the time of ovulation, resulting from leakage of blood or fluid from the graafian follicle. Sudden, sharp, well-localized peritoneal irritation is usually found without fever, hypotension, or signs of inflammation or infection. An adnexal mass is infrequent. Occasionally, symptoms can be severe and generalized, but they classically decrescendo and resolve within 24 to 48 hours. In some patients, midcycle pain is recurrent and predictable.

Ovarian Cyst Disease

Ovarian cyst disease may occur at any age. There are several types of cysts, including simple, functional cysts, which may contain follicular fluid or blood; corpus luteal cysts; and benign or malignant cysts, including dermoids, endometriomas, and serous and mucinous cysts. Corpus luteum cysts are extremely vascular. Rupture of a cyst may lead to a significant and life-threatening amount of hemoperitoneum.[23] Cysts are particularly common during pregnancy when differentiation of rupture from other catastrophic problems, such as EP, may be difficult. With cyst rupture, rapid onset is characteristic and local peritoneal irritation is common, but fever or systemic signs are rare. On physical examination, there is often a tender, unilateral, adnexal mass and focal peritonitis. Cervical motion tenderness due to adjacent pelvic irritation is common and should be differentiated from PID, TOA, EP, or even appendicitis. Ovarian cysts may also cause pain if the cyst distends rapidly, or cause severe ischemic pain if torsion occurs. Because most low-dose oral contraceptives do not prevent ovulation, cyst problems are also seen in patients taking birth control pills, although there remains a protective measure against cysts by oral contraceptives.

Visceral Pain with Progression

Some inflammatory and infectious conditions progress to peritoneal irritation as they extend beyond the confines of the original organ. PID and appendicitis are the common disorders that do not remain well contained within their visceral origins. PID (discussed earlier and in Chapter 82) and appendicitis (discussed in a later section and in Chapter 41) are most classic for this history. While each frequently presents with mild pain either in the right lower quadrant (more common in appendicitis) or bilaterally (more common in PID), peritoneal signs develop over time in each. This can be reflected in cervical motion tenderness, and even progression to guarding and percussion pain in the lower abdomen. The progression in appendicitis is usually over 12 to 24 hours, while that in PID may occur over several days or not at all.

Chronic Pelvic Pain

Pain of 6 months' or greater duration is a difficult diagnostic and management problem. Chronic pelvic pain has most commonly been associated with endometriosis and PID. The most common primary complaints in patients with chronic pelvic pain include dysmenorrhea, intermenstrual pain, deep dyspareunia, gastrointestinal and urologic symptoms, and pelvic tenderness. Cul-de-sac nodularity and a fixed, retroverted uterus are the most common physical findings and are characteristic of endometriosis and chronic PID. Chronic pelvic pain affects approximately one in seven U.S. women, with a prevalence rate of 14.7% in a study of more than 5263 women.[16] In a recent study of adolescent girls with chronic pelvic pain not responding to conventional therapies, such as nonsteroidal and hormonal therapies, more than 69% (two-thirds of the study population) were diagnosed with endometriosis.[15]

Pregnancy-Related Causes of Abdominal Pain

Once pregnancy has been established or is highly suspected, a differentiation must be made between pregnancy-related and non–pregnancy-related causes of acute pelvic or abdominal pain.

Miscarriage at any stage can cause pelvic pain. Examination of the cervical os may differentiate a threatened abortion (closed os) from an abortion in progress, with products of conception in the cervix or vagina. Septic abortion presents with a tender, boggy, palpable uterus and fever. Ruptured corpus luteum cysts are common in pregnancy, presenting with sudden unilateral pain that is usually mild and localized. In rare cases, pain may be diffuse if cyst fluid or blood contaminates the entire abdominal cavity. Adnexal torsion also occurs with increased frequency during pregnancy. Traction on the round ligament and other pelvic structures as the uterus grows can cause significant but transient pain.

Other causes of pelvic pain in pregnancy include appendicitis (the most common surgical emergency in pregnancy) and processes unrelated to the pregnancy. Pyelonephritis is more common in pregnancy and should always be considered. Diagnosis of most such diseases, including appendicitis, becomes more difficult as pregnancy progresses, because the uterus obscures the examination and distorts the location of the affected organ. Delays in surgical management in pregnancy result in increased morbidity for both the mother and the fetus.[2]

Gastrointestinal and Urologic Causes of Abdominal Pain

Appendicitis is a common cause of abdominal pain and should be considered along with gynecologic etiologies of abdominal pain in females. The classic presentation of appendicitis is pain that begins in the periumbilical or epigastric area and becomes more localized to the right lower quadrant, with anorexia. Appendicitis in women is particularly difficult to diagnose, reflected by the 35% false-negative appendectomy rate for women in reproductive years. Cervical motion tenderness may occur in either PID or appendicitis because organs are close to each other and movement of adjacent organs is frequently painful. Pyuria occurs in 10% to 20% of both PID and appendicitis because of the proximity of the ureter to both organs. The presence of significant bilateral adnexal tenderness and a longer symptom duration (greater than 3 days) may suggest PID, but laparoscopy may be required to differentiate the two. Ultimately, clinical differentiation may be difficult.[24]

Diverticulitis is characterized by alteration in bowel habits and left lower-quadrant, colicky, recurrent abdominal pain, particularly in middle-aged and older patients.

Cholecystitis must be differentiated from Fitz-Hugh–Curtis syndrome, because both can present with more severe, steady upper abdominal pain of relatively sudden onset. Ultrasound is useful to identify calculi in the gallbladder.

Urologic causes of pelvic pain include pyelonephritis and renal calculi. Pyelonephritis usually causes unilateral pain in the lower abdomen and flank. Suprapubic tenderness and costovertebral angle tenderness are frequently elicited. Evaluation of the urine specimen for bacteria and leukocytes is supportive. Renal calculi cause severe visceral pain that is colicky and unilateral. The patient may have a history of renal calculi. Hematuria is almost always present. An intravenous pyelogram or ultrasound is diagnostic.

EMERGENCY DEPARTMENT EVALUATION

History

An appropriate history includes a description of the pain—onset, progression, quality, character, intensity, and radiation—as well as the reason for the ED presentation. The menstrual history includes gravidity, parity, date, and duration of the last two menstrual periods; regularity; any recent menstrual abnormalities; as well as time of menarche and menopause, when applicable. A history of STDs, use and type of contraceptives, recent vaginal discharge, breast symptoms, dyspareunia, and urinary complaints should be obtained. Gastrointestinal complaints must also be evaluated, including nausea, vomiting, diarrhea, or constipation. A history of fever and chills should be noted.

Physical Examination

The physical examination should be directed but complete. General appearance may be helpful, although individual pain thresholds vary greatly. A patient writhing in pain may have severe visceral pain from renal colic, bowel obstruction, or ovarian torsion. The patient who avoids movement may have peritoneal irritation. Early pain of appendicitis may be dull, poorly localized, and similar to more benign diseases, such as gastroenteritis.[1]

Vital signs are useful in recognizing systemic infection, sepsis, or significant hypovolemia. The general examination should look for systemic and supradiaphragmatic etiologies, such as pneumonia and endocarditis. Abdominal, pelvic, and rectal examinations are mandatory in *all women* with pelvic pain.

The abdominal examination should address three important objectives: a search for masses or palpable organs, localized areas of tenderness by quadrant and location, and demonstrating peritonitis. The diagnosis of peritonitis is made by performing maneuvers that move the peritoneum but do not put pressure on visceral organs (heel tap, cough, light percussion, pelvic jarring, and general patient movement). "Rebound" tenderness has been the classic procedure for demonstrating peritoneal irritation, yet it is probably the least accurate for diagnosing peritonitis. Interobserver variability is substantial, and the test causes unnecessary pain in patients with potentially surgical disease.[24]

The pelvic examination should include inspection of the external genitalia as well as the introitus and cervix. In pregnancy, there is often a bluish hue to the cervix (Chadwick sign). The bimanual examination assesses uterine size, palpable masses, and cervical motion tenderness. The "chandelier sign" occurs when the patient is said to have grabbed the chandelier on movement of the cervix, and is considered a sign of PID. This test is, however, nonspecific and insensitive. Patients with other diseases, such as appendicitis, cyst rupture, and EP, also have pelvic peritoneal irritation and will demonstrate increased pain on movement of the cervix, while patients with mild clinical PID may have minimal cervical motion tenderness. A uterus that is fixed and poorly mobile often indicates adhesions secondary to endometriosis, tumor, or prior infection. Rectal examination involves palpation for masses, induration, nodularity, or blood.

Laboratory Studies

A complete blood count is not useful in the assessment of pelvic pain, but an increased white blood cell count may reflect systemic infection. Chronic blood loss may be suspected if a low hematocrit is obtained. A qualitative, sensitive pregnancy test screening for the beta subunit of human chorionic gonadotropin is essential for evaluation in all women of childbearing age. With a low threshold (less than 50 mIU/mL International Reference Preparation), false-negative pregnancy tests occur in less than 1% of patients, even with an abnormal pregnancy (ectopic or miscarriage).

An uncontaminated (usually catheterized) urinalysis is needed to diagnose a urinary tract infection; it may assist in differentiating renal colic from ovarian torsion. Vaginal wet mount suspension can indicate various causes of vaginitis (rarely a cause of pelvic pain, but possibly a marker for STD exposure). Cervical cultures or tests to detect *Neisseria gonorrhoeae* and *Chlamydia trachomatis* may assist in the diagnosis of PID.

Imaging Studies

Plain radiography is rarely useful in the evaluation of pelvic pain unless perforation, bowel obstruction, or abdominal calcifications are suspected clinically. An *intravenous pyelogram* is useful in providing evidence of obstructive uropathy or in ureteral calculi.

In most cases, *ultrasound* is the imaging modality of choice for pelvic pain. Transabdominal and endovaginal ultrasounds are being used more frequently as diagnostic adjuncts.

Ultrasound is useful to distinguish between intrauterine and ectopic pregnancies. A gestational sac with a fetal pole should be evident by 5 weeks after the last menstrual period, and a fetal heartbeat should be seen by the seventh to eighth week of gestation. While ultrasound can be exceptionally useful, it is less specific than laparoscopy.

Computed tomography (CT) may be useful in the diagnosis of pelvic pain of otherwise unclear etiology. However, as an initial screening examination, ultrasound is still recommended. Ultrasounds are increasingly being performed in the ED by emergency physicians. One study indicated that the ultrasounds performed by emergency physicians trained in the use of ultrasound have a specificity and sensitivity in ruling out EP and making an accurate diagnosis in most complicated first-trimester presentations to the ED that is comparable to those performed by radiology and obstetric personnel.[8] In addition, in a recent study of 115 patients, emergency physician–performed ultrasounds significantly reduced the length of stay in the ED.[21]

Other Diagnostic Procedures

Laparoscopy is the gold-standard study in the diagnosis of pelvic pain. It remains the procedure of choice to confirm the diagnosis in the patient who is acutely ill or has an uncertain diagnosis, or in whom surgical disease (e.g., appendicitis) cannot be excluded. In a study of laparoscopic examination of 316 women with acute pelvic pain, more than 76% had an abnormal laparoscopic examination, and 45% of those with abnormal laparoscopic examinations had ectopic pregnancy, while 15.4% had PID, 27% had ovarian cysts, 3.3% had appendicitis, and 13.7% had pelvic adhesions, fibroma uteri, or endometriosis.[18]

Culdocentesis in the patient with sudden peritoneal pain may also be helpful to the physician who needs to rapidly diagnose hemoperitoneum or serious infection. Aspiration of nonclotting blood indicates a ruptured EP or other source of bleeding in the pelvis or abdomen; purulent fluid may be indicative of PID or ruptured TOA; a normal culdocentesis yields straw-colored fluid. A dry tap occurs in 10% to 20% and is nondiagnostic.

EMERGENCY DEPARTMENT MANAGEMENT

Sepsis and significant hypovolemia often require urgent management before the diagnosis is clear. Fluid resuscitation begins with intravenous crystalloid in a hypovolemic patient. Broad-spectrum antibiotics for sepsis from a presumed pelvic source should include good anaerobic and gram-negative coverage.

Gynecologic and surgical consultation should be obtained promptly for the patient with peritonitis, hemoperitoneum, or presumed appendicitis. In addition, surgical intervention may be required in patients with severe pain due to ovarian or bowel ischemia, or bowel obstruction.

Traditionally, it is taught that the administration of pain medication sufficient to alleviate the pain may also eradicate the signs needed to determine surgical disease or perform serial examinations. However, studies indicate that pain medicine is safe and useful for patient comfort. Administration of pain medication to patients with acute abdominal pain may quantitatively blunt pain, but it does not qualitatively alter physical signs or interfere with diagnosis. Analgesics such as intravenous opiates may actually allow for more accurate evaluation.[4] Patients with potential surgical conditions should, ideally, receive an early surgical evaluation before administration of analgesics, but long delays for "observation" of a patient with significant pain should be discouraged.

DISPOSITION

Pelvic pain is caused by a spectrum of diseases. Uncommonly, patients with sudden peritonitis may require rapid stabilization, with laparotomy as a diagnostic and therapeutic tool. At the other end of the spectrum are patients in whom the diagnosis is not determined in the ED. Admission is necessary for potential surgical disease, including appendicitis, selected cases of PID, and ectopic pregnancy associated with significant symptoms. If surgical evaluation is necessary, it should be done in a timely and efficient manner.

Observation may be necessary if a surgical etiology is possible, pain remains severe, or vomiting and other signs of systemic toxicity are worrisome to the clinician. Observation is appropriate for patients with focal peritonitis secondary to presumed cystic rupture or for suspected early appendicitis. If patients are to be observed (increasingly done in EDs), strict criteria for admission should be established and serial examinations should be performed and recorded.

If a patient is discharged from the ED with abdominal pain in which the etiology is uncertain but the patient is stable, *instructions for appropriate and early follow-up are imperative*. Early reexamination should be arranged for those with suspected PID, because the diagnosis is often inaccurate. Any woman with abdominal pain who is discharged from the ED must be instructed to obtain a repeat evaluation if her pain continues or worsens.

Because many causes of pelvic pain, particularly when the pain is chronic, are not amenable to ED diagnosis, there will exist a population of patients for whom exclusion of surgical disease, short-term pain relief, and referral for definitive diagnosis are the appropriate actions in the ED.

COMMON PITFALLS

- Two critical pitfalls are failure to recognize abnormal vital signs, including hypotension and tachycardia, and failure to reasonably account for abnormal vital signs.
- A pregnancy test should be obtained on *all women* of childbearing age, because ectopic pregnancy or other pregnancy-related diseases must be considered. The exception is the woman who has had a hysterectomy.
- Surgical and nonsurgical diseases must be differentiated. The patient with severe pain may have surgical disease (e.g., bowel ischemia or ovarian disease) but lack the peritonitis of the "acute abdomen."
- Clinical presentations may vary for each disease. PID and ectopic pregnancy may present with varying patterns of pain, from very mild and nonspecific to severe peritonitis.
- Cervical motion tenderness is not specific or sensitive for PID. It can be seen with various pelvic diseases and nongynecologic etiologies.
- Pyelonephritis requires confirmation of an abnormal urine with a catheterized specimen to avoid overdiagnosis based on a contaminated urine specimen.
- Even with upper abdominal pain, the pelvic examination is an important part of the physical examination.

ACKNOWLEDGEMENT

The author gratefully acknowledges the contribution of Jean T. Abbott, who cowrote the previous version of this chapter.

References

1. Abbott J. Pelvic pain: lessons from anatomy and physiology. *J Emerg Med* 1990;8:441.
2. Abbott J, Emmans LS, Lowenstein S. Ectopic pregnancy: ten common pitfalls in diagnosis. *Am J Emerg Med* 1990;8:515.
3. Ali V, Lilja JF, Chuang AZ, et al. Incidence of perihepatic adhesions in ectopic gestation. *Obstet Gynecol* 1998;92(6):995.
4. Attard A, Corlett MJ, Kidner NJ, et al. Safety of early pain relief for acute abdominal pain. *BMJ* 1992;305:554.
5. Bider D, Mashiach S, Dulitzky M. Clinical surgical and pathologic findings of adnexal torsion in pregnant and nonpregnant women. *Surg Gynecol Obstet* 1991;173:363.
6. Brosens IA. Endometriosis: current issues in diagnosis and medical management. *J Reprod Med* 1998;43[Suppl 3]:281.
7. Dart RG, Kaplan B, Varaklis K. Predictive value of history and physical examinations in patients with suspected ectopic pregnancy. *Ann Emerg Med* 1999;33(3):283.
8. Durham B, Lane B, Burbridge L, et al. Pelvic ultrasound performed by emergency physicians for the detection of ectopic pregnancy in complicated first trimester pregnancies. *Ann Emerg Med* 1997;29(3):338.
9. Grabo T, Fahs PS, Nataupsky LG, et al. Uterine myomas: treatment options. *J Obstet Gynecol Neonatal Nurs* 1999;28(1):23.
10. Harlow DS, Park M. Longitudinal study of risk factors for occurrence, duration and severity of menstrual cramps in a cohort of college women. *Br J Obstet Gynaecol* 1996;103:1134.
11. Jamieson D, Steege F. The association of sexual abuse with pelvic pain complaints in a primary care population. *Am J Obstet Gynecol* 1997;177(6):1408.
12. Jossens MOR, Eskenazi B, Schachter J, et al. Risk factors for pelvic inflammatory disease: a case control study. *Sex Transm Dis* 1996;23(3):239.
13. Jonsson M, Karlson R, Rylander E, et al. The associations between risk behaviour and reported history of sexually transmitted diseases, among young women: a population-based study. *Int J STD AIDS* 1997;8:501.
14. Krivak T, Propst A, Horowitz ZG. Tubo-ovarian abscess: principles of contemporary management. *Fem Pat* 1997;27:22.
15. Laufer MR, Goitein L, Bush M, et al. Prevalence of endometriosis in adolescent girls with chronic pelvic pain not responding to conventional therapy. *J Pediatr Adolesc Gynecol* 1997;10(4):199.
16. Mathias SD, Kupperman M, Liberman RF, et al. Chronic pelvic pain: prevalence, health-related quality of life and economic correlates. *Obstet Gynecol* 1996;87(3):321.
17. McNeeley SG, Hendrix SL, Mazzoni MM, et al. Medically sound, cost effective treatment for pelvic inflammatory disease and tuboovarian abscess. *Am J Obstet Gynecol* 1998;1786:1272.
18. Mikkelson A, Felding C. Laparoscopy and ultrasound examination in women with acute pelvic pain. *Gynecol Obstet Invest* 1990;30:162.
19. Owens S, Yeko TR, Bloy R, et al. Laparoscopic treatment of painful adhesions in Fitz-Hugh-Curtis syndrome. *Obstet Gynecol* 1991;78(Pt 2):542.
20. Schenken RS. Modern concepts of endometriosis: classification and its consequences for therapy. *J Reprod Med* 1998;43[Suppl 3]:269.
21. Shih C. Effect of emergency physician–performed pelvic sonography on length of stay in the emergency department. *Ann Emerg Med* 1997;29(3):348.
22. Siemel DL, Rennie D. The clinical examination: an agenda to make it more rational. *JAMA* 1997;277:572.
23. Tarraza HM, Moore RD. Gynecologic causes of the acute abdomen and the acute abdomen in pregnancy. *Surg Clin North Am* 1997;776:1371.
24. Thomson W, Liddington MI. Rebound tenderness test. *Br J Surg* 1991;78:795.
25. Walker CK, Workowski KA, Washington AE, et al. Anaerobes in pelvic inflammatory disease: implications for the Centers for Disease Control and Prevention's guidelines for treatment of sexually transmitted diseases. *Clin Infect Dis* 1999;28[Suppl 1]:S29.
26. Wiesenfeld HC, Sweet RL. Progress in the management of tuboovarian abscesses. *Clin Obstet Gynecol* 1993;36:433.
27. Zhang J, Thomas AG, Leybovich E. Vaginal douching and adverse health effect: a meta-analysis. *Am J Publ Health* 1997;87(7):1207–1211.

CHAPTER 82
Pelvic Inflammatory Disease

Alfred Sacchetti

Pelvic inflammatory disease (PID) comprises a spectrum of inflammatory diseases of the upper genital tract in women. PID may include any combination of endometritis, salpingitis, tuboovarian abscess, or pelvic peritonitis.[2,6,7,12,19,28] In the majority of cases, sexually transmitted pathogens (*Neisseria gonorrhoeae* and *Chlamydia trachomatis*) are implicated. However, PID may also be caused by other organisms, including anaerobic bacteria, *Gardnerella vaginalis, Haemophilus influenzae,* enteric gram-negative rods, *Streptococcus agalactiae, Mycoplasma,* and *Ureaplasma urealyticum.*[5,23,25,31] Over 100 aerobic and anaerobic bacterial strains have been recovered from the pouch of Douglas or high cervical cultures in patients with PID.[8] Because this disease is sexually transmitted, the peak incidence is during the childbearing years, although PID may be found in female patients of any age. Child abuse must be suspected in any prepubertal female with the diagnosis of salpingitis.

PATHOPHYSIOLOGY

Most pelvic infections originate from colonization of the vagina or cervix. From this site, the pathogens ascend through the cervical os into the lower uterine segment and uterine cavity. Normal cervical mucus presents a natural barrier to vaginal organisms; however, both *N. gonorrhoeae* and *C. trachomatis* appear able to produce uterine infections despite this protection. Certain cervical conditions, including recent menses, surgical cervical procedures, foreign bodies (intrauterine devices), and various hormonal changes during a menstrual cycle decrease the defensive ability of the cervix. The hormonal changes induced by oral contraceptive agents enhance rather than reduce the bacteriostatic properties of the cervix if administered prior to colonization. There is recent evidence that indicates that oral contraceptives may mask the symptoms of chlamydial infection once it does become established.[6,10,17,25,37,39]

Once entry into the uterus has been gained, inflammation of the uterine lining results. In postpartum patients, the myometrium becomes infected, but in other patients, this inflammation is seldom invasive and is limited to the endometrium. The inflammation may produce uterine bleeding, but in the nongravid uterus, the infection is seldom clinically significant. The pathogens then continue their migration through the fallopian tubes. In the case of mycoplasmal infection, ascension may occur by way of parametrial structures rather than through the uterine cavity.

Initial tubal infection is limited to the mucosa of the lumen, but the inflammation rapidly extends through the full thickness of the tubes. This transmural reaction of the fallopian tubes often causes the early pain of pelvic infection. In severe cases, the purulent material from the fallopian lumens exudes through the open fimbriae into the abdominal cavity, producing peritonitis.[12]

The infection of the endometrium and fallopian tubes results in an inflammation of the surrounding parametrial structures. Even though they may not undergo actual infection by the invading pathogens, the proximity to the true infection produces a severe parametritis in many patients.

The inflammation initiated by *N. gonorrhoeae* or *C. trachomatis* frequently overwhelms the normal uterine defense mechanisms and results in infections from opportunistic pathogens, particularly *Bacteroides* species.[8,10,25,33,37]

Inflammation and stagnation of host defenses, particularly in the fallopian tubes, allow for the possibility of unchecked bacterial growth. A tuboovarian abscess may develop; originating in the fallopian tube, the abscess may extend to involve the fimbriae and ovary as well. The bacterial content of a tuboovarian abscess is mixed, with a preponderance of anaerobes.[20]

Localized pelvic infection is not the only result of infection with *N. gonorrhoeae* and *C. trachomatis.* Escape through the end of the right fallopian tube and ascent to the right colic gutter may result in inflammation around the liver. The *Fitz-Hugh-Curtis syndrome (perihepatitis)* is usually associated with *C. trachomatis* but may occur in 8% to 10% of all cases of salpingitis.

CLINICAL PRESENTATION

A clinical diagnosis of PID may be difficult due to the wide variation in signs and symptoms. Some authorities believe that the examination is notoriously inaccurate in the diagnosis of pelvic infections. No single historical, physical, or laboratory finding is both sensitive and specific for the diagnosis of acute PID. The Centers for Disease Control and Prevention (CDC) estimate that a clinical diagnosis of PID has a positive predictive rate of 65% to 90% for salpingitis.[6] Mild or nonspecific complaints may go unrecognized by the clinician (e.g., abnormal bleeding, dyspareunia, or vaginal discharge). Most authorities recommend a low threshold for diagnosis of PID because of the long-term effects and potential damage to the reproductive system of women.

Minimum criteria for diagnosis have been published[6] and appear in Table 82.1. Additional criteria for diagnosis are also listed.

Although attempts have been made to distinguish between features of infection caused by *N. gonorrhoeae* and *C. trachomatis,* they have not been consistent or reliable. *N. gonorrhoeae* salpingitis develops in the first few days after menses, producing a purulent vaginal discharge and severe pelvic pain. *C. trachomatis* infection may occur at any point in the menstrual cycle, and results in less cervical discharge and milder symptoms. Chlamydia is responsible for more significant fallopian tube damage.[5,26]

History

The patient with pelvic infection almost invariably presents to the emergency department with a complaint of lower abdominal pain. Inflammation of the endometrium, fallopian tubes, and parametrial structures usually produces diffuse bilateral pelvic pain. When questioned, most women describe a dull, constant, poorly localized pain. Because of the sensitive nature and social stigma of sexually transmitted diseases, physicians should be empathetic and tactful in eliciting the patient's history.[5] Pelvic pain is seldom the only presenting complaint. *N. gonorrhoeae* or *C. trachomatis* cervicitis results in a vaginal discharge in greater than 50% of patients, while abnormal vaginal bleeding is seen in 30%. Gastrointestinal complaints, including nausea and vomiting, are less common but may be present. Urinary tract symptoms are common, with 20% of laparoscopically proven pelvic infections associated with irritative voiding symptoms.[10] Pelvic infection should be suspected in patients who complain of *dysuria or suprapubic pain* that occurs only during micturition and is unaccompanied by frequency and urgency. The urinalysis is normal because the bladder urine is not infected.

Physical Examination

A temperature above 38°C (100.4°F) is found in only 33% of patients; fever supports the diagnosis but does not confirm it; nor

TABLE 82.1. Diagnosis of PID

MINIMUM CRITERIA FOR THE DIAGNOSIS OF PID
Empiric treatment of PID should be instituted on the basis of the presence of all of the following three minimum clinical criteria for PID and in the absence of an established cause other than PID: Lower abdominal tenderness Bilateral adnexal tenderness Cervical motion tenderness
ROUTINE CRITERIA
For women with severe clinical signs, more elaborate diagnostic evaluation is warranted because incorrect diagnosis and management may cause unnecessary morbidity. These additional criteria may be used to increase the specificity of diagnosis: Oral temperature >38.3°C Abnormal cervical or vaginal discharge Elevated erythrocyte sedimentation rate Elevated C-reactive protein Laboratory documentation of cervical infection with *N. gonorrhoeae* or *C. trachomatis*
ELABORATE CRITERIA FOR DIAGNOSING PID
Histopathologic evidence of endometritis on endometrial biopsy Tuboovarian abscess on sonography or other radiologic tests Laparoscopic abnormalities consistent with PID

From Centers for Disease Control and Prevention. 1998 Guidelines for treatment of sexually transmitted diseases. *MMWR* 1998;47(RR-1):1–111.

does its absence preclude the diagnosis of PID. The abdominal examination commonly reveals tenderness in both lower quadrants, although one side may be more tender. Peritoneal signs indicate a more severe infection, with free exudate in the pelvis or abdomen,[12] and intraperitoneal extension should be considered. If perihepatitis is also present, there may be tenderness in the right upper quadrant.

Pelvic examination must be approached carefully if meaningful information is to be gained. Because of pain or previous experience, many patients may not be cooperative.[4,10] Speculum examination may reveal a vaginal discharge. A markedly inflamed purulent cervix is indicative of an acute cervicitis and is supportive of some degree of pelvic infection. Bimanual examination begins with testing for cervical motion tenderness. Elicitation of pain with either lateral or anteroposterior motion of the cervix is sensitive but not specific for pelvic infection. The emergency physician must remember that other causes of pelvic irritation, including fluid from ruptured cysts and blood from ectopic pregnancies, can also produce this sign.[10,11] The uterus is frequently firm but tender. *Bilateral adnexal tenderness is one of the most consistent physical findings in studies evaluating diagnostic criteria for salpingitis.*[1,12,21,29] An adnexal mass may be appreciated but is not a consistent finding in the absence of a tuboovarian abscess. Findings on pelvic examination may be atypical in patients who have had multiple prior infections or tubal ligation. Obstruction of the fallopian tube may prevent extension of the infection beyond the proximal tube, limiting the degree of adnexal tenderness.

DIFFERENTIAL DIAGNOSIS

The differential diagnosis of abdominal pain in women should include three possibilities: (1) ectopic pregnancy, (2) PID, and (3) appendicitis. Ovarian cyst, urinary tract infection, hernia, and ovarian torsion should also be considered. Ectopic pregnancy is addressed in Chapter 74. *All women with pelvic pain, regardless of their menstrual history, should have a pregnancy test; the only exception is the woman who has had a hysterectomy.*[27] *Salpingitis* is the most common incorrect diagnosis in missed ectopic pregnancy and should be considered only after ectopic pregnancy has been ruled out.[1] The coexistence of infection and pregnancy is possible but unusual, because, after implantation, a mucous plug forms, preventing the spread of lower genital infections into the upper genital system. However, there is a brief window between insemination and mucous plug formation during which infection may occur. *Appendicitis* may be differentiated from PID by its unilateral nature, but this is by no means diagnostic. Only 82% of patients with clinical presentations consistent with PID actually had pelvic infections on laparoscopic examination.[12]

EMERGENCY DEPARTMENT EVALUATION

When PID is suspected, additional support for the diagnosis may be obtained through laboratory analysis. Although results are not immediately available, cervical cultures for *Chlamydia* and *N. gonorrhoeae* should be done on all patients during the speculum examination. Because results are not immediately available, a system must exist for follow-up of patients whose positive-culture results return to the emergency department after the patient has been discharged.[15]

Gonorrhea cultures are obtained by placement of a sterile swab 1 to 2 cm into the endocervical canal, with rotation of the swab for 10 to 30 seconds.[1] Following collection, the swab should be immediately plated on either chocolate agar or Thayer-Martin agar.[4] Gram stains, cervical mucus enzyme, and antibody detection tests may also be used in the identification of *N. gonorrhoeae,* although these tests are neither as sensitive nor as specific as cultures.[11,16]

Chlamydia detection techniques include culture, antibody detection (ELISA and fluorescent), and DNA probes.[9,24,26,32] In contrast to gonorrhea testing, nonculture techniques are the preferred detection procedures for the diagnosis of *C. trachomatis.* Both direct fluorescent antibody tests and ELISA-type antibody tests have been shown to be 70% to 90% sensitive and more than 90% specific in *Chlamydia* infections in women.[4] DNA probe tests that appear to be highly sensitive and specific have been developed, but their clinical applicability remains to be determined.[22,26,38]

Additional laboratory studies should include urinalysis to rule out urinary tract infection and a urine or serum pregnancy test.[11,27] A complete blood count may be obtained for use in some disposition decisions, but the clinician should recognize that the test has limited usefulness. In toxic patients with severe unilateral symptoms, pelvic ultrasonography is indicated to confirm a tuboovarian abscess, although laparoscopy is more accurate.[30] The CDC recommends serology for syphilis and the human immunodeficiency virus (HIV).

EMERGENCY DEPARTMENT MANAGEMENT

Treatment regimens are summarized in Table 82.2. The management of acute pelvic infection centers on prompt antibiotic therapy. The goal of treatment is to prevent continued or worsened infection; complications of PID, including ectopic pregnancy and infertility; and chronic infection.[5,14,18] Selection of the appropriate antimicrobial combination depends on the current recommendations of the local public health department and the CDC.

Alternate single-dose therapies have been described for the treatment of cervicitis or mild salpingitis. The clinician may consider these therapies more convenient; to date, however, none has been endorsed by the CDC. These regimens have not been advocated for established or severe pelvic infections and should be used cautiously with patients exhibiting more than minimal

TABLE 82.2. Antibiotic Therapy of PID

OUTPATIENT TREATMENT FOR PID
Regimen A
Cefoxitin 2 g i.m., plus probenecid 1 g PO
or
Ceftriaxone 250 mg IM
plus
Doxycycline 100 mg PO, b.i.d. for 14 d
Regimen B
Ofloxacin 400 mg PO b.i.d. for 14 d
plus
Metronidazole 500 mg PO q.i.d. for 14 d
INPATIENT TREATMENT FOR PID
Regimen A
Cefotetan 2 g i.v. q12h
or
Cefoxitin 2 g i.v. q6h
plus
Doxycycline 100 mg i.v. or orally q12h
Regimen B
Clindamycin 900 mg i.v. q8h
plus
Gentamicin (Load, 2 mg/kg i.v., maintenance 1.5 mg/kg q8h. Single daily dosing may be substituted.)
Alternate Parenteral Regimens
Ofloxacin 400 mg i.v. q12h
plus
Metronidazole 500 mg i.v. q8h
Ampicillin/sulbactam 3 g i.v. q6h
plus
Doxycycline 100 mg i.v. or orally q12h
Ciprofloxacin 200 mg i.v. q12h
plus
Doxycycline 100 mg i.v. or orally q12h
plus
Metronidazole 500 mg i.v. q8h

Note: ALL patients with suspected PID, gonorrhea, or chlamydial infection should have serologic testing for syphilis and should be offered confidential counseling and testing for HIV infection.

Special therapeutic considerations: Pregnant women with suspected PID should be hospitalized and treated with parenteral antibiotics. HIV patients are more likely to require surgical intervention and may have a leukopenia or lesser leukocytosis than non–HIV-infected women. Therefore, HIV-infected women who develop PID should be hospitalized and provided parenteral therapy.

Data from references 2, 6, 13, 19, 35.

symptoms. One regimen employing clindamycin 300 mg PO t.i.d., plus ciprofloxacin 250 mg PO b.i.d., for 14 days has been described for moderate PID, although this regimen has also not been advocated for severe infections.[3]

Practitioners should monitor public health service publications concerning recommendations for antimicrobial treatment of sexually transmitted diseases in their areas because the incidence of *N. gonorrhoeae* and *C. trachomatis* cervicitis and salpingitis varies in different areas. In all regions, however, the two often coexist.[4,31] Because concomitant infection is frequent and it is clinically difficult to distinguish one type of infection from the other, management includes empiric treatment with antibiotics active against both pathogens.[6,13,19,35,36]

DISPOSITION

Suggested criteria for admission are listed in Table 82.3. Hospitalization is indicated for pregnant patients. A combination of ceftriaxone and erythromycin is considered safe, although the estolate form of the erythromycin must be avoided

TABLE 82.3. Criteria for Which Hospitalization Should Be Considered in PID Patients

1. Toxic appearance[a]
2. Nausea and vomiting precluding oral therapy[a]
3. Suspected tuboovarian or pelvic abscess[a]
4. Pregnancy[a]
5. Uncertain diagnosis, particularly if other surgical emergencies cannot be ruled out (i.e., ectopic pregnancy, appendicitis)[a]
6. Intrauterine device
7. Nulligravida
8. Failure to improve with outpatient therapy within 72 hours[a,b]
9. Peritonitis, spread beyond pelvis[a]
10. Adolescent (unpredictable compliance)[a]
11. HIV infection or other immunocompromised conditions
12. Follow-up within 72 hours of initiating antibiotic therapy cannot be arranged.[a]
13. Patient is unable to follow or tolerate an outpatient regimen.[a]

Note: None of these criteria are absolute; all should be applied on an individual basis.

[a]Patients with these criteria should be strongly considered for admission. Patients with the above characteristics but who appear clinically well, are reliable, and can be followed closely as outpatients, need not be admitted to the hospital.

[b]Clinical criteria for improvement within 72 hours consist of defervescence, reduction in direct or rebound abdominal tenderness, and reduction in uterine, adnexal, and cervical motion tenderness within 3–5 days of initiation of therapy.

From Centers for Disease Control and Prevention. 1998 Guidelines for treatment of sexually transmitted diseases. *MMWR* 1998;47(RR-1):1–111.

because it may produce hepatitis. Women with HIV infection are also considered candidates for hospitalization.

Outpatient management is appropriate for those patients not meeting criteria for admission shown in Table 82.3. All discharged patients should receive follow-up care to ensure response to treatment. If cultures are obtained, a mechanism should be in place to ensure that patients and their physicians or the public health department are notified of positive results.[15]

COMMON PITFALLS

- The most serious problem is the general insensitivity of the history, physical examination, and laboratory results in the diagnosis of PID.
- All women with abdominal pain do not have PID; a differential diagnosis must be maintained, particularly in regard to ectopic pregnancy and appendicitis.
- If the clinical picture suggests PID, treatment should be initiated early.
- The clinician should question the diagnosis of pelvic infection in any patient with unilateral pelvic pain.
- Pregnancy must be ruled out.
- Urinary tract irritative voiding symptoms may confuse the picture in PID; a pelvic examination is mandatory to rule out PID.
- Serologic testing for syphilis and HIV testing are indicated for most women with sexually transmitted disease.

References

1. Abbott J, Emmans L, Lowenstein R. Ectopic pregnancy: 10 common pitfalls in diagnosis. *Am J Emerg Med* 1991;8:515.
2. American College of Obstetricians and Gynecologists. *Gonorrhea and chlamydia infections.* Technical Bulletin no. 190. Washington, DC: American College of Obstetrics and Gynecology, 1994.
3. Arredondo JL, Diaz V, Gaitan H, et al. Oral clindamycin and ciprofloxacin versus intramuscular ceftriaxone and oral doxycycline in the treatment of mild-to-moderate pelvic inflammatory disease in outpatients. *Clin Infect Dis* 1997;24:170.

4. Birnbaumer D. Diagnosis and management of sexually transmitted diseases, Part 1. *Crit Decis Emerg Med* 1993;7:256.
5. Cates W, Wasserheit JN. Genital chlamydial infections: epidemiology and reproductive sequelae. *Am J Obstet Gynecol* 1991;164:1771.
6. Centers for Disease Control and Prevention. 1998 guidelines for treatment of sexually transmitted diseases. *MMWR* 1998;47(RR-1):1.
7. Centers for Disease Control. Chlamydia trachomatis genital infections—United States, 1995. *MMWR* 1997;46:193.
8. Chaudhry R, Thakur R, Talwar V, et al. Anaerobic and aerobic microflora of pouch of Douglas aspirate vs. high vaginal swab in cases of pelvic inflammatory disease. *Ind J Pathol Microbiol* 1996;39:115.
9. Cunningham FG. Treatment and prevention of female pelvic infection: the quest for single agent therapy. *Am J Obstet Gynecol* 1987;157:485.
10. Deeney J, Sacchetti AD. Pelvic pain—part I. *Curr Top Emerg Med* 1983;1:4.
11. Deeney J, Sacchetti AD. Pelvic pain—part II. *Curr Top Emerg Med* 1983;1:5.
12. Eschenbach DA, Wolner-Hanseen P, Hawes DE, et al. Acute pelvic inflammatory disease: associates of clinical and laboratory findings with laparoscopic findings. *Obstet Gynecol* 1997;16:157.
13. Handsfield H, Ronald A, Corey L, et al. Evaluation of new anti-infective drugs for the treatment of sexually transmitted chlamydial infections and related clinical syndromes. *Clin Infect Dis* 1992;15[Suppl 1]:S131 (published errata appear in *Clin Infect Dis* 1993;16:346).
14. Joesoef MR, Westrom L, Reynolds G, et al. Recurrence of ectopic pregnancy: the role of salpingitis. *Am J Obstet Gynecol* 1991;165:46.
15. Kuhn GJ, Campbell A, Merline J, et al. Diagnosis and follow-up of chlamydia trachomatis infections in the ED. *Am J Emerg Med* 1998;16:157.
16. Manis RD, Harris B, Geiseler PJ, et al. Evaluation of Gonozyme, an enzyme immunoassay for the rapid diagnosis of gonorrhea. *J Clin Microbiol* 1984;20:742.
17. Mardh PA, Hoff V. Are oral contraceptives masking symptoms of chlamydial cervicitis and pelvic inflammatory disease? *Eur J Contracept Reprod Health Care* 1998;3:41.
18. Martin DH, Mroczkowski TF, Dalu ZA, et al. A controlled trial of a single dose of azithromycin for the treatment of chlamydial urethritis and cervicitis. *N Engl J Med* 1992;327:921.
19. McCormack WM. Pelvic inflammatory disease. *N Engl J Med* 1994;330:115.
20. McNeeley SG, Hendrix SL, Mazzoni MM, et al. Medically sound, cost-effective treatment for pelvic inflammatory disease and tuboovarian abscess. *Am J Obstet Gynecol* 1998;178:1272.
21. Morcos R, Frost N, Hnat M, et al. Laparoscopic versus clinical diagnosis of acute pelvic inflammatory disease. *J Reprod Med* 1993;38:53.
22. Paavonen J, Lehtinen M. Chlamydial pelvic inflammatory disease. *Hum Reprod Update* 1996;2:519.
23. Paavonen J, Teisala K, Heinonen PK, et al. Microbiological and histopathological findings in acute pelvic inflammatory disease. *Br J Obstet Gynaecol* 1987;94:454.
24. Peipert JF, Montagno AB, Cooper AS, et al. Bacterial vaginosis in adolescents: a review. *Am J Obstet Gynecol* 1997;177:1184.
25. Plummer DC, Garland SM, Gilbert GL. Bacteremia and pelvic infection in women due to Ureaplasma urealyticum and Mycoplasma hominis. *Med J Aust* 1987;146:135.
26. Potts J. Chlamydial infection. Screening and management update, 1992. *Postgrad Med* 1991;91:120.
27. Ramoska EA, Sacchetti AD, Nepp M. Reliability of patient history in determining the possibility of pregnancy. *Ann Emerg Med* 1989;18:48.
28. Reddy SPM, Yeturu SR, Slupik R. Chlamydia trachomatis in adolescents: a review. *J Pediatr Adolesc Gynecol* 1997;10:59.
29. Sellors J, Mahony J, Goldsmith C, et al. The accuracy of clinical findings and laparoscopy in pelvic inflammatory disease. *Am J Obstet Gynecol* 1991;164:113.
30. Soper D. Diagnosis and laparoscopic grading of acute salpingitis. *Am J Obstet Gynecol* 1991;164:1370.
31. Soper DE, Brockwell NJ, Dalton HP. Microbial etiology of urban emergency department acute salpingitis: treatment with ofloxacin. *Am J Obstet Gynecol* 1992;167:653.
32. Stamm WE. Diagnosis of *Neisseria gonorrhoeae* and *Chlamydia trachomatis* infections using antigen detection methods. *Diagn Microbiol Infect Dis* 1986;4:93S.
33. Sweet R. Pelvic inflammatory disease. *Hosp Pract* 1993;28:25(S-2).
34. Taylor-Robinson D, Furr PM. Genital mycoplasma infections. *Wien Klin Wochenschr* 1997;109:578.
35. Treatment of sexually transmitted diseases. *Med Lett Drugs Ther* 1999;36:913.
36. Wendel GD, Cox SM, Bawdon RE, et al. A randomized trial of ofloxacin versus cefoxitin and doxycycline in outpatient treatment of acute salpingitis. *Am J Obstet Gynecol* 1991;164:1390.
37. Westrom L, Wolner-Hanssen P. Pathogenesis of pelvic inflammatory disease. *Genitourin Med* 1993;69:9.
38. Witkin S, Jeremias J, Toth M, et al. Detection of *Chlamydia trachomatis* by the polymerase chain reaction in the cervices of women with acute salpingitis. *Am J Obstet Gynecol* 1993;168:1438.
39. Wolner-Hanssen P, Eschenbach DA, Paavonen J, et al. Decreased risk of symptomatic chlamydial pelvic inflammatory disease associated with oral contraceptive use. *JAMA* 1990;263:54.

CHAPTER 83

Non–Pregnancy-Related Vaginal Bleeding

Eric Anderson and H. Trent MacKay

Abnormal vaginal bleeding unrelated to pregnancy is a common gynecologic complaint and may occasionally present as a life-threatening emergency. Such bleeding can be categorized by the source as either uterine or extrauterine. Extrauterine bleeding may be caused by trauma, a foreign body, or a lesion involving the cervix, vagina, vulva, or urinary tract. Abnormal vaginal bleeding may be the first sign of a vaginal or cervical malignancy or may occur after cervical conization or hysterectomy. Postcoital bleeding may be due to a benign cervical lesion, such as a polyp or inflammation caused by an infection, or it may be caused by a previously undiagnosed cervical cancer.

Bleeding caused by a foreign body in the vagina is a relatively frequent presentation in premenarchal girls.[4] Postoperative bleeding most commonly occurs at the time absorbable sutures dissolve. The usual site of bleeding after hysterectomy is the vaginal cuff, and after cervical conization, bleeding may occur from the operative site. Occasionally, bleeding from urethral prolapse or hematuria may be confused with a gynecologic source.

Uterine bleeding may be either cyclic (menorrhagia) or unrelated to the menstrual cycle (metrorrhagia). It may be dysfunctional (hormonal) in origin, related to a benign or malignant lesion, or caused by a coagulopathy. Endometrial cancer, endometrial polyps, or submucous leiomyomata may cause abnormal bleeding. Bleeding may also be related to pelvic inflammatory disease, coagulopathies associated with leukemia, aplastic anemia, von Willebrand disease, or other hematologic disorders. Functioning ovarian tumors are a rare source of abnormal bleeding.

Dysfunctional uterine bleeding, which is defined as abnormal uterine bleeding in the absence of organic pathology on clinical pelvic examination, is usually related to anovulation with estrogen overstimulation of proliferative endometrium unopposed by the stabilizing influence of progesterone, leading to spontaneous breakdown of the endometrium. The bleeding is typically both excessive and prolonged. Treatment of dysfunctional bleeding is directed at stabilizing the endometrium with a progestational agent, combination oral contraceptive, or, if necessary, high-dose estrogen. Dysfunctional bleeding is most common in the adolescent and in the perimenopausal woman and less common in women aged 20 to 35.[1] Breakthrough bleeding due to oral contraceptives, Norplant, or Depo-Provera, or bleeding from an intrauterine device may also bring a woman into the emergency department.

CLINICAL PRESENTATION

Excessive vaginal bleeding may be defined as bleeding that soaks more than one tampon or pad an hour over several hours. Most women with abnormal bleeding are hemodynamically stable. However, the occasional patient may present with a life-threatening hemorrhage. This situation is particularly likely to occur with bleeding from cervical cancer, postoperative bleeding, and dysfunctional bleeding in adolescents. Many women with dysfunctional bleeding have a history of delayed menses with the onset of heavy, painless vaginal bleeding.

DIFFERENTIAL DIAGNOSIS

The differential diagnosis includes the many possible sources of both extrauterine and uterine bleeding listed in Table 83.1. Diagnosis is based on the patient's age, history, and pelvic examination findings. Pregnancy should always be ruled out in any woman of reproductive age.

EMERGENCY DEPARTMENT EVALUATION

The patient's history, including her menstrual history, contraceptive history, and any history of bleeding problems may lead to a diagnosis. A thorough pelvic examination is usually the key to diagnosis. The vulva, vagina, and cervix must be carefully examined for lesions. The size and shape of the uterus and the adnexal structures must be determined by bimanual examination. The anus should be inspected, and a rectovaginal examination, including a guaiac test, should be performed. Transvaginal ultrasound may be useful in identifying anatomic sources of bleeding, such as endometrial polyps or submucous leiomyomata.[3] Laboratory tests should include a pregnancy test and complete blood count. Clotting studies are usually not necessary unless suspicion of a bleeding diathesis exists.

EMERGENCY DEPARTMENT MANAGEMENT AND DISPOSITION

Although life-threatening non–pregnancy-related vaginal bleeding is unusual, patients who are hemodynamically unstable require rapid diagnosis and stabilization. Pelvic examination usually reveals the source of the bleeding. A large-bore intravenous line should be started and blood sent for complete blood count and type and crossmatch.

Mild-to-moderate bleeding from a cervical or vaginal lesion can usually be controlled by application of a silver nitrate stick or a cotton swab with Monsel's solution (ferric subsulfate). If control is not obtained, an obvious bleeding vessel or the lesion itself can be sutured with a figure-of-eight stitch of 0 chromic or 0 polyglycolic acid suture. Suturing is also the appropriate method of dealing with postoperative bleeding from the cervix or vaginal cuff or with traumatic lesions with significant bleeding. Consultation with the gynecologist should occur.

TABLE 83.1. Non–Pregnancy-Related Abnormal Vaginal Bleeding

Nonuterine Causes	Uterine Causes
Vulva	Endometrial polyp
Malignant neoplasm	Submucous leiomyoma
Benign neoplastic lesions	Endometrial hyperplasia
Trauma	Endometrial carcinoma
Ulcerative lesions	Chronic endometritis
Urethral caruncle	Intrauterine device
Condyloma acuminata	Coagulopathy
Vagina	Dysfunctional uterine bleeding
Vaginitis	Breakthrough bleeding
Trauma	
Malignant neoplasm	
Foreign body	
Condyloma acuminata	
Postoperative	
Cervix	
Malignant neoplasm	
Cervical polyps	
Cervicitis	
Ectropion	

If neither of these approaches controls the bleeding, a gauze pack soaked in acetone, phenylephrine hydrochloride 1:200,000, or epinephrine 1:200,000 often provides control. If none of these methods is effective, specialist consultation should be obtained rapidly. Other treatment alternatives include radiologically directed selective arterial embolization, emergency radiation therapy for malignant lesions, and hypogastric artery ligation.

Copious uterine bleeding in the hemodynamically unstable patient can often be rapidly controlled with dilatation and curettage. Gynecologic consultation should be sought for these procedures.

Pediatric patients with vaginal bleeding should have a vaginal examination with a small instrument, such as a nasal speculum, to search for foreign bodies. If the emergency physician is comfortable with this procedure, it can be performed in the emergency department. The presence of vulvar or vaginal trauma may suggest child abuse or sexual abuse, and requires follow-up by social services and law enforcement agencies.

Dysfunctional uterine bleeding in adolescents and women under age 35 can almost always be controlled with hormonal therapy. In this age group, dilatation and curettage should be reserved for cases not controlled with medication or for situations in which there is a high risk of endometrial hyperplasia. Premenopausal women over age 35 require endometrial sampling before they receive hormonal therapy because of their increased risk of endometrial hyperplasia. Hormonal control of heavy dysfunctional bleeding can be obtained in most cases with any combination oral contraceptive such as Ortho-Novum 1/35 or Ovcon 35, using one pill four times a day for 1 or 2 days until the bleeding slows, then two pills daily until day 5, and then one pill daily for an additional 20 days.

If bleeding is profuse, more rapid control may be obtained with intravenous conjugated estrogen (25 mg every 4 hours for three or four doses), followed by the previously described oral contraceptive regimen.[2] Patients should continue on combination oral contraceptives for an additional 2 or 3 months and should be referred for gynecologic follow-up before completing the course of medication. If these regimens fail to acutely control dysfunctional bleeding, dilatation and curettage must be performed.

All women over age 35 with dysfunctional bleeding and all postmenopausal women with bleeding other than withdrawal bleeding with estrogen replacement therapy should have an endometrial biopsy.[5] Although the initial diagnostic procedure may be performed in the emergency department, these patients should be referred for gynecologic consultation.

The occasional patient who presents in the emergency department with breakthrough bleeding on oral contraceptives, Norplant, or Depo-Provera may be reassured as to the benign nature of the bleeding. Control of breakthrough bleeding may be obtained with a 7-day course of conjugated estrogen 1.25 mg, or estradiol 2 mg.[6]

COMMON PITFALLS

- The most common pitfall in the treatment of abnormal bleeding is the unnecessary use of dilatation and curettage for the treatment of dysfunctional bleeding in women under age 35. Almost all adolescents and women under age 35 can be successfully treated with hormonal therapy.
- Pregnancy must be considered in all women of reproductive age.

References

1. Brenner PF. Differential diagnosis of vaginal bleeding. *Am J Obstet Gynecol* 1996;175:766.
2. DeVore GR, Owens O, Kase N. Use of intravenous Premarin in the treatment of dysfunctional uterine bleeding—a double-blind randomized control study. *Obstet Gynecol* 1982;59:285.

3. Goldstein SR, Zeltser I, et al. Ultrasonography-based triage for perimenopausal patients with abnormal uterine bleeding. *Am J Obstet Gynecol* 1996;177:102.
4. Paradise JE, Willis ED. Probability of vaginal foreign body in girls with genital complaints. *Am J Dis Child* 1985;139:472.
5. Petrozza JC, Polet K. Dysfunctional uterine bleeding. In: Curtis MG, Hopkins MP, eds. *Glass's office gynecology*, 5th ed. Baltimore: Williams & Wilkins, 1999.
6. Speroff L, Darney PD. *Clinical guide for contraception*, 2nd ed. Baltimore: Williams & Wilkins, 1996.

CHAPTER 84
Amenorrhea

Stuart P. Swadron and William K. Mallon

Unlike hemorrhage, amenorrhea is less likely to be perceived by a patient as an emergency. Despite this reality, patients do present to the emergency department with amenorrhea. *Primary amenorrhea* is defined as the absence of menses by age 16 or by age 14 if secondary sexual characteristics are also absent. *Secondary amenorrhea* is defined as the absence of menses for at least three cycle lengths or for 6 months in a previously menstruating woman.[2,16] From the point of view of the emergency physician, any delay in menses could be significant, and these definitions are less relevant. There is significant overlap in the workup of primary and secondary amenorrhea, and some authorities no longer utilize these traditional categories for clinical evaluation.[15] Furthermore, evaluation may be warranted in the absence of these somewhat arbitrary criteria in the patient with certain other important signs, such as galactorrhea, hirsutism, or weight loss.

CLINICAL PRESENTATION

While amenorrhea may be the principal reason for a visit to the emergency department, it is most often an important secondary aspect of another chief complaint. It is well established that both history and physical examination are unreliable in the detection of early pregnancy.[13] Women using various methods of contraception and even those who have had tubal ligation have been found to be pregnant.[13] It is imperative that pregnancy be eliminated from the differential diagnosis in all women of reproductive age. Pregnancy can be reliably detected using a sensitive blood or urine assay for β-human chorionic gonadotropin (β-hCG). In fact, many emergency departments incorporate a routine inquiry regarding menstruation during the triage process. These triage data serve to alert the emergency physician to the possibility of pregnancy so that radiographs and other potentially harmful diagnostic studies or treatments are not employed, particularly in the first trimester.[9] Emergencies related to pregnancy are discussed elsewhere in this text.

Due to the sensitivity of the modern pregnancy test (either urine or serum β-hCG), a positive test may be obtained even prior to missed menses. Commonly employed bedside pregnancy tests will become positive at a level between 10 and 50 IU, and a level of 100 U is typically found at the time of the expected but missed menses in a normal pregnancy.[15] Even in the absence of any menstrual irregularity, pregnancy testing may be warranted if potentially harmful procedures or treatments are to be employed. With pregnancy rates as high as 10% to 15% in women presenting to the emergency department with no history of menstrual irregularity, routine screening for pregnancy has been advocated by some authors.[9,13]

Common physiologic states other than pregnancy may result in amenorrhea. Constitutional delay, for example, may result in primary amenorrhea. The perimenopausal and postmenopausal periods are associated with secondary amenorrhea. Even when such a physiologic state is strongly suggested by the patient's presentation, the emergency physician should not be misled into a false sense of security—pregnancy should always be considered first in the evaluation. This error can easily be made during the period of amenorrhea associated with postpartum lactation. Although lactation provides a contraceptive effect, it is short-lived and unreliable.[15]

Patients receiving hormonal contraception may also experience amenorrhea. This is especially true of long-acting formulations such as intramuscular depot-medroxyprogesterone acetate (Depo-Provera) or implanted levonorgestrel (Norplant). Although women who remain amenorrheic throughout their use of these agents are unlikely to become pregnant,[15] pregnancy must again be the first consideration in the emergency department. After a negative pregnancy test, an explanation to the patient and referral back to the primary physician are appropriate.

"Post-pill" amenorrhea is a misnomer. Its incidence is actually similar to the rate of spontaneous secondary amenorrhea in patients with no history of hormonal contraception.[12,15,16] In addition, rates of fertility among women who have stopped hormonal contraception do not differ significantly from those of the general population.[15] Therefore, all patients who have not resumed normal menstrual function after discontinuation of hormonal contraception should be considered pregnant until otherwise proven. The remainder of the amenorrhea evaluation, however, may be delayed for 6 to 12 months after discontinuation of contraceptive therapy, after which time amenorrhea can no longer be ascribed to the therapy.[15]

DIFFERENTIAL DIAGNOSIS

Once pregnancy has been ruled out, the causes of amenorrhea can be divided into disorders of the four compartments that underlie the process of normal menstruation. These are disorders of the uterus and outflow tract, disorders of the ovaries, disorders of the anterior pituitary gland, and disorders of the hypothalamus and higher central nervous system (CNS) centers (Fig. 84.1).[3,15] Table 84.1 utilizes this four-compartment model to present the differential diagnosis of amenorrhea. Although many etiologies can result in either primary or secondary amenorrhea, their relative incidence as a cause of each clearly differs. Ovarian causes predominate in primary amenorrhea, whereas hypothalamic causes predominate in secondary amenorrhea.[3]

EMERGENCY DEPARTMENT EVALUATION

The diagnostic algorithm in the nonpregnant patient with amenorrhea varies only slightly among different authors and has not changed substantially in recent years. Figure 84.2 gives an abbreviated outline of such an algorithm. Clearly, most of the evaluation is not emergent and may be performed in the outpatient setting after specialist referral. However, several causes of amenorrhea in the nonpregnant patient may pose a serious threat to life and deserve special consideration by the emergency physician.

Anorexia Nervosa

Anorexia nervosa, characterized by low body weight, disordered eating habits, and distorted body image, may be heralded

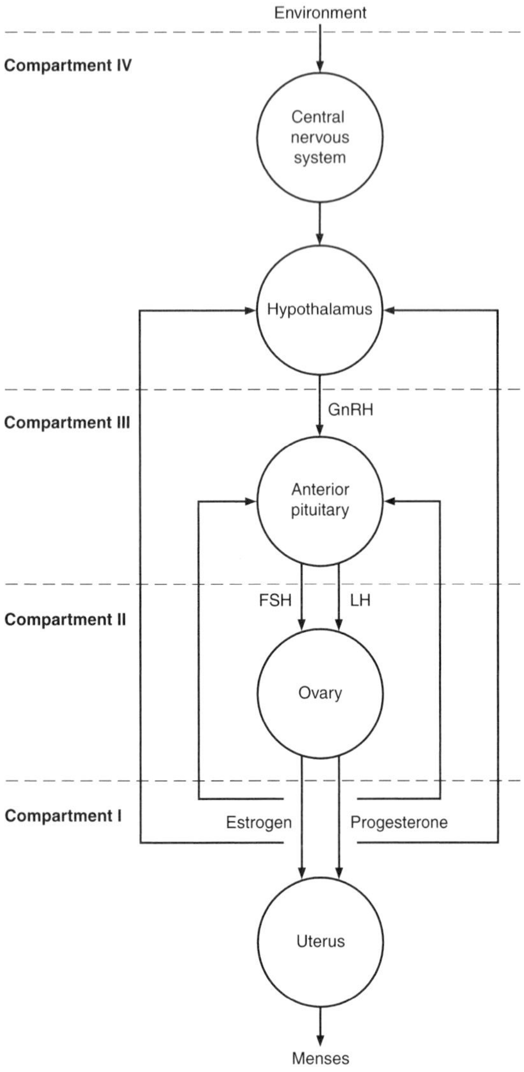

Figure 84.1. The four-compartment model for normal menstruation.

TABLE 84.1. Causes of Amenorrhea

PHYSIOLOGIC
Constitutional delay
Lactation
Perimenopausal and postmenopausal
Pregnancy
PATHOLOGIC
Disorders of the Uterus or Outflow Tract
Androgen insensitivity
Asherman syndrome
Mullerian agenesis or abnormalities
Disorders of the Ovary
Effects of radiation or antineoplastic drugs
Gonadal agenesis/dysgenesis
Mosaicism
Polycystic ovary syndrome
Polyglandular autoimmune endocrine disease
Premature ovarian failure
Resistant ovary syndrome
Disorders of the Anterior Pituitary
Pituitary tumors
Prolactinoma
Other
Sheehan syndrome
Disorders of the Hypothalamus and CNS
Anorexia nervosa
Drugs
α-Methyldopa
Heterocyclic antidepressants
Metoclopramide
Neuroleptics (phenothiazine and butyrophenone)
Opiates
Rifampin
Serotonin reuptake inhibitors
Steroid hormones
Exercise
Female athlete triad (amenorrhea, osteoporosis, eating disorder)[20]
Genetic (e.g., Kallman syndrome)
Hypoadrenalism and hyperadrenalism
Hypothyroidism
Infection (subacute, e.g., TB, syphilis)
Infiltrative (e.g., sarcoidosis, hemolytic anemias)
Neoplasm (e.g., craniopharyngioma)
Other systemic diseases
Psychosocial stress

by amenorrhea.[6] Common associated clinical symptoms and signs are constipation, abdominal pain, hypotension, hypothermia, dry skin, parotid enlargement, soft lanugo-type hair, and edema.[6,10] Although low body weight itself may be a major determinant of amenorrhea in these patients, amenorrhea may be present before significant weight loss occurs.[6,19] From a psychiatric standpoint, these patients are often secretive and deny their symptoms.[6,10] Therefore, a high level of vigilance is required so that this potentially fatal disorder may be recognized and referred at an early stage.

Bulimia

Bulimia is a syndrome of episodic binge eating followed by self-induced vomiting, fasting, or the use laxatives or diuretics.[10] It may occur together with anorexia nervosa. Clinical features are few but may include fluctuating weight, dental caries from repeated vomiting, and scars from self-mutilation. Although amenorrhea is less common in bulimics who are not underweight, the possibility of life-threatening electrolyte abnormalities must be considered, most notably hypokalemia.[6]

Intracranial Space-Occupying Lesions

The presence of headaches, galactorrhea, visual field changes, or any other neurologic symptoms or signs in association with amenorrhea may represent an intracranial space-occupying lesion, most commonly of the pituitary gland. In this instance, an imaging study in the emergency department (computed tomography [CT] or magnetic resonance imaging [MRI]) may prevent an undue delay of diagnosis. Although there has been a clear trend toward the use of MRI for the identification of subacute parenchymal lesions,[8] CT scanning is probably still preferable in the emergency department. Not only is CT more readily available and less expensive, but its increased sensitivity for detecting bleeding and bony pathology[8] underscores its utility for the emergency physician who treats an undifferentiated population. Once emergent pathology has been ruled out, MRI studies may be pursued on an outpatient basis.

Drug-Associated Amenorrhea

Certain medications may cause amenorrhea. Most exert this effect on a neuroendocrine basis, although certain agents are directly toxic to the ovaries. A list of commonly implicated prescription drugs is included in Table 84.1. Perhaps more important to the emergency physician, drugs of abuse have also been implicated. The causal relationship of heroin and other opiates to amenorrhea is well established.[1] Opiates, either en-

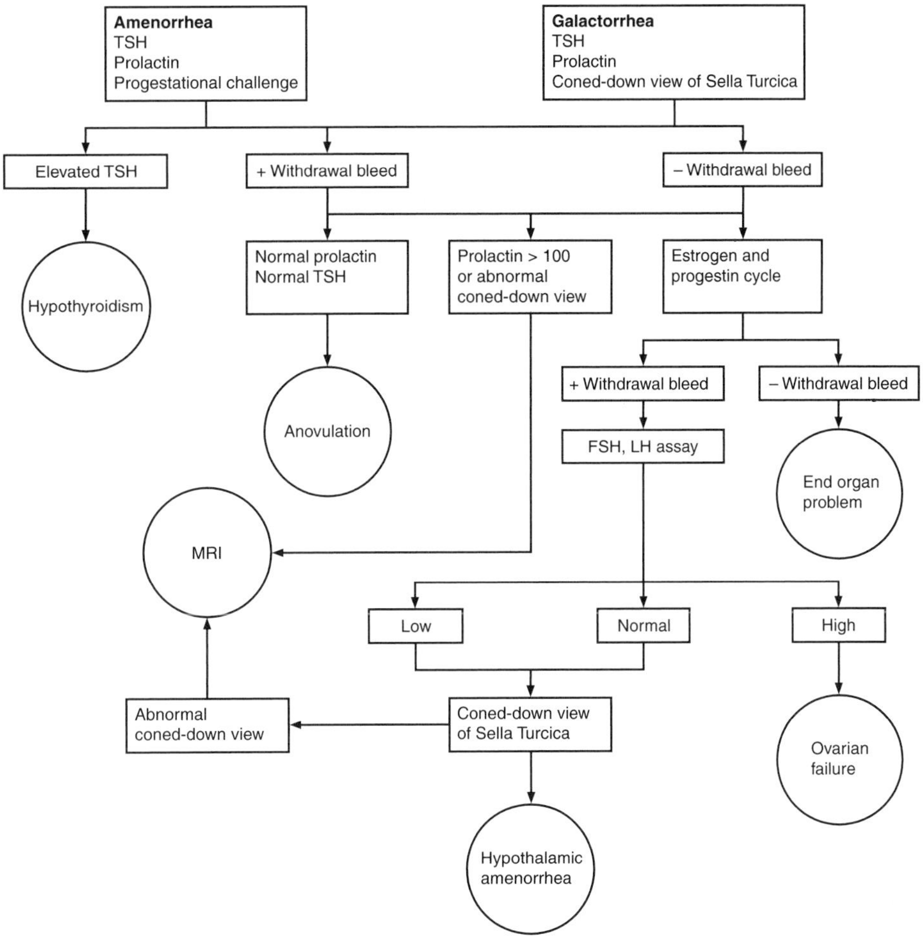

Figure 84.2. Diagnostic algorithm for the amenorrhea in the nonpregnant patient.

dogenous or exogenous, can suppress ovulation by inhibiting the hypothalamic release of gonadotropin-releasing hormone. The relationships with alcohol and sympathomimetics are less clear, with studies plagued by the confounding variables of nutritional and socioeconomic status.[7,17,18]

Serious Systemic Illnesses

There are a number of serious systemic illnesses that may present in association with amenorrhea. Systemic illness may interfere with normal menstruation at more than one of the four compartments mentioned earlier. For example, tuberculosis can cause amenorrhea centrally through weight loss and neuroendocrine effects, but it may also directly invade the uterus, causing end-organ damage. Many endocrine diseases disrupt the menstrual cycle at the hypothalamic–pituitary level. In the majority of these cases, there will be other clues, but the amenorrhea itself may enable the emergency physician to ultimately reach the diagnosis. With a list of potential causes so diverse as to include sarcoidosis,[14] type I diabetes mellitus,[14] and even possibly human immunodeficiency virus,[4,5] a compulsive and broad-minded approach is essential.

In the absence of any of these specific concerns, the evaluation of amenorrhea may be initiated in the emergency department with outpatient follow-up. History should be thorough with respect to menstruation, contraceptive use, and sexual function and should also include an assessment for weight loss, exercise level, and psychosocial stressors. Physical examination should include a pelvic examination in the postmenarchal patient, assessment for galactorrhea, and a screening examination for signs of endocrine or other systemic disease. As always, intimate examinations in the emergency department should be chaperoned and documented as such in the treatment record. After a pregnancy test, blood may be sent for thyroid-stimulating hormone and prolactin levels. If there are signs of virilization, tests for DHEA-S and testosterone levels may be added.

Amenorrhea itself is not necessarily benign. The associated underlying hormonal changes have important implications. Hypoestrogenemia affects mineral metabolism and can lead to significant bone loss and osteoporosis.[2,20] Young women may be at even greater risk as they are prevented from attaining their desired peak bone mass.[11] There also may be an increased risk of cardiovascular disease in such women. If unopposed estrogen underlies amenorrhea, there is an increased risk of uterine cancer.[11] Because of these implications for future health, it is indeed important for all patients presenting to the emergency department to receive follow-up and treatment for amenorrhea.

DISPOSITION

Nonpregnant patients with amenorrhea without evidence of serious systemic illness may be referred for outpatient gynecology follow-up within a week following the emergency department visit. Hospitalization may be required for an underlying systemic illness when identified. Hospitalization may be life-saving in cases of severe anorexia nervosa; however, its routine use in the initial presentation is disputed.[6]

COMMON PITFALLS

- The failure to consider the possibility of pregnancy is the most common pitfall in the evaluation of amenorrhea. All patients with amenorrhea should have a pregnancy test.

- Serious systemic illness should always be considered as a cause of amenorrhea in the nonpregnant patient.
- In the nonpregnant patient with amenorrhea and without symptoms or signs of serious illness, care should be taken to avoid the indiscriminate use of expensive endocrinologic tests or MRI, which can safely be performed during outpatient follow-up.
- All patients who are not admitted to the hospital who present with amenorrhea should be referred for appropriate follow-up. Failure to refer could result in the failure to diagnose a serious underlying pathology or the development of complications.
- Anorexia nervosa is a potentially life-threatening cause of amenorrhea that is easily overlooked. It should always be considered in the evaluation of the nonpregnant patient with amenorrhea.

References

1. Bai J, et al. Drug-related menstrual aberrations. *Obstet Gynecol* 1974;44:713.
2. Baird DT. Amenorrhoea. *Lancet* 1997;350:275.
3. Barbieri RL, Ryan KJ. The menstrual cycle. In: Ryan KJ, Berkowitz RS, Barbieri RL, eds. *Kirstner's gynecology: principles and practice,* 6th ed. St. Louis: Mosby, 1995.
4. Chirgwin KD, et al. Menstrual function in human immunodeficiency virus-infected women without acquired immunodeficiency syndrome. *J AIDS* 1996;12:489.
5. Ellerbrock TV, et al. Characteristics of menstruation in women infected with human immunodeficiency virus. *Obstet Gynecol* 1996;87:1030.
6. Foster DW. Anorexia nervosa and bulimia nervosa. In: Fauci AS, et al. *Harrison's principles of internal medicine,* 14th ed. New York: McGraw-Hill, 1998:462.
7. Gruber AJ, Pope HG Jr. Ephedrine abuse among 36 female weightlifters. *Am J Addict* 1998;7:256.
8. Hesselink JR, et al. MR imaging of brain contusions: a comparative study with CT. *AJR* 1988;150:1133.
9. Hirsh HL. Routine pregnancy testing: is it standard of care? *South Med J* 1980;73:1365.
10. Kaplan HI, Sadock BJ. *Synopsis of psychiatry,* 8th ed. Baltimore: Williams & Wilkins, 1998.
11. Mciver B. Evaluation and management of amenorrhea. *Mayo Clin Proc* 1997;72:1161.
12. Munster K, Helm P, Schmidt L. Secondary amenorrhoea: prevalence and medical contact—a cross-sectional study from a Danish county. *Br J Obstet Gynaecol* 1992;99:434.
13. Ramoska EA, et al. Reliability of patient history in determining the possibility of pregnancy. *Ann Emerg Med* 1989;18:48.
14. Reyes FI. Hypothalamic-pituitary disease. In: Gold JJ, Josimovich JB, eds. *Gynecologic endocrinology,* 4th ed. New York: Plenum Publishing, 1987.
15. Speroff L, Glass HG, Kase NG. *Clinical gynecologic endocrinology and infertility,* 5th ed. Baltimore: Williams & Wilkins, 1994.
16. Scommegna A, Carson SA. Secondary amenorrhea and the menopause. In: Gold JJ, Josimovich JB, eds. *Gynecologic endocrinology,* 4th ed. New York: Plenum Publishing, 1987.
17. Stoffer SS, et al. Effect of D-amphetamine on menstruation. *Am J Obstet Gynecol* 1969;105:989.
18. Teoh SK, et al. Hyperprolactinemia and macrocytosis in women with alcohol and polysubstance dependence. *J Stud Alcohol* 1992;53:176.
19. Vigersky RA, et al. Hypothalamic dysfunction in secondary amenorrhea associated with simple weight loss. *N Engl J Med* 1977;297:1141.
20. West RV. The female athlete. The triad of disordered eating, amenorrhea and osteoporosis. *Sports Med* 1998;26:63.

CHAPTER 85
Vaginitis

Constance S. Greene

Vaginal discharge is the most common gynecologic symptom in women during reproductive years, and many seek emergency care for the discomfort. Other symptoms of vaginal infection are unpleasant odor, pruritus, burning, superficial dyspareunia, and dysuria. In this age group, the vaginitis is usually due to one of three different causes: a fungus (*Candida* vulvovaginitis), a protozoan (*Trichomonas* vaginitis), or the replacement of the hydrogen peroxide (H_2O_2)–producing, gram-positive lactobacilli of natural vaginal flora with anaerobic bacteria and *Gardnerella vaginalis* in far greater concentrations than they are normally found (bacterial vaginosis). In postmenopausal women, these symptoms are most likely due to atrophic vaginitis. A careful history, pelvic (speculum) examination with pH determination, and microscopic examination of a wet mount slide of the discharge will yield a diagnosis in about 80% of cases (Table 85.1). While cultures were considered the gold standard for diagnosis in the past, polymerase chain reaction identification of the organisms may be more sensitive, but these methods are more suited to the gynecologist's practice than the emergency department (ED).[3]

CANDIDA VULVOVAGINITIS

The organism responsible for this infection is an airborne fungus, almost always *Candida albicans*. Its filamentous forms penetrate the mucosal surface, causing hyperemia and lysis of tissue locally. This infection occurs predominantly during reproductive years, with 75% of women experiencing at least one episode in their lifetimes. Fungi can be isolated from the vaginas of 20% to 40% of asymptomatic women and need not be treated. It is commensal until the ecosystem of the vagina is disturbed. Predisposing factors include hormonal shifts (pregnancy and just premenstrual), antibiotic or immunosuppressant (e.g., corticosteroid) use, diabetes mellitus, and immune suppression, such as with acquired immunodeficiency syndrome. Oral contraceptives, once thought to increase risk, do not in the present low-estrogen dosages. *Candida* infections do not occur simultaneously with bacterial vaginosis or *Trichomonas* infection, but may follow treatment. There is no evidence for sexual transmission, and routine treatment of partners is not recommended.

Recurrence is a major problem, occurring in 20% to 80% of women after an apparent cure. In some cases, this may be due to an unidentified host factor, possibly a subtle defect in cell-mediated immunity. Some women appear to be hypersensitive to a small number of organisms. There is a higher incidence of other fungal species in recurrent infections.

CLINICAL PRESENTATION

Patients primarily complain of vulvar itching, burning, external dysuria, and dyspareunia. The quantity of the discharge is variable. It does not have an odor and may not be a presenting symptom. Vulvar signs are erythema, edema, and traumatic excoriation. There may be satellite pustules at the periphery of inflammation. Insert the speculum gently, as the vagina may be very sore. The typically thick, clumpy discharge will be adherent to the walls or may look like thrush patches. The pH of the vagina is less than 4.5.

The most efficient diagnostic test in the ED is to put a small sample of the discharge or a scraping from a plaque or the erythematous border onto a slide and add 1 to 2 drops of a 10% or 20% solution of potassium hydroxide (KOH). This will dissolve the cellular elements (and the microscope lens as well, if a cover slip is not used!). Several fields may have to be scrutinized to identify the mycelia or pseudohyphae, which appear as tangled, branching chains, or the oval spores that are about one-fourth of the size of a white blood cell (WBC). Although the sensitivity of this method varies widely (from 22% to 80%, averaging 65%), the clinical picture coupled with either the patient's self diagnosis or the absence of a watery discharge or amine odor should prompt the ED physician to treat in most cases.[1]

TABLE 85.1. Features of Vaginal Discharge

Features of Discharge	Normal	Candidiasis	*T. vaginalis*	Bacterial Vaginosis
Color	Clear, white	White	Gray, green-yellow	Gray, white
Consistency	Floccular	Clumped, adherent to vaginal mucosa	Homogenous, occasionally frothy	Homogenous, occasionally frothy
Quantity	Variable; usually scant	Scant to moderate	Profuse	Moderate
pH	≤4.5	≤4.5	≥5.0	≥4.5
Amine odor with KOH	Negative	Negative	Usually positive	Positive
Wet mount	Epithelial cells, lactobacilli	WBCs, epithelial cells, spores, mycelia or pseudohyphae Recommend KOH to dissolve nonfungal cellular elements	WBC, motile trichomonads	Few WBCs, clue cells

TREATMENT

Candida albicans is almost uniformly sensitive to all azoles. Intravaginal agents are inexpensive, available over the counter, effective, and well tolerated by most women. They may be less acceptable to many women than the recently approved single dose (150 mg) of oral fluconazole, which has similar cure rates.[13] If fluconazole is used in diabetic patients on oral hypoglycemic agents, there may be significant hypoglycemia due to drug interaction. The Centers for Disease Control and Prevention (CDC) still recommends topical therapy as a first line.[5] Table 85.2 provides a listing of specific preparations and dosing.

Recurrence

As noted, recurrence of symptoms after a "cure" is particularly problematic in vulvovaginal candidiasis. The cause may be a hypersensitivity to the organism or to the vehicle in topical agents, noncompliance (more likely with topical preparations), infection with an uncommon fungus species, true azole resistance, reinfection from a symptomatic partner, or risk factors, possibly unidentified. Patients who report several episodes should have their urine checked for sugar, especially if they present before puberty or after menopause.

Sexual Partners

Many studies have found no evidence of sexual transmission, and routine treatment of partners does not reduce the incidence of reinfection; therefore, there is no rationale for treating them. About 10% to 27% of men have a balanoposthitis. They should be treated with either the same topical preparation as the patient or a dermatologic fungicide. Oral treatment has not been evaluated.

Pregnancy

The incidence of vulvovaginal *Candida* infection is increased 10- to 20-fold in pregnancy. Oral fluconazole is not recommended. Clotrimazole is effective and safe.

TABLE 85.2. Treatment of Vaginitis

Disorder	First Line	Alternative	Partner	In Pregnancy
T. vaginalis	*Metronidazole 2 g po single dose	*Metronidazole 500 mg b.i.d. for 7 days	*Metronidazole 2 g po single dose	Treat only if symptomatic but treat partner 1st trimester, clotrimazole 100 mg hs for 7 days After 1st trimester, 2 g *Metronidazole
Bacterial vaginosis	*Oral* *Metronidazole 500 mg b.i.d. for 7 days *or* Clindamycin 300 mg po b.i.d. for 7 days *or* *Intravaginal* 0.75% Metronidazole gel b.i.d. for 5 days *or* 2% clindamycin cream hs for 7 days	*Metronidazole 2 g po single dose *or* Amoxicillin/clavulinic acid 500 mg t.i.d. for 7 days	Exam for STD No Rx if normal	1st trimester, clindamycin vaginal cream 2%, one applicator vaginally for seven days if symptoms are distressing After 1st trimester, 2 g Metronidazole po once *or* 500 mg b.i.d. for 7 days po
Candidiasis	Butoconazole 2% cream 5 g intravaginally for 3 days *or* Fluconazole 150 mg po single dose	Clotrimazole 1% 5 g cream intravaginally for 7–14 days (OTC)	Candicidal cream if dermatitis present	Avoid fluconazole and ketoconazole. Treat for 7 days

*Patients should be warned to avoid alcohol for 24 hours after last dose.

TRICHOMONAS VAGINITIS

Approximately one-fourth of vaginal infections are caused by *Trichomonas vaginalis,* a unicellular protozoon that is sexually transmitted. It is found in the vagina and 90% of the time in the lower urethra and Skene's ducts. Male partners are usually asymptomatic, but may complain of the symptoms of urethritis. They harbor the organisms in the urethra and paraurethral glands and occasionally in the seminal vesicles, epididymis, and prostate. Trichomoniasis is often concurrent with bacterial vaginosis and gonorrhea, and probably other sexually transmitted diseases as well. Trichomonads are also suspected of being vectors in pelvic inflammatory disease. In any event, because the epidemiology of all sexually transmitted diseases is similar, the emergency physician should either do appropriate screening for gonorrhea, chlamydia, and syphilis or refer the patient for these and for human immunodeficiency virus (HIV) counseling regarding testing and safe sexual practice.

Trichomonads are often noted on urine microscopy in asymptomatic women. One-third of these women will become symptomatic within 3 months. It is prudent to treat them.

Polymerase chain reaction analysis of vaginal secretions has been shown to be very sensitive in identifying *T. vaginalis.* However, on-site wet mount slide microscopy still seems sensitive enough, inexpensive, and practical for ED diagnosis.[10,11]

CLINICAL PRESENTATION

The primary symptom of acute *Trichomonas* infection is profuse vaginal discharge. Patients often complain of feeling wet. The discharge is thin and may be white, gray, yellow, or green. It has been classically described as "frothy," but this is only present 10% to 20% of the time. It is often malodorous. Dysuria is present 20% of the time. Patients with chronic infection may complain only of a malodorous discharge. The examiner frequently notes the discharge on the vulva, which can also be erythematous and edematous. Unlike candidiasis, which can cause extensive involvement of the vulva and perineum, inflammation due to *Trichomonas* is usually limited to the vestibule and labia minora. The vaginal walls are inflamed and the discharge is copious in amount.

A saline wet mount of the discharge should be viewed under low power first to identify areas of relatively few WBCs. In fresh warm preparations, trichomonads will have a twitchy forward motion. They are slightly larger than WBCs. If the slide has an abundance of WBCs, or the typical movement is not seen, a higher power should be tried, dampening down the condenser to give better contrast. If WBCs are clumped on the protozoa or the preparation is cold, only the beating of the flagella may be seen. The wet mount is diagnostic up to 90% of the time. It is characteristic to see many WBCs (also seen in atrophic vaginitis and sexually transmitted diseases, but not in *Candida* or bacterial vaginosis). The pH, using colorimetric paper, will usually be above 5 and can be as high as 7. If KOH is added to the discharge, a "fishy" or amine odor may be present.

TREATMENT

Metronidazole 2 g orally in a single dose has been the standard first-line treatment, but recently 1.5 g has been shown to be equally effective.[14] A 7-day course of 500 mg daily has similar (95%) cure rates, but compliance is lower. Metronidazole affects the hepatic metabolism of alcohol in the same manner as disulfiram (Antabuse), so patients should abstain from alcohol for 24 hours after the last dose. Metronidazole vaginal gel does not appear to be as effective against *T. vaginalis* and is not recommended.[7] Patients who are allergic to metronidazole should be treated with topical clotrimazole.

Sexual Partners

It is necessary to treat all sexual partners. There is a 2.5-fold increase in reinfection rates if the sexual partner is not treated.

Pregnancy

Treatment of *T. vaginalis* infection in pregnancy is controversial. Metronidazole has both mutagenic and carcinogenic effects in animal studies. There is no evidence of either in human studies. A metaanalysis of the literature concluded that there is no relationship between metronidazole use in the first trimester and the incidence of birth defects.[2] That said, it is still prudent for the emergency physician to avoid metronidazole in the first trimester. Intravaginal clotrimazole will improve or relieve symptoms in about 80% of patients. Cure rates are low. Sexual partners should be treated with single-dose metronidazole.

T. vaginalis infection is associated with preterm and low-birth-weight births, particularly in Blacks.[8] Because pregnant patients will need prenatal care, it is appropriate to refer them for follow-up of both symptomatic *Trichomonas* infection and incidental identification of the organism on urinalysis.

Recurrent Infection

Recurrence is usually due to reinfection or noncompliance with therapy. There are resistant strains of *Trichomonas.* They usually respond to a 7-day course of metronidazole, 1 to 2 g daily.

BACTERIAL VAGINOSIS

The most common cause of an abnormal vaginal discharge is a change in the vaginal flora, which has undergone several name changes as our understanding of the pathogenesis has evolved. High concentrations of anaerobic bacteria replace the normal lactobacilli, especially those species that produce hydrogen peroxide. Anaerobes increase tenfold, and *Gardnerella* species even more. The anaerobic vibrios from the *Mobiluncus* group are seen in about 50% of symptomatic patients. Therefore, bacterial vaginosis is best understood as a syndrome of bacterial synergism in which the vaginal flora become predominantly anaerobic. It does not produce inflammatory changes, hence the term, *vaginosis,* rather than vaginitis.

CLINICAL PRESENTATION

The most uniform complaint of women with this condition is an unpleasant vaginal odor, particularly noted after intercourse, when alkaline semen triggers the release of aromatic amines. The odor may be described as "fishy" or "musty." The discharge is most often thin and adherent to the walls of the vagina. There is rarely any pruritus or erythema of the vulva or vagina unless concomitant *Trichomonas* infection is present. A wet mount of the discharge classically has "clue cells," which are epithelial cells that have bacteria "studded" all over the surface, obscuring the cell wall. Few WBCs or lactobacilli are noted, but clumps of bacteria may be seen. The pH of the discharge is 5 to 6. When KOH is added to the slide, a fishy odor is released, a positive "whiff test."

TREATMENT

Metronidazole 500 mg twice daily for 7 days is the treatment of choice. It results in 85% to 95% cure and a return of normal lactobacilli. Single-dose therapy is considerably less effective. Topical therapy with either metronidazole gel or clindamycin cream is also approved by the Food and Drug Administration and should have fewer side effects. Women who are allergic to metronidazole or who develop recurrence may be treated with clindamycin 300 mg every 12 hours for 7 days. Alternative therapy is listed in Table 85.2.

Sexual Partners

Sexual transmission is probable but not certain, and there is no consensus on treatment of partners.[6] The CDC does not recommend routine treatment, and no decrease in recurrence has been shown if partners are treated.

Pregnancy

Although there is an association between bacterial vaginosis and increased incidence of preterm labor, premature rupture of membranes, and endometritis, a causal etiology has not been established. If the patient is quite symptomatic and in the first trimester, 2% clindamycin vaginal cream daily for 7 days can be used. Minimally symptomatic patients may be referred to their obstetricians.[12]

Recurrence

Clindamycin 300 mg every 12 hours for 7 days is standard. Repeated regimens of metronidazole are not well accepted by patients. In one small study, recurrent infection was successfully (78%) treated with a 3-minute instillation of 3% hydrogen peroxide in the vagina.[9,15]

COMMON PITFALLS

- The patient with a chief complaint of vaginal discharge is never a high priority in a busy ED. The most common pitfall is failure to do a good history and methodical examination.
- Misdiagnosing urinary tract infection in patients who complain of dysuria that is actually external and due to *Candida* vulvovaginitis or *Trichomonas*
- Overlooking noninfectious causes of vaginal symptoms, such as chemical irritants (bubble bath, topical contraceptive and feminine hygiene products, scents, deodorants, and soaps) or hormone depletion in postmenopausal women
- Failure to provide or refer for counseling regarding behavior risks and testing for HIV and other sexually transmitted diseases for patients with *Trichomonas* infection

References

1. Abbott J. Clinical and microscopic diagnosis of vaginal yeast infection: a prospective analysis. *Ann Emerg Med* 1995;25(5):587–591.
2. Caro-Paton T, Carvajal A, Martin de Diego I, et al. Is metronidazole teratogenic? A meta-analysis. *Br J Clin Pharmacol* 1997;44(2):179–182.
3. Carr PL, Felsenstein D, Friedman RH. Evaluation and management of vaginitis. *J Gen Intern Med* 1998;13(5):335–346.
4. Centers for Disease Control and Prevention. HIV prevention through early detection and treatment of other sexually transmitted diseases—United States. Recommendations of the Advisory Committee for HIV and STD prevention. *MMWR* 1998;47(No. RR-12).
5. Centers for Disease Control and Prevention. 1998 Guidelines for treatment of sexually transmitted diseases. *MMWR* 1998;47(No. RR-1).
6. Colli E, Landoni M, Parazzini F. Treatment of male partners and recurrence of bacterial vaginosis: a randomized trial. *Gen Med* 1997;73(4):267–270.
7. duBouchet L, Spence MR, Rein MF, et al. Multicenter comparison of clotrimazole vaginal tablets, oral metronidazole, and vaginal suppositories containing sulfanilamide, aminacrine hydrochloride, and allantoin in the treatment of symptomatic trichomoniasis. *Sex Transm Dis* 1997;24(3):156–160.
8. Eschenbach DA, Edelman R, Carey JC, et al. Trichomonas vaginalis associated with low birth weight and preterm delivery. The Vaginal Infections and Prematurity Study Group. *Sex Transm Dis* 1997;24(6):353–360.
9. Ferris DG, Litaker MS, Woodward L, et al. Treatment of bacterial vaginosis: a comparison of oral metronidazole, metronidazole vaginal gel and clindamycin vaginal cream. *J Fam Pract* 1995;41(5):443–449.
10. Heine RP, Wiesenfeld HC, Sweet RL, et al. Polymerase chain reaction analysis of distal vaginal specimens: a less invasive strategy for detection of Trichomonas vaginalis. *Clin Infect Dis* 1997;24(5):985–987.
11. Madico G, Quinn TC, Rompalo A, et al. Diagnosis of Trichomonas vaginalis infection by PCR using vaginal swab samples. *J Clin Microbiol* 1998; 36(11):3205–3210.
12. McCoy MC, Katz VL, Kuller JA, et al. Bacterial vaginosis in pregnancy: an approach for the 90's. *Obstet Gynecol Surv* 1995;50(6):482–488.
13. Sobel JD, Brooker D, Stein GE, et al. Single oral dose fluconazole compared with conventional clotrimazole topical therapy of candida vaginitis. Fluconazole Vaginitis Study Group. *Am J Obstet Gynecol* 1995;172(4 Pt 1):1263–1268.
14. Spence MR, Harwell TS, Davies MC, et al. The minimum single oral metronidazole dose for treating trichomoniasis: a randomized, blinded study. *Obstet Gynecol* 1997;89(5 Pt 1):699–703.
15. Winceslaus SJ, Calver G. Recurrent bacterial vaginosis—an old approach to a new problems. *Int J STD AIDS* 1996;7(4):284–287.

CHAPTER 86
Gynecologic Cancers

Guy I. Benrubi, Robert C. Nuss, and Ann Harwood-Nuss

Approximately 81,000 new invasive cancers of the female reproductive tract are diagnosed annually in the United States.[14] These cancers eventually result in approximately 27,300 deaths each year.[14] The yearly incidence of these diseases is increasing. As the baby boom cohort in the population ages, more ovarian, vulvar, and endometrial cancers will develop. An increased prevalence of human papillomavirus infection will result in an increase in cervical dysplasia and, possibly, cervical cancer, particularly if cytologic surveillance is not aggressively encouraged.[10]

With the advent of cytologic screening, and the consequent decrease in invasive cervical cancer, the most frequently diagnosed cancer of the female reproductive tract currently is endometrial.[14] This condition is followed in incidence by ovarian, cervical, and vulvar cancer and, less frequently, gestational trophoblastic neoplasia and tubal and vaginal cancer. Although the most frequent cause of gynecologic cancer emergencies in the population at large is ovarian cancer, emergency physicians probably primarily see patients with cervical cancer. These patients typically belong to lower socioeconomic groups and are more likely to seek help in emergency department settings than from their primary physicians. This chapter's discussion of gynecologic cancer emergencies is organized according to their most frequent emergent clinical presentations, rather than according to the primary malignancies that cause these presentations.

VAGINAL BLEEDING

Patients who present to the emergency department with vaginal bleeding secondary to a gynecologic malignancy probably have either cervical or endometrial cancer.[7] Occasionally, other corpus malignancies, such as sarcomas and gestational trophoblastic disease, are the cause. Rarely, the cause is advanced vulvar cancer.

Women who present with vaginal bleeding due to cervical cancer have a mean age between 40 and 45 years.[20] This mean age has recently decreased because younger women have been contracting cervical cancer secondary to an increased incidence of human papillomavirus infection, increased sexual contacts, and increased smoking.[1] Essential points in the history of patients who present with vaginal bleeding due to cervical cancer include the following:

Painless vaginal bleeding, exacerbated or caused by coitus
Lack of previous cytologic screening, or a history of prior abnormal findings on cytologic screening
Lower socioeconomic status
Multiple sexual partners

Although the physical examination should assess extrapelvic spread of disease, such as supraclavicular or inguinal adenopathy, the main focus of the examination should be the pelvis. In a patient whose lesion is so advanced that vaginal bleeding is the presenting complaint, the lesion should be visible on speculum examination. The speculum should be inserted gently to avoid further trauma to the bleeding site. A careful inspection of the vulva, vagina, and cervical os should be performed. If there is no visible lesion on the cervix and the bleeding is coming through the cervical os, then cervical cancer is an unlikely cause of bleeding. Bimanual examination as well as a rectovaginal examination should be performed to assess possible involvement of the parametrial tissues. Laboratory studies should include a pregnancy test and a complete blood count. If the bleeding is not severe, the patient can be discharged from the emergency department once appropriate referral and prompt follow-up by a qualified gynecologist have been obtained. If the bleeding is severe or life-threatening, then supportive measures should be instituted and consultation obtained. Measures that are effective in control of vaginal bleeding include packing the vagina, after insertion of a Foley catheter; use of Monsel's solution; and application of Oxycel. When all else fails, the packing material can be impregnated with a solution of epinephrine (1:500,000). If the bleeding is unremitting, the patient may need to be admitted for hypogastric artery ligation, embolization, or high-dose radiation therapy.[5]

In vaginal bleeding caused by endometrial or other corpus cancers, the bleeding is usually not as severe as that caused by cervical cancer. Patients tend to be in an older age group; the mean age for patients with this disease is 60.[21] In approximately 5% of cases, endometrial cancers occur in women under age 40.[7] Essential points of the history in the older patient include use of unopposed exogenous estrogens and obesity. In younger women, obesity, nulliparity, and infertility may be predisposing factors. Although vaginal bleeding is the most common presenting complaint for this disease, it is seldom of sufficient magnitude to cause an emergency department visit, unless the patient lacks a primary physician. In women who present with postmenopausal vaginal bleeding, the diagnosis should be endometrial cancer until proved otherwise.

Careful examination should be performed to assess the size of the uterus and the presence of extrauterine tumor. On speculum examination, the bleeding will be from the cervical os. Occasionally, endometrial cancer presents with a visible lesion on the cervix. The bleeding is seldom life-threatening, and the patient can be discharged from the emergency department as long as adequate provisions are made for prompt referral to a qualified gynecologist.

Vaginal bleeding caused by gestational trophoblastic neoplasia occurs in women in either early or late reproductive age. With

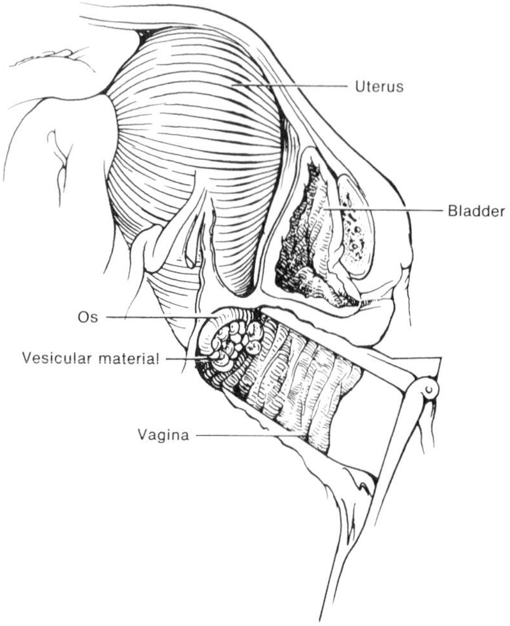

Figure 86.1. Gestational trophoblastic neoplasm.

increasing numbers of immigrants from Latin America and particularly from Asia, emergency physicians in inner-city situations may see this particular problem. Gestational trophoblastic neoplasia occurs in one out of 1200 pregnancies in the United States, but it is much more common in Asia and Latin America. In addition, as the pregnancy rate among inner-city teens burgeons, emergency physicians will see a steadily increasing incidence of this disease. Vaginal bleeding is the most common presentation for gestational trophoblastic neoplasia.[12] Salient points in the history include uterine enlargement greater than expected for gestational age, absence of fetal movements, repeated visits to medical facilities for bleeding (often the diagnosis is threatened abortion), and hypertension in early pregnancy.

Physical examination reveals a large-for-gestational-age fundal height; speculum examination shows bleeding coming from the os. Vesicular material also may be seen extruding through the os (Fig. 86.1). The definitive diagnosis is made by ultrasonography, which shows a distinctive multiechogenic pattern. The patient with gestational trophoblastic neoplasia should be admitted after a prompt obstetric consultation.

Bleeding caused by vulvar cancer is rare.[16] Women who present with this entity usually have an advanced lesion. Most are over age 60 and have other signs of neglect. Because of the possibility of either self- or institutional neglect, it is advisable to admit women who present with large, bleeding vulvar cancer lesions. Therapy can then be promptly instituted.

BOWEL EMERGENCIES

Bowel emergencies in patients with gynecologic malignancies are divided into two major subheadings: those that occur in nonradiated bowel and those with complications secondary to radiated bowel.

COMPLICATIONS OF NONRADIATED BOWEL

In the nonradiated bowel group, the most common bowel emergencies are bowel obstruction, colostomy problems, fistula formation, and perforation.

Bowel Obstruction

Small bowel obstruction, not in the perioperative period, is usually due to internal adhesions secondary to a previous surgical procedure or to gynecologic malignancy. In ovarian cancer, approximately 5% of patients have small bowel obstruction as the presenting complaint.[21] Ovarian cancer spreads on the serosal surfaces of the bowel and can cause either adhesive or bulk obstruction (Fig. 86.2). The presentation of small bowel obstruction secondary to ovarian cancer is similar to that of bowel obstruction caused by nongynecologic causes. Consequently, the reader is referred to the appropriate chapters in this text for emergency department management. Two important points are unique to gynecologic cancer: (1) in elderly patients with no history of prior abdominal surgery, small bowel obstruction is a harbinger of ovarian cancer; and (2) in patients with a history of pelvic malignancy, small bowel obstruction may be the first sign of recurrence. In both situations, appropriate consultation should be obtained. Frequently, patients with obstruction secondary to long-standing ovarian cancer should not have surgical intervention immediately on presentation, but be managed conservatively.

Large bowel obstruction can occur by direct extension of a cervical malignancy that blocks the rectum. It is also seen when a large tumor in the omentum causes compression at either the splenic or the hepatic flexure. The evaluation of the patient with large bowel obstruction secondary to gynecologic malignancy is the same as that in any other patient. However, emergency department management should include prompt consultation with a gynecologist. The most critical aspect of the evaluation is to rule out overdistention of the cecum; if in excess of 10 cm in diameter, prompt surgical decompression is necessary.[22]

Colostomy Emergencies

Colostomy complications occur in approximately 30% of patients. These complications include stenosis of the stoma, peristomal hernia, wound infection, and prolapse.[13] Most problems can be managed by a stomal therapist. However, some stomal complications require prompt initiation of care. Peristomal herniation of bowel requires admission for prompt surgical correction. Surgical or gynecologic consultation should be obtained, and the bowel should be kept moist in the emergency department. Mucosal prolapse of the stoma can be reduced by gentle digital pressure, but it should be done expeditiously to prevent infection and stomal damage.

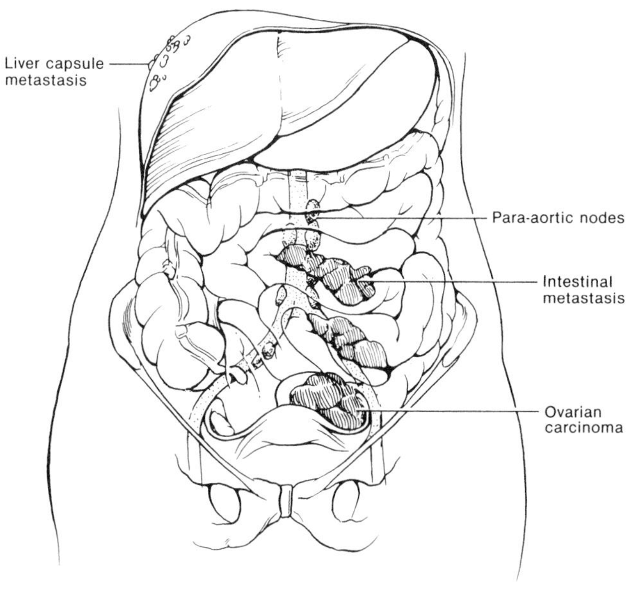

Figure 86.2. Pattern of spread of ovarian cancer.

Fistula Formation

Bowel fistulas in patients with gynecologic malignancies are usually enterocutaneous, enterovaginal, or rectovaginal. Rarely, these fistulas are the presenting sign of a gynecologic malignancy. More often they occur secondary to therapy. The patient with a new fistula should be admitted so that prompt evaluation can be done.

COMPLICATIONS OF RADIATED BOWEL

The role of radiation therapy in gynecologic malignancies is constantly changing. Radiation therapy is currently most frequently used for the primary treatment of advanced cervical cancer or cervical cancer in patients who are not operative candidates. It is also used with increasing frequency as adjuvant therapy for endometrial cancer and as adjuvant or consolidation therapy in ovarian cancer. Two stages of complications result from radiation therapy: early and late. An early bowel complication is radiation proctitis or enteritis with diarrhea. This injury can be seen during therapy (resulting in therapy interruption) or shortly after the completion of therapy. Patients with severe diarrhea secondary to radiation enteritis or proctitis can usually be treated conservatively and seldom need to be admitted. The diarrhea can be managed with diphenoxylate (Lomotil). Fluid resuscitation may be necessary secondary to severe diarrhea. The patient can be treated and discharged to her radiation oncologist or gynecologist for continuing care.

Late complications of radiation injury to the bowel are caused by endarteritis and progressive sclerosis of the smaller vessels.[2] This leads to several complications, including ulceration, infarction, enterofistulas, enteroenterofistulas, necrosis, and stenosis.[6] Usually, the patient presents with either intestinal obstruction or severe intractable abdominal pain. In the emergency department, the patient must be managed with fluid resuscitation, nasogastric suction, prompt gynecologic or surgical consultation, and admission.

Another common emergency presentation is rectal bleeding owing to radiation proctitis. If the bleeding is minimal, the patient can be discharged on Cort enemas (hydrocortisone) and a low-residue diet. Prompt arrangements should be made for follow-up with either the radiation therapist or the gynecologist. When the bleeding is severe or symptoms of shock exist, fluid resuscitation, transfusion, and prompt consultation should occur. When medical management fails, intervention may include angiographic embolization and colostomy.

UROLOGIC EMERGENCIES

Patients with genital tract cancer may present with urologic emergencies secondary to surgery, radiation therapy, or the malignancy itself.

URETERAL OBSTRUCTION

Ureteral obstruction may result from any of the three previously mentioned factors. It is seldom the presenting complaint in the emergency department, as most instances of this condition are diagnosed in nonacute settings. Ureteral obstruction most often presents as nonspecific flank pain, occasionally radiating to the pelvis and groin. Urinary infection is common, and may result in urosepsis. In rare cases in which there is bilateral obstruction, anemia and azotemia may result. Ureteral obstruction can occur at any time after surgery or radiation therapy, but it is usually seen during the first posttreatment year. It may be the first presenting sign of late recurrence of genital malignancy. It can also be an initial sign of cervical cancer (Fig. 86.3). The diagnosis is made on intravenous pyelography, computed tomography, renal nuclear scanning, or renal ultrasonography. Management depends on the severity of the obstruction. In patients with urosepsis, hospitalization should be arranged and antibiotics started after specimens for blood and urine cultures have been obtained. In patients who are stable and have insidious signs of ureteral obstruction, discharge may be contemplated once arrangements are made for continuing follow-up.

UROLOGIC FISTULAS

Most patients with gynecologic malignancies do not present to the emergency department because of urinary fistulas. Urinary fistulas occur either because of extensive primary disease or secondary to radical hysterectomy for cervical or endometrial cancer. Surgical fistulas occur from 7 to 21 days after surgery.[6] Occasionally, fistulas occur secondary to radiation therapy and are diagnosed 6 to 12 months after completion of treatment. The incidence of fistula formation after radical hysterectomy is approximately 1%.[4] There is a three- to fourfold increase in this rate when radiation is given in conjunction with surgery. Fistulas that occur in patients after radical surgery are usually diagnosed by the patient's surgeon and seldom present to the emergency department. However, in inner-city situations, it is possible that the presenting sign of the malignancy may be vesicovaginal fistula secondary to spread of the disease into the trigone of the bladder.

Fistulas can be diagnosed either by direct observation of urine in the vagina or by injecting indigo carmine intravenously and placing a tampon in the vagina.

HEMORRHAGIC CYSTITIS

Hemorrhagic cystitis can be due to either radiation therapy or chemotherapy. Hemorrhagic cystitis secondary to cyclophosphamide or ifosfamide chemotherapy is seen infrequently because cyclophosphamide is now given in combination with cisplatin as a bolus with maximal hydration. Hemorrhagic cystitis is not uncommon after radiation, and the pathophysiology is similar to that of radiated bowel. Management can usually be done in the emergency department with a three-way catheter, irrigation, and, possibly, a hydrocortisone-containing solution. Once clots are removed and if the bleeding is not severe, the patient may be discharged with follow-up. In severe hemorrhage, the patient will need to be admitted and managed either with cautery by way of cystoscopy or by instillation of a sclerosing agent such as formalin. In all situations, urologic and gynecologic consultation are necessary.

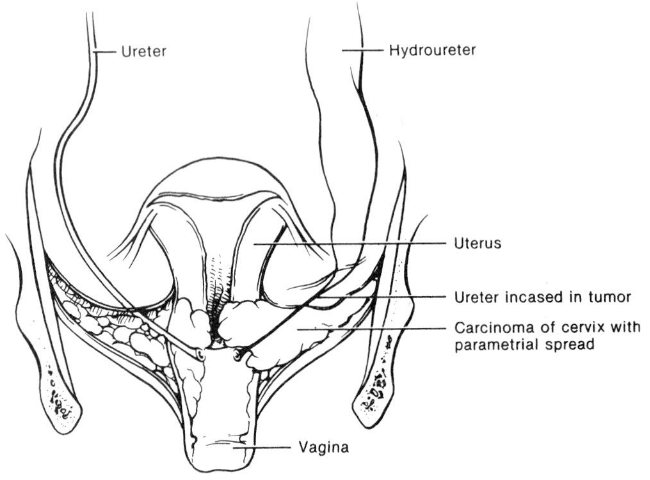

Figure 86.3. Cervical cancer: patterns of local spread.

URINARY CONDUIT COMPLICATIONS

Urinary conduits are either ileal or colon conduits. Complications include blockage of the ureteroconduit anastomotic site, with ureteral obstruction and possibly urosepsis; conduit necrosis; stomal necrosis secondary to avascularity; stomal problems, as described under the section on colostomy; and electrolyte imbalance owing to absorption of chloride in an overly long conduit, resulting in hyperchloremic acidosis.[11] Management in the emergency department is supportive. Admission considerations depend on the patient's overall electrolyte balance, the presence of urinary obstruction, and the patient's ability to return for follow-up care. Intravenous pyelography or ultrasonography usually defines the problem. If urinary obstruction has resulted in urosepsis, emergency percutaneous nephrostomy is necessary.[9] Appropriate consultation with the radiologist and gynecologist needs to be obtained.

POSTOPERATIVE COMPLICATIONS

The emergency physician is most likely to be involved with three types of postoperative complications: (1) bowel obstruction secondary to surgery, (2) urologic fistula secondary to surgery, and (3) postoperative infection. The first two have already been discussed.

In the vast majority of cases, postoperative infections are diagnosed while the patient is still in the hospital. This is particularly the case with ovarian cancer, in which the first course of chemotherapy is initiated in the hospital in the absence of postoperative infection. The postoperative infections most likely to be seen by the emergency physician are wound infection, wound dehiscence, and wound evisceration. Wound dehiscence occurs 5 to 7 days after surgery; in some situations, it may occur after discharge. The patient can usually be managed with debridement and dressing changes. The patient's surgeon should be consulted. In situations in which home care is inadequate, the patient may need to be admitted. If signs of necrotizing fasciitis (skin discoloration, skin necrosis, and crepitus) are present, the patient needs to be admitted for surgical debridement.[17] If there is fascial separation (evisceration), the patient must be admitted. The wound should be covered with sterile, moist towels and arrangements made for the patient to be taken to the operating room for fascial closure.

The other common postoperative infections in patients with gynecologic malignancies are vaginal cuff cellulitis and cuff abscess.[17] Vaginal cuff cellulitis occurs in 8% of those who receive antibiotic prophylaxis before a hysterectomy. The most common cause is a mixed infection of anaerobes endogenous to the vagina. Occasionally, gram-negative aerobic bacteria may be involved. When this diagnosis is made, the patient should be admitted and broad-spectrum antibiotic coverage should be started. If the diagnosis is certain, the antibiotics can be started in the emergency department. Appropriate drugs for anaerobic bacteria are metronidazole, ampicillin–sulbactam, and ticarcillin–clavulanate. If an abscess is identified, gynecologic consultation should be obtained and arrangements made for drainage in the operating room.

The emergency physician may see patients with complications secondary to outpatient therapy such as colposcopy, conization, and laser therapy. The most common problem with these procedures is postoperative cervical bleeding. This can usually be managed by the application of Monsel's solution or packing the vagina with a Neo-Synephrine- or epinephrine-impregnated pack. Occasionally, the cervix needs to be sutured. In that situation, gynecologic consultation should be obtained. If the patient is not severely bleeding and the bleeding is controlled with the previously outlined procedures, the patient may be sent home and told to avoid intercourse and to follow up promptly with her primary physician.

COMPLICATIONS OF CHEMOTHERAPY

Chemotherapy is used primarily in ovarian cancer and gestational trophoblastic disease and as an adjuvant in endometrial cancer. The most commonly used drugs in gynecologic oncology are cisplatin, carboplatinum, and paclitaxel. Complications caused by cisplatin are nausea and vomiting, which may be unremitting. In gynecologic oncology, cisplatin is given as a bolus medication. Most of the nausea and vomiting occur during the day of administration. Occasionally, the vomiting can be severe enough that the patient may come to the emergency department the day after chemotherapy instillation. Once fluid and electrolyte status are assured, the patient can often be managed by intravenous antiemetic medication as well as metoclopramide (Reglan). If nausea and vomiting are unremitting, the patient needs to be admitted for hydration. Elderly patients tend to have less nausea and vomiting on cisplatin.[3] Other drugs that are commonly used in gynecologic oncology are cyclophosphamide, methotrexate, fluorouracil, doxorubicin, dactinomycin, vinblastine, etoposide, and ifosfamide. The most common complication with these medications is bone marrow suppression. It is unusual for these patients to present to the emergency department; however, if the patient presents with a neutropenia of less than 500 granulocytes and fever, she should be admitted for antibiotic therapy. Rarely, the patient presents with a very low platelet count. If the platelet count is less than 20,000 and there is spontaneous bleeding, the patient needs to be admitted for transfusion as well as platelet therapy. Bleomycin, another commonly used drug, may cause pulmonary fibrosis. The patient may present with dyspnea, cough, and bibasilar rales. A chest radiograph usually shows basilar infiltrates. The patient needs to be admitted, particularly if there is an upper respiratory tract infection in addition to the bleomycin toxicity.

Paclitaxel (Taxol) is now used in induction chemotherapy in ovarian cancer chemotherapy protocols. In addition to its bone marrow toxicity, it also can cause cardiac toxicity manifested by sinus bradycardia (30%), bradyarrhythmia with AV blockade, and short lived ventricular tachycardia.[15] Although most of these side effects are noted while the patient is receiving chemotherapy, they can occasionally occur after discharge, particularly if the patient is given a 3-hour Taxol regimen.

COMPLICATIONS OF TOTAL PARENTERAL NUTRITION

In the past, the emergency physician seldom saw patients who presented with complications secondary to total parenteral nutrition (TPN). However, as home infusion services have increased, it is now more common to see extramural complications of TPN. The most likely complications secondary to home infusion TPN are infection and metabolic derangements.[19] The patient with signs and symptoms of sepsis should be managed aggressively and promptly admitted. Metabolic complications include acid–base and electrolyte abnormalities and abnormalities in glucose metabolism as well as hypokalemia, hypomagnesemia, hypophosphatemia, and hypocalcemia. Patients may present with muscle weakness, hyporeflexia or hyperreflexia, lethargy, and mental status change. It is imperative for the emergency physician to obtain adequate screening laboratory studies before deciding whether the patient can be discharged.

ORGAN FAILURE

Patients with gynecologic malignancies may experience organ failure because of either the primary disease or therapy. A gynecologic organ failure should be managed the same as organ failure from any other cause.

As discussed, renal failure can occur from ureteral obstruction, conduit anastomosis problems, or urosepsis. It may represent a primary presentation of cervical cancer with bilateral ureterovesical junction obstruction. Liver failure is most frequently due to metastasis from ovarian cancer and less frequently from gestational trophoblastic neoplasia and endometrial, vulvar, or cervical cancer. Pulmonary metastasis is seen most frequently in endometrial cancer or cervical cancer; parenchymal pulmonary metastasis is seen somewhat less frequently in ovarian cancer.[18] It is not infrequent, however, to see pleural effusions secondary to ovarian cancer in association with ascites. Brain metastasis is rare in gynecologic malignancies, except for gestational trophoblastic neoplasia. In the presence of gestational trophoblastic neoplasia, complaints of headache, seizure, visual disturbance, or mental status change should be evaluated with a computed tomographic scan of the head.[8]

COMMON PITFALLS

- In the presence of vaginal bleeding in a patient of reproductive age, pregnancy should be ruled out.
- If the cecum is dilated to 10 cm from large bowel obstruction, prompt decompression is mandatory.
- Necrotizing fasciitis requires prompt surgical debridement and admission.
- If any amount of ureteral obstruction is diagnosed, urosepsis must be ruled out before discharge from the emergency department.
- Febrile neutropenic patients must be admitted.

References

1. American College of Obstetricians and Gynecologists. 1999 Compendium of selected publications: Genital Human Papilloma Virus Infection (no. 193). Washington, DC: American College of Obstetrics and Gynecology, 1999.
2. Beer W, Fan A, Halsted C. Clinical and nutritional implications of radiation enteritis. *Am J Clin Nutr* 1985;41:85.
3. Benrubi G, Norvell M, Nuss R, et al. The use of methylprednisolone and metoclopramide in control of emesis in patients receiving cis-platinum. *Gynecol Oncol* 1985;21:306.
4. Chamberlain D, Hopkins M, Roberts J, et al. The effects of early removal of indwelling urinary catheter after radical hysterectomy. *Gynecol Oncol* 1991;43:98.
5. Dehaeck C. Transcatheter embolization of pelvic vessels to stop intractable hemorrhage. *Gynecol Oncol* 1986;24:9.
6. Delgado G, Smith J. *Management of complications in gynecologic oncology*. New York: John Wiley and Sons, 1982.
7. Disaia P, Creasman W. *Clinical gynecologic oncology*, 5th ed. St. Louis: Mosby, 1997.
8. DuBeshter B, Berkowitz R, Goldstein D, et al. Metastatic gestational trophoblastic disease: experience at the New England Trophoblastic Disease Center, 1965–1985. *Obstet Gynecol* 1987;69:390.

9. Dudley B, Gershenson D, Kavanaugh J, et al. Percutaneous nephrostomy catheter use in gynecologic malignancy: M.D. Anderson Hospital experience. *Gynecol Oncol* 1986;24:273.
10. Guijon F. Sexually transmitted disease and cervical neoplasia. *Curr Opin Obstet Gynecol* 1990;2:857.
11. Hancock K, Copeland L, Gershenson D. Urinary conduits in gynecologic oncology. *Obstet Gynecol* 1986;67:680.
12. Kim D, Park D, Boe S, et al. Subsequent reproductive experience after treatment for gestational trophoblastic disease. *Gynecol Oncol* 1998;71:108.
13. Kretschmer P. *The intestinal stoma.* Philadelphia: WB Saunders, 1978.
14. Landis S, Murray T, Bolden P, et al. Cancer statistics 1999. *CA* 1999;48:8.
15. McGuire W, Hopkins W, Brady M, et al. Cyclophosphamide and cisplatin compared with paclitaxel and cisplatin in patients with stage III and stage IV ovarian cancer. *N Engl J Med* 1996;334:1–6.
16. Morley G. Cancer of the vulva: a review. *Cancer* 1981;48:597.
17. Nichols D. *Reoperative gynecologic surgery.* St. Louis: Mosby–Year Book, 1991.
18. Peeples W, Inalsingh C, Tapan A, et al. The occurrence of metastasis outside the abdomen and retroperitoneal space in invasive carcinoma of the cervix. *Gynecol Oncol* 1976;4:307.
19. Rayburn W, Walk R, Roberts J. Parenteral nutrition in obstetrics and gynecology. *Obstet Gynecol Surv* 1986;41:200.
20. Rubin S, Hoskins W. Cervical cancer and pre-invasive neoplasia. Philadelphia: Lippincott–Raven Publishers, 1996.
21. Rubin S, Sutton G. *Ovarian cancer.* New York: McGraw-Hill, 1993.
22. Schwartz S. *Principles of surgery,* 6th ed. New York: McGraw-Hill, 1994:1213.

Bibliography

Harwood-Nuss AL, Benrubi G, Nuss RC. Emergencies of gynecologic cancer. *Emerg Med Clin North Am* 1987;5(3):577.

TABLE 87.1. Causes of Adnexal Mass

Gynecologic	Nongynecologic
OVARIAN—BENIGN	Distended bladder
Follicle cyst	Feces
Sclerocystic ovary	Pelvic kidney
Corpus luteum cyst	Urachal cyst
Cystadenoma	Urinoma
Endometriotic cyst	Diverticular abscess
Germinal inclusion cyst	Appendiceal abscess
Theca-lutein cyst	Lymphoma
Benign cystic teratoma	Lymphocyst
	Anterior sacral teratoma
OVARIAN—MALIGNANT	Retroperitoneal fibrosis or tumor
Germ cell tumor	Gastrointestinal tumor
Epithelial carcinoma	Metastatic carcinoma
Gonadal stromal tumors	Abdominal wall hematoma
FALLOPIAN TUBE	
Ectopic pregnancy	
Inflammatory mass	
UTERUS	
Pedunculated myoma	
Broad ligament rests	

CHAPTER 87
The Adnexal Mass

Robert C. Nuss

Adnexal masses are frequently seen in the emergency department and warrant evaluation in women of any age. Anatomically, the adnexal structures are defined in reference to the uterus, and they consist of the fallopian tubes, ovaries, uterine ligaments (round, cardinal, broad, and uterosacral), and structures within the broad ligament. In addition, other nongynecologic anatomic structures normally found in the pelvis may be confused as an adnexal mass (e.g., sigmoid colon).

A systematic approach must be taken to determine the cause of an adnexal mass. Ovarian enlargement—physiologic or pathologic, benign or malignant—is the most common cause of an adnexal mass. Other gynecologic and nongynecologic masses occur with enough frequency to warrant consideration. During the emergency department evaluation, consideration must be given to those entities listed in Table 87.1 and shown in Fig. 87.1. The list is most useful in considering the more unusual causes of an adnexal mass. The age of the patient is significant and should influence the differential diagnosis and selection of diagnostic studies. Patients can be categorized by age into three groups: infancy to puberty, puberty through menopause, and postmenopause. Within these groups, further subdivisions occur. In the first group, a prepubertal girl may develop an ovarian tumor. Although this type of tumor accounts for only 1% of new growths, it remains the most common genital neoplasm in this age group. Any palpable mass in this age group must be considered abnormal and evaluated promptly. Similarly, in the perimenopausal and postmenopausal woman, a malignant ovarian neoplasm should be a main concern and warrants prompt referral and evaluation. The second age group produces the most frequent diagnostic dilemmas and controversies in management. At the age extremes of group 2 (under age 15 and over age 40), consideration is given to neoplasia, with clear indications for prompt intervention. In the mid–age range of group 2, gynecologic disorders representing physiologic changes (functional cyst), inflammatory changes (salpingitis), and pregnancy abnormalities (ectopic pregnancy) occur with peak frequencies. It is at this mid-range of group 2 that most controversies in management occur.

Although the causes of adnexal masses may vary, awareness of the ovarian neoplastic potential is mandatory to fully appreciate the various possibilities. A woman at birth has a 5% to 7% chance of developing ovarian carcinoma.[3,11] In the prepubertal age group, this is usually of the germ cell variety. The most frequent cell type is a dysgerminoma, but embryonal cell carcinoma and endodermal sinus tumor must also be considered.[2,3] Gonadal stomal tumors, such as granulosa cell tumors or thecomas, may also occur, but these are less common and have a less malignant behavior. The exception to this is in the child who exhibits precocious puberty. Tumor markers such as α-fetoprotein, beta human chorionic gonadotropin (β-hCG), carcinoembryonic antigen (CEA), and CA-125 are of limited value, but occasionally they are helpful in diagnosis.[5,10] A negative test is of no significance. In the menstruating woman and the postmenopausal woman, epithelial malignancies represent 85% of all ovarian malignant neoplasms and continue to increase in incidence until age 80. Other cell types, such as germ cell and gonadal stromal tumors, metastatic tumors, lipid cell tumors, and mixed tumors, constitute the rest of the cell types. For a complete histologic classification of ovarian tumors, see Table 87.2.

Despite the malignant potential of the ovary and the devastating outcome when malignancy occurs, benign neoplasms and functional cysts occur far more frequently. A benign cystic teratoma (dermoid) is the most commonly occurring neoplasm in the age range of 1 to 20 years.[22] Serous and mucinous cystadenomas occur throughout the reproductive years as well as in the postmenopausal period. Mucinous cystadenomas may grow to more than 100 pounds.[13,26] Physiologic cysts, such as follicle cysts, corpus luteum cysts, germinal inclusion cysts, endometri-

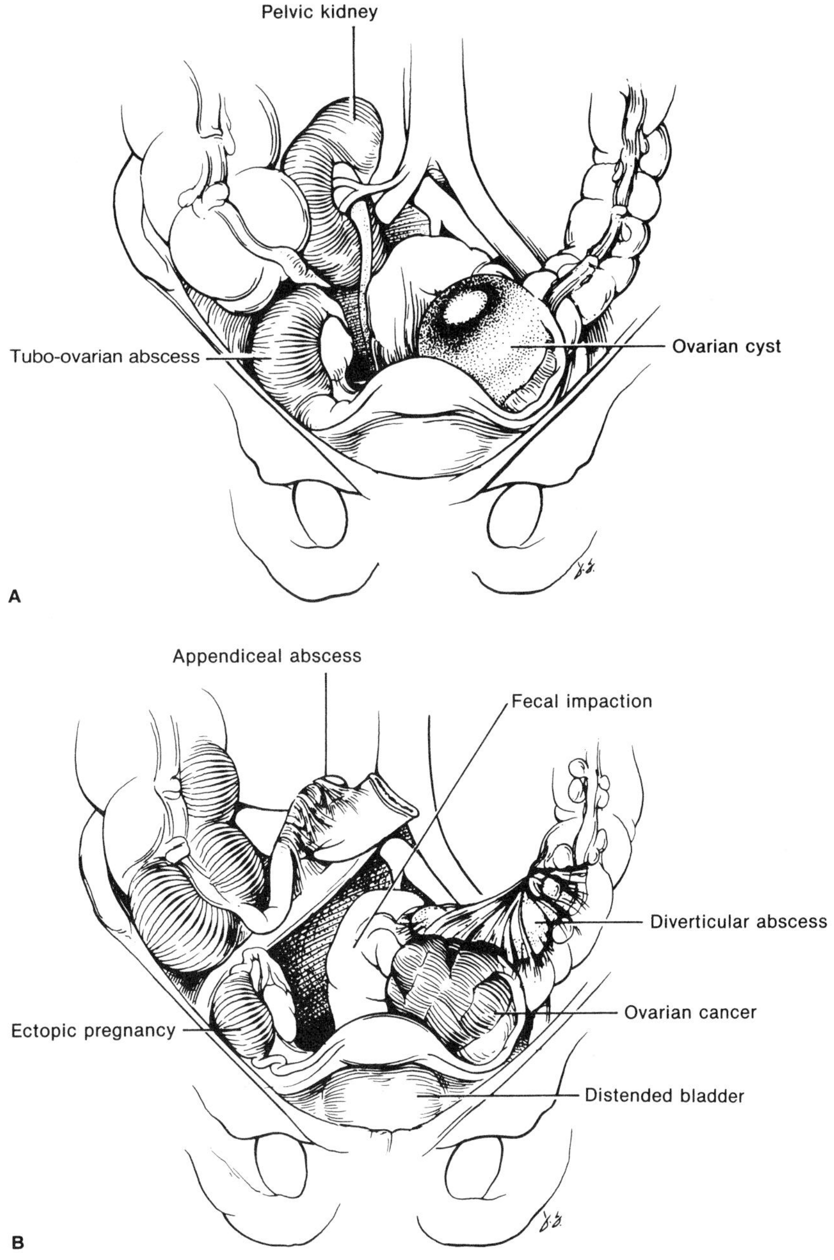

Figure 87.1. Adnexal mass.

omas, theca-lutein cysts, and sclerocystic ovaries (polycystic ovary), occur throughout the reproductive years and may masquerade as pregnancy, inflammatory masses, and neoplastic growths.

Discussion of the adnexal mass is incomplete without consideration of pelvic inflammatory disease and ectopic pregnancy. Pelvic inflammatory disease may present without the classic acute symptom complex. An inflammatory mass may be as hard and discrete as an ovarian carcinoma. Ectopic pregnancies are usually tubal (98%) in location and present as an adnexal mass approximately 50% of the time. These are discussed in detail in Chapter 74.

CLINICAL PRESENTATION

The presentation depends primarily on the cause of the adnexal mass. Initial signs and symptoms, which apply to all age groups, include pain, mass, and vaginal bleeding, or the patient may be asymptomatic. In children, ovarian enlargement presents as an abdominal mass, because the ovary does not become a pelvic organ until puberty. Pain is a variable symptom and depends on the rapidity of growth, capsular stretch, and complications such as torsion, rupture, infection, and infarction. A functioning ovarian tumor may result in signs of isosexual precocious puberty and vaginal bleeding. Menstrual disorders may be produced by most adnexal masses of gynecologic cause. Nongynecologic disorders are seldom associated with menstrual dysfunction unless there is a significant systemic manifestation of the disease. Myomas, specifically pedunculated myomas, are not associated with abnormal bleeding, but coexisting submucous or intramural myomas may be associated with menorrhagia or hypermenorrhea. Ectopic pregnancy is invariably associated with menstrual dysfunction. Parovarian cysts are nonfunctional and have no associated menstrual abnormalities. Ovarian functional cysts are often associated with menstrual irregularity manifested primarily by menstrual delay and subsequent hypermenorrhea. An ovarian carcinoma usually causes more menstrual dysfunction

TABLE 87.2. Modified World Health Organization Comprehensive Classification of Ovarian Tumors

I. COMMON "EPITHELIAL" TUMORS	
Serous	Benign, borderline, or malignant
Mucinous	Benign, borderline, or malignant
Endometrioid	Benign, borderline, or malignant
Clear cell	Benign, borderline, or malignant
Brenner	Benign, borderline, or malignant
Mixed epithelial	
Undifferentiated	
Mixed mesodermal tumors	
Unclassified	
II. SEX-CORD STROMAL TUMORS	
Granuloma stromal cell	
Granulosa cell	
Thecoma-fibroma	
Androblastomas; Sertoli-Leydig cell tumors	
Well-differentiated (Pick's adenoma, Sertoli cell tumor)	
Intermediate differentiation	
Poorly differentiated	
With heterologous elements	
Lipid cell tumors	
Gynandroblastoma	
Unclassified	
III. GERM CELL TUMORS	
Dysgerminoma	
Endodermal sinus tumor	
Embryonal carcinoma	
Polyembryoma	
Choriocarcinoma	
Teratomas	
Immature	
Mature (dermoid)	
Monodermal (struma ovarii, carcinoid)	
Mixed forms	
Gonadoblastoma	
IV. SOFT-TISSUE TUMORS NOT SPECIFIC TO THE OVARY	
V. UNCLASSIFIED TUMORS	
VI. SECONDARY (METASTATIC) TUMORS	
VII. TUMOR-LIKE CONDITIONS (e.g., PREGNANCY, LUTEOMA)	

Modified International Histologic Classification of Tumors, No. 9, World Health Organization, Geneva, 1973.

than a benign ovarian neoplasm. This may be manifested as amenorrhea, hypomenorrhea, or hypermenorrhea.

Ovarian neoplasms may be asymptomatic. A careful history may reveal nonspecific gastrointestinal symptoms such as anorexia, indigestion, belching, and dyspepsia. Pain and abdominal swelling are the most frequent signs of ovarian carcinoma. Pelvic fullness, abdominal swelling, ascites, bowel obstruction, and pain are indicative of advanced malignant disease.

The adnexal mass produced by gastrointestinal disease is usually associated with chronic symptom complex. Pain, alternating consistency of the stool, food intolerance, mucus and blood in the stool, and a left-sided mass are the most frequent signs and symptoms.

DIFFERENTIAL DIAGNOSIS

The differential diagnosis includes those diseases listed in Table 87.1. Age grouping and a careful history facilitate the evaluation. Chills and fever are associated with inflammatory disorders and seldom occur with ovarian neoplasms, benign or malignant. Ascites is usually a manifestation of ovarian malignancy, but it may be present[15] in benign situations (Meigs syndrome) associated with pleural effusion.[8] In evaluating the adnexal mass, signs that favor benignity are unilateral location, smooth surface, mobility, cystic consistency, and symmetric shape. Features of the mass that suggest malignancy are bilateral location, solid nodular and irregular surface, ascites, and nodular cul-de-sac. Extremely large masses that fill the entire abdomen are usually benign ovarian masses. A mass seen in a patient at either extreme of life must be considered malignant, and managed expeditiously. Tender masses associated with severe pain and peritoneal signs are usually of inflammatory origin. They may also represent complications of a noninflammatory process such as torsion, rupture, or hemorrhage. Masses that are located anterior to the uterus are most frequently benign cystic teratomas (dermoid) or endometriotic cysts.[10,16] If a gynecologic cause of the mass is excluded, the other major source of an adnexal mass is the gastrointestinal tract. A rectovaginal examination with Hemoccult examination of the stool is mandatory.

EMERGENCY DEPARTMENT EVALUATION

History and physical examination should permit a refining of the differential diagnosis, but diagnostic studies usually are necessary. These are dictated by the patient's age, symptom complex, physical findings, and general condition.

LABORATORY STUDIES

Complete blood count, urinalysis, erythrocyte sedimentation rate, and β-hCG determination should be done in all cases. Serum electrolytes, renal function studies, and type and crossmatch are performed according to the clinical situation. Sensitive, rapid urinary β-hCG tests are now available and are valuable in the evaluation of pregnancy-related complications. Quantitative methods are not required for initial management or evaluation. Occasionally, serum markers will be positive (e.g., α-fetoprotein in embryonal carcinomas and endodermal sinus tumors; β-hCG in the presence of trophoblastic tissue).

RADIOLOGIC STUDIES

Ultrasonographic evaluation of the palpable adnexal mass is of limited immediate value if complications of pregnancy are not under consideration. The ultrasonographic features of the mass, although suggestive, are not diagnostic in malignancy, and false-positive results frequently occur.[5,13,18] Ultrasonography may be helpful in the patient who is difficult to examine if a mass is thought to be present. Additional sonographic information, such as solid versus cystic, free peritoneal fluid, and additional masses, have little clinical value in the immediate management, although these findings are very helpful for later evaluation. Transvaginal (TV) ultrasonography, now readily available, is far superior to transabdominal (TA) ultrasound. TA ultrasound is diminished by poor spatial resolution, operator dependency, and patient body habitus. Although TV ultrasonography is considered superior in evaluating the adnexa for ectopic pregnancy,[2] this benefit does not extend to situations in nonpregnant patients. TV color Doppler sonography has become more readily available, but still has limited use. It does not appear to improve the diagnostic accuracy of TV ultrasonography in the areas of ovarian endometriomas[1] and is not as sensitive or nor as specific as TV ultrasonography in evaluating premenopausal patients.[23,25] Furthermore, color and pulsed ultrasound measuring pulsatility index (PI) and resonance index (RI) cannot reliably differentiate benign from malignant lesions.[6] Computed tomography (CT) and magnetic resonance imaging (MRI) offer similar advantages and disadvantages.[24] CT is far superior to ultrasonography in evaluating the pelvic retroperitoneum.[27,28] TV ultrasound appears to be superior to MRI for assessment of suspected pelvic masses and is less expensive and more accessible.[14] The role of MRI in evaluating pelvic masses remains to be determined, especially in differentiating between loops of bowel and masses.[11] Reports of the gynecologic applications of MRI suggest that MRI is of value in differentiating uterine from adnexal masses if unresolved by ultrasonography.[12] MRI is the preferred modality for confirming suspected endometriosis (endometrioma).[14,19] Currently, MRI of the pelvis should be reserved for resolution of indeterminate findings of TV ultrasonography.[20] Plain films are often helpful in evaluating the mass. Information may be seen on plain films, such as free intraperitoneal air and intestinal obstruction. Calcifications are seen on plain films of benign cystic teratomas, but they may also be present in other ovarian neoplasms, such as fibroadenoma, papillary serous tumors (psammoma bodies), gonadoblastoma, and Brenner tumors. Contrast studies of the lower gastrointestinal tract are often helpful. Upper gastrointestinal studies are often warranted when metastatic lesions are considered, but they are probably not indicated emergently. In premenopausal women, gastric carcinomas may metastasize to the ovaries. Intravenous pyelography (IVP) is one of the most useful diagnostic studies. It provides information about the location of the kidneys and the pathway of the ureter. Upper urinary tract obstruction requires prompt management to minimize subsequent renal damage. Abnormalities in the normal course of the ureter may suggest the origin of the mass and provide essential information if retroperitoneal exploration is later required.

EMERGENCY DEPARTMENT MANAGEMENT

The history and physical examination determine the urgency of both subsequent evaluation and emergency department intervention. In the course of the initial evaluation, specific information must be recorded regarding size, location, consistency, and tenderness of the mass. This is especially important if subsequent changes occur in the mass or clinical situation. Immediate emergency intervention is required primarily in the patient who presents with symptoms secondary to complications—specifically, ovarian rupture, torsion, infection, hemorrhagic shock, severe pain, gastrointestinal symptoms, peritoneal signs, and a febrile state. Vascular access should be established and intravascular volume expanded. In patients with peritoneal signs and vascular instability, culdocentesis should be considered. Ruptured structures with hemoperitoneum require immediate fluid resuscitation, blood therapy, supplemental oxygen, and cardiac monitoring. Intraperitoneal pus secondary to a ruptured pelvic abscess requires immediate fluid expansion along with intravenous antibiotics with activity against aerobic and anaerobic organisms. Although a number of antibiotics are known to be effective, the selection remains controversial among gynecologists. The emergency physician should discuss this with the consultant, if possible, before instituting therapy. Appropriate cultures should be taken from the blood, urine, cervix, and culdocentesis fluid before therapy is initiated.

DISPOSITION

Role of the Consultant

The urgency and type of consultation depend on the presenting situation. A ruptured ectopic pregnancy, tuboovarian abscess, or bleeding cyst requires hemodynamic stabilization and immediate evaluation by a gynecologist. Less acute situations require gynecologic evaluation, depending in part on patient reliability. Masses in children should be evaluated in the emergency department by a gynecologic oncologist or pediatric surgeon, as these masses are usually malignant ovarian neoplasms. Masses in postmenopausal women should be considered malignant, and consultation obtained from a gynecologic oncologist or gynecologist regarding further evaluation and management. In the menstruating woman, ectopic pregnancy should be ruled out. The size of the mass will influence subsequent management and timing of the consultation. Palpable masses found in individuals during the reproductive years that are between 5 cm and 10 cm in size may be managed expectantly, and consultation evaluation is not necessary in the emergency department.[4,7] Appropriate telephone consultation with a gynecologist must be obtained and the patient counseled regarding the possible complications and the necessity for expeditious follow-up. In appropriate situations, in which malignancy is of minimal concern, operative laparoscopists should be consulted for definitive management.[9,21] Pregnant women with adnexal masses not believed to be a simultaneous tubal ectopic pregnancy should be referred to operative laparoscopists who have advanced endoscopic skills.[17,29] General surgical consultation should be obtained in older patients with gastrointestinal symptoms associated with left-side adnexal masses that may represent a diverticular abscess.

Indications for Admission

All patients who present with evidence of ovarian rupture, torsion, infection, or hemorrhage should be admitted to the hospital. Because of the probability of malignant changes in the prepubertal girl and the postmenopausal woman, these patients should also be admitted for definitive studies and prompt surgical exploration. Women in the menstruating age group generate the most controversy in management. If the physical findings suggest features of malignancy as described earlier, admission is indicated on an urgent basis. A patient with a mass less than 10 cm in size, with benign features, may be treated as an outpatient.

Transfer Considerations

Most adnexal masses are of gynecologic origin. If the treating facility has no gynecologic surgeon, the patient should be transferred after stabilization. Children should be transferred to a facility with a gynecologic oncologist or pediatric surgeon. The patient with a mass suggestive of malignancy should, ideally, be transferred to a gynecologic oncologist. With the exception of hemodynamically unstable patients, most complications of an adnexal mass may be treated with appropriate fluids, analgesics, and antibiotics, and then transferred.

COMMON PITFALLS

- Spurious masses created by retained urine and feces must be considered. The bladder and rectum must be emptied. This may require catheterization and low rectal enemas.
- Ectopic pregnancy must always be considered in a fertile female with an adnexal mass.
- Ruptured tubal or ovarian abscesses may present without systemic febrile response. Culdocentesis is often diagnostic.
- Ovarian carcinoma is commonly associated with gastrointestinal symptoms and ascites. If this complex is present, serious consideration should be given toward the diagnosis.
- Ovaries decrease in size with advancing age, and a palpable,

normal-sized ovary (3.5 × 2.0 × 1.5 cm) in the postmenopausal woman is abnormal and must be evaluated.[3] Functional cysts do not occur in postmenopausal women.

- Ovarian cysts are often thin-walled, and examination must be gentle to avoid rupture, with subsequent potentially serious complications.
- Ultrasonographic examination in a nonpregnant female with an adnexal mass is of little value and may delay or confuse diagnosis or therapy.
- The location, size, and consistency of the mass are helpful in diagnosis, but only histologic diagnosis is definitive. Care must be exercised to provide the patient with expeditious referral to the appropriate specialist. There are no noninvasive procedures that are totally reliable.

References

1. Alcazar JL, Leparte C, Junado M, et al. The role of transvaginal ultrasonography combined with color velocity imagery and pulsed Doppler in the diagnosis of endometrioma. *Fertil Steril* 1997;67(3):487.
2. Athey PA, Lamki N, Matyas MA, et al. Comparison of transvaginal and transabdominal ultrasonography in ectopic pregnancy. *Can Assoc Radiol J* 1991;42:349.
3. Barber HRK. Diagnosing and managing the adnexal mass. In: Barber HRK, ed. *Ovarian carcinoma*, 2nd ed. New York: Masson, 1992.
4. Barber HRK, Graber EA. The PMPO syndrome (postmenopausal palpable ovary syndrome). *Obstet Gynecol Surv* 1973;28:357.
5. Benacerraf BR, Finkler NJ, Wojciechowski C, et al. Sonographic accuracy in the diagnosis of ovarian masses. *J Reprod Med* 1990;35:491.
6. Brown DL, Frates MD, Laing FC, et al. Ovarian masses: can benign and malignant lesions be differentiated with color and pulsed Doppler US? *Radiology* 1994;190:333.
7. DiSaia PJ, Creasman WT. *Clinical gynecologic oncology*, 5th ed. St. Louis: Mosby, 1997.
8. Disantis DJ, Scatarige JC, Kemp G, et al. A prospective evaluation of transvaginal sonography for detection of ovarian disease. *AJR* 1993;161:91.
9. Dottino PR, Levine DA, Reply DL, et al. Laparoscopic management of adnexal masses in premenopausal and postmenopausal women. *Obstet Gynecol* 1999;93(2):223.
10. Finkler NI, Bast RC, Knapp RC. Tumor markers in gynecologic cancer. *Contemp Obstet Gynecol* 1987;30:29.
11. Frank JA, Dwyer AJ, Doppman JL. Nuclear magnetic resonance imaging in oncology. In: DeVita VT Jr, Hellman S, Rosenberg SA, eds. *Important advances in oncology, 1987*. Philadelphia: JB Lippincott Co, 1987.
12. Jain KA, Friedman DL, Pettinger TW, et al. Adnexal masses: comparison of specificity of endovaginal ultrasound and pelvic MR imaging. *Radiology* 1993;186:697.
13. Luxman D, Bergman A, Sagi J, et al. The post menopausal adnexal mass: correlation between ultrasonic and pathologic findings. *Obstet Gynecol* 1991;77:726.
14. McCarthy S. Gynecologic applications of MRI. *Crit Rev Diagn Imaging* 1990;31:263.
15. Meigs JV, Cass JW. Fibroma of the ovary with ascites and hydrothorax with report of 7 cases. *Am J Obstet Gynecol* 1937;33:249.
16. Morrow CP, Townsend DE. Tumors of the ovary. In: Morrow CP, Townsend DE, eds. *Synopsis of gynecologic oncology*, 3rd ed. New York: John Wiley and Sons, 1987.
17. Nezhat FR, Tazuke S, Nezhat CH, et al. Laparoscopy during pregnancy: a literature review. *J Soc Laparoendosc Surg* 1997;1(1):17.
18. O'Brien WF, Buch DR, Nash JD. Evaluation of sonography in the initial assessment of the gynecologic patient. *Am J Obstet Gynecol* 1984;149:598.
19. Olson MC, Posniak HV, Tempany CM, et al. MR imaging of the female pelvic region. *Radiographics* 1992;12:445.
20. Outwater EK, Dunton CJ. Imaging of the ovary and adnexa: clinical issues and applications of MR imaging. *Radiology* 1995;194:1.
21. Parker WH. Management of adnexal masses by operative laparoscopy. Selection criteria. *J Reprod Med* 1992;37:603.
22. Parsons L, Sommers S. Tumors in childhood. In: Parsons L, Sommers S, eds. *Gynecology*, 2nd ed. Philadelphia: WB Saunders, 1978.
23. Riles A, Wein U, Lichtenegger W. Transvaginal color Doppler sonography and conventional sonography in the pre operative assessment of adnexal masses. *J Clin Ultrasound* 1997;25(5):217.
24. Sawyer RW, Vick CW, Walsh JW, et al. Computed tomography of benign ovarian masses. *J Comput Assist Tomogr* 1985;9:784.
25. Strigini FA, Gadducci A, Del Brane B, et al. Differential diagnosis of adnexal masses with transvaginal sonography, color flow imaging, and serum CA 125 assay in pre and post menopausal women. *Gynecol Oncol* 1999;61(1):68.
26. Symmonds RE, Spraitz AF, Koelshe GA. Large ovarian tumors. *Obstet Gynecol* 1963;22:473.
27. Wittenberg J. Computed tomography of the body. Part I. *N Engl J Med* 1983;19:1160.
28. Wittenberg J. Computed tomography of the body. Part II. *N Engl J Med* 1983;20:1224.
29. Yuan PM, Chang AM. Laparoscopic management of adnexal mass during pregnancy. *Acta Obstet Gynecol Scand* 1997;76(2):173.

CHAPTER 88
Sexual Assault

Gwendolyn L. Hoffman

An emergency physician confronts a great variety of medical emergencies. One of the more complex is sexual assault or rape. The legal definition of *sexual assault*, which is the gender-neutral term, may vary from state to state, but most definitions of *rape*, which is the legal term, include genital, anal, or oral penetration by a part of the accused's body or by an object, using force or without the victim's consent.[4] In 1996, the Bureau of Justice Statistics estimated there were 307,000 women who were the victims of rape, attempted rape, or sexual assault.[12,15] It is estimated that less than one in three assaults is reported and that one in five American women will be victims of rape or sexual assault.[5] The emergency physician must be adept at meeting the physical, emotional, and judicial needs of these patients.

CLINICAL PRESENTATION

The sexual assault victim may present to the emergency department immediately after the event. She is often accompanied by friends, family, or the police. She may have visible physical trauma and be emotionally distraught. On the other hand, it may be hours or days later before she presents. The victim may feel guilt, shame, humiliation, and embarrassment. She may not be immediately able to share her experience with anyone and may delay seeking treatment. The victim with physical trauma, such as airway compromise, severe laceration, or fracture, is most likely to obtain early medical intervention.

EMERGENCY DEPARTMENT EVALUATION

The emergency physician's first duty to the rape victim is to evaluate for any life threat. The ABCs—airway, breathing, and circulation—must be addressed appropriately. If specific treatment is administered, care must be taken not to destroy or alter any evidence on the patient's person or at the scene. If the patient herself calls the emergency department to say she has been sexually assaulted, she should be advised to come immediately for evaluation and treatment. She should be encouraged not to bathe, shower, douche, gargle, brush her teeth, eat, drink, urinate, defecate, take medicines, or change her clothing. If she has already changed clothes, she should be advised to place in a paper bag the clothes she took off and bring them to the hospital. If she has not notified the police, she should be advised to do so, or the emergency physician should offer to do it for her.

At the emergency department, the patient should be ushered into a private room where care can begin. Informed consent must be obtained in writing and witnessed before hospital personnel may perform the medical examination, collect and analyze specimens, take pictures, release information to legal authorities, or render treatment. If the hospital has a special sexual assault team, the team should initiate involvement with the victim at this point. An increasing number of institutions are associated with a sexual assault nurse examiner (SANE) program.[7]

Once consent has been obtained, the pertinent historical facts can be obtained if the patient is physically stable. The history need not be an exhaustive account of the details of the encounter. Information about minute details that the victim provides at a time of acute emotional strain may later prove confusing in court if any discrepancy is noted between the hospital and police reports. The history should include information necessary for medical treatment and for the collection of evidence, including time, date, and place of the event. This information may be important when trying to relate physical findings, such as a bruise, to the assault, or when looking for corroborating evidence, such as sand if the assault occurred at the beach. Threats of violence or reprisal made by the assailant should be noted. If any type of weapon, restraints, foreign bodies, alcohol, or drugs were involved, these facts should be noted, as well as the number of assailants; whether vaginal, oral, or anal penetration was attempted; and whether ejaculation occurred. If ejaculation occurred, seminal deposits must be carefully sought on clothing as well as on the patient's person. The patient should be asked if she has douched, bathed, urinated, or defecated since the assault. If she has, some evidence might have been destroyed.

A pertinent gynecologic history should include gravidity, parity, last menstrual period, contraceptive history, date of last consensual intercourse, history of recent sexually transmitted disease, and any recent gynecologic surgery. If the victim is taking birth control pills, she should be asked if she has missed taking any pills. All of this information will assist in deciding what type of medical treatment is necessary.

The medical history should include current medication, allergies, and tetanus immunization status. In some emergency departments, nurses take the history and collect specimens. It does not matter who gathers this evidence as long as it is done in a caring and professional manner. The important thing is that important information is not omitted and the chain of evidence is not broken. For this reason, most departments have specific protocols and prepared forms that should be used. The physician must be thoroughly familiar with department procedure.[1,11]

It does not matter whether the physical examination is performed by a female or male physician. It is important that the physician be understanding, supportive, and caring. The purposes of the physical examination are to determine the need for medical treatment, to gather specimens for analysis, and to make and document observations for corroboration of the assault. If the police are present and if the victim is wearing the clothes she wore during the attack, the police may want to take photographs before she undresses. In this case, the patient should be asked to place her clothes in a paper bag, or to place each item in a separate bag, depending on protocol. Paper bags are used instead of plastic bags, because plastic bags do not "breathe" and may promote molding of blood and seminal stains. The patient should put the clothes in the bag herself to avoid possible cross-contamination from blood group antigens in the sweat of hospital personnel.

When the patient has donned a hospital gown and is ready, the physician should thoroughly explain what the physical examination will entail. The skin should be inspected for scratches, lacerations, abrasions, contusions, and bite marks; special attention should be paid to the neck, mouth, breasts, wrists, and thighs. When the mouth is being examined for trauma, a saliva sample should be obtained. The sample can be used to determine the patient's status as a blood group antigen secretor or nonsecretor. The teeth should be swabbed for acid phosphatase and sperm analysis. In addition to noting evidence of trauma, the presence of any foreign material, such as hair, blood, or semen, should also be noted. Foreign material should be scraped from under the fingernails and placed in the appropriate envelope. This material may reveal bits of the assailant's hair, blood, or skin, if the victim were able actively to resist. Semen may appear as lightly crusted areas. A Wood light can help to identify these areas because they fluoresce in ultraviolet light.[9] Semen can be removed with a water-moistened swab. Fluorescence is not pathognomonic of semen because other stains and urine may fluoresce, but it may be helpful.

If photographs are not taken, the physician must be even more careful to document the findings completely and accurately. Documenting thoroughly at the time of the examination makes it easier to recall the examination accurately when called on in a court of law.

The pelvic examination should be performed next. The external genitalia should be checked for trauma and evidence of semen. If semen is present on the upper inner thighs, it can be swabbed as previously described. If it is present on pubic hair, the hairs should be trimmed. The patient's pubic hair should be combed to find strands of the assailant's hair, which can be analyzed to help identify the assailant's race and hair color.[6] In order to differentiate it from the victim's hair, some of her pubic hair must be plucked for analysis also. Each specimen should be placed in the appropriate envelope.

Small vaginal lacerations can be identified with the use of toluidine blue.[4] A small amount of the blue dye can be applied to the vaginal mucosa at the introitus. A positive test result is indicated by a linear blue stain, because the dye will be taken up by the nuclei of exposed submucosal cells. The dye is applied externally, not intravaginally. Therefore, it should not interfere with the collection of other evidence, but any excess should be wiped off before the speculum is inserted, just to be sure.

The hymen should be inspected to determine if it is present, intact, absent, or traumatized, with bleeding or fresh clots. In adolescent girls with an estrogenized hymen, the examination is more difficult. A Foley catheter (14F) inserted through the hymen orifice and inflated, using 40 cc of air, has been used successfully to assess the redundant hymen.[10] The speculum should be lubricated only with water; other lubricants may affect the acid phosphatase determination and sperm motility. The vaginal wall should be inspected for lacerations and for evidence of the penetration of any foreign objects. Any secretions that have pooled in the posterior fornix should be aspirated and placed in a sterile receptacle. These secretions can be used to determine the presence of sperm, acid phosphatase, and blood group antigens. If no secretions are present, the vagina should be washed with 5 to 10 mL of nonbacteriostatic sterile saline solution and followed with aspiration. If washing is not necessary, the posterior fornix should be swabbed with a cotton-tipped applicator and secretions smeared on two glass slides for later laboratory examination. One more swab should be obtained for wet mount examination. A Papanicolaou smear should be obtained from the cervix to help determine the presence of nonmotile sperm (the smear is useful up to several days after the assault). Cultures for gonorrhea, chlamydial infection, and herpes should be obtained, if indicated. A bimanual examination should be performed, and uterine size, adnexal masses, and tenderness noted. The rectal area should be examined carefully, especially if anal intercourse took place. Signs of trauma, semen stain, blood, and lubricant should be noted. Anal and rectal swabs can be obtained through the lumen of a water-lubricated anoscope; these are used to determine the presence of motile and nonmotile sperm and acid phosphatase. It is often difficult to document genital findings in sexual assault victims by gross visualization alone. Magnification with colposcopic examination and photography allows the examiner to document and characterize genital findings with more accuracy. Many emergency departments have a colposcope readily available.[8,14]

Blood should also be drawn for ABO analysis, syphilis serology, drug and alcohol screen, and beta human chorionic gonadotropin (β-hCG). Routine testing for hepatitis B virus and human immunodeficiency virus must also be considered. This is especially true in an area of high seropositivity or if the assailant is known to be in a high-risk group.[11] Pregnancy may be detected as early as 1 week after implantation by using the radioimmunoassay beta subunit of hCG or the Tandem Icon II hCG urine assay. If the test result is negative initially and positive at a follow-up visit, the pregnancy probably originated at the time of the assault.

The oral, vaginal, and rectal swabs obtained for the identification of sperm must be examined microscopically for motile and nonmotile sperm. Sperm are not usually found motile after 12 hours. The presence of motile sperm is a reliable indication that the assault occurred at some point during the 12 hours preceding the examination, provided consensual intercourse did not also take place during that period. Nonmotile sperm may be present for 72 hours or longer.

The acid phosphatase enzyme may also indicate sexual contact. This enzyme is present in vaginal secretions but is found in much greater quantities in prostatic secretions. A high concentration of acid phosphatase is an excellent indicator of the presence of seminal fluid, even in the absence of sperm. The presence of acid phosphatase may be a more accurate indicator of the postcoital interval than the presence of nonmotile sperm.

A major seminal plasma glycoprotein produced in the prostate, p30, has been identified as another semen-specific marker. This protein is male-specific; therefore, the finding of any p30 in vaginal fluid establishes the presence of semen. p30 is present in men who have had vasectomies as well as in men who have not, and it can be found for approximately 48 hours after the assault.

The forensic laboratory will also develop a specific genetic profile of the assailant to compare with that of the victim. Genetic typing can determine the blood group and type of both parties. Three genetic markers found in semen are phosphoglucomutase (PGM), the peptidase-A (Pep-A) enzyme marker, and the ABO blood group antigens. With electrophoretic analysis, PGM and Pep-A can be further subdivided into a total of 40 possible combinations. Reference markers for the victim must be obtained at the initial evaluation; these markers are also in vaginal secretions but in lower concentrations.

DNA typing or fingerprinting is the newest method used to identify the assailant. This method involves the extraction of DNA from a small sample of blood, semen, or other DNA-bearing cells. Through various procedures, a specific "DNA fingerprint" is developed. This "fingerprint" can be analyzed and compared with the assailant's to establish a positive identification. The chance that two unrelated persons having the same DNA fingerprint is one in a quadrillion.[3,14]

EMERGENCY DEPARTMENT MANAGEMENT

Physical trauma experienced by a sexual assault victim is treated like trauma in any other patient. In addition, the possibilities of psychological trauma, pregnancy, and venereal disease must be addressed.

Efforts to decrease the victim's distress can begin with her arrival at the emergency department. The staff must be attentive and encourage the victim to share her feelings. She has just experienced a threat to her life and must be helped to feel safe and secure. It is often helpful to have a rape crisis volunteer present to provide additional support and to make sure the patient understands the procedures explained to her by the physician and nurse. Her emotional trauma may be significant.

Rape is sudden and does not allow the victim to gather adequate defenses. Also, the victim feels trapped and often cannot fight back. The ability to trust is destroyed when the perpetrator is known.[13] Rape also often involves intentional cruelty and physical injury. The victim will feel most comfortable with hospital personnel who are capable of projecting both professional objectivity and personal concern.

The possibility of pregnancy should be explained to the patient. It is estimated that the risk of pregnancy without contraception is 2% to 4%. If midcycle (days 14 to 16), the risk is higher.[11] Pregnancy should be ruled out before prophylactic treatment is considered. The "morning-after pill" can be administered if prophylaxis is desired. Diethylstilbestrol (DES; 25 mg by mouth twice daily for 5 days) must be administered within 72 hours of sexual contact to be effective. If conception occurs despite DES prophylaxis, a female fetus is at risk for vaginal adenosis and cancer and a male fetus is at risk for penile and testicular lesions.[9] Birth control pills may be used instead of DES. A regimen that includes norgestrel plus oral ethinyl estradiol (two pills initially and two pills 12 hours later) is acceptable. Ethinyl estradiol (0.5 mg daily for 5 days) may also be used.[11] Premarin (25 mg), an oral conjugated estrogen, may be administered daily for 5 days. Good results and less nausea have been reported with the use of intravenous Premarin (50 mg for 2 days). One problem is ensuring that the patient return for the follow-up visit. All of the estrogen preparations may cause nausea and vomiting. To combat this problem, some physicians order an antiemetic to accompany the estrogen preparation. A history of pulmonary embolism, thrombophlebitis, estrogen-dependent tumor, or cardiovascular or liver disease is a contraindication to the administration of estrogens.

If the initial pregnancy test result is negative and a follow-up test result is positive, counseling is indicated, after which the patient may want to have a suction curettage or a therapeutic abortion.

The risk of contracting a sexually transmitted disease as the result of sexual assault is hard to estimate. Risk varies according to geographic area, the populations within that area, and whether the assault is reported. Some reports have indicated that the incidence of acquiring a sexually transmitted disease from a single sexual encounter is 5% to 10%.[11] Prophylaxis should be given if the patient requests it, if evidence of infection is present on examination, if follow-up is questionable, and if the assailant is suspected of being infected. The Centers for Disease Control and Prevention recommend prophylaxis for gonorrhea, chlamydia, and syphilis. Trichomoniasis should be treated with metronidazole 2 g PO if seen on wet mount.[2]

Patients are usually treated by using one of the following regimens[2]:

Ceftriaxone 125 mg i.m.
Cefixime 400 mg PO once
Ciprofloxacin 500 mg PO once
Ofloxacin 400 mg PO once
Spectinomycin 2 g i.m.
Azithromycin 1 g PO once
Doxycycline 100 mg PO twice a day for 7 days

Ciprofloxacin and ofloxacin are contraindicated in pregnancy. Spectinomycin is recommended only for use during pregnancy in patients allergic to beta-lactams. Erythromycin, except for erythromycin estolate, (500 mg PO four times a day for 7 days) can be used in pregnancy. Both doxycycline and erythromycin will cover early syphilis, but the drug of choice remains penicillin G benzathine (2.4 million units i.m. once).[2] Hepatitis B virus vaccine should be considered if the patient was previously unimmunized. A dose of 1.0 mL i.m. should be given acutely and repeated 1 and 6 months later. Hepatitis B immune globulin should be reserved for a high-risk exposure, such as if the assailant is an intravenous drug user or if multiple assailants were involved.[11] Victims may be particularly concerned about the transmission of human immunodeficiency virus (HIV). The risk is felt to be very low but appropriate counseling should be arranged as well as pretesting if deemed necessary. At this time there is no proven prophylactic intervention.[2]

DISPOSITION

A gynecologist may be called during the initial examination if the emergency physician deems it necessary, especially if an operative intervention is needed. The emergency physician should strongly recommend that the victim seek follow-up care from a gynecologist or family physician.

Most hospitals have rape crisis volunteers available to consult with the victim during the first 24 hours after the assault. Encourage the patient to talk to the volunteers or to seek counseling with psychologists or psychiatrists, if indicated.

Admission to the hospital may be required in the case of significant physical trauma. As a rule, the sexual assault victim may be discharged from the emergency department in the company of relatives or friends. Follow-up care for the victim must be arranged before discharge. She will need to return after 2 weeks and after 6 weeks to be reevaluated for pregnancy and venereal disease. Any physical injury, such as a laceration, will need follow-up care. Psychological trauma may necessitate long-term treatment.[1] The short-term phase, characterized by disorganization, may last from a few days to a few weeks. During this time, the victim may exhibit a wide range of emotional behavior, from being quiet and subdued to demonstrating anger and fear. The long-term phase, characterized by reorganization, may last for months or years. Many victims experience depression, flashbacks, anxiety, and sexual dysfunction.[4] These experiences may explain why 80% of rape victims end primary relationships within 1 year of the rape.[4] Because the rape victim may have a large spectrum of psychological needs and concerns, the emergency physician must be certain that follow-up evaluation will address them. The patient should be reevaluated psychologically approximately 1 to 2 weeks after the initial medical evaluation. At that visit, the need for further counseling should be discussed.

COMMON PITFALLS

- When treating a sexual assault victim, the physician and other involved personnel must be certain that the collection, disposition, and transfer of all specimens are documented at every stage, from collection to introduction into the courtroom. This legal protocol is the chain of evidence and safeguards the rights of the accused during the judicial process. All specimens must be correctly collected and labeled. Documentation must be made of each person who takes possession of the evidence—the physician or nurse who gathers the evidence, the police officer who transfers it to the forensic laboratory, and laboratory technicians. No break must occur in this process, or the evidence will not be admissible in court.
- Each institution and state may have some variation in their requirements and protocol, so the emergency physician must be familiar with the sexual assault kit and the forms and procedures of his or her institution.
- Another pitfall is lack of follow-up. Up to 94% of rape victims do not return for their follow-up visits.[4] Therefore, it is advisable that some member of the medical team, such as a social worker, contact the victim after discharge, to address concerns that arise later and to encourage follow-up care.

References

1. American College of Emergency Physicians. Management of the patient with the complaint of sexual assault. *Ann Emerg Med* 1995;25:728.
2. Centers for Disease Control and Prevention. 1998 Guidelines for treatment of sexually transmitted diseases. *MMWR* 1998;47:RR-1.
3. Dawkins R. Arresting evidence. *The Sciences* 1998;Nov-Dec:20.
4. DeLahunta E, Baram DA. Sexual assault. *Obstet Gynecol* 1997;40:648.
5. Department of Justice. Prevalence, evidence, and consequences of violence against women. Research-in-Brief 1998. http://www.ncjrs.org/victdv.htn#172837
6. Ferris LE, Sandercock J. The sensitivity of forensic tests for rape. *Med Law* 1998;17:333.
7. Ledray LE. Sexual assault: clinical issues. *J Emerg Nurs* 1998;24:197.
8. Lenahan LC, Ernst A, Johnson B. Colposcopy in evaluation of the adult sexual assault victim. *Am J Emerg Med* 1998;16:183.
9. Lynnerup N, Hjalgrim H. Routine use of ultraviolet light in medicolegal examinations to evaluate stains and skin trauma. *Med Sci Law* 1995;35:165.
10. Persaud DI, Squires JE, Rubin-Remer O. Use of Foley catheter to examine estrogenized hymens for evidence of sexual abuse. *J Pediatr Adolesc Gynecol* 1997;10:83.
11. Petter LM, Whitehill DL. Management of female sexual assault. *Am Fam Physician* 1998;58:920.
12. Rape, Abuse, and Incest National Network (RAINN). Washington, DC. E-mail: RAINNmail@aol.com
13. Rickert VJ, Wiemann CM. Date rape among adolescents and young adults. *J Pediatr Adolesc Gynecol* 1997;10:83.
14. Rogers D. Physical aspects of alleged sexual assaults. *Med Sci Law* 1996;36:117.
15. United States Department of Justice, Bureau of Justice Statistics. Crime and Victim Statistics 1999. http://www.ojp.usdoj.gov/bjs

SECTION III

Section Editor: Suzanne Moore Shepherd

Trauma

PART I
General Considerations

CHAPTER 89
General Principles of Trauma

Peter Rosen

Trauma is the leading cause of death in the first three decades of life.[4] Many of the 100,000 fatalities resulting from accidents each year could be prevented by expeditious transfer of the multiply injured patient to a trauma center that can provide high-quality trauma care in the first hour after injury.

CLINICAL PRESENTATION

The appropriate care of the major trauma patient is best achieved in an institution that has a dedicated mission for trauma. Although there is no completely accurate field system for appraising the patient with subtle but serious trauma, and there are great economic concerns about overtriage of minor trauma, it is not the obvious case of major trauma that is the problem; rather, the problem is the patient with a moderate mechanism of injury who appears to have an isolated orthopedic injury, but who is harboring a ruptured liver or spleen. It is far better to overtriage the less serious injury than to undertriage the subtle serious injury.

In rural areas, it may well be impossible to have a trauma center as a destination; there are no trauma centers in Wyoming, Idaho, or Montana, for example. There are variations in capabilities of communities, and it may make sense to take a patient past the nearest hospital to reach one with a general surgeon or one that has computed tomography (CT) scan capacity. It is often necessary to attempt to stabilize a patient before transferring him or her to a tertiary care center or a trauma center in another state. It is therefore wise to have the transfer agreements and routes as well as the mechanics of evacuation worked out well in advance of the individual patient's need.

The trauma center can assemble a more efficient team and has the experience and resources to achieve timely response to reparable injury, which will definitely lower morbidity and mortality. Even if the emergency physician has been well trained in trauma, if the institution is not committed to the total care of the trauma patient, the effectiveness of the prehospital care or emergency department resuscitation will be lost.

Patients assessed by prehospital personnel as having a major mechanism of injury, or those arriving on their own who are recognized as having a potentially serious injury, should be triaged immediately to a suitable treatment area capable of major resuscitation. Appropriate management must coordinate not only the entire institution in which the patient will receive definitive care, but also the field care. There must be a total system commitment to ensure that the injured patient is taken to the correct facility where there are properly trained and skilled emergency physicians, surgeons, and technical personnel. Laboratory and special diagnostic equipment and technicians must be readily available, as well as anesthesia and operating rooms. There must be good intensive care unit support and the psychological and rehabilitative functions that will restore the patient toward full health.

Appropriate personnel should accompany the patient from the emergency department entrance to the resuscitation room to ensure that adequate life-support measures are being accomplished en route. Whether or not prehospital communication has taken place, details regarding the mechanism of injury are important clues in predicting potential injuries (Table 89.1).

Triage must take into account the immediate threat to life or limb as well as patient discomfort and anxiety; the means to evaluation is an adequate history and physical examination. The triage officer must be capable of rapid decision making and must understand that the wrong decisions can have drastic consequences. Correct decisions require maturity, appropriate awareness, intelligence, and experience. In many hospitals, the triage function is fulfilled by an emergency department nurse. Larger centers may use a highly trained and experienced trauma nurse or a triage physician.

Seriously injured patients or those with a major mechanism of injury must be triaged to a major resuscitation room. Human nature is such that once a patient has been labeled "not serious," it is difficult to change that label and achieve appropriate care for the patient. Therefore, it is wise to overestimate the possible injuries. Fewer mistakes will be made by overresuscitation than by underresuscitation. Patients who are not overtly seriously injured may nevertheless be evaluated in the trauma resuscitation room if their injuries are potentially serious.

The trauma team must have a captain. The training and experience of this person may vary from place to place and should be appropriate to the specific hospital. Although the ideal may be impossible to achieve—a captain who is a physician with extensive experience in trauma management—an institution can no longer promote itself as a major trauma center without having that expertise. Increasingly, the captain is initially an emergency physician. In some settings, an emergency physician may be the only physician physically present in the emergency department (and, for that matter, in the hospital). Ideally, surgical support personnel are available within 10 to 15 minutes.

In trauma centers, surgical support is immediately available within the hospital. In this system, the emergency physician

TABLE 89.1. Important Details about Mechanism of Injury

BLUNT TRAUMA

Motor Vehicle Accident

1. Estimated speed of both vehicles on impact
2. Orientation of the vehicles (e.g., head-on, broadside)
3. Trajectory and extent of damage to patient's vehicle
4. Was there an explosion or fire?
5. Was the patient restrained?
6. Was the windshield intact?
7. Was the steering wheel intact?
8. Was there an initial loss of consciousness at the scene?
9. Were any alcohol or drugs recovered from the patient or car?
10. How long did it take to extricate the patient?
11. What is the ambient temperature (potential for hypothermia)?

Fall

1. Estimated height?
2. Possible reason for fall (e.g., electrocution, explosion)
3. Was there an initial loss of consciousness at the scene?
4. Were any alcohol or drugs recovered from the patient or scene?
5. How long was the patient down?
6. What is the ambient temperature (potential for hypothermia)?

PENETRATING TRAUMA

Stab Wound

1. Description of the weapon (e.g., length, width)
2. See 4 and 5 under "Fall."

Gunshot Wound

1. Description of the weapon (including caliber)
2. See 4 and 5 under "Fall."

may assume the role of trauma captain for the initial assessment and resuscitation. When the attending trauma surgeon arrives, a defined transition of leadership should occur. The team concept must be maintained at all times.

If the responsibility for the major orchestration is formally handed over to the trauma surgeon, it does not relieve the emergency physician of responsibility for the patient. The emergency physician should stay and assist until the patient physically leaves for the operating room, intensive care unit, or special diagnostic study. On occasion, the emergency department may be busy with other seriously injured patients who demand immediate attention. In this situation, the emergency physician may have to leave the trauma patient, but this departure should always be made in coordination with the team and the team leader. The team may summon subspecialty consultations, as needed, for stabilization, but there must be a single person in charge of the orchestration of total patient needs. Too often, resuscitation becomes chaotic, with multiple subspecialists tunneled into the concerns of their own specialty. The trauma surgeon or emergency physician must stay in command of the overall care.

Nurses who care for trauma patients should have the special knowledge and skills to serve the patient adequately. In the large urban center, there is usually no paucity of physicians to complete resuscitative procedures, but this is not the case in the rural emergency department, where the trauma nurse may need many technical skills ordinarily reserved for physicians. Field paramedics may need to stay in the emergency department so that their technical skills can be used, if they do not have to return to service or a field location immediately. Occasionally, they may be called on to initiate stabilization until a physician arrives. Protocols and guidelines should be available regarding expectations of nursing staff.

A coordinated, knowledgeable response from the blood bank, laboratory, respiratory therapy, and radiology department is key to an effective trauma system. Their direction and coordination for integral function with the trauma team are essential. Social workers, clergy, and lay support should be included in the team framework. The area of the radiology department designated for emergency patients should be located adjacent to the emergency department. Portable or built-in x-ray equipment in the trauma resuscitation room is also necessary for proper care of the seriously injured patient.

The radiologist must be considered a member of the trauma team; availability for consultation at all hours and adequate communication are essential. The radiology department should be integrated into the trauma team and should participate in planning.

The operating room must be immediately accessible to the emergency department for operative resuscitation of critically injured patients. Some centers have emphasized this relation by having an operating room as part of the emergency department or by reserving a single operating room for trauma use.

Ideally, potentially or obviously seriously injured patients are triaged either to a trauma resuscitation room or to an area where an appropriate history and physical examination can be carried out. Because of lack of space and personnel, sometimes triage must be consigned to the waiting room. Patients should not, however, be sent to a minor trauma room or the waiting room, to be forgotten. Adequate explanation of the need for delay and some show of concern and attention are required, for what the emergency department staff considers minor or nonurgent is almost never perceived as such by the patient.

EMERGENCY DEPARTMENT MANAGEMENT

The approach to the multiple-trauma patient begins with a rapid initial examination; this takes no longer than 1 minute and is done while vital signs are being assessed.[6] The patient is stripped of all clothing. If there is any hint of vital sign instability, the clothes should be cut away. Too many patients have been thrown into severe shock when someone tries to sit them up to remove a T-shirt or some other trivial item of clothing.

Immediately ascertain the patency of the airway. Examine the neck for direct trauma, carotid pulsation, tracheal position, and character of neck veins. Quickly observe the chest for sucking wounds or paradoxical motion; palpate for crepitus, and auscultate for the absence of breath sounds or the presence of adventitious sounds.

Palpate the extremities. If they are cool, moist, or pale, shock must be presumed. In the absence of any contraindications, roll the patient from side to side to ensure that there are no wounds on the back. In the field, it may be impossible to auscultate the blood pressure because of extraneous noise, but in the emergency department, an attempt should be made to auscultate the systolic and diastolic pressures.

Locating a palpable pulse provides much information about the perfusion pressure. For example, if a radial pulse is present, the patient must have a systolic blood pressure of at least 80 mm Hg. A palpable femoral pulse indicates a systolic blood pressure of at least 70 mm Hg, and a carotid pulse, a systolic blood pressure of 60 mm Hg.

When intravenous lines are placed, blood is drawn for blood typing and other tests. If the field system can draw blood, having field staff draw samples will save time for blood typing, but not every hospital laboratory accepts field blood samples. It is more efficient to use a large, 50-mL syringe and simultaneously draw all needed blood samples, as well as measure arterial blood gas from the femoral artery. This site gives a quick indication of subtle malperfusion and provides quick access to a good blood source for obtaining the specimen quickly. It is the trauma captain's responsibility to ensure that blood is obtained in a timely manner.

The cervical spine must remain immobilized until it is radiographically cleared of injury. Hyperextension or flexion of the neck should be avoided if neck injury is suspected or if the patient is unconscious from a head injury.

Delivery of oxygen to the tissues is of primary importance, and clearing the airway is the initial step. In the unconscious patient, use a finger to sweep vomitus, blood, teeth, bone, or other debris from the oral cavity. A suction apparatus may be used to clear the upper airway. The patient who has facial but no neck injuries may be turned to a lateral or prone position, or placed in a sitting position, leaning forward, to allow rapid clearing of the airway. If the condition of the spine is unknown, it may be necessary to leave a suction catheter in the patient's mouth while the cervical spine is being cleared. A chin lift or jaw thrust will usually relieve upper airway obstruction.

If necessary, grasping the tongue with a towel clip or placing a suture in the tongue and drawing it forward will open a difficult airway. In some cases of severe maxillofacial trauma or direct tracheal injury, cricothyrotomy is needed. Supplemental oxygen should be given. If the patient needs active airway management because of secretions, the kinds of injuries present, or respiratory distress, do not take time to obtain arterial blood gas analysis; instead, secure the airway. Once the airway is patent, recheck breath sounds.

If the patient is not breathing spontaneously or adequately, ventilation must be controlled. Initial control may be by bag-valve-mask ventilation with high-flow oxygen. Once the patient is oxygenated and hypercapnia has been corrected, intubation is less hazardous, but undertaking it must always be weighed against the risk of distending an already full stomach.

Major trauma victims often need active airway management, even if they are breathing spontaneously. There is a tremendous metabolic cost to breathing, especially with thoracic or abdominal injuries, and this can be overcome by taking over the work of breathing for the patient. Moreover, many patients have injuries that potentially can distort their airways (e.g., a gunshot wound to the neck). It is far better to intubate these patients before the anatomy becomes so distorted that intubation is impossible to perform, even with a fiberoptic bronchoscope. It will also be much harder, if not disastrous, to attempt a surgical airway when the neck is filled with a massive hematoma.

There is almost always some degree of head injury in the patient with multiple trauma, and it is worthwhile to try to prevent or contain cerebral edema by hyperventilation. Finally, because few trauma patients have an empty stomach at the time of the injury, intubation can help prevent the risk of the patient's vomiting and aspirating the vomitus.

For many years it was believed unsafe to intubate the trauma patient unless there were radiologic clearance of the integrity and stability of the spinal column. For this reason, there were long delays during attempts to clear the cervical spine, and many cricothyrotomies were performed. We now have more data and experience with the management of the trauma patient's airway, and the preferred approach is to keep the neck immobilized to prevent hyperflexion, hyperextension, or hyperdistraction, and to proceed with a rapid-sequence intubation (RSI) using sedation, prophylactic lidocaine, muscle paralysis, and oral intubation (Table 89.2).

In the presence of head injury, nasal intubation should be avoided, if possible. Not every helicopter or ground system is set up to manage the airway in this fashion, and one must work within the agreed-on field protocols, but in the emergency department, the optimal approach to the airway is via the oral route.

TABLE 89.2. Rapid-Sequence Induction

Crash intubation summary
Oxygenate the patient
Select appropriate endotracheal tube
Test the balloon
Insert stylette
Ensure suction is working
Apply tonsil tip to suction
Pretreat with lidocaine 1.5 mg/kg
In children, give atropine 0.01 mg/kg
Sedate the patient
Give succinylcholine 1.5 mg/kg
Perform Sellick's maneuver
Await fasciculations
Intubate quickly
Assess tube position
If correct, tie and tape in place
Assist ventilations
Obtain chest x-ray study

While oral intubation using an RSI has been very successful and has virtually eliminated the need for cricothyrotomy, the technique is important. While a second pair of hands other than those of the intubator stabilizes the head and neck, it is necessary to open the anterior portion of the cervical collar. It is almost never possible to intubate orally with the anterior collar closed, and it is safer and preferable to open it before making any intubation attempt.

While RSI oral intubation has largely replaced cricothyrotomy, some patients with midface crunches and severe oral trauma are best managed by placement of a surgical airway. A surgical airway is also necessary if there is extensive damage to the patient's larynx or if there is complete tracheal separation. In the latter instance, the trachea may not separate because it is held together by the cervical fascia. Before making an incision in the neck of a patient with this possible injury (as seen in motorcyclists who have run into a chain strung across their paths), it is prudent to grasp the distal stump of the trachea with a towel clip. Then, when the incision is made, this distal stump will not retract into the anterior mediastinum, where it cannot be reached without splitting the sternum. If the damage to the larynx is too great or if the separation is distal to the larynx, a tracheostomy will have to be performed.

The need for active airway management is the most critical question in the patient with multiple trauma; universally accepted criteria for mandatory intubation, however, have never been established. Table 89.3 lists mandatory and relative criteria that serve as guidelines for this decision.

Use direct pressure only to control external hemorrhage. Blind probing and clamping deep within a wound risk further injury to vessels and nerves.

Shock can be defined as inadequate perfusion of the tissues. Once oxygen has reached the alveolus and crossed into the blood, there must be a functional pump, adequate circulating volume, and an ample oxygen carrier before the oxygen can reach the tissues. Cool, pale, moist skin indicates shock.

In the treatment of shock, a Foley catheter is needed to monitor renal perfusion. A central venous catheter is also helpful in monitoring central volume. Vascular access is critical. Two large-bore (14- to 16-gauge) percutaneous catheters should be placed, avoiding, if possible, injured extremities. If veins are collapsed or sclerosed, cutdowns, either in the antecubital or saphenous veins, can be rapidly placed. A pediatric feeding tube or intravenous tubing works well as a large-bore catheter. Percutaneous central catheters inserted through the subclavian or internal jugular veins are more hazardous, particularly in the hypovolemic patient.

TABLE 89.3. Criteria for Active Airway Management

MANDATORY
Massive facial injuries
Head injury with Glasgow Coma Scale <8
Penetrating injury to the cranial vault
Missile penetrating injury to the neck
Blunt injury to the neck, with expanding hematoma, painful phonation, or alteration of the voice
Bilateral missile penetrating injuries of the thorax
Multisystem trauma with persistent shock
RELATIVE INDICATIONS
Upper airway obstruction from any cause
Any patient with injuries impairing ventilation
Flail chest with increasing respiratory rate or deteriorating blood gases
Any patient with one or more rib fractures who is going to need a ventilator or a general anesthetic
Bilateral pneumothorax
Expanding hemothorax that recurs or does not respond to thoracostomy
Any patient developing severe hypovolemic shock, extensive burns, pulmonary or facial or neck burns

Percutaneous femoral lines may be useful, and, in the child under age 3, intraosseous needles may be the only available route. There is no single answer to intravenous access: Each patient must be evaluated individually, and the cost–benefit ratio of the chosen routes weighed. In general, it is best to insert a minimum of two large-bore peripheral lines, adding more as necessary. Sometimes, this scenario is impossible to achieve, however, and it is necessary to proceed immediately to a central line or peripheral cutdown to gain access.

While most traumatized adults can tolerate generous fluid infusions, because they are usually young and in previous good health, if there is any question about underlying diseases, it is wise to give intravenous fluids under control. An initial dose of 20 mL/kg is always safe. If the patient still shows signs of volume deficit after administration of 50 mL/kg, type-specific or O-negative blood should be started. In the patient who has an injury that obviously will produce a major volume deficit (e.g., shotgun blast with marked tissue destruction and loss), blood should be given immediately.

In the adult, crystalloid can be continued while progress is being made, but if there is no response or only a partial restoration toward a normal pulse or blood pressure, do not exceed a dose of 50 mL/kg before initiating blood or blood products.[1,2,5,6]

When massive transfusions are necessary, one must remember the need for additional platelets and other clotting factors. Blood should be warmed whenever possible.

In children, fluids should be given as aliquots rather than run wide open. An aliquot of 20 mL/kg is safe as an initial bolus. This dose can be repeated once and then halved, at a dose of 10 mL/kg. At this time, blood is started at 10 mL/kg. In addition to an aliquot dose, the time must be specified. The first volume should be administered in 30 minutes or less, the second volume over the course of an hour.

In all cases, the amount of fluids given depends on continued losses, which should be minimized as much as possible through proper splinting, bandaging, and avoidance of probing large soft-tissue wounds. We often forget how much a soft-tissue injury, especially to the scalp, can bleed, and the best treatment of hypovolemia is to locate the source of bleeding and stop the blood loss. The degree to which long-bone and pelvic fractures bleed is also not generally appreciated, and it is far more effective to begin giving blood as soon as these injuries are recognized than to wait.

Noting the character of the neck veins of the trauma patient is invaluable in identifying the cause of shock. If the neck veins are collapsed, hypovolemia must be presumed. If they are distended, then cardiogenic shock, tension pneumothorax, or pericardial tamponade must be excluded. Most trauma patients in shock are hypovolemic. Tension pneumothorax causes shock by increasing intrathoracic pressure, shifting the mediastinum, and compressing the great veins, thereby preventing venous return. The diagnosis is possible in any patient in shock who has distended neck veins and an increased resistance to bagging. An ipsilateral decrease in breath sounds may be noted, as well as a contralateral tracheal shift. Unfortunately, these physical findings are often not present in the acute trauma situation, and the only clues to the presence of a correctable cause of patient collapse may be a sudden rise in pulse, a drop in blood pressure, and an increased resistance to ventilation. The neck veins may not even be distended if the patient is concomitantly hypovolemic.

If tension pneumothorax is suspected in the field, it should be immediately decompressed with a large-bore over-the-needle catheter in the second intercostal space–midclavicular line. Many air ambulance personnel can perform tube thoracostomies. This route should be chosen in field cases if personnel have been trained to do the procedure, and in the emergency department. A tension pneumothorax is what kills patients, not a simple collapse of the lung.

Do not waste time obtaining radiographic confirmation of a suspected tension pneumothorax, as the patient may well arrest while the film is being obtained. Perform thoracostomy by inserting a large-bore chest tube in the fifth intercostal space, in the midaxillary line, to evacuate any blood present, as well as any air.

Cardiac causes of shock must not be overlooked. Pericardial tamponade is rare with closed-chest injuries, and another source of the shock should probably be sought. It must always be considered with penetrating injuries, even if the entrance wound appears anatomically remote. The physiologic response to tamponade is to compensate for the fall in cardiac output by raising the pulse rate. The classic physical findings in this disorder may also be absent in the acute situation. Thus, one may not see distended neck veins if the patient is profoundly hypovolemic. Furthermore, heart sounds may be difficult to appreciate during a major resuscitation. If the patient still has vital signs, a pericardiocentesis can be performed. If, on the other hand, the patient has lost vital signs or has suddenly become bradycardic (an ominous sign in a patient with this potential pathology), an immediate thoracotomy should be performed.

Myocardial contusion, most commonly from blunt trauma, may cause dysrhythmias, often within the first hour after injury. An electrogram (ECG) should be obtained in patients with significant anterior blunt chest trauma. Continuous ECG monitoring is indicated. Myocardial infarction may occur as a result of the stress associated with blood loss and catecholamine release, or it may have preceded the traumatic injury. Coronary arterial air embolization occurs with penetrating neck and chest trauma or serious rib fractures after intubation and positive-pressure ventilation. Air passes from the airway into the pulmonary veins and embolizes to the arterial circulation, often involving the cerebral and coronary arteries. If air embolization is suspected, the patient should be immediately turned to the left lateral decubitus position (i.e., right side up); fluid infusion should be increased, and immediate thoracotomy with bypass arranged. It may be possible to salvage some of these patients with immediate femorofemoral bypass while preparing the operating room.

Possible sources of significant blood loss causing hypovolemic shock include the chest, abdomen (including the pelvis and retroperitoneum), and thighs. Head injuries seldom cause hypovolemia, even in children (except for extensive scalp lacerations), and other sites of occult blood loss must be excluded in a head-injured patient with shock. Spinal cord trauma with loss of sympathetic vascular tone can be assessed by rectal examination and examination of peripheral reflexes.

The diagnosis of intraabdominal hemorrhage is often difficult. Abdominal examination may be totally normal despite significant intraabdominal pathology. The pulse may not be rapid, especially if the bleeding has been sudden and profound, or if the patient has alcohol or other drugs in his or her system. Bowel sounds may be present, and no abdominal tenderness or guarding may be seen. Distention is a late finding that may be present even if there is no abdominal pathology, and does not predict the degree of blood loss.

The patient may also have other problems that interfere with an accurate diagnosis (e.g., intoxication, head injury, or competitive pain from another major injury). Few patients can perceive more than one major source of pain at a time. Unfortunately, the pain they may focus on may not be from the most serious injury.

The hemoglobin and hematocrit may not dilute, and may be normal right up to the time the patient arrests from hypovolemia.

One of the most important decisions in the management of the multiple-trauma patient is when to obtain an objective evaluation of the abdomen. With a major mechanism of injury (such as an automobile accident in which someone was killed), no matter how well a patient looks, it is wise to assess the abdomen for occult hemorrhage. The physical examination of the abdomen is extremely unreliable when there are multiple injuries, competing pain from skeletal (especially vertebral) trauma, or head injury, or if drugs or alcohol are involved. In the presence of any of these factors, objective evaluation must be obtained. Finally, in any patient who demonstrates vital sign instability without obvious source, it is important to evaluate the abdomen for hemorrhage.

The diagnostic peritoneal lavage (DPL) is one method to evaluate the abdomen. It is very accurate, being one of the few tests in medicine that has reliable significance when negative. It has largely been replaced by the CT scan as well as ultrasound (US), both of which are noninvasive. There are times, however, when performing DPL makes the most sense. If there is no institutional access to US or CT scanning, a DPL may provide information that will perhaps save a transfer to another institution or mandate a laparotomy prior to transfer. If the patient is unstable, the CT scan can accurately identify the intraperitoneal pathologies causing the hemorrhage, but the CT gantry is a very poor place to attempt to manage an unstable patient.

Ultrasonography can also be performed at the bedside, as is occurring with greater frequency in many institutions. It is reliable but may need to be performed more than once if the patient is seen very early after the trauma when there has been no time to produce visible bleeding. As with DPL, the US shows fluid in the abdomen, but not its source or the magnitude of injury.[3] Another advantage of US is that the heart can be assessed for pericardial effusion.

The abdominal CT scan has become more useful with the advent of the very rapid spiral CT scanner. If the patient is too ill for oral contrast, intravenous (i.v.) contrast is useful. Moreover, a head CT scan can be obtained before any contrast is given, and the i.v. contrast can be administered and the abdomen evaluated. Rectal contrast is rarely needed without some indication of colonic injury.

Military antishock trousers have fallen into disuse, except to stabilize lower extremity fractures or attempt to minimize hemorrhage from pelvic fractures. Antishock trousers are dangerous to use in the instance of penetrating chest injury and do not appear to convey any advantage in the penetrating abdominal injury. Moreover, if a combative patient or an inexperienced physician removes them abruptly, there may be severe hypotension or lethal dysrhythmias.

Blood from a traumatic hemothorax can safely be collected and reinfused. After reinfusion of autologous blood, there is a transient coagulopathy that resolves after several days. Platelet function is also depressed. Because increased bleeding may result, this procedure should be reserved for more serious hemorrhage and when banked blood is not readily available.

If the patient has a cardiac arrest from hypovolemia or pericardial tamponade, or has evidence of coronary air embolization, immediate emergency thoracotomy is indicated. Thoracotomy offers the only chance for salvage. The best results are obtained in the presence of penetrating injury to the chest, particularly the heart. It is probably of no benefit to perform a thoracotomy unless the surgical expertise and institutional resources to render definitive care are readily available.

Surgery is part of the resuscitation of the unstable trauma victim. In the patient who cannot be resuscitated from shock and who has no obvious source of blood loss, immediate exploration is indicated. A chest film determines whether the chest or the abdomen is the site of initial exploration.

The priorities of definitive management are still vigorously debated, and it is often necessary to perform invasive procedures without the luxury of confirming diagnostic studies. In general, one should attempt to approach the pathology that poses the most immediate threat to the patient's life—usually in the abdomen. Any rule or protocol will at times have to be modified or abandoned to fit a given patient, but, fortunately, most patients are not in such an unstable life dilemma that they cannot be efficiently and effectively managed.

In the patient who stabilizes during resuscitation, the next priority is a complete head-to-toe examination, which includes performing repeat cardiopulmonary and maxillofacial, abdominal, neurologic, and orthopedic examinations, as well as checking for occult blood loss. A rectal examination is very important to reveal potential displacement of the prostate, any gross blood, and the neurologic assessment of the anal sphincter tone and sensation. The absence of tone or sensation can point to a spinal cord injury in a patient who has been assessed to have only head injury. If the patient is unconscious, determining the level of brainstem function and the presence of a herniation syndrome is paramount. Most trauma victims die of central nervous system–related injuries.

It is necessary to immobilize the spinal column until its status can be ascertained, but it is unnecessary to spend long periods of time trying to clear the cervical or other spinal column before dealing with more life-threatening injuries. The patient can be maintained on a backboard or hard cart with a hard collar while more immediate life threats are determined and prevented. Then, special imaging studies can be obtained to determine the limits of spinal injury.

Open fractures should be cultured, gently irrigated (realizing that this procedure will not substitute for more effective and complete irrigation and debridement under anesthesia), and splinted to prevent further injury and reduce pain and bleeding. Open fractures should be covered with clean dressings, and i.v. antibiotics commenced with an antistaphylococcal drug. Definitive care must await the diagnostic elimination or the surgical treatment of more serious, life-threatening injuries.

If the patient remains unstable, the single most useful diagnostic study is the chest film. Additional films are obtained depending on specific injuries encountered. Intravenous pyelography may be the only diagnostic modality available to some rural institutions, but elsewhere, the abdominal CT scan with i.v. contrast has replaced the i.v. pyelogram (IVP). The ease of obtaining an abdominal CT scan has somewhat liberalized the workup of the kidney. Prior to the high-speed scans, the indication for IVP was gross hematuria, penetrating injury that could involve kidney or ureter (e.g., gunshot would of the flank), and decelerating flank trauma that might have produced an injury to the renal artery. With the abdominal CT scan, one obtains information about the other intraabdominal organs as well as the kidney. It does not replace a cystourethrogram, however, in those patients with straddle injuries or pelvic fractures.

Gross penile bleeding should be evaluated by retrograde urethrography before passage of a Foley catheter.

Aortography still has a role in the evaluation of the trauma patient, especially with some indication of blood vessel damage. For example, Doppler US may reveal a flow impairment in the carotid or vertebral vessels after a whiplash trauma to the neck. Most trauma surgeons will then wish to obtain an arteriogram to define the injury. Another place for angiography is in the patient with a penetrating wound near a large vascular structure. If the patient is unstable, it is more prudent to take the patient to the operating room, obtain vascular control, and perform the angiography intraoperatively.

The CT aortogram has largely replaced aortography. It will accurately demonstrate aortic transection and may provide information about injuries to other intrathoracic or intraabdominal injuries.

A transesophageal echocardiogram is also very accurate in the diagnosis of aortic transection and has the added advantages that it can be performed at the bedside and requires no contrast material.

Unfortunately, not all of these modalities are available 24 hours a day, especially in rural institutions, and the patient will need to be transferred to an appropriate institution to obtain the diagnostic information.

The indications for arteriography include penetrating neck injuries, possible thoracic aortic tears, penetrating wounds of the extremities in proximity to major vessels (if exploration is not mandatory), dislocations of the knee, fractures associated with abnormal pulses, a kidney that is not visualized by IVP, and selected pelvic fractures.

The sequencing of radiologic studies should be prioritized in the same manner as the other components of the resuscitation. Because the patient's airway is the primary concern, the cervical spine should be assessed if active airway management is indicated and the patient is stable. If the airway has already been secured in the field, then the cervical spine can be immobilized while other, more pressing studies are obtained (e.g., chest and pelvic films). However, if the patient is unstable and an airway has not been secured in the field, immediate airway management is indicated without the delay of obtaining radiographic studies.

Once the airway has been addressed, other studies may be obtained. In victims of blunt trauma, chest and pelvic films should be obtained next and, if necessary, extremity films obtained thereafter. Patients with penetrating wounds of the chest (stab or gunshot wounds) should have chest radiographs taken either before resuscitative procedures are performed (if stable) or afterward (if unstable). Abdominal series are of low yield in the evaluation of stab wounds, but they are useful in localizing gunshot fragments.

While the ranking of priorities with head, chest, and abdominal injuries is still very difficult, there are some advantages from the modern spiral CT scan speed. In general, the critical ordering is still abdomen, head, and then chest, but, obviously, decisions must be colored by the actual pathologies present. A US or DPL that shows blood in the abdomen does not reveal the organ damaged or the amount of damage, and the patient's brain may have been the actual target. While the CT scan requires transfer to the radiology suite, the speed of the procedure may enable a quick assessment of the head en route to the operating room for laparotomy. It also adds a little time to the assessment to take cuts of the chest and abdomen.

While head injury alone rarely causes hypotension, it is critical to avoid hypotension in the head-injured patient, and thus it is critical to find and manage the sources of hypotension outside the head. An often overlooked source of shock in the patient who actually has only a head injury is an extensive scalp laceration. The bleeding is often hidden by the neck-stabilizing devices. It is helpful to control the scalp laceration until it can be safely repaired either by the use of Raney clips (the neurosurgical skin clips that can be quickly applied to the scalp laceration edges) or by placement of a 2-0 Ethilon running locked stitch to the laceration.

Finally, it is imperative to recognize that the trauma patient needs definitive care. Time wasted in the field, the emergency department, or the radiology suite may lead to death. Sometimes, the trauma surgeon must proceed to the operating room with a paucity of diagnostic information rather than have the patient continue to lose massive amounts of blood.

Trauma in Children

The pediatric trauma patient is not a miniature adult, and many important anatomic differences must be kept in mind when caring for injured children. Children under age 6 months are obligate nose breathers, so nasal obstruction in these infants may have serious consequences. The infant's oral cavity is small, and the tongue is relatively larger than the adult's. The larynx is located more cephalad in the infant, and the vocal cords are more distensible. Moreover, the vocal cords are anterior and inferior to their usual location in the adult. If these differences are not appreciated, an endotracheal tube may become lodged in the anterior commissure or passed into the esophagus.

The trachea is short: If this is not remembered, right mainstem bronchial intubation or perforation may result. The infant has a large occiput, so the neck is already flexed and the head is slightly extended, even in the "neutral" position. Oral intubation is easier than nasal intubation in infants and young children, and cricothyrotomy is virtually impossible in children under age 8. Needle jet insufflation by way of the cricothyroid membrane may be an appropriate temporizing technique if there is no upper airway obstruction.

The normal systolic blood pressure of a young child should be about 80 plus twice the age in years; diastolic pressure should be about two-thirds of the systolic pressure.

The high ratio of body surface area to body mass in young children greatly affects their ability to regulate core temperature. Their lack of substantial subcutaneous tissue and the presence of thin skin contribute to an increased evaporative heat loss and caloric expenditure. The resulting hypothermia leads to catecholamine secretion and shivering, resulting in a metabolic acidosis. The young child who is hypothermic may be refractory to therapy for shock. Therefore, the child's temperature should be maintained at 37°C by overhead heaters.

The child's chest wall is very compliant and allows energy to transfer to the intrathoracic structures, frequently without any evidence of injury to the ribs. The result is a higher frequency of pulmonary contusion and intrapulmonary hemorrhage than in adults. Injury to the great vessels is infrequent, however.

Almost all infants and young children who are stressed and crying swallow a large amount of air, and it is particularly important to decompress the stomach by inserting a small nasogastric tube. The tenseness of the abdominal wall often decreases as the gastric distention is relieved. Avoid deep palpation at the onset of the examination, as the child will voluntarily guard against subsequent abdominal compression. When performing a diagnostic peritoneal lavage, use a fluid volume of 10 to 15 mL/kg of warmed normal saline solution.

Blood loss associated with long-bone and pelvic fractures is proportionately greater in the child than in the adult. Injuries near joints in children will usually lead to a fracture through the growth plate, which will often be undetectable radiographically.

Head injuries are much more common in children than in adults. However, long episodes of unconsciousness in children do not necessarily correlate with a poorer prognosis. Conversely, children may sustain a significant concussion without any loss of consciousness being observed. Children are also prone to have apneic episodes at the time of injury.

DISPOSITION

The stable trauma patient may spend a number of hours between the emergency department and the radiology department during the completion of diagnostic tests. There is a finite period of time that it takes to completely exclude multiple occult injuries, and this period also allows an observation period to recognize the development of neurologic, cardiac, or pulmonary pathologies. Someone from either the trauma service or the emergency department must monitor the patient during these procedures to ensure that instability is not occurring and that a quick transfer to the operating room has not become necessary. While in the emergency department, this person is often the emergency physician, because the surgeon may be busy arranging for an operating team or consulting with the other subspecialty surgeons in regard to the timing of their repairs.

The patient is an emergency department responsibility until he or she is admitted to an operating room or an intensive care unit. Even if the trauma team monitors the patient in the radiology department, when the patient returns to the emergency department it again becomes the emergency physician's responsibility to become involved with the patient.

Not every patient will need to be admitted to the hospital after careful evaluation and some period of observation. However, any patient who has had a significant mechanism of injury is likely to develop areas of pain and dysfunction that are not predictable in the emergency department. It is therefore prudent, although not mandatory, to provide 24 to 48 hours of observation and care in the hospital.

Transfer of the patient to another institution depends on multiple factors. If the patient is unstable, the only rationale for transfer is to achieve a level of care impossible at the original treating facility. It may be necessary to care for a threat to life (e.g., remove or salvage a torn spleen) and then transfer the patient for more sophisticated neurosurgical or thoracic observations and treatment.

COMMON PITFALLS

- Failing to ascertain details, or ignoring the severity of the mechanism of injury
- Ascribing positive physical findings to a benign cause
- Failing to set up for the patient before his or her arrival
- Failing to have a visible trauma captain throughout the resuscitation
- Failing to use a well-thought-out, systematic approach to the patient
- Chaotic and inefficient resuscitation because of poor use of team members or because too many physicians are trying to give orders
- Focusing on subspecialty need at the expense of real or potential life threats
- Overemphasizing diagnostic tests in an unstable patient.

References

1. Barkin RM, Rosen P, eds. *Emergency pediatrics,* 2nd ed. St. Louis: Mosby, 1986.
2. Davis JW, Hoyt DB, MacKersie RC, et al. Complications in evaluating abdominal trauma: diagnostic peritoneal lavage versus computerized axial tomography. *J Trauma* 1990;30:1506.
3. Healey MA, Simons RK, Winchell RJ, et al. A prospective evaluation of abdominal ultrasound in blunt trauma. Is it useful? *J Trauma* 1996;40:875.
4. Mattox DL, Moore EE, Feliciano DV. *Multiple trauma,* 3rd ed. East Norwalk, CT: Appleton & Lange, 1996.
5. Moore EE, Eiseman B, Van Way CW III, eds. *Critical decisions in trauma.* St. Louis: Mosby, 1984.
6. Rosen P, Baker FJ III, Barkin RM, et al., eds. *Emergency medicine, concepts and clinical practice,* 3rd ed. St. Louis: Mosby, 1992.

CHAPTER 90
Trauma Scoring Systems

Charles L. Emerman and Thomas E. Collins

Trauma scoring systems have been developed over the years to serve a multitude of purposes. In the prehospital setting, trauma scores are used to identify those patients requiring intervention and to aid in decisions regarding patient destination. In the emergency department, these same scoring systems are used to guide therapy, determine the level of response, and provide a means of monitoring changes in status.

Prehospital providers, emergency physicians, and inpatient trauma services use these scores for planning purposes and as a quality assurance screen to monitor performance of the system. Regional planners use these scoring systems to compare institutions and assess resource needs, and as a tool for performing research on the effects of intervention.

PREHOSPITAL SCORING SYSTEMS

Emergency physicians may be called on to choose trauma scores for their prehospital care systems. Several factors should be considered. First, the score that is chosen should be one that has been shown to be valid in a prehospital care system. Many trauma scores were developed by assessing their predictive value only for patients admitted to trauma services from the emergency department. Scores developed in this manner have a lower predictive value, as the patient population in which they were developed has a higher prevalence of serious injury than the general trauma population seen by an emergency medical services (EMS) system.

Second, the items that compose the score must be easily measurable by prehospital providers. For example, capillary refill may be easily assessed in the brightly lit emergency department but very difficult under field conditions.

Third, the components of the scale must have a high degree of interrater reliability. The observations must be easily made under field conditions and the criteria unambiguous. The score itself should be easily remembered and easily calculated.

Finally, scores are most useful when they can be used to assess changes in the patient's condition during the transition from prehospital care through the emergency department into the inpatient service. Ideally, the score that is chosen already has been demonstrated to be valid and reliable in several prehospital care systems. Consideration should also be made to prehospital scoring systems utilized by other EMS systems in the region. Use of a common scoring system would greatly facilitate quality monitoring among EMS agencies. Scores designed to determine the need for transport to a trauma center might also be employed to determine whether the surgery team needs to be present in the emergency department on the patient's arrival.

EMERGENCY DEPARTMENT SCORING SYSTEMS

Scores chosen for use in the emergency department will most likely be used to determine the patient's resource needs. For example, these scores may be chosen to assess the need for a trauma team response, the need for prophylactic intubation, the likelihood of occult injury, or the need for intensive care unit (ICU) admission.

A number of scores have been developed to assess injury severity. These scores use one or more of three predictive components: physiologic derangement, anatomic site of injury, or mechanism of injury. Many scoring systems use a combination of these factors. The comparison of these scores is complicated by the lack of an agreed upon "gold standard" against which the scores have been measured. These scores are commonly compared with regard to need for hospital admission, need for ICU admission, need for operative intervention, length of stay, injury severity score, or mortality.

Each of these end points has limitations. While it is clearly desirable to minimize death or missed injuries from trauma, the more subtle benefits of trauma center care, such as optimal resource use, low rate of missed injuries, and early return to functionality, are difficult to measure. The practicing physician considering the use of individual trauma scores should be aware of both the standard against which the score was developed and the setting in which it will be applied. A score that performs well in determining the need for trauma center transport by EMS may not be an appropriate score to use to assess the effects of new inpatient interventions. Similarly, a score developed in an urban environment with a high rate of serious injury may not be appropriate for another setting in which serious injuries are uncommon.

The advantages of using measures of physiologic derangement include the fact that these measures are part of routine clinical assessment, are unambiguous, and are easily measured. Additionally, these measures identify patients with substantial bleeding or major organ injury. Patients seen early after injury may not have indicators of physiologic derangement and may be mistriaged unless serial measurements are taken. Measures of anatomic injury are good predictors of the need for operative intervention. These measures are useful in retrospective reviews of trauma care, particularly when based on operative or autopsy information. Many of the factors that must be taken into account in these measures may not be available on initial clinical evaluation. Finally, mechanism of injury is generally sensitive in predicting the likelihood of injury. Experience has demonstrated, however, that reliance solely on mechanism of injury leads to a high rate of overtriaging.

The goal of a prehospital evaluation should be the timely transport of patients to appropriate hospitals. In doing so, two concepts conflict. Ideally, it is desirable to minimize the rate of undertriage, wherein patients who are seriously injured are transported to centers less prepared to care for them. Alternatively, it is also desirable to minimize overtriage, because it increases resource utilization, lengthens EMS transport times, and overloads trauma hospitals with patients with minor injuries. Unfortunately, as one increases the sensitivity of triage rules (thus minimizing undertriage), there is generally a concomitant fall in specificity (which increases overtriage). The best scores, therefore, are those that have a high sensitivity with an acceptable level of specificity. In general, one would expect an urban EMS system to consider approximately 5% to 10% of their trauma patients as having an injury serious enough to warrant transport to a trauma center.

Several studies have demonstrated that transport to designated centers has an effect on overall outcome. A study conducted in Orange County, California, reviewed 118 deaths from motor vehicle accidents, approximately half of which occurred prior to, and half of which occurred after, implementation of a regional trauma system.[5] Following implementation of the system, the proportion of deaths from injuries that were potentially salvageable decreased from 34% to 15%.

Most of the apparently salvageable cases occurred in patients treated in nontrauma facilities. Further, when the authors of the study compared the death rates in the region prior to implementation of the system with those after implementation, they found that the death rates were lower than would have been projected using linear regression. In another study, 73% of deaths due to causes other than central nervous system injury were judged to be preventable prior to implementation of a trauma care system.[26] After implementation of the system, the percentage of deaths from causes other than central nervous system injury were reduced to 9%.

Abbreviated Injury Scale

Early efforts at categorizing trauma patients focused on quantifying the extent of injury. The Abbreviated Injury Scale (AIS) was developed as part of an attempt to assess automotive safety. In the AIS, injuries to various body areas were graded from 0 to 6, with 6 representing fatal injury.[1] The problem with the AIS was the difficulty in accounting for the effect of multiple injuries. Because the AIS is a summation, injuries in patients with multiple minor injuries may have a higher score than ones with single, life-threatening injuries. The AIS was last revised in 1990, with an emphasis on improving its accuracy with children.

Injury Severity Score

The Injury Severity Score (ISS) was developed as an extension of the AIS.[1] The original ISS was devised by summing the squares of the highest AIS grade in each of the three most severely injured areas. This modified scale was shown to correlate with fatality from trauma. Death from trauma begins to rise significantly with ISSs above 15. Unfortunately, both the AIS and the ISS can be calculated accurately only after the full extent of the patient's injuries is known. The ISS is now commonly used as a quality assurance tool, but it has no role in decision making either in the emergency department or in EMS systems.

Trauma Index

One of the earlier trauma scores intended for prehospital use was the Trauma Index. This index was developed from a retrospective review of trauma patients.[4] Twenty-five variables were grouped under five categories related to site of anatomic injury, type of injury, and status of the cardiovascular, the central nervous, and the respiratory systems. The authors found that a high score (over 18) correlated with the occurrence of multiple injuries.

Triage Index

These concepts were further extended by Champion, in the development of the Triage Index.[7] The Triage Index was derived from a series of 1,084 patients. It was initially composed of 12 variables found to correlate with death following initial hospitalization. Using statistical techniques, these variables were condensed into five variables that included respiratory expansion, capillary refill, eye opening, verbal response, and motor response.

Trauma Score

The Trauma Score was based on a retrospective analysis of 2,000 patients, using death from trauma as the end point. It included respiratory state and effort, blood pressure, capillary refill, and the Glasgow Coma Scale as variables.[8] The Trauma Score was prospectively studied by Morris, who reviewed 1,106 patients admitted to the trauma center at San Francisco General Hospital. A trauma score less than 15 was significantly associated with mortality, the presence of closed head injuries, the need for immediate surgery, and length of both ICU and hospital stays. The trauma score predicted an ISS greater than 20 with a sensitivity of only 63%. More importantly, however, patients whose trauma score deteriorated from the initial value obtained in the field had a mortality rate of 26%, compared with a rate of 9% of those whose trauma scores improved and 4% of those whose trauma score remained the same.

Triage-Revised Trauma Score

The trauma score was revised in 1989, using data from the Washington Hospital Trauma Center and the Major Trauma Outcome Study. The revised trauma score was broken into three components: Glasgow Coma Scale, systolic blood pressure, and respiratory rate (Table 90.1). A Triage-Revised Trauma Score (T-RTS) less than 12 identified 97.2% of all fatally injured patients. As this score is based entirely on physiologic variables, there is the risk of inappropriate decision making when patients are seen early after injury. The authors recommended using a multistep approach in conjunction with the T-RTS. In another study, in which 4% (53 of 1,325) of patients were classified as having severe trauma using the ISS (ISS greater than 16), 11 of those 53 patients were missed using the T-RTS.

Trauma and Injury Severity Score

While the ISS accounts for patients' injuries, prediction of mortality should take into account factors that affect likelihood of survival. Trauma and Injury Severity Score (TRISS) methodology incorporates the patient's age and ISS into a prediction of survival. Patients with outcomes different from those predicted by the formula may be candidates for quality assurance review. TRISSs are heavily weighted toward head injury. The W statistics, derived by comparison of a hospital's results to those from the Major Outcome Trauma Study, portray the number of excess survivors per 100 patients. The misclassification rate for TRISS is around 4%.

TABLE 90.1. Revised Trauma Score Variable Breakpoints

Glasgow Coma Scale	Systolic Blood Pressure	Respiratory Rate	Coded Value
13–15	>89	10–29	4
9–12	76–89	>29	3
6–8	50–75	6–9	2
4–5	1–49	1–5	1
3	0	0	0

From Champion HR, Sacco WJ, Copes WS, et al. A revision of the trauma score. *J Trauma* 1989;29:623.

APACHE

The APACHE score takes into account acute vital signs, laboratory tests, age, and chronic health. Although it was intended for use in both medical and surgical patients, some communities use it for general hospital QA scoring. The APACHE II is limited by the relatively small number of trauma patients used for the derivation study. It tends to underestimate the risk of death for multiply injured patients with head trauma. APACHE III used a larger number of trauma patients and adjusts for head injury. Some studies have found that APACHE and TRISS perform in a similar, although limited, manner in predicting mortality in ICU patients.[25]

ASCOT

A severity characterization of trauma system was developed based on analysis of the shortcomings of TRISS seen in the Major Trauma Outcome Study. In addition to the revised trauma score variables, ASCOT adds scoring assignments for injury to three body regions, including brain/spinal cord, thorax/neck, and abdomen/major vessel. ASCOT adjusts for patients with very good or poor expected outcomes in order to improve prognostic power for patients with less certain outcome. In comparison, ASCOT seems to perform superior to TRISS for bluntly injured adults. Both TRISS and ASCOT appear adequate for pediatric patients.[6]

CRAMS

The CRAMS Scale (Table 90.2) was developed through a review of 500 trauma transports, of which only 12 had major trauma defined as death in the emergency department or immediate transport to the operating room.[14] The authors in the original study

TABLE 90.2. Field Categorization of Trauma—CRAMS Scale

CIRCULATION	
Normal capillary refill and BP > 100	2
Delayed capillary refill or 85 < BP < 100	1
No capillary refill or BP < 85	0
RESPIRATIONS	
Normal	2
Abnormal (labored or shallow)	1
Absent	0
ABDOMEN	
Abdomen and thorax nontender	2
Abdomen or thorax tender	1
Abdomen rigid or flail chest[a]	0
MOTOR	
Normal	2
Responds only to pain (other than decerebrate)	1
No response (or decerebrate)	0
SPEECH	
Normal	2
Confused	1
No intelligible words	0

Score ≤8—Major trauma
Score ≥9—Minor trauma

[a] "Penetrating wounds to the abdomen or thorax" has been added since the study.

From Gormican SP. CRAMS scale: field triage of trauma victims. *Ann Emerg Med* 1982;11:132.

TABLE 90.3. Prehospital Index[a]

Components	Value	Score
Blood pressure	>100	0
	86–100	1
	75–85	2
	0–74	5
Pulse	≥120	3
	51–119	0
	<50	5
Respirations	Normal	0
	Labored/shallow	3
	<10/min needs intubation	5
Consciousness	Normal	0
	Confused/combative	3
	No intelligible words	5
Total		0–20

[a]0 to 3, minor trauma; 4 to 20, major trauma.
(Penetrating abdominal or chest injuries are given 4 points in addition to the calculated PHI.)
From Koehler JJ, Baer LJ, Malafa SQ, et al. Prehospital Index: a scoring system for field triage of trauma victims. *Ann Emerg Med* 1986;15:178.

found that the CRAMS Scale has a higher sensitivity than the original Trauma Score. The CRAMS Scale was validated, with modifications, in 2,110 patients.[11] In the validation study, a score less than 7 identified all but one of the emergency department deaths.

Prehospital Index

Another widely used trauma score is the Prehospital Index (PHI) (Table 90.3).[15] The PHI was developed using 313 trauma patients, who were considered to have major trauma if they died within 72 hours of injury or required surgical intervention within 24 hours. As originally constituted, this trauma score utilized only physiologic parameters. The authors realized, however, that the addition of a measure of anatomic injury (penetrating injuries of the abdomen or chest) would improve the accuracy of their score. The PHI was validated in a multicenter study of 3581 patients.[20] In the validation study; the PHI had a positive predictive value of 52.1% and a negative predictive value of 99.4%.

Additional Methods

As mentioned previously, other authors have utilized mechanism of injury and anatomic injury as criteria for transport to trauma centers. A review of 2,057 patients compared various mechanisms and types of injuries with the ISS.[12] Combined with a trauma score greater than 12, the authors found that the likelihood of major injury was increased when the trauma score was combined with the presence of head, spine, chest, abdomen, or extremity injury. The prevalence of major trauma was also increased if it was caused by motor vehicle accident; a fall greater than 15 ft; penetrating injury to the head, chest, or abdomen; or Glasgow Coma Scale less than 10. In a similar vein, another study found that the addition of mechanism of injuries, including falls greater than 16 ft, motorcycle accidents greater than 20 mph, and automobile versus pedestrian accidents, increased the sensitivity of the various trauma scores.[18]

USE OF SCORING SYSTEMS

Scoring systems are among the many tools utilized to improve the quality and efficiency of care of the injured patient.

TABLE 90.4. Baxt Trauma Triage Rule

Patient meets the criteria for trauma center transport if any of the following are present:

1. Systolic BP <85 mm Hg
2. Motor component of Glasgow Coma Scale <5
3. Penetrating injury of head, neck, or trunk

Unfortunately, prehospital trauma rules, although they have been found to be good predictors of mortality, have not been found to be good predictors of other measures of major trauma.[2] The CRAMS Scale, Revised Trauma Score, and the PHI have been found to correlate poorly with ISSs.[21] One study found that, using trauma prediction rules, 30% of patients initially classified as major trauma victims would be misclassified, while 30% of patients initially designated as having minor injuries would be later found to have major injuries.

These findings led Baxt and colleagues to utilize a different gold standard in designing a trauma score (Baxt Trauma Triage Rule) (Table 90.4).[3] They classified major trauma patients as those who required operative intervention (other than orthopedic) within the first 48 hours, needed inhospital fluid resuscitation of at least 1 L, had placement of invasive central nervous system monitoring, or died of their injuries. The score developed utilized systolic blood pressure less than 85 mm Hg, a motor component of the Glasgow Coma Scale less than 5, or penetrating injury of the head, neck, or trunk as indicators of major trauma.

The American College of Surgeons has advocated a stepwise approach to trauma center triage (Fig. 90.1).[21] In this classification scheme, patients are first assessed with the T-RTS, Glasgow Coma Score, Pediatric Trauma Score, or measurement of the blood pressure or respiratory rate. If none of those factors is abnormal, then anatomic injury and mechanism of injury are considered. Lastly, patients also meet the criteria for transport to a trauma center if they are at the extremes of age or if they have complicating medical factors. The authors of this system consider an undertriage rate of 5% to 10% to be unavoidable, with an overtriage rate up to 50% necessary to minimize missed patients.

This stepwise approach was assessed in a prospective study.[4] The first step, involving physiologic parameters, was found to have a sensitivity of 46% and a specificity of 93%. The anatomic injury factors were found to have a sensitivity of 22% and a specificity of 98%. However, when mechanism of injury was added into the evaluation, the overtriage rate exceeded 92%.

Another study examined the individual American College of Surgeons trauma triage criteria and found that, individually, all criteria except speed greater than 20 mph or greater than 30-in. vehicle deformity had predictive value for hospital resource utilization.[13]

A few studies have been performed comparing the different scoring systems. One such study, performed in a rural population, found that the CRAMS Scale had a greater sensitivity than either the Trauma Score or the PHI.[15] Another study, however, found that neither the CRAMS Scale nor the Trauma Score adequately identified major trauma patients in the field. A comparison of the CRAMS Scale, Baxt Trauma Triage Rule, PHI, and T-RTS found that all of the scores predicted mortality with a sensitivity of 100%. The T-RTS appeared to predict death, or the need for emergency operation, to a lesser degree than the Trauma Triage Rule, the CRAMS Scale, or the PHI.[13] ASCOT performed better at predicting survival for adult blunt trauma when compared with TRISS.[6]

After reviewing the available scores and methodologies for triaging trauma patients, the practicing physician may wish to

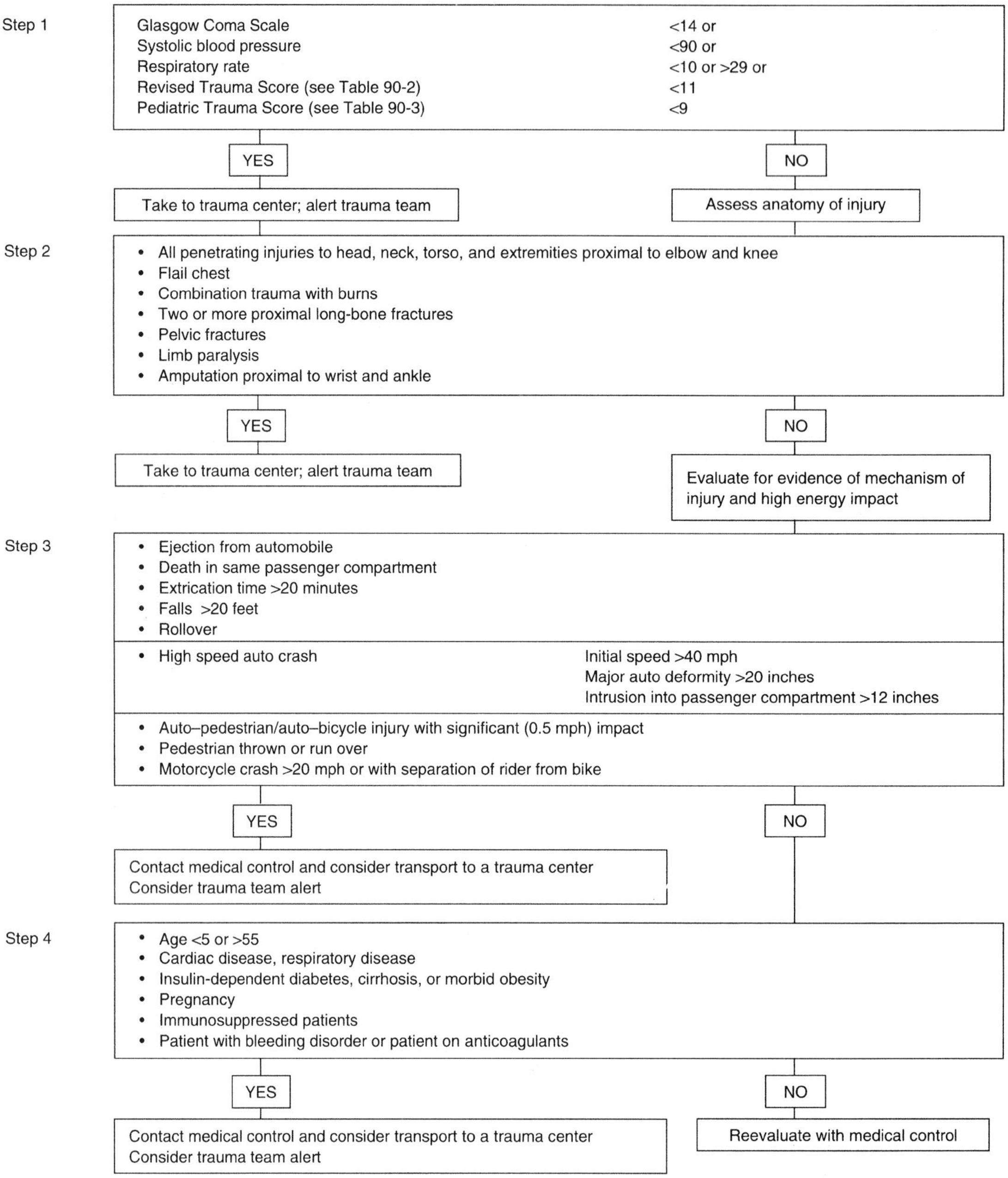
Step 1
Glasgow Coma Scale <14 or
Systolic blood pressure <90 or
Respiratory rate <10 or >29 or
Revised Trauma Score (see Table 90-2) <11
Pediatric Trauma Score (see Table 90-3) <9
YES
NO
Take to trauma center; alert trauma team
Assess anatomy of injury
Step 2
• All penetrating injuries to head, neck, torso, and extremities proximal to elbow and knee
• Flail chest
• Combination trauma with burns
• Two or more proximal long-bone fractures
• Pelvic fractures
• Limb paralysis
• Amputation proximal to wrist and ankle
YES
NO
Take to trauma center; alert trauma team
Evaluate for evidence of mechanism of injury and high energy impact
Step 3
• Ejection from automobile
• Death in same passenger compartment
• Extrication time >20 minutes
• Falls >20 feet
• Rollover
• High speed auto crash
Initial speed >40 mph
Major auto deformity >20 inches
Intrusion into passenger compartment >12 inches
• Auto–pedestrian/auto–bicycle injury with significant (0.5 mph) impact
• Pedestrian thrown or run over
• Motorcycle crash >20 mph or with separation of rider from bike
YES
NO
Contact medical control and consider transport to a trauma center
Consider trauma team alert
Step 4
• Age <5 or >55
• Cardiac disease, respiratory disease
• Insulin-dependent diabetes, cirrhosis, or morbid obesity
• Pregnancy
• Immunosuppressed patients
• Patient with bleeding disorder or patient on anticoagulants
YES
NO
Contact medical control and consider transport to a trauma center
Consider trauma team alert
Reevaluate with medical control

Figure 90.1. American College of Surgeons Guidelines for Optimal Care of the Injured Patient. (Adapted from Krantz B. *Field triage in resources for optimal care of the injured patient.* Chicago: American College of Surgeons, 1993.)

consider the role of clinical judgment. One study noted that inclusion of advanced emergency medicine technician (EMT) injury perception, in addition to standard out-of-hospital triage criteria, improved accuracy of field trauma triage.[24] In a large study evaluating the ability of urban EMTs to assess trauma, none of the scores were found to perform better than EMT judgment. Again, the physician considering the use of these scores will need to consider the setting in which the scores will be used. It would appear that most urban EMTs have the ability to recognize major trauma patients.[5] In the prehospital setting, trauma scores can be used to guide trauma patient destination and to help educate EMTs on the importance of various anatomic, physiologic, and mechanism of injury factors that can identify the potentially seriously injured patient, as well as on their significant use in quality monitoring.

Prehospital trauma scores have also been used in stratifying the level of trauma team response. One study separated trauma patients into two classifications. Category 1 patients were felt to have a high likelihood of injury, while category 2 patients had a low likelihood of injury. Category 1 patients were treated by the full trauma team, consisting of both emergency medicine residents and staff and trauma surgery residents and staff. Category 2 patients were initially treated by emergency medicine personnel, with a member of the trauma surgery service responding within 30 minutes to provide consultation. This system effectively predicted the likelihood of serious injury, mortality, and need for emergency surgery. Over the 6-month study period, an estimated 578 physician-hours were saved using the two-tiered system.[23]

New trauma-scoring systems continue to be devised. As discussed at the beginning of this chapter, until there is an agreement over a gold standard against which these scores can be measured, there is likely to be disagreement over the optimal scoring system. Hospital trauma services will likely continue to use both the T-RTS and the ISS because of their usefulness in assessing quality assurance through the TRISS methodology.

Depending on the purpose for which they are being used, emergency departments have a number of scoring systems available for their use. The T-RTS may be used to monitor changes in patient's condition during the course of the patient's initial resuscitation. Clearly, the use of mechanism of injury to activate the trauma team will lead to an overutilization of that resource, but, as mentioned earlier, a degree of overtriage is accepted in the effort to include all potentially injured trauma patients. EMS systems commonly use the PHI or the T-RTS. Medical directors may wish to consider the use of the Baxt Trauma Triage Rule because it has been demonstrated to be valid and easy to use.

References

1. Baker SP, O'Neill B. The injury severity score: an update. *J Trauma* 1976;16:882.
2. Baxt WG, Berry CC, Epperson MD, et al. The failure of prehospital trauma prediction rules to classify trauma patients accurately. *Ann Emerg Med* 1989;18:1.
3. Baxt WG, Jones G, Fortlage D. The trauma triage rule: a new, resource-based approach to the prehospital identification of major trauma victims. *Ann Emerg Med* 1990;19:1401.
4. Bickell WH, Sacra JC, Thompson CT. Prospective evaluation of field trauma triage. *Ann Emerg Med* 1993;22:208.
5. Cales RH. Trauma mortality in Orange County: the effect of implementation of a regional trauma system. *Ann Emerg Med* 1984;13:1.
6. Champion HR, Copes WS, Sacco WJ, et al. Improved predictions from a Severity Characterization of Trauma (ASCOT) over Trauma and Injury Severity Score (TRISS): Results of an independent evaluation. *J Trauma* 1996;40:42.
7. Champion HR, Copes WS, Sacco WJ, et al. The major trauma outcome study: establishing national norms for trauma care. *J Trauma* 1990;11:1356.
8. Champion HR, Sacco WJ, Carnazzo AJ. Trauma score. *Crit Care Med* 1981;9(9):672.
9. Champion HR, Sacco WJ, Hannan DS, et al. Assessment of injury severity: the triage index. *Crit Care Med* 1980;8(4):201.
10. Champion HR, Sacco WJ, Copes WS, et al. A revision of the trauma score. *J Trauma* 1989;29:623.
11. Clemmer TP, Orme JF, Thomas F, et al. Prospective evaluation of the CRAMS Scale for triaging major trauma. *J Trauma* 1985;25:188.
12. Cottington EM, Young JC, Shufflebarger CM, et al. The utility of physiological status, injury site, and injury mechanism in identifying patients with major trauma. *J Trauma* 1988;28:305.
13. Emerman CL, Shade B, Kubincanek J. Comparative performance of the Baxt Trauma Triage Rule. *Am J Emerg Med* 1992;10:294.
14. Gormican SP. CRAMS Scale: field triage of trauma victims. *Ann Emerg Med* 1982;11:132.
15 Hedges JR, Feero S, Moore B, et al. Comparison of prehospital trauma triage instruments in a semirural population. *J Emerg Med* 1987;5:197.
16. Henry MC, Hollander JE, Alicandro JA, et al. Incremental benefit of individual American College of Surgeons Trauma Triage Criteria. *J Trauma* 1996;3:992.
17. Kirkpatrick JR, Youmans RL. Trauma index. An aid in the evaluation of injury victims. *J Trauma* 1971;11(8):711.
18. Knudson P, Frecceri CA, DeLateur SA. Improving the field triage of major trauma victims. *J Trauma* 1988;28:602.
19. Koehler JJ, Baer LJ, Malafa SQ, et al. Prehospital Index: a scoring system for field triage of trauma victims. *Ann Emerg Med* 1986;15:178.
20. Koehler JJ, Malafa SA, Hillesiand J, et al. A multicenter validation of the prehospital index. *Ann Emerg Med* 1987;16:380.
21. Krantz B. *Field triage in resources for optimal care of the injured patient.* Chicago: American College of Surgeons, 1993.
22. Morris JA Jr, Auerbach PS, Marshall GA, Bluth RF, Johnson LG, Trunkey DD. The Trauma Score as a triage tool in the prehospital setting. *JAMA* 1986;256(10):1319.
23. Plaiser BR, Meldon SW, Jouriles NJ, et al. Effectiveness of a 2-specialty, 2-tiered triage and trauma team activation protocol. *Ann Emerg Med* 1998;32:436.
24. Simmons E, Hedges JR, Irwin L, et al. Paramedic injury severity perception can aid trauma triage. *Am Emerg Med* 1995;26:461.
25. Vassar MJ, Lewis FR Jr, Chambers JA, et al. Prediction of outcome in the intensive care unit trauma patients: a multicenter study of Acute Physiology and Chronic Health Evaluation (APACHE), Trauma and Injury Severity Score (TRISS), and a 24-hour intensive care unit (ICU) point system. *J Trauma* 1999;47(2):324.
26. West JG, Cales RH, Gazzaniga AB. Impact of regionalization. *Arch Surg* 1983;118:740.
27. Wong DT, Barrow PM, Gomez M, McGuire GP. A comparison of the Acute Physiology and Chronic Health Evaluation (APACHE) II score and the Trauma-Injury Severity Score (TRISS) for outcome assessment in intensive care unit trauma patients. *Crit Care Med* 1996;24(10):1642.

CHAPTER 91
Injury Prevention

B. Tilman Jolly

The science of injury prevention is both one of the oldest and one of the newest areas of medicine. During the first year of life, we learn about different forms of energy and the harm they can cause. Thermal energy from hot water causes burns. Kinetic energy caused by the typical fall of a new walker elicits cries of pain. Thus, injury prevention becomes one of our most basic instincts.

Basic as it may be, injury prevention as a science has lagged behind the analysis of other illnesses, both in research output and funding support. As recently as 1989, Baker[3] wrote of the "failure, until recently, of most health professionals and their institutions to give appropriate attention to the major cause of lost potential years of life before retirement."

The foundation for the current practice of injury prevention was laid by a small group of true pioneers. Hugh DeHaven described the elements of effective crash protection after he was involved in a midair collision in World War I.[22] Carl Clark developed early prototypes of air bags, also using himself as a demonstration subject.[3]

Among others, William Haddon stands out as the developer of a framework for analysis and prevention of injury. His matrix, now known as the "Haddon Matrix," allows for the placement of causative factors of injury into one of nine specific categories (Table 91.1).[12] This matrix, while originally designed for the analysis of motor vehicle crashes, can be easily applied to other types of injuries. Haddon also listed ten strategies available for reducing energy-damage losses (injuries) (Table 91.2).[12]

TABLE 91.1. The Haddon Matrix (with examples)

	Human	Vehicle	Environment
Pre-crash	Alcohol	Maintenance	Poor signage
Crash	Injury threshold (related to age, etc.)	Energy-absorbing frame	Poles and trees near roadway
Post-crash	First-aid knowledge	Gas tank rupture	Access to EMS

TABLE 91.2. Options for Reducing Injury Losses

1. To prevent the initial collection of the form of energy
2. To reduce the amount of energy collected
3. To prevent the release of energy
4. To modify the rate of spatial distribution of release of energy from its source.
5. To separate in space or time the energy being released from the susceptible structure.
6. To separate the energy being released from the susceptible structure by interposition of a material barrier.
7. To modify the contact surface, subsurface, or basic structure which can be impacted.
8. To strengthen the living or nonliving structure which might be damaged by the energy transfer.
9. To move rapidly in detection and evaluation of damage and to counter its continuation and extension.
10. All those measures which fall between the emergency period following the damaging energy exchange and the final stabilization of the process (including intermediate and long-term reparative and rehabilitative measures).

TABLE 91.3. Leading Causes of Death in the United States by Age Group — 1995

Rank	<1	1–4	5–9	10–14	15–24	25–34	35–44	45–54	55–64	65+	Total
1	Congenital Anomalies 20,537	Unintentional Injuries 7,387	Unintentional Injuries 4,806	Unintentional Injuries 5,712	Unintentional Injuries 41,706	Unintentional Injuries 40,909	HIV 53,148	Malignant Neoplasms 130,146	Malignant Neoplasms 267,834	Heart Disease 1,845,511	Heart Disease 2,213,432
2	Short Gestation 12,497	Congenital Anomalies 2,213	Malignant Neoplasms 1,648	Malignant Neoplasms 1,520	Homicide 23,824	HIV 35,310	Malignant Neoplasms 50,708	Heart Disease 100,798	Heart Disease 209,618	Malignant Neoplasms 1,128,877	Malignant Neoplasms 1,602,669
3	SIDS 12,139	Malignant Neoplasms 1,528	Congenital Anomalies 757	Homicide 1,283	Suicide 14,589	Homicide 20,328	Unintentional Injuries 41,040	Unintentional Injuries 26,058	Bronchitis Emphysema Asthma 30,994	Cerebro-vascular 404,653	Cerebro-vascular 461,405
4	Respiratory Distress Synd 4,386	Homicide 1,389	Homicide 507	Suicide 963	Malignant Neoplasms 5,120	Suicide 18,953	Heart Disease 39,967	HIV 22,302	Cerebro-vascular 28,937	Bronchitis Emphysema Asthma 261,951	Bronchitis Emphysema Asthma 305,604
5	Maternal Complications 3,948	Heart Disease 832	Heart Disease 388	Congenital Anomalies 611	Heart Disease 3,012	Malignant Neoplasms 15,010	Suicide 19,012	Cerebro-vascular 15,885	Diabetes 23,450	Pneumonia & Influenza 220,912	Unintentional Injuries 275,280
6	Placenta Cord Membranes 2,904	HIV 613	HIV 333	Heart Disease 536	HIV 1,879	Heart Disease 10,520	Homicide 13,186	Liver Disease 14,993	Unintentional Injuries 19,580	Diabetes 127,554	Pneumonia & Influenza 247,216
7	Unintentional Injuries 2,574	Pneumonia & Influenza 517	Pneumonia & Influenza 202	Bronchitis Emphysema Asthma 286	Congenital Anomalies 1,387	Cerebro-vascular 2,319	Liver Disease 11,159	Suicide 12,996	Liver Disease 16,499	Unintentional Injuries 85,197	Diabetes 169,840
8	Perinatal Infections 2,388	Perinatal Period 301	Benign Neoplasms 142	HIV 193	Bronchitis Emphysema Asthma 684	Liver Disease 2,058	Cerebro-vascular 8,008	Diabetes 11,134	Pneumonia & Influenza 10,667	Nephritis 59,591	HIV 122,496
9	Pneumonia & Influenza 1,581	Septicemia 267	Bronchitis Emphysema Asthma 122	Pneumonia & Influenza 164	Pneumonia & Influenza 679	Pneumonia & Influenza 1,993	Diabetes 5,326	Bronchitis Emphysema Asthma 7,926	Suicide 8,677	Alzheimer's Disease 54,869	Suicide 93,528
10	Intrauterine Hypoxia 1,561	Benign Neoplasms 210	Septicemia 92	Benign Neoplasms 136	Cerebro-vascular 563	Diabetes 1,898	Pneumonia & Influenza 4,539	Pneumonia & Influenza 5,943	HIV 6,349	Septicemia 50,184	Liver Disease 75,837

Reprinted from Reference 9, with permission.

Combinations of these strategies form the basis for injury prevention science as it is practiced today.

Others describe injury in terms of performance and task demand. Performance relates to how an individual accomplishes an action. Task demand describes the skill required to complete that action. Injury occurs when energy is transmitted because an individual task demand exceeds performance.[24] A toddler attempting to climb stairs may fall because she has not achieved the skills necessary to complete the climb. A driver may be able to operate a motor vehicle under normal circumstances, but may suffer from decreased performance with the same task demand while intoxicated.

Injury prevention professionals also speak of the three E's: Education, enforcement, and engineering, in various combinations, can be used to approach almost any injury problem. Education can include gun safety classes and public service announcements about the need for smoke detectors. Enforcement includes use of laws and regulations regarding fences around swimming pools (to prevent entrance of small children) to tougher drunk-driving standards. Engineering improvements range from roadside guardrails and antilock brakes to safety locks on guns. The "E's" must continue to be thought of as working together to reduce death and disability from injury.

COMPARATIVE EPIDEMIOLOGY

That injury is a major public health problem is well documented. In 1995, there were 37 million emergency department (ED) visits for injury and over 147,000 deaths due to injury. Injury accounted for 52% of all deaths among 5- to 14-year-olds and 77% of all deaths for 15- to 24-year-olds. Injury also accounted for 12% of all medical expenditures, with an estimated total cost of $260 billion.[15] Table 91.3 illustrates the leading causes of death by age group in the United States in 1995.[27] Deaths, while easiest to count, represent only a small part of the injury picture. Figure 91.1 illustrates the well-known injury pyramid, showing the relatively small number of deaths compared with the total number of injuries.[9]

Injury must compete with other diseases, both in the United States and around the world, for attention and research funding. Unintentional injuries are the leading cause of death in the United States from age 1 to age 34. Intentional injuries, either homicide or suicide, also play a major role in this age group. The Centers for Disease Control and Prevention (CDC) reports these

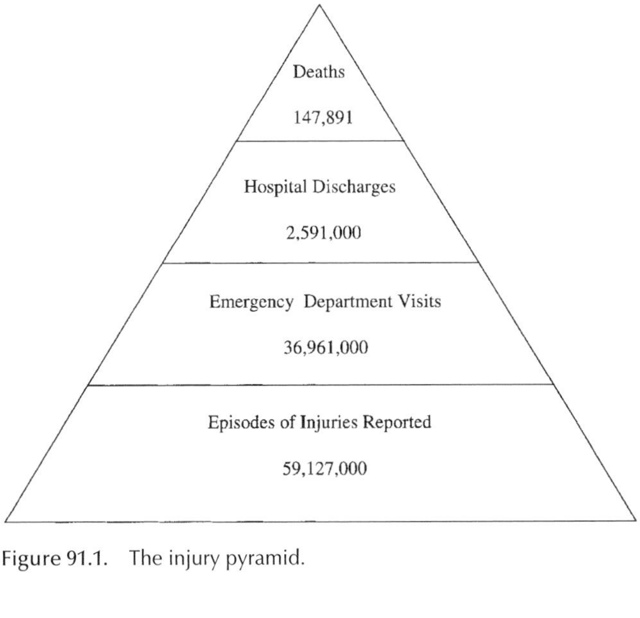

Figure 91.1. The injury pyramid.

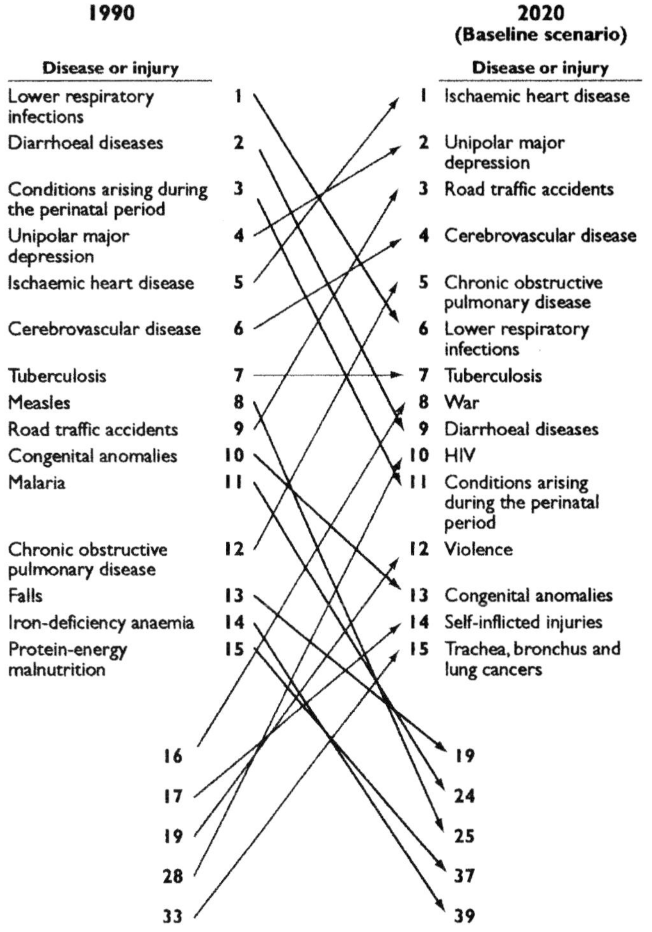

Figure 91.2. Change in the rank order of disease burden for 15 leading causes, world, 1990–2020 (Disease burden measured in Disability-Adjusted Life Years [DALYs]). (From The Global Burden of Disease (Summary), the World Health Organization, with permission.)

comparative statistics through the National Vital Statistics System.[8] The World Health Organization estimates that injury will increase significantly as a cause of death throughout the world by the year 2020 in comparison to other illnesses. Traffic crashes are projected to move from ninth to third as a cause of loss of disability adjusted life years (DALYs) worldwide. Violence is projected to move from nineteenth to twelfth on the same list (Fig. 91.2).[43]

As is shown by these statistics and the casual observation of a typical day in the ED, injury has a great impact on the practice of emergency medicine. The treatment model of medical practice places the role of emergency physician only in one box of the Haddon Matrix—postevent, environment. The prevention model expands the role of emergency medicine into all areas of the matrix, much in the way the medical community works to prevent heart disease, cancer, and acquired immunodeficiency syndrome (AIDS).

TERMINOLOGY

Injury is defined as "the result of a harmful event that arises from the release of specific forms of physical energy or barriers to normal flow of energy."[24] The term *accident* has been a source of much consternation in the injury prevention field. While some, particularly investigators in the United Kingdom, continue to use the term, others feel that *accident* implies random events or "acts of God," while *injuries* are caused by predictable and preventable events. A recent review of the issue by the Institute of Medicine (IOM) Committee on Injury Prevention and Control recommended against continued use of the word *accident*.[15]

The IOM also considered the terms *prevention, control,* and *treatment*. *Prevention* refers to preevent or event interventions that reduce the risk or severity of injury. *Treatment* refers to postevent measures (acute care and rehabilitation) that ameliorate the effects of injury. *Injury control* has gained common use as a term to encompass aspects of prevention and treatment. The IOM committee recommends against the term *injury control* as confusing, although it continues to be used extensively.[15]

DATA SOURCES

Adequate information about the injury problem and the effectiveness of interventions relies on adequate surveillance. How many injuries are happening, under what circumstances do they happen, and how are patterns changing, are all important questions to answer. Surveillance is basic to the planning and implementation of any public health intervention, including injury prevention.

Federal Sources

At the federal level, the National Center for Health Statistics maintains basic mortality data based on information from death certificates. This information is only as good as the quality of the death certificate information, which is influenced by the skill and interest of the person who completes the investigation. The National Hospital Discharge Survey collects and disseminates data on a probability sample of discharged patients. This data set can provide interesting information on patients injured enough to be hospitalized. The federal government also conducts periodic surveys on health behaviors and health-care expenditures.

The federal government also maintains data collection systems related to specific types of injuries. For motor vehicles, the Fatal Analysis Reporting System (FARS) collects data on nearly all crash fatalities. The National Automotive Sampling System (NASS) Crashworthiness Data System (CDS) provides for detailed analysis of a randomized area sample of tow-away crashes, which in many cases can be generalized to reflect national trends. The General Estimates System (GES) draws from a larger sample of police-reported crashes but also relies on police-reported injury data, which may not be sufficiently reliable for injury comparisons.

Injuries and deaths not related to motor vehicles are catalogued by multiple agencies. The Federal Bureau of Investigation (FBI) collects annual and frequently quoted data on homicides and assaults. The Bureau of Labor Statistics and the National Institute for Occupational Safety and Health collect data on occupational deaths and injuries, although reporting may be spotty. Emergency physicians may be familiar with a surveillance system maintained by the Consumer Product Safety Commission. This system is known as NEISS. The National Emergency Department Injury Surveillance System collects information on product-related injuries from a selected sample of EDs around the country. Rates and trends in product-related injuries (bicycles, tools, toys, childcare products, etc.) are obtained and disseminated from this system.[1]

State and Local Sources

States, local jurisdictions, and hospitals maintain injury data in various forms. The most basic data collected by states are mortality data, in the form of medical examiner reports and death certificates. Deaths are coded using ICD-9-CM (International Classification of Diseases), N-codes (Nature of injury), and E-codes (external cause of injury).[10] While in many cases medical examiners must investigate all unexpected deaths, specific information regarding the circumstances of the death and injuries sustained can be sketchy. This may be particularly true when death occurred at the scene, without the benefit of hospital data collection.

State and local morbidity data are usually based on hospital-acquired data. This information is available from discharge databases, trauma registries, ED surveillance, surveys, and specialized registries (burns, spinal cord injuries, etc.) Each of these systems has its own strengths and weaknesses, largely dependent on the purpose for which the method exists. For instance, if a discharge database was created to use ICD-9 codes to track financial and resource utilization information, it may not include important information necessary for epidemiologic research. Trauma registries, while highly specific, contain data on only the sickest patients. Improved ED surveillance systems hold promise for providing improved injury and cause of injury information on a broad subset of the population. The CDC has published initial guidelines for uniform ED injury data collection, which represents a first step toward improved ED injury surveillance.[33]

UNINTENTIONAL INJURY

Motor Vehicles

The motor vehicle is ubiquitous in U.S. society and the most common factor related to unintentional injury. The first U.S. motor vehicle fatality was a pedestrian struck by a taxicab on the streets of New York in 1899.[45] Since then, millions have died on the road. Currently, approximately 42,000 people die in roadway crashes every year. Of these, approximately 32,000 are vehicle occupants. The rest are pedestrians, bicyclists, and motorcyclists. While the absolute number of deaths has remained relatively constant over the past two decades, the rate of death per 100 million miles traveled has dropped dramatically, from 7.6 in 1950 to 1.7 in 1997. Just between 1987 and 1997, the rate dropped 32%.[30] These decreases can be attributed to a complex combination of changes in vehicle and roadway engineering and changes in human behavior.

Several federal agencies play a role in traffic safety. The lead agency is the National Highway Transportation Safety Administration (NHTSA), charged with reducing death and disability on the highways. Other agencies, including the Federal Highway Administration and the CDC, have an impact. State efforts are most commonly led by Governors' Highway Safety Representatives, with close affiliations with law enforcement, medicine, and public health.

Kinetic energy is the agent that causes injury in motor vehicle occupants. Occupant restraint is the most important factor in reducing injury risk. Different types of impact cause different injury patterns. The biokinetics of impact stretch across all types of impact. A crash typically consists of three collisions. First, a vehicle strikes an object. The velocity, direction, mass, and rigidity of the involved objects govern the dynamics of the crash. The second collision occurs when the occupant strikes the interior of the vehicle. Proper restraint use will frequently allow the occupant to "ride down" this collision, reducing the impact force. The third collision causes direct injury to the organs involved. Complex linear and angular accelerations are involved in producing organ injuries.

The most common type of impact is frontal. Many safety systems, including air bags, laminated windshields, and collapsible steering columns, were created to reduce the severity of frontal crashes for occupants.[23] The second most common type of crash involves a side impact. Injury mechanisms can be complex. From the standpoint of prevention, it is interesting to note that drivers over age 55 experience a greater risk of side-impact crashes, suggesting numerous prevention strategies targeted at this age group.[6] Rear impacts are very common, but typically less severe than other crashes. One area of particular interest to emergency physicians may be "whiplash," for which there is little consensus about diagnosis, treatment, or outcomes. Rollovers are complex random events that represent a very high injury risk, particularly in the absence of seat belt use. Patients should be aware that being thrown clear of the car is not the goal, and can lead to death or serious injury.

Motorcycles

In 1997, 2106 motorcyclists died in the United States, and another 54,000 were seriously injured.[40] The kinematics of motorcycle crash injuries are complex. Single-vehicle crashes may occur after loss of control of the vehicle, creating a random pattern of injuries that may include severe head, chest, and extremity injuries, along with the familiar abrasions (road rash). Motorcycle-to-vehicle impacts can also cause a constellation of injuries. First, the rider separates from the motorcycle, followed by significant contact with the other vehicle. The rider then strikes the road surface, causing a new set of major injuries.

There are numerous factors that contribute to effective injury prevention for motorcyclists. These include rider training programs, driver education about avoiding motorcycles, improved roadway design, and helmets and other safety equipment.

There is no doubt, however, that the most contentious and heavily researched area of motorcycle safety concerns helmets. Helmets work by absorbing energy that would otherwise be transmitted to the rider's head after a crash. Offner et al.[32] reported that the use of helmets reduced severity of head injury and overall resource utilization in a group of riders matched for overall severity of injury. Sosin et al.[37] documented that motorcycle head injury–related death rates increased when state helmet laws were weakened and rates decreased where helmet laws were strengthened. Advocates use these findings and others when discussing motorcycle helmet requirements with state legislatures.

Bicycles

Injured bicyclists frequently present to EDs for care. In the United States, there are 800 deaths and 500,000 ED visits annually for bicycling-related injuries.[34] Bicyclists may not develop the speed of motorcyclists, but they benefit from some of the same equipment, including helmets.

The motion of the cyclist after a bicycle crash can be very random. Cyclists become large projectiles early in the crash sequence. The most common body region injured is the shoulder joint.[31] Helmets clearly reduce the severity of the most potentially severe injury, brain injury.[39] Particularly among children, local programs to increase helmet use, combining education with enforcement, are having good results in reducing the incidence of bicycle-related brain injury.

Pedestrians

Approximately 6000 to 7000 pedestrians die annually in the United States.[34] Of the 500,000 annual worldwide traffic deaths, at least half are pedestrians.[22] The young and the old are especially at risk. Children cross into streets unexpectedly, increasing the risk of a collision outside an intersection. Multiple factors may be contributing to recent declines in childhood pedestrian deaths. Traffic-calming measures may be working to reduce vehicle speeds through susceptible areas. A decrease in walking as a means of childhood transportation may also be a factor.

Among older adults, performance, manifested by walking speed, may not meet the task demand of crossing a street. Older adults are unable to clear intersections as quickly as younger adults,[13] and may also perceive oncoming vehicle speeds differently. Younger adults have the added risk of alcohol consumption. In 1992, of fatally injured pedestrians over 14 years old, 43% had consumed alcohol. Of these, 55% had a blood alcohol concentration (BAC) of 20 g/dL or higher.[5]

The mechanism of injury of the pedestrian often relates to the relationship between the victim's center of gravity (CG) and the vehicle bumper height. Children with a lower CG may be "run over," sustaining a predictable pattern of head and torso injuries. Adults with a higher CG may be "run under," sustaining typical lower extremity fractures, followed by injuries to the pelvis, torso, and head.

Intervention strategies focus on at-risk populations. Neighborhood streets may be reengineered to calm traffic in areas frequented by children. Childhood education may focus on street-crossing technique. Areas populated by older adults may require retiming of crosswalk lights to allow for safe crossing.

Falls

While young people can suffer serious injury and death from falls, the most severe outcomes are concentrated in the older population. Emergency departments see typical patterns of children who fall from heights, and older persons who fall and suffer hip fractures and other debilitating injuries.

Pediatric falls are typically the result of a child falling down stairs or through windows where safety devices were not installed. The prime example of a pediatric fall prevention program is represented by "Kids Can't Fly" from New York in the early 1970s. Over a 4-year period, 123 children died in falls through windows in high-rise buildings. A citywide program to install window guards in at-risk buildings reduced these numbers dramatically, cutting the rate of falls by 50% in 2 years.[38]

Falls in the elderly constitute a major burden for society and a principal focus for local injury prevention programs. Hip fractures are a common complication of these events. Death rates as high as 21.7% at 1 year after hip fractures, compared with 4.7% in a control group, have been reported.[17] Local fall prevention programs include optimizing medical management of at-risk populations to prevent medical causes of falls, and direct examination of homes to look for loose throw rugs, poorly placed wires, and other tripping hazards and to install handles and railings to assist occupants. ED and emergency medical services (EMS) workers are ideally placed to identify those at risk for falls and to intervene.

Burns

One of the successes of injury prevention efforts has been in the area of burn prevention. Mortality from burns has decreased 80%, accompanied by a 74% decrease in injuries from residential fires. Smoke detectors and sprinkler systems have now become a standard part of building construction, both for reduction of property losses and for reduction of deaths and injuries. Burn deaths decreased from 6357 annually to 3700 annually from 1977 to 1997, respectively.[30] The most common cause of death in fires is not from burns, but from smoke inhalation and carbon monoxide poisoning. Unfortunately, scalding still remains a relatively common means of injury for children. Intervention programs have focused on public education aimed at reducing the set temperature for water heaters to 120°F.

Farm Injuries

In rural areas, agricultural injuries are frequent occurrences. In 1995, 679 deaths were reported related to farm work. As death certificates may not always include place of death, these numbers may be understated. Interestingly, each year approximately 50% of farm deaths are related to tractor overturns. While farm deaths and injuries have been dropping, the circumstances identified by available statistics may suggest educational and engineering interventions to make the farm a safer workplace.[30]

General Occupational Injuries

The workplace, defined in many ways, can be very dangerous. Fortunately, working is much safer now than at the beginning of the twentieth century. In 1912, there were 21 unintentional work deaths per 100,000 population, while, in 1997, that rate was only two per 100,000 population. Occupational injury and death risk can be measured in a number of ways. The leading overall circumstance involved in occupational death is motor vehicle crashes (21.7%), followed by assaults (14.9%). Of the major occupation divisions, mining and agriculture carry the highest death rates. When analyzed by a measure known as index of relative risk by specific occupation, fishing and timber cutting are at least twice as dangerous as the third occupation in line, aircraft pilots.[30]

Nonfatal occupational injuries can be generally divided into acute injuries and overuse (repetitive motion) injuries. Both of these categories are well known in the typical ED. While somewhat difficult to track, these injuries can be categorized using records of days lost from work or workers' compensation claims. Acute injuries are common in air and ground transportation, food service, and lumber and metal-related industries. Disorders associated with repeated trauma are most commonly reported in manufacturing industries. Leigh et al.[19] estimated total overall cost of occupational injury in the United States in 1992 as $171 billion. Intervention strategies in the workplace range include safe driving programs, equipment use in-service training, inspection of work sites by state and federal authorities, dispute resolution, and many others.[30]

INTENTIONAL INJURY

Intentional injury, most often related to interpersonal violence, is a frequent cause of ED visits in all settings—from the most urban to the most rural. Intervention programs abound, with various levels of success. Injuries not involving guns have a clear impact. However gun-related violence, by virtue of volume and lethality of the weapon, is the focus of the vast majority of public interest and research efforts now, and will continue to be for the foreseeable future.

Injury from penetrating objects, particularly bullets, is also governed by the laws of physics. However, because the impact is very localized, a missile impact causes a much greater amount of energy transmission, and thus injury potential, per volume of tissue involved than does a vehicular impact. Bullets wound by causing permanent cavities of roughly the diameter of the bullet and temporary cavities caused by stretching of the tissue as the bullet passes through.

Firearms can be thought of in two categories: rifled firearms and shotguns. Rifled bullets, used in rifles and handguns, have smooth grooves to help with stability during flight. Lower velocity bullets, such as those in handguns, travel at speeds less than 274 mi/s, causing less tissue damage than higher velocity weapons because of their decreased capacity to create temporary cavitation. Higher velocity bullets, in the range of 600 to 900 mi/s, are fired from rifles.

Bullets may also come in two broad categories: nonexpanding and expanding. Nonexpanding bullets are jacketed to maintain the shape of their leading edge as they pass through tissue. Expanding bullets (also known as soft-point or hollow-point) begin to deform quickly on contact, potentially causing more tissue damage by creating a larger permanent cavity.

Shotguns have smooth barrels and typically fire multiple projectiles, distinguishing these weapons from rifled weapons. The multiple projectiles begin to expand quickly during flight, causing a wide but not deep area of tissue destruction. Beyond a range of about 7 m, shotgun blasts typically do not cause any massive tissue destruction.[7]

SPECIFIC INJURY ISSUES

Air Bags

Air bags came into wide use in the motor vehicle fleet in the late 1980s. These devices act as supplemental restraint systems, meant to fill space between occupant and vehicle structure. Driver and passenger frontal air bags are now required to be present in every new car sold in the United States. In recent years, the benefits and risks have become a focus of interest of injury researchers and the public.

Air bags are rapidly inflating, multiple-component systems that deploy quickly after impact occurs above a preset threshold. For frontal bags, sensors are placed in various positions in the front portion of the car. Above a Δ V of between 12 and 18 mi/h, the sensor sends a signal to the inflator, which initiates a deployment, all within a period of milliseconds. The air bag vents hot inflation gases through specific vent holes, and then rapidly deflates. Optimal protection occurs when the occupant is properly restrained by a three-point seat belt.[20]

Air bags are regulated by federal safety standards. As technology has changed and data have been acquired, standards have changed. Several specific issues hold interest for clinicians. Because deaths and injuries related to air bags were increasingly reported, public interest in air bag disconnection began to grow. Prior to 1997, air bag disconnection was the only option for concerned vehicle owners, and this option required specific approval by the federal government based on medical or other need. As of November 1997, on–off switches may be obtained under specific conditions certified by the vehicle owner. Among the potential reasons are medical conditions of concern. An extensive analysis of medical conditions of potential concern to patients was published in connection with release of the on–off switch rule.[28]

Speed and power of air bag deployment may be directly related to injury potential. Occupants who are out of position may by killed or injured during deployment. Injuries to the upper extremities, face, eyes, and chest have been reported. In the cases resulting in death, there are three distinct patterns of injury. Adult drivers tend to be unbelted and suffer lethal chest injuries, including myocardial rupture. All infant deaths have occurred when the infants were placed rear-facing in infant seats in the front seat of vehicles with passenger-side air bags. These deaths occur when the deploying air bag creates a lethal brain injury. Older children killed have generally been unbelted or improperly belted in the front seat and have sustained lethal head and neck injuries after coming into close proximity to the air bag module. The NHTSA maintains a listing of investigations of air bag–related deaths on its World Wide Web site (http://www.nhtsa.gov).[20]

Frontal air bags continue to evolve. There has been much interest in "smart" air bags. In theory, advanced-generation air bags would be able to sense various types of impacts, along with specific information, such as size, position, and restraint status of the occupant. After the system processes this information, the inflator would deliver very quickly a graded response appropriate for the situation. While theoretically optimal, the technical achievement of truly "smart" air bags will be very difficult, given the multiple permutations of potential crash dynamics. Air bags other than frontal air bags are now being introduced into the fleet. Side air bags may deploy from the door, from an area between the doors, from the side of the vehicle seat, or from above (in the roof header). These bags are designed to protect vulnerable occupants from the significant forces generated in a side impact. These devices differ from frontal bags in that they must fill a smaller space (between occupant and door) in much less time. The injury reduction benefits, and the risks, of these devices remain to be fully quantified.

Motorcycle Helmets

One of the ongoing battles in injury control is waged over the issue of mandatory use of motorcycle helmets. Three states have no helmet law, 24 states and the District of Columbia have comprehensive helmet laws, and 24 states have something in between. Until 1996, state helmet laws were common, based on federal law that gave states financial incentives to pass such laws. This incentive system was then repealed by Congress.[16]

The political battles over motorcycle helmets follow predictable lines. Advocates point out the known benefits of reduction in brain injury and death in states with mandatory helmet use.[37] These advocates also cite literature documenting the economic benefits of helmet laws from reduced direct and indirect costs.[26] In answer to anticipated concerns, advocates also cite directed studies that document the lack of significant loss of peripheral vision or hearing while wearing a properly fitting helmet.[21]

Those who oppose helmet laws challenge advocates on scientific and personal freedom grounds. The scientific arguments cite potential concerns about an increased risk of cervical spine injuries while wearing helmets. Those in opposition to helmet laws may argue that a decreased death rate after a passage of a helmet law actually reflects decreased motorcycle use by those who would prefer not to ride with a helmet. However, the discussion concerning motorcycle helmets most frequently centers around the conflict between individual freedoms and societal regulation of behavior for the greater societal good. While this general issue is not unique to injury prevention, it pervades many controversial discussions. Helmet laws will continue to be major areas of contention in many state legislatures for the foreseeable future.

Alcohol

Alcohol plays a role in many types of injury. Assaults, domestic violence, falls, drowning, and pedestrian crashes have all been related to injury risk. Nowhere is alcohol abuse more of a issue than in the case of drunk driving. Each year, approximately 17,000 people die on the highways in crashes caused by a drunk driver. As a percentage of total motor vehicle deaths, drunk driving deaths have now dropped to 38%, the lowest rate in years.[29] Improvements are related to a number of factors, including improved public awareness, lower blood alcohol levels constituting drunkenness, tougher sanctions, and technology-based sanction programs. Intervention efforts in drunk driving span the range of possibilities suggested by basic injury prevention theory. The "designated driver" message is now widely known in society. While education has not solved the problem, even the casual observer will note behavioral changes among the drinking public in the past 20 years. Frequent public service announcements reinforce the message.

TABLE 91.4. International BAC Limits

BAC Limit	Countries
0.08	Austria, Canada, Denmark, France, Italy, New Zealand, Spain, Switzerland, United Kingdom, parts of Australia
0.05	Finland, Iceland, Japan, the Netherlands, Norway, parts of Australia
0.02	Sweden

Many efforts currently focus on enforcement. Drunkenness is defined by a combination of behavioral observations and serum alcohol levels. All of the complexities of drunk driving laws are beyond the scope of this text, but some of the key elements necessary for understanding the landscape are reviewed.

Most states recognize 0.10 mg/dL as a *per se* legal limit for defining *drunk driving*. In this case, *per se* in the law means that it is illegal to operate a car at that level, without any behavioral evidence being required. A growing number of states have revised this level to 0.08 mg/dL. In fact, one of the earliest levels set as law in the United States was 0.15 mg/dL. Many advocate lower standards because of the combination of the known physiologic effects of alcohol and the difficulty of operating a motor vehicle. Other countries in the developed world typically have lower *per se* limits than most of the United States[36] (Table 91.4).

Other aspects of drunk driving laws can be confusing for those not regularly working in the field. For example driving under the influence (DUI) and driving while intoxicated (DWI) carry different connotations. DWI occurs when a driver operates a motor vehicle in an unsafe manner after consuming alcohol, regardless of the level. In some states, a driver is presumed not to be intoxicated (no DWI) if the level is less than 0.05. DUI requires levels (either 0.08 or 0.10) of BAC to provide physiologic evidence of the influence of alcohol.[36] Administrative license revocation (ALR) is allowed in many states to immediately remove driving privileges for someone found to be operating a motor vehicle under the influence of alcohol. Ignition interlock devices are used in many states as a form of punishment, usually for repeat offenders. These devices are essentially breath alcohol sensors with which a driver must test himself before starting the vehicle ignition. Zero tolerance is a relatively new concept supported by Congress. Because it is illegal in all states to drink before age 21, many states have decreed that any measurable level of alcohol in an underage driver is evidence of drunk driving. These and other measures are in place to reduce drunk-driving incidence in the states. Optimal application of these countermeasures has yet to be achieved to reduce drunk-driving rates to levels set as national priorities.

Injuries in circumstances other than motor vehicle crashes are also commonly related to alcohol use. Two-thirds of partner abuse victims reported that alcohol was a factor in the abuse.[11] Other assaults are also strongly correlated with alcohol use by involved parties, either the victims or the perpetrators. In other areas of unintentional injury, alcohol also plays a major role. Pedestrians, while potentially victims of drunk drivers, are also likely to be intoxicated, as discussed previously.

Legislation aimed at reducing alcohol-related injury, particularly related to drunk driving, is not without controversy. The most recent major debate has concerned the 0.08 drunk-driving standard. Supporters of the standard note that several studies have shown or projected reductions in injuries because of this law, that other countries have even lower standards, and that the detrimental physiologic effects of alcohol are almost universally present at this level. Opponents question the methodology of the studies of this law, express concerns about the effects on the "social drinker," and feel that enforcement efforts should be directed at drivers with higher BAC levels. Alcohol-related legislation continues to be a regular focus of debate in state legislative sessions and has the potential to affect ED practices.

Gun-Related Violence

Gun-related injuries and death are indisputably a major problem in the United States. In nearly constant dispute are the root causes and solutions. Approximately 39,000 firearm-related deaths occur each year in the United States. This number has trended generally upward each year since 1983[14] (Fig. 91.3). Rates of firearm-related deaths in the United States are 20 to 30 times higher than those in Scotland, The Netherlands, and England and Wales, and two to seven times higher than those in other similarly developed nations. In the United States, 51% of firearm deaths are suicides, while 43% are homicides.[8]

Gun-related violence is clearly a disease of the young, and, quite disproportionately, a disease of young Black males[14] (Fig. 91.4). In 1993, the rate of firearm homicide among White adolescents was 12.8 per 100,000, while the rate among Black adolescents was 131.5 per 100,000. A 1993 survey showed that more than 13% of male teenagers had carried a gun within a 30-day period; a similar survey of inner-city gun carrying revealed a rate of 22%, with rates as high as 83% among juvenile offenders.[2]

Debates about guns and gun-related violence permeate political and social discussions. The IOM panel identified several priority areas for attention in gun discussions. Issues of personal freedom, issues of instrumentality and availability, and issues of child and adolescent vulnerability all warrant considerable attention as public health and politics collide over gun issues.

Issues of personal freedom are not unique to gun use in the injury prevention literature. However, in this case, the Second Amendment to the Constitution is specifically cited as pertaining to this issue. This amendment states, "A well-regulated militia, being necessary to the security of a free State, the right of the people to keep and bear Arms, shall not be infringed." Although all Supreme Court decisions have held that the Constitution does not protect an individual's right to private gun ownership, organizations such as the National Rifle Association (NRA) and a large proportion of the public feel otherwise. A 1991 poll showed that 60% of Americans thought that gun ownership was constitutionally protected, and a 1993 poll showed that 48% of Americans thought that stricter laws would violate the Constitution.[4] The landscape of attitudes regarding private gun ownership changes very rapidly, and is significantly influenced

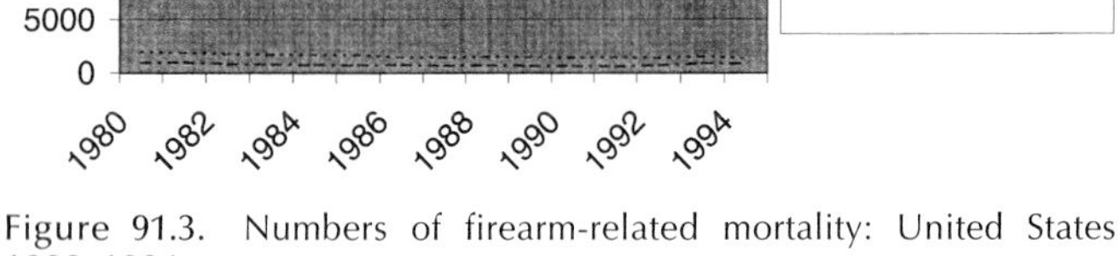

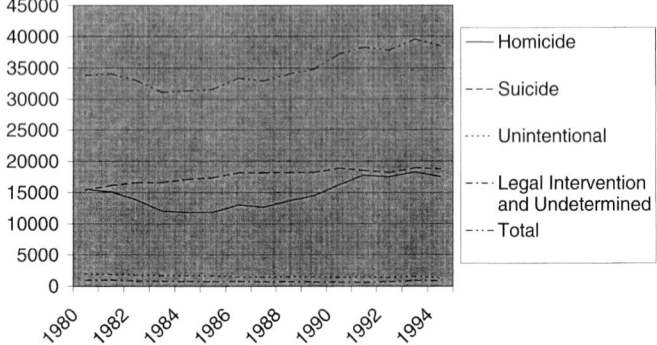

Figure 91.3. Numbers of firearm-related mortality: United States 1980–1994.

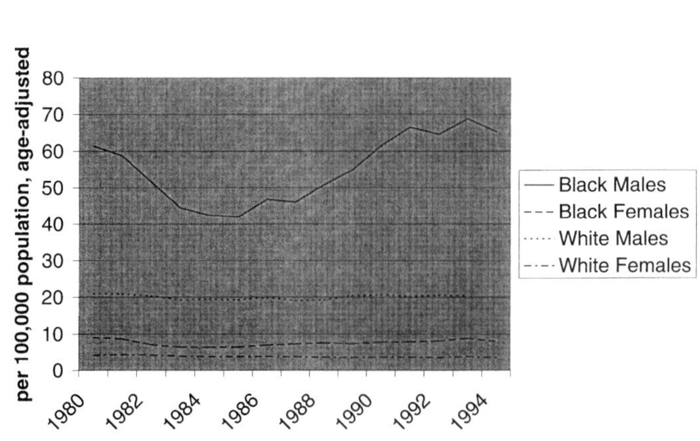

Figure 91.4. Rates of firearm-related mortality, by race and sex: United States 1980–1994.

by individual events, such as a 1998–1999 rash of school shootings, and changes in political realities.

Instrumentality and availability relate to the risk of firearm-related death and injury. Handguns and long guns (rifles, shotguns, etc.) are the two major types of weapons used in the United States. Handguns are generally divided into revolvers and semiautomatic pistols. Specific discussion of the mechanics of these types of weapons is beyond the scope of this text. Wintemute[42] has reviewed the subject of handgun types in great detail. Handguns are more frequently associated with violent acts than are long guns for a number of reasons. Long guns are most commonly used in sport and hunting, for which handguns are less effective. Handguns are lighter, easier to handle, and easier to conceal, all factors that make them more likely to be used in both planned and impulsive illegal acts. The concealability of handguns raises specific public policy questions, as many states consider and enact laws that allow private citizens to carry concealed weapons.[42] Public health and sociologic data are used on both sides of the thorny debate over concealed carry laws.

Specific issues of gun availability are raised by laws that attempt to introduce waiting periods and background checks for gun ownership, such as the "Brady Bill." Weil and Knox[41] determined that a law limiting handgun purchases in Virginia to one per month significantly disrupted the illegal interstate transfer of firearms. Wright et al.[44] found that among persons with felony convictions, denial of handgun purchases lowered the potential rate of violent and gun offenses. Those who favor this type of legislation feel that impulsive purchase of weapons leads to "crimes of passion" and that frequent and bulk purchases increase the risk of illegal transfer of weapons to criminals. Those who oppose restrictions on gun availability and purchase tend to argue that these restrictions are ineffective and impede the rights of law-abiding citizens. Restrictions on the frequency and volume of individual gun purchases will continue to be a focus of public debate.

Child and adolescent vulnerability to gun-related injury, both intentional and unintentional, is a specific area of increased concern. Highly publicized cases of children causing injury with guns taken from their own homes have raised the profile of this issue. Equally as alarming are concerns about suicide. One case-control study by Kellermann et al.[18] documented an increased risk for suicide across all age groups in homes where weapons were readily available. Data from the NEISS was used to calculate a rate of 2.6 per 100,000 unintentional, nonfatal firearm-related injuries annually in those under age 14. The rate of similar injuries for those ages 15 to 24 rises to 16.2 per 100,000.[35] News reports of deaths related to children playing with guns found in the home are particularly poignant. Educational programs that teach children to avoid guns and report their presence to adults, combined with legislation proposing mandatory child-safety devices, are in use to reduce the incidence of unintentional gun injury among children. Patient education materials related to gun safety are available from numerous sources for distribution in EDs.

Knives are also commonly used in assaults. While clearly dangerous and potentially deadly, knives do not pose the risk associated with guns. Mock et al.[25] reported reduced hospital charges and public costs associated with reduced severity of illness in a population of stabbing victims, compared with victims of gunshot wounds in the same institution. The authors calculated an annual savings of $981,000 in public funds in their institution if all of their gun assaults had taken place with knives instead.

Gun-related violence continues to occur at alarming rates. Politics will continue to play a major role in all facets of public discussion of this issue. The recent IOM report "recommends the development of a national policy on the prevention of firearm injuries directed toward reduction of morbidity and mortality associated with unintended or unlawful uses of firearms. An immediate priority should be a strategic focus on reduction of firearm injuries caused by children and adolescents." Public education about gun safety and proper storage, engineering of solutions directed at children, and enforcement of current and future laws will all work in concert to reduce the incidence of gun-related death and injury.

SUMMARY

Injury is a broad field about which volumes can and have been written. EDs are the point of presentation for many victims of injury, both intentional and unintentional. Many parts of this and other texts focus on methods for improving the acute and continuing care of those who are injured. Just as in other diseases, prevention is a major part of treating injury as a disease. Through understanding of the principles of surveillance, biomechanics, public policy, and patient education, the emergency physician can quickly develop skill and expertise in the field of injury prevention.

References

1. Annest JL, Conn JM, James SP. *Inventory of federal data systems in the United States for injury surveillance, research and prevention activities.* Atlanta: Centers for Disease Control and Prevention, National Center for Injury Prevention and Control, 1996.
2. Ash P, Kellermann AL, Fuqua-Whitley D, et al. Gun acquisition and use by juvenile offenders. *JAMA* 1996;275:1754.
3. Baker SP. Injury science comes of age. *JAMA* 1989;262:2284.
4. Blendon RJ, Young JT, Hemenway D. The American public and the gun control debate. *JAMA* 1996;275:1719.
5. Centers for Disease Control and Prevention. Alcohol involvement in pedestrian fatalities—United States 1982–1992. *MMWR* 1993;42:716.
6. Dischinger PC, Cushing BM, Kerns TJ. Injury patterns associated with direction of impact: drivers admitted to trauma centers. *J Trauma* 1993;35:454.
7. Edlich RF, Thacker JG, Rodeheaver GT. Wound management and skin closure: Appendix A—Ballistics. In: Harwood-Nuss AL, Linden CH, Luten RC, et al., eds. *The clinical practice of emergency medicine,* 2nd ed. Philadelphia: Lippincott–Raven Publishers, 1996.
8. Fingerhut LA, Cox CS, Warner M, et al. *International comparative analysis of injury mortality: findings from the ICE on injury statistics.* Advance data from vital and health statistics; no. 303. Hyattsville, MD: National Center for Health Statistics.
9. Fingerhut LA, Warner M. *Injury chartbook. Health United States, 1996–97.* Hyattsville, MD: National Center for Health Statistics.
10. Graitcer PL. The development of state and local injury surveillance systems. *J Safety Res* 1987;18:191.
11. Greenfield L. *Alcohol and crime: an analysis of national data on the prevalence of alcohol involvement in crime.* US Department of Justice, Office of Justice Programs, Bureau of Justice Statistics. Report no. NCJ-168632, Washington, DC, 1998.
12. Haddon W. A logical framework for categorizing highway safety phenomena and data. *J Trauma* 1972;12:193.
13. Hoxie RE, Rubenstein LZ. Are older pedestrians allowed enough time to cross intersections safely? *J Am Geriatr Soc* 1994;42:241.
14. Ikeda RM, Gorwitz R, James SP, et al. *Fatal firearm injuries in the United States, 1962–1994.* Atlanta: Centers for Disease Control and Prevention, National Center for Injury Prevention and Control, 1997. Violence Surveillance Summary Series, no. 3.
15. IOM (Institute of Medicine). *Reducing the burden of injury: advancing prevention and treatment.* Washington, DC: National Academy Press, 1999.
16. Insurance Institute for Highway Safety. Without a helmet there's no easy ride. *Status Report* 1998;33:1.
17. Katelaris AG, Cumming RG. Health status before and mortality after hip fracture. *Am J Publ Health* 1996;86:557.
18. Kellermann AL, Rivara FP, Somes G, et al. Suicide in the home in relation to gun ownership. *N Engl J Med* 1992;327:467.
19. Leigh JP, Markowitz SB, Fahs M, et al. Occupational injury and illness in the United States: estimates of costs, morbidity, and mortality. *Arch Intern Med* 1997;157:1557.
20. McKay MP, Jolly BT. A retrospective review of air bag deaths. *Acad Emerg Med* 1999;6:708.
21. McKnight AJ, McKnight AS. The effects of motorcycle helmets upon seeing and hearing. DOT HS 808 399 Washington DC, US Department of Transportation, National Highway Traffic Safety Administration, 1994.
22. Mackay M. Engineering in accidents: vehicle design and injuries. *Injury* 1994;25:615.
23. Mackay M. A review of the biomechanics of impacts in road accidents. In: Ambrosio JAC, et al., eds. *Crashworthiness of transportation systems: structural impact and occupant protection.* The Netherlands: Kluwer Academic Publishers, 1997:115.
24. Martinez R. Injury control: a primer for physicians. *Ann Emerg Med* 1990;19:72.
25. Mock C, Pilcher S, Maier R. Comparison of the costs of acute treatment for gunshot and stab wounds: further evidence of the need for firearms control. *J Trauma* 1994;36:516.
26. Muelleman RL, Mlinek EJ, Collicott PE. Motorcycle crash injuries and costs: effect of a reenacted comprehensive helmet use law. *Ann Emerg Med* 1992;21:266.
27. National Center for Injury Prevention and Control (CDC). Ten leading causes of death by age group—1995. (WWW document) URL http://www.cdc.gov/ncipe/images/101C95.gif
28. National Highway Traffic Safety Administration. National Conference on Medical Indication for Air Bag Disconnection. Final Report, October 1997, Washington, DC.
29. National Highway Traffic Safety Administration. Traffic Safety Facts 1997—Alcohol. DOT HS 808764, Washington, DC.
30. National Safety Council. *Accident facts, 1998.* Itasca, IL: National Safety Council, 1998.
31. Nekomoto JS, Hunting K, Jolly BT, et al. Bicycle couriers: a unique injury risk group. Forty-first Annual *Proceedings* of the Association for the Advancement of Automotive Medicine, 1997;41:157.
32. Offner PJ, Rivara FP, Maier RV. The impact of motorcycle helmet use. *J Trauma* 1992;32:636.
33. Pollack DA, Adams DL, Bernardo LM, et al. Data elements for emergency department systems, release 1.0 (DEEDS): a summary report. *Ann Emerg Med* 1998;31:264.
34. Rivara FP, Grossman DC, Cummings P. Injury prevention [first of two parts]. *N Engl J Med* 1997;337:543.
35. Sinauer N, Annest JL, Mercy JA. Unintentional, nonfatal firearm-related injuries: a preventable public health burden. *JAMA* 1996;275:1740.
36. Snyder MB. Driving under the influence: a report to Congress on alcohol limits. DOT HS 807 879. US Department of Transportation, National Highway Traffic Safety Administration, Washington, DC, 1992.
37. Sosin DM, Sacks JJ, Holmgreen P. Head-injury associated deaths from motorcycle crashes: relationship to helmet-use laws. *JAMA* 1990;264:2395.
38. Spiegel CN, Lindaman FC. Children can't fly: a program to prevent childhood morbidity and mortality from window falls. *Am J Publ Health* 1977;67:1143.
39. Thompson DC, Rivara FP, Thompson RS. Effectiveness of bicycle helmets in preventing head injuries: a case-control study. *JAMA* 1996;276:1968.
40. US Department of Transportation. *Traffic safety facts 1997.* DOT HS 808 806, Washington, DC, 1998.
41. Weil DS, Knox RC. Effects of limiting handgun purchases in interstate transfer of firearms. *JAMA* 1996;275:1759.
42. Wintemute GJ. The relationship between firearm design and firearm violence: handguns in the 1990s. *JAMA* 1996;275:1749.
43. World Health Organization. The global burden of disease (summary). In: Murray CJL, Lopez AD, eds. Boston: Harvard University Press, 1996.
44. Wright MA, Wintemute GJ, Rivara FP. Effectiveness of denial of handgun purchase to persons believed to be at high risk for firearm violence. *Am J Publ Health* 1999;280:2083.
45. Yanik AJ. The first 100 years of transportation safety: part 1. *Automotive Engineering* 1996;(January):33.

CHAPTER 92

Out-of-Hospital Care and Transport of the Trauma Patient

Juan A. March and C. Crawford Mechem

Out-of-hospital care for the trauma patient has evolved tremendously over the past two centuries. During the Napoleonic Wars, wounded soldiers in Europe were transported from the front line to the hospital in light, two-wheeled wagons called "flying ambulances."[2] In contrast, today highly trained medical personnel transport patients in fully equipped air and ground ambulances.

Emergency medical services (EMS) in its current form arose from the realization that the quality of medical care administered to wounded soldiers in Vietnam far surpassed that administered to civilians injured in automobile accidents back home. To help address this, the National Highway Safety Act of 1966 established an EMS division of the National Highway Traffic Safety Administration. It also set aside funds for training of hospital care providers and for ambulances and communication systems.[14] The Emergency Medical Systems Act of 1973 led to the establishment of 300 regional EMS systems across the United States and made the Department of Transportation (DOT) responsible for creating a formal training curriculum for emergency medical technicians (EMTs).[9] Since 1981, funding and oversight of the EMS system has shifted from the federal level to state and local levels.[22]

ADVANCES IN OUT-OF-HOSPITAL THERAPY

In 1995 the National Highway Traffic Safety Administration implemented a revised, national, standard EMT-Basic curriculum.[26] Adoption and implementation of the new curriculum is the choice of the lead EMS agency in each state. In some states, legislative changes will be required before full adoption of the new curriculum is possible. As a consequence, even today, individual state and local EMS systems continue to have levels of certification varying from EMT-Basic to EMT-Paramedic.[15]

Appropriate airway management is critical to the out-of-hospital care of the trauma patient. The new standards for the EMT-Basic curriculum include an optional session for endotracheal intubation, thus allowing for advanced airway intervention in EMS systems that otherwise might not be able to afford personnel trained to the paramedic level. While orotracheal intubation is the preferred method for ventilation and prevention of aspiration in patients with respiratory compromise, skills maintenance may be difficult in EMT-Basic systems or in smaller EMS systems with low call volumes.[11,20] The traditional alternative to intubation has been bag-valve-mask ventilation with an oral airway in place. Bag-valve-mask ventilation can be technically difficult, often resulting in inadequate tidal volumes, and may lead to aspiration of gastric contents. Other airway adjuncts that have proven successful in lower volume EMS systems include the Pharyngeal Tracheal Lumen Airway (PTL), the Laryngeal Mask Airway, and the Combitube. However, there are no data available regarding the morbidity or mortality associated with the use of these devices in the trauma patient.[19]

The role of out-of-hospital fluid resuscitation has been an area of controversy for numerous years. Whether fluids improve outcome and, if so, which fluid is best are questions that have been hotly contested. Deliberately delaying fluid resuscitation in hypotensive trauma patients until bleeding is surgically controlled has been referred to as "permissive hypotension." The rationale behind this practice is that giving fluids increases hemorrhage by increasing intravascular hydrostatic pressure. In addition, soft clots may be dislodged and clotting factors diluted.[8,16]

Clinical support for this comes from a prospective study of 598 hypotensive adults with penetrating thoracic trauma who were randomized to either receive intravenous fluids in the out-of-hospital setting or have a heplock placed but not given fluids. Those not given fluids had a higher survival rate.[5] However, it is unclear whether these results can be generalized to blunt trauma victims, to those with closed-head injuries, or to EMS systems with long transport times. Ultimately, the extent of out-of-hospital fluid resuscitation may be dictated by the specific injuries involved and the EMS location.[21]

The Pneumatic Anti Shock Garment (PASG), a modification of the jet aviator's G-suit, was in widespread use in the late 1970s and early 1980s to restore blood pressure in hypotensive trauma patients. Its mechanism of action was thought to involve increased preload and increased systemic vascular resistance.[12] This device has fallen into disfavor following the publication of studies questioning its theoretical mechanism of action and suggesting a lack of efficacy. In fact, a study of 911 hypotensive blunt and penetrating trauma victims who were randomized to PASG or no-PASG therapy demonstrated a worse outcome in the PASG group in patients with cardiac and thoracic vascular injuries.[4,13]

A position paper developed by the National Association of EMS Physicians reviewed the available clinical data on use of the PASG.[7] In the trauma setting, scenarios in which use of the PASG was acceptable, and probably helpful, included hypotension due to suspected pelvic fracture, uncontrollable lower extremity hemorrhage, and severe traumatic hypotension with a pulse but no obtainable blood pressure. The PASG was possibly helpful in the setting of penetrating abdominal trauma, pelvic fracture without hypotension, and spinal shock. The use of the PASG was felt to be inappropriate in case of diaphragmatic rupture, penetrating thoracic injury, abdominal evisceration, and as a splint of extremity fractures.

PATIENT TRANSPORT

Options for transport of trauma victims from the scene to definitive care include both ground and air ambulances. Air transport involves both helicopters and fixed-wing aircraft. In most cases, trauma victims will be transported by helicopter from the scene to definitive care. One distinct advantage of air ambulances over ground transport is the speed of transfer between two points. In addition, highly trained flight crews can perform life-saving interventions en route, such as rapid-sequence intubation, needle decompression of a tension pneumothorax, and cricothyroidotomy. Air travel is ideal in the rural setting, where there are often great distances to cover and transport time becomes a crucial factor.[10]

The first helicopter aeromedical program in the United States went into service in 1972 at St. Anthony's Hospital in Denver, Colorado.[23] In 1998 approximately 275 helicopter air medical programs were operating in the United States.[1] Helicopter staffing includes the pilot and generally two medical members, often two flight nurses or a nurse and a paramedic. However, physicians and respiratory therapists may also be used, as dic-

TABLE 92.1. NAEMSP Guidelines for Transport of Trauma Patients

A. SPECIFIC

Patients with critical injuries resulting in unstable vital signs require the fastest, most direct route of transport to a regional trauma center in a vehicle staffed with a team capable of offering critical care enroute. Often this is the case in the following situations:

a. Trauma Score <12
b. Glasgow Coma Score <10
c. Penetrating trauma to the abdomen, pelvis, chest, neck, or head
d. Spinal cord or spinal column injury, or any injury producing paralysis of any extremity or any lateral signs
e. Partial or total amputation of an extremity (excluding digits)
f. Two or more long bone fractures or a major pelvis fracture
g. Crushing injuries to the abdomen, chest, or head
h. Major burns of the body surface area; *or* burns involving the face, hands, feet, or perineum; *or* burns with significant respiratory involvement; *or* major electrical or chemical burns
i. Patients involved in a serious traumatic event who are less than 12 or more than 55 years of age
j. Patients with near-drowning injuries, with or without existing hypothermia
k. Adult patient with any of the following vital sign abnormalities:
   1. Systolic blood pressure <90 mm Hg
   2. Respiratory rate <10 or >35
   3. Heart rate <60 or >120 per min
   4. Unresponsive to verbal stimuli.

B. OPERATIONAL SITUATIONS IN WHICH HELICOPTER USE SHOULD BE CONSIDERED

1. Mechanism of injury
   a. Vehicle roll-over with unbelted passengers
   b. Vehicle striking a pedestrian at >10 miles per hour
   c. Falls from >15 feet
   d. Motorcycle victim ejected at >20 miles per hour
   e. Multiple victims
2. Difficult access situations
   a. Wilderness rescue
   b. Ambulance egress or access impeded at the scene by road conditions, weather, or traffic

Printed with permission by the National Association of Emergency Medical Service Physicians.

tated by the nature of the mission.[24] In the wake of a series of air medical tragedies, the Commission on Accreditation of Medical Transport Systems in 1991 established accreditation standards to ensure patient and flight crew safety. These address such issues as pilot and crew training and equipment maintenance. As of 1998 there were 62 accredited transport services.[6]

When applied appropriately, air medical transport can have a profound impact on trauma patient survival. A large study of 1273 blunt trauma victims transported by helicopter found a 21% reduction in predicted mortality.[3] Data involving air transport of traumatic cardiac arrest patients are less promising. In a study of 67 trauma patients in cardiac arrest at the scene, 47 were transported to hospital. None survived to hospital discharge.[25] Therefore, the benefits of air transport must be weighed against potential risks on a case-by-case basis.

Although helicopters attain much greater speeds than ground transport, flight team preparation usually requires 3 to 8 minutes prior to lift-off from the base, and patient loading in the vehicle may require more time than it would in a routine ground transport. In addition, helicopters may be limited by inclement weather and the need for a safe landing zone, which can often be difficult to find in an urban setting.[18] Thus, air transport is not appropriate in all cases. Guidelines developed by the National Association of Emergency Medical Services Physicians (NAEMSP) for trauma patient transport via helicopter are outlined in detail in Table 92.1.

PATIENT DESTINATION

Direct transport from the scene to a regional trauma center has obvious advantages. These include the immediate availability of highly trained medical staff, including but not limited to emergency physicians, trauma surgeons, neurosurgeons, and cardiovascular surgeons. In addition, the necessary ancillary equipment and personnel for such as blood bank, x-ray, computed tomography scanners, cardiopulmonary bypass, and surgery are readily available. The American College of Surgeons' Committee on Trauma (Table 92.2) has developed guidelines for transfer directly to a trauma center.

Frequently, for logistic reasons, victims of major trauma are initially transported to hospitals that are not trauma centers. The decision to transfer these patients to a regional trauma center must be based on the capabilities and limitations of the local institution. Guidelines provided by the American College of Surgeons recommend that patients identified as having a high risk of dying of their injuries should be transferred. Such injuries include but are not limited to major head and chest trauma, pelvic fractures, multisystem injury, or the presence of comorbid conditions. Table 92.3 provides a complete listing.

Patients not initially brought to a regional trauma center, but identified as requiring a trauma center referral, should be transferred as soon as possible following initial assessment and resuscitation. Early contact with the referral facility is necessary to optimize patient management en route and to facilitate the transport process, whether by ground or air ambulance. The Consolidated Omnibus Budget Reconciliation Act of 1985 (COBRA), also known as the Emergency Medical Treatment and Active Labor Act (EMTALA), requires that the physician at the receiving hospital be contacted and accept the patient prior to transport.

The receiving hospital must have the necessary facilities to care for the patient. The referring and receiving physicians share the medical and legal responsibilities of transferring a patient. Direct communication should occur between these physicians as frequently as necessary to ensure appropriate patient care en route. This initial contact should be made as soon as criteria indicating the transfer are identified. Communication should remain open to inform the receiving physician of details of the physical examination, pertinent diagnostic test results, or any changes in the patient's condition.[15,17]

Recently, there has been some controversy over air medical transport and the COBRA requirement for an emergency department evaluation of each patient by a physician. Is an evaluation at the local community hospital by a physician required, when the trauma patient is transported by ground ambulance from the scene directly to the helipad at the local community hospital and the patient never enters the emergency department doors at the local community hospital? Even when the sole purpose for ground transport to the local community hospital is to facilitate rendezvous with the flight team, is the local hospital required to perform a screening evaluation, which might include x-rays of the chest, pelvis, and cervical spine? This evaluation would only delay the patient's transport to definitive care at a regional trauma center, particularly since flight teams are capable of performing most of any critical emergency interventions required. No literature is currently available regarding this aspect of COBRA. Local policies should determine how these cases should be handled.

TABLE 92.2. ACS Trauma Center Transfer Guidelines

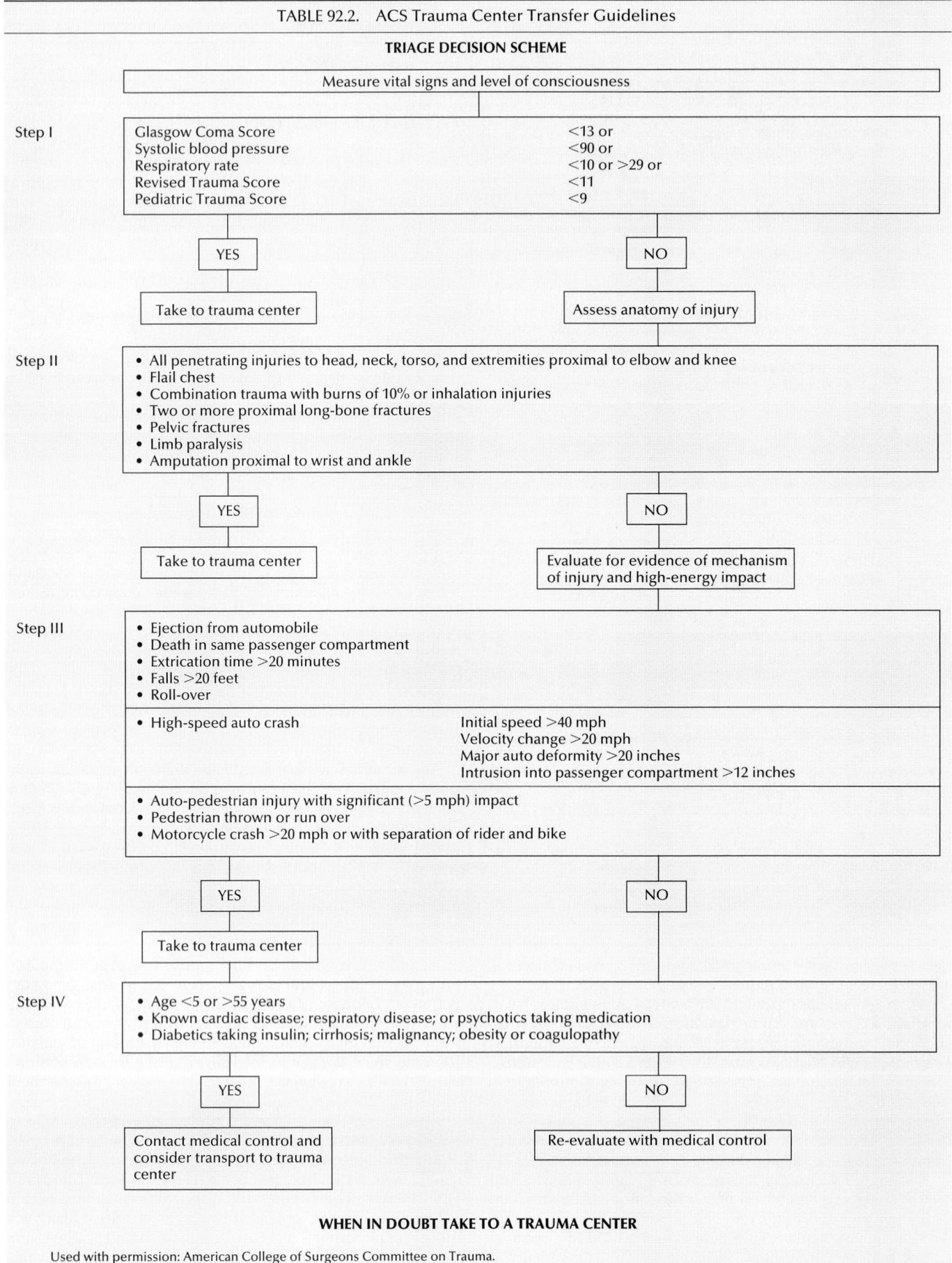

TRIAGE DECISION SCHEME

Measure vital signs and level of consciousness

Step I

Glasgow Coma Score	<13 or
Systolic blood pressure	<90 or
Respiratory rate	<10 or >29 or
Revised Trauma Score	<11
Pediatric Trauma Score	<9

YES → Take to trauma center

NO → Assess anatomy of injury

Step II

- All penetrating injuries to head, neck, torso, and extremities proximal to elbow and knee
- Flail chest
- Combination trauma with burns of 10% or inhalation injuries
- Two or more proximal long-bone fractures
- Pelvic fractures
- Limb paralysis
- Amputation proximal to wrist and ankle

YES → Take to trauma center

NO → Evaluate for evidence of mechanism of injury and high-energy impact

Step III

- Ejection from automobile
- Death in same passenger compartment
- Extrication time >20 minutes
- Falls >20 feet
- Roll-over

• High-speed auto crash	Initial speed >40 mph
	Velocity change >20 mph
	Major auto deformity >20 inches
	Intrusion into passenger compartment >12 inches

- Auto-pedestrian injury with significant (>5 mph) impact
- Pedestrian thrown or run over
- Motorcycle crash >20 mph or with separation of rider and bike

YES → Take to trauma center

NO → Step IV

Step IV

- Age <5 or >55 years
- Known cardiac disease; respiratory disease; or psychotics taking medication
- Diabetics taking insulin; cirrhosis; malignancy; obesity or coagulopathy

YES → Contact medical control and consider transport to trauma center

NO → Re-evaluate with medical control

WHEN IN DOUBT TAKE TO A TRAUMA CENTER

Used with permission: American College of Surgeons Committee on Trauma.

TABLE 92.3. Interhospital Triage Criteria

CENTRAL NERVOUS SYSTEM
Head injury
Penetrating injury or depressed skull fracture
Open injury with or without cerebrospinal fluid leak
Glasgow Coma Score (GCS) <13 or GCS deterioration
Lateralizing signs
Spinal cord injury
CHEST
Wide mediastinum
Major chest wall injury
Cardiac injury
Patients who may require protracted ventilation
PELVIS
Unstable pelvic ring disruption
Pelvic ring disruption with shock and evidence of continuing hemorrhage
Open pelvic injury
MULTIPLE SYSTEM INJURY
Severe face injury with head injury
Chest injury with head injury
Abdominal or pelvic injury with head injury
Burns with associated injuries
Multiple fractures
EVIDENCE OF HIGH-ENERGY IMPACT
Auto crash or pedestrian injury—velocity ≥25 mph
Rearward displacement of front axle or front of car (20 inches)
Ejection of patient or rollover
Death of occupant in same car
CO-MORBID FACTORS
Age <5 years or >55 years
Known cardiorespiratory or metabolic diseases
SECONDARY DETERIORATION (LATE SEQUELAE)
Mechanical ventilation required
Sepsis
Single or multiple organ system failure (deterioration in central nervous, cardiac pulmonary, hepatic, renal, or coagulation systems)
Major tissue necrosis

Printed with permission by: the American College of Surgeons Committee on Trauma. *Resources for optimal care of the injured patient.* American College of Surgeons, 1990.

In conclusion, management of the trauma patient by out-of-hospital care providers has changed tremendously over the past two centuries. This change has been even more dramatic in the past three decades, as new advances in emergency medicine research have continued to change out-of-hospital care.

References

1. Air Medical Physician Association (Web address: http//www.ampa.org/).
2. Barkley KT. *The ambulance.* Kiamesha Lake, NY: Load N Go Press, 1990.
3. Baxt WG, Moody P, Cleveland HC, et al. Hospital-based rotorcraft aeromedical emergency care services and trauma mortality: a multicenter study. *Ann Emerg Med* 1985;14:859–864.
4. Bickell WH, Pepe PE, Bailey ML, et al. Randomized trial of pneumatic anti-shock garments in the prehospital management of penetrating abdominal injuries. *Ann Emerg Med* 1987;16:653–658.
5. Bickell WH, Wall MJ, Pepe PE, et al. Immediate versus delayed fluid resuscitation for hypotensive patients with penetrating torso injuries. *N Engl J Med* 1994;331:1105–1109.
6. Commission on Accreditation of Medical Transport Systems (Web address: http://www.camts.org/).
7. Domeier RM, O'Connor RE, Delbridge TR, et al. Use of the pneumatic anti-shock garment (PASG). *Prehosp Emerg Care* 1997;1:32–35.
8. Dries DJ. Hypotensive resuscitation. *Shock* 1996;6:311–316.
9. Emergency Medical Services Systems Act of 1973. Public Law 93-154, Title XII of the Public Health Services Act. Washington, DC, U.S. Government Printing Office, 1973.
10. Gabram SGA, Jacobs LM. The impact of emergency medical helicopters on prehospital care. *Emerg Med Clin North Am* 1990;8:85–102.
11. Larmon B, Schriger DL, Snelling R, et al. Results of a 4-hour endotracheal intubation class for EMT-Basics. *Ann Emerg Med* 1998;31:224–227.
12. MacLeod BA, Seaberg DC, Paris PM. Prehospital therapy past, present, and future. *Emerg Med Clin North Am* 1990;8:57–74.
13. Mattox KL, Bickell W, Pepe PE, et al. Prospective MAST study in 911 patients. *J Trauma* 1989;29:1104–1112.
14. National Highway Safety Act of 1966. Public Law 89-564. Washington, DC, Congressional Register, 1966.
15. Ossmann EW, Bartkus EA, Olinger ML. Prehospital pearls, pitfalls, and updates. *Emerg Med Clin North Am* 1997;15:283–301.
16. Pepe PE, Eckstein M. Reappraising the prehospital care of the patient with major trauma. *Emerg Med Clin North Am* 1998;16:1–15.
17. Publication L. No. 99-272, 100 Stat. 82. Codified as amended at 42 USC 1395dd.
18. Rodenberg H, Blumen IJ. Aeromedical transport and in-flight medical emergencies. In: Rosen P, Barkin R, eds. *Emergency medicine: concepts and clinical practice,* 4th ed. St. Louis: Mosby, 1998:334–350.
19. Rumball CJ, MacDonald D. The PTL, Combitube, laryngeal mask, and oral airway: a randomized prehospital comparative study of ventilatory device effectiveness and cost-effectiveness in 470 cases of cardiorespiratory arrest. *Prehosp Emerg Care* 1997;1:1–10.
20. Sayre MR, Sakles JC, Mistler AF, et al. Field trial of endotracheal intubation by basic EMTs. *Ann Emerg Med* 1998;31:228–233.
21. Silbergleit RR, Satz W, McNamara RM, et al. Effect of permissive hypotension in continuous uncontrolled intra-abdominal hemorrhage. *Acad Emerg Med* 1996;3:922–926.
22. Tamkin GW. Emergency medical services systems. *Crit Decis Emerg Med* 1998;12:9–16.
23. Thomas F. The development of the nation's oldest operating civilian hospital-sponsored aeromedical service. *Aviat Space Environ Med* 1988;59:567–570.
24. Thomas S, Alson R. Aeromedical transport. In: Plantz S, Adler J, Collman D, et al., eds. *The emergency medicine on-line reference* (Web address: http//www.emedicine.com/). Boston: Boston Medical Publishing Company, 1997.
25. Wright SW, Dronen SC, Combs TJ, et al. Aeromedical transport of patients with post-traumatic cardiac arrest. *Ann Emerg Med* 1989;18:721–726.
26. United States Department of Transportation. 1994 Basic EMT National Standard Curriculum (Web address: http://www.nhtsa.dot.gov/people/injury/ems/).

CHAPTER 93
Trauma Airway Management

Kevin R. Ward

Expert management of the airway is the single most important skill that must be acquired and maintained by the emergency physician. Because of the potential diversity of patient population and presentations, acquisition of the skills and knowledge base necessary for optimal management of acute airway emergencies calls for multidisciplinary training unique to emergency medicine that includes anesthesia, critical care, pediatrics, surgery, and emergency medical services training. This chapter discusses the unique aspects of airway management in patients with multisystem trauma in the setting where the emergency physician may be the sole physician provider of resuscitative care.

PROBLEMS UNIQUE TO TRAUMA AIRWAY MANAGEMENT

Many victims of trauma will benefit from early control of the airway to ensure adequate oxygenation and ventilation, and to pro-

TABLE 93.1. Factors Complicating Trauma Airway Management

1)	Inability to position airway optimally for intubation secondary to possibility of C-spine injury.
2)	Presence of hypovolemic shock or occult hypovolemia
3)	Presence of full stomach and risk of aspiration
4)	Possibility of concomitant head injury
5)	Known or unknown pre-existing disease states

tect against aspiration. Contrary to popular belief, most trauma patients are not initially managed in the sophisticated environment of the trauma center, where ample expert assistance is readily available. Instead, these patients are managed by the community emergency physician who has little or no surgical, anesthesia, or additional emergency medicine assistance. Therefore, the chosen approaches must result in very rapid and safe acquisition of the airway in the majority of clinical scenarios.

Airway management in trauma victims is problematic for many reasons. The five most immediate concerns are listed in Table 93.1. It is wise to assume the presence of cervical spine (c-spine) injury in most blunt trauma victims. Because of altered mental or hemodynamic status, and difficulty in obtaining adequate c-spine radiographs rapidly, c-spine injury cannot be excluded in most patients requiring emergent intubation.

All well-known methods used to predict the difficulty of intubation, including the Mallampati classification, or measuring distances between various landmarks, require a cooperative patient or one who is able to fully extend his or her neck. The inability to optimally position the airway can be problematic in obtaining an adequate laryngeal view during intubation. Coexisting facial and penetrating neck trauma add to this problem. Therefore, the ability to predict the difficulty of intubation in the setting of trauma is minimal.

Hypovolemia complicates airway management because secondary hemodynamic deterioration can be caused by the drugs given to facilitate airway management. Occult hypovolemia or compensated shock is especially hazardous if not considered. Not until the patient has lost 30% to 40% of his or her blood volume does shock uniformly manifest itself. Occult myocardial dysfunction has also been found to exist in trauma victims.[12]

Because the timing of traumatic injuries is unpredictable, all trauma patients must be presumed to have a full stomach. The response to pain from injury and resuscitative maneuvers frequently causes nausea and vomiting, resulting in an increased risk of aspiration.

Concomitant head injury also alters the approach to airway management in the multiply injured patient. Issues of cerebral blood flow and intracranial pressure (ICP) must be considered together with volume status and cardiovascular function so that neither is compromised. The presence of a drug or alcohol-induced altered mental status further complicates the determination of the potential presence of closed-head injury requiring emergent airway management.

All of these concerns are aggravated by the presence of pre-existing disease. Elderly patients, for example, may be taking cardioactive medications that adversely affect the hemodynamic response to injury or intervention. All of these issues must be considered when selecting approaches to trauma airway management.

TECHNIQUES OF AIRWAY MANAGEMENT

Intubation of the trachea with a cuffed endotracheal tube is the standard of care when it is clear that the patient cannot protect his or her airway or is at the point of respiratory failure. Orotracheal intubation (OTI), blind nasotracheal intubation (NTI), and surgical cricothyrotomy are the major choices for definitive airway management. The act of intubation is not benign and may cause severe stress to the patient. The routine use of awake intubation is too stressful in all but the most severely injured patients who are deeply comatose and hypotensive.

Laryngoscopy and intubation result in circulatory responses that can cause bradycardia, tachycardia, hypertension, increased ICP, and disturbances in cerebral blood flow. Intubation in an awake patient that causes struggling may result in gagging, with profound spikes in ICP, vomiting and aspiration, and significant movement of the c-spine. Regardless of technique, proper preparation is essential. The use of the mnemonic SOAPME is helpful to ensure readiness (Table 93.2).[32]

Orotracheal Intubation and Rapid-Sequence Induction

OTI may be performed in several modes, ranging from having the patient totally awake to performing it in conjunction with rapid-sequence induction (RSI). RSI is a technique by which the physician quickly prepares the patient for intubation: Oxygen and various induction and paralytic agents are used to perform intubation in a manner that reduces the chance of aspiration and hemodynamic disturbances.

OTI with RSI has become the procedure of choice in managing the trauma airway. It is also meeting with a great deal of success in the prehospital setting. Although different pharmacologic agents may be chosen, the major components of this technique remain the same: preoxygenation, administration of agents that cause loss of consciousness, administration of paralytics, and administration of postintubation analgesia and sedation.

Preoxygenation is performed to prevent hypoxemia during the intubation process. It is achieved either actively, such as with use of a bag-valve-mask (BVM), or by letting the patient with spontaneous respiration (and adequate minute ventilation) inhale 100% oxygen. Active preoxygenation should be avoided, if possible, to reduce the risk of gastric insufflation, although arguments exists that a brief attempt should be made to assist the patient with a BVM to ensure the patient can be adequately ventilated prior to inducing paralysis. Regardless, application of cricoid pressure (Sellick maneuver) is essential during RSI, or any other active ventilation technique, to prevent gastric insuf-

TABLE 93.2. Preparation for Airway Management: Mnemonic

S:	Suction should be readily available with Yankauer or tonsil tip apparatus.
O:	High-flow oxygen (15 1/min) with appropriate methods of delivery such as bag-valve-mask device and nonrebreathing masks should be available.
A:	Airway supplies should be present in various sizes. These include naso- and oropharyngeal airways, endotracheal tubes with stylets and 10-mL syringes, and functioning straight- and curved-blade laryngoscopes. Consider having other airway adjuncts available for difficult airways. Adequate assistance to keep the airway positioned and to provide cricoid pressure is essential.
P:	Pharmacology in the form of induction, sedative, analgesic and neuromuscular blocking agents, as well as local anesthetics should be available for immediate administration.
ME:	Monitoring equipment such as ECG, pulse oximetry, end-tidal CO_2 monitoring, and stethoscopes should be applied and in working condition.

flation and regurgitation. This maneuver is applied until the endotracheal tube cuff is inflated and tube position is confirmed.

Unless lung or chest trauma exists, it should be possible to significantly denitrogenate the lungs within 30 seconds if the patient receiving 100% oxygen can take four maximally deep breaths or if the equivalent can be delivered actively with a BVM.[10] This reservoir of oxygen will last several minutes before desaturation of hemoglobin occurs. Although pulse oximetry should be used to detect desaturation, it should be remembered that it is essentially insensitive to PaO_2 levels above 90 mm Hg. In addition, pulse oximetry readings may lag behind true oxyhemoglobin changes by 1 to 2 minutes.

Induction refers to a rapid and controlled drug-induced loss of consciousness. Producing a state of controlled unconsciousness before intubation has many advantages. Even hypotensive trauma patients are often conscious and aware of their surroundings, making intubation both mechanically difficult and stressful for the patient. Induction is most commonly produced by such drugs as the sedative–hypnotics.[26–28,32]

Paralysis is performed during RSI for a number of reasons. It reduces the chance of regurgitation and aspiration by eliminating the efferent gagging and coughing response to the stimulus of laryngoscopy. Paralysis also totally relaxes the upper airway musculature to allow the physician an optimal view of the larynx. It also prevents spontaneous movements by the at-risk patient that might produce spinal cord injury during the periintubation period.

Because of the problem in predicting the degree of difficulty in intubating the trauma patient who has facial and neck injuries, inhalation injuries, or potential c-spine injuries, care must be taken in using paralytic agents if there is likely to be a problem in providing other forms of artificial ventilation.

Airway adjuncts, as well as cricothyrotomy equipment, must be immediately available at all times during RSI. In such cases, RSI may be modified to provide adequate sedation: An appropriate sedative–hypnotic is used in conjunction with topical or intravenous anesthesia, but the paralysis component is deleted. This combination may be the best alternative to reduce patient stress and to partially blunt the physiologic response to laryngoscopy and intubation. Paralytic agents may then be given immediately after proper endotracheal tube position is confirmed.

Although advocated by some, placement of a nasogastric tube prior to intubation can be extremely problematic, depending on the patient's level of consciousness at the time. Although gastric emptying prior to RSI would appear to offer advantages, many patients in distress will not tolerate its placement. The result is sometimes dangerous movement of the c-spine as well as gagging and vomiting, which may lead to aspiration or deleterious changes in cerebral hemodynamics.

Blind Nasotracheal Intubation

NTI has long been advocated as the method of choice for intubating patients with suspected c-spine injury and patients in whom sedation is contraindicated. It requires a patient who is spontaneously breathing and in whom the operator can recognize inspiration and expiration. Patients with significant midface trauma have not been considered candidates for NTI, although clinical studies demonstrate its safety in patients with demonstrated cribriform plate fractures.[16]

Although popular, NTI has drawbacks. Because optimal performance requires proper preparation of the nasal mucosa, it can be time consuming, taking several minutes to complete. NTI often requires multiple attempts. Even after mucosal preparation, significant epistaxis may occur, placing the patient at risk for aspiration and possibly making subsequent OTI more difficult. NTI is capable of causing intense cardiovascular stimulation, which along with any patient struggling may result in increasing ICP. In addition, struggling may cause significant c-spine movement in those at risk for cord injuries.

NTI has a place if time and circumstances do not permit preparation for OTI. If it is performed, oxygen should be given by high-flow delivery throughout the procedure to prevent desaturation. The largest nares should be chosen. The nasal mucosa should be prepared, using a topical anesthetic and vasoconstrictive agent (i.e., 4% lidocaine and 1% phenylephrine) if possible. Adequate sedation, as well as adjuncts such as intravenous lidocaine, may decrease the incidence of the previously discussed side effects. Attention should be paid to maintaining c-spine immobilization if indicated, as well as to the application of cricoid pressure.

Special endotracheal tubes have been designed in which the tip of the tube can be manipulated by a proximal trigger, thus enhancing the success of blind placement in the trachea (Endotrol, Mallinckrodt Medical Inc.). In addition, a technique has been described in which the endotracheal tube cuff is inflated in the oropharynx using 15 cc of air.[31] In patients with normal pharyngeal anatomy, this technique centers the tip of the tube and directs it anteriorly toward the larynx. When resistance is felt on advancement, this signifies contact with the vocal cords (breath sounds should still be heard). The cuff is then deflated and the tube is advanced into the trachea.

This technique has actually been demonstrated to have a high degree of success in nonbreathing, paralyzed patients. It has also been demonstrated to be as successful as the use of fiberoptic assistance in patients who require c-spine immobilization.[31] Still, in patients in whom secretions are minimum, fiberoptic assistance may be valuable but requires as higher degree of skill maintenance. In patients with shallow breathing, the use of capnography may be helpful in determining the exact onset of inspiration and expiration.

Surgical Airway Management

Surgical airway management, in the form of cricothyrotomy, was previously recommended as the procedure of choice in patients in whom a c-spine injury was suspected and NTI had failed or was impossible because of massive facial or upper airway injury. Despite the high success rates of RSI/OTI and NTI, cricothyrotomy continues to serve a role. Cricothyrotomy equipment must always be immediately available in any patient undergoing RSI. Even with the development of percutaneous kits, experience remains essential. Cricothyrotomy is often better performed after successful use of an airway adjunct (discussion follows) to allow for more control of the procedure while avoiding any intervening hypoxemia.

SPECIAL MANEUVERS AND INTUBATION ADJUNCTS

Displacement of the thyroid cartilage backward against the cervical vertebrae, upward or as superiorly as possible, and laterally to the right—the BURP maneuver (Fig. 93.1)—has been described and found to significantly improve the view of the glottis during laryngoscopy.[30] It is finding widespread acceptance as an aid in management of the difficult airway. The mechanism by which BURP improves visibility may lie in the ability to move the glottis back into the line of vision, as laryngoscopy itself tends to push the tongue and possibly the larynx toward the left.

The use of BURP in the setting of potential c-spine injury in which in-line immobilization of the neck is necessary has not been studied. It is, therefore, unknown if the laryngeal view in this set-

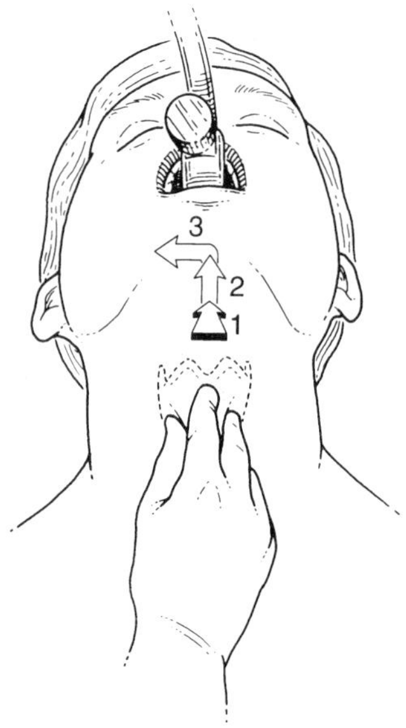

Figure 93.1. Diagram of application of the BURP maneuver in improving the glottic view during laryngoscopy. The thyroid cartilage is moved backward against the cervical vertebrae, upward or as superiorly as possible, and laterally to the right. See text for further explanation.

ting is significantly improved. It is also unknown how displacement of the thyroid cartilage might effect an unstable c-spine injury. However, its use in patients without suspected cervical spine injuries would seem to be advantageous and without contraindications. It should be remembered that BURP does not replace the need for cricoid pressure in any patient undergoing intubation.

Several airway adjuncts either aid in the intubation process or are designed to temporarily replace intubation if it cannot be performed (Table 93.3). As an adjunct is likely to be used after unsuccessful intubation in the most desperate of circumstances, the chosen adjunct would ideally provide adequate ventilation with some degree of airway protection when blindly placed, while resulting in little movement of the c-spine.

The esophageal tracheal Combitube (ETC) and the laryngeal mask airway (LMA) deserve comment. Each of these devices is gaining in popularity and each has its advantages and disadvantages. Both, however, require little training for proper use. Major advantages of the ETC include its double-lumen design (ability to ventilate regardless of esophageal or tracheal placement), ability to be placed blindly, the upper airway protection afforded by its pharyngeal balloon, and the ability to aspirate gastric contents from one of its lumens.[3] Once placed, other approaches to the airway (fiberoptic, surgical, etc.) may be attempted while avoiding hypoxemia. The LMA was originally designed for the outpatient surgery setting, but its use as a rescue airway device has become popular. Although more attention is required for specific placement, recent modifications of the device have resulted in an intubating version that allows passage of specially designed endotracheal tubes.[17]

The major disadvantage is that until an endotracheal tube is placed via the LMA, little airway protection is afforded, and decreases in chest wall compliance or increases in airway pressure may prevent adequate ventilation. Application of cricoid pressure has also been demonstrated to impede placement and ventilation through the LMA. Placement of both devices can be greatly enhanced by lubrication of the devices, use of paralytic agents, and use of a laryngoscope to reduce obstruction from the tongue. Use of these adjuncts earlier rather than later in the course of managing an airway may greatly reduce the incidence of hypoxemia or other complications.

Several new laryngoscopes and laryngoscopic blades have been marketed in an attempt to help improve the glottic view, especially during difficult intubation in which minimal or no movement of the c-spine is desired. These include the Bullard and McCoy laryngoscope and the Belscope blade.[8,9,34] The Bullard laryngoscope is rigid and uses fiberoptic technology to obtain an indirect view of the larynx. The McCoy laryngoscope has a blade with a hinged tip, allowing elevation of the epiglottis from a fulcrum deep within the pharynx. The Belscope blade is specially angulated, with a detachable prism allowing indirect visualization of the larynx. All have advantages and disadvantages; the Bullard and Belscope apparatus take more time to use and master. A large emergency department experience has not been reported with any of these devices.

TABLE 93.3. Intubation Alternatives and Adjuncts

Nasal
Use with audio assist device or capnography, or use with fiberoptic assistance.

Oral
1) Blind with tactile (digital) technique
2) Blind with use of lighted stylet
3) Use with fiberoptic assistance: Fiberoptic apparatus or Bullard laryngoscope
4) Use with other special laryngoscopes or blades: McCoy laryngoscope, Belscope blade
5) Blind with use of retrograde technique through trachea

Surgical
1) Needle cricothyrotomy and percutaneous translaryngeal jet ventilation
2) Cricothyrotomy using various cricotomes and percutaneous devices

Nondefinitive management alternatives
1) Esophageal tracheal Combitube
2) Pharyngotracheal lumen airway
3) Laryngeal mask airway
4) Intubating laryngeal mask airway

PHARMACOLOGIC ADJUNCTS

Pharmacologic agents may be chosen to accomplish several goals, including topical anesthesia, sedation, analgesia, amnesia, and paralysis. Judicious use of these agents may facilitate rapid intubation, while avoiding such complications as increased ICP and regurgitation. Selecting the wrong agent can cause life-threatening complications such as prolonged paralysis with an inability to ventilate or cardiovascular collapse. Unfortunately, there are no agents that are rapid acting, of short duration, and totally void of complications in all situations. Current suggestions are based on a combination of practical and theoretical considerations.

Local Anesthetics

Lidocaine is an amide that can be used topically, locally, or intravenously to aid in airway management. Maximum doses are 3 to 4 mg/kg. When applied topically in a 4% solution, lidocaine may be used with topical vasoconstrictors to aid in NTI. Nebulization of a 4% solution into a spontaneously breathing patient can produce complete topical anesthesia of the oro- and nasopharynx and the vocal cords in 5 to 7 minutes.[4] Although somewhat controversial, when given intravenously in a dose of 1.5 to 2.0 mg/kg 2 to 3 minutes before intubation, lidocaine may attenuate much of the hemodynamic and cough reflex–mediated rise in ICP.[24] As lidocaine is, for the most part, hemodynamically inert, its use in intubation as an aid in modulating the response to laryngoscopy, especially in cases of head injury, seems reasonable.

Induction Agents

Sedatives and hypnotics, as well as potent narcotic analgesics can be used as pharmacologic adjuncts to achieve states ranging from light sedation to loss of consciousness. There is a risk-to-benefit ratio for each of these agents in the trauma setting. Although adverse effects on respiration can be countered in most instances with artificial ventilation, there is no simple maneuver to counteract the cardiac dysfunction that may be produced by these agents in the trauma victim. The choice of agent should be based on the following:

- The agent's reliability of induction
- The need to maintain spontaneous respiration
- The patient's level of consciousness and risk of head injury
- The patient's hemodynamic or suspected hemodynamic status
- The patient's preexisting physiologic state, if known

The barbiturates thiopental and methohexital are very short-acting sedative and hypnotic agents that provide no analgesia. Their onset of action is within 1 minute; their duration of action is between 5 and 10 minutes.[26] The benefits of these agents are their induction reliability and rapidity of onset. The major disadvantage is that they can result in myocardial and respiratory depression.[26] Their use may cause sudden and profound hypotension in the presence of preexisting myocardial dysfunction or hypovolemia, although this is not a major factor in the normal host. Even in "normal" subjects, mild-to-moderate decreases in blood pressure and increases in heart rate may result. Thiopental doses, ranging from 3 to 5 mg/kg in the setting of normal hemodynamics, and 0.5 to 1.0 mg/kg in the unstable patient, have been recommended for induction.[26]

Barbiturates reduce ICP by reducing cerebral blood flow in a dose-dependent fashion. Concomitant matched reductions in the cerebral metabolic rate must also occur to prevent cerebral ischemia. Whether matched reductions occur after a single bolus or lower titrated doses in the injured area of brain is unclear. Although barbiturates may be safely used in victims of isolated head trauma in whom preexisting disease states are known, their widespread use in the multiply injured patient in whom volume status and history are unknown may be risky because of potential side effects.

Propofol is a substituted isopropylphenol; it is highly lipophilic and capable of producing profound sedation, hypnosis, and amnesia but is without innate analgesic properties.[28] Propofol's major unique characteristic is its rapid metabolic clearance and redistribution, which is approximately ten times faster than that of thiopental. Clinical recovery is extremely rapid (4 to 8 minutes), with little residual sedation apparent, even after prolonged administration. A large experience with the use of propofol as an induction agent in the initial resuscitation of the critically ill or injured patient is lacking. Its major drawbacks (due to its potency) are those of respiratory and cardiovascular depression even in healthy normovolemic individuals.[28] Extreme caution must, therefore, be exercised if propofol is used in the undifferentiated trauma patient. Favorable cerebral hemodynamics can be produced, similar to those seen with the barbiturates if decreases in mean arterial pressure can be minimized. Again, it is unclear if this extends to injured brain areas after single-dose use. Because trauma patients remain intubated for prolonged periods for resuscitation and diagnostic purposes, the advantages of propofol's rapid redistribution is limited in this setting. If used, slowly administered doses ranging from 1.5 to 2.5 mg/kg are recommended.

Etomidate is a nonbarbiturate, nonnarcotic sedative–hypnotic induction agent that exhibits no analgesic properties.[28] In doses of 0.2 to 0.3 mg/kg, induction is reliably produced in less than 1 minute, and the duration of action is between 4 and 6 minutes. This drug has several properties that make it attractive for use in the multisystem trauma victim. When given in single induction boluses, it evokes minimal changes in heart rate and cardiac output compared with equipotent doses of thiopental.[28] This advantage may be particularly useful in patients with hypotension or compensated shock, as well as in those patients with preexisting myocardial dysfunction.

Etomidate also causes significantly less respiratory depression than do barbiturate agents, although, when given rapidly, transient apnea, may induce.[28] Etomidate may in fact stimulate ventilation independent of action on the medullary respiratory centers. For this reason, it may be advantageous to choose etomidate when maintenance of respiration is desirable, such as during sedation with NTI or modified RSI. Like the barbiturates, etomidate can reduce ICP by causing a dose-dependent reduction in cerebral blood flow and cerebral metabolic rate. Whether consistent improvements in cerebral hemodynamics are obtained after a single induction bolus of etomidate remains to be determined.

Etomidate occasionally causes side effects, but none should contraindicate its use as a single injection in the unstable or potentially unstable patient (with or without head injury). Side effects include transient burning on injection, transient but potentially significant myoclonus after administration, and transient suppression of endogenous cortisol production.[28] Although a concern, this occasional temporary suppression of cortisol production has not been shown to affect outcome. Supplemental cortisol can be given if needed. The relatively inert hemodynamic profile of etomidate in the trauma setting outweighs these potential problems.

Ketamine is a phencyclidine derivative that produces dissociative anesthesia. It is the only agent that possesses sedative, hypnotic, analgesic, and amnestic properties.[28] It provides the most cardiovascular and respiratory support of any agent. Although it is a direct myocardial depressant, heart rate and blood pressure are usually maintained or increased because of centrally mediated sympathetic stimulation. Central sympathetic stimulation also results in transient bronchodilation. Unless it is given rapidly, apnea does not occur.

The major advantage of ketamine lies in the setting of the overtly hypovolemic patient, especially when the heart is directly involved, such as in pericardial tamponade.[28] Its onset of action is within 1 minute when given intravenously (1 to 2 mg/kg), and its duration of action ranges from 5 to 15 minutes. It may also be given intramuscularly (4 mg/kg), with the onset of action delayed by several minutes. This is advantageous when rapid control of the patient without venous access is needed.

The disadvantages of ketamine are few. Its use may result in worsening hypotension if given to patients who are either sympathetically depleted or who have severe coronary artery disease and may not tolerate increased myocardial oxygen demand. However, administration of any induction agent in this setting is hazardous. Use in hypertensive patients with suspected traumatic aortic injuries may also be problematic. Because it is a phencyclidine derivative, ketamine can cause an emergence delirium. While this is a concern during conscious sedation, this should never prohibit its use as an intubation adjunct in a critically ill trauma patient. Intubated trauma patients are usually kept sedated and paralyzed for many hours after their initial presentation, and emergence delirium at this time is rare.[28] Continued sedation with benzodiazepines virtually eliminates the occurrence of emergence delirium.

An additional concern regarding the use of ketamine is its potential to affect ICP, secondary to its ability to increase cerebral blood flow by 30% to 60%.[28] Even though the cerebral metabolic rate is increased with ketamine, cerebral blood flow is probably sufficient to meet demand. Evidence is accumulating that this increase in cerebral blood flow does not increase ICP.[14,15] In fact, there is evidence that ketamine is neuroprotective in the setting of head trauma.[22] Despite this evidence, there is still reluctance to use ketamine in the presence of potential head injury. Its use may still be warranted in the setting of head injury, however, when induction is needed in a hypotensive patient: Any reduction in mean arterial pressure has more potential to worsen cerebral ischemia than will a transient rise in ICP.

Benzodiazepines (diazepam and midazolam) have been used alone, and in combination with narcotics, as induction agents. They provide good anxiolysis and amnesia, but large doses are usually needed to produce states of induction that are equivalent to and similarly predictable as the previously discussed agents.[27] No analgesia is provided.

Midazolam is currently the most commonly used benzodiazepine for airway management. It is two to four times as potent as diazepam. An induction dose of midazolam (0.3 mg/kg) takes effect within 1 to 2 minutes and has a duration of action of between 30 and 60 minutes. Even at doses of 0.3 mg/kg, induction is not always predictable. This dose can be accompanied by side effects such as severe respiratory depression (even more so than equivalent doses of thiopental). Significant decreases in mean arterial pressure and cardiac contractility can also occur, especially in patients with hypovolemia or heart disease.[1] All of these effects are more pronounced when opioids are given simultaneously. Subinduction doses (0.03 to 0.05 mg/kg) of midazolam are not commonly associated with these complications and can serve as valuable adjuncts in providing continued sedation for patients after intubation, but they do not provide sufficient induction conditions.

The newer synthetic opioid agonists (fentanyl family), which include fentanyl, sufentanil, and alfentanil, are 100, 500 to 1000, and 20 times more potent than morphine, respectively.[25] They are fast acting, having an onset of action of less than 1 minute, and their duration of action is between 15 and 60 minutes. Fentanyl has gained widespread popularity in emergency medicine as a fast-acting analgesic used in conscious sedation. For reasons not entirely clear, it has also become used as an induction agent in emergency medicine. Although not an ideal induction agent in the trauma setting, fentanyl can induce states of unconsciousness. However, the doses required to induce it are extremely variable and if high enough may cause unwanted side effects in the critically ill patient. Depending on the existing state of consciousness and the presence of drugs such as alcohol, the dose necessary to produce unconsciousness can range from 2 to 20 μg/kg or more.

The effect of fentanyl on ventilation varies, but doses above 2 μg/kg result in a high incidence of respiratory depression in "normal" subjects.[2] This incidence is even higher when used with other agents. Fentanyl results in little or no histamine release, and its cardiovascular effects in the normal host are minimal. At higher doses, however, small but potentially significant decreases in blood pressure may occur.[25] Fentanyl has been touted as a valuable preinduction adjunct in intubation of the head-injured patient because of its ability to attenuate the hemodynamic response to intubation. Although effective, when given in sufficient doses to achieve this (at least 3 μg/kg, 2 to 3 minutes before laryngoscopy), increases in ICP result that possibly negate any advantage to its use in the setting of traumatic brain injury.[23]

This increase in ICP has also been shown with sufentanil and alfentanil administration. Coupled with their potential for producing premature hypoventilation and apnea, their routine use as induction or preinduction agents in this setting is controversial. The best roles for fentanyl in trauma airway management may be to provide postintubation titrated sedation and analgesia to attenuate hyperdynamic responses from pain and intubation and to make continued intubation and ventilation more tolerable.

The use of morphine in the management of the trauma airway is discouraged because of its effect on histamine release, which may result in hypotension. If used, carefully administered test doses should be given first.

Despite the most careful of evaluations and precautions, occasionally, the use of any induction agent may result in sudden and profound hypotension not responsive to simple fluid boluses. In cases of head injury, even transient hypotension can result in prolonged cerebral hypoperfusion whether or not blood pressure and oxygen delivery are restored to normal levels.[18] For this reason, it may be advisable to have an agent such as phenylephrine available for administration in bolus form (50 to 200 μg) to help immediately restore mean arterial pressure until the offending induction agent is sufficiently redistributed or metabolized. Phenylephrine is a synthetic noncatecholamine that stimulates principally alpha-1 adrenergic receptors by a direct effect. Its onset is very rapid and relatively short-lived when given in bolus form.

Neuromuscular Blocking Agents

The use of neuromuscular blocking agents (NMBAs) to facilitate intubation has become widespread in emergency airway management. They help provide ideal intubating conditions in many circumstances, as well as help to facilitate and control other aspects of patient management. They have no analgesic or sedative properties; their sole use without analgesia and sedation, except in the most hemodynamically tenuous or deeply comatose patients, is never indicated. These agents are classified as depolarizing and nondepolarizing.

The only depolarizing NMBA in use in the United States is succinylcholine. Succinylcholine (1.0 to 2.0 mg/kg) is the agent of choice during emergent RSI. No agent has a faster onset (less than 1 minute) or is of shorter duration (4 to 6 minutes). The disadvantages of succinylcholine are relatively minor and should never prohibit its use in the acutely injured patient. These include fasciculations, hyperkalemia, and transient rises in intragastric, intraocular, and intracranial pressure.[29] These side effects have caused some to disapprove of its use in patients with burns, crush injuries, and eye and head injuries. Succinylcholine-induced hyperkalemia in burns and crush injuries does not occur in the acute setting. If fasciculations and elevated intraocular, intragastric, and intracranial pressure are major concerns, administration of a defasciculating dose of a nondepolarizing agent (i.e., vecuronium 0.01 mg/kg) 2 to 3 minutes before succinylcholine administration may help prevent these occurrences.[29] If a defasciculating dose of a nondepolarizing agent is used, the dose of succinylcholine should be increased to 1.5 to 2.0 mg/kg to maintain its rapidity of onset. Unpredictably, a few patients may develop vagally mediated bradycardia, histamine-induced hypotension, and malignant hyperthermia with succinylcholine administration. Succinylcholine can also be given intramuscularly (4 mg/kg), but its onset is delayed by 2 to 4 minutes.

There are several nondepolarizing NMBAs in current use, with vecuronium and rocuronium the major agents in use in trauma airway management. The advantages of these agents are that they are longer acting, cause no fasciculations, and cause no reported increase in intraocular, intragastric, or intracranial pressure. They also have little effect on the cardiovascular system.[7,29] The major disadvantage of vecuronium is that it may take up to 2 to 3 minutes to take full effect. Time to onset can be reduced with the priming principle, in which an initial smaller subparalyzing dose is given 1 to 2 minutes before the paralyzing dose.[29] This method would appear to have no advantage in managing an emergent trauma airway, wherein time is the issue.

Priming and defasciculating doses of nondepolarizing agents may produce significant respiratory impairment in elderly patients, so meticulous care of the airway is necessary.[13] Large doses of vecuronium (0.25 mg/kg), used as an initial bolus, can achieve paralysis within 90 seconds but may last as long as 90 minutes. The onset of action of rocuronium (0.6 mg/kg) is similar to that of succinylcholine, although its duration of action is similar to that of vecuronium (25 to 40 minutes).[29] Nondepolarizing agents can be reversed to some extent by drugs that block cholinesterases, such as neostigmine, edrophonium, and pyridostigmine. Their routine use is not advised because of potential cardiovascular complications.

Because the peak onset of both succinylcholine and rocuronium approaches 1 minute and the onset of action of induction agents such as etomidate, thiopental, and ketamine essentially occurs in a one-arm-to-brain circulation time (less than 1 minute), it may be advantageous to administer the paralytic agent first, followed by the induction agent (timing principle).[21] Because clinical weakness will occur at approximately 30 seconds with both agents, administration of an induction agent such as etomidate 10 to 20 seconds after administration of either succinylcholine or rocuronium will produce adequate intubating conditions in approximately 1 minute after paralytic administration.

For patients who are not being actively oxygenated with a BVM prior to RSI, this helps to guard against premature apnea/hypoventilation (thus preserving the functional residual capacity of oxygen) while ensuring adequate induction at the time of laryngoscopy. Patients intubated with the timing principle do not demonstrate restlessness prior to loss of consciousness and do not report any dissatisfaction postoperatively.[21]

SPECIAL CONSIDERATIONS

Cervical Spine Injury

In most urgent situations, a detailed neurologic examination cannot be performed before the need to intubate is addressed. Even in the face of normal radiographs, the patient would need to be able to fully cooperate with a physical examination to exclude c-spine injury. The patient with a blunt trauma or penetrating neck injury requiring intubation is unlikely to be able to meet this criterion. The role of c-spine radiography before intubation is, therefore, controversial. Lateral c-spine radiography can miss up to 20% to 30% of c-spine injuries.

It has been estimated that a small but significant percentage (1.2%) of all blunt trauma victims will have an occult c-spine injury, given a 6% total incidence of injury and a 20% miss rate on lateral c-spine radiography.[33] If time permits, a lateral c-spine radiograph that reveals an unstable injury may cause the operator to choose a particular intubation technique. It is imperative to remember, however, that a negative radiograph does not exclude injury. Of interest, recent studies have indicated that certain populations traditionally intubated with c-spine precautions may not require such precautions, including victims of penetrating head trauma.[11]

Cadaveric studies of unstable c-spine injuries demonstrate no superiority of one method over the other when meticulous c-spine immobilization is practiced. However, even maneuvers such as jaw thrust, BVM ventilation, and cricoid pressure have been demonstrated to induce significant movement of unstable c-spine injuries if extreme care is not taken.[5]

OTI utilizing RSI is now the procedure of choice in achieving definitive airway control in patients with suspected c-spine injury.[19] Because the ability to position the airway in this setting is limited, it may be preferable to use a straight laryngoscope blade rather than a curved blade; the straight blade will lift the epiglottis directly.

Perhaps counterintuitive, removal of the front of the cervical collar while maintaining in-line immobilization (not traction) significantly improves the view of the larynx during intubation.[6] When manual immobilization is present, an intact c-collar offers no additional advantage. Regardless of approach, airway management in the setting of potential c-spine injury is optimally performed with at least three people: One is the intubator, one provides in-line immobilization of the c-spine, and one applies cricoid pressure (Fig. 93.2).

In cases of penetrating neck trauma with possible altered upper airway anatomy or signs of airway obstruction, OTI with RSI is still the procedure of choice in most circumstances.[20] Administration of paralytic agents may be strategically deleted if proper sedation and upper airway anesthesia are provided. Use of induction agents with less effect on ventilation (etomidate and ketamine), along with intravenous and/or nebulized lidocaine, will aid in reduction of gagging and further hemorrhage or distortion. Concomitant use of the lighted stylet or fiberoptic assistance may be helpful.

Head Injury

The pathophysiology of traumatic brain injury is complex and involves a combination of mechanical and biochemical events initiated by the trauma itself, followed by the potential of secondary injury in the form of ischemia. Traditional approaches to the head trauma victim who required intubation assumed that the brain had lost some degree of its ability to autoregulate its blood flow. Cerebral blood flow in this setting is determined by the mean arterial pressure minus the ICP. Emphasis has been placed on reducing ICP during intubation with the use of agents such as barbiturates, but little emphasis has been placed on ensuring maintenance of the mean arterial pressure during this critical time. Because ICP is not known at the time of initial resuscitation, a mean systemic arterial pressure between 80 mm Hg and 100 mm Hg should be maintained. Although an attempt to reduce ICP during intubation is of theoretical benefit, it has

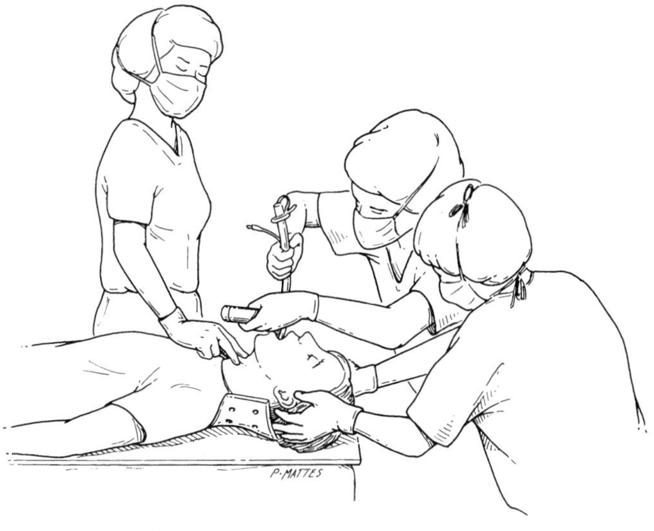

Figure 93.2. Demonstration of RSI OTI in victim of multisystem trauma. Note that three persons are participating. One is intubating, one is maintaining c-spine immobilization, and one is applying cricoid pressure. Also note that the front of the c-collar is removed to aid in viewing the larynx.

never been demonstrated to affect outcome. Because reductions in ICP are caused by reductions in cerebral blood flow, and must be matched by similar reductions in cerebral metabolic rate to avoid ischemia, it would appear that achieving this goal with the use of a single dose of an induction agent would be of very transient, if any, benefit.

More important, any advantage gained in reducing ICP would be lost if the mean arterial pressure were not maintained. Restoration of mean arterial pressure after transient hypotension does not ensure restoration of prehypotensive cerebral blood flow.[18] Titration of various cardioactive medications (barbiturates, beta blockers, and nitrates) for induction of head-injured patients to reduce ICP and blunt the cardiovascular effects of laryngoscopy has been suggested, but this strategy is unlikely to result in the desired effect of decreasing ICP and may still lower blood pressure, thus jeopardizing cerebral oxygen delivery.

In reality, probably no airway drug affects ICP more than the struggles of the patient or the procedures (many of them painful) performed during the initial examination and resuscitation. Because most head injuries occur in association with multisystem trauma, a more reasonable approach would be to administer agents that cause a predictable loss of consciousness, cause no increase in ICP, and maximize the chance to maintain mean arterial pressure. Use of paralytic agents and adjuncts such as lidocaine prevents the largest and most harmful increases in ICP caused by gagging and coughing during laryngoscopy. Cerebral hemodynamics are probably best managed immediately after intubation with limited hyperventilation and continued paralysis, along with concomitant sedation and analgesia guided by heart rate and blood pressure. An earnest attempt should be made to document the patient's Glasgow Coma Score and mental status prior to intubation.

PRESENTATIONS AND SUGGESTED APPROACHES

Despite the deluge of suggested techniques and approaches, the final decision on airway management depends primarily on the urgency of the situation and how comfortable the physician feels with a particular approach. In the end, the most immediate causes of mortality and morbidity are hypoxemia and hypotension that are not quickly reversed. In the most urgent of situations, use of rapid-acting paralytic agents followed by laryngoscopy with c-spine control, if needed, may be the best approach. Follow with sedation and analgesics as tolerated.

Assuming that the emergency physician is the sole physician provider of initial trauma care, examination and resuscitation roles cannot be split. It is difficult to spend long periods of time securing an airway by titrating therapy when other resuscitative maneuvers are also rapidly needed. Although each patient is unique, several assumptions should be made to prevent iatrogenic harm when faced with a patient who needs aggressive airway control. In trauma victims at risk for internal thoracic and abdominal injuries, one should assume that the patient is occultly hypovolemic, even if no signs of shock are present. In victims of blunt trauma or penetrating head injuries who require intubation, one should assume that intracranial injury exists until proven otherwise. In victims of blunt multisystem trauma or victims with penetrating neck trauma, one should assume that a c-spine injury exists.

Trauma patients can be grouped into three categories based on the possibility of their having head and neck injuries and hypovolemia. This grouping is helpful in choosing the approach to airway management (Table 93.4). Bearing these groups in mind, the following goals should be achieved during both the preparation period and during intubation:

TABLE 93.4. Major Presentations of Trauma Patients

1) Blunt trauma with suspected head, maxillofacial, neck, and multisystem injury involvement at risk for hypovolemic shock
2) Isolated blunt or penetrating head or neck trauma requiring c-spine control but not at risk for hypovolemia
3) Penetrating injury below the head and neck not at risk for c-spine and head injury but at risk for hypovolemia.

1. The patient does not experience further decreases in mean arterial pressure secondary to administration of medications or maneuvers.
2. The patient does not develop premature apnea or hypoventilation.
3. The patient does not develop large increases in ICP.

If these assumptions and goals are addressed, and airway and pharmacologic interventions are chosen accordingly, rapid and safe acquisition of an airway should be possible, and the physician will rarely be caught off guard by hemodynamic changes or neurologic deficits. Tables 93.5 and 93.6 demonstrate intubation sequences that should meet the needs of the majority of severely injured patients and result in few complications.

After intubation, most patients benefit from continued sedation and analgesia. Small and frequent aliquots of midazolam (1 to 3 mg) and fentanyl (50 to 100 μg), guided by cardiac moni-

TABLE 93.5. Example of RSI Protocol for Multiply Injured Patient with Suspected Hypovolemia and Head and Neck Injuries

1) Prepare and preoxygenate passively or actively with BVM. Use Sellick maneuver if using BVM. Manually immobilize c-spine but remove front of c-collar.
2) Lidocaine 1.5–2.0 mg/kg IV (2–3 minutes prior to laryngoscopy)
3) Sellick maneuver, and a defasciculating dose of nondepolarizing agent if using succinylcholine in step four. Give at least two minutes prior to succinylcholine administration. May be given simultaneously with lidocaine.
4) Succinylcholine 1.5–2.0 mg/kg IV
5) Etomidate 0.2–0.3 mg/kg IV (reduce to 0.1–0.2 mg/kg if hypotensive) 10–20 seconds after paralytic administration.
6) Intubate trachea, inflate cuff, confirm placement with auscultation and end-tidal CO_2. After placement is confirmed, release cricoid pressure.
7) Continue paralysis with nondepolarizing agent if desired. Provide appropriate sedation and analgesic as allowed.

If using rocuronium step 3 may be deleted (with exception of Sellick maneuver). Rocuronium administered in place of succinylcholine in step 4 at dose of 0.6 mg/kg followed by induction agent (step 5) 10–20 seconds later.

TABLE 93.6. Example of RSI Protocol for Patient at Risk for Shock but Not Head or Neck Injuries

1) Prepare and preoxygenate passively or actively if required. Apply Sellick maneuver if using BVM. Optimally position airway.
2) Ensure Sellick maneuver and give succinylcholine (1–2 mg/kg) or rocuronium (0.6 mg/kg) IV.
3) 10–20 seconds later administer etomidate 0.2–0.3 mg/kg (0.1 to 0.2 mg/kg if hypotensive) or ketamine 1–2 mg/kg (0.5–1.0 mg/kg if hypotensive).
4) Intubate trachea, inflate cuff, confirm placement with auscultation and end-tidal CO_2. Release Sellick maneuver after placement confirmed.
5) Continue paralysis if desired along with appropriate sedation and analgesia.

toring, blood pressure monitoring, and movement (if the patient is not paralyzed), are appropriate and devoid of major side effects.[12] After loading, carefully titrated, continuous infusions of the same may also be considered. Longer acting agents such as lorazepam and morphine may also be carefully used.

Continued or newly initiated paralysis simultaneous with provision of analgesia and sedation may be required to optimize resuscitation and diagnostics. It does little good to perform a meticulous neuroinduction for a brain-injured patient only to have the patient fight and buck the ventilator during the ensuing resuscitation. Early removal of patients from backboards, proper splinting of fractures, and application of local anesthetics to wounds will significantly decrease patient discomfort.

COMMON PITFALLS

- Failure to consider occult hypovolemia and shock and preexisting disease states when choosing induction agents
- Failure to provide cricoid pressure (Sellick maneuver) during intubation until proper endotracheal tube placement is confirmed
- Failure to maintain meticulous control of the c-spine during intubation in patients with suspected c-spine injuries
- Failure to have airway rescue adjuncts available for cannot intubate–cannot ventilate situations.
- Failure to provide adequate ongoing postintubation sedation and analgesia

References

1. Adams P, Gelman S, Reves JG, et al. Midazolam: pharmacodynamics and pharmacokinetics during acute hypovolemia. *Anesthesiology* 1985;63:140.
2. Bailey PL, Pace NL, Ashburn MA, et al. Frequent hypoxemia and apnea after sedation with midazolam and fentanyl. *Anesthesiology* 1990;73:826.
3. Blostein PA, Koestner AJ, Hoak S. Failed rapid sequence intubation in trauma patients: esophageal tracheal Combitube is a useful adjunct. *J Trauma* 1998;44:534.
4. Bourke DL, Katz J, Tonneson A. Nebulized anesthesia for awake endotracheal intubation. *Anesthesiology* 1985;63:690.
5. Donaldson WF, Heil B, Donaldson VP, et al. The effect of airway maneuvers on the unstable C1-C2 segment. *Spine* 1997;22:1215.
6. Heath KJ. The effect of laryngoscopy of different cervical spine immobilisation techniques. *Anaesthesia* 1994;49:843.
7. Hunter J. Drug therapy: new neuromuscular blocking drugs. *N Engl J Med* 1995;332:1691.
8. Gabbot DA. Laryngoscopy using the McCoy laryngoscope after application of a cervical collar. *Anaesthesia* 1996;51:812.
9. Gajraj NM, Chason P, Shearer VE. Cervical spine movement during orotracheal intubation: comparison of the Belscope and Macintosh blades. *Anaesthesia* 1994;49:772.
10. Gold MI, Duarte I, Muravchick S. Arterial oxygen in conscious patient after 5 minutes and after 30 seconds of oxygen breathing. *Anesth Analg* 1981;60:313.
11. Kaups K, Davis J. Patients with gunshot wounds to the head do not require cervical spine immobilization and evaluation. *J Trauma* 1998;44:865.
12. Khalil B, Scalea TM, Trooskin SZ, et al. Hemodynamic responses to shock in young trauma patients: need for invasive monitoring. *Crit Care Med* 1994;22:633.
13. Mahajan RP, Hennessy N, Aitken AR. Effect of priming dose of vecuronium on lung function in elderly patients. *Anesth Analg* 1993;77:1198.
14. Nimkoff L, Quinn C, Silver P, et al. The effects of intravenous anesthetics on intracranial pressure and cerebral perfusion pressure in two feline models of brain edema. *J Crit Care* 1997;12:132.
15. Rodriguez A, Sanchez L. Intravenous ketamine does not increase intracranial pressure in neurosurgical patients with normal or increased ICP. *Crit Care Med* 1994;24:A57(abst).
16. Rosen CL, Wolfe RE, Chew SE, et al. Blind nasotracheal intubation in the presence of facial trauma. *J Emerg Med* 1997;15:141.
17. Rosenblatt WH, Murphy M. The intubating laryngeal mask: use of a new ventilating-intubating device in the emergency department. *Ann Emerg Med* 1999;33:234.
18. Schmoker JD, Zhuang J, Shackford SR. Hemorrhagic hypotension after brain injury causes an early and sustained reduction in cerebral oxygen delivery despite normalization of systemic oxygen delivery. *J Trauma* 1992;32:714.
19. Shatney CH, Brunner RD, Nguyen TQ. The safety of orotracheal intubation in patients with unstable cervical spine fracture or high spinal cord injury. *Am J Surg* 1995;170:676.
20. Shearer VE, Giesecke AH. Airway management for patients with penetrating neck trauma. a retrospective study. *Anesth Analg* 1993;77:1135.
21. Sieber TJ, Zbinden AM, Curatolo M, et al. Tracheal intubation with rocuronium using the "Timing Principle." *Anesth Analg* 1998;86:1137.
22. Smith DH, Okiyama K, Gennarelli TA, et al. Magnesium and ketamine attenuate cognitive dysfunction following experimental brain injury. *Neurosci Lett* 1993;157:211.
23. Sperry RJ, Bailey PL, Reichman MV, et al. Fentanyl and sufentanil increase intracranial pressure in head trauma patients. *Anesthesiology* 1992;77:416.
24. Splinter WM, Cervenko F. Haemodynamic responses to laryngoscopy and tracheal intubation in geriatric patients: effects of fentanyl, lidocaine, and thiopentone. *Can J Anaesth* 1989;36:370.
25. Stoelting RK. Opioid agonist and antagonist. In: Stoelting RK, ed. *Pharmacology and physiology in anesthetic practice,* 2nd ed. Philadelphia: JB Lippincott Co, 1991:70.
26. Stoelting RK. Barbiturates. In: Stoelting RK, ed. *Pharmacology and physiology in anesthetic practice,* 2nd ed. Philadelphia: JB Lippincott Co, 1991:102.
27. Stoelting RK. Benzodiazepines. In: Stoelting RK, ed. *Pharmacology and physiology in anesthetic practice,* 2nd ed. Philadelphia: JB Lippincott Co, 1991:118.
28. Stoelting RK. Nonbarbiturate induction agents. In: Stoelting RK, ed. *Pharmacology and physiology in anesthetic practice,* 2nd ed. Philadelphia: JB Lippincott Co, 1991:134.
29. Stoelting RK. Neuromuscular blocking drugs. In: Stoelting RK, ed. *Pharmacology and physiology in anesthetic practice,* 2nd ed. Philadelphia: JB Lippincott Co, 1991:172.
30. Takahata O, Kubota M, Mamiya K, et al. The efficacy of the "BURP" maneuver during difficult laryngoscopy. *Anesth Analg* 1997;84:419.
31. Van Elstraete AC, Mamie JC, Mehdaoui H. Nasotracheal intubation in patients with immobilized cervical spine: a comparison of tracheal tube cuff inflation and fiberoptic bronchoscopy. *Anesth Analg* 1998;87:400.
32. Vanstrum GS. Airway. In: Vanstrum GS, ed. *Anesthesia in emergency medicine.* Boston: Little, Brown and Company, 1989:12.
33. Walls RM. Airway management in the blunt trauma patient: how important is the cervical spine? *Can J Surg* 1992;35:27.
34. Watts A, Gelb A, Bach D, et al. Comparison of the Bullard and Macintosh laryngoscopes for endotracheal intubation of patient with potential cervical spine injury. *Anesthesiology* 1997;87:1335.

CHAPTER 94
Traumatic Shock

James Manning and Samir M. Fakhry

Shock generally refers to inadequate tissue perfusion manifested clinically by hemodynamic disturbances and organ dysfunction. At the cellular level, shock indicates the insufficient delivery of required metabolic substrates, principally oxygen, to sustain cellular homeostasis. In the setting of trauma, shock is most often related to loss of circulating blood volume due to hemorrhage, although inadequate oxygenation, mechanical vascular obstruction, neurologic dysfunction, and cardiac dysfunction may be either primary or contributing factors.[3,6]

Traumatic shock may result from either blunt trauma (e.g., motor vehicle collisions, falls, assault) or penetrating trauma (e.g., gunshot wounds, stab wounds, impalements). Traumatic shock usually results from one or more of the following conditions: hemorrhage from solid-organ injury, major vascular injury, pelvic fracture, or multiple long-bone fractures; tension pneumothorax; hemothorax; pericardial tamponade; pulmonary contusion or hemorrhage; myocardial contusion and dysfunction; and neurologic injury that adversely affects ventilation or hemodynamics.

PATHOPHYSIOLOGY

The pathophysiology of traumatic shock relates largely to an imbalance in oxygen supply and demand. In the early phase of acute trauma, this imbalance is usually due to hypoperfusion, although low arterial blood oxygen saturation may be a significant contributing or even a predominant factor. Aggressive resuscitation with fluids having low oxygen-carrying capacity in the setting of severe and ongoing hemorrhage may lead to a critically low hemoglobin concentration that further contributes to tissue oxygen debt.

Acute blood loss elicits compensatory hemodynamic changes that serve to maintain vital organ perfusion. They include increased heart rate and vasoconstriction primarily in splanchnic vascular beds and the peripheral circulation. Compensated shock generally indicates varying degrees of tachycardia and peripheral vasoconstriction that maintain adequate vital organ perfusion. Arterial blood pressure in compensated shock states may be moderately low to within normal range. Uncompensated shock generally indicates significant hypotension with inadequate vital organ perfusion. It is important to recognize that "compensated shock" and "uncompensated shock" are imprecise designations along a continuum of progressive physiologic derangement.

Vasoconstriction in response to hemorrhage and hypovolemia is a protective response that preserves perfusion to the vital organs at the expense of peripheral and abdominal organ perfusion. In the hypoperfused tissues, however, oxygen demand exceeds oxygen delivery, and the numerous cellular processes that depend on oxidative metabolism and adenosine triphosphate (ATP) begin to fail. If the pathologic processes are not stabilized or corrected, cellular metabolism is depressed, resulting in loss of transmembrane ion gradients, membrane integrity, and enzyme activity. These processes lead to total cellular dysfunction and organ failure.

There are four general pathophysiologic types of shock: (1) hemorrhagic or hypovolemic, (2) cardiogenic, (3) neurogenic or vasogenic, and (4) septic.[3] *Hemorrhagic* or *hypovolemic shock* involves the loss of circulating intravascular volume caused by blood loss internally, externally, or both. *Cardiogenic shock* indicates a process that prevents the normal pumping of the heart and can be caused by pericardial tamponade that prevents normal ventricular filling, tension pneumothorax with vena caval compression and reduction in venous return to the heart, or direct cardiac damage with loss of contractile force (myocardial contusion).

Neurogenic or *vasogenic shock* may be caused by severe brain injury with loss of autonomic regulatory function or spinal cord injury with loss of peripheral vascular resistance. Major spinal cord injury results in acute vasodilatation but generally does not cause impaired tissue perfusion unless other injuries are present. *Septic shock* refers to the hyperdynamic responses (elevated cardiac output, tachycardia, and low systemic vascular resistance), followed by decreased cardiac output, increased systemic vascular resistance, and organ function deterioration associated with the metabolic demands and toxic mediators accompanying infection.

Although septic shock is seldom an emergency department concern in the trauma patient, traumatic shock may be caused by more than one of these pathophysiologic mechanisms. A complex, confusing clinical picture results in which important pathologic processes may be difficult to detect. If the acute stress of the traumatic shock state is sufficiently severe or prolonged, organ dysfunction may subsequently develop, including acute tubular necrosis (ATN), adult respiratory distress syndrome (ARDS), systemic inflammatory distress syndrome (SIRS), and multiple organ failure (MOF). These entities can develop within a few hours to several days after the acute injury.

CLINICAL PRESENTATION

The most common initial findings in a patient with traumatic shock are tachycardia, hypotension, signs of poor peripheral perfusion, and alteration in mental status. Loss of circulating blood volume eventually results in a decrease in blood pressure. In response to this blood pressure drop, heart rate increases to sustain normal cardiac output. Peripheral vasoconstriction and central venoconstriction shunt blood centrally and result in a narrowed pulse pressure. Decreases in peripheral perfusion are manifested by cool, pale, diaphoretic extremities, with prolongation of capillary refill.

The skin commonly becomes mottled in appearance, but cyanosis is relatively rare. The narrowed pulse pressure makes the pulse quality weak or thready. Alterations in mental status caused by hypoperfusion may be subtle initially and can be difficult to distinguish from associated head injury or intoxication. Therefore, altered mental status on presentation or a subsequent decline in mental status, especially in patients with no evidence of head trauma, should raise concern of systemic hypoperfusion and impending circulatory collapse.

Not all patients present with tachycardia, hypotension, and poor peripheral perfusion. Young, healthy patients with substantial blood loss may maintain a blood pressure within the normal range by compensatory vasoconstriction and increases in heart rate. Heart rate can even occasionally be in the upper normal range. In such patients, signs of peripheral hypoperfusion and subtle changes in mental status may be the only warning signs preceding rapid hemodynamic decompensation. Elderly patients may not develop a tachycardic response to blood loss because of heart disease or medications. A bradycardic response to abdominal trauma that may be vagally mediated has been described.[18] Conversely, hypotension and tachycardia may be exacerbated in a pregnant trauma patient for a given degree of blood loss due to compression of the inferior vena cava by the gravid uterus, resulting in decreased venous return.[12]

Decline in urine output due to renal hypoperfusion and renal fluid reabsorption is an important manifestation of shock physiology. Monitoring urine output may be useful in the emergency department and, later, it is a critical parameter for the trauma surgeon and intensivist. Therefore, a urinary catheter should be placed in patients who exhibit evidence of shock, and the bladder should be drained to begin urine output monitoring as well as to search for hematuria.

DIFFERENTIAL DIAGNOSIS

As stated, the most common cause of traumatic shock is hemorrhage-induced hypovolemia. However, several pathologic entities must be considered as either potential contributors or primary causes of shock (Table 94.1). These include cardiac tamponade, tension pneumothorax, pulmonary contusion or hemorrhage affecting oxygenation, myocardial contusion with dysfunction, myocardial infarction associated with trauma, autonomic dysfunction or spinal cord shock, and effects of toxicologic or pharmacologic agents. Other less common entities include pneumothorax, hemothorax, flail chest, air or fat embolism, and diaphragmatic rupture extensive enough to significantly affect oxygen saturation.

Pericardial tamponade is classically described as exhibiting Beck's Triad of hypotension, distended neck veins, and muffled heart sounds. A pulsus paradoxus of greater than 10 mm Hg may also be seen. All of these markers may not be present. In a hypovolemic patient, the neck veins may be flat. Muffled heart sounds may be difficult to distinguish in the busy trauma resuscitation arena, and detection of a pulsus paradoxus is not reliable. Thus, pericardial tamponade must be considered whenever a penetrating object might have reached the heart or there are rib fractures near the heart. The immediate availability of ultrasonography or echocardiography offers the best potential for rapid and accurate diagnosis.

TABLE 94.1. Differential Diagnosis and Treatment

Pathologic Process	Diagnosis	Signs and Diagnostic Studies	Therapeutic Options
HEMORRHAGE			
			Volume replacement to maintain vital organ perfusion, using crystalloid solutions and blood as needed Supplemental oxygen
Thoracic	Hemopneumothorax	Decreased breath sounds Chest x-ray	Chest tube Possible thoracotomy (<20%)
	Aortic transection	Widened mediastinum on chest x-ray Aortography Chest CT scan Transesophageal echocardiography	Thoracotomy (OR only)
Abdominal	Hemoperitoneum (many potential etiologies)	Abdominal distention Abdominal CT scan Diagnostic peritoneal lavage Abdominal ultrasonography	Exploratory laparotomy
Pelvic	Retroperitoneal and pelvic hemorrhage	Pelvic instability Pelvic x-ray CT scan	MAST External fixation Embolization of pelvic arterial vessels
Retroperitoneum	Renal vascular or parenchymal injury	"One-shot" IVP CT scan	Observation vs. surgery
Extremity	Long-bone fractures	Deformity, hematoma X-rays	Alignment/traction Circumferential pressure (without causing distal vascular compromise) Early open reduction and internal fixation
	Vascular injury	Hematoma Pulse or neurologic deficit Duplex scan Arteriography	Surgical repair
	Lacerations Avulsions, amputations	Physical examination	External pressure Surgical repair
BLOOD FLOW OBSTRUCTION			
Central vascular	Tension pneumothorax	Decreased breath sounds Distended neck veins Tracheal deviation	Needle decompression Chest tube
	Pulmonary embolism	Hypoxemia Tachypnea Ventilation–perfusion scan Pulmonary angiography	Consider anticoagulation Consider placing filter in the inferior vena cava
Cardiac	Pericardial tamponade	Diminished heart tones Distended neck veins Increased pulsus paradoxus Echocardiography	Pericardiocentesis Emergency thoracotomy
	Massive air embolism	Continuous cardiac murmur (turbulent in character) Echocardiography	Right heart catheterization and aspiration of air Left lateral positioning with head elevated
OXYGENATION–VENTILATION FAILURE			
			Supplemental oxygen Ventilatory support as needed
	Pulmonary contusion	Hypoxemia Chest x-ray	
	Tracheobronchial foreign body	Stridor, retractions Unequal breath sounds Hypoxemia Chest x-ray Bronchoscopy	Removal by rigid or flexible bronchoscopy

(continued)

TABLE 94.1. *Continued*

Pathologic Process	Diagnosis	Signs and Diagnostic Studies	Therapeutic Options
OXYGENATION–VENTILATION FAILURE (*cont.*)			
	Laryngotracheal trauma (fracture, collapse, or separation)	Stridor, altered voice Crepitus, SQ emphysema Loss of normal airway anatomy Airway obstruction Hypoxemia Fiberoptic laryngoscopy	Cautious endotracheal intubation (consider fiberoptic-guided) Surgical airway Cricothyrotomy (less severe injury or for isolated larynx injury) Tracheostomy (severe injury or for laryngotracheal separation)
	Bronchopleural fistula associated with bronchial injury	Mediastinal emphysema Large air leak with chest tube Bronchoscopy	Consider placing double-lumen endotracheal tube Consider additional chest tubes Surgical repair
CARDIAC PUMP FAILURE			
	Myocardial contusion	ECG abnormalities (usually right ventricular ischemic changes) Dysrhythmias Elevated cardiac enzymes Echocardiography	Inotropic agents if needed Telemetry or intensive care unit observation
	Myocardial infarction (may be primary or secondary to trauma)	ECG abnormalities Dysrhythmias Elevated cardiac enzymes Echocardiography Cardiac catheterization	Consider thrombolytics Nitroglycerin Intensive care unit Cardiology consultation
CENTRAL NERVOUS SYSTEM TRAUMA			
Intracranial	All major central nervous system injuries		Neurosurgery consultation Supplemental oxygen (aim for 100% O_2 saturation) Avoid hypercarbia (aim for arterial PCO_2 of 35–40 mm Hg) Intravenous fluids as needed to maintain normal perfusion Mild head elevation if possible
	If lateralizing, neurologic deficits or signs of impending herniation		Mild hyperventilation (aim for arterial PCO_2 of 30–35 mm Hg) Mannitol Consider ICP monitoring and vasopressors to maintain mean arterial pressure (optimize cerebral perfusion pressure)
	Epidural hematoma Subdural hematoma	Abnormal mental status Lateralizing neurologic examination	Surgical decompression
	Subarachnoid hemorrhage Intraparenchymal hemorrhage	Abnormal mental status Focal neurologic deficits	
	Diffuse axonal injury with parenchymal edema	Abnormal mental status Neurologic examination generally nonfocal	
Spinal	Spinal cord transection	Neurologic deficits with a dermatomal level Spine x-rays Spine CT or MRI scan	Spinal immobilization Traction (by neurosurgeon) High-dose steroids Neurosurgical consultation
	Partial	Unilateral or partial bilateral neurologic deficits Sacral sparing likely	
	Complete	Bilateral neurologic deficits without sacral sparing (absent rectal tone and bulbocavernosus reflex)	
	Vascular spinal cord syndrome Anterior cord syndrome Central cord syndrome	Neurologic deficits consistent with a vascular distribution	Spinal immobilization (until spine instability ruled out) High-dose steroids Neurosurgical consultation

CT, computed tomography; OR, operating room; MAST, military antishock trousers; IVP, intravenous pyelography; SQ, subcutaneous; ECG, electrocardiograph; ICP, intracranial pressure; MRI, magnetic resonance imaging.

A large pneumothorax or hemothorax can usually be detected by diminished breath sounds. Confirmation with a chest radiograph is usually prudent if the patient is not hypotensive. A tension pneumothorax may also result in deviation of the trachea away from the affected side, cardiac displacement, and hypotension related to inferior vena caval compression that limits venous return to the heart. However, tracheal deviation and cardiac displacement may be difficult to detect by physical examination, and hypotension associated with a pneumothorax may be caused by hemorrhage elsewhere. A chest radiograph usually demonstrates a tension pneumothorax well. Ultrasonography may also be beneficial. However, if a patient is hypotensive and has clinical evidence of a pneumothorax, placement of a chest tube or needle thoracostomy before diagnostic imaging is appropriate.

Myocardial contusion resulting in significant contractile dysfunction is a difficult diagnosis to ascertain during the emergency department phase of trauma evaluation, unless echocardiography is immediately available. Myocardial contusion should be suspected when blunt trauma involves the sternum and anterior left chest. Evidence of cardiogenic shock (hypotension, tachycardia, elevated central venous pressure) should be sought, although it may be difficult to distinguish when there is multisystem trauma. Myocardial contusion should be suspected in the presence of ventricular ectopy, dysrhythmias, or electrocardiographic demonstration of ST segment elevations (especially in the anterior precordial leads).

Head trauma with severe brain injury may result in autonomic dysfunction that manifests hypotension in the absence of significant hemorrhage, although this event usually does not occur acutely. Spinal cord trauma with neurogenic shock may present with hypotension due to loss of peripheral vascular resistance. In this setting, presence of neurologic deficits and lack of signs of peripheral vasoconstriction should arouse suspicion for this entity. Such patients generally have warm extremities and good urine output. Volume status must be carefully monitored, because excess fluid administration in patients with spinal shock may be detrimental.

Signs of shock in a trauma patient may not be a direct consequence of the injury. For example, a myocardial infarction in a patient may cause a motor vehicle collision, or the physiologic stress associated with trauma may cause a myocardial ischemic event in a patient with coronary artery disease. A history, examination, or electrocardiographic findings consistent with myocardial infarction arouse suspicion of combined medical and surgical processes. Pharmacologic agents such as beta-adrenergic blockers and recreational agents such as ethanol and cocaine may significantly affect the clinical picture in the setting of acute trauma.

EMERGENCY DEPARTMENT EVALUATION

Effective management of the acute trauma victim exhibiting shock requires that initial assessment and treatment begin simultaneously.[1] Assessment of airway patency, adequacy of ventilation (respiratory excursion and lung auscultation), hemodynamic status (pulse rate, central and peripheral pulse quality, blood pressure), and evidence of controllable hemorrhage should be immediately linked with interventions to (1) secure the airway while protecting the cervical spine, (2) enhance oxygenation, (3) provide ventilatory assistance, (4) limit further hemorrhage, (5) gain intravenous access, (6) initiate volume replacement, and (7) obtain blood for laboratory and blood bank testing (Fig. 94.1).

After the primary assessment and initiation of treatment, a thorough secondary assessment should be initiated to identify potential injuries to the head, neck, chest, abdomen, pelvis, back, extremities, and neurologic system. The patient's temperature should be determined and the patient should be kept normothermic. Hypothermia can markedly depress hemodynamics and should be aggressively treated. The potential for the presence of any of the entities listed under "Differential Diagnosis" should be considered, and clinical signs of these conditions should be sought. Acute trauma is a highly dynamic disease process that requires frequent and careful reassessment of ventilation and hemodynamic status, and physical examination, to optimally adjust therapeutic interventions and identify evolving pathologic processes.

Initial laboratory studies in patients with major trauma should include (1) CBC: white blood cell count, hemoglobin, hematocrit, platelets; (2) arterial blood gases: pH, PO_2, PCO_2, HCO_3, base balance, oxygen saturation; (3) electrolytes: Na, K, Cl, HCO_3, blood urea nitrogen (BUN), creatinine, glucose; (4) coagulation studies: prothrombin time (PT), partial thromboplastin time (PTT); (5) type and crossmatch for 4 to 8 U of blood; and (6) toxicologic studies (Table 94.2). Urine should be obtained and checked for blood. Lactate and ketone levels may be useful when there is metabolic acidosis. Initial radiographs should include the lateral view cervical spine, chest, and pelvis. Completion of the cervical spine series and other radiographs should be done after hemodynamics have stabilized and after determination that immediate surgery is not required.

Monitoring of heart rate, respiratory rate, blood pressure, temperature, and pulse oximetry are important. Placement of arterial pressure catheters and central venous pressure lines may be considered in patients who do not rapidly stabilize or are suspected of having cardiogenic or neurogenic shock components. Placement of a nasogastric or orogastric tube for decompression reduces the chances of aspiration and may improve ventilation if the stomach is distended with air. A urinary drainage catheter should be placed after a search for potential urethral injury has been performed.

Urethral injury should be suspected in patients with pelvic fractures in the area of the symphysis, anterior lacerations on rectal or vaginal examination, or abnormal position of the prostate gland. As noted, urine output becomes an important indicator of the adequacy of organ perfusion. Quantitative end-tidal carbon dioxide ($ETCO_2$) monitoring, if available, is useful in intubated patients. $ETCO_2$ can help avoid hypoventilation, prevent excessive therapeutic hyperventilation, and detect decreases in cardiac output. Pulmonary artery catheterization is useful in complex critical cases, but this is seldom performed in the emergency department phase of trauma care. Sequential assessment of hemoglobin/hematocrit and arterial blood gases during therapy for traumatic shock may be useful. These should be interpreted together in terms of oxygen-carrying capacity and blood oxygen content. For example, an O_2 saturation of 90% with a hematocrit of 35% may be more favorable than an O_2 saturation of 100% with a hematocrit of 20% in terms of actual tissue oxygen delivery. Serial lactate levels or base deficit assessments have been advocated.[13,14] In the trauma patient, the presence of metabolic acidosis in the early phase of resuscitation indicates poor tissue perfusion and should be considered an indicator of inadequate volume resuscitation or ongoing hemorrhage.

Constant reassessment of ventilation and oxygenation, hemodynamic response to volume replacement therapy, and physical examination findings is crucial to detect clinical deterioration, adjust therapy, and identify previously missed injuries. Trauma resuscitations involve multiple individuals performing numerous tasks. During the process of this activity, tubes and catheters can become dislodged or disconnected, pneumothoraces can develop or enlarge, external or internal injuries may

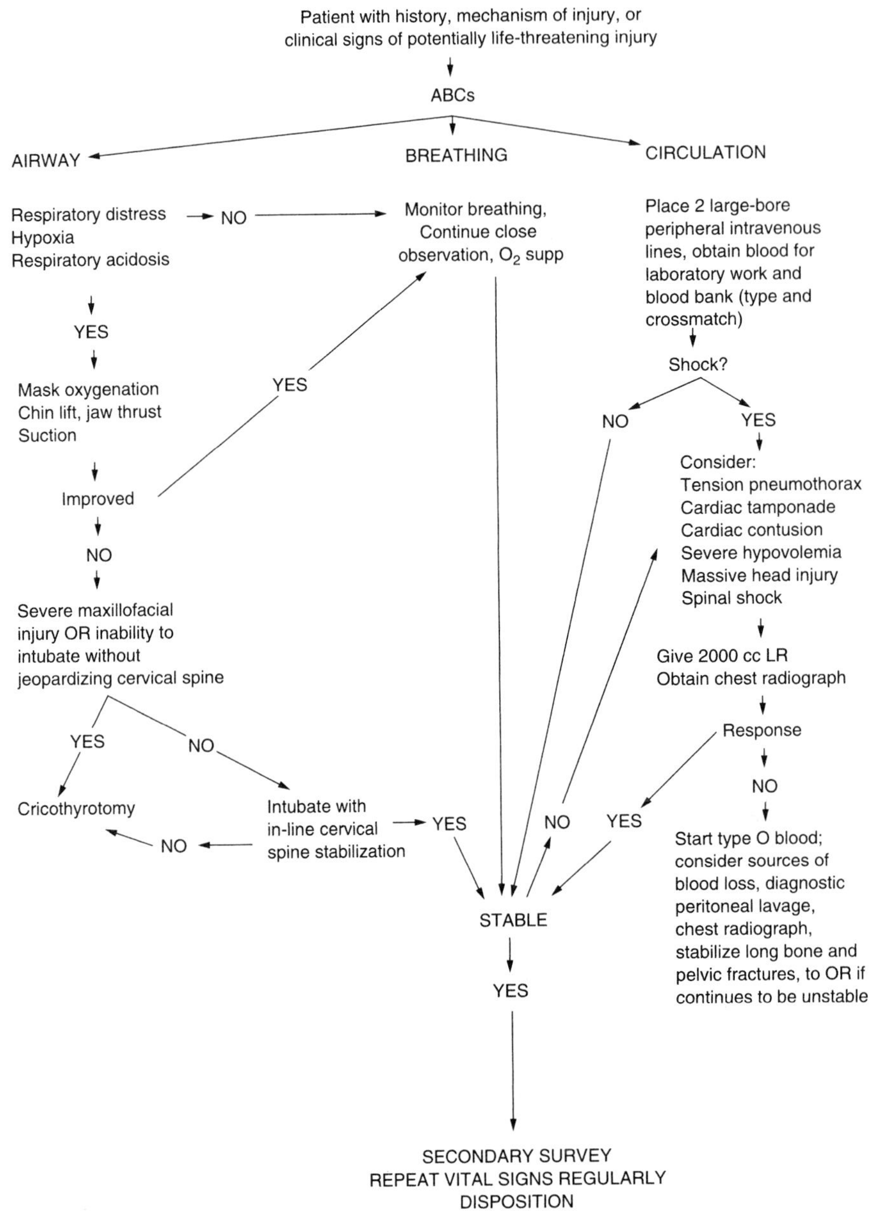

Figure 94.1. Treatment algorithm for traumatic shock.

bleed again as blood pressure increases, pulmonary congestion may develop in response to volume therapy, core temperature may drop substantially in an exposed patient receiving large amounts of intravenous fluids, or the previously unremarkable abdomen may become distended or rigid. These are examples of significant changes that can occur rapidly during the trauma resuscitation. Careful and constant attention with frequent reassessment is crucial to ensure optimal outcome.

TABLE 94.2. Initial Laboratory and Radiographic Studies in Major Trauma

LABORATORY
Complete blood count
Arterial blood gases
Electrolytes (including BUN, creatinine, glucose)
Coagulation studies (PT, PTT)
Type and crossmatch for 4–8 U of blood
Toxicologic studies (as indicated)
Urinalysis
RADIOGRAPHS
Chest x-ray, portable AP
Cross-table lateral cervical spine
Pelvis x-ray, AP view

EMERGENCY DEPARTMENT MANAGEMENT

As discussed, initial treatment in traumatic shock occurs concurrently with initial evaluation. Insertion of oral or nasal airways, assisted ventilation, endotracheal intubation, hemorrhage control, and vascular access are all essential components of the initial trauma resuscitation. Early control of the airway in the patient with traumatic shock may be lifesaving and should take priority over all other interventions.

Gaining intravenous access rapidly is essential to begin volume replacement and support the hemodynamics of the patient in traumatic shock. In the presence of obvious shock and impending circulatory collapse, establishing adequate intravenous access and initiating volume replacement is a higher priority than performing the secondary survey or obtaining such parameters as a blood pressure or pulse oximetry measurement. If a patient appears to be in profound shock, knowing the exact blood pressure does not change initial decision making regarding rapid volume replacement.

The antecubital fossa is an excellent site to initiate intravenous access. Large-bore catheters and high-flow intravenous tubing should be used to maximize delivery rate of fluids. At least two intravenous sites should be secured, and, if adequate intravenous access cannot be established within a few minutes, percutaneous femoral venous access, ankle venous cutdown, greater saphenous venous cutdown at the proximal thigh, or subclavian/jugular venous access should be considered. The intravenous sites should be above the diaphragm if a major vascular injury in the abdomen is suspected, as may occur with penetrating abdominal trauma and less commonly with blunt abdominal trauma.

Fluid therapy in trauma is an area of emerging controversy.[11] Intravascular volume replacement to compensate for blood loss and restore tissue perfusion has been accepted standard therapy for many years. Research, mostly laboratory investigations, has raised questions regarding the appropriate end point of fluid therapy. Briefly, these studies suggest that normalizing blood pressure with intravenous crystalloid solutions may be detrimental by increasing bleeding at sites of tissue injury.[4,16] These studies suggest that limited volume replacement, termed *hypotensive resuscitation,* that maintains minimally adequate organ perfusion may result in improved outcome. Although these studies raise very important questions, there are presently insufficient clinical data to support deviation from the guidelines for fluid therapy presently recommended by *Advanced Trauma Life Support* (American College of Surgeons Committee on Trauma).[1]

Volume replacement should initially begin with crystalloid solutions, such as normal saline or lactated Ringer's solution. Warmed fluids should be used to work against hypothermia. Fluids may be warmed ahead of time or administered through a fluid warmer. In an average-sized adult showing signs of shock, infusion of 2 L of crystalloid and immediate reassessment of hemodynamics is a reasonable course of action. The point in volume resuscitation at which blood transfusion is initiated is not defined. Factors that influence the decision to start blood transfusion include severity of shock, initial response to crystalloid, initial hemoglobin/hematocrit, and general health of the patient. In general, if hemodynamics do not respond adequately to 3 to 4 L of crystalloid (or about 40 to 50 mL/kg) given rapidly, further volume replacement with blood is indicated.

The value of colloids in the treatment of traumatic shock is uncertain. Colloids, such as albumin, hetastarch, and dextran, can effectively increase intravascular volume and maintain plasma oncotic pressure at more normal levels than can crystalloids. Substantial data, however, demonstrate that crystalloid and colloids are equally effective in resuscitation from hemorrhagic shock.[15,17] Because the cost of colloids is high and because their effectiveness is in doubt, use of colloids in this setting is not endorsed. Furthermore, evidence suggests that colloids may have deleterious effects in patients with hemorrhagic shock. Hypertonic saline has been extensively studied but has not become an accepted resuscitation fluid in clinical trauma care.

Typed and crossmatched blood is the best choice for blood transfusion. If the need for transfusion does not permit the time required for crossmatching, however, type-specific blood is an appropriate alternative. If traumatic shock is severe and immediate transfusion is critical, low-titer O-negative blood should be used until type-specific or typed and crossmatched blood is available.

If several units of blood are required to manage profound hypovolemia or ongoing hemorrhage, fresh-frozen plasma (FFP) and platelets may be needed to stabilize the coagulation system and limit further "nonmechanical" hemorrhage. In otherwise healthy individuals, FFP is rarely required until blood transfusion approaches 10 U. Empiric administration of FFP and platelets is not indicated.[8] Coagulation studies and platelet counts should be used to help guide such decisions.

Calcium therapy is controversial and is generally indicated only in the presence of documented hypocalcemia or cardiac dysfunction that is unresponsive to inotropic agents. Bicarbonate therapy in patients with traumatic shock should, in general, be avoided. Restoration of circulating volume and control of hemorrhage are the mainstays of therapy. When metabolic acidosis is profound, however, bicarbonate therapy might be considered as a temporary measure until hemodynamic stability can be obtained. As a general guideline, a pH of less than 7.10, despite aggressive volume replacement, has been suggested as an indicator of the need for bicarbonate therapy. Bicarbonate should not be administered if adequate ventilation has not been established.[7]

Pneumothorax or hemothorax should be managed by the placement of a large chest tube (32F or 36F) in the lateral chest with the tubes oriented toward the apicoposterior chest wall. If a tension pneumothorax is suspected and the patient is hypotensive, needle thoracostomy using a long, large-gauge angiocatheter or needle inserted at the second intercostal space in the midclavicular line is an appropriate measure until a chest tube can be inserted.

If pericardial tamponade is suspected and the patient is hypotensive and worsening despite volume resuscitation, pericardiocentesis is an appropriate intervention. A pericardiocentesis needle is inserted in the left subxiphoid area and directed 45 degrees toward the left shoulder or sternal notch while suction is maintained on an attached syringe. If possible, the needle should be hooked to an electrocardiographic lead to show evidence of needle contact with the myocardium. Blood in the pericardium often forms clots, thus precluding the value of pericardiocentesis. If the patient is profoundly hypotensive or has lost discernible blood pressure for only a few minutes, an emergency left lateral thoracotomy may be considered to open the pericardium. Patients who have not shown signs of life after sustaining blunt trauma are poor candidates for emergency department thoracotomy.[2]

Traumatic shock due to hemorrhage is most often caused by intraabdominal injury. The clinical presentation and response to initial therapy dictate the subsequent assessment of the abdomen. Hemodynamically unstable patients with physical examination evidence of abdominal injury should immediately undergo exploratory laparotomy. Patients with suspected abdominal trauma who have exhibited transient hemodynamic instability or patients with other injuries causing hemodynamic instability should undergo diagnostic peritoneal lavage (DPL) to rule out an intraabdominal source of bleeding. Focused abdominal (or assessment) sonography for trauma (FAST) is an acceptable alternative to DPL and will reliably identify free intraabdominal fluid, provided that the person performing the examination is adequately proficient.[5,9] Hemodynamically stable patients with potential abdominal trauma are reasonable candidates for abdominal computed tomography (CT) scanning.

The role of a pneumatic antishock garment (PASG) or military antishock trousers (MAST) is controversial.[10] The use of these devices is not a substitute for volume replacement, and their value in the emergency department and in the prehospital setting with short transport times is questionable. One generally accepted indication for the use of these devices is in the patient with pelvic fractures in whom these garments provide fracture stability and pelvic compression that limits further blood loss until the patient is surgically stabilized.

In general, vasopressors and inotropic agents are not used in the emergency department management of traumatic shock. In cases of neurogenic or vasogenic shock (e.g., spinal cord injury) in which peripheral vasodilatation causes or contributes to hemodynamic instability, however, vasopressors such as dopamine, phenylephrine, or norepinephrine may be useful. In cases of myocardial infarction associated with trauma or significant myocardial contusion, inotropic support with dobutamine, for example, may be appropriate.

Emergency Department Thoracotomy

Performing a thoracotomy in the emergency department is appropriate when it is unlikely that the patient will survive long enough to reach the operating room. Indications for an emergency department thoracotomy are (1) cardiac arrest in or just before arrival at the emergency department, (2) suspected pericardial tamponade with profound hypotension (extremis), and (3) uncontrollable, exsanguinating hemorrhage below the diaphragm.

The technique involves a left lateral chest incision at the level of the lower margin of pectoralis major muscle, extending from the costochondral junction to the posterior axillary line, curving in the general path of the ribs. The chest cavity is entered in the fourth or fifth intercostal space, using a scalpel or scissors to divide the intercostal muscles over the top of one of the exposed ribs. A rib spreader should be used to give adequate exposure. The pericardium should be examined for signs of tamponade. A dull reddish appearance of the heart without visible epicardial blood vessels indicates pericardial tamponade.

To avoid injury to the phrenic nerve, the pericardium should be opened in a cephalad-to-caudal direction, using the fingers after a small opening is made with scissors or a scalpel. Internal manual cardiac compression can be done with one hand pressing the heart upward against the sternum or with two hands cupped around the heart. The aorta can be identified by running the hand posteriorly along the ribs toward the spine. The aorta has a more rubbery texture than the esophagus. (A nasogastric tube in place greatly aids in distinguishing between the two.) The aorta should be cross-clamped with a vascular clamp after incising the overlying pleura. Penetrating cardiac injuries can be temporarily managed with finger pressure over the defect. Insertion and inflation of Foley catheters and temporary sutures have also been advocated.

DISPOSITION

Definitive management of the patient with traumatic shock often requires emergency surgery. Consultation with a surgeon (preferably a trauma surgeon) should be initiated as soon as possible in all victims of significant trauma who might require operative or critical care interventions. If information from prehospital care providers indicates potentially serious injury, the surgeon (or trauma team) should be notified before the patient arrives at the emergency department. If transfer to another hospital is required, early mobilization of resources (ambulance, staff, or air medical transport service) should be initiated concurrently with assessment and stabilization.

The criteria for transfer to a trauma center include lack of an experienced trauma surgeon, lack of adequate critical care or support services, and lack of adequate resources to manage a patient's injuries. The use of scoring systems such as the Trauma Score (TS), Revised Trauma Score (RTS), and the Glasgow Coma Score (GCS) for triage may be useful in identifying patients with severe injury. Patients with a TS less than 12, an RTS of 8 or less, or a GCS less than 10 generally have serious injuries and should be managed within an organized trauma system.

Criteria for emergency surgical intervention include evidence of internal abdominal hemorrhage (liver, spleen, vascular, bowel), intracranial hemorrhage (subdural hematoma, epidural hematoma), open skull fracture, penetrating cardiac injury, traumatic aortic disruption, complex pelvic fractures, or multiple trauma. Criteria for intensive care unit monitoring include neurologic injury, ventilatory support, hemodynamic instability, and potential for serious complications.

COMMON PITFALLS

- A common error in traumatic shock is not recognizing the severity of trauma. Vital signs, such as a relatively normal blood pressure or absence of tachycardia, can be misleading. Failure to recognize signs of decreased peripheral perfusion can lead to suboptimal management. An initial favorable response to volume replacement should not lull the emergency physician to be less vigilant in trauma management. Adequate resuscitation can temporarily mask ongoing significant hemorrhage. Careful monitoring and repeated examinations are important to detect changes in clinical status and to respond with appropriate interventions.
- Delays in surgical consultation or transfer to a trauma center can have adverse effects, especially when transfer is required. The emergency physician must determine which interventions and diagnostic studies are essential before transfer. These decisions are affected by mode of transport, distance to the trauma center, and the capabilities of the referring hospital. For example, delaying transfer to obtain a head CT scan, abdominal CT scan, or plain radiograph is of no benefit if there is no neurosurgeon, general surgeon, or orthopedist available or if no immediate intervention will take place at the referring hospital. On the other hand, if a head CT scan is indicated and can be obtained while waiting for transfer transport to arrive, and will not cause a delay in transport, it is optimal to proceed with the head CT scan.
- Missed injuries, especially in patients with severe multiple trauma, can have devastating effects. Frequently, repeated examinations can minimize such missed injuries.

References

1. American College of Surgeons Committee on Trauma. *Advanced trauma life support: providers' manual*. Chicago: American College of Surgeons, 1997.
2. Baker CC, Thomas AN, Trunkey DD. The role of emergency room thoracotomy in trauma. *J Trauma* 1980;20:848.
3. Baue AE. Physiology of shock and injury. In: Gelder ER, ed. *Shock and resuscitation*. New York: McGraw-Hill, 1993.
4. Bickell WH, Wall MJJ, Pepe PE, et al. Immediate versus delayed fluid resuscitation for hypotensive patients with penetrating torso injuries. *N Engl J Med* 1995;332:681.
5. Block EFJ. Diagnostic modalities in acute trauma. *New Horiz* 1999;7:10.
6. Britt LD, Weireter LJ, Riblet JL, et al. Priorities in the management of profound shock. *Surg Clin North Am* 1996;76:645.
7. Emergency Cardiac Care Committees and Subcommittees, American Heart Association. Guidelines for cardiopulmonary resuscitation and emergency cardiac care. III. Adult advanced cardiac life support. *JAMA* 1992;268:2199.
8. Fakhry SM, Sheldon GF. Blood transfusion and disorders of surgical bleeding. In: Sabiston DC, Lyerly HK, eds. *Textbook of surgery: the biological basis of modern surgical practice*. Philadelphia: WB Saunders, 1997:118.
9. Ma OJ, Mateer JR, Ogata M, et al. Prospective analysis of a rapid trauma ultrasound examination performed by emergency physicians. *J Trauma* 1995;38:879.
10. Mattox KL, Bickell WH, Pepe PE, et al. Prospective randomized evaluation of antishock MAST in posttraumatic hypotension. *J Trauma* 1986;26:779.
11. Mattox KL, Brundage SI, Hirshberg A. Initial resuscitation. *New Horiz* 1999;7:1.
12. Pearlman MD, Tintinalli JE, Lorenz RP. Blunt trauma during pregnancy. *N Engl J Med* 1990;323:1609.
13. Porter JM, Ivatury RR. In search of the optimal endpoints of resuscitation in trauma patients: a review. *J Trauma* 1998;44:908.
14. Rutherford EJ, Morris JA, Reed GW, et al. Base deficit stratifies mortality and determines therapy. *J Trauma* 1992;33:417.
15. Shierhout G, Roberts I. Fluid resuscitation with colloid or crystalloid solutions in critically ill patients: a systematic review of randomised trials. *BMJ* 1998;316:961.

16. Stern SA, Dronen SC, Birrer P, et al. The effect of blood pressure on hemorrhage volume and survival in a near-fatal hemorrhage model incorporating a vascular injury. *Ann Emerg Med* 1993;22:155.
17. Velanovich V. Crystalloid versus colloid fluid resuscitation: A meta-analysis of mortality. *Surgery* 1989;105:65.
18. Vayer JS, Henderson JV, Bellamy RF, et al. Absence of a tachycardic response to shock in penetrating intraperitoneal injury. *Ann Emerg Med* 1988;17:227.

CHAPTER 95
Wound Management

Judd E. Hollander and Adam Singer

Nearly 12 million patients with traumatic wounds are treated annually in emergency departments (EDs) in the United States.[36] The ultimate goals are to restore the physical integrity and function of the injured tissue in a cosmetically pleasing manner and to reduce the risk of infection. Treatment of these wounds involves a series of decisions that determine the methods of evaluation, wound preparation, wound closure, and postoperative care most likely to help attain these goals.

Experimental studies provided the basis for previous wound care recommendations. Over the last 5 years, clinical studies have helped refine and better delineate appropriate wound management strategies.

CLINICAL PRESENTATION

Evaluation of the patient with a traumatic wound begins with an expeditious, comprehensive assessment of the patient. This assessment can be divided into primary and secondary surveys, following Advanced Trauma Life Support Algorithms (see Chapter 89). Unless the wound compromises the ABCs, formal wound evaluation and management occurs during the secondary survey and management phase of the trauma evaluation.

Lacerations occur predominantly in young adults, although they span the spectrum from childhood until older adulthood; the majority of patients with lacerations are males.[21] Most wounds are located on either the head or neck (50%) or the upper extremity (35%), usually involving the fingers or hands. The most common mechanism of injury is application of a blunt force, such as bumping the head against a coffee table. Such contact crushes the skin against an underlying bone, causing the skin to split. Other causes of injury include sharp instruments, glass, and wooden objects.[21] While mammalian bites continue to receive much attention, they are a relatively infrequent cause of puncture wounds and lacerations.[21]

Most patients present within several hours of the injury and they may have already attempted to cleanse or care for their wounds. The emergency physician should identify conditions that place the patient at risk for infection or delayed healing after wound closure. Patients with diabetes mellitus, obesity, malnutrition, chronic renal failure, advanced age, and steroid use are at increased risk for wound infection.[10] Chemotherapeutic or other immunosuppressive agents may delay wound healing by affecting inflammation and the synthesis of new wound matrix and collagen.

Because anesthetic agents and antibiotics may be used, a detailed history of any allergies to these agents is essential. With the increased incidence of severe reactions to latex products, it is also vital to review any prior allergy to latex. Tetanus immunization status should be verified.

External bleeding can usually be controlled by applying direct pressure over the site of bleeding. When possible, skin flaps should be returned to their original position prior to application of pressure, to prevent vascular compromise of the injured area. Amputated parts should be cared for as outlined in the chapter on orthopedic emergencies (Chapter 120). Digits should be covered with a protective dressing, placed within a waterproof bag, and then placed in a container of ice water for preservation and consideration of future reattachment.

Most other aspects of wound management are not emergent and are addressed in the following sections.

EMERGENCY DEPARTMENT EVALUATION

Proper wound management begins with a thorough patient history. Particular emphasis should be placed on the various factors that can have adverse effects on wound healing. Host factors such as the extremes of age, diabetes mellitus, chronic renal failure, obesity, malnutrition, and the use of immunosuppressive medications such as steroids and chemotherapeutic agents all increase the risk of wound infection and can impair wound healing.[10] Wound healing can also be impaired in the presence of inherited and acquired connective-tissue disorders such as Ehlers-Danlos syndrome, Marfan syndrome, osteogenesis imperfecta, and protein and vitamin C deficiencies. The tendency of patients to form keloids should be ascertained; the formation of keloids can result in a scar with less than acceptable cosmesis. Black and Asian populations are more prone to keloid formation.[36]

Identification of the mechanism of injury is essential to help ascertain the presence of potential wound contaminants and foreign bodies that might result in chronic infection and delayed healing.[36] Failure to diagnose foreign bodies in wounds is the fifth leading cause of litigation against emergency physicians. Missed tendon and nerve injuries and failure to prevent infection are other common wound-related causes of litigation.

A careful history can also predict the likelihood of foreign bodies. Organic and inorganic components of soil can potentiate infection. Wounds contaminated by these fractions will become infected with lower doses of bacterial inoculum. The major inorganic particles that potentiate infection are the clay fractions, which reside in heaviest concentration in the subsoil rather than in the topsoil. Injuries that occur in swamps or excavations are at high risk of being contaminated by these fractions. Other soil contaminants, such as sand grains, are relatively innocuous. The black dirt on the surface of highways appears to have minimal chemical reactivity.

Knowledge of the types of forces applied at the time of injury also helps predict the likelihood of infection. Thus, crush injuries that tend to cause greater devitalization of tissue are more susceptible to infection than are wounds resulting from the more commonly seen shearing forces.[9] Impact injuries with low energy levels may not result in division of the skin; they can, however, disrupt vessels and produce an ecchymosis.

Disruption of vessels in the underlying tissue results in hematoma formation. Some hematomas spontaneously resorb. Those that become encapsulated usually require treatment to prevent permanent subcutaneous deformity. When still gelatinous, a hematoma may be treated by incision and drainage. As further liquefaction occurs, aspiration with a large-bore needle (18-gauge or larger) may be possible.

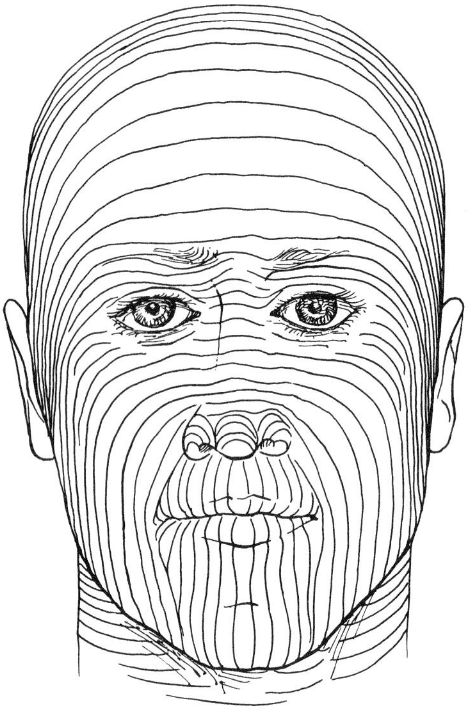

Figure 95.1. Langer's lines of least skin tension. Lacerations parallel to these lines will have less evident scarring.

Adequate wound examination should always be conducted under optimal lighting conditions in a field where bleeding has been controlled. Cursory examination under poor lighting conditions or when the depths of the wound are obscured by blood will ultimately result in underdetection of embedded foreign bodies and damage to important structures such as tendons, nerves, or arteries. One way to minimize the possibility of missing an injury to a vital structure is to start the wound examination with a careful neurovascular assessment of pulses, motor function, and sensation distal to the laceration. Finger tourniquets may then be used to obtain a bloodless field, but they should not be used for more than 30 to 60 minutes.

The anatomic location of the injury helps to predict the likelihood of infection. In general, the composition of the skin microflora allows subdivision of the body into separate anatomic areas. The first area comprises the torso, upper arms, and legs, in which the density of the bacterial population is low. Moist areas of the body, such as the axillae, perineum, toe webs, and intertriginous areas, harbor millions of bacteria per square centimeter. The exposed anatomic areas of the body constitute the third anatomic region, with a bacterial density in the millions per square centimeter. Organisms are normally sparse on the palms and dorsa of the hands, in the hundreds per square centimeter. The majority of organisms (10,000 to 100,000/cm^2) on the hands reside beneath the distal end of the fingernail plate or adjacent to the proximal or lateral fingernail folds. Lacerations of the oral cavity are usually heavily contaminated with facultative species and obligate anaerobes. Obviously, wounds with human or animal fecal contaminants run a high risk of infection despite therapeutic intervention.

TABLE 95.1. Recommendations for Tetanus Prophylaxis[36]

	Clean Minor Wounds		All Other Wounds[a]	
History of tetanus immunization	Td	TIG	Td	TIG
<3 or uncertain doses	Yes	No	Yes	Yes
≥3 doses				
Last dose within 5 years	No	No	No	No
Last dose within 5–10 years	No	No	Yes	No
Last dose : 10 years	Yes	No	Yes	No

[a]For example, contaminated wounds, puncture wounds, avulsions, burns, crush injuries.

Td, tetanus–diphtheria toxoid; TIG, tetanus immune globulin.

Anatomic variation in regional blood flow also plays a role in determining the likelihood of infection. Wounds located on highly vascular areas, such as the face and scalp, are less likely to be infected than are wounds located in less vascular areas.[21] The increased vascularity of the scalp more than offsets the high bacterial inoculum found in this area. As a result, lacerations of the scalp and face have a very low infection rate regardless of the intensity of cleansing.[22]

Wound location also contributes to the cosmetic appearance of the scar by affecting static and dynamic skin tensions (Fig. 95.1). Lacerations over joints are subject to large, dynamic skin tensions and will have a wider scar than will similar lacerations subject to less tension. Wounds that run perpendicular to the lines of minimal skin tension will also be prone to the development of wider and more visible scars.

Finally, the presence of allergies to local anesthetics, latex, and antibiotics should be determined. The tetanus status of all patients should be assessed, and patients should receive immunization in accordance with current Centers for Disease Control and Prevention recommendations (Table 95.1). Before inspecting the wound, the emergency physician must carefully question the patient regarding the time and mechanism of injury. The amount of time elapsed since the accident has considerable influence on treatment decisions.

EMERGENCY DEPARTMENT MANAGEMENT

Aseptic Technique

Practitioners should probably use sterile gloves for examination and repair of routine lacerations in the ED, despite the fact that their use has not been clearly demonstrated to reduce infection rates. Caps and gowns may be worn to for the protection of the practitioner, although they have not been shown to decrease the development of infection following laceration repair.[33] Likewise, the use of full sterile technique has not been shown to effect a lower infection rate than laceration repair using a surgically clean technique.[40] Nonetheless, the use of some type of gloves is necessary to comply with universal precautions.

The use of sterile gloves makes common sense, despite the lack of clinical evidence supporting their use. While more costly, use of powder-free gloves may reduce the risk of foreign-body reaction or infection that can theoretically occur from the introduction of talc particles into the wound. While the practice of universal precautions is recommended in all patients, double-gloving is recommended when caring for patients who can transmit serious infections to the health-care provider. Patients who harbor the human immunodeficiency virus or hepatitis are among those for whom the health-care provider may wish to take extra precautions, such as double-gloving.

Latex Allergy

Concerns have been raised about the safety of latex. Absorption of water-soluble proteins through intact mucosa or the surgical wound is believed to elicit an immunoglobulin-E (IgE)–mediated anaphylactic response in sensitive individuals. Severe reactions have resulted in fatalities. Populations that appear to be at increased risk for allergic reactions to latex include patients who have undergone multiple operations, patients with atopic disease, children with spina bifida, and medical personnel with frequent latex exposures.[28] Careful screening should identify patients who may be at increased risk for latex hypersensitivity.

Wound Examination

Wound examination should always be conducted under optimal lighting conditions and with bleeding in the field controlled. Wound examination should begin with a neurovascular assessment of pulses, motor function, and sensation distal to the laceration.

Bleeding should be controlled with direct pressure. When lacerations continue to bleed despite reasonable pressure, placement of a sphygmomanometer cuff proximal to the injury, with inflation to a pressure greater than the patient's systolic blood pressure, will help contain bleeding to allow proper examination. Palpation of the bones adjacent to the injured site may detect tenderness, a defect, or instability consistent with an underlying injury. Liberal use of radiography should be used to detect fractures. Detection of an open fracture will dictate a change from usual management. Carefully evaluate wounds occurring adjacent to a joint for joint violation. This condition requires meticulous cleaning and possibly debridement, usually in the operating room.

Complicated injuries involving most open fractures, joint penetration, flexor tendon injuries, nerve injuries, or arterial injuries are usually treated in the operating room. In most other cases, wound repair will occur in the ED.

The ultimate appearance and function of a scar can be predicted by the static and dynamic skin tensions on the surrounding skin. The static skin tensions are the forces that stretch the skin over the underlying bony framework when the body is motionless. The clinical relevance of these tensions can be ascertained by visualization of the gap between wound edges. The static skin tensions vary between different anatomic body sites. In some regions of the body, static skin tensions possess a directional orientation that has an effect on the ultimate cosmetic outcome (see Fig. 95.1). The most aesthetically pleasing scar occurs when the long axis of the scar is parallel to the direction of maximal skin tension, because the static skin tensions continually pull on the wound edges even after wound closure. The ultimate width of the scar is proportional to the magnitude of the static skin tensions. This information can be used to help answer the ubiquitous question, "Will I have a scar?"

The magnitude of static skin tension per unit length of wound is also considerably influenced by configuration of the wound. In uneven, jagged-edged wounds, the perimeter of the wound is considerably longer than that of linear incisions. Consequently, the magnitude of static tensions per unit length of a jagged-edged wound is less than that for a straight laceration. Meticulous reapproximation of the jagged edges of the wound yields a narrow scar. When jagged wound edges are converted into smoother edges, the potential benefits of the long wound perimeter are eliminated and a lenticular defect that is considerably wider than the initial wound may result. Knowledge of static tensions might alert the practitioner that certain unfavorable lacerations would benefit from the use of absorbable sutures beneath the surface of the skin. They may help reduce the tendency of the scar to widen as wound remodeling occurs.

Dynamic skin tensions may have considerable impact on the magnitude and extent of scar formation. These changing tensions are caused by a combination of forces that are associated with joint movement or mimetic muscle contraction. The clinical significance of dynamic tensions is particularly apparent in skin of changing dimensions in which elasticity is needed for normal function. In general, a linear scar intersecting the transverse axis of a joint or running perpendicular to the wrinkle lines can result in a serious contracture because the scar does not stretch or recoil like uninjured tissue. The patient should be warned that an unattractive scar may result. An appreciation of the effects of various dynamic tensions can be used to determine the need for absorbable sutures in addition to the nonabsorbable skin closure.

Wound Anesthesia

Most lacerations will require some form of anesthesia prior to wound closure. The administration of anesthesia prior to wound cleansing will enable more vigorous wound cleansing and possibly surgical debridement. All visibly contaminated wounds and wounds that will require anesthesia for closure should receive anesthesia prior to cleansing so that adequate mechanical removal of bacteria, soil, and other debris can be more readily accomplished.

Local Infiltration

The most common form of anesthesia for traumatic injuries is local infiltration. Unfortunately, local anesthesia is painful. In order to reduce the pain associated with local infiltration, several strategies can be employed. The addition of sodium bicarbonate to lidocaine (pK_a, 7.9) in a 1:9 ratio increases the ratio of uncharged to charged ions and results in more rapid diffusion of anesthetic agent into nerve endings. It reduces the pain associated with local infiltration without altering the ability of host defenses to prevent infection.[3] The use of warm anesthetic solutions, small needles, slow rates of infiltration, injection through the wound edges in noncontaminated wounds, and pretreatment with topical 1% tetracaine or LET are additional strategies that can be used to decrease the pain of infiltration.[4,7,23,25,18]

For injection of local anesthesia, use a 27- to 30-gauge needle attached to a 10-mL syringe. The needle should be passed into the subdermal tissue rather than the intradermal tissue because subdermal injections are less painful. Full anesthesia to pinprick is present 5 to 6 minutes after subdermal injection. The local anesthetic agent should be instilled slowly to decrease the pain that accompanies tissue infiltration.[25] The needle should be passed through the dermal tissue initially; then the anesthetic agent can be injected as the needle is slowly withdrawn. This technique minimizes distention and pain by providing a potential space for the anesthetic solution. Aspiration of the syringe before injection is recommended to prevent inadvertent intravascular injection.

The two major classes of local anesthetics are the esters and amides (Table 95.2). Because the amides cause less sensitivity and allergic reactions than the esters, lidocaine and bupivacaine are most commonly used for local anesthesia. These anesthetic agents do not damage tissue defenses, nor do they increase the risk of infection. Both classes of agents are similar with respect to the degree of pain upon subdermal injection, time to onset of anesthe-

TABLE 95.2. Classification of Local Anesthetics

Amides	Esters
Lidocaine	Procaine
Bupivacaine	Cocaine
Etidocaine	Tetracaine
Mepivacaine	Benzocaine
	Chloroprocaine

sia, and frequency of satisfactory anesthesia. Because the duration of local anesthesia induced by bupivacaine is nearly four times longer than that of lidocaine, bupivacaine (0.25%) should be used when longer durations of anesthesia are desirable (Table 95.3).

Vasoconstrictors such as epinephrine can be used as adjuncts to the local anesthetic agents. They will reduce bleeding and oozing within the laceration, which will make exploration and closure easier to accomplish. Clinical studies have not found that the vasoconstriction associated with epinephrine use results in differences in infection rates. The use of vasoconstrictors is generally discouraged in areas with end-organ blood supply, such as the fingers and toes.

Although patients may state that they have had an allergic reaction to local anesthetic agents in the past, careful review of this reaction will usually indicate the presence of either a vasovagal response associated with painful injection or evidence of minor toxicity from the anesthetic agent.[23] Rarely, patients may report a true allergy to one of the local anesthetics. Because there is little cross-reactivity between agents of the two classes, use of an agent from the other class should be considered (see Table 95.2). Some patients with "allergies" to lidocaine are really allergic to methylparaben, the preservative used in multidose vials. This preservative is similar in molecular structure to one of the ester anesthetic degradation products. As a result, the use of an ester in place of an amide may be problematic. Cardiac lidocaine is a single-use preparation that does not contain this preservative. As such, it represents a therapeutic alternative. Another option is to use an anesthetic agent unrelated to the "caines," such as diphenhydramine or benzyl alcohol.[5,14] Diphenhydramine is an effective local anesthetic, but its infiltration is more painful than with lidocaine. If diphenhydramine is used, it must be diluted to 1% in order to avoid risk of tissue necrosis. Benzyl alcohol is as effective as lidocaine and is less painful to inject than diphenhydramine.

Regional Anesthesia

When the nerve supply to a wound is easily accessible, a regional nerve block is a valuable alternative to local anesthesia. The use of regional nerve blocks will prevent distortion of the wound edges, facilitating approximation and increasing the likelihood of an excellent cosmetic result. Additionally, it is more useful than local anesthesia in areas with abundant sensory nerve supplies, such as the fingers, palms, and soles. Regional nerve blocks can be accomplished by only one or two needle passages through skin proximal to the injury site. Often these areas have a considerably higher threshold of pain. Regional nerve blocks of the supraorbital, infraorbital, and mental nerves are useful for facial lacerations. Median, radial, and ulnar nerve blocks may be useful for lacerations of the hand. Digital or metacarpal nerve blocks can be used for finger lacerations. Regional nerve blocks can also be used for lacerations of the feet. Field blocks can be considered for more proximal extremity injuries.

A 27- or 25-gauge needle is preferred to a 30-gauge needle for a regional nerve block, because either one is more resistant to deflection during passage through tissue. The duration of sensory analgesia can be significantly prolonged when epinephrine (1%) is added to the anesthetic solution. When the needle puncture site is the mucus membrane, anesthetizing the mucous membrane with a topical anesthetic agent makes the introduction of the needle painless.

Topical Anesthesia

Topical anesthesia eliminates needle use and the risk of inadvertent needle sticks while allowing the application of painless anesthesia. A combination of tetracaine, adrenaline, and cocaine (TAC) is an effective topical anesthetic in children and on the face and scalp.[19] However, improper use can result in serious adverse events (e.g., seizures and death).[19,36] Better alternatives include various combinations of lidocaine (1% to 4%), adrenaline (1:1,000 to 1:2,000), and tetracaine (0.5% to 2.0%).[17,18] EMLA cream (eutectic mixture of local anesthetics) can be used to decrease the pain associated with local infiltration, but it takes more than 30 minutes to develop significant anesthesia. Novel methods for enhancing the topical absorption of local anesthetics, such as iontophoresis and sonophoresis, are currently being studied. Their role has not yet been defined.

Preparation of Skin

Removal of the hair surrounding a laceration may facilitate meticulous wound closure. Because many bacteria normally reside in hair follicles, shaving the hair prior to repair may increase wound infection rates.[34] Reduced damage to hair follicles may be achieved by using hair clippers instead of a razor. Removal of the eyebrow hair should be avoided because it does not always grow back. Additionally, the presence of hair serves as a guide to approximation of wound edges during laceration repair.

The skin surrounding the wound should be disinfected; avoid contacting the wound itself with disinfectant. The ideal agent for disinfection must be a safe, fast-acting, broad-spectrum antimicrobial preparation that significantly reduces the number of microorganisms on intact skin, usually after a single application. Two groups of antiseptic agents, containing either an iodophor or chlorhexidine, may be used for preparation of the intact skin around the wound. Both agents have a long shelf life and no significant inactivation. Both exhibit a substantive effect on the skin microflora, suppressing the proliferation of a broad spectrum of microorganisms. Although these agents can reduce the bacterial concentration on intact skin, they appear to damage wound defenses, making it more susceptible to development of infection. Consequently, any contact of these agents with the wound should be avoided. Also take care to avoid antiseptic contact with the eyes.

Debridement

Appropriate debridement is an important factor in the management of contaminated wounds.[20] Retained devitalized soft tis-

TABLE 95.3. Properties of Commonly Used Local Anesthetics

Agent	Trade Name	Local Anesthetic Class	Concentration	Maximal Safe Dose	Onset	Duration
Procaine	Novocaine	Ester	0.5%–1.0%	7 mg/kg	2–5 min	15–45 min
With epinephrine				9 mg/kg		30–90 min
Lidocaine	Xylocaine	Amide	0.5%–2.0%	4.5 mg/kg	2–5 min	1–2 h
With epinephrine				7 mg/kg		2–4 h
Bupivacaine	Marcaine	Amide	0.125%–0.25%	2 mg/kg	2–5 min	4–8 h
With epinephrine				3 mg/kg		8–16 h

sue, fat, muscle, and skin can damage wound defenses and increase the likelihood of infection through the promotion of bacterial growth and the inhibition of phagocytosis. Identification of the exact limit of devitalized tissue in wounds may be difficult. Evaluation of the color, consistency, contraction, and circulation is useful.

In some anatomic sites, such as the trunk, debridement is best accomplished by complete excision of the skin and deep tissues. Heavily contaminated wounds with serpiginous defects in these regions can be converted to clean wounds by more generous tissue excision. When a heavily contaminated wound contains specialized tissues, such as the nerves for tendons, that perform important physical functions, complete excision often is not feasible. In such instances, mechanical wound cleansing followed by excision of all fragments of tissue that are not clearly viable is indicated.

The benefits of debridement must be weighed against the consequences of excision of the tissue. Debridement of skin and underlying tissue leaves a significant soft-tissue defect that makes reapproximation more difficult. The increased static skin tensions produced may result in a wider scar. In some cases, debridement may be best performed in the operating room, where sterile conditions, lighting, and assistants may offer an advantage.

Cleansing the Wound

Using Mechanical Forces

Mechanical forces are typically used to cleanse the wound of bacteria and other particulate matter retained on the wound surface by adhesive forces. For such forces to be successful, they must exceed the adhesive forces of the contaminant. The two basic methods of wound cleansing are hydraulic forces (irrigation) and direct contact (scrubbing).

Irrigation. Some debate exists over both the optimal method of irrigation and the preferred solution. The efficacy of wound irrigation can be correlated with the pressure at which the irrigant is delivered to the wound.[16] In irrigation, the hydraulic forces of the irrigating stream act on particulate matter in the wound. The magnitude of the hydraulic force is a function of the relative velocities and the configuration of the particle. When subjected to the same velocity of irrigating stream, particles with a smaller frontal surface area experience less force than particles with a similar configuration but with a greater surface area. Consequently, it takes significantly less hydraulic pressure to rid the wound of large foreign bodies than it does to remove bacteria.

In an experimental model involving a contaminated animal wound, high-pressure irrigation was more effective than low-pressure irrigation in reducing both bacterial wound counts and wound infection rates.[38] High-pressure irrigation successfully cleans wounds of small particulate matter, such as bacteria and soil. Such cleansing has reduced the infection rate of experimentally contaminated wounds. In contrast, low-pressure syringe irrigation, even with large volumes of fluid, demonstrates negligible capability for removing small particles (bacteria), but removes large particulate matter, such as detached devitalized tissue.

Wound impact pressures of more than 8 psi can be easily obtained using a 30- to 60-mL syringe and a 19-gauge needle[38] or Zerowet splash shield. However, it must be noted that sustained high-pressure irrigation can result in tissue damage. As a result, at very high pressures, infection rates actually increase.[16] Thus, the optimal irrigation pressure lies somewhere in between.

For individual wounds, the benefits of high-pressure irrigation should be weighed against the potential risks. Thus, for noncontaminated wounds in highly vascularized areas containing loose areolar tissue, such as the eyelid, high pressures should be avoided. In fact, high-pressure irrigation has not been found to offer any advantages for cleansing clean, noncontaminated facial lacerations. Infection rates and cosmetic appearance at the time of suture removal demonstrated comparable results when facial wounds were repaired with and without prior irrigation.[22] Conversely, high-pressure irrigation is clearly indicated for contaminated wounds of the lower extremity.

The choice of irrigation solution is relatively straightforward. Normal saline is the most cost-effective and readily available choice. It has compared favorably with more expensive, less easily available alternatives.[13] Because of their tissue toxicity, detergents, hydrogen peroxide, and concentrated forms of povidone–iodine should not be used to irrigate wounds.[16] Irrigation volume should be individualized based on patient and wound characteristics such as location and etiology. Use of a device designed to reduce splatter will minimize the health-care provider's risk of exposure to potentially infectious materials.

Scrubbing. Direct scrubbing of the wound with a sterile surgical brush helps remove both bacteria and particulate matter, which potentiate the risk of wound infection. However, scrubbing also contributes to the tissue damage and reduces the ability of the wound to resist infection. The magnitude of the damage to the local tissue resistance is correlated with the porosity of the sponge. Sponges with a low porosity (45 pores per inch [ppi]) are more abrasive and exert more damage to the wound than do sponges with a higher porosity (90 ppi). The addition of a nontoxic surfactant to a sponge minimizes the tissue damage it inflicts while maintaining the bacterial removal efficiency of mechanical cleansing. Because the use of high-porosity sponges and surfactant adds to the cost of wound care, their use is probably justified only for highly contaminated wounds.

Use of Drains

The potential benefits of the use of surgical drainage in a clinical setting must be weighed against its harmful effects. Drainage evacuates potentially harmful collections of pus and blood from wounds. When no definite localized fluid exists, drainage must be considered prophylactic, and its potentially harmful effects become more important. Drains act as retrograde conduits through which skin contaminants gain entrance into the wound. Placement of both Silastic and Penrose drains within experimental wounds exposed to subinfective inoculations of bacteria greatly enhanced the rate of infection compared with that observed in undrained controls.[26]

Open Wound Management

After wound cleansing, the physical integrity and function of the injured tissue must be restored. The technique of wound closure largely depends on whether the wound has lost tissue. If not, primary closure usually can be accomplished. For wounds with associated significant tissue loss, grafts or flaps are often required to close the defect. These procedures are usually performed in the operating room. They are relatively infrequent occurrences in the ED.

The timing of laceration closure is critical. Most wounds should be closed primarily in order to reduce patient discomfort and speed healing. While there is a direct relationship between the time interval from injury to laceration closure and the risk of subsequent infection, the length of this "golden period" is highly variable.[36] A study of forearm lacerations found that closure within 4 hours had a lower infection rate than later closure.[29] A large series of pediatric patients (2,834 patients) with lacerations did not find a difference in infection rate for lacerations closed within or greater than 6 hours from the time of injury.[2] Facial lacerations healed well regardless of the time to closure. In contrast,

TABLE 95.4. Advantages and Disadvantages of the Common Wound-Closure Techniques

	Advantages	Disadvantages
Suture	Time honored Meticulous closure Greatest tensile strength Lowest dehiscence rate	Requires removal Requires anesthesia Greatest tissue reactivity Highest cost Slowest application
Staples	Rapid application Low tissue reactivity Low cost Low risk of needlestick	Less meticulous closure May interfere with some older generation imaging techniques (CT, MRI)
Tissue adhesives	Rapid application Patient comfort Resistant to bacterial growth No need for removal Low cost No risk of needlestick	Lower tensile strength than sutures Dehiscence over high-tension areas (joints) Not useful on hands Cannot bathe or swim
Surgical tapes	Least reactive Lowest infection rates Rapid application Patient comfort Low cost No risk of needlestick	Frequently falls off Lower tensile strength than sutures Highest rate of dehiscence Requires use of toxic adjuncts Cannot be used in areas of hair Cannot get wet

trunk and extremity lacerations exhibited lower rates of healing if they were closed more than 19 hours from the time of injury (63% to 75%) as compared to earlier (75% to 91%).[6]

On the basis of these data, it seems appropriate to consider each individual laceration separately, taking the time from injury until presentation into account, along with laceration location, degree of contamination, risk of infection, and importance of cosmetic appearance, before deciding whether to perform primary wound closure. For example, a 19-hour-old laceration on the face of a healthy 5-year-old child may be closed primarily, while a deep laceration from a puncture in the dirty foot of a diabetic patient will be at very high risk of infection and should not be closed primarily. Thus, the timing during which wound closure is deemed safe must be individualized.[36] Wounds that are not closed primarily due to a high risk of infection should be considered for delayed primary closure after 3 to 5 days, when the risk of infection decreases.

Wound Closure

The ideal wound closure technique should allow a meticulous closure, be accomplished rapidly with ease, be painless, pose a low risk to the health-care provider, be inexpensive, result in minimal scarring, and involve a low infection rate. The optimal wound closure technique varies with the clinical situation. Sutures are the most commonly employed wound-closure technique. Tissue adhesives can be used in up to one-third of ED laceration repairs.[32] Staples and surgical tapes can be used in selected situations. The advantages and disadvantages of various wound-closure techniques are summarized in Table 95.4.

Sutures

The choice of suture technique should be determined by the configuration and biomechanical properties of the wound, in combination with an assessment of its risk of infection. Percutaneous sutures pass through the epidermal and dermal layers of the skin. They are used alone for low-tension lacerations and in combination with dermal (subcuticular) sutures for higher tension lacerations. The dermal suture reapproximates the divided edges of the dermis without penetrating the epidermis. Often, dermal and percutaneous sutures are used together.

Most often, percutaneous sutures are performed with nonabsorbable sutures (Table 95.5), such as nylon and polypropylene. Both nylon and polypropylene retain most of their tensile strength for more than 60 days and are relatively nonreactive.[36] Removal of nonabsorbable sutures is required. Percutaneous sutures of either monofilament nylon or polypropylene exert the least damage to the wound defenses. Polybutester suture has greater elasticity than other sutures, allowing the suture to return to its original length once tension is removed. Polybutester sutures are useful when sutures are subject to wound edema and may be expected to stretch. Nylon, polypropylene, and silk resist extension under low forces, thereby lacerating encircled tissue and creating unsightly marks on the skin.

Nonabsorbable sutures made from natural fibers potentiate infection more than synthetic nonabsorbable sutures, correlating with the reaction of tissue to these sutures in clean wounds. The use of silk and cotton should be avoided in wounds that have significant bacterial contamination. The incidence of infection in contaminated tissue containing monofilament sutures is lower than in those containing multifilament sutures. Although use of ab-

TABLE 95.5. Characteristics of Nonabsorbable Sutures

Suture	Knot Security	Tensile Strength	Tissue Reactivity	Workability
Nylon (Ethilon)	Good	Good	Minimal	Good
Polypropylene (Prolene)	Least	Best	Least	Fair
Silk	Best	Least	Most	Best

TABLE 95.6. Characteristics of Absorbable Sutures

Suture	Knot Security	Tensile Strength	Wound Security (50% Tensile Strength)	Tissue Reactivity
Surgical gut	Poor	Fair	5–7 d	Most
Chromic gut	Fair	Fair	10–14 d	Most
Polyglactin (Vicryl)	Good	Good	30 d	Minimal
Polyglycolic acid (Dexon)	Best	Good	30 d	Minimal
Polydioxanone (PDS)	Fair	Best	45–60 d	Least
Polyglyconate (Maxon)	Fair	Best	45–60 d	Least

sorbable sutures is generally reserved for dermal closures, more rapidly absorbing forms can be used to close skin in children and avoid the discomfort and inconvenience of suture removal.

Dermal closures are generally accomplished with absorbable sutures (Table 95.6). They increase the duration of time the wound retains 50% of its tensile strength from 1 week until as many as 8 weeks. Chromic gut lasts for up to 2 weeks, but it is associated with increased tissue reactivity. Polyglactin (Vicryl) and polyglycolic acid (Dexon) maintain tensile strength for 20 to 28 days and have less tissue reactivity. Some synthetic absorbable sutures, such as polydioxanone (PDS) and polyglyconate (Maxon), retain their tensile strength for as long as 2 months. They are particularly useful in areas with high static and dynamic tensions. These sutures should be used only in the deeper areas, because they can become extruded after long periods of time.

The use of dermal sutures relieves skin tension, decreases dead space and hematoma formation, and, theoretically, should improve cosmetic outcome. Research in experimental animal models has found that deep sutures increase the risk of infection in highly contaminated wounds, but they do not do so in clean, noncontaminated lacerations.[1,27] Sutures placed through adipose tissue do not reduce tension and they increase the infection rate. Deep sutures should not placed in adipose tissue and should not be used in contaminated wounds.[12]

Undermining the wound margin decreases the forces required for wound closure. Theoretically, it should limit the width of the ultimate scar. However, this benefit must be weighed against its potential damage to the skin blood supply, which may limit the patient's defenses, increasing the likelihood of infection. Consequently, undermining should be reserved for clean, noncontaminated wounds subjected to strong static and dynamic tensions.

The magnitude of the suture's damage to the local tissue defenses is related to the quantity of the suture within the wound. As a result, the narrowest diameter suture (50 or 60) that is strong enough to resist disruption of the skin should be used (Table 95.7). Approximation of the midportion of the laceration first, with subsequent bisection of the remaining portion, will enable the use of least amount of suture. Interrupted dermal sutures placed in each quadrant of the wound subjected to strong static and dynamic skin tensions provide sufficient strength to permit early suture removal.

TABLE 95.7. Suture Selection Based on Anatomic Location

Location	Suture Size[a]
Face	6-0 or 7-0
Scalp	5-0
Chest	3-0 or 4-0
Back	3-0 or 4-0
Forearm	4-0 or 5-0
Fingers	4-0 or 5-0
Hand	4-0 or 5-0
Lower extremity	4-0 or 5-0
Foot	4-0 or 5-0

[a]Larger suture sizes may need to be used for wounds with higher tension.

Tissue Adhesives

Tissue adhesives are cyanoacrylate polymers. Shorter alkyl chain molecules (methyl, ethyl) are more reactive and have greater histotoxicity and weaker tissue binding than longer alkyl chain cyanoacrylates. In large quantities, the shorter chain molecules result in tissue toxicity. The *n*-butyl-cyanoacrylates are less toxic than shorter chain cyanoacrylates and maintain a stronger bond. 2-Octylcyanoacrylate (Dermabond) is even more stable, has greater flexibility, and maintains a stronger bond. It has a breaking strength three to four times greater than the butylcyanoacrylates, and degrades much more slowly. It is considered nontoxic.

Observational studies of children with small scalp, face, or limb lacerations treated with Histoacryl Blue (Braun, Germany), a butyl-2-cyanoacrylate, found low infection rates (less than 2%) and low dehiscence rates (0.6% to 1.8%). Histoacryl Blue results in similar long-term cosmetic outcomes to 5-0 or 6-0 sutures when used for repair of small facial lacerations.[32,41]

Several clinical studies have compared the use of 2-octylcyanoacrylate to 5-0 and 6-0 sutures. Quinn et al.[42] found the long-term cosmetic outcomes to be equivalent. The use of 2-octylcyanoacrylate was faster and less painful than the use of sutures. The clinical trial that led to Food and Drug Administration approval of Dermabond enrolled 818 patients from a variety of office-based and ED sites. Patients were randomized to receive skin closure with either 5-0 or 6-0 sutures or 2-octylcyanoacrylate. Of the 818 patients enrolled, 333 had subcuticular or subcutaneous sutures placed prior to laceration closure.

Comparing the group of patients who received 2-octylcyanoacrylate with the group of patients who received skin closure with sutures, the 3-month cosmetic outcomes, short-term infection rates, and wound dehiscence rates were all similar. Again, the time to wound closure was reduced by more than 50% in the group treated with 2-octylcyanoacrylate. Results of the study in the ED patient subpopulation were analogous to the findings of the group as a whole.[37] Likewise, subgroup analysis of patients from the pediatric ED found equivalent 3-month cosmetic outcomes.[8] The use of octylcyanoacrylates for skin closure following elective facial plastic surgical procedures produced better long-term results than did the use of sutures.[39]

Although *in vitro* and *in vivo* studies have found that cyanoacrylate tissue adhesives possess gram-positive antimicrobial properties, it is imperative that clinicians adhere to standard wound preparation and wound-cleansing procedures. When tissue adhesives have been used without anesthesia, and wound cleansing is not performed in a thorough manner, an increased rate of wound infections has been observed.

The application of tissue adhesives is rapid and relatively painless. Adhesives also have the advantage that they do not require later removal, as do sutures. They will usually slough off in 7 to 10 days as the keratinized layer of epithelium sloughs. They should be used only topically. Tissue adhesives should not be placed within the wound or between wound margins. Octylcyanoacrylate tissue adhesives provide greater three-dimensional tensile strength than do butylcyanoacrylates. Both polymers are a needleless alternative to sutures for the closure of most facial lacerations, providing an excellent cosmetic appearance, comparable to that provided by sutures.

2-Octylcyanoacrylate is packaged in a sterile, single-use ampule and is colored with violet dye. After the inner glass portion of the ampule is manually crushed, the polymerization process begins. The adhesive should be painted on top of the skin as the laceration edges are manually approximated. If lacerations cannot be manually approximated and the skin edges cannot be held together without tension, the use of tissue adhesives is inappropriate. When 2-octylcyanoacrylate is painted on the laceration, the clinician should apply at least three to four coats to provide adequate strength to the wound closure. Take care to avoid applying too much tissue adhesive, because polymerization is associated with an exothermic reaction (heat release). Increased rates and amounts of polymerization may be associated with the perception of increased heat sensation by the patient.

2-Octylcyanoacrylates can be used in locations that could otherwise be closed with 5-0 or 6-0 nonabsorbable sutures. 2-Octylcyanoacrylates should be used in higher-tension areas only if subcutaneous or subcuticular absorbable sutures are placed to relieve tension on the skin. They should not be used over high-tension areas or areas with repetitive movement, such as joints. When tissue adhesive application leads to a suboptimal wound closure, antibiotic ointment, petroleum jelly, or bathing can be used to accelerate removal. Acetone can be used when more rapid removal is necessary.

The butylcyanoacrylates possess less tensile strength than 5-0 sutures and only approximately one-third the tensile strength of the octylcyanoacrylates.[36] They are not currently available in the United States, although clinical trials are ongoing. Studies have found that for the repair of very small facial lacerations, the butylcyanoacrylates are equivalent to 5-0 and 6-0 sutures or octylcyanoacrylates. They are packaged in nonsterile, multiuse vials and are applied in beads across the laceration. In general, the butylcyanoacrylates are more brittle and friable than octylcyanoacrylates and do not allow the same degree of movement and flexibility of the skin.

When 2-octylcyanoacrylate is used, take care to avoid picking or scrubbing of the area. For patients on whose skin tissue adhesives remain for prolonged periods, antibiotic ointment, petroleum jelly, or bathing may accelerate removal.

Staples

Staples can be applied more rapidly than sutures. Staples are associated with a lower rate of foreign-body reaction and a lower infection rate.[30] In general, staples are considered particularly useful for scalp, trunk, and extremity wounds.[36] They can also be used when time is limited, such as in situations of mass casualties or multiple trauma.[36] On the other hand, they do not allow as meticulous a skin closure as sutures, and their use is limited when cosmetic appearance is of utmost importance. They are slightly more painful to remove than sutures. In experimental animal models, staples have shown lower rates of bacterial growth and lower infection rates than sutures,[24] although these effects appear to have limited clinical significance.

Adhesive Tapes

The ideal adhesive tape should have the following performance characteristics.[31] It should be strong enough, even when wet, to withstand the forces disrupting the wound. Its adhesive should be sufficiently aggressive to securely adhere to the skin and maintain approximation of the wound edges. Although a secure bond to skin is necessary for wound security, it also appears to be beneficial for the tape to stretch slightly under constant stress. This ability to elongate under moderate loads reduces the shear forces on the underlying edematous skin, thereby preventing blister formation. The tape construction should provide an environment on the skin surface that is resistant to bacterial growth.

The ease with which wounds can be closed by tape varies according to the anatomic and biomechanical properties of the wound site. Linear wounds in skin subjected to minimal static and dynamic tensions are easily approximated by tape. The relatively lax skin of the face and abdomen is amenable to wound closure by tape. With tape closures, patients are spared the discomfort of suture removal and the development of suture puncture scars. An additional benefit of this technique is that patients need not be subjected to the painful injection of the local anesthetic agent required for suturing.

Surgical tapes are intrinsically less reactive than staples.[24] However, adhesive tapes require the use of adhesive adjuncts (e.g., tincture of benzoin), which are tissue toxic and increase local induration and wound infection rates. Adhesive adjuncts are toxic to wounds, and care should be taken so that they do not enter the wound. Although the various surgical tapes have different degrees of adhesion, porosity, breaking strength, and elasticity,[31] tapes alone will not maintain wound integrity in areas subject to tension.[36] They are seldom recommended for primary wound closure in the ED, but are often used after suture removal to decrease tension on the wound until they fall off.

Postoperative Wound Care

Postoperative wound care should optimize healing. It must be tailored to both the type of wound and method of wound closure. Sutured or stapled lacerations should be covered with a protective nonadherent dressing for 24 to 48 hours until enough epithelization takes place to protect the wound from gross contamination. Maintenance of a moist wound environment increases the rate of reepithelization. Additionally, pressure dressings minimize the accumulation of the intercellular fluid dead space. When possible, the site of injury should be elevated above the patient's heart to limit the accumulation of fluid in the wound interstitial spaces. The wound with little edema heals more rapidly than one with marked edema.

Topical antibiotic ointments may help reduce infection rates and prevent scab formation. Although white petrolatum may be as effective as bacitracin in ambulatory surgery patients, topical antibiotics result in lower infection rates than white petrolatum in traumatic lacerations.[15] Patients whose lacerations are closed with tissue adhesives should not have topical ointments applied. They will loosen the adhesive and result in dehiscence.

Prophylactic antibiotic administration should not be used as a regular adjunct to wound care. Several studies and a meta-analysis have found no benefit to prophylactic antibiotics for routine laceration repair.[11] Use of antibiotics should be individualized on the basis of the degree of bacterial contamination, the presence of infection-potentiating factors (e.g., soil), the mechanism of injury, and presence or absence of host predisposition to infection. In general, decontamination is far more important than antibiotics. Antibiotics should be used in most human, dog, and cat bites; intraoral lacerations; open fractures; and exposed joints or tendons.[36] Additionally, patients with soft-tissue lacerations who are prone to the development of infective endocarditis, patients with prosthetic joints and other permanent "hardware," and patients with lymphedema should receive antimicrobial therapy. Intravenous antibiotics should be given prior to wound care in patients at high risk for systemic complications of infected soft-tissue injuries.

Sutured or stapled wounds should be kept clean and gently cleansed after 24 to 48 hours. Patients with tissue adhesives may shower, but they should avoid bathing and swimming: Prolonged moisture will loosen the adhesive bond. Gentle blotting should be used to dry the area, as wiping could result in dehiscence. Elevation of the injured area decreases edema formation. Splinting may prove helpful in areas subject to high tension (e.g., in lacerations across joints). Patients should be instructed to observe the wound for erythema, warmth, swelling, and drainage, as these findings may indicate infection. Use of standardized wound-care instructions improves patient compliance and understanding.

Sutures or staples in most locations should be removed after approximately 7 days (Table 95.8). Facial sutures should be removed sooner (within 3 to 5 days) to avoid the formation of unsightly sinus tracts. Sutures subject to high tension (e.g., in joints, hands) should be left in for 10 to 14 days. When 2-octylcyanoacrylate is used, take care to avoid picking or scrubbing the area or exposure to water for more than brief periods until the previously noted times. When tissue adhesives remain on the skin for prolonged periods, antibiotic ointment, petroleum jelly, or bathing can accelerate removal. Acetone can be used when more rapid removal is required. Patients should be told when and with whom to follow up for suture removal or wound examinations.

Abraded skin may develop permanent hyperpigmentation after exposure to the sun.[35] Consequently, abraded skin should be protected with a sun-blocking agent for at least 6 to 12 months after injury.

Prevention of Tetanus

Two-thirds of the recent tetanus cases in the United States have followed lacerations, puncture wounds, and crush injuries. For every wounded patient, information about the mechanism of injury, the characteristics of the wound and its age, previous active immunization status, history of a neurologic or severe hypersensitivity reaction after a previous immunization treatment, and plans for follow-up should be recorded in a permanent medical record.

Proper immunization plays the most important role in tetanus prophylaxis. Recommendations on tetanus prophylaxis are based on the condition of the wound and the patient's immunization history. A summary guide to tetanus prophylaxis of the wounded patient, as recommended by the CDC, is outlined in Table 95.1. As noted, passive immunization with TIG is indicated only under specific conditions.

The only contraindication to tetanus and diphtheria toxoids is a history of neurologic or severe hypersensitivity reaction after a previous dose. Local side effects do not preclude repeated use. Local reactions, generally erythema and induration with or without tenderness, are common after the administration of vaccines containing diphtheria, tetanus, and pertussis antigens. These reactions are usually self-limited and require no therapy. If a systemic reaction is suspected to represent allergic hypersensitivity, immunization should be postponed until appropriate skin testing is undertaken. If the use of a tetanus toxoid is contraindicated, passive immunization against tetanus should be considered in a tetanus-prone wound. In those patients who have not completed a primary tetanus immunization series, appropriate follow-up should include referral to a physician who can complete active immunization.

TABLE 95.8. Optimal Time from Placement of Sutures until Suture Removal

Location	No. of Days
Face	3–5
Scalp	7
Chest	8–10
Back	10–14
Forearm	10–14
Fingers	8–10
Hand	8–10
Lower extremity	8–12
Foot	10–12

DISPOSITION

Role of the Consultant

The appropriate surgical specialist should be consulted for patients with open fractures of long bones, nerve or vascular injuries, flexor tendon disruptions, repair of specialized structures such as the parotid or lacrimal duct, replacement of skin loss by a flap or graft, or extensive debridement.

Indications for Admission

Few patients with lacerations will require admission to the hospital. Even those patients requiring surgical intervention can often be discharged with appropriate follow-up arrangements. Often, definitive repair can be accomplished via same-day surgery.

Transfer Considerations

If the initial receiving hospital does not have the appropriate emergency or surgical specialist, transfer is necessary. The patient should be transferred in the most expeditious manner possible.

COMMON PITFALLS

- Failure to detect sensory, motor, and vascular complications or injuries to specialized tissues
- Failure to detect and remove foreign bodies
- Vasoconstrictors in anesthetic agents should not be used in areas with terminal end-arteriole blood supply.
- Removal of hair by a razor may increase the infection rate.
- Antiseptic agents should not contact the wound.
- Drain placement should not be used as a replacement for meticulous hemostasis, but should be reserved for removal of harmful collections of fluid.
- Tetanus toxoid adsorbed should not be administered indiscriminately to all patients with traumatic wounds, but should be considered part of the recommended tetanus prophylaxis regimens for the patient with traumatic wounds.
- The use of tissue adhesives should not preclude appropriate cleansing and exploration.
- Tissue adhesives should not be used in high-tension wounds or over joints.
- Not understanding the different indications for the use of butyl- and cyanoacrylate tissue adhesives.

APPENDIX

BALLISTICS

A collision between a missile and the human body represents a considerably higher level of energy absorption per unit volume of tissue than that encountered in an automobile accident. As tissues are struck by a missile, a combination of shear, tensile, and compressive forces interact to produce a relatively reproducible amount of destruction.[24] The two mechanisms of tissue disruption caused by a penetrating missile are the permanent and the temporary cavities. The penetrating missile or fragment destroys tissue by crushing it during penetration and punching a hole through the tissue. This hole, or missile track, is the permanent cavity. The cross-sectional area of the missile track is similar to the presenting area of the missile, and its dimensions are comparable for all soft tissues tested.

After passage of the missile, the walls of the permanent cavity are stretched outward radially. The maximum lateral tissue displacement delineates the temporary cavity. Tissue stretch is responsible for the damage of temporary cavitation. The resistance of tissue to stretch depends on tissue elasticity. The same stretch that causes moderate contusion and functional changes in relatively elastic muscle, skin, lung, and bowel wall can cause catastrophic disruption of the liver, heart, and brain. Muscle, skin, lung, and bowel wall are flexible and elastic, having the physical characteristics of good energy absorbers.

These permanent and temporary cavities are the sole wounding mechanisms of missiles. The sonic shock wave generated by supersonic missiles does not cause either tissue displacement or detectable damage. In general, based on missile velocity in projectile–tissue interactions, there are a minimum of five variables: projectile mass, projectile shape, projectile construction, projectile fragmentation, and target tissue type. Projectile fragmentation can greatly enhance the effects of the temporary cavity by providing points of weakness on which the stretching effects of cavitation are focused, rather than being absorbed evenly by the tissue mass. A muscle, which tolerates a temporary cavity stretch from a nonfragmenting bullet with little gross disruption, is severely damaged when the stretch follows its penetration by a fragmenting bullet.

Firearms include two basic types: rifled firearms and shotguns. A rifled firearm (pistol and rifle) has spiral grooves in its barrel and discharges hot gases, soot, powder grains, and bullet. Rifled bullets are rotated around their long axes by the rifling of the barrel to give them a sufficient gyroscopic stability to maintain the point-forward position while traveling through air. Bullets fired from a properly designed rifle barrel yaw (the yaw angle is the angle between the long axis of the bullet and the line of flight) no more than a few degrees during flight. However, this gyroscopic rotation may be insufficient to stabilize bullet point-forward travel in tissue; the development of bullet yaw in tissue can be an important determinant of injury.

Most handgun projectiles strike tissue at a speed less than 274 m/s. At this velocity, the predominant mechanism of tissue injury is the permanent cavity. There is some temporary cavitation, but tissue displacement is so small that there is no clinically detectable damage. Bullet shape, construction, and yaw make little difference at this velocity.

Rifle bullets are available in nonexpanding and expanding types. The nonexpanding rifle bullets are designed primarily for military use and strike tissue at speeds between 610 and 914 m/s. No deformation of the bullet occurs unless bone is struck. Nonexpanding bullets make a 180-degree rotation around their short axes (yaw) and terminate by traveling in a base-forward position. The distance traveled by a particular bullet in tissue before it begins rotation around its short axis is a relatively constant characteristic. The increase in size of the permanent cavity caused by the yawing bullet is determined by how much tissue the bullet strikes while traveling sideways. As the bullet yaws, there is also a marked increase in the temporary cavitation.

Most bullets of the expanding variety (soft-point or hollow-point) that are used for hunting are designed to deform on striking the tissue. They produce a marked increase in the size of the permanent cavity that occurs at a shallower depth. The expanding bullet also causes a large temporary cavity for the same reason that the yawing bullet does. For expanding bullets striking at more than 762 m/s, bullet fragmentation causes the major part of the permanent tissue destruction. As pieces of the bullet break off, they are flung radially outward by the centrifugal force of bullet rotation. Each fragment crushes its own path through tissue, ending up as far as 8 cm from the original path. This tissue, perforated a number of times, is stretched by temporary cavitation. The synergy between fragmentation and the temporary cavity causes massive tissue destruction.

Shotguns differ from rifles and pistols in that they have a smooth barrel that discharges hot gases, wad, and either multiple projectiles or a single projectile (rifled slug). Shot charges containing multiple projectiles spread out from the muzzle in a conelike pattern. The distance from the muzzle of the shotgun to the point of impact of the projectiles is a key determinant of the magnitude of injury. At short range (less than 6 m), the shot charge containing multiple projectiles results predominantly in a single-hole inshoot wound (diameter of less than or equal to 6 cm) that communicates with a deep underlying wound with massive tissue destruction. At this short range, soft-tissue impact deforms the individual pellets, increasing their original cross section with a concomitant increase in tissue crush or hole size. The multiple pellets result in severe disruption between the multiple wound channels. A gradual decrease in the amount of pellet deformation and tissue destruction occurs as the distance of the impact range increases. When the impact range exceeds 7 m, the multiple projectiles result in numerous discrete wounds that are not associated with underlying massive tissue destruction.

Shotguns also can discharge rifled slugs that are designed for killing larger animals. The muzzle velocity of rifled slugs (487 m/s) is approximately half that of nonexpanding, fully jacketed rifle projectiles. The rifled slug does not hold the point orientation that it has as it is propelled from the muzzle of the gun, but drifts toward a sideways orientation as it moves toward the target. The rifled slugs experience a 25% decrease in velocity as the impact range increases from 5 to 45 m. At short range (less than or equal to 45 m), the slug deforms on striking the tissue, thereby enhancing the size of the permanent and temporary cavities.

ACKNOWLEDGMENT

Dr. Richard Edlich is acknowledged for his excellent contribution to *The Clinical Practice of Emergency Medicine*, Second Edition.

References

1. Austin PE, Dunn KA, Eily-Cofield K, et al. Subcuticular sutures and the rate of inflammation in noncontaminated wounds. *Ann Emerg Med* 1995;25:328.
2. Baker MD, Lanuti M. The management and outcome of lacerations in urban children. *Ann Emerg Med* 1990;19:1001.
3. Bartfield JM, Gennis P, Barbera J, et al. Buffered versus plain lidocaine as a local anesthetic for simple laceration repair. *Ann Emerg Med* 1990;19;1387.
4. Bartfield JM, Lee FS, Raccio-Robak N, et al. Topical tetracaine attenuates the pain of infiltration of buffered lidocaine. *Acad Emerg Med* 1996;3:1001.
5. Bartfield JM, Jandreau SW, Raccio-Robak N. Randomized trial of diphenhydramine versus benzyl alcohol with epinephrine as an alternative to lidocaine local anesthesia. *Ann Emerg Med* 1998;32:650.
6. Berk WA, Osbourne DD, Taylor DD. Evaluation of the "golden period" for wound repair: 204 cases from a third world emergency department. *Ann Emerg Med* 1988;17:496.
7. Brogan GX, Giarrusso E, Hollander JE, et al. Comparison of plain, warmed, and buffered lidocaine for anesthesia of traumatic wounds. *Ann Emerg Med* 1995;26:121.
8. Bruns TB, Robinson BS, Smith RJ, et al. A new tissue adhesive for laceration repair in children. *J Pediatr* 1998;132:1067.
9. Cardany CR, Rodeheaver G, Thacker J, et al. The crush injury: a high risk wound. *J Am Coll Emerg Physicians* 1976;5(12):965.
10. Cruse PJE, Foord R. A five-year prospective study of 23,649 surgical wounds. *Arch Surg* 1973;107:206.
11. Cummings P, Del Beccaro MA. Antibiotics to prevent infection of simple wounds: a meta-analysis of randomized studies. *Am J Emerg Med* 1995;13(4):396.

12. deHoll D, Rodeheaver G, Edgerton MT, et al. Potentiation of infection by suture closure of dead space. *Am J Surg* 1974;127:716.
13. Dire DJ, Welsh AP. A comparison of wound irrigation solutions used in the emergency department. *Ann Emerg Med* 1990;19:704.
14. Dire DJ, Hogan DE. Double-blinded comparison of diphenhydramine versus lidocaine as a local anesthetic. *Ann Emerg Med* 1993;22:1419.
15. Dire DJ, Coppola M, Dwyer DA, et al. A prospective evaluation of topical antibiotics for preventing infections in uncomplicated soft-tissue wounds repaired in the ED. *Acad Emerg Med* 1995;2:4.
16. Edlich RF, Rodeheaver GT, Morgan RF, et al. Principles of emergency wound management. *Ann Emerg Med* 1988;17:1284.
17. Ernst AA, Marvez-Valls E, Mall G, et al. 1% Lidocaine versus 0.5% diphenhydramine for local anesthesia in minor laceration repair. *Ann Emerg Med* 1994;23:1328.
18. Ernst AA, Marvez-Valls E, Nick TG, et al. LAT versus TAC for topical anesthesia in face and scalp lacerations. *Am J Emerg Med* 1995;13:151.
19. Grant SAD, Hoffman RS. Use of tetracaine, epinephrine, and cocaine as a topical anesthetic in the emergency department. *Ann Emerg Med* 1992;21:125.
20. Haury B, Rodeheaver G, Vensko J, et al. Debridement: an essential component of traumatic wound care. *Am J Surg* 1978;135:238.
21. Hollander JE, Singer AJ, Valentine S, et al. Wound registry: development and validation. *Ann Emerg Med* 1995;25:675.
22. Hollander JE, Richman PB, Werblud M, et al. Irrigation in facial and scalp lacerations: does it alter outcome? *Ann Emerg Med* 1998;31:73.
23. Hollander JE, Singer AJ. State of the art laceration management. *Ann Emerg Med* 1999;34:356.
24. Johnson A, Rodeheaver GT, Durand LS, et al. Automatic disposable stapling devices for wound closure. *Ann Emerg Med* 1981;10:631.
25. Krause RS, Moscatti R, Filice M, et al. The effect of injection speed on the pain of lidocaine infiltration. *Acad Emerg Med* 1997;4:1032.
26. Magee C, Rodeheaver GT, Golden GT, et al. Potentiation of wound infection by surgical drains. *Am J Surg* 1976;131:547.
27. Mehta PH, Dunn KA, Bradfield JF, et al. Contaminated wounds: infection rates with subcutaneous sutures. *Ann Emerg Med* 1996;27:43.
28. Merguerian PA, Klein RB, Graven MA, et al. Intraoperative anaphylactic reaction due to latex hypersensitivity. *Urology* 1991;308:301.
29. Morgan WJ, Hutchison D, Johnson HM. The delayed treatment of wounds of the hand and forearm under antibiotic cover. *Br J Surg* 1980;67:140.
30. Ritchie AJ, Rocke LG. Staples versus sutures in the closure of scalp wounds: a prospective, double-blind, randomized trial. *Injury* 1989;20:217.
31. Rodeheaver GT, Halverson JM, Edlich RF. Mechanical performance of wound closure tapes. *Ann Emerg Med* 1983;12:203.
32. Rothnie NG, Taylor GW. Sutureless skin closure. A clinical trial. *BMJ* 1963;(October 26):1027.
33. Ruthman JC, Hendricksen D, Miller RF, et al. Effect of cap and mask on infection rates. *Illinois Med J* 1984;165:397.
34. Seropian R, Reynolds BM. Wound infections after preoperative depilation versus razor preparation. *Am J Surg* 1971;121:251.
35. Ship AG, Weiss PR. Pigmentation after dermabrasion: an avoidable complication. *Plast Reconstr Surg* 1985;75:528.
36. Singer AJ, Hollander JE, Quinn JV. Evaluation and management of traumatic lacerations. *N Engl J Med* 1997;337:1142.
37. Singer AJ, Hollander JE, Valentine SM, et al. Prospective randomized controlled trial of tissue adhesive (2-octylcyanoacrylate) vs standard wound closure techniques for laceration repair. *Acad Emerg Med* 1998;5:94.
38. Stevenson TR, Thacker JG, Rodeheaver GT, et al. Cleansing the traumatic wound by high pressure syringe irrigation. *J Am Coll Emerg Physicians* 1976;5:17.
39. Toriumi DM, Ogrady K, Desai D, et al. Use of 2-octylcyanoacrylate for skin closure in facial plastic surgery. *Plast Reconstr Surg* 1998;102:2209.
40. Whorl GJ. Repairing skin lacerations: does sterile technique matter? *Can Fam Physician* 1987;33:1185.
41. Quinn JV, Drzewiecki A, Li MM, et al. A randomized, controlled trial comparing a tissue adhesive with suturing in the repair of pediatric facial lacerations. *Ann Emerg Med* 1993;22:1130.
42. Quinn JV, Wells GA, Sutcliffe T, et al. Tissue adhesive vs. suture wound repair at one year: randomized clinical trial correlating early, three-month, and one-year cosmetic outcome. *Ann Emerg Med* 1998;32:645.

PART II

System Considerations

CHAPTER 96

Head Injuries

Pierre Borczuk and Stephen H. Thomas

Data from the National Institute of Neurologic Disorders and Stroke estimate that there are 2,000,000 cases of traumatic brain injury (TBI) in the United States per year, with approximately 500,000 patients requiring hospitalization. There are many more patients who do not seek any medical attention after mild head trauma. A review of U.S. mortality data reveals that head injury is responsible for 26% of trauma-related deaths. TBI deaths are bimodal, with a peak in the 15- to 24-year age group due to motor vehicle collisions and a second peak due mostly to falls in the 75 year and older group.[15] The economic impact of head injury in the United States is estimated to exceed $25 billion annually.[15]

The nature of crucial interventions in the emergency department (ED) depends on the severity of the head injury. In patients with a moderate TBI (Glasgow Coma Scale [GCS] score of 9 to 12) (Table 96.1) and a severe TBI (GCS less than or equal to 8), the goal is to adequately resuscitate the patient to prevent further brain injury. In patients with mild head trauma (GCS 13 to 15), the initial challenge is to identify which patients harbor a significant intracranial lesion that may lead to neurologic deterioration and require neurosurgical intervention.[1]

TABLE 96.1. Glasgow Coma Scale

EYE OPENING	
Opens spontaneously	4
Opens eyes to verbal command	3
Opens eyes to pain	2
Does not open eyes	1
VERBAL RESPONSE	
Alert and oriented	5
Converses but disoriented	4
Speaking but nonsensical	3
Moans or makes unintelligible sounds	2
No response	1
MOTOR RESPONSE	
Follows commands	6
Localizes pain	5
Movement or withdrawal to pain	4
Abnormal flexion (decorticate)	3
Abnormal extension (decerebrate)	2
No response	1
	3–15

CLINICAL PRESENTATION

The clinical presentation of patients with head trauma has been arbitrarily divided into mild, moderate, and severe categories based on the GCS. Over 80% of patients seen by emergency physicians will have a GCS of 13 to 15. Alcohol and other drugs are the most common causes of a loss in a GCS speech point. Patients may complain of headache, nausea, or vomiting; have a history of loss of consciousness or amnesia; or have external signs of head trauma. The possibility of a coexisting cervical spine injury should be considered, and the patient should be placed in spine precautions until injury has been ruled out. In addition, the patient with an altered sensorium from TBI may require radiologic imaging and observation to determine whether there is coexisting intraabdominal injury. Concurrent medical conditions may need prompt identification and treatment.

DIFFERENTIAL DIAGNOSIS

The dramatic presentation of the trauma patient should not detract the physician from considering other medical conditions that could have contributed to the trauma or that may be causing a change in mental status. Myocardial infarction, arrhythmia, a cerebrovascular event, or a seizure may have been the primary insult that precipitated the head trauma. Causes of hypotension, including infection and sepsis, and gastrointestinal bleeding should also be considered. Secondary factors should especially be considered in patients involved in single automobile collisions or falls. The etiology of an altered sensorium in a patient with TBI may also be multifactorial. One should consider metabolic causes, including hypo- and hyperthermia and hypo- and hyperglycemia. Drugs, both legal and illicit, may also play a role in the patient with a change in mental status, with alcohol the most common ingestion noted. Frequently, a complete and reliable history cannot be obtained, and proper management by the clinician requires maintenance of a broad differential diagnosis and systematic exclusion of medical conditions through objective testing.

EMERGENCY DEPARTMENT EVALUATION

The general goal in the management of patients with head trauma is to minimize further brain injury from secondary insults such as hypotension, hypoxia, herniation, seizures, and infection.[5] Prehospital information such as mechanism of injury, speed of vehicle, airbag deployment, height of a fall, loss of consciousness, posttraumatic seizure(s), or alterations in neurologic function since the accident will determine the need for urgent neuroimaging and for neurosurgical consultation. Other important historical components include preexistent history of cardiac disease or stroke, diabetes mellitus, as well as conditions that suggest the patient may be coagulopathic (cirrhosis, hemophilia, or, more commonly, warfarin anticoagulation).

The crucial initial intervention will be based on the patient's general appearance and vital signs. All resuscitations begin with the ABCs. Both hypotension (systolic blood pressure less than 90) and hypoxia (PaO_2 less than 60) have been shown to be independent predictors of poor outcome. Hypotension has been associated with a doubling of mortality, even when controlled for trauma to extracranial organ systems.[4] As many as one-fourth of patients with severe brain injury are hypoxic and hypotensive. The emergency physician needs to be aggressive at volume resuscitating hypotensive head injury patients, without the fear that excess fluids will lead to brain swelling and herniation.

After the initial ABCs, the clinician will complete the primary and secondary surveys, with focus on pupillary size, symmetry, and motor function. Intervention will be necessary if there is evidence of increased intracranial pressure (ICP) or signs of herniation, or if the patient demonstrates seizure activity. Seizures increase the metabolic requirements of the brain and produce hypoxia and hypercarbia, which promote secondary injury. Herniation from a laterally based intracranial hematoma causes downward pressure on the uncus, which in turn causes compression of the ipsilateral third cranial nerve, and therefore produces pupillary dilation on the same side as the hematoma (Fig. 96.1). The presence of a palpable cranial defect, which may be depressed; a fracture near the middle meningeal artery groove; "raccoon" eyes; hemotympanum; or a penetrating object suggests the presence of more severe intracranial pathology. Open skull fractures serve as an entry site for bacteria, with the associated risk of secondary infection. The same risk applies to patients who exhibit leaks of cerebrospinal fluid (CSF) from the ears or nose, suggesting injury to the basilar skull or cribriform plate, respectively.

In patients with mild head injury, ED evaluation focuses on the selection of those patients who need urgent cranial computed tomography (CT) scans, as well as the evaluation of any other medical conditions that might have led to the trauma. The prevalence of positive a CT scan in the GCS 13 to 15 group is in the 7% to 18% range, while the prevalence of neurosurgical lesions is approximately 1%.[15] A subgroup of patients, called "talk and deteriorate," present to the ED with GCS speech scores of 4 and 5, but, within 24 hours, have a total GCS less than or equal to 8. In this group, mortality is high, and the remaining survivors tend to be severely disabled. The most common CT finding is a subdural hematoma (SDH), which causes a greater than 10-mm midline shift (Fig. 96.2).[9]

Many investigators have tried to elucidate risk factors that identify those of these apparently low-risk patients who harbor significant intracranial pathology; however, an adequate triage algorithm that addresses those who need CT scans remains elusive. Some clinicians use the presence of loss of consciousness or amnesia as a marker to screen patients for urgent cranial CT scan.[1,6,11,16] The alcoholic patient who experiences head trauma is a frequent visitor to the ED. A strategy of serial observation until sobriety is achieved is a common one, although, as previously stated, once the patient has undergone deterioration, the outcome is significantly worse. Elderly patients also compose a high-risk subgroup for acute intracranial pathology. The anticoagulated patient is also likely to be in a high-risk subgroup, although this has not been studied in a prospective fashion.

Skull films should not be used to rule out intracranial injury, as they can have a false-negative rate as high as 80%.[10] Skull fractures, however, should raise the suspicion for further intracranial injury; the range of associated injury is between 7% and 50%, depending on the study reviewed.

Specific Lesions

Epidural hematomas (EDHs) usually result from a blow to the head that fractures the skull immediately adjacent to the middle meningeal artery (Fig.96.3). The arterial pressure is able to dis-

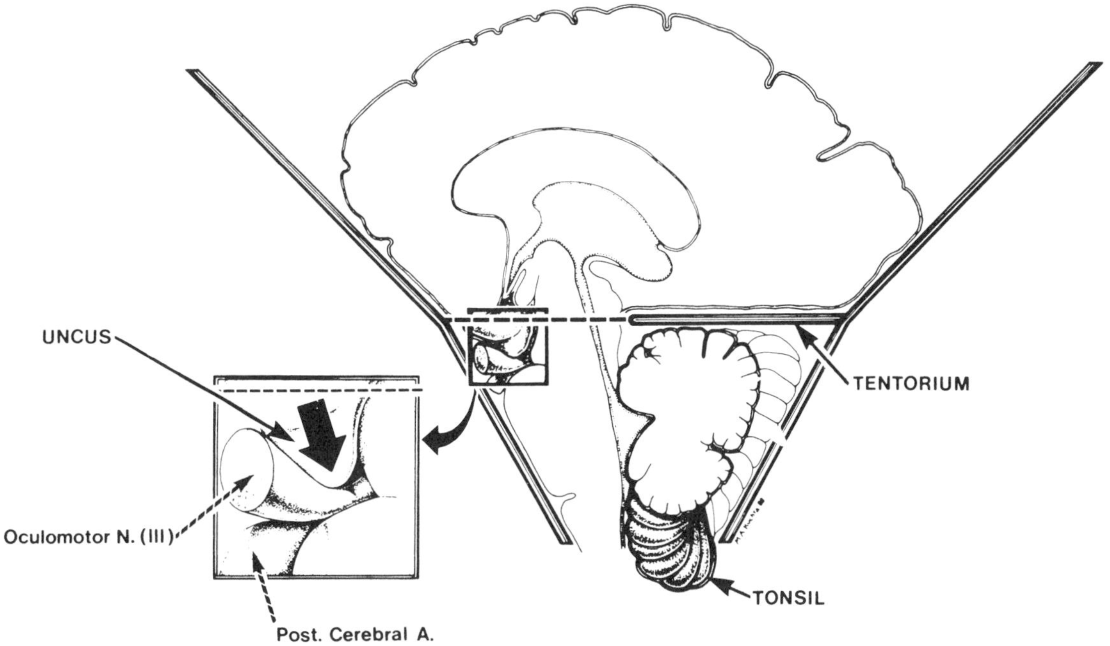

Figure 96.1. The intracranial cavity depicted as a funnel and subdivided by the tentorium into the supratentorial and the infratentorial compartments. Note herniation of the ipsilateral uncus with compression of the adjacent third cranial nerve and the posterior cerebral artery. Note also cerebellar tonsillar herniation with compression against the medulla.

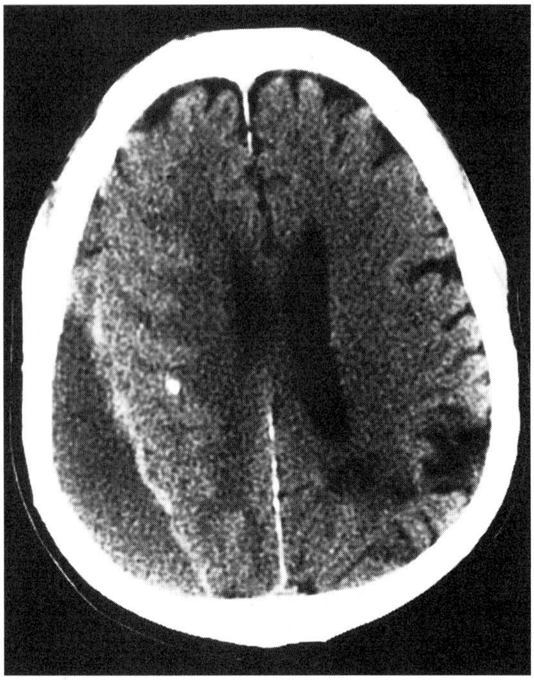

Figure 96.2. A male presents 3 weeks after a fall, with increased sleepiness and change in personality. Cranial CT scan demonstrates a chronic subdural hematoma.

sect the dura away from the inner skull table. This occurs less commonly in elderly patients, as the dura is more closely attached to the periosteum. The classic history of a blow to the head, loss of consciousness, lucid interval, and subsequent deterioration is seen in less than 30% of patients. EDH is an operative emergency: Prompt neurosurgical intervention is important, as operative patients who exhibit intact neurologic examinations have a mortality of close to 0. Mortality in unconscious operative patients is approximately 20%.[13] EDHs can also involve lower pressure dural structures, and these can develop over longer periods of time.

SDHs are more common than EDHs, and they can be present in as many as 70% of patients with moderate and severe head trauma. Individuals with brain atrophy (i.e., elderly and chronic alcoholic patients) are more susceptible to damage to bridging veins in the increased subdural space produced by rotational or acceleration–deceleration mechanisms. An SDH can be characterized by the time it takes for patients to become symptomatic after injury (Fig. 96.5). Acute SDH appears as a crescent-shaped, hyperdense (whiter than brain tissue) mass on CT scan. As the time to presentation increases, the SDH becomes less dense and can appear isodense when compared with brain tissue. Chronic SDHs are hypodense and become symptomatic more than 2 weeks after injury. In elderly patients, there may be no history of trauma, and patients may present with a more subtle change in cognition and mental status (Fig. 96.2). SDHs exhibit a higher mortality than do EDHs, which can approach 70%. Patients with signs of neurologic dysfunction usually require clot evacuation.

Cerebral contusions are the most common lesions seen on cranial CT scans in patients with mild head trauma. They are found in frontal, temporal, and occipital distributions and can frequently be seen on the inferior surfaces of these lobes (because the skull base has a rough interior). Contusions can vary from punctate (millimeters in size) to several centimeter collections of blood, necrotic brain tissue, and edema. Complications include worsening edema and rebleeding from injured vessels. Patients may exhibit focal neurologic deficits if contusions occur in the sensorimotor strip.

Penetrating Trauma

Penetrating head trauma most commonly results from firearm injuries. The projectile may traverse the skull or may ricochet intracranially, making anatomic prediction of injury clinically difficult. The overall mortality of patients who arrive in the ED is in excess of 60%. Cranial CT can demonstrate bleeding, skull fragments, bullet fragments, and intracranial air (pneumo-

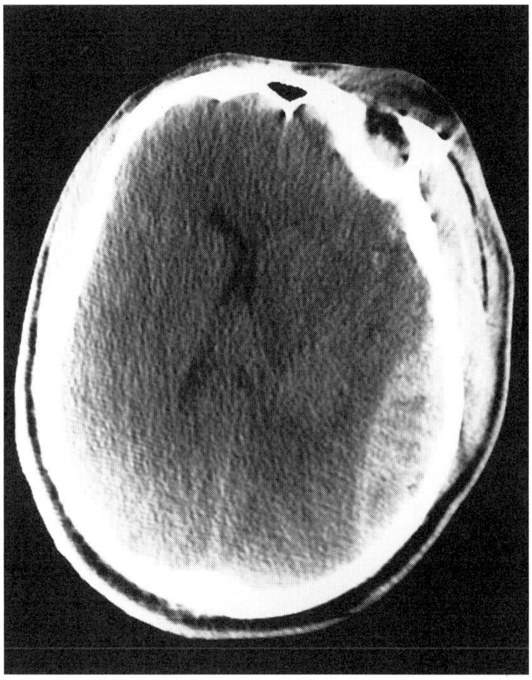

Figure 96.3. A case of an epidural hematoma. Note the classic biconvex, hyperdense lesion on the CT scan. This patient underwent urgent clot evacuation in the emergency department.

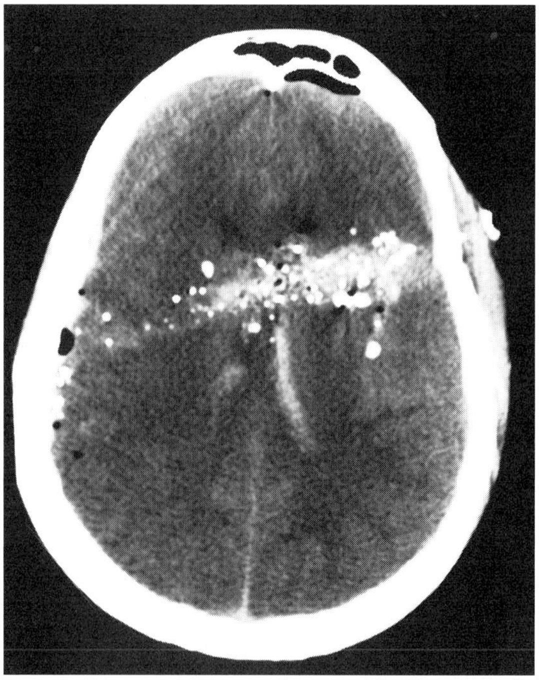

Figure 96.4. A self-inflicted wound from a handgun. CT scan reveals injury to the bilateral hemispheres and intracranial fragments of bone, bullet, and air.

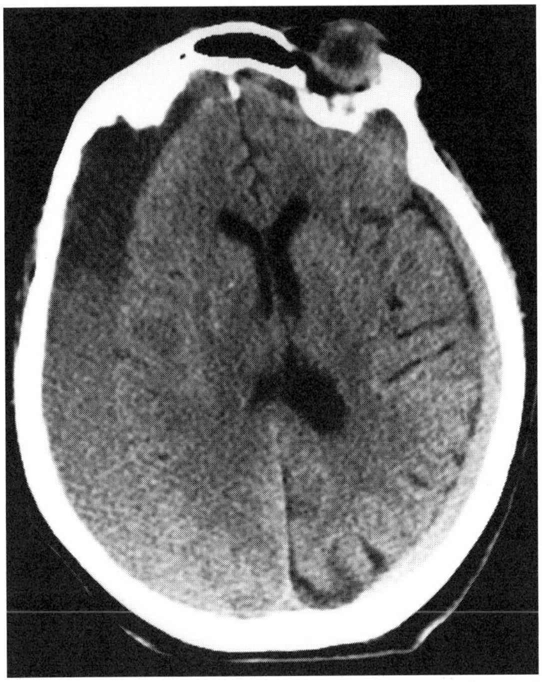

Figure 96.5. An elderly woman with change of mental status after a fall. Note the bilateral, subacute subdural hematoma, with varying densities and layering.

cephalus). Impaled objects should be left in place in the ED and removed in the operating room.

EMERGENCY DEPARTMENT MANAGEMENT

Prehospital

The prehospital phase begins secondary injury prevention. Airway management, intravenous (i.v.) access, and fluid resuscitation, as well as spinal immobilization, are initiated by trained paramedics. Determination of a scene GCS, detection and treatment of hypoglycemia, control of seizures, and "coma cocktail" administration can also begin in the prehospital phase. Prehospital personnel are frequently the sole source of information from scene witnesses regarding trauma mechanism or details regarding loss of consciousness.

Hospital

ED management begins with the primary survey and the ABCs. Managing the airway includes familiarity with rapid-sequence techniques.[17] Patients with an initial GCS less than or equal to 8 or a decreasing level of consciousness will be unable to protect their airway and will need intubation. As laryngeal stimulation can reflexively increase ICP, blood pressure, and heart rate, one should utilize drugs that blunt those increases (e.g., thiopental, fentanyl, and lidocaine) prior to intubation. One should be aware that the use of these drugs can also produce hypotension, especially in the patient who is hypovolemic from blood loss. The F_iO_2 should be set to 100%. A patient should not be hyperventilated unless signs of herniation exist. Shock needs to be treated aggressively with crystalloids and blood. Those studies that have suggested that patients with penetrating trauma have a better prognosis when managed with controlled hypotension did not include patients with head trauma. Patients must undergo frequent hemodynamic monitoring, cardiac monitoring, and pulse oximetry. Initial blood analysis, depending on both the degree of head injury and coexistent injury, may include complete blood count, including a platelet count, rapid glucose determination, blood urea nitrogen and creatinine, type and screen or cross, a coagulation profile, and a serum ethanol level. Urine screening for drugs of abuse may also be appropriate.

If the patient exhibits signs of intracranial hypertension, several therapeutic options are available.[4] Hyperventilation can decrease cerebral blood flow and decrease intracranial hypertension, as cerebral arteries constrict when there is a decrease in hydrogen ions in the CSF. A PCO_2 of 30 is the hyperventilation target. Because of regional imbalances in cerebral perfusion and loss of autoregulation in the early postinjury period, hyperventilation can worsen an ischemic insult. A growing body of evidence indicates that prophylactic hyperventilation in patients with TBI has been shown to be detrimental at 3 and 6 months postinjury.[12] Sedation, mannitol, and ICP bolt placement with direct drainage of CSF (if possible) demonstrate a lower risk-to-benefit ratio than hyperventilation.[3]

Osmotic diuresis is another modality used to reduce ICP.[3] Recommended doses of mannitol range from 0.25 to 1.0 g/kg. The duration of action of mannitol ranges from 90 minutes to more than 6 hours. Repeated mannitol use may allow it to concentrate within brain tissue, causing a reverse effect and a worsening of ICP. Like hyperventilation, mannitol should be used only in patients who exhibit signs of increased ICP. The patient's fluid status should be carefully monitored to avoid osmotic dehydration. When given as a rapid bolus, mannitol serves as a small-volume resuscitation fluid and will expand intravascular volume and cause an increase in cerebral blood flow.

While steroids can decrease edema in patients with intracerebral malignancies, they have no utility in head injury; this finding is supported by prospective randomized trials.[2] Active seizures are treated with either diazepam (0.1 mg/kg up to 5-mg bolus i.v. every 5 minutes) or lorazepam (0.05 mg/kg up to 2-mg bolus every 5 minutes), followed by i.v. phenytoin (13- to 18-mg/kg load). Seizure prophylaxis with phenytoin is also commonly used to prevent secondary injury in individuals with intracranial hematomas.

Once the patient's vital signs and neurologic function have been stabilized, the ED physician needs to complete the primary and secondary surveys. Patients with severe and moderate head injuries will require urgent cranial CT scanning. Any patient with a suspicion of significant intracranial injury will require prompt neurosurgical consultation. Severely compromised patients may go from the CT scanner directly to the operating room for hematoma evacuation. Emergency burr holes may be indicated in the patient who rapidly deteriorates despite the use of conventional ICP-lowering treatments. Neurologic intensive care management of patients with severe intracranial injury is based on the optimization of cerebral perfusion pressure (CPP). ICP and mean arterial blood pressure (MAP) are directly measured; then, using the relationship CPP = ICP − MAP, CPP is maintained at a minimum of 70 mmHg.

Magnetic resonance imaging (MRI) scans are generally more difficult to obtain and take longer to perform than cranial CT scans. They are useful in those instances when posterior fossa injuries, or nonhemorrhagic injuries, especially diffuse axonal injury, are suspected. Cranial CT scans are much better than MRI scans, however, for the detection of skull fractures.[14]

In the mild head trauma patient, the moderate risk factors listed in Table 96.2 may prompt the physician to order a cranial CT scan. Patients with cerebral contusions and nonoperative SDHs are generally admitted for observation with serial examinations, seizure prophylaxis, and follow-up imaging. Mild head trauma patients with negative CT scans who have a GCS of 15 and normal neurologic examinations are said to have suffered a concussion. Concussion is very common and ranks third high-

TABLE 96.2. Categorizations for Imaging Head Trauma Patients

LOW-RISK GROUP
Asymptomatic
Headaches
Dizziness
Scalp hematoma, laceration, contusion
MODERATE-RISK GROUP
History of altered consciousness
History of progressive headache
Alcohol or drug intoxication
Unreliable or inadequate history of injury
Age <2 yr (unless trivial injury)
Posttraumatic seizure
Vomiting
Posttraumatic amnesia
Multiple trauma
Serious facial injury
Signs of basilar skull penetration or depressed fracture
Possible skull penetration or depressed fracture
Suspected physical child abuse
HIGH-RISK GROUP
Depressed level of consciousness not clearly caused by alcohol or drug use or other causes
Focal neurologic signs
Decreasing level of consciousness
Penetrating skull injury or palpable depressed fracture

est in incidence among all neurologic diseases, behind migraine headache and herpes zoster. Symptoms include headache, nausea, blurry vision, unsteadiness, vertigo, and difficulty with concentration. The duration of symptoms noted after a head injury is related to the patient's age and the length of posttraumatic amnesia. Young patients with no loss of consciousness may have symptoms for days to weeks, while those who are 55 years old and older who exhibit prolonged posttraumatic amnesia may require months to clear, if they ever have a full recovery. Treatment options include analgesics, antiemetics, amitriptyline, as well as psychotherapy and neurorehabilitation.[18]

DISPOSITION

Patients who have documented intracranial pathology and depressed neurologic function (GCS less than or equal to 8) need to be managed in a facility with immediately available neurosurgical capability and an intensive care unit that can monitor ICP and CPP. This may require safe and expeditious transfer from facilities that lack these capabilities.

A negative cranial CT scan in patients with mild head trauma is useful in deciding who can be safely discharged home, even if a home observer is not available.[8] A patient with mild head trauma, in whom a cranial CT scan was not obtained, and who has a lack of risk factors for significant injury (e.g., minor mechanism, no loss of consciousness or amnesia), may be discharged home as long as the patient and a competent observer can understand and execute post–head injury discharge instructions. Patients with mild head injury, for whom a CT scan cannot be obtained, may be either transferred to an institution with CT capability or admitted for observation and frequent neurologic checks.

Protocols have been designed to help manage the patient with a sports-related head injury.[7] These management recommendations incorporate the concept and risk of the second impact (reports of severe neurologic sequelae after multiple minor concussions). Concussions are graded on the basis of duration of confusion (15 minutes is the threshold) or loss of consciousness (even if seconds). Depending on the number and grade of concussion, the physician may recommend that the athlete remain inactive for a day, a week, or the entire season.

COMMON PITFALLS

- Being concerned that fluid resuscitation in the hypotensive head-injured patient will worsen brain injury by increasing the risk for swelling. Persistent hypotension (systolic blood pressure less than or equal to 90) or hypoxia (PO_2 less than 60) is the greatest contributor to posttraumatic morbidity and mortality.
- Failing to consider that other conditions that contribute to changes in mental status, including stroke, hypoglycemia, or other drugs and toxins (including alcohol), may be present in the head-injured patient.
- Failing to remember that the use of hyperventilation and mannitol should be limited to patients with signs of intracranial hypertension. Prophylactic use of hyperventilation has been shown to be detrimental.
- Failing to remember that patients with mild head trauma may have an intracranial injury that can cause neurologic deterioration. Patient outcome is enhanced if these lesions can be identified before clinical decompensation.
- Failing to remember that skull films are not a substitute for a cranial CT scan, as skull films can have a false-negative rate of up to 80% for the detection of intracranial pathology.

References

1. Borczuk, P. Predictors of intracranial injury in patients with mild head trauma. *Ann Emerg Med* 1995;25:731.
2. Braakman R, Schouten HJ, Blaaw-van Dishoeck M, et al. Megadose steroids in severe head injury: results of a prospective double blind clinical trial. *J Neurosurg* 1983;58:326.
3. Bullock R, Chestnut RM, Clifton G, et al. *Guidelines for the management of severe head injury*. New York: Brain Trauma Foundation, 1996.
4. Chesnut R. Guideline for the management of severe head injury: what we know and what we think we know. *J Trauma* 1997;42(5)[Suppl]:19S.
5. Chesnut RM, Marshall LF, Klauber MR, et al. The role of secondary brain injury in determining outcome from severe head injury. *J Trauma* 1993;34:216.
6. Cheung DS, Kharasch M. Evaluation of the patient with closed head trauma: an evidence based approach. *Emerg Clin North Am* 1999;17:9.
7. Kelly J, Rosenberg JH. Diagnosis and management of concussion in sports. *Neurology* 1997;48:575.
8. Livingston DH, Loder PA, Koziol J, et al. The use of CT scanning to triage patients requiring admission following minimal head injury. *J Trauma* 1991;31:343.
9. Marshall LF, Toole BM, Bowers SA. The National Coma Data Bank. Part II. Patients who talk and deteriorate. Implications for treatment. *J Neurosurg* 1983;59:285.
10. Masters SJ. Evaluation of head trauma: efficacy of skull films. *Am J Radiol* 1980;135:539.
11. Miller EC, Derlet RW, Kinser D. Minor head trauma: is computerized tomography always necessary? *Ann Emerg Med* 1996;27:290.
12. Muizelaar JP, Marmarou A, Ward JD, et al. Adverse effects of prolonged hyperventilation in patients with severe head injury: a randomized clinical trial. *J Neurosurg* 1991;75:731.
13. Narayan RK. Closed head injury. In: Rengchary SS, Wilkens RH, eds. *Principles of neurosurgery*. London: Wolfe Publishing, 1994.
14. Orrison WW, Gentry LR, Stimac GK, et al. Blinded comparison of cranial CT and MR in closed head injury evaluation. *Am J Neuroradiol* 1994;15:351.
15. Sosin DM, Sacks JJ, Smith SM. Head injury—associated deaths in the United States from 1979–1986. *JAMA* 1989;262:2251.
16. Stein SC, Ross SE. Minor head injury: a proposed strategy for emergency management. *Ann Emerg Med* 1993;22:1193.
17. Walls RM. Rapid sequence intubation in head trauma. *Ann Emerg Med* 1993;22:1008.
18. Alexander MP. Mild traumatic brain injury: Pathophysiology, natural history, and clinical management. *Neurology* 1995;45:1253.

CHAPTER 97
Maxillofacial Injuries

Suzanne Moore Shepherd and Iris M. Reyes

Blunt and penetrating facial trauma are commonly seen in the emergency department. About 54% to 70% of all motor vehicle collision victims sustain facial injuries, accounting for an estimated 300,000 to 3 million maxillofacial injuries per year from this mechanism alone.[21] Blunt maxillofacial injuries have also been reported to occur with significant frequency in other settings, such as athletic events. Penetrating maxillofacial trauma is becoming increasingly common in the urban setting.[5,14] Unfortunately, up to one-fourth of women who sustain facial trauma do so in the setting of domestic violence.

The variety of mechanisms of injury and the complexity of the facial structures result in multiple potential injuries when the face is traumatized. In large series, the most frequently fractured facial bones are the zygoma, maxilla, and mandible; orbital, ethmoidal, and frontal injuries are less common.[4,9,21,23] As might be expected, the relative frequency of specific bony injuries is dependent on the setting of the injury and the likely destination of hospital: For example, community hospitals, where more minor vehicle crash victims and sporting and recreational injuries are more commonly seen, most frequently see blunt nose and mandible injuries; and urban trauma centers more commonly see midfacial and zygomatic injuries. These findings are generally consistent with the relative strength of individual bones of the face (Fig. 97.1).[22]

In the multiple trauma patient, the maxillofacial region is only one of many potential areas of injury, and the emergency physician must not allow the easily visible and often remarkable appearance of maxillofacial injuries to distract attention from more critical injuries. Maxillofacial injuries are rarely a proximate cause of death, and standard trauma priorities must not be altered because of an obvious facial abnormality. Underscoring the need to follow standard trauma care is the significant association of maxillofacial fractures with injuries to other body regions, most notably the head and neck.[3,4,9,22,23]

Both short- and long-term considerations are pertinent to the management of facial trauma. Facial injuries may require prompt attention early in the trauma resuscitation if disruption of bony integrity or hemorrhage results in airway compromise. Blood loss in the patient with maxillofacial trauma is rarely life-threatening, but the vascularity of the facial region can result, in some instances, in substantial hemorrhage. Timely planning of further evaluation and management of individual fractures is best discussed with the appropriate consultant. Cosmesis is likely to be a major concern of the patient and family, but discussion of further management and prognosis is best done by the surgical specialist in a more controlled setting.

CLINICAL PRESENTATION

The presentation of patients with significant maxillofacial trauma depends largely on the mechanism of injury. Patients who have sustained facial injuries as part of a significant blunt traumatic event (e.g., motor vehicle collision) are likely to present with multiple potentially injured body systems. The initial evaluation and stabilization of these patients should follow a standard multiple trauma resuscitation: Neglect of potentially serious chest or abdominal/pelvic injuries in the multiple trauma patient with distracting facial deformities is a dangerous error.

Victims of penetrating maxillofacial trauma are less likely to have sustained serious injuries to other organ systems (except the globe, head, and neck) but have a high likelihood (33%) of requiring urgent airway control.[14] In addition, the emergency physician must be particularly attuned to the possibility of central nervous system (CNS) injury, which has been reported to occur in about 20% of victims of penetrating facial trauma.[4,5,8,19] A patient who presents with decreased visual activity, visual field limitation, eye pain, limitation of extraocular movements, subconjunctival hemorrhage or lid laceration, diplopia, or infraorbital anesthesia should prompt a careful examination of the globe and periorbital area. Blindness occurs in 0.5% to 3.0% of patients who sustain facial fracture(s), particularly zygomatic, LeFort II, and LeFort III (2.2%).

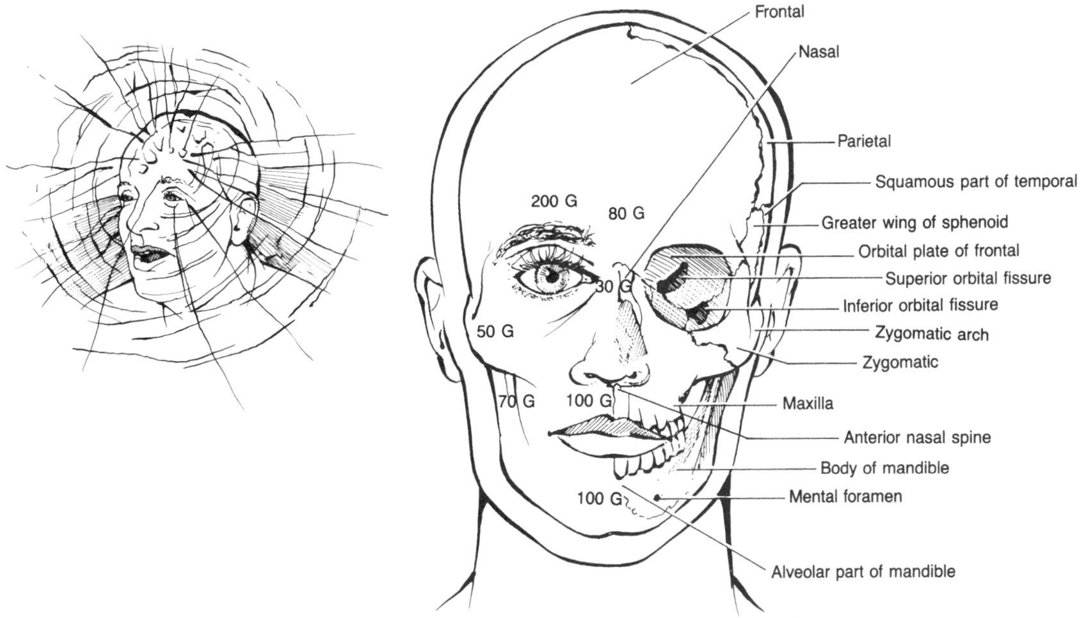

Figure 97.1. Relative strength of facial bones.

Maxillofacial injury becomes a treatment priority during evaluation of the multiple trauma patient primarily due to airway compromise. Airway problems may result from dislodged teeth or intraluminal hemorrhage, or from facial fractures, causing loss of structural support for the soft tissues surrounding the airway. Foreign bodies such as teeth, denture fragments, or other soft-tissue fragments may be aspirated, with resulting respiratory embarrassment.[11] In addition to the immediate risks of hemorrhage into the airway, edema and hematoma formation may compromise airway patency 24 to 48 hours after the injury.[17] This delayed risk of airway compromise has prompted some authors to recommend intubating patients who present with significant intraoral blood or moderate-size hematomas in the neck or face.[5]

The significant vascularity of facial structures may result in substantial blood loss with maxillofacial trauma, producing hypotension and, rarely, exsanguination. However, the tamponading effect of the facial musculature combined with the relative ease of application of direct pressure on most bleeding sites makes life-threatening hemorrhage relatively unlikely.[22]

DIFFERENTIAL DIAGNOSIS

The remarkable appearance of the patient with facial trauma sometimes distracts the examining physician from more serious injuries, but it also ensures that the diagnosis of severe facial trauma is rarely missed. The primary diagnostic goals in evaluating the facial trauma patient, once life-threatening injuries have been addressed, concern delineation of all bony and soft-tissue facial injuries.

Due to neurologic dysfunction from associated injuries or intoxication, the patient with facial trauma often cannot provide an adequate history. When confronted with the patient presenting with altered mental status and facial swelling, the physician should use the history provided by family or prehospital care providers, the initial physical examination, and screening laboratory tests to rule out other causative processes, including infection (e.g., cellulitis), immunologic reaction (e.g., angioedema, anaphylaxis), and atraumatic structural pathology (e.g., superior vena cava syndrome). The history should include the time of injury, the mechanism of injury, and possible loss of consciousness. Ocular complaints should be sought, in order not to miss important globe injuries and orbital fractures (see Chapter 99, "Eye Trauma"). The examining physician must always maintain a high index of suspicion for domestic violence and pediatric and elder abuse.

EMERGENCY DEPARTMENT MANAGEMENT

The initial evaluation of the patient with maxillofacial trauma should follow standard trauma resuscitation. The need for meticulous trauma evaluation in patients with facial fractures has been underscored by multiple series describing serious associated thoracic, abdominal, orthopedic, and neurologic injuries.[4,7,9,14] Maxillofacial injuries are seldom life-threatening, but other organ system injuries occur frequently and are associated with significant morbidity and potential mortality.[4,5,7,9,14,23]

Head injury is the most prevalent associated injury. This association has prompted the recommendation that routine head computed tomography (CT) be performed in all patients with blunt or penetrating maxillofacial injuries who have a suspicious mechanism of injury or neurologic deficit.[5,23] Studies have cast significant doubt on the classical association of maxillofacial trauma with cervical spine (c-spine) injury.[5,23] Until this issue is resolved, liberal use of plain c-spine radiography is recommended, in keeping with both routine trauma management and the need to clear the c-spine before performing certain facial imaging techniques.

The airway is the first consideration in patients with maxillofacial trauma. The potential for respiratory embarrassment in a patient with facial trauma is significant; many mechanisms and treatment strategies for airway compromise have been described.[11] Any portion of the airway may be blocked by hemorrhage or soft-tissue swelling or edema. Soft-tissue swelling and edema usually do not cause airway compromise until hours after the patient's initial presentation to the emergency department, but the significant risk of airway impingement by progressive swelling is one reason for the liberal use of early prophylactic airway control. In patients who exhibit continued blood loss from accessible vessels despite direct pressure, hemorrhage control may be achieved by packing open wounds or the nose. Major vessel embolization or ligation is sometimes needed to provide definitive control of facial bleeding.

Maxillofacial trauma can result in airway compromise at the nasal, oropharyngeal, or laryngeal level. Collapse of the nasal airway can result from posteroinferior displacement of maxillary fractures. In this instance, definitive control of the airway and hemorrhage may be achieved by correcting fracture fragment alignment by anterior traction on the maxilla.[8] The oropharyngeal airway may also be occluded by a prolapsing tongue, the anterior attachments of which have been disrupted by central mandibular fracture. Anterior traction on the tongue with a traction suture or towel clip should reestablish airway patency in these patients. Maxillofacial trauma may also be associated with direct trauma to the neck, causing airway collapse at the level of the larynx. Cricothyreotomy is possible if the level of injury is above the larynx. In patients with injuries at or inferior to the level of the larynx, endotracheal intubation may be attempted, but tracheostomy is often necessary. If tracheal injury is inferior to a level at which tracheostomy will provide an adequate airway, emergent consultation by a thoracic surgeon is warranted.[11,24]

Urgent airway control by oral endotracheal intubation or the creation of a surgical airway is reportedly needed in one-third of patients sustaining gunshot wounds to the face.[14] As such, early intubation is recommended for all patients who exhibit hemodynamic instability or who have significant intraoral bleeding or facial hematomas.[5] The justification for aggressive airway intervention in victims of penetrating trauma lies primarily in the potential for airway lumen compromise by expanding hematoma, intraluminal bleeding, or collapse of surrounding soft tissues.

Other factors support early, aggressive airway control in patients with significant blunt or penetrating facial trauma. Significant technical difficulties may be encountered in patients who deteriorate and require airway intervention on an emergent basis. In addition, stability of the airway should always be ensured in patients who will have a prolonged stay in the radiology suite. Anatomic distortion and the risk of tube misplacement preclude nasal endotracheal intubation in the patient with significant midface trauma. If there is any question concerning the ability to perform bag-valve-mask ventilation or rapid-sequence orotracheal intubation easily, jet insufflation or cricothyreotomy equipment should be immediately available. The intubating physician should first assess the degree of potential difficulty for both intubation and mask-valve ventilation (Mallinpati criteria). One alternative may be awake intubation. Fiberoptic intubation may provide another choice, depending on the injuries sustained and the comfort level of the operator. The c-spine should be cleared or adequately immobilized until clearance is possible. Certain diagnostic imaging, due to required patient positioning, may need to wait until c-spine immobilization is discontinued.

In the patient with facial trauma, the "B" of the trauma ABCs is much less of a problem than airway maintenance. Breathing is rarely problematic in patients with isolated maxillofacial injury. Patients with severe injury are usually intubated and mechanically ventilated. CNS injury is the most likely explanation for hypoventilation in the setting of facial trauma. Continuous pulse oximetry, which is indicated for any severely injured patient, is a helpful monitor of ventilatory adequacy in patients with facial trauma.

Circulation problems in the patient with maxillofacial trauma may be due to bleeding from traumatized vascular structures of the face. However, hypovolemic shock in such patients should be assumed to be due to other injuries until proven otherwise. Standard trauma resuscitation should identify and address hemorrhage from intrathoracic, abdominopelvic, or extremity trauma.

The general approach to hemorrhage should include direct pressure both externally and internally (such as with anterior and posterior nasal packing) where indicated. A steady flow of blood from the nasal or oral cavities, accompanied by bleeding into the soft tissues of the face, may be produced by closed fractures of the maxilla, nose, and ethmoids. If blood loss is not expeditiously addressed, ongoing hemorrhage may be sufficient to cause hypotension and coagulopathy. Blind vessel clamping is contradicted due to possible inadvertent damage to other major structures, such as the facial nerve or parotid duct. Manual reduction of fracture fragments may cease hemorrhage; this is especially helpful in some Le Fort fractures or dislocations. Urgent surgical consultation is indicated if the preceding steps do not control hemorrhage.

The initial examination should include assessment for basilar skull fracture and cerebrospinal fluid (CSF) leakage. Basilar skull fracture may be indicated by hemotympanum, or later by periorbital (raccoon eyes) or retroauricular ecchymosis (Battle's sign). CSF rhinorrhea may be found in patients with naso-orbito-ethmoid, frontal sinus, Le Fort, or orbital roof fractures. The CSF leak is created when a bony fracture (accompanied by interruption of the periosteum and mucosa) of the anterior cranial fossa causes disruption of the arachnoid and dural layers. Identification of CSF rhinorrhea is important as a diagnostic clue to underlying fractures and, depending on individual neurosurgical preferences, serves as an indication for prophylactic antibiotics. The filter paper ring sign and assessment of rhinorrhea fluid for glucose and protein may help determine whether CSF is present in nasal drainage. Definitive treatment for CSF rhinorrhea associated with facial fractures is open reduction and fixation of the bony injury.[6]

After the ABCs of trauma and any injuries to other organ systems are addressed, the emergency physician should perform a thorough and directed examination of the maxillofacial region. Performing an optimal physical examination of the face is challenging due to anatomic complexity, swelling, lacerations, pain, and altered level of consciousness. These difficulties, in addition to the often significant distraction produced by the impressive appearance of facial trauma, underline the importance of proceeding with an orderly physical examination.

Some general comments regarding the traumatized facial region should help organize the approach to physical examination. The first steps in evaluating patients with maxillofacial trauma are inspection and palpation; improved imaging techniques have not relegated physical examination to a minor role. Asymmetry, loss of contour, ecchymosis, and hemorrhage are important visual clues to soft-tissue and underlying bony injuries (Fig. 97.2). Remember to view the face from the superior, lateral, and inferior positions, as each may reveal injury not obvious from other views. Also examine for facial function; for example, have the patient smile. Palpation may reveal step-off, tenderness, crepitance, or bony mobility in patients with fractures. Subcutaneous crepitus is usually present in patients with fractures involving the sinuses.

Mandible Fractures

In several series, the mandible has been described as the most commonly fractured facial bone.[2,9,23] Figure 97.3 illustrates sites and incidence of mandible fractures.

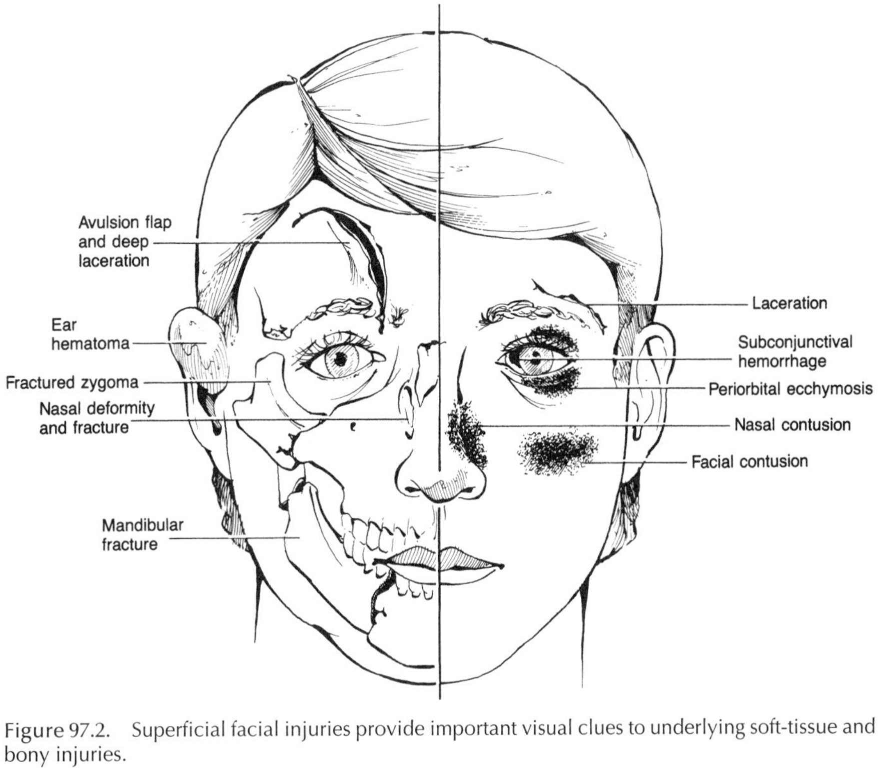

Figure 97.2. Superficial facial injuries provide important visual clues to underlying soft-tissue and bony injuries.

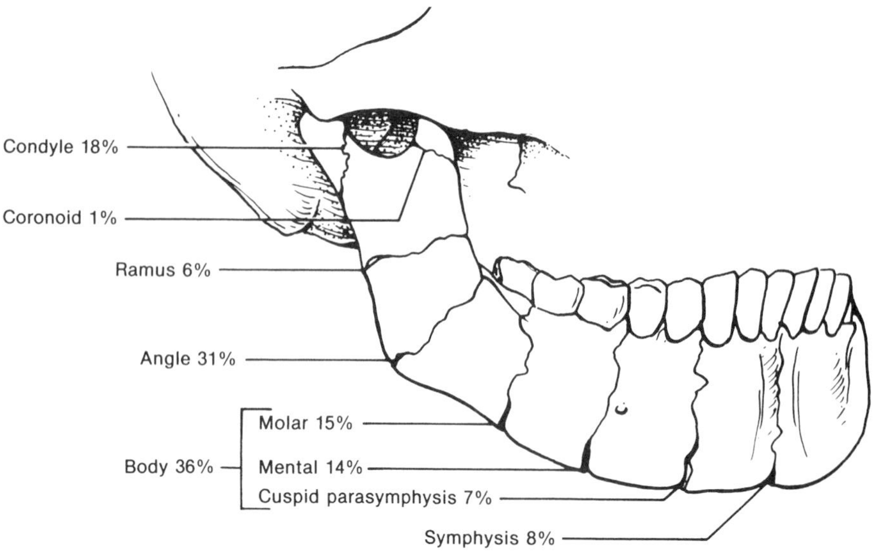

Figure 97.3. Mandible fractures: sites and incidence.

Evaluation

Inspection of the patient's jaw for asymmetry is the first step in the evaluation of possible mandibular fracture. When a fracture is present, the jaw is often deviated toward the injured side; with a unilateral dislocation, the mandible is deviated toward the contralateral side. Preauricular swelling or bleeding from the external auditory canal may indicate a condylar fracture, which can be notoriously difficult to identify on plain radiographs.[1]

The patient is asked whether occlusion feels normal, as bite discrepancy suggests mandibular or maxillary fracture. The sensitivity of the proprioceptive receptors of the teeth allows for detection of as little as 1 to 2 mm of bite discrepancy.[22] After inspection and palpation of the mandible, normal condylar excursion is assessed: The examiner's finger is inserted into the external ear canal and the patient is instructed to open and close the mouth. In the patient with pain and without obvious fracture, the tongue depressor test may prove useful. A positive test, suggestive of possible fracture, is elicited when the patient reflexly opens his mouth when a tongue depressor clenched between the teeth on the suspect side is twisted by the examiner. [22] Finally, the lower lip and mandibular dentition are assessed for sensory function. Abnormalities of sensation in these regions indicate mental nerve injury, possibly secondary to mandibular fracture.

If mandibular fracture is suggested by the history or physical examination, plain radiographs are indicated (Fig. 97.4). The posteroanterior view provides information on the symphysis and body of the mandible, and the lateral oblique view adds delineation of the mandibular rami. Towne's projection demonstrates the mandibular rami and condyles. The 180-degree panoramic view provides good visualization and definition of most of the mandible, except the symphysis.

The most frequently missed mandibular fracture is the condylar fracture. This is sometimes inadequately imaged with plain films. A facial CT scan is indicated when clinical suspicion of condylar fracture persists despite negative plain radiography.[14] Advanced imaging sometimes provides the surgeon with additional information to help plan the operative management of the fracture (Fig. 97.5).

Management

Open mandibular fractures require admission for surgical therapy and intravenous antibiotic coverage of oral pathogens. Penicillin is the drug of choice, with clindamycin and first-generation cephalosporins serving as alternatives. Mandible fractures secondary to penetrating trauma are, by definition, open fractures, and thereby also merit hospital admission. These fractures should probably undergo open reduction, because of the high rate of associated complications.[14] Many closed mandibular frac-

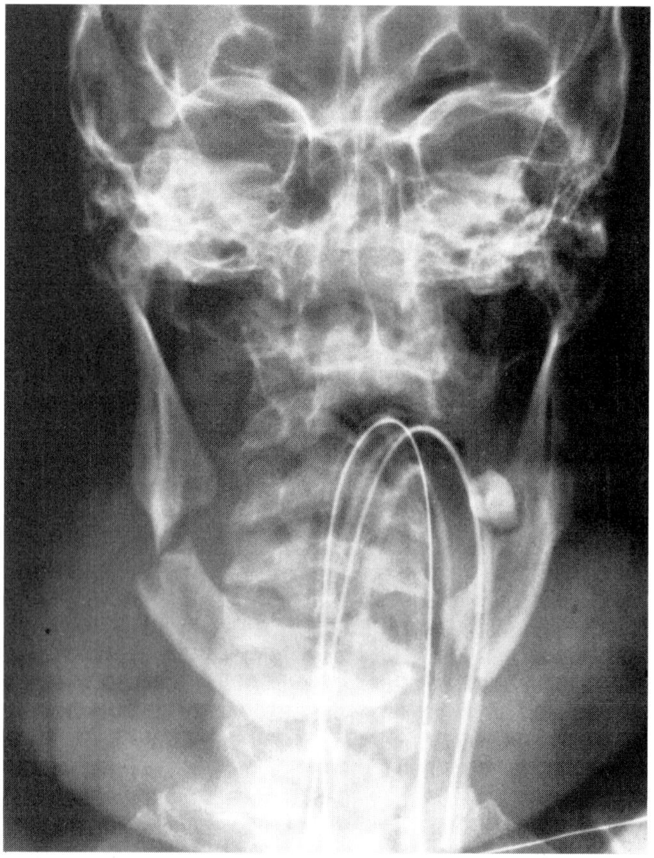

Figure 97.4. Plain PA radiograph of the mandible shows displaced fractures of the mandible. Illustrated are fractures near the right angle, one within the body, and one just to the left of the symphysis. There are also bilateral fractures of the maxillary antra, involving the lateral walls and anterior walls. There is a slightly displaced fracture involving the lateral wall of the right orbit at the zygomaticofrontal suture.

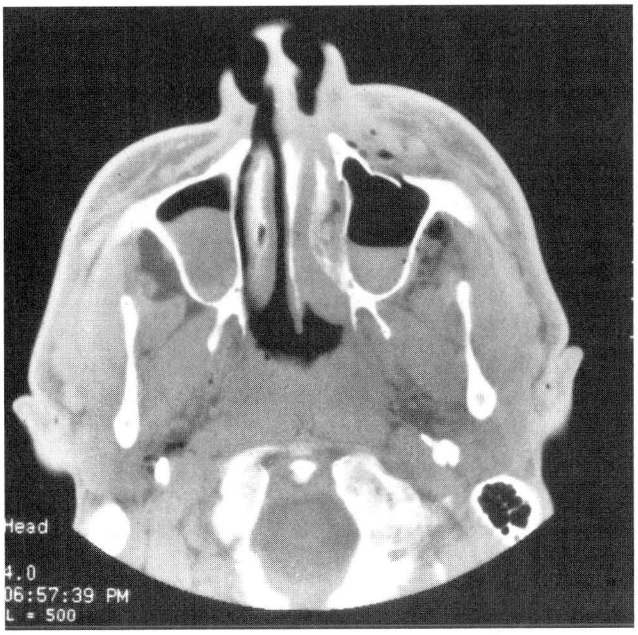

Figure 97.5. Facial CT image. There are multiple eggshell-like fractures involving the wall of both maxillary antra. Both maxillary antra are opacified with blood. The nasal passages are filled with soft-tissue density, suggesting blood and contused tissues.

tures can be treated on an outpatient basis with a Barton's bandage, pain medication, and a liquid diet. The specific treatment plan should be formulated with the appropriate consultant.

Maxillary Fractures

Maxillary fracture is the most common finding in patients sustaining penetrating facial trauma. These also occur quite frequently in victims of blunt trauma.[14,23]

Evaluation

Fractures of the maxilla may be detected by inspection but are usually more easily identified by palpation. Anterior and lateral inspection for symmetric contour of the midface may be the best means of identifying impacted (i.e., immobile) maxillary fractures, which are relatively common due to the large forces required to produce midface fractures.[22]

Palpation of the maxillary structures follows inspection. Special attention is given to crepitus, which indicates possible maxillary sinus fracture. Next, the examiner firmly grasps and exerts pressure on the upper alveolar ridge (not the teeth), checking for abnormal midface mobility (Fig. 97.6). In patients with facial mobility on maxillary manipulation, the fracture is further characterized by delineating the mobile portions of the midface.

In the patient with a Le Fort I fracture, the nose does not move with the abnormally mobile alveolar ridge. The Le Fort I fracture line is a transverse separation of the hard palate from the lower portion of the pterygoid plate and nasal septum (Fig. 97.7). The Le Fort II, or pyramidal, fracture is associated with mobility of the nose and the alveolar ridge of the maxilla. This fracture line separates the central maxilla and palate from the rest of the face. Craniofacial dysjunction (Le Fort III fracture) is associated with separation of the entire facial skeleton from the cranium; maxillary excursion reveals mobility of the entire face (including the inferior and lateral orbital rim). In actual practice, pure Le Fort fractures are much less common than unilateral or bilaterally mixed (e.g., left Le Fort I with right Le Fort II) maxillary fractures.

Physical findings with maxillary fractures are tenderness, loss of contour, and crepitus (with involvement of maxillary sinuses). Maxillary (or zygomatic) fracture may result in damage to the infraorbital nerve, manifested by paresthesias of the upper lip and central incisors. Facial nerve injury may also accompany maxillary fractures, with resultant facial muscle paralysis. When there is trauma to the lateral midface, especially if there is clinical suggestion of facial nerve injury, the physician should carefully examine cheek wounds for clear or pink fluid leakage, representing possible parotid duct damage.[11]

Management

Assuming the ABCs are assessed and stable, the clinician's next step is to order appropriate imaging of the face. In the patient with trauma sufficient to warrant cranial CT scanning, the answer is simple: Coronal scan the facial bones simultaneously.[16] For patients with physical findings consistent with facial trauma and no indication for cranial CT, the decision is more difficult, but specialists still recommend beginning the radiographic workup with coronal cut facial CT scanning and proceeding to three-dimensional CT scanning if needed.[20] The rationale for the direct use of facial CT scanning is that it delineates fractures clearly and is thus a prerequisite to preoperative surgical planning; also, plain films are time consuming to perform and usually add no additional information. This relatively recent change in the choice of radiographic imaging for patients with midface trauma is a result of evolution in the surgical therapy of these fractures. Closed reduction techniques required only plain radiographs to identify the presence of fractures. Current optimal surgical therapies require careful delineation of facial architecture, which can be achieved only with CT scanning.[1]

If the patient's condition permits, optimal management of maxillary fractures dictates that the midface should be imaged in the coronal plane.[1] This approach has the added benefit of allowing subsequent three-dimensional reconstruction of the image. Three-dimensional CT scanning offers superior fracture delineation and preoperative planning, and may reduce the time spent in the operating room. However, this procedure is currently too expensive to be used in every patient.[18,20] MRI has little role in the emergency department evaluation of the patient with suspected maxillary (or other facial) injuries, as CT scanning is more readily available and provides better information in a shorter period of time.[7] For patients whose history suggests significant facial trauma but who have no findings consistent with maxillofacial fracture, plain radiography provides a reasonable, cost-conscious screening examination.[13,22]

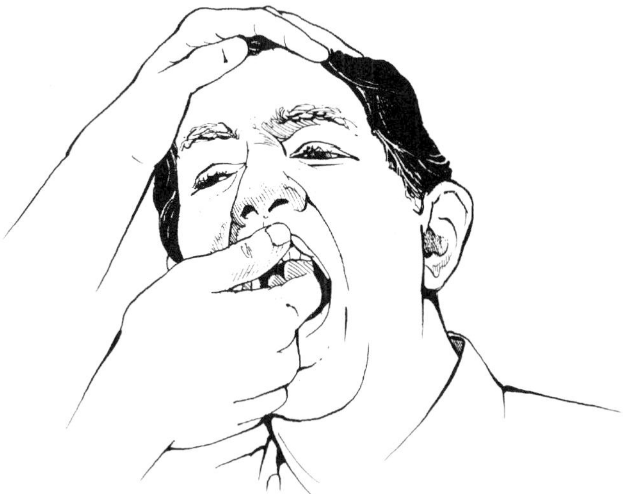

Figure 97.6. Checking for abnormal midface mobility.

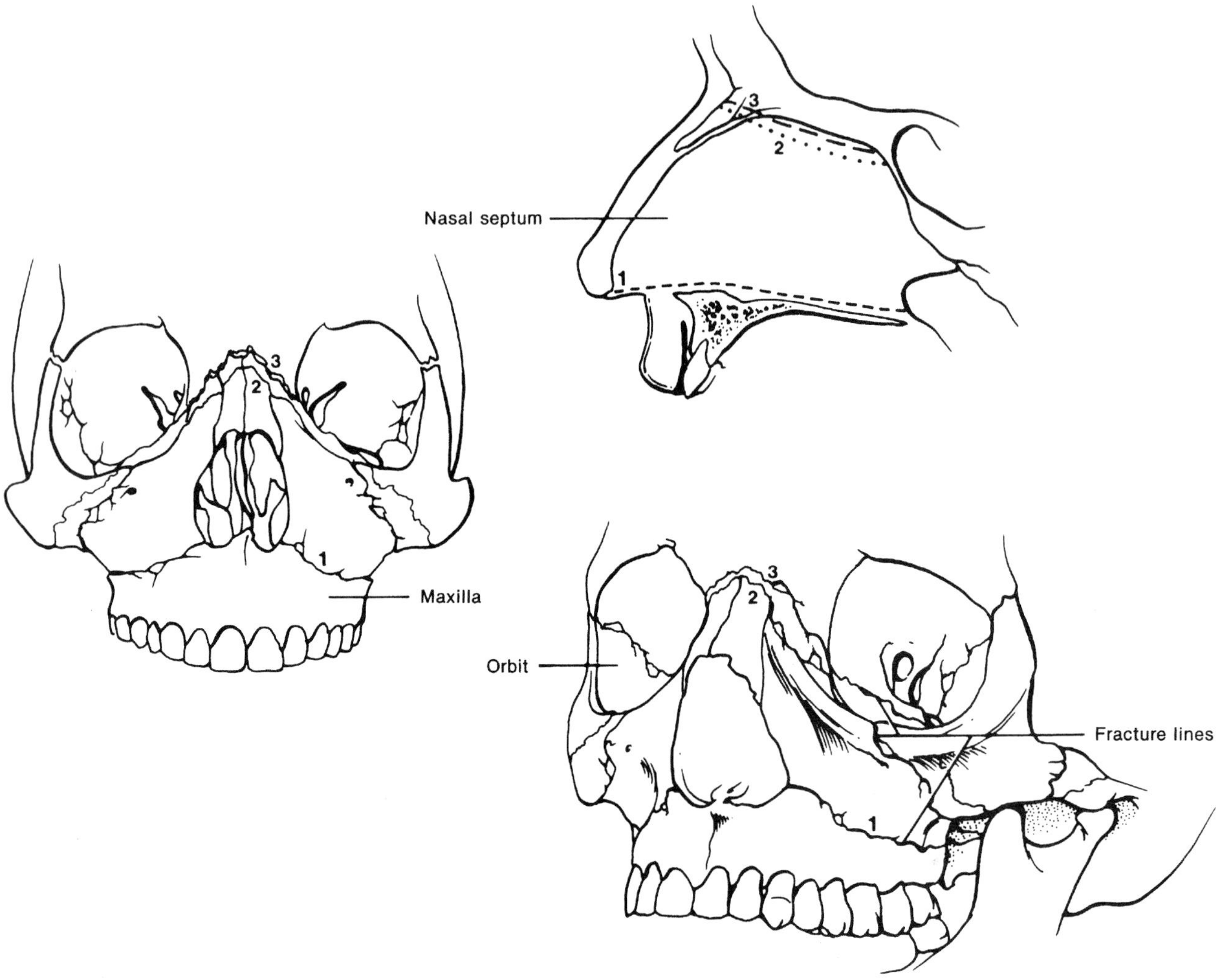

Figure 97.7. Lines of fracture in Le Fort I, Le Fort II, and Le Fort III. Fractures are shown from different views.

Surgical specialists should be consulted early when fractures are identified, as an increasing number of facial surgeons have correlated early management with improved outcome.[6,16,20] For patients with midface injuries secondary to penetrating injury, the need for early surgical consultation remains, but early open reduction is probably contraindicated due to the high risk of complications.[14]

Orbital Fractures

Trauma to the orbital regions may result in a number of injury patterns. Almost always, direct ocular trauma results in traumatic iritis. Injury to virtually any part of the eye may occur when the globe is impacted with sufficient force.[12] Injuries occurring as a result of trauma to the globe are discussed in detail in Chapter 99, "Eye Trauma." Relevant to the current discussion is the blowout fracture (Fig. 97.8). Orbital floor fractures, which may result in development of entrapment when intraorbital soft tissues herniate into the maxillary sinus, account for as many as one-fifth of facial fractures.[21]

Evaluation

Inspection of the patient's orbital region sometimes provides clues to the presence of fracture. Eyelid edema or ecchymosis, enophthalmos or hypophthalmos, or obvious inability of the patient to deviate the involved eye are pertinent findings on visual examination of the patient with orbital region fractures.[12,19]

Palpation of the orbital rims often reveals any fracture(s) present. The medial orbital rim may be palpated from both sides with the aid of a padded hemostat or alligator forceps very gently placed in the nares as the external orbital rim is palpated with the fingers; any movement elicited is abnormal.

Orbital blowout fracture associated with entrapment syndrome may also be identified by a patient complaint of diplopia or inability to deviate the eye upward. Infraorbital anesthesia or crepitus may be present in orbital fractures involving the infraorbital nerve or sinuses, respectively.

When there are findings consistent with fracture in the orbital region, the emergency physician's first step is a meticulous evaluation of the globe. The ocular examination takes precedence because certain injuries (e.g., globe rupture) benefit from early diagnosis and management, and because an adequate examination may be impossible to perform after a few hours of swelling and edema formation.

Once ocular injuries have been ruled out, or identified and appropriately managed, attention shifts to radiographic evaluation of the orbital region.

Blowout fractures most commonly involve the orbital floor, but the medial, lateral, and superior walls may also fracture (in that order).[17] The blowout fracture is said to be "pure" if the central area of the orbital wall is the only portion fractured; impure blowout fractures extend to the orbital rim. Impure fractures are often found in association with maxillary, nasoorbital, and frontal bone fractures.[17] The emergency physician identifying

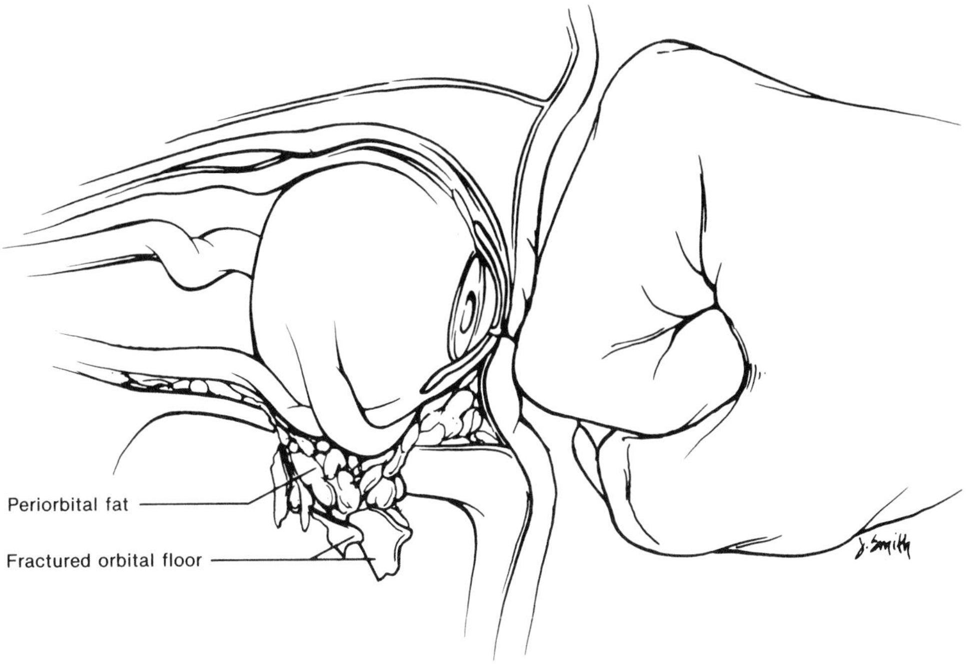

Figure 97.8. Blowout fracture.

one of these injuries should carefully search for an associated blowout fracture and entrapment syndrome. The orbital wall defect created by a blowout fracture may be filled with a variety of soft tissues; orbital fat is most commonly entrapped. However, the extraocular muscles may become involved, resulting in the entrapment syndrome. This syndrome, which almost always involves the inferior rectus muscle, is characterized by diplopia or failure of conjugate gaze. Muscle function is impaired, but the entrapment syndrome is usually caused by herniation, not of the muscles, but of fibrous septae that provide positional support for the extraocular muscles.[17]

Management

When a low index of suspicion exists, plain radiographs provide a cost-conscious screening examination for fractures in the orbital region. When there is significant question about the presence of a blowout fracture, CT scanning in the horizontal and coronal planes is the optimal imaging study.[17]

Management of orbital blowout fractures has been controversial, but guidelines for therapy provide a reasonable basis for decision making in the emergency department.[17] In cases associated with minimal displacement, no entrapment, and no diplopia, the patient may be treated as an outpatient with next-day surgical follow-up. Absolute indications for surgery include acute enophthalmos or hypophthalmos or muscular entrapment with mechanical gaze restriction. Contraindications for surgery include hyphema, retinal tears, and globe perforation, as soft-tissue injuries of the eye may be aggravated by surgery for blowout fractures. Patients with a single eye should not undergo surgical exploration and repair for blowout injuries, as the small but real risk of visual loss from the operation outweighs the potential benefits of the procedure. Timing of surgery for orbital blowout injuries is critical. If repair is attempted too soon, the outcome can be compromised by incomplete diagnosis, localized swelling, excess hemorrhage in tissues in the inflammatory phase of healing, or problems resulting from associated traumatic injuries. If surgery is delayed too long, however, bones will have fused and scarring may be established. A period of 7 to 10 days appears optimal. This decision is left to the consultant, who should see the patient the next day if the fracture is to be managed on an outpatient basis.[17]

Nasal Fractures

Many (if not most) significant fractures of the midface are associated with fractures of the nasal bones. Other than prompting evaluation for airway, hemorrhage, and septal hematoma, these fractures do not play a significant role in the emergent management of patients with significant facial trauma. Isolated nasal fractures are very common, however, and the emergency physician should be able to manage most patients with these injuries.

Evaluation

Inspection is the primary means to make the diagnosis of nasal fractures, which require no immediate treatment other than ice packs and analgesia if alignment is satisfactory. If radiography is required to make the diagnosis of nasal fracture, the fracture is unlikely to require significant therapy in the emergency department; x-rays are, therefore, not recommended in the initial evaluation of patients with suspected nondisplaced nasal fractures. Depression of nasal contour, with or without lateral deviation, usually indicates a fracture or dislocation of the nasal cartilage or bone.

After inspection, the most important part of the physical examination of the patient with nasal trauma is careful speculum examination of each naris to identify lacerations or septal hematomas and ability to breathe through each naris. A septal hematoma may appear as a bulging blue mass inside the septum, or it may be identified during palpation as a doughy area of the septum.

Management

If a fracture with malalignment is identified, the emergency physician can anesthetize the nose with cocaine or tetracaine-soaked pledgets and perform closed reduction. Some ear, nose, and throat (ENT) surgeons prefer to reduce the fracture themselves, however, either acutely or after swelling has subsided. The emergency physician and consulting plastic or ENT surgeon

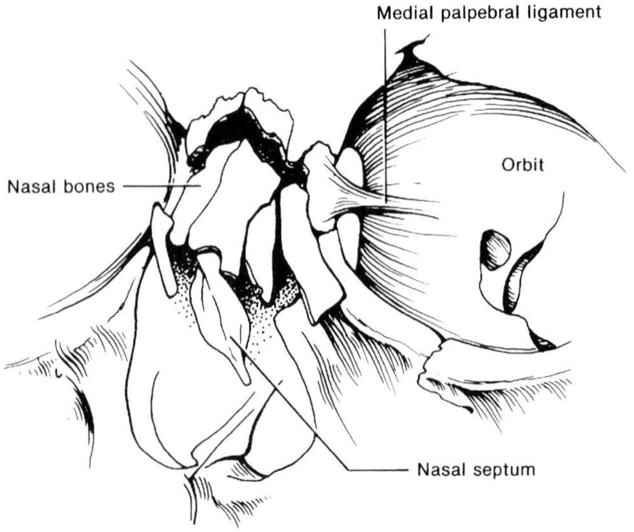

Figure 97.9. Nasoethmoidal fractures.

should prospectively discuss the management plan for their practice area. Those patients with significant swelling or deformity should be seen by the consultant in 5 to 7 days when swelling has resolved, in order to optimally time further reduction.

Septal hematomas, if not drained in the emergency department, can lead to abscess formation or necrosis of the nasal cartilage, with resultant saddle nose deformity. Drainage is performed through a mucosal incision. The area is subsequently packed with gauze, which is removed on next-day follow-up.[22] Patients who have difficulty breathing through the nose should be seen by the consultant in follow-up in the outpatient setting.

Ethmoid Fractures

Naso-orbito-ethmoid (NOE) fractures are produced by trauma to the bridge of the nose and involve the central portion of the midface (the nasal bones, frontal processes of the maxilla, and ethmoid bones) (Fig. 97.9). These often prove difficult to diagnose. The diagnostic challenge is emphasized by the fact that these fractures are fairly common, accounting for almost 40% of midface fractures in one series.[4]

Evaluation

A thorough history, especially regarding the mechanism of injury, combined with careful physical examination will help the emergency physician make the diagnosis of NOE fracture. If performed before the development of significant swelling and edema, inspection of the face may aid in the evaluation of patients for NOE injury. In the patient with NOE fracture, the intercanthal distance, normally about half the interpupillary distance, is usually widened enough to require open surgical repair. An intercanthal distance of 35 mm suggests a displaced NOE fracture; a distance of 40 mm is diagnostic.[6] Also characteristic of NOE fractures are a short and retruded nasal bridge, enophthalmos, shortened and blunted medial palpebral fissure, and epiphora. These findings are increasingly difficult to detect as swelling progresses. Palpation of the medial orbital rim may reveal crepitus or movement of bony fragments.[6]

Management

Because of the difficulty in detecting NOE fractures by physical examination or plain radiographic assessment, this diagnosis is usually made by facial CT scan. CT scanning should be the initial imaging modality for any patient with suspected NOE injury. Both axial and coronal sections are desirable, as reconstructed coronal sections are usually of insufficient quality to visualize properly the middle third of the orbit and the anterior cranial fossa.[6]

The emergency physician's role in management of the patient with NOE fracture is to make the diagnosis and to rule out associated lacrimal system injury or dural tear. These tasks may prove difficult but are very important: NOE fractures are difficult to repair if the diagnosis is delayed by more than 2 weeks.[6] The emergency physician must carefully search for NOE fractures. The consultant should be contacted regarding admission of the patient if NOE injury is identified.

Zygomatic Fractures

Zygomatic fractures, reported in some series[4,21] as the most common facial bony injury, are infrequently missed in the emergency department evaluation. The zygoma may fracture through its arch or body, or at one of its many attachments to the frontal, maxillary, or temporal bones. Fracture at the suture lines with the three adjacent bones is termed a *tripartite* or *tripod fracture* (Fig. 97.10).

Evaluation

Physical examination reliably detects most zygomatic fractures. Inspection of patients with zygomatic injuries may reveal flattening of the lateral facial contour, depression and tenderness of the orbital rim at the zygomaticomaxillary or zygomaticofrontal sutures, lateral orbital droop secondary to disruption of the lateral canthal ligament, lateral subscleral hemorrhage, or trismus. Further examination may reveal horizontal diplopia (damage to the lateral rectus muscle), vertical diplopia (damage to the inferior rectus or oblique muscle), or hypesthesia in the infraorbital nerve distribution.[22] Simultaneous palpation of both zygomatic arches allows easy detection of flattening due to fractures of these bones. Displacement of zygomatic fractures may interfere with excursion of the mandibular condyle, producing resultant occlusal impairment or trismus.[20,22]

Radiographic evaluation of patients with zygomatic fractures is managed in much the same way as for other facial injuries. If the index of suspicion is low based on history and physical examination, evaluation should be initially limited to plain radiographs. Standard x-rays (e.g., the submentovertex view or "bucket handle" for simple arch fractures) detect many zygomatic injuries. Facial CT scanning is necessary to determine the status of surrounding soft tissues (e.g., orbital contents) and sinuses and the existence of tripod fractures in patients with zygomatic body fractures.

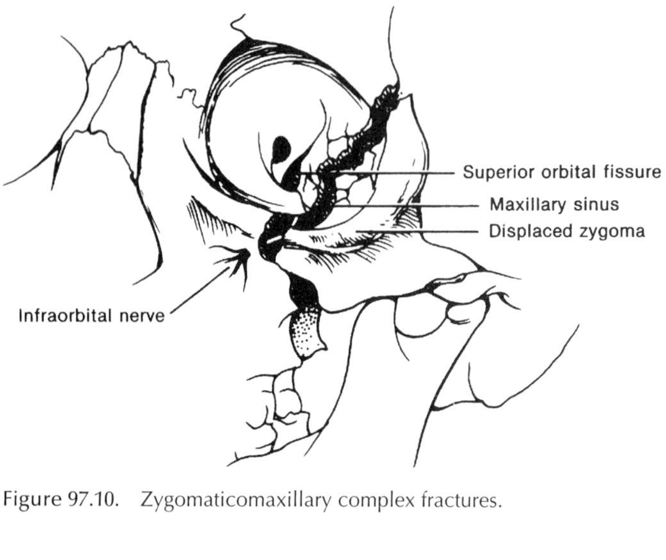

Figure 97.10. Zygomaticomaxillary complex fractures.

Management

The presence of a zygomatic fracture does not necessarily prompt further evaluation with CT scanning, as some nondisplaced fractures can be managed nonoperatively.[17] When tripod or other complex fractures are identified or suggested by plain radiography, CT scanning and surgical consultation are obtained. In patients with uncomplicated, nondisplaced fractures (e.g., the zygomatic arch), emergency department management is limited to providing antibiotics in patients with sinus disruption, analgesia, and surgical follow-up within 2 to 3 days.

Frontal Fractures

Figure 97.1, depicting the forces required to fracture the facial bones, shows why the frontal bones are relatively rarely fractured.[21,23] Due to the proximity of the frontal bone and sinus to the brain, and the significant forces required to fracture these bones, fractures in this area are associated with a high risk of intracranial injury.[22,23] The large forces required to produce frontal fractures usually cause other facial bony injuries as well; thus, any patient with a frontal bone fracture should undergo head CT scanning and meticulous evaluation for associated facial injury.

Evaluation

Frontal bone fractures may be apparent on inspection, which may reveal depression of the involved region of the forehead. Glabellar depression indicates fracture of the anterior wall of the frontal sinus.[22] Palpation of the frontal region may reveal crepitus if the sinus is involved, or tenderness or step-off due to other fractures.

Injuries involving the frontal sinus or nasal region, especially displaced nasofrontal fractures, may be clearly imaged with plain radiography.[15] If cranial CT scanning is performed on all patients with significant frontal injury, most frontal fractures will be identified on simultaneous frontal bone imaging. The improved delineation of soft tissues and sinus walls provided by CT imaging allows more accurate management. Assessment of the integrity of the posterior wall of the frontal sinus is particularly important, as fracture of this structure may be associated with frontal lobe contusions and lacerations, dural tears, and CSF rhinorrhea.[22]

Management

Antibiotic prophylaxis is indicated when the walls of the frontal sinus are fractured. The rest of the emergency department management of patients with frontal bone injuries includes evaluation of other parts of the face and the intracranial contents. Early consultation with neurosurgical and facial surgery specialists, in addition to the ophthalmologist, as necessary, is indicated in patients with frontal bone fractures.[15]

Soft-Tissue Injuries

Almost all patients with facial fractures have associated cutaneous injuries. These should not be closed in the patient who will undergo surgical evaluation in the emergency department, as the opening may be used for examination or repair. Laceration repair is discussed in Chapter 95. In addition to lacerations, oral, ocular, salivary, lacrimal, or neurologic injuries may also be associated with maxillofacial trauma (Fig. 97.11).

Evaluation and Management

Careful intraoral examination should be part of the evaluation of all patients with facial trauma. Attention should be given to airway and bleeding considerations; tongue, frenulum, and gingival lacerations; identification of alveolar or palatal fracture; and dentition. Any dental appliances present should be removed to prevent their aspiration from compromising the airway. These appliances should be saved: They are expensive and may provide important guides to pretraumatic oral alignment.

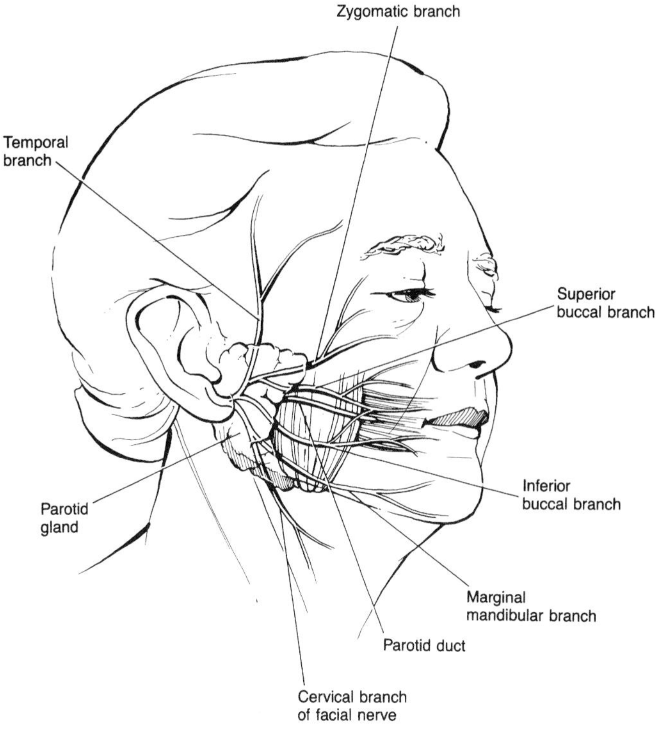

Figure 97.11. Important soft-tissue structures of the face.

The significant incidence of ocular injuries associated with various facial fractures necessitates meticulous ophthalmologic evaluation in all patients sustaining maxillofacial trauma. Injuries to the lacrimal system, with associated findings such as epiphora, may be present in patients with midface fractures. Lacrimal disruption is rare, however, even in patients with significant craniofacial trauma.[20] These injuries are discussed more fully in Chapter 99.

Maxillofacial trauma may damage the parotid gland or duct. Clear or pink-tinged fluid in a wound over the course of Stensen's duct or the parotid gland should prompt the examiner to evaluate the patient for these injuries. Glandular laceration does not require repair, as commonly occurring salivary fistulas resolve spontaneously in less than a month. Stensen's duct may be repaired by suturing the ends together over a stent; this is most appropriately performed by an oral and maxillofacial, ENT, or plastic surgery consultant.

Except for mandibular fractures, the classically emphasized risk of c-spine fractures occurring in association with facial injuries has been greatly overstated. However, there is sufficient risk to warrant c-spine imaging as the initial radiographic evaluation in patients with significant facial trauma.[4,9,10,22,23] If the incidence of c-spine injury occurring concurrently with facial fracture has been overstated, the significant association between maxillofacial trauma and brain injury merits special emphasis. As many as 85% of patients sustaining significant facial fractures have associated intracranial injury. Certain trends have been illustrated in published series (e.g., the high risk of intracranial injury with frontal bony injury), but no definite set of clinical parameters currently allows prediction of intracranial pathology based on fracture location.[23] As a result, all patients with significant facial fractures require cranial CT scanning.

DISPOSITION

Role of the Consultant

In the vast majority of patients with maxillofacial trauma, the emergency physician can perform the initial trauma resuscitation and stabilization without the need for consultation with maxillofacial specialists. The role of emergent surgical consultation in patients with airway compromise or refractory facial hemorrhage has been discussed.

Involvement of the appropriate surgical specialist is now recommended at an earlier time than had been standard in the past. Delays in treatment have been shown to result in suboptimal outcome in some facial injuries.[6,15,19] In patients with severe multisystem trauma, the maxillofacial surgeon should be consulted early for brief examination, wound closure, debridement of avulsive dentoalveolar injuries, and temporary stabilization of grossly unstable dentoalveolar or mandible fractures.[15]

Indications for Admission

Indications for admission of patients sustaining maxillofacial trauma may be related to concomitant injuries in adjacent or remote regions, or for management of the facial trauma itself. Patients with nondisplaced simple facial fractures can often be managed as outpatients after telephone consultation with the appropriate surgical specialist provides for disposition and follow-up planning. Any patient with significant airway compromise, hemorrhage, or complex facial trauma requires admission. In the patient with isolated facial fractures, a regular-floor bed should suffice; however, any patient with injuries prompting concern for airway compromise or hemorrhage should be observed in a monitored setting.

Patients with CSF leak must be evaluated by a neurosurgeon in addition to the specialist consulted for accompanying facial fractures. Many neurosurgeons consider CSF rhinorrhea an indication for prophylactic antibiotics, but this decision is left to the consultant.

Transfer Considerations

The surgical therapy of maxillofacial trauma is a rapidly evolving field. Patients with significant injuries should be transferred to referral centers if local consultants lack expertise in treating the injury in question. Before transfer, the patient who requires definitive care of maxillofacial injuries must be evaluated for other more potentially life- or limb-threatening injuries. Even in the setting of isolated maxillofacial trauma, the potential for airway deterioration is real, and pretransfer stabilization in these instances may reasonably include intubation. The potential for airway compromise, as well as the high frequency of significant associated injuries, dictates a high level of training for personnel involved in the prehospital or interhospital transport of the patient with significant maxillofacial trauma.

COMMON PITFALLS

- Failure to manage the airway aggressively with intubation or cricothyreotomy where indicated. Do not wait for swelling or hemorrhage to convert an elective procedure into an urgent one.
- Failure to consider the presence of injuries other than ones that are obvious. Pay particular attention to the neurologic and ophthalmologic examinations.
- Failure to order CT views where the index of suspicion is high, even if plain radiographs are negative.
- The historical emphasis on searching for c-spine injuries in patients with facial fractures is probably relevant only in patients with mandible fractures. Because of the potential need for endotracheal intubation for airway management and the patient positioning required for many facial imaging modalities, plain radiography of the c-spine remains the initial radiologic study.
- Frontal bone injuries are particularly likely to be associated with intracranial injury, but investigators have been unable to define rules allowing correlation of specific facial fractures with intracranial injury. All patients with significant facial fractures require cranial CT scanning.

References

1. Assael LA. Clinical aspects of imaging in maxillofacial trauma. *Radiol Clin North Am* 1993;31:209.
2. Azevedo AB, Trent R, Ellis A. Population-based analysis of 10,766 hospitalizations for mandibular fractures in California, 1991 to 1993. *J Trauma* 1998;45:1084.
3. Bayles SW, Abramson PJ. McMahon SJ, et al. Mandibular fracture and associated cervical spine fracture, a rare and predictable injury: protocol for cervical spine evaluation and review of 1382 cases. *Arch Otolaryngol Head Neck Surg* 1997;123:923.
4. Cook HE, Rowe M. A retrospective study of 356 midfacial fractures occurring in 225 patients. *J Oral Maxillofac Surg* 1990;48:574.
5. Dolin J, Scalea T, Mannor L, et al. The management of gunshot wounds to the face. *J Trauma* 1992;33:508.
6. Ellis E. Sequencing treatment for naso-orbito-ethmoid fractures. *J Oral Maxillofac Surg* 1993;51:543.
7. Gentry LR. Facial trauma and associated brain damage. *Radiol Clin North Am* 1984;27:435.
8. Greene D, Raven R, Carvalho G, et al. Epidemiology of facial injury in blunt assault: determinants of incidence and outcome in 802 patients. *Arch Otolaryngol Head Neck Surg* 1997;123:923.
9. Haug RH, Prather J, Indresano AT. An epidemiologic survey of facial fractures and concomitant injuries. *J Oral Maxillofac Surg* 1990;48:926.
10. Hills MW, Deane SA. Head injury and facial injury: is there an increased risk of cervical spine injury? *J Trauma* 1993;34:549.
11. Hutchison I, Lawlor M, Skinner D. Major maxillofacial injuries. *BMJ* 1990;301:595.
12. Joondelph BC. Blunt ocular trauma. *Emerg Med Clin North Am* 1988;6:147.
13. Kassel EE. Traumatic injuries of the paranasal sinuses. *Otolaryngol Clin North Am* 1988;21:455.
14. Kihtir T, Ivatury RR, Simon RJ, et al. Early management of civilian gunshot wounds to the face. *J Trauma* 1993;35:569.
15. Lee T, Ratzker PA, Galarza M, et al. Early combined management of frontal sinus and orbital and facial fractures. *J Trauma* 1998;44:665.
16. Marciani RD, Gonty AA. Principles of management of complex craniofacial trauma. *J Oral Maxillofac Surg* 1993;51:535.
17. Mathog RH. Management of orbital blowout fractures. *Otolaryngol Clin North Am* 1991;24:79.
18. Min YG, Dong HJ, Jung HW, et al. Clinical significance of three-dimensional computed tomography performed in maxillofacial trauma. *Rhinology* 1992;14:162.
19. Pelletier CR, Jordan DR, Braga R, et al. Assessment of ocular trauma associated with head and neck injuries. *J Trauma* 1998;44:350.
20. Rohrich RJ, Shewmake KB. Evolving concepts of craniomaxillofacial fracture management. *Clin Plast Surg* 1992;19:1.
21. Scherer M, Sullivan WG, Smith DJ, et al. An analysis of 1423 facial fractures in 788 patients at an urban trauma center. *J Trauma* 1989;29:388.
22. Shepherd SM, Lippe MS. Maxillofacial trauma. *Emerg Med Clin North Am* 1987;5:371.
23. Sinclair D, Schwartz M, Gruss J, et al. A retrospective review of the relationship between facial fractures, head injuries, and cervical spine injuries. *J Emerg Med* 1988;6:109.
24. Taicher S. Changing indications for tracheostomy in maxillofacial trauma. *J Oral Maxillofac Surg* 1996;54:292.

CHAPTER 98
Dental Injuries

Brigitte M. Baumann and Laura B. Thomas

Injuries to the teeth and their supporting structures occasionally present the emergency physician with a challenge in both diagnosis and treatment, in part because of the limited training physicians receive in dentistry and oral emergencies. Another problem is that in patients with multiple injuries, oral injuries are often overlooked once the airway is secured and more life-threatening injuries are addressed. Teeth have the lowest potential of any tissue for returning to a normal healthy state after injury; because the prognosis of some dental injuries is greatly enhanced by prompt initial treatment, rapid care is imperative.[15]

Dental trauma is best categorized as either intentional or unintentional, with injuries caused by domestic violence or assaults considered intentional and those caused by sporting events, motor vehicle crashes, falls, or collisions categorized as unintentional. Over 50% of all physical trauma from child abuse is inflicted on the child's head and neck region, with soft-tissue injuries predominating.[1,8,15] These types of injuries should alert the physician, and a complete physical examination must be undertaken to ascertain other injuries. In adult abuse (inflicted typically on women and the elderly), lip lacerations, fractured teeth and jaws, missing teeth, and bruises and burns of the palate, gingivae, and face predominate.[1,8,15]

Of the unintentional injuries, sporting injuries are most prevalent in teen-age males, and account for 13% to 39% of all dental trauma.[2] Motor vehicle crashes account for 11%, and motorcycle or bicycle crashes account for another 10% of dental trauma.[2] Finally, falls account for 17% to 69% of injuries, and occur most frequently in young children, the elderly, and the intoxicated.[2,8]

Predisposition to dental trauma involves the extremes of age (children and the elderly), patients prone to risk-taking behavior (teen-age males), and the debilitated. In children, predisposing anatomic factors for traumatic tooth injuries include postnormal occlusion, an overbite exceeding 4 mm, short upper lip, incompetent lips, and mouth breathing.

INITIAL EVALUATION

As with other injuries, the examiner should attempt to determine the exact time and mechanism of the injury. Any missing teeth or dental prostheses must be accounted for, to prevent them from compromising the airway or being retained in soft-tissue wounds. A comprehensive medical history helps determine if tetanus immunizations are up to date and whether antibiotics are indicated as a prophylaxis before any dental manipulation or as an aid to wound healing (e.g., if the patient has a history of rheumatic heart fever or diabetes).[1,11]

EXTRAORAL EVALUATION

The extraoral evaluation should assess for lacerations, abrasions, and contusions. In wounds under the chin, jaw fractures and condylar injuries must be excluded. If the patient has difficulty opening or closing the jaw or if there is asymmetry to these movements, fractures of the mandible or facial bones should be suspected. Assess midface stability by placing two fingers along the hard palate and pulling the alveolar process forward and backward gently. If there is crepitus or motion, the patient has, at minimum, a LeFort I fracture.[1]

INTRAORAL EXAMINATION

Next, evaluate intraoral bleeding sites and lacerations of the mucosa and gingival tissues. Contaminated or bleeding areas should be cleansed with dampened gauze or irrigated. Hemorrhage in the gingival crevice of the tooth may indicate subluxation, and the presence of traumatized gingivae or mucosa suggest underlying dentoalveolar injuries. This examination and the remainder of the intraoral examination is best performed with two tongue blades and a bright light. Once this examination is complete, bimanually palpate the cheeks and floor of the mouth for foreign bodies or tooth fragments.

Evaluate the dentition for cracks, chips, abnormal alignment, and missing or abnormally occluding teeth. If teeth are missing or chipped, look for fragments in soft-tissue wounds.[1,11] Changes in tooth coloration (red or greyish hue) may occur with pulpal necrosis or congestion. The horizontal and vertical mobility of teeth should be assessed using tongue blades rather than fingers, because the fingers can miss subtle findings.

Remember that deciduous teeth near the time of exfoliation normally exhibit mobility. If teeth move en bloc, a fracture of the alveolar process may be present.[1,11] Percussion of the occlusal edge of teeth may elicit extreme sensitivity or tenderness if periodontal tissues are traumatized. This sensitivity also supports the diagnosis of subluxation.[10]

Finally, if a partial denture or missing tooth cannot be located, it may be imbedded in soft-tissue wounds or the patient may have swallowed or aspirated it. The examiner should document all damaged or missing teeth (Fig. 98.1). Finally, injuries to the orofacial region are often not limited to the teeth and supporting soft tissues. In trauma patients, one must always suspect

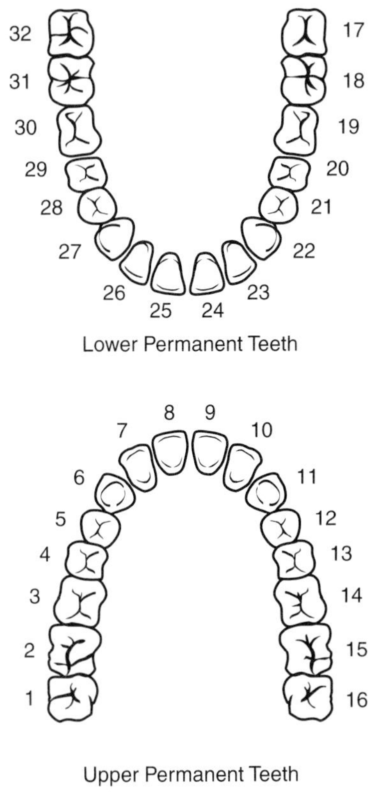

Figure 98.1. Upper and lower permanent teeth.

other bony injuries to the face as well as neurologic injury (discussed in depth in Chapters 96 and 97).

RADIOGRAPHIC EXAMINATION

Dental radiographs, such as panoramic, occlusal, or periapical films, are helpful in further diagnosis. Because most emergency departments are poorly equipped in this regard, standard mandible or facial films may be useful in certain circumstances to aid diagnosis.

TREATMENT OF DENTAL INJURIES

The treatment of dental injuries in the emergency department varies according to the facilities available and the examiner's expertise.

Concussed Teeth

Concussed teeth are those that, when examined, have no obvious injury other than a sensitivity to percussion.[5,18] These teeth may have sustained an injury sufficient to cause later pulpal (nerve) death and necrosis. Treatment consists of a soft diet and follow-up care.

Tooth Displacement

Subluxation

Subluxated teeth appear undamaged but demonstrate abnormal mobility on examination. Teeth may be sensitive to extremes of temperature and there may be some gingival bleeding. The patient may complain of not being able to bite all the way into his or her normal occlusion. This slight extrusion is due to edema at the apex of the root. Treatment consists of minor adjustment of occlusion or splinting.

Displaced Teeth

There may be intrusive, extrusive, buccal, or lingual displacement of the tooth; the tooth is in an abnormal position. For buccal, labial, and lingual displacements, the tooth is repositioned in its alveolar socket with the aid of a gloved hand and a gauze pad. Extruded teeth may be repositioned by having the patient gently bite down on a folded gauze pad. If gentle attempts at these maneuvers are too painful, dental anesthesia by infiltration or a nerve block may be necessary. Once reduced, the tooth should be splinted.

Occasionally, teeth sustain a blow sufficient to intrude or embed them into the alveolar bone.[5] These teeth are usually not mobile and present no interference to the patient's occlusion. These patients must be referred to a dentist as soon as possible. Primary teeth are allowed to reerupt or are extracted. Permanent teeth may reerupt on their own, but often require orthodontic or surgical eruption with stabilization. Subsequent root canal therapy is often necessary. All patients with displaced teeth should be prescribed analgesia and a soft diet. The use of straws should be avoided. Warm saline rinses three times a day may help promote gingival healing. Dental follow-up is required in 24 hours.[5,6,18]

Avulsed Teeth

Complete displacement of a tooth from its alveolar socket constitutes an avulsion. A permanent tooth that has been avulsed is a true dental emergency, with the prognosis for recovery greatly enhanced by prompt intervention.[5,20] Primary teeth are usually not replanted: Replanted teeth fuse to the alveolar bone and interfere with the eruption of the underlying permanent teeth. Most anterior primary teeth are present until age 6 or 7.

Avulsed permanent teeth must be replanted for both aesthetic and functional reasons. In adults, the open space is unaesthetic, and it is often difficult to match a false tooth to the remaining teeth. Functionally, the adult teeth will shift if the tooth is not replaced. This malalignment can lead to periodontal disease and temporomandibular joint pain and dysfunction.

The object of initial care is to ensure immediate replantation of the tooth to prevent or lessen the process of root resorption, which may cause loss of the tooth. Although early replantation is viewed as a temporary measure, it has been shown that teeth replanted within 30 minutes have a 90% retention rate without significant root resorption for up to 5 to 10 years. Conversely, 95% of the teeth replanted after 2 hours show root resorption.[5,11,18,19]

Proper handling of the tooth is equally important to ensure the long-term survival of the tooth and the periodontal ligament remnants attached to the root. These remnants are sensitive to damage by drying, and successful replantation depends on their survival.[1,5]

When the patient, parents, or emergency medical technicians contact the emergency department concerning treatment for an avulsed tooth, they should be told the following[1,5,18–20]:

- The root of the tooth may not be touched. Only the crown may be handled.
- If the caller is able to replace the tooth in its exact location, have him or her do so after thoroughly rinsing the tooth with tap water (advise the caller to stopper or close off the drain first). Debris *should not* be scrubbed from the root surface.
- If replantation in the field is unsuccessful or impractical, have the caller transport the tooth by placing it under the patient's tongue, if the patient is a coherent, responsible adult. Alternatively, the tooth may be wrapped in moist gauze or placed in a cup of saline solution, saliva, milk, or Hanks balanced salt solution[13] for immediate replantation by a physician or dentist.

If replantation was successful in the field, the physician must check for proper alignment and degree of mobility. Most teeth require some form of stabilization (see the later discussion on stabilization of traumatized teeth).

If replantation is done in the emergency department, follow these guidelines:

- Replantation should be questioned in patients with grossly neglected oral hygiene and severe periodontal disease. There is minimal chance of successful replantation.
- If the alveolus or socket is intact, replantation should be attempted.
- The tooth should be handled by the crown only. Saline solution is used to irrigate debris from the root.
- The socket should then be gently irrigated or swabbed free of clot. The socket should not be subjected to curetting, which damages the remaining periodontal ligaments.
- The tooth is reinserted using gentle pressure with the aid of gauze to provide a firm grip on the crown. Once the tooth is inserted, have the patient slowly bite down on folded gauze and seat the tooth into its proper position.
- If possible, the position of the tooth should be checked radiographically.
- Reimplanted teeth should be splinted.
- Tetanus immunization should be updated.
- Penicillin or clindamycin are prescribed for antibiotic coverage.
- Follow-up care is required within 24 hours.

Fractured Teeth

Fractures of the Enamel (Ellis Class I)

Fractured teeth may show minor chipping of superficial enamel surfaces, causing sharp edges that may be irritating. Referral to a dentist for follow-up care and smoothing of rough edges should be arranged.

Fractures of the Enamel and Dentin (Ellis Class II)

Fractures through enamel (white) and the underlying dentin (pale yellow) expose dentinal processes that communicate directly with the central nerve or pulp and make them susceptible to necrosis and abscess formation. The patient experiences pain to touch or percussion, and frequently the exposed free nerve endings cause exquisite pain when air passes over them.[1,11,18]

The dentist will cover the exposed dentin with a layer of calcium hydroxide, an inert substance that seals the dentinal tubules, commonly eliminating the pain.[1,2,5] This layer is then covered by a composite dental material by acid-etching the surrounding enamel to provide microscopic undercuts that aid in retention of the material on the tooth surface.[5] Emergency department treatment is limited to providing dental consultation or follow-up as soon as possible. A soft diet is prescribed, and the patient should avoid hot or cold foods.

Fractures of the Enamel and Dentin with Pulp (Nerve) Exposure (Ellis Class III)

When a pink or red color or fleshy substance is noted within the surrounding dentin (pale yellow) on inspection of a fractured tooth, a fracture involving the pulp (nerve) should be suspected. The relative size of the pulp chamber in an adult central incisor is shown in Fig. 98.2. The patient usually has pain with manipulation of the tooth, exposure to air, or exposure to hot or cold fluids. Most fractures that involve pulp exposure require root canal therapy by removing the remaining vital pulp as soon as possible to prevent later abscess formation.[5] However, more conservative measures of pulp capping, or covering the exposure with calcium hydroxide, followed by restoration, may be indicated in small exposures of healthy teeth.

Ideally, a dental consultant should see the patient in the emergency department. If unavailable, dental follow-up should be provided as soon as possible.

Root Fractures

Teeth with root fractures are difficult to diagnose by clinical examination alone. The only outward sign may be abnormal mobility or sensitivity to percussion. Dental films are mandatory to confirm the diagnosis, so immediate dental consultation is advisable.

In the acute setting, significantly displaced teeth must be reduced to their proper position and stabilized with a splint. Early intervention allows retention of the teeth without the need for root canal therapy in up to 80% of cases.[1]

Crown Root Fractures

While similar in appearance to crown fractures (described earlier), crown root fractures start above the gingival margin of the tooth and continue subgingivally within the tooth's alveolar socket. If the fracture fragments are nondisplaced, they are difficult to detect clinically. Management rests on determining the extent of damage to permanent teeth by removing the coronal portion of the tooth. Primary teeth generally require extraction. Immediate dental consultation is warranted.[18]

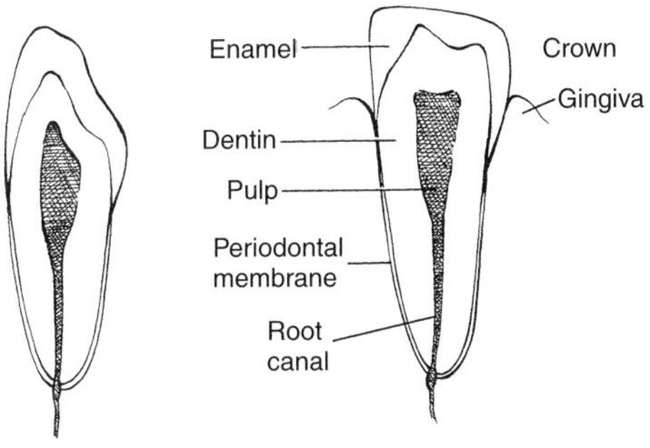

Figure 98.2. An adult central incisor.

Dentoalveolar Fractures

Fractures that involve the alveolus or tooth-bearing portion of the maxilla and mandible vary in their degree of displacement, mobility, and comminution and in the number of teeth affected. The patient usually complains of malocclusion, mobile teeth or alveolar segments, and local pain when biting. The examiner usually notes a displaced alveolar segment or group of teeth, a mobile segment on palpation, and malocclusion. Dental radiographs or facial films should be ordered. They may show fracture lines running between or just apical to the roots of the teeth.

Treatment of dentoalveolar fractures usually involves repositioning the displaced segment, possibly under local anesthesia or intravenous sedation, stabilization of the segment with rigid splinting, and follow-up care. Often these fractures require care that is unavailable in the emergency department. Therefore, urgent consultation should be sought from a qualified general dentist or oral and maxillofacial surgeon.[5]

Oral Soft-Tissue Injuries

Most soft-tissue injuries of the mouth can be managed by an emergency physician. Rapid closure in the emergency department results in decreased risk of infection, decreased healing time, and improved hemostasis and future cosmetic result. Final cosmetic result, however, depends on the rapidity of closure after injury (ideally within 12 hours), the degree of contamination, and the orientation of the injury to Langer's lines of skin tension. Favorable lacerations parallel Langer's lines. Unfavorable ones cross Langer's lines, and patients must be advised that they have a greater risk of contraction and scar formation. Scars can be revised by a plastic surgeon when they are mature (when fibrous elements dominate over vascular elements), 1 year after repair.

General Approach

All soft-tissue wounds require copious irrigation, assessment of retained foreign bodies, and, if grossly contaminated or devitalized, minimal debridement. A patient's tetanus immunization status must be assessed and updated if necessary. Penicillin is advocated for intraoral and puncture wounds, while clindamycin is utilized in patients who cannot tolerate penicillin. Through-and-through wounds require the addition of an antistaphylococcal antibiotic (dicloxacillin or cephalexin) for 5 days.[15] A soft diet and warm saline rinses four times a day are prescribed, and patients should see a dentist within 24 to 48 hours. Immediate medical attention must be sought in the case of fever, increasing edema, or erythema at a wound site, or if pus is noted.

Puncture Wounds

Animal bites, particularly dog bites, are the most common bites of the face in children. Wounds must be meticulously examined for foreign bodies, especially in cat bites, where the small, relatively brittle teeth can remain in the wound. Lacerations smaller than 2 cm and all puncture wounds should be left to heal by secondary intention. If the patient presents within 12 hours and the wound is minimally contaminated, however, it may be closed with as few interrupted sutures as possible to achieve approximation of wound edges.

Closure should be undertaken only if the defect is so great that secondary healing will result in a deformity. A drain may be placed for 24 to 48 hours in the setting of a deep laceration. Prophylactic and empiric therapy of bites is best achieved with amoxicillin–clavulanic acid for 5 days.[3,7] In addition to antibiotic coverage, all animal bites should be considered for rabies prophylaxis.

Human bites are highly prone to infection. As some *Bacteroides* species are resistant to penicillin because of their β-lactamase activity, penicillin and a penicillinase-resistant penicillin or amoxicillin–clavulanic acid are advocated.[3,7]

Tongue Lacerations

In treating tongue lacerations, anesthesia is achieved by using a 25-gauge needle filled with 1% lidocaine and inserting the needle posterior and medial to the most distal molar on the side of the tongue laceration. In children, advance the needle approximately 0.5 cm in depth, and in adults approximately 1 cm in depth; aspirate to check for intravascular needle placement; and then inject 0.5 to 1.0 mL of anesthetic agent. If the laceration is bleeding, local anesthesia with 1:100,000 epinephrine can be used to decrease the rate of bleeding. The only disadvantage to this mode of anesthesia is that the tissues may be distorted by the anesthetic bolus.

Interrupted absorbable sutures (3-0 or 4-0 chromic or Vicryl) approximate deep muscle, then submucosa, and finally the dorsal or ventral surface (or both). All knots are buried (inverted). Occasionally, placement of sutures is difficult because of the floppy nature of the tongue. Grasp the tongue between folded gauze or place a single suture at the tip, with the two long ends wrapped about your nondominant hand, and exert gentle outward traction; this technique generally provides adequate visualization.[16,19]

Buccal Mucosa

Anesthesia of the buccal mucosa is most easily achieved by local infiltration of 1% lidocaine with 1:100,000 epinephrine. Through-and-through lacerations should be closed in layers from the inside out. The inner layer should be approximated with an inverted 3-0 or 4-0 absorbable suture. If irrigation was difficult to achieve when both margins were open, the closure of the inner layer will now allow the irrigation solution to flow outward and not fill the mouth. The muscle layer is then closed with absorbable inverted sutures, and the skin is closed with interrupted sutures of 5-0 or 6-0 nylon.

Remove these sutures in 4 to 5 days. If there is any injury to Stensen's duct, the patient should be referred to an oral surgeon to avoid complications of fistula or mucocele formation and infection.[19] Lacerations or injury to Stensen's duct can be diagnosed in the following ways:

- Dry the inside of the cheek and exert gentle pressure on the parotid gland. If it is intact, a globule of saliva should appear at the ductal opening.
- On occasion, the severed ends of the duct can be localized in the wound.
- If the upper lip on the side of the injury is drooping: The buccal branch of the facial nerve runs slightly superior to the duct as it crosses anterior to the masseter. Injury to this nerve suggests injury to the duct as well.
- The patient complains of swelling of the cheek, particularly after meals. The swelling is the accumulation of saliva in the buccal tissues.

Injury to the parotid gland is repaired by closing the skin over the cut gland. Warn the patient that fluid may escape through the margins of the wound. This seepage should cease once scar tissue forms in the wound. If a fistula develops, the duct was either severed or obstructed and needs to be reexplored and repaired.[19]

Gingiva

Gingival lacerations are sometimes noted at the site of mandibular or maxillary fracture locations or at the site of avulsed teeth.[14] Rarely, patients present with gingival degloving, but treatment is the same.[2] The gingiva are repositioned and sutured in place with fine silk sutures. Given the friability of the gingiva, suturing may be best accomplished with an anchoring stitch on the opposite side of the tooth. Sutures are removed in 4 to 5 days.

Lip Lacerations

In lip lacerations, it is best to use nerve blocks rather than local infiltration in order to prevent distortion of the vermilion border. If local infiltration is used, the addition of epinephrine to the anesthetic solution decreases the amount of agent needed for anesthesia and will help maintain hemostasis. Blanching of the mucosa may occur, however, obliterating the vermilion border.

For injuries of the upper lip, an infraorbital block is used. In injuries of the lower lip, a mental block will provide anesthesia from the midline to the labial commissure. An inferior alveolar block will encompass the area of a mental block and also anesthetize the buccal mucosa, the lingual gingiva, the anterior two-thirds of the tongue, and the dentition on the side of the injection.

After anesthesia is achieved, minimal debridement of devitalized tissue and damaged minor salivary glands is undertaken. If salivary glands are incorporated in the repair, there is risk of mucocele formation.

Proper closure rests on first approximating the vermilion border. Place a stitch that aligns the two edges of the wound and then continue with local anesthetic infiltration or the closure itself. Needle scratches or marking the edges with a surgical marker are not recommended: The scratch or pen mark may be obliterated once the wound is prepped with Betadine, and the marker tips are often not fine enough to clearly demarcate the border.

Closure of a through-and-through laceration begins at the inner fibro-fatty layer. Using a 3-0 or 4-0 absorbable suture, place inverted, interrupted sutures starting inferiorly and continue upwards, stopping at the apex of the wound. Suture the outer fibro-fatty layer in a similar fashion, working inferiorly to the wound apex. Reapproximate the two fibro-fatty layers once the outer closure meets the inner closure at the apex of the wound. Close the epidermal–dermal layer last. Using the vermilion border as a starting point, place interrupted, 5-0 nonresorbable sutures (nylon) to the apex of the wound. If the laceration extends to the mucosa (wet inner surface) of the lip, 4-0 or 5-0 chromic is used to close this layer. Another option in this setting is to close both inner fibro-fatty layer and mucosa as a unit and to suture from the base to the apex.[16]

Another option is the use of isobutyl cyanoacrylate in the repair of both superficial and deep lip lacerations. In one case report, a deep wound that included the orbicular muscle was repaired by inserting isobutyl cyanoacrylate from the bottom of the wound toward the lip surface, while continuously approximating the margins of the wound. After application, the patient was asked to slowly open his mouth to control bonding and orbicular muscle position. Excess material was removed with wet gauze.[4]

Penetrating Intraoral Trauma

The incidence of intraoral trauma in children is unknown, but it is likely that most cases heal spontaneously without complications.[12] However, there is a sizable literature documenting complications from these injuries, including retropharyngeal and mediastinal abscesses, mediastinitis, widespread emphysema, internal carotid artery thrombosis, and airway obstruction.[9,12]

Most commonly, children sustain injuries after falling with sharp objects in their mouths.[9,17] The injuries tend to be on the posterolateral oropharynx, and initial symptoms are limited to mild erythema or slight bleeding at the site of injury.[9,17]

Management of these patients is controversial. Patients with obvious symptoms need hospital admission and aggressive management of the airway and infection. There is no consensus on the management of symptom-free patients.

Some authors advocate admission and observation for those with lateral or retropharyngeal injuries. Others recommend discharging patients with detailed instructions for prompt return.[9,17] Patients should return immediately if they have difficulty breathing, difficulty handling secretions, fever, change in mental status, or any change or worsening in condition. Finally, there is no consensus on the use of antibiotics for surgical exploration. However, the suturing of minor wounds should be resisted.[9,12,17]

STABILIZATION OF TRAUMATIZED TEETH

In teeth that are concussed, there is typically no displacement of the tooth; therefore, splinting is generally not required. In teeth that are subluxated a flexible splint should be placed if one or more teeth are mobile. However, if only one tooth is slightly mobile, a splint is not required. The splint stabilizes teeth during the healing phase and can be safely removed in 7 to 10 days,[6] ample time for healing of the periodontal ligament.

In both extrusive and buccal luxation, teeth are splinted and joined together by a wire or nylon line.[13] Intrusive luxation is the most severe form of luxation injury and the tooth frequently undergoes external root resorption. Treatment is difficult and may involve either repositioning and splinting or watchful waiting. Because most teeth that are repositioned have a greater likelihood of external root absorption, watchful waiting is now recommended.[13] Teeth that have been displaced long enough for blood to thoroughly clot should not be forced back into position because of the induction of root resorption.[4] As with intrusive luxation, better results are achieved with orthodontic therapy.

An avulsed tooth should also be splinted once reimplanted into the socket. This splint may be removed in 7 to 10 days as well. However, with a concurrent alveolar fracture, the splint is left in place for 4 to 8 weeks.[18]

Temporary stabilization can be achieved by crimping a piece of aluminum foil around the teeth or using cotton rolls placed between the lip and teeth. Another means of stabilization if a formal dental examination is imminent is by having the patient bite down on a piece of folded gauze. A periodontal dressing, such as Coe-Pak (COE Laboratories, Chicago, Illinois) can also be used. The teeth are first cleaned and dried. Equal lengths of two pastes are mixed on a paper pad and then the material is folded over and crimped around the teeth and soft tissues.[18]

Two other means of stabilization include splinting with wire or nylon fishing line (flexible fixation) and Erich arch bars (rigid fixation). Light ligature wire (28-gauge) or fishing line can be used with isolated avulsed teeth or multiple mobile teeth, as long as there is no concomitant dentoalveolar fracture. For rigid fixation in severe injuries, Erich bars are utilized.

In the case of a single maxillary subluxated tooth, the tooth is first brought back into position, as outlined earlier. Stabilization is achieved by including both teeth distal and mesial (lateral and medial) to the injured tooth. A large loop of wire is first placed, encompassing all three teeth and gently crimped on the labial surface at the posterior tooth. Smaller pieces of wire are then placed interdentally, passing over the original loop of wire superiorly on both labial and lingual surfaces. This second wire passes back inferiorly between the teeth, sandwiching the original loop of wire between it. It is then twisted and crimped on the labial side.

This process continues until all interdental areas are secured. Care must be taken not to break the wire at any point. If it does break, the entire procedure must be redone.[1,6] If available, the wire can be further stabilized by bonding it to individual teeth with acid etching. Small beads are placed on individual teeth and the wire is embedded in the material. If nylon fishing line is used, multiple ties are used instead of twisting and crimping.

An Erich arch bar is a semirigid wire, which is placed along the labial surface of the teeth and held in place with loops of wire, in a fashion similar to the previously described interdental technique. A similar splint, considered to be the splint of choice, is the acid-etched resin and arch wire splint. An arch wire is conformed to the labial surface of the teeth to be splinted. The middle third of each tooth is etched and the wire is attached with resin. At least two uninjured teeth are included in this splint, with the injured teeth sandwiched between them, and the arch is applied to these uninjured teeth first.[1,6,13,18] Because Erich arch bars require advanced dental techniques, the emergency physician should master ligature wire–nylon splinting. In all cases, patients should be advised to eat a soft diet and use oral rinses in place of brushing until dental follow-up can be obtained.

COMMON PITFALLS

- Improper handling and transport of avulsed teeth
- Delaying reimplantation of avulsed teeth
- Failure to radiographically rule out aspirated teeth in the comatose patient
- Failure to splint teeth that are subluxated, avulsed, or have root fractures
- Failure to first approximate the vermilion border in lip lacerations

References

1. Andreasen JO, Andreasen FM. *Essentials of traumatic injuries to the teeth.* Copenhagen: Munksgaard, 1990.
2. Andreasen JO, Andreasen FM. *Textbook and color atlas of traumatic injuries to the teeth,* 3rd ed. Copenhagen: Munksgaard, 1994.
3. Asseal LA. Infection in the maxillofacial trauma patient. In: Topazian RG, Goldberg MH, eds. *Oral and maxillofacial infections,* 3rd ed. Philadelphia: WB Saunders, 1994:430–447.
4. De Blanco LP. Lip suture with isobutyl cyanoacrylate. *Endod Dent Traumatol* 1994;10:15–18.
5. Diangelis AJ, Bakland LK. Traumatic dental injuries: current treatment concepts. *J Am Dent Assoc* 1998;129:1401.
6. Dumsha T. Luxation injuries. *Dent Clin North Am* 1995;39:79.
7. Goldstein EJC. Bites wounds and infection. *Clin Infect Dis* 1992;14:633.
8. Gutmann JL, Gutmann MS. Cause, incidence, and prevention of trauma to teeth. *Dent Clin North Am* 1995;39(1):1–13.
9. Hellman JR, Shott SR, Gootee MJ. Impalement injuries in the palate of children: review of 131 cases. *Int J Pediatr Otorhinolaryngol* 1993;26:157–163.
10. Josell SD, Abrams RG. Managing common dental problems and emergencies. *Pediatr Clin North Am* 1991;38:1325–1342.
11. Josell SD, Evaluation, diagnosis, and treatment of the traumatized patient. *Dent Clin North Am* 1995;39(1):15–24.
12. Law RC, Fouque CA, Waddell A, et al. Lesson of the week: penetrating intraoral trauma in children. *BMJ* 1997;314(7073):50–51.
13. McDonald N, Strassler HE. Evaluation for tooth stabilization and treatment of traumatized teeth. *Dent Clin North Am* 1999;43(1):135–149.
14. Oikarinen K. Clinical management of injuries to maxilla, mandible, and alveolus. *Dent Clin North Am* 1995;39:113.
15. Oyler R. Dental injuries. In: Harwood-Nuss AH, ed. *The clinical practice of emergency medicine.* Philadelphia: JB Lippincott Co, 1996.
16. Quinn PD, Loiselle J. Management of soft tissue injuries of the mouth. In: Henretig FM, King C, eds. *Textbook of pediatric emergency procedures.* Baltimore: Williams & Wilkins, 1997:741–750.
17. Radowski D, McGill TJ, Healy GB, et al. Penetrating trauma of the oropharynx in children. *Laryngoscope* 1993;103:991–994.

18. Serio FG. Clinical rationale for tooth stabilization and splinting. *Dent Clin North Am* 1999;43(1):1–6.
19. Shesser R, Smith M. Oral emergencies. *Top Emerg Med* 1984;6(3):48–65.
20. Trope M. Clinical management of the avulsed tooth. *Dent Clin North Am* 1995;39:93.

CHAPTER 99
Eye Trauma

William H. Shoff and Suzanne Moore Shepherd

Eye trauma is common, accounting for up to 10% of emergency department visits. In general, it is associated with 12 to 29% of facial fractures. Each year, over 2 million eye injuries occur at home, work, and play. Sixty thousand are admitted. Visual impairment occurs in 50,000. Children under 17 have a higher percentage of serious injuries. It is estimated that wearing protective lenses could prevent 90% of all eye injuries.[5]

The emergency physician (EP) is in an ideal position to diagnose, manage, and refer eye injuries. It is important that the EP be aware of conditions that threaten vision and perform a systematic examination to exclude those conditions. Many conditions that would have impaired vision in the past can now be preserved through advances in ophthalmologic therapy. Injuries to the eye occur by four mechanisms: abrasion, blunt force, penetrating object, and burns. This chapter presents an overview of the EP's approach to and management of eye trauma.

EMERGENCY DEPARTMENT EVALUATION

When confronted with eye trauma, the EP must conduct a systematic and comprehensive eye evaluation. Therapy is usually reserved until the evaluation is completed; however, there are two instances in which immediate action is imperative: the chemical burn and traumatic endophthalmitis. On arrival to the emergency department, the chemically burned eye must be irrigated immediately and continuously for at least 30 minutes with saline or another neutral solution (usually several liters), and preferentially until the measured pH reaches physiologic neutrality. This must happen before the completion of triage or any other portion of the evaluation. Traumatic endophthalmitis usually presents as pain and inflammation out of proportion to the penetrating injury that has led to the infection. It demands immediate ophthalmologic consultation to inject the eye with intravitreal antibiotics.

History

The history should establish four basic pieces of information: mechanism of injury, symptoms, eye history, and scene of the injury. The mechanism may involve an object striking the eye, a fall, a motor vehicle crash, an explosion, or a fire. Was the globe ruptured by blunt trauma or penetrated by an object? Symptoms referable to the globe include blepharospasm (involuntary lid closure), blurred vision, diplopia, eye pain, discharge from the eye, flashes of light, floaters, foreign-body (FB) sensation, halos, photophobia, redness of the eye, and tearing. The history includes visual acuity prior to the injury, eye disease, and past injury.

Visual Acuity

Visual acuity should be documented as soon as possible after the patient arrives, because it is the single most important predictor of visual outcome. Test one eye at a time, covering the opposite eye. Begin with the worst eye. Corrective lenses should be worn when possible; if they are missing, try using a piece of paper with multiple pinholes. Do not put contact lenses into an injured eye. The order of preference for testing acuity is as follows: far vision (20 ft from a Snellen chart), near vision (14 in. from a Rosenbaum card), reading print (note distance), counting fingers, hand motion, light perception, and no light perception. Children require some special consideration. From age 6 months to 3 years, fixing on a moving light source corresponds to 20/40 vision. From age 3 to 6 years, use Allen pictures. For those who cannot read, use the "E" chart.

Lids and Other Periorbital Structures

Examine the lids and periorbital structures. When there is any suspicion of an open globe secondary to blunt or penetrating trauma, *no pressure* should be applied to the globe thereafter for *any* part of the examination (see Emergency Department Management). Inspect for swelling, ecchymosis, proptosis, enophthalmos, ptosis, lacerations, and FBs. If the eye is swollen shut, lid retraction is necessary to view the globe and underlying structures. Ptosis suggests contusion or laceration of the levator palpebrae, Horner syndrome, or third-nerve palsy. Upper lid lacerations should be explored enough to note penetration of the tarsal plate, the muscle, or the entire lid (through-and-through). All three indicate significant force and raise the concern for injury to the globe. Any surface FBs that are noted should be removed. Penetrating FBs are always left for the surgeon to remove. Palpate the orbital rim and soft tissues and the zygomatic arch area, noting point tenderness, step-off, and subcutaneous emphysema.

Anterior Segment

The anterior segment of the eye includes the sclera, conjunctiva, cornea, anterior chamber, iris, and lens. To examine this part of the eye requires the use of a topical anesthetic, usually a minimum of 2 drops of anesthetic followed by 2 or more drops 20 seconds or more later. Inspect for globe laceration, FBs, subconjunctival hemorrhage (note extent), chemosis, limbal edema, lid laceration, and contact lens (remove when identified). Remove nonadherent FBs as soon as identified (see Emergency Department Management). Perform a slit-lamp examination to evaluate the globe (FBs, lacerations, and leaking vitreous), lid margins (lacerations), the cornea (FBs and abrasions), the anterior chamber (cell, flare, FBs, hyphema, and hypopyon), the iris (any disruption), and the lens (may be displaced partially or completely). Under a cobalt light, fluorescein dye is used to highlight abrasions on the cornea and to perform Seidel's test for leaking vitreous.

Pupils

The pupils provide information through size, shape, and reaction. Inspect the pupils, looking for anisocoria and distortion in the pupil. *Anisocoria* has been defined as a disparity in size greater than 0.3 to 1.0 mm. If the pupils react briskly and the degree of anisocoria is unchanged with and without bright light, the anisocoria is physiologic. A distorted pupil suggests globe rupture, iridectomy, or synechiae. In a ruptured globe, the pupil is tear-shaped, with the apex of the teardrop pointing toward the rupture. Test for relative afferent pupillary defect (RAPD) suggesting any of the following: efferent third-nerve damage, glaucoma, iris incarceration, massive internal derangement of the eye, optic chiasm or tract damage, optic nerve damage, retinal detachment, traumatic mydriasis, or vitreous hemorrhage. Observe the pupil symmetry and size in ambient light. Swing a bright light from eye to eye. When the light strikes the *unaffected* eye, both pupils constrict. When the light strikes the *affected* eye, both pupils paradoxically dilate. Verify the findings by swinging the light from eye to eye a few times.

Extraocular Muscles

Test the extraocular muscles in the six cardinal positions of gaze. With infants, use keys, a light, or toys. Binocular diplopia can be seen with an abscess, cellulitis, cranial nerve palsy, hematoma, orbital edema, orbital floor fracture with muscle entrapment, orbital wall fracture with muscle entrapment, or retrobulbar hemorrhage. Monocular diplopia can be seen with corneal irregularity, a dislocated lens (natural or implant), iridodialysis, or retinal detachment.

Posterior Segment

The posterior segment consists of the optic nerve, retina, and vitreous. The direct ophthalmoscopic examination yields limited but important information. It is not necessary to dilate the pupils. Absence of the red reflex or inability to visualize the fundus suggests cataract, hyphema, lens rupture, retinal detachment, or vitreous hemorrhage.[4] Visual field testing by confrontation is sufficient for the EP. Optic nerve function is assessed by testing for RAPD (see previous section on pupils). If the pupils are nonreactive or irregular, red desaturation testing is a suitable substitute. To test red desaturation, ask the patient to view a bright red object with each eye separately and compare the two images. If the optic nerve is damaged in one eye, the image coming from that eye will appear gray or washed out in comparison to the good eye.

Intraocular Pressure

The intraocular pressure (IOP) may be elevated above 22 mm Hg in several conditions: acute glaucoma (from angle recession), globe rupture, hyphema, lens dislocation, lens swelling, suprachoroidal hemorrhage, and retrobulbar hemorrhage. Normal pressure ranges from 10 to 20.[10] When the pressure is less than 5 mm Hg, penetration of the globe should be considered.

Imaging the Eye

When there is suspicion of injury to the orbit or globe, spiral computed tomographic (CT) scanning with axial and coronal cuts is the preferred study. Choroidal detachment, endophthalmitis, fractures, FBs, extraocular hemorrhage or hematoma (less than 3 days old), lens luxation or subluxation, globe rupture, orbital cellulitis, subperiosteal hematoma, vitreous hemorrhage (less than 3 days old), and, probably, retinal detachment can be identified. It can detect FBs as small as 0.6 to 1.5 mm, depending on the composition. Although ultrasound can detect FBs as small as 0.2 mm, operator dependence and the necessity of applying pressure to the globe limit its use.[9]

EMERGENCY DEPARTMENT MANAGEMENT

Blowout Fractures and Other Facial Fractures

When a ball, fist, or another object larger than the orbital rim strikes the eye, a blowout or other fracture may result. It is important to maintain a high index of suspicion, because the signs and symptoms can be minor. Suggestive signs and symptoms are diplopia, enophthalmos, epistaxis (medial orbital wall involvement), inferior displacement of the globe, ipsilateral numbness of the cheek and the upper lip (damage to the infraorbital nerve), periorbital ecchymosis, periorbital swelling, periorbital subcutaneous emphysema (sinus involvement), point tenderness of the orbital rim or maxilla, and palpable step-off.[11] Plain films have been used for diagnosis, but can be falsely negative (less than or equal to 60%) or falsely positive (less than or equal to 46%)[2]; therefore, a spiral CAT scan with coronal cuts is preferred for diagnosis. Most blowout fractures involve the inferior or medial walls of the orbit. Involvement of the roof of the orbit signals that considerably more force (about seven times) occurred and suggests violation of the cranial vault with associated injury to the brain.

LeFort fractures (I to III), tripod fractures, nasal fractures, and other fractures about the head and face may or may not have an associated eye injury, but it should be sought, given the forces involved. At the minimum for an apparently uninvolved eye, the visual acuity, extraocular movement, absence of obvious trauma, and absence of visual symptoms should be documented. See Chapter 97, "Maxillofacial Injuries," for further discussion of facial trauma.

Management consists of oromaxillofacial referral, ophthalmologic referral, antibiotics (cover *Staphylococcus* and *Streptococcus*) for 10 to 14 days, avoidance of blowing the nose, ice packs, and nasal decongestant spray (oxymetazoline). Surgical repair can be delayed for up to 14 days. Eighty-five percent of blowout fractures (even symptomatic) will resolve without necessitating surgical intervention.[1]

Burns

Five types of burns are considered here: chemical, electrical, infrared (IF), thermal and ultraviolet (UV). All eyes with chemical burns must be irrigated immediately with saline for at least 30 minutes. Check the pH 5 minutes after completing the irrigation. Repeat the irrigation until the pH is 7.0 to 7.4. Irrigation must not be held up for triage or registration. Time is sight. Irrigation at the scene is not an adequate substitute, because it is often inadequate. Contact the local poison control center for assistance in identifying the chemical in question, its pH, and its potential to cause damage to the eye. It is always a good idea to notify poison control so they can add the information to their record of exposures. After the irrigation is completed, the eye examination is conducted. *Alkali burns* are particularly devastating, because alkalis destroy and penetrate (liquefaction necrosis). Alkali damage is classified as four grades:

1. Corneal epithelial damage similar to a corneal abrasion with a good prognosis
2. Cornea is hazy, but the details of the iris are seen and up to one-third of the limbus is ischemic (whitened); the prognosis is still good.
3. Corneal epithelium is destroyed and the details of the iris are blurred; one-third to one-half of the limbus is ischemic; the prognosis is guarded.
4. Cornea is opaque, with the details of the iris and pupil obscured; more than half of the limbus is ischemic; the prognosis is poor.

Acid burns are classified in the same manner, but less often produce severe damage, because strong acids precipitate proteins, forming a barrier to further penetration (coagulation necrosis).

For severe chemical burns, the symptoms are dramatic. Pain is severe. The eye is reddened or white. The signs include anterior chamber reaction, chemosis, corneal edema or opacification, and vessel loss or ischemia (conjunctiva, limbus, and episclera). Prior to irrigation, remove all foreign matter by sweeping the fornices with a moistened cotton-tipped applicator. *Calcium hydroxide* tends to cake and may be easier to remove if the applicator is moistened with 10% EDTA. Minimal irritation and no symptoms after irrigation require no further follow-up. Moderate irritation with symptoms requires instillation of antibiotic ointment, and referral to an ophthalmologist in 24 hours. Any injury producing more than moderate irritation and significant change in vision mandates immediate consultation with an ophthalmologist.

Electrical burns are rare; however, the injury may be indirect. Nine percent of patients experiencing electrical injuries about the head develop cataracts 6 to 12 months after the injury. *Infrared radiation* can produce keratitis and "glassblower cataract" after prolonged exposure to heat. It can also result in macular damage or cataract formation. *Thermal burns* are rare. The light of a heat flash reaches the eye faster, producing the upward rotation reflex of the globe (Bell's phenomenon), which protects the cornea from damage. Thermal corneal injury occurs when hot objects, such as lighted matches, spitting grease, and car radiator steam, are propelled into the eye. These burns rarely involve more than the corneal epithelium and heal in a few days. Treatment involves the application of cold compresses (just cold enough to eliminate the pain) for up to 2 hours. Then, for partial thickness burns of the lids and surrounding skin, ophthalmic antibiotic ointment is applied. Minor burns of the cornea are managed similarly to a corneal abrasion. For more severe burns, an ophthalmologist should be consulted immediately. *Ultraviolet radiation* from the sun, tanning salons, and welder's arc produces acute, diffuse, superficial punctate keratitis (SPK) of the corneal epithelium about 6 to 12 hours after exposure. The amount of radiation is enhanced by reflection (water, rocks, snow) and altitude above 8000 ft. If the exposure is prolonged, damage may occur to the retina, particularly the fovea, and vision is affected 1 to 2 days later.[14] This injury is managed similarly to that of a corneal abrasion. A nonsteroidal antiinflammatory medication and a narcotic-containing analgesic are prescribed. Ophthalmologic follow-up for all burns of the eye is essential unless the injury is minimal.

Corneal and Conjunctival Injuries

The corneal epithelium is four to six cells thick, and abrasions thereof usually heal in 12 to 36 hours, and sometimes longer, depending on the injury. Wounds that extend through the basement membrane of the epithelium, and deeper, require surgical approximation. Infection is a risk with any wound, and a retained FB heightens that risk. Iron-containing FBs will leave a rust ring deposit after being in place for a couple of hours. Rust rings extrude to the surface over 2 days, where they are easily removed with an ophthalmic burr, similarly to an FB.

Corneal abrasions usually present with an FB sensation, whether or not there is an FB present on the cornea. Often, there is a history of something striking the eye. High-speed particles raise the suspicion for a penetrating eye injury. In addition to an FB sensation, symptoms include blepharospasm, blurred vision, eye pain, halos around lights, photophobia, red eye, and tearing. Occasionally, there is no report of pain. Visual acuity is mildly decreased. The eye is hyperemic, the eyelids are mildly swollen, and an anterior chamber reaction (cells and/or flare) is sometimes noted. Abrasions are highlighted by fluorescein and easily seen on slit-lamp examination or in a darkened room, using a hand-held cobalt light. Because fluorescein permanently stains a soft contact lens, remove the lens prior to fluorescein instillation. Low-mass, low-speed particles produce insignificant trauma without anterior chamber reaction; therefore, the IOP need not be measured. When larger objects, such as a finger, fist, or ball, strike the eye, the IOP should be measured. Treatment begins with instilling anesthetic ophthalmic drops (1 to 2 drops, followed in 20 seconds by 1 to 2 more drops). Removal of an FB is accomplished by using gentle irrigation; a saline-moistened, cotton-tipped applicator (brush off); an ophthalmic burr; or a 25-gauge needle held tangential to the corneal surface (pick off). Rust ring removal is accomplished with an ophthalmic burr. Instill a cycloplegic (homatropine 2% or cyclopentolate 2%, 1 to 2 drops) to reduce synechiae formation secondary to inflammation. Although controversial, some ophthalmologists would advocate patching the eye if there is considerable pain caused by blinking or the abrasion is greater than 2 mm in size. Antibiotic ointment is instilled and the patch (use two eye pads) is applied lightly, but firmly enough to keep the lids from opening under the patch. Patches are removed and the eye reexamined in 12 to 24 hours. Do not keep a patch in place for more than 24 hours because of increased risk of infection. If the eye is not patched, an ophthalmic antibiotic (drops q.i.d. or ointment b.i.d. or t.i.d.) is prescribed. Analgesics prescribed include a nonsteroidal antiinflammatory (daily dosing for 3 days) and a narcotic as needed. All corneal abrasions are followed closely, usually at a 1-day interval, until healed. EPs can manage corneal abrasions, but referral to an ophthalmologist the next day is a suitable option.

Contact lens usage can lead to numerous corneal problems. The symptom complex is similar to that of corneal abrasions. Contact lens–related corneal abrasions result from hypoxic injury (improper fit or overwear), toxic deposits under the lens, and trauma related to insertions or removal of the lens. Infectious keratitis can occur secondary to gram-negative bacterial organisms, particularly *Pseudomonas,* and protozoa, specifically, *Acanthamoeba* (soft contact lens wear, nonsterile saline rinsing solution made from salt tablets, and swimming while wearing the lenses). Chemical irritation occurs secondary to preservatives (thimerosal and chlorhexidine) and inadequate rinsing of lens after enzyme use. Tight lens syndrome occurs within 2 days of the fitting of the offending lens (usually a soft lens). The lens appears "sucked-on" and leaves a conjunctival imprint of the lens after lens removal. Other findings that may be seen with soft contact lens use include corneal ulceration, SPK, anterior uveitis, and hypopyon (infrequent).[14] Treatment begins with removal of the contact lens. Remember that fluorescein permanently stains the lens. The eye is not patched. An antipseudomonal ophthalmic antibiotic preparation is prescribed. A cycloplegic is instilled (see corneal abrasion management in previous paragraph). Refer to an ophthalmologist the next day.

Conjunctival and *subconjunctival* injuries are minor if the underlying sclera remains intact, because the conjunctiva do not provide any structural support to the eye. Often, there is no history of anything striking the eye. The visual acuity is usually unaffected. There may be an associated corneal injury, exhibiting the usual corneal symptoms. All conjunctival wounds, with or without an associated FB, must be examined under magnification for indications of scleral penetration. The eye is anesthetized in the usual manner (as noted under corneal abrasion management) and the wound is teased with a cotton-tipped applicator, while observing for white scleral tissue. Seidel's test can provide additional information. If there is any doubt about wound penetration of the sclera, the injury should be managed as though there has been violation of the globe, and an ophthalmologist should be consulted immediately. FBs are removed from the fornices by hand-held irrigation or forniceal sweeping with a saline-moistened, cotton-tipped applicator (eye must be anesthetized in the usual manner). If the wound solely involves the conjunctiva and there is no associated corneal injury, an ophthalmic antibiotic is prescribed, as noted with corneal abrasions. There is no need to patch the eye. Refer the patient to follow-up with an ophthalmologist the next day.

Eyelid Lacerations (Complex) and Other Penetrating Trauma

As soon as there is any evidence of globe penetration, either overt or suggestive, the visual acuity must be documented grossly, the eye shielded immediately from any further pressure, and an ophthalmologist consulted. All protruding objects penetrating the eye must be left alone and protected from manipulation until an ophthalmologic surgeon takes over the management of the injury. Any penetrating wound near the eye is assumed to have penetrated the globe until proven otherwise. Isolated lacerations of the conjunctiva are benign. Lacerations of the sclera, or the full thickness of the cornea, are considered a penetrating injury. When the cornea is penetrated, the iris plugs the wound and distorts the pupil into a teardrop shape, with the apex of the drop pointing at the wound (Fig. 99.1). When there is doubt regarding a penetrating wound, Seidel's test should be performed. Parenteral antibiotics (gentamicin plus vancomycin or clindamycin) should be administered prophylactically (see section on Endophthalmitis). All penetrating eye wounds demand an emergent ophthalmologic consultation.

An ophthalmologic surgeon should repair complex eyelid lacerations. These wounds are characterized by any of the following: exposed orbital fat, globe penetration, muscle laceration, nasolacrimal system damage, significant force involved, tarsal plate laceration, or through-and-through laceration. With any wound of the eyelid or near the eye, it is imperative that the lids be retracted to rule out globe penetration. The nasolacrimal duct system is located in the medial eyelids, extending laterally 5 to 7 mm from the medial canthus. Medial to the canthus, the system runs vertically to empty into the nose. A parenteral antibiotic (cover *Staphylococcus* and *Streptococcus*) should be administered prophylactically. All wounds should be covered with a sterile saline dressing to keep the tissues moist until the ophthalmologist arrives.

Eyelid Laceration (Simple) and Periorbital Contusion

Either an eyelid laceration or a periorbital contusion, isolated or in combination, mandates a thorough evaluation (as outlined under Emergency Department Evaluation) to eliminate involvement of the globe or other underlying structures. Periorbital contusion is managed with ice packs, concurrent intracranial injury must be evaluated, and instructions are given for the ensuing 48 hours. Resolution of a simple contusion can take 2 to 3 weeks, while hemorrhage into the levator palpebrae may produce ptosis that can last for months. A simple laceration of the eyelid involves neither underlying structures (see Complex Eyelid Lacerations) nor the lid margin. Simple eyelid lacerations can be repaired readily by an EP. Contaminated wounds must be irrigated without directing the force against the underlying globe. No tissue should be debrided, because of the excellent blood supply to the eyelid. Wound closure is accomplished with single interrupted 6-0 or 7-0 unabsorbable suture, which should be removed in 5 days. If the wound was contaminated, parenteral antibiotics (cover *Staphylococcus* and *Streptococcus*) are administered in the emergency department and oral antibiotics prescribed for the following 7 to 10 days. Unless the trauma was minimal, refer the patient to an ophthalmologist for follow-up evaluation.

Globe Luxation or Subluxation

This is rare. The visual acuity in the involved eye may vary from mildly reduced to no light perception. Reduction must be effected immediately, before the onset of orbital edema prevents reduction and to decrease tension on the optic nerve. If an ophthalmologist cannot be present within 20 minutes to reduce the globe, the EP should attempt reduction by applying gentle pressure to the globe while retracting the eyelids. Admission is mandatory for further ophthalmologic management.

Globe Rupture Secondary to Blunt Trauma

As soon as a ruptured globe is suspected, it is imperative to shield the globe, using a Fox shield, paper cup, Styrofoam cup, or similar device; and then to consult an ophthalmologist immediately (Fig. 99.2). Parenteral antibiotics (gentamicin plus vancomycin or clindamycin) should be administered prophylactically (see the section on Endophthalmitis). Additionally, bedrest, with the head of the bed elevated, and antiemetics are

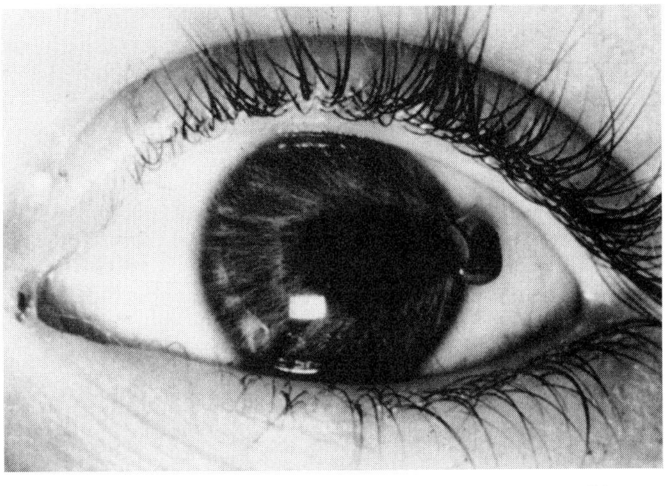

Figure 99.1. Penetrating corneal foreign body with entrapment of the iris, forming a teardrop pupil. This was a metallic chip projectile that resulted from hammering metal on metal.

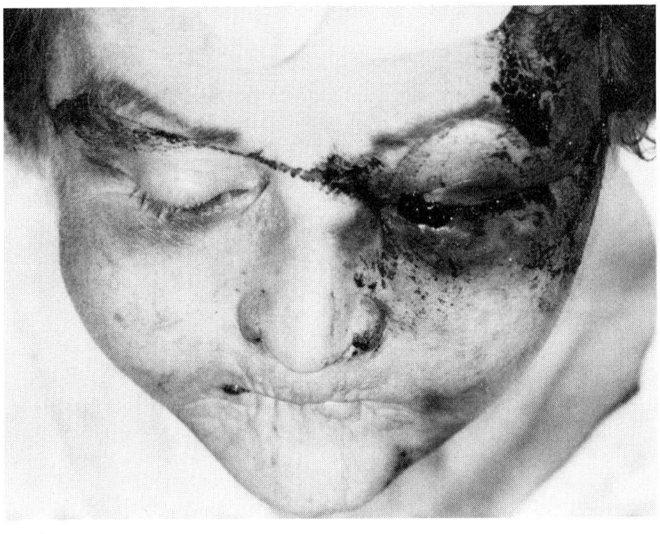

Figure 99.2. Ruptured globe from blunt trauma with prolapse of choroid, easily mistaken for clotted blood.

indicated to lessen the occurrence of stresses that might increase IOP. The globe is ruptured up to 3.5% of the time in blunt trauma.[3,7] Ruptures typically occur at the weakest areas of the globe: the equator, the limbus, or muscle insertions. Another site of rupture is that opposite to the point of impact. The conjunctiva often remain intact after rupture, and bleeding occurring beneath the conjunctiva produces circumferential bloody chemosis (Fig. 99.3). When severe eye hemorrhage (hemorrhagic chemosis, hyphema, vitreous hemorrhage) or severe periocular hemorrhage has occurred, the presence of one of four signs predicts rupture with a sensitivity of 100% and a specificity of 98.5%. Those signs are (1) a visual acuity that demonstrates light perception or less, (2) an anterior chamber that is abnormally deep or shallow, (3) an IOP of less than or equal to 5 mm Hg, and/or (4) a media opacity that prevents fundus visualization.[7] If intubation is necessary, the use of succinylcholine should be avoided, if possible, because it raises extraocular muscle tone.

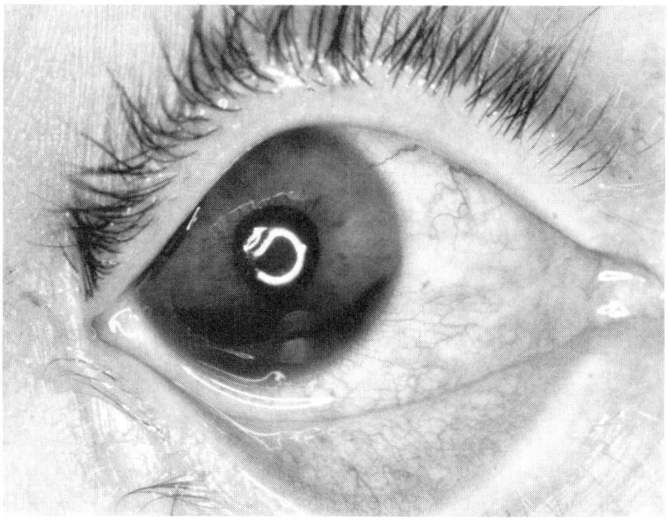

Figure 99.4. Traumatic hyphema (25%) with blood layering in the anterior chamber, subsequent to impact from a racquetball.

Hyphema and Other Anterior Segment Injuries

The forces of blunt and penetrating trauma contuse, cut, rupture, stretch, and tear the tissues of the anterior segment of the eye, resulting in hyphema, glaucoma, lens displacement, and cataracts. When any of these conditions are diagnosed or suspected, an ophthalmologist should be consulted immediately. *Hyphema* may be microscopic (cells visualized by slit lamp) or gross (gauged by the percentage of the anterior chamber that is filled). If blood fills the chamber entirely, it is called an "eight ball" hyphema (Fig. 99.4). Symptoms include pain, red eye, and blurred vision. Treatment begins by shielding the eye and elevating the head to 30 degrees. Medications, other than those for pain and nausea, are administered only at the direction of an ophthalmologist. Some microhyphemas are managed on an outpatient basis. When there is a history of sickle cell disease or trait and the IOP is greater than 25 mm Hg, the anterior chamber may need to be washed out. In general, rebleeding will occur in up to 37% of the cases.[6]

Traumatic glaucoma occurs if the trabecular meshwork is obstructed by blood and inflammatory products or is disrupted. Glaucoma may develop acutely over hours or be delayed for months or years, depending on the injury. Medications employed acutely include topical β-blockers, acetazolamide, mannitol, and, sometimes, miotics. Lens displacement varies in degree, as do its associated symptoms, which include myopia, monocular diplopia, and, most commonly, blurred vision. Several signs suggest this diagnosis, including decreased visual acuity, anterior chamber asymmetry, a displaced lens, quivering of the iris (iridodonesis) or the lens (phacodonesis) after rapid eye movement, visibility of the lens edge, and the presence of vitreous in the anterior chamber. *Traumatic cataracts* can occur secondary to blunt trauma alone (contusion cataracts) or secondary to penetrating trauma, irrespective of direct injury of the lens capsule. Violation of the lens capsule tends to accelerate the process. Traumatic cataracts also may occur after lightning injuries. They develop in hours to months. Symptoms include blurred vision, glare from lights (particularly headlights), and reduced color vision. Signs include decreased visual acuity, an indistinct retina, lens opacity, and a reduced red reflex. In acute trauma, the eye should be shielded as soon as any of these conditions are identified or suspected.

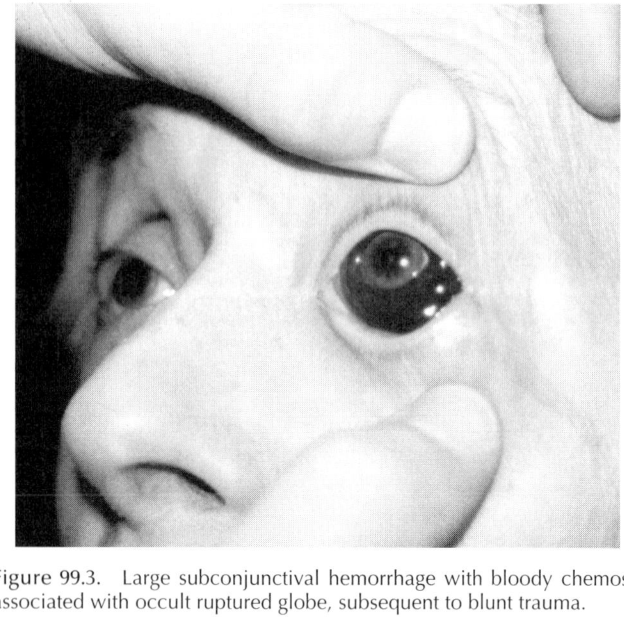

Figure 99.3. Large subconjunctival hemorrhage with bloody chemosis associated with occult ruptured globe, subsequent to blunt trauma.

Intraocular Foreign Bodies

Eighty percent of all intraocular FBs enter the eye through the cornea. The obvious penetrating FB of the eye is easy to diagnose. When not evident, they should be suspected in certain circumstances, including a history of hammering metal on metal (grinding usually does not lead to penetration), a child with eye pain and a history of something sharp being near the eye, and a history of head trauma with the eye(s) swollen shut. Metal splinters produced by hammering metal on metal and glass splinters produced by shattering glass can penetrate the eye painlessly.[8] Plain films can be helpful but do not differentiate intraocular from extraocular FBs. Some FBs are not intraocular but intraorbital. In this circumstance, damage to the globe must be ruled out. The imaging study of choice for detecting intraocular FBs is spiral CT.

Intraocular FBs that remain in the eye can produce varying degrees of inflammatory reaction. Copper, iron, steel, vegetable matter, and wood produce severe reactions. Aluminum, nickel, mercury, and zinc produce mild reactions. Carbon, coal, glass, gold, lead, plaster, plastic, platinum, porcelain, rubber, silver, and stone are inert. Iron, nickel, and steel are magnetic. Inflammatory reactions put the eye at risk for endophthalmitis.

Posterior Segment Injuries

The posterior segment consists of choroid, optic nerve, retina, and vitreous, and any indication of injury to it mandates an immediate ophthalmologic consultation. The choroid, retina, or vitreous may be detached, hemorrhagic, ruptured, or torn. The optic nerve may be injured along its course by direct or indirect mechanisms.

Symptoms are often lacking. When they occur, they are nonspecific: blurred vision, curtain of darkness, flashes of light, floaters, pain, and red eye. Important signs are blurring of fundus detail, decreased acuity, and RAPD. Anatomic findings are not necessarily apparent on direct funduscopy performed in the emergency department, even with dilatation. They are best identified by an ophthalmologist using dilated indirect funduscopy.

Retrobulbar Hematoma

This is a very rare condition. It is associated with intraoperative retrobulbar injections and occurs postoperatively. It is less often associated with trauma. Signs and symptoms include severe eye pain, nausea, vomiting, decreasing vision, diplopia, RAPD, decreased ocular motility, hemorrhagic chemosis, and proptosis. If it develops over minutes, the eye must be decompressed immediately by lateral canthotomy (Fig. 99.5). If it develops over hours, conservative management is appropriate and involves head elevation, ice packs, acetazolamide, mannitol, timolol, and serial measurements of IOP and pupillary responses. An ophthalmologist must be consulted as soon as this condition is suspected.

Subconjunctival Hemorrhage (Isolated)

Typically, an isolated subconjunctival hemorrhage is flat and involves a small portion of the bulbar conjunctiva without any break in the membrane. The history may reveal a related Valsalva maneuver or rubbing the eye, but often there is no history to explain the event. In addition, there is no history of anticoagulant use, blood dyscrasia, or recurrent subconjunctival hemorrhage. No treatment is necessary. The condition is not threatening to the eye and will resolve over approximately 14 days.

Traumatic Iritis

Any trauma to the eye may produce inflammation in the anterior segment of the eye, with symptoms of blurred vision, pain, photophobia, redness of the eye, and tearing. Other names for this condition are *anterior chamber reaction, anterior uveitis, uveitis,* and *iridocyclitis.* Iritis occurs in up to 18% of eye trauma.[12] Symptoms vary from mild to severe and include blurred vision, pain, photophobia, redness of the eye, and tearing. Visual acuity is usually mildly decreased, but can be significantly reduced. The pain of ciliary spasm is exacerbated by light shining in the eye, which increases ciliary muscle contraction (photophobia). When light strikes the unaffected eye, the consensual response exacerbates the pain (consensual photophobia). Protein and white cells are visible by slit lamp in the anterior chamber. The limbus is injected. In severe reactions, there may be hypopyon. The IOP may be increased or decreased. Treatment includes a cycloplegic (2% homatropine or 2% cyclopentolate), a nonsteroidal antiinflammatory medication (for 3 days), and a narcotic analgesic (as needed). The patient is referred to an ophthalmologist (usually within 36 hours), who, in some cases, will prescribe steroids.

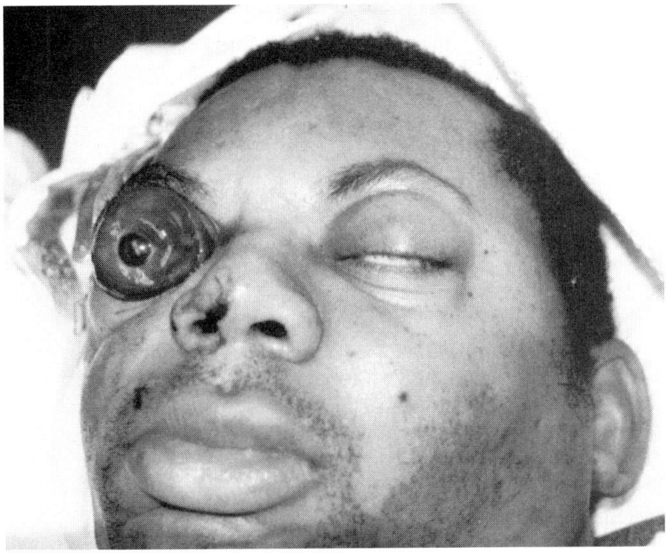

Figure 99.5. Retrobulbar hemorrhage demonstrating dramatic proptosis and subconjunctival hemorrhage after a fist strike in a man on warfarin.

SECONDARY CONDITIONS

Endophthalmitis

Eye trauma (25% of cases) and eye surgery (62% cases) predispose to endophthalmitis. It develops in 8% to 13% of eye trauma when there is a retained FB. The percentage rises to 26% if the FB is organic material from a rural setting. The onset is sudden and begins from hours to 2 months after the injury. *Bacillus cereus* infection has been reported to develop within 24 hours, streptococci within 2 days, and *Staphylococcus epidermidis* within 4 days.[13]

Delay in treatment of a few hours, particularly with *Bacillus* species, can lead to the loss of an eye. The symptoms are blurred vision, fever, a red eye, and severe pain. The signs are anterior chamber reaction, acuity decreased (marked), cells and opacities in the vitreous, conjunctival hyperemia, corneal ring abscess, decreased red reflex, hypopyon, increased IOP, and proptosis. There is a noted association between *B. cereus* infections, metallic intraocular FBs, and injuries related to soil. Early diagnosis is imperative for the best outcome; therefore, the EP must maintain a high index of suspicion for endophthalmitis.

Sympathetic Ophthalmia

The incidence is 0.2% after penetrating eye trauma and 0.01% after routine eye surgery. Sixty-five percent of cases begin between 2 and 8 weeks after the insult, and 90% within 1 year (range of 5 days to decades). The signs and symptoms in the sympathetic eye begin as a mild anterior uveitis, which progresses over time to anterior and posterior uveitis. In about 5% of the cases, only the posterior uveitis manifests (blurred vision, floaters, pain, photophobia, and possible redness). The condition of the injured eye (exciting eye) may worsen at the same time.

References

1. Catone GA, Morrissette MP, Carlson ER. A retrospective study of untreated blow-out fractures. *J Oral Maxillofac Surg* 1988;46:1033.
2. Crikelair GF, et al. A critical look at the "blowout" fracture. *Plast Reconstr Surg* 1972;49:374.
3. Emmanuella J, et al. Predictors of blinding or serious eye injury in blunt trauma. *J Trauma* 1992;33:19.
4. Gossman MD, Roberts DM, Rarr CC. Ophthalmic aspects of orbital injury. Clin Plast Surg 1992;19:71.
5. *Impact protection and polycarbonate lenses.* Schamburg, IL: Prevent Blindness America, 1995.
6. Kearns A. Traumatic hyphema: a retrospective study of 314 cases. *Br J Ophthalmol* 1991;74:137.
7. Kylstra JA, Lamkin JC, Runyan DK. Clinical predictors of scleral rupture after blunt ocular trauma. *Am J Ophthalmol* 1993;115:530.

8. Lubeck D. Penetrating ocular injuries. *Emerg Med Clin North Am* 1988;6:127.
9. Lustrin ES, et al. Radiologic assessment of trauma and foreign bodies of the eye and orbit. *Neuroimaging Clin North Am* 1996;6(1):219.
10. Martin XD. Normal intraocular pressure in man. *Ophthalmologica* 1992;205:57.
11. O'hare TH. Blow-out fractures: a review. *J Emerg Med* 1991;9:253.
12. Rothova A, et al. Clinical features of acute anterior uveitis. *Am J Ophthalmol* 1987;103:137.
13. Shemmer GB, Driebe WT Jr. Posttraumatic *Bacillus cereus* endophthalmitis. *Arch Ophthalmol* 1987;105:342.
14. Tso MM, LaPiana RG. The human fovea after sungazing. *Trans Am Acad Ophthalmol Otolaryngol* 1975;79:788.

Bibliography

Barr DH, Samples JR, Hedges JR. Ophthalmologic, otolaryngologic, and dental procedures. In: Roberts JR, Hedges JR, eds. *Clinical procedures in emergency medicine,* 3rd ed, Philadelphia: WB Saunders, 1991.
Catalano RA, ed. *Ocular emergencies.* Philadelphia: WB Saunders, 1992.
Cullom RD Jr, Chang B, eds. *The Wills eye manual.* Philadelphia: Lippincott–Raven Publishers, 1994.
MacCumber MW, ed. *Management of ocular injuries and emergencies.* Philadelphia: Lippincott–Raven Publishers, 1998.
Palay DA, Krachmer JH, eds. *Ophthalmology for the primary care physician.* St. Louis: Mosby, 1997.
Scott JL, Ghezzi KT, eds. Emergency treatment of the eye. *Emerg Med Clin North Am* 1995;13(3):521.
Shingleton BJ, Hersh PS, Kenyon DR, eds. *Eye trauma.* St. Louis: Mosby, 1991.

CHAPTER 100

Neck Injuries

Gerard R. Cox and Brigitte M. Baumann

The emergency management of the patient with a neck injury is one of the greatest challenges in trauma care. Neck wounds occur in 5% to 10% of all trauma victims, with associated mortality exceeding 10%. Either blunt or penetrating trauma can cause damage to multiple systems due to the close proximity of numerous vital structures in the neck. The occult nature of many of these injuries requires a thorough understanding of the anatomy of the neck and a systematic approach to evaluation and management. Whereas early surgical intervention was once the rule, growing experience with other diagnostic modalities and nonoperative management has led to reevaluation of traditional treatment approaches.[15]

This chapter focuses on the emergency department (ED) evaluation and management of blunt and penetrating neck trauma. The management of cervical spine injuries and hanging and strangulation injuries is reviewed elsewhere in the text.

ANATOMIC COMPLEXITY OF THE NECK

The neck contains components of the respiratory, gastrointestinal, vascular, musculoskeletal, endocrine, and central and peripheral nervous systems in closer proximity than in any other body region. These structures are partially protected by the mandible anteriorly and the cervical spine and thick paraspinous musculature posteriorly, but the lack of a surrounding skeletal or fibrous covering and the flexibility of the neck place them at risk of injury.

Discussions of surgical anatomy often divide the neck into either zones or triangles.[3] Zone I is the region between the clavicles and the inferior aspect of the cricoid cartilage (Fig. 100.1). This area includes the thoracic outlet; proximal portions of the common carotid, subclavian, and vertebral arteries; apices of the lungs; trachea; esophagus; thoracic duct; and thyroid gland. Mortality is highest for zone I injuries because of the risk to intrathoracic structures and the difficulty in attaining surgical exposure and proximal control of vascular injuries.

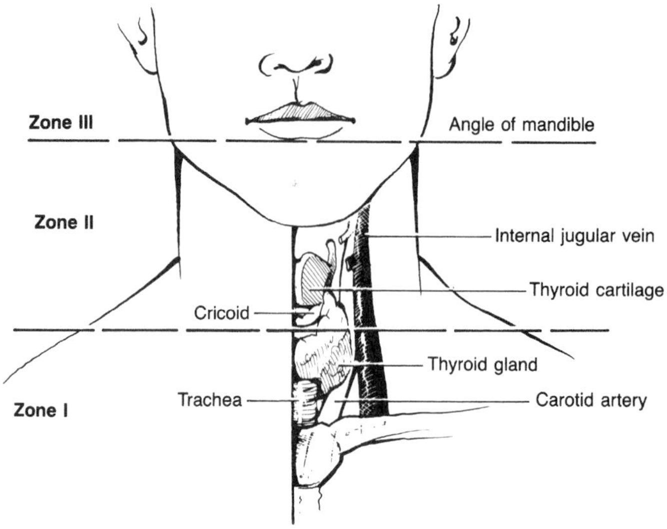

Figure 100.1. Anterior view of the neck. Significant structures and the zones of the neck are illustrated.

Zone II includes the territory between the cricoid and the angle of the mandible. This zone contains the carotid and vertebral arteries; jugular veins; larynx; trachea; esophagus; cervical spinal cord; and vagus and recurrent laryngeal nerves. The mortality rate for zone II injuries is the lowest of the three zones due to easier surgical access and the ability to control hemorrhage from bleeding vessels using direct pressure.

Zone III extends cephalad from the angle of the mandible. As in zone I, the difficult surgical approach and inability to control distal bleeding make management of injuries in this area more challenging than in zone II. The upper aerodigestive tract; salivary glands; distal carotid and vertebral arteries; and cranial nerves IX, X, XI, and XII are at risk in zone III injuries.

The boundaries of the anterior triangle are the anterior border of the sternocleidomastoid muscle, the underside of the mandible, and the midline anteriorly (Fig. 100.2). Wounds to this area are more likely to damage multiple structures but generally pose fewer problems in terms of surgical access.

Injuries to the posterior triangle of the neck, bounded by the posterior border of the sternocleidomastoid, the anterior border of the trapezius, and the middle third of the clavicle inferiorly, are particularly difficult to evaluate and are more likely to damage intrathoracic structures.[26]

The platysma is a thin superficial muscle that originates over the upper thorax, then extends superiorly across the clavicles and neck before blending into the superficial facial muscles. It is an important surgical landmark because wounds that penetrate this muscle mandate hospital admission and further diagnostic investigation. The deep cervical fascia underlies the platysma and is subdivided into investing, pretracheal, and prevertebral layers. The tight fascial compartments of the neck reduce the chance of exsanguination from vascular injuries but may lead to airway compromise from external compression of the larynx or trachea by a hematoma.[15]

The cartilaginous structures of the larynx, including the hyoid bone, thyroid cartilage, and cricoid cartilage, are held together by connective tissue attachments. The weakest of these is

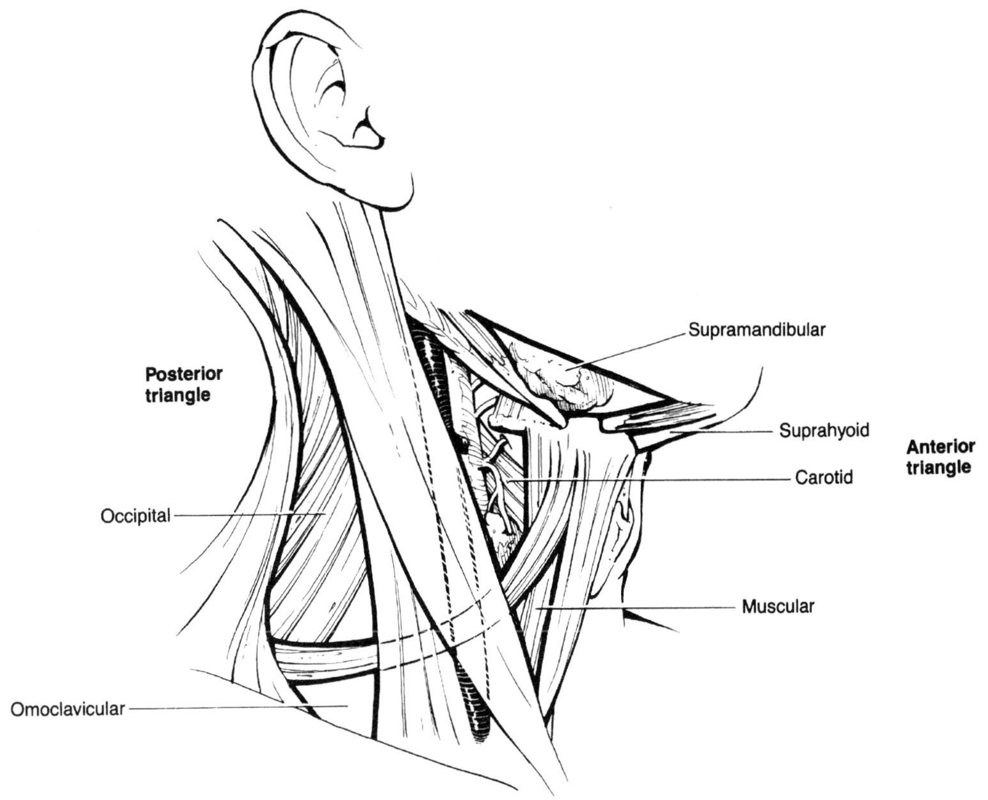

Figure 100.2. Lateral view of the neck demonstrating the anterior and posterior triangles.

the cricotracheal ligament; direct injury here may cause complete cricotracheal separation.[20] Just superior to the cricoid cartilage, the cricothyroid ligament is penetrated by the recurrent laryngeal nerve as it enters the larynx. Fractures in this location may result in unilateral or bilateral vocal cord paralysis.[18]

CLINICAL PRESENTATION

Penetrating Neck Injuries

Penetrating neck injuries are typically categorized as gunshot or stab wounds, but this division offers little in predicting the severity or extent of the injury. It is more useful to classify wounds based on the amount of energy imparted to tissues. Projectile injuries from handguns, rifles, shotguns, BB guns and explosions differ significantly according to the size and speed of the projectiles and their distance from the victim. For example, birdshot pellets are small (less than 3.5-mm diameter) and have a very short effective range; few serious injuries occur beyond 12 ft. Buckshot pellets are larger and behave more like individual bullets, with an effective range up to 150 ft.

Table 100.1 lists missile injuries in increasing order of severity and morbidity. It also presents a formula for estimating the range from the attacker, which may be more accurate than the estimate provided by the victim.[21]

Low-energy stab wounds may be inflicted by an imaginative array of objects, including knives, razors, broken glass, screwdrivers, ice picks, meat thermometers, scissors, and axes. Construction and sports equipment, including nails from a nail gun, chain saws, javelins, and golf clubs, have also been reported to cause penetrating neck injuries.

In adults, penetrating injuries to the neck occur most frequently in young males as a result of physical violence. There is a strong association with substance abuse, particularly alcohol intoxication. Knife and gun wounds also predominate among children in the United States, but dog bites and falls onto sharp objects cause a significant number of penetrating neck injuries in younger age groups.[12,19]

Blunt Neck Injuries

Blunt neck injuries may result from motor vehicle accidents, assaults, suicide attempts, or recreational and athletic activities such as boxing, karate, and team sports. Multiple system trauma involving the central nervous system, thorax, abdomen, or extremities occurs in 30% to 50% of cases. A common mechanism is the "padded dash" syndrome, a particular pattern of injury sustained by front-seat passengers in automobiles. The victim, often unrestrained or wearing only a lap restraint, is thrown forward at the moment of impact with the neck hyperextended, resulting in a direct blow to the anterior neck against the dashboard or rim of the steering wheel (Fig. 100.3). Another common

TABLE 100.1. Missile Injuries (In Increasing Order of Severity)

1. Stab wounds
2. Long-range (>12 m) birdshot shotgun injuries
3. Handgun injuries (low-velocity single bullets)
4. Buckshot shotgun injuries
5. Rifle injuries (high-velocity single bullets)
6. Close-range (<5 m) shotgun injuries (birdshot or buckshot)
7. Bomb or mortar fragment injuries (multiple high-velocity projectiles)

For shotgun weapons with a choke: estimated range (m) = 2 X radius of wound (in.).

For shotguns with cylinder bore: estimated range (m) = 4 X radius of wound (in.).

Source: Adapted from Ordog GJ. Penetrating neck trauma. J Trauma 1987;27:543.

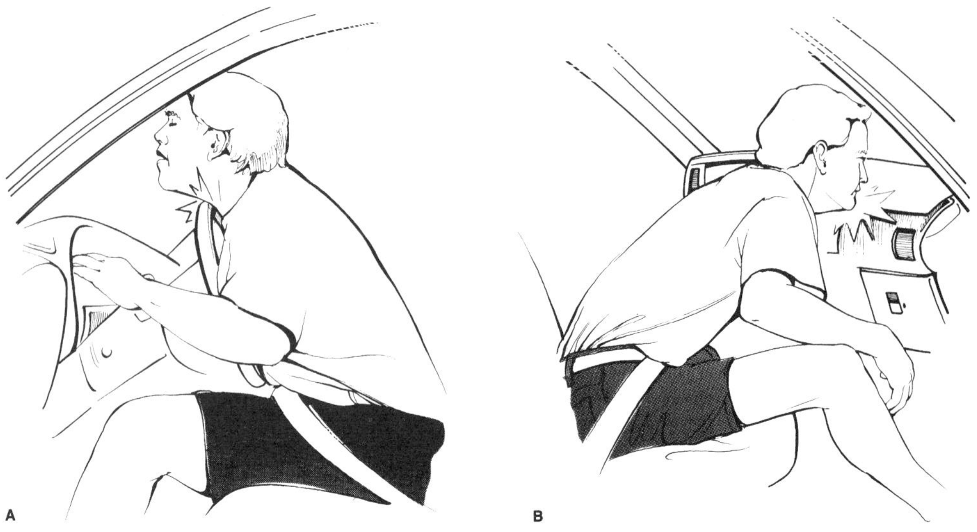

Figure 100.3. Mechanisms of laryngeal injury. **(A)** Unprotected larynx hits steering wheel. **(B)** The padded dash syndrome. Hyperextension of the head and neck places the larynx in an unprotected position.

scenario is the "clothesline" injury, which occurs when a victim riding a bicycle, motorbike, or snowmobile is struck in the anterior neck by a clothesline or other cable strung across the path of travel. These injuries carry an especially high risk of laryngeal trauma, including complete separation of the trachea at the cricoid cartilage.[20] In children, blunt neck trauma is usually a result of bicycle accidents (usually by striking the handlebars), motor vehicle accidents, and sports injuries.[12]

DIFFERENTIAL DIAGNOSIS

The signs and symptoms associated with wounds to various organ systems are listed in Table 100.2.

Airway Injuries

Injuries to the cervical airway range from minor to life-threatening (Table 100.3). Any patient who presents with hoarseness, subcutaneous emphysema, dysphagia or odynophagia, odynophonia, hemoptysis, or neck tenderness following anterior neck trauma must be considered to have sustained a laryngeal injury.[20] Figure 100.4 depicts several types of injury to the laryngotracheal skeleton. Rupture of the vocal folds or anterior dislocation of the arytenoid cartilage most commonly results from an anterior blow to the neck, with posterior displacement of the thyroid cartilage followed by springing forward of the lax cords and attached structures (Fig. 100.5). Even minor blunt impact in

TABLE 100.2. Signs and Symptoms of Specific System Injuries

LARYNGOTRACHEAL	VASCULAR
Respiratory distress	Hematoma
Stridor	Persistent hemorrhage
Cyanosis	Neurologic deficit
Hemoptysis	Pulse deficit
Tracheal deviation	Horner syndrome (carotid injury)
Subcutaneous emphysema	Hypovolemic shock
Mediastinal emphysema	Bruit or thrill over vessel
Pneumothorax	Altered sensorium
Sucking wound	**NEUROLOGIC**
Dysphonia, aphonia, hoarseness	Altered sensorium or coma
Cough	Hemiplegia/quadriplegia
Loss of palpable landmarks	Respiratory paralysis (spinal cord transection above C5)
Ecchymosis or abrasions over anterior neck	Brown-Séquard syndrome (spinal cord hemisection)
Tenderness over larynx	Diaphragmatic paralysis (phrenic nerve)
PHARYNGOESOPHAGEAL	Extremity paresis or sensory loss (brachial plexus)
Neck or substernal pain	Horner syndrome (stellate ganglion)
Subcutaneous emphysema	Hoarseness (recurrent laryngeal nerve)
Dysphagia	Airway obstruction (bilateral recurrent laryngeal nerves)
Odynophagia	Droop of corner of mouth (mandibular branch of CN VII)
Hoarseness	Trapezius weakness (CN XI)
Cough	Tongue deviation (CN XII)
Hematemesis	
Hemoptysis	
Persistent tachycardia	
Fever	

CN, cranial nerve.

TABLE 100.3. Types of Laryngeal Injuries

Mucosal edema
Endolaryngeal hematoma
Mucosal laceration
Hyoid bone fracture
Vocal cord rupture
Arytenoid cartilage dislocation
Thyroid cartilage fracture
Cricoid cartilage fracture
Cricotracheal separation

children can result in laceration of the posterior tracheal wall and pneumomediastinum with or without pneumothorax.[25]

Gastrointestinal Tract Injuries

Perforating injuries of the digestive tract are frequently occult and may be devastating if undiagnosed. Leakage of saliva, bacteria, gastric acid, and pepsin produces an intense necrotizing inflammatory reaction in the neck and mediastinum, with an attendant risk of upper airway obstruction, sepsis, and death.

Signs and symptoms suggestive of pharyngoesophageal injury include severe anterior neck pain, drooling, dysphagia or odynophagia, hematemesis, subcutaneous crepitus, and retropharyngeal air on lateral neck radiograph.[14,15] When the injury is to the lower esophagus, midthoracic or abdominal pain, upper abdominal rigidity, and splinted respirations may be noted.

Pharyngoesophageal perforation due to blunt external neck trauma is an extremely rare injury. It has been ascribed to hyperextension of the cervical spine; acceleration or deceleration injuries, such as falls and motor vehicle accidents; and assaults, such as strangulation injuries and blows to the neck. Perforation occurs when the esophagus is compressed between the laryngeal cartilages and the anterior osteophytes of the cervical spine.

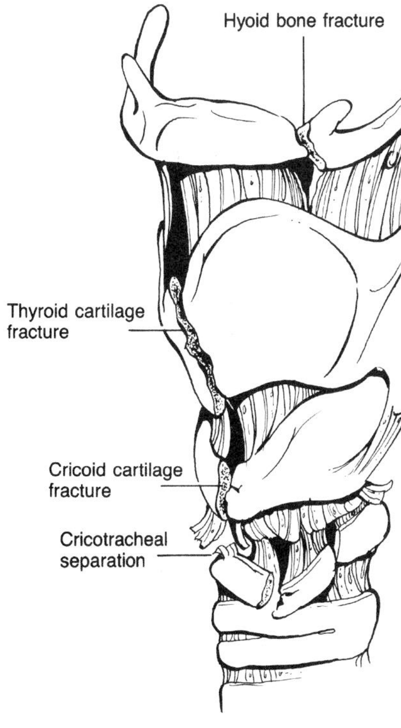

Figure 100.4. Types of laryngeal injuries: hyoid bone fracture; thyroid cartilage fracture; cricoid cartilage fracture; cricotracheal separation.

Iatrogenic injury may occur as a complication of instrumentation or inexpert intubation attempts.[14]

Vascular Injuries

Vascular structures are damaged in approximately 25% of penetrating neck injury victims. Careful physical assessment of cervical vascular injuries must include inspection for brisk bleeding from the wound site; palpation of radial, ulnar, temporal, and facial pulses; decreased breath sounds due to hemothorax; and signs of air embolism accompanying venous injury.[15] Obvious signs of injury to major vessels include hemorrhage or shock, an enlarging or pulsatile hematoma, absent distal pulses, and neurologic deficits.[3,16] A hematoma in the supraclavicular space that does not extend below the clavicle is usually due to a subclavian artery injury confined by the coracoclavicular fascia. Hematomas in the axilla are associated with both subclavian and axillary artery injury. Even benign-appearing lacerations may penetrate the carotid artery and lead to subsequent false aneurysm formation and delayed rupture.

Blunt carotid injury may be caused by a motor vehicle accident or by more trivial injury, such as a direct blow to the lateral neck. The usual mechanism of blunt injury to the carotid artery is rapid deceleration with hyperextension or lateral hyperflexion of the neck, which stretches the internal carotid artery over the upper cervical vertebrae, producing an intimal tear. This may result in dissection or pseudoaneurysm formation, with the risk of subsequent thrombosis or cerebral embolism. Blunt carotid injury is rarely diagnosed at the time of initial presentation because symptoms classically do not appear until 12 to 24 hours after injury; neurologic deficits may not appear for weeks or months after injury.[4] Only half of patients have external signs of neck trauma. The diagnosis should be suspected whenever a neurologic deficit cannot be explained by cranial computed tomography (CT) scan or by spinal cord or peripheral nerve injury. The presence of a lateral neck hematoma, Horner syndrome, transient ischemic attack, or hemiparesis, monoparesis, or aphasia in a patient with no evidence of head trauma should also stimulate a search for carotid injury.[4,11]

Isolated dissection of the subclavian artery has been attributed to shoulder harness injury following a high-speed motor vehicle accident. Vertebral artery injury has been documented after upper cervical spine fractures (where the artery courses through the transverse foramina), hyperflexion injuries, chiropractic manipulation, and yoga exercises.

Neurologic Injuries

The neck contains a variety of neural structures, including the spinal cord, cervical nerve roots and brachial plexus, cervical sympathetic ganglia, phrenic nerve, and cranial nerves IX through XII. Either blunt or penetrating trauma can injure one or more of these structures, producing the signs listed in Table 100.2.

Spinal cord injury resulting from stab wounds is unusual, but may be caused by an assailant wielding a knife from behind the victim. Most of these injuries do not cross the midline because of the protection afforded by the lateral and spinous vertebral processes. Hemisection of the spinal cord, or Brown-Séquard syndrome, presents as ipsilateral motor paralysis and contralateral sensory loss below the level of the injury. Complete cord transection above the level of C5 results in respiratory arrest due to diaphragmatic paralysis. Complete transection below C5 will result in paraplegia and possibly respiratory distress from paralysis of accessory respiratory muscles. Spinal cord injury may also lead to neurogenic shock.[15]

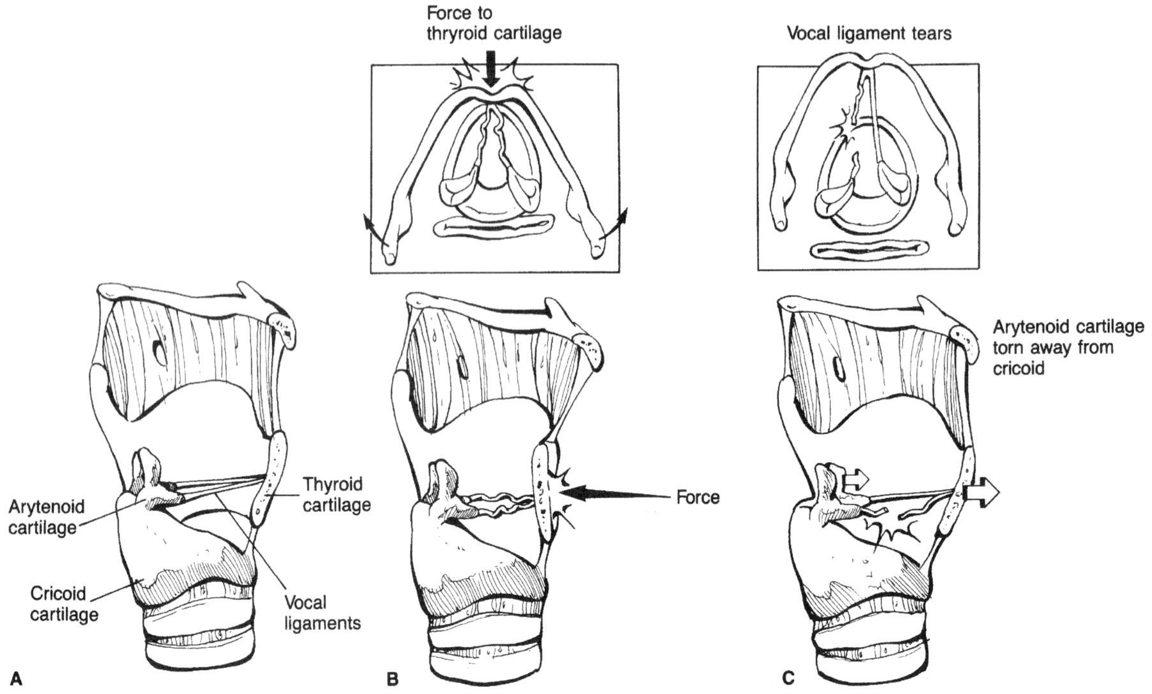

Figure 100.5. Mechanism of rupture of vocal folds and/or anterior displacement of arytenoid cartilage. **(A)** Larynx at rest. **(B)** Anterior blow displaces larynx posteriorly toward vertebral bodies, which splays the thyroid cartilage and releases all tension on the vocal ligaments. **(C)** With the anterior pressure removed, the thyroid cartilage springs forward, either avulsing the vocal fold or dislocating the arytenoid forward, where it hits the cricoid lamina and is trapped.

Injuries to Other Structures

Thyroid gland injuries often result in extensive hemorrhage, distorting anterior neck landmarks and complicating attempts to establish a surgical airway. Laceration of the thoracic duct by a knife or missile wound may cause chylothorax or chylous wound drainage, or may be discovered during surgical exploration.[28] Soft-tissue injuries, including lacerations, ecchymoses, and abrasions, are managed in standard fashion. Cervical spine injuries are considered elsewhere in the text.

EMERGENCY DEPARTMENT EVALUATION

The initial evaluation of a victim of neck trauma must be rapid, systematic, and thorough. Information gathered from prehospital care providers and law enforcement personnel, combined with meticulous physical examination, allow the emergency physician to plan further diagnostic and therapeutic maneuvers and develop an appropriate disposition from the ED. As with any trauma, initial evaluation of the patient with a neck injury should be conducted according to the ABCs of resuscitation, as outlined in Table 100.4.

Prehospital Care

Prehospital personnel should assess and document the mechanism of injury, type of weapons used, estimated blood loss, vital signs and other significant physical findings at the scene, scene time, and transport time. Transport should not be delayed to perform detailed examination or extensive stabilizing measures. In an urban setting, patients should be transported to the nearest level I trauma center without delay.

After basic airway-opening maneuvers have been applied, further immediate management may be required. Persistent stridor may indicate upper airway obstruction from mucosal edema, extrinsic compression by hematoma or other mass, or direct injury to the larynx or trachea.[26] Bag-valve-mask ventilation may be used as a temporizing measure but, in the face of penetrating neck injury, can cause dissection of air into surrounding tissues, with resultant airway or vascular complications.

Airway management in the prehospital setting can be extremely difficult if the airway is distorted by presence of blood or secretions, hematoma, edema, or laryngotracheal injury. For this reason, intubation should be attempted only in patients with stridor, severe respiratory distress, or cardiac or respiratory arrest, or if transport time is likely to be long. When prehospital intubation is indicated, the orotracheal route is preferred because it permits direct airway visualization and is associated with fewer complications. Use of neuromuscular paralytic agents should be avoided.

Prehospital cricothyroidotomy may be necessary when orotracheal intubation is unsuccessful or impossible due to massive facial trauma, suspected cervical spine injury, or patient position during entrapment. Cricothyroidotomy should be *avoided* if laryngeal trauma is suspected based on the mechanism of injury (e.g., clothesline injury) or the presence of an anterior neck hematoma or ecchymosis. Routine cervical spine precautions are indicated in blunt trauma victims but are rarely necessary in those with penetrating injury, unless neurologic signs or symptoms are present.

The primary survey continues with evaluation of breathing and circulatory status. Careful examination of the chest for evidence of intrathoracic trauma is critically important, particularly with zone I neck injuries. Emergency medical service personnel should assess the patient for signs of tension pneumothorax and perform needle thoracostomy as indicated. Intractable hemorrhagic shock is a greater risk with zone I injuries as well, because bleeding from innominate or subclavian vessels cannot be tamponaded using direct external pressure.

TABLE 100.4. Prehospital/Initial Emergency Department Management of Neck Injuries

1. *Secure the airway*
Head positioning; mandible/tongue maneuvers
C-spine protection (collar/sandbags/tape):
All blunt neck trauma
Penetrating neck trauma if loss of consciousness, obtunded, or neurologic deficit
Suction blood and secretions
100% O_2 via nonrebreather mask
Indications for urgent intubation:
Acute respiratory distress or persistent stridor
Altered mental status
Continued airway compromise from blood, secretions
Expanding neck hematoma or tracheal deviation
Suspected recurrent laryngeal nerve injury
Extensive subcutaneous emphysema
Evidence of direct laryngotracheal trauma
Method of intubation:
Fiberoptic-guided nasotracheal intubation if patient breathing
Orotracheal intubation if apneic and no neurologic deficit
Cricothyroidotomy if severe maxillofacial injuries or apneic with neurologic deficit except:
Avoid cricothyroidotomy, arrange for emergent tracheostomy if suspected cricotracheal separation or hematoma over cricothyroid membrane
2. *Assess breathing*
Beware intrathoracic injury with zone I wounds
Palpate chest wall for crepitus, subcutaneous emphysema
Thoracostomy for hemothorax or tension pneumothorax
3. *Assess circulation*
Control bleeding by direct pressure; avoid blind clamping
Hemorrhage from major vessels can be tamponaded by inserting 18- or 20-F Foley catheter into wound; inflate with 15–20 mL saline
Intravenous fluid resuscitation or blood transfusion; use arm opposite side of penetrating wound if feasible
Emergent left thoracotomy or median sternotomy may be necessary to control hemorrhage in zone I injury
If venous air embolism suspected: Place patient in Trendelenburg in left lateral decubitus position
4. *Brief neurologic assessment*
Level of consciousness
Examine for pupillary responsiveness, motor deficits
5. *Further evaluation and stabilization*
Radiographs: c-spine, soft tissue neck, and upright portable chest x-ray
CBC, type and cross match, coagulation studies
Examine wounds for penetration of platysma; avoid probing
Careful secondary survey for injuries to other systems (see Table 100.2), especially:
Skeletal
Laryngotracheal
Vascular
Pharyngoesophageal
Neurologic
If platysma intact and no other signs or symptoms of injury: local wound repair

All patients with penetrating neck trauma should have at least one large-bore intravenous line established en route to the ED. When feasible, it should be placed in the upper extremity opposite the side of the neck wound in case there is venous injury. Prehospital care providers should cover wounds with air sucking or bubbling through the site with Vaseline gauze and place the patient in the Trendelenburg position to reduce the risk of venous air embolism.[15]

Initial Emergency Department Evaluation

Airway, breathing, and circulatory status must be rapidly reassessed once the patient arrives in the ED (see Table 100.4). A secure airway must be established early in the management of any victim of neck trauma. Urgent intubation is mandated in the presence of an expanding neck hematoma, tracheal deviation, suspected recurrent laryngeal nerve injury, severe subcutaneous emphysema, or other external evidence of direct laryngotracheal trauma, in addition to the usual indications of airway compromise due to the presence of blood or secretions, respiratory distress, or altered mental status.[10] Failure to recognize these indications for early placement of an endotracheal tube may lead to both rapid deterioration and increasing difficulty in obtaining an airway. If a cervical collar is in place, remove the anterior half (while an assistant ensures manual immobilization of the head) to examine the front of the neck for signs of injury to the upper airway.[3]

Controversy persists regarding the optimal method of controlling the airway in cases of neck injury. Most authors recommend early endotracheal intubation when any sign of airway compromise is present, although others recommend early tracheostomy under local anesthesia as the initial intervention.[12,15] The method of choice for airway management depends on the physician's level of comfort and skill with each technique.

In the presence of significant respiratory distress, the initial attempt should usually be orotracheal intubation under direct view.[7] This route is associated with fewer complications and allows the physician to visualize the airway during intubation.

Orotracheal intubation with manual in-line cervical immobilization is widely accepted for the apneic patient who is neurologically intact, even when the status of the cervical spine is unknown. Rapid-sequence intubation using neuromuscular paralytic agents may be used in carefully selected patients, but bag-valve-mask ventilation may cause air to dissect into the neck, as previously discussed, while the decrease in muscle tone induced by these agents may lead to total airway obstruction.

In stable patients, fiberoptic nasotracheal intubation should be attempted first. Blind nasotracheal intubation is not recommended because it is associated with a higher rate of complications and a greater likelihood of causing further damage to the airway. Intubation over a fiberoptic bronchoscope not only permits careful, atraumatic intubation of the trachea with minimal neck movement, but also is extremely useful in the presence of excessive secretions, foreign bodies, or anatomic distortion.[7] Furthermore, endoscopic evaluation is the standard of care for assessing the degree of laryngotracheal injury.[12,20] Less frequently used intubation methods include placement of the tube through an open wound that communicates directly with the trachea or into the visible distal segment of the transected larynx or trachea.[15]

In all of these instances, the treating physicians should be ready to provide a surgical airway if intubation attempts are unsuccessful. Cricothyroidotomy may be necessary as the initial airway maneuver in the presence of known cervical spine instability, neurologic deficit, or severe maxillofacial injuries. It is contraindicated in the presence of bruising or hematoma over the cricothyroid membrane or suspected laryngotracheal injury; in these cases, emergency tracheostomy is mandated due to the risk of converting a partial to a complete cricotracheal disruption. The appearance of subcutaneous emphysema and a large air leak after positive-pressure ventilation is initiated indicates tracheal injury distal to the cuff of the endotracheal tube. This situation mandates immediate tracheostomy, and in some cases median sternotomy, to regain control of the distal tracheal segment.[5]

Identify open or actively bleeding wounds and observe for evidence that the platysma has been penetrated. Blind probing of wounds is *strictly contraindicated* because of the potential for damaging deep structures. Similarly, blind attempts to clamp bleeding vessels risk injury to nerves and other organs and should never be performed. External bleeding is controlled by direct pressure. If this is unsuccessful, tamponade of bleeding, using a Foley catheter balloon, may be attempted. Insert the catheter into the wound toward the estimated source of bleeding. Inflate the balloon with saline until the bleeding stops or moderate resistance is felt.[7] Patients with exsanguinating hemorrhage, shock unresponsive to resuscitative measures, or an expanding neck hematoma should be rapidly transferred to the operating room for immediate surgical exploration.

Careful physical examination is the basis of the ED evaluation of neck trauma victims and guides decision making regarding further diagnostic or therapeutic maneuvers. Once the patient has become hemodynamically stable, conduct a thorough secondary survey, giving special attention to the respiratory, digestive, vascular, and nervous systems. Signs and symptoms of injuries to these systems are listed in Table 100.2.

In the hemodynamically stable patient, radiographs of the cervical spine, the soft tissues of the neck, and the upright chest are obtained. Radiographic evidence of air in the soft tissues, due to injury to the airway or gastrointestinal tract, may precede the development of clinically evident subcutaneous emphysema by several hours.[5] Other possible findings on soft-tissue neck films include pretracheal or retropharyngeal soft-tissue swelling, distortion or interruption of the tracheal air column, and elevation or fracture of the hyoid bone. If the body of the hyoid bone is elevated above the level of the third cervical vertebral body, or if the greater cornu is located less than 2 cm from the angle of the mandible, complete tracheal transection should be suspected.[23] Obtain both anteroposterior and lateral chest films when possible, as mediastinal air may not be seen on an anteroposterior view alone in half of cases.

EMERGENCY DEPARTMENT MANAGEMENT

Blunt Neck Injuries

Any patient presenting with hoarseness, subcutaneous emphysema, hemoptysis, or neck tenderness following anterior neck trauma must be evaluated for laryngeal injury. Severe respiratory distress may not necessarily be present, especially in the young, healthy patient. Fiberoptic laryngoscopy has replaced direct laryngoscopy as the standard method of evaluating upper airway injuries. It is useful in assessing airway patency, vocal cord mobility, and the presence of endolaryngeal lacerations or hematoma without causing movement of the cervical spine. Fiberoptic bronchoscopy permits additional visualization of the subglottic airway and may be used to facilitate endotracheal intubation. Direct laryngoscopy may be performed when fiberoptic laryngoscopy is not available, but it requires general anesthesia, may exacerbate mucosal injury, and risks cervical spine movement. CT is the best study for evaluating the laryngeal skeleton and assists in planning the surgical repair.[20]

Minor airway injuries amenable to nonoperative management are minimal endolaryngeal edema, hematoma, or laceration seen on laryngoscopy with normal phonation or minimal hoarseness and no or minimal airway compromise. Provide humidified oxygen and elevate the patient's head, and reexamine frequently for signs of impending airway compromise. A tracheostomy tray should be immediately available in case of rapid deterioration. Otolaryngologic consultation and hospital admission are required.[26]

Contrast esophagography is indicated when pharyngoesophageal trauma is suspected based on odynophagia, hematemesis, or subcutaneous emphysema. The initial study should be performed using a water-soluble medium (Gastrografin), due to the irritating effect of barium on tissues. If negative, esophagography is then repeated with barium or followed by direct esophagoscopy, due to the high rate of false-negative results when water-soluble contrast is used.[17] Direct visualization using fiberoptic or rigid endoscopy identifies hypopharyngeal tears but may miss small injuries. CT with contrast is useful to determine the site and extent of the injury and help plan the surgical approach.[14]

Four-vessel cerebral arteriography is indicated when there are abnormal or evolving neurologic findings in the presence of a normal CT scan of the brain. Conventional angiography remains the standard method for diagnosing blunt carotid or vertebral arterial injury.[4] Duplex ultrasound (color flow Doppler) imaging is a noninvasive and less expensive alternative to angiography that is sensitive for detecting lesions at the carotid bifurcation (i.e., in suspected zone II carotid injuries) but not for detecting dissection or pseudoaneurysm high in the neck. In selected blunt neck trauma victims undergoing head or abdominal CT scanning for another indication, additional views of the cervical region with intravenous contrast can screen for suspected carotid injury. CT angiography in this setting adds minimal time to the diagnostic workup, can indicate the need for conventional angiography, and may increase the detection of blunt carotid trauma.[24] Magnetic resonance angiography could serve the same purpose, but there is little experience with its use in the acute trauma setting.

If signs of vascular trauma are obvious (e.g., enlarging hematoma, massive hematemesis or hemoptysis), the need for surgical intervention can usually be identified clinically. Although surgical management was previously advocated for the treatment of blunt carotid injuries, more recent studies have suggested that heparin anticoagulation is independently associated with improved survival and neurologic improvement with an acceptable rate of complications.[6,11,22]

Penetrating Neck Injuries

The optimal management of penetrating neck injuries remains controversial. There is no debate regarding the need for emergency surgery when obvious signs or symptoms of vascular of aerodigestive tract trauma are present. However, disagreement persists about the role of surgical exploration in those with no clinical sign of significant injuries.[7]

During World War II, combat victims whose injuries penetrated the platysma routinely underwent neck exploration, with a substantial reduction in mortality compared with the pre–World War II period. The success of this strategy led to the dictum of "mandatory exploration" for all penetrating neck injuries.[19] Proponents of routine exploration argue that physical examination is unreliable and that potentially dangerous injuries may be missed. However, high rates of negative exploration (30% to 89%) have led others to propose a more selective approach that uses physical examination findings to guide the use of subsequent diagnostic tests such as angiography, contrast esophagography, and endoscopy.[15] Advocates of a more selective approach cite a lower rate of unnecessary operation, shorter hospitalization, and decreased costs.[3,16]

Immediate surgery is indicated for any patient presenting with hemorrhagic shock, massive or expanding hematoma, airway compromise, evolving stroke, or deterioration during a diagnostic study.[3] Surgical exploration is also mandatory in the setting of wounds caused by high-velocity (i.e., rifle) bullets, explosives and shrapnel fragments, and shotguns at a range of less than 5 m.[21] Initially stable patients with other signs of injury, such as ongoing hemorrhage, stable hematoma, hemoptysis, dysphonia, subcutaneous emphysema, hematemesis, dysphagia, or peripheral neurologic deficit, may undergo diagnostic evaluation prior to definitive operative management (see Table 100.5).[3,9]

Four-vessel arteriography is routinely recommended in penetrating zone I injuries, where it may help guide the surgical approach, and in zone III injuries, where it may determine not only the optimal approach, but also the need for surgery. Angiographic embolization of bleeding vessels may also be possible, particularly for vertebral artery lesions.[7] High-velocity missile wounds, regardless of anatomic zone, are generally best evaluated using angiography because of the unpredictable course of the projectile and the potential for damage to deep vascular structures.[9] Less agreement exists regarding the role of angiography in zone II injuries due to other causes. Significant vascular injuries in this zone are usually detectable on physical examination, and those that are clinically occult tend to be small carotid intimal tears amenable to nonoperative treatment.[1,2,8,9] However, the incidence of asymptomatic vascular injuries requiring surgical repair diagnosed by angiography has been reported to be as high as 9%.[16]

Duplex ultrasonography has not been studied extensively in the setting of penetrating neck trauma. Early studies have reported the sensitivity and specificity of duplex ultrasound to exceed 95%.[7] It may be useful as a screening test in individuals with penetrating neck injuries in proximity to major vessels but no physical signs suggestive of vascular injury. Patients with negative duplex scans can probably be safely observed, while those with positive or equivocal results should undergo angiography.[9,13]

TABLE 100.5. Indications for Immediate Surgery or Further Studies Following Penetrating Neck Trauma

INDICATIONS FOR IMMEDIATE SURGERY
Stage III or IV shock
Stage II shock not responding to resuscitation
Positive findings on diagnostic studies (below)
Deterioration during diagnostic studies
High-velocity missile injuries
Close-range (<5 meters) shotgun injuries
INDICATIONS FOR FURTHER STUDIES
Active bleeding
Stable or enlarging hematoma
Dysphagia
Hemoptysis
Hematemesis
Subcutaneous emphysema
Absent or decreased carotid pulses
Respiratory distress
Dysphonia
Neurologic deficit
Coexisting injury requiring surgery
METHOD OF SELECTIVE MANAGEMENT OF PENETRATING NECK WOUNDS
Cervical spine radiographs
Soft-tissue neck radiographs
Chest radiograph
Water-soluble contrast swallow (followed by barium swallow if negative)
Aortography with four-vessel study
Direct and indirect laryngoscopy
Bronchoscopy (if indicated)
Esophagoscopy (if indicated)

Adapted from Ordog GJ. Penetrating neck trauma. J Trauma 1987;27:543.

In general, the approach to penetrating neck trauma must be tailored to the capabilities of the individual institution. If selective surgical management is considered, it should be undertaken only at a level I or II trauma center that possesses the necessary facilities and surgical and support staff to provide diagnostic studies and emergency surgery on a 24-hour basis.[9] In such institutions, hemodynamically stable asymptomatic or minimally symptomatic patients with stab wounds, injuries caused by low-velocity (i.e., handgun) bullets, or shotguns beyond a 5-m range may be selectively managed using a diagnostic approach such as the one outlined in Fig. 100.6.

DISPOSITION

Any trauma victim with a wound penetrating the platysma or suspected blunt injury to deeper structures requires admission and observation for at least 24 hours, in addition to further studies that may be indicated. Obtain early consultation in such cases with a trauma or head and neck surgeon. When one of these consultants is not immediately available, transfer the patient to a facility capable of providing comprehensive trauma care. Additional consultation with an anesthesiologist or vascular surgeon should be sought during the resuscitation phase when difficulty with airway management is anticipated or signs of vascular trauma are present.

Minor laryngeal injuries are best managed with voice rest, humidification of inspired air, elevation of the head, and close observation. Prophylactic broad-spectrum antibiotics and a short course of steroids are often recommended. Laryngeal frac-

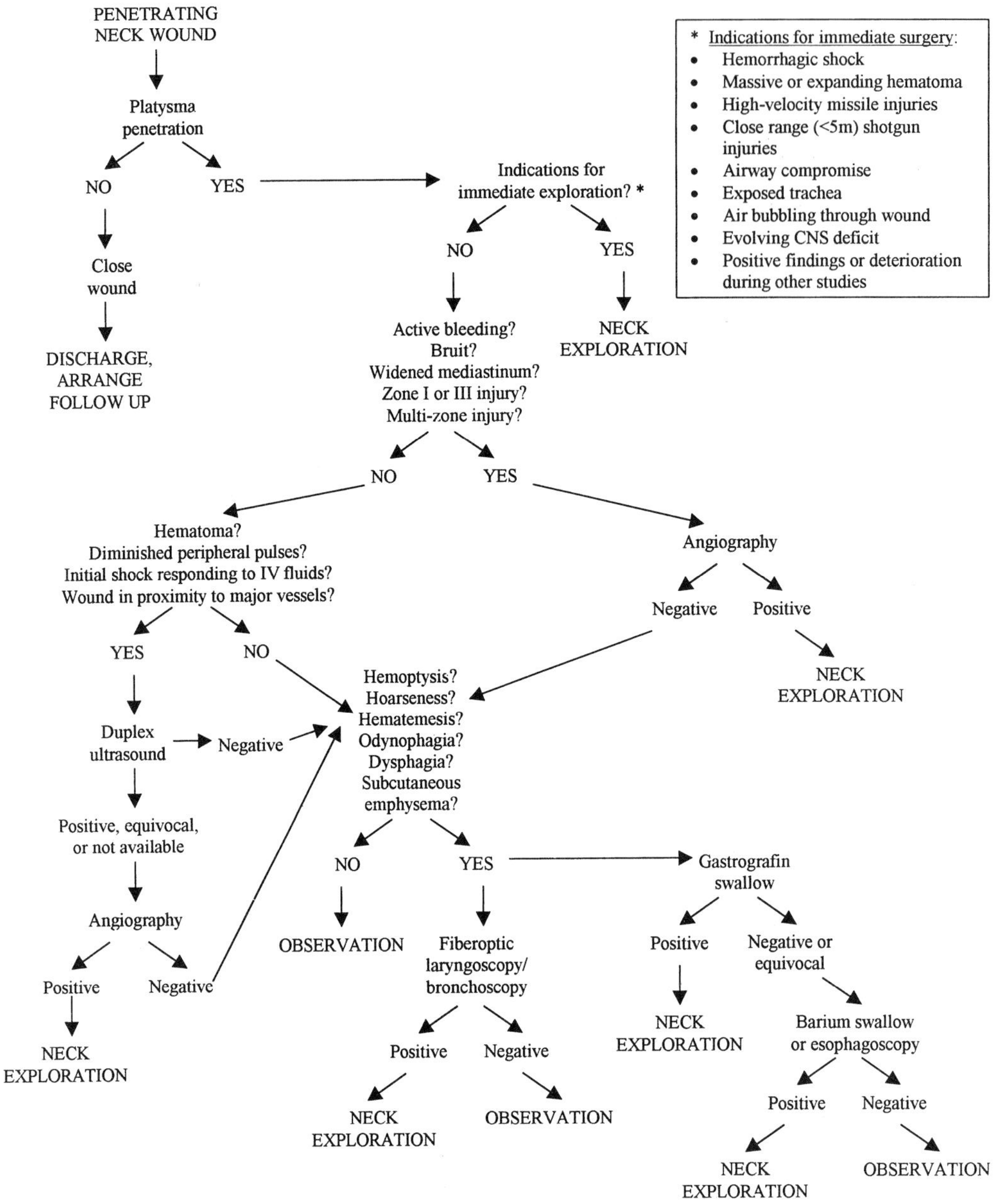

Figure 100.6. Algorithm for management of penetrating neck injuries.

tures or vocal cord injury must be repaired surgically. Delayed diagnosis of laryngeal trauma may lead to late morbidity, including permanent hoarseness, dysphonia, or aphonia; subglottic or tracheal stenosis; granulations on or paralysis of the vocal cords; and the need for permanent tracheostomy.[27]

Patients with demonstrated pharyngeal or esophageal perforation require admission and close monitoring. Initial treatment consists of intravenous fluid resuscitation, parenteral antibiotics, and restricted oral intake. Aqueous penicillin G is effective against the usual flora of the oropharynx and esophagus and is thus the drug of choice. An aminoglycoside should be added to the antibiotic regimen in elderly patients, in whom gram-negative colonization of the oropharynx is common. Pharyngeal perforations of less than 2 cm may be managed nonoperatively. Larger perforations or those involving the esophagus require surgical repair and drainage.[14]

The sequelae of vascular trauma include shock, persistent hemorrhage, neurologic deficits, and extremity ischemia. The role of surgical repair of the extracranial carotid artery is controversial when a preoperative neurologic deficit exists, because of fear of converting an ischemic to a hemorrhagic cerebral infarction once circulation is reestablished. Surgery is generally not advocated when the deficit is moderate or dense, but it may be indicated if the deficit is mild or absent.[26] Penetrating injuries to the spinal cord are initially managed with wound debridement and prophylactic antibiotics to prevent meningitis.

COMMON PITFALLS

- Avoid blind clamping to control bleeding from open neck wounds.
- Do not blindly probe penetrating neck wounds to determine their depth.
- Seek and recognize the indications for urgent intubation.
- Beware of inexpert blind intubation attempts or inadvisable attempts at cricothyroidotomy that may convert a partial tear to complete laryngotracheal separation.

References

1. Atteberry LR, Dennis JW, Menawat SS, et al. Physical examination alone is safe and accurate for evaluation of vascular injuries in penetrating zone II neck trauma. *J Am Coll Surg* 1994;179:657.
2. Beitsch P, Weigelt JA, Flynn E, et al. Physical examination and arteriography in patients with penetrating zone II neck wounds. *Arch Surg* 1994;129:577.
3. Biffl WL, Moore EE, Rehse DH, et al. Selective management of penetrating neck trauma based on cervical level of injury. *Am J Surg* 1997;174:678.
4. Cheatham ML, Block EFJ, Nelson LD. Evaluation of acute mental status change in the nonhead injured trauma patient. *Am Surg* 1998;64:900.
5. Cicala RS, Kudsk KA, Butts A, et al. Initial evaluation and management of upper airway injuries in trauma patients. *J Clin Anesth* 1991;3:91.
6. Cogbill TH, Moore EE, Meissner M, et al. The spectrum of blunt injury to the carotid artery: a multicenter perspective. *J Trauma* 1994;37:473.
7. Demetriades D, Asensio JA, Velmahos G, et al. Complex problems in penetrating neck trauma. *Surg Clin North Am* 1996;76:661.
8. Demetriades D, Charalambides D, Lakhoo M. Physical examination and selective conservative management in patients with penetrating injuries of the neck. *Br J Surg* 1993;80:1534.
9. Demetrides D, Theodorou D, Cornwall E, et al. Penetrating injuries of the neck in patients in stable condition: physical examination, angiography, or color flow Doppler imaging. *Arch Surg* 1995;130:971.
10. Eggen JT, Jorden RC. Airway management, penetrating neck trauma. *J Emerg Med* 1993;11:381.
11. Fabian TC, Patton JH, Croce MA, et al. Blunt carotid injury: importance of early diagnosis and anticoagulant therapy. *Ann Surg* 1996;5:513.
12. Ford HR, Gardner MJ, Lynch JM. Laryngotracheal disruption from blunt pediatric neck injuries: impact of early recognition and intervention on outcome. *J Pediatr Surg* 1995;30:331.
13. Ginzburg E, Montalvo B, LeBlang S, et al. The use of duplex ultrasonography in penetrating neck trauma. *Arch Surg* 1996;131:691.
14. Jacobs I, Niknejad G, Kelly K, et al. Hypopharyngeal perforation after blunt neck trauma: case report and review of the literature. *J Trauma* 1999;46:957.
15. Kendall JL, Anglin D, Demetriades D. Penetrating neck trauma. *Emerg Med Clin North Am* 1998;16:85.
16. Klyachkin ML, Rohmiller M, Charash WE, et al. Penetrating injuries of the neck: selective management evolving. *Am Surg* 1997;63:189.
17. Latimer EA, Clevenger FW, Osler TM. Tear of the cervical esophagus following hyperextension from manual traction: case report. *J Trauma* 1991;31:1448.
18. Levine RJ, Sanders AB, LaMear WR. Bilateral vocal cord paralysis following blunt trauma to the neck. *Ann Emerg Med* 1995;25:253.
19. Mutabagani KH, Beaver BL, Cooney DR, et al. Penetrating neck trauma in children: a reappraisal. *J Pediatr Surg* 1995;30:341.
20. Offiah CJ, Endres D. Isolated laryngotracheal separation following blunt trauma to the neck. *J Laryngol Otol* 1997;111:1079.
21. Ordog GJ. Penetrating neck trauma. *J Trauma* 1987;27:543.
22. Parikh AA, Luchette FA, Valente JF, et al. Blunt carotid artery injuries. *J Am Coll Surg* 1997;185:80.
23. Polansky A, Resnick D, Sofferman RA, et al. Hyoid bone elevation: a sign of tracheal transection. *Radiology* 1984;150:117.
24. Rogers FB, Baker EF, Osler TM, et al. Computed tomographic angiography as a screening modality for blunt cervical arterial injuries: preliminary results. *J Trauma* 1999;46:380.
25. Schoem SR, Choi SS, Zalzal GH. Pneumomediastinum and pneumothorax from blunt cervical trauma in children. *Laryngoscope* 1997;107:351.
26. Thal ER, Meyer DM. Penetrating neck trauma. *Curr Probl Surg* 1992;29:4.
27. Trone TH, Schaefer SD, Carder HM. Blunt and penetrating laryngeal trauma: a 13-year review. *Otolaryngol Head Neck Surg* 1980;88:257.
28. Whiteford MH, Abdullah F, Vernick JJ, et al. Thoracic duct injury in penetrating neck trauma. *Am Surg* 1995;61:1072.

CHAPTER 101
Spinal Cord Injuries

Brian D. Mahoney

The clinical spectrum of the patient with spinal cord injury varies from the awake patient complaining of pain, paresthesias, numbness, weakness, or paralysis to that of the unconscious patient, usually due to associated head injury, unable to give any clues about the severity of his or her injuries. In the United States, most spinal cord injuries are due to motor vehicle accidents, followed by falls, assaults, and, far less frequently, athletic injuries. Young men in their 20s are the largest single group suffering this tragic injury. Elderly patients frequently suffer compression fractures of the thoracolumbar spine, but these are rarely associated with any cord injury. A large northern California study found 53 spinal cord injuries per million population.[9] This extrapolates to over 14,000 new cases per year in the United States.

PATHOPHYSIOLOGY

Normally, the spinal column ensures stability and protects the cord, the spinal roots, and the cauda equina from injury. Panjabi and White[14] defined *spinal stability* as "the ability of the spine, under physiologic loads, to maintain the relationships between vertebrae such as there is neither damage nor irritation to the spinal cord or roots, nor incapacitating deformity nor pain due to structural changes." Injury can render the usually protective spinal column a threat to the cord and its roots. The cord can suffer injury through crush, laceration, penetration, stretch, or ischemia. In unusual circumstances, the spinal column can be rendered unstable due to infectious or inflammatory causes, such as the subluxation of C1 on C2 seen in rheumatoid arthritis or due to the inflammation associated with pharyngeal infections.[1]

The most mobile segments of the spinal column (C4, C5, C6, L1, L2) place the adjacent segments of the spinal cord at higher risk for injury. The ribs buttress the thoracic spinal column, providing a relatively safe environment for the cord. There are fewer fractures here, but when there is a fracture with bony displacement, the cord injury is usually devastating. The spinal medullary canal is relatively narrow here, and the thoracic cord is an area of watershed circulation.[16] In animal and human studies, there is roughly an 8-hour window of opportunity for mechanical or pharmacologic intervention to prevent ongoing secondary injury to the cord.

CLINICAL PRESENTATION

The patient may describe pain or tenderness at the level of injury and paresthesias distal to the injury level, either at the time of injury or at a later time. History and physical examination establish motor, reflex, or sensory deficits; fecal incontinence; or urinary retention[15] (Table 101.1). Careful mapping of the level of sensory loss, including attention to areas around the anus for lower segmental lesions and for sacral sparing, identifies the level of cord injury and the level at which radiologic studies need to focus (Fig. 101.1).

When the patient has no function of any segment of the cord below the level of injury, the injury is physiologically complete. Such a circumstance carries with it a grim but not hopeless prognosis for meaningful recovery. It is nearly impossible to diagnose accurately a physiologically complete cord injury in the emergency department, because spinal shock may be an intercurrent factor. Spinal shock is the temporary cessation of ascending and descending communication past the injured segment of cord (spinal neurogenic shock will be discussed further). Spinal shock lasts a variable amount of time, typically about 24 hours. Immediately after a severe cord injury, the patient usually exhibits flaccid paralysis. In the long term, a spastic paralysis typically develops. Termination of spinal shock is identified by the return of segmental reflexes. The earliest seg-

TABLE 101.1. Motor, Sensory, and Reflex Tests by Nerve Root Levels

Nerve Root Level	Motor	Sensory	Reflex
C3		Lower neck	
C4	Diaphragm	Clavicular area	
C5	Deltoid, biceps	Lateral upper arm	Biceps
C6	Extensor carpi radialis	Thumb and lateral forearm	Brachioradialis
C7	Triceps, wrist flexors, finger extensors	Middle finger	Triceps
C8	Finger flexors	Little finger	
T1	Hand intrinsics	Medial forearm	
T4	Intercostals	Nipples	
T10	Abdominals	Umbilicus	
T12		Suprapubic area inguinal ligament	
L1, L2	Iliopsoas	Upper thigh	
L3, L4	Quadriceps	Lower anterior thigh Medial calf	Quadriceps
L5	Extensor hallucis longus	Dorsal foot	
S1	Gastrosoleus, flexor hallucis longus	Little toe	Achilles tendon
S2, S3, S4	Anal sphincter Bladder	Perineum	Bulbocavernosus Anal wink

From Trafton PG. Spinal cord injuries. *Surg Clin North Am* 1982;62:64. Reprinted with permission.

mental reflexes to return are often those around the genitals and anus; for example, the bulbocavernosus reflex elicited when squeezing or tugging on the glans penis causes reflex contraction of the anal sphincter.

There are several important partial cord syndromes (Fig. 101.2). The anterior spinal cord syndrome (see Fig. 101.2B) is the result of either direct blunt injury to the cord itself or compression of the anterior spinal artery, causing ischemic damage to the anterior cord. The patient presents with a loss of motor and pain sensation bilaterally below the level of the lesion, but posterior cord function is preserved. Posterior cord function may be tested with a tuning fork for vibratory sensation or by plantarflexing and dorsiflexing the great toe for gross proprioception. After an appropriate attempt at reduction and reestablishment of the normal diameter of the spinal medullary canal, computed tomographic (CT) myelography should follow to assess for possible soft-tissue masses, such as an extruded disc or hematoma that may continue to exert extrinsic pressure on the spinal cord or anterior spinal artery. If found, these would be relieved by laminectomy. Unfortunately, the prognosis for recovery with this injury is poor.

The acute central cord syndrome (see Fig. 101.2C) usually afflicts patients with a narrowed spinal canal. This may be due to degenerative spine disease or to a congenital stenotic canal. The mechanism of injury is usually hyperextension. The hallmark of this lesion is greater damage to the central portion of the cord than to the periphery. This leads to a variable sensory loss but a predictable motor loss, with motor function of the upper extremities below the level of the lesion more impaired than those of the lower extremities. This is because the motor fibers in the lateral corticospinal tract lie in a laminar fashion, with cervical segments most medial and thoracic, lumbar, and sacral motor fibers progressively more lateral. Management of this injury is usually nonoperative. There is a relatively good prognosis for recovery of at least partial neurologic function, with three-fourths of these patients walking at 1 year.

The Brown-Séquard syndrome (see Fig. 101.2D) is a hemicord injury that presents with a crossed sensory and motor deficit. Motor function is lost ipsilateral to the cord lesion, but sensory function is preserved on this side. Sensory function is lost on the contralateral side, where motor function is preserved. The crossed lesion is explained by the decussation of motor fibers in the medulla and the decussation of sensory fibers about two segments above the segment at which their sensory root enters the spinal cord. Causes include penetrating injuries, tumor, and disc disease. The prognosis is poor with penetrating injuries.

The patient with a cervical or high thoracic cord injury may present with relative hypotension due to the sudden loss of sympathetic tone below the level of the lesion. The patient has warm, dry skin and normal capillary refill, but with a paradoxical bradycardia. Labeling this condition "spinal neurogenic shock" helps to differentiate it from the aforementioned spinal shock. Spinal neurogenic shock in the patient with signs or mechanisms of multiple injuries may be difficult to differentiate from other causes of shock. Hemorrhagic shock classically presents as hypotension; tachycardia; cool, moist skin; and delayed capillary refill. The hypotensive patient should be assumed to have hemorrhagic shock until all gross external bleeding is controlled and the search for occult hemorrhage in the chest, abdomen, and pelvis is complete. This search should include, at a minimum, chest x-ray, pericardial ultrasonography, pelvic x-ray, abdominal ultrasonography, peritoneal lavage, or abdominal CT. After this survey is complete and no other explanation for shock is found, the hypotension may be attributed to spinal neurogenic shock. At that point, fluid administration is reduced to maintenance levels and the hypotension is treated with dopamine as necessary to maintain perfusion of the brain and spinal cord. Unfortunately, the optimal blood pressure to maintain the patient is unknown.

DIFFERENTIAL DIAGNOSIS

Determination of a cord injury is straightforward in the patient with quadri- or paraplegia. It becomes more difficult in patients with partial cord syndromes, particularly in those with acute central cord syndrome. This is due to both the patchy nature of the sensory loss and preservation of at least some motor function in the lower extremities. Evaluation for cord injury is also difficult in the unconscious patient. Most patients who present to the emergency department with complaints of neck or back pain or tenderness are found to have muscular strains or ligamentous sprains and no associated cord injury. The clinician

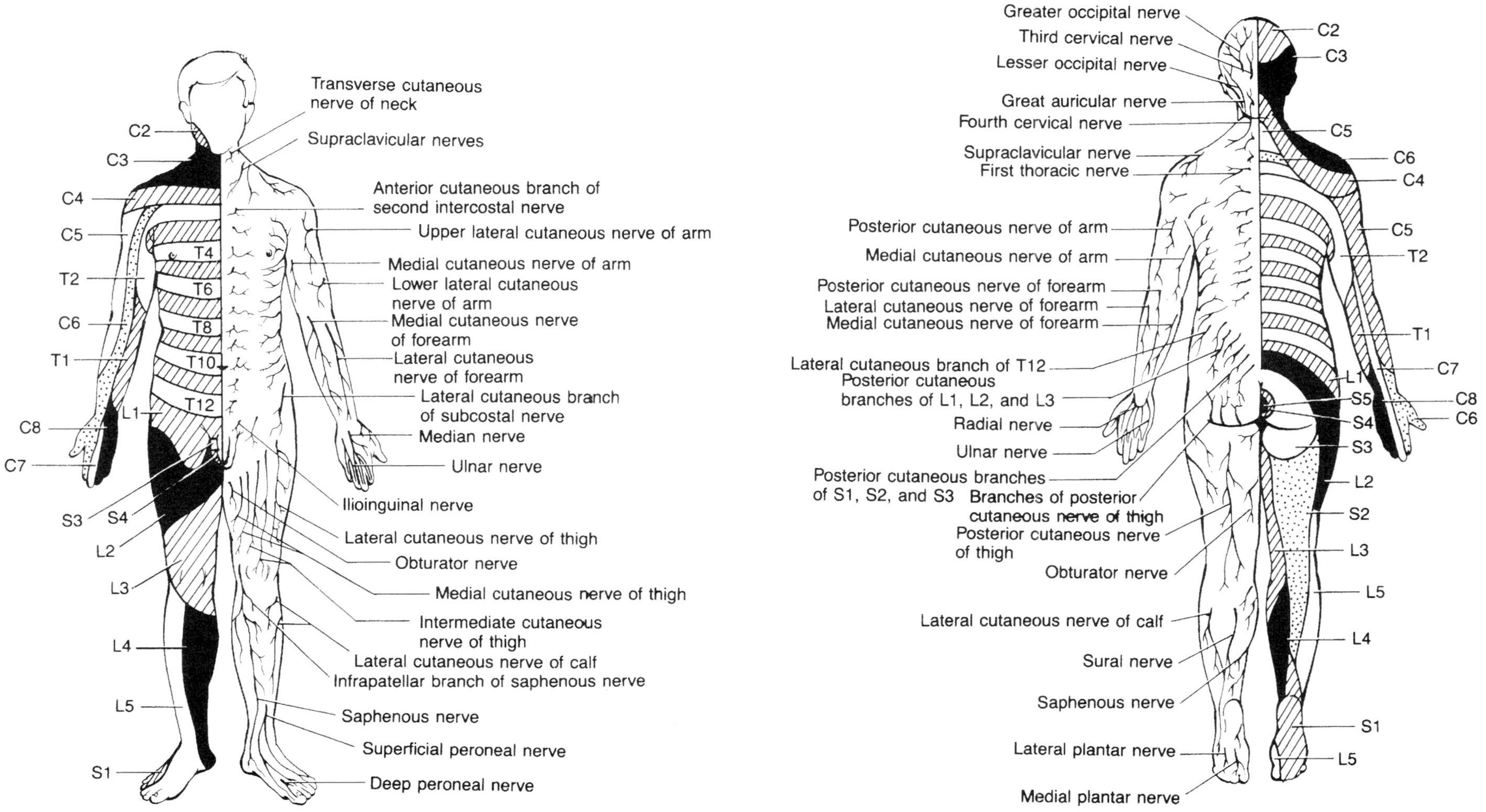

Figure 101.1. Sensory dermatomal segments. **(Left)** Anterior view. **(Right)** Posterior view.

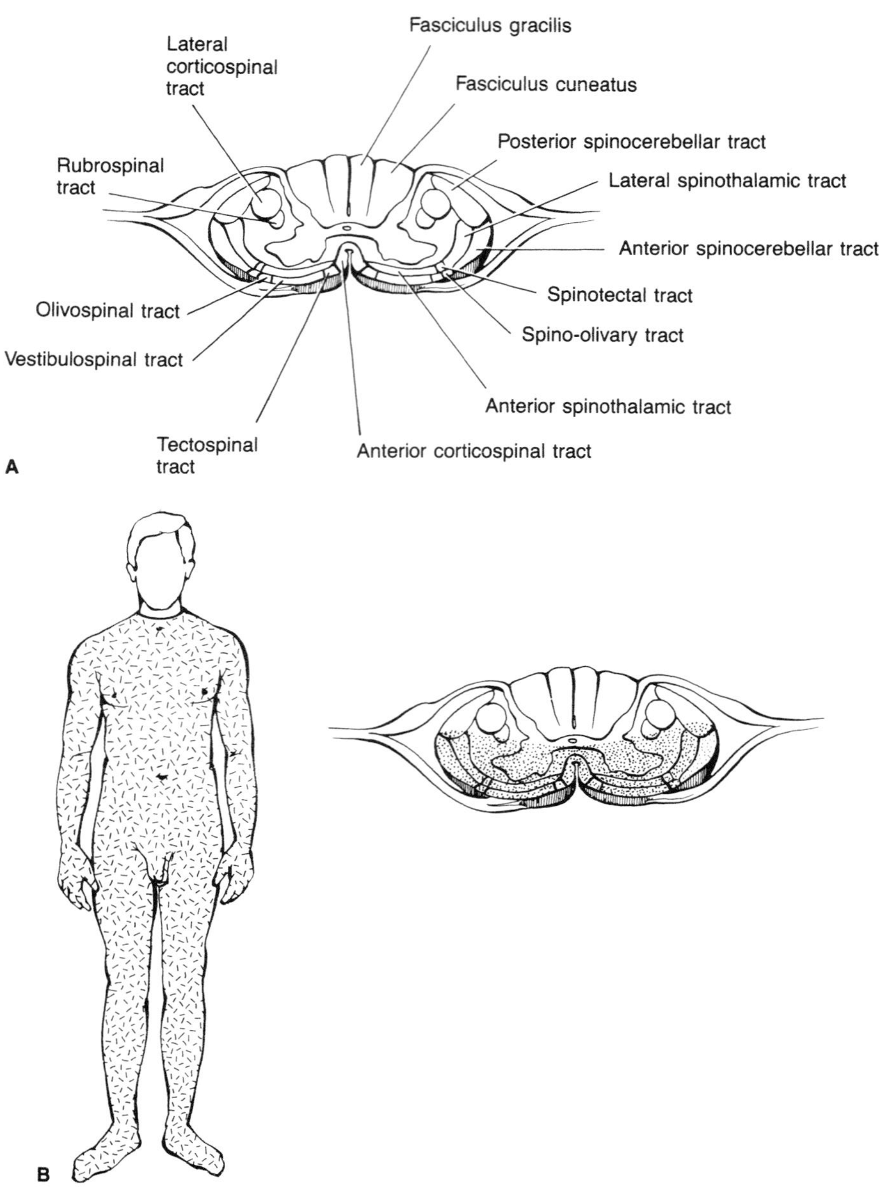

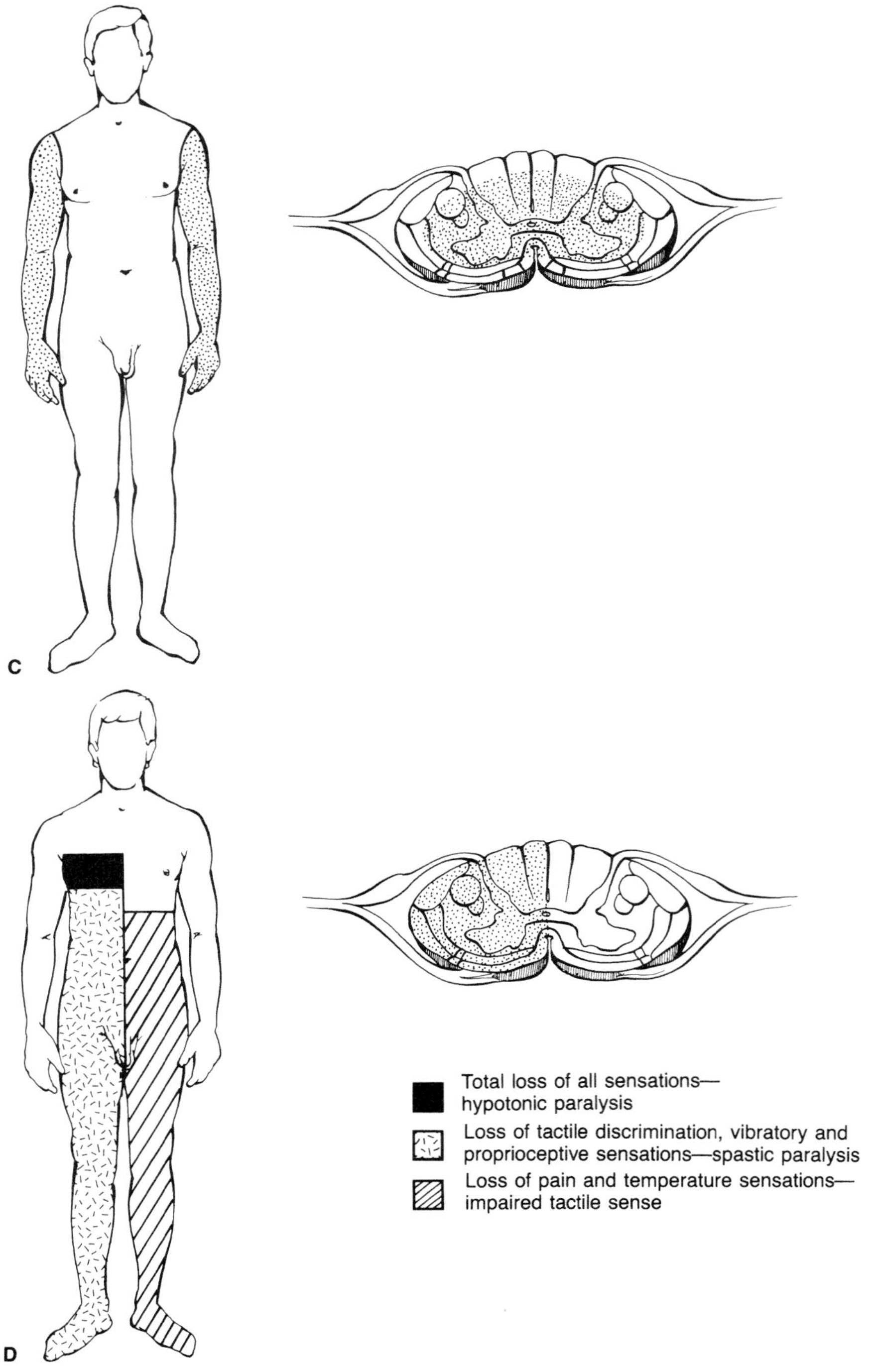

Figure 101.2. Transverse section of the spinal cord at the cervical level. **(A)** The ascending and descending tracts. **(B)** Tracts that may be damaged in the anterior spinal artery syndrome. **(C)** Tracts that may be damaged in the central cord syndrome. **(D)** Involved tracts and the superimposed areas of deficit from an injury at T4, resulting in the Brown-Séquard syndrome.

should not be fooled by the absence of a fracture: A third-degree ligamentous sprain can render the spinal column unstable, allowing motion between vertebral bodies and subsequent cord or spinal root injury.

EMERGENCY DEPARTMENT EVALUATION

The principles of evaluation are the same for all significantly injured patients. Initial attention should be paid to airway, breathing, circulation, disability, exposure, and environment (ABCDEs), with simultaneous resuscitation involving high-flow oxygen, two large-bore intravenous lines, a nasal or orogastric tube, a Foley catheter, and serial vital sign determinations. This primary survey should be followed by critical x-rays, including lateral cervical spine, chest, and pelvis films; ultrasound of the pericardium and abdomen; a secondary survey; definitive care; and, finally, appropriate disposition. During the secondary survey, a careful neurologic examination must be performed. This examination is carefully recorded so that an ascending lesion or deterioration in function can be identified by serial examinations. Motor function for all muscle groups is tested and recorded on a 0 to 5 scale (0 equals no function; 2, muscle activity apparent but cannot overcome gravity; 3, can overcome gravity; 4, diminished but can overcome more than gravity; 5, full normal). The level of sensory loss is plotted to identify the level on which to concentrate with radiographic imaging. This level should be drawn on the body in ink to identify any changes. Gross proprioception or vibratory function is measured to examine posterior column function. Deep tendon reflexes, anogenital reflexes (bulbocavernosus, anal wink), and perianal sensation are elicited to identify spinal shock or sacral sparing. Serial vital sign determinations must be made. Serial neurologic examinations are performed to identify any important change in functional status, which would have a profound influence on the management of the patient by the neurosurgeon or orthopedic surgeon. Deterioration of function implies the need for a CT myelogram to check for the presence of an extrinsic mass compressing the cord, which might be surgically correctable. No specific laboratory studies aid in this evaluation.

After the history and physical examination have identified the level of the lesion, plain films help characterize the lesion. A true lateral projection of the cervical spine identifies 90% of significant bony and ligamentous lesions. Specific attention should be paid to full visualization of all seven cervical vertebrae and the top of T1; atlantooccipital alignment (using the X method, a line drawn from the tip of the basion to midway on the spinolaminal line of C2 should intersect tangentially the edge of the odontoid, and a line drawn from the tip of the opisthion to the posteroinferior corner of the body of C2 should intersect tangentially the spinolaminal line of C1)[10]; a predental space 3 mm or less; prevertebral soft tissue that measures less than 5 mm anterior to C3; the spinal canal on 72-in. plain film, anteroposterior diameter 13 mm or greater; any horizontal subluxation of one vertebra on the next; fanning of the space between spinous processes; fracture of any bone; and incidental findings of the skull or mandible. The open-mouth odontoid view identifies most of the remaining 10% of significant lesions. This view should be examined for the alignment and equal spacing between C2 and the lateral masses of C1 and for fracture of these bones. The anteroposterior view rarely identifies injury not already suspected.

These three views compose the baseline cervical plain film series. The lateral and anteroposterior views form the baseline series for thoracolumbar injuries. Some advocate supine anterior oblique views of the cervical spine to better visualize the posterior elements.[6] These views show the neural foramina well in patients with radicular symptoms. They also clearly demonstrate the pedicles, as well as the lamina, which should stack like shingles on a roof.

Flexion and extension views are used carefully to demonstrate spinal column stability if the initial three views raise a question but would predict a stable spinal column (e.g., a small chip fracture of the anterior–inferior margin of the vertebral body, or a step-off of 1 to 2 mm with no other noted abnormalities). Flexion–extension views should be used when the initial three views are normal but the pain seems out of proportion, suggesting greater occult ligamentous damage. Instability should be suspected, and immobilization maintained, if there is more than a 3-mm step-off of one vertebra on the next or if there is an 11-degree or greater angulation between vertebral segments.[14] In questionable cases, the neurosurgeon will use CT scanning. The neurosurgeon may also use flexion–extension views to prove instability before fusion if the initial three views are suspicious but not diagnostic for instability.

In any case, for this study, the patient carefully and slowly flexes and later extends the head and neck; movement is stopped immediately if pain or paresthesias are elicited. Instability is confirmed if there is displacement of one vertebral body on another or if there is abnormal flaring between spinous processes. The physician should be present during this maneuver to ensure that no force is applied.

CT scanning is best for bony detail. CT is indicated when a fracture is identified on plain films, when neurologic injury is present, when pain seems out of proportion to the injury and findings on plain film, when instability is suspected based on plain films, and when there are questionable findings on plain film that cannot otherwise be determined. It frequently shows additional fractures, clarifies the extent of the fracture, and adds some information on soft-tissue injury. Neurosurgeons use CT myelography to identify an extrinsic mass pressing on the cord, as evidenced by inability of the dye to pass the level of the lesion. Magnetic resonance imaging (MRI) is better for soft-tissue injury but lacks bony detail. Early in management, the patient may be too unstable in a cardiovascular sense or too uncomfortable to stay still for the prolonged time needed for an MRI study.

The physician must avoid the common diagnostic error of relying on the lateral view alone before removing the semirigid collar. The semirigid collar is removed in a supine, immobilized patient, as needed, to examine the neck. When this examination is complete, the collar is replaced. It should otherwise be left on until the full series of cervical films shows the spine to be stable. Other common diagnostic errors are due to inadequate neurologic examination. One common problem is failing to examine for posterior column function (gross proprioception, vibratory sensation). A second error is failing to examine the sacral area for sparing, which is needed to differentiate a partial cord lesion from a physiologically complete injury.

It is impractical to leave every patient who presents on a spine board immobilized until a radiologist, neurosurgeon, or orthopedist examines the film and patient. The emergency physician must act on his or her interpretation of the films in the vast majority of cases. The physician must not accept inadequate x-rays. The most common problem is that the lateral view of the neck does not fully show the first seven-and-a-third vertebrae. C7-T1 injuries are not common, but nor are they rare. A swimmer's view may be used to see this junction on patients with large shoulders. The physician should not spend too much time obtaining adequate spine films; the patient may die of other injuries. The spinal cord and column should be protected with a long board and semirigid collar while attending to the ABCDEs of the primary survey and resuscitation. The patient can go to the operating room on the backboard if necessary. The surgeon can return to a careful spinal evaluation after surgery once the cardiorespiratory condition has been stabilized.

EMERGENCY DEPARTMENT MANAGEMENT

The pace of acute intervention for the patient with a spinal cord injury should be urgent. The focus should be on identifying and managing life-threatening injuries, while protecting the spinal column from unnecessary motion. Immobilize these patients; do not apply traction until after films carefully define the lesion. Traction that causes distraction on the cord or roots may cause severe, possibly irreparable neurologic damage. The first priority is to ensure that the patient survives, by attending to the ABCDEs. The second priority is to prevent secondary injury to the damaged spinal cord.

The physician must not allow, or cause, the patient to have unnecessary motion of the unstable spinal column. However, at times, such motion may be necessary to preserve the patient's life, such as in the patient with an obstructed airway who needs immediate management when initial maneuvers have proven unsuccessful. In-line immobilization should be used, allowing only as much motion as is needed to successfully control the airway. The physician should prepare to logroll and suction if the patient regurgitates, while maintaining the patient's spinal column as straight as possible. Although x-ray studies show that logrolling is associated with some motion of the thoracolumbar spinal column,[13] it must be done to prevent aspiration and obstruction in the patient who regurgitates without a protected airway. The backboard can be used to help logroll the patient, provided the straps are properly applied and have not been removed. Straps on the body may be released to remove clothing, while maintaining the head immobilized on the board. The body straps should be immediately reapplied after removing the clothing. A nasogastric tube is placed in the unconscious or intoxicated patient to decompress the stomach and reduce the risk of regurgitation.

The patient must be protected against unnecessary motion until the history, physical examination, and, if indicated, radiologic studies are complete and show that the spinal column is stable. The physician must not be fooled, by the fact that the patient was walking after the injury, into thinking films are unnecessary in a patient who has posttraumatic spinal pain, tenderness, paresthesias, neurologic findings, a high-energy mechanism, other painful distracting injuries, or a decreased level of consciousness. Timely reduction of the displaced column is vital to achieve decompression of the spinal cord. The physician is expected to preserve residual spinal cord function and not to cause a secondary injury to an already damaged cord while managing the patient. The cord can suffer devastating secondary injury if motion is allowed in the direction of instability. (Most injuries are unstable in flexion, but this is unknown until x-rays are obtained.)

The phrenic nerve, providing motor innervation to the diaphragm, arises from the C3 and C4 segments of the spinal cord. An otherwise healthy patient can maintain adequate long-term ventilation with diaphragmatic breathing alone. However, if a traumatic lesion affects C3 or C4, or if the level of the lesion ascends, as sometimes happens, the patient will become ventilator-dependent.

With blunt cord injury, very high doses of methylprednisolone are given early in treatment.[3–5] The patient being treated within 3 hours of blunt injury is loaded with 30 mg/kg as a bolus, followed by a continuous drip of 5.4 mg/kg/h for the subsequent 23 hours. The patient being treated from 3 to 8 hours following injury receives the same loading dose but then is maintained on the continuous drip for 48 hours, although this increases the severity of sepsis and pneumonia in this group. Although it is impossible to measure the direct effect on any one patient, this treatment has been shown to lead to a statistically significant improvement in neurologic outcome while not causing a statistically significant increase in wound complications or gastrointestinal bleeds.[3,4] Very high doses of methylprednisolone are considered the standard of care within 8 hours of blunt injury: Alternate drugs should be used only as part of an approved study protocol. This drug treatment is used on all patients, including the immunocompromised and elderly. Very high dose methylprednisolone is not indicated after penetrating spinal cord injury.[11]

DISPOSITION

Role of the Consultant

The emergency physician must decide if a spinal column or cord injury exists: Too many patients present with such potential injuries to rely on consultation. Next, the physician must decide whether the column is stable. Consultation should be requested if the emergency physician cannot decide whether an injury is stable or significant, when an unstable injury is found, or when cord or root injury is found. The timing of consultation is urgent—it should be done while the patient is in the emergency department—but not emergent in the sense of an airway problem. It should be requested after attention is focused on primary survey activities and initial resuscitation.

Indications for Admission

Patients are admitted if there is a cord injury or unstable column injury, for pain control, or for an anticipated complication such as the association of ileus with a thoracolumbar compression fracture. Patients with cord or unstable column injuries are admitted to the intensive care unit, and circle beds, rotating frames, or serial inflating devices are used to protect from pressure sores.

Early in their course, patients often have an atonic bladder. A Foley catheter is used to monitor urine output during the resuscitation and to prevent damaging distention of the bladder. Early in hospitalization, the Foley catheter is removed and replaced by intermittent catheterization to decrease the chance of developing an ascending urinary tract infection.

Patients with a stable spinal column injury may be managed on an outpatient basis. This includes the huge number of patients who carry the diagnosis of acute cervical strain or acute lumbar strain. Patients with isolated, stable thoracolumbar compression fractures of less than 40% of the anterior height of the vertebral body are often managed at home. Follow-up care of cervical sprains and strains should be arranged within 2 to 3 weeks to recheck for subacute instability.[7] The patient should return immediately for a recheck if there is any sign of worsening, such as the development of a cauda equina syndrome with urinary retention, fecal incontinence, or saddle hypoesthesia. Paresthesias are a sign of potential instability.

Transfer Considerations

The patient should be transferred to a specialized trauma facility if the trauma team cannot meet all the special requirements of the cord- or spinal column–injured patient, or for the extensive rehabilitation and specialized care of the cord-injured patient. Deteriorating or unstable internal injuries are best managed before transfer. The patient may be transferred by air or by ground; air transfer may provide a smoother ride. Transport personnel should be, at a minimum, advanced life support certified to ensure the continuous administration of intravenous methylprednisolone. For the emergent transfer, the patient should remain immobilized on a spinal board with a semirigid collar.

COMMON PITFALLS

- Evaluation errors include a neurologic examination inadequate to identify changes in the neurologic status. Change is a key parameter leading to CT myelography and possible decompressive surgery. It is vital to record an accurate baseline motor, sensory, posterior column, and rectal tone examination. This should be followed by serial examinations.
- Misreading x-rays or accepting inadequate films
- Missing other injuries in the anesthetic or hypoesthetic patient. The patient cannot feel pain or tenderness below the lesion, so common historical and physical examination findings will be absent. The patient requires a very thorough examination, and it is wise to x-ray all significant bruises.
- The most common early management error is applying cervical spine traction instead of immobilization.[2,8,12] The patient is at the highest potential risk for traction injury during prehospital placement on a spinal board or during intubation, when in-line immobilization, not traction, should be used.
- Failing to ensure survival by attending to the ABCDEs and initial resuscitation
- Blaming hypotension on spinal neurogenic shock without completing the search for occult injury
- Failing to follow a high-dose methylprednisolone protocol
- Serious medicolegal risk will arise if there is deterioration due to secondary injury. Such risk would be particularly high if the physician allowed unnecessary motion, or if there was deterioration after failure to identify an unstable segment.

References

1. Bicknell JM, Kirsch WM, Seigel R, et al. Atlantoaxial dislocation in rheumatic fever. *J Neurosurg* 1987;66:286.
2. Bivins HG, Ford S, Bezmalinovic Z, et al. The effect of axial traction during orotracheal intubation of the trauma victim with an unstable cervical spine. *Ann Emerg Med* 1988;17(1):25.
3. Bracken MB, Shepard MJ, Collins WF, et al. A randomized, controlled trial of methylprednisolone or naloxone in the treatment of acute spinal-cord injury. *N Engl J Med* 1990;322:1405.
4. Bracken MB, Shepard MJ, Collins WF, et al. Methylprednisolone or naloxone treatment after acute spinal cord injury: 1-year follow-up data (results of the Second National Acute Spinal Cord Injury Study). *J Neurosurg* 1992;76:23.
5. Bracken MB, Shepard MJ, Holford TR, et al. Administration of methylprednisolone for 24 or 48 hours or tirilazad mesylate for 48 hours in the treatment of acute spinal cord injury. Results of the Third National Acute Spinal Cord Injury Randomized Controlled Trial. National Acute Spinal Cord Injury Study. *JAMA* 1997;277(20):1597–1604.
6. Doris PE, Wilson RA. The next logical step in the emergency radiographic evaluation of cervical spine trauma: the five-view trauma series. *J Emerg Med* 1985;3:371.
7. Herkowitz HN, Rothman RH. Subacute instability of the cervical spine. *Spine* 1984;9:348.
8. Holley J, Jorden R. Airway management in patients with unstable cervical spine fractures. *Ann Emerg Med* 1989;18:1237.
9. Kraus JF, Franti CE, Riggins RS, et al. Incidence of traumatic spinal cord lesions. *J Chron Dis* 1975;8:471.
10. Lee C, Woodring JH, Goldstein SJ, et al. Evaluation of traumatic atlanto-occipital dislocations. *Am J Neuroradiol* 1987;8(1):19.
11. Levy ML, Gans W, Wijesinghe HS, et al. Use of methylprednisolone as an adjunct in the management of patients with penetrating spinal cord injury: outcome analysis. *Neurosurgery* 1996;39(6):1141–1149.
12. Majernick TG, Bieniek R, Hughes HG. Cervical spine movement during orotracheal intubation. *Ann Emerg Med* 1986;15:417.
13. McGuire RA, Neville S, Green BA, et al. Spinal instability and the logrolling maneuver. *J Trauma* 1987;27:525.
14. Panjabi MM, White AA. Basic biomechanics of the spine. *Neurosurgery* 1980;7(1):76.
15. Trafton PG. Spinal cord injuries. *Surg Clin North Am* 1982;62(1):61.
16. Trafton PG, Boyd CA. Computed tomography of thoracic and lumbar spine injuries. *J Trauma* 1984;24:506.

CHAPTER 102
Pulmonary and Pleural Injuries

C. Keith Stone and Ron Forrest Koury

When lung tissues or the pleural linings are injured, devastating effects on pulmonary function can quickly ensue. Thoracic trauma is involved in nearly one-third of acute admissions to trauma centers and accounts for 25% of all trauma-related deaths in the United States.[12] The initial emergency department treatment of injuries to the pleura and lung parenchyma is often lifesaving.

PNEUMOTHORAX

A pneumothorax is the abnormal accumulation of air between the visceral and parietal pleurae. Penetrating thoracic trauma can introduce air into the pleural space by violating the chest wall and parietal pleura, resulting in a transient or continuous communication of the pleural space with ambient air. Penetrating trauma can also violate the pulmonary parenchyma, resulting in the flow of bronchoalveolar air into the pleural space.

Blunt thoracic trauma can result in a pneumothorax due to visceral pleural and pulmonary parenchymal damage from thoracic shearing forces and from the sharp fracture lines of injured ribs. Barotrauma can also indirectly result in pneumothorax. The negative pressure differential of the intrapleural space, with respect to both atmospheric air and bronchoalveolar air, results in its filling. Traumatic pneumothorax occurs in 15% to 50% of patients with blunt chest trauma and is almost invariably present in those with transpleural penetrating wounds.[9]

CLINICAL PRESENTATION

Traumatic pneumothorax typically results in the complaints of chest pain and dyspnea. Patient presentation may range widely, depending on the size of the pneumothorax, the degree of prior pulmonary insufficiency, and the presence of other associated injuries. Diminished breath sounds with auscultation, and hyperresonance with percussion, on the side of injury may be appreciated. One patient may present with cyanosis and tachypnea and may appear acutely ill; another patient may have no symptoms or findings except that of mild chest discomfort. In the multiply injured patient, the signs and symptoms of the other injuries may overshadow those of pneumothorax; therefore, a high index of suspicion is mandatory.

DIFFERENTIAL DIAGNOSIS

A simple pneumothorax does not cause the hypotension and profound respiratory distress seen with tension pneumothorax. Hemothorax often demonstrates ipsilateral dullness to percussion as opposed to the hyperresonance seen with pneumothorax.

EMERGENCY DEPARTMENT EVALUATION

The evaluation of a suspected pneumothorax begins with a focused history and physical examination. Gather information from the patient and emergency medical service personnel to determine the mechanism of injury. Observe the chest for wounds or asymmetry. Palpate for crepitance associated with broken ribs, which are associated with pneumothorax in up to one-third of cases. Percuss for hyperresonance, and, most importantly, auscultate for decreased breath sounds on the injured side.

If patient stability warrants, the chest radiograph is the next primary evaluation technique. A supine chest radiograph is acceptable, but an upright view allows air in the pleural space to rise to the apices and makes the diagnosis easier. In a multiply injured trauma victim whose spinal evaluation and clearance may be delayed, clinical suspicion and a supine film may be the only immediately available information sources. Some emergency department stretchers allow Fowler positioning (head of bed up) without compromising spinal precautions, and thus aid in obtaining a more informative x-ray.

A pneumothorax appears on chest x-ray as an area devoid of lung markings (Fig. 102.1). The initial film should be at full inspiration. If this film does not show a pneumothorax but clinical suspicion remains high, an expiratory film can be obtained. Despite a thorough examination and a good-quality x-ray, pneumothoraces can be elusive. The noisy emergency department environment is often less than ideal to auscultate for breath sounds, and low oxygen saturations are often not evident because injured patients are immediately placed on 100% O_2.

Pneumothoraces also frequently may present anteriorly and not be evident on initial supine x-rays. Computed tomographic (CT) scanning of the chest is highly effective in locating intrapleural air.[8] Although chest x-ray is less sensitive in detecting injuries than is CT, the majority of injuries identified by CT alone are minor and require no treatment.[13]

Pneumothorax size has traditionally been reported as a percentage of lung collapse. A small pneumothorax corresponds to 15% collapse, a moderate pneumothorax to 15% to 60%, and a large pneumothorax to more than 60%. A less ambiguous and simpler system is to measure and report the distance on the chest radiograph of the visceral pleural reflection from the inside of the chest wall at the apex and laterally.

EMERGENCY DEPARTMENT MANAGEMENT

Tube thoracostomy is the definitive emergency department treatment for traumatic pneumothorax. A small pneumothorax in a patient who will not undergo general anesthesia or receive positive-pressure ventilation may be managed with observation while the pleural air collection spontaneously resorbs. All other patients with traumatic pneumothorax should have a large chest tube (36F to 40F in adults) placed. The tube is placed in the fourth or fifth intercostal space just anterior to the midaxillary line. The plane of dissection through the chest wall courses over the top of the rib in order that the neurovascular bundle is not traumatized. The tip of the chest tube is directed apically and posteriorly. All chest tube side holes must lie within the pleural space. Chest radiographs must be taken after tube thoracostomy placement to demonstrate adequate evacuation of the pneumothorax and proper tube placement.[16] It is imperative that emergency medicine physicians become highly skilled in the proper placement and management of tube thoracostomies, as complication rates as high as 14% have been reported.[5]

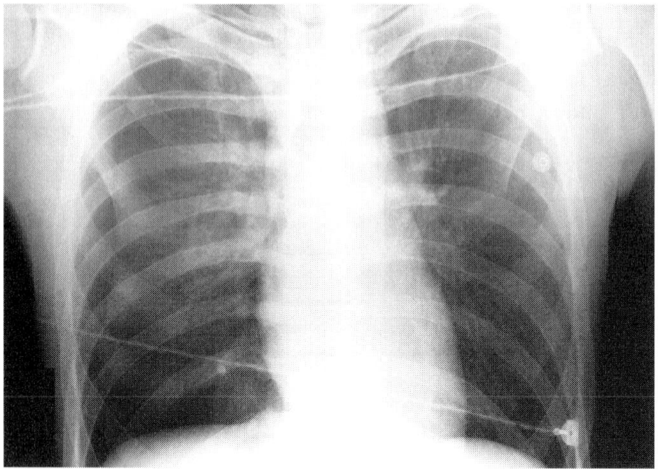

Figure 102.1. Chest film demonstrating a pneumothorax on the right.

The chest tube is attached to a three-bottle system, using a trap bottle to collect fluid drainage from the pleura, a water-seal bottle to prevent air from returning to the pleural space during inspiration, and a manometer bottle to generate the suction. These containers are currently combined into a single molded-plastic apparatus. The initial suction placed on this system is usually 20 cm H_2O in adults.

DISPOSITION

All patients with traumatic pneumothorax require surgical consultation and admission. If no other significant injuries are present, admission to a floor surgical bed is adequate.

Air transport of the patient with a pneumothorax poses special risks. As atmospheric pressure decreases with ascent, the trapped gas of an unevacuated pneumothorax expands, increasing the size and lethality of the pneumothorax. A tube thoracostomy must remain on suction or have a one-way seal in place before air transport. The safest air transport is in an aircraft pressurized to sea level.

COMMON PITFALLS

- If a patient has a mechanism of injury consistent with chest wall trauma, assume there is a potential pneumothorax, even if not visualized on initial x-ray.
- Because pneumothoraces are easy to miss on an initial supine film, maintain a high index of suspicion.
- Observe carefully for clinical signs suggesting *progression* of simple pneumothorax to tension pneumothorax.
- Do not allow a patient with a small pneumothorax to undergo positive-pressure ventilation or ascend in an aircraft before tube thoracostomy evacuation.
- Do not insert a chest tube without first inserting a finger to ensure that the tube will not be placed through the lung, diaphragm, liver, or spleen.

TENSION PNEUMOTHORAX

A tension pneumothorax is a critical condition that exists when the communication between the bronchoalveolar and pleural spaces results in a progressive accumulation of intrapleural air. A pulmonary injury can act as a one-way valve, allowing air to enter the intrapleural space with inspiration but preventing its escape with expiration. Intrapleural pressures can rise dramatically because forced inspiration can generate pressures of up to −80 mm Hg. The contralateral lung and the vena cava become compressed. The cavoatrial junction can become distorted, obstructing right ventricular filling.

CLINICAL PRESENTATION

The patient with a tension pneumothorax is extremely ill, with profound respiratory distress and impending vascular collapse. Classic signs include jugular venous distention, tachycardia, hypotension, and absent breath sounds ipsilateral to the injury. The patient may be cyanotic and restless, and the trachea may be shifted contralateral to the side of injury. The patient may have a hyperexpanded hemithorax (highly resonant to percussion), with one side of chest tangibly bigger than the other and immobile. The patient may even present with pulseless electrical activity.

DIFFERENTIAL DIAGNOSIS

A patient with simple pneumothorax will present with unilateral loss of breath sounds, but will not be in extremis from this injury alone. Pericardial tamponade presents with hypotension and central venous distention, but heart sounds are distant and breath sounds are normal unless a pneumothorax is coincident. The patient in hypovolemic shock may be difficult to distinguish from the patient with intravascular volume depletion who has a coincident tension pneumothorax.

EMERGENCY DEPARTMENT EVALUATION

The rapid lethality of tension pneumothorax does not allow the luxury of radiographic evaluation. If the diagnosis of tension pneumothorax is suspected based on the physical examination, the physician should institute immediate treatment. If a radiograph is obtained prior to correction of a tension pneumothorax, marked mediastinal shift contralateral to the affected side and flattening or even partial inversion of the ipsilateral hemidiaphragm are seen.[6]

EMERGENCY DEPARTMENT MANAGEMENT

Immediate intervention is indicated when this diagnosis is suspected. Rapid decompression of the pleural space can be accomplished by placing a large-bore needle (12-gauge) into the second or third interspace anteriorly, or in the fourth or fifth interspace laterally, on the affected side. The lateral approach (anterior axillary line behind body of pectoralis muscle) provides the easiest access, because there is less muscle there and fewer anatomic structures are at risk for injury.[19] This needle decompression reduces the deadly tension pneumothorax to the merely life-threatening communicating pneumothorax. This rapid technique can be easily accomplished in the prehospital setting. A standard tube thoracostomy must then be performed to evacuate the pleural space completely.

DISPOSITION

All patients with tension pneumothorax must be admitted to the hospital. The proper level of care is determined by the associated injuries. A patient who presented in shock with no other injuries and then stabilized with tube thoracostomy placement could be admitted to a standard floor surgical bed. Additional inpatient care is identical to that of simple pneumothorax.

COMMON PITFALLS

- In the patient with unilateral diminished breath sounds and shock, do not await radiographic confirmation of tension pneumothorax before placing the tube thoracostomy.
- After temporizing needle decompression, placement of a tube thoracostomy must follow as soon as possible.

HEMOTHORAX

The accumulation of blood in the intrapleural space is a hemothorax. This hemorrhage may originate from a pulmonary laceration, or injury to the intercostal vessels, internal mammary vessels, or great vessels of the thorax. Enough blood can accumulate to interfere with ventilatory function of the ipsilateral lung. Hypovolemic shock due to the large volume of blood that can fill the thorax is the predominant concern. Hemothorax is often associated with a pneumothorax.

CLINICAL PRESENTATION

The patient with a large hemothorax may present with the signs and symptoms of hypovolemic shock, including tachycardia, hypotension, pallor, and anxiety. Additionally, the patient may demonstrate respiratory compromise, including tachypnea and cyanosis due to diminished vital capacity. Dullness to percussion may be noted over one or both blood-filled hemithoraces. The symptoms of a small hemothorax may be completely overshadowed by other injuries. The signs and symptoms of a pneumothorax are more likely to predominate in the patient with a hemopneumothorax.

DIFFERENTIAL DIAGNOSIS

Tension pneumothorax presents with shock and unilateral diminished breath sounds. Pericardial tamponade presents with shock. Both of these conditions, however, may be accompanied by central venous distention, which would be absent in a large hemothorax.

EMERGENCY DEPARTMENT EVALUATION

Once primary resuscitation with restoration of intravascular volume has been completed, obtain a chest radiograph (Fig. 102.2). An upright chest radiograph will show blunting of the costophrenic angles when more than 250 mL of fluid is present. Often, because of hemodynamic instability or concern for cervi-

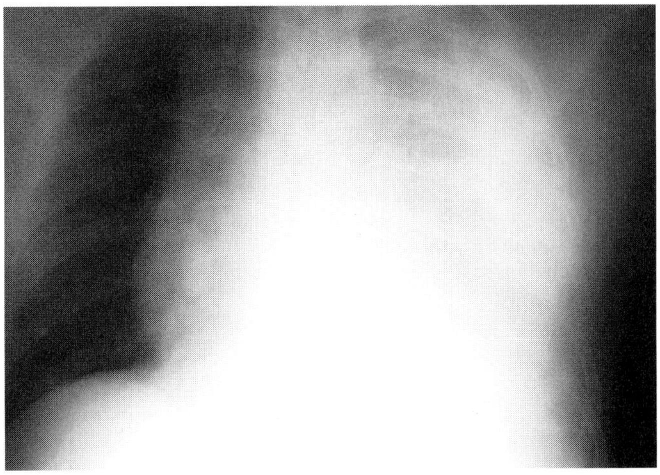

Figure 102.2. Chest film with massive hemothorax on the left.

cal spine injury, only a supine film is obtained. The supine film may show only a subtle haziness in the lung fields as the blood layers out posteriorly. Ultrasound and CT scan will also detect hemothoraces but are usually not as readily available as a portable film. Transesophageal echocardiograms can be used to evaluate the possible source of bleeding in patients with protected airways. The highest-yield study for evaluating the source of bleeding is an angiogram, but it requires that the patient be stable enough for transport to the angiography suite.

EMERGENCY DEPARTMENT MANAGEMENT

Once the diagnosis of hemothorax is made, a large-bore tube thoracostomy (at least 36F) should be placed in the fourth or fifth intercostal space just anterior to the midaxillary line and directed posteriorly to evacuate the blood and to monitor ongoing hemorrhage. This tube should be connected to the same suction apparatus previously described for pneumothoraces. Uncontaminated blood obtained from the intrapleural space with a cell-saver device can be reinfused into the hypovolemic trauma patient.

In most cases of hemothorax, tube thoracostomy is the definitive treatment. However, if more than 1500 mL of blood is initially obtained on placement of the tube thoracostomy, or if there is continued drainage of more than 200 to 300 mL/h, the tube should be clamped and an open thoracotomy may be required.[3] If there is clinical or radiographic evidence of aortic dissection or rupture, chest tube drainage can lead to rapid exsanguination.[20]

DISPOSITION

All patients with traumatic hemothorax must have prompt surgical consultation and admission. Patients with ongoing hemorrhage require emergent surgical consultation and intensive care unit (ICU) admission. If stable, they may be admitted to a floor surgical bed. As with pneumothorax, air transport of the patient with hemothorax is hazardous and should be done only with the tube placed on suction or with a one-way seal in place.

COMMON PITFALLS

- Intravascular volume must be replaced adequately.
- Because hemothoraces are easily missed on initial supine films, keep a high index of suspicion.
- A large chest tube must be used to evacuate the intrapleural space because of clotting in small-bore tubes.
- One must recognize that ongoing evacuation of blood may be an indication for open thoracotomy.

PULMONARY CONTUSION

The most common injury identified in blunt chest trauma is pulmonary contusion. Despite improvements in diagnostic imaging and critical care, the associated mortality has not appreciably changed over the last three decades and remains at 25% for blunt trauma.[1] The term *pulmonary contusion* loosely refers to a set of distinct injuries that may be sustained after high-impact blunt chest trauma: True pulmonary contusion is the most common and most serious injury. Pulmonary contusion, histologically, is the leakage of blood and protein into the alveoli and interstitial spaces of the lung, which stimulates increased secretions, resulting in atelectasis and consolidation. Pulmonary hematoma, a diagnosis that has been more clearly defined since the advent of the CT scan, represents an abnormal collection of blood. Pulmonary hematomas are initially seen as indistinct nodules on chest radiographs and usually resolve without sequelae. Pulmonary lacerations result from a shear force that disrupts the lung, parenchyma, and vessels. Pulmonary lacerations may cause bleeding or, less commonly, an air leak. Pulmonary contusions lead to hypoxia via the production of ventilation–perfusion mismatches.

Pulmonary contusion is a common sequela of blunt trauma in children. Previous reports suggest that children have more favorable outcomes than adults because of differences in mechanisms, associated injuries, and physiologic response. Recent studies have shown that although children and adults differ in regard to injury mechanism (automobile–pedestrian accidents versus motor vehicle accidents, respectively), their overall injury severity and outcomes are quite similar.[2] In contrast, elderly patients, who have a less compliant chest wall, are much more susceptible to injury and, as a group, have very poor outcomes after pulmonary contusions.[11]

CLINICAL PRESENTATION

The patient with a pulmonary contusion may initially demonstrate dyspnea and tachypnea. There may be tenderness or obvious ecchymosis and deformity over the affected chest wall. Large pulmonary contusions may be associated with tachycardia, hypotension, and cyanosis. Patients with multiple rib fractures or flail segments of the chest wall are likely to have associated pulmonary contusion. Within 4 to 6 hours, the chest radiograph will show a localized alveolar pattern, ranging from irregular patchy infiltrates to consolidation.[7]

DIFFERENTIAL DIAGNOSIS

The symptoms of adult respiratory distress syndrome are dyspnea, hypoxia, and diffuse radiographic infiltrates, but they typically appear later than contusion. Fat emboli syndrome can occur in the patient with severe long-bone fractures and causes similar symptoms, but is also evident much later than pulmonary contusion and with less focal x-ray findings. A simple pneumothorax can present with findings consistent with contusion and initially may be difficult to differentiate.

EMERGENCY DEPARTMENT EVALUATION

In the emergency department, pulmonary contusion is often a clinical diagnosis. The suspicion of pulmonary contusion is raised whenever there is significant trauma to the chest wall or bony thoracic cage. The chest radiograph can be critical in establishing the diagnosis. Clinical suspicion must initially be relied on because characteristic x-ray findings do not usually appear for 4 to 6 hours.

In a dog model of pulmonary contusion, the initial x-ray films failed to visualize the lung lesion in two-thirds of subjects, whereas 100% of the lesions were discernible by CT scan. At 6 hours, contusions were still not visible in 21% of chest x-rays.[7] It has been demonstrated that when more than 28% of the airspace is involved with contusion, all patients required mechanical ventilation.[7] The degree of pulmonary damage can also be evaluated by arterial blood gas analysis. An initially low PaO_2 and a wide alveolar–arterial oxygen gradient may be the first signs of pulmonary contusion. Deteriorating blood gas values predict a poorer prognosis.

EMERGENCY DEPARTMENT MANAGEMENT

Initial therapy includes aggressive pulmonary toilet. Early researchers suggested that fluid restriction would prevent lung edema associated with direct pulmonary contusion. Since then we have learned that mortality in patients with pulmonary contusion is not related to the use of crystalloid or to the volume of fluid used in resuscitation of these patients. Crystalloid should be used to improve end-organ perfusion and optimize tissue oxygen delivery.[14] Patients with pulmonary contusions must be monitored very closely for any signs or symptoms of respiratory decompensation, and early aggressive airway management to support ventilation is warranted.

Positioning the uninjured lung in the dependent position will increase pulmonary blood flow to the segments of the lung that are better perfused. Numerous studies suggest that between 30% and 60% of patients with pulmonary contusion will require intubation and some form of mechanical ventilatory assistance.[14] Patients with pulmonary contusions who have other injuries, such as flail chest with paradoxic movement, or severe pain are at high risk for CO_2 accumulation because of depressed central drive for breathing associated with splinting, hypoventilation, and narcotic sedation. Although volume-controlled ventilatory modes have been traditionally used, new data suggest that pressure-controlled modes are acceptable and probably should be preferred in patients with poorly compliant lungs and in young trauma victims who require high inspiratory flow rates.[17]

DISPOSITION

All patients require admission to a critical care bed, where ventilatory status and oxygen saturation can be frequently assessed. These patients usually have multiple serious injuries, which also require critical care monitoring and often prove a clinical challenge to the trauma team. Atelectasis and pneumonia are common complications. Patients with small pulmonary contusions, despite the lack of other apparent injury, should be admitted to a surgical bed for observation.

COMMON PITFALLS

- Realize that signs and symptoms will evolve over several hours and may be missed on the initial evaluation.
- Intervene early with intubation and mechanical ventilation before respiratory failure develops.
- Expect elderly patients to have very poor outcomes from pulmonary contusion, and admit them to an ICU bed.

TRACHEAL AND BRONCHIAL INJURIES

Disruptions of the trachea and bronchi are infrequent (incidence of 0.03%) but life-threatening injuries follow trauma. Because of their effects on ventilation, these injuries are often fatal; however, improved emergency services and transport have been cited as a reason for increasing numbers of patients reaching tertiary care centers. Several studies addressing both penetrating and blunt injuries show that 70% occur as a result of penetrating trauma, whereas 30% occur from blunt trauma.[10,15] Penetrating injuries involve the relatively unprotected cervical trachea in the majority of cases. Disruptions of the intrathoracic trachea and bronchi are less common. In contrast, the main bronchi are frequently involved in blunt trauma. The right main stem bronchus is involved twice as frequently as the left bronchus.[10]

CLINICAL PRESENTATION

Tracheal and bronchial injuries must be considered in any patient with a history of a significant mechanism, such as severe, sudden deceleration of any kind; penetration of neck or chest; or direct blow to neck or chest. Falls from heights over 18 ft cause high-energy impacts that may produce tracheobronchial injuries.[18] Occasionally, few clinical signs or symptoms are present, even with severe tracheobronchial injury. Dyspnea, hoarseness, and aphonia are common, as is hemoptysis. Subcutaneous emphysema is extremely likely to be present. Cervical emphysema, confined to the deep cervical fascia between the mandible and the clavicle, is highly suggestive. With a straddle injury of the mainstem bronchus, surrounding fascia and mediastinal tissue can maintain airflow with few signs and symptoms.[4]

DIFFERENTIAL DIAGNOSIS

Pneumothorax presents with unilateral decreased breath sounds and is corrected by tube thoracostomy. Pulmonary lacerations, hematomas, and contusions may cause hypoxia, abnormal pulmonary examination, and chest x-ray findings, but will not cause a persistent air leak.

EMERGENCY DEPARTMENT EVALUATION

Only a minority of patients with tracheobronchial injuries reach the hospital alive. Those that do are either in severe distress or in extremis, with obvious ventilatory problems, or exhibit other more obvious injuries that are attended to first during the initial resuscitation. All trauma patients require a chest x-ray once the ABCs have been addressed. Mediastinal emphysema may be massive if the pleura are intact. If a chest tube is already in place, tension pneumothorax with a massive air leak will be apparent if the pleura are ruptured. Any time a well-placed tube thoracostomy continues to demonstrate a significant air leak or is unable to reexpand the lung, tracheobronchial injury must be suspected. Rarely, a lobar bronchus is all that is injured, in which case the patient generally will have persistent atelectasis either with or without persistent air leak. Fiberoptic bronchoscopy is required for definitive diagnosis. Bronchoscopy should be mandatory in any patient with penetrating injuries near the trachea of major bronchi.

EMERGENCY DEPARTMENT MANAGEMENT

In a patient with obvious major airway or ventilatory problems, endotracheal intubation should be attempted; if successful, it may temporarily improve the problem. Bilateral tube thoracostomies should be placed if the patient remains in distress and there is any suspicion of a pneumothorax. Occasionally, emergent or urgent sternotomy or thoracotomy must be performed to obtain and secure an airway.[15] A stable patient who exhibits subcutaneous air without obvious pneumothorax should probably receive a tube thoracostomy if he or she will require ventilatory support. All tracheobronchial lacerations and disruptions require surgical repair.

DISPOSITION

All patients with suspected or confirmed tracheobronchial injury should be admitted to a surgical ICU.

COMMON PITFALLS

- If one does not think about the diagnosis of tracheobronchial injury early, the diagnosis will probably be made by the pathologist.
- Early intubation and aggressive airway management, as well as tube thoracostomy, cannot be delayed; they may be temporarily life-saving.
- As soon as the diagnosis is suspected, call a surgical colleague for immediate consultation or transfer to a trauma center.

References

1. Allen GS, Coates NE. Pulmonary contusion: a collective review. *Am Surg* 1996;62:895.
2. Allen GS, Cox CS, Moore FA, et al. Pulmonary contusion: are children different?. *J Am Coll Surg* 1997;185:229.
3. *Advanced trauma life support student manual: course for physicians,* 5th ed. Chicago: American College of Surgeons, 1993.
4. Calhoon JH, Grover FL, Trinkle JK. Chest trauma, approach and management. *Clin Chest Med* 1992;13(1):55.
5. Chan L, Reilly K, Henderson C, et al. Complication rates of tube thoracostomy. *Am J Emerg Med* 1997;15:4:368.
6. Chan O, Hiorns M. Chest trauma. *Eur J Radiol* 1996;23:23.
7. Cohn SM. Pulmonary contusion: review of the clinical entity. *J Trauma* 1997;42(5):973.
8. Collins JA, Samra GS. Failure of chest x-rays to diagnose pneumothoraces after blunt trauma. *Anesthesia* 1998;53:74.
9. Dann L. Acute pneumothorax. *Aust Fam Physician* 1994;23(2):144.
10. Huh J, Milliken J, Chen JC. Management of tracheobronchial injuries following blunt and penetrating trauma. *Am Surg* 1997;63(10):896.
11. Jackimczyk K. Blunt chest trauma. *Emerg Clin North Am* 1993;11(1):81.
12. Kollmorgan DR, Murray KA, Sullivan JJ, et al. Predictions of mortality in pulmonary contusion. *Am J Surg* 1994;168:659.
13. Marts B, Durham R, Shapiro M, et al. Computed tomography in the diagnosis of blunt thoracic injury. *Am J Surg* 1994;168:688.
14. Nelson LD. Ventilatory support of the trauma patient with pulmonary contusion. *Respir Care Clin North Am* 1996;2(3):425.
15. Richardson JD, Miller FB, Carrillo EH, et al. Complex thoracic injuries. *Surg Clin North Am* 1996;76(4):725.
16. Roberts JR, Hedges JR. *Clinical procedures in emergency medicine,* 3rd ed. Philadelphia: WB Saunders, 1998.
17. Sharma S, Mullins RJ, Trunkey DD. Ventilatory management of pulmonary contusion patients. *Am J Surg* 1996;171:529.
18. Song JK, Beaty CD. Diagnosis of pulmonary contusions and a bronchial laceration after a fall: trauma cases from Harborview Medical Center. Am J Radiol 1996;167:102.
19. Winchell RJ. Chest trauma. *Audio-Digest Emerg Med* 1998;15:23.
20. Yeam I, Sassoon C. Hemothorax and chylothorax. *Curr Opin Pulm Med* 1997;3:310.

CHAPTER 103

Blunt and Penetrating Cardiac Injuries

Lee W. Shockley

BLUNT CARDIAC INJURY

Blunt cardiac injury (BCI) refers to a spectrum of heart injuries, including BCI with septal rupture, BCI with free wall rupture, BCI with coronary artery thrombosis, BCI with cardiac failure, BCI with minor electrocardiogram (ECG) or enzyme abnormalities, and BCI with complex dysrythmias.[13,16] The terms *cardiac concussion* (*commotio cordis*) and *myocardial contusion* have been used, but lack a consensus for diagnostic criteria. BCI can occur when a moderate-to-severe force is applied to the chest or upper abdomen. Motor vehicle collisions (particularly those in which the driver hits the steering wheel), blast injuries, direct blows, falls from heights, and chest compression are the most common mechanisms. Seventy percent to 80% of blunt chest trauma victims are male, with a peak incidence in the third decade. Alcohol consumption and hazardous occupations are risks. Multiple trauma is associated in two-thirds of these patients. Mortality and morbidity are greater in patients over age 65.

Injuries to the heart occur in 8% to 71% of blunt chest trauma patients.[16] This wide range probably represents the difficulty in diagnosing and defining the problem, rather than representing the actual incidence. Eighty percent to 90% of lethal BCIs are immediately fatal (prehospital). These are usually from cardiac rupture or dysrhythmias (most commonly ventricular fibrillation). Mortality in patients who survive this initial period after BCI is related closely to their concomitant injuries.[9]

PATHOPHYSIOLOGY

By virtue of its location and suspension in the chest, the heart is susceptible to injury from compression of the chest wall or upper abdomen and from deceleration forces. The right ventricle is most commonly injured, probably due to its relatively vulnerable position immediately behind the sternum.

True cardiac chamber rupture is rare. The chamber ruptured most frequently, however, is the right atrium (50%), followed by the left atrium (25%), the right ventricle, and the left ventricle. Death is usually the result of tamponade (two-thirds of cases) or exsanguination (one-third).Less than 10% of patients with cardiac chamber rupture survive more than 30 minutes after injury.[17]

The heart valve most vulnerable to blunt trauma is the aortic. When mitral valve dysfunction is present, it is most commonly due to rupture of the chordae tendineae or papillary muscles.

CLINICAL PRESENTATION

Physical findings in BCI may be nonspecific. Seventy percent to 80% of patients with BCI have external signs of chest trauma, including contusions, abrasions, palpable crepitus, and flail segments.[9] The presence of a fracture of the sternum, once thought to be a marker for BCI, has been shown not to predict the presence of a BCI.[7] The most common vital sign abnormality is sinus tachycardia. Hypotension is a serious sign and should raise the possibility of cardiac tamponade, cardiac rupture, other noncardiac trauma with hypovolemia, valve rupture, or decreased cardiac output (pump failure). Chest pain is often present, but it is neither a sensitive nor specific symptom in the multiple trauma victim. Cyanosis of the upper torso, head, and neck may be present in up to 75% of patients with cardiac rupture.

Cardiac tamponade is a rare complication of blunt chest trauma (in contradistinction to penetrating trauma). Beck's triad of acute cardiac tamponade is hypotension, elevated jugular venous pressure (JVP), and muffled heart sounds. It is present in only about a third of patients with acute cardiac tamponade of any etiology. Pulsus paradoxus, although present in up to one-third of patients with tamponade, is not pathognomonic for tamponade. It is also present in chronic obstructive pulmonary disease, asthma, obesity, cardiac failure from many causes, constrictive pericarditis, pulmonary embolism, and cardiogenic shock.

New murmurs, or acute congestive heart failure, after chest trauma should raise the suspicion of a ruptured intraventricular septum, valve leaflet, or chordae tendineae. Traumatic ventricular septal rupture presents with a pansystolic murmur auscultable over the entire precordium, especially at the left lower sternal border. This may not be appreciated, however, until the patient has been resuscitated to euvolemia.

DIFFERENTIAL DIAGNOSIS

The differential diagnosis of blunt cardiac trauma includes pulmonary contusion, flail chest, simple pneumothorax, hemothorax, aortic injuries, extrathoracic hemorrhage, myocardial infarction, air embolism, and tracheal injuries. In the differential diagnosis of high central venous pressure (CVP) shock, tension pneumothorax is more common than cardiac tamponade.

EMERGENCY DEPARTMENT EVALUATION

There are no widely accepted criteria for making the diagnosis of BCI. No single test or combination of tests has proved useful in reliably confirming the diagnosis. The diagnosis could be entertained in any patient with a compatible mechanism of injury.

The admission ECG is the most important diagnostic tool in diagnosing BCI.[8] Almost every ECG abnormality has been described in BCI: Dysrhythmias, conduction blocks, axis shifts, ST and T wave changes, and injury patterns have all been described, but none of these changes are diagnostic. Total electrical alternans (both the P wave and QRS complex) is pathognomonic for pericardial tamponade, but this is a rare finding. The presence of abnormalities on the initial emergency department (ED) ECG, however, has the best correlation of any immediately available test with the risk of subsequent cardiac complications. If the initial ED ECG is abnormal, continuous cardiac monitoring for 24 to 48 hours is prudent. If the initial ED ECG is normal, the risk of having a BCI that requires treatment is very slight. Although many BCIs affect the right ventricle, right-sided ECG tracings have not been proven to be of value.

If the patient with a suspected BCI is hemodynamically unstable or has an elevated CVP, new heart murmurs, or significant dysrhythmias, echocardiography is indicated.[15] Transthoracic echocardiography has several advantages in the evaluation of these patients. This noninvasive test, which can be performed at the bedside, can quickly give information about wall motion abnormalities, pericardial fluid collections, ruptured valves, and ruptured septa, as well as an estimate of ejection fraction.[18] If the transthoracic echocardiogram is suboptimal, a transesophageal echocardiogram should be considered.[19]

Creatinine kinase (CK), CK-MB, and cardiac troponin-T (cTnT) determinations do not help in making the diagnosis. These tests lack sensitivity, specificity, and the ability to predict complications.[5,10] Cardiac troponin-I (cTnI) may be more accurate than CK-MB, but still lacks the ability to predict complications and appears to add no additional clinical value to the initial ED ECG.[1]

Chest radiographs are not helpful in diagnosing blunt cardiac trauma *per se,* but they are useful in identifying other thoracic injuries to narrow the differential diagnosis.

Radionuclide imaging studies, including MUGA scans, technetium scans, thallium-201 myocardial scintigraphy, thallium-201 single proton emission CT (SPECT) scans, and antimyosin scintigraphy have never been demonstrated to be superior to the initial ED ECG and echocardiogram in diagnosing BCI, nor in predicting complications.[5,8,11,12]

EMERGENCY DEPARTMENT MANAGEMENT

The chance that a patient has a BCI in the face of a normal initial ECG and an injury severity score less than 10 is less than 1%. Even in the presence of BCI, young, hemodynamically stable patients with normal ECGs on admission after chest trauma are very unlikely to suffer complications. Intravenous fluids may help support the blood pressure by supplying preload to an injured right ventricle. External cardiopulmonary resuscitation (CPR) in the victim of arrest from cardiac trauma is likely to be ineffective. Standard antidysrhythmics should be used to treat life-threatening dysrhythmias. There are no data to support the use of prophylactic antidysrhythmics. Monitoring the ECG and CVP helps identify patients with developing tamponade. A CVP line should be placed early in the persistently hypotensive patient with a suspected cardiac injury. The patient in shock may benefit from pulmonary artery pressure monitoring to optimize fluid resuscitation. Patients who remain hemodynamically compromised after volume repletion may benefit from pressor support (dobutamine). The last option for refractory cardiogenic shock is the use of intraaortic balloon counterpulsation.

The prognosis for patients with BCI is most closely correlated with the severity and number of other injuries. In patients with suspected tamponade, pericardiocentesis may be diagnostic and may buy some time by stabilizing the patient before surgery. However, false-negative taps can mislead the clinician. Survivors of cardiac rupture are most commonly patients with atrial involvement who undergo early thoracotomy. Some centers advocate thoracotomy in the ED for patients who have had vital signs (palpable pulse or recorded blood pressure) present in the prehospital environment and then lost their vital signs, realizing that the neurologically intact survival rate in blunt trauma arrest is much lower than in penetrating trauma (2.5% vs. 7%).[2,3] Only 10% of blunt cardiac rupture patients require extracorporeal bypass. Rarely, blunt cardiac trauma can cause coronary thrombosis. The clinical picture is similar to that of acute myocardial infarction. The treatment would be similar except that the use of thrombolytics is contraindicated.

DISPOSITION

Role of the Consultant

Patients with significant blunt chest trauma benefit from evaluation by a trauma center team. A cardiothoracic surgeon should be consulted for suspected myocardial rupture, pericardial rupture, or valve rupture. An echocardiographer or cardiologist may be necessary to aid in heart imaging.

Indications for Admission

Patients with operable blunt trauma to the heart (cardiac rupture, valve rupture, tamponade) need early and aggressive surgical treatment. Because the prognosis of patients with BCI is related to the magnitude of the initial trauma, the preexisting condition of the heart, the size and location of the cardiac injury, and the patient's other injuries, patients who have coronary artery disease, hemodynamic compromise, significant dysrhythmias, a major mechanism of injury, or multiple trauma and suspected blunt cardiac trauma are best cared for in the intensive care unit. A young, healthy patient with no hemodynamic instability, a normal ECG free of significant dysrhythmias, and no other significant extracardiac trauma could be safely discharged after a 6- to 12-hour period of observation in the ED. Such a patient should be observed at home by a reliable adult, with instructions to return for increasing chest pain, lightheadedness, dizziness, syncope, or shortness of breath.

Transfer Considerations

If the patient with blunt cardiac trauma arrives at a hospital that is not equipped to care for the injury, the patient should be rapidly stabilized while arrangements for transfer are made. Stabilizing maneuvers may include endotracheal intubation and mechanical ventilation, volume resuscitation, initiation of transfusion, pressor support, tube thoracostomy, pericardiocentesis, central venous monitoring, and ECG monitoring. Monitoring should continue en route to the receiving facility, and the patient should be accompanied by paramedics (with or without a physician).

COMMON PITFALLS

- Paramedics should not delay transport while attempting stabilizing procedures; these should be accomplished en route if possible.
- Do not ascribe hypotension to cardiogenic shock from BCI with pump failure without a search for hypovolemia.
- Do not wait for Beck's triad to be evident.
- Do not lose sight of the patient's other serious injuries in the search for a BCI.
- Do not allow attempts at pericardiocentesis to delay or cancel definitive surgery in patients with suspected tamponade.
- Do not overlook tension pneumothorax as a more likely cause of high CVP shock.
- Do not forget the utility of blood transfusion, including uncrossmatched blood in the severely hypovolemic blunt cardiac trauma patient.

PENETRATING CARDIAC INJURIES

Wounds that penetrate the heart include stab wounds, gunshot wounds, impalement injuries, and industrial accidents. Most of these injuries are the result of interpersonal violence. Nearly 90% of the victims are male, 75% are between ages of 16 and 35, and the overall mortality of patients transported to the hospital exceeds 50%.[6,14] Wounds directly over the precordium and epigastrium (the "cardiac box") are more likely to involve cardiac injury than those from more posterior or lateral locations. Due to its location, the right ventricle is the chamber most often injured, followed in frequency by the left ventricle, the right atrium, and the left atrium.[6]

The pericardial sac normally contains 30 to 40 mL of fluid. The fibrous pericardium is only minimally distensible, so after an accumulation of 80 to 120 mL of fluid, the pressure within the pericardium rises. This raises end diastolic pressure, decreases diastolic filling, decreases coronary artery perfusion, and decreases stroke volume and cardiac output. As the pressure continues to rise, compensatory mechanisms fail (tachycardia, increased peripheral vascular resistance, and enhanced contractility), cardiac output drops, and hypotension results. Eighty percent to 90% of patients with stab wounds to the heart and 20% of patients with gunshot wounds to the heart develop tamponade. Up to 70% of these present with "early tamponade" and appear "clinically stable."[4] The presence of tamponade is associated with a greater chance of survival, presumably because the pericardium prevents rapid exsanguination from the cardiac wound. The patient with a waxing and waning clinical status may have an intermittently decompressing cardiac tamponade with the concomitant accumulating hemothorax.

CLINICAL PRESENTATION

Beck's triad of tamponade—hypotension, elevated JVP, and muffled heart sounds—is present in only about a third of patients with tamponade. Pulsus paradoxus, although present in up to one-third of patients with tamponade, is not pathognomonic for tamponade. Pulsus paradoxus is also present in chronic obstructive pulmonary disease, asthma, obesity, cardiac failure from many causes, constrictive pericarditis, pulmonary embolism, and cardiogenic shock. In the setting of a gunshot wound to the heart, loss of an extremity pulse or focal neurologic deficits should raise the question of arterial embolization of the bullet, pellet, or fragment. New murmurs or acute congestive heart failure after chest trauma should raise the suspicion of intraventricular septum, valve leaflet, or chordae tendineae injuries. Ventricular septal lacerations present with a pansystolic murmur auscultable over the entire precordium, especially at the left lower sternal border. This may not be appreciated, however, until the patient has been resuscitated to euvolemia.

DIFFERENTIAL DIAGNOSIS

The differential diagnosis of penetrating cardiac trauma includes simple pneumothorax, hemothorax, aortic injuries, extrathoracic hemorrhage, air embolism, and tracheal injuries. In the differential diagnosis of high CVP shock, tension pneumothorax is more common than tamponade.

EMERGENCY DEPARTMENT EVALUATION

The most common vital sign abnormality is sinus tachycardia. Bradycardia or pulseless electrical activity (PEA) is often a preterminal sign. Hypotension is a serious sign and should raise the possibility of cardiac tamponade, massive hemothorax from the cardiac wound, other noncardiac trauma with hypovolemia, or valve injury. Measuring the CVP early in the course of resuscitation will help differentiate tamponade (high CVP) from hypovolemia (low CVP) in the patient with systemic hypotension. However, the CVP may not be elevated in the severely hypovolemic patient in tamponade until a reasonable circulating volume has been restored.

Chest radiographs are not very helpful in diagnosing penetrating cardiac trauma *per se*, but they are useful in identifying other thoracic injuries associated with penetrating cardiac injuries. The radiograph may demonstrate a hemothorax, pneumothorax, pneumopericardium, or the offending missile(s). The blurry image of a bullet overlying the cardiac silhouette should raise the question of an intracardiac location and "movement artifact" on the film.

Echocardiography has several advantages in the evaluation of these patients. A noninvasive test that can be performed at the bedside, it can quickly give information about pericardial fluid collections, valve injuries, and septal lacerations. This test probably gives the most clinically relevant information and is indicated in the evaluation of the patient at risk for a penetrating cardiac injury who exhibits signs of hemodynamic instability: persistent tachycardia, hypotension, elevated pulsus paradoxus, elevated CVP, new heart murmurs, or significant dysrhythmias.[18,19]

EMERGENCY DEPARTMENT MANAGEMENT

As in blunt trauma, monitoring the ECG and CVP will help identify patients with developing tamponade. A CVP line should be placed early in the persistently hypotensive patient with a suspected cardiac injury. Intravenous fluids may help support the blood pressure by supplying preload to the injured right ventricle.

In patients with suspected tamponade, pericardiocentesis may be diagnostic and may buy some time by stabilizing the patient before surgery. However, false-negative taps can be misleading.

External CPR in the victim of arrest from cardiac trauma is likely to be ineffective. Thoracotomy in the ED is indicated for patients with penetrating trauma to the chest who have a rapidly deteriorating clinical course, uncontrolled hemorrhage, or cardiac arrest. Only 10% of penetrating cardiac trauma patients require extracorporeal bypass.[4]

The role of prophylactic antibiotics has never been proven, but they may be of some benefit. There is no consensus about an antibiotic regimen. The use of a pneumatic antishock garment is contraindicated.

DISPOSITION

Role of the Consultant

Patients with suspected or potential penetrating cardiac injury should have a trauma surgeon involved early during their care.

Indications for Admission

Patients who develop cardiac tamponade following penetrating injuries require surgical intervention. In addition to tamponade, the risk of rapid exsanguination accompanies these injuries. Patients with any potential for cardiac injury should be observed in a monitored setting where any deterioration can be quickly detected.

Patients in whom penetrating cardiac trauma can be ruled out are candidates for discharge. These include patients with low-energy trauma (stab wounds), with no hemodynamic instability, and with normal CVP, normal ECG, normal vital signs, and stable hematocrit (all monitored serially over 8 to 12 hours). They should have no hemothorax, no pneumothorax, and no evidence of other significant trauma.

Transfer Considerations

If a patient with penetrating cardiac trauma arrives at a hospital that is not equipped to care for this injury, the patient should be rapidly stabilized while arrangements for transfer are made. Stabilizing maneuvers may include endotracheal intubation and mechanical ventilation, volume resuscitation, initiation of transfusion, pressor support, thoracostomy, pericardiocentesis, central venous monitoring, and ECG monitoring. Monitoring should continue en route and the patient should be accompanied by paramedics (with or without a physician).

COMMON PITFALLS

- Expedient prehospital transport is vital. Paramedics should not delay at the scene while attempting to perform stabilizing procedures; these should be performed en route, if possible.
- Completely undress the patient and examine the entire body (including the back, buttocks, and axilla) to search for other injuries.
- Minor-appearing exterior wounds (such as from an ice pick) can cause serious cardiac wounds.
- Do not try to predict a bullet's trajectory within the body based on the external wounds.
- Do not wait for Beck's triad to develop.
- Do not allow attempts at pericardiocentesis to delay or cancel definitive surgery in patients with suspected tamponade.
- Do not overlook tension pneumothorax as a more likely cause of high CVP shock.
- Become familiar with the technique of ED thoracotomy.
- Do not forget the utility of blood transfusion, including the use of uncrossmatched blood, in the severely hypovolemic cardiac trauma patient.
- Remember tetanus prophylaxis.

References

1. Adams JE III, Davila-Roman VG, Bessey PQ, et al. Improved detection of cardiac contusion with cardiac troponin I. *Am Heart J* 1996;131:308.
2. Attar S, Suter CM, Hankins JR, et al. Penetrating cardiac injuries. *Ann Thorac Surg* 1991;51:711.
3. Branney SW, Moore EE, Feldhaus KM, et al. Critical analysis of two decades of experience with postinjury emergency department thoracotomy in a regional trauma center. *J Trauma* 1998;45(1):87–94; discussion 94.
4. Buchman TG, Phillips J, Menker JB. Recognition, resuscitation and management of patients with penetrating cardiac injuries. *Surg Gynecol Obstet* 1992;174:205.
5. Cachecho R, Grindlinger GA, Lee VW. The clinical significance of myocardial contusion. *J Trauma* 1992;33:68.
6. Campbell NC, Thomson SR, Muckart DJ, et al. Review of 1198 cases of penetrating cardiac trauma. *Br J Surg* 1997;84(12):1737.
7. Chiu WC, D'Amelio LF, Hammond JS. Sternal fractures in blunt chest trauma: a practical algorithm for management. *Am J Emerg Med* 1997;15(3):252.
8. Christensen MA, Sutton KR. Myocardial contusion: new concepts in diagnosis and management. *Am J Crit Care* 1993;2:28.
9. Dowd MD, Krug S. Pediatric blunt cardiac injury: epidemiology, clinical features, and diagnosis. Pediatric Emergency Medicine Collaborative Research Committee: Working Group on Blunt Cardiac Injury. *J Trauma* 1996;40(1):61.
10. Ferjani M, Droc G, Dreux S, et al. Circulating cardiac troponin T in myocardial contusion. *Chest* 1997;111(2):427.
11. Hendel RC, Cohn S, Aurigemma G, et al. Focal myocardial injury following blunt chest trauma: a comparison of indium-111 antimyosin scintigraphy with other noninvasive methods. *Am Heart J* 1992;123:1208.
12. Maenza RL, Seaberg D, D'Amico F. A meta-analysis of blunt cardiac trauma: ending myocardial confusion. *Am J Emerg Med* 1996;14(3):237.
13. Mattox KL, Flint LM, Carrico CJ, et al. Blunt cardiac injury [Editorial]. *J Trauma* 1992;33:649.
14. Mittal V, McAleese P, Young S, et al. Penetrating cardiac injuries. *Am Surg* 1999;65(5):444.
15. Olsovsky MR, Wechsler AS, Topaz O. Cardiac trauma. Diagnosis, management, and current therapy. *Angiology* 1997;48(5):423.
16. Pasquale MD, Nagy K, Clarke J. *Practice management guidelines for screening of blunt cardiac injury*. EAST Practice Parameter Workgroup for Screening of Blunt Cardiac Injury, 1998; http://east.org/tpg/chap2body.html/
17. Powell MA, Lucente FC. Diagnosis and treatment of blunt cardiac rupture. *W V Med J* 1997;93(2):64.
18. Rozycki GS, Feliciano DV, Ochsner MG, et al. The role of ultrasound in patients with possible penetrating cardiac wounds: a prospective multicenter study. *J Trauma* 1999;46(4):543–551; discussion 551.
19. Weiss RL, Brier JA, O'Connor W, et al. The usefulness of transesophageal echocardiography in diagnosing cardiac contusions. *Chest* 1996;109(1):73.

CHAPTER 104
Great Vessel Injuries

Daniel S. Gabbay and Patrick M. Reilly

Vesalius first described great vessel injury in 1557, but today great vessel injuries are most commonly caused by rapid and sudden deceleration in the setting of a motor vehicle crash (MVC).[10] Typically, these injuries involve the aorta, but deceleration injuries to the brachiocephalic artery and inferior vena cava (IVC) have also been reported.[24,31] Nearly 15% of automobile fatalities, accounting for approximately 7,500 deaths yearly, occur secondary to traumatic disruption of the aorta.[14] Penetrating injury to the thoracic great vessels is less common, with an overall incidence of 4%.[8]

Disruption of a great vessel usually portends a poor outcome. The seminal work of Parmley and coworkers[20] in 1958 demonstrated that 80% of these patients exsanguinate quickly and do not survive to hospital admission. Weiman et al. confirmed this bleak statistic, reporting that most patients with major injuries of the thoracic outlet die of massive hemorrhage before they reach the hospital.[31] In 1961, Ochsner et al.[17] reported that 36% of patients sustaining IVC injuries would not survive to hospitalization. More recently, Rosengart and coworkers[24] also recorded a significant mortality from blunt IVC trauma.

Those who suffer from penetrating trauma often fare no better. With the exception of select patients who are fortunate enough to have small, contained penetrations or arteriovenous, fistulous communications, which favor hemodynamic stability, the literature is replete with studies demonstrating a poor outcome after penetrating thoracic aorta or subclavian injuries.[8] The subclavian vessels are the most commonly injured thoracic great vessels, with an overall incidence of 3.3% in patients with penetrating chest trauma. Venous injuries have a worse prognosis than arterial injuries, most probably due to air embolism or the inability of veins to contract to control exsanguination.[8]

Even with the advent of sophisticated prehospital and trauma systems, the early mortality of great vessel injury remains largely unchanged.[6,17] Victims of blunt aortic injury (BAI) who arrive hypotensive (systolic blood pressure less than 90 mm Hg), with an age greater than 55, have still been consistently shown to experience a bad outcome in great vessel injury.[10,17,18] Of the initial survivors of BAI, 30% die within 6 hours of presentation, and a further 20% will not live beyond 24 hours, should there be a significant delay in diagnosis or definitive repair.[12]

Demetriades[8] suggested that in patients with significant vascular injury, any delays of advanced life support on the scene may actually increase mortality. In penetrating torso injuries, Bickell et al.[3] similarly posited that some degree of hypotension may be protective by compensatorily serving to reduce bleeding. These authors implied that prehospital fluid resuscitation might have paradoxically led to a significantly higher mortality and longer hospitalization.

The recent literature is somewhat contradictory regarding mortality differences in BAI patients with delayed transport times, but differences between survivors and nonsurvivors do not appear to be related to the time between diagnosis and subsequent thoracotomy.[10,18] Similarly, Ochsner et al.[17] reported that time from admission to surgical intervention in the setting of IVC injury did not significantly differ between survivors and fatalities.[17] Burch et al. reported an increase in in-hospital mortality from IVC injuries; it was postulated that as more critically ill patients have survived to admission because of decreased emergency medical service transport times, the occurrence of preoperative shock, resuscitative thoracotomy, and death has subsequently increased.[17]

PATHOPHYSIOLOGY

Disruption of a great vessel is usually seen in high-speed motor vehicle or airplane crashes, falls from height, or crushing chest injury. Several mechanisms have been postulated to explain BAI. Foremost, rapid horizontal or vertical deceleration produces shearing forces at the aortic isthmus (the weakest and most susceptible portion of the aorta) just distal to the origin of the left subclavian artery, where the aorta changes from relatively mobility to a relatively fixed structure (Fig. 104.1).[2] Although the aorta may withstand intraluminal pressures of up to 350 mm Hg, this pressure may be surpassed in a high-speed MVC; a burst or "water-hammer" effect directly compresses the aorta and propagates a pressure wave, which can lead to aortic injury.[9,19] A direct shearing force secondary to vertebral fractures; a bending stress caused by chest compression, with subsequent flexion of the arch across the left lung hilum; or entrapment of the thoracic vasculature between the anterior chest wall and the thoracic spine have also been implicated in great vessel injury.[10,19]

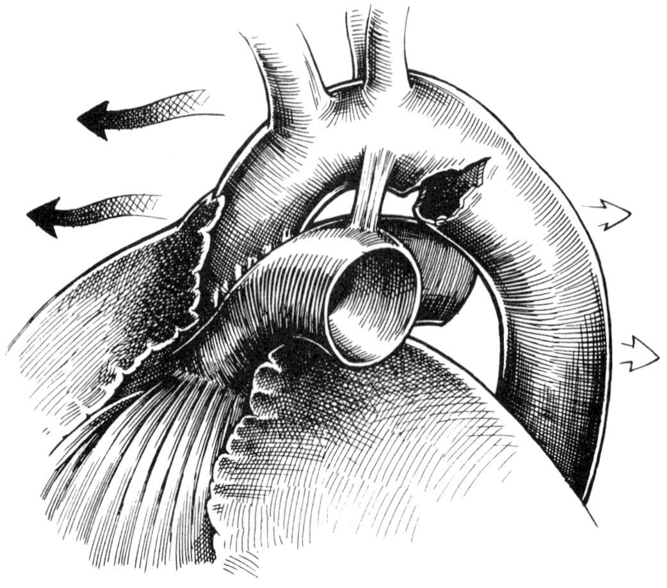

Figure 104.1. Rapid decelerative injury causing a tear in the thoracic aorta. The ascending (anterior) aorta tends to continue moving forward, while the more fixed descending aorta is held stationary. The rupture occurs just distal to the ligamentum arteriosum at the level of the isthmus.

In 70% to 90% of cases, the classic site of rupture is just distal to the left subclavian artery at the site of the ligamentum arteriosum.[7] Anatomically, this can be explained by the fact that the descending aorta is tethered by the ligamentum arteriosum and the intercostal arteries. The ascending aorta is relatively mobile, and, during deceleration, continues to move forward while the descending aorta is held in place. In seatbelted motor vehicle occupants, descending thoracic aortic tears are more common, while ascending aortic disruption tends to be seen more often in unrestrained drivers.[10]

The tear usually involves the anteromedial border of the aorta and is almost exclusively a circumferential transverse laceration that disrupts the physical integrity of one or more structural layers of the aorta.[19] If complete, a tear usually results in transmural extension and death due to immediate exsanguination. In survivors, the adventitia remains intact and blood is contained by a false aneurysm formed by the adventitia and surrounding mediastinal tissues. An overall mortality of 5.4% has been reported for this group.[18] If surgical or medical therapy is not initiated, mortality is 66% at 2 weeks and 98% 4 months after the injury.

Concomitant aortic branch vessel injuries occur in 4% to 10% of cases.[9,14,19] Brachiocephalic injuries, including complete avulsion from the aortic arch, probably result from the decreased space between the sternum and vertebral bodies.[31] This decrease in space causes the heart to shift to the left and posteriorly, with an increase in tension on the thoracic outlet vessels.

CLINICAL PRESENTATION

In penetrating trauma, physical findings are not insidious. Usually, there is overt bleeding from a visible wound, a massive hemothorax, or continuous bleeding from a thoracostomy tube. In the proper context, an absent or diminished pulse in the arm represents subclavian artery injury, while the presence of a murmur or bruit suggests an aneurysm or arteriovenous fistula.

In the setting of blunt trauma, diagnosis is more difficult and historic features suggestive of a major decelerative mechanism should be sought. Such characteristics are usually seen in victims of an MVC (with speeds greater than 30 mi/h), but may also be present in patients who have fallen from a height (generally greater than 10 ft) or have been struck by an automobile. Prehospital personnel may be able to provide indirect evidence of deceleration by noting the lack of restraint system use and the presence of steering wheel or dashboard damage.

Unfortunately, symptoms of traumatic great vessel injury are often absent or masked by coexisting injuries.[28] The most frequently recorded complaints are chest pain (26%), dyspnea (25% to 30%), and back pain (14%). Other symptoms include dysphagia, hoarseness, and ischemic pain of the extremities. Interestingly, half of the deaths after brachiocephalic and carotid artery injury were attributed to ischemic cerebral infarction. The neurologic and clinical symptomatology attendant with such pathophysiology may also be seen.[31]

Physical examination may reveal ecchymosis, abrasion, or tenderness of the anterior chest consistent with impact of this area on the steering wheel. Thirty-one percent of patients with an aortic disruption present with pseudocoarctation syndrome. In these cases, upper extremity hypertension is present, with decreased or absent femoral pulses. This may be due to compression of the aortic lumen by surrounding periaortic hematoma. Reflex stimulation by stretching of cardiac sympathetic fibers at the aortic isthmus may account for the observation that 72% of patients with an aortic rupture manifest a relative hypertension (average blood pressure, 152/98). A harsh systolic murmur over the precordium or interscapular area (thought to be due to turbulent flow across the area of transection) is present in 26% of cases.[14]

Less common signs include a diminished left radial pulse, transient anuria, and paraplegia. Some authors have reported swelling at the base of the neck, resulting from extravasation of blood from the mediastinum; however, this finding has not been confirmed clinically in antemortem studies.

Despite the severe nature of traumatic aortic injury, one-third to one-half of patients have no external evidence of chest injury on presentation to the emergency department. Furthermore, many patients have associated central nervous system, abdominal, or bony injuries that may distract the physician from considering great vessel injury promptly. Most often, the presence of great vessel injury cannot be confirmed or ruled out on the basis of physical examination in patients suffering blunt trauma.[1,14]

DIFFERENTIAL DIAGNOSIS

Ninety percent of patients who suffer from blunt thoracic aortic injury have coexisting lethal injuries. A high index of suspicion must be maintained to detect any of the host of possible injuries, including soft-tissue damage; clavicle, sternum, or rib fractures; hemothoraces or pneumothoraces; tracheobronchial injuries; diaphragmatic rupture; esophageal perforation; pericardial tamponade; coronary artery injury; or myocardial contusion or rupture.[19] Concomitant abdominal, orthopedic, and neurotraumatic injuries often are found. A higher Injury Severity Score has consistently been reported in nonsurvivors versus survivors.[10]

EMERGENCY DEPARTMENT DIAGNOSIS

Chest Radiography

Although a normal initial chest radiograph has been reported in 7% to 28% of cases,[10] an upright chest radiograph remains the investigative method of choice for screening for BAI in patients with an appropriate mechanism of injury.[5,11,14] In penetrating trauma, the chest radiograph may be helpful in identifying missiles or fragments, hemothorax, lung contusions, fractures, or mediastinal hematomas.[8] Ideally, this study is obtained as an upright posteroanterior chest radiograph, but the traumatized patient is often immobilized and cannot sit or stand for such a radiograph. Portable supine anteroposterior radiographs can be obtained in the emergency department, but technical differences between these two techniques make the radiographic features of traumatic aortic rupture more difficult to interpret.

TABLE 104.1. Radiographic Features of Great Vessel Injury

Widening of the superior mediastinum at the level of the aortic knob in an upright radiograph
Mediastinal width–chest width ratio of more than 0.25
Deviation of the trachea or endotracheal tube to the right
Deviation of the nasogastric tube (representing the esophagus) to the right
Narrowing of the carinal angle
Depression of the left mainstem bronchus
Irregularity of the aortic knob contour
Left apical cap
Opacification of a clear space between the aorta and pulmonary artery ("aortic pulmonary window")
Widening of the left or right paraspinous stripe
Hemothorax, sternum or rib fractures

Despite the many radiographic signs of traumatic aortic injury (Table 104.1, Fig. 104.2), no single radiographic criterion is diagnostic or can rule out the injury. A widened mediastinum has received the most attention of these radiographic criteria in the literature, but in 6% of cases it may develop late or not at all. Moreover, vertebral fracture or increased aortic tortuosity associated with age may produce mediastinal widening, making it a sensitive but nonspecific indicator of aortic rupture.[5,11,22,32]

Traditionally, great vessel injury has been thought to be associated with first or second rib fractures, given the close anatomic relation. However, several studies have shown that vascular injury does not correlate with the anatomic location or degree of displacement of rib fractures, although multiple rib fractures were more prevalent in the aortic injury group.[12,13] It has also been postulated that blood or fluid in a widened mediastinum secondary to acute traumatic aortic injury might track up into the neck and cause cervical prevertebral soft-tissue swelling. However, cervical soft-tissue swelling at the level of C3 and C6 did not correlate well with mediastinal width–chest width ratios and seems to be a poor marker of aortic injury.[21]

Despite these shortcomings, a chest radiograph interpreted in the proper clinical context can still form an effective strategy to screen for great vessel injury. Patients with a significant mechanism of injury or abnormalities on the chest radiograph mandate further study. However, in those patients in whom there is a low pretest probability of BAI, the upright chest radiograph has been shown to have a negative predictive value of 98%, making further investigation unnecessary.[19]

Computed Tomography

In the past, when the possibility of great vessel injury mandated additional study, aortography was clearly the procedure of choice. However, 80% to 92% of patients with blunt chest trauma who are triaged to angiography because of the mechanism of injury, clinical suspicion, and an abnormal chest radiograph will not have an aortic or brachiocephalic injury.[19] Consequently, this approach has undergone review since dynamic computed tomography (CT) scanning of the chest has become an option for the diagnosis of aortic rupture (Fig. 104.3).

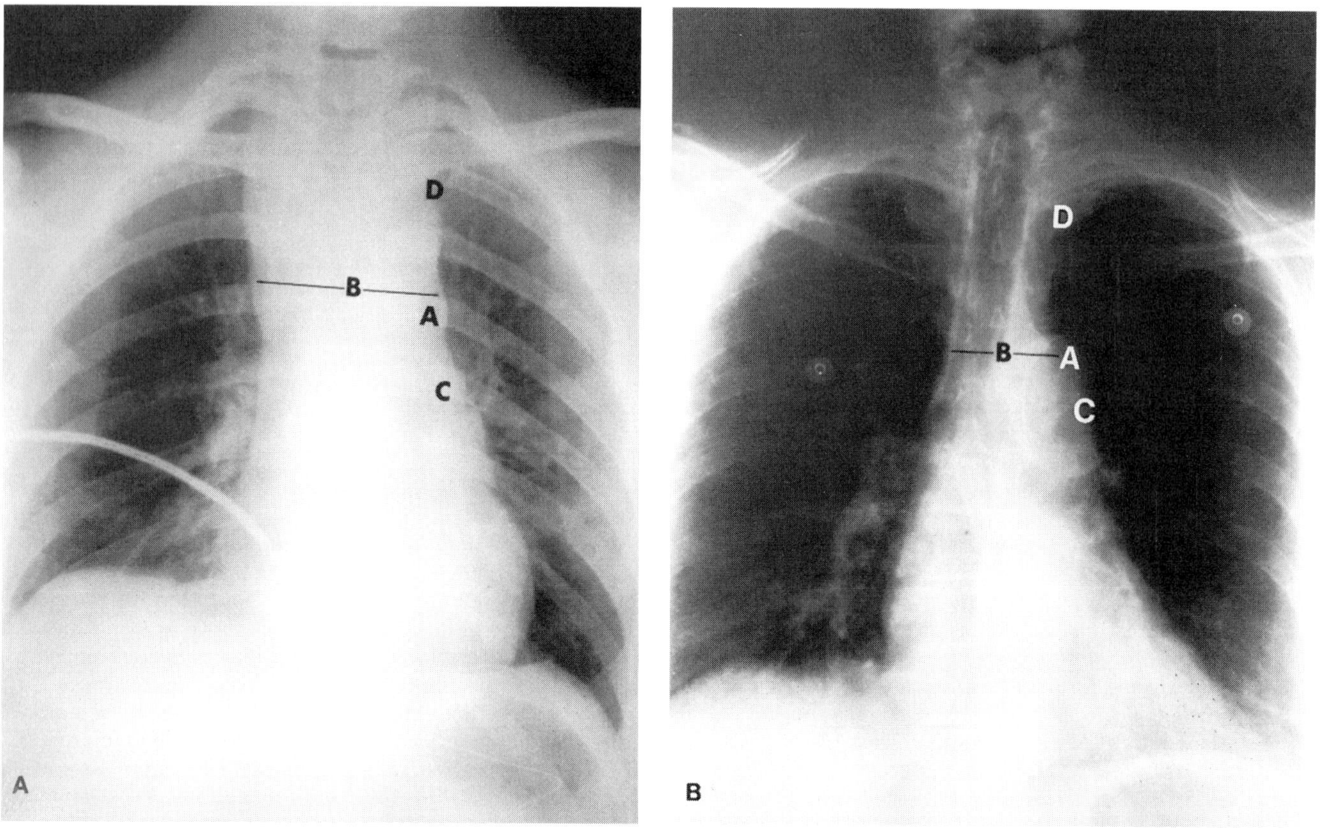

Figure 104.2. Upright posteroanterior chest radiographs of a 20-year-old man involved as a driver in a head-on motor vehicle accident **(A)** compared with that of a normal person **(B).** The first radiograph has several abnormalities suggestive of a great vessel disruption. *(A)* Loss of detail of aortic knob with blurring of the aortic outline. *(B)* Widened mediastinum (mediastinal width–chest width ratio greater than 0.28). *(C)* Opacification of the clear space between the aorta and pulmonary artery (aortopulmonary window). *(D)* Obliteration of the medial aspect of the left upper field. The aortogram revealed rupture of the aortic arch. (Radiographs courtesy of the Department of Radiology, St. Luke's Hospital, Milwaukee, Wisconsin.)

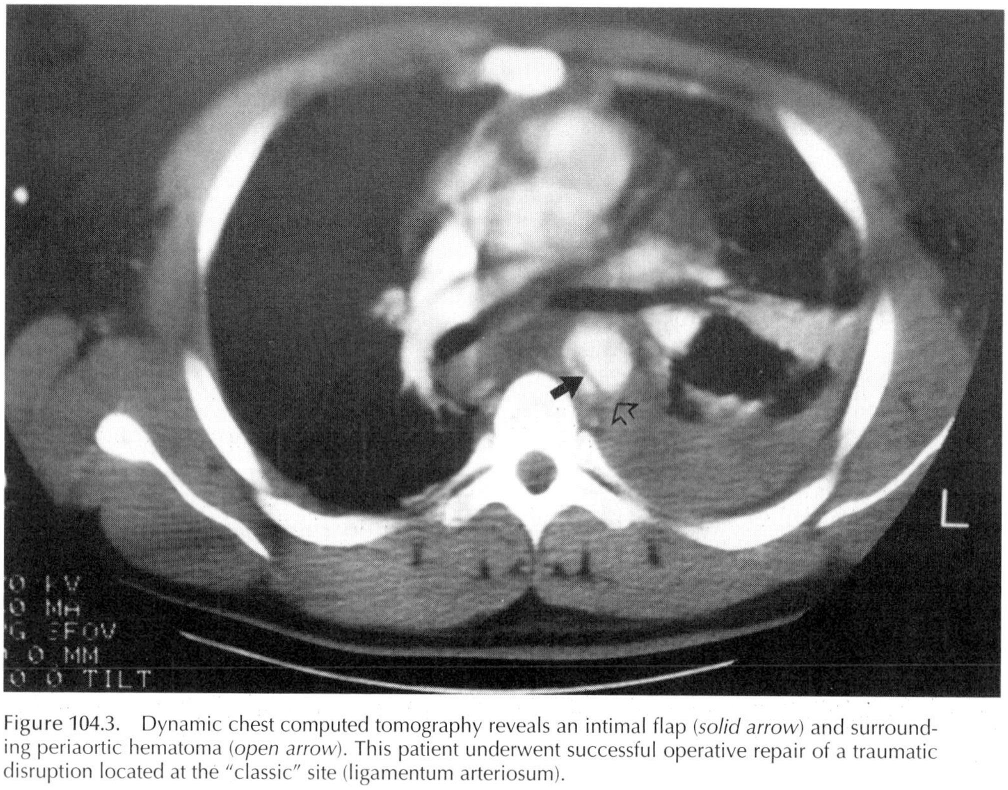

Figure 104.3. Dynamic chest computed tomography reveals an intimal flap (*solid arrow*) and surrounding periaortic hematoma (*open arrow*). This patient underwent successful operative repair of a traumatic disruption located at the "classic" site (ligamentum arteriosum).

CT scanning is noninvasive, requires less time for completion than aortography, and may actually be more cost effective than chest radiography for screening hemodynamically stable patients with blunt trauma.[19] There is also the added benefit of ruling out associated head and abdominal injuries without moving the patient from the CT table.

On the CT scan, positive criteria for the diagnosis of BAI include periaortic hematoma, an irregular aortic contour, change in caliber of the aorta, and intraluminal irregularity (intimal flap).[1] In some studies, mediastinal hemorrhage has not been shown to be as specific a finding as periaortic hematoma. However, when intravenous contrast was utilized in those patients with an equivocal or indeterminate screening chest radiograph, Patel et al.[19] found that mediastinal hematoma, as an indirect CT sign of BAI, had a sensitivity of 100%, was 87% specific, and had a negative predictive value of 100%.

When chest CT was performed without the use of intravenous contrast material, Harris and coworkers prevented unnecessary aortography in 63 of 100 patients with blunt trauma in whom equivocal or indeterminate screening radiographs were obtained.[19] On the basis of clinical outcome, no cases of acute traumatic aortic injury were missed and only six (17%) of the remaining 36 patients who had aortography performed were found to have significant injury.

Transesophageal Echocardiography

In the unstable, severely traumatized patient with an equivocal or indeterminate chest radiograph, transesophageal echocardiography (TEE) provides mobile, real-time imaging of the heart, thoracic aorta, and mediastinum and may offer an alternative to aortography. In at least one study, color flow Doppler has also been shown to be a reliable investigation in the evaluation of neck vessels, including the subclavian artery and vein.[8]

Technically, TEE is performed in a manner similar to flexible endoscopy of the esophagus. Because of the probe's close proximity to the thoracic vasculature, good visualization of both aortic wall disruptions and intimal irregularities such as intimal flaps is facilitated. While TEE shows the area of the ligamentum arteriosum well, it often does not visualize the proximal aortic branches adequately.

TEE findings of mediastinal hematoma include a distance of more than 3 mm between the probe and the aortic wall, a double contour of the aortic wall, or an "ultrasound signal" between the aortic wall and visceral pleura. LeBret et al. found that a distance of more than 3 mm between the probe and the aortic wall was the most accurate of these ultrasonographic signs.[19]

There have been several studies specifically evaluating the accuracy of TEE with respect to traumatic aortic injury.[12,25,26] The largest involved 69 patients (nine true positive) and showed 100% accuracy.[12] More recently, sensitivity and specificity for detecting mediastinal hematoma via TEE of 100% and 75%, respectively, with no false-negative results, were reported.[19] It is unclear, however, how many of these patients would have required operative intervention.

Most awake patients who undergo TEE require sedation to tolerate the examination.[12] Sedation may be problematic, because many multiple trauma patients are prone to hemodynamic instability and may have an increased risk of aspiration without airway protection. In addition, some intubated patients need to have the endotracheal tube cuff deflated so the echocardiography probe may pass; this again increases the risk of aspiration. In centers where TEE is available, its best application may be for patients in whom there is concern for great vessel injury, who are unstable, and who require immediate operative intervention for other life-threatening injuries (e.g., hemoperitoneum). In a situation like this, TEE can be performed intraoperatively to provide a rapid evaluation of the aorta.

Aortography

Irrespective of these other emerging diagnostic modalities, aortography remains the gold standard for depicting the extent of blunt or penetrating thoracic vascular injury.[8,11,19] With a complication rate of less than 1% in transfemoral examination, aortography has been consistently shown in the literature to have a sensitivity approaching 100% and a specificity of nearly 98%. This is largely because it is the only imaging modality that allows complete evaluation of the thoracic aorta from the aortic root to the diaphragmatic hiatus and the brachiocephalic arteries and their branches.[19] This need to accurately visualize the thoracic vasculature is critically important, because multiple disruptions occur in 18% to 20% of cases.[7]

Classically, findings of aortic intimal injury consist of an intimal irregularity, a linear defect, or a filling defect caused by an intimal flap. False-positive interpretations of atypical or equivocal aortographic findings for acute traumatic aortic injury have been attributed to congenital abnormalities such as a ductus diverticulum, anatomic variants, atheromatous plaques, syphilitic aortic aneurysms, or motion artifact.[19,23,27] There have been reports of CT and TEE demonstrating small aortic intimal tears not seen on angiography, but the need for surgical intervention for these tears is controversial.

Major trauma centers may perform several negative investigations to diagnose all aortic disruptions. Most strategies would use chest radiography and dynamic chest CT scanning as initial screening examinations, followed by aortography or TEE as definitive studies. In transmediastinal penetrating injuries, esophagography should be performed in stable patients prior to aortography because of the greater likelihood of esophageal injury in this setting.[8]

EMERGENCY DEPARTMENT MANAGEMENT

The role of the emergency department thoracotomy (EDT) has been questioned in recent years, in terms of both its overall efficacy and its potential risk of exposing hospital personnel to bloodborne pathogens. In a recent retrospective study involving 950 patients and spanning 23 years at a level I trauma center, a 2.5% neurologically intact survival rate was reported for blunt traumatic arrest when vital signs were present in the field.[4] Conversely, the literature is replete with data showing that patients who have sustained a blunt mechanism of injury, are without vital signs in the field, and demonstrate asystole on arrival should not receive an EDT.[4] Thus, blunt trauma should not be considered an absolute contraindication to the performance of EDT if the patient had vital signs at the time of initial paramedic contact.

In the setting of penetrating trauma, the EDT may be warranted for those patients who had vital signs in the field (regardless of cardiac rhythm on emergency department presentation) with a total prehospital time of 30 minutes or less.[4,16] Indeed, Branney and coworkers[4] reported a 16.4% survival rate for penetrating trauma victims with field vital signs. Most interestingly, they also reported a 3.6% survival rate for patients without field vital signs who accounted for 26.5% of the neurologically intact survivors. Four of these patients presented in asystole and went on to have functional survival. They attributed this remarkable statistic to relatively short transport times and on-scene times. Drawing from these data, it would be reasonable to terminate resuscitative efforts in those patients who present in asystole unless there is clinical evidence of penetrating thoracic trauma.

In the presence of a penetrating supraclavicular wound, balloon tamponade using one or two Foley catheters may be effective in controlling the bleeding until surgical control is achieved in the operating room. By inserting the catheter as far as it can go and then inflating the balloon, the physician may be able to compress the subclavian vessels against the clavicle and the first rib, helping to achieve hemostasis. For persistent bleeding, a second catheter may be inserted and the balloon inflated inside the wound tract superficial to the first balloon.[8]

The role for medical management of great vessel injury in the emergency department setting is rather limited, but in the recent literature this possibility, coupled with delayed surgical repair, has been raised. The use of beta-blocking and antihypertensive agents is integral to this management option and is frequently used in the subset of patients in whom there exists severe comorbid disease or other significant traumatic injuries. The decision to embark on nonoperative management should be made in consultation with the trauma or vascular surgeon. The use of magnetic resonance imaging is an emerging modality and may have an ideal role in monitoring these patients prior to surgical repair.[19]

As systemic hypertension may increase stress on any pseudoaneurysm that may be present and promote rupture, blood pressure and wall tension must be carefully controlled. This may best be done by initial use of a beta blocker such as propranolol, which reduces stress forces to the aortic wall.[18,30] Nitroprusside or other pure vasodilators may then be used to reduce the blood pressure appropriately. Hypotension usually indicates hemorrhage and should be managed with volume replacement and rapid transport to the operating room for definitive repair.[14]

DISPOSITION

Traumatic circumferential disruption of the great vessels is a surgical emergency; as soon as the diagnosis is suspected, a surgeon competent in vascular repair should be consulted while definitive investigations are being obtained. If appropriate personnel or technology, either to confirm the diagnosis or to definitively manage the injury, are unavailable, preparations for transfer must be made immediately.[29]

Methods of repair and operative intervention are beyond the scope of this text, but even in the best of circumstances, significant morbidity (including chronic thoracic aneurysm, renal failure, and paraplegia) and mortality (15% to 33%) are reported at major trauma centers.[7,15,29] The in-hospital surgical mortality rate is largely contingent on the degree of hemodynamic instability, the severity of associated injuries, and the magnitude of the aortic laceration.

COMMON PITFALLS

- Failing to pursue the diagnosis in a patient with a major mechanism of injury and a normal chest radiograph
- Delaying aggressive radiologic confirmation of the diagnosis
- Allowing more obvious injuries to delay pursuit of or obscure the diagnosis
- Failing to transfer the patient promptly to an appropriate trauma center if facilities and personnel necessary to diagnose or treat the patient are unavailable at the initial facility.

ACKNOWLEDGMENT

The authors gratefully acknowledge the contribution of Jedd Roe, MD, who wrote the previous version of this chapter.

References

1. Agee CK, Metzler MH, et al. Computed tomographic evaluation to exclude traumatic aortic disruption. *J Trauma* 1992;33:876.
2. BenMenachem Y. Rupture of the thoracic aorta by broadside impacts in road traffic and other collisions: further angiographic observations and preliminary autopsy findings. *J Trauma* 1993;35:363.
3. Bickell WH, Wall MJ, Pepe PE, et al. Immediate versus delayed fluid resuscitation for hypotensive patients with penetrating torso injuries. *N Engl J Med* 1994;331:1105–1109.
4. Branney SW, Moore EE, Feldhaus KM, et al. Critical analysis of two decades of experience with postinjury emergency department thoracotomy in a regional trauma center. *J Trauma* 1998;45(1):87–95.
5. Burney RE, Gundry SR, et al. Chest roentgenograms in diagnosis of traumatic rupture of the aorta. *Chest* 1984;84:605.
6. Camp PC, Shackford SR. Outcome after blunt traumatic thoracic aortic laceration: identification of a high risk cohort. *J Trauma* 1997;43(3):413–422.
7. Cernaianu AC, Cilley JH Jr, et al. Determinants of outcome in lesions of the thoracic aorta in patients with multiorgan system trauma. *Chest* 1992;101:331.
8. Demetriades D. Penetrating injuries to thoracic great vessels. *J Card Surg* 1997;12[Suppl]:173–180.
9. Feczko JD, Lynch L, et al. An autopsy case review of 142 nonpenetrating (blunt) injuries of the aorta. *J Trauma* 1992;33:846.
10. Frick E, Cipolle MD, Pasquale MD, et al. Outcome of blunt thoracic aortic injury in a level I trauma center: an 8-year review. *J Trauma* 1997;43(5):844–851.
11. Hunt MD, Schwab FJ. Chest trauma. In: Rosen P, Doris PE, et al., eds. *Diagnostic radiology in emergency medicine*. St. Louis: Mosby–Year Book, 1992.
12. Kearney PA, Smith W, et al. Use of transesophageal echocardiography in the evaluation of traumatic aortic injury. *J Trauma* 1993;34:696.
13. Livoni JP, Barcia TC. Fracture of the first and second rib: incidence of vascular injury relative to type of fracture. *Radiology* 1982;145:31.
14. Markovchick V, Duffens KR. Vascular and cardiac trauma. In: Rosen P, ed. *Emergency medicine concepts and clinical practice*. St. Louis: Mosby–Year Book, 1992.
15. Merrill WH, Lee RB, et al. Surgical treatment of acute traumatic tear of the thoracic aorta. *Ann Surg* 1988;207:699.
16. Mezghebe E. Is 30 minutes the golden period to perform emergency room thoracotomy (ERT) in penetrating chest injuries? *J Cardiovasc Surg* 1999;40: 147–151.
17. Ochsner JL, Crawford ES, DeBakey ME. Injuries of the vena cava caused by external trauma. *Surgery* 1961;49:397.
18. Pate JW, Fabian TC, Walker W. Traumatic rupture of the aortic isthmus: an emergency? *World J Surg* 1995;19:119.
19. Patel NH, Stephens KE, Mirvis SE, et al. Imaging of acute thoracic aortic injury due to blunt trauma: a review. *Radiology* 1998;209(2):335–348.
20. Parmley LF, Mattingly TW, Manion WC, et al. Nonpenetrating traumatic injury of the aorta. *Circulation* 1958;17:1086.
21. Plewa MC, Stavros M, Boorstein JM, et al. Cervical prevertebral soft-tissue measurements and chest radiographic findings in acute traumatic aortic injury. *Am J Emerg Med* 1997;15(3):256–259.
22. Raptopoulos V, Sheiman RG, et al. Traumatic aortic tear: screening with chest CT. *Radiology* 1992;182:667.
23. Rose SC, Moore EE. Angiographic artifacts that simulate arterial pathology in acute trauma. *Am J Emerg Med* 1990;8:109.
24. Rosengart MR, Smith DR, Melton SM, et al. Prognostic factors in patients with inferior vena cava injuries. *Am Surg* 1999;65(9):849–856.
25. Shapiro MJ, Yanofsky SD, et al. Cardiovascular evaluation in blunt thoracic trauma using transesophageal echocardiography (TEE). *J Trauma* 1991;31:835.
26. Sparks MB, Burchard KW, et al. Transesophageal echocardiography: preliminary results in patients with traumatic aortic rupture. *Arch Surg* 1991;126:711.
27. Sturm JT, Hankins DG, et al. Thoracic aortography following blunt chest trauma. *Am J Emerg Med* 1990;8:92.
28. Sturm JT, McGee MB, et al. An analysis of risk factors for death at the scene following traumatic aortic rupture. *J Trauma* 1988;28:1578.
29. Townsend RN, Colella JJ, et al. Traumatic rupture of the aorta—critical decisions for trauma surgeons. *J Trauma* 1990;30:1169.
30. Warren RL, Akins CW, et al. Acute traumatic disruption of the thoracic aorta: emergency department management. *Ann Emerg Med* 1992;21:391.
31. Weiman DS, McCoy DW, Haan CK, et al. Blunt injuries of the brachiocephalic artery. *Am Surg* 1998;64(5):383–387.
32. Woodring JH, King JG. Determination of normal transverse mediastinal width and mediastinal-width to chest-width (M/C) ratio in control subjects: implications for subjects with aortic or brachiocephalic arterial injury. *J Trauma* 1989;29:1268.

CHAPTER 105
Bony Thorax and Diaphragm Injuries

Vincent J. Markovchick and Joanne Edney

DIAPHRAGM

Traumatic injury of the diaphragm may result from either penetrating or blunt trauma to the chest or abdomen. The absence of distinct symptoms, combined with the high incidence of serious and more obvious associated injuries, may lead the physician to overlook these injuries. However, missed diaphragmatic injuries may lead to devastating sequelae acutely or years later.[4,19,20]

Traumatic diaphragmatic injuries were first described by Sennertus in 1541, when he reported a delayed visceral herniation through a ruptured diaphragm. In 1853, Bowditch published the first antemortem diagnosis of a diaphragmatic hernia. The first surgical repair was in 1886 by Riolfi.[11,14]

There are no reliable data to suggest the true incidence of this entity, because many cases go undiagnosed. However, it is estimated that diaphragmatic injuries are present in 3.0% to 5.8% of patients who undergo emergency surgery for thoracoabdominal trauma. The relative frequency of blunt versus penetrating injuries varies greatly with published reports.

Stab and gunshot wounds may affect any portion of the diaphragm, but there is a higher incidence of stab wounds to the left hemidiaphragm, theoretically because of the greater number of right-handed assailants. Blunt trauma also has a predilection for the left hemidiaphragm, because the right hemidiaphragm is partially protected by the liver,[11,16,21] and because the posterolateral portion of the left leaflet is structurally the weakest portion of the diaphragm. Figure 105.1 shows the relative position of the diaphragm with inspiration and expiration.

Blunt trauma typically produces defects greater than 10 cm on the average, and penetrating trauma an average of less than 2 cm. Blunt injuries have a higher mortality rate, directly related to the higher incidence of serious associated injuries.

Ruptures of the diaphragm, regardless of size, are unlikely to heal spontaneously because of the pleuroperitoneal pressure gradient. During quiet respirations, this is normally 7 to 20 cm H_2O, but it may increase to more than 100 cm H_2O during labored respirations. These pressure differentials inhibit or prevent the normal healing process.[13] In addition, this negative pressure causes inherniation of intraabdominal contents into the thoracic cavity and may result in subsequent strangulation of the abdominal viscera as well as respiratory embarrassment. The stomach is the abdominal structure that herniates most often, followed by the spleen, colon, small bowel, and omentum in variable order.[14,16]

CLINICAL PRESENTATION

Diaphragmatic injuries should be suspected with any penetrating wound between the lower chest and upper abdomen. Significant blunt trauma to the lower chest and upper abdomen is associated with diaphragmatic rupture, usually on the left side.

The signs and symptoms are highly variable, depending on the size of the defect, the mechanism, the viscus that is herniated, and the degree of cardiopulmonary compromise. Common symptoms include cough, dyspnea, nonspecific chest or abdominal pain radiating to the shoulder, and the perception of peristalsis in the chest. Signs include an immobile left hemithorax, decreased breath sounds, and tympany or borborygmi in the left chest. However, in the absence of herniation, a diaphragmatic tear may be completely asymptomatic and without overt signs.

Abdominal viscera may herniate into the thoracic cavity and dilate rapidly, resulting in severe respiratory distress. This condition may be difficult to distinguish from a tension pneumothorax. Therefore, great care should be taken when performing a thoracostomy, always verifying a free pleural space before inserting the chest tube. Intrapericardial rupture of the diaphragm (a rare entity) with herniation may result in a tamponade from compression by the herniating viscus.[11]

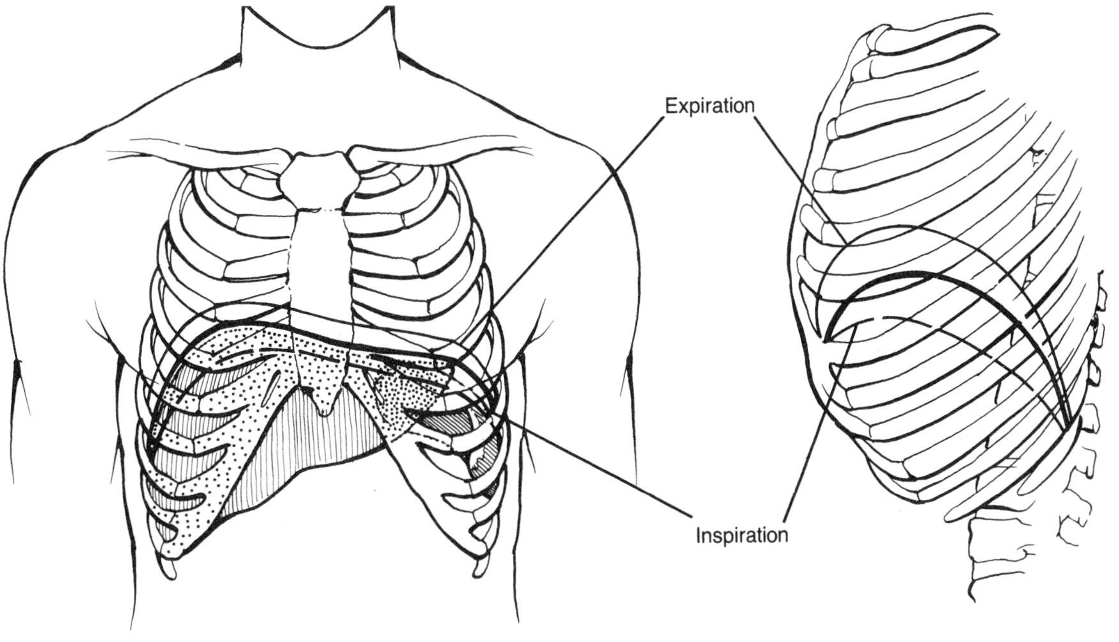

Figure 105.1. Location of the diaphragm with inspiration and expiration.

Delayed herniation has been reported in the immediate posttraumatic phase or as long as 40 years after the initial diaphragmatic injury. Delayed presentation is associated with a mortality as high as 20% after visceral incarceration, increasing to 80% after strangulation occurs. This occurs most commonly following unrecognized stab wounds to the diaphragm.

EMERGENCY DEPARTMENT EVALUATION

Serial examinations looking for signs of obstruction, strangulation, or cardiopulmonary compromise are performed. The chest radiograph is the single most important diagnostic tool. Although it is frequently nonspecific, the chest radiograph often arouses the initial suspicion of diaphragmatic disruption. Significant findings include lower rib fractures, pleural effusion, and a unilaterally elevated hemidiaphragm or difficulty in visualizing the hemidiaphragm. If herniation has occurred, one may see an intrathoracic abdominal viscus, a shift of the mediastinum away from the affected side, atelectasis at the base of the lungs, or the nasogastric tube positioned above the diaphragm.[8]

In stable patients, contrast studies are useful if there is herniation of hollow viscera. The position of the stomach, small bowel, and colon can be demonstrated using upper and lower gastrointestinal contrast studies. Findings may include contrast-filled viscera above the diaphragm, obstruction at the level of the diaphragm, and delayed gastric emptying. The entire gastrointestinal tract must be visualized before the study can be interpreted as normal.[8]

Diagnostic peritoneal lavage has a 25% false-negative rate in the detection of isolated diaphragmatic injury using the criteria of 100,000 red blood cells (RBCs)/μL.[2,5,8] Some authors advocate lowering the RBC count considered positive to 5000 RBCs/μL when evaluating injuries at high risk for diaphragmatic injury (i.e., lower chest or upper abdominal penetrating wounds).[1,6,13] Computed tomography (CT) scanning has a low sensitivity because the imaging plane is parallel to the dome of the diaphragm, and the dome is not well visualized. Radionuclide liver or spleen imaging can be of value in the presence of solid viscera herniation.[12] Laparoscopy and thoracoscopy have been utilized with mixed results.[15,17] Ultrasonography may be helpful in some patients.[9]

Magnetic resonance imaging (MRI) has shown promising results in isolated cases. Boulanger and associates[2] used MRI scanning to diagnose diaphragmatic rupture definitively in two patients and to rule it out in three other patients who had equivocal chest radiographs. However, further studies are needed to determine its utility and value in the diagnosis of diaphragmatic injury.

PREHOSPITAL AND EMERGENCY DEPARTMENT MANAGEMENT

In the prehospital setting, basic management consists of volume administration; high-flow oxygen; monitoring; active airway management, if there are signs of compromise; and rapid transport. In the emergency department, basic trauma management should proceed as usual, with early surgical consultation. If the diagnosis of herniation is suspected, a nasogastric tube should be placed for decompression as well as to aid in the diagnosis. The dilated intrathoracic abdominal viscus may masquerade as an atypical pneumothorax, so a chest tube is placed only after careful digital verification of the free pleural space.

Any patient suspected of having a diaphragmatic rupture should be hospitalized. Surgical treatment is mandatory once the diagnosis is established.

BONY THORAX

RIB FRACTURES

Rib fractures account for more than 50% of nonpenetrating chest trauma. Fractures typically occur at the site of impact or the posterior angle, where the rib is structurally the weakest. Fractures are more common in adults because of the relative inelasticity of the mature thorax. Although the fourth through ninth ribs are the most commonly involved, fractures of ribs 9 through 11 deserve special concern, as there is an increased incidence of associated abdominal injuries due to their location. Multiple rib fractures or the presence of a flail chest segment is often associated with intrathoracic injury, usually a pulmonary contusion.

Clinical findings typically include tachypnea, splinting, and point tenderness intensified by deep breathing or coughing, ecchymoses, crepitus, and muscle spasm. Compression over the rib anteriorly or posteriorly produces referred pain to the fracture site. The diagnosis of rib fractures should be made on clinical grounds, because 50% of these injuries are missed on the initial chest radiograph; 10% do not visualize radiographically for 7 to 14 days after the injury, regardless of the views taken. A chest radiograph is valuable, however, when looking for complications of rib fractures, such as hemothorax, pneumothorax, pulmonary contusion, telectasis, and pneumonia. Oxygen saturation should also be measured.

The principal goals in the treatment of simple rib fractures are pain control and maintenance of adequate pulmonary function. The patient should be encouraged to breathe deeply. Binders are not recommended, as they decrease ventilation and promote atelectasis. Mild-to-moderate pain relief may be achieved with oral pain medications, such as nonsteroidal or opioid analgesics. The most effective, but often temporary, relief for moderate-to-severe pain is a long-acting anesthetic such as bupivacaine (Marcaine) in an intercostal block. Hospitalization may be indicated for elderly patients and for those with preexisting pulmonary disease to ensure adequate pulmonary toilet while controlling pain.

Although delayed hemothorax or pneumothorax may develop 6 to 24 hours after the injury, most rib fractures heal uneventfully within 3 to 6 weeks.[18] Patients should be discouraged from engaging in vigorous contact sports during that time. Rarely, the long-term course is complicated by posttraumatic neuroma.

Costochondral separation presents with signs and symptoms similar to those of rib fractures. The chest radiograph is normal. Healing is delayed due to the poor vascularity of the cartilage, and pain may persist for months. Often there is a snapping sensation with deep breathing. An anterior flail chest may occur from massive costochondral separation, but this is uncommon.[17]

STERNAL FRACTURES

Sternal fractures usually result from high-energy direct trauma to the anterior chest wall, most commonly in motor vehicle accidents, in which the chest strikes the steering wheel, dashboard, or shoulder belt at high velocity. A tremendous amount of force is necessary to fracture the sternum; consequently, these injuries should be viewed as harbingers of severe thoracic trauma. There is a 25% to 45% mortality rate associated with sternal fractures, which is directly proportional to the high incidence of myocardial injury, cardiac tamponade, aortic trauma, pulmonary contusion, and other serious intrathoracic injuries.

The diagnosis is suspected in the patient with a compatible history who complains of point tenderness over the sternum that is intensified with respirations. External signs of trauma, such as crepitus, ecchymoses, swelling, or abrasions, are not always present. The lateral radiograph of the chest is the most useful diagnostic test.[3] Care should be taken not to misdiagnose as a fracture the nonossified intrasternal cartilage of young patients.

In the field and in the emergency department, these patients should have intravenous access, oxygen, and cardiac monitoring. Isolated sternal fracture is not an indication for active airway management, but this should be undertaken if there are signs of respiratory compromise from associated injuries.[7] A widened mediastinum should alert the physician to an associated aortic injury. Mechanical ventilation using positive end-expiratory pressure has been used as internal fixation for grossly unstable fractures. Operative fixation is often unsatisfactory. Occasionally, painful pseudarthroses and overflap deformities develop and require later reconstruction.

Admission should be seriously considered for serial electrocardiograms and cardiac monitoring for myocardial contusions. If transfer is necessary, advanced cardiac life-support personnel should accompany the patient, with continued oxygen, cardiac monitoring, and intravenous access. Particular attention should be paid to the possibility of dysrhythmias, pneumothorax, and pulmonary compromise. These are painful injuries that often require opioid analgesics.

FLAIL CHEST

A flail chest is a free-floating section of chest wall resulting from two or more adjacent ribs fractured in two or more places, or rib fractures in combination with either sternal fractures or costochondral separations. This is a serious injury that carries an 8% to 35% mortality rate, directly related to associated injuries (of which pulmonary contusions are the most common).[10]

These patients often present with pain, crepitus, and ecchymoses over the chest wall. The classically described paradoxical movement of the flail segment refers to its unexpected movement inward during inspiration and outward during expiration, in response to the intrathoracic pressure changes during the respiratory cycle. The paradox may not be seen initially because of muscle splinting, only to become dramatically apparent hours later as the underlying contused lung decreases in compliance and the patient tires. Muscle splinting with subsequent hypoventilation may result in focal atelectasis, decreased tidal volume and vital capacity, pulmonary arteriovenous shunting, hypoxemia, and decreased cardiac output.

The diagnosis is made clinically. The thorax is inspected and palpated in search of areas of tenderness and crepitus. Serial examinations using tangential lighting looking for paradoxical movement may be necessary. In the field, the flail chest may be stabilized by positioning the patient with the injured side down.

In the emergency department, a careful search for other injuries is made, and baseline arterial blood gas measurements, oxygen saturation, and chest radiographs are obtained. Continuous oxygen saturation monitoring is done. Tube thoracostomy is indicated if intrapleural air or blood is present, or prophylactically if the patient is mechanically ventilated, as such patients are at high risk for developing a tension pneumothorax.

The mere presence of a flail chest is not an indication for endotracheal intubation. There is debate regarding which patients benefit from mechanical ventilation. The following guidelines should be used in conjunction with the patient's overall status. Intubation should be considered if one or more of the following are present: shock, three or more associated injuries, previous pulmonary disease, fracture of eight or more ribs, age above 65 years, or PaO_2 less than 60 mm Hg (or decreasing O_2 saturation readings) on a nonbreather bag reservoir mask at sea level.

All patients with a flail chest should be admitted to an intensive care unit for aggressive pulmonary toilet, pain control, observation, and monitoring.

COMMON PITFALLS

- All patients with penetrating trauma below the tips of the scapula posteriorly or nipple level anteriorly should be considered at high risk for diaphragmatic perforation.
- Beware of the diaphragmatic hernia masquerading as a "high-riding" or "paralyzed" diaphragm on a chest radiograph.
- Never place a chest tube without first digitally verifying the free pleural space.
- Consider delayed diaphragmatic herniation when there is any history of previous thoracoabdominal trauma, acute signs and symptoms of intestinal obstruction, pulmonary complaints, or radiographic abnormalities.
- Consider the possibility of spleen or liver injury with fractures of ribs 9 through 12.

References

1. Aitken RJ, Immelman EJ. Traumatic diaphragmatic hernias—pitfalls in the barium meal. *Injury* 1986;17:224.
2. Boulanger BR, Mirvis SE, Rodriguez A. MRI in traumatic diaphragmatic rupture: case reports. *J Trauma* 1992;32:89.
3. Buckman R, Trooskin SZ, Flancbaum L, et al. The significance of stable patients with sternal fractures. *Surg Gynecol Obstet* 1987;164:261.
4. Feliciano DV, Cruse PA, Mattox KL, et al. Delayed diagnosis of injuries to the diaphragm after penetrating wounds. *J Trauma* 1988;28:1135.
5. Freeman T, Fisher RP. The inadequacy of peritoneal lavage in diagnosing acute diaphragmatic rupture. *J Trauma* 1976;16:538.
6. Gurney J, Harrison WL, Anderson JC. Omental fat stimulating pleural fluid in traumatic diaphragmatic hernia: CT characteristics. *J Comput Assist Tomogr* 1985;9:1112.
7. Harley DP, Mena I. Cardiac and vascular sequelae of sternal fractures. *J Trauma* 1986;26:553.
8. Kanowitz A, Marx JA. Delayed traumatic diaphragmatic hernia simulating acute tension pneumothorax. *J Emerg Med* 1989;7:619.
9. Kim HH, Shin YR. Blunt traumatic rupture of the diaphragm. *J Ultrasound Med* 1997;16:593–598.
10. Landercasper J, Cogbill TH, Lindesmith LA. Long-term disability after flail chest injury. *J Trauma* 1984;24:410.
11. McCollum C, Anyanwu CH, Umeh BUO, et al. Management of traumatic rupture of the diaphragm. *Br J Surg* 1987;74:181.
12. McHugh K, Ogilvie BC, Brunton FJ. Delayed presentation of traumatic diaphragmatic hernia. *Clin Radiol* 1991;43:246.
13. Moore JB, Moore EE, Thompson JS. Abdominal injuries associated with penetrating lower chest trauma. *Am J Surg* 1980;140:724.
14. Morgan AS, Flancbaum L, Esposito T, et al. Blunt injury to the diaphragm: an analysis of 44 patients. *J Trauma* 1986;26:565.
15. Murray JA, Demetriades D, et al. Occult injuries to the diaphragm: prospective evaluation of laparoscopy in penetrating injuries to the left lower chest. *J Am Coll Surg* 1998,6:626–633.
16. Rodriguez-Morales G, Rodriguez A, Shatney CH. Acute rupture of the diaphragm in blunt trauma: analysis of 60 patients. *J Trauma* 1986;26:438.
17. Rosen P, Barkin RM, et al., eds. *Emergency medicine: concepts and clinical practice,* 4th ed. Chapters 35, 37. St. Louis: CV Mosby, 1998.
18. Ross RM, Cordoba A. Delayed life-threatening hemothorax associated with rib fractures. *J Trauma* 1986;26:576.
19. Saber WL, Moore EE, Hopeman AR, et al. Delayed presentation of traumatic diaphragmatic hernia. *J Emerg Med* 1986;4:1.
20. Sharma OP. Traumatic diaphragmatic rupture: not an uncommon entity—personal experience with collective review of the 1980s. *J Trauma* 1989;29:678.
21. Wiencek RG, Wilson RF, Steiger Z. Acute injuries of the diaphragm. *J Thorac Cardiovasc Surg* 1986;92:989.

CHAPTER 106
Thoracic Esophageal Injuries

Brian Tiffany and Robert C. Jorden

Injuries to the esophagus are a major diagnostic challenge for the emergency physician. With the deep and well-protected location of the esophagus, signs of perforation or other serious esophageal injury are often subtle and frequently masked by injuries to adjacent structures. Because recognition is often delayed, a perforation occurring in the esophagus is more treacherous than in any other part of the gastrointestinal tract. Perforation can produce severe mediastinal and pleural infections due to contamination with bacterial-laden saliva and, occasionally, gastric contents. Left untreated, perforation nearly always results in mortality unless it is very small. There are five basic mechanisms of esophageal injury: penetrating trauma, blunt trauma, barotrauma, ingestions, and iatrogenic injury.

PENETRATING TRAUMA

Penetrating esophageal trauma can be caused by either an impaling or a projectile weapon. Both are generally the result of interpersonal violence, with impalements most frequently the result of domestic violence.[5] Reported series show a preponderance of cervical esophageal injuries, probably because penetrating trauma to the thoracic esophagus is associated with nonsurvivable injuries to the great vessels or heart. The peritoneal esophagus is relatively short and mobile, and thus is less likely to be injured. In all cases of penetrating esophageal injury, a careful evaluation to delineate the inevitable injuries to adjacent structures is mandatory. Gunshot wounds in particular can be quite complex. A round from a high-velocity military weapon can exert a blast effect well outside the direct path of the bullet, with delayed perforation from the devascularized and mural necrosis.[17]

BLUNT TRAUMA

Blunt injuries can occur from several mechanisms. A sharp blow to the upper abdomen can force air and gastric contents into the esophagus. If the proximal esophageal sphincter is closed when this occurs, a rise in esophageal pressure sufficient to cause perforation can result. The usual site of perforation is identical to that seen with a spontaneous rupture associated with vomiting (Boerhaave syndrome). It typically occurs in the left side of the distal esophagus, a physiologically weakened area due to the paucity of circular muscle fibers. Although falls and motor vehicle accidents account for most injuries by this mechanism, there have been several reported cases of perforation caused by the Heimlich maneuver.[14] Finally, cardiopulmonary resuscitation may be associated with a significant rate of esophageal injury.[13] In one autopsy series, 12% of patients who had undergone cardiopulmonary resuscitation (CPR) had a gastroesophageal perforation.[3] This potential complication should be considered in successfully resuscitated patients, particularly those with extended periods of CPR or those who were subjected to abdominal counterpulsation CPR techniques. Compression of the esophagus against the spine can produce longitudinal tears in the upper thoracic esophagus. These lesions are frequently accompanied by a laceration in the membranous (posterior) portion of the trachea, resulting in a traumatic tracheoesophageal fistula. These injuries can go undetected for days in critically injured patients who are intubated if the inflated endotracheal tube cuff seals off the trachea below the level of perforation. Finally, rapid deceleration can produce a traction injury, resulting in a segmental devascularization of the esophagus with delayed perforation.[6]

BAROTRAUMA

As a hollow, potentially air-containing organ, the esophagus is susceptible to barotrauma. While perforation via this mechanism can occur anywhere in the esophagus, the left lateral wall of the distal esophagus is the weakest area and by far the most common site of perforation by this mechanism.

The most well known barotrauma injury is Boerhaave syndrome, or postemetic esophageal rupture, in which a rapid rise in intraluminal pressure due to a forceful vomiting is the culprit. The classically described presentation of chest pain, respiratory difficulty, and subcutaneous emphysema may not be evident, and the diagnosis is often delayed or mistaken for perforated viscus myocardial infarction.[7]

An unusual mechanism for esophageal barotrauma is accidental insufflation of compressed air into the mouth. Air under pressure enters the mouth, overcoming the upper esophageal sphincter and entering the esophagus.[11] The cardiac sphincter does not open rapidly enough to dissipate the intraluminal pressure; the result is esophageal perforation. Experimental studies have shown that rupture occurs at 5 pounds per square inch of pressure,[12] a pressure easily achieved by common household items such as aerosol cans, air compressors, inflation devices, and vacuum cleaner exhausts. A remarkable variety of injuries due to this mechanism, including children biting tire inner tubes, eruption of bottled carbonated beverages, discharge of fire extinguishers, and mishaps with compressed air lines, have been reported.[8,9,15,20]

INGESTION-INDUCED INJURIES

Accidental or intentional ingestion of acids rarely produces significant esophageal injury,[19] while strong alkali (pH greater than 12) ingestions can produce devastating injury to the entire esophagus. The "sticky" nature of bases and the coagulative necrosis they produce allow very prolonged contact times and ongoing injury, while acids have short contact times in the esophagus and tend to produce their most significant injuries in the stomach and duodenum.[7] Impaction of food or medications can cause injuries ranging from mucosal irritation to frank perforation. Injury occurs as a result of direct chemical effects on the mucosa, pressure-induced necrosis, or both, depending on the composition of the impaction. Patients with strictures or esophageal motility disorders are particularly susceptible to impactions. Finally, any of a vast array of ingested foreign bodies can cause injury, whether from sharp points and edges or pressure-induced necrosis of the esophageal lining from an impacted object.

IATROGENIC INJURIES

The most common cause of esophageal perforation is iatrogenic, with most of these occurring in the thoracic esophagus.[16] The esophagus can be injured during nasogastric[1] or tracheal intubation, esophagoscopy, dilation of strictures, and sclerotherapy for the management of esophageal varices. Injuries due to CPR were discussed earlier in this chapter. Diagnosis of iatrogenic esophageal injuries is frequently delayed, and a high index of suspicion should be maintained in these patients.

CLINICAL PRESENTATION

Pain is the dominant symptom and is present in nearly all cases of thoracic esophageal rupture. Other common signs and symptoms are subcutaneous emphysema (especially in the neck or supraclavicular fossa), unexplained tachycardia, dyspnea, dysphagia, odynophagia, cyanosis, pneumomediastinum, pneumothorax, pleural effusion, and hematemesis.

Because of the nonspecific nature of these findings, it is easy to overlook esophageal perforation. The rarity of the injury, particularly from a blunt mechanism, also contributes to missed and delayed diagnosis. One must, therefore, consider the diagnosis whenever the trajectory of a wounding implement is proximate to the esophagus. In addition, whenever injury to an adjacent organ is apparent, esophageal injury should be presumed and investigated.

DIFFERENTIAL DIAGNOSIS

The differential diagnosis for esophageal injury is limited to trauma to the surrounding structures. Subcutaneous emphysema or pneumomediastinum can be a result of a respiratory tract injury.

Hematemesis or bloody regurgitation implicates gastric or pharyngeal injury. The other signs and symptoms of esophageal injury are so nonspecific that the differential includes all organ systems located in the chest.

EMERGENCY DEPARTMENT EVALUATION

Thoracic esophageal injury can be suspected but not diagnosed on clinical grounds alone. Once the suspicion is entertained, the diagnosis can be confirmed by several means, including esophagography, esophagoscopy, and exploration in the operating room. As a preliminary study, a plain chest film should be performed on all victims of suspected esophageal trauma, looking for subcutaneous and mediastinal air and concomitant chest wall and respiratory tract injuries. Furthermore, in gunshot victims, plain radiographs can be helpful in determining the risk of esophageal trauma. The diagnosis should be suspected and pursued whenever a transmediastinal trajectory is identified.

The choice of initial diagnostic procedure is somewhat controversial, with some authors advocating esophagography[1] and others esophagoscopy.[18] Contrast esophagraphy has the disadvantage of potentially introducing contrast material into the mediastinum or the tracheobronchial tree. For this reason, the study should first be performed with a water-soluble contrast material that has a much lower risk of mediastinitis or pneumonitis than does barium. If the water-soluble contrast study is negative, the study should be repeated using barium, which provides better detection of small perforations.[15] Both flexible and rigid esophagoscopy have been used in evaluating esophageal injuries, with sensitivities of 90% to 100%[4,10] and reported instances of esophagoscopic detection of perforations missed by contrast studies. Whatever initial diagnostic procedure selected, it seems prudent in the high-risk patient to use both modalities before declaring the patient free of esophageal injury.

Computed tomography (CT) scanning is not a primary diagnostic study for thoracic esophageal perforation, but it can reveal nonspecific findings suggestive of perforation, such as air in soft tissues or abscess cavities. CT scanning can also be helpful in detecting postoperative leaks and abscess formation.[11]

EMERGENCY DEPARTMENT MANAGEMENT

Management in the emergency department consists primarily of providing supportive care. Cardiorespiratory instability may result from the associated injuries that are invariably present, and should be addressed by appropriate stabilizing measures, such as airway management, volume replacement, and tube thoracostomy. Nasogastric intubation should also be performed to empty the stomach and lower the risk of gastric contents further contaminating the mediastinum. It may also be of diagnostic help if blood is recovered on aspiration.

Besides providing supportive care and pursuing diagnostic studies, initiation of antibiotic therapy is the only specific management required in the emergency department. Antibiotic coverage should be chosen in conjunction with the consulting surgeon. Infections that arise from esophageal perforations are normally polymicrobial, with gram-negative rods, *Streptococcus, Staphylococcus,* and oral flora as the dominant organisms. The antibiotic regimen chosen should be broad in spectrum and should include anaerobic coverage.

DISPOSITION

All patients with confirmed esophageal perforation require admission. Surgical consultation is obtained as soon as possible to coordinate the evaluation and final disposition. Nearly all patients with thoracic esophageal perforation require surgical intervention. Rarely, a patient with a small lesion and a localized infection may be successfully managed with antibiotics alone.[2] Most, however, require mediastinal drainage with esophageal repair and temporary esophageal exclusion (creation of a cervical esophagostomy and distal esophageal ligature). A few patients require esophagectomy with subsequent reconstruction using the stomach or colon. Surgical management is supplemented by hyperalimentation or tube feedings by way of an operatively placed jejunostomy tube and continuation of antibiotic therapy.

Patients should be transferred to an appropriate facility if resources for care are unavailable locally. Transfer should be effected as promptly as possible.

COMMON PITFALLS

- By far, the most common pitfall is failure to make the diagnosis. If the patient is severely injured, with other indications for surgery, the diagnosis is frequently made when operating. Patients who are managed nonoperatively and/or have isolated esophageal injuries are most likely to be missed, with worsening morbidity and mortality with the delay in the diagnosis. In fact, many authorities quote a twofold increase in mortality when the diagnosis is delayed beyond 24 hours.
- Always consider esophageal injury in patients with pneumomediastinum after blunt trauma. This finding should mandate further evaluation.
- Be sure to follow a negative water-soluble contrast study, with one performed with the more sensitive barium swallow.
- If the index of suspicion is high, consider esophagoscopy if contrast studies are negative.

References

1. Ahmed A, Aggarwal M, Watson E. Esophageal perforation: a complication of nasogastric tube placement. *Am J Emerg Med* 1998;16:64.
2. Altorjay A, Kiss J, Voros A, et al. Nonoperative management of esophageal perforations. Is it justified? *Ann Surg* 1997;225:415.
3. Anthony PP, Tatersfield AE. Gastric mucosal lacerations after cardiac resuscitation. *Br Heart J* 1969;31:72.
4. Armstrong WB. Diagnosis and management of external penetrating cervical esophageal injuries. *Ann Otol Rhinol Laryngol* 1994;103:863.
5. Bastos RBN, Graeber GM. Esophageal injuries. *Chest Surg Clin North Am* 1997;7:357.
6. Beal SL, Pottmeyer EW, Spisso JM. Esophageal perforation following external blunt trauma. *J Trauma* 1988;28:1425.
7. Brauer RB, Liebermann-Meffert D, Stein HU, et al. Boerhaavs syndrome: an analysis of the literature and report of 18 new cases. *Esophagus* 1997;10:64.
8. Conlan AA, Wessels A, Hammond CA, et al. Pharyngoesophageal barotrauma in children: a report of six cases. *J Thorac Cardiovasc Surg* 1984;88:452.
9. Guth AA, Gouge TH, Depan HJ. Blast injury to the thoracic esophagus. *Ann Thorac Surg* 1991;51:837.
10. Horowitz B. Endoscopic evaluation of penetrating esophageal injuries. *Am J Gastroenterol* 1993;88:1249.
11. Jones WG, Ginsberg RJ. Esophageal perforation: a continuing challenge. *Ann Thorac Surg* 1992;53:534.
12. Mackler SA. Spontaneous rupture of the esophagus: an experimental and clinical study. *Surg Gynecol Obstet* 1952;95:345.
13. McGrath RB. Gastroesophageal lacerations: a fatal complication of closed chest cardiopulmonary resuscitation. *Chest* 1983;83:570.
14. Merriedith M, Liebowitz R. Rupture of the esophagus caused by the Heimlich maneuver. *Ann Emerg Med* 1986;15:106.
15. Meyerovitch J, BenAmi T, Rozenman J, et al. Pneumatic rupture of the esophagus caused by carbonated drinks. *Pediatr Radiol* 1988;18:468.
16. Parischa PJ, Fleischer DE, Kalloo AN. Endoscopic perforations of the upper digestive tract: a review of their pathogenesis, prevention, and management. *Gastroenterology* 1994;106:787.
17. Popovsky J. Perforations of the esophagus from gunshot wounds. *J Trauma* 1984;24:337.
18. Richardson JD, Miller FB, Carrillo EH, et al. Complex thoracic injuries. *Surg Clin North Am* 1996;76:725.
19. Swann LA, Munter DW. Esophageal injuries. *Emerg Med Clin North Am* 1996;14:557.
20. Weissberg D, Kaufman M. Compressed air injury to the esophagus. *J Trauma* 1991;31:150.

CHAPTER 107
Blunt Abdominal Trauma

Kevin M. Curtis and Vicente H. Gracias

Blunt abdominal trauma remains an important source of morbidity and mortality, accounting for 10% of all deaths from trauma. It is seen most commonly in the context of motor vehicle crashes. A significant minority of injuries result from sports, assaults, falls, bicycle accidents, and injuries to pedestrians.[14]

In the face of frequent concomitant multisystem trauma, the early detection of intraabdominal injury is a challenge to the emergency physician. Unlike other more obvious causes of blood loss, such as hemothorax, external hemorrhage, and pelvic or femur fractures, intraabdominal bleeding may easily go unrecognized. Although injuries to the solid organs are most frequently involved after blunt abdominal trauma, a high clinical suspicion must be maintained for the more subtle injuries to the bowel, mesentery, and pancreas, such as in the "lapbelt syndrome" or from bicycle handlebars.

Many traumatic deaths, such as diffuse axonal injury, transection of the aorta, and cardiac rupture, are inevitable; but death due to abdominal injury may be prevented by early recognition. Therefore, after initial resuscitation, one of the primary objectives of the emergency physician is to decide which patients require early surgical consultation. Although the history and physical examination continue to be essential components of the assessment, the addition of the focused abdominal sonography for trauma (FAST) and helical computed tomography (CT) scanning to the previous armamentarium has significantly enhanced our diagnostic ability and therapeutic approach.

CLINICAL PRESENTATION

It is well recognized that abdominal injuries from blunt trauma can be difficult to diagnose by history and physical alone.[11] The presence of an altered sensorium from head injury or substance abuse, distracting injuries, spinal cord injuries, or shock can render the initial assessment unreliable. In addition, because patients with abdominal injuries are often victims of multisystem trauma, dramatic head, chest, and orthopedic injuries may distract the physician's attention.

Although initial vital signs may be helpful in patients with brisk internal bleeding secondary to disruption of the liver or spleen, in those with less profound injury, vital signs may be normal. Injuries that produce minimal bleeding, such as perforation of the bowel or diaphragm, and those that are isolated to the retroperitoneum typically result in a paucity of physical findings. In an effort to identify patients with significant abdominal injuries, one study of 16,000 blunt trauma victims identified seven factors associated with an increased risk of abdominal injuries: (1) gross hematuria, (2) admission hypotension, (3) lower rib fractures, (4) hemothorax or pneumothorax, (5) abdominal wall hematoma or abrasion, (6) HCO_3^- less than 21, and (7) pelvic fracture.[11]

DIFFERENTIAL DIAGNOSIS

Injury to the abdominal musculature may be confused with an intraperitoneal lesion. Contusions of the rectus muscle often produce greater pain when the abdomen is palpated during muscle contraction. To elicit this finding, ask the patient to lift the head or leg off the stretcher during the abdominal examination. Patients with intraperitoneal injury usually have less pain during this maneuver and greater pain on palpation of the relaxed abdomen, as the contracted muscles shield the intraabdominal organs. However, this finding is not absolute, and significant tenderness should always prompt further objective workup. Nausea and vomiting may occur after an injury and may be ascribed to head trauma or stress reaction; however, repeated emesis following abdominal trauma should prompt consideration of a duodenal hematoma, particularly in children.

EMERGENCY DEPARTMENT EVALUATION

As is true of any trauma patient, the assessment of the patient with abdominal trauma must be performed in light of the patient's overall status. Initial attention is directed toward the airway with cervical spine control, breathing, and circulation, with the rapid administration of 2 L of crystalloid to the hypotensive patient. The abdomen is fully examined during the secondary, not the primary, survey. Early categorization of the patient as stable or unstable should be made, and prioritization of resuscitation, evaluation, and diagnosis occurs accordingly. Among victims of motor vehicle crashes arriving in the emergency department without significant external bleeding, abdominal injuries are the most likely cause of hypotension.[14] Therefore, the diagnosis of intraabdominal hemorrhage should be considered in all cases of shock. Although T6 or higher paraplegia may produce neurogenic shock, hypotension in this setting should also be presumed to be secondary to intraabdominal injury until proven otherwise. In general, the more critically injured the patient, the more quickly the emergency physician must determine the need for laparotomy and obtain early surgical consultation.

History

A brief initial history is obtained using the AMPLE format (allergies, medications, past medical history, last meal, and events surrounding the injury). Potential sources of information include the patient, prehospital care providers, and witnesses. The paramedic report should include a description of the mechanism of injury, and, in the case of a vehicular accident, damage to the vehicle, use of seatbelts, air bag deployment, and deformity of the steering column. The paramedic report also must indicate loss of consciousness, initial mental status, vital signs, evaluation of the ABCs, interventions, and significant complaints. Of particular importance is a history of prehospital hypotension.

Physical Examination

The patient is completely undressed, and life threats are addressed before examining the abdomen. Evaluation of the abdomen should begin with inspection for abrasions or ecchymosis. Evidence of ecchymosis over the lower abdomen in a lapbelt distribution is suspicious for hollow viscus injury and warrants consideration for further evaluation, even in the absence of abdominal tenderness. Although Cullen's sign (ecchymosis around the umbilicus) and Turner's sign (ecchymosis of the flanks) are associated with retroperitoneal bleeding and often sought on examination, they are insensitive, often taking hours to manifest. Auscultation for bowel sounds adds little to the assessment, as patients often have multiple reasons for an ileus, as well as the possibility of normal bowel sounds despite significant hemoperitoneum.

Palpation of the abdomen begins with examination of the lower chest. Care should be taken to detect lower rib fractures, because up to 20% of patients with left lower rib fractures have associated splenic injury, and 10% of patients with right-sided injury have hepatic trauma.[9] The abdomen is carefully palpated, paying particular attention to the right and left upper quadrants. The finding of Kehr's sign (pain in either shoulder unrelated to shoulder tenderness or range of motion) indicates the presence of blood irritating the diaphragm and is often secondary to splenic or liver injury. Pelvic stability is assessed by applying distraction and compression forces over the iliac crest and over the symphysis pubis. Of patients found to have a major pelvic fracture, up to 50% of patients have an intraabdominal injury.[9]

Rectal examination may demonstrate a high-riding or boggy prostate in patients with urethral disruption. Blood on rectal examination may indicate gastrointestinal disruption and mandates surgical consultation. The patient should be log-rolled with palpation of the lumbar and thoracic area. Lumbar fractures, particularly those in conjunction with the seatbelt sign, are markers of hollow viscus injury.

Despite the necessity of a well-directed physical examination, the emergency physician must be aware of its limitations. One study found physical examination to be 65% accurate in the setting of blunt abdominal trauma,[29] and another trauma center reported abdominal examination alone as adequate in only 35% of patients.[4] The true value of the initial examination is to stratify patients into categories of those who need (1) immediate laparotomy, (2) additional diagnostic adjuncts, or (3) serial clinical examinations.

Plain Radiographic Evaluation

The plain film has limited utility in the evaluation of blunt abdominal trauma and contributes to operative decision making in less than 4% of patients.[9] Indirect evidence of abdominal injury includes the flank stripe and dog-ear signs secondary to intraabdominal blood. A splenic hematoma may displace the gastric air bubble to the right. However, because these signs are neither reliable nor consistent, and because therapeutic interventions are not made on the basis of the results, routine abdominal films are not warranted. A chest x-ray should be done and rarely may show evidence of free air or a ruptured diaphragm. Pelvic films should be obtained based on the reliability of the examination and on physical findings.

Laboratory Tests

Standard laboratory analysis of the blunt abdominal trauma victim includes a complete blood count, chemistry panel, type and crossmatch, and evaluation of the urine. Additional tests, such as coagulation factors, ethanol level, drug screens, and arterial blood gases (ABGs) should be obtained as appropriate. As is the case for plain films, initial results are often not particularly helpful, and the physician should never rely on a blood test to exclude intraabdominal injury. The most valuable laboratory investigation is a type and crossmatch.

The hematocrit level is influenced by many factors, including the rate of blood loss, dilutional effects of intravenous fluids, fluid shifts from the interstitium to the intravascular space, and preinjury level. Intravenous fluids alone may decrease the hematocrit by up to six points. In light of these confounding variables, most of the utility of hemoglobin and hematocrit levels lies in their use as serial tests over time. However, an initial hemoglobin level less than 8 g/dL in the presence of abdominal injury is a strong indicator of occult hemorrhage.[20] The white blood cell (WBC) count is often increased in multiple trauma and lacks diagnostic and prognostic significance. Although a serum amylase level is routinely obtained, several studies have demonstrated that it is neither sensitive nor specific for pancreatic injury.[8,27] The addition of pancreatic isoenzymes or lipase does not improve the accuracy. Ethanol levels and drug screens may provide additional information about the reliability of the examination.

Coagulation studies are useful in patients on anticoagulants, those with severe liver disease, pregnant patients who may have abruptio placentae and possible disseminated intravascular coagulation (DIC), and those receiving massive transfusions. The base deficit provided by ABG analysis accurately measures the severity of shock and the efficacy of fluid resuscitation. Base deficit or serum lactate is a more sensitive indicator of compensated shock than blood pressure or even invasive monitoring. A deficit of –6 or less (i.e., more negative) is a useful indicator of occult hemorrhage and should prompt further evaluation of the abdomen. Serial base deficits or serial lactates indicate trends in patient status.[12,13]

Diagnostic Peritoneal Lavage

Diagnostic peritoneal lavage (DPL) is an excellent test for determining the presence or absence of intraperitoneal blood, with a sensitivity of 94% to 96%, a specificity of 96% to 99%, a 1.4%

false-positive rate, a 1.3% false-negative rate, and a complication rate less than 1%.[15] DPL can be considered in the blunt abdominal trauma patient with (1) an unreliable examination, including those with altered sensorium, spinal cord trauma, or distracting injuries; (2) an abdominal examination suspicious for abdominal injury without frank peritoneal signs; (3) general anesthesia planned in the face of a possible abdominal injury; or (4) as a quick test in the unstable patient with unexplained hypotension. The only absolute contraindication for DPL is the need for emergency laparotomy.

One of the main drawbacks of DPL is its lack of specificity for identifying the underlying intraabdominal injury. DPL was originally popularized prior to the advent of the modern CT and trauma ultrasound, and before the current nonoperative management of many solid-organ injuries. It has been estimated that 30% of patients with a positive DPL have injuries amenable to conservative treatment.[34] In addition, although the complication rate is low, it is an invasive procedure that, unless the aspirate is positive, takes a minimum of 10 minutes to complete.[10] As a result, at many centers, CT and ultrasound have replaced DPL in the majority of blunt abdominal trauma victims. Other drawbacks of DPL are its inability to detect retroperitoneal injury and its relatively poor sensitivity for bowel and diaphragmatic injuries.

DPL does still have a significant role in the evaluation of blunt abdominal trauma in many emergency departments, however, particularly in the unstable patient and situations in which CT and ultrasound are unavailable. DPL can be performed open, semi-open, or closed. The closed Seldinger technique is fastest, as well as safe and accurate.[1,32] In all cases, gastric and bladder decompression must occur first with a nasogastric tube and Foley catheter. Criteria for a positive test after blunt trauma include an initial aspirate of more than 5 mL of blood or greater than 100,000 RBC/μL in the lavage fluid. Other lavage criteria based on WBC, amylase, and bile are rarely helpful and should not be relied on.

DPL can be falsely positive in patients with pelvic fractures[18] because of catheter placement through an abdominal wall hematoma or diapedesis of red cells into the peritoneum. In patients with significant pelvic fractures in whom the information from a DPL is needed, the open supraumbilical technique is recommended to decrease the incidence of false-positive results.

Computed Tomography Scanning

CT has become the gold standard for radiographic evaluation of the hemodynamically stable patient with blunt abdominal trauma. Accuracy has been reported as high as 97.6%.[27] By its ability to define injuries to the liver, spleen, and kidneys, CT has revolutionized the management of solid-organ injuries.[24,31] Abdominal CT after blunt trauma is indicated in patients in whom the physical examination has proven unreliable, including those with altered sensorium, spinal cord trauma, or distracting injuries. It is also indicated when an abdominal examination causes the examiner to suspect abdominal injury but there are no frank peritoneal signs, when general anesthesia is planned in the face of a possible abdominal injury, in the case of suspected retroperitoneal injury, or for delineation of a pelvic fracture. In addition, CT may demonstrate an occult pneumothorax or hemothorax, injuries to the spine and spinal cord, or vascular injuries. The current use of helical CT has resulted in increased speed, decreased artifact, improved parenchymal and vascular definition, as well as increased sensitivity for diaphragmatic injuries.[28]

One area of current controversy with respect to the use of CT for abdominal trauma is the need for oral contrast. Three case series suggest that it is unnecessary in this setting.[7,33,35] However, two of the reports were small, and a prospective study has yet to be performed. When oral contrast is administered, CT should not be subsequently delayed awaiting passage of the contrast material. Although complications of CT can include allergic reactions to the dye and, rarely, aspiration, the most serious potential complications are decompensation in the scanner (hypotension or respiratory arrest) and delay in necessary laparotomy.

Ultrasound

In the United States, which has lagged behind many parts of the world in the use of ultrasound in trauma, the role of ultrasound has increased rapidly over the last decade. The FAST examination is a directed assessment of the abdomen, with the goal of detecting hemoperitoneum. It has become the radiologic screening test of choice in many trauma centers in the United States, and has a sensitivity of 81% to 100% and a specificity of 94% to 98% for identifying intraperitoneal blood.[26] Although it has virtually replaced both CT and peritoneal lavage as the primary radiographic tool in at least one hospital,[17] in most centers, its use has been as a substitute for DPL. In this role, ultrasound has several advantages over lavage: It (1) is faster, (2) is noninvasive, (3) can be performed repeatedly, and (4) does not interfere with most other procedures or evaluations. In addition, many of the relative contraindications to DPL do not apply to FAST, such as prior abdominal surgery, coagulopathy, or pregnancy.

In a prospective study by Healey et al.[17] of patients with blunt abdominal trauma, of a total of 734 negative FAST examinations, only six were found to be false negatives. Of these, one was diagnosed by a repeat ultrasound and required splenorrhaphy; another patient had a positive DPL and an intestinal injury at laparotomy; a third patient had a CT showing omental and ileal injuries requiring surgical repair; three patients required nonoperative management. A study by McKenney et al.[25] included patients with suspected blunt abdominal trauma and initial hypotension. Initial FAST examination was normal in 856 patients. Within this group, 15 had a positive CT, but only one required a laparotomy for a colon injury. Ten patients with a negative ultrasound had a subsequent DPL, and, in all cases, the lavage was also normal.

The main advantages of FAST over CT scan are its speed and its location in the resuscitation suite, making it the test of choice in the hemodynamically unstable victim of blunt abdominal trauma. Ultrasound is clearly inferior to CT for identifying specific solid-organ injuries, for evaluating the retroperitoneum, and for identifying small amounts of blood. Therefore, in the stable patient who requires a radiologic evaluation of the abdomen, a CT scan is often performed regardless of the FAST results. FAST also shares some of the inadequacies of CT in that it lacks sensitivity for hollow viscus injuries, and for injuries to the pancreas and mesentery. The only contraindication to ultrasound in trauma is an indication for emergent laparotomy. Reports regarding the amount of hemoperitoneum required for detection by FAST have varied, with earlier studies indicating over 600 mL and more recent reports suggesting less than 200 mL.[5,19,36]

The FAST examination is performed with the patient supine and is designed to look for hemoperitoneum and for hemopericardium. Four locations are examined: (1) the right upper quadrant (RUQ), (2) the left upper quadrant (LUQ), (3) the suprapubic region, and (4) the pericardium. The RUQ view is generally done first, being the easiest, and the most sensitive for hemoperitoneum. This view is specifically designed to detect blood in Morison's pouch between the kidney and liver. Although this location has the greatest yield, the addition of the other two abdominal views has been found to increase the sensitivity from 51% to 87%.[22] The LUQ is examined next, specifically looking for blood in the splenorenal space. Either view of the upper quadrants may also reveal a hemothorax. The suprapubic view looks at the space between the rectum and bladder (the pouch of Douglas or rectovesicular pouch), and the heart and pericardium are examined by a subxiphoid view.

The ability of emergency physicians and surgeons to perform an accurate FAST examination has been demonstrated repeatedly.[22,30] Clearly, the accuracy of the examiner increases with experience. One study found that sensitivity stabilized after 100 examinations,[35] and another reported no false negatives after 200 examinations.[23] The 1994 curriculum guidelines from the Society for Academic Emergency Medicine recommend 40 hours of instruction and 150 examinations.[26] In addition to increased accuracy with repeated examinations, the time for completion of the four views has been noted to decrease from 4.7 to 2.5 minutes.[30]

EMERGENCY DEPARTMENT MANAGEMENT

In level I trauma centers, prehospital criteria such as vital signs, level of consciousness, and mechanism of injury will alert a trauma team before arrival of the patient. In most hospitals, however, the emergency physician is solely responsible for initial trauma management. The seriously injured patient with blunt abdominal trauma must undergo standard ATLS resuscitation.

First, address the airway with maintenance of cervical spine immobilization. Administer 12 L of oxygen by nonrebreather mask initially and continue until oxygenation can be assessed by pulse oximeter or ABG analysis. Obtain vascular access using two large-bore (14-gauge or 16-gauge) intravenous catheters connected to normal saline or lactated Ringer's, and place the patient on a cardiac monitor. Evaluate the neurologic status by pupils and the AVPU method or according to the Glasgow Coma Scale. The patient should be fully undressed, with subsequent prevention of hypothermia. Insert a nasogastric or orogastric tube, and, after ensuring no evidence of urethral injury, place a Foley catheter. By this point, the emergency physician should classify the victim of blunt abdominal trauma as stable or unstable.

Unstable Patients

In the hypotensive or tachycardic patient, administer 2 L of crystalloid wide open; surgical consultation is urgent. If the patient remains hypotensive, give packed RBCs. Because type-specific blood requires only 10 minutes to process, it is preferable to a full crossmatch in the unstable patient. In the massively injured trauma victim, it may be necessary to give O-negative blood.

Emergent laparotomy is indicated for those patients with obvious signs of peritoneal irritation or evisceration. Patients with hemodynamic instability in whom an abdominal injury is clearly the source should also be taken to the operating room. For unstable patients, particularly those with multisystem trauma, in whom intraabdominal injury is a possibility, management options include laparotomy, DPL, and FAST examination. A proposed algorithm is provided in Fig. 107.1.

The speed and sensitivity of the FAST examination for intraabdominal blood, if the immediate availability and expertise exist, make it possibly the best means of evaluation in the unstable blunt abdominal trauma patient. It can be performed in less than 2 minutes. A positive test in this setting mandates laparotomy. Management options of the unstable patient with a negative examination include a further search for nonabdominal sources of hemorrhage, DPL, a repeat FAST examination in

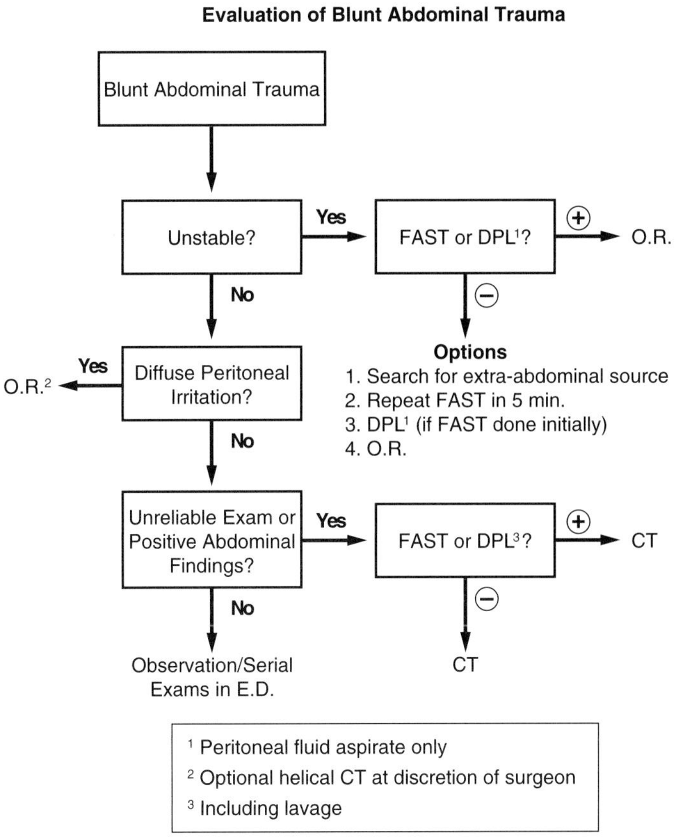

Figure 107.1. Evaluation of blunt abdominal trauma. *1,* peritoneal fluid aspirate only; *2,* optional helical CT at discretion of surgeon; *3,* including lavage.

5 minutes, or laparotomy. Obviously, these decisions must be made in concert with the surgeon.

For unstable patients in whom a FAST examination is not available, the peritoneal aspirate component of a DPL remains a useful tool. An initial aspirate of more than 5 mL of blood is an indication for surgery, and can be performed in a time frame similar to the FAST examination. In addition, Fabian and Croce[14] reported that in the presence of a negative aspirate, intraabdominal hemorrhage is an unlikely source of hemodynamic compromise.

In the truly unstable patient, it is impractical to continue with the complete lavage, because after a minimum of 10 minutes just to complete the procedure, definitive results must still await laboratory analysis. The physician's ability to estimate RBC counts based purely on visual inspection of lavage fluid has repeatedly been shown to be grossly inaccurate.[3,16] Despite the improved speed of the current generation of scanners, CT does not have a role in the persistently unstable victim of blunt abdominal trauma.

Stable Patients

For patients with blunt abdominal trauma and hemodynamic stability, either persistently or after initial resuscitation efforts, the approach to patient management is somewhat different (see Fig. 107.1). Victims of blunt abdominal trauma who are awake and alert, with a reliable, benign abdominal examination, can be followed clinically with serial examinations in the emergency department. For stable patients with positive abdominal findings, an unreliable examination, significant distracting injuries, possible retroperitoneal injury, or planned general anesthesia, abdominal CT is the diagnostic test of choice.[37]

Although an initial FAST examination can be done, a subsequent CT is indicated regardless of the results. If intraabdominal blood is visualized on FAST, CT will determine whether the underlying injury can be managed nonoperatively. CT of patients with a negative FAST examination may identify significant injuries that have not resulted in intraabdominal bleeding, particularly those in the retroperitoneum, pelvis, spine, and lower chest. In a situation in which there is no CT capability and no evidence of other injuries that would necessitate transfer, DPL should be performed. If transfer is inevitable, it should be arranged emergently and DPL performed at the discretion of the accepting surgeon. If DPL is done, it should not delay transfer, and the lavage fluid should accompany the patient.

Concomitant Head Injury

The greatest risk to a patient who has both a head injury and shock is death from uncontrolled intraabdominal bleeding. In patients who cannot be hemodynamically stabilized, diagnosis and management of uncontrolled intraabdominal hemorrhage takes precedence over neurosurgical imaging. Patients who are head injured with hypotension that is unresponsive to fluid administration should undergo a FAST examination (or DPL) in the emergency department. If the CT scanner is adjacent to the emergency department, and it is felt that the patient can tolerate a single cut through the lateral ventricles, this procedure may provide useful information to the neurosurgeon. If the patient's status, or the results of the FAST or DPL, warrant immediate laparotomy, the neurosurgeon should be present in the operating room to consider the placement of burr holes or an intraventricular bolt.

The patient with blunt abdominal trauma who is head injured but not hypotensive may undergo CT scanning of the head and abdomen. If the CT scan is positive for a neurosurgical lesion, surgery should not be delayed for a prolonged abdominal scan. In this case, a current generation spiral scanner may be used to perform an abdominal CT in less than 1 minute. If an older generation scanner is being used, the abdominal scan should be canceled. In this case, a FAST examination or DPL should be performed by the surgeon in the operating room as the patient undergoes craniotomy.

DISPOSITION

If there is no trauma team present and the patient is critically injured, the physician should notify the surgeon after performing the primary and secondary surveys and initiating resuscitative efforts. When in-house capability exists, the ultimate disposition of these patients with hemodynamic instability or significant injuries is straightforward. For stable patients who require evaluation by CT, although CT scanning is not 100% sensitive, two recent studies[6,21] indicate that patients with a normal CT scan and a brief period of observation in the emergency department can be safely discharged from the emergency department. However, it is worth noting that outcomes were measured only to 20 hours in one study and to 1 week in the other. Patients who are awake and alert, with a reliable, benign abdominal examination, can be followed clinically with serial abdominal examinations in the emergency department over a 4- to 6-hour period.

Transfer Considerations

Delay to operation is the primary cause of preventable deaths in patients with blunt abdominal trauma. At a very early stage, the emergency physician must determine whether a patient is a candidate for transfer. FAST examination or DPL may be the most expedient way to make this determination in a small rural hospital. However, the receiving institution may elect to have a patient transferred on the basis of the primary and secondary surveys alone, allowing the accepting surgeon to determine whether DPL, CT scanning, or further investigation is warranted.

If, on the basis of the initial assessment, the patient is a candidate for trauma center transfer, multiple investigative studies at the transferring hospital will only delay care. However, resuscitation efforts must be initiated prior to transfer, including attention to the ABCs, two large-bore intravenous lines, a Foley catheter, and a nasogastric or orogastric tube. A chest x-ray should be obtained and chest tubes placed for hemothorax or pneumothorax. The transferring physician must immobilize the neck and place the patient on a backboard. A cross-table lateral cervical spine film is helpful but not imperative, as patients should be immobilized during transport. Extremity x-rays are unnecessary prior to transfer; splint clinically apparent fractures, reduce dislocations if possible, and cover open fractures or dislocations with moist sterile gauze.

COMMON PITFALLS

- Failing to consult the surgeon early
- Attributing hypotension to extraabdominal causes, such as chest trauma, spinal shock, or external blood loss
- Failing to evaluate the abdomen in the patient with an unreliable examination
- Performing an abdominal CT scan in the hemodynamically unstable patient
- Delaying transfer while performing unnecessary studies

References

1. Adkinson C, Roller B, Clinton J, et al. A comparison of open peritoneal lavage with modified closed peritoneal lavage in blunt abdominal trauma. *Am J Emerg Med* 1989;7:352.
2. Amoroso TA. Evaluation of the patient with blunt trauma: an evidence based approach. *Emerg Med Clin North Am* 1999;17(1):63.
3. Bellows CF, Salomone JP, Nakamura SK, et al. What's black and white and red (read) all over? The bedside interpretation of diagnostic peritoneal lavage fluid. *Am Surg* 1998;64(2):112.
4. Boulanger BR, McLellan BA. *Emerg Med Clin North Am* 1996;14(1):151.
5. Branney SW, Wolfe RE, Moore EE, et al. Quantitative sensitivity of ultrasound in detecting free intraperitoneal fluid. *J Trauma* 1995;39(2):375.
6. Brasel KJ, Borgstrom DC, Kolewe KA, et al. Abdominal computed tomography scan as a screening tool in blunt trauma. *Surgery* 1996;120:780.
7. Breen DJ, Janzen DL, Zwirewich CV, et al. Blunt bowel and mesenteric injury: diagnostic performance of CT signs. *J Comput Assist Tomogr* 1997;21:706.
8. Buechter KJ, Arnold M, Martin L, et al. The use of serum amylase and lipase in evaluating and managing blunt abdominal trauma. *Am Surg* 1990;56:204.
9. Colucciello SA, Marx JA. Blunt abdominal trauma. In: Harwood-Nuss AL, et al., eds. *The clinical practice of emergency medicine,* 2nd ed. Philadelphia: Lippincott–Raven, 1996.
10. Cotter CP, Hawkins ML, Kent RB, et al. Ultrarapid diagnostic peritoneal lavage. *J Trauma* 1989;29:615.
11. Cushing BM, Clark DE, Cobean R, et al. Blunt and penetrating trauma—has anything changed? *Surg Clin North Am* 1997;77(6):1321.
12. Davis JW, Hoyt DB, Mackersie RC, et al. Complications in evaluating abdominal trauma: diagnostic peritoneal lavage versus computerized axial tomography. *J Trauma* 1990;30:1506.
13. Davis JW, Shackford SR, Holbrook TL. Base deficit as a sensitive indicator of compensated shock and tissue oxygen utilization. *Surg Gynecol Obstet* 1991;173:473.
14. Fabian TC, Croce MA. Abdominal trauma, including indications for celiotomy. *J Trauma* 1996;39:441.
15. Gomez GA, Alvarez R, Plasencia G, et al. Diagnostic peritoneal lavage in the management of blunt abdominal trauma: a reassessment. *J Trauma* 1987;27:1.
16. Gow KW, Haley LP, Phang PT. Validity of visual inspection of diagnostic peritoneal lavage fluid. *Can J Surg* 1996;39(2):114.
17. Healey MA, Simons RK, Winchell RJ, et al. A prospective evaluation of abdominal ultrasound in blunt trauma. Is it useful? *J Trauma* 1996;40:875.
18. Hubbard SG, Bivins BA, Sachatello CR, et al. Diagnostic errors with peritoneal lavage in parents with pelvic fractures. *Arch Surg* 1979;114:844.
19. Jehle D, Abrams B, Sukumvanich P, et al. Ultrasound for the detection of intraperitoneal fluid: the role of Trendelenburg position. *Acad Emerg Med* 1995;2(5):407.

20. Knottenbelt JD. Low initial hemoglobin levels in trauma patients: an important indicator for ongoing hemorrhage. *J Trauma* 1991;31:1396.
21. Livingston DH, Lavery RF, Passannante MR, et al. Admission or observation is not necessary after a negative abdominal computed tomography scan in patients with suspected blunt abdominal trauma: results of a prospective multi-institutional trial. *J Trauma* 1998;44:273.
22. Ma OJ, Mateer JR, Ogata M, et al. Prospective analysis of a rapid trauma ultrasound examination performed by emergency physicians. *J Trauma* 1995;38(6):879.
23. Mateer J, Plummer D, Heller M, et al. Model curriculum for physician training in emergency ultrasonography. *Ann Emerg Med* 1994;38:879.
24. Maull KI, Rozycki GS, Vinsant O, et al. Retroperitoneal injuries: pitfalls in diagnosis and management. *South Med J* 1987;80:1111.
25. McKenney MG, Martin L, Lentz K, et al. 1000 consecutive ultrasounds for blunt abdominal trauma. *J Trauma* 1996;40(4):607.
26. Melanson SW, Heller M. The emerging role of bedside ultrasonography in trauma care. *Emerg Med Clin North Am* 1998;16(1):165.
27. Mure AJ, Josloff R, Rothberg J, et al. Serum amylase determination and blunt abdominal trauma. *Am Surg* 1991;57:210.
28. Novelline RA, Rhea JT, Bell T. *Radiol Clin North Am* 1999;37(3):591.
29. Olsen WR, Hildreth DH. Abdominal paracentesis and peritoneal lavage. *J Trauma* 1971;11:824.
30. Rozycki GS, Ochsner MG, Jaffin JH, et al. Prospective evaluation of surgeons' use of ultrasound in the evaluation of trauma patients. *J Trauma* 1993;34(4):516.
31. Serck J, Shatney C, Sensaki K, et al. The accuracy of computed tomography in the diagnosis of blunt small bowel perforation. *Am J Surg* 1994;168:670.
32. Sherman JC, Delaurier GA, Hawkins ML, et al. Percutaneous peritoneal lavage in blunt trauma patients: a safe and accurate diagnostic method. *J Trauma* 1989;29:801.
33. Sriussadaporn S. CT scan in blunt abdominal trauma. *Injury* 1993;24:541.
34. Thal ER, May RA, Beesinger D. Peritoneal lavage: its unreliability in gunshot wounds of the lower chest and abdomen. *Arch Surg* 1980;115:430.
35. Thomas B, Falcone R, Vasquez D, et al. Ultrasound evaluation of blunt abdominal trauma: program implementation, initial experience and learning curve. *J Trauma* 1997;42:384.
36. Tiling T, Bouillon B, Schmid A, et al. Ultrasound in blunt abdominothoracic trauma. In: Border JR, et al., eds. *Blunt multiple trauma: comprehensive pathophysiology and care.* New York: Marcel Dekker Inc, 1990:415–433.
37. Wing VW, Federle MP, Morris JA, et al. The clinical impact of CT for blunt abdominal trauma. *AJR* 1985;145:1191.

CHAPTER 108

Penetrating Abdominal Trauma

Vicente H. Gracias and Kevin M. Curtis

The application of mandatory surgical exploration for penetrating abdominal injuries remains a firm surgical dictum, and was so for the greater part of this past century. Although occasionally performed by aggressive surgeons during the nineteenth century, laparotomy for penetrating wounds was infrequently used because of its uniformly poor outcome. Of note, during the U.S. Civil War, expectant management was the treatment of choice, with laparotomy reserved for penetrating wounds with evisceration.[16]

By the late 1800s, the folly of the noninterventional approach was better appreciated, yet surgical outcomes remained dismal.[3] During World War I, surgical exploration became more commonplace, and by World War II, surgical treatment had gained international acceptance,[1] with a survival rate of 75% for gunshot wounds to the abdomen.

The incidence of penetrating trauma continues to rise as our society becomes increasingly violent. A stab wound (SW) results from impalement by a sharp, narrow instrument, with injury depending on the depth and type of tissue traversed and being confined to the instrument's path.[10] A gunshot wound (GSW) carries significantly greater force, with injury and cavitation extending along, as well as radial to, the missile tract. The likelihood of peritoneal penetration is also dependent on the mode of injury. GSWs to the abdomen require surgical repair in 80% to 95% of patients, whereas SWs require laparotomy in only 25% to 33% of cases. Therefore, both mortality and the need for operative intervention are significantly higher for GSWs, which require a more aggressive management strategy.

The goal of triage and diagnosis in penetrating abdominal injury is expedience. Because of the wide range of scenarios and possible injuries, the emergency physician and trauma surgeon play critical roles in the treatment of these patients. The evaluation, resuscitation, and method of definitive diagnosis are dependent on the type of penetrating injury, the zone of penetration, and, most important, the hemodynamic status of the patient.

CLINICAL PRESENTATION

Although penetrating abdominal trauma is often considered relatively straightforward, its clinical patterns can be confusing. Not only is patient assessment frequently complicated by the presence of alcohol or drugs, but signs and symptoms can be lacking as well, despite the presence of major injury. The critical determinant in the initial assessment is the patient's overall status and hemodynamic stability. In the treatment of any patient with a penetrating traumatic injury and unstable vital signs, immediate surgical consultation must occur as resuscitation efforts are underway.

Evaluation of a penetrating injury to the abdomen requires an understanding of the anatomic zones of the abdomen, which aids in the prediction of underlying intraabdominal injuries.

Anterior abdomen: The zone demarcated by the costal margins to the inguinal ligaments and bordered by the anterior axillary lines is the anterior abdomen. This area of injury involves peritoneal structures in approximately one-third of cases. If the peritoneal cavity has been violated, one must assume internal injury has occurred, and steps should be taken to confirm or refute this assumption. Surgical consultation must be sought if peritoneal penetration has occurred.

Thoracoabdominal area: The zone demarcated by the nipples to the costal margin anteriorly and the scapular tips to the costal margin posteriorly is the thoracoabdominal region. Although the risk for intrathoracic injury in this area is obvious, it is equally important to recognize the possibility of intraabdominal and diaphragmatic injuries. All thoracoabdominal SWs should be evaluated with surgical consultation.

Flank: The zone demarcated by the costal margins to the iliac crests between the anterior and posterior axillary lines is the flank. Flank zone injuries are often difficult to evaluate because the physical examination can prove unreliable. In addition, there is often a delay from the time of injury to presentation. The higher risk of retroperitoneal injury and colonic injury necessitates the evaluation of flank wounds by means of computed tomography (CT) scan and possibly rectal contrast.

Back: The zone demarcated by the costal margins to the iliac crests between posterior axillary lines is the back. This area may be the most difficult to assess for intraperitoneal involvement. It is also more likely that there has been retroperitoneal injury in the event of penetrating back injury. As in flank wounds, the back zone often requires CT scanning for adequate assessment.

DIFFERENTIAL DIAGNOSIS

Unstable vital signs are typically the result of intracavitary hemorrhage, but tension pneumothorax, pericardial tamponade, or, in delayed presentation, sepsis can be causal factors. Rapid assessment as to zone of involvement, chest x-ray, and ultrasound are invaluable in delineating hemoperitoneum, tension pneumothorax, cardiac tamponade, and the likelihood of hypotension due to massive hemothorax. The main differential diagnosis depends on which structures are injured.

EMERGENCY DEPARTMENT EVALUATION AND MANAGEMENT

The principal tenet in the management of penetrating abdominal trauma is to discern the presence of organ injury that requires operation. Standard practices of resuscitation and stabilization prevail.

Stab Wounds

Peritoneal violation occurs in 50% to 70% of anterior abdominal SWs; laparotomy is required in approximately half of these cases. Therefore, only one-fourth to one-third of patients who sustain SWs to the anterior abdomen ultimately require operative intervention. Thus, diagnostic strategies are intended to separate those patients who require operation from those for whom expectant management will suffice. For this determination, serial clinical examinations, local wound exploration, diagnostic peritoneal lavage (DPL), CT, and laparoscopy are used as fundamental or complementary tools (Fig. 108.1).

Laparotomy Warranted

Certain clinical features portend a high likelihood of intraperitoneal pathology, but none is an absolute indicator of intraperitoneal injury.

Unstable vital signs: Patients with unstable vital signs are always surgical candidates. Surgical consultation is mandatory while proceeding with chest x-ray and ultrasound. Very few unstable patients with abdominal SWs are managed expectantly.

Gastrointestinal hemorrhage: Treat upper or lower gastrointestinal hemorrhage in the context of an abdominal SW with exploration of the abdomen. This finding usually signals perforation of the stomach or duodenum.

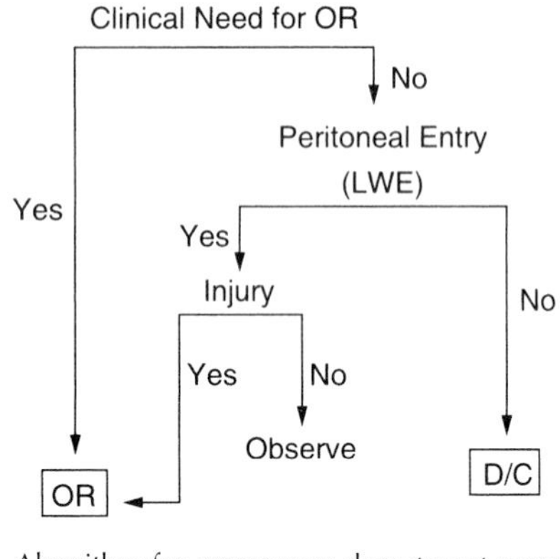

Figure 108.1. Algorithm for emergency department management of abdominal stab wounds. Most centers proceed to laparotomy if intraperitoneal injury is suspected. Further evaluation may be appropriate in selected cases. OR, operation; LWE, local wound exploration; D/C, discharge.

Evisceration: Coincident intraperitoneal injury requiring operation is found in approximately two-thirds of patients with omentum or bowel evisceration. Therefore, most institutions will explore evisceration on a mandatory basis. Some trauma centers with a large number of SW victims have managed these injuries with reduction of the evisceration in the emergency department and expectant observation. This approach should not be considered commonplace, nor attempted without surgical consultation.

Diaphragmatic injury: Thoracoabdominal SWs may cause injury to the diaphragm, which may or may not be seen on chest x-ray. If such injury is present, exploration is mandatory. Often, penetrating trauma inflicts small tears in the diaphragm, producing limited clinical or radiographic signs of injury.[4]

Peritoneal signs: The lack of sensitivity and specificity for peritoneal signs is well documented.

Implement in situ: The prevailing maxim is to remove implements *in situ* of the torso in the operating room.

Determination of Peritoneal Penetration

For those patients who do not satisfy any clinical requisites for laparotomy, the presence of peritoneal violation can be assessed by other means.

Free intraperitoneal air: The presence of free air on an upright chest or left lateral decubitus film establishes that the stabbing implement penetrated the peritoneal cavity and drew air in with it. It does not, however, establish that a hollow viscus injury has necessarily occurred.

Local wound exploration: Local exploration can be performed safely on the anterior abdomen only. A negative local wound exploration establishes that the end of an SW tract is anterior to rectus fascia, present only on the anterior abdominal wall. Such patients can be discharged from the emergency department after appropriate wound care.[5,19] An indeterminate local wound exploration must be considered positive. Patients who have multiple wounds or who pose technical obstacles, such as being massively obese, may not be candidates for this procedure.

CT scan: CT scans for SWs are particularly helpful in the case of injuries to the flank and back. In addition, after a penetrating abdominal wound, if CT reveals violation of the transversus abdominus muscle or the presence of a hematoma near the colon, surgical consultation and likely exploration are warranted.

Equivocal Findings of Peritoneal Penetration

At present, several diagnostic modalities are available to aid in the triage of patients who have sustained penetrating trauma with equivocal findings and possible intraperitoneal injury. Although the role of ultrasound is expanding rapidly, its primary use has been for visualization of the pericardial space in the rapid evaluation of upper abdominal and low chest penetration. As familiarity with this modality grows, it may become a more useful adjunct in other situations.

Diagnostic peritoneal lavage: DPL, although invasive, is rapid, generally considered safe, and carries a 90% to 95% accuracy rate for the discovery of intraperitoneal pathology.[6] Its main drawback is false-positive peritoneal aspiration results caused by drainage of free blood from the SW site into the peritoneal cavity. Debate remains as to the appropriate red blood cell (RBC) count to depict a positive study, with ranges from 5,000 to 25,000 RBCs.

Serial examination: Careful patient selection is required for serial examination. Although safely employed in trauma centers with large numbers of stabbing victims, it requires meticulous, ongoing observation, which may be impractical on a hectic trauma service.[8]

CT scan: The CT has become an integral diagnostic procedure following blunt trauma. It is excellent for detecting solid visceral injury, but is not as accurate in determining hollow viscus pathology, which predominates after penetrating trauma.[8] It is also insensitive for small diaphragmatic tears. As previously discussed, CT can be a valuable adjunctive tool where colorectal injury is more likely.[9]

Laparoscopy: Laparoscopy has been used with success as an intermediate step in discerning peritoneal penetration prior to formal exploratory laparotomy. Some trauma centers have espoused its usefulness for direct inspection of the diaphragm and certain solid viscera. Significant experience is required to render this approach reliable for hollow viscus injury, and only a limited number of centers have accepted this approach.[20]

Laparotomy: When there is any doubt as to the possibility of an internal injury, exploration by a surgical consultant should be sought.

Stab Wound—Special Cases

The chance of retroperitoneal injury is significantly greater after an SW to the flank and back than after one to the anterior wall. In addition, the risk of intraperitoneal organ injury ranges from 15% to 40% after SWs to these sites. Local wound exploration can be very difficult to perform in these areas because of the lack of a definite fascial plane of demarcation with the peritoneal cavity. DPL can discern the presence of intraperitoneal and diaphragmatic injury. The addition of rectal contrast to a standard double-contrast CT scan may be indicated for SWs to the low abdomen, flank, and back, where colorectal injuries are most likely. Because missed injuries to the diaphragm may eventually cause substantial morbidity and mortality, certain centers promote mandatory exploration to inspect the diaphragm when it is considered at risk, based on the wound entry site alone. Although exploratory laparotomy is the most sensitive technique of injury determination, it incurs the highest complication rate. Thus, laparoscopy, thoracoscopy, and DPL are more commonly employed to aid in diagnosing an injury prior to formal open laparotomy.

Gunshot Wounds

In most institutions, the determination of peritoneal violation by missile is enough to prompt laparotomy. A more comprehensive approach employs additional diagnostic tests, such as DPL, serial physical examinations, CT, and laparoscopy.[11,12] In contrast to SWs, multiple-organ and cavity entry is the rule in GSWs, with a mortality that is ten times greater. GSWs to the anterior abdomen incur peritoneal violation in 80% to 85% of patients, and, in this circumstance, laparotomy is required in 89% to 98%. Together, these data support a more conservative strategy, whereby laparotomy is the ultimate diagnostic procedure in most patients (Fig. 108.2).

Laparotomy Warranted

As with SWs to the abdomen, GSWs to the abdomen have accepted criteria for immediate surgical consultation and operation.

Unstable vital signs: Any victim of a GSW with unstable vital signs requires immediate surgical consultation. If the GSW is to the abdomen, there are relatively few cases that are managed outside the operating theater.

Gastrointestinal hemorrhage: As is true in the case of SWs, gastrointestinal bleeding in association with a GSW to the abdomen, flank, or back mandates surgical exploration.

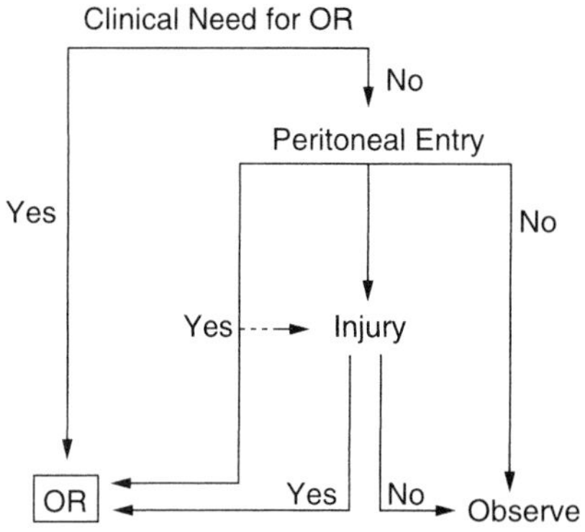

Figure 108.2. Algorithm for emergency department management of abdominal gunshot wounds. Most centers proceed to laparotomy if peritoneal entry is determined. Most centers proceed to laparotomy if intraperitoneal injury is suspected. Further evaluation may be appropriate in selected cases. OR, operation.

Evisceration: Because of the greater energy transference and cavitation that occurs with GSWs to the abdomen (compared with SWs), evisceration warrants surgical exploration.

Peritoneal signs: As with SWs, there is a well-documented lack of specificity of peritoneal signs with GSWs.

Determination of Peritoneal Penetration and Trajectory

Multiple studies have been conducted to assist with the determination of trajectory and thereby include or exclude peritoneal penetration following GSWs to the abdomen. Of these, CT and DPL have received the most attention, with a smaller number of studies evaluating laparoscopy.

CT scan: In patients with torso injuries, CT has been studied in an attempt to determine trajectory and avoid nontherapeutic invasive procedures.[4] There is evidence that, in this scenario, CT scan can be helpful in excluding peritoneal or transpelvic trajectories. This group of patients, however, is highly selective in that it accounts for less than 2% of all GSWs evaluated by the trauma service.[2] A more common use for CT, whether the standard or triple-contrast technique, is to provide information and assist in the management of select hemodynamically stable patients with penetrating trauma to the abdomen, flank, or pelvis.

Diagnostic peritoneal lavage: The use of DPL to exclude a transabdominal trajectory has been examined by Nagy et al.[13] at Cook County Hospital in Chicago. They retrospectively reviewed their use of DPL in 529 patients with GSWs in the vicinity of the abdomen and without a definite indication for surgery. Using a threshold of 10,000 RBC/μL to define a positive study, 150 patients were found to have a positive examination and underwent laparotomy, of which six had no evidence of peritoneal penetration or injury. Two patients had negative lavages but subsequently developed symptoms requiring surgical exploration. Both were found to have injuries that had been missed. With its limitations, DPL appears to offer adjunctive information in determining peritoneal penetration but is far from an ideal test for this diagnosis.

Laparoscopy: Likely indications for this procedure following penetrating trauma include determining peritoneal penetration and identifying injuries for either operative repair or those without need for further operative intervention. A minimally invasive exploration can proceed in a timely fashion, although it, too, has its liabilities. To date, laparoscopy's main use has been as a diagnostic procedure.[6,22]

Ultrasound: As familiarity grows with ultrasound in trauma, its use will invariably increase. There are currently at least two studies in progress in the United States that are looking into the role of ultrasound in penetrating abdominal trauma. At this point, there is no consensus as to its role, and it should probably not be employed outside of study protocols for abdominal GSWs.

Gunshot Wound—Special Cases

Nonoperative Management

As specific injury patterns are better understood and newer diagnostic modalities are incorporated into clinical practice, it is clear that not every patient with a penetrating abdominal injury requires surgery. A selective approach to nonoperative management for abdominal SWs was proposed a number of years ago[21] and has included a limited experience with a similar management protocol for abdominal GSWs.[15] This approach has received renewed interest,[14,17] partly because of improved understanding of the nontrivial morbidity associated with unnecessary abdominal explorations.[18] Patient physiology, reliability of examination, and availability of the patient and surgeon for reexamination all need to be factored in with immediate accessibility of an operating room. If these issues cannot be addressed satisfactorily, this method of management should not be attempted. GSWs of the low chest, flank, or back create the same issue as for SWs, and similar diagnostic strategies are in order.

DISPOSITION

Role of the Consultant

The earliest notification possible should be made to the on-call trauma surgeon, trauma team, and operating personnel. Information gleaned from prehospital communication alone can be sufficient to alert consultants.

Indications for Admission

After an SW, patients with a negative local wound exploration may be discharged after wound care and attention to toxicologic concerns. Patients who undergo an apparently negative DPL, CT, or laparoscopy should be held for 12 to 24 hours to ensure absence of injury resulting from the original mechanism or the diagnostic procedure.

It is rarely possible to determine with confidence that a low-velocity GSW is superficial. If there is doubt, a 12- to 24-hour observation period is necessary. High-velocity GSWs impose tremendous energies and can cause serious intraperitoneal damage despite an extraperitoneal course.

Transfer Considerations

Optimally, all patients with an SW or a GSW are triaged from the point of injury directly to a level I or a level II trauma center. When this does not occur, transfer to such a center at the earliest opportunity is advised. Only life-saving maneuvers such as endotracheal intubation, tube thoracostomy, pericardial aspiration, and fluid resuscitation are indicated before initiating transfer.

COMMON PITFALLS

- Failure of recognition. All patients with suspected trauma must be completely undressed and scrupulously examined. In penetrating trauma in particular, the scalp, axilla, and perineum easily hide narrow but deep and dangerous wounds. The examiner should not be swayed by prehospital or patient testimony or by the identification of a single site of penetration.
- Minimizing the injury. "It's probably OK," should never be stated. One must determine the severity of the injury and never assume it.
- Unnecessary delay. The speed with which operation is undertaken depends on the patient's clinical status. It may be appropriate to wait for serial examinations or the results of peritoneal lavage. However, transport to the operating suite must immediately follow resuscitation measures when a patient's status is precarious.
- Blind probing. Plunging digits and instruments into wound tracts is inaccurate and hazardous.
- Failure to observe. No patient should be summarily discharged without a complement of careful, repeated examinations, necessary diagnostic studies, or both. Presumption that a "negative" study, notably DPL or CT, warrants immediate discharge is incorrect. If the test was necessary, then an appropriate period of observation is necessary.
- Delay to consultation. It is wise to give an early warning to consultants. A timely operation should never be delayed because of a failure to notify consultants.
- Radiology. The most precarious place for a trauma patient is the radiology department. Be assured of proper monitoring and, if needed, recruit personnel to assist in observing patients in the radiology department and CT scanner.

ACKNOWLEDGMENT

The authors gratefully acknowledge the contribution of John A. Marx and Stephen Collucciello, who wrote the previous version of this chapter.

References

1. Bailey H, ed. *Surgery of modern warfare,* 3rd ed, vol. 2. Baltimore: Williams & Wilkins, 1944.
2. Ginzburg E, Carillo EH, Kopelman T, et al. The role of computed tomography in selective management of gunshot wounds to the abdomen and flank. *J Trauma* 1998;45:1005.
3. Grant HH. The practical management of bullet wounds of the abdominal viscera. *Trans South Surg Gynecol Assoc* 1899;2:37.
4. Grossman MD, May AK, Schwab CW, et al. Determining anatomic injury with computed tomography in selected torso gunshot wounds. *J Trauma* 1996;45:446.
5. Henneman PL, Marx JA, Moore EE. Diagnostic peritoneal lavage: accuracy in predicting necessary laparotomy following blunt and penetrating trauma. *J Trauma* 1990;30:1345.
6. Ivatury I, Simon RJ, Weksler B, et al. Laparoscopy in the evaluation of the intrathoracic abdomen after penetrating injury. *J Trauma* 1992;33:101.
7. Madden MR, Paull DE, Finkelstein JL, et al. Occult diaphragmatic injury from stab wounds to the lower chest and abdomen. *J Trauma* 1989;29:292.
8. Mariadason JG, Parsa MH, Ayuyao A, et al. Management of stab wounds to the thoracoabdominal region. *Ann Surg* 1988;207:335.
9. McAllister E, Perez M, Albrink MH, et al. Is triple contrast computed tomographic scanning useful in the selective management of stab wounds to the back? *J Trauma* 1994;37:401.
10. McCarthy MC, Lowdermilk GA, Canal DF, et al. Prediction of injury caused by penetrating wounds to the abdomen, flank and back. *Arch Surg* 1991;126:962.
11. Moore EE, Moore JB, Van Duzer-Moore S, et al. Mandatory laparotomy for gunshot wounds penetrating the abdomen. *Am J Surg* 1980;140:847.
12. Muckart DJJ, Abdool-Carrim ATO, King B. Selective conservative management of abdominal gunshot wounds: a prospective study. *Br J Surg* 1990;77:652.
13. Nagy KK, Krosner SM, Joseph KT, et al. A method of determining peritoneal penetration in gunshot wounds to the abdomen. *J Trauma* 1997;43:242.
14. Nance ML, Nance FC. It is time we told the emperor about his clothes. *J Trauma* 1996;40:185.
15. Nance F, Wennar M, Johnson L, et al. Surgical judgment in the management of penetrating wounds of the abdomen. *Ann Surg* 1974;179:639.
16. Otis GA. The medical and surgical history of the war of the rebellion, part 2, vol II. In: *Surgical history.* Washington, DC: U.S. Government Printing Office, 1877.
17. Renz BM, Feliciano DV. Gunshot wounds to the right thoracoabdomen: a prospective study of nonoperative management. *J Trauma* 1994;37:737.
18. Renz BM, Feliciano DV. The length of hospital stay after an unnecessary laparotomy for trauma: a prospective study. *J Trauma* 1996;40:187.
19. Rosenthal RE, Smith J, Walls RM, et al. Stab wounds to the abdomen: failure of blunt probing to predict peritoneal penetration. *Ann Emerg Med* 1987;16:172.
20. Salvino CK, Esposito TJ, Marshall WJ, et al. The role of diagnostic laparoscopy in the management of trauma patients: a preliminary assessment. *J Trauma* 1993;34:506.
21. Shaftan GW. Indications for operation in abdominal trauma. *Am J Surg* 1960;99:657.
22. Zantut LF, Ivatury RR, Smith RS, et al. Diagnostic and therapeutic laparoscopy for penetrating abdominal trauma: a multicenter experience. *J Trauma* 1997;442:825.

CHAPTER 109
Genitourinary Trauma

B. Tilman Jolly and Scott D. Weir

The approach to genitourinary (GU) trauma is an essential although frequently misunderstood component of the evaluation of blunt and penetrating trauma. GU injuries occur infrequently; when they do occur, they are usually associated with other multisystem trauma. It is frequently quoted that as many as 10% of acutely injured patients may have associated GU injuries.[27,32] Large-scale studies, however, have demonstrated an incidence of 1.5%[15] to 3.1%.[18]

GU injuries frequently may be overlooked because of their relative rarity and failure of the clinician to consider the diagnosis. The injury may be occult, and clues to suggest the possibility of GU trauma may lie in the mechanism of injury, or a constellation of associated injuries and physical findings identified during the secondary survey. Furthermore, GU injuries may be overshadowed by more dramatic and immediately life-threatening injuries. A systematic approach and thorough understanding of the available diagnostic modalities are necessary to efficiently and effectively evaluate GU injuries and provide complete information to urologic consultants.

This chapter focuses on trauma to both the upper (kidney and ureters) and lower (bladder and urethra) urinary tracts. Evaluation and management of upper and lower tract injuries are discussed separately because the mechanisms of injury and diagnostic modalities employed are unique to each. Considerations for both blunt and penetrating injuries are included.

UPPER URINARY TRACT

CLINICAL PRESENTATION

The kidneys and ureters lie in an anatomically sheltered vantage, secured in the retroperitoneum, beneath the lower ribs and musculature of the back. Therefore, injuries to the upper urinary tracts typically occur in the setting of high-energy multisystem trauma. Blunt force to the back, flank, or abdomen; falls from height; or, less commonly, rapid deceleration may result in injuries to the kidneys or ureters.[26] While hematuria may reveal an injury, it is not a reliably sensitive marker in isolation. Penetrating injury may be suggested by transaxial wounds or wounds in anatomic proximity. Penetrating injuries may account for 20% of renal injuries.[17]

DIFFERENTIAL DIAGNOSIS

Upper urinary tract injuries must be differentiated from myriad other blunt and penetrating injuries to the abdomen and pelvis. Upper tract injuries may occur alone. Much more commonly, however, the high-energy mechanisms that result in renal injuries concurrently produce associated bony, vascular, and visceral injuries that directly contribute to the observed morbidity and mortality.[15] In addition to aortic, splenic, and liver trauma, renal pedicle injuries must be considered as a cause of refractory hypotension following a fall from height or rapid-deceleration injury.[26] Traumatic injury to the ureters and kidneys may be suggested on the basis of the mechanism of injury, hematuria, or location of penetrating wounds.

Classification of upper tract injuries is by anatomic involvement and severity. This classification system reflects differences in clinical management. Eighty-five percent of patients suffering blunt renal trauma have only minor injuries that may be managed expectantly. Renal contusion is the most common of these minor injuries. Hematuria (microscopic or, less commonly, gross hematuria) and a normal renal outline, intact collecting system, in the absence of a perirenal hematoma, identify patients with renal contusions. Other minor injuries include ruptures of the renal fornix and shallow cortical lacerations not extending into the collecting system or deep medulla.[27,30]

Intermediate injuries comprise segmental vascular infarcts and deep lacerations of renal parenchyma. The depth of the laceration correlates with the risk of hemorrhage or extensive perirenal hematoma. Major injuries constitute only 5% of blunt injuries but as many as 50% of penetrating renal injuries. These include renal rupture, fractured or shattered kidney, renal pedicle injury, and avulsion of the renal pelvis.

Vascular pedicle injuries are more commonly associated with blunt trauma (75%) than with penetrating trauma (25%). Pedicle injuries typically imply an extremely high-energy mechanism, and are associated with multisystem trauma and a higher injury severity score.[7,26] Injuries include intimal tears and partial or complete tearing of the renal artery, vein, or segmental branches.

EMERGENCY DEPARTMENT EVALUATION

The emergency department evaluation of a multiply injured trauma patient begins with the standard advanced trauma life-support assessment and resuscitation. In this manner, immediately life-threatening injuries are identified and treated. Identifying and staging injuries to the upper urinary tracts within this high-risk population requires adjunctive radiographic studies. The emergency physician must determine the necessity of further evaluation and which diagnostic modalities to employ.

The first task is to identify those patients at risk for significant renal trauma requiring further evaluation. Mee et al.[28] published the influential article establishing criteria for the evaluation of blunt renal trauma. Their 10-year prospective study of 1,007 consecutive blunt trauma patients who underwent radiographic evaluation established markers associated with increased risk of major renal lacerations. Those were gross hematuria, microscopic hematuria (greater than 5 red blood cells [RBC]/HPF) with shock either in the prehospital setting or in the emergency department, or, less commonly, a history of significant deceleration without hematuria or shock. The authors concluded that if radiographic evaluation were limited to those patients, no significant renal injuries would have been missed. These guidelines have been supported by subsequent studies and have become the criteria defining the population of patients who require further radiographic evaluation.[7,12,18,29] It should be noted, however, that this schema is based on the assumption that patients with microscopic hematuria in the absence of any hemodynamic instability or high-energy mechanism are likely to have minor injuries that would be managed by simple observation.

Almost all authors advocate radiographic imaging in the setting of penetrating trauma to evaluate for upper urinary tract injuries, as a substantial percentage of patients may have significant injury in the absence of hematuria[2,6] (Table 109.1).

It has become convention that urine dipstick analysis for blood is used as a screening test for traumatic hematuria to identify those patients requiring further evaluation. This practice is based largely on the work of Daum and associates,[11] who demonstrated urine dipstick analysis to be 100% sensitive in

TABLE 109.1. Indications for Radiographic Evaluation

Penetrating trauma
Blunt trauma with gross hematuria
Blunt trauma with microscopic hematuria and hemodynamic instability (hypotension or tachycardia)
High-energy mechanism or suspected associated intraabdominal injuries

identifying patients with greater than 5 RBC/HPF by spun urine microscopy. Although the specificity was only 58%, these characteristics support the use of a urine dipstick as a screening test for hematuria. Other authors and subsequent studies have confirmed these findings.[19]

Computed tomography (CT) scan has largely supplanted intravenous pyelography (IVP) as the preferred diagnostic modality for evaluating the hemodynamically stable patient with blunt or penetrating trauma (Fig. 109.1). Several characteristics make CT the preferred modality. CT clearly defines parenchymal lacerations, hematomas, and the presence of urinary extravasation and may identify renal vascular injuries. Furthermore, the findings of IVP, when abnormal, are frequently nonspecific and require CT scan to better define the extent of the renal injury.[4,6,15,18,27] Finally, as previously described, patients at risk for blunt or penetrating injuries to the upper GU tract have incurred a high-energy mechanism and have a high incidence of associated bony, visceral, and vascular injury. These associated injuries may have direct bearing on the operative or nonoperative management. CT scan is required to adequately assess and stage these associated injuries.

IVP still has a distinct role in the evaluation of the unstable patient requiring resuscitation or immediate operative intervention who is not a candidate for CT scan. It may be done during the acute resuscitation or in the operating room. A bolus of contrast media is injected intravenously (2 mL/kg to a maximum of 100 mL). An anterior–posterior (AP) abdominal radiograph is then obtained 5 minutes after contrast bolus. In this setting, IVP may confirm the presence of bilateral kidneys, and may suggest the extent of the injury.

The most significant findings are either nonfunctional renal unit or extravasation of urine. Nonfunction suggests extensive trauma to the kidney, pedicle injury, or severely shattered kidney. Extravasation of contrast material implies trauma involving the capsule, parenchyma, and collecting system. Other findings are less reliable and require additional evaluation and staging.[2]

Arteriography is reserved for stable patients requiring further clarification of pedicle injuries, following equivocal CT findings. Arteriography may demonstrate intimal tears and complete or partial disruption of the renal vasculature. CT findings requiring further evaluation by arteriography include large perirenal hematoma, major renal fractures, or segmental areas of nonenhancement. Penetrating trauma with renal laceration or retroperitoneal hematoma requires arteriography because of the high risk of associated renal vascular injury.[13] Small hematomas do not require further evaluation. A hypotensive patient requires surgical intervention, and further studies may be delayed until the patient is stabilized. Nonenhancement of the kidney on CT scan is diagnostic of renal artery thrombosis and is sufficient indication for surgery without additional studies.[7,8]

The role of magnetic resonance imaging (MRI) and ultrasound remains limited. Several studies have suggested that the performance of MRI approximates that of CT scan. The additional time and expense required limit its clinical application.[20,21] Ultrasound has performed poorly in the evaluation of patients with suspected injuries to the upper GU tract[35] (Table 109.2).

Ureteral injury remains a diagnostic dilemma. A third of ureteral injuries are not identified on initial evaluation. Hematuria was present in only 63% of patients with no other GU injuries. This underscores the lack of reliability of hematuria in identifying isolated ureteral trauma. The most successful means of identification were surgical exploration and retrograde pyelography. IVP and CT were diagnostic in only a third of cases.[5]

EMERGENCY DEPARTMENT MANAGEMENT

The principles of care for the patient with multisystem trauma apply equally to the patient with trauma to the upper GU tract. Crystalloid and blood products are indicated for hemodynamic instability.

The most contentious issue remains which patients require operative intervention and which may be managed nonopera-

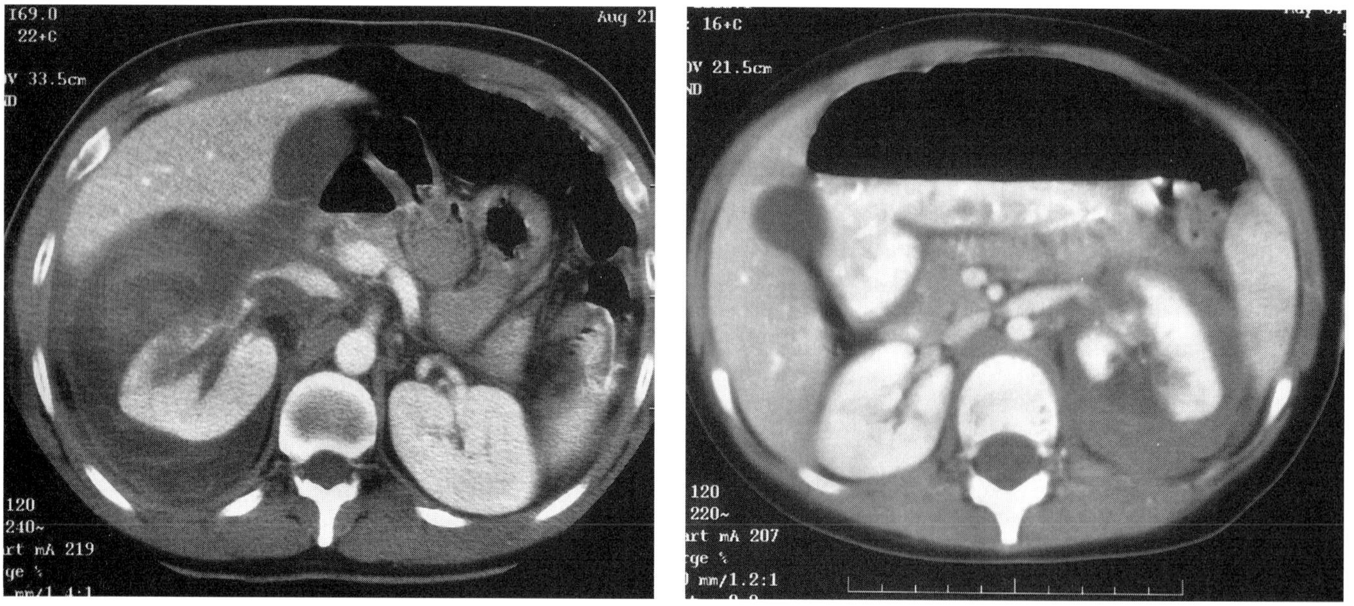

A B

Figure 109.1. **(A, B)** Renal laceration with perirenal hematoma.

TABLE 109.2. Diagnostic Modalities for Evaluating Upper Tract Injuries

Diagnostic Modalities	Advantages	Disadvantages
CT scan	Study of choice in blunt trauma Most sensitive/specific Better staging information Evaluation for other associated injuries	Requires stable patient Commonly misses ureteral injury May incompletely identify vascular pedicle injuries
IVP	Rapid and readily available for unstable patients Useful as screening test in patients with isolated renal trauma	Nonspecific findings require additional studies Hypotension may preclude adequate visualization Commonly misses ureteral injury May miss minor injuries
Angiography	Gold standard for vascular pedicle injuries	Requires stable patient Invasive and time consuming
MRI	Performance may equal that of CT scan Can be used in iodine-allergic patients	Time consuming Expensive

tively (Table 109.3). It is generally accepted that patients with minor injuries (grades I and II) may be managed nonoperatively. It is generally accepted that patients with renovascular injuries, shattered kidneys, extensive urinary extravasation, or an unconfined, expanding, or pulsatile hematoma require early surgical intervention (grade V).

There is less universal agreement concerning other major injuries (grades III and IV). There is an increasing trend toward nonoperative management. Several authors have reported series of selective nonoperative management of major renal injuries.[15,24,26,27] In general, the majority of blunt renal trauma may be managed nonoperatively. Delayed interventions may be necessary in a subset of patients managed nonoperatively. Those most likely to require delayed intervention include those demonstrating extravasation of urine, devitalized renal segments, or both, on initial CT scan. Recent advances in percutaneous and endourologic techniques have decreased the morbidity of these complications.[24,32]

There is a lower threshold for operative exploration and intervention in penetrating trauma. Most penetrating injuries are explored and repaired. Ureteral injuries are repaired surgically and stented, or repaired in a staged fashion.[1,2]

DISPOSITION

Patients with microscopic hematuria in the absence of any hemodynamic instability, or an isolated renal contusion demonstrated on CT scan without other injuries, may be discharged with follow-up repeat urinalysis. An isolated renal injury is, however, uncommon. Most patients with blunt renal injuries will have associated injuries requiring admission. All patients with penetrating renal or ureteral trauma require admission or transfer to a facility capable of providing definitive diagnostic and therapeutic care.

TABLE 109.3. Grading System for Renal Injuries[a]

MINOR INJURIES
Grade I: Contusions and contained subcapsular hematomas Grade II: Nonexpanding perirenal hematomas and cortical lacerations
MAJOR INJURIES
Grade III: Parenchymal lacerations into the corticomedullary junction and thrombosis of a segmental artery without an associated parenchymal laceration Grade IV: Renal lacerations involving segmental renal vessels, lacerations violating the collecting system, and contained injuries to the renal vessels Grade V: Avulsion of the renal hilum, thrombosis of the main renal artery, shattered kidney

[a]American Association for the Surgery of Trauma Grading System.

COMMON PITFALLS

- In the setting of acute traumatic injury, remember to consider kidney and ureteral trauma as potentially concurrent or occult injuries.
- In the absence of hematuria, upper tract injury must not be ruled out on that basis alone. While most patients with significant blunt injury requiring intervention will demonstrate gross hematuria or microscopic hematuria with hypotension, patients with renal pedicle injury or penetrating trauma resulting in ureteral injury may not demonstrate hematuria.
- In the setting of penetrating trauma, ruling out significant injury based on a suboptimal local flank wound exploration. If the wound is suspicious and in anatomic proximity, the patient requires further diagnostic evaluation.

LOWER URINARY TRACT

CLINICAL PRESENTATION

Blunt trauma to the lower urinary tract (bladder and urethra) is usually associated with pelvic rami fractures and symphyseal diastasis. Anterior urethral injuries (penile and bulbous urethra below the urogenital diaphragm) are associated with self-instrumentation, falls, and straddle injuries. Posterior urethral injuries (membranous and prostatic urethra above the urogenital diaphragm) commonly accompany pelvic fractures. As the urinary continence mechanism and autonomic innervation responsible for erection are contained in the posterior urethra, posterior urethral injuries may result in permanent incontinence and erectile dysfunction. Signs of anterior urethral injury depend on the integrity of Buck's fascia. If this fascial layer is torn, blood and urine may pass into the penis, scrotum, and abdominal wall.

A mechanism of injury suggestive of pelvic ring disruption, pelvic tenderness, or instability, or radiographic findings further define the population at risk for lower tract injury. Clinical signs such as blood at the urethral meatus, high-riding prostate, scrotal hematoma, hematuria, or difficulty voiding may be directly suggestive of lower tract injury. These signs may be absent in as many as 57% of patients with urethral injury.[23]

Extraperitoneal bladder injuries are most commonly associated with pelvic fractures and bladder laceration by bony fragments. Extraperitoneal bladder injury less commonly may occur alone. Intraperitoneal bladder injuries result from compressive forces in the presence of a full bladder, and rupture occurs at the dome of the bladder.

As with penetrating trauma to the upper GU tract, penetrating injuries to the lower tract are suggested by location of wounds. Any penetration of the lower abdominal wall in the region of the pelvis raises the possibility of urinary tract injury. Given the variability of projectile tract, any gunshot wound in the region should include consideration of GU tract injury.

DIFFERENTIAL DIAGNOSIS

The primary differential of lower urinary tract injury is that of hematuria due to upper tract injury. The emergency physician, trauma surgeon, or urologist must determine whether the bleeding originates from the urethra, bladder, ureter, kidneys, or some combination of sources.

EMERGENCY DEPARTMENT EVALUATION

The fundamental principle in the approach to traumatic GU injuries dictates that the urinary tract be evaluated from lower to upper sequentially. Therefore, once the potential for injury has been identified based on mechanism of injury, physical findings, and/or radiographic evidence of associated high-risk injuries, the urethra should be evaluated first. It is important that the presence of urethral injury be ruled out prior to catheter placement, because catheter placement may potentially convert a partial urethral tear to a complete urethral disruption. The diagnostic modality for evaluating the urethra is the retrograde urethrogram.

The study is done with the patient supine to avoid moving the patient (oblique views, advocated by some authors, add little and risk disrupting a retroperitoneal hematoma). A preinjection KUB is obtained for comparison. A Foley catheter is then passed approximately 1 to 2 cm to the fossa navicularis, and the balloon is inflated with 1 to 2 mL of saline. Alternatively a 60-cc Toomey syringe with Christmas tree or Cooke adapter may be gently inserted until snug. Lateral traction is applied to the penis to avoid the column effect, and 60 mL of water-soluble contrast material is injected over 30 to 60 seconds. The radiograph is exposed as the last 10 mL of contrast material is injected.[38]

Extravasation of contrast material or failure of contrast material to reach the bladder is diagnostic of urethral injury, mandates urologic consultation, and precludes the passage of a urethral catheter by the emergency physician (Fig. 109.2).

If a team member places a urinary catheter prior to adequate evaluation for urethral injury, *do not remove it*. It is not necessary to remove the catheter to perform a retrograde urethrogram. Instead, document the presence or absence of urethral injury by passing a small feeding tube beside the catheter and performing a modified retrograde urethrogram.[38]

Following assessment of the urethra, evaluate the bladder. Extraperitoneal bladder rupture is more common and is typically associated with pelvic fracture. Intraperitoneal bladder rupture may result from compressive forces in the presence of a distended bladder. The retrograde cystogram is the most reli-

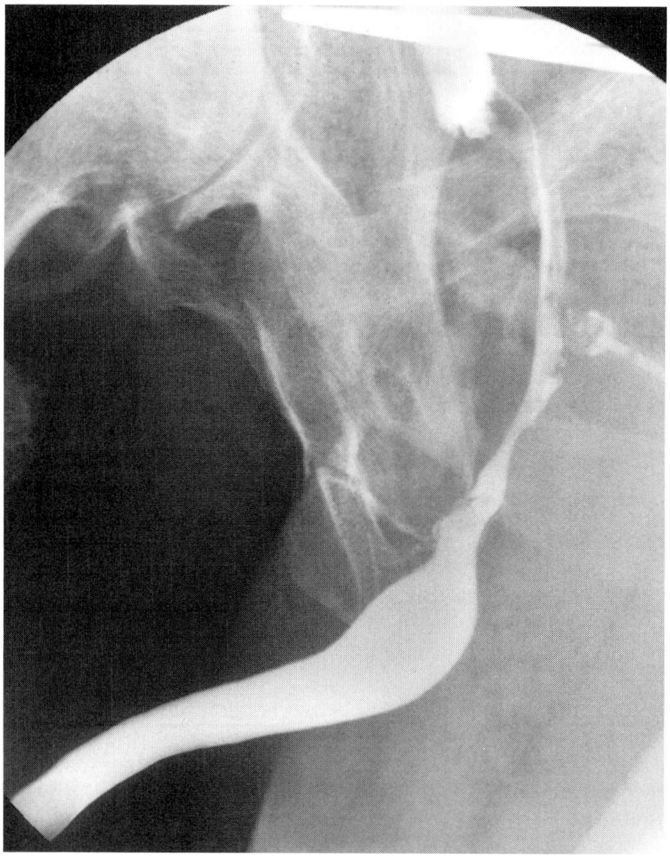

Figure 109.2. Retrograde urethrogram with partial tear of membranous urethra.

able study for evaluating bladder injuries. After exclusion of urethral injury and placement of catheter, retrograde cystography is obtained as follows: Obtain a precontrast KUB for comparison. Then instill radiocontrast dye under gravity through the catheter until a total of 400 mL of contrast is instilled. Then clamp the Foley catheter and obtain a full-bladder AP radiograph.

If bladder contraction occurs prior to administration of 400 mL, contrast refluxes into the Toomey syringe. Simply wait a few minutes and then reintroduce the contrast material to the volume that stimulated contraction previously. Then gently administer an additional 50 mL, clamp the catheter, and similarly obtain a full-bladder AP radiograph.[38]

Then allow the bladder to empty, and obtain postvoid radiographs. In the presence of intraperitoneal rupture, contrast material will extravasate, outlining intraperitoneal structures. In the presence of extraperitoneal rupture, contrast material will extravasate at the pubic symphysis or pelvic outlet.

Take care to avoid spillage of contrast externally, which may produce false-positive findings or obscure the findings. Multiple studies have demonstrated false-negative cystography due to insufficient contrast material (less than 400 cc), particularly in penetrating trauma, in which inadequate distension of the bladder may allow a tenuous seal of a penetrating wound, thereby failing to demonstrate extravasation of contrast.[3,38]

Cystography remains the standard for evaluating the bladder, although a CT scan with retrograde contrast may be useful in patients undergoing CT for other indications (Fig. 109.3).This is simply done by instilling contrast in a similar retrograde fashion prior to imaging. Intraperitoneal rupture results in contrast dye within the peritoneum. Extraperitoneal rupture may be more difficult to visualize but may be evident on pelvic cuts.[3,14]

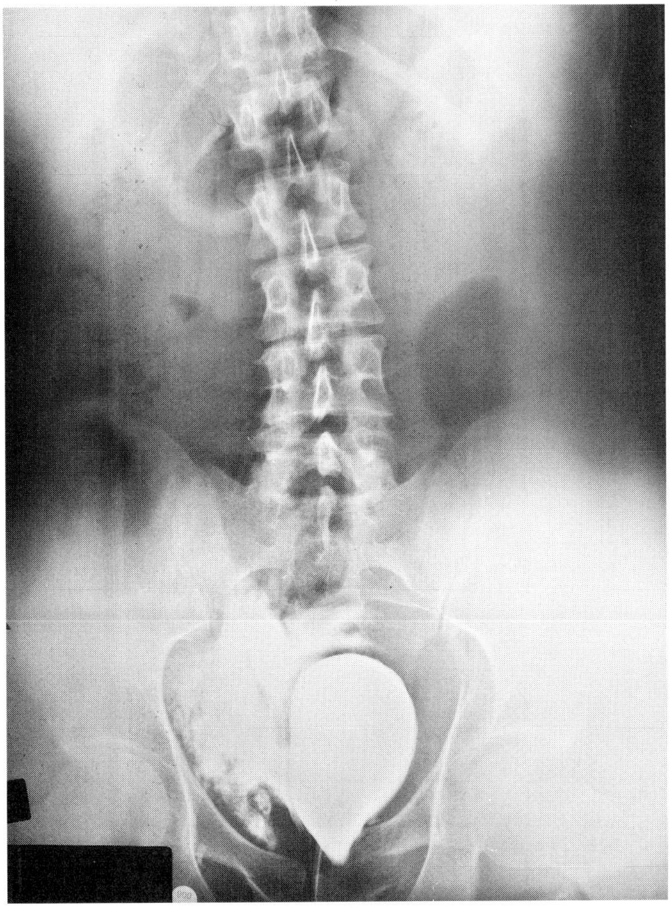

Figure 109.3. Cystogram with extraperitoneal bladder rupture.

Penetrating trauma to the pelvis presents numerous therapeutic challenges, but the diagnostic approach is relatively straightforward. Any and all structures at risk because of their anatomic proximity to the injury need to be evaluated, including the bladder, the urethra, the vasculature, and the gastrointestinal tract.

EMERGENCY DEPARTMENT MANAGEMENT

Once a urethral or bladder injury is identified, the emergency physician must take steps to manage the injury while continuing to address immediate life-threatening injuries. Patients subject to high-energy mechanisms responsible for urinary tract injury are also at risk for serious intraabdominal injuries.

If a urethral disruption is identified, a suprapubic cystostomy should be performed to allow drainage of the bladder. This may be done in the resuscitation bay if the patient is stable. If the patient is unstable and requires operative intervention for associated injuries, it may be done in the operating room. If a catheter was placed prior to identifying the injury, it should be left in place. Occasionally, a catheter may be placed through a partial urethral tear. Once the partial disruption is identified, however, any gentle and limited attempts at urethral catheterization should be done by a urologist.

The acute management of bladder rupture is bladder drainage via Foley catheter. Patients with intraperitoneal bladder rupture undergo primary surgical repair. Those patients with extraperitoneal bladder rupture are typically managed nonoperatively, with simple urinary drainage by Foley catheter or cystostomy. If, however, the patient is undergoing exploratory laparotomy for another indication, some authors advocate primary repair at that time.[3,10,36]

DISPOSITION

All patients with injuries to the lower GU tract require hospital admission or transfer to a facility capable of managing these injuries and their potential complications. Early involvement of urologic consultants and good communication between the emergency physician, urologic consultant, and trauma surgeons are essential to the global management of the patient. It is also worth remembering that extremely painful injuries, such as pelvic fractures, may mask other serious injuries, including cervical spine and thoracoabdominal injuries.

COMMON PITFALLS

- Placing a Foley catheter before adequately ruling out urethral injury risks converting a partial tear to a complete disruption. However, if the catheter was placed before radiographic evaluation, to rule out urethral injury, do not remove the catheter to perform a urethrogram.
- Insufficient contrast dye administered during retrograde cystogram may fail to adequately distend the bladder to demonstrate extravasation.
- Allowing spillage of contrast dye externally may obscure radiographic findings on retrograde cystogram.

INJURIES TO THE MALE GENITALIA

Intentional amputation of the penis has been reported and has received a great deal of media attention. There have been several reported cases of successful microvascular reimplantation. Successful repair depends on the condition of the severed part and ischemic time. In the prehospital and emergency setting, the amputated penis should be preserved in a manner similar to that for other amputated parts. Prompt urologic and microvascular consultation is imperative for successful reimplantation.[40]

The incidence of penetrating trauma to the external genitalia resulting from gunshot wounds and stabbing has been increasing (Fig. 109.4). Penetrating trauma to the external genitalia mandates early surgical exploration and conservative debride-

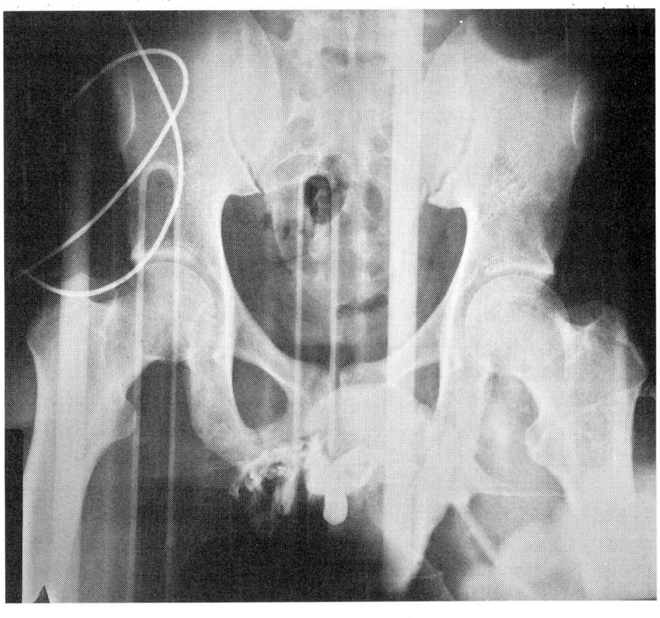

Figure 109.4. Gunshot wound—retrograde urethrogram with extravasation at penile urethra.

ment, followed by, in most cases, primary repair. Most patients require a retrograde urethrogram to rule out urethral injury. Some patients with minimal injury may be candidates for nonoperative management, but delayed complications are not uncommon. The majority of patients with penile trauma will retain erectile and urinary function.[9,16]

Penile fracture most commonly occurs during overzealous vaginal intercourse, although several other mechanisms have been reported. The fracture involves rupture of the tunica albuginea of the corporal body. Authors have advocated operative repair, proposing that it may decrease the incidence of erectile deformity and may speed recovery. There is, however, no accepted standard of treatment.[37] Entrapment of the penis in a zipper occurs most often in uncircumcised young boys. Nolan and associates[33] described the successful atraumatic removal by cutting the median bar of the zipper with bone cutters. The upper and lower shields of the zipper device separate, releasing the skin with minimal injury. Penile incarceration may be managed by the string technique, similar to that described for removal of rings from fingers.[39]

The evaluation of blunt scrotal trauma can be clinically challenging. Suspicion of testicular rupture should prompt timely urologic consultation, as surgical repair within 72 hours dramatically improves the salvage rate. Several studies have suggested that ultrasound may be useful in the evaluation of acute scrotal trauma, by identifying patients for surgical exploration.[22,25,34] A small series has questioned its diagnostic accuracy, although a normal scrotal ultrasound had a high negative predictive value in a high-risk population.[31] The role of ultrasound in the evaluation of blunt scrotal trauma requires further study.

References

1. Azimuddin K, Ivantury R, Porter J, et al. Damage control in a trauma patient with ureteric injury. *J Trauma* 1997;43:977.
2. Baniel J, Schein M. The management of penetrating trauma to the urinary tract. *J Am Coll Surg* 1994;178:417.
3. Bodner DR, Selzman AA, Spirnak JP. Evaluation and treatment of bladder rupture. *Semin Urol* 1995;13:62.
4. Bretan PN, McAnnich JW, Federle MP, et al. Computerized tomographic staging of renal trauma: 85 consecutive cases. *J Urol* 1986;136:561.
5. Campbell EW, Filderman PS, Jacobs SC. Ureteral injury due to blunt and penetrating trauma. *Urology* 1992;40:216.
6. Carlin CI, Resnick M. Indications and techniques for urologic evaluation of the trauma patient with suspected urologic injury. *Semin Urol* 1995;13:9.
7. Carroll PR, McAninch JW. Staging of renal trauma. *Urol Clin North Am* 1989;16:193.
8. Cass AS, Luxenberg M. Accuracy of CT in diagnosing renal artery injuries. *Urology* 1989;34:249.
9. Cline KJ, Mata JA, Venable DD, et al. Penetrating trauma to the male external genitalia. *J Trauma* 1998;44:492.
10. Corriere JN, Sandler CM. Management of extraperitoneal bladder rupture. *Urol Clin North Am* 1989;16:275.
11. Daum GS, Krolikowski FJ, Reuter KL, et al. Dipstick evaluation of hematuria in abdominal trauma. *Am J Clin Pathol* 1988;89:538.
12. Eastham JA, Wilson TG, Ahlering TE. Radiographic assessment of blunt renal trauma. *J Trauma* 1991;31:1527.
13. Federle MP, Brown TR, McAninch JW. Penetrating renal trauma: CT evaluation. *J Comput Assist Tomogr* 1987;2:1026.
14. Gay SB, Sistrom CL. CT evaluation of blunt abdominal trauma. *Radiol Clin North Am* 1992;30:367.
15. Goff CD, Colin GR. Management of renal trauma at a rural, level 1 trauma center. *Am Surg* 1998;64:226.
16. Goldman HB, Dmochowski RR, Cox CE. Penetrating trauma to the penis: functional results. *J Urol* 1996;155:551.
17. Guerriero WG. Etiology, classification, and management of renal trauma. *Surg Clin North Am* 1988;68:1071.
18. Herschorn S, Radomski SB, Shoskes DA, et al. Evaluation and treatment of blunt renal trauma. *J Urol* 1991;146:274.
19. Kennedy TJ, McConnell JD, Thal ER. Urine dipstick vs. microscopic urinalysis in the evaluation of abdominal trauma. *J Trauma* 1988;28:615.
20. Leppaniemi A, Lamminen A, Tervahartiala P, et al. Comparison of high-field magnetic resonance imaging with computed tomography in the evaluation of blunt renal trauma. *J Trauma* 1995;38:420.
21. Leppaniemi A, Lamminen A, Tervahartiala P, et al. MRI and CT in blunt renal trauma: an update. *Semin Ultrasound CT MR* 1997;18:129.
22. Lewis CA, Michell MJ. The use of realtime ultrasound in the management of scrotal trauma. *Br J Radiol* 1991;64:792.
23. Lowe FC, Fishman EK, Oesterling JE. CT in diagnosis of bladder rupture. *Urology* 1989;33:341.
24. Mansi MK, Alkhudair WK. Conservative management with percutaneous intervention of major blunt renal injuries. *Am J Emerg Med* 1997;15:633.
25. Martinez-Piñeiro L, Cerezo E, Cozar JM, et al. Value of testicular ultrasound in the evaluation of blunt scrotal trauma without haematocele. *Br J Urol* 1992;69:286.
26. Matthews LA, Smith EM, Spirnak JP. Nonoperative treatment of major blunt renal lacerations with urinary extravasation. *J Urol* 1997;157:2056.
27. Matthews LA, Spirnak JP. The nonoperative approach to major blunt renal trauma. *Semin Urol* 1995;13:77.
28. Mee SL, McAninch JW, Robinson AL, et al. Radiographic assessment of renal trauma: a 10-year prospective study of patient selection. *J Urol* 1989;141:1095.
29. Miller KS, McAnnich JW. Radiographic assessment of renal trauma: our 15 year experience. *J Urol* 1995;154:352.
30. Moore EE, Shockford SR, Pachter HL, et al. Organ injury scaling: spleen, liver and kidney. *J Trauma* 1989;29:1664.
31. Mulhall JP, Gabram SG, Jacobs LM. Emergency management of blunt testicular trauma. *Acad Emerg Med* 1995;2:639.
32. Nguyen HT, Carroll PR. Blunt renal trauma: renal preservation through careful staging and selective surgery. *Semin Urol* 1995;13:83.
33. Nolan JF, Stillwell TJ, Sands JP Jr. Acute management of the zipper-entrapped penis. *J Emerg Med* 1990;8:305.
34. Pantil MG, Onora VC. The value of ultrasound in the evaluation of patients with blunt scrotal trauma. *Injury* 1994;25:177.
35. Perry MJ, Porte ME, Urwin GH. Limitations of ultrasound evaluation in closed renal trauma. *J R Coll Surg Edinb* 1997;42:420.
36. Peters PC. Intraperitoneal rupture of the bladder. *Urol Clin North Am* 1989;16:279.
37. Ruckle HC, Hadley HR, Lui PD. Fracture of penis: diagnosis and management. *Urology* 1992;40:33.
38. Schneider RE. Genitourinary trauma. *Emerg Med Clin North Am* 1993;11:137.
39. Vahasarja VJ, Hellstrom PA, Serlo W, et al. Treatment of penile incarceration by the string method: two case reports. *J Urol* 1993;149:372.
40. Wells MD, Boyd JB, Bulbul MA. Penile replantation. *Ann Plast Surg* 1991;26:577.

CHAPTER 110
Peripheral Vascular Injuries

Peter T. Pons

Prompt recognition and management of peripheral vascular injuries are crucial to limb salvage and preservation of function. Penetrating trauma accounts for approximately 85% of vascular injuries; blunt trauma and iatrogenic causes are responsible for the rest. Until the advent and widespread use of antibiotics, these wounds were treated by ligation or amputation. Once infection could be controlled, the already developed methods of primary vessel repair were used and are now the mainstay of management.

Vascular injury may result from direct or indirect trauma. Direct injury may produce partial or complete transection, contusion, laceration, or arteriovenous fistula. Indirect injury may cause spasm, external compression, mural contusion, thrombosis, or aneurysm formation. The vessels most often involved are the brachial and axillary arteries in the upper extremity and the femoral and popliteal arteries in the lower extremity.

Vascular damage should be suspected in penetrating trauma when the penetrating object has traversed the path of a vessel or is in proximity to one. Blunt vascular injury may be subtler in presentation. Stretching, tearing, or shearing forces may damage a vessel, yet leave little external evidence. The classic example is dislocation of the knee, with associated popliteal artery injury. Failing to recognize this complication frequently leads to amputation of the leg, which can be prevented by appropriate evaluation. The emergency physician must obtain a careful, complete history and be aware of the mechanics that may produce vascular injury, even if there are no or few physical findings that suggest vessel damage.

CLINICAL PRESENTATION

The most obvious sign of arterial injury is profuse, spurting red blood. Venous laceration may be manifested by a continuous flow of dark blood, which also may be profuse. Significant blood loss may produce shock. However, many vascular injuries, either blunt or penetrating in origin, appear relatively innocuous at first glance. Penetrating wounds of an extremity can present with a small entrance site that harbors significant underlying vascular damage. Blunt injury may be quite misleading because of few obvious external signs. The vessel wound, either arterial or venous, may produce a significant hematoma. Occasionally, a pulsatile mass is felt.

The absence of a palpable pulse distal to the site of injury in a normotensive patient is pathognomonic of vessel injury. However, the presence of a pulse does not exclude a significant wound. Collateral circulation or transmitted pressure waves through a small clot or intimal flap can produce a distal pulse, misleading the unwary physician. A patient in shock must have repeated examinations to assess vascular status, as the physical findings may change as the patient is resuscitated. The presence of a palpable thrill or bruit suggests an arteriovenous fistula. Comparison of blood pressure using a Doppler in the injured and uninjured extremities, or in the injured extremity compared with an arm, can be helpful.[9] If the ratio of the blood pressures is less than 0.9 to 1.0, vascular injury is suggested.[9,12] In addition, an arm/ankle (ABI) blood pressure comparison is also useful: the ankle blood pressure should be equal to or greater than the arm (brachial) pressure. If these blood pressure comparisons are abnormal, arteriography is indicated.

Classic signs of arterial compromise of an extremity have been described as "the five P's": pallor, pulselessness, pain, paresthesias, and paralysis. Additional findings may include tenseness of the extremity, coolness to touch, and delayed capillary refill (greater than 3 seconds). Unfortunately, some of these signs require a patient who can relate these complaints, and many multiply injured patients cannot. In addition, concomitant neurologic injury of the extremity may present with similar findings. Careful examination is necessary to differentiate the paresthesias of vascular insufficiency from those of neurologic injury. As many as 70% of upper and 30% of lower extremity vascular injuries have associated nerve damage, of which 40% to 45% result in permanent deficit.

Doppler examination of distal blood flow can assist in the evaluation of patients with swelling, hematoma, displaced fractures, or obesity. Pulse deficits and limb comparisons can be performed with greater sensitivity using the Doppler device.

Finally, the structural integrity of the skeletal system must be evaluated. About 18% of patients with peripheral vascular injuries have an associated fracture.

A growing body of literature documents the importance and value of the physical examination in determining the presence or absence of a peripheral vascular injury.[4,5,8]

EMERGENCY DEPARTMENT EVALUATION

The mainstay of evaluation and diagnosis has been contrast arteriography. However, if the peripheral pulse is absent, obvious signs of major vessel injury are present (i.e., pulsatile hemorrhage), or the location of the injury is apparent from physical examination, immediate surgery is indicated and should not be delayed for radiographic imaging unless the location of the vessel injury cannot be determined clinically. Angiography has been used in patients with so-called soft signs of vascular injury and in those with wound trajectories in proximity to a major vessel but without obvious signs of damage. Arteriography is 97% to 99% sensitive in detecting arterial injury.

Digital subtraction angiography has been used with significant success to evaluate vascular injuries. This study may be performed by either intravenous or intraarterial injection. This technique appears to be more sensitive in detecting extravasation of contrast material, whereas conventional arteriography is better for subtle findings, such as intimal disruption. Digital subtraction studies require a cooperative patient who can remain still, as it is very sensitive to motion artifact.

Studies have focused on the need for angiography in patients without obvious physical signs of vessel injury and in those with "proximity" wounds.[1–6,8,9,11,13,14] Several studies have shown that surgically important lesions in these patients are rare and that most of these patients do not need surgery. Instead of angiography, serial physical examination with measurement of blood pressures in the injured extremity compared with an uninjured extremity[3–6,8–10] and evaluation with color-flow duplex Doppler ultrasonography[1,2,7,11,13] have been advocated as the primary methods of evaluation in this select group of patients.

Shotgun wounds to an extremity have a much higher incidence of vascular injury due to the nature of the weapon (i.e., multiple missiles and multiple trajectories).[3,13] Therefore, more of these patients are likely to undergo an angiographic study.

Each institution should determine in advance how it plans to evaluate patients with potential peripheral vascular trauma by having in place protocols agreed on by the emergency medicine and surgery physician staffs.

EMERGENCY DEPARTMENT MANAGEMENT

Prehospital and emergency department management priorities include control of hemorrhage, fluid resuscitation, and assessment and management of other life threats.[10]

Hemorrhage should be controlled by direct pressure over the bleeding site. Blind clamping of vessels deep in a wound is to be condemned, as adjacent structures such as nerves and tendons may be crushed in the attempt to stop bleeding.[10] If a bleeding vessel can be identified and isolated, it may be clamped using a noncrushing vascular clamp. Fluid restoration is accomplished by initiating one or more intravenous lines (as the trauma mechanism and vital signs dictate) and infusing crystalloid. After bleeding is controlled and resuscitation started, a careful examination for other life-threatening injuries is performed. As with all trauma patients, a patent airway and adequate ventilation must be ensured while circulation is being addressed. Vascular injuries are treated after other potential life threats have been assessed and managed.

Angulated fractures associated with pulse deficits should be anatomically repositioned and splinted. This may restore perfusion to an ischemic extremity.

Blood for type and crossmatch should be sent to the laboratory, and appropriate preparations made for transfusion if blood loss or anticipated surgical needs indicate. Unless indications for immediate surgery are present, rapid diagnosis by means of arteriography should follow.

Tetanus immunization status should be ascertained and the patient immunized, if necessary. Prophylactic antibiotics are indicated when operative repair or vascular grafts are to be undertaken. Anticoagulants should generally not be given until surgical consultation has been obtained, the absence of other major injuries has been determined, and the patient is ready to undergo arterial repair.

DISPOSITION

Surgical consultation must be obtained as early as possible, as the amount of time elapsed from injury until operative repair is a crucial determinant of successful repair and decreased morbidity. Endovascular embolization may be an option for treatment of nonessential vessels in select situations. Observation for a period of 12 to 24 hours is appropriate for patients without obvious signs of vessel injury and normal ABIs. If surgical intervention or arteriography is unavailable in the primary receiving institution, the patient should be transferred, as soon as possible after appropriate stabilizing procedures have been performed, to a facility capable of providing the necessary therapy.

COMMON PITFALLS

Vascular injuries may be subtle in origin and misleading on physical examination. Failure to appreciate injury mechanics or vessel proximity to a penetrating wound may lead to misdiagnosis. Up to 25% of patients may have normal pulses distal to the site of injury, and 16% may have normal physical examinations. Delay in diagnosis of vascular compromise may lead to permanent deficit or loss of the limb.

References

1. Bergstein JM, Blair JF, Edwards J, et al. Pitfalls in the use of color-flow duplex ultrasound for screening of suspected arterial injuries in penetrated extremities. *J Trauma* 1992;33:395.
2. Bynoe RP, Miles WS, Bell RM, et al. Noninvasive diagnosis of vascular trauma by duplex ultrasonography. *J Vasc Surg* 1991;14:346.
3. Dennis JW, Frykberg ER, Crump JM, et al. New perspectives on the management of penetrating trauma in proximity to major limb arteries. *J Vasc Surg* 1990;11:85.
4. Dennis JW, Frykberg ER, Veldenz HC, et al. Validation of nonoperative management of occult vascular injuries and accuracy of physical examination alone in penetrating extremity trauma: 5- to 10-year follow-up. *J Trauma* 1998;44:243.
5. Francis H, Thal ER, Weigelt JA, et al. Vascular proximity: is it a valid indication for arteriography in asymptomatic patients? *J Trauma* 1991;31:512.
6. Frykberg ER, Dennis JW, Bishop K, et al. The reliability of physical examination in the evaluation of penetrating extremity trauma for vascular injury: results at 1 year. *J Trauma* 1991;31:502.
7. Gagne PJ, Cone JB, McFarland D, et al. Proximity penetrating extremity trauma: the role of duplex ultrasound in the detection of occult venous injuries. *J Trauma* 1995;39:1157.
8. Johansen K, Lynch K, Paun M, et al. Non-invasive vascular tests reliably exclude occult arterial trauma in injured extremities. *J Trauma* 1991;31:515.
9. Lunch K, Johansen K. Can Doppler pressure measurement replace "exclusion" arteriography in the diagnosis of occult extremity arterial trauma? *Ann Surg* 1991;214:737.
10. Modrall JG, Weaver FA, Yellin AE. Diagnosis and management of penetrating vascular trauma and the injured extremity. *Emerg Med Clin North Am* 1998;16:129.
11. Ordog GJ, Balasubramanium S, Wasserberger J, et al. Extremity gunshot wounds. Part 1: identification and treatment of patients at high risk of vascular injury. *J Trauma* 1994;36:358.
12. Schwartz MR, Weaver FA, Bauer M, et al. Refining the indications for arteriography in penetrating extremity trauma: a prospective analysis. *J Vasc Surg* 1993;17:116.
13. Schwartz M, Weaver F, Yellin A, et al. The utility of color-flow Doppler examination in penetrating extremity arterial trauma. *Am Surg* 1993;59:375.
14. Weaver FA, Yellin AE, Bauer M, et al. Is arterial proximity a valid indication for arteriography in penetrating extremity trauma? *Arch Surg* 1990;125:1256.

PART III
Orthopedic Considerations

CHAPTER 111
Approach to Musculoskeletal Injuries

David F. Gaieski and Joseph Bernstein

Musculoskeletal injuries represent a significant percentage of all emergency care rendered. In a recently completed study by the authors in the emergency department (ED) of a large, urban, teaching hospital, musculoskeletal problems accounted for at least 11% of total patient visits. Clearly, a coherent and systematic approach to patients with orthopaedic injuries and other musculoskeletal complaints is essential. These injuries range from tendinitis, trivial sprains, and contusions to life- and limb-threatening trauma. Often, but not always, acute trauma is responsible for the presenting complaints; and often, but not always, the primary impairment is an inability to move a part of the body without pain or discomfort. The mechanisms of trauma are protean, ranging from sports injuries to assaults to motor vehicle accidents to falls in the home to industrial catastrophes. When acute trauma is absent, overuse syndromes or repetitive movements are often the culprit.

The immediate tasks of the emergency physician evaluating a patient with a musculoskeletal complaint include:

- Correctly determining injuries that need only symptomatic care and those that require more complex, timely intervention
- Differentiating injuries that can be handled solely by an emergency physician (the vast majority of musculoskeletal injuries) from those that require emergent consultation with, or timely referral to, an orthopedic surgeon (e.g., open fractures, compartment syndrome, acute meniscal tears in the young to middle-aged patient, and flexor tendon injuries)
- Formulating a logical, cost-effective algorithm for the diagnosis and management of each patient
- Managing pain early and effectively, recognizing, for example, that "a mere contusion" can be the source of exquisite pain
- Recognizing that care is not complete when emergency care has been delivered; rather, successful management of the patient is only complete when appropriate follow-up has been arranged, as a large percentage of acute musculoskeletal injuries require reevaluation and ongoing care (e.g., physical therapy and rehabilitation) for optimal recovery.

TYPES OF INJURY

Sprain

A sprain is a ligamentous injury. Ligaments link bone to bone. Damage to the fibers of the ligament range from microscopic damage to complete disruption. A sprain can result from an abnormal (nonbiomechanical) force vector applied to a joint, an excessive force applied along a normal vector, or a combination of the two mechanisms. The phrase "just a sprain" is probably best relegated to the past; it is possible to sustain a sprain that is significantly more severe than an analogous fracture. For example, a complete lateral ankle ligament rupture and a transverse avulsion fracture of the distal fibula cause the same pattern of instability, but, because bone regenerates without scarring, the outcome for the latter injury is usually much better. The grading of sprains is based on the severity of the damage:

- *Grade I sprain:* A grade I sprain (in older terminology, "first-degree") represents microscopic tears of the ligament, which lead to localized hemorrhage and inflammation as the healing process evolves. Active range of motion is usually preserved but painful. Abnormal movement of the joint stabilized by the sprained ligament is not elicited by stress maneuvers, but these maneuvers may produce focal pain and the area overlying the sprained ligament is tender to palpation.
- *Grade II sprain:* In a grade II sprain "second-degree", or partial tear, the overall architecture of the ligament is preserved, with the majority of fibers still in continuity, but some of them have been completely ruptured. Hemorrhage is more extensive and swelling is pronounced. Loss of function secondary to decreased and painful range of motion is the hallmark. When the joint that the ligament stabilizes is stressed, there may be some gapping of the joint, or abnormal motion. However, frank instability does not occur and a clearly defined end point is reached.
- *Grade III sprain:* A grade III sprain "third-degree" denotes a complete tear of the ligament and is synonymous with a complete rupture. Hemorrhage is more extensive and healing involves the formation of scar tissue in the area between the fragments of the ligament. Stressing the joint reveals greater gapping than in the case of a grade II sprain, and frank instability without a well-defined end point may be elicited. This frank instability can be summed up by the examiner's thought, "I should stop stressing this joint, as it isn't going to resist my efforts."

Common ligament sprains seen in the ED include lateral ankle sprains, injuries to the anterior cruciate and collateral ligaments of the knee, and ligamentous injuries of the shoulder, associated with either glenohumeral dislocations or acromioclavicular separations.

The clinical signs of a sprain typically include point tenderness to palpation, swelling, painful and/or decreased range of motion, and ecchymosis. A complete sprain, with no fibers in continuity, may be completely pain-free when stressed. Often, athletes will continue play after a grade III sprain of the medial collateral ligament of the knee, but it is rare that they continue activities after a grade II sprain. In fact, pain may be inversely proportional to the severity of the injury: A grade I sprain is extremely painful when stressed, as there are many intact but damaged and inflamed fibers that will be stretched, triggering the discharge of pain fibers as the ligament is loaded with force; with a grade III sprain, the same maneuver does not cause any stretching of the ligament, as it cannot be loaded by force and the only pain fibers triggered by the stress maneuver will lie in surrounding soft tissue. Bone can be injured at the same time as a ligament is damaged; for example, grade III sprains of the medial, deltoid ligament of the ankle are often accompanied by fibula fractures. Bony evidence of sprains on x-ray includes small avulsion fractures at the point of insertion of the ligament into the bone, impaction injuries, and simple joint-space widening. Thus, in many instances, radiographs are appropriate when a ligamentous injury is suspected.

Strains

Tendons connect muscles to bone. A strain is an injury to the musculotendinous unit, which can range from mild "pulled muscles" to complete tendon ruptures. The mechanisms of injury are twofold: (1) stretching a muscle beyond its normal range of motion by forced extension (an "overstretching injury") and (2) tearing of muscle or tendon fibers by a violent, uncontrolled contraction or repetitive, prolonged contractions, often in attempted compensation for an unexpected change in direction of movement, unanticipated variations in terrain, or a sudden force applied to the antagonist muscle group (an "overexertion injury").

Strains are graded from first-degree to third-degree, reflecting the severity of damage:

- In a first-degree strain, microscopic damage occurs to the muscle or tendon, with associated localized hemorrhage, inflammation, and tenderness to palpation. Active range of motion is often unrestricted, but pain can be elicited by resisted contraction or forced extension of the muscle group.
- A second-degree strain involves more severe damage, with rupture of some fibers of the muscle or tendon. Hemorrhage is usually visible, swelling more severe, and range of motion limited by pain.
- In a third-degree strain, the muscle or tendon is completely ruptured. The rupture can occur in the muscle belly, at the musculotendinous junction, within the tendon itself, or at the point of insertion of the tendon into bone.

Common strains seen in the ED include those to the quadriceps, hamstring, and rotator cuff muscles; "groin pulls"; and Achilles tendon ruptures.

The clinical signs of a strain include pain, ecchymosis, edema, and decreased or painful range of motion. With complete disruption of the muscle or tendon, a palpable defect is often present. Physical examination should include inspection of the injured area, observation of active and passive range of motion, palpation of the affected area, and provocative maneuvers—either resisted contraction or passive stretching—to elicit the location and extent of injury. In addition, with certain suspected injuries, specific tests should be performed. For example, if an Achilles' tendon rupture is suspected, then Thompson's test is performed. While the patient lies prone with his or her foot and ankle hanging off the end of the examination bed, the examiner squeezes the calf on the affected side and observes whether the foot plantar-flexes in response to the calf being squeezed), the presence of plantar flexion indicates an Achilles' tendon that is at least partially intact.

Contusions

A contusion is a bruise caused by a direct blow to a body part. Contusions can occur to bone, with significant pain from periosteal bruising, or, more commonly, to soft tissue, especially fat and muscle. In these crush injuries, the degree of injury is proportional to the force of the blow and the surface area of impact; tissue damage occurs as the energy transmitted by the impact dissipates into or is absorbed by surrounding structures.

Fundamentally, *the diagnosis of contusion is one of exclusion,* with fracture, sprain, and strain being the most important diagnoses that must be eliminated. Common contusions seen in the ED include bruised quadriceps muscles, rib cage contusions, contusions of the ulnar aspect of the forearm in "defensive maneuvers" during an assault, and direct blows to the anterior tibia.

Either the blow itself or the body's reaction to it causes signs and symptoms that prompt the patient to seek emergency care. Typically, they include pain, swelling, ecchymosis, and decreased range of motion of the affected part.

Usually, the entities that are ruled out (e.g., fracture, sprain, and strain) are potentially more serious than the diagnosis of contusion itself, but the clinician must remember that contusions can lead to serious complications, including severe pain, rhabdomyolysis, compartment syndrome, and *myositis ossificans.*

- *Severe pain:* One of the most common reasons that patients seek reevaluation in an emergency room is inadequate analgesia following a soft-tissue injury. Initial attention to adequate analgesia ensures patient comfort and decreases the incidence of reevaluation.
- *Rhabdomyolysis:* Severe muscle breakdown can occur after strenuous exercise without an acute, isolated injury or after a significant contusion to an extremity. Rhabdomyolysis consists of the destruction of the integrity of the cell membranes of myocytes. The subsequent release of intracellular contents, including potassium, myoglobin, uric acid, phosphate, and the enzyme creatine kinase, into the bloodstream results in a number of systemic complications, including metabolic abnormalities and acute renal failure. The emergency physician must assess the extent of tissue involvement, the degree of tissue destruction, and the potential for systemic complications. If rhabdomyolysis is suspected, urinalysis for evidence of myoglobinuria (dipstick positive for blood without microscopic evidence of erythrocytes) should be performed and the level of serum creatine kinase checked. (Please see Chapter 179 for details.)
- *Compartment syndrome:* Compartment syndrome occurs when pressure within soft tissues in a fixed body compartment increases to the point at which it compromises venous blood flow and limits capillary perfusion, leading to muscle ischemia and necrosis. Most commonly associated with long-bone fractures, it can occur in the setting of severe contusion or excessive exertion and must be considered in any patient with pain out of proportion to physical findings or with swelling causing obvious tautness in a nonexpansible compartment, such as the anterior tibial compartment. When this diagnosis is considered, it must be objectively ruled out by manometry. (Please see Chapter 122 for details.)
- *Myositis ossificans:* Severe hemorrhage into a muscle can initiate a cascade of "healing," which can lead to the formation of ectopic bone within the muscle. A large number of these cases have occurred in athletes treated with early, aggressive nonsteroidal antiinflammatory drugs (NSAIDs), heat, mas-

sage, and physical therapy in the hope of facilitating early return to athletic competition. This is of concern to the emergency physician for a number of reasons. If severe quadriceps tear and resultant hemorrhage and ecchymosis are suspected, the initial management should include ice, a brief period (24 hours) of immobilization in a stretched position (knee flexed to 120 degrees for severe quadriceps contusion), and acetaminophen, instead of NSAIDs, for pain control. This regimen limits the ongoing bleeding and inflammation in the area. These patients must be referred for appropriate long-term follow-up care. In addition, a patient's complaint of decreased range of motion, ongoing pain, and a mass or firmness in soft tissue weeks to months after sustaining a contusion should suggest the possibility of *myositis ossificans*. A soft-tissue x-ray is the best way to evaluate for heterotopic bony formation. If heterotopic bone is present, the patient should be referred to an orthopaedic surgeon for close follow-up care and potential resection of the bone when it has matured (usually at 9 to 12 months).

Fractures

Most fractures require urgent medical attention, and without appropriate emergency care, many will not heal properly or healing will be accompanied by unnecessary complications. A *fracture* is defined as a partial or complete break in a bone. Bone is unique in that it is the only tissue in the human body, other than the liver, that heals by regeneration, not by scarring. For regeneration to occur, however, the bone must be immobilized to allow uninterrupted formation of new bone. Ensuring appropriate immobilization is one of the fundamental tasks of the emergency physician when dealing with musculoskeletal problems.

The process of new bone formation begins with hematoma bridging the realigned fracture fragments. Hematopoietic cells in the hematoma secrete growth factors, which stimulate the formation of granulation tissue at the fracture ends, resulting in slow resorption of the hematoma. Over the next several weeks, a primary callus is formed, beginning as a soft callus and progressing to a hard callus. The final phase of healing is remodeling, during which the bone reassumes its original architecture as it is exposed to the normal stresses of weight bearing and movement.

Fractures also require immediate attention for several other reasons: Virtually all fractures are painful; the vast majority of them result from high-energy trauma (relative to sprains, strains, and contusions) and, because of force vectors, are accompanied by well-known associated injuries (e.g., 15% of calcaneal fractures sustained in a fall from height have associated lumbar vertebral fractures); and many fractures place the patient at risk for specific complications (e.g., compartment syndrome in long-bone fractures, blood loss in pelvic fractures, avascular necrosis in scaphoid fractures of the hand).

A working knowledge of the nomenclature of fractures is essential to the successful management of fractures in the ED, and to clear communication with radiologists and consulting orthopaedic surgeons. Adequate description of a fracture includes whether it is open or closed, the bone(s) involved, the location within the bone, the direction of the main fracture line, the number of fragments, the alignment of the fracture fragments, the displacement of the fragments, various additional descriptive modifiers, and notation of associated complications.

Closed Versus Open Fractures

The old terminology of simple (closed) and compound (open) is best abandoned. In a closed fracture, the skin and soft tissue overlying the fracture have not been violated; therefore, no communication exists between the outside environment and the fracture fragments. Any break in the skin overlying a fracture must be considered an open fracture until proven otherwise. It may be difficult to tell whether there has been actual communication between the bone and the environment or whether the patient has simply sustained an abrasion (from the trauma that caused the fracture) to the skin overlying the fracture.

Open fractures are traditionally classified into three types based on the size of the wound and the amount of soft-tissue injury. Type I wounds are less than 1 cm long, the energy dissipated by the mechanism of injury is low, and there is minimal soft-tissue trauma. Type II wounds are less than 10 cm long, the mechanism of injury has dissipated a low or moderate amount of energy, and there is moderate soft-tissue trauma but no gross contamination of the wound, major crush injury, or soft-tissue defects or flaps. Type III wounds are greater than 10 cm long. These include high-velocity gunshot wounds, close-range shotgun wounds, open fractures with major vascular injuries, fractures more than 8 hours old, or open fractures sustained in environments where exposure to fecal contents is a concern (e.g., barnyard accidents), or extensive soft-tissue or periosteal stripping of bone, or evidence of gross contamination or significant crush injury.

Open fractures are orthopedic emergencies and require immediate control of hemorrhage; splinting, with reduction if neurovascular compromise exists; copious irrigation; early administration of sufficient analgesia and appropriate antibiotics; tetanus prophylaxis; and emergent consultation with orthopedic surgery for definitive irrigation, debridement, reduction, and fracture repair. Early intervention is the best way to prevent complications; the incidence of infection following open fracture is directly proportional to the time from injury to definitive irrigation and debridement.

Bone Involvement and Location within Bone

The description of the injury should include the side of the body, the specific bone, and the location within the bone. By convention, long bones are divided into proximal, middle, and distal thirds, and these divisions are used to describe the fracture location. If the fracture lies at the junction of any two thirds of the bone, it should be described as such.

Direction and Description of Nature of Fracture

The *direction* of a fracture refers to the configuration of the fracture—the way the fracture disrupts the bone. Convention stipulates that this descriptive modifier communicates the direction of the fracture in relation to the long axis of the involved bone (Fig. 111.1). A *transverse* fracture disrupts the bone perpendicular to its long axis; an *oblique* fracture lies at an angle to the long axis of the bone; a *spiral* fracture results from a rotational force and spirals around the center of the long axis of the bone.

Additional terms used to describe the configuration of a fracture include *comminuted,* referring to a fracture in which there are three or more fragments; *segmental,* referring to the presence of two or more fractures in a bone, creating at least one segment of bone that is not connected to either end of the bone; *avulsion,* referring to a piece of bone that is pulled off at the site of insertion of a tendon or ligament; *impacted,* referring to the fractured surfaces of the bone being forced into each other, foreshortening the bone; *compression,* referring to a fracture in which the trabeculae of the bone are compressed, decreasing the overall volume of the affected part of the bone. Avulsion fractures are usually the result of traction injuries. Their presence indicates potential instability at the joint, which is caused by the loss of stabilization normally provided by the avulsed ligament or tendon. On computed tomography (CT) scan, impacted fractures are often comminuted with numerous small fragments wedging across the main fracture line.

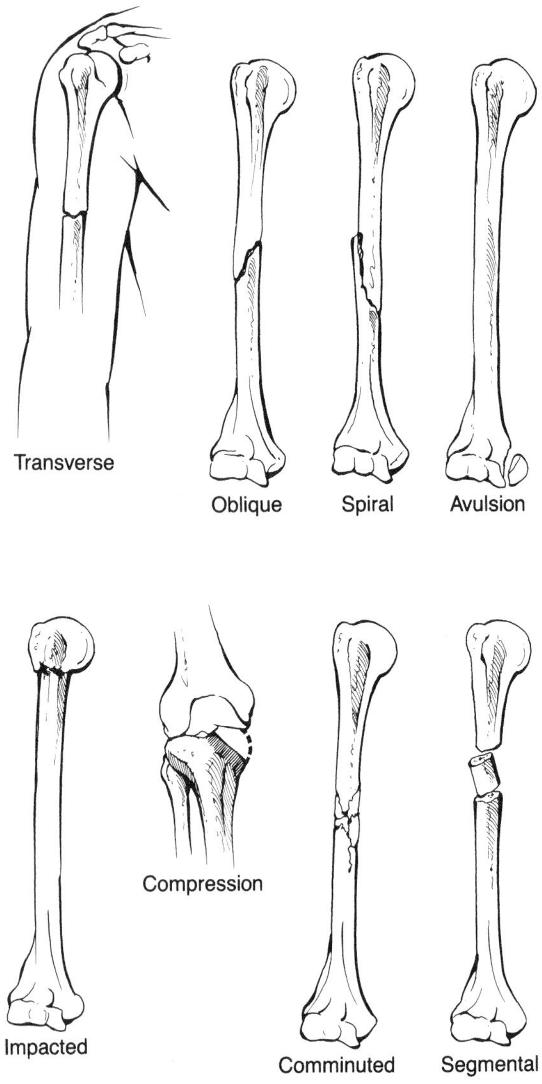

Figure 111.1. Fracture configuration.

Alignment of Fracture

A fracture is also described in terms of its alignment—the relationship of the fracture fragments to each other. The fracture may be *displaced, angulated,* or *rotated.*

A fracture is *displaced* if the fragments are offset in a transverse or longitudinal plane. The position of the distal fragment in relation to the proximal fragment is described, and the distal fragment may be displaced anteriorly, posteriorly, medially, laterally, radially, ulnarly, proximally, or, less frequently, distally, among other possibilities. The amount of displacement is commonly measured in terms of the width of the fractured shaft, using fractions of the width in the description.

A fracture is *angulated* if there is a deviation from the normal relationship of the bony fragments along the longitudinal axis of the bone (Fig. 111.2). The direction of angulation may be described in two ways. It may be described in terms of the direction of the apex of the angle formed at the fracture site by the two main fracture fragments: The apex may point anteriorly, posteriorly, laterally, or medially. The direction of the apex may also be described by other adjectives, including ulnarly, radially, dorsally, or volarly, depending on the involved bones. A second way to describe the angulation of the fracture is in terms of the relation of the distal fragment to the proximal fragment. If the distal fragment is angled away from the midline of the body, there is *valgus* angulation (the fracture is in valgus); if the distal fragment angles toward the midline, the fracture is in *varus* (there is varus angulation to the distal fragment).

Rotation refers to twisting of the distal fragment in relation to the proximal fragment around the center of the long axis of the fractured bone. When viewed along the long axis of the bone from the most distal point on the bone, if the distal fracture fragment has rotated toward the midline in relation to the proximal fragment, it is *medially rotated;* if it has rotated away from the midline, it is *laterally rotated.*

Other Descriptive Modifiers

An *incomplete* fracture involves only one cortex of the bone; a *complete* fracture disrupts both cortices. A *pathologic* fracture occurs in an area of abnormal bone, weakened by disease or prior trauma, and is often the result of apparently trivial trauma or a biomechanically routine force applied along a natural vector. Pathologic fractures occur at sites of old fractures, through primary osteosarcomas, at sites of tumor metastases, near cysts, and in bone weakened by Paget disease, rickets, osteomalacia, tuberculosis, osteomyelitis, chronic steroid therapy, anorexia, and many other disease processes. A *stress* fracture is the result of the bony cortex becoming fatigued by repeated low-level

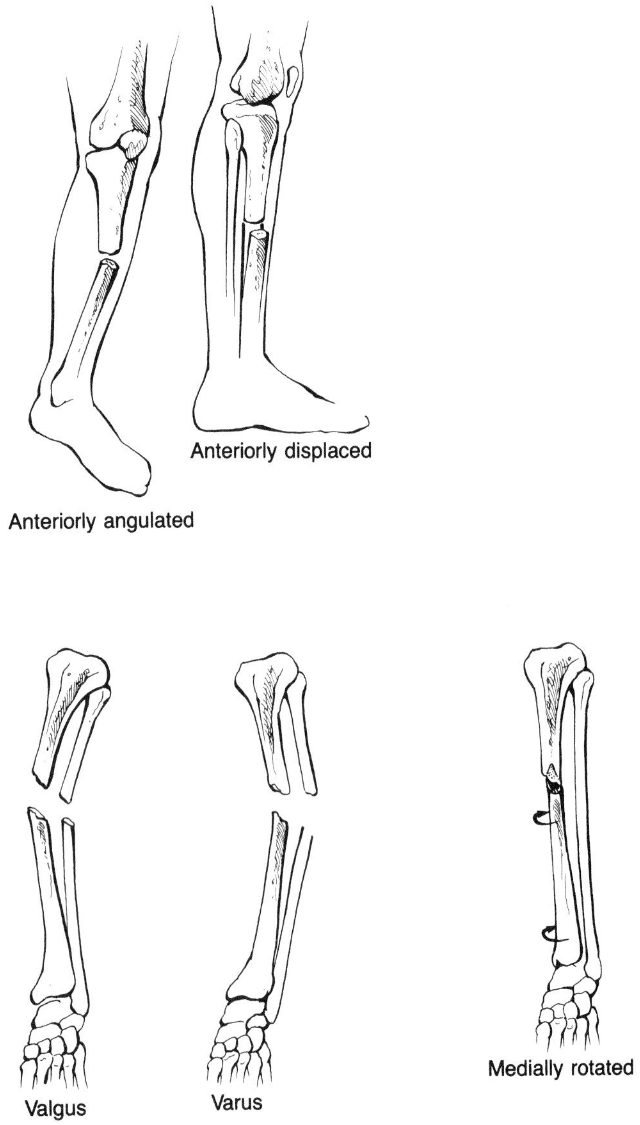

Figure 111.2. Fracture alignment.

loading rather than disrupted by one acute episode of trauma. The repeated stress to the cortex causes bone resorption, is manifest clinically as pain with activity and tenderness to palpation over the affected bone, and may result in overt fracture if adequate healing is not allowed. Eating disorders and amenorrhea predispose to stress fractures in female athletes. Stress fractures are most common in the proximal tibia but have also been described in the spine, pelvis, femur, tarsal navicular, metatarsals, and sesamoid bones, among other sites.

Complications of Various Fractures

No assessment and description of a fracture is complete without a thorough assessment for, and identification of, possible associated complications (Table 111.1). Well-recognized complications of fractures are suggested by the site of the fracture and the mechanism of injury.

Blood Loss and Shock. Bone has a generous blood supply, and fractures can disrupt the blood vessels, causing localized bleeding. If this bleeding results in the loss of a significant percentage of the patient's blood volume, hypovolemic shock can result. Rarely, exsanguination occurs. An isolated long-bone fracture is rarely the cause of shock, with a unilateral tibia and fibula fracture typically resulting in loss of around 500 mL of blood; certain femoral fractures can have 3 or 4 U of blood loss into the thigh, producing class III shock. Hemorrhagic shock can occur with pelvic fractures, in which typical blood loss is between 1,500 and 3,000 mL. If a bleeding disorder such as hemophilia A, thrombocytopenia, or marked anemia is present, a fracture that typically results in modest blood loss may be the source of life-threatening hemorrhage. This is also true in patients on anticoagulation therapy, and the occasional, isolated long-bone fracture will require the administration of vitamin K, fresh-frozen plasma, and transfusion of packed red blood cells.

Vascular Injuries. Vascular injuries occur most commonly in open fractures, widely displaced fractures, or fracture-dislocations, and at sites where the vessels lie close to the bone or are held in a relatively fixed position. Vulnerable sites include the popliteal artery at the knee, which may be injured in supracondylar fractures of the distal femur or in fracture–dislocations of the knee; the axillary artery at the shoulder, injured in fractures of the proximal humerus and humeral head; and the brachial artery at the elbow, which is at risk in supracondylar fractures of the distal humerus (Fig. 111.3). Even at the most vulnerable sites, these injuries are rare, but if they are not diagnosed in a timely fashion, the consequences can be devastating.

The classic signs of vascular injury are the "Five P's": pain, pallor, pulselessness (or diminished pulse), paresthesia, and paralysis. The Five P's are present only in a complete injury to the vessel. A partial injury can have subtle clinical signs and symptoms or be completely asymptomatic. In addition, collateral circulation may maintain distal flow around a vascular injury. Vascular compromise may also be delayed, as in the case of

TABLE 111.1. Complication of Fractures and Dislocations

Vascular injuries	Ischemic necrosis
Nerve injuries	Delayed union
Compartment syndrome	Nonunion
Infection	Malunion
Shock	Joint stiffness
Cast-induced injuries	Posttraumatic arthritis
DVT	Reflex sympathetic dystrophy
Fat embolism	

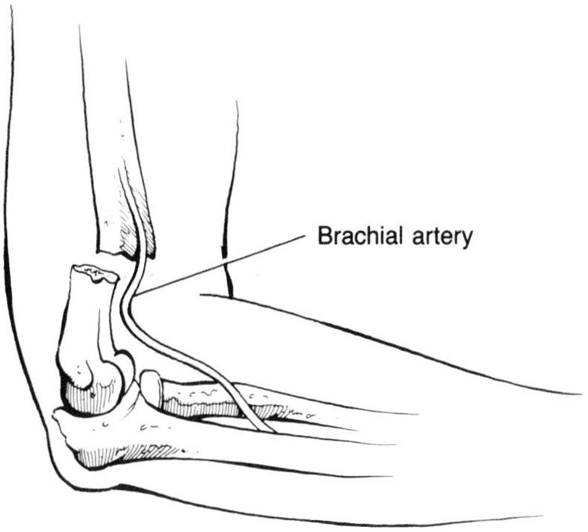

Figure 111.3. Fracture-associated vascular injury.

an initial vascular intimal injury leading to progressive thrombosis. Therefore, the location of the fracture and the mechanism of injury determine the need to assess for a potential vascular injury in the asymptomatic patient. Initial evaluation should involve assessment of pulses, evaluation with a Doppler stethoscope if palpable pulses are diminished or absent, observation of the color of the distal extremity, and assessment of capillary refill. If vascular injury is suspected, further evaluation with angiogram, magnetic resonance angiography (MRA), or surgical exploration is usually warranted. Complications of fracture-associated vascular injuries include *in situ* thrombosis, false aneurysms, true aneurysms, compartment syndrome, arteriovenous fistulas, and distal limb ischemia with mechanical dysfunction.

Nerve Injuries. Nerves are more frequently injured than vessels in association with fractures and can be damaged by blunt trauma, along the trajectory of penetrating trauma causing an associated fracture, or by the fracture fragments themselves. Nerves are at increased risk of injury when they are superficial to the skin, lie close to the bone, or span the joint, making them susceptible to stretch injury.

The most frequently injured nerves in association with specific fractures include the axillary and musculocutaneous nerves in shoulder fracture–dislocations; the radial nerve in fractures of the distal third of the humerus; the radial, median, and/or ulnar nerves in supracondylar elbow fractures; the median nerve in fracture-dislocations about the wrist; the peroneal and tibial nerves in knee fracture-dislocations; and the peroneal nerve in fractures of the fibular head or proximal fibula (see Fig. 111.4).

Nerve injuries are classified based on the amount of damage to the nerve according to Seddon's staging system:

- *Neuropraxia:* The most minor injury, neuropraxia involves a contusion to the nerve, with minor injury to the myelin sheath. Sensory loss and transient paralysis may occur, but spontaneous and complete recovery occurs over a period of several days to weeks to, at most, a few months.
- *Axonotmesis:* In axonotmesis, more severe crush injury to the nerve occurs with axonal breakdown followed by distal wallerian degeneration. The epineurium and the continuity of Schwann tubes are maintained. Prolonged paresthesias and muscle weakness are the clinical hallmarks. Recovery can be complete but takes months to years, as the axon has to regenerate proximally to distally, and for functional conduction to occur, the myelin sheath must be fully repaired. Often, recovery is incomplete or spotty.

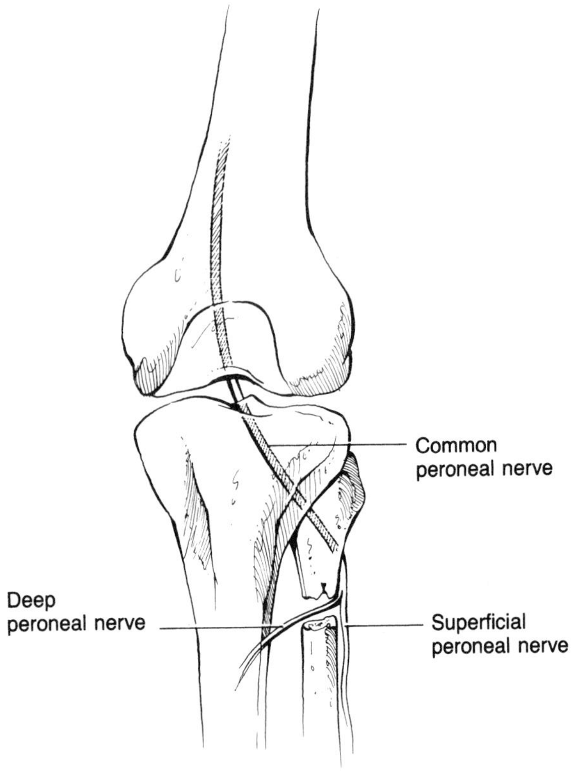

Figure 111.4. Peroneal injury in a knee fracture.

- *Neurotmesis:* The most severe form of nerve damage is neurotmesis, with disruption of the axon, epineurium, and Schwann cell sheath or complete severance of the nerve. When complete disruption occurs, all functions controlled by the injured nerve are interrupted.

The emergency evaluation of a nerve injury should involve assessment of motor strength, deep tendon reflexes, light touch, and two-point discrimination. Formal testing can be done by electromyogram (EMG); however, this is rarely necessary in the ED.

Compartment Syndrome. Compartment syndrome (fully discussed in Chapter 122) should be suspected in long-bone fractures and fractures associated with significant vascular injuries or pronounced swelling, especially when the patient has pain out of proportion to physical examination findings or when paresthesias occur. Manometry must be performed if compartment syndrome is suspected, as the clinical signs are variable and may be delayed.

Infection. Infections occur primarily in open fractures, especially in those in which there is a delay in treatment. Infection can also occur with extensive hematoma, after open reduction, and after internal fixation repair, and may be seen independent of fracture in cases of osteomyelitis, septic arthritis, and abscesses eroding to bone. Septic arthritis should be suspected in the patient with monoarticular arthritis and ruled out in those patients with rheumatoid arthritis or gout who present with a swollen, erythematous, hot joint. Aspiration for crystal analysis, Gram stain, cell count, and culture is the standard of care. Many orthopedic surgeons recommend aggressive arthroscopic lavage to prevent destruction of the joint space by bacteria and inflammatory-mediated damage. Lavage can be performed in the emergency room if other options are not available, utilizing an influx catheter for the delivery of sterile saline and an outflow catheter for the removal of the irrigation fluid along with the pathologic contents of the joint space.

Casts and Splints. Immobilization devices may cause postinjury problems. They may become too tight as swelling increases during the first 24 to 48 hours postinjury and cause pain and impair circulation. Pressure sores may occur on the skin in areas where a cast or external fixation device exerts localized excessive pressure (e.g., over the heel in a patient with a bimalleolar fracture). Immediate steps should be taken to correct the problem. A cast that is too tight can be split lengthwise; the underlying padding can then be cut and the cast spread open. A cast that is pressing on a particular site can have a window cut out. The window may be replaced more loosely with plaster or covered with soft dressing. An ill-fitting splint can be trimmed.

Deep Venous Thrombosis. A deep venous thrombosis (DVT) is a clot that forms in one of the deep veins of an extremity, usually a leg. When a lower extremity DVT propagates above the popliteal fossa, the patient is at risk for having a piece of clot break free and flow up the inferior vena cava to the pulmonary circulation, with the potential to cause respiratory distress, hypoxia, pleuritic chest pain, circulatory compromise, syncope, and death. (Upper extremity DVTs are responsible for a much lower incidence of pulmonary emboli [PEs], and the clot burden associated with these PEs is much lower. Nevertheless, upper extremity DVTs should be diagnosed and treated aggressively, usually with anticoagulation therapy.) When a patient develops signs and symptoms suggestive of a DVT or PE, including calf or arm swelling, erythema, induration, pain on ambulation, a palpable cord in the calf, shortness of breath, tachycardia, hypoxia, or pleuritic chest pain, duplex Doppler of the affected extremities, impedance plethysmography (IPG), and ventilation–perfusion scanning (V/Q scan) should be performed as indicated.

Fat Emboli Syndrome. Single or multiple long-bone fractures in the young and hip fractures in the elderly predispose to fat emboli. Twenty percent of patients with pelvic or long-bone fractures have detectable fat droplets in their blood. The vast majority of these patients remain asymptomatic. Fat emboli syndrome is the most common form of nonthrombotic embolism and has a characteristic clinical course. Its etiology is unclear, but three main hypotheses have been postulated: (1) After fat droplets enter the bloodstream, the liberation of free fatty acids from marrow fat by circulating lipase causes a toxic vasculitis and capillary leak syndrome; (2) it is the end result of extensive platelet–fibrin thrombosis; and (3) it results from direct obstruction of distal vascular lumen by fat emboli. Clinically, a fracture is sustained, and the patient often remains asymptomatic, other than the fracture and associated pain, for 12 to 36 hours before suddenly and unexpectedly developing a life-threatening syndrome characterized by rapid cardiopulmonary and neurologic deterioration, including agitation, hallucinations, delirium, coma, hypoxia, dyspnea, tachypnea, and tachycardia. If this deterioration is not quickly reversed, refractory hypotension, anemia, thrombocytopenia, disseminated intravascular coagulopathy (DIC), and adult respiratory distress syndrome (ARDS) often ensue, with an associated high morbidity and mortality.

Ischemic or Avascular Necrosis. Ischemic or avascular necrosis is characterized by bone death that occurs following the interruption of blood supply to bone. Avascular necrosis is most frequently associated with carpal scaphoid fractures, lunate dislocations, hip dislocations, femoral neck fractures, and complex fractures of the talus.

Delayed Complications. Other complications of fractures may occur some time after the initial injury is seen by the emergency physician. Many fractures require reduction of the displaced fracture fragments in the ED or the operating room. The goal in reduction is always to reestablish anatomic position; eliminate displacement, angulation, and other forms of malalignment; and immobilize the broken bone in the reestablished anatomic position to promote healing. Sometimes, this ideal condition is not achieved and the systematic progression from hematoma to callus formation to bony union is delayed or interrupted. *Delayed unions* are fractures that take longer than usual to heal; *malunions* are fractures that heal in a faulty position; *nonunions* occur when the process of fracture healing stops before the fracture is united.

Joint stiffness, posttraumatic arthritis, and *reflex sympathetic dystrophy* (RSD) may also occur as delayed complications of extremity trauma. For example, any intraarticular fracture of a weight-bearing joint predisposes the patient to early degenerative changes, and the patient may present to the ED years after a fracture, complaining of *perceived* sudden onset of joint pain and decreased range of motion. Radiographs typically demonstrate extensive *osteoarthritis.*

RSD, formerly known as causalgia, is a three-stage, posttraumatic syndrome of unclear etiology, the development of which has no correlation to the severity of the initial injury. The first, or early, stage, characterized by continuous burning and aching in the posttraumatic extremity, is exacerbated by weight bearing and by movement. After a variable period of time, the middle, or dystrophic, stage ensues, characterized by the development of shiny, cool skin over the affected extremity and a progressively decreased range of motion. In the final, or atrophic, stage, the skin atrophies, the muscles waste, and flexion contractures develop.

In 1992, Gibbons and Wilson, in the *Clinical Journal of Pain,* developed an RSD score, which was proposed as a strict system for the clinical diagnosis of RSD. The scoring system consists of nine criteria and has more than academic interest, as early diagnosis improves outcome, interrupting the progression from burning to dystrophy to atrophy. The nine criteria are (1) allodynia—the phenomenon whereby pain is increased by stimuli that activate the involved nerve, such as a breeze blowing on the area, temperature changes, or emotional outbursts—or hyperpathia; (2) burning pain; (3) edema; (4) change in color or hair growth in the affected area; (5) change in sweating; (6) change in temperature; (7) demineralization of bone in the involved limb, as documented in radiographs; (8) quantitative measurements of vasomotor disturbances; and (9) a triple-phase bone scan consistent with RSD. A score of five points qualifies as a clinical diagnosis of RSD, with one point being given for each positive criterion, zero points for each negative criterion, and one-half point for each equivocal criterion. Application of heat or cold, exercises, early sympathetic blockade, or sympathectomy to the affected limb can halt the progression to atrophy. A minority of patients have been helped by a short course of high-dose prednisone (a 3-week taper) in conjunction with heat, cold, and exercise therapy.

Subluxations and Dislocations

Acute or chronic ligamentous laxity or tearing can result in subluxation or dislocation of a joint. Chronic ligamentous laxity is usually the result of an overuse syndrome, in which repetitive microtrauma leads to an attenuation of the static restraints of the joint; acute ligamentous tears are the result of excessive or abnormal forces applied to the joint. The classic example is subluxation or dislocation of the glenohumeral joint. Subluxation occurs when one bone becomes partially disarticulated from the other bone that forms the joint. The articular surfaces forming the joint remain partially intact. Dislocation occurs when the bones are completely disarticulated and no parts of their articular surfaces are in contact. Dislocations can occur in isolation or with an associated fracture (Fig. 111.5). Often, the fracture is anatomic evidence of the direction of the pathologic force vector resulting in the dislocation. For example, 90% to 95% of shoulder dislocations occur anteriorly, disrupting the continuity of the anterior capsule and the labrum. Sometimes, these structures resist the forces producing dislocation to the point that a fracture occurs, avulsing a piece of bone from the anterior glenoid rim, known as a bony Bankart lesion.

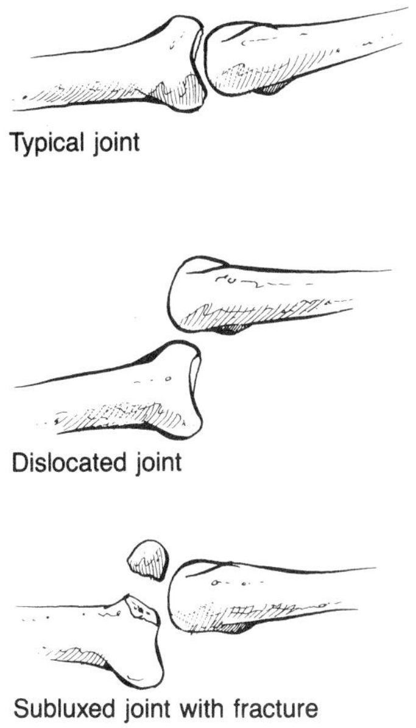

Figure 111.5. Joint subluxation and dislocation.

The nomenclature of subluxations and dislocations is straightforward. Most subluxations and dislocations occur at a joint formed by two bones, and the subluxation or dislocation is named after the affected joint (e.g., posterior dislocation of the distal interphalangeal (DIP) joint of the fourth finger of the right hand). If a joint is formed by three bones, and the two major bones are disarticulated, the subluxation or dislocation is named after the joint involved (e.g., posterior dislocation of the knee). If the joint is formed by three bones, and the minor bone is subluxed or dislocated, the abnormality is named after the minor bone (e.g., lateral dislocation of the patella). As for fractures, direction is assigned referential to the distal segment.

Specific subluxations and dislocations are frequently seen in the ED and need to be skillfully and efficiently reduced, with restoration of anatomic position, by the emergency physician. These include anterior and posterior dislocations of the shoulder joint; anterior and posterior dislocations of the sternoclavicular joint; posterior dislocations of the elbow joint; posterior dislocations of the proximal interphalangeal (PIP) and DIP joints, often with accompanying avulsion fractures; posterior dislocations of the hip joint; posterior dislocations of the knee joint; lateral dislocations of the patella; and fracture–dislocations of the ankle.

The hallmarks of subluxations and dislocations are pain, deformity, and decreased range of motion. Certain dislocations are associated with specific complications, and these must be ruled out in the evaluation and treatment of the injury. For example, the aorta and trachea are at risk in posterior dislocations of the sternoclavicular joint, and injury to them can lead to rapid respiratory compromise or intrathoracic hemorrhage; the axillary nerve and, less commonly, the musculocutaneous nerve are at risk in anterior shoulder dislocations, and their function must be clearly assessed prior to any attempted reduction and then reassessed after the reduction is complete; the popliteal artery can be stretched, torn, or completely disrupted in a posterior dislocation of the knee, and many experts recommend angiogram followed by close observation in any knee dislocation. Radiographs should be obtained prior to attempts at reduction, and after the reduction has been achieved, to document the position of the bones, restoration of anatomic position, and the presence of associated fractures.

Techniques for the reduction of specific joints are discussed in the chapters dedicated to those joints, but certain principles hold true for all subluxations and dislocations: Increasing length of time between injury and relocation corresponds proportionally to the severity of spasm and swelling that will occur and the difficulty involved in reducing the joint; adequate pain control and sedation facilitate smooth reduction; excess force applied during the reduction can result in fractures, nerve damage, and vascular injury; the technique used to reduce the dislocation should initially replicate the mechanism of injury to release the dislocated bone from the anatomic structure that is keeping it dislocated; in certain dislocations, the incidence of delayed complications is directly proportional to the time from injury to relocation. For example, avascular necrosis of the femoral head occurs in 10% to 20% of hip dislocations, and the rate is directly proportional to the total time from injury to successful reduction; similarly, myositis ossificans is a well-recognized complication of posterior dislocation of the elbow, and its incidence is directly related to three variables: the number of attempts at reduction, the length of time from injury to successful reduction, and whether the joint is adequately immobilized after reduction.

TENDINITIS

Tendinitis can be viewed as a subset of strain because it is an injury to the musculotendinous unit, but it is better viewed as a separate entity. Tendinitis differs from strain in that the inflammation is *isolated* to the tendon and *involves the insertion of the tendon into the bone,* which occurs via a transitional, calcified fibrocartilage known as Sharpey's fibers. Tendinitis can result from chronic use or from one acute episode of overuse. In acute inflammation, the tendon is irritated and an acute inflammatory response occurs, initiated by fibroblasts within the tendon and perpetuated by the migration of macrophages into the tendon tissue and their fundamental role in the prostaglandin-mediated healing process; with repeated irritation, signs of chronic inflammation develop, including the continued migration of macrophages to the site of injury, influx of plasma cells into the tendon matrix, phagocytosis of debris, and a cellular predominance of lymphocytes within the tendinous fibers occurs. If this cycle is not interrupted, permanent changes in the architecture of Sharpey's fibers and atrophy of the tendon fibers occur.

Common tendons involved in acute or chronic tendinitis presenting to the ED include patellar tendinitis, quadriceps tendinitis, rotator cuff tendinitis, Achilles' tendinitis, lateral epicondylitis of the elbow, and de Quervain's stenosing tenosynovitis of the first dorsal compartment of the wrist (the abductor pollicis longus and extensor pollicis brevis tendons).

Clinically, tendinitis presents with pain during active range of motion, loss of function, point tenderness over the affected tendon near its insertion in bone, and, often, localized edema and erythema. Forced contraction of the affected muscle against resistance elicits pain, which is exacerbated by pressure over the point of insertion. Pain can also be elicited by forced extension of the tendon, stretching the inflamed fibers. Calcific tendinitis is a different entity. It is usually associated with chronic inflammation and consists of calcium deposition within the body of the tendon. It is often an indication of tendinous degeneration altering the macrostructure of the tendon. Calcific tendinitis has a characteristic radiographic appearance, revealing the calcium depositions within the tendon; for example, a band of calcification can be seen passing over the bicipital groove in calcific biceps tendinitis at the shoulder.

Chronic Musculoskeletal Pain Syndromes

In a recent study conducted in the emergency room of a tertiary care hospital in an urban setting, 10% of all patients presenting for evaluation and treatment of a musculoskeletal complaint sought treatment for a chronic musculoskeletal pain syndrome. These patients accounted for 1% of total ED visits; the primary reason for their presentation to the ED was dissatisfaction with their current level of pain control. In some instances, patients such as those in the study are obviously undermedicated and can be easily helped; in other cases, they are already on one or more powerful analgesics, and addressing their complaints can be a difficult, potentially frustrating therapeutic encounter for the emergency physician; and another group of patients will raise concerns about physical and psychologic dependence on narcotics—they often have multiple drug allergies and often present to the ED late at night or on weekends when their regular doctors are "unavailable."

When patients with chronic musculoskeletal pain syndromes are followed at your institution and their x-rays, reports of other imaging studies, laboratory values, and management plans can be reviewed, their ED management is often straightforward. If they are followed at outside institutions, it can be a daunting challenge to adequately assess their pathology; decide when repeat imaging studies are necessary; ensure that they have not been misdiagnosed, that a complication has not been overlooked, or that a significant progression in their pathology has not occurred; and successfully treat their pain while continuing to orchestrate patient flow in a busy ED. Often, allowing them *a reasonable but finite period of uninterrupted time to "tell their story"* is the most efficient way to approach a new patient presenting with chronic pain. Knowing when to redirect their thoughts and concerns is a learned art that requires sensitivity and confidence.

Muscle Spasms

Muscle spasms are a poorly understood phenomenon in which a voluntary muscle undergoes sustained involuntary contraction, leading to depletion of stored glycogen, localized build-up of lactic acid, and severe pain. The causes of muscle spasm are not known, but hypotheses include localized alterations in blood flow, regional or systemic electrolyte imbalances (especially sodium and calcium; less often, potassium), and postural abnormalities that place a bone in a nonanatomically neutral position, causing attached musculature to fire continuously. For example, overdevelopment of the muscles on one side of the body in a racquet-sports athlete can cause latissimus dorsi spasm, as the proprioceptors present in the latissimus sense that the arm is out of the neutral position and cause repetitive muscle contraction in attempted compensation.

Muscle spasms typically seen in the ED include spasms of the gastrocnemius, levator scapulae, trapezii, rhomboids, and latissimus dorsi. Rectus abdominus muscle spasm can mimic an acute abdomen and will respond best to intravenous benzodiazepine therapy.

Treatment includes freezing the muscle belly with fluoroethane spray, followed by passive, gentle, forced range of motion to "break the spasm"; massage; treatment with muscle relaxants, including diazepam and other benzodiazepines; pain control with acetaminophen, NSAIDs, or opioid analgesics; and laboratory evaluation of serum electrolytes, including calcium, sodium, and potassium (which are low yield in most situations).

Muscle spasm must be distinguished from myoclonus, as the implications of the two conditions are very different.

EMERGENCY DEPARTMENT MANAGEMENT

The ED management of any injured patient begins with the basic ABCs: airway, breathing, and circulation. In the conscious, cooperative patient who, for example, sprained his ankle playing basketball, evaluation of the ABCs is routinely done in triage by asking the patient, "Why did you come to the emergency room today?"; listening to his response; noting that his voice is normal and his speech is unlabored; watching him breathe in and out in a symmetric, unlabored fashion; and taking his vital signs—pulse, blood pressure, and respiratory rate. *In other words, in most instances, a simple, human interaction encompasses an adequate primary trauma survey.* When the patient is reliable, not intoxicated, and has an isolated injury, and the mechanism of injury does not suggest other possible injuries that are being ignored by the patient because he or she is distracted by the pain of the obvious injury, evaluation and treatment can be limited to the injured joint along with the joints immediately proximal and distal to the injury (and the contralateral partner of the injured joint or limb for comparison of range of motion, anatomy, and laxity).

In patients with multiple injuries, head trauma, amnesia, intoxication, or medical illnesses resulting in their musculoskeletal injury (e.g., a distal radial fracture after syncope), a complete physical evaluation is mandatory and should follow basic trauma guidelines, beginning with a primary survey, assessing the ABCs; evaluating neurologic disability, including a formal grading of their Glasgow Coma Scale; then continuing with complete exposure of the patient, searching for any accompanying injuries, before systematically evaluating the underlying medical problem that could have produced the trauma (unless it is of significant severity, e.g., a myocardial infarction or arrhythmia, that it is addressed earlier in the primary survey). If a problem is identified, it should be addressed before moving on to the next step in the systematic evaluation. For example, the motorcyclist thrown from the cycle, who presents with an open fracture of the tibia and fibula and flail chest, needs breathing stabilized before the leg is further evaluated. In extremity wounds, hemorrhage can often be rapidly but temporarily controlled with a direct-pressure dressing, ensuring continued circulatory stability until the source of bleeding can be systematically evaluated. After the primary survey, each joint should be palpated and ranged systematically, and the integrity of long bones assessed by inspection, palpation, and range of motion.

As alluded to previously, certain extremity injuries are true orthopedic emergencies, meriting expeditious evaluation and management. These include vascular injuries, compartment syndromes, open fractures and dislocations, and certain dislocated joints (Table 111.2). They should be addressed immediately after the ABCs have been evaluated, stabilized, and recorded on a trauma flow sheet. To reiterate, if vascular compromise is suspected, immediate consultation with the orthopedic or vascular surgeon is advised. When vascular insufficiency is caused by stretching of the vessel across the site of a dislocation or displaced fracture, reduction of the fracture or dislocation may correct the problem. Pulses must be documented after the reduction. If an injury to the vessel itself is suspected, arteriography, MRA, or surgical exploration may be indicated. In certain instances, Doppler evaluation, followed by close observation with serial neurovascular examinations, is a standard of care. These decisions should be left to the consulting surgeon. Blood flow to an ischemic extremity should, ideally, be reestablished within 6 to 8 hours to prevent permanent injuries, including ischemia and necrosis.

Similarly, if compartment syndrome is suspected, it must be ruled out by manometry. This is usually done through emergent consultation with an orthopedic surgeon. If compartment pressures are elevated, emergent fasciotomy is mandatory.

The initial management of open fractures and joints should be directed toward reducing the chances of infection. Gross particulate debris in the wound should be removed. Exposed bone *should not be replaced in the wound,* because this may further introduce contamination. A sterile dressing should be applied. The extremity is splinted to prevent further tissue and neurovascular injury. Intravenous antibiotic therapy, usually with a first- or second-generation cephalosporin, is instituted (if not contraindicated by drug allergies), and tetanus prophylaxis (sometimes including tetanus immune globulin) given when indicated. (A macrolide antibiotic or trimethoprim–sulfamethoxazole is a good choice for the penicillin-allergic patient.) After these initial management steps have been taken, orthopedic consultation should be obtained. Most open fractures and dislocations require formal debridement in the operating room, which should be performed within 8 hours of the injury. The incidence of infection is directly proportional to the length of time from injury until copious irrigation and formal debridement.

Dislocated hips may later develop ischemic necrosis, and dislocated elbows may later develop Volkmann's ischemic contracture (compartment syndrome, decreased blood flow, necrosis, and contracture following a dislocation). Avascular necrosis of the hip is thought to be caused by damage to the vessels supplying the femoral head. In general, these vessels are not completely torn in the dislocation; rather, they are stretched and blood flow through them is compromised. Therefore, the incidence of avascular necrosis is directly related to the length of time from injury to adequate relocation of the hip. Similar principles apply to the development of Volkmann's ischemic contracture following elbow dislocation. Therefore, reduction should be accomplished as soon as is feasible.

After all life- and limb-threatening injuries have been addressed, attention can be directed toward the management of individual injuries—fractures, dislocations, sprains, strains, tendinitis, and spasm. In the majority of cases presenting to the ED, a brief confirmation of stable ABCs will be followed immediately by an evaluation of the injured joint or extremity. This evaluation begins with a *thorough history,* ascertaining the mechanism of injury, previous injury to the limb, handedness where applicable, and medical problems potentially contributory to current disability. It is not a sufficient history to note that a patient sustained a puncture wound "on the job." Was it from a nail gun? A high-pressure grease gun? Or a sewing machine? Different mechanisms of injury imply different potential problems. What was the timing of the injury? Has the patient experienced associated symptoms of pain, paresthesia, or weakness, or signs of pallor, deformity, and so forth? *Inspection follows.* Does the injured area appear normal? Is it deformed, swollen, erythematous, ecchymotic? Is exposed bone visible? Is a spot of grease visible at a minute puncture wound? Is purulent fluid draining from a wound? Is there an obvious abrasion, laceration, or puncture wound over the injured area? *Palpation follows.* Is there a palpable deformity? Is tenderness focal or diffuse? Is there edema? Calor? Induration? Palpation must include a care-

TABLE 111.2. Orthopedic Emergencies

Vascular injuries
Compartment syndrome
Open fractures
Open joints
Dislocated hip

ful assessment of neurovascular integrity. Is the injured area dusky or mottled? Are distal pulses intact? Symmetric with the unaffected side? Is capillary refill normal? Is sensation to light touch unaffected? Hypesthesia often occurs over an area of acute injury. Active range of motion should be tested. In the majority of acute injuries, the patient is not enthusiastic about actively ranging the joint, and passive range of motion and provocative maneuvers are of limited utility secondary to pain.

Radiographs are the cornerstone of further evaluation and management of most musculoskeletal complaints. Many fractures can be diagnosed clinically, but, in the vast majority of cases, the diagnosis should be supported radiographically. Radiographs frequently determine the need for operative reduction, the length of time the fracture needs to be immobilized, and potential complications during the rehabilitation process. Criteria for obtaining radiographs of specific injuries are formalized but constantly evolving, and are beyond the scope of this chapter. They are addressed in the chapters on injuries to specific joints. The goals of objective criteria for obtaining radiographs include reduction in unnecessary imaging, increased efficiency of patient flow in the ED, decreased exposure to radiation, and containment of health-care costs. For example, the "Ottawa Ankle Rules" are objective criteria for obtaining an ankle series after an ankle injury, and state that ankle films are required in patients over 18 years old if pain in the malleolar area is accompanied by inability to bear weight (defined as walking four steps) immediately after the injury and in the ED, or by bony tenderness over the posterior aspect of the distal 6 cm of the medial or lateral malleolus. In a study in the *Journal of the American Medical Association* in 1993, by Stiell et al., strict implementation of the Ottawa Ankle Rules was shown to reduce the number of ankle series ordered by 28%, increase ED efficiency, and decrease ED costs without increasing the percentage of missed fractures.

When the decision is made to obtain roentgenograms, the correct views must be obtained, they need to be of sufficient quality to competently evaluate for fracture, and they need to be read thoroughly, in an unharried fashion. Poor-quality films should never be accepted. Many fractures have been missed because of technically inadequate films. In addition, thorough examination of the soft tissue and every bone in the x-ray is essential to avoid missing subtle findings that may indicate fracture or dislocation. For example, the fat pad sign on an elbow x-ray may be the sole indication of a radial head fracture.

Other pitfalls in interpretation include the following:

- Misinterpretation of a nutrient foramen, housing a nutrient artery, as a fracture. A nutrient foramen will appear less radiolucent than a fracture (very smooth-edged) and will angle obliquely from the edge of the bone through the cortex, and then terminate without involving the cortex on the other side of the marrow.
- Confusing sesamoid bones or accessory ossicles with fractures. These anatomic variants usually have smooth edges and are well corticated, and no defect in the adjacent bone will be noted. In some instances, a comparison view can help clarify the structure in question. For example, the patient with pain over the patella following a dashboard injury, who is found to have a two-part patella on x-ray in the area corresponding to his clinical pain, may have bipartite patella, which is confirmed by its presence on an x-ray of the unaffected knee.
- Misinterpretation of fat folds, clothing folds, casts, or splints as fractures; misinterpretation of jewelry or body piercings as foreign bodies.

Every x-ray series should include a minimum of two views that are *shot at right angles to each other*. If the plane of the fracture is at 90 degrees (perpendicular) to the plane of the x-ray beam, the fracture may not be evident on that view but would be readily visible on an x-ray taken in a plane parallel to the plane of the fracture line.

Fractures in the shaft of long bones are often accompanied by additional fractures in that bone proximal or distal to the main fracture site or by dislocations at the joints at either end of the bone. Therefore, all long-bone shaft fractures require imaging of the entire length of the bone, including adequate views of its joints. For example, a midshaft femur fracture requires x-rays of the entire shaft, a two-plane knee series, and a two-plane hip series.

Fractures to paired long bones, such as the radius and ulna or the tibia and fibula, present with different associated fractures: A fracture to one bone is sometimes accompanied by a distant fracture to the other bone in the pair. For example, medial malleolar ankle fractures resulting from a lateral twisting mechanism sometimes have an associated proximal fibular or fibular head fracture or dislocation. The mechanism of injury explains this association: The twisting force that breaks the medial malleolus is transmitted up the shafts of the tibia and fibula and is dissipated at the weakest point, the proximal fibula, resulting in either fracture or dislocation. Thus, more complex ankle fractures require imaging of the entire shafts of the fibula and tibia and a two-way series of the knee. For an additional example, certain forearm fractures are commonly associated with a fracture–dislocation of the other bone of the forearm, such as a radial shaft fracture and distal radioulnar joint dislocation, known as a Galeazzi fracture (Fig. 111.6).

Additional views are sometimes helpful. A dedicated scaphoid view can aid in the detection of a subtle scaphoid fracture. An axial view of the calcaneus can reveal a fracture missed on standard ankle and foot series. Many posterior dislocations of the shoulder are not evident, except on an axillary view of the glenohumeral joint, clearly depicting the relationship between the humeral head and the glenoid fossa. In certain instances, comparison views to the patient's other side are helpful. For example, in distal clavicle osteolysis, characterized by pain and os-

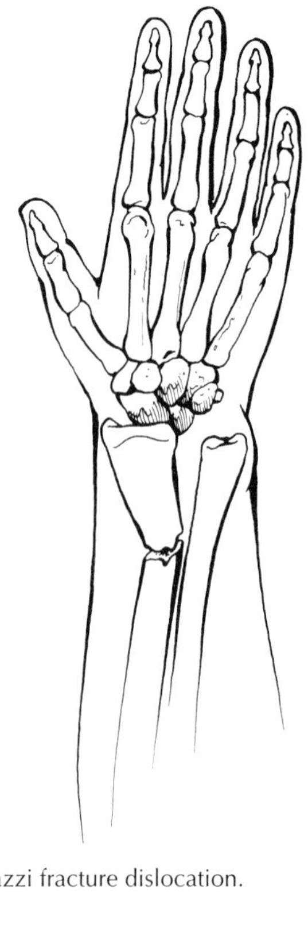

Figure 111.6. Galeazzi fracture dislocation.

teolysis of the distal clavicle—seen in power lifters and in contact athletes suffering significant blunt trauma to the point (acromion) of the shoulder—bilateral clavicle views help confirm the diagnosis when a larger separation is seen at the affected acromioclavicular joint compared with the unaffected one.

Adequate films, correctly interpreted, are not 100% sensitive for fractures. Nondisplaced, or hairline, fractures often become visible, or radiolucent, only on roentgenograms 7 to 10 days after injury, as bone resorption widens the fracture line, hematoma develops, and new bone formation proceeds. If there is potential morbidity associated with a missed fracture on plain x-rays, a clinically fractured joint should be treated as a fracture, or more sophisticated imaging studies should be obtained, if possible. A patient with a story and an examination consistent with a femoral neck fracture, who has normal plain radiographs and remains non–weight bearing in the ED, needs to be treated as having a nondisplaced hip fracture, kept non–weight bearing, and seen in orthopedics follow up in 7 to 10 days. On the other hand, MRI scan may reveal the fracture, and bone scan can be diagnostic. Similarly, snuff box tenderness (the space on the radial side of the wrist between the extensor pollicis longus tendon and the paired extensor pollicis brevis and adductor pollicis longus tendons) following a *fall on an outstretched hand* (FOOSH) needs to be treated as a scaphoid fracture, *even if the radiographs are normal.* If the radiographs show no fracture, immobilization in a thumb spica with follow-up examination and repeat radiographs in 10 days is mandatory.

DISPOSITION

ED care is not complete when the diagnosis is made. Appropriate immobilization needs to be instituted, and instructions for immediate care and follow-up given. These need to be tailored to the specific injury but, in general, involve rest, ice, and elevation. These simple, cost-effective steps are often overlooked in the rush to discharge patients from the ED and can, in some cases, affect more than the patient's comfort. For example, the simple application of ice to a lateral ankle sprain during the first 24 hours after injury has been shown to decrease time to return of full function by 50%.

Depending on the injury, the patient may be instructed to remain non–weight bearing or keep the injured joint immobilized; in other cases, activity as tolerated is appropriate and may speed recovery (e.g., low-back strain). Pain control must be achieved in the ED, and the pain medications given for the outpatient setting need to be commensurate with the injury. For example, the patient who requires morphine in the ED for a rib cage contusion is mismanaged if he or she is discharged with instructions to take acetaminophen as needed for pain. Adequate postinjury pain control improves outcome and decreases repeat visits to the ED.

Patients should be instructed to return to the ED if they experience any signs or symptoms of neurovascular compromise, excessive pain, coldness, erythema, fevers, chills, cough, pleuritic chest pain, or a cast or splint that feels too tight or causes pain. Appropriate follow-up depends on the nature and extent of the injury and can range from a visit to the patient's primary care doctor in 2 weeks, to orthopedic referral in 10 days' time, to being seen by a hand surgeon in the next few days for operative repair of a flexor tendon laceration.

COMMON PITFALLS

- Ordering the wrong x-ray because of an inadequate physical examination. For example, an x-ray of the ankle might be ordered when the tenderness is actually over the base of the fifth metatarsal.
- Not recognizing all injuries because the physician's (and often the patient's) attention is focused on one specific injury. For example, the patient who falls off a ladder and presents with a grade II lateral ankle sprain may have a calcaneal fracture from the initial impact, which goes unnoticed because of the obviousness of the ecchymosis and edema accompanying the lateral sprain.
- Acceptance of poor-quality x-rays or relying on a single view without an accompanying view shot at 90 degrees to the initial view. There are well-defined criteria for the radiographic evaluation of different injuries, and these must be strictly adhered to if the physician wants to avoid missed diagnoses.
- In the case of long-bone fractures, failure to include the length of the bone, the joint above, and the joint below in adequately exposed radiographs.
- Failure to rule out infection in a patient presenting with a swollen joint or similar condition, such as olecranon bursitis. It is a mistake to assume that the swollen joint in the patient with a history of gouty arthritis is another flare of gout. With rare exceptions, in a patient presenting with monoarthritis, fluid should be obtained, analyzed for crystals, and sent for cell count, Gram stain, and culture, to confirm the diagnosis and to rule out concomitant infection. In most cases, antibiosis should be initiated until infection is excluded, unless this can be done over the course of a few hours in the emergency room.
- Failure to realize that drops of blood or small abrasions on the skin in the area of a fracture connotes an open fracture until clearly proven otherwise.
- Not checking, or documenting, a complete neurovascular examination on initial presentation and after any procedures to reduce a fracture or a dislocation.
- Not obtaining radiographs prior to and/or after the reduction of a fracture or a dislocation to rule out accompanying avulsion fracture from the dislocation or from the reduction procedure. X-rays should not be obtained only when the delay created by x-raying the dislocation or fracture–dislocation could contribute to morbidity. If x-rays are only obtained post-reduction, there is no way to know whether the bony Bankart lesion accompanying the reduced anterior shoulder dislocation was caused by the dislocation or the reduction procedure.
- Attributing pain in an extremity to an unrelated injury. Frequently, when patients develop extremity pain, they try to think of any injury that they have recently sustained and attribute the pain to that injury. The examiner may then be misled into believing that the pain, actually due to an independent condition, such as tumor or septic arthritis, was caused by some unrelated injury. If a patient describes being struck by a vacuum cleaner nozzle over the carpal bones on the dorsum of the hand, but physical examination reveals a boggy, erythematous, warm carporadial joint and tenosynovitis, disseminated gonococcal infection must be explicitly ruled out, despite the conflicting history.
- Attributing pain noted after a fracture to the fracture itself, rather than thoroughly investigating other potential sources of pain, such as a cast problem, neurovascular compromise, or compartment syndrome.
- Considering compartment syndrome in the differential of a patient's pain but not formally evaluating for it. Once the physician considers the diagnosis of compartment syndrome, it must be excluded, explicitly, by manometry.
- Suspecting a fracture clinically but not pursuing additional studies when the plane radiographs are normal or not treating the clinical fracture as a fracture on discharge.

Assessment of a patient's ability to ambulate is essential prior to discharge, and the inability to ambulate can further confirm the presence of an occult lower extremity fracture.

- Not providing patients with printed or clearly written, simply worded discharge instructions for the immediate management of their injuries and for post-ED follow-up care. Instructions should include specifics about the application of ice, elevation of the injured extremity, analgesia, and weight bearing. Some orthopedic injuries heal well with benign neglect; many have suboptimal outcomes when treated apathetically.

Bibliography

Brighton CT. Principles of fracture healing: part I: the biology of fracture repair. In: Murray JA, ed. *American Academy of Orthopedic Surgery Instructional Course Lecture XXXIII*. St. Louis: CV Mosby, 1984.

Connoly JF. *DePalma's management of fractures and dislocations*. Philadelphia: WB Saunders, 1983.

Gibbons JJ, Wilson PR. RSD score: a criteria for the diagnosis of reflex sympathetic dystrophy and causalgia. *Clin J Pain* 1992;8:260.

Hocutt JE, Jaffe R, Rylander R, et al. Cryotherapy in ankle sprains. *Am J Sports Med* 1982;10(5):316.

Keats TE. *An atlas of normal roentgen variants that may simulate disease*, 3rd ed. Chicago: Year Book, 1984.

Marder RA, Chapman MW. Principles of management of fractures in sports. *Clin Sports Med* 1990;9:1.

McKibbin B. The biology of fracture healing in long bones. *J Bone Joint Surg* 1978;60:150.

Miller MD. *Review of orthopaedics*, 2nd ed. Philadelphia: WB Saunders, 1996.

Patzakis MJ, Narvey JP, Ivler D. The role of antibiotics in the management of open fractures. *J Bone Joint Surg* 1974;56A:532.

Proctor MT. Non-union of the scaphoid: early and late management. *Injury* 1994;25:15.

Rockwood CA, Green DP. *Fractures*. Philadelphia: JB Lippincott Co, 1975.

Schultz RJ. *The language of fractures*, 2nd ed. Baltimore: Williams & Wilkins, 1990.

Scuderi GR, McCann PD, Bruno PJ. *Sports medicine: principles of primary care*. St. Louis: Mosby, 1997.

Snell R, Smith M. *Clinical anatomy for emergency medicine*. St. Louis: CV Mosby, 1993.

Stiell IG, Greenberg GH, McKnight RD, et al. A study to develop clinical decision rules for the use of radiography in acute ankle injuries. *Ann Emerg Med* 1992;21:384.

Stiell IG, Greenberg GH, McKnight RD, et al. Decision rules for the use of radiography in acute ankle injuries: refinement and prospective validation. *JAMA* 1993;269:1127.

Walls RM, Rosen P. Traumatic dislocation of the knee. *J Emerg Med* 1984; 1:527.

CHAPTER 112
Shoulder Injuries

Jeffrey Schaider and Robert Simon

The shoulder joint is composed of three bones and three joints. The bones are the humeral head, clavicle, and scapula; the joints are the sternoclavicular (SC), acromioclavicular (AC), and glenohumeral. Figures 112.1 and 112.2 demonstrate the essential osseous and ligamentous anatomy of the shoulder, respectively. The rotator cuff surrounds the glenohumeral joint and is composed of the teres minor, infraspinatus, and supraspinatus muscles attaching to the greater tuberosity of the humerus, and the subscapularis muscle attaching to the lesser tuberosity of the humerus. Superficial to these muscles is the deltoid muscle.

The glenohumeral joint and scapulothoracic articulation function as a unit in abducting the humerus. The ratio of scapular to glenohumeral movement is 1:2; therefore, for every 30 degrees of abduction of the arm, the scapula moves 10 degrees and the glenohumeral joint moves 20 degrees. If the glenohumeral joint is completely immobilized, the scapulothoracic articulation can provide 65 degrees of abduction.

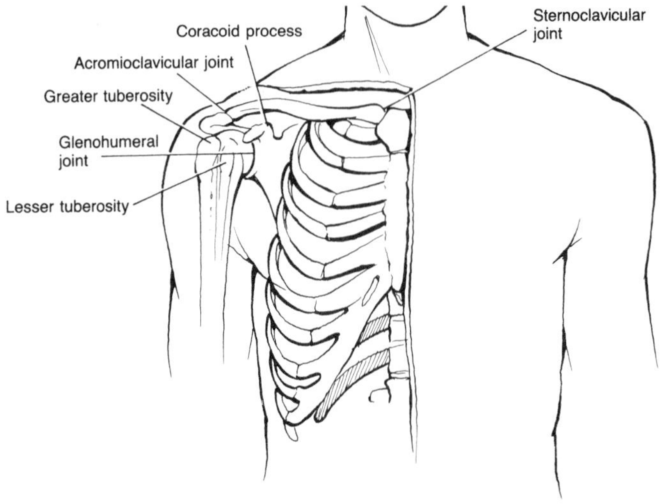

Figure 112.1. The essential anatomy of the shoulder. (Adapted from Simon RR, Koenigsknecht SJ. *Emergency orthopedics*. Norwalk, CT: Appleton & Lange, 1994.)

GENERAL EVALUATION

The clavicle is anchored to the scapula by the AC and coracoclavicular ligaments. The SC and costoclavicular ligaments anchor the clavicle medially. The SC joint is palpable immediately lateral to the suprasternal notch. The AC joint is palpated by pushing in a medial direction against the distal end of the clavicle as it protrudes above the flattened acromion process.

The greater tuberosity of the humerus lies lateral to the acromion process, and can easily be palpated by following the acromion process to its lateral edge and then sliding the fingers inferiorly. The bicipital groove, which contains the biceps tendon, is located anterior and medial to the greater tuberosity and is bordered laterally by the greater tuberosity and medially by the lesser tuberosity. External rotation places the groove in a more exposed position for palpation, and permits the examiner to palpate the greater tuberosity first, then the bicipital groove, and finally the lesser tuberosity by moving from a lateral to a medial position. The articular surface of the proximal humerus articulates with the glenoid, forming the glenohumeral joint. Because the articular surface ends at the anatomic neck, fractures located proximal to the anatomic neck are considered articular surface fractures. The surgical neck is the narrow portion of the proximal humerus distal to the anatomic neck.

The examiner must consider injury to proximate structures. The subclavian vessels and the brachial plexus lie in close proximity to the clavicle, so displaced clavicular fractures can be associated with injuries to these structures. The brachial plexus, axillary nerve, and axillary artery lie in close proximity to the proximal humerus, and injuries to these structures frequently accompany proximal humerus fractures.

The scapula covers ribs 2 through 7 posteriorly. It is covered with thick muscles over its entire body and spine. The scapula is connected to the axial skeleton solely by the AC joint. The examiner should test function of the associated muscles and range of motion of this joint.

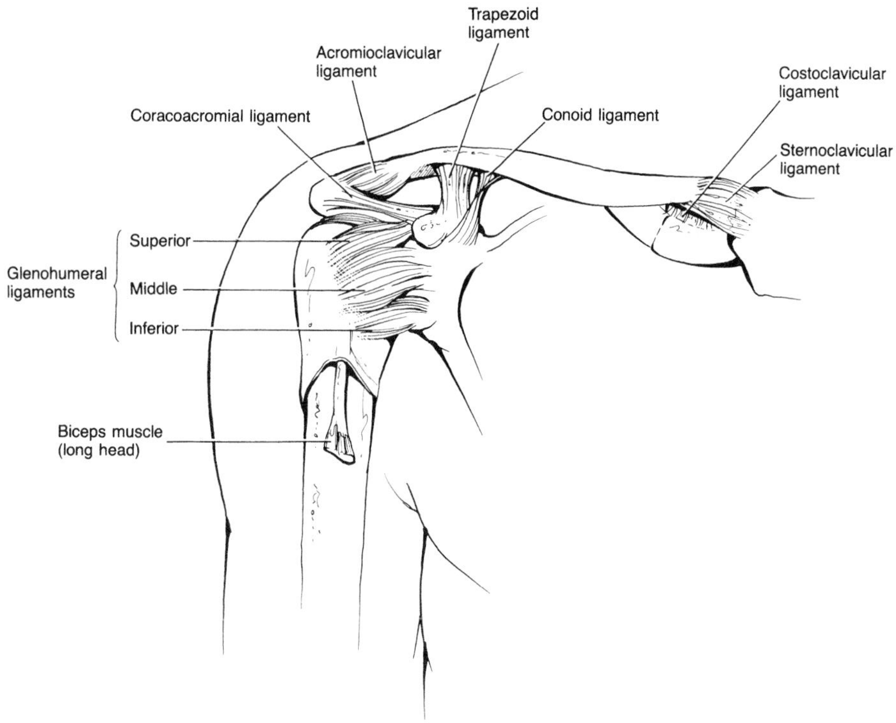

Figure 112.2. The ligaments around the shoulder.

Routine clavicular radiographs include an anteroposterior (AP) view of the upper thorax to define the structures. Occasionally, an AP view with the tube directed 45 degrees cephalad (apical lordotic) is needed to detect medial-third fractures. At times, cone-down views, upper rib radiographs, and tomograms may be necessary to delineate fractures adequately.

Four views of the shoulder are optimal to evaluate the proximal humerus and glenoid joint for fractures and dislocations. The trauma series recommended by Neer[12] includes an AP view of the shoulder in addition to a transscapular projection commonly known as the Y view. The transscapular view is obtained by placing the radiographic film along the lateral side of the humerus, with the beam projected along the length of the scapula. This view is helpful in identifying shoulder dislocations. In addition to the two-view trauma series, an AP internal rotation view of the humerus and an axillary view permit full evaluation of the shoulder and proximal humerus, including the articular surface.

FRACTURES

Clavicular Fracture

Clavicular fractures are the most common childhood fracture. They are often encountered in newborns secondary to birth trauma. Clavicular fractures account for 5% of all fractures seen for all age groups. Two mechanisms are commonly responsible: (1) force applied directly to the clavicle and (2) force applied to the outer end of the clavicle, which can push the shoulder inward toward the chest, causing a shearing force and fracture of the clavicle.[14]

Evaluation

Most patients have swelling and tenderness over the fracture site. Middle-third clavicular fractures usually result in a downward and inward slump of the involved shoulder due to loss of support.

Management

Eighty percent of all clavicular fractures occur in the middle third. Nondisplaced middle-third fractures in adults have an intact periosteum. These require a sling for support and ice to reduce swelling. Figure-of-eight splints can be used for reduction and maintenance of position for displaced middle-third clavicular fractures in adults and children; however, they show no benefit over a simple sling for fractures in children. Complications of middle-third clavicular fractures include malunion; excess callus formation, resulting in cosmetic defect; and neurovascular compromise. Rarely, nonunion occurs in fractures treated with open reduction and internal fixation.

Fifteen percent of clavicular fractures occur in the distal third. Nondisplaced fractures of the distal clavicle are splinted by the surrounding intact ligaments and muscles. They are usually treated symptomatically with ice, analgesics, a sling, and early motion. Complications include delayed union of displaced fractures treated conservatively, and degenerative arthritis with intraarticular involvement.

Medial-third fractures represent only 5% of all clavicular fractures. Considerable force is required to fracture the medial clavicle, so associated injuries, such as vascular injuries, should be sought. Management includes ice, analgesics, and a sling for support. Displaced fractures require orthopedic referral for reduction. Degenerative arthritis frequently accompanies these fractures.

Proximal Humerus Fracture

Proximal humeral fractures account for 5% of all fractures. They are most common in the elderly.[19] Anatomically, proximal humeral fractures include all humeral fractures proximal to the surgical neck.

Evaluation

Two mechanisms of injury commonly produce proximal humeral fractures: (1) a direct blow on the lateral aspect of the arm and (2) a fall on an outstretched arm. Patients present with tenderness and swelling over the upper arm and shoulder. Most commonly, the arm is held adducted. Patients who present with the arm abducted have a much higher incidence of neurovascular injury.

Using the Neer classification system for proximal humerus fractures, the proximal humerus is divided into four segments: greater tuberosity, lesser tuberosity, anatomic neck, and surgical neck.[12,13] This classification system has both prognostic and therapeutic implications, and depends on the relation of the bone segments involved and their displacement. The Neer system divides the fractures into one-part, two-part, three-part, and four-part fractures, depending on the displacement and angulation of the fracture (Fig. 112.3).

Management

If all the proximal humeral fragments are nondisplaced and without angulation (less than 45 degrees), the injury is classified as a one-part fracture. The humeral fragments are held in place by the periosteum, rotator cuff, and joint capsule. Examples of one-part fractures are a surgical neck fracture with less than 45 degrees of angulation, a nondisplaced anatomic neck fracture, and a nondisplaced greater tuberosity fracture. Therapy for one-part fractures requires immobilization in a sling and swathe and orthopedic referral. Circumduction exercises should begin as soon as tolerated, and should be followed by passive exercise of the elbow and shoulder at 2 to 3 weeks. Shoulder motion exercises can usually be started within 3 to 4 weeks.

Two-part fractures have either a fragment with more than 1 cm of displacement or one with over 45 degrees of angulation to the intact proximal humerus. Surgical neck fractures with over 45 degrees of angulation, and displaced anatomic neck fractures, require immobilization with a sling and swathe and emergent orthopedic referral for reduction. Anatomic neck fractures have a high incidence of avascular necrosis.

The insertions of the supraspinatus, infraspinatus, and teres minor on the greater tuberosity complicate fractures in this region. Displaced greater tuberosity fractures (two-part fractures) are always associated with a tear of the rotator cuff. Greater tuberosity fractures are also seen in about 15% of all anterior shoulder dislocations.[5,17] Therapy for displaced greater tuberosity fractures depends on the patient's age. Young patients require internal fixation or excision of the fragment, with repair of the torn rotator cuff. Older patients are usually not candidates for surgical repair and require ice, immobilization with a sling and swathe, and early orthopedic referral. Complications of greater tuberosity fractures include impingement on the long head of the biceps, resulting in chronic tenosynovitis and eventually tendon rupture; nonunion; and myositis ossificans.

Lesser tuberosity fractures commonly occur in conjunction with posterior shoulder dislocations, due to intense contraction of the subscapularis muscle, which inserts on the lesser tuberosity. Management of these fractures includes sling and swathe immobilization. Most orthopedic surgeons recommend 3 to 5 days of immobilization, followed by gradually increasing range-of-motion exercises. Some orthopedists prefer surgical fixation, so early consultation is advised.

Combination fractures—Neer three- and four-part fractures—result from severe forces. Three-part fractures involve two fragments that are individually displaced from the proximal humerus. Four-part fractures involve three fragments individually displaced from the remaining proximal humerus. Combined proximal humeral fractures are associated with shoulder dislocations, rotator cuff injuries, and neurovascular compromise. Therapy includes sling immobilization and emergent orthopedic referral. These complex injuries usually require admission. Virtually all combined fractures require surgical repair. Many four-part fractures require the insertion of a prosthesis, as a high incidence of avascular necrosis of the humeral head occurs secondary to compromised blood supply.

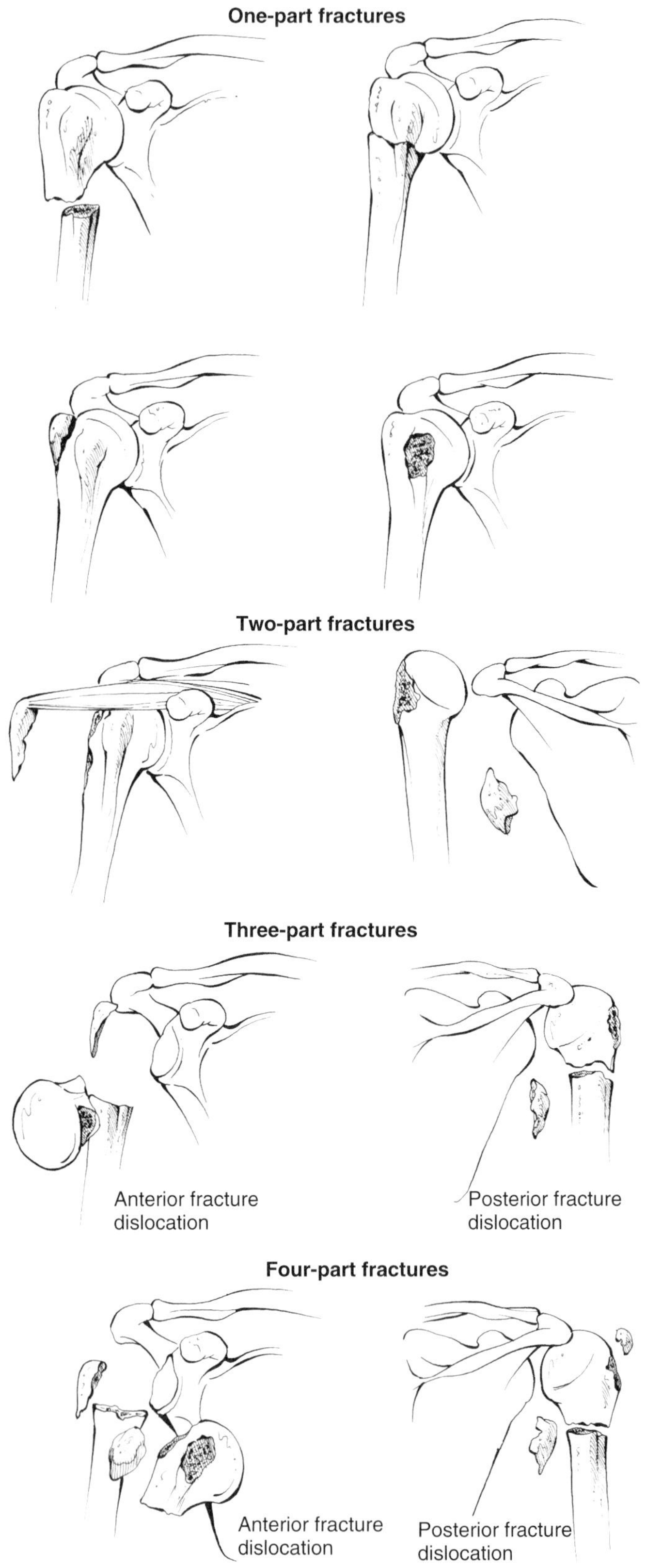

Figure 112.3. Examples of one-, two-, three-, and four-part fractures as described by Neer.

Articular surface fractures, also referred to as impression fractures, often result from direct trauma to the lateral arm. Fractures that involve less than 20% of the joint surface can be treated with sling and swathe immobilization in external rotation and early referral. Fractures involving more than 20% of the joint surface require surgical repair, and possibly prosthesis insertion. Complications of these fractures include joint stiffness, arthritis, and avascular necrosis with severely comminuted fractures.

Scapular Fractures

Scapular fractures represent only 1% of all fractures, and 5% of fractures involving the shoulder.[7] Many fracture patterns are associated with scapular fractures.

Management

Because a great deal of force is usually required to fracture the body or spine of the scapula, these fractures are often associated with much more serious injuries. Typically, there is little displacement, due to the support of the investing muscles and periosteum. Treatment includes sling and swathe immobilization, early limited exercise, and orthopedic referral.

Acromion fractures result from a direct downward blow to the shoulder. Due to the large amount of force required to produce these fractures, they are often accompanied by associated injuries, including brachial plexus injuries, rotator cuff tears, and superior shoulder dislocations. Nondisplaced fractures may be treated with sling immobilization in conjunction with an elastic circular dressing that pushes the elbow up and the lateral clavicle down. Displaced fractures require internal fixation.

Glenoid rim fractures are associated with two mechanisms of injury. A direct blow may result in a stellate fracture. An upward force, secondary to a fall on the flexed elbow, may cause a displaced glenoid rim fracture. Therapy for fractures with small fragments consists of sling immobilization, ice, and analgesia. Large or widely displaced fragments and stellate fractures require surgical fixation.

Coracoid process fractures may occur from a direct blow to the superior part of the shoulder, or from violent contraction of one of the inserting muscles, causing an avulsion fracture. The patient presents with tenderness to palpation over the coracoid process. Radiographs should include an axillary lateral view for delineation of any displacement of the fragment. Coracoid fractures are usually treated symptomatically with a sling, ice, and analgesics.

SHOULDER DISLOCATIONS

Anterior Shoulder Dislocation

Anterior shoulder dislocation is one of the most common dislocations, accounting for half of all dislocations presenting to the emergency department. This injury occurs when a blow to an abducted, externally rotated arm disrupts the anterior capsule and the glenohumeral ligaments.[5] There are three types of anterior dislocations: subclavicular, subcoracoid, and subglenoid.

Evaluation

The patient presents with the arm held to the side. The acromion is prominent, and there is loss of the normal rounded contour of the shoulder. Axillary nerve injury is the most common associated neurologic injury in anterior shoulder dislocations, occurring in about 12% of cases. Nerve injury is assessed by testing pinprick sensation over the lateral aspect of the deltoid. A defect in the posterior lateral portion of the humeral head is often seen on radiographs: This impaction fracture of the humeral head is known as the Hill-Sachs deformity.

Management

Adequate analgesia and muscle relaxation improves patient comfort and the success rate of reduction. There are numerous reduction techniques.

Scapular Manipulation Technique. The patient lies prone on the table, with the affected arm hanging off the table and suspended with about 5 to 10 lb of weight, similar to the Stimson technique (discussion follows). The physician pushes the tip of the scapula medially and the superior aspect of the scapula laterally.[11] This technique may be performed on an upright patient, with an assistant grasping the patient's arm and applying mild traction while the physician rotates the scapula in a similar fashion. For patients immobilized in the supine position due to multiple trauma, the scapular manipulation technique involves placing the affected extremity in adduction and 90-degree flexion at both the shoulder and elbow joints. Steady, gentle, upward traction is applied on the arm while the inferior tip of the scapula is gently manipulated with a force directed medially.[4]

Hennepin Technique. The external rotation requires little manipulation and permits the shoulder muscles to reduce the dislocation with minimal analgesia. The patient is seated upright or at 45 degrees. One of the physician's hands supports the elbow, and the other hand slowly externally rotates the patient's arm (Fig. 112.4). The arm is externally rotated to 90 degrees. The rotation must be performed gradually, and the patient must remain relaxed. After reaching 90 degrees, the shoulder may have reduced spontaneously. If not, the arm is slowly elevated, and the humeral head is lifted into the socket if it does not spontaneously reduce on elevation. Each of the aforementioned techniques requires little or no sedation or anesthesia and can be successfully performed within a few minutes.[6]

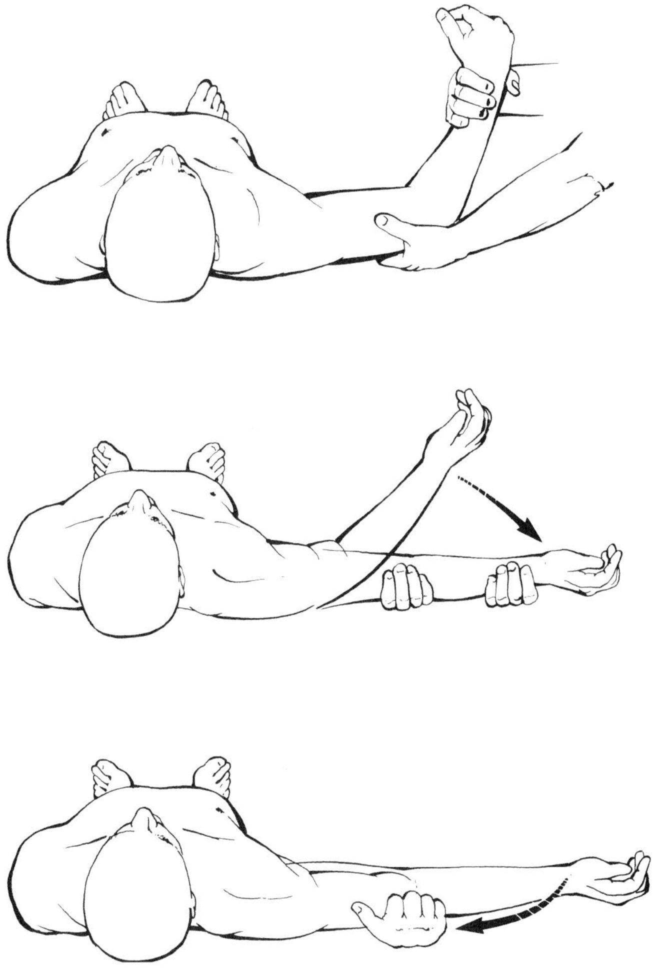

Figure 112.4. Hennepin technique for anterior shoulder dislocation reduction. (Adapted from Simon RR, Koenigsknecht SJ. *Emergency orthopedics.* Norwalk, CT: Appleton & Lange, 1994.)

Stimson Technique. The patient is placed in the prone position, with the arms dependent over a pillow or folded sheet and hanging over the side of the stretcher. A strap is added to the wrist and weights are applied (10 to 15 lb) over 20 to 30 minutes.[13,19,20] If unsuccessful, the examiner may rotate the humerus gently, externally and then internally with mild force, which usually reduce the dislocations.

Traction and Countertraction. With the patient lying in the supine position, an assistant applies countertraction with a folded sheet around the upper chest while the examiner applies traction to the arm (Fig. 112.5). Additional lateral traction may be added with a second sheet applied to the proximal portion of the humerus, with lateral force applied to this area. To prevent avulsion injuries[8] when using this maneuver, the patient must have good muscle relaxation. Alternatively, traction can be applied with the patient seated in an upright position of a chair. The patient sits as straight as possible. Traction is provided by a 3-ft loop of 4-in.-wide cast stockinette placed around the proximal forearm of the involved extremity, with the elbow flexed at 90 degrees. Countertraction is proved by the chair. An assistant maintains the patient upright by standing adjacent to the unaffected shoulder and clasping his or her hands around the chest in the axilla of the affected side. The physician places a foot in the stockinette loop to provide firm downward traction.[3]

If the dislocation cannot be reduced by these methods, general anesthesia should be considered and reduction attempted in the operating room. Irreducible dislocations are usually due to soft-tissue interposition.

For patients less than 30 years old, after reduction the shoulder is immobilized for 3 weeks, followed by gentle active range-of-motion exercises. The patient should avoid abduction and external rotation for an additional 3 weeks. For patients over age 30, the shoulder is immobilized for 1 week, followed by active range-of-motion exercises, avoiding abduction and external rotation.[18] The shoulder may be kept immobilized for circumduction exercises. The older the patient, the earlier the mobilization should be instituted to avoid stiffness. Exercises forcing internal rotation of the arm strengthen the subscapularis muscle, helping to prevent recurrent anterior shoulder dislocations.

Complications of anterior shoulder dislocations include tears of the rotator cuff, avulsion of the greater tuberosity, axillary nerve injury, and fracture of the humeral head. Operative repair is indicated in patients who have sustained more than three dislocations.

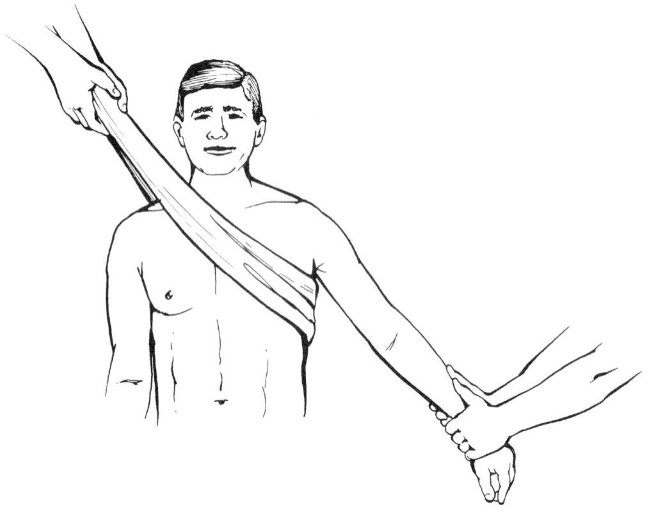

Figure 112.5. Traction–countertraction technique for reducing anterior shoulder dislocations. (Adapted from Simon RR, Koenigsknecht SJ. *Emergency orthopedics*. Norwalk, CT: Appleton & Lange, 1994.)

Postreduction radiographs are not necessary if the reduction was performed smoothly and postreduction physical examination shows no suspicion of unsuccessful reduction.[8]

Posterior Shoulder Dislocations

Posterior dislocations are less common than anterior dislocations and are the most frequently missed major dislocation. There are three types of posterior dislocations: subacromial, subglenoid, and subspinous. Almost all dislocations are the subacromial type. The mechanisms involved in this injury include violent internal rotational force occurring during a fall on the forward-flexed, internally rotated arm; and internal rotational force following a generalized tonic–clonic seizure.

Evaluation

On physical examination, the arm is held in adduction and internal rotation, with abduction severely limited. External rotation of the shoulder is blocked. There is a prominence in the posterior aspect of the shoulder, accompanied by a flattening of the normal anterior shoulder contour.

Radiographically, there is loss of the normal elliptic pattern produced by overlap of the humeral head and the posterior glenoid rim. The greater tuberosity is internally rotated. Isolated fractures of the lesser tuberosity are associated with posterior shoulder dislocations.

Management

Posterior shoulder dislocations may be reduced using the Stimson method, or other techniques that push the posteriorly displaced humeral head forward. If there is severe pain or muscle spasm, general anesthesia may be necessary to reduce the dislocation. Surgical intervention is needed for major displacement of the lesser tuberosity that cannot be reduced on reduction of the dislocation. Neurovascular compromise is uncommon.

Inferior Dislocations (Luxatio Erecta)

Inferior dislocations of the shoulder are uncommon, and occur due to hyperabduction. These injuries are always associated with detachment of the rotator cuff.

Evaluation

On physical examination, the patient is in severe pain and holds the arm at 180 degrees of elevation. The humeral head can be palpated along the lateral chest wall. Compression of the axillary artery and brachial plexus may occur as the humeral head tears through the inferior capsule. Vascular injury is more common with inferior dislocations than with any other form of shoulder dislocation.[11] Associated fractures of the acromion, inferior glenoid rim, and greater tuberosity may occur.[10]

Management

To reduce the dislocation, the physician applies traction in the longitudinal axis of the humerus while an assistant applies countertraction with a folded sheet wrapped around the supraclavicular region. With traction maintained, the arm is rotated inferiorly in an arc toward a position of complete adduction. After reduction, the shoulder is immobilized for 2 to 4 weeks. Occasionally, general anesthesia may be required to reduce the dislocation and repair the torn rotator cuff.

ACROMIOCLAVICULAR JOINT INJURY

The AC joint functions to elevate and abduct the arm. Stability is provided by two ligaments: the AC and the coracoclavicular.

Most injuries of the AC joint are caused by a direct force applied to the point of the shoulder.

Evaluation

The diagnosis of an AC joint injury is made by examining the patient in the upright position and looking for a deformity at the tip of the shoulder. This deformity represents a prominence of the distal clavicle, created by a tear of the AC ligament, and possibly the coracoclavicular ligament. Coracoclavicular ligament injury may involve the conoid ligament, the trapezoid ligament, or both.

For suspected AC joint injury, stress views taken in the AP position with 5 to 10 lb of weight should be obtained only when one cannot clinically demonstrate the classical features of third-degree injury. Hand-held weights temper the actual degree of separation, so weights should be suspended from the arm or wrist for full effect.

Management

The therapy for AC joint injuries depends on the degree of AC and coracoclavicular ligament injury. The traditional three-part *Aliman classification* of AC joint injuries has been expanded to a six-part classification system.

Type I injuries are a simple sprain of the AC ligament and involve an incomplete tear of that structure. The patient complains of tenderness over the joint. Swelling is minimal and no subluxation is present. Radiographs are negative, even with stress views. Therapy includes rest, ice, and a sling, with early range of motion.

Type II injuries involve disruption of the AC ligament, with sprain of the coracoclavicular ligament (Fig. 112.6). There is a partial subluxation of the distal end of the clavicle from the acromion. The patient experiences tenderness to mild palpation, and moderate swelling is present. Routine radiographs are usually normal, although subluxation with stress views is noted. The pathognomonic radiographic finding is a separation of the distal clavicle by no more than half its diameter from the acromion on stress films. Separation of the clavicle by more than half its diameter indicates a type III injury. Type II injuries are treated conservatively with ice, rest, and immobilization in a sling. Additional measures for reducing the clavicle and holding it in place with a brace-strap (Kenny-Howard sling) may be used, but clavicular support has not been shown to produce superior improvement in long-term function over that produced by a sling.

Type III injuries result in complete dislocation at the AC joint, with upward displacement of the clavicle and disruption of both the AC and coracoclavicular ligaments (see Fig. 112.6). Controversy exists regarding therapy. In the past, type III injuries were treated surgically in young patients. However, conservative treatment similar to type II therapy has been shown to produce results as good as those after surgical intervention.[12,15] Immobilization in the Kenny-Howard sling should be used for 3 weeks. Type III injuries require orthopedic referral. In *type IV* injuries, the clavicle is displaced posteriorly into or through the trapezius muscle.

Type V injuries are severe injuries that involve disruption of all ligaments above the joint. The clavicle is displaced far cephalad toward the base of the neck.

In *type VI* injuries, the clavicle is dislocated inferiorly, with the lateral end displaced under the acromion or the coracoid process. Type VI injuries are associated with clavicle fractures, rib fractures, or brachial plexus injuries.

Types IV, V, and VI injuries require surgical intervention.

STERNOCLAVICULAR JOINT INJURIES

The SC joint is stabilized by the SC ligament and the costoclavicular ligament. The most common mechanism of injury to this joint is a force that thrusts the shoulder forward.

Evaluation and Management

First-degree SC joint injury is a sprain of the SC joint and involves incomplete tears of the SC and costoclavicular ligaments. The

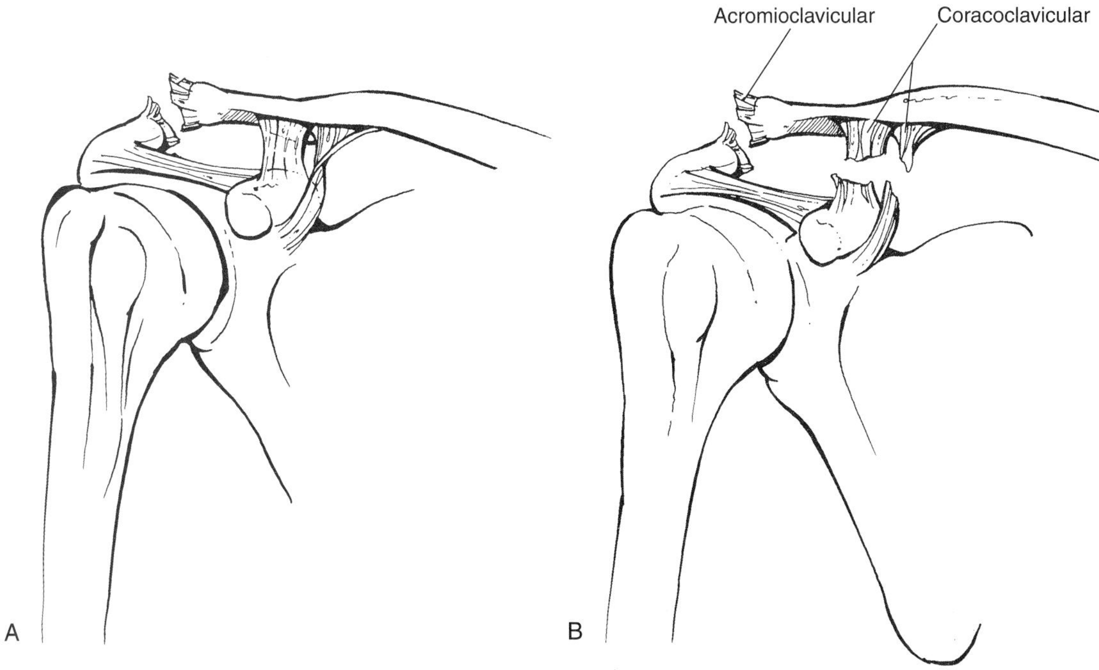

Figure 112.6. Acromioclavicular subluxation and dislocation. **(A)** A grade II sprain with tear of the acromioclavicular ligament. **(B)** A grade III sprain with tear of both the acromioclavicular and coracoclavicular ligaments.

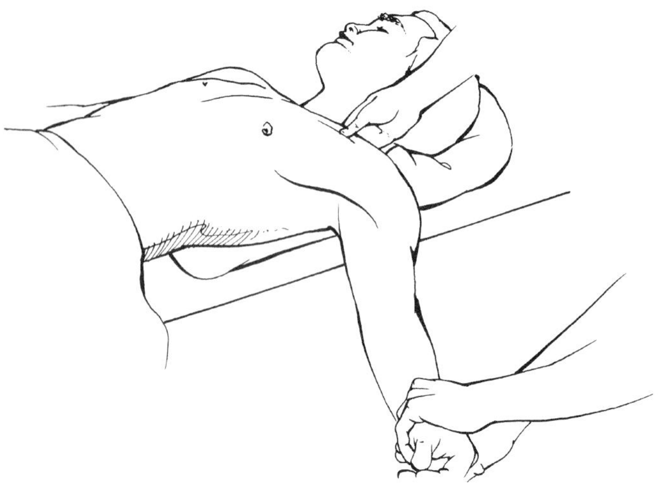

Figure 112.7. Reduction of a displaced sternoclavicular joint injury. The arm is abducted and traction is applied. With traction maintained, an assistant pushes the clavicle back into its normal position for anterior dislocations (*not shown*). With posterior dislocations, the clavicle is pulled back into its normal position. In difficult cases, the clavicle can be grasped with a towel clip. (Adapted from Simon RR, Koenigsknecht SJ. *Emergency orthopedics*. Norwalk, CT: Appleton & Lange, 1994.)

patient experiences minimal swelling and complains of tenderness over the joint. Therapy includes ice, analgesics, and a sling for 3 to 4 days.

Second-degree SC joint injury involves subluxation of the clavicle from its manubrial attachment: Complete rupture of the SC ligament and partial rupture of the costoclavicular ligament occur. There is pain on abduction of the arm, and swelling is noted over the joint. Treatment includes 6 weeks of immobilization with a figure-of-eight clavicle strap and a sling to hold the clavicle in its normal position. This immobilization permits ligamentous healing.

Third-degree SC joint injury involves complete rupture of the SC and costoclavicular ligaments, permitting the clavicle to dislocate from its manubrial attachment. Anterior dislocations are much more common, but posterior dislocations result in much more serious injuries. Patients experience severe pain, increased by any motion of the shoulder. Posterior dislocations may constitute a true orthopedic emergency, for respiratory embarrassment may occur secondary to tracheal compression or a pneumothorax, or venous congestion may occur secondary to compression of vessels in the neck. These associated injuries necessitate emergency reduction of the SC joint dislocation by the physician in the emergency department.

Reduction is accomplished by placing a folded sheet between the shoulders, with the patient supine, which serves to separate the clavicle from the manubrium. The arm is abducted and traction is applied. For anterior dislocation, while traction is maintained, the clavicle is pushed in place (Fig. 112.7). For posterior dislocations, using the same maneuver, the clavicle should be grasped near its medial border with a towel clip (following the instillation of local anesthesia) and pulled out of its posterior position. General anesthesia may be required to relocate a posterior dislocation of the SC joint.

Complications of an anterior SC dislocation are cosmetic, with chronic swelling around the joint. About 25% of posterior dislocations are associated with complications, including pneumothorax, laceration of the superior vena cava, occlusion of the subclavian artery or vein, and rupture or compression of the trachea.

ROTATOR CUFF INJURY

Tears of the rotator cuff are more common in the elderly because of degenerative changes that occur with advancing age. In young patients, a tear requires much more trauma. The mechanism of injury is a sudden forceful elevation of the arm against resistance in an attempt to cushion a fall, heavy lifting, or a direct impact to the shoulder. The most common area of disruption of the cuff is at its anterior superior portion, at the attachment of the supraspinatus muscle. At this point, the tendon is worn down by the compressive forces between the humeral head and the coracoacromial arch.

Evaluation

Patients complain of pain, aggravated by activity, that radiates to the anterior aspect of the arm. Abduction of the arm is painful and weak. Tenderness is present over the insertion at the greater tuberosity.

The *drop arm test* is positive in patients with significant tears. This is performed by horizontally elevating the arm to the 90-degree position and asking the patient to continue to hold the arm in this position. Slight pressure on the distal forearm will cause the patient to drop the arm suddenly. In addition, the patient cannot bring the arm from the abducted position to the side in a slow fashion, but drops it precipitously.

Thirty percent or more of the tendon must be ruptured to produce a significant reduction of strength. The extent of the tear is directly related to the limitation of shoulder abduction.[2] Arthrography may be used to detect the location and extent of the tear.

Management

Emergency treatment includes ice, immobilization, and orthopedic referral. Conservative therapy results in a good outcome in only 50% of patients. Arthroscopic treatment can be performed in a number of rotator cuff tears, particularly in the young. Anterior tears have been shown to have the best outcome with arthroscopic repair.[9] Patients with large posterior rotator cuff tears are poor candidates for arthroscopy. In the young, early surgical repair is indicated for complete tears of the rotator cuff.[1] In the elderly patient who has a more sedentary life, repair may not be indicated.

COMMON PITFALLS

- Not obtaining a transscapular radiographic view (Y view) when assessing the shoulder for dislocation
- Forgetting that lesser tuberosity fractures are often associated with posterior shoulder dislocations
- Not searching for other injuries in patients with scapular fractures
- Forgetting that posterior sternoclavicular joint dislocations may constitute a true orthopedic emergency due to impingement on the trachea, transection of subclavian vessels, or a pneumothorax.

References

1. Burkhart SS. Arthroscopic treatment of massive rotator cuff tear. *Clin Orthop* 1991;267:45.
2. Cofield RF. Current concepts review: rotator cuff disease of the shoulder. *J Bone Joint Surg Br* 1981;63B:198.
3. Craig DW, Gill EA, Noyes ME, et al. Anterior shoulder dislocation, a simple and rapid method for reduction. *Am J Sports Med* 1995;23:369–371.
4. Doyle WL, Ragar. Use of the scapular manipulation method to reduce an anterior shoulder dislocation in the supine position. *Ann Emerg Med* 1996;27:92–94.
5. Flatlow EL, Cuomo F, Maday MG, et al. Open reduction and internal fixation of two-part displaced fractures of the greater tuberosity of the proximal part of the humerus. *J Bone Joint Surg Am* 1991;73:1213.
6. Graeme KA, Jackimczyk KC. The extremities and spine. *Emerg Med Clin North Am* 1997;15:365–379.

7. Herscovici D, Fiennes AG, Allgower M, et al. The floating shoulder: ipsilateral clavicle and scapular neck fractures. *J Bone Joint Surg Br* 1992;74:362.
8. Kaufman D, Leung J. Evaluation of the patient with extremity trauma: an evidence based approach. *Emerg Med Clin North Am* 1999;17:77–95.
9. Lyons AR, Tomlinson JE. Clinical diagnosis of tears of the rotator cuff. *J Bone Joint Surg Br* 1992;74B:414.
10. Mallon WJ, Bassett FH, Goldner RD. Luxatio erecta: the inferior glenohumeral dislocation. *J Orthop Trauma* 1990;4:19.
11. McNamara RM. Reduction of anterior shoulder dislocation by scapular manipulation. *Ann Emerg Med* 1993;21:1140.
12. Neer CS II. Displaced proximal humeral fractures. Part I: classification and evaluation. *J Bone Joint Surg* 1970;52:1077.
13. Neer CS II. Fractures about the shoulder: a classification. *J Bone Joint Surg* 1970;52:1081.
14. Post M. Current concepts in the treatment of fractures of the clavicle. *Clin Orthop* 1989;245:89.
15. Press J, Zuckerman JD, Gallagher, M et al. Treatment of grade III acromioclavicular separations, operative versus nonoperative management. *Bull Hosp Jt Dis* 1997;56:77–83.
16. Riebel GD, McCabe JB. Anterior shoulder dislocation: a review of reduction techniques. *Am J Emerg Med* 1991;9:180.
17. Rockwood CA, Green DP. eds. *Fractures.* Philadelphia: JB Lippincott Co, 1991.
18. Simon RR, Koenigsknecht SJ. *Emergency orthopedics.* Norwalk, CT: Appleton & Lange, 1994.
19. Stimson BB. *A manual of fractures and dislocations,* 2nd ed. Philadelphia: Lea & Febiger, 1947.

CHAPTER 113
Elbow Injuries

Jefferson D. Bracey and Alok Saxena

The elbow is a synovial hinge joint consisting of three articulations between the distal humerus, radius, and ulna. The humerus widens distally to form the lateral and medial condyles. The capitellum is a spheroidal cartilaginous structure of the lateral condyle that articulates with the radial head, permitting pronation and supination. The trochlea is a spoon-shaped cartilaginous projection of the medial condyle that articulates with the deep trochlear notch of the ulna, permitting flexion and extension at the elbow. The articulating surfaces of the head of the radius and ulna are held together by the annular ligament. The anterior capsule combined with the radial and ulnar collateral ligaments provide stability at the elbow joint.

The wrist flexor and pronator muscles originate from the medial epicondyle. The wrist extensor and supinator muscles attach to the lateral epicondyle. The brachial artery is palpable medial to the biceps tendon in the antecubital space. The median nerve transverses deep in the antecubital fossa medial to the brachial artery. The ulnar nerve courses posteriorly in the cubital tunnel between the medial epicondyle and olecranon process. The radial nerve passes between the heads of the triceps in the posterior humerus and may be injured in humeral shaft fractures.

There are several bursal structures in the elbow. The superficial olecranon bursa lies beneath the skin over the olecranon process and is particularly vulnerable to traumatic and infectious processes.

EMERGENCY DEPARTMENT EVALUATION AND MANAGEMENT

The assessment of elbow injuries should include a detailed history of the mechanism of injury. The most common complaints are pain, restriction of movement, and swelling. A description of the location and duration of pain, aggravating factors, and presence of paresthesias or loss of movement is important. Elbow pain may also be referred from injuries to the shoulder, forearm, or wrist. An occupational history may provide a clue to the diagnosis in patients presenting with chronic pain.

Inspection of the involved extremity for swelling, open wounds, deformities, effusions, and discoloration is the first step in the physical examination of the patient with elbow pain. The involved joint should not be extensively manipulated until radiographs have been obtained to exclude fracture and dislocation. The shoulder, forearm, wrist, and hand should be examined. Laceration over the medial epicondyle should raise suspicion of an ulnar nerve injury. Any abnormality noted in the involved extremity should be compared with the contralateral extremity.

An effusion is best palpated over the soft-tissue area lateral to the radial head. The bony prominences of the medial and lateral condyles, olecranon, and radial head should be palpated for tenderness. The radial head is best palpated with the thumb of one hand while pronating and supinating the forearm with the examiner's other hand. With the elbow flexed to 90 degrees, the medial and lateral condyles and the olecranon should form a triangle. In an elbow dislocation, this triangle is disrupted with displacement of the olecranon. A posterior dislocation or extension-type fracture is suggested by a prominent olecranon. Loss of the olecranon prominence suggests an anterior dislocation or supracondylar fracture. The triangular relationship is maintained in supracondylar fracture. Each of the muscle groups should be tested against resistance and the muscle belly palpated during contraction.

Careful neurovascular examination is of critical importance. Brachial, radial, and ulnar pulses should be palpated and capillary refill assessed. The brachioradialis, biceps, and triceps reflexes should be elicited. The radial nerve is tested by evaluating wrist and finger extension. Wristdrop results from radial nerve injury. Flexion of the wrist and digits and pronation of the forearm are the functions of the median nerve. Inability to flex and abduct the thumb is diagnostic of median nerve injury. Loss of strength of the interossei muscles and adduction of the thumb suggests ulnar nerve paralysis. The sensory component of the radial nerve innervates the dorsum of the hand and is best tested in the web space between the thumb and index finger. Median nerve sensation is tested over the palmar aspect of the thumb and the digits to the radial one-half of the ring finger. The ulnar nerve is tested over the fifth digit. The neurovascular examination of the extremity should be repeated after manipulation and at regular intervals for increased edema and potential neurovascular compromise.

Radiography of the Elbow

The radiographic examination of the elbow should consist of a minimum of two views: the anteroposterior and lateral. Oblique views may provide additional information. Specialized views, such as the radial head–capitellum view, are indicated when a high index of suspicion for particular injury exists.

On the lateral radiograph, a line parallel to the anterior border of the humerus should intersect the anterior portion of the middle third of the capitellum (Fig. 113.1).[10] If this intersection is displaced, usually anteriorly, a supracondylar fracture should be suspected.

The radiocapitellar line extends from the center of the radius and should intersect the middle third of the capitellum on the lateral view.[10] Disruption of this line suggests radial head dislocation or fracture and is most useful in evaluating subtle fractures in children.

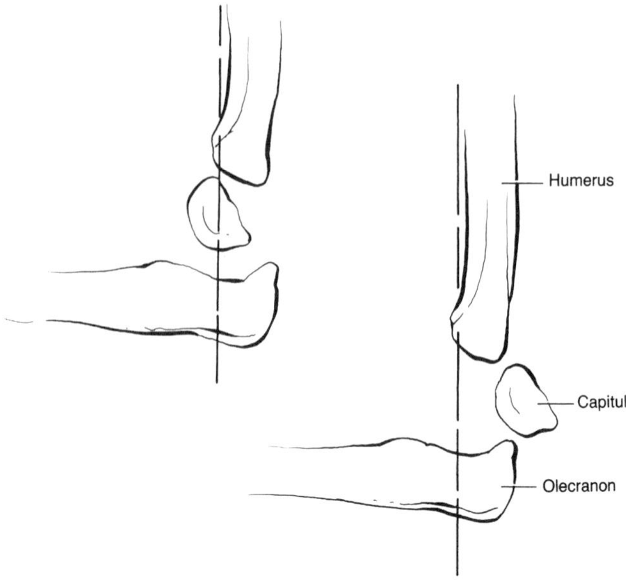

Figure 113.1. Anterior humeral line. The anterior humeral line is a line drawn on the lateral radiograph along the anterior surface of the humerus through the elbow. Normally this line transects the middle of the capitellum **(left)**. With an extension fracture of the supracondylar region, this line will either transect the anterior third of the capitellum or pass entirely anterior to it **(right)**. (Adapted, with permission, from Simon RR, Koenigsknecht SJ. *Emergency orthopedics: the extremities,* 2nd ed. Norwalk, CT: Appleton & Lange, 1987.)

Fat pad signs are helpful in diagnosing occult fractures within the joint capsule. The anterior fat pad is a combination of fat in the coronoid and radial fossa. This radiolucent fat overlaps and appears as a triangular area over the distal humerus on a lateral radiograph of the elbow. The posterior fat pad is located in the olecranon fossa and is normally hidden by the overlying humeral condyles on a lateral radiograph.

When an effusion is present, it distends the joint capsule and displaces the fat pads (Fig. 113.2). The anterior fat pad displaces anteriorly and superiorly and appears as a "ship's sail." The posterior fat pad becomes visible on radiography and is highly indicative of intraarticular disease. In the setting of elbow trauma, a positive fat pad sign in the absence of visible fracture should mandate a search for occult fracture, most commonly of the radial head.

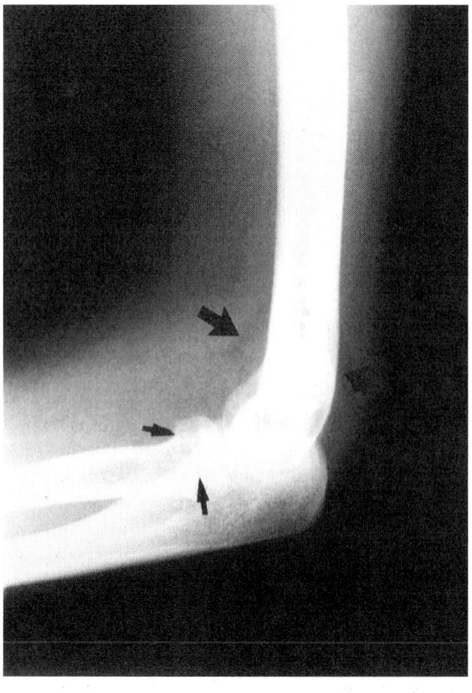

Figure 113.2. Anterior and posterior fat pad signs are indicated by the *large arrows*. *Small arrows* indicate the radial head fracture that produced the effusion displacing the fat pads.

Positive fat pad signs can also be present with any intraarticular disease process and are not pathognomonic for fracture. Fat pad signs may be seen with arthritis, gout, pseudogout, infection, neoplasia, or other disease process causing an intraarticular fluid collection.[8] A fat pad sign may not be present with severe injury causing disruption of the joint capsule.

Computed tomography (CT) scanning may be useful in delineating complex fractures in adults. Magnetic resonance imaging has become the procedure of choice for evaluating soft tissues, cartilaginous surfaces, joint space, and trabecular bone.[6]

Fractures of the Elbow

Supracondylar Fractures

Supracondylar fractures occur in the distal humerus proximal to the epicondyles and are most commonly seen in children. In adults, because of their stronger bones, elbow dislocations from ligamentous disruption are more common. These fractures most commonly result from a fall on the outstretched hand with the elbow in extension.

Twenty-five percent of supracondylar fractures are nondisplaced. Treatment of nondisplaced fracture is a posterior splint from axilla to palm, with the elbow flexed to 90 degrees. These patients should be referred to an orthopedic surgeon. A child with elbow tenderness and swelling should be splinted, even without a demonstrable radiographic fracture, because of the possibility of occult fracture.

In displaced fractures, the distal fragment is usually displaced posteriorly (extension injury), and an abnormal anterior humeral line will be visualized on the lateral radiograph. Anterior displacement of the distal fragment (flexion injury) occurs less frequently and is caused by a direct blow to the posterior aspect of the flexed elbow.

Assessment of neurovascular function is essential, especially with extension injuries, because occult injury to the brachial artery may occur. A strong pulse does not rule out arterial injury, and an arteriogram should be performed if injury is suspected. Closed reduction of displaced fractures should be attempted if neurovascular compromise is present.

Displaced fractures require internal fixation or percutaneous pinning if good alignment is not maintained with closed reduction. Patients with displaced fractures should be admitted because of the risk of delayed swelling and neurovascular compromise, including Volkmann ischemia and, eventually, contracture. Flexion fractures may also require internal fixation and should be splinted in extension. Range-of-motion exercises after internal fixation are encouraged and should be started within 1 to 2 weeks.

A common complication of supracondylar fracture is an abnormal carrying angle. The normal carrying angle is 10 degrees to 15 degrees of valgus. Measurement of the Baumann angle, formed by a line perpendicular to the humeral shaft and a line through the lateral humeral condyle, is predictive of an acceptable carrying angle.[14] This angle normally measures about 75 degrees. A discrepancy of greater than 5 degrees to 10 degrees, compared with the uninjured extremity, is an unacceptable reduction.

Intercondylar Fractures

Intercondylar fractures usually occur in older patients as a result of direct trauma to the flexed elbow. They usually occur in "T and Y" configurations, and treatment is based on the displacement of the humeral condyles from each other and the proximal humerus. Neurovascular complications are so uncommon that these fractures rarely require manipulation by the emergency physician.

Nondisplaced fractures are treated in a posterior splint for 3 weeks, and then active range of motion is begun. Displaced fractures are treated with internal fixation and early range of motion beginning after 1 week. Severely comminuted fractures may be treated with olecranon traction for 3 to 4 weeks if operative repair is not possible.

Humeral Condyle Fractures

Isolated humeral condyle fractures are caused by a fall on the outstretched hand, by direct trauma, or by avulsion of bone from the pull of the flexor or extensor muscles from the medial and lateral condyles, respectively. Lateral condyle fractures are more common than medial fractures and frequently involve the joint surface.

Nondisplaced lateral condyle fractures are immobilized in a posterior splint, with the elbow flexed to 90 degrees and the forearm in supination with the wrist extended. The forearm should be in pronation and the wrist flexed for medial condyle fractures. Active range of motion is begun as early as 2 to 3 weeks after injury. Operative fixation is required for displaced fractures, owing to instability caused by the pull of the forearm muscles. All of these patients should be treated in consultation with an orthopedic surgeon.

Epicondyle Fractures

Epicondyle fractures in adults are usually caused by a direct blow. The medial epicondyle is involved more commonly than is the lateral, and ulnar nerve function should be evaluated.

Nondisplaced fractures may be treated with immobilization and early range of motion. If displacement of more than 10 mm is present, then surgical fixation is required. Intraarticular fragments may impede joint mobility and are difficult to visualize radiographically. Entrapment of the ulnar nerve is a possible complication.

Articular Surface Fractures

Fractures of the capitellum and trochlea usually occur as a result of a posterior elbow dislocation. Isolated fractures are rare, and joint stability is maintained because the condyles remain intact, but motion may be impeded.

Nondisplaced fractures with normal anatomic alignment can be treated with immobilization for 2 to 3 weeks. Displaced small fragments may be excised, whereas larger fragments require internal fixation with early range of motion. Common complications of capitellar fractures include restriction of motion and, rarely, nonunion and avascular necrosis.

Olecranon Fractures

Olecranon fractures are usually intraarticular and may result from a direct blow or an avulsion injury from the pull of the triceps muscle. On examination, the patient is unable to extend the elbow against resistance. Because of its proximity, the ulnar nerve may be injured, and its function should be assessed.

Treatment of these injuries varies with the amount of displacement and requires orthopedic consultation. Nondisplaced fractures may be splinted with the elbow in a semiflexed position and with early range of motion begun in 2 to 3 weeks. Complete healing generally occurs in 6 to 8 weeks. If greater than 2 mm of displacement is present, then operative intervention is indicated. Treatment options include tension band wiring, olecranon screws, or plates.[5] Range-of-motion exercises may be started in 1 week. Management of severely comminuted fractures is controversial and may require removal of the loose fragments.

Radial Head Fractures

Radial head fractures are the most common elbow injuries in adults. They usually occur as a result of a fall on the outstretched hand, which drives the radial head into the capitellum. On examination, patients have tenderness to palpation over the radial head and pain with pronation and supination of the forearm.

Fractures are classified as nondisplaced, displaced, or comminuted. Nondisplaced fractures may be difficult to visualize on standard radiographs. Any disruption of the normally smooth, concave cortical contour of the radial head suggests fracture. A positive fat pad sign on a lateral radiograph without evidence of fracture should raise suspicion for an occult radial head fracture. This fracture may be better visualized radiographically with a radial head–capitellar view.

Nondisplaced fractures are treated with a posterior splint or sling, with early range of motion in a few days. Aspiration of the hemarthrosis in the emergency department may provide pain relief and expedite mobilization. Minimally displaced fractures may be treated in a similar manner. Fractures displaced more than 3 mm or involving more than one-third of the joint surface should be treated with operative fixation using small screws. These patients should begin early range of motion postoperatively.

Comminuted fractures may be treated with a sling and early range of motion in 1 to 2 weeks. Joint aspiration and injection of a local anesthetic will aid in assessing joint mobility. The treatment of severely comminuted and displaced fractures is controversial and may include excision of fragments or complete radial head excision, with or without prosthetic implants.

Any patient with a radial head fracture should also be examined for wrist tenderness. The Essex-Lopresti lesion, a radial head fracture with disruption of the distal radioulnar joint ligaments and forearm interosseous membrane, must be recognized early for internal fixation to produce the best results.[1]

Nursemaid's Elbow

Subluxation of the radial head is most commonly seen in children 1 to 3 years of age. The mechanism of injury is a sudden longitudinal pull of the forearm, causing fibers of the annular ligament to become stuck between the capitellum and the radial head. The child is unwilling to move the arm, and the elbow is held in slight flexion with pronation of the forearm.

When a child presents with the characteristic history for radial head subluxation, radiographs are not necessary. However, the presence of swelling or deformity, or the child's refusal to resume normal use of the arm after reduction, is an indication for a radiograph.

Treatment is supination and flexion of the forearm in one continuous motion. The examiner's thumb can be used to apply pressure over the radial head. With successful reduction of a nursemaid's elbow, the child will resume using the arm normally within several minutes, and no further treatment is necessary.

Monteggia Fracture

Fracture of the proximal one-third of the ulna with dislocation of the radial head is a Monteggia fracture (Fig. 113.3). Based on the position of the radial head, there are four types of Monteggia fractures. The radial head dislocates anteriorly in 60% of cases, with posterolateral, lateral, and posterior dislocations being less common. The mechanism of injury involves direct trauma, forced hyperpronation, or hyperextension. The most commonly associated injury is paralysis of the radial nerve. The usual treatment is open reduction with internal fixation.

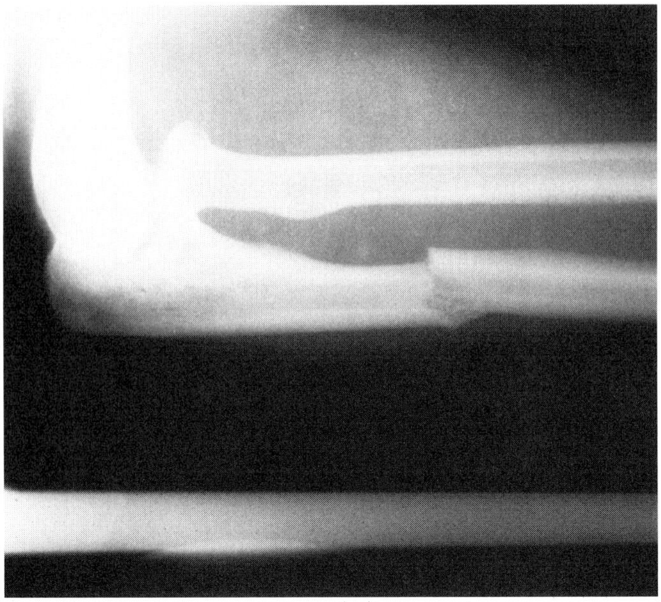

Figure 113.3. Monteggia fracture. The first component is fracture of the proximal one-third of the ulna; the second component is dislocation of the radial head.

Aspiration of the Radiohumeral Joint

Aspiration of the radiohumeral joint is indicated to relieve pain, promote early range of motion, and assess joint mobility with radial head fractures. It is also indicated to diagnose a septic joint. The aspiration should be performed over the lateral elbow in the center of the triangle that connects the radial head, lateral epicondyle, and olecranon process (Fig. 113.4).[12] No neurovascular structures are located in this area, and the joint capsule is present beneath the skin and the thin anconeus muscle.

Under sterile technique, the skin over this area is anesthetized with a local anesthetic. An 18-gauge needle on a 10- to 20-mL syringe is directed into the center of the triangle and perpendicular to the skin. Aspiration of up to 5 mL of blood from the joint and injection of 1 to 2 mL of a long-acting anesthetic provide relief of pain and allow assessment of joint mobility.

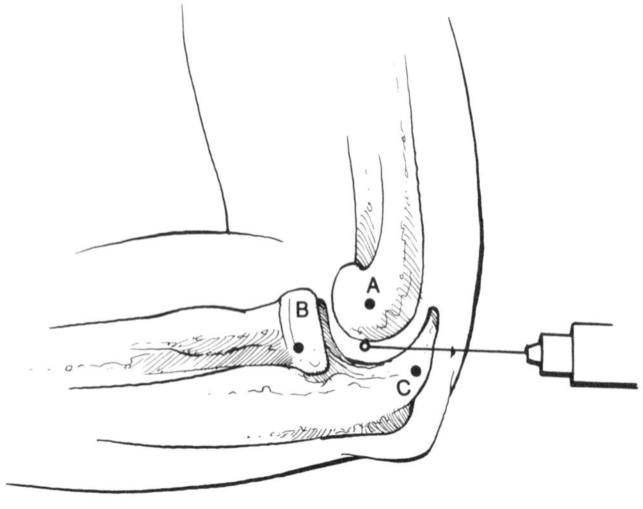

Figure 113.4. Elbow aspiration. The safest place to aspirate the elbow is in the center of a triangle produced by connecting *(A)* the lateral epicondyle of the humerus, *(B)* the radial head, and *(C)* the olecranon. (Adapted, with permission, from Simon RR, Koenigsknecht SJ. *Emergency orthopedics: the extremities,* 2nd ed. Norwalk, CT: Appleton & Lange, 1987.)

Elbow Dislocation

Dislocation of the elbow accounts for 20% of all dislocations and is described by the direction in which the forearm is displaced in relationship to the distal humerus. Posterior and posterolateral dislocations account for 90% of all elbow dislocations. Dislocation may also occur between the radius and ulna. Posterior dislocations are caused by a fall on an extended and abducted arm. Patients present with significant swelling, tenderness, and deformity, with the elbow held in flexion and prominence of the olecranon. Anterior dislocation is the result of a blow to the olecranon while the elbow is held in extension with the forearm supinated and is associated with loss of the olecranon prominence.

Radiographs should be obtained before reduction to exclude associated fractures, which occur in up to 60% of patients with elbow dislocation. Supracondylar fractures in the younger patient and avulsion fractures of the medial epicondyle are the most common. A complete neurovascular examination must be done on presentation. Neuropraxia is present in 20% of patients, most commonly involving the ulnar and median nerves. As with most nerve injuries associated with dislocations and fractures, these deficits are usually transient.[9] Brachial artery injury is most commonly associated with open dislocations and those with concomitant fractures. The incidence of vascular injury is greater with anterior dislocations.

Analgesia and muscle relaxation are required for closed reduction. Posterior, medial, and lateral dislocations are reduced using the same technique. With the patient lying supine, the area of the wrist and forearm is grasped and traction is applied along the long axis of the forearm. An assistant provides countertraction to the upper arm. Any medial or lateral displacement is corrected. While forearm traction is continued, the elbow is flexed and a palpable clunk should be felt as the elbow is reduced. Downward pressure over the proximal forearm may aid in disengaging the coronoid from the olecranon fossa (Fig. 113.5). After reduction, the neurovascular examination should be repeated and postreduction films obtained. The elbow should be flexed to 90 degrees as long as good pulses are maintained and then immobilized in a posterior splint. All patients should follow up with an orthopedic surgeon within 1 week to begin early range-of-motion exercises and help prevent contractures.

Indications for open reduction include an associated fracture, open dislocation, neurovascular injury, or inability to accomplish a closed reduction. Long-term complications include stiffness, contractures, neurovascular injury, heterotropic bone formation, and ankylosis. Recurrent elbow dislocations are rare.

Epicondylitis

Tennis elbow, or lateral epicondylitis, is an "overuse syndrome" characterized by inflammation at the radiohumeral joint or the lateral epicondyle. It is believed to represent a failure of the extensor carpi radialis brevis attachment to bone in this region.[11] It is most commonly seen in athletes or adults with occupations requiring repeated rotary motion, as in twisting or grasping (e.g., tennis players, pipefitters, and carpenters).[3] The gradual onset of a dull ache appears over the lateral epicondyle and radiates into the forearm. Dorsiflexion of the wrist and supination of the forearm against resistance with the elbow extended will reproduce the pain. Radiographs should be obtained to exclude an associated fracture. In chronic conditions, calcification may be seen over the lateral epicondyle.

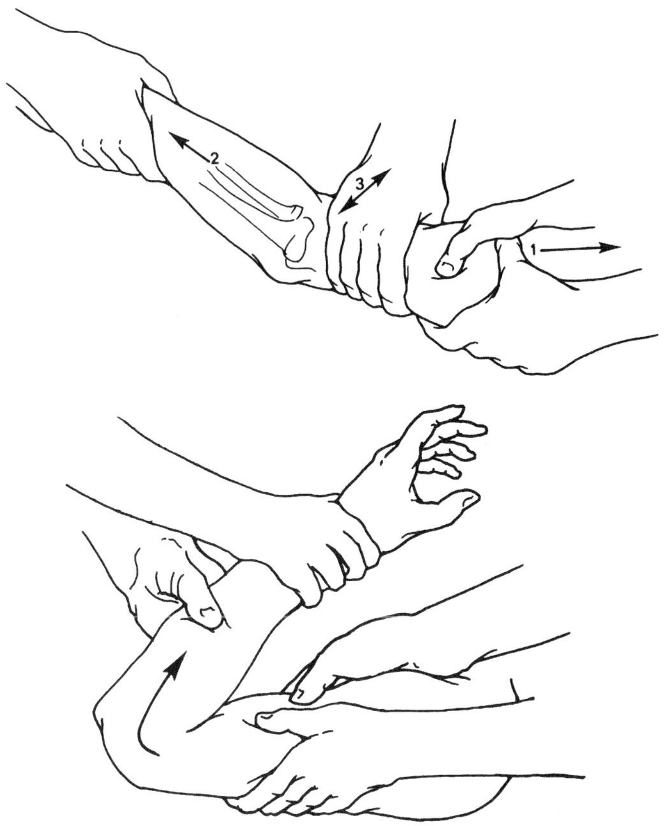

Figure 113.5. Technique for reduction of posterior dislocation of the elbow.

The mainstay of treatment is avoidance of the offending activity and immobilization. A posterior splint is applied with the elbow flexed 90 degrees, the forearm supinated, and the wrist slightly dorsiflexed. Moist heat, nonsteroidal antiinflammatory agents, and physical therapy may be helpful. Local infiltration of the affected area with 1 to 2 mL of a corticosteroid and anesthetic mixture will give dramatic relief. All patients should have an orthopedic referral.

Medial epicondylitis is similar to tennis elbow and involves the common flexor origin at the medial epicondyle of the humerus. It is seen in golfers but occurs more frequently in people who routinely perform household chores, manual labor, and other tasks involving repetitive movements. Maximal tenderness is localized over the medial aspect of the elbow and medial epicondyle. Treatment is similar to that of lateral epicondylitis, and orthopedic follow-up is essential.

Olecranon Bursitis

Olecranon bursitis is most commonly caused by a direct blow to the olecranon process. Patients present with erythematous, warm, and painful swelling over the posterior aspect of the elbow. Flexion of the elbow may be slightly restricted, owing to tightening of the skin over the inflamed bursa. Repetitive trauma can result in a chronic inflammatory process and a thickened, rubbery, and usually painless bursa.

Aspiration of the bursa is essential for both diagnostic and therapeutic purposes if infection is suspected. The aspirated fluid should be analyzed for crystals, cell count (greater than 1000 white blood cells/μL in septic bursitis), Gram stain, and cultures. *Staphylococcus aureus* is the most commonly identified organism in septic olecranon bursitis, and high resistance to penicillin has been reported.[4] Intravenous antibiotics, drainage of bursal fluid, moist heat, and splinting are the recommended treatment measures.

In traumatic olecranon bursitis, the mainstays of treatment are a compression dressing after drainage, nonsteroidal antiinflammatory agents, and protective measures to prevent recurrence.

Distal Rupture of the Biceps or Triceps Tendon

Distal rupture of the biceps tendon may be the result of degenerative changes or sudden, forceful flexion of the elbow against resistance. Patients present with a history of a painful snap at the elbow. Flexion of the elbow and supination of the forearm are weakened. On flexion, the belly of the biceps retracts, producing a bulbous swelling in the upper arm. The treatment is surgical if significant motor weakness is present, and should occur within 2 weeks postinjury.[13]

Avulsion of the triceps tendon should be considered in patients with pain, swelling, and weakness with arm extension. A defect is often palpable just proximal to the olecranon. Associated injuries include radial head and neck fractures and wrist fractures. The diagnosis is confirmed radiographically when a bony avulsion is seen on the lateral view of the elbow. Orthopedic consultation should be obtained, and surgical treatment is recommended.

Osteochondritis Dissecans

Osteochondritis dissecans is a process of avascular necrosis of the subchondral bone and the overlying articular cartilage, and is most common in males and adolescents. There is usually a history of trauma or sports-related activities. Patients may complain of the gradual onset of dull, aching pain; limited extension; intermittent swelling; and catching, locking, or clicking of the affected elbow.[7] The capitellum is the most common site of involvement, and joint effusion may be present. Treatment consists of immobilization with a sling or cast, avoidance of all throwing activities, and nonsteroidal antiinflammatory agents. Loose bodies within the joint may restrict movement of the elbow and should be surgically removed. Prognosis is usually good.

COMMON PITFALLS

- Radiographs are most commonly misread because a true lateral view of the elbow is not obtained. In one university emergency department setting, the incidence of missed elbow fractures was 12%.[2]
- Injuries to the elbow may refer pain to the wrist. Identification of one injury should not preclude the search for other injuries.
- The most common injury that is overlooked is an occult radial head fracture. A high index of suspicion is needed when a positive fat pad sign is present on radiography without demonstrable fracture. Several oblique views of the radial head may need to be taken to visualize the fracture.
- Any fracture of the proximal ulna should prompt the examiner to assess the radial head for dislocation. Monteggia fractures require internal fixation, whereas isolated ulna fractures are treated with immobilization.
- Patients with radial head fractures should have their wrist examined for the Essex-Lopresti lesion. These patients require internal fixation, whereas radial head fractures are usually treated conservatively.
- One should never assume that a negative radiograph rules out elbow injury. Injuries to cartilaginous and ligamentous

structures, as well as the soft tissues, may be present. Splinting of the elbow and orthopedic referral should be considered when a significant mechanism of injury is present.

- Radiographs should always be obtained before the reduction of dislocations to exclude associated fractures. Postreduction films should always be obtained.
- A potential medicolegal pitfall is missing the diagnosis of neurovascular injury. A careful neurovascular examination should be documented, in addition to interval reexamination.
- A commonly missed injury is avulsion of the biceps muscle from the bicipital tuberosity of the radius. The patient will still be able to flex the elbow with the brachialis muscle.
- Another commonly overlooked injury is the supracondylar fracture in children. Measure the anterior humeral line to aid in diagnosing these fractures. Splint the arm if a significant mechanism of injury or swelling exists, and refer for orthopedic consultation.

References

1. Edwards GS, Jupiter JB. Radial head fractures with acute distal radioulnar dislocation: Essex-Lopresti revisited. *Clin Orthop Rel Res* 1988;234:61.
2. Freed HA, Shields NN. Most frequently overlooked radiographically apparent fractures in a teaching hospital emergency department. *Ann Emerg Med* 1984;13:900.
3. Gellman H. Tennis elbow (lateral epicondylitis). *Orthop Clin North Am* 1992;23:75.
4. Ho G, Tice AD, Kaplan SR. Septic bursitis in the prepatellar and olecranon bursae: an analysis of 25 cases. *Ann Intern Med* 1978;89:21.
5. Horne JG, Tanzer TL. Olecranon fractures: a review of 100 cases. *J Trauma* 1981;21:469.
6. Miller TT. Imaging of elbow disorders. *Orthop Clin North Am* 1999;30:21.
7. Mitsunaga MM, Adishian DA, Bianco AJ. Osteochondritis dissecans of the capitellum. *J Trauma* 1981;22:53.
8. Murphy WA, Siegel MJ. Elbow fat pads with new signs and extended differential diagnosis. *Radiology* 1977;124:659.
9. Nelson AJ, Izzi JA, et al. Traumatic nerve injuries about the elbow. *Orthop Clin North Am* 1999;30:91.
10. Pitt MJ, Speer DP. Imaging of the elbow with an emphasis on trauma. *Radiol Clin North Am* 1990;28:295.
11. Putnam MD, Cohen M. Painful conditions around the elbow. *Orthop Clin North Am* 1999;30:109.
12. Quigley TB. Aspiration of the elbow joint in the treatment of fractures of the head of the radius. *N Engl J Med* 1949;240:915.
13. Strauch RJ. Biceps and triceps injuries of the elbow. *Orthop Clin North Am* 1999;30:95.
14. Worlock P. Supracondylar fractures of the humerus: assessment of cubitus varus by the Baumann angle. *J Bone Joint Surg Br* 1986;68:755.

Additional Readings

Hildebrand KA, Patterson SD, King GJ. Acute elbow dislocations: simple and complex. *Orthop Clin North Am* 1999;30:63.
Hurley JA. Complicated elbow fractures in athletes. *Clin Sports Med* 1990;9:39.
Karasick D, Burk DL, Gross GW. Trauma to the elbow and forearm. *Semin Roentgenol* 1991;26:318.
Kuntz DG, Baratz ME. Fractures of the elbow. *Orthop Clin North Am* 1999,30:37.
Watson JT. Fractures of the forearm and elbow. *Clin Sports Med* 1990;9:59.

CHAPTER 114
Hand, Wrist, and Elbow Injuries

Suzanne Moore Shepherd, Jeffrey Desmond, Carl R. Chudnofsky, and William H. Shoff

Hand Injuries

The hand is the primary organ with which we manipulate objects and interact with our environment. Damage to the complex and intricate structure of the hand from injury, infection, or disease may cause a loss of function, resulting in severe disability. Hand injuries are a common problem in the emergency department, accounting for 10% to 20% (1.4 million) of emergency department visits, most commonly for lacerations (42%) and least commonly for infections (5%).[6,10,19] Hand infections are covered separately in Chapter 55.

Emergency physicians must be skilled in the evaluation and management of hand injuries; the outcome depends on accurate assessment of the injury, appropriate initial management, and prompt recognition of those injuries that require immediate specialty consultation or outpatient referral.

ANATOMY AND TERMINOLOGY

An understanding of the anatomy and terminology of the hand is crucial for the diagnosis and treatment of hand injuries. The surfaces of the hand and digits are referred to as dorsal, volar (or palmar), ulnar, and radial. The palmar surface is divided into the thenar (overlying the thumb metacarpal), hypothenar (overlying the little finger metacarpal), and midpalm areas. The digits are named thumb, index, middle (or long), ring, and little fingers. Each digit has a metacarpophalangeal (MCP) joint and interphalangeal (IP) joints. The thumb has one IP joint, while the fingers have a proximal interphalangeal (PIP) joint and a distal interphalangeal (DIP) joint. Motion of the hand at the wrist is described as radial or ulnar deviation and extension or flexion. Finger motion is described as extension, hyperextension (i.e., MCP or IP joints greater than 180 degrees), flexion, and abduction and adduction (as related to the midline of the long finger). In addition, the thumb can perform opposition to touch the pads of all the fingers.

There are 27 separate bones of the hand and wrist, including 5 metacarpals, 14 phalanges, and 8 carpal bones. The carpal bones are arranged in two concentric arches or rows. The proximal row from radial to ulnar consists of the scaphoid, which contributes structurally to both rows and forms the floor of the anatomic snuffbox, the lunate, the triquetrum, and the pisiform. The distal row from radial to ulnar is the trapezium, trapezoid, capitate, and hamate, which has a hooklike process that forms a fibroosseous tunnel through which the ulnar artery and nerve travel (i.e., Guyon canal). The flexor retinaculum is a dense band of fibrous tissue that attaches to the hook of the hamate and pisiform bone on the ulnar aspect and the trapezium and scaphoid radially. This structure forms the roof of the "carpal tunnel," through which pass the tendons of the flexor digitorum superficialis, flexor digitorum profundus, and flexor pollicis longus and the median nerve.

The carpal bones are stabilized by three ligamentous bands, two volarly and one dorsally, and by numerous interosseous ligaments. The volar ligaments are the strongest and form two concentric rows extending from the radial styloid to the distal ulna. The distal ligamentous complex arches across the proximal capitate, while the proximal band crosses and stabilizes the lunate. The space between these ligamentous bands is an inherent weak spot and accounts for the injury patterns seen with lunate and perilunate dislocations. Because these ligaments have their attachment on the radial styloid, fracture of the radial styloid can be an unstable fracture.

Muscles that control hand motions are divided into flexors and extensors, each of which may be intrinsic or extrinsic to the hand. The extrinsic muscles have their origins in the forearm and exert their effect on hand motion by means of tendinous insertions in the hand (Table 114.1). The intrinsic muscles have

TABLE 114.1. Muscles That Control Hand Motions

Muscle	Nerve	Insertion	Functional Test
EXTRINSIC FLEXORS			
Palmaris longus	Median	Palmar aponeurosis and flexor retinacuium	Wrist flexion with thumb and little finger opposition; palpate tendon
Flexor carpi radialis	Median	Base of metacarpal 2 and 3	Wrist flexion with radial deviation, palpate tendon
Flexor digitorum profundus	Median ($^1/_2$—FDP) Ulnar ($^1/_2$—FDP)	Distal phalanges of index, long, ring, and little fingers	DIP flexion with PIP held in extension
Flexor digitorum superficialis	Median	Middle phalanges of index, long, ring, and little fingers	PIP flexion with adjoining fingers held in extension at DIP and PIP
Flexor pollicis longus	Median	Distal phalanx of thumb	DIP flexion of thumb
Flexor carpi ulnaris	Ulnar	Pisiform, hook of hamate, base of metacarpal 5	Wrist flexion with ulnar deviation; palpate tendon
EXTRINSIC EXTENSORS			
Extensor carpi radialis brevis	Radial	Base of metacarpal 3	Wrist extension with closed fist; palpate tendons
Extensor carpi radialis longus	Radial	Base of metacarpal 2	Wrist extension with closed fist; palpate tendons
Extensor digitorum	Radial	Middle and distal phalanges of index, long, ring, and little fingers	MCP extension with PIP flexed, index long, ring and little fingers
Extensor digiti minimi	Radial	Extensor expansion of little finger	DIP and PIP extension of little finger with closed fist
Extensor carpi ulnaris	Radial	Base of metacarpal 5	Wrist extension and ulnar deviation with closed fist; palpate tendon
Abductor pollicis longus	Radial	Base of metacarpal 1	Radial deviation of thumb MCP; palpate tendons (radial side of anatomic snuffbox)
Extensor pollicis brevis	Radial	Base of proximal phalanx of thumb	Radial deviation of thumb MCP; palpate tendons (radial side of anatomic snuffbox)
Extensor pollicis longus	Radial	Base of distal phalanx of thumb	Elevate thumb of flat surface; palpate tendon (dorsal tendon of anatomic snuffbox)
Extensor indicis	Radial	Extensor expansion of index finger	DIP and PIP extension of index finger with closed fist
INTRINSIC MUSCLES			
Flexor pollicis brevis	Median	Base of proximal phalanx of thumb	Opposition of thumb and little finger; palpate thenar muscles for contraction
Abductor pollicis brevis	Median	Base of proximal phalanx of thumb	Opposition of thumb and little finger; palpate thenar muscles for contraction
Opponens pollicis	Median	Shaft of metacarpal 1	Opposition of thumb and little finger; palpate thenar muscles for contraction
Adductor pollicis	Ulnar	Base of proximal phalanx of thumb	Forcibly oppose thumb and radial aspect of index finger. IP flexion of thumb denotes weak adductor pollicis
Lumbricals	Median—I & II: Ulnar—III & IV	Extensor expansion of index, long, middle, and little fingers	DIP and PIP extension with MCP flexion
Interossei	Ulnar	Base of proximal phalanges of fingers; extensor expansion	All flex MCP and extend IP
4 palmar			Adduction of index, ring, and little fingers (long finger midline)
4 dorsal			Abduction of index, ring, and little fingers (long finger midline)
Abductor digiti minimi	Ulnar	Base of proximal phalanx of little finger	Abduction of little finger from hand; palpate hypothenar muscles for contraction; hypothenar skin dimpling
Flexor digiti minimi	Ulnar	Base of proximal phalanx of little finger	Abduction of little finger from hand; palpate hypothenar muscles for contraction; hypothenar skin dimpling
Opponens digiti minimi	Ulnar	Shaft of metacarpal 5	Abduction of little finger from hand; palpate hypothenar muscles for contraction; hypothenar skin dimpling

DIP, distal interphalangeal: PIP, proximal interphalangeal: MCP, metacarpophalangeal; IP, interphalangeal.

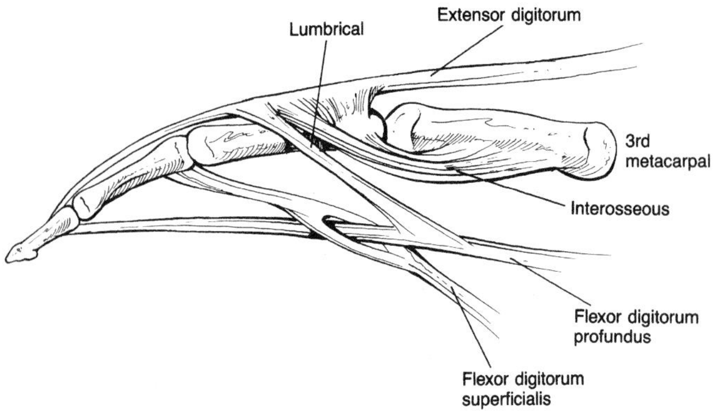

Figure 114.1. Musculotendinous anatomy of the finger.

their origins and insertions within the hand. The lumbricals are four small intrinsic muscles of the hand that originate from the flexor digitorum superficialis tendons and insert on the radial aspect of the extensor expansion of the extensor digitorum. The eight interossei (four dorsal and four palmar) originate from the lateral metacarpals and insert on the base of the proximal phalanxes and extensor expansion (Fig. 114.1; see Table 114.1).

The median, radial, and ulnar nerves provide sensory and motor innervation to the hand. The median nerve supplies motor function to the extrinsic flexors of the hand (only the radial portion of the flexor digitorum profundus), the intrinsic thenar muscles (abductor pollicis brevis, a portion of the flexor pollicis brevis, and the opponens pollicis), and first and second lumbricals. The ulnar nerve innervates the flexor carpi ulnaris and the ulnar portion of the flexor digitorum profundus; it then travels through the Guyon canal to innervate all the remaining intrinsic muscles of the hand. The radial nerve innervates those muscles of the forearm that provide extension of the wrist and digits and extension and abduction of the thumb. The radial nerve does not innervate any of the intrinsic hand muscles. The sensory innervation of the hand is detailed in Fig. 114.2.

The arterial supply to the hand is provided by the radial and ulnar arteries, which arise from the brachial artery in the antecubital fossa. The radial artery passes through the anatomic snuffbox and terminates as the deep palmar arch. The ulnar artery passes into the hand through the Guyon canal superficial to the flexor retinaculum to form the superficial palmar arch. A deep branch of the ulnar artery anastomoses with the deep palmar arch, and a superficial branch of the radial artery anastomoses with the superficial palmar arch. The four common digital arteries arise from the superficial palmar arch and then divide to form the proper digital arteries.

The thick palmar skin is adherent to the underlying palmar aponeurosis by numerous fibrous bands, which may produce a gritty sensation when lacerated. The palmar aponeurosis is the triangular, thick, deep fascia of the palm. It is attached to the distal flexor retinaculum, where it receives the insertion of the pal-

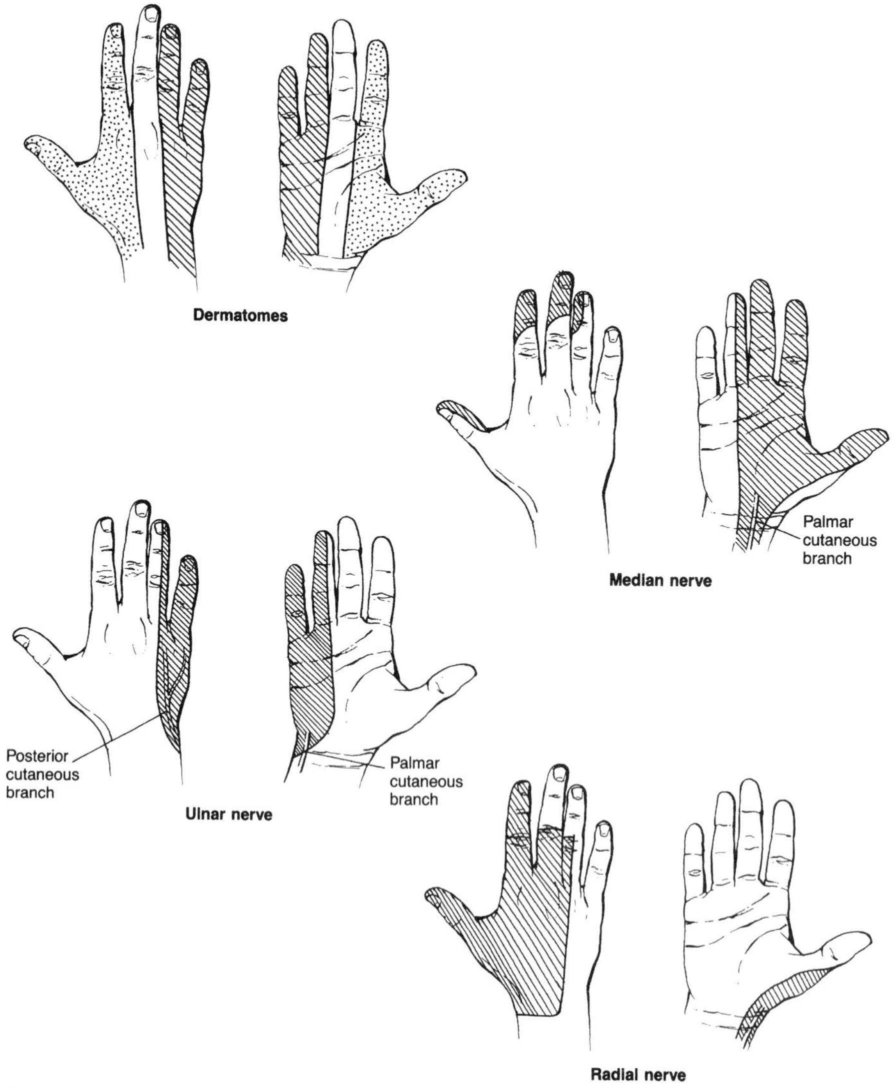

Figure 114.2. Sensory innervation of the hand.

maris longus tendon and spreads distally to the base of the four fingers. In contrast to that of the palm, the dorsal skin of the hand is thin and supple, with little underlying adipose or fibrous tissue. For this reason, edema from hand injuries is often more pronounced on the dorsal surface.

CLINICAL PRESENTATION

Most patients with acute hand injuries present with varying degrees of pain, swelling, loss of function, and laceration or puncture after either blunt or penetrating injury. Obvious deformity may or may not be present or may be obscured by associated swelling. In contrast, injuries resulting from repetitive motions or systemic or bone diseases usually present more insidiously, with chronic waxing and waning symptoms.

EMERGENCY DEPARTMENT EVALUATION

In the appropriate clinical setting, initial emergency department evaluation should focus on the need for resuscitation, followed by a general assessment of the patient to detect other significant injuries and control hemorrhage. Rarely will more than direct pressure and hand elevation be required to control bleeding from a hand wound; in such situations, the careful and intermittent use of a tourniquet (i.e., proximal blood pressure cuff) will usually gain control of the bleeding and allow adequate visualization of the wound. Blind clamping of bleeding vessels should be avoided, because adjacent nerves and tendons may be injured.

A focused, but thorough history is essential in the evaluation and treatment of the injured hand. Important historic information includes the patient's age, dominant hand, occupation and avocations (e.g., musician, typist, mechanic), other patient activities that require special use of the hands, smoking status (particularly for replantation candidates), prior hand injuries, preinjury hand function, medical history (e.g., diabetes mellitus, immunosuppression), time of the injury, mechanism and circumstances of injury (e.g., power tools, contaminated environment, associated burn or chemical exposures, potential for foreign bodies), position of the hand at the time of injury, treatment administered before arrival, and previous tetanus immunization.

A systematic and careful examination of the hand is also of paramount importance to the accurate diagnosis of hand injuries. Initially, the hand should be observed at rest, completely exposed. All rings should be removed because swelling may become diffuse and create a tourniquet effect, even on apparently uninjured fingers. The location and type of wounds, skin loss, ecchymosis, pallor, swelling, and resting attitude of the digits should be noted. The normal resting cascade of the fingers reveals progressive flexion of the digits from the index to the little finger, which is generally symmetric.

Alterations in this stance may indicate an underlying tendon injury. For example, a flexor tendon injury may appear as an extended digit on account of unopposed extensor tone, while an extensor tendon injury may reveal a flexion deformity. In addition, the hand can be observed during passive flexion and extension of the wrist. With wrist extension, the fingers naturally assume a flexed posture, and with wrist flexion, the fingers will passively extend.[17] Knowledge of this may be particularly helpful in evaluating children or patients who are uncooperative because of intoxication or pain.

The hand should be carefully palpated to identify areas of tenderness, bony step-off, and crepitus. Finally, in patients with phalangeal or metacarpal fractures the presence of rotational malalignment must be sought. Clinically, rotational deformity may be diagnosed by having the patient make a fist. Normally, all of the fingers point to the same spot on the scaphoid (Fig. 114.3). Scissoring of the digits and loss of the usual parallel relationship of the fingernails are additional signs of rotational deformity. Radiographically, there is asymmetry of the diameters of the shafts on each side of the fracture (Fig. 114.4).

Nerve integrity is assessed by testing both sensory and motor function. Sensation should always be evaluated before the administration of any anesthetic agent. Digital nerve sensory function is best assessed by two-point tactile discrimination. This test is easily performed with any number of devices, such as a paper clip bent into a U shape, electrocardiographic calipers, or a device specifically designed for this purpose. It is helpful to first explain and demonstrate the technique on the noninjured hand. The volar lateral aspects of the digits are lightly stroked in a longitudinal direction with the two points. Normal discrimination is 2 to 5 mm at the fingertips but may vary between individuals and appears to worsen with age.[21] Comparison with the opposite hand may be helpful.

In young children or uncooperative patients, it can be difficult to convincingly perform two-point tactile discrimination. In these circumstances, nerve integrity can be assessed through the presence of sympathetically mediated skin wrinkling and skin sweating. Soaking the hand in warm water for 30 minutes should cause wrinkling of the normally innervated skin. Skin sweating can be assessed by stroking the digit with a smooth ob-

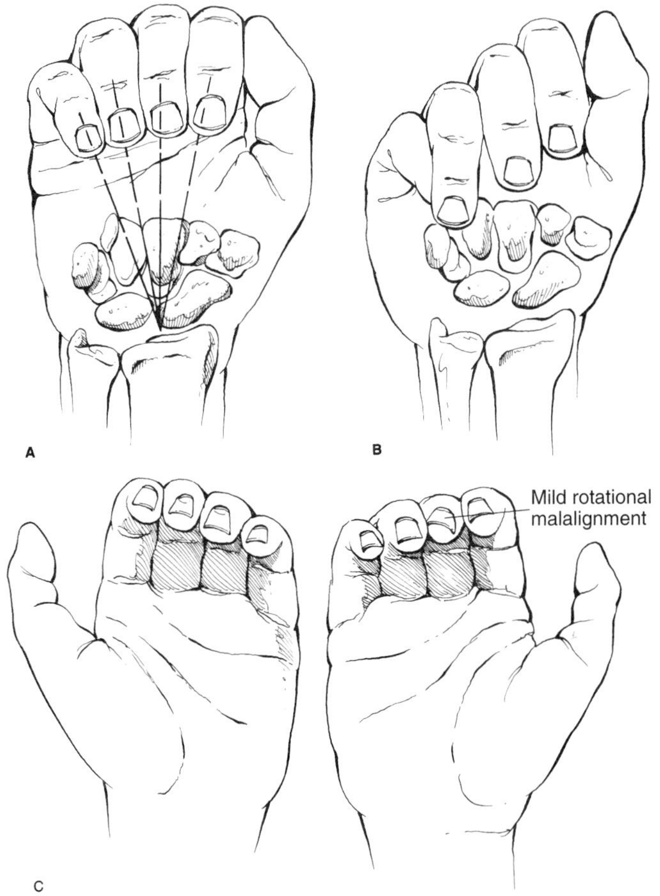

Figure 114.3. Clinical signs of rotational malalignment. **(A)** Normally, all fingers point to the same spot on the scaphoid when making a fist. **(B)** With rotational malalignment, the affected finger does not point to the scaphoid. **(C)** Loss of the usual parallel relationship of the finger nails with rotational malalignment. (Redrawn from Simon RR, Koenigsknecht SJ. *Emergency orthopedics: the extremities,* 3rd ed. Norwalk, CT: Appleton & Lange, 1995: 64.)

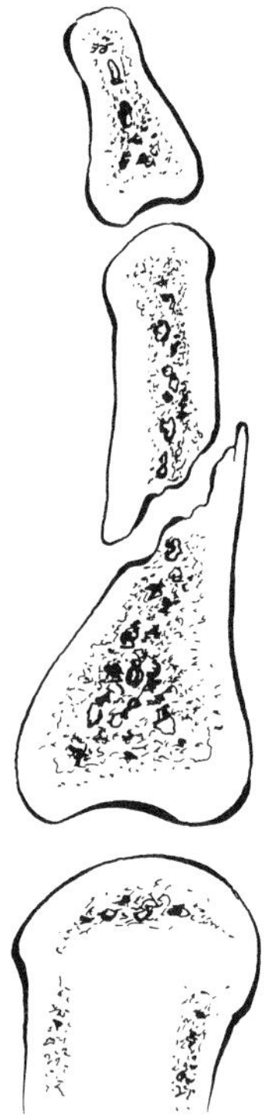

Figure 114.4. Radiographic sign of rotational malalignment. Note the asymmetry of the diameters of the shafts on each side of the fracture.

ject (e.g., the barrel of a pen). Less resistance (due to loss of sweating) should be noted over the denervated area. Alternatively, the hand can be painted with povidone–iodine solution, allowed to dry completely, then placed in a sterile glove. Normal digital sweating will moisten the povidone–iodine and cause the talc in the glove to turn black.

Vascular integrity of the hand is evaluated by noting cyanosis or pallor, noting skin temperature, assessing capillary refill (normal is less than 2 seconds), and assessing palpation of the ulnar and radial artery at the wrist.[17] The Allen test is used to test the patency of the radial and ulnar arteries and the palmar arches. The test is performed by having the patient clench the fist to exsanguinate the hand while the examiner occludes the radial and ulnar arteries. When the hand is blanched, pressure over one of the arteries is released. Normal hand color should return in 3 to 5 seconds.[17] The test is then repeated releasing the other artery. A digital Allen test performed in a similar fashion has also been described.[17]

Testing for musculotendinous integrity of both the extrinsic and intrinsic hand muscles is another important aspect of the hand examination (see Table 114.1). It should be noted that a significant portion of the population does not have independent function of the flexor digitorum superficialis to the small finger, and the ring finger PIP joint may also need to flex for an accurate examination.[22]

When evaluating finger lacerations, the digit should be moved through a full range of motion against light resistance, because a tendon laceration may be proximal or distal to the skin wound, depending on the position of the hand when the injury occurred. A high index of suspicion must be maintained, because partial tendon lacerations are easily missed (see Tendon Lacerations). In addition, the action of the lumbricals and interossei to independently extend the IP joints and flex the MCP joints may mask a tendon laceration. Furthermore, a bloodless field may be necessary to adequately assess the wound for foreign body or subtle tendon laceration. The tourniquet should not be left in place for more than 20 minutes. The digit is milked proximally and then a local tourniquet or Penrose drain is applied at the base of the finger and held in place by a hemostat.

Radiographs of the hand or wrist should be obtained whenever the mechanism could cause bony disruption, joint instability, or a retained foreign body. Standard views of the hand and fingers include posteroanterior (PA), lateral, and external oblique views. When evaluating an injured finger, a true lateral view is needed to adequately evaluate the DIP and PIP joints for volar lip injuries, and a frontal view of the hand is recommended to avoid overlooking an adjacent fracture. An internal oblique view may be helpful in visualizing phalangeal or metacarpal fractures after an initially nondiagnostic standard radiographic series.[9,24] Hand radiographs differ in technique from wrist radiographs, so both series must be obtained for the adequate evaluation of both hand and wrist symptoms. If there is suspicion of a foreign body despite negative plain radiographs, xeroradiography, ultrasonography, or computed tomography (CT) scanning may be required to localize the object.[13]

EMERGENCY DEPARTMENT MANAGEMENT

Emergency department management of hand injuries includes ice application and elevation of the extremity to reduce swelling. The liberal use of oral or parenteral analgesics is also recommended. Intravenous antibiotics are indicated for open fractures and dislocations and for severely contaminated or infected wounds. Tetanus immunization status should be assessed and updated appropriately. Open wounds should be covered with a sterile, moist gauze dressing pending radiographs, surgical consultation, or wound closure. In addition, fractures (or suspected fractures) should be temporarily immobilized with a bulky hand dressing or an appropriate splint while awaiting radiographs, reduction, or surgical consultation.

The disposition of patients with a hand injury depends on the nature and severity of the injury. A hand surgeon should be consulted in the case of suspected or actual nerve and tendon injuries, one who may examine such injuries in the emergency department directly. Alternatively, the injury can be vigorously irrigated and cleaned, the skin closed, and the hand splinted, with follow-up in 1 to 3 days for definitive management.

Important discharge instructions for all patients include elevation of the extremity and the use of ice for the initial 24 to 48 hours. Instructions regarding signs of infection, the timing of return visits for complications, wound checks, and suture removal are mandatory. Patients with injuries that are splinted should also receive instructions regarding splint care and signs or problems that should prompt an immediate return to the emergency department. Appropriate and timely follow-up arrangements should be provided for all patients treated in the emergency department. There will be institutional and regional variations in the specialty background of hand surgery consultants. In this chapter, we refer to hand surgeons or surgical consultants, recognizing that this category may include orthopedic surgeons, plastic surgeons, and surgeons who limit their practice to hand surgery.

Anesthetic Techniques

Anesthesia for the evaluation and repair of hand injuries can be provided by local infiltration (dorsum of the hand and superficial wounds of the palm), digital nerve block, or regional nerve block at the wrist. In addition, a hematoma block is useful for the reduction of metacarpal fractures.[15] Lidocaine without epinephrine should be used in 2% concentration for nerve blocks and in 1% or 2% concentration for infiltration. Use of a 25-

to 30-gauge needle, slow injection, and buffering with bicarbonate (1:10 dilution) will help reduce injection pain. A longer acting agent (i.e., bupivacaine) can also be used if prolonged anesthesia is required.

A digital block can be performed by injecting 2 to 3 mL of local anesthetic either at the medial and lateral aspect of the base of the proximal phalanx or at the level of the metacarpal head. Some authors prefer to perform a digital block at the metacarpal head because there is more space for tissue distention.[10] With either technique, infiltration of the proximal dorsal surface of the digit is also required to anesthetize the dorsal digital nerves and complete the block. Complete anesthesia usually requires 5 to 10 minutes. Circumferential infiltration of the digit is not recommended because it may result in distal necrosis.

Regional nerve blocks at the wrist can anesthetize the median, ulnar, and radial nerves. A median nerve block is performed by injecting 5 to 7 mL of local anesthetic 1 cm proximal to the distal wrist flexion crease radial and deep to the palmaris longus tendon, or deep to the ulnar aspect of the flexor carpi radialis tendon in those individuals lacking a palmaris longus tendon. An ulnar nerve block is accomplished by injecting 5 to 7 mL of local anesthetic 1 cm proximal to the distal wrist flexion crease just radial and deep to the flexor carpi ulnaris tendon. The ulnar artery at this level lies in close proximity to the ulnar nerve, and aspiration before injection is important to avoid intravascular injection of the anesthetic. The dorsal sensory branch of the ulnar nerve is blocked by subcutaneous infiltration of anesthetic just distal to the ulnar styloid. A radial nerve block is performed by subcutaneous infiltration of 5 mL of anesthetic agent just distal to the radial styloid. If paresthesias are elicited during insertion of the needle, it should be withdrawn before injection, because direct injection into the nerve may cause neuritis. Ten to 15 minutes is often required before complete anesthesia occurs. A hematoma block is performed by injecting a local anesthetic into the hematoma surrounding a fracture. A 27- to 30-gauge needle is inserted over the fracture site. When blood is aspirated into the syringe, indicating correct needle placement, 5 to 10 mL of anesthetic is injected. Up to 15 minutes may be needed for full anesthetic effect.

SPECIFIC INJURIES

Carpal Injuries

Most carpal injuries are caused by a fall on an outstretched hand (i.e., FOOSH injury), resulting in forced dorsiflexion of the wrist, or by a direct blow or crush injury to the wrist. Carpal fractures account for 7% to 10% of all hand and wrist injuries and are among the most frequently missed fractures in the emergency department.[5] The scaphoid is fractured most commonly (60% to 70% of carpal fractures), followed by the triquetrum, lunate, trapezium, pisiform, hamate, capitate, and trapezoid. Carpal dislocations are less common but are associated with severe sequelae if not diagnosed and treated appropriately.

CLINICAL PRESENTATION

Patients will complain of pain, swelling, and a limited range of motion in the wrist. However, the presentation will vary, depending on the nature and severity of the injury.

DIFFERENTIAL DIAGNOSIS

Carpal injuries may include fractures, dislocations, or a combination of the two. Fractures of the distal radius or ulna may be confused with, or accompanied by, a carpal injury. De Quervain tenosynovitis often presents with wrist pain, though there is commonly a more protracted history of pain with repetitive motions.

EMERGENCY DEPARTMENT EVALUATION

As discussed previously, emergency department evaluation begins with a careful history and physical examination. Radiographs are indicated in all but trivial injuries. In addition to standard x-ray review, the frontal radiograph should be examined for abnormalities of the carpal joint spaces (normally 1 to 2 mm), the shape of the scaphoid (normally elongated), the radiolunate articulation (at least one-half of the articular surface of the lunate should be in contact with the radius), and the radial slope (normally 15 to 30 degrees). The navicular fat stripe, normally seen on the frontal radiograph as a radiolucent line on the radial side of the scaphoid near the distal radius may be obliterated with a scaphoid fracture.[12] On the lateral projection, the normal linear alignment of the radius, lunate, and capitate should be carefully evaluated. The lunate appears as a "cup in a saucer" articulating with the distal radius. The capitate articulates with the distal concavity of the lunate and creates an angle of 10 to 20 degrees. The scaphoid and lunate should form an angle of 30 to 60 degrees. Additional radiographs that may be helpful include frontal views with maximum radial and ulnar deviation, lateral views with maximum flexion and extension, and carpal tunnel views for suspected hamate fractures. The presence of unfused epiphyses in children and adolescents can make interpretation of radiographs difficult. In this situation, comparison views may be helpful. Radiographs of the joint above or below the injury are indicated for pain, tenderness, or limitation of motion in those joints or in the presence of a fracture of the distal radius or ulna.

Scaphoid Fractures

The blood supply to the scaphoid is through ligamentous attachments, primarily to its distal pole. Blood supply to the proximal pole is, therefore, dependent on continuity with the upper pole. As a result, scaphoid fractures have a high incidence of delayed union, nonunion, avascular necrosis, and pseudoarthrosis.[2] On examination, anatomic snuffbox tenderness and swelling, pain with axial compression of the thumb, and pain with supination of the wrist against resistance are sensitive signs of a scaphoid fracture.[14,25] Unfortunately, 10% to 20% of scaphoid fractures will not be apparent on initial four-view radiographs. For this reason, patients with suspicion of a scaphoid fracture have historically had their injuries immobilized and reevaluated in 10 to 14 days. However, one study has demonstrated a 100% sensitivity for initial detection of scaphoid fractures using six-view radiographs (PA, lateral, extreme ulnar deviation, radial deviation, 25-degree pronation and supination views).[14] The authors of this study suggest that an initially negative six-view radiographic series may obviate the need for immobilization and follow-up. However, the number of patients in this study was small and a larger corroborating study is needed before this can be recommended as a standard of care. Until then, patients with clinical signs of a scaphoid fracture, despite negative radiographs, should be placed in a thumb spica splint, with the forearm in midposition and the wrist in approximately 25 degrees of extension, and referred for follow-up in 10 to 14 days.

Patients with nondisplaced fractures may be treated initially with immobilization in a thumb spica splint (with the forearm and wrist positioned as just described) and timely follow-up.

Immobilization of the elbow, using a long-arm versus a short-arm thumb spica splint, is controversial; therefore, discussion with the on-call hand surgeon is advised. Interestingly, evidence exists to support both practices.[25] As many as 95% of nondisplaced fractures will heal with simple immobilization. Unstable fractures or those displaced 1 mm or more require consultation with a hand surgeon. These fractures should be immobilized in a thumb spica splint pending definitive care, which usually involves open reduction and internal fixation. Prognosis is dependent on the location of the fracture and the presence of any displacement; oblique and proximal pole fractures are associated with a worse prognosis.

Triquetrum Fractures

The majority of triquetrum fractures are dorsal chip (avulsion) fractures due to a FOOSH injury. Less often, a direct blow to the wrist may cause a fracture of the body of the triquetrum. Body fractures are frequently associated with other carpal injuries (e.g., perilunate dislocation), but an isolated fracture of the body is rare. Triquetrum fractures are best seen on lateral or oblique radiographs of the wrist. Emergency department management involves immobilizing the wrist in a short-arm volar splint and close surgical follow-up.

Triquetrum fractures generally heal well with proper immobilization but may be complicated by damage to the deep branch of the ulnar nerve, with subsequent motor impairment.

Lunate Fractures

Isolated lunate fractures are relatively rare, accounting for only about 3% of traumatic wrist injuries.[16] More commonly, lunate fractures occur in association with other wrist injuries. Similar to the scaphoid, the blood supply to the lunate is through ligamentous attachments primarily to the distal pole; hence these injuries have a high incidence of avascular necrosis, leading to Kienbock disease, nonunion, and subsequent carpal instability. The lunate is located distal to the Lister tubercle, and a fracture of the lunate results in marked tenderness and swelling in this area. In addition, axial compression of the third metacarpal usually causes marked discomfort. Unfortunately, initial plain radiographs of the wrist often fail to demonstrate the fracture. Therefore, if there is clinical suspicion of a fracture (or diagnostic radiographs), the wrist should be immobilized in a long-arm thumb spica splint and the patient referred for prompt surgical follow-up.

Kienbock Disease

Kienbock disease, or osteonecrosis of the lunate, is a disabling affliction resulting from avascular necrosis of the lunate. The pathogenesis is thought to be a combination of vascular predisposition, mechanical risk, and loading forces on the lunate that result in vascular compromise, bony degeneration, and eventual collapse. A shortened ulna (a normal variant known as ulna minus variant) may also be a predisposing factor to the development of Kienbock disease. Patients present with pain localized in the area of the lunate, stiffness, occasional swelling, and marked loss of grip strength. A history of significant wrist trauma is often lacking, but carpal tunnel syndrome may be the presenting symptom in some cases.[1] Diagnosis is usually confirmed by plain radiographs that demonstrate sclerosis, collapse, and, ultimately, fragmentation of the lunate. However, radiographs may be normal early in the course of the disease. Patients suspected of having Kienbock disease should be immobilized in a short-arm volar splint and referred to a hand specialist.

Scapholunate Dissociation

Scapholunate dissociation is a subtle injury often misdiagnosed as a simple wrist sprain. The mechanism of injury is forced dorsiflexion resulting in a torn scapholunate ligament. Patients usually present with pain, swelling, and a clicking sensation in the wrist.[4] The diagnosis should be suspected when there is tenderness over the area of the scapholunate ligament, located just distal and radial to the Lister tubercle, and painful motion of the scaphoid. A gap of greater than 3 mm between the scaphoid and the lunate on the frontal view of the wrist is diagnostic. Other helpful radiographic signs include volar angulation of the scaphoid (e.g., a radioscaphoid angle greater than 60 degrees), lack of parallelism of the articular surfaces of the scaphoid and lunate, and V-shaped notching of the normally smooth C-shaped line formed by the volar surfaces of the scaphoid and radius.[9] Emergency department management includes immobilization in a thumb spica splint and prompt referral. Although some controversy exists regarding optimal treatment, most hand surgeons favor open reduction and repair of the scapholunate ligament.

Lunate and Perilunate Dislocations

Lunate and perilunate dislocations can be viewed as similar injuries.[8] With extreme dorsiflexion, forces transmitted through the wrist dorsally displace the capitate and disrupt the capitolunate joint. Disruption of this joint allows volar or, rarely, dorsal displacement of the lunate, resulting in lunate dislocation. Perilunate dislocation results from the same mechanism, although the lunate remains aligned with the distal radius, and the capitate and metacarpals are dislocated, usually dorsally. Perilunate dislocations can be associated with carpal bone fractures and are described as transradial, transscaphoid, transcapitate, or transtriquetrum perilunate dislocations, depending on which carpal bones are fractured. In both perilunate and lunate dislocations, the frontal radiograph may reveal increased carpal bone overlap, shortening of the scaphoid, or other carpal bone fractures. In addition, with lunate dislocations, the normally rectangular lunate appears triangular on the frontal view.

In evaluating the lateral view, an imaginary straight line should be drawn through the distal radius, lunate, and capitate. If this line does not pass through the centers of the lunate or capitate, a lunate or perilunate dislocation should be suspected, respectively. In addition, on the lateral radiograph, a perilunate dislocation demonstrates disarticulation of the capitolunate joint, with the capitate dorsally displaced and the lunate remaining in normal alignment with the distal radius. With a lunate dislocation, the capitate has a near linear alignment with the radius, but the lunate is volarly rotated and displaced (i.e., "spilled teacup" sign). Emergency department management of a lunate or perilunate dislocation includes immobilizing the wrist in the neutral position in a volar splint and immediate consultation with a hand surgeon for reduction. Some surgeons believe that if reduction is not accomplished and maintained easily, open reduction and internal fixation with repair of the damaged ligaments is required.[8]

DISPOSITION

Patients with closed, nondisplaced carpal bone fractures can be discharged from the emergency department with prompt (24 to 72 hours) referral to a hand surgeon. In most cases, discussion with the follow-up physician is recommended before discharge. Patients with displaced fractures and lunate or perilunate dislocations should be evaluated by a hand surgeon in the emergency department. All patients with open fractures or dislocations will require intravenous administration of an antibiotic (e.g., cefazolin) and operative lavage and debridement.

COMMON PITFALLS

- Failure to diagnose an associated injury when confronted with a clinically or radiographically obvious carpal injury
- Misdiagnosing a scaphoid fracture or scapholunate dissociation as a wrist sprain and not providing adequate immobilization and follow-up
- Failure to appreciate radiographic evidence of a lunate or perilunate dislocation and obtain hand surgery consultation
- Failure to provide adequate analgesia and sedation for patients requiring fracture or joint reduction
- Failure to provide adequate discharge instructions regarding splint and/or cast care, extremity elevation, and specific precautions regarding splint and/or cast complications

METACARPAL INJURIES

CLINICAL PRESENTATION

Patients with metacarpal injuries generally present with pain, swelling, deformity, and limitation of movement after a direct blow to the hand, a crush injury (e.g., industrial press), a missile injury, or striking an object with a closed fist. The location of maximal tenderness and the presence of crepitus and deformity will help localize the area of injury. Furthermore, in patients with a metacarpal head fracture, axial compression of the extended digit causes severe discomfort; in patients with a metacarpal base fracture, flexion or extension of the wrist or longitudinal compression exacerbates the pain. Metacarpal fractures are classified according to which bone is injured, as well as the fracture site. Fractures of metacarpals 2 through 5 are classified together and divided into head, neck, shaft, and base fractures. First metacarpal fractures are classified as extraarticular base and shaft fractures and intraarticular base fractures.

DIFFERENTIAL DIAGNOSIS

Metacarpal injuries include fractures, dislocations, or combinations of the two. Carpal–metacarpal dislocations may accompany or be confused with proximal metacarpal injuries, while proximal phalangeal injuries and MCP joint dislocations must be included in the different diagnosis of distal metacarpal injuries.

EMERGENCY DEPARTMENT EVALUATION

Evaluation should include a detailed history and physical examination and standard radiographs, as outlined earlier. Diagnosis and correction of rotational malalignment (see Figs. 114.3 and 114.4) is particularly important with metacarpal injuries.

EMERGENCY DEPARTMENT MANAGEMENT

Nondisplaced metacarpal fractures are managed by immobilization in an ulnar gutter splint (metacarpals 4 and 5), radial gutter splint (metacarpals 2 and 3), or thumb spica splint (metacarpal 1) and by prompt referral. It is imperative that malalignment, especially rotational malalignment, is excluded by radiographs and careful physical examination (see Figs. 114.3 and 114.4). The wrist should be splinted in 20 degrees of extension, the MCP joints near 90 degrees' flexion, and IP joints in extension. All open fractures, unstable fractures, multiple metacarpal fractures, and fractures that cannot be reduced by closed technique require surgical consultation for open reduction and internal fixation.

Metacarpal Neck Fractures

Most commonly seen in the fifth metacarpal (i.e., boxer fracture), neck fractures are usually the result of striking an object with a closed fist. Metacarpal neck fractures are easily reduced, but reduction is often difficult to maintain due to comminution of the volar cortex. Furthermore, because metacarpals 2 and 3 are relatively fixed and immobile, reduction of these fractures must be near anatomic. Any volar angulation will project the metacarpal head into the palm and impair grip strength. Greater angulation is acceptable in metacarpals 4 and 5 because they have greater mobility and can move dorsally without impairment of grip strength. Most hand surgeons will allow up to 40 degrees of angulation in fractures of the fifth metacarpal neck and 20 degrees of angulation in fractures of the fourth metacarpal neck. In contrast, as little as 10 degrees of angulation is unacceptable for metacarpals 2 and 3. Reduction of a metacarpal neck fracture is accomplished by taking advantage of the fact that the MCP joint collateral ligaments are taut in flexion and the proximal phalanx can be used as a lever to manipulate the distal fracture fragment. Reduction techniques are the same regardless of which metacarpal is fractured; however, surgical consultation is recommended before reduction of metacarpals 2 and 3, because some surgeons prefer operative fixation. After adequate anesthesia has been obtained, the MCP and PIP joints are flexed to 90 degrees and pressure is applied to the PIP joint in a dorsal direction to force the metacarpal head into its normal position. Stabilizing volar pressure should be applied with the physician's other thumb just proximal to the fracture site (Fig. 114.5). If reduction is difficult, longitudinal distraction may be needed to disimpact the fracture before attempting reduction. A gutter splint incorporating the adjacent finger should be placed while carefully keeping the MCP joint flexed to maintain reduction. The wrist should be splinted in 20 degrees' extension, the MCP near 90 degrees' flexion, and the IP joints in extension. It is very important to immobilize the MCP

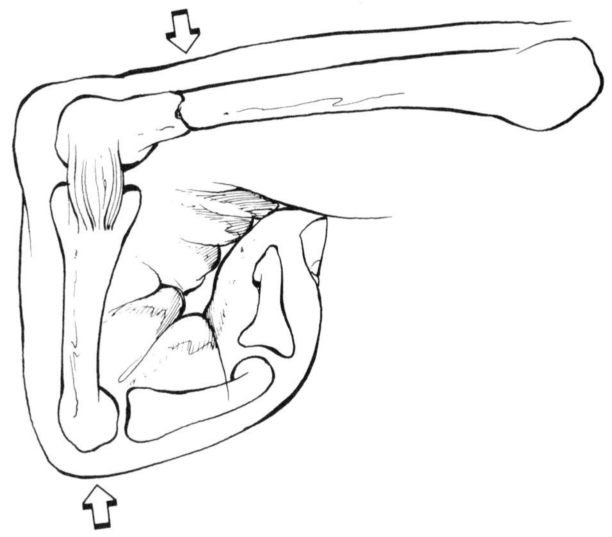

Figure 114.5. The 90–90 method of reduction for metacarpal neck fractures.

joint as close to 90 degrees as possible, because the metacarpal head is cam shaped, causing the collateral ligaments to be taut in flexion and relaxed in extension. Shortening of the collateral ligaments from immobilization in extension can permanently limit flexion of the MCP joint. Furthermore, the "90–90" splint that maintains both the MCP and PIP joints at 90 degrees should never be used, because it may cause skin sloughing over the PIP joint and PIP joint stiffness.[7] Follow-up should be arranged within 5 to 7 days; if loss of reduction occurs, operative fixation may be needed.

Metacarpal Head Fractures

Usually the result of a direct blow or crush injury, metacarpal head fractures are often comminuted and may be complicated by rotational malalignment. Management consists of temporary immobilization in a bulky hand dressing or well-padded volar splint. Emergency department evaluation by a hand surgeon is indicated for most metacarpal head fractures because anatomic reduction, which is essential to prevent loss of function, frequently requires operative intervention. Even with optimal management, severe metacarpal head fractures may have a poor functional outcome. Extensor tendon damage and fibrosis and interossei muscle fibrosis are complications of metacarpal head fractures.[3]

Metacarpal Shaft Fractures

Metacarpal shaft fractures usually result from a direct blow to the hand, resulting in a transverse or comminuted fracture, or from a rotational force to a digit, causing an oblique or spiral fracture. The action of the interossei muscles usually causes transverse fractures to angulate dorsally, while oblique or spiral fractures tend to shorten and rotate.[3] Nondisplaced transverse fractures are treated by immobilization in a gutter splint, with the wrist in 20 degrees of extension, the MCP joint in 60 to 90 degrees of flexion, the PIP joint in 20 to 30 degrees of flexion, and the DIP joint in 10 to 15 degrees of flexion.[23] Whenever possible, displaced transverse metacarpal shaft fractures should be reduced by a hand surgeon. However, if consultation is not available, reduction may be attempted by the emergency physician by applying volar force over the dorsal apex of the fracture and dorsal pressure on the flexed MCP joint. It is essential that any rotational deformity be corrected. If reduction is successful, the hand is splinted as described earlier and the patient is referred for follow-up in 3 to 5 days. If a transverse fracture cannot be reduced, or if an oblique, spiral, or comminuted fracture is present, consultation with a hand surgeon for operative repair is indicated.

Metacarpal Base Fractures

Base fractures of the metacarpals are generally stable, but even slight rotational deformity will be greatly amplified at the fingertip.[7] Nondisplaced fractures without rotational deformity may be treated by immobilization in a gutter or volar splint and by surgical referral. Displaced or intraarticular base fractures require hand surgery consultation for open reduction and internal fixation.

First Metacarpal Fractures

First metacarpal fractures are usually the result of a direct injury to the thumb. These fractures usually occur at or near the base and may be either extraarticular or intraarticular. Extraarticular fractures are more common and are usually transverse or, less often, oblique. Because of the mobility of the first metacarpal, as much as 20 to 30 degrees of angulation may be present without loss of mobility or function. Transverse fractures with less than 30 degrees of angulation are treated with immobilization in a short-arm thumb spica splint and prompt follow-up. A transverse fracture with greater than 30 degrees of angulation requires reduction, which involves manipulation of the fracture, using the thumb for distraction. After reduction, the thumb is splinted as described earlier, and the patient is referred for follow-up. Oblique fractures are often unstable and frequently require percutaneous pinning for adequate immobilization; therefore, consultation is advised before manipulation or discharge.

There are two types of intraarticular fractures: Bennett fracture and Rolando fracture. In a Bennett fracture, the fracture line extends through the articular surface and creates a fragment off the volar lip of the metacarpal base. Because of the pull of the abductor pollicis longus, the metacarpal base is subluxed or dislocated proximally and radially. A Rolando fracture is a T- or Y-shaped intraarticular fracture of the base of the first metacarpal—in essence, a comminuted Bennett fracture. Both fractures result from an axial blow to the metacarpal, commonly sustained by striking an object with a closed fist. Emergency department management includes immobilization in a bulky hand dressing and hand surgery consultation. If surgical consultation is not readily available, the thumb may be immobilized in a short thumb spica splint and follow-up arranged within 24 hours. Definitive therapy for a Bennett fracture frequently requires pinning for a stable anatomic reduction. A Rolando fracture often requires open reduction and has a poor prognosis, even with optimal management.[7]

Metacarpal Dislocations

Dislocations involving the metacarpals are either carpometacarpal (CMC) or metacarpophalangeal (MCP). CMC dislocations require a significant force and are usually caused by a crush injury; a direct blow, causing a longitudinal force along the metacarpals; or a levering, dorsiflexion force. These dislocations are generally dorsal and often associated with metacarpal or carpal fractures and significant soft-tissue trauma. The presence of a displaced proximal metacarpal fracture should prompt a careful search for an associated CMC dislocation. The lateral view is usually the most helpful for diagnosing CMC dislocations. However, overlapping densities on standard wrist radiographs (PA, oblique, and lateral) may make the detection of CMC dislocations difficult. Special views (e.g., anteroposterior [AP] in supination, 30-degree radial, and ulnar obliques) may also be useful in detecting CMC dislocations. Emergency department care is supportive pending hand surgery consultation. CMC dislocations are easily reduced with the patient under general anesthesia or brachial plexus block, but operative fixation (i.e., Kirschner pinning) is usually required to maintain reduction, particularly if multiple fractures or dislocations are present. Complications of CMC dislocations are ulnar and median nerve injuries, extensor tendon injuries, and circulatory compromise.

MCP dislocations are usually dorsal, occasionally lateral, and rarely volar. They are generally well visualized on standard radiographs of the hand. Dorsal MCP dislocations are classified as simple (reducible) or complex (irreducible). Simple dorsal dislocations are the most common and are usually readily reduced in the emergency department. Complex dorsal dislocations are irreducible by closed techniques because the volar plate is forced between the metacarpal head and the proximal phalanx, trapping the metacarpal head between the flexor tendons and the lumbricals (Fig. 114.6). On examination, complex dislocations often appear less deformed than simple dislocations (because of overlap of the proximal phalanx on the metacarpal head) and are associated with puckering of the palmar skin overlying the metacarpal head. Radiographically, the presence of a sesamoid bone within the MCP joint space is pathognomonic of a complex

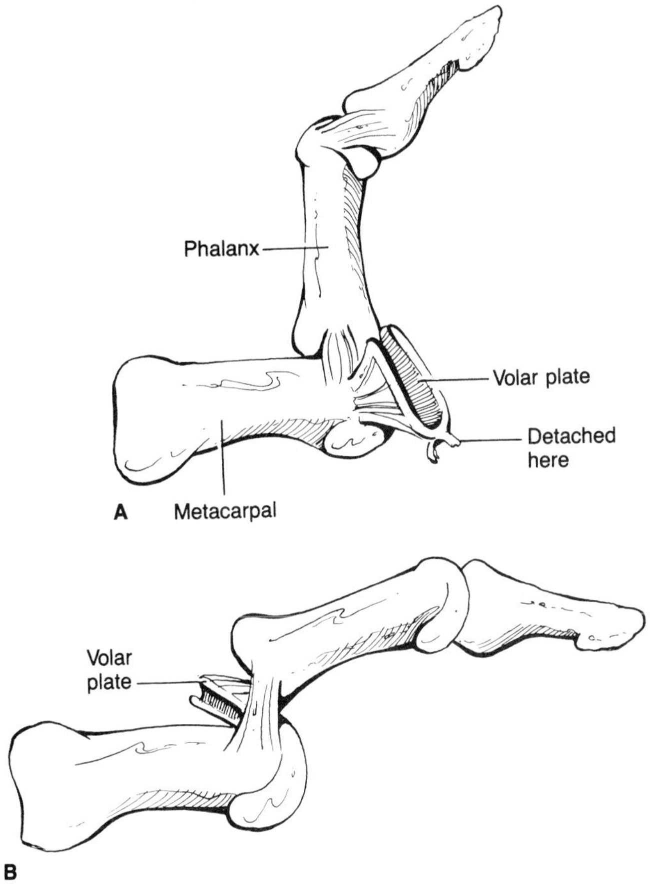

Figure 114.6. Dorsal dislocation of the MCP joint. **(A)** Simple dorsal dislocation. **(B)** Complex dorsal dislocation; note entrapment of the volar plate.

dislocation.[7] Simple dorsal dislocations are reduced by slight flexion of the wrist to relax the extrinsic flexors, followed by gentle hyperextension of the MCP joint (not beyond 90 degrees) and firm pressure on the dorsal aspect of the proximal phalanx. Longitudinal traction and extreme hyperextension are to be avoided, because this may interpose the volar plate, converting a simple dislocation to a complex one. After reduction, the hand is immobilized, with the wrist in 20 degrees of extension, the MCP joint in 50 to 70 degrees of flexion, the PIP joint in 20 to 30 degrees of flexion, and the DIP joint in 10 to 15 degrees of flexion. One attempt at reduction of a possible complex dislocation may be warranted, but multiple attempts should be avoided. These patients require open reduction and repair of the volar plate injury.

Collateral MCP ligament injuries occur infrequently and are often missed acutely. The presence of an avulsion fracture from the metacarpal head or corner fracture of the base of the proximal phalanx suggests an MCP collateral ligament injury. Consultation with a hand surgeon is recommended for patients with a collateral ligament injury, because some surgeons prefer operative reduction and repair of these injuries, especially if the fracture involves greater than 20% of the articular surface or is displaced more than 2 to 3 mm.[7] Emergency department care involves immobilization in a gutter splint, with the MCP in at least 50 degrees of flexion, and appropriate referral.

Gamekeeper Thumb (Skier Thumb)

Initially described as a chronic laxity of the thumb MCP joint ulnar collateral ligament in British gamekeepers (a result of the technique by which they killed wounded rabbits), the term *gamekeeper thumb* has come to include all injuries to the thumb ulnar collateral ligament. Today, acute rupture of the ulnar collateral ligament caused by sudden abduction of the thumb is much more common and is most often due to falls while skiing, earning the eponym *skier thumb*.

Plain radiographs may be normal or may reveal an avulsion fracture from the base of the proximal phalanx. If plain radiographs do not reveal a fracture, stressing the ligament may help determine the degree of injury (e.g., partial vs. complete tear). The joint should be stressed in slight flexion to reduce the stabilizing effect of the volar plate. A difference of greater than 10 degrees between the injured and uninjured thumb is considered positive. Unless the joint is grossly unstable, local anesthesia may be needed for a reliable examination. In equivocal cases, stress radiographs of both sides may be diagnostic.[7]

Emergency department management includes immobilization in a thumb spica splint and early (i.e., 24 to 48 hours) referral. A frequent complication of ulnar collateral ligament rupture is chronic laxity of the MCP joint due to interposition of the adductor aponeurosis between the ends of the torn ligament that prevents healing.[7,11] As a result, many surgeons prefer operative repair of the torn ligament. The presence of a fracture involving greater than 25% of the articular surface or of a displaced avulsion fracture is also an indication for open repair.[7]

DISPOSITION

Most patients with metacarpal injuries can be discharged from the emergency department with appropriate immobilization and instructions. Those patients with open fractures, irreducible fractures or dislocations, or circulatory compromise should be evaluated by a hand surgeon in the emergency department. Patients with stable fractures, anatomically reduced dislocations, and ligamentous injuries can be discharged with early follow-up, because operative repair or fixation can be performed 3 to 5 days after the injury.

COMMON PITFALLS

- Failure to appreciate volar angulation of fractures of metacarpals 2 and 3
- Failure to diagnose associated or multiple hand injuries
- Failure to appreciate and correct rotational deformity in metacarpal fractures
- Failure to appreciate CMC dislocation due to overlapping densities
- Improper splinting of the hand. In most circumstances, the hand should be splinted, with the wrist in 20 degrees of extension, the MCP joint in 60 to 90 degrees of flexion, and the IP joints in 10 to 15 degrees of flexion.

PHALANGEAL INJURIES

Phalangeal injuries are commonly thought of as trivial, but they can result in significant functional disability if not recognized and treated appropriately. Injuries to the fingers are usually a result of direct trauma to the digit.

CLINICAL PRESENTATION

Patients present with varying degrees of pain, swelling, and tenderness; limited or complete loss of function; and deformity of the involved digit.

DIFFERENTIAL DIAGNOSIS

The differential diagnosis of acute phalangeal injuries includes fractures, fractures–dislocations, and ligamentous injuries. Associated metacarpal injuries must always be excluded, especially in the presence of a proximal phalanx injury.

EMERGENCY DEPARTMENT EVALUATION

As with all hand injuries, a detailed history and physical examination are essential. The presence of rotational deformity must be carefully sought (see Figs. 114.3 and 114.4) and corrected, particularly with proximal phalangeal fractures. Radiographs are indicated in most injuries. It is important to accept only high-quality radiographs, because subtle injuries may be missed on lesser-quality films.

EMERGENCY DEPARTMENT MANAGEMENT

Treatment of closed phalangeal injuries depends on the nature of the injury (discussion follows). Open phalangeal fractures, with the exceptions of distal amputations and distal phalanx fractures, are managed in a fashion similar to that for other open fractures.

Proximal and Middle Phalangeal Fractures

Stable, nondisplaced middle and proximal phalangeal fractures without angulation or rotational deformity can be managed with dynamic splinting (i.e., "buddy taping") to an adjacent normal digit. An absorbent material (e.g., felt, gauze, lamb's wool) should be placed between the digits for padding and to prevent maceration of the skin. The patient should bend the fingers normally and use the hand as comfort allows. Radiographs are obtained in 7 and 14 days to assess angulation and healing. Unstable fractures of the proximal and middle phalanges (e.g., oblique, condylar, displaced, or angulated transverse fractures) and displaced intraarticular fractures generally require operative reduction or fixation. Emergency department management of these fractures includes immobilization in a gutter splint and surgical consultation.

Of special note are avulsion fractures off the dorsal aspect of the base of the middle phalanx. If not recognized and treated appropriately, these fractures can result in a boutonniere deformity (i.e., fixed flexion of the PIP joint and fixed hyperextension of the DIP joint). This deformity is caused by avulsion of the central slip of the extensor tendon, with loss of extensor function at the PIP joint, and unopposed force from the flexor digitorum superficialis. With time, the lateral bands of the extensor expansion sublux laterally and volarly, becoming PIP joint flexors and DIP joint extensors; contractures make this a fixed deformity. These fractures should be immobilized in a volar splint, with the PIP joint in extension, followed by prompt referral. Avulsion fractures from the volar aspect of the base of the middle phalanx can be indicative of a volar plate injury. These injuries should be immobilized in a volar splint in 15 degrees of flexion, followed by appropriate referral. Unrecognized or improperly managed volar plate injuries at the PIP joint may result in a swan-neck deformity, characterized by hyperextension of the PIP joint and flexion of the DIP joint.[18]

Distal Phalanx Fractures

Distal phalanx fractures are divided into intra- and extraarticular fractures. Extraarticular fractures usually result from a direct blow to the distal phalanx. These injuries are frequently associated with a subungual hematoma and nail bed laceration. Nondisplaced extraarticular fractures are managed with a protective splint for 3 to 4 weeks, elevation, and appropriate analgesia. A U-shaped splint can be constructed using commercially available aluminum and foam splints and positioned in either a sagittal or a coronal plane. Displaced extraarticular fractures are reduced by applying dorsal traction to the distal fragment. If reduction is successful, the digit is immobilized in a volar splint and the patient is referred to a hand surgeon; otherwise, hand surgery consultation is indicated.

Intraarticular fractures most commonly involve the dorsal surface of the joint and are often referred to as a mallet finger. This injury is frequently caused by a ball striking the tip of an extended finger. The mechanism of injury is forced flexion of the distal phalanx with the finger in taut extension, resulting in injury to the extensor tendon (e.g., stretching, rupture) or an intraarticular avulsion fracture of the dorsal aspect of the distal phalanx with loss of extensor function. Patients typically present with tenderness and swelling over the dorsal aspect of the DIP joint and loss of extension at the DIP joint. Emergency department management includes immobilization using a Stack splint or a padded dorsal aluminum splint with the DIP joint in extension. If the fracture involves less than 25% of the articular surface, immobilization is maintained for 6 to 8 weeks to coapt the tendon or fracture segments. If the fracture involves more than 25% of the articular surface, the patient should be referred for surgical fixation. Open distal phalanx fractures are treated by copious irrigation and wound closure, ensuring complete soft-tissue coverage of exposed bone. Prophylactic antibiotics generally are administered but are likely of benefit only in high-risk cases (e.g., gross contamination, delayed presentation, immunosuppression).

Proximal Interphalangeal Joint Dislocations

Dislocation of the PIP joint is the most common dislocation of the hand. Dorsal dislocations result from hyperextension forces, such as occurs when the outstretched finger is struck by a ball, and are accompanied by partial or complete rupture of the volar plate or collateral ligaments. Volar dislocations occur less often but are associated with complete rupture of the volar plate and collateral ligaments, as well as the central slip of the extensor mechanism. Patients usually present with pain, swelling, and deformity of the PIP joint. Rarely, severe swelling will mask an otherwise obvious deformity. The presence of pain and a locking sensation with flexion suggests a volar plate injury. Radiographs are diagnostic for acute dislocations, but small avulsions of the volar plate may not be visible or are seen only on the lateral postreduction view. Most dorsal dislocations are easily reduced, but the volar plate may become interposed in the joint space, preventing reduction by closed techniques. If this occurs, open reduction is required. For closed reduction, a digital nerve block will provide adequate anesthesia. The distal portion of the digit is firmly grasped and slightly hyperextended; then, with gentle traction parallel to the middle phalanx, the base of the middle phalanx is pressed back into position and the PIP joint is flexed. The PIP joint should be immobilized using a volar splint, in 15 to 20 degrees of flexion for 2 to 5 weeks.

Some authors recommend dynamic splinting (buddy taping) for 3 to 6 weeks if the collateral ligaments are stable and there is no evidence of a fracture.[7,24] Volar dislocations can be reduced by traction with both the MCP and PIP joints flexed. Consultation with a hand surgeon before reduction is recommended, because some surgeons prefer to treat these dislocations operatively to prevent a boutonniere deformity. Joint stiffness is a common complication after both volar and dorsal dislocations.

Distal Interphalangeal Joint Dislocations

Dislocations of the DIP joint are relatively uncommon injuries. They are almost exclusively dorsal and often associated with an open wound. DIP joint dislocations can usually be reduced with digital block anesthesia and simple traction. After reduction, the DIP joint should be immobilized in extension using a dorsal splint and the patient referred to a hand surgeon in 3 to 7 days.

DISPOSITION

Patients with stable, anatomically reduced phalangeal injuries can be discharged from the emergency department with appropriate follow-up. Patients with open fractures or nonreducible or unstable fractures or dislocations require consultation with a hand surgeon.

COMMON PITFALLS

- Failure to diagnose subtle fractures due to inadequate radiographic studies, including lack of true lateral views of injured digits, and both pre- and postreduction views
- Failure to recognize a volar plate disruption that may lead to a swan-neck deformity
- Failure to appreciate and correct rotational deformity in a phalangeal fracture
- Inadequate splinting or lack of appropriate surgical referral
- Inadequate instructions regarding cast or splint care or indications that should prompt an immediate return to the emergency department

HAND LACERATIONS

The objectives of emergency department care of hand lacerations are to preserve function, prevent infection, minimize scar formation, and provide the optimal wound environment for rapid healing. Simple lacerations (clean, less than 6 hours old, and not involving tendons, joints, or neurovascular structures) are managed in the same manner as lacerations elsewhere (see Chapter 95). However, in many areas of the hand, vital structures are extremely superficial, and injuries to these structures are not always readily apparent. Therefore, great care must be taken in the evaluation of hand lacerations to identify associated injuries, particularly injuries to tendons, nerves, or arteries.

CLINICAL PRESENTATION

Hand lacerations may range from clean, superficial wounds to severely contaminated crush injuries or amputations. Associated tendon injuries may cause a partial or complete loss of motor function, and injury to surrounding nerves may result in loss of both motor and sensory function. Due to their close proximity, digital nerve and flexor tendon injuries frequently occur together.

DIFFERENTIAL DIAGNOSIS

The diagnostic challenge of hand lacerations lies in the detection of underlying injuries that may threaten function of the hand. Tendon lacerations and injury to bones, joints, nerves, and arteries must be excluded by examination, radiography, and/or direct exploration of the wound.

EMERGENCY DEPARTMENT EVALUATION

Evaluation of a hand laceration begins with a pertinent history and meticulous examination. Adequate exploration of the wound requires a clean, bloodless, well-illuminated field and adequate anesthesia. Hemostasis can generally be obtained by direct pressure over the wound. A proximal blood pressure cuff (for hand and wrist wounds) or finger tourniquet (for digit wounds) may be needed to control hemorrhage. Blind clamping of bleeding vessels may injure adjacent nerves or tendons and should be avoided. Anesthesia may be obtained by direct infiltration of a local anesthetic or regional nerve block but should never be attempted until a complete sensory examination has been performed. When a complex injury requiring hand surgery consultation is apparent from the initial evaluation, the instillation of local anesthetic should await examination by the consultant. Pain control can be provided with systemic analgesics. Radiographs are indicated in any case in which the mechanism of injury could produce a fracture, dislocation, joint capsule injury, or retained foreign body.

EMERGENCY DEPARTMENT MANAGEMENT

All hand lacerations, regardless of the depth, must be carefully explored, because injury to significant underlying structures can occur with even very small surface wounds. In addition, exploration should be carried out through a full range of motion, otherwise injury to underlying structures, particularly tendon lacerations, may be missed. Simple lacerations are cleaned, irrigated, and repaired in the same fashion as in other areas of the body. Deep sutures should be avoided. After repair, lacerations over areas of motion should be splinted until the skin edges are well adherent. In addition, lacerations that cross the flexor surface of joints may create a flexion contraction as they heal. This can be prevented by performing a Z-plasty, which creates a transverse scar. Antibiotics are generally not required for simple hand lacerations in otherwise healthy patients.

Clenched-Fist Injuries

Lacerations over the MCP joints are often a result of striking an object (e.g., an opponent's teeth during an altercation) with a clenched fist and may be associated with extensor tendon injury, joint capsule violation, or metacarpal neck fracture. Because of the devastating consequences of inadequate treatment (wound infection, septic arthritis), any laceration over the MCP joints must be approached with suspicion and assumed to be a human bite wound until proven otherwise. Treatment includes copious irrigation, immobilization and elevation, intravenous antibiotics (penicillin G 2 million units, and cefazolin 1 g), and hand surgery consultation for admission and possible debridement in the operating room. These wounds are not closed, owing to the high incidence of infection.

Tendon Lacerations

Tendon injuries are frequently associated with hand lacerations. A high index of suspicion combined with a detailed examination and careful wound exploration are essential in detecting these injuries. There are a number of reasons that tendon injuries are missed on initial presentation. Discomfort and anxiety may reduce patient cooperation, making a reliable examination difficult. This problem can be overcome by the judicious use of local anesthesia. Frequently, the tendon is only partially cut, allowing limited or even complete function. In this case, only a high index of suspicion and meticulous wound exploration will prevent the complications associated with a missed partial tendon laceration (i.e., adhesions, delayed rupture, triggering, bow-stringing). Once identified, management of a tendon laceration depends on the type of tendon injured, the cross-sectional area of tendon involved, and the location of the laceration.

Because of their complex structure (tendon sheaths, pulley system), deep location, and high complication rate after injury (10% to 30%), all suspected flexor tendon lacerations (partial and complete) require consultation and repair by a hand surgeon. In circumstances in which a hand surgeon is not immediately available, the wound can be copiously irrigated and the skin closed primarily without tendon repair. The hand is then immobilized in a volar splint, with the wrist in 20 to 30 degrees of flexion, the MCP joint in 60 to 70 degrees of flexion, and the IP joints in 10 to 15 degrees of flexion; and the patient is referred to a hand surgeon for delayed repair within 7 to 10 days. Broad-spectrum antibiotic coverage (i.e., first-generation cephalosporin) is generally recommended for tendon lacerations.

In contrast to flexor tendons, extensor tendons are anatomically less complex, have a more superficial location, and are associated with fewer complications after repair. As a result, emergency department repair of many simple extensor tendon lacerations has become an accepted practice. Tendon lacerations at or distal to the DIP joint (open mallet finger) and lacerations over the metacarpals, middle phalanges, and proximal phalanges (not involving the PIP joint) are amenable to emergency department repair. Lacerations over the PIP joint may involve the lateral bands or the central slip of the extensor mechanism, which, if not repaired correctly and followed closely, can result in a boutonniere deformity. Therefore, these patients are best referred to a hand surgeon for repair. Partial extensor tendon lacerations involving greater than 10% of the cross-sectional area of the tendon should also be repaired.

Tendon lacerations at the level of the wrist and distal forearm require repair in the operating suite, because proximal extension of the wound is often needed to search for retracted tendons. Multiple tendon lacerations or injuries with underlying fractures will also require operative repair. Moreover, because increased attention is now being given to recovery and rehabilitation after extensor tendon repairs, particularly dynamic splinting and early mobilization, timely hand surgery referral should be arranged for all patients undergoing tendon repair in the emergency department.

Technique of Repair

Wound preparation of a hand injury is similar to that for injuries of other areas of the body (see Chapter 95). However, the entire hand should be sterilely prepped and draped so that the laceration and digits distal to it can be manipulated during exploration. An alternative is to place a sterile surgical glove over the patient's hand and cut away a portion of the glove to expose the wound. This is especially useful in repairing digital lacerations, in which a tourniquet can be created by removing the fingertip of the glove and rolling the remainder of the glove finger proximally. As always, copious irrigation with normal saline is essential. Extension of the wound may be necessary to visualize the tendon laceration or locate the proximal tendon slip. Extending incisions should start from one corner of the wound and generally follow the course of the involved tendon, avoiding obvious veins. Scar contractures are less problematic on the dorsum of the hand than on the palm. Once the involved tendon is identified, a holding stitch can be placed through the proximal tendon for traction during repair. The tendon can then be repaired with 4-0 or 5-0 simple, interrupted sutures or a horizontal mattress suture with the knot "buried" between the ends of the tendon. Nylon or polyglycolic acid, either braided or monofilament, is an acceptable material for tendon repair. More reactive or less long-lasting material (e.g., silk, plain gut, chromic gut) should be avoided. Sutures should be placed 5 to 10 mm from the cut edge of the tendon to avoid the suture tearing through the end of the tendon.

The hand or digit should be splinted in a position with the extensor mechanism relaxed. Tendon repairs at or distal to the DIP joint can be treated with a Stack or mallet finger splint, leaving the PIP joint mobile. Injuries at or proximal to the PIP joint should be splinted with the wrist in 30 degrees of extension, the MCP joint in 10 to 20 degrees of flexion, and the IP joints in slight flexion. Splinting may be required for up to 6 weeks, although some surgeons prefer to allow early protected motion. It is advisable to reevaluate patients for signs of wound infection 36 to 48 hours after tendon repair.

Nerve Injuries

The emergency physician should be proficient in the diagnosis of hand injuries complicated by nerve injury, because outcome is improved with early diagnosis. It is imperative that a careful examination of the hand is performed before the instillation of any local anesthetics; and if suspicion of a peripheral nerve injury exists, anesthetics should be withheld until consultation with the hand surgeon. Nerve repair requires microsurgical techniques and can be performed down to the level of the digital nerve proximal to the DIP flexor crease.[21] Reapproximated peripheral nerves will regenerate at a rate of 1 to 4 mm/d. When nerve injuries occur in fresh, clean, well-perfused tissue, most surgeons prefer immediate repair. However, when necessary, repair can be delayed for 2 weeks to 3 months.[21]

Arterial Injuries

Arterial injuries may complicate either blunt or penetrating trauma and are frequently associated with nerve injuries due to their close proximity to peripheral nerves. However, because the hand has a dual blood supply, ischemia is uncommon with a single artery injury. Wound exploration is important, because even complete arterial lacerations may spasm and stop bleeding by the time the patient is evaluated. Arterial injuries with distal ischemia or associated nerve injury usually require surgical repair. However, isolated injury to the radial or ulnar artery without distal ischemia or sensory impairment is often managed by simple ligation. If a severed digital artery is not repaired, both the proximal and distal ends should be ligated to avoid rebleeding.

DISPOSITION

Patients with simple hand, or extensor tendon, lacerations repaired in the emergency department can be discharged. Reevaluation in 36 to 48 hours for signs of wound infection is advisable for all but minor lacerations. Surgical referral should be made for any complex injury. Discharge instructions should include strict hand elevation, application of ice for the first 24 hours, and splint precautions. Patients should receive written instructions on specific signs or symptoms for which to return to the emergency department.

COMMON PITFALLS

- Failure to suspect a tendon injury because of a small skin wound
- Failure to recognize a partial tendon laceration due to inadequate wound exploration

- Failure to identify a foreign body in a wound as a result of inadequate exploration or omission of a radiograph
- Inadequate splinting or lack of hand surgery referral when indicated
- Inadequate discharge instructions, particularly not explaining the signs of infection or need for immediate return should these signs develop

FINGERTIP LACERATIONS, AVULSIONS, AND AMPUTATIONS

Fingertip injuries are classified according to the extent and level of injury. Simple lacerations and small avulsion injuries are easily managed by the emergency physician. However, injuries that involve significant tissue loss or bony exposure should be referred to a hand surgeon for repair.

CLINICAL PRESENTATION

Patients may present with a minor laceration or a severe injury with significant tissue loss or destruction. There may be considerable discomfort, particularly with crush injuries and amputations. Bleeding is usually not severe unless there is associated injury to a digital artery.

EMERGENCY DEPARTMENT EVALUATION

Evaluation should include a focused history and careful hand examination. Standard radiographs of the injured hand should also be performed.

EMERGENCY DEPARTMENT MANAGEMENT

Crush injuries, amputations, and avulsion injuries in which there is significant soft-tissue or bone loss or bone exposure require evaluation and repair by a hand surgeon. These injuries frequently necessitate split- or full-thickness skin grafts or the use of skin flaps for adequate coverage. Pending consultation, emergency department care includes administration of a parenteral antibiotic (e.g., cefazolin), appropriate analgesia, wound cleansing, and elevation. Avulsion injuries with minimal soft-tissue loss (wound area less than 10 mm^2) and no bone loss or exposure may be allowed to heal by secondary intention, with excellent cosmetic and functional results. This is particularly true in children, who have excellent regenerative capacity. The technique consists of debriding all dead and devitalized tissue, followed by copious irrigation. The digit is then bandaged with a nonadherent dressing (e.g., Xeroform) and gauze and splinted for comfort and protection. The patient or family member is then instructed on how to perform daily dressing changes. Healing will occur in 14 to 21 days, and the patient is often able to return to work within 1 month. Complications include cold intolerance, hypersensitivity in the area of the scar, and a volar curving of the nail at the amputation site.

DISPOSITION

Patients with simple lacerations and minor avulsion injuries may be discharged from the emergency department. A follow-up visit at 48 hours to check for infection is advised. Patients with more significant injuries require surgical consultation.

NAIL BED INJURIES

Subungual Hematoma

A subungual hematoma is a collection of blood under the nail plate. It commonly occurs after a direct blow to the fingertip and may be associated with a nail bed laceration or distal phalanx fracture.

CLINICAL PRESENTATION

Patients frequently complain of severe throbbing pain. A variable amount of blood will be visible beneath the nail plate and appears as a blue or black discoloration. There may also be associated injury to the nail bed and surrounding nail folds.

EMERGENCY DEPARTMENT EVALUATION

Evaluation should include a focused history and careful hand examination. Standard radiographs of the injured digit should also be performed.

EMERGENCY DEPARTMENT MANAGEMENT

One study has shown that all subungual hematomas, regardless of size or the presence of a distal phalanx fracture, may be treated by simple nail trephination as long as the nail plate and surrounding nail folds are intact.[20] The use of a hand-held, portable, high-temperature cautery device is recommended as a safe, effective, and painless method to drain a subungual hematoma. Heated paper clips may introduce carbon particles known as "lampblack" into the nail bed. These particles act as foreign bodies and can delay wound healing. Use of a needle, drill, or scalpel can be very painful and often requires the use of a digital block. Furthermore, the opening produced by these instruments is small and will frequently be occluded by clotted blood. After trephination, the digit should be dressed with absorbent gauze and splinted if a distal phalanx fracture is present. If there is disruption of the nail plate or surrounding nail folds, the nail plate should be removed and proper alignment of the nail bed assured through careful wound repair (see Nail Bed Lacerations).

NAIL BED LACERATIONS

Nail bed lacerations include simple lacerations, stellate lacerations, crush injuries, and avulsions. Failure to properly repair lacerations can result in a split nail deformity, irregular nail surface, or failure of the nail to adhere to the nail bed; these deformities are significant from both a cosmetic and a functional standpoint.

CLINICAL PRESENTATION

Presentation varies from innocuous-appearing injuries to those with severe deformity and tissue loss. There is usually throbbing pain, swelling, and tenderness. The nail plate may be intact, broken, partially avulsed, or completely torn away. Bleeding is usually not significant, but if a digital artery is injured, it can be profuse.

EMERGENCY DEPARTMENT EVALUATION

Evaluation should include a focused history and careful hand examination. Standard radiographs of the injured digit are also indicated.

EMERGENCY DEPARTMENT MANAGEMENT

Management depends on the type and severity of the injury. Crush and avulsion injuries often require a grafting procedure and are best repaired by a hand surgeon. However, management of simple and stellate lacerations may be performed in the emergency department under digital block anesthesia and tourniquet hemostasis using a 1-in. sterile Penrose drain placed securely around the proximal portion of the finger. If present, a broken nail can be removed using a small hemostat or iris scissors by gently opening and closing the instrument beneath the distal free edge of the nail until the nail plate is loose. The distal end of the nail is then grasped with a Kelly clamp and gently removed. The lacerations should be explored carefully for foreign bodies and then irrigated copiously. Debridement of the wound margins should be conservative, because removal of even small amounts of tissue can increase tension on the wound edges, leading to enhanced scar formation. Simple lacerations should be closed with interrupted 6-0 chromic sutures (or other adsorbable suture material) on an atraumatic needle. The use of loop magnification aids in accurate approximation of the wound edges. The sutures should be tied with only three to four knots so that they do not interfere with nail replacement. Stellate lacerations are repaired in a similar manner, keeping in mind that accurate approximation of each arm of a stellate laceration is essential for normal nail growth.

After repair, the involved nail (if available) should be used as a protective covering for the injured nail bed. Replacing the nail has many advantages, including reduced postoperative pain, less adherence of the gauze dressing, the ability to mold the healing nail bed, minimization of formation of granulation tissue or adhesions between the eponychium and the nail bed, and the ability to splint fractures of the distal phalanx. The nail should be inspected for debris or foreign matter and rinsed in normal saline before replacement. No squamous tissue should be removed from the undersurface of the nail, because replacing the nail in its normal position often replaces avulsed tissue as well. This tissue acts as a free graft that reduces nail bed scarring. A hole should be placed in the center of the nail to permit blood drainage. The proximal end of the nail is inserted under the eponychium until the nail is in its normal position on the nail bed. A 5-0 monofilament nylon suture placed through the fingertip and the distal free border of the nail secures the nail plate. The suture is cut in 2 to 3 weeks, allowing growth of the new nail to push out the old one. If the nail is missing or damaged, various materials can be used to cover the injured nail bed and keep the nail fold open. These include an INRO surgical nail splint, metal foil, polyurethane foam sponge, silicone sheeting adaptic, Xeroform, or sterile urine cup trimmed to fit under the nail fold and over the nail bed. An absorbent gauze dressing and application of a splint for comfort and protection are important adjunctive measures.

DISPOSITION

Patients with a subungual hematoma may be discharged from the emergency department. If a fracture was detected on the radiograph, the digit should be immobilized as described previously under distal phalanx fractures. In addition, all patients should be informed about the possibility of nail loss or deformity. Follow-up in 2 to 3 days is recommended for patients with a distal phalanx fracture, to check for infection. Similarly, those with a simple or stellate laceration may be discharged with a wound check arranged in 48 hours. Antibiotics are unnecessary in immunocompetent patients with clean, fresh wounds. For high-risk patients (e.g., immunosuppressed, delayed care, contaminated wound), many practitioners still recommend prophylactic use of an antibiotic, such as cephalexin or dicloxacillin, for 3 days.

References

1. Amadio PC. Scaphoid fractures. *Orthop Clin North Am* 1992;23:7.
2. Barton NJ. Twenty questions about scaphoid fractures. *J Hand Surg [Br]* 1992;17:289.
3. Bowman SH, Simon RR. Metacarpal and phalangeal fractures. *Emerg Med Clin North Am* 1993;11:671.
4. Chin HW, Visotsky J. Ligamentous wrist injuries. *Emerg Med Clin North Am* 1993;11:717.
5. Chin HW, Visotsky J. Wrist fractures. *Emerg Med Clin North Am* 1993;11:703.
6. Clark DP, Scott RN, Anderson IW. Hand problems in an accident and emergency department. *J Hand Surg [Br]* 1985;10:297.
7. Green DP, Rowland SA. Fractures and dislocations in the hand. In: Rockwood CA, Green DP, Bucholz RA, eds. *Rockwood and Green's fractures in adults,* 3rd ed. Philadelphia: JB Lippincott Co, 1991:441.
8. Green DP. Carpal dislocations and instabilities. In: Green DP, ed. *Operative hand surgery,* 3rd ed. New York: Churchill Livingstone, 1993:901.
9. Harris JHJ, Harris WH, Novelline RA. *The radiology of emergency medicine,* 3rd ed. Baltimore: Williams & Wilkins, 1993:435.
10. Jarvik JG, Dalinka MK, Kneeland JB. Hand injuries in adults. *Semin Roentgenol* 1991;26:282.
11. Kahler DM, McCue F. Metacarpophalangeal and proximal interphalangeal joint injuries of the hand, including the thumb. *Clin Sports Med* 1992;11:57.
12. Kirk M, Orlinsky M, Goldberg R, et al. The validity and reliability of the navicular fat stripe as a screening test for detection of navicular fractures. *Ann Emerg Med* 1990;19:1371.
13. Lammers RL. Soft tissue foreign bodies. *Ann Emerg Med* 1988;17:1336.
14. Mehta M, Brautigan MW. Fracture of the carpal navicular: efficacy of clinical findings and improved diagnosis with six-view radiography [see comments]. *Ann Emerg Med* 1990;19:255.
15. Melone CJ, Isani A. Anesthesia for hand injuries. *Emerg Med Clin North Am* 1985;3:235.
16. Omer GJ. Injuries to nerves of the upper extremity. *J Bone Joint Surg Am* 1974;56:1615.
17. Overton DT, Uehara DT. Evaluation of the injured hand. *Emerg Med Clin North Am* 1993;11:585.
18. Phair IC, Quinton DN, Allen MJ. The conservative management of volar avulsion fractures of the P.I.P. joint. *J Hand Surg Br* 1989;14:168.
19. Redmon HA. Acute hand injuries: emergency room management. *J Fla Med Assoc* 1989;76:633.
20. Seaberg DC, Angelos WJ, Paris PM. Treatment of subungual hematomas with nail trephination: a prospective study. *Am J Emerg Med* 1991;9:209.
21. Sloan EP. Nerve injuries in the hand. *Emerg Med Clin North Am* 1993;11:651.
22. Stein A, Lemos M, Stein S. Clinical evaluation of flexor tendon function in the small finger. *Ann Emerg Med* 1990;19:991.
23. Stern PJ. Fractures of the metacarpals and phalanges. In: Green DP, ed. *Operative hand surgery,* 3rd ed. New York: Churchill Livingstone, 1993:695.
24. Street JM. Radiographs of phalangeal fractures: importance of the internally rotated oblique projection for diagnosis. *AJR* 1993;160:575.
25. Waeckerle JF. A prospective study identifying the sensitivity of radiographic findings and the efficacy of clinical findings in carpal navicular fractures. *Ann Emerg Med* 1987;16:733.

Injuries to the Wrist

ANATOMY AND TERMINOLOGY

The ulna is essentially a straight bone, while the radius has outward bowing; these configurations allow the relatively mobile radius to rotate around the relatively fixed ulna during supination and pronation. A fibrous interosseous membrane joins these bones along their entire length. They become proximate only at the ends to form the complex distal and proximal radioulnar joints. Because of this close relationship, injury to one bone usually disrupts the other or causes a dislocation of either the distal or proximal joint (Galeazzi or Monteggia fracture–dislocations) (Figs. 114.7 and 114.8). These bones are under the influence of multiple muscle groups, including the supinators and pronators such as the biceps brachii. Neurologic innervation of the wrist extensors is provided by the radial nerve, which traverses the lateral epicondyle. The radial nerve then gives off the posterior interosseous nerve, which traverses the proximal radius and innervates the muscles that extend the thumb and fingers. The distal portion of the radial nerve is sensory, innervat-

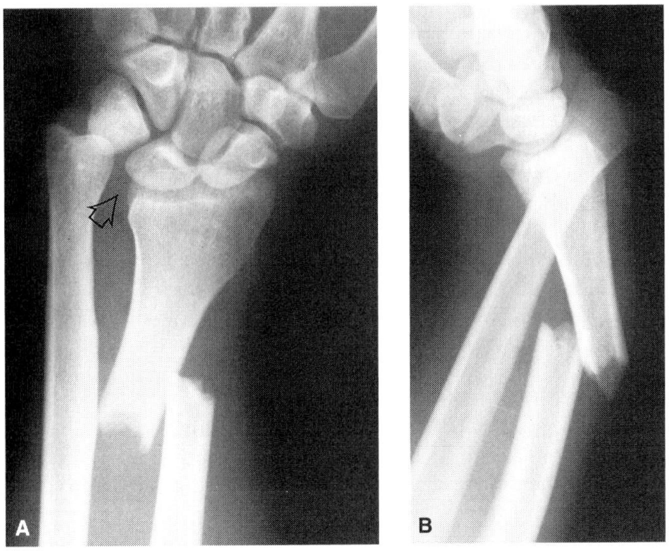

Figure 114.7. Severely displaced Galeazzi fracture–dislocation in frontal **(A)** and lateral **(B)** projections. The distal radioulnar dislocation (*open arrow*) is secondary to the marked shortening of the radius caused by the severe ulnar displacement and dorsal angulation of the distal radial fragment. (From Harris JH Jr, Harris WH. *The radiology of emergency medicine*, 3rd ed. Philadelphia: Lippincott–Raven, 2000:390, with permission.)

ing the posterior radial aspect of the hand. Therefore, injury level in the forearm dictates which functions of the radial nerve will be disturbed. The proximal median nerve controls basic wrist flexion and the wrist flexor nerve. In addition, the previously described hand flexion and palmar hand sensation from the radial aspect of the ring finger to the thumb are provided by the distal median nerve. The ulnar nerve provides innervation to a few forearm muscles.

The wrist is commonly injured, but specific diagnosis may be subtle. It is mandatory to understand the mechanics of the injury, the functional anatomy of the wrist unit, and utilize proper clinical assessment so as to appropriately recognize and manage important injuries. The wrist includes the area from the carpometacarpal joints to the distal radius and ulna. This is a complex structure, with multiple articulations among the distal radius and ulna and the eight carpal bones.

The distal radius is the only forearm bone that directly articulates with the carpal bones, specifically the lunate and scaphoid. This distal radius has three articular surfaces: the distal radioulnar; the radiocarpal, which is tilted in two planes; and the triangular fibrocartilage, which is the main stabilizing unit of the distal radioulnar joint. The distal radioulnar joint is also stabilized by volar and dorsal radioulnar ligaments, which merge with the triangular fibrocartilage. The distal radius has a concave notch on its ulnar aspect, which articulates with the curved surface of the ulnar head, allowing wrist rotation. The triangular fibrocartilage complex separates the ulna from the carpal bones and supports the triquetrum and lunate on the distal ulna. The proximal carpal row functions as an intercalated segment, or mobile link, between the distal row and the radius, making it potentially unstable.

The scaphoid serves as the stabilizing link between the distal and proximal carpal rows, placing it at greater risk for injury. The carpal bones are stabilized to the bones of the forearm by the two volar arcades and one dorsal arcade of extrinsic ligaments. The apex of one volar arch inserts on the lunate and supports the proximal carpal row, while the other arch attaches to the capitate of the distal carpal row. The space of Poirier, an inherently weak spot, lies at the junction of the capitate and lunate between these two palmar arches and widens with wrist dorsiflexion. Because of the mobile nature of the proximal carpal row, the intrinsic ligaments of this row—the triquetrolunate and scapholunate—are particularly prone to injury. Forearm muscles that insert on the base of the metacarpals produce wrist movement. Except for the pisiform, a sesamoid of the flexor carpi ulnaris, there are no direct tendon insertions on the carpal bones. These bones move passively as a function of hand position. Wrist motion is equivalently produced by midcarpal and radiocarpal joint movement.

CLINICAL PRESENTATION

Injuries most often occur to the wrist because of falls on the outstretched hand (FOOSH). If the thenar eminence is impacted, the scaphoid and its supporting ligaments are more commonly injured, while hypothenar impact most commonly injures the pisiform or triquetrum and supporting ligaments. The age of the individual affects the maturity of the bones in the wrist and therefore directly influences the type of injury seen. Carpal injuries are rare in children. Injuries in the pediatric patient often involve the immature, relatively weak metaphysis of the radius or epiphyseal plate. The carpus in children is primarily cartilage. Young adults are more likely to injure the wrist with significantly greater force, and fracture either the distal radial metaphysis or the carpi. In the elderly, the distal radial metaphysis is injured most commonly because of its increased osteoporosis.

Injuries may be localized by careful inspection and palpation of the anatomic landmarks of the wrist for tenderness. The most

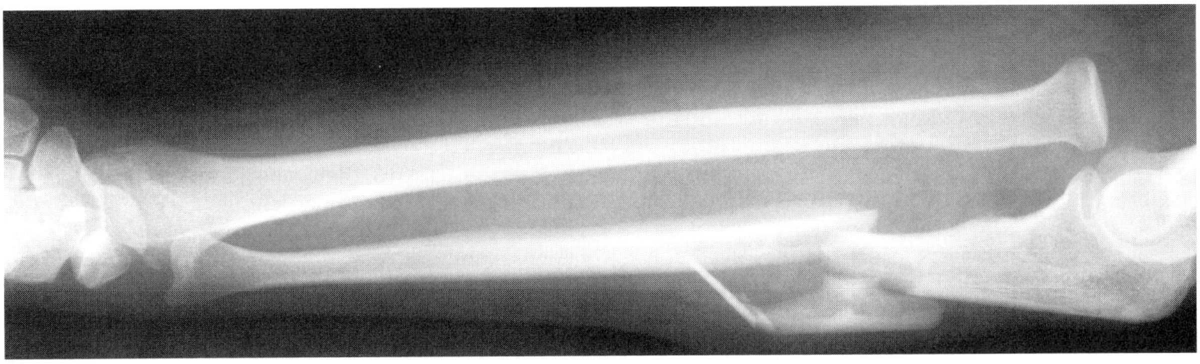

Figure 114.8. In this variation of the Bado I Monteggia injury, the fracture site is comminuted and the volar angulation less than usual. The volar dislocation of the radial head and the ulnar fracture make this a Bado I fracture–dislocation. (From Harris JH Jr, Harris WH. *The radiology of emergency medicine*, 3rd ed. Philadelphia: Lippincott–Raven, 2000:365, with permission.)

clearly visible landmark on the volar wrist is the crease that marks the proximal carpal row. At the base of the thenar eminence lies the scaphotrapezial joint. The most important landmark on the dorsal surface is the anatomic snuffbox, with the radius styloid at the proximal base and the scaphoid at the apex of the triangle.

A palpable indentation in the middle of the wrist, immediately ulnar to the scapholunate joint, overlies the capitate and the lunate. With flexion of the wrist, the lunate is palpable at this location. Just distal to it lies the triangular fibrocartilage and the triquetrum.

Standard radiologic evaluation of the wrist includes a posteroanterior (PA) view, a lateral view, and oblique views. Additional special views may be required to identify more specific carpal injuries. Key positioning of the hand is integral to these examinations. On the PA view, three smooth arcs should outline the articular surfaces at the midcarpal and radiocarpal joints. Any disruption of these lines suggests a possible subluxation, dislocation, or fracture. The ulna and adjacent radius should appear of equal length, and the distal radius should articulate with at least one-half of the lunate at the distal radioulnar joint. With injury to the triangular fibrocartilage, the ulna may translocate and will not appear to contact the radius to the usual degree. On this same view, the radial styloid should project 8 to 18 mm beyond the distal radioulnar joint and create a 15- to 25-degree ulnar inclination of the distal radius. Distal radius fractures will alter these. The lateral view provides important information regarding the alignment of the carpi and the degree of fracture angulation present. The "three C's"—the capitate, lunate, and radius—should be colinear on this view. Actual measurement of the scapholunate and capitolunate angles will provide a more accurate view of carpal alignment. The scaphoid axis should form an angle that is between 30 degrees and 60 degrees with the lunate on this view, because of its normal palmar flexion on lateral view. Oblique views are performed in either supination or partial pronation. They project the pisiform or scaphotrapezium joint away from the adjacent overlapping carpal bones.

FRACTURES

Fractures of the carpal bones are discussed in the Hand Injuries section of this chapter.

ULNAR FRACTURES

Isolated ulnar fractures result most often from direct blows to the forearm, most commonly to ward off an assailant's blow (nightstick fracture). Undisplaced fractures are immobilized in a long-arm cast or splint, depending on the amount of initial swelling, and closely monitored for displacement or further significant swelling. Displaced fractures, those with greater than 10 degrees' angulation or with greater than 50% displacement of the width of the bone, usually require open reduction and internal fixation with a compression plate and screw to prevent length loss, angulation, or rotation. Again, these injuries should be examined carefully for evidence of associated radial dislocation or fracture.

Ulnar styloid fractures may be produced by forced radial dorsiflexion, radial deviation, and rotary stress. These styloid fractures may occur solely or accompany other fractures, such as the Colles fracture. Displace ulnar styloid fractures may be accompanied by important injury to the triangular fibrocartilage. Often, individuals with this accompanying injury will complain of a painful locking sensation or clicking sensations in the wrist. Delineation of accompanying triangular cartilage injury may require wrist arthrography or magnetic resonance imaging. Ulnar styloid fractures are treated with casting or splinting in the neutral position of the wrist and slight ulnar deviation.

Fracture of the ulnar shaft with associated radial head dislocation is referred to as the Monteggia fracture–dislocation (see Fig. 114.8). This is usually a diaphyseal fracture in the proximal one-third of the ulna, with an associated anterior dislocation of the radial head. Occasionally, posterolateral or anterolateral radial head dislocation or a metaphyseal ulnar fracture may be seen. Clinically, the forearm may appear angulated and shortened. The ulnar fracture is clearly noted. Although less obvious than the ulnar findings, there is usually pain and swelling at the elbow, and the radial head may be palpated in the posterior or anterior location. On plain radiography, the apex of the ulnar fracture points toward the radial head dislocation, and the radial head may not point toward the capitellum on all views. In adults, these are treated with open reduction internal fixation (ORIF) of the ulna and closed reduction of the radial head dislocation. In children, adequate reduction may be achieved by closed reduction of both bones and long-arm casting. Complications of this fracture–dislocation include redislocation, infection, paralysis of the posterior interosseous nerve, and nonunion.

DISTAL RADIUS FRACTURES

Fractures of the distal one-third of the radial shaft are produced by either a direct blow or FOOSH in forced pronation. A force directed along the radial side of the hand can produce an oblique or transverse fracture of the radial styloid. This is most easily seen on an anteroposterior (AP) radiograph as a thin, lucent line proximal to the radial styloid. Displacement of this fracture can produce carpal instability because of the major carpal ligaments of the radial side of the wrist on this styloid. A displaced fracture may often require ORIF. Accompanying scapholunate dislocation should be sought. Posttraumatic arthritis may be worsened if the examiner fails to recognize associated intercarpal ligament tears.

FOOSH most often produces a dorsally angulated and displaced distal radial metaphyseal fracture called a Colles fracture (Fig. 114.9). Due to compression forces on the dorsal surface, dorsal bone comminution is often seen. The fracture line may also extend into the radiocarpal or radioulnar joint and comminute. A fracture of the radial styloid is often seen, which may suggest associated injury to the triangular fibrocartilage. On clinical examination, the wrist will appear in the classic "silver fork" or dorsiflexion deformity. Associated pressure on the median nerve may produce palmar paresthesias. On an AP radiograph, the dorsum may appear shortened, due to the angulation or comminution of the bone.

Stable fractures may be either reduced by the orthopedic surgeon, utilizing traction via finger traps and pushing the distal and palmar fracture fragment against the firmly held forearm, or treated with a splint and compression dressing until they can be evaluated by the consulting orthopedic surgeon. Particularly in younger patients, the goal is to restore normal radial inclination, volar tilt, and proper length to the radius. Unstable fractures, recognized radiologically by angulation greater than 20 degrees, intraarticular involvement, more than a centimeter of shortening, or marked comminution, often require ORIF or casting with external fixation, pinning, and possible bone grafting. In addition, any neurovascular compromise or an open fracture requires immediate hand surgery, plastic surgery, or orthopedic consultation. Complications of Colles fractures include median nerve injuries, radioulnar and radiocarpal instability, triangular cartilage injury, arthritis, and malunion.

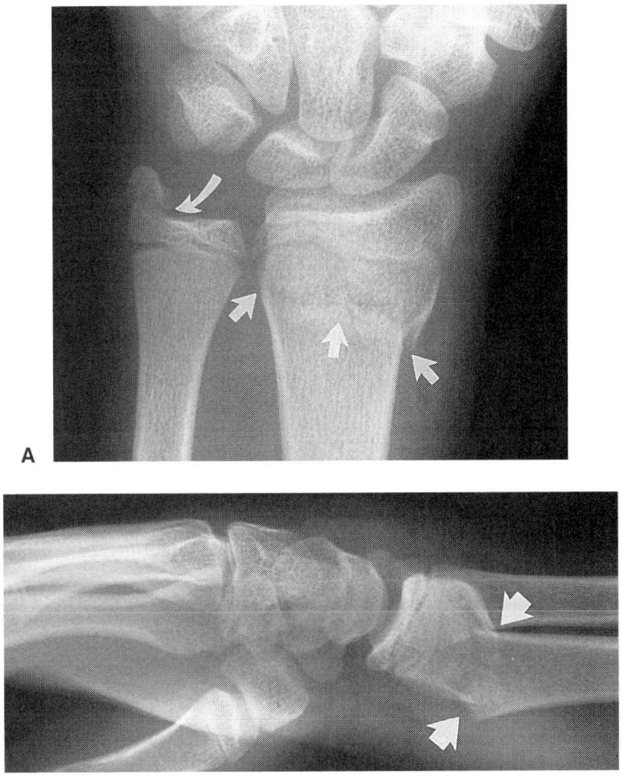

Figure 114.9. Extraarticular (Colles) distal radial fracture (*arrow*) in frontal **(A)** and lateral **(B)** projections associated with a fracture of the base of the ulnar styloid (*curved arrow,* **A**). (From Harris JH Jr, Harris WH. *The radiology of emergency medicine*, 3rd ed. Philadelphia: Lippincott–Raven, 2000:386, with permission.)

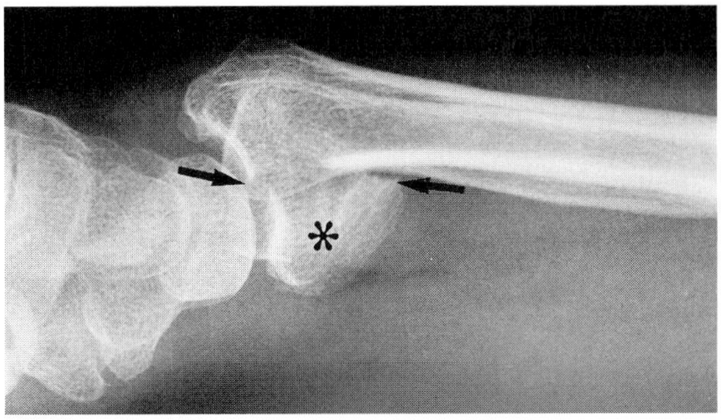

Figure 114.11. Classic volar Barton fracture. The oblique intraarticular fracture (*arrows*) involves the volar aspect of the distal radius. The separate fragment (*asterisk*) and the bones of the wrist and hand are volarly and proximally displaced. (From Harris JH Jr, Harris WH. *The radiology of emergency medicine*, 3rd ed. Philadelphia: Lippincott–Raven, 2000:388, with permission.)

A reverse Colles fracture or Smith fracture (Fig. 114.10) is a volarly angulated fracture of the distal radius. This injury is produced by a blow to or fall onto the dorsum of the hand and wrist or a FOOSH in supination. The hand is palmarly displaced in the so-called garden spade deformity. AP radiographs appear similar to those seen with a Colles fracture, with a distal metaphyseal fracture that may be either comminuted or shortened. On a lateral radiograph, the fracture is volarly angulated and displaced. The complications and treatment are similar to those for a Colles fracture, but the angulation is in the opposite direction.

A Barton fracture (Fig. 114.11) is a volar or dorsal rim fracture of the distal radius. The more common dorsal rim fracture results from forced pronation and dorsiflexion of the wrist, while the less common volar rim fracture results from a fall on the supinated outstretched hand. Often, initially subtle subluxations or fracture–dislocations are seen, because the hand is frequently displaced in the direction of the fracture and associated ligamentous injuries produce radiocarpal instability. On AP radiography, a comminuted fracture of the distal radial metaphysis is often seen. On a lateral view, an intraarticular fracture of the dorsal or volar rim of the radius is seen, often with accompanying carpal subluxation in the same direction. Fractures with minimal displacement can be treated with closed reduction and a splint or cast until they are reevaluated with the consulting orthopedist. Unstable fractures, which involve more than 50% of the radioarticular surface or have associated carpal subluxation, require reduction and immobilization by the consulting hand specialist, orthopedist, or plastic surgeon, as they frequently require open reduction and fixation.

A distal radial shaft fracture is often complicated by a distal radioulnar joint dislocation (Galeazzi or reverse Monteggia fracture). The radius fracture is usually short oblique or transverse with dorsolateral angulation. Localized tenderness is seen over the wrist and distal radius. AP-view plain films may exhibit only a slight increase in the distal radioulnar joint space. The lateral view will exhibit dorsal displacement of the ulna. This injury is managed by the consultant with ORIF, with compression plating and screws of the radius fracture. Reduction of the distal radioulnar joint is maintained with either immobilization of the forearm in supination or K-wire fixation for 6 weeks.

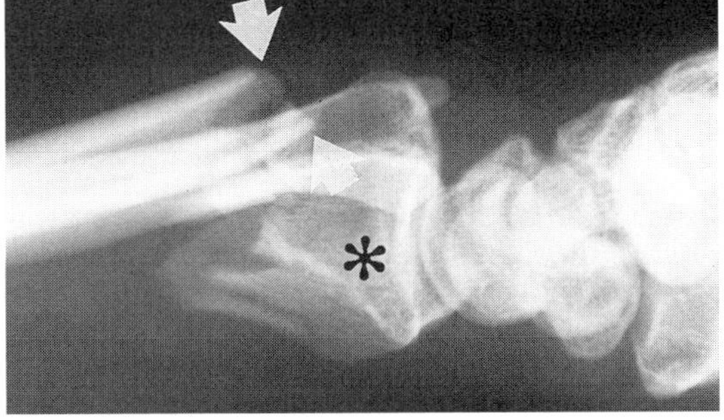

Figure 114.10. Smith fracture characterized by a transverse fracture (*arrows*) of the distal radius, with volar and proximal displacement of the distal radial fragment (*asterisk*). (From Harris JH Jr, Harris WH. *The radiology of emergency medicine*, 3rd ed. Philadelphia: Lippincott–Raven, 2000:386, with permission.)

LIGAMENTOUS INJURY

Radioulnar disruption is usually seen with fractures of both bones of the forearm, or intraarticular or distal radial shaft fractures. Isolated injury is uncommon and may go unrecognized in 50% of cases. Unfortunately, these often more obvious injuries may cause the examiner to miss associated radioulnar joint disruption, with the injury discovered later because of pain and decreased wrist movement. Volar dislocation, which is rare, is produced by forced hypersupination of the wrist. The more commonly seen dorsal dislocation is usually produced by falls on the wrist in hyperpronation. The presentation is one of wrist pain and restricted range of motion, with an occasional palpable prominence of the head of the ulna. Appropriately positioned lateral radiography shows either dorsal or volar displacement of the ulna. AP radiography demonstrates overlap and narrowing of the distal radioulnar joint. Computed tomography scanning may be required to establish the diagnosis. The wrist should be immobilized in supination to reduce dorsal dislocation, while pronation will reduce volar dislocation. These injuries require consultation with a hand or orthopedic surgeon or a plastic surgeon because they have a high recurrence rate and may require reconstructive surgery.

COMMON PITFALLS

- Failure to appropriately position the wrist and hand for radiography
- Failure to recognize associated ligamentous or triangular cartilage injury with fracture
- Failure to recognize the complex of Galeazzi or Monteggia fractures
- Failure to appropriately and expeditiously consult the hand surgeon, orthopedist, or plastic surgeon.

The reader is referred to any of the commonly used orthopedic texts for a more specific discussion of the anatomy, evaluation, and management of each of the aforementioned injuries.

Bibliography

Bradway JK, Amadio PC, Cooney WP. Open reduction and internal fixation of displaced, comminuted intraarticular fractures of the distal end of the radius. *J Bone Joint Surg Am* 1989;71A:839.

Breckenbraugh RD. Accurate evaluation and management of the painful wrist following injury. *Orthop Clin North Am* 1984;15:289.

Cooney WP, Bussey R, Dobyns JH. Difficult wrist fractures. *Clin Orthop* 1987;214:136.

Johnson R. The acutely injured wrist and its residuals. *Clin Orthop* 1980;149:55.

Linscheid RL. Kinematic considerations of the wrist. *Clin Orthop* 1986;202:27.

Malone CP. Open treatment for displaced articular fractures of the distal radius. *Clin Orthop* 1986;202:104.

Propp DA, Chin HW. Forearm and wrist radiology. *J Emerg Med* 1989;7:393.

CHAPTER 115
Back Pain and Injury

Robert S. Hockberger and Martin O'Bryan

Low back pain (LBP) is one of the most common and expensive medical disorders. Almost 80% of adults experience at least one incapacitating episode of LBP during their lifetime. LBP is the most common cause of restricted activity in people younger than 45 years of age and the third most common cause of disability in people older than 45 years, following heart disease and arthritis. The cost of diagnosis, treatment, disability, worker's compensation, and litigation approaches $50 billion annually, making LBP the third most expensive medical problem in the United States after heart disease and cancer.[9]

Many patients with LBP present to the emergency department for evaluation. An emergency physician should identify those patients with LBP who harbor underlying organic disease, determine the presence of intervertebral disc herniation, suspect when patients may be malingering, know when to obtain appropriate diagnostic tests, recognize the indications for emergent orthopedic or neurosurgical consultation, initiate appropriate treatment for nonemergent patients, and maximize patient satisfaction.

CLINICAL PRESENTATION

Low back strain, the most common cause of LBP, results from injury to the ligaments and muscles of the lower back. Pain and stiffness secondary to inflammation and subsequent muscle spasm begin minutes to hours after the initiating event but may not reach peak intensity until several hours or several days later. Occasionally, patients with nonmusculoskeletal disease, structural skeletal disorders, and skeletal malignancies; infections; or inflammatory disorders may present in a similar fashion.

Approximately 75% of patients with low back strain recover without residual symptoms within 1 to 4 weeks. Patients with symptoms persisting for more than 4 to 6 weeks should be evaluated for underlying organic disease and for psychosocial problems that might be inhibiting recovery.[1] Approximately 7% of patients have symptoms that persist longer than 6 months. At this point, the term *chronic LBP* is employed; patients with this designation rarely become asymptomatic, often experience recurrences, and rarely return to a normal lifestyle. The pathophysiology or psychopathology underlying chronic LBP is not well understood.

DIFFERENTIAL DIAGNOSIS

Nonmusculoskeletal Disorders

Disorders that can present as LBP include pleural effusions, pancreatic disease, perforated peptic ulcer, retrocecal appendicitis, large-bowel obstruction, renal disease, pelvic disease, prostatic disorders, retroperitoneal bleeding, and abdominal aortic aneurysm.[9] History and physical examination exclude these disorders in most instances.

Malignancy

Malignancy that is either primary or metastatic to the vertebral column should be suspected in patients with known malignancy (particularly breast, lung, and prostate cancers) and in patients older than 50 years of age who have LBP associated with unexplained weight loss, pain lasting longer than 1 month, or failure of symptoms to improve with conservative therapy. High-risk patients should be evaluated with spinal radiographs and an erythrocyte sedimentation rate (ESR).[7]

Spinal Infections

Spinal infections, including osteomyelitis, disc space infection, and epidural abscess, are usually blood-borne from other sites, particularly the skin and urinary tract. Patients at highest risk include children, immunosuppressed patients, and intravenous drug users. Only 50% to 80% of patients with spinal infections have a fever at the time of presentation but almost all have significant pain and local spinal tenderness at the infection site. High-risk patients should be evaluated with spinal radiographs and an ESR.[3]

Ankylosing Spondylitis

Ankylosing spondylitis should be suspected in patients younger than 40 years of age who complain of the slow onset of LBP persisting longer than 3 months, with a daily pattern of morning stiffness followed by improvement with exercise. Patients at risk should be evaluated with an ESR and a pelvic radiograph to evaluate the sacroiliac joint.[2]

Fractures

Fractures of the thoracolumbar region of the vertebral column can be broadly classified as either minor or major injuries. Minor injuries (isolated fractures of the spinous process, transverse processes, or articular processes) are uncommon, usually result from direct blows, and have little clinical significance except for patient discomfort. Major injuries (fractures of the vertebral body or posterior elements) usually result from motor vehicle accidents or falls from heights, are easily overlooked due to their occurrence in the setting of major multisystem trauma, and may result in permanent neurologic dysfunction, particularly when the bony injury is unstable. Pathologic fractures, even in the absence of a history of trauma, may be seen in cancer patients with bony spinal metastases, patients receiving chronic corticosteroid treatment, and patients who are chronically bedridden or are older than 70 years of age.

Spinal Stenosis

Spinal stenosis is the progressive narrowing of the distal spinal canal or vertebral foramina, sometimes associated with nerve compression, that can occur in elderly patients. Patients present with slowly progressive symptoms, usually over several years, characterized by pain in the lower back and legs after walking (termed *neurogenic claudication*). There may be neurologic deficits in the lower extremities, particularly after the onset of symptoms following a period of walking. Neurologic and vascular examination of the lower extremities usually differentiates neurogenic claudication from arterial ischemic claudication.[5]

Intervertebral Disc Herniation

Disc herniation occurs in 20% to 30% of adults, but most disc herniations cause minimal or no symptoms. Clinically significant disc herniation should be suspected in patients with LBP that radiates to a lower extremity (termed *sciatica*). Patients with sciatica may have pain that is referred down a leg as the result of inflammation of the sciatic nerve or that radiates down a leg as the result of nerve root impingement (usually from a herniated lumbar disc or narrowing of a vertebral foramina from spinal stenosis). Referred pain is usually dull and poorly localized, does not radiate distal to the knee, and is not associated with a positive straight-leg-raising (SLR) test or neurologic impairment of the lower extremities. Alternatively, nerve root impingement results in sharp, well-localized radicular pain that frequently (but not always) radiates distal to the knee, is invariably associated with a positive SLR test, and may be associated with neurologic impairment.[12,13]

Cauda Equina Syndrome

The cauda equina syndrome is usually caused by a massive midline disc herniation impinging on multiple nerve roots within the distal spinal cord. It is characterized by severe LBP that develops acutely or over days to weeks in association with unilateral or bilateral sciatica, evidence of bowel or bladder dysfunction, a positive SLR test, and neurologic deficits. The most common sensory deficit involves the buttocks and perineal region (termed *saddle anesthesia*); the most common motor deficits are diminished rectal sphincter tone and urinary retention.

Malingering

Malingering is occasionally seen in patients presenting with LBP who are seeking drugs, worker's compensation, litigation, increased attention from loved ones, or other sources of secondary gain. Malignancy should be suspected in the presence of nonorganic signs and symptoms, as discussed in the following section. However, nonorganic signs are also seen in patients with psychiatric disorders, chronic pain syndromes, and occasionally in individuals with underlying organic disease.[13] As a result, the diagnosis of malingering should rarely, if ever, be made in the emergency department.

EMERGENCY DEPARTMENT EVALUATION

Patient history should be directed at raising or lowering suspicion for disorders other than simple low back strain. In addition, the medical record should note whether an injury was work-related, the nature and duration of symptoms (particularly muscle weakness and bowel or bladder dysfunction), and the patient's impression of the severity of symptoms.

Physical examination should include a general description of the patient's degree of distress and limitation of movement. Chest and abdominal examinations should be performed routinely. Depending on the history, rectal and pelvic examinations may be indicated. Musculoskeletal examination should note areas of maximal tenderness and the presence or absence of muscle spasm. In the setting of major multisystem trauma, the signs and symptoms of spinal injury may be subtle or nonexistent due to alterations in mental status or the presence of other painful, distracting injuries.

Neurologic examination should document neurologic deficits (Table 115.1) and the results of SLR tests. The SLR test is performed by placing the patient supine and slowly elevating the involved leg until the patient experiences pain. A positive test occurs when the patient complains of a sharp pain that radiates down the involved leg, indicating nerve root impingement. However, only 60% to 80% of patients with a positive SLR test are ultimately found to have a disc herniation. The crossed-SLR test is performed by slowly elevating the opposite (asymptomatic) leg, until the patient experiences pain. A positive test occurs when the patient complains of a sharp pain that radiates down the contralateral (symptomatic) leg. The crossed-SLR test is less sensitive than the SLR test, but it is highly specific for nerve root impingement.[9]

Nonorganic signs, which may connote malingering or a psychogenic component to a patient's symptoms, include the following: pain that does not follow an organic pattern, endorsement of false symptom suggestions, cogwheel weakness, sensory deficits with a stocking-glove distribution, weakness to manual tests not seen in other activities, disablement disproportionate to objective findings, and overreaction during the examination. However, as previously noted, the presence of nonorganic signs does not necessarily exclude the existence of true underlying disease and discomfort.

Ancillary tests used to assess patients with LBP include lum-

TABLE 115.1. Pain Distribution and Neurologic Abnormalities Seen with Common Lumbar Disc Herniations

Disk	L4	L5	S1
Pain	Front of leg	Side of leg	Back of leg
Weakness	Extension of leg at knee	Dorsiflexion of foot	Plantar flexion of foot
Sensory loss	Knee	Lateral lower leg and web space of great toe	Back of calf and lateral foot
Reflex loss	Knee jerk	None	Ankle jerk

bar spinal radiographs, ESR, and computerized tomography (CT) or magnetic resonance imaging (MRI). Spinal radiographs are indicated in cases of significant trauma, when neurologic deficits are present, or when a spinal malignancy or infection is clinically suspected.[1,8] An ESR should be obtained when a malignancy, infection, or inflammatory disorder is suspected. CT or MRI is indicated in the acute setting for the following indications: suspected cauda equina syndrome; suspected disc herniation, causing significant and progressive motor weakness; and suspicion for the presence of either a spinal epidural abscess or metastasis causing any neurologic deficit.[3] A CT scan is also indicated in victims of major trauma when routine spinal radiographs identify a major injury, to both fully evaluate the extent of injury (particularly the posterior elements) and assess the integrity of the neural canal.

EMERGENCY DEPARTMENT MANAGEMENT

Most patients with symptoms severe enough to bring them to the emergency department benefit from parenteral treatment with either an opioid analgesic or a nonsteroidal antiinflammatory drug (NSAID). Pain relief appropriate for a patient's degree of discomfort should be provided as soon as possible. Early symptom management facilitates accurate patient assessment and improves patient satisfaction with care. Patient satisfaction is further optimized when physicians perform more than a superficial examination (the "laying on of hands" effect) and when they spend time with patients, explaining the cause of symptoms and their treatment recommendations. When this is done, unnecessary spinal radiographs do little to improve overall patient satisfaction.

DISPOSITION

Emergent surgical intervention may be indicated for patients with severe cauda equina syndrome, disc herniation associated with severe and progressive motor weakness, and spinal epidural abscess in the presence of any neurologic impairment. Patients with suspicion for these disorders should receive an emergent CT or MRI scan in addition to immediate orthopedic or neurosurgical consultation. Emergent treatment with parenteral steroids and radiation therapy is indicated for patients with spinal epidural metastasis causing acute neurologic impairment. The decision to hospitalize patients other than those just described depends on multiple factors, including a patient's degree of distress and disability, the presence and extent of neurologic deficits, the patient's home environment, and the local practice of orthopedic and neurosurgical consultants.

Outpatient treatment of low back strain should include analgesics, bed rest, and follow-up evaluation. All patients with symptoms severe enough to bring them to the emergency department should receive a prescription for an analgesic appropriate for their degree of distress. NSAIDs should be prescribed for patients with mild-to-moderate distress, whereas opioid analgesics may be a necessary adjunct for patients with moderate-to-severe symptoms.[10] Opioid analgesics should not be required after the first 2 to 3 days. Muscle relaxants, when used in combination with analgesics, cause increased analgesia, increased drowsiness, and increased cost. Their major benefit may come from improved patient compliance with instructions for bed rest due to sedation. Bed rest, in the supine position on a flat and firm surface, may be of benefit to some patients, but should not be prescribed for more than 2 to 3 days.[17] Follow-up with the patient's physician of choice, particularly for work-related low back strain, is important to identify patients with persistent or worsening symptoms. Early, aggressive rehabilitation may prevent such patients from developing chronic LBP.

The outpatient management of patients with suspected lumbar disc herniation, particularly if associated with a neurologic deficit, should consist of NSAIDs and opioid analgesics, 7 to 10 days of bed rest, and follow-up with an orthopedic surgeon or neurosurgeon. Fortunately, conservative management is effective in most instances, and only 2% to 5% of patients eventually require surgical treatment.[11]

Patients with thoracolumbar fractures are almost invariably hospitalized for further evaluation and treatment. Patients with minor fractures resulting from direct blows may be treated as outpatients when there are no other associated injuries, when there is no suspicion of involvement of the posterior elements (this frequently requires CT scan), and when patient distress does not require treatment with parenteral narcotics.

Numerous studies have touted the benefits of heat or cold application, steroids or other medications, traction, corsets or braces, flexion or extension exercises, acupuncture, and the use of transcutaneous nerve stimulation for the treatment of LBP. None are of proven benefit.[11] Both spinal manipulation and back schools appear to benefit patients with symptoms that persist for 1 to 6 weeks, but their effectiveness appears to diminish thereafter.[4]

COMMON PITFALLS

- Failure to perform an abdominal examination. Numerous abdominal disorders, including abdominal aortic aneurysm, can present with LBP.
- Failure to recognize the potential for underlying pathology in high-risk patients (children, elderly patients, immunosuppressed patients, and intravenous drug users) who present with apparent low back strain.[6] Normal spinal radiographs and ESR exclude underlying disease in most instances.
- Failure to diagnose thoracolumbar fractures in the setting of major multisystem trauma. Examination of the back may be deferred while more immediately life-threatening injuries are addressed. In addition, the signs and symptoms of spinal injury may be subtle or nonexistent due to an alteration in mental status or other painful injuries that distract the patient. A complete examination of the spine should be performed in trauma patients once they are hemodynamically stable. Spinal radiographs should be obtained in patients who cannot be assessed clinically when the mechanism of injury suggests the possibility of a spinal injury.
- Failure to practice cost-effective medicine. Studies have repeatedly shown that 40% to 80% of spinal radiographs performed to evaluate LBP are unnecessary.[8]
- Failure to practice the "art" of medicine. Patient satisfaction is determined by a physician's attitude and willingness to examine and talk to patients, not by the number of radiographs and other tests that are performed.

References

1. Bigos SJ, Bowyer OR, Braen GR, et al. Acute low-back pain problems in adults. Clinical practice guidelines no. 14. Rockville, MD: Agency for Health Care Policy and Research Publication No. 95-0642, December 1994.
2. Blackburn WD, Alarcon GS, Ball GV. Evaluation of patients with back pain of suspected inflammatory nature. *Am J Med* 1988;85:766.
3. Byrne TN. Spinal cord compression from epidural metastases. *N Engl J Med* 1992;327(9):614.
4. Cherkin DC, Deyo RA, Battie M, et al. A comparison of physical therapy, chiropractic manipulation, and provision of an educational booklet for the treatment of patients with low back pain. *N Engl J Med* 1998;339:1021.
5. Ciricillo SF, Weinstein PR. Lumbar spinal stenosis. *West J Med* 1993;158:171.
6. Combs JA, Caskey PM. Back pain in children and adolescents: a retrospective review of 648 patients. *South Med J* 1997;90(8):789.
7. Deyo RA. Cancer as a cause of back pain: frequency, clinical presentation and diagnostic strategies. *J Gen Intern Med* 1988;3(3):230.

8. Deyo RA. Diagnostic imaging procedures for the lumbar spine. *Ann Intern Med* 1989;111(11):865.
9. Deyo RA, Rainville J, Kent DL. What can the history and physical examination tell us about low back pain? *JAMA* 1992;268(6):760.
10. Deyo RA. Drug therapy for back pain: which drugs help which patients? *Spine* 1996;21:2840.
11. Deyo RA. Nonoperative treatment of low back disorders: differentiating useful from useless therapy. In: Frymoyer JW, ed. *The adult spine: principles and practice,* 2nd ed., Vol 2. New York: Raven Press, 1997:1777.
12. Frymoyer JW. Back pain and sciatica. *N Engl J Med* 1988;318(5):291.
13. Frymoyer JW. Radiculopathies: Lumbar disc herniation. In: Frymoyer JW, ed. *The adult spine: principles and practice,* 2nd ed., Vol 2. New York: Raven Press, 1997:1937.

CHAPTER 116
Pelvic Fractures

Paula S. Wadbrook and Charles V. Pollack, Jr.

Pelvic fractures are among the most common significant injuries of motor vehicle accident victims. Because of the pelvis's bony and ligamentous stability, a force that results in a fracture should alert the emergency physician to the possibility of adjacent as well as anatomically distant injuries. Although the mortality of blunt multiple trauma with pelvic fracture reaches 20%, in some reports, up to 80% of pelvic fractures are relatively minor injuries from which patients typically recover without sequelae.[6] The widely varying figures for morbidity and mortality associated with pelvic trauma reflect the use of multiple classification schemes. (Some classifications include these minor injuries, while others do not.) Regardless of variability, the emergency physician should remain cognizant of the fact that for any patient who presents with a pelvic fracture and who is hypotensive, the mortality is 40% to 50%.[1]

Vehicular and automobile-versus-pedestrian accidents account for 60% of pelvic fractures; falls from a height are responsible for another 30%.[9] The last 10% is largely composed of two disparate groups: elderly osteoporotic women who fall from a sitting or standing position, and young, otherwise healthy athletes who sustain avulsion fractures of the ischium and iliac wings. Although the mechanism of injury may help predict optimal overall emergency management of each patient, the bony pelvis and its contents may be evaluated in a systematic fashion. After reviewing the anatomic and radiographic considerations of pelvic trauma, we will outline such a management scheme. Related injuries will be considered, but a detailed discussion of trauma to the pelvic contents is found in other chapters.

CLINICAL PRESENTATION

The bony pelvis supports the trunk and lower extremities and protects the lower abdominal viscera. As such, it absorbs much of the impact transmitted to the long or transverse axis of the body; injuring forces directed toward the pelvic bones are, in turn, often transmitted to the contents of the pelvis. The pelvis is a ring of two identical innominate bones (each consists of the fused ilium, ischium, and pubis) joined to the sacrum posteriorly by the sacroiliac complex ligaments and to each other anteriorly at the symphysis pubis (Fig. 116.1).

Because the bony pelvis derives its strength from its ringlike structure, pelvic fractures are best differentiated according to the extent of ring disruption: stable or unstable fractures—one or two or more disruptions, respectively. Because this distinction is generally apparent clinically and radiographically, it provides a useful reference point for the emergency physician. Also, because specific mechanisms of injury are predictably associated with stable or unstable fractures, it provides the most practical scheme for evaluating, categorizing, and managing pelvic trauma. This system is presented in Table 116.1 and will be followed for discussion purposes.

Avulsion fractures are among the most trivial of pelvic fractures and are often sustained by athletes who stress muscular or ligamentous insertions onto the bony pelvis (Fig. 116.2). Avulsions of the anterior superior iliac spine generally occur in adolescent hurdlers and long jumpers and reflect forceful contraction of the sartorius muscle or abdominal musculature transmitted to the iliac epiphysis.[11] Less commonly, the anterior inferior iliac spine may be avulsed by intense contraction of the straight head of the rectus femoris muscle; this injury may occur in athletes playing sports that involve kicking (e.g., soccer and rugby).[6]

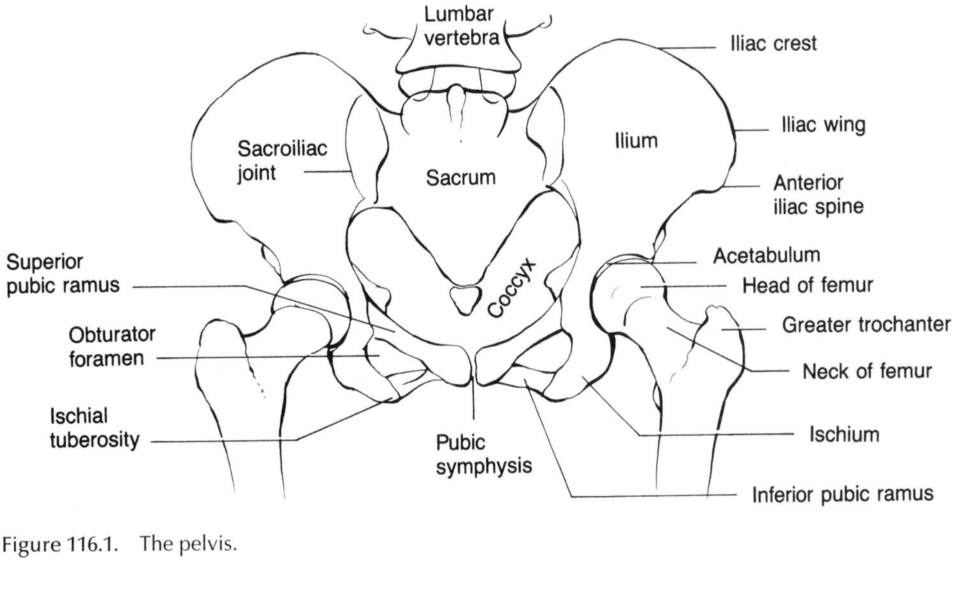

Figure 116.1. The pelvis.

TABLE 116.1. Pelvic Fractures Categorized by Mechanism

Mechanism	Typical Pelvic Fracture	Typical Associated Injuries	Typical Presentation
Athletic injuries without contact	*Stable:* avulsion fractures of anterior superior or inferior iliac spine, ischial tuberosity	None	Pain; restricted motion of muscle that inserted on avulsed fragment; stable pelvis
Fall from standing height or direct blow	*Stable:* bony prominence fracture (iliac spines, ischial tuberosities, superior pubic rami, coccyx)	None	Pain; ecchymosis; localized tenderness with stable pelvis
Lateral compression force	*Stable:* isolated fracture of pelvic wing; pubic ramus fracture; transverse sacral fracture *Unstable:* "bucket handle fracture"	Usually minimal; mild bowel contusion; occasional sacral nerve root contusion; rare hemorrhage	Pain; localized tenderness with stable pelvis
AP compression force	*Stable:* pubic ramus fracture or simple diastasis *Unstable:* complete ligamentous disruption at symphysis and SI joints ("sprung pelvis" or open-book pelvis")	Lower urinary tract; pudendal vessel injury; rare sacral nerve injury	Pain; hematuria; occasional ischemic injury
Straddle injuries	*Unstable:* bilateral double pubic ramus fractures	Lower GU and GI tracts; hemorrhage	Pain; ecchymosis; bony crepitus; hematuria or inability to void
Vertical shear force	*Unstable:* Malgaigne fracture, with anterior rami fractures or pubic diastasis and ipsilateral SJ joint disruption	20% mortality; local nerve or vessel injury; hemorrhage	Bony instability; hypotension
Crush, fall from great height	*Unstable:* any combination of above injuries with or without acetabular fracture	High morbidity and mortality; hemorrhage; visceral injury	Bony instability; hypotension; hematuria hematochezia; open fracture
Various	Acetabular fractures: are themselves STABLE (not in the ring) but may be associated with unstable pelvic fractures	Femoral head, sciatic nerve injury; hip dislocation	Hip dislocation or fracture; nerve deficit

Rarer still is an avulsion fracture of the ischial tuberosity. This injury usually results from strenuous stretching of the pelvic ring, as in hurdling or pole vaulting.[6] Patients with avulsion fractures generally present with a characteristic history and local tenderness. In isolated trauma, there are usually no associated complaints or injuries. These are stable fractures because the integrity of the pelvic ring remains intact.

A fall from a standing height frequently presents as pelvic pain localized to the bony prominences. Areas such as the iliac spine, ischial tuberosities, superior pubic rami, and coccyx are particularly susceptible to direct trauma. These fractures are stable injuries and are particularly common in elderly osteopenic patients. Presentation involves localized pain, swelling, and ecchymosis. There are usually no associated injuries.

Lateral compressive force to the bony pelvis may result in any of several fracture patterns: pelvic wing fractures, pubic rami fractures, "bucket handle" fractures, or transverse sacral fractures. Although these are generally stable injuries, the forces required to cause them (e.g., broadside impact in a motor vehicle crash) are significantly greater than those previously considered. Therefore, the potential for associated injuries with lateral compressive force is higher.

The "stove-in," or *pelvic wing fracture* (Fig. 116.3), was first described by Duverney in 1751. It may produce an unstable fragment off the iliac crest, but the load-bearing stability of the pelvic ring is not jeopardized. The patient with ipsilateral fracture of both pubic rami from lateral compressive force presents with pelvic or hip pain; there may be trauma to the bladder or

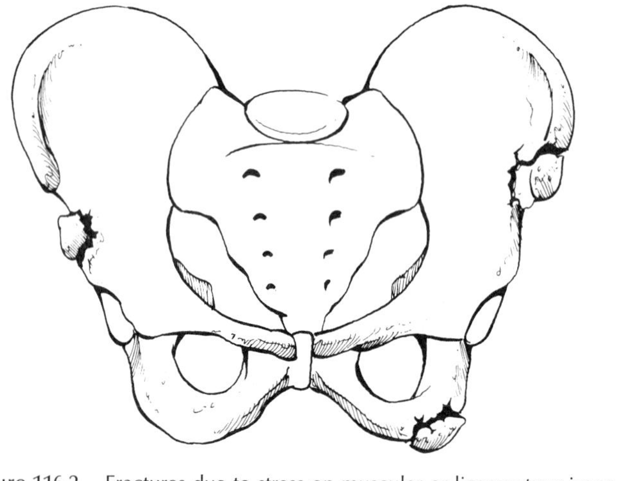

Figure 116.2. Fractures due to stress on muscular or ligamentous insertions onto the bony pelvis.

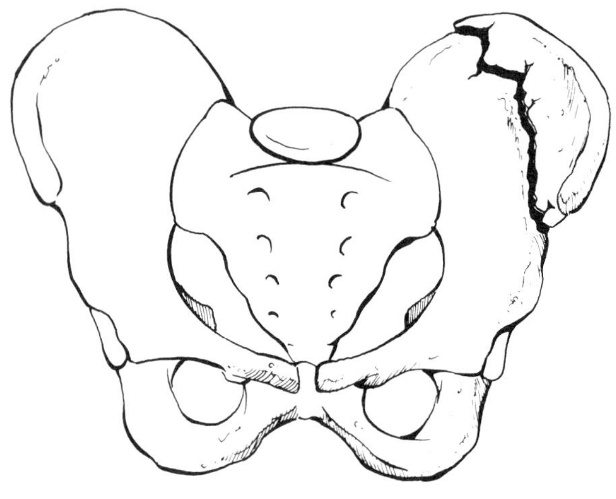

Figure 116.3. Duverney fracture. Pelvic wing or "stove-in" fracture.

proximal urethra. This injury may be stable or may be associated with disruption of the sacroiliac complex, rendering the pelvic ring unstable. Rami fractures due to lateral force injuries are typically horizontally oriented.

A *bucket handle fracture* (Fig. 116.4) occurs when lateral force is sustained in combination with upward rotatory force.[6,9] Generally, there is a fracture or disruption of the sacroiliac complex ipsilateral to the impact and a double pubic ramus fracture contralaterally. The hemipelvis that absorbed the blow is medially and superiorly rotated, presenting a recognizable clinical and radiographic picture. Because there are fractures on both sides of the pelvic ring, these are unstable injuries. Lateral compression of the pelvis can also transfer force to the sacrum. This force may fracture the bone and can separate the ilium from its ligamentous connections unilaterally or bilaterally.

Sacral fractures occur in transverse upper, transverse lower, and vertical planes and are associated with different presentations. Upper sacral fractures are frequently difficult to recognize both radiographically and clinically, often presenting only as buttock and perianal pain. These fractures may injure sacral nerve roots, resulting in decreased anal sphincter tone and loss of perineal sensation. Lower sacral fractures are equally painful but are rarely complicated by neurologic injury. Vertical sacral fractures occur as a result of vertical shear injury and are discussed later.

Anteroposterior compressive force is most commonly applied from the front; typical examples are the pedestrian struck head-on by a car and the front-seat passenger who hits the dashboard. Patients injured by the former mechanism manifest injury of the anterior (symphysis pubis) or posterior (sacroiliac complex) pelvic stabilizers. Those injured by the latter mechanism manifest injuries from transmission of the force through the femurs into the acetabula. (Acetabulum fractures are considered later.) Anteroposterior-force pelvic injuries include pubic ramus fractures, simple symphysis diastasis, and the more severe and potentially unstable "open-book" or "sprung pelvis" injuries. As discussed, *isolated ipsilateral double pubic ramus fractures* are stable injuries, but they require careful clinical and radiographic examination to exclude further injury to the posterior pelvic elements.

Diastasis of the symphysis pubis can occur as an isolated, stable injury; however, the posterior urethra and pudendal vessels are at risk. Symphyseal separation of more than 2.5 cm on the anteroposterior pelvic radiograph indicates injury to the posterior sacroiliac ligaments.[2] When both the symphysis and sacroiliac complex are disrupted by anteroposterior force, the result is an open-book or sprung pelvis (Fig. 116.5). The stability of these injuries depends on the remaining integrity of the posterior sacroiliac ligaments[9] and may not be discernible on plain radiography alone. Bladder rupture is relatively common in connection with this injury.

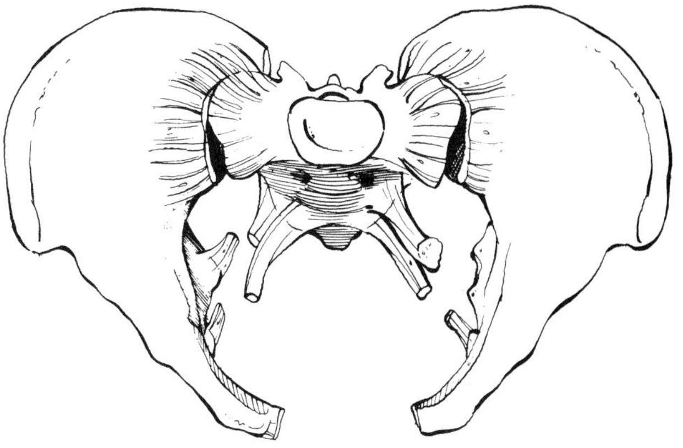

Figure 116.5. "Open-book" or "sprung" pelvis.

Straddle injuries (Fig. 116.6) are characterized by bilateral double pubic ramus fractures and are, by definition, unstable. The lower genitourinary tract is particularly susceptible to injury by this mechanism. Classically, as the name implies, this fracture is caused by falling while straddling a solid object between the legs. However, both lateral and anteroposterior compressive forces can cause straddle injuries as well. These are usually closed fractures; patients present with perineal tenderness, ecchymosis, and frank hematuria (or sometimes, in males, inability to void). The incidence of hemorrhage and bowel injury is greater than 33%.[9]

Vertical shear mechanisms create pelvic fractures that are also unstable. First described by Malgaigne in 1859, these injuries still bear his name. They are the least common of the major fractures and generally result from a fall from a height onto the lower extremities. The resulting fractures are longitudinally oriented through the anterior and posterior pelvis (Fig. 116.7); they are usually unilateral but may be bilateral. The acetabulum is frequently involved, but even when it is not, the patient has diminished motion of the ipsilateral lower extremity. If the sacrum fractures vertically, it may be occult radiographically. This is considered the posterior component of a Malgaigne fracture. Vertical shear injuries are associated with significant intraabdominal and concomitant thoracic injuries and hemorrhage; morbidity and mortality rates are high.

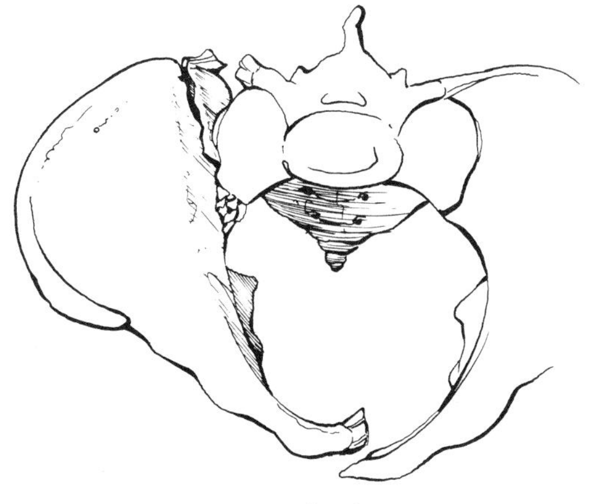

Figure 116.4. "Bucket handle" fracture.

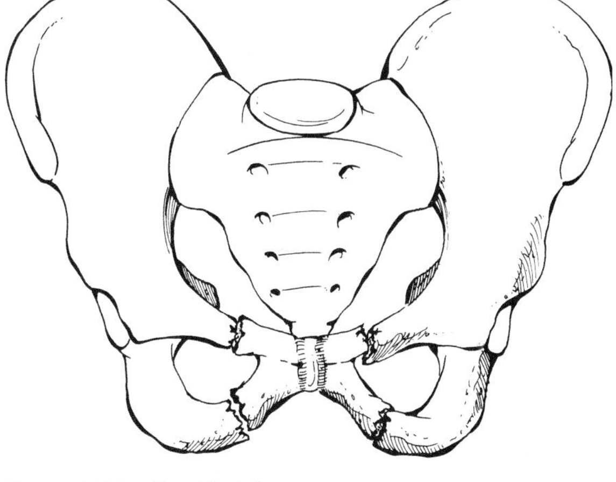

Figure 116.6. Straddle injury.

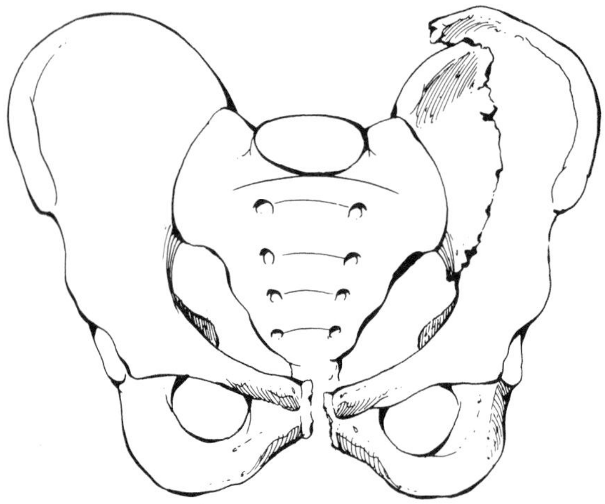

Figure 116.7. Vertical shear (Malgaigne) fracture.

Crush injuries of the pelvis result from a combination of these mechanisms or from extreme force in one direction (e.g., a 70-mi/h motor vehicle crash). If they are open fractures, they carry a high mortality rate. Hemorrhage, intraabdominal injury, thoracic injuries, and head injuries are common, due to the magnitude of the injuring force. These patients typically present in frank hypovolemic shock and require immediate resuscitation.

Acetabular fractures result from one of two mechanisms. They are caused by indirect forces transmitted around the pelvic brim or from forces applied directly to the femur. Both forces cause disruption of the acetabular cup. The classification schemes for these fractures are beyond the typical scope of practice for the emergency physician. The major point of reference is the mechanism of injury; in addition, the presence and type of associated hip dislocation are important. Posterior acetabular fractures, which result from direct trauma to the flexed knee and hip, present with posterior hip dislocations. If the knee and thigh are flexed and the thigh is abducted, trauma to the knee is transmitted to the medial acetabulum, resulting in an ilioischial column fracture and a central hip dislocation.

When force is applied to the greater trochanter posteroanteriorly or lateromedially with the hip flexed, the acetabulum fractures transversely, also resulting in a central hip dislocation. If the hip is externally rotated and the injuring force strikes lateromedially, the anterior lip and iliopubic column of the acetabulum are fractured; the hip joint is usually maintained but may dislocate anteriorly. A history of significant injuring force and a typical lower extremity posture of dislocation should prompt consideration of acetabular fracture. Acetabular fractures are complicated by sciatic nerve injury and disruption of blood supply to the femoral head.

EMERGENCY DEPARTMENT EVALUATION

Once airway, breathing, and circulation are addressed, complete evaluation of the multiply injured patient may proceed. Pelvic injury must be excluded; this is particularly important if there is hemodynamic instability. Examination of the unresponsive patient should parallel that of the awake patient who specifically complains of symptoms in the pelvic region.

Whenever possible, a thorough history is obtained. Mechanism of injury and direction of forces are crucial details. In motor vehicle accident victims, a description of the vehicular damage is also useful. The ability to ambulate after the incident excludes unstable injuries but does not eliminate the possibility of stable fractures. Patients should be asked about the presence of back, buttock, pelvic, groin, perineal, hip, or thigh pain. Symptoms such as lower extremity numbness, paresthesias, or weakness are sought. Bladder and rectal sensation and function should be subjectively assessed in the conscious patient.

The physical examination of both the conscious and unconscious patient, symptomatic or not, begins with inspection over bony prominences for ecchymosis or abrasion. Perineal or scrotal hematomas (Destot sign) or blood at the anus or urethral meatus should be noted. Retroperitoneal bleeding may be apparent from the Grey Turner sign (flank ecchymosis). Any evidence of open fracture is sought.

Palpation for tenderness and instability begins with the iliac crests, then progresses medially toward the symphysis. A "pelvic rock," or exertion of pressure over the iliac wings, should detect instability, but this should be preceded by assessment for localized tenderness. The back examination should include the lower lumbar spine, both sacroiliac regions, and the coccyx. Abdominal, rectal, and scrotal or vaginal examinations are also necessary. The rectal examination must include an assessment of anal sphincter tone, prostate position and tenderness, evidence of bony intrusion into the rectum, and presence of blood; palpation of a fracture line or pelvic hematoma may be possible (Earle sign). The lower extremities are evaluated for pulses (by palpation or Doppler stethoscope), strength, sensation, and deep tendon reflexes. Leg-length discrepancy should be noted.

There are physical examination findings that are specific for certain types of injury. Pain due to an avulsion fracture is worsened by range of motion of the inserting muscle and direct tenderness to palpation over the involved bony prominence. Palpating over a Duverney fracture often yields false motion of the iliac wing. The FABER test is positive with pubic ramus fractures: Pain occurs when the ipsilateral foot is placed on the contralateral knee and the ipsilateral hip is *f*lexed, *ab*ducted, and *e*xternally *r*otated.[6] Any tenderness over the symphysis should prompt close study and measurement of the width of the anterior connection.

Radiographs are also obtained as part of the evaluation in both the conscious and unconscious trauma patient. In the unconscious victim, an anteroposterior radiograph of the pelvis is done routinely secondary to the patient's inability to contribute symptoms of pain on examination. Even in the conscious patient, empiric pelvic radiography remains standard practice; in one study, however, this policy is questioned for patients who are normotensive, alert, and sober and have no physical findings suggestive of pelvic, femoral, or lower urinary injury.[7] The anteroposterior film has a reported accuracy of 88% in detecting ring instability.[4] If the anteroposterior pelvic x-ray is suggestive or diagnostic of a fracture, or if the physical examination suggests instability or localized injury, further studies may be indicated.

Ring instability may be detected by fracture pattern or joint diastasis. The hemipelves should appear symmetric. The physician should look for sacroiliac (greater than 4-mm) and symphyseal (greater than 5-mm) widening. There should be careful evaluation for fractures of the iliac wings and pubic rami, as well as for avulsion fractures of the iliac spines and ischial tuberosities. Transverse fractures of the sacrum are frequently difficult to delineate and must be carefully sought. The arcuate lines of the neural foramina should be followed and examined for irregularity or asymmetry (Fig. 116.8). Acetabular fractures may also be difficult to recognize and can be found by following the iliopectineal and ilioischial lines (Fig. 116.9).

Even though the standard anteroposterior pelvic radiograph will accurately assess pelvic stability in 88% of cases, other imaging modalities are useful for particular injuries.[2] If an acetabular, sacral, or sacroiliac fracture is suspected, adjunctive

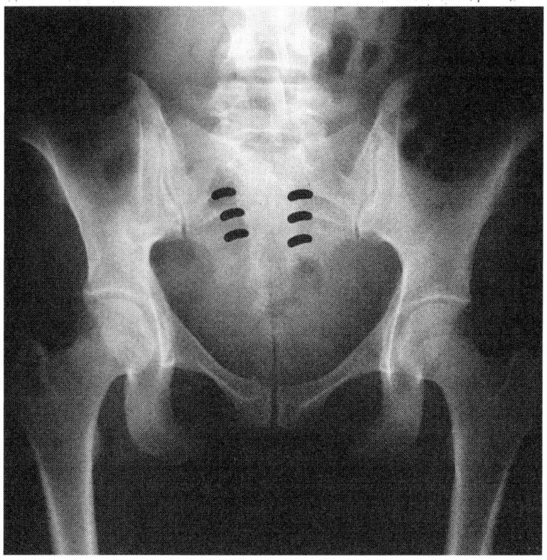

Figure 116.8. Anteroposterior x-ray of the sacrum. The arcuate lines (*highlighted*) that outline the sacral neural foramina should be symmetric and smooth. Sacral fractures are usually more evident on the lateral x-ray view. Any suspicion of fracture or disruption of the arcuate lines on the anteroposterior view should prompt further studies.

studies are often indicated; these areas are difficult to visualize solely by the anteroposterior radiograph secondary to position and overlying structures. A computed tomography (CT) scan usually demonstrates these areas clearly and is superior to plain films at delineating the sacrum and the axial relationships of the sacroiliac joint.[2] In a study by Berg et al.,[2] the anteroposterior pelvic radiograph missed posterior pelvic ring injuries of the sacrum, sacroiliac joints, and posterior ilium in 47% of cases. If a scanner is not available, other plain radiographs may be useful: Pelvic inlet views for the posterior arch, pelvic outlet or tangential views for the sacrum and sacroiliac complex, and Judet views for focusing on the acetabulum.

Associated injuries must also be addressed. Multiply injured patients should have blood counts, appropriate chemistry studies, and type and crossmatch performed in the emergency department. A pregnancy test is done on all women of childbearing age. All patients with detected pelvic injury should also have a urinalysis. A retrograde urethrogram (with cystogram, if indicated) should be done before Foley catheter insertion in patients with blood at the urethral meatus. Major trauma patients

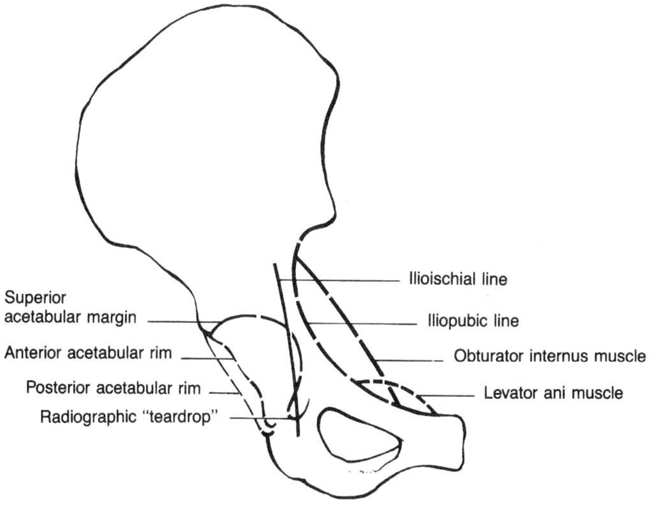

Figure 116.9. Iliopectineal and ilioischial lines.

who are hypotensive, have a compromised sensorium, or have abdominal injuries or symptoms are assessed for concomitant intraperitoneal injury or hemorrhage. Diagnostic peritoneal lavage (performed by the open technique through a supraumbilical approach to minimize the possibility of inadvertently entering a pelvic hematoma[1]) is performed, depending on the patient's stability, the physician's preference, and the institution's capability.

EMERGENCY DEPARTMENT MANAGEMENT

The initial management of a patient with possible pelvic trauma proceeds with the same ABCs of trauma care. With airway and breathing secured, circulation and hemorrhage become important considerations in these patients. *The only immediately life-threatening aspect of pelvic trauma is hemorrhage.* Unfortunately, such bleeding is typically internal, and the usual measures of quantification and suppression are difficult. There are four primary and often overlapping methods of managing hemorrhage from pelvic fracture: emergency department resuscitation, application of an external fixation device, open reduction and external fixation, and angiography with direct embolization of bleeding vessels. Any unstable trauma patient will receive emergency department resuscitation. The management method choices that follow will depend on the institution and its orthopedic surgeons.

Hypotensive patients with pelvic trauma should receive intravenous crystalloid through two large-bore peripheral lines. A central venous pressure monitoring line can be useful but is usually unnecessary. If the patient remains unstable after 3 to 4 L of crystalloid, type-specific or fully crossmatched blood is given. In addition, pelvic trauma with hypotension may be the final bona fide indication for the prehospital and emergency department use of the pneumatic antishock garment (PASG or MAST). Hemorrhage from pelvic fractures is lessened with immobilization and reapproximation of bony fragments; inflating all three compartments of the PASG may accomplish this. The PASG may also tamponade bleeding from smaller vessels and exposed raw surfaces of cancellous bone.

There are many reports of experience with external fixation, operative fixation, and arteriography with embolization in the control of exsanguinating hemorrhage after pelvic fracture.[1,3,8,10] No study has directly compared these modalities. External fixation is relatively rapid and can be performed in the emergency department. Internal fixation, although more definitive, is associated with the usual operative risk and the added consideration of loss of tamponade and sudden profound shock when the pelvic cavity is entered. Selective embolization is technically challenging and relatively time consuming and does not address venous blood loss, which may be significant. Angiographic embolization is, however, the currently recommended method for controlling arterial bleeding from pelvic fractures.[1,3,8]

Pelvic fracture hemorrhage presents as a multispecialty challenge. The decision making regarding management modalities in the face of ongoing bleeding is shared among emergency physicians, surgeons, and orthopedists. The role of the emergency physician in the later stages of management is often limited, but he or she should be thoroughly familiar with the facility's and consultant's respective capabilities. Clinical picture and availability often dictate management choices and imaging modalities. While much has been written of the relative merits of CT and angiography for the detection and localization of pelvic hemorrhage, several facts remain apparent: First, not every facility has an angiography suite or interventional radiologist readily available, and second, CT scanning can detect pelvic hemorrhage with 90% accuracy and is less invasive to perform.[1,3,8,10]

Lastly, pelvic fractures often present with associated injuries that must be managed accordingly. Hip dislocations must be reduced promptly to prevent neurovascular compromise. Urethral injuries may require placement of a suprapubic cystostomy. Abdominal injuries are generally addressed operatively, and genital injuries may require surgical or plastic reconstruction. Patients with open fractures or any penetrating pelvic trauma should receive tetanus prophylaxis and an empiric dose of a broad-spectrum antibiotic. Finally, the possible occurrence of fat embolism, and the often devastating pulmonary and cardiovascular consequences of such, must be remembered.

DISPOSITION

Patients with simple avulsion fractures or isolated stable fractures can be managed conservatively with bed rest, analgesia, and arrangements for physical therapy; many do not require hospital admission. Patients with more significant pelvic injuries must be assessed for related trauma and admitted. Extremes of age and overall physical condition are also important considerations. Patients with unstable fractures and multiple trauma usually require urgent or emergent operative intervention.

COMMON PITFALLS

- Remember that all unconscious patients with blunt multiple trauma require an anteroposterior pelvic radiograph.
- Use the history of the injuring mechanism to help predict the type and severity of pelvic injury.
- Always respect the hemorrhagic potential of unstable pelvic fractures. Vigorous fluid resuscitation, early blood transfusion, consideration of PASG application, and prompt orthopedic consultation are mandatory.
- Associated injuries to the intra- and retroperitoneal organs, the sacral nerves, and the pudendal blood vessels must be suspected and investigated as early as possible.

References

1. Ben-Menachem Y, Coldwell DM, Young JWR, et al. Hemorrhage associated with pelvic fractures: causes, diagnosis, and emergent management. *AJR* 1991;157:1005.
2. Berg EE, Chehubar C, Bell RM. Pelvic trauma imaging: a blinded comparison of computed tomography and roentgenograms. *J Trauma* 1996;41:994.
3. Cerva DS, Mervis SE, Shanmuganathan K, et al. Detection of bleeding in patients with major pelvic fractures: value of contrast-enhanced CT. *AJR* 1996;166:131.
4. Edeiken-Monroe BS, Brunner BO, Jackson H. The role of standard roentgenograms in the evaluation of instability of pelvic ring disruption. *Clin Orthop Rel Res* 1989;240:63.
5. Gens DR. Imaging priorities in the admitting area. In: Mirvis SE, Young JWR, eds. *Imaging in trauma and critical care.* Baltimore: Williams & Wilkins, 1992:1.
6. Jerrard DA. Pelvic fractures. *Emerg Med Clin North Am* 1993;11:147.
7. Koury HI, Peschiara JL, Welling RE. Selective use of pelvic roentgenograms in blunt trauma patients. *J Trauma* 1993;34:236.
8. Panetta T, Selafami S, Goldstein A. Percutaneous transcatheter embolization for massive bleeding from pelvic fractures. *J Trauma* 1985;25:1021.
9. Pitt MJ, Ruth JT, Benjamin JB. Trauma to the pelvic ring and acetabulum. *Semin Roentgenol* 1992;27:299.
10. Shanmuganathan K, Mirvis SE, Sover ER. Value of contrast-enhanced CT in detecting active hemorrhage in patients with blunt abdominal or pelvic trauma. *AJR* 1993;161:65.
11. Young JWR, Resnik CS. Fractures of the pelvis: current concepts of classification. *AJR* 1990;155:1169.

CHAPTER 117
Hip Injuries

Norberto Adame, Jr. and Timothy Seay

Injuries to the hip are a major cause of morbidity and mortality, a problem that has worsened, and will continue to worsen, as the population ages. Injuries to the hip are a major health hazard. For the elderly, as many as 37% of hip fractures result in death within 1 year, and half of these deaths are thought to be directly due to the fracture.[6] Causes of hip fractures are primarily pathologic (from osteopenia) and due to falls (primarily a disease of the elderly), whereas motor vehicle crashes account for the majority of dislocations (primarily a disease of the young). The frequency of traumatic hip dislocations and proximal fracture–dislocations of the femur has declined with the use of seatbelts. Although this decline is encouraging, early recognition of hip dislocations and proximal femur fractures will minimize the likelihood of developing avascular necrosis of the femoral head. In traumatic hip dislocations, the incidence of associated osteoarthritis is 26%.[1,7,10] For avascular necrosis, the incidence ranges from 8% to 30%, depending on the degree of displacement.[7] The incidence of these complications can be minimized by prompt diagnosis, evaluation, and definitive treatment in the emergency department (ED).

Anatomically, the hip is an articulation between the femoral head and the acetabulum, joined together by the ligamentum teres and the capsular ligament of the hip joint. It is a very stable articulation, requiring violent injury to dislocate. Primary sources of blood flow for the femoral head are the retinacular branches of the circumflex femoral artery. These enter the femur

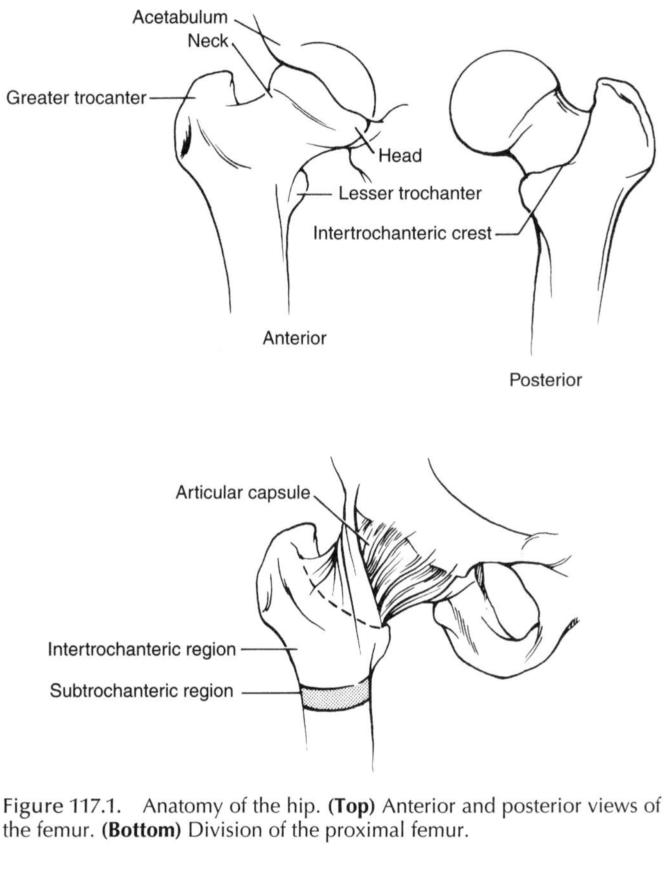

Figure 117.1. Anatomy of the hip. **(Top)** Anterior and posterior views of the femur. **(Bottom)** Division of the proximal femur.

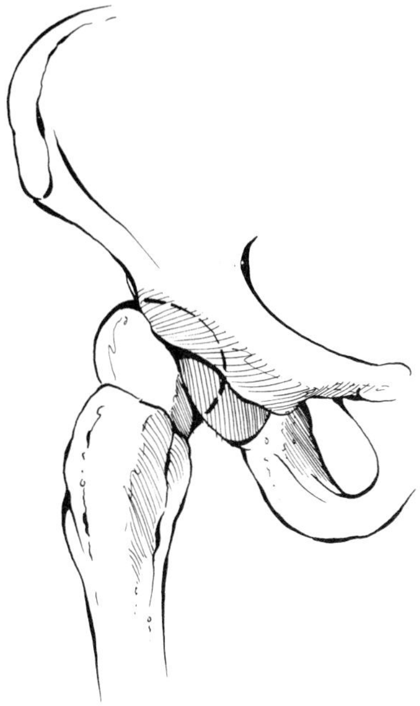

Figure 117.2. Posterior dislocation of the hip.

in the region of the femoral neck, and fractures proximal to their entry can result in disruption of blood flow and cause avascular necrosis of the femoral head. The other source of blood for the femoral head comes from the artery of the ligamentum teres. Often, this artery is absent or vestigial, and its loss is rarely of clinical significance. Avascular necrosis of the femoral head is a common *early* complication of fracture of the femoral neck. It is identified on x-ray films as an increase in density in the region of the femoral head, thought to be new bone deposition onto necrotic spicules.

In addition to the capsule, the hip joint is reinforced by the hip abductor muscles (gluteus medius and miminus, obturator, gamelli, and piriformis) attached to the greater trochanter and flexor (iliopsoas), which is attached to the lesser trochanter (Fig. 117.1).

HIP DISLOCATIONS

Posterior Hip Dislocations

Posterior hip dislocations are the most common type of dislocation and result from force applied to a flexed knee and hip. When the knee hits the dashboard during a motor vehicle crash, the hip is forcefully adducted and flexed while simultaneously pushed posteriorly. This is prevented by the use of a lap belt.

EMERGENCY DEPARTMENT EVALUATION

In posterior hip dislocations, the limb is flexed, adducted, and internally rotated, with limb shortening. If the patient is thin, the femoral head can often be palpated in the buttocks region (Figs. 117.2 and 117.3). Examination of the leg should ensure vascular function (rarely compromised) and include neurologic evaluation for possible sciatic nerve injury. The sciatic nerve lies posterior to the femoral head, separated from it by the capsule and by the obturator and gamelli muscles. Up to 50% have an associated acetabular or femoral head fracture (discussion follows).

EMERGENCY DEPARTMENT MANAGEMENT

Posterior dislocations optimally need reduction within 6 hours to minimize the risk for avascular necrosis,[4,9] which should be

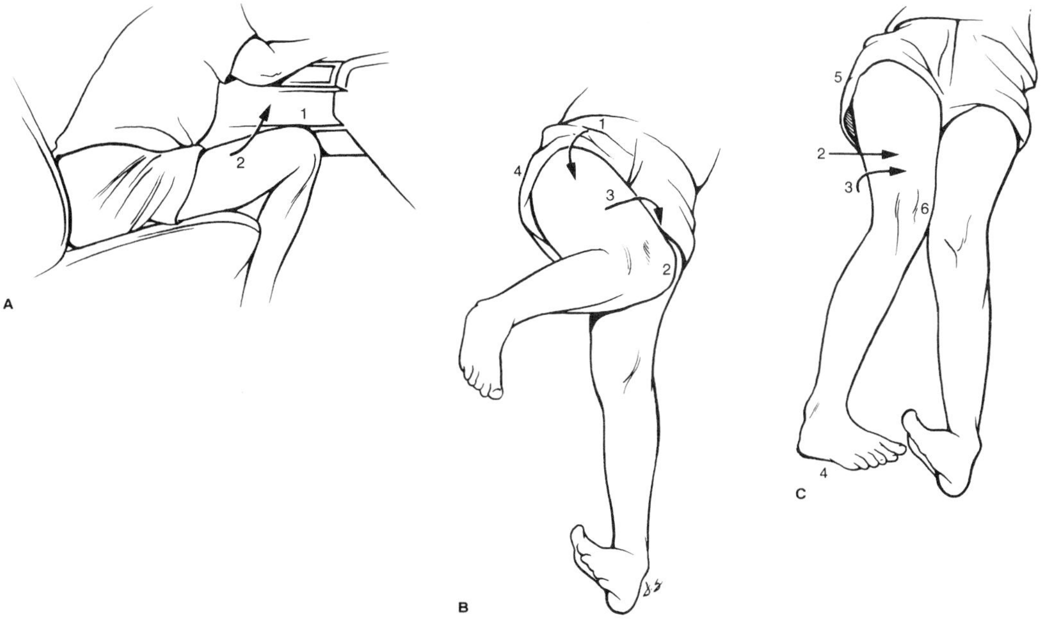

Figure 117.3. Posterior dislocation of the hip. **(A)** Mechanism of injury. The knee *(1)* strikes the dashboard. The thigh *(2)* is forced into flexion and adduction, and the femoral head is driven backward out of the acetabulum. **(B)** Ischial dislocation. The hip *(1)* is flexed. The hip is markedly adducted so that the knee *(2)* of the affected limb lies on the opposite thigh. The limb *(3)* is in extreme internal rotation. The greater trochanter and buttock *(4)* on the affected side are unusually prominent. **(C)** Iliac dislocation. As in **(B)**, the hip is flexed and is adducted *(2)*. It is internally rotated *(3)*. The affected extremity *(4)* appears shortened. The greater trochanter and buttock *(5)* on the affected side are unusually prominent. The knee *(6)* of the affected extremity rests on the opposite thigh.

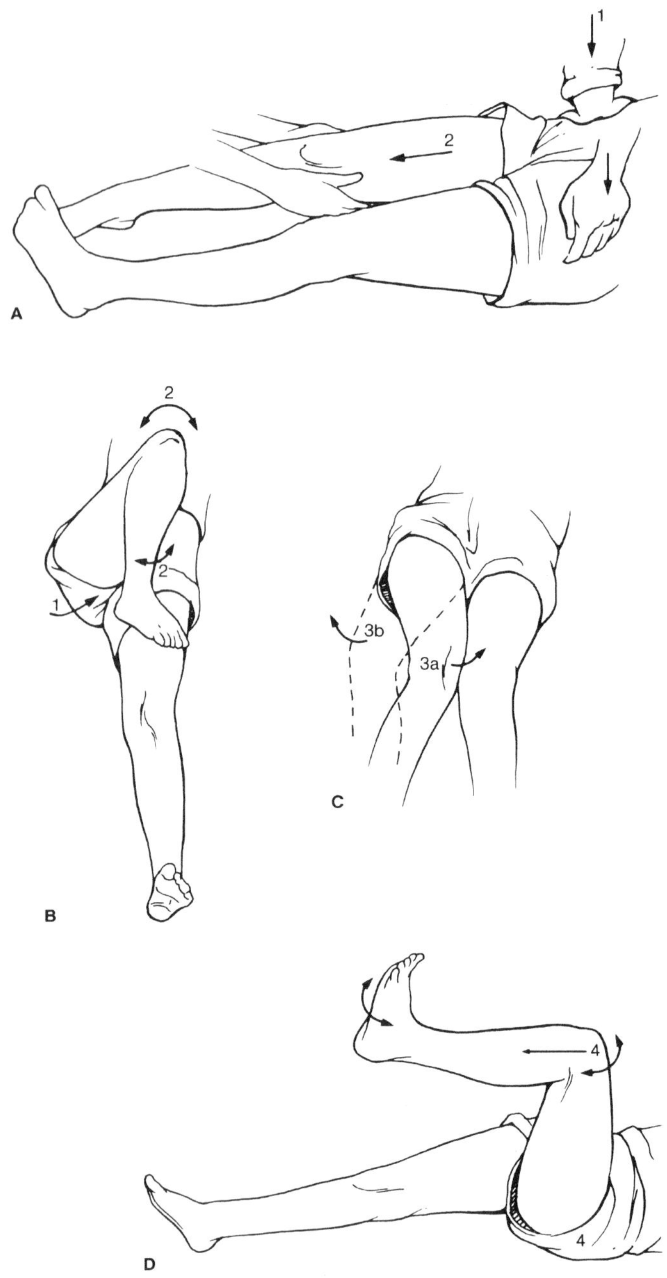

Figure 117.4. Posterior dislocation of the hip: method of manipulative reduction. **(A)** The assistant makes downward pressure *(1)* on the anterior–superior iliac spine. With the knee flexed *(2),* the operator pulls on the limb in the line of deformity. **(B)** The assistant slowly brings the thigh *(1)* to 90 degrees of flexion. The assistant gently rotates the thigh internally and externally and rocks the thigh *(2)* backward and forward to disengage the head from the external rotator muscles and the posterior capsule. **(C)** The assistant relocates the femoral head by further internal rotation and extension of the thigh *(3a),* or external rotation and extension of the thigh *(3b).* **(D)** The assistant pushes firmly on the trochanter to direct the femoral head into the acetabulum while the limb is rotated and extended *(4).* Forceful rotation should be avoided, because it can readily fracture the femoral neck. If the reduction is not accomplished with two adequate attempts, open reduction is indicated.

attempted in the ED (Fig. 117.4). Adequate analgesia and muscle relaxation must be obtained by using a short-acting narcotic (e.g., fentanyl) and a short-acting benzodiazepine (e.g., midazolam) with proper conscious sedation monitoring. After the patient is adequately relaxed, an assistant should apply pressure to the iliac crests, stabilizing the pelvis from lifting off the board. At this time, the physician should apply traction in line with the deformity and gently begin to flex the hip to 90 degrees. The reducing physician must stand on the gurney astride the patient. Successful reduction is often felt by a dull click. General anesthesia is occasionally necessary, and orthopedic consultation is always necessary. After reduction, the extremity should be placed in extension and neurovascular function of the extremity reassessed. Postreduction radiographs should be obtained. The patient should be admitted to the hospital and be kept from bearing weight on the extremity for 10 to 14 days.

Anterior Hip Dislocations

Anterior hip dislocations occur most commonly from a direct blow to the abducted hip. A distally applied force causes the femoral head to tear through the anterior capsule. Anterior dislocations may be classified as obturator, iliac, and pubic (Fig. 117.5). Obturator-type hip dislocations occur when the hip is abducted and in flexion. The pubic and iliac types occur most commonly when the hip is abducted and in extension.

EMERGENCY DEPARTMENT EVALUATION

Careful neurovascular examination is mandatory, owing to the risk of arterial damage and venous thrombosis.[8] Anterior obturator dislocations present as abduction, external rotation, and flexion of the involved extremity. Anterior iliac and pubic dislocations present as slight abduction, external rotation, and extension of the involved extremity (Fig. 117.6).

EMERGENCY DEPARTMENT MANAGEMENT

Anterior dislocations are best treated with closed reduction with the patient under general anesthesia. Emergent orthopedic consultation for early reduction is extremely important because of associated vascular injuries. This will minimize major sequelae, such as avascular necrosis of the femoral head.

COMMON PITFALLS

- Failure to look for associated acetabular, femur, and knee injuries (especially ligamentous) with hip dislocations; computed tomography (CT) or magnetic resonance imaging (MRI) may be necessary.
- Failure to obtain early closed reduction, which lowers the risk of avascular necrosis and posttraumatic osteoarthritis; less than 6 hours is ideal.
- Failure to realize that persistent pain after reduction may indicate the possibility of entrapment within the joint of neurologic or vascular components
- Failure to recognize sciatic nerve injury with posterior hip dislocation

HIP FRACTURES

Fractures of the hip are one of the common injuries seen in the ED, especially among elderly patients. It is estimated that 5% to 10% of those reaching their 80s will have a femoral neck fracture. The increasing elderly population could double the number of hip fractures seen over the next 20 years. A third of those over age 65 who live at home, and half of institutionalized individuals, are estimated to fall yearly. Morbidity in this age group is staggering, with a third dying within 1 year.[6] Thirty percent of those who were independently ambulatory prefracture require

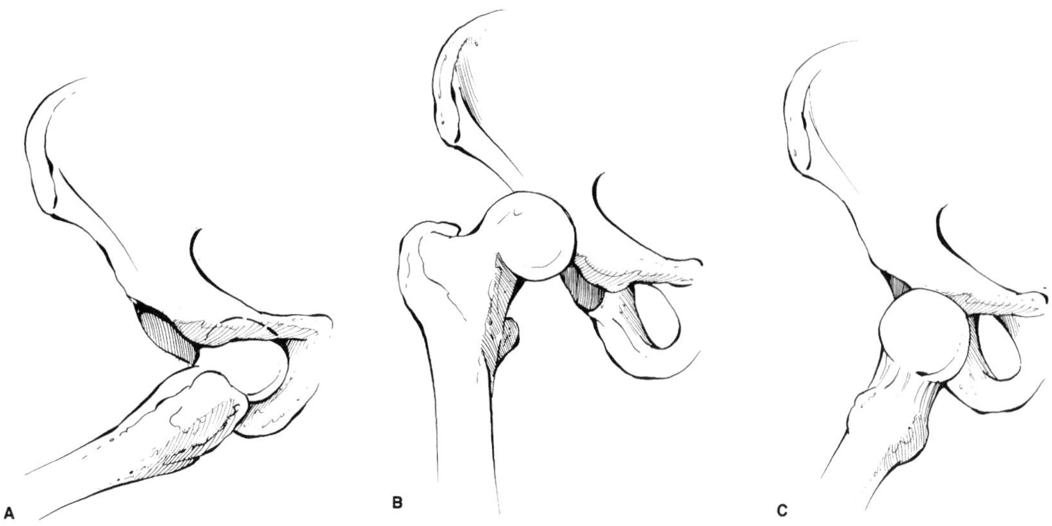

Figure 117.5. Anterior hip dislocations. (**A**) Anterior obturator hip dislocation. (**B**) Anterior iliac hip dislocation. (**C**) Anterior pubic hip dislocation.

permanent postinjury crutches or a walker, and 7% of them become permanently bedridden.[2] For the emergency physician, the diagnosis becomes the important step, as, almost invariably, these patients are repaired intraoperatively with an Austin-Moore–type femoral head prosthesis. The emergency physician should determine prior level of function, including the degree of independent ambulation, mental status, and any associated illnesses, as they are important factors in the ED and in the definitive management of these patients.

The term *hip fracture* refers to a fracture of the femur proximal to the subtrochanteric region. Hip fractures are broadly classified into six anatomic groups: femoral head and neck fractures, intertrochanteric fractures, subtrochanteric fractures, and isolated fractures of greater or lesser trochanters. Pertinent anatomy is shown in Figure 117.1.

Femoral Head Fractures

Isolated fractures of the femoral head are relatively uncommon. These fractures usually occur in conjunction with dislocations of the femoral head (unlike most other types of hip fractures).

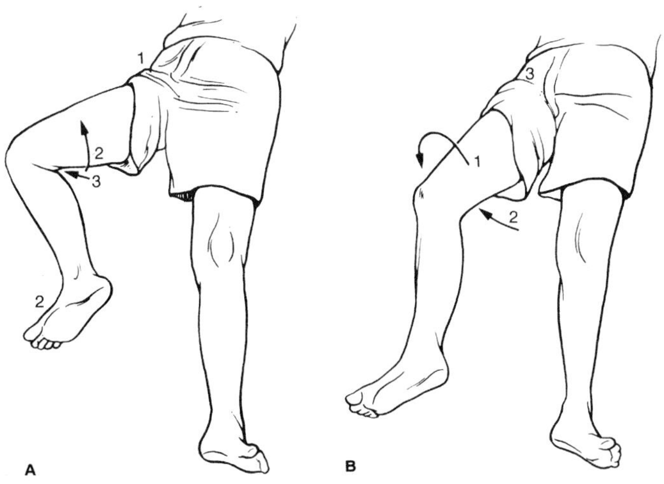

Figure 117.6. Anterior dislocations of the hip. (**A**) Obturator dislocation. The hip *(1)* is slightly flexed. The limb *(2)* is externally rotated. The thigh *(3)* is abducted. (**B**) Pubic dislocation. The extremity *(1)* is in severe external rotation (90 degrees). The extremity *(2)* is abducted only slightly (15 to 20 degrees), and it is slightly flexed. The femoral head *(3)* can readily be palpated in the inguinal region.

Three-fourths are due to motor vehicle crashes, generally in younger patients. As with dislocations of the hip, acetabular fracture may also be seen, and should be sought.

EMERGENCY DEPARTMENT EVALUATION

Femoral head fractures may not be noted on routine radiographs; additional studies, such as tomography, radionuclide scans, CT, or MRI may be required. Persistent pain in the absence of radiographic findings should prompt further investigation. In one report, one in seven changes in the femoral head noted after trauma, which were typically thought to be due to avascular necrosis, were actually due to impaction of the femoral head.[3]

These fractures may be subdivided into two types: single fragment (type I) and comminuted (type II). The site of fracture and the accompanying complications are also related to the type of dislocation associated with the fracture.[5] Posterior dislocations are more likely to result in fracture of the inferior aspect of the femoral head and may have concomitant sciatic nerve injury. Anterior dislocations tend to result in fracture of the anterior femoral head and may have associated vascular injury.

EMERGENCY DEPARTMENT MANAGEMENT

Precise and early reduction are important to maximize range of motion and subsequent function and to minimize complications such as avascular necrosis or degenerative joint disease. Unfortunately, complications occur regardless of proper intervention and result in the need for prosthetic replacement. Urgent orthopedic consultation is mandatory.

Femoral Neck Fractures (Transcervical or Intracapsular Fractures)

These fractures occur below the femoral head and above the greater trochanter and are much more common than femoral head fractures. They are located within the joint capsule and include subcapital fractures (which occur through the fused epiphyseal plate). In the elderly, these fractures are pathologic, occurring with little or no trauma, while in younger patients they are usually the result of violent, unrestrained motor vehicle trauma. Osteoporosis is a major risk factor, making the injury

TABLE 117.1. Garden Classification of Femoral Neck Fractures	
Type	Definition
Type I	Impaction or incomplete fracture
Type II	Complete transcervical fracture with displacement
Type III	Complete fracture with partial displacement of the distal fragment
Type IV	Fracture with total displacement or comminution

four times more common in women than in men. Indeed, the fracture may sometimes occur due to angular or torsional forces placed on the neck before a fall.[1]

EMERGENCY DEPARTMENT EVALUATION

Classifications of these fractures have been based on both patient and fracture characteristics. The system proposed by Garden is one of the most commonly used (Table 117.1). In type I, there is impaction or incomplete fracture. Type II is complete transcervical fracture with displacement. Type III is a complete fracture with partial displacement of the distal fragment, and type IV is fracture with total displacement or comminution. Ambulation does not imply absence of a fracture, because patients with types I and II fractures commonly walk after these injuries. Individuals with types III and IV are unable to ambulate and usually present with a shortened, externally rotated extremity and an abducted hip.

Stress Fractures

Stress fractures represent a unique type of femoral neck fracture. They most commonly occur in young, athletic individuals, but also occur in those with pathologic bone, such as in rheumatoid arthritis, renal osteodystrophy, and chronic steroid use. They may be bilateral and are usually the result of repetitive abnormal stress on normal bone or repetitive normal stress on abnormal bone. The pain is often gradual in its onset. Ambulation is common, with weight-bearing pain. The usual signs of fracture are missing both clinically and radiographically. Bone scan and MRI is indicated in any high-risk individual who cannot bear weight. Treatment centers on the degree of the injury and the state of the underlying bone. The range is from resting the affected hip to prosthetic hip replacement.

EMERGENCY DEPARTMENT MANAGEMENT

Type I fractures may be nonoperatively managed, but patient compliance is mandatory, and the likelihood of complications make operative management the preferred modality (pinning, most commonly). Types II, III, and IV fractures require open reduction and internal fixation (compression screw and plate or Austin-Moore–type femoral head prosthesis). Early and precise anatomic reduction, within 12 hours, reduces the risk of avascular necrosis. Prompt recognition and orthopedic consultation in the ED may help minimize avascular necrosis and the other sequelae associated with these types of fracture.

Intertrochanteric Fractures

These are the most common type of hip fracture. They are usually extracapsular, and the vast majority are due to falls in the elderly (they are pathologic fractures). DeLee[1] found these to be four times as common as femoral neck fractures. X-ray findings usually show

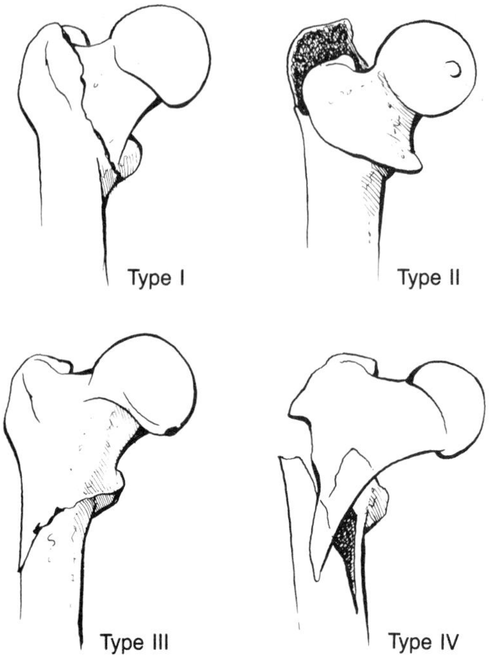

Figure 117.7. Boyd and Griffin classification of intertrochanteric hip fractures. (Adapted from Rockwood CA Jr, Green DP, Bucholz RW. *Rockwood and Green's factures in adults,* 3rd ed. Philadelphia: Lippincott Co., 1991.)

comminution, with only 20% composed of two pieces, 65% composed of three or four fragments, and 15% highly comminuted.[7]

EMERGENCY DEPARTMENT EVALUATION

Emergency diagnosis is usually straightforward. Any movement causes extreme pain, and the hip may be tender to palpation. The affected leg is shortened and externally rotated, and weight bearing is not possible. The diagnosis is usually confirmed radiographically with a single anteroposterior (AP) view of the hip. A lateral or groin view may be necessary to evaluate the degree of comminution.

The intertrochanteric fracture is extraarticular, but transarticular forces clearly play a major role in its occurrence. The fracture typically extends in a relatively straight line between the greater and lesser trochanters (Fig. 117.7). A variety of classifications are used to describe these fractures, and there is no universal agreement. As seen in Fig. 117.7, the Boyd and Griffin classification uses four categories. Type I is nondisplaced. Type II fracture lines parallel those in type I, but there is displacement. Types III and IV fracture lines run nearly perpendicular to types I and II. Type III is nondisplaced, whereas type IV is displaced. Another system uses stability and comminution as criteria. When obtaining orthopedic consultation, precise anatomic description may be more useful than a specific classification type.

EMERGENCY DEPARTMENT MANAGEMENT

Initial management consists of immobilization with sandbags or Buck's traction (2 to 4 kg). This helps to decrease blood loss until definitive therapy can be performed. Intravenous volume placement, with crystalloid or blood, may be necessary, because patients can lose 1 to 2 L of blood with these fractures. Many of these patients have concomitant chronic medical problems. These should be addressed, including the cause of the fall, and will help to establish whether the patient is an operative candidate. Laboratory evaluation should include the standard preoperative laboratory assessment, as well as other analysis necessary to ascertain the cause of the fall. This may include neurologic and cardiovascular evaluations. Avascular necrosis is an uncommon complication.

Operative repair has historically been considered safer than conservative therapy. This is due to the morbidity and mortality associated with extended immobilization. As a result, the treatment of choice is surgical (variety of procedures). Surgical reduction and fixation should be considered urgent rather than emergent, and all patients should have a thorough preoperative evaluation. Selected fractures may be managed by splinting, traction, or spica immobilization, as determined by the consulting orthopedist and the patient's underlying medical condition. Complications are common after these injuries and reflect the frail status of most of these patients; about a third of these patients will die within 1 year of injury.

Greater Trochanter Fractures

These injuries are quite uncommon. They occur as a result of direct trauma (generally adults, including the elderly), and in those with preepiphyseal plate fusion (ages 7 to 17), secondary to avulsion of the apophysis as a result of forceful muscular contraction. If due to direct trauma, they are rarely displaced and can be difficult to see on routine radiographic views. Radiographic imaging frequently requires comparison views.

EMERGENCY DEPARTMENT EVALUATION

In both, tenderness to palpation is usually present over the greater trochanter. Patients are usually ambulatory, frequently with a limp. The fracture in adults, due to a direct blow, is usually comminuted without significant displacement. The epiphyseal avulsion type of injury is usually displaced but not comminuted.

EMERGENCY DEPARTMENT MANAGEMENT

Management varies from adduction splint and bed rest, to open reduction and internal fixation. In most instances, the prognosis is good, regardless of the method used. DeLee[1] recommends ORIF for greater than 1-cm displacement of either a large isolated fragment for the direct trauma (adult) type or the entire apophysis in the epiphyseal avulsion (youth) type.

Lesser Trochanteric Fractures

Lesser trochanteric fractures usually occur in the young, with 85% occurring before age 20.[1] They usually occur from forceful contraction of the iliopsoas muscle during strenuous activities. The lesser trochanter can be displaced up to 1 cm. This type of injury in an adult mandates a search for pathologic bone.

EMERGENCY DEPARTMENT EVALUATION

Patients will have pain and tenderness in the femoral triangle. There will be the inability to lift the affected extremity when in the sitting position if there is complete avulsion (Ludloff's sign). Radiographic imaging frequently requires comparison views.

EMERGENCY DEPARTMENT MANAGEMENT

Treatment is usually bed rest, unless there is significant displacement. Some orthopedists favor nonoperative management, regardless of the degree of separation, because the outcome is uniformly good.[1]

Subtrochanteric Fractures

Subtrochanteric fractures are defined as fractures occurring between the lesser trochanter and a point 5 cm (or 2 in.) distally. They account for one in ten hip fractures and are associated with more severe trauma, or are in pathologic bone (such as severe osteoporosis, Paget disease or cancer metastasis).

EMERGENCY DEPARTMENT EVALUATION

Clinical presentation is similar to that of intertrochanteric fractures. The forces of the muscles extending across this region frequently result in abduction, flexion, and external rotation. Young patients with these fractures are subject to violent forces; associated injuries are common and should be sought. Blood loss can be substantial in fractures of the midshaft femur, and these fractures fall into this subset. Subtrochanteric fractures may occur in combination with other hip fractures: Classification is varied and complex. Accepted anatomic description is best used when describing these fractures.

EMERGENCY DEPARTMENT MANAGEMENT

Treatment involves immobilization, analgesia, volume replacement (if indicated), and timely orthopedic intervention. Associated neurovascular injuries should be identified. Prompt vascular surgery consultation should be obtained, if indicated. Operative reduction and fixation (usually some type of intramedullary nail) is used based on specific patient and fracture characteristics.

COMMON PITFALLS

- The ability to walk does not rule out fracture of the hip.
- Failure to evaluate an elderly patient with a history of a recent fall and a complaint of knee pain for hip fracture
- Failure to carefully examine patients with impaired mental status due to dementia, intracranial injury, or substance abuse for fractures
- Failure to evaluate young, athletic adults with pain in the femoral triangle for lesser trochanteric fracture
- Failure to realize that pain in the hip, in the absence of trauma, does not rule out fracture; radiographs should be obtained.

ACETABULAR FRACTURES

Acetabular fractures should be considered in both types of femoral head dislocations and, more commonly, in pelvic fractures. The force of injury applied to the femur from impact onto the dashboard is transmitted to the acetabulum.

EMERGENCY DEPARTMENT EVALUATION

There are four types of acetabular fractures. The posterior lip fracture is the most common and is associated with posterior hip dislocations. The transverse acetabulum fracture is best seen on AP view as it crosses the acetabulum. The third is the anterior fracture, which disrupts the arcuate or iliopubic line. The fourth is the ilioischial, or posterior, fracture. In type IV fractures, the entire posterior column (the bone extending from the ilium to the ischium) becomes separated from the pelvis. An occult acetabular fracture should be suspected when the patient gives a history of a recent fall, but the pelvic radiograph is normal. Always consider the use of oblique views to diagnose these fractures, as the first films generally do not visualize the injury. It is frequently necessary to consider CT scan, MRI, and nuclear medicine to image these patients' injuries.

EMERGENCY DEPARTMENT MANAGEMENT

Acetabular fractures are managed in consultation with the orthopedic surgeon. ED management involves immobilization, analgesia, volume replacement, if necessary, and identification of associated injuries.

COMMON PITFALLS

- Failure to look for acetabular fractures in patients with hip dislocations and inferior pubic rami fractures
- Failure to suspect occult acetabular fracture when the patient gives a history of a recent fall, the pelvic radiograph is normal, and there is persistent hip pain

References

1. DeLee JC. Fractures and dislocations of the hip. In: Rockwood CA Jr, Green DP, Bucholz RW. *Rockwood and Green's fractures in adults,* 3rd ed. Philadelphia: JB Lippincott Co, 1991:1481.
2. Finsen V, Borset M, Rossvoll I. Mobility, survival and nursing-home requirements after hip fracture. *Ann Chir Gynaecol* 1995;84(3):291–294.
3. Gruen GS, Mears DC, Tauxe WN. Distinguishing avascular necrosis from segmental impaction of the femoral head following an acetabular fracture: preliminary report. *J Orthop Trauma* 1980;2(1):5.
4. Jasulka RA, Fischer G, Fenzl G. Dislocation and fracture-dislocation of the hip. *J Bone Joint Surg Br* 1991;73(3):465–459.
5. Meislin RJ, Zuckermann JD. Case report: bilateral posterior hip dislocations with femoral head fractures. *J Orthop Trauma* 1989;3:358.
6. Parker MJ, Anad JK. What is the true mortality of hip fractures? *Publ Health* 1991;105(6):443–446.
7. Rogers, LF. *The radiology of skeletal trauma,* 2nd ed. New York: Churchill Livingstone, 1992.
8. Simon RR, Koenigsknecht SJ. *Emergency orthopedics—the extremities,* 3rd ed. Norwalk CT: Appleton & Lange, 1995.
9. Vecsei V, Schwendenwein E, Berger G. Hip dislocation without bone injuries. *Orthopade* 1997;26(4):317–326.
10. Yang RS, Tsuang YH, Hang YS, et al. Traumatic dislocations of the hip. *Clin Orthop Rel Res* 1991;265:218.

CHAPTER 118
Knee Injuries

John E. Gough and Nicholas H. Benson

ANATOMY

The knee is a synovial hinge joint with a complex architecture of bone, ligament, muscle, and cartilage (Fig. 118.1). The three bones that make up the knee are the distal femur, patella, and proximal tibia. The femoral condyles articulate with the proximal tibia (tibial plateau) to form the weight-bearing portion of the knee joint. The femoral condyles also articulate with the posterior portion of the patella in the trochlear groove. The patellofemoral articulation does not function in weight bearing; the patella provides protection to the femur, however, as well as improved stability and strength of the extensor mechanism. The proximal fibula is not part of the knee joint proper, although it does serve as the site of attachment of the lateral collateral ligament (LCL).

The bony structures of the knee offer the joint little stability; the knee relies on fibrinous soft-tissue components for stability and proper function. Stability of the medial aspect of the knee is provided mainly by the medial collateral ligament (MCL). The MCL has a superficial and deep layer. The superficial portion originates from the medial femoral epicondyle and inserts on the medial aspect of the tibia just distal to the tibiofemoral joint and provides most of the resistance to valgus forces. The deep portion of the MCL helps stabilize the medial meniscus. The LCL protects the knee from varus stresses and originates from the lateral femoral epicondyle.

The cruciate ligaments are located within the intercondylar notch. The anterior cruciate ligament (ACL) originates from the posterior aspect of the lateral femoral epicondyle and inserts into the anterior tibia at the tibial spine. The posterior cruciate ligament (PCL) arises from the medial femoral condyle, crosses behind the ACL, and inserts on the posterior tibial spine. The ACL prevents anterior displacement of the tibia relative to the femur; the PCL helps prevent posterior displacement. Both cruciate ligaments also play a minor role in resisting varus and valgus rotation within the knee.

The menisci are cartilages positioned on the articulating surface of the tibia. They provide a contact surface between the tibia and femur and distribute and dissipate forces within the knee. The menisci also aid in stabilizing the knee by preventing abnormal motion of the tibia and femur. They have only peripheral vasculature, which is of clinical importance in the healing process following injury.

The muscles involved with normal knee function can be divided into extensors and flexors. Extension is primarily provided by the quadriceps muscles, composed of the vastus medialis, vastus intermedius, vastus lateralis, and rectus femoris. The tendons of these muscles combine to form the quadriceps tendon, which inserts into the superior patella and the medial and lateral retinaculum of the joint capsule. The tendon then becomes the patellar tendon, which connects the inferior portion of the patella to the tibial tubercle.

The hamstring muscles of the posterior thigh are the primary flexors of the knee. The four muscles of the hamstring are the semimembranosus, semitendinosus, and the two heads of the biceps femoris. The biceps femoris attaches to the proximal fibula. The semitendinosus and semimembranosus form the medial aspect of the hamstrings and insert into the tibia and medial joint capsule of the knee.

The major vascular structures around the knee pass posteriorly and are of extreme clinical importance. The popliteal artery is fixed proximally at the hiatus of the adductor magnus and distally at the tendinous arch of the soleus muscle.[7] This tethering makes it susceptible to injury by traction forces, as seen with dislocations. The popliteal artery is also at risk of disruption by fractures or penetrating wounds. The collateral circulation is generally poor, so significant damage to the popliteal artery places the viability of the lower limb in jeopardy.

Proximal to the knee, the sciatic nerve separates into the tibial and peroneal nerves. The tibial nerve passes posteriorly and is therefore susceptible to the same mechanisms of injury as the popliteal artery. The peroneal nerve courses superficially around the lateral aspect of the knee to the proximal fibula. Because of its superficial location, the peroneal nerve may be injured in trauma involving less significant forces than those needed to affect the deeper tibial nerve.

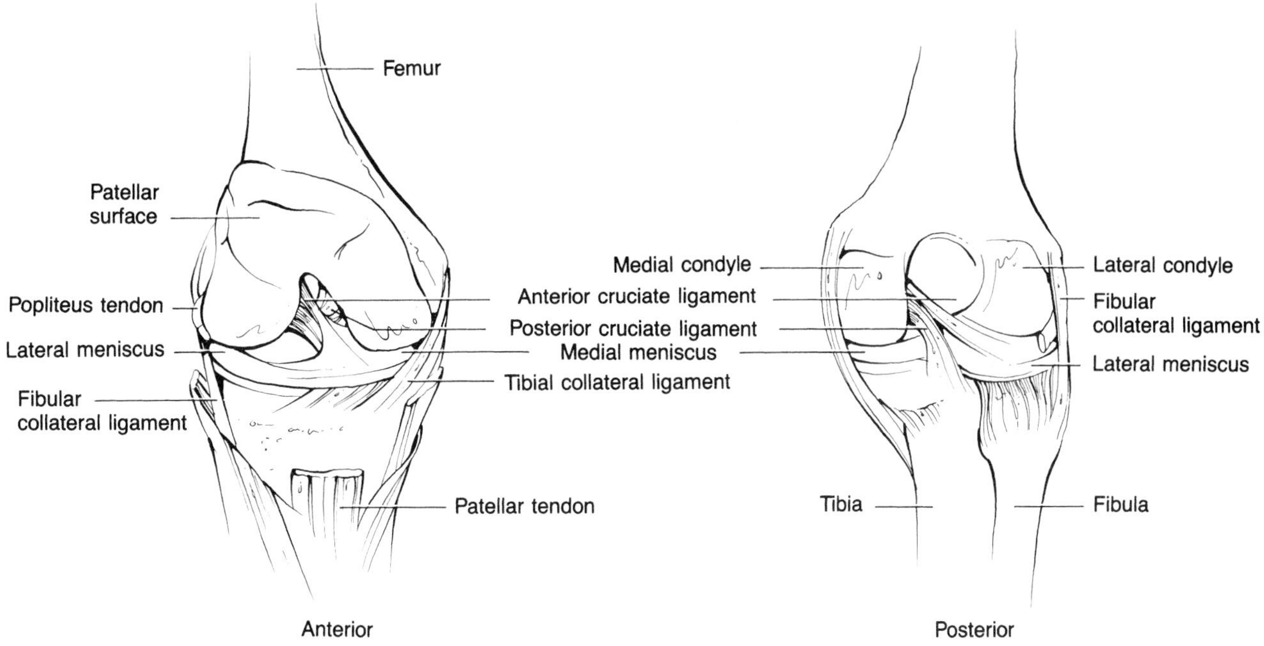

Figure 118.1. Anatomy of the knee.

EMERGENCY DEPARTMENT EVALUATION

The history is extremely helpful in directing the evaluation of a knee injury. The chief complaint, mechanism of injury, and the nature and duration of symptoms help differentiate acute trauma from chronic problems or reinjury.

The mechanism of injury is a key piece of the history. The force, direction, and placement of traumatic stresses, as well as the position of the knee at the time of injury, should be identified. Associated complaints, such as locking of the joint, effusions (and how quickly the fluid accumulated), popping sensations, and ability to ambulate, should be elicited. Any associated injuries, particularly to the hip and ankle, should be evaluated.

The physical examination begins with inspection of the knee and entire limb for obvious deformity, ecchymosis, erythema, edema, or cutaneous lesion. The presence of scars should be noted, as they may indicate previous trauma or surgery. Careful palpation will identify tenderness, crepitus, abnormal skin temperature, or the presence of an effusion.

At this point, if a fracture is suspected, obtain appropriate radiologic studies before performing extensive manipulation of the knee. Recently several clinical decision rules for the use of radiographs in the acutely injured knee have been developed. The Pittsburgh rules classify mechanism of injury (blunt trauma, falls), patient age (less than 12 years, greater than 55 years), and inability to walk (at least four weight-bearing steps) as predictors of fractures.[16] The Ottawa knee rules identify five factors; the presence of any of them indicates that radiographs should be obtained. These are age greater than 55, tenderness at the head of the fibula, isolated tenderness of the patella, inability to flex to 90 degrees, and inability to transfer weight for four steps either immediately after the injury or in the emergency department (ED).[17] Both sets of rules have been demonstrated to be highly sensitive in predicting the presence of fractures and may prove useful for the ED physician in the evaluation of an acute knee injury.

If radiographs are not indicated or are negative, continue assessment of potential injuries, using a systematic examination of the soft tissues, as well as determination of weight-bearing gait. When possible, the unaffected knee should be examined for comparison. Often, it is useful to examine the uninjured joint first to assess normal variability for the patient: Discrepancies between the patient's joints are more important than absolute laxity.[15] Examining the uninjured knee also permits the physician to demonstrate the maneuvers that will be performed, ideally allaying the patient's fears and improving cooperation.

The presence of excessive tenderness and joint effusions may make the examination difficult. Effusions and tensing of the musculature secondary to pain may give the impression of more joint stability than is actually present. Therefore, although it is important to evaluate the patient acutely, it is often necessary in the ED to immobilize the injured knee and provide for a follow-up examination.

Specific Tests for Soft-Tissue Injuries

During each of the following tests, the patient should be as relaxed as possible. Explain the examination to the patient and compare the findings with those of the uninjured knee. If the patient cannot cooperate because of pain, appropriate analgesia or sedation may be necessary. In certain cases, it may be necessary to have the orthopedist perform these tests with the patient under general anesthesia.[15]

Collateral Ligaments

Examine the knee in both full extension and at 30 degrees of flexion (Fig. 118.2).[15] Stabilize the tibia and femur with your hands while applying varus and valgus stresses to the knee, testing the stability of the LCL and MCL, respectively. With a first-degree sprain, there is no laxity at either extension or flexion. A second-degree sprain demonstrates some laxity in flexion (with a solid end point) but no laxity in extension. With a third-degree sprain, there is some laxity in extension and significant laxity in flexion, without a solid end point. Marked opening of the joint in both extension and flexion indicates the possibility of a cruciate ligament disruption in addition to the collateral ligament injury.[15]

Cruciate Ligaments

The Lachman test is the best way to evaluate the ACL clinically.[15] Position the patient supine; stabilize the tibia and femur

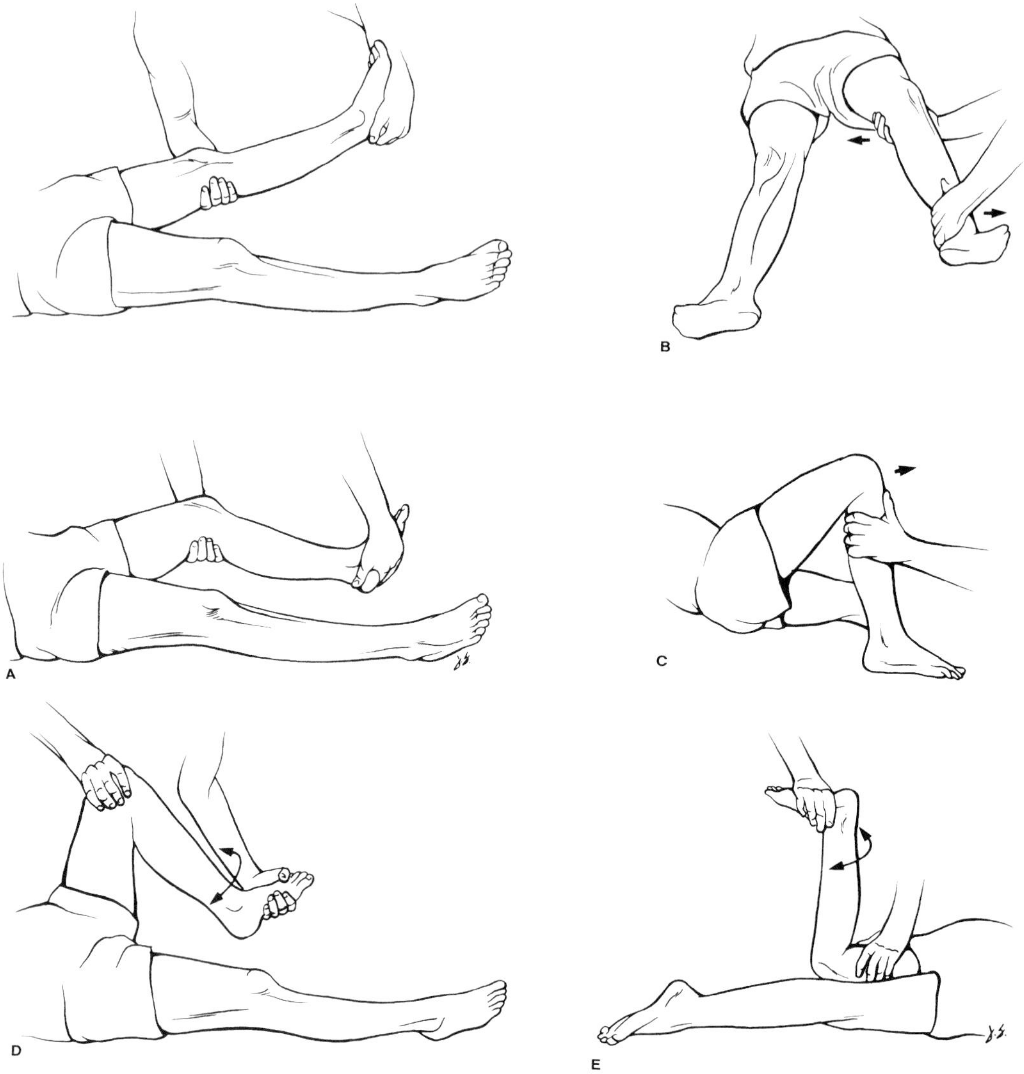

Figure 118.2. Examination of the knee. **(A)** Valgus stress at 0-degree and 30-degree flexion, as viewed from the side. **(B)** Valgus stress at 0-degree flexion, as viewed from above. **(C)** Anterior drawer test. **(D)** McMurray test. **(E)** Apley test.

with your hands and the knee flexed to 20 to 30 degrees. Then pull the tibia anteriorly. Excessive anterior displacement of the tibia relative to the femur and a lack of a distinct end point indicate an ACL rupture.

Although not as sensitive as the Lachman test, the anterior drawer test may also be utilized to evaluate the ACL. Flex the knee to 90 degrees with the foot flat on the stretcher in a neutral position and stabilized (see Fig 118.2). Place anterior force on the tibia. Significant displacement of the tibia anteriorly (compared with the unaffected knee) suggests ACL rupture.[15] This test can also be performed with the foot in 15 degrees of external rotation (Slocum test) and 15 degrees of internal rotation.

Another test of ACL injury is the pivot shift. With the knee in full extension, the leg is lifted by the distal tibia. With an ACL rupture, the tibia is subluxed anteriorly in this position. Then apply a mild valgus force while the knee is carefully flexed to 20 to 40 degrees. At this point, the tibia jumps into a reduced position. Pain may hinder the performance of this test in the acutely injured knee.[8]

The posterior drawer test, the reverse of the anterior drawer, is used to evaluate the PCL. Flex the knee to 90 degrees and secure the foot in a neutral position. Then apply posterior force to the tibia. If the tibia moves posterior to the femoral condyles, the test is positive, representing PCL injury.[15]

An alternative test of PCL injury is the posterior sag. Hold the knee in mild flexion with the thigh supported by a pillow and the foot secured. In this position, the tibia will displace posteriorly, or sag, if the PCL is ruptured.[15]

Meniscus

The McMurray test is used to identify meniscal injury. Hold the knee in one hand, the lower leg or foot in the other. Then apply internal and external rotation to the lower leg while flexing and extending the knee (see Fig. 118.2). Palpate the knee for catching or clicking sensations. Suspect a medial meniscal tear if clicking occurs as the leg is extended and externally rotated after being completely flexed. Clicking with internal rotation during extension is used to help identify a lateral meniscal injury. While a positive test does not guarantee a meniscal injury, it does suggest an intraarticular injury warranting further evaluation.[6]

Another test used to identify meniscal injury is the Apley test. Position the patient prone and flex the knee to 90 degrees. Apply upward force to the tibia while it is rotated and the knee is extended (see Fig. 118.2). Pain and clicking in the joint suggest a meniscal injury.[15]

Patellar Subluxation

The apprehension sign is seen with patellar subluxation. The knee is in extension and the examiner attempts to displace the patella laterally. With patellar subluxations, this manipulation is painful, and the patient, who is typically anxious and apprehensive about this maneuver, will contract the quadriceps.[15]

Other Tests

Plain radiographs are indicated in many knee injuries. Standard anteroposterior and lateral views should be supplemented with sunrise (skyline) and tunnel views to evaluate the patellofemoral joint and intercondylar notch, respectively.[3] Plain films help diagnose fractures, effusions, dislocations, foreign bodies, and calcified loose bodies. Fluid–fluid levels seen on plain radiographs have traditionally been thought to represent lipohemarthrosis (fat floating on synovial fluid) and are thought to be an indication of an occult fracture. While not all fluid–fluid interfaces seen on plain films represent lipohemarthrosis, the presence of such a finding warrants further evaluation utilizing tomography, computed tomography (CT) scanning, or magnetic resonance imaging (MRI).[10]

Plain radiographs give little information on soft-tissue structures, but stress views and arthrography may be used to evaluate soft-tissue injuries. More recently, MRI scanning has become the test of choice for evaluating the soft tissues of the knee. Although more expensive than plain films, MRI scanning has many advantages over plain radiography. MRI scanning involves no ionizing radiation and clearly defines soft-tissue structures. It can also identify subtle injuries, such as bone contusions and occult fractures, not seen on plain films.[10]

Angiography, utilized to evaluate the presence of vascular injury, is indicated in the presence of any penetrating trauma in proximity to vascular structures. Furthermore, it is frequently indicated in the presence of a knee dislocation to rule out an occult injury to the popliteal artery.

Arthrocentesis and joint fluid analysis can be helpful in determining the etiology of a knee effusion. It may be difficult to differentiate hemarthrosis from an infective or inflammatory effusion clinically, particularly if the history is difficult to obtain. Analysis of the joint fluid may point to a diagnosis: For instance, an acute hemarthrosis may suggest an ACL tear, and the presence of lipid droplets in a bloody effusion may signify an occult fracture. The presence of white blood cells may indicate inflammatory or infectious processes. White counts in the range of 20,000 to 60,000 are associated with inflammatory processes; higher counts (greater than 100,000) usually represent infection.[15]

Further studies, such as Gram stain, cultures, crystal analysis, and glucose and protein determinations, are generally performed and provide clues to the etiology of the effusion. Some authors advocate arthrocentesis of acute hemarthrosis for pain relief; others, however, note that after evacuation of an acute hemarthrosis, it may quickly reaccumulate. Therefore, it may be preferable to utilize arthrocentesis in a diagnostic rather than a palliative role.

FRACTURES

Distal Femur

The distal femur is the lower third of the bone. Fractures in this area are typically described relative to the femoral condyles and are separated into supracondylar or intercondylar (Fig. 118.3).

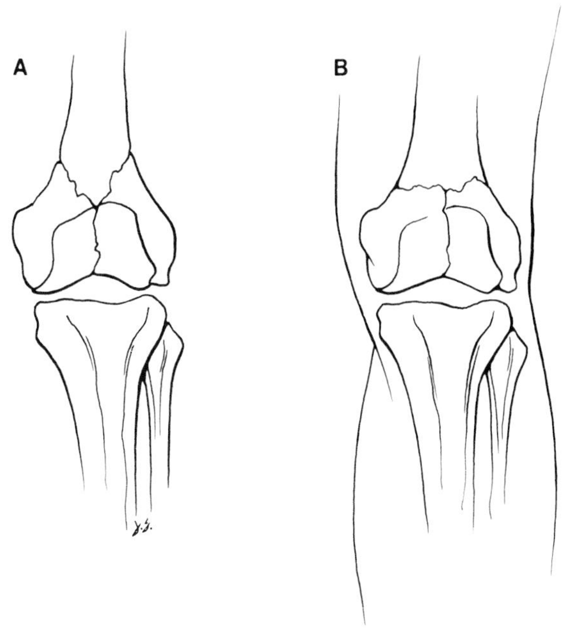

Figure 118.3. Distal femur fractures. **(A)** Y-shaped intercondylar. **(B)** T-shaped intercondylar.

Distal femur fractures account for 4% to 7% of all femur fractures (31% if hip fractures are excluded). They are most often associated with high-energy trauma (e.g., knee to dashboard in high-speed motor vehicle crashes [MVCs]), but they may occur with less violent forces, particularly in the elderly.

EVALUATION

The physical examination typically demonstrates a tender, edematous knee and distal femur. Obvious deformity may be present, and crepitus may accompany movement. If a fracture is suspected, the knee should be immobilized and radiographs obtained. Although neurovascular injuries are uncommon, the proximity of the femoral artery and peroneal nerves to the bone requires that the neurovascular status of the extremity be evaluated and documented. Differential diagnoses include patellar fractures, knee dislocations, and soft-tissue injuries with resulting effusions. Associated injuries, such as hip fractures and dislocations, acetabular fractures, knee dislocations, and proximal tibial fractures, should be suspected and evaluated.

Standard diagnostic tests include anteroposterior and lateral radiographs. Oblique views and tomography help evaluate intracondylar and intraarticular injuries. If vascular trauma is suspected, arteriography should be performed.

MANAGEMENT

Initial management includes immobilization, pain management, and evaluation of concomitant injuries. Early orthopedic consultation is indicated for definitive care (skeletal traction or surgical repair).

Proximal Tibia

Tibial plateau fractures occur as a result of varus–valgus forces, from axial loads, or both. Fractures of the tibial plateau may cause a major impairment in the stability and function of the knee joint. The lateral portion of the tibial plateau is most commonly involved (approximately 80% of cases).[3]

EVALUATION

Clinical findings vary with the severity and type of fracture. There may be gross or only minimal deformity. The knee is usually swollen and tender. The potential for neurovascular injuries is much higher in proximal tibial fracture than in distal femoral fracture. The physician should maintain a high level of suspicion for such injuries and carefully evaluate neurovascular status.[2] The potential for the development of a compartment syndrome is also significant. Paresthesias and paralysis from compartment syndromes may be mistaken for a primary nerve injury. Injuries to the menisci, as well as to the collateral and cruciate ligaments, should be suspected. Deep venous thrombosis (DVT) is another common complication seen with tibial plateau fracture.[1]

Diagnostic tests include plain radiographs, tomography, and CT scans. If a vascular injury is suspected, an arteriogram should be obtained. Doppler studies and venograms may be indicated to exclude DVT. If compartment syndrome is clinically suspected, compartment pressures should be measured.

MANAGEMENT

In addition to the standard management of immobilization and evaluation of other injuries, orthopedic consultation is indicated. Simple fractures may be treated with immobilization; depressed fractures require surgical reduction.

Tibial Spine Fractures

Fractures of the tibial spines generally represent avulsion injuries caused by trauma to the cruciate ligaments. Tibial spine fractures are more common in children, as their ligaments are stronger than their bone. The anterior spine is most commonly affected.[4]

EVALUATION

Clinical examination generally reveals a swollen, tender knee. Because there is a high correlation with ACL injuries, hemarthrosis is common. The most common diagnostic test needed is a plain radiograph. Fractures are usually seen on plain films, but MRI scanning or arthroscopy may be needed to identify associated injuries.

MANAGEMENT

Management involves immobilization and orthopedic referral. Some fractures may be treated nonsurgically, but if significant displacement is present, surgical intervention may be necessary.

Tibial Tuberosity

A fracture of the tibial tuberosity represents an avulsion injury caused by the patellar tendon. This uncommon fracture occurs with either strong flexion or extension of the knee against resistance. It most commonly occurs before closure of the epiphysis.[4]

EVALUATION

Examination reveals tenderness and possible deformity at the site of injury. As this is an extraarticular injury, joint effusion is rare. The differential diagnosis must include Osgood-Schlatter disease in adolescents. Osgood-Schlatter disease is a traction injury to the apophysis of the tibial tuberosity.[11] Although most common in boys ages 10 to 13, it may be seen in girls, usually ages 8 to 13.[4] It is thought that repetitive trauma to the epiphysis results in incomplete separation of parts of the cartilaginous and chondroosseous portions of the tibial tuberosity.[4] Diagnosis is based on the history and physical examination. The tubercle is painful, tender, and usually enlarged. Pain is exacerbated by extension of the knee, particularly against resistance.

The diagnosis of a tibial tuberosity fracture is generally made on plain radiographs. If Osgood-Schlatter disease is suspected, plain radiographs may be difficult to interpret, as fragments of the tuberosity may be a normal variant.[4]

MANAGEMENT

Tibial tuberosity fractures may require open reduction but are usually treated with immobilization.[4] Osgood-Schlatter disease is treated with rest, sometimes plaster cast immobilization, and, rarely, surgical excision of loose ossicles to relieve symptoms.[13]

Patellar Fractures

Patellar fractures may result from direct or indirect forces. Direct forces, as seen with falls and MVCs, are most common. Less common are fractures resulting from severe tension placed on the patella by strong contraction of the quadriceps; the usual result is a transverse fracture, which may disrupt the extensor mechanism.

EVALUATION

Examination generally reveals pain and tenderness over the patella, inability to walk, and, commonly, a joint effusion. If the fracture is significantly displaced, a defect may be palpable. Diagnosis is generally made with plain radiographs. Tomograms and CT scans may identify an occult fracture. A bipartite patella may be confused with a fracture. Often, the margins of a bipartite patella are rounded, but in the setting of acute trauma, it may be difficult to differentiate from an acute fracture.[3]

MANAGEMENT

Therapy is based on the type of fracture, degree of separation, and condition of the extensor mechanism. Orthopedic referral is indicated. Simple fractures are treated with immobilization, but surgery may be indicated in severe cases. As with all fractures about the knee, posttraumatic arthritis is a significant complication.

DISLOCATIONS

Tibiofemoral Joint

Dislocation of the tibiofemoral joint is rare. It is generally associated with high-energy trauma but may be seen with low-energy forces (e.g., stepping in a hole, jumping on a trampoline).[7] The dislocation is described as anterior, posterior, medial, lateral, or rotary based on the position of the tibia relative to the femur. For a dislocation to occur, significant trauma to the surrounding soft tissue is generally seen, including the collateral ligaments, cruciate ligaments, menisci, joint capsule, and neurovascular structures.[2]

EVALUATION

Physical examination may be difficult. Some dislocations spontaneously reduce before the patient arrives at the ED. The patient may relate a history of abnormal position of the joint before reduction. Tenderness, swelling, joint effusion, and deformity may be present. Because of a high incidence of peroneal nerve and popliteal artery injury, specific attention should be devoted to this aspect of the physical examination.[5] The absence of distal pulses highly correlates with significant vascular injury; the presence of pulses, however, does not eliminate the possibility of vascular damage.[12] Considering the common high-force mechanisms of injury and the potential for vascular damage, compartment syndrome is a significant potential complication.

Diagnosis is based on history, physical examination, and plain radiographs. CT scanning may be useful. MRI scanning will identify intraarticular injuries, but it is not commonly used in the acute setting.

For years, arteriography has been used in evaluating knee dislocations. If distal pulses are absent or abnormal, the need for arteriography is obvious. Recently, however, some have advocated the selective use of arteriography. These authors argue that although some patients with intact normal pulses may demonstrate arteriographic evidence of injuries, such as intimal tears, these lesions rarely need surgical intervention.[7,18] Other authors suggest that arteriography is indicated in all patients[2] because of the devastating complications of missed injuries that can lead to limb ischemia and amputation.

MANAGEMENT

Emergency management involves rapid reduction of the dislocation, especially if vascular compromise is evident. It can be accomplished by longitudinal traction (Fig. 118.4). If the clinical status permits, intravenous sedation and analgesia may facilitate the reduction. The limb's neurovascular status must be reassessed periodically, particularly after manipulation. If the patient is stable, appropriate diagnostic tests and orthopedic and vascular surgery consultations should be quickly obtained.

Patella

The patella may be completely dislocated or subluxed from the intercondylar groove as a result of a direct blow or by hyperflexion of the knee joint. The patella almost always displaces laterally. This injury is common in adolescent girls.[11] The patient often reports previous episodes in which subluxations spontaneously reduced.

EVALUATION

The physical examination generally reveals an inability to extend the knee and obvious deformity. A joint effusion is commonly present. The subluxed patella may often reduce spontaneously. The apprehension sign may suggest this injury. Plain

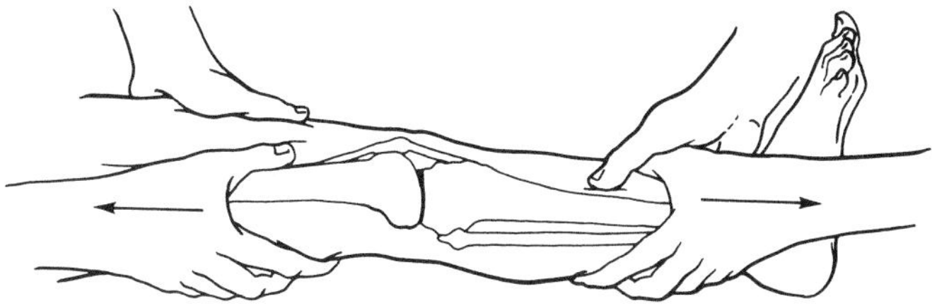

Figure 118.4. Technique for reduction of knee dislocation.

radiographs help confirm the diagnosis if it is not apparent on clinical examination. If the patella has spontaneously reduced, plain films will confirm proper placement and identify any bony injury. If subluxations are recurrent, plain films may assist in the evaluation of the anatomy of the patellofemoral joint and help direct further treatment.

MANAGEMENT

Emergency management of subluxations involves acute reduction. It is usually done by applying medial force to the patella while the knee is being extended. Appropriate sedation and analgesia are often necessary. Once reduced, the knee is immobilized and the patient treated with elevation, ice, and crutches. Complete dislocations often require surgical repair to decrease the incidence of recurrence or subluxation.[14]

SOFT-TISSUE INJURIES

Collateral Ligaments

The collateral ligaments protect the knee from varus and valgus stresses. The MCL is the most commonly injured ligamentous structure in the knee.[11] It is typically injured in sporting events when a direct valgus force is applied to the knee while the foot is relatively stationary. The LCL can also be injured, but injury to it is less likely to occur secondary to athletic events. LCL injuries are more commonly seen with falls and MVCs. MCL and LCL tears are associated with cruciate ligament injuries, with the LCL injury less likely to occur as an isolated event.[11]

EVALUATION

The patient generally presents with tenderness along the distribution of the ligament. There is often a history of "popping" and abnormal bending of the knee. The physical examination should include the previously listed diagnostic tests, with varus and valgus forces applied to the knee at extension and 30 degrees of flexion. The presence of an associated effusion may complicate the examination, warranting a few days of elevation and immobilization prior to reexamination.

MANAGEMENT

Treatment is based on the severity of the injury. First- and second-degree sprains are treated with immobilization, ice, and crutches. Follow-up examination by an orthopedist is required to reevaluate the patient's progress and the need for further intervention (e.g., arthroscopy, surgical repair).

Cruciate Ligaments

Injuries to the cruciate ligaments are common with low-velocity trauma (e.g., football, basketball) as well as with high-energy forces. The patient usually reports a direct anterior or posterior blow to the knee. The cruciates can also be injured by rotational forces, usually in association with other soft-tissue trauma (e.g., collateral ligaments, menisci). The ACL is weaker than the PCL and is more commonly injured.[11]

EVALUATION

The patient often presents with a swollen, tender knee. Seventy percent of patients presenting with an acute, traumatic hemarthrosis have a tear of the ACL. Because the cruciate ligaments are located deep in the articular surface and are associated with a high incidence of joint effusions, clinical diagnosis is often difficult.

Tests for ACL injuries include the Lachman, anterior drawer, and pivot shift tests. The Lachman test is the most sensitive. PCL stability is evaluated by the posterior drawer and posterior sag tests. Plain radiographs are of little value. MRI scanning is the best imaging test to evaluate the cruciate ligaments.

MANAGEMENT

Arthroscopy is used for both diagnosis and treatment. Definitive treatment is based on factors such as the patient's age, level of activity, and the severity of the injury. Initially, immobilization and orthopedic consultation are necessary.

Meniscal Tears

Meniscal injuries generally occur with a twisting force applied to the knee. The twisting may result from relatively minor forces, such as those produced when rising from a squatting position. Patients frequently complain of hearing a "snap" or "pop," which is common but not specific to meniscal injuries. Often, the patient reports locking of the knee, usually a result of a "bucket handle" tear of the meniscus, with a free central portion of the cartilage becoming lodged in the intercondylar notch. The medial meniscus is most commonly affected.

EVALUATION

The patient usually presents with a joint effusion. Unlike the hemarthrosis seen with an ACL rupture, the effusion accumulates much more slowly, generally over 12 to 24 hours. Pain is usually localized to the side of the knee where the tear is located. A decrease in the range of motion is often noted and may be related to the effusion or a loose body. Diagnostic tests include the McMurray and Apley tests. MRI scanning is very helpful in defining the anatomy of the meniscus and in pinpointing injuries.

MANAGEMENT

Arthroscopy is generally reserved for treatment, as the accuracy of the MRI is well documented. Initial treatment consists of immobilization, analgesia, and orthopedic referral. Definitive treatment is based on clinical evaluation. If symptoms persist, meniscectomy is generally performed arthroscopically.

Tendon Injuries

The extensor mechanism includes the quadriceps tendon, the patella, and the patellar tendon. Injuries to these structures, or with avulsion of the tibial tubercle, can disrupt the extensor mechanism. Disruption may result from high-energy or penetrating trauma, but is also seen with low-energy forces. Tendon ruptures associated with low-energy trauma commonly occur when the tendons are weakened (e.g., by gout, arthritis, infection, metabolic diseases, tenosynovitis, previous trauma). If the tendon is already weakened, rupture may occur with forceful contraction of the quadriceps.

Generally, the patellar tendon is least likely to rupture. The quadriceps tendon is more commonly ruptured, and this is usually seen in elderly patients.[9] The quadriceps tendon usually ruptures just proximal to the patella. The patellar tendon frequently ruptures at the insertion into the patella.[9]

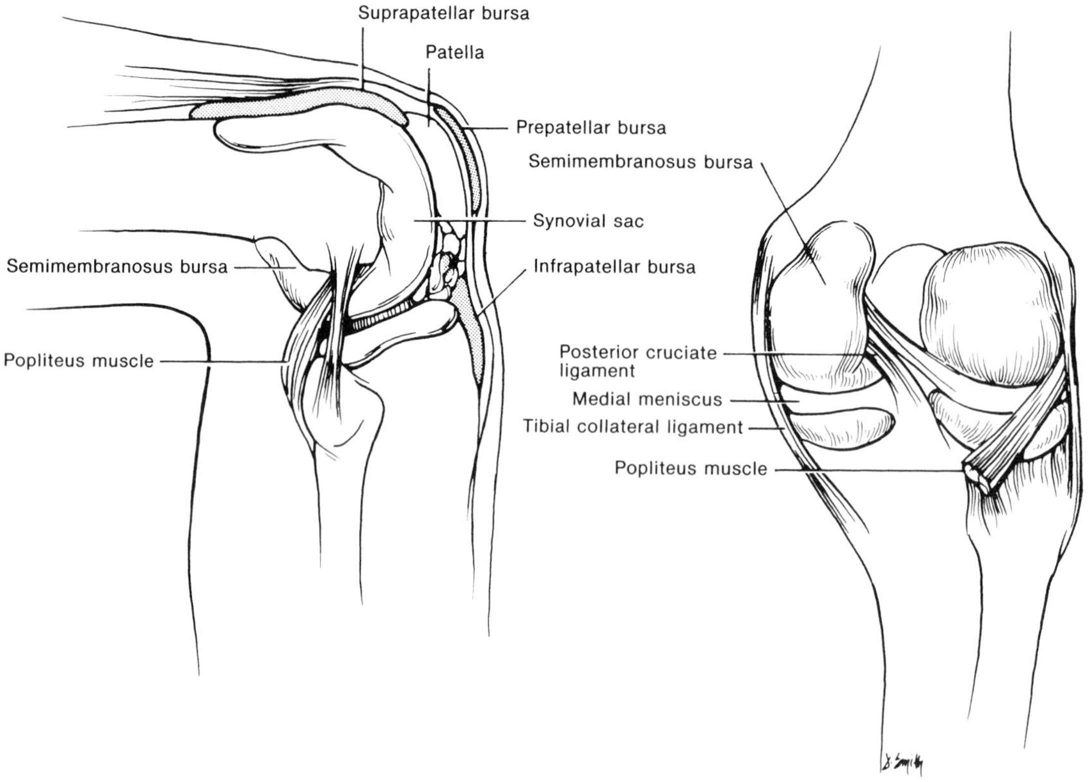

Figure 118.5. Bursae of the knee

EVALUATION

The physical examination generally reveals a swollen, tender knee. A palpable deficit may be present. Tenderness is usually identified at the site of injury. To evaluate the tendons properly, the patient's ability to extend the knee fully against resistance must be tested. The diagnosis is usually suspected clinically; CT and MRI scanning may be used for definitive diagnosis of tendon ruptures.

MANAGEMENT

A complete rupture requires surgical repair. Incomplete ruptures necessitate orthopedic referral for definitive management.

Bursitis

Local inflammation and subsequent bursitis may be a complication of knee trauma. The bursae of the knee are illustrated in Figure 118.5.

EVALUATION

The physical examination often reveals a swollen, tender knee with a localized effusion that is warm to the touch. Other causes of knee swelling (hemarthrosis, infection) should be considered and evaluated. Arthrocentesis and joint fluid analysis are performed if an effusion is present.

MANAGEMENT

If bursitis is suspected, rest, ice, and nonsteroidal antiinflammatory medications are prescribed. The patient is referred to an orthopedist for follow-up.

COMMON PITFALLS

- Failing to examine the hip carefully. Knee pain is often referred from the hip, and knee trauma may precipitate hip injuries.
- Performing a soft-tissue examination in the face of joint effusion and muscle guarding. A period of immobilization and reexamination is indicated after the effusion resolves.
- Mistaking bipartite patella for a patellar fracture
- When evaluating the extensor mechanism, failing to examine the knee in full extension, against resistance
- Overlooking the possibility of proximal fibula fractures and dislocations resulting from ankle injuries
- Failing to consider Osgood-Schlatter disease in an adolescent with knee pain

References

1. Abelseth G, Buckley RE, Pineo GE, et al. Incidence of deep-venous thrombosis in patients with fractures of the lower extremity distal to the hip. *J Orthop Trauma* 1996;10(4):230.
2. Ciottone GR. Upper and lower extremity trauma. In: Aghababian RV, ed. *Emergency medicine. The core curriculum.* New York: Lippincott–Raven Publishers, 1998:1250.
3. Cooper JR, Barrington NA. Pitfalls in radiologic diagnosis of lower limb injuries. *Br J Hosp Med* 1997;58(10):524.
4. Davids JR. Pediatric knee. Clinical assessment and common disorders. *Pediatr Clin North Am* 1996;43(5):1067.
5. Harrell DJ, Spain DA, Bergamini, et al. Blunt popliteal artery trauma: a challenging injury. *Am Surg* 1997;63(3):228.
6. Kim SJ, Min BH, Han DY. Paradoxical phenomena of the McMurray test. *Am J Sports Med* 1996;24(1):83.
7. Kwolek CJ, Sundaram S, Schwarcz TH, et al. Popliteal artery thrombosis associated with trampoline injuries and anterior knee dislocations in children. *Am Surg* 1998;64(12):1183.
8. LaPrade RF, Terry GC. Injuries to the posterolateral aspect of the knee. Association of anatomic injury patterns with clinical instability. *Am J Sports Med* 1997;25(4):433.
9. Levine RJ. Patellar tendon rupture. The importance of timely recognition and repair. *Postgrad Med* 1996;100(2):241.
10. Lugo-Olivieri CH, Scott WW, Zerhouni EA. Fluid-fluid levels in injured knees: do they always represent lipohemarthrosis? *Musculoskel Radiol* 1996;198:499.
11. Maffulli N, Chan KM, Miao, et al. Athletic knee injuries. *Clin Orthop Rel Res* 1996;323:98.
12. Moniz MP, Ombrellaro MP, Stevens SL, et al. Concomitant orthopedic and vascular injuries as predictors for limb loss in blunt lower extremity trauma. *Am Surg* 1997;63(1):24.
13. Nowinski RJ, Mehlman CT. Hypenated history: Osgood-Schlatter disease. *Am J Orthop* 1998;27(8):584.
14. Sallay PI, Poggi J, Speer KP, et al. Acute dislocation of the patella. *Am J Sports Med* 1996;24(1):52.
15. Schenck RL, Heckman JD: Injuries of the knee. *Clin Symp* 1993;45(1):2.
16. Seaburg DC, Yealy DM, Lukens T, et al. Multicenter comparison of two clinical decision rules for the use of radiography in acute, high-risk knee injuries. *Ann Emerg Med* 1998;32(1):8.
17. Steill IG, Wells GA, Hoag RH, et al. Implementation of the Ottawa knee rule for the use of radiography in acute knee injuries. *JAMA* 1997;278(23):2075.
18. Wascher DC, Dvirnak PC, DeCostner TA. Knee dislocations: initial assessment and implications for treatment. *J Orthop Trauma* 1997;11:525.

CHAPTER 119
Injuries of the Ankle and Foot

Daniel R. Martin and Wenzel Tirheimer

LIGAMENTOUS INJURIES OF THE ANKLE

Ankle sprains are the most common sports-related injury,[1] and they comprise 75% of all ankle injuries. They are caused by eversion or inversion of the ankle, usually while the ankle is plantar flexed. More than 90% of all ankle sprains involve the lateral ligaments. Eversion injuries are much less common, often resulting in a avulsion fracture of the medial malleolus.

Ligaments stabilize the talus between the tibia and fibula. Three ligaments provide lateral ankle support: the anterior talofibular, the calcaneofibular, and the posterior talofibular. The anterior talofibular ligament is injured 90% of the time. The broad deltoid ligament supports the medial aspect of the ankle (Fig. 119.1).

EMERGENCY DEPARTMENT EVALUATION

The patient's history can help to differentiate the injury. Several important questions should be asked: How did the injury occur? Has the ankle been injured previously? Is the patient able to ambulate?

The injured ankle should be examined systematically, beginning with the unaffected areas. The ankle is inspected for swelling and ecchymosis. The entire extremity, including the hip and the knee, is palpated for tenderness. The patient's neurovascular status distal to the injury site, including dorsalis pedis and posterior tibial pulses and capillary refill, is assessed. The lateral and medial ligaments are palpated for tenderness. The proximal

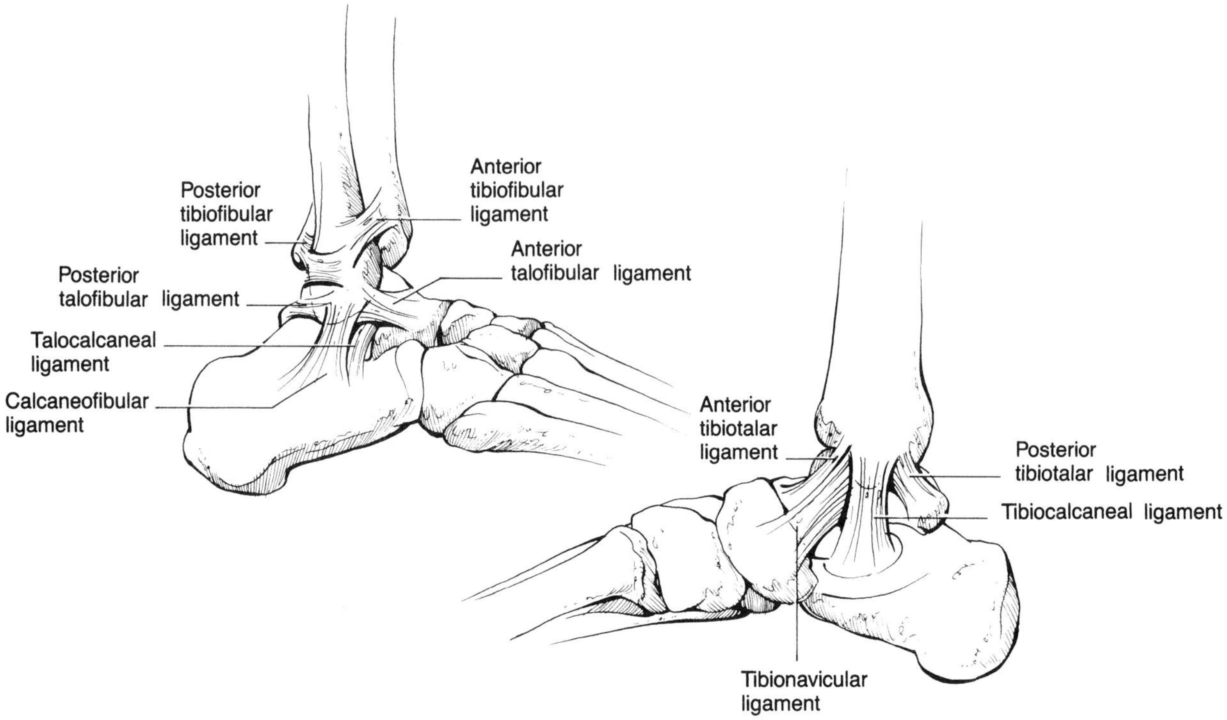

Figure 119.1. Ligaments of the ankle.

fibula and the base of the fifth metatarsal and the navicular bone are palpated to evaluate for an associated fracture.

Provocative Tests for Ankle Stability

The *anterior drawer test* evaluates the anterior talofibular ligament. With the ankle in a neutral position, the lower leg is immobilized with one hand. The physician's other hand holds the hindfoot in slight external rotation and distracts the hindfoot anteriorly. A positive test, greater than 1 cm anterior talar movement or the lack of a distinct end point, indicates anterior talofibular ligament disruption. The *talar tilt test* evaluates whether the ankle mortise opens up medially or laterally. With the ankle again in a neutral position, the ankle is inverted and everted while holding onto the hindfoot. If the talar joint opens as little as 5 degrees radiographically or there is greater than 10 degrees of difference between the injured and unaffected ankles, injury to the calcaneofibular ligament may have occurred. Pain elicited when the tibia and fibula are squeezed together 15 cm below the knee is a positive *squeeze test* and may indicate interosseous membrane disruption. The calf should also be squeezed in all patients with an ankle injury (Thompson test; see section below, Achilles Tendon Rupture) to be certain an Achilles tendon rupture has not occurred. Although the patient's pain and ankle swelling may limit the usefulness of provocative testing, such testing should be attempted in all patients.

Grading Ligamentous Injuries

Although grading remains controversial, it helps to establish criteria for treating ankle sprains. In a grade I injury, the ankle has localized swelling and tenderness, without loss of function or stability. A grade II injury involves more marked swelling and tenderness, as well as significant pain with weightbearing. The anterior drawer test may be positive. A grade III injury involves disruption of at least two of the lateral ligaments. The anterior drawer and talar tilt tests are often positive, and the patient will be unable to bear weight.

Radiographic Evaluation

Routine radiologic views of the ankle include an anteroposterior (AP) view to evaluate for talar shift and malleolar fractures, a mortis view to look for widening of the tibial–talar joint from ligamentous rupture, and a lateral view. Stiell and associates[7] have developed criteria (the Ottawa rules) to assist in determining which patients with acute ankle or midfoot pain require radiographic evaluation. According to these criteria, ankle films are indicated if there is pain near the malleoli and either (1) an inability to bear weight (four steps) both immediately after the injury and in the emergency department or (2) bone tenderness at the posterior edge or inferior tip of the malleolus. Foot films are indicated if there is midfoot pain and (1) an inability to bear weight both immediately after the injury and in the emergency department or (2) bone tenderness over the navicular or base of the fifth metatarsal. Prospective and pooled trials have demonstrated the usefulness of these criteria in reducing the need for radiographic evaluation.[3,5]

EMERGENCY DEPARTMENT MANAGEMENT

The goal of initial treatment is to minimize pain and ankle inflammation. Therapy should include the following, easily remembered by the acronym RICE: *r*est, *i*ce, *c*ompression, and *e*levation. Instruct the patient to rest the ankle and to avoid activities that aggravate the injury. Cryotherapy, 20 minutes four times a day, and compression from an elastic wrap or ankle brace will help reduce pain and swelling. The patient should elevate the involved extremity whenever sitting or lying down.

Treatment of mild-to-moderate sprains centers around early mobilization.[9] Early mobilization encourages stronger and faster soft-tissue healing and less muscle atrophy, inflammation, and inconvenience. Pneumatic compression braces and other marketed supports prevent recurrent ankle inversion or eversion but do not impede dorsiflexion or plantarflexion.

Although grade I and II sprains are treated with immobilization and protected weightbearing, grade III injuries may require cast immobilization for 3 to 6 weeks. All grade III ankle sprains should be splinted and immediately referred to an orthopedist for follow-up.

DISPOSITION

All ankle sprains can be discharged home with appropriate follow-up. Orthopedic or sports medicine consultation should be considered for all ankle sprains. Grade I and II sprains should be treated with compression, such as a pneumatic brace and early mobilization, including exercise recommendations. Referral to the patient's primary care physician or to a specialist within 7 days should be arranged if pain persists or if the patient has not returned to normal activity. Grade III sprains should be referred to an orthopedist within 1 to 2 weeks to change the splint to cast immobilization, if indicated. Other recommended reasons for orthopedic referral, according to Swain and Holt,[8] include (1) a "pop" that is felt or heard, (2) prolonged recovery, (3) a history of several previous injuries, (4) medial ankle tenderness, or (5) a positive squeeze test or other stress test.

FRACTURES OF THE ANKLE

The ankle can be conceptualized as a closed "ring" surrounding the hindfoot. If this ring is disrupted in two or more places, instability occurs. A fracture of the ankle may indicate severe coexistent ligamentous disruption or dislocation, and a thorough neurovascular examination must be performed. The ankle should be properly splinted until such consultation is possible. Open fractures and neurovascular compromise necessitate emergent orthopedic consultation. Although not well supported in the literature, it is widely recommended that open fractures receive intravenous antibiotics. Stable, uncomplicated fractures should have outpatient follow-up within 7 days.

DISLOCATIONS OF THE ANKLE

Ankle dislocations require a large degree of force, owing to the bony anatomy of the ankle.[4] They are commonly associated with ankle fractures. The talus most commonly dislocates posteriorly on the distal tibia.

EMERGENCY DEPARTMENT EVALUATION

Skin tenting and evidence of neurovascular compromise are indications for immediate reduction. In uncomplicated dislocations, radiographs should precede attempts at reduction.

EMERGENCY DEPARTMENT MANAGEMENT

The examining physician may require two assistants to perform closed reduction of ankle dislocations. For posterior dislocations, the first assistant flexes the knee to 45 degrees and applies countertraction over the calf. The second assistant pushes down on the front of the lower leg. The physician applies traction to the heel and forefoot, first plantarflexing the foot and then lifting the heel (Fig. 119.2). For anterior dislocations, the first assistant flexes the knee to 45 degrees and applies countertraction over the calf. The second assistant lifts up on the lower leg. The physician dorsiflexes the foot initially to disengage the talus and then pushes downward on the foot (Fig. 119.3). For lateral dislocations, the physician applies longitudinal traction to the foot, with one hand on the heel and the other on the dorsum of the foot. With assistants applying counteraction to the leg, the physician then manipulates the foot medially.

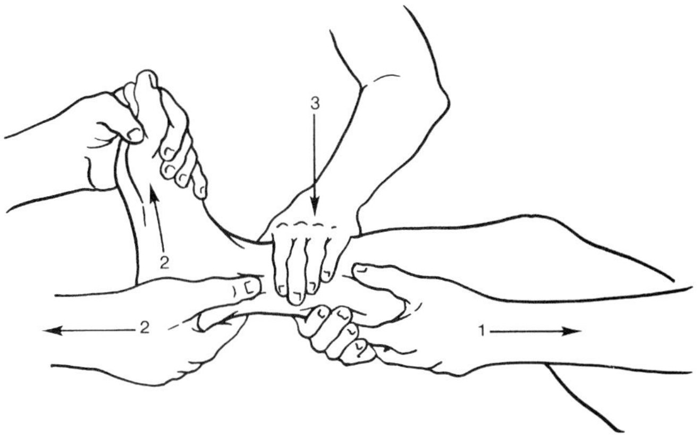

Figure 119.2. Technique of reduction of posterior dislocation of the ankle.

Most patients require open reduction and internal fixation to effect reduction of either anterior or posterior dislocations. If closed reduction is successful, a posterior splint should be initially applied and replaced with a short leg cast once swelling has decreased. The patient should be admitted. The patient should not bear weight on that extremity for approximately 6 weeks.

DISPOSITION

Dislocations or fracture–dislocations that cause neurovascular compromise require emergent reduction by the emergency medicine physician to restore proper anatomic alignment. It is important that such injuries be reduced prior to transferring the patient to another facility. Open injuries or fracture dislocations without neurovascular compromise require emergent orthopedic consultation for an attempt at closed reduction or open reduction and internal fixation, if needed. These injuries should be properly splinted prior to transfer. Closed fractures without neurovascular compromise and good anatomic alignment should be splinted, and arrangements should be made for orthopedic consultation within 48 to 72 hours.

MISCELLANEOUS ANKLE INJURIES

Other possible soft-tissue and bony injuries must also be considered. Injury to the deltoid ligament is usually accompanied by either a proximal fibula fracture (Maisonneuve fracture) or a

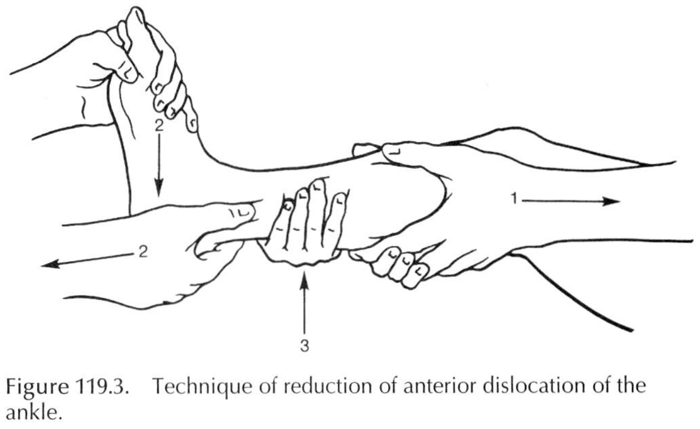

Figure 119.3. Technique of reduction of anterior dislocation of the ankle.

disruption of the tibiofibular syndesmosis. These injuries are especially common with eversion injuries. Patients with a syndesmotic injury often prefer to walk on their toes, and the squeeze test will elicit pain. These injuries require proper splinting and orthopedic consultation within 48 to 72 hours.

Achilles Tendon Rupture

Rupture of the Achilles tendon may present somewhat similarly to an ankle injury. The patient may recall hearing a "pop" and subsequently being unable to bear weight on the leg. Achilles tendon rupture often affects middle-aged men involved in an athletic endeavor. The tendon rupture generally occurs at the narrowest portion of the tendon, about 5 cm above its calcaneal attachment. The left Achilles tendon ruptures more frequently than the right. Tendinitis or steroid injections may be risk factors for tendon rupture.

EMERGENCY DEPARTMENT EVALUATION

On examination, the patient may exhibit weakened plantarflexion. There may be an obvious defect in the tendon 2 to 6 cm proximal to its insertion on the calcaneus. Failure of the foot to plantarflex when the physician squeezes the calf, with the patient prone and the knee flexed to 90 degrees, indicates a positive Thompson test and probable Achilles tendon rupture.

EMERGENCY DEPARTMENT MANAGEMENT

Emergency department management consists of placing the leg in a posterior splint, with the foot in passive equinus. An orthopedist should be consulted.

DISPOSITION

Once this injury is properly splinted, orthopedic consultation should be accomplished within 48 to 72 hours, as there is evidence that early surgical repair of this injury results in a better outcome.

FOOT INJURIES

The foot is divided anatomically into the hindfoot, midfoot, and forefoot. The hindfoot includes the calcaneus and talus; the midfoot includes the navicular, cuboid, and cuneiforms; and the forefoot includes the metatarsals and phalanges. The Chopart joint separates the hindfoot from the midfoot, and the Lisfranc joint separates the midfoot from the forefoot (Fig. 119.4).

Plantar Fasciitis

The plantar fascia extends from the os calcis to the flexor apparatus of the toes. Overuse, as from hill running or sprinting; poor arch support; and poor foot mechanics may contribute to cause inflammation and thus, plantar fasciitis.

PRESENTATION AND EMERGENCY DEPARTMENT EVALUATION

Patients with plantar fasciitis often note pain in the sole and heel of the foot that is worse in the mornings or when climbing stairs. Pain may be elicited by palpation of the plantar fascia. Radiographic evaluation is usually not indicated unless the pain is localized, significant trauma has occurred, or a stress fracture is suspected.

EMERGENCY DEPARTMENT MANAGEMENT

The pain of plantar fasciitis subsides with rest, ice, and antiinflammatory drugs. Referral to an orthopedist, sports medicine physician, or physical therapist is appropriate to evaluate the patient for an orthotic device or exercise program.

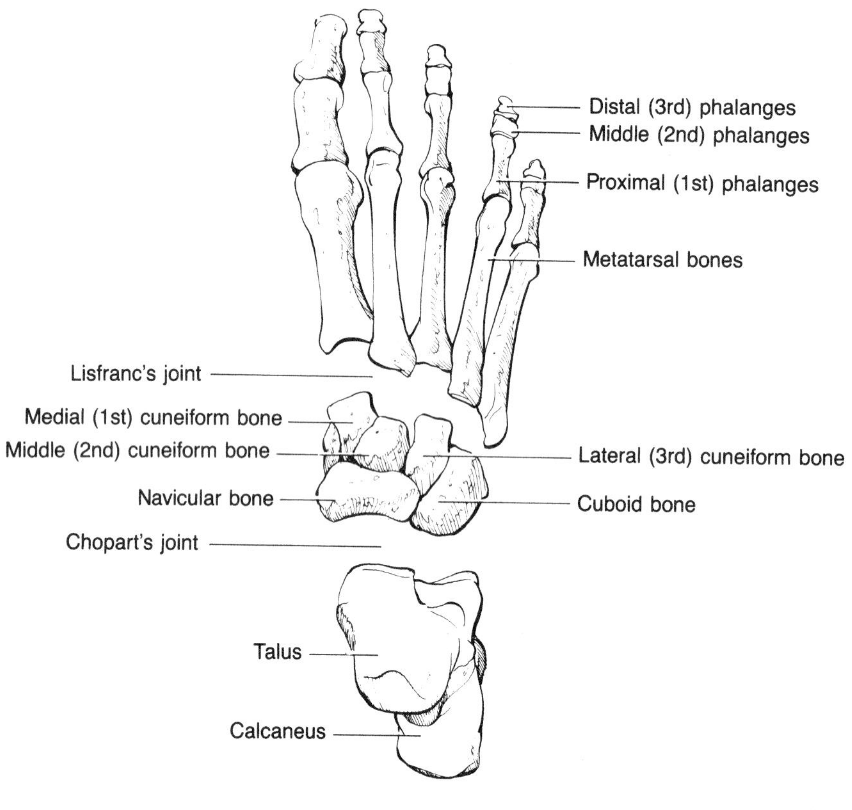

Figure 119.4. Bones of the foot.

DISPOSITION

Although crutches and decreased weightbearing are rarely indicated, consultation, as previously outlined, should be arranged within 1 to 2 weeks.

Turf Toe

Turf toe refers to a sprain of the great toe's metatarsophalangeal joint. Pushing off a severely dorsiflexed great toe causes the injury.

EMERGENCY DEPARTMENT EVALUATION AND MANAGEMENT

The area over the metatarsophalangeal joint is painful, swollen, and tender. Radiographic evaluation to rule out fracture may be indicated. A stiff-soled shoe that limits dorsiflexion at the metatarsophalangeal joint provides significant relief.

DISPOSITION

These patients respond well to rest, ice, and antiinflammatory agents. Orthopedic or sports medicine consultation may be needed if symptoms persist for more than 1 to 2 weeks.

Calcaneal Fractures

Calcaneal fractures account for 1% to 2% of all fractures. The calcaneus is the tarsal bone that is most often fractured. Calcaneal fractures occur in persons aged 30 to 50 years old, with men being affected five times more often than women. The calcaneus fractures under vertical compression. Typically, this occurs in a fall. These fractures are commonly (10%) associated with compression fractures of the dorsolumbar spine, and 25% are associated with other lower extremity fractures.

EMERGENCY DEPARTMENT EVALUATION

If a calcaneal fracture is suspected, three radiographic views of the heel should be obtained: AP, lateral, and axial. On the lateral radiograph, the angle formed by a line extending along the superior aspects of the os calcis and another line extending from the dome to the anterior tubercle, which is referred to as Böhler's angle, should be measured. A normal angle ranges from 20 degrees to 40 degrees. An angle of less than 20 degrees indicates a calcaneal fracture.

EMERGENCY DEPARTMENT MANAGEMENT

A minimum-to-severe disability may result from calcaneal fractures, and the degree of residual symptoms does not always correlate with the degree of subtalar joint disruption. Postinjury pain may result from a number of sources. These injuries are best managed in consultation with an orthopedic surgeon because of the potential for complications.

DISPOSITION

These injuries are best managed with emergent orthopedic consultation. They should be splinted, and the patient should do no weightbearing until such consultation can be accomplished.

Talus Fractures

Fractures of the talus are the second most common foot fractures. The talus fractures as a result of midfoot hyperdorsiflexion. Such a mechanism often occurs in motor vehicle accidents, when the foot is braced against the brake pedal. The tenuous blood supply to the talus makes it vulnerable to avascular necrosis when injured, especially if the fracture occurs through the neck.

Lisfranc Fracture–Dislocation

The midfoot is the least mobile portion of the foot, making it the most susceptible to direct trauma. A fracture–dislocation through the Lisfranc joint, usually involving a fracture of the second cuneiform with dislocation of the lateral four metatarsals, may result from a motor vehicle accident. Hyperdorsiflexion of the forefoot on the midfoot causes the forefoot to dislocate dorsally. Lisfranc fractures are rare (one in 55,000 per year), but delays in treatment, caused by a 20% rate of missed diagnoses, may result in significant morbidity.

PRESENTATION AND EMERGENCY DEPARTMENT EVALUATION

The foot is usually very swollen and painful. Ross and associates[6] describe a consistent physical finding of a well-defined plantar ecchymosis in Lisfranc fractures. A fracture through the second metatarsal base may indicate disruption at a Lisfranc joint. The oblique radiograph may demonstrate widening between the first and second metatarsal bases, which suggests subluxation. In more subtle injuries, abduction stress radiographs may reveal disruption of the medial column line (a line tangential to the medial aspect of the navicular and medial cuneiform that should intersect the base of the first metatarsal).[2] Figure 119.5 illustrates a Lisfranc dislocation.

EMERGENCY DEPARTMENT MANAGEMENT

Most tarsometatarsal dislocations require open reduction and internal fixation to effect accurate reduction and stabilization. Closed reduction in the emergency department should be considered only when marked displacement and neurovascular compromise are present.

DISPOSITION

These injuries require splinting, no weightbearing, and emergent orthopedic consultation.

Fifth Metatarsal Fractures

The most common metatarsal fracture occurs through the base of the fifth metatarsal. Two distinct fractures may occur at the proximal end of the fifth metatarsal. An avulsion fracture by the peroneus brevis tendon results from plantarflexion and inversion of the foot. Another commonly seen fracture through the base of the metatarsal is a transverse fracture through the tuberosity. This fracture is common in athletes. Both of these fractures are relatively stable and can be treated conservatively with a hard-soled shoe, unless the fracture fragment is markedly displaced. A Jones fracture differs from the other two fractures in that it occurs at the metatarsal diaphysis distal to the tuberosity. Jones fractures have a higher incidence of nonunion or delayed union in comparison with avulsion fractures.

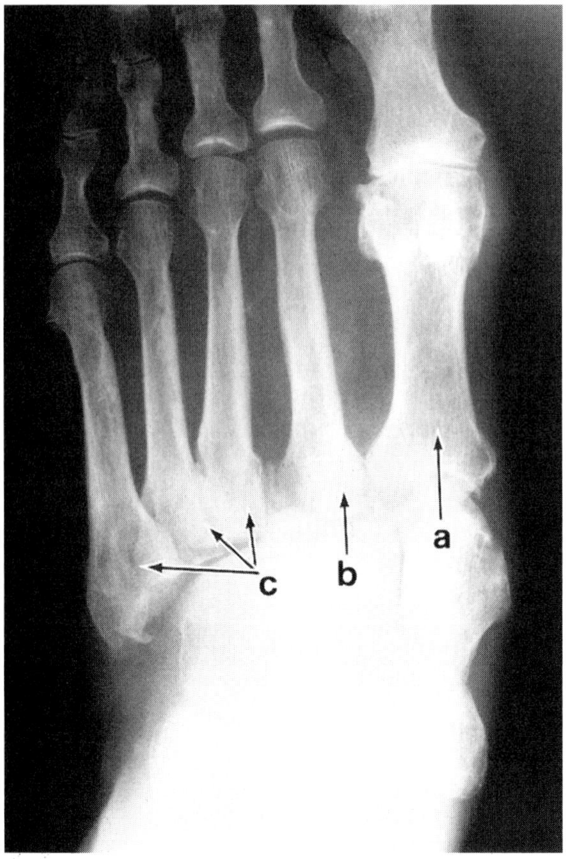

Figure 119.5. Radiograph of a Lisfranc dislocation: **(a)** first metatarsal; **(b)** second metatarsal; **(c)** third, fourth, and fifth metatarsals, which have been dislocated laterally.

DISPOSITION

Orthopedic consultation should be obtained when a Jones fracture is identified, because athletic patients are usually managed operatively. In the nonathlete, this injury is treated with a walking cast for 4 to 6 weeks and then the wearing of a hard-soled shoe. Sports participation is avoided until a secure union is achieved. If nonunion or a recurrent fracture occurs, screw fixation is the preferred treatment.

Second and Third Metatarsal Fractures

Because of the stresses incurred while pushing off, the second and third metatarsals are particularly prone to stress fractures. Initial radiographs may not reveal the fracture line. Radiographs performed 2 to 3 weeks later will likely show callus formation and periosteal reaction. If the fracture is not evident on follow-up films but symptoms persist, a bone scan should be considered. Radionuclide scanning is sensitive for stress fractures but not highly specific, because tumors and infections also result in positive scans.

DISPOSITION

Stress fractures require close orthopedic follow-up. Initial management includes cessation of any pain-producing activity, followed by a rehabilitation program and biomechanics evaluation.

Metatarsophalangeal and Interphalangeal Dislocations

In metatarsophalangeal dislocations, the phalanx commonly dislocates dorsal to the metatarsal. In interphalangeal dislocations, the distal phalanx may dislocate either volar or dorsal to the proximal phalanx. Dislocation is usually clinically evident, but radiographs should be obtained to rule out associated fracture. If no fracture is coexistent, the dislocation can usually be reduced by applying longitudinal traction in the direction of the dislocated phalanx with either dorsal or volar pressure (Fig. 119.6).

DISPOSITION

With successful reduction, the toe is "buddy-taped" to the adjacent toe for 3 to 4 weeks. If reduction is unsuccessful, the flexor tendon or joint capsule may be entrapped. Open reduction may be necessary.

COMMON PITFALLS

- Failure to palpate the base of the fifth metatarsal and navicular bone to evaluate for associated fracture when addressing ankle sprains
- Failure to evaluate for Maisonneuve fracture and syndesmotic injury with deltoid ligament injuries or ankle sprains
- Prolonged immobilization of grade I and II ankle sprains rather than early mobilization and exercises
- Failure to consider Achilles tendon rupture in the patient with "ankle pain"

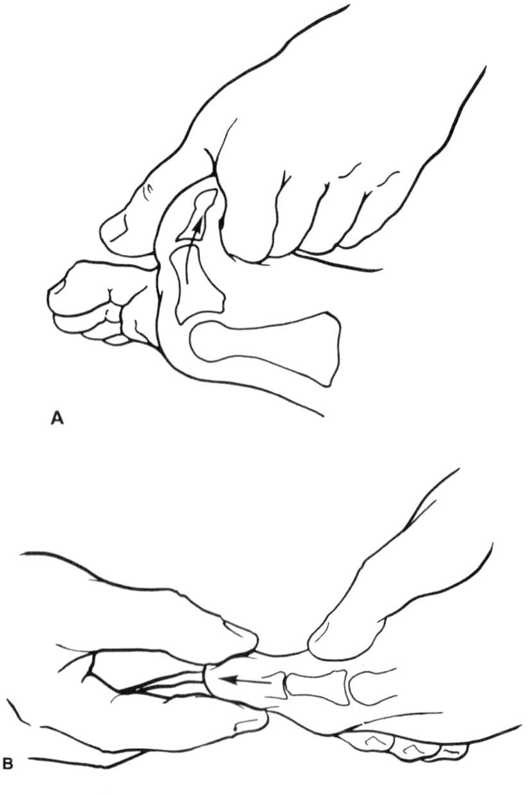

Figure 119.6. Technique of reduction of metatarsophalangeal dislocation of the great toe.

- Failure to differentiate a Lisfranc fracture–dislocation from a simple metatarsal fracture
- Failure to differentiate a Jones fracture from a simple proximal fifth metatarsal fracture

References

1. Balduini FC, Vegso JJ, Torg JS, et al. Management and rehabilitation of ligamentous injuries to the ankle. *Sports Med* 1987;4:364.
2. Coss HS, Manos RE, Buoncristiani A, et al Abduction stress and AP weightbearing radiography of purely ligamentous injury in the tarsometatarsal joint. *Foot Ankle* 1998;19(8):537.
3. Leddy JJ, Smolinski RJ, Lawrence J, et al. Prospective evaluation of the Ottawa ankle rules in a university sports medicine center. *Am J Sports Med* 1998;26(2):158.
4. Linscott MS. Joint dislocations. In: Harwood-Nuss A, ed. *Clinical practice of emergency medicine,* 2nd ed. Philadelphia: Lippincott–Raven Publishers, 1996.
5. Markert RJ, Walley ME, Guttman TG, et al. A pooled analysis of the Ottawa ankle rules used on adults in the ED. *Am J Emerg Med* 1998;16(6):564.
6. Ross G, Cronin R, Hauzenblas J, et al. Plantar ecchymosis sign: a clinical aid to diagnosis of occult Lisfranc tarsometatarsal injuries. *J Orthop Trauma* 1996:10(2):119.
7. Stiell IG, Greenberg GH, McKnight RD, et al. Decision rules for the use of radiography in acute ankle injuries. *JAMA* 1993;269:1127.
8. Swain FA, Holt WS. Ankle injuries, tips from sports medicine physicians. *Postgrad Med* 1993;93:91.
9. Wilkerson GB. Treatment of ankle sprains with external compression and early mobilization. *Phys Sportsmed* 1985;13:83.

PART IV

Special Considerations

CHAPTER 120
Replantation

Steven C. Larson and Iris M. Reyes

Replantation is defined as the reattachment of a completely amputated body part, while *revascularization* is the reconstruction of a partially or incompletely amputated part. With the advent of refined instrumentation and surgical techniques, success rates approaching 90% have been reported for both the replantation of complete amputations and the revascularization of partial amputations.[16] As a result, emergency department physicians should consider all patients with complete amputations potential candidates for replantation, and all patients with partial amputations candidates for revascularization.

Partial and complete amputations occur equally often. Distal amputations are more common than proximal amputations. Sharp, guillotine-type injuries suffer less tissue destruction, devitalization, and contamination and heal better than crushing and degloving injuries. Most amputations and crush injuries of the extremities occur in patients between the ages of 20 and 40, with males predominating over females by a margin of 4:1.[1,9] Up to 65% of these amputations are characterized as local crush wounds; the rest are divided between sharp injuries and diffuse crush wounds.

While advances in microvascular surgery have permitted surgical subspecialists to replant fingers, toes, extremities, ears, noses, penises, and virtually any musculoskeletal tissue, the media have propagated unrealistic expectations among the public about the success of replanting amputated body parts. The cost to the patient in dollars, repeated surgery, prolonged rehabilitation, and time lost from productive activity can be great. A replanted body part has little functional value to the patient if it is disfiguring or has unsatisfactory neurologic function, cold intolerance, or pain. Anticipation of good functional recovery has become the critical factor when considering revascularization of a severed body part. The cost of replanting a single distal phalanx may be excessive when disability and rehabilitation costs are included.[8]

Although the success rate in children is somewhat less than in adults, replanted limbs that remain viable have better return of function and usually have less pain and cold intolerance and better two-point discrimination than in adults. About 80% of continued longitudinal bone growth can be expected in children with replanted extremities.[4]

EMERGENCY DEPARTMENT EVALUATION

Indications for Replantation

While the final decision regarding microvascular repair rests with the surgical team and the patient, the emergency physician must be aware of the factors that influence the decision to perform replantation or revascularization (Table 120.1). There are no absolute indications for microvascular repair; however, general indications and contraindications are listed in Table 120.2. The decision to operate on patients with one or more relative contraindications is made on an individual basis. Contraindications are weighed by the treating surgeon and are considered when attempting to predict outcome. As a rule, even if the possibility of replantation seems remote, the treating emergency physician should manage the stump and amputated tissue as if they were suitable for replantation or revascularization.

Classically, the indications for replantation of upper extremity amputations include multiple digits, thumb, wrist or forearm, sharp amputations with minimum-to-moderate avulsion proximal to the elbow, single digits amputated between the proximal interphalangeal joint and the distal interphalangeal joint (distal to the flexor digitorum superficialis insertion), and amputations in children.[16]

Injuries to the distal phalanx less than 1 cm^2 may be allowed to heal by secondary intention. Granulation tissue and wound contraction will yield satisfactory functional and cosmetic results. Advancement flap skin grafts or pinch skin grafts may be used to cover larger wounds.

A solitary digit is less likely to be restored sufficiently to improve hand function (excluding the thumb) and is often not a candidate for replantation.[2] An exception is noted with amputations of digits distal to the insertion of the flexor digitorum superficialis (between the proximal interphalangeal and distal interphalangeal joints). With amputations at this level of the middle phalanx, an undisturbed superficial flexor tendon will provide up to 82 degrees of proximal interphalangeal joint motion.[2,16]

Multiple-digit injuries, unlike single-digit amputations, mandate attempted repair to maximize functional recovery.

TABLE 120.1. Predictors of Replantation Outcome

Favorable Outcome	Poor Outcome
Young age	Elderly
Healthy	Systemic disease
Sharp injury	Diffuse crush injury
Short ischemic time	Long ischemic time
Appropriate ED care	Proximal injury
Motivated patient	Poorly motivated

TABLE 120.2. Indications and Contraindications for Replantation

INDICATIONS
Young, healthy patient
Thumb or multiple digits
Sharp, guillotine injury
Upper extremity
RELATIVE CONTRAINDICATIONS
Single digit, except thumb
Avulsion injury
Prolonged ischemia
Gross contamination
Previous injury or surgery to part
Emotionally unstable
Lower extremity amputations
ABSOLUTE CONTRAINDICATIONS
Associated life threats
Severe crush injury
Unable to tolerate anesthesia or surgery

From Dalsey WC. Management of amputated part. In: Robert JR, Hedges JR, eds. *Clinical procedures in emergency medicine*. Philadelphia: WB Saunders, 1985.

Toe-to-hand transfers may improve opposition and grasping mechanisms for mutilating injuries of the hand involving the thumb or fifth digit. The thumb is the most important digit of the hand, and only the carpometacarpal joint is required to preserve functional opposition.[16] An injured thumb is usually replanted or revascularized.[6] Revision of the thumb amputation, pollicization of other digits, and toe-to-hand transfers may be acceptable alternatives if reimplantation is not an option.[6,12]

Proximal amputations at the metacarpal or wrist levels are associated with devastating loss of hand function; replantation often yields suprisingly good results.[2] Amputations of the hand at the midpalm or carpal tunnel level may be successfully replanted up to 70% of the time.[9,18] Conversely, amputations proximal to the distal forearm and elbow are often complicated by severe avulsion or crush injury components, making them prone to muscle necrosis, infection, and functional failure.[16] Functional recovery is less satisfactory the more proximal the injury. Nevertheless, some surgeons have reported successful upper extremity replantation rates as high as 90%.[17]

Traumatic amputations of the lower extremities are rare. Successful replantation of the legs has been performed with acceptable functional recovery.[3] Russian surgeons successfully replanted both lower legs of a 3-year-old girl that were severed in a mower accident.[5] Seven years after the injury, and after additional surgery to correct leg-length discrepancy, the girl enjoyed all of her usual activities.

Successful replantations of the penis, ears, nose, and avulsed scalp have been reported.[11,14,19] Cosmetic results are improved with the preservation of tissue. Penile replantation provides urethral competence in most cases, but sexual dysfunction is common.

EMERGENCY DEPARTMENT MANAGEMENT

Resuscitation and Initial Assessment

The initial evaluation and management of patients presenting with upper extremity amputations is aimed at stabilization of the patient and preservation of the limb and its components.[16] Patients with amputated limbs are treated with urgency. Although these injuries are dramatic, they cannot be allowed to distract the treating physician from more severe life-threatening injuries. Airway management, when indicated, and the placement of two large-bore intravenous lines are imperative. Hemodynamic instability is aggressively corrected with crystalloid solution or blood. Coexistent life threats are addressed before attention is directed toward the injured extremity.

Bleeding may be profuse in partially amputated limbs but minimal in guillotine-type injuries, owing to vessel retraction and spasm. Direct pressure and elevation are usually sufficient to control hemorrhage. The blind use of ligature, clamps, hemostats, or occlusive tourniquets must be avoided; these maneuvers may damage nerve tissue and blood vessels, rendering a limb unsuitable for replantation. If bleeding is uncontrollable, a blood pressure cuff placed on the proximal limb and inflated to 30 mm Hg above the systolic blood pressure may allow direct pressure and elevation to become effective.

The history explores the factors that will affect the decision to attempt replantation. The time and mechanism of injury, the inflicting agent, and the onset of cooling are noted. Medical history, last meal, allergies, tetanus status, and smoking history are recorded. Vocations, hobbies, handedness, lifestyle, and attitudes or religious beliefs toward replantation may influence the decision to amputate or replant.

Broad-spectrum antibiotics, such as first-generation cephalosporins, are given intravenously as soon as feasible.[10] Wound cultures may be obtained before starting antibiotics, if warranted. Preoperative laboratory studies are ordered and tetanus toxoid is given, if indicated.

Evaluation and Initial Care of the Limb

The stump and amputated part are irrigated with copious quantities of normal saline or lactated Ringer's solution to remove gross contaminants. No amputated part should be discarded until carefully inspected by the surgical team; a completely amputated body part, even if not suitable for replantation, may serve as a donor source for skin, bone, or vessel grafts.[16] Alcohol, povidone–iodine, or formaldehyde-containing solutions are avoided. The limb is handled as little as possible; exploration, debridement, and dissection are deferred to the microvascular surgeon. All constricting bands, tourniquets, and jewelry are removed. The proximal stump (as well as the amputated part, in the case of partial amputations) is evaluated for distal pulses, capillary refill, motor and reflex function, sensation, and two-point discrimination.

The absolute length of time an amputated limb can tolerate ischemia and still undergo successful replantation is unknown. The longer the ischemic time, the greater the likelihood of failure, particularly when rapidly necrosing muscle and connective tissue are involved. When amputated parts are preserved at or near room temperature, it is referred to as "warm ischemia," which may be tolerated for 6 to 8 hours. Cold preservation, or "cold ischemia," may extend the time an amputated part remains viable up to 12 to 24 hours.[13] Intracellular ATP is preserved and cellular acidosis delayed when tissue is cooled to 10°C, although no further benefit is gained by cooling amputated parts to 1°C.[15] One hour of warm ischemia is approximately equal to 6 hours of cold ischemia.[16] Cold ischemia has allowed amputated digits to be replanted 30 hours after injury.[9] The ischemic time is one of many factors that should influence the success of replantation surgery and should not be considered the sole predictor of viability (see Table 120.1).

Amputated tissue is wrapped in sterile, saline-moistened dressings and placed in a sealed plastic bag immersed in an "ice-and-water slurry" (Fig. 120.1). The tissue must not be placed directly on ice and must not be allowed to freeze. Partial amputa-

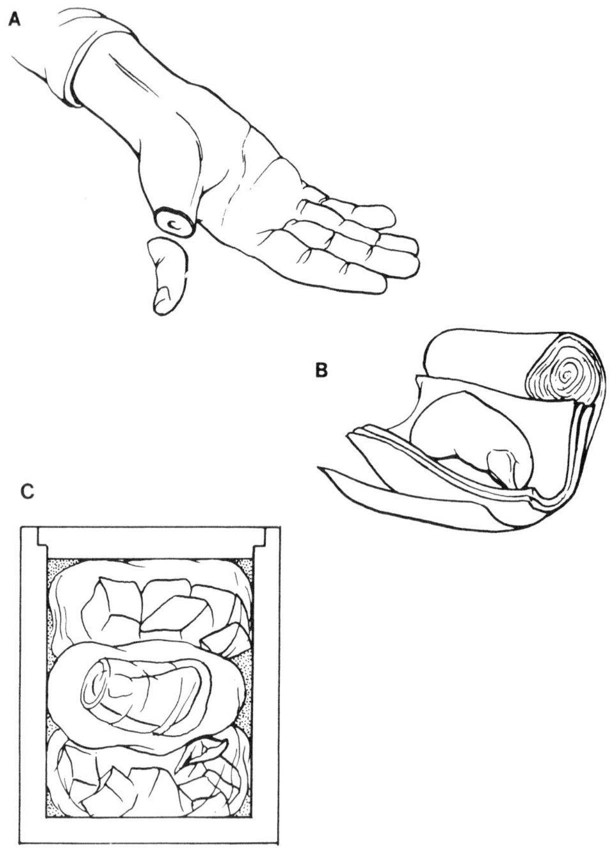

Figure 120.1. Replantation. Evaluate the patient's condition to ensure that he or she does not need to be resuscitated before transfer. **(A)** The wound should be rinsed with saline solution. *Do not scrub or apply antiseptic solution to the wound.* Apply dry sterile dressing, wrap in Kling or Kerlix for pressure, and elevate. **(B)** The amputated part should be rinsed with saline. *Do not scrub or apply antiseptic solution to the amputated part.* Wrap it in moist, sterile gauze or a towel, depending on size, and place it in a plastic bag or plastic container. **(C)** The part is then put in a container, preferably Styrofoam, and cooled by separate plastic bags containing ice.

tions are more cumbersome but are also cooled when possible. Tissue bridges must not be divided, as they may carry enough venous or lymphatic drainage to make replantation possible. Partially amputated limbs are "splinted as they are found" (Fig. 120.2). Attempting to place the limb in the anatomically correct position may twist a neurovascular bundle 360 degrees, totally occluding any remaining blood flow.[9] The stump is also wrapped in sterile, saline-moistened dressings.

After the initial stabilization of the patient is complete and the limb evaluated and dressed, radiographs of the entire extremity are obtained to define fractures.

DISPOSITION

Timely notification of the replantation team is the responsibility of the emergency physician. If transfer to another facility is required, arrangements must be completed by the time the patient is stable for transfer. It is prudent to treat every mangled or amputated limb as though it will be replanted or revascularized. The decision to perform microsurgery rests with the surgeon and the patient. Only after the surgeon has evaluated the extremity can a frank, thorough discussion about limb viability and functional recovery be entertained. It is inappropriate for the emergency physician to reassure the patient or the patient's family that limb salvage is possible or that replantation will be attempted.

COMPLICATIONS

Complications of microvascular reanastomosis are many and can be divided into early and late complications.[7] Ongoing ischemia requiring reexploration, reanastomosis, revision, debridement, or completed amputation can occur at any time during the postoperative period. Systemic acidosis, hyperkalemia, and rhabdomyolysis may be seen during major limb replantation when ischemic times are prolonged. Because muscle tolerates ischemia poorly and may swell after revascularization, replanted limbs containing large amounts of muscle may be subject to compartment syndrome. Systemic and local infection may occur due to the many factors that hinder wound healing. Late complications include scar contracture, tendon rupture or adhesion, poor or dysfunctional nerve regeneration, and osteomyelitis. Surgery resulting in a poorly functioning or frankly dysfunctional limb is the most feared complication. Sometimes, complete amputation with stump revision may be the best alternative.

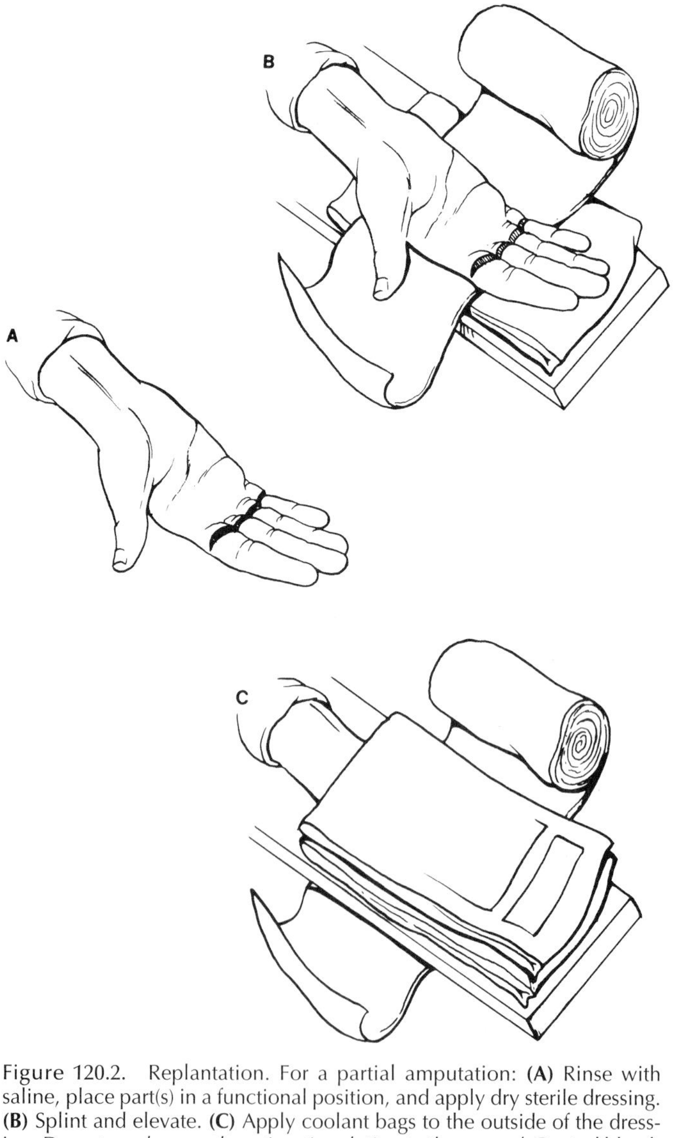

Figure 120.2. Replantation. For a partial amputation: **(A)** Rinse with saline, place part(s) in a functional position, and apply dry sterile dressing. **(B)** Splint and elevate. **(C)** Apply coolant bags to the outside of the dressing. *Do not scrub or apply antiseptic solution to the wound.* Control bleeding with pressure. If a tourniquet is necessary, place it close to the amputation site.

COMMON PITFALLS

- Aggressively resuscitate the patient and address other life-threatening injuries first.
- Do not clamp or ligate blood vessels in the emergency department.
- Do not sever tissue bridges between the proximal stump and amputated part.
- Splint the stump and injured extremity to prevent further injury.
- Treat all amputated limbs as though they will be replanted or revascularized.
- Do not discard any body parts; consider all a possible donor source for skin, bone, and vessels.
- Rapidly cool, but do not freeze, amputated body parts.
- Give antimicrobial agents as soon as possible.
- Rapidly consult the microvascular surgeon to minimize total ischemic time.

References

1. Bondurant FJ, Cotler HB, Buckle R, et al. The medical and economic impact of severely injured lower extremities. *J Trauma* 1988;28:1270.
2. Boulas HJ. Amputations of the fingers and hand: indications for replantation. *J Am Acad Orthop Surg* 1998;6:100.
3. Chen ZW, Zeng BF. Replantation of the lower extremity. *Clin Plast Surg* 1983;10:103.
4. Daigle JP, Kleinert JM. Major limb replantation in children. *Microsurgery* 1991;12:221.
5. Datiashvili RO. Simultaneous replantation of both lower legs in a child; a long-term result. *Plast Reconstr Surg* 1993;91:541.
6. Goldner RD, Howson MP, Nunley JA, et al. 111 thumb amputations: replantation vs. revision. *Microsurgery* 1990;11:243.
7. Idler RS, Steichen JB. Complications of replantation surgery. *Hand Clin* 1992;8:427.
8. Lukash FN, Greenburg BM, Gallico GG, et al. A socioeconomic analysis of digital replantation resulting from home use of power tools. *J Hand Surg* 1992;17A:1041.
9. May JW, Gallico GG. Upper extremity replantation. *Curr Probl Surg* 1980;17:632.
10. McAndrew MP, Lantz BA. Initial care of massively traumatized lower extremities. *Clin Orthop* 1989;23:20.
11. Niazi Z, Lee TC, Eadie P, et al. Succesful replantation of nose by microsurgical technique, and review of the literature. *Br J Plast Surg* 1990;43:617.
12. O'Brien BM, et al. Hallux-to-hand transfer. *Hand* 1975;7:128.
13. Razaboni R, Shaw WW. Preservation of tissue for transplantation and replantation. *Clin Plast Surg* 1983;10:211.
14. Sanger JR, Matloub HS, Yousif NJ, et al. Penile replantation after self-inflicted amputation. *Ann Plast Surg* 1992;29:579.
15. Sapega AA, Hepenstall RB, Sokolow DP, et al. The bioenergetics of preservation of limbs before replantation. *J Bone Joint Surg Am* 1988;70A:1500.
16. Schlenker JD, Koulis CP. Amputations and replantations. *Emerg Med Clin North Am* 1993;11:3.
17. Tamai S. 20 years' experience of limb replantation—review of 293 upper extremity replants. *J Hand Surg* 1982;7:549.
18. Tark KC, Kim YW, Lee YH, et al. Replantation and revascularization of hands: clinical analysis and functional results of 261 cases. *J Hand Surg* 1989;14A:17.
19. Zhou S, Chang T, Guan W, et al. Microsurgical replantation of the avulsed scalp: a report of six cases. *J Reconstr Microsurg* 1993;9:121.

CHAPTER 121
High-Pressure Injection Injuries of the Hand

Paul Blackburn

To the unwitting physician, a high-pressure injection injury of the hand may at first appear innocuous, but clinical sequelae are devastating if the initial recognition or management is delayed or inadequate. The emergency physician can significantly diminish morbidity with prompt recognition, initiation of treatment, and immediate referral.

An injury of the industrial age, the first reported case by Rees in 1937 described a patient injured while working on the fuel-injection system of a diesel engine.[24] The clinical course described was classic: marked pain with edema of the digit, vascular compromise noted with a resultant amputation. As this type of machinery has entered numerous work environments, case reports and reviews have corroborated this clinical scenario and led to consensus concerning initial treatment. Few systematic studies of high-pressure injection injuries have been undertaken because of the low incidence of this type of injury in comparison with all hand injuries. However, the consensus among clinicians is that prompt recognition with aggressive treatment, including surgical debridement, is the only course that avoids a disastrous clinical outcome.[2,9,11,15,20,23,26–28]

PATHOPHYSIOLOGY

It has been shown that a pressure of approximately 100 pounds per square inch (psi) is required to breach the skin.[25] The nozzle does not have to be in contact with the skin in order to cause injury. The pressures involved allow for injury even centimeters from the orifice.

Three types of industrial equipment (grease guns, spray guns, and diesel injectors) have accounted for most injection injuries.[14,27] The air-compressed grease gun used to lubricate motor vehicles accounted for 57% of injuries in one review. Injection occurs as the operator uses a finger to wipe the plugged nozzle. The suddenly open orifice extrudes grease into the extremity at 5,000 to 10,000 psi. Hydraulic-pressured spray guns (3,000 to 7,000 psi) accounted for 18% of injuries. Spray guns are ubiquitous in industry and deliver fluids of varying viscosity: paints and lacquers, petroleum products, solvents (including paint thinner), animal vaccines, gases (Freon, oxygen), and semifluid mud, cement, and sand, for example. Diesel-fuel injectors accounted for 14% of cases reported. For diesel fuel to spontaneously ignite in the pressure chamber, the fuel must pass through an injector mechanism, which compresses the fuel between 2,000 and 12,000 psi. Injuries are most often sustained when the injection mechanism is being tested.[15,24,27]

Numerous other types of pressure-related injuries may occur, and the hand need not necessarily be the only anatomic site involved. Defects of pneumatic hoses, valves from tractor greaseboxes, oil rig drilling and pipeline equipment, and hydraulic lines of sandblasters can lead to high-pressure injuries of other body parts.[15,24] It should also be noted that some industrial equipment is capable of generating higher psi than the previously mentioned three examples.

The injury demographics are typical. It is an injury of the workplace, is usually due to operator inexperience or careless-

TABLE 121.1. Factors Influencing the Type and Degree of High-Pressure Injection Injury
Type of material
Amount of material
Location of injection site
Velocity of injection

ness,[13] and occurs most often with attempts to clean the pressure nozzle. Men between ages 16 and 65 are most commonly affected[26] on the nondominant hand. The most common site of injection is the distal volar surface of the index finger, followed by the distal volar long finger, then the palm.[15,26] At the time of the injury, the patient may feel temporary stinging or no pain at all, which, unfortunately, may result in delay in seeking treatment.[14,15,27]

Four factors determine the type and degree of high-pressure injection injury (Table 121.1).[23] The *type of material* is the most important element in determining the subsequent morbidity, owing to each material's propensity to create tissue inflammation and the resultant fibrosis that develops during healing. Paint and paint thinner create the greatest tissue inflammatory response and result in a high rate of amputation. Conversely, grease gun injuries do not create much inflammation. The morbidity from grease is due to eventual development of fibrosis, oleomas, and draining sinuses.[12,15,20,26,28] It should be noted that both paint thinner and grease (and most injectates) are nearly bacteriostatic *in vivo*. Although infection is not usually a primary concern, empiric administration of broad-spectrum antibiotics is indicated.

The *amount of material* injected determines tissue distention, compression, and mechanical distortion of blood flow. Simple compression of arterial and venous structures may impede venous outflow or arterial perfusion. Others feel that thrombosis and vasospasm are important components of vascular interruption.[15,23,27] Whatever the precise etiology of impaired circulation, tissue viability is threatened, and necrosis with superimposed bacterial infection may occur.

The *location of the injection* determines the direction of injectate dispersion. Cadaveric studies using a mixture of turpentine and green-stained wax permitted controlled observation of the spread of materials.[15] The substance under pressure travels in a direct line, with little lateral spread, until it encounters a resistance structure. Injection lateral to the bones of the finger leads to through-and-through penetration, with extensive spread around the dorsal surface. The fibrous tendon sheaths in the middle of a phalanx prevent direct penetration, and material travels laterally, encompassing the digital neurovascular bundles. However, at their thinnest area over the interphalangeal joints, the tendon sheaths allow penetration. If the sheath is penetrated, retrograde contamination may occur, including the radial and ulnar bursae if the thumb or little finger is involved.[14,27] Isolated involvement of the thenar and hypothenar muscles (sparing the palm) can occur.[27] Palmar injection may involve deep structures if the aponeurosis is violated.

The *velocity* of the material injected does not lead to direct tissue damage, but determines the amount of material dispersion. While not a factor in creating direct tissue injury, broader spread of material will lead to more tissue damage.[23]

CLINICAL PRESENTATION

The clinical appearance is determined by the time elapsed between injury and presentation. The clinical course can be divided into three stages: acute, intermediate, and late.[19] At the time of high-pressure injection, the patient may feel a stinging sensation at the site of penetration, or nothing at all. The examiner may note a small puncture wound, which may or may not have a droplet of the injected material at the site. Instantaneous swelling of the digit may be noted if sufficient material was injected.[15]

Within 1 to 2 hours, discoloration occurs, accompanied by increasing swelling, numbness, and pain. Within several hours, increased discoloration and swelling occur, accompanied by pain severe enough to be unrelieved by narcotics. This may appear similar to an infectious process, but conservative therapy consisting of antibiotics, elevation, and heat will doubtlessly prove catastrophic.[15,27] Continued conservative treatment will almost certainly lead to the need for amputation of the affected part.[27]

The *intermediate* stage is characterized by development of oleogranulomas, or oleomas around the site of injection, a foreign-body reaction to the injected material. The *late* stage is defined by ulceration of the oleomas, which discharge a sterile, amorphous material of grease and epithelium that may become secondarily infected. The skin becomes thickened and pitted, leading to functional disturbance and a poor cosmetic appearance. A possible late complication is squamous cell malignancy of the chronically irritated sinus tracts.[15]

In addition to the local effects, generalized constitutional symptoms may be present. Presumably because of the foreign material injected, the patient may develop a low-grade fever, leukocytosis, lymphadenitis, renal impairment, and blood chemistry alterations.[15,16,27]

DIFFERENTIAL DIAGNOSIS

Taking a thorough history and performing a complete physical examination greatly limits the differential diagnosis. If the patient presents immediately following the injection, the puncture wound may not be evident, and a presumption of no injury might be inappropriately entertained. If a wound is noted, a mistaken clinical conclusion would be to treat it as a simple puncture wound. If the patient presents later in the acute stage, the appearance of the discolored and swollen involved part may mislead the physician to suspect an infectious condition.

EMERGENCY DEPARTMENT EVALUATION

The patient usually presents to the emergency department in significant pain within hours of the injury. Systemic manifestations are few. There may be abnormal vital signs: tachycardia or increased blood pressure due to pain, or low-grade fever.

The affected area must be meticulously inspected to find the site of injection in order to anticipate dispersion of injected material. The amount and location of swelling, tendon function, and joint range of motion are evaluated. The degree of vascular compromise, as assessed by discoloration, temperature, and capillary refill of the nailbed, is vital information for the consultant. Pulse oximetry of the affected part (with comparison with its contralateral partner) may give additional information.

Laboratory studies have little bearing on the emergency department evaluation and treatment. However, because of reports of temporary renal dysfunction from systemic absorption of injected material, urinalysis and baseline blood urea nitrogen and creatinine levels should be obtained.[16] Drawing of routine preoperative studies may be considered. The clinician may consider the potential organ-specific toxicity of the material injected and add appropriate studies.

Plain films of the involved extremity are useful in determin-

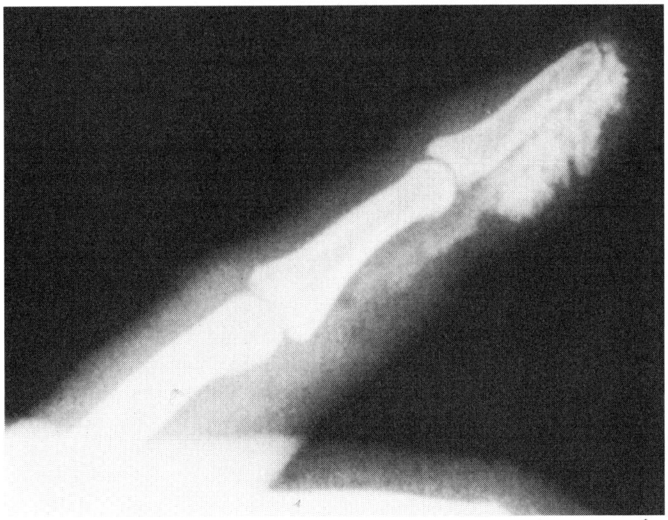

Figure 121.1. Radiographic appearance of high-pressure injection injury of the digit. The extent of dispersal of the radiopaque material (lead-based paint) is demonstrated. (From Proust AF. Special injuries of the hand. *Emerg Med Clin North Am* 1993;11:770, with permission.)

ing the extent of the dispersed material and may help guide the extent of surgical debridement. Material can be dispersed a considerable distance from the site of penetration.[21] Therefore, imaging to the elbow is mandatory. Some recommend imaging the entire upper extremity.[27]

The x-ray appearance of injected substances may be characteristic (Fig. 121.1). The silica from sandblasting injuries is easily seen, as is the deposition of lead-based paint from a spray gun.[21,27] The opacities of lead-based paint must not be confused with calcifications.[21] Grease may appear as a radiolucency within the tissue and be mistaken for subcutaneous emphysema. Xeroradiography may better show the extent of grease injection.[21] The use of magnetic resonance imaging has not been studied,[23,27] nor has angiography.

EMERGENCY DEPARTMENT MANAGEMENT

Emergency department treatment must be rapid and definitive if a catastrophic outcome is to be avoided (Table 121.2). The time from injury to proper treatment is the prime determinant of prognosis.[28] Some authors feel that amputation is more likely if debridement is not done within 10 hours,[27] although others are of the opinion that there is no safe time window and all require urgent surgical decompression.[18]

Emergency department care must include elevation of the extremity, administration of broad-spectrum antibiotics, tetanus prophylaxis, and general preparation for surgery. Empiric broad-spectrum antibiotics are indicated, even though most injected materials show antibacterial activity or are bacteriostatic. Pain control is provided through opiates or proximal extremity (preferably brachial plexus) nerve blocks. Digital nerve blocks are absolutely contraindicated because of the additional fluid volume and tissue compression added to the already compromised digit.[12,15,23,27,28] Warm soaks also are contraindicated. The increased blood flow into the extremity adds further volume and tissue compression.

Corticosteroid administration is controversial. Some argue that steroids are useful if an intense inflammatory response develops, if a delay in treatment has occurred, or if there is a systemic reaction.[9,13] Others note that because wound infection is rarely a complication, and considering the high likelihood of poor outcome due to tissue inflammation, steroids (along with broad-spectrum antibiotics) should be administered to all.[18] Data are currently insufficient to recommend the use of heparin or dextran.[23]

The high-pressure injection injury is a true surgical emergency. Immediate surgical consultation is mandatory. The entire involved area must be operatively debrided and copiously irrigated with normal saline. Wounds are left open postsurgically, with Penrose drains in place to facilitate drainage. Wounds are closed at a later date, using split-thickness skin grafts. Early and aggressive treatment may preserve some function of a hand that otherwise would require amputation.[27] However, it must be noted that some advocate proceeding directly to amputation if there is vascular compromise.[18] Reconstruction of the hand can occur at a later date.

The emergency physician should be made aware that there are case reports of conservative management of some injection injuries. One must be cognizant that the majority of reports involve gases,[1,5,7,8,10,17,22] but isolated examples of water to the dorsum of the thumb[6] and small volumes of nonirritating material (2-PAM chloride[3]) exist. In addition, the authors of a report relating to injection of veterinary vaccines notes that, with poultry vaccine (0.2 mL of injectate), the surgeon may attempt conservative or "minimally invasive" management. They go on to state that all other veterinary products must be treated entirely as high-pressure injections.[4] One must take into account that this conclusion is based on a case series of four patients, two of whom had surgical procedures that involved opening and lavage of portions of the hand and the carpal tunnel.

Emergency physicians must realize that any decision concerning therapy beyond the initiation of treatment (antibiotics, tetanus prophylaxis, pain control, preparation for surgery) and surgical referral is not theirs to make. They must approach all high-pressure injection injuries in a similar fashion, with immediate surgical referral.

TABLE 121.2. Emergency Department Management of Injection Injuries

1. Recognition of injury and physical examination
2. Plain films of the extremity
   a. Consider preoperative lab draw
3. Broad-spectrum antibiotics, tetanus prophylaxis
4. Pain control
   a. Opiates
   b. Proximal nerve blocks as *digital blocks are contraindicated.*
5. Immediate surgical consultation

Use of steroids, heparin, and dextran is controversial.
Esmarch bandages and compressive dressings are contraindicated.

DISPOSITION

The only appropriate disposition for the patient with a high-pressure injection injury is immediate surgical consultation, with expectation of wide debridement and copious irrigation of all involved areas. Alteration from this course of action is solely the surgeon's determination.

COMMON PITFALLS

- The most common error is not to suspect or not to recognize the injury. The patient may have felt only a transient stinging sensation, and the entrance wound may be minuscule or absent. A drop of material may or may not be present at the injection site.
- Early after injury, the clinician may be faced with a puncture-

like wound and a discolored, swollen, painful extremity. An infectious process may be considered if a thorough history is not obtained. Conservative treatment with antibiotics, heat, or localized incision and drainage will have predictably disastrous results.

- Digital blocks are absolutely contraindicated. The injected material has already compressed the normally nondistensible tissues of the finger. The added volume of local anesthetic will cause further compression of tissue and vascular compromise.
- Warm soaks increase blood flow to the compromised extremity and, like the added volume of injected local anesthetics, cause increased tissue compression.
- Esmarch or other compressive dressings to reduce swelling or create a bloodless field must be avoided. Their use serves only to distribute the injected material further throughout the tissue.

References

1. Caspi I, Lin E, Nerubay J, et al. Subcutaneous emphysema following high-pressure injection injury of inert gas. *J Trauma* 1987;27:1305.
2. Chung-Ho P, Wei DC, Hou SP. High-pressure injuries of the hand. *J Trauma* 1991;31:110.
3. Combs J, Hise L. High-pressure injection injury involving a 2-PAM chloride autoinjector. *Milit Med* 1992;157:434.
4. Couzens G, Burke FD. Veterinary high-pressure injection injuries with inoculations for larger animals. *J Hand Surg* 1995;20B:497.
5. Craig EV. A new high-pressure injection injury of the hand. *J Hand Surg* 1984;9A:240.
6. Curka PA, Chisholm DC. High-pressure water injection injury to the hand. *Am J Emerg Med* 1989;7:165.
7. Eyres KS, Morley T. Subcutaneous emphysema of the upper limb: an air gun injury. *J Hand Surg* 1993;18B:251.
8. Geller E, Gursel E. A unique case of high-pressure injection injury of the hand. *J Trauma* 1986;26:483.
9. Gillespie CA, Rodeheaver GT, Smith S, et al. Airless paint gun injuries: definition and management. *Am J Surg* 1974;128:383.
10. Goetting AT, Carson J, Burton BT. Freon injection injury to the hand: a report of four cases. *J Osteopath Med* 1992;34:775.
11. Harrison R. Grease-gun injury. *Br J Surg* 1959;46:514.
12. Harter BT, Harter KC. High-pressure injection injuries. *Hand Clin* 1986;2:547.
13. Herrick RT, Godsil RD, Widener JH. High-pressure injection injuries to the hand. *South Med J* 1980;73:896.
14. Kaufman HD. High-pressure injection injuries of the hand. *Hand* 1970;2:63.
15. Kaufman HD. The clinicopathological correlation of high-pressure injection injuries. *Hand* 1970;2:63.
16. Kaufman HD, Williams HO. Systemic absorption from high-pressure spray-gun injuries. *Br J Surg* 1966;53:57.
17. Klareskov B, Gebuhr P, Rordam P. Compressed air injuries of the hand. *J Hand Surg* 1986;11B:436.
18. Lewis HG, Clarke PC, Kneafsey B, et al. A 10-year review of high-pressure injection injuries to the hand. *J Hand Surg* 1998;23B:479.
19. Mason ML, Queen FB. Grease gun injuries to the hand. *Q Bull Northwest Med School* 1941;15:122.
20. Neal NC, Burke FD. High-pressure injection injuries. *Injury* 1991;22:467.
21. O'Reilly RJ, Blatt G. Accidental high-pressure injection gun injuries of the hand. *J Trauma* 1975;15:24.
22. Pinto MR, Turkula-Pinto LD, Cooney WP, et al. High-pressure injuries of the hand: review of 25 patients managed by open wound technique. *J Hand Surg* 1993;18A:125.
23. Proust AF. Special injuries of the hand. *Emerg Med Clin North Am* 1993;11:767.
24. Rees CE. Penetration of tissue by fuel oil under high pressure from a diesel engine. *JAMA* 1937;109:866.
25. Scott AR. Occupational high-pressure injection injuries: pathogenesis and prevention. *J Soc Occup Med* 1983;33:56.
26. Shoo MJ, Scott FA, Boawick JA. High-pressure injection injuries to the hand. *J Trauma* 1980;20:229.
27. Sirio CA, Smith JS, Graham WP. High-pressure injection injuries of the hand. *Am Surg* 1989;55:714.
28. Stark HH, Ashworth CR, Boyle JH. Paint-gun injuries of the hand. *J Bone Joint Surg Am* 1967;49:637.

CHAPTER 122
Acute Compartment Syndrome

Steven C. Larson

Acute compartment syndrome is the term used to describe the constellation of clinical symptoms and signs associated with a pathologic elevation in tissue pressure within anatomic "compartments" of the body.[7] Left undiagnosed and untreated, this elevated pressure leads to muscle ischemia and death. Clinically, the result is the muscle contracture and deformity referred to as Volkmann's ischemic contracture. In the late 1800s Richard von Volkmann described a progressive, posttraumatic muscle contracture (which had previously been attributed to neurologic injury) that he believed was secondary to the ischemia caused by trauma, swelling, and tight bandaging.[6] Volkmann postulated,[22]

> . . . The paralysis is caused by the death of primitive muscle fibers deprived of oxygen. The contractile substance coagulates, falls into pieces, and is afterwards absorbed. The following contracture may be considered simply as a condition closely akin to rigor mortis, and indeed the limbs, if, as is usually the case, all muscles of a part are equally affected by the ischemia, assume the well known position as after death . . . .

Today, our understanding of acute compartment syndrome and Volkmann's ischemic contracture is more detailed and sophisticated; and yet, at the core of the issue is a simple appreciation of anatomy. Basically, muscle groups and neurovascular structures are surrounded and encased in fascial sheaths, which create compartmentalized anatomic space. These compartments afford little room to accommodate swelling.[21] When swelling occurs within this limited space or when externally applied forces such as constrictive dressings cause increased intracompartmental pressures, circulation is compromised. The resulting ischemia produces abnormal muscle function, followed by abnormal neurovascular function, and this process has come to be termed *compartment syndrome*. Matsen and associates[12] defined *compartment syndrome* as "a condition in which increased pressure within a limited space compromises the circulation and function of the tissues within that space."

The incidence of compartment syndrome is unknown because of inconsistencies in diagnostic criteria, as well as the prophylactic fasciotomy often performed to prevent development of this syndrome.[18] The disorder is most common in the calf or forearm, but the hand, foot, and upper portions of limbs may also be affected.[8] In one study, the incidence of lower-limb compartment syndrome in adults was 6% in open fractures of the tibia and 1.2% in closed tibial fractures.[1,25] Trauma associated with vascular injury markedly increases the likelihood of compartment syndrome. In another study, the incidence of compartment syndrome was 30% with arterial injuries and 14% with significant venous injuries.[17,22] The incidence of compartment syndrome in children is not well documented.[22]

PATHOPHYSIOLOGY

Two mechanisms produce acute compartment syndrome. The first is an increase in volume within a closed space. The second is a decrease in the size of a body space.[6] Both of these events result in a rise in intracompartmental pressure, a prerequisite for the development of compartment syndrome.[14] Clinically, elevated intracompartmental pressure may result from an increase in the contents of the compartment due to edema, hemorrhage, or intravenous fluid infiltration, or from a decrease in compartment size produced by constriction from casts, pneumatic garments, and eschar formation.[4,18]

Table 122.1 provides a complete list of etiologies. Trauma is the most common cause of compartment syndrome.[3,13,18,19] Of traumatic events, fractures are the most common cause.[13] In addition, pressure applied to a limb for prolonged periods, such as in the intoxicated patient whose body weight rests on the limb[13] or in a patient undergoing a long operation in the lithotomy position,[13,16] may precipitate a compartment syndrome.

Although hemorrhage or trauma can lead to an abrupt rise in compartment pressures, the development of compartment syndrome is more often delayed and follows a period of ischemia.[18] Ischemia may be local and related to increased tissue pressures,[11,13,14] or it may result from factors that limit blood flow to the involved region, such as systemic hypotension, arterial injury, venous obstruction, or elevation of the extremity.[13,14]

Compartment syndrome occurs in many locations, but it is most common in the anterior compartment of the leg (Table 122.2).[21] It is not surprising that the extremities are most frequently involved. In the upper extremities and lower extremities, the arm, forearm, hand, thigh, leg, and foot all have muscle groups and neurovascular bundles surrounded by strong fascial boundaries. In addition, the extremities are frequently injured and are common sites for intravenous fluid administration, dialysis grafts, and catheterization procedures (Fig. 122.1).

Many theories have been proposed to explain the relationship between increased tissue pressure and decreased tissue perfusion. Experimental studies have shown an inverse linear correlation between muscle blood flow and compartment pressures in animals.[14] Matsen argued that the "the increased tissue pressure in a given compartment decreases the overall arterial–venous pressure gradient by increasing local venous pressure." [21] A decrease in the arterial–venous pressure gradient decreases flow.[14] This theory is currently widely accepted.[4,14,19,24] The pressure within the compartment is not great enough to compress the major arterial structures; thus, pulses are usually present in acute compartment syndrome.[24]

Newer pathophysiologic explanations for compartmental hypertension also take into account the "ischemia–reperfusion" theory for cellular injury. Essentially, ischemia results in the depletion of intracellular energy stores. Following reperfusion and the generation of toxic oxygen radicals, a cascade of pathophysiologic consequences results, including activation and adhesions of leukocytes and platelets, calcium influx, disruption of cellular membrane ion pumps, and transudation of fluid in the aggregate, producing both cellular swelling and edema formation.[7]

Regardless of the etiology, raised intracompartmental pressure results in venous outflow obstruction. The increasing capillary pressure worsens fluid transudation and cellular swelling, thus perpetuating a vicious cycle. Ultimately, when intracompartmental pressure equals capillary pressure, nutrient blood flow is reduced to zero.[7]

At rest, the normal compartment pressure approaches 4 to 8 mm Hg in the recumbent position.[6] An absolute value for a compartment pressure at which cellular metabolism and subsequent tissue infarction occur is unclear. Elevated pressures ranging from 30 to 45 mm Hg have been considered indications for emergent fasciotomies.[6] However, recent work suggests that such threshold pressure measurements are inadequately sensitive or specific for the diagnosis of compartment syndrome.[7] The physiologic issues of greatest relevance are the arterial perfusion pressure and the interstitial pressure, which of course is a function of systemic arterial pressure.[7]

Heppenstall and colleagues[5] demonstrated that "the threshold for cellular metabolic derangement in skeletal muscle subjected to increased tissue pressure was more closely associated with the difference between mean arterial blood pressure and compartment pressure than with the absolute compartment pressure alone." They termed this difference *delta P* and noted that the lowest delta P at which a normal metabolic state could be maintained was about 30 mm Hg in normal muscle and 40 mm Hg in moderately traumatized muscle. Thus, these authors argue that compartment pressures must be viewed in relation to the amount of trauma sustained and the overall clinical picture.

The earliest symptoms of compartment syndrome are neurologic, relating to the fact that the tissue most sensitive to hypoxia is the nonmyelinated, type C sensory fiber that transmits fine touch and mediates symptoms such as paresthesias.[7] Tissue hy-

TABLE 122.1. Common Etiologies of Compartment Syndromes Seen in Emergency Medicine

INCREASED COMPARTMENT CONTENT
Infiltrated infusion
Bleeding
• Vascular injury
• Coagulation defect
Increased capillary permeability
• Reperfusion after ischemia
• Trauma
• Fracture
• Contusion
• Intensive use of muscles
• Exercise
• Seizures
• Eclampsia
• Tetany
• Burns
• Cold
• Snakebite
Increased capillary pressure
• Venous obstruction
Diminished serum osmolarity
• Nephrotic syndrome
EXTERNALLY APPLIED PRESSURE
• Casts, dressings, splints, pneumatic garment
• Lying on limb

From Matsen FA. *Compartmental syndromes.* New York: Grune & Stratton, 1980, with permission.

TABLE 122.2. Common Locations of Compartment Syndromes

Upper Limb Compartments	Lower Limb Compartments
Arm	Buttock
• Deltoid	• Gluteal
• Biceps	Thigh
Forearm	• Quadriceps
• Dorsal	Leg
•Volar	• Anterior
Hand	• Lateral
• Interosseous	• Superficial posterior
	• Deep posterior

From Matsen FA. *Compartmental syndromes.* New York: Grune & Stratton, 1980, with permission.

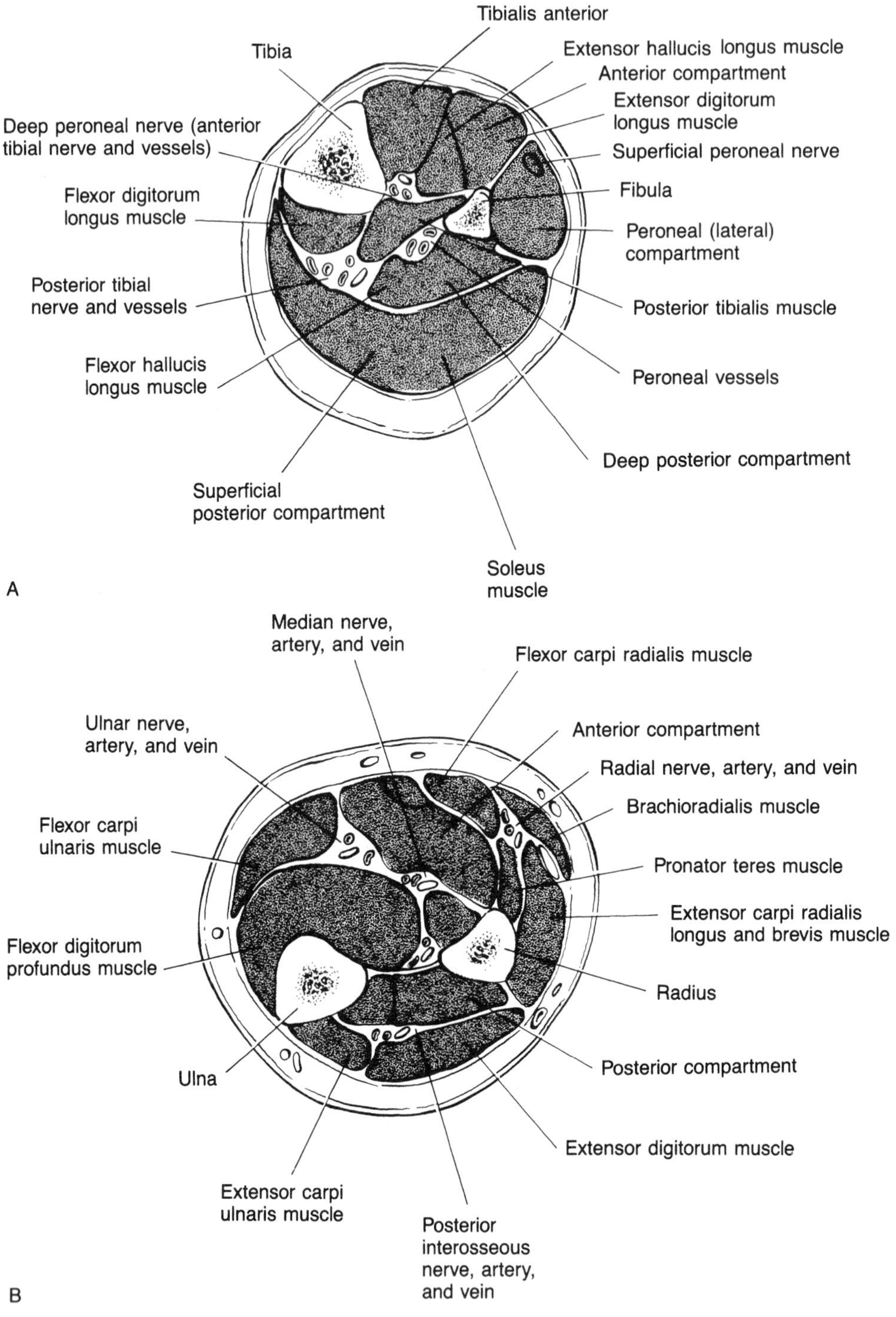

Figure 122.1. Compartments of the leg **(A)** and forearm **(B)**.

poxic tolerance increases from nonmyelinated to myelinated nerves, skeletal muscle, and (most resistant to hypoxia) skin and bone.[7,12,15,18] The length of time muscle and nerve can tolerate elevated pressure is unclear. Extrapolating from data related to acute arterial insufficiency, a 6-hour "grace period" appears to be the upper limit of successful revascularization before muscle injury is irreversible.[6,7]

CLINICAL PRESENTATION

As in many clinical circumstances, the diagnosis of acute compartment syndrome is facilitated by the "prepared mind," which takes into account the patient's history, symptoms, and clinical findings.[7] The best possible outcome for acute compartment syndrome depends on early diagnosis and intervention. In the past, the "Five P's (pulselessness, pallor, paralysis, paresthesia, and pain) were advocated as clinical signs of a developing compartment syndrome. Unfortunately, these are late signs and symptoms associated with an established compartment syndrome, and fasciotomies performed utilizing these guidelines have been inconsistent in maintenance of limb function.[6]

The earliest and most important symptom of an impending acute compartment syndrome is the perception of pain "out of proportion" to the clinical findings on examination.[3,12–14,18,21,24] Other important symptoms are those of distal motor and sensory dysfunction, characteristically weakness and paresthesias in the distribution of nerves passing through the compressed tis-

TABLE 122.3. Compartment Syndromes and Associated Physical Signs

Compartment	Painful Passive Movement	Location of Tenseness	Muscles Weakened	Sensory Loss
FOREARM				
Dorsal	Thumb and finger flexion Thumb and finger extension	Dorsal forearm Volar forearm	Thumb and finger extensors Thumb and finger flexors	— Ulnar and median nerves
HAND				
Interosseous	Adduction, abduction of metacarpophalangeal joints	Dorsum of hand between metacarpals	Interosseous	—
LEG				
Anterior	Toe flexion	Anterior aspect of leg	Toe extensors and tibialis anterior	Deep peroneal nerve
Lateral	Foot inversion	Lateral aspect of leg over fibula	Peroneal muscles	Superficial and deep peroneal nerves
Superficial posterior	Foot dorsiflexion	Calf	Soleus and gastrocnemius	—
Deep posterior	Toe extension	Distal medial leg between Achilles tendon and tibia	Toe flexors and tibialis posterior	Posterior tibial nerve

From Matsen FA. Compartmental syndromes. *Clin Orthop* 1975;113:8.

sue compartments.[7] There are, however, reports of compartment syndrome with little pain,[13] and a substantial diagnostic dilemma is presented by the patient who is unconscious, intubated, intoxicated, paraplegic, or quadriplegic, or who, for some other reason, cannot sense or communicate sensations of pain.[7]

The most reliable clinical signs of compartment syndrome are weakness, pain on passive stretching of muscles, tenseness and pain on palpation of the involved compartment, and hypoesthesia in the distribution of nerves in the compartment (Table 122.3).[3,4,12–14,18,21,24] These signs may be evident within 2 hours of the inciting event or may appear as late as 6 days after the injury.[21] Increased pain on active movement or passive stretch of the muscles in the compartment is an early finding. Hypoesthesia is always a late finding.[3,18] Both the two-point discrimination and light touch tests are more sensitive than the pinprick test.[9,21] Pulses are most often present,[3,4,12–14,18,21,24] and absence of pulses should widen the differential diagnosis to include arterial occlusion or injury.[4,12–14] Other diagnoses must also be considered in the differential, including deep vein thrombosis, cellulitis, neuropraxia, osteomyelitis, tenosynovitis, and synovitis.[14]

EMERGENCY DEPARTMENT EVALUATION

Laboratory studies are not helpful in diagnosing compartment syndrome. Hyperkalemia, elevated creatinine phosphokinase level, and myoglobinuria suggest muscle destruction, a nonspecific finding in compartment syndrome.[13,14,18] The best diagnostic test is measurement of intracompartmental pressures.[13] Elevated tissue pressure may occur before the onset of clinical signs and symptoms and may lead to early diagnosis.[25] In addition, measurement of pressures is extremely helpful in patients in whom examination is unreliable.[10,12,17] Many techniques are available to measure pressures, including the needle manometer technique,[13,21] the wick catheter method,[13,14,24] and the portable Stryker hand-held monitor.[13,14]

Normal intramuscular pressures may range from 0 to 8 mm Hg and may be as high as 20 mm Hg in the lower leg.[14,18] There is no consensus as to an absolute pressure above which fasciotomy must be performed.[5,13,14,18] Rorabeck and associates[20] suggest decompression at pressures above 30 to 35 mm Hg; Matsen,[10,18] at pressures above 45 mm Hg; and Whitesides and colleagues,[23] when the intracompartmental pressure falls within 10 to 30 mm Hg of the diastolic blood pressure.[14] Many authors emphasize that compartmental pressures should be evaluated only in conjunction with the diastolic pressure and clinical examination, and stress that both hypotensive and hypertensive patients may show different susceptibility to damage from elevated tissue pressures.[5,10,23]

Transcutaneous Doppler measurement of tibial venous blood flow may be helpful in supporting the diagnosis of compartment syndrome in the anterior compartment of the leg. As tissue pressure exceeds venous pressure (normally 7 to 16 mm Hg), the tibial venous flow is reduced.[18] Current trauma research utilizing near-infrared wavelength reflection to measure muscle oxyhemoglobin levels may prove useful in providing noninvasive, continuous monitoring, but further clinical studies are warranted.[2]

Nerve conduction studies may help to differentiate local nerve damage due to compartment syndrome from more proximal nerve injury, but are usually unavailable to the emergency physician in a timely manner.[12,18] Arteriography may be required to evaluate the origins of ischemia.[18] Intracompartmental pressure measurements remain the best objective test for possible compartment syndrome, but much value is placed on a thorough clinical examination.

EMERGENCY DEPARTMENT MANAGEMENT

The emergency physician must maintain a high index of suspicion and be knowledgeable about the clinical presentation of, and predisposing factors for, compartment syndrome. Management should include thorough, repeated clinical examinations, with special attention to the early signs and symptoms of compartment syndrome. Appropriate laboratory studies, including preoperative evaluation, should be sent. Any constrictive dressing, casts, or pneumatic garments must be removed as soon as possible and the limb placed in a neutral position, as elevation of the limb has been shown to be harmful.[3,4,13] Circulation is aggressively supported with intravenous crystalloid and blood products, where indicated.[13]

Compartment syndrome is truly a limb-threatening condition. Surgical consultation should take place immediately. The definitive treatment of compartment syndrome is fasciotomy, which relieves pressure elevation within the compartment(s).[13,14,18,24] Fasciotomy must be performed early, ideally less than 6 hours after the onset of symptoms.[21] Other treatment, such as vasodilating drugs or sympathetic nerve blocks, have not been shown to be effective.[14]

Mannitol is controversial; recent data suggesting the important role of oxygen radicals in the pathogenesis of acute compartment syndrome has raised interest in the use of mannitol to scavenge toxic oxygen species (reducing ischemia–reperfusion injury) in addition to its known hyperosmolar capabilities (reducing tissue edema).[7] Hyperbaric oxygen therapy has been used as an adjunct early in the course of a developing compartment syndrome, but in light of the "ischemia–reperfusion" theory, it remains debatable whether its use is indicated in an established acute compartment syndrome.[14]

COMMON PITFALLS

- Lack of clinical suspicion
- Failing to recognize early symptoms
- Attributing the signs and symptoms of compartment syndrome to other types of injury
- Failing to do a thorough extremity and neurologic examination, especially in intoxicated patients or in patients with an unreliable history

References

1. Delee JC, Stiehl JB. Open tibia fracture with compartment syndrome. *Clin Orthop Rel Res* 1981;160:175.
2. Garr JL, Gentilello LM, Cole PA, et al. Monitoring for compartment syndrome using near-infrared spectroscopy: a noninvasive, continuous, transcutaneous monitoring technique. *J Trauma* 1999,46:613.
3. Goldman FD, Dayton PD, Hanson CJ. Compartment syndrome of the foot. *J Foot Surg* 1990;29(1):37.
4. Greenberg M. Compartment syndromes. In: Harwood-Nuss A, ed. *The clinical practice of emergency medicine*. New York: JB Lippincott Co, 1990:412.
5. Heppenstall RB, Sapega AA, Scott R, et al. The compartment syndrome: an experimental and clinical study of muscular energy metabolism using phosphorus nuclear magnetic resonance spectroscopy. *Clin Orthop* 1988;226:138.
6. Heppenstall RB. An update in compartment syndrome investigation and treatment. *Univ Penn Orthop J* 1997;10:49.
7. Johansen K, Watson J. Compartment syndromes: new insights. *Semin Vasc Surg* 1998;11:294.
8. Kalb RL. Preventing the sequelae of compartment syndrome. *Hosp Pract* 1999;(Jan 15):105.
9. Matsen FA. Compartmental syndromes. *Clin Orthop* 1975;113:8.
10. Matsen FA. *Compartmental syndromes*. New York: Grune & Stratton, 1980.
11. Matsen FA. A practical approach to compartmental syndromes, part 1. *AAOS Inst Course Lect* 1983;32:88.
12. Matsen FA, Winquist RA, Krugmire RB. Diagnosis and management of compartmental syndromes. *J Bone Joint Surg Am* 1980;62:286.
13. McGee DL, Dalsey WC. The mangled extremity, compartment syndrome and amputations. *Emerg Med Clin North Am* 1992;10:783.
14. Moore RE, Friedman RJ. Current concepts in pathophysiology and diagnosis of compartment syndromes. *J Emerg Med* 1989;7:657.
15. Mubarak SJ, Hargens AR. Acute compartment syndromes. *Surg Clin North Am* 1983;63:539.
16. Neagle CE, Schaffer JL, Heppenstall RB. Compartment syndrome complicating prolonged use of the lithotomy position. *Surgery* 1991;110:566.
17. Patman RD, Thompson JE. Fasciotomy in peripheral vascular surgery. *Arch Surg* 1970;101:663.
18. Perry MO. Compartment syndromes and reperfusion injury. *Surg Clin North Am* 1988;68:853.
19. Quinn RH, Ruby ST. Compartment syndrome after elective revascularization for chronic ischemia: a case report and review of the literature. *Arch Surg* 1992;127:865.
20. Rorabeck CH, Castle GSP, Hardie R, et al. Compartmental pressure measurements: an experimental investigation using the slit catheter. *J Trauma* 1981;21:446.
21. Simon RR, Koenigknecht SJ. Complications. In: *Emergency orthopedics: the extremities*, 2nd ed. Norwalk, CT: Appleton & Lange,1987.
22. Trice M, Colwell C. A historical review of compartment syndrome and Volkmann's ischemic contracture. *Hand Clin North Am* 1998;14:335.
23. Whitesides TE, Haney TC, Morimoto K, et al. Tissue pressure measurements as a determinant for the need for fasciotomy. *Clin Orthop* 1975;113:43.
24. Willis RB, Rorabeck CH. Treatment of compartment syndrome in children. *Orthop Clin North Am* 1990;21:401.

CHAPTER 123

Blast Injuries

J. Stephan Stapczynski

Blast injury is a general term used to describe the harmful effects produced by the sudden change in environmental pressure originating from an explosion. Blast injuries were first identified during World War II when aerial bombing of large cities produced many casualties.[5] Blast injuries were also common among civilians during war conditions in Vietnam, Afghanistan, Lebanon, Croatia, and Bosnia.[1] In the United States, blast injuries commonly result from terrorist bombings and the rare civilian industrial accident.[8] Injuries produced by explosions can be divided into four categories. Primary blast injuries are caused by the sudden change in environmental pressure as the explosion-produced shock wave passes by. Secondary blast injuries result from the victim being struck by flying debris. Tertiary blast injuries are sustained when the victim is hurled against a stationary object. Both secondary and tertiary blast injuries are due to the accelerative force imparted to loose objects by the shock wave. Although the duration of an explosion-produced shock wave is brief, the accelerative force is significant. For a 70-kg adult, a shock wave with a peak overpressure of 15 pounds per square inch (psi) produces an instantaneous acceleration of 450 ft per second squared or about 14 *g*. Miscellaneous blast injuries include exposure to dust, direct thermal burns, and burns from blast-ignited fires.

PATHOPHYSIOLOGY

There are four energy sources for explosions.

1. Mechanical (alternatively, hydraulic): Due to sudden structural failure of a pressurized container
2. Electrical: As an electrical arc passes through the air, intense heat is generated that produces a sudden increase in pressure.
3. Nuclear: Intense heat generated by the process of fission or fusion
4. Chemical
   a. Diffuse reactants: Flammable gases or particulate matter mixed with air
   b. Condensed reactants: Liquid or solid, which can be either low-order (e.g., black powder) or high-order (e.g., TNT) explosives

Chemical explosions are the most common cause of accidental or intentional blast injuries. Once ignited, a solid or liquid explosive undergoes a chemical decomposition into a gas. The space previously occupied by the explosive is now filled with gas under high pressure and temperature. This pressure is transmitted through the surrounding medium and propagates outward as a shock wave at speeds of 6 to 8 km/s. As measured at a position away from the explosion, the passing shock wave produces a rapid increase in environmental pressure to a peak above the ambient pressure (the peak overpressure), followed by a slow decline back to baseline. The peak overpressure can be very intense but brief, especially close to an explosion; at a distance of 10.2 m (33 ft), from 0.364 kg (0.8 lb) of TNT, the peak overpressure is about 45 kPa (6.5 psi), with a duration of about 2 ms.[5]

As the shock wave expands, the overpressure decreases, the duration lengthens, and the velocity of propagation diminishes. For free field air blast, the peak pressure of the shock wave falls off as the inverse of the distance from the explosion to the third power. This translates into a rough formula to use to the scaling factor in explosive science: For a bomb to produce twice the damage, it must be eight times as large. In denser media, such as water, explosions produce shock waves that have a much higher peak overpressure and a shorter duration, and propagate at a faster velocity than comparable explosions in air. In addition, the overpressure is less just below the surface than at greater depths. Parts of the body submerged to a greater depth are correspondingly more damaged than body parts submerged just below the surface or those that are above the surface.

If the explosion is contained within a closed space, reflections of the shock wave lead to greater overpressure, longer duration, and an increased incidence of primary blast injuries and death.[12]

Primary blast injuries are unique to this form of trauma. As the shock wave passes through biologic tissue, the injury is greatest at the interface between tissues of different densities, such as the lungs (which contain both blood and air), the tympanic membrane (which separates two air-filled cavities), and the bowel (which contains a slurry of solid and gas).[14] The potential for primary blast injuries correlates with both the height and duration of the peak overpressure. The likelihood of primary blast injury can be illustrated for a specific clinical outcome (e.g., threshold for lung damage or 50% lethality [LD50]) by pressure-duration graphs. By the last 1960s, the Lovelace Foundation of Albuquerque, New Mexico, had assembled enough animal data to make an estimate of human tolerance to shock waves using pressure-duration graphs.[10] The most vulnerable organ to primary blast injury is the tympanic membrane, followed by the lungs.[14]

The most common primary blast injury is a linear tear in the inferior portion of the tympanic membrane.[6] Depending on the orientation of the external auditory canal in relation to the source of the shock wave, tympanic membranes may rupture at pressures as low as 2 to 5 psi. Explosions also commonly produce damage to the cochlea, which results in sensorineural hearing loss and tinnitus.[6]

In the lungs, primary blast injury produces a diffuse lung contusion; damage to the alveolar parenchyma leads to edema and hemorrhage into the interstitial and interalveolar spaces.[14] The threshold for lung damage is about 15 psi of peak overpressure, and moderate-to-severe lung damage can be seen with 50 psi.[5] Lacerations of the delicate parenchyma may occur in many locations, rupturing alveolar walls, tearing visceral pleura, and creating fissures between the alveolar spaces and the pulmonary veins. The latter allows air to enter into the pulmonary venous system, which can then travel to the left side of the heart and enter the systemic circulation. Systemic air emboli are the likely cause of sudden death, abnormal neurologic findings, and myocardial ischemia seen in some victims in the immediate postblast period.

Primary blast injury of the bowels requires even higher peak overpressures. Such injuries are relatively rare in air explosions, but are more common in water explosions, where the victim is completely or partially submerged. The most common injuries are serosal tears, subserosal and intramural hemorrhages, as well as bowel perforations, usually involving the ileocecal region.[14]

CLINICAL PRESENTATION

Casualty analysis of terrorist bombing incidents has found that secondary, tertiary, and miscellaneous injuries account for the vast majority of victims.[9,12,13] The following principles are important to remember.

1. Terrorist explosions often occur within a populated and confined space, producing a large number of casualties.
2. The most common type of injury from terrorist bombs is superficial soft-tissue damage to exposed areas of the body from flying debris. The nonaerodynamic shape of most debris fragments means that they have marked air resistance and limited range for serious injury.
3. Serious injuries from terrorist bombings are usually major soft-tissue damage, flash burns, fractures, and eye injuries. Most of these victims are within 10 to 15 m of the source of the explosion.
4. While flash burns commonly injure exposed skin, the temperature content of gas is low and the duration of exposure is brief so that skin underlying clothing and the upper respiratory tract are rarely burned. However, burns and smoke from blast-ignited fires can, of course, be more damaging.
5. Other than tympanic membrane rupture, primary blast injuries are uncommon and account for less than 10% of the victims in open-air explosions but up to 38% in closed-space (e.g., bus) explosions.[9,12]

A triad of hypotension, bradycardia, and apnea has been observed in experimental animals exposed to moderate thoracic blast injury.[7] The first two responses—hypotension and bradycardia—have been observed in human victims immediately after the explosion.

The clinical presentation of patients with primary blast injuries is usually the result of damage to the ears, lungs, brain, and bowel. The most common respiratory symptoms are dyspnea, chest pain, and hemoptysis. Physical examination will disclose rales, rhonchi, and, occasionally, the presence of a pneumothorax or pneumomediastinum. Frothy, blood-tinged sputum is seen in severe cases. Radiographic progression of pulmonary injury can occur during the first 48 hours after the explosion, corresponding to the clinical development of respiratory failure.

Tympanic membrane rupture usually presents with decreased hearing occasionally accompanied by bleeding into the external auditory canal. Perforations are usually small and located in the inferior portion of the membrane.[6,11] The degree of associated conductive hearing loss is related to the size of the perforation. Sensorineural hearing loss can occur from damage to the sensory structures in the cochlear basal membrane.[15]

Concussion with amnesia is common in blast-injured victims. Focal neurologic findings usually result from cerebral air emboli. If the victim was exposed to underwater blast, concussion of the spinal cord may present as lower extremity weakness, paralysis, or paresthesias lasting from seconds to minutes.

Bowel injuries are more common in victims exposed to underwater explosions, compared with those exposed to air blasts. Clinical symptoms include acute abdominal pain, tenderness, nausea, vomiting, and an urge to defecate.

Systemic air emboli may be difficult to detect, and the diagnosis depends on clinical suspicion. Definite diagnosis of systemic air emboli can made if air emboli are visualized in retinal vessels or on computed tomography of the brain. Air embolism usually develops immediately or very soon after the explosion.

However, delayed cases can occur when positive-pressure ventilation is initiated in patients with pulmonary blast injury.

DIFFERENTIAL DIAGNOSIS

The key to diagnosis is to obtain a history of injury associated with an explosion. Finding a tympanic perforation may be a clue to potential blast injuries, but the absence of tympanic membrane perforation does not exclude potential blast injury. Nonexplosive blast injury to the ear can occur from a blow that seals the external auditory meatus and causes a sudden increase in air pressure.[3] Tympanic membrane perforations and conductive hearing loss are common. Such perforations almost always heal with improvement in the conductive hearing loss.

EMERGENCY DEPARTMENT EVALUATION

Initial evaluation is similar to that of any multiple trauma victim, with initial evaluation of the ABCs, followed by the secondary survey and ongoing monitoring, including vital signs, electrographic monitoring, and pulse oximetry. The focus of the examination is the detection of primary blast injury, which may be obscured by secondary and tertiary injury. After the primary and secondary patient assessments, further examination is directed toward identifying emergent life-threatening arterial emboli. A chest radiograph is indicated because of pulmonary susceptibility to primary blast injury. Radiographic injuries seen with primary blast injury include pneumothorax, pneumomediastinum, hemothorax, subcutaneous emphysema, pulmonary interstitial emphysema, interstitial infiltrates, and alveolar edema.

Laboratory studies should be ordered if clinically indicated, but routine arterial blood gas analysis is particularly useful. In blast-injured patients, the arterial blood gas may be the first sign of lung damage, preceding radiographic changes.

All patients exposed to blast explosions need to be observed to exclude delayed manifestations of primary blast injuries. For patients with only soft-tissue injuries, the observation period can be as short as the time it takes for evaluation of such injuries in the emergency department or treatment center.

EMERGENCY DEPARTMENT MANAGEMENT

Evaluation, resuscitation, and ongoing management should proceed as it would for any other victim of multiple trauma in both the prehospital setting and the emergency department. For prehospital personnel, it is important that the scene be secured and declared safe before approaching the victims. Accurate triage is an important determinant of survival for critically injured casualties from terrorist bombings and industrial accidents. High-flow oxygen should be administered, because injury to the lungs may not be initially recognized and hypoxemia may develop insidiously. Because excessive fluid accumulation may occur in damaged lungs, fluid resuscitation should be carefully monitored to avoid exacerbation of pulmonary insufficiency.

For victims with systemic air emboli, hyperbaric oxygen therapy is the treatment of choice. It can be dramatically effective for cerebral air emboli, even up to 12 hours after the acute event. Although unproved, the Trendelenburg position is sometimes advocated to reduce embolization to the brain. However, experimental models and anecdotal reports find no clear benefit to this position, as compared with the standard and supine position for assessment and treatment of the trauma patient.

Primary blast lung injury requires careful management.[2] For trauma patients with respiratory failure, the standard approach is endotracheal intubation and positive-pressure ventilation. However, positive-pressure ventilation in patients with blast-injured lungs may produce or exacerbate pneumothorax, increase the alveolar-to-pulmonary vein pressure gradient, and potentiate systemic air embolization. The immediate use of mechanical ventilation during the first 2 hours in a dog model of blast-injured lungs produced increased air embolism and mortality. In addition, general anesthesia is poorly tolerated in patients with primary blast injury during the first 24 to 48 hours; therefore, regional or spinal anesthesia should be used, if possible. Intravenous fluid management needs to be carefully monitored, and pulmonary artery and arterial catheters may be required to manage fluids appropriately. For patients with severe pulmonary blast injuries, a regimen of volume-controlled, synchronized, intermittent, mandatory ventilation with small tidal volumes and permissive hypercapnia ($PaCO_2$ 57 mm Hg) appears beneficial.[16]

Abdominal blast injury is managed just like that of any other blunt-force trauma to the abdomen. Lacerations, abrasions, fractures, and burns resulting from secondary and tertiary blast injury can be managed the same as trauma caused by other mechanisms. Fragments generated by small explosions (e.g., from a hand grenade) tend to produce wounds with little damage and can usually be managed without extensive wound exploration and fragment removal.[4] However, high-velocity fragment wounds (e.g., from a terrorist bomb incident) should have as many fragments excised as possible and the wound left open for delayed primary closure.

Tympanic membrane perforation has a high rate of spontaneous healing, especially if it is small and marginal in location.[11] For large and central perforations, immediate paper patching has been advocated.[11] If a perforation (large or small) does not heal after 10 months, tympanoplasty should be performed. In general, the external auditory canal should be kept clean and dry; there is no need for routine irrigation or use of topical solutions. One potential long-term sequela to bear in mind is the development of cholesteatoma. The ruptured tympanic membrane can distribute small pieces of keratinizing squamous epithelium throughout the middle ear and mastoid sinuses, viable fragments of which may grow into a mass of keratinous debris known as a cholesteatoma. Cholesteatoma may lead to varying degrees of sensorineural or conductive hearing loss and may erode into surrounding structures.

DISPOSITION

Blast injuries that result in multiple trauma require consultation with the hospital trauma service or referral and transfer to the regional trauma center. If systemic air embolism is suspected, urgent consultation with a hyperbaric specialist is required for definitive therapy. Patients with signs of blunt-force trauma and those with tympanic membrane rupture should be observed for occult injuries during the first 24 hours. Outpatient management is acceptable for patients who were a distance from the blast origin and received relatively minor lacerations, abrasions, fractures, or burns.[13]

Patients with serious blast injuries should be transferred to a regional trauma center. Those with suspected systemic air embolism may require transfer to a hyperbaric therapy facility. If air transport is used, pressurized aircraft or flights at low altitude are important to prevent further exacerbation of air emboli or pneumothoraces from barometric changes during flight.

COMMON PITFALLS

- Accurate triage at the scene is an important determinant of survival for critically injured victims of explosions.
- The tympanic membrane should always be checked as an indicator of the potential for primary blast injuries to the lungs.
- The most lethal problem in blast injuries is air emboli affecting the brain or the heart. Symptoms suggestive of cerebral emboli or myocardial ischemia need to be carefully addressed for this potential.
- Positive-pressure ventilation poses a significant risk of worsening pneumothorax or producing systemic air embolization.

References

1. Aboutanos MB, Baker SP. Wartime civilian injuries: epidemiology and intervention strategies. *J Trauma* 1997;43:719.
2. Argyros GJ. Management of primary blast injury. *Toxicology* 1997;121:105.
3. Berger G, Finkelstein Y, Avraham S, et al. Patterns of hearing loss in non-explosive blast injury of the ear. *J Laryngol Otol* 1997;111:1137.
4. Coupland RM. Hand grenade injuries among civilians. *JAMA* 1993;270:624.
5. Elsayed NM. Toxicology of blast overpressure. *Toxicology* 1997;121:1.
6. Garth RJ. Blast injury of the ear: an overview and guide to management. *Injury* 1995;26:363.
7. Guy RJ, Kirkman E, Watkins PE, et al. Physiologic responses to primary blast. *J Trauma* 1998;45:983.
8. Karmy-Jones R, Kissinger D, Golocovsky M, et al. Bomb-related injuries. *Milit Med* 1994;159:536.
9. Katz E, Ofek B, Adler J, et al. Primary blast injury after a bomb explosion in a civilian bus. *Ann Surg* 1989;209:484.
10. Kokinakis W, Rudolph RR. An assessment of the current state-of-the-art of incapacitation by air blast. *Acta Chir Scand* 1982;508[Suppl]:135.
11. Kronenberg J, Ben-Shoshan J, Wolf M. Perforated tympanic membrane after blast injury. *Am J Otol* 1993;14:92.
12. Leibovici D, Gofrit ON, Stein M, et al. Blast injuries: bus versus open-air bombings—a comparative study of injuries in survivors of open-air versus confined-space explosions. *J Trauma* 1996;41:1030.
13. Mallonne S, Shariat S, Stennies G, et al. Physical injuries and fatalities resulting from the Oklahoma City bombing. *JAMA* 1996;276:382.
14. Mayorga MA. The pathology of primary blast overpressure injury. *Toxicology* 1997;121:17.
15. Patterson JH, Hamerik RP. Blast overpressure induced structural and functional changes in the auditory system. *Toxicology* 1997;121:29.
16. Sorkine P, Szold O, Kluger Y, et al. Permissive hypercapnia ventilation in patients with severe pulmonary blast injury. *J Trauma* 1998;45:35.

CHAPTER 124
Trauma in Pregnancy

Andy Jagoda and Stu G. Kessler

Trauma is the most frequent cause of nonobstetric maternal and fetal death during pregnancy.[15] The incidence of trauma in pregnancy is 7% to 8%.[1] Diagnosis and treatment follows the same general guidelines as for the nonpregnant trauma victim. The initial treatment must be directed toward stabilizing maternal hemodynamics. However, due to the altered anatomy and physiology of the gravid female, several critical differences exist. Knowing these differences and applying this knowledge in the critical minutes following trauma will have an important impact on the life and health of both mother and fetus.

PHYSIOLOGY AND ANATOMY OF PREGNANCY

Pregnancy is a high-flow, low-resistance state of cardiovascular homeostasis (Table 124.1). Heart rate increases until the end of the second trimester, when it plateaus at 10 to 15 beats above baseline. Meanwhile, systolic and, to a greater degree, diastolic blood pressures decrease 5 to 15 mm Hg during the first and second trimesters, returning to prepregnancy baseline levels during the third trimester. Cardiac output increases 40% by the end of the first trimester and persists at this level, causing a systolic flow murmur in 90% of pregnant women. By the third trimester, there is increased vascular congestion in the pelvis and a 50% decrease in the velocity of venous flow in the lower limbs associated with a 10-mm Hg increase in venous pressure.[3] These changes predispose the gravida to deep vein thromboses, as well as increased bleeding with lower extremity trauma.

The diaphragm is gradually pushed up 3 to 4 cm, causing the QRS axis on the electrocardiogram to shift an average of 15 degrees to the left. Other pregnancy-related electrocardiographic changes include Q waves in leads III and aVF and flattened or inverted T waves in lead III.

Elevation of the diaphragm causes a 25% decrease in functional residual capacity, resulting in decreased maternal oxygen reserve. Pulmonary function is further compromised by increased oxygen consumption. Starting in the first trimester, stimulation of the medullary respiratory center by progesterone gradually increases minute ventilation by up to 50% (a result of increased tidal volume). This is accompanied by a 10-mm Hg increase in PO_2, a 10-mm Hg decrease in PCO_2, and a compensatory decrease in bicarbonate to about 19.5 mEq/L, producing a net slight respiratory alkalosis.

Progesterone also causes smooth muscle relaxation in the gastrointestinal tract, which leads to decreased motility and decreased gastroesophageal sphincter competence, producing a greater risk of aspiration.

Urologic changes begin at the end of the first trimester. The bladder becomes hyperemic and rises out of the pelvis, and the ureters dilate and become laterally displaced.

After the third month, the uterus is no longer protected by the pelvis. Uterine blood flow increases tenfold by term. The uterine vascular bed has no autoregulatory capability and is completely dependent on maternal blood pressure for perfusion.

Several hematologic changes accompany pregnancy. A 50% increase in blood volume, accompanied by only a 20% to 30% increase in red blood cell mass, results in a 3% to 6% drop in hematocrit. The white blood cell count increases to 12,000 to 18,000/μL by the second trimester and may increase to 25,000/μL with stress. Neutrophils predominate. The prothrombin and partial thromboplastin times are somewhat shortened. Coagulation factors rise gradually and, by the third trimester, exceed fibrinolytic activity.

The fetus has a higher hemoglobin concentration than the mother, and fetal hemoglobin has a greater affinity for oxygen. As a result, fetal oxygen consumption does not decrease until oxygen delivery decreases by 50%.[21] This allows the fetus to tolerate brief periods of maternal hypoxia and hypoperfusion. Furthermore, late in pregnancy, the fetus is capable of the mammalian diving reflex by which blood can be redistributed to the heart and brain.[21]

PREHOSPITAL CARE

The best outcome is ensured by prevention of maternal hypoxia and hypotension. The airway should be aggressively managed

TABLE 124.1. Anatomic and Physiologic Changes in Pregnancy

			Trimester		
System	Change	Effect	1st	2nd	3rd
CARDIOVASCULAR					
	↑ cardiac output		Increased	6–7 L/min	6–7 L/min
	↑ heart rate		↑	↑	80–95 beats/min
	↑ blood volume	↓ initial response to hemorrhage	↑ 50% →	→	→
	↓ PVR	↓ BP	↓ BP	↓ BP	↑ to normal
		↑ skin temp.	(0–15 mm Hg)		
	↓ uterine perfusion	↑ fetal risk			↑ to normal
	Aortocaval compression	↑ supine hypotension syndrome with progressive increased uterine size			
PULMONARY					
	↑ tidal volume	↑ minute ventilation	↑	↑	↑ 50%
		↓ serum bicarbonate			
		↓ acidosis tolerance			
	↑ diaphragm elevation	↑ excursion	↑	↑	↑ 4 cm
		↑ anteroposterior chest diameter			
		↓ FRC (↑ sensitivity to inhalational anesthesia agents)			
	↑ O_2 consumption	↓ tolerance to hypoxia →	→	→	→
	↑ fetal O_2 demand				
HEMATOLOGIC					
	Minimal ↑ red blood cell mass	Dilutional anemia		↓ 3–6%	↓ 3–6%
	↑ leukocytosis		5–12K	12–18K	12–18K
	↑ hypercoagulability	↑ risk deep venous thrombosis →	→	→	→
GASTROINTESTINAL					
	↓ motility	↑ risk aspiration →	→	→	→
	↓ gastric emptying				
GENITOURINARY					
	Dilation of ureters and kidneys	Abnormal intravenous pyelogram			
		Can overestimate hydration	7–10 mg/dL →	→	→
	↓ BUN and creatinine	↑ risk injury		↑	↑
	Displacement of bladder				

PVR, pulmonary vascular resistance; BP, blood pressure; FRC, functional residual capacity; BUN, blood urea nitrogen.

and supplemental oxygen liberally utilized. A low threshold for volume replacement should exist. Maternal blood loss of 30% to 35% can cause a 10% to 20% decrease in uterine blood flow without a detectable change in maternal vital signs.[27] After the twentieth week, transport should be done, with the patient in the left lateral decubitus position or with the right hip elevated. If the patient is fully immobilized, the backboard should be tilted 15 degrees to the left. This will help keep the uterus off the descending aorta and inferior vena cava and prevent a number of adverse hemodynamic effects collectively known as the supine hypotension syndrome (Fig. 124.1). Uterine compression of the inferior vena cava can cause up to a 30% decrease in cardiac output, due to decreased preload.[3] Maternal hypotension resulting either from this or from hypovolemia leads to uteroplacental insufficiency, increased risk of placental abruption, and possible cardiopulmonary arrest.[12] If possible, vasopressors should be avoided, because they decrease uterine blood flow. Pneumatic antishock garments (PASGs) are not well studied in pregnancy. Their use is controversial and generally contradicted, although there has been some support for their role as an adjunct to stabilize pelvic fractures in patients in extremis in the first trimester.

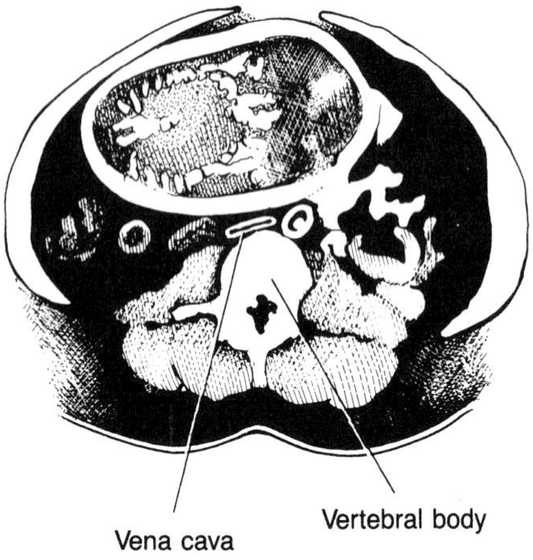

Figure 124.1. Cross section of the lower abdomen in a supine pregnant patient. Note the vena caval compression against the vertebral body.

Transport should proceed without delay and with early notification of the receiving hospital, so that all involved services and resources can be mobilized.

EMERGENCY DEPARTMENT EVALUATION

An appropriate patient history should determine the date of the last menstrual period, estimated date of delivery, problems with present and previous pregnancies, ultrasound results, and time of last fetal movement. Initial evaluation and therapy must be directed primarily at the case of the mother and should not be

TABLE 124.2. Estimated Radiation Dose to Fetus Per Radiograph

Cervical spine	<1 mrad
Chest	1–3 mrad
Abdomen	200–500 mrad
Pelvis	200–500 mrad
Lumbar spine	600–1,000 mrad
Hip/femur	100–450 mrad
CT head/chest with shielding	<1,000 mrad
CT abdomen	3,000 mrad
CT pelvis	3,000–9,000 mrad

delayed or compromised because of pregnancy. Fetal survival is largely dependent on maternal condition and resuscitation. After the primary survey has been completed, uterine size is estimated, bearing in mind that if the fundus is above the umbilicus, fetal age is probably more than 20 weeks and there is potential viability. Uterine tenderness, irritability, contractions, and fetal movement should be sought. Fetal heart rate is auscultated. A careful speculum examination is performed if no frank bleeding exists. Abdominal examination is less reliable, due to the blunted response to peritoneal irritation caused by stretching of the abdominal wall.[27,30]

Monitoring is the best way to determine the functional and anatomic viability of the fetal–placental unit. External cardiotocographic monitoring should be instituted as soon as is practical. Contractions may portend abruption or the start of labor. Fetal tachycardia (rate greater than 160) or bradycardia (rate less than 120) or loss of accelerations, and particularly late or prolonged decelerations, may represent fetal distress or occult maternal shock. Real-time ultrasonography provides important information about fetal age and movement, amniotic fluid volume, and the position and integrity of the placenta.

Radiation is potentially hazardous to the fetus throughout pregnancy. This is particularly true in the first 7 weeks following conception, during organogenesis, when the fetus is sensitive to radiation's teratogenic, growth-retarding and postnatal neoplastic effects. It is reassuring, however, that significant risk is unlikely with exposures of less than 10 rads[30] (Table 124.2). If the fetus is outside the radiographic field, radiation dose is limited to that delivered by leak and scatter. The dose drops off rapidly with fetal distance from the radiographic field. Appropriate radiographs are obtained as necessary for the proper care of the patient, without delay, but the pelvis is shielded and care taken to minimize the dose of radiation to the lower abdomen.[27,30]

EMERGENCY DEPARTMENT MANAGEMENT

The evaluation and resuscitation of the seriously, or potentially seriously, injured pregnant trauma patient often benefit from a multidisciplinary team approach. In addition to the emergency physician and nursing staff, trauma surgeons and, when available, physicians and nurses from obstetrics and gynecology, pediatrics or neonatology, and possibly anesthesia may offer specific expertise. The first priorities are airway, breathing, and circulation. Hypoxia, acidosis, and alkalosis all decrease uterine blood flow and oxygen delivery to the fetus. Oxygen saturation is kept greater than 90%.[30] Extra care is warranted during intubation because of smaller maternal oxygen reserve and increased risk of aspiration. Hemodynamics should be maximized using standard protocols for crystalloid and blood infusion, with central venous monitoring as needed. Vasopressors are withheld until appropriate fluid resuscitation is accomplished. The supine hypotension syndrome is avoided by proper patient positioning.

Maternal head trauma is managed as in the nonpregnant patient. If there is a history of a seizure before the accident, eclampsia must be considered in the differential diagnosis. Hypertension may be masked by hypovolemia.

In late pregnancy, if a chest tube is necessary to manage thoracic injury, it should be placed one to two interspaces higher than usual to avoid the elevated diaphragm present at this stage of pregnancy.

Pelvic fractures may prove especially serious in the pregnant patient, due to increased pelvic vascularity and the proximity of the fetus. There is a 25% incidence of associated fetal death,[29] due to shock, abruption, and direct fetal injury.

Tetanus prophylaxis may be given without fetal ill effects. Antibiotics considered safe to use in pregnancy include penicillins, cephalosporins, and erythromycin (except the estolate salt).

The risk of thromboembolic disease in the third trimester and immediately postpartum is five to six times that of the general population.[3] Subcutaneous heparin or pneumatic compression devices may be used for prophylaxis.

Disseminated intravascular coagulation is associated with several sequelae of trauma in pregnancy, including abruptio placentae, amniotic fluid embolism, and fetal death in utero. Baseline coagulation studies, including prothrombin time and partial thromboplastin time, fibrinogen level, and fibrin split products, should be obtained in any gravid patient sustaining significant trauma.

Anesthesia is safe as long as adequate oxygenation and perfusion are maintained.[30] Laparotomy risks for the mother are not increased with pregnancy, and labor and abortion will not be precipitated,[3,8,27] although uterine manipulation should be minimized. When contemplating the need for emergent cesarean section, one should first consider the mother's ability to tolerate the procedure and then weigh the risk of fetal distress against the risk of immaturity. Survival with normal development has been achieved at 22 weeks.[31] By 24 weeks, 50% survival can be achieved, but morbidity remains high.[15]

In the event of cardiopulmonary arrest, rapid airway access should be gained and aggressive fluid resuscitation ensured. One member of the team should be assigned to deflect the uterus to the left. The fetus should be monitored. Defibrillation, lidocaine, and bretylium tosylate are safe to administer. After a few minutes of unsuccessful resuscitation with standard cardiopulmonary resuscitation, and if not already performed for other indications, one should consider a perimortem emergent cesarean section.[14,17]

Based on knowledge of fetal and maternal physiology and a review of case reports, one study recommends that perimortem cesarean delivery be initiated after 4 minutes and completed within 5 minutes of unsuccessful cardiopulmonary resuscitation.[11] These reports document decreased fetal survival as time from maternal death to delivery increases. If not already accomplished, simultaneous open cardiac massage and aortic cross-clamping (after delivery of the fetus) should be considered. A midline incision is made from the epigastrium to the pubis. The uterus is vertically incised from the fundus to the bladder reflection. An anterior placenta is incised as necessary and the cord promptly clamped and cut. Successful outcome depends on the interval between maternal death or arrest and fetal delivery, cause of maternal death, fetal age, and extent of direct fetal injuries. In addition, the ability to provide immediate and adequate neonatal resuscitation is imperative. No physician has been found liable in performing this operation, and there is unanimous consensus among legal authorities that, regardless of outcome, judgment would not be found against this physician.[11]

BLUNT TRAUMA

The most common causes of blunt trauma during pregnancy are motor vehicle crashes, falls, and direct assaults. Motor vehicle injuries account for the majority of severe obstetric trauma.[32] However, direct assaults, including cases of domestic violence, are likely underreported.[18,23,28] Falls occur more frequently in women at greater than 20 weeks' gestation, due to pelvic laxity and imbalance. Most cases involving minimum-to-mild trauma have good maternal and fetal outcomes; however, instances of abruption and fetal death have been reported in cases of minimal maternal injury. Maternal death is most often due to head injury or hemorrhagic shock. The most common causes of fetal death are maternal death (fetal mortality greater than 90%) and maternal shock (fetal mortality approaches 80%), followed by significant maternal injury, placental abruption, and direct fetal injury.[15] Fetal deaths are not uncommon, however, even when maternal injuries are not life-threatening.

As in the nonpregnant trauma victim, the most frequently injured abdominal organs are the spleen, liver, and kidney. Bowel injuries are less frequent. Diaphragm and serious retroperitoneal injuries occur more often.

EMERGENCY DEPARTMENT EVALUATION

Diagnostic peritoneal lavage is safe and accurate with the supraumbilical open technique.[21] Indications for lavage and criteria for a positive lavage are similar to those for the nongravid trauma patient. Ultrasound has the potential to evaluate both mother and fetus and, in experienced hands, can identify hemoperitoneum and injuries to the spleen, liver, and kidney (Fig. 124.2). Computed tomography (CT) is not well studied in pregnancy, and the additional dose of radiation must be considered. However, CT may be indicated to evaluate the retroperitoneal space due to the increased risk of significant retroperitoneal hemorrhage following lower abdominal and pelvic trauma in pregnant women.

EMERGENCY DEPARTMENT MANAGEMENT

Patients with significant blunt abdominal trauma are admitted to the hospital and managed as inpatients. Fetal monitoring is indicated. Operative indications are the same as in the nongravid patient.

Pregnant patients with minor injuries, who are beyond 20 weeks of gestation, should undergo observation and fetal monitoring.[30] The optimal length of in-hospital observation and fetal monitoring remains controversial, with suggestions ranging from 2 to 48 hours.[5,20] Fetal heart rate and uterine contractions and patterns are evaluated, along with any evidence of vaginal bleeding, rupture of membranes, or uterine tenderness. If this period of evaluation does not reveal significant findings, and if the mother is otherwise stable and the mechanism of injury was not significant, the patient can likely be discharged home. Any abnormal findings warrant admission and further evaluation. If discharged, the mother should be instructed to record fetal movements over 1 week and return to the hospital immediately for a nonstress test if she notes fewer than four fetal movements per hour or any bleeding, preterm labor, rupture of membranes, or uterine or abdominal pain. Serial ultrasound evaluations and monitoring should be scheduled for a few days after the trauma and periodically for the remainder of the pregnancy.

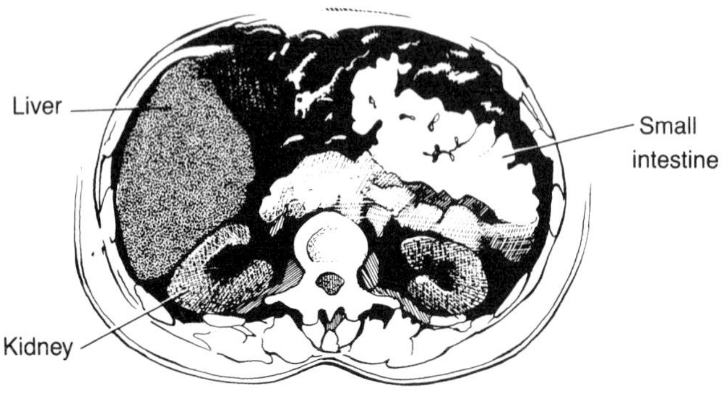

Figure 124.2. Cross section of the upper abdomen in a pregnant trauma patient. Crowding and upper displacement of the small intestine may increase the likelihood of missing mesenteric and hollow viscus injuries.

SPECIAL CONSIDERATIONS

Placental abruption occurs in 1% to 5% of minor trauma and in 40% to 50% of major trauma.[21,30] It is initiated by a direct blow or deceleration force and may be propagated by increased amniotic fluid pressure or elevated pressure in the vena cava. The clinical consequences are proportional to the amount of placenta involved.

Clinical signs and symptoms of abruption include vaginal bleeding, abdominal cramps, contractions, uterine tenderness, and fetal distress. It is important to note, however, that abruption may be present in the absence of vaginal bleeding in up to 20% of cases. In some cases, up to 2 L of blood can be sequestered in uterine tissue without external bleeding. Ultrasound may fail to identify abruption in up to 50% of cases; often, cardiotocographic monitoring is more sensitive. Pearlman and associates[20] detected all abruptions in the first 4 hours of monitoring. Fewer than four contractions an hour ensured a good outcome in all cases. Abruption of less than 25% is consistent with fetal survival but may induce premature labor. A 50% or greater abruption uniformly results in fetal demise. The maternal death rate is less than 1%.[15]

Heavy vaginal bleeding, evidence of coagulopathy, and fetal distress are indications for cesarean section. Management of mild abruption is controversial and is determined by the obstetric consultant.

Uterine injury is common. Contractions are the most frequently seen obstetric problem caused by trauma. Any damage to the myometrium or placenta can cause contractions. Ninety percent will stop spontaneously.[20] The use of tocolytics in the setting of trauma is controversial: Tocolysis has been successfully employed,[31] but many researchers believe that regular uterine contractions after trauma suggest abruption until proven otherwise.[1,20]

Rupture of membranes can lead to early labor or infection. Obstetric consultation should be obtained and the patient should undergo observation and fetal monitoring in labor and delivery.

Uterine rupture is devastating but, fortunately, rare. It is associated with major trauma, especially fractures of the anterior pelvic ring.

The clinical presentation of uterine rupture is usually dramatic and may include shock, severe abdominal pain, difficulty palpating the fundus, and easily palpable fetal parts. Diagnosis is readily confirmed with ultrasound. Treatment is immediate cesarean section. Fetal mortality is nearly 100%.

Fetal injuries are minimized in blunt trauma by the cushioning provided by the uteroplacental unit. Fetal injuries, when they do occur, usually involve intracranial hemorrhage and skull fracture secondary to maternal pelvic fractures when the fetal head is engaged. The nonvertex fetus may sustain intracranial trauma even in the absence of significant maternal trauma, presumably due to deceleration forces.[30]

PENETRATING ABDOMINAL TRAUMA

Penetrating abdominal trauma is rare during pregnancy: Gunshot wounds are more common than stab wounds. In late pregnancy, the gravid uterus is the most commonly injured intraperitoneal structure with penetrating trauma.

EMERGENCY DEPARTMENT EVALUATION AND MANAGEMENT

Controversy regarding evaluation and management may be divided into two broad categories: injuries above the fundus and those below the fundus.

Gunshot wounds above the fundus, or suspicious for intraperitoneal violation, require exploration. Management of upper abdominal stab wounds remains somewhat controversial. Local wound exploration can frequently exclude peritoneal penetration. Because the bowel is displaced superiorly, and there is a high incidence of reported bowel injury with stab wounds during pregnancy, most of the literature supports mandatory exploration when peritoneal penetration cannot be excluded.[24,26,27] Recommendations for exploration are based on the lack of sensitivity of diagnostic peritoneal lavage in picking up bowel injuries, the delayed peritoneal response to these injuries, the difficulty in clinically evaluating the pregnant abdomen, and the fact that diagnostic peritoneal lavage has not been specifically studied for stab wounds in pregnancy (see Fig. 124.2).

Although there has been support for selective observation of gunshot wounds to the uterus,[9] most now agree that these wounds should be explored.[24,26,30] The viable fetus should be delivered by cesarean section to decrease the risk of delayed death from fetal and placental injury. The dead fetus should be left in utero,[9,10,27] sparing the mother unnecessary blood loss and operating time. Labor proceeds uneventfully despite the injured uterus and laparotomy scar.[10,26,27] If labor does not ensue in a few days, it can be induced.[10] Lower abdominal contents are relatively shielded from stab wounds by the gravid uterus. Stab wounds to the uterus are more controversial, with advocates of both mandatory surgery[24,27] and diagnostic peritoneal lavage–guided observation under certain circumstances.[26,30] There have been no reported maternal deaths with uterine stab wounds, but the incidence of fetal injury is very high.[24] Any sign of fetal distress on external fetal monitoring warrants immediate cesarean section for a potentially viable fetus.

BURNS

Pregnancy does not affect maternal outcome in burns.[2] Fetal survival is related to gestational age and the extent of burn. In the first trimester, there is high fetal wastage, while premature labor is common in the third trimester.[26] Pregnancy is usually unaffected by a less than 20% total body surface area (TBSA) burn. Burns between 20% and 50% TBSA show increasing risk of fetal loss and premature labor, as well as maternal complications and death. With a more than 50% TBSA burn, there are few maternal or fetal survivors. Burn criteria for inpatient versus outpatient management do not differ in the pregnant patient. The fetus should be monitored continuously in all cases of moderate-to-severe burns. Hemodynamic monitoring is the best guide to fluid replacement.[26] Silver sulfadiazine should be used sparingly in the last trimester, due to the risk of kernicterus.[6] Delivery of the fetus should be considered at the first sign of septic shock or other significant burn complications, due to the high risk of abortion.[2]

ELECTRICAL INJURIES

Reports of electrical injury by household current are rare in pregnancy. Lieberman and coworkers[16] reviewed six cases. No maternal morbidity was noted, but two mothers noticed decreased fetal movements and experienced stillbirths within 1 week of injury. One exposure resulted in intrauterine growth retardation and, later, stillbirth. The remaining three cases had normal outcomes, but two of these were complicated by oligohydramnios. Regardless of how minor the exposure, women should seek medical care and carefully monitor fetal movements for the remainder of their pregnancy.

Pierce and associates[22] reviewed 12 cases of pregnant lightning-strike victims. No maternal deaths resulted, but one cardiac arrest was successfully resuscitated. There were five immediate fetal deaths, one from uterine rupture. Three strikes resulted in spontaneous labor; all victims were at greater than 34 weeks' gestation. Five infants were normal at birth. This review by Pierce et al. would suggest that lightning causes either an immediate problem or no problem at all.

PREVENTING MORBIDITY FROM MOTOR VEHICLE ACCIDENTS

The use of three-point restraints can significantly reduce both maternal and fetal morbidity and mortality from motor vehicle accidents.[25] The lap belt should be worn snug and low over the anterior iliac spines. The shoulder belt should be worn above the gravid uterus without touching the neck. The pregnant woman should sit upright and use the headrest.

FETAL–MATERNAL HEMORRHAGE

Fetal–maternal hemorrhage (FMH), or the occurrence of fetal bleeding into the maternal circulation, occurs in 2% to 8% of normal pregnancies.[15] The incidence is believed to increase to 8% to 30% of pregnant women involved in trauma.[21,30] The incidence and extent of bleeding is likely higher with more significant trauma; however, the relationship is not linear.

All Rh-negative trauma victims should receive 300 μg of Rho(D) immune globulin (RhIG or RhoGAM) no more than 72 hours after trauma to prevent Rh sensitization. This covers hemorrhages up to 30 mL. Larger hemorrhages are quantitated using the Kleihauer-Betke test or similar techniques. An additional 300 μg of RhoGAM is given for each additional 30 mL of hemorrhage. Kleihauer-Betke testing may also be useful in guiding intervention for other complications of FMH, such as fetal and neonatal anemia.

AMNIOTIC FLUID EMBOLISM

Amniotic fluid embolism is occasionally associated with trauma and abruption. Amniotic fluid and debris enter the maternal venous circulation and lodge in the lung.

This is a clinical diagnosis based on sudden dyspnea, hypoxia, and hypotension. The chest radiograph is consistent with pulmonary edema or adult respiratory distress syndrome. Disseminated intravascular coagulation develops in 30%.

Treatment is supportive and includes oxygen, maximizing hemodynamics, and correcting coagulopathy. Mortality is 80%.

COMMON PITFALLS

- Failure to diagnose pregnancy in the trauma patient
- Failure to appreciate the anatomic and physiologic changes of pregnancy in interpreting physical, laboratory, and radiologic data
- Failure to aggressively treat maternal hypovolemia and hypoxia
- Neglecting proper patient positioning
- Inadequate fetal monitoring
- Failure to obtain indicated radiographic studies
- Failure to consider and treat FMH
- Failure to appreciate the increased risk to the fetus with maternal burns, carbon monoxide exposure, and electrical shock
- Delay in performing perimortem cesarean section during maternal cardiopulmonary arrest
- Delay in assembling the appropriate multidisciplinary team

References

1. Ali J, Yeo A, Gana TJ, et al. Predictors of fetal mortality in pregnant trauma patients. *J Trauma* 1997;42:782.
2. Amy BW, McManus WF, Goodwin CW, et al. Thermal injury in the pregnant patient. *Surg Gynecol Obstet* 1985;161:209.
3. Barron WM. The pregnant surgical patient: medical evaluation and management. *Ann Intern Med* 1984;101:683.
4. Caravati EM, Adams CJ, Joyce SM, et al. Fetal toxicity associated with maternal carbon monoxide poisoning. *Ann Emerg Med* 1988;17:714.
5. Connolly AM, Katz VL, Bash KL, et al. Trauma and pregnancy. *Am J Perinatol* 1997;14:331.
6. Deitch EA, Rightmire DA, Clothier J, et al. Management of burns in pregnant women. *Surg Gynecol Obstet* 1985;161:1.
7. Elkharrat D, Raphael JC, Korach JM, et al. Acute carbon monoxide intoxication and hyperbaric oxygen in pregnancy. *Intensive Care Med* 1991;17:289.
8. Esposito TJ. Trauma during pregnancy. *Emerg Med Clin North Am* 1994;12:167.
9. Franger AL, Buchsbaum HJ, Peaceman AM. Abdominal gunshot wounds in pregnancy. *Am J Obstet Gynecol* 1989;160:160.
10. Goff BA, Muntz HG. Gunshot wounds to the gravid uterus. *J Reprod Med* 1990;35:436.
11. Katz VL, Dotters DJ, Droegemueller W. Perimortem cesarean delivery. *Obstet Gynecol* 1986;68:571.
12. Katz VL, Hansen AR. Complications in the emergency transport of pregnant women. *South Med J* 1990;83:7.
13. Kloeck W, Cummins RO, Chamberlain D, et al. Special resuscitation situations: an advisory statement from the international liaison committee on resuscitation. *Circulation* 1994;95:2196.
14. Lanoix R, Akkapeddi V, Goldfeder B. Perimortem cesarean section: case reports and recommendations. *Acad Emerg Med* 1995;2:1063.
15. Lavery JP, Staten-McCormick M. Management of moderate to severe trauma in pregnancy. *Obstet Gynecol Clin North Am* 1995;22:69.
16. Leiberman JR, Mazor M, Molcho J, et al. Electrical accidents during pregnancy. *Obstet Gynecol* 1986;67:861.
17. Morris JA, Rosenbower TJ, Jurkovitch GJ, et al. Infant survival after cesarean section for trauma. *Ann Surg* 1996;223:481.
18. Parker B, McFarlane J, Soeken K. Abuse during pregnancy: effects on maternal complications and birth weight in adult and teenage women. *Obstet Gynecol* 1994;84:323.
19. Pearlman MD, Tintinalli JE. Evaluation and treatment of the gravida and fetus following trauma during pregnancy. *Obstet Gynecol Clin North Am* 1991;18:371.
20. Pearlman MD, Tintinalli JE, Lorenz RP. A prospective controlled study of outcome after trauma during pregnancy. *Am J Obstet Gynecol* 1990;162:1502.
21. Pearlman MD, Tintinalli JE, Lorenz RP. Blunt trauma during pregnancy. *N Engl J Med* 1992;323:1609.
22. Pierce MR, Henderson RA, Mitchell JM. Cardiopulmonary arrest secondary to lightning injury in a pregnant woman. *Ann Emerg Med* 1986;15:597.
23. Poole GV, Martin JN, Perry KG, et al. Trauma in pregnancy: the role of interpersonal violence. *Am J Obstet Gynecol* 1996;174:1873.
24. Sakala EP, Kort DD. Management of stab wounds to the pregnant uterus: a case report and a review of the literature. *Obstet Gynecol Surv* 1988;43:319.
25. Schoenfield A, Ziv E, Stein L, et al. Seat belts in pregnancy and the obstetrician. *Obstet Gynecol Surv* 1987;42:275.
26. Sherer DM, Schenker JG. Accidental injury during pregnancy. *Obstet Gynecol Surv* 1989;44:330.
27. Sherman HF, Scott LM, Rosemurgy AS, et al. Changes affecting the initial evaluation and care of the pregnant trauma victim. *J Emerg Med* 1990;8:575.
28. Smikle CB, Sorem KA, Satin AJ. Physical and sexual abuse in a middle-class obstetric population. *South Med J* 1996;10:983.
29. Speer DP, Peltier LF. Pelvic fractures and pregnancy. *J Trauma* 1972;12:474.
30. *Trauma during pregnancy: ACOG technical bulletin.* Washington, DC: American College of Obstetricians and Gynecologists, November 1991.
31. Williams JK, McClain L, Rosemurgy AS, et al. Evaluation of blunt abdominal trauma in the third trimester of pregnancy: maternal and fetal considerations. *Obstet Gynecol* 1990;75:33.
32. Wolf ME, Alexander BH, Rivara FP, et al. A retrospective cohort study of seatbelt use and pregnancy outcome after a motor vehicle crash. *J Trauma* 1993;34:116.

CHAPTER 125
Burns

Janet Talbot-Stern

In 1992, more than 1 million Americans sustained thermal burns; of these, at least 75,000 were hospitalized and 5,500 died.[3] Over the past decades, major strides have been made in burn care. These include improvements in fluid management, infection prevention, surgical management (in the form of early excision),[15] and nutritional support. Survival has significantly improved: In 1952, half of patients with a 50% burn survived; by 1996, the same survival rate was seen in those with a 70% burn.[15] Patients now die of respiratory complications or sepsis rather than of "burn shock."

Fifty percent of burn patients are younger than 20 years old, and 30% (of all burn patients) are younger than 10 years old.[20] The median age of burn patients is 22 years, and males predominate.[17] Interestingly, in one study,[2] 75% of drug-positive and 58% of ethanol-positive fatalities were aged 21 to 50 years. Ninety-three percent of burns occur in the home, with more than half due to flames.

For patients older than 65 years, burns are the fourth leading cause of death (they represent 28% of fire-related deaths in all age groups). Mortality is directly proportional to the extent of injury and patient age.[15] With a 15% burn, the mortality is 50%, while for a 30% burn, it is 75%; 50% burns are generally fatal.

Elderly patients have a poorer prognosis than do younger ones. Their burns are generally more extensive because of slow reaction time and thin skin. Their thin skin regenerates poorly, particularly in donor sites.[15] When two or more preinjury health problems are present, there is a higher incidence of complications and death. The most common site of infection is the lower respiratory tract.[6]

PATHOPHYSIOLOGY

Burns threaten the ability of the skin, the largest organ of the body, to prevent water and heat losses and to be a barrier to infection. Damage occurs sequentially: The initial direct cellular injury is followed by later injury from continued dermal ischemia.[20] Three concentric zones have been proposed: (1) the central zone of coagulation closest to the heat source (where there is irreversible death and avascularity); (2) the zone of stasis, where injury can continue for 24 to 48 hours if not arrested (blood flow is impaired secondary to the release of local mediators)[22]; and (3) the zone of hyperemia, or minimal injury, which will recover unless there is another insult.[10]

The amount of penetration through the epidermis and the

dermis also determines the extent of injury. Damage to the integrity of the epidermis and to the capillary membrane causes patients with significant burns to lose fluids, with most lost in the first 8 to 12 hours. Capillary integrity is generally restored by 24 hours. Dermal burns may damage or destroy the sensory, vascular, and endocrine functions of the skin.

The severity of thermal injuries is determined by several factors: the character and temperature of the agent, the duration of exposure, and the character of skin at the site of injury.[14] The type of agent involved helps to determine the potential severity. Scalds tend to be more superficial, while chemical and electrical burns are very deep. An exposure of 40°C will not injure the skin. At temperatures in excess of 40°C, the higher the temperature and the longer the period of exposure, the greater the damage that is produced. Associated inhalation injury, trauma, and the presence of preexisting medical problems put the patients at increased risk. Burns tend to be deeper where the skin is thinner. Patients younger than 3 years and older than 65 years appear to be particularly at risk.[4] It has also been shown that intoxication at the time of the injury is an important predictor of complications in adult patients.[11] Chronic alcoholics have a higher mortality rate, die of smaller burns than do nonalcoholics, and have longer hospital stays.[13]

PREHOSPITAL CARE

The patient should be removed from the scene and any flames extinguished. Jewelry and clothing should be removed or cut away. Embedded material may remain until hospital evaluation. No topical agents should be applied during transport, just clean sterile sheets or dressings to cover the burns. If there is any suspicion of inhalation injury, 100% oxygen should be given by facemask. Place large-bore intravenous lines for burns greater than 15% total body surface area (TBSA); run them wide open unless transport time is prolonged. With prolonged transport, it is possible to administer excessive fluids with lines running wide open. As such, total fluids infused should be carefully tracked and titrated to the patient's response. Transport to the receiving facility should occur as expeditiously as possible. In areas where a burn center is nearby and easily accessible by ground transport, the American Burn Association advises that patients with significant burns be taken there rather than to the closest facility, unless the patient is in near arrest.[1]

EMERGENCY DEPARTMENT EVALUATION

Information that needs to be expeditiously obtained includes (1) the circumstances of the injury, (2) the specific agent or agents involved, (3) the anatomic location and extent and depth of the burns, (4) the possibility of inhalation injury, (5) factors that may affect long-term prognosis (such as age), and (6) previous medical problems. A rapid determination needs to be made in the emergency department, if it was not made in the prehospital environment, as to the level of expertise that will be required to manage the patient appropriately.

Evaluation of the percentage of burn can be done a number of ways. The "rule of nines" is the most popular and consists, in the adult patient, of assigning 9% TBSA to each of the following: the head, each upper extremity, and each half of each lower extremity. The front and back of the torso are 18% TBSA apiece, and the genitalia are 1% TBSA (Fig. 125.1). Superficial partial-

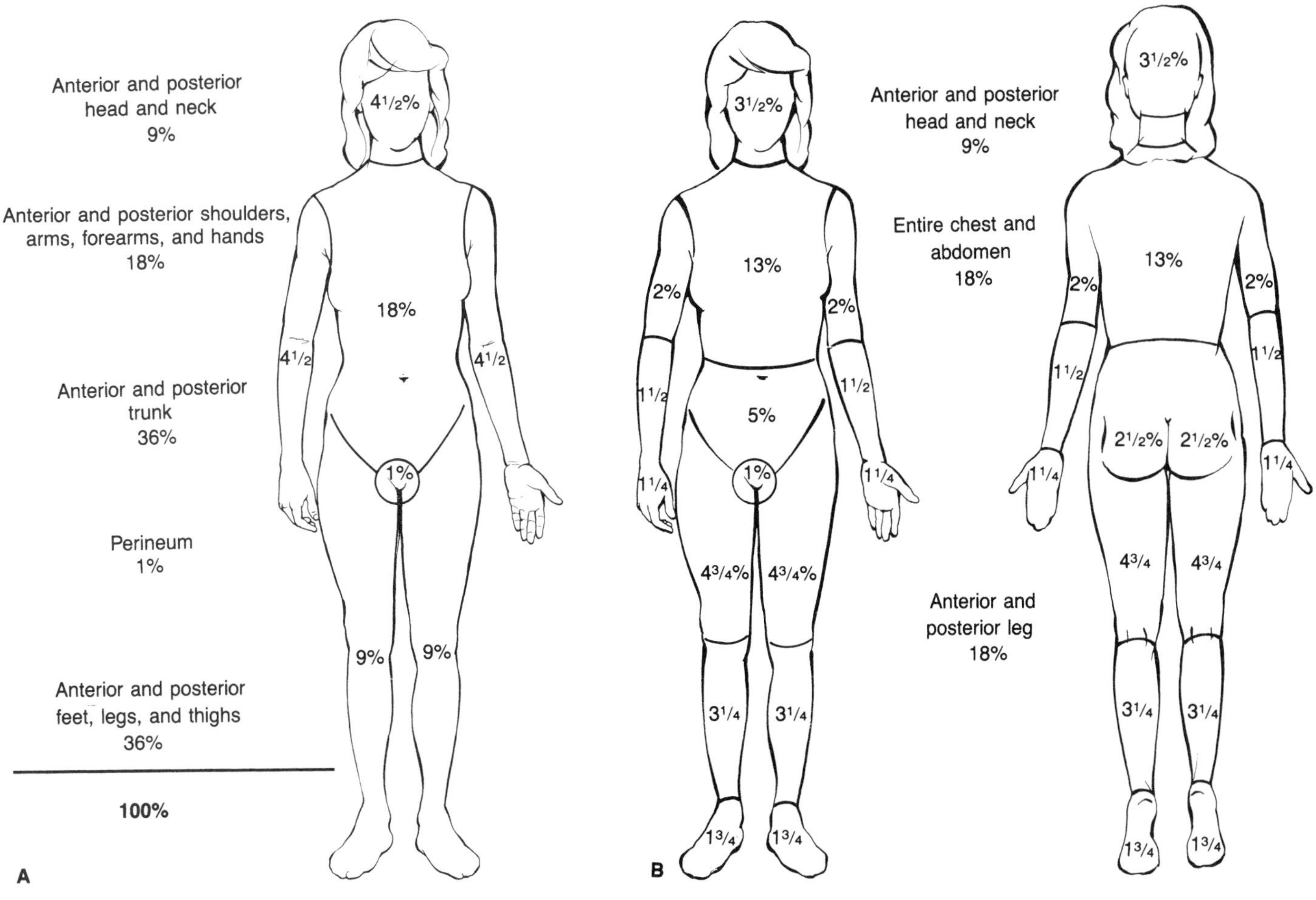

Figure 125.1. Methods to evaluate the percentage of burn. **(A)** Rule of nines. **(B)** Lund and Browder chart.

thickness burns are not included in this system.[14] This evaluation is good for a rough estimate but can lead to overestimation and inappropriate transfer. In children, as the proportion of body surface areas changes with growth, an age-appropriate Lund and Browder chart should be used. The Lund and Browder chart is more accurate in all age groups and should be used after the initial resuscitation is completed. A third method designates the palm of the patient's hand as approximately 1% TBSA.

The full extent of the burn is categorized as minor, moderate, or major (Table 125.1).[1] A minor burn encompasses less than 15% TBSA in adults (less than 10% in children and the elderly) and less than 2% TBSA full-thickness. These patients can be managed as outpatients. A moderate burn covers 15% to 25% mixed partial- and full-thickness in adults, 10% to 20% in children and those older than age 40 years, and less than 10% TBSA full-thickness. A major burn covers more than 25% TBSA in adults, more than 20% in children and patients older than age 40 years, and 10% TBSA full-thickness. Patients with inhalation injury, high-voltage injury, associated fractures, or major trauma, as well as patients at high risk because of underlying medical problems, are also considered to have major burns.

Estimation of the depth of the burn is often difficult in the first few hours. Repeated evaluations must be done at least daily. The designation of first-, second-, and third-degree burns has been replaced by that of superficial partial-thickness, deep partial-thickness, and full-thickness burns. Very superficial burns (first-degree), such as those from sunlight or very short flash, involve the superficial epidermal layers. They are erythematous, are painful, lack blisters, are sensate, and heal without scars.

Second-degree burns have been divided into superficial and deep partial-thickness burns. Superficial partial-thickness burns, from scalds or short flashes, involve the full epidermis and cause varying levels of destruction in the dermis but spare important structures. They are red, blistered, weeping, and painful, and they generally heal without scarring in 3 weeks. Deep partial-thickness burns are usually caused by flames, oil, or grease; involve deeper areas of the dermis; and also spare dermal structures. Such burns may have, in addition to blisters, areas that are waxy and dry, and they can be difficult to distinguish from full-thickness burns. In fact, they can be converted to full-thickness burns by coincidental trauma or infection. They usually scar on healing.

Full-thickness burns caused by flames, scalds, and chemical and electrical contact destroy dermal structures (third-degree) or underlying tendons, muscle, and bone (fourth-degree). The skin appears white or charred, is inelastic, and exhibits thrombosed vessels. The patient notes no pain on palpation. These wounds will scar with contracture.[18]

Laboratory evaluation should include a complete blood cell count; determination of electrolytes, glucose, blood urea nitrogen, and creatinine; urinalysis (including myoglobin when suspected); arterial blood gas analysis; measurement of carboxyhemoglobin level; and type and screen and coagulation studies. An electrocardiogram and a chest radiograph should be obtained.

EMERGENCY DEPARTMENT MANAGEMENT

The ultimate philosophy of burn management is to "do no harm."[4] A sterile environment should be provided to decrease the risk of secondary infection. The patient's airway, breathing, and circulation (ABCs) are attended to primarily. If available, an additional provider should be designated to place cool, sterile compresses on all burned areas. This treatment retards the process of cell death by inhibiting the release of toxic metabolites in cells in the zone of stasis, preventing leukocyte adhesion and increasing perfusion to the burned area.[20] Ice causes vasoconstriction and can worsen the extent of the burn; it should not be applied.[9]

As with all emergency patients, the physician should consider the ABCs as part of the initial assessment. If there has been associated trauma, immobilize the neck until a cervical spine injury has been ruled out. Until a good history about the circumstances of the injuries is obtained, significantly burned patients should be given humidified 100% oxygen by a nonrebreathing mask.

With severely burned patients, an expeditious decision must be made regarding potential airway damage. Intubation should be performed *before* the airway is lost. Intubation must be performed immediately in unconscious patients with a history of prolonged smoke or fire exposure in a confined space and in those with a high clinical probability of airway edema (stridor, increasing respiratory distress, hypoxia despite 100% oxygen, high carbon monoxide level, and poor peak flow). Nasotracheal intubation may be attempted in the awake, cooperative patient who is still breathing; otherwise, rapid-sequence orotracheal intubation should be performed. Performing emergency surgery to open an airway, particularly if the neck is burned, places the patient at great risk for later infection. After intubation, the head should be elevated 30 degrees to decrease edema and increase venous return. Many patients may require positive end-expiratory pressure to keep the distal airways open; begin with 5 cm H_2O. Bronchodilators may be effective if secretions or particulate inhalation leads to bronchospasm. Concurrent carbon monoxide exposure may require hyperbaric oxygen therapy.

In the more stable patient, whose clinical examination is suggestive of the potential for airway damage (burned nasal hair, carbonaceous deposits in the pharynx and sputum), immediate nasolaryngoscopy or bronchoscopy is warranted. If no injury is present, the patient may not need admission to the intensive care unit.[19] Early airway visualization may be negative, however, despite severe injury.

If the patient is in severe respiratory distress and has sus-

TABLE 125.1. American Burn Association Grading System

Minor Burns	*Moderate Burns*	*Major Burns*
Outpatient	Inpatient	Burn Center
First degree <15% TBSA Second degree <15% TBSA Third degree <2% TBSA	Second degree 15%–25% Third degree <10%	Second degree >25% Third degree >10% All listed below[a]

TBSA, total body surface area.

[a]Burns of hands, face, eyes, ears, feet, or perineum; inhalation burns; electrical burns; those associated with major trauma and in poor-risk patients (previous medical illness, head injury, cerebrovascular accident, psychiatric illness, closed space injury).

tained circumferential burns to the chest, an immediate escharotomy may be necessary. Incision should be made in the anterior axillary line connected by a third incision in the form of an inverted V (Fig. 125.2).[4] The lower respiratory tract can be further evaluated in the inpatient environment with xenon scans, but there is a high incidence of false-positive results. If patients exhibit persistent acidosis despite adequate fluid resuscitation, normal carbon monoxide level and, absent other major injuries, the possibility of cyanide toxicity should be addressed.

Place two large-bore intravenous lines through unburned skin, if possible. Crystalloid remains the intravenous fluid of choice for the first 24 hours. Calculation of fluid requirement should begin at the time of the burn, *not* when the patient arrives in the emergency department. Most institutions managing burns of greater than 15% TBSA use the Parkland formula (4 mL/kg of lactated Ringer's solution × percentage TBSA burn) as an estimate of the total fluid required during the first 24 hours: One half is given during the first 8 hours, and the remainder during the next 16 hours. Because lactated Ringer's solution has 80 to 100 mL/L of free water, additional maintenance fluids are not necessary in the adult.[12] In certain cases, patients have increased fluid requirements: inhalation or electrical injury, escharotomies, delayed resuscitation, or associated trauma.[22] Some authors have recommended the use of hypertonic saline, particularly in patients with underlying cardiac disease, pulmonary hypertension, and renal disease. After 24 hours, the fluid is changed to dextrose 5% in water, and colloids may be given to replace plasma volume deficiency.[9] Some burn units start fresh-frozen plasma for burns greater than 50%, elderly patients, and those with inhalation injury at 8 to 10 hours after the burn.[22] Neither of these has been demonstrated to improve patient outcome, while colloid has been associated with increased lung water and decreased glomerular nitration rate, and hypertonic saline has been associated with renal failure and death.

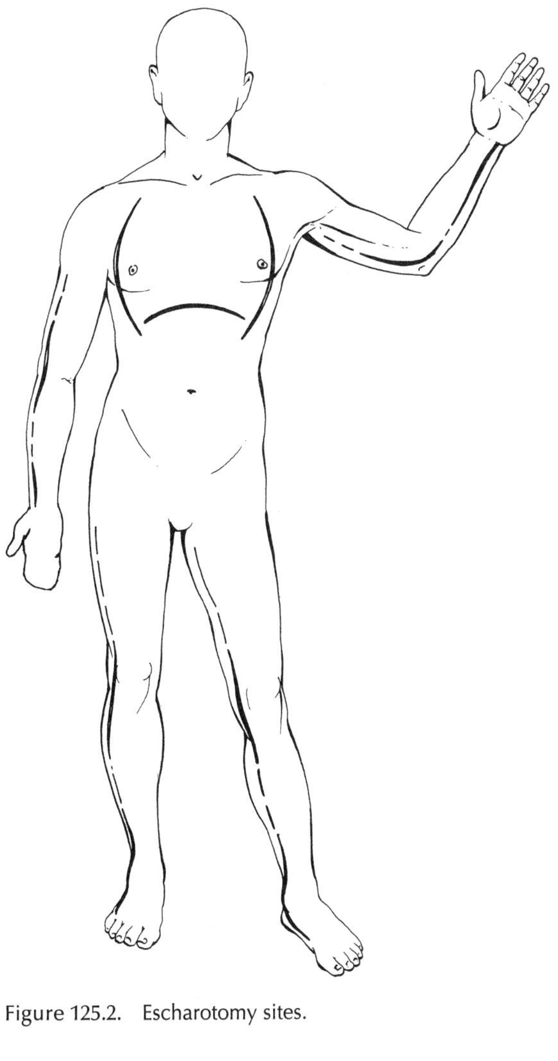

Figure 125.2. Escharotomy sites.

In elderly patients who have more than 5% burns, it is recommended to give intravenous fluids at 3 mL/kg/TBSA burn. In some pediatric burn centers, the fluid resuscitation formula is based on body surface area rather than on weight, with D5LR being used as the fluid.[22] Such formulas are established as guidelines; fluid management should be guided by pertinent clinical parameters, including pulse rate, blood pressure, capillary refill time, urine output, and mental status. Urine output is a very sensitive indicator of adequate resuscitation in the first 24 hours and should be 0.5 to 1.0 mL/kg/h.

A sinus tachycardia that develops within a few hours of a large burn injury is considered a desirable physiologic response, and patients who do not develop it have a higher mortality.[9] Base deficit may also be used very effectively to monitor the appropriateness of resuscitation.[8]

Hemodynamic monitoring is frequently used; however, central venous pressure monitors are not necessary routinely during the first 24 hours, except in those patients who require twice the usual amount of fluid or in those who have cardiac disease. Patients with deep burns (including electrical burns), associated trauma, or inhalation injuries will generally require more fluid resuscitation. Intravenous lines should be changed every 3 days because of the risk of suppurative thrombophlebitis.

Patients with electrical injuries should be carefully monitored for 24 hours if there was loss of consciousness at the scene or any evidence of arrhythmias in either the prehospital phase or the emergency department.

All clothing should be removed as soon as possible. If clothing adheres tightly to the skin, however, forcible removal can inflict even more damage. Many synthetic materials significantly increase the skin temperature while burning. Application of topical ointment may facilitate later removal.[9] Hypothermia can contribute to coagulopathy, decrease circulation to the wound, and, if less than 33°C, can actually increase metabolic rate.[14] Hypothermia should, therefore, be prevented during resuscitation.

Patients who have sustained a burn greater than 25% should have a nasogastric tube placed. These patients will develop an ileus secondary to splanchnic vasoconstriction.[20] This ileus usually resolves by 24 to 48 hours: Most burn units begin enteral feedings as early as the first day postburn to satisfy caloric needs,[22] regulate the microflora of the gastrointestinal tract, and maintain the integrity of the mucosal barrier.[7]

A Foley catheter should be placed in patients with severe burns (greater than 20%).[22] A majority of patients with deep burns and electrical injuries will filter the hemochromogens hemoglobin and myoglobin into the urine.[12] If myoglobinuria is present, additional fluid resuscitation may be necessary to prevent acute tubular necrosis and resultant renal failure. Mannitol and bicarbonate may also be employed to maintain urine output and prevent precipitation of pigments, respectively.[12]

If tetanus prophylaxis is not up to date, it should be given. Tetanus toxoid is usually sufficient, but if there is any doubt as to primary immunization status, tetanus immunoglobulin should also be administered, and the patient will require the remainder of the immunization series at appropriate intervals.

Pain can be severe, particularly in patients with partial-thickness burns; full-thickness burns tend to be painless because nerve endings have been destroyed. All pain medication should be given intravenously in small, frequent aliquots, titrated to pain relief, after fluid resuscitation has been accomplished; otherwise, the vasodilatory effect of the narcotics may negatively affect the patient's blood pressure. Intramuscular pain medications may have erratic absorption. Morphine remains the narcotic of choice. Fentanyl and nitrous oxide are acceptable alternatives. If the patient is extremely anxious, and is not hypoxic or hypovolemic, small doses of intravenous diazepam or lorazepam may be used.

Escharotomy may be indicated on extremities in the case of distal pain, paresthesias, decreased pulses, or cyanosis, suggesting the development of a compartment syndrome. The most reliable way of checking arterial flow is by an ultrasonic flow meter.[14] Compartment pressure measurement can be helpful, if it is readily available. Incisions should be made on the radial and ulnar borders of the arm and forearm and along the midaxial lines of the digits. Incisions are made on the medial and lateral borders of the lower extremities. Escharotomy may lead to significant soft-tissue bleeding, which may require electrocautery to control (see Fig. 125.2).

Burns are at risk for infection for several reasons: The skin no longer serves as a barrier to microorganisms, the exudate from the burn is an ideal culture medium, the host's immune system is impaired, and many sick patients require the performance of invasive procedures. Antibiotics made a great difference in mortality with their discovery in the 1940s. At first, gram-positive organisms, such as group A β-hemolytic *Streptococcus*, predominated, and penicillin G was often given prophylactically. Indiscriminate parenteral antibiotic use over the ensuing decades, however, has tended to select out resistant gram-negative organisms, such as *Pseudomonas*. This selection occurs in the gastrointestinal tract, where antibiotics overwhelm the normal mucosal anaerobes and allow the overgrowth of gram-negative organisms and yeast.[7] As a result of this process, systemic antibiotics are generally not given prophylactically at this time. Topical antimicrobials, such as 1% silver sulfadiazine, and aggressive early excision of eschar are used to prevent the development of infection. If a patient returns to the emergency department with burns that appear infected, admission may be warranted.

If the patient is to be transferred, no wound care (except for emergency escharotomy) should be performed unless discussed with the accepting burn center. The burns should be covered with cool, sterile compresses (small areas) and then sterile drapes. Cooling produces vasoconstriction, appears to reduce histamine release and thromboxane B2 and kinin formation, and stabilizes mast cells. Transfer should not be delayed by burn debridement. If the patient's burns are such that hospitalization is not necessary, they should be irrigated with sterile saline and cleaned with mild soap. Necrotic skin should be sharply debrided, and broken blisters should be unroofed and debrided. Blisters over joints and large blisters should be debrided. Some controversy exists about the management of small intact blisters in compliant patients: Some authorities believe that the intact blister provides protection for the new skin; others believe that the fluid contains toxic products of the inflammatory reaction (e.g., thromboxane) and recommend debridement of bullae larger than 2 cm,[14] or sterile aspiration of the fluid[20] to improve normal neutrophil function, to decrease production of arachidonic acid metabolites, and to allow normal fibrinolytic processes to occur.[21] Shaving hair (except the eyebrows) 3 to 4 in. from the wound border has also been recommended by some.[14]

Outpatient management can be summarized by the five C's: cut, cool, clean, chemoprophylaxis, and cover. The ideal burn dressing is one that is inexpensive, safe, and painless; prevents infection; promotes rapid wound healing; promotes functional and cosmetic results; and requires infrequent dressing changes that can be done at home.[10] For very superficial, small burns, some use only nonadherent dressings with simple antibiotics, such as bacitracin,[16] or no antibiotics at all. The final covering is absorbent gauze and stockinette, which is changed twice daily while the burn weeps and once daily thereafter.

For the remainder of outpatient burns, topical antibiotic ointments are applied after cleansing. The most commonly used topical therapy is silver sulfadiazine, which is broad spectrum and nontoxic. It does have a 5% to 7% incidence of allergic reaction,[17] however, and is expensive. It should not be used in pregnant patients or nursing mothers and should not be used on the face because of staining. Mafenide, Furacin, and silver nitrate are not used in the outpatient setting.

The burn is then covered with a nonadherent dressing and, finally, a gauze dressing. Dressing changes must be done twice a day while the burn weeps. Each time, the old silver sulfadiazine should be completely washed off. Several trials have compared synthetic occlusive dressings (Biobrane, DuoDerm, OpSite, and Inerpan) with silver sulfadiazine. These dressings were found to have a decrease in the frequency of dressing changes, better compliance, and marginally faster healing, but none was found to produce superior healing.[5]

Outpatient management of burns of the face and neck consists of the use of bacitracin ointment, no dressing, and thrice-daily washing.[10] In an interesting study from India,[24] 100% of burns treated with pure unprocessed honey healed in 15 days, compared with 50% healing in the same time period with boiled potato peel. Separate dressings should be used for each finger. The hand should be immobilized in the position of function (wrist extension, metaphalangeal flexion, interphalangeal extension),[18] which is opposite of the position assumed by the burned hand.[25] Ideally, the extremity should be elevated and joints must be exercised, particularly in the case of burns that cross joints.[23] Patients should be cautioned that burned skin is sun-sensitive for up to a year,[18] and that they should protect the skin by using SP25 sunning agents and, in the case of head and neck burns, by also wearing a hat. Aspirin should not be used for pain control, because antiplatelet effects may worsen blood loss if skin grafting becomes necessary.[5]

If a deep burn heals untreated, new collagen is formed randomly, with a piling up of excessive tissue and hypertrophic scar formation. Two approaches exist for the management of deep partial- and full-thickness burns: early excision and grafting versus delayed grafting after the eschar separates.[25] The former approach appears to be the most accepted at the present time. When wounds are greater than 60%, use of growth hormone has decreased donor-site healing.[22]

DISPOSITION

Most patients who sustain minor burns can be managed as outpatients. Burns should be rechecked within 24 to 48 hours. Beyond that period, further management depends on the mechanisms available in an individual's particular setting. Some emergency departments manage their own follow-up burn care. Patients with deep partial-thickness or full-thickness burns should be referred to a plastic surgeon or other burn-care specialist in 2 to 4 days for consideration of skin grafting and physical therapy. Hospitalization should be considered, even for minor burns, in those patients who are immunocompromised, including the very young and the old, and in those with poor home situations or possible abuse.

Recommendations for transfer to a burn center are as follows: any person with a burn of more than 20% TBSA; patients older than 50 years or younger than 10 years with a burn greater than 10% TBSA; patients with full-thickness burns greater than 5%; patients with burns to the face, hands, feet, perineum, or major joints; patients with electrical or chemical burns or associated inhalation injuries; patients with multiple trauma; and patients with circumferential injuries of the chest or extremities.[9] A BURN PLAN is a simple acronym (airway, breathing, urine output, resuscitation, nasogastric tube, pulses, lines, accurate documentation, and notify unit) that is used to ensure documentation and communication of all required treatment and information.[9] In making the decision to transfer a patient to a higher level of care, an important question must be asked: Can the patient tolerate the evacuation? In transfers up to 150 miles, a helicopter can be used; greater distances require fixed-wing aircraft.

A flowsheet containing a complete record of initial findings, ongoing resuscitation, and patient response by appropriate clinical parameters, consultations, and the results of pertinent laboratory, radiologic, and other testing should be maintained on any significantly burned individual. A copy of this record must accompany all transferred individuals.

COMMON PITFALLS

- Failure to calculate fluid requirements from the time of the burn
- Using the pulse to determine if an extremity is compromised
- Waiting too long to intubate a patient with a compromised airway
- Overestimating or underestimating the size of the burn
- Using blood pressure as a guide to fluid requirements and not adjusting fluid resuscitation by physiologic parameters such as urine output

References

1. American Burn Association. Hospital and prehospital resources for optimal care of patients with burn injury: guidelines for development and operation of burn centers. *J Burn Care Rehabil* 1990;11:97.
2. Barillo DJ, Goode R. Substance abuse in victims of fire. *J Burn Care Rehabil* 1996;17:71.
3. Brigham P, McLoughlin E. Burn incidence and medical care use in the United States: estimates, trends, and data sources. *J Burn Care Rehabil* 1996;17:95.
4. Calistro AM. Burn care basics and beyond. *RN* 1993;56(3):26.
5. Clayton MC, Solem LD. No ice, no butter: advice on management of burns for primary care physicians. *Postgrad Med* 1995;97(5):151.
6. Covington DS, Wainwright DJ, Parks DH. Prognostic indicators in the elderly patient with burns. *J Burn Care Rehabil* 1996;17:222.
7. Epstein MD, Benducci DR, Manders EK. The role of the GI tract in the development of burn sepsis. *Surgery* 1992;90:3.
8. Gerding RL, Emerman CL, Effron D, et al. Outpatient management of partial-thickness burns: Biobrane versus 1% silver sulfadiazine. *Ann Emerg Med* 1990;19:2.
9. Gordan M, Goodwin CW. Initial assessment, management and stabilization in burn management. *Nurs Clin North Am* 1997;32(2):237.
10. Griglak MJ. Thermal injury. *Emerg Med Clin North Am* 1992;10:2.
11. Grobmyer SR, Maniscalco SP, Purdue GR, et al. Alcohol, drug intoxication, or both at the time of burn injury as a predictor of complications and mortality in hospitalized patients with burns. *J Burn Care Rehabil* 1996;17:532.
12. Hunt JL, Purdue GF. The elderly burn patient. *Am J Surg* 1992;164(5):472.
13. Jones JD, Barber B, Engrav L. Alcohol use and burn injury. *J Burn Care Rehabil* 1991;12:148.
14. Jordan BS, Harrington DT. Management of the burn wound in burn management. *Nurs Clin North Am* 1997;32(2):251.
15. Mann R, Heimbach D. Prognosis and treatment of burns. *West J Med* 1996;165:215.
16. Mertens DM, Jenkins MF, Warden GD. Outpatient burn management. *Nurs Clin North Am* 1997;32(2):343.
17. Osguthorpe JD. Head and neck burns: evaluation and current management. *Arch Otolaryngol Head Neck Surg* 1991;117.
18. Peate WF. Outpatient management of burns. *Am Fam Physician* 1992;45(3):1321.
19. Purdue GR, Hunt JF. Inhalation injuries and burns in the inner city. *Surg Clin North Am* 1991;71:2.
20. Robson MC, Burns BR, Smith DJ. Acute management of the burned patient. *Plast Reconstr Surg* 1992;89:6.
21. Rockwell WB, Erlich HP. Should burn blister fluid be evacuated? *J Burn Care Rehabil* 1990;11(1):93.
22. Rose JK, Barrow RE, Desai MH. Advances in burn care. *Adv Surg* 1997;30: 71.
23. Smith S, Duncan M, Mobley J, et al. Emergency room management of minor burn injuries: a quality management evaluation. *J Burn Care Rehabil* 1997;18(1):77.
24. Subrahmanyam M. Honey dressing versus boiled potato peel in the treatment of burns: a prospective randomized study. *Burns* 1996;22(6):491.
25. Yakuboff KP, Kurtzman LC, Stern PJ. Acute management of thermal and electrical burns of the upper extremity. *Orthop Clin North Am* 1992;23:1.

CHAPTER 126
Hanging and Strangulation Injuries

Yevgeniy Gincherman and Edward T. Dickinson

Strangulation injuries are broadly categorized as either hanging, manual ligature strangulation (choking), or throttling. Hanging is the most common form of strangulation injury. Hanging occurs when pressure is exerted on the neck by an external force, usually a rope, with the degree of external force increased by the weight of the victim. In complete hanging, the point of suspension is placed over the occiput. In manual ligature strangulation or choking, the ligature is tied around the victim's neck and the weight of the body is not used to increase the pressure on the neck structures. In throttling, the force is applied to the victim's neck by the assailant's hand or arm.

EPIDEMIOLOGY

Adult

Hanging and strangulation injuries are quite common in the United States and the rest of the world. Among all suicide deaths reported in the United States in 1989, 4484 were due to hanging or strangulation. Hanging was the most common mechanism of suicide after firearms and poisonings.[33]

In a recent article, a disturbing increase in frequency of suicides by hanging was found in young Australians.[5] Among all deaths by hanging in Western Australia during the 1988–1992 period, 88% occurred in males.[7] There was one homicide, 14 cases were thought to be accidental, and the remainder were suicides. Alcohol was the most commonly detected drug at autopsy. In one-third of the cases, there was a positive history of psychiatric illness. An increasing number of hangings was reported in a review of methods of suicide in Denmark over a 70-year period.[2] In developing countries, hanging is frequently the most common mechanism of suicide.[16,23,35]

The elderly are particularly at risk for suicide by hanging.[21,27,32] Psychiatric inpatient populations are also at risk for suicide, with hanging noted to be the method of choice. Nearly half of these suicides occur outside of the hospital setting.[28] Prison inmates are also at increased risk, with reported rates of death from hanging up to nine times higher than in the general population.[24]

Pediatric

Causes of strangulation injuries vary in pediatric populations relative to age. Infants are often strangled intentionally by cords, or unintentionally by clothing becoming tangled in cribs. Strollers as causes of accidental strangulation have also been reported.[4] Toddlers to early-school children tend to be injured by window cords, plant holders, or looped rope swings. Older children and adolescents are at risk for strangulation during play and by suicide.[6,9,10,14] A number of potentially dangerous sleeping environments at risk for accidental strangulation in infants and toddlers have been identified,[3,26] which include large spaces between bed sides and wall, beds with plastic bed covers, and co-sleeping with adults.

Special Cases: Autoerotic

Autoerotic asphyxiation is defined as induction of hypoxia by hanging or strangulation in an attempt to achieve sexual arousal. Autoerotic behavior is associated with significant mortality rates.[8] Mortality estimates are two to four deaths per million in the United States and one to two deaths per million in Scandinavian countries.[18,30] Fatalities resulting from autoerotic behavior are most commonly encountered in males 12 to 25 years of age.[8,13] Individuals engaged in such behavior often use a number of safety devices, which include a slipknot to loosen the ligature, knives to cut cords, and more involved self-rescue mechanisms that are activated if a person faints. However, these safety devices frequently fail, leading to significant morbidity and mortality.[8]

PATHOPHYSIOLOGY

Bony Injuries

It is estimated that as many as 16,000 judicial hangings have occurred in the United States.[19] In classic judicial hanging, no injury to the spinal cord, spine, or base of skull was usually noted. Death resulted from asphyxiation. With longer judicial drops, disjointing of second and third cervical vertebrae occurred, with resulting hangman's fracture.[25] Associated spinal cord injury was usually seen in such cases.[22] Some evidence suggests that the frequency of neck fractures increases with longer hanging time.[25] Decapitation, as a result of extreme distracting force leading to cervical spine fracture in conjunction with complete severance of other neck structures, has also been reported.[29] Decapitation appears to occur with longer drops and when single-twist ropes are used.

Injuries to Vascular Structures

Almost all strangulation causes obstruction of venous flow, with resultant petechial hemorrhages seen on the neck surface. Significant injury to deep vascular structures may also occur. The vertebral arteries are most commonly injured. Injuries to the bifurcation of the common carotid arteries are less frequently encountered.[19] Most injuries are intimal tears. Vascular injuries often lead to cerebral anoxia, which causes most immediate deaths in hanging victims. Autonomic nervous system instability, secondary to stimulation of deep neck vascular structures, also contributes to immediate mortality as a result of profound bradycardia.[20,22]

Injuries to Laryngotracheal Apparatus

Injuries to the laryngotracheal apparatus in strangulation victims are common; however, most such injuries are rarely life-threatening. They are usually observed in drops from longer heights and when the ligature is tied lower down the neck. Injuries to the thyroid cartilage occur almost 50% of the time, whereas injuries to the hyoid bone occur in 20% of strangulations. Cricoid cartilage injuries are uncommon.[19] Interestingly, one series failed to document any injuries to the laryngotracheal structures.[12] Injuries to the laryngotracheal apparatus are less common in the pediatric population, secondary to increased flexibility of the larynx in this age group.[31]

Pulmonary Sequelae

Immediate and delayed pulmonary complications following near-fatal hanging are routinely encountered.[15] The pathophysiology of such injuries is multifactorial. Patients often develop pulmonary edema or pneumonia. Adult respiratory distress syndrome following near-fatal hanging has also been reported. Pulmonary edema may be secondary to the increased airway pressures produced with inhalation against a closed airway, or due to neurogenic causes. Aspiration pneumonias are also common. Iatrogenic volume overload from overly aggressive resuscitation may also occur.

Neurologic Sequelae

Both immediate and delayed neurologic sequelae have been documented. Case reports document patients whose neurologic function continued to deteriorate, resulting in death. Deaths secondary to global hypoxic encephalopathy or vascular intimal tears, with resultant, later cerebral infarction, have been recorded.[11,17] Reports also document patients who completely recover, with no long-term sequelae, despite the presence of agonal respirations and posturing on presentation to the emergency department.[34]

NATURAL HISTORY AND PROGNOSIS

The natural history of strangulation victims is unpredictable. The degrees of injury seen vary from minor injuries to superficial neck structures to life-threatening pulmonary, airway, and neurologic sequelae. Immediate neurologic prognostication is of little value. Patients who fail to resume spontaneous breathing and circulation with first aid measures appear to carry a worse prognosis.[14] In one study, 22 of the 24 hanging patients who died experienced either prehospital or emergency department cardiopulmonary arrest. In the same study, all treated patients who died required intubation prior to death.[1]

CLINICAL PRESENTATION

A wide variety of clinical presentations are encountered in strangulation victims. Patients often present with severe cyanosis. Grunting respirations may be observed, and patients may exhibit severe stridor. Tachypnea is common. Subcutaneous emphysema is more common in victims of throttling injuries. The presenting neurologic status can vary widely from complete normalcy to unconsciousness and posturing. Ligature marks and subconjunctival and facial petechiae are usually present.

EMERGENCY DEPARTMENT MANAGEMENT

As with any potentially severe injury to the neck structures, airway management is a first priority. The method of endotracheal intubation chosen depends on the clinician's experience. Any approach to airway control in a strangulation victim must presume that a cervical spine injury exists. As such, in-line stabilization of the cervical spine during intubation is mandatory. Once the airway is adequately controlled, the use of positive end-expiratory pressure should be considered because of the high incidence of pulmonary complications associated with the initial injury. In hypotensive patients, fluid resuscitation may result in delayed pulmonary edema and adult respiratory distress syndrome. The cervical spine should continue to be immobilized at all times, despite the fact that associated spine injuries are uncommon. Radiographic investigation of the cervical spine and the soft tissues of the neck is indicated. In the face of neurologic deterioration, intracranial pressure monitoring should be employed. Gentle hyperventilation, as well as osmotic and nonosmotic diuresis, may be utilized in the presence of increased intracranial pressure.

Once immediately life-threatening injuries are addressed, a detailed history should be obtained. The distance of fall, estimated time to initiation of rescue efforts, condition of the patient at the scene, and response to initial resuscitation are particularly important predictors of outcome. Evidence of associated suicidal injuries, including ingestions, should be sought.

DISPOSITION

All strangulation victims should be admitted for at least a 24-hour observation period to an area where adequate monitoring for potential airway, pulmonary, and neurologic sequelae is available. The airway should be secured via endotracheal intubation if transfer is deemed necessary. Early neurosurgical and/or otolaryngologic consultation should be considered if severe neurologic and/or laryngeal injuries are suspected. In conscious patients, psychiatric consultation should be obtained. "One-to-one" patient supervision, to prevent further attempts at self-destructive behavior, is mandatory in all intentional hanging victims.

COMMON PITFALLS

- Attempting to predict outcome based on the initial condition
- Failure to control airway in a timely fashion
- Failure to institute early, aggressive positive end-expiratory pressure
- Failure to maintain cervical spine immobilization
- Failure to consider early neurosurgical and otolaryngologic consultation
- Failure to consider early psychiatric consultation
- Failure to institute precautions against further attempts at self-destructive behavior
- Failure to definitively control the airway via endotracheal intubation prior to transfer of the patient to another facility
- Premature discharge (especially in hanging victims who are incarcerated)

References

1. Aufderheide TP, Aprahamian C, Mateer JR, et al. Emergency airway management in hanging victims. *Ann Emerg Med* 1994;24:879.
2. Bille-Brahe U, Jessen G. Suicide in Denmark, 1922–1991: the choice of method. *Acta Psychiatr Scand* 1994;90:91.
3. Byard RW, Beal SM, Simpson A, et al. Accidental infant death and stroller-prams. *Med J Aust* 1996;165:140.
4. Byard RW, Beal S, Bourne AJ. Potentially dangerous sleeping environments and accidental asphyxia in infancy and early childhood. *Arch Dis Child* 1994;71:497.
5. Cantor CH, Baume PJM. Access to the methods of suicide: what impact? *Aust N Z J Psychiatry* 1998;32:8.
6. Chin N, Berns SD. Near-hanging causes by a toy necklace. *Ann Emerg Med* 1995;26:522.
7. Cooke CT, Cadden GA, Margolius KA. Death by hanging in Western Australia. *Pathology* 1995;27:268.
8. Cooper AJ. Auto-erotic asphyxiation: three case reports. *J Sex Marital Ther* 1996;22:47.
9. Cummings P, Theis MK, Mueller BA, et al. Infant injury death in Washington State, 1981 through 1990. *Arch Pediatr Adolesc Med* 1994;148:1021.
10. Digeronimo RJ, Mayes TC. Near-hanging injury in childhood: a literature review and report of three cases. *Pediatr Emerg Care* 1994;10:150.
11. Dooling EC, Richardson EP. Delayed encephalopathy after strangling. *Arch Neurol* 1976;33:196.
12. Elfawal MA, Awad OA. Deaths from hanging in the Eastern Province of Saudi Arabia. *Med Sci Law* 1994;34:307.
13. Emson HE. Accidental hanging in auto-eroticism: an unusual case occurring outdoors. *Am J Forensic Med Pathol* 1983;4:337.
14. Feldman KW, Simms RJ. Strangulation in childhood: epidemiology and clinical course. *Pediatrics* 1980;65:1079.
15. Fischman CM, Goldstein MS, Gardner LB. Suicidal hanging: an association with adult respiratory distress syndrome. *Chest* 1977;71:225.
16. Fisher AJ, Parry CDH. Suicide in South Africa. *Acta Psychiatr Scand* 1994;90:348.
17. Hausmann R, Betz P. Delayed death after attempted suicide by hanging. *Int J Legal Med* 1997;110:164.
18. Innala SM, Ernuff KE. Asphyxiophillia in Scandinavia. *Arch Sex Behav* 1989;18:181.
19. Iserson KV. Strangulation: a review of ligature, manual, and postural neck compression injuries. *Ann Emerg Med* 1984;13:179.
20. Kaki A, Crosby ET, Lui ACP. Airway and respiratory management following non-lethal hanging. *Can J Anaesth* 1997;44:445.
21. Kelleher MJ, Keohane B, Corcoran P, et al. Elderly suicides in Ireland. *Irish Med J* 1997;90:72.
22. Lachmamm E. Anatomy of judicial hanging. *Resident Staff Phys* 1972;18:46.
23. Lester D. Suicide and homicide in Costa Rica. *Med Sci Law* 1995;35:316.
24. Marcus P, Alcabes P. Characteristics of suicides by inmates in an urban jail. *Hosp Commun Psychiatr* 1992;44:256.
25. Morild I. Fractures of neck structures in suicidal hanging. *Med Sci Law* 1996;36:80.
26. Nixon JW, Kemp AM, Levene S, et al. Suffocation, choking, and strangulation in childhood in England and Wales: epidemiology and prevention. *Arch Dis Child* 1995;72:6.
27. Obafunwa JO, Busuttil A. A review of completed suicides in the Lothian and Borders region of Scotland (1987–1991). *Soc Psychiatry Psychiatr Epidemiol* 1994;29:100.
28. Proulx F, Lesage AD, Grunberg F. One hundred in-patient suicides. *Br J Psychiatry* 1997;171:247.
29. Raja U, Sivaloganathan S. Decapitation—a rare complication in hanging. *Med Sci Law* 1997;37:81.
30. Rosenblum S, Faber MM. The adolescent sexual asphyxia syndrome. *Am Acad Child Psychiatry* 1979;18:546.
31. Sabo RA, Hanigan WC, Flessner K, et al. Strangulation injuries in children. Part 1. Clinical analysis. *J Trauma Inj Inf Crit Care* 1996;40:68.
32. Scott KWM. Suicides in Wolverhampton (1976–1990). *Med Sci Law* 1994;34:99.
33. *Statistical Abstracts of the United States,* 112th ed. Washington, DC: US Bureau of the Census, 1992:89.
34. Vande Krol L, Wolfe R. The emergency department management of near-hanging victims. *J Emerg Med* 1994;12:285.
35. Yip PSF. Suicides in Hong Kong, Taiwan, and Beijing. *Br J Psychiatry* 1996;169:495.

CHAPTER 127
Trauma in the Elderly

Suzanne Moore Shepherd and William H. Shoff

Trauma in the elderly is a growing concern. The elderly (above age 65 years) have increased in number and now make up about 12% of our population (Fig. 127.1). They are expected to represent 13% of the U.S. population by the year 2005.[28] In 1990, a staggering 977,000 elders required care for fractures.[25] The elderly account for 25% of hospitalizations for trauma and 25% of all trauma costs.[21] Unfortunately, when the elderly are injured, they are more likely to suffer complications and to die than their younger counterparts, and they exhibit different injury patterns.[12,24]

PATHOPHYSIOLOGY

Many elderly patients seem to function very well, but the aging process limits the physiologic reserve needed to respond adequately to injury. The following is an overview of the physiologic derangements of aging that increase the morbidity and mortality of trauma in this group.

Cardiovascular

Functional losses in the cardiovascular system result from a loss of normal elasticity and changes in tissue collagen. As the heart

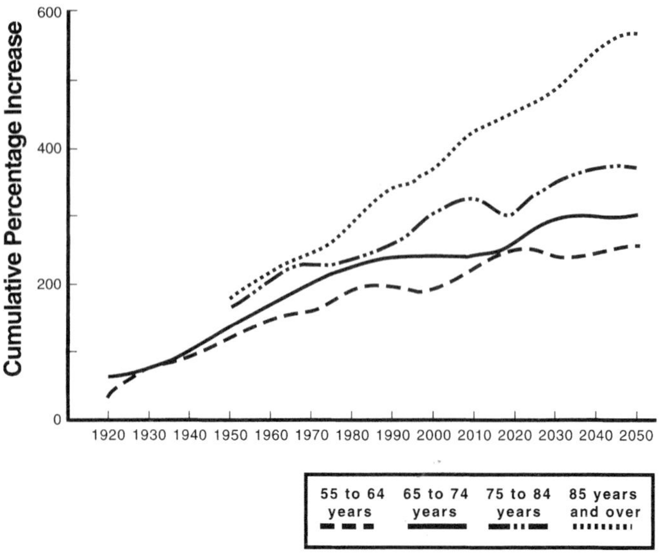

Figure 127.1. Percentage increase of elderly population, 1920–2050. (Redrawn from Eliastam M. Elderly patients in the emergency department. *Ann Emerg Med* 1989;18:1222.)

and pericardium stiffen, resting cardiac output and stroke volume begin to fall.[6,9] This effect may progress to overt congestive heart failure in up to 10% of patients over age 75 years.[7] Although the resting heart rate often does not change, fibrosis of the conduction system and the loss of specialized conduction cells impede the heart's ability to increase its rate when necessary.[5] Also, aging is often accompanied by the development of atherosclerotic coronary disease. The combination of fixed coronary artery lesions, decreased cardiac compliance, increased wall tension, and the inability to raise heart rate limits myocardial oxygen delivery. Because cardiac output often needs to increase after injury or blood loss, these patients are at risk for developing myocardial ischemia. Ischemia, in turn, may further impair cardiac output. The accompanying increase in pulmonary pressure also tends to decrease cardiac output. Dysrhythmias may also occur, further complicating the situation.

Many elderly patients are on prescription medications that tend to limit the heart's ability to respond to stress (i.e., beta blockers, calcium channel blockers, clonidine). Afterload-reducing agents and diuretics may limit preload, thereby decreasing blood pressure under stress. Diuretic-induced electrolyte abnormalities (e.g., hypokalemia, hypomagnesemia), as well as medications such as digoxin and theophylline, may precipitate dysrhythmias.

The changes in the vascular system are similar to those in the heart. Loss of compliance tends to make vessels more easily injured by shearing forces, producing vascular rupture, occlusion from intimal disruption, or aneurysm formation.[6,22]

Pulmonary

As the lungs age, they undergo numerous changes, none of them helpful. The same loss of elasticity that impedes the cardiovascular system tends to occur in the lung. As the lungs stiffen, forced vital capacity and maximal expiratory flow are reduced. Residual volume rises and vital capacity decreases as the total lung capacity does not change. These alterations, combined with a decrease in lung surface area due to emphysematous changes (remarkably common in the elderly), contribute to a decrease in ventilation.[27] As perfusion does not change, ventilation–perfusion mismatch occurs, characterized by a fall in Po_2.

Loss of elasticity also occurs in the muscle and connective tissue of the chest wall. Combined with osteoporosis of the ribs (discussion follows) and the pulmonary parenchymal changes, this condition makes the elderly much more prone to rib fractures and pulmonary contusion, which may occur even with seemingly minor forces. These patients often require mechanical ventilation; thus, these injuries may prove lethal.

Renal

With aging, kidneys lose both structure and function due to a loss of both glomeruli and nephrons, in both number and function. Renal blood flow falls secondary to decreases in cardiac output and the development of renal artery atherosclerosis. Progressive fibrosis occurs in the remaining parenchyma. All of this produces the well-recognized decrease in creatinine clearance that accompanies aging.[13] We lose an estimated 8 to 10 mL/min of creatinine clearance per decade of life after the 20s. Diminution of renal function is characterized by an inability to concentrate urine, as the kidneys cannot retain free water.

Serum creatinine and urine output are two of the clinical tools often used to estimate renal function, but this is potentially disastrous in the elderly. Older patients progressively lose lean muscle mass, so they do not produce as much creatinine. The loss of concentrating ability means they may continue to produce seemingly adequate amounts of dilute urine, even in the face of significant hypovolemia. Patients with an impaired myocardium may also not make adequate amounts of urine in response to a fluid challenge, again making urine output an unreliable indicator of intravascular volume. Because these normally reliable indices cannot be used in the elderly, our approach must be changed, especially when we use nephrotoxic agents, such as antibiotics, or contrast agents.

Osteoporosis

Osteoporosis is present to some degree in almost every elderly patient. The loss of histologically normal bone produces a significant loss of bone strength, making these bones much more susceptible to fractures. Osteoporosis accounts for an estimated 1.5 million fractures in the United States every year.[4,15] The most common osteoporotic fractures in the elderly are vertebral compression fractures and fractures of the wrist, hip, pelvis, and skull.

Osteoporotic fractures have tremendous clinical implications. Fractures often require operative fixation, subjecting the elderly patient to myriad postoperative complications. Nonoperative therapy puts the patient at risk for skin breakdown, pulmonary embolus, and pneumonia. Narcotics used to treat pain may cause marked decreases in mental status. A seemingly straightforward fracture may carry substantial morbidity and mortality in the elderly patient.

Central Nervous System

The central nervous system undergoes substantial changes with aging. The brain progressively loses volume, and the dura becomes more tightly adherent to the skull, limiting the occurrence of epidural hematoma. The smaller brain is allowed more angular movement in the skull. This increased space could potentially protect the brain from contusions, but the loss of volume also stretches the parasagittal bridging veins, making them prone to rupture. This stretching makes the elderly patient particularly prone to the development of subdural hematoma. The increased space around the brain can also hold a remarkable amount of blood before the hematoma produces clinical signs. Neurotrauma is second only to shock as a predictor of death in the traumatized elderly patient.[12]

CLINICAL PRESENTATION AND DIFFERENTIAL DIAGNOSIS

Traumatized elderly patients present a special problem for the emergency physician. Because of the inability of the elderly patient to respond to injury, seemingly minor trauma can result in major complications; preventing these complications requires alert, accurate assessment.

Trauma in the elderly, as in younger patients, is classified by mechanism of injury. When an elderly person is traumatized, the emergency physician must rapidly determine that a medical emergency did not lead to the traumatic event (i.e., syncope, seizure). Falls are a common consequence of such medical emergencies in elderly patients, as are motor vehicle crashes.

Falls are relatively insignificant in younger people but are a source of considerable morbidity and mortality in older patients, in part because 50% of these individuals fall repeatedly.[26] The careful emergency physician must evaluate an elderly person who has fallen not only for potential injuries, but also for the underlying factors causing the fall. The causes of falls are divided into three categories: environmental (chairs, stairs, rugs), gait disturbances, and medical problems unrelated to gait. Clearly, these etiologies are interrelated. For instance, nocturia and urinary or fecal incontinence are common in the elderly. The urgency to avoid soiling oneself, combined with postural hypotension, an unsteady gait, and a slippery rug, may result in a fall. In patients older than 85 years, 20% of such falls occur in nursing homes.[26]

A host of common medical problems may manifest as syncope, near-syncope, dizziness, or vertigo, and can lead to falls. Tables 127.1 and 127.2 outline the most common etiologies and the minimum evaluation needed to rule them out. Many of these etiologies are immediately life-threatening.

It is unacceptable to learn that a patient is hypoglycemic 2 hours after he or she arrives at the emergency department, when a serum glucose value finally returns from the laboratory. It is equally unacceptable to send to radiology an unmonitored patient having bouts of ventricular tachycardia. It is safest to assume that an elderly person who has fallen is hypoglycemic, is having dysrhythmias, has multiple chronic medical problems, is on a host of medications, and has simultaneously suffered a stroke, myocardial infarction, or pulmonary embolus.[19]

Falls need not be an inevitable consequence of aging, and the elderly person who has fallen is not necessarily doomed to do so repeatedly. Rubenstein and associates[16] demonstrated the value of assessing falls in the elderly. They performed a randomized study in which patients were given routine care or a detailed postfall study (detailed physical examination, environmental assessment by a nurse practitioner, laboratory studies, electrocardiogram, and 24-hour Holter monitoring). The probable cause of the fall, risk factors, and therapeutic recommendations were then passed on to the patient's primary physician. At the end of a 2-year follow-up period, the intervention group had 26% fewer hospitalizations, a 52% reduction in hospital days, 9% fewer falls, and 17% fewer deaths.

TABLE 127.1. Emergency Department Evaluation of the Patient Who Has Fallen

ATLS protocol
Cardiac monitoring (continue for at least 24 h)
Transcutaneous oxygen saturation monitoring
Rapid glucose assessment (give D50W if equivocal)
Arterial blood gas analysis
CBC, serum electrolytes, glucose, BUN, creatinine
Serum calcium, magnesium, phosphorus (low levels promote seizures)
12-lead ECG (should be performed serially to help rule out myocardial infarction)
Consider serum cardiac enzymes
Consider naloxone (Narcan) administration if mental status is altered and there is no evidence of head injury
Give i.v. or i.m. thiamine (100 mg)
Careful history and physical examination, particularly neurologic
Consider head CT scan, particularly if no obvious cause for the fall is identified

TABLE 127.2. Internal Causes of Falls Unrelated to Gait[a]

Vasovagal syncope
Cardiac dysrhythmia
Cardiac valvular stenosis
Postural hypotension
Vasomotor insufficiency
Carotid sinus syndrome
Hypovolemia/dehydration
Hypoxemia
Pulmonary embolism
Anemia
Hemorrhage
Cerebrovascular accident
Subarachnoid hemorrhage
Inner ear disturbances
Defecation/micturition
Hypoglycemia
Focal/partial seizures
Generalized seizure
Medications

[a]Common causes of syncope, near-syncope, dizziness, and seizures.

Referrals from the emergency department to gerontologists, neurologists, physiatrists, and social workers may be of significant benefit to an elderly person who has fallen but who does not require admission. Caregivers can decrease a person's risk of future falls by identifying people at high risk for falls, modifying their environments, aiding the hearing and vision, improving their footwear, and getting them to exercise the legs and trunk to improve strength.

Motor vehicle crashes are another source of tremendous morbidity and mortality in the elderly. Although the number of miles driven each year decreases with advancing age, the risk of crash involvement increases significantly. Many of the etiologic factors responsible for falls should also be considered in the elderly crash victim. Crashes among the elderly are more likely to involve intersections, traffic sign violations, right-of-way decisions, and two-car accidents than are those in younger drivers, and are more often fatal.[8,10,21] This fact suggests that there are real problems with cognitive and perceptual functions, as well as impaired reaction times. Dementia, attention deficits, sensory and motor slowing, loss of motor strength, arthritis, decreases in peripheral vision, prescription drug use, and concurrent medical conditions all contribute to the increased crash rate per mile seen in the elderly.[14]

All of these impairments also put elderly pedestrians at risk for being hit by a motor vehicle.[23] They do not readily perceive threats or react to them. They have lost their ability to evade an onrushing accident. In particular, the elderly have difficulty at crosswalks. Add to their problems kyphoscoliosis (restricting upward gaze at traffic lights and signs), decreased hearing, and a slow gait, and one can see why the crosswalk is too often an insurmountable obstacle.[15] Of motor vehicle accidents in general, elderly pedestrians struck may have the highest morbidity and mortality rates.

Finally, the elderly patient's injury may have been intentionally inflicted. Emergency physicians must maintain the same grim alertness for elder abuse that they do for child and spousal abuse. The abuse may be obvious (penetrating trauma, burns, or head injuries) or subtle (poor hygiene, dehydration, weight loss, or unexplained bruising). Because it can escape notice, elder abuse is often unrecognized and, therefore, underreported. Dementia, fear of abandonment, and cultural mores may cause the elderly patient to deny the abuse.[2] The elderly are also at increased risk to be the victims of violent robbery.[21]

EMERGENCY DEPARTMENT EVALUATION AND MANAGEMENT

The principles governing the emergency department evaluation and management of traumatized geriatric patients are identical to those for younger patients. Follow the usual guidelines for trauma management,[3] with some modifications for elderly patients. The two most important differences are that no one is stable, and every minute counts.

Some elderly trauma victims are obviously in extremis at the time of initial evaluation. These badly injured patients almost always die, particularly if they have suffered a head injury.[12] Of more concern are patients who have sustained a significant mechanism of injury but seem relatively stable at the initial evaluation.

One group of patients is at high risk for dying or developing significant complications after the injury (Table 127.3). Although the patient is relatively normotensive in the emergency department, the combination of soft-tissue injury, long-bone fractures, and head injuries produces tissue oxygen deficits that the elderly patient has trouble meeting. If these oxygen delivery deficits are not met in a timely fashion, the patient develops an oxygen debt that cannot be repaid, and he or she will expire early from heart failure or late from multiorgan failure.[20] Failing to recognize this oxygen debt is one of the main reasons for the high mortality rate in the traumatized elderly patient. Invasive monitoring can be extremely helpful in guiding resuscitation in these patients.[18]

Because many emergency departments cannot yet provide this level of critical care monitoring, the period of time elderly trauma victims spend in the emergency department must be minimized. When Scalea et al.[20] cut the time from emergency department presentation to intensive care unit monitoring from 5.5 to 2.2 hours in this high-risk group, survival rose from 7% to 53%. The initial period in the emergency department is the window of opportunity, a window that closes when poor oxygen delivery is not addressed.

Therefore, emergency department diagnostics must be limited to only those that are necessary. Evaluation should begin with a rapid primary survey. If there is any question about airway integrity, it is controlled by means of endotracheal intubation, as the injured elderly patient will often not tolerate even transient hypoxemia. Remember to check for dentures in the elderly patient with airway obstruction or pending intubation. Also, remember that the increased presence of arthritis in the cervical spine further prohibits neck extension during intubation attempts.[17]

The history is of significant importance in the elderly patient, as current medical problems or medications may significantly affect the patient's presentation, response to injury, and response to therapy. The patient's family or physician or emergency medical service personnel may provide vital information regarding the injury, the patient's current level of functioning, and the patient's medical problems, medications, and use of alcohol or drugs.

TABLE 127.3. High-Risk Geriatric Patients

Pedestrian vs. motor vehicle mechanism
Initial systolic blood pressure <130 mm Hg
Acidosis (pH <7.35)
Multiple long-bone fractures
Head injury

Limit initial radiographs to films of the cervical spine, chest, and pelvis. Evaluate the abdomen by ultrasound (which is much quicker than computed tomography [CT] scanning) or by CT scanning.[11] Long-bone films that cannot be obtained as stat portables may need to be deferred, and obvious fractures splinted. Only patients with clinically serious head injuries (markedly depressed mental status or lateralizing neurologic signs) may need to have head CT scanning emergently.

Patients then undergo invasive monitoring. Unless an intensive care unit bed is immediately available, initiate invasive monitoring in the emergency department or trauma resuscitation area. Although a detailed description of hemodynamic optimization is beyond the scope of this chapter, general guidelines are that fluid and blood are used to optimize preload; inotropes are used to increase oxygen delivery further if it remains inadequate after volume loading. Scalea et al.[19,20] successfully used dobutamine and amrinone. These agents are also vasodilators and do not markedly increase myocardial oxygen demand as they increase cardiac output. Augment oxygen delivery until oxygen consumption plateaus and the serum lactate level normalizes.[1]

This approach may seem radical to some, but it follows the basic principles of trauma resuscitation. The clinician has not adequately evaluated the "C" of the ABCs of the primary survey until the patient is invasively monitored. Unfortunately, no noninvasive measures, especially the normally followed signs (i.e., vital signs, urine output, central venous pressure), are adequate to determine the adequacy of tissue oxygen delivery. Hypotension is a late sign of shock and a grim prognostic indicator of survival in the elderly.[29]

Early, aggressive trauma care increases survival in the elderly.[19] It is risky to assume that a normotensive, traumatized, elderly patient in the high-risk group is stable: Multiple organ failure and death may occur from unrecognized, inadequate cardiovascular response to injury. Although complete skeletal surveys are necessary to complete the trauma evaluation, they almost never affect the immediate treatment plan and almost always take much longer than planned. The same is true for studies such as precautionary head CT scans or the evaluation of microscopic hematuria. These are of lower priority than invasive monitoring and should be deferred until the patient's cardiovascular status has been clearly optimized.

Because the elderly have such limited cardiac reserve, a rapid search for all sources of blood loss is mandatory. In addition to loss from abdominal trauma, the elderly are at risk for blood loss from all other injuries. As with younger patients, fractures—in particular, pelvic fractures—can be the source of significant blood loss. The loss of tissue turgor that accompanies aging may limit the tamponade effect that the skin and connective tissue provide in younger patients, which puts the elderly patient at an even higher risk for blood loss at fracture sites. As coronary artery disease limits myocardial oxygen delivery, even at rest, the consequences of anemia may be devastating in the elderly patient. Elderly trauma patients should be transfused more liberally than their younger counterparts, because the blood's oxygen-carrying capacity may be more critical to myocardial oxygen delivery, and crystalloid administration may reduce volume overload, in this setting of diminished compliance of the ventricles.

Because hematocrit determinations require time for equilibration, they are inaccurate in determining acute blood loss. Scalea et al.[19–21] routinely empirically transfused elderly pa-

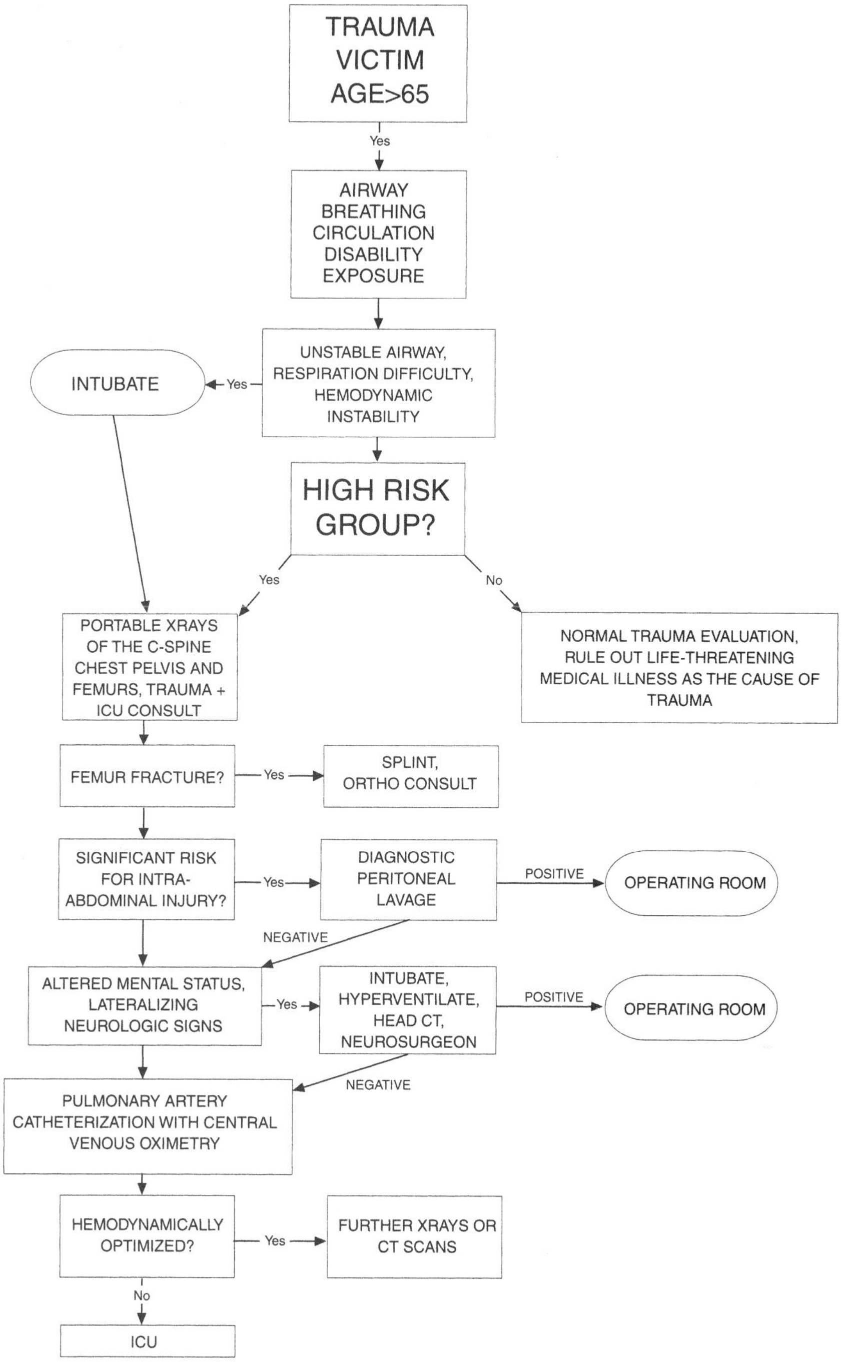

Figure 127.2. Algorithm showing management strategy used for the injured elderly.

tients at high risk for blood loss, such as those with multiple fractures (particularly pelvic), without waiting for a fall in the hematocrit.

Figure 127.2 outlines one basic strategy for the management of the injured elderly patient.

DISPOSITION

Due to the complexities inherent in the management of elderly trauma patients, the trauma surgeon, orthopedist, neurosurgeon, and intensivist must be involved early in their care. Good communication is essential to maximize functional outcome in these difficult patients. All patients in the high-risk group require invasive monitoring and, therefore, admission to the intensive care unit. Elderly patients suffering falls should be evaluated for the need for cardiac monitoring, either in the coronary care unit or in the telemetry department. Transfer criteria for traumatized elderly patients are the same as for their younger counterparts, with one caveat. Because significantly injured elderly patients require invasive monitoring, transfer to a level I trauma center should be considered, particularly if those resources are unavailable at the referring institution.

Despite the best efforts, some elderly patients do not return to their preinjury levels of functional activity. A number of markers for poor outcome in this population have been described, including (1) a Glasgow Coma Score greater than or equal to 7, (2) age greater than 75 years, (3) severe head injury, (4) presence of shock on admission, and (5) the development of sepsis during the admission for the traumatic event. However, early, aggressive resuscitation and evaluation are essential to limit long-term disability.[28] Referring the elderly person who has fallen to a gerontologist or rehabilitation specialist may help prevent recurrent falls.

COMMON PITFALLS

- "Stable vitals" do not necessarily mean a stable patient.
- Do not delay hemodynamic monitoring and optimization for nonurgent studies (e.g., distal extremity x-rays) in patients in the high-risk group.
- Do not rely on urine output to guide resuscitation.
- Do not rely on central venous pressure measurements to guide resuscitation (except early in the resuscitation, when finding a low central venous pressure can be helpful).
- Delaying transfusion can lead to the development of an unrecoverable oxygen debt. Elderly patients should be transfused early.
- Allowing a period of observation to see how an elderly patient responds risks closing the window of opportunity.

ACKNOWLEDGMENT

The authors wish to acknowledge the contribution of Lewis Kohl and Thomas M. Scalea, who wrote the previous version of this chapter.

References

1. Abramson DA, Scalea TM, Hitchcock R, et al. Lactate clearance and survival following injury. *J Trauma* 1993;35:584.
2. Appleton W. Elder abuse: diagnose, treat, cure. *Ann Emerg Med* 1988;17:1006.
3. American College of Surgeons Committee on Trauma. *Advanced trauma life support course for physicians*. Chicago: American College of Surgeons, 1993.
4. Berg RL, Cassels JS, eds. *Osteoporosis in the second 50 years: promoting health and preventing disability*. Washington DC: National Academy Press, 1990:76.
5. Darr KC, Basset DR, Morgan BJ, et al. Effects of age and training status on heart rate recovery after peak exercise. *Am J Physiol* 1988;254:H340.
6. Davies MJ. Pathology of the aging heart. In: Brocklehurst JC, Tallis RC, Fillit HM, eds. *Textbook of geriatric medicine and gerontology*. Edinburgh: Churchill Livingstone, 1992:181.
7. Gibson TC, White KL, Klainer LM. The prevalence of congestive heart failure in two rural communities. *J Chronic Dis* 1966;19:141.
8. Hakamies-Blomquist LE. Fatal accidents of older drivers. *Accid Anal Prev* 1993;25:19.
9. Lakatta EG. Determinants of cardiovascular performance: modification due to aging. *J Chronic Dis* 1983;36:15.
10. Li G, Baker SP, Langlois JA, et al. Are female drivers safer? An application of the decomposition method. *Epidemiology* 1998;8:379.
11. Ma OJ, Mateer JR, Ogata M, et al. Prospective analysis of a rapid trauma ultrasound examination performed by emergency physicians. *J Trauma* 1995;38:875.
12. Osler T, Hales K, Baack B, et al. Trauma in the elderly. *Am J Surg* 1988;156:537.
13. Papper S. The effects of age in reducing renal function. *Geriatrics* 1973;28:83.
14. Retchin SM, Anapolle J. An overview of the older driver. *Clin Geriatr Med* 1993;9:279.
15. Riggs BL, Melton LJ III. Involutional osteoporosis. *N Engl J Med* 1986;314:1676.
16. Rubenstein LA, Robbins AS, Josephson DR, et al. The value of assessing falls in an elderly population: a randomized clinical trial. *Ann Intern Med* 1990;15:113.
17. Ryan MD, Henderson JJ. The epidemiology of fractures and fracture dislocations of the cervical spine. *Injury* 1992;23:38.
18. Scalea TM, Holman M, Fuortes M, et al. Central venous blood oxygen saturation: an early, accurate measurement of volume status during hemorrhage. *J Trauma* 1988;28:725.
19. Scalea TM, Kohl L. Geriatric trauma. In: Feliciano DV, Moore EE, Mattox KL, eds. *Trauma*. Norwalk, CT: Appleton & Lange (*in press*).
20. Scalea TM, Simon HM, Duncan AO, et al. Geriatric blunt multiple trauma: improved survival with early invasive monitoring. *J Trauma* 1990;30:129.
21. Schwab CW, Kauder DW. Trauma in the geriatric patient. *Arch Surg* 1992;127:701.
22. Schlag G, Krosl P, Heinz R. Cardiopulmonary response of the elderly to traumatic and septic shock. In: *Perspectives in shock research*. Vienna: Ludwig Boltzman Institute for Experimental Traumatology, 1988:223.
23. Sklar DP, Demarest GB, McFeeley P. Increased pedestrian mortality among the elderly. *Am J Emerg Med* 1989;7:387.
24. Smith DP, Enderson BL, Maull KI. Trauma in the elderly: determinants of outcome. *South Med J* 1990;83:171.
25. Strange GR, Chen EH, Sanders AB. Use of emergency departments by elderly patients: projections from a multicenter data base. *Ann Emerg Med* 1992;21:819.
26. Tinetti ME, Speechley M. Prevention of falls among the elderly. *N Engl J Med* 1989;320:1055.
27. Tockman MS. Aging of the respiratory system. In: Hazzard WR, Bierman EL, Blass JP, et al., eds. *Principles of geriatric medicine and gerontology*. New York: McGraw-Hill, 1994:555.
28. U.S. Senate Special Committee on Aging. *Aging America: trends and projections, 1987–1988*. Washington, DC: U.S. Department of Health and Human Services, 1988.
29. Van Aalst JA, Yates HK, Miller RS, et al. Severely injured geriatric patients' return to independent living: a study of factors influencing function and independence. *J Trauma* 1991;31:1096.

PART V

Special Procedures

CHAPTER 128
Ultrasound

Sarah A. Stahmer and Verena T. Valley

The real and potential clinical applications of ultrasonography in the emergency department (ED) setting have greatly expanded over the past decade, and no discussion of its clinical applications will remain current for more than a few years. Ultrasound (US) provides real-time information about anatomic structures and cardiac activity, provides guidance for invasive procedures, and localizes areas of pain. It has been incorporated into the clinical practice of a number of specialties outside of radiology, by virtue of its ability to provide immediate clinical information to the assessing physician at the patient's bedside.

Over the past decade, the use of US by emergency physicians has become increasingly widespread, and there is a growing body of literature describing its use by emergency medicine (EM) physicians in a variety of clinical contexts. It is still not routinely incorporated into the practice of most EM physicians, and so this chapter attempts to address the role of US for physicians with and without ultrasonographic capabilities in their ED.

BASIC PRINCIPLES OF ULTRASOUND

For clinicians either requesting a US or performing one on a patient, there are some basic principles of physics and instrumentation that must be appreciated. US imaging uses sound waves to provide images of structures within the body. The sound waves are nonionizing forms of energy that are propagated in waves of variable frequencies. The sound waves are emitted from the transducer with frequencies typically ranging from 2.5 to 10 million hertz (MHz).

The sonographer selects the desired frequency by choosing a transducer or probe that is designed to emit sound waves at a given frequency. Higher frequencies improve image resolution; lower frequencies allow greater penetration and visualization of deeper structures. In general, the sonographer will select a high-frequency probe for superior resolution of a superficial structure such as a subcutaneous foreign body or vein, and a low-frequency probe for imaging of larger subjects or retroperitoneal structures such as the aorta. For most routine imaging in the ED, a range of 3.5 to 5.0 MHz will visualize most intraabdominal structures, with higher frequencies (7.5 to 10.0 MHz) reserved for endovaginal and subcutaneous imaging and testicular and vascular structures.

The ability of a US machine to visualize a structure is dependent on a number of variables, specifically the body habitus of the patient, the ability of the organ and surrounding tissues to transmit sound waves, and, finally, the skill of the sonographer. The limitations of sonography are usually due to inability to obtain good-quality images. Simply stated, if you cannot see the organ or cavity in question well, you cannot accurately interpret the image.

It is always more difficult to obtain high-resolution images on larger patients, because lower frequency waves are needed to penetrate deeper structures. For example, the obese individual in whom you suspect an abdominal aortic aneurysm (AAA) may be better screened with abdominal computed tomography (CT), owing to the difficulty of obtaining good-quality images of retroperitoneal structures with US.

Image resolution of specific organs is greatly affected by the fluid content of the organ and surrounding structures. Fluid transmits sound waves well, and organs containing fluid (e.g., blood, bile, urine) or those adjacent to fluid-filled structures will usually be readily visualized. One of the reasons the gallbladder is so easily visualized by US is its proximity to the liver, which is filled with blood, and the fact that the gallbladder is filled with bile. Conversely, air and bone transmit sound waves poorly, and images containing or adjacent to air-filled or bony structures may be difficult to image well. For this reason, US is a less reliable tool to use for imaging intraabdominal structures because of gas contained within the bowel.

TERMINOLOGY

It is important that clinicians appreciate the terminology used to describe images, in order to interpret radiology reports and, in addition, to describe their own findings when performing bedside US. Images are described with respect to the orientation of the transducer beam to the organ being imaged. When the transducer is aligned in a sagittal or cephalad–caudad orientation, this is termed a *long-axis* or *longitudinal view*. When the transducer is rotated 90 degrees from the longitudinal view, a *transverse view* of the organ is obtained. When the transducer beam is aligned to separate the body into anterior–posterior (AP) sections, the image is described as a *coronal view*.

The US machine has a number of controls that allow the sonographer to modify the image and the signal. Through manipulation of these variables, the signal that returns to the transducer can be altered to obtain optimal images. Images are usually obtained while in *B-mode (brightness) scanning*. The B mode electronically converts US signals to intensity-modulated dots on the display screen. B-mode scanning provides a real-time cross-sectional image. *M-mode (motion) scanning* is a one-dimensional display of motion, usually of the walls and valves of the heart. It takes a one-dimensional signal from the B-scan image and displays it over time.

Gain refers to the echo signal that is received by the transducer. Increasing the gain is roughly equivalent to turning up the volume of a radio, and it increases the number of incoming signals. Too much gain can result in increased scatter and generation of artifacts. Because the strength of the returning image is often attenuated as the depth of imaging is increased, *the time gain compensation control (TGC)* is often used to create a more uniform image. Gain at varying depths can be increased or decreased without affecting overall gain.

Echogenicity refers to the ability of the organ being imaged to reflect sound waves. *Hyperechoic, hypoechoic,* and *anechoic* describe the relative echogenicity of a structure or space. Stones and calcified structures are hyperechoic, appearing bright or white on the screen. Hypoechoic structures have a higher fluid content, are less reflective, and appear darker on the screen. Fluid-filled areas are echo-free, or anechoic, and appear dark or black on the screen.

Artifacts are commonly encountered, which can produce either misleading or clinically relevant imaging effects, depending on the artifact and the clinical scenario. *Shadowing* is an artifact that results from a highly echogenic structure blocking further transmission of the beam to distal structures. The image on the screen will reveal a relatively hypoechoic area, compared with surrounding tissues, immediately beyond a brightly reflective structure. The classic example of this is a stone or calculus, either biliary or renal (Fig. 128.1). When searching for stones, the shadow may be the only clue to their presence, particularly when the stones are small.

Lateral cystic shadowing results from bending of the signal when it comes in contact with a large curved structure (Fig. 128.2). It can be easily misinterpreted as posterior shadowing, except that it can be made to "disappear" by altering the direction of the signal. *Enhancement* refers to the fact that structures that lie below a fluid-filled structure appear brighter than objects in the near field. This phenomenon is due to the disparity

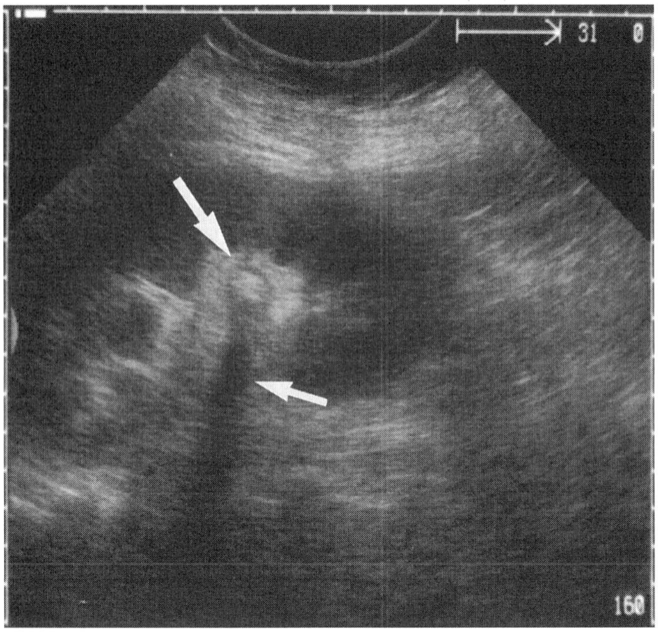

Figure 128.1. Posterior shadowing: A stone within the renal pelvis *(large arrow)* casts a posterior shadow *(small arrow)*.

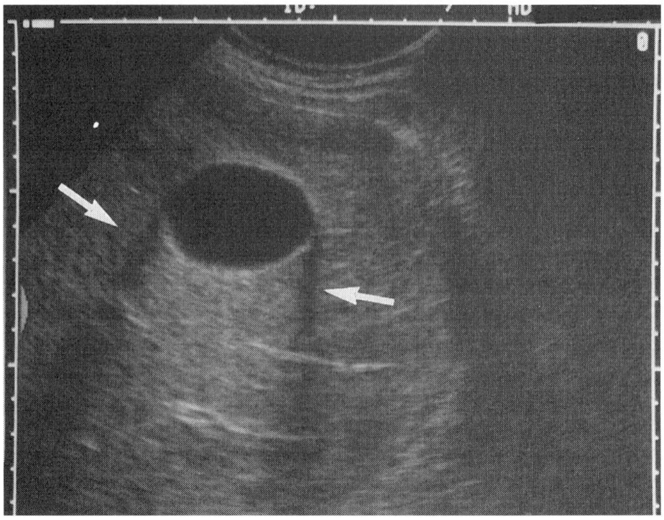

Figure 128.2. Lateral cystic shadowing: This transverse cystic image reveals a lateral cystic shadowing artifact *(arrows)*. This is caused by refractive defocusing of the sound beam on the edges of the cystic structure (gallbladder).

in attenuation that occurs when adjacent signals pass through tissue or fluid. Those that pass through tissue are attenuated and appear "dimmer." Those that pass through fluid are enhanced and appear brighter when they make contact, compared with the shadows from the surrounding structures (Fig. 128.3).

Sonographers frequently make use of this artifact to obtain high-quality images of deep structures, and refer to it as an *acoustic window*. A classic example is imaging of the female pelvis, where a full bladder provides an ideal acoustic window for the pelvic organs.

CLINICAL USES OF ULTRASOUND

Evaluation of the Patient with Suspected Cholelithiasis

The role of ultrasonography is to screen those patients presenting with right upper quadrant or epigastric pain for gallstones and evidence of cholecystitis. The predictive value of history, physical examination, and laboratory studies for cholecystitis are poor, particularly in the elderly and diabetic patient.[18,20] Ultrasonography can accurately identify those patients with acute cholecystitis as the cause of their symptoms, and is complementary to hepatobiliary scanning in distinguishing between acute and chronic cholecystitis.

The gallbladder is uniquely suited for evaluation with ultrasonography because of its location beneath the liver, which serves as an ideal acoustic window. The normal gallbladder appears as a thin-walled, fluid-filled structure located adjacent to the liver. It is best evaluated when the patient has been fasting for at least 6 hours, because the postprandial gallbladder will be contracted and difficult to evaluate. A number of ED examinations will be suboptimal due to insufficient fasting periods and may need to be repeated at a later time.

Gallstones appear as a brightly echogenic structure located within the dependent portion of the gallbladder. The stones do not transmit sound waves, and so the image generated is the reflection of the sound waves from the surface of the stones and the posterior shadowing that results from their reflection. The shadow is quite distinct and may be the only visible sign that a stone is present (Fig. 128.4). The presence of gallstones does not always mean that they are the cause of the patient's symptoms,

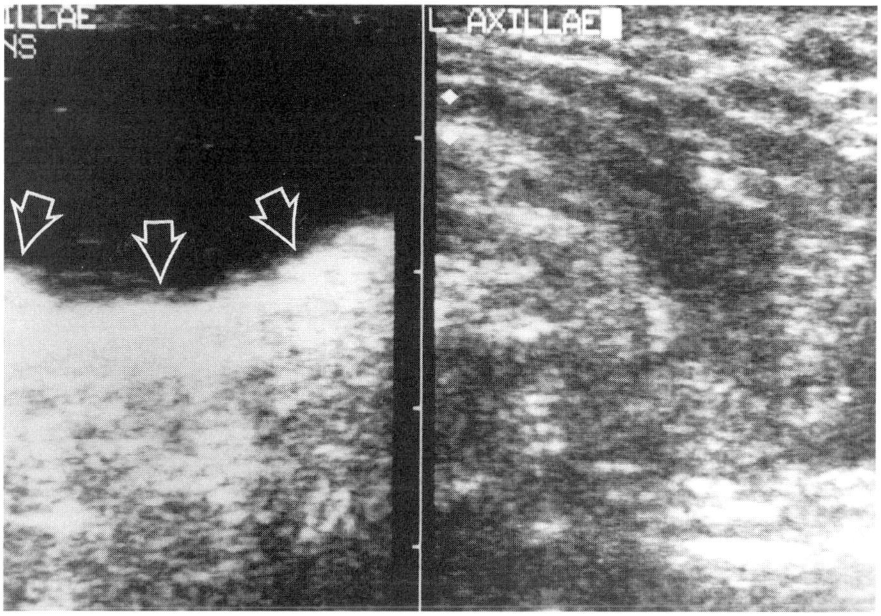

Figure 128.3. Posterior acoustic enhancement: These transverse views of the bilateral axillae reveal a fluid-filled structure in the right that is consistent with an abscess *(arrows)*. The contralateral side **(left)** is examined for comparison. The bright distal echoes are secondary to posterior acoustic enhancement. This enhancement artifact helps in differentiating solid from fluid-filled masses.

and the sonographer should note whether the stones are mobile or fixed by imaging the patient in more than one position. Mobility can be ascertained by turning the patient onto the left side and seeing if the stones move. A stone that does not move, particularly when located in the neck of the gallbladder, suggests that it is impacted and likely to be the cause of the patient's symptoms.

Stones are not always readily visualized, owing to large body habitus, nonfasting states, or location of the stone within the biliary tree. In this situation, the sonographer can use other aspects of the examination to suggest the presence of stones. A large, distended gallbladder, greater than 4 cm in diameter in the transverse view, is suggestive of an obstructing stone in the gallbladder neck or cystic duct. The common bile duct in non–disease states is usually difficult to image, located adjacent and anterior to the portal vein. A duct that is easily visualized and measures greater than 4 mm in internal diameter should be considered obstructed.

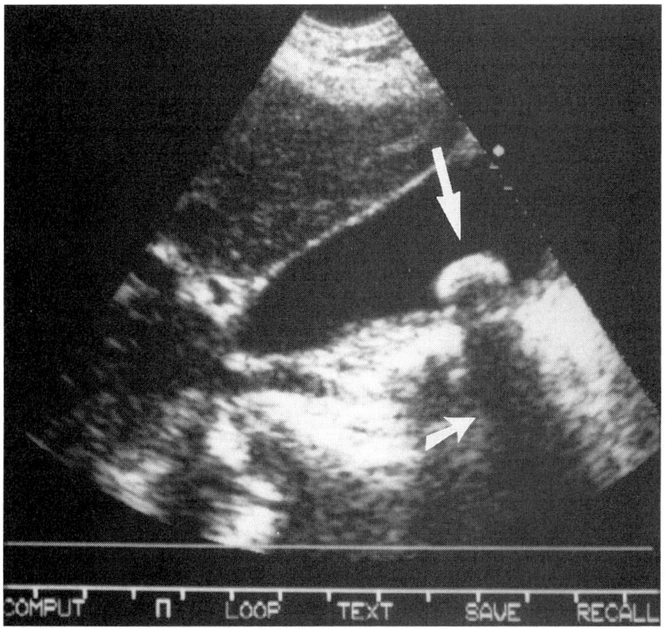

Figure 128.4. Gallstone: There is a hyperechoic stone *(large arrow)* in the dependent portion of the gallbladder, with a posterior shadow *(small arrow)*. There is no thickening of the gallbladder wall or fluid around the gallbladder.

The most useful clinical finding is the presence or absence of the sonographic Murphy sign. Application of pressure with the US probe directly over the gallbladder should elicit pain if the patient's symptoms are due to gallstones. The absence of this important sign should lead the clinician to consider alternative causes of the patient's pain, even when gallstones are visualized.

The ultrasonographic diagnosis of acute cholecystitis is based on the presence of stones, a positive ultrasonographic Murphy sign, and one or more signs of gallbladder obstruction or inflammation. These may include thickening of the gallbladder wall (greater than 3 mm, but usually in excess of 4 mm), fluid around the gallbladder (pericholecystic fluid), intramural gas, or a tense, distended gallbladder (Fig. 128.5). These findings are highly suggestive of acute cholecystitis when supported by the appropriate clinical presentation.

The sensitivity of US alone for revealing changes consistent with cholecystitis has been reported as approaching 90%, but the specificity is closer to 50%.[20] Gallbladder wall thickening is seen in a number of other conditions, including hepatitis, congestive heart failure, renal disease, and ascites. The gallbladder will also appear enlarged and may be tender to palpation in other conditions that cause nausea, vomiting, and epigastric pain. Because of these confounding features, the US examination must be interpreted in the appropriate clinical context.

Evaluation of the Patient with Blunt or Penetrating Thoracoabdominal Trauma

US is routinely incorporated into the clinical practice of many traumatologists and EM physicians when evaluating patients with blunt and penetrating thoracoabdominal trauma. The ultrasonographic examination of the traumatized patient has been standardized to include a minimum of four views. These are (1) the subcostal view of the heart, which rapidly assesses the pericardial space for fluid and cardiac wall motion; (2) the right upper quadrant view, which visualizes the right costophrenic angle and Morison's pouch for fluid within the pleural space and peritoneum, respectively; (3) the left upper quadrant, which vi-

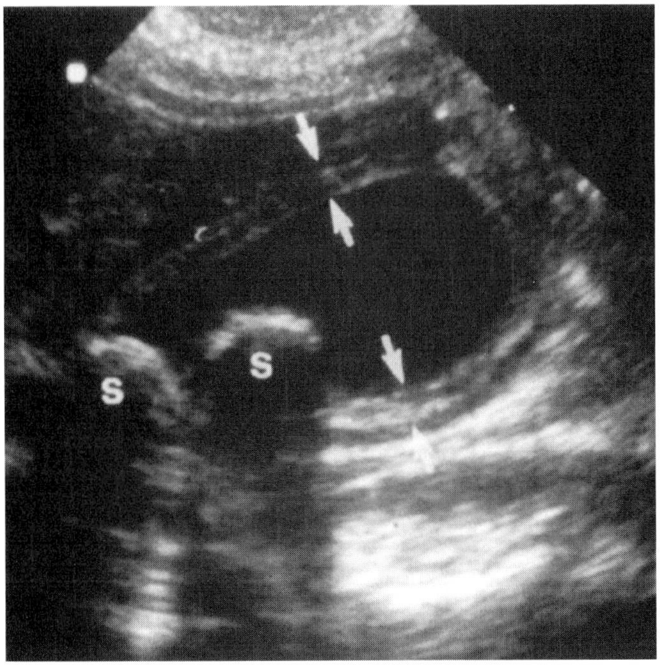

Figure 128.5. Acute cholecystitis: There are two stones within the gallbladder, in addition to thickened gallbladder walls *(arrows)*.

sualizes the left costophrenic angle and potential space between the left kidney and spleen for fluid within the pleural space and peritoneum, respectively; and (4) the suprapubic view, which looks for fluid within the retrovesicular space (Fig. 128.6).

In the hands of experienced sonographers, it is comparable to CT and direct peritoneal lavage (DPL) in detection of free intraperitoneal fluid, with sensitivity and specificity ranges of 80% to 95% and 96% to 99%, respectively.[11,14,15] The diagnostic sensitivity is improved with increasing sonographer experience, increased number of views, placing the patent in a supine position, and repeating negative examinations after short periods of observation.

It has also been shown to be comparable to chest radiographs in the detection of hemothorax.[9] The sensitivity and specificity

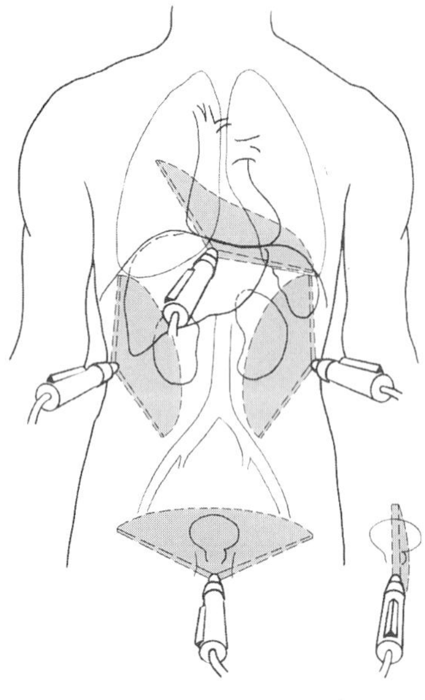

Figure 128.6. Trauma scan: This illustration demonstrates probe positioning to obtain the four quadrant views of the chest, abdomen, and pelvis.

for detection of hemoperitoneum for pediatric patients are similar those for adults, with superior ability to detect specific organ injury due to their small body size and minimal subcutaneous fat.[4,8] Ultrasonography is limited in its inability to detect fluid (blood) within the retroperitoneal space, and injuries to specific organs, particularly the pancreas and bowel. When injuries to these regions are suspected, CT is a superior imaging modality.

There are relatively few contraindications to US. Massive obesity and subcutaneous emphysema may limit the sonographer's ability to obtain high-quality images. The presence of ascites will compromise the clinical interpretation of free fluid, and may result in a falsely positive study. Prior abdominal surgery can limit the free flow of fluid within the peritoneal or pleural cavities. It is the initial study of choice in traumatized pregnant patients, particularly with respect to its ability to rapidly assess fetal viability.

The role of US in assessing the traumatized patient has evolved into a screening examination performed shortly after arrival. It can rapidly detect free fluid within the pericardial sac, pleural space, and peritoneal cavity (Figs. 128.7 through 128.9). For the low-risk individual, US is an excellent screening tool for intraperitoneal bleeding when combined with close clinical monitoring and serial examinations. In the moderate- or high-risk patient, it rapidly identifies acute bleeding and the need for emergent laparotomy. For patients who can be stabilized in the ED, CT scanning provides important additional information about parenchymal, retroperitoneal, and hollow viscus injury.

The Patient with Suspected Kidney Stone

The typical patient with ureteral colic is between the ages of 20 and 50 years and presents with acute onset of flank pain, vomiting, and hematuria. The choices of imaging studies available to evaluate such a patient include plain abdominal radiographs, intravenous urography (IVU), helical CT, and ultrasonography. Which study, or combination of studies, used is dependent on the ability of each study to answer the following questions: (1) Is this the correct diagnosis, (2) what is the likelihood of this stone's passing spontaneously, and (3) what are the risks to the patient?

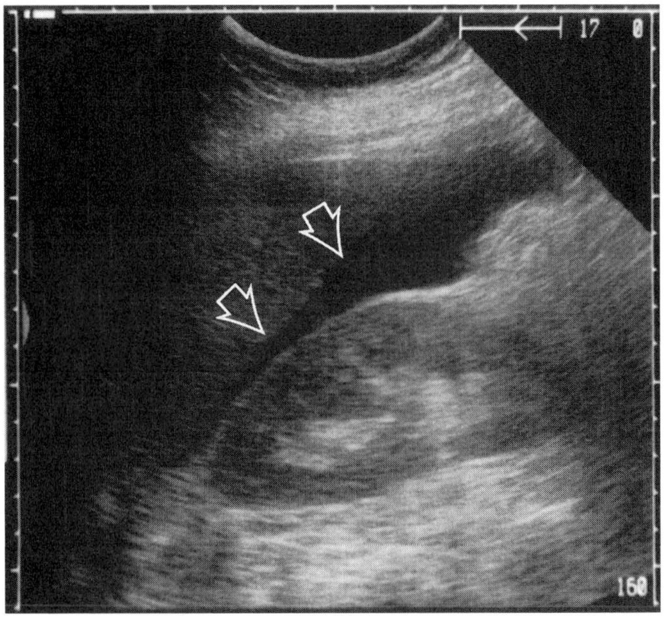

Figure 128.7. Intraperitoneal fluid: This image demonstrates free fluid within the peritoneal cavity. Fluid is seen as a black anechoic stripe in Morison's pouch *(arrows)*, which is the potential space between the liver and the kidney.

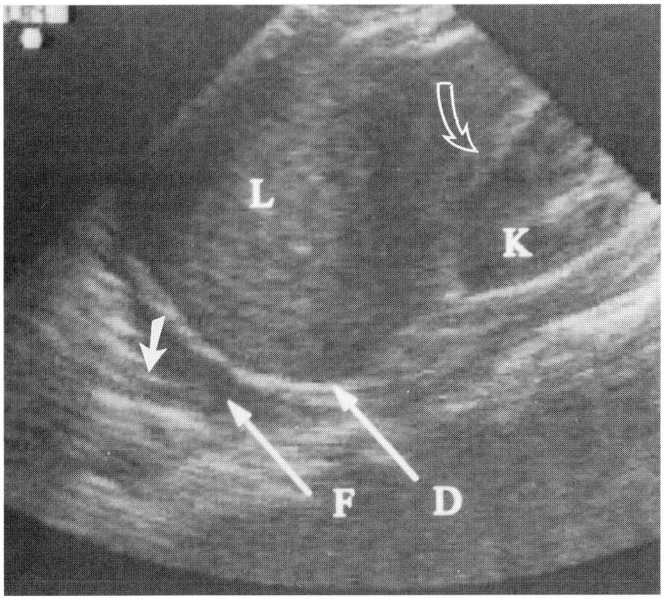

Figure 128.8. Pleural effusion: This right upper quadrant view reveals a pleural effusion. There is loss of the mirror image artifact above the diaphragm *(D)*, and a wedge of lung *(small arrow)* can be seen within the fluid *(F)*. The liver *(L)* and kidney *(K)*, in addition to Morison's pouch *(hollow arrow)*, are seen in this view. There is no fluid in Morison's pouch.

The advantage of bedside ultrasonography is that it is quick and noninvasive and does not expose the patient to ionizing radiation or contrast. The sonographic diagnosis of kidney stones relies on the fact that most symptomatic stones cause some degree of obstruction, which can be seen as hydronephrosis (Fig. 128.10). Rarely can the sonographer visualize the stone itself. The sensitivity of ultrasonography for detecting hydronephrosis, when present, is over 90%. When combined with plain radiographs of the abdomen, ultrasonography has a sensitivity for diagnosing stones that approaches 100%.[2]

There are a number of important caveats to this statement. The first is that approximately one-fourth of patients with obstructing stones have no evidence of hydronephrosis on presentation. Repeat examination after a period of hydration and observation greatly increases the sensitivity of the ultrasonographic examination.

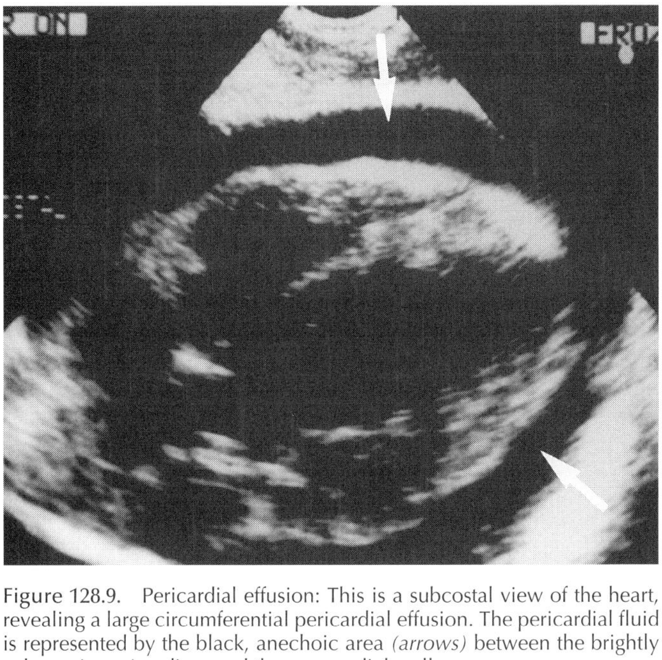

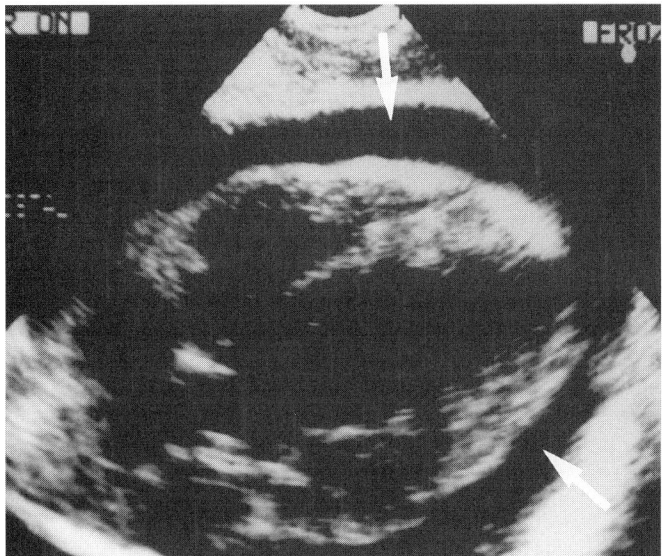

Figure 128.9. Pericardial effusion: This is a subcostal view of the heart, revealing a large circumferential pericardial effusion. The pericardial fluid is represented by the black, anechoic area *(arrows)* between the brightly echogenic pericardium and the myocardial wall.

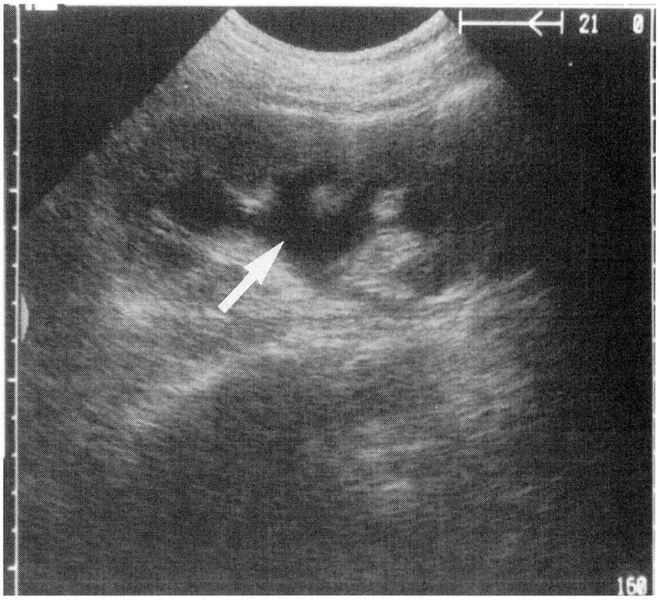

Figure 128.10. Hydronephrosis: This is a longitudinal view of the right kidney. There is moderate hydronephrosis, which is seen as separation of the pelvic calyces by fluid *(arrow)*.

Second, not all hydronephrosis is due to kidney stones, and approximately 20% of patients with suspected renal colic do not have stones. Commonly encountered confounding disorders include extrinsic compression of the ureters due to tumor, urologic tumors, papillary necrosis, congenital abnormalities of the genitourinary system, polycystic kidney disease, and processes causing obstruction or impaired emptying of the bladder. Ultrasonography is inferior to CT or IVU in identifying many of these alternative causes of hydronephrosis.

Finally, ultrasonography cannot describe the amount of functional impairment secondary to the stone or predict the likelihood that the stone will pass spontaneously. Stone size is the major determinant of whether the stone will pass spontaneously, and the degree of hydronephrosis seen on US correlates poorly with either stone size or extent of obstruction. Both CT and IVU can offer superior information regarding the anatomy of the genitourinary system in addition to functional information regarding the level and degree of obstruction.

So, what is the role of ED ultrasonography? Most EM physicians with access to bedside US have found that in the patient with a classic presentation, the presence of unilateral hydronephrosis is a reassuring adjunct to their clinical impression. When combined with a KUB radiograph showing a calcification on the side of the hydronephrosis, the diagnosis of kidney stones can be made with excellent accuracy. Many of these patients can be safely discharged from the ED and scheduled for either IVU or CT at a later time. In those patients with normal examinations, either the US examination should be repeated after a period of hydration, or an alternative imaging modality (CT or IVU) chosen, if clinically indicated. In patients with contraindications to either contrast or radiation, ultrasonography remains the initial study of choice.

When alternative causes of flank pain, such as an AAA, are clinically suspected, ultrasonography can also be a useful initial screening tool. Negative studies should be followed up with a more definitive imaging study, such as CT or magnetic resonance imaging (MRI), if AAA is clinically suspected, or CT or IVU when renal calculus remains the primary clinical diagnosis.

First-Trimester Bleeding

US is invaluable in the evaluation of the patient with vaginal bleeding or pain in the first trimester of pregnancy. The primary goal is to rapidly identify those patients with ectopic pregnancy, and, secondarily, to assess fetal viability. Emergency physician use of bedside pelvic ultrasonography has been shown to significantly improve detection of ectopic pregnancies on initial presentation to the ED.[10]

Two sonographic techniques exist for imaging of pelvic structures. The transabdominal approach utilizes a low-frequency probe (2.5 to 3.5 MHz), and the endovaginal method employs a higher frequency, endocavitary probe (5.0 to 7.5 MHz). The two techniques of imaging the pelvis are complementary, with advantages and limitations directly related to the principles of high- versus low-frequency sonography. The transabdominal approach offers an overall view of the uterus and pelvis and is the best technique for identifying free fluid within the pelvis. The higher frequency, endovaginal probe provides a detailed, high-resolution view of the uterus, ovaries, and cul-de-sac.

Most ED-based protocols focus on using US to confirm the *presence* of an intrauterine pregnancy (IUP) in the patient with pain or bleeding in the first trimester. Endovaginal imaging has greatly enhanced the ability to visualize an IUP within 5 weeks of gestation. The first sonographic indicator of pregnancy is the gestational sac at 4.5 to 5.0 weeks; however, the yolk sac is the earliest *reliable* sign of an IUP (Fig. 128.11). A fetal pole can be seen adjacent to the yolk sac, and as early as 6 weeks the presence of embryonic cardiac activity can be readily visualized.

When there is no evidence of an IUP on US, subsequent clinical management depends on the quantitative beta human chorionic gonadotropin (beta-hCG) and the presence or absence of high-risk clinical findings. If the serum beta-hCG is above the discriminatory zone, the patient has an ectopic pregnancy until proven otherwise. A discriminatory zone is a cut-off level for serum beta-hCG above which an IUP should be seen.[7] The actual value may vary by institution, with a conservative discriminatory level for endovaginal imaging being 2,000 mIU/mL (IRP). Ectopic pregnancies have been seen on US at levels below

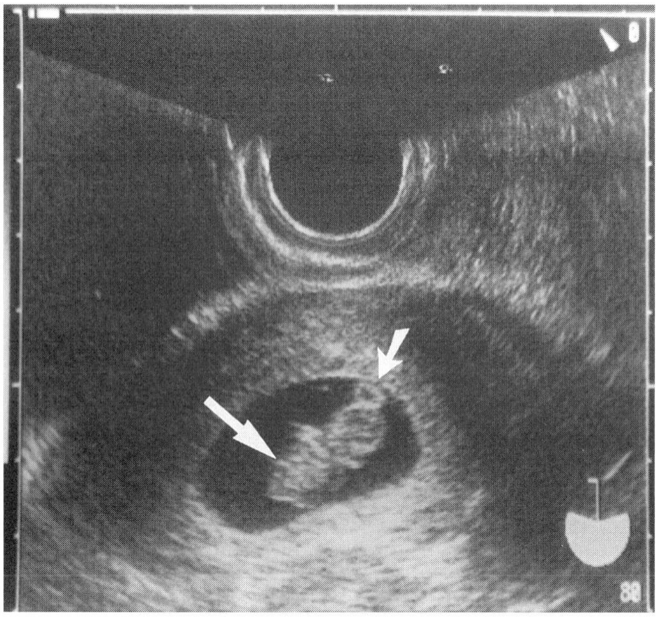

Figure 128.11. Intrauterine pregnancy with yolk sac and fetal pole: This is a transvaginal view of an intrauterine gestational sac with fetal pole *(large arrow)* and yolk sac *(small arrow)*.

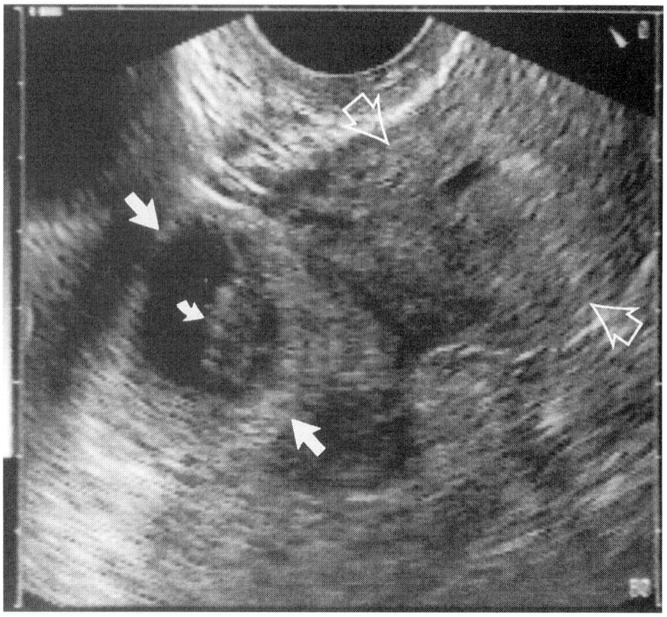

Figure 128.12. Ectopic pregnancy: This is an endovaginal view of a right adnexal ectopic pregnancy with a gestational sac *(large arrows)* and fetal pole *(small arrow)*. The uterus is seen to the right of the image, with a small amount of endometrial fluid *(hollow arrows)*.

1,000 mIU/mL, and clinical management should not be based solely on the quantitative hCG.[1]

There is a spectrum of sonographic findings of ectopic pregnancy. A very early extrauterine pregnancy may have the appearance of an echogenic (or tubal) ring surrounding a hypoechoic area. Other sonographic findings include an empty extrauterine gestational sac, a ruptured ectopic with hemoperitoneum, or a mass within the adnexa. A true or definite ectopic pregnancy (defined as a thick, brightly echogenic structure outside of the uterus with a gestational sac containing a fetal pole or yolk sac) is seen in less than 5% of all patients with ectopic pregnancies[10] (Fig. 128.12). The presence of an abnormal adnexal mass, free cul-de-sac fluid, and severe adnexal tenderness with probe pressure are additional worrisome findings, irrespective of the beta-hCG.

In view of the spectrum of sonographic findings in the diagnosis of an ectopic pregnancy, it is an appropriate initial approach to *rule in* an IUP. If an IUP is not visualized and the beta-hCG is greater than the discriminatory zone *or* there are additional clinical or sonographic findings suggestive of an ectopic pregnancy, obstetric or radiologic consultation is indicated.

Potential pitfalls in the sonographic diagnosis of ectopic pregnancy include (1) failure to image patients with low beta-hCG levels, (2) failure to determine the exact location of a gestational sac, (3) mistaking an ectopic pregnancy for a corpus luteum cyst or bowel, and (4) misdiagnosing an advanced ectopic (interstitial) pregnancy as an IUP. The best way to avoid these potential pitfalls is to scan the entire pelvis, even when an IUP is identified.

When the pregnancy is determined to be intrauterine, sonography can be helpful in determining viability. One of the best indicators of fetal viability is the presence of embryonic cardiac activity. The rate of spontaneous abortion is very low (2% to 4%) if normal embryonic cardiac activity is observed. Sonographic findings suggestive of a nonviable pregnancy include (1) an irregular gestational sac, (2) a gestational sac greater than 25 mm on transabdominal US or greater than 16 mm on endovaginal US without a yolk sac or embryo, (3) an embryo that measures over 5 mm in length without a heart beat, and (4) abnormal echogenic material within the uterine cavity. The lack of embryonic cardiac activity after 8 weeks (as determined by crown rump length) is highly indicative of embryonic demise.

The presence of maternal anatomic abnormalities may occur in 10% to 15% of women with recurrent spontaneous abortion. These anatomic abnormalities include a bicornuate or septate uterus and leiomyomas, all of which are readily identified on US. Other entities that can be diagnosed with US in patients with pelvic pain, bleeding, and a positive pregnancy test include retained products of conception and hydatidiform moles.

The Nonpregnant Patient with Pelvic Pain

The nonpregnant female patient presenting with pelvic pain is a common ED complaint. The differential diagnosis is broad and includes tuboovarian abscesses (TOAs), ovarian cysts, torsion, and masses such as fibroids and teratomas. US is the primary diagnostic imaging tool used to differentiate among these disorders. Uterine fibroids are common and appear as moderately echogenic masses distorting the shape of the uterus. A degenerating fibroid can often be the source of severe lower abdominal pain, and will appear as a heterogenous mass with fluid filled areas within or adjacent to the uterus.

Ovarian cysts are frequently seen on routine pelvic scanning. When accompanied by the presence of tenderness with palpation of the probe or pelvic fluid, the diagnosis of a leaking or ruptured cyst becomes likely. Complex ovarian masses may be noted on US, and may be due to a TOA or tumor. Although ovarian neoplastic disease is beyond the scope of this discussion, consultation with gynecology is recommended to determine further evaluation and treatment. If an ovarian torsion is suspected, endovaginal color flow sonography is recommended to determine intrinsic ovarian arterial flow.

In the evaluation of *right-sided* pelvic pain, it is important to remember that the appendix can occasionally be seen on US. In appendicitis, the appendix appears on US as a noncompressible tubular structure with a diameter greater than 7 mm. An appendicolith, which appears as a highly echogenic structure with distal shadowing, may be seen within the distended appendix. US is not the ideal screening examination for suspected appendicitis, especially when the clinical suspicion is either very high or low. In those cases, the patients should undergo either exploratory laparotomy or CT scanning. For borderline cases, ultrasonography may reveal a nonappendiceal cause of the patient's symptoms, particularly those due to gynecologic disorders.

The Patient with Suspected Deep Venous Thrombosis

The diagnosis of an acute deep venous thrombosis (DVT) often is clinically challenging because the clinical signs and symptoms are unreliable. US is the imaging modality of choice in the evaluation of suspected lower extremity DVT. Even when the study reveals no clot, it can identify other etiologies of a swollen lower extremity, such as pseudothrombophlebitis or Baker's cyst. The examination is performed with the patient in the supine position and the leg turned slightly outward. The reverse Trendelenburg position allows blood to pool into the leg veins. Most scanning is performed in the transverse orientation. The vein is compressed in the transverse orientation and repeated in increments of 1 to 2 cm. The sonographer should use only the force needed to bring the walls together. The walls must touch completely for the test to be diagnostic.

The common femoral vein should be imaged first, and is easily identified distal to the inguinal ligament. The greater saphenous vein takes off from the common femoral vein. The course of the common femoral vein extends distally under the superficial femoral artery and then divides into the superficial and deep femoral veins. Imaging should include the popliteal vein and popliteal fossa, which is territory for a Baker cyst. A large Baker cyst may cause swelling of the lower extremities by either compression of the deep veins or rupture of the cyst itself.

The best-studied diagnostic criterion for an acute DVT is loss of vein wall compressibility. Arteries are noncompressible and pulsatile. The presence of echogenic material within a noncompressible vein is further supportive evidence of a thrombus. An acute DVT is usually found centrally in the lumen. When the thrombus is obstructing, the vein is usually large and easily imaged proximate to the obstruction. Color flow imaging is helpful in distinguishing a partially obstructed vein from a total obstruction. Emergency physicians can perform color flow Doppler US to diagnosis acute DVT with reasonable accuracy.[6] Potential pitfalls include (1) the edematous leg, (2) obesity, and (3) nonvisualization of a venous segment containing clot. Negative or nondiagnostic studies should be followed up with definitive imaging studies (venography, MRI) if there is a high clinical suspicion for DVT.

The Patient with a Pulsatile Abdominal Mass

US is a highly accurate imaging procedure for patients with an AAA. For the patient with a symptomatic AAA due to acute expansion or leakage, timely diagnosis and early surgical consultation are crucial. Ultrasonography has clear advantages over other imaging modalities as an initial screening tool when this diagnosis is clinically suspected. It can be performed at the bedside, obviating the need to take a potentially unstable patient out of the department. If a normal-sized aorta is visualized through its entire abdominal course, it is unlikely that this is the cause of a patient's symptoms. When performed immediately on arrival in the ED in patients with suspected AAA, US can rapidly confirm the diagnosis and shorten times to surgical consultation.[17]

The normal sonographic appearance of the abdominal aorta is that of a tapering, echogenic, and pulsatile vessel just left of midline in longitudinal orientation. It can be distinguished from the inferior vena cava by its posterior course along the lumbar spine, lack of change with respiration (sniff test), and echogenic walls. The aorta should be scanned in its entirety from the diaphragm to the bifurcation. The proximal common iliac arteries should be viewed if an aneurysm is present.

The most accurate measurement is in the AP diameter, with measurement made from outer wall to outer wall. The abdominal aorta should be no larger than 3 cm in diameter, and the aorta should taper proximate to the iliac bifurcation to a diameter of 1.0 to 1.5 cm. Loss of this taper, which is often the earliest sign of AAA, or a diameter greater than 3 cm is diagnostic of AAA. Thrombus is often noted within the lumen of the aneurysm (Fig. 128.13). Approximately 90% of AAAs are infrarenal. Identification of a normal sized aorta within 2 cm (distal) of the origin of the superior mesenteric artery should exclude involvement of the renal arteries. Potential pitfalls include (1) bowel gas obscuring the abdominal aorta; (2) tortuosity of the aorta, in which case, oblique views are often helpful; (3) obesity; and (4) failure to identify a mural thrombus.

The role of bedside US is to confirm or exclude the presence of AAA. US is not useful in making the diagnosis of dissection or rupture, and alternative imaging studies should be obtained when these complications of AAA are suspected. For those patients with hemodynamic instability and AAA on US, the diagnosis of rupture can be inferred, and urgent surgical consultation is indicated. Approximately one-fourth of all aneurysms

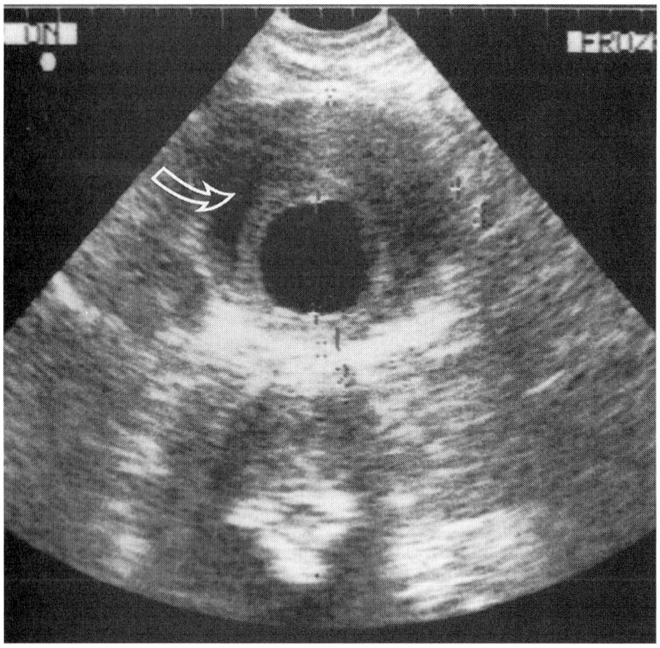

Figure 128.13. Abdominal aortic aneurysm: This is a transverse image of a large AAA with mural thrombus *(arrow)*. The spine is well outlined posteriorly.

will rupture intraperitoneally, and a rupture can be seen on bedside sonography as free intraperitoneal fluid.

ULTRASOUND-ASSISTED PROCEDURES

US-assisted procedures include identification and localization of abscesses and foreign bodies and identification and staging of hematomas, paracentesis, pericardiocentesis, and joint aspiration, as well as vascular access.[16]

Abscess

US may assist in determination and localization of an abscess, depending on the stage of the process. A variety of echogenic patterns have been described, including an anechoic, hypoechoic, or hyperechoic mass or diffuse echogenicity with no demonstrable mass. The presence of posterior acoustic enhancement is very helpful diagnostically in the determination of an abscess or liquid-filled mass versus a solid mass (see Fig. 128.3).

Foreign Body

Emergency physicians are commonly faced with the problem of extracting soft-tissue foreign bodies that are complicating wounds, and US may have a role in identification and removal.[16] Foreign bodies as small as 0.5 mm can be readily identified on US, with wooden foreign bodies (acutely) best visualized, then glass, plastic, and metal. Secondary signs, such as hematoma, abscess formation, or air trails (acutely), may assist in localization.

Hematomas

Hematomas can be sonographically identified and staged. The initial appearance is hypoechoic. After several hours, a fluid level appears and the echogenic clot will be in the dependent portion of the hematoma. Within several days, the fluid appears anechoic. Hematoma formation is the hallmark of muscle rupture.

Nontraumatic Intraperitoneal Fluid

US can readily identify and localize intraperitoneal fluid collections. Ascites may be loculated, depending on the presence of adhesions. US may provide assistance in localizing the optimum approach to fluid collections prior to paracentesis. In addition, patient positioning and the effects of abdominal palpation may be viewed. In a similar manner, pleural fluid can be identified prior to and following aspiration.

Pericardiocentesis

Blind pericardiocentesis is often accompanied by complications, with an associated mortality of up to 6%. Echocardiography-guided pericardiocentesis is now performed routinely in many EDs and is considered the procedure of choice for removal of hemodynamically significant pericardial effusions. Under US guidance, the site of needle entry is the point at which the largest amount of fluid is closest to the body surface, without injuring vital structures. The left chest wall has become the preferred site of needle entry instead of the subcostal approach.[19] A 3.5- to 5.0-MHz transducer held in the subcostal position is recommended. The probe is held under a transparent plastic surgical sheet, thus allowing US imaging and a sterile field.

Joint Aspiration

Joint aspiration is routinely performed in the ED. US can identify joint effusions and demonstrate enhanced patient positioning for fluid aspiration[16] (Fig. 128.14). In addition, US can demonstrate the presence of synovial proliferation, especially in inflammatory arthritis, and predict success or failure of joint aspiration.

Central Vein Cannulation

US-assisted internal vein catheterization in the ED has been described as particularly useful in patients with no visible or palpable anatomic landmarks. US has been associated with an increased rate of successful internal jugular cannulation in at least one prospective trial.[3]

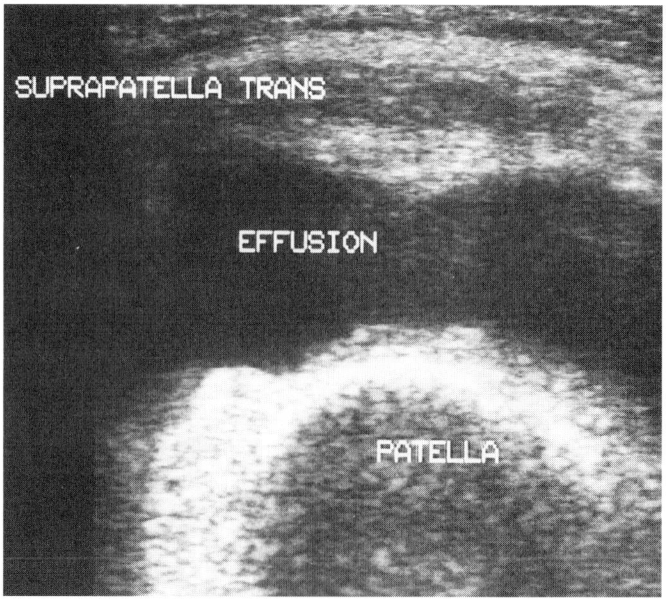

Figure 128.14. Knee joint effusion: This transverse suprapatellar view of the knee reveals a large joint effusion. The patella is well outlined inferiorly.

SUSPECTED SEPTIC, HEMOPHILIC, OR INFLAMMATORY ARTHRITIS

US has proven accuracy in the determination and characterization of joint effusions and hence in the diagnoses of septic, hemophilic, or inflammatory arthritis. It can detect as little as 1 mL of intraarticular fluid and is more sensitive than blind aspiration. Although not commonly performed in the ED, imaging of the joints has distinct clinical promise. Large joints are readily imaged with a variety of sonographic windows. The affected joint is identified and compared with the normal side by use of the split-screen function on the US machine. The most commonly utilized probe for this application is a linear array probe (5 to 10 MHz).

Simple joint effusions are typically anechoic or hypoechoic in appearance (see Fig. 128.14). In septic arthritis, the fluid frequently has a hypoechoic appearance, with internal echoes in addition to synovial irregularity and joint capsule thickening. However, a septic arthritis cannot be ruled out solely based on the sonographic appearance. Hemarthrosis can be difficult to distinguish from a simple effusion. Lipohemarthrosis has the sonographic appearance of a two-layer effusion, with the superior layer being fat and the inferior layer blood.

CARDIAC APPLICATIONS

One of the more useful clinical applications of US is the assessment of the patient who presents with acute hemodynamic instability or pulseless electrical activity (PEA). PEA is defined as the absence of a discernible pulse in the presence of electrical activity observed on a cardiac monitor. The causes are multifactorial and can be broken down into those that compromise cardiac filling (hemorrhage, pneumothorax, and tamponade) and those that are due to poor myocardial contractility (cardiogenic shock). The resuscitation efforts depend on the physician's interpretation of history and physical findings on presentation, which are often unreliable and nonspecific.

Immediate application of US can quickly sort out these very distinct clinical entities. When performed by EM physicians, the use of echocardiography has been shown to reduce time to identification and treatment of clinically significant pericardial effusions due to trauma and cardiac rupture, with significant improvements in overall mortality.[12,13] Bedside sonography can not only assist in differentiation among the various causes of PEA[5], but also allow the clinician to continuously assess the response, or lack of response, to interventions. The sonographer typically utilizes a subcostal or long-axis parastomal view. The benefit of the subcostal view is that it can be performed simultaneously while other chest procedures and tests are being performed. Both views rapidly identify a large pericardial effusion and grossly assess vigor of cardiac wall motion (see Fig. 128.9). The parasternal long-axis view provides superior views of the left ventricle wail, valve motion, and posterior pericardium.

Clinically significant pericardial effusions are easily visualized with ultrasonography. The pericardial sac is a fibrous, echogenic structure that surrounds the heart, and there is normally a small amount of pericardial fluid within the dependent portion of the sac. Greater amounts of fluid are easily seen as an anechoic space between the pericardium and the heart. Small amounts of fluid usually collect in the dependent portion of the heart, but clinically significant effusions are circumferential. In large effusions, there may be echogenic material due to fibrin or clot formation within the pericardial space. The presence of fluid alone does not indicate tamponade physiology. The echocardiographic diagnostic criteria for tamponade are often subtle and not within the purview of most EM sonographers. The most important finding is the presence of a large circumferential effusion, a hyperdynamic heart, and collapse of the right atria and ventricle during diastole.

Other clinically significant findings that can be helpful in guiding therapy include the inability to visualize the heart, suggesting the presence of air within the pleural space, as in a pneumothorax. The presence of a hyperdynamic heart without fluid in the pericardial sac leads the clinician to search for signs of hemorrhage and suggest volume resuscitation as an initial step. A large, dilated right ventricle in the setting of hypotension and hypoxia is suggestive of a large pulmonary embolus.[5] Poor or absent cardiac contractility indicates a primary cardiac cause and suggests the need for inotropic therapy. Bedside sonography can provide immediate confirmation of the patient's response to resuscitative measures. Patients with poor or absent cardiac activity have a poor prognosis, and lack of response to therapy can support termination of resuscitative efforts.

If a primary cardiac cause of instability cannot be readily identified, US can be used to search for other potential reversible causes, specifically evidence of acute blood loss. Fluid within the pleural cavity can be identified with excellent sensitivity,[9] and often before the chest radiograph can be performed. Large amounts of free fluid within the peritoneal cavity may indicate spontaneous splenic rupture or ruptured ectopic pregnancy. Identification of a large aortic aneurysm in the setting of hypotension suggests a leaking aneurysm, and surgery should be consulted immediately. Fluid above or below the diaphragm can appear as pericardial fluid, and the sonographer should make all efforts to confirm the location of the fluid. The subcostal view will not show fluid within the pleural space. Fluid within the peritoneal cavity will not follow the contours of the heart, and imaging from a number of positions will usually clarify its location.

The limitations of US are largely related to operator experience, patient body habitus, and suboptimal imaging conditions—the sonographic imaging is usually being performed in the midst of a major resuscitative effort. Identification of clinically significant pericardial effusions and a gross assessment of cardiac wall motion can be readily achieved under these conditions. Further clinical information regarding cardiac wall motion, valve function and chamber size, and aortic caliber should be performed only by those with sufficient imaging experience.

SUMMARY

The clinical applications for US within the ED will continue to expand as both experience and technology improve. EM physicians will play an increasingly central role in the performance and interpretation of examinations used to answer discrete and directed clinical questions. In particular, EM physicians are uniquely positioned to play a key role in the performance of ultrasonographic examinations in those clinical situations that require immediate assessment, such as patients with acute instability, both traumatic and atraumatic. EM physicians performing US for less urgent situations must work collaboratively with the radiologists, cardiologists, and other subspecialists with ultrasonographic expertise in their institution to ensure that this exciting technology is being used to ensure both rapid and expert patient care.

References

1. Counselman FL, Shaar GS, Heller RA, et al. Quantitative B-hCG levels less than 1000 mIU/ml in patients with ectopic pregnancy: pelvic ultrasound still useful. *J Emerg Med* 1998;16:699.
2. Henderson SO, Hoffner RJ, Aragona JL, et al. Bedside emergency department ultrasonography plus radiography of the kidneys, ureters, and bladder vs intravenous pyelography in the evaluation of suspected renal colic. *Acad Emerg Med* 1998;5:66.

3. Hrics P, Wilber S, Blanda MP, et al. Ultrasound-assisted internal jugular vein catheterization in the ED. *Am J Emerg Med* 1998;16(4):401.
4. Ingeman JE, Plewa MC, Okasinski RE, et al. Emergency physician use of ultrasonography in blunt abdominal trauma. *Acad Emerg Med* 1996;3:931.
5. Johnson ME, Furlong R, Schrank K. Diagnostic use of emergency department echocardiogram in massive pulmonary emboli. *Ann Emerg Med* 1992;21:760.
6. Jolly BT, Massarin E, Pigman EC. Color Doppler ultrasonography by emergency physicians for the diagnosis of acute deep venous thrombosis. *Acad Emerg Med* 1997;4(2):129.
7. Kadar N, DeVore G, Romero R. Discriminatory hCG zone: its use in the sonographic evaluation for ectopic pregnancy. *Obstet Gynecol* 1981;58:156.
8. Luks FI, Lemire A, St.-Vil D, et al. Blunt abdominal trauma in children: the practical value of ultrasonography. *J Trauma* 1993;34:607.
9. Ma OJ, Mateer JR. Trauma ultrasound examination versus chest radiographs in the detection of hemothorax. *Ann Emerg Med* 1997;29:312.
10. Mateer JR, Valley VT, Aiman EJ, et al. Outcome analysis of a protocol including bedside endovaginal sonography in patients at risk for ectopic pregnancy. *Ann Emerg Med* 1996;27:283.
11. Nordenholz KE, Rubin ME, Gularte GG, et al. Ultrasound in the evaluation and management of blunt abdominal trauma. *Ann Emerg Med* 1997; 29:357.
12. Plummer D, Brunette D, Asinger R, et al. Emergency department echocardiography improves outcome in penetrating cardiac injury. *Ann Emerg Med* 1992;21:709.
13. Plummer D, Dick C, Ruiz E, et al. Emergency department two-dimensional echocardiography in the diagnosis of nontraumatic cardiac rupture. *Ann Emerg Med* 1994;23:1333.
14. Porter RS, Nester BA, Dalsey WC, et al. Use of ultrasound to determine need for laparotomy in trauma patients. *Ann Emerg Med* 1997;29:323.
15. Rozycki GA, Ochsner MG, Jaffin JH, et al. Prospective evaluation of surgeons' use of ultrasound in the evaluation of trauma patients. *J Trauma* 1993;34:516.
16. Schlager D. Ultrasound for the detection of foreign bodies and procedure guidance. *Emerg Med Clin North Am* 1997;15(4):895.
17. Shuman WP, Hastrup W Jr, Kohler TR, et al. Suspected leaking abdominal aortic aneurysm; use of sonography in the emergency room. *Radiology* 1988;168:117.
18. Singer AJ, McCracken G, Henry MC, et al. Correlation among clinical, laboratory and hepatobiliary scanning findings in patients with suspected acute cholecystitis. *Ann Emerg Med* 1996;28(3):267.
19. Tsang TS, Freeman WK, Sinak LJ, et al. Echocardiographically guided pericardiocentesis: evolution and state-of-the-art technique. *Mayo Clin Proc* 1998;73:647.
20. Vasilescu C, Jovin GH, Popescu I, et al. Decision analysis in the clinical and imaging diagnosis of acute cholecystitis. *Med Interna* 1990;28:329.

SECTION IV

Section Editor: Allan B. Wolfson

General Medical Emergencies

PART I

Cardiovascular Disease

CHAPTER 129

Cardiac Arrest and Resuscitation

Arthur B. Sanders

The modern era of cardiopulmonary resuscitation (CPR) has been marked by the development of closed-chest cardiac massage, artificial respiration, and electrical defibrillation into a practical set of techniques for the treatment of patients in cardiac arrest. After its introduction in 1960, closed-chest CPR was shown to be successful in resuscitating approximately 25% of patients from in-hospital cardiac arrests. However, it was soon realized that the vast majority of patients suffered cardiac arrest outside a hospital and that most patients who die of myocardial infarction succumb to arrhythmias within the first hour after the infarction. The concept of extending treatment into the community was developed in the 1970s. Pioneering studies in Belfast, New York, Seattle, and other cities demonstrated that emergency medical services (EMS) providing advanced cardiac life support (ACLS) by trained paramedics could significantly improve resuscitation and survival in patients suffering cardiac arrest. Thus an effective approach to cardiac arrest required the development of new concepts for bringing emergency care into the community.[6,15]

Improvements in the treatment of patients in cardiac arrest have generally come by evaluating cardiac arrest as a systems problem that requires new solutions beyond the traditional medical model. Advances have come with community solutions such as the development of an out-of-hospital community emergency medical care system and the training of laypersons to deliver CPR.[16] More recently, the development of the automatic external defibrillator further extends the possibilities for community treatment. Public-access defibrillation holds the promise of providing early defibrillation in the community by trained persons, such as security guards and flight attendants, prior to the arrival of the EMS medics.[6,15,16]

BASIC CARDIOPULMONARY RESUSCITATION

The function of basic CPR is to provide some blood flow to vital organs until more definitive treatment, such as defibrillation, can be initiated. There has been some debate about the efficacy of CPR in the resuscitation of patients in cardiac arrest. Although studies from one city with a rapid-response EMS system have failed to show the benefit of layperson CPR in the resuscitation of victims of cardiac arrest, other studies from several cities have demonstrated that the earlier CPR is applied, the better is the outcome.[6,15] It is important to remember, however, that CPR itself usually does not resuscitate patients from cardiac arrest. CPR must be accompanied by the early institution of advanced life support.

The importance of early defibrillation is emphasized by the concept of "phone first," in which laypersons are taught to activate the EMS system before CPR is started in adults in cardiac arrest.[15] This concept recognizes the importance of getting the defibrillator to the scene as soon as possible. The standard technique of CPR includes chest compression and ventilation. It is designed to provide some blood flow to vital organs until more definitive therapy, such as defibrillation, is available.

There has also been much debate about the mechanism of blood flow during closed-chest compression. Some authorities believe that the thorax acts as a pump when the chest is compressed and that pressure gradients are generated between the intrathoracic and extrathoracic structures. Other authorities believe that the heart itself is compressed during chest massage and that pressure gradients are developed between intracardiac and extracardiac structures. If the mechanism of blood flow during CPR were known, techniques could be developed to increase blood flow to vital organs. For example, if the thorax-pump mechanism of blood flow predominates, techniques that maximize thoracic pressure differences, such as simultaneous ventilation and compression, or abdominal binding, might improve cardiac output during CPR. On the other hand, if the heart acts as the pump during chest compression, one could improve cardiac output by increasing the number of chest compressions per minute. Although studies investigating these alternative forms of CPR have yielded encouraging results in specific laboratories or animal models, there are not yet enough data in humans to determine which mechanism of blood flow predominates. There may even be a dimorphic population, meaning that thorax compression may predominate in some persons and cardiac compression in others.

Thus far, no alternative CPR techniques have yielded improved resuscitation or survival rates in clinical studies. Therefore, the standard technique of CPR has changed little over the past decade.

Airway

In approaching the victim of cardiac arrest, one must assess unresponsiveness, activate the system for initiating advanced life support, and position the patient on the floor or a backboard to assess the airway. The tongue may fall back and obstruct the airway. Rescuers may open the airway by using the head tilt–chin lift maneuver (Fig. 129.1). The rescuer places backward pressure

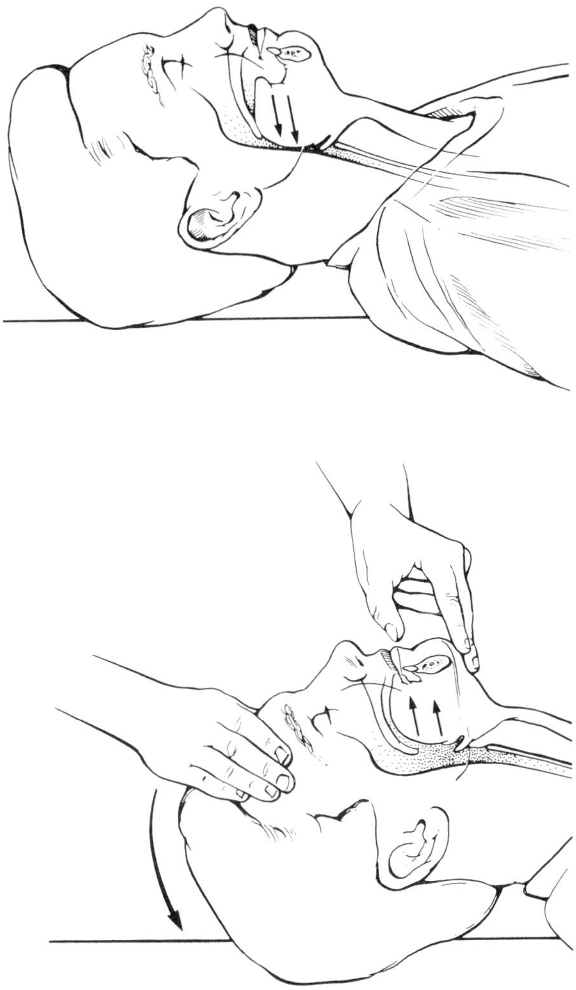

Figure 129.1. Opening the airway. **(Top)** Airway obstruction produced by tongue and epiglottis. **(Bottom)** Obstruction is relieved by head tilt–chin lift. (Emergency Cardiac Care Committee and Subcommittees, American Heart Association. Guidelines for cardiopulmonary resuscitation and emergency cardiac care, I: introduction. *JAMA* 1992;268:2172.)

on the patient's forehead while lifting the chin anteriorly. This maneuver pushes the tongue and epiglottis forward, removing the obstruction.

The head tilt–chin lift maneuver should not be used if neck injury is suspected for any reason. In patients with possible neck injury, the jaw thrust maneuver is used. Pressure applied to the angles of the mandible moves the jaw anteriorly, opening the airway.

Breathing

Once the airway is open, the rescuer looks, listens, and feels for an exchange of air. If the patient is not breathing, mouth-to-mouth respirations are administered by pinching the victim's nostrils and blowing slowly into the mouth for two breaths. The rescuer watches for the rise and fall of the chest during ventilation. The patient receives ten to 12 breaths per minute, with each ventilation lasting 1.5 to 2.0 seconds. Slow ventilations, with time for complete exhalations, may result in less gastric distention and less potential for regurgitation and aspiration. The patient should be intubated and ventilated with oxygen as soon as it is practical in the ACLS sequence. After endotracheal intubation, the rescuers do not need to pause between compressions for ventilation to be given.

Obstructed Airway

If the rescuer has optimally positioned the jaw, chin, and tongue and still cannot detect adequate air exchange, one must be concerned about an obstructed airway. The Heimlich maneuver, or subdiaphragmatic abdominal thrust, is the recommended procedure for clearing the obstructed airway of a foreign body (Fig. 129.2). The rescuer's hand is positioned between the patient's xiphoid and navel, and several quick thrusts are administered in an attempt to relieve the foreign-body obstruction. In the unconscious victim, the Heimlich maneuver may be accompanied by attempts to visualize the foreign body in the pharynx and by finger sweeps to remove the foreign body. Complications of the Heimlich maneuver include regurgitation, aspiration, and traumatic injury to the abdomen.[15]

Circulation

The rescuer determines pulselessness through palpation of the carotid. If no pulse is detected, chest compressions should be in-

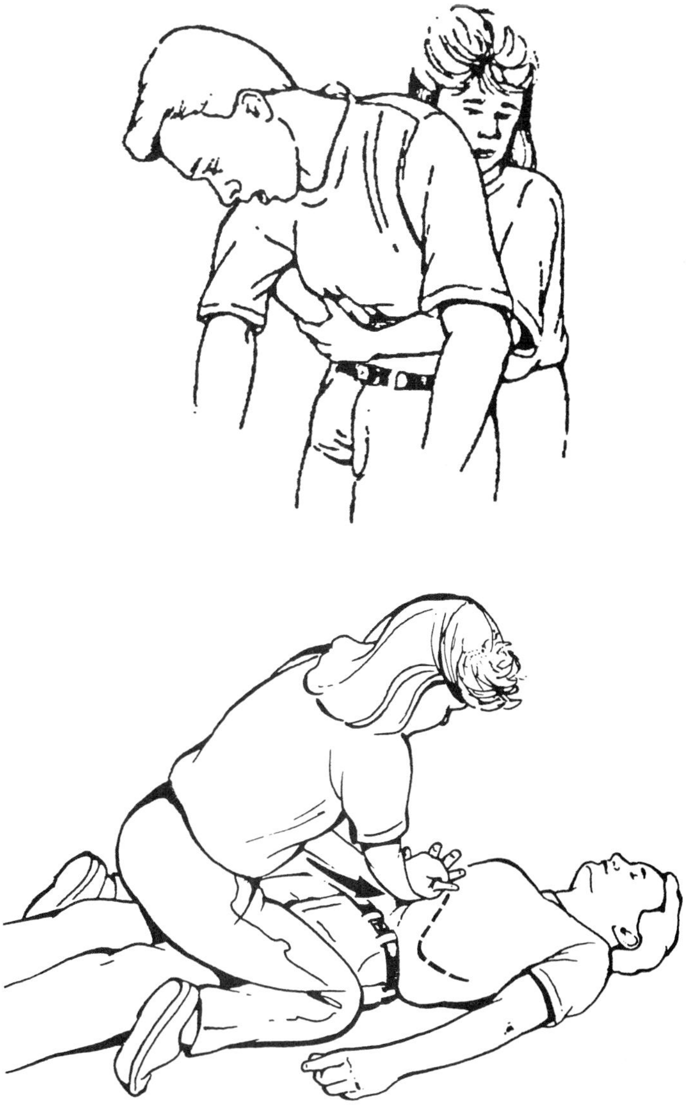

Figure 129.2. **(Top)** Administration of Heimlich maneuver to *conscious* victim of foreign-body airway obstruction. **(Bottom)** Administration of Heimlich maneuver to *unconscious* victim of foreign-body airway obstruction. (Emergency Cardiac Care Committee and Subcommittees, American Heart Association. Guidelines for cardiopulmonary resuscitation and emergency cardiac care, I: introduction. *JAMA* 1992;268:2172.)

stituted. After placing the victim on a backboard or firm surface, the heel of the hand is placed on the lower half of the sternum and depressed 1.5 to 2.0 in. The recommended compression rate is 80 to 100 times per minute.[15] The duration of compression should be 50% of the entire compression–release cycle. A 5:1 ratio of compression to ventilation is used when there are two or more rescuers. When there is only one rescuer, the ratio should be 15 compressions to two ventilations.[15]

Closed-chest compression can provide 10% to 30% of normal cardiac output. The key hemodynamic parameter that predicts whether resuscitation will be successful is the aortic diastolic pressure. Animal studies have shown that if an aortic diastolic pressure of 40 mm Hg can be generated during CPR, there is an excellent chance of successful resuscitation, presumably because it is during diastole that the coronary arteries are filled.

Mechanical resuscitators are commercially available that deliver standard American Heart Association chest compression and ventilation. These resuscitators have been shown to produce pressures comparable to manual CPR. Once applied, the resuscitators deliver standard CPR throughout the resuscitation effort, freeing personnel to perform ACLS.

Alternative Cardiopulmonary Resuscitation Techniques

A number of alternatives to the standard CPR technique have been proposed, based on theoretical advantages in achieving higher cardiac output during CPR. Although many of the techniques have shown promise in laboratory investigations and limited clinical studies, none has yielded improved survival from cardiac arrest when compared with standard CPR. The most promising techniques include interposed abdominal compression CPR (IAC-CPR), active compression–decompression CPR (ACD-CPR), simultaneous ventilation compression CPR (SVC-CPR), and high-frequency CPR.

IAC-CPR involves compression of the abdomen by a second rescuer during the relaxation phase of chest compression. IAC-CPR has been shown to improve the aortic systolic and diastolic pressure, as well as cardiac output and myocardial profusion pressures, when compared with standard CPR in experimental models. Clinical studies comparing IAC-CPR with standard CPR have shown some promise.[13] The technique requires an additional rescuer, however, and compression of the abdomen may predispose to complications such as abdominal injury and aspiration if used in patients with unprotected airways. The role of IAC-CPR needs to be defined by future clinical studies.

ACD-CPR makes use of a suction device that is applied to the anterior thorax and creates negative intrathoracic pressure during the relaxation phase of CPR. Studies in experimental models and humans in cardiac arrest have demonstrated improvement in some hemodynamic parameters but not in others. Clinical trials of the device have demonstrated mixed results.[4]

SVC-CPR attempts to use the entire thorax as the pump to produce forward blood flow. Chest compression is applied at full inspiration to maximize the gradient between intrathoracic and extrathoracic structures. A newer circumferential vest CPR has shown improved hemodynamics in limited clinical trials.[8] High-frequency or rapid-compression-rate CPR has been shown in experimental models to improve cardiac output, myocardial perfusion pressures, and 24-hour survival compared with standard CPR. Clinical studies are limited, but there is some evidence for improved hemodynamics using rapid manual compression rates.[9]

Other studies have questioned the role of ventilation as a standard part of layperson CPR. In experimental models of cardiac arrest, chest-compression-only CPR provides outcomes comparable to conventional CPR. While professional health-care providers will continue to provide ventilation with basic life support, further clinical trials are needed before any recommendations can be made regarding the option of chest-compression-only CPR for lay rescuers.[2]

Studies evaluating these alternative techniques of CPR appear to show benefits in some groups of patients but not in others. One explanation may be that certain physiologic characteristics may be more important in some subsets of patients than in others. For example, patients who are obese or have large anterior–posterior chest diameters probably receive no direct cardiac compression during standard CPR but might benefit from techniques designed to take advantage of the thorax mechanism of forward blood flow, such as SVC-CPR. Patients with a thin body habitus, for whom cardiac compression may be the primary mechanism of forward blood flow, might benefit from techniques such as rapid-compression-rate CPR. It may be that the use of one standard method of CPR for all patients in cardiac arrest is inappropriate. At the present time, however, these alternative techniques of CPR should be considered experimental.

ADVANCED CARDIAC LIFE SUPPORT

Because the recommended treatment protocols are based on the patient's underlying rhythm, it is important that electrocardiographic (ECG) monitor leads be placed early and followed throughout the resuscitation attempt. If the patient is in ventricular fibrillation, immediate defibrillation is recommended even before CPR, intubation, and other interventions. As soon as possible, the patient is endotracheally intubated and an intravenous line is placed. Peripheral lines may be placed in the antecubital area, or central lines through the internal or external jugular veins. Peripheral lines should not be placed in the lower half of the body, because external chest compression results in retrograde blood flow through the vena cava (because there are no valves in the inferior vena cava).[15]

Defibrillation

Early defibrillation is the one intervention that has been repeatedly shown to be efficacious for patients in pulseless ventricular tachycardia or ventricular fibrillation. The longer the patient remains in fibrillation, the more likely it is that defibrillation and resuscitation will be unsuccessful.[6,15] It is the current passing directly through the heart that allows defibrillation. Current is directly related to the energy set on the defibrillator and inversely related to the transthoracic impedance. The transthoracic impedance can be minimized by attention to several factors, including position of the defibrillation paddles, firm pressure on the paddles, the use of conductive material between the skin and paddles, employing sets of shocks (pairs or triplets), and coordinating the shock with the end-expiratory phase of ventilation.[15]

A precordial thump generates 0.5 to 1.0 joule of energy. Rarely, when applied early to a patient in cardiac arrest, a precordial thump can convert ventricular fibrillation to a perfusing rhythm; pulseless ventricular tachycardia may be converted to a perfusing rhythm in 11% to 25% of cases. However, a thump can also convert ventricular tachycardia to a more malignant dysrhythmia, such as ventricular fibrillation, asystole, or pulseless electrical activity (PEA). The precordial thump may be used for patients with witnessed cardiac arrest while another rescuer is preparing the defibrillator. It should, however, never delay the definitive treatment—electrical defibrillation.

The automatic external defibrillator (AED) is capable of analyzing the rhythm of a patient in cardiac arrest and shocking the patient per ACLS protocols. Semiautomatic external defibrillators analyze the rhythm and advise the rescuer to attempt defibrillation through the sensing electrodes.[19] These devices extend the capability of EMS systems to reach victims of cardiac arrest earlier. Rescue workers and even spouses of high-risk patients can be trained to operate the AED. Some communities have trained basic emergency medical technicians (EMTs) in the recognition of ventricular fibrillation and the use of defibrillators, providing for early defibrillation in communities in which paramedics cannot respond to cardiac arrests within a few minutes.[15] AEDs have also been advocated for use by other professionals who may come in contact with patients in cardiac arrest. These include security guards, airline flight attendants, and police officers in situations in which EMS responders might not be immediately available. The use of AEDs might help some communities solve the difficult issue of prompt defibrillation. The place of public access defibrillation in community EMS systems remains to be determined by future clinical studies and individual community needs and resources.

Pressor Agents

Epinephrine, a mixed α- and β-adrenergic agent, is the pressor drug of choice for patients in cardiac arrest.[15] Epinephrine increases peripheral vascular resistance and raises aortic diastolic pressure, thus augmenting coronary blood flow. It also increases cerebral blood flow during cardiac arrest. The recommended dose is 1 mg initially, with repeated doses every 3 to 5 minutes,[15] but the optimal dose has not been established. Although there is some evidence that higher doses of epinephrine may increase myocardial and central nervous system blood flow, several outcome studies have failed to demonstrate any difference in survival to hospital discharge with standard-dose compared with high-dose epinephrine.[3] In fact, there is some evidence that high doses of epinephrine may result in worse neurologic outcome.[1,7] Thus, after the initial 1-mg dose, subsequent doses may be higher based on the treating physician's discretion. Epinephrine can also be given through the endotracheal tube; the dose is two to two and one-half times the intravenous dose. Vasopressin is a potent vasopressor that has been shown to improve cardiac as well as cerebral blood flows in cardiac arrest. The role of vasopressin as an alternative to epinephrine is being investigated in larger clinical trials.[12]

Acid–Base Abnormalities

The optimal treatment of acidosis during cardiac arrest is hyperventilation. The role of bicarbonate administration is controversial. The patient in cardiac arrest develops lactic acidemia from poor tissue perfusion, but lactic acid does not accumulate significantly until relatively late in the course (20 or more minutes of total arrest time). Many patients in cardiac arrest also develop a venous respiratory acidosis because they are unable to transport CO_2 to the lungs where it may be excreted.[20] This CO_2 readily crosses membranes and may worsen intracellular and central nervous system acidosis. If bicarbonate is given to a patient in cardiac arrest, CO_2 is generated by the buffering of metabolic acids and P_{CO_2} increases locally. Thus, bicarbonate may actually worsen the acid–base status. In addition, overzealous administration of bicarbonate can produce alkalosis and hyperosmolarity, both of which are associated with a poor prognosis. Clearly, however, there are patients in cardiac arrest in whom aggressive treatment with bicarbonate can be life-saving. These include patients with hyperkalemia and those with tricyclic antidepressant overdosage. In addition, patients with other drug overdosages and those with preexisting metabolic acidosis may benefit from early treatment with bicarbonate. Arterial and central venous blood gases may be useful in assessing acid–base status and the advisability of administering bicarbonate for patients in cardiac arrest.

Antiarrhythmic Agents

No studies have shown that antiarrhythmics improve survival from cardiac arrest. Many of the antiarrhythmic agents raise the fibrillation threshold, however, and are thus useful in preventing recurrent ventricular fibrillation in patients who have been successfully defibrillated. Antiarrhythmic agents that may be beneficial in the treatment of patients in ventricular fibrillation include amiodarone, lidocaine, bretylium, magnesium sulfate, and procainamide. Amiodarone may be an important drug for the treatment of patients in persistent ventricular fibrillation or pulseless ventricular tachycardia resistant to electrical defibrillation. In one study,[11] it improved the rate of return of spontaneous circulation and admission to the hospital for patients with out-of-hospital ventricular fibrillation unresponsive to electrical defibrillation. Studies assessing the effects of amiodarone on the rate of discharge from the hospital and on long-term survival will determine the place of amiodarone in ACLS algorithms. Lidocaine has been used in the treatment of patients in cardiac arrest for many years. In clinical studies, no difference in overall resuscitation or survival has been seen when lidocaine and bretylium are compared in patients with ventricular fibrillation. In general, when antiarrhythmic agents are administered, they should be followed by immediate attempts at electrical defibrillation so that the sequence of drug-shock-drug-shock is maintained.

Atropine

Atropine may be useful in some patients with asystolic cardiac arrest who have an excess of parasympathetic stimulation. Studies in the prehospital use of atropine have shown improved resuscitation rates but not improved overall survival in patients in asystolic arrest.[17] Atropine is also useful in patients with symptomatic bradycardia.

Pacemakers in Cardiac Arrest

The wide adoption of transcutaneous cardiac pacing has extended the availability of pacemakers to many patients. Transcutaneous pacing capability is often a feature of newer defibrillators. Pacing is indicated in patients with hemodynamically unstable bradycardia and may also be useful for overdrive pacing patients with tachycardia unresponsive to pharmacologic therapy. Although the successful use of pacing for patients in asystolic cardiac arrest has been reported anecdotally, most studies have failed to show significant improvements in resuscitation rates. Thus, pacemakers cannot be recommended for routine use in asystolic cardiac arrest. If pacing is used in the management of patients in cardiac arrest, however, it should be applied early.

GUIDELINES FOR CARDIAC ARREST

Guidelines for the treatment of patients in cardiac arrest have been developed by the American Heart Association.[15] They are updated every few years; clinicians should be aware of the updated versions. Although the ACLS treatment for patients in cardiac arrest is based on the ECG monitor rhythm, the clinician must always consider the etiology of the arrest in developing a treatment plan. Cardiac arrest is the end point of a physiologic process that results in the loss of circulation or ventilation. Etiologies such as respiratory failure, asthma, medication toxicity, hypovolemia, pulmonary embolism, sepsis, trauma, acute myocardial infarction, anaphylaxis, metabolic abnormalities, and others may be treated specifically while going through the ACLS algorithm.[10]

Patients in cardiac arrest present with either ventricular fibrillation–pulseless ventricular tachycardia (Fig. 129.3), asystole (Fig. 129.4), or PEA (Fig. 129.5). Treatment modalities have been classified by a consensus of experts based on the scientific evidence of their efficacy and safety, as follows:

Class I: Definitely helpful
Class IIA: Acceptable, probably helpful
Class IIB: Acceptable, possibly helpful
Class III: Not indicated, may be harmful

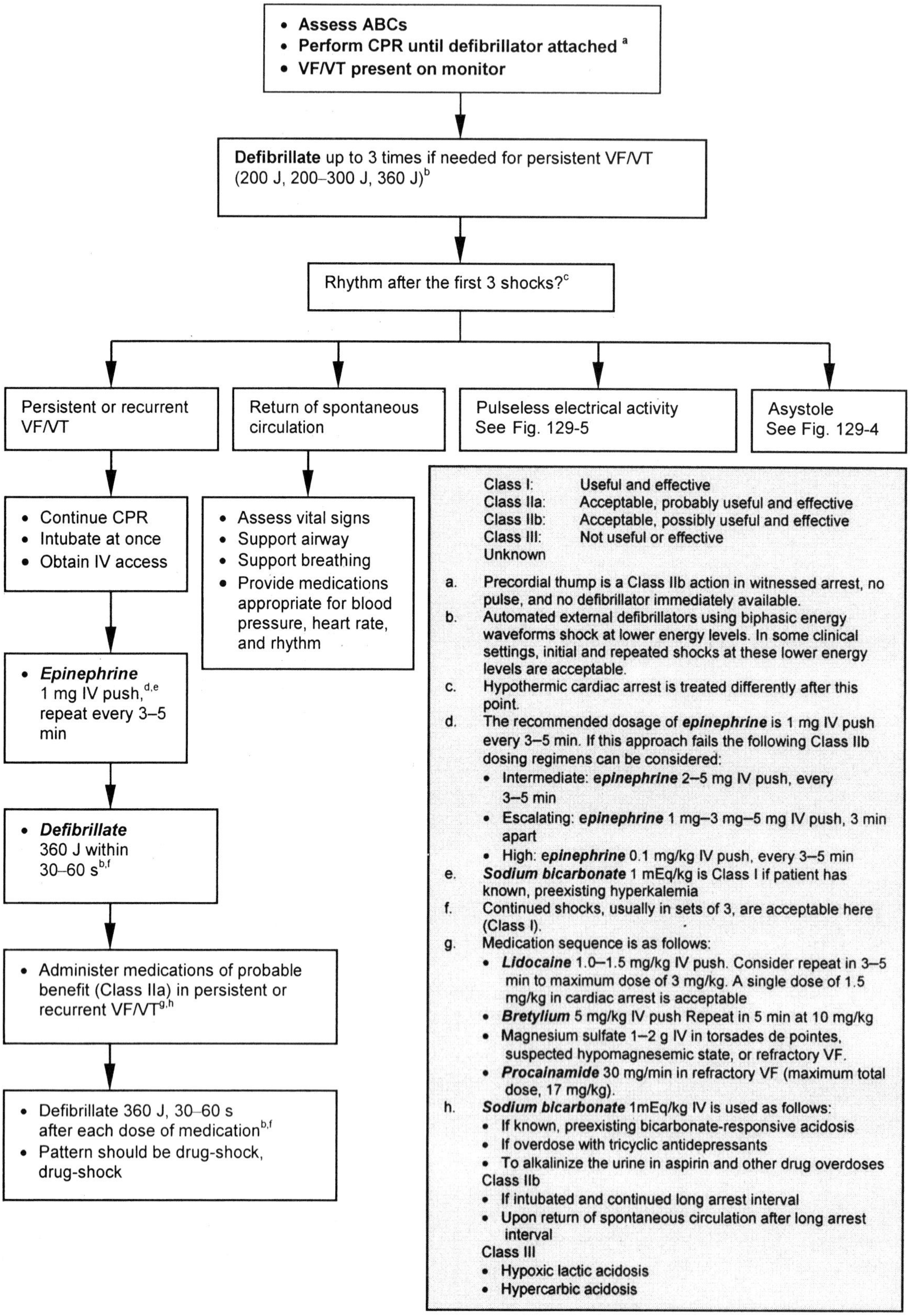

Figure 129.3. Ventricular fibrillation–pulseless ventricular tachycardia (VF/VT) algorithm. (*1997–99 Handbook of emergency cardiovascular care for healthcare providers*. American Heart Association, Dallas, 1997.)

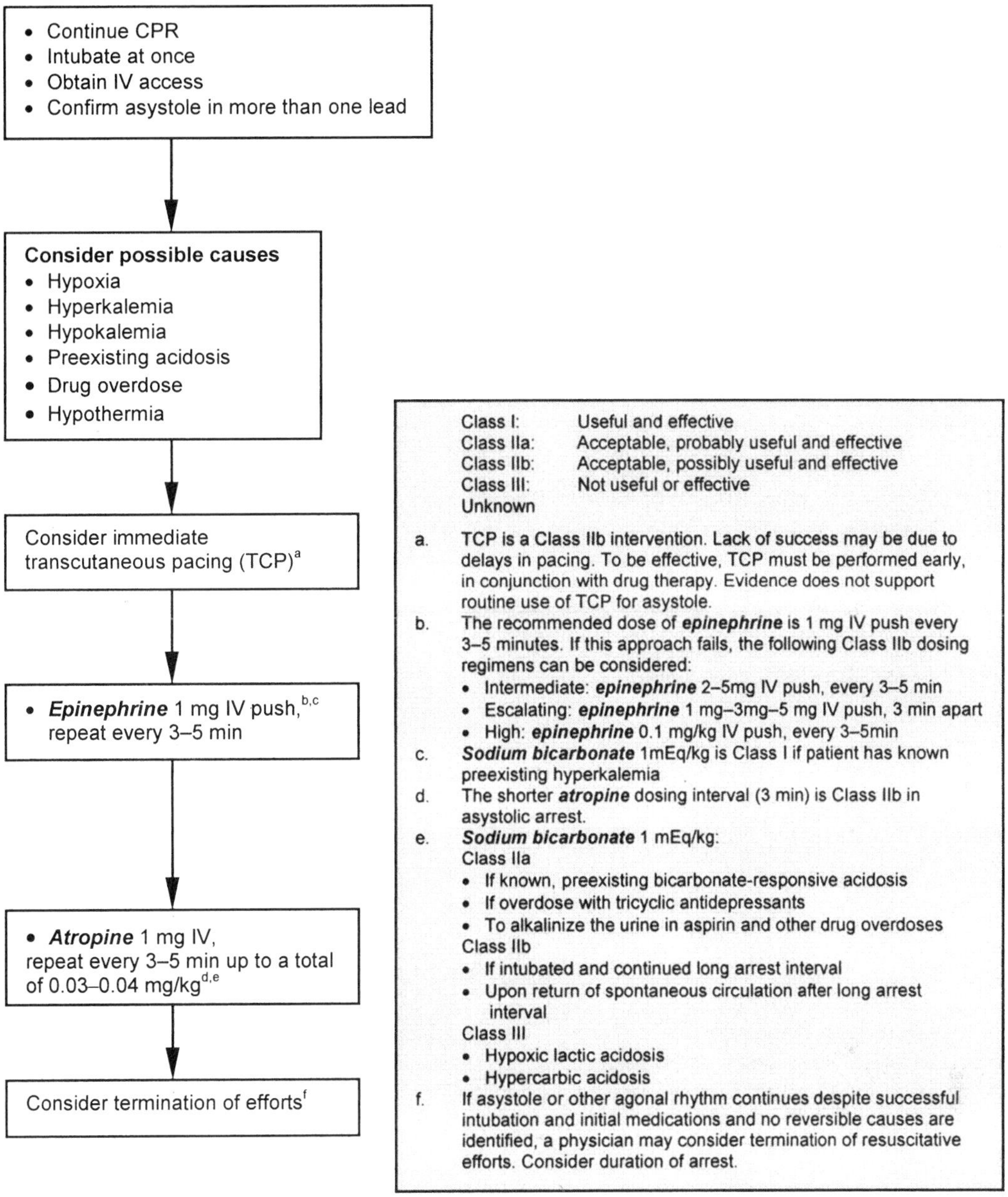

Figure 129.4. Asystole algorithm. (*1997–99 Handbook of emergency cardiovascular care for healthcare providers*. American Heart Association, Dallas, 1997.)

Ventricular Fibrillation and Pulseless Ventricular Tachycardia

The key to the treatment of patients with ventricular fibrillation or pulseless ventricular tachycardia is to remember that successful resuscitation depends on electrical defibrillation. All other treatments, including CPR, intubation, and drugs, are merely attempts to prepare the patient for successful defibrillation. Defibrillation should be attempted with up to three shocks as soon as the diagnosis is made.[15] Shocking the patient several times in a row decreases the transthoracic impedance and increases the chances for successful defibrillation. If defibrillation attempts are unsuccessful, CPR is initiated, the trachea is intubated, and an intravenous line is placed as soon as possible. Epinephrine is the first recommended pharmacologic agent; repeat doses should be given every 3 to 5 minutes until defibrillation is successful. Each administration of drug should be followed by attempts at electrical defibrillation. Antiarrhythmic drugs may be useful in preventing refibrillation once the patient has been electrically defibrillated. Lidocaine is frequently given as the first antiarrhythmic agent. In the future, amiodarone may be the first antiarrhythmic drug recommended. If this is ineffective, treatment with bretylium, magnesium sulfate, and procainamide may be considered. Treatment with bicarbonate should be initiated if there is any clinical suspicion of hyperkalemia, tricyclic antidepressant, or preexisting acidosis.[15]

Asystole

The asystolic patient has a poor prognosis for resuscitation. However, because some patients who appear to be asystolic are actually in fine ventricular fibrillation, the diagnosis of asystole must be confirmed by checking for a straight-line rhythm on three leads. If there is any suspicion that ventricular fibrillation is present, one should proceed with defibrillation as in the ventricular fibrillation protocol. For asystole, one must consider possible causes such as hypoxia, drug overdose, hypothermia, and electrolyte imbalance. As noted previously, transcutaneous pacing has not generally been efficacious for patients in asystole. If it is used in selected patients, however, it should be applied

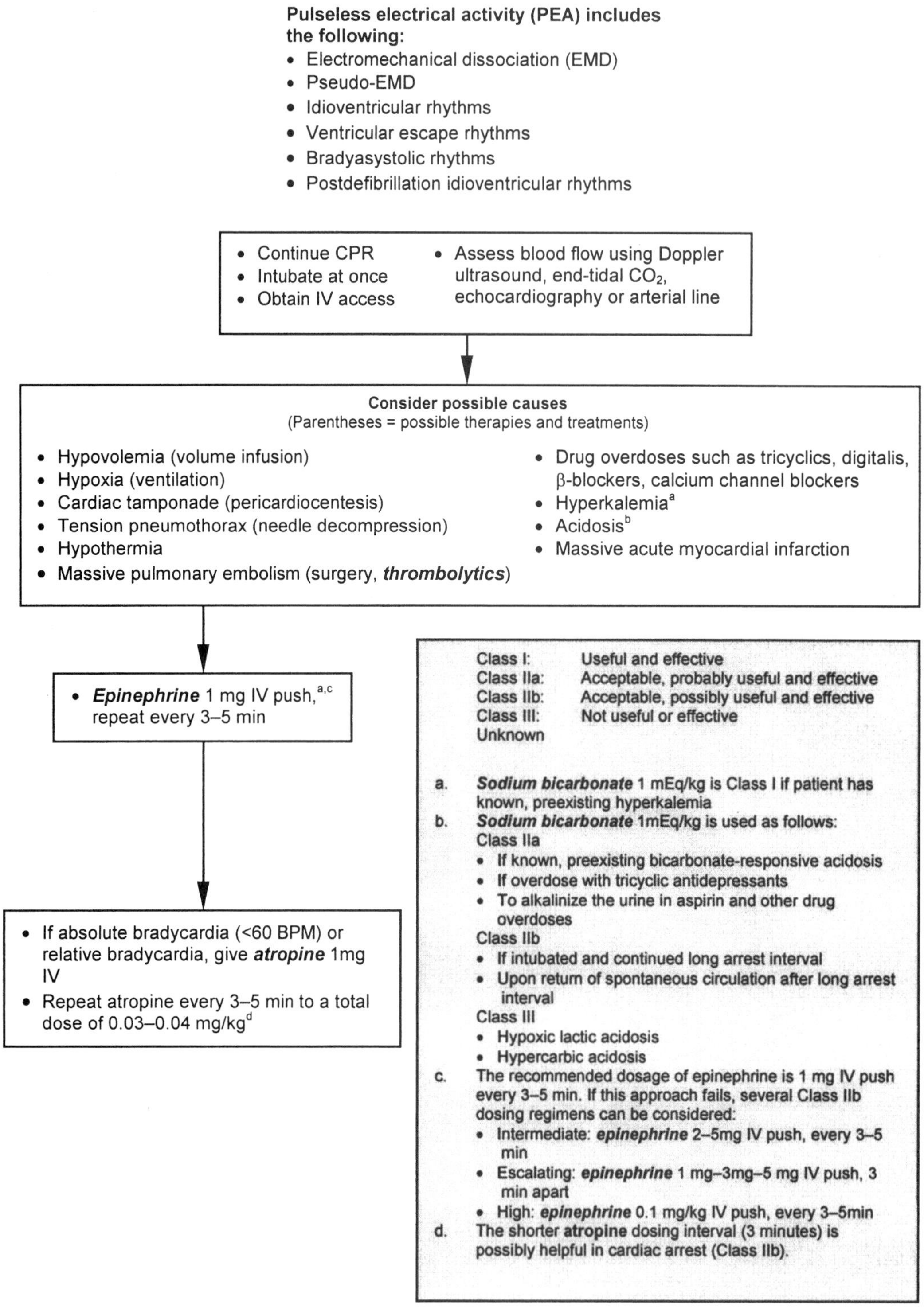
Pulseless electrical activity (PEA) includes the following:
• Electromechanical dissociation (EMD)
• Pseudo-EMD
• Idioventricular rhythms
• Ventricular escape rhythms
• Bradyasystolic rhythms
• Postdefibrillation idioventricular rhythms
• Continue CPR
• Intubate at once
• Obtain IV access
• Assess blood flow using Doppler ultrasound, end-tidal CO2, echocardiography or arterial line
Consider possible causes
(Parentheses = possible therapies and treatments)
• Hypovolemia (volume infusion)
• Hypoxia (ventilation)
• Cardiac tamponade (pericardiocentesis)
• Tension pneumothorax (needle decompression)
• Hypothermia
• Massive pulmonary embolism (surgery, thrombolytics)
• Drug overdoses such as tricyclics, digitalis, β-blockers, calcium channel blockers
• Hyperkalemia[a]
• Acidosis[b]
• Massive acute myocardial infarction
• Epinephrine 1 mg IV push,[a,c] repeat every 3–5 min
• If absolute bradycardia (<60 BPM) or relative bradycardia, give atropine 1mg IV
• Repeat atropine every 3–5 min to a total dose of 0.03–0.04 mg/kg[d]
Class I: Useful and effective
Class IIa: Acceptable, probably useful and effective
Class IIb: Acceptable, possibly useful and effective
Class III: Not useful or effective
Unknown
a. Sodium bicarbonate 1 mEq/kg is Class I if patient has known, preexisting hyperkalemia
b. Sodium bicarbonate 1mEq/kg is used as follows:
Class IIa
• If known, preexisting bicarbonate-responsive acidosis
• If overdose with tricyclic antidepressants
• To alkalinize the urine in aspirin and other drug overdoses
Class IIb
• If intubated and continued long arrest interval
• Upon return of spontaneous circulation after long arrest interval
Class III
• Hypoxic lactic acidosis
• Hypercarbic acidosis
c. The recommended dosage of epinephrine is 1 mg IV push every 3–5 min. If this approach fails, several Class IIb dosing regimens can be considered:
• Intermediate: epinephrine 2–5mg IV push, every 3–5 min
• Escalating: epinephrine 1 mg–3mg–5 mg IV push, 3 min apart
• High: epinephrine 0.1 mg/kg IV push, every 3–5min
d. The shorter atropine dosing interval (3 minutes) is possibly helpful in cardiac arrest (Class IIb).

Figure 129.5. Pulseless electrical activity (PEA) algorithm. (*1997–99 Handbook of emergency cardiovascular care for healthcare providers*. American Heart Association, Dallas, 1997.)

early in the treatment protocol. Pharmacologic treatment of asystole involves the use of epinephrine to improve myocardial and cerebral blood flow during CPR, and atropine to antagonize parasympathetic stimulation.[15]

Pulseless Electrical Activity

PEA describes a situation in which there is an electrical rhythm other than ventricular tachycardia or fibrillation, but no palpable pulses. This condition may be due to true electromechanical dissociation (EMD), in which the heart muscle itself is not contracting despite the presence of electrical activity. True EMD has a very poor prognosis. However, PEA may also be due to states of severely decreased flow, so patients must be evaluated for cardiac and extracardiac causes of severe shock. Bedside ultrasonography may allow the treating physician to determine whether the heart is beating and whether pericardial fluid is present. Alternatively, the placement of an arterial line can be used to differentiate severe shock states from true EMD. In cases in which these modalities are not available, the clinician must consider causes such as hypovolemia, hypoxia, cardiac tamponade, tension pneumothorax, hypothermia, pulmonary embolism, drug overdose, acidosis, and electrolyte imbalance. A thorough reevaluation of the respiratory system is also critical. This may involve reintubation of the patient or confirmation of endotracheal tube placement both visually and with capnometry. The possibility of pneumothorax should be evaluated by listening to breath sounds bilaterally; if necessary, needle decompression can be performed to rule out a tension pneumothorax. Pericardiocentesis may help to identify cardiac tamponade if bedside ultrasonography is not available. Arterial blood gases may be particularly useful in patients with PEA to determine oxygen and acid–base status. Empiric treatment with a fluid bolus while evaluating for acute blood loss from gastrointestinal hemorrhage, ruptured aortic aneurysm, or other causes for hypovolemia may also be useful. Once extracardiac causes of EMD are ruled out, treatment recommendations include epinephrine to improve myocardial and cerebral blood flow during cardiac arrest, and atropine if the ECG shows bradycardia.

Initiating and Discontinuing Resuscitation Efforts

CPR should be instituted for all patients in cardiac arrest, except in two circumstances:

1. The patient made it clear, while competent and informed, that he or she did not want resuscitation efforts to be instituted.
2. Successful resuscitation would be futile because the patient has clear signs of irreversible death, such as rigor mortis, dependent lividity, or decapitation.

Emergency physicians and paramedics are obligated to respect patients' wishes regarding resuscitation. In most cases, these wishes may be known through documentation on advance directives. Many EMS communities throughout the United States have developed a standardized "do not attempt resuscitation"' (DNAR) form that patients and their physicians can fill out, documenting their wishes, and present to paramedics. Portable or prehospital DNAR orders are likely to become more commonplace over the next decade and should be respected by emergency health-care professionals.

Once undertaken, resuscitation efforts are generally continued until it is clear that the patient is not responding to them. The longer the patient remains in cardiac arrest without response, the worse the prognosis for survival. There is, however, no definitive time interval that can predict the impossibility of survival after cardiac arrest. Indeed, special circumstances, such as hypothermic arrest in a child, may dictate prolonged resuscitation efforts. Thus, clinicians must use their judgment in going through the ACLS protocols and determining unresponsiveness to resuscitation.

INVASIVE CARDIOPULMONARY RESUSCITATION

Studies in animal models have shown that techniques of invasive CPR, such as open chest CPR and cardiopulmonary bypass, and the use of direct mechanical assist devices improve hemodynamics, resuscitation, and the chances of surviving cardiac arrest. It has also been demonstrated that when invasive CPR is applied late in the treatment protocol (after more than 15 to 20 minutes of total arrest time), there is no improvement in resuscitation. At the present time, however, these techniques should be used only in the context of well-defined experimental protocols and should not be used as last-ditch efforts for patients who do not respond to standard ACLS protocols.

QUALITY OF RESUSCITATION EFFORTS

How well CPR is performed and ACLS delivered does make a difference in the outcome for patients in cardiac arrest. Unfortunately, the performance of CPR is frequently not optimal.[18] Ideally, the quality of resuscitation efforts might be best assessed by monitoring pressures during CPR so that the diastolic pressure gradient could be maximized, but this is clearly impractical except under special circumstances. The use of capnometry to monitor end-tidal CO_2 levels during CPR gives clinicians a noninvasive assessment of the cardiac output generated by CPR.[14] The quality of resuscitation efforts should also be assessed retrospectively by systematically tracking key variables and the outcome of resuscitation efforts in both the in-hospital and out-of-hospital setting.[5]

PROGNOSIS

The prognosis for survival of cardiac arrest depends on many factors. These include patient variables such as the etiology of the arrest and comorbid diseases, arrest variables such as initial rhythm, and system variables such as time to CPR and defibrillation.[5] None of these variables, by themselves or in combination, can accurately predict survival or neurologic outcome. However, it has been demonstrated in several studies that the longer the patient remains in cardiac arrest, the poorer the chances for successful resuscitation.[6]

The presenting rhythm is the most important factor in overall prognosis. Rhythms that are amenable to treatment with electrical defibrillation (ventricular tachycardia and ventricular fibrillation) have a relatively good prognosis, whereas asystole and EMD usually have poor outcomes. Resuscitation success for patients in ventricular fibrillation depends on the time elapsed before the patient is defibrillated; the longer the patient remains in ventricular fibrillation, the less likely is successful defibrillation.[6,15] In units where staff are prepared to treat cardiac patients for ventricular arrhythmias promptly, successful defibrillation is nearly universal.

Another important factor in predicting resuscitation is the time that elapses before CPR is initiated. By providing some blood flow to the heart and other vital organs, one can extend the time in which defibrillation is effective. For example, data from Seattle show that if ACLS is started within 8 minutes of cardiac arrest, there is a successful outcome in 27% of patients. For those patients who have CPR started within 4 minutes in addition to having ACLS within 8 minutes, successful resuscitation is increased to 43%.[6]

Finally, the cause of the cardiac arrest is another factor important for prognosis.[5] In cardiac arrest due to extracardiac causes such as pulmonary embolism and hypovolemia, the prognosis is very poor. In addition, specific pathophysiologic entities, such as complete thrombosis of the left main coronary artery, have poor prognoses, because providing adequate coronary blood flow is impossible no matter how quickly CPR and ACLS are provided.

COMMON PITFALLS

- It is important to remember that resuscitation efforts require a well-disciplined team in which each member plays a role. Often, cardiac arrests are managed in a chaotic, undisciplined environment that is not conducive to optimal patient care. Well-disciplined teams develop through frequent drills and critique. Each resuscitation should be carefully reviewed. Hospitals and prehospital care systems should constantly monitor the success of their resuscitation efforts and compare them with studies in the literature.

- After the placement of an endotracheal tube, bilateral equal breath sounds should be heard in the axilla. Correct placement of the tube can be confirmed by quantitative capnometry. Breath sounds heard anteriorly may be transmitted from the stomach. Breath sounds and capnometry readings should be checked repeatedly during the resuscitation. Asymmetry of breath sounds or a sudden absence of CO_2 excretion mandates prompt evaluation—the endotracheal tube may have slipped out or down into the right bronchus or the patient may have developed a pneumothorax secondary to the trauma of chest compressions. Either of these serious conditions can be easily treated if recognized early.
- Intracardiac medications should be avoided. If an intravenous line cannot be started, many standard advanced life-support medications, including epinephrine, atropine, and lidocaine (*but not bicarbonate*), can be administered through the endotracheal tube.
- Hyperkalemia should be suspected as the cause of cardiac arrest in any patient with renal failure. The ECG may show a characteristic sine wave pattern, which should not be mistaken for ventricular fibrillation. Patients with hyperkalemia will not respond until the potassium level is lowered. Vigorous treatment with bicarbonate and calcium is indicated when hyperkalemia is suspected.
- Most patients in ventricular fibrillation can be defibrillated. Repeated unsuccessful defibrillation attempts may be due to poor technique. Successful defibrillation involves the depolarization of a critical mass of left ventricular myocardium. One paddle should be placed to the right of the sternum below the right clavicle, and the other in the midaxillary line at the level of the nipple. If the paddles are too close together, the skin, rather than the heart, may be getting the current. Alternatively, the anteroposterior position may be used over the left precordium. Firm pressure of approximately 25 lb should be applied to each paddle, and the appropriate contact gel must be used. The chest should be in full expiration when shocks are administered, because air in the lungs can significantly add to transthoracic impedance. Repeated shocks decrease the transthoracic impedance and improve the chances of successful defibrillation; therefore, the shocks may be delivered in pairs or triplets, with only a short pause between shocks to check for a pulse and the rhythm on the monitor.
- Torsades de pointes can be mistaken for ventricular tachycardia or fibrillation. The ECG reveals cycles of QRS complexes "twisting around" the isoelectric point of the ECG. It is associated with a congenital or drug-induced prolonged QT interval, most frequently due to quinidine. Although antiarrhythmic drugs are commonly ineffective in terminating torsades, electrical cardioversion is usually successful. Further treatment with magnesium sulfate, isoproterenol, or overdrive pacing decreases the QT interval and prevents recurrence.[15]
- There are no good parameters that can be used to assess the effectiveness of ongoing CPR or to guide treatment during the resuscitation effort. Femoral pulsations may reflect venous rather than arterial blood flow. Carotid pulsations may reflect some blood flow but cannot be used as a guide to decision making during resuscitation. The longer the patient remains in cardiac arrest, the worse is the prognosis for resuscitation. After 30 minutes of resuscitation attempts, the prognosis is very poor, although there are case reports of successful resuscitation after hours of CPR. Therefore, no clear guidelines can be given as to when resuscitation efforts should be stopped.
- In patients who are hypothermic, as in near-drowning victims, resuscitation efforts should continue until the patient has been adequately warmed. Strong consideration should be given to cardiopulmonary bypass for these patients. In other patients, resuscitation efforts should be continued until the patient is unresponsive to ACLS protocols as outlined.

References

1. Behringer W, Kittler H, Sterz F, et al. Cumulative epinephrine during cardiopulmonary resuscitation and neurologic outcome. *Ann Intern Med* 1998;129:450–456.
2. Berg RA, Kern KB, Sanders AB, et al. Bystander cardiopulmonary resuscitation: is ventilation necessary? *Circulation* 1993;88:1907–1915.
3. Brown CG, Martin DB, Pepe PE, et al. A comparison of standard-dose and high-dose epinephrine in cardiac arrest outside-the-hospital. *N Engl J Med* 1992;327:1051.
4. Callaham M, Schwab I, Shultz JJ, et al. A randomized prospective trial of active compression-decompression CPR versus manual CPR in prehospital cardiac arrest. *Ann Emerg Med* 1993;22:885.
5. Cummins RO, Chamberlain D, Hazinski MF, et al. Recommended guidelines for reviewing, reporting, and conducting research on in-hospital resuscitation: the in-hospital "Utstein style." *Circulation* 1997;95:2213–2239.
6. Eisenberg MS, Bergner L, Hallstrom A. Cardiac resuscitation in the community: importance of rapid provision and implications for program planning. *JAMA* 1979;241:1905.
7. Gueuhniaud PY, Mols P, Goldstein P, et al. A comparison of repeated high doses and repeated standard doses of epinephrine for cardiac arrest outside the hospital. *N Engl J Med* 1998;339:1595–1601.
8. Halperin HR, Tsitlik JE, Gelfand M, et al. A preliminary study of cardiopulmonary resuscitation by circumferential compression of the chest with use of a pneumatic vest. *N Engl J Med* 1993;329:762.
9. Kern KB, Sanders AB, Raife J, et al. A study of chest compression rates during cardiopulmonary resuscitation in humans: the importance of rate-directed chest compressions. *Arch Intern Med* 1992;152:145.
10. Kloeck W, Cummins RO, Chamberlain D, et al. Special resuscitation situations. *Circulation* 1997;95:2196–2210.
11. Kudenchuk PJ. Report at the 70th Scientific Sessions of the American Heart Association, Orlando, Florida, November 12, 1997.
12. Lindner KH, Dirks B, Strohmenger HU, et al. Randomized comparison of epinephrine and vasopressin in patients with out-of-hospital ventricular fibrillation. *Lancet* 1997;349:535–537.
13. Sack JB, Kesselbrenner MB, Bregman D. Survival from in-hospital cardiac arrest with interposed abdominal counterpulsation during cardiopulmonary resuscitation. *JAMA* 1992;267:379.
14. Sanders AB, Kern KB, Otto CW, et al. End-tidal carbon dioxide monitoring during cardiopulmonary resuscitation: a prognostic guide for survival. *JAMA* 1989;262:1347–1351.
15. Standards and guidelines for cardiopulmonary resuscitation and emergency cardiac care. *JAMA* 1992;268:2171.
16. Stiell IG, Wells GA, Field BJ, et al. Improved out-of-hospital cardiac arrest survival through inexpensive optimization of an existing defibrillation program. *JAMA* 1999;281:1175–1181.
17. Stueven H, Tonsfeldt DJ, Thompson BM, et al. Atropine in asystole: human studies. *Ann Emerg Med* 1984;13:815.
18. Van Hoeyweghen RJ, Bossaert LL, Mullie A, et al. Quality and efficacy of bystanders CPR. *Resuscitation* 1993;26:47–52.
19. Weaver WD, Hill D, Fahrenbruch CE, et al. Use of the automatic external defibrillator in the management of out-of-hospital cardiac arrest. *N Engl J Med* 1988;19:661.
20. Weil MH, Ruiz CE, Trevino R, et al. Difference in acid–base state between venous and arterial blood during cardiopulmonary resuscitation. *N Engl J Med* 1986;315:153.

CHAPTER 130
Acute Respiratory Insufficiency

Paul E. Pepe

Acute respiratory insufficiency usually implies a failure of the breathing apparatus to maintain an adequate systemic arterial O_2 tension (PaO_2) so that hemoglobin (Hgb) in the red blood cells becomes significantly desaturated (less than 92%) or when CO_2 levels rise enough to result in significant arterial acidosis (pH less than 7.30). To some, the term may simply mean severe respiratory distress, with a respiratory rate (RR) at rest greater than 30 to 35 breaths per minute. However, it must also be emphasized that respiration refers not only to the act of breathing, but also to cellular respiration (O_2 consumption and CO_2 production).

Cellular respiration depends on systemic O_2 delivery, which, in turn, depends on an adequate Hgb level, an adequate Hgb O_2 saturation, and an adequate cardiac output. Thus, the need to maintain adequate tissue O_2 delivery directs us to the basics of emergency care: (1) Stop the bleeding or provide definitive surgical care and transfuse as necessary (preserve Hgb); (2) ensure an airway and adequate lung inflation with O_2 (facilitate an adequate PaO_2); and (3) when appropriate, provide intravascular volume or assure circulation through the use of appropriate interventions such as cardiovascular drugs and, if necessary, external cardiac compressions (to maintain cardiac output). In essence, the ABCs of emergency resuscitation (airway, breathing, and circulation) are directed at maintaining adequate cellular respiration. Therefore, acute respiratory insufficiency can be viewed as a failure of an integrated systemic mechanism to maintain tissue O_2 delivery and consumption.

In turn, if CO_2 is not cleared by the lungs as quickly as it is produced, the arterial CO_2 tension ($PaCO_2$) rises, the acidity of the blood increases, and, readily crossing the blood–brain barrier, the elevated $PaCO_2$ results in cerebral acidosis, depressing the level of consciousness and dilating the cerebral vessels. This last event, in turn, may significantly elevate intracranial pressure (ICP), a potentially serious effect in patients with serious head injury or a cerebrovascular insult. Unlike impaired O_2 delivery, however, a high $PaCO_2$ in itself may not always constitute a major acute problem. For example, patients who are chronic CO_2 retainers usually have compensated for chronic respiratory acidosis by renal bicarbonate retention and tolerate a high $PaCO_2$ quite well. A pounding headache (caused by cerebral vasodilatation) may be their only manifestation of further CO_2 retention during acute exacerbations of underlying pulmonary disease.

The removal of CO_2 is a relatively simple process in the normal lung. Simply flushing the alveoli with fresh breaths causes CO_2 to leave the bloodstream because of the significant concentration gradient. However, the more O_2 is consumed, the more CO_2 is produced. With increased CO_2 production (exercise, stress, and metabolic alterations), more fresh ventilation needs to be introduced. A shivering, awake patient undergoing the stress of acute injury or illness may require extraordinary ventilatory support to adequately remove CO_2 from the body. On the other hand, a comatose patient with a phenobarbital overdose or a hypothermic patient whose oxygenation and circulation are properly supported usually requires little ventilation because of very low metabolic rates. In apneic, pulseless patients who are receiving cardiopulmonary resuscitation (CPR) efforts, O_2 delivery to the tissues is severely compromised.[1] In turn, there eventually is diminished systemic CO_2 production, and markedly diminished venous return to the lungs, and thus a markedly decreased need for ventilation. As long as such patients receive an adequate lung inflation (10 to 15 mL/kg) with each breath, they may only require five to eight breaths per minute. If and when spontaneous circulation is restored, CO_2 production and return to the lungs will increase significantly, and the delivered RR should be increased accordingly (e.g., ten to 15 breaths per minute).

From a pragmatic viewpoint, the key aspects of emergency care can be targeted by the emergency physician by answering the following questions:

1. Does the patient need ventilatory support (a certain number of manual or mechanical breaths to remove CO_2)?
2. Does the patient need oxygenation support (hemorrhage control or transfusion, supplemental O_2, positive-pressure lung inflations, or even positive end-expiratory pressure), with or without circulatory support?
3. What are the potential complications of these interventions (e.g., barotrauma and circulatory compromise)?

Although oxygenation and ventilation are undeniably intertwined, a critically ill or injured patient should be approached by specifically distinguishing between the need for ventilatory support and that for oxygenation support. That is, some patients may require mechanical ventilatory support for one and not the other. For example, if unoxygenated blood is shunted through gas exchange units that are not being adequately inflated, resulting in a low PO_2, alveoli that remain well inflated still pro-

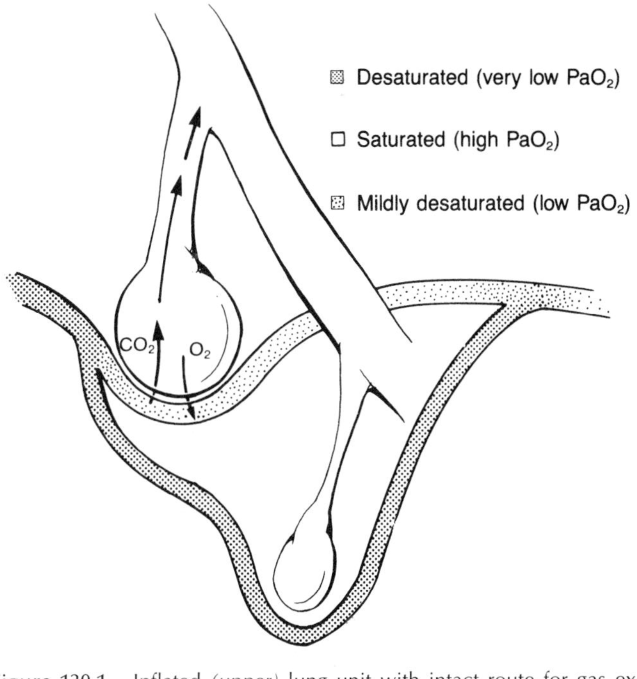

Figure 130.1. Inflated *(upper)* lung unit with intact route for gas exchange (CO_2 clearance and O_2 saturation of red blood cells), while deflated or consolidated *(lower)* lung unit leads to shunting of desaturated *(blackened)* red blood cells to the arterial side. An increased RR allows additional clearing of CO_2 in the upper zone to maintain a normal (or even low) CO_2 tension in the systemic arterial blood, but still does not achieve O_2 saturation of red blood cells when a large enough number of air spaces are closed in the lower zone. Thus, shunting may lead to significant decreases in arterial O_2 content, even when the patient is hyperventilating (i.e., low $PaCO_2$).

vide a route for clearance of CO_2 (Fig. 130.1). On the other hand, despite their ability to maintain adequate oxygenation, some patients may need ventilatory support for CO_2 retention (chronic lung patients) or to purposefully lower $PaCO_2$ to decrease ICP (severe head injury).[6,7,17]

In summary, respiratory support involves the preservation of adequate Hgb levels and adequate circulation, adequate lung inflation and O_2 supplementation, and appropriate clearance of CO_2.

VENTILATORY SUPPORT

Minute ventilation (V_E) is the product of tidal volume (V_T) and respiratory rate (RR). From a clinician's point of view, the patient's immediate "V_E demand" can be considered the V_T and RR required to maintain a normal blood pH. Thus, need for ventilatory support usually arises when a patient is unable to ventilate adequately to remove enough CO_2 to maintain a normal blood pH. The removal of CO_2 to compensate for excess production of metabolic acids can be considered part of the immediate demand as well. V_E demand can be increased by (1) augmented CO_2 production by body tissues, (2) metabolic acidosis, and (3) an increased amount of wasted ventilation because of an increased ratio of dead space to tidal volume (V_D/V_T).

Most critically ill or injured patients are stressed and have an increased V_E demand, especially when there is shock and anaerobic acidosis. Most patients can briefly tolerate even large stresses in V_E demand. But like prolonged exercise, prolonged increases in V_E demand owing to injury may lead to respiratory muscle fatigue and eventual ventilatory failure, even in the healthiest of patients. All severely ill and injured patients, particularly those with respiratory system impairment, are potential (if not immediate) candidates for ventilatory support. The third mechanism of increased V_E demand, an acute increase in dead space (wasted ventilation), is usually the result of extremely shallow breathing (high V_D/V_T) or pulmonary embolism (air or thromboemboli).

Meeting ventilatory demand requires an intact bellows system, including open airways; an intact, tightly sealed chest wall; and respiratory muscles capable of generating enough negative (outward-pulling) pleural pressure to expand the lungs into an inflated state. The chest wall is a particularly important component because it anchors the respiratory muscles, including the diaphragm. The signal generator is the central nervous system, which determines the required V_E and signals adjustments in V_T and RR by way of the brainstem and spinal cord. In patients with cerebral insults or severe injuries, all of these elements may be compromised or malfunctioning, but even when these elements are intact, ventilatory support may be necessitated by overwhelming demands. Active ventilatory intervention may also be considered in cases of severe head injury to lower $PaCO_2$ in an intentional attempt to decrease ICP acutely.[6,7,17]

Common reasons for inadequate ventilation are airway obstruction, high spinal cord injury, flail chest, and open pneumothorax (sucking chest wound). In the latter, air preferentially enters the thorax through the path of least resistance (the chest wound that is larger than the tracheal orifice) during inspiration. Underlying medical problems such as acute asthma or chronic lung disease can cause expiratory phase air-flow obstruction and may also result in CO_2 retention, as may narcotic and other sedative drug overdoses, stroke, head injury, and neuromuscular disorders. Hemodynamic compromise (extreme blood loss, tension pneumothorax, and pericardial tamponade) may eventually result in ventilatory failure because of inadequate perfusion of the respiratory apparatus.

OXYGENATION SUPPORT

In the absence of severe anemia or circulatory compromise, the need for tissue oxygenation support normally arises from pulmonary failure to oxygenate the bloodstream, usually when a critical number of the lung's gas exchange units fail to remain inflated.[14] Although inadequate ventilation can lead to hypoxemia (by increasing the partial pressure of CO_2 relative to O_2 in the alveoli), the degree of hypoxemia is usually not great and is readily reversible once ventilatory support or supplemental O_2 is administered. On the other hand, *hypoinflation* is more likely to result in serious hypoxemia (PaO_2 less than 60 mm Hg) as blood perfuses across collapsed alveolar beds. This arterial hypoxemia may be refractory to even a high inspired O_2 fraction (FiO_2). This is a common mechanism of respiratory insufficiency in the critically ill or injured patient. Thus, tidal volume (V_T) size plays an important role in the maintenance of an adequate PaO_2 in these patients. For example, it is estimated that without intervention, 60% to 70% of patients with severe head injury have relative hypoxemia and 30% to 40% have critical hypoxemia (PaO_2 less than 60 mm Hg), despite apparently normal respiratory patterns and the absence of signs of respiratory distress.[4,5,8,9] The reasons may include aspiration of gastric contents or concomitant lung contusion, but more often, hypoxemia occurs because of clinically inapparent changes in the respiratory pattern. This hypoxemia can often be reversed by the initiation of effective positive-pressure lung inflations alone (e.g., with V_T equal to 10 to 15 mL/kg lean body weight).[1,2,12,17,22] The critically ill patient is recumbent in most situations and may also have a significant decrease of functional residual capacity, owing to thoracic muscle weakness and a decrease in total thoracic compliance.

Cardiac arrest patients rapidly deflate their lungs, and lung compliance diminishes by fivefold or more.[12] Endotracheal (ET) intubation is often required to guarantee reinflation, particularly after 1 or 2 minutes of CPR.[12] In patients who are conscious, lung deflation is normally not a problem; even in obtunded patients, stimulation or commands such as "take a deep breath" can often substitute for more invasive support. However, most unconscious patients must also be considered to be at high risk for aspiration (unprotected upper airway) or progressive closure of the smaller airways.

Alveolar closure can also result from physical compromise by increased abdominal pressure, a collapsed or paralyzed chest wall, or hemothorax or pneumothorax. Filling of alveoli with blood, vomitus, pus, or edema fluid blocks the movement of O_2 from the airways to the blood and also causes atelectasis. Obstruction of larger airways with distal collapse of airspaces can occur from foreign bodies. Less obvious is the diffuse alveolar closure that occurs after prolonged hypoinflation. Although V_E demand may be met by increasing RR and the flow in and out of remaining open alveoli (see Fig. 130.1), specific support measures may still be required to reverse hypoxemia (i.e., ET intubation and provision of V_T of 15 mL/kg).

Although the need for active ventilatory support and the need for active oxygenation support should be addressed independently, the means to provide these two types of support often overlap. For example, while a patient's V_E demand may be met by various combinations of mechanically delivered V_T and RR, hypoxemia secondary to shallow breaths will probably be reversed by 10 to 15 mL/kg V_T. Thus, the selected V_T could be used for both ventilatory and oxygenation support. If the V_T is increased for purposes of oxygenation, the effect on $PaCO_2$ and pH must then be taken into account and the RR tailored appropriately. A logical approach is to first choose an adequate delivered V_T and then adjust the RR to meet V_E demands. The need for additional oxygenation support, such as increased FiO_2 and positive end-expiratory pressure, can then be judged independently.

Although such guidelines are useful, experience and clinical judgment are still the keys to proper management. In some situations, early intervention may be warranted, despite normal arterial blood gas (ABG) analysis and clinical appearance. For example, elderly patients with rib fractures or head-injured patients with unstable neurologic status may benefit from early ET intubation and positive-pressure mechanical ventilation, particularly before undergoing extensive evaluations such as radiologic examination, peritoneal lavage, or computed tomographic scans. Such patients may experience fatigue, and their condition may deteriorate after the initial evaluation while these diagnostic studies are carried out. The same applies to patients with chronic obstructive pulmonary disease (COPD), chronic musculoskeletal disorders, pneumonia, or asthma, who may experience fatigue before other therapy (e.g., antibiotics and bronchodilators) can take full effect.

IDENTIFYING WHO NEEDS VENTILATORY AND OXYGENATION SUPPORT

In identifying which patients require ventilatory and oxygenation support, four considerations should be kept in mind: (1) Certain immediately life-threatening problems (e.g., airway obstruction, inadequate respirations or apnea, and open or tension pneumothorax) require urgent attention before other assessments; (2) some urgent problems, not obvious at first, can be detected by repeated assessments (e.g., simple pneumothorax and flail chest); (3) the risk of late pulmonary complications (e.g., adult respiratory distress syndrome [ARDS] and pneumonia) can often be predicted by initial assessments; and (4) underlying conditions (e.g., asthma, COPD, heart failure, and overdose) must be promptly addressed.

Whether a patient is breathing spontaneously or receiving manual ventilation, certain respiratory problems require immediate attention. Auscultation of the upper anterior chest bilaterally should be performed with simultaneous inspection for apnea, cyanosis, tracheal deviation, engorged neck veins, retractive respirations, accessory muscle use, ecchymoses, flail segments, and sucking wounds. With auscultation, the following observations can be made: (1) lack of air movement (obstruction or respiratory arrest); (2) tachypnea or agonal respirations (impending arrest); (3) the presence of stridor (inspiratory obstruction); (4) prolonged expiration or wheezing (expiratory obstruction); (5) asymmetric breath sounds (large hemopneumothorax or lung collapse); and (6) abnormal quality or pattern of respirations (retractive, shallow). The initial screening is best performed over the anterior chest because the larger airways can be heard best there. Once the presence of reasonable ventilation has been ascertained by auscultation and visualization, the assessment of other systems and secondary assessments of the respiratory system can be accomplished. It must be remembered that upper airway obstruction may not be obvious at first in a patient who has had blunt trauma to the head, neck, and chest. However, the trachea may become progressively compromised by mechanical compression from an expanding hematoma deep in the throat, and such an obstruction may not be discovered until stridor develops (a late sign) or, in some cases, until the unintubated unconscious patient becomes cyanotic and apneic. Repeated assessments are the key; one must always keep one's index of suspicion high in the context of the overall picture.

Abnormal chest findings on chest examination may be perceived in the heat of an emergency, while normal examinations do not guarantee that active ventilatory and oxygenation support will not be necessary. Again, a high degree of suspicion and repeat examinations are the best tools of respiratory assessment. This rule also applies to chest radiography and ABG analysis. For example, many patients at high risk of developing ARDS after trauma have reasonable arterial oxygenation at first. Many cases of ARDS are not confirmed until several hours after injury, but physiologic (ABG) changes can evolve rapidly (usually within 3 to 4 hours), and thus close monitoring is essential in those with associated risk.[3,11,13] Contusions, pneumothorax, and atelectasis can also have a delayed onset (6 to 48 hours after injury)[3,10,11,15,19–21,23] and can occur without early signs of respiratory distress or change in physical examination. In severely ill or injured patients, ABG measurements should probably be repeated every 1 or 2 hours, at least in the early stages, and particularly in those who are already receiving early ventilatory and oxygenation support or are noncommunicative. In those with frank shock, ABG analysis should be performed frequently. Whenever an adjustment in ventilatory therapy is made or when there is an adverse change in the patient's assessment (decreased breath sounds, new infiltrate on chest radiograph), ABG analysis should be performed promptly, but preferably after 4 to 5 minutes of equilibration time on new ventilator settings.

Pulse oximetry is now available in most ambulances and emergency facilities. It is a very useful tool for detecting desaturation of red cells, although false-positive "normal saturations" can occur (e.g., CO poisoning). On the other hand, deterioration of overall respiratory status may not always be detected by pulse oximetry, especially when supplemental O_2 is in use. For example, while O_2 saturation may be maintained in an asthma patient on supplemental O_2, a rising $PaCO_2$ may go undetected. Likewise, worsening oxygenation (e.g., PaO_2 of 210 mm Hg falling to 150 mm Hg), despite the same amount of supplemental O_2, will not be detected by the pulse oximeter (which will show 100% saturation at both readings). False-positive *desaturations* are more common. Hypoperfusion, excess vasoconstriction, cool skin, and mechanical problems can cause falsely low readings.

The use of an end-tidal CO_2 (E_TCO_2) detector can be helpful in both the assessment and management of patients with acute respiratory insufficiency.[27,28] E_TCO_2 detection is best suited for patients who have received ET intubation. Detection of expired CO_2 can be accomplished through either a colorimetric E_TCO_2 device (capnometer) or an E_TCO_2 electronic graphic monitor (capnograph). *Capnometers* can be easily attached to the end of the ET tube and are commonly used to confirm proper ET tube placement by demonstrating tidal CO_2 expulsion (rising and falling of the CO_2 level with each breath). When CO_2 is not detected, this generally indicates inappropriate tube placement (e.g., in the esophagus). However, a false-negative reading (i.e., proper ET tube placement with low or no CO_2 detection) can occur. For example, patients with inadequate circulation (little CO_2 returning to the lungs) or significantly increased dead space (e.g., massive pulmonary embolus) may not show CO_2 detection despite proper tube placement.

Capnography can also be used for confirmation of proper ET tube placement, but it requires a more sophisticated electronic monitoring device (Fig. 130.2). The capnographic tracing does provide additional information, however. Even if a low CO_2 level is detected, the tidal waxing and waning of the CO_2 curve can indicate appropriate ET tube placement. The tracing can provide other important diagnostic and management information. For example, patients with severe expiratory obstruction (e.g., COPD, asthma) do not show a quick rise in the CO_2 level during expiration, but rather a more gradual upslope (Fig. 130.3). The tracing improves (quicker upslope) with improvements in airway obstruction. The E_TCO_2 tracing can also be useful in CPR. For example, E_TCO_2 levels may fall gradually over several minutes during CPR, indicating fatigue of the person performing chest compressions and the need to rotate rescuers (Fig. 130.4). Conversely, a sudden rise in CO_2 production during CPR may herald the return of spontaneous circulation (Fig. 130.5). Many practitioners consider capnography to be the stan-

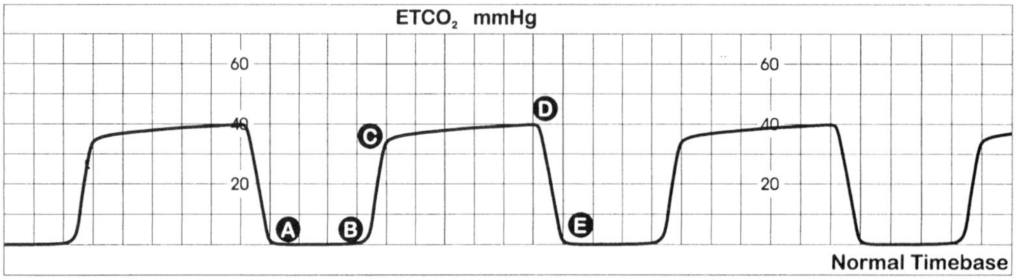

Figure 130.2. Normal capnograph indicating exhalation of the dead-space gas (no CO_2) in the first phase of exhalation *(A-B)*; exhalation of mixed dead-space and alveolar gas from the air spaces with the shortest transit time *(phase B-C)*; the alveolar plateau *(phase C-D)*, exhalation of primarily alveolar gas; and, finally, inhalation *(phase D-E)*, in which there is inspiration of fresh gas. Point *D* represents the end-tidal CO_2 value.

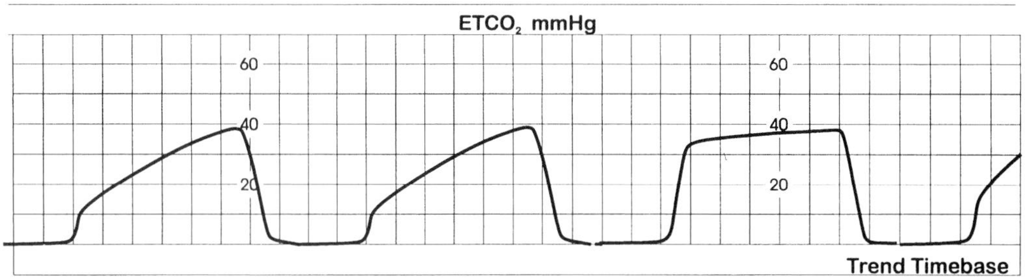

Figure 130.3. A capnograph of a patient with severe expiratory obstruction, showing a delay in reaching the alveolar gas plateau as reflected by a more gradual upstroke of phase B-C (see Fig. 130.2). Improvements in air-flow obstruction are reflected by a normalization of the tracing.

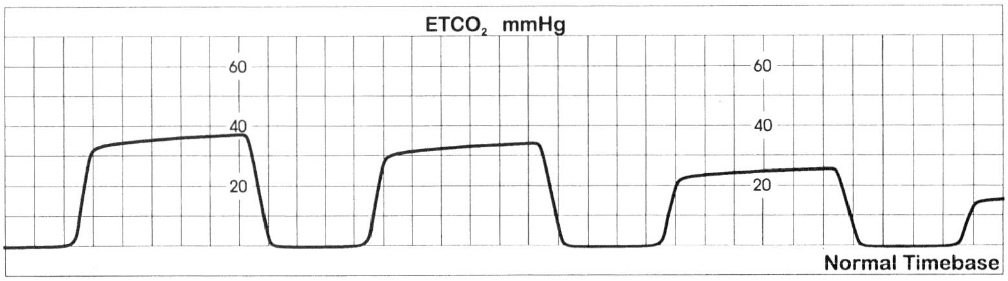

Figure 130.4. Capnograph indicating a gradual decrease in circulation (relatively normal tracing, but of decreasing magnitude over time).

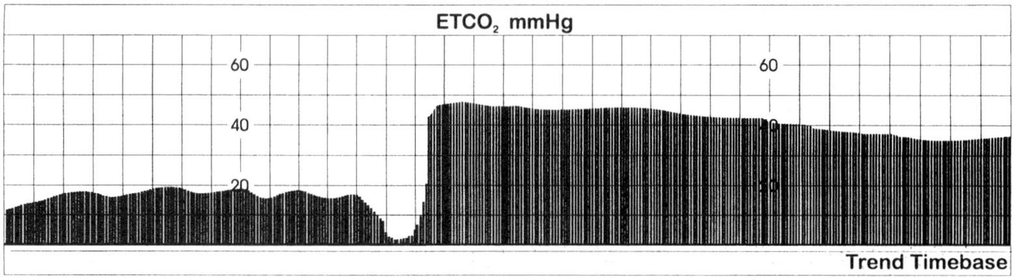

Figure 130.5. Capnograph over an extended period of time (trended timebase), showing a low magnitude of end-tidal CO_2 during CPR, then increasing dramatically, indicating a sudden return of spontaneous circulation, with an increase in CO_2 production and a return of CO_2 via the circulation to the lungs.

dard of care, at least for those greater than 2 to 3 years of age. E_TCO_2 devices are more complex in infants and are thus less useful in that population.

DIFFERENTIAL DIAGNOSIS

When faced with a patient with difficulty breathing or signs of respiratory insufficiency, the clinician should always keep an open mind, even after formulating an initial working assessment, and should continue to reassess the patient and review a mental differential diagnostic list. Above all, one should think in terms of O_2 transport; thus, the differential diagnosis includes both pulmonary and circulatory processes (Table 130.1). Such a mental list helps the physician to better direct historical queries and the physical examination to cover all pertinent areas. It also must be remembered that multiple processes may be occurring simultaneously. For example, an exacerbation of COPD may be associated with a pulmonary embolus or pneumonia.

The chest radiograph is a critical tool in the evaluation of respiratory status. It usually reveals the source of any intrapulmonary shunt detected by ABG analysis (e.g., pulmonary edema, pneumonia, atelectasis, main-stem intubation, or pneumothorax). Aside from cardiac right-to-left shunts (congenital and traumatic), pulmonary emboli, and early hypoinflation, hypoxemia unresponsive to low levels of FiO_2 (less than 0.3) usually can be identified by a chest radiographic finding. If not obvious on initial films, in most cases follow-up films show the source or infiltrate progression within a few hours. However, while radiographic infiltrates are usually present in the patient with severe hypoxemia, the severity of hypoxemia does not necessarily correspond to the amount of infiltrate seen. The clinical picture, associated findings, ET secretions, ABG analyses, and response to positive-pressure ventilation can aid in the delineation of the causes of infiltrates seen on chest radiographs.[10,11,14]

EMERGENCY DEPARTMENT EVALUATION AND MANAGEMENT

ABG values are the immediate end point of early respiratory support: The traditional aim is to deliver the V_E that will maintain normal blood pH (7.35 to 7.45) and to maintain adequate saturation of Hgb (preferably greater than 97%) by maintaining adequate arterial O_2 tensions (PaO_2 greater than 70 mm Hg).

Acutely, pH rather than $PaCO_2$ should be the focus of ventilatory interventions; an abnormal $PaCO_2$ is not necessarily harmful in itself, except for its effect on pH and ICP. The usual normal range for $PaCO_2$ is 35 to 40 mm Hg, but in a patient with shock whose $PaCO_2$ is 38 mm Hg, the pH may be less than 7.10, owing to excessive production of lactic acid. In such cases, the $PaCO_2$ can be temporarily lowered by increasing V_E enough to return the pH toward normal (until the underlying metabolic disturbance can be corrected). In a patient who has received excess sodium bicarbonate (e.g., during cardiac resuscitation) or in a patient with chronic CO_2 retention, a high $PaCO_2$ should be left untreated as long as the pH is normal. Attempts to lower $PaCO_2$ acutely will raise the pH and increase the risk of life-threatening complications from alkalosis.[11] "Permissive hypoventilation" is now considered an optional therapy to diminish mean airway pressure in selected patients, including those with "auto-PEEP" (diminished venous return and cardiac output due to overzealous positive-pressure ventilation).

Because misinterpretation of ABG values can have serious consequences, during the early hours after acute illness or injury, *trends* in PaO_2 (rather than a single result) should guide therapy. The variability of duplicate PaO_2 analysis can be as much as $\pm 10\%$.[24] Artifacts in technique can affect PaO_2 measurements, such as inadvertent venous sampling (or mixed arteriovenous sampling when the needle tip is moved), laboratory error (technician error or miscalibration of the machine), and misreporting (misunderstanding over the phone, misplaced decimal point, or poor handwriting). If the sample is run within 10 or 15 minutes, air bubbles and failure to place the sample on ice are not significant problems. However, longer delays can lead to unreliable analyses. Furthermore, if too much liquid heparin is in the syringe, the measurement will be inaccurate; this seldom affects PaO_2 significantly but may cause artifactual lowering of the measured $PaCO_2$ (as well as pH).

Finally, one's interpretation of the ratio of PaO_2 to FiO_2 should clearly consider the O_2 delivery system and the temporally related activities surrounding the sampling. Even 100% O_2 given by a loosely fitting mask usually does not achieve much more than 50% to 70% inspired O_2; when sampling takes place during or soon after a transient removal of supplemental O_2 for transport or suctioning or when the patient continually removes the O_2 facemask, the interpretation of the degree of respiratory insufficiency will be inaccurate. When in doubt, maintaining a high FiO_2 and repeating the sampling is the safest approach.

Even when the PaO_2 is sampled, measured, and reported correctly, other factors can still interfere with oxygenation of the tissues. Above a PaO_2 of 70 to 80 mm Hg, the red blood cells are almost completely saturated. Thus, in a patient with an adequate hematocrit, a PaO_2 of 500 mm Hg does not add much to O_2 delivery. However, in a patient whose hematocrit is 15% or less, the amount of O_2 dissolved in the blood with PaO_2 equal to 500 mm Hg (about 1.5 mL O_2 per 100 mL blood) may be significant. Therefore, if severe anemia is even a slight possibility, maintaining a high FiO_2 (greater than 0.6) may be temporarily advisable to achieve the highest possible O_2 tensions, even when lung function appears adequate.

Even with an acceptable hematocrit, good cardiac output, and adequate PaO_2, adequate tissue oxygenation and utilization are not guaranteed. For example, in cyanide or CO poisoning, PaO_2 that would normally saturate Hgb would no longer be adequate. Not only are O_2-binding sites blocked on Hgb, but the poisons also interfere with O_2 utilization in the mitochondria. In addition, in CO poisoning, O_2 binds tighter than usual to Hgb, thus diminishing release at the tissues. Although CO poisoning

TABLE 130.1. Differential Diagnosis of Acute Respiratory Problems

CARDIAC OUTPUT PROBLEMS
Bleeding, myocardial ischemia, sepsis, pericardial tamponade, tension pneumothorax, etc.
PULMONARY PROBLEMS
Airway obstruction (upper airway problems such as anaphylaxis, foreign body, inflammation, infection, trauma)
Bronchial obstruction (asthma, bronchitis, COPD)
Congestive heart failure and other forms of pulmonary edema
Drug-induced (stimulants, e.g., cocaine, vs. depressants, e.g., narcotics)
Emboli (air, thrombi)
Fractures (with or without underlying contusions)
Gross hemoptysis (usually from bronchial circulation fed from the aorta)
Hemothorax and pneumothorax (spontaneous and traumatic)
Inhalation injuries (CO, toxic fumes, near-drowning, aspiration)
"Junky" lungs (pneumonia, cancer, empyema)
"Compensation" for metabolic acidosis (shock, ketoacidosis, renal failure, toxins)
Lower (subdiaphragmatic) problems and restrictive breathing (tense ascites, pain, injury)
Muscle weakness (Ca^{2+}, PO_4^-, K^+, Mg^{2+}, myasthenia, dystrophies)
Neurologic impairment (spinal or central lesion, Guillain-Barré syndrome)

leads to anoxic lactic acidemia, attempts to lower $PaCO_2$ to compensate for the acidosis should be avoided, as O_2 release to the tissues is better in an acidemic environment. PaO_2 should be kept as high as possible to compete with CO-Hgb binding and decrease the half-life of carboxyhemoglobin and also to dissolve a certain amount of O_2 in the blood for tissue oxygenation. Hyperbaric O_2 therapy should be considered in severe cases.

In the patient with chronic lung disease who retains CO_2 and has lost the usual stimulus to breathe from elevated CO_2 levels, the much weaker "hypoxic" stimulus to breathe helps to maintain the respiratory drive to some extent. It is commonly taught that one should give these patients *only* low-flow O_2 (1 to 2 L/min). This consideration may be applicable if there is no acute exacerbation of lung disease, but when dyspnea, increasing respiratory distress, or disorientation is involved, one should not withhold liberal O_2 flows while gauging the PaO_2. During acute exacerbations, in fact, these patients are more likely to be critically hypoxic while on low-flow O_2. A pragmatic resolution may be to monitor O_2 saturation with pulse oximetry and titrate O_2 supplementation to maintain a satisfactory O_2 saturation (e.g., greater than 92%).

Even without a specific indication, supplemental O_2 should be considered in all ill or injured patients, because it provides a small but possibly critical margin of tissue PO_2 in a patient who has a sudden, unexpected setback (e.g., sudden airway obstruction, hemorrhage, or arrest). The basic modes of O_2 administration include nasal cannula, facemask, and ET tube. As discussed earlier, the use of ET intubation should be emphasized in critically ill and injured patients.[12,18] In cases in which ET intubation or 100% inspired O_2 is not specifically indicated, low-flow O_2 (i.e., approximately 2 L/min) should be administered, preferably by nasal prongs in alert or semialert patients without obvious nasopharyngeal injury. Patients who are short of breath often become apprehensive when masks cover their faces, and they tend to pull the masks off. Communication is somewhat hampered by a mask and may also promote aspiration by the supine obtunded patient. Nasal cannulas can deliver up to 35% inspired O_2 at 6 L per minute, a level that should suffice in most noncritical cases, but may be inadequate if there is a significant intrapulmonary shunt (greater than 15%) or if nasal inhalation is impaired. In cases in which a very high FiO_2 is indicated but ET intubation cannot be readily performed, an O_2 mask should be considered along with available suction and close observation. A mask with an attached reservoir can supply nearly 100% inspired O_2 at high-flow rates. Assisted ventilation with bag-valve-mask, oral airways, and proper positioning is a mandatory adjunct to ET tube placement attempts.

Because most pH abnormalities can be controlled immediately by adaptations in ventilation, it is more advantageous in patients with severe injuries and acid–base abnormalities to manipulate acid–base status acutely by effecting changes in ventilation. Alkali should be administered only if ventilatory support is inadequate or if acidosis is persistent or refractory to transfusion, intravascular volume restoration, and other primary modes of oxygenation support.

Many clinicians have traditionally attempted to "hyperventilate" patients they believe to be acidotic or in need of lowered ICP.[23] However, more recent practices have deemphasized the use of early, aggressive hyperventilation for patients with severe head injuries.[8] Rather, maintenance of O_2 saturation and prevention of hypoventilation have become the primary focus. In fact, overzealous ventilation may diminish cardiac output significantly, particularly in those with severe COPD and/or hypovolemia.[16] This effect is difficult to recognize and may be responsible for continued cardiovascular impairment or even "pulseless electrical activity" during CPR. Transient suspension of ventilation (e.g., for 10 seconds) may be helpful in detecting its presence. Permissive hypoventilation may even be useful in such cases until the underlying problem (e.g., hypovolemia, asthma, bronchospasm) can be improved.

COMMON PITFALLS

- Assuming that an initially stable respiratory status will remain that way, particularly in the very young and the elderly
- Providing overzealous positive-pressure ventilation, which can lead to profound circulatory compromise, particularly in hypovolemic patients and those with severe COPD
- Failing to consider multiple processes in assessing respiratory failure. For example, an acute exacerbation of chronic obstructive lung disease could be caused or accompanied by a concurrent pneumonia, pneumothorax, or pulmonary embolus.
- Assuming a stable respiratory status because of a high pulse oximetry reading. Pulse oximetry does not measure CO_2 levels, nor does it always indicate worsening oxygenation when supplemental O_2 is in use.
- Failing to appreciate that patients with severe head injury may appear to be breathing normally and may even be "hyperventilating" (low $PaCO_2$) but still have significant hypoxemia, even while on supplemental O_2

References

1. Becker LB, Berg RA, Pepe PE, et al. A re-appraisal of mouth-to-mouth ventilation during bystander-initiated cardiopulmonary resuscitation. *Ann Emerg Med* 1997;30:654–666.
2. Brown AS. Intermittent positive pressure ventilation in the management of severe head injuries. In: *Head injuries: proceedings of an international symposium.* Edinburgh, Churchill Livingstone, 1971:266.
3. Cooper KR, Boswell PA. Reduced functional residual capacity and abnormal oxygenation in patients with severe head injury. *Chest* 1983;84:29.
4. Fowler AA, Hamman RF, Good JT, et al. Adult respiratory distress syndrome: risk with common predispositions. *Ann Intern Med* 1983;98:593.
5. Frost EAM, Arancibia CU, Shulman K. Pulmonary shunt as a prognostic indicator in head injury. *J Neurosurg* 1979;50:768.
6. Gildenberg PL, Makela M. The effect of early intubation and ventilation on outcome following head trauma. In: Winn WR, Rimel R, Jane JA, eds. *Recent advances in neurotrauma.* New York, Raven Press, 1985:79.
7. Jones PW. Hyperventilation in the management of cerebral oedema. *Intensive Care Med* 1981;7:205.
8. Marion DW, Firlik A, McLaughlin MR. Hyperventilation therapy for severe traumatic brain injury. *New Horiz* 1995;3:439–447.
9. McGillicuddy JE. Cerebral protection: pathophysiology and treatment of intracranial pressure. *Chest* 1985;87:85.
10. Miller JD, Butterworth JF, Guderman SK, et al. Further experience in the management of severe head injury. *J Neurosurg* 1981;54:289.
11. Miller JD, Sweet RC, Narayan R, et al. Early insults to the injured brain. *JAMA* 1978;240:439.
12. Pepe PE. Infections in the traumatized lung. *Curr Concepts Trauma Care* 1983;6:4.
13. Pepe PE. The clinical entity of adult respiratory distress syndrome: definition, prediction, and prognosis. *Crit Care Clin* 1988;2:377.
14. Pepe PE, Copass MK, Joyce TH. Prehospital endotracheal intubation: rationale for training emergency medical personnel. *Ann Emerg Med* 1985;14:1085.
15. Pepe PE, Holtman Reus D, et al. Clinical predictors of the adult respiratory distress syndrome. *Am J Surg* 1982;144:124.
16. Pepe PE, Hudson LD. Acute respiratory failure. In: Callaham ML, ed. *Current therapy in emergency medicine (1986–1987).* Toronto: BC Decker, 1986:33.
17. Pepe PE, Hudson LD, Carrico CJ. Early application of positive end-expiratory pressure in patients at risk for the adult respiratory distress syndrome. *N Engl J Med* 1984;311:282.
18. Pepe PE, Marini JJ. Occult positive end-expiratory pressure in mechanically ventilated patients with airflow obstruction: the auto-PEEP effect. *Am Rev Respir Dis* 1982;126:166.
19. Pepe PE, Stewart RD, Copass MK. Prehospital management of trauma. *Ann Emerg Med* 1986;15:1484.
20. Pepe PE, Zachariah BS, Chandra N. Invasive airway techniques in resuscitation. *Ann Emerg Med* 1993;22(II):393.
21. Robertson HT, Lakshminarayan SI, Hudson LD. Lung injury following a 50 meter fall into water. *Thorax* 1978;33:175.
22. Shackford SR. Selective use of ventilator therapy in flail chest injuries. *J Thorac Cardiovasc Surg* 1981;81:194.
23. Shin B, McAshlan TC, Hankins JR, et al. Management of lung contusion. *Am Surg* 1979;45:168.

24. Sinha RP, Ducker TB, Perot PL. Arterial oxygenation: findings and its significance in central nervous system trauma patients. *JAMA* 1973;224:1258.
25. Thomas AN. Management of the injured patient: thoracic injuries. In: Way LW, ed. *Current surgical diagnosis and treatment.* Los Altos, CA: Lange Publishing, 1983:221.
26. Thorson SH, Marini JJ, Pierson DJ, et al. Variability of arterial blood gas values in stable patients in the I.C.U. *Chest* 1984;84:14.
27. Ward KR, Yealy DM. End-tidal carbon dioxide monitoring in emergency medicine. Part 1: basic principles. *Acad Emerg Med* 1998;5:628–636.
28. Ward KR, Yealy DM. End-tidal carbon dioxide monitoring in emergency medicine. Part 2: clinical applications. *Acad Emerg Med* 1998;5:637–646.

CHAPTER 131

Ischemic Heart Disease, Angina Pectoris, and Myocardial Infarction

James T. Nieman

More than 65 million Americans live with cardiovascular disease, including hypertension, coronary artery disease, rheumatic heart disease, and stroke. Approximately 45% of all deaths in the United States are due to cardiovascular disease, and nearly half of these deaths are in patients younger than age 65. More than 1.5 million patients with suspected acute ischemic heart disease (IHD) are admitted to coronary care units (CCUs) in the United States each year. At least 250,000 patients with IHD experience prehospital cardiac arrest each year, and only approximately 6% of these patients survive to be discharged from the hospital. IHD is thus a major national health concern as well as a common problem encountered in the emergency department.

Of increasing importance is the effective triage of patients with symptoms suggestive of acute IHD. Unnecessary admission to the hospital of patients with chest pain is estimated to cost more than $12 billion annually.[13]

The coronary arterial lesion most commonly encountered in the patient with typical, stable angina pectoris is a smooth-surfaced atherosclerotic plaque that may permit sufficient coronary arterial flow at rest or with minimal exercise to meet the metabolic demands of the myocardium. The determinants of myocardial oxygen supply and the factors that determine myocardial oxygen demand are listed in Table 131.1. During physical exertion or emotional stress, myocardial oxygen demand increases due to an increase in heart rate and blood pressure (the double product). To meet an increase in oxygen demand, either coronary arterial flow or myocardial oxygen extraction must increase. Because myocardial oxygen extraction is near maximal under normal circumstances, the only way to balance myocardial oxygen supply and demand is to increase coronary flow. If a fixed obstructive lesion is present, flow cannot increase sufficiently to meet augmented demands. Supply–demand imbalance ensues, with the development of ischemia, contractile dysfunction, and the classic symptoms of angina.[23] When supply and demand are equalized, the supply–demand imbalance ceases and symptoms subside. This pathophysiologic substrate is the basis for medical management of chronic stable angina. Nitroglycerin preparations, beta blockers, and calcium channel blockers either increase myocardial oxygen supply or decrease demand.

TABLE 131.1. Determinants of Myocardial Oxygen Supply and Demand

Oxygen Demand	Oxygen Supply
Frequency of pressure development (heart rate)	Diastolic time
Rate of pressure development (contractility)	Extravascular resistance
Ventricular volume (preload)	Perfusion pressure
Pressure developed (afterload)	Collateral resistance
	Coronary arterial tone

TABLE 131.2. Causes of Nonatherosclerotic Myocardial Ischemia

VALVULAR HEART DISEASE
Aortic stenosis
Aortic regurgitation
Pulmonary stenosis (right ventricular ischemia)
Mitral stenosis with pulmonary hypertension (right ventricular ischemia)
CONGENITAL HEART DISEASE
Congenital valvular disease
Coarctation of the aorta
Cyanotic heart disease
NONATHEROSCLEROTIC CORONARY DISEASE
Coronary artery spasm, spontaneous or drug-induced (e.g., from use of cocaine)
Coronary artery embolus
Congenital coronary disease (anomalous anatomic origin)
Coronary dissection
Coronary artery vasculitis

Unstable coronary artery syndromes encompass unstable angina pectoris and acute myocardial infarction (MI). The pathologic substrate is a complex, irregular, and thrombogenic atherosclerotic plaque that may not be flow-limiting, even during activities that increase the double product. The occurrence of chest pain is thought to result from intermittent flow limitations caused by platelet or fibrin thrombi, an increase in coronary vasomotor tone (i.e., vasospasm), or a combination of both, in the area of the unstable arterial plaque. Myocardial supply–demand imbalance, therefore, occurs because of a decrease in oxygen supply rather than an increase in demand, as in the stable coronary syndrome. Such patients may present with a history of chest pain and may have had a normal exercise stress test or coronary angiography that demonstrated noncritical coronary obstruction.[6,31]

Myocardial ischemia can also occur in the absence of coronary atherosclerosis. Common causes of nonatherosclerotic myocardial ischemia are listed in Table 131.2.

CLINICAL PRESENTATION

History of Present Illness

No single presenting symptom is uniformly diagnostic of IHD. Chest pain or chest discomfort is the most common chief complaint. Such pain or discomfort may be described as a burning, tightness, squeezing, or heaviness, and as dull, sharp, or knife-like in character. Substernal or retrosternal chest pain may radiate to the left shoulder or to the arm, neck, or jaw due to convergence of sympathetic and somatic afferent pathways at the spinal level. Patients with IHD may also complain of similar types of abdominal discomfort. Chest pain caused by IHD is of visceral origin and is poorly localized. Chest pain that can be localized with a fingertip is unlikely to be of ischemic cardiac origin.[21]

Chest pain caused by IHD usually occurs abruptly, increases in intensity over time, and reaches peak intensity within 2 to 5 minutes of onset. If the pain occurs during or immediately after exertion, it typically resolves gradually within minutes of cessation of physical activity. Chest discomfort that lasts for only seconds or chest pain that is constant and lasts for hours to days is not consistent with IHD. Similarly, chest pain that is pleuritic, reproduced by palpation, and is sharp, stabbing, or positional has a low likelihood of being due to IHD[25] (Table 131.3).

Patients with IHD, usually the elderly or those who also have diabetes mellitus or hypertension, may present with symptoms other than chest pain during acute ischemia. Such patients may complain of dyspnea, early fatigue, or declining exercise tolerance, symptoms that are caused by diastolic myocardial dysfunction. Decreased ventricular compliance leads to an increase in left ventricular (LV) end-diastolic pressure and pulmonary artery pressure, resulting in an increase in pulmonary interstitial fluid.

Patients with a history of chest pain or with known medically controlled angina pectoris may present with new symptoms, such as chest pain at rest, chest pain associated with previously tolerated levels of exertion, chest pain unrelieved by a previously effective dose of a nitrate preparation, or chest pain of increasing severity, duration, or frequency. These patients should be considered to have unstable angina. Patients with typical exertional angina of less than 2 months' duration that is severe or frequent (three or more episodes per day) should also be considered to have unstable angina.[31]

Coronary artery vasospasm may produce symptoms that are atypical for classic angina pectoris. Episodes of chest pain or discomfort may occur at rest, pain may persist longer than is common for typical angina, and symptoms more commonly occur during the early morning. Such patients may also relate no risk factors for IHD.

The symptoms of an acute MI may not be distinguishable from those of a severe stable anginal episode or of unstable angina, although patients with acute MI usually have chest pain of typical anginal quality for at least 30 minutes. This consideration has served as a major entry criterion in studies of the efficacy of thrombolytic agents in acute MI.

TABLE 131.3. Characteristics of Chest Pain Typical and Atypical for Ischemic Heart Disease

Typical
Substernal in location
Squeezing, heavy, or burning sensation
Precipitated by exertion
Promptly (within 2–3 min) relieved by nitroglycerin
Lasting minutes (typically 5–15 min; longer with acute infarction)

Atypical
Pain described as sharp or stabbing
Fleeting (lasting seconds) or prolonged (>24 h)
Unrelated to exercise
Not relieved by rest or nitroglycerin
Positional or related to respiration ("pleuritic")
Characterized by palpitations without chest pain
Well localized to a specific point

TABLE 131.4. Physical Signs That Occur during Ischemia

Physical Sign	Underlying Pathophysiology
Soft S1	Decreased LV dp/dt or first-degree AV block
Paradoxically split S2	Prolonged LV ejection time
S3 and/or S4	Decreased LV compliance
Mitral regurgitation	Papillary muscle ischemia
Palpable precordial systolic bulge	Anterior or lateral dyskinesis
Bibasilar rales	Increased preload

LV, left ventricular; dp/dt, rate of pressure rise; AV, atrioventricular.

Based on a number of epidemiologic studies, major and minor risk factors for coronary artery disease have been defined. Major risk factors include family history (MI in a first-degree relative of age less than 55 years), smoking, hypertension, hypercholesterolemia, diabetes mellitus, and male sex.

Physical Examination

Most patients with chest pain caused by IHD have one or more abnormal physical findings, but these are not specific for IHD and may occur in patients with valvular or congenital heart disease, or cardiomyopathy. If the finding of an S_4 is excluded, about 25% of patients with symptomatic IHD have a normal physical examination.

Common physical findings during myocardial ischemia are noted in Table 131.4 with their respective pathophysiologic explanations. The clinician should also seek evidence of risk factors for IHD, for example, hypercholesterolemia (xanthomas and arcus senilis) and hypertension (elevated arterial blood pressure and funduscopic changes).

DIFFERENTIAL DIAGNOSIS

A detailed discussion of the differential diagnosis of chest pain is included elsewhere in this volume. Diseases that are life-threatening and which may be confused with IHD include aortic dissection, pulmonary thromboembolism, pneumothorax, and esophageal rupture. Pneumonia, mitral valve prolapse, pericarditis, reflux esophagitis, esophageal spasm, peptic ulcer disease, and chest wall pain should also be included in the differential diagnosis. Particular attention to the character of the pain, precipitating factors, associated symptoms, and the physical examination usually allows the clinician to rule out a number of these other causes for chest pain.

EMERGENCY DEPARTMENT EVALUATION

The emergency department evaluation, management, and triage of patients suspected of having chest pain caused by myocardial ischemia have changed dramatically in the past decade. These changes are the result of cost-containment concerns as well as the demonstration that early administration of thrombolytic agents in the setting of acute MI significantly decreases mortality.[5,27,35]

Annually, about 1.5 million patients are hospitalized in CCUs in the United States for suspected acute MI. Only about 30% of these patients subsequently have an acute MI diagnosed by conventional standards during hospitalization. Large-scale studies have shown that emergency department chest pain units (CPUs) can quickly identify and stratify patients with chest pain of suspected ischemic origin into low- and high-risk groups in an effort to more effectively use the resources uniquely available in the CCU setting.[35] Diagnostic efforts in the emergency department should be directed toward *ruling in* acute IHD, not just ruling out acute MI. In nearly all instances, patients with suspected acute IHD, not just those with acute infarction, require hospitalization.

Acute transmural MI is caused by complete occlusion of the infarct-related coronary artery by thrombus. Numerous large-scale, multicenter trials have demonstrated that dissolution of the thrombus by intravenous administration of thrombolytic agents and early reperfusion of the occluded coronary artery can preserve ventricular function and reduce mortality from acute MI by nearly 30%. This beneficial effect depends on the time from onset of symptoms to reperfusion.[5,11,14,34] Diagnostic techniques for the early recognition of acute MI in patients who are likely to benefit from thrombolytic therapy are an active area of investigation.[28]

Electrocardiography

The electrocardiogram (ECG) and clinical history are the major screening methods available in most emergency departments when acute IHD is suspected. It has been stated that the emergency department ECG is often "normal" in patients subsequently diagnosed as having acute MI. Recent data indicate that the admission ECG is rarely normal but that nonspecific findings are frequent in this group of patients.

The early ECG signs of MI are ST-segment and T-wave changes that may also be seen with transient reversible ischemia or in patients with an established diagnosis of coronary artery disease. ST-segment elevation of more than 1 mm (0.1 mV) in two contiguous limb leads or 2 or more mm in two contiguous precordial leads is reported in the setting of acute transmural (Q-wave) MI. ST-segment elevation is seen in approximately 40% to 50% of patients with chest pain and acute MI at the time of initial evaluation. This population of patients is most likely to benefit from early administration of thrombolytic agents.

ST-segment depression of a similar degree (greater than or equal to 1 mm) or T-wave inversion is most commonly seen in nontransmural (non-Q-wave) infarction. Approximately 75% of patients with non-Q-wave infarction present with ST-segment depression. As a corollary observation, about one-third of patients with chest pain who have ST-segment depression or T-wave inversion subsequently evolve a non-Q-wave infarction.

ST-segment and T-wave changes are not always due to acute IHD. Common nonischemic causes for ST and T-wave changes suggestive of acute IHD are listed in Table 131.5. Although the presence of new nonspecific ECG changes increases the likelihood that chest pain is due to myocardial ischemia, the predictive value of such a finding is only about 50%.

Nonconventional surface ECG recordings are of value in some patients with suspected acute MI. The right coronary artery supplies the inferior wall of the LV as well as the right ventricle (RV) in 90% of patients. In the setting of inferior MI, a right precordial electrogram should be recorded to detect RV infarction. The right precordial electrogram is obtained by placing the V leads over the anterior right chest in a pattern that is the mirror image of the standard left-sided placement. RV infarction occurs in about 60% of patients who suffer an inferior MI and is detected by ST-segment elevation of greater than 1 mm in lead V_{3R} or V_{4R}, or both. Although RV infarction commonly accompanies infarction of the inferior wall of the LV, RV contractile dysfunction becomes hemodynamically significant in only about 10% of patients. Patients with hemodynamically significant RV infarction typically present with arterial hypotension and jugular venous distention, but clear lung fields. RV involvement with inferior infarction is associated with a greater 1-year mortality than inferior wall infarction alone.

The optimal time interval at which to perform a repeated emergency department ECG in patients with initial nondiagnostic findings has not been determined. Repeated ECGs are most commonly performed in patients who experience recurrent chest pain during emergency department observation or in those who have received a thrombolytic agent and are being monitored for ST-segment changes suggestive of reperfusion.

TABLE 131.5. Nonischemic Causes of Precordial ST-Segment Elevation

Left bundle-branch block
Left ventricular hypertrophy
Pericarditis
Paced ventricular rhythm
Hypothermia (Osborne J waves)
Hyperkalemia
Drug-induced (e.g., tricyclic antidepressants)
Left ventricular aneurysm

Chest Radiography

The most common chest film abnormality in patients with IHD is cardiomegaly, usually associated with prior infarction or chronic arterial hypertension. Additional radiographic signs of LV dysfunction may also be found (e.g., pulmonary venous hypertension, Kerley B lines, and chronic pleural effusions).

The primary value of the chest radiograph in the evaluation of the patient with chest pain and suspected IHD is in the detection of other causes of chest pain (e.g., pneumothorax, pneumonia, or a widened mediastinum suggesting aortic dissection).

Biochemical Markers

After the clinical history and 12-lead ECG, the third tool readily available to assist in the diagnosis of an acute ischemic cardiac event is the serial measurement of enzymes and proteins released into the blood during myocardial ischemia.[8] When myocytes are damaged, there is loss of cell membrane integrity, and these macromolecules diffuse into the interstitium and subsequently into the intravascular space and lymphatics. Their patterns of appearance in blood depends on the intracellular location, molecular weight (heavier molecules diffuse more slowly), local blood and lymph flow, and rate of elimination from the blood. The enzyme creatine kinase (CK), its myocardial subunit (CK-MB), and the proteins troponin I and T are the most readily available and most commonly used biochemical markers of cardiac ischemia. CK is typically reported as total enzyme activity (units per liter) and CK-MB as a concentration (CK-MB mass, nanograms per milliliter) or as a percentage of total CK (CK-MB activity). The former measurement of CK-MB is now available as a microparticle enzyme immunoassay based on monoclonal antibody technology. It is analytically and clinically more sensitive than the CK-MB percentage activity measured by electrophoresis. Elevations above the reference range or normal value for total CK and CK-MB mass are not specific for myocardial injury. CK and CK-MB are also present in skeletal muscle, and elevations may be seen after vigorous exercise, rhabdomyolysis, skeletal muscle trauma, dermatomyositis or polymyositis, renal failure, and cardiac contusion. Interpretation of total CK and CK-MB mass values must take this nonspecificity into consideration. Elevations of total CK and CK-MB mass are detectable 4 to 6 hours after acute infarction. Peak CK-MB mass is typically observed 12 to 18 hours after ischemia, while the peak of total CK occurs slightly later (12 to 24 hours). Both measurements return to normal values 24 to 36 hours after the ischemic event; a secondary rise suggests reinfarction. Time to peak levels of total CK and CK-MB mass vary, depending on the extent of myocardial injury. Peaks generally occur earlier with non-Q-wave or subendocardial infarction and later with Q-wave or transmural infarction.

The troponins (troponin [Tn] I and T) are proteins that regulate calcium-dependent interactions between myosin and actin. The cardiac troponins (cTnI, CTnT) are highly specific for myocardial tissue and are immunologically distinct from the skeletal muscle troponins. Due to this specificity, the concomitant use of a troponin measurement and CK-MB mass assists in differentiating myocardial from skeletal muscle injury in the presence of an elevated CK-MB measurement. Elevated cardiac Tn levels are detectable in serum within 4 to 6 hours following acute cardiac ischemia, reach peak concentrations in approximately 12 hours, and remain elevated after an ischemic event for 3 to 10 days. This temporal pattern allows detection of an acute cardiac event days after it has occurred and should replace lactate dehydrogenase (LDH) isoenzyme determinations for the diagnosis of "remote" acute myocardial injury. Due to its lower molecular weight, TnT appears earlier in the plasma than TnI. This advantage may be offset by the fact that TnT can be artificially elevated in the setting of renal failure.

At present, there is an indeterminate range of Tn values (typically 0.4 to 2.0 ng/mL) that are not normal yet are below the levels accepted for the diagnosis of acute MI. Such values may be seen in the clinical settings of unstable angina (presumably due to "microinfarction"), chronic congestive heart failure, and myocarditis, and after cardiac surgery.

A single measurement of total CK, CK-MB mass, and Tn has a low sensitivity (30% to 40%) in ruling out acute MI, despite a specificity of 80% to 99%. Because of this low sensitivity, single normal values cannot be relied on to eliminate acute infarction as a diagnostic possibility in a patient with chest pain. Measurements should be performed serially, usually at 3- to 6-hour intervals for 12 to 18 hours. The reported sensitivities, specificities, and positive and negative predictive values for the various biochemical markers vary considerably in the literature (Table 131.6).[8] This variation is due to the reported timing of blood sampling (from onset of symptoms or from time of emergency department arrival), the use of one marker or a panel of markers, and the populations studied (e.g., patients with diagnostic vs. nondiagnostic ECGs). In general, sensitivity increases over this time period (0 to 6 hours), while specificity remains relatively constant (greater than 90%). Within 8 to 10 hours after the ischemic event, the sensitivity of CK-MB mass and the troponins is approximately 90%.[36]

Other biochemical markers for acute MI may facilitate the earlier diagnosis of acute infarction, particularly in the patient with a nondiagnostic ECG. Myoglobin is released from the myocardium within 2 to 4 hours of the onset of ischemia and appears earlier in the plasma than CK-MB. Serial measurements of myoglobin using newer rapid assays have been shown to be 100% sensitive, but with a specificity of approximately 80%, in detecting acute MI within 6 hours of symptom onset. Similarly, measurement of CK-MB isoforms (MB1 and MB2) has a sensitivity and specificity of greater than 90% of detecting acute MI within 6 hours of onset of symptoms. These latter markers are currently not widely used.

Noninvasive Assessment of Myocardial Perfusion and Cardiac Function in the Emergency Department

Patients who present with chest pain suggestive of acute cardiac ischemia, a nondiagnostic ECG or an ECG demonstrating "nonspecific" ST-segment or T-wave changes, and normal total CK, CK-MB, and Tn on serial measurements present a diagnostic problem. This patient population is the one most likely to have acute MI and unstable angina ruled out after hospital admission to a CCU or intensive care unit, at a cost of billions of dollars annually. These patients are also those most likely to benefit from extended observation in a CPU. The CPU has been shown to be a cost-effective alternative to hospital admission for these patients and to result in a decrease in the incidence of "missed" MI. Standard treadmill exercise stress testing (EST), myocardial scintigraphy at rest and during exercise, and stress echocardiography are standard diagnostic tests performed in patients with suspected coronary artery disease. The sensitivities, specificities, and positive and negative predictive values of these tests have been defined largely in the population of patients with a moderate-to-high probability of coronary artery disease (Table 131.7). These tests are now being applied to the broader group of patients who present to the emergency department with a chief complaint of chest pain. The diagnostic accuracy of these tests in this population has not been well established and is likely to be different from those with a greater probability of having significant coronary artery disease due to selection criteria or bias. It is likely that these tests will be more useful in risk stratification than in diagnosis.

Acute myocardial ischemia depletes adenosine triphosphate stores, resulting in ventricular contractile dysfunction and ventricular wall motion abnormalities that may occur in the absence of diagnostic ECG changes. Two-dimensional echocardiography with the patient at rest is sensitive in detecting regional wall motion abnormalities that accompany acute ischemia, and has been used in the screening of patients with chest pain and suspected acute ischemia. However, echocardiography cannot reliably differentiate prior infarction (with myocardial scarring) from a new ischemic event. The sensitivity and specificity of the test appear to depend on whether the test is performed during chest pain or after its resolution. Based on limited studies, it is estimated that the sensitivity of standard echocardiography in the emergency department for acute cardiac ischemia or infarction is approximately 50% to 90%, with a specificity of 50% to 100%.[28,35]

Technetium-99m–labeled sestamibi is a radionuclide agent that is taken up by the myocardium in proportion to regional blood flow and is therefore capable of demonstrating myocardial perfusion defects. With ECG-gating, the technique can also detect wall motion abnormalities. Limited studies indicate that

TABLE 131.6. Sensitivity and Specificity of Biochemical Markers of Ischemia at 0 to 6 Hours

	Myoglobin (%)	CK Total	CK-MB Mass (%)	CK-MB Isoforms (%)	Troponin T (%)	Troponin I (%)
Sensitivity	50–100	NR	15–65	90–95	50–60	6–45
Specificity	75–95	NR	90–100	95–100	75–95	90–100

NR, not reported.
Adapted from Char et al.[8]

TABLE 131.7. Reported Sensitivity and Specificity of Noninvasive Diagnostic Tests for Coronary Artery Disease (CAD) in Patients with a High Pretest Probability of CAD

	EST (%)	2D-Echo (%)	Nuclear Imaging (%)
Sensitivity	67–69	83–87	70–94
Specificity	76–78	74–80	43–97

EST, treadmill exercise stress test.
2D-echo includes exercise, dobutamine, and dipyridamole studies.
Imaging includes thallium and sestamibi.
Adapted from Garber and Solomon[15] and Kuntz et al.[22]

this method of perfusion imaging is greater than 90% sensitive for detecting coronary artery disease in an emergency department population, with a specificity of approximately 70%. The accuracy of the test does not appear to be affected by the presence or absence of chest pain at the time of imaging.[35]

Standard treadmill EST has also been used for evaluation and risk stratification in this patient population. EST can be safely performed, requires less technical expertise than does echocardiography, and is less expensive that radionuclide imaging. Based on limited studies, EST in the emergency department assessment of chest pain has a sensitivity ranging from 29% to 90% for detecting coronary artery disease, with a specificity of 50% to 99%.[16a,35a] As clinical experience with EST in the emergency department increases, it is likely that the reported range of sensitivity and specificity will narrow.

EMERGENCY DEPARTMENT MANAGEMENT

The initial management of all patients with chest pain and suspected acute IHD should include administration of low-flow oxygen, establishment of vascular access, and continuous cardiac rhythm monitoring combined with frequent blood pressure determinations. Continuous pulse oximetry should also be employed, if available.

Interventions in the Patient with Chest Pain and Suspected Unstable Angina Pectoris or Non-Q-Wave Infarction

Unstable angina is generally defined as a clinical syndrome falling between stable angina and acute MI. Typical presentations of unstable angina are presented in Table 131.8. Clinical features usually include a history of typical chest pain or a history of stable angina or MI and two or more risk factors for coronary artery disease. The ECG may be normal, nonspecific (ST-segment depression, 0.05 mm; T-wave flattening or inversion of less than 1 mm in leads with dominant R waves), or highly suggestive (ST-segment depression greater than or equal to 1 mm or marked symmetrical T-wave inversion in multiple leads) of ischemia. Therapeutic interventions in this clinical setting are directed toward decreasing myocardial oxygen demand and stabilizing thrombogenic atherosclerotic plaques.[2,31]

TABLE 131.8. Clinical Presentations of Unstable Angina

- Angina at rest within 1 wk of presentation
- New-onset angina of Canadian Cardiovascular Society Classification (CCSC) class III (pain when walking < two blocks or climbing < one flight of stairs) or IV (inability to carry on any physical activity without discomfort) within 2 months of presentation
- Angina increasing in CCSC class to at least class III or IV
- Non-Q-wave MI
- Postinfarction angina (>24 h after acute MI)

Adapted from Braunwald et al.[7]

Nitroglycerin

Sublingual nitroglycerin decreases myocardial oxygen demand by decreasing ventricular preload, improves myocardial perfusion by dilating the coronary vascular bed, and has antiplatelet properties. This combination of pharmacologic effects often results in relief of chest pain. The usual starting dose is 0.3 to 0.4 mg of nitroglycerin sublingually via a tablet or spray. If chest pain persists, this dose may be repeated every 5 minutes if the systolic blood pressure remains greater than 100 mm Hg. If chest pain persists after three to five sublingual doses, the administration of intravenous nitroglycerin should be considered (50 mg of nitroglycerin in 250 mL of dextrose 5% in water). The initial infusion rate is 10 to 20 μg/min and can be increased in increments of 5 to 10 μg/min at 5- to 10-minute intervals until chest discomfort resolves or mean arterial pressure decreases by 10%. Most patients respond to infusion rates of 50 to 200 μg/min. At low doses, nitroglycerin acts principally as a venous and coronary vasodilator. At high doses, it acts as an arterial vasodilator as well, thereby affecting an additional component of myocardial oxygen demand.

The major complication of nitrate therapy, whether sublingual or intravenous, is hypotension. This is most likely to occur in patients who are hypovolemic at the time of emergency department presentation or in those who have suffered an RV infarction complicating inferior wall infarction. If hypotension occurs, nitrate therapy should be discontinued and intravenous normal saline administered, with careful monitoring of vital signs and lung sounds. Hemodynamically significant bradyarrhythmias have been reported during nitrate therapy; these should be treated with atropine.

Morphine Sulfate

Intravenous morphine may be administered if chest pain is not relieved with sublingual or intravenous nitroglycerin. The usual dose is 2 to 4 mg administered every 5 to 30 minutes if systolic blood pressure remains greater than 100 mm Hg.[1] Morphine may decrease venous tone and decrease ventricular preload, but the required dose for these desired pharmacologic effects may produce respiratory depression. In addition, morphine may relieve pain but not necessarily reverse or modify the pathophysiologic processes involved in acute myocardial ischemia. Other potential complications of morphine therapy are hypotension and bradycardia, which may be treated with normal saline and atropine, respectively.

Antiplatelet and Antithrombin Agents

Aspirin prevents platelet aggregation and platelet-induced coronary vasoconstriction via acetylation of platelet cyclooxygenase and prevention of the formation of thromboxane A_2. All patients with suspected acute ischemic heart disease who have no contraindications to the use of aspirin (such as allergy or active gastrointestinal hemorrhage) should receive a dose of 80 to 325 mg as soon as possible after the onset of symptoms.[11] Concomitant aspirin and heparin therapy have been shown to be more effective than either agent alone.[24]

Unfractionated heparin is a heterogeneous mixture of polysaccharides, which activates antithrombin III, which in turn inhibits thrombin and coagulation factors X to XII. It also inhibits platelet aggregation, platelet vascular adhesion, and leukocyte chemotaxis.[11] Heparin is often administered intravenously as a 5,000-U bolus, followed by an infusion of 1,000 U/h. The infusion rate is adjusted based on periodic measurement of the partial thromboplastin time (goal, 45 to 75 seconds).

Low-molecular-weight heparin can also be used. It does not require monitoring of coagulation times, is associated with fewer clinically significant bleeding complications, and may be more effective than unfractionated heparin in preventing infarction, recurrent pain, and the need for early revascularization.[10,19] Similarly, the glycoprotein IIb/IIIa inhibitors, although not extensively evaluated in the emergency department, may offer benefit in preventing recurrent symptoms or acute infarction in this patient group.[16,33]

Beta Blockers

Beta blockers reduce myocardial oxygen demand by decreasing ventricular contractility (dP/dt), heart rate, and afterload (blood pressure). These agents also have antiarrhythmic properties (class III antiarrhythmics) and may counteract the effects of catecholamines of the myocardium. These agents should be administered in the setting of suspected unstable angina or acute MI if contraindications to their use are not present.[2] (Dosing and contraindications are discussed later.)

Patients with chest pain suggestive of acute cardiac ischemia who have ST-segment depression or T-wave inversions on the ECG are usually treated as if they are having a non-Q-wave (subendocardial) infarction. This diagnosis is supported if the ECG findings are new or "dynamic" (change in depth or amplitude over time). These patients are treated the same as patients with unstable angina. Thrombolytic agents have not been shown to improve survival in this patient population.[2,32]

Specific Interventions in Patients with Suspected Acute Transmural Myocardial Infarction (Q-Wave Infarction)

Acute MI is most commonly caused by abrupt thrombotic occlusion of a coronary artery at the site of a "thrombogenic" atheromatous plaque (i.e., one that is ulcerated or fissured).[5] Clot dissolution using thrombolytic agents in acute MI is safe and effective. A number of large prospective, controlled clinical trials comparing an intravenous thrombolytic agent with placebo have shown significant reductions in mortality with minimal risk (25% to 30% mortality reduction when used early).[5,11,34] Other trials[10,24] have compared thrombolytic agents with and without other adjunctive interventions (e.g., aspirin, beta blockers). The latter studies have resulted in controversies regarding the thrombolytic agent of choice and the timing or method of administration. However, it is generally agreed that (1) the promptness of administration of a thrombolytic agent after the onset of symptoms is more important than the choice of agent and (2) adjunctive drugs add to the mortality reduction observed with thrombolysis alone.

The generally accepted ECG criteria for thrombolytic therapy are ST-segment elevation of more than 1 mm in two or more contiguous limb leads or greater than 2 mm of elevation in two or more contiguous precordial leads, either persisting after sublingual nitroglycerin administration. It is well recognized that left bundle-branch block (LBBB) may obscure the diagnosis of acute MI because of the secondary ST-segment and T-wave changes that accompany altered ventricular depolarization. Criteria have been reported to identify acute MI in the presence of an LBBB, but although generally highly specific, they are insensitive in making this diagnosis.[29,30] Due to this problem with recognition of acute MI in the setting of LBBB (either old or new) and the high mortality encountered when LBBB develops during the course of acute infarction, thrombolytic administration is recommended in patients with a history suggestive of acute cardiac ischemia and LBBB, regardless of whether it is new or old.[14,30]

The time to administration of thrombolytic therapy is critical for achieving maximum benefit. The best outcomes have been observed when the thrombolytic agent is administered within 4 to 6 hours of symptom onset. There still may be some benefit if the agent is given later (up to 12 hours), especially if symptoms have had a "stuttering" character (i.e., an intermittent resolution and recurrence of chest pain).

The patient who is a candidate for thrombolytic therapy but has a contraindication to its use (Table 131.9) should be considered for immediate coronary angiography and percutaneous transluminal angioplasty (PTCA).

Patient age alone should not be a consideration in the decision to administer a thrombolytic agent. Mortality with acute MI increases with age, and it can be reduced significantly with thrombolytic therapy.[14]

Choice of Thrombolytic Agent

Although thrombolytic agents have been shown unequivocally to reduce mortality from acute MI when compared with placebo or therapy previously considered "standard," the best agent to use in the setting of acute MI is undecided; the choice remains with each practitioner (Table 131.10). Tissue plasminogen activator (TPA) is, however, generally preferred in patients who have previously received streptokinase to avoid the risk of allergic reactions. Streptokinase is associated with a lower incidence of stroke and central nervous system hemorrhage in the elderly. An accelerated regimen of TPA (alteplase) administration is now routinely used in most centers (see Table 131.10).[12] Reteplase (a mutant wild-type TPA that lacks several of the

TABLE 131.9. Thrombolytic Therapy in Acute Myocardial Infarction

INDICATIONS
Chest pain of >30 min and <12 h duration
ST elevation ≥1 mm in two or more contiguous limb leads
ST elevation ≥2 mm in two or more contiguous precordial leads
New bundle-branch block
CONTRAINDICATIONS
Absolute (consider for immediate PTCA or CABG)
Altered level of consciousness
Suspected aortic dissection
History of hemorrhagic cerebrovascular accident, known intracranial aneurysm, arteriovenous malformation, or central nervous system neoplasm
Spinal or intracranial surgery within 2 mo
Active internal bleeding (e.g., gastrointestinal)
Persistent uncontrolled hypertension (systolic >200 mm Hg, diastolic >120 mm Hg)
Trauma or surgery that could result in bleeding in a closed space, within 2 wk
Recent head trauma
Known bleeding disorder
Pregnancy
Prolonged or traumatic CPR during current MI
Diabetic hemorrhagic retinopathy
Allergy to streptokinase (not a contraindication to use of other agents)
Relative
Active peptic ulcer disease
History of ischemic or embolic cerebrovascular accident
Current use of oral anticoagulants
Major trauma or surgery within previous 2 wk to 2 mo
History of chronic, uncontrolled hypertension (diastolic >100 mm Hg), treated or untreated
Recent subclavian or internal jugular venous cannulation

Data from Theroux P, Waters D, Qui S, et al. Aspirin versus heparin to prevent myocardial infarction during the acute phase of unstable angina. *Circulation* 1993;88:2045.

TABLE 131.10. Thrombolytic Agents

STREPTOKINASE
Administer 1.5 million U over 1 hour, and heparin 5,000–7,500 U i.v. bolus and 1,000 U/h (keep PTT 1½ to 2 times normal).
TPA
Standard regimen Administer 10-mg i.v. bolus, then 90 mg over 3 h. Administer heparin as for streptokinase. Accelerated regimen Administer 15-mg bolus, then 0.75 mg/kg (up to 50 mg) over 30 min, then 0.5 mg/kg (up to 35 mg) over 60 min. Administer heparin as for streptokinase.
ANISOYLATED PLASMINOGEN–STREPTOKINASE ACTIVATOR COMPLEX
Administer 30 U over 3 min. Administer heparin as for streptokinase, 4 to 6 h later.

i.v., intravenous; PTT, partial thromboplastin time; TPA, tissue plasminogen activator.

molecular "domains" of alteplase, resulting in a longer plasma half-life) can be administered as a double bolus but has not been shown to be more effective than alteplase.[17] Approximately 25% of patients receiving a thrombolytic agent will not recanalize the obstructed coronary artery, and approximately 20% will reocclude after successful reperfusion. ECG and biochemical marker changes after thrombolytic administration have been shown to be relatively reliable noninvasive markers of thrombolytic effect.[9,26]

Primary PTCA (i.e., used as the initial intervention to achieve coronary reperfusion) has been the subject of much recent investigation and appears to be at least as effective as, and possibly superior to, thrombolytic therapy. It is the reperfusion method of choice when acute MI is complicated by cardiogenic shock.[4]

Adjunctive Therapy with Thrombolysis

In addition to heparin, aspirin, and thrombolytics, beta blockers and the angiotensin converting enzyme (ACE) inhibitors have been shown to decrease both short- and long-term mortality after acute MI.[18] Although a metaanalysis of published studies suggested that nitroglycerin and magnesium also were beneficial in the setting of acute MI, benefit has not been demonstrated in a large clinical randomized clinical trial.[18,20] Nitroglycerin use for pain relief in acute MI is given according to the same regimen for the management of pain in unstable angina and non-Q-wave infarction (see previous discussion).

There have been a number of randomized trials of intravenous beta blockade initiated early in the course of acute MI.[2,18] A metaanalysis of such studies indicates that early intravenous beta blockade reduces mortality by 13% by day 7 of treatment. Continued chronic oral therapy decreases long-term mortality. Beta blockers are contraindicated in the setting of obstructive airway disease (asthma or chronic obstructive pulmonary disease), atrioventricular (AV) block, hypotension, congestive heart failure, or known allergy. Esmolol, a beta blocker with an ultrashort half-life, may be administered by infusion and titrated to effect if beta blockade is necessary in patients with airways disease or depressed MI. Typical dosing schedules are shown in Table 131.11.

The ACE inhibitors (captopril, enalapril, and lisinopril have been most extensively studied) have also been shown to improve survival after acute MI. Patients with large infarctions or a history of LV dysfunction appear to derive the most benefit

TABLE 131.11. Dosing of Beta Blockers

ATENOLOL
Administer 10 mg i.v. (5 mg i.v. every 10 min). After 15 min, give 50 mg orally.
METOPROLOL
Administer 5 mg every 5 to 10 min to a total dose of 15 mg. After 15 min, give 100 mg orally.

i.v., intravenously.

from this intervention. The mechanism of benefit is related to the vasodilator and neurohumoral effects of these drugs. The ACE inhibitors appear to modify maladaptive ventricular remodeling, thereby decreasing LV volume, and to attenuate the effects of activation of the renin–angiotensin system during the early infarct period, and may improve collateral coronary flow.[1] Although early use of these drugs (within 24 hours) is recommended, particularly in selected populations, they are rarely given in the emergency department.

Complications of Acute Ischemia or Infarction

Arrhythmias

Cardiac rhythm disturbances are common during unstable angina or acute infarction.[3] The most common arrhythmias are of ventricular origin. Premature ventricular contractions (PVCs) are noted in 80% to 100% of patients who experience an acute MI. Ventricular ectopy should be treated with intravenous lidocaine. One regimen consists of an initial bolus of 1 mg/kg followed by an infusion of 1 to 4 mg/min. The major side effect of lidocaine is neurotoxicity, typically manifested as altered mental status and seizures. In low cardiac output states, lidocaine metabolism is decreased, and usual therapeutic doses may be toxic. Thus, in this setting, the initial intravenous loading dose should be halved and the continuous infusion should be started at 1 mg/min.

Lidocaine should not be used prophylactically. Such use does not improve mortality and may actually contribute to the morbidity and mortality of acute MI. Indications for the use of lidocaine include frequent PVCs (more than 6 per minute), closely coupled PVCs (R-on-T phenomenon), multiform PVC, and nonsustained ventricular tachycardia.

Bradyarrhythmias or tachyarrhythmias that compromise systemic or myocardial perfusion require immediate therapy (see Chapters 134 and 135).

Conduction Disturbances

Second- and third-degree AV block may occur during either inferior or anterior infarction. In the setting of inferior MI, these conduction disturbances are normally associated with an increase in vagal tone and are usually transient and responsive to atropine. The abrupt occurrence of complete heart block is rare. In anterior MI, high-degree AV block is due to ischemia of the conduction pathways, and complete heart block may occur abruptly. Bundle-branch blocks are usually associated with anterior infarction. The indications for temporary artificial pacing in the setting of acute ischemia are listed in Table 131.12.

Cardiogenic Shock

LV pump failure begins to occur when approximately 40% of the ventricular muscle mass has been lost. Severe contractile dysfunction results and necessitates the use of a number of therapeutic interventions (see Chapter 132). Studies suggest that PTCA may improve both short- and long-term outcome; this in-

TABLE 131.12. Indications for Temporary Pacing in Acute Myocardial Infarction

INDICATED
Mobitz II AVB
Complete AVB
New RBBB in anterior MI
RBBB plus LAFB
RBBB plus LPFB
LBBB plus first-degree AVB
Drug-resistant symptomatic bradycardia
NOT INDICATED
First-degree AVB
Wenckebach second-degree AVB
Old LBBB
Old RBBB
CONTROVERSIAL
New LBBB
New RBBB in infenor MI

AVB, atrioventricular block; LBBB, left bundle-branch block; RBBB, right bundle-branch block; LAFB, left anterior fascicular block; LPFB, left posterior fascicular block; MI, myocardial infarction.

tervention should be considered early in the course of management in selected patients.[4]

DISPOSITION

All patients with suspected acute myocardial ischemic syndromes should be admitted to the hospital, typically to an intensive care unit or CCU. Recent studies have shown that a low-risk group of patients may be identified, based on clinical and ECG findings, that could be cared for in an intermediate care unit or a monitored short-term emergency department observation unit.[27,35]

When acute MI is suspected, the consulting cardiologist should be contacted as soon as possible to facilitate intervention therapy with intravenous thrombolytic or emergent PTCA, as indicated.

Patients in the acute phase of infarction or with unstable angina should not be transferred to another facility unless definitive care cannot be given at the institution where the initial evaluation is performed. In such an instance, transfer in an appropriately equipped vehicle is justified after initial treatment and stabilization. The transport team should include personnel trained in advanced cardiac life support. It has been demonstrated that patients having an acute MI can be safely transported to a referral center for thrombolytic or interventional therapy.

Patients discharged from the emergency department with a diagnosis of stable angina or atypical chest pain should be referred to a cardiologist for further evaluation (e.g., EST and ambulatory ECG monitoring).

COMMON PITFALLS

- Missed MI is the fourth most common cause of malpractice suits filed against emergency physicians, and it ranks first with respect to monetary awards.
- For patients in whom the diagnosis is uncertain, the threshold for admission should be low. Due to the limited diagnostic tools available in the emergency setting, only a minority of patients admitted to the hospital with suspected acute IHD ("rule out MI") actually have an acute infarct.
- A single ECG or CK-MB determination cannot be used to rule out the diagnosis of acute MI.
- Comparison of a current ECG to a prior or baseline ECG should not be relied on to exclude acute IHD.
- If the patient meets appropriate criteria, reperfusion therapy should be administered as soon as possible. Every institution needs to address the issues of appropriate early triage of ambulatory patients with chest pain and rapid access to 12-lead electrocardiography.

References

1. ACE Inhibitor Myocardial Infarction Collaborative Group. Indications for ACE inhibitors in the early treatment of acute myocardial infarction. Systemic overview of individual data from 100,000 patients in randomized trials. *Circulation* 1998;97:2202.
2. A Report of the American College of Cardiology/American Heart Association Task Force on Practice Guidelines (Committee on Management of Acute Myocardial Infarction). ACC/AHA guidelines for the management of patients with acute myocardial infarction: Executive summary. *Circulation* 1996; 94:2341.
3. Aufderheide TP. Arrhythmias associated with acute myocardial infarction and thrombolysis. *Emerg Med Clin North Am* 1998;16:583.
4. Berger PB, Tuttle RH, Holmes DR, et al. One-year survival among patients with acute myocardial infarction complicated by cardiogenic shock, and its relation to early revascularization. Results from the GUSTO-I Trial. *Circulation* 1999;99:873.
5. Boersma E, Mass AC, Deckers JW, et al. Early thrombolytic treatment in acute myocardial infarction: reappraisal of the golden hour. *Lancet* 1996;348:771.
6. Braunwald E. Unstable angina. An etiologic approach to management. *Circulation* 1998;98:2219.
7. Braunwald E, Mark DB, Jones RH, et al. *Diagnosing and managing unstable angina. Quick reference guide for clinicians, number 10 (amended).* AHCPR Publication No. 94-0603. Rockville MD, 1994.
8. Char DM, Israel E, Ladenson J. Early laboratory indicators of acute myocardial infarction. *Emerg Med Clin North Am* 1998;16:1998.
9. Christenson RH, Ohman EM, Topol EJ, et al. Assessment of coronary reperfusion after thrombolysis with a model combining myoglobin, creatine kinase-MB, and clinical variables. *Circulation* 1997;96:1776.
10. Cohen M, Demers C, Gurfinkel EP, et al. A comparison of low-molecular-weight heparin with unfractionated heparin for unstable coronary artery disease. *N Engl J Med* 1997;337:447.
11. Collins R, Peto R, Baigent C, et al. Aspirin, heparin, and fibrinolytic therapy in suspected acute myocardial infarction. *N Engl J Med* 1997;336:847.
12. Continuous Infusion Versus Double-Bolus Administration of Alteplase (COBALT) Investigators. A comparison of continuous infusion of alteplase with double-bolus administration for acute myocardial infarction. *N Engl J Med* 1997;337:1124.
13. *DRG Handbook.* Washington, DC: Academic Press, 1997.
14. Fibrinolytic Therapy Trialists' (FTT) Collaborative Group. Indications for fibrinolytic therapy in suspected acute myocardial infarction: collaborative overview of early mortality and major morbidity results from all randomized trials of more than 1000 patients. *Lancet* 1994;343:311.
15. Garber AM, Solomon NA. Cost-effectiveness of alternative test strategies for the diagnosis of coronary artery disease. *Ann Intern Med* 1999;130:719.
16. Gibler WB, Wilcox RG, Bode C, et al. Prospective use of glycoprotein IIb/IIIa receptor blockers in the emergency department setting. *Ann Emerg Med* 1998;32:712.

16a. Gibler WB, Runyon JP, Levy RC, et al. A rapid diagnostic and treatment center for patients with chest pain in the emergency department. *Ann Emerg Med* 1995;25:1.

17. Global Use of Strategies to Open Coronary Arteries (GUSTO III) Investigators. A comparison of reteplase with alteplase for acute myocardial infarction. *N Engl J Med* 1997;337:1118.
18. Hennekens CH, Albert CM, Godried SL, et al. Adjunctive drug therapy of acute myocardial infarction—evidence from clinical trials. *N Engl J Med* 1996;335:1660.
19. Hirsh J. Low-molecular-weight heparin. A review of the results of recent studies of the treatment of venous thromboembolism and unstable angina. *Circulation* 1998;98:1575.
20. ISIS-4 (Fourth International Study of Infarct Survival) Collaborative Group. ISIS-4: a randomized factorial trial assessing early oral captopril, oral mononitrate, and intravenous magnesium sulphate in 58,050 patients with suspected acute myocardial infarction. *Lancet* 1995;345:669.
21. Jesse RL, Kontos MC. Evaluation of chest pain in the emergency department. *Curr Probl Cardiol* 1997;22:149.
22. Kuntz KM, Fleischmann KE, Hunink MGM, et al. Cost-effectiveness of diagnostic strategies for patients with chest pain. *Ann Intern Med* 1999;130:709.
23. Muller JE, Kaufman PG, Leupker RV, et al. Mechanisms precipitating acute cardiac events. Review and recommendations of an NHLBI workshop. *Circulation* 1997;96:3233.
24. Osler A, Whooley MA, Oier J, et al. Adding heparin to aspirin reduces the incidence of myocardial infarction and death in patients with unstable angina. A meta-analysis. *JAMA* 1996;276:811.

25. Panju AA, Hemmelgarn BR, Guyatt GH, et al. Is this patient having a myocardial infarction? *JAMA* 1998;280:1256.
26. Purcell IF, Newall N, Farrer M. Change in ST segment elevation 60 minutes after thrombolytic initiation predicts clinical outcome as accurately as later electrocardiographic changes. *Heart* 1997;78:465.
27. Roberts R, Fromm RE. Management of acute coronary syndromes based on risk stratification by biochemical markers. An idea whose time has come. *Circulation* 1998;98:1831.
28. Selker HP, Zalenski RJ, Antman EM, et al. An evaluation of technologies for identifying acute cardiac ischemia in the emergency department: executive summary of a National Heart Attack Alert Program Working Group Report. *Ann Emerg Med* 1997;29:1.
29. Sgarbossa EB, Pinski SL, Barbagelata A, et al. Electrocardiographic diagnosis of evolving acute myocardial infarction in the presence of left bundle-branch block. *N Engl J Med* 1996;334:481.
30. Shilipak MG, Lyons WL, Go AS, et al. Should the electrocardiogram be used to guide therapy for patients with left bundle-branch block and suspected acute myocardial infarction? *JAMA* 1999;282:714.
31. Theroux P, Fuster V. Acute coronary syndromes. Unstable angina and non-Q-wave myocardial infarction. *Circulation* 1998;97:1195.
32. TIMI IIIB Investigators. Effects of tissue plasminogen activator and a comparison of early invasive and conservative strategies in unstable angina and non-Q-wave myocardial infarction. Results of the TIMI IIIB Trial. *Circulation* 1994;89:1545.
33. Topol EJ. Toward a new frontier in myocardial reperfusion therapy. Emerging platelet preeminence. *Circulation* 1998;97:211.
34. White HD, Van de Werf FJJ. Thrombolysis for acute myocardial infarction. *Circulation* 1998;97:1632.
35. Zalenski RJ, Shamsa F, Pede KJ. Evaluation and risk stratification of patients with chest pain in the emergency department. Predictors of life-threatening events. *Emerg Med Clin North Am* 1998;16:495.
35a. Zalenski RJ, McCarren M, Roberts R, et al. An evaluation of a chest pain diagnostic protocol to exclude acute cardiac ischemia in the emergency department. *Arch Intern Med* 1997;157:1085.
36. Zimmerman J, Fromm R, Meyer D, et al. Diagnostic Marker Cooperative Study for the diagnosis of myocardial infarction. *Circulation* 1999;99:1671.

CHAPTER 132
Cardiogenic Shock

Brian R. Tiffany and Robert C. Jorden

The clinical definition of cardiogenic shock is hypotension with evidence of impaired perfusion in the setting of acute myocardial infarction (AMI). Specifically, a blood pressure less than 90 mm Hg (or a drop of more than 80 mm Hg in systolic pressure in a known hypertensive patient) with accompanying confusion; cold, moist skin; cyanosis; and oliguria defines the syndrome. [7,22] Approximately 7.5% of all patients with AMI develop this complication, which, in historic series, carried a mortality of 80% to 90%.[3] Today, despite diagnostic and therapeutic advances, cardiogenic shock remains the leading cause of death in AMI.[7]

A variety of other causes, such as myocardial contusion, myocarditis, and cardiomyopathy, can produce cardiogenic shock, but the majority of cases result from coronary atherosclerosis and AMI. Infarction can cause shock in several ways. Papillary muscle dysfunction or rupture can result in severe mitral insufficiency. An infarcted interventricular septum can rupture, resulting in a hemodynamically significant left-to-right shunt. Transmural infarction can cause rupture of the ventricular wall into the pericardium with cardiac tamponade. A right ventricular infarction can be extensive enough to impair left ventricular filling.

By far, the most common cause of cardiogenic shock, however, is extensive myocardial necrosis. When more than about 40% of the left ventricle is infarcted, the ability to maintain the systemic circulation is impaired. [8,22] This amount of damage can result from a single massive infarction or from an acute infarction superimposed on a previous one. The compensatory mechanisms that normally act to prevent hypotension can worsen the situation. Specifically, catecholamine release produces tachycardia, vasoconstriction, and increased cardiac contractility, all of which increase the workload of the left ventricle and increase myocardial oxygen demand, potentially causing extension of the infarct and further compromising left ventricular function.

CLINICAL PRESENTATION

Often, the clinical presentation is straightforward: clinical shock associated with the characteristic pain and associated symptoms of ischemia. In some patients, however, the diagnosis may be obscured, as, for example, when the patient has an altered sensorium and cannot communicate effectively, or when chest pain is not severe or is overshadowed by other symptoms. Depending on the degree of decompensation, physical findings vary from minimal signs of shock to stupor, cyanosis, and florid pulmonary edema. Not only can signs and symptoms vary from patient to patient, but they can also rapidly deteriorate in a given patient. Hence, close observation and repeated examinations are needed whenever the diagnosis is suspected.

DIFFERENTIAL DIAGNOSIS

Massive pulmonary embolism complicated by hypotension should be considered in the differential diagnosis of cardiogenic shock, although the nature of the pain of pulmonary embolism is not commonly characteristic of ischemia. The presence of cyanosis and tachypnea could support either diagnosis, but the absence of auscultatory findings favors pulmonary embolism over a cardiac etiology. Arterial blood gas analysis is probably not helpful in distinguishing the two entities, but an electrocardiogram (ECG), a chest radiograph, and an echocardiogram may prove valuable.

Thoracic aortic dissection may be mistaken for cardiogenic shock under certain circumstances. Although hypertension is the rule with dissection, hypotension can occur if the dissection extends retrograde into the pericardial sac and causes tamponade. Rupture of the dissection into the chest or abdominal cavity also produces shock, but this complication is usually an abrupt, terminal event. Pulmonary edema is not often present with aortic dissection but can occur from aortic insufficiency induced by dissection of the aortic root and distortion of the annulus. A chest film and ECG should help to distinguish the two diagnoses; ultimately, an aortic angiogram or a transesophageal echocardiogram confirms or rules out dissection.

Esophageal perforation can cause many of the signs and symptoms of cardiogenic shock, including retrosternal chest pain, diaphoresis, and respiratory distress, but shock is not universally present. When shock does occur, it is due to septic complications, which can occur within hours but are usually more delayed in onset. Absence of pulmonary edema and the presence of a fever and precordial crunch favor esophageal perforation over cardiogenic shock. Pleural effusion with or without pneumothorax also supports the diagnosis.

Pericarditis complicated by effusion and tamponade can mimic cardiogenic shock. The more insidious course of pericarditis, the absence of pulmonary edema, and the typical ECG findings help to distinguish it from cardiogenic shock. An echocardiogram can establish or exclude the diagnosis.

Acute bacterial endocarditis complicated by severe mitral or aortic insufficiency is also a potential diagnosis. Fever, if present, and perhaps a more indolent course, support endocarditis over cardiogenic shock, but distinguishing between the two entities may be difficult. An echocardiogram showing valve vegetations can establish a diagnosis of endocarditis, but normal findings do not rule it out.

Other, less specific conditions should also be considered in the differential diagnosis. Shock of any etiology that results in coronary insufficiency and ischemic chest pain could be mistaken for cardiogenic shock. Similarly, noncardiogenic pulmonary edema with hypoxemia and secondary myocardial oxygen deprivation could suggest an early phase of cardiogenic shock before hemodynamic decompensation has occurred. A rapid response to treatment directed at the true underlying cause should distinguish these conditions from cardiogenic shock.

EMERGENCY DEPARTMENT EVALUATION

As in any critically ill patient, diagnostic evaluation of patients with cardiogenic shock is initiated during stabilization. Depending on the degree of decompensation on presentation, a variety of diagnostic investigations should be undertaken, but performing a detailed history and physical examination is an important first step. A history of pain consistent with myocardial ischemia should direct the physical examination toward findings that support a diagnosis of cardiogenic shock, such as pulmonary congestion, jugular venous distention, a mitral insufficiency murmur, decreased level of consciousness, and poorly perfused skin. The examination should be repeated frequently to detect deterioration.

Important studies to perform include an ECG (with a V_{4R} lead to detect right ventricular infarction), a portable chest radiograph, arterial blood gas analysis, and baseline complete blood count and electrolyte determination. Cardiac isoenzymes should be measured. The ECG can be helpful if it is diagnostic of an acute infarction, but it may show only a nonspecific pattern. The chest film may show early changes of congestive failure or a more fulminant picture of pulmonary edema. Cardiomegaly may or may not be present, depending on whether the patient has preexisting congestive heart failure or cardiomyopathy. Arterial blood gas values can help gauge the severity and progression of decompensation. Although they are not helpful in establishing a specific diagnosis, they can be invaluable in directing therapeutic interventions such as endotracheal intubation.

Bedside echocardiography is of enormous value in the evaluation of the shock patient.[17] Identification of an akinetic or dyskinetic area of the left ventricle that corresponds to an area of ischemia or infarction on the ECG, although not specific, supports a diagnosis of cardiogenic shock. Conversely, normal results all but rule out acute transmural infarction and cardiogenic shock. The echocardiogram can also effectively diagnose surgically correctable causes of cardiogenic shock, such as ruptured interventricular septum or ruptured papillary muscle.

EMERGENCY DEPARTMENT MANAGEMENT

The management of cardiogenic shock consists of three components: prevention, supportive care, and myocardial reperfusion. The basis for these measures is the fact that an area of infarction is not homogeneous. Rather, necrotic tissue is surrounded by and intermingled with ischemic yet potentially viable tissue. Preservation of this periinfarction zone can save enough myocardial function to prevent pump failure. Thus, interventions that favorably affect myocardial oxygen supply and demand should prove beneficial.

The most effective way to treat cardiogenic shock is to prevent it. Measures should be taken to minimize infarct size in all patients with acute infarction. Tachyarrhythmias, symptomatic bradycardia, and hypertension, conditions that increase myocardial oxygen consumption, should be aggressively treated. The routine use of beta blockers such as atenolol and metoprolol is of proven value. Large, well-controlled studies have documented the efficacy of beta blockers in limiting infarct size and improving survival.[12,13] Even so, data from the National Registry of Myocardial Infarction suggest that a surprisingly low number of AMI patients receive beta blockers early in their treatment.[16]

Supportive care is geared toward maintaining oxygenation and vital organ perfusion. In the early stages, supplemental oxygen may be sufficient to accomplish the first goal. However, if the patient deteriorates and tires, active airway management may be necessary. The usual clinical and blood gas parameters are used to determine when intubation is indicated.

Maintaining an adequate blood pressure is far more complex. The measures normally used to restore pressure can adversely affect myocardial oxygen consumption, and thus worsen the underlying problem. To complicate matters further, emergency physicians do not usually have ready access to measurements of cardiac output and left heart pressures. As a result, the clinician must decide between administering empiric therapy that could be deleterious, taking the time to place a Swan-Ganz catheter, or transferring an unstable patient to an intensive care unit. The patient's condition, however, may force the issue and mandate immediate treatment without the benefit of hemodynamic measurements. Newer noninvasive modalities, such as measurement of cardiac output by thoracic electrical bioimpedance, may be of great value in making these decisions.[20]

Under these circumstances, it is reasonable to attempt volume expansion by giving small boluses of normal saline solution. Some patients in cardiogenic shock have normal or low left ventricular end-diastolic pressures, and although most do not respond to volume expansion, it is nevertheless acceptable to initiate careful incremental saline infusions as a first step. If the patient is already in pulmonary edema, one can presume an elevated wedge pressure and avoid a fluid bolus.

If fluid challenge is ineffective, a vasopressor is used. Dobutamine, considered the drug of choice by many authorities, has the advantage of increasing cardiac output and lowering left ventricular filling pressure while not increasing the pulse rate or otherwise increasing oxygen demand. Dobutamine decreases vascular resistance, improving cardiac output without increasing blood pressure. This property is problematic at lower pressures, when coronary blood flow is jeopardized. If the blood pressure remains low despite adequate doses of dobutamine, dopamine is added to the regimen. Both vasopressors are titrated to the desired clinical effect. Amrinone and milrinone, bipyridine derivatives that cause vasodilation and have positive inotropic effects, have also been effective in improving cardiac output. Published experience with these drugs in cardiogenic shock to date is limited, however.

If a Swan-Ganz catheter and arterial line can be inserted, more precise management is possible. An optimal filling pressure of 18 to 24 cm H_2O should be achieved through volume expansion before considering vasopressors. Vasodilators such as intravenous nitroglycerin and nitroprusside can be added to decrease afterload, and thus left ventricular work and oxygen consumption. Extreme caution must be exercised when using these potent drugs because of their hypotensive effects. All hemodynamic parameters must be monitored continuously and drugs titrated carefully.

Furosemide and morphine may also be of help. The anxiolytic effect of morphine relieves apprehension and may help to reduce tachycardia. However, the preload and afterload reduction caused by morphine, although potentially helpful, may be detrimental. Similarly, furosemide may cause deterioration by reducing preload excessively through venodilatation and diuresis. Because of these hazards, it is probably wise to avoid these drugs unless left-sided heart pressures can be monitored.

For patients who remain hemodynamically unstable despite all of these interventions, insertion of an intraaortic balloon pump (IABP) can be considered. IABP supports the diastolic blood pressure, thus improving coronary perfusion, and it reduces afterload and therefore myocardial oxygen consumption. However, in spite of the widespread acceptance and use of this modality, only limited evidence supports its benefit in cardiogenic shock patients,[1] unless in conjunction with a revascularization strategy.[18]

Other circulatory assist devices, such as the Hemopump (a device placed by means of the femoral artery and threaded across the aortic valve into the left ventricle), percutaneous cardiopulmonary bypass, and various surgically implantable ventricular assist devices, have also been used as temporizing measures.[19] Unfortunately, neither pharmacologic manipulation nor the use of these devices has lowered the mortality of AMI complicated by cardiogenic shock.[9] Nevertheless, both interventions can be helpful or even essential in maintaining patients until more definitive treatment can be instituted.

Although data are equivocal, it appears that reperfusion of the infarct zone is the only therapy that improves survival.[14] Toward that end, thrombolytic therapy has had disappointing results in patients who develop cardiogenic shock in the setting of AMI, showing no significant reduction in mortality.[5,6,11] The reason appears to be a low rate (less than 50%) of reestablishing patency of the infarct-related vessel.[5] The low reperfusion rate is probably related to the low perfusion pressure inherent in the shock state.[6] Patients in whom thrombolysis is successful demonstrate a substantial reduction in mortality.

In contrast to thrombolysis, percutaneous transluminal coronary angioplasty (PTCA) has been more effective. Several studies have demonstrated a reperfusion rate of about 70% to 90% and a 6-month mortality rate in the range of 30% to 50% when the procedure is successful.[2,11] This is a vast improvement over the 80% mortality rate for noninvasive management. A large-scale, randomized trial of PTCA and emergency coronary bypass grafting in cardiogenic shock is underway (the SHOCK trial).[10]

In summary, cardiogenic shock is a highly lethal condition, with an 80% mortality rate that is usually unaffected by supportive measures. Reestablishing perfusion to the infarcted area is the only intervention with demonstrated efficacy. The role of emergency physicians in salvaging these critically ill patients lies in early recognition, prompt application of stabilizing and supportive measures, administration of thrombolytic agents where appropriate, and early involvement of a cardiologist to consider revascularization strategies.

DISPOSITION

Role of the Consultant

The role of the cardiology consultant in patients with cardiogenic shock is crucial. Difficult decisions must be made quickly about additional resuscitative efforts, invasive monitoring, and the feasibility of coronary angiography and reperfusion. Therefore, once the diagnosis is seriously considered, consultation should be requested immediately.

Indications for Admission

There is no difficulty in deciding whether admission is needed for these patients, but determining disposition within the hospital is more challenging. Depending on the resources and policies of the institution, the patient should go either to the cardiac care unit or directly to the cardiac catheterization laboratory. Regardless of the destination, transport must be expeditious, and the patient must be monitored and accompanied by appropriate resuscitative equipment and capable physician personnel.

Transfer Considerations

Transfer of patients from one institution to another is hazardous and doomed to failure unless some hemodynamic stability has been achieved. Ideally, transport should be done by a specialized team, including physicians capable of transporting and inserting a balloon pump and of instituting and maintaining supportive care and invasive monitoring. Transport under less favorable conditions carries a significant risk of a less favorable outcome.

COMMON PITFALLS

- Failing to diagnose cardiogenic shock promptly in its early stages is probably the most significant management error. Not recognizing the diagnosis until decompensation is severe may preclude any meaningful intervention, due to irreversible deterioration in cardiac function.
- Failing to recognize right ventricular infarction or surgically correctable causes of cardiogenic shock is also a serious error. The former condition requires more vigorous volume expansion; the latter ones require surgery. Because the prognoses for both entities, however, are better than for shock related to extensive left ventricular necrosis, patient survival is seriously affected if these conditions are not accurately diagnosed.
- Liberal use of morphine and diuretics, as might be implemented for patients with pulmonary edema, may produce untoward hemodynamic effects. Morphine can also cause respiratory depression or a deterioration in mental status, which makes aspiration more likely. These drugs should be used cautiously, preferably while monitoring left-sided heart pressures and cardiac output.
- Applying medical antishock trousers (MAST trousers) to treat cardiogenic shock should be avoided. MAST trousers cause an increase in afterload that further taxes the compromised left ventricle.

References

1. Bates ER, Topol EJ. Limitations of thrombolytic therapy for acute MI complicated by congestive heart failure and cardiogenic shock. *J Am Coll Cardiol* 1991;18:1077.
2. Becker RC. Hemodynamic, mechanical, and metabolic determinants of thrombolytic efficacy: a theoretic framework for assessing the limitations of thrombolysis in patients with cardiogenic shock. *Am Heart J* 1993;125:919.
3. Bengtson JR, Kaplan AJ, Pieper KS, et al. Prognosis in cardiogenic shock after acute MI in the interventional era. *J Am Coll Cardiol* 1992;20:1482.
4. Eckman MH, Wong JB, Salem DN, et al. Direct angioplasty for acute MI: a review of outcomes in clinical subsets. *Ann Intern Med* 1992;117:667.
5. Gacioch GM, Ellis SG, Lee L, et al. Cardiogenic shock complicating acute MI: the use of coronary angioplasty and the integration of the new support devices into patient management. *J Am Coll Cardiol* 1992;19:647.
6. Goldberg RJ, Gore JM, Alpert JS, et al. Cardiogenic shock after acute MI: incidence and mortality from a community-wide perspective, 1975–1988. *N Engl J Med* 1991;325:1117.
7. Gruppo Italiano per lo Studio della Streptokinase nell'Infarto Miocardio (GSSI). Effectiveness of intravenous thrombolytic treatment in acute MI. *Lancet* 1986;1:397.

8. Guyton RA, Arcidi JM, Langford DA, et al. Emergency coronary bypass for cardiogenic shock. *Coron Artery Surg* 1987;76:22.
9. International Collaborative Study Group. Reduction of infarct size with the early use of timolol in acute MI. *N Engl J Med* 1984;9:310.
10. International Study of Infarct Survival. Randomized trial of intravenous atenolol among 16,027 cases of suspected acute MI: ISIS-1. *Lancet* 1986;2:57.
11. Klein LW. Optimal therapy for cardiogenic shock: the emerging role of coronary angioplasty. *J Am Coll Cardiol* 1992;19:654.
12. Klocke RK, Mager G, Kux A, et al. Effects of a 24-hour milrinone infusion in patients with severe heart failure and cardiogenic shock as a function of the hemodynamic initial condition. *Am Heart J* 1991;121:1965.
13. Lee L, Erbel R, Brown TM, et al. Multicenter registry of angioplasty therapy of cardiogenic shock: initial and long-term survival. *J Am Coll Cardiol* 1991;17:599.
14. Massachusetts Medical Society. Reducing mortality in patients with extensive MI. *N Engl J Med* 1991;325:1166.
15. McGhie AI, Goldstein RA. Pathogenesis and management of acute heart failure and cardiogenic shock: role of inotropic therapy. *Chest* 1992;102:626.
16. Miami Trial Research Group. Metoprolol in acute myocardial infarction (MIAMI): a randomized placebo-controlled international trial. *Eur Heart J* 1985;6:199.
17. Moosvi AR, Khaja F, Villanueva L, et al. Early revascularization improves survival in cardiogenic shock complicating acute MI. *J Am Coll Cardiol* 1992;19:9074.
18. Mueller HS. Inotropic agents in the treatment of cardiogenic shock. *World J Surg* 1985;9:3.
19. Mueller HS, Cohen LS, Braunwald E, et al. Predictors of early morbidity and mortality after thrombolytic therapy of acute MI: analyses of patient subgroups in the Thrombolysis in Myocardial Infarction (TIMI) trial, phase II. *Circulation* 1992;85:1254.
20. O'Connor CM, Mark DB, Califf RM. Combined thrombolysis and angioplasty in acute MI: clinical results. In: Califf RM, Mark DB, Wagner GS, eds. *Acute coronary care in the thrombolytic era*. Chicago: Year Book, 1988.
21. Phillips SJ, Zeff RH, Kongtahworn C, et al. Benefits of combined balloon pumping and percutaneous cardiopulmonary bypass. *Ann Thorac Surg* 1992;54:908.
22. Rackley CE, Russell RO, Mantle JA, et al. Cardiogenic shock. *Cardiovasc Clin* 1981;11:15.
23. Richard C, Ricome JL, Rimailho A. Combined hemodynamic effects of dopamine and dobutamine in cardiogenic shock. *Circulation* 1983;67:620.
24. Seydoux C, Goy JJ, Beuret P, et al. Effectiveness of percutaneous transluminal coronary angioplasty in cardiogenic shock during acute MI. *Am J Cardiol* 1992;69:968.
25. Tan LB, Littler WA. Measurement of cardiac reserve in cardiogenic shock: implications for prognosis and management. 1990;121.
26. Wampler RK, Frazier OH, Lansing AM, et al. Treatment of cardiogenic shock with the Hemopump left ventricular assist device. *Ann Thorac Surg* 1991;52:506.

CHAPTER 133

Congestive Heart Failure and Cor Pulmonale

James T. Nieman

CONGESTIVE HEART FAILURE (LEFT HEART FAILURE)

Congestive heart failure (CHF) is not a single disease but a symptom complex. The pathophysiologic definition of heart failure is "that condition or state in which an abnormality of cardiac function is responsible for failure of the heart to pump blood at a rate commensurate to meet the requirements of the metabolizing tissues." The clinical definition is broader in its scope; that is, it is "a condition in which ventricular dysfunction is accompanied by reduced exercise capacity." The latter definition incorporates less severe forms of ventricular dysfunction that are manifest only during exercise.[22]

The incidence and prevalence of CHF have increased in recent years, despite an overall decrease in cardiovascular mortality in the United States. It has been estimated that more than 3 million Americans have CHF. Approximately 30% to 40% of patients with CHF are hospitalized every year, and CHF is the leading diagnostic-related group among hospitalized patients over the age of 65.[9] CHF is associated with increasing age, and these numbers are likely to increase as the number of elderly persons in the United States continues to increase. Prognosis after onset of clinical symptoms and signs of CHF is poor.[19] When all New York Heart Association (NYHA) classes are considered, the 5-year mortality rate after diagnosis is approximately 60% in men and 45% in women. However, the 1-year mortality rate for NYHA class IV is about 50%. The cause of death may be the result of disease progression or may be the sudden result of ventricular arrhythmias. In the overwhelming majority of these studies, CHF was attributed to left heart failure (LHF). In this section, only LHF is discussed.

The symptoms and signs of LHF are produced by a variety of primary heart diseases as well as systemic diseases that alter left ventricular (LV) anatomy and result in mechanical dysfunction, myocardial contractile failure, or impaired LV filling. The causes of LHF are listed in Table 133.1. Systolic dysfunction, characterized by a low ejection fraction, is the most common form of CHF. Diastolic dysfunction with impaired LV filling has been increasingly recognized as a cause of LHF and is present in 30% to 40% of patients with CHF.[21]

With the advent of early and effective therapy for hypertension in the 1970s, ischemic heart disease (IHD) has become the major cause of acute or chronic LHF in the United States. LHF caused by IHD may have multiple causes, such as loss of ventricular muscle, intermittent ischemia and contractile dysfunction (e.g., papillary muscle dysfunction), ventricular aneurysm formation with paradoxical expansion and increased wall stress, and decreased ventricular diastolic compliance. The cardiomyopathies (dilated, hypertrophic, and restrictive) of both primary (idiopathic) and secondary origin are also becoming an increasingly more frequent cause of heart failure, especially among younger patients.

TABLE 133.1. Functional Classification and Causes of Left Heart Failure

CONTRACTILE DYSFUNCTION
Ischemic heart disease
Idiopathic cardiomyopathy
Myocarditis
SYSTOLIC PRESSURE OVERLOAD
Aortic stenosis
Systemic hypertension
SYSTOLIC VOLUME OVERLOAD
Aortic regurgitation
Mitral regurgitation
RESTRICTED DIASTOLIC FILLING
Mitral stenosis
Left atrial myxoma
Hypertrophic cardiomyopathy
HIGH-OUTPUT STATES
Hyperthyroidism
Anemia
Arteriovenous fistula

TABLE 133.2. Neuroendocrine Changes in Left Heart Failure

Increased circulating catecholamines
Increased angiotensin
Increased aldosterone
Increased arginine vasopressin
Increased atrial natriuretic factor
Increased prostaglandin E2 and prostacyclin

A decrease in effective cardiac output (CO) at normal LV filling pressures is the hemodynamic hallmark of LHF. When CO falls because of such factors as loss of muscle and obstruction to outflow, there are three principal compensatory mechanisms that maintain systemic perfusion: (1) the Frank-Starling principal relating preload to contractile force or CO, (2) ventricular hypertrophy, and (3) central neural and peripheral neurohumoral responses to maintain systemic perfusion pressure and effective intravascular volume.[7]

An increase in systemic vascular resistance and maintenance of effective intravascular volume are accomplished by means of complex neurohumoral compensatory mechanisms. Hormonal changes that occur during LHF are summarized in Table 133.2. Based on measurements of neurohumoral agents in LHF, hemodynamic profiles of LHF patients, and the response to pharmacologic agents that attenuate neurohumoral responses to a decrease in CO, it has become evident that compensatory mechanisms may be maladaptive; that is, reflex responses further impede ejection of blood from the compromised ventricle. Manipulating the compensatory response to a fall in CO (e.g., use of vasodilators and angiotensin converting enzyme inhibitors) has become a therapeutic focus in the management of chronic CHF.[4,5]

CLINICAL PRESENTATION

The typical patient with LHF presents with dyspnea at rest, decreased exercise tolerance, shortness of breath when supine (orthopnea or paroxysmal nocturnal dyspnea), and ankle swelling and weight gain.[11] In acute LHF (acute pulmonary edema), shortness of breath is the major presenting symptom. Clinical findings usually include (1) rales, caused by pulmonary venous hypertension and extravasation of fluid into the pulmonary interstitium and alveoli; (2) a third heart sound, caused by decreased LV compliance; (3) a fourth heart sound, caused by forceful atrial contraction to overcome the rise in LV diastolic pressure (not heard in atrial fibrillation); (4) peripheral edema, the consequence of renal sodium and water retention initiated by hormonal responses; and (5) jugular venous distention (JVD), owing to pulmonary venous hypertension, restricted right ventricular (RV) output, and fluid retention.[18]

No single feature or physical examination finding reliably distinguishes patients with CHF due to systolic dysfunction (decreased ejection fraction, typically less than 40%) from those with dystolic dysfunction (increased left heart filling pressures, pulmonary capillary wedge pressure [PCWP] typically greater than 18 mg Hg). Patients with systolic dysfunction often have increased filling pressures due to a decrease in compliance as well as a decrease in ejection fraction. In addition, many of the clinical symptoms of LHF (e.g., exercise intolerance and pedal edema) may be caused by isolated right heart failure, primary pulmonary disease, obesity, or poor physical conditioning.[3]

Four highly specific clinical findings suggesting a cardiac cause for dyspnea and pedal edema are pulsus alternans; reduced proportional blood pressure (BP) (defined as [systolic BP − diastolic BP]/systolic BP less than 0.25); abnormal BP response to the Valsalva maneuver; and jugular venous distention at rest or during the hepatojugular reflex test.[2,21]

TABLE 133.3. Causes of Dilated Cardiomyopathy

Idiopathic
Connective tissue disease (e.g., systemic lupus erythematosus, scleroderma)
Neuromuscular disorders (muscular dystrophies)
Infection (viral, parasitic, bacterial)
Metabolic (e.g., beriberi, hyperthyroidism or hypothyroidism)
Toxic (alcohol, daunorubicin, cocaine)
Miscellaneous (postpartum)

DIFFERENTIAL DIAGNOSIS

Common causes of LHF are listed in Table 133.1. Constrictive pericarditis and cardiac tamponade are also characterized by impaired diastolic filling and can mimic LHF.

Although systemic hypertension and coronary artery disease are the major causes of LHF in the United States, valvular heart disease (see Chapter 137), especially aortic stenosis and mitral regurgitation, should be considered in the elderly and immigrant populations.

Cardiomyopathies are becoming an increasingly recognized cause of LHF. Patients with a dilated or restrictive cardiomyopathy most commonly present with progressive symptoms. Cardiomegaly is noted on chest radiograph, and electrocardiogram (ECG) findings of four-chamber enlargement and intraventricular conduction defects are commonly seen. Only about 10% of patients with dilated cardiomyopathy have an underlying cause determined after extensive evaluation. Most patients are classified as idiopathic; secondary causes of dilated cardiomyopathy are listed in Table 133.3. Common causes for restrictive cardiomyopathy are listed in Table 133.4; this entity is also commonly idiopathic in origin.[17] In both dilated and restrictive cardiomyopathy, definitive diagnosis typically requires an extensive evaluation, which often includes endomyocardial biopsy. These distinctions are unimportant in acute management, however, if the patient's presentation is that of acute LHF.

Patients with hypertrophic cardiomyopathy rarely present with LHF. Dyspnea on exertion, chest pain that may be anginal in character, palpitations, and syncope are the major symptoms and are caused by a combination of diastolic dysfunction, functional outflow obstruction, and a propensity to dysrhythmias. If LHF does occur, it is most commonly the result of a tachyarrhythmia.

Myocarditis is an uncommon cause for LHF but should be considered in the patient who presents with subacute signs and symptoms of heart failure and who relates a history of an antecedent "viral infection." Coxsackievirus A and B are most commonly implicated. These patients often have elevated serum creatine kinase MB levels because of active myocardial inflammation and necrosis.[15]

TABLE 133.4. Causes of Restrictive Cardiomyopathy

Idiopathic
Amyloidosis
Hemachromatosis
Sarcoidosis
Scleroderma
Metastatic malignancy
Hypereosinophilic syndrome

TABLE 133.5. Exacerbation of Chronic Congestive Heart Failure: Precipitating Factors

Lack of medications (noncompliance)
Dietary indiscretion (increased sodium intake)
Arrhythmias
Myocardial infarction
Infection (increased metabolic demand)
Pulmonary embolism
Anemia
Thyroid disease

Common causes of sudden worsening of symptoms in patients with chronic stable CHF are listed in Table 133.5.

EMERGENCY DEPARTMENT EVALUATION

Other than a carefully obtained history and physical examination, there are few other diagnostic aids available to the emergency physician. The posteroanterior chest radiograph is usually the only readily available ancillary test of value.[2] Radiographic stages that reflect the severity of LHF have been described, but the classic radiographic progression is not always seen. In addition, the chest radiograph may not correlate temporally with the patient's immediate condition; that is, there may be as long as a 12-hour diagnostic lag from the onset of LHF, and a posttherapeutic lag of up to 4 days after clinical resolution.

The earliest radiographic finding is redistribution or "cephalization" of flow. Normally, more blood flow occurs to the dependent portions of the lungs. When PCWP increases to 12 to 18 mm Hg, flow to the lower lung fields is reduced because of the vasoconstriction, and flow to the upper lung fields increases. Redistribution is best detected on an upright film and is most commonly seen in the setting of chronic LHF. When the PCWP is 18 to 25 mm Hg, fluid accumulates in the interstitial spaces, producing Kerley B lines, and the pulmonary vessels are enlarged and their radiographic shadows become blurred. Alveolar edema occurs when the PCWP acutely rises above 25 mm Hg and is recognized by the classic butterfly pattern of bilateral perihilar infiltrates. In all stages, the cardiac silhouette is typically enlarged (cardiothoracic ratio more than 50%), and, in chronic LHF, pleural effusions are common.

The ECG is of limited diagnostic value. In chronic LHF, the ECG usually shows enlargement or hypertrophy of one or more chambers. Intraventricular conduction defects are frequent, and secondary ST-T wave changes caused by ventricular hypertrophy or bundle-branch blocks often preclude accurate diagnosis of acute ischemia or infarction.

Arterial blood gas analysis predictably shows hypoxemia caused by ventilation–perfusion mismatch, but it is of no value in diagnosis and of limited use in guiding therapy. Other blood tests show typical but nondiagnostic abnormalities (e.g., abnormal liver function tests caused by passive hepatic congestion, and hyponatremia caused by retention of excess free water).

EMERGENCY DEPARTMENT MANAGEMENT

All patients with LHF should receive supplemental oxygen, an intravenous line should be placed, heart rate and rhythm should be continuously monitored, and the head of the bed should be elevated. Continuous pulse oximetry should also be used, if available. Treatment is directed primarily toward reducing LV preload or filling pressure, and secondarily toward improving myocardial contractility or decreasing afterload. The sequence of drug therapy and the pace of acute intervention depend on the severity of symptoms.

Patients with mild-to-moderate LHF usually have typical symptoms of varying duration. On examination, patients are normotensive or hypertensive and have bibasilar rales, JVD, third and fourth heart sounds, and pedal edema. Murmurs caused by underlying valvular disease may also be heard. Emergency department therapy would include intravenous furosemide (80 mg) to decrease preload and induce diuresis and sublingual (0.8 to 1.2 mg) or oral (20 to 40 mg) nitroglycerin to increase venous capacitance and lower preload. Urine output and BP should be monitored to detect the response to diuresis as well as any complications of excessive preload reduction (e.g., hypotension). Due to renal vasoconstriction caused by decreased CO, an increase in urine output after diuretic administration may not be immediate and may be delayed for 30 to 60 minutes. If a supraventricular tachyarrhythmia other than sinus tachycardia is present, controlling the ventricular response rate to facilitate ventricular filling also decreases preload and improves CO. The most common supraventricular tachyarrhythmia encountered in LHF is atrial fibrillation, which probably occurs because of atrial distention. In most instances, immediate cardioversion is not necessary, and the ventricular response rate can be controlled quickly with an intravenous calcium channel blocker (e.g., diltiazem).[20] If premature ventricular contractions (PVCs) are present and treatment is indicated, lidocaine can be given (1 mg/kg intravenous bolus, followed by a continuous infusion at a rate of 1 mg/min). A low infusion rate is recommended because of depressed CO and the resulting decrease in the hepatic clearance of lidocaine. Mild hypertension caused by neural and hormonal compensatory responses is common in the mildly to moderately symptomatic patient and usually responds to diuresis and preload reduction alone. Aggressive afterload reduction (e.g., nitroprusside infusion) is usually required only when acute CHF is the result of a hypertensive crisis.

Acute pulmonary edema is LHF in its most extreme form and is a life-threatening emergency. The typical patient is anxious, severely dyspneic, diaphoretic, pale, cool, and clammy. Inspiratory rales and wheezes may be heard over all lung fields. A summation gallop may be heard on cardiac auscultation, and JVD is common. Hypertension is usual and is due to intense vasoconstriction. Other peripheral signs (e.g., pedal edema and hepatomegaly) may be present if acute decompensation is superimposed on chronic LHF.

Immediate therapy in the normotensive or hypertensive patient should include furosemide (80 mg intravenously) and intravenous nitroglycerin (5 to 200 μg/min).[6,16] The transdermal route (e.g., nitroglycerin paste or patch) should not be used, because there is limited skin perfusion in acute pulmonary edema. Morphine sulfate administered in small intravenous doses (2-mg increments) is a time-honored therapeutic agent in acute pulmonary edema. Although morphine is a venodilator, its effects on venous capacitance have not been well established in the setting of acute pulmonary edema caused by LHF, and respiratory depression may occur at doses that do not affect hemodynamic variables. An inhaled selective beta agonist can be used if severe bronchospasm is present. Theophylline preparations should be avoided because of their arrhythmogenicity. If BP remains severely elevated after initial improvement in symptoms, afterload reduction with nitroprusside, infused at a rate titrated to desired response, or enalaprilat, 1.25 mg every 6 hours, can be used.[1] If the patient is hypotensive at the time of presentation, inotropic agents should precede the use of venodilators and diuretics.[16] Dopamine (initial infusion rate of 10 μg/kg/min) or a combination of dopamine and dobutamine (each infused at an initial rate of 7.5 μg/kg/min) can be used. If a sustained supraventricular tachyarrhythmia (e.g., atrial fibrillation) is present and is judged to be a major cause of hypotension, electrical cardioversion should be attempted. PVCs can be treated with lidocaine, as discussed. Endotracheal intubation may be required if pulmonary edema is accompanied by severe hypoxemia that does not improve during early treatment. The most reliable indication of life-threatening hypoxemia is a decreasing level of consciousness, although it is a relatively insensitive sign. Continuous or bilevel positive airway pressure (CPAP, BiPAP) may reduce the need for intubation.[14]

DISPOSITION

Role of the Consultant

Acute pulmonary edema is a medical emergency, and therapy should be instituted immediately, even before consultation with the patient's personal physician or the on-call cardiologist. Initial therapy and symptomatic response should be carefully documented to assist the admitting physician in planning further therapy. In the patient with mild-to-moderate LHF, early consultation after initial assessment is appropriate.

Indications for Admission

All patients with acute pulmonary edema should be admitted to an intensive care unit. Invasive hemodynamic monitoring may be required in patients who do not respond to emergency department therapy. Patients with chronic LHF and a mild worsening of symptoms who respond to intravenous diuretics may be discharged after adjustments in the chronic drug regimen (e.g., an increase in the furosemide dose), consultation with the patient's physician regarding medication changes, and assurance of follow-up within 24 to 48 hours. Patients with more severe symptoms or other complicating factors (e.g., new rhythm disturbances, poorly controlled hypertension, or a suspected acute myocardial ischemic event) should be admitted for observation, evaluation, and optimization of drug therapy.[12] All patients with new onset of LHF of uncertain origin should be admitted for evaluation. If an interfacility transfer is required, the patient should be stabilized first.

COMMON PITFALLS

- The signs and symptoms of cor pulmonale and acute respiratory failure are similar to those of LHF, and, in some cases, it may not be possible to distinguish between them by physical examination alone.
- In the patient with CHF atrial fibrillation with a rapid ventricular response, digoxin alone should not be used. Slowing of the ventricular response rate is usually not seen for approximately 8 hours after administration.
- RV infarction should always be considered in the patient with an acute inferior wall infarction who has clear lung sounds, JVD, hypotension, and a normal heart rate and rhythm. Increasing venous capacitance in this setting decreases RV filling pressures and further decreases CO. RV infarction can be diagnosed with a right precordial ECG. ST-segment elevation is typically seen in leads V_{3R} and V_{4R} (see Chapter 131).
- If the cardiac silhouette is not enlarged, but other radiographic findings of LHF are seen, the failure is most likely to be of acute onset and caused by valvular disease (e.g., aortic insufficiency due to endocarditis, papillary muscle rupture in patients with mitral valve prolapse, valvular dysfunction in patients with prosthetic valves, or acute myocardial infarction). Noncardiogenic pulmonary edema should also be considered.
- CHF is a complex physiologic state. There are a number of drugs that can alleviate symptoms, improve quality of life, and increase long-term survival. However, these drugs have well-described complications. Altering a patient's medical regimen by adding a new medication prior to discharge from the emergency department should not be undertaken without consultation with the patient's primary physician, in order to assure follow-up monitoring of drug effect.

CHRONIC COR PULMONALE (PULMONARY HEART DISEASE)

Chronic cor pulmonale has been defined as a combination of RV hypertrophy and dilatation caused by increased resistance of the pulmonary circulation due to intrinsic pulmonary disease, inadequate function of the chest bellows, or inadequate ventilatory drive from the respiratory centers. Implicit in this definition is the exclusion of congenital heart disease and LHF as causes.[8] Although cor pulmonale may be acute (most commonly caused by pulmonary thromboembolism), only the chronic form is discussed. Causes of chronic cor pulmonale are listed in Table 133.6. In the United States, chronic bronchitis and emphysema are the major causes of chronic cor pulmonale, and the yearly incidence of these diseases is approximately ten per 1 million persons. At autopsy, cor pulmonale is estimated to occur in 40% of patients with emphysema or bronchitis. Cor pulmonale is estimated to account for 7% to 10% of all heart disease.

The hemodynamic hallmark of cor pulmonale is pulmonary hypertension (elevated pulmonary artery pressure), which may either manifest at rest and worsen with exercise or occur only during exercise. Increased pulmonary vascular resistance is the result of a reduction in the size of the effective cross-sectional area of the pulmonary vascular bed because of obstruction or destruction and is usually combined with active vasoconstriction. Hypoxemia is a potent pulmonary vasoconstrictor, and concurrent hypercapnia and acidemia are synergistic. Most causes of cor pulmonale are accompanied by these gas exchange and acid–base abnormalities. The rise in pulmonary vascular resistance impedes RV ejection, and a compensatory response results in hypertrophy or dilatation and increased preload.

TABLE 133.6. Causes of Chronic Cor Pulmonale

DISEASES THAT PRIMARILY AFFECT AIR PASSAGES
Chronic bronchitis/emphysema
Bronchial asthma
Pulmonary fibrosis (e.g., pneumoconiosis)
Granulomas and infiltrates (e.g., sarcoid)
Pulmonary resection
Congenital cystic disease
High-altitude hypoxia
DISEASES THAT PRIMARILY AFFECT CHEST BELLOWS
Kyphoscoliosis
Thoracoplasty
Pleural fibrosis
Chronic neuromuscular weakness
Obesity
DISEASES THAT PRIMARILY AFFECT PULMONARY VASCULATURE
Primary pulmonary hypertension
Pulmonary embolism
Polyarteritis nodosa
Other arteritides

CLINICAL PRESENTATION

The clinical manifestations of cor pulmonale are largely determined by the underlying disease process, and symptoms of pulmonary dysfunction most often precede manifestations of right heart failure.

Common symptoms include dyspnea at rest or with minimal exertion, weight gain, ankle swelling, and, in severe cases, abdominal swelling due to ascites. Physical signs usually include bibasilar crackles and scattered wheezes (caused by lung disease, not interstitial fluid accumulation) on auscultation. The pulmonic component of the second heart sound may be palpable, and the jugular vein may fill paradoxically during inspiration or exhibit no respiratory fluctuations. Tricuspid insufficiency may be present, manifested by a systolic murmur heard best at the lower left sternal border and increasing with inspiration; this is often accompanied by the finding of a pulsatile liver edge.

DIFFERENTIAL DIAGNOSIS

The signs and symptoms of cor pulmonale may mimic those of LHF, constrictive pericarditis, and cardiac tamponade. Severe and advanced mitral stenosis may present with predominant right heart failure or "silent mitral stenosis." When signs and symptoms of cor pulmonale are of abrupt onset, acute pulmonary thromboembolism should be considered.

EMERGENCY DEPARTMENT EVALUATION

The chest radiograph usually shows only evidence of the underlying pulmonary disorder, but it may be helpful in diagnosing the cause of an acute exacerbation (e.g., pulmonary infiltrate). The ECG is not a sensitive test for detecting RV hypertrophy or dilatation, but some findings are reasonably specific. These include a P-pulmonale pattern (P-wave amplitude of at least 2.5 mm in lead II), right-axis deviation, R/S amplitude ratio in V_1 of greater than 1, low-voltage QRS, and right bundle-branch block pattern.[10] Failure to detect radiographic or ECG evidence of RV hypertrophy or dilatation does not rule out the diagnosis. Arterial blood gas analysis usually shows some combination of hypoxemia, hypercapnia, and acidemia. Liver function tests may be abnormal because of passive hepatic congestion. Pulmonary function tests are always abnormal, and the typical patient has a forced expiratory volume in 1 second of less than 1 L.

EMERGENCY DEPARTMENT MANAGEMENT

Most patients who present with an acute exacerbation of chronic cor pulmonale have acute respiratory failure caused by the worsening or progression of the underlying lung disease. Therapeutic efforts should be directed toward reversing reactive pulmonary vasoconstriction (i.e., improving oxygenation, decreasing hypercarbia, and normalizing pH). Therapy is usually the same as that employed in acute respiratory failure resulting from emphysema or chronic bronchitis. Such therapy should include administration of low-flow oxygen, corticosteroids, and antibiotics and inhaled and systemic bronchodilation (see Chapter 147).

DISPOSITION

Role of the Consultant

An acute worsening of chronic cor pulmonale is usually caused by acute respiratory failure. Acute respiratory failure is a life-threatening emergency, and immediate treatment should be instituted before consultation.

Indications for Admission

Indications for admission for an exacerbation of chronic cor pulmonale are usually the same as for acute respiratory failure (see Chapter 130).

COMMON PITFALLS

- The clinical symptoms and signs of LHF and cor pulmonale overlap. Administering high-flow oxygen to a patient with suspected LHF who has cor pulmonale may result in worsening of clinical status, because the hypoxic drive is suppressed and hypercapnia worsens.
- The diagnosis of cor pulmonale cannot be ruled out simply by the absence of ECG or radiographic findings of RV hypertrophy or dilatation.[10]
- Emergency treatment should be directed toward improving pulmonary function and decreasing pulmonary vascular resistance, rather than toward alleviating signs of right heart failure (e.g., aggressive diuresis, which may decrease RV preload and worsen left heart outflow).
- Patients with obstructive sleep apnea typically present with manifestations similar to those of chronic cor pulmonale.[13] A careful history is helpful in suggesting the diagnosis and appropriate referral.

References

1. Annane D, Bellissant E, Pussard E, et al. Placebo-controlled, randomized, double-blind study of intravenous enalaprilat efficacy and safety in acute cardiogenic pulmonary edema. *Circulation* 1996;94:1316.
2. Badgett RG, Lucey CR, Mulrow CD. Can the clinical examination diagnose left-sided heart failure in adults? *JAMA* 1997;277:1712.
3. Blankfield RP, Finkelhorn RS, Alexander JJ, et al. Etiology and the diagnosis of bilateral leg edema in primary care. *Am J Med* 1998;105:192.
4. Cohn JN. The management of chronic heart failure. *N Engl J Med* 1996;335:490.
5. Coodley E. Newer drug therapy for congestive heart failure. *Arch Intern Med* 1999;159:1177.
6. Cotter G, Metzkor E, Kaluski E, et al. Randomized trial of high-dose isosorbide dinitrate plus low-dose furosemide versus high-dose furosemide plus low-dose isosorbide dinitrate in severe pulmonary edema. *Lancet* 1998;351:389.
7. Eichorn EJ, Bristow MR. Medical therapy can improve the biological properties of the chronically failing heart. *Circulation* 1996;94;2285.
8. Fishman AP. Pulmonary hypertension and cor pulmonale. In: Fishman AP, ed. *Pulmonary disease and disorders,* 3rd ed. New York: McGraw-Hill, 1998:1261.
9. Goldberg RJ, Konstam MA. Assessing the population burden from heart failure. *Arch Intern Med* 1999:159:15.
10. Incalzi RA, Fuso L, De Rosa M, et al. Electrocardiographic signs of chronic cor pulmonale. A negative prognostic finding in chronic obstructive lung disease. *Circulation* 1999;99:1600.
11. Karon BL. Diagnosis and outpatient management of congested heart failure. *Mayo Clin Proc* 1995;70:180.
12. Konstam MA, Dracup K, Baker DW, et al. Heart failure: evaluation and care of patients with left-ventricular systolic dysfunction. *Clinical Practice Guideline, No. 11.* Rockville, MD: Agency for Health Care Policy and Research, June 1994. (Publication No. AHCPR 94-0612).
13. Kramer NR, Cook TE, Carlisle CC, et al. The role of the primary care physician in reorganizing obstructive apnea. *Arch Intern Med* 1999;159:965.
14. Pang D, Keenan SP, Cook DJ, et al. The effect of positive pressure airway support on mortality and the need for intubation in cardiogenic pulmonary edema. A systematic review. *Chest* 1998;114:1185.
15. Pisani B, Taylor DO, Mason JW. Inflammatory myocardial diseases and cardiomyopathies. *Am J Med* 1997;102:459.
16. Report of the American College of Cardiology/American Heart Association Task Force on Practice Guidelines (Committee on Evaluation and Management of Heart Failure). Guidelines for the evaluation and management of heart failure. *Circulation* 1995;92:2764.
17. Report of the 1995 World Health Organization/International Society and Federation of Cardiology Task Force on the Definition and Classification of Cardiomyopathies. *Circulation* 1996;93:841.
18. Sacchetti AD, Harris RH. Acute cardiogenic pulmonary edema. *Postgrad Med* 1998;103:145.
19. Senni M, Tribouilloy CM, Rodeheffer RJ, et al. Congestive heart failure in the community. Trends in incidence and survival in a 10-year period. *Arch Intern Med* 1999;159:29.

20. Statement for Healthcare Professionals from the Subcommittee on Electrocardiography and Electrophysiology, American Heart Association. Management of patients with atrial fibrillation. *Circulation* 1996;93:1262.
21. Vasn RS, Benjamin EJ, Levy D. Congestive heart failure with normal left ventricular systolic function. *Arch Intern Med* 1996;156:146.
22. Young JB. Contemporary management of patients with heart failure. *Med Clin North Am* 1995;79:1171.

CHAPTER 134
Bradyarrhythmias

Mary B. Staten-McCormick and
David Overton

The cardiac conduction system consists of pacemaker cells, conducting cells, and contractile cells. *Pacemaker cells* possess the capacity to spontaneously depolarize. The sinus (sinoatrial) node, normally the predominant pacemaker of the heart, is located at the junction of the right atrium and the superior vena cava and has an intrinsic basal rate of 60 to 100 beats per minute.

The atrioventricular (AV) node, located beneath the right atrial endocardium above the insertion of the septal leaflet of the tricuspid valve, can also function as a pacemaker, with an intrinsic rate of 45 to 60 beats per minute. It fires in the absence of sinus node impulses, or it may itself usurp control from the sinus node. Other cells in the bundle branches and Purkinje network can function as pacemakers as well, but their intrinsic rate is quite low, approximately 30 to 40 beats per minute.

Electrical impulses in the heart travel over a network of *conducting cells*. Impulses normally originate in the sinus node. Passage through the AV node is relatively slow, accounting for a normal physiologic delay in ventricular depolarization. The AV node blends into the bundle of His, which divides into bundle branches. They, in turn, arborize into a network of Purkinje fibers that transmit impulses to the ventricular myocardial *contractile cells*. Contractile cells in the atria and the ventricles do not spontaneously depolarize.

The electrocardiographic (ECG) P wave represents atrial depolarization. The P-R interval (normally 0.12 to 0.20 second in the adult) reflects intraatrial, AV nodal, and His-Purkinje conduction. The QRS complex, representing ventricular depolarization, has a normal duration of 0.04 to 0.10 second, and the following T wave represents ventricular repolarization. The U wave is seen in a variety of circumstances, such as hypokalemia. Its electrophysiologic basis is uncertain.

Two basic pathophysiologic mechanisms underlie the production of both tachyarrhythmias and bradyarrhythmias: disorders of impulse formation and disorders of impulse conduction. Depressed *automaticity* may result in bradyarrhythmias such as sinus bradycardia or sinus arrest. If sinus node automaticity is sufficiently depressed, escape rhythms originating elsewhere in the heart may assume control. Depressed *impulse conduction* may lead to AV or fascicular blocks.

EMERGENCY DEPARTMENT EVALUATION AND MANAGEMENT

In the approach to the patient with bradyarrhythmia, as with any patient, the priorities of airway, breathing, and circulation must be addressed first. The urgency and means of treating bradyarrhythmias depend on how symptomatic the arrhythmia is, the clinical setting in which the arrhythmia occurs, the propensity for the arrhythmia to progress, and concurrent drug therapy.

Bradyarrhythmias may produce light-headedness, dizziness, fatigue, syncope, or even convulsions. Prompt therapy is required for these symptoms and for hypotension, congestive heart failure, mental status changes, and angina. However, many arrhythmias are asymptomatic and require no treatment. An arrhythmia that occurs during an acute myocardial infarction often mandates a different treatment approach than an arrhythmia that is incidentally discovered during a routine physical examination. Electrolyte imbalances and the use of certain drugs (e.g., digitalis, beta blockers, and calcium channel blockers) may also be the cause of bradyarrhythmias, and each has its own implications for treatment. General supportive measures, such as oxygenation, ventilation, and correction of electrolyte abnormalities, are usually the first step. Specific drug therapy or artificial cardiac pacing are also required in many instances.

Among drug therapy, the cornerstone is atropine sulfate, a vagolytic agent that enhances sinus node automaticity and AV nodal conduction. The usual adult dose is 0.5 to 1.0 mg intravenous push every 3 to 5 minutes to a total maximum dose of 0.04 mg/kg (3 mg) in the adult. Atropine is effective when administered by the endotracheal route; the suggested dose is 2.0 to 2.5 times the recommended intravenous dose diluted in 10 mL of normal saline.[3] Because it can increase myocardial oxygen consumption, atropine should be used with caution in the presence of myocardial ischemia. Adverse effects include sinus tachycardia, ventricular tachycardia, or ventricular fibrillation, as well as manifestations of anticholinergic toxicity. In the patient with high-degree AV block, one may see, in rare instances, a marked reduction in the heart rate after atropine use.[3]

Isoproterenol, a beta-adrenergic sympathomimetic drug with potent inotropic and chronotropic effects, may be useful as a temporary measure in the treatment of bradycardia unresponsive to atropine. It is, however, gradually being relegated to a position behind pacing in this situation.[4] It is administered as an infusion at a rate of 2 to 10 μg/min. Isoproterenol markedly increases myocardial oxygen demand and, like atropine, may cause significant adverse effects, including ventricular tachycardia or fibrillation.

Glucagon has been found to be beneficial in treating bradyarrhythmias secondary to beta-adrenergic blocking agents and calcium antagonists. The drug appears to be effective in both the toxic and nontoxic patient. Glucagon has been shown to stimulate the sinoatrial node, resulting in a modest increase in the heart rate. It increases automaticity at the AV node, which may be helpful in slow junctional rhythms. It has also been shown to increase cardiac contractility, thereby increasing coronary perfusion. The peak action of glucagon occurs approximately 5 to 10 minutes after intravenous administration. Suggested initial dosing ranges are 0.05 to 0.10 mg/kg in children and 0.05 to 0.15 mg/kg in adults. This may be repeated based on the clinical situation and the characteristics of the offending medication.[1]

When drug therapy is ineffective artificial pacing should be instituted.

DISORDERS OF IMPULSE FORMATION

ATRIAL BRADYARRHYTHMIAS

Sinus arrhythmia is a physiologic finding commonly seen in healthy young people in which the sinus discharge rate decreases with expiration and increases with inspiration. It is

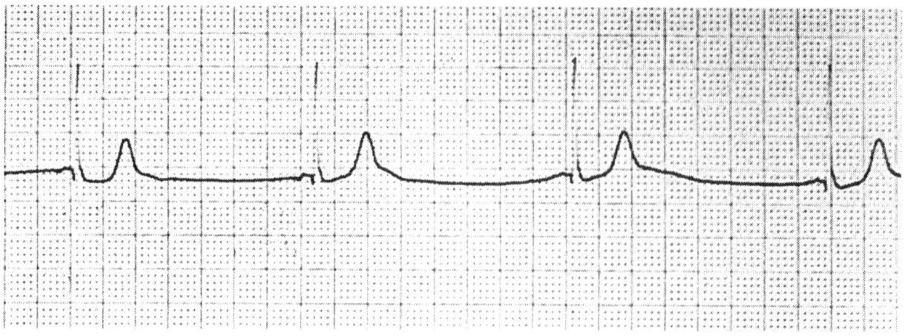

Figure 134.1. Junctional escape rhythm.

thought to be due to changes in vagal tone during respiration. P-wave morphology and P-R intervals are usually constant. No treatment is indicated.

Sinus bradycardia, arbitrarily defined as a sinus rhythm of less than 60 beats per minute, may be the result of organic heart disease, and may cause symptoms, but is also a common finding in healthy patients and particularly in conditioned athletes. Studies have found that 50% to 85% of conditioned athletes have benign sinus bradycardia, compared with 23% in the general population.[2] The significance of sinus bradycardia depends on the clinical setting. It is common during drug therapy with digitalis and beta blockers, and may not warrant intervention. The following findings should suggest possible nonphysiologic vagotonia: (1) profound bradycardia in an individual not engaged in strenuous endurance training, (2) sinus pauses longer than 3 seconds on a Holter monitor, or (3) syncope or near-syncope at rest or after strenuous exercise.[2] When sinus bradycardia is associated with symptoms, treatment with atropine is usually successful. Use of cardiac pacing and other drug therapies is sometimes necessary.

The *sick sinus syndrome* encompasses a spectrum of conditions, including severe sinus bradycardia, sinoatrial block, sinus arrest, and the bradycardia–tachycardia syndrome. The latter refers to the intermittent occurrence of bradyarrhythmias and tachyarrhythmias (e.g., atrial fibrillation, flutter, or paroxysmal supraventricular tachycardia) in the same patient. Bradyarrhythmia typically occurs immediately after resolution of an episode of tachycardia. Symptoms such as syncope or chest pain may result from either the tachycardia or the bradycardia. Effective pharmacologic therapy for tachycardia can exacerbate the bradycardia, so cardiac pacing must often be initiated before pharmacologic therapy.

ATRIOVENTRICULAR NODAL BRADYARRHYTHMIAS

An *AV junctional rhythm* may be a physiologic escape rhythm initiated by the AV node in the absence of an adequate sinus stimulus, or may result from an abnormally rapid AV junctional focus that usurps control from the sinus node (e.g., accelerated junctional rhythm). Junctional rhythms usually exhibit the same QRS morphology as the patient's sinus rhythm. The P waves are usually inverted if they are conducted in a retrograde manner, and can fall before, during, or after the QRS complex, depending on the location of the focus within the AV junction and the degree of retrograde AV block. When the P wave occurs before the QRS complex, the P-R interval is, usually, less than 0.12 second. The absence of P waves may be due to obliteration by the QRS complex or to retrograde block.

AV junctional escape beats occur singly or multiply in the absence of stimuli arriving at the AV node (Fig. 134.1). Their hallmark is occurrence *after* an interval longer than the dominant cycle. The underlying disorder may be sinus bradycardia, sinus arrest, sinus exit block, or AV block. Digitalis or beta-blocker therapy may also be responsible. Junctional escape rhythms may also be incidental findings in otherwise healthy people with increased vagotonia. Treatment is not indicated for asymptomatic patients with infrequent escape beats. If symptoms occur, the clinician should treat the underlying rhythm rather than attempt to obliterate the escape beats. Treatment involves withholding offending drugs or using atropine, artificial pacing, or isoproterenol.

VENTRICULAR BRADYARRHYTHMIAS

A ventricular rhythm with a rate of less than 50 beats per minute is termed a *ventricular escape rhythm,* or idioventricular rhythm. Ventricular escape rhythm represents a physiologic safety mechanism that arises in the absence of stimuli from above, as in sinus bradycardia, sinus arrest, or, more commonly, AV block. Most patients with ventricular escape are symptomatic, because the heart rate is low. Treatment is directed at the underlying arrhythmia (i.e., use of atropine, isoproterenol, or, most often, cardiac pacing). Lidocaine, which may abolish the ventricular rhythm, is contraindicated, because it has the potential for causing cardiac standstill.

Also known as idioventricular tachycardia or slow ventricular tachycardia, *accelerated idioventricular rhythm* has a rate of 50 to 100 beats per minute. It is one cause of isorhythmic dissociation, with occasional fusion beats demonstrating the continued presence of an intact AV node (Fig. 134.2). It may be associated with acute myocardial infarction (particularly after thrombolysis,[12] but may also be seen in otherwise healthy patients. In the absence of symptoms, specific therapy is not warranted.

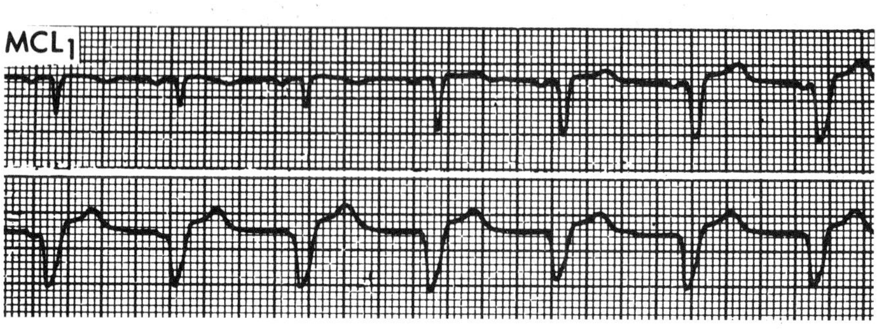

Figure 134.2. Idioventricular rhythm, with isorhythmic dissociation and fusion beats.

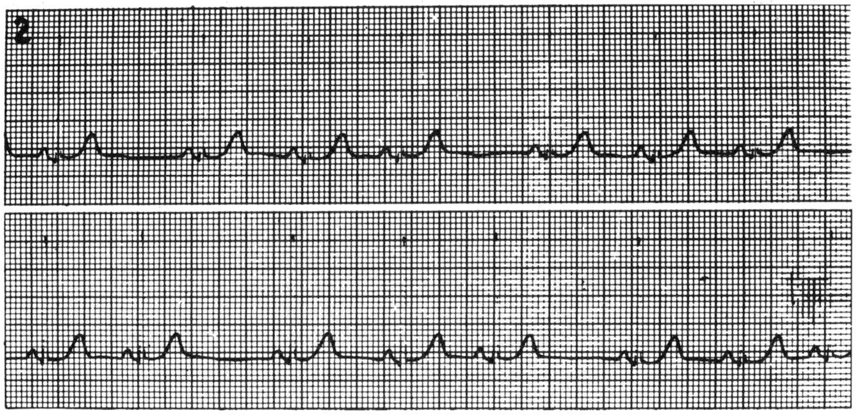

Figure 134.3. Type I (Wenckebach) sinoatrial block.

DISTURBANCES OF CONDUCTION

DISORDERS OF SINOATRIAL CONDUCTION

The tissue surrounding the sinus node may delay or prevent conduction of sinus node impulses to the atria and AV node. Such conduction disorders are termed *sinoatrial block* and are classified in a manner analogous to AV block. However, because of the limitations of the surface ECG, their precise diagnosis is more difficult than the varieties of AV block.

In *first-degree sinoatrial block,* there is a delay in the propagation of the sinus node impulse out to the atrial myocardium. Every beat is transmitted, however, and no abnormality is detected on the surface ECG.

Like AV block, *second-degree sinoatrial block* may be divided into types I and II. In *type I* (Wenckebach), there is, with each succeeding beat, a progressive delay in conduction from the sinus node to the atria, until conduction is totally blocked and a P wave is dropped (Fig. 134.3). The P-P interval progressively shortens before the dropped P wave, analogous to the situation in second-degree AV block, in which the R-R interval shortens before the dropped QRS complex.

In *type II* second-degree sinoatrial block, there is intermittent failure of the sinus impulse to reach the atria, resulting in a missing P wave and a sudden lengthening of the P-P interval. The resulting P-P interval is usually a multiple of the previous one, which is doubled in the case of 2:1 block (Fig. 134.4). This disorder can be mimicked by blocked premature atrial contractions, in which the P wave is obscured by the preceding T wave (Fig. 134.5).

Third-degree sinoatrial block, in which there is a failure of any sinus node impulses to be conducted to the atria (Fig. 134.6), is usually indistinguishable from sinus arrest, in which there is a failure of impulses to arise from the sinus node.

DISORDERS OF ATRIOVENTRICULAR CONDUCTION

Traditionally, AV blocks have been divided into first, second, and third degree. However, AV block is a relative phenomenon, and the physiologic delay normally present in the AV node is one end of a continuum. For example, in the patient with atrial flutter "normal" AV conduction usually results in 2:1 block. In addition, the degree of block is rate dependent. One patient with mild AV disease may exhibit second-degree block at a particular supraventricular rate, while another patient with more advanced AV nodal disease may exhibit 1:1 conduction if the supraventricular rate is slower.

A P-R interval of more than 0.20 second defines *first-degree AV block*. All P waves are conducted, 1:1 AV conduction is maintained, and the P-P and R-R intervals are consistent. Most commonly, the delay in AV conduction is within the AV node, and the QRS complex is of normal duration. Delays within the His bundle or His-Purkinje system are less common and are usually associated with widened bundle-branch block QRS patterns, but can be localized conclusively only by intracardiac recordings.

First-degree AV block may be associated with electrolyte disturbances or the use of digitalis, beta blockers, or calcium channel blockers. It may be a finding during acute myocardial infarction, particularly inferior myocardial infarction. Treatment includes correction of electrolyte abnormalities or removal of an inciting agent. During acute myocardial infarction, close observation is warranted to detect progression to higher degrees of block. Otherwise, specific treatment is not indicated.

Second-degree AV block can be divided into Mobitz types I and II. Interestingly, Wenckebach distinguished between these two in the pre-ECG era, using only physical observation.[12]

Mobitz type I (Wenckebach) second-degree AV block is characterized by repeated cycles of progressively slowing AV conduction until conduction is totally blocked. This pattern is manifested electrocardiographically by a progressive prolongation of successive P-R intervals, until there is a nonconducted P wave, after which the cycle repeats itself (Fig. 134.7). The cycle is referred to by the ratio of P waves to QRS complexes (i.e., 4:3. 3:2, and so on). Classically the R-R interval shortens as the P-R interval lengthens.

Type I block usually results from conduction delay in the AV node, although delays may occur in the bundle of His, bundle branches, or Purkinje system. For this reason, the QRS complex in type I block is most often of normal duration. It may be asso-

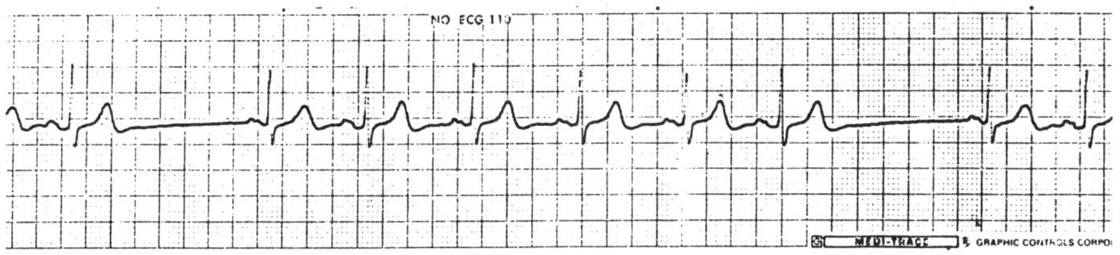

Figure 134.4. Type II sinoatrial block 2:1.

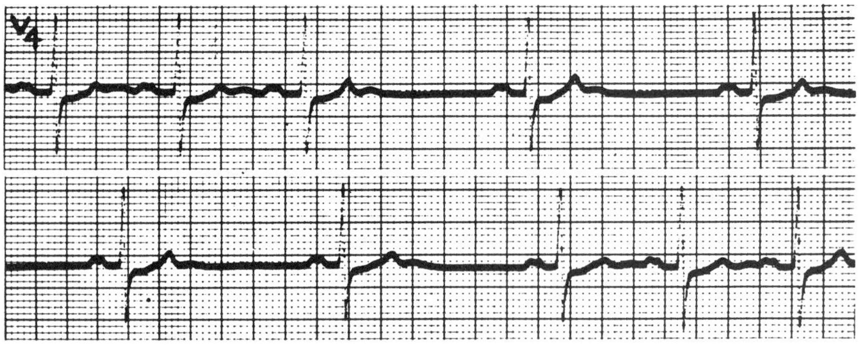

Figure 134.5. Blocked premature atrial contractions mimicking AV or sinoatrial block.

ciated with inferior myocardial infarction or the use of digitalis, beta blockers, and calcium channel blockers. Mobitz type I AV block is usually transient and asymptomatic and has a good prognosis. If it is symptomatic, atropine can be given to enhance AV nodal conduction, but pacing is usually not necessary. Offending drugs may need to be withheld.

Mobitz type II second-degree AV block is less common. The site of blockage is usually within the His-Purkinje system, and, thus, a bundle-branch block QRS pattern is usually seen. In type II block, the P-R intervals are constant until single or multiple beats are suddenly dropped (Fig. 134.8).

Type II block is usually symptomatic and has a high likelihood of progressing to complete AV block. If associated with acute anterior myocardial infarction, it carries an ominous prognosis. Most authorities agree that Mobitz type II second-degree AV block requires permanent cardiac pacing. Because emergency treatment with atropine or isoproterenol is often ineffective, temporary pacing may be necessary as a stabilizing measure.

A particular clinical problem is presented by the patient with 2:1 AV block. Although it is often assumed that such patients have type II block, type I block can, and does, present as 2:1 block, and, in fact, is more common than type II. The distinction is important, given the difference in prognosis and treatment between the two entities. Although definitive proof may require intracardiac recordings, the following principles may aid in the clinical distinction[5]:

- Type I block is more common than type II.
- A narrow QRS complex usually reflects a type I block (although not all type I blocks have a narrow QRS complex). Type II block usually has a wide QRS complex.
- Coexistent acute inferior myocardial infarction suggests type I block, while anterior myocardial infarction suggest type II.
- Digitalis, beta-blocker, or calcium channel blocker therapy tends to be associated with type I block.
- Other areas of the rhythm strip may reflect other patterns of type I conduction, such as 3:2 or 4:3.

In *third-degree (complete) AV block,* no atrial impulses reach the ventricles, and a subsidiary, escape pacemaker usually emerges. AV dissociation results, with constant but independent P-P intervals and R-R intervals. The P-R interval is variable, and P waves have no discernible relation to QRS complexes (Fig. 134.9). The site of block may be within the AV node, His bundle, bundle branches, or Purkinje system. In general, the lower the site of the block, the more severe the symptoms.

Third-degree AV block may be intermittent or self-limited. If it complicates digitalis, beta-blocker, or calcium channel blocker therapy, it usually resolves on withdrawal of the offending agent. It may be associated with acute myocardial infarction, but, occasionally, it is an asymptomatic finding in an otherwise healthy person.

Like other bradyarrhythmias, the emergent treatment of third-degree AV block depends on symptomatology and clinical setting. Symptomatic patients may improve with atropine, particularly if the block is within the AV node. Symptomatic patients who are unresponsive to pharmacologic therapy require emergent pacing. Stable patients with acute inferior infarction may require only a prophylactic pacemaker. Acute anterior infarction complicated by third-degree AV block is more ominous and requires emergent pacing.

The term *AV dissociation,* although commonly used interchangeably with the term *third-degree AV block,* encompasses a much broader range of rhythms. AV dissociation implies that the atria and ventricles are beating independently, a situation that includes not only complete AV block, but also accelerated junctional and idioventricular rhythms (including ventricular tachycardia). In *isorhythmic dissociation* (Fig. 134.10), the sinus rate and the escape or ectopic rate are nearly identical, producing an ECG pattern characterized by varying P-R intervals as the sinus and ectopic foci slowly change their relative firing rates.

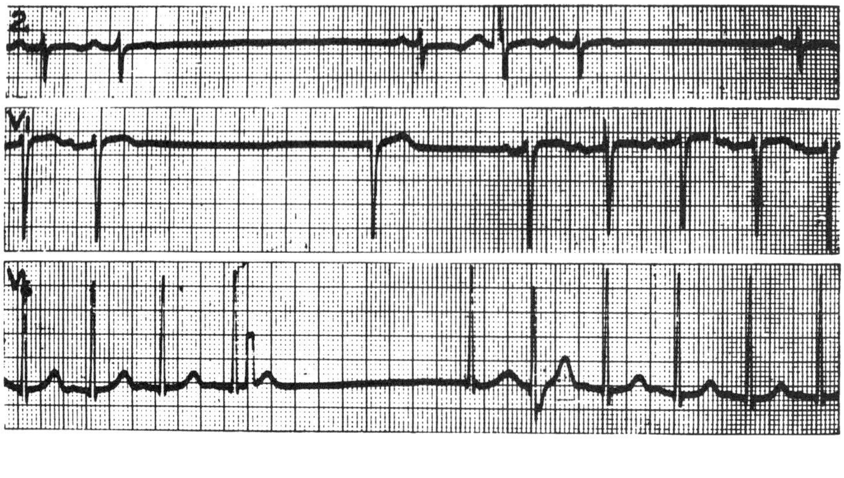

Figure 134.6. Third-degree sinoatrial block, with escape rhythm.

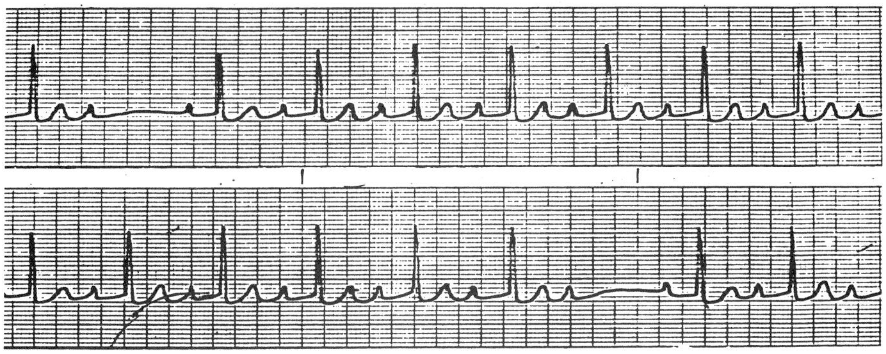

Figure 134.7. Mobitz type I (Wenckebach) second-degree AV block.

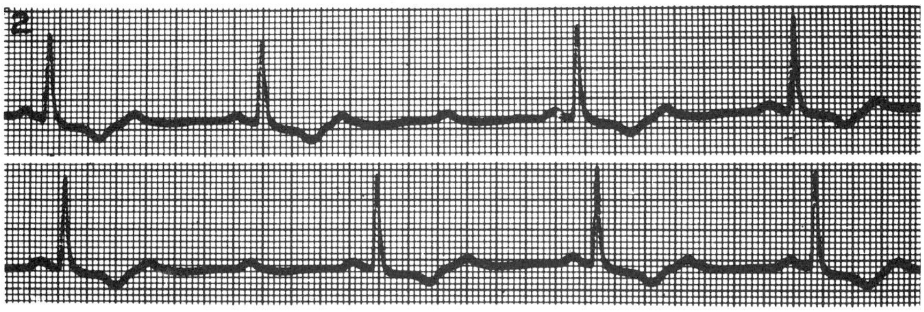

Figure 134.8. Mobitz type II second-degree AV block.

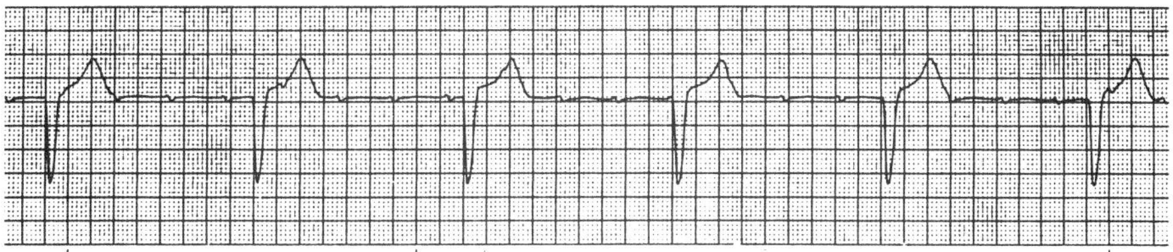

Figure 134.9. Third-degree AV block.

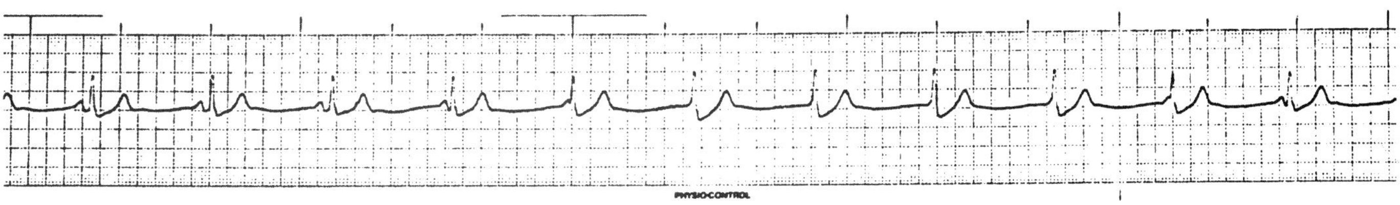

Figure 134.10. AV dissociation, with isorhythmic dissociation due to a junctional focus.

Occasional fusion beats are an indication that the cause is not complete AV block.

ARTIFICIAL PACEMAKERS

Temporary cardiac pacemakers are normally used in emergent or urgent circumstances, whereas most permanent pacemakers are placed electively. The emergency physician should be familiar with the indications and use of temporary pacemakers, and with the principles of permanent pacemakers and their complications.

TEMPORARY PACEMAKERS

Therapeutic emergent cardiac pacing is indicated in any hemodynamically unstable bradycardia that fails to respond to pharmacologic therapy. In addition, prophylactic emergent cardiac pacing may be indicated, even without symptoms, for patients with acute myocardial infarction in the following circumstances:

- First-degree AV block with new-onset bundle-branch block
- Second-degree AV block type II
- Third-degree AV block
- Right bundle-branch block with left anterior fascicular block or left posterior fascicular block (either new or old)
- Left bundle-branch block (old or new) and placement of a Swan-Ganz catheter (because of the risk of inducing iatrogenic right bundle-branch block, and hence complete block)

Emergent pacing may also be indicated in bradyasystolic cardiac arrest, if initiated early. It appears that pacing is of no benefit if it is initiated more than 20 minutes after arrest.[3]

Transcutaneous cardiac pacing involves the application of cutaneous electrodes to the chest and delivery of electrical impulses through the chest wall to the myocardium. Interestingly, transcutaneous pacemakers, developed in the early 1950s, were the first modern cardiac pacemakers. They were largely replaced by other devices until "rediscovered" in the early 1980s.[6,10] Transcutaneous pacing is now the technique of choice for emergent pacing in the emergency department, and it is the only option available for prehospital use.

The advantages of transcutaneous pacing are its ease and speed of use and the absence of serious side effects. Its disadvantages include an inability to capture in some patients and the discomfort experienced by conscious patients due to chest wall contractions. The latter can usually be treated satisfactorily with analgesics or sedation. Because the possibility of myocardial tissue damage from prolonged transcutaneous pacing has not been extensively investigated, the transcutaneous pacer should be considered a stabilizing device, to be replaced by another pacing technique when possible.

Transthoracic cardiac pacing involves the placement of a pacing wire through the skin directly into the right ventricular cavity. Because significant complications have been reported, such as pericardial tamponade, pneumothorax, and coronary vessel injury, transthoracic pacing should usually be considered only if transcutaneous pacing is unsuccessful or unavailable. *Transvenous cardiac pacing* involves the placement of the pacing electrode into the right ventricle by way of a central vein, often the subclavian or internal jugular. Thus, it carries the risk of central venous catheterization, but it is the temporary modality that most closely approximates the function of a permanent pacemaker. It does not involve painful muscle contractions or the hazard of direct cardiac puncture, and it can be used for relatively prolonged periods. Unfortunately, emergent transvenous pacemaker placement in the emergency department setting is often a lengthy and unsuccessful procedure associated with a high incidence of noncapture. Ideally, transvenous pacemaker placement is performed under fluoroscopic guidance. With the advent of transcutaneous pacing, transvenous pacing has been relegated to those situations in which fluoroscopy is available, in which stabilization has been achieved by another modality, or in which attempts at transcutaneous pacing have been unsuccessful.

Once capture has been achieved, regardless of the device used, the pacemaker settings will be dependent on the clinical situation. An initial rate of 80 to 100 beats per minute is appropriate for the majority of the patients. The mode should initially be asynchronous (sensitivity off) in those patients requiring emergency pacing for cardiac arrest. The initial output setting should be at maximum and then decreased after capture is achieved.

PERMANENT PACEMAKERS

Permanent cardiac pacemakers (see also Chapter 136) are classified using a three-letter code. The first letter (A, V, or D) indicates the chamber being paced (atrium, ventricle, or dual). The second letter indicates the chamber being sensed. The third letter (I, T, D, or O) indicates the mode of response (inhibited, triggered, dual, or not applicable). Optional fourth and fifth letters can indicate programmability and antitachycardia functions. Patients often carry identification cards indicating the type and settings of their particular unit.

Many permanent pacemakers currently in use are of the VVI type, which pace the ventricle, sense intrinsic ventricular activity, and inhibit pacemaker output if ventricular complexes are sensed at a rate greater than that of the pacemaker setting. Increasingly common are AV sequential (DDD) units and units that are externally programmable.

Owing to improvements in pacemaker design and function, pacemaker malfunction requiring emergency intervention is uncommon but still occasionally occurs. Pacemaker malfunction can be classified as failure to pace, failure to capture, or failure to sense.

Failure to pace is indicated by a lack of appropriate pacer spikes on the ECG. Apparent failure to pace may be caused by the presence of a faster intrinsic rate than that of the pacemaker or by problems with the ECG recording equipment. True failure to pace is the result of battery or lead wire problems or of oversensing (e.g., sensing T waves as QRS complexes, or mistakenly sensing external, noncardiac activity).

Failure to capture is indicated by appropriate pacer spikes without corresponding QRS complexes. This may be due to fibrosis about the electrode tip, local myocardial changes (such as infarction), migration or displacement of the lead tip, battery malfunction, or lead wire malfunction.

Failure to sense is indicated by the inappropriate delivery of pacer spikes, usually during the patient's intrinsic cardiac complexes. Such undersensing may be due to battery or lead failure or to a decrease in the intrinsic QRS amplitude, as may occur with infarction or electrolyte disturbance.

Most pacemakers may be temporarily converted to the nonsynchronized firing mode by placing a magnet directly over the subcutaneous generator. This maneuver is particularly helpful when pacemaker malfunction is suspected in the patient whose intrinsic rhythm is, for the moment, fast enough to suppress pacemaker activity.

With improvements in technology, most forms of pacemaker malfunction do not require emergent treatment. However, the emergency physician should still be able to recognize dysfunction in order to arrange appropriate management.

DISPOSITION

Virtually all patients with symptomatic bradyarrhythmia require admission to the hospital. Patients with type II second-degree AV block and complete AV block warrant admission even if asymptomatic. Admission should be to a monitored bed in a unit with the capability of initiating emergent pacing.

If transfer to another facility is necessary, pacing should first be initiated, if indicated and available. En route, the patient should have continuous cardiac monitoring and access to advanced cardiac life support. Transcutaneous pacing capability en route is also desirable.

COMMON PITFALLS

- Automatically assuming that a 2:1 second-degree AV block is of the Mobitz type II variety, possibly leading to unnecessary treatment and intervention
- Not taking rate into account when evaluating AV and fascicular blocks
- Misdiagnosing blocked premature atrial contractions as significant AV block, possibly leading to unnecessary treatment and intervention
- Mistakenly blocking an escape rhythm, with the potential for causing cardiac standstill

References

1. Brady WJ, Harrigan RA. Evaluation and management of bradyarrhythmias in the emergency department. *Emerg Med Clin North Am* 1998;16:361.
2. Bryan G, Ward A, Rippe JM. Athletic heart syndrome. *Clin Sports Med* 1992;11:259.
3. Dalsey WC, Syverud SA, Hedges JR. Emergency department use of transcutaneous cardiac pacing for cardiac arrest. *Crit Care Med* 1985;13:399.
4. Emergency Cardiac Care Committee and Subcommittees, American Heart Association. Guidelines for cardiopulmonary resuscitation and emergency cardiac care, I: introduction. *JAMA* 1992;268:2172.
5. Gomes JAC, El-Sherif N. Atrioventricular block: mechanisms, clinical presentation, and therapy. *Med Clin North Am* 1984;68:955.
6. Jeffrey K. The invention and reinvention of cardiac pacing. *Cardiol Clin* 1992;10:561.
7. Love JN, Howell JM. Glucagon therapy in the treatment of symptomatic bradycardia. *Ann Emerg Med* 1997;29:181.
8. Ng L, Nikolic G. Atropine bradycardia. *Heart Lung* 1991;20:414.
9. Ornato JP, Peberdy MA. The mystery of bradyasystole during cardiac arrest. 1996;27:576.
10. Syverud S. Cardiac pacing. *Emerg Med Clin North Am* 1988;6:197.
11. Trigano JA, et al. Noninvasive transcutaneous cardiac pacing: modern instrumentation and new perspectives. *PACE* 1992;15:1937.
12. Walsh DG, Kaplan LR, Burney RE, et al. Use of tissue plasminogen activator in the emergency department for acute myocardial infarction. *Ann Emerg Med* 1987;16:243.
13. Wenckebach KF. Zur analyse des unregelmassigen pulses. *Z Klin Med* 1899;37:475.

CHAPTER 135
Tachyarrhythmias

Scott R. Votey, Mel Herbert, and Jerome R. Hoffman

The truism that we must treat patients and not electrocardiograms (ECGs) or laboratory results is perhaps nowhere more relevant than in the emergency management of tachyarrhythmias. Decisions must be guided principally by the clinical presentation, and rhythm interpretation should be subservient to the goal of prompt appropriate management. Hemodynamic abnormalities are more typically dependent on the heart rate produced by any arrhythmia than they are on the arrhythmia's source. Ventricular tachycardia (VT), for example, conjures up images of imminent catastrophe, and supraventricular tachycardia (SVT) is usually assumed to be benign. However, some patients with VT are relatively stable, at least in the short run, whereas, in other patients, SVT can be acutely life-threatening.

Types of Tachyarrhythmias

Under normal circumstances, the sinoatrial (SA) node is the pacemaker for the heart. Depolarization is initiated in the SA node, and the impulse is conducted down the atrium to the atrioventricular (AV) node. Atrial depolarization corresponds to the P wave on the ECG. Conduction is slowed in the AV node, which provides a measure of protection against hemodynamically unstable tachycardias, because even in the presence of atrial tachycardias, ventricular rates will remain relatively slow. The normal slowing in the AV node is seen on the ECG as the PR interval. After the impulse traverses the AV node, it is conducted first down the His bundle, followed by the left and right bundle branches, and is then dispersed to the ventricular myocardium via the Purkinje fibers. Ventricular depolarization corresponds to the QRS wave on the ECG. The His-Purkinje system is made up of specialized myocardial cells that conduct impulses very rapidly. Normal impulse conduction thus produces a narrow QRS complex. Disease of the AV node causes heart blocks; disease of the His-Purkinje system produces bundle-branch blocks.

Tachycardias can be generated from any focus in the heart, because essentially all myocardial tissue has intrinsic pacemaker activity. There are two principal mechanisms by which tachyarrhythmias arise: reentry and enhanced automaticity. *Reentry* is a phenomenon in which an initial depolarizing impulse travels a closed-loop path that returns cyclically to its point of origin, and, in doing so, generates a regular sustained tachyarrhythmia.

The requirements for a reentrant tachyarrhythmia are (1) a closed-loop conduction path; (2) slower conduction and prolonged refractoriness in one limb of the loop; (3) propagation of the initiating impulse down the faster limb of the loop, with antegrade conduction down the slower limb blocked; and (4) retrograde excitation of the initially blocked slower limb, returning the impulse to its point of origin, where depolarization is reinitiated. Repetition of this cycle sustains the arrhythmia. A premature beat is the typical precipitant. Reentry can occur at a microscopic or a macroscopic level. Most reentry circuits occur with both limbs within the AV node, producing paroxysmal supraventricular tachycardia (PSVT). Reentry is often a common mechanism in VT as well, with the reentrant circuit typically contained entirely in a local area of abnormal ventricular tissue.

Enhanced automaticity is an increase in the rate of the spontaneous depolarization of myocardial cells above their electrical threshold. Sinus tachycardia is the physiologic response to enhanced automaticity of the SA node. When enhanced automaticity results in more rapid depolarization of extranodal myocardial cells, these foci can produce ectopic tachyarrhythmias. Examples include paroxysmal atrial tachycardia (PAT) and junctional tachycardia. Enhanced automaticity often occurs as a result of increased sympathetic tone (e.g., with fever, thyrotoxicosis, or sympathomimetic overdose). Treatment of these arrhythmias generally should be directed at removing the underlying stressor.

In adults, SVT generally does not generate a ventricular response of more than 180 beats per minute because of the damping effect of the AV node. In the presence of a bypass tract, however (e.g., the atrial tissue bundle of Kent found in Wolff-Parkinson-White [WPW] syndrome), rates of 200 or more beats per minute may be attained. VT, on the other hand, particularly when due to a reentry mechanism, may reach rates as high as 250 to 300 beats per minute, but is usually less than 220 beats per minute.

Tachycardias that originate below the AV node produce wide QRS complexes; therefore, any tachycardia with a narrow QRS complex can be presumed to originate from the AV node or above. On the other hand, SVTs and nodal tachycardias can produce wide QRS complexes in several circumstances: underlying bundle-branch block, rate-related bundle-branch block induced by the tachycardia itself, and anterograde conduction from the atrium to the ventricle through a bypass tract that circumvents the AV node. Thus, wide-complex tachycardias can be of either ventricular or supraventricular origin.

Although VT is more likely than SVT to produce hemodynamic decompensation, and thus more likely to initiate an episode of ventricular fibrillation (VF), VT is not always immediately life-threatening, nor is every episode of SVT benign.[21] VT tends to be more worrisome, both because of the lack of atrial systole and, more important, the generally faster ventricular rate it produces. However, very rapid atrial or junctional tachycardias can produce hemodynamic instability, and efforts to distinguish between SVT and VT based purely on symptomatic effects produced by the arrhythmia are frequently inaccurate.[21] The configuration of the QRS complexes seen during an episode of tachycardia is less important as a clue to the origin of the rhythm disturbance than as a guide to choosing between several possible therapeutic approaches.

TREATMENT MODALITIES

Electrical Cardioversion

With the exceptions of sinus tachycardia and multifocal atrial tachycardia (MFAT), any tachycardia that produces significant end-organ hypoperfusion can be treated in the same manner, regardless of its mechanism. Patients with tachyarrhythmia and hypotension, altered mental status, significant chest pain, or significant congestive heart failure generally require emergency electrical cardioversion. Expeditious sedation and analgesia should precede electrical cardioversion in awake patients.

The amount of electrical energy required depends on the mechanism of the tachycardia. Fibrillatory rhythms, including both atrial fibrillation (AF) and VF, normally require significantly more energy than tachycardias such as PSVT or VT. Atrial flutter is the most electrosensitive rhythm and usually responds to energies in the range of 10 to 50 J. PSVT and VT both respond in at least 80% of cases to energies of 10 to 20 J; an initial energy of 50 J achieves successful conversion in more than 90% of cases. By contrast, AF and VF often require 100 to 200 J, or more. Initial doses should be as low as can reasonably be expected to succeed in converting the rhythm. If conversion fails on the initial attempt, energy levels can be serially increased until cardioversion is achieved.

Antiarrhythmic Agents

Drug therapy (Table 135.1) is reserved for patients who are clinically stable despite the tachyarrhythmia (or in whom cardioversion is either not indicated [MFAT, torsade de pointes] or has been tried unsuccessfully). The standard classification of antiarrhythmic agents provides a useful scheme for the treatment of tachycardias. Class I agents stabilize cell membranes and decrease the slope of phase zero of the action potential. Class II agents, the beta-adrenergic blockers, depress the SA and AV nodes. Class III agents decrease the entire duration of the action potential in all cardiac tissues, and thus have effects on all types of arrhythmias. Class IV agents, the calcium channel blockers, affect primarily the SA and AV nodes.

Three subclasses of class I are distinguished by their independent effects on repolarization. Although all these drugs slow phase zero of the action potential, and thus indirectly lengthen repolarization, the clinical effects of the various subclasses differ because they each have separate direct effects on repolarization. Class IA drugs directly prolong repolarization, class IB drugs independently shorten it, and class IC drugs have little independent effect on repolarization. The total effect on repolarization is thus minimal for class IB drugs, whereas prolongation of repolarization is moderate for class IC agents and pronounced with class IA drugs.

These properties are clinically important, because delayed repolarization (which is reflected on the ECG as a prolonged QT interval) can result in reentrant-type ventricular arrhythmias. This is of particular concern in the presence of ischemia, when the difference between the refractory periods of normal and ischemic cells is enhanced. Clinically, prolonged QT intervals associated with class IA antiarrhythmic agents are linked to the development of VT of the torsade de pointes variety. Class IA agents are contraindicated if the tachycardia manifests a prolonged QT interval.

The most important class IA agent is *procainamide*. Procainamide is probably more effective for the treatment of VT than is lidocaine, and it is also effective for many SVTs. In cases of regular wide-complex tachycardias of uncertain type, it is particularly useful because it treats both VT and SVT with aberrancy. It is also of use in patients with WPW and AF because it reduces conduction speed in the accessory pathway. It does, however, increase conduction through the AV node, so it should be used in conjunction with an AV node blocking agent in these cases. It is given in a dose of 17 mg/kg at not more than 50 mg/min. Procainamide may cause hypotension and QRS widening, particularly if given rapidly, and serial assessment of the ECG is required. Long-term therapy is associated with a lupus-like syndrome.

Quinidine and *disopyramide* are class IA agents seldom used in the emergency department (ED). Tricyclic antidepressants share the same electrophysiologic properties, and tricyclic antidepressant poisoning is associated with prolonged QT intervals (as well as prolonged QRS complexes). Emergency physicians should be familiar with these drugs, because many patients use them and because, in some patients, tachyarrhythmias may be due to their proarrhythmic effects.[19] *Lidocaine,* the prototype parenteral class IB agent, has long been considered the drug of first choice in the acute treatment of ventricular arrhythmias. More recent studies suggest that it is not as effective in this role as previously believed; conversion rates for VT may be as low as 30%.[8] It continues to be used, however, in the ED in the treatment of VT in clinically stable patients (i.e., those without signs of end-organ hypoperfusion), to protect against recurrent VF after resuscitation from cardiac arrest, and to treat significant ventricular ectopy in acute ischemia. However, there is no evidence that lidocaine is valuable in the primary prophylaxis of ventricular arrhythmias in acute myocardial infarction, and its utilization in this manner is widely discouraged.[3] Lidocaine is safe when used appropriately. Toxicity, which is primarily related to the central nervous system, can be avoided if appropriate total

TABLE 135.1. Drugs for Tachyarrhythmias

Drug	Dosage	Contraindications	Side Effects	Comments
Adenosine	6 mg i.v. rapid push Repeated doses of 12 or 18 mg may be used	• Known VT • AV node block • AF with WPW	Hypotension: transient Prolonged AV block: rare Chest pain Flushing	Reduce dose in patients taking carbamazepine or dipyridamole (start at 3 mg) or heart transplant patients (start at 1–2 mg) or administration via central line (start at 1–2 mg)
Amiodarone	150 mg over 10 min 1 mg/min for 6 h 0.5-mg/min maintenance infusion 150-mg boluses for breakthrough VT/VF	• AV block • Renal failure	Hypotension: Rx fluid bolus AV block: Rx decrease dosage	Amiodarone has many side effects when given chronically, but not acutely. Amiodarone should be considered in stable VT, because it is probably much more effective than lidocaine. Amiodarone is expensive.
Atenolol/ metoprolol	5 mg i.v. over 1–2 min; repeated up to 15 mg if required	• Asthma/COPD • Hypotension • AF with WPW	Hypotension: Rx with fluids, glucagon 1 mg i.v.; if severe, 1 mg and repeated	Secondary choice for most tachyarrhythmias due to negative inotropic effects
Diltiazem	5–10 mg i.v. slowly for AF Repeated to total of 50 mg in first 30 min, if required Infusion: 5–15 mg/min	• Regular wide-complex tachycardias • AV node block • Hypotension • Digoxin toxicity • AF in WPW • Age <2 yr	Hypotension: Rx with fluid and calcium High-degree AV bock: Rx with calcium or atropine. May require temporary pacing	Consider calcium pretreatment Studies in class IV heart failure in patients with AF and noted to be safe in small series
Esmolol	500-μg/kg/min bolus 50–300-μg/kg/min infusion	• As for other beta blockers	Hypotension: Rx with fluids, glucagon 1 mg i.v.; if severe, 1 mg and repeated	A very short half-life makes this a good choice when one is unclear whether the patient can tolerate beta blockers. May be particularly useful in AF in patients with thyrotoxicosis.
Lidocaine	1 mg/kg i.v., repeated at 0.5–0.75 mg/kg i.v. to a total of 3 mg/kg, if required. Infusion of 1–4 mg/h	• AF (increases AV conduction)	Seizures, confusion, lethargy, but only in overdose	Used for stable VT but only 20% effective. May reduce recurrent VT/VF but not helpful for primary prophylaxis
Magnesium	2–4 g i.v. over 5 min Infusion of 1–2 g/h	• AV block • AF with WPW • Renal failure (infusion)	Hypotension Flushing Respiratory and muscle weakness at high dose	Patients with infusions running should be checked every few hours to determine respiratory status and reflexes. Decreasing reflexes suggest magnesium toxicity, and infusion should be stopped
Procainamide	17 mg/kg loading at no more than 50 mg/min	• Hypotension (relative contraindication)	Hypotension: Rx with fluids QRS widening: If $>50\%$ widening, stop infusion, as torsade may result	More effective than lidocaine for VT. Effective in SVT with aberrancy. Reduces conduction though accessory pathways but may increase conduction through the AV node.
Verapamil	5–10 mg i.v. at 2 mg/min for PSVT	• As for diltiazem	As for diltiazem	May cause more hypotension than diltiazem. Not extensively studied in patients with congestive heart failure

doses (typically less than 225 mg in adults) are given at rates no faster than 50 mg/min for the initial 1-mg/kg bolus and 50 mg/5 min for further loading doses.

Phenytoin is another class IB drug, but like several newer oral lidocaine analogues, such as mexiletine and tocainide, it is seldom used in the ED as an antiarrhythmic agent.

Class IC agents, including *encainide* and *flecainide,* effectively suppress premature ventricular complexes (PVCs). They are not as effective at preventing propagation of whatever ectopic beats continue to occur, and thus are not useful in the suppression of ventricular tachyarrhythmias. They have powerful proarrhythmic effects and actually increase mortality when given chronically to patients who have suffered myocardial infarction.[7] Although class IC agents have little current role in the ED, there have been sporadic reports of utility in the initial treatment of AF.

Class II agents (beta blockers) play only a secondary role in the acute treatment of tachycardias. They have negative dromotropic and chronotropic effects, and thus are sometimes used to treat sinus tachycardia when the elevated heart rate is associated with significant hemodynamic consequences. They are also occasionally used as adjunctive therapy for tachycardias involving the AV node.[23] Because of the superior efficacy and safety of adenosine and calcium channel blockers, however, even esmolol, a very short acting beta blocker, is, in most cases, only a second-line agent in this circumstance. A possible exception to this general rule is the presence of an acute coronary syndrome, in which the use of beta blockers is generally beneficial, and where there are concerns about the overall effects of calcium channel blocking agents. Although these concerns probably do not apply to the long-acting nondihydropyridine agents such as verapamil and diltiazem, some experts believe that beta blockers should be preferred over calcium channel blockers in this setting.

Sotalol is a noncardioselective beta-adrenergic blocker that, unlike other beta blockers, prolongs the duration of the action potential, increases the refractory period, and lengthens the QT interval. As a result, sotalol is an effective antidysrhythmic agent and has been marketed for the treatment of life-threatening ventricular dysrhythmias. Although sotalol also has demonstrated efficacy in the prophylaxis and treatment of AF and PSVT, its role in the emergency management of these conditions remains poorly defined.

Class III agents include *amiodarone* and *bretylium,* as well as *ibutilide,* which is not yet approved in the United States but has been studied in Europe. Amiodarone is a complex antiarrhythmic with multiple effects. Although previously available only in oral form, an intravenous preparation of amiodarone was approved by the Food and Drug Administration in 1996 for the treatment of refractory VT and VF. Amiodarone is probably superior to lidocaine and bretylium for this indication, as well as for the treatment of stable VT. Amiodarone has also been moderately effective in the treatment of AF for rate control and conversion to sinus rhythm. Amiodarone can cause hypotension, heart block, and QT prolongation leading to torsade de pointes. Usual doses for VT and VF are 150 mg intravenously (i.v.) over 10 minutes, followed by 1 mg/min for 6 hours and then 0.5 mg/min. An additional bolus of 150 mg can be given for breakthrough arrhythmias. Similar doses can be used for unstable AF.[17]

Bretylium has been widely used in emergency medicine, particularly in the setting of cardiac arrest. However, in light of the greater safety and efficacy of other agents, bretylium should be considered, at best, a second- or third-line option.

Calcium channel blockers, particularly *diltiazem* and *verapamil,* continue to have a role in the therapy of tachycardias that involve the AV node. These drugs, which constitute class IV, dramatically decrease conduction through the AV node, thus slowing the ventricular response in conditions such as AF and interrupting reentry in PSVT (both when the circuit is contained entirely in the AV node and when one of its limbs is in the AV node and the other is in a bypass tract, such as occurs with WPW syndrome). Despite the popularity of adenosine, verapamil remains an excellent choice for the treatment of stable patients with regular narrow QRS complex tachycardia (usually PSVT), although it is contraindicated when the QRS complex is wide.[13] VT is the most common cause of a regular wide-complex tachycardia, and it cannot be ruled out with certainty on clinical or electrocardiographic grounds; calcium channel blockers may cause fatal degeneration to VF if given to patients with VT. Diltiazem has effects on the AV node similar to those of verapamil, but fewer vasodilatory and negative inotropic effects. The primary indication for intravenous diltiazem is for prompt control of the ventricular response rate in patients with rapid AF, particularly in the presence of mild-to-moderate congestive heart failure.[11]

Because of their vasodilatory and negative inotropic effects, calcium channel blocking agents can cause significant hypotension. They are contraindicated in the presence of severe hypotension and should also be used with caution in the presence of significant congestive heart failure. They are contraindicated in the presence of SA and AV nodal disease. Intravenous calcium blocking agents should be used cautiously in the presence of oral beta blockade, and are relatively contraindicated when intravenous beta blockers have recently been used. They are also relatively contraindicated in the presence of digitalis toxicity (but not merely because a patient is on digitalis) because of their effect on the AV node. Calcium, in doses as low as 100 mg of calcium chloride, can ameliorate the vasodilatory and negative inotropic effects of verapamil without diminishing its negative dromotropic effects on the AV node.[12]

Several drugs with important antiarrhythmic effects do not fit easily into this classification scheme. *Adenosine* is a naturally occurring nucleotide, which, like verapamil and diltiazem, exerts its principal antiarrhythmic effects by slowing conduction at the AV node. Adenosine also shares the potentially adverse cardiovascular effects of vasodilation, negative inotropy, and potentially excessive blockade of the AV node. The unique pharmacokinetic properties of adenosine, however, which has a serum half-life of less than 10 seconds, set it apart from the calcium channel blockers. In the treatment of reentrant AV nodal tachycardia (which makes up the vast majority of cases of PSVT), in which only a transient slowing of AV nodal conduction is necessary to interrupt the reentrant impulse and thus effect conversion to sinus rhythm, the shorter duration of action is particularly attractive, because side effects, even when momentarily severe, resolve so quickly that they are typically of minimal clinical consequence. On the other hand, the short half-life may also be responsible for the higher rate of recurrence of PSVT that is seen following conversion with adenosine than with verapamil.[5] The ultrashort duration of action also precludes the use of adenosine for control of the ventricular response in AF or atrial flutter.

In addition to its use in the termination of PSVT, adenosine is probably safe in regular wide-complex tachycardias of uncertain origin, and has been used diagnostically in this patient group. This practice should not be routine in patients with a high likelihood of VT (known coronary artery disease, ECG with evidence of AV dissociation) in whom benefit is unlikely. Adenosine is contraindicated in patients with an irregular wide-complex tachycardia (often due to AF with WPW) in whom VF may be induced.

Although the side effects of adenosine are generally too transient (less than 10 to 30 seconds) to be clinically significant, the drug is uniquely capable of causing brief but sometimes severe chest pain. The cause of this pain, which mimics myocardial ischemia, is uncertain, but it may be related to cardiac afferent innervation. It is not a sign of myocardial ischemia. Reassuring the patient of the benign nature of the pain is the only treatment necessary.

Because of its rapid degradation, adenosine must be given by rapid bolus injection, preferably in a more proximal venous access site (e.g., antecubital fossa), followed by a flush of normal saline. In the treatment of PSVT, an initial dose of 6 mg (0.01 mg/kg) can be followed by a 12-mg dose if the first dose is ineffective. Heart transplant patients are very sensitive to adenosine and require reduced doses, starting at 1 to 2 mg. Adenosine is potentiated by carbamazepine and dipyridamole and is antagonized by the methylxanthines (theophylline and caffeine). Contraindications include AV block, significant hypotension, and known WPW with AF.

Digoxin slows conduction through the AV node and has long been used for the control of the ventricular response in acute and chronic AF. Although digoxin may still have a role in the long-term management of AF, it has largely been supplanted by diltiazem for acute rate control. Digoxin is no more effective than placebo in converting AF to sinus rhythm, and it is less effective in this regard than a number of other drugs. Digoxin has a low toxic–therapeutic index and can induce arrhythmias at concentrations only minimally above therapeutic.

Magnesium appears to be an effective antiarrhythmic agent, although clinical and research experience with it is relatively limited. Magnesium is a necessary cofactor in the energy-dependent transmembrane sodium–potassium adenosine triphosphatase pump, and it is important in correcting intracellular hypokalemia (which greatly increases the risk of serious arrhythmias in the setting of acute ischemia). It also has antiarrhythmic effects in a variety of circumstances in which repolarization abnormalities exist. Clinically, magnesium has been demonstrated to be effective in the treatment of ventricular arrhythmias, particularly torsade de pointes, for which it is the drug of choice, and stable monomorphic VT.

Magnesium slows the ventricular rate in AF by blocking the AV node and may increase the rate of conversion to sinus rhythm. Magnesium can terminate MFAT and is marginally effective in PSVT. Usual doses of magnesium are 2 to 4 g i.v. over 5 minutes, followed by an infusion of 1 g per hour. At these dosages, magnesium is a safe agent that produces few side effects. At excessive doses or rates of administration, hypotension, loss of reflexes, and respiratory depression can occur. Infusions should be avoided in patients with renal failure, as accumulation can result in respiratory failure.

Automated Implantable Cardioverter–Defibrillators

Automated implantable cardioverter-defibrillators (AICDs) are being used in a growing number of patients with recurrent ventricular tachyarrhythmias who are at increased risk of sudden death. These devices have a computerized pulse generator, typically implanted in the abdominal wall, and both afferent and efferent cardiac leads. They are designed to recognize malignant rhythms and deliver a countershock to the heart.[24]

AICD failure can take several forms, each of which may result in emergent problems. The device may fail to fire when necessary, or may fire inappropriately (randomly, or in response to a nonmalignant tachycardia). When the AICD fails to fire, a patient can present in cardiac arrest (in VT or VF) or with recurrent bouts of tachycardia-related symptoms (palpitations, lightheadedness, syncope). During an arrest, the AICD should be deactivated by placing a standard pacemaker magnet over the upper right corner of the pulse generator for at least 30 seconds, until the QRS-synchronous beeps are replaced by a single continuous tone. Although the AICD poses no threat to the resuscitation team, it can interfere with the resuscitation. A cardiologist expert in the use of these devices should analyze the reason for AICD failure (sensing problems, lead problems, or pulse generator failure) in an intensive care unit.

Patients may present because the AICD has fired. This could represent an appropriate (and lifesaving) response to a malignant arrhythmia, or an inappropriate shock due to device malfunction. These patients should be seen by their cardiologist in the ED, and almost all (even those in whom the shock was ostensibly appropriate) should be admitted to a monitored setting to evaluate the underlying arrhythmia, to monitor antiarrhythmic drug therapy, and to ensure that the AICD is working properly. If the device continues to fire intermittently in the ED in the absence of malignant arrhythmic stimuli, it must be deactivated. This should be done only after ensuring that appropriate resuscitation equipment is immediately available; all such patients require admission to an intensive care unit.

EMERGENCY DEPARTMENT MANAGEMENT

In the ED, where diagnostic data are often limited and the patient's condition warrants prompt action, tachyarrhythmias are most successfully managed using an algorithmic diagnostic and therapeutic schema that is easily remembered and applied. The following approach is broadly applicable to the emergency management of tachyarrhythmias.

Step 1. Be Prepared for a Cardiopulmonary Arrest

Any patient with a tachyarrhythmia is at risk for deterioration, due either to the arrhythmia or to its treatment. Being prepared for a cardiopulmonary resuscitation by having advanced airway equipment and a defibrillator at the bedside minimizes the patient's risk.

Step 2. Determine Stability

Determine what hemodynamic effect the rhythm is having on the patient. In this context, *unstable* is defined as a heart rate and blood pressure inadequate to maintain vital organ perfusion and function, manifested clinically by significant chest pain, pulmonary edema, altered mental status, syncope, or severe hypotension. Categorizing a patient as stable or unstable is complicated by the innumerable gradations on the continuum from asymptomatic health to cardiopulmonary arrest. The most important feature in determining a patient's stability is the state of perfusion. Altered mental status and ischemic chest pain with ECG changes of ischemia are convincing evidence of instability. Electrical cardioversion should be used to treat unstable patients with any tachyarrhythmia except sinus tachycardia and MFAT.

It is important to note that although up to 70% of patients with a tachyarrhythmia complain of chest pain, the majority of these people do not have myocardial ischemia and are not really unstable. Chest pain associated with a tachyarrhythmia in a young healthy patient, in the absence of other evidence of hypoperfusion, is rarely clinically important. On the other hand, if the patient has a reasonable chance of underlying coronary artery disease, the chest pain must be taken seriously. Similarly, arbitrary blood pressure cut-offs for defining stable or unstable do not take into account the patient's baseline blood pressure. A systolic blood pressure of 80 mm Hg is of far more concern in a hypertensive elderly patient than in a young and healthy 20-year-old. It should be emphasized that stability is subject to change on a minute-to-minute basis, and therapy must be adjusted accordingly.

After clinical stability is assessed, the ECG should be rapidly and systematically evaluated. Although most therapeutic decisions can be made on the basis of a rhythm strip, a rapid search for evidence of acute ischemia (particularly ST-segment elevation or depression) is necessary and appropriate.

Step 3. Determine the Rate

The more extreme the ventricular rate, the more likely the patient is to become unstable. Sinus tachycardia rarely reaches 160 to 80 beats per minute in adults. Although SVTs typically have rates slower than 180 beats per minute, they can be faster in the presence of a bypass tract. VT is not slowed by passage through the AV node and can thus be much faster (250 to 300 beats per minute), but is usually less than 220 beats per minute.

Step 4. Determine the QRS Complex Width

When emergent cardioversion is not required, subsequent decisions can be based on the duration of the QRS complex. In an adult, a QRS width of greater than 0.12 milliseconds is considered "wide." In many adults with a wide-complex tachyarrhythmia, the QRS duration is substantially greater than 0.12 milliseconds. In children, the QRS duration is age-dependent, but any QRS duration over 0.10 milliseconds is considered prolonged.[1] It is usually possible to determine if a rhythm is wide or narrow from a rhythm strip alone, but if there is uncertainty, the widest QRS complex in the 12-lead ECG should be used as the measure.

Narrow-complex tachycardias can be assumed to be supraventricular. Wide-complex tachycardias are the result of any of three distinct pathophysiologic processes:

1. The rhythm originates in the ventricle and does not use the normal conduction pathway.
2. There is a block of the normal conduction pathway below the AV node (bundle-branch block).

3. The origin of the tachycardia is supraventricular, but there is an accessory conduction pathway that bypasses the normal conduction pathway.

With rare exceptions, a wide-complex tachycardia should be treated as VT for three reasons: (1) VT is the most common cause of a wide-complex tachycardia; (2) despite the existence of diagnostic criteria, VT cannot be reliably distinguished from SVT with aberrancy in the clinical setting, and treating VT as SVT can be fatal (while treating SVT as VT is not harmful); and (3) even if the tachycardia has a supraventricular origin, there may be an associated bypass tract, in which case, standard SVT treatment (e.g., verapamil) is contraindicated. It is never safe to assume that a wide-complex tachycardia is due to aberrancy.

Most important treatment decisions can be made on the basis of the foregoing process. Some, usually less critical, decisions require the following steps as well.

Step 5. Assess the Regularity of the RR Intervals

An irregular narrow-complex tachycardia is usually caused by AF, although it can occasionally be due to MFAT. Because VT is usually regular except during the first few beats, an irregular wide-complex tachycardia should raise the suspicion of AF with a bypass tract, for which the treatment of choice is cardioversion, even in a stable patient.

Step 6. Determine the Presence or Absence of P Waves

Determine whether P waves are present, their morphology, whether they are regular, and how they are related to the QRS complexes. Regular uniform P waves preceding the QRS complex help distinguish sinus tachycardia from other SVTs. Although similar P waves may be present with the much rarer PAT, an abnormal P-wave axis or morphology should alert one to the ectopic origin of that rhythm. An irregular narrow QRS complex rhythm with more than three P wave morphologies is indicative of MFAT. One should, in addition, look for the regular sawtooth deflections of the ECG baseline that characterize atrial flutter waves.

Application of this scheme organizes arrhythmias into a limited number of categories, each with a specific management strategy. Unstable patients sometimes need treatment initiated before analysis of the rhythm can be completed. Once the rhythm is stabilized, the patient may require additional pharmacologic treatment to prevent recurrent arrhythmias.

NARROW-COMPLEX TACHYCARDIAS

Regular, P Waves Present

Sinus tachycardia makes up the vast majority of these cases. PAT is a rare alternative diagnosis. Therapy for sinus tachycardia is usually directed at the rhythm's underlying cause rather than at the rhythm itself. However, there are exceptions. In the setting of acute myocardial ischemia, slowing the heart rate with beta blockers diminishes myocardial oxygen demand and improves mortality.[25] Beta blockers are also important in thyroid storm to counteract the adverse consequences of extraordinary increases in sympathetic drive. In cocaine overdose, beta blockade may be appropriate for control of heart rate, but only once simultaneous alpha blockade has been begun to avoid the greater danger of unopposed alpha-adrenergic stimulation.

Regular, No P Waves

PSVT (Fig. 135.1) makes up the majority of cases in this category. Although the rhythm strips of patients having atrial flutter with a consistent degree of AV nodal block can appear similar, careful inspection of a 12-lead ECG usually reveals flutter waves. Patients with PSVT who have severe signs of end-organ hypoperfusion should be cardioverted; more than 90% convert with small doses of electrical energy (10 to 50 J).

Treatment of PSVT, typically a reentrant tachycardia in which the AV node is part of the circuit, is directed at blockade of the AV node. Vagal maneuvers may be tried first: carotid massage, the Valsalva maneuver, and ice-water immersion work well in many patients. However, because many patients with recurrent PSVT are familiar with vagal maneuvers, they often present for treatment only when these maneuvers have failed; thus, these maneuvers are often not useful in the ED.

Pharmacotherapy for stable patients with PSVT involves blockade of the AV node. Treatment options include adenosine, verapamil, diltiazem, and beta blockers. Adenosine, due to its brief duration of action and its resultant lack of sustained hemodynamic effect, has become the drug of choice. The recommended initial dosage of adenosine is a 6-mg bolus over 1 to 3 seconds, followed by a 20-mg flush of normal saline. If there is no response in 1 to 2 minutes, a 12-mg dose can be administered in the same manner. It is important that the drug be given as a rapid bolus, so as to achieve high levels in the heart.

In the absence of any of the standard contraindications to calcium channel blockers (hypotension, congestive heart failure, sinus or AV nodal disease, or the previous use of i.v. beta blockers), verapamil is a safe and effective alternative. The standard initial dose is 0.075 to 0.150 mg/kg. In adults, an initial dose of 5 mg is usually appropriate. Most patients convert to sinus rhythm within about 2 minutes, and incremental doses to a maximum of 15 to 20 mg are usually successful in those who do not. Diltiazem is also effective in a dose of 10 mg i.v., repeated up to a total of 50 mg in the first 30 minutes. Calcium may be used to prevent or treat the hypotensive effects of verapamil and probably diltiazem.

Verapamil is safe when used in patients with narrow QRS complex tachycardias, particularly when calcium is used to prevent or treat transient hypotension. Nevertheless, there is a substantial incidence of adverse effects when contraindications are present, so they should not be ignored.[13] Many pediatric cardiologists consider it unsafe to use verapamil in children under 1 year of age, and so use adenosine exclusively in this age group.

Esmolol, an extremely short-acting beta-blocking agent with a half-life of less than 10 minutes, is moderately effective in treating PSVT, although success rates are significantly lower than with either adenosine or verapamil and the incidence of hypotension is higher. Esmolol is, therefore, a secondary drug in the treatment of PSVT.[23]

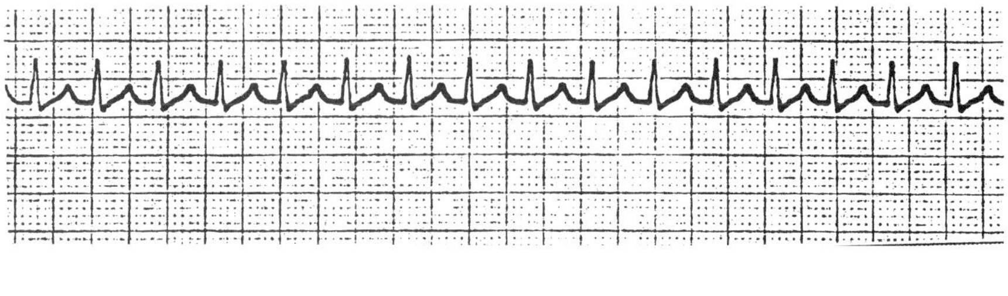

Figure 135.1. Paroxysmal supraventricular tachycardia.

Atrial Flutter

Atrial flutter is the most electrosensitive tachycardia, and electrocardioversion is the treatment of choice in most cases. The calcium channel blockers (verapamil and diltiazem), as well as digitalis, are capable of slowing the ventricular response in atrial flutter, and verapamil will convert perhaps 15% to 20% of cases to sinus rhythm.[2] Adenosine, while capable of slowing conduction for a few seconds, rarely results in cardioversion and has no role in the management of atrial flutter, although it can occasionally be of diagnostic value in distinguishing atrial flutter and PSVT. Unless cardioversion is contraindicated, pharmacologic therapy to slow heart rate is a secondary approach. Cardioversion, which occasionally results in AF rather than sinus rhythm, can be done semielectively in most patients in flutter. Given the small amount of current needed and the availability of excellent sedative agents, cardioversion should be possible with minimal discomfort.

While the diagnosis of atrial flutter is often fairly easy, some patients with flutter at first glance appear to be in other rhythms. Therefore, it is important to consider and exclude flutter before using any drug (such as procainamide) that speeds conduction through the AV node. This is because atrial activity in flutter is typically much faster than ventricular response, and such drugs can change the conduction from 2:1 or 3:1 to 1:1, with serious hemodynamic consequences. Vagal maneuvers can sometimes slow the ventricular rate enough to bring out flutter waves (if they are present), but adenosine is particularly effective in this regard.

Irregular, P Waves Present

Multifocal Atrial Tachycardia. MFAT is characterized by P waves of varying morphologies and by changing PR intervals. Because it originates in the atria, it is associated with narrow QRS complexes, except in the presence of underlying bundle-branch block. MFAT occurs primarily in patients with chronic lung disease, and within this group it is most common in patients with high or toxic levels of theophylline.

Because MFAT has been thought to occur due to the hypoxic effects of the underlying lung disease, treatment has been considered futile. The recognition that theophylline toxicity may contribute to this arrhythmia,[14] and several small series demonstrating slowing or conversion of MFAT with magnesium or verapamil, suggest that a nihilistic approach is inappropriate. Although MFAT is seldom life-threatening, the ability to control it can provide symptomatic benefit.

Irregular, No P Waves

Atrial Fibrillation. An irregular narrow-complex tachycardia is almost invariably AF or atrial flutter with variable block (Fig. 135.2). Occasionally, the P waves of MFAT are overlooked and that rhythm is confused with AF.

Although many patients with AF are seen in the ED, not all require emergency therapy. For example, those with chronic AF whose ventricular response rate is well controlled do not require immediate treatment. At the other extreme are patients with extremely rapid heart rates associated with hemodynamic deterioration, who require emergent cardioversion regardless of whether the AF is new or old. Because chronic AF is much less likely to convert to (or remain in) sinus rhythm regardless of the therapy used,[15] pharmacologic intervention to control the ventricular response rate is extremely important. Nevertheless, if there is evidence of severe end-organ hypoperfusion, cardioversion should always be tried.

For patients presenting with AF and a rapid ventricular response, treatment is directed at slowing the ventricular rate, and conversion to sinus rhythm is, at best, a secondary consideration. In the majority of these patients, the tachycardia itself (which profoundly decreases the time available for diastolic filling of the ventricles as well as coronary artery perfusion), rather than the loss of atrial systole, is responsible for the hemodynamic consequences. Patients with hypertrophic cardiomyopathy, as well as other patients with significant diastolic dysfunction of the heart, are an exception, because their stiff ventricles fill slowly and poorly during the passive phase of early diastole, and they thus rely on active atrial systole for an inordinate proportion of their end-diastolic ventricular volume.

At the other extreme, a slow ventricular response in new-onset AF is worrisome (unless the patient is already taking medications that slow conduction in the AV node), because it implies sinus node or AV node dysfunction (the "tachy–brady syndrome"). Such patients are rarely acutely unstable and may not require immediate treatment at all. In fact, attempted cardioversion may lead to asystole or prolonged bradycardia, and even if successful, it is typically followed by early reversion to AF.[4] Patients with spontaneously slow ventricular response to new-onset AF generally need to be admitted for consideration of long-term measures, including, in some cases, insertion of a permanent pacemaker.

Calcium channel blockers, in particular diltiazem, have supplanted digoxin as the drug of choice for AF with a rapid ventricular response in stable patients. This change in practice is the result of evidence that, although digoxin is no more effective than placebo in slowing ventricular response[18] in the first few hours, calcium channel blockers slow ventricular response within the first few minutes of i.v. administration. Neither digoxin nor calcium channel blockers are particularly effective at producing cardioversion to sinus rhythm. In stable patients, diltiazem can be given at a dose of 5 to 10 mg over 2 minutes, repeated as necessary every 5 minutes to a total dose of 50 to 60 mg in the first 30 minutes. To reduce hypotension, patients can be pretreated with calcium as described earlier. Following bolus injection, rate control can be maintained with an i.v. infusion of 5 to 15 mg per hour.

Alternative agents include verapamil, magnesium, beta blockers, and digoxin. Verapamil and magnesium are given in the same doses as for regular tachyarrhythmias. Beta blockers such as atenolol or metoprolol can be given in doses of 5 mg intravenously, repeated up to a total of 15 mg. Beta blockers are about as effective as calcium channel blockers for rate control, but are seldom used because of a higher incidence of hypotension. Beta blockers are indicated for rapid AF associated with thyrotoxicosis, a catecholamine excess state for which calcium channel blockers are minimally effective. Digoxin may be given as 0.5 mg i.v. or orally, followed by 0.25 mg 4 and 8 hours later. Even when using these loading regimens, rate control is no better than with placebo for at least several hours. Diltiazem or verapamil may be given i.v. at the same time as digoxin, in the absence of other contraindications. There may be some advantage to diltiazem in patients with mild hypotension or congestive

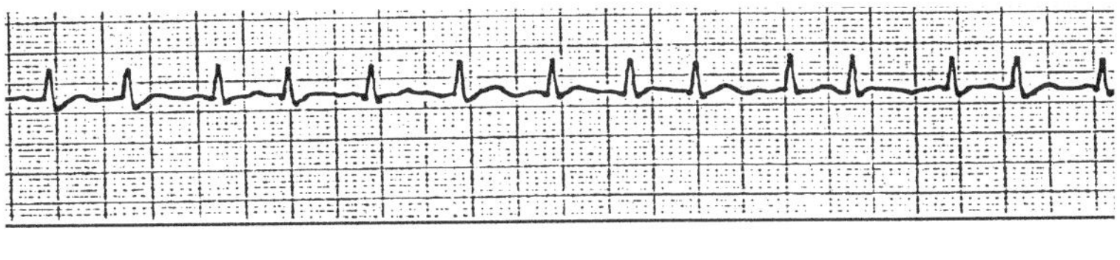

Figure 135.2. AF or atrial flutter with variable block.

heart failure, because of its less pronounced negative inotropic effect.[11] Calcium channel blockers should be avoided in the presence of digitalis toxicity.

The therapy of unstable patients with narrow-complex AF is one of the most challenging situations in all of arrhythmia management. Many AF patients have dilated atria and decreased ejection fractions. These patients do not easily cardiovert to sinus rhythm or remain in sinus rhythm if converted. In addition, cardioversion to sinus rhythm does not produce mechanical atrial contraction for hours to days. For this reason, cardioversion should be considered a form of rapid rate control and not a therapy that immediately restores atrial systole. Finally, if the patient has been in AF for more than 2 to 3 days, intraatrial thrombus may have formed and may embolize following cardioversion. For these reasons, cardioversion is considered by many a therapy of last resort.

If the patient is truly unstable, however, electrical cardioversion is required. Although some authorities suggest higher levels, 100 J is the usual starting dose, increasing to 200 J and 300 J as required. For unstable patients in whom electrical cardioversion fails and for somewhat more stable patients, rate control can be achieved by using repeated small boluses of diltiazem following pretreatment with calcium. Intravenous magnesium is a reasonable alternative. Amiodarone has been used in unstable atrial fibrillation in a number of small case series and in one randomized trial in which it was found to be inferior to magnesium.[17] Amiodarone slows ventricular rate and increases the frequency of conversion to sinus rhythm. In rare cases, the cautious use of dopamine may be required to maintain blood pressure. The seriousness of this clinical situation cannot be overemphasized, and no therapy is without significant risk.

New-onset AF has many causes, from the benign to the extremely serious. It has long been standard practice to admit almost all patients with new-onset AF in order to evaluate the possibility of serious underlying disease (e.g., acute myocardial infarction, mitral valve disease, pulmonary embolism, thyrotoxicosis, or drug effect) as its cause. However, 80% to 95% of stable patients with new-onset AF do not prove to have an acutely critical etiology, and those who do almost always have other worrisome clinical findings besides the arrhythmia itself.[20] Thus, the traditional policy is being questioned. Nevertheless, given the limited data on this subject to date, it remains reasonable to discharge only those patients with new-onset AF who do not have evidence of underlying heart disease or other acute instability, who convert easily in the ED back to sinus rhythm, and who are reliable and have good follow-up. Patients with chronic AF should be admitted to the hospital if they have signs of hemodynamic decompensation that requires cardioversion, or if hemodynamic effects and rapid ventricular response are not easily controlled.

Several agents have been the subject of limited testing in the pharmacologic cardioversion of new-onset AF, and they may prove to be of use in the future. These include flecainide, amiodarone, sotalol, clonidine, ibutilide, dofletanide, propafenone, and magnesium. The earlier rates of conversion of these drugs are offset by a high rate of proarrhythmia and hypotension and the fact that by 8 hours there is little difference from placebo in conversion rates.[6] For these reasons, the chemical conversion of recent-onset AF in the ED remains controversial. Magnesium given as an i.v. bolus of 2 to 4 g over 5 minutes, followed by an infusion of 1 to 2 g per hour, has been associated with a prompt reduction in heart rate and a 64% rate of conversion to sinus rhythm.[17] The fact that risks and benefits must be carefully explained to the patient, and that a trial of "time" may be very effective by itself, has led some authorities to suggest that attempts at chemical conversion should be performed only in the inpatient setting. The exact roles, if any, that these agents will play in the future management of new-onset AF await further study.

Anticoagulation is an important management issue for patients with AF. Not only are patients with AF that lasts more than several days at risk for systemic embolization, but recent evidence suggests that even shorter periods of AF may carry a risk of embolization, particularly following conversion to sinus rhythm. Even if accurate, a history of a brief duration of AF may fail to preclude the possibility of embolization due to intraatrial clot formation during the period of atrial stand-still that follows conversion to sinus rhythm. For this reason, some authorities suggest that all patients with acute AF be anticoagulated at the time of diagnosis and for 12 to 24 hours after conversion to sinus rhythm.

On the other hand, recent studies of transesophageal echocardiography (TEE) in ruling out an intraatrial thrombus prior to conversion of AF suggest that a negative TEE reduces the risk of embolization enough to obviate the need for anticoagulation. However, until additional studies more fully define the risks and benefits of these new management strategies, the standard of care is to anticoagulate all patients with AF of more than 72 hours' duration prior to elective electrical or chemical cardioversion. Of course, if it is necessary, cardioversion should never be withheld because of hemodynamic instability. In addition, all patients with chronic AF, except, perhaps, those less than 60 years old who have no other evidence of heart disease, should be on maintenance anticoagulant therapy unless there are substantial contraindications.[22]

Patients with chronic AF are usually taking antiarrhythmic medications. Digitalis has long been used for chronic rate control. Cardioversion in patients taking digoxin is a risk because of the potential for asystole. If cardioversion is required due to extreme hemodynamic compromise, it should initially be attempted at lower energy levels, such as 50 J. Many experts now prefer calcium channel blockers to digoxin for chronic rate control, because they control rate not only at rest, but also during exercise. There are also several recent reports suggesting a role for other drugs, including, particularly, amiodarone and sotalol, in chronic AF, although the overall safety of long-term therapy has been questioned.

WIDE-COMPLEX TACHYCARDIAS

As with narrow-complex tachycardias, tachycardias manifesting wide QRS complexes must be managed primarily according to their hemodynamic effects. Patients with wide-complex tachycardias are more likely to require cardioversion, because most have VT, which is more likely to be associated with end-organ hypoperfusion. Nevertheless, many such patients are relatively stable at presentation and respond to pharmacologic therapy.[21]

Regular, No P Waves

Diagnostic possibilities include VT, PSVT with aberrancy (bundle-branch block), and antidromic WPW syndrome. Several clinical and ECG criteria have been devised to enable clinicians to distinguish between VT and SVT when the QRS complex is wide. Useful indictors that make VT more likely include a history of heart disease, fusion and capture beats, and the presence of AV dissociation. Although such criteria are relatively accurate in predicting the source of tachycardia in series of patients, no single sign or combination of signs can definitively identify the origin of tachycardia.[10] For this reason, wide-complex tachycardia should virtually always be treated as VT. Thus, drugs contraindicated in VT (e.g., verapamil) are almost never used to treat wide-complex tachycardia.[16,21] Adenosine may be used to treat regular wide-complex tachycardia of uncertain etiology, because it is probably safe (if only very rarely effective) in VT and will convert most episodes of PSVT, including antidromic WPW syndrome.

Ventricular Tachycardia. VT is usually a life-threatening medical emergency. Although some patients have intermittent asymptomatic bouts of VT (usually episodes of less than 10 beats), patients who present to an ED with VT are usually either suffering from significant hemodynamic effects or experiencing other acute cardiac problems, including, particularly, myocardial ischemia, that require emergent treatment. Essentially, all patients with VT require consultation with a cardiologist and admission after ED therapy of the arrhythmia.

The typically very rapid heart rate of sustained VT usually causes hemodynamic deterioration.[16] Such patients require emergent electrical cardioversion. Fifty joules is a reasonable initial energy, because about 90% of episodes of VT respond to 10 to 50 watt-seconds of energy. Cardioversion is performed in the synchronized mode to avoid precipitating VF. Lidocaine, procainamide, and bretylium are standard agents used to prevent recurrence of VT after successful cardioversion or to treat patients with recurrent VT. Recent evidence suggests that magnesium and amiodarone may also be efficacious.

Sometimes, patients with sustained VT show no signs of hemodynamic instability in the short term. These patients can be treated with lidocaine, procainamide, magnesium, or amiodarone. The medical literature does not provide a clear basis for preferring one agent over another. Lidocaine, which is only moderately effective for VT, is given as an initial 100-mg i.v. bolus and may be repeated in 75-mg boluses up to 3 mg/kg. Procainamide, an effective therapy for both VT and PSVT, is given as a 17-mg/kg i.v. bolus at a rate of not more than 50 mg/min. Procainamide can cause QRS widening and hypotension. Magnesium is effective for VT and moderately effective for PSVT. Usual doses of magnesium are 2 to 4 g i.v. over 5 minutes, followed by an infusion of 1 g per hour. Amiodarone can be given as 150 mg i.v. over 10 minutes, followed by an infusion of 1 mg/min over the next 6 hours. An additional 150-mg i.v. bolus can be given for breakthrough VT. Amiodarone can cause hypotension (treated with fluid bolus) and AV nodal block.

Wide-Complex PSVT. PSVT can manifest with wide QRS complexes when bundle-branch block (either underlying or rate-related) is present (Fig. 135.3). The duration of the QRS complex in this circumstance is not likely to exceed 0.14 second, and heart rates usually range between 130 and 200 beats per minute. Nevertheless, it is virtually impossible to be certain that a wide-complex tachycardia represents PSVT with bundle-branch block, rather than VT; therefore, treatment should almost never be based on this assumption.[10]

Wide QRS complexes are also seen in PSVT in association with the WPW syndrome when anterograde conduction occurs down the bundle of Kent and retrograde conduction occurs through the AV node. It may be possible to make this diagnosis from the ECG in patients with known WPW syndrome, although confusion with VT may still occur. When faced with a stable patient with a regular wide-complex tachycardia of uncertain etiology, adenosine is the preferred antiarrhythmic. Neither verapamil nor digoxin is recommended in this circumstance.

When adenosine fails to convert regular wide-complex tachycardia or when VT is considered more likely, procainamide is a rational choice. Procainamide has antiarrhythmic effects on both atrial and ventricular tissue, and it is safe and useful in most cases of wide-complex tachycardia, whether VT or PSVT with anterograde conduction through the bundle of Kent. Wide-complex tachycardia in the setting of possible drug overdose, however, suggests cyclic antidepressant toxicity, in which case, procainamide is absolutely contraindicated. Lidocaine, the first-line pharmacologic agent for treatment of known VT (in the absence of hemodynamic consequences), can occasionally speed conduction through bypass tracts in experimental models; thus, lidocaine is less attractive than procainamide when wide-complex tachycardia is suspected to be due to WPW-related PSVT.

Irregular, No P Waves

Diagnostic possibilities include AF with bundle-branch block, AF with the WPW syndrome, torsade de pointes, and VF.

Wide-Complex AF. A few patients with AF present with wide QRS complexes, owing to an underlying or rate-related bundle-branch block or to the WPW syndrome. In the presence of known underlying bundle-branch block, treatment can be similar to that for routine narrow-complex AF (i.e., cardioversion for unstable patients and a calcium channel blocker for rate control in stable patients).

Patients with rate-related bundle-branch block often demonstrate both wide complexes (in beats that follow short RR intervals) and narrow complexes (in beats that follow longer RR intervals), but patients with AF and the WPW syndrome may also have both wide and narrow QRS complexes, depending on the conduction path followed by each depolarization. It is critical to recognize this latter entity, because agents that slow conduction through the AV node are absolutely contraindicated.[9]

WPW is a relatively rare syndrome that involves accessory pathway connections between the atrium and the ventricles. The presence of these rapidly conducting pathways predisposes to a number of arrhythmias, of which AF is the most dangerous. AF generates impulses at 300 to 600 per minute. The accessory pathways of WPW, which bypass the AV node and its protective slowing, conduct impulses to the ventricle at rates exceeding 250 beats per minute. The ventricle will fail or undergo fibrillation if these excessively rapid atrial impulses are conducted for more than a short time. Many patients are aware that they have WPW. Among patients who give no history of WPW, the possibility should be considered when the irregular rhythm is wide and very fast, and the QRS complexes are variable and bizarre.

Drugs such as verapamil, diltiazem, and digitalis are contraindicated in WPW syndrome with wide-complex AF, because they can actually increase the speed of conduction through the bypass tract. More importantly, relative blockade of the AV node causes preferential conduction through the bypass tract, resulting in much higher ventricular response rates; an extremely rapid ventricular response to AF can then deteriorate

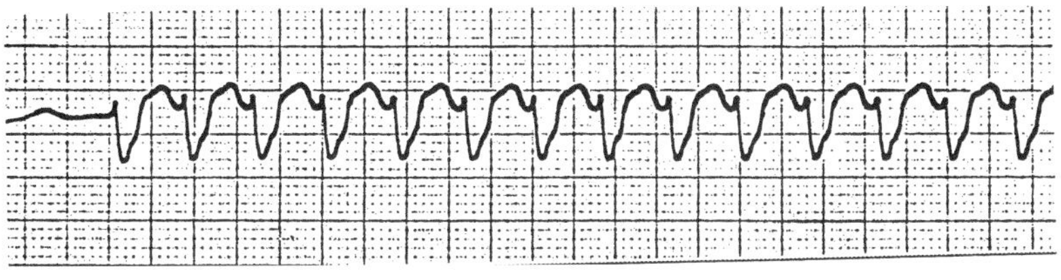

Figure 135.3. Wide-complex paroxysmal supraventricular tachycardia.

into VF. With calcium channel blockers, other hemodynamic effects, such as decreased inotropy and vasodilation, in the absence of any therapeutic effect, can add to the potentially catastrophic consequences of such therapy.

Although procainamide is unlikely to be harmful in WPW-related AF, it may not be particularly effective in the acute setting. Therefore, even in the absence of acute hemodynamic deterioration, patients with WPW-related AF are best treated with electrical cardioversion. After cardioversion, procainamide is given to prolong the refractoriness of the accessory pathway and to prevent recurrence of AF. Because procainamide can increase AV nodal conduction, some authorities suggest the addition of an AV node blocking agent.

Torsade de Pointes. Torsade de pointes is an unusual form of polymorphic VT characterized by the peculiar spiral pattern it produces on the surface ECG. The most common cause is the use of type IA antidysrhythmic agents (e.g., quinidine, procainamide, and disopyramide) that prolong the QT interval, a factor central to the development of this dysrhythmia. Other drugs (most prominently, the phenothiazines), drug interactions, and many other conditions (especially hypocalcemia and hypokalemia) are also associated with torsade.

Although most episodes of torsade are self-limited, they are nevertheless life-threatening, because any episode can precipitate VF. Because torsade usually converts spontaneously to sinus rhythm but then recurs, treatment is directed at preventing recurrences rather than terminating a given episode. In the long term, this often requires only withdrawal of the offending agent. In the ED, however, antidysrhythmic therapy is mandatory.

Magnesium, given as an i.v. infusion of 2 to 4 g over 30 minutes to 1 hour, is highly effective and is the treatment of choice for torsade. Alternately, overdrive electrical pacing can be used to speed the heart rate and thus decrease the dispersion of refractoriness that is the underlying basis for this arrhythmia. Infusions of isoproterenol have also been used with the same goal, although the proarrhythmic effect of isoproterenol is worrisome.

Ventricular Fibrillation. VF is the chaotic firing of the ventricle from multiple foci and never results in effective myocardial contraction. It is the most common rhythm found early in cardiac arrest. The only therapy proven to improve the outcome of patients with VF is electrical defibrillation. When a defibrillator is available, no other activity should take precedence: No time should be spent starting i.v. lines, securing an airway, performing cardiopulmonary resuscitation, or giving drugs, as these delay the performance of electrical defibrillation. Immediate defibrillation in the nonsynchronized mode with a dose of 200 J provides the greatest likelihood of success. Increasing energy levels probably does not improve the likelihood of defibrillation and may, in fact, be detrimental. Good contact with the chest, use of conduction gel, and firm pressure are all important to reduce transthoracic impedance and improve energy transfer to the heart.

Several adjunctive drugs are widely used when initial defibrillation is not successful. Although these drugs are considered standard therapy in this situation, it is important to remember that none of them has been definitively shown to increase the success of defibrillation or to improve long-term outcome in human beings with cardiac arrest. Thus, administration of these agents should never interfere with the rapid use of electrical defibrillation, the only intervention that has been definitively shown to affect outcome.

Specifically, no study has confirmed a positive effect of epinephrine use at either standard or high doses. Indeed high-dose epinephrine use is associated with increased costs from the small but significant increase in severely neurologically impaired survivors. Similarly, there is little evidence that lidocaine, bretylium, or amiodarone significantly improves outcome in refractory VF. Lidocaine remains the drug of choice in the current American Heart Association advance cardiac life-support guidelines, but there is evidence that amiodarone may be marginally more effective.

Intravenous lidocaine, bretylium, or amiodarone is used, however, to help prevent recurrence of VF after successful defibrillation. Comparative studies have failed to show any major differences between lidocaine and bretylium in this regard, but trends in several studies have favored lidocaine, which probably has fewer adverse effects. The role of amiodarone in arrhythmia prophylaxis following successful cardioversion is, as yet, undefined.

Although sodium bicarbonate and calcium chloride may worsen outcome if used routinely in cardiac arrest, they still have a role in specific circumstances. Sodium bicarbonate may be lifesaving in tricyclic antidepressant overdose, and i.v. calcium is often an effective antidote for calcium channel blocker overdose.

DISPOSITION

In most cases, the disposition of patients with tachyarrhythmia is obvious. The patient resuscitated from cardiac arrest due to VF obviously must be admitted to the intensive care unit. Similarly, there should be little controversy about discharging a healthy young patient with a brief, minimally symptomatic episode of PSVT that readily converted to sinus rhythm. In the few patients with a problematic disposition, the physician should remember that ED care involves only initial therapy and not definitive management of the tachyarrhythmia. Several categories of patients should be admitted:

- Patients who are symptomatic after acute onset of tachycardia and who have failed appropriate therapy or responded only transiently
- Patients who were clinically unstable as a result of a tachycardia, including all patients who require cardioversion because of end-organ hypoperfusion
- Patients who were treated successfully before the development of serious symptoms but who have the potential for decompensation if the tachyarrhythmia recurs

The basis of the arrhythmia also plays a role in disposition decisions: Any patient with a realistic likelihood of a dangerous etiology (e.g., possible acute myocardial infarction) should be admitted, even if the arrhythmia itself was benign.

Finally, it may be appropriate to admit a stable patient for continuous ECG monitoring during initiation of chronic drug therapy.

COMMON PITFALLS

- Failure to be prepared for deterioration of the patient's condition. All arrhythmias and their therapies have the potential to cause the patient to decompensate. A defibrillator and advanced airway equipment should be ready at the bedside.
- Failure to use a systematic approach to tachyarrhythmias based on the clinical status at presentation
- Being overly concerned with "diagnosis." One should concentrate more on the hemodynamic effects of the rhythm than on its origin. An apparently benign narrow-complex rhythm should not be treated conservatively in the face of end-organ hypoperfusion. Patients who are unstable in the

face of any very rapid tachycardia (except for sinus tachycardia or MFAT) require electrical cardioversion. Conversely, stable patients can often be managed without electrical cardioversion, even if their tachycardia appears ominous from the standpoint of its cause or morphology.

- Reliance on ECG and clinical findings to identify the likely source of an arrhythmia. ECG and clinical findings are suggestive but not infallible guides.
- Use of verapamil to treat a wide-complex tachycardia. Verapamil is appropriate for many narrow-complex tachycardias but can precipitate VF in wide-complex tachycardias. This is true not only when the rhythm is VT, but also for other wide-complex tachycardias originating above the AV node, such as AF with anterograde conduction down a bypass tract in WPW.
- Treatment of symptoms rather than the tachyarrhythmia precipitating those symptoms. In patients having symptoms related to a very rapid tachycardia, controlling the ventricular rate usually ameliorates the symptoms.
- Failure to seek and, if possible, correct the factors that precipitated a tachyarrhythmia. Examples of specific precipitants include hypoxemia, infectious or inflammatory processes (e.g., endocarditis, myocarditis, pericarditis), and endocrine or metabolic abnormalities (e.g., thyrotoxicosis, hypokalemia or hyperkalemia, hypomagnesemia). Arrhythmias can also be caused by intoxications, such as intentional overdose (e.g., tricyclic antidepressants), drug abuse (e.g., cocaine, alcohol), or therapeutic misadventure with prescribed medications (e.g., digoxin, theophylline). In patients taking antidysrhythmic agents, an acute dysrhythmia may be the result of subtherapeutic drug levels, a dysrhythmogenic effect of the drug at therapeutic or toxic levels, or simply a failure of the drug to prevent a preexisting dysrhythmia.
- Failure to consider myocardial ischemia in all patients. Myocardial infarction must be ruled out whenever it seems a reasonably likely cause of the arrhythmia, or when the arrhythmia has itself produced a substantial period of ischemia as suggested by ECG changes or symptoms.

References

1. Alander SW, Hulse JE. Pediatric ECG's and rhythm disturbances. *Pediatr Emerg Med Rep* 1999;4(7):63.
2. Aronow WS, et al. Verapamil in atrial fibrillation and atrial flutter. *Clin Pharmacol Ther* 1979; 26:578.
3. Berntsen RF, Rasmussen K. Lidocaine to prevent ventricular fibrillation in the pre-hospital phase of suspected acute myocardial infarction: The North Norwegian Lidocaine Intervention Trial. *Am Heart J* 1992;124:1478.
4. Bigger JT Jr. Management of arrhythmias. In: Braunwald E, ed. *Heart disease. A textbook of cardiovascular medicine.*. Philadelphia: WB Saunders, 1980:724.
5. Cairns CB, Niemann JT. Intravenous adenosine in the emergency department treatment of paroxysmal supraventricular tachycardia. *Ann Emerg Med* 1991;20:717.
6. Donovan KD, Power B, Hockings EF, et al. Intravenous flecainide versus amiodarone for recent onset atrial fibrillation. *Am J Cardiol* 1995;75:693.
7. Echt DS, Liebson PR, Mitchell LB, et al. Morbidity and mortality in patients receiving encainide, flecainide, or placebo. The Cardiac Arrhythmia Suppression Trial. *N Engl J Med* 1991;324:781.
8. Griffith MJ, Linker NJ, Garratt CJ, et al. Relative efficacy and safety of intravenous drugs of the termination of sustained ventricular tachycardia. *Lancet* 1990;336:670.
9. Gulamhusein S, Ko P, Carruthers SG, et al. Acceleration of the ventricular response during atrial fibrillation in the Wolff-Parkinson-White syndrome after verapamil. *Circulation* 1982;65:348.
10. Herbert ME, Votey SR, Morgan MT, et al. Failure to agree on the ECG diagnosis of VT. *Ann Emerg Med* 1996;27:35–38.
11. Heywood JT, Graham B, Marais GE, et al. Effect of intravenous diltiazem on rapid atrial fibrillation accompanied by congestive heart failure. *Am J Cardiol* 1991;67:1150.
12. Kuhn M, Schriger DL. Low-dose calcium pretreatment to prevent verapamil-induced hypotension. *Am Heart J* 1992;124:231.
13. Kuhn M, Schriger DL. Verapamil administration to patients with contraindications: is it associated with adverse outcomes? *Ann Emerg Med* 1991;20:1094.
14. Levine JH, Michael JR, Guarnieri T. Multifocal atrial tachycardia: a toxic effect of theophylline. *Lancet* 1985;1(8419):12.
15. Mancini GBJ, Goldberger AL. Cardioversion of atrial fibrillation: consideration of embolization, anticoagulation, prophylactic pacemaker, and long term success. *Am Heart* 1982;104:617.
16. Morady F, Shen EN, Bhandari A, et al. Clinical symptoms in patients with sustained ventricular tachycardia. *West J Med* 1985;142:341.
17. Moran JL, Gallagher J, Peake SI, et al. Parenteral magnesium sulfate versus amiodarone in the therapy of atrial tachyrhythmias: a prospective, randomized study. *Crit Care Med* 1995;23(11):1816.
18. Roberts SA, Diaz C, Nolan PE, et al. Effectiveness and costs of digoxin therapy for atrial fibrillation. *Am J Cardiol* 1993;72:567.
19. Ruskin JN, McGovern B, Garan H, et al. Antiarrhythmic drugs: a possible cause of out of hospital cardiac arrest. *N Engl J Med* 1983;309:1302.
20. Shlofmitz RA, Hirsch BE, Meyer BR. New onset atrial fibrillation: is there a need for emergent hospitalization? *J Gen Intern Med* 1986;1:139.
21. Stewart RB, Bardy GH, Greene H. Wide complex tachycardia. Misdiagnosis and outcome after emergent therapy. *Ann Intern Med* 1986;104:766.
22. Stroke Prevention in Atrial Fibrillation Investigators. Preliminary report of the Stroke Prevention in Atrial Fibrillation Study. *N Engl J Med* 1990;322:863.
23. Sung RJ, Blanski L, Kirshenbaum J, MacCosbe P, et al. Clinical experience with esmolol, a short acting beta adrenergic blocker in cardiac arrhythmias and myocardial ischemia. *Clin Pharmacol* 1986;26[Suppl A]:A15.
24. Winkle RA. State-of-the-art of the AICD. *Pacing Clin Electrophysiol* 1991;14:961–966.
25. Yusuf S, Sleight P, Rossi P, et al. Reduction in infarct size, arrhythmias, and chest pain by early intravenous beta blockade in suspected acute myocardial infarction. *Circulation* 1983;67[Suppl 1]:132.

CHAPTER 136
The Patient with a Pacemaker or Implantable Cardioverter–Defibrillator

Robert M. Rodriguez

THE PATIENT WITH A PACEMAKER

The first permanent cardiac pacemakers were implanted in the late 1950s, and since that time, advances in microprocessor technology have led to the production of compact pacemakers that adapt to changes in patient physiology.[11] While the earliest models had only single-chamber, asynchronous pacing capability, with less than a 2-year battery life, current dual-chamber pacemakers are rate-responsive to increased patient activity and are powered by lithium batteries that may last more than 10 years.[3]

Given that over 1 million Americans currently have pacemakers,[11] the emergency physician will undoubtedly care for many patients with these devices. While detailed knowledge of the myriad complexities of pacemaker programming and operation is unnecessary, the emergency physician must understand the basics of pacemaker terminology and function and must be familiar with the presentation, evaluation, and treatment of the common pacemaker-related problems.

Central to the understanding of basic pacemaker function are the five-letter codes used by the North American Society of Pacing and Electrophysiology–British Pacing and Electro-

TABLE 136.1. NASPE/BPEG (NBG) Codes

1st position indicates the chamber paced:
- V = ventricle
- A = atrium
- D = dual
- O = no pacing

2nd position indicates the chamber sensed:
- V = ventricle
- A = atrium
- D = dual
- O = no sensing

3rd position indicates the response to a sensed event:
- I = inhibited
- T = triggered/tracking
- D = dual
- O = no response

4th position indicates programmability & rate response:
- O = not programmable
- P = simple programming (three functions or less)
- M = multiprogrammable (more than three functions)
- C = communicating (M + telemetry capabilities)
- R = rate responsive

5th position indicates anti-tachyarrhythmia functions:
- O = none
- P = pacing
- S = shock
- D = dual (shock and pacing)

From Love C, ed. *Handbook of Cardiac Pacing*. Georgetown, TX: Landes Bioscience, 1998, with permission.

physiology Group (NASPE/BPEG) to characterize the modes of operation of current pacemakers (Table 136.1). In everyday practice, description of the mode of pacing is limited to use of the first three code letters: position I, chamber(s) paced; position II, chamber(s) sensed; and position III, pacemaker response to sensing. A VVI pacemaker thus paces the ventricle only, senses only ventricular depolarizations, and inhibits pacemaker output in response to a sensed ventricular depolarization. The more versatile DDD pacemaker, which is currently the most frequently implanted type of pacemaker,[11] may pace the atria, the ventricles, or both; sense atrial depolarizations, ventricular depolarizations, or both; and either inhibit or trigger pacemaker output to the atria and ventricles in response to sensed depolarizations. Intrinsic ventricular depolarizations will inhibit both atrial and ventricular output; intrinsic atrial depolarizations will inhibit atrial pacemaker output and will trigger ventricular output if the ventricle itself does not respond after a programmed time interval.

CLINICAL PRESENTATION AND DIFFERENTIAL DIAGNOSIS

Syndromes of pacemaker malfunction can generally be divided into those that cause underpacing, with associated bradycardia, hypotension, light-headedness, and syncope; and those that produce overpacing, manifested by tachycardia and palpitations with or without ischemia or hypotension symptoms. The differential diagnosis of these nonspecific presenting complaints is broad, however, encompassing multiple other disorders, including dysrhythmias, vasovagal phenomena, anemia, hypovolemia, and non–rate-related syndromes of low cardiac output. Before attributing presenting symptoms to pacemaker malfunction, the physician must first determine whether the device is truly malfunctioning. Patient history, electrocardiogram (ECG) analysis, and determination of the current programming and specifications of the pacemaker are the keys to making this evaluation.

EMERGENCY DEPARTMENT EVALUATION

In addition to elucidating standard history about the symptoms, time course, and precipitants related to the presenting complaint(s), the physician should also seek the following information regarding the pacemaker: pacemaker model, current programming, date of implantation, indication for implantation, history of pacemaker malfunction, and dates of last interrogation and battery check. Some of this vital information may be obtained from the pacemaker identification card, which the patient should carry at all times. If this card is unavailable, a chest x-ray may reveal the pacemaker's identifying serial number or code.[12] For technical support or to find out other information about the pacemaker, the physician may call the pacemaker manufacturer's assistance department.

The emergency physician should also ask about exposure to potential sources of environmental electromagnetic interference with pacemaker function. While most everyday appliances and devices pose virtually no risk to current pacemakers, electric toothbrushes, cellular telephones, induction ovens, and stove plates can markedly alter their operation. Most modern airport security gates pose minimal risk, but antitheft systems in stores emit signals of variable intensity, with unpredictable effects on pacemaker function.[8]

Because right ventricular (RV) pacemakers produce left bundle-branch block (LBBB) patterns of depolarization, the ECG diagnosis of myocardial ischemia or infarction (MI) may be difficult. Discordant T waves after paced beats are the norm; minor ST-segment evaluations inferiorly and anteriorly (leads V_1 to V_3) and ST-segment depression leads 1, V_1, V_5, and V_6 also commonly occur in the absence of ischemia.[2] Pacing may even induce marked ST-segment and T-wave abnormalities when the patient's native, spontaneous rhythm emerges.[2]

Applying the criteria used in the evaluation of patients with intrinsic LBBB, however, the physician may still occasionally diagnose MI in the patient with a pacemaker.[2] Concordant ST-segment elevations and markedly elevated (greater than 5 mm) discordant ST-segments are highly indicative of MI, especially when the T waves associated with these segments are of opposite polarity.[2,16] ST-segment depression in leads V_1, V_2, and V_3 also suggests ischemia or infarction, as does late notching of the ascending QRS limb in the left precordial leads.[2,16] A qR pattern after the pacemaker spike in leads 1, V_1, and V_5 has low sensitivity but very high specificity for anteroseptal MI.[2] Finally, serial ECGs may demonstrate progressive ST-segment and T-wave changes that lead to the diagnosis of MI. The emergency physician should certainly look for these patterns, but their absence does not, by any means, rule out ischemia or infarction.

Evaluating the utility of an ECG algorithm based on these patterns for the detection of MI in patients with intrinsic LBBB, investigators found that the algorithm had poor sensitivity (less than 10%) for MI prediction.[18] If the results of this study can be generalized to pacemaker patients with LBBB depolarization patterns, then the emergency physician must not base decisions about thrombolysis and other interventions for pacemaker patients with suspected ischemia or infarction solely or even primarily on the ECG.

Pacemaker Malfunction and Pacemaker-Associated Disorders

Pacemaker malfunction leading to a slow pulse arises from noncapture, pacemaker output failure, and/or pacemaker oversensing. *Noncapture* refers to an absence of ventricular or atrial depolarization after a pacemaker spike (Fig. 136.1). The most common cause of this condition is pacemaker lead dislodgement, which typically occurs within a few weeks of implanta-

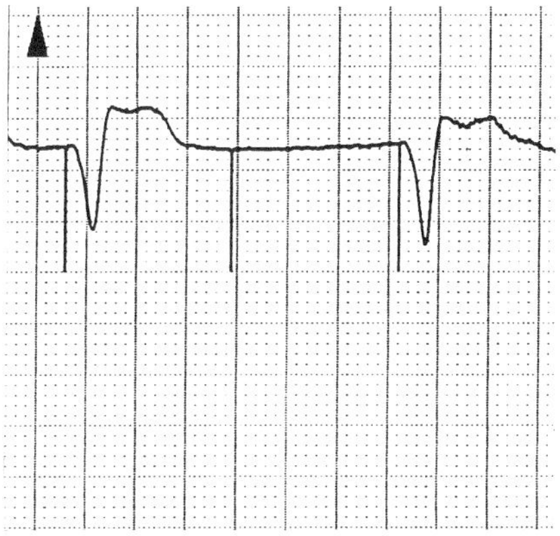

Figure 136.1. Noncaptured pacemaker spike between two captured spikes.

tion.[8] Other mechanical causes include insulation breaks, lead fracture, and inflammatory reaction at the lead tip.[8] Reversible metabolic abnormalities, such as hyperkalemia, and drug effects should also be considered. Of note, if a pacemaker spike occurs within 300 milliseconds of a prior ventricular depolarization, the ventricle may be in its refractory period and lack of capture is expected.[6] The pacemaker may be firing early because of undersensing of the prior depolarization, but it is not truly malfunctioning with regard to pacing (Fig. 136.2).

Absent or inappropriately delayed ventricular pacemaker spikes on the ECG of a bradycardic pacemaker patient indicate primary pacemaker output failure, battery depletion, or output failure secondary to oversensing (reading other signals as ventricular depolarizations).[8] Causes of primary output failure include lead fracture or disconnection and various pulse generator component failures. Oversensed signals may be of cardiac (P and T waves) or extracardiac (myopotentials) origin and lead to inappropriate inhibition of pacemaker ventricular output.[8]

These causes may be distinguished by performing a magnet test of the pacemaker. Application of a ring magnet over a normally functioning pacemaker disables sensing and induces asynchronous pacing at model-specific rates, which may be determined by checking the patient's records or calling the pacemaker manufacturer.[8,12] If the problem is oversensing, the magnet will induce asynchronous pacing at that model's characteristic rate. If battery depletion is the cause, asynchronous pacing will occur at a different, generally slower rate.[8] If the malfunction is due to lead displacement or some other primary cause, no pacing response to the magnet will be seen.

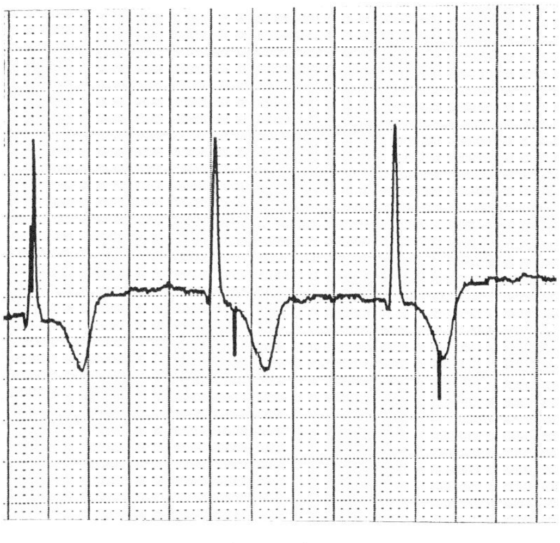

Figure 136.2. Pacemaker undersensing.

Pacemakers may produce inappropriate tachycardia by several mechanisms. When a pacemaker fails to sense intrinsic ventricular depolarizations, it will fail to inhibit pacemaker output, potentially causing a pacemaker-driven tachycardia; that is, "undersensing leads to overpacing."[12] In dual-chamber systems, the pacemaker circuit may act like an accessory pathway similar to those seen in Wolff-Parkinson-White syndrome, thus propagating a reentrant tachycardia known as pacemaker-mediated tachycardia or "endless-loop tachycardia."[12] This dysrhythmia may be terminated by vagal maneuvers, external magnet suppression of sensing, intravenous adenosine, or external cardiac pacing with 10 to 20 mA of output.[6,12]

A final pacemaker-related tachycardia that occurs only rarely with current pulse generators is "runaway pacemaker," a potentially lethal disorder in which battery depletion or other component failure causes extremely rapid pacing, with rates restricted only by the pacemaker's upper rate limit.[9] This disorder generally does not respond to conservative treatment measures, and, in the setting of hemodynamic instability, the emergency physician should attempt to disable the runaway pacemaker by incising over the pacemaker pocket and disconnecting the pulse generator leads.[6,9]

Pacemaker syndrome, a classic example of a pacemaker operating correctly according to its programming yet still causing bothersome symptoms, results from a loss of atrioventricular synchrony in the VVI pacing mode.[12] Fatigue, light-headedness, and syncope due to decreased cardiac output (loss of atrial kick), and disturbing neck pulsations related to regurgitant cannon A waves (atria contracting against closed atrioventricular valves) are the predominant symptoms. While this disorder is largely limited to patients with VVI pacemakers and is usually ameliorated with a change to synchronized dual-chamber pacing, it can occasionally occur in patients who have DDD pacemakers.[17]

In addition to the rhythm and hemodynamic problems associated with pacemakers, foreign-body–related complications also occur. Infections of pacemakers and associated hardware occur in approximately 6% to 15% of patients, with staphylococcal species being the most common pathogens.[6] In the patient presenting with fever and redness and tenderness over the pulse generator pocket, the diagnosis of pacemaker infection is obvious.

Subtler presentations are common, however, and the emergency physician should consider pacemaker-related infection as a potential cause of unexplained fever in any patient with a pacemaker. Notably, without superimposed endocarditis, embolic phenomena and murmurs are generally absent. Nuclear medicine scans may provide ancillary evidence of infected pacemaker hardware. Confirmed pacemaker infection mandates a course of parenteral antibiotics, and most authorities agree that removal of the device is indicated.[13]

Pacemaker-associated thrombosis of the upper extremity vessels is uncommon (less than 5% by venography), but it should be considered in the patient with unilateral arm swelling, erythema, and/or pain.[5] Ultrasound or venography may be used to distinguish this entity from similar-appearing arm cellulitis. Anticoagulation without pacemaker removal has been reported to successfully treat the thrombosis.[5]

EMERGENCY DEPARTMENT MANAGEMENT

As with other emergency department (ED) problems, patient stability determines the urgency of intervention in the patient with a pacemaker. The cardiac arrest patient should receive standard advanced cardiac life support (ACLS)–guided resuscitation. During defibrillation or cardioversion, however, the physician should avoid placing pads or paddles directly over the pulse generator.[7] Pacemakers of resuscitation survivors should be evaluated for damage and/or reprogramming arising from countershocks. In nonsurvivors, the pacemaker may continue to produce ECG spikes without associated ventricular capture, which represents isolated pacemaker activity and not true pulseless electrical activity.

The pacemaker patient with hypotensive bradycardia requires the usual emergent therapeutic measures (chronotropic support with medications, external pacing, and/or transvenous pacing). The physician may attempt to temporarily asynchronously pace the patient's rate with higher current by placing a ring magnet over the pacemaker, as described earlier in this chapter.[8] This maneuver may be helpful if the pacemaker is oversensing, and thereby suppressing output (absent or inappropriately slow pacemaker spikes on ECG), or if low pacemaker current is leading to noncapture.

During the ED management of pacemaker patients, the physician must recognize the multiple potential sources of electromagnetic interference with pacemaker function, especially magnetic resonance imaging (MRI) and electrocautery. Given that MRI may induce complete block of pacemaker output, severe pacemaker-driven tachycardias, and other potentially disastrous effects on pacemaker operation, MRI is contraindicated for patients with pacemakers.[8] If MRI is absolutely essential to patient management, some authorities have suggested switching the pacemaker to its "off" mode, turning pacemaker output down so that it will not capture, or surgically removing the device.[1,3] These maneuvers must be undertaken with the help of an electrophysiologist, and patient informed consent should be obtained. Electrocautery may also induce any of a number of hazardous abnormalities in pacemaker function; precautions and steps to minimize risk during surgical procedures may be found in other reference texts.[3]

DISPOSITION

Disposition of the patient with a pacemaker-related problem largely depends on the severity of signs and symptoms, and should be determined collaboratively with the patient's electrophysiologist. Patients with pacing malfunction, such as failure to capture or battery depletion, should be admitted to monitored settings. Patients requiring a higher level of care may occasionally need interhospital transfer. ACLS units should be used, and the patient's rhythm and hemodynamics obviously must be stabilized prior to transfer; backup pacing modalities (transthoracic and/or transvenous) should be in place during transit.

THE PATIENT WITH AN IMPLANTABLE CARDIOVERTER–DEFIBRILLATOR

The first implantable cardioverter-defibrillator (ICD) was placed in 1980, and, as with pacemakers, technologic improvements have produced smaller, "smarter" defibrillators that are more easily placed.[4] Early models were nonprogrammable shock or no-shock devices that required open thoracotomy for epicardial patch placement. Current programmable devices have defibrillator leads that are inserted transvenously and utilize improved rhythm analysis algorithms to deliver tiered therapy.

For example, slow ventricular tachycardia (VT) may be first treated with overdrive pacing; if it fails to convert the VT, low-energy shocks are delivered. If they also fail, higher energy shocks are given.[12] Some new ICDs also incorporate antibradycardia (pacing) functions that may be activated if cardioversion or defibrillation results in a bradycardic or asystolic rhythm. Major trials demonstrating increased mortality with pharmacologic antiarrhythmic therapy and markedly decreased mortality with ICDs have led to broader indications for ICD use.[4] Currently, there are approximately 400,000 ICDs in operation worldwide.[15]

NASPE/BPEG descriptive codes also characterize the types and functions of ICDs[12]: position I, chamber(s) shocked; position II, chamber(s) for antitachycardia pacing; position III, method of tachycardia detection; and position IV, chamber(s) for bradycardia pacing (Table 136.2). However, in everyday practice, these codes are less commonly used than are pacemaker codes.

TABLE 136.2. NBD Codes (for Implantable Defibrillators)

1st position indicates the chamber shocked:
V = ventricle
A = atrium
D = dual
O = no shock therapy
2nd position indicates the chamber for antitachycardia pacing:
V = ventricle
A = atrium
D = dual
O = no antitachycardia pacing
3rd position indicates the method of tachycardia detection:
E = electrogram
H = hemodynamic
4th position indicates chambers for bradycardia pacing*
V = ventricle
A = atrium
D = dual
O = no bradycardia pacing.

*Alternatively the three or four letter NBG pacing code may be used following the first three letters of the NBD code (e.g., VVE-VVIR indicating ventricular shock, ventricular ATP, electrogram detection and VVIR pacing capability).

From Love C, ed. *Handbook of Cardiac Pacing*. Georgetown, TX: Landes Bioscience, 1998, with permission.

CLINICAL PRESENTATION AND DIFFERENTIAL DIAGNOSIS

Patients with ICD malfunction generally present with either defibrillation–cardioversion failure or frequent ICD discharge. Defibrillation–cardioversion failure may result from failure to deliver a shock, analogous to pacemaker output failure, or from failure of delivered shock(s) to convert the dysrhythmia, analogous to pacemaker noncapture. ICD discharge for rhythms other than ventricular fibrillation (VF) or VT is common, occurring in 22% of patients over 2 years of follow-up in one case series.[10] Although the potential lethality of inappropriate ICD discharge is lower than that of ICD failure to discharge, repeated shocks may cause myocardial injury, temporary ventricular dysfunction, and rapid battery depletion.[14] Furthermore, they may be very painful and anxiety-provoking. The most common causes of recurrent discharges are dysrhythmias (supraventricular tachycardias and nonsustained VT) that fall into the ICD's window of treatment.[12]

PATIENT EVALUATION AND EMERGENCY DEPARTMENT MANAGEMENT

When treating the patient in cardiac arrest or with unstable hemodynamics, determination of the exact cause of ICD failure is, at least initially, unimportant. Resuscitation is the obvious priority and should generally follow ACLS protocols.[14] Most ICDs analyze and shock VF or VT within 30 seconds; therefore, if a patient presents in these rhythms, the physician should assume that ICD defibrillation–cardioversion has been unsuccessful and should immediately proceed with external countershocks.[7] However, to prevent ICD absorption of current, defibrillator pads or paddles should not be placed directly over the device and, when feasible, should be positioned anteroposteriorly.[7] Chest compressions should be given in the standard fashion. Without rubber gloves, the rescuer may feel a slight, harmless shock if an ICD discharges during compressions.[7]

After successful resuscitation, the emergency physician should investigate the events surrounding the arrest, focusing on the few causes of ICD failure (electrolyte imbalance, myocardial ischemia or MI, and drug effects) that may be treated without ICD reprogramming or surgery. When feasible, the physician should ask the patient if he or she recalls chest pain, palpitations, or ICD discharges. As with the pacemaker patient, the emergency physician should use direct history, the patient's ICD card, medical records and telephone calls to the ICD manufacturer to gather information about reasons for and date of ICD implantation, most recent ICD interrogation, and prior ICD malfunction. The emergency physician should ask about exposures to the sources of environmental electromagnetic interference described earlier in regard to pacemakers. There are many etiologies of ICD malfunction, and these may be explored later by the electrophysiologist, who may interrogate the ICD for detailed analysis of dysrhythmias and ICD response. Additionally, referral to an electrophysiologist is essential to evaluate the ICD for lead fracture or displacement caused by chest compressions and for pulse generator damage or reprogramming arising from external countershocks.[14]

When rapid atrial fibrillation triggers frequent ICD discharge, the physician should attempt to slow the ventricular rate with the usual pharmacologic agents.[14] If, after a period of close monitoring, it is determined that frequent ICD discharges are not occurring as appropriate responses to significant dysrhythmias, or if frequent ineffective ICD discharges are interfering with resuscitation, the physician may disable the ICD by applying a ring magnet to the chest wall over the device.[14] Occasionally, two magnets, stacked one on top of the other, are required to deactivate the ICD in markedly obese patients.[14] While the magnet suspends all antitachycardia functions (i.e., the ICD will not deliver a shock for VT), back-up pacing functions of the ICD may persist. Attention to hemodynamics, close monitoring, and sedation or analgesia for the anxious patient are other keys to ED management of frequent ICD discharges. The emergency physician must understand that although a ring magnet generally causes changes in pacemaker function only during application of the magnet (i.e., the pacemaker resumes its normal function after removal of the magnet), a magnet may reset some ICD models to the "off" mode indefinitely.[14] Thus, if a magnet is either intentionally or inadvertently applied to an ICD, the physician should assume the device has been deactivated and should arrange for ICD interrogation and reprogramming.

The presentation and management of infectious and thrombotic complications of ICDs parallel those of pacemakers, except that ICD infections may be more serious and difficult to treat.[13] Hospital admission for administration of parenteral antibiotics and hardware removal is recommended for all infected ICDs.[13] If the patient has an older model with epicardial patches, computed tomography imaging of the heart and mediastinum is warranted to determine the extent of mediastinal involvement.

DISPOSITION

Given the potentially catastrophic consequences of ICD failure, urgent referral to an electrophysiologist is recommended for essentially all types of ICD malfunction. ICD patients should be observed in or admitted to monitored settings until specialist evaluations are completed. If specialist evaluation or higher level of care issues mandate transfer to another facility, ACLS units should be used, and transthoracic (anteroposterior) defibrillation and pacing pads should be applied to the patient prior to transit.

COMMON PITFALLS

- Misdiagnosing pacemaker or ICD malfunction because of inadequate information about the current programming and operation of the device. The physician should gather as much information about the pacemaker or ICD as possible from patient history, device identification cards, pacemaker or ICD registration departments, and patients' cardiologists or electrophysiologists.
- When evaluating the pacemaker patient for MI, failing to understand both the utility and the limits of 12-lead ECG interpretation. Several ECG patterns are reliable indicators of ischemia or infarction during RV pacing, but a normal LBBB pattern of pacing does not rule out infarction or ischemia.
- In a patient with cardiac arrest, allowing the presence of a pacemaker or ICD to change resuscitation procedures. Other than anteroposterior positioning of paddles and avoiding shocks over the devices, resuscitation should generally follow the usual ACLS protocols.
- Assuming that, after magnet application over an ICD or after cardioversion or resuscitation of a patient with an ICD or a pacemaker, the device has reverted to its normal programming and operation. The ICD or pacemaker must be reevaluated after these procedures.
- Failing to make disposition decisions for most pacemaker problems and for essentially all cases of ICD malfunction in collaboration with an electrophysiologist.

References

1. Atlee JL, ed. *Arrhythmias and pacemakers: practical management for anesthesia and critical care medicine.* Philadelphia: WB Saunders, 1996.
2. Barold SS, Zipes DP. Cardiac pacemakers and antiarrhythmic devices. In: Braunwald E, ed. *Heart disease.* Philadelphia: WB Saunders, 1997:705–738.
3. Bourke ME. The patient with a pacemaker or related device. *Can J Anaesth* 1996;43:R24–R32.
4. Cannom DS, Prystowsky EN. Management of ventricular arrhythmias: detection, drugs and devices. *JAMA* 1999;281:172–179.
5. Ciocon JO, Galindo-Ciocon D. Arm edema, subclavian thrombosis, and pacemakers. *Angiology J Vasc Dis* 1998;49:315–319.
6. Coppola M, Yealy DM. Transvenous pacemakers. *Emerg Med Clin North Am* 1994;12:633–643.
7. Cummins RO, ed. *Advanced cardiac life support.* Dallas: American Heart Association, 1997.
8. Fischer W, Ritter PH, eds. Cardiac pacing in clinical practice. Berlin: Springer-Verlag, 1998.
9. Hayes DL, Vlietstra RE. Pacemaker malfunction. *Ann Intern Med* 1993;119:828–835.
10. Grimm W, Flores BF, Marchlinski FE. Complications of implantable cardioverter defibrillator therapy: follow up of 241 patients. *PACE* 1993;16:218–222.
11. Kusumoto FM, Goldschlager N. Cardiac pacing. *N Engl J Med* 1996;334:89–97.
12. Love C, ed. *Handbook of cardiac pacing.* Georgetown, TX: Landes Bioscience, 1998.
13. Molina JE. Undertreatment and overtreatment of patients with infected antiarrhythmic implantable devices. *Ann Thorac Surg* 1997;63:504–509.
14. Pinski SL, Trohman RG. Implantable cardioverter-defibrillators: implications for the nonelectrophysiologist. *Ann Intern Med* 1995;122:770–777.
15. Santucci PA, Haw J, Trohman RG, et al. Interference with an implantable defibrillator by an electronic antitheft-surveillance device. *N Engl J Med* 1998;339:1371–1374.

16. Sgarbossa EB, Pinski SL, Barbagelata A, et al. Electrocardiographic diagnosis of evolving acute myocardial infarction in the presence of left bundle-branch block. *N Engl J Med* 1996;334:481–530.
17. Schuller H, Brandt J. The pacemaker syndrome: old and new causes. *Clin Cardiol* 1991;14:336–340.
18. Shlipak MG, Lyns WL, Go AS, et al. Should the electrocardiogram be used to guide therapy for patients with left bundle-branch block and suspected myocardial infarction? *JAMA* 1999;281:714–719.

CHAPTER 137
Valvular Heart Disease

Joseph P. Ornato

A wide variety of common diseases and conditions can affect the heart valves (Table 137.1). In the 1950s, virtually all patients with clinically significant valvular disease suffered from complications of acute rheumatic fever or syphilis, or congenital heart disease. Since then, the pattern of disease responsible for valvular dysfunction in adults has changed dramatically.[1,22,24] The major reasons for this shift are a marked decline in the incidence and better early treatment of acute rheumatic fever and syphilis; the wide availability of invasive and noninvasive testing to detect valvular heart disease; the development and perfection of surgical techniques for the repair or replacement of diseased valves; the increased longevity of the general population, allowing even normal valves to be subjected to more years of wear and tear; and sociocultural changes in our society (e.g., intravenous drug abuse).

Regardless of the cause, significant acute or chronic valvular dysfunction has predictable hemodynamic consequences. Regurgitant lesions (e.g., mitral or aortic regurgitation) cause volume overload of the affected atrium or ventricle. Although massive acute regurgitation can lead to shock and pulmonary edema rapidly, mild-to-moderate volume overload is usually well tolerated until after months or years, when the ventricle will often dilate and fail, leading to signs and symptoms of heart failure. Stenotic lesions above, at, or below the valve can cause pressure overload of the affected atrium or ventricle. Pressure overload is metabolically more costly to the myocardium than volume overload, and leads to myocardial hypertrophy and eventual heart failure.

The combined hemodynamic effect of multiple valvular lesions is often complex.[16] Some compound lesions (e.g., combined aortic regurgitation and stenosis) impose a tremendous burden on the myocardium by producing both volume and pressure overload of a single chamber (in this example, the left ventricle). Other combination lesions may be "protective" of a given chamber (e.g., in aortic stenosis combined with mitral stenosis, the volume of blood reaching the left ventricle is decreased, thereby "protecting" it from heart failure). However, the net effect may be to decrease forward, and thus net, cardiac output.

Some valvular lesions produce a rapidly downhill course. For example, acute, severe mitral or aortic regurgitation can lead rapidly to pulmonary edema, shock, or both, which can usually be remedied only by immediate valve replacement.[6,8,17,28] Other lesions, such as chronic mitral or aortic regurgitation, can be tolerated well for decades.[1,15,17] A structurally abnormal valve puts the patient at increased risk of developing infective endocarditis, which can further impair valvular function. Other concomitant diseases (e.g., coronary atherosclerosis, myocarditis), arrhythmias (e.g., atrial fibrillation), or valvular calcification can also unfavorably influence the patient's symptoms and length of survival.

COMMON CLINICAL PRESENTATIONS

Patients with valvular heart disease may present to the emergency department (ED) with a complication of previously known disease, or they may challenge the emergency physician to evaluate a previously undetected and undiagnosed heart murmur. If complex congenital heart disease, such as tetralogy of Fallot, is excluded, complications of adult valvular heart disease are most often the result of left heart lesions (Table 137.2).

When a patient with a heart murmur presents to the ED with symptoms that could be due to valvular heart disease, an immediate question is whether the heart murmur is *causing, unrelated to,* or *caused by* the symptom complex. For example, if a 70-year-old man with dyspnea and moderate pulmonary edema on chest x-ray has a grade 3/6 systolic ejection murmur at the left upper sternal border and cardiac apex, the murmur may be due to aortic stenosis or mitral regurgitation, either of which could cause heart failure. The patient's heart failure could be caused by an unrelated problem, such as ischemic heart disease, cardiomyopathy, myocarditis, or a congenital shunt lesion (e.g., atrial septal defect). Finally, left ventricular (LV) failure and dilatation could be causing a "functional" murmur due to dilatation of the mitral valve and its supporting structures (papillary muscle dysfunction).

Myocardial ischemia (e.g., during angina) can also increase the murmur of papillary muscle dysfunction. "Functional" tricuspid regurgitation can be caused by right ventricular dilatation secondary to left heart failure. In practice, it is sometimes impossible to determine the relationship between the murmur and the patient's symptoms without further diagnostic evaluation, such as echocardiography or cardiac catheterization.

TABLE 137.1. The Most Common Causes of Valvular Heart Disease in Adults

Cause	Specific Disease	Valves Affected	Murmur
Congenital	Bicuspid valve	A	S, R
Rheumatic	Rheumatic fever	M>A>T>P	S, R
Infectious	Endocarditis	A, M (rheumatic) A, M, T, P (i.v. drugs)	R
Myxomatous degeneration	Prolapse	M:T	R
	Aortic root dilatation	A	R
Degenerative aging	Sclerosis	A	S

A, aortic; M, mitral; P, pulmonic; T, tricuspid; S, stenotic; R, regurgitant; i.v., intravenous.

TABLE 137.2. Common Complications of Left Heart Valvular Disease in Adults

Valvular Lesion	Common Complication(s)
Mitral stenosis	Pulmonary edema, atrial fibrillation, systemic embolism
Mitral regurgitation	Heart failure, endocarditis
Aortic stenosis	Angina, syncope, heart failure, arrhythmias, sudden death, endocarditis
Aortic regurgitation	Heart failure, endocarditis

The most frequent pathologic conditions affecting the heart valves in adults presenting to the ED are (1) mitral valve prolapse (MVP); (2) aortic valve sclerosis in the elderly, with or (more typically) without significant stenosis; (3) valvular aortic stenosis due to congenital bicuspid aortic valve; (4) mitral regurgitation due to papillary muscle dysfunction, rheumatic heart disease, infectious endocarditis, or ruptured chordae tendineae; (5) aortic regurgitation due to rheumatic fever, infectious endocarditis, bicuspid aortic valve, or aortic root disease; and (6) mitral stenosis due to rheumatic fever.

EMERGENCY DEPARTMENT EVALUATION

A careful cardiovascular physical examination, beginning with the pulse and blood pressure, often identifies the cause of a heart murmur.[4] A wide pulse pressure accompanied by a brisk (often bifid) carotid upstroke and a bounding ("water-hammer") peripheral pulse is common in moderate-to-severe aortic regurgitation; a narrow pulse pressure with a slow, delayed carotid upstroke ("pulsus parvus et tardus") is seen in severe aortic stenosis. When a harsh systolic murmur suggesting valvular aortic stenosis is accompanied by a brisk carotid upstroke (and *no* aortic regurgitation), idiopathic hypertrophic subaortic stenosis (IHSS) should be suspected. In a young person (especially male), hypertension in the upper extremities and a *lower* arterial pressure in the legs with a weak femoral pulse and a basal systolic murmur suggests coarctation of the aorta (which is associated with congenital bicuspid aortic valve in 40% to 80% of cases).

All normal and abnormal heart sounds should be carefully noted. A loud first heart sound (S_1) at the apex and/or an opening snap after the second heart sound halfway between the left sternal border and apex are clues to the presence of mitral stenosis with a mobile valve. Paradoxical splitting of the second heart sound (S_2) (i.e., widening of the split on *expiration*) is seen in moderate-to-severe aortic stenosis. A widely ("fixed") split S_2 that fails to close fully during normal expiration in the upright position suggests atrial septal defect.

A high-pitched, early systolic click that is heard best along the left sternal border and that is followed by a systolic murmur usually signifies valvular pulmonic or aortic stenosis with a pliable, noncalcified valve. Systolic clicks heard later than the carotid upstroke or multiple systolic ("machine gun") clicks suggest mitral valve prolapse.

A third heart sound (S_3) is often heard in normal, healthy children, adolescents, and young adults without heart or valvular disease. When the heart rate is rapid, the third heart sound is usually termed an *S_3 gallop*. In a person with heart disease, it usually indicates left ventricular failure. Chronic or acute mitral regurgitation is often accompanied by an S_3,[6] but its presence in this condition does *not necessarily* indicate heart failure, because its presence may indicate only the torrential inflow of blood from the left atrium into the left ventricle in early diastole.

A fourth heart sound (S_4) is abnormal in a young person; it can occur with hypertension or aortic stenosis.[4,18] A loud S_4 accompanying mitral regurgitation indicates that the lesion is acute and substantial, the sound being caused by the left atrium's valiant attempt to cope with overwhelming volume overload. With time, the left atrium dilates and the S_4 disappears.

The timing of heart murmurs should be studied carefully and characterized as systolic, diastolic, or continuous (Table 137.3). Innocent murmurs are virtually *never* accompanied by a thrill. In an older individual, a harsh, musical, vibratory murmur with a thrill at the base is usually due to valvular aortic stenosis. A similar murmur with the thrill at the apex can be seen with mitral regurgitation. A new-onset musical "cooing-dove" murmur at the apex is almost always caused by rupture of the mitral valve chordae tendineae due to underlying mitral valve prolapse, Marfan syndrome, or trauma.[4] It is interesting that, although mitral valve prolapse occurs slightly more often in young women than men, most complications (infective endocarditis, mitral regurgitation, and ruptured chordae), though unusual, occur disproportionately more often in men.[7]

The response of murmurs to "provocative" maneuvers, spontaneously occurring extrasystoles, change in body position, brief exercise, and pharmacologic intervention can help emergency physicians to differentiate among causative entities.[4] Virtually all systolic murmurs—except that caused by IHSS—get softer or disappear during the strain phase of the Valsalva maneuver (Table 137.4). After the Valsalva strain is released, right-sided systolic heart murmurs (such as pulmonic stenosis and many innocent murmurs) usually return during the next 1 to 4 beats as blood rushes back into the right side of the heart. Left-sided systolic heart murmurs (mitral regurgitation, valvular aortic stenosis) are usually not well heard for 8 to 10 heartbeats, until the right heart and pulmonary circulation have refilled.

The isometric handgrip (squeezing two of the examiner's fingers tightly for 30 to 60 seconds) increases the systemic vascular resistance and typically increases the intensity and duration of mitral or aortic regurgitation. If the patient has extrasystoles or an irregular rhythm as in atrial fibrillation, the murmur of valvular aortic stenosis usually becomes much louder in the

TABLE 137.3. Classification of Common Murmurs by Timing

SYSTOLIC MURMURS
Aortic stenosis (valvular, supravalvular, and subvalvular)
Mitral regurgitation, including MVP
Tricuspid regurgitation
Pulmonic stenosis
IHSS
Coarctation of the aorta
Ventricular septal defect
Atrial septal defect
Innocent systolic murmur
DIASTOLIC MURMURS
Mitral stenosis
Tricuspid stenosis
Aortic regurgitation
Pulmonic regurgitation
CONTINUOUS MURMURS (EXTENDING THROUGH S2 WITHOUT RELATIONSHIP TO AORTIC OR PULMONIC VALVE CLOSURE)
Patent ductus arteriosus
Mammary souffle
Ruptured sinus of Valsalva aneurysm

TABLE 137.4. Differentiation of Common Heart Murmurs in Adults

Valve Lesion	Timing	Pattern	Pitch	Location	Valsalva Strain	Other
AS	Systolic	CD	High	Base, neck	Decr	Slow carotid
IHSS	Systolic	CD	High	Base	Incr	Bifid carotid with rapid upstroke
AR	Diastolic	D	High	LSB	Decr	Water hammer pulse
MS	Diastolic	Rumble	Low	Apex	Decr	OS
MR, rheumatic	Systolic	CD or Pan	High	Apex, axilla	Decr	Increase
MR, MV prolapse	Systolic	CD or Pan	High	Apex, axilla	Decr	Systolic click(s)
PS	Systolic	CD	Med or high	Pulmonic area	Decr	May have systolic ejection click
PR	Diastolic	D	High	Base, LSB	Decr	Slight delay from S_2 to murmur
TS	Diastolic	Rumble	Low	LSB or RSB	Decr	Increase on inspiration
TR	Systolic	CD or Pan	High	LSB	Decr	Systolic pulsation of jugular pulse

A, aortic; M, mitral; T, tricuspid; P, pulmonic; V, valve; S, stenosis; R, regurgitation; Med, medium; C, crescendo; D, decrescendo; Pan, pansystolic; Decr, decrease; Incr, increase; LSB, left sternal border; RSB, right sternal border; OS, opening snap; IHSS, idiopathic hypertrophic subaortic stenosis.

beat following a long pause because of increased LV stroke volume and flow across the valve. In contrast, the murmur of mitral insufficiency generally does not change in intensity with the change in cardiac cycle length.

Listening to murmurs with the patient in different body positions may also be helpful. For example, most innocent systolic murmurs decrease or disappear in the sitting or standing position. These murmurs are often soft and blowing in quality, are heard best along the left sternal border without radiation, and are unaccompanied by any other abnormal clinical findings or symptoms. The diastolic rumble of mitral stenosis is heard best in the left lateral decubitus position with the bell of the stethoscope placed lightly over the apex (see Table 137.4). The high-pitched, early diastolic decrescendo murmur of aortic insufficiency is heard best along the left sternal border with the patient leaning forward and holding a maximal expiration. This murmur is virtually always louder to the left of the sternum when aortic regurgitation is due to rheumatic heart disease or a bicuspid valve. If it is louder to the right of the sternum, one should suspect that aortic regurgitation is due to aortic root dilatation caused by aortic dissection, hypertension, syphilis, ruptured sinus of Valsalva aneurysm, or Marfan syndrome.

Prosthetic Valves

Surgically implanted prosthetic valves present special diagnostic problems in the ED.[23,26] Patients with such devices are at risk for (1) endocarditis (which may present with fever, chills, or peripheral embolic complications, including stroke[12,13,27]); (2) embolization due to clot formation (which may present as a new stroke, transient ischemic attack, or occluded peripheral artery); and (3) prosthetic valve dysfunction due to dehiscence of suture lines, thrombosis of the valve, valve degeneration (porcine heterografts or human homografts), hemolysis, or structural failure (disc devices). Patients with prosthetic valve dysfunction may gradually develop heart failure or fatigue, or may present suddenly with syncope or pulmonary edema.

The sounds and murmurs that should be heard after valve replacement vary from device to device.[13,14,23,26] Mechanical disc valves should produce clicking or metallic opening and/or closing sounds. Most implanted mechanical valves are relatively stenotic compared with native valves, so it is common and permissible to have a short systolic murmur with a prosthetic aortic valve or a short diastolic rumble with a prosthetic mitral valve. Short whiffs of aortic regurgitation, common after aortic valve replacement, are often due to a small periprosthetic leak at the suture line. Prominent mitral regurgitant murmurs are usually not present following mitral valve replacement unless there is a mechanical problem with the valve.

Because severe mitral or aortic regurgitation due to prosthetic valve dysfunction occasionally produces no audible murmur, the development of heart failure or the appearance of other potential indicators of valve failure always warrants immediate investigation as to the valve's integrity, even in the absence of a murmur. Thrombolysis is a highly effective treatment in resolving prosthetic thrombosis. However, because it carries a significant risk of embolization, it should be limited to patients with hemodynamic deterioration in whom surgery could also entail a significant risk of death.[25]

Catheter balloon valvuloplasty[20] is now being performed for pulmonary, mitral, and aortic valve stenosis. Following a successful procedure, it is common to have a persistent stenotic murmur or a new murmur due to valve regurgitation. Complications of this procedure include valve regurgitation, inadequate opening of the stenosis, endocarditis, arrhythmias, embolization, or atrial septal defect (mitral valvuloplasty only).

EMERGENCY DEPARTMENT MANAGEMENT

All patients with a previously undiagnosed heart murmur should, of course, receive a thorough cardiovascular physical assessment, as described previously. A high-quality posteroanterior and lateral chest x-ray and an electrocardiogram (ECG) complement the physical examination. Specific chamber enlargement (e.g., LV dilatation due to aortic or mitral regurgitation, left atrial enlargement due to mitral stenosis, regurgitation, or both) or poststenotic dilatation of the aorta or pulmonary artery on x-ray, or chamber hypertrophy on ECG (LV hypertrophy in aortic stenosis, left atrial enlargement in mitral stenosis, right ventricular hypertrophy in pulmonic stenosis) can help to disclose the cause of a murmur. Cardiomegaly, pulmonary vascular congestion, pulmonary edema, and/or pleural effusions on chest x-ray can detect or confirm heart failure.

Two-dimensional echocardiography with Doppler is a sensitive and precise means of detecting and evaluating the severity of valvular lesions noninvasively.[2,3,19] It should be performed in the ED or ordered electively on any patient who is being referred to a cardiologist for follow-up evaluation of a murmur that is suspected to be due to valvular disease. It can often detect vegetations or intracardiac thrombi in patients with suspected endocarditis and/or evidence of systemic embolization[12,13,26,27] and can be used to evaluate prosthetic valve motion and function.[12–14,23,26] If transthoracic echocardiography cannot provide clear enough resolution to adequately define the anatomy, transesophageal echocardiography can be performed. The latter technique can produce spectacular images of the heart and great vessels.

Specific complications of valvular heart disease, such as heart failure, cardiogenic shock, embolization, or arrhythmias, should be managed in the normal fashion.[1,6,8,16,17] Severe heart failure, hypotension, and shock due to massive acute aortic or mitral regurgitation may be refractory to medical therapy.[1,6] In such cases, it is often preferable to use dobutamine or low-to-medium doses (5 to 15 μg/kg/min) of dopamine, or both, rather than potent alpha vasoconstrictors (e.g., high-dose dopamine or norepinephrine), because increases in afterload will only worsen valvular regurgitation. Intraaortic balloon counterpulsation or other LV mechanical assist devices may be required for stabilization prior to cardiac catheterization and/or surgery.

In general, antibiotic prophylaxis against infective endocarditis should be offered to all patients with significant valvular lesions who are about to undergo procedures that may result in bacteremia.[10] It is not clear whether all patients with MVP, which occurs in approximately 5% of the population, require such prophylaxis,[9] but those patients who have a systolic murmur or echocardiographic evidence of mitral regurgitation are 35 times more likely to develop endocarditis than are those who have no systolic murmur or other evidence of mitral regurgitation.[11] Thus, all patients with prolapsing and leaking mitral valves, evidenced by audible clicks and murmurs of mitral regurgitation or by Doppler-demonstrated mitral insufficiency, should receive prophylactic antibiotics.[5] Whether to provide coverage to other MVP patients is a decision that should be made, in most cases, by the patient's cardiologist.

DISPOSITION

Absolute indications for immediate ED consultation by a cardiologist while hospital admission is being arranged include (1) known or suspected valvular lesions that are accompanied by hemodynamic instability (heart failure and/or shock), fever, arrhythmia, or embolization; and (2) new onset or progression of these symptoms; or (3) significant hemolysis following valve surgery or valvuloplasty. Admission to the intensive care unit is usually indicated for significant arrhythmia (particularly in new-onset cases and/or those causing hemodynamic compromise), pulmonary edema, hypotension, or when there are other concomitant life-threatening medical problems. Immediate cardiac catheterization and surgical intervention are indicated for new-onset severe valvular regurgitation, prosthetic valve malfunction, systemic embolization in the face of adequate anticoagulation, valve ring abscess, intractable heart failure, or shock.

If transfer to another facility is required, the emergency physician should consult by telephone with the receiving cardiologist to get advice on initial treatment and stabilization and to discuss the appropriate means of transportation and the patient's care en route. If available, an advanced cardiac life-support team with monitoring and resuscitation equipment should always accompany the patient. Air transport by helicopter or pressurized fixed-wing aircraft may be indicated if the patient is in need of urgent cardiac catheterization and operative intervention.

Most asymptomatic patients in whom a previously undetected heart murmur is found incidentally should be referred electively to a cardiologist for further evaluation. Pregnant patients with newly detected murmurs or abnormal heart sounds should also be referred for further cardiac evaluation if there is any question of the finding not being physiologic during pregnancy, or if there is the slightest possibility that the patient may have structural heart disease.

COMMON PITFALLS

- It is easy to be misled by the physical findings when a patient is seen for the first time. For example, the severity of valvular disease is always underestimated during periods of severe heart failure, shock, or tachycardia, because the decreased cardiac output leads to a decrease in the intensity of heart murmurs under such conditions.[8,15,16,18] The elderly patient presents a special problem, because the presence of concomitant atherosclerosis with rigid vessels may either mask or amplify pulse or blood pressure changes due to valvular disease. In addition, the location and radiation of murmurs are notoriously unreliable diagnostic indicators in older patients.
- A common error is to mistake a normal heart sound (such as the physiologic S_3) or an innocent murmur in a young person for the presence of structural heart disease. Children or young adults may have a cervical venous hum, heard best in the upright position, at the base of the neck and occasionally in the upper chest. The murmur is continuous, extending throughout the second heart sound, and can mimic a patent ductus arteriosus murmur. It can be correctly diagnosed by proving that it can be obliterated by having the patient lie down, applying pressure at the base of the neck with the stethoscope while listening, and by turning the patient's head away from the examiner.
- Murmurs are difficult to evaluate during pregnancy.[4,21] They may suddenly appear or disappear as the cardiac output, blood volume, and vascular resistance change during each trimester and in the postpartum period. A continuous, innocent "mammary souffle" murmur can often be heard along the right or left chest during late pregnancy or during lactation following delivery. This murmur is caused by the increased flow of blood through the mammary arteries due to the hypertrophied breast tissue. It can often be eliminated by direct chest wall pressure or with changes in body position.
- Finally, perhaps the most important pitfall is the failure to consider infectious endocarditis as a possibility in a patient with known or suspected heart valve pathology who presents with suspicious signs or symptoms (e.g., unexplained fever, anemia, heart failure, hypotension, signs of systemic embolization). Emergency physicians should maintain a relatively high index of suspicion in such cases. When in doubt, consider infectious endocarditis to be present until proven otherwise.

References

1. Alpert JS, Dalen JE. Changing concepts in the diagnosis and management of patients with valvular heart disease. *Kardiologia* 1987;76:81–84.
2. Borow KM. The need for an integrated noninvasive approach to valvular heart disease. *Am Heart J* 1983;106:1177–1180.
3. Carabello BA. Assessment of cardiac hemodynamics and valvular function by Doppler echocardiography. *Bull N Y Acad Med* 1987;63:762–796.
4. Constant J. *Bedside cardiology,* 2nd ed. Boston: Little, Brown and Company, 1976.
5. Dajani AS, Taubert KA, Wilson W, et al. Prevention of bacterial endocarditis: recommendations by the American Heart Association. *Circulation* 1997; 96:358–366.
6. DePace NL, Nestico PF, Morganroth J. Acute severe mitral regurgitation: pathophysiology, clinical recognition, and management. *Am J Med* 1985; 78:293–306.
7. Devereux RB, Hawkins I, Kramer-Fox R, et al. Complications of mitral valve prolapse: disproportionate occurrence in men and older patients. *Am J Med* 1986;81:751–758.
8. Janz TG. Valvular heart disease: clinical approach to acute decompensation of left-sided lesions. *Ann Emerg Med* 1988;17:201–208.
9. Jeresaty RM. Mitral valve prolapse: an update. *JAMA* 1985;254:793–795.
10. Kaye D. Prophylaxis for infective endocarditis: an update. *Ann Intern Med* 1986;104:419–423.
11. MacMahon SW, Hickey AJ, Wilcken DEL, et al. Risk of infective endocarditis in mitral valve prolapse with and without precordial systolic murmurs. *Am J Cardiol* 1986;58:105–108.
12. Mayer KH, Schoenbaum SC. Evaluation and management of prosthetic valve endocarditis. *Prog Cardiovasc Dis* 1982;25:43–54.
13. McClung JA, Stein JH, Ambrose JA, et al. Prosthetic heart valves: a review. *Prog Cardiovasc Dis* 1983;26:237–270.
14. McGoon DC, Fuster V. Prosthetic valves. In: Brandenburg RO, Fuster V, Giuliani ER, et al., eds. *Cardiology: fundamentals and practice.* Chicago: Year Book, 1987.

15. Nishimura RA, McGoon MD, Schaff HV, et al. Chronic aortic regurgitation: indications for operation—1988. *Mayo Clin Proc* 1988;63:270–280.
16. Nitter-Hauge S, Horstkotte D. Management of multivalvular heart disease. *Eur Heart J* 1987;8:643–646.
17. O'Rourke RA, Crawford MH. Mitral valve regurgitation. *Curr Probl Cardiol* 1984;9:1–52.
18. Olson LJ, Edwards WD, Tajik AJ. Aortic valve stenosis: etiology, pathophysiology, evaluation, and management. *Curr Probl Cardiol* 1987;12:455–508.
19. Pearlman AS, Scoblionko DP, Saal AK. Assessment of valvular heart disease by Doppler echocardiography. *Clin Cardiol* 1983;6:573–587.
20. Rahimtoola SH. Catheter balloon valvuloplasty of aortic and mitral stenosis in adults: 1987. *Circulation* 1987;75:895–901.
21. Raymond R., Underwood DA, Moodie DS. Cardiovascular problems in pregnancy. *Cleve Clin J Med* 1987;54:95–104.
22. Rose AG. Etiology of acquired valvular heart disease in adults. *Arch Pathol Lab Med* 1986;110:385–388.
23. Schoen FJ, Kujovich JL, Levy RJ, et al. Bioprosthetic valve failure. *Cardiovasc Clin* 1988;18:289–317.
24. Selzer A. Changing aspects of the natural history of valvular aortic stenosis. *N Engl J Med* 1987;317:91–98.
25. Serafini O, Bisignani G, Plastina F. Acute disfunction from thrombosis of a prosthetic mitral valve: thrombolysis with rt-PA in the clinical emergency phase. *G Ital Cardiol* 1998;28:387–391.
26. Silver MD, Butany J. Complications of mechanical heart valve prostheses. *Cardiovasc Clin* 1988;18:273–288.
27. Sugarman B. Infections and prosthetic devices. *Am J Med* 1986;81:78–84.
28. Weinstein L. Life-threatening complications of infective endocarditis and their management. *Arch Intern Med* 1986;146:953–957.

CHAPTER 138

Acute Pericarditis and Cardiac Tamponade

Franklin D. Pratt and Howard A. Bessen

Acute pericarditis is a diagnostic challenge because its presentation is similar to that of several other disorders, and it may have life-threatening complications. Management ranges from symptomatic, supportive treatment to lifesaving invasive procedures.

The common causes of acute pericarditis are listed in Table 138.1. In many cases, the cause is unclear (idiopathic pericarditis). Viral pericarditis is frequently diagnosed presumptively in a patient who presents with pericarditis after a virus-like syndrome. Other infectious causes (bacterial, fungal, and parasitic) are less common, but pericarditis may occur as a complication of another systemic or intrathoracic infection.

TABLE 138.1. Causes of Acute Pericarditis

Idiopathic	Connective tissue disease
Infectious	Rheumatoid arthritis
Viral	Systemic lupus erythematosus
Bacterial	Scleroderma
Tuberculosis	Drug-related
Fungal	Anticoagulants
Parasitic	Procainamide
Malignancy	Hydralazine
Metastatic disease	Methyldopa
Radiation-induced	Cardiac injury
Uremia	Postmyocardial infarction
	Postsurgical
	Postinstrumentation
	Cardiac trauma
	Aortic dissection

Patients with human immunodeficiency virus (HIV) infection may develop pericarditis and pericardial effusions.[3] A wide variety of viral, bacterial, mycobacterial, and other opportunistic infections can cause pericarditis in these patients. Pericarditis may also be associated with acquired immunodeficiency disease syndrome (AIDS)–related malignancies such as Kaposi's sarcoma.

Pericarditis is the most prominent cardiac complication of neoplastic disease, and nontraumatic pericardial tamponade is usually of metastatic origin.[9,15] Lymphoma, leukemia, melanoma, and breast or lung carcinoma cause most pericardial metastases. Patients receiving radiation treatment may develop postirradiation pericarditis.

Pericarditis may occur as a complication of chronic renal failure, or of connective tissue diseases such as systemic lupus erythematosus, scleroderma, or rheumatoid arthritis. Medications, including anticoagulants and those associated with a drug-induced lupus syndrome (e.g., hydralazine, methyldopa, and procainamide), may also be implicated.

Pericarditis frequently occurs during the first few days after acute myocardial infarction[4,22]; it is unclear whether there is also a late-onset postinfarction pericarditis syndrome.[13] Aortic dissection, cardiac trauma, invasive procedures that involve the great vessels and the heart (central venous pressure catheter insertion and cardiac catheterization), and intrathoracic surgery may also cause pericarditis and pericardial tamponade within hours to weeks.

CLINICAL PRESENTATION

Most patients with acute pericarditis present with chest pain. The pain is usually sharp and often pleuritic, but it may also be dull, constrictive, or aching. It may radiate to any part of the chest and back and to the trapezius ridge.[11] Typically, the chest discomfort is eased by sitting up and leaning forward. The pain is frequently associated with shortness of breath, which may be caused by coexisting pleuritis or by cardiac tamponade. Patients may also present with hypotension and other signs and symptoms of tamponade.

DIFFERENTIAL DIAGNOSIS

The differential diagnosis includes other conditions that cause chest pain and dyspnea, such as acute myocardial infarction (MI), congestive heart failure (CHF), pulmonary embolism, pneumonia, pneumothorax, pneumomediastinum, pleuritis, and aortic dissection. Cardiac tamponade may be confused with CHF and cardiogenic shock.

Acute pericarditis is frequently mistaken for acute MI. In contrast to MI patients, patients with pericarditis may present with fever and typically have sharper pain that increases with body motion and varies with position. The ST-segment elevation in patients with acute MI is typically focal, with ST-segment depression in reciprocal leads. In pericarditis, ST-segment elevation is more diffuse, without reciprocal ST depression,[2] and the Q waves often seen in acute infarction do not develop. Patients with pericarditis (even with tamponade) have clear lung fields, as opposed to those with CHF or pneumonia.

On the electrocardiogram (ECG), a normal early repolarization variant may mimic pericarditis (discussion follows).

EMERGENCY DEPARTMENT EVALUATION

Initial assessment and therapy consist of measures appropriate for any patient who presents with shortness of breath and chest pain: supplemental oxygen administration, intravenous access placement, cardiac monitoring, and a 12-lead ECG.

The classic diagnostic physical finding is the pericardial friction rub, which may consist of one, two, or three components. Frequent careful auscultation allows recognition of a rub in most patients with pericarditis.[21] The rub may be transient or intermittent, and can be confused with a heart murmur. The ECG can be virtually diagnostic. Typically, the ECG changes of acute pericarditis evolve through four stages[2,20]:

- Stage 1 is the most characteristic and will probably be seen when the patient presents with acute symptoms. Concave–upward ST-segment elevation is seen in most of the leads; PR segment depression may also be seen (Fig. 138.1).
- In stage 2, the ST segments return to baseline, and the T-wave amplitude decreases; the PR segment may be depressed.
- T-wave flattening and then inversion in the leads with previous ST-segment elevation defines stage 3.
- In stage 4, the ECG normalizes.

The ECG findings in acute pericarditis are diffuse changes that are seen in most leads, rather than the focal abnormalities seen in acute MI.[2,20]

Although the ECG is usually abnormal, diagnostic changes may be absent in patients with clinically evident pericarditis.[14,20] Patients with post-MI pericarditis (diagnosed by the presence of a pericardial friction rub) frequently have no ECG changes.[14]

Early repolarization, a normal ECG variant characterized by ST-segment elevation, can be difficult to distinguish from pericarditis.[2,18] If the clinical presentation suggests pericarditis, serial ECGs may be required to differentiate pericarditis from the benign early repolarization variant. On a single ECG, an ST/T ratio (the amount of ST-segment elevation divided by the height of the T wave) of 0.25 or more in lead V_6 suggests pericarditis, not early repolarization.[8]

The chest radiograph is often normal. The cardiac silhouette may be enlarged secondary to a pericardial effusion, but the heart size may be normal, even if an effusion is present.[6] In addition, radiographic cardiomegaly is a nonspecific finding, and may represent significant myocarditis or many other types of heart disease.

The white blood cell count can range from normal to markedly elevated, and is usually not helpful in making or excluding the diagnosis. Similarly, the erythrocyte sedimentation rate is usually elevated, but this is a nonspecific finding. Cardiac enzyme levels are often normal or minimally elevated, but may be significantly elevated because of associated myocarditis.[12]

Echocardiography can provide useful information in suspected pericarditis. In the absence of significant associated myocarditis, most patients with pericarditis have normal cardiac wall motion. In contrast, patients with chest pain caused by cardiac ischemia often have focal wall motion abnormalities. Echocardiography is also the best method for detecting and monitoring pericardial effusions (discussion follows).

COMPLICATIONS

The major complications of acute pericarditis are pericardial effusion (potentially leading to cardiac tamponade), recurrent pericarditis, and chronic constrictive pericarditis. Dysrhythmias are unusual in pericarditis but may occur in patients with associated myocarditis or other underlying heart disease.

Cardiac tamponade is an acutely life-threatening complication. The presentation may be subtle, potentially leading to a delayed or missed diagnosis and a poor outcome. Close attention to physical findings is essential to make the diagnosis.

Cardiac tamponade results from the accumulation of fluid within the pericardial space, causing an impairment of cardiac filling and thus a decrease in cardiac output. Tamponade is often mistaken for CHF because patients present with dyspnea, orthopnea, jugular venous distention, and hepatic enlargement.

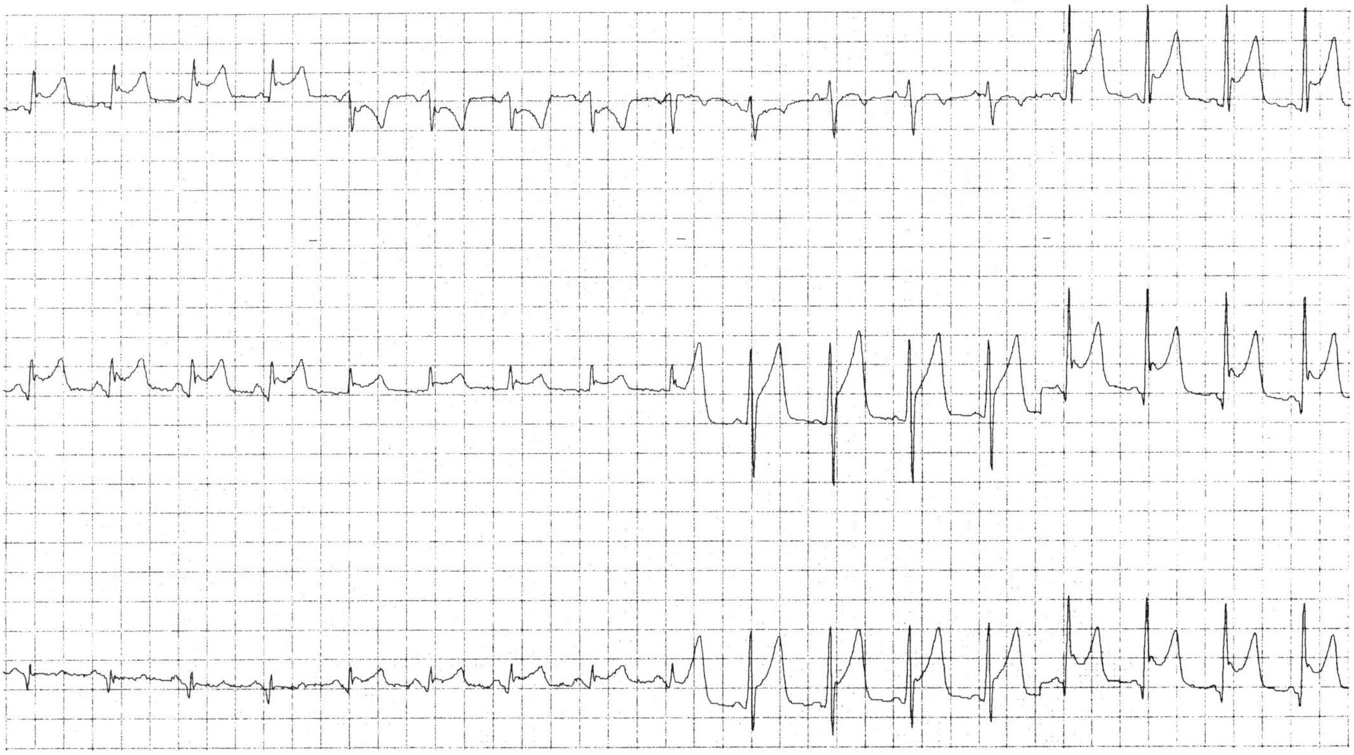

Figure 138.1. Electrocardiogram of a 35-year-old man with acute pericarditis. Note the diffuse, concave–upward ST-segment elevation.

The classic findings of cardiac tamponade are muffled heart sounds, diminished arterial pressure, and elevated venous pressure. However, these findings are seen only with fully developed tamponade and are much more likely to occur when pericardial fluid accumulates quickly, precluding pericardial distention.[7,9]

An important clue to the diagnosis is the presence of pulsus paradoxus, an inspiratory decrease in systolic blood pressure of more than 10 mm Hg.[5,16] Other clinical entities associated with pulsus paradoxus include emphysema, asthma, obesity, pulmonary embolism, cardiogenic shock, right ventricular infarction, and restrictive cardiomyopathy. Patients with acute traumatic tamponade may not have a pulsus paradoxus.

Patients with tamponade may have relatively normal ECGs. With large effusions, reduction of the QRS amplitude or electrical alternans (alternating beat-to-beat variation in QRS amplitude) may be seen. Central venous pressure measurements reveal an elevation of right-sided pressures and help confirm the diagnosis.

Clinical decompensation can be rapid. If time allows, definitive diagnosis using echocardiography is indicated. Echocardiography can detect small amounts of pericardial fluid; in cardiac tamponade, it may demonstrate diffuse hypokinesis, right atrial collapse, and right ventricular diastolic collapse.[7,11,19] If possible, echocardiography should be performed emergently in any patient with suspected tamponade, because delays in evaluating the presence and size of a pericardial effusion can be disastrous.[15]

The diagnosis of tamponade can also be definitively established by measuring pressures in the cardiac chambers. Right atrial, right ventricular diastolic, pulmonary artery diastolic, and pulmonary capillary wedge pressures are equalized in this condition.

Occasionally, after recovering from the acute illness, patients suffer one or several episodes of recurrent *pericarditis,* weeks to months after the initial episode.[1] Evaluation and management of recurrences are, for the most part, the same as for a first presentation of acute pericarditis.

Constrictive pericarditis, an uncommon complication of acute pericarditis, results when healing of acute pericarditis leads to encasement of the heart in fibrous tissue, impeding ventricular filling.[11,17] Patients often present with dyspnea on exertion, ascites, peripheral edema, and hepatic enlargement. The lung fields are clear, in contrast to patients with CHF. The presence of distended neck veins in constrictive pericarditis helps to separate these patients from those with severe liver disease, who may appear clinically similar. Pericardial calcification on the chest radiograph and pericardial thickening on echocardiography may also provide clues to this diagnosis. The definitive treatment is resection of the pericardium.

EMERGENCY DEPARTMENT MANAGEMENT AND DISPOSITION

Once the diagnosis of acute pericarditis is made or strongly suspected, most patients should be admitted. The admitting consultant can coordinate the diagnostic evaluation, perform echocardiography and pericardiocentesis, as needed, and arrange proper follow-up care.

Whether all patients with acute pericarditis require admission is controversial. Some young patients with uncomplicated idiopathic or viral pericarditis may be appropriately managed as outpatients. However, pericarditis may occur as a complication of MI, and, in any patient with pericarditis, development of a pericardial effusion and cardiac tamponade may be subtle. Obtaining an echocardiogram before discharge ensures that a pericardial effusion is not missed. Patients who are not admitted require close, careful follow-up.

The therapy for uncomplicated pericarditis is largely symptomatic, but specific therapy is available for a few causes of pericarditis. Nonsteroidal antiinflammatory agents give excellent results in viral and idiopathic pericarditis. Recurrent pericarditis may respond to colchicine.[1] Bacterial pericarditis must be treated with drainage and appropriate antimicrobial therapy. Uremic pericarditis is usually an indication for dialysis.

The definitive treatment of pericardial tamponade is pericardiocentesis. However, to "buy time" until pericardiocentesis can be performed, volume infusion is the treatment of choice. Ideally, pericardiocentesis should be done with echocardiographic and ECG guidance, but emergent "blind" pericardiocentesis may be necessary for hypotensive patients who do not respond to volume infusion.

The procedure for emergent pericardiocentesis is fully described elsewhere.[10] The pericardium may be approached by a left parasternal or subxiphoid puncture. In the parasternal approach, the needle is inserted perpendicular to the skin in the fifth intercostal space, just lateral to the sternum. In the subxiphoid approach, the puncture is made about 2 cm below and 1 cm to the left of the xiphoid process; the needle enters the skin at a 30-degree to 45-degree angle and is aimed toward the sternal notch or the left shoulder. The needle is advanced with constant syringe aspiration. As much fluid is aspirated as is needed to improve the clinical condition or to obtain specimens for diagnostic use.

After completing the procedure, a chest radiograph is obtained to look for complications such as pneumothorax or pleural effusion secondary to laceration of the lung or myocardium. Serial physical examinations and central venous pressure monitoring are done to detect reaccumulation of fluid. The admitting consultant may choose to observe the patient for fluid reaccumulation, place a soft catheter in the pericardial space for continued drainage, or perform surgical drainage in the operating room.

COMMON PITFALLS

- Failing to consider pericarditis in the differential diagnosis of chest pain
- Mistakenly diagnosing pericarditis in patients with other causes of chest pain, such as MI, pulmonary embolism, or aortic dissection
- Misdiagnosing acute pericarditis as acute MI, potentially leading to the inappropriate administration of thrombolytics.
- Failing to consider the etiology of pericarditis. Many of the causes listed in Table 138.1 require specific therapy.
- Failing to rule out the presence of a pericardial effusion in patients with pericarditis
- Failing to consider cardiac tamponade in the differential diagnosis of hypotension, especially in patients with cancer

References

1. Adler Y, Finkelstein Y, Guindo J, et al. Colchicine treatment for recurrent pericarditis: a decade of experience. *Circulation* 1998;97:2183.
2. Chan TC, Brady WJ, Pollack M. Electrocardiographic manifestations: acute myopericarditis. *J Emerg Med* 1999;17:865.
3. Chen Y, Brennessel D, Walters J, et al. Human immunodeficiency virus–associated pericardial effusion: report of 40 cases and review of the literature. *Am Heart J* 1999;137:516.
4. Correale E, Maggioni AP, Romano S, et al. Pericardial involvement in acute myocardial infarction in the post-thrombolytic era: clinical meaning and value. *Clin Cardiol* 1997;20:327.
5. Curtiss EI, Reddy PS, Uretsky BF, et al. Pulsus paradoxus: definition and relation to the severity of cardiac tamponade. *Am Heart J* 1988;115:391.
6. Eisenberg MJ, Dunn MM, Kanth N, et al. Diagnostic value of chest radiography for pericardial effusion. *J Am Coll Cardiol* 1993;22:588.

7. Fowler NO. Cardiac tamponade: a clinical or an echocardiographic diagnosis? *Circulation* 1993:87:1738.
8. Ginzton LE, Laks MM. The differential diagnosis of acute pericarditis from the normal variant: new ECG criteria. *Circulation* 1982;65:1004.
9. Guberman BA, Fowler NO, Engel PJ, et al. Cardiac tamponade in medical patients. *Circulation* 1981;64:633.
10. Harper RJ, Callaham ML. Pericardiocentesis. In: Roberts JR, Hedges JR, eds. *Clinical procedures in emergency medicine,* 3rd ed. Philadelphia: WB Saunders, 1998:231.
11. Hoit BD. Pericardial heart disease. *Curr Probl Cardiol* 1997;22:357.
12. Karjalainen J, Heikkila J. "Acute pericarditis": myocardial enzyme release as evidence for myocarditis. *Am Heart J* 1986;111:546.
13. Kossowsky WA, Lyon AF, Spain DM. Reappraisal of the postmyocardial infarction Dressler's syndrome. *Am Heart J* 1986;102:954.
14. Krainin FM, Flessas AP, Spodick DH. Infarction-associated pericarditis: rarity of diagnostic ECG. *N Engl J Med* 1984;311:1211.
15. Markiewicz W, Borovik R, Ecker S. Cardiac tamponade in medical patients: treatment and prognosis in the echocardiographic era. *Am Heart J* 1986;111:1138.
16. McGregor M. Pulsus paradoxus. *N Engl J Med* 1979;301:480.
17. Mehta A, Mehta M, Jain AC. Constrictive pericarditis. *Clin Cardiol* 1999;22:334.
18. Mehta M, Jain AC, Mehta A. Early repolarization. *Clin Cardiol* 1999;22:59.
19. Reydel B, Spodick DH. Frequency and significance of chamber collapses during cardiac tamponade. *Am Heart J* 1990;119:1160.
20. Spodick DH. Electrocardiogram in acute pericarditis: distributions of morphologic and axial changes by stages. *Am J Cardiol* 1974;33:470.
21. Spodick DH. Pericardial rub: prospective, multiple observer investigation of pericardial friction in 100 patients. *Am J Cardiol* 1975;35:357.
22. Sugiura T, Iwasaka T, Takehana K, et al. Clinical significance of pericardial effusion associated with pericarditis in acute Q-wave anterior myocardial infarction. *Chest* 1993;104:415.

CHAPTER 139

Deep Venous Thrombosis and Thrombophlebitis

Edward A. Panacek and J. Douglas Kirk

Deep venous thrombosis (DVT) of the lower extremity is a relatively common diagnosis made in the emergency department (ED), and up to 600,000 Americans are hospitalized with this diagnosis each year. However, because DVT is often occult, the true incidence is unknown.[3] Thromboembolic disease is responsible for an estimated 200,000 deaths annually in the United States, and millions more suffer from sequelae such as stasis dermatitis and venous ulcers. The elderly are at highest risk, and DVT is associated with a 21% mortality rate in this age group.[10] Subsets of children are also at risk, particularly those with spinal cord injuries or hypercoagulable conditions.

The risks for development of DVT were first described by Virchow in his description of the famous triad that includes stasis, hypercoagulability, and endothelial injury. It is now known that there are other "multifactorial" conditions that either cross categories or separately place patients at risk (Table 139.1). These risk factors are additive in nature, and it is important for the emergency physician (EP) to be familiar with them in order to evaluate patients appropriately. However, 25% to 50% of patients with DVT do not have obvious risk factors[4]; a substantial proportion of them have been found to have the so-called Leiden variant of Factor V. The proportion appears to be even higher in patients with recurrent DVT.

TABLE 139.1. Risk Factors for Deep Venous Thrombosis

Stasis
Immobility
Bed rest (≥ 3 days)
Long ride (plane, car, or train)
Paralysis
CNS injury
Cast
Endothelial Injury
Intravenous drug abuse
Vascular trauma
Recent surgery
Central lines
Hypercoagulability
Malignancy
Previous thromboembolic disease
Inflammatory conditions (e.g., SLE)
Nephrotic syndrome (loss of antithrombin III)
Coagulation disorders
Protein S deficiency or resistance
Protein C deficiency
Antithrombin III deficiency
Factor V Leiden
Increased estrogen
Pregnancy
Postpartum <3 mo
Oral contraceptives
Disorders of fibrinogen or plasminogen
Antiphospholipid antibodies (lupus anticoagulant and anticardiolipin)
Multifactorial
Recent trauma
Recent surgery
Age >60 yr
Cardiac disease (especially CHF)
Obesity
Venous insufficiency
Smoking

Assessment of risk factors is somewhat subjective, but there are some guidelines. Bed rest is generally considered to be "prolonged" if it occurs for 3 or more days. Immobility from long rides is considered to be significant if it is of at least 12 hours' duration. The period of risk after surgery and trauma (incriminated in up to 40% of cases of DVT) probably extends for a few weeks. Increased estrogen causes a fall in protein S (and cigarette smoking increases this tendency), yet the risk of DVT is only slightly increased with low-estrogen contraceptives, progesterone-only pills, or Norplant. Patients with three or more risk factors or specific examination findings are generally considered high-risk. Those with one or two factors are considered medium-risk, and those with no factors, low-risk.[18]

The initiating stimulus for thrombus formation is often an intimal defect. The dynamic interplay of coagulation and fibrinolytic forces then results in clot propagation or dissolution. Conditions affecting the balance of these forces are what place patients at increased risk for symptomatic thrombus formation. If the process is of sufficient severity or duration, the associated vein can become inflamed; the condition is then referred to as *thrombophlebitis.*

The vast majority of significant DVTs develop in the deep iliofemoral system. Although isolated superficial thrombophlebitis does not pose a risk for significant embolization, 25% of patients with symptoms of superficial thrombophlebitis have been shown to have involvement of the deep system as well.[9] In addition, patients with isolated calf vein involvement are also at risk. In up to 20%, these thrombi have been shown to propagate proximally and also embolize.

Although embolization to the lung is the most serious complication of DVT, it can also result in a number of other complicating conditions. Venous hypertension and persistent clot can destroy valves, leading to the postphlebitic syndrome in perhaps half of patients. Others can develop recurrent edema. Occasionally, acute cases can even develop a compartment syndrome of the thigh or lower leg. Most importantly, even in patients without any respiratory symptoms, at least 40% of patients with DVT have clinically silent pulmonary emboli (PEs).[15]

CLINICAL PRESENTATION

Patients with DVT can present with a symptom complex that ranges from completely occult to obvious. Most commonly, they present with lower extremity pain or swelling that may worsen with standing or walking. Manifestations are almost always unilateral, except in the rare and life-threatening case of inferior vena cava (IVC) involvement. Generally, DVT symptoms develop over a period of several days, whereas sudden severe pain is more likely to be related to an injury. Associated symptoms, such as chest pain or dyspnea, may also be present, particularly as they relate to the presence of PE. Risk factors can be identified in the majority of patients.

DIFFERENTIAL DIAGNOSIS

Many medical conditions can present with symptoms suggestive of DVT (Table 139.2). Most of these conditions generally cause *bilateral* leg swelling due to either increased production of edema fluid or an IVC obstructive process. However, if prior DVT has resulted in damage to the venous valves, these conditions can result in asymmetric swelling. In addition, abdominal masses (e.g., a gravid uterus) can occasionally compress a single iliac vein, resulting in unilateral venous stasis. One of the most difficult conditions to distinguish from DVT is the postphlebitic syndrome. Patients with prior DVT can develop recurrent unilateral pain and swelling that is clinically indistinguishable from acute DVT. The other conditions that are most often confused with DVT are superficial phlebitis and cellulitis. There is significant clinical overlap among many of these conditions, and a low threshold for objective diagnostic testing is required.

EMERGENCY DEPARTMENT EVALUATION

The clinical evaluation of the patient with possible DVT focuses both on identifying findings consistent with DVT and on identifying other conditions that explain the patient's presentation. It is important to question the patient about risk factors for DVT, including a family history (see Table 139.1). Perhaps one-fourth of patients with acute DVT have a history of prior DVT.[3]

TABLE 139.2. Differential Diagnosis of Deep Venous Thrombosis

Postphlebitic syndrome
Cellulitis/abscess
Muscle injury/hematoma
Popliteal cyst (Baker's cyst)
Superficial phlebitis
Congestive heart failure
Lymphedema
Malignancy (obstructive)
Capillary leak syndrome
Fracture
Sciatica
Acute arthritis
Myositis
Pregnancy
Superior vena cava syndrome (upper-extremity DVT)

The physical examination can provide useful findings, but must be interpreted with caution. Though patients with cellulitis and other infections often have a fever, DVT can also result in temperature elevations, although usually only low-grade. Unilateral warmth and erythema are common with DVT, but also with cellulitis. The presence of an abscess, enlarged lymph nodes, and ulcerations can be clues to an infectious etiology. A difference of 1 cm in the circumference of the calves, or 2 cm in the thighs, measured from a reference point such as the patella, is clinically significant and one of the most specific findings for DVT. The presence of palpable "cords" is generally thought to be fairly specific but quite insensitive for thrombosis. In the popliteal fossa, they can be confused with Baker's cysts. Homan's sign was classically taught as being important in the evaluation of DVT, but it is now well known that its sensitivity and specificity are only about 50%.

DVT is a difficult diagnosis to make clinically; between 50% and 75% of patients suspected of having DVT will not have the diagnosis confirmed by objective tests. Therefore, patients in whom the diagnosis is expected must undergo further diagnostic studies. The only blood test of relevance is the serum D-dimer level, which is elevated in the presence of clot breakdown. Early enthusiasm for this test has been tempered with time, however. The test is 93% to 98% sensitive for DVT, but only 40% to 80% specific.[2,12] False negatives are particularly common in chronic or recurrent DVT. The D-dimer should not be used to replace imaging studies in patients in high- or medium-risk groups. In patients without significant comorbidity and in a "low-risk" group, a negative D-dimer result may be sufficient evidence to avoid further studies.[18] Only the sensitive but more time-consuming ELISA test or the SimpliRed test should be used, not the less sensitive latex agglutination.

The primary imaging study for patients with DVT is now ultrasonography. It is relatively inexpensive, noninvasive, and widely available. Though a number of techniques are used, B-mode looking at compressibility of the vein is the standard for confirming the diagnosis. Ultrasound is considered 95% to 99% sensitive for acute thrombi above the knee, and it can also occasionally identify other conditions, such as tumor, cysts, aneurysms, and so forth. However, scans can be reader-dependent, and some institutions lack individuals with sufficient expertise or experience. In addition, the test is less accurate in the second half of pregnancy and for suprainguinal vein thrombus, in which case, the Doppler mode of the duplex ultrasound scan can be helpful. In these situations, or in patients felt to be at high risk for DVT, it may not be appropriate to end the evaluation with a single negative ultrasound examination. Use of additional tests or close follow-up with serial outpatient studies is recommended.[5]

Although venography is considered the gold standard for the diagnosis of DVT, it has a number of problems. Approximately 10% of the studies are technically inadequate, and radiologists often disagree on interpretation. Some patients develop phlebitis from the procedure, and there are occasional cases of anaphylaxis from the radiographic contrast material. Patients often report the procedure to be painful. For all of these reasons, the role of venography has largely been supplanted by ultrasound. Its main role is in patients with a history of prior DVT in whom ultrasound is equivocal. It can better distinguish between acute and chronic changes.

Impedance plethysmography (IPG) measures changes in lower extremity venous volume in response to selected maneuvers and draws comparisons between the legs. Though relatively inexpensive and noninvasive, IPG has been shown to be very operator-dependent, and its sensitivity is only 65% to 85%.[11] It is not recommended for use in ED patients. Likewise, radiolabeled fibrinogen studies, which are designed to identify growing thrombus, are relatively insensitive, take prolonged periods to perform, and are not useful in ED patients.

Magnetic resonance imaging (MRI) is developing a growing role in the evaluation of DVT. Its sensitivity (97%) and specificity (95%) are the equal of ultrasound. In addition, it is particularly useful in identifying thrombus in the pelvis, an area where ultrasound has limitations. It is also approved as safe for use during pregnancy and is the test of choice in that population.[17] It can distinguish mature from recent clot and also has applications for identifying pulmonary thrombi. However, it is relatively expensive, not widely available, and requires greater patient cooperation, somewhat limiting its use.

Though much less common, DVT can also develop in the upper extremities, usually in the subclavian or axillary veins.[1] The use of diagnostic imaging studies in such cases is less well studied. Because of differences in the anatomy, ultrasound may not be as sensitive as it is in the thigh, but it is still recommended as the first-line study. However, inadequate examinations or negative examinations in high-risk patients should be followed with contrast venography.

EMERGENCY DEPARTMENT MANAGEMENT

Patients with isolated DVT rarely require immediate lifesaving interventions. However, many of these patients have occult PEs, and all are at risk for new emboli. In patients in whom PEs are strongly suspected, starting heparin prior to imaging studies is appropriate. In addition, occasional patients can present with complete venous obstruction and the condition referred to as "phlegmasia dolens." These patients should also undergo immediate heparinization and fluid resuscitation prior to imaging studies when the diagnosis is suspected. They also often require thrombolytics and, occasionally, urgent thrombectomy (Table 139.3).

In the vast majority of patients, the initial treatment for DVT is anticoagulation with heparin. Those with absolute contraindications to anticoagulation require vena caval interruption, usually with an IVC filter.[6] Filters are approximately 95% effective in preventing further PEs, but they have a 10% complication rate on insertion. However, this complication rate is not appreciably higher than that of full anticoagulation.

Heparin blocks extension of thrombus and reduces the risk of further emboli. It does not actively break down clot, but allows the body's own fibrinolytic mechanism to operate over a period of several days to weeks.[8] Heparin has a relatively narrow therapeutic index and is noteworthy as the most common cause of drug-related deaths in the hospital. Significant bleeding occurs in up to one-fourth of patients; the elderly and those on aspirin are at greatest risk. However, these complications rarely occur during the first few hours of treatment or during the time the patient is in the ED. Though heparin is commonly given as a 5,000-U bolus (often 10,000 U if PE is expected), this "standard dosing regimen" often results in inadequate anticoagulation at 24 hours. It has been shown that more accurate dosing occurs when heparin is given as an 80-U/kg bolus and then as a drip of 18 U/kg/h.[16] The rate is then titrated, with the goal of prolonging the partial thromboplastin time by 1.5 to 2.5 times that of normal. Contraindications to heparin include active internal bleeding, malignant hypertension, central nervous system neoplasm, very recent surgery or significant trauma, or a history of heparin-induced thrombocytopenia. Relative contraindications include gastrointestinal bleeding or prior hemorrhagic stroke. Once heparin has been initiated, warfarin (10 mg PO) may be begun, although this is generally not administered in the ED.

Recently, there has been growing interest in the low-molecular-weight heparins (LMWHs) for the treatment of DVT. These are fractionated versions of standard heparin that have a more predictable effect (and therefore do not require close monitoring) and fewer side effects or complications. Most studies comparing these with standard heparin show that LMWHs have advantages but higher costs for the drug itself. Because they can be given subcutaneously once a day, however, and do not require repeated blood tests, home treatment of DVT is possible.[13] Some health systems have protocols for discharge from the ED of selected stable patients with DVT for home LMWH therapy.

Although occasionally recommended, there is no clear role for thrombolytic therapy in patients with isolated DVT, and it should not be initiated independently by the EP. There is some weak evidence that thrombolytics may decrease the incidence of subsequent complications, but these are balanced by an increased rate of acute complications. Therefore, its routine use is not recommended.[7]

There is some controversy regarding recommended management of DVT below the knee. Historically, most of these cases have been treated conservatively, with elevation and antiinflammatory drugs. More recently, however, it has been recognized that these DVTs often propagate and, in as many as one-third of patients, eventually embolize. Therefore, it is generally recommended that these DVTs be treated in a manner similar to that for iliofemoral DVTs. For those patients in which the decision is not to acutely anticoagulate, there should be close follow-up and serial noninvasive studies to document clot regression and absence of propagation, generally with ultrasound.

Similarly, there has been some controversy regarding the ideal treatment of superficial thrombophlebitis of the leg. Here, the danger of acute embolism is less than for calf DVT. However, it must be confirmed that propagation to the deep system has not occurred at the time of the ED visit, and, again, close follow-up must be arranged. Compression bandages, antiinflammatory drugs, and elevation are standard recommendations. If the patient is an intravenous drug user or appears toxic, septic thrombophlebitis must be ruled out. Treatment guidelines are outlined in Table 139.3.

TABLE 139.3. Disposition and Treatment

Deep Venous Thrombosis
Heparin load (80 U/kg) and infusion (18 U/kg/h)
Warfarin on first day
Admit to hospital (floor bed)
Consider outpatient protocol using LMWH in selected patients
IVC filter if heparin contraindicated or fails anticoagulation therapy
Superficial Venous Thrombosis
Ultrasound to exclude DVT
Outpatient care with elevation, NSAIDS; consider compression
Calf Thrombi
Same as DVT
Or treat like superficial phlebitis, but with serial outpatient studies to detect propagation
Phlegmasia Dolens
Immediately heparinize
Fluid resuscitate
Admit to ICU
Consider thrombolysis
Vascular surgery consult

NSAIDs, nonsteroidal antiinflammatory drugs; ICU, intensive care unit.

DISPOSITION

Historically, all patients with proximal lower extremity or upper extremity DVT required admission to the hospital. However, some institutions have now initiated protocols by which a select subset of patients (stable symptoms, no comorbid diseases, and reliable compliance) are being discharged directly home from the ED on a subcutaneous LMWH protocol with close outpatient follow-up. This should not be initiated by the EP, other than as part of a hospital or health-care system protocol.

Conversely, the treatment of patients with DVT distal to the knee was historically similar to that of superficial thrombophlebitis. Now, with increasing concerns that these patients have risks for embolization that are only moderately lower than those with proximal DVT, it is recommended they be hospitalized or entered into a close follow-up protocol.

There is one group of patients that requires a more aggressive approach, namely those with phlegmasia dolens. This condition represents a life-threatening emergency and requires admission to an intensive care unit. These patients also require vascular surgery consultation for consideration of thrombectomy in those situations in which there is risk of loss of the limb without urgent intervention. Fortunately, phlegmasia dolens is a very uncommon complication, but, in this situation, the lack of vascular surgery capability would be the one indication for transport to a higher level of care.

COMMON PITFALLS

- Patients with a painful or swollen leg should be considered to have DVT until proven otherwise. Clinical evaluation alone is not sufficient to rule out the diagnosis.
- The traditional physical examination findings of DVT are notoriously inaccurate. The Homan test should be abandoned, and the presence of a palpable cord should not be relied on.
- A negative D-dimer test is useful only in patients with a clinical low risk of DVT. It should not be used to exclude the diagnosis in moderate- or high-risk patients.
- Although ultrasound examination is generally an excellent test for DVT, it is somewhat operator-dependent, and there are false negatives. Patients with a very high clinical suspicion for DVT but a negative ultrasound should either undergo additional studies or be admitted for serial evaluations.
- Traditional loading doses of heparin result in under-anticoagulation of many patients. Weight-based dosing is more effective.
- Isolated DVT distal to the knee is not as benign as previously thought. It should be treated more like proximal DVT in terms of therapeutic aggressiveness.

References

1. Black MD, French GJ, Rasuli P, et al. Upper extremity deep venous thrombosis. Underdiagnosed and potentially lethal. *Chest* 1993;103:1887–1890.
2. Bounameaux H, de Moerloose P, Perrier A, et al. Plasma measurement of D-dimer as diagnostic aid in suspected venous thromboembolism. An overview. *Thromb Haemost* 1994;72:488–490.
3. Carter CJ. The natural history and epidemiology of venous thrombosis. *Prog Cardiovasc Dis* 1994;36:423–438.
4. Cogo A, Bernardi E, Prandoni P, et al. Acquired risk factors for deep-vein thrombosis in symptomatic outpatients. *Arch Intern Med* 1994;151:164–168.
5. Cronan JJ. Venous thromboembolic disease: the role of US. *Radiology* 1993;186:619–630.
6. Ferris EJ, McCowan TC, Carver DK, et al. Percutaneous inferior vena caval filters: follow-up of seven designs in 320 patients. *Radiology* 1993;188:851–856.
7. Ginsberg JS. Management of venous thromboembolism. *N Engl J Med* 1996;335:1816–1828.
8. Hirsh J, Dalen JE, Deyken D, et al. Heparin: mechanism of action, pharmacokinetics, dosing considerations, monitoring, efficacy and safety. *Chest* 1992;104:337S–3351S.
9. Jorgensen JO, Hanel KC, Morgan AM, et al. The incidence of deep venous thrombosis in patients with superficial thrombophlebitis of the lower limbs. *J Vasc Surg* 1993;18:70–73.
10. Kniffin WD Jr, Baron JA, Barrett J, et al. The epidemiology of diagnosed pulmonary embolism and deep venous thrombosis in the elderly. *Arch Intern Med* 1994;154:861–866.
11. Kristo DA, Perry ME, Kollef MH. Comparison of venography, duplex imaging, and bilateral impedance plethysmography for diagnosis of lower extremity deep vein thrombosis. *South Med J* 1994;87:55–60.
12. Lee AYY, et al. Clinical utility of a rapid whole-blood D-dimer assay in patients with cancer who present with suspected acute deep venous thrombosis. *Ann Intern Med* 1999;131:417–423.
13. Lensing AW, Prins MH, Davidson BL, et al. Treatment of deep venous thrombosis with low-molecular-weight heparins: a meta-analysis. *Arch Intern Med* 1995;155:601–607.
14. Lohr JM, Kerr TM, Lutter KS, et al. Lower extremity calf thrombosis: to treat or not to treat? *J Vasc Surg* 1991;14:618–623.
15. Moser KM, Fedullo PF, LitteJohn JK, et al. Frequent asymptomatic pulmonary embolism in patients with deep venous thrombosis. *JAMA* 1994;271:223–225.
16. Raschke RA, Reilly BM, Guidry JR. Weight-based heparin dosing nomogram compared with a standard care nomogram: a randomized controlled trial. *Ann Intern Med* 1993;119:874–881.
17. Spritzer CE, Evans AC, Kay HH. Magnetic resonance imaging of deep venous thrombosis in pregnant women with lower extremity edema. *Obstet Gynecol* 1995;85:603–607.
18. Wells PS, Anderson DR, Bormanis J, et al. Value of assessment of pretest probability of deep-vein thrombosis in clinical management. *Lancet* 1997; 350:1795–1798.

CHAPTER 140

Infectious Endocarditis

Corey M. Slovis and Rebecca R. Roberts

Infectious endocarditis (IE) is an infection of the endothelial lining of the heart, usually including the valvular endothelium. The disease has been described since the 1600s and continues to evolve and change. Because of a dramatic surge in intravenous (i.v.) drug use and the increased use of prosthetic heart valves, the number of cases of IE is increasing.

IE has classically been divided into two forms: a relatively insidious, chronic disease—subacute bacterial endocarditis (SBE)—and a more abrupt-onset, fulminant form—acute bacterial endocarditis (ABE).

Endocarditis is now more likely to be encountered in patients with prosthetic heart valves, i.v. drug users and the elderly, and less likely to be seen in patients with a history of rheumatic heart disease.[1,2] (Table 140.1). The most common organisms causing IE have also changed. As IE has evolved, the frequency of *Streptococcus viridans* has decreased, while the incidence of *Staphylococcus* species has risen.[1,9,13,14]

There are four steps in the development of SBE: (1) A hemodynamically defective valve produces turbulent blood flow and endothelial disruption; (2) a sterile platelet–fibrin thrombus forms on the damaged valve lining; (3) transient bacteremia infects the thrombus; and (4) high titers of antibodies to the infecting organism are produced. Bacterial endocarditis may also

TABLE 140.1. Emergency Department Patients at Highest Risk for Endocarditis

Patients with valvular or structural heart disease
Intravenous drug abusers
Patients with prosthetic heart valves
Patients with indwelling devices, especially hemodialysis shunts
Elderly patients who have recently undergone an invasive procedure

develop on previously normal native and prosthetic heart valves. In these cases, the only necessary measure is an inoculum of a highly invasive organism.[1,2]

Once endocarditis develops on a valve, the clinical manifestations are attributable to the following series of events: (1) local destruction and malfunction of the cardiac valve; (2) invasive infection of contiguous structures in the heart; (3) continuous bacteremia, leading to distant infections; (4) embolization of vegetations that break off from the valve; and (5) an antigen–antibody response, leading to immune-mediated complications.

IE is often classified into one of four distinct clinical groups: (1) patients with a damaged native valve; (2) i.v. drug abusers (IVDAs); (3) patients with prosthetic valves who develop early-onset prosthetic valve IE (PVE); and (4) patients with late-onset PVE.[7] Early-onset PVE is defined as infection that presents less than 2 months after valve replacement surgery; late-onset PVE presents more than 2 months after surgery.[7]

TABLE 140.2. Most Common Causes of Infectious Endocarditis

	Percentages[a]
NATIVE VALVE INFECTIOUS ENDOCARDITIS	
Streptococcus	
viridans	25–43
bovis	7–15
fecalis	10–16
Staphylococcus	
Coagulase-positive	21–38
Coagulase-negative	5
Gram-negative rods	<5
Fungi	<5
Culture negative	3–15
INTRAVENOUS DRUG ABUSER	
Streptococcus	
viridans	5
fecalis	8
Staphylococcus	
Coagulase-positive	50
Coagulase-negative	<5
Gram-negative rods	5
Fungi	5
Culture negative	<5
EARLY-ONSET PROSTHETIC VALVE INFECTIOUS ENDOCARDITIS	
Staphylococcus (all groups)	10
Streptococcus	
Coagulase-positive	20
Coagulase-negative	25–14
Gram-negative rods	20–38
Fungi	10
Diphtheroids	10
Culture negative	<5
LATE-ONSET PROSTHETIC VALVE INFECTIOUS ENDOCARDITIS	
Streptococcus viridans	25–41
Staphylococcus	
Coagulase-positive	3–10
Coagulase-negative	20–35
Gram-negative rods	15–31
Fungi	<5
Culture negative	<5

[a]Approximations based on multiple prior studies: references 2, 4, 7, 13, 18, and 23; Molavi A. Endocarditis: recognition, management and prophylaxis. *Cardiovasc Clin* 1993;23:139; Robbins MJ, Soeiro R, Frishman WH, et al. Right-sided valvular endocarditis: etiology, diagnosis and approach to therapy. *Am Heart J* 1986;111:128: and Robbins N, DeMaria A, Miller MH. Infective endocarditis in the elderly. *South Med J* 1980;73:1336.

Damaged Native Valve

Any condition causing cardiac valve damage (e.g., rheumatic, degenerative, and congenital cardiac abnormalities) can predispose the patient to IE. Patients with rheumatic valvular disease and those with mitral valve prolapse with documented valvular redundancy and incompetence are, by far, the two highest risk groups for native valve IE.[9] Patients with native valve IE are most likely to develop a syndrome similar to the classic SBE, a relatively chronic infection with only left-sided cardiac involvement, often with a streptococcal organism.[1,2] The mitral valve is the most common valve to be infected in the native valve group. Isolated mitral involvement occurs in 35% to 45% of cases, isolated aortic valve involvement in 15% to 35%, and involvement of both valves in 15% to 30%.[4] Tricuspid valve IE is unusual in this group and accounts for only 1% to 5% of cases.[4] Pulmonic involvement is rare in native valve IE, occurring in less than 1% of cases.[1,2,7]

Native valve IE is caused by streptococcal pathogens in approximately two-thirds of cases (Table 140.2).[1,2,7] *S. viridans* is by far the most common *Streptococcus* species causing IE.[1,7,13] *S. viridans* bacteremia and subsequent valvular seeding traditionally have been attributed to dental procedures in patients with preexisting valvular heart disease.[18] This presumed cause-and-effect relationship has been questioned, and it is no longer clear whether dental procedures are the cause of a significant number of cases of IE.[20] *Streptococcus bovis* (up to 15% of cases of native valve IE) and *Streptococcus fecalis* (more than 10%) are more commonly introduced by bowel and urologic infections or procedures, especially in the elderly.[5,23] Coagulase-positive *Staphylococcus* (up to one-third of all cases of native valve IE) and coagulase-negative *Staphylococcus* (less than 5%) are probably introduced via the skin and are most likely to cause infection in patients who have diabetes or chronic obstructive pulmonary disease, and in those who are elderly or are otherwise debilitated.[23] Central venous and arterial catheterizations are relatively high-risk procedures for causing IE.[16] Indwelling devices, especially hemodialysis shunts, also increase the risk for IE.[19] Gram-negative organisms, fungi, and diphtheroids seldom occur in native valve IE.[3]

Intravenous Drug Abusers

Drug abusers have become one of the leading high-risk groups for developing IE.[14,18] Because cocaine abusers inject themselves so frequently, as compared with other IVDA groups, they appear to have the highest risk of developing IE.[18] Their increased relative risk may also be due to such factors as lack of heating of the drug before injection and direct valvular damage caused by cocaine.[18] Right-sided IE is more common than left-sided involvement in IVDAs, and the tricuspid valve is involved in 50% to 70% of cases.[1,7,16] Left-sided disease may be seen in conjunction with right-sided involvement, or may occur alone. Pulmonic valve involvement is seen in less than 1% of IVDAs.[16]

Patients who inject illicit drugs often are infected with organisms that are normal skin flora. *Staphylococcus aureus* is the most common causative agent in this group of patients, accounting for approximately 50% to 80% of cases[1,2,16]; *Streptococcus* species are the next most common.[14] Gram-negative bacilli, fungi, and diphtheroids are seen only slightly more often in IVDA-associated IE than in native valve IE.[7,18]

Early-Onset Prosthetic Valve Infectious Endocarditis

Patients with early onset PVE either are contaminated intraoperatively or develop infection in the perioperative period.[1,2,4] *Staphylococcus* species, especially the otherwise rare coagulase-negative *Staphylococcus*, are the most commonly incriminated organisms.[1,4] Gram-negative organisms and fungi are also seen more commonly in this group.[3,21]

Late-Onset Prosthetic Valve Infectious Endocarditis

Late PVE shares characteristics of nosocomial infection and native valve IE. The organisms responsible for late PVE fall midway between those seen in early PVE and those common in native valve IE.[1,2,4] *S. viridans* and staphylococci, both coagulase-positive and -negative, are most frequent, but gram-negative bacteria and fungi also cause a significant number of infections.[3,21]

Mechanical valves and tissue valves have an approximately equal incidence of infection (overall incidence, 2.2% to 4.4%), but mechanical valves are more likely to develop early-onset PVE.[4] Mechanical valves tend to develop paravalvular abscesses, myocardial abscesses with conduction delays, pericarditis, and regurgitation caused by paravalvular leaks.[4,7] An acute regurgitant murmur caused by partial dehiscence of the valve is an emergency, because severe heart failure can develop rapidly or the valve can undergo total dehiscence.[4] Tissue valves, however, are more likely to develop leaflet tears, also resulting in new regurgitant murmurs and heart failure.[4] Valvular stenosis is also a potential complication with tissue valves.

CLINICAL PRESENTATION

Patients with IE may present acutely with fulminant heart failure and sepsis, with a chronic, indolent, nonspecific disease process, or with a syndrome intermediate between the two extremes. Because of the overlap, the artificial separation of ABE versus SBE is usually not clinically helpful. Table 140.3 lists the historical and physical findings seen most often in IE.

Complications

Cardiac

Cardiac complications of IE may involve any of the three layers of the heart. Endocardial damage of the valve may result in valvular destruction and variable degrees of congestive heart failure.[24] Severe failure is usually due to aortic insufficiency.[24] Myocarditis or myocardial abscess results when the infecting organism invades the contiguous myocardium. Infection involving the conduction system may result in conduction delays, bundle-branch block, or complete heart block. Ruptured myocardial abscesses may result in a purulent pericarditis.[7,24] Large emboli to the coronary arteries can cause acute myocardial infarction or sudden death.[6] Intracranial catastrophes may occur if thrombolytics are used in cases in which complications of IE cause electrocardiogram (ECG) changes that mimic those of acute ischemia due to coronary artery disease (CAD).[7]

Central Nervous System

Central nervous system complications not only occur in 20% to 40% of patients with IE, but also may be the presenting complaint in a significant number of cases.[6,12] Embolic cerebral infarction or stroke is the most common event and usually involves the middle cerebral artery or its branches.[12] Cerebral mycotic aneurysms, also resulting from emboli to either the vessel lumen or to one of its vasa, may remain asymptomatic or may enlarge and leak or rupture, with disastrous outcome.[24] Septic emboli give rise to cerebral abscesses or, if meningeal or cortical vessels are involved, signs and symptoms consistent with classic bacterial meningitis.[12,20] A syndrome consisting of headache, delirium, hallucinations, and confusion (i.e., a toxic encephalopathy) may occur.[1,12] When this is accompanied by a stiff neck and cerebrospinal fluid consistent with aseptic meningitis, the patient has meningoencephalitis. The cause is not clear, but multiple microinfarcts or microabscesses may be responsible.

Emboli and Immunologic Responses

Besides the brain and heart, other important areas of embolization are the splenic, renal, mesenteric, and extremity vasculature. The emboli result in endarteritis, mycotic aneurysm, local infection, and distal infarction. It is not clear how many of the signs and complications of IE are immune complex–mediated. It is thought that glomerulonephritis, aseptic arthritis, and most of the classic skin manifestations are immune-related.[1,2,7]

EMERGENCY DEPARTMENT EVALUATION

Patients with IE often have numerous nonspecific complaints. Most complain of fever, malaise, anorexia, and weakness.[2,23] Approximately one-half of patients report headache, weight loss, nightsweats, arthralgias, and myalgias.[1,2,7] A history of back pain, rash, dyspnea, or a spectrum of neuropsychiatric symptoms is not uncommon in IE.[1,2,7] Clinicians seldom initially

TABLE 140.3. Historical and Physical Findings Suggestive of Endocarditis

	History	Physical Examination
General	Fever, chills, malaise, weakness, anorexia, weight loss, back pain, myalgia, arthralgia	Acute or chronically ill appearance, fever, diaphoresis, pallor, splenomegaly, arthritis
Cardiopulmonary	Chest pain, dyspnea, edema	Murmurs, especially valvular insufficiency; signs of congestive heart failure
Neurologic	Headache, stiff neck, mental status changes, focal neurologic complaints, extremity pain or paresthesia	Meningismus, abnormal mental status, focal deficits
Other	Hematuria, abdominal pain	Skin: petechiae, Osler nodes, Janeway lesions, splinter hemorrhages
Risk factors	Intravenous drug abuse; heart disease; recent gastrointestinal, genitourinary, or dental procedure; poor dental hygiene	Embolic: mycotic aneurysm, visceral or extremity infarct or ischemia Other: pneumonia, skin abscess, urinary tract infection

attribute these less common symptoms to IE, however. Patients should be asked about recent dental, gastrointestinal, and urologic procedures. Elderly patients in particular may not volunteer or may forget to relate these high-risk procedures. Young patients who are being evaluated "for the flu" seldom volunteer information about i.v. drug use unless specifically questioned.

Physical findings suggestive of endocarditis are listed in Table 140.3. Patients with IE may appear acutely or chronically ill. Nearly all nonimmunosuppressed patients have fever.[9] Other abnormal vital signs, especially tachycardia, are relatively common.[23]

A careful cardiac examination is important in patients suspected of having IE. Approximately 85% of patients with IE have a murmur.[7] Patients most likely to lack murmurs are those with acute IE. Thus, lack of a murmur in an IVDA should never decrease the suspicion of IE. On the other hand, a new regurgitant murmur in a febrile patient is very strong evidence for the disease.[9] Rarely, a large (usually fungal) vegetation may block the outflow tract, resulting in a new stenotic murmur.[21] The cardiac examination should also seek any findings suggestive of heart failure.

A variety of skin lesions are considered classic for IE, but are relatively uncommon. Petechial lesions may be found in different locations. Splinter hemorrhages are tiny red, purple, brown, or black splinter-like lesions that appear under the fingernails. They are seen in up to 20% of patients with IE, but are also found in approximately 8% of all hospitalized patients.[7] Osler's nodes are small, painful, tender erythematous nodules that are most commonly seen in the distal finger pads; they occur in 5% to 20% of patients.[7,9] Janeway lesions are small, flat, nontender red spots on the palms and soles; they occur in only about one in ten patients with IE.[9] Conjunctival petechiae may occur in approximately 10% of patients. Roth spots are retinal petechial hemorrhages with central pallor, which may be seen in 10% to 25% of patients with IE.[6,9]

The remainder of the physical examination may reveal abnormal abdominal or neurologic findings. Splenomegaly is a common finding, and a tender, enlarged liver is often noted. Neurologic examination may reveal signs consistent with meningitis, encephalitis, embolic stroke, or a leaking aneurysm.[12] Some patients present with subtle mental status changes or behavioral symptoms that appear to be psychiatric in nature.

There are numerous nonspecific laboratory findings in IE (Table 140.4). Normochromic, normocytic anemia occurs in up to 75% of patients, and microscopic hematuria in nearly 50%.[14,16] Leukocytosis is seen in about half of cases, and, thus, its absence should not be used to rule out the diagnosis. An elevated sedimentation rate is typical, but it may be normal in up to one-third of patients.[23]

The most important part of the laboratory evaluation is the blood culture. Approximately 20 mL of blood (not 5 to 10 mL) should be drawn for each set of blood cultures and sent for aerobic and anaerobic cultures. The diagnosis of "possible endocarditis" should appear on the specimen label so that the laboratory will hold the specimen for at least 3 weeks to ensure detection of slow-growing organisms. If at all possible, blood cultures should be from three separate sites and should be drawn over a period of approximately 1 hour.

Blood cultures may be positive in up to 98% of patients with IE.[16] Unfortunately, some recent series have reported positivity rates as low as 60% to 80%.[9,14] To maximize the chances of a positive culture and to minimize the confusion caused by contaminants, three to five sets of cultures drawn at least 1 hour apart should be obtained before antibiotics are initiated. Recent antibiotic use by the patient and infection with fastidious or slow-growing organisms are the two major reasons for negative IE cultures.[23] The patients that most commonly have negative cultures are drug abusers, patients with prosthetic valves, and those who have recently received antibiotics.[3]

TABLE 140.4. Laboratory Findings in Endocarditis

BLOOD	ECHOCARDIOGRAM
Positive blood cultures Anemia Microscopic or gross hematuria Leukocytosis Uremia	Vegetations Valve dysfunction Chamber enlargement Pericardial effusion
CHEST RADIOGRAPH	**V/Q SCAN**
Cardiomegaly Pulmonary infiltrates Pulmonary infarcts Pulmonary effusions Chamber enlargement Abnormal movement of prosthetic valve Stimson's sign	Multiple pulmonary infarcts
	CEREBROSPINAL FLUID
	Purulent meningitis Aseptic meningitis Bloody leaking aneurysm
ELECTROCARDIOGRAM	**COMPUTED TOMOGRAPHY**
Conduction defect Acute myocardial infarction Pericarditis	Mycotic aneurysm Cerebral abscess Subarachnoid hemorrhage

The chest radiograph of patients with IE is usually normal. Signs of congestive heart failure, including cardiomegaly, isolated chamber enlargement, and abnormal vascular patterns, provide valuable information regarding abnormal valvular or cardiac function. The chest radiograph may also reveal pneumonia, especially in IVDA patients. Multiple pulmonary infarcts or nodules suggest right-sided disease, usually tricuspid valve endocarditis.[16] In PVE, a double shadow of a mechanical valve, known as Stimson's sign, indicates movement of a valve that has undergone partial dehiscence.[4]

Although usually normal, the ECG should always be carefully examined for evidence of pericarditis, ischemia, infarction, conduction delay, or any degree of heart block. These changes may be indirect evidence for the coexistence of myocarditis, myocardial abscess, pericarditis, or coronary artery embolism.[25]

Echocardiograms are almost always performed in patients who are suspected of having IE. The finding of a vegetation is very strong evidence for the diagnosis of IE.[9] However, a negative echocardiogram should never be used as the definitive test to rule out IE, as up to one-third of patients with IE have nondiagnostic echocardiograms.[15] Transesophageal echocardiography (TEE) is more sensitive than transthoracic echocardiography (TTE), though it is probably more appropriate to begin with a TTE.[11] Echocardiographic detection of valve malfunction, chamber enlargement, or an associated pericardial effusion may also be helpful in the clinical management of IE. Mechanical valves are too echo-dense for TTE to be of significant value, and valvular function should instead be evaluated by either TEE or cinefluorosopy.[4,15]

EMERGENCY DEPARTMENT MANAGEMENT

Definitive therapy for IE is guided by the infecting organism's sensitivity to specific antimicrobial agents. Once blood culture and sensitivity data are available, optimal therapy can usually be decided on easily. The choice of optimal empiric therapy for presumed IE prior to culture results is guided by the expected sensitivity of the bacteria that cause infection in a specific type of patient.

Antibiotics Based on Known Organism

Most experts recommend a combination of aqueous penicillin (12 to 18 million U/d) and gentamicin (1 mg/kg i.v. q8h) for IE in native valve endocarditis due to *S. viridans* or *S. bovis*.[10,26] Single daily dosing of gentamicin is not appropriate in treating IE.[10,26] A combination of high-dose penicillin and gentamicin is also recommended for enterococcal IE.[7,10,26] Nafcillin (2 g i.v. q4h) and gentamicin are often recommended for *S. aureus* infections on native valves.[10,26] Vancomycin is recommended when *Staphylococcus* species are methicillin-resistant.[26] Because *Staphylococcus* is the single most common organism in IVDAs, broad antistaphylococcal coverage is essential in this population.[17,18] Routine antipseudomonal coverage is not routinely recommended in IVDAs because of the rarity of this once more common organism.[10,18,26]

PVE occurring within 1 to 2 months of valve surgery is due to *S. aureus* in approximately 50% of cases and to *Staphylococcus epidermidis* in another 20%.[4,7] Gram-negative organisms and fungi are also common in patients who develop IE soon after surgery. Thus, coverage usually includes vancomycin, gentamicin, and rifampin.[7,10,26] PVE occurring more than 2 months after valve replacement is similar to native value IE, in that *S. viridans, S. bovis,* and *S. aureus* are the most common organisms.[7] Most experts recommend the same initial coverage for early and late PVE, as coagulase-negative *Staphylococcus* species and gram-negative organisms may also be the causative agents.[7,10,26]

If a stable patient presents to emergency department (ED) with the possibility of IE, it is best to obtain at least three sets of blood cultures from separate sites over a period of 1 hour. The patient should then be admitted to an inpatient area and subsequent care and additional culturing performed at the direction of the patient's physician or infectious disease consultant. Antibiotics should, however, be started in the ED if the patient appears septic; is elderly, debilitated, or immunocompromised; has concomitant pneumonia; is in heart failure; or is hemodynamically unstable.

Empiric Antibiotic Coverage

There is no universal agreement on optimal therapy. However, ED physicians can begin therapy by choosing an antibiotic regimen that provides broad-spectrum bactericidal coverage for the most common organisms causing IE. The authors' recommendations for empiric therapy to be begun in the ED appears in Table 140.5.

The recommendations attempt to provide broad coverage divided into two regimens: one for presumed IE in a seriously ill patient with native valves, and a second for presumed IE in a patient with one or more prosthetic valves. The regimens are designed to be easily remembered, and do not address whether the patient may have developed IE in association with i.v. drug abuse or how long ago the prosthetic valve was implanted. In addition, *Staphylococcus* species are assumed to have the potential to be of the methicillin-resistant type. Thus, patients with the possibility of IE should receive nafcillin, gentamicin, and vancomycin. Patients with prosthetic valves who require that therapy be initiated on an emergent basis should receive rifampin, gentamicin, and vancomycin. The regimen should be adjusted after the patient is admitted to the hospital, based on inpatient physician preference and culture and sensitivity data. Consultation with the patient's physician should be accomplished at the earliest possible time.

Anticoagulants

Anticoagulation is contraindicated in patients with native valve IE because of the greatly increased risk of intracranial bleeding that occurs in patients with IE who have cerebral emboli.[1,7] The exception is the patient who develops massive life-threatening pulmonary emboli.[7] Patients with PVE who are already maintained on anticoagulation should probably continue the medication and be closely monitored for complications.[4]

Surgery

Valve replacement has become much more widely accepted as a therapy for complicated IE.[4] Although there is agreement on the indications for surgery, the timing and specific details are debated. The following are general indications for valve replacement: heart failure as a result of new valve malfunction, major embolic complications, continued infection despite administration of appropriate antibiotics, arrhythmia or new conduction defect, or a fungal cause.[1,2,4,7] It is not clear to what extent the size of the vegetations seen on the echocardiogram determines the prognosis and need for valve replacement.

DISPOSITION

Because of the frequency of serious complications and the need for parenteral antibiotic therapy, all patients who are strongly suspected of having IE should be admitted to the hospital. Patients with overwhelming sepsis, serious embolic complications, or any degree of heart failure or conduction block require admission to an intensive care setting. In addition, intensive care unit admission is mandatory for PVE patients with any evidence of paravalvular leak.

Two to three sets of blood cultures (20 mL of blood for each set) should be obtained in patients suspected of having IE, but in whom the diagnosis is thought to be unlikely. Outpatient follow-up for these patients is appropriate if the patient is reliable and can be readily contacted and if the patient's private physician agrees.

TABLE 140.5. Empiric Emergency Department Therapy for Presumed Endocarditis prior to Culture Results

Patients with Native Valves (Including Intravenous Drug Abusers)		Patients with Prosthetic Valves	
Nafcillin[a]	2 g i.v. q4h	Rifampin	300 mg PO q8h
and		and	
Gentamicin[b]	1 mg/kg i.v. q8h	Gentamicin[b]	1 mg/kg i.v. q8h
and		and	
Vancomycin	1 g i.v. q12h (or 15 mg/kg)	Vancomycin	1 g i.v. q8h

[a]Consider ceftriaxone 2 g i.v. in penicillin-allergic patients.
[b]Use g8h dosing and not single daily dosing in infective endocarditis.

TABLE 140.6. Prophylaxis in Certain Cardiac Conditions

HIGH RISK
Prosthetic valves: all types
History of infectious endocarditis
Complex cyanotic heart disease
Surgically constructed pulmonary vasculative
MODERATE RISK
Most other congenital cardiac malformations
Acquired valvular dysfunction, including rheumatic heart disease
Hypertrophic cardiomyopathy
Mitral valve prolapse *with* regurgitation
PROPHYLAXIS NOT RECOMMENDED
Prior coronary artery bypass surgery
Mitral valve prolapse *without* valvular regurgitation
Cardiac pacemakers
Physiologic murmurs
History of rheumatic fever without valvular dysfunction
History of Kawasaki disease without valvular dysfunction
Surgically repaired ASD, VSD, or PDA
Isolated secundum-type ASD

ASD; atrial septal defect; VSD, ventricular septal defect; PDA,[???].
From Dajani AS, Taubert KA, Wilson W, et al. Prevention of bacterial endocarditis: recommendations by the American Heart Association. *JAMA* 1997;277:1794–1801.

When IE is strongly suspected, a cardiologist should be consulted for possible echocardiographic examination. TEE must be done as soon as possible in any patient with a prosthetic valve in whom the possibility of IE is considered. Patients with PVE or those who may need valve replacement should have a cardiac surgeon involved early to ensure that the timing of surgery is optimal. For patients with possible brain abscess or aneurysm, a neurosurgeon should be consulted promptly.

ENDOCARDITIS PROPHYLAXIS

The aim of antibiotic prophylaxis is to prevent bacteremia from occurring during procedures in patients who have conditions that predispose them to IE. Decisions regarding appropriate prophylaxis depend on knowing which patients are at risk, which procedures predictably cause bacteremia, and which are the most common organisms involved in each organ system (Tables 140.6 and 140.7).[5]

There is increasing debate over the efficacy of prophylactic antibiotics in preventing IE caused by instrumentation or other outpatient procedures. Prophylactic antibiotics may, in fact, not confer any significant protection from IE.[22] More importantly, dental procedures and perhaps most other outpatient procedures may not be significant causes of IE.[8,22]

The American Heart Association has revised its recommendations for prophylactic antibiotic administration.[5] The 1997 recommendations are simpler and much easier to follow. Now, only a single oral dose of amoxicillin is recommended 60 minutes prior to dental procedures. For patients who cannot take oral medications, a single i.v. dose of antibiotics within 30 minutes of the procedure is recommended. Previous, more complicated regimens were followed by only about one in four physicians.[8]

Patients with heart disease at highest risk for developing IE are listed in Table 140.6. Table 140.7 lists the prophylactic regimen for dental, oral, and upper respiratory procedures required for these patients.[5] Guidelines for preprocedure prophylaxis for gastrointestinal and genitourinary tract procedures are provided in Table 140.8.[5]

COMMON PITFALLS

- Not asking about risk factors in patients who present with nonspecific symptoms consistent with IE
- Missing the diagnosis in the elderly by attributing a cardiac murmur to chronic heart disease
- Failing to remember that IVDAs are at high risk for endocarditis
- Not asking specifically about i.v. drug use in patients who present with nonspecific symptoms consistent with endocarditis
- Failing to remember that IE in drug abusers often presents without a murmur
- Failing to consider the embolic and immune-mediated complications of IE as the underlying cause of stroke, meningitis, myocardial infarction, septic arthritis, or renal failure

TABLE 140.7. Prophylaxis for Dental, Oral, Respiratory, and Esophageal Procedures

	Antibiotic	Dosage	Timing
Oral	Amoxicillin	2 g PO (50 mg/kg PO in children)	1 h before procedure
	or		
Intravenous	Ampicillin	2 g i.v. or i.m. (50 mg/kg i.v. in children)	30 min before procedure
IF PENICILLIN-ALLERGIC			
Oral	Clindamycin	600 mg PO (20 mg/kg PO in children)	1 h before procedure
	or		
	Cephalixin	2 g PO (50 mg/kg in children)	1 h before procedure
	or		
	Azithromycin	500 mg PO (15 mg/kg in children)	1 h before procedure
Intravenus	*or*		
	Clindamycin	600 mg i.v. (20 mg/kg i.v. in children)	30 min before procedure

From Dajani AS, Taubert KA, Wilson W, et al. Prevention of bacterial endocarditis: recommendations by the American Heart Association. *JAMA* 1997;277:1794–1801.

TABLE 140.8. Prophylaxis for Genitourinary and Nonesophageal Gastrointestinal Procedures

Antibiotic	Dosage	Timing
ANTIBIOTICS FOR HIGH-RISK PATIENTS		
Ampicillin plus Gentamicin	2 g i.m. or i.v. (50 mg/kg up to 2 g in children) 1.5 mg/kg i.m. or i.v. (Max, 120 mg)	Within 30 min of procedure
And 6 h later: Ampicillin or Amoxicillin	1 g i.m. or i.v. (25 mg/kg in children) 1 g PO (25 mg/kg in children)	Six hours later
ANTIBIOTICS FOR MODERATE-RISK PATIENTS		
Amoxicillin	2 g PO (50 mg/kg in children)	1 h prior to procedure
or Ampicillin	2 g i.v. or i.m. (50 mg/kg in children)	Within 30 min of procedure
HIGH-RISK PATIENTS ALLERGIC TO PENICILLIN		
Vancomycin plus Gentamicin	1 g i.v. over 1–2 h (20 mg/kg in children) 1.5 mg/kg i.v. or i.m. (Max, 120 mg)	Complete infusion/injection within 30 min of procedure
MODERATE-RISK PATIENTS ALLERGIC TO PENICILLIN		
Vancomycin	1 g i.v. over 1–2 h (20 mg/kg in children)	Complete infusion/injection within 30 min of procedure

[a]See Table 140.6 for risk class.
From Dajani AS, Taubert KA, Wilson W, et al. Prevention of bacterial endocarditis: recommendations by the American Heart Association. *JAMA* 1997;277:1794–1801.

- Failing to recognize that, in patients with a mechanical valve, a regurgitant murmur is a sign of impending heart failure or valve dehiscence
- Failing to consult a cardiac surgeon in cases of IE that have only mild-to-moderate heart failure
- Forgetting that mild degrees of heart block and conduction delays are signs highly suggestive of myocardial abscess or myocarditis
- Not asking about risk factors for IE in patients about to undergo a procedure prone to cause bacteremia
- Failing to learn the new, simplified single-dose amoxicillin regimen for prophylaxis prior to dental procedures

References

1. Bansal RC. Infective endocarditis. *Med Clin North Am* 1995;79:1205–1240.
2. Bayer AS. Infective endocarditis. *Clin Infect Dis* 1993;17:313.
3. Berbari EF, Cockerill FR III, Steckelberg JM. Infective endocarditis due to unusual or fastidious microorganisms. *Mayo Clin Proc* 1997;72:532–542.
4. Cowgil LD, Addonzio VP, Hopeman AR, et al. Prosthetic valve endocarditis. *Curr Probl Cardiol* 1986;11:617.
5. Dajani AS, Taubert KA, Wilson W, et al. Prevention of bacterial endocarditis: recommendations by the American Heart Association. *JAMA* 1997; 277:1794–1801.
6. DiSalvo TG, Tatter SB, O'Gara PT, et al: Fatal intracerebral hemorrhage following thrombolytic therapy of embolic myocardial infarction in unsuspected infective endocarditis. *Clin Cardiol* 1994;17:340–344.
7. Durack DT. Infective and noninfective endocarditis. In: Hurst JW, ed. *The heart,* vol 2, 9th ed. New York: McGraw-Hill, 1998:2205–2239.
8. Durack DT. Antibiotics for prevention of endocarditis during dentistry: time to scale back? *Ann Intern Med* 1998;129:829–831.
9. Durack DT, Lukes AS, Bright DK, and the Duke Endocarditis Service. New criteria for diagnosis of infective endocarditis: utilization of specific echocardiographic findings. *Am J Med* 1994;96:200–209.
10. Gilbert DN, Moellering RC, Sande MA, eds. *The Sanford guide to antimicrobial therapy,* 29th ed. Antimicrobial Therapy, Inc., 1999
11. Irani WN, Grayburn PA, Afridi I. A negative transthoracic echocardiogram obviates the need for transesophageal echocardiography in patients with suspected native valve active infective endocarditis. *Am J Cardiol* 1996;78:101–103.
12. Kanter MC, Hart RG. Neurologic complications of infective endocarditis. *Neurology* 1991;41:1015.
13. King JW, Shehane RR, Leirl J. Infectious endocarditis at three hospitals in the same city: two study periods a decade apart. *South Med J* 1986;79:151.
14. Kjerulf A, Tvede M, Aldershvile J, et al. Bacterial endocarditis at a tertiary hospital—how do we improve diagnosis and delay of treatment? *Cardiology* 1998;89:79–86.
15. Lindner JR, Case RA, Dent JM, et al. Diagnostic value of echocardiography in suspected endocarditis. *Circulation* 1996;93:730–736.
16. Mathew J, Addai T, Anand A, et al. Clinical features, site of involvement, bacteriologic findings, and outcome of infective endocarditis in intravenous drug users. *Arch Intern Med* 1995;155:1641–1648.
17. Mortara LA, Bayer AS. *Staphylococcus aureus* bacteremia and endocarditis: new diagnostic and therapeutic concepts. *Infect Dis Clin North Am* 1993;7:53.
18. Roberts RR, Slovis CM. Infectious endocarditis in the intravenous drug abuser. *Emerg Med Clin North Am* 1990;8:665.
19. Robinson DL, Fowler VG, Sexton DJ, et al. Bacterial endocarditis in hemodialysis patients. *Am J Kidney Dis* 1997;30:521–524.
20. Roder BL, Wandall DA, Espersen F, et al. Neurologic manifestations in *Staphylococcus aureus* endocarditis: a review of 260 bacteremic cases in nondrug addicts. *Am J Med* 1997;102:379–386.
21. Rubenstein E, Lang R. Fungal endocarditis. *Eur Heart J* 1995;16[Suppl B]:84–89.
22. Strom BL, Abrutyn E, Berlin JA, et al. Dental and cardiac risk factors for infective endocarditis. *Ann Intern Med* 1998;129:761–769.
23. Terpenning MS, Buggy BP, Kauffman CA. Endocarditis: clinical features in young and elderly patients. *Am J Med* 1987;83:626.
24. Weinstein L. Life-threatening complications of infective endocarditis and their management. *Arch Intern Med* 1986;146:953.
25. Weinstein L, Schlesinger JJ. Pathoanatomic, pathophysiologic and clinical correlations in endocarditis. I. *N Engl J Med* 1974;91:832.
26. Wilson WR, Karchmer AW, Dajani AS, et al. Antibiotic treatment of adults with infective endocarditis due to streptococci, enterococci, staphylococci, and HACEK microorganisms. *JAMA* 1995;274:1706–1713.

CHAPTER 141
Syncope

Jay M. Goldman and Thomas P. Martin

Syncope, defined as *the sudden transient loss of consciousness associated with an inability to maintain postural tone and resolving without intervention,*[10] is the presenting complaint in 1% to 3% of emergency department visits.[3] The approach to the patient with syncope is problematic in that the signs and symptoms that led the patient to seek evaluation have, by definition, resolved before arrival in the emergency department. Furthermore, syncope is a symptom rather than a disease.

The differential diagnosis of syncope covers a spectrum that ranges from benign causes to life-threatening arrhythmias, with the potential to cause sudden death. The diagnostic effort, therefore, concentrates on identifying patients who are likely to benefit from further inpatient evaluation and therapy. As is common in the practice of emergency medicine, this group of high-risk patients represents only a small fraction of the entire population who present with syncope. The challenge of accurately identifying this small group is formidable.[17]

The incidence of syncope depends on the population studied. The Framingham study evaluated 5209 men and women aged 30 to 62 years on entry to the study. Over the next 26 years, 172 persons (3.3%) reported at least[23] one episode of syncope. In contrast, in an elderly institutionalized population, 23% had an episode of syncope.[16]

While prior epidemiologic studies frequently labeled significant proportions of patients as having "unexplained syncope" or "syncope of unknown origin," broader use of event monitoring, tilt-table testing, and psychiatric evaluation, as well as recognition that syncope is often multifactorial in the elderly, have substantially reduced the number of patients without a diagnosis.

TABLE 141.1. Differential Diagnosis of Syncope

CARDIAC CAUSES
Arrhythmias
Bradyarrhythmias: second- and third-degree heart block, sinus node dysfunction, pacemaker malfunction
Tachyarrhythmias: ventricular tachycardia, ventricular fibrillation, SVT, torsade de pointes
Pump failure
Myocardial infarction, cardiac ischemia
Obstruction to flow
Aortic stenosis, hypertrophic cardiomyopathy, pulmonary hypertension, pulmonary embolism, prosthetic valve dysfunction
Impairment of venous return
Pericardial tamponade
Other cardiovascular causes
Aortic dissection
REFLEX-MEDIATED
Vasovagal/vasodepressor syncope
Situational syncope
Micturition, defecation
Other
Carotid sinus hypersensitivity
ORTHOSTATIC HYPOTENSION
Hypovolemia, acute blood loss, dehydration, medications
NEUROLOGIC
Subarachnoid hemorrhage, posterior circulation TIA, subclavian steal, peripheral and autonomic neuropathies
MEDICATIONS
Vasodilators, calcium channel blockers, beta blockers, nitrates, diuretics, antiarrhythmics, ACEIs
PSYCHIATRIC DISEASE
Major depression, somatization disorder, panic disorder, substance abuse

SVT, supraventricular tachycardia; TIAs, transient ischemic attacks; ACEI, angiotensin converting enzyme inhibitors.

PATHOPHYSIOLOGY AND DIFFERENTIAL DIAGNOSIS

The pathophysiology common to most causes of syncope is a sudden, transient reduction in cerebral blood flow (Table 141.1). Impaired function results either in the area of the brainstem thought to be responsible for the conscious state (reticular activating system) or in both cerebral hemispheres simultaneously. In the few causes of syncope in which cerebral blood flow is not markedly reduced, substrate is either not available to the brain (hypoglycemia) or not used because of a sudden, dramatic reduction in cerebral metabolism secondary to acute brain injury or subarachnoid hemorrhage.

The sudden increase in intracranial pressure associated with these conditions may limit cerebral blood flow as well, and may also deform the neural structures involved in the maintenance of consciousness. In generalized seizures, the pathophysiology of loss of consciousness is related to widespread electrical discharge.

Transient tachyarrhythmias (ventricular or supraventricular) may produce syncope by decreasing ventricular filling and stroke volume, resulting in systemic hypotension and decreased cerebral blood flow. Loss of consciousness may also occur as a result of transient bradyarrhythmias. Although bradyarrhythmias are often an incidental finding and asymptomatic, some episodes of syncope are related to sinus node dysfunction, particularly in the elderly. Medications can also produce an inappropriate bradycardia and depressed left ventricular output. In pacemaker-dependent patients, pacemaker malfunction has been reported to produce syncope as a result of bradyarrhythmias or pacemaker-induced tachycardia. Of note, studies in patients with chronic bifascicular block and syncope have shown that in fewer than 20% are the two related and that, in fact, ventricular tachycardia is responsible for more episodes of syncope in these patients than are bradyarrhythmias.

Syncope may also be a manifestation of cardiovascular disease producing an obstruction to blood flow. Exertional syncope may be the first clue to a diagnosis of aortic stenosis or hypertrophic cardiomyopathy. In these disorders, the conventional explanation of decreased cardiac output as a result of left ventricular outflow obstruction has been supplemented by findings that tachyarrhythmias occur frequently in these patients and may be particularly compromising to those who depend on adequate ventricular filling to overcome the obstruction. In addition, paradoxical vasodilation has been shown to occur in patients with aortic stenosis and may contribute to the syncopal episodes common to this disease.

Mitral valve disease may also cause syncope. Severe mitral stenosis may be associated with syncope, most commonly during periods of atrial fibrillation. Various tachyarrhythmias and neuropsychiatric complaints occur in patients with mitral valve prolapse, which may be associated with syncope. Left atrial myxoma is a rare tumor that causes an abrupt decrease in cardiac output, often when a change in position causes the tumor to occlude the mitral orifice.

Acute pulmonary hypertension causes functional acute obstruction to pulmonary flow, and thus abruptly decreases left ventricular preload and cardiac output. This event may occur with massive pulmonary embolism. In patients with chronic pulmonary hypertension, activities that acutely raise intrathoracic pressure, such as coughing or the Valsalva maneuver during defecation, produce the same phenomenon. Air embolism may produce syncope by obstructing flow through the heart, lungs, or carotids, causing myocardial infarction by occluding coronary flow or by inducing ventricular arrhythmias.

Other causes of cardiac-related syncope include sudden left ventricular dysfunction or ventricular arrhythmias associated with myocardial ischemia or infarction,[2] and impairment of venous return, leading to decreased left ventricular output, as seen in pericardial tamponade, constrictive pericarditis, and constrictive myocardial disease.

Reflex-mediated syncope is a common cause of syncope in all populations. Vasovagal syncope (precipitated by painful or emotional situations), carotid sinus hypersensitivity, and situational syncope (with micturition or defecation) may share components of a common pathophysiologic mechanism.[21] Until recently, the explanation for the findings of hypotension or bradycardia was anchored in a cardiac mechanoreceptor mechanism.

The orthostatic stress of upright posture, causing an underfilled left ventricle, or the emotional stress of phlebotomy, for example, leads to vigorous left ventricular contraction and stimulation of arterial and cardiopulmonary mechanoreceptors. Stimulation of these receptors leads to the transmission of vagal afferent signals to the ventral lateral medulla. The result is a withdrawal of sympathetic efferents (producing peripheral vasodilation and hypotension) and increased vagal efferents to the heart (producing bradycardia) in susceptible individuals.[7,21]

The finding that vasovagal syncope occurs in individuals following cardiac transplantation, as well as information from animal studies, has led to recognition that a purely cardiac mechanoreceptor mechanism is inadequate to explain the physiologic changes of reflex-mediated syncope. Increasingly, the importance of neurohumoral factors, including the renin–aldosterone–angiotensin system, vasopressin, serotonin, pancreatic polypeptides, endogenous opioids, and nitric oxide, is being recognized. The exact contributions of each of these factors and the nature of their interaction remain to be elucidated.[7,21]

Syncope may be a manifestation of psychiatric illness. Studies have documented a high prevalence of psychiatric illness among patients with syncope, particularly patients with syncope of unknown origin. Psychiatric disorders included somatoform disorders, mood disorders (including major depressive disorder), anxiety disorders (including panic attacks), and substance abuse.

Psychiatric disease may be associated with syncope by several mechanisms, including exacerbation of coexisting medical illness, by leading to hyperventilation, by triggering a vasovagal response, or as a presenting complaint in a somatic disorder. Syncope may also be the result of volume depletion or cardiac ischemia produced by alcohol or cocaine abuse, respectively.[22]

True seizures also cause a transient loss of consciousness. Distinguishing a seizure disorder from other causes of syncope is usually straightforward by history. Postictal disorientation is the most reliable discriminator, occurring in most patients with seizures and very rarely in patients with syncope. Brief (usually less than 10 seconds) tonic–clonic seizure activity can accompany syncope of any etiology, especially vasodepressor syncope. This activity is not accompanied by postictal disorientation, and it does not represent true seizure activity.

Transient ischemic attacks and stroke rarely cause syncope.[14] For cerebrovascular disease to cause a loss of consciousness, either both cerebral hemispheres or the brainstem must be deprived of blood flow. In a patient with a prior hemispheric infarction, marked ischemia or infarction on the contralateral side may cause a loss of consciousness, but it is unlikely that this alteration in consciousness would be transient and resolve spontaneously. Similarly, vertebrobasilar ischemia may cause syncope, but not in isolation. Other manifestations of brainstem dysfunction (diplopia, vertigo, or nausea) are required to make this rare diagnosis. Most investigators agree that syncope is rarely a manifestation of neurologic disease, except for seizures.[14]

Subarachnoid hemorrhage can produce syncope, presumably as a result of a sudden increase in intracranial pressure and a sudden transient decrease in cerebral metabolism. The complaint of headache or the appearance of focal neurologic findings in a patient with syncope raises this possibility.

Medications can produce syncope by several mechanisms: by producing volume depletion, causing orthostasis, promoting gastrointestinal hemorrhage, or depressing left ventricular function, or by virtue of having proarrhythmic effects. Medications and the interaction of multiple medications, particularly in the elderly, are important considerations in the evaluation of syncope.

Other causes of syncope include orthostasis secondary to acute blood loss, dehydration, and third-spacing of fluid, as well as disorders of autonomic function, including peripheral neuropathies and central nervous system disease.

EMERGENCY DEPARTMENT EVALUATION

The emergency physician should have several goals in the evaluation of patients presenting with syncope. First, the clinician must identify the subgroup of syncope patients presenting with life-threatening or other causes of syncope requiring emergent or urgent diagnosis and treatment (e.g., subarachnoid hemorrhage, abdominal aortic aneurysm, myocardial infarction). Second, the clinician must be able to identify other recognizable causes of syncope that will benefit from specific treatment or other intervention (e.g., volume depletion, adverse effects of medications). Third, in the patients who remain without a diagnosis despite a thorough emergency department evaluation, the emergency physician must identify those who require further evaluation. Finally, the physician must determine whether the most appropriate setting for that evaluation is as an inpatient or outpatient.

History, physical examination, and the initial electrocardiogram (ECG) are the crucial elements in determining a cause of syncope and in stratifying the risk of those patients in whom it is not possible to make a diagnosis during the emergency department visit. These three components established the diagnosis in 88% of patients who eventually received a diagnosis in two large studies.[3,11] In addition, specific abnormalities revealed in this evaluation led to the performance of other tests, which established the diagnosis in another 5% of patients, resulting in a net yield of 93% from a directed emergency department evaluation. A history of exercise-induced syncope, for example, suggests hypertrophic cardiomyopathy or aortic stenosis and justifies echocardiography, while a history of sudden-onset headache with syncope suggests an intracranial hemorrhage and justifies computed tomography of the brain and lumbar puncture.

Physical examination may reveal asymmetric upper extremity blood pressures and lead to consideration of aortic dissection or subclavian steal. Similarly, dysrhythmias on ECG direct the evaluation down another path. Screening laboratory studies have been shown to add little in establishing a cause of syncope (hypoglycemia was clinically suspected, abnormal electrolytes never accounted for a loss of consciousness, and anemia from bleeding was clinically evident).[3,17] There is, therefore, no "standard" emergency department workup for syncopal patients beyond history, physical examination, and ECG; further studies are indicated only for selected patients as determined by the initial evaluation.

The history should focus on the events and sensations before, during, and after the syncopal episode, as well as on the medical and medication histories. Physical examination focuses on vital signs and a careful cardiovascular (murmurs, pulses, signs of congestive heart failure) and neurologic evaluation. The ECG is analyzed for arrhythmias, conduction abnormalities, and signs of ischemia or infarction.

Although orthostatic vital signs are a part of the physical examination for a patient with syncope, there is little agreement on the definition of orthostatic hypotension. An increase in the heart rate of 30 beats or more on standing correlates with an acute blood loss of 1000 mL, but smaller degrees of volume loss do not reliably correlate with orthostatic changes.[1,13,19–21] Even symptoms of dizziness on standing correlate poorly with orthostatic changes or volume depletion. Thus, the diagnosis of postural syncope is probably best made by a history of syncope on arising (unless hypovolemia is profound, in which case the orthostatic vital signs will be reliably abnormal).

Although there are reports of syncope as the initial complaint of elderly patients with acute myocardial infarction, there are no convincing reports of acute myocardial infarction presenting solely with syncope.[2] Of ten patients whose painless infarction was "ushered in by a syncopal attack," all had other symptoms or signs (acute severe dyspnea or cardiovascular collapse) or ECG changes that were diagnostic of myocardial infarction at the time of their first evaluation.

More recent reports of syncope as the initial symptom of myocardial infarction in the elderly have also stressed that these patients are often pain-free on presentation. Diagnoses were made nevertheless on the basis of other symptoms, signs, and ECG findings available to the initial examining physician. Thus, admission to the hospital to "rule out myocardial infarction" for the patient whose syncope is unexplained is not warranted (unless indicated for other reasons).

Somewhat similarly, syncope has been described as the initial symptom in patients with aortic dissection, ruptured aortic aneurysm, pulmonary embolism, subarachnoid hemorrhage, and ruptured ectopic pregnancy. However, careful evaluation directed by findings on initial history, examination, and ECG was sufficient to make the diagnosis in all cases.

Attributing syncope to transient arrhythmias, unless they are identified on the initial ECG or monitor strip, can be problematic. Long-term, continuous ECG (Holter) monitoring has inadequate specificity to provide useful results; the vast majority of abnormalities detected cause no symptoms and are of no particular significance.[6,11] Invasive electrophysiologic studies may be indicated for a small group of patients who are at high risk for sudden death (those with a history of ventricular tachycardia or fibrillation, myocardial infarction, congestive heart failure, or valvular or hypertrophic heart disease).[4,12] Consultation with a cardiologist is desirable when deciding on disposition in this setting.

Upright tilt-table testing has become a useful adjunct in the further evaluation of patients with suspected vasovagal or neurocardiogenic syncope. Tilt-table testing reveals abnormalities in 20% to 70% of patients whose ED evaluation leaves them without a diagnosis. A positive test in patients with a recurrent syncope may guide therapy with a beta blocker, anticholinergic agent, or fludrocortisone. Treatment has been shown to be effective in preventing recurrence of syncope in the majority of patients with positive tests.

EMERGENCY DEPARTMENT MANAGEMENT AND DISPOSITION

As with the emergency department evaluation, the management of patients with syncope also requires a tiered approach. For patients presenting with symptoms that allow identification of a cause of the syncopal episode, management is directed toward that entity. For patients who remain without a diagnosis at the end of the emergency department visit, disposition is predicated on an assessment of risk.

Large cohort studies in the 1980s stratified risk based on the etiology of syncope. Patients eventually found to have cardiac causes of syncope were found to have increased rates of mortality, cardiovascular mortality, and sudden death, compared with patients who had syncope of noncardiac origin or in whom an explanation for syncope was not found.[3,5,11] Often, however, this information is of little help to the emergency physician when the etiology of syncope remains undefined.

The job of the emergency physician is further complicated by other deficiencies in the available medical literature. First, no information is available concerning the risk of adverse outcome (significant arrhythmia or cardiovascular mortality) in the time typically covered by hospitalization surrounding an acute syncopal episode. Second, no literature supports the conclusion that hospital admission results in a benefit to patients or a change in outcome.

Despite these shortcomings, some guidance is available concerning the question of disposition in patients with syncope. Left ventricular function is a clear determinant of outcome. Studies have documented left ventricular function as a significant predictor of arrhythmia, cardiovascular mortality, and sudden death.[18–20] In populations matched for age and comorbid illnesses, syncope was not a risk factor for overall and cardiac mortality or for cardiovascular events. Rather, age, male sex, and congestive heart failure were the factors predictive of these end points.[9]

More recently, one emergency department study[18] found that the risk of arrhythmia and 1-year mortality could be stratified by the presence of the following: (1) age greater than 45 years, (2) a history of congestive heart failure, (3) a history of ventricular ectopic activity, and (4) an abnormal ECG, defined as any finding other than sinus tachycardia, sinus bradycardia, or nonspecific ST and T-wave changes. Arrhythmias and death within 1 year occurred in 4% to 7% of patients without any risk factors and in 57% to 80% of patients with three or four risk factors.[18] However, no combination of variables available to the emergency physician identifies a cohort of patients with syncope who have no risk of an adverse outcome.

Given this perspective, it becomes apparent that the decision to hospitalize a patient presenting to the emergency department with syncope, in whom the history, physical examination, and initial ECG are unrevealing, must be made on a case-by-case basis. This decision must be predicated on a careful assessment of the risk of adverse outcome and the potential benefit to the patient of inpatient evaluation. Factors that should be considered include (1) a history of congestive heart failure or left ventricular dysfunction; (2) a history of ventricular arrhythmias; (3) historical factors, physical examination findings, or ECG findings suggestive of structural heart disease, left ventricular dysfunction, arrhythmia, or conduction system disease; (4) the patient's age; (5) the use of medications that may predispose to arrhythmia; and (6) the occurrence of syncope related to exertion.[15,18]

A clear recommendation for admission can be made for any patient with syncope and known or suspected left ventricular dysfunction or a history of ventricular arrhythmias. Patients with no suspicion of structural heart disease and a single episode of syncope may often be closely followed without other testing, while those with recurrent episodes should be referred for tilt-table testing, event monitoring, or psychiatric evaluation.[15]

In patients for whom emergency department discharge is considered, the ability of the patient to provide for basic needs, the safety of ambulation, and the availability of necessary supports following discharge should be assured.

COMMON PITFALLS

- Attributing syncope to a vasovagal or unknown cause because of a failure to take a detailed history of the syncopal event
- Attributing syncope to an incidentally found, asymptomatic arrhythmia
- Attributing syncope to a transient ischemic attack
- Attributing syncope to any finding when the causal relation is tenuous
- Failure to take seriously the finding of an aortic outflow murmur in a patient with syncope
- Admission of patients with isolated syncope of unknown cause to "rule out myocardial infarction"
- Failure to recognize the following catastrophic scenarios: syncope with headache (subarachnoid hemorrhage), syncope with chest pain (myocardial infarction, aortic dissection, pulmonary embolism, pulmonary hypertension), syncope with exertion (aortic stenosis, hypertrophic cardiomyopathy), and syncope with abdominal pain (leaking aortic aneurysm, ruptured ectopic pregnancy)

References

1. Atkins D, Hanusa B, Sefcik T, et al. Syncope and orthostatic hypotension. *Am J Med* 1991;91:179.
2. Bayer AJ, Chadha JS, Farag RR, et al. Changing presentation of myocardial infarction with increasing age. *J Am Geriatr Soc* 1986;34:263.
3. Day SC, Cook EF, Funkenstein H, et al. Evaluation and outcome of emergency room patients with transient loss of consciousness. *Am J Med* 1982;73:15.
4. Dennis AR, Rodd DL, Richards DA, et al. Electrophysiologic studies in patients with unexplained syncope. *Int J Cardiol* 1992;35:211.
5. Eagle KA, Black HR. The impact of diagnostic tests in evaluating patients with syncope. *Yale J Biol Med* 1983;56:1.
6. Gibson TC, Heitzman MR. Diagnostic efficacy of 24-hour electrocardiographic monitoring for syncope. *Am J Cardiol* 1984;53:1013.
7. Kapoor WN. Using a tilt table to evaluate syncope. *Am J Med Sci* 1999;317(2):110.
8. Kapoor WN, Cha R, Peterson JR, et al. Prolonged electrocardiographic monitoring in patients with syncope. *Am J Med* 1987;82:20.
9. Kapoor WN, Hanusa BH. Is syncope a risk factor for poor outcome? Comparison of patients with and without syncope. *Am J Med* 1996;100:646.
10. Kapoor WN, Karpf M, Maher Y, et al. Syncope of unknown origin. *JAMA* 1982;247:2687.
11. Kapoor WN, Karpf M, Wieand S, et al. A prospective evaluation and follow-up of patients with syncope. *N Engl J Med* 1983;309:197.
12. Kapoor WN, Snustad D, Peterson J, et al. Syncope in the elderly. *Am J Med* 1986;80:419.
13. Koziol-McLain J, Lowenstein S, Fuller B. Orthostatic vital signs in emergency department patients. *Ann Emerg Med* 1991;20:606.
14. Linzer M. Syncope. *South Med J* 1987;80:545.
15. Linzer M, Yang EH, Estes M, et al. Diagnosing syncope. Part 2: unexplained syncope. *Ann Intern Med* 1997;127(1):76.
16. Lipsitz LA, Wei JY, Rowe JW. Syncope in an elderly, institutionalized population: prevalence, incidence and associated risk. *Q J Med* 1985;55:45.
17. Martin GJ, Adams SL, Martin HG, et al. Prospective evaluation of syncope. *Ann Emerg Med* 1984;13:499.
18. Martin TP, Hanusa BH, Kapoor WN. Risk stratification of patients with syncope. *Ann Emerg Med* 1997;29:459.
19. Middlekauff HR, Stevenson WG, Saxon LA. Prognosis after syncope: impact of left ventricular function. *Am J Heart* 1993;125:121.
20. Middlekauff HR, Stevenson WG, Stevenson LW, et al. Syncope in advanced heart failure: high risk of sudden death regardless of the origin of syncope. *J Am Coll Cardiol* 1993;21:110.
21. Morillo CA, Ellenbogen KA, Pava LF. Pathophysiologic basis for vasodepressor syncope. *Cardiol Clin* 1997;15(2):233.
22. Oh JH, Kapoor WN. Psychiatric illness and syncope. *Cardiol Clin* 1997;15(2):269.
23. Savage DD, Corwin L, McGee DL, et al. Epidemiologic features of isolated syncope: the Framingham study. *Stroke* 1985;16:626.

CHAPTER 142
Hypertension

Katerina T. Parmele and Alison J. McDonald

Although the acute complications of hypertension are less common today than in previous years, they must be recognized and treated promptly and effectively when they occur.[15,20] Elevations of blood pressure may be divided into hypertensive emergencies, in which the blood pressure must be lowered within hours, and asymptomatic hypertension, in which the blood pressure can be lowered over a period of days to weeks.

A true hypertensive emergency is a severe elevation in arterial blood pressure that represents a threat to life or vital organ function unless treatment is initiated immediately.[3,23] The diagnosis of hypertensive emergency should never be made solely on the basis of the blood pressure measurement; rather, the patient's response to the blood pressure and the immediate risk to the cardiovascular system are of primary importance.[9] Many patients with hypertension tolerate high blood pressure levels chronically without acute end-organ damage.[3,9] In more recent years, the terms *nonemergent hypertension* and *asymptomatic hypertension* have come into favor. Generally, a systolic blood pressure greater than 140 mm Hg and a diastolic blood pressure greater than 90 mm Hg for two or more readings are considered significant and help define asymptomatic hypertension.[1,18]

HYPERTENSIVE EMERGENCIES

EMERGENCY DEPARTMENT MANAGEMENT

The goal of therapy in hypertensive emergencies is to control the blood pressure to a level that will prevent end-organ damage. The exact level depends on the clinical situation. It is important not to lower the blood pressure too quickly or to levels that produce cerebral or myocardial ischemia, especially in patients with atherosclerosis.[3] If the patient has been hypertensive and poorly controlled for years, the cerebral autoregulation curve may be shifted to the right, and rapid reduction of blood pressure may not be well tolerated. A safe goal is to bring the diastolic blood pressure down to 100 to 110 mm Hg over a period of hours, with the higher level being more appropriate in atherosclerotic or elderly patients.[9,17] The patient should be closely monitored for symptoms of cerebral or coronary insufficiency.

True hypertensive emergencies require parenteral therapy, ideally in an intensive care setting where cardiac and blood pressure monitoring are available. Diuretics should be avoided unless necessary to treat fluid overload. Intravenous furosemide is a relatively ineffective antihypertensive when used alone; moreover, patients with malignant hypertension may be volume contracted and may deteriorate when given diuretics because of stimulation of the renin–angiotensin system and increased sodium retention. In addition, diuretics can cause hypotensive episodes, especially when given in the presence of vasodilating drugs.

The agents most commonly used in hypertensive emergencies are either direct vasodilators (e.g., nitroprusside, nitroglycerin, hydralazine) or inhibitors of the sympathetic or adrenergic system (e.g., labetalol, phentolamine, esmolol).[18] Table 142.1 provides a guide to pharmacologic management. The agent chosen depends on the clinical situation, the availability of immediate close monitoring, and the physician's familiarity and experience with the drugs available.

Nitroprusside is the drug of choice in many hypertensive emergencies, including malignant hypertension, hypertensive encephalopathy, and aortic dissection (combined with a beta blocker). Nitroprusside is a direct arteriovenous vasodilator that decreases both preload and afterload. Its onset of action is 1 to 2 minutes, and its effect lasts for only 2 to 5 minutes after the drug is discontinued. It is given as an intravenous drip, starting at a dosage of 0.2 to 0.5 μg/kg/min and increasing every 5 minutes to a maximum of 8 μg/kg/min, or until the desired effect is achieved. Nitroprusside should be given with close hemodynamic monitoring of the blood pressure and pulse to prevent inadvertent hypotension. There is no tachyphylaxis, but thiocyanate toxicity may occur if the drug is used over a period of days, particularly in patients with renal failure. It is contraindicated in pregnancy. Nitroprusside is light-sensitive, so bottles and tubing must be kept covered. Because there is no oral form, the patient must be switched to another antihypertensive once control is achieved.[3,15]

Nitroglycerin functions via stimulation of the cyclic GMP pathway and is a potent peripheral arterial and venous vasodilator. It has both afterload and preload reducing properties. As such, it is especially useful in pulmonary edema and states of high peripheral resistance. Nitrates are also thought to effect coronary artery vasodilatation, making them first-line agents in the treatment of hypertension with associated cardiac ischemia. Nitrates can be administered sublingually in bolus doses of 0.4 mg as tablets or sprays. Nitroglycerin drips start at 5 μg/min and are titrated upwards to effect. The usual dose ranges from 5 to 200 μg/min.[18]

Labetalol, a combined alpha and beta blocker, has been used in certain hypertensive emergencies as an alternative to nitroprusside. In certain instances, such as aortic dissection, it can be used in conjunction with nitroprusside; its beta-blocking effects reduce the abrupt rise in pressure during early systole, helping to decrease shear forces at the dissection site. Labetalol is also useful in acute cocaine-associated hypertension because its alpha-blocking effects prevent the unopposed alpha vasoconstriction that may occur when pure beta antagonists are given. Labetalol can be given either intravenously or orally and has the advantage of not causing reflex tachycardia.[8] The ratio of alpha- to beta-blocker activity is 1:7, but the antihypertensive effects of alpha blockade are felt first. The onset of action averages 30 minutes, and its duration is 3 to 4 hours. Labetalol can be given intravenously in 10- to 20-mg boluses every 5 to 10 minutes. An alternative is to infuse 2 mg/min to a total dose of 300 mg. Patients already taking other antihypertensive agents may require a smaller dose of labetalol to control the blood pressure. Advantages of labetalol include the absence of reflex tachycardia and the ease of converting to the same agent orally once blood pressure is controlled. Labetalol should not be used in patients with contraindications to beta blockade.

Esmolol is a beta-blocking agent with a very rapid onset and offset. It is used in similar situations as labetalol but can be more easily titrated, and can be used as a drip. The initial dose is a bolus of 500 μg/kg, and the drip is titrated between 50 and 200 μg/kg/min. As with labetalol, esmolol should not be used in patients with asthma, chronic obstructive pulmonary disease (COPD), or other contraindications to beta blockade.[18]

Hydralazine as an agent for immediate blood pressure control has found application principally in eclampsia, because it has been shown to be safe in pregnancy. Using a dose of 10 to 20 mg, the onset of action is 10 to 30 minutes when given intravenously; its duration of action is 3 to 8 hours.[3,14] The drug produces marked reflex tachycardia. The advantage of hydralazine over beta blockers is that it can be used in bradycardic patients without concern about further decreases in heart rate.

Phentolamine, an alpha-receptor blocker, is particularly useful in pheochromocytoma, monoamine oxidase (MAO) inhibitor reactions, and antihypertensive drug withdrawal states. The dose is 5 to 10 mg intravenously, and the effect lasts only 15 minutes, requiring repeated dosing. Once the patient is adequately alpha blocked, oral phenoxybenzamine can be begun. Beta blockers should be used only for tachycardia and dysrhythmias, and only after alpha blockade has been achieved.[15]

CLINICAL PRESENTATIONS

Malignant Hypertension

Malignant hypertension, the prototype of the hypertensive emergency, occurs in 2% of patients with essential hypertension. It is more common in young Black men and in patients with underlying renal parenchymal disease or renovascular disease. The diagnosis is usually a clinical one based on the marked ele-

TABLE 142-1. Pharmacologic Management of Hypertensive Emergencies

Drugs	Indications	Dose/Route	Pitfalls
Nitroprusside	All hypertensive emergencies except pregnancy	0.2–0.5 μg/kg/min up to 8 μg/kg/min i.v.	Avoid in pregnancy
Nitroglycerin	Myocardial infarction/ischemia, acute left ventricular failure	5–200 μg/min i.v.	Predominant use in CHF or MI
Esmolol	All hypertensive emergencies	500 μg bolus, 50–200 μg/kg/min	Avoid in asthma, COPD, heart block
Labetalol	All hypertensive emergencies	10–20 mg q 5 min I.v. or 2 mg/min i.v. drip	Avoid in asthma, COPD, heart block
Hydralazine	Eclampsia	5–20 mg i.v./i.m. q 6 h	Use with magnesium sulfate
Phentolamine	Pheochromocytoma, MAO inhibitor crisis	5–10 mg i.v.	Use alpha blocker before Beta blocker

CHF, congestive heart failure; MI, myocardial infarction; COPD, chronic obstructive pulmonary disease; MAO, monoamine oxidase.

vation of the blood pressure and characteristic eyeground changes, including papilledema, which most authors believe is a *sine qua non* of the diagnosis.

Pathologically, malignant hypertension is a physical vasculitis.[21] Flame-shaped hemorrhages occur around the optic disk due to the high intravascular pressure; "soft" exudates are due to ischemic infarction of the nerve fibers secondary to occlusion of supplying arterioles. However, eyeground changes of increased arteriolar light reflex, arteriovenous nicking, arteriolar tortuosity, and hard exudates are all chronic changes and cannot be used to establish the diagnosis of malignant hypertension.

Common symptoms of malignant hypertension are headache (85%), visual blurring (55%), nocturia (38%), weakness (30%), and weight loss (25%).[21] Laboratory evaluation reveals progressive azotemia, proteinuria, microscopic or gross hematuria, and cylindruria. Additional findings are microangiopathic hemolytic anemia, thrombocytopenia, and increased fibrin degradation products. Hypokalemia and metabolic alkalosis commonly result from stimulation of the renin–angiotensin system.[21]

If untreated, malignant hypertension carries a 90% 1-year mortality, usually from uremia, cerebrovascular accident (CVA), or congestive heart failure (CHF). With treatment, 1-year survival is increased to 85%.

Hypertensive Encephalopathy

Hypertensive encephalopathy is characterized by significant alteration in cerebral function that improves with lowering of the blood pressure.[21] It is believed to be due to a loss of normal cerebrovascular autoregulation that results in overperfusion and forced dilatation of the cerebral vessels and the development of multiple areas of cortical edema. Patients complain of headache, nausea, vomiting, confusion, and blurred vision.[15,21] On physical examination, there is a marked elevation of blood pressure (usually greater than 130 mm Hg diastolic), altered mental status, and, commonly, papilledema. Focal neurologic deficits are sometimes noted, as are seizures.[15]

The differential diagnosis is vast, but no other condition resolves with lowering of the blood pressure. Cerebral infarction usually has a more rapid onset (minutes to hours); the headache is typically mild, and neurologic deficits are fixed. Cerebral embolism has a sudden onset, and usually causes minimal or no headache or mental status change. With intracerebral or subarachnoid hemorrhage, neurologic deficit or alteration of consciousness is also of rapid onset; sudden severe headache is also characteristic, particularly with subarachnoid hemorrhage. To differentiate among these entities, a computed tomography (CT) scan of the head must be done immediately while other supportive measures are being initiated.

Lowering the blood pressure is the key to managing hypertensive encephalopathy, but if it is lowered too rapidly, hypoperfusion may result. A rough guideline is that the diastolic blood pressure should be lowered only 20% to 30% during the first 24 hours. The patient's mental status should be followed closely. Any medications that may change the neurologic examination are to be avoided. Drugs of choice include nitroprusside, labetalol, and esmolol.

Aortic Dissection

Aortic dissection usually presents with sudden, severe, tearing chest pain that radiates into the midscapular region of the back. CT scan of the chest with intravenous contrast, transesophageal echocardiography, or aortography can show the intimal flap. More than 90% of patients with aortic dissection are hypertensive by history, even if they are not hypertensive on presentation. Patients with known aortic dissection must have their blood pressure aggressively managed. Stabilization and control of the blood pressure is crucial, because propagation of the dissection depends on the instantaneous slope of the intraaortic pressure curve and the resulting stress on the aortic wall. The goal of therapy is to lower the blood pressure to 100 to 120 mm Hg systolic over a few hours in order to decrease this pressure head. This is accomplished with medications that decrease cardiac inotropy and chronotropy and decrease peripheral resistance. The typical emergency department (ED) regimen includes nitroprusside in conjunction with a beta blocker such as esmolol or labetalol.[15] Medications that cause reflex tachycardia, such as hydralazine, should be avoided. Surgery is the definitive treatment for proximal dissections, whereas distal dissections can often be managed medically.

Ischemic Heart Disease and Myocardial Infarction

In patients with severe coronary artery disease, hypertension may have an immediately deleterious effect by increasing resistance to left ventricular emptying, leading to increased ventricular wall tension and increased myocardial oxygen demand. Excessive blood pressure reduction should be avoided so as not to compromise coronary artery perfusion. The degree of blood pressure reduction should be based on the hemodynamic effect rather than on a predetermined blood pressure end point, and hemodynamic monitoring should be available to avoid excessive pressure lowering. To control ischemic pain, the usual antianginal drugs should be used first because they are often effective in treating the hypertension as well. Intravenous nitroglycerin is an excellent immediate agent. Beta blockers such as metoprolol, atenolol, or propranolol are indicated in the tachycardic patient, as decreasing the heart rate reduces myocardial oxygen demand and has been shown to decrease morbidity and mortality following myocardial infarction. As mentioned previously, hydralazine causes reflex tachycardia and should be avoided.

Acute Left Ventricular Failure

Untreated hypertension can lead to acute CHF. More commonly, however, acute pulmonary edema triggers a catecholamine release, which increases peripheral vascular resistance and further reduces forward flow. The initial therapy for pulmonary edema with hypertension is to treat the pulmonary edema in the usual manner; nitroglycerin is the drug of choice. Nitroprusside can be added in individuals who have low cardiac output in conjunction with high peripheral vascular resistance. Both drugs decrease peripheral vascular resistance and therefore help to increase cardiac output. Hydralazine should be avoided because of reflex stimulation of myocardial contractility and heart rate.

Hypertension with Cerebrovascular Accident

In managing patients with hypertension and CVA, the major concern is to avoid hypoperfusion of already ischemic tissue. For a chronically hypertensive patient, the mean arterial blood pressure necessary to maintain cerebral blood flow is higher than normal. If the blood pressure is brought below the lower limit of autoregulation, cerebral blood flow will fall, possibly leading to further neurologic damage.[9,15,19] Thus, cautious lowering of the blood pressure may be indicated, and the use of a short-acting, titratable agent such as nitroprusside or labetalol is advised.[6] A reasonable target is to lower the diastolic pressure to 100 to 110 mm Hg. A rapid rise in blood pressure can increase the intracranial pressure, while a rapid fall can cause brain tissue ischemia. Therefore, it is safer to aggressively control fluctuations in blood pressure and to aim for blood pressure stability rather than simply lowering the rapid blood pressure rapidly.

Some experts advocate not treating hypertension in patients with nonhemorrhagic CVAs.[9] This is based on a lack of data showing a benefit of acutely reducing blood pressure in these patients, as well as case reports of morbidity and mortality that have resulted from this practice.[2,17] In the case of patients with subarachnoid hemorrhage, treating with the calcium channel blocker nimodipine during the first 2 days may improve outcomes. This is thought to be a result of the antivasospastic effects and not specifically due to the antihypertensive effects of this medication.[11,12]

Catecholamine Excess

Hypertension due to catecholamine excess occurs in patients with pheochromocytoma, in patients taking MAO inhibitors who eat tyramine-containing foods or ingest sympathomimetic drugs, and in patients who are withdrawing from certain antihypertensive agents.

Pheochromocytoma is rare and typically presents with a history of paroxysms of headache, anxiety, diaphoresis, pallor, palpitations, nausea, and abdominal discomfort. The blood pressure can be markedly elevated (systolic greater than 300 mm Hg),[15] although only 50% of cases have sustained hypertension. In suspected cases, therapy should be started before a biochemical diagnosis is made. The drug of choice is intravenous phentolamine, an alpha-adrenergic blocker. Beta blockers should be used only after alpha blockade to avoid paradoxical hypertension; they are usually necessary only if tachyarrhythmias are present.[15]

In patients taking MAO inhibitors, severe hypertension can be precipitated by the ingestion of tyramine-containing foods and drinks (e.g., unpasteurized cheeses, certain beers, wines, pickled herring, chicken liver, broad beans, and certain milk products). Drugs such as ephedrine, phenylpropanolamine, and amphetamines can cause a similar elevation. The onset of symptoms is within 15 minutes to 2 hours of ingestion; the peak effect is normally in 2 to 4 hours, and symptoms usually abate by 6 hours. The drug of choice is phentolamine, which should be continued until hypertension and symptoms resolve.[15]

Rapid withdrawal from clonidine can cause a syndrome consisting of nausea, palpitations, anxiety, sweating, and headaches, similar to that seen with pheochromocytoma. These effects are thought to be due to enhanced sympathetic activity after discontinuing the drug.[15]

Hypertension in Pregnancy

Because blood pressure normally falls during pregnancy, the threshold for the diagnosis of hypertension in pregnancy is at a lower level than in the nonpregnant person. A pressure above 140/90 mm Hg or an increase of more than 30/15 mm Hg from baseline is abnormal. Intravenous magnesium sulfate is first-line therapy. It has smooth muscle relaxation properties and increases the seizure threshold. As such, it has mild antihypertensive effects as well as tocolytic and antiepileptic properties. If the diastolic pressure remains over 100 mm Hg despite adequate magnesium therapy, hydralazine can be used. Nitroprusside should be avoided because of possible resulting cyanide toxicity in the fetus,[3] and diuretics should be avoided because of their volume-depleting effect. The definitive treatment for medication-resistant preeclampsia and eclampsia is delivery of the fetus.

ASYMPTOMATIC HYPERTENSION

A common problem facing the emergency physician is the chronically hypertensive patient who presents to the ED for an unrelated reason and is found to have a significant but asymptomatic elevation of blood pressure. Not uncommonly, the patient has run out of medications, and usually has minimal or no complaints.[1,13,18] The physical examination may reveal signs of chronic hypertension but no evidence of acute end-organ damage in the cardiovascular, neurologic, and renal systems. On funduscopic examination, there may be evidence of retinopathy, but there are no acute changes of papilledema or flame hemorrhages.

If the blood pressure is significantly elevated (greater than 120 to 130 mm Hg diastolic), many clinicians prefer to initiate a treatment regimen for chronic blood pressure control in the ED and have the patient follow up in 2 to 3 days to continue management. The goal is often to begin the process of chronic blood pressure control, while avoiding a potentially dangerous precipitous drop. Oral medications are usually sufficient.

Controversy has arisen as to the need to treat asymptomatic hypertension acutely. There is no scientific basis for believing that immediately reducing an asymptomatic blood pressure elevation reduces complications. There is, on the other hand, a finite risk associated with rapid correction of asymptomatic hypertension. Several case reports document the occurrence of cerebral infarction, myocardial ischemia or infarction, or deterioration in renal function with rapid correction of the blood pressure in patients with asymptomatic hypertension.[2,10,22] The frequent use of sublingual nifedipine in the early 1990s, and the subsequent criticism of this practice because of such case reports, highlights this problem.[5,10,22] In addition, the current widespread use of sildenafil citrate (Viagra) has resulted in significant symptomatic hypotensive episodes and cases of hemodynamic collapse after antihypertensive therapy is instituted by practitioners who are unaware their patients are taking this drug.[4,16] Finally, there is no proof that initiation of maintenance therapy in the ED leads to sustained reductions in blood pressure or better long-term outcomes.[2]

EMERGENCY DEPARTMENT MANAGEMENT

Because asymptomatic hypertension does not represent a threat to life or vital organ function, it does not require the aggressive therapy appropriate for hypertensive emergencies. Before receiving any medications, the patient with elevated blood pressure should be placed in a quiet room for 30 to 60 minutes. The pressure should then be rechecked to ensure that hypertension is still present, because many people have labile blood pressures ("white coat hypertension") that respond readily to such nonpharmacologic interventions.[1,7] In addition, hypertensive patients tend to experience a spontaneous decline in their blood pressures because of "regression to the mean."[1,13] Nonpathologic causes of elevated blood pressure include stress, anxiety, pain, and drug withdrawal. If the blood pressure remains elevated and it is judged that long-term therapy will be necessary (e.g., in a patient with a well-defined history of hypertension who has run out of medications), it is reasonable to begin oral treatment with an agent that is judged to be appropriate as part of the patient's long-term blood pressure regimen.

The emergency physician can choose from several oral antihypertensive agents in this situation. (Table 142.2.) The choice of medication should be tailored to the patient's medical history. Generally, diuretics and beta blockers are considered the primary initial agents. Beta blockers have been shown to reduce morbidity and mortality in patients with coronary artery dis-

TABLE 142-2. Antihypertensive Agents for Asymptomatic Patients

Drug Class	Appropriate Patient Groups	Avoid In
Diuretics (thiazides, loop diuretics)	CHF Elderly Blacks	Gout (thiazide: hyperuricemia)
Calcium channel blockers	Coronary heart disease Atrial fibrillation	Heart block Patients already on beta-blockers
Beta blockers	Coronary artery disease Atrial fibrillation Migraines	CHF COPD/asthma Severe depression IDDM Heart block
Alpha and beta blockers	Same as for beta blockers	Same as for beta blockers
ACE-inhibitors	CHF Coronary artery disease Renal insufficiency Blacks	Bilateral renal artery stenosis[a] Hyperkalemia
Central alpha-blockers (clonidine)	Clonidine withdrawal Drug-resistant patients with ESRD	Non-compliant patients Not a first-line agent

[a]contraindicated

ease. They may also help in patients with migraines. They should be avoided in patients with asthma or COPD, depression, and, possibly, insulin-requiring diabetes mellitus because of the risk of blunting the hypoglycemic catecholamine response. Diuretics such as thiazides are useful in that they offer blood pressure reduction with little change in heart rate. They should be used in CHF. Blacks tend to be more responsive to diuretics and angiotensin converting enzyme (ACE) inhibitors than beta blockers or calcium channel blockers. ACE inhibitors have beneficial effects in patients with CHF and mild-to-moderate renal insufficiency. They are contraindicated in the rare patient with bilateral renal artery stenosis. Certain patients cannot tolerate the side effect of cough, and ACE inhibitor–associated angioedema is well documented. Calcium channel blockers are effective in patients with atrial fibrillation to help control ventricular response, and they also have antianginal properties. They should be used with caution in patients already on AV nodal blocking agents such as beta blockers. The centrally acting alpha antagonist clonidine should not be a first-line agent in the ED for asymptomatic hypertension. It is a potent antihypertensive than can cause significant hypertension in withdrawal states in poorly compliant patients. It is indicated in clonidine withdrawal syndromes.

Patients with asymptomatic hypertension do not require any acute therapy in the ED. In patients who have documented elevated blood pressures on more than one visit, the ED physician may choose to begin an antihypertensive regimen and refer them to their primary physicians. Effective long-term treatment of hypertension requires intensive patient education, the prescription of an appropriate medical regimen, compliance with that regimen, and reliable follow-up. Acutely lowering the blood pressure of chronically hypertensive patients does little to change their morbidity and mortality and, in fact, may cause cardiovascular morbidity. A more gradual lowering of the blood pressure allows the resetting of the cerebral autoregulation curve.[9]

DISPOSITION

All hypertensive emergencies require admission to an intensive care setting or a monitored bed. Close blood pressure monitoring, preferably with an arterial line, is indicated. Patients with hypertensive encephalopathy or a CVA may require neurologic consultation if the diagnosis is in question. Aortic dissection requires immediate cardiothoracic surgical evaluation while blood pressure is acutely controlled. Eclamptic patients require emergent obstetric consultation.

Patients with asymptomatic hypertension do not require hospital admission. Blood pressure control can be initiated, and close medical follow-up is required.

COMMON PITFALLS

- Diagnosing a hypertensive emergency when one does not exist. Many patients who present to the ED have blood pressure elevations related to stress, anxiety, drug withdrawal, or pain, or have chronic asymptomatic hypertension. Patients with hypertensive emergencies have evidence of acute end-organ dysfunction.
- When treating a hypertensive emergency, reducing the blood pressure too quickly or to too low a level. In patients with chronic hypertension whose autoregulation curve has been reset, this can lead to cerebral or cardiac ischemia.
- In patients with CHF and hypertension, failing to treat fluid overload first.
- Failing to diagnose hypertension in pregnant patients with blood pressures above 140/90 mm Hg, or with an increase in blood pressure of more than 30/15 mm Hg. These patients should be referred urgently for obstetric care.
- Attempting to decrease the blood pressure to a certain absolute number in every patient, or attempting to normalize the blood pressure completely in the ED. This often leads to many episodes of hypotension and the sequelae of hypoperfusion.

References

1. Chiang WK, Jamshahi B. Asymptomatic hypertension in the ED. *Am J Emerg Med* 1998;16:701.
2. Fagan TC. Acute reduction of blood pressure in asymptomatic patients with severe hypertension: an idea whose time has come and gone. *Arch Intern Med* 1989;149:2169.
3. Ferguson RK, Vlasses PH. Hypertensive emergencies and urgencies. *JAMA* 1986;255:1607.
4. Goldenberg MM. Safety and efficacy of sildenafil citrate in the treatment of male erectile dysfunction. *Clin Ther* 1998;20:1033.
5. Grossman E, et al. Should a moratorium be placed on sublingual nifedipine capsules given for hypertensive emergencies and pseudoemergencies? *JAMA* 1996;276:1328.

6. Lavin P. Management of hypertension in patients with acute stroke. *Arch Intern Med* 1986;146:66.
7. Lebby T, Paloucek F, Cruz FD, et al. Blood pressure decrease prior to initiating pharmacological therapy in nonemergent hypertension. *Am J Emerg Med* 1990;8:27.
8. Llebel M, Langlois S, Belleau LJ, et al. Labetalol infusion in hypertensive emergencies. *Clin Pharmacol Ther* 1985;37:615.
9. Murphy C. Hypertensive emergencies. *Emerg Med Clin North Am* 1995;13:973.
10. O'Mailia J, Sander G, Giles T. Nifedipine-associated myocardial ischemia or infarction in the treatment of hypertensive urgencies. *Ann Intern Med* 1987;107:85.
11. Petruk KC, et al. Nimodipine treatment in poor-grade aneurysm patients. *J Neurosurg* 1988;68:505.
12. Pickard JD, et al. Effect of oral nimodipine on cerebral infarction and outcome after subarachnoid haemorrhage: British aneurysm nimodipine trial. *BMJ* 1989;298:636.
13. Pitts SR, Adams RP. Emergency department hypertension and regression to the mean. *Ann Emerg Med* 1998;31:214.
14. Ram CVS. Management of hypertensive emergencies—changing therapeutic options. *Am Heart J* 1991;122:356.
15. Ram CVS. Immediate management of severe hypertension. *Cardiol Clin* 1995;13:579.
16. Reed DB, et al. Prehospital consideration of sildenafil-nitrate interactions. *Prehosp Emerg Care* 1999;3:306.
17. Reed WG, Anderson RJ. Effects of rapid blood pressure reduction on cerebral blood flow. *Am Heart J* 1986;111:226.
18. Thach AM, Schultz PJ. Nonemergent hypertension. *Emerg Med Clin North Am* 1995;13:1009.
19. Tietjen CS, et al. Treatment modalities for hypertensive patients with intracranial pathology: options and risks. *Crit Care Med* 1996;24:311.
20. Varon J, Fromm RE Jr. Hypertensive crises. *Postgrad Med* 1996;99:189.
21. Vaziri ND. Malignant or accelerated hypertension. *West J Med* 1984;140:575.
22. Wachter R. Symptomatic hypotension induced by nifedipine in the acute treatment of severe hypertension. *Arch Intern Med* 1987;147:556.
23. Zampaglione B, et al. Hypertensive urgencies and emergencies. *Hypertension* 1996;27:144.

PART II

Pulmonary Disease

CHAPTER 143

Adult Respiratory Distress Syndrome

Darryl J. Macias and Joe Alcock

Adult respiratory distress syndrome (ARDS; noncardiogenic pulmonary edema) results from the nonspecific response of the lung to various noxious insults. The clinical presentation depends on the underlying cause. The most common antecedent is sepsis, but ARDS must be considered in any patient with acute respiratory failure who has sustained any of a number of local or systemic insults associated with development of the condition (Table 143.1).

ARDS is a form of pulmonary edema, but, unlike cardiogenic pulmonary edema, is not caused primarily by increased pulmonary capillary hydrostatic pressure. Rather, ARDS results from a disequilibrium among all the factors that affect total lung water, including pulmonary arterial tone, osmotic pressure, alveolar epithelial permeability, surfactant integrity, and the efficiency and rate of lymphatic drainage.[9] This disequilibrium is due to the influence of toxic agents from exogenous sources (such as inhaled gases), bacterial toxins, endogenous mediators, or any of these combined. These agents or mediators are responsible for increased pulmonary microvascular permeability, major disruption in alveolar epithelial integrity, and interstitial edema. Air spaces become filled with edema fluid, causing loss of surfactant and microatelectasis. Airway closure, decreased alveolar ventilation, shunting of blood flow, and hypoxia follow.

Studies indicate that the mortality rate for ARDS ranges from 40% to 60%.[10] Only 15% of patients die of respiratory failure; most die of multisystem organ failure.[13]

CLINICAL PRESENTATION

The ARDS patient may already be acutely ill, with respiratory failure a prominent component of the clinical condition, or may be a previously healthy person with rapidly progressive respiratory failure. Clinical criteria for the diagnosis of ARDS include a ratio of the partial pressure of arterial oxygen (PaO_2) to the fraction of inspired oxygen (F_IO_2) of less than 200, regardless of the amount of positive end-expiratory pressure (PEEP) used; new diffuse bilateral infiltrates (all lung fields involved) on chest x-ray; a pulmonary arterial wedge pressure below 18 mm Hg; and the absence of other entities that might be responsible for these findings (i.e., no evidence of congestive heart failure, pleural effusion, atelectasis, or bacterial pneumonia).[2] A decrease in static lung compliance is also noted.

Initially, patients complain of shortness of breath and exhibit mild tachypnea. Scattered rales may be heard, and arterial blood gas values reflect an increased alveolar–arterial oxygen gradient. As the course progresses, the patient becomes more tachypneic, dyspneic, and cyanotic, and diffuse rales are noted on auscultation. Serial arterial blood gas values usually reveal progressive hypoxemia refractory to increasing levels of inspired oxygen.

Table 143.1 lists conditions that predispose to or have been associated with the development of ARDS. Clinical symptoms usually become evident with 2 to 24 hours of the inciting event.

Sepsis

Sepsis and the systemic inflammatory response syndrome SIRS, especially with gram-negative organisms, is the most common—and the most commonly fatal—cause of ARDS. Although there is a 20% incidence of clinically evident lung injury after sepsis, it is unknown why sepsis results in ARDS in some patients and not in others, or why some patients with ARDS recover and others do not. ARDS is thought to result from toxic effects of neutrophil-based inflammatory mediators in the lung. Sustained hypotension and thrombocytopenia place a septic patient at greater risk for lung injury. Most often, in the septic patient with ARDS, death does not result from respiratory failure but from the underlying illness.

Trauma

The association of trauma and pulmonary dysfunction has long been recognized, although the exact mechanisms involved are not well understood. ARDS has been noted in 5% to 10% of patients with multiple fractures and in 5% to 34% of patients receiving multiple transfusions.[12] Hemorrhagic shock alone probably does not result in ARDS, and massive blood transfusions, especially when given through micropore filters, do not necessarily result in pulmonary dysfunction.[5] Still, a clear relation between the injury severity score and the likelihood of developing ARDS has been consistently noted.[4] Respiratory dysfunction after trauma is probably the consequence of a variety of insults, including direct pulmonary trauma, embolism, and associated soft-tissue injury.[3]

Aspiration

Aspiration of liquids can disrupt surfactant (freshwater and petroleum distillates), produce an osmotic gradient favoring

TABLE 143.1. Agents and Conditions Predisposing to the Development of ARDS

INFECTIOUS
Sepsis
Pneumonia (bacterial, viral, fungal)
TRAUMA
Lung confusion
Fat embolism/long-bone fractures
Shock
Head injury
Crush injury
Burns
ASPIRATION
Gastric contents
Near-drowning
Petroleum distillates/organic solvents
Turpentine
INHALATIONAL INJURY
Smoke
Corrosives (phosgene, sulfur dioxide, ammonia, chlorine, nitrogen dioxide)
Oxygen
Paraquat
DRUG ASSOCIATED
Aspirin
Opiates
Ethchlorvynol
Nitrofurantoin
Colchicine
Hydrochlorothiazide
Tricyclic antidepressants
Iron
ENVIRONMENTAL
High altitude
Hypothermia
Radiation pneumonitis
Snake venom
CIRCULATING AGENTS
Hematologic (TTP, DIC)
Tumor lysis
Emboli (pulmonary, fat, air)
Pancreatitis
Massive blood transfusion
Hemodialysis
Cardiopulmonary bypass
Obstetric
Eclampsia
Postpartum endometritis
Amniotic fluid embolism
Miscellaneous
Neurogenic
Reexpansion after pneumothorax
Radiation pneumonitis
Intravenous freebase cocaine
Gastrografin
Uremia
Seizure

TTP, thrombotic thrombocytopenic purpura; DIC, disseminated intravascular coagulation.

fluid movement into the lungs (saltwater), or cause an inflammatory response in the alveoli (water, saline solution, gastric contents). The inflammatory response to acidic gastric contents is particularly rapid and severe. Patients who are unconscious or chronically debilitated or who have neurologic lesions are those most likely to aspirate gastric contents.

The diagnosis of aspiration rests on the clinical history of drowning or ingestion, or on the sudden onset of choking, coughing, or shortness of breath while eating or during emesis. An overt history of the aspiration event may not be obtained. Clinically, the patient may appear well or may be coughing, choking, or wheezing. Respiratory dysfunction usually becomes symptomatic within the first hour, but may take up to 24 hours to develop. The degree of hypoxemia is quite variable initially and should be assessed by arterial blood gas analysis. Respiratory function may improve spontaneously or may rapidly deteriorate as inflammation and pulmonary edema develop.

Inhalation Injury

Inhalation injuries can produce pulmonary dysfunction by thermal damage and by direct chemical irritation or destruction of lung tissue. Steam can reach the parenchyma of the lung and cause direct thermal injury. Some gases (e.g., nitrogen dioxide, ammonia, chloramine, sulfur dioxide, hydrochloric acid fumes) liberated from the combustion of building materials and fabrics are direct pulmonary irritants. Pulmonary edema may occur immediately or days later.

Phosgene has been used by the military and by industry. Exposure results in irritation of the mucous membranes, chest pain, nausea, and vomiting, but these initial symptoms do not correlate with the potentially fatal pulmonary edema that may develop hours to days later.[3] Ammonia, nitrous oxides, and chlorine are also used in manufacturing and can cause severe pulmonary edema.

Drugs

Various drugs cause pneumonitis and pulmonary hypersensitivity reactions that result in ARDS. These include methotrexate, cytarabine, mitomycin, protamine, hydrochlorothiazide, nitrofurantoin, lidocaine, haloperidol, chlordiazepoxide, terbutaline, and amphotericin B.[6,8] Opiates, aspirin, colchicine, iron, and ethchlorvynol cause pulmonary injury only after overdose.[6] Symptoms occur within minutes to hours and can result from any route of exposure.[8] The prognosis in drug-induced pulmonary edema is better than for many other causes of ARDS, presumably because the presence of the offending agent is temporary.

Neurogenic Causes

Neurogenic pulmonary edema has long been recognized as a cause of death in the head-injured patient. With all head injuries, there is an increase in extravascular lung water. Pulmonary edema has been noted to result from head trauma, intracranial infection, acute hydrocephalus, subarachnoid hemorrhage, brain tumor, cerebrovascular accident, and seizures, and has also been noted after hanging.[6] Neurogenic pulmonary edema may be mediated by way of alpha-adrenergic pathways, and can develop acutely within minutes to hours after a central nervous system insult, or in a delayed manner over 12 hours to several days.[6]

High-Altitude Pulmonary Edema

Rapid ascent without acclimatization results in the development of high-altitude pulmonary edema (HAPE) in about 5% to 10% of persons. It is currently believed that exaggerated pulmonary vasoconstriction, coupled with pulmonary capillary membrane leaks, is responsible for the development of HAPE.[1] Symptoms occur 1 to 4 days after ascent to altitudes above 8,000 ft. The onset is often insidious and commonly occurs at night. The patient complains of dyspnea, a dry cough, weakness, fatigue, headache, nausea, and vomiting. As pulmonary edema progresses, the patient may produce frothy or blood-tinged sputum. Symptoms are worsened by exercise, which increases pulmonary vascular resistance.

Supplemental oxygen is the most rapid treatment for HAPE, but descent is the definitive treatment; nifedipine has been used if descent is delayed.[1] The prognosis is good if the patient is brought down from altitude, and pulmonary dysfunction may resolve without requiring aggressive intervention.

DIFFERENTIAL DIAGNOSIS

Because the signs and symptoms of respiratory distress may initially be quite subtle, the clinician must have a high index of suspicion to identify respiratory compromise before it develops into frank pulmonary edema. A detailed history may prompt the physician to consider the possibility of ARDS, as well as the more common entities in the differential diagnosis of respiratory failure, such as pneumonia and cardiogenic pulmonary edema.

The diagnosis is relatively easy when a clear history of an insult to the lung, such as near-drowning or exposure to high altitude, is known. Other patients may present a greater problem. In the septic patient, one must determine whether tachycardia and tachypnea are due to hypoxia secondary to bacterial pneumonia, or secondary to early ARDS. Patients with ARDS do not normally have purulent sputum or a localized infiltrate on chest radiography. Diagnosis is also difficult in the hypoxic patient with diffuse pulmonary infiltrates, when cardiogenic pulmonary edema must be differentiated from ARDS. The ARDS patient usually does not have a history of cardiac disease, orthopnea, paroxysmal nocturnal dyspnea, nocturia, or chest pain, nor will signs of heart failure such as pedal edema, jugular venous distention, hepatojugular reflex, or S_3 gallop be present on examination.

In the trauma patient, pulmonary contusion is usually symptomatic within minutes of injury. It is often apparent on the initial chest radiograph and is commonly confined to one area of the lung fields. It should begin to clear by 48 hours. ARDS, in contrast, develops 24 to 72 hours after trauma and involves the lungs diffusely.

The chest radiograph is an extremely valuable tool for differentiating ARDS from other entities. Full progression to diffuse, bilateral alveolar infiltrates can take place within 4 to 24 hours after the first abnormal radiographic signs appear.[10] In contrast to the patient with pulmonary contusion, aspiration, or bacterial pneumonia, the ARDS patient has more diffuse infiltrates on chest radiograph. Radiographic evidence of enlargement of the right-sided heart chambers and pulmonary artery often appears early in ARDS, and is presumably related to the increased pulmonary vascular resistance that is a common feature of the syndrome. The heart may be of normal size, however. Enlargement of only the left-sided heart chambers, as is often seen in cardiogenic pulmonary edema, is not noted in ARDS. Hilar blurring, an early sign of cardiogenic pulmonary edema, occurs only late in ARDS. A peripheral distribution of edema is specific for ARDS and is more common early in its course. Other signs of interstitial fluid accumulation, such as peribronchial and perivascular cuffing and septal lines, which are common in cardiac failure, are uncommon in patients with ARDS, as is pleural effusion. Rarely, differentiating cardiogenic pulmonary edema from ARDS requires pulmonary artery catheterization.

The radiographic appearance of ARDS has been correlated with its clinical severity: Peripheral or extensive white density of the lung field on chest radiograph indicates severe lung involvement.

Computed tomography (CT) in ARDS often reveals more patchy areas of infiltrate interspersed with normal lung. The degree of lung involvement on CT correlates with gas exchange efficiency and compliance of the lung. It can reveal barotrauma and localized empyemas or abscesses not evident on plain films.[10]

EMERGENCY DEPARTMENT EVALUATION

Emergency department evaluation has two goals. The first is to establish the presence of respiratory distress and determine its magnitude. If possible, the patient must be questioned about the severity of respiratory distress, the nature of its onset, the duration of symptoms, the presence of sputum, and any medical history. On physical examination, attention is directed to the vital signs and cardiopulmonary system. The chest radiograph and arterial blood gas analysis add important information.

The second priority is to establish a specific cause. The clinician must be aware of the wide range of predisposing conditions and events. Although investigation directed toward establishing a specific cause for ARDS may be initiated in the emergency department, it is usually accomplished after the patient has been admitted.

Pertinent laboratory tests include a complete blood count with white cell differential and a coagulation profile. Serum chemistries and a blood lactate level may be helpful as well. A urinalysis, chest radiograph, and electrocardiogram are obtained. Blood gases may guide treatment. Measurement of cytokines in a bronchoalveolar lavage specimen predicts ARDS with good specificity,[7] but it is impractical in the emergency department.

EMERGENCY DEPARTMENT MANAGEMENT

Close observation of the patient's respiratory status is the essential component. Because the hallmark of this syndrome is hypoxemia that is increasingly refractory to increased concentrations of inspired oxygen, supplemental oxygen is mandatory. However, the progressive derangement of respiratory function limits the value of increasing percentages of inspired oxygen (F_IO_2). As extravascular lung water accumulates, lung compliance decreases and the work of breathing increases. With progressive atelectasis, pulmonary arterial blood is shunted through nonventilated alveoli. Because of the danger of oxygen toxicity and of absorption atelectasis, the F_IO_2 should be limited to 0.5 if possible. Intubation and mechanical ventilation are indicated when signs of clinical respiratory fatigue supervene. Other indicators are a ratio of PaO_2 to an F_IO_2 of less than 200, or a $PaCO_2$ above 50 mm Hg and a pH below 7.3. An arterial line may be placed to facilitate monitoring of arterial oxygen tension.

The use of PEEP may initially decrease the oxygen requirement in ARDS, but it has not improved the mortality rate, even if used prophylactically.[10] Although PEEP increases functional residual capacity, allowing alveoli to remain open and to participate in gas exchange, it may also depress cardiac output, overdistend alveoli, and cause pulmonary barotrauma. The optimum level of PEEP is usually between 0 and 15 cm H_2O, but, in each patient, it may need to be defined by hemodynamic indices obtained during intensive care monitoring.[13] Adding PEEP in small increments (2 to 3 cm H_2O) allows careful titration. The use of PEEP in neurogenic pulmonary edema is limited by its deleterious effect on intracranial pressure.[6]

Other oxygenation strategies currently being used or studied include pressure control ventilation,[11] inverse-ratio ventilation, high-frequency jet ventilation, permissive hypercapnia (allowing gradual increases in $PaCO_2$ in order to improve oxygenation),[10] extracorporeal membrane oxygenation,[4] and lateral decubitus or prone positioning of ARDS patients.[10]

Steroids are not recommended in the treatment of ARDS. Several clinical trials have demonstrated that steroids are of no benefit in reversing respiratory failure or improving survival in ARDS; in fact, steroid-treated groups had a greater incidence of subsequent infections.[3,10] Other agents, such as nonsteroidal antiinflammatory drugs and antiendotoxin antibodies, have not been shown to be of benefit.[10,13] Ibuprofen is of some overall benefit in the sepsis syndrome but does not improve oxygenation.[9,10,13] Surfactant replacement therapy is not currently recommended.[10] The use of vasodilators or vasoconstrictors should be limited to patients with hemodynamic instability.[10] Pentoxifylline ketoconazole, inhaled nitric oxide, and cytokine inhibitors are being studied and may show promise.[9,10,13]

DISPOSITION

The diagnosis of ARDS should be entertained, if only briefly, in all patients with a condition known to be associated with ARDS. Asymptomatic patients (e.g., those with a narcotic overdose, HAPE, mild near-drowning, or possible aspiration) may be observed for 6 to 12 hours in the emergency department; if they are asymptomatic after this period, they may be discharged, with follow-up scheduled for the next day. Patients with other indications for admission (e.g., head trauma) must have their respiratory status followed closely while in the hospital.

All symptomatic patients must be admitted, because they are at greatest risk for rapid deterioration. Most require intensive care, and an intensivist should be involved early in their care.

If transfer to another facility is necessary to provide the required level of care, transport should be expeditious and the transferring personnel must be skilled in advanced life-support techniques, including airway management. Associated illnesses make the transfer of a patient with possible or proven ARDS even more hazardous.

COMMON PITFALLS

- Failing to associate certain conditions with the potential for the development of ARDS
- Failing to appreciate these risks in emergency department patients may lead to their premature or inappropriate discharge, or may lead the physician to disregard early signs of pulmonary dysfunction.
- Failing to recognize the degree of respiratory insufficiency in the frankly symptomatic patient exposes the patient to the risks of prolonged unsuspected hypoxemia and delays the institution of mechanical ventilation, if necessary.
- Failing to appreciate the potential for rapid progression
- Failing to pick up subtle early cases
- Failing to intubate early enough

References

1. Bartsch P. High altitude pulmonary edema. *Med Sci Sports Exerc* 1999;31:523.
2. Bernard GR, Artigas A, Brigham KL, et al. The American-European Consensus Conference on ARDS: definitions, mechanisms, relevant outcomes, and clinical trial coordination. *Am J Respir Crit Care Med* 1994;149:818.
3. Bernard GR, Luce JM, Sprung CL, et al. High-dose corticosteroids in patients with ARDS. *N Engl J Med* 1987;317:1565.
4. Bone RC. The ARDS lung: new insights from computed tomography. *JAMA* 1993;269–216.
5. Carrico CJ, Mileski WJ, Kaplan HS. Transfusion, autotransfusion, and blood substitutes. In: Feliciano DV, Moore EE, Mattox KL, eds. *Trauma,* 3rd ed. Stanford, CT: Appleton & Lange, 1996.
6. Colice GL. Neurogenic pulmonary edema. *Clin Chest Med* 1985;6:315.
7. Connelly KG, Repine JE. Markers for predicting the development of acute respiratory distress syndrome. *Annu Rev Med* 1997;48:429.
8. Cooper JA, Matthay RA. Drug-induced pulmonary diseases. *Dis Mon* 1987;33:61.
9. Gommers D, Van Daal GJ, Lachmann B. Oxygen uptake in the lungs under pathological conditions and its therapeutic efforts. In: Erdmann W, Bruley DF, eds. *Oxygen transport to tissue.* New York: Plenum Publishing, 1992:47.
10. Kollef MH, Schuster DP. The acute respiratory distress syndrome. *N Engl J Med* 1995;332:27.
11. Marik PE, Krikorian J. Pressure-controlled ventilation in ARDS: a practical approach. *Chest* 1997;112:1102.
12. Maunder RJ. Clinical prediction of ARDS. *Clin Chest Med* 1985;6:413.
13. Rinaldo JE. ARDS. In: Rippe JM, Irwin RS, Alpert JS, et al., eds. *Intensive care medicine,* 2nd ed. Boston: Little, Brown and Company, 1991.

CHAPTER 144
Pneumonia

Gregory J. Moran and David A. Talan

In the United States, more than 3 million persons contract community-acquired pneumonia annually, resulting in about 500,000 hospital admissions. Pneumonia is the sixth leading cause of death in the United States, and the most common infectious cause. Most deaths occur in the elderly or immunosuppressed, but pneumonia occurs in otherwise healthy persons as well. To manage patients with pneumonia successfully, the emergency physician must be knowledgeable about a number of constantly changing factors, including an expanding spectrum of pathogens, changing antibiotic-resistance patterns, and the availability of newer antimicrobial agents. Although several noninfectious diseases may cause pneumonia, this discussion focuses on infectious etiologies, because they are by far the most common in emergency medicine practice.

Traditional pathogens such as *Streptococcus pneumoniae, Haemophilus influenzae, Mycoplasma pneumoniae,* and viruses continue to be important causes of community-acquired pneumonia. Less common etiologies include *Staphylococcus aureus,* gram-negative bacilli, and oral anaerobes. Organisms such as *Legionella* species and *Chlamydia pneumoniae* are being increasingly recognized as pathogens in a significant number of cases of community-acquired pneumonia. *Pneumocystis carinii* and *Mycobacterium tuberculosis* are important as pathogens related to pulmonary infections in acquired immunodeficiency disease (AIDS) patients. Knowledge of local prevalence patterns for pathogens of community-acquired pneumonia is important to make appropriate choices regarding evaluation and treatment.

CLINICAL PRESENTATION

"Typical" and "Atypical" Pneumonias

Pneumonia is often divided into "typical" (pyogenic bacterial) and "atypical" categories, but this division is somewhat artificial. Prediction of these etiologies based on clinical and radiographic findings is inaccurate.[7] The classic presentation of typical pyogenic bacterial pneumonia is the abrupt onset of fever and chills, followed by development of cough that is productive of purulent sputum and pleuritic chest pain. Elderly or debilitated patients may present with nonspecific complaints, such as altered mental status. Tachypnea and tachycardia are usually present. Examination of the chest may reveal signs of consolidation, such as dullness to percussion, coarse rales, bronchial breath sounds, or increased tactile fremitus.

The atypical pneumonia syndrome is caused by organisms such as *M. pneumoniae, C. pneumoniae,* viruses, *Legionella,* or rickettsial organisms such as *Coxiella burnetii.* Patients with this type of pneumonia generally present with a subacute onset of systemic complaints, such as fever, headache, malaise, and myalgias, associated with cough that is often nonproductive. Although mucopurulent sputum generally indicates the presence of pyogenic bacterial pneumonia or bronchitis, it may also be present with mycoplasmal or viral pneumonia. Chest examination often reveals scattered rhonchi or rales. Signs of consolidation are less common.

The high degree of overlap between the clinical and radiographic features of typical pyogenic and atypical pneumonia makes it impossible to definitively identify a specific type of pneumonia without the results of microbiologic or serologic tests. Typical and atypical pathogens sometimes coexist in the same patient, and bacterial infections often follow viral respiratory infections. Although one may not be able to determine with certainty the specific etiology of pneumonia within the time frame of an emergency department evaluation, certain clinical factors may suggest a likely etiology and can help guide empiric therapy. The clinical characteristics of several types of pneumonia are noted next.

Common Etiologies

S. pneumoniae is the single most common etiologic agent in community-acquired pneumonia. About 40% of healthy adults carry this organism in the nasopharynx. Patients with a history of diabetes, cardiovascular disease, alcoholism, or malignancy, or with other immunosuppressing illness, are at increased risk of pneumococcal infection. The classic presentation of pneumococcal pneumonia is the abrupt onset of a single shaking chill, followed by fever, cough productive of rust-colored sputum, and pleuritic chest pain. Not all patients exhibit this pattern. Many have had a preceding upper respiratory illness, and the onset of pneumonia may be insidious, especially among the elderly or those with underlying lung disease. Patients with a history of asplenia, sickle cell disease, AIDS, multiple myeloma, or agammaglobulinemia are at increased risk of pneumococcal bacteremia and sepsis. Extrapulmonary complications such as meningitis, endocarditis, or arthritis occasionally develop.

H. influenzae is a common pathogen in adults with chronic obstructive pulmonary disease (COPD), alcoholism, malnutrition, malignancy, or diabetes. The organism is a pleomorphic gram-negative rod that can be encapsulated; among serotypes a through f, type b most commonly leads to serious illness with bacteremia. In several studies, *H. influenzae* has been found to be the second most frequently isolated organism in community-acquired pneumonia among adults. Nontypeable strains (once thought to be benign) are a frequent cause of lower respiratory tract infection in patients with chronic lung disease. Such patients typically present with an insidious worsening of baseline cough and sputum production, and bacteremia is rare. *Moraxella catarrhalis* is another gram-negative rod that can be found in patients with COPD, but it appears to be associated with exacerbations of chronic bronchitis much more frequently than it is associated with pneumonia.

Intravenous (i.v.) drug users may develop hematogenous spread of *S. aureus* that involves both lungs and presents as multiple small infiltrates. This type of pneumonia is often associated with tricuspid valve staphylococcal endocarditis. *S. aureus* may also cause a primary bacterial pneumonia that may be clinically indistinguishable from other bacterial pneumonias. Staphylococcal pneumonias are often necrotizing, with cavitation and pneumatocele formation. An increased incidence of staphylococcal pneumonia has been noted during epidemics of influenza.

Klebsiella pneumoniae rarely causes disease in the normal host and accounts for a very small percentage of community-acquired pneumonias, but it may cause severe pneumonia in debilitated patients with alcoholism, diabetes, or other chronic illness. Sputum is often described as resembling currant jelly because of the necrotizing, hemorrhagic nature of the infection. Abscess formation, empyema, and bacteremia are common, and mortality is high. A chest radiograph characteristically demonstrates a dense lobar infiltrate with a bulging appearance of the fissure, but this finding is nonspecific and most cases present as a more subtle bronchopneumonia. Because the organism is often hospital-acquired, there is a high incidence of antibiotic resistance. *Pseudomonas aeruginosa* is also uncommon as an etiology of community-acquired pneumonia, but it may be present in patients with underlying lung disease, such as bronchiectasis or cystic fibrosis, or in patients who have recently been in a hospital or nursing home.

Seroprevalence studies demonstrate that virtually everyone is infected with *C. pneumoniae* at some time, and that reinfection is common. Most infections in young adults cause a minor, self-limited upper respiratory illness that is subacute in onset. This organism has also been associated with bronchitis, wheezing, sinusitis, pharyngitis, and atherosclerosis. Development of radiographically evident pneumonia is more common in the elderly, in contrast to the common perception that atypical pneumonias occur in the young.[9] *C. pneumoniae* is a relatively common etiology of community-acquired pneumonia, accounting for at least 8% of cases; however, this is probably an underestimate, due to the difficulty in diagnosing infection with this organism.

M. pneumoniae is regarded as one of the most common causes of community-acquired pneumonia in previously healthy patients less than 40 years of age. Although most studies have found it to be uncommon among hospitalized pneumonia patients, one study found it to be a common etiology among hospitalized older adults.[11] Infection usually begins as a flulike illness with headache, malaise, and fever. Cough is usually nonproductive, but may sometimes produce clear or even purulent sputum. Skin lesions, including maculopapular, vesicular, urticarial, or erythema multiforme-type rashes, are not uncommon, especially in younger patients. Many patients complain of sore throat or ear pain, but the classic finding of bullous myringitis is less common and is also nonspecific. Common physical findings include pharyngeal erythema, cervical adenopathy, and scattered rales and rhonchi. Rare extrapulmonary manifestations include pericarditis, glomerulonephritis, aseptic meningitis, and Guillain-Barré syndrome. Patients generally do not appear toxic, and the vast majority can be treated as outpatients.

At least 30 species of *Legionella* have been isolated since the 1976 outbreak in Philadelphia from which the organism derives its name. Up to 20% of community-acquired pneumonia cases may be due to this organism.[2] *Legionella* is an intracellular organism that lives in aquatic environments. There is no person-to-person transmission. Although it has often been implicated in point-source outbreaks related to cooling towers and similar aquatic sources, the organism also lives in ordinary tap water and has probably been underdiagnosed as an etiology of community-acquired pneumonia. It may account for as much as 19% of community-acquired pneumonia. Some patients present with a mild, self-limited atypical pneumonia, but older patients, smokers, and those with chronic disease or immunosuppression are at risk for developing the more acute manifestations of a severe systemic illness, with malaise, lethargy, and high fever. There is usually a dry cough, which is accompanied by pleuritic chest pain in 25% to 30% of patients. Purulent sputum often develops later. Gastrointestinal symptoms such as diarrhea and abdominal cramping are often prominent. Patients may appear toxic, with high fever and altered mental status.

Viral pneumonia is common in infants and young children, and has been recognized as an important cause of pneumonia in adults as well. Respiratory syncytial virus (RSV) and parainfluenza viruses are the most common seasonal causes of pneumonia in small children. Influenza viruses are the most common cause of viral pneumonia in adults. Winter influenza outbreaks, usually due to influenza type A, cause an average of 20,000 deaths yearly in the United States, mostly among persons age 65 or older.[4] Symptoms of upper respiratory infection, such as rhinitis or sore throat, usually precede the onset of viral pneumonia in adults. The onset of pneumonia may be insidious. Cough is usually nonproductive, and pleuritic chest pain is less common than with bacterial pneumonia. Cytomegalovirus (CMV) can cause pneumonia in persons with severe immunosuppression (e.g., transplant recipients). Varicella zoster virus (chickenpox) may cause pneumonia; this appears to be more common in adults, and factors such as smoking or pregnancy are predisposing conditions.

Although *P. carinii* does not cause pulmonary disease in normal hosts, the possibility of opportunistic infection and unrecognized AIDS must always be considered. *P. carinii* pneumonia (PCP) is the most common presentation leading to a diagnosis of AIDS, and many patients who present with this pneumonia are unaware of their human immunodeficiency virus (HIV) status. *All* patients who present with pulmonary complaints should be questioned about HIV risk factors, and clinicians should search for signs of HIV-related immunosuppression, such as weight loss, lymphadenopathy, and oral thrush. PCP typically presents subacutely with fatigue, exertional dyspnea, nonproductive cough, pleuritic chest pain, and fever.

Lower respiratory infection due to anaerobic organisms generally results from the aspiration of oropharyngeal contents. These infections are typically polymicrobial, including *Peptostreptococcus* spp., *Bacteroides* spp., *Fusobacterium* spp., *Prevotella* spp., and several other organisms. Presentation is often subacute or chronic, and may be difficult to distinguish clinically from other etiologies of pneumonia. Clinical factors that suggest an anaerobic infection include risk factors for aspiration (e.g., central nervous system depression or swallowing dysfunction), severe periodontal disease, fetid sputum, and radiographic appearance (e.g., location in posterior segment of right upper lobe or superior segment of lower lobe, lung abscess).

Fungal infections due to organisms such as *Histoplasma capsulatum, Blastomyces dermatitides,* and *Coccidioides immitis* commonly present as pulmonary disease. These organisms are present in the soil in various geographic areas of the United States: *H. capsulatum* in the Mississippi and Ohio river valleys, *B. dermatitides* in a poorly defined area extending beyond that of *H. capsulatum,* and *C. immitis* in desert areas of the Southwest. These infections should be considered in persons in appropriate geographic areas, especially in persons who are near activities that disturb the soil (e.g., construction, dirtbike riding). The clinical presentation ranges from an acute or chronic pneumonia to an incidental finding of asymptomatic granulomas on chest radiography.

Unusual Causes of Pneumonia

Q fever is an acute febrile illness, caused by the rickettsial organism *C. burnetii,* that may present as pneumonia. It is most common in persons with occupational exposure to animals. Fever is present in all patients, and a severe headache occurs in about 75% of cases. This infection is rarely fatal.

Plague (caused by *Yersinia pestis*) is endemic in many parts of the world. It occurs in the southwestern states of the United States in persons bitten by fleas from infected rodents or carnivores. Hematogenous spread may lead to pneumonia that is highly contagious and has a high mortality. It typically presents with cough, chest pain, purulent sputum, and hemoptysis, and is associated with fever and adenopathy.

Hantaviruses have recently been associated with a syndrome of severe respiratory distress and shock that has occurred in persons in several areas of the United States. Infection appears to occur from inhalation of aerosols of material contaminated with rodent urine and feces. Patients typically present with a prodrome of fever, myalgia, and malaise, followed in several days by the onset of respiratory distress. Hypoxia may progress rapidly, requiring ventilatory support. Chest radiographs demonstrate bilateral interstitial lung infiltrates that are more pronounced in dependent areas.

Tularemia is a febrile illness, caused by the bacterium *Francisella tularensis,* that is spread by contact with body fluids of infected mammals (especially rabbits) or the bite of an infected arthropod. The illness usually begins with an ulcerated skin lesion and painful regional lymphadenopathy. Some patients have a typhoidal form, with only fever, malaise, and weight loss. Pneumonia may occur with either form, presenting as a nonproductive cough and patchy infiltrates on the chest radiograph.

Psittacosis is a chlamydial infection that can be spread to humans from infected birds. It may occur in owners of pet birds, petshop employees, or others exposed to birds, or workers in poultry-processing plants. Illness often begins rapidly with chills, high fever, myalgias, and malaise; severe headache is often the major complaint. Cough is usually nonproductive. Splenomegaly is often present. Radiographic findings are variable, but patchy perihilar or lower lung field infiltrates are most common.

DIFFERENTIAL DIAGNOSIS

Several noninfectious etiologies may result in inflammatory lung processes. These include exposure to mineral dusts (e.g., silicosis), chemical fumes (e.g., chlorine, ammonia), toxic drugs (e.g., bleomycin), radiation, thermal injury, or oxygen toxicity. Immunologic diseases such as sarcoidosis, Goodpasture syndrome, Wegener's granulomatosis, collagen vascular disease, or hypersensitivity to environmental agents (e.g., farmer's lung) may also result in pneumonia. Tumors may sometimes be confused with pneumonia radiographically, or may present initially as a postobstructive infection or adenopathy with peripheral infiltrates. Pulmonary embolism must be considered in patients who present with tachypnea, hypoxia, tachycardia, or chest pain in the appropriate clinical setting. Cardiac illness often presents with respiratory complaints such as dyspnea. Aspiration of a foreign body must also be considered as an etiology of pulmonary infiltrates, especially in younger children.

In many studies of community-acquired pneumonia, no microbial etiology can be determined in one-third to one-half of cases, even after thorough investigation. To a great extent, the likely etiologies must be predicted based on epidemiologic considerations and prevalence of pathogens in careful research studies. In general, the likelihood of *S. pneumoniae* is related to the severity of illness, having been identified in as many as 50% of intensive care unit (ICU)–admitted and fatal cases. In studies of adults with community-acquired pneumonia who were hospitalized, traditional pathogens such as *S. pneumoniae* and *H. influenzae* accounted for about one-fourth of cases. *Legionella, M. pneumoniae,* and *C. pneumoniae* together accounted for 15% to 40%.[7,11] Another large study, in which serologic testing was done for common viral agents, revealed a viral etiology in about 17% of cases, with influenza and parainfluenza viruses the most common.[10] Studies of patients with more severe illness who required ICU admission have shown the prevalence of *S. pneumoniae* to be as high as 38% and that of *Legionella* to be as high as 22%, although the "unknown" category still accounts for 30% to 50% of cases.[15,17] Atypical organisms such as *Mycoplasma* appear to account for a relatively higher proportion of pneumonias in those who have milder illness amenable to outpatient therapy. Nevertheless, it is important to be aware of how frequently atypical organisms are identified in patients with severe illness requiring hospitalization.

EMERGENCY DEPARTMENT EVALUATION

The emergency department evaluation should focus on establishing the diagnosis of pneumonia, determining the presence of clinical features associated with specific infectious etiologies, and identifying host factors that will influence decisions regarding the need for hospitalization and choice of antibiotics.

Chest Radiograph

The chest radiograph is generally the most important test to determine the presence of pneumonia. A number of predictive models have been developed to optimize chest x-ray use in patients with cough in whom pneumonia is suspected. Factors found to be associated with a positive chest x-ray are fever, tachycardia, and tachypnea; rales or decreased breath sounds, sputum production, and absence of rhinorrhea or sore throat have also been predictive in some models. Although use of predictive models may reduce the number of unnecessary chest x-rays, they appear to be less sensitive than physician judgment.[6] Because of its relatively low cost and risk, chest x-ray is appropriate when management will be affected by the result (e.g., hospital admission, antimicrobial use, exclusion of other diagnoses). Chest x-ray may be particularly useful in groups such as the elderly (who may have subtle clinical signs of pneumonia), patients with serious underlying disease or severe illness, or those at risk for tuberculosis (TB) (to quickly establish the need for isolation). Young healthy adults who will receive outpatient treatment with empirical antimicrobials may have the chest radiograph deferred unless there is suspicion of immunosuppression or other unusual features of disease. Routine chest radiography for patients with exacerbation of chronic bronchitis or COPD has been shown to be of low yield and can be limited to those with other signs of infection or congestive heart failure.[19]

Although the causative agent cannot be determined solely by the results of chest radiography, certain radiographic patterns tend to be associated with specific pathogens. In pyogenic bacterial pneumonias, radiographs usually show an area of segmental or subsegmental infiltration and air bronchograms. Lobar consolidation is present in a minority of cases of bacterial pneumonia, and is often due to pneumococcus or *Klebsiella*. Bronchopneumonia resulting from spread of infection along the intralobular airway causes fluffy or patchy infiltrates in the involved areas of the lung. A wide variety of bacteria may cause this pattern, as well as agents such as *C. pneumoniae, M. pneumoniae, Legionella,* and even viruses. An interstitial pattern on the chest radiograph is typically caused by *M. pneumoniae,* viruses, or *P. carinii*. Tiny nodules disseminated throughout both lungs represent a miliary pattern typical of granulomatous pneumonias such as TB or fungal disease. The location of infiltrates may also give a clue to the etiology. Aspiration pneumonia occurs in dependent areas of the lung, most commonly the superior segments of the lower lobes or the posterior segments of the upper lobes.[3] Pneumonia produced by hematogenous spread (such as staphylococcal) tends to be multifocal and peripheral. Apical infiltrates suggest TB.

Additional radiographic features associated with infiltrates may suggest specific etiologies. An infiltrate associated with hilar or mediastinal adenopathy suggests the presence of TB or fungal disease, or may indicate pneumonia associated with a neoplasm. Cavitation is most commonly present with infections caused by anaerobes, gram-negative organisms, fungi, or *S. aureus;* cavitation may also be present in fungal disease or TB. Pneumatoceles or spontaneous pneumothorax may be seen in AIDS patients with PCP. Pleural effusions can be seen with a wide variety of organisms, including many types of pyogenic bacterial pneumonia, *C. pneumoniae, Legionella,* and TB. Anaerobic infections associated with an effusion are especially prone to the development of empyema.

Radiographic findings are nonspecific for a particular infectious etiology. For example, *M. pneumoniae* pneumonia may present with a dense infiltrate, and pneumococcal pneumonia with diffuse interstitial infiltrates. Immunocompromised patients are particularly likely to have atypical radiographic appearances. Occasionally, patients with a clinical picture strongly suggestive of pneumonia have a normal chest radiograph. The absence of findings on the chest radiograph should not preclude the use of antimicrobial therapy in patients thought to have pneumonia on clinical grounds.[13]

Other Tests

Laboratory studies are also nonspecific for identifying the etiology of pneumonia. Although an elevated peripheral white blood cell (WBC) count may increase the likelihood of a pyogenic bacterial etiology, this finding is of limited value in making decisions regarding therapy in an individual patient and must be considered in light of other clinical features. A WBC count may be helpful if it yields evidence of immunosuppression, such as neutropenia, or if it reveals lymphopenia that may indicate immunosuppression from HIV infection.[3] Serum chemistry studies may be helpful in identifying patients with metabolic acidosis or renal–hepatic dysfunction associated with sepsis or with underlying disease. Such findings may be helpful in predicting a complicated course and may influence decisions regarding disposition, choice of antimicrobial agents, and dosages. These ancillary tests are not necessary in patients with mild illness.

Assessment of respiratory function with arterial blood gas measurements or pulse oximetry must also be part of the evaluation. Hypoxia is a clear indication for hospital admission.

Although a Gram stain of the sputum is often recommended as a means to identify a bacterial pathogen, the use of the Gram stain as a basis for empiric therapy in the emergency department can be problematic for several reasons. Many patients cannot provide an adequate sputum specimen. Induction of sputum without adequate isolation facilities can put patients and staff at risk if sputum is induced from persons with unrecognized TB. Moreover, the correlation between the identification of pneumococcus on Gram stain and by sputum culture is often poor, even when commonly used criteria for an adequate sputum specimen are applied (fewer than five squamous epithelial cells and more than 25 WBCs per high-power field).[18] The Gram stain is even less likely to demonstrate gram-negative pathogens such as *H. influenzae,* and should not be relied on to rule out a gram-negative etiology. Sputum Gram stains are less accurate when done by less experienced physicians outside the microbiology laboratory and may lead to erroneous conclusions regarding which pathogens are present. Effective empiric antimicrobial therapy can be selected on the basis of clinical information, even if a sputum Gram stain is not done.

The utility of routine blood cultures has been questioned, because studies of nonimmunocompromised adults with pneumonia have demonstrated a low prevalence of noncontaminant bacteremia, and management is rarely changed based on the results.[5] Blood cultures should be obtained from immunocompromised patients, those with severe sepsis or shock, or those with risk factors for endovascular infection (e.g., prosthetic valves or i.v. drug use). When positive, blood cultures reflect the etiologic agent more accurately than do sputum cultures. Bacteremia occurs in about 25% to 30% of cases of pneumococcal pneumonia. Routine blood cultures are not indicated for outpatients.

Serologic tests are available for the diagnosis of a number of organisms, including *C. pneumoniae, Legionella,* and fungi. Serologic tests to determine the etiology of pneumonia may be helpful retrospectively, but both acute and convalescent serum titers are usually required, and are therefore of little use to the emergency physician. *M. pneumoniae* pneumonia is associated with the presence of serum cold hemagglutinins in up to 60% of cases, but they may also be present in a number of viral infections. The diagnosis of the exact etiology of viral pneumonia is made difficult by the nonspecific nature of the presentation and the lack of widely available rapid tests. Rapid diagnostic tests for viral antigens are available for several viruses, including RSV and influenza. Improvements in therapy for specific viral pneumonias (such as newly developed neuraminidase inhibitors for influenza) are likely to make these tests more useful. In the future, rapid testing, using technology such as the polymerase chain reaction, may provide emergency physicians with a reliable method for determining the specific etiology of pneumonia.

EMERGENCY DEPARTMENT MANAGEMENT

As with any seriously ill patient in the emergency department, initial attention should focus on ensuring adequate ventilation, oxygenation, and perfusion. Hypoxic patients with pneumonia should receive supplemental oxygen. Those with severe respiratory compromise may require endotracheal intubation. Patients with underlying asthma or COPD who present with wheezing may benefit from bronchodilator therapy. Seriously ill patients who present with volume depletion or septic shock will require fluid resuscitation and may require vasopressors.

It is usually necessary to begin empiric antimicrobial therapy for pneumonia before a definite microbiologic etiology is established. Antimicrobials should be started in the emergency department for patients who are being admitted to the hospital; deferring treatment until arrival on the ward can sometimes cause significant delays. Mortality has been shown to be reduced among elderly pneumonia patients who receive initial antimicrobials within 8 hours of presentation, as compared with later.[12] The antibiotics chosen must provide coverage of the likely etiologies based on clinical, laboratory, radiologic, and epidemiologic information. Though care must be taken not to miss possibly dangerous pathogens, the regimen should be as selective as possible to avoid problems with drug toxicity, emergence of resistance to broad-spectrum agents, and excessive cost.

The prevalence of drug-resistant *S. pneumoniae* (DRSP) has increased steadily over the past decade. In the United States, among outpatient pneumococcal sputum isolates collected between 1997 and 1998, approximately 36% were resistant to penicillin, with 14% having high-level resistance.[20] Isolates that are resistant to penicillin are also very likely to be resistant to other β-lactams as well as macrolides, tetracyclines, and trimethoprim–sulfamethoxazole (TMP/SMX). A number of extended-spectrum fluoroquinolones have been introduced, such as levofloxacin, grepafloxacin, sparfloxacin, and trovafloxacin, and others such as moxifloxacin, clinafloxacin, and gatifloxacin, are expected. These agents have enhanced activity against DRSP as well as other typical and atypical organisms that commonly cause pneumonia, and may offer additional alternatives to vancomycin if DRSP is a concern. However, it is not clear that *in vitro* resistance is related to adverse clinical outcome; in one study, patients infected with resistant pneumococcal isolates had no greater mortality than those with susceptible organisms, even when treated with antibiotics to which the organism was resistant.[16]

Guidelines have been issued for empirical antibiotics for patients with community-acquired pneumonia.[1,14] For patients whose illness is severe enough to require hospital admission and parenteral antibiotics, options include a combination of a second- or third-generation cephalosporin and a macrolide (e.g., i.v. erythromycin or azithromycin, or oral azithromycin), or an extended-spectrum fluoroquinolone alone. These regimens will treat the most common bacterial pathogens, such as *S. pneumoniae, M. catarrhalis,* and *H. influenzae,* as well as atypical pathogens such as *Mycoplasma, Chlamydia,* and *Legionella.* Intravenous azithromycin alone is another option, though this drug does not achieve significant serum levels and lacks significant activity against many aerobic gram-negative bacilli and DRSP. Azithromycin alone might be an appropriate choice for persons with milder illness who are less likely to be bacteremic. If anaerobic organisms are suspected (e.g., aspiration), clindamycin or metronidazole could be added to the regimen, or a β-lactam–β-lactamase inhibitor antibiotic such as ampicillin–sulbactam or piperacillin–tazobactam could be used. Some of the newer quinolones, such as moxifloxacin, clinafloxacin, and gatifloxacin, are also active against anaerobes.

Severely ill and compromised patients (e.g., neutropenic, recent nursing home or hospital stay) are at relatively greater risk of infection due to *S. pneumoniae,* aerobic gram-negative bacilli, *S. aureus,* and, in some areas, *Legionella* spp. Empirical therapy should include extended gram-negative activity, including P. *aeruginosa* with drugs such as ceftazidime, piperacillin–tazobactam, ciprofloxacin, or an aminoglycoside. Vancomycin and erythromycin may be combined with these agents for DRSP and *Legionella* spp., respectively, or an extended-spectrum fluoroquinolone may be included.

For patients with AIDS, it is important to treat *P. carinii* as well as bacterial pathogens such as *S. pneumoniae.* TMP/SMX is the treatment of choice; the usual regimen is 20 mg/kg of TMP and 100 mg/kg of SMX in four divided doses (3 amps i.v. q6h for most adults), to be continued for 21 days. For patients allergic to sulfa, pentamidine can be given in a dose of 4 mg/kg over 1 hour. Because pentamidine has no activity against *S. pneumoniae* or other bacterial pathogens, it is important to add a cephalosporin or other antibacterial agent to the initial empiric regimen. Other options include clindamycin 900 mg i.v. q8h plus primaquine 15 mg PO qd, TMP plus dapsone, atovaquone, or trimetrexate. The addition of steroids (prednisone 40 mg PO b.i.d.) has been shown to reduce mortality and clinical deterioration in patients with PaO_2 less than 70 or A-a gradient greater than 35.

A number of antimicrobials are available for outpatient therapy of community-acquired pneumonia. Appropriate agents for outpatient treatment of adults include macrolides (erythromycin, clarithromycin, azithromycin), fluoroquinolones with enhanced activity against *S. pneumoniae,* or doxycycline. Alternative options that would be appropriate in those patients with a higher likelihood of a "typical" bacterial etiology include amoxicillin–clavulanate or a second-generation cephalosporin such as cefuroxime axetil, cefpodoxime, or cefprozil. These β-lactam agents do not have activity against atypical pathogens. In patients properly identified at low risk for complications and who are evaluated for careful outpatient follow-up, use of a macrolide or doxycycline is reasonable, even when there is concern over DRSP. Use of more expensive agents, such as the newer fluoroquinolones, may be justified based on convenience, avoidance of side effects and drug interactions, or concern over DRSP in patients with a higher likelihood of bacterial etiology. Use of ampicillin or amoxicillin is not generally recommended due to the high incidence of β-lactamase production in pneumonia pathogens, although these have been used successfully in higher doses (e.g., amoxicillin 1 g t.i.d.) in other conditions with a high prevalence of DRSP. TMP/SMX has also been largely abandoned for treatment of pneumonia because of concern about increasing resistance. Except for the administration of fluoroquinolones, these recommendations also apply to school-aged children and adolescents, in whom *Mycoplasma* is common.

The antiviral agents amantadine and rimantadine can decrease the duration and severity of influenza A if started within 48 hours of symptom onset.[4] They are also useful as prophylaxis to control outbreaks within families or group settings such as nursing homes. Because they are not effective against other respiratory viruses, they should be used only if influenza A virus is confirmed with a rapid test or is highly likely based on the season and epidemiology. The usual adult dose for both amantadine and rimantadine is 100 mg PO b.i.d. Dosage should be reduced to 100 mg once daily for debilitated or elderly patients to reduce side effects such as confusion (less common with rimantadine). New antiviral agents are being developed that may improve the treatment of influenza. Neuraminidase inhibitors

TABLE 144.1. Empiric Therapy for Pneumonia

Clinical Setting	Antibiotic Regimen	Comments
PARENTERAL REGIMENS		
Community-acquired, nonimmunocompromised	Second- or third-generation cephalosporin ± macrolide	Third-generation cephalosporin more likely to be active against DRSP. Add macrolide to treat atypical pathogens.
	Extended spectrum fluoroquinolone (e.g., levofloxacin)	Treats most common bacterial as well as atypical pathogens. Active vs. DRSP.
	Azithromycin (alone)	Treats most common typical as well as atypical pathogens. High tissue levels, but low serums levels and poor CSF penetration.
	β-lactam/β-lactamase inhibitor (e.g., ampicillin-sulbactam) ± macrolide	Superior activity vs. anaerobes. Piperacillin-tazobactam more active vs. gram-negative pathogens, including *P. aeruginosa.*
Suspected aspiration	Cefoxitin or cefotetan	Best anaerobic activity among cephalosporins
	β-lactam/β-lactamase inhibitor	
	Clindamycin ± aminoglycoside	
	Metronidazole + second- or third-generation cephalosporin	
Severe pneumonia (ICU)	Cefotaxime, ceftriaxone, or β-lactam/β-lactamase inhibitor plus macrolide or fluoroquinolone	Consider adding aminoglycoside if septic shock is present. Use extended-spectrum fluoroquinolone or add vancomycin if DRSP is suspected.
Neutropenic, bronchiectasis, recent hospitalization	Antipseudomonal β-lactam (e.g., piperacillin, ceftazidime, cefepime, imipenem) + macrolide or fluoroquinolone ± aminoglycoside	Add aminoglycoside if neutropenic or in septic shock. Choice of antipseudomonal aminoglycoside is based on local antibiotic-resistance patterns.
ORAL REGIMENS		
Age <60, otherwise healthy (atypical pathogens likely)	Erythromycin	Poor activity vs. *H. influenza;* GI upset common.
	Doxycycline	Preferred for adolescent or young adult when likelihood of *Mycoplasma* is high; variable activity vs. *S. pneumoniae.*
	Clarithromycin	Treats common typical bacterial and atypical pathogens; active vs. DRSP.
	Azithromycin	5-day course, treats common typical bacterial and atypical pathogens.
	Extended-spectrum fluoroquinolone	Treats common typical bacterial and atypical pathogens; active vs. DRSP.
Age ≥ 60, COPD, purulent sputum (pyogenic bacterial etiology likely)	Second- or third-generation cephalosporin (e.g., cefuroxime axetil, cefpodoxime, cefprozil)	No activity vs. atypical pathogens or some resistant *S. pneumoniae.*
	Amoxicillin-clavulanate	Better activity vs. anaerobes; frequent diarrhea. No activity vs. atypical pathogens or some resistant *S. pneumoniae.*
	Extended-spectrum fluoroquinolone	Treats common typical bacterial and atypical pathogens; active vs. DRSP

DRSP, drug-resistant *Streptococcus pneumoniae;* CSF, cerebrospinal fluid; GI, gastrointestinal.

have been shown to be effective against both influenza A and B viruses and appear to have fewer side effects.

Many emergency departments initiate outpatient therapy in moderately ill patients, who previously might have been hospitalized, with an initial parenteral dose of a long-acting antibiotic such as ceftriaxone, and employ extended observation (i.e., 12 to 24 hours) while administering supportive care such as hydration, antipyretics, and bronchodilators before discharge on an oral regimen. Certain patients may also be brought back to the emergency department for follow-up in 24 hours and receive a second parenteral or observed oral dose of antibiotics. Extended-spectrum fluoroquinolones are another option that may be employed in this strategy, and they have additional activity against atypical pathogens and DRSP. Oral administration of these agents results in blood and tissue levels similar to those with i.v. therapy, provided that normal intestinal absorption exists.

Empiric therapy for pneumonia is summarized in Table 144.1.

DISPOSITION

The disposition of patients with pneumonia is dictated by the patient's underlying medical conditions, the severity of illness and likelihood of clinical deterioration, and the feasibility of home care and outpatient follow-up. Outpatient treatment is 15 to 20 times less expensive than inpatient treatment, and most patients prefer the home environment. The decision to hospitalize a patient with pneumonia is not necessarily a commitment to prolonged inpatient care. Twelve- to 24-hour emergency department or hospital ward observation may allow the early discharge of certain moderate-risk patients.

A prospectively validated prediction rule for mortality among immunocompetent adults with community-acquired pneumonia suggests a two-step approach to assess risk.[8] Patients in the lowest risk class are those less than age 50, without significant comorbid conditions (neoplasm, congestive heart failure, cerebrovascular disease, renal disease, liver disease), and without the following findings on physical examination: altered mental status, pulse greater than or equal to 30 beats per minute, systolic blood pressure less than 90, and temperature less than 35°C or greater than or equal to 40°C. Patients who do not fit the lowest risk category are classified into categories based on a scoring system that accounts for age, comorbid illness, physical examination findings, and laboratory abnormalities. Hospitalization is recommended for those in moderate- to high-risk categories. Although this method of assessing the likelihood of successful outpatient management is helpful in establishing general guidelines, it has not been modeled to predict acute life-threatening events, does not take into account dynamic evaluation over time, and has not been prospectively compared with physician judgment. Additional discharge criteria could include improving and stable vital signs over a several-hour observation period, ability to take oral medications, an ambulatory pulse oximetry greater than 90%, home support, and ability to follow-up.

Most patients with community-acquired pneumonia do not need respiratory isolation. Those who are suspected of having an etiology of pneumonia that could pose a threat of transmission to other patients (e.g., influenza, varicella, TB, plague) should be isolated. Neutropenic patients are generally placed in reverse isolation. HIV-infected patients who present with pneumonia ideally should be isolated until TB can be ruled out by sputum AFB smears, particularly those with other risk factors for TB. The chest radiograph cannot be relied on to rule out TB in AIDS patients, because it often does not have the typical appearance of TB. Isolation should be strongly considered for others at high risk for TB, such as inner-city homeless persons or i.v. drug users.

COMMON PITFALLS

- Failure to recognize pneumonia in a patient with exacerbation of underlying lung disease, such as asthma or COPD
- Delaying initiation of antibiotics for seriously ill patients
- Failure to question patients who present with respiratory complaints about HIV risk factors
- Failure to consider other possible etiologies of lung infiltrates, such as aspiration of foreign body
- Failure to recognize TB and initiate respiratory isolation in a patient with HIV infection or other TB risk factors

References

1. Bartlett JG, Breiman RF, Mandell LA, et al. Community-acquired pneumonia in adults; guidelines for management. The Infectious Diseases Society of America. *Clin Infect Dis* 1998; 26:811–838.
2. Bates JH, Campbell GD, Barron AL, et al. Microbial etiology of acute pneumonia in hospitalized patients. *Chest* 1992;101:1005–1012.
3. Blatt SP, Lucey CR, Butzin CA, et al. Total lymphocyte count as a predictor of absolute CD4+ count and CD4+ percentage in HIV-infected persons. *JAMA* 1993;269:622–626.
4. Centers for Disease Control and Prevention. Prevention and control of influenza: recommendations of the Immunization Practices Advisory Committee (ACIP). *MMWR* 1999;48(RR-4):1–28.
5. Chalasani NP, Valdecanas MA, Gopal AK, et al. Clinical utility of routine blood cultures in adult patients with community-acquired pneumonia without underlying risks. *Chest* 1995;108:891–936.
6. Emerman CL, Dawson N, Speroff T, et al. comparison of physician judgment and decision aids for ordering chest radiographs for pneumonia in outpatients. *Ann Emerg Med* 1991;20:1215–1219.
7. Fang GD, Fine M, Orloff J, et al. New and emerging etiologies for community-acquired pneumonia with implications for therapy: a prospective multicenter study of 359 cases. *Medicine* 1990;69:307–316.
8. Fine MJ, Auble TE, Yealy DM, et al. A prediction rule to identify low-risk patients with community-acquired pneumonia. *N Engl J Med* 1997;336:243–250.
9. Grayston JT. Infections caused by Chlamydia pneumoniae strain TWAR. *Clin Infect Dis* 1992;15:757–763.
10. Marrie TJ, Durant H, Yates L. Community-acquired pneumonia requiring hospitalization: 5-year prospective study. *Rev Infect Dis* 1989;11:586–599.
11. Marston BJ, Plouffe JF, File TM Jr, et al. Incidence of community-acquired pneumonia requiring hospitalization: results of a population-based active surveillance study in Ohio. *Arch Intern Med* 1997;157:1709–1718.
12. Meehan TP, Fine MJ, Krumholz HM, et al. Quality of care, process, and outcomes in elderly patients with pneumonia. *JAMA* 1997;278:891–936.
13. Melbye H, Berdal BP, Straume B, et al. Pneumonia—a clinical or radiographic diagnosis? *Scand J Infect Dis* 1992;24:647–655.
14. Niederman MS, Bass JB, Campbell GD, et al. Guidelines for the initial management of adults with community-acquired pneumonia: diagnosis, assessment of severity, and initial antimicrobial therapy. American Thoracic Society. *Am Rev Respir Dis* 1993;148:1418–1426.
15. Pachon J, Prados MD, Capote F, et al. Severe community-acquired pneumonia: etiology, prognosis, and treatment. *Am Rev Respir Dis* 1990;142:369–373.
16. Pallares R, Linares J, Vadillo M, et al. Resistance to penicillin and cephalosporin and mortality from severe pneumococcal pneumonia in Barcelona, Spain. *N Engl J Med* 1995;333:474–480.
17. Potgieter PD, Hammond JM. Etiology and diagnosis of pneumonia requiring ICU admission. *Chest* 1992;101:199–203.
18. Reed WW, Byrd GS, Gates RH, et al. Sputum Gram's stain in community-acquired pneumococcal pneumonia: a meta-analysis. *West J Med* 1996; 165:197–204.
19. Sherman S, Skoney JA, Ravikrishnan KP. Routine chest radiographs in exacerbations of chronic obstructive pulmonary disease: diagnostic value. *Arch Intern Med* 1989;149:2493–2496.
20. Thornsberry C, et al. In: Abstracts of the 38th Interscience Conference on Antimicrobial Agents and Chemotherapy, 1998; Abstract E22.

CHAPTER 145
Pleural Effusion

Robert Sigillito and Peter M. C. DeBlieux

A pleural effusion is an abnormal collection of fluid within the pleural space. An acute or previously undiagnosed effusion presents the emergency physician with a diagnostic challenge. A pleural effusion that is chronic and previously diagnosed presents therapeutic considerations.

The pleural space is bordered by the visceral pleura lining the lung and by the parietal pleura lining the mediastinum, diaphragm, and inner surface of the thoracic wall. A small amount of fluid (a few milliliters) is normally present in this space. As with all capillary beds in the body, there is a dynamic balance between fluid production and absorption in both the parietal and visceral pleura.

Only at the parietal pleura, however, do the net forces favor accumulation of fluid, accounting for physiologic pleural fluid, which is normally cleared from the pleural space via the lymphatic vessels of the parietal pleura.[1,7] Pathologic amounts of pleural fluid accumulate when pleural fluid formation increases beyond the capacity of lymphatic clearance, or when the lymphatic clearance is impaired (Table 145.1).

CLINICAL PRESENTATION

Patients with pleural effusions commonly present with complaints related to the underlying disease process rather than to the pleural effusion itself. Small effusions are often asymptomatic. Symptoms directly attributable to an effusion result from either pleural inflammation (pain), compromised pulmonary mechanics (dyspnea), impaired gas exchange (altered mental status with hypoxia or hypercarbia), or compression of the lung with collapse of bronchial structures (nonproductive cough).

TABLE 145.1. Causes of the Impairment of Pleural Fluid Clearance

1. Diffusion of fluid across the visceral pleura due to increased pulmonary interstitial fluid (e.g., secondary to ventricular failure, pneumonia, hypoalbuminemia, or pulmonary embolus)
2. Increased hydrostatic pressure gradient across the parietal and visceral pleural capillary membranes due to diminished pleural pressure (e.g., with postobstructive pulmonary atelectasis)
3. Increased hydrostatic pressure gradient across the parietal and visceral pleural capillary membranes due to increased capillary pressure (right ventricular failure, left ventricular failure, and superior vena cava syndrome)
4. Increased oncotic pressure gradient across the pleural capillary membranes secondary to increased pleural fluid protein concentration (malignancy)
5. Increased peritoneal fluid with transit across the diaphragm (ascites, peritoneal dialysis)
6. Hemorrhage into the pleural space (malignancy, trauma, iatrogenic)
7. Disruption of the thoracic duct (trauma, iatrogenic)
8. Urine diffusion from the retroperitoneum into the pleural space (a rare condition resulting from trauma, urinary obstruction, or disruption of the collecting system)

Pleural fluid clearance may be impaired by two mechanisms:

1. Obstruction of the lymphatic system, which drains the parietal pleura (malignancy)
2. Elevation of the systemic venous pressure (right ventricular failure, superior vena cava syndrome)

Parietal pleural inflammation causes pain referred to the overlying chest wall. Central diaphragmatic irritation causes pain referred to the ipsilateral shoulder. The visceral pleura is not innervated, and visceral pleuritis does not result in pain.

The predominant findings on physical examination likewise often reflect the underlying disease process. Vital sign abnormalities and hemodynamic instability may be consequences of the primary disease or the result of impaired cardiopulmonary function. In the extreme, the right or left ventricle may collapse during diastole[6,16,18] because of an elevated pleural pressure ("effusion under tension").

The chest should be inspected for asymmetry. As the pleural space fills with fluid, the involved hemithorax increases in total volume, and the lung decreases in volume. Markedly elevated or negative pleural pressure may be evidenced by bulging or retraction of the intercostal spaces, tracheal deviation, or displacement of the cardiac apical pulse. Percussion of the chest may reveal dullness; diminished tactile fremitus, however, is easier to detect. Auscultation of the chest is often revealing. A pleural rub indicates an irregular pleural surface, due either to a mass or to inflammation. An audible rub suggests that the effusion is small or loculated, because a rub will disappear as an enlarging effusion separates the visceral and parietal pleura. Diminished breath sounds are frequently appreciated. Abnormalities of the character of the breath sounds reflect pulmonary parenchymal disease. The remainder of the physical examination should include a meticulous search for clues to the underlying disorder.

DIFFERENTIAL DIAGNOSIS

The most common causes of pleural effusion in adults, in order of decreasing approximate frequency, are congestive heart failure (CHF) (37%), pneumonia (22%), malignancy (15%), pulmonary embolus (11%), viral disease (7%), and ascites (3.5%). Collagen vascular disease, tuberculosis, and other diseases account for a minority of cases.[7] In contrast, the relative frequencies in children are pneumonia (50%), postoperative with congenital heart disease (14%), malignancy (10%), renal disease (9%), trauma (7%), and CHF secondary to congenital heart disease (3%). Effusions are further classified as either transudative or exudative (Table 145.2).

CHF may lead to the development of a pleural effusion in several ways. Increased pulmonary interstitial fluid may diffuse directly into the pleural space, and right and left ventricular failure elevate the hydrostatic pressures within the pleural capillaries of the parietal and visceral pleura, respectively. When the hydrostatic pressures exceed the opposing oncotic pressures, there is net pleural fluid production. Right ventricular failure also leads to elevation of the pressure within the lymphatic vessels, impeding drainage of the pleural space.

There are three stages in the development of a parapneumonic effusion and empyema. First, there is an accumulation of sterile pleural fluid characterized by low lactate dehydrogenase (LDH), normal pH and glucose level, and low white blood cell (WBC) count. If this is not treated, or if therapy fails, bacteria invade the pleural space; bacteria, WBCs, debris, and large pleural effusions accumulate. Fibrin sheets line the pleural surfaces, with a tendency to form loculations. The pleural fluid LDH concentration, and WBC count rise, while the pH and glucose level fall. Finally, fibroblasts grow into the exudate to form an inelastic pleural coating, or peel, encasing the lung and causing pulmonary restriction.[7,8]

TABLE 145.2. Etiology of Pleural Effusion

Transudate	Exudate
Congestive heart failure	Asbestosis
Cirrhosis with ascites	Chylothorax
Glomerulonephritis	Collagen vascular diseases
Meig syndrome	Rheumatoid arthritis
Myxedema	Systemic lupus erythematosus
Nephrotic syndrome	Drug-induced pleural disease
Peritoneal dialysis	Esophageal rupture
Pulmonary atelectasis	Hemothorax
Pulmonary embolus	Chest trauma
Sarcoidosis	Aortic dissection
Superior vena cava obstruction	Iatrogenic
Urinothorax	Intraabdominal inflammatory processes
	Cholecystitis
	Hepatitis
	Pancreatitis
	Perihepatitis
	Peritonitis
	Pyelonephritis
	Splenic abscess
	Subphrenic abscess
	Pulmonary or pleural infection
	Empyema
	Parapneumonic effusion
	Tuberculosis
	Viral
	Fungal
	Parasitic
	Neoplasm
	Pericarditis
	Pleuritis
	Pulmonary embolus
	Uremia

Various authors have developed criteria for the definition of *empyema*. Light[7] suggests that the term *complicated parapneumonic effusion* be used to designate those that do not resolve without tube thoracostomy. *Empyema* is reserved for describing those effusions that have the gross appearance of pus.[7,8]

Young, otherwise healthy, patients with parapneumonic effusion or empyema most often have *Staphylococcus aureus, Streptococcus pneumoniae,* or *Streptococcus pyogenes* infection. Elderly and infirm individuals with aspiration pneumonia more often have anaerobic infection. Postoperative thoracotomy patients are more likely to be infected with *S. aureus*.[3] In children, *S. pneumoniae* and *S. aureus* are the most common causes, with *Haemophilus influenzae* now the third most common.[2,3,5] Other pathogens include enteric gram-negative organisms, *Klebsiella, Enterococcus, Pseudomonas, Legionella, Mycobacterium tuberculosis, Chlamydia, Mycoplasma,* viruses, rickettsiae, and fungi. Infection with *Pneumocystis, Nocardia,* and *Cryptococcus* may cause effusion in the immunocompromised patient.

Other infectious processes may also lead to pleural effusion. Virtually any abdominal infection or inflammatory process may lead to a sympathetic effusion. Such processes include pancreatitis, hepatitis, perihepatitis, cholecystitis, hepatic amebiasis, splenic abscess, pyelonephritis, glomerulonephritis, peritonitis, and abdominal abscess.

The most common types of malignant effusions are those due to lung, breast, lymphoma, ovarian, and stomach tumors.[17] This type of effusion may be secondary to lymphatic obstruction, superior vena cava syndrome, postobstructive atelectasis, or pleural metastases.

A pulmonary embolus may produce either a transudative or an exudative effusion. The mechanism is probably infarction of a portion of lung and visceral pleura, with resultant loss of interstitial fluid across the membrane.

EMERGENCY DEPARTMENT EVALUATION

Effusions are most frequently diagnosed by chest radiography. Because freely flowing fluid follows gravity to the most dependent region of the thorax, small effusions manifest as blunting of the costophrenic angle on the upright posteroanterior (PA) film. Experimentally, at least 175 mL of fluid is required to produce this appearance.[4] Larger effusions appear to assume a meniscus configuration (a purely radiographic phenomenon).[7] The lateral upright radiograph will reveal a smaller effusion than the PA film, with an air–lung interface evident in the posterior costophrenic recess.

Effusion is more difficult to detect on supine anteroposterior (AP) films. The only evidence that fluid is present may be a diffuse homogeneous density of the affected hemithorax, compared with the contralateral side. Bilateral lateral decubitus films should be a routine part of the evaluation of every patient with newly diagnosed or suspected effusion. This aids in differentiation between effusion and pulmonary infiltrate, tumor, pleural thickening, or eventration or rupture of a hemidiaphragm. With the affected side down, fluid layers along the lateral wall of the thorax. More than 10 mm of fluid thickness in this view is considered significant.[7] With the opposite side dependent, the fluid layers along the mediastinum, allowing clearer visualization of the underlying lung parenchyma and allowing one to exclude pulmonary infiltrate, atelectasis, or mass.

Once the presence of a pleural effusion is confirmed, further emergency department (ED) evaluation should be directed at answering the following questions:

1. Is the effusion new or previously diagnosed?
2. If new, is the effusion a transudate or an exudate?
3. Is the effusion causing respiratory compromise such that therapeutic thoracentesis is indicated?
4. Is chest tube thoracostomy indicated?

In general, a previously diagnosed effusion does not require a new diagnostic workup, unless there is evidence that a complication has arisen (e.g., a patient with a known effusion secondary to CHF who presents with sepsis and is suspected of having an infected effusion).

To narrow the differential diagnosis, a new effusion should be characterized as a transudate or an exudate. (The exception to this rule is effusion in the setting of CHF. In that scenario, the underlying CHF should be treated, and thoracentesis should be performed only if the effusion does not resolve with therapy.) Although several sets of criteria have been proposed for such differentiation, Light's criteria are the most reliable[9] (Table 145.3). Fluid that meets any one of the three following criteria is an exudate:

1. Pleural fluid–serum protein ratio greater than 0.5
2. Pleural fluid–serum LDH ratio greater than 0.6
3. Pleural fluid LDH greater than two-thirds of the upper limit of normal for serum LDH

If the effusion proves to be a transudate, therapy is directed at the underlying process. Exudates, however, require further fluid analysis, including glucose, pH, amylase, fluid hematocrit, cell count with differential, Gram stain, culture, and cytology (Table 145.4). (Pleural biopsy may be necessary for the diagnosis of malignancy or tuberculosis. Pleural biopsy should be considered at the time of initial thoracentesis, because it is best accomplished before complete evacuation of the pleural fluid.)

A pleural fluid glucose level less than 60 mg/dL, although

TABLE 145.3. Light's Criteria

Pleural fluid-serum protein ratio >0.5
Pleural fluid-serum LDH ratio >0.6
Pleural fluid LDH >two-thirds of upper limit of normal for serum LDH

Source: From Light R, MacGregor M, Luchsinger P, et al. Pleural effusions: the diagnostic separation of transudates and exudates. Ann Intern Med 1972;77(4):507-513.

not a sensitive indicator of any particular etiology, suggests either a parapneumonic effusion–empyema or malignancy, rheumatoid disease, or tuberculosis.[7,10] A pleural fluid pH less than 7.0, or a glucose less than 40 mg/dL, indicates a complicated parapneumonic effusion–empyema, and the need for chest tube thoracostomy.[7,11] An elevation of the pleural fluid amylase narrows the differential diagnosis to pancreatitis, malignancy, and esophageal rupture.[7,10] A pleural fluid hematocrit greater than half that of the patient's blood defines a hemothorax and indicates the need for a chest tube.[7]

Additional routine workup should include a complete blood count, urinalysis, and serum electrolyte, blood urea nitrogen, and creatinine levels. If diagnostic thoracentesis is anticipated, serum glucose, protein, LDH, and amylase levels should be ordered to allow calculation of the necessary indices. If there is a history of coagulopathy, a prothrombin time can help to assess the risk associated with the invasive procedure. Continuous pulse oximetry should be used to monitor oxygenation status, particularly during thoracentesis.

An electrocardiogram may reveal an associated pericarditis or manifestations of underlying heart disease, or may suggest pulmonary embolus. Extreme QRS deviation mimicking myocardial infarction has been reported with pleural effusion.[14] Additional diagnostic tests (e.g., liver or thyroid function tests, tests for collagen vascular disease, ventilation–perfusion scan, or arteriography) may be ordered as indicated by findings on the history, physical examination, and initial laboratory evaluation.

Ultrasound can be used as a guide to thoracentesis in order to decrease the risk of complications. Computed tomography may also help to localize effusion and can identify pleural masses

EMERGENCY DEPARTMENT MANAGEMENT

As for all patients who present with acute signs or symptoms, the first priority is evaluation and stabilization of the airway, optimization of oxygenation and ventilation, and circulatory support. Treatment of life-threatening conditions such as pulmonary edema should be initiated.

Diagnostic evaluation of a pleural effusion, as described, is often undertaken on an inpatient basis. For some patients (e.g., those who are likely to have parapneumonic effusion–empyema, esophageal rupture, or sepsis), ED thoracentesis may be indicated for rapid diagnosis, drainage, and institution of specific treatment. Patients with chronic pulmonary disease and the elderly may have diminished cardiopulmonary reserve, and are likely to require urgent therapeutic thoracentesis. It is wise to obtain specialty consultation early in the course, to determine whether thoracentesis is best performed in the ED or after admission to the hospital.

A number of techniques for thoracentesis have been described. The size and location of the effusion should be determined by radiography and by physical examination. Examining for tactile fremitus and percussion of the chest determine the upper limit of the fluid level. The patient is usually placed in a seated position, leaning slightly forward. For small effusions, or if the patient cannot tolerate sitting, the lateral decubitus position may be used. A small or loculated effusion is best evacuated under fluoroscopy or ultrasound guidance. If a difficult thoracente-

TABLE 145.4. Fluid Analysis of Exudates

Cause	Appearance	WBC Count	Glucose	pH	Comments
Asbestosis	Serous or serosanguinous	Elevated (may be >25 K)	Normal	7.4	Chronic/recurrent; 25%-50% have eosinophilia
Chylothorax	Milky	Variable	Normal		Centrifuged specimen supernatant cloudy with elevated triglycerides; lymphoma in 75% of nontraumatic cases
Rheumatoid arthritis	Green	Variable	<60 mg/dL	<7.2	Pleural fluid LDH and rheumatoid factor titer high
	Yellow or serosanguinous	Variable	>80 mg/dL	>7.2	Pleural fluid ANA titer >1:320
Hemothorax	Bloody				Pleural fluid/whole blood hematocrit >0.5
Empyema	Purulent	High	<40 mg/dL	<7.0	Centrifuged specimen supernatant clear; chest tube indicated
Pancreatitis	Serosanguinous to bloody	Highly variable (1-50 K)	Equal to serum		Elevated fluid amylase
Parapneumonic effusion	Variable clear to turbid	Variable	>40 mg/dL	>7.2	pH 7.0-7.2 may require repeat thoracentesis
Tuberculosis	Yellow or serosanguinous	<10 K	Variable	Variable	Cell differential >50% lymphocytes; protein often >5.0 g/dL; pleural biopsy 90% sensitive
Neoplasm	Serous to bloody	Variable (1-10K)	Variable	Variable	Low pH and glucose suggest high tumor load; cytology more reliable than pleural biopsy
Pulmonary embolus					All indices highly variable; thoracentesis used to exclude other diagnoses
Uremia	Serosanguinous to bloody	Variable	Normal	Normal	Cell differential lymphocyte predominance

sis is anticipated, early consultation with an invasive radiologist or pulmonologist may be the most appropriate course of action.

Clotting abnormalities and anticoagulant therapy represent relative contraindications to thoracentesis, although safe thoracentesis is reported with thrombocytopenia (platelet count as low as 50,000/μL), or prolonged prothrombin time and partial thromboplastin time (up to twice the midrange of control) in the absence of active bleeding.[15] Likewise, chest wall infection is a contraindication unless the infected site can be avoided. Thoracentesis should also be avoided when there is diaphragmatic rupture on the side of effusion.

After sterile preparation of the aspiration site, local anesthesia is injected. A small-gauge needle, a catheter and needle, a commercial thoracentesis apparatus, or a pigtail catheter using the Seldinger technique may be used. The usual site for the insertion of the needle is in the midscapular line posteriorly, in the highest appropriate intercostal space. The needle is directed over the inferior rib to avoid the intercostal vessels. The catheter is advanced into the chest, and the fluid is removed under sterile conditions. In most cases, removal of the largest possible amount of fluid, until respiratory distress is alleviated or a limit of 1,500 mL is reached, is advisable. Removing larger amounts of fluid may increase the likelihood of developing postexpansion pulmonary edema,[12] a syndrome that can carry a mortality rate as high as 20%.[13] Less fluid should be withdrawn in the hypoalbuminemic patient.

After evacuation of the effusion, the catheter is removed and a chest radiograph is obtained to rule out iatrogenic pneumothorax. If a moderate or large pneumothorax has been inadvertently created, a thoracostomy tube is usually necessary. Other complications of thoracentesis include hemothorax, hemoperitoneum, shearing of the catheter tip, and infection.

DISPOSITION

The presence of a pleural effusion, in and of itself, does not necessitate admission. A patient with a stable effusion of known etiology may be sent home if the clinical situation allows. For most other cases, however, discussion of the timing and setting of thoracentesis with the primary physician or pulmonologist is appropriate. A clear exception is when the clinical situation demands urgent drainage. If thoracentesis is performed, hospital admission is usually indicated for further treatment of the underlying disease and for observation for procedural complications. In all other cases, the patient's condition and underlying disease process dictate the need for admission. Patients may be admitted to a bed on a regular floor or observation unit, unless cardiovascular or respiratory instability warrants admission to a monitored bed.

When definitive care is available only at another institution, patient transfer may be indicated. If thoracentesis was performed, transfer can be accomplished safely once a follow-up chest radiograph reveals no complications and provided the usual criteria for stability are satisfied.

COMMON PITFALLS

- Failure to recognize the presence of an effusion by failing to order a chest radiograph or, once taken, by misreading it. Effusion may be misdiagnosed as thickened pleura or infiltrate. This leads to inadequate or delayed evaluation and treatment, which might be particularly critical in cases of empyema, esophageal rupture, or intrathoracic hemorrhage.
- An incorrect presumptive diagnosis of the cause of the effusion or an incorrect presumption that an effusion is old and unchanged can likewise result in an inadequate evaluation or treatment. Comparison with old radiographs is essential.
- A misdiagnosis of pleural effusion may lead to inappropriate attempts at thoracentesis, with complications such as puncture of an intrathoracic mass (e.g., malignancy) or abdominal contents (in diaphragmatic rupture).
- Failure to recognize the potential need for pleural biopsy before thoracentesis. This makes subsequent biopsy more difficult if only a small effusion remains.
- Complications such as pneumothorax (from piercing the lung parenchyma or from leaving the needle or catheter hub exposed to the air); laceration of the liver, spleen, or intercostal vessels; and shearing of the catheter tip by withdrawing it incorrectly through the needle may be best avoided by careful attention to technique.
- The risk of postexpansion pulmonary edema is diminished by avoiding removal of very large quantities (e.g., more than 1000 mL) of pleural fluid and by using very low negative evacuation pressures.
- Transient hypoxia during thoracentesis may be avoided by the routine administration of oxygen and by continuous pulse oximetry.

References

1. Agostoni E, Zocchi L. Mechanical coupling and liquid exchanges in the pleural space. *Clin Chest Med* 1998;19(2):241–260.
2. Alkrinawi S, Chernick V. Pleural fluid in hospitalized pediatric patients. *Clin Pediatr* 1996;35(1):5–9.
3. Bryant R, Salmon C. Pleural empyema. *Clin Infect Dis* 1996;22:747–764.
4. Collins J, Burwell D, Furmanski S, et al. Minimal detectable pleural effusions. *Radiology* 1972;105:51–53.
5. Givan D, Eigen H. Common pleural effusions in children. *Clin Chest Med* 1998;19(2):363–371.
6. Kisanuki A, Shono H, Kiyonaga K, et al. Two-dimensional echocardiographic demonstration of left ventricular diastolic collapse due to compression by pleural effusion. *Am Heart J* 1991;122:1173–1175.
7. Light RW. *Pleural diseases,* 3rd ed. Baltimore: Williams & Wilkins, 1995.
8. Light R, Rodriguez R. Management of parapneumonic effusions. *Clin Chest Med* 1998;19(2):373–382.
9. Light R, MacGregor M, Luchsinger P, et al. Pleural effusions: the diagnostic separation of transudates and exudates. *Ann Intern Med* 1972;77(4):507–513.
10. Light R, Ball W. Glucose and amylase in pleural effusions. *JAMA* 1973;225(3):257–260.
11. Light R, Girard W, Jenkinson S, et al. Parapneumonic effusions. *Am J Med* 1980;69:507–512.
12. Light R, Jenkinson S, Minh VD, et al. Observations on pleural fluid pressures as fluid is withdrawn during thoracentesis. *Am Rev Respir Dis* 1980;121:799–804.
13. Mahfood S, Hix W, Aaron B, et al. Reexpansion pulmonary edema. *Ann Thorac Surg* 1988;45:340–345.
14. Manthous C, Schmidt G, Hall J. Pleural effusion masquerading as myocardial infarction. *Chest* 1993;103:1619–1620.
15. McVay P, Toy P. Lack of increased bleeding after paracentesis and thoracentesis in patients with mild coagulation abnormalities. *Transfusion* 1991; 31:164–171.
16. Negrus R, Chachkes J, Wrenn K. Tension hydrothorax and shock in a patient with a malignant pleural effusion. *Am J Emerg Med* 1990;8:205–207.
17. Sahn S. Malignancy metastatic to the pleura. *Clin Chest Med* 1998; 19(2):351–361.
18. Vaska K, Wann S, Sagar K, et al. Pleural effusion as a cause of right ventricular collapse. *Circulation* 1992;86:609–617.

CHAPTER 146
Asthma

Rita K. Cydulka and Michael A. Kaufman

Asthma is characterized by increased airway responsiveness to various stimuli. It is manifested by bronchoconstriction, widespread bronchial wall edema, and thick, tenacious secretions.[1] The characteristic that differentiates asthma from other airway diseases is its reversibility: Acute exacerbations of asthma are interspersed with symptom-free intervals.

Asthma affects about 5% of adults in the United States. About half of all cases are diagnosed before the patient reaches age 10, and another one-third are detected before age 40. The male–female ratio of this disease is 2:1 in childhood but equalizes during early adulthood.

The natural course of asthma has not been investigated thoroughly, but studies suggest that 50% to 80% of patients have a good prognosis, especially those with mild disease or disease that develops in childhood. Nevertheless, asthma has a high morbidity rate. The average asthmatic has 15 days of restricted activity each year and spends 5.8 days in bed. In the United States, over 4000 deaths per year are attributable to asthma.

Asthma is a heterogeneous disease. Clinically, it can be separated into two groups: allergic or extrinsic asthma, and nonallergic or intrinsic asthma. Many patients have components of both types. *Extrinsic asthma* accounts for less than 10% of patients and tends to develop early in life. It is associated with a well-defined sensitivity to inhaled allergens, a family history of allergic diseases, increased serum levels of immunoglobulin E (IgE), positive immediate skin tests, and blood eosinophilia. It may be seasonal (trees, grasses, spores) or perennial (animals, gardens, house dust). A good response to bronchodilator therapy is usually observed.

Intrinsic asthma is the more common type. An inciting allergen cannot be identified, a family history of allergies is less common, IgE levels may be normal or low, and skin tests are negative. Intrinsic asthma is perennial, tends to be more severe than extrinsic asthma, and has a limited response to bronchodilator therapy.

All asthmatics have hyperresponsive airways that narrow when exposed to various stimuli: allergic, infectious, pharmacologic, environmental, occupational, exercise-related, and emotional.

Allergic asthma occurs when inhaled allergens bind to IgE molecules bound to mast cells in the lining of the tracheobronchial tree. During the early response, various mediators are released, causing increased vascular permeability, mucosal edema, and bronchial smooth muscle contraction. A second wave of reaction, the late response, is seen hours to days later and involves the accumulation of inflammatory cells in the bronchial mucosa, thus perpetuating the reaction.

Although several theories attempt to explain the pathophysiologic changes that occur in nonallergic asthma, none adequately explains all clinically observed phenomena. Current hypotheses include the following:

- The cholinergic reflex theory, which suggests that asthmatics have increased parasympathetic reactivity
- The beta-adrenergic blockade theory, which proposes that asthmatics have defective adrenergic receptors, thus permitting unopposed intrinsic parasympathetic activity
- The alpha-adrenergic hyperresponsiveness theory
- The heat flux theory, which states that airway cooling is the primary stimulus for bronchoconstriction[16]

Research suggests that even patients without atopy have the same pathophysiology as atopic patients.[20]

Respiratory infections, particularly viral infections, commonly precipitate bronchospasm. Viruses cause mucosal inflammation and lower the firing threshold of the subendothelial vagal receptors, resulting in enhanced airway reactivity. This hyperactivity may last up to 8 weeks, even in nonasthmatic persons.

Pharmacologic agents also may induce acute asthma. The agents most frequently implicated are aspirin and nonsteroidal antiinflammatory compounds, coloring agents, and beta-adrenergic antagonists.

Up to 10% of adult asthmatics suffer from the triad of aspirin-induced bronchospasm, nasal polyps, and eosinophilia. Ingestion of aspirin, nonsteroidal antiinflammatory compounds, and tartrazine (FDC yellow dye no. 5) and other dyes may induce severe asthma in these patients, possibly by diverting arachidonic acid metabolism toward the lipoxygenase pathway and causing the production of leukotrienes, which are potent bronchoconstrictors.

Sulfating agents are used widely as food preservatives and antioxidants in pharmaceutical products. Exacerbation of asthma has been reported after food ingestions and after the use of sulfite-containing drugs, including some inhalation bronchodilators.

A large variety of occupational dusts and fumes may provoke acute airway obstruction. Patients with occupational asthma classically give a cyclic history. They are symptom-free during weekends, vacations, and on arrival at work. As the workday progresses, wheezing develops. A history of similar symptoms in fellow employees may be noted. Three mechanisms are involved in occupational asthma: immunologic reactions (e.g., animal handlers), direct liberation of bronchoconstrictors (e.g., cotton workers), and direct irritant effects (e.g., meat wrappers).

Exercise also may stimulate an asthma attack. Exercise-induced bronchospasm is usually noted within 5 to 20 minutes after the completion of exercise and is related to thermal changes in the respiratory tree. Exercising in a cold, dry environment causes a more marked response than exercising in a warm, humid environment.

Endocrine factors have been recognized as yet another cause of airway hyperresponsiveness. Normal variations in progesterone and estradiol levels are believed to modulate airway reactivity.

Psychological factors also influence asthma exacerbations, probably through modification of vagal efferent activity. The extent to which psychological factors participate in the induction and continuation of an asthma attack is unknown but probably varies from patient to patient and from episode to episode.[1,2]

Regardless of the underlying precipitant, airway narrowing, bronchial wall edema, bronchial smooth muscle contraction, and mucosal plugging ensue. These changes result in increased airway resistance, decreased forced expiratory volumes and flow rates, lung hyperinflation, increased work of breathing, and ventilation–perfusion mismatch.

CLINICAL PRESENTATION

Asthma attacks frequently occur at night. The classic triad of symptoms is cough, dyspnea, and wheezing. Chest tightness and nonproductive cough may precede dyspnea and wheezing. As airway obstruction worsens, the expiratory phase becomes prolonged. Asthmatic patients coming to the emergency department are frequently anxious, tachypneic, tachycardic, and mildly hypertensive. Lung hyperinflation, accessory respiratory muscle use, muscle retraction, and pulsus paradoxus may be noted.

Patients may attempt to sit upright or lean forward in an effort to ease the work of breathing. These signs may be absent despite severe airway obstruction, however.[4] A silent chest indicates insufficient air movement or extensive mucous plugging and is an ominous sign. Cyanosis may appear only immediately before respiratory arrest and should not be relied on as an indication of the severity of the attack. The termination of an exacerbation is often marked by a cough productive of thick mucus plugs and bronchial casts (Curschmann spirals).

A subset of asthmatic patients experiences the sudden onset of severe symptoms. These individuals tend to respond rapidly to treatment but appear to be at significant risk for a fatal outcome.

Occasionally, an asthmatic patient may complain of intermittent dyspnea or cough on exertion. Patients with cough-equivalent asthma tend to have normal breath sounds on examination, even during an exacerbation, but reversible bronchospasm may be demonstrated on pulmonary function testing.

Complications of asthma include pneumothorax, pneumomediastinum, and subcutaneous emphysema. These may require insertion of a chest tube for evacuation. Mild atelectasis may occur as a result of bronchial mucous plugging, but rarely requires intervention other than conventional bronchodilator therapy. In addition, rib fractures and costochondral strain may occur as a result of excessive coughing. Cough syncope, a rare complication of asthma, is noted most frequently in moderately obese, middle-aged asthmatic men. Finally, dysrhythmias may occur as a result of hypoxia, especially in patients who have received oral adrenergic agents.[8]

DIFFERENTIAL DIAGNOSIS

Wheezing, coughing, and dyspnea are present in many conditions. Common problems include pneumonia, bronchitis, croup, bronchiolitis, chronic obstructive lung disease, congestive heart failure, pulmonary embolism, allergic reactions, and upper airway obstruction from edema or a foreign body. Less common problems include cystic fibrosis, hypersensitivity pneumonitis, carcinoid syndrome, and exposure to odors, dust, and gas. A careful history and physical examination should help differentiate asthma from these other conditions.

EMERGENCY DEPARTMENT EVALUATION

The ability to perform a thorough history and physical examination before initiating treatment is often limited by the patient's dyspnea. Aggressive therapy directed at relieving airway obstruction begins as soon as a diagnosis of asthma is established. Meanwhile, an attempt is made to obtain a history from family members or the patient. Important points to establish include the following:

- Duration and onset of the current attack
- Identification of precipitating causes
- Type and amount of medications used before arrival in the emergency department
- Response to prior therapy, including current or previous use of steroids
- Frequency of emergency department visits and hospitalizations
- Previous need for intubation or ventilation
- History of concurrent medications and allergies
- History of concurrent medical problems

Immediate attention is also directed to the patient's appearance, vital signs, chest examination, and heart examination. The presence of a pulsus paradoxus is noted.

Judging the state of a patient's ventilatory status and pulmonary function on clinical grounds alone can be misleading. The degree of tachycardia and tachypnea often do not correlate well with the degree of airway obstruction. Pulsus paradoxus may be absent in up to one-third of severe asthmatics. Furthermore, wheezing is absent if airflow is minimal.[3] To complicate matters, all of the aforementioned clinical parameters can normalize with even minimal improvement in pulmonary function.[3,17] Therefore, quantification of airway changes must be assessed using either the forced expiratory volume in 1 second (FEV_1) or the peak expiratory flow rate (PEFR). An initial FEV_1 of less than 1 L (less than 30% predicted) or a PEFR of less than 100 L/min (less than 20% predicted) indicates severe obstruction.[22]

Hypoxemia is common during acute exacerbations.[20] Pulse oximetry may be useful in assessing and following oxygenation. A saturation of less than 91% generally correlates with severe hypoxemia. Arterial blood gas measurements (ABGs) need to be obtained only in patients experiencing severe or prolonged attacks. In general, hypercapnia, severe hypoxemia, or metabolic acidosis does not occur until the PEFR or FEV_1 is less than 25% of predicted values,[20] but young children and elderly patients commonly present exceptions to this rule. The degree of hypoxemia determined by the ABG generally reflects the extent of ventilation–perfusion mismatch. A normal or increased pCO_2 indicates severe airway obstruction and impending ventilatory failure.

Expectorated sputum may appear purulent because of the presence of eosinophils, but this finding may not reflect infection. A wet preparation of sputum may contain Charcot-Leyden crystals (eosinophilic granules), Curschmann spirals (mucus casts), and bacteria.

Chest radiographs may demonstrate hyperinflation and atelectasis but are usually nondiagnostic. A chest radiograph is necessary only if pneumonia, pneumothorax, or pneumomediastinum is suspected or if the patient fails to respond to aggressive bronchodilator therapy.[11]

The electrocardiogram, although it occasionally reveals evidence of right ventricular strain, is generally not helpful, except to rule out concurrent cardiac problems. All older patients, especially those with cardiac disease, should be monitored during therapy.[8]

Blood tests, including a complete blood count, are unlikely to help guide the acute management of an asthma attack. A theophylline level, however, should be obtained to guide therapy if theophylline is used.

Asthma scores that incorporate subjective and objective criteria (pulse, respiratory rate, pulsus paradoxus, subjective dyspnea, accessory muscle use, wheezing, PEFR) should not be relied on for predicting emergency treatment or disposition.[5,26]

EMERGENCY DEPARTMENT MANAGEMENT

Emergency department interventions are guided by pulmonary function tests (FEV_1, PEFR), vital signs, chest and heart examinations, and the patient's subjective assessment of dyspnea. The goal of emergency treatment is to ensure adequate oxygenation and to relieve airflow obstruction.

Unfortunately, no ideal therapy is available, and the use of multiple drug regimens is common. Supplemental humidified oxygen, inhaled beta-adrenergic agonists, oral or intravenous corticosteroids, and, to a lesser extent, inhaled anticholinergic agents are the mainstays of asthma treatment in the emergency

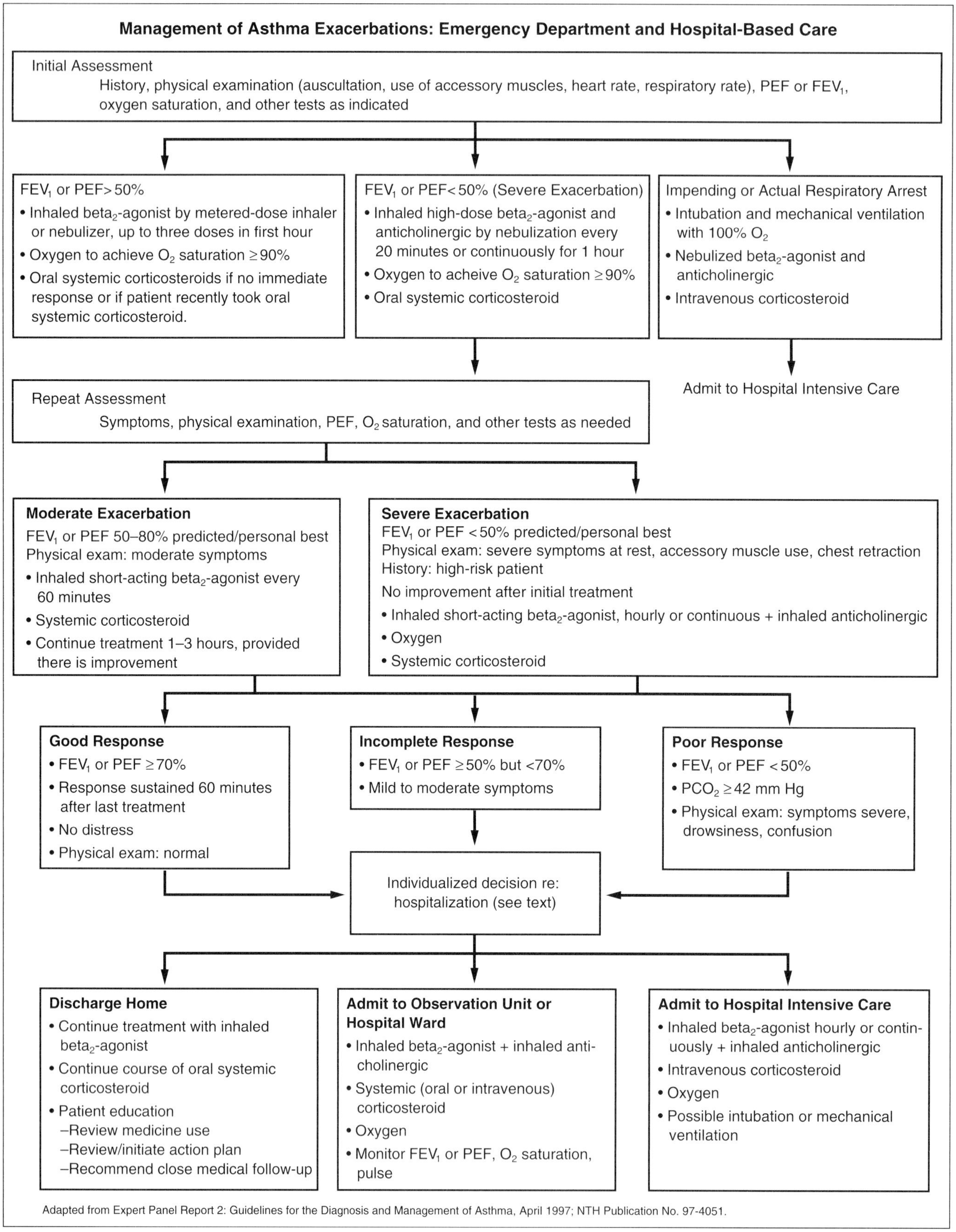

Figure 146.1. Management of asthma exacerbations: Emergency department and hospital-based care. (Adapted from *Expert Panel Report 2: Guidelines for the diagnosis and management of asthma, April 1997;* NIH Publication No. 97-4051. Bethesda, MD: Department of Health and Human Services, 1997.)

department. The methylxanthines (e.g., theophylline) have only a minor role in emergency management; the chromones are reserved for maintenance therapy only. The role of leukotriene modifiers, ketamine, and halothane remains to be further defined. Guidelines for the diagnosis and management of acute exacerbations of asthma have been established by the National Asthma Education Program Expert Panel (Fig. 146.1).[19]

Acute pharmacologic therapy can be divided into three categories: beta-adrenergic agonists, glucocorticoids, and anticholinergics. A fourth category of drugs, the methylxanthines, has only a minor role in the emergency department. A fifth category of drugs used to treat asthma, the chromones (e.g., cromolyn sodium), has no place in emergency treatment.

Beta-Adrenergic Agonists

Beta-adrenergic agonists are the drugs or choice for the management of acute bronchospasm. They produce bronchodilation by stimulating beta receptors, resulting in the formation of cyclic AMP, which results in relaxation of bronchial smooth muscle, inhibition of mediator release, and increase in mucociliary clearance. Drugs in this category include resorcinols, saligenins, and catecholamines (Table 146.1).

Resorcinols and saligenins available in the United States include metaproterenol, terbutaline, albuterol (salbutamol), and bitolterol mesylate. Aerosol forms are available for metaproterenol and albuterol. Metaproterenol, bitolterol mesylate, and albuterol are available in metered-dose inhalers. Aerosol agents and metered-dose inhalants are rapid-acting, are theoretically long-lasting, and may be repeated every 20 to 30 minutes in the acute situation. Salmeterol is a chemical derivative of albuterol with an extended duration of action and a bronchodilator effect ten times that of albuterol. Formoterol is similar, but is even longer acting than salmeterol. Neither has been studied for use in acute exacerbations of asthma.[17] Albuterol, metaproterenol, and terbutaline also are available in oral form. Terbutaline is available for subcutaneous injection.

The resorcinols and saligenins are highly $beta_2$ selective and are virtually devoid of cardiac side effects when given in inhaled or aerosol form. A frequent noncardiac side effect is tremor. Inhaled or aerosolized beta agonists rapidly promote bronchodilation comparable with that produced by parenteral agents, appear to be longer lasting, and cause fewer side effects. Treatments given every 20 to 30 minutes or in a continuous fashion result in more effective and sustained improvement of pulmonary function than treatments given less frequently.[21,23] The use of spacer devices improves drug delivery when patient technique is suboptimal.

Subcutaneous administration of beta agonists may be of use in the treatment of asthmatics who cannot use inhalation devices effectively, in patients in extremis, in patients who fail initial treatment with aerosol beta-adrenergic agents, or when preparation of aerosol or metered-dose agents for acute use risks delaying the initiation of therapy.[2]

The catecholamines (epinephrine, isoproterenol, isoetharine) have largely been supplanted by their more selective and longer acting derivatives. Epinephrine, a nonselective alpha- and beta-adrenergic agonist, may be given by oral inhalation (in a nonprescription preparation) or subcutaneously. The usual subcutaneous dose in adults is 0.3 to 0.5 mL of a 1:1000 solution, which may be repeated every 20 minutes to a total of three doses. Epinephrine reaches peak blood levels 20 to 40 minutes after injection, and its bronchodilating effects last up to 4 hours. Side effects include increased myocardial irritability, dysrhythmias, and nervousness. Although some studies suggest that epinephrine may be safely used in asthmatics over age 40, extreme caution should be used in patients with coronary artery disease.[8] Epinephrine is also available in a thioglycolate 1:200 preparation (Sus-Phrine) used for subcutaneous injection, with effects lasting up to 6 hours. Its side effects are similar to those of the 1:1000 preparation.

TABLE 146.1. Adrenergic Agents Used to Treat Acute Bronchospasm

Preparation	Dosage	Dosing[a]	Side Effects
Albuterol	5% solution 0.5 mL diluted in 2.5 mL saline, aerosolized inhalation	Every 20–30 min, up to 3 doses, then hourly	Uncommon, tremor
	4 puffs (90 μg/puff), metered-dose inhaler	Every 20–30 min, up to 3 doses, then hourly	Uncommon, tremor
Bitolterol mesylate	4 puffs (370 mg/puff), metered-dose inhaler	Every 20–30 min, up to 3 doses, then hourly	Tremor (musculoskeletal)
Epinephrine hydrochloride	0.3–0.5 mL 1:1000 aqueous solution, subcutaneous injection	Every 20 min up to a total of 3 doses	Myocardial irritability, dysrhythmias, nervousness, hypertension, tremor (CNS)
Epinephrine in thioglycolate	0.15–0.25 mL 1:200 aqueous solution, subcutaneous injection	Every 6 h	Myocardial irritability, dysrhythmias, nervousness
Isoetharine	1% solution, 0.5 mL diluted in 1.5 mL saline, aerosolized inhalation	Every 20–30 min, up to 3 doses, then hourly	Uncommon
	4 puffs (34 mg/puff), metered-dose inhaler	Every 20–30 min, up to 3 doses, then hourly	
Isoproterenol	0.5% solution 0.5 mL in 2.5 mL saline, aerosolized inhalation		Paradoxical bronchospasm
	2 puffs (131 μg/puff), metered-dose inhaler	Every 3 h	Paradoxical bronchospasm
	0.5–5 μg/min, 1 mg 1:5000 diluted in 500 mL 5% dextrose solution, intravenous drip		Myocardial necrosis, dysrhythmias, hypotension
Metaproterenol	5% solution, 0.3 mL diluted in 2.5 mL saline, aerosolized inhalation	Every 20–30 min, up to 3 doses, then hourly	Uncommon, tremor
	4 puffs (0.65 mg/puff), metered-dose inhaler	Every 20–30 min, up to 3 doses, then hourly	Uncommon, tremor
Terbutaline sulfate	0.25–0.50 mg, subcutaneous injection	Every 30–60 min, up to a total of 3 doses	Tachycardia, hypertension, tremor (CNS)

[a] Doses and dosing frequencies during acute exacerbation; maintenance doses and dosing intervals may vary from the acute situation.

Isoetharine is more $beta_2$ selective than epinephrine and is as effective a bronchodilator as albuterol.[10] It is supplied as a 1% aerosol solution or in a metered-dose inhaler preparation. Its duration of action is 30 to 90 minutes. Doses may be repeated every 20 to 30 minutes during an acute attack.

Isoproterenol is a potent selective beta-adrenergic agent. It is available in aerosol form, in a metered-dose inhaler, and as an intravenous solution. The duration of action of the inhaled form is 3 hours, and inhalations may be repeated every 3 hours. Use of isoproterenol inhalants was associated with a number of asthmatic deaths in England and Wales in the 1960s, suggesting that it should be used cautiously, although a cause-and-effect relation was not demonstrated. In addition, inhaled isoproterenol may cause paradoxical bronchospasm. Intravenous isoproterenol should be reserved for dire emergencies, and strict monitoring of heart rate, rhythm, and blood pressure is a must.

Glucocorticoids

Glucocorticoids should be administered to all patients whose acute airway obstruction is not promptly relieved by an inhaled beta-adrenergic agent. Patients who receive glucocorticoids early require fewer hospital admissions and sustain fewer relapses after discharge from the emergency department.[6] Corticosteroids are thought to exert their effect on acute asthma by reducing airway inflammation. The initial dose is 60 to 125 mg of intravenous methylprednisolone or 40 to 80 mg of oral methylprednisolone, or the equivalent dose of prednisone.[27] Doses of 60 to 80 mg intravenous or oral methylprednisolone (or the equivalent dose of prednisone) every 6 to 8 hours should follow. Oral administration of corticosteroids is equivalent to intravenous administration. Because the effects of steroids are not noted for 4 or more hours, vigorous concomitant bronchodilator therapy must be continued. There is no place for inhaled steroids in the emergency department.

Anticholinergic Agents

There has been a resurgence of enthusiasm for the use of anticholinergic agents to treat acute bronchoconstriction. These medications, including ipratropium bromide and glycopyrrolate, antagonize the neuromuscular transmitter acetylcholine at the postganglionic parasympathetic receptor, reducing vagally mediated bronchoconstriction in the larger central airways. There may be an additive effect when beta-adrenergic agents and anticholinergic agents are used together, although this finding is not securely established.[9,14a] Peak anticholinergic bronchodilation is achieved within 1 to 2 hours. Aerosolized atropine sulfate and glycopyrrolate, although effective, have fallen out of favor because of the high incidence of anticholinergic side effects (tachycardia, restlessness, irritability, dry mouth, thirst, and difficulty swallowing).

Methylxanthines

Theophylline and its salts have been used to treat acute bronchospasm for over 50 years. Studies suggest that the methylxanthines, when used alone or in combination with beta agonists during an acute episode, are associated with an increased incidence of side effects but do little to relieve bronchospasm. Methylxanthines have a narrow therapeutic–toxic window and are subject to many interactions with other drugs. Toxicity may result in life-threatening cardiac dysrhythmias or seizures.

Patients on chronic theophylline therapy who present with acute bronchospasm and a subtherapeutic theophylline level may benefit from oral theophylline or intravenous aminophylline, but methylxanthines otherwise should play no significant role in the acute treatment of airflow obstruction. There is controversy over the utility of aminophylline in patients requiring hospitalization.[15]

Other Agents

Magnesium sulfate, a physiologic regulator of intracellular calcium flux, is an effective bronchodilator. In addition to preventing histamine release from mast cells and opposing the action of acetylcholine, magnesium directly inhibits bronchial smooth muscle contraction. Both aerosolized magnesium (0.66 g in 10 mL of saline) and intravenous magnesium solutions (1.2 g over 20 minutes) have been used investigationally to treat asthmatics who have failed maximal standard therapy, although neither form is currently approved for this indication in the United States. Bronchodilation is observed within 2 to 5 minutes after administration, but it disappears rapidly after treatment is discontinued; thus, additional bronchodilator therapy must accompany the use of magnesium. Side effects include hypotension, malaise, and a warm sensation. Cardiac rhythm, blood pressure, pulse, neurologic status, and renal function must be monitored closely.[26]

Nedocromil and cromolyn inhibit the release of inflammatory cytokines from mast cells, but they have no role in acute management. Likewise, leukotriene inhibitors, although useful in long-term management, are not indicated for emergency department treatment.

Heliox, an 80:20 mixture of helium and oxygen, should be considered in patients with respiratory acidosis who fail conventional therapy. Helium is a low-density, biologically inert gas that lowers airway resistance and decreases respiratory work. Significant improvement may be noted within 10 to 20 minutes of initiating therapy.[12]

If the patient deteriorates or fails to improve despite intensive therapy, intubation and mechanical ventilation must be considered. Although there are no absolute criteria other than respiratory arrest and coma, the following patients should be considered for intubation and mechanical ventilation:

- Those with worsening pulmonary function tests despite vigorous bronchodilator therapy
- Those with decreasing pO_2, increasing pCO_2, or progressive respiratory acidosis
- Those with declining mental status or increasing fatigue.

Noninvasive respiratory therapies such as continuous positive airway pressure (CPAP) and biphasic positive airway pressure (BiPAP) have been shown to reduce the work of breathing and to improve oxygenation in some causes of respiratory failure. At this time, no clinical studies have been performed to evaluate these therapies in the treatment of acute asthma.

Expiratory airflow obstruction can result in air trapping and higher lung volumes in mechanically ventilated asthmatics. This condition may result in "auto-PEEP," a continuously increased intrathoracic pressure that may decrease venous return and cause hypotension. Auto-PEEP may be avoided by using a rapid inspiratory flow rate, a reduced respiratory frequency, and a prolonged expiratory phase. This type of mechanical ventilation is commonly referred to as "permissive hypercapnia." An acute deterioration can be treated by simply disconnecting the patient from the ventilator and allowing the lungs to deflate completely before reconnecting it.

The anesthetic agent halothane and the dissociative agent ketamine are potent bronchodilators. Both have a rapid onset of action and a rapid decay of effects. Although both are direct myocardial depressants, ketamine indirectly stimulates catecholamine release. Although the optimal dose for ketamine has not been established, a dose of up to 2 mg/kg has produced bronchodilation in critically ill asthmatics.[16] Ketamine is contraindicated in patients with ischemic heart disease, severe hypertension, preeclampsia, or increased intracranial pressure; increased secretions are common, and hallucinations ("emergence reaction") are not uncommon. Side effects of 1% halothane include cardiac dysrhythmias and increased intrapulmonary shunting. Close monitoring of heart rate, ABGs, and blood pressure is essential when using either agent.[20,24]

Narcotics, sedatives, and tranquilizers should be avoided in acute asthma, because respiratory arrest may occur after their use. Mucolytics, expectorants, and hydration do not aid in the treatment of asthma. Antibiotics are advisable only when the sputum Gram stain or wet preparation show evidence of bacterial infection.

Asthma in Pregnancy

About 0.4% to 1.3% of pregnant women suffer from asthma. One-third improve during pregnancy, one-third remain unchanged, and one-third become worse. Asthma therapy during pregnancy is directed at providing adequate oxygenation for both mother and fetus. The management of pregnant asthmatics is essentially the same as for nonasthmatics. The use of subcutaneous or inhaled beta-adrenergic agents, theophylline, and corticosteroids appears to be safe during pregnancy.[7,13]

DISPOSITION

Several asthma-scoring indices have been proposed to predict the need for hospitalization, but all have proven disappointing.[5,22] The following patients should be considered for hospital admission:

- Those whose condition deteriorates in the emergency department
- Those who return for further therapy within several days after emergency department discharge
- Dyspneic patients with significant hypoxemia (pO_2 less than 60), hypercapnia, or acidosis
- Patients with a pretreatment FEV_1 less than 1.0 L (less than 30% predicted) or a PEFR less than 100 L/min (less than 20% predicted), and a posttreatment FEV_1 less than 2.1 L (less than 60% predicted) or a PEFR less than 300 L/min (less than 60% predicted)
- Patients who remain subjectively dyspneic after aggressive therapy
- Patients with continued abnormal vital signs after therapy
- Unreliable patients

Even patients who improve enough to be discharged from the emergency department have residual airway obstruction for up to several weeks after the acute episode subsides.[19] Therefore, arrangements must be made for ongoing treatment and early follow-up. An 8- to 10-day course of oral corticosteroids (40 to 60 mg/d methylprednisolone and, in the practice of many clinicians, tapered) and a 10-day treatment regimen of a beta$_2$-adrenergic metered-dose inhaler (two puffs as needed, up to every 4 to 6 hours) should be prescribed. In addition, the role of chronic aerosolized steroids or cromolyn sulfate should be discussed with the patient. Instruction in the proper use of the inhaler is essential. Patients on chronic theophylline therapy should be continued on a long-acting preparation. If oral theophylline is used, the serum level must be monitored.

COMMON PITFALLS

- Failure to recognize that a silent chest or a normal pCO_2 is a sign of severe obstructive disease and may result in respiratory arrest.
- Withholding beta-agonist therapy in the emergency department because of beta-agonist use at home. This approach has no scientific basis and is extremely dangerous.
- Failure to use measurements of pulmonary function, in addition to clinical and subjective parameters of dyspnea, when judging the adequacy of bronchodilator therapy.
- Failure to give glucocorticoids to all but the mildest asthmatics, especially in those who fail to respond to one or two doses of beta agonists.

References

1. American Thoracic Society. Definition and classification of chronic bronchitis, asthma, and pulmonary emphysema. *Am Rev Respir Dis* 1987;134:225.
2. Appel D, Karpel JP, Sherman M. Epinephrine improves expiratory flow rates in patients with asthma who do not respond to inhaled metaproterenol sulfate. *J Allergy Clin Immunol* 1989;84:90.
3. Bray WR, Gilman MJ, Slovis C. A comparison of aerosolized glycopyrrolate and metaproterenol in acute asthma. *Am Rev Respir Dis* 1986;133:320.
4. Carden DL, Nowak RM, Sarkar D, et al. Vital signs including pulsus paradoxus in the assessment of acute bronchial asthma. *Ann Emerg Med* 1983;12:80.
5. Centor RM, Yarbrough B, Wood JP. Inability to predict relapse in acute asthma. *N Engl J Med* 1984;310:577.
6. Chapman KR, Verbeek PR, White JG, et al. Effect of a short course of prednisone in the prevention of early relapse after the emergency room treatment of acute asthma. *N Engl J Med* 1991;324:788.
7. Coutts II, White RJ. Asthma in pregnancy. *J Asthma* 1991;28:433.
8. Cydulka R, Davison R, Grammer L. The use of epinephrine in the treatment of older adult asthmatics. *Ann Emerg Med* 1988;17:322.
9. Cydulka RK, Emerman CE. Effects of combined treatment with glycopyrrolate and albuterol in acute exacerbation of asthma. *Ann Emerg Med* 1994;23:270.
10. Emerman CL, Cydulka RK, Effron DE, et al. A randomized, controlled comparison of isoetharine and albuterol in the treatment of acute asthma. *Ann Emerg Med* 1991;20:1090.
11. Findley LJ, Sahn SA. The value of the chest roentgenogram in acute asthma in adults. *Chest* 1981;80:535.
12. Gluck EH. Helium-oxygen mixtures in intubated patients with status asthmaticus and respiratory acidosis. *Chest* 1990;98:693.
13. Greenberger PA, Patterson R. Management of asthma during pregnancy. *N Engl J Med* 1985;312:897.
14. Harrison BD, Stokes TC, Hart GJ, et al. Need for intravenous hydrocortisone in addition to oral prednisolone in patients admitted to hospital with severe asthma without ventilatory failure. *Lancet* 1986;1:181.

14a. Karpel JP, Schacter EN, Fanta C, et al. A comparison of ipratropium and albuterol vs albuterol alone for the treatment of acute asthma. *Chest* 1996;110:611–616.

15. Kelly HW. Should we stop using theophylline for the treatment of the hospitalized patient with status asthmaticus? *Ann Pharmacother* 1989;23:995.
16. L'Hommedieu CS, Arens JJ. The use of ketamine for the emergency intubation of patients with status asthmaticus. *Ann Emerg Med* 1987;16:568.
17. Lofdahl CG. Formoterol fumarate, a new beta$_2$-adrenoreceptor agonist. *Allergy* 1989;44:264.
18. McFadden ER, Gilbert IA. Asthma. *N Engl J Med* 1992;327:1928.
19. Management of exacerbations of asthma. In: *Guidelines for the diagnosis and management of asthma: National Asthma Education Program Expert Panel Report*. Bethesda, MD: Department of Health and Human Services, 1991 (NIH publication 91-3042).
20. Martin TG, Elenbaas RM, Pingleton SH. Use of peak expiratory flow rates to eliminate unnecessary arterial blood gases in acute asthma. *Ann Emerg Med* 1982;11:70.
21. Nelson MS. Frequency of inhaled metaproterenol in the treatment of acute asthma exacerbation. *Ann Emerg Med* 1990;19:21.
22. Nowak RM, Pensler MI, Sarkar DD. Comparison of peak expiratory flow and FEV_1, admission criteria for acute bronchial asthma. *Ann Emerg Med* 1982;11:64.
23. Olshaker J. The efficacy and safety of a continuous albuterol protocol for the treatment of acute adult asthma attacks. *Am J Emerg Med* 1993;11:131.
24. O'Rourke PP, Crone RK. Halothane in status asthmaticus. *Crit Care Med* 1982;10:341.
25. Self TH. Inhaled albuterol and oral prednisone therapy in hospitalized adult asthmatics: does aminophylline add any benefit? *Chest* 1990;98:1317.
26. Skobeloff EM, Spivey WH, McNamara RM. Intravenous magnesium sulfate for the treatment of acute asthma in the emergency department. *JAMA* 1989;262:1210.
27. Webb JR. Dose response of patients to oral corticosteroid treatment during exacerbation of asthma. *BMJ* 1986;292:1045.

CHAPTER 147
Chronic Obstructive Pulmonary Disease

Erica E. Remer and David S. Howes

Chronic obstructive pulmonary disease (COPD) comprises a spectrum of chronic respiratory diseases characterized by cough, sputum production, dyspnea, airflow limitation, and impaired gas exchange. The mortality rate is greater than 50% within 10 years of diagnosis.[7] Affecting at least 15 million Americans, COPD is the fourth leading cause of death and costs more than $15 billion dollars for treatment annually.[6,7]

The term *COPD* includes conditions, other than asthma, that have the common feature of airflow obstruction. Chronic bronchitis is characterized clinically by a chronic productive cough that is due to excessive bronchial mucus production and airway inflammation. To be called *chronic bronchitis,* the cough must be present for 3 months a year in at least two successive years. *Pulmonary emphysema,* in contrast, is defined pathologically by an irreversible enlargement of the alveolar air spaces, with associated destruction of the alveolar wall and pulmonary capillary bed. Patients suffering from pure forms of each condition are the exception, and most patients exhibit characteristics of both.

The predominant risk factor for COPD is tobacco use.[5,17] However, 5% to 10% of patients with COPD have never smoked, implicating other casual factors.[3] Other risk factors include environmental pollution, passive smoke inhalation, occupational exposure, and repeated respiratory infections.[5,17] There may also be genetic factors, the best defined being α_1-antitrypsin deficiency.[17] Regardless of the inciting etiology, the ultimate outcome is irreversible airflow limitation.

The natural course of COPD is one of progressively worsening dyspnea, hypoxemia, and diminished exercise tolerance, with recurrent exacerbations. Many COPD patients have a component of reversible airway obstruction,[7] but the fixed component seems to be the major determinant of outcome. In fact, the FEV_1 is the best prognostic indicator of disability and mortality.[4,14,17] Chronic hypoxemia leads to progressive clinical deterioration due to cor pulmonale, which worsens already diminished lung function. Recurrent episodes of infection and respiratory failure ultimately result in death. Long-term ambulatory oxygen therapy is the only treatment that has been demonstrated to prolong life in patients with advanced COPD.[4,6]

CLINICAL PRESENTATION

All patients with COPD exhibit airflow obstruction, but the pure forms of emphysema and chronic bronchitis have distinctive clinical features. Patients with emphysema tend to hyperventilate to compensate for the lungs' decreased ability to oxygenate the blood. These classic "pink puffers" work hard to establish a near-normal pO_2, and they appear barrel-chested, dyspneic, and tachypneic. They use pursed-lip breathing to create positive end-expiratory pressure in order to prevent early airway closure. Breath sounds are markedly diminished, with a prolonged expiratory phase.[15]

In contrast, patients with chronic bronchitis tolerate hypoxemia well and make no effort to hyperventilate. Chronic hypoxia induces a secondary polycythemia that, combined with the cyanosis of marked desaturation of hemoglobin, produces a plethoric appearance. These patients tolerate an elevated pCO_2 and have a less labored respiratory pattern. With the decreased work of breathing, the chronic bronchitic does not suffer from muscle wasting like the emphysematous patient. These features produce the picture of the "blue bloater." Lung examination reveals rhonchi, rales, and variable wheezing.[15]

Most patients presenting with an acute exacerbation of COPD do not fit either picture precisely. Patients typically complain of dyspnea and chest tightness and often note a change in the character of their sputum. Physical examination may reveal tachypnea and a variable degree of respiratory distress, as evidenced by accessory muscle use, retractions, and cyanosis. On auscultation, one may hear diminished breath sounds, a prolonged expiratory phase, wheezing, rales, or rhonchi. Signs of cor pulmonale should be sought: a centrally displaced point of maximal impulse, heart gallop, tricuspid murmur, peripheral edema, jugular venous distention or hepatojugular reflux, and hepatomegaly. This complication of long-standing hypoxemia is associated with substantial mortality.[15]

The causes of exacerbation include respiratory infection, noncompliance with (or underdosing of) medications, changes in weather, exposure to certain drugs (e.g., sedatives or beta-blockers), cardiac dysrhythmias, left ventricular dysfunction, and environmental exposure to pollens, fumes, allergens, or other irritants. Patients typically present with a gradual, but progressive, deterioration over hours to days.

Acute decompensation may be the result of a number of other conditions. Spontaneous pneumothorax in COPD carries a significantly higher complication and mortality rate than in patients with a more normal cardiorespiratory status. The chronic bronchitic patient is predisposed to embolic and thrombotic phenomena due to the hyperviscosity associated with polycythemia. Other disorders, such as congestive heart failure (CHF), pneumonia, acidosis, or renal or hepatic failure, may also overwhelm the COPD patient's limited reserves, resulting in respiratory failure.

DIFFERENTIAL DIAGNOSIS

COPD is a clinical diagnosis; it is usually made after extended observation of a patient at risk (most commonly due to cigarette smoking) who demonstrates progressive lung dysfunction. Because those at risk are likely to have sedentary lifestyles, they may present only when an acute event precipitates dyspnea at rest, unmasking previously undiagnosed lung disease.

Other conditions must also be considered in the patient who presents to the emergency department with wheezing, cough, dyspnea, or respiratory failure. Pneumonia or acute bronchitis may present with varying degrees of shortness of breath, cough, and bronchospasm with wheezing. Previously undiagnosed COPD may be discovered after the acute pneumonic process has resolved. Dyspnea and hypoxemia may also be seen in pulmonary embolism. An acute onset of respiratory symptoms and pleuritic chest pain, associated with risk factors such as recent surgery, malignancy, or immobility, or a swollen leg suggestive of deep venous thrombosis, strongly suggest consideration of this entity. It is often a challenge to diagnose or rule out left ventricular dysfunction in the face of COPD.[20] CHF may present with cough, dyspnea, and hypoxemia. Some patients exhibit wheezing, referred to as "cardiac asthma." Orthopnea, paroxysmal nocturnal dyspnea, and cardiomegaly are suggestive of CHF, but COPD patients with cor pulmonale may well demonstrate jugular venous distention. The chest radiograph may assist in distinguishing the two: Lack of cardiomegaly and pulmonary venous redistribution, and the presence of bullae and hyperinflation of the lungs suggests COPD. Many patients have histories of both conditions, and, if the clinical presentation and chest x-ray are not conclusive, it may be prudent to initiate therapy for both conditions.

EMERGENCY DEPARTMENT EVALUATION

If the patient's respiratory status allows a brief history to be taken, attention should be directed to the rapidity of onset and duration of symptoms, any precipitating factors, and the dosage and timing of medications. Information should be sought regarding the character of the sputum, the course of previous exacerbations, and any history of concomitant disease processes.

The physical examination focuses on the patient's mental status and the degree of respiratory distress. Hypercapnia and hypoxia can cause confusion, irritability, and somnolence. The cardiac and pulmonary examinations are vital, and repeated examinations are mandatory after therapeutic interventions in order to monitor the response to treatment.

Pulse oximetry is useful in monitoring the oxygen saturation and the effectiveness of oxygen supplementation. Arterial blood gas (ABG) analysis provides information on the $PaCO_2$, reflecting the adequacy of ventilation. Baseline or prior blood gas results may be useful for comparison; in general, hypercapnia with acidemia suggests acute respiratory failure.

The chest radiograph is usually done portably at the bedside, unless the patient is stable and can tolerate being transported to the radiology suite for posteroanterior (PA) and lateral films. Its primary utility is not in demonstrating changes consistent with COPD, but in ruling out other disease processes, such as pneumothorax, atelectasis, infiltrate, lung mass, or CHF.

Measurements of airflow do not always yield accurate assessments of the severity of illness, but may be more useful in judging the response to therapy. The peak expiratory flow rate (PEFR) is the marker most commonly used in the emergency department setting, but, in contradistinction to the asthmatic's response, it does not typically demonstrate a marked change in COPD.

Laboratory studies are generally of limited value. A serum theophylline level should be obtained in patients who are taking the medication, as it has a narrow therapeutic window and myriad drug interactions.[13] β-agonists may cause hypokalemia, although this is rarely clinically significant. A complete blood count may reveal anemia, which can compound the problem of hypoxemia, or a high white blood cell count, which may be a clue to pneumonia or another systemic infection. Other tests may be indicated if other disease processes are being investigated.

A twelve-lead electrocardiogram (ECG) may suggest right atrial enlargement, low voltage, or right ventricular hypertrophy or strain (cor pulmonale). Acute ischemic patterns must be appreciated to identify an acute coronary event that may be triggering or complicating the acute COPD attack. Continuous ECG monitoring may be useful in revealing dysrhythmias, which may be the cause or effect of the acute exacerbation.

EMERGENCY DEPARTMENT MANAGEMENT

The effective management of the acutely decompensated COPD patient depends on rapid estimation of the severity of illness, aggressive therapy, frequent reevaluation, and recognition of treatable entities that may have precipitated or complicated the patient's course. As with any critically ill patient, the patient should be placed on a cardiac monitor and have intravenous access established. It is difficult to determine whether dysrhythmias, such as atrial fibrillation and ventricular dysrhythmias, reflect coexisting heart disease or are caused by the COPD exacerbation and hypoxemia. Current evidence suggests that most patients exhibiting ventricular dysrhythmias have underlying left ventricular diastolic dysfunction.[8]

Treatment with oxygen is critical because hypoxemia is the major immediate threat to life. The goal is to maintain a PO_2 greater than 60 mm Hg, corresponding to an oxygen saturation of approximately 90%. A controlled oxygen delivery system is preferable; a Venturi mask system can deliver a precise oxygen concentration ranging from 24% to 50%. If the patient cannot tolerate a mask, low-flow oxygen (2 to 4 L/min) by nasal cannula may be utilized. Adjustments in oxygen delivery should be guided by continuous pulse oximetry and ABG determinations as needed. Although there is a concern of eliminating the hypoxic drive in chronic CO_2 retainers by administering oxygen, the percentage of patients at risk is small and the danger of hypoxemia far outweighs the potential hazard from hypercarbia.

Sympathomimetics, specifically β_2 agonists, are the agents of choice for acute COPD exacerbations, with maximal effectiveness noted in patients who have a reversible bronchospastic component.[5,7,10,19] Undesirable side effects include tremor, agitation, insomnia, headache, cardiac tachyarrhythmias, and hypokalemia.[19] Although bronchodilatation is equivalent when delivered by a metered-dose inhaler (MDI) coupled with a spacer device or by nebulizer aerosolization, the latter delivery method is generally used in the emergency department because dyspneic patients may have difficulty effectively performing the MDI procedure.[10,17] Although there are many β_2 agonists available, albuterol, 2.5 mg, is the most widely used agent. It is used either in repeated treatments every 20 to 60 minutes or by continuous nebulization in severe cases.

Although anticholinergics are considered by some investigators to be the bronchodilators of choice in the management of chronic disease,[3,11] their slower onset of action makes them a second-line treatment in the acute setting.[10,20] Ipratropium bromide, a congener of atropine, which has little systemic absorption when inhaled, minimizing undesirable anticholinergic effects,[10] has been shown to have an additive effect when combined with a β_2 agonist.[2,7,10] Anticholinergics are considered by some investigators to be the bronchodilators of choice in the management of chronic disease.[3,11]

Corticosteroids are considered useful in acute exacerbations of COPD,[5,17,20] but are not reliably beneficial when used long-term. Thus, patients who do not respond to steroids when stable may still benefit from them during acute attacks.[5,17] Because steroid use may suppress the adrenal–pituitary axis, patients with current or recent use may require steroids for the stress of any acute illness. High-dose parenteral methylprednisolone or oral prednisone appear to be equally effective. Inhaled steroids are not currently used in the acute setting.

Prior to the widespread availability of oral or inhaled, β_2 agonists, methylxanthines, most commonly theophylline preparations, were used as monotherapy for COPD. Symptomatic improvement of dyspnea and exercise tolerance is presumed to be at least partially due to mild bronchodilatation and positive inotropic effects on the diaphragm.[13] However, theophylline has a narrow therapeutic window and is associated with frequent adverse effects. Nausea, vomiting, cardiac dysrhythmias, and seizures can be seen even at therapeutic levels. Although current recommendations do not support instituting methylxanthine therapy in acute exacerbations, if a patient is maintained on theophylline, one might continue intravenous therapy as guided by drug levels. The therapeutic range is 10 to 20 mg, and a 1-mg/kg bolus of aminophylline can be expected to raise the serum level by approximately 2 mg/dL.

Other medications may be utilized in the management of acute COPD. Magnesium sulfate has modest bronchodilatory effects, and may be given a trial as adjunctive therapy to patients with severe exacerbations who have normal renal function.[18,20] There is no compelling evidence that mucolytics such as acetylcysteine are efficacious.[5] Inhibitors of neutrophilic inflammation, proteinases, and prostaglandins are currently under investigation, but there are, as yet, no data suggesting their utility in COPD.[1,3]

Although it is not typically addressed in the emergency department, cessation of tobacco use may well be the most important therapeutic intervention for COPD.[4,6,17] Bupropion and nicotine replacement therapy may be very useful in assisting patients to stop smoking.[3] COPD patients in the emergency department are also candidates to receive polyvalent pneumococcal and influenza vaccines in order to decrease the risk of future exacerbations.[1]

It is estimated that only half of acute COPD exacerbations are due to bacterial infection, with the predominant species being *Haemophilus influenzae, Moraxella catarrhalis,* and *Streptococcus pneumoniae*.[16] If dyspnea is associated with a change in the volume or purulence of sputum, or if a new infiltrate is noted on chest x-ray, antibiotics should be instituted.[1,6,10] A Gram stain of the sputum may aid in the selection of an antimicrobial, and adjustments may be needed according to geographic location and local resistance patterns. For less severe cases, oral therapy with tetracycline or doxycycline, a second- or third-generation cephalosporin, trimethoprim–sulfamethoxazole, or a β-lactam–β-lactamase inhibitor combination, with or without a macrolide, is appropriate.[1,6] In hospitalized patients with pneumonia or toxicity, parenteral therapy should be instituted with a second- or third-generation cephalosporin, or a β-lactam–β-lactamase inhibitor, possibly in conjunction with a macrolide.[6] Several of the newer fluoroquinolones, such as sparfloxacin and levofloxacin, may also see an expanded role in the treatment of acute COPD.[16]

In patients who do not respond to acute interventions and begin to show signs of respiratory failure, such as deterioration of mental status, worsening hypoxemia (PaO_2 less than 50 mm Hg), or worsening respiratory acidosis (pH less than 7.3), assisted ventilation is indicated.[10,20] BiPAP or CPAP may prevent the need for invasive airway management, and may result in fewer complications and shorter hospital stays.[12,20] However, in patients who are not candidates for these modalities, or in whom noninvasive ventilation has failed, endotracheal intubation and mechanical ventilation is the treatment of choice.

DISPOSITION

Most patients presenting with an acute exacerbation of COPD require admission to the hospital. However, if the patient responds to therapy and the vital signs and pulmonary function tests approach baseline, discharge may be considered if good follow-up is assured. The bronchodilator regimen should be maximized, and steroids should be continued for a short course. Antibiotics should be prescribed for exacerbations of chronic bronchitis. It should be recognized that approximately 15% of COPD patients who are discharged from the emergency department require readmission.[20]

Accepted criteria for hospitalization of patients with COPD include poor response to outpatient therapy, severe limitation of function, inability to eat or sleep due to dyspnea, presence of significant comorbid conditions, worsening respiratory failure, new or progressive cor pulmonale, and the need for invasive procedures, especially those requiring analgesics or sedatives.[4,20] Guidelines for admission to the intensive care unit are not as well defined. Treatment in an intensive care unit is indicated when the close observation, monitoring, and therapeutic interventions (including assisted ventilation) required by these patients cannot be provided elsewhere.

If transfer to another institution is required, it must be done carefully, because transfer is often associated with an interruption in treatment and increased patient fatigue. The transport team must be capable of managing the airway if decompensation occurs .

COMMON PITFALLS

- The COPD patient should not be expected to have as rapidly reversible disease as the asthmatic patient. Look for a slower course of improvement, and have a lower threshold for admission.
- Precipitating or complicating conditions may be overlooked when treating only the exacerbation of COPD. Thorough evaluation is mandatory.
- Oxygen should never be withheld due to concern about respiratory depression. If inadequate ventilation occurs, ventilatory support should be provided.
- It is easy to underestimate the severity of illness in patients with chronic dysfunction. Utilize radiography, pulse oximetry, ABG analyses, and pulmonary function tests liberally. Respect the patient's estimation of severity of illness.

References

1. Aboussouan LS. Acute exacerbations of chronic bronchitis. *Postgrad Med* 1996;99(4):89–90, 95–98, 101–102.
2. Anonymous. Routine nebulized ipratropium and albuterol together are better than either alone in COPD. The Combivent Inhalational Solution Study Group. *Chest* 1997;112(6):1514–1521.
3. Barnes PJ. New therapies for chronic obstructive pulmonary disease. *Thorax* 1998;53(2):137–147.
4. Celli BR. Standards for the optimal management of COPD: a summary. *Chest* 1998;113[4 Suppl]:283S–287S.
5. Ferguson GT. Management of COPD. Early identification and active intervention are crucial. *Postgrad Med* 1998;103(4):129–134, 136–141.
6. Fiel SB. Chronic obstructive pulmonary disease. Mortality and mortality reduction. *Drugs* 1996;52[Suppl 2]:55–60.
7. Friedman M. Changing practices in COPD. A new pharmacologic treatment algorithm. *Chest* 1995;107[5 Suppl]:194S–197S.
8. Fuso L, Incalzi R, Pistelli R, et al. Predicting mortality of patients hospitalized for acutely exacerbated chronic obstructive pulmonary disease. *Am J Med* 1995;98(3):272–277.
9. Hoyt JW. Debunking myths of chronic obstructive lung disease [Editorial; comment]. *Crit Care Med* 1997;25(9):1450–1451.
10. Ikeda A, Nishimura K, Izumi T. Pharmacological treatment in acute exacerbations of chronic obstructive pulmonary disease. *Drugs Aging* 1998; 12(2):129–137.
11. Levin DC, Little KS, Laughlin KR, et al. Addition of anticholinergic solution prolongs bronchodilator effect of beta 2 agonists in patients with chronic obstructive pulmonary disease. *Am J Med* 1996;100(1A):40S–48S.
12. Poponick JM, Renston JP, Emerman CL. Successful use of nasal BiPAP in three patients previously requiring intubation and mechanical ventilation. *J Emerg Med* 1996;15(6):785–788.
13. Ramsdell J. Use of theophylline in the treatment of COPD. *Chest* 1995;107[5 Suppl]:206S–209S.
14. Rennard SI. COPD: overview of definitions, epidemiology, and factors influencing its development. *Chest* 1998;113[4 Suppl]:235S–241S.
15. Rochester D. Respiratory muscles and ventilatory failure: 1993 perspective. *Am J Med Sci* 1993;305(6):394–402.
16. Schentag JJ, Tillotson GS. Antibiotic selection and dosing for the treatment of acute exacerbations of COPD. *Chest* 1997;112[6 Suppl]:314S–319S.
17. Senior RM, Anthonisen NR. Chronic obstructive pulmonary disease (COPD). Am *J Respir Crit Care Med* 1998;157(4 Pt 2):S139–S147.
18. Skorodin MS, Tenholder MF, Yetter B, et al. Magnesium sulfate in exacerbations of chronic obstructive pulmonary disease. *Arch Intern Med* 1995;155(5):496–500.
19. Ziment I. The beta-agonist controversy. Impact in COPD. *Chest* 1995;107[5 Suppl]:198S–205S.
20. Zuege DJ, Whitelaw WA. Management of acute respiratory failure in chronic obstructive pulmonary disease. *Curr Opin Pulm Med* 1997;3(3):190–197.

CHAPTER 148
Lung Cancer

Marc Borenstein

Lung cancer is the leading cause of cancer-related death in both men and women in the United States. The marked rise in the incidence of lung cancer closely parallels the increase in cigarette smoking by men during World War I and, subsequently, by women in the 1950s and 1960s. Occupational carcinogens for lung cancer have also been identified; they include asbestos, metal fumes, hydrocarbons, and radiation. Radon exposure in homes is an environmental risk factor for lung cancer in many regions of the United States. Cigarette smoking and occupational or environmental risk factors act synergistically to increase the risk of developing lung cancer markedly.[2,6]

Lung cancer is divided into four main histologic types: large-cell carcinoma, adenocarcinoma, squamous cell (epidermoid) carcinoma, and small-cell (formerly called oat-cell) carcinoma. Although cigarette smoking has been implicated in all four types, the strongest association is with squamous cell and small-cell carcinomas.

Lung cancer is staged using an internationally accepted T (tumor), N (node), M (metastases) system. Five basic stages are recognized[5,8]:

Stage 0: carcinoma *in situ*
Stage I: no lymph node involvement
Stage II: spread to immediately adjacent nodes
Stage III: large tumor or localized nodal spread
Stage IV: any distant metastasis

Patients are carefully staged on the basis of physical examination, laboratory findings, radiographs, and results of scans and biopsy to determine whether the tumor is localized. Operative therapy is determined based on the patient's ability to tolerate the stress of surgery and the diminished pulmonary function that results from a surgical lobectomy or pneumonectomy. Operative candidates are then evaluated as to whether the tumor is resectable or unresectable. Often, resectability can be determined with thoracic computed tomography, but, for many patients, a surgical procedure is required to establish it.

CLINICAL PRESENTATION

Clinical presentations of lung cancer in the emergency department are highly varied and depend on the histologic type as well as the extent of the cancer. Patients may present with symptoms related to local extension, distant spread of the tumor, paraneoplastic effects, or the complications of treatment.

The diagnosis of lung cancer should be considered in patients with persistent cough or hoarseness, recurrent bronchitis, unresolving or recurrent pneumonia, and hemoptysis.[1] A background of smoking or environmental exposure should greatly raise the physician's concern. The risk of developing lung cancer increases disproportionately with the duration and amount of smoking. A symptomatic patient with a history of previously treated lung cancer should be evaluated carefully for tumor recurrence or the development of a second primary tumor.

Local tumor extension can produce superior venal caval obstruction (SVC syndrome) or tracheal or esophageal compression. Symptoms such as cough, dyspnea, hoarseness, chest pain, and thoracic pain are frequently encountered. Tumor in the lung apex (superior sulcus) can be associated with a brachial plexopathy, Horner syndrome, and pain in the shoulder (Pancoast syndrome). Jaundice usually results from extrinsic nodal compression of the biliary tree.

The symptoms of metastatic disease are protean.[1,3] Central nervous system metastases may present as altered mental status, headache, or seizures. Bony pain may result from osseous metastases or pathologic fractures and typically precedes the development of clinically apparent neurologic deficits for weeks to months in patients with underlying spinal cord compression. Dyspnea may result from tumor infiltration, superimposed pneumonia, or complications of treatment. The patient may seek medical evaluation for a "lump" that has not gone away. Hepatic metastases usually present with right upper quadrant abdominal pain, anorexia, or nausea.

Paraneoplastic syndromes are frequent and are usually seen in association with small-cell carcinoma. Some of the more commonly encountered ones include the syndrome of inappropriate secretion of antidiuretic hormone, ectopic production of adrenocorticotropic hormone, and the Eaton-Lambert syndrome. Hypercalcemia is associated only with squamous cell carcinoma and can be used as a marker that reflects the persistence or regression of tumor. Migratory thrombophlebitis, nonbacterial thrombotic endocarditis, and disseminated intravascular coagulation (DIC) have all been described in association with lung cancer.[7]

Complications of treatment include nausea, vomiting, electrolyte abnormalities, neutropenia, fever, and sepsis. A dilated cardiomyopathy with congestive heart failure may occur secondary to anthracycline toxicity. Acute radiation pneumonitis may manifest as cough, dyspnea, and fever.

The specific histologic types of lung cancer are characteristically associated with a number of distinct clinical manifestations. Squamous cell (bronchogenic) carcinoma and small-cell carcinoma both occur centrally, leading to complications from compression of mediastinal structures such as the recurrent laryngeal nerve (hoarseness, voice changes) and the trachea (respiratory distress). Pancoast syndrome is most often associated with squamous cell carcinoma. SVC syndrome is typically caused by small-cell carcinoma. Adenocarcinoma and large-cell carcinoma tend to occur as peripheral tumors and do not usually produce local obstruction.

In contrast to other histologic types, small-cell lung cancer is highly responsive to chemotherapy, in part because of its characteristically rapid cell division. Small-cell carcinoma is likely to metastasize early, however, and a thorough workup is necessary to ensure accurate staging of this cancer. Bone marrow biopsy is positive in approximately 50% of patients with small-cell lung carcinoma, making this test an essential part of the initial staging workup.

DIFFERENTIAL DIAGNOSIS

All patients suspected of having cancer should have the diagnosis proven by biopsy. This principle also applies to a suspected first recurrence of cancer after curative surgery, radiation therapy, or chemotherapy. Although biopsy and tissue diagnosis are not germane to the immediate evaluation of the cancer patient in the emergency department, it is essential to understand this concept and to recognize its importance when arranging for appropriate follow-up for the emergency department patient suspected of having lung cancer.

The differential diagnosis of the most frequent emergency department presentations includes the following:

Cough: bronchitis, pneumonia, obstruction
Dyspnea: chronic obstructive pulmonary disease, congestive heart failure, pneumonia, pleural effusion
Chest pain: pleurisy, pneumonia, myocardial infarction, pneumothorax, pulmonary embolism
Thoracic pain: musculoskeletal, degenerative joint disease
Lymphadenopathy: inflammatory, infectious

If a pulmonary nodule is discovered on a chest radiograph, the differential diagnosis should include tuberculosis, fungal infection, and vascular abnormality.[4]

EMERGENCY DEPARTMENT EVALUATION

Although the range of potential presentations in lung cancer is broad, general guidelines can be used effectively in emergency management.

In the patient without a prior diagnosis of lung cancer, the emergency physician should ask about risk factors. A chest radiograph is the most useful test in most cases. It should be obtained in patients at risk: smokers, miners who present with persistent cough, and patients complaining of progressive hoarseness, voice changes, unresolved "bronchitis," recurrent pneumonias, or nontraumatic persistent chest pain.

In the patient with an established diagnosis of lung cancer (either in remission or under active treatment), the emergency physician must rule out serious complications, such as spinal cord compression, SVC syndrome, central nervous system metastasis, osseous metastasis, cytopenias, infection, and metabolic abnormalities. Complaints of cough, dyspnea, chest pain, bone pain, back pain, fever, headache, and changes in mental status must be regarded seriously. Laboratory testing should generally include a complete blood cell count; platelet count; determination of electrolytes, blood urea nitrogen, creatinine, and glucose; and chest radiograph. Skeletal radiographs, urinalysis, oximetry, arterial blood gases, and computed tomography may be indicated as well, depending on the specific clinical setting.

A common diagnostic error in the setting of known lung cancer is the failure to obtain adequate historical information regarding the type of lung cancer, the specific treatments received, and the dates of treatment. In some cases, the patient may not mention a history of lung cancer and may not have an understanding of the risks associated with microscopic residual disease. The patient may think that therapy was curative and fail to realize that there is a small but real risk of recurrence that requires ongoing surveillance.

EMERGENCY DEPARTMENT MANAGEMENT

The patient with lung cancer may present with life-threatening oncologic emergencies. These include airway compromise, respiratory insufficiency, fever with neutropenia, SVC compression, cardiac tamponade, seizures, hypercalcemia, hyponatremia, DIC, massive hemoptysis, altered mental status, pulmonary embolism, and overdose (accidental and intentional). Specific management principles are outlined in detail elsewhere in this text. The emergency physician must distinguish between those situations in which resuscitative measures are appropriate and those in which supportive and symptomatic care is indicated in lieu of endotracheal intubation, cardiopulmonary resuscitation, and ventilatory support. The patient may have a living will, an advance directive, or a do not resuscitate (DNR) order in place. The specific legal guidelines in this arena vary from state to state. Close communication with the patient's family and personal physician, if available, can be helpful. Seek it whenever possible.

DISPOSITION

Patients with cancer are frequently treated with complex regimens involving oncology, radiation therapy, surgery, and medical subspecialties. Care is usually coordinated by an oncologist, with close involvement of the patient's personal physician. After emergency assessment and stabilization, oncologic consultation is often invaluable to the emergency physician in determining further management and ultimate disposition. In some cases, the patient may be receiving investigational chemotherapy, and early consultation can provide important information regarding adverse reactions not readily available in general textbooks.

Patients with lung cancer who present with serious, life- or limb-threatening complications require urgent evaluation, treatment, and admission. Such complications include fever with neutropenia, pneumonia, sepsis, respiratory insufficiency (typically secondary to decompensated chronic obstructed pulmonary disease, irradiation, or chemotherapy), suspected spinal cord compression, and symptomatic SVC compression. They also include symptomatic or severe hyponatremia, symptomatic hypercalcemia, airway compromise, moderate hemoptysis, altered mental status, stroke, raised intracranial pressure, neurologic impairment (often secondary to paraneoplastic syndromes), coma, overdose (accidental or intentional), coagulopathy, and DIC.

Most patients who present *de novo* with symptoms suggestive of an underlying lung cancer can be evaluated and discharged from the emergency department with an emphasis on timely follow-up. Similarly, patients who have a history of previously treated lung cancer can often be managed on an outpatient basis, provided their presentation does not fall into one of the previously mentioned categories.

In general, few patients with lung cancer require transfer to another facility unless the hospital cannot provide a level of care consistent with the patient's needs. Alternatively, some patients may request transfer to another hospital where they have been receiving ongoing cancer care, particularly if they are receiving investigational treatment.

COMMON PITFALLS

- Failure to obtain a chest radiograph in the patient at risk for lung cancer or its recurrence
- Failure to recognize the high incidence of complications in the lung cancer patient population
- Failure to recognize the urgency and importance of back pain in the patient with lung cancer as potentially caused by spinal cord compression
- Failure to take a history thoroughly detailing the type, stage, and treatment of lung cancer
- Failure to obtain and thoroughly review medical records
- Failure to obtain oncology consultation for treatment planning

References

1. Anderson HA, Prakash UBS. Diagnosis of symptomatic lung cancer. *Semin Respir Med* 1982;3:165.
2. Frank AL. Epidemiology of lung cancer. In: Roth J, Ructersall J, Weisenburger T, eds. *Thoracic surgery*. Philadelphia: WB Saunders, 1989.

3. Grippi MA. Clinical aspects of lung cancer. *Semin Roentgenol* 1990;25:12.
4. Karsell PR, McDougall JC. Diagnostic tests for lung cancer. *Mayo Clin Proc* 1993;68:288.
5. Mountain CF. A new international staging system for lung cancer. *Chest* 1986;89[Suppl]:225.
6. Pastorino U, Berrino F, Gervasio A, et al. Proportion of lung cancers due to occupational exposure. *Int J Cancer* 1984;33:231.
7. Patel Am, Davilla DG, Peters SG. Paraneoplastic syndromes associated with lung cancer. *Mayo Clin Proc* 1993;68:278.
8. Sobin LH, Hermanek P, Hutter RVP. TNM classification of malignant tumors: a comparison between the new (1987) and the old editions. *Cancer* 1988;61:2310.

CHAPTER 149

Spontaneous Pneumothorax and Pneumomediastinum

Susan M. Dunmire

Spontaneous pneumothorax and pneumomediastinum are not infrequently encountered in emergency medicine. These entities should be considered in any individual who presents with the acute onset of shortness of breath, chest pain, or subcutaneous emphysema.

Pneumothorax is defined as the presence of gas within the pleural space. A pneumothorax occurring in the absence of penetrating or blunt injury to the chest wall is termed a *spontaneous pneumothorax*. This can be classified either as primary (idiopathic), in which there is no underlying pulmonary disease, or as secondary to any of a wide variety of causes. With large accumulations of air in the pleural space, a *tension pneumothorax* may develop, which leads to hypotension due to impaired venous return.

Although most authorities agree that a primary spontaneous pneumothorax is the result of rupture of small subpleural cysts or blebs, the etiology of these structural abnormalities (congenital vs. acquired) is still controversial. Spontaneous pneumothorax recurs in up to 50% of patients within 2 years. The recurrence is much more likely to be on the same side as the initial pneumothorax.

Another less common but interesting entity is *catamenial pneumothorax*. It is a spontaneous pneumothorax occurring in young girls at the time of menstruation. Although its etiology is multifactorial, in some patients it is due to small implants of endometrial tissue in the pleural lining.[3,5,11]

Spontaneous *pneumomediastinum* is the result of alveolar rupture, with dissection of air along the bronchus and into the mediastinum. Although it is usually a benign entity, serious causes, such as esophageal rupture, must be ruled out. The cause of pneumomediastinum often cannot be identified. It can occur in patients with a history of vigorous vomiting or in those who use repetitive and prolonged Valsalva maneuvers to enhance the effects of inhaled, pipe-smoked cocaine.[10]

CLINICAL PRESENTATION

Primary (idiopathic) spontaneous pneumothorax commonly occurs in young adults (male-to-female ratio, 5:1) between the ages of 20 and 40.[8] Affected individuals tend to be tall and thin and frequently have a history of cigarette smoking.[2] There is also a strong association with Marfan syndrome.[9]

Patients with spontaneous pneumothorax typically present with the sudden onset of constant ipsilateral chest or shoulder pain that may or may not increase with inspiration. The majority of patients complain of dyspnea, although the severity of that symptom depends on the size of the pneumothorax. Most patients have the onset of symptoms at rest or during sleep. Rarely, spontaneous pneumothorax can present as a tension pneumothorax with severe cardiopulmonary compromise.

Symptoms in adults with spontaneous pneumomediastinum include retrosternal chest pain and, less frequently, subcutaneous emphysema due to tracking of air into the chest wall, neck, face, abdominal wall, and scrotum. If enough air accumulates in the mediastinum, the pleura can rupture, resulting in an associated pneumothorax. Spontaneous pneumomediastinum in infants is a much more serious entity and can cause cardiopulmonary compromise by compression of the hilum.[13]

DIFFERENTIAL DIAGNOSIS

Pulmonary embolism, exacerbation of chronic obstructive pulmonary disease (COPD) or asthma, pneumonia, and myocardial ischemia should all be in the differential diagnosis of a patient with shortness of breath and chest pain. Often, the entity of spontaneous pneumothorax is not considered until the chest radiograph is obtained.

Spontaneous pneumomediastinum usually presents as substernal chest pain. The differential diagnosis includes myocardial ischemia, gastroesophageal reflux, pulmonary embolism, and pneumonia.

Once the diagnosis of pneumothorax has been made, the physician is obligated to search for the underlying cause. In the case of spontaneous pneumothorax, it is important to reevaluate the history and physical examination to ensure that there is no sign of blunt or penetrating trauma. An elderly person may have forgotten a recent fall, resulting in rib fractures and an underlying pneumothorax. A puncture site in the neck or supraclavicular area can easily be missed in an unsuspected drug abuser who has penetrated the pleural space. In patients with spontaneous pneumomediastinum, it is also essential that esophageal rupture be ruled out.

One of the most common causes of secondary pneumothorax is COPD with rupture of bullae through the visceral pleura. The presentation can be misleading, in that patients may report only a worsening of chronic dyspnea. The unsuspected pneumothorax is often found on chest radiography during the evaluation of a COPD exacerbation. Because these patients already have compromised pulmonary function, the pneumothorax is usually treated aggressively and the patient monitored closely.

Pneumocystis carinii pneumonia has become an increasingly common cause of secondary pneumothorax as the population of patients with acquired immunodeficiency disease rises. A subgroup of patients with *Pneumocystis* pneumonia have an accelerated inflammatory response, with spontaneous rupture of necrotic lung tissue, resulting in pneumothorax.[1]

Other less common causes of secondary pneumothorax include malignancy, asthma (sometimes presenting as sudden severe respiratory compromise), pulmonary infarction, histiocytosis X, and Hamman-Rich syndrome (acute interstitial pulmonary fibrosis). Because, as previously noted, patients with significant underlying lung pathology may have respiratory decompensation with a relatively small pneumothorax, they require aggressive therapy and close monitoring.

EMERGENCY DEPARTMENT EVALUATION

Physical examination is often not very helpful in making the diagnosis of spontaneous pneumothorax. Patients often exhibit mild resting tachycardia and tachypnea. Depending on the extent of the pneumothorax, breath sounds may be diminished unilaterally. The presence of hypotension, tachycardia (more than 140 beats per minute), or tracheal deviation should immediately alert the emergency physician to the possibility of a tension pneumothorax requiring emergent decompression.

The diagnosis of pneumothorax is usually made by chest radiography, which reveals a peripheral lucent area containing no lung markings. Films taken in maximal expiration with the patient in an upright position optimize visualization of small pneumothoraces. The size of a pneumothorax may be roughly gauged from the plain chest film, but such estimates are notoriously unreliable. Algorithms that yield more accurate estimates of size are available but are relatively complicated to apply.[7]

Patients with a significant (greater than 25%) pneumothorax have an increase in the alveolar–arterial oxygen gradient, although an arterial blood gas is rarely necessary.[6] The electrocardiogram is not helpful for diagnosis. Nonspecific changes, including T-wave inversion in the precordial leads, decreased amplitude of the R wave, and left axis deviation, are often noted.

The diagnosis of a spontaneous pneumomediastinum is often overlooked and requires a thorough examination and a high index of suspicion. On physical examination, auscultation of the heart may reveal a crunching sound during systole (Hamman sign).[4] Rarely, subcutaneous air may be present. On chest radiography, a very thin lucent stripe can be seen outlining the heart and mediastinum. A lateral neck radiograph may reveal subcutaneous air. The electrocardiogram is useful only in helping to rule out ischemia in the patient presenting with substernal chest pain.

EMERGENCY DEPARTMENT MANAGEMENT

Most patients with primary spontaneous pneumothorax do not have significant cardiopulmonary compromise. Any hemodynamic instability should suggest the presence of tension pneumothorax requiring immediate needle decompression, followed by tube thoracostomy.

Invasive treatment of a spontaneous pneumothorax can be accomplished by several methods. Many simple pneumothoraces (greater than 25% or symptomatic) can be treated by placement of a pigtail catheter. Using the Seldinger technique, a pigtail catheter can be inserted at the anterior axillary line between the fourth and fifth ribs (nipple line). Care should be taken when the wire is introduced into the pleural space, and the clinician must be certain that all of the side holes of the catheter are within the pleural space. The pigtail catheter is then attached to suction. These patients should be admitted for observation overnight.

A pneumothorax that occurs in the setting of chest wall trauma should be treated with a tube thoracostomy to drain a possible coexisting hemothorax. These patients also require admission to the hospital and close monitoring.

The major controversy in the management of spontaneous pneumothorax arises when there is less than 25% collapse, and revolves around whether to allow the air to reabsorb spontaneously or to actively remove the air. It is estimated that pleural air is spontaneously reabsorbed at a rate of 1.0% to 1.5% of the volume of the hemithorax per day. Therefore, a small pneumothorax (less than 15%) would be expected to be reabsorbed within 10 to 15 days. A conservative approach would be to allow spontaneous reabsorption in asymptomatic young patients with a primary spontaneous pneumothorax of 15% or less. Some less conservative practitioners would increase this threshold for more active treatment to 25%. Those with three or more recurrences of a spontaneous pneumothorax are usually considered candidates for thoracoscopic surgery.

Management of pneumomediastinum is conservative. It is essential, however, to exclude potentially catastrophic causes such as Boerhaave syndrome (esophageal rupture), which has a high mortality. A contrast-medium–enhanced esophagram is usually recommended in all patients with spontaneous pneumomediastinum,[12] although many clinicians choose to observe patients who are minimally symptomatic, appear well, and have developed pneumomediastinum after straining or vigorous Valsalva maneuvers.

DISPOSITION

Appropriate disposition of patients with spontaneous pneumothorax depends on the size of the pneumothorax, the therapeutic approach chosen, the reliability of the patient, and the availability of outpatient follow-up.

Patients with a small primary spontaneous pneumothorax, for which the physician has opted for conservative management (i.e., observation and spontaneous reabsorption), should have a follow-up radiograph within 24 hours to make sure the pneumothorax has not enlarged. If it has not, a follow-up radiograph should be performed in 7 to 10 days. Patients should be instructed to return for any increase in shortness of breath or chest pain or the development of fever.

Patients who have undergone placement of a pigtail catheter or a tube thoracostomy must be admitted to the hospital. The catheter or thoracostomy tube is connected to continuous suction. These patients do not require monitoring and do not require admission to an intensive care unit unless there is significant underlying pulmonary or cardiac disease.

Patients with spontaneous pneumomediastinum and a negative contrast-medium–enhanced esophagram may be discharged as long as they are highly reliable and have close outpatient follow-up arranged. Antibiotics are unnecessary if the esophagram is normal.

COMMON PITFALLS

- Spontaneous pneumothorax and spontaneous pneumomediastinum are diagnoses of exclusion. It is essential to consider other causes, including trauma, underlying pulmonary disease, infection, and malignancy.
- Management of spontaneous pneumothorax by observation alone can save hospitalization and health-care costs only if employed in the appropriate circumstances and only if the patient is compliant and receives appropriate discharge instructions.

References

1. Beers MF, Sohn M, Swartz M. Recurrent pneumothorax in AIDS patients with *Pneumocystis* pneumonia: a clinicopathologic report of three cases and review of the literature. *Chest* 1990;98:266.
2. Bense L, Eklund G, Odont D, et al. Smoking and the increased risk of contracting spontaneous pneumothorax. *Chest* 1987;9:1009.
3. Carter EJ, Ettensohn DB. Catamenial pneumothorax. *Chest* 1990;98:713.
4. Collins RK. Hamman's crunch: an adventitious sound. *J Fam Pract* 1994;38:284.
5. Gray R, Cormier M, Yedlicka J, et al. Catamenial pneumothorax: case report and literature review. *J Thorac Imaging* 1987;2:72.

6. Norris RM, Jones JG, Bishop JM. Respiratory gas exchange in patients with spontaneous pneumothorax. *Thorax* 1965;23:427.
7. Rhea JT, Deluca SA, Greene RE. Determining the size of pneumothorax in the upright patient. *Radiology* 1982;144:733.
8. Saha S, Arrants JE, Kossa A, et al. Management of spontaneous pneumothorax. *Ann Thorac Surg* 1975;91:561.
9. Sensenig DN, LeMarch P. Marfan syndrome and spontaneous pneumothorax. *Am J Surg* 1980;139:602.
10. Shesser R, David C, Edelstein S. Pneumomediastinum and pneumothorax after inhaling alkaloidal cocaine. *Ann Emerg Med* 1981;10:213.
11. Shiraishi T. Catamenial pneumothorax: a report of a case and review of the Japanese and non-Japanese literature. *Thorac Cardiovasc Surg* 1991;39:304.
12. Smith BA, Ferguson DB. Disposition of spontaneous pneumomediastinum. *Am J Emerg Med* 1991;9:256.
13. Versteegh FG, Broeders JA. Spontaneous pneumomediastinum in children. *Eur J Pediatr* 1991;150:304.

CHAPTER 150
Pulmonary Embolism

Susan M. Dunmire

Identifying and diagnosing the patient with pulmonary embolism (PE) remains one of the greatest challenges facing the emergency physician. Approximately 10% of patients with PE die within the first hour. Of the remaining patients, only about one-third are correctly diagnosed. The mortality of undiagnosed PE is estimated to be 30%.

The patient who has suffered a PE often presents with nonspecific signs and symptoms that may mimic a long list of both benign and life-threatening illnesses. The absence of a definitive noninvasive diagnostic test and the consequences of a missed diagnosis make evaluation a formidable challenge. Consequently, the emergency physician must always consider PE in any patient presenting with chest pain, shortness of breath, syncope, or unexplained hypoxemia or tachycardia. Once the possibility of a PE enters the differential diagnosis, it is the responsibility of the emergency physician to pursue the diagnosis until it can be adequately confirmed or ruled out. In the past several years, diagnostic tests have been added to aid in diagnosing PE and newer treatment modalities are now available.

CLINICAL PRESENTATION

PE occurs when a substance (usually thrombus, air, fat, or amniotic fluid) lodges in the pulmonary vasculature, resulting in an obstruction of blood flow to that particular portion of the lung. Virchow's triad of hypercoagulability, venostasis, and intimal damage to the blood vessel wall remains the basis for all risk factors for pulmonary thromboembolism (Table 150.1). However, it is important that the clinician recognize that 10% to 15% of patients with PE have no demonstrable risk factors at the time of presentation. The single most important risk factor is a history of deep venous thrombosis (DVT) or PE, which increases the incidence of PE 15- to 30-fold.[3] Another important risk factor is hypercoagulability. A family history of DVT or PE at a young age may be suggestive of an inherited disorder of coagulation or thrombolysis. All three trimesters of pregnancy place the mother at increased risk for PE due to hypercoagulability, but it is often forgotten that this risk extends for a 3-month period postpartum. Central venous catheters in all locations are another important source of thromboemboli. One study of femoral catheters found a 25% incidence of lower extremity thrombus after the catheter was removed. While the presence of a risk factor may elevate the clinician's level of suspicion of a PE, it is important to reiterate that the absence of risk factors should not lower this level of suspicion.

TABLE 150.1. Risk Factors for Pulmonary Embolism

Hypercoagulable state
Pregnancy or recently postpartum
Estrogen therapy
Protein C or S deficiency
Malignancy
Antithrombin III deficiency
Prolonged immobilization
Recent surgery
History of PE or DVT
Trauma (pelvis and lower extremities)
Burns
Obesity
Congestive heart failure
Central venous catheters
Intravenous drug abuse
Systemic lupus
Ulcerative colitis

The presenting signs and symptoms of PE depend on the size of the thrombus load and the extent of preexisting cardiopulmonary disease. Healthy patients are often asymptomatic, whereas a patient with significant cardiopulmonary disease may not tolerate a relatively small embolus and may experience syncope or cardiac arrest.

Stein and Henry[24] have noted that patients with angiographically documented PE tend to have one of three basic clinical presentations. The first group has massive PE and presents with circulatory collapse. The second group has small emboli and resultant pulmonary infarction. These patients complain of pleuritic chest pain and hemoptysis and frequently have a higher PaO_2 than the other groups. The third group presents with unexplained dyspnea. These patients experience larger emboli, resulting in a higher incidence of hypoxemia and electrocardiogram (ECG) changes, and are more likely to have a positive ventilation–perfusion (V/Q) scan.[24]

Among patients with angiographically proven PE, the most common symptoms are dyspnea (81%), pleuritic chest pain (73%), and cough (60%). Chest wall tenderness reproducing the patient's chest pain is not uncommon in PE and should not mislead the clinician into concluding that the pain is musculoskeletal in origin.[4] Syncope is a common presentation of PE in the elderly.[7]

DIFFERENTIAL DIAGNOSIS

The differential diagnosis of PE is extensive. The chest pain associated with PE can vary from the more typical pleuritic pain to reproducible pain with palpation of the chest wall to a substernal heaviness mimicking myocardial infarction. The ECG and cardiac isoenzymes may help to differentiate a myocardial infarction from a PE, but not in all cases. Electrocardiographic changes associated with PE include tachycardia and, less commonly, right heart strain (right axis deviation and/or the classic S1Q3T3 pattern).

Pneumonia is the most common "misdiagnosis" in autopsy-proven PE. Fever is present in more than 40% of patients with PE and, in some cases, may be quite high (39°C to 40°C). Common abnormalities found on chest x-ray include atelectasis, pleural effusions, and infiltrates.

The clinician should be particularly careful in making a diagnosis of "pleurisy" or "musculoskeletal chest pain." To diagnose musculoskeletal chest pain, a specific injury must be identified, and the pain should not only be reproducible with both palpation and motion, but also be attributable to a particular muscle group. Pleurisy is a diagnosis of exclusion once PE has been ruled out. A sudden onset of pleuritic chest pain should be worrisome to the clinician and mandate further investigation.

EMERGENCY DEPARTMENT EVALUATION

Evaluation of the patient with suspected PE begins with a careful history and investigation of potential risk factors. Initial clinical testing should include an ECG and a chest x-ray. An ECG can help to eliminate other diagnostic possibilities, such as myocardial infarction and pericarditis. A chest x-ray can rule out pneumothorax or pneumomediastinum, but PE is often associated with many nonspecific findings. The chest x-ray is also necessary for interpretation of a V/Q scan.

The value of an arterial blood gas in the workup of suspected PE is debatable. Although hypoxemia is present in the majority of patients with PE, a normal PaO_2 does not exclude the diagnosis. A retrospective study of patients with proven PE found that 29% of patients under 40 years of age (but only 3% of patients over 40) had a PaO_2 of greater that 80 mm Hg.[12] Nor does a normal A-a gradient rule out the diagnosis of PE. One study found that 35% of patients with a documented PE had a normal PaO_2 and a normal A-a gradient.[14]

There has been great interest in the use of D-dimer levels in the evaluation of suspected PE. Plasma D-dimers are degradation products of cross-linked fibrin, and levels are elevated in diseases with thrombus formation. Several rapid quantitative D-dimer tests have become available, and some have been reported to be as accurate as the more time-consuming and expensive standard ELISA.[6,17] An elevated D-dimer level is a nonspecific finding. The potential utility of a normal D-dimer level (less than 500 ng/mL) lies, however, in its negative predictive value.[5,18] That is, a normal D-dimer level in a patient with a low clinical suspicion of PE may make further testing for PE (e.g., V/Q scan) unnecessary.

V/Q scanning remains the initial diagnostic test for PE in most medical centers. The perfusion scan is performed by injecting an infusion of radioisotope-labeled microaggregates of albumin. Normally, there is an even distribution of blood flow throughout the lungs. The ventilation scan is performed by having the patient inhale a radioactive gas or aerosol. PE initially causes a perfusion defect with minimal changes in ventilation (V/Q mismatch). As splinting and air-space collapse occur, ventilation also decreases in the affected area.

V/Q scans are generally read as normal, low probability, intermediate probability, or high probability. The PIOPED (Prospective Investigation of Pulmonary Embolism Diagnosis) study delineated the importance of combining the clinician's level of clinical suspicion for PE with the result of the V/Q scan (Table 150.2).[26] Only 2% of patients with a normal V/Q scan and a low clinical suspicion of PE were found to have PE on pulmonary angiography, whereas 96% of patients with a high-probability V/Q scan and a high clinical suspicion had PE.[26] A more recent study of 536 patients with a low clinical suspicion of PE and a low-probability V/Q scan revealed no deaths attributed to PE at 6-month follow-up.[19]

However, the difficulty with the V/Q scan lies in the fact that a substantial proportion of patients have low-probability or intermediate-probability V/Q scans. In the PIOPED study, these patients had an overall incidence of angiographically documented PE of 14% and 30%, respectively. Among those with a low-probability scan, the incidence of PE was 4% to 40%, depending on the estimated clinical likelihood of PE; the corresponding figures for patients with an intermediate-probability scan were 16% to 66%. Thus, in individuals with these "indeterminate" V/Q results, other diagnostic modalities are required to either establish or exclude the diagnosis. Duplex Doppler ultrasound of the lower extremities may be helpful at this point if it is positive. However, if the ultrasound is negative, the clinician must proceed with pulmonary angiography.

Pulmonary angiography remains the "gold standard" diagnostic test for PE against which all other tests are measured. The disadvantages of this test are its invasive nature and administration of iodinated contrast. The morbidity rate for pulmonary angiography is approximately 4% and consists of contrast allergy, cardiac arrhythmias, and cardiac perforation. The mortality rate is approximately 0.3% and is largely limited to patients with pulmonary hypertension.[16]

The diagnostic approach to suspected PE can thus be summarized as follows: If the clinician has a low clinical suspicion for PE and the V/Q scan is read as either normal or low probability, PE can be effectively ruled out. Similarly, if there is an intermediate or high clinical suspicion for PE and the V/Q scan is read as high probability, the likelihood of PE is generally high enough to initiate treatment. For other combinations of clinical likelihood and V/Q scan results, further testing is indicated. The role of D-dimer testing and other newer diagnostic modalities in this scheme remains to be investigated.

Helical computed tomography (CT) scanning has shown considerable promise as a diagnostic tool for suspected PE. It is noninvasive and is reported to have a sensitivity and specificity for the diagnosis of PE that approaches that of V/Q scanning.[11,21] However, the sensitivity of helical CT in detecting subsegmental emboli is significantly worse.[15] The clinical significance of these small emboli is not known. Other limitations of helical CT include variability of its reported sensitivity and specificity (de-

TABLE 150.2. Probability of Pulmonary Embolism Based on Clinical Suspicion and Results of Ventilation-Perfusion Scan

	V/Q Results			
Clinical Suspicion	High	Interm.	Low	Normal or Near-Normal
High	96%	66%	40%	N/A
Intermediate	88%	28%	16%	6%
Low	56%	16%	4%	2%
All patients	87%	30%	14%	4%

NA, not applicable.

Adapted from The PIOPED Investigators. Value of the ventilation perfusion scan in acute pulmonary embolism: results of the prospective investigation of pulmonary embolism diagnosis (PIOPED). *JAMA* 1990;263:2753-2759.

pending on the level of expertise of the radiologist), a requirement for iodinated contrast, and the necessity for the patient to breath-hold for 20 seconds. Helical CT is particularly valuable in ruling out other disease processes that can mimic PE, such as pneumonia and thoracic aortic dissection. Some centers use the V/Q scan as the diagnostic tool of choice in the young patient with a normal chest x-ray, but prefer helical CT in the older patient or in the patient with an abnormal chest x-ray.

Transesophageal echocardiography (TEE) is useful in the diagnosis of massive PE. It has the advantage of being able to be performed at the bedside in a hemodynamically unstable patient. Findings on TEE that are suggestive of massive PE include right ventricular dysfunction, right ventricular dilatation, and, possibly, visualization of the thrombus.[22,25]

EMERGENCY DEPARTMENT MANAGEMENT

Heparin remains the cornerstone of therapy for PE. Prompt anticoagulation with heparin has been shown to reduce mortality from PE to less than 10%.[1,2] In patients with a moderate-to-high clinical suspicion of PE and no contraindication to anticoagulation, heparin should be initiated while awaiting diagnostic studies. Weight-based dosing of heparin has been shown to be optimal[20]:

Heparin loading dose: 80 U/kg
Heparin maintenance dose: 18 U/kg/h

Low-molecular-weight heparin has been shown in several studies to be as effective as heparin in the treatment of DVT and PE.[13,23] Its advantages over heparin include the possibility of home therapy and reduced hospitalization costs. Currently, enoxaparin (Lovenox) is the only low-molecular-weight heparin preparation approved by the Food and Drug Administration . It is approved for treatment of DVT with or without PE, but it is not yet approved for therapy of PE alone. The recommended dosage is 1 mg/kg subcutaneously every 12 hours.

Thrombolytic therapy should be initiated in any hemodynamically unstable patient with PE. In a patient with clinically suspected PE who is too unstable to undergo V/Q scanning or helical CT, bedside echocardiography is an ideal diagnostic tool. If it is unavailable, the clinician must weight the potential risk of thrombolysis against that of progressive cardiopulmonary compromise from a massive pulmonary embolus. While heparin can prevent further clot formation, it is ineffective in dissolving already existing clot and therefore will not provide hemodynamic improvement in cases of massive PE. Streptokinase, urokinase, and recombinant tissue plasminogen activator (r-TPA) are all approved for the treatment of massive PE, but r-TPA is recommended because it produces a faster improvement in hemodynamic parameters than do the other two (usually within 2 hours).[8,10] The usual dosage of r-TPA is 100 mg over 2 hours, but studies have investigated a rapid "bolus" protocol aimed at improving hemodynamic parameters as rapidly as possible.[9]

DISPOSITION

Any patient with an intermediate- or high-probability V/Q scan or a positive helical CT scan should be anticoagulated and admitted to the hospital. Warfarin therapy should be initiated as soon as possible, and patients can be discharged to home once the INR is in the therapeutic range. Patients who qualify for low-molecular-weight heparin therapy may be given the first dose of low-molecular-weight heparin and warfarin in the emergency department and discharged to home. These patients require instruction for self-administration of the low-molecular-weight heparin and careful follow-up.

Patients who are hemodynamically unstable and require thrombolytic therapy may require transfer to a tertiary level facility for intensive care monitoring. It is important to initiate thrombolytic therapy in the hemodynamically unstable patient prior to transfer.

COMMON PITFALLS

- Failing to consider PE in any patient presenting with unexplained tachycardia, tachypnea, and/or hypoxemia. The clinical presentation of PE is quite variable and often nonspecific.
- Dismissing chest wall tenderness as musculoskeletal in origin when there are other clinical findings that suggest PE. PE can present with chest wall tenderness.
- Failing to recognize that PE commonly presents atypically in the elderly (often with syncope).
- Dismissing the possibility of PE because the patient has no identifiable risk factors Assuming that a normal PaO_2 and A-a gradient rule out PE.
- Failing to initiate heparin therapy before diagnostic testing when there is a clinical suspicion of PE and no contraindication to anticoagulation.
- Failing to initiate thrombolytic therapy as early as possible in the hemodynamically unstable patient when there is a strong clinical suspicion of PE. Bedside echocardiography is the fastest and easiest diagnostic test for massive PE.

References

1. Barritt DW, Jordan SC. Anticoagulant drugs in the treatment of pulmonary embolism: a controlled trial. *Lancet* 1960;1:1309–1311.
2. Carson JL, Kelley MA, Duff A, et al. The clinical course of pulmonary embolism. *N Engl J Med* 1992;326:1240–1243.
3. Coon WW. Venous thromboembolism—prevalence: risk factors and prevention. *Clin Chest Med* 1984;5:391.
4. Dreyfuss AI, Weiland DS. Chest wall tenderness as a pitfall in the diagnosis of acute pulmonary embolism. *Arch Intern Med* 1984;144:2057.
5. Duet M, Benelhadj S, Kedra W, et al. A new quantitative D-dimer assay appropriate in emergency: reliability of the assay for pulmonary embolism exclusion diagnosis. *Thromb Res* 1998;91(1):1.
6. Freyburger G, Trillaud H, Labrouche S, et al. D-dimer strategy in thrombosis exclusion: a gold standard study in 100 patients suspected of deep venous thrombosis or pulmonary embolism: 8DD methods compared. *Thromb Haemost* 1998;79(1):32–37.
7. Gisselbrecht M, Diehl JL, Meyer G, et al. Clinical presentation and results of thrombolytic therapy in older patients with massive pulmonary embolism: a comparison with non-elderly patients. *J Am Geriatr Soc* 1996;44:189–193.
8. Goldhaber SZ. Thrombolytic therapy in venous thromboembolism: clinical trials and current indications. *Clin Chest Med* 1995,16:307–311.
9. Goldhaber SZ, Feldstein ML, Sors H. Two trials of reduced bolus alteplase in the treatment of pulmonary embolism. *Chest* 1994;106:725.
10. Goldhaber SZ, Kessler CM, Heit J, et al. Randomized controlled trial of recombinant tissue plasminogen activator versus urokinase in the treatment of acute pulmonary embolism. *Lancet* 1988;2:293.
11. Goodman LR, Curtain JJ, Mewissen MW, et al. Detection of pulmonary embolism in patients with unresolved clinical and scintigraphic diagnosis: helical CT versus angiography. *AJR* 1995;164:1369–1374.
12. Green RM, Meyer TJ, Dunn M, et al. Pulmonary embolism in younger adults. *Chest* 1992;101:1507–1511.
13. Hull RD, Raskob GE, Peneo GF, et al. Subcutaneous low molecular weight heparin compared with continuous intravenous heparin in the treatment of proximal vein thrombosis. *N Engl J Med* 1992;326:975–978.
14. Jones JS, Neff TL, et al. Use of alveolar-arterial oxygen gradient in the assessment of acute pulmonary embolism. *Am J Med* 1998;16(4):333–337.
15. Mayo JR, Remy Jardin M, Muller NL, et al. Pulmonary embolism: prospective comparison of spiral CT with ventilation-perfusion scintigraphy. *Radiology* 1997;205:447–452.
16. Mills SR, Jackson DC, Older RA, et al. The incidence, etiologies and avoidance of complications of pulmonary arteriography. *Radiology* 1980;136:295.
17. Oger E, Leroyer C, Bressollette L, et al. Evaluation of a new, rapid, and quantitative D-dimer test in patients with suspected pulmonary embolism. *Am J Respir Crit Care Med* 1998;158(1):65–70.
18. Perrier A, Desmarais S, Miron MJ, et al. Non-invasive diagnosis of venous thromboembolism in outpatients. *Lancet* 1999;353(9148):190–193.
19. Rajendran JG, Jacobson AF. Review of 6 month mortality following low-probability lung scans. *Arch Intern Med* 1999;159(4):349–352.

20. Raschke RA, Reilly BM, Guidry JR, et al. The weight-based heparin dosing nomogram compared with a standard care nomogram: a randomized controlled trial. *Ann Intern Med* 1993;119:874–881.
21. Remy-Jardin M, Remy J, Deschildre F, et al. Diagnosis of acute pulmonary embolism with spiral CT; comparison with pulmonary angiography and scintigraphy. *Radiology* 1996;200:699–706.
22. Simarro E, Iglesias G, Segovia E, et al. Diagnosis of pulmonary embolism by tranesophageal echocardiography. *Acta Cardiol* 1998;53(2):105–107.
23. Simmoneau G. Subcutaneous fixed dose of enoxaparin versus intravenous adjusted dose of unfractionated heparin in the treatment of deep venous thrombosis. *Thromb Haemost* 1991;65[Suppl]:754–756.
24. Stein PD, Henry J. Clinical characteristics of patients with acute pulmonary embolism stratified according to their presenting symptoms. *Chest* 1997;112(4).
25. Tapson VF. Massive pulmonary embolism. Diagnosis and therapeutic straegies. *Clin Chest Med* 1995;16:329–340.
26. The PIOPED Investigators. Value of the ventilation perfusion scan in acute pulmonary embolism: results of he prospective investigationof pulmonary embolism diagnosis (PIOPED Investigators. Value of the ventilation perfusion scan in acute pulmonary embolism: results ofthe prospective investigation of pulmonary embolism diagnosis (PIOPED). *JAMA* 1990;263:2753–2759.

CHAPTER 151
Hemoptysis

Steven J. Parrillo

Few complaints bring a patient to medical attention as readily as the coughing up of blood. Hemoptysis is a common symptom in adults, but it is quite uncommon in children. Etiologies and presentations are diverse. Adding to the diagnostic challenge is the fact that many cases of presumed hemoptysis are actually due to ear, nose, and throat (ENT) or gastrointestinal bleeding, so-called pseudohemoptysis. Although typically indicative of primary pulmonary pathology, hemoptysis can also result from numerous systemic illnesses. The severity of bleeding often does not correlate with the gravity of the underlying disease. As a matter of fact, the majority of major bleeding occurs in patients with bronchiectasis and bleeding diatheses, while minor bleeding is usually the case with cancer and bronchitis.

Many pathophysiologic mechanisms account for the bleeding. Primary bleeding sources include bronchial and nonbronchial arteries. The direct cause of bleeding varies greatly, depending on underlying etiology. Table 151.1 lists the cause or causes of bleeding for several common problems. Several mechanisms may be responsible for bleeding in any given patient. Exsanguination is rarely the ultimate cause of death in hemoptysis. Rather, blood fills alveoli, impairing gas exchange. Death is secondary to hypoxemia.

TABLE 151.1. Mechanisms of Bleeding in Hemoptysis

Malignancies: invade vessels, or the tumor itself may become necrotic
Inflammatory and infectious problems: vascular engorgement of the tracheobronchial mucosa
Bronchiectasis: associated with abnormal vascular anastomoses between bronchial and pulmonary arteries
Lung abscesses: bronchial ulceration and necrosis
Mycetomas of cavitary TB: rupture and cause life-threatening hemorrhage
Left ventricular failure or mitral stenosis: increased intravascular pressure with capillary and venous rupture
Pulmonary embolism: infarction of lung parenchyma
Goodpasture syndrome: breakdown of the alveolocapillary basement membrane
Aortic aneurysm: erosion into adjacent vascular structures
Coagulopathy: exacerbation of an underlying reason for bleeding
Cocaine: intense vasoconstriction with cell injury

CLINICAL PRESENTATION

The overall picture of hemoptysis has changed in recent years. The most common causes are infections, malignancy, bronchiectasis, bronchitis, and cardiovascular disorders.[5,8,17] Although tuberculosis (TB) was once a leading infectious cause, it is now much less common than pneumonia and bronchitis, except in areas of high TB prevalence, such as New York City.[8,12] Only time will tell if the new multidrug-resistant strains will bring about a resurgence of TB.

In children, cystic fibrosis, congenital heart disease, and trauma head the list of causes of hemoptysis, not vascular abnormalities and neoplasms, as was once believed.[5,6] Cystic fibrosis may be associated with recurrent, severe bleeding in both children and young adults. A case presentation reported significant hemoptysis in two children with bronchiolitis obliterans organizing pneumonia.[13]

The prevalence of immunocompromised patients has prompted study of common causes in that population. Although many of the data come from hospitalized patients, it appears that the vast majority of cases are infectious, mostly due to bacterial pneumonias. Even in that group, TB is not a common cause of respiratory tract bleeding.[15]

With the advent of thrombolytic therapy, researchers have sought to determine whether hemoptysis is a common problem. It appears that it is not.[4]

Goodpasture syndrome may present with hematuria and hemoptysis, as may vasculitis. Occult malignancy should always be considered in a cigarette smoker, even with a normal physical examination and chest radiograph.[9,11]

Table 151.2 lists the common causes of hemoptysis by category.

DIFFERENTIAL DIAGNOSIS

Hemoptysis must be confirmed before the broad differential diagnosis can be considered. An appropriate, focused history and physical examination should eliminate gastrointestinal and otolaryngologic sources. Gastrointestinal bleeding can usually be identified by its dark red color, the presence of clots and food particles, and an acid pH. True hemoptysis is typically bright red, frothy, and normal to alkaline in pH. Mouth, throat, and nasopharyngeal sources of bleeding can usually be visualized, sometimes with direct, indirect, or fiberoptic laryngoscopy.

EMERGENCY DEPARTMENT EVALUATION

Whenever bleeding is an issue, hemodynamic stabilization takes precedence over efforts to make a definitive diagnosis. For that reason, the first question that needs to be answered concerns the rate and quantity of bleeding.

"Massive" hemoptysis is usually defined as bleeding of 600 mL within 24 to 48 hours, or at a rate of 100 mL/h or more. Differentiating massive from "submassive" or minor bleeding carries both diagnostic and prognostic implications, but may not be easy to do in the emergency department (ED). Mortality for

TABLE 151.2. Common Causes of Hemoptysis

INFLAMMATORY
Bronchitis
Bronchiectasis
Lung abscess
Pneumonia (viral, bacterial, fungal)
Tuberculosis
Parasites (e.g. ascariasis, schistosomiasis)
NEOPLASTIC
Bronchial adenoma
Bronchogenic carcinoma
CARDIOVASCULAR
Arteriovenous malformation
Arteriovenous fistula
Congestive heart failure
Aneurysm
Pulmonary thromboembolism
Primary pulmonary hypertension
Mitral stenosis
Vascular injury (e.g., foreign body)
CONGENITAL
Cystic fibrosis
IMMUNOLOGIC
Collagen vascular disease
Vasculitis
Goodpasture syndrome
EXTRAPULMONARY DISEASE
Thrombocytopenia
Coagulopathies
Trauma
DRUGS
Anticoagulants
Cocaine
Thrombolytics

the massive bleeding group is high (12% to 50%).[8] Causes of mortality include asphyxiation (due to airway obstruction with blood) and exsanguination. Most series list TB and bronchiectasis as the most common causes of massive hemoptysis in adults. Other diseases associated with massive bleeding include lung abscess, malignancy, and aspergilloma. In children, massive bleeding is a predictor of mortality in congenital heart disease.[5]

Next, baseline cardiopulmonary status and overall physical condition must be determined. History, physical, and laboratory studies can help evaluate the patient's ability to respond to the physiologic stress of hemoptysis and the therapy it necessitates. To the patient with limited cardiopulmonary reserve or significant underlying disease, almost any amount of bleeding may prove detrimental. Indeed, a more useful definition of *massive hemoptysis* may be bleeding into the tracheobronchial tree at a rate that poses a threat to life.[14]

Finally, efforts to determine the cause should begin. "Baseline" ED evaluation includes history, physical examination, and chest radiograph. Depending on the clinical scenario, many clinicians would also do a complete blood count, urinalysis, arterial blood gas analysis, coagulation studies, electrocardiogram, and sputum evaluation (Gram stain, AFB, cultures). Definitive diagnosis may require a ventilation–perfusion scan, high-resolution[12] or standard computed tomography scans, bronchoscopy, bronchography, sputum cytology, pulmonary function testing, angiography, or specialized sputum studies. Most of those tests will not be done in the ED. Aggressive management must occur at the same time as evaluation. Some diagnostic modalities, most notably bronchial artery embolization, are both diagnostic and therapeutic.[3,7]

It is worth noting that up to 22% of cases will have no identifiable etiology, even after exhaustive study.[17] Those patients might then be classified as having idiopathic or cryptogenic hemoptysis. It is presumed that subtle airway or parenchymal disease is responsible for bleeding.

EMERGENCY DEPARTMENT MANAGEMENT

The primary goals of therapy are prevention of asphyxia and exsanguination, termination of bleeding, and treatment of the underlying cause.

Airway control and adequate oxygenation are the first priorities. Endotracheal intubation, which may be technically challenging, is the procedure of choice. Large tubes facilitate suctioning. Bag-valve-mask ventilation may be problematic in the patient who is briskly bleeding, because it may spread blood further through the tracheobronchial tree. Separate intubation of left and right main-stem bronchi may be achieved by someone skilled in the use of either the Carlens or Robertshaw tube. Intubation over a fiberoptic laryngoscope may allow selective intubation of one bronchus but requires skills that most emergency physicians have not learned. Empiric intubation of a main-stem bronchus will probably be necessary in that uncommon patient with severe hemorrhage.

In cases involving significant hemoptysis, the patient is placed in the Trendelenburg position, with the suspected bleeding source dependent. This position may protect the uninvolved lung from filling with blood and, in so doing, maximize gas exchange.

Isotonic fluids and blood products should be infused, as indicated, through large-bore intravenous lines, recognizing that some authors question the wisdom of initiating infusion before bleeding has been controlled. All patients with significant hemoptysis should be placed on a cardiac monitor. Some will require continuous hemodynamic monitoring.

Although most causes of bleeding require definitive therapy beyond the scope of emergency medical practice, there are times when treatment should begin in the ED. Examples include some coagulopathies and some infectious etiologies.

Pulmonary, ENT, and surgical consultants will soon attempt to localize the bleeding site, especially if surgery is being considered. Techniques including bronchoscopy and angiography may be both diagnostic and therapeutic.[14] Consultants may employ topical vasoconstrictors and catheter tamponade to control bleeding. Intravenous pitressin therapy and bronchial artery embolization have been used successfully in patients with cystic fibrosis.[2,7] Selective embolization carries the risk of systemic embolization. Although success rates of 80% are frequently cited, spontaneous recanalization may occur and may cause more bleeding. Flexible endoscopy may be done at bedside. Rigid endoscopy is usually performed in the operating room (OR).

Hemoptysis may be best controlled by dealing with the source of the problem: mitral valve surgery for stenosis or nephrectomy plus steroids in Goodpasture syndrome. Bleeding associated with cystic fibrosis may respond to intravenous pitressin therapy.[2]

There are times when surgery is the only way to control bleeding. The patient and the operating surgeon will benefit from accurate localization, identification of cause, and preoperative stabilization.[10]

DISPOSITION

Patients with significant bleeding should be admitted to an intensive care unit setting, preferably on the service of the surgeon who will go to the operating room. As in all situations of potentially exsanguinating hemorrhage, the OR must be readily available. Transfer to an appropriate facility must be arranged when definitive care is not available at the presenting institution. Stabilization must address airway control and hemodynamic needs. Given the difficulties of trying to establish an airway in a bleeding patient, consideration should be given to prophylactic intubation before transfer. At the very least, personnel effecting the transfer must be competent in emergency airway management.

Patients in the "submassive" group require an individualized approach. Many can be referred to an appropriate physician after the initial ED evaluation and institution of therapy when appropriate. It would be prudent to suggest to discharged patients that bronchoscopy may be an important part of the diagnostic process, especially in males, smokers, patients over 40, those with a localized abnormality on chest radiograph, and those in whom bleeding has lasted more than 7 days.[16] Hemoptysis is a frightening symptom requiring patient reassurance.

Follow-up instructions must be specific. They should include the name of the physician and the time frame required. Patients must be reliable and hemodynamically stable. A conversation between the emergency physician and the primary care physician or consultant would be wise.

Patients at high risk for deterioration—those with limited pulmonary reserves or respiratory compromise—should be hospitalized. Those with mycetomas or cavitary TB are also at high risk.[1] Patients with significant underlying disease should be admitted. Immunocompromised patients may need to be admitted if the cause of bleeding is infectious. The possible public health risk of blood-borne diseases may also be a factor in the disposition decision.

COMMON PITFALLS

- Hemoptysis must be recognized and differentiated from nasopharyngeal or gastrointestinal bleeding.
- The bleeding rate must be estimated as accurately as possible. Dismissing a few ounces of hemoptysis as trivial during a brief evaluation is a potentially lethal error.
- Each patient's cardiopulmonary reserve and overall clinical status must be evaluated. Even a small amount of hemoptysis may have potentially devastating consequences for a patient with significant underlying disease.
- The patient must be closely monitored. Clinical deterioration may respond to such simple measures as repositioning the patient or performing endotracheal intubation, thereby preventing the further spread of blood through the lungs.
- In situations requiring transfer to a higher level of care, patient stability may require attention not only to hemodynamic status, but also to the airway. Prophylactic intubation should be considered.
- Radiographic lesions may be subtle. The emergency physician must obtain the radiologist's final report on all patients with hemoptysis and relay that report to the patient or consulting physician.

References

1. Athayde J, Shore E. Invasive pulmonary *Aspergillosis* presenting as massive hemoptysis in a nonimmunocompromised host. *Chest* 1993;103:961.
2. Bilton D, Webb A, Foster H, et al. Life-threatening hemoptysis in cystic fibrosis: an alternative therapeutic approach. *Thorax* 1990;45:976.
3. Brinson G, Noone P, Mauro M, et al. Bronchial artery embolization for the treatment of hemoptysis in patients with cystic fibrosis. *Am J Respir Crit Care Med* 1998;157:1951.
4. Chang YC, Patz EF, Goodman PC, et al. Significance of hemoptysis following thrombolytic therapy for myocardial infarction. *Chest* 1996;109(3):727.
5. Coss-Bu JA, Sachdeva RC, Bricker JT, et al. Hemoptysis: a 10 year retrospective study. *Pediatrics* 1997;100(3):E7.
6. Fabian MC, Smitheringale A. Hemoptysis in children: the Hospital for Sick Children experience. *J Otolaryngol* 1996;25(1):44.
7. Fernando H, Stein M, Benfield J, et al. Role of bronchial artery embolization in the management of hemoptysis. *Arch Surg* 1998;133:862.
8. Hirshberg B, Biran I, Glazer M, et al. Hemoptysis: etiology, evaluation and outcome in a tertiary referral hospital. *Chest* 1997;112(2):440.
9. Jackson C, Savage P, Quinn D. Role of fiberoptic bronchoscopy in patients with hemoptysis and a normal chest roentgenogram. *Chest* 1985;87:142.
10. Jones D, Daries R. Massive hemoptysis. *BMJ* 1990;300:889.
11. Lederle F, Nichol K, Parenti C. Bronchoscopy to evaluate hemoptysis in older men with nonsuspicious chest roentgenograms. *Chest* 1989;95:1043.
12. McGuiness G, Beacher J, Harkin T, et al. Hemoptysis: prospective high resolution CT/bronchoscopic correlation. *Chest* 1994;105:1155.
13. Mroz B, Sexauer W, Meade W, et al. Hemoptysis as the presenting symptom in bronchiolitis obliterans organizing pneumonia. *Chest* 1997;111(6):1775.
14. Metzdorff M, Vogelzang R, LoCicero J, et al. Transcatheter bronchial artery embolization in the multimodal management of massive hemoptysis. *Chest* 1990;97:1494.
15. Nelson J, Fornan M. Hemoptysis in HIV-infected patients. *Chest* 1996; 110(3):737.
16. O'Neill K, Lazarus A. Hemoptysis: indications for bronchoscopy. *Arch Intern Med* 1991;151:171.
17. Santiago S, Tobias J, Williams A. A reappraisal of the causes of hemoptysis. *Arch Intern Med* 1991;151:2449.

CHAPTER 152
Sarcoidosis

Steven J. Parrillo and Christopher C. Rose*

Sarcoidosis is a multisystem, chronic granulomatous disease with diverse manifestations and a variable clinical course. It is characterized by a heightened cellular immune response at sites of disease activity; the lungs are the primary target organ and are involved in most cases.[8] A number of etiologies have been postulated, including exposure to infectious agents (especially *Mycobacterium tuberculosis*), noninfectious environmental agents (especially beryllium), and autoantigens.[8] Curiously, as of 1995 only nine human immunodeficiency virus (HIV)–infected patients had been reported to have coexistent sarcoidosis[4,6]

In the United States, the prevalence of sarcoidosis is about five per 100,000 in the White population and about 40 per 100,000 in the Black population. Among Black patients, women usually outnumber men 2 to 1. Although the peak incidence is in the middle years of life (20 to 40 years of age), the disease has been reported in children and the elderly. Sarcoid has also been identified in twins (monozygotic more commonly than dizygotic) and in husband–wife pairs.[3] The vast majority of cases resolve spontaneously, with or without treatment. Indicators of a favorable prognosis include acute manifestations of inflammation, such as erythema nodosum, polyarthritis, fever, and bilateral lymphadenopathy. Poor prognostic indicators include Black race, lupus pernio, and chronic bone, lung, or nasopharyngeal involvement.[7]

* Deceased

TABLE 152.1. Characteristics at Clinical Presentation[3]

Characteristic	Incidence (%)
Age	
<40	75
>40	25
May occur in the elderly	
Gender	
Male	60
Female	40
Race	
Black	90
Caucasian	10
Asymptomatic	10–20
Acute/subacute (fever, fatigue, malaise, anorexia, weight loss, respiratory symptoms)	20–40
Insidious (respiratory complaints without constitutional symptoms)	40–70

CLINICAL PRESENTATION

In the United States, approximately 20% of sarcoidosis patients are asymptomatic, the diagnosis being suspected only because hilar adenopathy is seen on a chest film (Table 152.1). This group may need only to be referred to confirm the diagnosis. For the emergency physician, however, the more important issue is when to suspect and treat active disease.

In 20% to 40% of cases, acute or subacute sarcoidosis develops over a period of several weeks. The symptoms are usually mild and may include fever, malaise, anorexia, and weight loss. Most patients develop a more indolent form that develops over months. Most have vague respiratory complaints. Unfortunately, it is this group that is more likely to develop chronic disease with significant organ damage.

As a multisystem disease, sarcoidosis can present with symptoms referable to a variety of organ systems. The lungs, however, are almost always almost involved, and the clinical presentation is often dominated by the presence of interstitial lung disease. These patients are dyspneic, especially on exertion, and have a dry cough. Physical examination may reveal nothing more than dry rales, but wheezing suggestive of reactive airway disease may be heard. Ninety percent have an abnormal chest radiograph.

The radiographic findings of sarcoid are characteristic, with bilateral mediastinal lymphadenopathy being the classic, as well as the most common, finding (Fig. 152.1).

Radiographic evaluation is helpful to define pulmonary involvement, rather than stage the disease. There are three or four types of involvement shown on chest films (Table 152.2). Type I radiographs show bilateral hilar adenopathy without parenchymal changes. Type II films demonstrate bilateral hilar adenopathy plus diffuse parenchymal changes, but no fibrosis. In type III, there are diffuse parenchymal changes but no adenopathy. Some authors add a IV, showing fibrotic changes, whereas others subdivide III.

Radiographic typing has some limited prognostic significance, in that type I changes usually resolve, while changes in the other types are chronic. It is important to recognize that these are not stages of the disease, but represent different manifestations.[3]

Although myocardial sarcoidosis is found in 25% of autopsied cases, in only about 10% has there been an abnormal electrocardiogram (without clinical symptoms). Conduction disturbances, including complete heart block, are the most common cardiac presentations and may be the cause of death. Life-threatening ventricular dysrhythmias are also seen. As many as 25% of those with cardiac dysfunction die of congestive heart failure.[9]

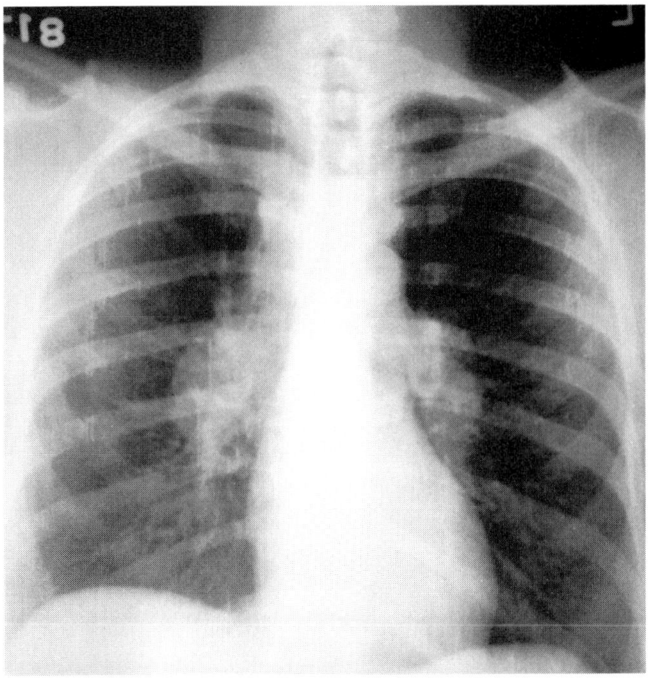

Figure 152.1. Typical type I radiograph. (Courtesy of K. Murray and M.D. Dalinka, Department of Radiology, Hospital of the University of Pennsylvania, Philadelphia.)

Both hypercalciuria (30%) and hypercalcemia (10%) are common and may lead to nephrocalcinosis and nephrolithiasis. Glomerular disease and renal arteritis may occur, and hypertension is common. Primary renal infiltration with sarcoid granulomas is rare.[3]

Hypercalcemia may arise from increased intestinal calcium absorption due to overproduction of 1,25-dihydroxyvitamin D_3 by activated macrophages. Corticosteroids can control hypercalcemia by inhibiting the action of this hormone, but severe hypercalcemia in sarcoidosis is unusual. Hypercalcemia needs to be corrected, and treatment begins with conservative measures, such as decreasing oral calcium intake before corticosteroids are considered.[11]

Approximately 25% of patients have eye involvement, most commonly anterior uveitis. Uveitis may develop rapidly and may become chronic. Other lesions include posterior uveitis, conjunctivitis, cataracts, and retinal hemorrhages.

Superficial lymphadenopathy is a frequent finding. Only 20% to 40% of patients have hepatomegaly or abnormalities of liver function. Portal hypertension is rare. Splenomegaly is seen in only 10%. Clinical disease is uncommon.

Skin lesions occur in about one-fourth of patients. Specific lesions include lupus pernio (Fig. 152.2), plaques, and symmetric maculopapular eruptions. The most common lesion is erythema nodosum, a hypersensitivity reaction most commonly seen in women of childbearing age but not specific to sarcoidosis.[9]

TABLE 152.2. Radiographic Stage and Prognosis in Sarcoidosis

Stage	% of Patients	Prognosis (Likelihood of Resolution) (%)
0	5–10	—
I	50	60
II	25–30	46
III	15	12

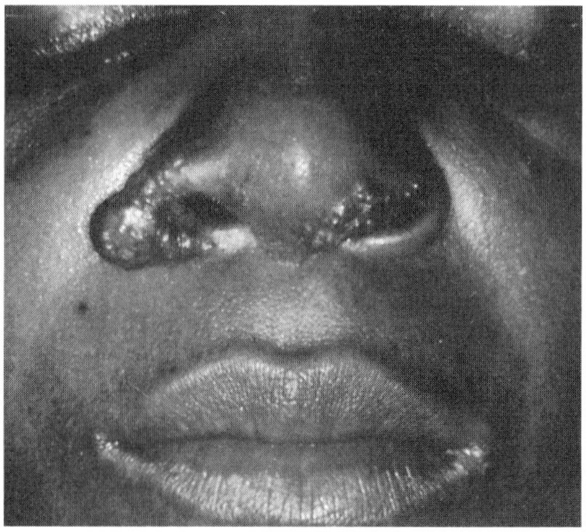

Figure 152.2. Lupus pernio. (Courtesy of Gerald S. Lazarus, MD, Department of Dermatology, Hospital of the University of Pennsylvania, Philadelphia.)

Joint involvement is very common in sarcoidosis, with 25% to 50% of patients suffering from arthralgias or true arthritis, mostly in larger joints. Both can be migratory and are usually transient. The arthritis associated with erythema nodosum can be incapacitating and may require corticosteroid therapy. Chronic arthritis is associated with chronic persistent disease and is most frequently seen in Black patients with skin involvement.[3]

Nasal and laryngeal involvement occurs infrequently but may cause severe airway compromise.

Only 5% of patients have neural involvement, with multiple cranial neuropathy (e.g., peripheral seventh nerve palsy) being most frequent. Aseptic meningitis and peripheral neuropathy occur occasionally. Seizures are infrequent. Neurologic symptoms usually improve with corticosteroid therapy.[7]

Two other syndromes have been described. Lofgren syndrome includes erythema nodosum and radiographic findings of bilateral hilar adenopathy, and may also be associated with arthritis of small and medium joints. Patients with the Heerfordt-Waldenstrom syndrome have fever, anterior uveitis, facial nerve palsy, and parotid enlargement.[3]

It is worth noting that sarcoidosis usually improves during pregnancy.[3]

DIFFERENTIAL DIAGNOSIS

If there were to be a "classic" presentation of sarcoidosis, it would be of a young adult suffering from a combination of fever, dyspnea, blurred vision, and erythema nodosum, with a chest radiograph showing bilateral hilar adenopathy. Most cases, of course, are not that typical. Virtually all of the diseases to be considered in the differential diagnosis have the propensity to occur in almost any anatomic location. Sarcoidosis is most likely to be confused with tuberculosis (or other mycobacterial infections), lymphoma, and some fungal disorders (e.g., coccidioidomycosis). Other diseases to be considered include leprosy, berylliosis, and hypersensitivity pneumonitis.

HIV infection must also be considered in patients suspected of having sarcoidosis. Patients with HIV commonly have several of the features found in sarcoid, including chest radiograph abnormalities, lymphocytopenia, and a positive gallium-67 chest scan.[6]

A definitive diagnosis of sarcoidosis cannot be made with certainty on initial clinical presentation in an emergency setting, although the clinical suspicion may be high. The patient who already carries the diagnosis of sarcoidosis, however, may present with a complication of the disease or a concurrent, perhaps unrelated, illness and should be evaluated accordingly.

EMERGENCY DEPARTMENT EVALUATION

The initial history should be directed to ascertain the duration and severity of the patient's symptoms, a previous diagnosis of sarcoidosis, and any previous need for corticosteroid therapy.

The major complications of systemic sarcoidosis include upper airway obstruction from laryngeal involvement; cardiac dysrhythmias and conduction disturbances (especially heart block); congestive heart failure; advanced pulmonary fibrosis with cor pulmonale, superimposed tuberculosis, or bacterial infection; sudden loss of vision from ocular complications; incapacitating arthritis or arthralgias; space-occupying lesions of the brain and hydrocephalus; and hypercalcemia with its attendant cardiac, neurologic, and renal sequelae. Severe thrombocytopenia may occur. Abrupt corticosteroid withdrawal may cause the signs and symptoms of adrenal insufficiency.[2,9–11]

Physical examination should focus first on the airway and cardiopulmonary systems, but attention should be given to all organ systems that potentially may be involved, as well as to the possibility of relative adrenal insufficiency secondary to rapid withdrawal of corticosteroid therapy.

Ocular, neurologic, skin, or joint complaints dictate the need for more specialized testing or examination. Funduscopic examination is essential in patients with altered mental status or abnormal neurologic findings.

Diagnostic studies in the emergency department should be directed toward detecting the potential problems associated with sarcoidosis. All patients should have a 12-lead electrocardiogram. Consideration should be given to ordering Holter monitoring for discharged patients. Chest radiography, pulse oximetry, and arterial blood gas analysis may be indicated in those who have respiratory complaints. Renal function studies, electrolytes, and calcium and platelet counts should be routine.

Strict criteria must be satisfied to make the diagnosis of sarcoidosis. The emergency physician must establish compatible clinical presentations or radiographic findings, or both; histologic evidence of noncaseating granuloma; and negative special stains and cultures for other entities (e.g., acid-fast bacilli or fungi on sputum or tissue biopsy specimens). A diagnosis based on only one of these features may be misleading.[5]

Outpatient evaluation often includes serum and cerebrospinal fluid (CSF) studies, isotopic imaging studies, biopsy, and bronchoalveolar lavage. Advances in gallium scanning have improved diagnostic accuracy, but this test is not diagnostic of sarcoidosis.[12] The Kveim-Siltzbach skin test is also helpful, but requires and biopsy at 6 weeks. Most patients will eventually have a 24-hour urinary calcium determination.[3] Serum and CSF angiotensin converting enzyme levels are elevated in up to 50% of patients. Bronchoalveolar lavage reveals cells consistent with the diagnosis in the majority of those with pulmonary sarcoid.[10]

EMERGENCY DEPARTMENT MANAGEMENT

Incapacitating disease interfering with normal life activities merits serious consideration for corticosteroid therapy. Conversely, relatively asymptomatic disease warrants an optimistic outlook and conservative management without corticosteroids. Causes of symptoms or signs other than progression of sarcoidosis must be excluded to avoid inappropriate management. Systemic corticosteroids (e.g., prednisone 40 mg/d) remain the safest and best form of treatment.

Strong indications for steroid treatment include significant pulmonary parenchymal disease, hepatic disease, hypercalcemia, myocardial disease, incapacitating arthritis, severe thrombocytopenia, posterior ocular disease, neurologic disease, laryngeal involvement, or any other vital organ impairment. Weaker indications are persistent constitutional symptoms and abnormal results of liver function tests.[13] Local corticosteroids are used for anterior ocular and skin disease.[2,3,7,9,11]

Patients with cardiac conduction abnormalities due to granulomatous infiltration are usually refractory to conventional pharmacotherapy and often need to be admitted to the hospital to determine the most appropriate pharmacologic or electrical therapy. Cardiac transplantation has been performed successfully in younger patients with severe heart failure. Ventricular aneurysm resection may be required to eliminate refractory dysrhythmias.[7,9] Lung transplantation has been performed for end-stage pulmonary disease.[7]

Hypercalcemia, if severe or symptomatic, may be treated in the normal fashion while high-dose corticosteroid therapy is initiated. Milder elevations of serum calcium levels may be treated with corticosteroids alone, with frequent monitoring.[1]

Although corticosteroids remain the mainstay of treatment, a number of other agents have also been used. They include methotrexate, azathioprine, cyclophosphamide, chlorambucil, cyclosporine, nonsteroidal antiinflammatories, chloroquine, and hydroxychloroquine.

Sarcoidosis clears spontaneously in half of all patients.[3]

DISPOSITION

The emergency physician may require the advice and assistance of a variety of specialty consultants in diagnosing and managing the patient with suspected sarcoidosis. Pulmonary, ophthalmologic, dermatologic, and neurologic consultation may be necessary before any definitive therapy is undertaken.

Patients for whom hospitalization should be considered are those with cardiac or neurologic disease, hypercalcemia, severe thrombocytopenia, or any degree of airway compromise. Hospital admission should be considered strongly for diagnostic purposes at initial presentation.

Because frequent and long-term care is usually required, the family physician, internist, or pulmonary specialist is most commonly called on to provide primary outpatient therapy for sarcoidosis.

COMMON PITFALLS

- Sarcoidosis is frequently asymptomatic and should be included in the differential diagnosis of patients with eye findings, suggestive skin lesions, hypercalcemia, persistent cough, or unexplained fever and weight loss.
- The emergency physician should resist the temptation to announce a firm diagnosis or prognosis to the patient, yet it is essential that follow-up be arranged so that a definitive diagnosis can be made and appropriate treatment begun.
- Most cases of sarcoid resolve without treatment. Specialty consultation should be obtained before treating with systemic corticosteroids and when dealing with cardiac, neurologic, or ocular disease.
- Serum calcium level should be checked in all patients with suspected or previously diagnosed sarcoidosis.
- As a rule, hypercalcemia should not be treated on an outpatient basis.
- Patients with sarcoid should have an electrocardiogram, and most should have Holter monitoring.
- The presence of wheezing may incorrectly suggest reactive airway diseases. Corticosteroids may not be indicated in this setting.

References

1. Bascom R, Johns CJ. The natural history and management of sarcoidosis. In: Stollerman GH, ed. *Advances in internal medicine,* vol 31. London: Year Book Medical, 1986.
2. Berkman YM. Radiologic aspects of intrathoracic sarcoidosis. *Semin Roentgenol* 1985;4:356.
3. Crystal RG. Sarcoidosis. In: *Harrison's principles of internal medicine,* ed. 14, 1998:1922.
4. Graniem J. Sarcoid myopathy in a patient with HIV infection. *South Med J* 1995;88(5):591.
5. James DG, Sharma OP. Overlap syndromes with sarcoidosis. *Postgrad Med J* 1985;61:767.
6. Lowery WS, Whitlock WL, Dietrich RA, et al. Sarcoidosis complicated by HIV infection: three case reports and a review of the literature. *Am Rev Respir Dis* 1990;142:887.
7. Lynch JP, Kazerooni EA, Gay SE. Pulmonary sarcoidosis. *Clin Chest Med* 1997;18(4):755.
8. Moller DR. Etiology of sarcoidosis. *Clin Chest Med* 1997;18(4):695.
9. Sharma OP. *Sarcoidosis: a clinical approach.* Springfield, IL: Charles C Thomas Publisher, 1975.
10. Sharma OP. Sarcoidosis: clinical, laboratory and immunologic aspects. *Semin Roentgenol* 1985;4:340.
11. Sharma OP. Vitamin D, calcium, and sarcoidosis. *Chest* 1996;109(2):535.
12. Slovik SB, Spencer RP, Palestro CJ, et al. Specificity and sensitivity of distinctive chest radiographs and/or ^{67}Ga images in the noninvasive diagnosis of sarcoidosis. *Chest* 1993;103:403.
13. Winterbauer RH, Kirtland SH, Corley DE. Treatment with corticosteroids. *Clin Chest Med* 1997;18(4):843.

PART III
Gastrointestinal Disease

CHAPTER 153
Esophageal Disease

Charles M. Seamens and Allan B. Wolfson

Patients with esophageal disease generally present to the emergency department in one of four ways: (1) with odynophagia, (2) with heartburn or chest pain, (3) with dysphagia, or (4) with gastrointestinal (GI) bleeding. There is often a great deal of overlap in these symptoms, however. For example, disorders causing mucosal destruction may result not only in odynophagia, but also in dysphagia, whereas certain motor disorders may cause both dysphagia and chest pain. Esophageal disease that causes bleeding is usually due to varices (see Chapter 154). Esophageal perforation is discussed in Chapter 106.

ODYNOPHAGIA

CLINICAL PRESENTATION

Odynophagia refers to pain on swallowing and implies mucosal disease of the oropharynx or esophagus. Inflammation of adjacent structures may produce symptoms indistinguishable from mucosal inflammation. The pain may be described as a retrosternal ache, a burning sensation, or a stabbing pain with radiation to the back. Esophagitis typically presents as odynophagia, with or without dysphagia. Other common complaints include atypical chest pain, a sensation of feeling each bolus of food as it passes down, heartburn, or, occasionally, anorexia and weight loss. The most important immediate consequences of esophagitis are local pain and impaired oral alimentation. Rarely, the initial manifestation of esophageal disease is GI bleeding.

Infectious esophagitis should always be a consideration in immunocompromised individuals. In esophageal candidiasis, odynophagia is usually relatively mild. If symptoms are so severe that the patient consciously limits oral intake, ulcerative esophagitis of some other etiology is likely. Oropharyngeal candidiasis is noted in many patients with candidal esophagitis, but it is not a very good predictor of its presence, except in patients with the acquired immunodeficiency syndrome (AIDS).

Herpetic esophagitis is the most common viral infection affecting the esophagus, and presents with odynophagia that is typically abrupt in onset. It is also suspected when symptoms of dysphagia or odynophagia do not improve with typical antifungal medications in immunocompromised patients.[6] Immunocompetent patients often give a history of an upper respiratory tract infection before the onset of swallowing problems, and most have skin or oral lesions of herpes simplex virus (HSV) infection. In contrast, oropharyngeal and perioral lesions are frequently absent in immunosuppressed patients.

Cytomegalovirus (CMV) esophagitis presents in a similar fashion, with odynophagia, dysphagia, and variable degrees of substernal chest pain, but nausea and vomiting seem to be more common in CMV esophagitis.

Complications of candidal or viral esophagitis are uncommon; they include hemorrhage, perforation, esophageal narrowing with stricture formation, and dissemination of infection.

The true incidence of *medication-induced* esophageal injury is unknown, because many cases are not reported in the literature and many more go unrecognized. Tablets and capsules can adhere to the esophageal wall and dissolve locally in spite of normal esophageal function. Although patients with structural abnormalities and motility disorders are more likely to develop medication-induced esophagitis, most patients have normal esophageal motility.

Patients with pill esophagitis typically report retrosternal pain, odynophagia, and dysphagia that are temporally related to ingestion of medication. A significant proportion give a history of taking the medication with little or no water. Symptoms generally improve within a couple of days, provided the medication is discontinued, but complete resolution may take several weeks, and there are no sequelae. Pill esophagitis affects the proximal esophagus, usually at the level of the aortic arch or left atrium, in contrast to reflux esophagitis, which affects the distal esophagus. The most common complication is stricture formation.

Odynophagia is usually not a prominent component of *reflux esophagitis,* which is discussed elsewhere in this chapter.

DIFFERENTIAL DIAGNOSIS

The differential diagnosis of odynophagia includes diffuse infectious causes and localized trauma or inflammation.

Candidal esophagitis is increasing in incidence, probably because of aggressive immunosuppressive therapy in patients with cancer and the emergence of AIDS. HSV esophagitis is much less common, and CMV is recognized as an important cause of infectious esophagitis in patients with AIDS as well as in bone marrow transplant patients.

Pill-induced esophagitis may be confused with other causes of esophagitis if the patient does not relate the ingestion of medication with symptoms. As with other causes of esophageal pain, cardiac disease must be excluded. The age and sex of patients with drug-induced esophagitis reflects the population group most likely to receive commonly prescribed drugs. Doxycycline (the most frequent offender in the United States) and tetracycline are more commonly prescribed in younger patients for *Chlamydia* and respiratory infections. Potassium chloride and quinidine tablets, which also cause a large number of cases of pill-induced esophagitis, are more frequently used in elderly patients. Ferrous sulfate, aspirin, and nonsteroidal antiinflammatory agents are used by patients of all ages.

Odynophagia localized to the posterior pharynx may be due to a pharyngitis or abscess. Epiglottitis is another potential concern. The patient should also be asked about the possibility of ingestion of foreign bodies or food impaction.

EMERGENCY DEPARTMENT EVALUATION

The initial history should focus first on the duration and severity of the symptoms and on the patient's ability to maintain normal oral intake. The patient should be asked about a history of diagnosed human immunodeficiency virus (HIV) infection, risk factors for HIV, or other conditions associated with an immunosuppressed state. Patients should be further questioned about a possible association of symptoms with pill ingestion or possible foreign bodies, as well as any symptoms suggestive of esophageal reflux.

Esophageal candidiasis is common in patients with AIDS and immunosuppressed individuals, but severe odynophagia that results in diminished oral intake or dehydration is uncommon in patients with candidal esophagitis alone. More than one potential pathogen may be identified in severely symptomatic patients.

The physical examination should concentrate initially on the patient's state of hydration. Blood pressure, pulse, and orthostatic changes should be noted, as well as skin turgor and the condition of the mucous membranes.

The oropharynx should be examined for oral candidal or herpetic lesions, and signs of cancer or AIDS or other possible opportunistic infections should be sought. A soft-tissue lateral neck radiograph should be obtained if a retropharyngeal or prevertebral abscess or epiglottitis is a consideration. If hydration is adequate and the patient does not otherwise appear ill, evaluation may continue on an outpatient basis.

Two options are available for further evaluation of odynophagia: barium swallow and esophagoscopy. The advantages of the barium swallow are its lower cost, lesser degree of invasiveness, and decreased risk to health-care workers and other patients. However, findings on barium swallow are often nonspecific, making endoscopy necessary. Air–contrast barium studies also provide more sensitivity, but patients with severe odynophagia are often unable to perform these tests. Endoscopy allows one to obtain tissue samples for cytology or culture and is thus usually more useful in making a specific diagnosis. Other parts of the upper GI tract can be examined at the same time, increasing diagnostic ability without adding much to the cost, duration, or risk of the procedure.

Serologic tests for CMV and HSV, although commercially available, play little role in the diagnosis of acute esophageal disease.

EMERGENCY DEPARTMENT MANAGEMENT

A number of antifungal agents have been used to treat oral and esophageal candidiasis in patients with AIDS. Ketoconazole or one of its congeners is the drug of choice. Clinical experience with local therapy, such as nystatin and clotrimazole lozenges, suggests some efficacy against oropharyngeal candidiasis, but these are generally considered inadequate for esophageal candidiasis. Symptoms may clear and oropharyngeal candidiasis may be eradicated, even in the presence of persistent endoscopically visible esophageal disease. High doses of ketoconazole may be required in patients with AIDS. The usual starting dose is 200 mg twice daily, increased to 200 mg three times a day if needed. Fluconazole is more expensive but has more reliable oral absorption, a longer half-life, and less toxicity, and it is better tolerated. Fluconazole is also associated with a higher cure rate than other antifungal agents, such as itraconazole.[1] The combination of itraconazole and flucytosine may be an effective alternative if fluconazole cannot be used.[2] Patients who are granulocytopenic or who are otherwise at high risk for disseminated candidiasis are candidates for intravenous amphotericin B, as are those who are not at high risk but cannot take oral medications.

Foscarnet and ganciclovir appear to be similarly effective and safe in the treatment of AIDS-related CMV esophagitis. Consequently, the choice of the anti-CMV agent should be tailored to the individual patient according to side-effect profiles.[13] HSV esophagitis may be self-limited in the immunocompetent host, but therapy with oral or intravenous acyclovir should be instituted in immunocompromised patients.

In patients presenting with mild esophageal symptoms that do not limit oral intake, an empiric trial of antifungal therapy with ketoconazole or fluconazole is reasonable regardless of the presence or absence of oral candidiasis. If symptoms improve after 7 to 10 days of treatment, a presumptive diagnosis of esophageal candidiasis may be made and the patient is continued on chronic suppressive therapy. If symptoms have not responded to a short course of empiric therapy, the patient should proceed to endoscopy to investigate the possibility of other causes.

If *medication-induced esophagitis* is recognized early and is treated appropriately, it is generally reversible. The offending medication should be discontinued or changed to liquid form when possible. Because swallowing and salivation occur less during sleep, patients should be instructed not to take medications immediately before bedtime. Other commonsense caveats apply: Small tablets are swallowed more quickly than larger ones, oval pills better than round ones, and coated pills faster than uncoated pills. Patients should also be instructed to take medications with plenty of water and to avoid lying down shortly after ingesting their pills. Symptomatic resolution and endoscopic healing of pill esophagitis is usually evident in 3 days to 6 weeks.[16]

DISPOSITION

Immunocompetent patients with mild symptoms may be treated as outpatients. Referral and follow-up are appropriate for these patients, as well as for those who do not respond to initial therapy.

Patients who are experiencing severe difficulty with swallowing and are unable to maintain hydration require hospital admission. Patients at risk for disseminated infection should be admitted for intravenous therapy.

Patients with pill esophagitis should be referred to their primary care physician to ensure that timely resolution of symptoms occurs.

COMMON PITFALLS

- Pain on swallowing is not always due to pharyngitis. Severe and potentially life-threatening conditions, including

epiglottitis and retropharyngeal and prevertebral space abscesses, should be excluded. A careful history should be taken to ascertain the likelihood of an immunosuppressed state and a susceptibility to infectious esophagitis.
- Foreign bodies and food impaction are not uncommon, especially in the elderly and the alcoholic, whose oropharyngeal tactile sense is blunted. Pill esophagitis is likewise a probably underappreciated condition.

ESOPHAGEAL CHEST PAIN

CLINICAL PRESENTATION

The two most common esophageal disorders in patients presenting with angina-like chest pain are gastroesophageal reflux and esophageal motility disorders.

Symptomatic gastroesophageal reflux disease (GERD) is common. It is estimated that 10% of the general population has daily heartburn and that at least one-third of the population experiences heartburn once a month. Acid reflux can be detected in the distal esophagus for up to 75 minutes a day in healthy individuals, and many patients who suffer complications of acid reflux never experience heartburn or reflux.[15] It has been widely held that nocturnal reflux is the most important factor in the pathogenesis of reflux disease. Twenty-four-hour esophageal pH has shown, however, that, in the majority of patients (those who have mild erosive esophagitis or no endoscopic abnormality), most reflux occurs in the daytime postprandial periods, and especially in the early evening, with relatively little reflux during the night. More severe esophagitis, which is due to greater acid exposure, is, however, associated with an increase in nocturnal reflux.

There has also been much debate about the relationship between the presence of hiatal hernia and GERD. Hiatal hernias seen on routine chest radiography do not correlate well with clinical reflux disease. However, approximately 80% of patients with hiatal hernia have an abnormal reflux frequency (as measured with 24-hour pH monitoring), compared with only about 40% of those without hernias.

The primary determinant of GERD is the structural and functional integrity of the lower esophageal sphincter (LES). The most important factor contributing to GERD is transient relaxation of the esophagogastric junction.[6,19] The incidence of GERD rises dramatically after age 40. Factors that influence the degree of reflux injury include the volume and pH of the gastric refluxate, the efficiency of gastroesophageal clearance, and the resistance and restorative repair capabilities of the esophageal epithelium. Patients with severe complications of GERD generally have an incompetent LES.[19] Esophagitis results from excessive reflux of gastric juice rather than excessive gastric secretion.[9]

Patients typically suffer from GERD for years before seeking medical help. The predominant complaint is that of pyrosis, or "heartburn," which is due to mucosal irritation caused by refluxed gastric contents. The discomfort is usually described as a burning pain felt behind the sternum, often seeming to ascend from the epigastrium toward the throat, where a bitter taste may be sensed, and sometimes radiating to the back. There may be radiation of the discomfort to the neck or left arm. The intensity is variable, ranging from a dull ache to severe pain; the duration of discomfort may be minutes or hours. Symptoms may occur spontaneously and are rarely precipitated by swallowing, although they may also seem to be brought on by exercise, bending, or lying down. A large meal, as well as certain foods, such as chocolate, peppermint, alcohol, onions, and fat, increase esophageal acid exposure, while cola, beer, and milk increase gastric acid secretion. Orange juice, tomato juice, and coffee have a direct irritative effect on the esophagus.[19] Heartburn often disappears quickly on drinking liquids or antacids.

Interestingly, only 30% to 40% of patients who complain of heartburn have demonstrable mucosal injury of the esophagus, and, conversely, reflux disease can occur without heartburn.

Strictures, manifested clinically by dysphagia, are the most common complication of reflux esophagitis. They appear to be caused by a combination of deep esophageal mural inflammation, fibrosis, spasm, and edema.

Motility disorders comprise the second group of esophageal disorders presenting predominantly as chest pain. *Achalasia*, a disorder characterized by the absence of peristalsis throughout the esophagus and, usually, deficient LES relaxation during swallowing, is associated with chest pain in about one-half of patients with the condition. The pain is rarely severe and may vary in quality. Chest pressure may be due to esophageal dilation from delayed emptying of food; heartburn or odynophagia may be due to stasis esophagitis and bacterial overgrowth or to esophageal pill retention. Reflux esophagitis is distinctly unusual, because LES pressure is high. Achalasia is eventually diagnosed in up to 10% of patients with noncardiac chest pain.

The primary neurologic defect responsible for achalasia remains unknown. The most consistent pathologic finding is a decrease of ganglion cells in the myenteric plexus at the LES. The disorder may occur at any age, but its exact incidence and prevalence are unknown. The disease typically follows an indolent course; at the time of presentation, symptoms have usually been present for an average of about 7 years. Longitudinal population studies of patients with achalasia suggest the disease does not affect life expectancy.

Diffuse esophageal spasm is characterized by simultaneous contractions in the body of the esophagus occurring with at least 30% of swallows. The contractions are frequently repetitive, spontaneous, of prolonged duration, or of high amplitude. Patients present with dysphagia or intermittent chest pain. The chest pain is not necessarily related to eating, although it may be triggered by the ingestion of very hot or very cold liquids. The diagnosis of diffuse esophageal spasm requires that both clinical and manometric criteria be fulfilled, because asymptomatic individuals can display similar manometric features. No organic lesion is demonstrable radiographically, endoscopically, or histologically.

In *nutcracker esophagus*, motility is ordered and peristaltic, but the waves are of longer duration and higher amplitude than normal.

DIFFERENTIAL DIAGNOSIS

A cardiac etiology must always be excluded when a patient presents with burning substernal chest pain. Chest pain of esophageal origin may be impossible to distinguish from angina by history alone. One must remember that the administration of an antacid or "GI cocktail" is a therapeutic intervention and not a diagnostic procedure. It has been well documented that cardiac chest pain can respond to these preparations, for reasons that are open to speculation.

Even among patients with a history that is classic for cardiac ischemia, a significant percentage (approaching 30% in some studies) undergoing cardiac catheterization have normal or clinically nonsignificant occlusions.[3,6] Unfortunately, there are no characteristic features of chest pain that are pathognomonic of esophageal disorders, including response to antacids, nitroglycerin, or calcium channel blockers. Even pain that is associated with dysphagia and is unrelated to exertion may be ischemic in origin.

EMERGENCY DEPARTMENT EVALUATION

If a cardiac cause can be excluded and the patient gives a history of heartburn without dysphagia, weight loss, or GI bleeding, no laboratory or imaging studies are needed in the emergency department.

Further evaluation is needed if heartburn persists after treatment or if it recurs when treatment is stopped. Heartburn refractory to treatment, or heartburn accompanied by dysphagia, odynophagia or GI bleeding, requires endoscopy to exclude other causes.[9] However, endoscopy shows no evidence of ulcerations in most patients who seek treatment for uncomplicated reflux symptoms.[15] The most useful tests for diagnosing reflux disease are barium swallow, endoscopy, and 24-hour gastric pH monitoring, all of which are performed on an outpatient basis.

Evaluation of esophageal motility disorders usually employs esophageal manometry and is also carried out on an outpatient basis (see subsequent chapter section, "Dysphagia").

EMERGENCY DEPARTMENT MANAGEMENT

Mild symptomatic esophagitis can usually be managed empirically with lifestyle and dietary modifications, antacids, and nonprescription H_2-antagonists.[9,12]

Lifestyle modifications alone are rarely sufficient to relieve symptoms of mild GERD, but they can be an adjunct to pharmacologic management.[4] Patients are often advised to raise the head of the bed approximately 6 in. or to elevate their shoulders with a wedge. The effects of these maneuvers on esophageal acid exposure are modest and appear to be greater when the patient has severe disease. This is consistent with pH monitoring studies that show that, in the majority of patients, most acid exposure occurs during the daytime. The nonpharmacologic measures most likely to benefit the patient are a reduction in fat intake, elimination of tobacco use, and elevation of the head of the bed.[15]

Antacids provide rapid relief and are useful in controlling daytime symptoms, but they are inadequate for patients with moderate-to-severe symptoms, who require around-the-clock therapy. For mild reflux esophagitis, H_2-antagonists, prokinetic agents, or sucralfate may be used initially. Superior healing rates of erosive esophagitis have been noted with H_2-blockers. However, because H_2-antagonists at higher doses than those used in peptic ulcer disease are needed for more severe esophagitis, proton pump inhibitors (PPIs) are usually a more cost-effective alternative. In general, they result in faster healing rates and greater symptom relief than H_2-antagonists.[7,16,19] The dose of omeprazole is 20 mg/d, and the dose of lansoprazole is 30 mg/d.[4,7] Therapy is usually continued for 6 to 8 weeks. All patients who do not respond to a 4-week trial of PPIs for typical GERD symptoms should be considered for endoscopy to establish a diagnosis.[10,19]

Sucralfate, which inhibits pepsin, as well as absorbs and inactivates bile salts, has been shown to be superior to placebo and comparable to antacids and H_2 blockers. Cisapride increases LES tone, accelerates gastric emptying, and has similar efficacy to H_2-antagonists in the treatment of mild esophagitis.[9,19] Metoclopramide increases LES pressure and accelerates gastric emptying in retention states. Its effectiveness is not clear-cut, and it has a relatively high side-effect profile; it is not recommended as first-line therapy.

The treatment of esophageal motility disorders is discussed in the next section.

DISPOSITION

If the diagnosis of GI chest pain is not in doubt, the patient can be discharged and referred to the primary care physician. For resistant symptoms or suspected complications of reflux esophagitis, the patient may be referred to a gastroenterologist for endoscopy or 24-hour pH monitoring.

COMMON PITFALL

Chest pain due to coronary artery disease may be misdiagnosed as GI in origin, especially when substernal burning or atypical chest pain appears to be relieved by antacids or a "GI cocktail."

DYSPHAGIA

CLINICAL PRESENTATION

Dysphagia refers to difficulty or impairment in swallowing. Difficulty in moving a food bolus from the mouth to the upper part of the esophagus is termed *oropharyngeal dysphagia,* whereas a problem with the passage of food or liquid down the esophagus to the stomach is referred to as *esophageal dysphagia.* Whenever the esophagus does not empty in a coordinated, sequential manner, dysphagia may be accompanied by odynophagia, heartburn, GI chest pain, or nausea and vomiting. Globus hystericus is the constant sensation of a lump in the throat, associated with the need to swallow with no identifiable cause. In contrast to true dysphagia, there is no difficulty when swallowing is actually performed.[20]

Dysphagia is often the principal presenting symptom of esophageal motility disorders, which usually present during middle age and are more common in women.[16] These include primary esophageal disorders, such as achalasia, diffuse esophageal spasm, and nutcracker esophagus, as well as esophageal dysfunction secondary to other conditions, most notably scleroderma. Although patients with these disorders frequently experience dysphagia, not all patients with abnormal motility have symptoms.

Achalasia, discussed previously and characterized by deficient peristalsis and failure of the LES to relax on swallowing, is the best studied disorder of esophageal motility. Dysphagia to both liquids and solids is present in nearly all patients with achalasia, but is usually intermittent at first and typically worsens with time. The site of obstruction is often correctly located by the patient in the xiphoid area. Patients with achalasia learn maneuvers to assist esophageal emptying, such as throwing the shoulders back, extending the neck, or performing a Valsalva maneuver.[16]

Food eventually empties into the stomach as gravity aids in its passage through the nonrelaxing sphincter, but stagnant undigested food may also be regurgitated. This occurs most commonly at night because of the recumbent position; vomitus may be noted on the pillow on awakening in the morning. Not surprisingly, aspiration is a complication of achalasia and may present as cough, pneumonia, or lung abscess. Weight loss is also a feature of the motility disorders and is due not only to the physical difficulty of swallowing, but also to decreased oral intake because of fear of dysphagia and chest pain.

Nutcracker esophagus and diffuse esophageal spasm, also discussed previously, are also characterized by dysphagia and intermittent chest pain but are much less well studied than achalasia.

Obstructive dysphagia may be due to *benign* structural lesions of the esophagus, including esophageal webs and rings and intramural hematomas and dissections.[18] Webs are squamous mucosal protuberances that are either congenital or acquired, usually single, and located in the proximal 2 to 4 cm of the esophagus. Rings could easily be called distal esophageal webs; however, these terms are entrenched in the literature. The typical ring lies within the LES at the squamocolumnar junction. Like a web, it is a mucosal lesion. Its cause is unknown, but a hiatal hernia is usually present. Rings more than 20 mm in diameter are rarely symptomatic; those less than 13 mm in diameter almost always cause dysphagia.[16,20] Rings are probably congenital, but the elasticity of the ring decreases with age, explaining why symptoms rarely occur before age 40.[8]

Intramural hematomas and dissections are rare submucosal lesions of the esophagus. Esophageal hematomas and dissections present in much the same manner as esophageal perforations. Nonbloody emesis followed acutely by chest pain, often radiating to the back, dominates the clinical picture of both. Patients with perforations, however, appear more toxic, and their condition deteriorates rapidly. Esophageal carcinoma is a very important cause of dysphagia and is important to recognize early in its course, because the prognosis is dismal by the time a patient presents with progressive dysphagia. Squamous cell carcinoma accounts for 98% of malignant lesions of the esophagus; adenocarcinoma arising from Barrett's esophagus comprises the remainder. Squamous cell tumors are equally distributed among the upper, middle, and lower thirds of the esophagus. Heavy alcohol intake and smoking significantly increase the likelihood of squamous cell carcinoma of the esophagus, while adenocarcinoma tends to occur in patients with a long history of GERD.[20]

The symptoms of esophageal carcinoma are usually insidious in onset. Initially, substernal discomfort and slight alterations in eating habits may go unrecognized. Patients may complain of substernal burning that mimics reflux esophagitis. Carcinoma should be suspected if reflux esophagitis is refractory to therapy or if symptoms change. In addition to dysphagia, anorexia and weight loss are other common manifestations. As the esophageal lumen progressively narrows, clearance of liquids and, eventually, even secretions becomes difficult, leading to recurrent aspiration pneumonia. As with other esophageal disorders, physical examination is unrevealing except for signs of malnutrition. Laboratory evaluation may reveal anemia secondary to blood loss from the tumor.

DIFFERENTIAL DIAGNOSIS

Oropharyngeal dysphagia should first be distinguished from esophageal dysphagia. Patients with *oropharyngeal dysphagia* describe difficulty in passing food from the mouth to the esophagus. Associated manifestations may include drooling, nasal regurgitation, inability to initiate swallowing, coughing during swallowing, aspiration pneumonia, and dysarthria or nasal speech. There may be weight loss due to fear of eating.[11]

In 80% of cases, the underlying cause is neuromuscular, including central, peripheral, and motor end-plate disorders. Central neuromuscular causes include cerebrovascular accidents or tumors (usually in the region of the brainstem), Parkinson disease, multiple sclerosis, and amyotrophic lateral sclerosis.

If the history suggests *esophageal dysphagia,* the distinction must be made between motor disorders and obstructive lesions. The two are easily confused, because both present as esophageal dysphagia. The history is often helpful, because chest pain is a more significant and more frequent complaint in patients with motility disorders. The dysphagia associated with achalasia tends to occur with solids and liquids from the outset, whereas progressive, obstructive lesions present as difficulty swallowing solids, which then progresses to difficulty swallowing solids, liquids, and secretions.

EMERGENCY DEPARTMENT EVALUATION

The evaluation of dysphagia should begin, as always, with attention to the airway, breathing, and circulation and particularly to hydration status. A basic history and physical examination should be performed. Just as when evaluating patients with symptoms suggestive of reflux, a cardiac cause of chest pain should first be considered before implicating the esophagus. If, after initial questioning, esophageal dysphagia is suspected, a chest radiograph should be obtained once the patient's condition has been stabilized. Radiographic hints that achalasia may be present include a widened mediastinum (caused by a dilated esophagus), the presence of an air–fluid level in the posterior mediastinum (caused by the dilated, fluid-filled esophagus), and the absence of a gastric air bubble (because swallowed air cannot get into the stomach). A chest radiograph may also reveal an extrinsic mass causing compression of the esophagus.

The remainder of the diagnostic evaluation can generally take place on a nonemergent outpatient basis. Double-contrast barium esophagography provides excellent visualization of structural lesions and should be the initial test performed in patients with esophageal dysphagia or odynophagia.[17] An upper GI series is not a suitable substitute for a barium esophagram, because this study focuses on the stomach.[16,20]

Patients with suspected motility disorders are better studied with dynamic techniques or cinefluorography. In achalasia, these reveal a paucity of peristaltic movements and a dilated, fluid-filled esophagus tapering to a characteristic "bird's beak" narrowing at the LES. Patients with diffuse esophageal spasm demonstrate diffuse, powerful contractions, appearing as "curling," that obliterate normal peristaltic contractions.[10]

Esophageal manometry is the gold standard for diagnosing motility disorders. However, it will provide a diagnosis in only 25% of patients and is normal in half of those patients referred for dysphagia. Provocative testing during manometry, using edrophonium, esophageal balloon distention, or acid perfusion, may further clarify the diagnosis.[20]

Obstructive lesions can be further evaluated by barium swallow under fluoroscopy, which can usually be performed as an outpatient. Esophageal rings, webs, and carcinoma may be seen; occasionally, some findings, such as proximal dilation with rapid tapering at the LES, may mimic achalasia. More typical findings of mass lesions are asymmetric stenosis, distinct mucosal irregularities, strictures, and masses. If any suspicious abnormality is seen after the barium study, the patient should undergo upper GI endoscopy for biopsy and cytologic brushings.

Endoscopy is indicated in all patients suffering from food impaction, whether the food bolus is eventually passed or not, because this may be the first sign of an obstructive lesion.

EMERGENCY DEPARTMENT MANAGEMENT

In patients in whom normal alimentary intake has been prevented, attention should initially focus on hydration and nutritional status.

Pharmacologic options for managing painful motility disorders are directed principally at reducing smooth muscle spasm or decreasing LES pressure. Treatment of diffuse esophageal spasm is aimed at decreasing the amplitude of esophageal contractions by the use of nitrates and calcium channel blockers. Patients who fail medical therapy can be treated with myotomy or dilations.[11,21,27] Treatments for achalasia include sublingual isosorbide dinitrate and calcium channel blockers with meals or on a prn basis for pain and dysphagia. Other medications, such as anticholinergics, psychotropics, and analgesics, may also be tried.[3,5,6,16] Botulinum toxin administered by endoscopic injection may give relief of dysphagia for up to 1 year.[6,14,16] Pneumatic dilation is a final therapeutic avenue.

Although some squamous cell carcinomas are responsive to chemotherapy, most esophageal cancers are incurable. Esophageal dilation is an integral part of most palliative treatment programs. A small amount of bleeding is commonly seen after dilation, but massive bleeding is unusual. The major risk of esophageal dilation is perforation, which occurs at a rate of one in every 400 to 1000 dilations. Management of esophageal perforation depends on the degree of spillage, the time to diagnosis, and the patient's fitness for surgery. In the past, surgical treatment was considered the only management option, but there has been some experience with a conservative approach using antibiotics and parenteral alimentation, always in conjunction with a thoracic surgery consultation. The surgeon's opinion should be sought early on.

DISPOSITION

Patients with dysphagia whose hydration and nutritional status are adequate may be discharged home and should be referred to their primary care physician or gastroenterologist for further evaluation and treatment. If coronary artery disease cannot be ruled out, the patient should be admitted to a monitored bed; a cardiac evaluation must be undertaken before a GI workup is launched.

COMMON PITFALLS

- Failure to consider cardiac ischemia in patients who describe chronic, intermittent, nonspecific chest discomfort
- Failure to evaluate and refer patients with mild dysphagia, in whom a potentially treatable obstructive lesion may be the cause
- Attribution of persistent symptoms of dysphagia to "globus hystericus" or anxiety without referring the patient for further testing

References

1. Barbaro G, Barbarini G, Calderon W. Fluconazole vs itraconazole for candida esophagitis in acquired immunodeficiency syndrome. *Gastroenterology* 1996;111:1169–1177.
2. Barbaro G, Barbarini G, DiLorenzo G. Fluconazole vs itraconazole-flucytosine association in the treatment of esophageal candidiasis in AIDS patients: a double blind, multi-center placebo-controlled study. *Chest* 1996;110:1507–1514.
3. Bremner RM, DeMeester TR. Current management of patients with esophageal motor abnormalities. *Adv Surg* 1996;30:349–384.
4. Boyce HW. Therapeutic approaches to healing esophagus. *Am J Gastroenterol* 1997;92[4 Suppl]:S22–S27.
5. Clement DJ. Achalasia management: difficult no matter how you slice it [Letter]. *Am J Gastroenterol* 1998;93:478–480.
6. Domenech E, Kelly J. Swallowing disorders. *Med Clin North Am* 1999;83:97–113.
7. Franko TG, Richter JE. Proton-pump inhibitors for gastric acid-related disease. *Cleve Clin J Med* 1998:65:27–34.
8. Johnson DA. Medical therapy for gastroesophageal reflux disease. *Am J Med* 1992;92[Suppl 5A]:88S.
9. Kahrilas PJ. Gastroesophageal reflux disease. *JAMA* 1996;276:983–988.
10. Malagelada JR, Distrutti E. Management of gastrointestinal motility disorders. *Drugs* 1996;52:494–506.
11. Mathog RH, Reming SM. A clinical approach to dysphagia. *Am J Otolaryngol* 1992;13:133.
12. Minocha A, Joseph AS. Pathophysiology and management of noncardiac chest pain. *Korean Med Assoc J* 1995;93:196–201.
13. Parente F, Bianchi PG. Treatment of cytomegalovirus esophagitis in patients with acquired immune deficiency syndrome: a randomized controlled study of foscarnet versus ganciclovir. *Am J Gastroenterol* 1998;93:317–322.
14. Patti MG, Way LW. Evaluation and treatment of primary esophageal motility disorders. *West J Med* 1997;166:263–269.
15. Reynolds JC. Influence of pathophysiology, severity, and cost on the medical management of gastroesophageal reflux disease. *Am Health Syst Pharm* 1996;53:S5–S12.
16. Richter JE. Practical approach to the diagnosis and treatment of esophageal dysphagia. *Compr Ther* 1998;24:446–453.
17. Shapiro J. Evaluation and treatment of swallowing disorders. *Compr Ther* 1992;18:17–21.
18. Shay SS. Benign structural lesions of the esophagus. *Gastroenterol Clin North Am* 1991;20:673.
19. Steele GH. Cost-effective management of dyspepsia and gastroesophageal reflux disease. *Gastroenterology* 1996,23:561–576.
20. Trate DM, Parkman HP, Fisher RS. Dysphagia. *Gastroenterology* 1996; 23:417–441.

CHAPTER 154
Upper Gastrointestinal Bleeding

Edward A. Panacek

Over 2% of all hospital admissions in the United States, and over 5% of admissions from emergency departments, are related to acute gastrointestinal bleeding. In the vast majority of these patients, the bleeding source is in the upper gastrointestinal tract.[6] Although bleeding stops spontaneously in up to 80% of patients, approximately 10% of those admitted require intervention to control their hemorrhage. Despite advances in diagnostic and therapeutic care, the overall mortality of admitted patients is 8% to 10% and has remained relatively unchanged for the past 40 years.[6,7,10] For this reason, gastrointestinal bleeding should always be considered potentially life-threatening until proven otherwise.

The source of gastrointestinal bleeding is generally divided into three anatomic regions. *Upper gastrointestinal bleeding* (UGIB) is defined as occurring proximal to the ligament of Treitz. This anatomic site is important, in that bleeding distal to the ligament of Treitz rarely regurgitates back into the duodenum or stomach. Exceptions are seen in patients with bowel obstruction or massive bleeding, such as in aortoenteric fistula. *Middle gastrointestinal tract bleeding* is from the ligament of Treitz to the ileocecal valve (i.e., the jejunum and the ileum). *Lower gastrointestinal tract bleeding* is that which occurs in the colon or rectum.

The most common causes of UGIB are listed in Table 154.1; up to 30% of patients may have multiple causes or numerous anatomic sites involved. UGIB can occur in people of any age but is most common in adults older than 40, and it is more common in males than in females (2:1 ratio). Elderly patients have less ability to compensate for acute hemorrhage, and the majority of deaths occurs in elderly patients.[3,7]

TABLE 154.1. Causes of Upper Gastrointestinal Tract Bleeding

MOST COMMON (90%)	
Peptic ulcer (duodenal two-thirds, gastric one-third)	40%
Erosive gastritis	25%
Varices (esophageal and gastric)	20%
Mallory-Weiss tear	5%
UNCOMMON (10%)	
Epistaxis, hemoptysis	
Aortoenteric fistula	
Boerhaave syndrome	
Carcinoma	
Vascular anomalies	
Caustic ingestion	
Anastomotic ulcer	

CLINICAL PRESENTATION

Most patients with acute UGIB have obvious related signs or symptoms, but there are also more subtle presentations. Thus, these patients can present primarily with severe tachycardia, angina, acute myocardial infarction, hypotension, syncope, weakness, confusion, or even full cardiac arrest.

The classic presentation, however, is with hematemesis. Another common presentation is with abdominal pain or cramps, usually with a change in bowel habits. The character of the pain varies depending on the underlying disorder, but it is most often described as "burning" or "sharp" and is located in the epigastrium. Although it is often assumed that hematochezia (the passage of obviously bloody stools) is a result of lower gastrointestinal hemorrhage, UGIB is still a common cause. Maroon, burgundy, currant-jelly, and melanotic stools differ from each other in that they contain varying amounts of metabolized hemoglobin. Stool appearance alone generally does not help to localize the site of hemorrhage and is more dependent on the volume and timing of the bleeding. One exception to this rule is that the black, tarry stool of melena requires substantial digestion of the blood during its passage through the gastrointestinal tract, and therefore almost always represents a bleeding source proximal to the right colon.

When severe, UGIB can result in varying degrees of hemodynamic compromise. An acute blood loss of 10% of normal volume can usually be compensated through contraction of the venous compartment, with minimal physiologic change. Greater degrees of blood loss (10% to 20%) initiate reflex sympathetic mechanisms, resulting in peripheral vasoconstriction, tachycardia, widened pulse pressure, and orthostatic hypotension. Such patients often complain of thirst, apprehension, weakness, or light-headedness. When blood loss exceeds 20%, reflex mechanisms can no longer fully compensate; hypotension develops and organ perfusion is impaired. This can result in oliguria, mental confusion or coma, metabolic acidosis, and dyspnea.

DIFFERENTIAL DIAGNOSIS

The exact anatomic site or cause for bleeding in the upper gastrointestinal tract cannot always be determined in the emergency department, but the differential diagnosis can usually be narrowed to the most likely causes. In fact, 90% of UGIBs are the result of only four causes (see Table 154.1).

The single most common cause is *peptic ulcer disease* involving the duodenum or stomach. The usual history is that of persistent burning, sharp, or aching pain in the epigastrium that develops 1 to 2 hours after eating. However, bleeding peptic ulcers are sometimes painless, and melena can be the sole presentation. Predisposing factors for peptic ulcers include cigarette smoking, ingestion of alcohol, and hereditary factors. It is now also felt that many ulcers are related to infections with *Helicobacter pylori*.[17]

Erosive gastritis is also a common cause of UGIB. The resultant bleeding can range from minimal to massive. The clinical presentation is often indistinguishable from that of peptic ulcer, and suspicion of the diagnosis is generally based on the clinical setting and history. The most common predisposing factor is the use of nonsteroidal antiinflammatory drugs. Other risk factors include use of alcohol, prolonged corticosteroid use, and major trauma, burns, or head injury.

Patients with bleeding esophageal or gastric *varices* can be among the most difficult to manage. Because varices result from portal hypertension, this diagnosis should be suspected in patients with a history of cirrhosis or other stigmata of severe hepatic dysfunction. Bleeding can be sudden and massive. Complicating the evaluation, however, is the fact that up to 50% of episodes of UGIB in patients with known varices are not due to the varices (they are usually due to gastritis or peptic ulcer disease). Patients with variceal hemorrhage have a very poor prognosis, with a mortality rate of 70% within 1 year of the first bleeding episode. They account for one-third of all deaths from UGIB.

Mallory-Weiss tears are longitudinal lacerations or ruptures of the gastroesophageal junction, usually caused by recurrent forceful vomiting or retching. They are uncommon in children. The history of sudden hematemesis of bright red blood after retching is characteristic, but it is present in only half of patients. Risk factors include alcohol, hiatal hernia, and underlying esophagitis. The amount of bleeding can range from mild to massive, but, in the absence of complicating medical conditions, the course is usually benign.

A number of other less common conditions account for the remaining 10% of episodes of UGIB (see Table 154.1). *Aortoenteric fistula* typically carries a high mortality, with patients generally presenting with extremely massive bleeding resulting from erosion of an aortic aneurysm or a synthetic aortic graft into the distal duodenum. There is usually no time for diagnostic studies, and the patient must be moved rapidly to the operating room. Some patients experience a "herald" bleed of smaller volume within a week before the massive hemorrhage, but this is not usual.

Massive *epistaxis* and, occasionally, *hemoptysis* can sometimes be misinterpreted as UGIB when patients cannot provide a clear history.

EMERGENCY DEPARTMENT EVALUATION

Stabilization takes precedence over comprehensive evaluation in patients with potential UGIB. Patients who are hemodynamically or otherwise unstable must undergo rapid resuscitation and initial treatment concurrent with a brief, focused history and examination.

The history and physical examination often help to localize the bleeding source and indicate the severity of hemorrhage, but they have their limitations. Patients can be misled by food products or medications that look very much like blood. Only 10 mL of blood can turn all of the water in a toilet bowl red. Estimates regarding the amount of blood lost are notoriously inaccurate, whether reported by patients or prehospital personnel.

The history should focus on the following areas:

Onset of bleeding (specifically, was the onset before or after vomiting?)
Amount of blood loss

Relevant medical history (e.g., prior bleeding episodes, history of hepatic disease, aortic graft repair or known aneurysm, alcohol use, use of nonsteroidal antiinflammatory agents)
Associated symptoms (e.g., abdominal pain, peritoneal symptoms, change in bowel habits)
Complicating symptoms (e.g., chest pain, dyspnea, light-headedness, or syncope)

The goals of the initial physical examination are to assess the patient's hemodynamic status, estimate the severity of bleeding, search for clues to the bleeding source, and identify evidence of other organ complications. A supine systolic blood pressure of less than 100 mm Hg or an orthostatic pulse increase of more than 20 to 30 beats per minute suggests an acute blood loss of at least 1 L in an adult. However, changes in vital signs are less specific at the extremes of age, and, conversely, some patients can tolerate substantial volume losses with minimal changes in the vital signs. Findings of flat neck veins; cold, mottled extremities; altered mental status; or diaphoresis can contribute to the clinical assessment, but they are too subjective to be relied on primarily. Occasionally, blood in the gastrointestinal tract can induce nausea, with an increase in vagal tone resulting in a paradoxical bradycardia despite profound hypovolemia.

Underlying hepatic disease can be suggested by spider angiomas, gynecomastia, jaundice, or palmar erythema. Portal hypertension is suggested by ascites, splenomegaly, or a caput medusae. Purpuric lesions or petechiae suggest an underlying coagulopathy. Findings consistent with arthritis suggest an underlying rheumatic disorder for which the patient may be on nonsteroidal antiinflammatory agents.

The nose and oropharynx should be examined for potential bleeding sources, particularly in atypical or confusing cases. The abdominal examination focuses on areas of tenderness, or evidence of ascites, but should also determine whether peritoneal signs are present. Iron and bismuth can make the stools appear melenic, so the stool should be formally tested to confirm the presence of blood. Of note, stools can test positive for occult blood for 2 weeks after a single episode of bleeding. False-positive results have been associated with iron preparations, ingestion of red meats, and bromide preparations. False-negative results can be caused by magnesium-containing antacids, ascorbic acid, and activated charcoal, as well as a number of other medications and food substances. As such, test results should be interpreted with skepticism if they conflict with the clinical picture.

A nasogastric tube should be placed in all patients in whom gastrointestinal bleeding is suspected, regardless of the presumed source or degree. There is no evidence that passage of a nasogastric tube in a patient with esophageal varices results in variceal trauma or increases bleeding. Even if the patient has obvious hematemesis, a tube should be placed to assess ongoing bleeding and to decrease the risk of aspiration. Flecks of red blood that accompany initial gastric intubation can be ignored. Testing of nonbloody aspirates for occult blood is of little clinical use. If blood is found, the nasogastric tube should be capable of fully evacuating the stomach; a large evacuator tube is necessary when large amounts of blood or clots are present. Lavage should be carried out, ideally with the patient in the left lateral decubitus position, until the gastric contents become clear, but large volumes of tap water lavage should be avoided, as they can induce hyponatremia. Either normal saline or tap water can be used for the lavage. Iced fluids should be avoided because they may interfere with normal coagulation function and can also induce hypothermia. There is no advantage to the addition of vasoconstrictors or antacids to the lavage fluid. A negative nasogastric tube aspirate does not exclude UGIB, because it does not reliably sample material past the pylorus. The nasogastric tube aspirate may be negative in up to 25% of patients with a bleeding duodenal ulcer, although this percentage is lower if the aspirate contains bile.

Initial laboratory evaluations should include a complete blood cell count; determination of electrolyte, blood urea nitrogen, and creatinine levels; and tests of coagulation. An elevated blood urea nitrogen value is frequently seen in the setting of an UGIB or small intestinal hemorrhage, particularly when there is hypovolemia or some degree of renal insufficiency. A chest radiograph is indicated in patients in whom aspiration is clinically suspected. Abdominal films are indicated in the subset of patients in whom there is concern about perforation, obstruction, or abdominal aortic aneurysm. Barium contrast studies have limited indications in the emergency setting and can interfere with subsequent endoscopy and angiographic studies.

EMERGENCY DEPARTMENT MANAGEMENT

Patients transported by emergency medical services should have a large-bore (14- to 18-gauge) intravenous catheter placed and normal saline infused at a rate dependent on the patient's stability. They should also be placed on a cardiac monitor. Low-flow oxygen supplementation is suggested, especially for elderly or symptomatic patients. Transport should not be delayed.

Once the patient reaches the emergency department, acute resuscitative interventions and stabilization assume the highest priority. The overall approach to the emergency department management of UGIB is outlined in Table 154.2. In practice, the first three steps are usually executed simultaneously. Definitive localization of the bleeding site and identification of the cause are not always possible, nor necessary, in the emergency department setting.

If not already initiated by prehospital personnel, patients with any degree of compromise should be immediately placed on a cardiac monitor and be given supplemental oxygen. Intravenous access should be established with one or two large-bore (14- to 18-gauge) catheters, depending on the severity of the patient's condition and the presence of active bleeding. Initial laboratory studies should be sent at the same time, including a sample for type and crossmatch for at least 4 U of blood. One or 2 L of crystalloid is infused initially, or until the patient is stable. The hematocrit is rechecked after each 2 L of intravenous fluid or every 2 to 4 hours. If the clinical condition has not substantially improved after 2 L of fluid, and there is clinical evidence of ongoing hemorrhage or severe anemia, blood product transfusions should be considered. Of note, the hemoglobin and hematocrit values are difficult to interpret in the setting of acute bleeding, because compensatory hemodilution may not fully occur for 6 to 12 hours. Therefore, a normal blood cell count does not rule out an acute massive hemorrhage. Even when an upper source is obvious, a nasogastric tube must be inserted to assess for ongoing mild bleeding.

TABLE 154.2. Emergency Department Management of Upper Gastrointestinal Bleeding

1. Assess the patient's overall clinical status and hemodynamic stability.
2. Resuscitate and replete intravascular volume.
3. Localize the general anatomic location of bleeding (i.e., upper, middle, or lower).
4. In ongoing bleeding, determine the cause or source.
5. If bleeding is persistent, initiate interventions.
6. Make decisions concerning patient disposition and the use of consultants.

When active bleeding continues, or the patient's condition otherwise remains unstable, other diagnostic options must be considered. These include acute endoscopy, radionuclide imaging, and arteriography. Of these, endoscopy is the most valuable and the most available. In many situations, these studies would best be performed not in the emergency department but on the inpatient service. In other situations, the emergency department is the most appropriate setting for further study, particularly when the patient's condition remains unstable.

Emergent endoscopy is indicated in any patient with active bleeding that does not clear with lavage, or in patients who present with hemodynamic instability in the setting of liver disease (portal hypertension).[13] Urgent endoscopy may also be indicated when an aortoenteric fistula is suspected, although the patient's clinical condition in such cases usually does not allow time for endoscopy. In preparation for endoscopy, the patient's stomach must be fully evacuated to allow for optimal visualization. This is best performed with a large gastric lavage tube.

Emergent endoscopy provides potential therapeutic options for treatment of persistent UGIB. Cauterization of actively bleeding ulcers or "visible vessels" with a bipolar heater probe or laser can significantly reduce further bleeding, the need for surgery, and subsequent mortality. Injection sclerosis of visible vessels is also an option.[5] However, except in patients with variceal bleeding or other persistent hemorrhage, emergency endoscopy has not been shown to provide any advantage in reducing mortality, morbidity, or transfusion requirement. In stable patients, endoscopy can be safely delayed for 1 to 2 days.[4]

The administration of histamine-2 (H_2) antagonists and similar medications has been shown to prevent bleeding from stress ulcers in high-risk patients in the intensive care unit (ICU) and to speed the healing of peptic ulcers. However, none of these agents has been proven to be of benefit in controlling the bleeding in the acute setting.[10] Only omeprazole (40 mg intravenously q12h) has been shown to be beneficial for patients with recent UGIB, but not active bleeding.[8] Nonetheless, unless there is a specific contraindication, it is recommended to initiate therapy with an H_2 antagonist by giving an initial bolus dose in the emergency department (e.g., cimetidine 300 mg, or ranitidine 50 mg intravenously). If early endoscopy is indicated, antacids and sucralfate should be withheld to avoid interfering with endoscopic visualization.

The therapeutic approach to patients with acute hemorrhage from esophageal varices is substantially different from that employed with other types of UGIB. The presence of hepatic disease, portal hypertension, or even prior variceal hemorrhage does not reliably predict a variceal source for the bleeding. As noted previously, in up to 50% of such patients, bleeding is due to peptic ulcer disease or gastritis. For this reason, emergent endoscopy is necessary both diagnostically and therapeutically in these patients.[4] In the acute setting, emergent endoscopic therapy is often used in combination with pharmacologic agents, and the rate of initial control of bleeding is 90% to 95%.[4]

Endoscopic therapy is divided into two types: endoscopic variceal sclerotherapy and band ligation. With the first, sclerosing agents are injected into the esophageal vessels, causing thrombosis and eventual necrosis. Up to 30% of patients can have complications, including ulcerations and fibrosis.[13] Band ligation involves endoscopic placement of a rubber band around the varix, inducing obstruction and eventual tissue necrosis that obliterates the varix. This has recently become the therapy of choice, due to lower complication rates, for acute variceal hemorrhage at most centers.[16] However, the technique is more difficult technically, and active bleeding can preclude adequate visualization.

Another therapeutic option for variceal hemorrhage is intravenous vasopressin, a potent nonselective vasoconstrictor, which can be used in conjunction with endoscopic therapy or as the sole therapy when sclerotherapy is unsuccessful or unavailable. The dosage is 0.2 to 0.4 U/min by constant infusion. Vasopressin must be used with caution in patients with coronary artery or other vascular disease; a reduction in dosage or the concurrent use of nitroglycerin decreases the risk of adverse effects such as myocardial or extremity ischemia.[4] Studies have shown that somatostatin and its analogues are as effective as vasopressin, with fewer side effects.[2] Although somatostatin remains investigational, a long-acting analogue, octreotide, is available; the dosage is 25 to 50 μg/h intravenously.[4]

When sclerotherapy and vasoconstrictor therapy have been unsuccessful, balloon tamponade is the next therapeutic option. The Sengstaken-Blakemore tube (with three lumens) and the Minnesota tube (with four lumens) are among a number that are available. They are less successful than sclerotherapy but can control bleeding acutely in up to 80% of cases.[4] However, the use of these tubes is associated with a number of major complications, including esophageal necrosis and rupture, pulmonary aspiration, and airway compromise. The tubes come with an explicit list of instructions that should be reviewed in detail before their use, and they are best placed by an experienced practitioner.

Although the vast majority of patients with UGIB never require surgery, early surgical consultation is advisable for any patient who has been hemodynamically unstable or who requires early blood transfusions. Most of the indications for surgical intervention are defined by the patient's clinical course during the initial 24 hours of hospitalization. However, for patients who present with hypotension or shock and massive uncontrollable hemorrhage that is not from varices, immediate surgery should be considered. For variceal bleeding, acute endoscopic therapies and balloon tamponade should be considered before turning to surgical intervention.[4]

DISPOSITION

Historically, all patients with UGIB were admitted to the hospital, but it is now accepted that there is a subset of patients who can safely be discharged from the emergency department with close follow-up.[3,12,14,15] Of patients requiring hospitalization, about half meet high-risk criteria for rebleeding or other complications that necessitate admission to a monitored ICU or telemetry bed.[7,9]

Though each study has used different thresholds or predictive factors, the general criteria for outpatient management are listed in Table 154.3. Some investigators recommend an age cutoff of 60 years, but the majority use an age of 75.[1,9] Candidates for outpatient management must have reliable access to close outpatient follow-up and a demonstrated history of compliance with medical instructions, and they must have remained stable during 4 to 6 hours of emergency department observation.

TABLE 154.3. Criteria for Outpatient Management of Acute UGIB

Age younger than 75 years
No unstable comorbid illness
No evidence of portal hypertension or ascites on examination
Normal coagulation function
Systolic blood pressure > 100 mm Hg and no orthostatic changes within 1 hour of presentation to emergency department
Nasogastric aspirate free of fresh blood after initial lavage
Hemoglobin at least 10 g/dL
Patient compliant with reliable access to close follow-up

TABLE 154.4. Intensive Care Unit Admission Guidelines for Patients with UGIB

Unstable vital signs in the emergency department
Persistent bleeding that does not clear with lavage
Advanced age (older than 75 years)
Presence of coagulopathy
Portal hypertension or ascites
Severe anemia (e.g., hematocrit <20%)
Large drop in hematocrit (>8%)
Unstable comorbid disease (e.g., unstable coronary artery disease, chronic obstructive pulmonary disease, renal insufficiency, peripheral vascular disease, cerebrovascular disease)
Endoscopic findings of a "visible vessel" or an "overlying clot" or a variceal source
Use of vasopressin drip or esophageal tamponade balloon

The specific criteria for admission to an ICU are listed in Table 154.4. Patients should be admitted to an ICU or monitored bed if their condition is unstable in the emergency department, if bleeding persists, or if they are at high risk for rebleeding or associated complications. Patients with UGIB who do not meet criteria for discharge or for admission to the ICU are appropriately admitted to a nonmonitored ward bed.

A number of recent studies have shown that early endoscopy performed in the emergency department can identify a subset of up to 25% to 50% of patients who would otherwise be admitted, but who can safely be managed as outpatients. It is argued that this aggressive approach can provide overall cost savings.[11,12,15]

Those who are discharged with outpatient follow-up should be placed on H_2 blockers (e.g., cimetidine 300 mg four times a day or 800 mg two times a day) and prescribed liquid antacids as needed. The advantages of a bland diet are controversial, but known gastric stimulants such as alcohol, tobacco, and caffeine are best avoided. Frequent small meals may also be beneficial. Follow-up should be arranged within 3 to 7 days, with instructions to return earlier for recurrence of bleeding, worsening of pain, or any orthostatic symptoms.[17]

Emergency consultation with a gastroenterologist or endoscopist is indicated for patients who remain clinically unstable despite resuscitative efforts and for those whose bleeding persists after initial gastric lavage. This is particularly true if the patient may have a variceal bleeding source. Patients who remain unstable or have persistent bleeding also require early surgical intervention and early surgical consultation.[3,17]

Patients who require ICU admission or emergency consultation should be considered for transfer to a referral hospital if either general surgery or endoscopy consultants are not available. Because UGIB patients often have encephalopathy and recurrent vomiting, transport personnel must be skilled in airway management and resuscitation. The patient must have multiple large-caliber intravenous lines in place, and crossmatched blood should be sent with the patient, if available.

COMMON PITFALLS

- Because a number of foods, medications, or other substances can be mistaken for blood in the gastrointestinal tract, the presence of blood in the gastrointestinal tract should be confirmed by testing.
- Despite new developments in diagnosis and therapy, the mortality rate in acute UGIB remains at 8% to 10%. Therefore, all such patients should be considered to have a potentially life-threatening medical problem until proven otherwise.
- Although it is uncommon, patients may exsanguinate into the gastrointestinal tract, with no acute external evidence of blood.
- Accurate assessment of hemodynamic status is critically important. Some patients can lose up to 20% to 30% of their blood volume and still maintain a normal blood pressure in a supine position.
- The nasogastric aspirate may be falsely negative in up to 25% of patients with acute UGIB. These are usually patients with a duodenal bleeding source.
- Among patients with acute UGIB and a known history of variceal hemorrhage, only about half have recurrent bleeding from varices.
- Using specific criteria, a subset of patients with UGIB can be safely managed as outpatients.
- Aortoenteric fistula typically presents as sudden massive hematemesis. This entity is notoriously difficult to diagnose premorbidly, and diagnostic studies are often not helpful or are unavailable. Emergent surgical intervention is the only treatment.

References

1. Ahmed A, Aggarwal M, Watson E. Esophageal perforation: a complication of nasogastric tube placement. *Am J Emerg Med* 1998;16:1.
2. Avgerinos A, Armonis A, Raptis S. Somatostatin or octreotide versus endoscopic sclerotherapy in acute variceal hemorrhage: a meta-analysis. *J Hepatol* 1995;22:247–251.
3. Corley DA; Stefan AM, Wolf M, et al. Early indicators of prognosis in upper gastrointestinal hemorrhage. *Am J Gastroenterol* 1998;93(3):336–340.
4. Grace ND. Diagnosis and treatment of gastrointestinal bleeding secondary to portal hypertension. *Am J Gastroenterol* 1997;92:1082–1090.
5. Gralnek IM, Jensen DM, Kovacs TO, et al. An economic analysis of patients with active arterial peptic ulcer hemorrhage treated with endoscopic heater probe, injection sclerosis, or surgery in a prospective, randomized trial. *Gastrointest Endosc* 1997;46:105–112.
6. Gupta PK, Fleischer DE. Nonvariceal upper gastrointestinal bleeding. *Med Clin North Am* 1993;77:973–992.
7. Katschinski B, Logan R, Davies J, et al. Prognostic factors in upper gastrointestinal bleeding. *Dig Dis Sci* 1994;39(4):706–712.
8. Khuroo MS, Yattoo GN, Javid G, et al. A comparison of omeprazole and placebo for bleeding peptic ulcer. *N Engl J Med* 1997;336:1054–1058.
9. Kollef MH, O'Brien JD, Zuckerman GR, et al. BLEED: a classification tool to predict outcomes in patients with acute upper and lower gastrointestinal hemorrhage. *Crit Care Med* 1997;25:1125–1132.
10. Laine L, Peterson WL. Bleeding peptic ulcer. *N Engl J Med* 1994;331:717–727.
11. Lee JG, Turnipseed S, Romano PS, et al. Endoscopy-based triage significantly reduces hospitalization rates and costs of treating upper GI bleeding: a randomized controlled trial. *Gastrointest Endosc* 1999;50:755–761.
12. Longstreth GF, Feitelberg SP. Successful outpatient management of acute upper gastrointestinal hemorrhage: use of practice guidelines in a large patient series. *Gastrointest Endosc* 1998;47:219–222.
13. Roberts LR, Kamath PS. Pathophysiology and treatment of variceal hemorrhage. *Mayo Clin Proc* 1996;71:973–983.
14. Rockall TA, Logan RFA, Devlin HB, et al. Risk assessment after acute upper gastrointestinal hemorrhage. *Gut* 1996;38:316–321.
15. Rockall TA, Logan RF, Devlin HB, et al. Selection of patients for early discharge or outpatient care after acute upper gastrointestinal hemorrhage. *Lancet* 1996;347:1138–1140.
16. Schoenfeld PS, Butler JA. An evidence-based approach to the treatment of esophageal variceal bleeding. *Crit Care Clin* 1998;14:441–455.
17. Soll AH. Consensus conference. Medical treatment of peptic ulcer disease. Practice guidelines. Practice Parameters Committee of the American College of Gastroenterology. *JAMA* 1996;275(8):622–629.

CHAPTER 155
Peptic Ulcer Disease

Dale S. Birenbaum and David J. Vukich

Peptic ulcer disease (PUD) eventually affects one of every ten Americans. The prevalence of PUD in the population, between 1.7% and 2.9%, implies that there are 4 to 8 million active cases at any given time.[9] Despite these disconcerting numbers, there has been a significant decline in the total number of cases since the 1960s. Interestingly, the disease is becoming less common in developed countries and more common in developing nations.[11]

Duodenal ulcer is more common than gastric ulcer (5:1), and men are afflicted more commonly than women (1.8:1). The incidence is increased in patients with renal failure and transplants, alcoholic cirrhosis, and chronic obstructive pulmonary disease (COPD). The stereotypes of young or middle-aged affluent men developing duodenal ulcers and the elderly or poor developing gastric ulcers are grossly inaccurate. Among the elderly, gastric or duodenal ulceration is an increasing problem. Although mortality rates for PUD have generally declined over the past 30 years, they remain amazingly high for the elderly—50 to 100 times greater at age 75 than at age 35.[11,20]

MECHANISMS OF FORMATION

The mechanisms of peptic ulcer formation in the stomach and in the duodenum are not thought to be the same, but they do share some elements. There appears to be an imbalance between the production of acid and the ability of the mucosa to prevent itself from being damaged (Table 155.1). Acid secretion has been considered the key to ulcer formation, and indeed, ulcers will not form without it. Furthermore, reduction of acid secretion or acid neutralization promotes ulcer healing.

Because duodenal and gastric ulcers develop in patients who are not acid hypersecretors, acid production is not the sole factor involved; weakened defensive factors also play a role in ulcerogenesis. Healthy gastric or duodenal mucosa is an impressive barrier to the diffusion of hydrogen ions and can maintain a gradient of 3 million to 1 between lumen and blood. It also secretes bicarbonate and mucus, which form a buffering gel over the mucosa. Mucosal gel thickness is increased by the E prostaglandins and diminished by aspirin and nonsteroidal antiinflammatory drugs (NSAIDs). Maintenance of normal blood flow to the mucosa is an essential component of resistance to injury.

TABLE 155.1. Factors Acting On or in Gastric Mucosa

Endogenous Aggressive Factors	Endogenous Defensive Factors
Acid	Mucosal barrier
Pepsin	Mucus
Bile	Bicarbonate
Lysolecithin	Cell renewal
	Mucosal blood flow
	Prostaglandins

From Emas S. Medical principles for treatment of peptic ulcer. *Scand J Gastroenterol* 1987;137:28–32.

When ulceration does occur, pain results from direct chemical irritation by hydrochloric acid and disordered motor activity of the stomach and duodenum.

Research has focused on the small microaerophilic gram-negative spiral bacterium *Helicobacter pylori,* which is strongly linked to the formation of duodenal ulcers. This agent increases antral gastrin production, causes chronic gastric metaplasia and duodenitis, and decreases mucosal integrity. The most compelling evidence for the role of *H. pylori* in peptic ulcer disease is that the 1-year relapse rate for duodenal ulcers is less than 15% following eradication therapy but 70% to 80% after H_2-receptor antagonist therapy alone. Its eradication from the gastrointestinal (GI) tract on first presentation has been routinely advocated; this strategy has been associated with accelerated ulcer healing, a reduced rate of ulcer recurrence, and cure of the disease.

Regimens in current use include "standard triple therapy" with bismuth subsalicylate, metronidazole, and tetracycline for 2 weeks, combined with an H_2-receptor antagonist for 4 weeks. "Dual therapy" combines a proton pump inhibitor such as omeprazole 40 mg/d plus clarithromycin 500 mg t.i.d. for 2 weeks. Other current Food and Drug Administration (FDA)–approved regimens for the eradication of *H. pylori* include combinations of one or two antibiotics with either ranitidine, a bismuth salt, or a proton pump inhibitor (Table 155.2).[3,4,7,10,12–17,19,21] Eradication of *H. pylori* does not affect symptoms of nonulcerative gastritis or symptoms of dyspepsia.

In some patients with duodenal ulcer, there is an increase in the number of acid-producing gastric parietal cells and a direct relation between acid hypersecretion and the severity of ulcer disease. However, 50% of ulcer patients have normal acid secretion and show no relation between the severity of illness and the level of acid secretion. Other explanations of duodenal ulcer formation involve the delivery of a large, unbuffered acid load to the duodenum with subsequent mucosal damage, as occurs, for example, in the Zollinger-Ellison syndrome, in which serum gastrin levels are astronomic and normal feedback inhibition does not occur. More than 90% of duodenal ulcers occur within 3 cm of the junction of the pyloric and duodenal mucosa, and most are small (less than 1 cm).

Gastric ulcers are larger and more extensive, and the majority are found on the lesser curvature of the stomach at the junction of the body and antral mucosa. Formation is probably related to an abnormality of the gastric mucosal barrier. Although their role in ulcer formation is yet to be proved, human bile, aspirin, and ethanol increase the permeability of the gastric mucosa to hydrogen ions. Pyloric dysfunction, bile reflux, and gastritis have been proposed to lead to gastric ulceration by weakening the normal mucosal defense mechanisms. Many factors may predispose to the development of ulcers (Table 155.3). Of these factors, cigarette smoking plays a major role both in ulcer formation and in recurrence through several mechanisms (Table 155.4). Of the other predisposing factors, aspirin and NSAIDs cause anatomic and physiologic alterations of the gastric mucosa, but there is still no conclusive evidence that they actually produce ulceration. Despite popular opinion, alcohol and caffeine ingestion have not been conclusively linked to ulcer disease. Diet also is not clearly related to PUD, and, at present, the only reasonable dietary recommendation for ulcer patients is to avoid foods that produce symptoms.[9]

COMPLICATIONS

PUD continues to produce major complications despite the introduction of several apparently effective pharmacologic agents. However, the type of surgical procedure performed for complications of PUD has changed since the introduction of H_2

TABLE 155.2. Current FDA-Approved Therapeutic Regimes for *Helicobacter pylori* Infection

Therapy	Regimen (dosage × no. of days)	Eradication Rate (%)
Bismuth-based triple therapy with H_2-receptor antagonist		
Bismuth subsalicylate	2 tabs q.i.d. × 14	
Metronidazole	250 mg q.i.d. × 14	
Tetracycline	500 mg q.i.d. × 14	
Rantidine (or equivalent)	150 mg b.i.d. × 28	77–82
H_2-receptor antagonist-based therapy	(or equivalent)	
Ranitidine bismuth citrate	400 mg b.i.d. × 28	
Clarithromycin	500 mg t.i.d. × 14	73–84
Proton pump inhibitor-based dual therapy		
Clarithromycin	500 mg t.i.d. × 14	
Omeprazole	40 mg q.d. × 14, then 20 mg q.d. × 14	64–74
Lansoprazole	30 mg t.i.d. × 14	
Amoxicillin	1 g t.i.d. × 14	66–77
Proton pump inhibitor-based triple therapy		
Lansoprazole	30 mg b.i.d. × 14	
Amoxicillin	1 g b.i.d. × 14	
Clarithromycin	500 mg b.i.d. × 14	86–92

Adapted from Peura D. *Helicobacter pylori:* rational management options. *Am J Med* 1998;105(5):424-430, with permission.

blockers. Fewer elective procedures are performed in the relatively fit, younger population, and more emergent operations are performed on older and sicker patients who are less able to tolerate surgery.[18]

Perforation continues to occur in peptic ulcer patients despite the availability of reasonably effective medical treatment.[18] Perforation is heralded by a dramatic change in the pain pattern. Either severe pain and a surgical abdomen develop rapidly secondary to release of air and secretions into the peritoneal cavity, or a constant, deeper pain increases gradually with the slower development of surgical signs as a result of posterior penetration or a partially occluded perforation. Whether presenting suddenly or gradually, perforation is a surgical emergency requiring rapid diagnosis, resuscitation, and operation.

Hemorrhage from peptic ulcers is usually self-limited but is occasionally massive and life-threatening; it accounts for 20% to 30% of patients who require surgery for PUD.[6] It is a common complication of PUD, with presentations ranging from melena alone to frank hypovolemic shock. Upper GI bleeding should be anticipated in any ulcer patient.

TABLE 155.3. Risk Factors for Peptic Ulcer

DEFINITELY RELATED
Family history
Associated disease (COPD, cirrhosis, chronic renal failure)
Male gender
Advanced age
Smoking
POSSIBLY RELATED
Use of certain drugs (e.g., ASA, NSAIDS)
Psychological profile
NOT RELATED
Diet (caffeine, spicy or fatty foods)
Alcohol

Modified from Ruoff GE. Peptic ulcer disease. The role of the primary care physician in therapeutic intervention. *Postgrad Educ* 1987;81(5):86.

Gastric outlet obstruction, the result of scarring from repeated episodes of ulceration and fibrous healing, is usually associated with duodenal ulcer. It may also be caused by edema from an active ulcer. Fluid and gas accumulate in the stomach, causing fullness or distress that is often relieved by vomiting. Massive distention of the stomach can occur; volume depletion and electrolyte disturbances may be dramatic. In the emergency department, fluid resuscitation should be performed and the stomach should be decompressed by means of a nasogastric tube, but surgery may be necessary for definitive treatment. Gastric outlet obstruction may be the indication for as many as 30% of ulcer operations.[6]

Nonhealing, the failure of a gastric ulcer to improve with medical treatment, is suggestive of malignancy.

CLINICAL PRESENTATION

Peptic ulcer is a chronic but not necessarily life-long disease, frequently running a course of 10 to 15 years and marked by periods of acute exacerbation and remission. Pain may develop without obvious cause and persist for several days or weeks, but rarely longer. Because these episodes sometimes resolve with over-the-counter preparations, many patients do not seek medical assistance. Most ulcer patients experience a benign course, except for occasional symptomatic periods, but 10% to 20% develop some complication of the disease.

Most patients present to the emergency department for relief from a constant burning, gnawing, or aching pain. The pain of PUD is primarily epigastric, but it can be localized anywhere in

TABLE 155.4. Effects of Smoking on Peptic Ulcer Disease

Increased rate of gastric emptying
Diminished pancreatic bicarbonate secretion
Decreased duodenal luminal pH
Reduced mucosal blood flow
Inhibition of mucosal prostaglandin synthesis

From Eastwood GL. Current therapy for recurrent ulcer. *J Clin Gastroenterol* 1987;9 [Suppl 1]:14.

the upper abdomen. With perforation of a posterior duodenal ulcer, pain often begins in the epigastrium and moves to the back. If pneumoperitoneum develops, pain may be referred to the shoulder as well.

The description and location of the pain is not as important in diagnosis as is its timing and any exacerbating and ameliorating factors. Gastric ulcer usually produces pain immediately after eating, when acid production increases in response to food. The pain of duodenal ulcer is most common between or just before meals and at night, when the upper GI tract is empty. Ingestion of food or antacids may bring rapid relief. Pain at 2 or 3 a.m. is classic for duodenal ulcer, probably because acid production is high and unbuffered by food. Acid production is at its lowest later in the morning, and pain is rarely present at this time. The classic history of a repetitive pain–food–relief sequence remains one of the better clinical diagnostic clues to PUD.

Asymptomatic peptic ulcer is not uncommon; an estimated 20% to 25% of all ulcers may be silent.[8] In fact, nearly a third of patients with ulcer perforation and a fifth of those with upper GI hemorrhage have no previous symptoms of ulcer disease.

Uncomplicated PUD does not produce remarkable physical findings. Epigastric tenderness may be noted, but guarding and rebound are not present. Bowel sounds are most often normal, and there is no organomegaly. Rectal examination may show guaiac-positive stool if there has been unrecognized bleeding. The purpose of the physical examination is to exclude complications and other diseases, rather than to confirm the presence of peptic ulcer. Thus, examination of the heart and lungs is indicated to help rule out cardiac or pulmonary disease masquerading as an abdominal process.

Guarding, rebound, and a tense abdomen signal perforation of an ulcer. There may be slight improvement immediately following perforation, but, within hours, shock ensues. Patients with perforation usually lie perfectly still, because the slightest movement produces intense peritoneal pain. In the elderly, findings may be minimal or absent, tending to delay the diagnosis in the group least able to tolerate delay.

Hemorrhage from PUD may cause surprisingly few physical findings on examination. A history of melenic stools should be sought, and orthostatic vital signs may help uncover clinically important but nonobvious bleeding. Frequently, significant bleeding presents with hematemesis; a nasogastric tube can be inserted to determine whether blood or "coffee grounds" are present in the stomach.

Gastric outlet obstruction usually produces some degree of bloating and a tympanitic epigastrium or succussion splash secondary to a distended stomach.

DIFFERENTIAL DIAGNOSIS

Myocardial infarction and angina are perhaps the most important diagnoses to consider in the differential diagnosis. They may present atypically as midepigastric pain, with complaints of nausea, bloating, and burning surprisingly similar to those of PUD, but without the typical periodicity and ameliorating factors. Moreover, many ulcer patients also have coronary artery disease. A careful history and electrocardiographic (ECG) examination can usually differentiate heart disease, however.

Gastritis usually produces a constant feeling of bloating and may not be relieved by antacids. Gastroenteritis produces colicky or crampy abdominal pain associated with diarrhea and vomiting. Biliary tract disease causes upper abdominal pain (classically after ingestion of fatty foods), but typically there is no history of early-morning pain or improvement with antacids. Esophagitis as a complication of hiatal hernia may be associated with intense pain immediately or shortly after swallowing. The constant, boring pain of pancreatitis frequently radiates to the back and is associated with elevated serum amylase levels.

A host of other conditions can produce pain in the upper abdomen, but, for the most part, these conditions are readily ruled out by history and physical examination.

EMERGENCY DEPARTMENT EVALUATION

A careful history and physical examination remain the most important methods for evaluating uncomplicated peptic ulcer. However, because other diseases may also present with epigastric distress, and because some complications of PUD may not be immediately apparent, additional diagnostic interventions are recommended.

For any patient in the age group at risk for coronary artery disease, an ECG should be performed and cardiac monitoring used, at least initially. A nasogastric tube should be passed if bleeding or obstruction is suspected, but routine use is probably unnecessary. Chemical tests for the presence of occult gastric blood are available, but their value is questionable because clinically insignificant iatrogenic bleeding often accompanies nasogastric tube insertion.

The chest x-ray is a useful adjunct for detecting free air from perforation and for ruling out thoracic disease. The patient is placed in an upright sitting position for 10 to 15 minutes before the x-ray to allow time for any free air to rise to the diaphragm; insufflating 100 to 200 mL of air through the nasogastric tube may enhance the chances of detecting free air radiographically. Unfortunately, pneumoperitoneum is seen on x-ray in less than 50% of patients with perforation, and the absence of this finding is often associated with delayed diagnosis and significantly increased mortality.

Abdominal x-rays can also be useful but are not routinely necessary. If the chest x-ray does not show free air, but suspicion of perforation is still high, an upright abdominal or left lateral decubitus view can be ordered. Contrast studies are also not a routine part of emergency department evaluation, but they are sometimes performed (using water-soluble contrast material) in an effort to identify suspected perforation. Likewise, endoscopy in the emergency department for uncomplicated PUD is not warranted.

A complete blood count is justified in most emergency department patients who complain of abdominal pain. Low red cell and hematocrit values may reveal significant recent blood loss, and the red cell indices can suggest that anemia is from chronic blood loss. The white cell count is usually normal in uncomplicated PUD, but it may help to differentiate upper abdominal pain of other causes. The white count rises with perforation. Serum amylase or lipase determinations are helpful if pancreatitis is a possibility, but they are not of much value for uncomplicated PUD.

Electrolytes, blood urea nitrogen, serum creatinine, and type and screen are useful for critically ill patients and those who are bleeding, vomiting, or "third-spacing" fluids. Liver function tests, including alkaline phosphatase and bilirubin levels, may be useful when a hepatobiliary process remains in the differential diagnosis. Hypochloremic hypokalemic metabolic alkalosis may be noted with intractable vomiting or gastric outlet obstruction.

Relief with antacids is a strong part of the classic peptic ulcer history and can be a helpful indicator, but it is not diagnostic of PUD. As many as one-fourth of ulcer patients may have concomitant coronary artery disease; thus, it is often difficult to ascribe symptoms or relief of symptoms to one or the other.[18] The indiscriminate use of "GI cocktails" consisting of various combinations of antacids, anticholinergics, barbiturates, and viscous lidocaine, particularly as a diagnostic maneuver, should be discouraged.

EMERGENCY DEPARTMENT MANAGEMENT

Most patients with PUD have normal vital signs, are in minimal distress, and do not require any major intervention. These patients may be given antacids to help relieve pain. Because salicylates and other NSAIDs are associated with the development of peptic ulcer, these agents should be discontinued if in use.

With the recognition that *H. pylori* therapy plays a central role in the pathogenesis of peptic ulcer, the objective of therapy is now eradication and cure. Thus, patients with documented peptic ulcer disease by upper GI contrast radiography or endoscopy should be treated for *H. pylori*. This should be done with appropriate consultation to guide the decision on the most effective antibiotic regimen. Detection of *H. pylori* can be confirmed on histologic mucosal biopsies, by culture, serologically by ELISA, and urea breath test.[2] Serology is now widely used for routine detection and to monitor treatment. Caution should be used for those patients who display signs and symptoms of gastric hypersecretory state, recent antibiotic therapy, and recent use of NSAIDs. If there is nothing to suggest that complications have occurred, specific diagnostic testing for *H. pylori* may be unnecessary, and treatment for eradication may begin as discussed.[3,4,7,10,12–17,19,21]

Traditional agents for peptic ulcer disease are used in an adjunctive role and for symptomatic relief of peptic ulcer. Additionally, these agents neutralize or reduce acid secretion, accelerate the rate of ulcer healing, and prevent recurrence and complications.

H_2-receptor antagonists competitively inhibit the action of histamine on H_2 receptors located in gastric parietal cells and dramatically reduce basal acid secretion as well as secretion in response to feeding, gastrin, hypoglycemia, and vagal stimulation. They are generally safe and effective. Currently, four H_2 antagonists are available in the United States: 800 mg of cimetidine is equivalent to 300 mg of ranitidine, 40 mg of famotidine, or 300 mg of nizatidine. A single bedtime dose of 800 mg of cimetidine (or equivalent doses of the other three H_2 blockers) appears to be roughly as effective as several doses given throughout the day. When used primarily for exacerbations of PUD, low-dose maintenance therapy with H_2-receptor antagonists may also be safe and effective.

Sucralfate is an aluminum salt of sucrose that forms a polymer in the acid environment of the stomach. This polymer adheres selectively to the ulcer crater, forming a physiologic dressing for the damaged mucosa and protecting it from acid; other mechanisms may be at work as well. Sucralfate appears to heal ulcers as effectively as H_2 blockers. It is nonabsorbable and has a very low incidence of side effects. The usual initial dose is 1 g four times a day or 2 g twice a day.

Anticholinergics have been used for PUD for many years and are available in a number of formulations. They decrease acid production, but they also produce dry mouth, urinary retention, and other anticholinergic side effects.

Other agents now available have been found to be at least as efficacious as the H_2 blockers. These include the prostaglandin congeners, such as misoprostol, which increase the cytoprotective properties of the gastric mucosa, and proton pump inhibitors, such as omeprazole, which effectively reduce gastric acid secretion.[1,5]

Patients with complications of PUD require more intensive management, including intravenous infusion of crystalloid or blood, supplemental oxygen, cardiac monitoring, and more specific endoscopic or surgical intervention.

Transfusion is indicated for bleeding patients who fail to stabilize after receiving 2 L of crystalloid, have known coronary artery disease, or are experiencing angina. Trends in hemoglobin and hematocrit values are more useful than a single value; any significant decrease should be considered an indication for transfusion.

DISPOSITION

Patients who are obviously critically ill, have unstable vital signs, or are suffering from a complication of PUD require prompt consultation with a specialist. Other patients may need admission for pain control, gastric decompression, or fluid resuscitation, and do not necessarily require monitoring. Cases of apparently uncomplicated PUD may be referred to a family physician or internist. Initiation of PUD therapy in the emergency department does not obviate the need for outpatient referral, to identify patients who do not respond and may be candidates for endoscopy.

Ulcer patients who require admission may need to be transferred to another institution for endoscopy, critical care services, or surgery. Potentially unstable patients should be transported by an advanced life-support unit.

COMMON PITFALLS

- Failure to consider other life-threatening etiologies for epigastric pain, especially myocardial infarction or abdominal aortic aneurysm
- Failure to recognize sudden changes in symptomatology that herald the onset of a serious complication
- Failure to place a nasogastric tube when indicated
- Failure to refer the patient to an appropriate specialist for evaluation of response to therapy and the need for further diagnostic workup

References

1. Ballinger A. Cytoprotection with misoprostol: use in the treatment and prevention of ulcers. *Dig Dis* 1994;12:37.
2. Chen Y. Comparison of two rapid urease tests for detection of *Helicobacter pylori* infection. *Dig Dis Sci* 1998;43(8):1636–1640.
3. Cotton P. NIH consensus panel urges antimicrobials for ulcer patients, skeptics concern with caveats. *JAMA* 1994;271:808.
4. Fennerty MB. *Helicobacter pylori*. *Arch Intern Med* 1994;154:721.
5. Florent C. Progress with proton pump inhibitors in acid peptic disease: treatment of duodenal and gastric ulcer. *Clin Ther* 1993;15[Suppl B]:14.
6. Hermann RE. Obstructing duodenal ulcer. *Surg Clin North Am* 1976;56:1403.
7. Hosking SW, Ling TK, Chung SC, et al. Duodenal ulcer healing by eradication of *Helicobacter pylori* without antiacid treatment: randomized controlled trial. *Lancet* 1994;343:508.
8. Jorde R, Burhol PG. Asymptomatic peptic ulcer disease. *Scand J Gastroenterol* 1987;22:129.
9. Kurata JH, Haile BM. Epidemiology of peptic ulcer disease. *Clin Gastroenterol* 1984;13:289.
10. Labenz J, Ruhl GH, Bertrams J, et al. Medium or high-dose omeprazole plus amoxicillin eradicates *Helicobacter pylori* in gastric ulcer disease. *Am J Gastroenterol* 1994;89:726.
11. Langman MJS. Peptic ulcer treatment now and tomorrow. *J Clin Gastroenterol* 1987;9[Suppl 2]:2.
12. Logan RP, Gummett PA, Schaufelberger HD, et al. Eradication of *Helicobacter pylori* with clarithromycin and omeprazole. *Gut* 1994;35:323.
13. Maniatis AG, Brazer SR. Omeprazole/amoxicillin versus ranitidine/triple therapy for duodenal ulcer: when is the same the same? *Am J Gastroenterol* 1994;89:947.
14. NIH Consensus Conference. *Helicobacter pylori* in peptic ulcer disease. *JAMA* 1994;272;65.
15. Nomura A, Stemmermann GN, Chyou PH, et al. *Helicobacter pylori* infection and the risk for duodenal and gastric ulceration. *Ann Intern Med* 1994;120:977.
16. Peura D. The report of the Digestive Health Initiative International Update Conference in *Helicobacter pylori*. *Gastroenterology* 1997;113:S4–S8.
17. Peura D. *Helicobacter pylori:* rational management options. *Am J Med* 1998;105(5):424–430.

18. Scheeres DE, DeKryger LL, Dean RE. Surgical treatment of peptic ulcer disease before and after introduction of H_2 blockers. *Ann Surg* 1987;53:392.
19. Sung JJ, Chung SC, Ling TK, et al. One-year follow-up of duodenal ulcers after 1-week triple therapy for *Helicobacter pylori*. *Am J Gastroenterol* 1994;89:199.
20. Walt RP, Katschinski B, Logan R, et al. Rising frequency of ulcer perforation in elderly people in the United Kingdom. *Lancet* 1986;i:489.
21. Wilhelmsen I, Weberg R, Berstad K, et al. *Helicobacter pylori* eradication with bismuth subnitrate, oxytetracycline and metronidazole in patients with peptic ulcer disease. *Hepatogastroenterology* 1994;41:43.

CHAPTER 156

Gastrointestinal Foreign Bodies

Valerie C. Norton

Gastrointestinal (GI) foreign bodies present a diverse set of challenges to the emergency physician. Presentations range from the obvious to the occult, from the mundane to the bizarre, and from the benign to the life-threatening. Management options are accordingly diverse as well, ranging from watchful waiting to emergent endoscopy or surgery.

Physicians must be familiar with the signs and symptoms of ingested foreign bodies, especially in patients such as small children or psychiatric patients who have no obvious history of ingestion. They must have a good understanding of various removal techniques for foreign bodies in the esophagus or rectum. They must also know which situations require emergent intervention and whom to consult when intervention is necessary.

About 80% of cases involve ingestion of foreign bodies by a child (see Chapter 271). Children tend to ingest coins, toys, and other small objects left within their reach. Adult patients at highest risk include psychiatric patients, prisoners, those with impaired mental status or intoxication, those with underlying esophageal abnormalities (e.g., strictures), and denture wearers, who have reduced sensation of the palate.[16] Adults most commonly have trouble with boluses of meat and animal bones, though psychiatric patients and prisoners may intentionally ingest unusual objects, such as razor blades or open safety pins.

Ingested foreign bodies frequently become lodged in the esophagus, often requiring urgent removal. Much more rarely, objects fail to pass the pylorus or the ileocecal valve. Over 80% of ingested foreign bodies that pass into the stomach will traverse the rest of the gut uneventfully.[15] Objects that are less likely to pass spontaneously are those longer than 6 cm; sharp objects, such as pins and toothpicks; and blunt objects wider than 2.5 cm.[1]

Of primary concern are objects lodged in the esophagus, because these are at highest risk for complications such as mucosal erosions, perforation, or airway compromise. Objects typically lodge at the level of the cricopharyngeus muscle, the level of the aortic arch, or the lower esophageal sphincter. High esophageal impactions are most common in children; adults most often have obstructions at the lower esophageal sphincter.[15] Foreign bodies with toxic contents, such as button batteries and packages of cocaine, represent special cases (discussed in Chapters 333 and 326, respectively). A button battery lodged in the esophagus is a true emergency requiring immediate endoscopic removal.

Rectal foreign bodies are usually the result of sexual misadventure or assault, though occasionally a patient will present with an ingested foreign body, such as an animal bone, that has passed through the entire gut only to become lodged in the rectum.[2,17] Men are at least 28 times more likely than women to present with rectal foreign bodies.[15] Objects inserted into the rectum include vibrators, vegetables, broomsticks, drugs or other contraband, and even live animals, such as gerbils. Many objects are not visible on x-ray, though most are low-lying and palpable on rectal examination. Mucosal lacerations and rectal perforations are fairly common, especially in assault victims, and may result in life-threatening sepsis.

CLINICAL PRESENTATION

Healthy adults with ingested foreign bodies often give a clear history of the inciting incident and may report a foreign-body sensation if the object is lodged in the upper esophagus, where somatic nerve endings are present. If a meat bolus or other object is impacted in the lower esophagus, they usually complain of more visceral-type chest pain, odynophagia, and difficulty handling secretions. Objects that have passed into the stomach or beyond frequently cause no symptoms, unless obstruction or perforation has ensued.

Small children and adults with impaired mentation may not give a clear history of foreign-body ingestion. Clinicians may have to rely on symptoms of obstruction, such as drooling if the object is in the esophagus, or vomiting and distension if it is impacted below the stomach. Patients may also present with GI bleeding or signs and symptoms of peritonitis due to perforation. Small children often display indirect symptoms such as gagging and choking, refusal to eat, irritability, or respiratory distress if the object is compressing the trachea or causing aspiration of saliva.

Patients with rectal foreign bodies usually state clearly that something is in the rectum, though they may be very vague as to how it got there. These patients or their partners have often made multiple prior attempts to remove the object.[15] Occasional patients may be unaware of the object if intoxicated at the time of insertion, or may be too embarrassed to admit to it, complaining instead of rectal pain or bleeding. Patients with extraperitoneal rectal perforation may present with sepsis, while those with intraperitoneal perforation present with peritonitis.

DIFFERENTIAL DIAGNOSIS

In the absence of a history of ingestion or insertion of a foreign body, the differential diagnosis is difficult. It should include all processes that can obstruct, irritate, erode, or perforate the GI tract. Other organ systems may initially be the focus of concern, because esophageal pain can mimic cardiac angina, and children with esophageal obstruction may present with stridor or other respiratory symptoms that may be mistaken for croup or asthma.

Subacute and chronic presentations do not rule out foreign bodies. A wealth of literature has reported objects dwelling in the stomach or intestines for years before causing symptoms. Esophageal foreign bodies have been impacted for a month or more in some children, without serious sequelae.[4,7,9] Clinicians should also be aware that even when there is a clear-cut history of foreign-body ingestion or insertion, other unsuspected pathologies may be present, such as a second foreign body, a mucosal laceration, or underlying esophageal disease.[1,2,14]

EMERGENCY DEPARTMENT EVALUATION

Initial assessment should aim at immediate detection and treatment of those with frank airway compromise, sepsis, or perforation. In more stable patients, the physical examination may find signs of esophageal obstruction, such as drooling or gagging; signs of lower intestinal obstruction; or evidence of GI bleeding. In the majority of patients with upper GI foreign bodies, the physical examination is unrevealing. By contrast, rectal foreign bodies are usually palpable on rectal examination. Some authors advise against a digital rectal examination prior to obtaining radiographs, because examiners may injure themselves if an unexpectedly sharp object is present.[15]

Imaging studies are often very helpful, though a negative study does not rule out a radiolucent foreign body. For suspected esophageal foreign bodies, both anteroposterior and lateral radiographs of the neck and chest are recommended to avoid missing a second foreign body located behind the first or one lower in the esophagus. Both views also help to rule out a tracheobronchial foreign body.[14,15] Flat objects in the esophagus, such as coins, typically appear "en face" on anteroposterior views and "on end" on lateral views, because the easily compressible esophagus typically lies somewhat flattened between the trachea and the spine. Tracheal coins, by contrast, typically appear "on end" on anteroposterior views, because the more rigid tracheal rings have their widest diameter in the sagittal plane.[15]

Some authors have advocated the use of a hand-held metal detector in lieu of plain films to evaluate the presence and location of metallic foreign bodies.[12] Accuracy appears to be good for coins, but not for smaller metal objects, making this modality of questionable utility unless one is certain that the object is a coin.[11] In addition, the number of patients studied so far has been too small to know whether metal detectors can make the crucial distinction between the lower esophagus and the stomach when localizing a coin.

Objects below the esophagus may be evaluated with standard plain films or contrast radiography if necessary. In most cases, the primary reasons to obtain radiographs are to determine (1) whether an ingested object has passed beyond the esophagus and (2) whether the object has any physical characteristics that will make passage or extraction more difficult, such as a sharp edge.

EMERGENCY DEPARTMENT MANAGEMENT

Patients with signs of airway compromise require definitive airway management and emergent endoscopic consultation to remove the foreign body. Those with signs of hollow viscus perforation, massive bleeding, or sepsis require immediate resuscitation, intravenous antibiotics, and emergent surgical consultation.

The management of stable patients depends on the type, location, and duration of impaction of the foreign body. Management guidelines are summarized in Fig. 156.1. In the esophagus, sharp objects and button batteries require immediate endoscopic removal. Blunt esophageal foreign bodies are typically objects in the midesophagus to upper esophagus, objects at the lower esophageal sphincter, or food boluses. Objects in the upper half of the esophagus are unlikely to pass spontaneously, mandating intervention. The standard of care at most large institutions is prompt endoscopic removal.[1,15,16] If endoscopy is not readily available, it may be postponed briefly if the patient is able to handle secretions. Most experts recommend removal within 12 to 24 hours.[1,5,16]

Objects lodged at the lower esophageal sphincter are often managed with a trial of watchful waiting with or without measures to relax the sphincter, because many of these objects will pass spontaneously. Glucagon may be given to help relax the lower esophageal sphincter in a dose of 1.0 to 2.0 mg intravenously, though its use is controversial and may cause vomiting.[15,16] This dose may be repeated once in 20 to 30 minutes if unsuccessful. If passage has not resulted in 12 to 24 hours, most authors recommend endoscopic removal.[1,4,16]

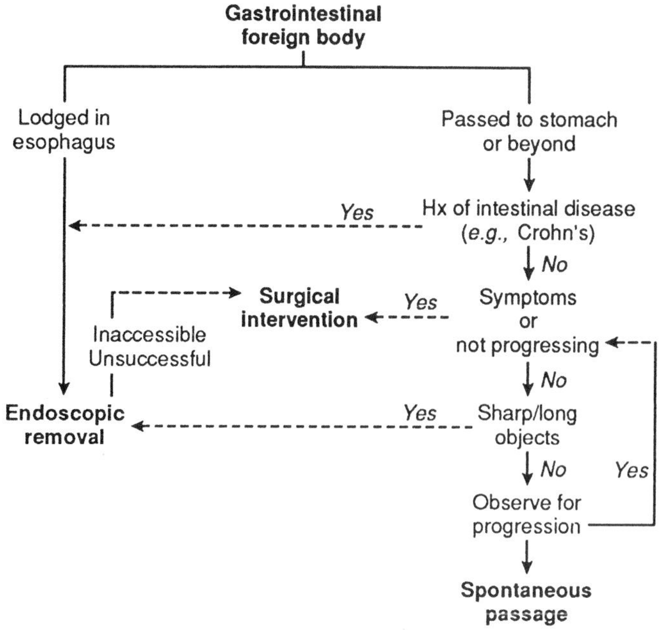

Figure 156.1. Management of gastrointestinal foreign bodies.

The management of esophageal food boluses depends on the degree of symptoms experienced by the patient as well as the composition of the bolus. Boluses causing high-grade obstruction and inability to handle secretions require emergent endoscopic removal.[1,16] Most authors also recommend prompt endoscopic removal of boluses that are seen radiographically to contain sharp bones, because these are more likely to cause esophageal perforation. Other boluses may be managed by watchful waiting with or without glucagon, with removal in less than 24 hours if passage does not occur.[1,16] The use of gas-producing liquids such as carbonated beverages to aid in break-up and passage of the bolus has been reported[8] but remains controversial. Proteolytic enzymes are contraindicated, as they can cause severe damage to the esophageal mucosa.

Although endoscopic removal of esophageal foreign bodies is standard at many institutions, the choice of technique is controversial in some areas because of cost concerns. A number of authors have advocated the alternative, less costly techniques of fluoroscopic Foley catheter extraction and esophageal bougienage (advancement of the foreign body with an esophageal dilator).[3,5–7,9,13] In experienced hands and in selected patients, these techniques have success and complication rates comparable to those of endoscopy. These alternative techniques should be limited to patients with a blunt foreign-body (usually a coin) impaction of less than 24 hours' duration, no history of esophageal disease, and no signs of respiratory distress or airway compromise.[3,6,9]

Patients with radiographic signs of esophageal edema or underlying esophageal disease are not ideal candidates and will have lower success rates.[7,13] Advanced airway management should be immediately available at all times. The procedure should be terminated if resistance is met or multiple attempts are needed, as serious complications have occurred in these settings.[3,13]

Cost is becoming less of an issue as flexible endoscopy under conscious sedation in the emergency department increasingly replaces rigid endoscopy under general anesthesia in the operating room,[16] resulting in lower charges and shorter recovery times. In many institutions, flexible endoscopy may now be comparable to catheter extraction or bougienage in terms of cost and convenience.

Objects in the stomach and small intestine are much less problematic than those in the esophagus, because the vast majority will pass spontaneously. The exceptions are sharp objects, which may cause perforation in up to 35% of patients; they should be removed endoscopically if still in the stomach or duodenum.[1,15] Some authors also recommend endoscopic removal of objects more than 6 cm long or 2.5 cm wide that are found in the stomach or duodenum, as these are less likely to pass.[1,16] Small, blunt objects can be followed clinically, with repeat x-rays weekly if passage in the stool is not noted. A high-fiber diet may aid passage of the foreign body. Blunt objects should be given 3 to 4 weeks to pass out of the stomach before resorting to endoscopic removal.[1,16] Objects may be given 2 to 3 weeks to traverse the rest of the gut. The development of symptoms or the failure of the object to progress mandates surgical consultation.

Rectal foreign bodies frequently require surgical consultation to bring about removal, although various authors report being able to remove 20% to 60% of objects in the emergency department.[2,17] Removal in the emergency department is dependent on the ability to achieve adequate relaxation of the anal sphincter and adequate purchase on the foreign body. Many patients with long histories of rectal stimulation have lax anal tone and may require only lidocaine gel, with or without conscious sedation, to relax the sphincter. Other patients may require infiltrative local anesthesia, and some may only achieve adequate relaxation with spinal or general anesthesia in the operating room.

Soft, low-lying objects with an edge can often be grasped and removed manually or with forceps. Some objects create suction on the rectal mucosa with downward traction, which can be overcome by passing a Foley catheter beyond the object and insufflating air into the rectum.[10,15] Sigmoidoscopy after removal is mandatory to look for complications such as abscesses or mucosal lacerations, as these are very common.[2,15,17] Hard, smooth-edged, or high-lying objects usually cannot be removed manually and require surgical consultation for removal by flexible sigmoidoscopy in the operating room or endoscopy suite.[17] Laparotomy is a last resort for foreign bodies in which sigmoidoscopy is unsuccessful.

DISPOSITION

Asymptomatic patients with uncomplicated, blunt foreign bodies in the stomach or small intestine can be discharged from the emergency department with observation of the stools and radiographic follow-up at appropriate intervals to ensure progress of the object through the gut. All others require consultation with an endoscopist or a surgeon, depending on the type and location of the foreign body and the presence of any complications. Following the uncomplicated removal of a foreign body in the emergency department, asymptomatic patients who have fully recovered from any sedation can be sent home with close follow-up by their primary care provider or an appropriate consultant. Patients who remain symptomatic or who develop complications after a procedure require admission.

COMMON PITFALLS

- Failure to consider an esophageal foreign body in patients without a foreign-body history but with suggestive symptoms, such as gagging, drooling, wheezing, or refusal to eat
- Failure to obtain immediate endoscopy for patients with high-grade esophageal obstruction, sharp esophageal foreign bodies, or button batteries in the esophagus
- Inappropriate use of Foley catheter or other removal techniques in patients with sharp or irregularly shaped esophageal foreign bodies, prolonged impactions, signs of respiratory compromise, or when initial attempts meet resistance—all of these may lead to serious complications.
- Inappropriate, repeated attempts to remove hard, smooth, or high-lying rectal foreign bodies in the emergency department. This may lead to further mucosal damage or even rectal perforation.
- Failure to obtain sigmoidoscopy after removal of rectal foreign bodies to rule out mucosal lacerations

References

1. Anonymous. Guideline for the management of ingested foreign bodies. American Society for Gastrointestinal Endoscopy. *Gastrointest Endosc* 1995;42:622–625.
2. Cohen JS, Sackier JM. Management of colorectal foreign bodies. *J R Coll Surg Edinb* 1996;41:312–315.
3. Conners GP. A literature-based comparison of three methods of pediatric esophageal coin removal. *Pediatr Emerg Care* 1997;13:154–157.
4. Conners GP, Chamberlain JM, Ochsenschlager DW. Symptoms and spontaneous passage of esophageal coins. *Arch Pediatr Adolesc Med* 1995;149:36–39.
5. Dokler ML, Bradshaw J, Mollitt DL, et al. Selective management of pediatric esophageal foreign bodies. *Am Surg* 1995;61:132–134.
6. Emslander HC, Bonadio W, Klatzo M. Efficacy of esophageal bougienage by emergency physicians in pediatric coin ingestion. *Ann Emerg Med* 1996;27:726–729.
7. Harned RK, Strain JD, Hay TC, et al. Esophageal foreign bodies: safety and efficacy of Foley catheter extraction of coins. *AJR* 1997;168:443–446.
8. Karanjia ND, Rees M. The use of Coca-Cola in the management of bolus obstruction in benign oesophageal stricture. *Ann R Coll Surg Engl* 1993;75:94–95.
9. Kelley JE, Leech MH, Carr MG. A safe and cost-effective protocol for the management of esophageal coins in children. *J Pediatr Surg* 1993;28:898–900.
10. Kouraklis G, Misiakos E, Dovas N, et al. Management of foreign bodies of the rectum. *J R Coll Surg Edinb* 1997;42:246–247.
11. Ros S, Cetta F. Detection of ingested foreign bodies with a metal detector. *J Pediatr* 1992;121:837–838.
12. Sacchetti A, Carraccio C, Lichenstein R. Hand-held metal detector identification of ingested foreign bodies. *Pediatr Emerg Care* 1994;10:204–207.
13. Schunk JE, Harrison AM, Corneli HM, et al. Fluoroscopic Foley catheter removal of esophageal foreign bodies in children: experience with 415 episodes. *Pediatrics* 1994;94:709–714.
14. Smith SA, Conner GP. Unexpected second foreign bodies in pediatric esophageal coin ingestions. *Pediatr Emerg Care* 1998;14:261–262.
15. Stack LB, Munter DW. Foreign bodies in the gastrointestinal tract. *Emerg Med Clin North Am* 1996;14:493–521.
16. Webb WA. Management of foreign bodies of the upper gastrointestinal tract: update. *Gastrointest Endosc* 1995;41:39–51.
17. Yaman M, Deitel M, Burul CJ, et al. Foreign bodies in the rectum. *Can J Surg* 1993;36:173–177.

CHAPTER 157

Pancreatitis and Pancreatic Cancer

David C. Seaberg and Allan B. Wolfson

Pancreatitis is a frequently encountered problem in most emergency departments. Its incidence varies with patient population and geographic location, but it has been estimated to affect up to 0.5% of the general population in the United States. Pancreatitis can be divided somewhat arbitrarily into two types: acute and chronic. Acute pancreatitis, although commonly a relatively mild disease, may be a life-threatening illness characterized by infection and necrosis of pancreatic tissue and potentially lethal manifestations in other organ systems. The mortality associated with acute pancreatitis may be as high as 5%.[2] Chronic pancreatitis, typically manifested by recurrent episodes of acute pancreatitis superimposed on a chronically damaged pancreas, is fatal only rarely.

TABLE 157.1. Causes of Acute Pancreatitis

METABOLIC
Ethyl alcohol and methyl alcohol
Hyperlipoproteinemias
Medications (azathioprine, estrogens, corticosteroids, tetracycline, diuretics, sulfonamides, valproic acid, didanosine)[13]
Hypercalcemia
Scorpion envenomation
Amanita phalloides ingestion
Cystic fibrosis
Pregnancy
Heredity
MECHANICAL
Biliary tract disease
Abdominal surgery
Trauma
Iatrogenic (e.g., endoscopic retrograde cholangiopancreatography, upper gastrointestinal endoscopy)
Sphincter of Oddi dysfunction
Carcinoma of the pancreas
Duodenal obstruction
Posterior penetrating ulcer
VASCULAR
Vasculitis
Thrombosis
Atheroembolism
Surgery
Ischemia or shock
INFECTIOUS
Coxsackievirus
Mumps
Mycoplasma
Legionella
Campylobacter
IDIOPATHIC

Adapted from Geokas MC, Baltaxe HA, Banks PA, et al. Acute pancreatitis. *Ann Intern Med* 1985;103:86; and Ranson JHC. Etiologic and prognostic factors in human acute pancreatitis: a review. *Am J Gastroenterol* 1982;77:633.

Table 157.2. Complications of Acute Pancreatitis

Local	Systemic
Necrosis	Shock
Sterile tissue	Coagulopathy
Infected tissue	Respiratory failure
Pancreatic fluid collections	Acute renal failure
Pseudocyst	Hyperglycemia
Abscesses	Hypocalcemia
Necrotizing obstruction or fistulization of colon	Subcutaneous nodules
Gastrointestinal hemorrhage	Retinopathy
Ulceration	Psychosis
Gastric varices	
Rupture of pseudoaneurysm	
Right-sided hydronephrosis	
Splenic rupture or hematoma	

The major causes of acute pancreatitis are shown in Table 157.1. In the United States, alcoholism and cholelithiasis account for 80% to 90% of all cases.[8,18] Alcohol-associated acute pancreatitis is clinically recognized in 1% to 10% of alcoholics; episodes usually occur only after a prolonged period (generally at least 6 to 8 years) of heavy alcohol abuse. In nonalcoholic patients with acute pancreatitis, gallstones can be demonstrated in 60%.

In 15% to 20% of cases of acute pancreatitis, no underlying cause can be identified. Studies have found, however, that occult biliary microlithiasis and biliary sludge may be the cause of perhaps two-thirds of cases of "idiopathic" acute pancreatitis.[12]

The pathologic mechanism responsible for the development of acute pancreatitis is believed to be autodigestion by inappropriate intrapancreatic activation of proteolytic enzymes (primarily trypsin) and release of other substances, such as elastase, phospholipase A, lipase, and vasoactive polypeptide.[8] These events result in coagulation necrosis and vascular injury, causing hemorrhage, edema, and pain. Severe cases of acute pancreatitis are associated with systemic effects in a wide variety of organ systems, presumably due to release of vasoactive factors into the circulation. These systemic manifestations can include cardiac dysfunction, acute renal failure, central nervous system dysfunction, and disseminated intravascular coagulation (Table 157.2).[24] Significant pulmonary complications, such as pleural effusion, hypoxemia, and the adult respiratory distress syndrome, occur in an appreciable proportion of patients.[24] Subcutaneous fat necrosis occurs in some individuals. Severe hypocalcemia is another systemic effect; although it has been attributed to the formation of soaps by necrotic pancreatic tissue, other factors, such as hypoalbuminemia, appear to be at least as important.[8] As acute pancreatitis resolves, it may be complicated by the development of pancreatic pseudocyst or pancreatic abscess.

Chronic pancreatitis is a destructive inflammatory disorder commonly characterized by recurrent attacks of acute pancreatitis and often leading to pancreatic exocrine and endocrine dysfunction. Excessive alcohol consumption is, by far, the most common cause, accounting for 75% of cases.[14] The remaining cases are attributed to idiopathic causes, congenital anatomic predispositions, neoplasia, trauma, or metabolic disease, such as hyperlipidemia, cystic fibrosis, or hyperparathyroidism. Gallstones are believed not to play a major etiologic role.

The risk of pancreatic cancer appears to be elevated in patients with chronic pancreatitis.[13] Other risk factors include smoking, chronic familial pancreatitis, and occupational exposure to the metal mining, sawmill, chemical, and coke industries.[25] The incidence of this malignancy increases with age, peaking in the sixth to eighth decades. Patients with pancreatic cancer often present with recurrent abdominal pain and exocrine or endocrine dysfunction similar to that seen in chronic pancreatitis. Pancreatic cancer has the lowest 5-year survival rate (3%) of any gastrointestinal malignancy.[7] Tumor has often spread beyond the pancreas by the time symptoms develop.

CLINICAL PRESENTATION

Although no clinical finding is pathognomonic of acute pancreatitis, abdominal pain is almost always its most striking clinical feature. The pain is often localized to the epigastrium or left upper quadrant and often radiates through to the back, presumably because of retroperitoneal irritation. It is often severe and constant and is typically exacerbated by recumbency and relieved by sitting up and flexing forward. Nausea and vomiting are noted in the majority of cases.

On physical examination, there is usually abdominal tenderness and guarding, often with signs of peritoneal irritation. Fever, tachycardia, and diaphoresis may also be noted, depending on the severity of the case. An elevation of the serum amylase activity is often incorrectly considered to be diagnostic of acute pancreatitis. Because amylase is found in a variety of extrapancreatic locations (including the salivary glands, the small intestine, and the female genital tract), reliance on the amylase level alone may be misleading.

Necrotizing acute pancreatitis is a systemic disease. Intravascular volume loss due to massive edema and exudation of fluid into the peritoneal cavity, due to systemic effects of released vasoactive substances, or due to pancreatic hemorrhage may lead to frank hypovolemic shock.[3] Two classic signs of retroperitoneal hemorrhage are the Cullen sign (periumbilical ecchymosis) and the Grey Turner sign (flank ecchymosis), but these are uncommon. In fact, the term *hemorrhagic pancreatitis* has been abandoned because hemorrhage is not usually a major component of acute pancreatitis.[2] In some cases, the clinical picture is dominated by manifestations of remote organ system dysfunction or by the systemic effects of pancreatic abscess.

The hallmarks of *chronic pancreatitis* include abdominal pain, weight loss, steatorrhea, exocrine and endocrine dysfunction, and pancreatic calcification.

Patients with chronic pancreatitis often present to the emergency department with recurrent attacks of abdominal pain, although, in some patients, pain is overshadowed by weight loss and the effects of pancreatic endocrine or exocrine dysfunction (i.e., diabetes mellitus or malabsorption and steatorrhea).

More than 90% of the gland must be destroyed before exocrine insufficiency results in clinically significant malabsorption of protein, fat, and fat-soluble vitamins. Pancreatic endocrine dysfunction, with deficient insulin and glucagon secretion, may result in diabetes mellitus that is occasionally "brittle" and associated with frequent episodes of hypoglycemia.

Pancreatic cancer, which is most often ductal in origin, can simulate the pain and glandular damage seen in patients with chronic pancreatitis. More than 90% of patients have pain, jaundice, or weight loss at the time of diagnosis. Clinical pancreatitis and diabetes mellitus are noted in up to 14% and 33% of patients, respectively.

DIFFERENTIAL DIAGNOSIS

The most common conditions confused with acute pancreatitis are acute cholecystitis and peptic ulcer disease, but essentially any intraabdominal emergency may be mimicked. The pain of cholecystitis is located more often in the right upper quadrant, tends to be more gradual in onset, and is not always constant. Ultrasound examination and radionuclide scanning are useful in establishing the diagnosis of biliary tract disease. An elevation of the alkaline phosphatase level in the absence of a comparable elevation in serum transaminase levels is also suggestive. Although simple acute cholecystitis may be complicated by acute pancreatitis, the serum amylase value may be elevated in both conditions. Gallstones should be excluded early in all patients with acute pancreatitis, because their presence is associated with increased morbidity and mortality.[5]

Alcoholic gastritis is commonly present in association with alcohol-induced pancreatitis, and distinguishing between the two entities clinically is often difficult or impossible. Tenderness and peritoneal signs are more likely to represent pancreatitis, but a posterior penetrating ulcer may produce features of both illnesses. Other serious disorders may be responsible for significant abdominal pain in association with elevated serum amylase levels, and failure to recognize this fact may lead to a dangerous misdiagnosis. These disorders include intestinal obstruction, ruptured ectopic pregnancy, mesenteric infarction, dissecting aortic aneurysm, peritonitis, acute appendicitis, and diabetic ketoacidosis. The differential diagnosis of upper abdominal pain must also include myocardial infarction, pneumonia, and renal colic.

The diagnosis of chronic relapsing pancreatitis is primarily a clinical one. Diagnosing pancreatic cancer against a background of chronic pancreatitis may be difficult, however. Chronic pancreatitis can produce all of the symptoms of pancreatic cancer and can cause focal or diffuse enlargement of the gland as well.

Calcific deposits are fairly specific for chronic pancreatitis, however, while jaundice is much more common with carcinoma of the head of the pancreas. Endoscopic retrograde cholangiopancreatography (ERCP) is often useful in identifying pancreatic cancer, although an identical picture can be seen in both entities[7]; ERCP also allows the collection of pancreatic secretions for cytologic examination.[7]

EMERGENCY DEPARTMENT EVALUATION

The challenge of the emergency department evaluation of unsuspected pancreatitis is to make the diagnosis and to exclude other causes of abdominal distress, yet to keep in mind the fact that other serious illness may occur in combination with pancreatitis. Once the diagnosis is made, one must assess the severity of the pancreatitis to make an appropriate disposition.

The diagnosis of pancreatitis is based primarily on the history and physical examination and is *supported* by laboratory studies, most notably the serum amylase level. The "gold standard" of diagnosis is direct inspection or pathologic examination of the pancreas; all other diagnostic modalities are indirect tests. Thus, it is often stated that pancreatitis should remain a "working diagnosis" that one should feel free to modify in the face of a changing clinical picture.

Because the serum amylase value is a reasonably sensitive test, the diagnosis should be questioned if the level is normal. Nevertheless, a normal amylase value was found in about one-third of patients with clinical pancreatitis in one series, and there is no correlation between the severity of pancreatitis and the degree of amylase elevation.[15] There are several possible reasons for this. Renal clearance of amylase is rapid, and the serum amylase level in pancreatitis may remain elevated for only up to 72 hours; thus, in a patient who presents a few days after the onset of symptoms, the level may be only minimally elevated or normal.[15] Moreover, in some individuals who have had many episodes of acute pancreatitis, extensive scarring may result in a "burned out" pancreas that releases little amylase. One other cause for spuriously low serum amylase measurements is severe hypertriglyceridemia, in which there may be a circulating amylase inhibitor; this laboratory artifact may be corrected for by measuring the serum amylase activity on serial dilutions of plasma.

Despite the reasonably good sensitivity of the serum amylase test, it is nonspecific, at least when the conventional upper limit of normal is employed.[22] (Interestingly, elevated serum total amylase in patients with clinical pancreatitis was noted in one series to be due to the salivary isoenzyme in 26% of individuals.[23]) Using a higher cut-off level greatly increases the specificity of the total amylase determination, while sensitivity appears to be maintained.[21] The urinary amylase–creatinine clearance, although recommended as a more specific test for acute pancreatitis, particularly to distinguish it from biliary tract disease, appears to offer no advantage.[15]

Because of its availability and high specificity (99%), the serum lipase level is the confirmatory test that is most widely used when the diagnosis of pancreatitis is in doubt.[21] Because the pancreas is the only major source of lipase, an increased level (and particularly a level more than three times the upper limit of normal) is very specific for acute pancreatic inflammation. Other confirmatory tests, such as measurements of amylase isoenzymes (pancreatic and salivary), trypsinogen, serum elastase, and phospholipase A_2, have been investigated, but they are less widely available for use in emergency department patients.[15,21,24] A number of these tests not only are more specific (about 85%) than the total amylase (at least using its conventional upper limit of normal), but also are reported to remain abnormal for significantly longer (7 to 14 days) than the total serum amylase level.[11,21]

Plain radiographs of the chest and abdomen should be obtained primarily to rule out other entities, such as pneumoperitoneum, small bowel obstruction, and aortic aneurysm.[15] The abdominal radiograph in acute pancreatitis may show regional or localized ileus ("sentinel loop"), gallstones, widening of the duodenal sweep, blurring of the left renal outline and psoas margin, elevation of one or both hemidiaphragms, or pleural or pericardial effusion.[8] These radiographic findings are caused initially by motility disturbances in the surrounding bowel and later by pancreatic edema and peripancreatic fluid collection. The finding of pancreatic calcifications is an indication that previous episodes of acute pancreatitis have occurred, and it is essentially diagnostic of chronic pancreatitis.

Other diagnostic imaging studies are sometimes extremely helpful. Ultrasonography can identify pancreatic edema as well as such complications as pancreatic pseudocyst or abscess. It is also useful in identifying the presence of gallstones or dilatation of the biliary tree, findings that have obvious diagnostic and therapeutic implications.[19] A practice guideline for acute pancreatitis recommends that an abdominal ultrasound should be part of the evaluation of the initial episode of acute pancreatitis and should be performed during the initial 24 to 48 hours of hospitalization.[2] Its most important use among patients with additional episodes of pancreatitis is to determine whether the cause is gallstones. Ultrasound visualization is difficult, however, if the pancreas is surrounded by large amounts of adipose tissue or if there are overlying distended loops of bowel.

In recent years, dynamic, contrast-enhanced computed tomography (CECT) has become the imaging gold standard for evaluating the presence and extent of pancreatic necrosis and other local anatomic sequelae of acute pancreatitis, such as pseudocyst, abscess, or fistula. As such, it has become a routine part of the diagnostic workup of most patients. CECT assessment of disease severity is based on semiquantitative estimation of pancreatic and peripancreatic inflammation, presence and degree of necrosis, and associated abnormalities, such as pleural effusion or ascites.[6]

Table 157.3 lists the CT severity index developed by Balthazar and Ranson.[1] The practice guideline for acute pancreatitis by the American College of Gastroenterology recommends that CECT be performed among patients that are clinically demonstrated to have severe pancreatitis. Magnetic resonance imaging has not been shown to be superior to CT.[15,20]

ERCP should be considered for patients in whom the cause of pancreatitis remains unclear after initial evaluation. ERCP may be helpful in elucidating the cause of pancreatitis in up to half of such individuals,[22] revealing small pancreatic tumors, pancreatic ductal stricture, gallstones, pancreas divisum, choledochocele, or sphincter of Oddi dysfunction.

After establishing the diagnosis of acute pancreatitis, the second priority is to determine its severity. Five percent to 10% of patients develop serious complications or die of the disease. Severe cases are indicated by the presence of organ failure (in-

TABLE 157.3. Balthazar CECT Scoring System

CT Grade	Grade Score	Definition
A	0	Normal pancreas
B	1	Focal or diffuse pancreatic enlargement
C	2	Intrinsic pancreatic abnormality + haziness/streaky densities in peripancreatic fat
D	3	Single, ill-defined fluid collections
E	4	Multiple, ill-defined fluid collections or pancreatic or peripancreatic gas

Gland Necrosis (%)	Necrosis Score	Definition
None	0	Uniform pancreatic enhancement
<30	2	Nonenhancement of region(s) of gland equivalent in size to the pancreatic head
30–50	4	Nonenhancement of 30%-50% of the gland
>50	6	Nonenhancement of over 50% of the gland

Severity index = Necrosis score + Grade score.

Mild pancreatitis = severity index of 1–3.
Moderate pancreatitis = severity index of 4–6.
Severe pancreatitis = severity index of 7–10.

Adapted from Balthazar EJ, Freeny PC, van Sonnenberg E. Imaging and intervention in acute pancreatitis. *Radiology* 1994;193:297.

cluding shock, pulmonary insufficiency, and renal failure) and/or local complications (especially pancreatic necrosis).[2,4]

An increased risk of major complications has been associated with a number of clinical features, the so-called Ranson criteria or their modifications (Table 157.4).[2,18] Among them are age greater than 55; leukocytosis (reflecting the degree of inflammatory response); elevated serum lactate dehydrogenase and aspartate aminotransferase levels (suggesting hepatic and other tissue injury or necrosis); marked hyperglycemia (reflecting possible pancreatic endocrine dysfunction); hypocalcemia (from the formation of soaps by necrotic pancreatic tissue or other poorly defined mechanisms); rising blood urea nitrogen levels (secondary to third-space fluid losses or renal impairment); a falling hematocrit (reflecting both initial hemoconcentration and hemorrhagic necrosis); arterial hypoxemia (due to pleural effusion or adult respiratory distress syndrome from systemic effects of severe pancreatic damage); and the development of metabolic acidosis or marked fluid retention.

The APACHE-II score is based on 12 physiologic variables, the patient's age, and any history of severe organ system insufficiency or immunocompromised state. Studies indicate that measurement of the APACHE-II score on the day of admission has high sensitivity and specificity in distinguishing mild from severe pancreatitis, and is superior to other grading systems for this purpose.[2] An advantage of the APACHE-II system is that it can be done at presentation and can be followed daily, whereas other systems (including Ranson's signs) rely, to a degree, on data points collected at 48 hours. When the APACHE-II score is less than 8 during the first 24 to 48 hours, the patient usually survives. One study found the APACHE-II score to be superior to CT grading in the initial evaluation of the severity of acute pancreatitis.[6] The practice guideline for acute pancreatitis recommends that a formalized severity index be generated for each patient (Table 157.5). The APACHE-II score and/or Ranson's criteria score should be generated on the day of admission to help identify patients with severe pancreatitis.[2,3]

Emergency department evaluation of chronic pancreatic disease should focus on both functional and structural components. Clinical examination should seek evidence of endocrine and exocrine manifestations such as hyperglycemia or hypoglycemia, hyperlipidemia, steatorrhea, and nutritional deficiencies.

Structural abnormalities in chronic pancreatitis or cancer can be identified by imaging or endoscopy. Plain abdominal radiographs show diffuse calcification of the pancreas in about 20% of cases of chronic pancreatitis. Ultrasonography, CT, and ERCP can all be used to diagnose ductal abnormalities, pancreatic tumors, pseudocyst, abscess, or phlegmon.

TABLE 157.4. Ranson Criteria for Predicting the Severity of Acute Pancreatitis

ON ADMISSION
Age >55 yr
WBC >16,000/mm^3
Blood glucose >200 mg/dL
Lactate dehydrogenase >350 IU/L
Aspartate transaminase >250 U/L
WITHIN 48 HOURS
BUN >5 mg/dL
PaO_2 <60 mm/Hg
Serum calcium <8 mg/dL
Hematocrit fall >10%
Base deficit >4 mEq/L
Fluid sequestration >6 L

Mortality is based on number of prognostic signs: 0–2, 1%; 3–4, 15%; 5–6, 40%; >6, 100%.

Adapted from Ranson JHC. Etiologic and prognostic factors in human acute pancreatitis: a review. *Am J Gastroenterol* 1982;77:663.

TABLE 157.5. Prognostic Factors for Severe Pancreatitis

EARLY PROGNOSTIC SIGNS
Ranson's signs ≥3
APACHE-II score ≥8
ORGAN FAILURE
Shock: systolic blood pressure <90 mm Hg
Pulmonary insufficiency: PaO_2
Renal failure, creatinine >2 mg/dL
Gastrointestinal bleeding >500 mL/24 h
LOCAL COMPLICATIONS
Necrosis
Abscess
Pseudocyst

Adapted from Banks PA. Practice guidelines in acute pancreatitis. *Am J Gastroenterol* 1997;92:377.

EMERGENCY DEPARTMENT MANAGEMENT

Ninety percent of all cases of acute pancreatitis may be treated with supportive measures only. The aim of medical therapy is generally held to be "to place the pancreas at rest." Although it is commonly recommended that oral intake should be withheld, it appears that the oral intake of clear liquids is not harmful, at least in mild to moderately severe cases. Intravenous fluids should be administered as needed, and electrolyte abnormalities such as hypokalemia, hypocalcemia, and hypomagnesemia corrected. In patients with moderate-to-severe pain, meperidine has traditionally been the analgesic of choice because it is thought to cause less spasm of the ampulla of Vater than morphine.[11] Antiemetics such as prochlorperazine or hydroxyzine may be given to control vomiting. Nasogastric suction, long thought to be a necessary component of management, has not been shown to offer any additional benefit in mild-to-moderate pancreatitis if ileus is not present.[17] Likewise, anticholinergics are no longer believed to be of value. Although it was speculated that H_2 blockers might serve to decrease the severity or the duration of episodes of acute pancreatitis by decreasing the acid stimulus to pancreatic secretion, several studies have shown them to have no benefit.[17]

About 5% of cases of acute pancreatitis result in serious complications or death (see Table 157.2). These patients commonly require large amounts of fluid replacement (and sometimes colloid) because of retroperitoneal sequestration of pancreatic exudate and remote systemic effects of released vasoactive substances. A central venous or Swan-Ganz catheter and an indwelling urinary catheter may be needed to monitor intravascular volume status and to guide fluid replacement. In patients with ileus or intractable vomiting, a nasogastric tube should be inserted. Surgical consultation is indicated for patients with clinically severe pancreatitis or evidence of large peripancreatic fluid collections, abscess, or pancreatic necrosis on CT. Antibiotic administration should be reserved for those patients with evidence of established infection.

In patients with chronic pancreatitis or pancreatic cancer, the overall goals of therapy are symptom relief and prevention or correction of local and systemic complications. Pancreatic enzyme supplementation and balanced nutritional intake are the basics of therapy for pancreatic exocrine insufficiency.[9]

Provision of adequate amounts of supplemental oral pancreatic enzymes (pancreatin or pancrelipase) can lead to relief of pain, presumably by a process of negative feedback inhibition.[9] Diabetes mellitus as a consequence of endocrine insufficiency requires obsessive attention to insulin administration and diet to avoid ketoacidosis and other complications.

Control of chronic abdominal pain is also of prime importance. Impaired absorption of orally administered medications because of pancreatic disease may necessitate the use of parenteral analgesics. Surgery may be necessary for the treatment of regional complications of chronic pancreatitis (e.g., drainage of a pseudocyst, decompression of the biliary tree, or alleviation of duodenal obstruction).[16]

DISPOSITION

Patients with mild pancreatitis, in whom the likelihood of biliary tract disease is believed to be low, may be managed on an outpatient basis if they are able to tolerate clear liquids in the emergency department and have no evidence of systemic complications. For these individuals, a clear-liquid diet and oral analgesics should be prescribed, and close follow-up should be arranged. Patients with alcohol-associated pancreatitis should be encouraged to stop drinking.

All other patients must be admitted to the hospital. If severe or necrotizing acute pancreatitis is suspected, admission to an intensive care unit is mandatory for critical care monitoring of cardiac, pulmonary, and renal function. In the patient with unremitting fulminant or infected pancreatitis, a surgeon should be consulted for possible laparotomy to debride the necrotic pancreas and to ensure that there is no other cause amenable to surgical treatment. Prompt surgery is indicated when there are signs of sepsis or pancreatic abscess.[8] For patients who do not respond to initial supportive measures, peritoneal lavage has been recommended to help remove the toxic pancreatic exudate from the abdominal cavity. Individuals with gallstone-induced pancreatitis may benefit from early endoscopic papillotomy.

For patients with chronic pancreatitis or pancreatic cancer, indications for hospital admission include uncontrollable pain, severe nutritional deficiencies, or complications requiring surgery. Any adjustments in the regimen for analgesia or pancreatic enzyme supplementation should be carried out in consultation with the patient's primary care physician.

COMMON PITFALLS

- No clinical or laboratory finding is pathognomonic of pancreatitis. The serum amylase value is not a specific test, nor is an elevated serum amylase value a *sine qua non* for making the diagnosis. Because many disorders can cause abdominal pain and an elevated serum amylase concentration, these entities must be actively excluded before the diagnosis of pancreatitis can be definitively made. In addition, acute pancreatitis and another serious intraabdominal disorder may be present simultaneously.
- Another potential pitfall in the evaluation of the patient with acute pancreatitis is underestimating the severity of an attack. Measurements of APACHE-II and/or Ranson's criteria should be made to estimate severity. The criteria in Tables 157.4 and 157.5 are helpful in providing objective guidelines by which the clinician can identify patients with a high likelihood of clinical deterioration.
- Pancreatic cancer can mimic the pain and glandular damage encountered in cases of chronic pancreatitis.

References

1. Balthazar EJ, Freeny PC, van Sonnenberg E. Imaging and intervention in acute pancreatitis. *Radiology* 1994;193:297.
2. Banks PA. Practice guidelines in acute pancreatitis. *Am J Gastroenterol* 1997;92:377.
3. Baron TH, Morgan DE. Acute necrotizing pancreatitis. *N Engl J Med* 1999;340:1412.
4. Blamey ST, Imrie CW, O'Neill J, et al. Prognostic factors in acute pancreatitis. *Gut* 1984;25:1340.
5. Blamey SL, Osborne DH, Gilmour WH, et al. The early identification of patients with gallstone-associated pancreatitis using clinical and biochemical factors only. *Ann Surg* 1983;198:574.
6. DeSanctis JT, Lee MJ, Gazelle GS, et al. Prognostic indicators in acute pancreatitis: CT vs APACHE II. *Clin Radiol* 1997;52:842.
7. Fernandez-del Castillo C, Warshaw AL. Diagnosis and preoperative evaluation of pancreatic cancer, with implications for management. *Gastroenterol Clin North Am* 1990;19:915.
8. Geokas MC, Baltaxe HA, Banks PA, et al. Acute pancreatitis. *Ann Intern Med* 1985;103:86.
9. Isaksson G, Ihse I. Pain reduction by an oral pancreatic enzyme preparation in chronic pancreatitis. *Dig Dis Sci* 1988;28:97.
10. Isenhower H, Mueller BA. Selection of narcotic analgesics for pain associated with pancreatitis. *Am J Health Syst Pharm* 1998;55:480.
11. Kolars JC, Ellis CJ, Levitt MD. Comparison of serum amylase, pancreatic isoamylase and lipase in patients with hyperamylasemia. *Dig Dis Sci* 1984;29:289.
12. Lee SP, Nicholls JF, Park HZ. Biliary sludge as a cause of acute pancreatitis. *N Engl J Med* 1992;326:589.
13. Lowenfels AB, Misonneuve P, Cavallini G, et al. Pancreatitis and the risk of pancreatic cancer. *N Engl J Med* 1993;328:1433.
14. Mergener K, Baillie J. Chronic pancreatitis. *Lancet* 1997;350:1379.
15. Moossa AR. Diagnostic tests and procedures in acute pancreatitis. *N Engl J Med* 1984;311:639.
16. Moossa AR. Surgical treatment of chronic pancreatitis: an overview. *Br J Surg* 1987;74:661.
17. Navarro S, Ros E, Aused R, et al. Comparison of fasting, nasogastric suction and cimetidine in the treatment of acute pancreatitis. *Digestion* 1984;30:224.
18. Ranson JHC. Etiologic and prognostic factors in human acute pancreatitis: a review. *Am J Gastroenterol* 1982;77:633.
19. Silverstein W, Isikoff MB, Hill MC. Diagnostic imaging of acute pancreatitis: prospective study using CT and sonography. *Am J Radiol* 1981;137:497.
20. Stark DD, Moss AA, Goldberg HI, et al. Magnetic resonance and CT of the normal and diseased pancreas: a comparative study. *Radiology* 1984;150:153.
21. Steinberg WM, Goldstein SS, David ND, et al. Diagnostic assays in acute pancreatitis. *Ann Intern Med* 1985;102:576.
22. Steinberg WM, Tenner S. Acute pancreatitis. *N Engl J Med* 1994;330:1199.
23. Swensson EE, King ME, Malkpour A, et al. Serum amylase isoenzyme alterations in acute abdominal conditions. *Ann Emerg Med* 1985;14:421.
24. Tenner S, Banks PA. Acute pancreatitis: nonsurgical management. *World J Surg* 1997;21:143.
25. Wanebo HJ, Verzeridis MP. Pancreatic carcinoma in perspective. *Cancer* 1996;78:580.

CHAPTER 158
Hepatitis

Joel M. Geiderman and Mark J. Ault

Viruses are responsible for the majority of cases of acute hepatitis. The primary hepatotropic viruses include hepatitis A virus (HAV); hepatitis B virus (HBV); hepatitis C virus (HCV); hepatitis D virus (HDV, also called the delta agent); hepatitis E virus (HEV); and the non–A through E hepatitis viruses. In addition, Epstein-Barr virus (EBV), cytomegalovirus (CMV), and other viruses are known to cause hepatitis as part of a systemic infection, as are a variety of bacteria, rickettsiae, and protozoal organisms (Table 158.1). A similar histopathologic picture can result from a variety of toxic and anoxic processes.

TABLE 158.1. Infectious Agents Known to Cause Hepatitis

PRIMARY HEPATITIS VIRUSES
Hepatitis A (HAV)
Hepatitis B (HBV)
Hepatitis C (HCV)
Hepatitis D (HDV)
Hepatitis E (HEV)
Non-A through E
SECONDARY HEPATITIS VIRUSES
Epstein-Barr
Cytomegalovirus
Herpes simplex
Varicella-zoster
Rubella
Rubeola
Mumps
Adenovirus
Coxsackievirus B
Yellow fever
NONVIRAL INFECTIOUS AGENTS
Brucellosis
Ehrlichiosis
Gram-negative sepsis
Gram-positive toxic shock syndromes
Legionellosis
Leptospirosis
Malaria
Mycoplasma disease
Plague
Q fever
Salmonellosis
Syphilis
Toxoplasmosis
Tularemia
Tuberculosis

CLINICAL PRESENTATION

The clinical manifestations of hepatitis, regardless of cause, are protean and vary from individual to individual with respect to severity of symptoms, duration of illness, and outcome. The ultimate course of the illness is thought to depend on the nature of the etiologic agent, the extent of preexisting or underlying liver disease, and, with infectious causes, the interaction between host factors and the pathogen.

In its classic presentation, viral hepatitis has a highly characteristic clinical picture that is easily recognizable in its various stages. After a variable incubation period, a "prodromal phase" of illness occurs, with symptoms such as anorexia, low-grade fever, malaise, and lassitude. Often characterized as "flulike" symptoms, they are nonspecific constitutional complaints typical of a variety of viral illnesses. Gastrointestinal symptoms may predominate, particularly in the adult patient, and abdominal discomfort representing hepatic, and occasionally splenic, enlargement may be reported. Within days to weeks after the onset of symptoms, the patient who enters the "icteric phase" of the illness first notes discoloration of the urine, representing the early rise of direct-reacting bilirubin and the spillage of bilirubin pigment into the urine. Subsequently, light (clay-colored) stools develop, scleral icterus may be noted, and clinical jaundice may become evident both to the patient and to the clinician as the serum bilirubin level exceeds 3 to 4 mg/dL. At this point, particularly in hepatitis A, symptoms may begin to resolve, heralding the convalescent phase of the illness.

Physical findings are highly variable in that the examination may be completely normal or may reveal frank jaundice and evidence of hepatic dysfunction. Liver enlargement and tenderness are common, and splenomegaly and lymphadenopathy may be present in 15% to 20% of cases.

Hampered frequently by unfamiliarity with the patient; by misleading, confusing, vague, or nonspecific historical details; and by multiple etiologic possibilities, the emergency physician may not recognize hepatitis when it does not present as the classic textbook picture. This may occur, for example, when surreptitious toxin ingestion is involved or when the patient is reluctant to reveal specific risk factors for viral hepatitis.

If the patient is frankly jaundiced, hepatitis is usually readily considered. Recognition of the more subtle findings of scleral discoloration, sublingual yellowing, or evidence of excoriations, which may be evident only on careful head-to-toe examination, also may lead to the discovery of hepatic disease.

When frank jaundice is absent, however—the rule rather than the exception in viral hepatitis—a higher index of suspicion is necessary. When present, constitutional symptoms alone are not at all specific for hepatitis but nonetheless are usually a sensitive marker for active hepatic disease and may provoke initial preliminary laboratory screening.

Extrahepatic manifestations are particularly prevalent in hepatitis B and are generally considered to be due to formation of immune complexes, with deposition in various extrahepatic sites. They include urticaria and morbilliform rashes, arthralgias and frank arthritis, hematuria and proteinuria, and, less commonly, vasculitis of the mixed cryoglobulinemia or polyarteritis nodosa types.[11] Other extrahepatic manifestations are not believed to be immunologically mediated. Pancreatitis, pneumonitis, and myocarditis are thought to be due to direct viral involvement.

Occasionally, a patient presents with advanced hepatic failure and no history of previous hepatitis. This may occur in the context of progressive chronic hepatitis, a toxic insult, or acute-on-chronic hepatitis. Unexplained encephalopathy (which may be as subtle as a personality change), coagulopathy, hypoglycemia, or respiratory alkalosis should prompt consideration of a hepatic disorder and a diligent search for confirmatory evidence.

DIFFERENTIAL DIAGNOSIS

Viral Hepatitis

Acute viral hepatitis is characterized by four stages: the incubation period, the preicteric phase, the icteric phase, and convalescence. During the incubation period, there are no clinical manifestations of disease, but viral replication is occurring, and serologic and chemical markers of this activity and the host response to it can be measured. Clinical manifestations appear only if and when enough hepatocytes are invaded.

The etiologic agent causing hepatitis cannot be determined from the clinical presentation; all of the hepatotropic viruses are capable of producing a similar clinical picture. Therefore, in evaluating the patient with presumed viral hepatitis and attempting to determine the cause, it is imperative to understand the significance of the serologic markers associated with the various types.

Hepatitis A

HAV is spread primarily by the fecal–oral route, although the virus can be found in the blood as well as in the liver, bile, and stool during the later part of the incubation period. The 2-week period before the onset of jaundice is the time of greatest infectivity; viremia, fecal shedding in the stool, and infectivity diminish markedly by the time the icteric phase begins (Fig. 158.1). Source outbreaks are the result of fecal contamination of

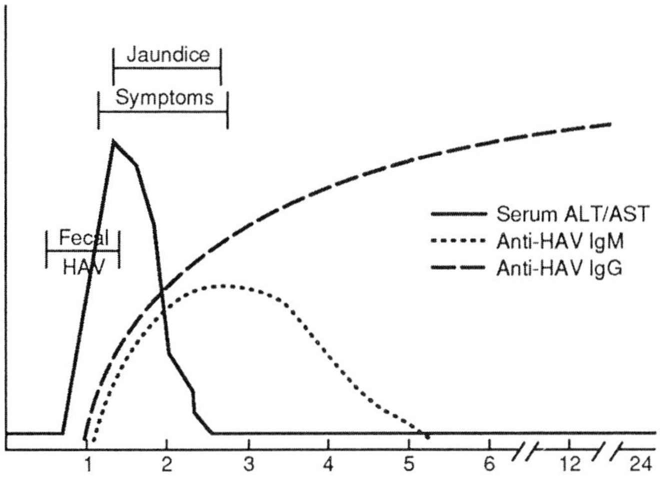

Figure 158.1. Serologic course of viral hepatitis A. Children usually have only mild symptoms with no jaundice. Adults more often develop jaundice. (Adapted from Hoofnagle JH. Serologic diagnosis of acute and chronic hepatitis. In: Hepatology Update/Portal Hypertension: Viral Hepatitis [postgraduate course of the American Association for the Study of Liver Diseases]. *Hosp Med* 1988;6:26.)

water supplies (e.g., with poor sanitation or during disasters), or when food becomes contaminated. The disease may also be spread by oral–anal contact.

The incubation period is short: 2 to 7 weeks. The "preicteric" phase of hepatitis A, usually lasting 4 to 14 days, presents nonspecifically with weakness, malaise, anorexia, nausea, and vomiting. There may be pain in the right upper quadrant and a characteristic loss of taste for cigarettes. Rash, urticaria, and joint pain occur infrequently, but the diagnosis of acute hepatitis should be considered in patients with these complaints. The term *preicteric* is presumptive, because not all patients go on to have clinically evident jaundice. Children with hepatitis A typically present with gastroenteritis and commonly do not develop jaundice.

The presence of dark urine frequently heralds the onset of the icteric phase and is often what prompts the patient to seek medical attention. Most of the other symptoms, with the exception of malaise, resolve shortly after the appearance of jaundice, which may persist for up to a month. Jaundice appears in the minority of patients infected with HAV.

The convalescent period is variable; weakness and malaise may last for months. This tends to be true less often with hepatitis A than with the other viral hepatitides, but such an observation is of little use in making the initial diagnosis. The onset of hepatitis A is usually more abrupt and less insidious than of the other types of viral hepatitis, but this observation is not useful in the individual case.

Figure 158.1 depicts the usual serologic and biochemical course of hepatitis A. The alanine aminotransferase (ALT, formerly serum glutamic pyruvic transaminase [SGPT]) level begins to rise late in the incubation phase, just before the onset of symptoms. Fecal shedding has peaked before this time and is abating. During the symptomatic period, about 4 to 5 weeks after exposure, immunoglobulin-M (IgM) antibodies to HAV (anti-HAV IgM) begin to rise. Because this antibody usually becomes undetectable after 4 to 5 months, its presence implies recent infection; HAV itself is not measured. Antibodies of the IgG variety (anti-HAV IgG) rise a little later and remain detectable for life. The presence of such antibodies in the serum of at least 50% of adults reflects the high incidence of asymptomatic or unrecognized disease early in life, and is responsible for the effectiveness of pooled serum in preventing disease in exposed individuals.

Hepatitis B

HBV is spread by the parenteral route, including exposure to blood or certain blood products, contaminated needles and syringes (both in drug abusers and accidentally in health-care workers), infected excretions or saliva, sexual contact, and perinatal contact. Its prevalence is high among homosexual men, intravenous drug abusers, dialysis patients, and patients and staff of institutions for the mentally retarded, and in certain endemic regions of the world.

Hepatitis B has an incubation period of 45 to 160 days. During this phase, the virus is actively replicating and is present not only in the hepatocyte, but also in virtually all body fluids, including blood, saliva, semen, and vaginal secretions. The implications of this fact are important: Patients can transmit disease during this incubation period, biochemical and serologic markers can be measured before disease becomes clinically apparent, and appropriate immunoprophylactic measures given after exposure, but before the onset of symptoms, may prevent or ameliorate the disease.

Acute hepatitis B usually follows a course similar to that of hepatitis A. Infrequently, a serum sickness–like illness occurs with the onset of symptoms. Jaundice is more likely to occur in hepatitis B than in hepatitis A, but still occurs in a minority of cases. Eighty percent to 85% of cases resolve completely, leaving the patient immune to hepatitis B. One percent to 3% of cases evolve into fulminant hepatitis, with a mortality rate of 90%; the remaining 5% to 10% of cases become chronic.

The serologic and biochemical course of acute hepatitis B is depicted in Fig. 158.2. The first marker to appear in the serum is the hepatitis B surface antigen (HBsAg), indicating infection with hepatitis B. Next, DNA polymerase, HBV DNA, and the hepatitis B e antigen (HBeAg) appear in the serum. These reflect active HBV replication and infectivity and appear well before the onset of biochemical damage to the liver. Of this group, only HBeAg can be measured easily; the presence of antibody to the HBeAg (anti-HBe) suggests low infectivity. In patients who become symptomatic, the ALT level rises and, in some, jaundice appears. Most patients seen at this time will still be HBsAg-positive.

Acute type B hepatitis

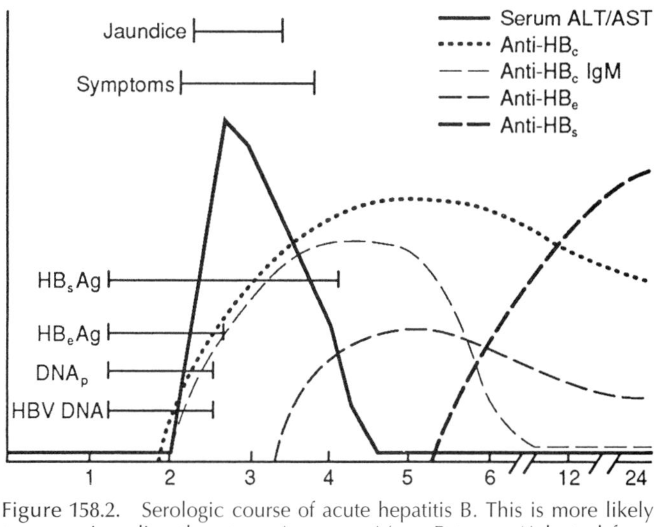

Figure 158.2. Serologic course of acute hepatitis B. This is more likely to cause jaundice than type A or non-A/non-B types. (Adapted from Hoofnagle JH. Serologic diagnosis of acute and chronic hepatitis. In: Hepatitis Update/Portal Hypertension: Viral Hepatitis [postgraduate course of the American Association for the Study of Liver Diseases]. *Hosp Med* 1988;6:33.)

It is important to understand the significance of the next immunologic event—the appearance of antibody to the hepatitis B core antigen (anti-HBc), first of the IgM class and then IgG. This rise precedes the rise in antibodies to the surface antigen (anti-HBs). (In Fig. 158.2, note the gap between the box labeled *HBsAg* and the line labeled *anti-HBs*.) Therefore, in some patients recently infected with HBV who are seen during this gap or, "window," the sole specific marker of recent infection with HBV is the presence of anti-HBc IgM.

Anti-HBsAg is a neutralizing antibody; therefore, its rise correlates with abatement of symptoms and the return of ALT to normal levels and signifies immunity to HBV. Thereafter, the patient will test positive only for Anti-HBs, Anti-HBc IgG, and Anti-HBe.

The *carrier state* occurs when HBsAg remains positive for 6 months or more in the absence of clinical or laboratory features of acute infection. Some carriers represent a source of infection (those with circulating HBV particles and HBeAg). The carriage rate in the United States is only 0.1% to 0.5%, although, in some parts of the world, it is 5% to 20%.

Chronic persistent hepatitis (CPH) and *chronic active hepatitis* (CAH) are two distinct forms of chronic liver disease that may be due to hepatitis B or a variety of other causes. Although each has reasonably distinct clinical presentations and biochemical profiles, the diagnosis can be made on histologic grounds only. In CPH, there is chronic inflammatory infiltration but minimal fibrosis, and the lobular architecture is preserved. In CAH, there is a far more aggressive histologic picture, with piecemeal necrosis and intralobular fibrous septa. Symptomatology and biochemical abnormalities tend to be less severe with CPH, and the long-term prognosis is generally good. Biochemical abnormalities and clinical manifestations, both hepatic and extrahepatic, commonly are more severe in CAH, and the long-term prognosis tends to be poor, with progression to cirrhosis and end-stage liver disease. Treatment with immunosuppressive agents such as prednisone and azathioprine may be beneficial in the patient with CAH unrelated to hepatitis B. The role of the emergency physician is to identify those individuals who would benefit from workup and evaluation of these entities, as well as to appreciate the long-term clinical implications and the potential complications in patients with these forms of chronic liver disease.

Figure 158.3 depicts the serologic course of chronic HBV disease. Note that the HBsAg remains positive, antibodies (anti-HBs) are lacking, and the patient remains susceptible to further liver damage or to superinfection with hepatitis D.

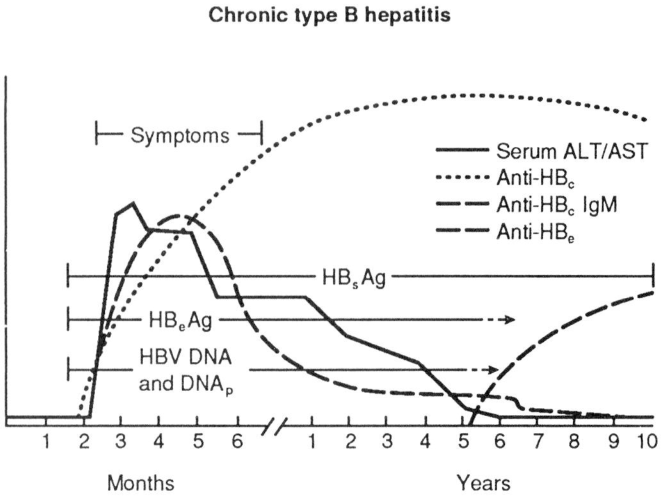

Figure 158.3. Serologic course of chronic HBV disease. (Adapted from Hoofnagle JH. Serologic diagnosis of acute and chronic hepatitis. In: Hepatitis Update/Portal Hypertension: Viral Hepatitis [postgraduate course of the American Association for the Study of Liver Diseases]. *Hosp Med* 1988;6:33.)

Hepatitis C

After the introduction of donor screening for HBV infection, posttransfusion hepatitis continued to be a significant problem. This led to the conclusion that most posttransfusion hepatitis was caused by another blood-borne pathogen, which was designated non-A, non-B (NANB) hepatitis. After the discovery of HCV in 1989 and the routine screening of the blood supply in the United States since 1990, it became clear that 80% to 90% of parenterally transmitted NANB hepatitis was caused by HCV.

HCV is an RNA virus of the Flaviviridae family. Extensive genetic heterogeneity of this virus may explain variations in clinical course, difficulties in vaccine development, and variations in response to therapy.[1] It may also explain why the virus so frequently escapes immunosurveillance, leading to chronic infection.

The incidence of newly acquired HCV infection has fallen dramatically since 1989 due to the effectiveness of blood donor screening.[1] Currently, the risk of transfusion-related hepatitis C is in the range of one in 100,000 U transfused. Aside from blood transfusion, other parenteral sources of HCV infection include intravenous drug use, noninjection illegal drug use (sharing instruments for intranasal cocaine use), hemodialysis, organ transplantation, and occupational exposure. Low levels of transmission occur in sexual and household contacts and perinatally, (i.e., vertical transmission). There is no evidence that breast feeding transmits HCV from mother to baby. Sporadic cases also occur.

Hepatitis C viral RNA can be detected in blood within 1 to 3 weeks of exposure. Anti-HCV can be detected in 50% to 70% of patients at the onset of symptoms and in approximately 90% of patients 3 months after onset of infection. However, the majority of infected patients are asymptomatic and anicteric.

The symptoms of HCV—malaise, weakness, and anorexia—are similar to those seen with other types of hepatitis; however, compared with hepatitis B, the acute disease is usually milder, the peak ALT level lower, and the patient less likely to be icteric. Serum transaminase levels fluctuate and may even normalize during the course of both acute and chronic disease and may not indicate resolution of disease. Acute HCV infection rarely causes fulminant disease.

Chronic disease, with persistent although sometimes intermittent viremia, occurs in 85% of infected patients.[10] Most patients with chronic disease are clinically well, with a small minority (20% or fewer) experiencing mild intermittent fatigue and malaise.

Unfortunately, approximately 20% of patients with chronic human immunodeficiency virus (HIV) infection experience a slow, insidious course that results in cirrhosis. Concomitant alcohol use may hasten such an eventuality. Currently, hepatitis C is the leading reason for liver transplantation in the United States. Chronic hepatitis C infection also leads to an incidence of hepatocellular carcinoma of 1% to 5% after 20 years. In the presence of cirrhosis, the rate of acquiring hepatocellular carcinoma rises to 1% to 4% per year.

A commercially available enzyme immunoassay (EIA) is routinely used to detect antibodies to regions of the HCV genome. The test detects anti-HCV in approximately 90% of infected patients. Antibody is detectable 5 to 6 weeks after the onset of clinical hepatitis in 80% of patients, but seroconversion may take as long as 32 weeks in some individuals. The limitations of anti-HCV screening are that (1) anti-HCV is not detected in 10% of infected persons; (2) assays do not distinguish among acute, chronic, and past infection (i.e., positive titers do not reflect either infectivity or immunity); (3) there is a prolonged interval between onset of illness and seroconversion in some cases; and (4) positive tests are frequently false-positive in populations with a low prevalence of infection.

The more specific recombinant immunoblot assay (RIBA) may be used to screen out false-positive results. Future development of a test for IgM would help in determining the time of onset of disease. Polymerase chain reaction (PCR)–band assays have been developed to detect the RNA virus directly, but these are mainly of research interest.

It appears that passive immunization with immune serum globulin derived from patients with previous HCV infection is unlikely to prevent disease, and no active vaccine is presently on the horizon. Patients with chronic hepatitis C have been treated with α-interferon, but, unfortunately, only 25% show long-term improvement as measured by a reduction in clinical and virologic markers. Ribavirin may prove to be useful adjunctive therapy. It is not known whether combination treatment with α-interferon can prevent the development of cirrhosis and hepatocellular carcinoma.

Hepatitis D

Hepatitis D, or delta hepatitis, is caused by a defective virus, the replication of which is dependent on the presence of HBsAg synthesis. The virus consists of the delta-antigen–bearing core encapsulated by an HBsAg coat.

It should not be surprising that a virus that requires HBV for its replication follows a similar transmission pattern. The clinical course of HDV infection depends on whether it is acquired at the same time as HBV (coinfection) or whether HDV infects a patient with chronic HBV infection (superinfection).

In coinfection, the fate of HDV parallels that of HBV. Because most cases of acute HBV are subsequently cleared, HDV, which requires the presence of HBV for replication, is also cleared. The clinical course of HDV is similar to that described for hepatitis B, although it is often more severe.

Because patients with HDV superinfection, by definition, have not been able to mount an immunologic response sufficient to clear their HBV infection, in these individuals, HDV replication may go unchecked, resulting in fulminant hepatitis in a large proportion. Rarely, acute delta superinfection results in clearance of HBV in a chronically infected patient, a phenomenon attributed to nonspecific stimulation of the immune system by a new antigen. This apparently occurs in only about 3% of patients.[11] It is important to remember that immunity to hepatitis B renders one immune to hepatitis D infection.

Bearing in mind the serologic courses of acute and chronic HBV infection, it is simple to predict the serologic courses of HDV coinfection and superinfection. Table 158.2 lists the serologic features of HBV/HDV coinfection and HBV/HDV superinfection. The antidelta IgM rises within 5 weeks of HDV infection and then persists in low titer, whereas the antidelta IgG continues to rise as long as HBV infection persists. Thus, IgG antibody to delta does not indicate immunity, but it is consistent with ongoing infection if associated with the presence of HBsAg.[3]

Hepatitis E

Hepatitis E, formerly called enterically transmitted non-A, non-B hepatitis (ET-NANB), is responsible for more than 50% of acute viral hepatitis occurring in some developing countries.[5] It is generally of little concern in the United States, although "imported" cases have occurred in patients who have traveled to endemic areas, such as India, Nepal, Pakistan, and parts of the former Soviet Union and Mexico.

As its former name suggests, hepatitis E is enterically spread. The incubation period is 2 to 9 weeks (average, 6 weeks), with an icteric phase that lasts 3 to 6 weeks. Nausea, vomiting, and diarrhea, which are frequent, usually resolve with the onset of jaundice. Fulminant disease occurs in 5% of cases, with a predilection for pregnant women. A carrier state has not been demonstrated.

A fluorescent antibody-blocking assay to detect hepatitis E infection is available experimentally through the Centers for Disease Control and Prevention. Patients who receive pooled immune globin in the United States before travel to endemic areas are unlikely to be protected against hepatitis E because anti-HEV antibodies are not present in the American population. Travelers to endemic areas should be advised as to enteric precautions, whether they are immunized or not.

Non–A through E Hepatitis

There remains a small population of patients exposed to blood or blood products and of other individuals with clinical hepatitis in whom all serologic studies on both the donor and the recipient patients are negative. Acute or chronic hepatitis in which both nonviral causes and infection with any of the five hepatitis viruses have been excluded is described as non–A through E hepatitis.[2] With the discovery of new viruses and the development of new serologic tests, these patients will undoubtedly be further differentiated.

Other Viruses

The discovery of two new viruses has raised questions concerning their role in the etiology of viral hepatitis.

One of these, independently discovered and named hepatitis G virus (HGV) and hepatitis GB virus C (HGBV-C), is an RNA virus of the Flaviviridae type. It appears to be blood-borne and has been found in as many as 10% of patients with non–A through E hepatitis. Its role has been questioned, and its definition as a true hepatotropic cause of acute or chronic hepatitis is yet to be determined.[6]

Similarly, hepatitis F virus has been isolated from the stool of a patient with hepatitis and transmitted to primates. As with hepatitis G, the role of this virus as a significant cause of non–A through E hepatitis is unclear.

TABLE 158.2. Serologic Factors in HBV/HDV Coinfection and HBV/HDV Superinfection

HBV/HDV Coinfection		HBV/HDV Superinfection	
HbsAg + [a] anti-HBcIgM+	Implies recent HBV infection	Anti–HBc IgM − Anti–HBc IgG +	Implies chronic HBV infection
Anti–delta IgM+	Implies recent HDV infection	Anti–delta IgM +	Implies recent HDV infection

[a]Unless in window period.

Infectious, Nonviral Causes

Although uncommon, hepatitis can accompany a wide variety of bacterial, rickettsial, and protozoal diseases. Included in this list are legionellosis, salmonellosis, tularemia, leptospirosis, brucellosis, plague, syphilis, gram-negative sepsis, gram-positive toxic shock syndromes, Q fever, mycoplasmal disease, tuberculosis, toxoplasmosis, ehrlichiosis, and malaria (see Table 158.1).

Autoimmune Hepatitis

Autoimmune hepatitis is a chronic inflammatory liver disorder of uncertain etiology. A standardized definition and diagnostic criteria have been developed.[7] The diagnosis relies heavily on the exclusion of viral etiologies, lack of exposure to alcohol and other hepatotoxic agents, and hypergammaglobulinemia with gamma globulin levels greater than 1.5 times the upper limits of normal.

Clinically, the presentation may be extremely variable and difficult to differentiate from viral hepatitis. Two types have been described based on the presence of circulating autoantibodies. Type I (classic) autoimmune hepatitis has been associated with antinuclear and anti–smooth muscle antibodies, and type II has been characterized by the presence of autoantibodies against liver–kidney microsome type I (anti-L K M-1). Both types are more prevalent in young females, and appropriate diagnosis is crucial, as they may be treated with prednisone and immunosuppressive therapy.

Toxic and Metabolic Causes

Liver injury from toxic or metabolic causes may result from direct hepatocellular toxicity or from idiosyncratic injury due to a hypersensitivity-type reaction.[8] Toxic exposures also may manifest as cholestasis, in which elevations of alkaline phosphatase and bilirubin levels predominate.

Pharmacologic and chemical agents produce a diverse spectrum of hepatic insults, including both acute and chronic liver disease (Table 158.3). Although any evidence of hepatic dysfunction should prompt a diligent search for both intentional and inadvertent exposure to any of a number of chemical agents, several agents deserve specific mention because of the inherent likelihood of hepatocellular injury, because of their widespread use, or because of their particular relevance to the practice of emergency medicine.

Acetaminophen is among the more common agents encountered in the acute setting that are likely to be responsible for what may be striking liver enzyme elevations. Toxicity is dose dependent, but several factors have been shown to contribute in a synergistic way to toxicity even at relatively low doses. These include concomitant alcohol ingestion, chronic phenobarbital use, or chronic exposure to moderately large doses of acetaminophen.

Hepatitis due to *isoniazid* clinically resembles acute viral hepatitis and may occur in as many as 20% of patients taking the drug, with the risk and severity of injury increasing with the age of the patient. Clinical toxicity generally occurs in the first few months of therapy, but transaminase elevations greater than two to three times normal at any time must be considered potentially serious, because progression to fulminant hepatitis may occur.

Lovastatin, a cholesterol-lowering agent, is generally well tolerated but has been associated with severe hepatocellular injury. Moreover, there is concern that concomitant use of nicotinic acid (also widely used for the treatment of hypercholesterolemia) may promote additional toxicity.

TABLE 158.3. Drug-Induced Hepatitis

Clinical/Morphologic Presentation	Examples
Hepatitis (acute)	α-Methyldopa
	Isoniazid
	Phenytoin
	Chlorothiazide
	Nonsteroidal antiinflammatory agents
	Lovastatin
Cholestasis	Anabolic steroids
	Flutamide
	Oral contraceptive agents
	Erythromycin estolate
	Methimazole
	Chlorpropamide
	Chlorpromazine
Hepatic necrosis	Carbon tetrachloride
	Amanita phalloides mushrooms
	Acetaminophen
	Yellow phosphorus
Hepatitis (chronic)	α-Methyldopa
	Arsenic
	Isoniazid
	Halothane

While overt hepatotoxicity to *phenytoin* is unusual, use of the drug is particularly common, and prevention of serious toxicity requires an awareness of the nature and mechanisms of injury. Hepatic injury is believed to be caused by toxic metabolites; current evidence has implicated a heritable metabolic defect that may predispose to a viral hepatitis–like hypersensitivity reaction within weeks of starting therapy at usual therapeutic doses. Like the other toxic exposures, early detection and interruption of therapy can result in complete resolution and the avoidance of serious hepatic injury.

Troglitazone (Rezulin) is a newer oral agent used in the treatment of patients with type 2 diabetes mellitus. The U.S. Food and Drug Administration has received numerous postmarking reports of hepatotoxicity, with some patients experiencing fatal hepatic failure.[9] The basis for this idiosyncratic reaction is unknown and therefore unpredictable. It is now recommended that ALT levels be monitored during therapy and that any patients with ALT levels more than three times the upper limit of normal discontinue the drug immediately. The drug is no longer being distributed in some European countries.

Flutamide is an antiandrogen drug used in the treatment of metastatic prostate cancer. Well-documented cases of serious hepatotoxicity have been reported. Although the toxicity appeared to be reversible, several patients have died with massive hepatic necrosis, emphasizing the need for prompt consideration and diagnosis.

Hepatitis has been reported to be associated with the use of several of the *nonsteroidal antiinflammatory drugs* (NSAIDs). Because of the frequency with which NSAIDs are used, emergency physicians should be aware of their potential for causing hepatic toxicity. Sulindac has received special attention because it has been well established as a cause of hepatitis, including fatal hepatic necrosis.

Well described as causes of fulminant hepatic failure, *halothane* and *methoxyflurane* are unusual causes of hepatitis. Patients may present with fevers and jaundice 1 to 2 weeks postoperatively. Specific risk factors may include obesity, multiple exposures to halothane over a brief period, and previous untoward reactions to halothane. Although no specific therapy is indicated, the emergency physician may be in the position of evaluating the postoperative patient who returns to the emergency department after discharge from the hospital. Recognition of this entity may avoid a fruitless search for other causes and, more importantly, will prevent reexposure.

Another cause of elevated transaminase levels (transaminitis) that should be considered in the differential diagnosis is *hepatobiliary disease*. Elevated ALT and aspartate transferase (AST, formerly serum glutamic oxaloacetic transaminase [SGOT]) levels should not lead one on a fruitless search for infection or toxic causes of hepatitis when the chemistry patterns suggest hepatobiliary obstruction (i.e., elevated serum bilirubin, alkaline phosphatase, and γ-glutamyl transpeptidase levels [GGTP]).

EMERGENCY DEPARTMENT EVALUATION

Evaluation of suspected hepatitis may be divided into several steps. The first step is to make the diagnosis, which, in light of the previous discussion, may not be entirely straightforward. Clearly, a reasonable index of suspicion is necessary in most cases, and the physician must consider the relative likelihood of illness in each particular patient compared with the risk of excessive testing in the many patients with nonspecific symptomatology.

If the likelihood of hepatitis is present but low, as in a patient followed serially for development of hepatocellular disease after a needlestick, a reasonable approach is initially to order a serum AST level as a preliminary screen. The AST is a cytoplasmic enzyme that is released with hepatocellular injury. Although nonspecific, this is a sensitive screen, and a normal AST value virtually excludes hepatocellular disease.

In the patient in whom hepatic disease is believed to be more likely or who has an abnormal AST on the preliminary screen, more extensive laboratory testing is necessary. This should consist of indices of necrosis (AST and ALT) as well as indices of cholestasis (alkaline phosphatase, total bilirubin, or GGTP). Although they lack diagnostic specificity, certain patterns may be helpful in limiting the differential diagnosis and directing further evaluation. For instance, a transaminase elevation of greater than ten times normal strongly suggests acute viral or toxic injury and essentially excludes chronic hepatitis. Elevation of alkaline phosphatase and bilirubin values suggests intrahepatic or extrahepatic obstruction. Transaminase elevations of two to three times normal, with the AST higher than the ALT, suggest alcoholic injury.

In the second step of the workup, after the diagnosis of liver disease has been made, specific tests of hepatic synthetic function are necessary. Tests of serum protein, albumin, and glucose levels should be ordered routinely and can be used in conjunction with the serum bilirubin level to assess the extent of hepatocellular dysfunction. If central nervous system involvement is suspected, or if unexplained lethargy, psychiatric symptoms, or other indicators of encephalopathy are present, an arterial ammonia level may be obtained that can serve as a useful baseline for further serial evaluations.

At the third step, other evaluations are performed to define more specifically the cause of the illness. If hepatocellular necrosis is the dominant picture, detailed serologic studies (anti-HAV IgM, HBsAg, anti-HBs, anti-HBc, anti-HCV, and Monospot test) are warranted, as well as a diligent historical search for foreign travel to hepatitis E–endemic regions and drug or toxic exposures. If cholestasis is the dominant picture, ultrasound examination should be performed to exclude mechanical obstruction. If none is found, a search for drug or toxic exposures is warranted.

EMERGENCY DEPARTMENT MANAGEMENT

Patients with acute viral hepatitis may present to the emergency department because of signs and symptoms typical of a viral syndrome that may include prostration, nausea, vomiting, and dehydration. Treatment for these patients is symptomatic and is usually limited to intravenous fluids, acetaminophen, and antiemetics. Metoclopramide (Reglan) is the antiemetic agent of choice, because phenothiazines can impair hepatic excretory function and may produce cholestasis.

Patients who present without symptoms or present because they have noticed jaundice require no specific therapy.

For patients with diagnosed viral hepatitis, there is no specific therapy indicated beyond routine supportive care and symptomatic treatment. If the prothrombin time is prolonged, the patient should receive intravenous vitamin K. Immune glob-

TABLE 158.4. Immunoprophylaxis of Viral Hepatitis

Type	Persons at Risk	Immunoprophylaxis
A	Household and sexual contacts[a] Staff and attendees of daycare centers Staff and residents of custodial institutions	Immune globulin, 0.02 mL/kg i.m.
B	Sexual contacts	Hepatitis B immune globulin, 0.06 mg/kg i.m.
	Percutaneous or transmucosal exposure	Begin active immunization (Heptavax or Recombivax)
C	Intravenous drug abusers, intranasal cocaine abusers, homosexuals, multiple sexual partners, perinatal exposure, household contacts	None
D	Same as B	Protection against hepatitis B
E	Travelers to endemic areas	None in serum pooled from U.S. donors
Non-A through E	Percutaneous exposure to blood or certain products of patients with no serologic evidence or HAV, HBV, or HCV	None

[a]Residents of dormitories and barracks are frequently considered in this group.

ulin is of no use in the patient who has already contracted hepatitis. Corticosteroids are probably harmful rather than beneficial.

Patients who present because they have been exposed, or think they have been exposed, to hepatitis present a different management problem. (For needlestick patients, see Chapter 198.) Immunoprophylaxis is highly effective if given under the proper circumstances. Because this treatment should be guided in part by serologic studies, it is often not initiated in the emergency department.

If results of serologic testing are not available, or not available in a timely fashion, therapy must be empiric and, as such, must be based on probabilities. The discussion that follows and the material in Table 158.4 should help guide immunoprophylactic therapy.

Patients considered to be at risk for contracting hepatitis A include household and sexual contacts of persons with hepatitis A; staff and attendees at daycare centers; and staff and residents in close contact at custodial care institutions. Immune globulin, which is derived from pooled human serum but treated so as not to be capable of transmitting HIV infection or other diseases, is given as a single intramuscular dose of 0.02 mL/kg as soon as possible within the first 2 weeks after exposure. Casual contacts need not be treated; such patients need little more than education and reassurance.

Postexposure prophylaxis for hepatitis B is indicated for sexual contacts of persons with hepatitis B, or after percutaneous or transmucosal exposure to HBsAg-positive blood. Treatment is with hepatitis B immune globulin, 0.06 mL/kg intramuscularly; active immunization is begun at the same time. This recommendation assumes that serologic data are available on the index patient with hepatitis and that the immune status of the exposed patient is known. If the data are not available but can be obtained within 5 to 7 days, it is reasonable to wait. If not, one must make a decision based on lifestyles and risk factors; the history obviously should include information regarding sexual contacts and intravenous drug use.

Immunoprophylaxis has not proven useful in patients who have been exposed to hepatitis C or in those suspected of being exposed to non–A through E hepatitis.

DISPOSITION

Most patients with hepatitis do not require hospital admission, because there is nothing that can be done for them in the hospital that cannot be done at home. Hospitalization is recommended under the following circumstances: persistent nausea and vomiting that is unresponsive to treatment; dehydration or electrolyte imbalance that cannot be corrected in the emergency department during a reasonable length of stay; or signs of hepatic deterioration, as evidenced by changes in sensorium or prolongation of the prothrombin time (50% activity is commonly used as a criterion). Obviously, patients with signs or symptoms suggesting a fulminant course require admission. The absolute levels of serum transaminase values should not be a criterion for admission.

Patients with acute viral hepatitis who are discharged should be prescribed antiemetic agents and instructed to ensure adequate caloric intake. It is best to allow patients to eat small meals of foods of their choice rather than insist they follow some of the high-calorie or high-protein dietary regimens that have been proposed. Prolonged bed rest, once a staple of care, has been shown to be of no value and has its own risks.[6] Most patients will limit their physical activities as needed. Alcohol consumption should be avoided during the acute illness. After complete recovery, alcohol consumption has not been shown to be any more harmful than for the general population.[4] Estrogen-based oral contraceptives may be continued during hepatitis.

Patients with acute hepatitis should be seen by an internist or gastroenterologist for follow-up within a few days; it is sensible to wait for the results of serologic tests before this visit. Patients with any prolongation of the prothrombin time are often admitted to the hospital, but those who are not should probably be seen the next day. Instructions should include an admonition to return if food and fluids cannot be kept down or if there is any change in sensorium.

Finally, it is the duty of the emergency physician in many locales to notify public health authorities of cases of acute hepatitis.

COMMON PITFALLS

Diagnostic Errors

- Missed toxic ingestion or exposure, with possible continued or recurrent exposure
- Failure to recognize hepatitis B or hepatitis C by performing serologic tests during "window periods" between infection and seroconversion
- Missed hepatobiliary disease, with failure to diagnose surgically correctable lesions
- Diagnosis of viral or alcoholic hepatitis as hepatobiliary disease, with operative intervention in a patient with excessive anesthetic risks
- Failure to recognize atypical presentations as secondary phenomena of liver disease and not primary events (e.g., coagulopathy, altered mental status, psychiatric abnormalities, hypoglycemia)

Evaluation Errors

- Failure to recognize the distinction between liver tests and liver function (e.g., patients with cirrhosis may have nearly normal enzyme levels; patients with "sky high" transaminase levels may have reasonably intact synthetic capability)
- Failure to distinguish between acute and chronic disease in patients who are anti-HCV positive
- Inappropriate admission of patients with uncomplicated hepatitis and markedly elevated ALT or AST levels without evaluation of synthetic factors or clinical status, or inappropriate discharge of patients with early evidence of synthetic failure
- Excessive emergency department evaluation because of inappropriate use of strategies and preliminary laboratory results

Inappropriate Follow-Up

- Failure to follow up contacts for recommended prophylaxis
- Inappropriate restrictions: Patients with hepatitis need not be excluded from school or work simply because of the diagnosis of hepatitis; education regarding precautions is indicated.

Failure to Consider the Pharmacokinetic Role of the Liver

- Administration of hepatotoxic drugs for symptomatic treatment in patients with hepatic injury (e.g., phenothiazines for nausea or NSAIDs for pain)
- Administration of hepatically cleared drugs, with resultant decrease in clearance and unexpectedly high serum levels or duration of action

References

1. Alter M. Epidemiology of hepatitis C. *Hepatology* 1997; 62S–65S.
2. Alter M, et al. Acute non-A-E hepatitis in the United States and the role of hepatitis G virus infection. *N Engl J Med* 1997;336:741–754.
3. DeCock KM, Govindarajan S, Chin KP, et al. Delta hepatitis in the Los Angeles area: a report of 126 cases. *Ann Intern Med* 1986;105–108.
4. Gardner HT, Rovelstad RA, Moore DJ. Hepatitis among American occupation troops in Germany. *Ann Intern Med* 1948;30:1009.
5. Herrera JL. Hepatitis E as a cause of acute non-A, non-B hepatitis. *Arch Intern Med* 1993;153:773.
6. Koffs RS, Galambos JT. Viral hepatitis. In: Schiff L, Schiff ER, eds. *Diseases of the liver*, 6th ed. Philadelphia: JB Lippincott Co, 1987.
7. Krawitt EL. Autoimmune hepatitis. *N Engl J Med* 1996;334:897–903 .
8. Lee WM. Drug-induced hepatotoxicity. *N Engl J Med* 1995;1118–1127.
9. Misbin RI. Troglitazone-associated hepatic failure. *Ann Intern Med* 1999;330.
10. National Institutes of Health Consensus Development Conference Panel Statement: Management of hepatitis C. *Hepatology* 1997;26(3):2S–10S.
11. Ockner RK. Acute viral hepatitis. In: Wyngaaden JB, Smith LH, eds. *Cecil's textbook of medicine*, 8th ed. Philadelphia: WB Saunders, 1998.

CHAPTER 159

Hepatic Failure and Cirrhosis

David M. Cline and E. Jackson Allison, Jr.

Acute hepatic failure differs clinically, prognostically, and therapeutically from an exacerbation of chronic liver failure, but the priorities for the management of both entities are similar. Despite significant recent advances in the management of hepatic encephalopathy, the exact mechanism for the widespread neural inhibition seen in this condition continues to elude investigators. Ammonia, a substance liberated from the intestinal flora and known to accumulate in hepatic failure, is a key factor in the development of hepatic encephalopathy.[11] However, ammonia accumulation causes an excitable state rather than neural inhibition, and the severity of hepatic coma does not correlate well with blood ammonia levels.[2] Although several other theories have been proposed, no single mechanism has explained all the features of this disorder.

Viral hepatitis has traditionally been regarded as the most common cause of fulminant hepatic failure (FHF) worldwide.[18] An analysis of six studies found acetaminophen overdose to be the single most common cause of acute hepatic failure in industrialized countries.[9] In 23% of cases, the cause could not be determined. Acute and chronic ingestion of the antituberculous drugs isoniazid and rifampin and Reye syndrome are other important causes of FHF. Less common causes include fatty degeneration of pregnancy, heat stroke, *Amanita phalloides* mushroom poisoning, cancer metastatic to the liver,[17] and the illicit drug ecstasy.[5]

Hepatic cirrhosis most commonly is caused by alcoholism; chronic active hepatitis is the second most common cause. Typically, there is progressive destruction of the normal sinusoidal architecture over several years, with resulting fibrosis. Progressive hepatocellular dysfunction results in impaired glycogen storage, coagulopathy, and loss of detoxifying capability. Continued fibrosis shunts blood away from the hepatic artery directly into the portal vein, resulting in secondary portal hypertension and esophageal varices.

CLINICAL PRESENTATION

The presentation of FHF is, to some degree, dependent on the specific etiologic agent, but the majority of patients have altered mentation, coagulopathy with clinical bleeding, jaundice (especially in children), motor dysfunction, and fetor hepaticus, a sweetish, musty, or pungent odor on the breath.

The manifestations of hepatic encephalopathy in both FHF and cirrhosis are similar, but the onset is generally slower with cirrhosis. FHF may present with rapid deterioration of mental status, with progression over several hours from slowed response times to frank coma. Patients with cirrhosis commonly present with euphoria, depression, or muscular incoordination, or may demonstrate more obvious mental status changes. Symptoms such as malaise, lethargy, fluid retention, loss of libido, and pruritus are common, and typical physical findings include hepatomegaly, spider nevi, ascites, and jaundice. Asterixis, a flapping tremor best seen with the patient's arms outstretched and wrists hyperextended, is a classic symptom that is not present in all cases. The factors most commonly precipitating hepatic encephalopathy in cirrhotics are gastrointestinal bleeding, use of tranquilizing drugs or alcohol, overuse of diuretics, and infection.

Complications of Hepatic Failure and Cirrhosis

Cerebral edema is a universal feature of acute hepatic failure and the most common cause of death in untreated cases. Early warning signs include systemic hypertension and increased muscle tone, which progresses to decerebrate posturing and eventual respiratory arrest if left untreated.[3] Hypoglycemia, thought to be secondary to inefficient degradation of insulin, impaired glycogen storage, or reduced hepatic metabolic capacity, may be profound and recurrent. More than 50% of patients demonstrate clinical evidence of coagulopathy, usually in the form of gastrointestinal, nasopharyngeal, or bronchial tree bleeding. Hypotension secondary to decreased systemic vascular resistance may occur in the absence of hemorrhage. Patients typically are tachypneic, with a respiratory alkalosis. Artificially increasing the pCO_2 toward normal leads to deterioration. Hypoxia and noncardiogenic pulmonary edema are common. Prerenal azotemia, acute tubular necrosis, or renal failure of unknown cause may occur. Hypokalemia and hypocalcemia are common.

Spontaneous bacterial peritonitis, pneumonia, urinary tract infection, bacteremia, or other bacterial infection complicates the hospital course of 80% of patients in FHF, and these infections account for 25% of deaths.[16] Febrile cirrhotics with abdominal pain and tenderness should be considered to have spontaneous bacterial peritonitis until proven otherwise.

Because of portal hypertension and secondary esophageal varices, death from gastrointestinal bleeding is more common with cirrhosis than with FHF. In the later stages of cirrhosis, ascites may become markedly symptomatic and limit ventilation and atrial filling.[12] The hepatorenal syndrome, or functional renal failure, occurs in advanced cirrhosis and is usually fatal despite treatment.

DIFFERENTIAL DIAGNOSIS

The differential diagnosis of jaundice includes hemolysis, obstructive jaundice, viral hepatitis, hepatotoxic ingestions, septicemia, and numerous minor causes. The association of mental status changes with jaundice should alert the emergency physician to the possibility of hepatic encephalopathy. In the patient without chronic liver disease, the differential diagnosis of hepatic encephalopathy includes viral hepatitis, fatty degeneration of pregnancy, Reye syndrome, and hepatotoxic ingestions such as acetaminophen, isoniazid, rifampin, *A. phalloides* mushrooms, carbon tetrachloride, or ecstasy. Historical information, such as pre-illness activity, previous suicidal behavior, and the presence of fever or malaise, may help to differentiate among potential causes. There are few clinical features that help to differentiate hepatic encephalopathy from other causes of acute mental status change, with the exception of fetor hepaticus. Unfortunately, fetor hepaticus is commonly mistaken for simple halitosis. The coexistence of jaundice and altered mental status should always alert the clinician to the possibility of hepatic failure.

Patients with hepatic cirrhosis may have chronic jaundice and may sustain acute mental status changes for reasons other than hepatic encephalopathy. Because alcoholic patients are at greater risk for accidents as well as for bleeding, subdural hematoma must be ruled out in cirrhotics with an altered sensorium. Patients with renal failure from other causes may present with features suggestive of severe liver disease—an altered sensorium, fluid retention, and coagulopathy. Alcoholics may develop pancreatitis or alcoholic hepatitis, with severe dehydration and associated mental status changes that may mimic hepatic encephalopathy.

EMERGENCY DEPARTMENT EVALUATION

The validity of information from the patient should be questioned, and additional information should be sought from prehospital personnel, family, the patient's private physician, and previous medical records. The conjunctiva and skin should be examined for the presence of jaundice. The respiratory system should be carefully assessed for the possibility of aspiration or pulmonary edema in advanced cases. Although an enlarged liver is common in alcoholic liver disease, the liver is usually small in FHF or advanced cirrhosis. A rectal examination is necessary to check for evidence of gastrointestinal bleeding. A careful neurologic examination should be done with attention to subtle changes in mental status, using serial sevens or formal psychometric testing. Asterixis, alterations in motor tone, or abnormal posturing should be noted.

The diagnosis of hepatic encephalopathy is largely clinical; no single laboratory test can confirm the diagnosis with certainty. Hypoxemia and hypoglycemia should be ruled out. A serum ammonia level should be measured, but patients may be encephalopathic before an elevation in the serum ammonia is observed.[3] A complete blood count, serum electrolyte determination, and coagulation studies should be performed to determine proper treatment. Serum aminotransferases, bilirubin, serologic tests, and serum amino acid levels may aid in diagnosis but do not alter management acutely. An electrocardiogram is advisable, especially in patients with preexisting heart disease.

EMERGENCY DEPARTMENT MANAGEMENT

The treatment of hepatic encephalopathy in patients with acute hepatic failure requires a more aggressive approach than in those with an exacerbation of chronic liver disease. Hepatic encephalopathy in acute hepatic failure develops rapidly and is almost always complicated by cerebral edema, with possible central herniation of the brain.[13]

Immediate attention should be given to securing a patent airway and initiating artificial ventilation if the patient is comatose or lacks an active gag reflex. Supplemental oxygen should be given, even in the absence of pulmonary edema. Fluid resuscitation should be aggressive in hypotensive or bleeding patients and should be undertaken despite the possibility of pulmonary edema. Pulmonary capillary wedge pressure measurements may be needed to guide therapy in patients who do not respond to boluses of less than 1 L of normal saline. Persistent hypotension signals the need for vasopressors. Dopamine (2 to 20 μg/kg/min) is recommended for initial treatment, but norepinephrine (0.5 to 30 μg/min) may be required.[3] Dopamine is useful in attempting to preserve urine flow and renal function.

Patients should be placed on a cardiac monitor and quickly assessed for cardiac manifestations of electrolyte imbalance. Patients with altered mental status or a blood glucose level below 100 mg/100 dL should receive 50% dextrose and thiamine intravenously, followed by an infusion of 10% or 20% dextrose solution.[3] Patients who demonstrate clinical signs of significant, increased intracranial pressure, such as abnormal posturing or unreactive pupils, should receive mannitol 0.5 g/kg intravenously over 10 minutes.[13] Arterial pCO_2 should be maintained at about 25 mm Hg. Ventilated patients often require sedation; fentanyl (2 μg/kg) and atracurium (0.4 mg/kg) are recommended to prevent surges in intracranial pressure related to agitation.[13] Consideration should be given to monitoring intracranial pressure with an extradural monitor, which, however, carries some risk and may be problematic if clinical bleeding is present.[8]

Fresh-frozen plasma (2 to 4 U) should be given when the prothrombin time is more than 1.5 times normal and there is evidence of active bleeding.[9] Platelet infusions (2 to 4 U) are recommended when thrombocytopenia is severe or there is active bleeding unresponsive to correction of clotting factor abnormalities. Administration of cimetidine or ranitidine can reduce the incidence of gastrointestinal bleeding.[10]

Proven or suspected infection should be treated promptly, using cultures to modify empiric therapy. The responsible organisms are usually gram-negative; cefotaxime (1 to 2 g i.v.) or a similar broad-spectrum cephalosporin is recommended.[18] Aspiration pneumonia also should be considered in these patients, and if suspected, should be treated with pulmonary toilet, ventilatory support as needed, and broad-spectrum antibiotics. Urinary tract infection requires treatment with intravenous antibiotics providing good gram-negative coverage. A large prospective trial showed that prophylactic antibiotics (cefuroxime 1.0 g i.v.) significantly reduced the incidence of infection in FHF.[15]

Lactulose, which increases intestinal motility and lowers colonic pH, accelerates recovery from hepatic coma, but its exact mechanism of action is not known. Oral lactulose can be given as a syrup, 50 cc every 1 to 2 hours until results are obtained, or can be given as an enema, 300 cc in a liter of saline.[4] Oral neomycin, 2 to 4 g/d, also has been shown to be effective, but should be withheld if an aminoglycoside is being considered for treatment of a coexisting infection. Metronidazole, 800 mg/d, is an alternative.[13] Acetylcysteine improves survival from acetaminophen overdose, even late in its course,[7] and may have benefits in the treatment of FHF from other causes.[6]

The management of gastrointestinal bleeding in patients with cirrhosis is much more difficult than in those with FHF. After initial resuscitation with necessary fluid and blood components, endoscopic sclerotherapy appears to be the best method to manage acute variceal bleeding. Patients ultimately may require a portacaval shunt to prevent rebleeding.

There has been promising work in the area of artificial liver support.[14,20] Decisions concerning liver support measures are best made by a gastroenterology consultant. In many cases of severe acute hepatic failure, transplantation is the only means of increasing the chance of survival.[1]

When patients with hepatic cirrhosis present to the emergency department with non–life-threatening conditions, care must be taken to avoid interventions (e.g., medications) that may cause clinical deterioration. Sedatives may trigger clinical hepatic encephalopathy. Nonsteroidal antiinflammatory drugs may induce renal failure in cirrhotic patients. Even acetaminophen may be harmful in cirrhotic patients. For the management of symptomatic ascites in cirrhotic patients, paracentesis has fewer side effects than diuretics and a comparable rate of fluid reaccumulation. Cirrhotics with recurrent variceal hemorrhage are now being routinely treated with a transjugular intrahepatic portosystemic shunt, which has an associated 25% incidence of chronic hepatic encephalopathy.[19] In some cases, the only means of correcting the encephalopathy is to reverse the shunt by transhepatic embolization.

DISPOSITION

Because patients with chronic liver disease commonly respond poorly to intermittent illness or other stress, indications for their admission to the hospital are generally less stringent than for other patients. For example, because cirrhotics have a limited ability to fight off infection, admission for intravenous antibiotic treatment should be considered for most infections.

Patients with advanced hepatic encephalopathy require admission to an intensive care setting, and immediate consultation with a gastroenterologist or a hepatologist is indicated. For severe cases, consideration should be given to transporting the patient to a facility capable of liver transplantation, provided intensive care transport is available.

COMMON PITFALLS

- Failing to consider a hepatotoxic drug as the cause of the patient's symptoms. Patients who have ingested a hepatotoxic drug may be unwilling to give an adequate history and may present early in the course of their illness, before there is obvious clinical evidence of hepatic failure. Teenagers ingesting acetaminophen are a common example.
- The diagnosis of hepatic encephalopathy cannot be ruled out on the basis of a serum ammonia level.
- Hypoglycemia should be treated empirically in patients with altered mental status. One bolus of 50% dextrose may not be adequate therapy because of depleted glycogen stores; maintenance infusions of D_{10} or D_{20} should be administered.
- It is essential that the emergency physician attempt to identify causes of coma other than hepatic encephalopathy in patients with cirrhosis. In particular, subdural hematoma, drug overdose, and meningitis should be ruled out.

References

1. Bismuth H, Samuel D, Castaing D, et al. Liver transplantation in Europe for patients with acute liver failure. *Semin Liver Dis* 1996;16:415.
2. Blom HJ, Ferenci P, Grimm G, et al. The role of methanethiol in the pathogenesis of hepatic encephalopathy. *Hepatology* 1991;13:445.
3. Caraceni P, Van Thiel DH. Acute liver failure. *Lancet* 1995;345:163.
4. Cordoba J, Blei AT. Treatment of hepatic encephalopathy. *Am J Gastroenterol* 1997;92:1429.
5. Ellis AJ, Wendon JA, Protmann B, et al. Acute liver damage and ecstasy ingestion. *Gut* 1996;38:454.
6. Harrison PM, Wendon JA, Gimson ES, et al. Improvement by acetylcysteine of hemodynamics and oxygen transport in fulminant hepatic failure. *N Engl J Med* 1991;324:1852.
7. Keays R, Harrison JA, Wendon JA, et al. Intravenous acetylcysteine in paracetamol induced hepatic failure: a prospective controlled trial. *BMJ* 1991;303:1026.
8. Keays RT, Alexander GJ, Williams R. The safety and value of extradural intracranial pressure monitors in fulminate hepatic failure. *J Hepatol* 1993;18:205.
9. Lidofski SD. Fulminant hepatic failure. *Crit Care Clin* 1995;11:415.
10. Martin LF, Booth FV, Karlstadt RG, et al. Continuous intravenous cimetidine decreases stress-related upper gastrointestinal hemorrhage without promoting pneumonia. *Crit Care Med* 1993;21:19.
11. Mousseu DD, Butterworth RF. Current theories on the pathogenesis of hepatic encephalopathy. *Proc Soc Biol Med* 1994;206:329.
12. Panos MA, Moore K, Vlavianos P, et al. Single total paracentesis for tense ascites: sequential hemodynamic changes and right atrial size. *Hepatology* 1990;11:662.
13. Riordan SM, Williams R. Treatment of hepatic encephalopathy. *N Engl J Med* 1997;337:473.
14. Roger V, Balladur P, Honiger J, et al. Internal bioartificial liver with xenogenic hepatocytes prevents death from acute liver failure: an experimental study. *Ann Surg* 1998;228:1.
15. Rolando N, Gimson A, Wade J, et al. Prospective controlled trial of selective parenteral and enteral antimicrobial regimen in fulminant liver failure. *Hepatology* 1993;17:196.
16. Rolando N, Harvey F, Brahm J, et al. Prospective study of bacterial infection in acute liver failure: an analysis of fifty patients. *Hepatology* 1990;11:49.
17. Rowbotham D, Wendon J, Williams R. Acute liver failure secondary to hepatic infiltration: a single center experience of 18 cases. *Gut* 1998;42:576.
18. Sherlock S. Fulminant hepatic failure. *Adv Intern Med* 1993;38:245.
19. Somberg KA, Riegler JL, LaBerge JM, et al. Hepatic encephalopathy after transjugular intrahepatic portosystemic shunts: incidence and risk factors. *Am J Gastroenterol* 1995;90:549.
20. Watanabe FD, Mullon CJ, Hewitt WR, et al. Clinical experience with a bioartificial liver in treatment of severe liver failure. A phase I clinical trial. *Ann Surg* 1997;225:484.

CHAPTER 160
The Patient with a Liver Transplant

Eric Savitsky, Scott R. Votey, and Don Mebust

Since the first human orthotopic liver transplant (OLT) in 1963, progressive improvements in surgical technique, immunosuppressive regimens, and medical care of these patients now result in 5-year survival rates approaching 80%.[3,5,14] Currently, over 100 centers perform more than 4,000 OLT operations each year in the United States. With improved survival rates and more centers performing liver transplantation, the number of OLT recipients presenting to the emergency department (ED) with complications continues to rise.

TRANSPLANT ANATOMY

The donor graft is prepared for implantation by undergoing a cholecystectomy.[6] The OLT recipient undergoes a bilateral subcostal incision, which is extended cephalad in the midline, creating a characteristic "Mercedes Benz" incision pattern. The recipient may be placed on femoral to axillary venovenous bypass, permitting clamping of the recipient portal vein and inferior vena cava (IVC). After vascular clamping, a hepatectomy is performed and the donor graft is inserted. Hepatic artery, portal vein, and both suprahepatic and infrahepatic IVC anastomoses are performed. Vascular clamps are released and reperfusion of the graft occurs. Immediate intraoperative production of bile by the newly transplanted liver is an excellent indicator of graft function.

Biliary reconstruction most commonly consists in an end-to-end reanastomosis (choledochocholedochostomy) with or without T-tube placement. T-tube placement affords direct monitoring of bile production, as well as access for evaluation of the biliary system by T-tube cholangiography. Despite these advantages, T-tube use has recently declined due to a high rate of postoperative complications. A Roux-en-Y loop with a choledochojejunostomy is an alternative form of biliary reconstruction. While choledochocholedochostomy is the preferred technique for biliary reconstruction in most adults, children and adults requiring repeat transplantation or having intrinsic biliary system disease undergo choledochojejunostomies. Pneumobilia is a normal result of choledochojejunostomy.

TYPICAL POSTTRANSPLANT COURSE

Following surgery, OLT recipients spend several days in an intensive care unit, during which time their liver function indices are closely monitored. The patient continues on an aggressive immunosuppressive regimen, begun intraoperatively, designed to minimize immune-mediated graft rejection. A two-drug regimen consisting of tacrolimus and prednisone is increasingly replacing the previously common triple-drug regimen of cyclosporine, azathioprine, and prednisone.

Early postoperative complications of transplantation include bleeding and primary graft failure. Systemic coagulopathy, thrombocytopenia, and portal hypertension–induced abdominal venous collaterals render OLT candidates susceptible to bleeding complications. Postoperative bleeding is usually the result of dehiscence of a vascular anastomosis; patients present with intraperitoneal hemorrhage before discharge from the hospital. Emergency physicians are much more likely to encounter OLT patients with upper gastrointestinal tract bleeding from peptic ulcer disease.[18] Upper and lower gastrointestinal tract bleeding in OLT patients is managed in the standard fashion.

Graft failure is a multifactorial process. Graft harvest technique, ischemia time, and reperfusion injury all influence graft viability. Early bile production, restoration of normal clotting function, and the absence of lactic acidosis are signs of good graft function. Profound hypoglycemia, progressive coagulopathy, metabolic acidosis, progressive encephalopathy, and hemodynamic instability clinically characterize graft failure.

In the absence of graft dysfunction, the OLT recipient is transferred to a ward bed and remains an inpatient for 1 to 2 weeks. Close outpatient care at the transplant center continues for an additional 1 to 2 months, during which time patients undergo careful adjustments of their immunosuppressive regimens. Patients are then followed on a monthly basis for the remainder of the first year after transplantation. The follow-up interval after 1 year is decided on a case-by-case basis.

CLINICAL PRESENTATION

OLT patients present to the ED with a wide variety of illnesses. Emergency physicians encounter vascular and biliary complications, rejection, infectious and metabolic complications, and medication-related adverse effects in OLT patients.[17,10,15,16]

Vascular Complications

Vascular complications include hepatic artery thrombosis (HAT), portal vein thrombosis (PVT), and hepatic artery rupture.[4] Together they account for about 10% of graft failure in adults and 30% of graft failure in children. The vascular supply to the donor common bile duct is dependent on the newly reconstructed hepatic artery. The graft, in contrast to the native liver, has no collateral arterial blood supply, and any disruption to hepatic artery blood flow inevitably leads to bile duct necrosis, with resultant bile duct leaks, graft dysfunction, abscess formation, and sepsis.

Although both HAT and PVT tend to occur within the first month and most often within the first week following transplantation, either may occur later, usually in association with episodes of acute rejection. The incidence of HAT varies from 4% to 25%, and it accounts for about 75% of post-OLT vascular complications. Patients with HAT or PVT typically have clinical (jaundice, dark urine, clay-colored stools) and laboratory (elevated transaminase and bilirubin levels) evidence of graft dysfunction, varying degrees of right upper quadrant abdominal pain, and fever. HAT is rare, and patients with it typically present acutely ill, in hypovolemic shock.

Biliary Complications

The incidence of biliary complications, including bile leaks and obstructions to bile flow, is 17% to 28%.[8,17] Patients typically complain of abdominal pain, jaundice, or fever, and evidence of cholangitis or peritonitis may be present. Unfortunately, some patients with biliary complications present with isolated fever or elevated liver enzymes without jaundice or abdominal pain. The abdomen may even be soft and nontender. Emergency physicians should strongly consider the possibility of a biliary complication whenever faced with an OLT patient presenting with any combination of abdominal complaints, fever, or evidence of graft dysfunction.

Immune-Mediated Disease

Immune-mediated disease in organ transplant recipients consists of hyperacute, acute, and chronic forms of rejection, as well as graft-versus-host disease. Acute and chronic rejection are the most clinically relevant immune-mediated diseases in OLT patients, because the liver is relatively resistant to hyperacute rejection and graft-versus-host disease.[16] Acute and chronic rejection are classified on the basis of time of occurrence and histology. Between 60% and 80% of patients in some published series have at least one episode of acute rejection. Chronic allograft rejection develops in approximately 5% to 9% of OLT recipients and may cause graft failure.

Acute rejection commonly manifests as malaise, generalized weakness, progressive jaundice, right upper quadrant pain, and, often, fever. Occasionally, acute rejection may be clinically asymptomatic, with elevation of liver enzymes the only clue to the diagnosis. A pattern of early alkaline phosphatase and bilirubin elevation, followed shortly by a rise in aspartate aminotransferase (AST) and alanine aminotransferase (ALT) levels, is typical of acute rejection. Although suggestive, this pattern is not specific for acute rejection, and may occur with cholestasis, cholangitis, drug toxicity, and other states of hepatic dysfunction.

The clinical presentation of chronic rejection is similar to that of an acute rejection. Patients may report low-grade fever, fatigue, progressive jaundice, right upper quadrant pain, clay-colored stools, and dark urine. Patients with chronic rejection usually experience a more gradual clinical deterioration compared with patients suffering acute rejection. Laboratory findings of chronic rejection are persistently elevated transaminase levels, increasing cholestasis, and declining hepatic synthetic function.

Infectious Complications

Infection continues to be a major source of morbidity and mortality in OLT patients.[2,12] Up to 67% of recipients have at least one serious infection following OLT. Approximately 50% to 60% of these infections are bacterial, 15% are fungal, 5% to 15% are viral, and less than 10% are caused by *Pneumocystis carinii* or

Toxoplasma species. Most infections occur during times of peak immunosuppression. Specifically, OLT recipients are at high risk for serious infections in the first several months following transplantation.

Patients maintained on high levels of immunosuppressive medications following acute rejection episodes, patients with indwelling central lines, and patients with biliary complications (e.g., biliary strictures) also remain at high risk for serious infections irrespective of duration posttransplantation. Emergency physicians should bear in mind that OLT recipients are immunocompromised and may present to the ED appearing well and complaining only of isolated fever, only to deteriorate rapidly during their subsequent hospital course.

Metabolic Complications and Medication-Related Adverse Effects

The immunosuppressive regimens that make graft survival possible are a frequent source of adverse effects. In addition to promoting infection, immunosuppressive medications may result in metabolic, renal, neurologic, hematologic, dermatologic, and bone disorders. Drug–drug interactions may precipitate these events, and the potential for adverse drug interactions should always be considered (Table 160.1).

The corticosteroids OLT patients receive result in all of the typical complications of chronic steroid excess, including adrenal suppression, cushingoid appearance, and osteoporosis. Osteoporosis-related fractures, especially vertebral body compression fractures, are a common problem in OLT patients because of preexisting hepatic osteodystrophies coupled with the osteopenic effects of corticosteroids.[9]

Dose-dependent cyclosporine or tacrolimus nephrotoxicity is common. Initial presentation may be occult, with azotemia and a rise in creatinine occurring with minimal symptoms. Corticosteroids, cyclosporine, and tacrolimus all induce insulin resistance, and OLT recipients may develop diabetes mellitus with hyperglycemic symptoms. Additionally, the immunosuppressive regimens OLT patients require have been associated with a variety of neurologic (tremors, headaches, altered mental status, seizures) and gastrointestinal symptoms (nausea, vomiting, and diarrhea).[19,20]

TABLE 160.1. Significant Drug Interactions

MEDICATIONS THAT *LOWER* CYCLOSPORINE (NEORAL, SANDIMMUNE) AND TACROLIMUS (PROGRAF) LEVELS	
Nafcillin	
Phenobarbital	
Carbamazepine	
Phenytoin	
Rifampin	
Valproic acid	
MEDICATIONS THAT *ELEVATE* CYCLOSPORINE (NEORAL, SANDIMMUNE) AND TACROLIMUS (PROGRAF) LEVELS	
Cimetidine	Clarithromycin
Diltiazem	Erythromycin
Fluconazole	Imipenem
Itraconazole	Ketoconazole
Methylprednisolone	Metoclopramide
Verapamil	

Avoid nonsteroidal antiinflammatory drugs, as they may further compromise renal function in patients taking either tacrolimus or cyclosporine.

Oral contraceptives are contraindicated, due to the increased risk of a thrombotic event (e.g., hepatic artery thrombosis).

No live virus vaccinations should be administered to OLT recipients or any of their close household contacts.

TABLE 160.2. Final Diagnoses for Common Presenting Complaints[a]

	Percentage
FEVER	
Bacterial illness	38
Viral illness	21
Fever of unclear origin	16
Immune-mediated illness	8
NAUSEA/VOMITING	
Gastroenteritis	14
Nausea/vomiting of unclear etiology	13
Bacteremia	11
Gastroesophageal reflux/gastritis	10
Biliary obstruction/leak	10
Medication effect	8
Immune-mediated illness	8
Pneumonia	6
Pancreatitis	5
ABDOMINAL PAIN	
Abdominal pain of unclear etiology	30
Biliary obstruction/leak	20
Gastroenteritis/colitis	9
Pancreatitis	9
Bowel obstruction	6
LETHARGY	
Bacterial illness	31
Hepatic dysfunction	14
Medication effect	11
JAUNDICE	
Immune-mediated illness	36
Biliary obstruction	29
ALTERED MENTAL STATUS	
Medication effect	46
Hepatic encephalopathy	36

[a]Because only the most common final diagnoses are included in this table, the listed percentages for each presenting-complaint subset do not add up to 100%.

Adapted from Savitsky EA, Mebust D, Schwartz E, et al. A descriptive analysis of 290 orthotopic liver transplant patient visits to an emergency department (In press).

Late Complications

Late complications are defined as those that occur more than 1 year after transplantation. The most common causes of late deaths are chronic rejection and new malignancies.[1] Major nonfatal late complications include biliary stricture, renal impairment, and infection.[13]

DIFFERENTIAL DIAGNOSIS

The differential diagnoses for some of the more common presenting complaints are provided in Table 160.2. The frequently nonspecific presentations of the major complications usually preclude making a specific diagnosis on clinical findings alone.[10,11] In addition, multiple diagnoses are common, owing to the interrelationship between many of the complications (e.g., HAT causing bile duct necrosis, leading to bile leakage and abscess formation).

EMERGENCY DEPARTMENT EVALUATION

ED evaluation of OLT patient begins with a thorough history and physical examination. Important historic factors include etiology of liver failure, date of transplant, history of postoperative complications, recent diagnostic studies, and current medications. A review of systems should determine the presence of fever, nausea, vomiting, abdominal pain, jaundice, acholic stools, and dark urine. Emergency physicians should bear in mind that serious OLT complications may present with deceptively nonspecific symptoms and normal initial physical examinations.

Because the presentations of many important complications of OLT are nonspecific, patients presenting to the ED generally require extensive laboratory testing.[11] Laboratory tests should include a complete blood count and platelet count to screen for overimmunosuppression related to medications. Electrolytes and serum creatinine concentrations are useful to detect the nephrotoxic effects of either tacrolimus or cyclosporine. Total bilirubin, AST, ALT, alkaline phosphatase, and prothrombin time levels are used to evaluate graft function. Patients presenting with a fever should have blood and urine cultures and a urinalysis (Table 160.3).

When suspicion of vascular complications arises, several diagnostic modalities may be useful. Duplex ultrasonography and spiral computed tomography (spiral CT) are noninvasive modalities that have a reported sensitivity of more than 90% for detecting vascular complications. Angiography is helpful in equivocal cases. Emergency physicians should have a low threshold for using ultrasonography or spiral CT to evaluate OLT patients for vascular complications in the presence of abdominal complaints or laboratory evidence of graft dysfunction.

Although ultrasound or CT imaging may suggest biliary complications, definitive diagnosis is made by visualization of the biliary tract with T-tube cholangiography, endoscopic retrograde cholangiopancreatography, percutaneous transhepatic cholangiography, or operative exploration.

Rejection is definitively diagnosed by liver biopsy. The histologic triad of portal tract inflammation and mononuclear cell involvement of portal vein branches and small bile ducts is diagnostic for acute rejection. Liver biopsy in chronic rejection reveals destruction and loss of interlobular bile ducts, mononuclear portal inflammation, arteriopathy, centrilobular cholestasis, and varying degrees of hepatocellular damage.

EMERGENCY DEPARTMENT MANAGEMENT

A majority of OLT patients with vascular complications require surgical intervention for definitive therapy, and management of their cases should be done in concert with the liver transplant team.

Patients diagnosed with bile leaks require parenteral antibiotics, percutaneous drainage of any abscess, and, occasionally, surgical intervention for refractory cases. Bile leaks occurring earlier in the post-OLT period tend to be more severe and are often unresponsive to conventional therapy, probably because the higher initial level of immunosuppression renders patients incapable of eradicating infection. Infections tend to be polymicrobial and include the typical biliary tract bacterial pathogens (*Enterobacter, Enterococcus, Bacteroides,* and *Clostridium* species). Broad-spectrum gram-positive, gram-negative (including *Pseudomonas aeruginosa*), and anaerobic coverage is recommended pending culture results. Many patients diagnosed with biliary strictures may be nonoperatively managed with stents or balloon dilation of their strictures.

Treatment of acute rejection involves the administration of high-dose intravenous methylprednisolone. Therapy is rarely initiated in the ED, because the definitive diagnosis of rejection is usually made later in the patient's hospital course by liver biopsy. Corticosteroids are effective in reversing 65% to 80% of acute rejection episodes. Patients who do not respond to glucocorticosteroids are treated with regimens using muromonab-CD3 (Orthoklone OKT3), with an 85% salvage rate. Chronic rejection does not respond to immunosuppressive regimens as uniformly as do acute rejection episodes. OLT recipients in whom chronic rejection is suspected should be referred to a liver transplant center for evaluation, because many patients with chronic rejection will suffer eventual graft failure and require retransplantation.

Emergency physicians should remember that rapid deterioration might occur in clinically stable OLT patients with acute

TABLE 160.3. Time of Occurrence and Management of Infections in OLT Recipients

Infectious Disease	Time of Presentation after OLT	Diagnostic Evaluation	Treatment[a]
Bacterial infections	Peak in months 1–2, progressive decline in incidence. Rare after 12 mo, unless patient is still taking high-dose immunosuppressive regimen, indwelling line, etc.	Blood, urine, and sputum cultures.[b] Culture all indwelling lines and biliary tube fluid if T-tube still present.	Empiric broad-spectrum antibiotic coverage pending culture results (e.g., ceftazidime 1 g i.v. q8h and ampicillin/sulbactam 3 g i.v. q6h)
Fungal infections	Peak in months 1–2. Rare after 2 mo, unless patient is still taking high-dose immunosuppressive regimen	Blood, urine, and indwelling line cultures.	Amphotericin B or fluconazole.[c]
Viral infections	Most common in month 2 after OLT; rare after 2 mo. Cytomegalovirus is most common infection.	Blood, urine, and indwelling line cultures.[d]	Ganciclovir or foscarnet
Protozoal infections	Rare, but occasionally occur months 1–6. P. *carinii* pneumonia is the most common pathogen.	Chest radiograph and sputum culture. Most require bronchoalveolar lavage; diagnosis is not usually made in ED.	Trimethoprim-sulfamethoxazole, 20 mg/kg i.v. divided q.i.d. for 14–21 days

[a]Medication dosages must be adjusted based on patient's renal function.
[b]Obtain sputum cultures and chest radiograph when clinically appropriate (e.g., patient with fever and cough). Consider stool cultures and *Clostridium difficile* toxin assay if infectious colitis is suspected.
[c]Antifungal and antiviral therapy are not routinely indicated in the ED. They are usually reserved for the OLT patient's hospital course when fungal infection has been documented or the patient's condition fails to improve with antibacterial therapy.
[d]Definitive diagnosis of clinically significant viral disease is difficult. Further diagnostic testing, such as polymerase chain reaction, serologic studies, and tissue histologic analysis, is performed later in the patient's hospital course and is not an immediate priority during the ED visit.

infections, particularly during times of peak immunosuppression. High-risk OLT patients presenting with fever, including recipients within 6 months of transplant, should receive empiric broad-spectrum antibiotic therapy pending definitive culture results. Antibiotic coverage should include gram-positive organisms, gram-negative organisms (including *P. aeruginosa*), and anaerobic organisms. Specific therapy against fungal, viral, and protozoal pathogens is rarely instituted in the ED.

DISPOSITION

Serious illness is common in OLT patients presenting to the ED. Not surprisingly, OLT recipients typically undergo extensive diagnostic evaluations and are frequently hospitalized. Much of the diagnostic testing these patients require is time-consuming and beyond the scope of everyday emergency medicine practice. Appropriate ED goals are assessing the severity and possible causes of an acute illness, stabilization, and transfer of care to the primary liver transplant team. Emergency physicians should involve the liver transplant team early in the decision-making process to help coordinate the timing and location of the evaluation, especially if transfer to a tertiary care center is necessary.

New-onset graft failure mandates admission. The causes of graft failure are diverse, and their evaluation is best performed in the inpatient setting.

In general, febrile OLT patients that are less than 1 year posttransplantation and are without an obvious source of infection are admitted. Febrile patients that are more than 1 year posttransplantation but are still maintained at a high level of immunosuppression (e.g., chronic rejection patients) should also be hospitalized. Well-appearing, febrile patients that are more than 1 year posttransplantation, with an uncomplicated post-OLT course, and whose immunosuppressives have been tapered, may be managed on an individual basis. Because maintaining a desired level of immunosuppression is vital in preventing rejection episodes, admission is mandatory if compliance with the immunosuppressive regimen is in doubt (e.g., because of intractable vomiting).

COMMON PITFALLS

- Failure to appreciate the complex and fragile nature of OLT patients
- Failure to coordinate the ED evaluation of OLT recipients with their liver transplant team
- Forgetting that OLT recipients are immunocompromised hosts and failing to manage fever aggressively, especially in the early post-OLT period
- Using the leukocyte count as a marker for severity of infection. Over 50% of OLT patients with serious bacterial infections have a normal leukocyte count.
- Assuming that a soft and nontender abdominal examination excludes hepatobiliary complications
- Forgetting that OLT patients are predisposed to adverse effects of medications because of the complexity of their drug regimens. One must ensure that medications prescribed to OLT patients in the ED do not have adverse interactions with the medications the patient is already taking.

References

1. Asfar S, Metrakos P, Fryer J, et al. An analysis of late deaths after liver transplantation. *Transplantation* 1996;61:1377–1381.
2. Chang FY, Singh N, Gayowski T, et al. Fever in liver transplant recipients: changing spectrum of etiologic agents. *Clin Infect Dis* 1998;26:59–65.
3. Jain A, Reyes J, Kashyap R, et al. Liver transplantation under tacrolimus in infants, children, adults, and seniors: long-term results, survival, and adverse events in 1000 consecutive patients. *Transplant Proc* 1998;30:1403–1404.
4. Langnas AN, Marujo W, Stratta RJ, et al. Vascular complications after orthotopic liver transplantation. *Am J Surg* 1991;161:76–83.
5. NIH consensus development conference statement: liver transplantation. June 20–23, 1983. *Hepatology* 1984;4[Suppl]:107–110.
6. Patenaude YG, Dubois J, Sinsky AB, et al. Liver transplantation: review of the literature. Part 1: anatomic features and current concepts. *Can Assoc Radiol J* 1997;48:171–178.
7. Patenaude YG, Dubois J, Sinsky AB, et al. Liver transplantation: review of the literature. Part 3: medical complications. *Can Assoc Radiol J* 1997;48:333–339.
8. Rabkin JM, Orloff SL, Reed MH, et al. Biliary tract complications of side-to-side without T tube versus end-to-end with or without T tube choledochocholedochostomy in liver transplant recipients. *Transplantation* 1998;65:193–199.
9. Rodino MA, Shane E. Osteoporosis after organ transplantation. *Am J Med* 1998;104:450–469.
10. Savitsky EA, Uner AB, Votey SR. Evaluation of orthotopic liver transplant recipients presenting to the emergency department. *Ann Emerg Med* 1998;31:507–517.
11. Savitsky EA, Mebust D, Schwartz E, et al. A descriptive analysis of 290 orthotopic liver transplant patient visits to an emergency department (In press).
12. Singh N, Gayowski T, Wagener MM, et al. Predictors and outcome of early-versus late-onset major bacterial infections in liver transplant recipients receiving tacrolimus (FK506) as primary immunosuppression. *Eur J Clin Microbiol Infect Dis* 1997;16:821–826.
13. Slapak GI, Saxena R, Portmann B, et al. Graft and systemic disease in long-term survivors of liver transplantation. *Hepatology* 1997;25:195–202.
14. Starzl TE, Marchioro TL, Von Kaulla KN, et al. Homotransplantation of the liver in humans. *Surg Gynecol Obstet* 1963;117:659–676.
15. Starzl TE, Demetris AJ, Van Thiel D. Liver transplantation—first of two parts. *N Engl J Med* 1989;321:1014–1022.
16. Starzl TE, Demetris AJ, Van Thiel D. Liver transplantation—second of two parts. *N Engl J Med* 1989;321:1092–1099.
17. Stratta RJ, Wood RP, Langnas AN, et al. Diagnosis and treatment of biliary tract complications after orthotopic liver transplantation. *Surgery* 1989; 106:675–684.
18. Tabasco-Minguillan J, Jain A, Naik M, et al. Gastrointestinal bleeding after liver transplantation. *Transplantation* 1997;63:60–67.
19. Van Thiel DH, Iqbal M, Jain A, et al. Gastrointestinal and metabolic problems associated with immunosuppression with either CyA or FK506 in liver transplantation. *Transplant Proc* 1990;22:37–40.
20. Walker RW, Brochstein JA. Neurologic complications of immunosuppressive agents. *Neurol Clin* 1988;6:261–278.

CHAPTER 161

Nonsurgical Causes of Abdominal Pain

Darrell C. Sandel and Sheldon Jacobson

Abdominal pain is the presenting symptom in 4% to 8% of adult emergency department (ED) visits.[3,17] Appropriately, much of the emergency physician's effort is focused on ruling out surgically correctible disease. Of patients with abdominal pain not due to obstetric or gynecologic problems, approximately 8% to 10% have obvious surgical disease. Of the remaining, most have self-limited abdominal pain, and some have an undiagnosed surgical or inflammatory disorder. These and other less common entities are listed in Table 161.1. In general, undertake evaluation for one of these disorders only if there has been recurrent or persistent pain lasting for a period of days and if a preliminary workup, including abdominal computed tomography (CT) imaging, has been negative. Additional factors that should be considered include the patient's age, ethnicity, and family history, or a known history of one of the diseases in question.

TABLE 161.1. Nonsurgical Causes of Abdominal Pain

Acute intermittent porphyria
Heavy-metal poisoning
Abdominal tabes (Dietl crisis)
Abdominal epilepsy
Abdominal migraine
Black widow spider bite
Vasculitis
Abdominal angina
Intestinal pseudoobstruction
Sickle cell crisis
Right-sided colonic diverticulitis
Meckel's diverticulitis
Familial Mediterranean fever
Massive intravascular hemolysis
Narcotic withdrawal
Factitious or drug-seeking behavior
Psychogenic abdominal pain
Addisonian crisis
C1′ esterase inhibitor deficiency
Spastic colon
Irritable bowel syndrome
Inflammatory bowel disease

FAMILIAL MEDITERRANEAN FEVER

Familial Mediterranean fever (FMF) is a disease that is most common in non-Ashkenazi Jews, Turks, Armenians, and Middle Eastern Arabs, but generally not in other Mediterranean populations.[13,18] It is characterized by bouts of abdominal pain with signs of peritonitis. Fever and pleuritis are very common, and arthritis and migratory skin lesions can also occur. It can mimic an acute abdomen and be accompanied by an elevated white cell count with a left shift and a high erythrocyte sedimentation rate. Episodes of the disease generally last 24 to 72 hours. The diagnosis is usually made by the second decade of life, and very rarely after the age of 40. A family history cannot always be obtained, as the transmission is autosomal recessive. Diagnosis is clinical, although work on genetic markers may someday make a laboratory diagnosis possible.[13]

FMF can be treated with oral colchicine 0.6 mg q1h for three doses, and then 0.6 mg q2h for an additional dose. Intravenous colchicine is not recommended unless the patient is unable to tolerate oral medications. Long-term prophylactic treatment with colchicine reduces the rate of recurrence and also helps prevent amyloidosis, the long-term complication of FMF. Opiates can be used to treat the pain. Patients should be admitted for observation, and surgical consultation obtained. A diagnosis of FMF should never be definitively made in the ED.

Patients with suspected FMF should be admitted and observed, given the possibility of misdiagnosis.

PORPHYRIA

The porphyrias affect the biosynthesis of heme and result in the accumulation of excessive porphyrins and their precursors. They are inherited enzyme disorders, almost always autosomal dominant with poor penetrance. They are characterized by abdominal pain with or without manifestations of autonomic dysfunction or neuropsychiatric symptoms. Other presenting conditions in patients with porphyria include demyelinating syndromes, SIADH, hypertensive crisis, and acute psychosis. There are many variants, depending on the particular enzyme deficiency and the heme precursor accumulated. The most common porphyria that causes abdominal pain is acute intermittent porphyria.[7,19]

TABLE 161.2. Potentially Toxic Drugs in the Treatment of the Acute Porphyrias

Barbiturates	Succinimides
Sulfonamide antibiotics	Carbamazepine
Meprobamate	Valproic acid
Glutethimide	Pyrazolones
Methyprylon	Griseofulvin
Ethchlorvynol	Ergots
Phenytoin	Danazol
Mephenytoin	Alcohol
Chlorpropamide	Estrogens and progestins

From *Cecil Textbook of Medicine*, 19th ed, Chap. 191. Philadelphia: WB Saunders, 1992.

The diagnosis is difficult, given the low prevalence. The pain of porphyria is usually out of proportion to physical signs, and fever is usually absent. A family history is helpful but not always present. Although not totally sensitive or specific, a Watson-Schwartz urine test should be ordered to look for porphobilinogen.[7,19] The urine dipstick for urobilinogen yields a strong false-positive result. The diagnosis is made by a finding of elevated 24-hour levels of urine and stool porphyrins.

Management is largely supportive. Intravenous glucose infusion may abort attacks. Intravenous hematin also may be helpful, although studies have not been large enough to prove its efficacy.[11] Many drugs can precipitate attacks; potentially harmful drugs are listed in Table 161.2.[17]

ABDOMINAL VASCULITIS

Abdominal vasculitis occurs in several disease processes, but polyarteritis nodosa, systemic lupus erythematosus, and Henoch-Schönlein purpura are probably the most common. The spectrum of presentation varies from acute severe ischemia to mild pain, malabsorption, and abdominal angina.

Patients with abdominal vasculitis may have peripheral manifestations of vasculitis as well. The abdominal pain may be epigastric or periumbilical, reflecting ischemia of the foregut or midgut, respectively. Fever is prominent in some cases. The key issue in these conditions is considering the diagnosis and then obtaining appropriate tests, such as angiography. Abdominal vasculitis should always be considered in patients with abdominal pain who also have a history of rheumatologic disease.

ANGIOEDEMA

Hereditary angioneurotic edema is transmitted as an autosomal dominant trait. Symptomatic patients have low levels of C1′ esterase inhibitor (type 1), or they have a dysfunctional inhibitor (type 2); either condition allows activation of the complement system.[1] Initial symptoms usually arise in adolescence but can have their onset in later life.

Classically, patients with angioedema do not have urticaria. Angioneurotic edema of the skin involves the deeper portions of the dermis and the subcutaneous layers, as well, and does not cause pruritus, whereas urticaria results from edema in the superficial layers of the skin and is pruritic.

Attacks of hereditary angioneurotic edema may begin with abdominal pain due to angioedema of the bowel wall. The pain is often colicky and is associated with nausea and vomiting, but there are scant physical findings in the abdomen. Fever is usually absent, and white blood cell counts are normal. During an attack, serum levels of C2 and C4 are low. Between attacks, the diagnosis can be established by assaying for the presence of the C1′ esterase inhibitor.

Use of angiotensin converting enzyme inhibitors (ACE inhibitors) has also been associated with angioedema.[10] There have been case reports of individuals presenting with small bowel angioedema thought to be secondary to ACE inhibitors.[4] Strong consideration should be given to withholding ACE inhibitors in patients with persistent, unexplained abdominal pain.

Attacks are self-limited but generally last 24 to 72 hours. Because the upper airway can be involved acutely, a major clinical concern is sudden upper airway obstruction requiring epinephrine administration, intubation, or cricothyrotomy.

C1′ esterase inhibitor concentrate has been successful in small randomized trials in patients with known functional C1′ esterase inhibitor deficiency and angioedema. It may be used in cases of facial, laryngeal, or severe abdominal angioedema,[14,21] but it is not indicated for minor subcutaneous attacks.[5] It should not be used in patients with ACE inhibitor–associated angioedema.

Anabolic steroids, which increase production of the inhibitor, are effective in reducing the frequency of attacks, but they are not used acutely. Management is otherwise supportive. Admission is usually advisable because of the risk of upper airway involvement.

INTESTINAL PSEUDOOBSTRUCTION

Intestinal pseudoobstructions are a group of diseases that present as bouts of recurrent abdominal distention, obstipation, and, on occasion, colicky abdominal pain. The presentation can be identical to that of small bowel mechanical obstruction. Pseudoobstruction can be caused by a primary disorder of the myenteric plexus or the smooth muscle itself, or may be secondary to a host of systemic diseases (Table 161.3). The diagnosis is made by ruling out other causes of abdominal pain and motility disorders, including adult Hirschsprung disease and mechanical obstruction. The differential diagnosis also includes toxic megacolon, typhlitis, and idiopathic colonic dilation of the elderly (Ogilvie syndrome). Definitive diagnosis requires manometric and electrophysiologic testing, as well as biopsy.

TABLE 161.3. Causes of Secondary Intestinal Pseudoobstruction

COLLAGEN DISEASES
Progressive systemic sclerosis
Dermatomyositis, polymyositis
Systemic lupus erythematosus
ENDOCRINE DISORDERS
Myxedema
Diabetes mellitus
Pheochromocytoma
Hyperparathyroidism
NEUROLOGIC DISORDERS
Myotonic dystrophy
Parkinson disease
Familial autonomic dysfunction
Psychosis
MISCELLANEOUS
Jejunoileal bypass
Jejunal diverticulosis
Amyloidosis
Chagas disease
Sclerosing mesenteritis
Drugs

SICKLE CELL DISEASE

It is not uncommon to see patients with sickle cell disease and vasoocclusive painful crisis in many emergency practices. These patients can present with pain almost anywhere in the body, including the abdomen. What is not commonly appreciated is that a few patients with homozygous sickle cell disease have their first painful crisis in their late teens or early 20s, frequently presenting with cryptogenic abdominal pain. Patients with established sickle cell disease can also pose a diagnostic challenge because their abdominal pain can be caused by a vasoocclusive event involving any of the abdominal viscera or the abdominal wall.

In addition, almost all patients with sickle cell disease have gallstones; acute cholecystitis, common duct obstruction, and ascending cholangitis are ever-present dangers in these immunocompromised patients. Abdominal pain also can develop for reasons unrelated to sickle cell disease, but the primary process may be misdiagnosed as crisis pain.

The laboratory evaluation of sickle cell patients with abdominal pain is often misleading. Many vasoocclusive crises are not associated with fever, and the white blood cell count is typically chronically elevated in these patients, commonly with a left shift. In addition, many sickle cell disease patients are icteric because of chronic hemolysis. Many have intrinsic liver disease as well, but liver function test abnormalities are not helpful unless there is a significant deviation from baseline values. For patients presenting with right upper quadrant pain, diagnosis can be assisted by the use of abdominal ultrasonography, nuclear scans of the biliary system, or abdominal CT scanning.

CHRONIC LEAD INTOXICATION

Chronic lead intoxication can present as a painful abdominal crisis (lead colic). Abdominal pain can be slowly progressive or subacute in onset. There is abdominal tenderness with voluntary guarding, but true peritoneal findings are rare. Patients commonly complain of fatigue, weakness, musculoskeletal pains, irritability, and constipation. Hemolytic anemia is usually evident, and the red blood cells show basophilic stippling. An occasional patient may have the triad of lead nephropathy, "saturnine" gout, and hypertension. The diagnosis is made by determining blood lead and erythrocyte protoporphyrin levels. Chelation therapy is often successful in relieving manifestations outside the central nervous system.

ADDISON DISEASE

Addison disease can present as a dramatic acute syndrome with vasomotor collapse, altered mental status, and characteristic electrolyte abnormalities. A subacute-to-chronic form of the disease, however, can present with recurrent abdominal pain, often associated with nausea and vomiting and usually with a negative abdominal examination.

The most common cause of primary adrenal insufficiency is idiopathic or autoimmune destruction of the gland. Patients with the acquired immunodeficiency syndrome (AIDS) have a high incidence of adrenal gland involvement from a number of mechanisms. Other presenting complaints include salt craving, anorexia, weight loss, and generalized weakness. Characteristic physical findings include orthostatic hypotension, freckling and hyperpigmentation of the skin, and surgical scars. Classic laboratory findings include hyperkalemia, hyponatremia, mild azotemia, mild metabolic acidosis, and hypoglycemia.

If the diagnosis of Addison disease is suspected, a serum cortisol level should be ordered and, if the patient's condition permits, a 1-hour ACTH stimulation test (see Chapter 172). Treatment should begin immediately with administration of intravenous corticosteroids (hydrocortisone 60 mg q6h, or dexamethasone if awaiting an ACTH stimulation test), glucose, and saline.

NARCOTIC WITHDRAWAL

Narcotic withdrawal frequently produces crampy abdominal pain, often associated with nausea, vomiting, and diarrhea. Diagnosis of this syndrome is frequently difficult unless the patient admits to narcotic addiction. Other signs and symptoms of narcotic withdrawal (e.g., mydriasis, rhinorrhea, piloerection) may be present, but these features are rarely prominent.

Patients often ask specifically for an analgesic medication or name a specific narcotic agent they have successfully used for their problem in the past. If narcotic withdrawal is suspected, confrontation in the ED is not helpful. These patients should be referred to a primary care physician and should have early psychiatric evaluation. The use of methadone detoxification or clonidine to relieve the patient's symptoms must be considered on an individual basis.

PSYCHOGENIC ABDOMINAL PAIN

Psychogenic abdominal pain involves a diverse group of psychiatric disturbances, including somatoform disorders, eating disorders, conversion reactions, depression, and hypochondriacal neurosis. Abdominal pain can also occur as a somatic delusion or as an hallucinatory phenomenon, but it generally is found in association with bizarre symptoms and evidence of underlying thought disorder. Women represent a disproportionately large percentage of patients with psychogenic abdominal pain in several studies. As noted previously, early psychiatric consultation is important, but it must be kept in mind that psychogenic abdominal pain must always remain, to some degree, a diagnosis of exclusion.

ABDOMINAL PAIN IN ACQUIRED IMMUNODEFICIENCY SYNDROME

The diagnosis of abdominal pain in patients with human immunodeficiency virus (HIV) infection and AIDS is challenging. There are no large ED-centered studies looking at this problem, but a number of studies have reviewed the outcome for specific disease entities, and data exist from large case series of patients admitted to subspecialty services.[1,20] Although the exact prevalence is not known, a number of entities are fairly common.

The differential diagnosis of abdominal pain in AIDS is summarized in Table 161.4. HIV-positive patients without AIDS probably have disease incidences similar to those of HIV-negative patients. As the disease progresses, however, the differential diagnosis expands and reliance on typical cues and laboratory tests becomes problematic.

For instance, one large case series of appendicitis in HIV-positive patients with and without AIDS showed leukocytosis and fever to be absent in more than 50% of patients.[9] As AIDS progresses, the differential diagnosis becomes skewed toward uncommon diseases. For example, in patients with right upper quadrant pain, the incidence of sclerosing cholangitis increases dramatically, and acalculous cholecystitis can be seen. Cytomegalovirus (CMV) colitis tends to be associated with diffuse pain and with diarrhea, often bloody. This symptom is of special concern, as it is associated with perforation and poor survival. Cryptosporidial disease can cause abdominal pain but is associated with profuse, unrelenting diarrhea.

TABLE 161.4. Differential Diagnosis of Abdominal Pain in Acquired Immunodeficiency Syndrome

Sclerosing cholangitis
Calculous cholecystitis
Acalculous cholecystitis
Pancreatitis
CMV enterocolitis
C. difficile colitis
Mycobacterium avium-intracellulare enteritis
Lymphoma
Renal stone disease (with ddI)
Appendicitis
Cryptosporidial infection
Gastrointestinal Kaposi's sarcoma
Intussusception (rare)

Pancreatitis is another vexing problem in AIDS. It is associated with the use of drugs, including pentamidine, indinavir (ddI), and, uncommonly, trimethoprim–sulfamethoxazole. CMV, herpes simplex virus, *Mycobacterium avium* complex, and *Cryptococcus* have also been implicated. Treatment is supportive and includes withholding of offending agents.[8] Asymptomatic hyperamylasemia has also been noted in AIDS patients.

Patients with HIV and/or AIDS have somewhat higher rates of operative complications, but this fact should not preclude surgical consultation where indicated. Studies have shown good results when patients with appendicitis or cholecystitis undergo operation.[9,15] Small case series of laparoscopy have also been encouraging.[2]

References

1. Borum ML, Howard DE. Hereditary angioedema. Complex symptoms can make diagnosis difficult. *Postgrad Med* 1998;103(4):251, 255–256.
2. Box JC, Duncan T, et al. Laparoscopy in the evaluation and treatment of patients with AIDS and acute abdominal complaints. *Surg Endosc* 1997; 11:1026–1028.
3. Brewer R, Golden F, Hitch D, et al. Abdominal pain: an analysis of 1000 consecutive cases in a university hospital emergency room. *Am J Surg* 1976; 131:219–223.
4. Brown NJ, Snowden M, Griffin MR. Recurrent angiotensin-converting enzyme inhibitor-associated angioedema. *JAMA* 1997;278(3):232–233.
5. Cicardi M, et al. Hereditary angioedema. *N Engl J Med* 1996;334(25):1666–1667.
6. Drossman DA. Patients with psychogenic abdominal pain: six years' observation in the medical setting. *Am Psychiatry* 1982;139:1549.
7. Elder GH, Hill RJ, Meissner PN. The acute porphyrias. *Lancet* 1997; 349:1613–1617.
8. Feldman M, et al. *Sleisenger & Fordtran's gastrointestinal and liver disease,* 6th ed. Philadelphia: WB Saunders, 1998:387–409.
9. Flum DR, Steinberg SD, et al. Appendicitis in patients with acquired immunodeficiency syndrome. *J Am Coll Surg* 1997;184:481–486.
10. Gregory KWP, Davis RC. Angioedema of the intestine. *N Engl J Med* 1996;334(25):1641.
11. Herrick AL, McColl KEL, Moore MR, et al. Controlled trial of haem arginate in acute hepatic porphyria. *Lancet* 1989;i:1295–1297.
12. Jenkins PL. Psychogenic abdominal pain. *Gen Hosp Psychiatry* 1991;13:27.
13. Koopman WJ. *Arthritis and allied conditions,* 13th ed. Baltimore: Williams & Wilkins, 1997:1280–1287.
14. Kunschak M, Engl W, et al. A randomized, controlled trial to study the efficacy and safety of C1 inhibitor concentrate in treating hereditary angioedema. *Transfusion* 1998;38(6):540–549.
15. Leiva JI, Etter EL, et al. Surgical therapy for 101 patients with acquired immunodeficiency syndrome and symptomatic cholecystitis. *Am J Surg* 1997;174:414.

16. Parente F, Cernuschi S, et al. Severe abdominal pain in patients with AIDS: frequency, clinical aspects, causes, and outcome. *Scand J Gastroenterol* 1994;29:511.
17. Powers RD, Guertler AT. Abdominal pain in the ED: stability and change over 29 years. *Am J Emerg Med* 1995;13(3):301–303.
18. Samuels J, Aksentijevich I, et al. Familial Mediterranean fever at the millennium. Clinical spectrum, ancient mutations, and a survey of 100 American referrals to the National Institutes of Health. *Medicine* 1998;77(4):268–297.
19. Tefferi A, Colgan JP, Solberg LA. Acute porphyrias: diagnosis and management. *Mayo Clin Proc* 1994;69:991–995.
20. Thulhvath RJ, Connolly GM, Forbes A. Abdominal pain in HIV infection. *Q J Med* 1991;78(287):275–285.
21. Waytes AT, Rosen FS, Frank MM. Treatment of hereditary angioedema with a vapor-heated C1 inhibitor concentrate. *N Engl J Med* 1996;334:1630.

CHAPTER 162

Inflammatory Bowel Disease

Howard A. Werman

Inflammatory bowel disease (IBD) comprises two chronic intestinal disorders: ulcerative colitis and regional enteritis or Crohn disease. Both are characterized by recurrent episodes of gastrointestinal disturbances separated by periods of remission, and both are associated with a variety of systemic manifestations. The emergency physician must be familiar with IBD for two reasons. First, these two disorders must be considered in the differential diagnosis of patients with gastrointestinal complaints, particularly if they are recurrent. Second, patients with well-established diagnoses of IBD often present to the emergency department (ED) for management of acute exacerbations and complications of their disease.

The cause of both disorders remains unknown. Immunologic, infectious, genetic, dietary, and psychological factors have all been implicated.[8] For both diseases, there is a bimodal distribution in the age at onset, with peaks at 15 to 25 years and at 55 to 60 years.[7] Ten percent to 15% of patients with IBD have relatives who are also affected. The incidence of Crohn disease has been rising over the past 20 years; the incidence of ulcerative colitis, which had been stable, has also risen in the past few years.

Ulcerative colitis tends to remain localized to the colon; in the majority of patients, the disease is found in the rectum and left colon only. The entire colon is affected (pancolitis) in the most severe cases. Ulcerative colitis is usually limited to the intestinal mucosa and submucosa. Diffuse involvement producing a finely granular, friable mucosa explains the propensity for bloody diarrhea noted in these patients. Crohn disease can be found along the entire gastrointestinal tract. In 30% of cases, only the terminal ileum is involved; 20% of patients have colonic disease only. Both small and large bowels are affected in the remaining 50%. Disease of the mouth, esophagus, and stomach is found in less than 1% of patients. The lesions of Crohn disease tend to involve all of the bowel wall layers and extend into the mesentery. Deep ulcerations, which often penetrate the bowel wall, are common and account for the development of fissures, fistulas, and abscesses. About one-third of patients with Crohn disease will manifest perianal complications such as abscesses, fistulas, fissures, and skin tags.

CLINICAL PRESENTATION

The most common signs and symptoms in patients with Crohn disease are chronic diarrhea, abdominal pain, fever, anorexia, and weight loss. The presentation characterizes 75% to 80% of patients with this disease, but the symptoms are so nonspecific, there is typically a long delay (weeks to months) in establishing the diagnosis. The presentation of cases seen in the ED varies, depending on the site of involvement of Crohn disease. Patients with primary ileal disease present with right lower quadrant abdominal pain that is associated with fever, abdominal distention, vomiting, and either profuse watery diarrhea or decreased output of stool and gas. Severe cases of Crohn colitis are characterized by abdominal pain associated with fever and massive diarrhea. Less common causes of emergent presentations include severe epigastric pain similar to peptic ulcer disease, acute pancreatitis, and large aphthous ulcers of the mouth.

As in Crohn disease, the presentation of ulcerative colitis is quite variable. In fact, separation of these disorders on the basis of clinical findings alone can be very difficult. In mild cases, occasional constipation and rectal bleeding may be the only complaints. In the more severe forms, patients have more than six to eight bloody diarrheal stools per day, as well as crampy abdominal pain, tenesmus, fever, tachycardia, and anemia. Ulcerative colitis is more commonly associated with rectal bleeding, whereas abdominal pain, abdominal masses, and perianal lesions are more common in patients with Crohn disease.

A common reason for patients with well-established IBD to present to the ED is complications of their underlying disease.[2] The major intestinal complications of Crohn disease and ulcerative colitis include intraabdominal abscess formation, bowel perforation, massive hemorrhage, intestinal obstruction, dehydration, perianal complications (fissures, fistulas, and perirectal abscesses), and toxic megacolon. Complications such as massive hemorrhage and toxic megacolon are more commonly seen in ulcerative colitis, whereas abscesses, obstruction, and perianal complications are far more common in Crohn disease. In addition to recognizing these complications, the emergency physician must also be aware that medications taken by patients with IBD, particularly corticosteroids, may mask the findings typically associated with complications.

Toxic megacolon is perhaps the most dramatic complication seen in patients with IBD. This process is the result of a loss of muscular tone in the patient with advanced disease. Toxic megacolon should be suspected in patients with active colitis who report a decrease in stool output, particularly if they are on antidiarrheal agents or have undergone a recent colonoscopy. Affected patients appear toxic; the abdomen is distended, tender, and tympanitic. Fever, tachycardia, and signs of volume depletion are noted. Other findings include leukocytosis, anemia, electrolyte disturbances, and an abdominal radiograph demonstrating a long, continuous dilated segment of bowel (greater than 6 cm in width). The mortality associated with this complication can be as high as 50% if perforation occurs.

Ten percent to 20% of patients with IBD have extraintestinal manifestations of their disease.[5] Occasionally, these symptoms actually appear before gastrointestinal ones, particularly in children. The most common of these manifestations are erythema nodosum, pyoderma gangrenosum, nongranulomatous anterior uveitis, polyarthritis, ankylosing spondylitis, and hepatobiliary disease.[1] In Crohn disease with small bowel involvement, malabsorption syndromes and fluid and electrolyte disturbances can occur. Gallstones are found in up to 33% of patients with Crohn disease. Calcium oxalate nephrolithiasis is also common. Patients with IBD may also develop a hypercoagulable state, resulting in deep venous thrombosis, pulmonary embolus, and, occasionally, arterial occlusion. Patients with thromboembolic complications have a mortality rate of approximately 25%. Pneumaturia and recurrent urinary tract infection occasionally occur with Crohn disease, because of enterovesical fistula.

A long-term complication, particularly of patients with ulcerative colitis, is colon carcinoma. Patients with ulcerative colitis have ten to 30 times the risk of developing colon cancer when compared with the general population, and patients with Crohn disease have a threefold increase in risk. Symptoms of a new colon cancer may overlap considerably with those of IBD, often making diagnosis difficult.

DIFFERENTIAL DIAGNOSIS

The major challenge for the emergency physician is to differentiate IBD as a cause of diarrhea, vague abdominal pain, malaise, and low-grade fever from other treatable causes of these symptoms. Several other entities present with similar complaints. Acute infectious diarrheal illness due to *Shigella*, *Salmonella*, *Campylobacter jejuni*, cytomegalovirus, or *Yersinia* must be considered. Parasitic disease such as amebiasis can also masquerade as IBD. Stool cultures and examination of stool for ova and parasites are necessary to identify an infectious cause of the patient's symptoms. In addition, serologic tests can be used to rule out invasive amebiasis, but in up to 50% of cases of infectious diarrhea, no pathogen can be identified. When the symptoms primarily involve the rectum, anal intercourse–associated bowel syndrome should be considered. Symptoms of chronic diarrhea, low-grade fever, and cachexia are also consistent with human immunodeficiency virus infection.

Antibiotic-induced colitis attributable to the overgrowth of *Clostridium difficile* must also be considered. Ischemic colitis and diverticulitis, generally seen in older patients, and radiation colitis may present, with a clinical and pathologic pattern similar to that of IBD.

When abdominal pain is the major complaint, IBD must be distinguished from other causes of the acute abdomen, including appendicitis, cholecystitis, other causes of intestinal obstruction, abdominal aortic aneurysm, and mesenteric occlusive disease. These entities can often be distinguished from IBD on the basis of history and physical examination. Abdominal radiographs, a complete blood cell count, serum amylase and lipase determination, and urinalysis can also be helpful. The emergency physician should consider IBD as a cause of abdominal complaints only after these other potentially serious causes of abdominal pain have been excluded.

EMERGENCY DEPARTMENT EVALUATION AND MANAGEMENT

In evaluating the patient with known IBD, the physician must first be concerned with identifying any significant complications of IBD, particularly gastrointestinal hemorrhage, intestinal obstruction, bowel perforation, and toxic megacolon. Particular attention should be given to patients on corticosteroids, whose symptoms may be masked by these drugs. Physical examination should be focused on the abdomen, evaluating for tenderness, rigidity, distention, rebound, and the presence of a mass.

The stool should be examined for the presence of blood. Other diagnostic aids include a complete blood cell count and abdominal radiographs. Patients with significant hemorrhage, obstruction, or perforation as a result of IBD are managed in the same manner as other patients with these conditions. Aggressive fluid management, gastrointestinal decompression, blood product administration as necessary, and surgical consultation are indicated. Antibiotic coverage of gram-negative and anaerobic bacteria is appropriate in cases of suspected perforation. In patients maintained on corticosteroids, stress doses of intravenous corticosteroids (hydrocortisone 300 mg/d) are also administered to prevent symptoms of adrenal insufficiency.

Patients with toxic megacolon are given a 24- to 48-hour trial of intensive medical therapy for the disease before surgical intervention is undertaken. Such therapy includes aggressive fluid and electrolyte replacement, gastrointestinal decompression, and antibiotic coverage for bowel pathogens (enteric bacilli and anaerobes). The use of corticosteroids is somewhat controversial in cases of toxic megacolon; stress doses are typically given in patients already maintained on corticosteroids.

Patients with an acute or subacute exacerbation of their IBD may present to the ED without any evidence of an emergent complication requiring surgical intervention. A careful history should ascertain the frequency of bowel movements, associated symptoms, severity of abdominal pain, and history of hospitalizations. The physical examination should assess signs of toxicity, dehydration, and metabolic imbalance and should include a careful abdominal examination. Laboratory evaluation should include a complete blood cell count and blood chemistry profile. If there is suspicion of liver involvement, liver function studies should be ordered. Abdominal radiographs are useful to detect clinically inapparent intestinal perforation, obstruction, or toxic megacolon. An abdominal computed tomography scan may be helpful in identifying intraabdominal abscesses, mesenteric inflammation, and fistulas.[4]

For patients who do not require hospital admission, arrangements should be made for follow-up with a gastroenterologist or internist. Continuing management, which usually includes dietary adjustment, bowel rest, antibiotics, and medications such as sulfasalazine and steroids, should be planned in discussion with the consulting physician. Typical outpatient medications include oral prednisone 40 to 60 mg/d, sulfasalazine 4 to 6 g/d, and antidiarrheal agents such as loperamide (Imodium) or diphenoxylate (Lomotil).

Patients admitted to the hospital usually require intravenous fluids, corticosteroids, and sulfasalazine. The exact medication regimen is best determined by the hospital consultant but typically includes methylprednisolone 60 mg/d intravenously, sulfasalazine 4 to 6 g/d, and, in some cases, hyperalimentation. Other agents, such as metronidazole, 6-mercaptopurine, cyclosporine, and corticosteroid enemas, may also be used.[3,6] Because of the toxicity profile associated with sulfasalazine, 5-aminosalicylic derivative agents are now available for either oral or topical use.

DISPOSITION

Fortunately, most cases of IBD can be managed in an outpatient setting. Patients who should be considered for hospital admission include those with severe manifestations (more than six bowel movements daily, severe abdominal pain, grossly bloody stool); those with systemic toxicity (fever, tachycardia, weight loss, cachexia); those with dehydration or metabolic disturbances; those with acute complications (intestinal obstruction, bowel perforation, gastrointestinal hemorrhage, toxic megacolon); and those who are refractory to outpatient therapy.

Surgical consultation is indicated in those patients with complications of the disease, including intestinal obstruction or hemorrhage, perforation, abscess or fistula formation, toxic megacolon, and perianal disease.

COMMON PITFALLS

- There is commonly a delay of several months from the onset of symptoms of IBD to the time the diagnosis is established. Thus, failure to suspect IBD and refer patients appropriately is not uncommon. Patients with previous episodes of similar symptoms, with a family history of IBD, with perirectal disease, or with any extraintestinal manifestations (rashes, back pain, arthritis, iritis) that might suggest the diagnosis should be referred to an appropriate specialist for endoscopic evaluation or barium examination.
- Severe abdominal pain, fever, tachycardia, and dehydration can be primary manifestations of IBD, yet these symptoms and signs are also associated with such complications as perforation, abscess formation, and peritonitis. Thus, the physician may fail to consider and recognize these serious complications. In addition, corticosteroids can mask abnormal findings in some patients, making the diagnosis of these serious complications even more difficult and problematic.

References

1. Balan V, LaRusso NF. Hepatobiliary disease in inflammatory bowel disease. *Gastroenterol Clin North Am* 1995;24:647–669.
2. Bitton A, Peppercorn MA. Emergencies in inflammatory bowel disease. *Crit Care Clin* 1995;11:513–529.
3. Bonner GF. Current medical therapy for inflammatory bowel disease. *South Med J* 1996;89:556–566.
4. Gore RM, Balthazar EJ, Ghahremani GG, et al. CT features of ulcerative colitis and Crohn's disease. *Am J Radiol* 1996;167:3–15.
5. Levine JB, Lukawski-Turbish D. Extraintestinal considerations in inflammatory bowel disease. *Gastroenterol Clin North Am* 1995;24:633–647.
6. Robinson M. Optimizing therapy for inflammatory bowel disease. *Am J Gastroenterol* 1997;92:12S–17S.
7. Russell MGVM, Stockbrugger RW. Epidemiology of inflammatory bowel disease: an update. *Scand J Gastroenterol* 1996;31:417–427.
8. Wills JS, Lobis IF, Denstman FJ. Crohn disease: state of the art. *Radiology* 1997;202:597–610.

CHAPTER 163
Diarrhea and Proctitis

Philip N. Salen and Michael B. Heller

DIARRHEA

The patient with diarrhea presents emergency physicians with a problem that is not only physical, but also social and personal. *Diarrhea* is defined as the passage of a greater number of stools of decreased form than usual. The term *gastroenteritis* should be reserved for those diarrheal diseases in which the patient also exhibits nausea and vomiting; *dysentery* refers to diarrhea containing blood and pus.

Almost 100 million cases of gastroenteritis and acute diarrheal episodes occur annually in the United States; half of these cause restriction of activity for more than a full day. Physicians are consulted in 8.2 million cases, and 250,000 people require hospitalization.[9] In the United States, mortality is rare and occurs mainly in the elderly and in young children.[12]

The most common causes of acute diarrhea, by far, are infectious agents. Less commonly implicated causes are drugs and toxins, chemotherapy, fecal impaction (overflow diarrhea), and psychosocial stress. Among infectious causes of diarrhea, viruses account for 50% to 70% of all cases, bacteria for 15% to 20%, and parasites for 10% to 15%. When patients present to the emergency department (ED) for evaluation, the complaint is either an acute onset of diarrhea or an acute exacerbation of chronic diarrhea. Diarrhea is especially problematic in particular settings: children in daycare settings, travelers to tropical and semitropical regions, homosexual males, immunocompromised individuals, people living in unhygienic environments, and those exposed to contaminated water or food.

Although an enormous number of stimuli may produce diarrhea, the four basic pathophysiologic mechanisms are alterations in mucosal morphology, alterations in ion secretion from the intestinal villi, alterations in intestinal motility, and osmotic diarrhea. The majority of diarrheal illnesses are noninflammatory, usually arising in the upper small bowel from the action of an enterotoxin or other process that specifically alters the absorptive function of the villus tip. Dysentery usually arises in the colon from an invasive process, with or without a cytotoxin.[4] Along with stabilizing the patient hemodynamically, the goal of the emergency physician is to determine whether the patient's diarrhea is inflammatory, which usually signifies a more severe diarrheal illness, and whether specific therapy is warranted.

CLINICAL PRESENTATION

Diarrhea is both a symptom and a sign. As a symptom, diarrhea can be described as an increase in stool frequency, an increase in stool volume, and a decrease in stool consistency. Possible associated gastrointestinal symptoms are nausea, vomiting, abdominal discomfort, abdominal cramps, bloating, tenesmus (constant urge to defecate), rectal urgency, perianal discomfort, intestinal gas–related complaints, and incontinence. As a sign, diarrhea is defined objectively as an increase in watery stool excretion to an amount greater than 200 mL every 24 hours.[4]

Depending on the etiology, the diarrhea may be liquid or soft, nonbloody or bloody, mucoid, and voluminous or scant. Physical examination may reveal fever, tachycardia, abdominal tenderness, or dehydration. When fever and bloody stool are present, the patient usually has intestinal inflammation due to invasive bacteria. From the standpoint of functional impairment from the illness, diarrhea may be categorized as mild (no change in normal activities), moderate (forced change in activities), or severe (disability with confinement to bed).[6]

When evaluating complaints of diarrhea, the physician should first distinguish whether the diarrhea is truly diarrhea or nondiarrheal rectal discharge, rectal bleeding, or abnormally colored stools. When seeking care in the ED for diarrhea, many patients do so out of concern about other issues in addition to the diarrhea. Once the diagnosis of diarrhea is confirmed, the clinician must decide whether the patient is seriously ill; what diagnostic workup is necessary; whether an etiology can be identified; whether any specific treatment is necessary; and what the health implications are for the family and the community. The severity of illness is directly correlated with the patient's volume and electrolyte status and whether the diarrhea has an inflammatory origin.

DIFFERENTIAL DIAGNOSIS

Although there are hundreds of causes of acute diarrhea, most cases presenting to the emergency physician are infectious.

Viral Diarrhea

The most common cause of diarrhea in most EDs, virus-induced diarrhea is characterized by destruction of villus mucosa. Shortened villi decrease the intestinal surface area available for fluid absorption and alter ion secretion.[20] Norwalk virus and rotavirus are responsible for more than 50% of viral enteric infections.[11]

Rotavirus is responsible for more diarrheal disease–associated morbidity than any other single agent, in developed as well as developing countries. Hallmarks of viral diarrhea are the absence of high fever and the occurrence of many nonbloody stools per day. Concomitant upper gastrointestinal distress with or without nausea is common, but severe abdominal pain is not characteristic. While improved hygiene has reduced bacterial diarrheal illness in the developed world, it has had less effect in preventing spread of viral gastroenteritis, in particular, rotavirus.[11]

Bacterial Diarrhea

Compared with viral diarrhea, bacterial enteritis causes more severe alterations of the mucosal morphology by invasion of the mucosa and submucosa of the terminal ileum and colon, resulting in inflammation. Edema, bleeding, and leukocytic infiltration of the colonic wall typically occur, which results in the appearance of red blood cells and white blood cells in the stool. Common etiologies are *Salmonella, Shigella, Escherichia coli, Yersinia,* and *Campylobacter*. A characteristic feature is fever, which may be quite marked, especially in the pediatric patient.[6] Passage of many stools per day, particularly when they are bloody and explosive in character, suggests bacterial enteritis. Special care must be taken when evaluating patients with suspected dysentery to eliminate the possibility that they may have a surgical cause (such as diverticulitis, appendicitis, or ischemic colitis) for their diarrhea, abdominal pain, or toxic appearance.

Food Poisoning

Although any toxin-produced gastrointestinal syndrome can be called *food poisoning,* this term is most commonly applied to gastroenteritis syndromes in which upper gastrointestinal symptoms predominate. Food poisoning occurs when infectious agents within the gut produce enterotoxin or when the enterotoxin is ingested from contaminated food. Depending on the type of organism that produces it, the enterotoxin can cause upper or lower gastrointestinal symptoms. The distinguishing feature of these conditions is not the characteristics of the diarrhea itself, but the typical clinical picture of nausea, vomiting, diarrhea, and a history of ingestion of a suspicious food. Concurrent illness in other persons exposed to the same food strongly suggests food poisoning.

Staphylococcal food poisoning is the most common form and typically occurs when food is contaminated by *Staphylococcus aureus* and then not cooked at a temperature sufficient to kill the bacteria. It is manifested by nausea, vomiting, abdominal cramps, and diarrhea 2 to 6 hours after eating food contaminated by the heat-stable, preformed enterotoxin. *Bacillus cereus* causes two distinct food-poisoning syndromes. In one, a heat-stable toxin produces primarily vomiting and abdominal cramping 2 hours after eating contaminated rice. The diarrheal syndrome results from ingestion of meat products contaminated with an enterotoxin produced by *B. cereus*. Scombroid fish poisoning is a food poisoning that causes a histamine-like reaction after ingestion of heat-stable toxins produced by bacterial action on dark-meat fish (tuna, mackerel, and related species). Ciguatera food poisoning results from the ingestion of a neurotoxin that accumulates in fish species that frequent coral reefs (e.g., red snapper, sea bass). Affected patients develop gastroenteritis and a potpourri of neurologic symptoms, such as paresthesias, dysesthesias, weakness, and even altered mental status.

E. coli 0157:H7

E. coli 0157:H7 is a common cause of bloody and nonbloody diarrhea and is estimated to cause more than 20,000 infections each year. The organism produces a Shiga-like toxin, which causes colonic vascular damage and allows inflammatory mediators to gain access to the circulation, at times initiating the hemolytic–uremic syndrome.[5] Transmission can be either from ingestion of contaminated beef or water or from person to person. Symptoms and signs that distinguish *E. coli 0157:H7* from other bacterial enteric diseases are the absence of fever in the presence of other symptoms and signs of inflammatory colitis, such as abdominal pain and bloody stool.

Hemolytic–uremic syndrome occurs in 6% of affected patients, usually 6 days after onset of the diarrhea, and it is the most common cause of acute renal failure in children. Clinical features of hemolytic–uremic syndrome include hemolytic anemia, thrombocytopenia, and acute renal failure. Once an isolate has been identified, the local health department should be notified so that, if the infected child attends daycare, the facility can increase its surveillance for diarrheal illness.

Protozoan Diarrhea

Giardia lamblia is neither rare nor exotic. Travel history, sexual history, pregnancy, and drinking well water are important risk factors. When evaluating patients suffering from persistent nonspecific complaints of chronic diarrhea, such as bloating and excessive flatulence, it is important to consider *G. lamblia* as the cause. Giardiasis presents similarly to a functional bowel disorder. Typically, the diarrhea is noninflammatory and does not contain blood, pus, or eosinophils.

Entamoeba histolytica predominantly affects individuals of lower socioeconomic status who live in developing countries. *E. histolytica* is an enteric protozoan that exists in either cyst or trophozoite form and causes infection after ingestion of the cysts.[14] Amebiasis causes an inflammatory colitis by invasion of the colonic epithelium by trophozoites that disrupt tissue planes. This occurs in 10% of asymptomatic carriers of the cysts. Hepatic infection results from the organism ascending the portal venous system; hepatic necrosis may result from obstruction of portal vessels. The diagnosis remains dependent on the morphologic identification of cysts in the affected patient's diarrhea.[14]

Traveler's Diarrhea

Traveler's diarrhea is a self-limited illness that usually resolves spontaneously within a few days, but it has the potential for wrecking a meticulously planned business trip or vacation. *Traveler's diarrhea* is usually defined as the passage of at least three unformed stools in a 24-hour period, together with nausea, vomiting, abdominal pain or cramps, fecal urgency or tenesmus, or the passage of bloody or mucoid stools, in a person who lives in an industrialized region and who has traveled to a developing semitropical or tropical country.[18] Among the 35 million people who travel from industrialized countries to a developing country annually, traveler's diarrhea has an incidence rate of 20% to 50% per 2-week stay. Although different organisms predominate in different regions, the principal agents in most of the high-risk areas are, in decreasing order of frequency, enterotoxigenic *E. coli, Rotavirus, Salmonella,* and *Campylobacter*.[18] The most common sources of traveler's diarrhea are contaminated food and water.

Antibiotic-Associated Diarrhea

Although some antibiotics are much more strongly associated with the development of a pseudomembranous colitis, virtually every antibiotic has been implicated. An overgrowth of *Clostridium difficile,* which occurs when native bowel flora are killed by antibiotics, is responsible for elaborating the enterotoxin. The enterotoxin induces a severe colitis with a pseudomembranous appearance that is bloody and positive for fecal leukocytes. The onset of the disease can be delayed considerably, even after the antibiotic has been stopped. In recently hospitalized patients in whom infectious diarrhea develops, *C. difficile* appears to be the pathogen most often encountered.[16]

Diarrhea in Acquired Immunodeficiency Syndrome

Diarrhea is a common and distressing symptom in acquired immunodeficiency syndrome (AIDS) patients, occurring in over 90% of individuals at some time during the course of their illness. AIDS patients are at risk for all the infectious causes of diarrhea in the immunocompetent population and are also at risk from other pathogens as well. A significant amount of morbidity and mortality of late AIDS is associated with gastrointestinal disease.[15] Enteric protozoal infections are the most common causes of diarrhea in AIDS patients, followed by cytomegalovirus and *Mycobacterium avium-intracellulare*. Microsporidia, *Isospora belli,* and *Cryptosporidium parvum,* the most common causes of protozoal diarrheal illness in AIDS patients, cause disruption of small intestinal villus architecture and severe malabsorption, maldigestion, and diarrhea.[15] Cytomegalovirus-induced colitis produces diarrhea that can be persistent or intermittent, lower abdominal pain, fever, and weight loss.[17] *M. avium-intracellulare* infects the small intestine and is characterized by diarrhea, abdominal pain, fever, nausea, weight loss, and malabsorption. The frequency of unexplained diarrhea in AIDS patients remains approximately 20%, even after extensive evaluations are performed. Many factors have been implicated in this idiopathic diarrhea, among them an alteration in intestinal villus architecture, undetectable infections, and human immunodeficiency virus (HIV)–induced cellular infection.[17]

Inflammatory Bowel Disease

Inflammatory bowel disease must be considered as an explanation for complaints of disordered bowel function in the patient with known disease, but first presentations of Crohn disease and ulcerative colitis are rare causes of acute diarrhea in the ED. Typically, patients presenting with inflammatory bowel disease give a history of weight loss during the preceding weeks or months. Other clinical and laboratory expressions of an ongoing inflammatory process can often be found, such as fever, elevated erythrocyte sedimentation rate, and anemia. If no infectious process is identified for persistently bloody stool, endoscopy and contrast studies should be considered to determine whether inflammatory bowel disease is present.

EMERGENCY DEPARTMENT EVALUATION

Most cases of diarrhea are managed, without the need for medical attention, by the affected patient or by a family member. Medical evaluation should occur for a subset of patients with more severe illness. Assessment of the severity of illness, presence of dehydration, character of stool patterns, and presence of fever, vomiting, or dysentery help to focus the evaluation to determine the likely cause of the illness. A detailed history, including travel, sexual practices, or immunocompromised status, is crucial, because it often points to the etiology. On physical examination, special attention is given to abdominal examination, which is most notable for generalized tenderness and increased bowel sounds but no peritoneal signs. Specific indications for further medical evaluation of patients with diarrhea are dehydration, dysentery, significant abdominal pain, suspicion of a concurrent systemic illness, and disease in the very young, the elderly, and the immunocompromised.

Fecal leukocytes are found in some patients with diarrhea and are caused either by organisms or by any factor that provokes inflammation and ulceration of the intestinal wall. Normal feces should have few or no white blood cells. The fecal sample can be examined as a wet preparation under the high-dry lens or as a Wright stain or Gram stain under the oil lens. Some authorities consider hemoccult-positive diarrhea in patients with acute enteric illness to be clinically equivalent to numerous fecal leukocytes.[22] The most commonly identified bacterial pathogens in patients with fecal leukocytes include *Shigella, Salmonella, Campylobacter, Aeromonas, Yersinia, Vibrio parahaemolyticus,* and *C. difficile*. Fecal leukocytes can also be seen in other conditions, such as appendicitis and inflammatory bowel disease. This finding is important because it identifies an inflammatory process that merits treatment and follow-up. Table 163.1 lists the infectious agents that produce fecal leukocytes.

Relatively well-appearing patients presenting with signs and symptoms of bacterial enteritis can be treated empirically with antibiotics, and stool cultures need not be sent. In the patient with symptoms of hypovolemia, red or white cells in the stool, or an abnormal abdominal examination, selected investigation may be warranted. Table 163.2 lists specific indications for sending diarrhea for culture and sensitivity. Clinicians should be wary of resistant infections because of the recent emergence of multidrug-resistant bacterial diarrheal illnesses.[21] If the patient has been on antibiotics before the onset of diarrhea, *C. difficile* must be considered and stool should be sent for *C. difficile* toxin assay. The emergency physician should rarely send stool for ova and parasites. However, illnesses lasting longer than 14 days should prompt an examination for parasites, particularly in immunocompromised patients and in travelers who have returned from areas where untreated water is consumed. In immunocompromised patients, endoscopy and biopsy are indicated when the illness persists, routine stool cultures are unrevealing, and a course of empiric antibiotics has not led to resolution.[14]

EMERGENCY DEPARTMENT MANAGEMENT

The assessment and treatment of dehydration and the relief of symptoms remain the cornerstones of ED care.

Fluid and Electrolyte Resuscitation

The most important intervention is fluid and electrolyte repletion. For mildly dehydrated individuals, resuscitation with oral fluids having sodium concentrations in the range of 45 to 75 mEq/L is recommended (Pedialyte or Rehydralyte solutions).[6] For moderately dehydrated individuals, the ideal formulation of oral fluids

TABLE 163.1. Infectious Agents that Produce Fecal Leukocytes

Bacterial Agent	Major Food Source	Primary Enterotoxins	Focal Leukocytes	Antimicrobial Therapy	Clinical Pearls
Norwalk Agent	Water, food	No	No	Bismuth subsalicylate	Highly effective vaccine available
Rotavirus	Person-person via fecal oral route	No	No	None	Most common cause of severe diarrhea in infants
Vibrio parahaemolyticus; vulnificus	Raw seafood; undercooked meat and poultry	Yes	Yes	None	History of seafood ingestion
Campylobacter jejuni	Raw milk	No	Yes	Macrolides	*C. jejuni* resistance to fluoroquinolones increasing
Yersinia enterocolitica	Pork, raw milk	No	Yes	Quinolones	Often presents with RLQ pain
Shigella species	Food contaminated during preparation	No	Yes	Quinolones	Explosive bloody diarrhea; only a small inoculum
Salmonella enteritidis	Raw eggs, incompletely cooked meat and poultry	No	Yes	Quinolones	Symptomatic patients with positive cultures should always be treated
E. Coli 0157:H7	Ground beef	No	Yes	None	Treatment with antibiotics may increase likelihood of HUS
Enterotoxigenic E. coli	Contaminated water, ice, leafy vegetables, unpeeled fruit	Yes	No	Bismuth subsalicylate	Most common cause of traveler's diarrhea
Staphylococcus aureus	Undercooked meat	Yes	No	None	Reheated foods; poor food storage for long periods
Clostridium botulinum	Preserved meat, fish, vegetables	Yes	No	None	Very difficult to culture organism
Clostridium difficile	Bacterial overgrowth from antibiotic use	Yes	Yes	Metronidazole; Vancomycin po	Cause of pseudomembranous colitis
Clostridium perfringens	Incompletely cooked meat and poultry	Yes	No	Metronidazole	Reheated foods; unrefrigerated food sitting out for long periods
Vibrio cholerae	Raw seafood	Yes	No	Doxycycline	Causes profound diarrhea, particularly in children
Bacillus cereus	Rice	Yes	No	None	Primarily an emetic syndrome
Bacillus cereus	Meat products; vegetables	Yes	No	None	Primarily a diarrheal syndrome
Giardia lamblia	Fecally contaminated water	No	No	Metronidazole	Common cause of persistent diarrhea; sometimes endoscopy required to make diagnosis
Entamoeba histolytica	Fecally contaminated food and water	No	Yes	Asympt. Cyst passer; Paromomycin Toxic; Metronidazole	Many infected but not symptomatic; travelers to 3rd world at risk
Cryptosporidia parvum/ Isospora belli	Fecal-oral, contaminated water	No	No	Paromomycin possible; no proven therapy	Most common cause of diarrhea in AIDS patients; can cause epidemics when water supply affected

is Na 60 to 90 mEq/L, K 20 mEq/L, Cl 80 mEq/L, citrate 30 mEq/L, and glucose 20 g/L; the World Health Organization's oral rehydration therapy contains these substances. Sports drinks, diluted fruit juices, and flavored soft drinks augmented with saltine crackers, broths, and soups can meet fluid and salt needs in nearly all nondehydrated, otherwise healthy persons with acute diarrhea. A homemade version of oral rehydration solution is made by preparing two separate glasses that are consumed alternately. The first contains 8 oz of orange juice or other potassium-containing fruit juices, one-half teaspoon of honey, and 1 pinch of table salt; the second glass contains 8 oz of clear water plus one-fourth teaspoon of baking soda.[6]

Dietary Advice

During a bout of acute diarrhea, calories facilitate enterocyte renewal. Boiled starches (potatoes), cereals (rice, noodles) with salt, saltines, bananas, yogurt, broths, steamed vegetables, and fruits are ideal foods during episodes of diarrhea. Although clinical lactose intolerance is uncommon in cases of acute diarrhea, many authorities recommend avoidance of dairy products in the first few days of illness.

Antimotility Agents

Codeine, diphenoxylate with atropine (Lomotil), and loperamide (Imodium) reduce urgency, frequency of bowel movements, and stool volume in diarrheal illness. They work by slowing the intraluminal flow of liquid, facilitating intestinal absorption. Loperamide is generally the recommended agent when antimotility agents are prescribed, due to its safety and efficacy; stool quantity has been reported to be reduced by approximately 80%.[8] Loperamide is the recommended treatment for AIDS patients in the absence of inflammatory disease of the colon and when diarrhea persists in the face of empiric antimicrobial and antiparasitic therapy. Antimotility agents may be

TABLE 163.2. Indications for Stool Culture in Patients with Acute Diarrhea

Immunocompromised individuals
Travel history to 3rd world
Homosexual activity
Failure to respond to empiric antibiotic therapy
Individuals with close contact to others where fecal–oral spread can occur (daycare workers, healthcare workers, food handlers)
"Toxic" appearance
Persistent diarrhea
Suspicion of antibiotic-resistant bacteria

used in patients with infectious enteritis of mild-to-moderate severity, but their use may be hazardous in the setting of severe dysentery. These agents should be used with caution in children and should not be used in infants.

Bismuth Subsalicylate and Attapulgite

Bismuth subsalicylate is effective therapy for acute diarrhea, either bacterial or viral, reducing the number of stools passed by approximately 50%.[7] The antidiarrheal effect is mediated by an antisecretory salicylate effect rather than by adsorption of toxin. It is also effective in relieving the vomiting associated with enteric viral infections. Additionally, it has antibacterial properties, which may explain its value in the prevention of traveler's diarrhea. The dose is 30 to 60 mL every 30 minutes for eight doses. An important caveat is to warn patients that this medication will turn their feces black. Attapulgite (Kaopectate), a clay-like material, may make stools more formed by absorbing intracolonic water. It is very safe.

Antibiotics in Acute Diarrhea

Patients with signs and symptoms of acute dysentery and patients with traveler's diarrhea should be treated empirically with antibiotic therapy. A majority of patients with numerous fecal leukocytes respond favorably to antimicrobial therapy and can therefore be treated empirically. Table 163.1 lists the antimicrobial therapy of choice for different pathogens. Patients with traveler's diarrhea are characteristically infected with bacterial pathogens, and their illness is shortened by antimicrobial therapy. Generally, a quinolone antibiotic is recommended as empiric therapy for 3 to 5 days, unless diarrheal culture results are available to tailor therapy.

After appropriate evaluation, AIDS patients with acute diarrhea can be started on empiric therapy with quinolone antibiotics for 10 days. As in infections outside the gut in immunocompromised patients, curative treatment requires prolonged therapy.

Patients with diarrhea lasting 2 to 4 weeks without systemic symptoms or dysentery may be treated empirically for *Giardia* with metronidazole, which is also effective against the small bowel bacterial overgrowth associated with persistent diarrhea. Metronidazole is also an effective agent of choice for *C. difficile* colitis and intestinal amebiasis.[6]

Special Advice to Travelers

Educating travelers about the prevention and treatment of diarrhea is important, because it is estimated that 25% to 40% of travelers in the developing world develop diarrhea.[18] Travelers committed to preventing diarrhea should be advised to follow the old British colonial axiom, "Cook it, boil it, peel it—or forget it." Instructions should include methods of diarrhea prevention, use of prophylactic agents, and methods of replenishing fluid and electrolytes. Bismuth subsalicylate, quinolone antibiotics, and vibramycin are effective prophylactically and as self-administered treatment of traveler's diarrhea.

DISPOSITION

The emergency physician can manage almost all cases of diarrhea presenting to the ED. Patients with diarrhea who are significantly dehydrated and who remain unable to tolerate oral fluids should be considered for admission. Situations in which there is a possible pathologic process, such as inflammatory bowel disease or ischemic bowel, require medical or surgical consultation. Moderately ill patients who are sent home, patients with traveler's diarrhea, and AIDS patients should have follow-up arranged with their primary care providers.

COMMON PITFALLS

- Overdiagnosing viral gastroenteritis. There is a temptation to label all diarrheal illnesses of uncertain cause as viral. Particularly in older patients, the diagnosis of viral gastroenteritis is statistically less likely, and many serious causes of diarrhea are more likely. If there are white blood cells or red blood cells in the stool or if the abdominal examination is abnormal, diarrhea should not be attributed to a viral cause.
- Failing to examine the stool. There are few truly useful tests in emergency medicine; examination of the stool is one of them.
- Failing to watch for antibiotic-resistant bacterial enteric infections. The incidence of multidrug-resistant infections is on the rise.
- Many surgical problems, including small bowel obstruction, inflammatory bowel disease, mesenteric infarction, and cancer, can present with diarrhea. The emergency physician must be vigilant to distinguish between these diseases and infectious diarrhea.

PROCTITIS

Proctitis is formally defined as inflammation of the rectal mucosa. Alternatively, it can be defined as anorectal symptoms associated with sigmoidoscopic findings limited to the distal 15 cm of the rectum. Proctitis should be distinguished from *proctocolitis,* which has different infectious etiologies. *Acute proctitis* is a nonspecific term that refers to several specific disease conditions that include inflammatory bowel disease, infections, venereal disease, antibiotics, radiation, and chemotherapy.[1]

The epidemiology of proctitis in ED patients varies with demographics. In urban areas with large populations of homosexual males, high rates of sexually transmitted infectious proctitis are seen; in facilities treating more elderly populations, proctitis is more frequently the sequela of other gastrointestinal disorders, exemplified by radiation proctitis or ulcerative proctitis.

CLINICAL PRESENTATION

Most patients have similar nonspecific symptoms of rectal discomfort, tenesmus (urge to defecate), and hematochezia. Other symptoms are pain with defecation, disordered bowel function (typically constipation), lower abdominal pain and pelvic pain, mucopurulent rectal discharge, and feelings of incomplete evacuation. Infectious and inflammatory conditions that involve the anal mucosa are typically very painful. Rectal mucosal erythema, friability, and a mucopurulent discharge are noted on physical examination. Patients with proctitis attempt frequent fecal evacuation that typically produces bloody mucus and little fecal matter.[19] Symptoms of fever, weight loss, abdominal pain, nausea, and vomiting indicate that proctitis may be manifestation of a more generalized process.

DIFFERENTIAL DIAGNOSIS

Before diagnosing symptoms of rectal pain and discharge as proctitis, the clinician must first exclude other entities that can cause these symptoms, such as perirectal abscess, rectal polyps, and anal fissures. The causes of proctitis are divided into infectious causes, most typically venereal diseases, and noninfectious causes.

Infectious Proctitis

Both homosexual and heterosexual anal intercourse have the potential for transmitting enteric pathogens and venereal infections, especially when people have multiple sexual partners and fail to use condoms. The most common infectious cause, and by far the most common cause in sexually active homosexual men, is gonorrhea.[13] In symptomatic gonococcal proctitis, the usual presenting complaint is rectal discharge, often noted as staining of the underwear. Additionally, scant bloody discharge and rectal pain may be noted spontaneously or with rectal intercourse. Gonococcal infection of the rectum occurs commonly in conjunction with gonococcal urethritis. Gonococcal infection of the female rectum is most commonly the result of anal intercourse, but may be caused by the spread of the organisms through vaginal secretions. Perhaps 10% to 20% of all patients with genital gonorrhea have positive rectal cultures for the organism.

Along with gonorrhea, chlamydia should be considered in patients with proctitis that appears to be sexually transmitted.[13] Infections with lymphogranuloma venereum (LGV) types are more severe but much less frequent than those due to the other strains of chlamydia. Although some patients are asymptomatic, anorectal pain, tenesmus, left lower quadrant abdominal tenderness, constipation, and a bloody mucopurulent discharge can be noted. Chlamydial proctitis may have a subacute or even chronic presentation, with regional adenopathy and fibrosis and stricture of the rectum. Granulomatous rectal changes with LGV chlamydial strains resemble Crohn disease, especially when perirectal abscesses and fistulas are present.[13]

Proctitis due to herpes simplex virus (HSV) infection, either type 1 or 2, is a common cause of proctitis; however, HSV-2 infections are more severe and recur more frequently. The predominant complaints are severe anorectal pain, discharge, and change in bowel habits (constipation being more frequent than diarrhea). Systemic symptoms are fever, chills, and malaise. Vesicles, in clusters surrounded by an erythematous base, hemorrhage, vascular congestion, and pus may extend as high as 15 cm up the rectal mucosa. With severe HSV proctitis, urinary dysfunction, impotence, neuralgia, and paresthesias in the buttocks and thighs may occur secondary to viral infection of the sacral plexus. Persistent herpes proctitis is seen almost exclusively in AIDS patients.

Noninfectious Proctitis

Patients who have signs and symptoms of rectal disease and histories of anal erotic activity may manifest primarily noninfectious consequences of their sexual behavior. Foreign objects inserted into the anus may cause mucosal damage and allow penetration by normal colonic organisms, with secondary inflammation. Anal and lower rectal mucosal inflammation due to the trauma of sexual activity may be extremely difficult to differentiate from inflammatory changes secondary to infectious agents.

Allergic proctitis occurs when substances used as lubricants during anal intercourse sensitize through abraded anal skin or intact mucosa. When used as lubricants, soaps, shampoos, cooking oil, suntan preparations, or medicinal creams may be directly irritating and can reduce the protective effectiveness of condoms. Even lubricating jelly has been associated with allergic contact sensitivity due to the propylene glycol vehicle.

Ulcerative colitis is a chronic inflammatory bowel disorder of unknown origin that is characterized by inflammation of the bowel. The proximal extent of the colonic mucosal inflammation varies among individuals, but the rectum is almost always involved. With predominantly rectal involvement, constipation and tenesmus are typical complaints. Patients with ulcerative proctitis usually have milder manifestations of inflammatory bowel disease and typically do not have the systemic manifestations of the disease.

Radiation proctitis is caused by pelvic irradiation for gynecologic or prostate malignancies. Symptoms of anorectal pain and bloody discharge can be severe. Proctoscopic findings are erythematous and edematous mucosa in the acute phase and characteristic telangiectasias and ulcerations in the chronic phase. Large ulcerations can result in distal rectal strictures or rectovaginal fistulas.[2]

EMERGENCY DEPARTMENT EVALUATION

An accurate diagnosis can be made by use of a careful history, anoscopy, culture, rectal biopsy, and stool analysis.[1] A sexual history is important in the evaluation of anorectal complaints. The patient may not volunteer a sexual history because of embarrassment or fear of a hostile response from health-care personnel. Patients with a history of receptive anal sex are at risk for a variety of sexually transmitted infections, including HIV infection.[3] Also important to obtain is a history of previous treatment for sexually transmitted disease, because it may have been ineffective in eradicating unrecognized rectal infection. Anoscopy with appropriate cultures identifies most sexually transmissible intestinal infections and should be carried out in all those who practice receptive anal intercourse who present with symptoms suggestive of proctitis.

Although specimens can be obtained with a pledget blindly inserted 2 cm into the canal and rotated, swabbing under direct anoscopic visualization raises the positive yield on Gram stains from 34% to 79%.[3] Cultures for sexually transmitted disease should be obtained not only from the rectum, but also from the urethra and the cervix. Immunofluorescence stains and viral cultures for HSV should be carried out, even when no lesions are grossly visible. Whenever patients have proctitis secondary to sexually transmitted disease, they should also be tested for concomitant infections such as syphilis and AIDS.

EMERGENCY DEPARTMENT MANAGEMENT

The ED management of infectious proctitis is analogous to that of urethritis. When sexually transmitted disease is suspected based on patient history, empiric therapy for gonorrhea and chlamydia is recommended, because they commonly cause infectious proctitis and antibiotic therapy does not compromise subsequent evaluation. Third-generation cephalosporins and quinolones are the preferred treatment for gonococcal infections. Doxycycline or macrolide antibiotics should be prescribed to treat chlamydial infections. Occasionally, rectal LGV requires several courses of antibiotic therapy.

Systemic therapy of herpetic proctitis with acyclovir is indicated when the diagnosis is suspected. Oral acyclovir effectively reduces the duration of symptomatic lesions, rectal pain, discharge, and the period of viral shedding. In immunocompetent hosts, the dosage is 400 mg five times daily for 10 days. AIDS patients require intravenous acyclovir for longer courses of therapy.[3] Patients with symptoms or signs of severe herpes proctitis, such as severe pain or urinary retention, should be admitted for aggressive pain control and intravenous acyclovir.

Even when a new presentation of proctitis does not appear to be due to infection, it is wise to treat empirically for common infectious etiologies. Pseudoinfectious and allergic proctitis are best treated by removal of the agents causing the disease. Ulcerative proctitis is responsive to oral, parenteral, and rectal administration of corticosteroids. Treatment should also be aimed at treating the perianal discomfort, which can be severe. Sitz baths for 20 minutes three to four times daily are helpful.

DISPOSITION

Most patients with proctitis can be managed in the ED without consultation or admission. Consultation is advisable when there is a problem with the diagnosis of an unusual mucosal appearance, a question of perirectal infection, systemic symptoms or local signs suggesting malignancy, or a suspicion of inflammatory bowel disease. If outpatient therapy is elected, these patients require close follow-up. Worsening of symptoms or failure to improve on antibiotic therapy and Sitz baths within 48 hours necessitates admission and further endoscopic evaluation. All patients should be referred to an appropriate physician for follow-up endoscopy and evaluation of culture results.

COMMON PITFALLS

- Failure to elicit a sexual history
- Failure to question a sexual history once elicited; many patients do not at first admit to rectal intercourse.
- Failure to visualize the mucosa by anoscopy and to examine and culture any exudate
- Failure to consider sexually transmitted disease, which can occur in men, women, and children
- Failure to arrange for proper identification and treatment of contacts
- Failure to consider or identify other rectal lesions that mimic proctitis, such as anal fissure, anal fistula, and perirectal abscess

References

1. Babb RR. Evaluation of acute proctitis. *JAMA* 1980;244:358.
2. Bartelsman JF, Tytgal GN. Extra-ordinary forms of proctitis. *Neth J Med* 1990;37:552.
3. Bassford J. Treatment of common anorectal disorders. *Am Fam Physician* 1992;45:1788.
4. Binder HJ. Pathophysiology of acute diarrhea. *Am J Med* 1990;88:6A-25S.
5. Boyce JH, Swerdlow DL, Griffin PM. *Escherichia coli* and the hemolytic-uremic syndrome. *N Engl J Med* 1995;333:364.
6. Dupont HL. Guidelines on acute infectious diarrhea in adults. *Am J Gastroenterol* 1997;92:1962.
7. Dupont HL, Sanchez JT, Ericsson CD. Comparative efficacy of loperamide hydrochloride and bismuth subsalicylate in the management of acute diarrhea. *Am J Med* 1990;88:6A-15S.
8. Ericsson CD, Johnson PC. Safety and efficacy of loperamide. *Am J Med* 1990;88:6A-10S.
9. Garthright WE, Archer DL, Kvenberg JE. Estimate of incidence and costs of intestinal infectious diseases in the United States. *Public Health Rep* 1988;103:107.
10. Hanauer SB. Inflammatory bowel disease. *N Engl J Med* 1996;334(13):841–848.
11. Kapikian AZ. Viral gastroenteritis. *JAMA* 1993; 69:627.
12. Lew JF, Glass RI, Gangarosa RE, et al. Diarrheal deaths in the United States; 1979 through 1987. *JAMA* 1991;265:3280.
13. Quinn TC, et al.. *Chlamydia trachomatis* proctitis. *N Engl J Med* 1981; 305(4):195–200.
14. Ravdin JI. Amebiasis. *Clin Infect Dis* 1995;20:1453.
15. Sharpstone D, Gazzard B. Gastrointestinal manifestation of HIV infection. *Lancet* 1996;348:379.
16. Siegel D, Edelstein PH, Nachamkin I. Inappropriate testing for diarrheal disease in the hospital. *JAMA* 1990;263:979.
17. Simon D, Brandt LJ. Diarrhea in patients with the acquired immunodeficiency syndrome. *Gastroenterology* 1993;105:1238.
18. Steffen R, Collard O, Tornieporth N, et al. Epidemiology, etiology and impact of traveler's diarrhea in Jamaica. *JAMA* 1999;281:811.
19. Tytgat GNJ, Fookens RH, Schotborgh RH, et al. Proctitis. *Neth J Med* 1990;37:537.
20. Vesikari J. Rotavirus vaccines against diarrhoeal disease. *Lancet* 1997;350:1538.
21. Villar RG, Macek MD, Simons S, et al. Investigation of multidrug-resistant *Salmonella* serotype typhimurium DT104 infections linked to raw-milk cheese in Washington State. *JAMA* 1999;281(10):1811–1816.
22. Vogtlin J, Stalden H, Loosli J. Modified guaiac test may replace search for faecal leucocytes in acute infectious diarrhoea. *Lancet* 1983; 1204.

CHAPTER 164

Lower Gastrointestinal Bleeding

Daniel T. Schelble and David J. Peter

The chief complaint of "rectal bleeding" includes symptoms ranging in severity from minor anorectal bleeding, to severe bleeding that has stopped, to massive persistent hemorrhage with shock. The evaluation, management, and disposition of each case are determined by the severity of the patient's symptoms. The bleeding stops spontaneously in about 80% of cases, with recurrent bleeding in about 25%.[3,10,16] In one database report of patients undergoing colonoscopy for lower gastrointestinal bleeding, 66% were hospitalized, 35% required transfusion, and 15% required surgery.[15]

Lower gastrointestinal bleeding has a hospitalization incidence of 20 to 25 episodes per 100,000 population per year and a mortality of 4% to 10%.[10,11,14] The incidence increases 200-fold from the third to ninth decade of life, and most episodes occur in the elderly.[1,10] As a group, the elderly have decreased cardiovascular reserve in the face of hemorrhage, often have comorbid disease, and have decreased tolerance for major surgery.[2,14] Lower gastrointestinal bleeding is a common problem in the emergency department that will increase in incidence with the aging of our population.

CLINICAL PRESENTATION

By definition, lower gastrointestinal bleeding occurs *distal* to the ligament of Treitz, including the small intestine, large intestine, rectum, and anus. It is generally intermittent and encompasses an extensive range of etiologies, severity of bleeding, and clinical significance. Large bleeds with rapid intestinal transport present with the bright red or maroon stools of hematochezia. With slower intestinal transport or less bleeding volume, the stools are darker or black and tarry (melena). Hematochezia is the chief complaint in up to 90% of patients with lower gastrointestinal bleeding. It is about six times more likely to be due to lower gastrointestinal bleeding than to upper gastrointestinal bleeding, while melena is about four times more likely to be due to an upper gastrointestinal source.[15] Minor anorectal bleeding commonly presents with traces of blood on the stool, undergarments, or toilet tissue, or within the toilet bowl. Occult bleeding is that detected by screening or coincidental guaiac stool testing or during the evaluation of iron-deficiency anemia, without other apparent etiology.

The severity of the clinical presentation is directly related to the volume and rate of blood loss. Rapid and severe losses present with rectal bleeding and cardiovascular decompensation, which may be manifested by near-syncope, syncope, myocardial infarction, stroke, or shock (pallor, tachypnea, tachycardia, hypotension, confusion). Slower, prolonged losses may present with the symptoms of anemia (fatigue, weakness, dyspnea, heart failure) or asymptomatic melena.

The loss of as little as 60 mL of blood can produce a black or melanotic stool. Rectal bleeding with symptoms of hypovolemia (weakness, orthostatic dizziness, near-syncope) is associated with the relatively rapid loss of at least 1000 mL of blood and usually causes the patient to seek medical attention immediately. The sudden loss of 2000 mL of blood (40% of circulating volume) can be fatal, and about 10% of unattended adults who sustain such a loss will die. In a series patients with lower gastrointestinal bleeding evaluated by colonoscopy, 19% presented with positive orthostatic changes or shock, and 35% required transfusion.[15]

DIFFERENTIAL DIAGNOSIS

The differential diagnosis of lower gastrointestinal bleeding is broad (Table 164.1).

Diverticulosis has historically been described as the most common cause of severe lower gastrointestinal bleeding in adults,[2,18] but angiodysplasia has been identified as nearly as frequent or more frequent cause as diagnostic capabilities have improved.[3,6] Diverticulosis should be considered in all patients older than age 40, and the prevalence increases in each succeeding decade of life. More than 50% of patients have diverticula by age 60.[2,3]

Diverticular bleeding is often arterial, sudden, and severe, and is usually dark red or maroon; pain is usually absent or mild.[3] Bleeding tends to occur in right colon diverticula, and accompanying symptoms of diverticulitis are uncommon. Bleeding stops spontaneously in 99% of patients who require transfusion of less than 4 U of blood, while most patients requiring 4 or more units usually continue to bleed.[12] The chance of recurrent diverticular hemorrhage is in the range of 20% to 40%, and surgery is required in up to 25% of cases.[2,12,18]

TABLE 164.1. Sources of Lower Gastrointestinal Bleeding in Adults

Diverticulosis
Angiodysplasia
Neoplasm, including polyps
Inflammatory bowel disease
Upper gastrointestinal bleeding
Anorectal disorders
Infectious
Postpolypectomy and iatrogenic
Less common sources (trauma, colonic varices in portal hypertension, mesenteric ischemia, aortoenteric fistula, endometriosis, radiation enteritis, coagulopathy)

Angiodysplasia (vascular ectasia) produces degenerative vascular abnormalities, primarily of the colon. Like diverticulosis, angiodysplasia can cause painless major hemorrhage with red or maroon stools, depending on location and volume of the bleeding. Bleeding due to angiodysplasia tends to be venous and more commonly recurrent than that due to diverticulosis. The prevalence increases with age, and up to 25% of all elderly patients are found to have angiodysplasia during colonoscopy. Rebleeding occurs in up to 85%. Therapeutic interventions such as colonoscopic coagulation, angiographic therapy, or surgery may be required.[6]

Neoplasms, whether benign or malignant, usually present with occult or mild chronic bleeding. Some authors state that neoplasms and polyps rarely or only occasionally cause severe lower gastrointestinal bleeding,[3,6] while others report an incidence ranging from 6% to 33% in severe gastrointestinal bleeding.[1,11,18] A change in stool or bowel habits, weight loss, obstructive symptoms, or detection of a mass on abdominal or digital rectal examination should alert one to the possibility of malignancy. Adenocarcinoma is a common cause of minor, intermittent bleeding.

Inflammatory bowel disease, including Crohn disease and ulcerative colitis, is usually associated with minor bleeding and diarrhea. Younger adults are most commonly affected. There is often a history of previous episodes, and the diagnosis is usually known by the patient. The incidence of massive bleeding is usually reported in the range of 3% to 9%.[1,18] Rebleeding occurs in up to 35%. Urgent surgery is often recommended after life-threatening hemorrhage.

Upper gastrointestinal bleeding accounts for hematochezia in 10% to 15% of cases and must be included in the differential for apparent lower gastrointestinal bleeding.[15] It is usually accompanied by a history of peptic ulcer disease, gastritis, varices, epigastric pain, hematemesis or coffee-ground emesis, nonsteroidal antiinflammatory drug use, or liver disease. It is important to place a nasogastric tube in all patients with suspected lower gastrointestinal bleeding and also to recognize that a negative nasogastric aspirate does not completely rule out an upper gastrointestinal source. Ten percent to 16% of patients with upper gastrointestinal bleeding will have a negative nasogastric aspirate.[17] It should also be noted that *small intestinal bleeding* may account for 3% to 5% of lower gastrointestinal bleeding cases.[18]

Anorectal disorders (hemorrhoids, fissures, fistula, proctitis, prolapse, impaction) usually cause minor bleeding and accounted for about 28% of rectal bleeding patients seen in one general practice study.[4] Up to 11% of patients, however, may have an anorectal source, accounting for "significant" bleeding. Hemorrhoids are the most common cause of rectal bleeding, especially in patients under the age of 50.[8] Hemorrhoids may present with pain and swelling consistent with thrombosis or with painless minor bleeding. Fissures usually result from the passage of hard stool and are usually painful, again with only minor bleeding. Radiation proctitis, infectious proctitis, fecal impaction, and rectal prolapse are associated with mucosal bleeding and are usually minor. Nevertheless, the presence of anorectal disease does not rule out the possibility of a more significant proximal source.

Infectious diarrhea usually causes minor bleeding in the face of predominant diarrhea and other gastroenteritis-related symptoms (nausea, abdominal pain and cramping, fever). Bacterial dysentery is a common cause of bloody diarrhea and pain in some settings.

Other less common causes of gastrointestinal bleeding include trauma, colonic varices in portal hypertension, mesenteric ischemia, aortoenteric fistula, endometriosis, radiation enteritis, and coagulopathy.[1] Overall, these entities account for a small percentage of cases.

Postpolypectomy bleeding occurs in 0.1% to 0.4% of patients following endoscopic polypectomy.[1] This bleeding usually presents in the first 2 weeks following the procedure and can be significant.

No definite etiology is identified in about 10% of cases of acute lower gastrointestinal bleeding, despite current diagnostic techniques.[3]

EMERGENCY DEPARTMENT EVALUATION

The initial priority in the evaluation of lower gastrointestinal bleeding is to identify hypovolemia and institute treatment, if necessary. A finding of hypotension or tachycardia should alert the emergency physician to the significance of the hemorrhage in terms of blood loss and continued rate of bleeding. Frequent reevaluation, especially of vital signs, including orthostatics, is imperative.

Orthostatic testing has been variably defined in the literature. A decrease in systolic blood pressure of 10 mmHg or an increase in heart rate of 20, two minutes after postural change to standing, has been used in upper gastrointestinal bleeding studies and is associated with an increase in mortality from 8.7% to 13.6%.[14] Positive orthostatic testing occurred in 30% of patients with "significant" lower gastrointestinal bleeding in one study.[16] Although orthostatic testing is recommended for all patients with lower gastrointestinal bleeding who can tolerate standing for 2 minutes without experiencing syncope, significant bleeding can occur in spite of normal vital signs and negative orthostatic testing.

If these are signs of hypovolemia or shock, intravenous fluid resuscitation with a minimum of two large-bore catheters must be immediately initiated. The patient should be placed on a monitor, given oxygen, and moved into an area of the department where close monitoring is available. Immediate and ongoing resuscitation, with crystalloid fluids and blood products as indicated, is the most important emergency department intervention in these unstable patients.

Specimens should be drawn for baseline laboratory studies, including a complete blood count, coagulation profile, liver function tests, chemistry profile, and a type and screen (if stable) or type and crossmatch (if unstable) for 4 to 6 U of packed red blood cells. An electrocardiogram is recommended for all elderly patients, patients with severe anemia, and those with cardiopulmonary complaints.

Abdominal x-rays are not indicated. An upright chest radiograph or supine chest and lateral decubitus radiographs are helpful in assessing pulmonary status and ruling out free air. Laboratory testing is used to define the severity and ongoing activity of bleeding, as well as underlying comorbidities and cardiovascular reserve.

Serial hemoglobin determinations often confirm the accuracy of the initial clinical assessment and also give an indication of the severity and activity of bleeding. Although the initial hematocrit may be normal, a decrease after volume replacement suggests significant initial blood loss or continued significant bleeding. An elevated blood urea nitrogen-to-creatinine ratio suggests volume depletion and possibly a greater likelihood of upper gastrointestinal bleeding.[14] Urine output, as measured by a Foley catheter, is a quick and useful indicator of the effectiveness of fluid replacement and may serve as an indirect indicator of the adequacy of fluid replacement. Saline or tapwater enemas have never been proven effective at diminishing or stopping lower gastrointestinal bleeding.

After the institution of resuscitative measures, the history should be obtained, with an emphasis on establishing the duration and intensity of bleeding, the nature and color of the stools, and the character of any pain. Patients often present with problems other than gastrointestinal bleeding (fatigue, dizziness, confusion, shortness of breath, chest pain, shock, cardiopulmonary arrest), and gastrointestinal bleeding should be considered in the differential diagnosis of these entities. A history of previous bleeding, gastrointestinal disorders (e.g., cirrhosis, peptic ulcer disease, inflammatory bowel disease), retching, tenesmus, weight loss, near-syncope or syncope, chest pain, shortness of breath, altered mental status, alcohol use, and medications may be helpful. Syncope has been noted in 10% of patients with significant lower gastrointestinal bleeding. Any medical history of unstable or potentially unstable comorbid disease should be elicited.[7]

Physical examination may reveal jaundice, abdominal wall varices ("caput medusae"), abdominal distention, or a palpable mass. Abdominal rigidity, guarding, rebound, or the absence of bowel sounds suggests peritonitis or perforation. Again, the examination should specifically try to identify unstable comorbid disease, such as congestive heart failure, angina, and stroke.

A digital rectal examination should be performed to detect masses or other rectal pathology and to obtain a stool specimen for direct observation and testing for occult blood (Hemoccult or Hematest). Aside from gastrointestinal bleeding, black stools can be caused by iron, charcoal, bismuth, food dyes, beets, Jello, Kool-Aid, and some antibiotic syrups. Testing for occult blood by either Hemoccult or Hematest method detects hemoglobin in stool. False-positive results can be produced by red meat, raw fruits and vegetables, some iron preparations, iodide, and bromide preparations. False-negative results can occur as a result of small hemorrhages in which the hemoglobin has lost its peroxidase activity in transit. Peroxidase activity loss is enhanced by magnesium-containing antacids and ascorbic acid.

A nasogastric tube should be placed in all patients with suspected significant lower gastrointestinal bleeding in which the rectal examination did not reveal an obvious source. The aspirate should be examined for red blood, "coffee-ground" material consistent with partially digested blood, and bile to help evaluate for an upper gastrointestinal source. As previously stated, a clear aspirate does not completely rule out upper gastrointestinal bleeding. Testing for occult blood in the gastric aspirate is unnecessary and often false-positive, due to blood from nasopharyngeal trauma during insertion. In any case, the gross appearance of the gastric aspirate provides the clinician with the needed information.

If active bleeding originates from the anorectum or lower sigmoid colon up to 25 cm from the anus, anoscopy and rigid proctosigmoidoscopy usually reveal the source. It is also helpful to document blood coming from proximal to the limits of the scope. Blood above the scope does not necessarily mean the source is more proximal, as blood may have refluxed back up the colon. A barium enema should not be used in the evaluation of lower gastrointestinal bleeding, because it may prevent the later use of colonoscopy or angiography.

EMERGENCY DEPARTMENT MANAGEMENT

Further management in the emergency department setting usually involves consultation with a variety of specialists while stabilization procedures and serial examinations are continued.

Colonoscopy has become the procedure of choice in acute lower gastrointestinal bleeding that has stopped. Its use in the setting of active bleeding is controversial. It offers the advantages of both diagnosis and endoscopic therapy. Urgent colonoscopy identifies the bleeding site in about 75% to 94% of cases,[1,16] and endoscopic therapy is successful in up to 80% or 90% of cases.[1] Shock is the only absolute contraindication. If bleeding is massive and ongoing, colonoscopy is not possible; the patient requires angiography.

Angiography is used for continuous, severe, or massive lower gastrointestinal bleeding, or when other modalities have failed to reveal a source. Diagnostic yields are in the range of 40% to 85%.[3,9,18] Continuous bleeding rates as low as 0.5 mL/min can be detected.[13] Therapeutic intervention with vasopressin infusion or arterial embolization with autologous clots, metal coils, or absorbable gelatin can be provided as well. Complications of angiography include hematomas, arterial embolization and dissection, renal failure, contrast reactions, and bowel ischemia and infarction. The complication rate is about 2% to 9%.

Radionuclide scanning with technetium-99m–labeled red blood cells or technetium-99m sulfur colloid is the least invasive but most controversial of the modalities available for the evaluation of lower gastrointestinal bleeding. The technique provides rough localization, distinguishing the right from left colonic bleeding sites, or proximal from more distal sources. Slow bleeding (rates as low as 0.1 mL/min) and intermittent bleeding can both be detected. Reported false-positive rates range from 0% to 48%, and prospective localization of the bleeding site for angiography or surgery is reported to be correct in 39% to 95% of cases.[5,14] Radionuclide scanning may be used for screening before angiography, but its use is controversial. It is especially valuable for patients who cannot tolerate angiography or other procedures because of underlying medical problems. However, bleeding scans should not delay therapy in patients with massive bleeding.

Surgical consultation should be considered when there has been massive initial bleeding, when bleeding continues, when the source of bleeding has been detected and is amenable to surgery, or when perforation is identified or strongly suspected.

DISPOSITION

Admission is indicated for patients with any lower gastrointestinal bleeding (excluding minor bleeding), for patients with continued bleeding, for patients with significant associated or underlying comorbid disease or injury, and for those with poor social support or questionable reliability for follow-up. Patients with stable vital signs and no significant comorbidity can go to the floor. Admission to an intensive care unit can be guided by the BLEED classification tool.[7] Any one positive criterion indicates the need for intensive care unit admission, including (1) ongoing *b*leeding, (2) *l*ow systolic blood pressure (less than 100), (3) *e*levated prothrombin time, (4) *e*rratic mental status, and (5) presence of unstable comorbid *d*isease. The majority of patients with minor lower gastrointestinal bleeding amenable to surgical or medical treatment, stable vital signs, good social support, and reliability for follow-up care can be sent home, but all cases of lower gastrointestinal bleeding require follow-up.

COMMON PITFALLS

- Failure to appreciate the significance and volume of lower gastrointestinal bleeding, leading to delays in therapy
- Failure to consider gastrointestinal bleeding as a precipitant for near-syncope or syncope, angina, dyspnea, fatigue, anemia, altered mental status, or shock. The rectal examination should be performed early in the evaluation of these presentations.
- Failure to place a nasogastric tube early in the evaluation of significant bleeding to help rule out an upper gastrointestinal source
- Failure to consider the possibility of coexisting serious causes of bleeding once a relatively benign, treatable source of bleeding has been established. Beware of the diagnosis of hemorrhoids in lower gastrointestinal bleeding.
- Failure to perform and record serial laboratory and clinical evaluations
- Failure to recognize that it may take several hours for the hematocrit to reflect the magnitude of blood loss
- Failure to consider other clinical entities (e.g., infarction, pulmonary embolism) when vital signs remain abnormal despite adequate volume replacement and when there is no further evidence of bleeding
- Failure to appreciate the possibility of perforation, especially when there has been previous instrumentation
- Reliance on the color of the stool as an indicator of the source or location of bleeding. The color of the stool is unreliable because of variability in degradation and transit time.

References

1. Billingham RP. The conundrum of lower gastrointestinal bleeding. *Surg Clin North Am* 1997;77:241.
2. Bokhari M, et al. Diverticular hemorrhage in the elderly—is it well tolerated? *Dis Colon Rectum* 1996;39:191.
3. DeMarkles MP, Murphy JR. Acute lower gastrointestinal bleeding. *Med Clin North Am* 1993;77:1085.
4. Fijten GH, et al. The incidence and outcome of rectal bleeding in general practice. *Fam Pract* 1993;10:283.
5. Garafalo TE, Abdu RA. Accuracy and efficacy of nuclear scintigraphy for the detection of gastrointestinal bleeding. *Arch Surg* 1997;132:196.
6. Jensen DM, Machicado GA. Colonoscopy for diagnosis and treatment of severe lower gastrointestinal bleeding: routine outcomes and cost analysis. *Gastrointest Endosc Clin North Am* 1997;7:477.
7. Kollef MH, et al. BLEED: a classification tool to predict outcomes in patients with acute upper and lower gastrointestinal hemorrhage. *Crit Care Med* 1997;25:1125.
8. Korkis AM, McDougall CJ. Rectal bleeding in patients less than 50 years of age. *Dig Dis Sci* 1995;40:1520.
9. Leitman IM, Paull DE, Shires GT. Evaluation and management of massive lower gastrointestinal hemorrhage. *Ann Surg* 1989;209:175.
10. Longstreth GF. Epidemiology and outcome of patients hospitalized with acute lower gastrointestinal hemorrhage: a population based study. *Am J Gastroenterol* 1997;92:419.
11. Makela JT, Kiviniemi H, et al. Diagnosis and treatment of acute lower gastrointestinal bleeding. *Scand J Gastroenterol* 1993;28:1062.
12. McGuire HH. Bleeding colonic diverticula: a reappraisal of natural history and management. *Ann Surg* 1994;220:653.
13. Pennoyer WP, Vignati PV, Cohen JL. Mesenteric angiography for lower gastrointestinal hemorrhage: are there predictors of a positive study? *Dis Colon Rectum* 1997;40:1014.
14. Peter DP, Dougherty JM. An evidence based approach to the evaluation of gastrointestinal bleeding. *Emerg Med Clin North Am* 1999;17:239.
15. Peura DA, Lanza FL, Goustout CJ, et al. The American College of Gastroenterology Bleeding Registry: preliminary findings. *Am J Gastroenterol* 1997;92:924.
16. Richter JM, Christensen MR, Kaplan LM, et al. Effectiveness of current technology in the diagnosis and management of lower gastrointestinal hemorrhage. *Gastrointest Endosc* 1995;41:93.
17. Talbot-Stern JK. Gastrointestinal bleeding. *Emerg Med Clin North Am* 1996;14:173.
18. Vernava AM, Moore BA, Longo WE, et al. Lower gastrointestinal bleeding. *Dis Colon Rectum* 1997;40:846.

PART IV

Renal, Metabolic, and Endocrine Disease

CHAPTER 165

Acid–Base Disturbances

Robert Shesser

Severe acid–base abnormalities, although potentially life-threatening in themselves, also serve as important indicators of serious underlying conditions or disorders. Precise identification of the cause of an acid–base disturbance is rarely required for proper immediate treatment, but the abnormality often provides a critical clue for the identification of an underlying disturbance. A thorough understanding of the principles of acid–base pathophysiology permits the physician to expand the diagnostic considerations and makes it possible to proceed promptly with appropriate interventions.

BASIC PHYSIOLOGY

The hydrogen ion concentration or its negative logarithm (pH) is a fundamental measure of the character of all organic solutions. Because cellular enzyme systems function over a very narrow range of hydrogen ion concentrations, maintaining a stable internal milieu is important for normal function. Three homeostatic systems help to maintain pH close to baseline.

Soluble buffer systems effect an immediate response to changes in pH. In the extracellular space, these include the carbonic acid, phosphoric acid, hemoglobin, and plasma protein systems. These extracellular buffers account for one-third of the body's acute buffering capacity. Intracellular tissue proteins are responsible for the remaining two-thirds.

Through a *rapid* or *respiratory response*, changes in ventilation can promptly cause hydrogen ions to be excreted or retained by changing the concentration of components of the carbonic acid buffer system.

Renal mechanisms mediate a slower response to changes in the total body hydrogen ion load by causing net excretion or generation of hydrogen ions.

For the clinician, the carbonic acid system is the single most important buffer system, for two reasons. First, changes in respiratory rate permit the rapid excretion (or retention) of large quantities of hydrogen ions by changing the P_{CO_2}, which in turn affects the serum bicarbonate and pH. Because of the effect of ventilatory changes on its constituents, the carbonic acid buffer system is said to be open-ended.

Second, the carbonic acid system's components are easily measured. Although inferences concerning systemic acid–base balance can be made by analyzing any buffer system, ease of measurement makes the carbonic acid system the most attractive for clinical use. In fact, common clinical terminology relies exclusively on the carbonic acid system's components to define acid–base status.

PATHOPHYSIOLOGY

Pathologic processes can modify the body's acid–base equilibrium in two fundamental ways: Disease can either increase or decrease the body's soluble hydrogen ion activity (a metabolic disturbance), and disease can either increase or decrease ventilation (a respiratory disturbance).

The disruption of acid–base equilibrium by a single disease process is termed a *primary disturbance*. This disruption initiates a series of compensatory responses that tend to return the pH toward normal. The compensatory response rarely returns the pH to the normal range and never overshoots the normal range.

The body responds to a primary metabolic disturbance by adjusting the respiratory rate and, thus, the P_{CO_2} (*respiratory compensation*), and it responds to a primary respiratory disturbance by increasing or decreasing renal hydrogen ion excretion (*metabolic compensation*) (Table 165.1).

A disease process causing a single primary acid–base abnormality is termed a *simple acid–base disturbance*. When two or more primary acid–base abnormalities occur simultaneously, possibly as a result of more than one disease process, the abnormality is termed a *mixed acid–base disturbance*.

Although the degree and rapidity of compensatory responses to simple acid–base disturbances vary from patient to patient, empiric data have defined a range of what can be considered the expected compensatory response for each type of simple disturbance. Table 165.2 lists the anticipated compensatory responses for the different types of primary simple acid–base disturbances.[18] Patients with acid–base profiles falling outside the range for a simple acid–base disturbance with its anticipated compensation should be suspected of having a mixed disorder.

Tables 165.3 and 165.4 list the causes of the simple or mixed acid–base disturbances most common in the emergency department. The emergency physician must be able to recognize simple and mixed acid–base abnormalities to identify all the disease processes operative in a given patient, although their differentiation rarely is necessary for treatment of the hydrogen ion disturbance *per se*.

TABLE 165.1. Primary Disturbances and Compensatory Responses in Terms of Changes in Carbonic Acid Constituents

	Usual pH	Hydrogen Ion Concentration	Serum Bicarbonate (Measured as Total CO_2 Content)	P_{CO_2}
Metabolic acidosis	<7.38	Primary increase	Immediate decrease	Rapid compensatory decrease
Metabolic alkalosis	>7.42	Primary decrease	Immediate increase	Variable compensatory increase
Acute respiratory acidosis	<7.38	Secondary increase	Immediate small compensatory increase	Primary increase
Chronic respiratory acidosis	<7.38	Secondary increase	Slow larger compensatory increase	Primary increase
Acute respiratory alkalosis	>7.42	Secondary decrease	Immediate small compensatory decrease	Primary decrease
Chronic respiratory alkalosis	7.40–7.42	Secondary decrease	Slow larger compensatory decrease	Primary decrease

EMERGENCY DEPARTMENT EVALUATION AND MANAGEMENT

The physician often must begin the laboratory evaluation before completing the history and physical examination. Acid–base disturbances should be suspected in patients who appear critically ill, are experiencing extreme dyspnea, have an abnormal mental status, or complain of vomiting or diarrhea. Arterial blood gas and serum electrolyte determinations provide enough data for the initial metabolic assessment.

The physician should attempt to interpret acid–base abnormalities only after completing the initial evaluation and formulating a set of preliminary hypotheses about the most likely cause or causes. To identify acid–base abnormalities accurately, the physician should then ask three questions:

1. Does the patient have an acidemia or an alkalemia? *Acidemia* is defined as a pH less than 7.38, and *alkalemia* as a pH greater than 7.42. An *acidosis* is any process that causes acid to accumulate; an *alkalosis* is a process that causes hydrogen ion depletion. If the patient is acidemic, at least one of the processes present must be an acidosis.
2. Is the disturbance respiratory or metabolic? Look at the serum bicarbonate and arterial P_{CO_2} (Table 165.5).
3. Is the acid–base disturbance simple or mixed? When the appropriate formula (see Table 165.2) is applied, a significant deviation from the parameters expected for a simple disturbance indicates the presence of a mixed disorder.

TABLE 165.2. Formulas Describing Expected Compensatory Response to Primary Acid–Base Disturbances

SIMPLE METABOLIC ACIDOSIS
Predicted decreased (P_{CO_2}) mm Hg = 1.2 · $\Delta(HCO_3^-)$ mEq/L
Predicted P_{CO_2} mm Hg = 1.5 (HCO_3^-) mEq/L + 8 ± 2
Anticipated P_{CO_2} approximates last two digits of arterial pH
SIMPLE METABOLIC ALKALOSIS
Predicted increased $\Delta(P_{CO_2})$ mm Hg = 0.67 · $\Delta(HCO_3^-)$ mEq/L
SIMPLE ACUTE RESPIRATORY ACIDOSIS
Predicted decreased Δ(pH) units = 0.8 $\Delta(P_{CO_2})$ mm Hg
Predicted increased $\Delta(HCO_3^-)$ mEq/L = .1 $\Delta(P_{CO_2})$ mm Hg
SIMPLE CHRONIC RESPIRATORY ACIDOSIS
Predicted decreased Δ(pH) units = 0.3 · $\Delta(P_{CO_2})$ mm Hg
Predicted increased $\Delta(HCO_3^-)$ mEq/L = .35 $\Delta(P_{CO_2})$ mm Hg
SIMPLE ACUTE RESPIRATORY ALKALOSIS
Predicted increased Δ(pH) units = 0.8 · $\Delta(P_{CO_2})$ mm Hg
Predicted decreased $\Delta(HCO_3^-)$ mEq/L = .2 · $\Delta(P_{CO_2})$ mm Hg
SIMPLE CHRONIC RESPIRATORY ALKALOSIS
Predicted increased Δ(pH) units = 0.17 · $\Delta(P_{CO_2})$ mm Hg
Predicted decreased $\Delta(HCO_3^-)$ mEq/L = .5 · $\Delta(P_{CO_2})$ mm Hg

Simple Metabolic Acidosis

This is the most common acid–base disturbance in hospitalized patients and is often present in emergency department pa-

TABLE 165.3. Causes of Simple Acid–Base Disturbances

SIMPLE METABOLIC ACIDOSIS
Elevated Anion Gap
Diabetic ketoacidosis
Alcoholic ketoacidosis
Starvation
Lactic acidosis
Renal failure
Methanol, ethylene glycol
Normal Anion Gap
Renal tubular acidosis
Diarrhea
Early renal failure
Carbonic anhydrase inhibitor therapy
Hydronephrosis
SIMPLE METABOLIC ALKALOSIS
Vomiting/gastric suction
Volume depletion
Diuretic therapy
Corticosteroid therapy
RESPIRATORY ACIDOSIS
CNS lesion
Sedative therapy/overdose
Neuropathies
Myopathies
Chest wall abnormalities
Trauma
Kyphosis
Pleural disease
Obstructive airways disease
SIMPLE RESPIRATORY ALKALOSIS
Anxiety
Progesterone therapy/increased exogenous progesterone
Sympathomimetic therapy
Fever
Hyperthyroidism
Hypoxia
Liver disease

TABLE 165.4. Mixed Acid–Base Disturbances

METABOLIC ACIDOSIS–RESPIRATORY ALKALOSIS

Salicylate ingestion
Liver disease
Sepsis
Pulmonary embolism or pulmonary edema with hypotension
Pulmonary–renal syndrome

METABOLIC ACIDOSIS–RESPIRATORY ACIDOSIS

Cardiopulmonary arrest
Pulmonary edema
Drug overdose

METABOLIC ALKALOSIS–RESPIRATORY ALKALOSIS

Critical illness
Pregnancy
Mechanically ventilated chronic hypercapnea

METABOLIC ALKALOSIS–RESPIRATORY ACIDOSIS

Chronic hypercapnea with:
Diuretic overuse
Dehydration
Hypokalemia

METABOLIC ACIDOSIS–METABOLIC ALKALOSIS

Diarrhea/vomiting
Organic acidosis/vomiting
Metabolic acidosis with excessive bicarbonate administration

tients.[7] The diagnosis of the underlying cause is aided by considering the *anion gap,* defined as serum sodium − (chloride + CO_2 content).[25] The normal range for the anion gap has been reduced to 6 ± 3 mEq/L from its previously accepted range of 12 ± 4 mEq/L, because the normal range of the serum chloride is slightly higher with newer analytic methods.[24] This gap represents anions that are present in the serum but not routinely measured.[9] A normal anion gap in an acidotic patient indicates the presence of excess hydrochloric acid; an anion gap greater than 14 mEq/L may indicate an excess of organic acids.

Table 165.3 classifies the causes of metabolic acidosis according to the presence or absence of an abnormal anion gap.[8] The emergency physician is likely to evaluate many patients with an increased anion gap. When using the anion gap diagnostically, several factors must be kept in mind:

1. A moderate increase in the anion gap (12 to 20 mEq/L) is noted in many situations in which a metabolic acidosis is not present. These include dehydration, alkalosis, spurious laboratory values, and treatment with citrate, lactate, or certain antibiotics.
2. An anion gap greater than 25 mEq/L is seen only with lactic acidosis, ketoacidosis, and the toxin-associated acidoses.[11]
3. Common sense indicates that in a pure, high anion gap metabolic acidosis, the degree to which the anion gap exceeds normal limits should be matched by an equal decrease in the serum bicarbonate level. This does not occur for several reasons. Nonbicarbonate intracellular buffers accept hydrogen ions, blunting the decrease in serum bicarbonate. The longer the duration of acidosis, the greater the contribution from intracellular buffers.[24] The unmeasured anions associated with different acidoses have different volumes of distribution. The greater the added anion's capacity to diffuse into cells, the lower the drop in the serum bicarbonate and the lower the anion gap. Also, acidemia itself decreases the anion gap by decreasing the negative charge on serum proteins that makes a major contribution to the normal anion gap.[24] Finally, variable clearance rates of the added anions can alter the anion gap. If an organic anion is rapidly cleared, the anion gap will be lower for any degree of acidosis.[6]

TABLE 165.5. Respiratory vs. Metabolic Acidosis/Alkalosis

	pH	P_{CO_2}	HCO_3
Metabolic acidosis	Decrease	Decrease	Decrease
Metabolic alkalosis	Increase	Increase	Increase
Respiratory acidosis	Decrease	Increase	Increase
Respiratory alkalosis	Increase	Decrease	Decrease

Several conditions tend to lower the anion gap. These include hypoalbuminemia (there is a decrease in the anion gap of about 3 mEq/L for every 1-g/L decrease in the serum albumin), hypercalcemia, lithium intoxication, paraproteinemia secondary to multiple myeloma, and hypertriglyceridemia, which can spuriously elevate the serum chloride determination.[13] Organic acidoses in these patients may thus result in a smaller anion gap than otherwise predicted.[24]

The serum potassium level must be closely monitored in patients with suspected metabolic acidosis.[1] The emergency physician should perform a rapid assessment of the serum potassium level (by seeking electrocardiographic evidence of hyperkalemia) in patients with suspected acidosis. In general, the serum potassium level increases as the patient becomes more acidemic. This increase may result from the interaction of the excess hydrogen ion with intracellular buffer systems.[19] Animals made acidemic by the addition of mineral acids such as HCl experience a greater increase in serum potassium per unit decrease in pH than do those made acidemic by organic acids such as lactate.[19] There is no reliable formula by which to estimate the expected change in serum potassium arising from a given change in pH.[1]

Simple Metabolic Alkalosis

Metabolic alkalosis is a common condition that should be suspected in patients with very high values for the total serum CO_2 content. Most metabolic alkaloses are initiated by primary volume depletion, potassium depletion, or both. Patients with this disorder rarely present with a pH in the life-threatening range (greater than 7.60), but they may require vigorous fluid administration or potassium repletion.

The compensatory responses to metabolic alkalosis are weak. The ventilatory response (which would require hypoventilation to increase the P_{CO_2}) is limited by systemic defenses against hypoxia, and the kidney cannot alkalize the urine if the patient is hypokalemic or significantly volume-depleted.[21] Metabolic alkalosis, therefore, tends to be self-perpetuating if untreated.[18]

Primary Respiratory Disturbances

Primary respiratory abnormalities are classified as acute or chronic according to their duration. Because the renal compensatory process becomes effective only with the passage of time (48 to 72 hours), patients with primary acute respiratory disturbances have a pH further from normal than patients with chronic disturbances. In chronic respiratory alkalosis, alone among the primary acid–base disturbances, compensation can be so effective that the pH may return to normal.[2]

The immediate treatment of a severe primary respiratory disturbance is mechanical intervention, such as increasing ventilation for respiratory acidosis or adding dead space to the upper airway for respiratory alkalosis. Longer-term treatment involves identifying and treating the underlying cause. The physician must avoid treatment that suddenly normalizes the P_{CO_2} in a patient with chronic respiratory disturbance. In these instances (when renal compensatory mechanisms have previously normalized the pH), rapid normalization of the respiratory parameters risks a dangerous overshooting of normal pH.

Patients with respiratory acidosis require the most emergent intervention, because the P_{CO_2} can rise quickly to cause both a life-threatening acidosis and serious encephalopathy (CO_2 narcosis).[7] An arterial blood gas determination is mandatory for patients with abnormal mental status, especially if they manifest any clinical evidence of ventilatory dysfunction.

Acute respiratory alkalosis is common in emergency practice, particularly in the hypoxic or febrile patient. Although most cases of this acid–base abnormality do not require treatment, it should lead to a search for a specific underlying cause.

Mixed Acid–Base Disturbances

When a mixed disorder is present, the patient may be acidemic or alkalemic, or may have a normal pH. Any two primary acid–base disturbances (other than acute respiratory acidosis and acute respiratory alkalosis) can coexist. Knowing the patient's history permits the physician to make a more accurate assessment of the underlying processes.

Metabolic acidosis with respiratory acidosis or alkalosis is diagnosed when the P_{CO_2} deviates significantly from that predicted (see Table 165.2) in a simple metabolic acidosis. Combined metabolic acidosis and respiratory acidosis is seen in situations such as cardiac arrest or the postictal state, in which ventilation is inadequate for the degree of metabolic acidosis. Combined metabolic acidosis and respiratory alkalosis is commonly noted in salicylate poisoning, in which salicylate induces metabolic acidosis and also directly stimulates ventilation in excess of that induced by the acidosis.

One should be cautious in diagnosing mixed disturbances in patients with a rapidly changing clinical status, because the formulas for the expected response to simple metabolic acidosis were derived from P_{CO_2} levels in patients who had achieved a steady state. Thus, there is an increased chance of overdiagnosing a mixed disorder in many acutely ill patients.[18]

The combination of *metabolic acidosis and metabolic alkalosis* often manifests with a relatively normal pH and an anion gap elevation significantly exceeding the decrease in total CO_2 content.[20] A common setting for this mixed disturbance is the patient with alcoholic ketoacidosis who has been vomiting. If combined metabolic acidosis and metabolic alkalosis occurs in a patient with a normal anion gap acidosis, however, there is no anion gap elevation to serve as a marker for the disturbance.

An example would be a patient with severe diarrhea (metabolic acidosis caused by loss of sodium bicarbonate in the stool) associated with vomiting (metabolic alkalosis caused by loss of gastric hydrochloric acid). Unless this disturbance is suspected because of the clinical setting, the presence of two acid–base abnormalities may become evident only when one of the deficits is corrected. In the vomiting and diarrhea example, rapid volume correction with normal saline but without concomitant bicarbonate replacement might unmask the normal anion gap acidosis, with the serum bicarbonate decreasing as volume is restored.

CONTROVERSIES IN MANAGEMENT

Diabetic Ketoacidosis

Insulin administration, rehydration, and close monitoring (and replacement) of potassium are the mainstays of emergent therapy of diabetic ketoacidosis (DKA). Judicious administration of bicarbonate may be useful in patients with severe acidosis and cardiovascular compromise.[17] Although bicarbonate has traditionally been recommended for patients with DKA whose pH is below 7.1, even patients with a pH between 6.9 and 7.1 do not benefit from receiving bicarbonate.[14] Bicarbonate is still recommended in patients with a pH below 6.9, however.[16]

Adverse effects of excessive bicarbonate administration in DKA include tissue hypoxia from bicarbonate's leftward shifting of the oxyhemoglobin dissociation curve; augmentation of hepatic ketogenesis; hypertonicity and sodium overload; hypokalemia; and late alkalemia, when bicarbonate is regenerated from keto acids.[10] Some patients have reportedly deteriorated after aggressive bicarbonate treatment; this deterioration has been attributed to either a "paradoxical" central nervous system acidosis[12,14] that occurs after vigorous bicarbonate administration (which does not cross the blood–brain barrier) or cerebral edema from activation of a membrane Na^+–H^+ exchanger by the organic acidosis.[28]

Lactic Acidosis

This common acidosis is defined as a pH below 7.35 and a serum lactate level greater than 6 mmol/L, but because serum lactate measurements are unavailable to most emergency physicians, the diagnosis is often made by excluding other causes of acidemia in patients with a compatible history and clinical picture.[15] Most patients with lactic acidosis have some degree of tissue hypoxia leading to overproduction and underuse of tissue-generated lactate. The treatment of patients with lactic acidosis should center around improvement of tissue oxygenation and identification and treatment of its underlying cause.[2,26,27] A bicarbonate infusion of 1 to 2 mEq/kg may be considered as a temporizing measure in the presence of severe academia.

Cardiac Arrest

A common emergency department setting in which the use of bicarbonate is considered is cardiac arrest. Classically, the arrest victim would be expected to manifest a combined metabolic and respiratory acidosis, although the actual acid–base status varies depending on the cause and duration of the cardiac arrest. Neither animal nor human data have demonstrated the effectiveness of bicarbonate in increasing survival after cardiac arrest, and there have been reports of severe hyperosmolality, alkalosis, hypernatremia, and even pediatric intracerebral hemorrhage from injudicious bicarbonate administration.[3,4,22,23] The 1997 American Heart Association *Advanced Cardiac Life Support* guidelines[5] unequivocally support the use of bicarbonate in cardiac arrest associated with hyperkalemia, in tricyclic or phenobarbital overdose, and in patients with preexisting bicarbonate-responsive metabolic acidosis. Bicarbonate therapy may also be considered during prolonged cardiopulmonary resuscitation in which the patient has been adequately ventilated but is not responding to standard resuscitative measures. When bicarbonate is used, the initial dose should be 1 mEq/kg, with subsequent doses and timing determined by the arterial pH.

Toxin-Induced Acidosis

Methanol and ethylene glycol are two low-molecular-weight alcohols that can produce severe metabolic acidosis when ingested. If treatment begins promptly, recovery can be excellent despite severe acidemia. Parenteral sodium bicarbonate is an effective interim treatment. In contrast with other high anion gap acidoses, the organic anions generated in these poisonings cannot be converted back to bicarbonate by the liver. The physician should administer 1 mEq/kg of bicarbonate if the pH is below 7.20 and gauge the quantity and frequency of further doses by the response. Additional treatment includes administration of ethanol or 4-methylpyrazole to delay the formation of toxic intermediates, and hemodialysis for removal of native toxin.

Use of Alternative Alkalinizing Agents

A number of alternatives to bicarbonate for the treatment of metabolic acidosis have been investigated. These include dichloroacetate (a stimulator of the enzyme pyruvate dehydrogenase), Carbicarb (a mixture of sodium bicarbonate and sodium carbonate that generates less carbon dioxide during the buffering process), and THAM, a commercially available solution of tromethamine that buffers both metabolic and respiratory acids. None of these bicarbonate alternatives is currently recommended for emergency department use.[2]

COMMON PITFALLS

- Emergency physicians must be proficient in differentiating simple from mixed acid–base disturbances. They should search for and aggressively treat any underlying causes of significant disturbances. The limitations of the standard formulas that assist in the categorization of acid–base disturbances must be understood.
- There is significant controversy about the indications for and appropriate doses of sodium bicarbonate in several common emergency conditions. Bicarbonate should be used in hyperkalemia, toxin-induced metabolic acidosis, or severe DKA, and can be used for alkalization after appropriate overdoses. In selected cases of suspected lactic acidosis, bicarbonate can be given cautiously and with close monitoring. Bicarbonate should be avoided in hypoxic lactic acidosis. In metabolic acidosis of unknown cause, bicarbonate should not be withheld if there is cardiovascular compromise and a pH below 7.0.

References

1. Adrogue HJ, Ledeier ED, Suki WW, et al. Determinants of plasma potassium levels in DKA. *Medicine* 1986;65:165.
2. Adrogue HJ, Madias NE. Management of life-threatening acid–base disorders. *N Engl J Med* 1998;338:26-33.
3. Bishop RL, Weisfelt ML. Sodium bicarbonate administration during cardiac arrest. *JAMA* 1976;235:506.
4. Chazan JA, Stenson R, Kurland GS. The acidosis of cardiac arrest. *N Engl J Med* 1968;278:360.
5. Cummins Richard O. *Advanced cardiac life support*. Dallas: American Heart Association, 1997:7–15.
6. DiNubile MJ. The increment in the anion gap: overextension of a concept? *Lancet* 1988;2:951.
7. Dulfano MJ, Ishikawa S. Hypercapnia: mental changes and extrapulmonary complications. *Ann Intern Med* 1963;63:829.
8. Elkington JR. Clinical disorders of acid–base regulation. *Med Clin North Am* 1966;50:1325.
9. Emmet M, Narins RG. Clinical use of the anion gap. *Medicine* 1977;56:38.
10. Fleckman AM. DKA. *Endocrinol Metabol Clin North Am* 1993;22:181.
11. Gabow PA, Kaehny WD, Fennessey PV, et al. Diagnostic importance of an increased serum anion gap. *N Engl J Med* 1980;303:854.
12. Hale PJ, Crase J, Nattras M. Metabolic effects of bicarbonate in the treatment of DKA. *BMJ* 1984;289:1035.
13. Jurado RL, Del Rio C, Nassar G, et al. Low Anion Gap. *South Med J* 1998;91:624.
14. Kreisberg RA. DKA: new concepts and trends in pathogenesis and treatment. *Ann Intern Med* 1978;88:681.
15. Mizack B. Controversies in lactic acidosis. *JAMA* 1987;258:497.
16. Morris LR, Murphy MB, Kitabchi AZ. Bicarbonate therapy in severe DKA. *Ann Intern Med* 1986;105:836.
17. Narins RG, Cohen JJ. Bicarbonate therapy for organic acidosis: the care for its continued use. *Ann Intern Med* 1987;106:615.
18. Narins RG, Emmett M. Simple and mixed acid–base disorders: a practical approach. *Medicine* 1980;59:161.
19. Oster JR, Perex GO, Vaamonde CA. Relationship between blood pH, potassium, and phosphorus during acute metabolic acidosis. *Am J Physiol* 1978;135:F345.
20. Paulson WD. Anion gap—bicarbonate relation in DKA. *Am J Med* 1986;81:995.
21. Pierce NF, Fedson DS, Brighton KL, et al. The ventilatory response to acute acid–base deficit in humans. *Ann Intern Med* 1970;72:633.
22. Redding JS, Pearson JW. Resuscitation from ventricular fibrillation. *JAMA* 1968;203:93.
23. Redding JS, Pearson JW. Metabolic acidosis: a factor in cardiac resuscitation. *South Med J* 1967;601:926.
24. Salem MM, Mujais SK. Gaps in the anion gap. *Arch Intern Med* 1992;152:1625.
25. Smithline N, Gardner KD. Gaps—anionic and osmolal. *JAMA* 1976;236:1594.
26. Stacpoole PW. Lactic acidosis: the case against bicarbonate therapy. *Ann Intern Med* 1986;105:276.
27. Stacpoole PW. Lactic acidosis. *Endocrinol Metab Clin North Am* 1993;22:221.
28. Van der Meulen JA, Klip A, Grinsten S. Possible mechanism for cerebral edema in DKA. *Lancet* 1987;2:306.

CHAPTER 166
Diabetic Ketoacidosis

Micheal D. Rush and Robert A. Schwab

Diabetic ketoacidosis (DKA) is a syndrome of hyperglycemia, ketonemia, and acidosis resulting from absolute or relative insulin deficiency. It occurs most commonly in insulin-dependent diabetics, but it may also be seen in patients with non–insulin-dependent diabetes.[29] DKA is the presenting illness in approximately 15% to 26% of patients with newly diagnosed diabetes, particularly in those with type 1 diabetes.[7]

DKA is a common illness. According to 1990 Centers for Disease Control (CDC) surveillance data, DKA was a listed diagnosis on 104,000 hospital discharge summaries.[5] Precipitating factors include noncompliance with medication, infection, myocardial infarction, alcohol use, pregnancy, trauma, and emotional stress.[6] Inadequate diabetic education and training may be a significant contributing factor in patients with recurrent episodes of DKA. The overall mortality rate is about 5%; despite intensive research and advances in treatment, mortality rates have not declined significantly in the past 20 years.[3] Death may result from metabolic derangements attributable to DKA itself or to complications of treatment. Most often, however, death in DKA is due to associated concurrent illness.[3,15]

The pathophysiology of DKA involves physiologic derangements induced by insulin deficiency. Hyperglycemia occurs as a result of decreased peripheral use of glucose.

Catecholamines, cortisol, and growth hormone, released in response to the stress of precipitating illness, contribute to glucose overproduction.[18] In the absence of adequate insulin, however, glucose is unavailable as a substrate for cellular energy production, and changes in hepatic metabolism occur to produce alternative energy sources. Triglyceride synthesis is inhibited in favor of lipolysis, which produces the ketoacids acetoacetate (AcAc) and beta-hydroxybutyrate (BHBA). These ketoacids can be used as substrate by the brain and other tissues, but they cause ketonemia and metabolic acidosis.

The combination of hyperglycemia and ketoacidosis results in a hyperosmolar state leading to osmotic diuresis, volume depletion, and electrolyte losses, all of which contribute to the clinical picture of DKA.

CLINICAL PRESENTATION

The most common presenting signs and symptoms of DKA can be predicted on the basis of an understanding of the precipitating factors and pathophysiology of the disease. Early on, the clinical picture may be dominated by the underlying cause, such as symptoms of infection or pancreatitis. Most often, however, the metabolic derangements of DKA tend to obscure the precipitating factors.

Hyperglycemia leads to blurred vision, polyuria, polydipsia, and polyphagia; ketoacidosis causes nausea, vomiting, and the characteristic fruity odor of acetone on the breath. Respiratory compensation for the acidosis manifests initially as tachypnea, and results in Kussmaul breathing as acidosis becomes more severe. As the syndrome progresses, volume depletion becomes significant; patients commonly complain of dizziness and weakness, and manifest tachycardia, dry mucous membranes, and poor skin turgor. A full-blown shock picture can be seen in severe cases.

The presenting mental status correlates most closely with serum osmolality.[18] Roughly one-third of patients presents stuporous or comatose, one-third has normal mentation, and the remaining third is somewhere between these extremes. Hypothermia has been described in DKA and is frequently associated with an underlying infection and a higher mortality rate.[12] Abdominal pain and tenderness are common, and have been attributed to gastric distention or stretching of the liver capsule.[19] Appropriate treatment of the metabolic derangements usually leads to prompt resolution of the pain. Persistent pain should prompt a search for underlying abdominal pathology.

DIFFERENTIAL DIAGNOSIS

The differential diagnosis of DKA depends on the patient's presentation. In known diabetics presenting with changes in mental status, the primary diagnostic concern is distinguishing between hypoglycemic and hyperglycemic states, including DKA and hyperglycemic hyperosmolar nonketotic coma (HHNC). This distinction can be made rapidly using bedside glucose assessments, which should be done in all patients presenting with altered mental status.

HHNC generally occurs in older, non–insulin-dependent diabetic patients, and is associated with higher blood glucose levels and greater volume deficits than in DKA. Urine and serum ketone analysis may assist in differentiating between DKA and HHNC, but the distinction is not always clear initially. Significant ketosis may be the result of starvation, alcoholic ketoacidosis (AKA), or isopropyl alcohol ingestion, in addition to DKA. The history, coupled with a blood glucose determination, should assist in sorting through the diagnostic possibilities.

In most cases, a diagnosis is made based on arterial blood gas (ABG) analysis or electrolyte determinations, which demonstrate a metabolic acidosis with increased anion gap. The differential diagnosis includes toxin ingestion (methanol, ethylene glycol, or salicylates), uremia, lactic acidosis, or drug effect (iron, isoniazid, paraldehyde), in addition to AKA or DKA. A careful history and determination of glucose, electrolytes, blood urea nitrogen (BUN), creatinine, lactate, and specific toxin levels direct the clinician to the proper diagnosis.

EMERGENCY DEPARTMENT EVALUATION

Regardless of the patient's presentation, evaluation must begin with an assessment of airway, breathing, and circulation. Most patients with DKA maintain a patent airway; comatose patients, however, may require intubation for airway protection. Assessment of ventilation, oxygenation, and acid–base status commonly requires ABG analysis. Pulse oximetry should be utilized to ensure adequate oxygenation pending ABG results.

Supplemental oxygen should be administered if the saturation is low, or if oximetry is unavailable. The circulatory assessment reveals significant volume depletion in most cases; large-bore, peripheral venous access should be obtained, and volume resuscitation begun with normal saline. Cardiac monitoring and urinary catheter insertion should be considered for patients who appear significantly ill.

A bedside glucose determination should be done on all patients with altered mental status to determine the need for dextrose administration. Naloxone and thiamine can be administered as well, as indicated. Blood loss should be ruled out with a quantitative hemoglobin determination and stool analysis for occult blood. Urinalysis should be performed as soon as a specimen is available; urine dipsticks can detect glucosuria and ketonuria rapidly and accurately. Blood should be sent for glucose, electrolytes, BUN, and creatinine, in addition to the tests mentioned previously.

Once initial stabilization has been accomplished, the physician should elicit a thorough history and perform a careful physical examination, looking for precipitating causes. A detailed review of the timing and dosages of recent insulin administration, as well as a dietary history, are often revealing, as are symptoms identifying recent or intercurrent precipitating illness. Further laboratory evaluation should be guided by the findings of the history and physical examination.

The typical patient with DKA presents with hyperglycemia, glucosuria and ketonuria, and an elevated anion gap metabolic acidosis. A mildly elevated BUN and hematocrit are consistent with volume depletion, and electrolyte values may reflect volume depletion as well.

Many patients, however, do not present with this "typical" picture, and the clinician must recognize the possible variations in laboratory results in order not to miss the diagnosis. Although initial glucose levels in DKA average 600 mg/dL or more, marked hyperglycemia may be absent if urine flow is adequate to allow glucose to be excreted.[24] In addition, many diabetics are also hyperlipidemic, which may result in spurious lowering of glucose levels as well as falsely elevated or depressed electrolyte levels.[16]

The degree of acid–base disturbance depends somewhat on the patient's volume status. The classic elevated anion-gap acidosis results from an accumulation of organic acids and an increase in unmeasured anions such as AcAc and BHBA, which cannot be excreted as urine flow decreases. If fluid intake maintains adequate renal perfusion, however, ketoacids are excreted, and chloride is retained to compensate for loss of the bicarbonate buffer, leading to a hyperchloremic, non–anion-gap acidosis.[11,25] In some cases, when vomiting and volume depletion are severe, loss of hydrogen chloride from the stomach and aldosterone-mediated renal bicarbonate resorption can cause a hypochloremic metabolic alkalosis and can actually result in alkalemia.[13] The sum of these effects may be a mixed metabolic picture that obscures the diagnosis.

The absence of detectable ketonuria and ketonemia may also confound the physician. Despite consistent increases in blood ketoacid levels, the relative ratio of AcAc and BHBA, which are mutually interconvertible, depending on the patient's redox state, varies from patient to patient. Because the nitroprusside test for qualitative ketones in serum and urine detects AcAc but not BHBA, patients with a high BHBA/AcAc ratio may appear not to be ketotic, and the diagnosis of DKA may be missed.[22]

EMERGENCY DEPARTMENT MANAGEMENT

Once the diagnosis is established, treatment requires correction of hypovolemia, reversal of ketoacid production, enhancement of glucose and ketoacid metabolism, replacement of electrolyte losses, and treatment of precipitating causes. Normalization of the metabolic state should occur gradually to avoid complications such as volume overload, hypoglycemia, hypokalemia, and cerebral edema.[24]

Volume replacement should begin as soon as hypovolemia is recognized. Fluid resuscitation should thus be underway before a definitive diagnosis is established. Fluid deficits in DKA average 5 L[28]; normal saline effectively restores intravascular volume while avoiding a rapid fall in extracellular osmolality. The initial rate of infusion should be rapid, but moderate rates of infusion (500 mL/h) appear to allow metabolic acidosis to be corrected more rapidly than higher rates (1 L/h).[1]

Giving smaller volumes of bicarbonate-free solutions tends to lessen the dilutional effect on existing bicarbonate and avoids excessive washout of ketone bodies, which, if retained, are metabolized to bicarbonate in the presence of insulin. An initial rate of 500 mL/h for 4 hours, followed by 250 mL/h for the next 4 hours, has been shown to be effective in patients without extreme volume deficit.[1] Ultimately, the initial infusion rate is dictated by the patient's hemodynamic stability and response to therapy, as reflected by urine output. Decisions to change to half-normal saline may be left to the admitting physician.

Volume replacement lowers serum glucose and ketone levels and helps correct metabolic acidosis, but insulin must be given for ketogenesis to be reversed, for ketone bodies to be metabolized back to bicarbonate, and for glucose to be utilized as a substrate for cellular energy production. Treatment should begin with a bolus dose of regular insulin, 0.1 U/g. A subsequent continuous infusion of 0.1 U/kg/h lowers serum glucose concentrations reliably and predictably, is as effective as high-dose insulin regimens in decreasing serum glucose and ketone body concentrations, and carries a lesser risk of hypokalemia and hypoglycemia. Continuous intravenous infusion achieves effective steady-state concentrations of insulin more reliably than does intermittent bolus therapy.[27] Intramuscular and subcutaneous injections are not recommended in volume-depleted patients.[9,17,20]

The osmotic diuresis associated with hyperglycemia produces clinically significant deficits in total body potassium, sodium, phosphate, and bicarbonate. Acidosis, insulin deficiency, and hyperosmolality all shift potassium and phosphate extracellularly, often masking the total body deficits.[2] Whether the initial serum potassium is high, normal, or low, all patients in DKA require potassium replacement. Patients whose potassium levels are elevated initially should receive replacement when the serum potassium level falls to 5. Patients with normal or low serum potassium levels should receive replacement as soon as urine output is confirmed. The administration of fluids and insulin, as well as the correction of acidosis, tend to lower the serum potassium level, placing patients with initially low serum potassium levels at considerable risk for respiratory arrest and cardiac dysrhythmias. An infusion rate of 10 to 40 mEq/h can substantially correct a total body deficit of 300 to 600 mEq within 24 hours.

Most patients in DKA present with hyperphosphatemia, despite total body phosphate depletion.[30] With appropriate restoration of volume and administration of insulin, phosphate levels fall, reaching a nadir 24 to 48 hours after the initiation of insulin therapy. Phosphate administration can be associated with undesirable side effects, such as hypocalcemia, and, more importantly, has not been shown to affect the outcome of patients with DKA.[8,30] Phosphate replacement should be reserved for patients with severe hypophosphatemia, and is not routinely indicated in the initial management of DKA.

Sodium deficits, although significant, are generally corrected by the administration of normal saline. The use of bicarbonate to correct base deficit is controversial. Although systemic acidosis has deleterious effects on cellular function throughout the body, it has been demonstrated that, during DKA, the central nervous system maintains a higher pH than the rest of the body, through a poorly understood buffering mechanism.[23] The administration of bicarbonate increases systemic levels of CO_2, which diffuses freely across the blood–brain barrier and combines with water to form carbonic acid. Because bicarbonate crosses the blood–brain barrier much less readily than does CO_2, cerebrospinal fluid (CSF) acidosis ensues.

Other cellular membranes exhibit this differential permeability to CO_2 and bicarbonate as well, suggesting that bicarbonate administration may cause a paradoxical intracellular and CSF acidosis. Although this paradoxical acidosis has never been demonstrated in clinical investigations involving patients in DKA, it has been shown that the administration of bicarbonate confers no therapeutic benefit in patients with a presenting pH of 6.9 or greater, and may actually increase ketone-body formation or delay the metabolism of ketoacids to bicarbonate.[10,14,23,26]

Other potential hazards of bicarbonate therapy include tissue hypoxia through shifting of the oxyhemoglobin dissociation curve, hypokalemia, and rebound alkalosis. Overall, it appears that bicarbonate administration, although it may transiently increase serum pH, does not improve clinical outcome and may actually be deleterious in the patient with DKA. Adjunctive bicarbonate therapy should be considered only for those patients presenting with a pH less than 6.9, in order to prevent complications of decreased cardiac contractility, cardiac dysrhythmias, and peripheral vasodilatation commonly associated with severe acidemia.

Initially, the patient's blood glucose should be monitored at least every 1 to 2 hours during treatment. Serum electrolytes should also be monitored closely to ensure that metabolic derangements are being corrected. A fall in blood glucose of 75 to 100 mg/dL/h is a reasonable goal, and insulin infusions should be adjusted accordingly. The serum potassium level generally reaches a minimum 1 to 4 hours after the initiation of therapy.[2] Although ABG measurement may be necessary to diagnose mixed acid–base disorders in DKA, repeated arterial sampling may not be necessary, because venous pH correlates well with arterial values. Many patients can be followed using venous samples alone.[4]

Ketone monitoring is not helpful and may demonstrate a paradoxical increase in quantitative ketones despite clinical improvement, which occurs as BHBA is oxidized to AcAc (with which nitroprusside reacts) in the presence of insulin.[22] While initial blood gas measurement may be necessary to diagnose coexisting acid–base disorders in DKA, repeated arterial sampling is usually unnecessary.[4] Patients who present with hemodynamic instability or hypokalemia should have continuous cardiac monitoring. Urinary output should be monitored closely. A careful search for underlying precipitating factors should be undertaken, with appropriate diagnostic studies utilized as indicated. The possibility of silent myocardial infarction should be considered in patients without an obvious precipitating cause.

Insulin therapy must be continued for ketonemia and acidemia to be corrected. To avoid hypoglycemia and to reduce osmotic gradients between blood and brain, 5% dextrose should be added to the intravenous infusion (usually half-normal saline at this point) when the blood glucose level reaches 250 mg/dL.[2] The insulin infusion also is reduced by half at this point.

Complications of therapy for DKA include hypoglycemia,[21] hypokalemia, and hypophosphatemia, as well as fluid overload and cerebral edema. Careful electrolyte and fluid monitoring and the use of 5% dextrose, as described, reduce the risk of these complications substantially. Vascular thrombosis, rhabdomyolysis, and disseminated intravascular coagulation are rare but often fatal complications of DKA.[3,15,30]

DISPOSITION

Proper management of DKA requires careful monitoring of vital signs and fluid status, as well as repeated assessment of pH, glucose, and electrolytes. The therapeutic plan may have to be altered frequently, especially in the early phase of treatment, and complications tend to occur rapidly, with potentially severe consequences. For these reasons, many patients with DKA require admission to an intensive care setting.

Specialty ward units with monitoring capability and low patient-to-nurse ratios have also been used safely and effectively.[15] These units provide a cost-effective alternative to the intensive care unit for patients who do not require cardiorespiratory support. In very unusual circumstances, patients may be treated in the emergency department and released. Such patients should have a mild presentation that responds rapidly to therapy; have no precipitating illness requiring hospitalization; have normal vital signs, pH, and anion gap; have a blood glucose level less than 300 mg/dL and a bicarbonate level greater than 15 mEq/L; should be taking oral fluids well; should be reliable and have good family support; and should have follow-up scheduled with their primary physician within 24 hours.

If needed, transfer to another facility should occur only after vital signs have been stabilized and volume resuscitation is well underway. Personnel capable of providing advanced life support should accompany the patient, who should have continuous cardiac monitoring. The transferring physician should provide a detailed flowsheet of fluid and electrolyte therapy, in addition to the usual transfer documentation.

COMMON PITFALLS

- Failure to administer dextrose to diabetic patients presenting in coma
- Failure to diagnose DKA in patients who are euglycemic, have a negative nitroprusside test, or do not present with a high anion-gap acidosis
- Failure to initiate potassium replacement in patients with normal or high initial potassium levels
- Failure to maintain insulin infusion until the anion gap is normal
- Failure to monitor glucose frequently and add dextrose to the infusion when the blood glucose level reaches 250 mg/dL
- Failure to search diligently for precipitating causes

References

1. Adrogue HJ, Barrero J, Eknoyan G. Salutary effects of modest fluid replacement in the treatment of adults with DKA. *JAMA* 1989;262:2108.
2. Alberti KGMM, Hockaday TDR. Diabetic coma: a reappraisal after 5 years. *J Clin Endocrinol Metab* 1977;6:421.
3. Basu A, Close CF, Jenkins D, et al. Persisting mortality in DKA. *Diabet Med* 1993;10:282.
4. Brandenburg MA, Dire DJ. Comparison of arterial and venous blood gas values in the initial emergency department evaluation of patients with diabetic ketoacidosis. *Ann Emerg Med* 1998;31:459–465.
5. Centers for Disease Control. *Diabetes surveillance, 1993.* Atlanta: U.S. Department of Health and Human Services, Public Health Service, 1993.
6. Davoren PM, Bowen KM. Precipitating factors in DKA [Letter]. *Med J Aust* 1991;154:855.
7. Faich GA, Fishbein HA, Ellis SE. The epidemiology of diabetic acidosis: a population-based study. *Am J Epidemiol* 1983;117:551.
8. Fisher JN, Kitabchi AE. A randomized study of phosphate therapy in the treatment of diabetic ketoacidosis. *J Clin Endocrinol Metab* 1983;57:177–180.
9. Fisher JN, Shahshahani MN, Kitabchi AE. Diabetic ketoacidosis: low-dose insulin therapy by various routes. *N Engl J Med* 1977;297:238–241.
10. Gamba G, Oseguera J, Castrejon M, et al. Bicarbonate therapy in severe diabetic ketoacidosis. A double blind, randomized, placebo controlled trial. *Rev Invest Clin* 1991;43:234–238.
11. Gamblin GT, Ashburn RW, Kemp DG, et al. DKA presenting with a normal anion gap. *Am J Med* 1986;80:758.
12. Guerin JM, Meyer FP, Segrestaa JM. Hypothermia in diabetic ketoacidosis. *Diabetes Care* 1987;10:801–802.
13. Goldman JM, Chiriboga M. DKA with alkalemia. *J Emerg Med* 1989;7:369.
14. Hale PJ, Crase J, Nattrass M. Metabolic effects of bicarbonate in the treatment of diabetic ketoacidosis. *BMJ* 1984;289:1035–1038.
15. Hamblin PS, Topliss DJ, Chosich N, et al. Deaths associated with DKA and hyperosmolar coma, 1973–1988. *Med J Aust* 1989;151:439.
16. Kaminska ES, Pourmotabbed G. Spurious laboratory values in DKA and hyperlipidemia. *Am J Emerg Med* 1993;11:77.
17. Kitabchi AE, Ayyagari V, Guerra SMO, Medical House Staff. The efficacy of low-dose versus conventional therapy of insulin for treatment of diabetic ketoacidosis. *Ann Intern Med* 1976;84:633–638.
18. Kitabchi AE, Murphy MB. DKA and hyperosmolar hyperglycemic nonketotic coma. *Med Clin North Am* 1988;72:1545.
19. Knight AH, Williams DN, Ellis G, et al. Significance of hyperamylasaemia and abdominal pain in DKA. *BMJ* 1973;3:128.
20. Luzi L, Barret EJ, Groop LC, et al. Metabolic effects of low-dose insulin therapy on glucose metabolism in diabetic ketoacidosis. *Diabetes* 1988;37: 147–1477.
21. Malone ML, Klos SE, Gennis VM, et al. Frequent hypoglycemic episodes in the treatment of patients with DKA. *Arch Intern Med* 1992;152:1470.
22. Marliss EB, Ohman JL, Aoki TT, et al. Altered redox state obscuring ketoacidosis in diabetic patients with lactic acidosis. *N Engl J Med* 1970;283:978.
23. Morris LR, Murphy MB, Kitabchi AE. Bicarbonate therapy in severe DKA. *Ann Intern Med* 1986;105:836.
24. Munro JF, Campbell IW, McCuish AC, et al. Euglycemic diabetic ketoacidosis. *BMJ* 1973;2:578.
25. Oh MS, Carroll HJ, Goldstein DA, et al. Hyperchloremic acidosis during the recovery phase of diabetic acidosis. *Ann Intern Med* 1978;89:925.
26. Okuda Y, Adrogue HJ, Field JB, et al. Counterproductive effects of sodium bicarbonate in diabetic ketoacidosis. *J Clin Endocrinol Metab* 1996;81:314–320.
27. Page MM, Alberti KGMM, Greenwood R, et al. Treatment of diabetic coma with continuous low-dose infusion of insulin. *BMJ* 1974;2:687.
28. Waldhausl W, Kleinberger G, Korn A, et al. Severe hyperglycemia: effects of rehydration on endocrine derangements and blood glucose concentration. *Diabetes* 1979;28:577.
29. Westphal SA. The occurrence of diabetic ketoacidosis in non-insulin dependent diabetes and newly diagnosed diabetic adults. *Am J Med* 1996;101:19–24.
30. Wilson HK, Keuer SP, Lea AS, et al. Phosphate therapy in DKA. *Arch Intern Med* 1982;142:517.

CHAPTER 167

Hyperosmolar Hyperglycemic Nonketotic Coma

Dana Pope and Leslie S. Zun

Hyperosmolar hyperglycemic nonketotic coma (HHNC) is a syndrome of profound dehydration that develops insidiously as a consequence of prolonged osmotic diuresis. Also known as the hyperglycemic nonketotic syndrome, it is commonly defined by a plasma osmolarity greater than 350 mOsmol/kg water, a serum glucose concentration greater than 600 mg/dL, and an absence of ketoacidosis in a patient with a depressed level of consciousness.[1,9,13,17] In the following discussion, a number of caveats should be kept in mind. The range of serum glucose values seen in HHNC is wide, usually far wider than that seen with diabetic ketoacidosis (DKA).[14] The absence of ketoacidosis or ketonuria is not absolute, and ketones may be present in small amounts.[1,12,16,25] The patient may not actually be comatose but is more likely to be drowsy or confused.[4] HHNC is associated with a high mortality[1,4,9,14] and should be considered a medical emergency.

CLINICAL SETTING

The patient most at risk for developing HHNC is elderly, with an average age of about 60 years.[1,4,8,14,17] The age range is wide, however, and case reports appear in the pediatric literature.[14,20,21]

Usually a diabetogenic stress is implicated in precipitating the hyperosmolar state. Chronic renal insufficiency, pneumonia, gram-negative sepsis, myocardial infarction, pancreatitis, and gastrointestinal bleeding are frequently associated with HHNC and contribute to its high mortality. The following have also been implicated in the development of HHNC: thiazide diuretics, corticosteroids, phenytoin, propranolol, chlorthalidone, furosemide, ethacrynic acid, diazoxide, cimetidine, chlorpromazine, *l*-asparaginase, immunosuppressive agents, loxapine, hyperalimentation, peritoneal dialysis and hemodialysis, cardiac surgery, stroke, severe burns, pancreatitis, and heat stroke.[1,2,4,6,9,16]

There is no history of diabetes mellitus in two-thirds of patients who develop HHNC.[1,9] The remaining one-third generally have a history of type II, or non–insulin-dependent, diabetes; a few patients are insulin dependent. On recovery, most patients prove to have mild type II diabetes.[4,13]

Patients with HHNC often have severe concurrent illnesses, which are commonly the precipitating cause of HHNC.[1]

HHNC has a reputation for being underrecognized. The high mortality rate of HHNC (20% to 60%)[1,9,14] is variously explained by delay in establishing the diagnosis,[13] by failure to treat aggressively from the outset,[1] and by the high incidence of serious underlying disease.[1,13]

Pancreatic endocrine insufficiency is thought to be an age-related process of progressive cell senescence, the effect of which is exaggerated by circulating catecholamines and adrenergic stimulation at the time of metabolic stress, such as trauma or infection. Furthermore, peripheral resistance to insulin has been demonstrated in HHNC, and hypertonicity itself inhibits secretion of pancreatic insulin.[7,19] With a decline in renal function, due to age or dehydration, the ability to excrete glucose is impaired and severe hyperglycemia may occur.[5] Continued osmotic diuresis causes progressive dehydration, which further impairs pancreatic beta-cell function, further decreases glomerular filtration rate, and sets in motion a worsening spiral of metabolic events.

To conceptualize the events that occur in response to hyperglycemic hypertonicity and dehydration due to osmotic diuresis, it is helpful to review the distribution of body water in the intracellular and extracellular spaces. Total body water is about 60% of normal body weight (perhaps 50% in the elderly).[23] Intracellular fluid comprises two-thirds of total body water, and extracellular fluid, one-third. The extracellular space is further subdivided into interstitial fluid, comprising three-fourths of the extracellular space, and plasma, occupying the remaining one-fourth. Because water is freely permeable between the various compartments, total solute concentration in all of the compartments is identical (normal osmolarity is 280 to 300 mOsmol/kg water; however, the solute composition is different).

Extracellular solute is composed primarily of sodium and its anions, and intracellular solute is composed primarily of potassium, magnesium, and phosphate. Unlike a substance such as urea, which is freely permeable across cell membranes and does not create an osmotic gradient, glucose is located only in the extracellular space and is osmotically active. Thus, with hyperglycemia, water moves from the intracellular to the extracellular space. The expanded extracellular space may be reflected in a dilution of the serum sodium concentration but without actual hypotonicity.[14] The serum sodium concentration typically falls 1.3 to 1.6 mEq/L for every 100-mg/dL rise of the serum glucose level above normal.[7] Sodium is also lost through osmotic diuresis as tubular sodium reabsorption is inhibited, and water is lost in greater amounts than sodium, further increasing the tonicity of the extracellular space and drawing free water from the intracellular space to compensate.[14]

Patients presenting with HHNC may have a slight degree of ketosis. In fact, the wide spectrum of glucose and ketoacid concentrations that is seen in practice blurs the distinction between DKA and HHNC.[1,12,24] The absence of ketosis is most often explained by the production of insulin sufficient to inhibit the release of free fatty acid from adipose tissue, yet insufficient to cause glucose uptake by cells.[1,10,14] This concept has been questioned. Investigators have found no difference in initial plasma insulin levels between patients with HHNC and DKA. The lack of ketosis has also been explained by the effect of hyperosmolarity itself in suppressing ketone formation and by the finding of lower levels of lipolytic hormones (i.e., growth hormone and cortisol) in HHNC patients compared with those with DKA.[9]

CLINICAL PRESENTATION

Most patients who develop HHNC experience polyuria and polydipsia for days or weeks before seeking medical attention. In these patients, insidious dehydration progresses until mental status is altered. Unresponsiveness has been cited as the most common reason patients are brought for medical attention.[1] In contrast, patients with DKA rapidly develop signs and symptoms from acidosis, bringing them to medical attention before dehydration becomes as severe. One study found that the average duration of symptoms before presentation was 12 days for HHNC and 3 days for DKA.[9]

A few notes of caution are in order when these patients are to be assessed. The standard signs of dehydration (poor skin turgor, dry mucous membranes) are not reliable in elderly patients, and it is not always possible to estimate fluid deficits by clinical or laboratory findings. Neither the serum sodium nor the plasma osmolarity has been found to correlate with the volume of replacement fluid required by patients with HHNC.[1] The advanced state of dehydration may be underestimated if urine output is maintained by osmotic diuresis.[16] On the other hand, renal dysfunction due to diabetic nephrosclerosis or other causes may prevent polyuria from occurring, even with progressively increasing levels of serum glucose.[5]

The severity of mental status changes in HHNC has been found to correlate with the degree of hyperosmolarity and the rate at which hyperosmolarity develops.[8,17,18] In addition to altered mental status, HHNC can cause a variety of other neurologic findings: seizures, Babinski reflexes, bilateral or unilateral focal deficits, aphasia, muscle fasciculations, central hyperthermia, hemianopsia, nystagmus, visual hallucinations, visual loss, acute quadriplegia, acute urinary retention, and severe dysphagia.[5,11,16]

As mentioned earlier, HHNC may be found in patients who

present with a number of serious associated illnesses, the most frequent being chronic renal insufficiency, pneumonia, gastrointestinal hemorrhage, and gram-negative sepsis.[1]

DIFFERENTIAL DIAGNOSIS

The differential diagnosis of HHNC includes DKA; other causes of altered mental status, such as hepatic failure, uremia, cerebrovascular accident, and drug ingestion; and other causes of severe dehydration.

In patients with altered mental status, early diagnosis requires a high index of suspicion. Blood glucose measurement must be performed routinely and immediately in all patients with altered mental status to identify hypoglycemia or hyperglycemia. Patients with DKA often display Kussmaul respirations, and the fruity odor of acetone may be detected on the breath. An elevated anion-gap acidosis, ketosis, and mild-to-marked hyperglycemia are diagnostic. Lactic acidosis is often suspected when patients are gravely ill and display signs of shock. Blood pH determination reveals severe metabolic acidosis, and the anion-gap and lactic acid levels are elevated.

EMERGENCY DEPARTMENT EVALUATION

Basic laboratory evaluation for a patient suspected of having HHNC should include determination of levels of serum electrolytes, glucose, blood urea nitrogen, and creatinine; a complete blood cell count; urinalysis; and arterial blood gas analysis. A search should be made for serious underlying illness. A chest radiograph, electrocardiogram, blood and urine cultures, serum amylase value, liver enzyme studies, coagulation studies, and, in some cases, cardiac enzyme tests should be ordered.

The blood glucose concentration in HHNC is typically greater than 600 mg/dL and may be as high as 4800 mg/dL, with average values of about 1000 mg/dL.[8,9,14,17] Caution must be exercised in the interpretation of rapid fingerstick readings when the blood sugar concentration is this high.[9]

Serum sodium and potassium concentrations may be low, normal, or high, and the values do not reflect total body losses.[17] If the serum sodium concentration initially is not low, but normal or elevated, significant water loss can be assumed to have occurred.[14] Potassium depletion is the rule, and profound deficits (on the order of 400 to 1000 mEq) may be encountered. If the initial serum potassium concentration is low, profound total body potassium depletion is undoubtedly present.[17]

All patients with HHNC are initially azotemic due to both prerenal and renal causes.[17] The blood urea nitrogen–creatinine ratio may exceed 30:1.[14] In one series, the average initial blood urea nitrogen and creatinine values were 87 mg/dL and 5.5 mg/dL, respectively. After treatment, the average values had fallen to 24 mg/dL and 2.0 mg/dL, respectively.[1]

The serum osmolarity can be calculated using the following formula:

$$\text{Osmolarity (mOsmol/kg water)} = 2(\text{serum Na}) + (\text{blood glucose})/18 + (\text{blood urea nitrogen})/2.8$$

Although the measured and calculated osmolarity values follow similar trends, there is not always a reliable correspondence between the values.[8,22]

Because urea is freely permeable across cell membranes, it does not create an osmotic gradient between the intracellular and extracellular spaces. The *effective* osmolarity should also be calculated (by excluding the blood urea nitrogen value from the equation), because azotemia may mask actual hypotonicity of the extracellular fluid. If a patient presents with hyperglycemia and a normal or low effective plasma osmolarity, it is potentially dangerous to administer hypotonic fluids or insulin, because lowering the tonicity of the extracellular fluid too rapidly might lead to cerebral edema.[14]

About half of patients with HHNC have a mild metabolic acidosis, with an anion gap about twice normal.[1] Various explanations of the acidosis are offered: accumulation of lactic acid or β-hydroxybutyric acid (not measured by Acetest or Ketostix tests) or acute or chronic renal insufficiency with accumulation of acid metabolites.

The complete blood cell count may show an elevated white blood cell count suggestive of a serious underlying infection. Because of profound dehydration, hemoconcentration can be expected to elevate the hemoglobin and hematocrit, so a patient with an initially normal hematocrit should be suspected of being anemic.[17]

The urinalysis may show only modest glycosuria, and ketonuria need not be absent to make the diagnosis of HHNC.[17]

EMERGENCY DEPARTMENT MANAGEMENT

The first priority in the treatment of HHNC is to replace volume (sodium) deficits, then to correct hyperosmolarity, and, finally, to manage any underlying illness.

Patients who are hypotensive or who have signs of shock need immediate fluid resuscitation with normal saline.[10,17] Because average fluid deficits are on the order of 9 to 12 L, it is reasonable to begin emergency treatment of all HHNC patients with normal saline. Central venous pressure monitoring should be considered.[13,17] One to 2 L of normal saline should be infused rapidly until the patient's blood pressure and urine output are acceptable or the central venous pressure begins to rise. It is then reasonable to switch to 0.5 normal saline, with the goal of replacing half of the estimated volume deficit during the first 12 hours and the remaining estimated deficit during the second 12 hours.[1]

Because all patients with HHNC have total body potassium deficits, potassium should be administered as soon as it is certain that the patient is neither hyperkalemic nor oliguric. An intravenous infusion of about 10 mEq/h may be begun even prior to insulin therapy.[3,17]

The use of insulin in the initial management of HHNC may not be necessary.[13,25] West and colleagues[25] have shown that blood glucose levels decrease by about 25% because of dilution from fluid replacement alone. After volume status has improved, the remaining hyperglycemia may resolve through the metabolism and renal excretion of excess glucose. Insulin should be given, however, if the patient is acidotic, hyperkalemic, or in renal failure.

When insulin is given for HHNC, a low-dose regimen is appropriate: A reasonable approach is to give 0.15 U of regular insulin per kilogram of body weight intravenously as an initial bolus, followed by a continuous intravenous infusion of about 0.1 U/kg/h. This therapy is stopped when the blood glucose concentration has fallen to about 250 mg/dL or the osmolarity has reached 315 mOsmol/kg water.[10] At this point, 5% dextrose should be added to the infusion to avoid hypoglycemia. Another suggested insulin regimen is 14 to 20 U of regular insulin intramuscularly, followed by 5 U intramuscularly every hour until the blood glucose level is about 300 mg/dL.[17]

If fluid resuscitation does not improve the urine output, treatment with furosemide should be initiated after making certain that fluid volume has been restored. Initial management may also involve empiric phosphate repletion, anticoagulation with subcutaneous heparin, and broad-spectrum antibiotic prophylaxis.[13,15,17]

DISPOSITION

All patients with HHNC should be admitted to an intensive care setting. Because of the need for immediate and closely monitored treatment for at least the first 24 hours, it is usually preferable to avoid transfer to another facility until after fluid deficits and hyperosmolarity have been corrected and treatment for any serious underlying illness has been initiated.

COMMON PITFALLS

- Measuring the blood glucose level in all patients with new neurologic abnormalities will avoid a misdiagnosis of cerebrovascular accident and a potentially lethal delay in proper treatment.
- Because there is at least a theoretical concern that treatment of HHNC with hypotonic fluids can cause cerebral edema, it is safest to initiate therapy with normal saline while monitoring central venous pressure.[11,13,17]
- Giving insulin before fluid deficits are restored may decrease the hypertonicity of the extracellular fluid abruptly and place the patient at risk for cerebral edema, systemic hypoperfusion, and cerebral infarction.[1,5] Initial therapy should be consistent with the degree of hyperglycemia and the calculated effective osmolarity. Iatrogenic hypokalemia may result from insulin therapy if potassium replacement is not adequate and the serum potassium level carefully monitored.[9,17]
- Phenytoin should not be used in treating seizures associated with HHNC. It is ineffective in this setting and inhibits the release of endogenous insulin.[17]

References

1. Arieff AI, Carroll HJ. Nonketotic hyperosmolar coma with hyperglycemia: clinical features, pathophysiology, renal function, acid–base balance, plasma–cerebrospinal fluid equilibria and the effects of therapy in 37 cases. *Medicine* 1972;51:73.
2. Asplund K, Eriksson S, Hagg E, et al. Hyperosmolar nonketotic coma in diabetic stroke patients. *Acta Med Scand* 1982;212:407.
3. Bendezu R, Wieland RG, Furst BH, et al. Experience with low-dose insulin infusion in diabetic ketoacidosis and diabetic hyperosmolarity. *Arch Intern Med* 1978;138:60.
4. Bivans BA, Hyde GL, Sachatello CR, et al. Physiopathology and management of hyperosmolar hyperglycemic nonketotic dehydration. *Surg Gynecol Obstet* 1982;154:534.
5. Cahill GF. Hyperglycemic hyperosmolar coma: a syndrome almost unique to the elderly. *J Am Geriatr Soc* 1983;31:103.
6. Dibendetto RJ, Crocco JA, Soscia JL. Hyperglycemic nonketotic coma. *Arch Intern Med* 1965;116:74.
7. Feig PU, McCurdy DK. The hypertonic state. *N Engl J Med* 1977;297:1444.
8. Fulop M, Rosenblatt A, Kreitzer SM, et al. Hyperosmolar nature of diabetic coma. *Diabetes* 1975;24:594.
9. Gerich JE, Martin MM, Recant L. Clinical and metabolic characteristics of hyperosmolar nonketotic coma. *Diabetes* 1971;20:228.
10. Kitabchi AE, Matter R, Murphy MD. Optimal insulin delivery in diabetic ketoacidosis (DKA) and hyperglycemic hyperosmolar nonketotic coma (HHNC). *Diabetes Care* 1982;5[Suppl 1]:78.
11. Maccario M, Messis CP. Cerebral edema complicating treated nonketotic hyperglycemia. *Lancet* 1969;2:352.
12. Malchoft CD, Pohl SL, Kaiser DL, et al. Determinants of glucose and ketoacid concentrations in acutely hyperglycemic diabetic patients. *Am J Med* 1984;77:275.
13. Mather HM. Management of hyperosmolar coma. *J R Soc Med* 1980;73:145.
14. McCurdy DK. Hyperosmolar hyperglycemic nonketotic diabetic coma. *Med Clin North Am* 1970;54(3):683.
15. McCurdy DK, Feig PU. Hyperosmolar coma. *N Engl J Med* 1977;15:855.
16. Podolsky S. Hyperosmolar nonketotic coma; death can be prevented. *Geriatrics* 1979;70:29.
17. Podolsky S. Hyperosmolar nonketotic coma in the elderly diabetic. *Med Clin North Am* 1976;4:815.
18. Popli S, Leehey DJ, Daugirdas JT, et al. Asymptomatic, nonketotic, severe hyperglycemia with hyponatremia. *Arch Intern Med* 1990;150:1962.
19. Rosenthal NR, Barrett EJ. An assessment of insulin action in hyperosmolar hyperglycemic nonketotic diabetic patients. *J Clin Endocrinol Metab* 1985;60:607.
20. Rubin HM, Kramer R, Drash A. Hyperosmolarity complicating diabetes mellitus in childhood. *J Pediatr* 1969;74:177.
21. Stevenson RE, Bowyer FP. Hyperglycemia with hyperosmolar dehydration in nondiabetic infants. *J Pediatr* 1970;77:818.
22. Tomkins AM, Dormandy TL. Osmolal pattern during recovery from diabetic coma. *Lancet* 1971;1:952.
23. Trangenquada RE, Grant WJ, Peterson CR. Lactic acidosis. *Arch Intern Med* 1966;117:192.
24. Wachtel TJ, Tetu-Mouradjian LM, Goldman DL, et al. Hyperosmolarity and acidosis in diabetes mellitus: a three year experience in Rhode Island. *J Gen Intern Med* 1991;6(6):495.
25. West ML, Massden PA, Singer GG, et al. Quantitative analysis of glucose loss during acute therapy for hyperglycemia hyperosmolar syndrome. *Diabetes Care* 1986;9:465.

CHAPTER 168
Diabetes Mellitus

Scott R. Votey and Anne L. Peters

Diabetes mellitus currently affects approximately 16 million Americans, and this number is likely to reach 20 million by the year 2010. It is a disproportionately expensive disease; patients diagnosed with diabetes accounted for 4.6% of the United States population, yet were responsible for 14.6% of all direct care expenditures in 1994. This chapter focuses on the emergency department evaluation and treatment of the acute and chronic complications of diabetes other than those directly associated with hypoglycemia and severe metabolic disturbances.

Diabetes is a chronic disease that requires long-term medical attention to limit the development of its devastating complications and to manage them when they do occur. Approximately 90% of diabetics have type 2 (or ketosis-resistant) diabetes (DM2), and the remainder have type 1 (ketosis-prone) diabetes (DM1). Although the frequency of the acute and chronic complications of diabetes differs between the two types of patient, both groups are at risk for the microvascular, macrovascular, and neuropathic complications of diabetes.

Microvascular complications of diabetes include retinopathy and nephropathy. Macrovascular complications are peripheral vascular, cerebrovascular, and coronary artery disease. Hypertension eventually occurs in approximately 50% of diabetic patients. Chronic, poorly controlled hyperglycemia, in addition to the metabolic consequences associated with glycosuria, can lead to impaired immune function and delayed wound healing. The development of complications is related to the duration of diabetes and the degree of glycemic control.

EMERGENCY DEPARTMENT EVALUATION

A diabetes-related history is important in assessing any patient with diabetes who presents to an emergency department. The first fact to be determined is which type of diabetes the patient has (Table 168.1). DM1 generally occurs in younger, lean patients and is characterized by the marked inability of the pancreas to secrete insulin. The distinguishing characteristic of a patient with DM1 is that if insulin is withdrawn, ketosis, and eventually ketoacidosis, develops. These patients are therefore insulin-dependent (i.e., insulin is life-sustaining), because they produce no endogenous insulin.

TABLE 168.1. Metabolic and Clinical Characteristics of the Two Major Types of Diabetes Mellitus

Characteristic	Type 1 Diabetes (DM1)	Type 2 Diabetes (DM2)
Synonyms	Juvenile-onset diabetes, IDDM	NIDDM
Age of onset	Usually <30 yr; sometimes in older adults	Usually >40 yr; sometimes in younger persons, even children
Genetic predisposition	Moderate (requires environmental factor[s] for expression); only 50% of identical twins develop DM1 if one sibling affected	Strong; 80%–100% of identical twins develop DM2 if one sibling is affected. More common among Native Americans, Hispanic, African Americans.
Precipitating factors	Viral/toxic/other trigger precipitating autoimmune response	Obesity, age
Findings at diagnosis	80% ICA-positive at diagnosis	Most patients had asymptomatic diabetes for 4–7 yr prior to "diagnosis"
Endogenous insulin levels	Very low to none	Present
Insulin resistance	Only present when blood glucose levels high	Almost always present
Response to prolonged fast	Hyperglycemia, ketoacidosis	Normal blood glucose levels
Response to stress, withdrawal of insulin	Ketoacidosis	Hyperglycemia without ketosis
Response to diet alone	Negligible	Always present to some degree
Response to sulfonylurea agents	Absent	Present

IDDM, insulin-dependent diabetes mellitus; NIDDM, non-insulin-dependent diabetes mellitus; ICA, islet cell antibody.

DM2 typically occurs in older (greater than 40 years of age) patients who have a family history of diabetes. Patients who develop DM2 have a genetic predisposition to do so and develop peripheral insulin resistance along with insufficient pancreatic β-cell secretion of insulin. Most patients (90%) who develop DM2 are obese, and obesity itself is associated with insulin resistance, which further worsens the diabetic state. Because patients with DM2 retain the ability to secrete some endogenous insulin, those who take insulin rarely develop diabetic ketoacidosis (DKA) when insulin is stopped. Therefore, they are considered insulin-requiring, not insulin-dependent. Moreover, patients with DM2 often do not require treatment with oral antidiabetic medication or insulin if they lose weight or do not eat.

Previously, differentiating between the two types of diabetes was relatively straightforward: If patients developed diabetes in childhood, especially if accompanied by DKA, they were considered to have DM1. Now, however, some patients are developing DM2 at younger ages (sometimes as young as age 6 or 7), and, to make matters more confusing, some present in DKA only to ultimately be controlled on diet or oral antidiabetic agents. Conversely, 30% of patients presenting with new-onset DM1 are more than 30 years old. Defining the type of diabetes can, therefore, be challenging, but a good clinical history often allows one to make the distinction. A lean Caucasian patient without a family history of diabetes who developed diabetes in childhood is likely to have DM1. A history of DKA or the presence of significant ketosis (greater than trace positive urine ketones) at the time of diagnosis of diabetes helps to identify DM1.

A strong family history of DM2, obesity, and Hispanic, African-American, or Native-American heritage all make the diagnosis of type 2 diabetes more likely, regardless of age. Patients who require insulin after a several-year history of treatment with oral agents are much more likely to have DM2. However, no definitive test exists for differentiating between the two types.

The duration of the diagnosis of diabetes is important also, because the chronic complications of diabetes are related to the length of time the patient has had the disease. Patients with DM2 have often had diabetes for 5 to 7 years before the diagnosis is made, however, and can present with the complications of diabetes at the time of diagnosis.[17]

Patients should be asked if they self-monitor their blood glucose levels, what their usual blood glucose levels are, and what the recent values have been. Patients should be asked about the types and doses of their diabetes medications. A sense of patients' level of knowledge about managing their diabetes is useful, as is a sense of their degree of compliance with diet and medications. The date and value of the most recent glycosylated hemoglobin determination is a useful indicator of both the quality of glycemic control and the patients' monitoring of their disease.

Symptoms of hypoglycemia and hyperglycemia (polyuria, polydipsia, nocturia, weight loss) should be elicited, with their time course and severity.

Although complications are often diagnosed by physical examination or by laboratory testing, the presence of known complications of diabetes should also be assessed in the patient history. Specifically, a history of retinopathy, nephropathy, vasculopathy (hypertension and coronary, peripheral, and cerebrovascular disease), neuropathy, or diabetic foot complications (ulcers and amputations) should be sought.

A diabetes-focused physical examination includes the following components: vital signs, funduscopic examination, limited vascular and neurologic examinations, and a foot assessment. Other organ systems should be examined as indicated by the patient's clinical situation.

Vital signs are useful for several reasons. Obviously, it is important to note whether the patient has hypertension or hypotension. Orthostatic vital signs may be useful in assessing volume status, as well as in suggesting the presence of an autonomic neuropathy. If the respiratory rate and pattern suggest Kussmaul respiration, DKA must be immediately considered and appropriate tests ordered.

The funduscopic examination should include a careful view of the retina, including both the optic disc and the macula. If hemorrhages or exudates are seen, the patient should be seen by an ophthalmologist as soon as possible, because nonophthalmologists tend to underestimate the severity of retinopathy, especially if the pupils have not been dilated.

The dorsalis pedis and posterior tibialis pulses should be palpated and their presence or absence noted. This is particularly important among patients with foot infection, because poor lower extremity blood flow can delay healing and increase the risk of amputation.

Documenting lower extremity sensory neuropathy is useful among patients who present with foot ulcers, because decreased sensation limits the patient's ability to protect the feet and ankles. If peripheral neuropathy is found, the patient should be made aware that foot care (including daily foot examinations) is very important for the prevention of foot ulcers and possible subsequent lower extremity amputation.

Diabetes Medications

In addition to sulfonylurea agents and insulin, a variety of new drugs have become available for the treatment of DM2.[30] These drugs allow for the use of combination oral therapy, often with improvement in glycemic control. The sulfonylurea agents (e.g., glyburide and glipizide) and meglitinides (e.g., repaglinide) increase insulin secretion. Their most common serious adverse reaction is hypoglycemia. The biguanides (e.g., metformin) decrease hepatic glucose production and insulin resistance. These drugs commonly cause gastrointestinal symptoms such as nausea, abdominal cramping, and diarrhea. Rarely, they can cause severe lactic acidosis, especially among patients with renal insufficiency. The α-glucosidase inhibitors (e.g., acarbose and miglitol) decrease intestinal absorption of carbohydrate, often producing flatulence and, rarely, causing small bowel obstruction. The newest class of drugs are the thiazolidinediones (troglitazone, rosiglitazone, and pioglitazone), which act as insulin sensitizers. Troglitazone has been associated with hepatotoxicity that is usually reversible but has resulted in fulminant hepatic failure. Patients on troglitazone should have monthly measurements of liver enzymes for the first year of use, and the medication should be stopped if transaminases exceed three times the upper limits of normal.

Abnormalities Caused by Hyperglycemia

Acute hyperglycemia, even when not associated with DKA or the hyperglycemic nonketotic syndrome (HNKS), is harmful for a number of reasons. If the blood glucose level exceeds the renal threshold for glucose (greater than 240 mg/dL in a healthy person, but diminished with advancing age, renal insufficiency, and pregnancy), an osmotic diuresis ensues, with loss of glucose, electrolytes, and water. Hyperglycemia impairs leukocyte function through a variety of mechanisms.[22] Patients with diabetes have an increased rate of wound infection,[8] and hyperglycemia may also independently impair wound healing.

Chronic hyperglycemia is associated with an increased risk for the development of the microvascular and neuropathic complications of diabetes, as elegantly demonstrated in the Diabetes Control and Complications Trial (DCCT) for DM1[12] and the United Kingdom Prospective Diabetes Study (UKPDS) for DM2.[25,26] In the DCCT, intensive therapy designed to maintain normal blood glucose levels greatly reduced the development and progression of retinopathy, microalbuminuria, proteinuria, and neuropathy as assessed over a 7-year period. Intensive therapy was not associated with increased mortality or major macrovascular events and did not decrease the quality of life, although it did increase the likelihood of severe hypoglycemic episodes. In the UKPDS, aggressive treatment of blood glucose levels and hypertension was shown to decrease the risk of microvascular complications in patients with DM2.

Among patients with known diabetes that is poorly controlled, there is no absolute level of blood glucose elevation that necessitates admission to the hospital or the administration of insulin. Patients with DM1 who cannot tolerate oral fluids require hospitalization. Likewise, if the patient is severely symptomatic or the precipitating cause of hyperglycemia cannot be adequately treated in the emergency department, the patient needs to be admitted. Generally, lowering the blood glucose level in the emergency department does not correct the underlying cause of hyperglycemia and has no long-term impact on the patient's blood glucose levels. Therefore, a plan must be formulated as to how the patient's blood glucose level will be lowered and how it will subsequently be monitored. The adequacy of follow-up is an extremely important consideration. Whether to give insulin in the emergency department is of lesser consequence and can be decided on an individual basis.

EMERGENCY DEPARTMENT MANAGEMENT

New-Onset Diabetes

Most patients with diabetes have DM2, and most of those are asymptomatic at diagnosis. The initial treatment for patients with newly discovered, asymptomatic diabetes is a trial of diet therapy. Therefore, if an asymptomatic patient is noted incidentally to have an elevated blood glucose level in the emergency department, this can be followed up by the patient's outpatient physician. Patients who have mild-to-moderate symptoms of poorly controlled diabetes but have not previously been diagnosed can usually be treated on an outpatient basis, often with the initiation of low-dose oral antidiabetic agent therapy.

Controversy exists over the management of markedly symptomatic patients with newly discovered DM2 and blood glucose levels over 400 mg/dL. If close follow-up can be arranged, these patients can be started on maximal doses of a sulfonylurea agent and treated as outpatients. Generally, the patient feels better within 1 to 2 days, and, within a week, the blood glucose levels are markedly lower. These patients can often have their sulfonylurea agent dose tapered as they comply with diet therapy, and, in some cases, diabetes can subsequently be controlled by diet alone. However, patients who cannot drink adequate amounts of fluid, who have serious coexisting medical conditions (e.g., myocardial infarction [MI] or systemic infection), or who do not have reliable follow-up should generally be hospitalized for initiation of therapy.

Patients with new-onset DM1 need to be started on lifelong insulin therapy. Many present in DKA. An occasional patient with new-onset DM1 who presents with mild manifestations and is judged to be very compliant can begin on insulin as an outpatient. This kind of treatment, however, requires close follow-up and the capability to provide immediate and thorough education concerning the use of insulin; the signs, symptoms, and treatment of hypoglycemia; and self-monitoring of blood glucose levels.

Management of Hyperglycemia during Medical Illness and Surgery

Serious medical illness and surgery produce a state of increased insulin resistance and relative insulin deficiency. Hyperglycemia can occur, even in nondiabetic patients, because of stress-induced insulin resistance plus the administration of dextrose-containing intravenous fluids.[3,18,22] Increases of glucagon, catecholamines, cortisol, and growth hormone antagonize the effects of insulin, and insulin secretion is itself inhibited by the α-adrenergic effect of increased catecholamine levels. The counterregulatory hormones also directly increase hepatic gluconeogenesis.

To maintain normal blood glucose levels, treatment regimens must be modified to compensate for both the decreased caloric intake and increased physiologic stress. Near-normal blood glucose levels should be maintained in medical and surgical patients with diabetes for four basic reasons:

1. To prevent the development of ketosis in patients with DM1
2. To prevent electrolyte abnormalities and volume depletion secondary to osmotic diuresis

TABLE 168.2. Suggested Intravenous Insulin Infusion Adjustment during Surgery

A. Start infusion of a solution containing 5% dextrose at a rate of 125 ml/hr.
B. Start intravenous insulin infusion as follows:

Whole Blood Glucose (mg/dL)	Insulin infusion Rate (U/hr)
≤100	None
101–150	1
151–250	2
251–350	3
>350	4[a]

C. Measure blood glucose level with a glucose meter every 2 hours before and after surgery and hourly during surgery.
   a. Do not change insulin infusion rate if blood glucose level ranges between 100 and 180 mg/dL.
   b. Increase insulin infusion rate by 0.5 U/h if blood glucose level is >180 mg/dL.
   c. Hold dextrose infusion if blood glucose level >350 mg/dL. Restart once blood glucose level ≤250 mg/dL.
   d. Decrease insulin infusion rate by 0.5 U/h if blood glucose level is <100 mg/dL, and increase dextrose infusion rate by 50 mL/h. Once blood glucose level increases to >100 mg/dL decrease dextrose infusion rate back to 125 mL/h.

[a]Dextrose infusion is held until blood glucose level ≤250 mg/dL.
From Peters AL. Prevention and treatment of glucose emergencies. *Infertil Reprod Med Clin North Am* 1992;3:947.

3. To prevent the development of impaired leukocyte function that occurs when blood glucose levels are elevated
4. To prevent the impaired wound healing that occurs when blood glucose levels are elevated

A variety of approaches have been described for the management of patients with diabetes who undergo surgery[18,22] or are otherwise unable to maintain oral caloric intake. Patients with DM1 must have insulin and carbohydrate given at all times to prevent the development of ketosis. For seriously ill patients and those undergoing general anesthesia, the optimal regimen involves continuous intravenous infusions of dextrose and insulin. This technique requires that the blood glucose level be measured with a glucose meter every hour, and that the insulin and dextrose infusion rates be adjusted accordingly to prevent hypoglycemia or persistent hyperglycemia (Table 168.2).

Frequent blood glucose monitoring is not always possible for every patient, and patients with less serious illness or those undergoing minor surgery may do just as well with subcutaneously injected insulin. In patients going to surgery who have not received a dose of intermediate-acting insulin that day, an injection of half of the patient's total daily dose as NPH insulin before surgery is often effective. At the same time, an intravenous infusion containing 5% dextrose should be started at a rate of 125 mL/h. Blood glucose levels should be checked every 2 hours during surgery, and small doses of regular or lispro (Humalog) insulin given if values are greater than 250 mg/dL.

The same principles of providing a constant source of insulin and carbohydrate apply to patients with DM1 who are not going to surgery but who must remain NPO due to other medical reasons. One approach is to give sliding-scale regular insulin every 4 hours, the dose based on the patient's blood glucose level. To avoid hypoglycemia, the regular insulin should not be given more frequently than every 3 to 4 hours, because the previous dose will peak in 2 to 4 hours and last up to 6 hours. Lispro insulin can be given every 3 hours.

Patients with DM2 who are on insulin can follow similar guidelines. However, because patients with DM2 secrete some endogenous insulin and do not develop ketosis, they can often be managed for brief periods without either insulin or dextrose. However, if the blood glucose is less than 80 mg/dL, or more than 250 mg/dL, appropriate treatment is required.

Patients who have been taking sulfonylurea agents or other oral antidiabetic agents should have their blood glucose levels monitored when oral intake is not allowed, and intravenous dextrose with or without insulin should be given to keep blood glucose levels between 100 and 250 mg/dL.

The presence of cardiovascular disease and renal dysfunction increases surgical morbidity and mortality in patients with and without diabetes.[29] In addition, diabetic autonomic neuropathy increases the likelihood of cardiovascular instability.[5] The emergency physician caring for the diabetic patient who requires emergent surgery must notify the surgeon and the anesthesiologist of the patient's condition, obtain medical consultation when appropriate, and promptly initiate a thorough medical evaluation so as not to delay surgery.

Acute Disturbances

Infections

Infections cause considerable morbidity and mortality among patients with diabetes. Infections may precipitate metabolic derangements, and, conversely, the metabolic derangements of diabetes may facilitate infection. Depending on the population studied, infections have been identified as the precipitant in 26% to 77% of cases of DKA.[6] A few infections, such as malignant otitis externa, rhinocerebral mucormycosis, and emphysematous pyelonephritis, occur almost exclusively in patients with diabetes. Certain infections, such as staphylococcal sepsis, occur more frequently and result in greater mortality among patients with diabetes, while others, such as pneumococcal pneumonia, affect diabetic patients no differently than the general population.

Although diabetes can compromise all aspects of host defenses against infection, all diabetic patients are nevertheless not equally susceptible to infection. Impairments in humoral immunity and polymorphonuclear leukocyte and lymphocyte function[3,22] are exacerbated by hyperglycemia and acidemia but are substantially, if not entirely, reversed by normalization of pH and blood glucose levels. Although the exact level above which impaired leukocyte function occurs has not been well defined, *in vitro* evidence suggests that glucose levels above 250 mg/dL impair leukocyte function.[2]

Patients with long-standing diabetes also tend to develop microvascular and macrovascular disease, with resulting poor tissue perfusion and an increased risk of infection. The ability of skin to act as a barrier to infection may also be compromised when the diminished sensation of diabetic neuropathy results in unnoticed injury.

Ear, Nose, and Throat Infections. Two head and neck infections that are associated with high morbidity and mortality, malignant otitis externa and rhinocerebral mucormycosis, are seen almost exclusively in diabetic patients.

Malignant or necrotizing otitis externa principally occurs in diabetic patients older than 35 years of age and is almost always caused by *Pseudomonas aeruginosa*. The infection starts in the external auditory canal and spreads to the adjacent soft tissue, cartilage, and bone. Patients typically present with severe ear pain and otorrhea; and although they often have a preexisting otitis externa, the progression to invasive disease is usually rapid. Examination of the auditory canal may reveal granulation tissue, but spread of infection to the pinna, the preauricular tissue, and the mastoid often makes the diagnosis apparent. Involvement of cranial nerves, particularly the facial nerve, is common; when there is extension to the meninges, the outcome is often fatal. Computed tomography (CT) is useful to define the extent of disease.

Prompt surgical consultation is mandatory for malignant otitis externa, because surgical debridement is often an essential part of therapy. Intravenous antipseudomonal antibiotic therapy should be started at once in patients with invasive disease. Diabetic patients with severe otitis externa but no evidence of invasive disease can be treated with an otic antibiotic drop and oral ciprofloxacin, but they require close follow-up.

Mucormycosis is the name given collectively to the infections caused by various ubiquitous molds. Invasive disease occurs in poorly controlled diabetic patients, especially in conjunction with DKA. In these patients, the organism colonizes the nose and paranasal sinuses, spreading into adjacent tissues by invading blood vessels and causing soft-tissue necrosis and bony erosion. Patients usually present with periorbital or perinasal pain and various degrees of swelling and induration. There may be a bloody nasal discharge. Involvement of the orbits, with lid swelling, proptosis, and diplopia, is common. The nasal turbinates may appear dusky red or frankly necrotic. The appearance of black necrotic tissue is an important visual clue. As the illness progresses, there is invasion of the cranial vault through the cribriform plate, which may result in cerebral abscess, cavernous sinus thrombosis, or internal carotid artery thrombosis. Wet smears of the necrotic tissue often reveal broad hyphae and distinguish mucormycosis from a severe facial cellulitis.

CT helps to delineate the extent of disease. Treatment consists of control of the predisposing hyperglycemia and acidemia, intravenous amphotericin B, and immediate surgical debridement. Until the diagnosis is confirmed, treatment with antistaphylococcal antibiotics is appropriate.

Urinary Tract Infection. Patients with diabetes have an increased risk for cystitis and, more importantly, for serious upper urinary tract infection. Intrarenal bacterial infection should be considered in the differential diagnosis of any patient with diabetes who presents with flank or abdominal pain.

The treatment of cystitis is essentially the same as in nondiabetic patients, although individuals with a neurogenic bladder due to diabetic neuropathy may not empty the bladder well and may require urologic referral. Sulfonamide antibiotics can cause hypoglycemia among patients taking sulfonylurea agents by displacing the sulfonylurea agents from their binding sites and increasing their hypoglycemic effect.

The principles of treatment of pyelonephritis do not differ for diabetic patients, but a lower threshold for hospital admission is appropriate for at least two reasons. First, pyelonephritis makes control of diabetes more difficult by causing insulin resistance; in addition, nausea may limit the patient's ability to maintain normal hydration. The ensuing hyperglycemia further compromises the immune response. Second, diabetic patients are more susceptible to the complications of pyelonephritis, including renal abscess, emphysematous pyelonephritis, renal papillary necrosis, and gram-negative sepsis.

In one series, 36 of 52 patients with renal abscess had diabetes, and more than 70% of cases of emphysematous pyelonephritis occur in patients with diabetes.[7] The latter is an uncommon necrotizing infection of the kidney caused by *Escherichia coli, Klebsiella pneumoniae,* or other organisms capable of fermenting glucose to carbon dioxide. The presentation is usually similar to that of uncomplicated pyelonephritis. The diagnosis is established by identifying renal gas on plain radiography, ultrasonography, or noncontrast helical CT urography, and surgical intervention is indicated once the diagnosis is made.

Skin and Soft-Tissue Infection. Sensory neuropathy, atherosclerotic vascular disease, and hyperglycemia all predispose diabetic patients to skin and soft-tissue infections. These can affect any skin surface but most commonly involve the feet. Even the smallest wound can be complicated by cellulitis, lymphangitis, and, more ominously, staphylococcal sepsis. Minor wound infections and cellulitis are typically caused by *Staphylococcus aureus* or hemolytic streptococci and can be treated with a penicillinase-resistant synthetic penicillin or a first-generation cephalosporin.[15]

Outpatient treatment of minor infections is appropriate if the patient is reliable, performs self-monitoring of blood glucose levels (and urine ketones for DM1 patients), and has close follow-up available. Wounds and, in particular, cutaneous ulcers can also be complicated by necrotizing infections of the skin, subcutaneous tissues, fascia, or muscle. These infections are typically polymicrobial, involving group A streptococci, enterococci, *S. aureus,* Enterobacteriaceae, and various anaerobes. Radiographs should be taken of any spreading soft-tissue infection in a diabetic patient to look for the soft-tissue gas that characterizes these infections. Surgical debridement is necessary for necrotizing infections. Gram stains and surface cultures are not helpful; antibiotic coverage should reflect the range of potential pathogens.

Osteomyelitis. Contiguous spread of a polymicrobial infection from skin ulcer to adjacent bone is common in diabetic patients. In one study, osteomyelitis was found underlying 68% of diabetic foot ulcers, and physical examination and plain radiographs each failed to make the diagnosis in one half of patients.[21] Unfortunately, these are typically the only diagnostic modalities available in the emergency department, and, often, the diagnosis is suspected but cannot be established. If osteomyelitis is apparent by radiograph or physical examination (e.g., if wounds are deep enough to expose tendons or bone), the patient should be admitted for intravenous administration of antibiotics. If osteomyelitis is suspected but admission is not necessitated by the soft-tissue infection or metabolic disturbances, the patient can be discharged to have an outpatient workup.

Other Infections. Although cholecystitis is probably no more common in patients with diabetes than in the general population, severe fulminating infection, especially with gas-forming organisms, is. The early clinical manifestations of emphysematous cholecystitis are indistinguishable from those of usual cholecystitis. The diagnosis can be made by finding gas in the gallbladder lumen, wall, or surrounding tissues. Even with immediate surgery, mortality is high. Clostridial species are found in over 50% of cases.

Diabetic patients have a greater incidence of staphylococcal and *Klebsiella* pneumonia than do persons without diabetes. Diabetes is also a risk factor for reactivation of tuberculosis. Cryptococcal infections and coccidioidomycoses are more virulent in diabetic patients.

Ophthalmologic Abnormalities

Diabetes is the leading cause of blindness in the United States; therefore, visual complaints by diabetic patients should be taken very seriously. Diabetes can affect the lens, the vitreous, and the retina, causing visual symptoms that may prompt the patient to come to the emergency department. Visual blurring may develop acutely as the lens changes shape with marked changes in blood glucose concentrations.[9] This effect, which is caused by osmotic fluxes of water into and out of the lens as the blood glucose concentration varies, usually occurs as hyperglycemia increases, but it may also be seen when high blood glucose levels are lowered rapidly. In either case, recovery to baseline visual acuity can take up to a month, and some patients are almost completely unable to read small print or do close-up work during this period.

Rarely, patients with DM1 who are in extremely poor control (e.g., those with frequent episodes of DKA) can acutely develop a "snowflake" (or "metabolic") cataract. Named for their snowflake or flocculent appearance, these cataracts can progress rapidly and create total opacification of the lens within a few days. Surgery is often required to restore vision. Patients with diabetes also tend to develop senile cataracts at a younger age than do persons without diabetes, although not in relation to the degree of glycemic control.

Some degree of diabetic retinopathy can be expected to develop in more than 90% of patients with DM1 and in 40% to 60% of patients with DM2 who have had the disease for 15 years or more. Patients with DM2 may already have diabetic retinopathy at the time their diabetes is diagnosed.[17] There are five stages in the progression of diabetic retinopathy:

1. Dilation of the renal venules and formation of retinal capillary microaneurysms
2. Increased vascular permeability
3. Vascular occlusion and renal ischemia
4. Proliferation of new blood vessels on the surface of the retina
5. Hemorrhage and contraction of the fibrovascular proliferation and the vitreous

Patients with DM2 do not develop proliferative retinopathy as often as those with DM1.

The first two stages of diabetic retinopathy are known as "background" or nonproliferative retinopathy. Initially, there is dilatation of the renal venules, followed by the appearance of microaneurysms, which appear as tiny red dots on the retina and cause no visual impairment. However, as the microaneurysms or retinal capillaries become more permeable, hard exudates appear, reflecting the leakage of plasma. These are sharply defined yellow deposits composed mostly of lipid material. Rupture of intraretinal capillaries results in hemorrhage. If these ruptures occur deep in the retina, they appear as "dot blot" hemorrhages that can be difficult to distinguish from microaneurysms. If a more superficial capillary ruptures, a flame-shaped hemorrhage appears. Hard exudates are often found in partial or complete rings (circinate pattern), which usually include multiple microaneurysms. These rings usually mark an area of edematous retina.

Many patients with macular edema are unaware of its presence. No change in visual acuity may be noted by the patient, unless the center of the macula is involved. Macular edema can cause visual loss, however, so it is extremely important to refer patients with suspected macular edema to an ophthalmologist for evaluation and possible laser therapy. Laser therapy is very effective in decreasing macular edema and preserving vision, but it is less effective in restoring vision once it is lost.

Preproliferative and proliferative diabetic retinopathy are the next stages in the progression of the disease. Cotton-wool spots can be seen in preproliferative retinopathy. These represent retinal microinfarcts due to capillary occlusion and are off-white to gray patches with poorly defined margins.

Proliferative retinopathy is characterized by neovascularization, the development of networks of fragile new vessels that are often seen on the optic disc or along the main vascular arcades. The vessels undergo cycles of proliferation and regression. During proliferation, fibrous adhesions develop between the vessels and the vitreous. Subsequent contraction of the adhesions can result in traction on the retina and retinal detachment. Contraction also tears the fragile new vessels, which hemorrhage into the vitreous.

Often, the first hemorrhage is small and is noted by the patient as a fleeting, dark area, or "floater," in the field of vision. Because subsequent hemorrhages can be larger and more serious, the patient should be referred immediately to an ophthalmologist for possible laser therapy. Patients with retinal hemorrhage should be advised to limit their activity and keep their head upright (even while sleeping), so that the blood settles to the inferior portion of the retina, thus obscuring less central vision.

Patients with active proliferative diabetic retinopathy are at increased risk for retinal hemorrhage if they receive thrombolytic therapy, so this is a relative contraindication to the use of thrombolytic agents.

Diabetic Nephropathy

Diabetic nephropathy occurs eventually in 30% to 40% of patients with DM1 (and, although less well studied, probably occurs with the same prevalence in patients with DM2).[28] All patients with diabetes should be considered to have the potential for renal impairment unless proven otherwise. Thus, extreme care should be exercised when using any nephrotoxic agent in a patient with diabetes. The use of contrast media can precipitate acute renal failure in patients with underlying diabetic nephropathy, and, although most recover within 10 days, some develop irreversible renal failure. Patients with diabetes who must undergo contrast medium–enhanced studies should be well hydrated before, during, and after the procedure and should have careful monitoring of renal function.[20] A better solution is to get equivalent clinical information by using an alternative study that does not require contrast medium administration (e.g., ultrasonography or noncontrast helical CT urography).

Potentially nephrotoxic drugs should be avoided whenever possible. Renally excreted or potentially nephrotoxic drugs should be given at reduced dosage as appropriate to the patient's serum creatinine level or creatinine clearance.

Because chronic blood pressure elevation contributes to the decline in renal function, it is extremely important that patients with diabetes who are found to be hypertensive be referred for chronic blood pressure management. If antihypertensive therapy is to be started in the emergency department, an angiotensin converting enzyme (ACE) inhibitor is a good choice,[19] because these agents have been found to reduce the rate of decline in renal function, independent of their effect on blood pressure. They also decrease proteinuria among patients with diabetic nephropathy. It should be kept in mind, however, that ACE inhibitors tend to increase the serum potassium level and should thus be used with caution in patients with renal serum insufficiency or somewhat elevated serum potassium levels.

Diabetic Neuropathy

Diabetic neuropathy is common. Distal symmetric sensorimotor polyneuropathy (in a "glove and stocking" distribution) is the most frequent pattern.[27] In addition to the pain often experienced in its early stages, this type of neuropathy eventually leads to loss of sensation. The combination of decreased sensation and peripheral arterial insufficiency often leads to foot ulceration and eventual amputation.

A variety of acute-onset neuropathies occur in diabetic patients, including acute cranial mononeuropathies, mononeuropathy multiplex, focal lesions of the lumbosacral plexus, and radiculopathies. Among cranial neuropathies, third oculomotor nerve palsy is the most common, followed by sixth (abducens) and fourth (trochlear) nerve palsies. All can present with diplopia and eye pain. In diabetic third-nerve palsy, the pupil is usually spared, whereas in third-nerve palsy due to intracranial aneurysm or tumor, the pupil is affected in 80% to 90% of cases.

It is important to consider nondiabetic causes for cranial nerve palsies, because 42% have been found to be due to causes other than diabetes. Evaluation should therefore include either nonenhanced and contrast medium–enhanced CT or magnetic resonance imaging of the optic nerve. Neurologic consultation is generally recommended. Acute cranial nerve mononeuropathies usually resolve within 2 to 9 months. These neuropathies are thought to be caused by acute thrombosis or ischemia of the blood vessels supplying the nervous system structure involved.

Autonomic dysfunction can involve any part of the sympathetic or parasympathetic chains and produces myriad manifestations. Patients likely to seek care in the emergency department include those with diabetic gastroparesis and vomiting, those with severe diarrhea, and those with bladder dysfunction and urinary retention. Symptoms tend to wax and wane over time. Treatment is only symptomatic. Patients with gastroparesis may benefit from the use of metoclopramide, cisapride, or erythromycin. Alleviating the functional abnormalities associated with the autonomic neuropathy is often difficult and frustrating for both doctor and patient. The patient's primary physician, and often an appropriate subspecialist, should be involved in devising a long-term treatment plan.

The Diabetic Foot

Fifty percent to 70% of all nontraumatic lower extremity amputations occur in diabetic patients.[4] At one clinic, however, the rate of amputation was halved after the institution of a program that ensured that patients removed their shoes for a foot examination at every clinic visit.[4] Although foot care is a lifelong challenge for the diabetic patient, the emergency physician can play an important role in this process. This is most obvious in the case of the acutely injured or infected limb, but extends to the recognition of feet at risk and appropriate referral for podiatric care.

The insensate, poorly perfused foot is at risk for ulcers from pressure necrosis or inflammation from repeated skin stress and unnoticed minor trauma. Either can evolve into cellulitis, osteomyelitis, or nonclostridial gangrene and end in amputation.

Wounds, infections, or ulcers of the feet demand particular attention in the diabetic patient. In addition to appropriate use of antibiotics, it is mandatory to avoid further trauma to the healing foot through use of crutches, a wheel chair, or bed rest. If bone or tendon is visible, osteomyelitis is present, and hospitalization for intravenous antibiotics is often necessary. Many patients need a vascular evaluation in conjunction with local treatment of the foot ulcer, because, in some cases, a revascularization procedure may be required to provide adequate blood flow for wound healing. For patients who may be discharged, every attempt should be made to ensure frequent follow-up or, if necessary, home nursing visits. If such follow-up is not available, hospitalization may be necessary for initial treatment. Follow-up care by a podiatrist or an orthopedist with experience in the care of a diabetic foot is optimal.

Because curing ulcers and foot infections is so difficult, it is better to prevent them. The emergency physician can facilitate this by briefly inspecting the feet of each patient with diabetes and educating the patient about the need for proper foot care. Patients with distal sensory neuropathy to pinprick or light touch, decreased peripheral pulses, moderate-to-severe onychomycosis, or impending skin breakdown deserve referral to a podiatrist for foot care.

Macrovascular Complications

Macrovascular disease is the leading cause of death in patients with diabetes. It is responsible for approximately 75% of deaths in patients with diabetes, compared with approximately 35% of deaths in the general population.[31] The presence of diabetes causes a twofold increase in MI in males and a fourfold increase in females that is in addition to the other known risk factors. The risk of stroke is doubled, and the risk of developing peripheral vascular disease is increased fourfold. Although the disease process itself is the same as in patients without diabetes, atherosclerosis develops earlier and follows a more malignant course among patients with diabetes. Patients with DM1 are predisposed to develop coronary artery disease at a younger age than are patients without diabetes; it is not rare for patients in their 30s and 40s to die of ischemic heart disease. Hypertension is twice as common among patients with DM2, which also increases the risk of atherosclerosis. *In fact, it has been shown that patients with DM2 who have never had an MI have the same risk of having an MI as nondiabetic patients who have had a prior MI.*[16] Patients with diabetes must therefore have their hypertension and lipid abnormalities treated aggressively to lessen their risk of developing atherosclerotic vascular disease.

Patients with diabetes have been said to have an increased incidence of silent ischemia. However, silent ischemia is common in many patients with coronary artery disease, and the apparent higher incidence among patients with diabetes may simply be related to the fact that they are more likely to have coronary artery disease to begin with. Nevertheless, it is prudent to order an electrocardiogram on patients with diabetes who have a serious illness or who present with generalized weakness, malaise, or other nonspecific symptoms that are not generally expected to be due to myocardial ischemia.

COMMON PITFALLS

- Failure to provide patients who have DM1 with a continuous source of insulin and glucose when they are unable to receive oral intake
- Failure to keep the blood glucose levels of patients with wounds or active infections below 250 mg/dL, which leads to poor healing
- Underestimating the severity of diabetic retinopathy on funduscopic examination through undilated pupils. Any patient with lesions near the macula should be referred urgently to an ophthalmologist.
- Failure to provide adequate hydration to patients with mild diabetic nephropathy before contrast material is given, precipitating acute renal failure
- Failure to examine the feet; overlooking small ulcers or underestimating their seriousness
- Failure to consider myocardial ischemia in patients with nonspecific symptoms

References

1. Airaksinen KEJ, Koistinen MJ. Association between silent coronary artery disease, diabetes and autonomic neuropathy—fact or fallacy? *Diabetes Care* 1992;15:288.
2. Bagdade JD, Root RK, Bulger RJ. Impaired leukocyte function in patients with poorly controlled diabetes. *Diabetes* 1974,23:9.
3. Bagdade JD, Segreti J. The infectious emergencies of diabetes. *Endocrinologist* 1991;1:155.
4. Brand PW, Coleman WC. The diabetic foot. In: Rifkin H, Porte D, eds. *Diabetes mellitus—theory and practice,* 4th ed. New York: Elsevier, 1990:792.
5. Burgos LG, Ebert TJ, Asiddao C, et al. Increased intraoperative cardiovascular morbidity in diabetics with autonomic neuropathy. *Anesthesiology* 1989;70:591.
6. Casey JL. Host defense and infections in diabetes mellitus. In: Rifkin H, Porte D, eds. *Diabetes mellitus—theory and practice,* 4th ed. New York: Elsevier, 1990:617.
7. Cook DJ, Achong MR, Dobranowski J. Emphysematous pyelonephritis. *Diabetes Care* 1989;12:229.
8. Cruse PJE, Foord R. A five-year prospective study of 23,649 surgical wounds. *Arch Surg* 1973,107:206.

9. Davidson MB. *Diabetes mellitus, diagnosis and treatment*, 4th ed. New York: Churchill Livingstone, 1998.
10. Davidson MB. Successful treatment of markedly symptomatic patients with type II diabetes mellitus using high doses of sulfonylurea agents. *West J Med* 1992;157:199.
11. Davis MD. Diabetic retinopathy: a clinical overview. *Diabetes Care* 1992 15:1844.
12. Diabetes Control and Complications Trial Research Group. Epidemiology of severe hypoglycemia in the Diabetes Control and Complications Trial. *Am J Med* 1991;90:450.
13. Diabetes Control and Complications Trial Research Group. The effect of intensive treatment of diabetes on the development and progression of long-term complications in insulin-dependent diabetes mellitus. *N Engl J Med* 1993,329:977.
14. Edwards TH, Braunstein GD, Davidson MB. Glyburide-induced hypoglycemia in an elderly patient: similarity of first-generation and second-generation sulfonylurea agents. *Mt Sinai J Med* 1985;52:644.
15. Gavin LA. A comprehensive approach to sidestep diabetic foot problems. *Endocrinologist* 1993;3:191.
16. Haffner SM, Lehto S, Ronnemaa T, et al. Mortality from coronary heart disease in subjects with type 2 diabetes and in nondiabetic subjects with and without prior myocardial infarction. *N Engl J Med* 1998;339:229–234.
17. Harris ML, Klein R, Welborn TA, et al. Onset of NIDDM occurs at least 4–7 years before clinical diagnosis. *Diabetes Care* 1992;15:815.
18. Hirsch IB, McGill JB. Role of insulin in management of surgical patients with diabetes mellitus. *Diabetes Care* 1990;13:980.
19. Kasiske BL, Kalil RSN, Ma JZ, et al. Effect of and hypertensive therapy on the kidney in patients with diabetes: a meta-regression analysis. *Ann Intern Med* 1993;118:129.
20. Manske CL, Sprafka JM, Strony JT, et al. Contrast nephropathy in azotemic diabetic patients undergoing coronary angiography. *Am J Med* 1990;89:615.
21. Newman J, Wallis J, Palesstro CJ, et al. Unsuspected osteomyelitis in diabetic foot ulcers: diagnosis and monitoring by leukocyte scanning with indium. *JAMA* 1991;266:1246.
22. Peters AL. Prevention and treatment of glucose emergencies. *Infertil Reprod Med Clin North Am* 1992;3:947.
23. Singer DE, Nathan DM, Fogel HA, et al. Screening for diabetic retinopathy. *Ann Intern Med* 1992;116:660.
24. Slama G, Traynard PY, Desplanque N, et al. The search for an optimized treatment of hypoglycemia. *Arch Intern Med* 1990;150:589.
25. United Kingdom Prospective Diabetes Study (UKPDS) Group. Intensive blood-glucose control with sulphonylureas or insulin compared with conventional treatment and risk of complications in patients with type 2 diabetes (UKPDS 33). *Lancet* 1998;352:839–855.
26. United Kingdom Prospective Diabetes Study (UKPDS) Group. Effect of intensive blood-glucose control with metformin on complications in patients with type 2 diabetes (UKPDS 34). *Lancet* 1998;352:856–867.
27. Vinik AI, Holland MT, Le Beau JM, et al. Diabetic neuropathies. *Diabetes Care* 1992;15:1926.
28. Vora JP, Anderson S. Diabetic renal disease: an overview with therapeutic implications. *Endocrinologist* 1992;2:223.
29. Walsh DB, Eckhauser FE, Ramsburgh SR, et al. Risk associated with diabetes mellitus in patients undergoing gallbladder surgery. *Surgery* 1982;91:254.
30. White JR. The pharmacological reduction of blood glucose in patients with type 2 diabetes mellitus.. *Clin Diabet* 1998;16:58–67.
31. Wittels EH, Gotto AM. Clinical features of ischemic heart disease in diabetes mellitus. In: Alberti KGMM, DeFronzo RA, Keen H, et al., eds. *International textbook of diabetes.* New York: John Wiley and Sons, 1992:1487.

CHAPTER 169

Hypoglycemia

Scott R. Votey and Anne L. Peters

Hypoglycemia is defined as a plasma glucose value less than 50 mg/dL, accompanied by signs and symptoms of adrenergic excess (sweating, nervousness, tachycardia, shakiness) or alterations in mental status, or both, that are relieved by the administration of carbohydrate. The glucose concentration at which clinical hypoglycemia occurs varies. Completely healthy women may have glucose levels less than 45 mg/dL during a fast without symptoms of hypoglycemia. Conversely, adrenergic symptoms of "hypoglycemia" may occur in patients without low blood glucose levels. Therefore, the diagnosis of hypoglycemia must be based on the presence of both biochemical hypoglycemia and concomitant hypoglycemic symptoms.

Although there are many causes of hypoglycemia, the vast majority of episodes encountered in the emergency department (ED) occurs as complications of the treatment of diabetes with insulin or an oral antidiabetic agent. Hypoglycemia is an important and growing concern for the approximately 16 million individuals with diabetes in the United States. The publication of the Diabetes Treatment and Control Trial (DCCT)[4] in 1993 and the United Kingdom Prospective Diabetes Study (UKPDS)[13] in 1998 have proven that tight control of blood glucose delays the development and progression of complications in patients with both type 1 and type 2 diabetes. From these has come a greater emphasis on maintaining euglycemia.

Unfortunately, tight control also increases the frequency of hypoglycemia, especially in patients treated with insulin.[5] Although mild episodes of hypoglycemia (defined as episodes recognized and treated by the patient) are not harmful and should not dissuade patients from adequately treating their diabetes, recurrent severe episodes (involving altered mentation and requiring assistance to treat) may be associated with progressive cognitive decline.[8] Goals for emergency physicians in the management of hypoglycemia are (1) recognition of each episode of hypoglycemia, (2) prompt and adequate treatment, (3) identification of the cause of the episode, and (4) establishment of a plan to prevent future episodes.

A balance between glucose utilization and production maintains normal blood glucose levels. In health, preprandial blood glucose levels are usually 70 to 100 mg/dL, with a small postprandial rise peaking 1 hour after eating and returning to baseline within 4 hours. The major glucose-requiring tissues are the brain, muscle, and red blood cells. During fasting, glucose production occurs through hepatic glycogenolysis (breakdown of glycogen) and gluconeogenesis. Insulin levels are high in the postprandial period and fall with fasting.

Glucoreceptors in the hypothalamus sense low blood glucose levels and cause the secretion of counterregulatory hormones. Glucagon is the primary counterregulatory hormone in nondiabetic patients. Patients with type 1 diabetes lose their glucagon response to hypoglycemia within the first 5 years of disease.

The onset of action of glucagon is rapid, and it acts by enhancing glycogenolysis and gluconeogenesis. If glucagon is not present, epinephrine serves as the major counterregulatory hormone. It also has a rapid onset of action, and acts by inhibiting glucose utilization by muscle, increasing gluconeogenesis, and inhibiting insulin secretion. Cortisol and growth hormone are secreted as part of normal hypoglycemic counterregulation, but their release is delayed and they do not contribute to the acute recovery from hypoglycemia.

CLINICAL PRESENTATION

The signs and symptoms of hypoglycemia fall into two categories: adrenergic (those caused by increased activity of the sympathetic autonomic nervous system) and neuroglycopenic (those caused by depressed activity of the central nervous system [CNS]) (Table 169.1). Although there is much individual variation, the adrenergic symptoms of hypoglycemia typically start at approximately 60 mg/dL, and evidence of neuroglycopenia occurs at approximately 50 mg/dL. Symptoms vary from person to person but, within an individual, remain fairly constant from episode to episode.

Not all patients experience the adrenergic symptoms of hy-

TABLE 169.1. Signs and Symptoms of Hypoglycemia

Adrenergic	Neuroglycopenia
Weakness	Headache
Tremor	Mental dullness
Sweating and warmth	Confusion
Tachycardia and palpitations	Amnesia
Nervousness	Incoordination
Irritability	Visual disturbances
Tingling of face and fingers	Seizures
Hunger	Coma
Nausea	Focal neurologic deficits

poglycemia.[7] Autonomic neuropathy, which occurs in more than 25% of patients with long-standing (more than 10 years) type 1 diabetes, can diminish adrenergic symptoms.[3] Patients who are chronically hypoglycemic, particularly patients with tightly controlled type 1 diabetes, accommodate to hypoglycemia and may not have adrenergic symptoms until the blood glucose is less than 50 mg/dL and neuroglycopenic symptoms develop. This phenomenon, termed *hypoglycemia-associated autonomic failure,* is the combined result of a downregulation of the adrenergic response to hypoglycemia, due to intensive insulin therapy or recent hypoglycemia, and autonomic dysfunction. Patients who lack adrenergic symptoms often fail to recognize impending hypoglycemia and are at increased risk for severe neuroglycopenia.

Because the CNS is almost entirely glucose-dependent for function, hypoglycemia manifests neurologically within minutes. Measurable cognitive deficits commonly begin at blood glucose levels less than 50 mg/dL, but some patients remain awake and alert at much lower levels.[9] Patients may fail to perceive their cognitive dysfunction and deny having any CNS symptoms. The blood glucose at which seizures occur varies, but a seizure at a glucose greater than 40 mg/dL should prompt investigation for an alternative cause. Focal neurologic deficits, including hemiparesis, are the presenting symptoms in a small percentage of patients.

Long-term cognitive deterioration is a function of the severity, duration, and number of hypoglycemic episodes.[8] Mild episodes consisting only of adrenergic symptoms do not result in CNS injury. Severe episodes, particularly those resulting in loss of consciousness or seizures, are damaging. Time to recovery and completeness of recovery depend on the severity and duration of hypoglycemia. Elderly patients and those with a history of prior CNS injury, such as a stroke, appear to be at higher risk for a prolonged or incomplete recovery.

DIFFERENTIAL DIAGNOSIS

Although chronic treatment of diabetes with insulin or a sulfonylurea agent is the root cause of the vast majority of hypoglycemic episodes encountered in the ED, there is invariably an acute precipitant perturbing the patient's usual glucose homeostasis. The key to preventing future hypoglycemic episodes is the identification of the precipitant of the current episode. A good history is the principal tool in achieving this goal, and will identify the precipitant in approximately 50% of cases. Common precipitants can be grouped according to their physiologic mechanisms (Table 169.2). Inadequate glucose availability is the most commonly identified cause of hypoglycemia, followed by increased caloric utilization, medication error, and diminished excretion.

Patients who take oral sulfonylurea agents can have prolonged periods of hypoglycemia (sometimes lasting up to a

TABLE 169.2. Precipitants of Hypoglycemia in Patients with Diabetes

INADEQUATE GLUCOSE AVAILABILITY
Decreased caloric consumption: missed or delayed meal, fasting
Decreased hepatic gluconeogenesis: suppression by alcohol, hepatic failure
Insufficient counterregulatory hormones: glucagon, epinephrine, cortisol
INCREASED CALORIC UTILIZATION
Exercise
Illness and injury
MEDICATIONS: INCREASED INSULIN EFFECT
Accidental overdose: poor vision, misunderstanding, change in syringe size, change in insulin concentration, pharmacy error
Intentional overdose
MEDICATIONS: DIMINISHED EXCRETION OR METABOLISM
Renal insufficiency: insulin and sulfonylurea agents are renally excreted.
Hepatic failure: sulfonylureas undergo hepatic metabolism

week) because of the long elimination half-life of many of these agents; this phenomenon occurs particularly in elderly patients and those with renal insufficiency or hepatic failure.[12] The possibility of declining renal function should be assessed in any patient who develops recurrent unexplained episodes of hypoglycemia while taking these agents. These individuals often require admission to the hospital, continuous intravenous administration of dextrose, and frequent blood glucose monitoring until blood glucose levels stabilize. In addition, even small doses of sulfonylurea agents may produce severe hypoglycemia in young children, and any sulfonylurea ingestion in this age group should be taken seriously.[11]

Replaginide (Prandin) is a new short-acting oral agent of the meglitinide class that, like the sulfonylurea agents, increases insulin secretion and may cause hypoglycemia. The hypoglycemia associated with repaglinide is expected to be of shorter duration than that caused by the sulfonylurea agents. On the other hand, metformin (Glucophage), the α-glucosidase inhibitors (acarbose [Precose], miglitol [Glyset]), and the thiazolidinediones (troglitazone [Rezulin], rosiglitazone [Avandia], and pioglitazone [Actose]) do not increase insulin secretion and rarely cause hypoglycemia when used alone. In combination with insulin or a sulfonylurea, however, these drugs may exacerbate an episode of hypoglycemia.

Some patients, particularly the elderly, are not aware that they are being treated for diabetes. Therefore, it is helpful to review all medications the patient is currently taking when investigating the cause of an unexplained episode of hypoglycemia. Surreptitious use of medication is a consideration in healthy-appearing patients with unexplained hypoglycemia, especially if it is severe or recurrent.

Aside from insulin and sulfonylurea agents, a number of other drugs can precipitate hypoglycemia, either at therapeutic doses or in overdose (Table 169.3). Patients taking β blockers are at increased risk for severe hypoglycemia both because of a blunted counterregulatory response and diminished adrenergic symptoms when hypoglycemia does develop. Salicylate overdoses occasionally precipitate hypoglycemia, particularly in children.

Many serious illnesses may result in hypoglycemia; the most common are renal failure, hepatic failure, malnutrition (including anorexia nervosa), and sepsis.[6] Others include severe right heart failure and malignancy. The etiology is often multifacto-

TABLE 169.3. Selected Causes of Hypoglycemia

FASTING
Healthy-Appearing Individuals
Drugs
Exogenous insulin
Oral hypoglycemic agents: sulfonylurea agents, replaginide
β-Adrenergic blocking agents
Salicylates
Disopyramide
Quinine
Pentamidine
Others
Ethanol and other alcohols
Insulinomas and non-β-cell tumors
Inherited disorders of metabolism
Ill-Appearing Individuals
Hepatic failure: depleted glycogen stores and impaired gluconeogenesis
Renal failure
Adrenal insufficiency
Sepsis
Shock
Malnutrition, including anorexia nervosa
Congestive heart failure, especially severe right heart failure
Pregnancy
FED (REACTIVE)
Impaired glucose tolerance
Alimentary
Idiopathic reactive

rial. Adrenal insufficiency itself rarely causes symptomatic hypoglycemia, but it may be a contributing factor during times of physiologic stress. Cortisol is necessary for gluconeogenesis, and, without it, glucose levels (especially fasting levels) fall (see Chapter 172).

Ethanol ingestion can precipitate hypoglycemia in patients with or without diabetes by suppressing gluconeogenesis, usually in association with inadequate intake of food. This phenomenon occurs most commonly in children, malnourished chronic alcoholics, binge drinkers, and diabetics who neglect to eat adequately when consuming alcohol.

Insulinomas are a rare cause of hypoglycemia. Patients with these tumors have recurrent episodes of hypoglycemia, typically presenting with neuroglycopenic rather than adrenergic symptoms; insulinomas often go undiagnosed for years. Weight gain from eating large amounts of food to self-treat the hypoglycemia is common. Non–β-cell tumors, including mesenchymal tumors, hepatocellular carcinomas, adrenal carcinomas, and others, can also produce hypoglycemia.

Newborns, especially premature infants, are at risk for hypoglycemia during times of physiologic stress due to small glycogen stores and limited hepatic gluconeogenesis. In addition, several inborn errors of metabolism can cause hypoglycemia in children. These include glucose-6-phosphatase deficiency, galactosemia, hereditary fructose intolerance, and carnitine deficiency. Inborn errors of metabolism usually present in the first year of life. Infants experiencing unexplained hypoglycemia should be hospitalized and evaluated for these disorders.

Although hypoglycemia occurs most commonly in the fasting state, there are several causes of fed or reactive hypoglycemia. Alimentary hypoglycemia occurs in patients who have undergone gastrointestinal surgery, most commonly gastrectomy. Patients have symptoms of hypoglycemia 30 to 120 minutes after eating. The hypoglycemia is thought to occur because of a more rapid emptying of food into the duodenum, leading to both an accelerated absorption of glucose and an exaggerated insulin response.

Some patients with "mild" diabetes, including patients treated with diet alone and those with risk factors for type 2 diabetes but who have not yet been diagnosed as having diabetes, experience postprandial hypoglycemia. The insulin response to food is initially delayed; the enhanced insulin secretion that follows produces postprandial hypoglycemia.

Idiopathic reactive hypoglycemia is a rare disorder that is substantially overdiagnosed, particularly in young women. In general, patients with this diagnosis have adrenergic symptoms on fasting or postprandially, but are rarely documented to have a glucose less than 50 mg/dL.

EMERGENCY DEPARTMENT EVALUATION

In the ED, the biochemical diagnosis of hypoglycemia is usually made by using a bedside glucose meter. A blood glucose level should be checked immediately on any patient presenting with adrenergic or neuroglycopenic symptoms, including behavioral abnormalities, decreased level of consciousness, and acute focal deficits. An immediate check should be done on patients with syncope and trauma patients in whom hypoglycemia as a precipitant may be overlooked.

Whole blood levels are approximately 5% to 10% lower than plasma levels, although some newer meters are calibrated to report a higher value that is equivalent to the plasma level. In addition, arterial blood has a glucose level 5% to 10% higher than that of venous blood. Test strips and meters are highly sensitive for the diagnosis of hypoglycemia, but may give falsely *high* readings in the setting of severe anemia and acetaminophen overdose.[2,10,15] Test strip accuracy also deteriorates with prolonged storage, so strips should not be used beyond their printed expiration date.

Laboratory confirmation of hypoglycemia diagnosed by bedside testing is usually not necessary, however. Laboratory glucose levels measured by the glucose oxidase method (and presumably test strips and meters, which also rely on this reaction) may be falsely low in the setting of high levels of ascorbic acid, levodopa, tolbutamide, and bilirubin.[10]

When the patient has recovered adequately, a focused history should be taken, investigating the cause of the episode, including the timing and doses of medications, food eaten, and activity. For diabetic patients, the history should include an assessment of diabetic control, whether home glucose monitoring is performed, usual values, and the frequency and severity of hypoglycemic episodes. The presence of comorbidities, including renal insufficiency and liver disease, should be ascertained.

Additional laboratory testing, including measurements of the serum creatinine or hepatic transaminases, is necessary only if the history fails to reveal the cause of the episode and contributory comorbidities are suspected.

Nondiabetic patients who are suspected of having hypoglycemia, but for whom the diagnosis was not established in the ED, can be referred for an outpatient diagnostic workup.

EMERGENCY DEPARTMENT MANAGEMENT

Hypoglycemia should be considered in every patient with an altered sensorium or any acute neurologic deficit. Ideally, a fingerstick blood glucose level should be obtained to confirm the diagnosis before treatment with glucose is initiated, but glucose should be given empirically if the level cannot be obtained immediately. Although animal studies and retrospective human studies have found a correlation between hyperglycemia and poor neurologic outcome among patients with stroke and severe brain injury, there is no evidence that the doses of glucose given to correct hypoglycemia are harmful. Only 15 to 20 g of carbohydrate is generally required to restore euglycemia, although, occasionally, more is required. Glucose can be administered orally or intravenously, depending on the patient's level of consciousness.

The initial treatment for a confused or comatose adult with hypoglycemia is a 50-mL bolus of 50% glucose intravenously. Less concentrated glucose solutions are recommended for children (25%) and neonates (10%) due to concerns about hyperosmolality. The mean increase in the serum glucose level following this bolus is 150 mg/dL, but it varies greatly and is not predictable.[1] The bolus should be followed by the continuous infusion of 5% or 10% glucose at a rate sufficient to keep the glucose level over 100 mg/dL until the patient is capable of eating. If there is any reason to suspect thiamine deficiency, thiamine 100 mg intravenously should be given concomitantly with glucose to avoid precipitating Wernicke-Korsakoff syndrome.

Patients who are alert enough to eat may be treated with glucose tablets or paste, orange juice, hard candy, or any form of concentrated sugar. If a patient is taking an α-glucosidase inhibitor, absorption of oral carbohydrate may be inhibited. These patients must be treated with dextrose (which is in glucose tablets) as opposed to sucrose (which is in table sugar). They can also be effectively treated with milk, because the drug does not inhibit lactase.

Adults with hypoglycemia who are unable to eat and in whom intravenous access cannot be secured can be given glucagon 1 mg intramuscularly.[14] Children should receive 0.5 mg. Available data have shown glucagon to be safe and effective in restoring euglycemia, with neurologic recovery occurring generally within 10 minutes.

Adrenergic symptoms respond to glucose therapy within minutes. The time to recovery of neuroglycopenic symptoms is more variable, ranging from minutes to (in rare cases) days.[9] A patient failing to show clear signs of neurologic recovery within 10 minutes should have the glucose level rechecked to verify that euglycemia has been restored, because an additional bolus of glucose is occasionally needed. Alternative etiologies should be considered if there are no signs of neurologic recovery within 30 minutes.

To prevent recurrence, a meal or snack should be given after treatment. The simple carbohydrate given to raise the blood glucose level quickly does not produce a sustained elevation of blood glucose (50 mL of D50 and an 8-oz glass of orange juice contain only about 100 calories each), so a more complete meal, containing protein, fat, and complex carbohydrate, should be given to produce a more sustained rise in blood glucose levels. If hypoglycemia is due to administration of a long-acting insulin or an oral hypoglycemic drug, low glucose levels will typically last for an extended time. It is important to continue treatment and close observation to prevent relapse.

Long-term therapy depends on the cause of the hypoglycemia. If the hypoglycemia is secondary to a disorder such as hepatic failure or adrenal insufficiency, treatment of the underlying disorder is necessary to prevent recurrent hypoglycemia.

Dietary therapy is the treatment of choice for reactive and alimentary hypoglycemia. Patients should avoid sugars and eat frequent small snacks that contain a mixture of carbohydrate, fat, and protein. Restricting carbohydrate intake to 40% of total calories also may help.

In insulin-treated patients who become hypoglycemic, whether the usual insulin dose should be adjusted depends on the severity of the reaction. If the reaction is minor (easily detected and treated by the patient) and there is an explanation for the reaction (e.g., a missed meal or increased exercise), no insulin dose adjustment is indicated. However, if the reaction is more severe or is unexplained, or if there is a pattern of hypoglycemia occurring at the same time each day, the insulin dose should be decreased. Close monitoring of blood glucose levels is necessary to prevent hypoglycemia or hyperglycemia when the insulin dose has been changed.

TABLE 169.4. Discharge Criteria Following a Symptomatic Hypoglycemic Episode

Brief episode
Full neurologic recovery
Able to eat
No major comorbidities that require hospital admission
Cause of the episode found and addressed
Treatment plan to prevent future episodes understood by the patient
Hypoglycemia accidental
Relapse unlikely—no long-acting insulin or oral agent, nor prolonged excretion or metabolism
Ability to do home glucose monitoring[a]
Responsible person to be with the patient[a]
Follow-up arranged[a]

[a]Imperative for severe episodes requiring assistance for recovery.

Recurrent hypoglycemia acutely downregulates the adrenergic response to additional episodes of hypoglycemia. A moderately severe episode of hypoglycemia on day 1 will induce hypoglycemia unawareness on day 2, resulting in a more severe episode on the second day. Therefore, on the day following a moderate-to-severe hypoglycemic episode, the insulin dose should be reduced by 25%.

DISPOSITION

Most patients seen in the ED for hypoglycemia meet discharge criteria (Table 169.4). Hospital admission is indicated for patients failing to meet these criteria.

Patients who are discharged should receive specific instructions on how best to avoid recurrent episodes (most commonly by increasing caloric intake or decreasing the insulin dose), should be instructed to perform self-monitoring of blood glucose, and should carry some form of oral glucose at all times. Family members of patients who have experienced a severe episode requiring assistance should be instructed in how to recognize and treat hypoglycemia.

COMMON PITFALLS

- Failure to consider hypoglycemia in all patients with acute neurologic or psychiatric symptoms, regardless of any history of diabetes
- Failure to consider hypoglycemia in any physiologically stressed infant
- Waiting for laboratory results before administering glucose
- Failure to feed the patient following a response to intravenous glucose
- Failure to follow a bolus of intravenous glucose with a continuous glucose infusion in patients who remain unable to eat
- Failure to administer glucagon to any hypoglycemic patient with neuroglycopenic symptoms who is unable to take oral glucose and in whom intravenous access has failed
- Prematurely discharging a patient whose episode of hypoglycemia is due to a long-acting insulin or a sulfonylurea agent
- Failure to consider intentional overdose as the cause of hypoglycemia

- Failure to reinforce the need for self-monitoring of blood glucose and, in particular, failure to discuss the need for monitoring blood glucose levels prior to driving
- Discharging a patient following an episode of hypoglycemia without establishing that the patient understands how to avoid future episodes

References

1. Adler PM. Serum glucose changes after administration of 50% dextrose solution: pre- and in-hospital calculations. *Am J Emerg Med* 1986;4:504.
2. Cartier LJ, Leclerc P, Pouilet M, et al. Toxic levels of acetaminophen produce a major positive interference on Glucose Elite and Accu-Chek Advantage glucose meters. *Clin Chem* 1998;44:893.
3. Davidson MB. *Diabetes mellitus, diagnosis and treatment*, 3rd ed. New York: Churchill Livingston, 1991.
4. Diabetes Control and Complications Trial Research Group. The effect of intensive treatment of diabetes on the development and progression of long-term complications in insulin-dependent diabetes mellitus. *N Engl J Med* 1993;329:977.
5. The Diabetes Control and Complications Trial Research Group. Hypoglycemia in the Diabetes Control and Complications Trial. *Diabetes* 1997;46:271.
6. Fischer KF, Lees JA, Newman JH. Hypoglycemia in hospitalized patients. N Engl J Med 1986;315:1245.
7. Heller SR, MacDonald IA, et al. Influence of sympathomimetic nervous system on hypoglycemia warning symptoms. *Lancet* 1987;2:359.
8. Langan SJ, Deary IJ, Hepburn DA, et al. Cumulative cognitive impairment following recurrent severe hypoglycemia in adult patients with insulin treated diabetes mellitus. *Diabetologia* 1991;34:337.
9. Malouf R, Brust JCM. Hypoglycemia: causes, neurologic manifestations, and outcome. *Ann Neurol* 1985;17:421.
10. Pointer JE. Glucose analysis: indications for ordering and alternatives to the laboratory. *Ann Emerg Med* 1986;15:372.
11. Quadrani DA, Spiller HA, Widder P. Five year retrospective evaluation of sulfonylurea ingestion in children. *J Toxicol Clin Toxicol* 1996;34:267.
12. Shorr RI, Ray WA, Daugherty JR, et al. Incidence and risk factors for serious hypoglycemia in older persons using insulin or sulfonylureas. *Arch Intern Med* 1997;157:1681.
13. UK prospective Diabetes Study (UKPDS) Group. Intensive blood-glucose control with sulphonylureas or insulin compared with conventional treatment and risk of complications in patients with type 2 diabetes (UKPDS 33). *Lancet* 1998;352:839.
14. Vukmir RB, Paris PM, Yealy DM. Glucagon: prehospital therapy for hypoglycemia. *Ann Emerg Med* 1991;20:375.
15. Wattoo MA, Liu HH. Alternating transient dense hemiplegia due to episodes of hypoglycemia. *West J Med* 1999;170:170.

CHAPTER 170
Alcoholic Ketoacidosis

Stephen L. Adams and Laura J. Bontempo

Alcoholic ketoacidosis (AKA) is characterized by a metabolic acidosis with an elevated anion gap due to an accumulation of ketone bodies. Typically, it occurs after an episode of binge drinking, followed by a period of abstinence and starvation.[5–7,15] Ketosis is attributed to multiple factors: direct damage of hepatic mitochondria by alcohol, diminished hepatic glycogen stores, a relative insulin deficiency, increased hepatic ketone formation, decreased gluconeogenesis, rapid lipolysis with increased free fatty acid formation (subsequently serving as a substrate for ketones), and decreased peripheral ketone utilization.[4–8,11,15]

In addition to the metabolic acidosis, there may be a concurrent metabolic alkalosis, respiratory alkalosis, or other acid–base disturbances.[6,7,16] AKA is reversible and is associated with a low mortality rate.[5,7] If death occurs, it is generally related to associated disorders rather than to AKA itself.[15,16]

CLINICAL PRESENTATION

AKA generally occurs in people with a history of chronic alcohol abuse. The patient is typically a binge drinker who has recently stopped drinking.[6,15] There may be alcohol detectable on the breath or in the serum, dependent on the amount of alcohol ingested and how recently intake was discontinued before the patient's presentation to the emergency department (ED). In one series, 40% of patients in whom the blood alcohol level was measured had levels consistent with intoxication.[16]

There is usually no history of diabetes, and men and women are affected equally.[7,11] The most common presenting symptoms include nausea, vomiting, and abdominal pain.[7] Cessation of alcohol intake is usually occasioned by the onset of these symptoms rather than an effort to abstain from alcohol.[6] There is typically also a history of anorexia, with poor fluid and caloric intake.[7] The abdominal pain may be due to liver disease, pancreatitis, alcoholic gastritis, or other diseases that may or may not be related to alcohol intake.[1,7,8,12] There is a broad spectrum of severity.

On physical examination, the odor of ketones is almost always present.[10] There may be profound orthostasis and other signs of volume depletion resulting from vomiting, decreased oral intake, and diaphoresis. Tachycardia and tachypnea are common, and the respirations may be deep and rapid (Kussmaul).[5] Patients may complain of dyspnea.[11]

Fever is not usually a part of the syndrome, even in patients who eventually prove to have a significant infection.[16] Mental status is usually normal, but an abnormality in orientation or level of consciousness has been reported in up to 15% of patients and may be attributable to a concomitant problem, such as alcohol intoxication, severe infection, hypoglycemia, or cerebrovascular accident.[7,16] Obtundation and coma have, however, been reported.[14]

The abdominal examination may reveal diffuse tenderness.[7] Distention, diminished bowel sounds, ascites, and rebound are uncommon, and are usually seen only when other processes, such as pancreatitis or sepsis, also are present. Other associated conditions include alcohol withdrawal, upper gastrointestinal bleeding, seizure, myopathy, hepatitis, chronic liver disease, gastritis, and small bowel obstruction. Physical examination may also reveal spider angiomas, as well as other markers of liver disease and chronic alcohol abuse.[1,7,8,14]

DIFFERENTIAL DIAGNOSIS

The differential diagnosis of AKA includes the other causes of an elevated anion-gap metabolic acidosis (see Chapter 165).[1,13] Of the several causes of ketoacidosis to be considered, the most common is diabetic ketoacidosis (DKA). It may be difficult to distinguish AKA from DKA based on clinical signs and symptoms alone. Polydipsia and polyuria are variable but may be present in both groups.[7,9] However, an elevated HbA1c level is consistent with ketosis due to diabetes mellitus.[9]

Methanol and ethylene glycol ingestions must also be considered in the chronic alcoholic with an elevated anion-gap metabolic acidosis. Patients with methanol ingestion may complain of visual changes and central nervous system (CNS) symptoms, including headache and vertigo.[7] Ethylene glycol ingestion may be suggested by the presence of calcium oxalate crystals in the urine.[7] Other entities that may cause a ketotic state include hyperemesis gravidarum and starvation.[1] Cyanide poisoning has also been associated with ketonemia.[1] Isopropyl alcohol (rubbing alcohol) causes ketosis by being metabolized to acetone, but does not cause an acidosis.[1]

The many causes of abdominal pain that could be associated with the patient's symptom complex must also be considered, including such disorders as pancreatitis, gastritis, gastrointestinal bleeding, hepatitis, cirrhosis, and urosepsis, among others.[16]

EMERGENCY DEPARTMENT EVALUATION

In addition to the clinical history, the diagnosis hinges on the laboratory finding of an elevated anion-gap metabolic acidosis. Hyperchloremic acidosis had been reported, and the presence of concomitant lactic acidosis is also common.[16] Metabolic alkalosis (due to persistent vomiting and volume depletion) and respiratory alkalosis (as a result of liver disease, alcohol withdrawal, or infection) may be present as well.[6–8,12] Some series note that between one-sixth and one-third of patients with AKA are actually alkalemic.[6,16] Due to a mixed acid–base disturbance or a compensatory hyperventilation, arterial blood gas analysis may show less severe acidemia than would be expected on the basis of the anion gap.

By definition, patients with AKA are ketotic. There are three types of ketone bodies: acetone and the ketoacids beta-hydroxybutyrate (BHB) and acetoacetate (AcAc). The nitroprusside reaction, which is commonly used to detect ketones in blood and urine, may be misleading in indicating the degree of ketosis, because only AcAc and acetone cause a positive reaction, whereas BHB does not.[6,7,15]

The ratio of BHB to AcAc depends on the ratio of reduced to oxidized nicotinamide adenine dinucleotide (NADH/NAD). In AKA, this ratio is high because the metabolism of ethanol generates NADH; the BHB/AcAc ratio averages 6:1.[7,15] A negative or trace-positive nitroprusside reaction may thus be inappropriately interpreted as indicating the absence of ketones. Therefore, the diagnosis of AKA should not be eliminated on the basis of an initially negative or minimally positive nitroprusside reaction.

As the patient is treated and AKA begins to resolve, the NADH/NAD ratio changes to favor the conversion of more BHB to AcAc, and the test for ketones may become more strongly positive.[7] A similar phenomenon has been described in the course of treatment of severe DKA, when, as the patient clinically improves with the administration of insulin and fluids, the test for ketones "worsens."[7] In one series of patients in whom ketones were measured, 4% had a negative semiquantitative reaction for serum AcAc and 10% had negative ketones on urine dipstick testing. This occurred more commonly in patients with higher blood alcohol levels.[16]

Although the classic presentation of AKA is one of ketoacidosis without marked hyperglycemia, the glucose concentration may be low, normal, or minimally elevated.[7–10,14] Ten percent of patients in one series had a serum glucose value of more than 250 mg/dL, but there was no history of diabetes mellitus, and no subsequent clinical evidence of glucose intolerance was found after treatment.[9,16] However, in another study, patients with ketoacidosis, hyperglycemia, and an elevated HbA1c were likely to have concurrent diabetes.[9]

Electrolyte disorders are common. These may include hyponatremia, hypokalemia, hypophosphatemia, hypocalcemia, and hypomagnesemia.[7] Hyperkalemia is seen in 15% of patients and is correlated with low pH.[16] Hyperphosphatemia, if present, resolves rapidly with therapy.[7,16] Liver enzymes, amylase, blood urea nitrogen, and false-positive creatinine levels may be elevated, but reflect dehydration and underlying chronic medical problems rather then being a direct result of AKA.[7,14]

An increased osmolar gap, even after accounting for any ethanol or other toxic alcohols, has been described in some patients with AKA.[2,3] Although the nature of the gap is unclear, it appears to be attributable, at least partly, to the presence of acetone, its metabolite acetol, 1,2-propanediol, and glycerol.[2,3]

Anemia and thrombocytopenia are common in AKA but are usually mild. Leukocytosis appears to be primarily a marker of volume depletion and demargination due to physical stress, rather than an infection, although leukopenia is often a marker of a severe underlying disease.

EMERGENCY DEPARTMENT MANAGEMENT

The treatment of AKA is relatively straightforward. Volume repletion and provision of glucose are the mainstays of therapy.[7,11] Saline, besides normalizing volume status, promotes the renal excretion of the ketone bodies BHB and AcAc.[14] The volume of saline required depends on the initial degree of dehydration and the patient's underlying clinical condition.[7] Glucose stimulates endogenous insulin secretion, decreasing the generation of ketone bodies.[5,7,12,15]

In the absence of shock or severe hepatic insufficiency, BHB and AcAc are rapidly converted back to bicarbonate in the liver, and acidosis resolves quickly. In a controlled study that compared the use of normal saline alone with that of saline plus glucose, patients in the glucose-treated group corrected their acidosis within 12 hours. The administration of exogenous bicarbonate or insulin was not necessary. Patients treated with normal saline alone also had favorable outcomes, although not as rapidly.[12]

Dextrose-containing solutions should probably be avoided in those patients who present with severe hyperglycemia.[16] Appropriate doses of insulin should be provided for patients who are known to be diabetic. However, insulin does not appear to play a role in the treatment of the normoglycemic patient with AKA.

Potassium repletion should be initiated in patients who are hypokalemic and in those with normokalemia who are acidemic, assuming there is no problem with renal function. This should be done with appropriate monitoring and frequent reassessments. Magnesium repletion is indicated, in the absence of renal insufficiency, not only to restore calcium homeostasis, but also to forestall alcohol withdrawal. Hypophosphatemia occurs in approximately 20% of patients with AKA, but routine repletion does not appear to improve morbidity and mortality.[10,16]

The use of bicarbonate in this disease, as in many others marked by acidosis, has been controversial.[1,8,11,12,16] However, in the absence of complicating features, the response of *even severe* AKA to volume repletion and glucose is such that the administration of bicarbonate is usually not necessary.[11]

Thiamine should be administered for the prevention of Wernicke's encephalopathy.[6,7,11] Vitamin supplements should be administered as indicated.

DISPOSITION

Many patients with AKA can be discharged home from the ED after receiving appropriate treatment. One series reported only a 54% admission rate.[16] Patients should not be discharged until they have demonstrated the ability to tolerate fluids, have had their volume status normalized, and have shown resolution of metabolic abnormalities. Underlying or precipitating illness must have resolved or been ruled out.

Admission is indicated for those who cannot tolerate oral hydration because of persistent nausea and vomiting, for those in whom a significant metabolic acidosis or electrolyte abnormality persists, and for those in whom the cause of abdominal pain is unclear or an associated illness complicated the picture. Admitted patients can often be treated on a general medical floor or in a short-term observation unit.

Close follow-up after discharge should be arranged. Many patients may benefit from referral to an alcohol rehabilitation program.

COMMON PITFALLS

- Misdiagnosis of AKA as DKA in the patient with ketosis, Kussmaul respiration, and minimally elevated blood glucose level
- Failure to consider AKA in the patient presenting with complaints of abdominal pain who does not offer a history of ethanol ingestion or binge drinking
- Failure to make use of the olfactory clue of a strong ketotic odor
- Assuming a patient is not ketotic because a serum or urine nitroprusside reaction is negative or only trace-positive
- Failure to appreciate the presence of a mixed acid–base disorder
- Failure to treat with dextrose-containing solutions
- Failure to consider other causes of nausea, vomiting, and abdominal pain in the alcoholic patient. Because the alcoholic is predisposed to a multitude of diseases, a careful history and physical examination must be done in even the most apparently straightforward of cases.

References

1. Adams SL. Alcoholic ketoacidosis. *Emerg Med Clin North Am* 1990;8:749.
2. Almaghams AM, Yeung CK. Osmolal gap in alcoholic ketoacidosis. *Clin Nephrol* 1997;48:52.
3. Braden GL, Strayhorn CH, Germain MJ, et al. Increased osmolal gap in alcoholic acidosis. *Arch Intern Med* 1993;153:2377.
4. Brinkmann B, Fechner G, Karger B, et al. Ketoacidosis and lactic acidosis—frequent causes of death in chronic alcoholics? *Int J Legal Med* 1998;111:115.
5. Fumeaux T, de Werra P. Acute metabolic acidosis in chronic alcoholism: ketoacidosis as differential diagnosis. *Intensive Care Med* 1996;22:1462.
6. Harper JP. Alcoholic ketoacidosis. *N Z Med J* 1997;110:18.
7. Hojer J. Severe metabolic acidosis in the alcoholic: differential diagnosis and management. *Hum Exp Toxicol* 1996;15:482.
8. Jenkins DW, Eckel RE, Craig JW. Alcoholic ketoacidosis. *JAMA* 1971;217:177.
9. Lu WT, Chen KW, Lin JD, et al. Ketoacidosis with hyperglycemia in heavy drinkers: a report of 12 cases. *Chang Gung Med J* 1997;20:34.
10. Machiels JP, Dive A, Donckier J, et al. Reversible myocardial dysfunction in a patient with alcoholic ketoacidosis: a role for hypophosphatemia. *Am J Emerg Med* 1998;16:371.
11. Marinella MA. Alcoholic ketoacidosis presenting with extreme hypoglycemia. *Am J Emerg Med* 1997;15:280.
12. Miller PD, Heining RE, Waterhouse C. Treatment of alcoholic acidosis: the role of dextrose and phosphorus. *Arch Intern Med* 1978;138:67.
13. Oh MS, Carroll HJ. The anion gap. *N Engl J Med* 1977;297:814.
14. Palmer JP. Alcoholic ketoacidosis: clinical and laboratory presentation, pathophysiology and treatment. *J Clin Endocrinol Metab* 1983;12:381.
15. Pounder DJ, Stevenson RJ, Taylor KK. Alcoholic ketoacidosis at autopsy. *J Forensic Sci* 1998;43:812.
16. Wrenn KD, Slovis CM, Minion G, et al. The syndrome of alcoholic ketoacidosis. *Am J Med* 1991;91:119.

CHAPTER 171
Thyroid Emergencies

T. Eugene Ragland and Robert C. Urbanic

THYROID FUNCTION TESTS

In the emergency department, the diagnosis of hyperthyroidism or hypothyroidism depends on clinical assessment and is supported and confirmed by thyroid function testing.

Thyroid hormone concentration depends on the rate of production by the thyroid gland and on utilization or metabolism at extrathyroidal sites (Fig. 171.1).[19] Thyroid hormone is secreted in response to stimulation of the thyroid gland by thyroid-stimulating hormone (TSH) produced in the anterior pituitary gland. TSH release, in turn, is promoted by thyrotropin-releasing hormone (TRH) derived from the hypothalamus, and is further modulated by intrapituitary T_3 concentration.

Thyroxine, T_4, is produced solely by the thyroid gland and is deiodinated in various parts of the body to the biologically active triiodothyronine, T_3, or to the inactive reverse T_3. In addition, small amounts of T_3 are produced by the thyroid gland. The vast majority of thyroid hormone is carried by various proteins; the most important clinically is thyroxine-binding globulin, TBG. Changes in the amount of carrier proteins or in their binding capacity can alter the concentration of total and free thyroid hormones. Free unbound T_4 and T_3 are physiologically active fractions and best correlate with the clinical status.

The best means of assessing thyroid hormone activity is measurement of the free T_4 level. Generally, the degree of reduction of the free T_4 below normal levels is proportionate to the severity of hypothyroidism, and the degree of elevation above normal levels is proportionate to the severity of thyrotoxicosis. Direct measurement of free T_4 is technically demanding and not readily available, but the commonly available free T_4 assays are accurate in most clinical situations and are less expensive. Free T_4 can also be assessed by using the less reliable free T_4 index, which is the product of the *total* T_4 concentration and the T_3 resin uptake. The latter reflects alterations in protein binding of hormone due to nonthyroidal illness and other conditions. Unfortunately, the term is sometimes confused with total T_3.

Sensitive assays of TSH have become the single most helpful measurements of thyroid function. The level of TSH reflects the pituitary's perception of thyroid hormone action. In thyroid gland failure (primary hypothyroidism), the basal TSH level is elevated. The TSH is suppressed with almost all causes of thyrotoxicosis, but now TSH assays are sensitive enough to distinguish euthyroid patients from those with hyperthyroidism.[2,12,15] Sensitive TSH assays have eliminated the need to perform TRH stimulation tests to evaluate questionably thyrotoxic patients and have made possible more precise thyroid hormone-replacement therapy.

The combination of free T_4 assay and a sensitive TSH assay is the primary means of assessing thyroid status in all patients. A single TSH assay may be an effective screening tool in some settings, but both tests are needed in the emergency department or in acutely ill patients. When the clinical picture suggests thyrotoxicosis, the finding of an elevated free T_4 and a suppressed (unmeasurable) TSH confirms the diagnosis.

Additional thyroid function tests are rarely used to establish a diagnosis of thyrotoxicosis in the emergency setting. Total T_3 and free T_3 assays are available. Their major use is in identifying

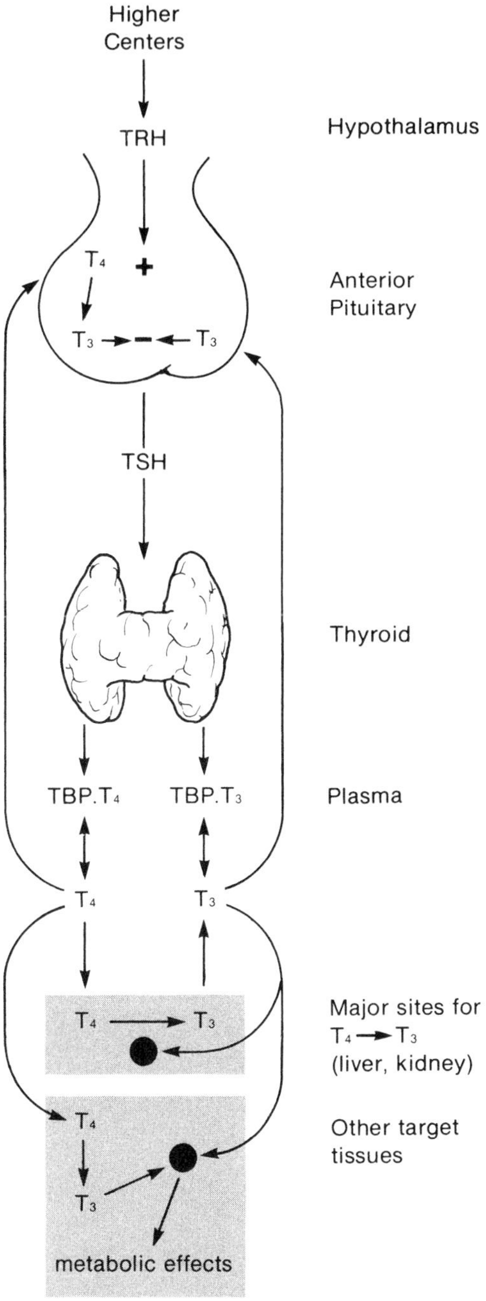

Figure 171.1. Major features of the hypothalamic–anterior pituitary–thyroid–target tissue axis. TBP, thyroid hormone–binding protein.

so-called T_3-toxicosis, an unusual condition in which T_3 rather than T_4 is responsible for hyperthyroid effects and in which, as might be expected, TSH is suppressed but free T_4 is low or normal.

Direct assessment of increased thyroid gland function can be obtained by measurement of thyroid radioactive iodine uptake. This nuclear medicine test quantitates the uptake of iodine by the thyroid gland and generally reflects thyroid hormone production. Because this test is strongly influenced by the patient's total iodine pool, recent exposure to iodine-containing contrast agents or medications may confuse the interpretation of test results. An exogenous iodine load expands the iodine pool and dilutes the radioactively labeled iodine, producing a spuriously low radioactive iodine uptake. The test is used chiefly to determine the etiology of hyperthyroidism. It has no place in the evaluation of the hypothyroid patient.

COMMON PITFALLS

- Thyroid function tests can be influenced by nonthyroidal illness, drugs, and a variety of other clinical states, such as pregnancy. Acute illness can affect the secretion and metabolism of thyroid hormone and can alter the equilibrium between free and protein-bound hormone, making interpretation of thyroid testing extremely difficult. Acutely ill hospitalized patients do not benefit from routine thyroid function testing.[7]
- Although by far the most common cause of a low TSH is thyrotoxicosis, TSH levels can be suppressed in hypopituitary or hypothalamic disease, in the first trimester of pregnancy, in acute psychiatric illness, in patients with nonthyroidal illness, and in patients receiving dopamine or high doses of glucocorticoids.[4] The most sensitive assays can distinguish some of these entities from ordinary thyrotoxicosis, in which the TSH is unmeasurable.[18] Conversely, the TSH can be elevated from causes other than hypothyroidism. Levels have been reported to be increased in the recovery stage after nonthyroidal illness and after the use of certain cholecystectographic contrast agents.[4] Nevertheless, when the TSH is combined with a free T_4 assay and a knowledge of the clinical setting, it is possible to make a correct interpretation in the majority of patients.
- Severe systemic illness, as well as the use of a number of medications, can lead to a confusing array of thyroid function test abnormalities in which patients may have a biochemical picture of either hyper or hypothyroidism.[3] In addition, patients with the "sick euthyroid syndrome" may appear to be clinically hypothyroid in the setting of acute nonthyroidal illness, but have normal free T_4 and a decreased T_3 level due to decreased peripheral conversion of T_4 to T_3. Thus, emergency department patients with mild or questionable signs and symptoms of either hyperthyroidism or hypothyroidism are best managed without immediate treatment.

THYROID STORM

Thyroid storm is a rare, life-threatening complication of thyrotoxicosis. It occurs most often in patients with undiagnosed or undertreated thyrotoxic Graves disease and, occasionally, in patients with toxic multinodular goiter. It is reported in 1% to 2% of patients who are hospitalized for hyperthyroidism. Although thyroid storm occurs in both sexes and at any age, it is more common in women during the middle decades. Its pathogenesis is unknown.

The onset of thyroid storm is usually abrupt. If untreated, it is usually fatal. The overall mortality is 10% to 20%, with underlying illness being the cause of death in many instances.

A precipitating event can be identified in 50% to 75% of cases. The causes most commonly implicated are infection (especially pulmonary), trauma, vascular accident, diabetic complications, and nonthyroidal surgery. Preoperative preparation of hyperthyroid patients and the use of antithyroid drugs, iodine, and propranolol in treatment have virtually eliminated thyroid storm in patients undergoing thyroid surgery for hyperthyroidism.

CLINICAL PRESENTATION

The criteria for a diagnosis of thyroid storm are a temperature higher than 37.8°C (100°F); tachycardia out of proportion to the fever; dysfunction of the central nervous system (CNS), cardiovascular system, and/or gastrointestinal (GI) system; and exaggerated peripheral manifestations of thyrotoxicosis.

Thyroid storm is a clinical diagnosis. The presence of thyrotoxicosis is a prerequisite for the development of storm, but determining the point at which thyrotoxicosis becomes thyroid storm is a matter of judgment and semantics.

Fever is an invariable finding and may be as high as 41.1°C (106°F), with or without concurrent infection. Marked diaphoresis is also present and can lead to significant insensible fluid loss.

CNS dysfunction occurs in 90% of patients with thyroid storm. Symptoms range from restlessness, anxiety, and emotional lability to delirium, obtundation, and coma. Neuromuscular manifestations include tremor and muscle weakness.

Cardiovascular abnormalities are present in 50% of patients. Sinus tachycardia is usual. Atrial fibrillation, premature ventricular contractions, and, rarely, complete heart block can occur. The pulse pressure is characteristically widened (one series reported an average pulse pressure of 80 mm Hg), with increased stroke volume, cardiac output, and myocardial oxygen consumption. Congestive heart failure is common in thyroid storm and may be the presenting manifestation. Progressive cardiac dysfunction leads to pulmonary edema and cardiogenic shock as terminal events.

GI dysfunction is also prominent in most patients with storm. Marked weight loss has often occurred in the preceding weeks or months, and storm may be heralded by diarrhea and hyperdefecation. During storm, anorexia, nausea, vomiting, and crampy abdominal pain may simulate an acute abdomen. Jaundice and tender hepatomegaly are occasionally additional GI manifestations.

TABLE 171.1. Differential Diagnosis of Thyroid Storm

Disease Entity	Manifestations
Anxiety states	Agitation, sleeplessness, emotional lability, weight loss
Psychosis	CNS dysfunction, tachycardia
Cocaine toxicity	Agitation, confusion, tachycardia, arrhythmias, weight loss, hyperthermia
Pheochromocytoma	Sweating, palpitations, nervousness, tremor, weight loss, heat intolerance
Heat stroke	Confusion, tachycardia, hyperthermia, prostration
Neuroleptic malignant syndrome	Hyperthermia, tachycardia, CNS dysfunction
Diabetes mellitus, out of control	Confusion, vomiting, weight loss, abdominal pain, tender hepatomegaly
Chronic obstructive pulmonary disease, end-stage	Confusion, cachexia, tachycardia, arrhythmias, pulmonary infection
Acute abdomen	Vomiting, abdominal pain, hyperthermia
Congestive heart failure	Cardiovascular dysfunction, arrhythmias, tender hepatomegaly
Alcoholic complications	Confusion, vomiting, restlessness, tremor, fever, jaundice, abdominal pain, tender hepatomegaly

DIFFERENTIAL DIAGNOSIS

The diagnosis of thyroid storm is a clinical one.[17] In general, storm should be suspected in any thyrotoxic patient with either a fever or the other cardinal manifestations discussed previously. Additional factors to consider include a history of Graves disease, a palpable goiter, or any eye signs suggestive of Graves ophthalmopathy.

Exaggerated symptoms of hyperthyroidism distinguish storm from routine thyrotoxicosis. When thyroid storm is suspected, therapy should generally be initiated immediately.

Additional disease entities that may be confused with thyroid storm are those that manifest with a hyperkinetic state, hyperpyrexia, or dysfunction of the previously described organ systems (Table 171.1).

EMERGENCY DEPARTMENT EVALUATION

Some historic information, if available, can be of great help in making the diagnosis. A history of goiter, increased sweating, rapid heart rate, severe weakness, heat intolerance, or weight loss despite an increased appetite suggests antecedent thyrotoxicosis. A history of eye complaints (stare, bulging eyes, conjunctivitis, periorbital swelling, corneal ulceration, diplopia, decreased visual acuity) suggests Graves disease. The medication history may provide important clues; the patient should be asked about thyroid hormone preparations, iodine-containing compounds, and recent radiographic studies with iodine-containing contrast materials.[9]

The physical examination is of increased importance when a history is unobtainable. Fever, tachycardia, widened pulse pressure, and CNS dysfunction are evident from the outset. Cardiovascular examination often shows arrhythmias, especially atrial fibrillation, or signs of congestive heart failure. Eye signs such as stare, lid lag, and Graves ophthalmopathy may be found. Examination of the thyroid gland almost always reveals a goiter, often with a thrill or a bruit. Muscle tremor and evidence of weakness, especially of the proximal muscle groups, should be sought.

Thyroid function tests do not distinguish uncomplicated thyrotoxicosis from thyroid storm because of an overlap in values,[3] and, in any event, these laboratory values are not normally available to the emergency physician quickly enough to affect initial management.

Nonspecific laboratory abnormalities of the complete blood count, electrolytes, and liver function studies are often noted, and hyperglycemia is common. Hypercalcemia may occur in 25% of patients with storm. Plasma cortisol levels have been observed to be inappropriately low for the degree of stress.

EMERGENCY DEPARTMENT MANAGEMENT

The treatment of thyroid storm must not be delayed once the diagnosis is suspected. The thyrotoxic patient who is treated unnecessarily for thyroid storm should do well. Specific therapeutic goals can be divided into five areas: general supportive care, inhibition of thyroid hormone synthesis, retardation of thyroid hormone release, blockade of peripheral thyroid hormone effects, and identification and treatment of precipitating events.

General Supportive Care

Adequate hydration with intravenous fluids and electrolytes must be ensured in order to replace GI and insensible losses. Supplemental oxygen should be provided because of increased oxygen consumption. Continuous cardiac monitoring to identify cardiac arrhythmias is indicated. Fever should be controlled with antipyretics and a cooling blanket.

Congestive heart failure must be treated in the usual fashion. Congestive heart failure due to thyrotoxicosis may be refractory to digitalis, however. Glucocorticoids equivalent to 300 mg of hydrocortisone per day should be administered intravenously. Occasionally, specific therapy is required to reduce unacceptably high levels of blood glucose or calcium. Finally, the patient's clinical status and response to treatment must be followed closely by frequent monitoring of vital signs and repeated physical examination.

Inhibition of Thyroid Hormone Synthesis

The antithyroid drugs propylthiouracil (PTU) and methimazole block the synthesis of thyroid hormone through inhibition of the organification of tyrosine residues. PTU (900 to 1200 mg orally as an initial loading dose, followed by 300 to 600 mg/d) should be administered until thyrotoxicosis is controlled. Methimazole is an alternative to PTU (dose: 90 to 120 mg orally initially, followed by 30 to 60 mg/d). A nasogastric tube may be required, because these medications are available only in oral form.

Antithyroid drugs begin to act during the first hour after administration, but full therapeutic effect is not achieved for 3 to 6 weeks. PTU is preferred over methimazole, because it produces a more rapid clinical response and also inhibits the peripheral conversion of T_4 to T_3.

Inhibition of Thyroid Hormone Release

Iodide administration immediately retards the release of stored thyroid hormones from the thyroid gland. Iodide should not be administered until 1 hour after the loading dose of an antithyroid drug to avoid worsening hyperthyroidism by increasing the pool of iodine available for incorporation into thyroid hormone before organification has been inhibited. It may be given as Lugol's solution, 30 drops orally per day, or as sodium iodide, 1 g every 8 to 12 hours by slow intravenous infusion. An alternative is lithium carbonate, 300 to 450 mg orally three times a day as an initial dose and then titrated by blood lithium level. Although lithium effectively blocks thyroid hormone release, it has a narrow margin of therapeutic safety.

Blockade of Peripheral Thyroid Hormone Effects

Adrenergic blockade is a mainstay of therapy for thyroid storm. Propranolol is the drug of choice. Given intravenously (1 mg/min to a total dose of 10 mg), it begins to control the cardiac and psychomotor manifestations of thyroid storm within minutes. Oral propranolol (20 to 120 mg or more every 4 to 6 hours) begins to be effective in about 1 hour.

Intravenous propranolol has been associated with cardiac arrest in rare instances, and the usual precaution of avoiding use of the drug in patients with bronchospastic disease and heart block should be considered. To detect the latter problem, electrocardiographic findings should be checked before the drug is administered.

In patients with thyrotoxic congestive heart failure, the use of propranolol is controversial.[8] Heart failure can be caused by tachycardia, especially in the presence of atrial fibrillation. The benefit of slowing the ventricular response in atrial fibrillation must be weighed against the risk of depressing myocardial contractility. Digitalis should be administered before propranolol in this clinical setting.

Guanethidine and reserpine also provide effective autonomic blockades and are alternatives to propranolol. Both act to deplete catecholamine stores, and guanethidine also blocks their release. Guanethidine can be given in a dose of 1 to 2 mg/kg/d orally. Reserpine is administered in an initial dose of 1 to 5 mg intramuscularly, followed by 1.0 to 2.5 mg every 4 to 6 hours.

Other Therapeutic Modalities

Symptomatic improvement should occur within hours of the initiation of therapy, but resolution of thyroid storm requires the degradation of circulating thyroid hormones. Because the biologic half-life of T_4 is 6 days and that of T_3 is 22 hours, thyroid storm may persist for days. Alternative therapeutic modalities such as exchange transfusion, plasmapheresis, and charcoal hemoperfusion have been used in the treatment of thyroid storm refractory to other measures.

DISPOSITION

Patients suspected of having thyroid storm require admission to an intensive care unit. An endocrinologist or an internist should be consulted. Treatment of thyroid storm should not be delayed pending consultation, however. When it is necessary to transfer a patient to another facility, transport must be effected by an advanced life-support unit with an intravenous line, supplemental oxygen, and continuous cardiac monitoring.

COMMON PITFALLS

- The most common pitfalls for the emergency physician center around diagnosis of this endocrine emergency. Because of the rarity and variable presentation of thyroid storm, the clinician may fail to consider it as the diagnosis. The diagnosis must be suspected based on the constellation of the patient's presenting signs and symptoms. Fever in a thyrotoxic patient does not necessarily imply thyroid storm. It is the exaggerated symptoms of hyperthyroidism that distinguish thyroid storm from routine thyrotoxicosis.
- Apathetic thyrotoxicosis is a distinct form of thyrotoxicosis that most often occurs in the elderly without the usual hyperkinetic manifestations. This diagnosis is frequently missed and should be considered in the elderly patient who presents with weight loss, proximal muscle weakness, slowed mentation, placid facies, congestive heart failure, or atrial fibrillation. Undiagnosed and untreated, these patients may quietly lapse into a coma and die. When signs and symptoms referable to dysfunction of one organ system dominate and obscure the underlying diagnosis of thyrotoxicosis, "masked" thyrotoxicosis is said to exist.

MYXEDEMA COMA

Myxedema coma is the ultimate life-threatening expression of severe hypothyroidism. It occurs most often during the winter months in elderly women who have long-standing hypothyroidism that is undiagnosed or undertreated. A precipitating stressful event can be discovered in most patients who develop this complication of hypothyroidism.

Myxedema coma is rare. It occurs in patients with hypothyroidism, which is usually a result of surgical or radioiodine ablative therapy for Graves disease, idiopathic hypothyroidism, or Hashimoto thyroiditis.[14] The pathophysiology of myxedema coma is unknown, but metabolic complications, intercurrent illness, and thyroid hormone deficiency *per se* have been implicated.

Hypothyroidism is generally a progressive, insidious disease.[14] Patients who develop hypothyroidism after subtotal thyroidectomy most often do so 12 to 15 months following surgery. Of patients treated with radioactive iodine, 40% to 70% develop hypothyroidism within 10 years. A patient with undiagnosed hypothyroidism may present with coma as the initial manifestation of the disease. More often, the disease progresses over a period of years, and coma occurs when the patient is stressed with an additional precipitating event. Of these, infection, especially pulmonary infection, is the most common. Exposure to a cold environment, cerebrovascular or cardiovascular events, hemorrhage, and trauma have also been identified as precipitants. In addition, because hypothyroid patients metabolize drugs slowly, even normal doses of sedatives, analgesics, or anesthetics can induce prolonged coma in a patient with severe hypothyroidism. More than 50% of patients who develop myxedema coma do so after admission to the hospital. Drugs, nosocomial infections, and the rigors of diagnostic and therapeutic procedures are the most likely causative factors. If untreated, myxedema coma is fatal.

CLINICAL PRESENTATION

All patients who develop myxedema coma are hypothyroid and have signs and symptoms of hypothyroidism. Patients with moderate-to-severe hypothyroidism develop myxedema—a nonpitting, dry, waxy swelling of the skin and subcutaneous tissues due to accumulation of mucopolysaccharides, resulting in characteristic puffy facies (Fig. 171.2). Additional cutaneous clues to the diagnosis include thinning of the eyebrows and scant body hair. Other frequent complaints are fatigue, weakness, cold intolerance, muscle cramps, constipation, and weight gain. Women often have a history of menometrorrhagia. A deepened voice and a thick, enlarged tongue may be noted.

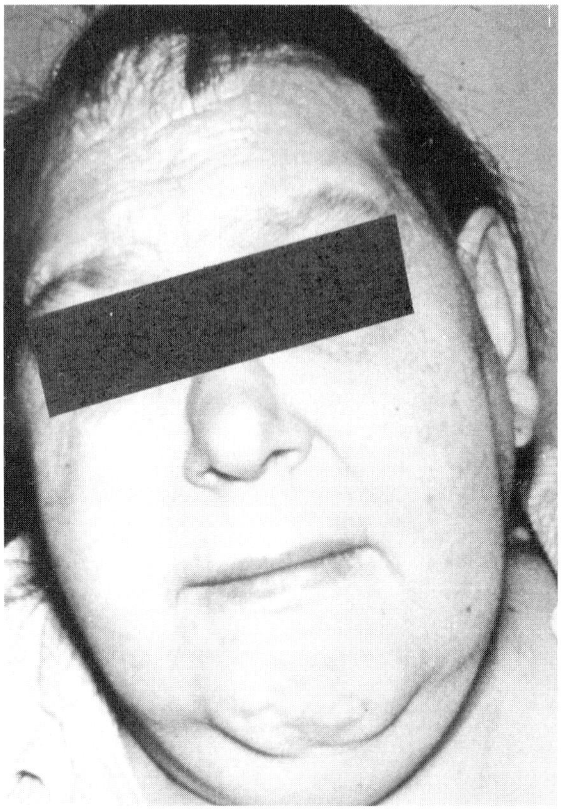

Figure 171.2. Myxedema.

DIFFERENTIAL DIAGNOSIS

The differentiation of myxedema coma from other entities rests on the clinical recognition of myxedema. Severely ill, elderly patients with hypothermia, respiratory failure, hyponatremia, or hypoglycemia may have myxedema coma or precoma. Because T_3 and T_4 may be depressed in an acutely ill euthyroid patient, and, in any event, are not usually available to the emergency physician, treatment must be based on a history and physical examination that clearly support the diagnosis of myxedema.

The clinical picture of myxedema superficially resembles that of chronic renal failure and nephrotic syndrome. Chronic renal failure can present with mental impairment or coma, sallow complexion, puffy face and extremities, seizures, and hyponatremia, but the patient with renal failure has an elevated serum creatinine. Patients with nephrotic syndrome may present with normal renal function but often appear pale and have anasarca. The serum T_4 may be low in these patients because of a loss of TBG in the urine, but the free T_4 and TSH are normal. Although mild proteinuria may occur with hypothyroidism, it is of a much lesser degree than in nephrotic syndrome.

EMERGENCY DEPARTMENT EVALUATION

A history of hypothyroidism, treatment for Graves disease, or discontinuation of replacement thyroid hormone therapy is helpful, if elicited.

Paresthesias, ataxia, and delay of the relaxation phase of the deep tendon reflexes may occur with hypothyroidism. Seizures (in 25% of those who develop myxedema coma) and mental disturbances are more severe neurologic manifestations. Coma is a terminal expression of neurologic dysfunction in myxedema.

Cardiovascular clues to hypothyroidism are bradycardia, cardiomegaly, and low voltage on electrocardiogram (ECG). Systolic blood pressure is usually less than 100 mm Hg, but mild hypertension may be observed. Pericardial effusion is present in up to 30% of patients; echocardiography is often required to confirm the presence of effusion.

Patients with severe hypothyroidism commonly have abdominal distention that may be due to ascites, paralytic ileus, or fecal impaction. Acquired megacolon is almost uniformly observed; bowel obstruction and pseudoobstruction have been reported.

Normal thermogenesis is impaired in hypothyroidism; hypothermia, unassociated with sweating or shivering, is a typical finding. A normal or elevated temperature in this clinical setting may indicate underlying infection.

Respiratory failure is common in myxedema coma.[20] Respiratory assistance may be required to treat hypercapnia and hypoxemia. Serum sodium levels of less than 120 mEq/L occur in up to two-thirds of patients with myxedema coma.[5,16]

Seventy percent of patients with myxedema coma have a temperature less than 37°C (98.6°F), and 15% less than 29.5°C (85°F). The systolic blood pressure is less than 100 mm Hg in 50% of cases, and bradycardia is common. A scar may be seen over the thyroid area. A distended urinary bladder is sometimes noted.

Thyroid function tests confirm the diagnosis of hypothyroidism but are not usually available during emergent evaluation. The free T_4 is low. The TSH level is elevated in primary hypothyroidism but may be low or normal in pituitary–hypothalamic disease. Hyponatremia, hypochloremia, and hypoglycemia may be present on routine laboratory testing. Additional laboratory abnormalities include hypercholesterolemia and occasional striking elevations of muscle enzymes such as creatine kinase, serum glutamic-oxaloacetic transaminase, and lactate dehydrogenase. When lumbar puncture is performed, the cerebrospinal fluid (CSF) pressure may be increased, and the CSF protein level is usually elevated.

Radiographic abnormalities in hypothyroidism may include an enlarged cardiac silhouette on chest radiograph or ileus on abdominal flat plate. Typical ECG findings consist of sinus bradycardia, low voltage, prolongation of the PR interval, and inversion of the T waves. The presence of a myocardial effusion may be confirmed by echocardiography.

EMERGENCY DEPARTMENT MANAGEMENT

The diagnosis of myxedema coma must be based on a clinical impression, and treatment should not be delayed once the diagnosis is made. However, the decision to treat must be made with extreme caution, because the administration of large doses of thyroid hormone can be fatal to the euthyroid or mildly hypothyroid patient. Every attempt to attribute coma to its proper cause should be made first.

Respiratory failure should be treated with oxygen administration and ventilatory support as needed. Hypothermic patients should be gradually rewarmed passively with blankets; hypothermic patients typically respond quite slowly. Aggressive rewarming techniques are hazardous.[11] Drugs that may further depress respiratory or metabolic function should be avoided. Hyponatremia should be treated with water restriction or, when hyponatremia is severe, with hypertonic saline and furosemide.[1] Hypoglycemia requires intravenous glucose infusion. Hypotension should be treated with isotonic fluid administration and thyroid hormone replacement. Vasopressors should be used only when hypotension is refractory to initial therapy. Glucocorticoids equivalent to 300 mg of hydrocortisone per day should be given to ensure adequate cortisol activity, because adrenal insufficiency may be a concomitant finding. Frequent vital signs, cardiac monitoring, and sequential physical examination are important to monitor the patient's status and response to treatment.

Thyroid hormone replacement is the most critical and specific aspect of therapy for myxedema coma. L-thyroxine is the recommended preparation.[13] An initial dose of 400 to 500 μg is given by slow intravenous infusion. (If cardiac arrest following intravenous L-thyroxine has occurred, the dose should be reduced in the face of cardiac ischemia.) The initial dose should be followed by 50 to 100 μg/d intravenously. Once the patient is able to take an oral dose, 100 to 200 μg/d can be started orally. Initiation and adjustment of this oral dose depend on the results of thyroid function testing.[6]

Triiodothyronine (T_3) is four times as potent pharmacologically as thyroxine (T_4). However, it was previously available only in tablet form, and its use was not favored because it had to be crushed and given by a nasogastric tube in many patients. There was also concern that absorption would be reduced because of myxedema-induced gastrointestinal dysfunction. Intravenous L-triiodothyronine is now available.[10] An initial intravenous dose of 25 to 50 μg is recommended for emergent treatment of myxedema coma or precoma in adults. The dose should be lowered to 10 to 20 μg for patients with known or suspected cardiovascular disease. Subsequent dosage is 65 to 100 μg per 24 hours in three to four divided doses, or half of this amount in patients with cardiovascular disease. Contraindications and drug interactions of intravenous T_3 are identical to those of T_4. With either drug, clinical improvement should be apparent within 24 to 36 hours.

A final aspect of treatment of myxedema coma is the identification and treatment of any precipitating event. Those factors previously mentioned should be sought and treated when present. Care should be taken not to place any additional metabolic demands on these precariously compensated patients.

DISPOSITION

All patients treated for myxedema coma require admission to an intensive care unit. Consultation with an endocrinologist or an internist should be arranged. Patients who require transfer to another facility should be transported in an advanced life-support unit in which supplemental oxygen and continuous cardiac monitoring are available.

COMMON PITFALLS

- Failure to consider the diagnosis of myxedema coma is a common pitfall. Because myxedema coma is rare and because the associated metabolic problems may distract attention from the underlying diagnosis, coma may be attributed to hypothermia, CO_2 narcosis, hyponatremia, hypoglycemia, drug overdose, or other causes. Unless the underlying thyroid failure is diagnosed and treated, therapeutic efforts will not be successful.
- Fever can occur in a patient with myxedema coma who has an underlying infection. The absence of hypothermia does not preclude a diagnosis of myxedema coma.

References

1. Ayns JC, Krothapalli RK, Arieff AI. Treatment of symptomatic hyponatremia and its relation to brain damage. *N Engl J Med* 1987;317:1190.
2. Borst GC, Eil C, Burman KD. Euthyroid hyperthyroxinemia. *Ann Intern Med* 1983;98:366.
3. Brooks MH, Waldstein SS. Free thyroxine concentration in thyroid storm. *Ann Intern Med* 1980;93:694.
4. Cavalieri RR. The effects of nonthyroid disease and drugs on thyroid function tests. *Med Clin North Am* 1991;75:27.
5. Derubertis FR, Michelis MF, Bloom ME, et al. Impaired water excretion in myxedema. *Am J Med* 1971;51:41.
6. Fish LH, Schwartz HL, Cavanaugh J, et al. Replacement dose, metabolism, and bioavailability of levothyroxine in the treatment of hypothyroidism. Role of triiodothyronine in pituitary feedback in humans. *N Engl J Med* 1987;316:764.
7. Hefland M, Crapo LM. Screening for thyroid disease. *Ann Intern Med* 1990;112:840.
8. Ikram H. Haemodynamic effects of beta-adrenergic blockade in hyperthyroid patients with and without heart failure. *BMJ* 1977;1:1505.
9. Leger AF, Massin JP, Laurent MF, et al. Iodine-induced thyrotoxicosis: analysis of eighty-five consecutive cases. *Eur J Clin Invest* 1984;14:449.
10. MacKerrow SD, Osborn LA, Levy H, et al. Myxedema-associated cardiogenic shock treated with intravenous triiodothyronine. *Ann Intern Med* 1992; 117:1014.
11. Maclean D, Griffiths PD, Browning MCK, et al. Metabolic aspects of spontaneous rewarming in accidental hypothermia and myxoedema. *Q J Med* 1974;171:371.
12. Nicoloff JT, Spencer CA. The use and misuse of the sensitive thyrotropin assays. *J Clin Endocrinol Metab* 1990;71:553.
13. Ridgway EC, McCammon JA, Benotti J, et al. Acute metabolic responses in myxedema to large doses of intravenous L-thyroxine. *Ann Intern Med* 1972;77:549.
14. Sawin CT. Hypothyroidism. *Med Clin North Am* 1985;69:989.
15. Seth J, Beckett G. Diagnosis of hyperthyroidism: the newer biochemical tests. *Baillieres Clin Endocrinol Metab* 1985;14:373.
16. Skowsky WR, Kikuchi TA. The role of vasopressin in the impaired water excretion of myxedema. *Am J Med* 1978;64:613.
17. Spaulding SW, Lippes H. Hyperthyroidism. Causes, clinical features, and diagnosis. *Med Clin North Am* 1985;69:937.
18. Spencer CA, LoPresti JS, Patel A, et al. Applications of a new chemiluminometric thyrotropin assay to subnormal measurement. *J Clin Endocrinol Metab* 1990;70:453.
19. White GH. Recent advances in routine thyroid function testing. *Crit Rev Clin Lab Sci* 1987;24:315.
20. Zwillich CW, Pierson DJ, Hofeldt FD, et al. Ventilatory control in myxedema and hypothyroidism. *N Engl J Med* 1975;292:662.

CHAPTER 172
Adrenal and Pituitary Disorders

Clare T. Sercombe and Louis J. Ling

ADRENAL INSUFFICIENCY

Adrenal insufficiency results when the adrenal cortices fail to produce adequate quantities of cortisol and aldosterone.[1,5] The disorder results from a primary failure of hormone production because of loss of adrenal tissue (Addison disease) or from a failure of the pituitary to produce sufficient adrenocorticotropic hormone (ACTH) to stimulate the adrenal glands.

Primary adrenal insufficiency is an uncommon disorder, affecting approximately 100 persons per million.[13] Over 90% of the gland must be destroyed before symptoms become apparent. The most important cause is "idiopathic autoimmune adrenalitis," with lymphocytic infiltration of the adrenal gland and antiadrenal antibodies. This disorder is more common in women, usually arising between the third and fifth decades, and is sometimes associated with other autoimmune diseases, such as early ovarian failure, hyperthyroidism and hypothyroidism, insulin-dependent diabetes, hypoparathyroidism, vitiligo, and pernicious anemia.

Various other causes of primary adrenal insufficiency are listed in Table 172.1. Primary adrenal insufficiency is also seen in patients with the acquired human immunodeficiency virus (HIV),[6,10] usually due to disseminated cytomegalovirus (CMV) infection. Up to 84% of patients with CMV show evidence of CMV adrenalitis,[7,12,16] which can be treated with ganciclovir.[14,18] Other causes of adrenal insufficiency in patients with HIV include Kaposi's sarcoma or drug therapy. Drugs such as metyrapone, mitotane, aminoglutethimide, ketoconazole, fluconazole, and possibly rifampin may also decrease adrenal steroidogenesis.[9]

TABLE 172.1. Causes of Primary Adrenal Failure

Metastatic cancer
Lung
Breast
Leukemia
Infectious bacterial diseases
Meningococcemia
Pneumococcemia
Infectious granulomatous diseases
Tuberculosis
Blastomycosis
Coccidioidomycosis
Histoplasmosis
Viral diseases
Cytomegalovirus (especially in HIV patients)
Herpes simplex virus
Infiltrative diseases
Sarcoidosis
Amyloidosis
Hemochromatosis
Hemorrhage
Anticoagulant therapy
Abdominal trauma
Congenital adrenal hyperplasia
Adrenalectomy
Adrenal infarction
Catheterization of adrenal veins
Overwhelming sepsis (Waterhouse-Friderichsen syndrome)

In an otherwise healthy person, acute primary adrenal failure is exceedingly rare. Most primary adrenal insufficiency appears to result from diseases that develop over a period of years and progresses slowly to complete destruction of the adrenal glands.

The most common cause of *secondary* adrenal insufficiency (inadequate pituitary ACTH reserve) is suppression of the hypothalamic–pituitary–adrenal (HPA) axis by exogenous glucocorticoids. This suppression occurs after as little as 1 to 2 weeks of glucocorticoid therapy, with rapid withdrawal of glucocorticoids precipitating signs of adrenal insufficiency. Depending on the dose and duration of therapy, it may require several months to 1 year after withdrawal of glucocorticoids before the HPA axis again functions normally.

Secondary adrenal insufficiency is otherwise caused by disorders that destroy or compromise pituitary or hypothalamic integrity, such as pituitary or parasellar tumors (prolactinoma, acromegaly, meningioma, craniopharyngioma), hypothalamic tumors, head trauma, infarction ("pituitary apoplexy"), infiltrative or inflammatory processes, and hemorrhage (Sheehan syndrome). With the exception of trauma, infarction, and hemorrhage, pituitary and hypothalamic disease tends to result in gradual rather than sudden loss of function. Aldosterone secretion is usually normal in secondary adrenal insufficiency.

CLINICAL PRESENTATION

The clinical presentation of adrenal insufficiency depends on how rapidly adrenocortical function is lost. Acute adrenal failure ("addisonian crisis") is a medical emergency that requires rapid intervention. It usually occurs in an individual with underlying chronic adrenal insufficiency that experiences an acute stress, such as severe infection, sepsis, alcohol withdrawal, trauma, surgery, or myocardial infarction. Thus, it is important that the physician try to identify an intercurrent illness that could have precipitated the acute episode. There may also be a history of other autoimmune disorders.

The clinical syndrome includes weakness, fatigue, anorexia, nausea and vomiting, abdominal pain, diarrhea, dizziness, musculoskeletal pain, and weight loss. The patient may be disoriented, confused, or comatose. There is tachycardia, as well as hypotension with orthostatic changes. The skin is cool and dry, and the urine output is decreased. The patient may have a low-grade fever but can also be hypothermic. The classic physical finding in primary adrenal failure is hyperpigmentation, which is present in 98% of patients and is described as "suntan that doesn't fade." There is pigmentation of skin creases or folds that are not exposed to the sun; the nails, buccal mucosa, and gingiva may also be hyperpigmented. In Blacks, the tongue may appear darker. Vitiligo may be present, the scalp hair may be prematurely gray, and calcification of the ear lobes may be noted. Commonly, the presenting complaint is related to the gastrointestinal tract (e.g., constipation, nausea and vomiting, vague abdominal pain). Personality changes, irritability, and restlessness can also be noted.

Patients with secondary adrenal insufficiency may have additional symptoms and signs related to hypothalamic or pituitary disease, such as loss of sexual performance and libido, menstrual disturbances, headache, visual disturbances, galactorrhea, features of acromegaly, or evidence of head trauma. Hyperpigmentation is rare, because circulating levels of ACTH and related peptides are low. Loss of ACTH is often accompanied by loss of thyroid-stimulating hormone (TSH) secretion, so signs of hypothyroidism may be present. In patients with HIV, the most common complaint is fatigue.[15]

The most sensitive laboratory finding of adrenal insufficiency is hyperkalemia, although, classically, hyponatremia, hypercalcemia (with a normal ionized fraction), mild metabolic acidosis, and hypoglycemia are described. The hyperkalemia is secondary to aldosterone deficiency, whereas the hyponatremia results from renal sodium loss and free water retention. The blood cell count may show lymphocytosis or eosinophilia. The urine sodium value is inappropriately high for a state of hypoperfusion. In secondary adrenal failure, the potassium level may be normal because mineralocorticoid function is intact and aldosterone is present. However, hyponatremia may still be present.

TABLE 172.2. Corticosteroid Coverage for Surgery

1. Correct electrolyte levels, blood pressure, and hydration if necessary.
2. Give hydrocortisone phosphate or succinate, 100 mg i.m., on call to operating room.
3. Give hydrocortisone phosphate or succinate, 50 mg i.m. or i.v. in recovery room and every 6 hours for the first 24 hours.
4. If progress is satisfactory, reduce dosage to 25 mg every 6 hours for 24 hours; then taper to maintenance dosage over 3 to 5 days. Resume previous 9α-fluorocortisol dose when patient is taking oral medications.
5. Maintain or increase cortisol dosage to 200 to 400 mg/24 h if fever, hypotension, or other complications occur.

From Felig P, et al. *Endocrinology and metabolism*, 2nd ed. New York: McGraw-Hill, 1987:596.

DIFFERENTIAL DIAGNOSIS

Acute adrenal failure may present as hypovolemic shock, hypoglycemia, or both. The diagnosis should be pursued in any patient with a history of chronic glucocorticoid use, because medication may be stopped or an intercurrent stress may arise to precipitate the crisis. The differential diagnosis of acute adrenal crisis includes other causes of cardiovascular collapse and shock: myocardial infarction, heart failure, hypovolemia, sepsis, pulmonary embolism, and so forth. The diagnosis should be considered in all patients with dehydration, hypotension, orthostasis, or obtundation. Hyperpigmentation and typical laboratory abnormalities suggest adrenal insufficiency.

Chronic adrenal insufficiency is difficult to diagnose because the symptoms may develop over months to years. It is often confused with a "flulike" illness because many of the complaints are nonspecific: fatigue, weakness, abdominal discomfort, poor appetite, and musculoskeletal complaints. The examination is often unremarkable. Laboratory evaluation may not be particularly revealing in all cases, especially with secondary insufficiency.

EMERGENCY DEPARTMENT EVALUATION AND MANAGEMENT

After attention has been given to the ABCs, a thorough history and physical examination should be performed, noting altered mental status, fever, tachycardia, hypotension or orthostatic changes, abdominal discomfort, cutaneous and oral hyperpigmentation, or vitiligo.

The first step of treatment is to reverse shock. Normal saline and vasopressors are administered as needed. Central venous lines for hemodynamic monitoring may be necessary, and cardiac monitoring should always be instituted. Laboratory studies are ordered as necessary, including electrolytes, glucose, creatinine, and baseline plasma ACTH, and serum cortisol. Because plasma ACTH is extremely labile, the blood sample must be placed on ice before being transported to the laboratory. The results of these tests can often take days to become available, so if adrenal insufficiency is suspected, treatment should be initiated promptly, particularly because the condition can progress rapidly to circulatory collapse and death. If no apparent cause for cardiovascular collapse is apparent, blood cultures, urine culture, and chest radiography should be performed to seek evidence of occult infection.

In severe cases, it may be necessary to treat the hyperkalemia immediately. The total body potassium level is often low, however, and the serum potassium value can be expected to decrease after glucocorticoids are administered. Symptomatic hyponatremia should also be treated. The next step is to administer glucocorticoids (e.g., dexamethasone, 6 to 8 mg i.v.). Dexamethasone is recommended because it will not interfere with the cosyntropin test, which may be used to try to establish the diagnosis. If the cause of adrenal insufficiency is pituitary failure, treatment with levothyroxine is also indicated. Desmopressin may also be necessary if diabetes insipidus is present.

Patients with known chronic adrenal insufficiency require three to four times their normal glucocorticoid replacement dose during illness and stress. Patients with illnesses severe enough to require hospitalization may need an even higher dose. Those receiving exogenous steroids as therapy for other illnesses must be given adequate doses during surgery, illness, or stress (Table 172.2).

Although not necessary in the emergency department, evaluation of adrenocortical function may be performed with the short ACTH (cosyntropin) test. Immediately after a baseline serum cortisol and plasma ACTH level are drawn, ACTH 0.25 mg is administered intravenously, and a serum cortisol value is obtained 60 minutes later. If prednisone or hydrocortisone has been administered, it will interfere with this test; however, dexamethasone does not interfere with the assay and, furthermore, has no acute effect on the response of the adrenal gland to ACTH.

After the short ACTH test, glucocorticoid replacement is continued with hydrocortisone (100- to 200-mg i.v. bolus, then 20 to 25 mg/h as a continuous infusion). Alternatively, one may give 100 to 200 mg of hydrocortisone every 6 hours as an intravenous infusion over 30 minutes (Table 172.3). Fluids and vasopressors are administered as needed. The clinical picture of shock should improve within 6 to 12 hours. When the acute adrenal crisis resolves, the infusion can be replaced with an oral regimen of hydrocortisone, 20 mg at 8 a.m. and 10 mg at 2 p.m. Three to four times this dose is needed for patients under continuing stress. Replacement of mineralocorticoid, if necessary, is accomplished with fludrocortisone acetate (Florinef), 0.1 mg daily.

TABLE 172.3. Treatment of Acute Adrenocortical Insufficiency (Adrenal Crisis)

1. Cortisol, 100 mg i.v., every 6 hours for 24 hours. Reduce to 50 mg every 6 hours if progress is satisfactory, and then taper to oral maintenance dose by day 4 or 5. Maintain or increase dosage to 200 to 400 mg/24 h if complications persist or occur.
2. Intravenous saline and glucose
3. Correction of precipitating factors
4. General supportive measures

From Felig P, et al. *Endocrinology and metabolism*, 2nd ed. New York: McGraw-Hill, 1987:594.

The hallmark of adrenal insufficiency is loss of adrenal reserve, and the diagnosis cannot always be made on the basis of a single cortisol level, which may be in the normal range. A low baseline cortisol level, especially in the presence of physiologic stressors, however, suggests adrenal failure: primary adrenal insufficiency if the ACTH level is high, and secondary adrenal insufficiency if both cortisol and ACTH levels are low.

DISPOSITION

After treatment for shock and glucocorticoid deficiency is begun in the emergency department, all patients with *acute* adrenal insufficiency should be admitted to an intensive care unit. Subspecialty consultation should be requested. The short ACTH test may be performed at this time. Patients in whom *chronic* adrenal insufficiency is suspected should be admitted to the hospital for evaluation.

COMMON PITFALLS

- Because adrenal insufficiency is uncommon and the symptoms are often nonspecific, the emergency physician may fail to consider the diagnosis.
- Patients may be potassium depleted even when the serum potassium concentration is high. The serum potassium value may drop substantially with glucocorticoid replacement and must be monitored closely during treatment.
- Patients with pituitary failure may not show evidence of diabetes insipidus until after deficiencies of glucocorticoids and thyroid hormone have been corrected.
- Patients receiving exogenous steroid therapy should always have the dose increased (to two to four times the usual replacement regimen) when there is intercurrent illness or stress.
- The clinician should not fail to institute appropriate fluid resuscitation and steroid replacement while performing the ACTH stimulation test.

CUSHING SYNDROME

Cushing syndrome, also known as hypercortisolism, occurs whenever there is symptomatic glucocorticoid excess, regardless of the cause of that excess. The syndrome as originally described by Harvey Cushing in 1932 includes truncal obesity, hypertension, weakness, and edema. The most common cause of Cushing syndrome is prolonged exogenous steroid administration.

Cushing disease refers to the situation in which this syndrome is specifically due to excessive ACTH secretion from the pituitary; this accounts for 70% of individuals with naturally occurring Cushing syndrome.[22] Cushing disease typically occurs in women between 20 and 40 years of age, is of gradual onset and slowly progressive, and produces only mild symptoms. Most of these patients have pituitary microadenomas; macroadenomas can develop, however, and may present as headaches or visual changes due to pressure on the optic chiasm.

Cushing syndrome can also be caused by an ACTH-secreting carcinoma (e.g., small-cell bronchogenic carcinoma, pancreatic cancer, bronchial carcinoid, or carcinoma of the thymus). The peak incidence is in men between the ages of 40 and 60; the typical course is very rapid, and the tumor is usually advanced when discovered.

Adrenal neoplasms are another cause of Cushing syndrome, comprising about 20% of cases. Typically, these tumors produce signs and symptoms of glucocorticoid excess, but not of androgen excess; they are usually unilateral, and approximately 50% are malignant. Adrenal carcinoma has a rapid onset and rapid progression, with hypokalemia and abdominal pain as common symptoms. Benign adrenal tumors have a slow, progressive course.

CLINICAL PRESENTATION

Obesity and weight gain are the main symptoms. Seventy-five percent of patients have deposition of fat in the face, described as "moon facies," and around the neck and shoulders, known as a "buffalo hump." Other fat accumulation occurs within the mesentery, producing truncal obesity. There also may be atrophy of the skin; half of patients have abdominal striae. The face can appear red and flushed. Patients also complain of fatigue and weakness; a proximal myopathy can be detected in about 60% of patients.

Osteoporosis develops from mobilization of calcium, resulting in vertebral compression and pathologic fractures. Glucose intolerance and insulin resistance are other features, but overt diabetes is seen in only about 20% of patients. Delayed wound healing and cutaneous fungal infections may also be noted. Hypertension is common. Women show signs of increased androgens: increased facial hair, acne, and amenorrhea, with the latter present in 75% of premenopausal women (Table 172.4).

Laboratory findings are generally nonspecific in the patient with Cushing syndrome. There may be glucose intolerance due to insulin resistance. The hemoglobin and hematocrit are high-normal, and the white blood cell count usually shows a leukocytosis that is predominantly a neutrophilia. Electrolytes are often normal, but a hypokalemic metabolic acidosis may be present in cases of extreme excess. In some elderly patients, the diagnosis is made in the workup for persistent hypokalemia, with no other signs or symptoms present.[3]

DIFFERENTIAL DIAGNOSIS

Because many features of Cushing syndrome, such as obesity, hypertension, amenorrhea, and weakness, are common for other reasons, and thus nonspecific, the diagnosis can be diffi-

TABLE 172.4. Clinical Features of Cushing's Syndrome

Feature	%
Obesity	94
Facial plethora	84
Hirsutism	82
Menstrual disorders	76
Hypertension	72
Muscular weakness	58
Back pain	58
Striae	52
Acne	40
Psychological symptoms	40
Bruising	36
Congestive heart failure	22
Edema	18
Renal calculi	16
Headache	14
Polyuria/polydipsia	10
Hyperpigmentation	6

From Felig P, et al. *Endocrinology and metabolism*, 2nd ed. New York: McGraw Hill, 1987:606.

cult to make. Random measurements of serum cortisol have little diagnostic value, because the serum cortisol exhibits substantial diurnal variation, but the diagnosis can be made using low-dose and high-dose dexamethasone suppression testing. Because the performance and interpretation of the dexamethasone suppression test is complicated, it is important to refer these patients to their primary care physician or to an endocrinologist for testing and follow-up.

EMERGENCY DEPARTMENT MANAGEMENT AND DISPOSITION

One should not expect to make a firm diagnosis of Cushing syndrome in the emergency department, but should promptly refer those patients with a constellation of symptoms consistent with the syndrome to an endocrinologist.

Treatment of Cushing syndrome requires reversal of hypersecretion of hormone, whether it is at a pituitary or an adrenal level. The treatment for microadenomas and macroadenomas is partial hypophysectomy or irradiation of the sella turcica. Complications of this treatment that may be seen in the emergency department include postoperative diabetes insipidus and hypothyroidism; however, hypothyroidism may take some time to present. Patients who undergo bilateral adrenalectomy may develop Nelson syndrome, the effect of an enlarging pituitary tumor that secretes high levels of ACTH; this syndrome presents as visual changes due to tumor encroachment on the optic chiasm. Ten percent to 20% of patients undergoing bilateral adrenalectomy develop Nelson syndrome within 10 years of surgery.

COMMON PITFALLS

- Because the symptoms are common and nonspecific, the clinician may fail to consider the diagnosis of Cushing syndrome.
- Excess glucocorticoid activity may permit the dissemination of viral disease such as herpes and chickenpox and may allow reactivation of tuberculosis and fungal infections. Most important, fever and other systemic signs of infection may be masked.

PHEOCHROMOCYTOMA

Chromaffin cells in the adrenal medulla are responsible for the release of epinephrine and norepinephrine into the circulation. These cells may form tumors called pheochromocytomas. The pheochromocytoma is known as the "10% tumor": 10% are bilateral, 10% are extraadrenal, and 10% are malignant. Most pheochromocytomas produce norepinephrine as the predominant catecholamine, but epinephrine, dopamine, and other vasoactive substances can also be secreted.

The incidence of pheochromocytoma is less than 1% in hypertensive patients. However, the diagnosis is important because it is a potentially treatable cause of hypertension. Moreover, the tumor can be malignant or may result in fatal paroxysms of hypertension. In one autopsy series, as many as 75% of cases were not correctly diagnosed before death, demonstrating the difficulty of making the diagnosis.[20] Pheochromocytomas are also associated with multiple endocrine neoplasia (MEN) syndromes. MEN-2a, the best known, is Sipple syndrome (pheochromocytoma, medullary carcinoma of the thyroid, and parathyroid adenoma).

CLINICAL PRESENTATION

When these tumors secrete norepinephrine and epinephrine, they are responsible for signs and symptoms of catecholamine excess. The most common of these effects is hypertension, occurring in 90% of patients.[11] The hypertension may be persistent but is reported as episodic in approximately 50% of patients. The sudden paroxysms of hypertension may cause the patient to feel a throbbing palpitation or headache. These symptoms may be transient, lasting minutes or several hours, or they may occur once a month or several times a week, but they usually increase in frequency as the tumor grows. Actions that put pressure on the tumor, such as the Valsalva maneuver or exercise, may precipitate attacks. Bladder wall tumors may produce symptoms with micturition. The 10% to 15% of patients who do not have hypertension are thought to have tumors that secrete dopamine or other vasodilating substances.[2]

Other symptoms of catecholamine excess may be more subtle and persistent. These may include heat intolerance, increased sweating, weight loss, and hyperglycemia. Chronic constriction of the arterial and venous beds may decrease the total intravascular volume, resulting in orthostatic symptoms despite the baseline increase in blood pressure. The heart rate may be increased, but most patients have a reflex bradycardia secondary to hypertension.[2]

DIFFERENTIAL DIAGNOSIS

Approximately one in 1000 hypertensive patients harbors a pheochromocytoma.[2] Unusual lability of blood pressure may provide a clue. Episodic symptoms thought to be hot flashes in perimenopausal women or preeclampsia during pregnancy may be due to pheochromocytoma. Other causes of hypertensive crisis may be in the differential diagnosis, especially in patients with refractory hypertension. Ninety percent of patients with pheochromocytoma report spells of headache, palpitations, or sweating.[8] The combination of uncontrolled hypertension and orthostatic hypotension should suggest the diagnosis.

The definitive diagnosis is established by demonstration of increased catecholamines and their metabolites in a 24-hour urine collection. The urine should be collected for vanillylmandelic acid (VMA), metanephrines, and free catecholamines. A wide variety of drugs (most antihypertensives) and common foods (e.g., bananas, caffeine, and chocolate) can interfere with the test, however. Because results will not be readily available in the emergency department, these tests have no place in emergency department evaluation and management.

EMERGENCY DEPARTMENT EVALUATION AND MANAGEMENT

The major priority for the emergency physician is treatment of hypertensive emergency, if present, and volume expansion. Initial management with sodium nitroprusside (starting at 1 to 3 μg/kg/min) helps to control hypertension through its arterial and venous dilating effects. If pheochromocytoma is suspected or hypertension is resistant to treatment with nitroprusside, alpha blockade can be achieved with intravenous phentolamine (1- to 4-mg bolus, followed by a continuous infusion titrated to effect). Beta blockade is used to treat arrhythmias and resistant hypertension but should be used only after alpha blockade has been accomplished, to avoid paradoxical hypertension from unopposed alpha effects. Low doses usually suffice. Both nifedipine (10 to 20 mg) and labetalol (20 mg) are useful in treating hypertensive crisis in these patients as well.[17]

DISPOSITION

Typically, patients with uncontrolled hypertension and symptoms suggesting hypertensive crisis require admission. Stable patients who are asymptomatic should be referred for prompt follow-up with an endocrinologist for further evaluation and testing.

The recurrence rate after surgical resection is less than 10%; the 5-year survival rate after surgery is approximately 95%. Approximately 25% of patients continue to have hypertension after removal of the pheochromocytoma; the cause is believed to be irreversible vascular damage from previous uncontrolled catecholamine excess or underlying essential hypertension. Hypertension in these patients is usually readily controlled with standard antihypertensive regimens.

COMMON PITFALLS

- A number of commonly used medications can cause catecholamine release and may result in uncontrolled hypertension in patients with pheochromocytoma.[4,19] These medications include glucagon, droperidol, histamine, tyramine, metoclopramide, saralasin, tricyclic antidepressants, phenothiazines, and naloxone.
- Pheochromocytoma should be considered in patients who complain of transient symptoms that have resolved by the time of emergency department evaluation. These patients may benefit from appropriate referral and outpatient evaluation.
- Because patients with pheochromocytoma are often hypovolemic, sudden blood loss or sudden loss of vascular tone can result in precipitous and severe hypotension.

HYPOPITUITARISM

Any lesion that destroys the pituitary or hypothalamus or that interferes with releasing and inhibiting factors that act on the anterior pituitary can result in pituitary insufficiency, or hypopituitarism. The pituitary hormones potentially involved include growth hormone, prolactin, the gonadotropic hormones follicle-stimulating hormone and luteinizing hormone, TSH, and ACTH. If the neurohypophysis is involved, vasopressin may also be decreased. The causes of hypopituitarism are summarized in Table 172.5.

TABLE 172.5. Causes of Hypopituitarism

Idiopathic
Infectious diseases
Bacterial abscess
Bacterial or viral meningitis
Granulomatous diseases
Infiltrative diseases
Sarcoidosis
Histiocytosis X
Hemochromatosis
Vascular
Hemorrhage (including pituitary apoplexy)
Thrombosis
Aneurysm
Vasculitis
Postpartum necrosis (Sheehan syndrome)
Neoplastic
Primary tumor
Metastatic tumor
Leukemia and lymphoma
Iatrogenic
Operation
Irradiation
Trauma
Blunt
Surgical
Congenital
Aqueductal stenosis
Arachnoid cyst
Intrasellar cyst
Basal encephalocele

CLINICAL PRESENTATION

The presentation of hypopituitarism depends on which pituitary hormone or combination of hormones is affected; the clinical manifestations are those of end-organ hypofunction, such as hypothyroidism, hypogonadism, or adrenal insufficiency.

Acute loss of pituitary function can be dramatic. Patients with pituitary apoplexy, necrosis, or hemorrhage into an existing pituitary tumor may present with headache, visual field defects, meningismus, or decreased level of consciousness from increased intracranial pressure.

Hypopituitarism occurring in the postpartum patient after an episode of hypotension or shock is known as Sheehan syndrome. These patients may fail to lactate in the postpartum period and may develop amenorrhea, gonadal atrophy, and symptoms of hypothyroidism and adrenal insufficiency. Some, however, remain undiagnosed until a later exposure to stress triggers an adrenal crisis.

Hypopituitarism in the elderly is a difficult diagnosis. Most tumors are nonfunctioning microadenomas. Although the most common presenting complaint in the elderly is visual field loss[21], incidental radiologic diagnosis is common.[1]

Most hypopituitarism, however, is chronic and partial. The signs and symptoms of single hormone deficiency or incomplete hormone deficiencies can be extremely subtle. Destruction of at least 90% of the pituitary is required before complete panhypopituitarism becomes clinically apparent. When a patient with known hypopituitarism presents to the emergency department because of an intercurrent illness unrelated to the endocrine system or the central nervous system, little further needs to be done other than ensuring that the patient continues to receive his or her usual hormonal replacement therapy, including stress doses of corticosteroids, if necessary.

EMERGENCY DEPARTMENT EVALUATION AND MANAGEMENT

The initial diagnosis of hypopituitarism is generally made after somewhat extensive testing by an endocrinologist, including measurement of specific hormone levels and magnetic resonance imaging of the pituitary. The treatment of hypopituitarism consists of lifelong hormone replacement. Suspected adrenal crisis should be treated promptly, even when a diagnosis has not been confirmed, because the patient's condition may deteriorate quickly if not treated. Patients with suspected pituitary apoplexy should be intubated and hyperventilated, and prompt neurosurgical consultation obtained.

Emergency hormone replacement is rarely needed in the emergency department. If hormones are given, however, blood samples should be sent for measurement of plasma cortisol, prolactin, ACTH, and TSH levels and thyroid function studies. Glucocorticoid replacement should precede administration of levothyroxine, because thyroxine accelerates the metabolism of cortisol and can precipitate an adrenal crisis.

Patients with chronic hypopituitarism usually have longstanding, vague, nonspecific complaints such as weakness, nausea, vomiting, and abdominal pain. Electrolyte abnormalities and hypotension may be noted.

DISPOSITION

Patients with evidence of shock or hemodynamic instability should be admitted to an intensive care unit setting for observation and prompt endocrine evaluation. Other patients should be referred to an endocrinologist for further testing and diagnosis.

COMMON PITFALLS

- Most hypopituitarism is chronic and difficult to diagnose. Some patients may have been given psychiatric diagnoses.
- Acute loss of pituitary function is also difficult to diagnose unless apparent on an imaging study.

References

1. Baxter JD, Tyrell JB. The adrenal cortex. In: Felig P, et al., eds. *Endocrinology and metabolism*. New York: McGraw-Hill, 1995.
2. Benowitz NL. Pheochromocytoma—recent advances in diagnosis and treatment (medical staff conference). *West J Med* 1988;148:561.
3. Berwaerts, JJ, Verhelst, JA, Verhaert GC, et al. Corticotropin-dependent Cushing's syndrome in older people: presentation of five cases and therapeutic use of ketoconazole. *J Am Geriatric Soc* 1998;46(7):880.
4. Boulox P, Grossman A, Besser GM. Naloxone provokes catecholamine release in pheochromocytoma and paraganglioma. *Clin Endocrinol* 1986;24:319.
5. Dunlop D. Eighty-six cases of Addison's disease. *BMJ* 1963;2:887.
6. Etzel JV, Brocavich JM, Torre M. Endocrine complications associated with human immunodeficiency virus infection. *Clin Pharmacol* 1992;11:705.
7. Geusau A, Stingl G. Primary adrenal insufficiency in two patients with the acquired immunodeficiency syndrome associated with disseminated cytomegaloviral infection. *Wien Klin Wochenschr* 1997;109(21):845.
8. Gifford RW, Kvale WF, Maher FT. Clinical features, diagnosis, and treatment of pheochromocytoma. *Mayo Clin Proc* 1964;39:281.
9. Gradon JD, Sepkowitz DV. Fluconazole-associated acute adrenal insufficiency. *Postgrad Med J* 1991;67:1084.
10. Greene LW, et al. Adrenal insufficiency as a complication of the acquired immunodeficiency syndrome. *Ann Intern Med* 1984;101:497.
11. Hermann H, Mornex R. *Human tumors secreting catecholamines.* New York: Macmillan, 1964.
12. Hilton CW, Harrington PT, Prasad C, et al. Adrenal insufficiency in the acquired immunodeficiency syndrome. *South Med J* 1988;81:1493.
13. Kong MF, Jeffcoate W. Eighty-six cases of Addison's disease. *Clin Endocrinol* 1994;41:757.
14. Muhlhofer A, Jung C, Gross M. Successful treatment with ganciclovir of an HIV endstage patient with adrenal insufficiency. *Eur J Med Res* 1997;2:469.
15. Piedrola G, Casado JL, Lopez E, et al. Clinical features of adrenal insufficiency in patients with acquired immunodeficiency syndrome. *Clin Endocrinol* 1996;45:97.
16. Pulakhandam U, Dincsoy HP. Cytomegaloviral adrenalitis and adrenal insufficiency in AIDS. *Am J Clin Pathol* 1990;93:651.
17. Reuler JB, Magarian GJ. Hypertensive emergencies and urgencies. *J Gen Intern Med* 1988;3:64.
18. Sanhes L, Michez E, Essig M, et al. Successful treatment of CMV-induced adrenal insufficiency by ganciclovir in a patient with the acquired immunodeficiency syndrome. *Nephrol Dial Transplant* 1995;10:704.
19. Sheps SG, Nai-Siang J, Klee GG, et al. Recent developments in the diagnosis and treatment of pheochromocytoma. *Mayo Clin Proc* 1990;65:88.
20. St. John Sutton MG, Sheps SG, Lie LJ. Prevalence of clinically unsuspected pheochromocytoma. *Mayo Clin Proc* 1981;56:354.
21. Turner HE, Wass JA. Pituitary tumours in the elderly. *Baillieres Clin Endocrinol Metab* 1997;11:407.
22. Tyrell JB, Aron DC, Forsharm PH. Glucocorticoids and adrenal androgens. In: Greenspan FS, ed. *Basic and clinical endocrinology*. Norwalk, CT: Appleton & Lange, 1997.

CHAPTER 173

Disorders of Sodium and Water Metabolism

Sandra A. Craig and John A. Marx

The serum sodium concentration and serum osmolality are normally maintained within a narrow range by homeostatic mechanisms involving thirst, antidiuretic hormone (ADH), and renal handling of sodium.

Sodium and chloride ions are normally separated from the glomerular filtrate in the ascending limb of the loop of Henle, leaving behind a hypotonic filtrate and resulting, in the absence of ADH, in the net excretion of free water. Increases in serum osmolality above the normal range of 280 to 300 mOsmol/kg are detected by osmoreceptor neurons in the hypothalamus and cause an increase in thirst and in circulating levels of ADH. ADH acts on the collecting ducts of the renal tubules, increasing free-water reabsorption from the glomerular filtrate into the hypertonic interstitium of the renal medulla; this results in the excretion of low volumes of urine of relatively high osmolality and a return of the serum osmolality toward normal. ADH is also secreted in response to decreases in intravascular volume and (although to a lesser degree) in response to noxious stimuli such as pain, fear, nausea, and hypoxia.[2]

Sodium balance is regulated independently of ADH by changes in the degree of sodium reabsorption in the proximal tubule. Hypovolemic states such as those caused by hemorrhage or dehydration are associated with increased sodium absorption in the proximal tubule and decreased delivery of sodium to the tubular diluting sites. Conversely, increases in intravascular volume and glomerular filtration rate suppress proximal tubular sodium reabsorption, resulting in increased delivery of sodium to diluting sites.

Disorders of water balance can be traced to abnormalities of thirst or water acquisition, glomerular filtration rate, renal sodium transport, or ADH metabolism.

HYPONATREMIA

CLINICAL PRESENTATION

Hyponatremia is physiologically significant only insofar as it reflects a state of extracellular hypoosmolality in which free water shifts from the vascular space to the intracellular space. Although the resulting cellular edema is well tolerated by most tissues, the brain is very sensitive to changes in cell volume. The clinical manifestations of hyponatremia, usually associated with serum sodium levels below 130 mEq/L, are therefore related primarily to cerebral edema. Symptoms include headache, difficulty in concentrating, confusion, lethargy, agitation, nausea, vomiting, and seizures. Anorexia and muscle cramps are also common.

The incidence and severity of manifestations increase not only with the degree of hyponatremia, but also with the rate at which it develops. When the serum sodium level falls gradually over a period of days or weeks, the brain can compensate by extruding solutes and fluid into the extracellular space.[12] Serum sodium values as low as 110 mEq/L may thus be reached with minimal symptomatology. However, a *rapid* fall in the serum sodium level, from a normal level to levels below 125 mEq/L, exceeds the capacity of these compensatory mechanisms and can lead to profound cerebral edema, to the point of coma or brainstem herniation.[2]

DIFFERENTIAL DIAGNOSIS

The diagnosis of hyponatremia rests entirely on the ability to obtain and measure accurately the concentration of sodium in the patient's serum. Therefore, the possibility of erroneous sampling should always be considered, especially when the reported value does not seem consistent with the clinical situation. Was the specimen properly labeled? Was it drawn from a venous site proximal to an infusion of hypotonic saline or dextrose 5% in water (D5W)? Is there an error in laboratory measurement or recording? When an error of some kind is suspected, a fresh sample should be obtained and tested before diagnostic or therapeutic procedures are initiated.

There are several clinical conditions in which an accurately measured, low serum sodium concentration does not represent a true hypoosmolar state. The most common is moderate-to-severe hyperglycemia. Extracellular glucose accumulation causes movement of free water into the extracellular space, resulting in hyponatremia yet a normal or even increased serum osmolarity. The serum sodium value decreases by approximately 1.6 mEq/L for each 100-mg/dL increase in the serum glucose value.[3] This hyponatremia is not physiologically significant, and it resolves as normoglycemia is reestablished. This phenomenon, termed *hypertonic hyponatremia,* is also noted in patients treated with mannitol or glycerol to control intracranial hypertension or acute glaucoma.

Pseudohyponatremia refers to a falsely low serum sodium measurement in patients whose plasma contains excessive amounts of lipid or protein. In this situation, the plasma water in which sodium is dissolved occupies a smaller proportion of the blood specimen. Laboratory methods that measure sodium content per unit of plasma thus report low sodium levels, even though the concentration of sodium in serum water is normal. This situation occurs when the serum sodium concentration is measured by the flame emission spectrophotometry or indirect potentiometry method, but not with direct potentiometry.[3] Because the serum osmolarity is normal, water metabolism is completely undisturbed. Hyperlipidemia severe enough to produce pseudohyponatremia is almost always associated with a lipemic appearance of the serum. Hyperproteinemia of a sufficient degree to cause pseudohyponatremia is most commonly due to multiple myeloma or administration of intravenous immune globulin.[7]

EMERGENCY DEPARTMENT EVALUATION

The emergency department evaluation of true hyponatremia has two goals. The first is to define the chronicity of the hyponatremic state, which must be based primarily on historic clues. In general, patients with a paucity of symptoms despite sodium levels less than 125 mEq/L are very likely to have chronic hyponatremia. Acute hyponatremia is much less common than chronic hyponatremia and should be suspected in patients with a history of sudden free-water loading (e.g., patients with psychogenic polydipsia, infants given only tap water for 1 to 2 days, and postoperative patients who have been given hypotonic intravenous fluids or who have absorbed hypotonic bladder irrigation fluids).[1]

The second goal in the evaluation of the hyponatremic patient is to establish the cause. Hyponatremia can be classified as hypovolemic, euvolemic, or hypervolemic based on the history and physical examination (Fig. 173.1). Hypovolemic patients demonstrate signs of volume depletion, such as tachycardia, orthostasis, dry mucous membranes, diminished skin turgor, oliguria, or azotemia. A low fractional excretion of sodium (less than 0.5%) plus low fractional excretion of urea (less than 55%) may be helpful in identifying subtle cases of hypovolemia.[9] Hypervolemia is manifested by the presence of congestive heart failure, peripheral edema, or ascites. Patients who appear neither volume depleted nor volume overloaded are classified as having euvolemic hyponatremia.

Hypovolemic Hyponatremia

Patients with hypovolemic hyponatremia have decreased total body sodium stores. Nonrenal causes of sodium depletion include vomiting, diarrhea, fistulas, gastrointestinal drainage tubes, excessive sweating, and third-spacing of fluids from peritonitis, pancreatitis, or burns. Renal causes of sodium loss include osmotic diuresis and salt-wasting nephropathies such as medullary cystic disease and obstructive uropathy. Thiazide diuretics are one of the most common causes of severe hyponatremia, especially in the elderly population, but hyponatremia appears more often to be the result of significant potassium depletion and of inhibition of free-water generation in the loop of Henle than of volume depletion *per se*.[5]

In general, the nonrenal causes of hypovolemic hyponatremia are associated with a urine sodium value of less than 20 mEq/L, while renal causes are associated with a urine sodium value of more than 20 mEq/L. As a general principle, hyponatremia does not develop unless free-water intake exceeds free-water excretion. In these hypovolemic conditions, hyponatremia is maintained by low glomerular filtration rates that preclude adequate free-water excretion and by high levels of ADH secreted in response to hypovolemia.

Hypervolemic Hyponatremia

Hyponatremic patients with clinical signs of total body sodium excess, usually as evidenced by the presence of edema, are classified as having hypervolemic hyponatremia. Two situations are associated with inappropriate increases in body sodium stores. The first is renal retention of sodium in response to states of decreased effective intravascular volume (e.g., congestive heart failure, cirrhosis, and the nephrotic syndrome). The second is an inability of the kidney to excrete ingested sodium loads because of acute or chronic renal insufficiency.

In patients with hypervolemic hyponatremia, the evaluation should include a search for signs of decreased cardiac output, increased portal vein pressure, nephrotic range proteinuria, or renal insufficiency. Patients with decreased effective vascular volume due to heart failure, cirrhosis, and nephrotic syndrome typically have urine sodium values that are less than 20 mEq/L; those with renal insufficiency typically have values greater than 20 mEq/L.

Euvolemic Hyponatremia

Patients who appear neither dehydrated nor edematous are considered to have euvolemic hyponatremia. As with the other types of hyponatremia, the low serum sodium concentration implies that free-water intake has occurred at a rate that exceeds the kidneys' ability to excrete it. This can occur in patients with psychogenic polydipsia (who, if renal function is normal, must drink at least 15 L of water per day), but it has also been noted in patients who have been given tap water enemas, in infants

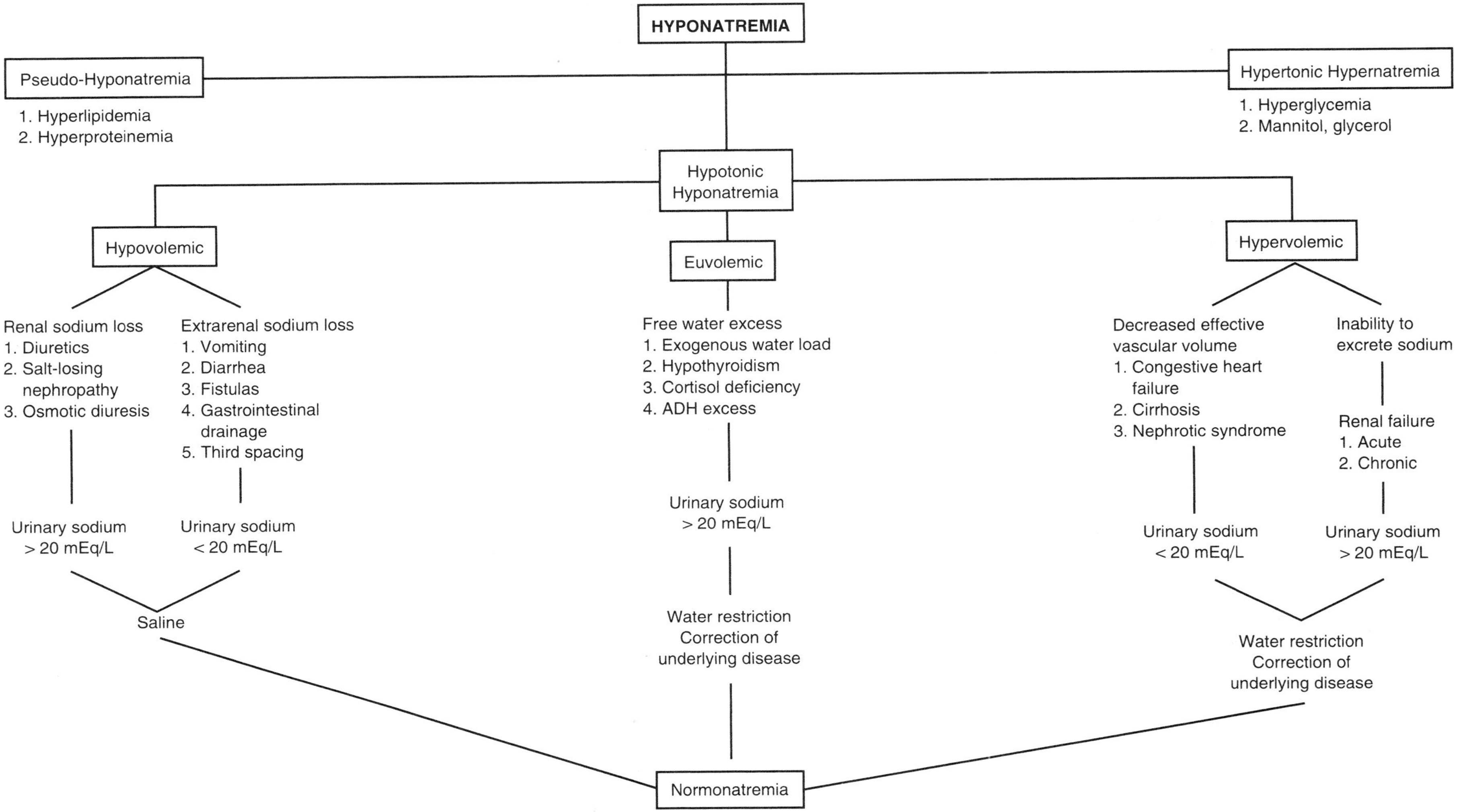

Figure 173.1. Algorithm for diagnosis and treatment of hyponatremia.

TABLE 173.1. Causes of SIADH

DISEASES OF THE CENTRAL NERVOUS SYSTEM	METABOLIC
Infection Trauma Neoplasm Vascular Degenerative diseases Psychosis	Acute porphyria
	NEOPLASMS
	Lung Pancreas Duodenum Lymphoma Ureter Ewing sarcoma Prostate
PULMONARY DISEASE	**STRESS**
Pneumonia Active tuberculosis Abscesses Asthma	Trauma
	DRUGS
	See Table 173.2
	IDIOPATHIC

given tap water bottle feedings, and in hospitalized patients who have been given large amounts of hypotonic fluids. This group is identified by the history of excessive free-water administration and by a urine osmolality that is appropriately low, generally less than 100 mOsmol/L.[2] Hyponatremia in association with a grossly normal volume status may also be seen in some patients with renal failure who have ingested more free water than can be promptly excreted, given their decreased glomerular filtration rate.

An often considered but somewhat uncommon cause of euvolemic hyponatremia is the syndrome of inappropriate ADH secretion, or SIADH (Table 173.1), in which ADH is secreted in excessive amounts despite the presence of hyponatremia and adequate intravascular volume. This syndrome is associated with a variety of pulmonary and central nervous system conditions, with malignancy, with the acquired immunodeficiency syndrome (AIDS), and with the use of a number of medications (Table 173.2).[11] The diagnostic criteria for SIADH are

Hypotonic hyponatremia
Inappropriately concentrated urine (UOsmol greater than 100 mOsmol/L)
Normal renal excretory function
Normal adrenal and thyroid function
Absence of hypovolemia and dehydration
Absence of edema

TABLE 173.2. Drugs Associated with Hyponatremia

ENHANCED EFFECT OF ANTIDIURETIC HORMONE (ADH)
Chlorpropamide Tolbutamide
INCREASED RELEASE OF ADH
Chlorpropamide Clofibrate Carbamazepine Vincristine Cyclophosphamide Opiates ? Thiazides
IMPAIRED WATER EXCRETION INDEPENDENT OF ADH
Thiazides Oxytocin Desmopressin

Interestingly, measurement of ADH levels is not helpful in making the diagnosis, because the ADH level is also commonly elevated when hyponatremia is due to other causes.

Two additional causes of euvolemic hyponatremia must be ruled out before one makes the diagnosis of SIADH or exogenous water toxicity–hypothyroidism and cortisol deficiency. Hyponatremia due to cortisol deficiency is rarely associated with a serum sodium level less than 120 mEq/L, and it corrects promptly after glucocorticoid replacement. Hypothyroidism has been associated with sodium levels as low as 110 mEq/L and is treated by thyroid hormone replacement. The mechanism of hyponatremia in these conditions remains incompletely understood.

EMERGENCY DEPARTMENT MANAGEMENT

The treatment of hyponatremia depends on the severity of symptoms and the rate at which hyponatremia has developed. It is important to distinguish between acute and chronic hyponatremia, because the pathophysiology and appropriate treatment are quite different.

Patients with acute hyponatremia (i.e., developing in less than about 48 hours) are at risk for severe central nervous system effects, such as obtundation and seizures, at levels of 125 mEq/L or less. Cerebral edema develops as free water shifts from the vascular space to the intracellular space within a period too short to allow the neurons to compensate by extruding cellular solutes. Cardiopulmonary arrest may occur secondary to brainstem herniation.[2] First, the source of excess free water must be identified and eliminated. Patients with obtundation or seizures should receive hypertonic (3%) saline to increase the serum sodium rapidly, but only enough to arrest the progression of symptoms. An increase of 4 to 6 mEq/L is usually sufficient to stop hyponatremic seizures. Further correction, using normal saline, should proceed at an overall rate of no more than 0.5 mEq/L/h, and serum sodium levels should be closely monitored. In theory, *acute* hyponatremia can be corrected more rapidly without risk of adverse consequences, but, in practice, it is usually difficult to be certain of the time course over which hyponatremia developed and the degree of cellular compensation that may already have occurred.

Chronic hyponatremia must be managed especially carefully. Overaggressive therapy is potentially more dangerous than the condition itself. In these patients, the brain cells have had time to reduce their solute content to match that of the hypoosmotic serum and are relatively protected from cerebral edema. When patients such as these have the serum sodium concentration increased rapidly, a significant number develop central pontine myelinolysis (CPM), an entity characterized by focal myelin destruction in the pons and extrapontine areas.[6] Symptoms begin 1 to 3 days after rapid correction of the serum sodium and consist of dysarthria, dysphagia, seizures, altered mental status, quadriparesis, and hypotension.[6] The condition is typically associated with permanent sequelae. The risk of CPM appears to be quite low in patients whose *chronic* hyponatremia is corrected at a rate of less than 0.5 mEq/L/h until levels in the normal range are reached.[6] Myelinolysis is not associated with rapid correction of hyponatremia of less than 24 hours' duration.[5]

Hypertonic saline is indicated only for the initial correction of severely symptomatic acute or chronic hyponatremia. The appropriate volume of hypertonic saline required to produce a given change in the serum sodium level may be calculated using the following formula:

$$\text{Required volume} = \frac{(\text{Na}_{\text{desired}} - \text{Na}_{\text{current}})(\text{TBW})}{(\text{Na}_{\text{IV fluid}} - \text{Na}_{\text{current}})}$$

Thus, for a 50-kg woman with 60% total body water and serum sodium of 113 mEq/L, the volume of 3% NaCl (513 mEq/L) required to raise the serum sodium by 4 mEq/L would be

$$\frac{(4\ \text{mEq/L})(50\ \text{kg} \times 0.6)}{(513 - 117)} = 0.3\ \text{L or } 300\ \text{mL}$$

One might give 300 mL of 3% NaCl over the first 1 to 2 hours until resolution of seizures and then proceed with other steps to increase the serum sodium by a total of less than 12 mEq/L over the first 24 hours. Furosemide may be given in addition to hypertonic saline to produce a net negative water balance, as well as to lessen the risk of sodium overload.

In patients *without* severe manifestations, such as seizures or coma, the treatment of hyponatremia should be directed at the underlying cause. Hypovolemic hyponatremia should be treated with normal saline. Hypervolemic hyponatremia is often difficult to treat, because the underlying disorders are usually not readily reversible. Sodium and water restriction is usually the best alternative. Diuretics may result in transient loss of sodium and water but may ultimately decrease glomerular filtration rate and thereby limit free-water excretion. Patients with euvolemic hyponatremia should have their free-water intake restricted, and any identifiable underlying cause should be treated. Diuretic-induced hyponatremia responds to withdrawal of the offending medication, liberalized sodium intake, and repletion of total body potassium.

COMMON PITFALLS

- Do not overlook the possibility of sampling error, hyperglycemia, hyperlipidemia, or hyperproteinemia before making the diagnosis of hypotonic hyponatremia.
- Always consider the diagnosis in groups at high risk for severe hyponatremia, including elderly patients on diuretics, psychiatric patients, infants given only tap water, postoperative patients receiving hypotonic intravenous fluid therapy, and patients with malignancy or AIDS.
- Acute symptomatic hyponatremia should be recognized and treated quickly in order to avoid cerebral edema and brainstem herniation syndrome. Chronic hyponatremia should be corrected at an overall rate less than 0.5 mEq/L/h or 12 mEq/L/d in order to minimize the risk of central pontine myelinolysis.

HYPERNATREMIA

Hypernatremia is considerably less common than hyponatremia, because even a small increase in the serum sodium concentration is a potent stimulus to thirst. Elevated serum sodium levels develop only in patients who are unable to experience thirst or are unable to gain access to water. Hypernatremia is most often seen at extremes of age.

CLINICAL PRESENTATION

Hypernatremia reflects a state of intravascular hyperosmolarity that results in the efflux of water from the intracellular space to the extracellular space. Signs and symptoms are primarily related to central nervous system dehydration. Mental status changes range from irritability to lethargy, confusion, delirium, seizures, and coma. Muscle tone tends to be increased, as are deep tendon reflexes. Central nervous system hemorrhage into the subarachnoid, intracerebral, or subdural space is seen in severe cases and is thought to be caused by tearing of bridging veins as they are stretched by shrinkage of brain tissue.[4]

As with hyponatremia, the severity of symptoms correlates both with the severity of hypernatremia and the rate at which it develops. When the serum sodium value increases gradually over several days or weeks, neurons respond by retaining excess quantities of osmotically active solutes. This minimizes the efflux of free water from the cells and delays the onset of symptoms until relatively extreme levels of hypernatremia are achieved. When hypernatremia develops rapidly (in less than 48 hours), this adaptive mechanism is overwhelmed, and symptoms develop.

EMERGENCY DEPARTMENT EVALUATION

It is helpful to classify hypernatremia as hypovolemic, hypervolemic, or euvolemic on the basis of clinical signs of dehydration or volume overload. Classification helps to narrow the list of causes and aids in the selection of therapy (Fig. 173.2).

Hypovolemic Hypernatremia

Patients with hypovolemic hypernatremia exhibit signs of dehydration such as tachycardia, orthostasis, dry mucous membranes, diminished skin turgor, oliguria, and azotemia. Hypovolemia implies that total body sodium stores are decreased, and hypernatremia implies that free water has been lost to a greater degree than sodium. There are nonrenal and renal causes. Nonrenal causes of hypovolemia include excessive sweating, protracted vomiting, diarrhea (hyperosmotic nasogastric feedings, acute gastroenteritis, lactulose), and gastrointestinal drainage tubes; the urine sodium concentration is less than 10 mEq/L. Renal causes include postobstructive, osmotic, or therapeutic diuresis; the urine sodium is greater than 20 mEq/L. Notably, to achieve a hypernatremic state, the loss of hypotonic fluids must be coupled with inadequate free-water replacement.

Hypervolemic Hypernatremia

Patients with signs of fluid overload (e.g., pulmonary edema or peripheral edema) are classified as having hypervolemic hypernatremia. This group has increased total body sodium stores, with a smaller increase in total body free water. The differential diagnosis includes acute renal failure, use of hypernatremic dialysate solutions, seawater ingestion, and excessive administration of sodium in the form of hypertonic saline, sodium bicarbonate, or saline enemas or emetics. An enteral overdose of as little as 4 teaspoons of table salt can result in a serum sodium concentration of 160 mEq/dL in the average adult. Patients who have taken an overdose of table salt but have had no intake of water may not have overt signs of hypervolemia. The urine sodium value is more than 20 mEq/L in these cases.

Euvolemic Hypernatremia

Patients who appear neither dehydrated nor edematous are considered to have euvolemic hypernatremia, implying appropriately normal total body sodium stores and an isolated loss of free water. This may occur in comatose or intubated patients whose insensible free-water losses are not adequately replaced. It is especially common in those whose insensible losses are accelerated because of tachypnea or fever. Euvolemic hypernatremia is also seen in infants whose powdered formula is inadequately diluted or, rarely, in persons with an intrinsic defect in

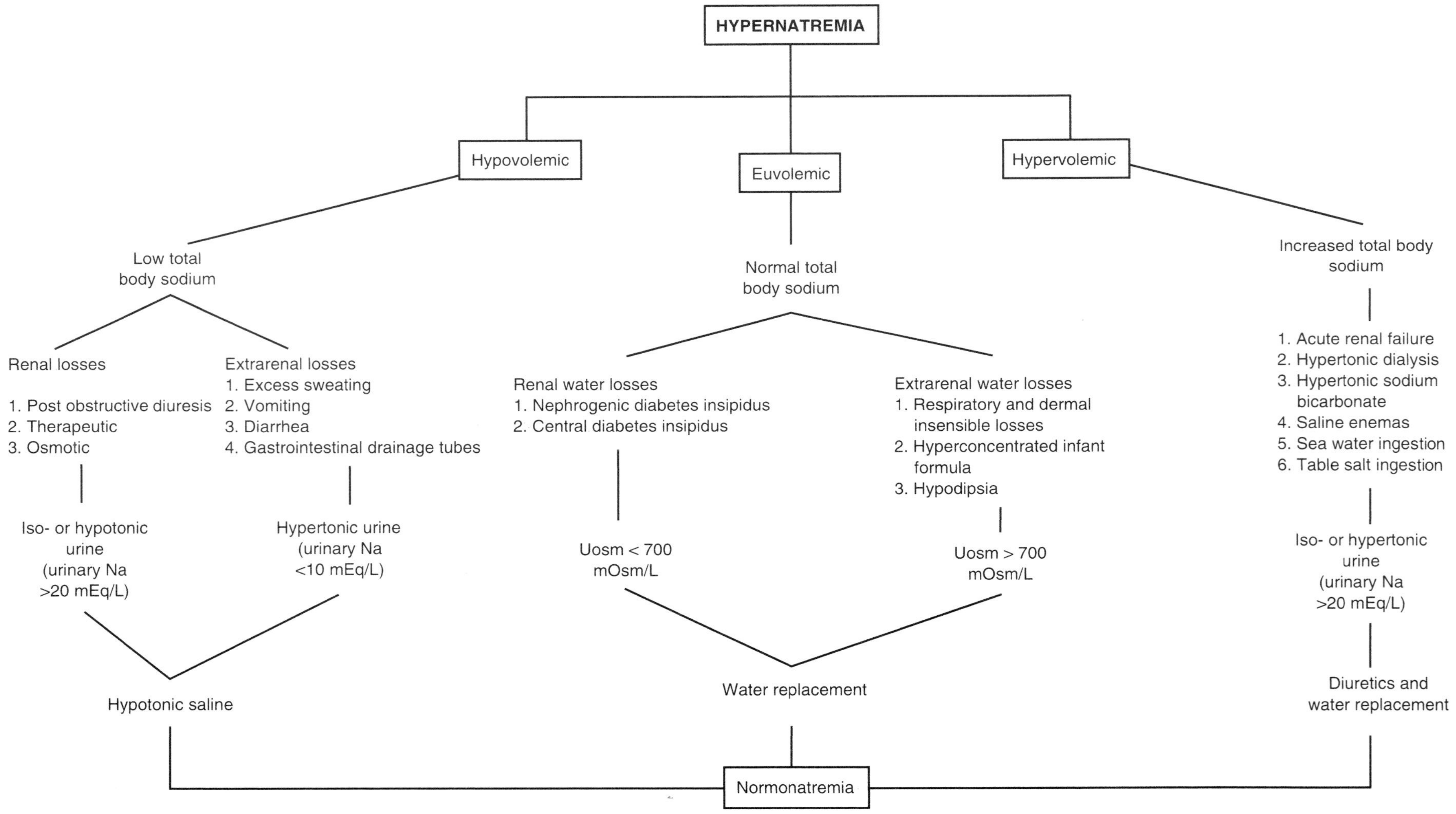

Figure 173.2. Algorithm for diagnosis and treatment of hypernatremia.

the hypothalamic thirst drive, a condition known as essential hypernatremia. In all of these cases, the urine osmolarity is appropriately greater than 700 mOsmol/L during water deprivation.

Diabetes insipidus causes euvolemic hypernatremia due to inappropriate loss of free water in the urine. In this condition, there is an inability to maximally concentrate urine during periods of water deprivation. This inability may be due to inadequate hypothalamic secretion of ADH (central diabetes insipidus) or an inability of the kidneys to respond adequately to circulating ADH (nephrogenic diabetes insipidus). In either case, hypernatremia is accompanied by inappropriately dilute urine (UOsmol less than 700 mOsmol/L^3), even during water restriction.

EMERGENCY DEPARTMENT MANAGEMENT

As with the treatment of hyponatremia, it is important to distinguish between acute hypernatremia (less than 48 hours' duration) and chronic hypernatremia (greater than 48 hours' duration), because cell physiology and the response to therapy are quite different.

Acute hypernatremia is much less common and usually develops in the setting of inadvertent sodium administration. Severe neuronal dehydration develops and the cells are unable to rapidly adapt by retention of additional cellular osmoles. Subarachnoid, intracerebral, and subdural hemorrhage may occur. Therefore, acute hyponatremia should be corrected rapidly, using D5W or oral administration, until acute manifestations begin to improve. Diuretics should be added for patients with clinical signs of volume overload.

More commonly, hypernatremia develops over several days or even weeks because of slower loss of hypotonic fluid or insensible free-water loss. The neurons adapt by retaining cellular solutes, minimizing movement of free water out of the cell. Rapid administration of hypotonic saline or D5W in these patients carries a risk of cerebral edema. Chronic hypernatremia should normalized at a steady rate over 48 to 72 hours.[10]

The free-water deficit can be calculated using the following formula:

$$\text{Water deficit} = \text{TBW}\,\frac{(\text{Na}_{\text{actual}} - \text{Na}_{\text{desired}})}{\text{Na}_{\text{actual}}}$$

where total body water is 60% of the usual body weight. This can be administered as D5W or oral water, with 30% given over the first 24 hours and 70% over the next 48 hours.[9] Hypovolemic patients should receive 0.9% normal saline (154 mEq/L) until they are euvolemic and can then be started on hypotonic fluids. Hypervolemic patients with chronic hypernatremia may require diuretic therapy in addition to free-water replacement.

COMMON PITFALLS

- Always consider the possibility of hypernatremia in high-risk patients: infants and demented, comatose, or intubated patients without access to free-water replacement.
- Chronic hypernatremia should be corrected gradually over 48 to 72 hours in order to minimize the risk of cerebral edema.

References

1. Arieff AI. Management of hyponatremia. *BMJ* 1993;307:305.
2. Fraser CL, Arieff AI. Epidemiology, pathophysiology, and management of hyponatremic encephalopathy. *Am J Med* 1997;102:67.
3. Fried LF, Palevsky PM. Hyponatremia and hypernatremia. *Med Clin North Am* 1997;81:585.
4. Hee Lee J, Arcinue E, Ross BD. Brief report: organic osmolytes in the brain of an infant with hypernatremia. *N Engl J Med* 1994;331:439.
5. Kumar S, Berl T. Sodium. *Lancet* 1998;352:220.
6. Laurento R, Karp BI. Myelinolysis after correction of hyponatremia. *Ann Intern Med* 1997; 126:57.
7. Lawn N, Wijdicks EFM, Burritt MF. Intravenous immune globulin and pseudohyponatremia. *N Engl J Med* 1998;339:632.
8. Liu BA, Mittmann N, Knowles SR, et al. Hyponatremia and the syndrome of inappropriate secretion of antidiuretic hormone associated with the use of selective serotonin reuptake inhibitors: a review of spontaneous reports. *Can Med Assoc J* 1996;155:519.
9. Musch W, Thimpont J, Vandervelde D, et al. Combined fractional excretion of sodium and urea better predicts response to saline in hyponatremia than do usual clinical and biochemical parameters. *Am J Med* 1995;99:348.
10. Palevsky PM. Hypernatremia. *Semin Nephrol* 1998;18:20.
11. Tang WW, Kaptein EM, Feinstein EI, et al. Hyponatremia in hospitalized patients with the acquired immunodeficiency syndrome (AIDS) and the AIDS-related complex. *Am J Med* 1993;94:169
12. Videen JS, Michaelis T, Pinto P, et al. Human cerebral osmolytes during chronic hyponatremia: a proton magnetic resonance spectroscopy study. *J Clin Invest* 1995;95:788.

CHAPTER 174

Disorders of Potassium Metabolism

Frank G. Walter and Elisabeth F. Bilden

Normally, total body potassium amounts to about 50 mEq/kg, or 3500 mEq in a person weighing 70 kg.[8] Ninety-eight percent of it is within the intracellular space, and 2% is in the extracellular space. The normal serum potassium concentration is between 3.5 and 5.0 mEq/L in most laboratory assays. Because of the relatively small percentage of total body potassium in the extracellular space, the serum potassium level does not always reflect total body potassium. The average 70-kg person has a total extracellular potassium content of only 70 mEq; therefore, potentially dangerous hyperkalemia may occur during overly rapid potassium administration because of a delay in the redistribution of potassium from the extracellular to the intracellular space.

PHYSIOLOGY AND PATHOPHYSIOLOGY AT THE CELLULAR LEVEL

The ratio of extracellular to intracellular potassium concentration is the major determinant of the cellular membrane resting potential, which affects the function of neurons, cardiac myocytes, smooth muscle cells of the gut, and skeletal muscle cells. Dysfunction of these cells causes most of the clinical manifestations of hyperkalemia and hypokalemia. Table 174.1 outlines the factors that affect transcellular potassium distribution.[1,2,4–6,10,23]

PHYSIOLOGY AND PATHOPHYSIOLOGY AT THE ORGAN AND SYSTEM LEVEL

Total body potassium content is determined by the difference between potassium intake and potassium excretion. About 90% of potassium excretion occurs in the urine, about 10% in feces, and a very small amount in sweat. Therefore, renal potassium

TABLE 174.1. Extrarenal Factors Affecting Transcellular Potassium Distribution

FACTORS INCREASING SERUM POTASSIUM CONCENTRATIONS	FACTORS DECREASING SERUM POTASSIUM CONCENTRATIONS
Acidemia	Alkalemia
Insulin deficiency	Insulin
Beta blockers	Beta-adrenergic agonists
Alpha-adrenergic agonists	Sodium–potassium–ATPase activity (cellular sodium–potassium pump)
Hyperosmolarity	Aldosterone
Aldosterone deficiency	

excretion is the major determinant of the total body potassium content and potassium homeostasis. Table 174.2 outlines the factors that affect renal potassium excretion.

HYPERKALEMIA

CLINICAL PRESENTATION

Hyperkalemia is most common in patients with chronic renal insufficiency. Clinical manifestations of hyperkalemia are most evident in the cardiovascular and neuromuscular systems.[20] Cardiac manifestations of hyperkalemia (Table 174.3) are most common and are often not heralded by any other symptoms before the onset of life-threatening dysrhythmias and cardiac arrest.[20] Neuromuscular manifestations are rarely clinically evident but can include decreased deep tendon reflexes, weakness, and respiratory muscle insufficiency. The clinical manifestations of hyperkalemia are potentiated by concomitant hyponatremia or hypocalcemia and tend to be more severe when the serum potassium concentration has risen rapidly.

DIFFERENTIAL DIAGNOSIS

There are four general causes of a high serum potassium level: artifactual hyperkalemia, excessive potassium intake, decreased renal potassium excretion, and transcellular maldistribution. Table 174.4 outlines the differential diagnosis and etiologies of hyperkalemia.[3,7,10,12–14,18,20]

EMERGENCY DEPARTMENT EVALUATION

The diagnosis of hyperkalemia should be suspected in patients with any of the predisposing conditions listed in Table 174.4, especially chronic renal insufficiency or acute renal failure. The

TABLE 174.2. Factors Affecting Renal Potassium Excretion

FACTORS INCREASING RENAL POTASSIUM EXCRETION	FACTORS DECREASING RENAL POTASSIUM EXCRETION
High-potassium diet	Low-potassium diet
Aldosterone and other mineralocorticoids	Aldosterone deficiency
Natriuresis	Oligoanuria
Chronic metabolic alkalosis	
Chronic metabolic acidosis	
Chronic respiratory acidosis	
Glucocorticoids	
Anions such as penicillin salts	

TABLE 174.3. Electrocardiographic Manifestations of Hyperkalemia[a]

EARLY CHANGES

Tall peaked (tented) T waves
Shortened QT interval

LATER CHANGES

Widened QRS complex
Increased PR interval
Low-amplitude P waves
Elevation or depression of ST segment

ADVANCED CHANGES

Absent P waves
Marked QRS complex widening
Sine wave pattern
Ventricular fibrillation
Asystole

[a]There is only a rough correlation of ECG changes with serum potassium concentration. Life-threatening dysrhythmias can occur at even mildly elevated serum potassium concentrations.

TABLE 174.4. Etiologies and Differential Diagnosis of Hyperkalemia

ARTIFACTUAL HYPERKALEMIA

Hemolysis *in vitro* or due to venipuncture
Extreme leukocytosis or thrombocytosis
Mild forearm exercise during venipuncture
General exercise within 20 minutes of venipuncture
Laboratory error
Cold agglutinins

INCREASED POTASSIUM LOADS

Oral or intravenous potassium supplements
Penicillin potassium salts
Massive blood transfusion
Intravascular hemolysis
Burns
Crush injuries
Mesenteric or muscular infarction
Tumor lysis due to chemotherapy or radiation

DECREASED RENAL POTASSIUM EXCRETION

Acute renal failure
Chronic renal insufficiency
Hypoaldosteronism
Drugs
- Nonsteroidal antiinflammatory drugs
- Cyclosporine
- Heparin
- Angiotensin converting enzyme inhibitors
- Potassium-sparing diuretics
- Trimethoprim
- Pentamidine

TRANSCELLULAR MALDISTRIBUTION

Acidemia
Hyperkalemic periodic paralysis
Succinylcholine
Massive digitalis overdose
Insulin deficiency
Beta blockers
Hypertonic agents
- Mannitol
- Hyperglycemia (endogenous or exogenous)

presumptive diagnosis of hyperkalemia is based on electrographic (ECG) changes (see Table 174.3) in a clinical setting that predisposes to hyperkalemia (see Table 174.4). If these presumptive diagnostic criteria are met, continuous cardiac monitoring and specific emergent therapy for hyperkalemia should be instituted before laboratory confirmation. The definitive diagnosis of hyperkalemia is established by determining a serum, plasma, or whole blood potassium concentration.

Artifactual hyperkalemia should be suspected in an appropriate clinical setting (see Table 174.4) when the patient does not have symptoms, signs, or ECG changes compatible with hyperkalemia. Continuous cardiac monitoring should be maintained while the potassium concentration is measured on a second blood sample.

Measurement of the plasma potassium level may be needed to confirm artifactual hyperkalemia that is due to extreme leukocytosis or thrombocytosis; the elevated *serum* potassium concentration in this case is due to release of potassium from platelets or leukocytes during clotting.[3,11]

EMERGENCY DEPARTMENT MANAGEMENT AND DISPOSITION

Because ECG changes correlate only roughly with serum potassium levels, continuous cardiac monitoring is advisable whenever the serum potassium level is elevated, although dangerous effects usually do not occur below a level of 6.5 mEq/L. Specific therapy is indicated when associated ECG changes are present.[13,17,20,21]

For mild potassium elevations in the absence of clinical and ECG manifestations of hyperkalemia, management should be directed at determining the most likely etiology of hyperkalemia and taking steps to correct any identified predisposing factors. This might include, for instance, discontinuing oral potassium supplements or drugs known to produce hyperkalemia. Spurious hyperkalemia should, of course, be ruled out. Provided there is no reason to believe that the serum potassium level will rise further, the patient can be discharged and outpatient follow-up arranged for a repeat potassium determination and further evaluation within 48 to 72 hours. In other cases, however, admission to the hospital is advisable. Patients with greater elevations of the serum potassium level require admission to a monitored bed.

When ECG or clinical manifestations of hyperkalemia are present, continuous cardiac monitoring and specific emergent therapy are indicated. These patients should be admitted to an intensive care unit with continuous cardiac monitoring.

Except in the setting of digoxin toxicity, calcium is the first-line therapy for severe hyperkalemia because its therapeutic effect is almost immediate, with a duration of about 30 to 60 minutes. Calcium does not alter the extracellular or total body potassium content but acts by electrophysiologically stabilizing cell membranes.[13,20] The adult dose is one ampule (10 mL) of a 10% calcium gluconate solution (4.6 mEq/10 mL),[13,20] or one ampule (10 mL) of a 10% calcium chloride solution (13.6 mEq/10 mL). This is given over at least 2 minutes by a peripheral vein and repeated in 5 to 10 minutes if necessary.[13,20] Intravenous calcium should be reserved for treatment of severe hyperkalemia and cardiac manifestations requiring immediate intervention. It is relatively safe, although it may cause transient hypercalcemia with its attendant adverse effects.

Intravenous sodium bicarbonate has a therapeutic effect that begins within minutes and lasts about 2 hours.[9,17] Like calcium, it is a temporizing measure, causing a shift of potassium from the extracellular to the intracellular space without altering total body potassium. The dose is one or two ampules (about 50 mEq per ampule) given intravenously over about 5 minutes and repeated after 15 minutes, if necessary.[9,17] Potential complications of $NaHCO_3$ include significant alkalemia, hypernatremia, hyperosmolality, hypervolemia, shift of the oxyhemoglobin dissociation curve to the left, and precipitation of hypocalcemic tetany.

Glucose and insulin act together to shift potassium from the extracellular to the intracellular space, but also do not change the total body potassium content. They thus provide another means of buying time until definitive therapy can be instituted. Therapeutic effects begin within 30 to 60 minutes and last 4 to 6 hours.

Unless the patient is hyperglycemic, glucose and insulin should be used in combination, even in the nondiabetic patient, because one cannot always depend on an adequate endogenous insulin response to a glucose load.[20] A common bolus dose is 10 U of regular insulin and 25 to 50 g of glucose.[13,17,20] Because bolus therapy causes an acute change in blood osmolality, which may transiently worsen hyperkalemia, some prefer administration by infusion. A typical infusion is 500 mL of $D_{10}W$ with 10 U of regular insulin, infused over 30 to 60 minutes. Potential complications of glucose and insulin therapy include hyperglycemia, hypoglycemia, and hyperosmolality.

Beta-adrenergic stimulation results in movement of potassium into cells, and both epinephrine and albuterol have been investigated for their potassium-lowering effects.[1,5] Inhaled nebulized albuterol reliably decreases the serum K^+ for at least 2 hours in hyperkalemic dialysis patients, with essentially no significant side effects.[1] A dose of 10 to 20 mg (four to eight times that usually given in a standard nebulizer treatment for asthma) causes the potassium to fall by 0.5 to 1.0 mEq/L. Further investigation may provide more information as to optimal dosing intervals and any adverse effects.

Definitive therapy for hyperkalemia actually removes potassium from the body and decreases the total body potassium burden. Available modalities include stimulation of renal potassium excretion, administration of cation exchange resins, and dialysis.

If renal function is adequate, the most straightforward way of removing potassium from the body is by increasing renal excretion. The glomerular filtration rate should be maximized by correcting volume depletion, if present, and potassium excretion can be augmented by giving a loop diuretic such as furosemide. If renal function has not been preserved (as in most clinical contexts associated with severe hyperkalemia), other means of removing potassium from the body must be used.

Sodium polystyrene sulfonate (Kayexalate), which removes potassium from the body by exchanging sodium ions for potassium ions, is one such measure. Kayexalate can be given by the oral or rectal route. About 1 mEq of potassium is removed for each gram of orally administered Kayexalate. Given rectally, Kayexalate acts more quickly, but total potassium removal is less. Orally, 15 to 30 g of Kayexalate is given with 50 to 100 mL of 20% sorbitol (or with 15 to 30 mL of 70% sorbitol) and may be repeated every 4 hours.[9,20]

Contraindications to the oral route include ileus, complete or partial bowel obstruction, and anticipated or recent gastrointestinal (GI) surgery. Kayexalate is given as a retention enema in a dose of 50 g in 200 mL of 20% sorbitol (or 150 mL of tap water with 50 mL of 70% sorbitol), which may be repeated every 4 hours.[9,20] Potential complications of Kayexalate therapy include hypervolemia due to the sodium load and hypokalemia due to excessive administration.

Dialysis is the most efficient way of removing potassium from the body. It is indicated when severe hyperkalemia has failed to respond to the aforementioned measures, and it is the definitive therapy for hyperkalemia in patients with acute or chronic renal failure. Dialysis is especially helpful when the serum potassium concentration is rising rapidly, such as in rhabdomyolysis. Hemodialysis is preferred over peritoneal dialysis for emergency therapy because it removes potassium more rapidly and effectively.[13]

The patient being treated emergently for severe hyperkalemia requires continuous cardiac monitoring, frequent serial examinations, and serum electrolyte determinations every 2 hours until out of danger. Admission, generally to an intensive care setting, is mandatory. If the patient must be transferred to another facility, or if the patient needs admission and the facility cannot provide the necessary level of care, transport must be by a vehicle and staff equipped to perform advanced cardiac life-support interventions. Airway, breathing, and circulation, including the cardiac rhythm, must be stabilized before transport.

COMMON PITFALLS

- Failing to recognize patients at risk for hyperkalemia (see Table 174.4)
- Failing to check the serum potassium level
- Treating the serum potassium level rather than the patient
- Waiting for laboratory confirmation to institute therapy for patients with hyperkalemic ECG changes (see Table 174.3) and hyperkalemic risk factors (see Table 174.4)
- Instituting vigorous emergent therapy for an elevated potassium level in a patient with a normal ECG and no hyperkalemic risk factors

HYPOKALEMIA

CLINICAL PRESENTATION

Hypokalemia (K^+ less than 3.5 mEq/L) is the most common electrolyte abnormality. The manifestations of hypokalemia are generally mild, but serious effects can occur, particularly when potassium depletion is severe (Table 174.5).[15,16] Hypokalemia should be suspected in patients taking certain diuretics, in those with chronic or severe diarrhea, and in those with chronic volume depletion, among others. Alkalemia, insulin, beta-adrenergic agonists, and hyperaldosteronism cause potassium to shift into the intracellular space.

TABLE 174.5. Manifestations of Hypokalemia

NEUROMUSCULAR
Weakness, areflexia, paralysis
Respiratory insufficiency due to severe weakness
Rhabdomyolysis
Paresthesia
CARDIOVASCULAR
U-wave prominence
T-wave flattening or inversion
ST-segment depression
Potentiation of digitalis toxicity
Orthostatic hypotension
GASTROINTESTINAL
Ileus
RENAL
Polyuria
Metabolic alkalosis
Increased renal ammonia production
ENDOCRINE
Glucose intolerance

TABLE 174.6. Etiologies and Differential Diagnosis of Hypokalemia

DECREASED POTASSIUM INTAKE
INCREASED POTASSIUM EXCRETION
Increased Renal Potassium Excretion
Drugs
Non–potassium-sparing diuretics
Amphotericin B
Aminoglycosides
Renal tubular acidosis
Magnesium deficiency
Diuretic phase of recovery from postobstructive nephropathy or acute tubular necrosis
Primary hyperaldosteronism
Secondary hyperaldosteronism
Hyperreninemic states
Hypovolemia
Nephrotic syndrome
Congestive heart failure
Cirrhosis
Bartter syndrome
Osmotic diuresis
Increased GI Potassium Loss
Protracted emesis or nasogastric suction
Diarrhea
Villous adenoma
Chronic laxative abuse
TRANSCELLULAR MALDISTRIBUTION
Alkalemia
Insulin excess
Beta-adrenergic agonists
Acute theophylline toxicity
Poisoning with soluble barium salts
Vitamin B_{12} therapy of megaloblastic anemia
Rapid malignant cell growth and multiplication
Hypokalemic periodic paralysis

DIFFERENTIAL DIAGNOSIS

The causes of hypokalemia fall into three general categories: decreased potassium intake, increased potassium excretion, and transcellular potassium shifts. Table 174.6 outlines the differential diagnosis and etiologies.[19,21,22]

The urine potassium concentration is sometimes helpful in differentiating among the etiologies of hypokalemia. A urine potassium concentration above 20 mEq/L suggests recent hypokalemia or excessive renal potassium loss; a concentration below 20 mEq/L is most compatible with decreased potassium intake or excessive GI potassium loss.

EMERGENCY DEPARTMENT EVALUATION

Hypokalemia should be suspected in patients with any of the predisposing conditions listed in Table 174.6, especially in those taking a non–potassium-sparing diuretic. An ECG with prominent U waves in multiple leads supports the diagnosis but is nonspecific. Hypokalemia is established by determining a serum, plasma, or whole blood potassium concentration.

The combination of hypokalemia and hypertension in the absence of other obvious predisposing factors suggests primary hyperaldosteronism.

EMERGENCY DEPARTMENT MANAGEMENT AND DISPOSITION

It is reasonable to admit patients with serum potassium concentrations less than 2.5 mEq/L. A serum potassium concentration of 2.5 mEq/L generally reflects a total body potassium deficit of 200 to 400 mEq[9,17,20] Patients with mild hypokalemia (2.5 to 3.5 mEq/L) can usually be managed as outpatients with gradual oral potassium repletion, provided they do not manifest cardiac dysrhythmias, ileus, profound muscle weakness, or other serious effects.

Emergency department management should focus on determining the etiology of hypokalemia, confirming that the patient can tolerate oral potassium repletion, and excluding other serious conditions or complications. Patients who can be sent home with oral potassium supplementation should have follow-up within 48 to 72 hours to check the potassium level and to undergo further diagnostic evaluation, as necessary.

In mild hypokalemia, the oral route for potassium repletion is preferred because of its ease, safety, and economy. Potassium chloride (KCl) at a daily dosage of 40 to 80 mEq, with no more than 40 mEq given as a single dose, is usually effective. KCl may be given as a liquid, in enteric-coated tablets, or in wax matrix tablets. KCl solution is the preparation of choice because it is generally well tolerated and inexpensive. Enteric-coated KCl tablets can cause GI ulceration. Wax matrix KCl tablets cause less GI ulceration and are the preferred alternative for the patient who finds oral KCl solution unacceptable because of its taste.

When metabolic acidosis accompanies hypokalemia (as may occur with severe diarrhea), potassium bicarbonate, potassium citrate, or potassium gluconate is preferred over KCl. Potassium-sparing diuretics do not, in themselves, replete total body potassium deficits, and they should generally not be used concurrently with oral potassium supplements, because severe hyperkalemia can result.

For more severe hypokalemia (K^+ less than 2.5 mEq/L), the total body potassium deficit can be profound, and potassium repletion is more urgent. Patients should have an intravenous line and should be monitored for rhythm disturbances or the development of other symptoms. In the absence of clinical or ECG manifestations, potassium repletion can be accomplished by the oral route while close observation and continuous cardiac monitoring are continued. Otherwise, repletion generally should begin with combined intravenous and oral administration of KCl.

Intravenous KCl should not be given at a rate greater than 40 mEq/h through a peripheral intravenous line, but it may be given through a femoral line at a rate of up to 60 mEq/h for emergent treatment of hypokalemia-induced paralysis or malignant ventricular arrhythmias.[9,13–15,20] For rates above 10 mEq/h, continuous cardiac monitoring and a constant infusion pump should be used to avoid accidental overinfusion.

Because intravenous KCl can cause local vein irritation and phlebitis, some clinicians recommend infusion into a central vein, but this practice seems to increase the potential for cardiac dysrhythmias. Simultaneous oral and intravenous potassium repletion, although effecting improvement more rapidly, carries a higher risk of hyperkalemia.

Patients with gastric acid loss from persistent vomiting often develop "hypokalemic contraction alkalosis." The dehydration and metabolic alkalosis from gastric acid loss cause the kidney to conserve sodium and chloride and to increase potassium and bicarbonate excretion. In addition to potassium supplementation, these patients require rehydration, usually with intravenous sodium chloride, to correct their hypokalemia.

Hypokalemic patients with any of the following conditions should be admitted to an intensive care unit with continuous cardiac monitoring: malignant cardiac dysrhythmias, digitalis toxicity, profound weakness with impending respiratory insufficiency, a serum potassium concentration below 2.0 mEq/L, rhabdomyolysis, or hepatic encephalopathy.

COMMON PITFALLS

- Replacing potassium too rapidly without appropriate cardiac and laboratory monitoring
- Overcorrecting hypokalemia into the hyperkalemic range by excessive potassium administration, especially when hypokalemia is due to transcellular maldistribution rather than a total body potassium deficit (e.g., hypokalemic periodic paralysis)

References

1. Allon M, Dunlay R, Copkney C. Nebulized albuterol for acute hyperkalemia in patients on hemodialysis. Ann Intern Med 1989;110:426.
2. Bia MJ, Tyler KA, DeFronzo RA. Regulation of extrarenal potassium homeostasis by adrenal hormones in rats. *Am J Physiol* 1982;242:641.
3. Bronson WR, Devita VT, Carbone PP, et al. Pseudohyperkalemia due to release of potassium from white cells during clotting. *N Engl J Med* 1966;274:369.
4. Burnell JM, Villamil MF, Uyeno BT, et al. The effects in humans of extracellular pH change on the relationship between serum potassium concentration and intracellular potassium. *J Clin Invest* 1956;35:935.
5. DeFronzo RA, Bia M, Birkhead G. Epinephrine and potassium homeostasis. *Kidney Int* 1981;20:83.
6. DeFronzo RA, Sherwin RS, Dillingham M, et al. Influence of basal insulin and glucagon secretion on potassium and sodium metabolism. *J Clin Invest* 1978;61:472.
7. Edes TE, Sunderrajan EV. Heparin-induced hyperkalemia. *Arch Intern Med* 1985;145:1070.
8. Forbes GB, Lewis AM. Total sodium, potassium, and chloride in adult man. *J Clin Invest* 1956;35:596.
9. Gibbs MA, Wolfson AB, Tayal VS. Electrolyte disturbances. In: Rosen P, Barkin RM, eds. *Emergency medicine: concepts and clinical practice,* 4th ed., vol 3. St. Louis: Mosby–Year Book, 1998:2435.
10. Goldfarb S, Strunk B, Singer I, et al. Paradoxical glucose-induced hyperkalemia. *Am J Med* 1975;59:744.
11. Hartman RC, Auditore JV, Jackson DP, et al. Studies on thrombocytosis: hyperkalemia due to release of potassium from platelets during coagulation. *J Clin Invest* 1958;37:699.
12. Hlavacek JR, Restifo R, Stone D, et al. Laboratory false-positive hyperkalemia in a patient with cold agglutinins. *Anesth Analg* 1986;65:1245.
13. Kamel KS, Halperin ML. Treatment of hypokalemia and hyperkalemia. In: Brady HR, Wilcox CS, eds. *Therapy in nephrology and hypertension: a companion to Brenner and Rector's the kidney.* Philadelphia: WB Saunders, 1999:270.
14. Kruse JA, Carlson RW. Rapid correction of hypokalemia using concentrated intravenous potassium chloride infusions. *Arch Intern Med* 1990;150:613.
15. Manary MJ, Keating JP, Hirshberg GE. Quadriparesis due to potassium depletion. *Crit Care Med* 1986;14:750.
16. Narins RG, Heilig CW, Kupin WL. The patient with hypokalemia or hyperkalemia. In: Schrier RW, ed. *Manuel of nephrology,* 4th ed. Boston: Little, Brown and Company, 1995:37.
17. Peterson LN, Levi M. Disorders of potassium metabolism. In: Schrier RW, ed. *Renal and electrolyte disorders,* 5th ed. Philadelphia: Lippincott–Raven Publishers, 1997:192.
18. Schlanger LE, Kleyman TR, Ling BN. K+-sparing diuretic actions of trimethoprim: inhibition of Na+ channels in A6 distal nephron cells. *Kidney Int* 1994;45:1070.
19. Shin B, MacKenzie CF, Helrich M. Hypokalemia in trauma patients. *Anesthesiology* 1986;65:90.
20. Singer GG. Fluid and electrolyte management. In: Carey CF, Lee HH, Woeltje KF, eds. *Washington manual of medical therapeutics,* 29th ed. Philadelphia: Lippincott–Raven Publishers, 1998:48.
21. Tannen RL. Hypokalemia and hyperkalemia. In: Massry SG, Glassok RJ, eds. *Textbook of nephrology,* 3rd ed, vol 1. Baltimore: Williams & Wilkins, 1995:313.
22. Whang R, Flink EB, Dyckner T, et al. Magnesium depletion as a cause of refractory potassium repletion. *Arch Intern Med* 1985;145:1686.
23. Williams ME, Rosa RM, Silva P, et al. Impairment of extrarenal potassium disposal by alpha-adrenergic stimulation. *N Engl J Med* 1984;311:145.

CHAPTER 175

Disorders of Calcium, Magnesium, and Phosphorus

Daniel R. Martin and Marc B. Schnapper

Disorders of calcium, magnesium, and phosphorus metabolism can result in life-threatening emergencies that have nonspecific presentations resembling those of many other disease processes. However, emergency department (ED) testing for the presence of these disturbances must be selective. Such testing must be guided by an understanding of the pathophysiology of these disorders and the clinical settings in which they are likely to occur. Once a diagnosis is made, this same understanding makes it possible for the physician to choose effective and appropriate therapy.

CALCIUM

About 40% of the serum calcium is protein-bound, an additional 10% to 15% is chelated with other anions, and the physiologically active, ionized component makes up the remaining 45% to 50%. Serum calcium levels are regulated primarily by interactions between parathyroid hormone (PTH) and vitamin D. PTH increases bone resorption and renal tubular calcium resorption. Vitamin D is responsible for regulating intestinal calcium absorption, and has an additional bone resorptive effect.

The normal total serum calcium level ranges from 8.5 to 10.5 mg/dL, and the free ionized level from 4.0 to 4.8 mg/dL. Raising the pH increases calcium binding to serum proteins, lowering the free ionized fraction without altering the total plasma calcium level. Ionized calcium changes by about 1.7 mg/dL for every change of 0.1 pH units. Alterations in serum protein also affect the measured Ca^{2+}; that is, decreasing the serum albumin by 1 g/dL lowers the total serum calcium by about 0.8 mg/dL.[1] Measurement of ionized Ca^{2+} may be warranted in patients with suspected hypocalcemia who are hypoalbuminemic or alkalotic.

Hypercalcemia

CLINICAL PRESENTATION, EMERGENCY DEPARTMENT EVALUATION, AND DIFFERENTIAL DIAGNOSIS

The severity of the manifestations of hypercalcemia depends on the serum calcium level, the rate of rise from normal values, and the presence of concurrent medical conditions.[4] Central nervous system (CNS) manifestations, ranging from weakness, lethargy, depression, and confusion to obtundation or coma, are prominent. Gastrointestinal (GI) manifestations such as anorexia, nausea, vomiting, abdominal pain, and constipation are also typical. In the kidney, hypercalcemia causes an inability to concentrate the urine, leading to polyuria and dehydration. Chronic hypercalcemia may be associated with nephrocalcinosis and renal failure.[1]

TABLE 175.1. Causes of Hypercalcemia

ENDOCRINE DISORDERS
Hyperparathyroidism
Hyperthyroidism
Adrenal insufficiency
Pheochromocytoma
MALIGNANCY
Solid tumors
Breast, lung, colon, stomach, cervix, ovary, kidney, bladder, head, and neck
Hematologic
Multiple myeloma
Lymphoma
GRANULOMATOUS DISEASES
Sarcoidosis
Tuberculosis
Histoplasmosis, coccidioidomycosis
DRUGS
Thiazides
Lithium
Vitamin D intoxication
Vitamin A intoxication
MISCELLANEOUS
Dehydration or prolonged immobilization
Excess calcium ingestion
Milk-alkali syndrome

ED evaluation should include at least serum electrolytes, calcium (total and ionized), and an electrocardiogram (ECG). The most common ECG correlate of hypercalcemia is shortening of the Q-T interval, but more severe effects include dysrhythmias and heart block; ultimately, asystole can occur. Hypercalcemia can also exacerbate digoxin toxicity.

The major causes of hypercalcemia are listed in Table 175.1. Among these, primary hyperparathyroidism and malignancy (especially carcinoma of the breast and lung) are the most common. The combination of CNS and GI symptoms and shortened QT in the setting of existing malignancy should suggest hypercalcemia. However, other causes of multisystem dysfunction, such as infection, or primary CNS or GI system dysfunction, should also be considered.

EMERGENCY DEPARTMENT MANAGEMENT AND DISPOSITION

Symptomatic hypercalcemia or a serum calcium level above 15 mg/dL requires immediate intervention. Forced saline diuresis is the first-line treatment; 1 to 2 L of isotonic saline is given initially, followed by 200 to 500 mL/h, depending on the level of volume depletion. Intravenous furosemide (20 to 40 mg every 6 to 8 hours) is given to enhance urinary output and decrease calcium reabsorption in the loop of Henle once intravascular volume has been repleted.[4,20]

Additional treatment should be considered when the serum calcium level does not respond rapidly to saline diuresis. Calcitonin (2 to 4 IU/kg intramuscularly or subcutaneously every 12 hours) causes a rapid fall of the serum calcium level in most patients and is appropriate for those who respond suboptimally to saline diuresis or for whom saline loading and diuresis are not practical (e.g., patients with congestive heart failure).[4,18]

Although mithramycin (25 μg intravenously) can also be used to lower the serum calcium level, the effect is not apparent for at least 12 hours.[4] Dialysis is occasionally necessary if rapid control of the serum calcium level is critical.[5,9]

Hydrocortisone (100 to 150 mg intravenously every 12 hours) is effective mainly in hypercalcemia due to hematologic malignancy.[16] Several other agents, among them gallium nitrate, etidronate, and pamidronate, have controlled the hypercalcemia of malignancy; all act by inhibiting bone resorption, but because of the slow onset of effect, they are inappropriate for emergency therapy.

Intravenous phosphate can decrease serum calcium levels rapidly, but should not be given because of the risk of metastatic calcification and resulting organ damage, including dysrhythmias. Intravenous sodium EDTA should also be avoided because of dangers associated with its use.[7]

The disposition of patients from the ED depends on the presence or absence of symptoms. Patients with symptomatic hypercalcemia need close monitoring in a telemetry unit to continually assess for cardiovascular complications, especially pulmonary edema. Serum calcium, potassium, and magnesium levels must also be checked regularly. In patients with asymptomatic hypercalcemia, discharge with close outpatient follow-up (less than 1 week) is appropriate. Prior to discharge from the ED, obtaining a serum PTH level may facilitate the outpatient workup.

COMMON PITFALLS

- Common complications of saline diuresis include congestive heart failure and fluid overload.
- A common error is to give a loop diuretic before intravascular volume repletion; this tends to deplete volume further, decreasing the glomerular filtration rate, and may exacerbate hypercalcemia.
- Frequent monitoring of calcium, magnesium, and potassium levels (and appropriate replacement) is necessary during treatment.
- Thiazide diuretics should be discontinued, because they can increase the serum calcium level.[20]

TABLE 175.2. Causes of Hypocalcemia

HYPOPARATHYROIDISM
Neck surgery
Neck irradiation
RENAL FAILURE
MEDICATIONS
Anticonvulsants
Colchicine overdose
Chemotherapeutic agents
GASTROINTESTINAL
Malabsorption syndromes
Vitamin D deficiency
Acute pancreatitis
OVERDOSE
Calcium channel blocker
Beta blocker
MISCELLANEOUS
Hyperphosphatemia
Massive transfusion
Ethylene glycol
Hydrofluoric acid
Neonatal (prematurity, rickets, lactic acidosis)
Rhabdomyolysis
Magnesium deficiency
Hypoalbuminemia (normal ionized fraction)

Hypocalcemia

CLINICAL PRESENTATION, EMERGENCY DEPARTMENT EVALUATION, AND DIFFERENTIAL DIAGNOSIS

Hypocalcemia should be considered in patients who have renal failure, chronic malabsorption, or a history of neck surgery or neck irradiation (Table 175.2). It should also be considered in those who display the cardinal signs or symptoms of hypocalcemia, primarily neuromuscular irritability. Hypocalcemia is also a feature of disorders in which intravascular calcium is chelated by any of a number of anions, such as rhabdomyolysis (phosphates), ethylene glycol poisoning (oxalate), hydrofluoric acid exposure (fluoride), and pancreatitis (fats). Lastly, it is found in settings of overdoses of two frequently used medications: beta blockers and calcium channel blockers.

Clinical symptoms depend on both the ionized calcium level and the rapidity of its fall from normal values. Patients with hypocalcemia frequently complain of circumoral and distal extremity paresthesias, although nonspecific symptoms such as weakness, fatigue, irritability, or altered mental status may predominate. The classic manifestations of carpopedal spasm, hyperreflexia, muscle cramping, and tetany are more troubling, and laryngospasm, seizures, or precipitation of congestive heart failure can be life-threatening. Trousseau's sign (carpopedal spasm after arterial occlusion of the arm for 3 minutes) and Chvostek's sign (contraction of the facial muscles after percussion over the facial nerve) may indicate subclinical hypocalcemia.

The typical ECG manifestation of hypocalcemia is prolongation of the Q-T interval. Inverted T waves, sinus bradycardia, complete heart block, ventricular dysrhythmias, and ventricular fibrillation have also been reported.

Hypocalcemia must be differentiated from other conditions presenting in a similar manner, including hypomagnesemia, severe alkalosis, strychnine poisoning, and tetanus.

EMERGENCY DEPARTMENT MANAGEMENT AND DISPOSITION

$CaCl_2$ is the drug of choice for acutely symptomatic patients with severe hypocalcemia, as 1 ampule (10 cc) delivers 13.6 mEq (272 mg) of Ca^{2+}, compared with 4.6 mEq (93 mg) provided by 10 cc of Ca^{2+} gluconate. Some clinicians recommend the routine use of calcium gluconate, as opposed to calcium chloride, in the absence of cardiovascular collapse, because it is less irritating to veins. Standard doses are 5 to 10 cc of $CaCl_2$ or 5 to 10 cc of calcium gluconate, up to a total one-time dose of 20 cc. In special situations (e.g., severe calcium channel blocker overdose), repeating the $CaCl_2$ may be beneficial. Furthermore, an infusion of 1 to 2 mg/kg/h is often necessary after bolus dosing. Continued cardiac monitoring and serial calcium levels are indicated. The infusion should be terminated if bradycardia or a shortening of the QT interval develops.

All symptomatic patients require admission to a telemetry or intensive care unit. For asymptomatic patients, oral calcium (1 to 4 g/d in divided doses), with or without vitamin D, is appropriate. Outpatient follow-up should be emphasized to evaluate the underlying etiology.

COMMON PITFALLS

- Refractory hypocalcemia that does not respond to intravenous calcium may be due to hypomagnesemia.[1]
- Calcium should be given cautiously to patients on digitalis, as digitalis toxicity may be precipitated or exacerbated.[24]
- If hyperphosphatemia is present, calcium administration may result in calcium phosphate precipitation in soft tissues.
- Calcium should not be given in the same intravenous line as sodium bicarbonate, or precipitation will occur.[1]

MAGNESIUM

Like calcium, serum magnesium is made up of fractions that are protein-bound (30%) and chelated (15%); the rest is the physiologically active, ionized component. The normal serum magnesium concentration is 1.5 to 2.5 mEq/L.

Hypermagnesemia

CLINICAL PRESENTATION, EMERGENCY DEPARTMENT EVALUATION, AND DIFFERENTIAL DIAGNOSIS

Because the kidney is efficient in excreting excess magnesium, hypermagnesemia is uncommon, except in the presence of renal insufficiency or severe dehydration. In patients with normal renal function, hypermagnesemia has been reported after parenteral administration of magnesium in the therapy of toxemia,[13] magnesium salt enemas, bladder irrigation with hemiacidrin,[8] and oral ingestion of magnesium preparations in the presence of a perforated viscus.[25]

Hypermagnesemia causes cardiac and neuromuscular depression. Lethargy, nausea, vomiting, flushing, and mental confusion are common but nonspecific manifestations. Depression of deep tendon reflexes is often noted as levels exceed 4 mEq/L. At higher levels, marked muscle weakness, paralysis, and respiratory insufficiency develop; dysrhythmias and cardiac arrest occur at even higher levels. The ECG manifestations of hypermagnesemia include prolongation of the P-R interval, QRS complex, and the Q-T interval, but these findings are variable and nonspecific.

EMERGENCY DEPARTMENT MANAGEMENT AND DISPOSITION

The treatment of hypermagnesemia begins with removal of the source of exogenous magnesium. In symptomatic patients, 10 mL of 10% calcium gluconate or calcium chloride solution can be given intravenously[1]; calcium transiently reverses hypermagnesemia effects by acting as a direct membrane antagonist. In patients with adequate renal function, intravenous normal saline and furosemide are given to promote a brisk diuresis and enhance urinary magnesium excretion. In patients with very high magnesium levels or in those with renal failure, emergency peritoneal dialysis or hemodialysis may be necessary.

ED disposition will vary based on the level of supportive care required. Relatively asymptomatic patients should be monitored on telemetry if renal function is abnormal or if ECG changes are evident. Magnesium levels below 5 mEq/L do not usually require aggressive treatment, and patients are generally asymptomatic. Such patients may be discharged with outpatient follow-up once dehydration is corrected and any source of supplemental magnesium is eliminated.

COMMON PITFALLS

- Magnesium-containing antacids and laxatives should be avoided in patients with renal failure and in those with a decreased glomerular filtration rate.
- Hypermagnesemia should be suspected in patients presenting with neuromuscular depression in a clinical setting potentially associated with hypermagnesemia. This is unlikely to occur unless there has been rapid and massive magnesium administration or renal function is impaired.

Hypomagnesemia

CLINICAL PRESENTATION, EMERGENCY DEPARTMENT EVALUATION, AND DIFFERENTIAL DIAGNOSIS

Hypomagnesemia can result from many causes (Table 175.3), but is most commonly seen in the ED in association with alcoholism, diuretic use, or malnutrition. The measured serum magnesium concentration may not accurately reflect the patient's total body magnesium status. Alcoholics and patients with renal disease may have depleted total body magnesium stores but a normal or even an elevated serum level. Up to 40% of patients with other electrolyte deficiencies are magnesium-deficient as well, whether or not symptoms are present.[22]

Hypomagnesemia may be responsible for a variety of psychiatric, neuromuscular, GI, and cardiovascular effects.[6,16] Many of the symptoms and signs may be due to other associated disorders, such as hypocalcemia and hypokalemia.[22] Psychiatric complaints can range from apathy and depression to delirium and coma. Neuromuscular effects are similar to those of

TABLE 175.3. Causes of Hypomagnesemia

DIETARY
Alcoholism
Malnutrition
GASTROINTESTINAL
Malabsorption syndromes
Chronic diarrhea
RENAL
Tubular dysfunction
DRUGS
Diuretics
DRUGS CAUSING INTRACELLULAR SHIFT
Insulin treatment of diabetic ketoacidosis
ENDOCRINE/METABOLIC
Diabetic or alcoholic ketoacidosis
Hypokalemia
Burns
Sepsis

hypocalcemia, ranging from extremity tremors to convulsions.[21] Nausea, anorexia, and abdominal pain may be noted. Cardiovascular effects, including atrial and ventricular dysrhythmias (especially torsades de pointes), are potentially immediately life-threatening.[21]

The ECG changes associated with hypomagnesemia may be related to an interaction with other abnormalities of calcium and potassium.[22] Although acute changes in magnesium levels may result in peaked or flattened T waves, chronic changes are associated with P-R prolongation, QRS widening, and, most commonly, Q-T prolongation.

EMERGENCY DEPARTMENT MANAGEMENT AND DISPOSITION

Emergent therapy and hospitalization are warranted when severe hypomagnesemia is associated with cardiac dysrhythmias, marked CNS manifestations, or other severe symptoms. ECG monitoring is mandatory, and there should be frequent evaluation of the deep tendon reflexes.

Magnesium therapy is indicated for arrhythmias associated with a prolonged Q-T interval. It is the drug of choice for torsades de pointes, in a dose of 2 g pushed intravenously. For other cardiac indications, the data are less clear. Although several studies appeared to show decreased mortality when Mg^{2+} was used in the treatment of myocardial infarction, this was not confirmed by the largest prospective study, the ISIS 4 trial.[3] Mg^{2+} may be helpful for supraventricular arrhythmias, if associated with hypokalemia, hypomagnesemia, or alcohol withdrawal.

For seizures, tetany, or malignant ventricular dysrhythmia, 2 g of magnesium sulfate may be given intravenously over several minutes, followed by 5 g intravenously over 6 hours. Dysrhythmias due to hypomagnesemia may be unresponsive to conventional antidysrhythmic therapy, but they respond well to intravenous magnesium.

In general, patients with serum magnesium levels below 1 mEq/L should be hospitalized: Most are symptomatic, and repletion typically takes several days. Repletion can be initiated with intravenous doses of 2 to 5 g given over several hours, followed by oral supplementation of up to 6 g/d until stable normal serum levels are restored. Most administered magnesium is rapidly excreted in the urine, and only a fraction is taken up by the cells. Doses should be withheld if the serum level rises above 1.5 mEq/L at any time, or if deep tendon reflexes are lost, indicating hypermagnesemia. Magnesium supplementation is also appropriate for patients with alcohol withdrawal and for those with hypokalemia or hypocalcemia that is unresponsive to the usual corrective measures.

Recent studies, however, do not support the routine use of Mg^{2+} for alcoholic patients presenting to the ED.[11] Nevertheless, intravenous Mg^{2+} is recommended for those being treated for withdrawal, as it has been shown to decrease the risk of seizures, as well as decrease arrhythmias during withdrawal. It takes 5 to 7 days to replete total body stores.

Other clinical settings in which treatment with magnesium may be indicated are digitalis toxicity, eclampsia, and cocaine-induced myocardial infarction. Mg^{2+} opposes the effect of digitalis on the resting membrane potential of myocardial cells, thereby decreasing spontaneous depolarizations. Mg^{2+} is the treatment of choice for eclampsia, because it blocks Ca^{2+}-mediated vasospasm. This may also be the mechanism for its beneficial effect in cases of cocaine-induced myocardial ischemia.

Patients with mild or chronic hypomagnesemia can be treated with oral supplementation (magnesium oxide or enteric-coated magnesium chloride[17]) and an adequate diet. These patients generally exhibit minimal symptoms and can be discharged from the ED with outpatient follow-up (less than 1 week). Oral magnesium can cause diarrhea, however, and the dose should be decreased if this occurs. Treatment should always include correction of the underlying cause of the hypomagnesemia.

COMMON PITFALLS

- The degree of hypomagnesemia generally correlates only roughly with the degree of total body magnesium depletion.
- Most administered magnesium is rapidly excreted in the urine, so correction of magnesium depletion requires days to weeks of supplementation.
- Hypokalemia or hypocalcemia refractory to the usual corrective measures may be due to underlying hypomagnesemia, correction of which allows correction of the other electrolyte disorder(s).

PHOSPHORUS

Eighty percent to 85% of total body phosphorus is found in bone; almost all of the remainder is in skeletal muscle and soft tissue.[9] Because most of the body's phosphorus is intracellular, serum phosphate concentrations do not necessarily reflect total body stores. Normal serum levels in adults range from 2.7 to 4.5 mg/dL. Fifteen percent of the phosphorus in serum is protein-bound; the remaining 85% is in the form of $HPO_4^{(-2)}$ and $H_2PO_4^{(-)}$ in a molar ratio of 4:1 at a pH of 7.4.

Phosphate homeostasis is under the control of vitamin D and PTH. The former stimulates bone resorption in some mineral-deficiency states and stimulates phosphate absorption in the GI tract; the latter acts in the proximal renal tubule to increase phosphate excretion.[15] Other hormones, such as insulin, estrogen, and thyroid hormone, may also modify renal tubular handling of phosphate.

Hyperphosphatemia

CLINICAL PRESENTATION, EMERGENCY DEPARTMENT EVALUATION, AND DIFFERENTIAL DIAGNOSIS

The most common cause of hyperphosphatemia is acute or chronic renal failure,[19] and severe hyperphosphatemia is rare unless renal function is at least moderately impaired. Other etiologies include hypoparathyroidism, excess human growth hormone, rhabdomyolysis, and cytotoxic therapy (as part of the tumor lysis syndrome). Exogenous causes of hyperphosphatemia include overtreatment of hypophosphatemia and the use of phosphate-containing laxatives and enemas (Table 175.5).

The clinical manifestations of hyperphosphatemia, if any, result from its effect on calcium homeostasis.[19] If phosphate and calcium concentrations reach levels at which the solubility product is exceeded, calcium–phosphate crystal deposition can occur in the heart, kidney, lungs, and other soft tissues. Acute hypocalcemic symptoms can also occur .

EMERGENCY DEPARTMENT MANAGEMENT AND DISPOSITION

Treatment of hyperphosphatemia *per se* should rarely be necessary in the ED. Any treatment these patients receive is directed

TABLE 175.4. Key Magnesium Conversions

1 g $MgSO_4$ = 8.12 mEq Mg
1 mEq Mg = 0.5 mmol Mg = 12.3 mg
1 mEq/dL Mg = 1.2 mg/dL
1 g $MgSO_4$ = 98 mg of elemental Mg
1 Mg oxide tablet = 111 mg = 9 mEq Mg
1 10-cc ampule of 50% $MgSO_4$ = 5 g of Mg or 40.6 mEq Mg

Not all ampules contain the same amount of Mg^{2+}.

at the underlying associated illness. For refractory hyperphosphatemia, hemodialysis may be required.

Phosphate-binding antacids containing calcium are used chronically by renal failure patients to control serum phosphate levels; oral phosphate intake is also restricted.[15]

COMMON PITFALL

Specific treatment for hyperphosphatemia *per se* is rarely indicated. Instead, therapy is directed at the underlying associated disorders.

Hypophosphatemia

CLINICAL PRESENTATION, EMERGENCY DEPARTMENT EVALUATION, AND DIFFERENTIAL DIAGNOSIS

As with magnesium and calcium, altered states of phosphate homeostasis often go unrecognized. The causes of hypophosphatemia are varied (Table 175.6); those related to alcohol and diabetes are most commonly seen in the ED.[15] Alcoholism is associated with hypophosphatemia because of dietary insufficiency and urinary phosphate losses, as well as several other postulated mechanisms.[15]

Patients with diabetic ketoacidosis (DKA) are usually hyperphosphatemic on initial presentation, although their total body phosphate level is depleted due to urinary losses.[10] After treatment with fluids and insulin, phosphate falls due to transcellular shifts and continuing urinary losses. Although the benefit of phosphate repletion in DKA remains controversial,[24] phosphate administration is recommended if hypophosphatemia is moderate (less than 1.5 to 2.0) or severe (less than 1.0 mg/dL).[23]

Unless hypophosphatemia is severe, most patients remain asymptomatic. With severe hypophosphatemia, which is associated with chronic total body phosphate depletion, there may be clinical effects on neurologic, pulmonary, and cardiac function.

TABLE 175.5. Causes of Hyperphosphatemia

ENDOGENOUS
Renal failure
Hypoparathyroidism
Excess growth hormone
Tumor lysis syndrome
Rhabdomyolysis
EXOGENOUS
Phosphate enemas
Phosphate laxatives
Overtreatment of hypophosphatemia

TABLE 175.6. Causes of Hypophosphatemia

DECREASED INTAKE OR ABSORPTION
Decreased dietary phosphate intake
Diarrhea, malabsorption
Vitamin D deficiency
Phosphate-binding antacid therapy for renal failure
INCREASED LOSS
Hyperparathyroidism
Renal tubular defects
Prolonged diuresis
TRANSCELLULAR MOVEMENT
Insulin administration
Respiratory alkalosis
Alcohol withdrawal
Treatment of diabetic ketoacidosis

Patients may present with paresthesias, weakness, dysarthria, depressed reflexes, or altered mental status.[15] Severe hypophosphatemia affects diaphragmatic contractility[2] and can therefore contribute to respiratory failure. Cardiomyopathy has been described in severely hypophosphatemic patients,[14] as have rhabdomyolysis and hemolytic anemia.

EMERGENCY DEPARTMENT MANAGEMENT AND DISPOSITION

Mild-to-moderate hypophosphatemia is asymptomatic and can be corrected with 1 to 3 g of phosphate supplementation daily.[15] Oral preparations such as skim milk, Neutra-Phos, or Phospho-Soda can be used. Severe or symptomatic hypophosphatemia is rarely encountered in ED patients; if it is, intravenous phosphate salts are required.[12] In these rare severe cases, therapy can be begun with 0.5 to 1.0 mL/h of K_2PO_4 for the average 70-kg patient, where 1 mL of K_2PO_4 contains 4.4 mEq K^+ and 3 mmol (93 mg) PO_4^-. A simple way to administer this is to put 2 cc K_2PO_4 in 1: of fluid and run it at 250 cc/h.

The rare patient with severe symptomatic hypophosphatemia needs intensive care monitoring.

COMMON PITFALL

The administration of intravenous phosphate is rarely required. Its use may be associated with hypocalcemia and tissue deposition of phosphate salts, and thus is strongly discouraged.

References

1. Agus ZS, Wasserstein A, Goldfarb S. Disorders of calcium and magnesium homeostasis. *Am J Med* 1982;72:473.
2. Aubier M, Murgiano D, Lecocguic Y, et al. Effect of hypophosphatemia on diaphragmatic contractility in patients with acute respiratory failure. *N Engl J Med* 1985;313:420.
3. Baxter GF, et al. Infarct size and magnesium: insights into LIMIT 2 and ISIS-4 from experimental studies. *Lancet* 1996;348:1424.
4. Belezikian JP. Management of acute hypercalcemia. *N Engl J Med* 1992; 326:1196.
5. Cardella CJ, Birkin BL, Rapoport A. Role of dialysis in the treatment of severe hypercalcemia: report of two cases successfully treated with hemodialysis and review of the literature. *Clin Nephrol* 1979;12:285.
6. Chernow B, Smith J, Rainy TG. Hypomagnesemia: implications for the critical care specialist. *Crit Care Med* 1982;10:193.
7. DeCristofaro JD, Tsang RC. Calcium. *Emerg Med Clin North Am* 1986;4:207.
8. Fassler CA, Rodriguez RM, Badesch DB, et al. Magnesium toxicity as a cause of hypotension and hypoventilation. *Arch Intern Med* 1985;145:1604.
9. Heyburn PJ, Selby PL, Peacock M, et al. Peritoneal dialysis in the management of severe hypercalcemia. *BMJ* 1980;280:525.

10. Kebler R, McDonald FD, Cadnappaphornachai P. Dynamic changes in serum phosphorus levels in diabetic ketoacidosis. *Am J Med* 1985;79:571.
11. Krishel S, Safranek D, Clarke RF. Intravenous vitamins for alcoholics in the emergency department: a review. *J Emerg Med* 1998;16:419.
12. Lentz RD, Brown DM, Kjellstrand CM. Treatment of severe hypophosphatemia. *Ann Intern Med* 1989;89:941.
13. McCubbin JH, Sibai BM, Abdella TN, et al. Cardiopulmonary arrest due to acute maternal hypermagnesemia. *Lancet* 1981;1:1058.
14. O'Conner LR, Wheeler WS, Bethune JE. Effect of hypophosphatemia on myocardial performance in man. *N Engl J Med* 1977;297:901.
15. Peppers MP, Gehelo M, Desai T. Hypophosphatemia and hyperphosphatemia. *Crit Care Clin* 1991;7:201
16. Percival RC, Yates AJP, Gray RES, et al. Role of glucocorticoids in the management of malignant hypercalcemia. *BMJ* 1984;289:287.
17. Reinhart RA. Magnesium deficiency: recognition and treatment in the emergency medicine setting. *Am J Emerg Med* 1992;10:78.
18. Silva OL, Becker KL. Salmon calcitonin in the treatment of hypercalcemia. *Arch Intern Med* 1973;132:337.
19. Slatopolsky E, Rutherford WE, Rosenbaum R, et al. Hyperphosphatemia. *Clin Nephrol* 1977;7:138.
20. Suki WM, Yium JJ, Von Minden M, et al. Acute treatment of hypercalcemia with furosemide. *N Engl J Med* 1970;283:836.
21. Topol EJ, Lerman BB. Hypermagnesemia and torsades de pointes. *Am J Cardiol* 1983;52:1367.
22. Whang R, Osei TO, Aikawa JF, et al. Predictors of clinical hypomagnesemia. *Arch Intern Med* 1974;144:1794.
23. Wilson JJ, Keuer SP, Lea AS, et al. Phosphate therapy in diabetic ketoacidosis. *Arch Intern Med* 1982;142:1114.
24. Zaloga GP, Chernow B. Hypocalcemia in critical illness. *JAMA* 1986;256:1924.
25. Zwanger ML. Hypermagnesemia and perforated viscus. *Ann Emerg Med* 1986;15:1219.

CHAPTER 176
Azotemia and Acute Renal Failure

Todd C. Rothenhaus and Samuel A. McLean

Normal kidney function depends on adequate renal perfusion, efficient filtration of plasma at the glomeruli, nearly complete reabsorption of filtered solutes by the renal tubules, and the unhampered passage of formed urine from the body. In addition to the elimination of wastes, the kidney is also involved in maintaining volume status and electrolyte balance.

Acute renal failure (ARF), defined as a recent (over hours to days) decline in renal function, accounts for about 1% of patients admitted to the hospital.[21] The hallmark of ARF is azotemia, in which nitrogenous wastes such as creatinine and urea accumulate in the blood. A decrease in urine output may or may not accompany ARF. Because about 400 to 600 mOsmol of solute is created by the body every 24 hours, and because maximum urine osmolality is approximately 1200 mOsmol/L, urine output must be at least 300 to 500 mL/d to maintain adequate solute clearance from the body. Oliguria is thus defined as urine output less than 400 mL/d, and anuria as urine output less than 100 mL/d.

Renal function is most often measured by determining the clearance of creatinine (C_{cr}), a clinical estimate of the glomerular filtration rate (GFR). Creatinine is released continuously from skeletal muscle as a by-product of the metabolism of creatine, and is completely filtered at the glomerulus. Thus, blood creatinine concentration is proportional to muscle mass and inversely proportional to GFR.[13] The Cockroft-Gault formula provides an estimate of creatinine clearance from a single measurement of serum creatinine (S_{cr})[4]:

$$C_{cr}\,(\text{mL/min}) = (140 - \text{age})\,(\text{lean body weight in kg})/72 \times S_{cr}\,(\text{mg/dL})$$

The result is multiplied by 0.85 in women, to correct for approximately 15% less muscle mass in proportion to body weight. These calculated results are only accurate in the steady state. For example, sudden bilateral ureteral obstruction would cause true GFR to fall to 0, but GFR calculated from the previous equation would only slowly decline, as serum creatinine increased at the rate of 1 to 3 mg/dL per day, as expected from ongoing endogenous production.

ARF can lead to life-threatening complications such as pulmonary edema, hyperkalemia, acidemia, severe hypertension, and uremic pericarditis with effusion and tamponade. The goal of the emergency physician is to recognize these complications and to halt any further decline in renal function by correcting any reversible underlying cause.

CLINICAL PRESENTATION

No presenting symptom or sign is pathognomonic of ARF, which most often occurs in the setting of other illness.[19] Patients may present in critical condition, or asymptomatic azotemia may be discovered on routine blood screening. Most symptoms, such as fatigue, weakness, shortness of breath, or peripheral edema, are nonspecific. The diagnosis is thus established only after laboratory studies are performed. Patients rarely present because of oliguria unless it is accompanied by pain from obstruction. However, bladder outlet obstruction may be suggested by complaints of urinary frequency, incontinence, and urgency. Volume overload eventually becomes apparent in oliguric patients, but the severity of symptoms depends significantly on the patient's prior cardiovascular status.

It may be difficult to distinguish clinically between acute and recently identified chronic renal failure. A careful history, as well as laboratory evaluation, can often help.[7] Patients with chronic renal failure generally have anemia, hypocalcemia, and hyperphosphatemia, as well as small kidneys and increased parenchymal echogenicity on ultrasound examination.[3]

Uremia refers to the clinical syndrome resulting from the adverse effects of renal failure on other organ systems. These include the cardiovascular (pericarditis with or without effusion), nervous (somnolence, coma, seizures), gastrointestinal (nausea, vomiting, ileus), hematologic (anemia, coagulopathy, platelet dysfunction), and immunologic (impaired defenses and response to infection) systems.[12,19] Only a minority of patients with ARF present with full-blown uremia.

DIFFERENTIAL DIAGNOSIS

ARF is classically divided into three broad etiologic categories (Table 176.1): prerenal failure (inadequate renal perfusion), intrinsic renal failure (disorders of the renal parenchyma), and postrenal failure (obstructive uropathy). Prerenal failure is most common in both adults and children, followed by acute tubular necrosis (ATN) in adults[19] and the hemolytic uremic syndrome (HUS) in children.[8,16] Other causes of ARF are less frequently seen.

Prerenal failure (azotemia) is characterized by decreased renal perfusion with intact tubular function. Hypoperfusion stimulates tubular reabsorption of sodium and free water and leads to the formation of concentrated urine, with a urinary sodium often less than 20 mEq/L.[12] Because the kidneys are essentially

TABLE 176.1. Common Causes of Acute Renal Insufficiency

PRERENAL AZOTEMIA (DECREASED RENAL PERFUSION)
Hypovolemia
Hemorrhage
Excessive diuresis
Vomiting or diarrhea
Heat losses
Burns
Decreased cardiac output
Myocardial diseases
Pulmonary hypertension
Altered systemic vascular resistance
Sepsis
Cirrhosis
General anesthesia
Impaired renal autoregulation
NSAIDs
Angiotensin converting enzyme inhibitors
INTRINSIC RENAL INSUFFICIENCY
Acute tubular necrosis
Ischemic injury secondary to shock, hemorrhage
Aminoglycosides
Intravenous contrast agents
Pigment nephropathy secondary to trauma
Acute interstitial nephritis
Drugs
Infections
Acute glomerulonephritis
Vascular disease
Malignant hypertension
Vascular occlusion
POSTRENAL OCCLUSION
Urethral obstruction
Prostatic hypertrophy or carcinoma
Cervical carcinoma
Urethral stricture
Ureteral obstruction
Blood clots
Intraabdominal tumor
Bilateral calculi
Retroperitoneal fibrosis
Retroperitoneal malignancy
Neurogenic bladder

normal, microscopic urinalysis is usually unremarkable.[19] Prerenal azotemia is seen in conditions of hypovolemia, decreased cardiac output, and altered systemic or intrarenal vascular resistance. Nonsteroidal antiinflammatory drugs (NSAIDs) and angiotensin converting enzyme (ACE) inhibitors are increasingly common causes of prerenal azotemia, especially in the elderly, who are predisposed to this condition by decreased renal function and a high incidence of coexisting disease.[18] If the underlying hemodynamic disorder can be corrected, prerenal failure is, by definition, reversible.

Intrinsic renal failure may be divided into disorders affecting the glomeruli (e.g., acute glomerulonephritis), the renal interstitium (e.g., acute interstitial nephritis [AIN]), the renal vasculature (e.g., malignant hypertension), or the tubules (e.g., ATN).[19]

ATN accounts for up to 85% of intrinsic renal failure in adults.[19] It is frequently self-limited and often reversible. Etiologies include ischemic insults to the kidney (e.g., shock, hemorrhage), administration of drugs (e.g., aminoglycosides, intravenous contrast agents), and pigment nephropathy (e.g., myoglobinuria occurring secondary to limb ischemia, cocaine use, hyperthermia, or crush injuries). In ATN, the tubules lose the ability to concentrate urine and to reabsorb sodium. The urine tends to have a specific gravity similar to that of serum (1.010), and the urinary sodium concentration tends to be greater than 40 mEq/L.[19] On microscopic urinalysis, granular casts and tubular epithelial cells are noted in about 80% of patients.[12] ATN may be either oliguric or nonoliguric, the nonoliguric variety having a better prognosis.[19]

AIN accounts for about 10% of intrinsic renal failure in adults.[19] It is usually caused by a drug hypersensitivity reaction, but can also be due to infection, immune-mediated disease, or other causes.[15] Many drugs have been implicated in AIN, including beta-lactam antibiotics, sulfonamide drugs, and NSAIDs.[15] Patients with AIN may present with fever, rash, arthralgias, eosinophilia, and eosinophiluria (the latter detectable by Hansel's stain of the urine). However, these findings are frequently absent, making differentiation of AIN from other causes of ARF difficult.[15]

Postrenal azotemia results from obstruction of the renal collecting system at the level of the ureters, bladder, or urethra. For renal failure to develop, ureteral obstruction must be bilateral (except in patients with a single functioning kidney). Among the common causes of obstruction are prostatic hypertrophy or carcinoma, cervical carcinoma, neurogenic bladder, and urethral stricture. Ureteral obstruction may also occur as a result of blood clots, tumors, calculi, retroperitoneal fibrosis, or malignancy.[10] It is important to note that patients with obstructive, postrenal failure may present with anuria, oliguria, or normal urinary output. Because the renal parenchyma is unaffected, microscopic urinalysis may reveal hematuria but is otherwise essentially normal.

EMERGENCY DEPARTMENT EVALUATION

The emergency department (ED) evaluation of the patient with ARF requires a two-step approach. The physician should immediately determine whether life-threatening complications exist, and then attempt to determine the cause of ARF so that potentially reversible causes can be corrected.

A detailed history should be obtained, including recent exposure to new medications (especially diuretics, NSAIDs, and ACE inhibitors), intravenous contrast material, chemicals, animal venoms, unusual plants or foods, or illicit drugs.[2,19] A history of recent hospitalization, surgery, or other intercurrent illness that might be associated with renal hypoperfusion (e.g., cirrhosis, aortic or vascular disease, or congestive heart failure) should also be sought. A history of malignancy is especially important, as these patients are at risk of ARF from obstruction, radiation nephritis, or chemotherapy. Urinary retention in such patients, especially in conjunction with back pain or neurologic symptoms, should prompt immediate evaluation for spinal cord compression. Bone pain in the elderly should suggest multiple myeloma. Recent onset of paroxysmal nocturnal dyspnea or orthopnea may suggest volume overload.

Physical examination should begin with an assessment of volume status. Hypertension, rales, peripheral edema, or jugular venous distention suggests fluid overload. Resting tachycardia, orthostatic hypotension, dry mucous membranes, or poor skin turgor points to hypovolemia. Signs of uremia should be sought, including asterixis, alteration in mental status, and pericardial friction rub. Skin examination may reveal generalized rash in AIN, livedo reticularis in atheroembolic renal failure, or palpable purpura with vasculitis.

Laboratory analysis should include a complete blood count, electrolytes, glucose, calcium, phosphorus, blood urea nitrogen (BUN), and creatinine. The urine should be sent for microscopic analysis, specific gravity, osmolality, and sodium and creatinine concentrations. Urine specific gravity, rapidly available in the ED, is a reasonable estimate of urine osmolarity, except when solutes such as glucose or radiocontrast media are present. Anemia and thrombocytopenia may suggest thrombotic thrombocytopenic purpura (TTP) or HUS. A pregnancy test should be done in women of childbearing age because of the unusual but important causes of ARF that are associated with pregnancy, including preeclampsia and septic abortion,[14] and because radiography may be used during the workup. A chest x-ray aids in the determination of volume status. An electrocardiogram (ECG) should be performed to evaluate for hyperkalemia. An arterial blood gas (ABG) analysis may be helpful, especially if acidosis, reflected in a low serum bicarbonate, is severe.

After ruling out immediately life-threatening complications, the patient should be evaluated for evidence of urinary tract obstruction. A prostate examination in men and a pelvic examination in women are mandatory. Percussion of the suprapubic area, or bedside ED ultrasonography, may reveal an enlarged bladder. Costovertebral angle tenderness may suggest ureteral obstruction. A Foley catheter should be passed to exclude bladder outlet obstruction and to monitor urine output, even in patients without oliguria.

If bladder catheterization does not reveal evidence of distal obstruction and another etiology for ARF is not readily apparent, attention must be directed at ruling out bilateral ureteral obstruction. Renal ultrasound can detect hydronephrosis with a sensitivity of 98% to 99% and a specificity of 75% to 80%.[5] Despite this high sensitivity, nondilated obstructive uropathy can occur early after obstruction, in cases due to malignancy or retroperitoneal fibrosis and in patients who are severely dehydrated.[12] Noncontrast computed tomography (CT) of the renal collecting system may be helpful if ultrasonography is inconclusive or if the etiology of the obstruction is unclear.[5]

The gold standard for diagnosing obstruction is retrograde pyelography, which avoids contrast-induced nephrotoxicity but requires urologic consultation. Intravenous pyelography (IVP) is contraindicated because of the real risk of nephrotoxicity due to contrast agent.[3]

If obstruction is not the cause of ARF, urinary electrolytes should be evaluated to determine whether renal failure is prerenal or renal.[7] As previously noted, urinary sodium is frequently less than 20 mEq/L in prerenal azotemia,[12] while, in intrinsic renal failure, tubular reabsorption of sodium is compromised and the urinary sodium concentration often exceeds 40 mEq/L.[19] In addition, in prerenal failure, enhanced sodium and water reabsorption results in increased passive reabsorption of urea, elevating the BUN out of proportion to the serum creatinine. Hence, a BUN/creatinine ratio greater than 20:1 suggests prerenal azotemia. The most accurate index for differentiating between prerenal and renal failure is the fractional excretion of sodium (FE_{Na}),[7] which measures the percentage of sodium presented to the renal tubules that is not reabsorbed:

$$FE_{Na} = [U_{Na}/P_{Na}]/[U_{cr}/P_{cr}]$$

In prerenal azotemia, the FE_{Na} is usually much less than 1%, whereas in ATN or AIN, it is elevated, often to above 3%. Urinary sodium and FE_{Na} are increased in patients who have received diuretics.

Microscopic urinalysis provides further information.[19] In prerenal azotemia, the urinalysis is unremarkable; occasional hyaline casts may be all that is noted. With intrinsic renal causes of ARF, one can expect to see a more "active" sediment. In ATN, the urine contains granular casts and tubular epithelial cells, individually or in casts.[12] In AIN, there is often eosinophiluria and white cell casts. Patients with acute glomerulonephritis often have dysmorphic red cells and red cell casts.[19] Table 176.2 lists laboratory features useful in distinguishing between prerenal azotemia and ATN.

EMERGENCY DEPARTMENT MANAGEMENT

Volume overload and hyperkalemia are the most common causes of early death in ARF patients. Fluid overload is best avoided by accurate initial assessment of volume status, judicious administration of fluids, and constant reassessment of oliguric or anuric patients. Patients who present in pulmonary edema benefit from traditional therapy (i.e., oxygen, morphine, and diuretics, with particular attention paid to the use of nitrates to reduce preload) until hemodialysis is available.[9]

Hyperkalemia is a life-threatening emergency that may become manifest abruptly in ARF, particularly in patients whose renal failure is due to rhabdomyolysis. The management of this entity is discussed in Chapter 179.

Hypertension requiring immediate treatment may be managed with intravenous nitrates or sodium nitroprusside.[11] The latter agent should be used for only relatively brief periods in patients with renal failure due to the risk of thiocyanate toxicity. Adjuvant oral medications with a relatively rapid onset of action include labetalols, β blockers, α_2 agonists, and calcium channel blockers.[11]

Once potentially life-threatening complications of renal failure have been addressed, the next priority is to identify the cause of renal dysfunction and to reverse it, if possible. If the etiology appears to be postrenal, prompt relief of the obstruction can prevent further renal injury. Bladder outlet obstruction is almost always relieved by passage of a Foley catheter. Clamping the Foley catheter when large volumes of urine are released from the bladder, once a common practice, is unnecessary, even if the patient develops gross hematuria.[10] If obstruction persists after bladder catheterization, or if a Foley catheter cannot be placed, urologic imaging and consultation are indicated.

If the cause of renal insufficiency appears to be prerenal, intravascular volume should be replenished with intravenous crystalloid or blood. If prerenal azotemia occurs in the face of normal or increased total body sodium (e.g., congestive heart failure), efforts must be made to correct the underlying disorder to improve renal perfusion. Invasive monitoring may be necessary to monitor volume status.

The efficacy of diuretics and dopamine in oliguric patients with ARF is the subject of controversy.[6,12,17,19,21] There are no

TABLE 176.2. Distinguishing between Prerenal Azotemia and Acute Tubular Necrosis

	Prerenal Azotemia	Acute Tubular Necrosis
BUN/creatinine ratio	>20:1	<20:1
Urinary sodium	<20 mEq/L	>40 mEq/L
Urinary osmolarity	>500	<350
Urine specific gravity	>1.020	<1.010
FE_{Na}	<1%	>2%
Urinalysis	Normal sediment or hyaline casts	Granular casts, tubular epithelial cells

data to support the routine use of dopamine (which can cause tachyarrhythmias, cardiac ischemia, and digital and gut necrosis) in patients with adequate cardiac output.[6,17,19–21] Similarly, there is no evidence that diuretics decrease morbidity, mortality, or progression to end-stage renal disease in patients with ARF.[17,19,21] Moreover, the routine use of diuretics in the initial care of ARF patients poses a number of risks. Administering a diuretic to a patient who is already volume contracted may precipitate ischemic ATN, and administering a diuretic to a patient with obstructive uropathy might increase hydrostatic damage to the kidneys. Administering mannitol to an anuric patient can cause intravascular volume expansion and pulmonary edema. For patients with myoglobinuric renal failure, however, mannitol is recommended, in combination with volume replacement and sodium bicarbonate.[1]

A number of life-threatening emergencies associated with ARF may require emergent dialysis. Nevertheless, treatments or temporizing measures are available for each and should be instituted while arrangements are made for dialysis or transfer. The indications for acute dialysis can be remembered using the mnemonic AEIOU: severe *a*cidosis, *e*lectrolyte abnormalities (especially hyperkalemia and hyponatremia), *i*ngestions (ethylene glycol, methanol, lithium, theophylline, salicylate, and others), volume *o*verload, and *u*remia. Central venous access with a large-bore catheter is required for hemodialysis, and percutaneous peritoneal access must be secured for peritoneal dialysis. Should emergent dialysis be necessary, direct consultation with a nephrologist is essential to coordinate timely intervention.

DISPOSITION

Although the initial evaluation and management of the patient with ARF can generally be performed in the ED, the patient with ARF is best managed in the hospital. If the etiology is clearly postrenal, consultation with a urologist is mandatory, as emergent surgical decompression may be indicated. For metabolic or uremic complications of renal failure, whether acute or chronic, nephrology consultation in the ED is prudent.

Most patients presenting to the ED with ARF should be admitted to the hospital for further evaluation. A possible exception is the patient with prerenal azotemia secondary to an easily correctable cause such as diarrhea or diuretic therapy. Such a patient can sometimes be discharged with close follow-up if fluid resuscitation is carried out in the ED and urine output is reestablished. Nonazotemic patients with acute urinary outflow tract obstruction corrected by bladder catheterization can, in many cases, also be discharged with an indwelling catheter. In this case, urine should be cultured and close urologic follow-up arranged.

Transfer to a tertiary care facility should be considered for any patient with renal failure if dialysis is not available at the primary facility. Because potentially life-threatening complications of renal failure can develop rapidly, the emergency physician should not wait until complications appear before arranging for transfer. In rare cases, the patient must be transferred to an out-of-hospital dialysis unit. In these cases, the ED physician must ensure that the accepting physician will be immediately available upon the patient's arrival. All available and appropriate modalities should be instituted before transfer, and the patient should be transported by an advanced life-support unit.

COMMON PITFALLS

- Failing to recognize and initiate therapy for life-threatening complications before continuing with any workup. An ECG should always be checked if hyperkalemia is possible.
- Failing to assess volume status adequately. Fluid replacement may be all that is necessary in order to reverse prerenal insufficiency.
- Forgetting the simple things: a prostate examination in men and a pelvic examination in women, and insertion of a Foley catheter to rule out bladder outlet obstruction, which can occur even in the patient who is voiding.
- Failing to appreciate that the serum creatinine is not an accurate measure of renal function in the ARF patient.
- Giving diuretics to the hypovolemic oliguric patient, which only further increases volume contraction, potentially worsening renal perfusion.
- Delaying appropriate transfer to a center where dialysis can be performed, even though most life-threatening uremic complications can be treated before emergency dialysis is initiated.

ACKNOWLEDGMENT

The authors gratefully acknowledge the work of Dr. Robert Rosenthal, who contributed significantly to this chapter in previous editions.

References

1. Abassi ZA, Hoffman A, Better OS. Acute renal failure complicating muscle crush injury. *Semin Nephrol* 1998;18(5):558.
2. Abuelo JG. Renal failure caused by chemicals, foods, plants, animal venoms, and misuse of drugs: an overview. *Arch Intern Med* 1990;150:505.
3. Brown DF, Rosen CL, Wolfe RE. Renal ultrasonography. *Emerg Med Clin North Am* 1997;15(4):877.
4. Cockcroft DW, Gault MH. Prediction of creatinine clearance from serum creatinine. *Nephron* 1976;16:31.
5. Cronan JJ. Contemporary concepts in imaging urinary tract obstruction. *Radiol Clin North Am* 1991;29:527.
6. Denton MD, Chertow GM, Brady HR. "Renal-dose" dopamine for the treatment of acute renal failure: scientific rationale, experimental studies and clinical trials. *Kidney Int* 1996;50:4.
7. Espinel CH. Diagnosis of acute and chronic renal disease. *Clin Lab Med* 1993;13(1):89.
8. Flynn JT. Causes, management approaches, and outcome of acute renal failure in children. *Curr Opin Pediatr* 1998;10(2):184.
9. Gehm L, Propp DA. Pulmonary edema in the renal failure patient. *Am J Emerg Med* 1989;7:336.
10. Gulmi FA, Felsen D. Management of post-obstructive diuresis. *AUA Update Series* 1998, Volume XVII, Lesson 23.
11. Joint National Committee on Detection, Evaluation, and Treatment of High Blood Pressure. The sixth report of the Joint National Committee on Detection, Evaluation, and Treatment of High Blood Pressure. *Arch Intern Med* 1997;157:2413.
12. Klahr S, Miller SB. Acute oliguria. *N Engl J Med* 1998;338:671.
13. Levey AS, Bosch JP, Lewis JB, et al. A more accurate method to estimate glomerular filtration rate from serum creatinine: a new prediction equation. *Ann Intern Med* 1999;130:461.
14. Maikranz P, Katz AI. Acute renal failure in pregnancy. *Obstet Gynecol Clin North Am* 1991;18(2):333.
15. Michel DM, Kelly CJ. Acute interstitial nephritis. *J Am Soc Nephrol* 1998;9(3):506–515.
16. Moghal NE, Brocklebank JT, Meadow SR. A review of acute renal failure in children: incidence, etiology and outcome. *Clin Nephrol* 1998;49(2):91.
17. Paller MS. Acute renal failure: controversies, clinical trials, and future directions. *Semin Nephrol* 1998;18(5):482.
18. Pascual J, Liano F, Ortuno J. The elderly patient with acute renal failure. *J Am Soc Nephrol* 1995;6:144.
19. Thadani R, Pascual M, Bonventre JV. Acute renal failure. *N Engl J Med* 1996;334:1448.
20. Thompson BT, Cockrill BA. Renal-dose dopamine: a siren song? *Lancet* 1994;344:7.
21. Vijayan A, Miller SB. Acute renal failure: prevention and nondialytic therapy. *Semin Nephrol* 1998;18(5):523.

CHAPTER 177
Chronic Renal Failure and Dialysis-Related Emergencies

Allan B. Wolfson

Patients with *acute* renal failure have, by definition, a relatively rapid loss of renal function and tend to develop clinical manifestations requiring prompt attention. In contrast, patients with *chronic* renal disease have usually experienced a slow decrease in renal function over a period of months to years; they commonly present to the emergency department with subacute or chronic symptoms, often of a progressive nature, or with acute problems due to a superimposed illness or stress.

Chronic renal failure is characterized by irreversible nephron loss and scarring. *Chronic renal insufficiency* is a condition in which renal function has been reduced to a moderate degree but not enough to cause clinical symptoms; in general, the glomerular filtration rate (GFR) has been reduced by no more than 75%. *End-stage renal disease* (ESRD) denotes a chronic condition in which the GFR is decreased to a very low level and in which clinical symptoms begin to be prominent. Serious, life-threatening manifestations can be expected to develop in the absence of dialysis treatments or renal transplantation.

The causes of chronic renal failure are numerous; as with acute renal failure, they can be classified as prerenal (vascular), intrinsic renal (glomerular and tubulointerstitial), and postrenal (obstructive) (Table 177.1). About one-third to one-half of ESRD is due to glomerular disease, with diabetic nephropathy accounting for the largest single group. Hypertensive nephrosclerosis is another major cause, particularly among Blacks. The history, physical examination, and laboratory and imaging studies may provide clues to other specific etiologies. Although determining the exact etiology of chronic renal failure allows the underlying cause to be treated in some cases, this is the exception rather than the rule.

Progressive loss of renal function eventually results in a syndrome termed *uremia*. Clinical manifestations are not usually evident unless the GFR has decreased to approximately 25% of normal, despite the fact that laboratory abnormalities may be impressive, because the remaining functioning nephrons are able to compensate reasonably well for those that have been lost. Beyond a certain point, however, significant amounts of metabolic by-products are retained. These poorly defined substances appear to be responsible for many of the clinical manifestations of uremia.

Uremia is associated with derangements in homeostasis and metabolism and results in specific defects in multiple organ systems (Table 177.2). Many of these manifestations are corrected or relieved by dialysis, but others are not. All tend to develop gradually in patients with chronic renal failure, although some result in dysfunction that may present acutely.

APPROACH TO THE PATIENT

Patients with chronic renal failure, particularly if they are not yet on dialysis, most commonly present to the emergency department with nonspecific complaints such as generalized weakness, poor appetite, or increasing confusion. These symptoms are typically of insidious onset. The first clue to the diagnosis may be a laboratory finding of a reasonably well tolerated but rather severe anemia. Elevated blood urea nitrogen and serum creatinine levels can then confirm the diagnosis.

Once it has been ascertained that the patient is in no immediate danger (e.g., from life-threatening hyperkalemia), the next step is to establish that renal failure is indeed chronic rather than acute. A well-documented history of chronic renal disease, either from medical records or from the patient or family, may provide the most reliable confirmation, but one should consider the possibility of a previously overlooked correctable cause. A finding of bilaterally small kidneys on plain radiography or ultrasonography is good evidence for chronic renal disease, although normal-sized or large kidneys do not rule out chronic renal failure. Ascertaining history of familial kidney disease, such as polycystic kidney disease or Alport syndrome, may also be helpful.

Laboratory abnormalities such as anemia, acidosis, hyperkalemia, hypocalcemia, and hyperphosphatemia can occur with *acute* renal failure as early as 10 days after its onset, but they tend to be better tolerated in patients with chronic renal disease. Findings on urinalysis are usually not helpful. Attention must be directed toward potentially reversible factors (e.g., volume depletion or obstruction), as they may represent the only opportunity to reverse the patient's disease rather than simply to manage its effects (Table 177.3).

TABLE 177.1. Major Causes of Chronic Renal Failure

VASCULAR
Renal arterial disease
Hypertensive nephrosclerosis
GLOMERULAR
Primary Glomerulopathies
Focal sclerosing glomerulonephritis
Membranoproliferative glomerulonephritis
Membranous glomerulonephritis
Crescentic glomerulonephritis
IgA nephropathy
Secondary Glomerulopathies
Diabetic nephropathy
Collagen vascular disease
Amyloidosis
Postinfectious
Heroin nephropathy
TUBULOINTERSTITIAL
Nephrotoxins
Analgesic nephropathy
Hypercalcemia/nephrocalcinosis
Multiple myeloma
Sickle nephropathy
Reflux nephropathy
Chronic pyelonephritis
Tuberculosis
OBSTRUCTIVE
Nephrolithiasis
Ureteral tuberculosis
Retroperitoneal fibrosis
Retroperitoneal tumor
Prostatic obstruction
Congenital
HEREDITARY
Polycystic kidney disease
Alport syndrome
Medullary cystic disease

TABLE 177.2. Major Manifestations of Uremia

DERANGEMENTS OF HOMEOSTASIS
Sodium balance
Water balance
Hyperkalemia
Metabolic acidosis
Hypercalcemia
Hyperphosphatemia
Hypermagnesemia
DERANGEMENTS OF METABOLISM
Azotemia
Decreased glucose tolerance
Hyperlipidemia
SPECIFIC ORGAN SYSTEM EFFECTS
Cardiovascular
Hypertension, volume overload, pericarditis
Pulmonary
Pulmonary edema, pleuritis
Neurologic
Lethargy, difficulty concentrating, altered mental status, seizures, myoclonic twitching, asterixis, hiccups, cramps, peripheral neuropathy
Gastrointestinal
Anorexia, nausea, vomiting, gastrointestinal ulceration, pancreatitis
Musculoskeletal
Secondary hyperparathyroidism, renal osteodystrophy, crystal-induced arthritis, myopathy, spontaneous tendon rupture, carpal tunnel syndrome
Hematologic
Anemia, altered immunity, qualitative platelet abnormality

DIALYSIS

Patients with ESRD are often sustained on chronic hemodialysis or chronic ambulatory peritoneal dialysis (CAPD). Although usually seen regularly by their nephrologists and nurse specialists, they continue to be relatively frequent visitors to emergency departments, being subject to those complications of chronic renal failure that are not corrected by dialysis, to the manifestations of underlying systemic diseases, and to complications of the dialytic therapy itself.[7,18–20]

TABLE 177.3. Reversible Factors and Treatable Causes of Chronic Renal Failure

REVERSIBLE FACTORS
Hypovolemia
Congestive heart failure
Pericardial tamponade
Severe hypertension
Catabolic state/protein loads
Nephrotoxic agents
Obstructive disease
Reflux disease
TREATABLE CAUSES
Renal artery stenosis
Malignant hypertension
Acute interstitial nephritis
Hypercalcemic nephropathy
Multiple myeloma
Vasculitis (e.g., systemic lupus erythematosus, Wegener granulomatosis, periarteritis nodosa)
Obstructive nephropathy
Reflux nephropathy

Compared with other patients, dialysis patients are less able to tolerate the stresses of intercurrent illness or trauma. Moreover, there is a significant potential for iatrogenic illness due to inappropriate fluid or drug administration. Even apparently innocuous agents, such as antacids and enemas, can cause serious problems. Physicians caring for patients with ESRD should thus have ready access to a reference compendium containing guidelines for the adjustment of drug dosages in renal failure.[2]

A number of serious problems are commonly encountered both in dialysis patients and in those with chronic renal failure who have not yet undergone dialytic therapy. The approach is similar in the two patient groups. The two major dialysis modalities, hemodialysis and CAPD, are themselves associated with specific complications with which the emergency physician should be familiar.

Hemodialysis

In hemodialysis, the patient's heparinized blood passes through an extracorporeal dialyzer circuit in which it is in contact with an artificial dialysis membrane. Water and solutes from the blood diffuse across this membrane to normalize blood volume and correct metabolic abnormalities. The amount of fluid transferred depends on the pressure under which blood is pumped through the dialyzer. Hemodialysis is usually performed several times a week for 3 to 5 hours per treatment. The high blood-flow rates that are necessary to make this an efficient process necessitate special access to the patient's circulation, generally through a surgically created arteriovenous fistula or through an artificial vascular graft, both of which are usually placed in the arm.

The vascular access device must be treated with care to avoid causing thrombosis or bleeding or introducing infection. The blood pressure should never be taken in the involved arm, and a tourniquet should never be applied. Unless absolutely essential, one should avoid drawing blood from the access or placing an intravenous line in it. However, if no other site is available and it is essential to obtain blood samples (e.g., if blood is needed immediately for crossmatch in a patient with serious bleeding), the fistula or graft can be used. Careful skin cleansing and sterile technique are mandatory, and firm but nonocclusive pressure should be applied to the site for 10 minutes after the puncture. The presence of a thrill both before and after the procedure should be documented.

Likewise, if intravenous access is critical but otherwise impossible, an intravenous line may be placed in the access, but with similar infection precautions and continuous observation during the infusion. Special care should be taken not to puncture the back wall of the access. An automated infusion pump is necessary to control the infusion rate, particularly when using the relatively high-pressure vessels in artificial arteriovenous grafts. With the low pressure typical of mature dilated fistulas, an infusion pump is still advisable.

Hemodialysis patients may present to the emergency department with a variety of complaints relating to the vascular access. Hemorrhage from a recent puncture site is usually easily managed with continuous, firm, but nonocclusive pressure over the site. Thrombosis, signaled by the loss of the thrill in the access, requires immediate consultation with a vascular surgeon, who may elect to perform a radiocontrast fistulogram, to infuse a thrombolytic agent, or to revise the access surgically. Forceful irrigation attempts are inadvisable.

The most common access-related problem is access infection, which is a serious concern in these patients because of the associated risk of bacteremia and metastatic infection, as well as the risk that the access may have to be removed because of persistent infection or impaired function. Infection is more likely to occur in an artificial graft than in a native fistula.

Most access infections are staphylococcal; contamination with skin flora at the time of puncture is believed to be the most likely cause. The diagnosis of access infection is not always obvious. When there is warmth, redness, tenderness, or local induration over the area and the patient is febrile, there is little cause for confusion, but some patients lack definite local signs and may present with repeated episodes of bacteremia or with fever and no obvious source of infection. In this situation, one should suspect access infection, draw blood cultures, and begin antibiotic therapy promptly.

A commonly used regimen is vancomycin 1 g, given intravenously as a single loading dose. Vancomycin is not hemodialyzable and needs to be given only once every 5 to 7 days, making it an attractive choice for staphylococcal coverage; in addition, its major toxicity is renal. A third-generation cephalosporin or an aminoglycoside can be added to this regimen if infection with a gram-negative organism is suspected. Local practice may vary, however, and emergency physicians should be familiar with the regimens in common use in their own institutions. Although a febrile illness may prove to be of viral etiology, it is prudent to treat such patients on the presumption of bacterial illness, because they can deteriorate rapidly and do have a high risk of access infection.

Not all febrile dialysis patients need to be admitted to the hospital. After intravenous antibiotic loading, a reliable patient who otherwise feels and looks relatively well may be sent home with careful instructions to return if there is any clinical deterioration. This decision is best reached in conjunction with the consulting nephrologist.

Peritoneal Dialysis

In CAPD, the patient's own peritoneum serves as the membrane across which diffusion of water and solutes occurs. Sterile dialysis fluid is infused into the peritoneal cavity through a surgically implanted Tenckhoff catheter; after a dwell period of 4 to 8 hours, it is exchanged for fresh fluid. Exchanges are performed by the patient at home, usually four times a day, 7 days a week, using a sterile exchange technique. Osmotic forces generated by high concentrations of glucose in the dialysis fluid ensure adequate removal of fluid volume from the blood; this is in contrast to hemodialysis, in which the amount of fluid removed is controlled by adjusting the pressure under which blood is introduced into the dialyzer coil. CAPD offers several advantages over hemodialysis: greater patient independence, smoother control of excess volume and hypertension, and avoidance of rapid solute shifts and intermittent anticoagulation.

As with hemodialysis, many of the emergency problems encountered by the patient on CAPD are related to access devices, in this case the peritoneal catheter. By far, the most common problem is peritonitis, caused by inadvertent contamination of the peritoneal cavity when exchanges are performed or by direct invasion of organisms from an infected catheter exit site. Peritonitis in these patients is, as a rule, less severe than other types of peritonitis. In fact, these infections are usually treated on an outpatient basis, despite the fact that they involve the presence of a foreign body. Occasionally, if infection cannot be eradicated with antibiotic therapy, the catheter must be removed surgically and hemodialysis initiated pending placement of a new catheter after the infection has cleared.

About two-thirds of episodes of peritonitis are due to gram-positive organisms, predominantly staphylococci. In most of the remainder, assorted gram-negative organisms are responsible; a small percentage are due to fungal infection, which is usually considered an indication for catheter removal. Polymicrobial infection suggests a communication with the bowel or genitourinary tract.

The diagnosis of peritonitis is usually based on the patient's observation of cloudiness in the dialysate effluent at the time an exchange is performed. This is generally the earliest sign of peritonitis; thus, patients are instructed to seek medical attention immediately when they notice it. Abdominal pain and fever often develop if treatment is not initiated promptly. Hospital admission becomes necessary if there is high fever, hypotension, severe abdominal pain, or nausea and vomiting, or if the patient cannot continue to carry out exchanges at home.

In the emergency department, the diagnosis of peritonitis is confirmed by the finding of organisms on Gram stain of the peritoneal fluid or of a cell count of more than 100 white blood cells/μL (predominantly neutrophils). This cell count corresponds approximately to the level at which cloudiness begins to be grossly detectable. Even in patients who have not noted cloudiness of the peritoneal effluent but who have fever, abdominal pain, or vague malaise, it is advisable to obtain a sample of fluid for examination, because the presentation of peritonitis can initially be subtle.

The fluid is obtained using meticulous sterile technique. Some is put into an open Vacutainer tube and sent for cell count and differential. The remainder, still in the syringe, should be sent to the microbiology laboratory for Gram stain and culture.

CAPD-related peritonitis can usually be treated on an outpatient basis.[8] In general, treatment decisions should be made in conjunction with the patient's nephrologist or the CAPD nurse specialist, because these individuals usually are aware of the patient's overall medical condition, the types of infection recently experienced, and any psychosocial considerations that might affect outpatient management.

A common treatment regimen is vancomycin 30 mg/kg intraperitoneally at the time of diagnosis, followed by once-weekly intraperitoneal dosing. Heparin 1000 U may be added to each bag for the first few days of treatment in an effort to decrease the risk of fibrin's obstructing the catheter. A third-generation cephalosporin or an aminoglycoside can be added to the regimen for gram-positive coverage if there is reason to suspect infection with gram-negative organisms (e.g., positive Gram stain, recent gram-negative infection). These are typically given as an intraperitoneal loading dose, followed by a once-daily intraperitoneal maintenance dose. Arrangements should be made for the patient to be seen within 2 days to make sure the infection is responding to treatment and to check culture results and adjust therapy accordingly. Again, because practice may vary in different settings, emergency physicians should be familiar with the regimens in common use in their own institutions.

Several important caveats should be noted regarding the diagnosis of peritonitis. Other acute abdominal processes, such as pancreatitis, diverticulitis, or ruptured viscus, may present with a picture similar to that expected for peritonitis, and thus may not be diagnosed if the physician's suspicion is not aroused.[16] To confuse the picture further, the finding of intraabdominal free air on radiograph may be the result of its inadvertent introduction during dialysis exchanges and does not necessarily indicate perforation.[9] (The finding of brownish or fecal material in the dialysate mandates immediate surgical consultation.)

Several other problems related to the peritoneal dialysis procedure occasionally bring the CAPD patient to the emergency department. An exit site infection or an infection of the subcutaneous catheter tunnel may present as tenderness, warmth, or induration or simply as a painless purulent exudate. Any exudate should be subjected to Gram stain and culture. Treatment can be started with an oral antibiotic active against skin flora, but intensive local cleansing and skin care are also a critical part of management. Closed infections of the subcutaneous tunnel may be difficult to appreciate, and they respond poorly to medical therapy unless they are drained. If the patient should develop a leak of dialysis fluid from the tubing, bag, or catheter, or from around the catheter, evaluation and treatment should proceed as with peritonitis. The leaking elements must be replaced, if possible, or surgical intervention arranged.

Difficulties with inflow or outflow of the dialysis fluid also occur occasionally. After ruling out straightforward problems such as kinked tubing or closed clamps, the physician must consider more troublesome mechanical causes, including obstruction of the catheter lumen, in which case, surgical or nephrologic consultation is necessary. Radiographic visualization with a contrast catheterogram may help to direct specific intervention. Fibrinolytic agents are sometimes helpful with obstructed catheters, but catheter replacement is often required.

CLINICAL PRESENTATION

Infection

Infections are a major cause of death in dialysis patients, and vascular access infection and peritonitis are the most common infections in hemodialysis patients and CAPD patients, respectively. Most infections are due to usual pathogens rather than to opportunistic organisms. The challenge for the clinician arises from the fact that classic findings may not be obvious.

Some manifestations of infections may be attributed to chronic renal failure *per se,* to the effects of dialysis, or to other underlying medical illness. For instance, pneumonia may present as dyspnea alone, which is easily attributed to volume overload or to the effects of chronic anemia. Urinary tract infection can occur even in patients who are essentially anuric[4]; upper urinary tract infection, presenting as renal colic or with symptoms typical of pyelonephritis, is most common in patients with polycystic kidney disease. These and other infections are generally treated according to the same principles that apply to other patients,[15] but antibiotic dosages must be adjusted for ESRD and the dialysis modality.

Hypotension

Hypotension commonly occurs in hemodialysis patients during or immediately after the dialysis procedure, but it usually resolves spontaneously or responds readily to fluid infusion. It is usually the result of rapid fluid and electrolyte shifts. CAPD patients are not subject to this cause of hypotension, but they, too, can become volume depleted if intake does not keep up with fluid losses that occur through dialysis. Other potentially lethal causes of hypotension must also be considered. Sepsis, drug effects, myocardial dysfunction, dysrhythmia, myocardial infarction, and pericardial tamponade are important considerations in patients treated by either dialysis modality; acute electrolyte disturbances, vascular instability, anaphylactoid reaction, and air embolism are considerations primarily in hemodialysis patients.

Pericardial tamponade may develop acutely when there is bleeding into the pericardial sac or when volume depletion allows a previously subclinical effusion to produce significant circulatory compromise. Although tamponade in this setting generally presents with the expected physical findings, coexistent cardiac or pulmonary disease may make the diagnosis difficult. Echocardiography is useful in detecting pericardial fluid; the size of an effusion does not correlate well with the presence of tamponade, however.

Many dialysis patients have effusions (of varying size) that do not appear to cause clinical difficulties. Echocardiographic demonstration of right ventricular collapse is a much better indicator of tamponade. Emergency pericardiocentesis may be necessary if the patient's condition deteriorates rapidly and tamponade is thought likely; it can establish the diagnosis and buy time until definitive surgical therapy can be undertaken. Another temporizing measure that is useful when tamponade has been precipitated by volume depletion is intravenous saline infusion to raise filling pressures.

Dyspnea and Volume Overload

Dyspnea in the dialysis patient is most commonly due to volume overload. In the hemodialysis patient, it usually develops during the interval between dialyses. Physical examination is not always reliable in detecting volume overload in these patients; even chest radiographic findings may be misleading.[10] The most reliable clue is a history of recent weight gain.

The definitive treatment of volume overload is dialysis, but several temporizing measures are available (Table 177.4).[6,13] Oxygen should be administered and the patient kept in the sitting position. Sublingual nitroglycerin can be administered quickly and does not require intravenous access; it often provides very rapid relief by reducing preload and afterload. Intravenous nitroglycerin and nitroprusside are additional useful options and can be titrated to effect; thiocyanate toxicity can result from prolonged use of nitroprusside in patients with renal failure, however.

Oral afterload reducers such as nifedipine provide a simpler option in patients who can get by without aggressive intravenous therapy.[13] Morphine can also be given, as in nondialysis patients. Intravenous furosemide produces rapid pulmonary venodilation but, of course, has a minimal diuretic effect in most dialysis patients.[14] Finally, the use of continuous positive airway pressure devices may make it possible to avoid intubation in some patients who would otherwise require it.

Although volume overload is the most likely cause of shortness of breath in the dialysis patient, dyspnea can also be the result of cardiac impairment of any cause, hypotension, infection, pleural or pericardial effusion, or any of the other causes of dyspnea in nondialysis patients.

Another potentially adverse effect of volume overload is severe hypertension, because, in most dialysis patients, blood pressure is at least partly volume dependent. For hypertensive crisis (i.e., hypertension, usually severe, with evidence of acute end-organ dysfunction), therapy should include not only sodium nitroprusside by intravenous infusion, but also prompt initiation or intensification of dialysis to lower blood volume.

Chest Pain

Chest pain in a dialysis patient should always suggest coronary artery disease. A significant proportion of dialysis patients die of

TABLE 177.4. Treatment of Pulmonary Edema in Renal Failure

Dialysis
Hemodialysis
Hemofiltration
Peritoneal dialysis
Oxygen
Nitroglycerin (sublingual or intravenous)
Nitroprusside
Nifedipine
Morphine
Loop diuretics

cardiovascular causes,[3] and most patients have risk factors such as hypertension, hyperlipidemia, and carbohydrate intolerance. Added to this are the effects of chronic anemia and intermittent or chronic volume overload. The hemodialysis procedure itself is often the occasion for additional ischemic stress to the myocardium because of transient hypoxemia and hypotension.

Initial interventions for suspected ischemic chest pain are similar to those for other patients, but particular attention should be directed toward such correctable factors as volume overload, hypertension, and anemia. The diagnosis of myocardial infarction by standard electrocardiographic and enzyme criteria is generally not affected by the abnormalities of ESRD.[11,12] Although baseline cardiac enzyme levels may be somewhat higher than in the nondialysis population, when infarction occurs, the pattern of enzyme changes is not affected. Decisions as to the most appropriate reperfusion therapy for dialysis patients with acute coronary syndromes should be made in concert with a cardiologist and the patient's nephrologist.

Chest pain may, of course, be due to any of the other commonly incriminated causes, but pericarditis should always be a consideration in the dialysis patient once myocardial ischemia has been excluded. Pericarditis (and tamponade) may occur even in well-dialyzed patients. The signs and symptoms are the same as those noted in nondialysis patients. Based on experience in undialyzed uremic patients, it has traditionally been taught that increased or intensified dialysis hastens resolution of pericarditis or prevents the development of tamponade or pericardial constriction, although this remains an open question. For many patients with pericarditis, indomethacin provides prompt relief of pain. Intrapericardial instillation of corticosteroids, or pericardial stripping, is ultimately necessary in others.

Bleeding

Bleeding is relatively common in dialysis patients; it is, at least in part, related to platelet dysfunction (which is not completely corrected by dialysis) and, in hemodialysis patients, to transient anticoagulation. It is important to ascertain what the bleeding patient's usual hemoglobin level has been. Erythropoietin is now administered routinely to almost all dialysis patients, but untreated, the baseline hemoglobin level may be 6 to 7 g/dL. Moderately severe anemia may present with increased angina or dyspnea. Other symptoms, sometimes life-threatening ones, may be caused by occult bleeding into particular anatomic sites; spontaneous intracranial, intraocular, pericardial, and retroperitoneal bleeding have been reported.

Treatment of acute bleeding episodes follows standard principles. It should also be established that dialysis has been adequate. Because correction of severe anemia (hematocrit less than 25%) improves bleeding time (probably by a rheologic effect), red cell transfusion should be considered, and additional acute treatment with desmopressin (0.3 μg/kg intravenously or subcutaneously) or conjugated estrogens (0.6 mg/kg intravenously) should be begun. For life-threatening bleeding, cryoprecipitate infusion and platelet transfusions are recommended.[5]

Neurologic Dysfunction

Neurologic dysfunction in the form of *disequilibrium syndrome* is common during and just after the hemodialysis procedure. Typical mild manifestations are headache, nausea, and muscle cramps; more severe cases may cause altered mental status and grand mal seizures. Disequilibrium is presumed to be due to the rapid fluxes of fluid and solutes that occur with dialysis: It coincides with the removal of large volumes of fluid or the correction of marked metabolic and electrolyte abnormalities with hemodialysis (it does not occur with CAPD); it usually resolves within a few hours after the treatment is completed; and symptoms often respond promptly to intravenous infusion of mannitol or hypertonic saline during dialysis.

However, because there are many other potential causes for neurologic dysfunction in these patients (not the least of which are intracranial bleeding, hypertensive encephalopathy, infection, and untoward drug effects), it is unwise to attribute any acute neurologic abnormality to the disequilibrium syndrome without carefully considering other causes. If findings are focal, appear suddenly, or fluctuate or become worse after a reasonable period of observation, attention should be directed to all of the other potential causes. Similarly, the presence of fever, papilledema, or severe hypertension should suggest more serious etiologies.

Electrolyte Abnormalities

Hyperkalemia is a common life-threatening emergency in undialyzed patients with acute or chronic renal failure, but it is seldom a serious problem in the dialyzed patient. When hyperkalemia does occur, it is usually due to noncompliance with dietary restrictions or dialysis treatments. On occasion, it may also be the result of intercurrent disorders such as rhabdomyolysis, sepsis, or severe acidosis. Hyperkalemia is particularly dangerous because it is generally completely asymptomatic until dangerous cardiac effects develop. Although many dialysis patients chronically tolerate moderate hyperkalemia (6 to 7 mEq/L) with no apparent problem, a potassium level in this range must still be considered potentially dangerous, because severe effects can develop fairly rapidly. Moreover, the electrocardiogram is occasionally completely normal even when hyperkalemia is severe,[17] and it cannot be relied on to exclude any danger of serious hyperkalemic complications developing. Thus, the serum potassium level should always be checked.

The treatment of hyperkalemia is outlined in Chapter 174. The guidelines for treatment in dialysis patients follow those for treatment in other patients, but particular attention must be directed to avoiding volume overload, symptomatic hypocalcemia, or other potential complications of therapy and to instituting or reinstituting dialysis as promptly as possible. A particularly convenient and effective method of decreasing the serum potassium level is by the administration of nebulized albuterol in a dose four to eight times as great as that used in the typical asthmatic. This intervention provides rapid and sustained improvement in the serum potassium concentration for at least several hours and appears to be associated with few side effects.[1]

A dialysis patient in cardiac arrest should be presumed to be hyperkalemic and should receive intravenous calcium and intravenous bicarbonate (through separate lines to prevent precipitation). This is one group of patients to whom these two drugs should still be administered routinely despite the recent revisions of advanced cardiac life-support guidelines.

Other electrolyte abnormalities can occur in ESRD patients under a variety of conditions, but the most important and the most common are hypocalcemia and hypermagnesemia. Hypocalcemic symptoms may occur in patients who have not been treated with vitamin D and calcium supplementation, particularly when intravenous bicarbonate is given to treat hyperkalemia or severe acidosis. Symptomatic hypocalcemia should be treated with intravenous calcium gluconate or calcium chloride.

Mild hypermagnesemia is common in ESRD, but symptoms do not usually occur until magnesium levels are high, generally over 4 mg/dL. Symptomatic hypermagnesemia is almost always due to inadvertent ingestion of magnesium-containing

TABLE 177.5. Indications for Emergency Dialysis

Pulmonary edema
Severe uncontrollable hypertension
Hyperkalemia
Other severe electrolyte or acid–base disturbances
Some overdoses
? Pericarditis

antacids or laxatives. Intravenous calcium acts as a direct antagonist to the neuromuscular effects of hypermagnesemia, but in the absence of the renal route of excretion, removal of excess magnesium from the body requires emergent dialysis.

DISPOSITION

A critical decision commonly facing the emergency physician is whether emergency dialysis is necessary for patients presenting to the emergency department with acute clinical problems. Some patients may have deteriorated between hemodialysis treatments or despite continuing CAPD; others may have failed to undergo scheduled dialyses. The most common indication for emergency dialysis (Table 177.5) is severe volume overload or pulmonary edema; available temporizing measures for managing the patient until dialysis can be effective have already been described. Appropriate temporizing measures also may be employed to manage malignant hypertension, severe electrolyte disturbances, or severe acidosis while awaiting the definitive treatment afforded by dialysis.

Uremic symptoms (e.g., lethargy, confusion, asterixis, nausea, and vomiting) indicate that dialysis is needed but are not, in themselves, indications for *emergency* dialysis. Similarly, serum creatinine and blood urea nitrogen levels correlate only roughly with uremic symptoms or life-threatening metabolic disturbances and do not, in themselves, indicate an urgent need for dialysis. The appearance of pericarditis, with or without pericardial tamponade, is often considered an indication for urgent or intensified dialysis, but pericarditis can occur even in well-dialyzed patients and it is not clear that there is an increased risk of clinical deterioration if it is not treated aggressively.

A key component of the emergency department management of all types of problems in the dialysis patient must always be consultation with the patient's nephrologist or dialysis nurse, both to take advantage of these specialists' expertise in caring for these patients' complicated problems and to ensure optimal continuity of care. However, the emergency physician has a responsibility to be familiar with the evaluation of and therapy for acute problems in dialysis patients so that emergency interventions can be performed promptly when necessary.

COMMON PITFALLS

- Failing to identify treatable factors in patients who may have a reversible component of their chronic renal insufficiency
- Causing iatrogenic illness through inappropriate fluid or drug administration
- Allowing the vascular access to be used for taking blood pressure or drawing blood, or for intravenous infusion
- Failing to consider vascular access infection in hemodialysis patients, or peritonitis in CAPD patients, because of lack of specific findings on history and physical examination
- Failing to consider the diagnosis of tamponade because the patient does not demonstrate all of the classic signs and symptoms
- Failing to treat volume overload because of a lack of specific findings
- Overlooking anemia as a cause of increased angina or shortness of breath
- Inappropriately attributing any neurologic dysfunction to disequilibrium syndrome
- Failing to seek evidence of hyperkalemia by blood test or electrocardiogram
- Inducing symptomatic hypocalcemia by ill-advised bicarbonate therapy

References

1. Allon M, Dunlay R, Copkney C. Nebulized albuterol for acute hyperkalemia in patients on hemodialysis. *Ann Intern Med* 1989;110:426.
2. Bennett WM, Aronoff GR, Golper TA, et al. *Drug prescribing in renal failure: dosing guidelines for adults*, 4th ed. Philadelphia: American College of Physicians, 1999.
3. Bleyer AJ, Russell GB, Satko SG. Sudden and cardiac death rates in hemodialysis patients. *Kidney Int* 1999;55:1553.
4. Chaudhry A, Stone WJ, Breyer JA. Occurrence of pyuria and bacteriuria in asymptomatic hemodialysis patients. *Am J Kidney Dis* 1993;21:180.
5. Eberst ME, Berkowitz LR. Hemostasis in renal disease: pathophysiology and management. *Am J Med* 1994;96:168.
6. Gehm L, Propp DA. Pulmonary edema in the renal failure patient. *Am J Emerg Med* 1989;7:336.
7. Hodde LA, Sandroni S. Emergency department evaluation and management of dialysis patient complications. *Am J Emerg Med* 1992;10:317.
8. Keane WF, Alexander SR, Bailie GR, et al. Peritoneal dialysis-related peritonitis treatment recommendations: 1996 update. *Perit Dial Int* 1996;16:557.
9. Kiefer T, Schenk U, Weber J, et al. Incidence and significance of pneumoperitoneum in continuous ambulatory peritoneal dialysis. *Am J Kidney Dis* 1993;22:30.
10. Kohen JA, Opsahl JA, Kjellstrand CM. Deceptive patterns of uremic pulmonary edema. *Am J Kidney Dis* 1986;7:456.
11. Lee TH, Goldman L. Serum enzyme assays in the diagnosis of acute myocardial infarction. *Ann Intern Med* 1986;105:221.
12. Martin GS, Becker BN, Schulman G. Cardiac troponin-I accurately predicts myocardial injury in renal failure. *Nephrol Dial Transplant*. 1998;13:1709.
13. Sacchetti A, McCabe J, Torres M, et al. ED management of acute congestive heart failure in renal dialysis patients. *Am J Emerg Med* 1993;11:644.
14. Schneider RE, Messerli FH, deCarvalho JGR, et al. Immediate hemodynamic response to furosemide in patients undergoing chronic hemodialysis. *Am J Kidney Dis* 1987;9:55.
15. Sklar AH, Caruana RJ, Lammers JE, et al. Renal infections in autosomal dominant polycystic kidney disease. *Am J Kidney Dis* 1987;10:81.
16. Steiner RW, Halasz NA. Abdominal catastrophes and other unusual events in continuous ambulatory dialysis patients. *Am J Kidney Dis* 1990;15:1.
17. Szerlip HM, Weiss J, Singer I. Profound hyperkalemia without electrocardiographic manifestations. *Am J Kidney Dis* 1986;7:461.
18. Wolfson AB. End-stage renal disease: emergencies related to dialysis and transplantation. In: Wolfson AB, Harwood-Nuss AH, eds. *Renal and urologic emergencies*. New York, Churchill Livingstone, 1986.
19. Wolfson AB, Singer I. Hemodialysis-related emergencies: I. *J Emerg Med* 1987;5:533.
20. Wolfson AB, Singer I. Hemodialysis-related emergencies: II. *J Emerg Med* 1988;6:61.

CHAPTER 178

The Patient with a Renal Transplant

Louis G. Graff

The kidney is the most commonly transplanted organ in the United States: More than 10,000 are transplanted each year.[14] In contrast to dialysis, transplantation allows the patient to live a normal life and has thus become the preferred treatment for patients with end-stage renal disease. Transplant patients do not need a treatment (dialysis) three times a week, need not restrict their diets (potassium, sodium, and fluid intake), and can have children.[15]

The transplanted kidney is obtained from a living related donor or from a cadaver. At surgery, it is connected to the common iliac vein and artery in the pelvic fossa, and the ureter is anastomosed to the bladder. The transplanted kidney is placed in the pelvic area not only because it is anatomically convenient for anastomosis to the vasculature and the bladder, but also because it is accessible there for direct palpation, biopsy, or removal. The patient and transplanted organ are matched for the human leukocyte antigen major histocompatibility gene complex to minimize the risk of transplant rejection, and the patient is given immunosuppressive drugs (e.g., corticosteroids, azathioprine, cyclosporine, tacrolimus). Graft survival is 95% at 1 year for properly matched, living related donors and 90% for cadaveric donors.[7,10,14] Patient survival is higher (greater than 98% at 1 year for living related donors and 95% for cadaveric donors), as the patient can go back on dialysis if the transplant fails.

The unique aspects of caring for the patient with a transplanted kidney must be kept in mind when such a patient presents to the emergency department. Evaluation and management of even minor problems is often complicated by the patient's immunosuppressed state and the presence of a transplant. Transplant patients often have a limited ability to tolerate intercurrent illness, trauma, or other physiologic stresses. Moreover, chronic immunosuppression places them at increased risk for severe infectious disease, and often makes it difficult to evaluate emergent problems such as abdominal pain or fever. The status of the transplanted kidney must always be a concern as well. Patients may present with complications of the transplant surgery or with subtle signs and symptoms of graft rejection.

MEDICATIONS

Once a problem is identified, treatment is often more complicated in the transplant patient, because certain medications may have adverse effects or be frankly contraindicated in these patients (Table 178.1). For example, potassium-sparing diuretics can cause severe hyperkalemia in patients on cyclosporine. Nephrotoxic drugs can act synergistically with cyclosporine and contribute to renal dysfunction. Lovastatin can cause a severe myopathy in patients taking cyclosporine. Also, a number of medications can increase or decrease cyclosporine and tacrolimus levels[2] and thus affect drug effectiveness and toxicity (see Table 178.1).

Emergency physicians should be familiar with the adverse effects of medications routinely prescribed to the transplant patient. Cyclosporine, tacrolimus, and azathioprine increase the patient's susceptibility to infection, particularly by opportunistic organisms. The patient's risk of cancer (especially lymphoma, cervical cancer, and skin cancer) is 3% or 4%.[6] Because azathioprine causes leukopenia in more than 50% of patients, close monitoring of the blood count is necessary. Both drugs can also cause hepatotoxicity, so liver enzymes should be checked in patients with symptoms consistent with hepatitis. Also, liver failure can decrease the metabolism of cyclosporine and cause cyclosporine nephrotoxicity. Corticosteroids can contribute to the development of peptic ulcer disease, hypertension, accelerated coronary artery disease, diabetes, osteoporosis, aseptic necrosis of the hip, impaired healing, cataract, hemorrhagic pancreatitis, and candidal pharyngitis. Additional immunosuppressive agents (e.g., mycophenolate mofetil, rapamycin, anti–interleukin-2 receptor monoclonal antibodies) are being developed and brought into clinical practice. These agents have their own side effects and adverse interactions with other medications.[20]

TABLE 178.1. Some Drugs to Avoid in the Renal Transplant Patient

NEPHROTOXINS
Gentamicin, tobramycin, vancomycin, cimetidine, ranitidine, diclofenac, amphotericin B, ketoconazole, melphalan, trimethoprim-sulfamethoxazole, azapropazone
DRUGS THAT DECREASE CYCLOSPORINE EFFECTIVENESS
Rifampin, phenobarbital, phenytoin, carbamazepine, isoniazid
DRUGS THAT INCREASE CYCLOSPORINE EFFECTIVENESS AND TOXICITY
Diltiazem, nicardipine, verapamil, danazol, bromocriptine, metoclopramide, ketoconazole, fluconazole, itraconazole, erythromycin, methylprednisolone, oral contraceptives
DRUGS THAT INCREASE TACROLIMUS EFFECTIVENESS AND TOXICITY
Diltiazem, nicardipine, nifedipine, verapamil, clotrimazole, fluconazole, itraconazole, ketoconazole, clarithromycin, erythromycin, imipenem, cisapride, metoclopramide, bromocriptine, cimetidine, cyclosporine, danazol, methylprednisolone, protease inhibitors
DRUGS THAT DECREASE TACROLIMUS EFFECTIVENESS
Carbamazepine, phenobarbital, phenytoin, rifabutin, rifampin, nafcillin, valproic acid
DRUGS THAT INHIBIT AZATHIOPRINE METABOLISM
Allopurinol
POTASSIUM-SPARING DIURETICS
Amiloride, spironolactone, triamterene
LOVASTATIN (MAY CAUSE MYOPATHY)

COMPLICATIONS OF TRANSPLANT SURGERY

Early after transplantation, complications of the surgery may bring patients to the emergency department. There may be acute tubular necrosis, especially if the graft preservation time before surgery was prolonged. Vascular complications, such as renal artery stenosis or thrombosis or renal vein thrombosis, can cause graft dysfunction or localized pain. Ureteral stenosis can cause decreased graft function as well.

Local hematoma or lymphocele can cause pain or compromise graft function by mass effect. The immunosuppressive drugs given to prevent graft rejection also inhibit wound healing and the normal response to infection. At least 20% of patients develop a wound infection, and many others develop other infections. Most patients with surgical complications present within days or weeks of transplantation, although some complications (e.g., ureteral stenosis, smoldering infection) may have a delayed presentation.

RENAL DYSFUNCTION

Evidence of renal dysfunction should always be sought in the patient with a renal transplant, and any reversible cause of renal failure must be identified and treated promptly (Table 178.2). Apparently, small changes in the serum creatinine level may indicate important changes in renal function. For example, an increase in the serum creatinine level from 1 to 2 mg/dL represents a 50% decrease in renal function. During the first days after transplant surgery, the most common causes of renal failure are acute tubular necrosis, hyperacute rejection, urinary tract obstruction, urine leak, compression of the graft or renal artery by hematoma, and hypovolemia. During the first 12 weeks after transplant surgery, the patient may experience acute rejection, renal artery stenosis, or urinary tract obstruction. Renal failure more than 3 months after surgery is usually due to acute rejection, chronic rejection, recurrence of underlying renal disease, or new renal disease.

All patients with renal dysfunction must be evaluated for obstruction. There are often no clues to this; the urinalysis is negative and urine output may be unchanged. Ultrasound, however, can show hydronephrosis and confirm the diagnosis of obstruction.

Prerenal causes are often responsible for decreased renal function in transplant patients (see Table 178.2). The patient may be volume-depleted or have widespread arteriosclerotic disease.

The anastomosis to the native artery may be a site of particular vulnerability to stenosis. A high blood urea nitrogen (BUN)–creatinine ratio and a low urine sodium are consistent with this cause of renal failure. If the stenosis is not severe, the only sign or symptom may be severe hypertension. Percutaneous transluminal angioplasty has been successful in reversing hypertension and renal failure,[18] but surgical reconstruction may be necessary. Radioisotope scanning using technetium or hippuran can identify renal artery stenosis; complete occlusion can result in irreversible infarction unless blood flow is restored within 2 hours.

Renal vein thrombosis can also occur. Patients may present with graft pain and tenderness, fever, hypertension, and proteinuria. The treatment is long-term anticoagulation.

Clues to the presence of intrinsic renal disease (see Table 178.2) may be found in the urinalysis. Red blood cell casts or proteinuria is seen in glomerulonephritis and vasculitis. Consideration should be given to recurrence of the disease that originally caused renal failure,[23] especially with systemic diseases such as diabetes mellitus or vasculitis. Glomerulonephritis may recur in the graft if the disease is still active in the original kidneys at the time of transplantation.

Patients with kidney transplants are always at risk for transplant rejection. Acute rejection usually occurs within 4 weeks of transplantation but can occur many months later, and can result in complete loss of graft function. The precipitant is usually unknown, but the clinician should be circumspect in exposing the transplant patient to antigens, whether in the form of drugs or blood transfusions.[3] The clinical findings are often those of prerenal or intrinsic renal disease (i.e., low urine sodium level and high BUN/creatinine ratio). The kidney is enlarged and tender, and there may be fever, hypertension, or oliguria. An increased serum level of β_2-microglobulin supports the diagnosis of acute rejection, but the diagnosis must usually be confirmed by percutaneous renal biopsy.[22] The prognosis is poor when acute rejection occurs more than 6 months after transplantation or shows evidence of increased severity (by histologic grade or change in the serum creatinine).[12] Treatment is hospitalization and administration of a combination of immunosuppressive drugs, including high-dose corticosteroids (e.g., methylprednisolone 500 to 1000 mg/d). Chronic rejection, which cannot be treated, occurs months to years after transplantation and is manifested by a gradual deterioration of renal function.

Cyclosporine and tacrolimus are low-molecular-weight fungal metabolites that are very effective at preventing transplant rejection by depleting circulating T lymphocytes. Unfortunately, they produce nephrotoxicity in up to 50% of patients,[20] which usually occurs more than 6 weeks after transplantation. Some centers change from these drugs to azathioprine at 4 to 6 months after transplantation to avoid the risk of nephrotoxicity. The BUN/creatinine ratio tends to reflect a prerenal process. The graft is not tender or swollen, and ultrasound examination is normal. A reduction in the dose of immunosuppressives can lead to return of renal function. In practice, the question often is whether a decrease in renal function is due to transplant rejection, requiring an increase in the dose of drug, or to drug nephrotoxicity, requiring a decrease in the dose. Assays for blood drug levels can help differentiate rejection from drug nephrotoxicity.[1]

TABLE 178.2. Differential Diagnosis of Renal Failure in the Patient with a Renal Transplant

PRERENAL
Hypovolemia
Renal artery stenosis
Renal artery thrombosis
Renal vein thrombosis
RENAL (INTRINSIC DISEASE)
Recurrence of disease (e.g., diabetes mellitus, systemic lupus erythematosus, focal glomerulosclerosis, Goodpasture syndrome. Wegener's granulomatosis, glomerulonephritis)
Acute rejection
Chronic rejection
Acute tubular necrosis
Cyclosporine toxicity
POSTRENAL (OBSTRUCTION)
Prostate
Abscess
Urinoma
Lymphocele
Ureteral stenosis at the anastomosis

FEVER OR INFECTION

Kidney transplant patients are at increased risk of infection (Fig. 178.1). Organ transplantation became possible because of the development of immunosuppressive agents to prevent organ rejection, but at the cost of greatly increased infectious complications. An aggressive approach to identifying and treating infection has been the primary factor responsible for today's high survival rates for all transplant patients.

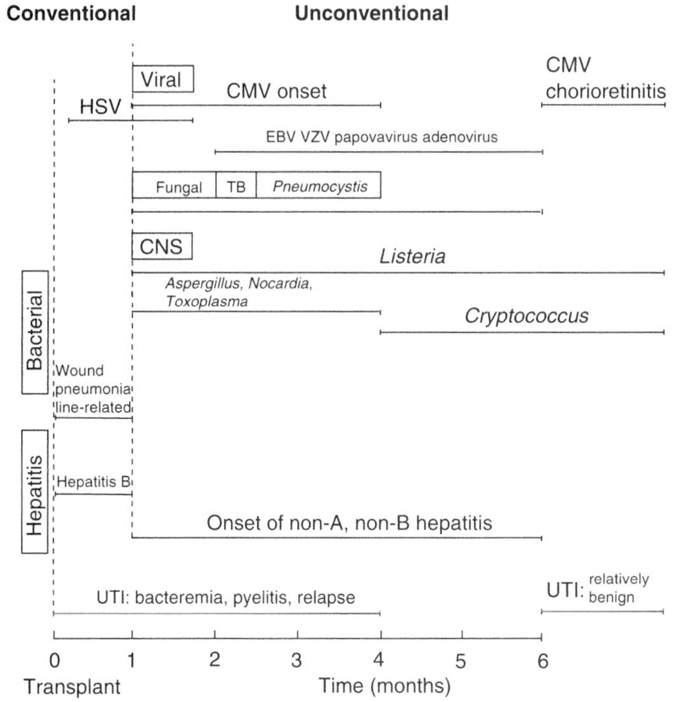

Figure 178.1. Timetable for the occurrence of infection in renal transplant recipients. HSV, herpes simplex virus; CMV, cytomegalovirus; EBV, Epstein-Barr virus; VZV, varicella zoster virus; TB, tuberculosis; CNS, central nervous system; UTI, urinary tract infection. (Redrawn after Rubin RH. Infectious disease complications of renal transplantation. *Kidney Int* 1993;44:224.)

As is the case with other immunosuppressed patients, the signs and symptoms of infection in renal transplant patients may be masked, and opportunistic infections may require specialized diagnostic and treatment modalities.[19] In contrast to the usual approach to the nonimmunosuppressed patient with fever, in whom treatment can generally be instituted on the basis of clinical criteria, aggressive efforts to identify a responsible organism are usually justified in transplant patients. Twenty percent of transplant patients develop urinary tract infections that are readily diagnosed on urinalysis. Ten percent develop clear-cut surgical wound infection. Sepsis, which may be evidenced only by positive blood cultures, occurs in 5%; occult abscess is found in another 5%.[5] Two percent to 4% develop systemic fungal infections, and 9% to 10%, local fungal infections.

Because the signs and symptoms of serious infection may be masked, blood cultures should be done for any transplant patient with fever, and hospital admission should be considered when the source of infection cannot be identified. Uncomplicated urinary tract infections and wound infections may be treated with conventional antibiotics on an outpatient basis.

Five percent to 12% of renal transplant patients develop cytomegalovirus (CMV) infection, which includes symptoms of fever, adenopathy, leukopenia, and myalgias. Complications include retinitis, pneumonitis, hepatitis, fungal and parasitic superinfection, and transplant rejection. Preoperative administration of CMV immunoglobulin or ganciclovir significantly reduces the risk of postoperative CMV infection.[17,21]

Meningitis can present very subtly in the transplant patient. Classic signs of meningitis (e.g., fever or meningismus) may not be present. Headache, which may suggest other serious disease, such as temporal arteritis or subarachnoid hemorrhage,[9] is the most common symptom. Opportunistic organisms such as *Cryptococcus* are more likely to cause disease than are the usual pathogens.[13] The emergency physician must have a high level of suspicion and a low threshold for performing a diagnostic lumbar puncture.

Trimethoprim–sulfamethoxazole prophylaxis has become the standard in renal transplant patients because of the high risk of infections.[8] *Pneumocystis carinii* pneumonia ordinarily develops in up to 12 % of patients, but it is eliminated with prophylaxis. In addition, prophylaxis with trimethoprim–sulfamethoxazole for the first 6 months reduces the risk of urinary tract infection from greater than 50% to 5%.[8]

ABDOMINAL PAIN

Evaluation of abdominal pain in the transplant patient is challenging because immunosuppressive medications can mask the signs and symptoms of disease. In one series of transplant patients with abdominal pain, 10% developed an acute abdomen, and half of them required surgery for perforation or bowel obstruction.[11] Of those who required surgery, only 29% had fever and only 29% had leukocytosis. Because of the subtle presentation and difficulty in diagnosis, delays before surgery were substantial (ranging from 18 to 96 hours), and 71% of patients had suffered perforation by the time of surgery. Notably, 43% had signs of perforation on plain abdominal radiographs.

The most common causes of an acute abdomen in transplant patients are similar to those in the general population: gastroduodenal bleeding or perforation, colonic bleeding or perforation, bowel obstruction, appendicitis, cholecystitis, volvulus, and ovarian torsion.[4,11] Patients with polycystic kidney disease may have abdominal pain because of hemorrhage or infection in the cysts, if their own kidneys have not been removed. Ultrasound may be helpful in evaluating these patients. Because both azathioprine and cyclosporine can cause hepatitis with abdominal pain, liver enzymes should be measured in transplant patients with abdominal pain. The transplant patient has an increased risk of developing lymphoma, probably because of chronic immunosuppression. Abdominal computed tomography scanning can identify enlarged retroperitoneal nodes or tumor mass.

Pancreatitis occurs infrequently (1%) in renal transplant patients. When it does occur, it is quite serious, with 80% to 100% mortality.[16]

IMMUNIZATIONS

Killed and antigen-based vaccines (tetanus, diphtheria, rabies, influenza, and pneumococcal vaccines) can be safely used in transplant patients. There is no contraindication to treatment with immunoglobulin. Live or attenuated vaccines are contraindicated in the immunosuppressed patient, because they can cause serious infection.

DISPOSITION

The threshold for hospitalizing the transplant patient should be very low. One must always suspect a pathologic process, even in patients who seem to have only minor complaints. When a transplant-related problem is identified, the emergency physician should not hesitate to seek appropriate consultation or to arrange transfer of the patient to a facility with the resources to manage transplant patients. Nevertheless, the emergency physician can manage most acute problems in renal transplant patients if a thorough and meticulous approach is used.

COMMON PITFALLS

- Prescribing potentially nephrotoxic drugs in the renal transplant patient
- Failing to realize that a small rise in the transplant patient's creatinine level may represent a relatively large decrement in renal function, necessitating aggressive evaluation
- Assuming that a normal urine output excludes obstruction as the cause of acute renal failure
- Failing to remember that the immunosuppressed transplant patient often does not show classic signs or laboratory findings of infection
- Failing to remember that certain drugs may decrease cyclosporine or tacrolimus levels and lead to transplant rejection; likewise, certain drugs may increase these drug levels and lead to toxicity
- Failing to provide increased doses of steroids when transplant patients taking corticosteroids undergo major stress, such as surgery, myocardial infarction, major trauma, or sepsis
- Giving a blood transfusion without a clear indication, because stimulation by exogenous antigens may lead to rejection
- Overlooking the fact that the transplant patient may have three kidneys (two original, one transplanted), all of which may become infected or be injured

References

1. Beutler D, Molteni S, Zeugin T, et al. Evaluation of instrumental, nonisotopic immunoassays (fluorescence polarization immunoassay and enzyme-multiplied immunoassay technique) for cyclosporine monitoring in whole blood after kidney and liver transplantation. *Ther Drug Monit* 1992;14:424.
2. Bottiger Y, Brattstrom C, Tyden G, et al. Tacrolimus whole blood concentrations correlate closely to side-effects in renal transplant recipients. *Br J Clin Pharmacol* 1999;48:445–448.
3. Burlingham WJ, Stratta R, Mason B, et al. Risk factors for sensitization by blood transfusions. *Transplantation* 1989;47:140.
4. Chan MK, Wilcox DT, Trompeter RS. Acute appendicitis in children after renal transplantation. *Arch Dis Child* 1999;81:372.
5. Dempsey J, Scott R. Duplex Doppler examination of a perinephric abscess in a renal transplant. *South Med J* 1990;83:1213.
6. Feczko BJ, Mezwa DG. Gastrointestinal carcinomas in renal transplant recipients. *Gastrointest Radiol* 1991;16:351.
7. Fischel RJ, Payne WD, Gillingham KJ, et al. Long-term outlook for renal transplant recipients with 1-year function. *Transplantation* 1991;51:118.
8. Fishman JA, Rubin RH. Infection in organ-transplant recipients. *N Engl J Med* 1998;338:1741–1751.
9. Fontanarosa PB. Recognition of subarachnoid hemorrhage. *Ann Emerg Med* 1989;18:1199.
10. Gentil MA, Rocha JL, Rodriguez-Algarra G, et al. Impaired kidney transplant survival in patients with antibodies to hepatitis C virus. *Nephrol Dial Transplant* 1999;14:2455–2460.
11. Hubbard SG, Bivins BA, Lucas BA, et al. Acute abdomen in the transplant patient. *Am Surg* 1980;46(2):116.
12. Humar A, Kerr S, Gillingham KJ, et al. Features of acute rejection that increase risk for chronic rejection. *Transplantation* 1999;68:1200–1203.
13. Kong NC, Shaariah W, Morad Z, et al. Cryptococcosis in a renal unit. *Aust N Z J Med* 1990;20:645.
14. Renal Data System. *USRDS 1999 annual report*. Bethesda, MD: National Institute of Diabetes and Digestive and Kidney Diseases, 1999.
15. Robinson TW, Wilkerson SA, Joyce MR. Pregnancy in renal transplant recipients: case report. *Am J Perinatol* 1992;9:52.
16. Slakey DP, Johnson CO, Cziperle DJ, et al. Management of severe pancreatitis in renal transplant recipients. *Ann Surg* 1997;225:217–222.
17. Snydman DR, Werner BG, Heinze-Lacey B, et al. Use of cytomegalovirus immune globulin to prevent cytomegalovirus disease in renal transplant recipients. *N Engl J Med* 1987;317:1049.
18. Thomas CP, Riad H, Johnson BF, et al. Percutaneous transluminal angioplasty in transplant renal artery stenosis: a long-term follow-up. *Transpl Int* 1992;5(3):129.
19. Tilney NL, Stom TB, Yineyard GC, et al. Factors contributing to the declining mortality rate in renal transplantation. *N Engl J Med* 1978;299:1321.
20. VanBuskirk AM, Pidwell DJ, Adams PW, et al. Transplantation immunology. *JAMA* 1997;278:1993–1999.
21. Walton T, Kankari B, Wyner L. Comparison of ganciclovir and immune globulin containing regimens in preventing cytomegalovirus infection in patients with renal transplants. *Am J Health Syst Pharm* 1999;56:1831–1834.
22. Wilczek HE. Percutaneous needle biopsy of the renal allograft: a clinical safety evaluation of 1129 biopsies. *Transplantation* 1990;50:790.
23. Ylinen K, Gronhagen-Riska C, Honkanen E, et al. Outcome of patients with secondary amyloidosis in dialysis treatment. *Nephrol Dial Transplant* 1992;7:908.

CHAPTER 179
Rhabdomyolysis

Mark T. Steele

Rhabdomyolysis is a clinical syndrome resulting from injury to skeletal muscle. The most common causes are alcohol and drug abuse, seizures, crush injury, muscle compression, and infection, but it is not uncommon for there to be multiple causes of a single episode (Table 179.1).[7] The final common pathway of all these etiologies is damage to the muscle cell membrane, or sarcolemma, with liberation of intracellular contents such as creatine phosphokinase (CPK), myoglobin, glutamic oxaloacetic transaminase, lactic dehydrogenase (LDH), aldolase, potassium, and phosphorus.

CLINICAL PRESENTATION

The presenting symptoms and signs of rhabdomyolysis are variable and generally reflect the underlying cause. Because the history can be very nonspecific, a high index of suspicion should be maintained, particularly in the setting of seizures, unconsciousness, or agitation. The prehospital history may be helpful, particularly if the patient has an altered mental status: There may be a history of suspected overdose, seizure, or prolonged immobilization. There may be a history of drug abuse or recent strenuous exercise or a family history of muscle dysfunction. Rarely, patients may report that their urine is dark reddish-brown. This symptom can occur if myoglobin levels exceed 100 mg/dL.

The physical examination may be of limited value in making the diagnosis. The classic triad of muscle weakness, tenderness, and swelling is rarely found. For example, in one series, only 50% of patients complained of myalgia or muscle weakness.[7]

The major complications of rhabdomyolysis are listed in Table 179.2. Hyperkalemia is the most serious complication, because it can result in cardiac arrest if not diagnosed and treated promptly. A review of earthquake survivors showed that hyperkalemic cardiac arrests were a significant cause of mortality, particularly in early deaths (less than 5 days).[13] Some degree of hyperkalemia is found in up to 40% of patients with rhabdomyolysis.[7] Hyperkalemia generally correlates with decreased renal function, rather than with the quantity of muscle injured.[5]

Hyperphosphatemia, hypocalcemia, hyperuricemia, and hypoalbuminemia are also potential complications. Hypocalcemia, the most commonly encountered metabolic abnormality, is felt to be caused by deposition of calcium in damaged muscle tissue. Hyperuricemia is related to the release of intracellular purines from damaged muscle tissue, and hypoalbuminemia from leakage of protein from injured muscle vessels.

Acute renal failure is a major complication of rhabdomyoly-

TABLE 179.1. Causes of Rhabdomyolysis

DIRECT TRAUMA
Crush injury
Burns
Electrical injury
MUSCLE OVERUSE/PROLONGED EXERTION
Jogging/contact sports
Seizures
Status asthmaticus
Delirium tremens
Psychosis
DRUGS AND TOXINS
See Table 179.3
INFECTIONS
See Table 179.4
METABOLIC ABNORMALITIES
Diabetic ketoacidosis
Nonketotic hyperosmolar coma
Hypokalemia
Hypo- or hypernatremia
Hypophosphatemia
Hypo- or hyperthyroidism
MUSCULAR ISCHEMIA
Prolonged immobility with external compression
Vascular obstruction (e.g., emboli, thrombosis)
Shock
Sickle cell disease
HYPO- OR HYPERTHERMIA (INCLUDING MALIGNANT HYPERTHERMIA, NEUROLEPTIC MALIGNANT SYNDROME, HEAT STROKE)
IMMUNE DISORDERS
Dermatomyositis
Polymyositis
GENETIC DISORDERS
Abnormal Carbohydrate Metabolism
Myophosphorylase deficiency (McArdle syndrome)
Alpha-glucosidase deficiency
Amylo-1,6-glucosidase deficiency
Phosphohexose isomerase deficiency
Phosphofructokinase deficiency
Abnormal Lipid Metabolism
Carnitine deficiency
Carnitine palmitoyltransferase deficiency
IDIOPATHIC

sis, the incidence ranging from 4% to 33% in retrospective studies.[18] In this setting, there is decreased glomerular filtration rate (GFR), presumably secondary to toxic exposure or an ischemic event. There appears to be increased renal vascular resistance secondary to vasoconstriction, which may be due to microthrombi, activation of the renin–angiotensin system, vasopressin, or prostaglandins. Most experts do not believe that

TABLE 179.2. Major Complications of Rhabdomyolysis

Hyperkalemia/cardiac dysrhythmias
Acute renal failure
Compartment syndrome
Disseminated intravascular coagulation
Respiratory dysfunction

TABLE 179.3. Drug- and Toxin-Induced Rhabdomyolysis

DRUGS OF ABUSE
Opioids
Cocaine
Amphetamines
Phencyclidine hydrochloride (PCP)
Lysergic acid diethylamide (LSD)
Barbiturates/sedative hypnotics
ALCOHOLS
Ethanol
Isopropyl alcohol
Ethylene glycol
PSYCHIATRIC DRUGS
Neuroleptics
Cyclic antidepressants
NEUROMUSCULAR BLOCKING AGENTS
Succinylcholine
OVER-THE-COUNTER PREPARATIONS
Aspirin
Phenylpropanolamine
Antihistamines
LIPID-LOWERING AGENTS
Clofibrate
Lovastatin
Simvastatin
Gemfibrozil
POISONOUS INSECT/REPTILE BITES
Snake bites
Spider bites
Massive bee stings
OTHER
Epsilon aminocaproic acid
Peanut oil
Theophylline
Caffeine
Carbon monoxide
Toluene
Mercuric chloride
Quail eating
Haff disease
Steroids
Colchicine

tubular obstruction by myoglobin, uric acid, and other muscle breakdown products is causative. The role of myoglobin is unclear,[11] but it is known that hypovolemia and acid urine are required for myoglobin to result in renal injury.[5] Likely predictors of renal failure in rhabdomyolysis include the degree of elevation of serum CPK, potassium, and phosphate; the degree of depression of serum albumin; and the presence of sepsis or dehydration.[19]

Compartment syndrome may be either a cause or a complication of rhabdomyolysis. In the latter case, fluid accumulates in the interstitial space, resulting in an increased size and pressure of the intracompartmental contents. Compartment syndrome should be anticipated in patients with rhabdomyolysis, and compartment pressures measured if suspected. Fasciotomy should be strongly considered in patients with pressures greater than 35 mm Hg.

There are other potential complications. Disseminated intravascular coagulation is believed to be the result of the liberation of activating substances such as thromboplastin from

TABLE 179.4. Infectious Etiologies of Rhabdomyolysis

BACTERIAL
Legionnaire's disease (most common)
Staphylococcus toxin
Streptococcus
Shigellosis
Salmonellosis
Tetanus
Gas gangrene
Septic shock
VIRAL
Influenza (most common)
Epstein-Barr virus
Cytomegalovirus
Echovirus
Coxsackievirus
Herpes virus
Adenovirus
Hepatitis
Human immunodeficiency virus
RICKETTSIAL
Rocky Mountain spotted fever
PARASITIC
Trichinosis
OTHER
Reye syndrome

necrotic muscle. Respiratory dysfunction can occur as a result of involvement of the respiratory musculature. Myocardial damage can also occur, resulting in manifestations ranging from isolated electrocardiographic (ECG) changes to heart failure and death.[5] Hepatic dysfunction has been described with severe rhabdomyolysis; it may result in hepatic failure and necessitate liver transplantation.

DIFFERENTIAL DIAGNOSIS

Rhabdomyolysis should be considered in patients with muscle injury (direct trauma, burns, or compartment syndrome), known muscle disease, or exceptional muscular activity.[16] A number of diseases are associated with one or more of the abnormalities seen with rhabdomyolysis, but no other entity is associated with the characteristic CPK elevation. In addition, rhabdomyolysis must always be part of the differential diagnosis of acute renal failure.

Drugs and toxins[5] (Table 179.3) are common causes of rhabdomyolysis. Ethanol, the most commonly implicated of these, has a direct toxic effect on the muscle cell membrane. More importantly, severe intoxication with alcohol or sedative–hypnotic drugs can result in prolonged immobilization and compression of the extremities, with resulting compromise of the blood supply to muscle. Metabolic complications of alcoholism, such as hypokalemia, hypophosphatemia, and hypomagnesemia, may also increase the risk of rhabdomyolysis. Alcohol withdrawal seizures and delirium tremens can cause excessive muscular activity, with resultant rhabdomyolysis.

Cocaine-induced rhabdomyolysis is not uncommon.[3,20] At least some degree of skeletal muscle injury and CPK elevation appears to be common in emergency department patients who present after using cocaine.[6] The exact etiology is unclear but may be related to excessive energy demands placed on the muscle cell, direct toxicity to the cell membrane, or seizure activity associated with cocaine toxicity. Moreover, cocaine-intoxicated patients with hyperthermia are more likely to develop rhabdomyolysis than are nonhyperthermic cocaine-intoxicated patients.[4] Phencyclidine hydrochloride and amphetamine toxicity cause similar toxicity.

Other toxins, such as carbon monoxide, snake venom, and mercuric chloride, are directly toxic to the muscle cell membrane. The eating of quail fed with hemlock has been associated with outbreaks of rhabdomyolysis.[14] Sickle cell trait has been associated with exertional rhabdomyolysis; several fatalities have been reported.[9] Haff disease is a syndrome of unexpected rhabdomyolysis related to the consumption of certain types of fish. All recent U.S. cases have been associated with buffalo fish (*Ictiobus cyprinellus*), a bottom-feeding species found mostly in the Mississippi River and its tributaries.[1] In immunologically mediated diseases (e.g., polymyositis and dermatomyositis), muscle cells may be injured by inflammation.

Any condition resulting in muscle cell hypoxia can lead to cellular injury and rhabdomyolysis, as can rigorous physical training, particularly in hot environments. Similarly, hypophosphatemia can result in severe depletion of adenosine triphosphate, an energy source required to maintain cell membrane integrity and function. Infections (Table 179.4) may induce rhabdomyolysis by direct muscle injury or by inducing tissue hypoxia. Influenza is the most common viral etiology, followed by human immunodeficiency virus infection and enteroviral infection. *Legionella* species are the most common bacterial organisms, followed by streptococcus species, *Francisella tularensis,* and *Salmonella* species.[17]

Finally, certain genetic defects, such as McArdle syndrome (absence of muscle phosphorylase) or carnitine palmitoyltransferase deficiency, prevent the effective use of carbohydrates or lipids as energy substrates. Up to one-fourth of patients with recurrent, unexplained rhabdomyolysis may have one of these enzyme deficiencies. Another 20% may have muscular dystrophy or a myopathy.[12]

EMERGENCY DEPARTMENT EVALUATION

Evaluation, as always, begins with confirmation of hemodynamic stability. The history should be directed at identifying any possible etiologic factors, including, especially, exposure to alcohol, cocaine, or other toxins. On physical examination, look for signs of focal or generalized muscular tenderness or swelling, and note any obvious trauma. Laboratory evaluation should include electrolytes, blood urea nitrogen (BUN), creatinine, glucose, CPK, calcium, and phosphate. Serum albumin, uric acid, LDH, SGOT, and coagulation studies may be helpful in some instances.

CPK is the most sensitive test for rhabdomyolysis. Five times the upper limit of normal is often considered the threshold for the diagnosis.[14] CPK is an excellent marker, because it is present almost immediately following injury, is easily measured, and is not rapidly cleared. Elevations are seen 2 to 12 hours following muscle injury; levels peak in 1 to 3 days and generally fall off within 3 to 5 days after muscle injury ceases.[14] Although early studies failed to establish a clear correlation between CPK levels and morbidity,[19] more recent investigations of cocaine-related rhabdomyolysis suggest a relationship between CPK level and severity of disease.[3,20] Mortality and acute renal failure in crush injuries have also been shown to be higher in the presence of markedly elevated CPK levels (greater than 75,000).[13] Although patients with very high levels of CPK appear to have more complications, patients with moderate levels may also develop significant problems.

Serum and urine myoglobin determinations have also been used to diagnose rhabdomyolysis. Myoglobin typically rises more quickly than CPK, so it may be helpful in the diagnosis of early rhabdomyolysis, but because its half-life in plasma is only 1 to 3 hours, it can also be unreliable. Urine tests that use guaiac, orthotolidine, or similar agents can detect myoglobin or hemoglobin in the urine but cannot distinguish between the two. False-negative tests for myoglobinuria can occur because of rapid clearance of myoglobin from the urine. In one large series, one-fourth of patients with proven rhabdomyolysis had a negative urine dipstick test.[7]

EMERGENCY DEPARTMENT MANAGEMENT

The goals of management are to treat the underlying cause or causes of rhabdomyolysis, to identify and treat complications, and to prevent acute renal failure.

Rhabdomyolysis may continue to proceed or may be exacerbated by excessive exertion, agitation, fighting of restraints, seizures, or abnormal posturing. These should be controlled by aggressive sedation, with a benzodiazepine, in order to prevent further muscle breakdown. Rarely, pharmacologic paralysis with nondepolarizing neuromuscular agents and intubation may be required. Hyperthermia, if present, should also be aggressively treated.

Patients with hyperkalemia require continuous cardiac monitoring and aggressive intervention. Hypocalcemia is generally self-limited and rarely requires specific treatment; the same is true of hyperphosphatemia. As noted previously, the patient should be monitored for the development of compartment syndrome. Coagulopathy can generally be addressed by treating the underlying disease process.

Several uncontrolled studies suggest the efficacy of early, aggressive isotonic fluid administration in preventing acute renal failure in crush-related or traumatic rhabdomyolysis.[2,10,15] This treatment results in increased renal tubular flow rates, which facilitate the excretion of substances that may injure or obstruct the renal tubules. A target urine flow rate of 200 to 300 cc/h has been suggested.

Many experts also recommend the use of intravenous sodium bicarbonate to alkalinize the urine, because myoglobin is toxic to the kidneys in acid urine. There have been no prospective randomized studies, however. Retrospective, uncontrolled trials suggesting benefit have been confounded by the concurrent use of saline loading. One small nonrandomized study has questioned the benefit of bicarbonate (and mannitol), suggesting that saline expansion alone is sufficient to prevent renal failure.[8]

The role of diuretics such as mannitol and furosemide is also unclear. Mannitol should probably be considered if urine output is inadequate despite saline infusion, because it may convert oliguric renal failure to nonoliguric renal failure, which has a better prognosis. Acute renal failure unresponsive to the aforementioned measures may require dialysis, but the prognosis for ultimate recovery is good.

DISPOSITION

Patients with rhabdomyolysis generally require admission to the hospital, as it is not possible to predict which individuals will develop complications. Patients with hyperkalemia, metabolic acidosis, or evidence of renal failure, and those with other serious comorbid conditions, require hospital admission. Patients with hyperkalemia require admission to a monitored setting, and nephrology consultation is indicated if renal insufficiency develops or if metabolic abnormalities are unresponsive to usual medical treatment. Dialysis is required for some individuals. If renal consultation and dialysis are not available at the treating institution, transfer to a facility with those capabilities should be initiated.

COMMON PITFALLS

- Failure to consider rhabdomyolysis in patients with alcoholism, unconsciousness, prolonged immobilization, seizures, hyperthermia, or infection
- Failure to identify and treat hyperkalemia associated with rhabdomyolysis
- Failure to pharmacologically control agitation, seizures, or abnormal posturing in patients who are at risk for rhabdomyolysis
- Failure to evaluate for compartment syndrome
- Failure to realize that the diagnosis of rhabdomyolysis cannot be ruled out on the basis of the serum or urine myoglobin alone
- Failure to provide adequate hydration and to prevent or treat acidosis in patients with rhabdomyolysis

References

1. Anonymous. Haff disease associated with eating buffalo fish—United States, 1997. *MMWR* 1998;47:1091.
2. Better OS, Stein JH. Early management of shock and prophylaxis of acute renal failure in traumatic rhabdomyolysis. *N Engl J Med* 1990;322:825.
3. Brody SL, Wrenn KO, Wilber MM, et al. Predicting the severity of cocaine-associated rhabdomyolysis. *Ann Emerg Med* 1990;19:1137.
4. Callaway CW, Clark RF. Hyperthermia in psychostimulant overdose. *Ann Emerg Med* 1994;24:68.
5. Curry SC, Chang D, Connor D. Drug- and toxin-induced rhabdomyolysis. *Ann Emerg Med* 1989;18:1068.
6. Counselman FL, McLaughlin EW, Kardon EM, et al. Creatine phosphokinase elevation in patients presenting to the emergency department with cocaine-related complaints. *Am J Emerg Med* 1997;15:221.
7. Gabow PA, Kaehny WD, Kelleher SP. The spectrum of rhabdomyolysis. *Medicine* 1982;61:141.
8. Homsi E, Barreiro MF, Orlando JM. Prophylaxis of acute renal failure in patients with rhabdomyolysis. *Ren Fail* 1997;19:283.
9. Kimmick G, Owen J. Rhabdomyolysis and hemolysis associated with sickle cell trait and glucose-6-phosphate dehydrogenase deficiency. *South Med J* 1996;89:1097.
10. Knottenbelt JD. Traumatic rhabdomyolysis from severe beating—experience of volume diuresis in 200 patients. *J Trauma* 1994;37:214.
11. Laios ID, Clark R, Wult B. Myoglobin clearance as an early indicator for rhabdomyolysis-induced acute renal failure. *Ann Clin Lab Sci* 1995;25:179.
12. Lofberg M, Jankala H, Paetau A, et al. Metabolic causes of recurrent rhabdomyolysis. *Acta Neurol Scand* 1998;98:268.
13. Oda J, Tanaka H, Yoshioka T, et al. Analysis of 372 patients with crush syndrome caused by the Hanshin-Awaji earthquake. *J Trauma* 1997;42:470.
14. Poels PJ, Gabreels FJ. Rhabdomyolysis: a review of the literature. *Clin Neurol Neurosurg* 1993;95:175.
15. Shimazu T, Yushioka T, Nakata Y, et al. Fluid resuscitation and systemic complications in crush syndrome: 14 Hanshin-Awaji earthquake patients. *J Trauma* 1997;42:641.
16. Sinert R, Kohl L, Rainone T, et al. Exercise-induced rhabdomyolysis. *Ann Emerg Med* 1994;23:1301.
17. Singh U, Scheld M. Infectious etiologies of rhabdomyolysis: three cases and a review. *Clin Infect Dis* 1996;22:642.
18. Slater MS, Mullins RJ. Rhabdomyolysis and myoglobinuric renal failure in trauma and surgical patients: a review. *J Am Coll Surg* 1998;186:693.
19. Ward MM. Factors predictive of acute renal failure in rhabdomyolysis. *Arch Intern Med* 1988;148:1553.
20. Welch RD, Todd K, Krause GS. Incidence of cocaine-associated rhabdomyolysis. *Ann Emerg Med* 1991;20:155.

CHAPTER 180
Hematuria

James P. d'Etienne and Steven A. Godwin

Hematuria is defined as the presence of an abnormal number of red blood cells in the urine. Specifically, more than 3 to 5 red blood cells per high-powered field on microscopic examination of a spun urine specimen is considered abnormal.

CLINICAL PRESENTATION

Gross hematuria can be quite startling and often brings the patient immediately to the emergency department for examination. Microscopic hematuria is usually discovered as an incidental finding during an evaluation for an unrelated complaint.

Rapid screening can be done simply with a urine dipstick analysis. Dipstick urinalysis is reported to have a sensitivity of 86% to 100%, a specificity of 65% to 99%, a false-negative rate of 3% to 24%, and a false-positive rate of 10% to 15% for detecting hemoglobin and myoglobin in urine.[2,5,16] The dipstick test depends, however, on lysis of intact erythrocytes to release free hemoglobin and does not differentiate between hemoglobin and myoglobin.[7]

False-positive reactions may also occur as a result of oxidizing contaminants (e.g., bacterial peroxidases, povidone). More commonly, false-positive results are due to menstrual blood, traumatic catheterization, and improper collection techniques. Pigments in the urine from medications (e.g., Pyridium) and bilirubin, as well as improper handling of the urine specimen, may also result in inaccurate readings. False-negative reactions are often due to reducing agents (e.g., ascorbic acid).

DIFFERENTIAL DIAGNOSIS

The differential diagnosis of hematuria is broad. Studies evaluating men age 50 or older for hematuria have found that the most common diagnoses, excluding trauma and exercise-induced hematuria, are benign prostatic hypertrophy (BPH), neoplasm, infection, nephrolithiasis, and unknown causes.[8,9,15,16] Neoplasm is a prime concern in adults. Population-based studies suggest that patients over 40 with hematuria should be aggressively investigated.[3,4,6]

In pediatric patients, the reported incidence of gross hematuria is approximately one in 1000 emergency visits. A cause can be found in approximately 60% of cases, the most frequent diagnoses (in descending order) being urinary tract infection, perineal irritation, meatal stenosis with ulceration, trauma, recent surgical procedure, clotting abnormalities, nephrolithiasis, and glomerulonephritis.[12]

Hemorrhagic cystitis should be suspected when hematuria is accompanied by dysuria, urinary frequency, suprapubic pain, leukocytosis, or pungent-smelling urine. Severe flank pain that radiates to the groin may indicate a ureteral calculus. Although hematuria is often associated with renal colic, up to 15% of cases may be dipstick-negative for hematuria.[11] Exercise-induced hematuria, trauma, neoplasm, prostatic hypertrophy, and hemorrhagic cystitis present as lower tract disease devoid of proteinuria and casts. Hematuria may also be caused by trauma to the flaccid posterior bladder wall, transient renovascular vasoconstriction, or direct renal trauma.[1]

Hematuria is symptomatic of a variety of systemic diseases. Poststreptococcal glomerulonephritis occurs 1 to 2 weeks after a sore throat; it may present solely with hematuria or as a florid nephritic syndrome with hematuria, edema, hypertension, and renal insufficiency. Immunoglobulin A (IgA) nephropathy (Berger disease), thought to be an immune-complex–related disorder, is often asymptomatic, presenting with hematuria and proteinuria several days after an upper respiratory tract infection. Hematologic conditions such as sickle cell disease, sickle-thalassemia, and bleeding dyscrasias; autoimmune disorders; and vasculitides may also present with hematuria. Symptoms of Henoch-Schönlein purpura include arthritis, rash, hematuria, and abdominal pain in children. Goodpasture syndrome, primarily a pulmonary disease, may present as gross hematuria associated with symptoms of hemoptysis, dyspnea, cough, and fatigue in a young adult man. Schistosomiasis, the most common cause of hematuria worldwide, may be present in patients who have lived in or traveled to Africa or the Middle East.

Anticoagulant therapy alone should not be considered a cause of hematuria. One prospective study found that 30% of anticoagulated patients who presented with hematuria had significant urinary tract disease.[18] Similarly, BPH may result in hematuria but should not be assumed to be the cause of bleeding, as many patients have other associated urologic problems of potentially greater significance.[6]

EMERGENCY DEPARTMENT EVALUATION

A common error in the evaluation of hematuria is failing to obtain a complete history and perform a thorough physical examination. The importance of a thorough evaluation is highlighted by the broad list of causes illustrated in Fig. 180.1. The large number of diagnostic possibilities makes the diagnosis of hematuria difficult if it is not approached in a systematic fashion.

As noted, dipstick evaluation is a fast, reliable method to screen for hematuria. Both myoglobinuria and hemoglobinuria present with heme-positive dipstick findings but no red cells on microscopic examination. Hemoglobinuria is usually associated with a characteristic pink color of the serum, whereas myoglobin tends to be cleared from the blood very rapidly. Microscopic urinalysis should be performed to look for formed red and white blood cells and casts. Hematuria of renal origin is classically associated with red cell casts and significant proteinuria; dysmorphic red cells may also be noted. Hematuria arising from the ureters, bladder, and urethra results in the presence of formed erythrocytes in the urine and no proteinuria or casts.

Proteinuria of 100 to 300 mg/dL or more, corresponding to 2+ to 3+ on dipstick analysis, should not be attributed to simple hematuria. It requires evaluation for glomerulonephritis.[2]

The history should address the onset and duration of symptoms, preceding illnesses, level of physical activity, travel history, medication history, and family history of renal, urologic, or hematologic disorders. Hematuria noted on initiation of the urinary stream indicates a possible urethral source, while hematuria only late in the stream suggests a source in the bladder or prostate. Blood noted throughout the entire stream indicates a renal, ureteral, or bladder source. The patient's blood pressure and history of hypertension should be noted, as hypertension is a common indicator of occult renal disease. An abdominal examination should be done to look for suprapubic or flank tenderness, masses, and bruits.

A history and physical examination consistent with renal colic may prompt further evaluation. Available diagnostic modalities include an intravenous pyelogram (IVP), a non–contrast-enhanced helical computed tomography (CT) scan, or an ultrasound to search for calculi, obstruction, or dilatation of the ureter or renal pelvis. Non–contrast-enhanced helical CT has

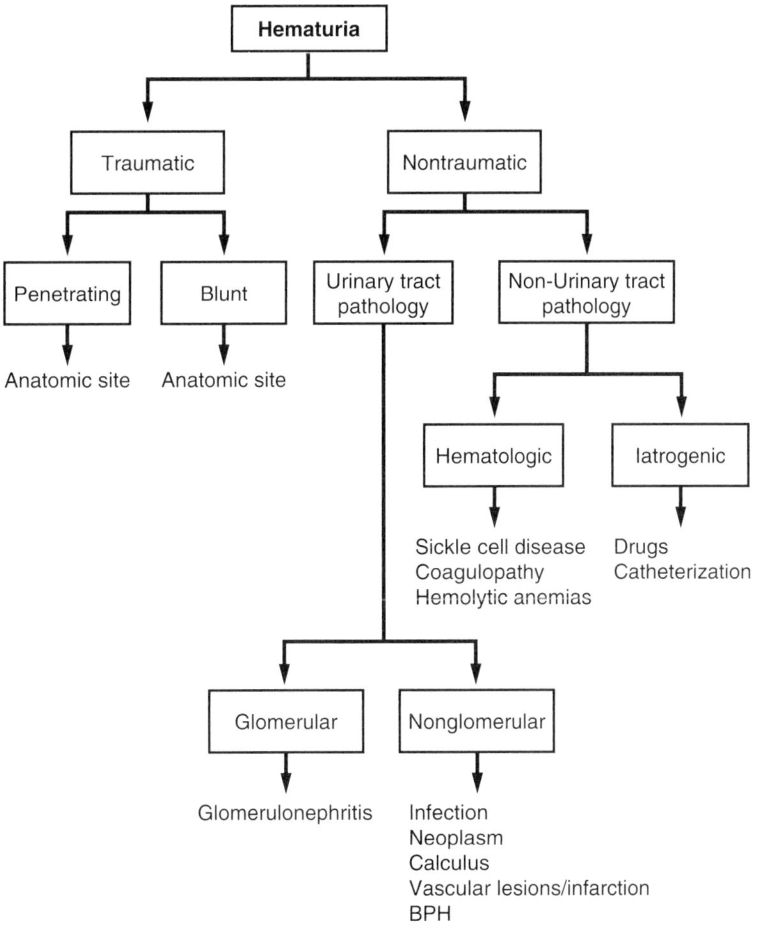

Figure 180.1. Causes of hematuria.

been shown to be an excellent tool for the evaluation of nephrolithiasis. The potential nephrotoxicity associated with intravenous contrast material is eliminated, making this the imaging study of choice in patients with renal disease. CT can also define other abdominal abnormalities, such as abdominal aortic aneurysm or masses involving the kidneys or urinary tract.[17,19] CT can delineate renal vascular pathology, but the definitive diagnosis usually requires arteriography or venography.

EMERGENCY DEPARTMENT MANAGEMENT AND DISPOSITION

The need for acute management of hematuria is limited. Nontraumatic hematuria does not cause life-threatening bleeding, with the rare exception of spontaneous rupture of a renal artery aneurysm or renal infarction secondary to an arterial embolus.[4] In these two conditions, aggressive fluid resuscitation and close hemodynamic monitoring are necessary.

Further evaluation, necessary for patients with asymptomatic hematuria, can usually be performed on an elective basis in consultation with a primary care physician, urologist, or nephrologist. The emergency department evaluation may be supplemented later by cystoscopy, IVP, CT scanning, and renal biopsy, depending on the laboratory and clinical presentation.[12] The patient should be counseled on the risk of significant disease, particularly with increasing age. Management of patients at risk for neoplasm may change dramatically, as rapid immunochromatographic qualitative assays for detection of transitional cell tumors become readily available.[10,13]

Patients in pain, like that due to renal calculi, should be given parenteral analgesics before the diagnosis is established. Patients with renal calculi should be admitted if they have uncontrolled pain, protracted vomiting, obstruction of a solitary kidney, or evidence of significant associated infection.[14] Relative indications for admission include high-grade ureteral obstruction, a large calculus, or preexisting impaired renal function. Urologic consultation should be requested for these patients.

When uncomplicated infection is the cause of hematuria, patients may be treated on an outpatient basis. For more seriously ill patients, intravenous antibiotics should be started promptly. Admission should be strongly considered for infected patients with malignancy, diabetes mellitus, in-dwelling Foley catheters, or known stone disease.

Patients with newly diagnosed or suspected disease of the renal vessels should be admitted to an intensive care unit, with surgical consultation. Patients with hematuria associated with glomerulonephritis are often admitted if the diagnosis is new or if the risk of complications (e.g., severe hypertension, oliguria, volume overload, pulmonary edema, or electrolyte imbalance) is thought to be significant.

COMMON PITFALLS

- Attributing hematuria to a benign condition that may be an incidental finding (e.g., BPH) may result in a serious misdiagnosis, particularly in patients over age 40.
- Ruling out nephrolithiasis because of a negative urine dipstick examination

- Failing to perform a complete history and physical examination to identify possible systemic causes of hematuria
- Failure to ensure follow-up for patients with hematuria, particularly those over age 40

References

1. Arbarbanel J, et al. Sports hematuria. *J Urol* 1990;143:887.
2. Brenner CB. Evaluation of the urologic patient history, physical examination and urinalysis. In: Walsh PL, et al., eds. *Campbell's urology,* 7th ed. Philadelphia: WB Saunders, 1998.
3. Britton JP, et al. A community study of bladder screening by the detection of occult urinary bleeding. *J Urol* 1992;148:788.
4. Driscoll CE. Hematuria. *Emerg Decis* 1985;1:35.
5. Gleeson MJ, et al. Comparison of reagent strip (dipstick) and microscopic haematuria in urologic out-patients. *Br J Urol* 1993;72:594.
6. Golin AL, Howard RS. Asymptomatic microscopic hematuria. *J Urol* 1980;124:389.
7. Kasiske BL, Keane WF. Laboratory assessment of renal disease: clearance, urinalysis, and renal biopsy. In: Brenner BM, ed. *Brenner & Rector's the kidney,* 5th ed. Philadelphia: WB Saunders, 1996.
8. Messing EM, et al. Home screening for hematuria: results of a multi-clinic study. *J Urol* 1992;148:289.
9. Messing EM, et al. Hematuria home screening: repeat testing results. *J Urol* 1995;154:57.
10. Pode D, et al. Noninvasive detection of bladder cancer with the BTA Stat test. *J Urol* 1999;161:443.
11. Press SM, Smith AD. Incidence of negative hematuria in patients with acute urinary lithiasis presenting to the emergency room with flank pain. *Urology* 1995;45:753.
12. Roy S. Hematuria. *Pediatr Rev* 1998;19(6):209.
13. Soloway MS. Do we have a prostate specific antigen for bladder cancer [Editorial]? *J Urol* 1999;161:147.
14. Stewart C. Nephrolithiasis. *Emerg Med Clin North Am* 1988;6:617.
15. Sultana SR, et al. Microscopic haematuria: urological investigation using a standard protocol. *Br J Urol* 1996;78:691.
16. Sutton JM. Evaluation of hematuria in adults. *JAMA* 1990;263:2475.
17. Takahashi N, et al. Ureterolithiasis: can clinical outcome be predicted with unenhanced helical CT? *Radiology* 1998;208:97.
18. Van Savage JG, Fried FA. Anticoagulant associated hematuria: a prospective study. *J Urol* 1995;153:1594.
19. Vieweg J, et al. Unenhanced helical computerized tomography for the evaluation of patients with acute flank pain. *J Urol* 1998;160:679.

PART V
Infectious Disease

CHAPTER 181
Skin and Soft-Tissue Infections

Alexander T. Trott

FOLLICULITIS AND CUTANEOUS ABSCESS

Folliculitis is an inflammation of hair follicles due to infection, overhydration, chemical irritation, or physical injury of the skin.[16] The most common sites of involvement are the apocrine areas of the upper back, chest, buttocks, hips, and axillae, but folliculitis can occur in any hair-bearing region of the body. The most common infecting organism is *Staphylococcus aureus,* but streptococci and gram-negative organisms are implicated in many cases. *Pseudomonas aeruginosa* has been reported after exposure to hot tubs as well as ordinary baths and showers.[3] The individual lesion of folliculitis is a 2- to 5-mm dome-shaped pustule with a central hair shaft surrounded by a rim of erythema. Superficial folliculitis is often primarily pruritic rather than painful, and heals without scarring. If inflammation progresses deeper into the follicle, pain and tenderness develop, and scar formation is more likely to occur with healing.

Pseudofolliculitis is a foreign-body reaction caused by close shaving in persons of African descent. The hair shaft becomes trapped below the follicle exit, and, because of its propensity for tight curling, grows into the follicular wall. Sycosis barbae is a deep infectious progression of pseudofolliculitis that, if untreated, can lead to significant facial scarring.

An untreated follicular infection, or one that does not resolve on its own, can evolve into a *furuncle* or *carbuncle*.[8] Furuncles are single, deep cutaneous nodules involving the hair follicle. These nodules often go on to suppurate. The bacteriology is the same as that of folliculitis. Carbuncles are formed by multiple interconnecting furuncles that drain through several skin openings. Common locations of carbuncles include the chin, back of the neck, and scalp.

Cutaneous *abscesses* can originate in any part of the body through local breaks in the skin. Patients with conditions such as diabetes, inflammatory bowel disease, and immune disorders are at greater risk. Involvement of the head and neck is often due to obstruction and infection of a sebaceous gland or cystic acne. Pure *S. aureus* is cultured in 25% of abscesses; streptococci, gram-negative organisms, and anaerobes are recovered in other cases, often as polymicrobial cultures.[3] Approximately 5% of abscesses are sterile, most commonly in association with parenteral drug abuse.[14]

A cutaneous abscess presents as a red, painful, usually fluctuant mass. The patient typically experiences discomfort and swelling for several days before presentation for care. Systemic symptoms (fever, chills, tachycardia, malaise) are unusual but can occur if the abscess is extensive, is surrounded by significant cellulitis, or extends along a mucous membrane such as the rectum or oral cavity.

Cutaneous abscesses are frequently associated with other conditions. Hidradenitis suppurativa is a recurrent, suppurative, and scarring disease of the apocrine glands, most commonly involving the axillae and pubic regions of persons of African descent. Their greater concentration of apocrine glands leaves these persons more susceptible to infection from chemicals (deodorants, depilatories), trauma (shaving), or poor hygiene. Hidradenitis can be divided into acute and chronic phases. In the acute phase, when burning and itching predominate, single abscesses can develop. In the chronic phase, sinus formation and honeycombed scarring can be seen. Multiple and recurring abscesses are not uncommon.

Abscesses of the buttock and perineum can arise from multiple sources.[1,3] An abscess in the proximal buttock crease is often associated with pilonidal disease. This condition generally afflicts hirsute young males, but its origins are unclear.[16] Ingrown hair or, possibly, congenital remnants of hair follicles and squamous epithelium at the sacrococcygeal junction predispose to abscess formation.

When an abscess arises close to the anus, careful differentiation has to be made between a true perianal and a simple buttock lesion. Perianal abscesses originate from anal crypts, are very painful on rectal examination, and are often associated with systemic symptoms such as fever, malaise, and anorexia.[13] If left untreated, they can dissect proximally into the ischiorectal space and become perirectal abscesses. Recurrent or persistent buttock and perianal abscesses can originate from fistulous tracts created by inflammatory bowel disease.

Bartholin gland abscess is a common problem that can arise from duct obstruction and infection with vaginal flora. The Bartholin glands are located within the vaginal vestibule at the 4 o'clock and 8 o'clock positions. A cyst or infection manifests as a mass medial to and often including the labium minus. The predominant organisms are anaerobic, including *Bacteroides fragilis* and peptostreptococci, and are associated with a variety of gram-negative enteric organisms in mixed culture. Ten percent to 15% of these abscesses are due to *Neisseria gonorrhoeae*.[9]

DIFFERENTIAL DIAGNOSIS

When considering folliculitis, the differential diagnosis includes impetigo, cutaneous fungal infections, skin infestations (scabies), insect bites, and viral disorders (herpesvirus). The lesions of a systemic bacterial infection (*P. aeruginosa* and *N. gonorrhoeae*) can appear like scattered follicular disease. Abscesses have to be differentiated from other nodular lesions, such as uninfected cutaneous cysts, malignant tumors, nodular fungal lesions, and foreign-body granulomas.

EMERGENCY DEPARTMENT EVALUATION

When assessing a patient for folliculitis, furuncles, or a cutaneous abscess, the most important differentiation is between those lesions that contain pus and those that do not. Folliculitis and early furuncles are nodular, whereas abscesses have a soft or "fluctuant" center. Fluctuance indicates the presence of pus and, therefore, usually the need for incision and drainage. Buttock and breast abscesses are often mistaken for simple cellulitis because the large amount of fibrous tissue can obscure the presence of fluctuance. Whenever there is doubt, the lesion should be aspirated with an 18-gauge needle attached to a small syringe (3 to 10 mL). If pus is discovered, incision and drainage should follow.

An assessment of underlying conditions is necessary to determine the overall risk to the patient. Patients with diabetes, immunosuppression, blood dyscrasia, altered white blood cell function, or valvular heart disease are at greater risk from cutaneous infections. The presence of systemic signs such as malaise, fever, and tachycardia indicates a more widespread involvement of the cutaneous infection and requires a somewhat more extensive emergency department evaluation.

Gram stain and culture are unnecessary in healthy patients with simple cutaneous abscesses. A stain and culture may be useful, however, in managing patients who are at higher risk, who have systemic signs, or to whom systemic antibiotics have been administered. The results can guide future management decisions, particularly if resolution is slow or inadequate.

EMERGENCY DEPARTMENT MANAGEMENT AND DISPOSITION

Treatment for folliculitis depends on the extent and depth of follicular involvement. For uncomplicated common folliculitis, hot tub folliculitis, and pseudofolliculitis, removing the offending agent and a gentle regimen of once or twice-daily skin cleansing with a mild hand soap often suffices.[15] This regimen can be supplemented by topical applications of antibiotics such as bacitracin and polymyxin B (Polysporin) or mupirocin (Bactroban). If the offending agent is a razor, special commercially available razors (PFB foil-guarded razor, Remington and Norelco electric razors for men of African descent) can be recommended.

If the folliculitis is painful or more extensive and involves the deep portions of the follicle, a 5- to 7-day course of oral antibiotics is added to the aforementioned measures (Table 181.1). Patients with recurrent folliculitis should seek follow-up for consideration of prophylactic measures, such as the prolonged administration of an oral antibiotic or intranasal mupirocin to eliminate an *S. aureus* carrier state.[5]

Untreated folliculitis can progress to a furuncle. If the furuncle has yet to suppurate, as demonstrated by the inability to obtain pus on needle aspiration, a regimen of warm soaks and antibiotics is recommended (see Table 181.1). For the buttock and perineal area, warm soaks or sitz baths are recommended at least twice a day. Patients should be seen within 48 to 72 hours for follow-up, at which time, surgical drainage can be performed if the furuncle has suppurated. Carbuncles are more likely to present as obvious suppuration that will require surgical drainage.

Incision and drainage is indicated for most cutaneous abscesses. Appropriate analgesia, sedation, and anesthesia should be provided. For most small (less than 5 cm) superficial abscesses, local anesthesia of the skin over the abscess usually suffices. For very small abscesses, ethyl chloride spray can be followed by immediate incision. Local anesthesia can be supplemented by administering a parenteral opioid before intervention. For large or deep abscesses or those located in particularly sensitive areas, such as the perineal region, consideration can be given to intravenous administration of short-acting sedative and analgesic agents with appropriate monitoring.

Before incision, the abscess is cleansed with povidone–iodine or a similar skin cleanser. The incision is made with a no. 11 surgical blade attached to a knife handle. To provide for maximum drainage and access, the length of the incision should be at least two-thirds the diameter of the actual cavity to allow for digital or gentle instrument probing and disruption of loculations and pockets in the irregularly shaped cavity. Probing is followed by saline irrigation with a soft-tipped catheter attached to a syringe. Probing and irrigation are terminated when the effluent is pus free and blood tinged.

The cavity is lightly packed with gauze tape (one-fourth or one-half in.) to encourage further drainage. Excessive packing can result in obstruction of drainage. A bulky dressing is usually necessary to absorb continuing secretions. The packing can most often be removed at follow-up in 48 to 72 hours. This is followed by a regimen of warm soaks or sitz baths at least two times a day until drainage ceases. An abscess cavity takes 10 to 14 days to heal. Large abscesses take longer to heal and may need to be repacked once or twice at 48-hour intervals.

Special considerations apply to the management of Bartholin abscess. The incision is made on the medial portion of the abscess, close to the vaginal introitus, to avoid excessive bleeding. Instead of gauze packing, a small balloon-tipped (Word) catheter is recommended for drainage.[18] This is followed by once- or twice-daily sitz baths. The catheter is left in place for 4 to 6 weeks to produce epithelialization of the incision and drainage site and to reduce the risk of abscess recurrence.

Early consultation should be considered for patients with facial, perianal, pilonidal, and Bartholin abscesses, as well as infection secondary to parenteral drug abuse. For cosmetic reasons, the approach to drainage of facial abscesses (e.g., needle aspiration, mucosal approach) should be discussed with a consultant. Perianal abscesses often require general anesthesia in an operative setting. Patients with pilonidal and Bartholin disease require appropriate follow-up because of the potential for recurrence. Soft-tissue infections in parenteral drug users can be deceptively extensive and involve the deep soft tissue; these patients are also at risk for systemic and cardiac valvular disease. They often require hospital admission for evaluation and treatment.

Ordinarily, cutaneous abscesses need not be treated with systemic antibiotics.[11] Antibiotics are indicated, however, under certain conditions. Relative indications include systemic toxicity as manifested by fever and chills; cellulitis extending well beyond the abscess cavity; underlying comorbid conditions (e.g., diabetes, immunosuppression); location (e.g., facial, Bartholin gland); and failure to respond to incision and drainage.[1] Table 181.1 lists the possible antibiotic choices for oral outpatient ther-

TABLE 181.1. Oral Antibiotic Regimens for Adults with Uncomplicated Cutaneous Infections

Condition	Antibiotic	Dose	Interval
Folliculitis, furuncles, abscesses, localized cellulitis/ erysipelas	Cephalexin	250–500 mg	q6h
	Dicloxacillin	250–500 mg	q6h
	Erythromycin	250–500 mg	q6h
	Azithromycin	500 mg (day 1); 250 mg (days 2–5)	q24h
Hot tub folliculitis	Ciprofloxacin	250–500 mg	q12h
Bartholin abscess	Ceftriaxone	250 mg IM *plus*	
	Doxycycline	100 mg	b.i.d.

TABLE 181.2. Intravenous Antibiotic Regimens for Adults with Serious or Complicated Cutaneous Infections

Condition	Antibiotic	Dose	Interval
Abscesses	Ampicillin/sulbactam	1.5–3 g	q6h
Cellulitis			
Suspected *Streptococcus/ Staphylococcus*	Cefazolin	1–2 g	q6h
	Erythromycin	500–1,000 mg	q6h
Suspected *Haemophilus influenzae*	Ampicillin/sulbactam	1.5–3 g	q6h
	Cefuroxime	0.75–1.5 g	q8h
	Trimethoprim/sulfamethoxazole	8 mg/kg[a]	q8h
Suspected gram-negative bacteria, diabetes	Ticarcillin/clavulanate	3.0 g	q4–6h
	Clindamycin plus ciprofloxacin	300–900 mg	q8h
		200–400 mg	q12h
Deep cutaneous infections (also, clostridial infections, diagnosis unconfirmed)	Ampicillin/sulbactam	1.5–3 g	q6h
	Ticarcillin/clavulanate	3.0 g	q4–6h
	Clindamycin plus gentamicin	300–900 mg	q8h
		1–1.7 mg/kg	q8h
Clostridial infections (diagnosis confirmed)	Penicillin	4 mU	q4h
	Chloramphenicol	25 mg/kg	q6h

[a]Based on trimethoprim content.

apy. Intravenous antibiotic regimens for patients who require hospitalization are summarized in Table 181.2. The duration of treatment is usually 5 to 7 days.

Manipulation of an abscess can cause bacteremia in 30% of cases but is most relevant in patients with preexisting cardiac valve disease. These patients must be given adequate antibiotic prophylaxis, as recommended by the American Heart Association guidelines, before intervention.[2]

COMMON PITFALLS

- Mistaking an abscess for a small area of cellulitis or a furuncle and failing to carry out needle aspiration
- Making an abscess incision that is too small to permit adequate drainage
- Mistaking a perianal abscess for a buttock abscess
- Removal of the catheter prematurely from a Bartholin abscess
- Failure to consider the possibility of coexisting cardiac valve disease and to provide antibiotic prophylaxis when draining an abscess
- Failure to refer patients with recurrent cutaneous infections for consideration of prophylaxis

CUTANEOUS CELLULITIS

Cellulitis is an acute, spreading infection of the skin and subcutaneous tissue characterized by warmth, swelling, and erythema. It is most often caused by group A *Streptococcus* and *S. aureus*.[15,16] The first sign of common cellulitis is local skin discomfort, which is followed by frank tenderness and erythema. Within 24 hours, there is noticeable expansion of the process, even though the margins themselves are indistinct. The terms *very hot, red,* and *swollen* apply. In many cases, lymphangitis or "streaking" can be observed proximally from the site of cellulitis. Soon afterward, there is involvement of local and regional lymph nodes that become swollen and tender. Ultimately, systemic symptoms such as fever, malaise, and tachycardia can occur. In the preantibiotic era, this progression was known as "blood poisoning" and not uncommonly led to death.

Erysipelas is a distinctive form of cellulitis caused almost exclusively by group A streptococci, although occasional cases are due to *S. aureus*. Erysipelas is most common in infants and young children, but it occurs in adults as well.[17] It can begin as a result of minor skin trauma, surgical intervention, or a preexisting skin condition. In adults, it is likely to occur in the setting of venostasis, lymphedema, diabetes, or alcohol abuse. In contrast to common cellulitis, the lesion of erysipelas is sharply demarcated, indurated, and easily palpable. Characteristically, it is also shiny red. It is usually associated with fever and an elevated white blood cell count. Untreated lesions can form bullae that break down and leave raw, weeping surfaces.

A serious form of cellulitis seen in children, and occasionally in adults, is caused by *Haemophilus influenzae* type B. Although most commonly involving the face and the periorbital tissues, *H. influenzae* cellulitis can also involve the arms and legs. In adults, it may originate as a respiratory infection and then involve the neck and chest. In children, the cellulitis often takes on a blue-red to purple-red appearance. In both adults and children, *H. influenzae* cellulitis is associated with systemic toxicity and a significant risk of sepsis and secondary site involvement.

Aeromonas hydrophila and *Vibrio vulnificus* are two water-related organisms that can cause uncommon forms of cellulitis.[4,6] The skin infection of *A. hydrophila* follows local trauma and exposure to fresh water; early infections are indistinguishable from streptococcal cellulitis but often progress to bullae, abscess formation, and foul-smelling exudate. *V. vulnificus* cellulitis occurs after trauma and exposure to salt water. The infection can range from mild cellulitis to an aggressive infection associated with vesicles, bullae, and myositis that can mimic gas gangrene.

DIFFERENTIAL DIAGNOSIS

Cellulitis can be difficult to distinguish from other cutaneous conditions. The most serious condition to be considered is thrombophlebitis, particularly when the lower extremity is involved. Cellulitis can be differentiated by the presence of fever, lymphangitic streaking, an advancing margin, and an elevated white blood cell count, although these findings are not consistently present.

Viral and drug-related exanthems can be localized, but usually are associated with recognizable precipitants and specific syndromes.

Dermatitis can appear red and somewhat warm but is usually associated with considerable itching and scaling. Secondary infection of dermatitic lesions, however, is not uncommon.

Insect stings, particularly due to *Hymenoptera,* can cause significant local reactions that can be confused with cellulitis, and these reactions can persist up to 7 days.[19] As compared with cellulitis, insect stings produce more pain than tenderness, cause more edema and less erythema, and are pruritic.

Fungal infections of the skin, particularly with *Candida,* appear in characteristic locations (often intertriginous), have a distinctive appearance (moist, bright red), and can be identified by potassium hydroxide staining.

EMERGENCY DEPARTMENT EVALUATION

Common cellulitis and erysipelas, when localized to a small area in an otherwise healthy patient, need no invasive or laboratory testing. With more extensive cellulitis, a white blood cell count is performed to check for signs of systemic involvement and to gauge the severity of infection. Because of the low bacterial count in the lesions of cellulitis, aspiration of the advancing margin for Gram stain and culture yields an organism in only 25% of cases.[12] In any event, these tests do not aid in immediate treatment decisions.

In compromised hosts and in patients in whom *H. influenzae* infection is suspected, a more extensive workup is indicated. The incidence of bacteremia ranges from 5% in toxic streptococcal cellulitis to 90% in *H. influenzae* cellulitis. Gram stain and culture, while of low yield, can be performed in an attempt to identify the causative organism. Older patients and those with underlying conditions such as diabetes or immunocompromised states should be evaluated for metabolic derangements and any evidence of other sites of involvement. Outlining the margins of the cellulitis with a marker can aid in the monitoring and follow-up of patients with cellulitis by indicating lesion progression or regression.

EMERGENCY DEPARTMENT MANAGEMENT AND DISPOSITION

Common, localized cellulitis and mild, uncomplicated erysipelas in patients without risk factors can be treated as outpatients. Oral antibiotics (see Table 181.1) are begun, and close (48- to 72-hour) follow-up is arranged. Antibiotics are continued for 3 days after the resolution of clinical findings (i.e., a total course of 6 to 10 days). (Because of its unique pharmacology, azithromycin is given only for 5 days, however.) Although oral ciprofloxacin is often prescribed as a first-line agent for cellulitis, it has only moderate activity against streptococcal organisms and poor activity against *S. aureus*.

Hospital admission and infectious disease consultation should be considered under the following conditions: when there are signs of systemic toxicity; underlying illnesses such as diabetes; specific involvement of areas such as the face, orbit, hand, perineum, or lower extremity (particularly with preexisting edema); presumed *H. influenzae* infection; or suspected gram-negative organisms or mixed infections. Patients who require admission should be treated with intravenous antibiotics (see Table 181.2).

COMMON PITFALLS

- Failure to instruct the patient about elevation and care of the involved area
- Misdiagnosing deep vein thrombosis as lower extremity cellulitis
- Failure to arrange follow-up in 48 to 72 hours for patients with cellulitis
- Unnecessarily treating insect stings with antibiotics

DEEP CUTANEOUS AND NECROTIZING SOFT-TISSUE INFECTIONS

Deep cutaneous and necrotizing soft-tissue infections often constitute a threat to life and limb, yet they can be deceptively benign in appearance.[10] Early in their clinical course, attempts at separating the various types of infections into discrete syndromes are made difficult by the fact that they share many characteristics. However, it is recognition of these characteristics that alerts the clinician to a potentially emergent condition:

1. These infections occur in settings that include trauma, foreign-body penetration, contamination with soil, surgical intervention, ischemia, or diabetes.
2. Tissue involvement is extensive, but classic signs of common cellulitis (heat, redness, induration) are often not present.
3. As the infection progresses, blebs, maceration, and exudate appear.
4. The hallmark of these infections, which, however, is not always present, is crepitance secondary to gas formation.

Specific deep cutaneous infections are summarized in Table 181.3.

Crepitant cellulitis occurs most commonly in the setting of preexisting, lower extremity, peripheral arterial disease; decubitus ulcer; or a moderately severe traumatic wound. Also known as nonclostridial anaerobic cellulitis, this is a gas-forming infection that results from the synergistic interaction of anaerobic bacteria (*Bacteroides* species and peptostreptococci) and of gram-negative bacteria of enteric origin. In spite of its seriousness, it is usually gradual in onset, with mild local tenderness, and is not likely to cause serious systemic toxicity. In the area of involvement, the skin is minimally discolored and may appear grayish to brown, depending on local vascularity. The exudate, if present, is dark and foul smelling. The hallmark of this infection is crepitance and abundant gas formation, as seen on radiographs. The infection remains localized to the skin and subcutaneous tissues without extending to muscle.

Synergistic necrotizing cellulitis has also been called nonclostridial gangrene and nonclostridial anaerobic myonecrosis. Fournier gangrene of the male genitalia and perineum is a variant of this condition. Synergistic necrotizing cellulitis occurs most often in older patients with serious underlying disease, such as diabetes, congestive heart failure, or renal failure, and in the setting of obesity and perirectal infections. Gram-positive streptococci (both aerobic and anaerobic), gram-negative enteric bacilli, and anaerobes (*B. fragilis*), interacting synergistically, have been implicated in this infection. The onset can be acute or subacute, but the infection rapidly progresses to severe local and systemic toxicity with high fever. There is often severe pain at the site of infection, and the skin is blue-gray. Necrosis of the fascia and muscle occurs. Twenty-five percent of cases have clinical crepitance and gas evident on radiographs. The exudate is thin and foul smelling and has the appearance of dish water. Bacteremia occurs in 50% of cases, and mortality has been reported to be as high as 75%.

Necrotizing fasciitis is predominantly a disease of the subcutaneous tissue and fascia, with early sparing of the skin and very late involvement of the muscle.[17] This condition can occur after trauma or abdominal surgery, or with perirectal infections, cutaneous ulcers, intravenous drug abuse, and infections of the

TABLE 181.3. Deep Cutaneous and Necrotizing Soft-Tissue Infections

Characteristics	Crepitant Cellulitis	Synergistic Necrotizing Cellulitis	Necrotizing Fasciitis	Clostridial Cellulitis	Clostridial Myonecrosis
Predisposing conditions	Wounds, decubiti, peripheral vascular disease, diabetes	Diabetes, obesity, advanced age	Postoperative wounds, perianal infection, chronic cutaneous ulcers, intravenous drug use	Contaminated wound	Devitalized tissue, focal contamination
Onset	Gradual	Subacute, over several days	Variable, indolent to fulminant	Gradual, 4–5 days	Acute, 1–3 days
Pain	Mild	Severe	Minimal, sometimes hypesthesia	Mild	Severe, early
Systemic toxicity	Mild to moderate	Moderate to severe	Marked	Mild to moderate	Marked, early
Overlying skin	Minimal, discoloration brown to gray	Blue-gray, necrosis	Initially spared, then pale followed by gangrene	Minimal change, occasional blebs	Initially normal, then pale bronze discoloration followed by necrosis
Exudate	Minimal, dark	Thin, reddish brown ("dishwater pus")	Rare, serous	Thin, dark	Serosanguinous
Odor	Foul	Foul	Foul	Rarely foul	"Mousy," slightly sweet
Gas formation	Abundant	Mild, up to 25%	Little	Abundant	Initially minimal, eventually moderate
Muscle involvement	No	Prominent feature, moderate spread	Rare, late	No	Prominent
Common pathogens	Anaerobes, Enterobacteriaceae	*Bacteroides fragilis*, streptococci, Enterobacteriaceae	Enterobacteriaceae, streptococci, *Bacteroides*, peptostreptococci	*C. perfringens*, *C. septicum*, *C. novyi*	*C. perfringens*, *C. septicum*, *C. novyi*

From Brillman JC, Quinzer RW, eds. *Infectious disease in emergency medicine*. Boston: Little, Brown and Company. 1992:822–823, with permission.

head and neck. A wide range of organisms, including gram-negative enteric bacilli, gram-positive streptococci (aerobic and anaerobic), and other anaerobes, has been implicated. Although the infection is usually mixed, it can also be caused by single organisms, such as group A *Streptococcus.* The onset is acute, and the patient develops severe systemic toxicity. In the early stages, the skin appears erythematous and is minimally painful. Later, as the subcutaneous tissue becomes involved, there is mottling, discoloration, marked edema, and bleb formation as a result of interruption of the blood supply to the skin. The exudate is foul smelling and seropurulent, but not abundant. Although gas can be seen on radiographs, clinical crepitance is unusual.

Clostridial cellulitis, also known as clostridial anaerobic cellulitis, is most commonly a result of traumatic wounds. The presence of foreign debris, soil, and necrotic tissue allows rapid growth of clostridial organisms, including *C. perfringens, C. septicum,* and *C. novyi.* It is distinguished from clostridial myonecrosis (gas gangrene) by the lack of muscle involvement. Unlike gas gangrene, the onset is gradual, and systemic toxicity is only mild to moderate. Skin changes are minimal, but there is a thin, dark, occasionally foul-smelling exudate at the site of the wound. The most prominent feature of the wound site is crepitance and gas formation that often extends well beyond the actual area of cellulitis. The gas tends to appear on a radiograph as aggregates of bubbles in the subcutaneous tissues.

Clostridial myonecrosis, or gas gangrene, almost always results from a deep injury to skeletal muscle that causes ischemia and tissue necrosis. The same organisms that cause clostridial cellulitis are responsible for this disorder. The incubation period can range from 7 hours to 6 weeks,[10] but once symptoms begin, severe deterioration can occur within 6 hours. Muscle swelling and severe pain are prominent features. Systemic toxicity, as a result of the many toxins elaborated by the clostridial organisms, is profound and leads to tachycardia and an altered sensorium, although fever is not a prominent feature. The involved skin has a yellow or bronze appearance, and the skin involvement progresses to bulla formation and green or black patches of necrosis. A serosanguineous discharge can develop with a characteristic "mousy" odor. Gas formation is minimal at the onset but extends throughout the muscle in a feathery pattern as it dissects through muscle fibers and bundles. Intravascular hemolysis, with thrombocytopenia, is often present. *These patients can die within hours.*

DIFFERENTIAL DIAGNOSIS

There is little difficulty in recognizing the picture of full-blown deep cutaneous and necrotizing soft-tissue infections. Occasionally, they can be confused with such conditions as dry ischemic vascular gangrene, pressure necrosis of a limb, acute deep venous thrombosis, and preexisting changes of venous insufficiency. Air can be introduced into the skin by traumatic lacerations and occasionally can cause some diagnostic concern.

It is important to emphasize, however, that these infections can be missed when they are not full blown. This is where difficulty can arise for the patient presenting to the emergency department in the early stages of infection.

EMERGENCY DEPARTMENT EVALUATION

The presence of a suspected deep cutaneous infection mandates an extensive and aggressive evaluation. This must be initiated promptly and carried out while any resuscitative or stabilizing interventions are in progress. Standard hematologic, biochemical, and clotting profiles are obtained, as well as arterial blood gas studies, a chest radiograph, and an electrocardiogram. A type and crossmatch may be indicated to correct blood loss or anemia.

A wound culture is taken and a Gram stain performed immediately, particularly if a clostridial etiology is suspected. The presence on Gram stain of gram-positive rods with few white blood cells indicates a clostridial infection. A finding of many white blood cells on the smear is more suggestive of a synergistic or mixed bacterial infection. Radiographs of anatomic areas of concern are obtained to look for soft-tissue gas. Because the infection can advance up to 6 in. an hour, the area of involvement should be outlined with a marker and checked at frequent intervals.

EMERGENCY DEPARTMENT MANAGEMENT AND DISPOSITION

Because it can progress so rapidly, clostridial myonecrosis is a true emergency. Concurrent with emergency department evaluation, planning and execution of intervention is carried out in consultation with a surgeon. A combination of hyperbaric oxygen (HBO), surgery, and antibiotics provides optimal treatment.[7] If immediately available, HBO is initiated to arrest the advance of the hemolytic, necrotizing, and potentially lethal tissue toxins. HBO produces a tissue level of 300 mm Hg, which is 50 mm Hg in excess of that required to cause bacteriostasis and halt production of tissue toxins. HBO significantly reduces the need for extensive debridement and amputation and assists the surgeon in demarcating clearly necrotic from viable tissue. If necessary, however, a fasciotomy can be performed before HBO is done in order to relieve compartmental swelling and pressure.

In clear cases of clostridial myonecrosis or cellulitis, high-dose penicillin is still the antibiotic of first choice. Chloramphenicol can be used in β-lactam–sensitive patients. If the diagnosis is uncertain, the antibiotics listed in Table 181.2 are also appropriate choices. Antitoxin therapy has never proven efficacious.

The primary treatment for other deep cutaneous infections consists of antibiotics and surgical intervention.[10] Patients with an immunocompromised state or rapidly spreading infection can significantly benefit from adjunctive HBO; this intervention should be considered for all patients with these infections, especially Fournier gangrene.[7] Broad-spectrum antibiotics are usually initiated empirically in the emergency department (see Table 181.2).

COMMON PITFALLS

- Failure to recognize a deep cutaneous infection because of a lack of classic skin changes of cellulitis
- Failure to perform a Gram stain in the emergency department
- Failure to take radiographs and thus missing subcutaneous gas
- Initiating only limited-spectrum antibiotics
- Delaying surgical consultation
- Failure to consider HBO therapy early in the patient's management

References

1. Centers for Disease Control. 1998 Guidelines for treatment of sexually transmitted diseases. *MMWR* 1998;47(RR-1):53.
2. Dajani AS, Taubert KA, Wilson, et al. Prevention of bacterial endocarditis: recommendations by the American Heart Association. *JAMA* 1997;274:1794.
3. Feingold FS, Hirschmann JV, Leyden JJ. Bacterial infections of the skin. *J Am Acad Dermatol* 1989;20:469.
4. Gold WL, Salit IE. Aeromonas hydrophila infections of the skin and soft tissue: report of eleven cases. *Clin Infect Dis* 1993;16:69.
5. Hedstrom SA. Treatment and prevention of recurrent staphylococcal furunculosis: clinical and bacteriologic follow-up. *Scand J Infect Dis* 1985;17:55.
6. Howard RJ, Lieb S. Soft tissue infections caused by halophilic marine vibrios. *Arch Surg* 1988;123:245.
7. *Hyperbaric oxygen therapy: a committee report.* Camporesi M, chairman. Bethesda, MD: Undersea and Hyperbaric Medicine Society, 1996:10, 31.
8. Ko WT, Adal KA, Tomecki KJ. Infectious diseases. *Med Clin North Am* 1998;82:1001.
9. Lee YH, Rankin JS, Alpert S, et al. Microbiological investigation of Bartholin's gland abscesses and cysts. *Am J Obstet Gynecol* 1977;129:150.
10. Lewis RT. Soft tissue infections. *World J Surg* 1998;22:146.
11. Llera J, Levy RC. Treatment of cutaneous abscesses: a double-blind study. *Ann Emerg Med* 1985;14:57.
12. Lutomski DM, Trott AT, Runyon JM, et al. Microbiology of adult cellulitis. *J Fam Pract* 1988;26:45.
13. Marcus R, Stine R, Cohen M. Perirectal abscess. *Ann Emerg Med* 1995;25:597.
14. Meislin HW. Pathogen identification of abscesses and cellulitis. *Ann Emerg Med* 1986;15:329.
15. O'Dell M. Skin and wound infections: an overview. *Am Fam Physician* 1998;57:2424.
16. Sadick NS. Current aspects of bacterial infections of the skin. *Dermatol Clin* 1997;15:341.
17. Stone DR, Gorbach SL. Necrotizing fascitis: the changing spectrum. *Infect Dis Dermatol* 1997;15:213.
18. Woodruff JD, Friedrick EG. The vestibule. *Clin Obstet Gynecol* 1985;28:134.
19. Zuckerberg AL, Schweich PJ. An arm red and hot: infection or not? *Pediatr Emerg Care* 1990;6:275.

CHAPTER 182
Tetanus

James J. Mathews and Kaveh Ilkhanipour

Tetanus is a rare disease in the United States, having an incidence of less than one case per million per year. The current rate may increase in the future, as more than 10% of the population is not adequately immunized, including immigrants from underdeveloped countries, elderly patients who have lost immunity, and an increasing population of immunocompromised patients who do not have an adequate response to routine immunization.[1,4,5,8]

Many countries do not mandate routine immunization, and, in these areas, this disease remains a major public health problem. Most deaths in underdeveloped areas result from the neonatal form of tetanus, and are secondary to unhygienic practices involving the umbilical stump and circumcision.[2,12] When immunization is mandated and hygienic practices are used, this disease is virtually eliminated.[11,15]

Tetanus is caused by *Clostridium tetani,* an organism with worldwide distribution in soil and feces.[7] *C. tetani* is a gram-positive, spore-forming organism with a characteristic drumstick appearance. The organism is motile and is an obligate anaerobe. Although *C. tetani* is killed by heat and various antiseptic agents, its spores are highly resistant and survive in extremely hostile environments.

The clinical syndrome of tetanus develops when *C. tetani* is introduced into the body and the spores germinate and multiply. Proliferation occurs only in anaerobic conditions. Tetanus-prone wounds are wounds with foreign debris or necrotic tissue, or wounds that have been heavily contaminated with soil or feces.

Once established, *C. tetani* releases two exotoxins, tetanolysin and tetanospasmin. Tetanolysin causes hemolysis *in vitro*, but appears to have little clinical effect. Tetanospasmin produces the signs and symptoms of tetanus, and is one of the most potent neurotoxins known. This toxin diffuses into local tissue and eventually into the bloodstream. Tetanospasmin is taken up preferentially by motor neurons, with little initial effect on neuronal function. When the toxin crosses the cleft to presynaptic spinal inhibitory interneurons, decreased amounts of inhibitory substances are released. This effect results in increased muscle tone, decreased coordination, and simultaneous contractions of agonist and antagonist muscle groups, producing tetanic spasms.

CLINICAL PRESENTATION

Tetanus is clinically divided into four separate types. Generalized tetanus, the most common, presents with generalized skeletal muscle spasm. Localized tetanus is associated with persistent localized muscle rigidity at the site of spore inoculation. This can often be a prodrome to the development of generalized tetanus. Cephalic tetanus is characterized by localized involvement of the cranial musculature. Finally, neonatal tetanus presents within the first several weeks of life as generalized tetanus secondary to infection of the umbilical stump.

Tetanus generally occurs 10 to 15 days after injury, and the clinical signs arise over a 2- to 5-day period.[7] The length of time between the initial symptoms and the development of the first generalized spasm is a reliable prognostic indicator. Patients tend to have severe disease if the time of onset of generalized spasms is less than 48 hours. The most common presenting symptom is trismus. Associated complaints may be pain or stiffness of the neck, excessive pain in the injured area, and dysphagia. Rarely, tetanic spasms are the initial manifestation.

As the disease progresses, more muscle groups are involved, and the spasms become exquisitely painful. The effect on the back muscles is extremely profound; tetanic spasms of this muscle group produces opisthotonos, in which only the back of the head and the heels rest on the bed. The violence of these spasms can be so severe as to completely rupture the rectus abdominalis muscles and to fracture vertebrae. Spasms may involve the muscles of respiration, producing a fixed chest wall and eventual asphyxia.

Systemic symptoms in mild cases are often minimal, but, in severe cases, marked autonomic disturbances are seen, with tachycardia, wide swings in blood pressure, hyperpyrexia, and cardiac dysrhythmias. These manifestations appear to be due to excessive catecholamine release and are the most common cause of death from tetanus.[7,13] Trivial stimuli may trigger not only severe spasms, but also wide swings in vital signs.

DIFFERENTIAL DIAGNOSIS

The only differential diagnosis for the established case of tetanus is strychnine poisoning. Muscle spasms associated with strychnine poisoning may resemble those of tetanus, but there are several important differences. The muscles of the jaw are not involved early in the course of strychnine poisoning or may be spared completely. In tetanus, the jaw muscles are involved early in the course, and trismus is almost always present. Also, in a patient with strychnine poisoning, muscle rigidity disappears completely between spasms.

The early stages of tetanus may be confused with psychoneurotic complaints and with dystonic reactions from such agents as phenothiazines. Dystonic reactions can be rapidly and safely treated, and therefore ruled out, by the administration of benztropine or diphenhydramine. Dental infections may produce trismus, but there is no progression, and signs of local infection are almost always present.

EMERGENCY DEPARTMENT EVALUATION

Laboratory testing is of little value in diagnosing tetanus.[9] Routine studies should be obtained, including blood cell counts, electrolyte levels, a chest x-ray, an electrocardiogram (ECG), arterial blood gases, and a vital capacity. Vital capacity and arterial blood gas analysis should be done at frequent intervals to ensure that the patient does not progress to ventilatory failure. If the vital capacity is less than 50% of predicted, paralysis and mechanical ventilation are indicated.[13]

The site of infection should be located, and appropriate treatment initiated. It must be remembered that a skin wound is not required for tetanus to occur. In underdeveloped countries, otitis media is a common source of *C. tetani* infection. Other sources include the tonsillar crypts, the lower gastrointestinal tract, septic abortion, and chronic wounds. Superficial abrasions and burns, and even corneal lesions, have been implicated in the development of tetanus.

EMERGENCY DEPARTMENT MANAGEMENT

The management of tetanus is supportive and symptomatic.[7,13,14] Initial attention should always be directed toward the establishing and supporting of an adequate airway, which may require rapid-sequence orotracheal intubation using a sedative and a paralytic agent. Benzodiazepines should be initiated in an aggressive fashion to help minimize muscle spasm and rigidity.[3] Large doses of intravenous (i.v.) diazepam, lorazepam, or midazolam are generally required. When benzodiazepines are not effective in controlling muscle spasms, generalized motor paralysis with nondepolarizing neuromuscular blocking agents such as pancuronium or vecuronium should be considered.

Autonomic instability secondary to sympathetic overactivity should also be monitored and treated aggressively. Agents providing both α- and β-adrenergic blockade (e.g., labetalol) are optimal in this setting.[6] Hypertension refractory to labetalol can be treated with a titratable agent such as sodium nitroprusside. Patients who are hypotensive should receive i.v. crystalloids and pressors, as needed. Bradydysrhythmia should be treated with cardiac pacing.

Human tetanus immunoglobulin (TIG) should be given (1,000 U i.v. and 2000 U intramuscularly). Antibiotic therapy with penicillin (4 million U i.v. every 6 hours), tetracycline (250 mg i.v. every 6 hours), metronidazole (500 mg orally every 6 hours), or erythromycin (500 mg i.v. every 6 hours) should be initiated. Wounds should be surgically debrided after i.v. instillation of TIG so that any toxin that is released by debridement is bound. An attack of tetanus does not provide immunity. Active immunization should be done during the recovery period.

DISPOSITION

Any patient with tetanus should be admitted to the intensive care unit. Although mild cases can be managed in the community setting, the patient with moderate-to-severe disease should be transferred to a tertiary care facility. As the degree of severity is difficult to predict in the early stages of the disease, it is reasonable to transfer all patients with this diagnosis to a tertiary care center. In a review of 106 cases of tetanus in Victoria, Australia, the most important element identified in the management of these patients was the level of nursing care and expertise,[13] especially for those patients with long-term paralysis requiring mechanical ventilation.

Where this practice has been instituted, the mortality rate from tetanus has been reduced to 10%. Patients with suspected tetanus should be accompanied during transport by personnel skilled in advanced cardiac life support and airway management. The airway should be secured before transfer if the patient is showing a decreasing vital capacity or if transfer is delayed or will be of long duration.

PREVENTION

The most important factors in the reduction of tetanus have been the enforcement of mandated immunization, improved hygiene, and better wound management.[10,15] The emergency physician can affect all of these areas. All wounds should be carefully cleansed and debrided. Antibiotic prophylaxis should be given when indicated. Patients should receive careful instructions as to wound management and how to avoid wound contamination.

Appropriate tetanus prophylaxis should be given (Fig. 182.1). In many patients, particularly those who have migrated to the United States from underdeveloped countries, it is safest to give both the toxoid and TIG. Immunocompromised and certain elderly patients should also receive both agents.

Many patients claim that they are allergic to the toxoid because they previously experienced a local reaction at the site of the injection. This type of reaction is not an allergic response, and it is safe to administer the toxoid. Patients with a true allergy to the toxoid should be given TIG and antibiotic prophylaxis. This treatment does not impart lasting immunity, but it will prevent the development of tetanus. The allergic patient should be referred to an allergist for desensitization and immunization.

Some patients may refuse to receive tetanus toxoid because they have read of severe neurologic disorders occurring after injection of it, either alone or in combination with other products. Careful epidemiologic studies have not conclusively demonstrated this association.[16] If, after discussion, the patient remains unwilling to receive the toxoid, TIG and appropriate prophylaxis should be given and referral made to the patient's personal physician to discuss adequate immunization.

COMMON PITFALLS

- It is unlikely that a full-blown case of tetanus will go unrecognized. Early cases may be misdiagnosed as a psychoneurotic disorder or dystonic reaction. Careful history and physical examinations will avoid this error.
- Even though tetanus is a rare disorder in the United States, the causative organism, *C. tetani*, is ubiquitous in the environment. Every wound must be considered as possibly contaminated.
- Prevention of tetanus is a responsibility of the emergency physician. Tetanus immunization status should be documented on all patients with wounds, and appropriate prophylaxis given (see Fig. 182.1).

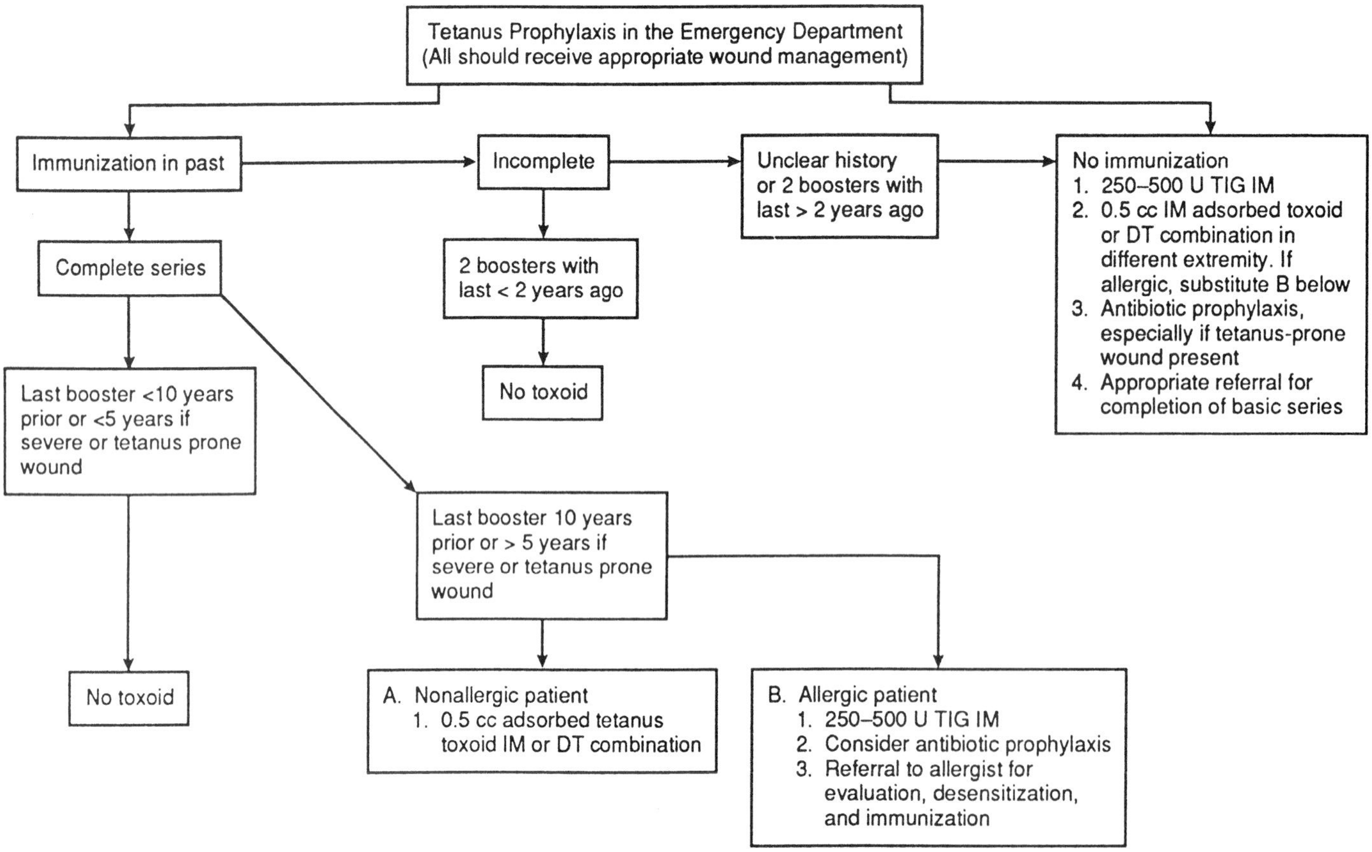

Figure 182.1. Appropriate tetanus prophylaxis.

References

1. Aggerbeck H. Vaccination against diphtheria and tetanus. Assays, antigens, adjuvants and application. *APMIS Supplementum* 1998;81:1.
2. Alemu W. Neonatal tetanus mortality survey, north and south Omo administrative regions, Ethiopia. *Ethiop Med J* 1993;31(3):99.
3. Bleck TP. Tetanus. *Dis Mon* 1991;37:547.
4. Cutts FT. Advances and challenges for the expanded programme on immunization. *Br Med Bull* 1998;54(2):445.
5. Dietz V, Galazka A, van Loon F, et al. Factors affecting the immunogenicity and potency of tetanus toxoid: implications for the elimination of neonatal and non-natal tetanus as public health problems. *Bull World Health Organ* 1997;75(1):81.
6. Domenghetti GM, Savary S, Striker H. Hyperadresurgic syndrome in severe tetanus responsive to labetalol. *BMJ* 1984;288:1483–1484.
7. Ernst ME, Klepser ME, Fouts M, et al. Tetanus: pathophysiology and management. *Ann Pharmacother* 1997;31(12):1507.
8. Groleau G. Tetanus. *Emerg Med Clin North Am* 1992;10:351.
9. Henderson SO, Mody T, Grotg DE, et al. The presentation of tetanus in an emergency department. *J Emerg Med* 1998;16(5):705.
10. Kanegaye JT. A rational approach to the outpatient management of lacerations in pediatric patients. *Curr Probl Pediatr* 1998;28(7):205.
11. Kessler ER. Vaccine-preventable diseases in health care. *Occup Med* 1997;12(4):731.
12. Kurtoglu S, Caksen H, Ozturk A, et al. A review of 207 newborn with tetanus. *J Pakistan Med Assoc* 1998;48(4):93.
13. Newton-John HF. Tetanus in Victoria, 1957–1980. *Med J Aust* 1984;140:1.
14. Sanders RK. The management of tetanus. *Trop Doct* 1996;26(3):107.
15. Thayaparan B, Nicoll A. Prevention and control of tetanus in childhood. *Curr Opin Pediatr* 1998;10(1):4.
16. Wentz KR, Marcuse EK. Diphtheria-tetanus-pertussis vaccine and seroneurologic illness: an updated review of the epidemiologic evidence. *Pediatrics* 1991;87:287.

CHAPTER 183
Meningitis and Encephalitis

Raymond J. Roberge and Richard Mark Kaplan

Meningitis and encephalitis are infectious and inflammatory processes occurring in the leptomeninges (meningitis), brain structures (encephalitis), or both (leptomeningitis). These disorders are discussed together because of considerable clinical and etiologic overlap.

By convention, meningitis is classified as either bacterial or, when due to any other cause, the aseptic meningitis syndrome. Untreated bacterial meningitis carries a mortality rate of greater than 90%. The aseptic meningitis syndrome, a generally self-limited symptom complex of fever, headache, and nuchal rigidity with characteristic cerebrospinal fluid (CSF) findings (lymphocytosis, variable protein elevation, and normal glucose), is primarily of viral origin. Aseptic meningitis may have many other causes, however, including certain bacteria (*Mycobacterium tuberculosis, Leptospira* species, *Treponema pallidum, Borrelia* species, *Nocardia,* and partially treated pyogenic infections), fungi, rickettsiae, *Mycoplasma,* parasites, parameningeal infections, malignancy, autoimmune diseases, and miscellaneous causes, such as intrathecal injections, heavy metal poisonings, nonsteroidal antiinflammatory agents, and antibiotics. With the advent of the acquired immunodeficiency syndrome (AIDS) epidemic and the growing numbers of other immunosuppressed individuals in the population, emergency physicians are more likely to see meningitis secondary to some of these previously rarer causes.

Although rapid diagnostic tests and effective antimicrobial agents are available, case fatality rates of greater than 20% are noted for bacterial meningitis in the United States, and significant residual neurologic deficit is noted in many survivors.[19] Early diagnosis and the rapid institution of appropriate antimicrobial therapy are the keys to decreasing this significant morbidity and mortality. Emergency physicians are often the first clinicians to evaluate the patient with meningitis, and their diagnostic acumen may have a significant impact on the ultimate clinical course of this disorder. Nonetheless, a review by a major medical malpractice insurance carrier has identified the missed diagnosis of bacterial meningitis as accounting for 9.4% of all malpractice dollar claims against emergency physicians.[9]

Two bacterial species, *Streptococcus pneumoniae* and *Neisseria meningitidis,* currently account for approximately three-fourths of all cases of bacterial meningitis.[19] *S. pneumoniae* is the most common agent in adults. *N. meningitidis,* responsible for up to 30% of cases of meningitis, is most frequently noted in children and adolescents but accounts for only 10% of bacterial meningitis in patients older than 45 years of age. *Listeria monocytogenes* is implicated in 5% of cases and is generally found in elderly or immunocompromised individuals. *Haemophilus influenzae,* previously a significant cause of childhood meningitis prior to institution of type B vaccine, is responsible for 1% to 3% of adult meningitis. Staphylococcal species and gram-negative bacilli are rarer causes of meningitis in adults. Meningitis due to anaerobic species is quite rare; its presence should suggest brain abscess.[16]

Although the aseptic meningitis syndrome remains overwhelmingly a disorder of viral etiology, with enteroviruses and the mumps virus accounting for more than 85% of reported cases,[18] it is important to bear in mind the numerous other causes of this syndrome, because many are amenable to antimicrobial therapy. With polioviruses and herpes simplex as notable exceptions, most viral meningitides are relatively benign, whereas some nonviral causes of the aseptic meningitis syndrome (e.g., syphilis, tuberculosis) are capable of causing significant morbidity and mortality.

Risk factors associated with meningitis include age (the very old and the very young), gender (men more often than women), nasopharyngeal colonization, chronic disease, immunosuppression, and lower socioeconomic status. Specific host risk factors may offer a clue to likely pathogens. For pneumococcal meningitis, risk factors include certain infectious processes (e.g., otitis, sinusitis, pneumonia), trauma (head injury), and immunocompromised states (e.g., sickle cell disease, Hodgkin disease, immunoglobulin deficiency, renal or bone marrow transplantation).

Overcrowded living conditions (e.g., college dormitories, military barracks, skid rows) and poverty increase the risk of contracting meningococcal meningitis. Close association with victims of meningococcal meningitis increases the risk of developing this illness by a factor of 500 to 800. Risk factors for listerial meningitis include the immunocompromised state and the ingestion of *Listeria*-contaminated foods. Adults who develop *H. influenzae* meningitis should be evaluated for anatomic defects such as dermal sinus tracts, previous head trauma with CSF leaks, or infectious processes (e.g., otitis, sinusitis).

Staphylococcal infection should be suspected in patients who have sustained penetrating skull injuries or who have undergone neurologic or otolaryngologic procedures. Gram-negative meningitis is noted after neurosurgical procedures or in association with other nosocomial infections. Chronic immunosuppression from a variety of causes, including human immunodeficiency virus (HIV) infection and organ transplantation, is an increasingly recognized risk factor for fungal meningitis. Because the majority of reported cases of viral meningitis are due to enteroviruses, and because these are spread by the oral–fecal route, poor hygienic habits are associated with an increased risk. The viral inoculum size is also an important risk factor.[25]

Acute encephalitis is generally a viral-related illness in which the brain matter (cerebral hemispheres, brainstem, or cerebellum) is injured either as a direct result of viral invasion or as a hypersensitivity reaction to a systemic viral illness. Occasionally, encephalitis occurs shortly after vaccination for measles, rubella, chickenpox, or rabies and is thought to represent a disordered immune reaction.

Although the list of viral agents capable of causing encephalitis is extensive, in North America enteroviruses, arboviruses, herpes simplex, mumps, and lymphocytic choriomeningitis account for the overwhelming majority of cases. Many other agents (e.g., rickettsiae, bacteria, fungi, parasites) and disorders (e.g., neoplasia, vascular disease, sarcoid, Behçet syndrome) can also cause encephalitic syndromes.

Increasingly, HIV encephalitis is being recognized. In 1991, 1103 cases of encephalitis were reported to the Centers for Disease Control,[5] but these figures reflect such factors as underreporting or the inherent difficulty in differentiating mild acute encephalitis from aseptic meningitis. The diagnosis of encephalitis should be considered in all patients who present with fever, headache, nuchal rigidity, and such neurologic findings as altered level of consciousness, seizures, or focal neurologic signs. The overall mortality rate for acute viral encephalitis ranges from 5% to 20% of afflicted individuals, and approximately 20% more suffer some residual neurologic deficit. However, some specific viral encephalitides (e.g., herpes simplex, eastern equine) carry mortality rates as high as 40% to 50%. Timely diagnosis is therefore essential, because specific therapies are available for some agents causing encephalitis (e.g., herpes simplex, syphilis).

CLINICAL PRESENTATION

The triad of fever, headache, and nuchal rigidity constitutes the classic presentation of meningitis, and any patient with these findings warrants a prompt evaluation for the presence of central nervous system (CNS) disease. This same triad is generally noted with encephalitis, coupled with signs and symptoms of brain parenchymal involvement (e.g., altered level of consciousness, seizures, and focal neurologic signs).

Focal findings reflect the portion of the brain that is involved (e.g., hemiparesis, cranial nerve abnormalities, aphasia, ataxia). Any of the encephalitides may demonstrate hypersomnia as an acute symptom. Fever is commonly noted with either condition but is not invariably present, especially in the elderly and the immunocompromised, as a result of decreased immune responses to circulating bacterial and viral antigens. Headache is occasionally absent early in the course of disease and in elderly patients. Nuchal rigidity, noted in more than 80% of patients with bacterial meningitis,[4] is considered the most characteristic finding in patients with meningeal irritation and is observed in patients with encephalitis in which there is concurrent meningeal involvement (meningoencephalitis). Nausea and vomiting, reflecting CNS inflammation and raised intracranial pressure, can be observed in either condition.

Three clinical signs are characteristic of meningeal irritation but cannot always be elicited. The Brudzinski sign occurs when flexion of the neck results in flexion of the knees and hips. The Kernig sign is elicited by extending the knee with the hip flexed; stretching of the lumbar roots causes pain in the hamstring and paraspinal muscles. The contralateral Brudzinski sign is described as flexion of the contralateral hip and knee during examination for the Kernig sign.

Petechiae, purpura, and morbilliform rash are commonly noted in association with meningococcal meningitis.[15] Similar rashes may be noted occasionally in association with meningitis due to *Staphylococcus, H. influenzae,* and *S. pneumoniae,* as well as some viral meningitides, especially echoviruses.

An in-depth neurologic examination is obviously of paramount importance in the evaluation of any patient thought to harbor a CNS infectious process. Mental status or behavioral changes (sometimes quite subtle) are commonly noted with encephalitis and occasionally are the only clues to meningitis in the elderly patient. Seizures noted in association with encephalitis are most commonly focal; either focal or generalized seizures may be noted in as many as 30% of patients with meningitis and may reflect the infectious process itself or associated complications (e.g., fever, electrolyte imbalances, hypoxia).

Seizures are uncommon in meningococcal meningitis, whereas they may be the sole presenting sign of encephalitis. Cranial nerve abnormalities, especially the ocular variety, are often a feature of viral encephalitides and occur in 10% to 20% of cases of meningitis. A careful funduscopic examination may reveal papilledema, the presence of which should arouse suspicion of a brain abscess or encephalitis. Acute deafness is occasionally the presenting complaint of adults with meningitis. Neurologic sequelae of meningitis are not uncommon, and some forms of viral encephalitis (e.g., herpes simplex, eastern equine) result in serious neurologic deficits in as many as of 50% of cases.

DIFFERENTIAL DIAGNOSIS

The differential diagnosis of meningitis and encephalitis includes infectious, neurologic, toxicologic, metabolic, environmental, and behavioral disorders. Infectious disorders include encephalopathy without actual invasion of the brain substance, brain abscesses, septic emboli, and cortical septic thrombophlebitis. Various noninfectious neurologic disorders, such as migraine and other vascular headaches, prolonged postictal states, and new-onset seizures, share some features common to both encephalitis and meningitis.

Drug ingestion (e.g., phencyclidine, salicylates) often presents in the form of febrile, mind-altered states and must be considered in the differential diagnosis. Metabolic disturbances (e.g., electrolyte imbalances, hypoglycemia, and hyperglycemia) and acute environmental toxicity (e.g., heat stroke) must also be considered. Behavioral alterations (e.g., psychosis, mania) should never be considered to be purely of psychological origin without an evaluation for the possibility of underlying organic causes such as meningitis and encephalitis.

EMERGENCY DEPARTMENT EVALUATION

The majority of patients with meningitis or encephalitis who present to the emergency department display classic complaints of severe headache and fever. Nuchal rigidity can be noted with meningitis and meningoencephalitis, and patients with encephalitis generally demonstrate some symptoms and signs of direct brain involvement. The astute emergency physician is aware that up to 20% of cases of meningitis may present in an atypical fashion and that the key to diagnosis in groups likely to display an atypical presentation (e.g., the elderly or immunocompromised) is a high index of suspicion coupled with a low threshold for performing a lumbar puncture.

Identification of risk factors may aid in the diagnosis of meningitis and assist in directing antibiotic therapy. Most risk factors can be identified with a few questions guided by the six I's:

*I*nfection (e.g., antecedent or concomitant upper or lower respiratory tract infection, sinusitis, otitis)
*I*mmunosuppression (e.g., splenectomy, sickle cell disease, corticosteroids, Hodgkin disease, myeloma, organ transplant, AIDS)
*I*njury (head trauma, neurologic or otolaryngologic procedures)
*I*ndwelling (catheters, shunts, ventricular reservoirs)
*I*mbiber (alcoholic)
*I*dentification (close contacts, such as spouses, roommates, and paramedics)

Many of the more common viruses causing outbreaks of encephalitis demonstrate characteristic seasonal and geographic distributions. For example, arbovirus and enterovirus infections tend to occur in summer and early fall, mumps in winter and spring, and lymphocytic choriomeningitis in fall and winter. Eastern equine encephalitis occurs in the eastern United States, and Venezuelan equine encephalitis is generally found in Florida and the southwestern United States, whereas herpes simplex encephalitis demonstrates no characteristic geographic pattern. Some important data to be elicited in suspected cases of encephalitis can be summarized through the use of the six V's:

*V*acation/travel (to endemic areas, foreign or domestic)
*V*eterinary or other animal contact (rabies)
*V*ectors (recent mosquito or tick bites)
*V*iral infections (recent or concurrent)
*V*accinations (recent for measles, varicella, rubella, rabies)
*V*ital statistics (contact local or national health agencies regarding outbreaks)

The physical examination should focus on likely sites of infection, namely, the oropharynx, ears, and sinuses in the case of meningitis. Similarly, the chest examination should focus on evidence of pulmonary or cardiac sources of infection. The entire body should be scrutinized for the presence of any rashes. Funduscopy is mandatory to rule out papilledema. The neurologic examination must be performed in a timely, but meticulous, fashion. With encephalitis, only subtle clues of neurologic dysfunction (e.g., inattention or drowsiness) are sometimes found.

If papilledema or other evidence of increased intracranial pressure is noted, control measures (e.g., mannitol, hyperventilation) should be undertaken, and the patient should undergo computed tomography of the brain. If meningitis is suspected, but the patient is unable to undergo computed tomography, or if a space-occupying lesion is noted on computed tomography, cultures should be obtained from blood and infectious sites, and antibiotics administered without delay. In cases of suspected encephalitis, antibody titers, cultures, polymerase chain reaction, or fluorescent antibody studies should be obtained, and stool cultures ordered.

Computed tomography or magnetic resonance imaging may also demonstrate changes consistent with disorders such as herpes encephalitis and HIV encephalitis. Suspicion of herpes simplex encephalitis mandates rapid institution of intravenous acyclovir. Intravenous access should be obtained and blood sent for a complete blood cell count, glucose analysis (preferably an initial bedside glucose determination), electrolyte determinations, and liver function studies. Urine and sputum cultures are also warranted. Consideration should also be given to obtaining a toxicology screen. After this, if not contraindicated, lumbar puncture is carried out.

Lumbar Puncture

Lumbar puncture, a safe and rapidly performed procedure with a low complication rate, is the key to confirming the diagnosis of meningitis and many treatable cases of encephalitis. Although there has been concern over the possibility of inducing meningitis by the lumbar puncture itself,[23] the differentiation of spontaneously occurring meningitis from that induced by the procedure is difficult, if not impossible.[10]

Two definite contraindications to lumbar puncture are infection at the site of the puncture and evidence of obstructive (noncommunicating) hydrocephalus. Papilledema, anticoagulant use, and the presence of a space-occupying lesion in the brain are relative contraindications. In the event that lumbar puncture is required in a patient with papilledema, a small-bore (22- or 24-gauge) needle should be employed and only a small amount of fluid withdrawn. Whether it is always necessary to perform computed tomography of the head before lumbar puncture is an ongoing controversy.

Cerebrospinal Fluid Parameters

Gram Stain

The visualization of the responsible organism on a Gram stain of fresh CSF is pathognomonic of bacterial meningitis or some nonviral causes of encephalitis. Gram-stained, centrifuged samples of CSF demonstrate bacterial organisms in 80% to 90% of culture-proven cases of bacterial meningitis.[1] CSF counts are highest in pneumococcal and *H. influenzae* meningitis. Patients with listerial meningitis or those who have received previous antimicrobial therapy demonstrate bacteria on Gram stain approximately 60% of the time.[3] *L. monocytogenes* is occasionally identified on the Gram stain as a "diphtheroid" contaminant.[1,3]

In patients with fungal meningitis or encephalitis, successful detection of pathogens requires the examination of a large volume of fluid, because only a small number of fungal organisms are typically present in the CSF. India ink preparations for the detection of fungal elements in CSF are positive in as few as one-half of cases. Similarly, acid-fast smears of CSF for diagnosing tuberculous meningitis are not consistently sensitive. In any event, tests for fungal or tuberculous meningitis or for encephalitis should not be routinely ordered unless there is a good clinical indication for doing so.

Glucose

Normally, the ratio of CSF to serum glucose concentration is 0.60. Hypoglycorrhachia—a CSF glucose level of less than 50 mg/dL, or a CSF/serum glucose ratio of less than 0.50—is noted in more than 50% of cases of bacterial, fungal, and tuberculous meningitis, and is not uncommon in mumps encephalitis and meningitis, lymphocytic choriomeningitis, and herpes simplex meningitis. Normal CSF glucose levels are generally noted in most viral meningitides and encephalitides, as well as in the early stage of pyogenic or tuberculous meningitis.

Protein

Normal protein levels in the CSF range from 15 to 45 mg/dL. Subarachnoid space infection results in increased protein permeability of the choroid plexus, ependyma, and pia mater. Marked protein elevations are observed in bacterial, fungal, and tuberculous meningitis. Viral meningitides or encephalitides generally manifest normal or only moderately elevated levels of protein.[17] Levels of 1000 mg/dL or more must raise the serious suspicion of impending or actual subarachnoid block. Blood (e.g., subarachnoid bleed, traumatic lumbar puncture) increases the CSF protein by 1 mg for each 1000 red blood cells if the protein and cell counts are measured from the same tube.

Cell Count and Differential

Normal CSF contains no red blood cells and has a white blood cell count of less than 5 cells/μL, all of which are mononuclear. Red blood cells, at times numbering in the thousands, and xanthochromia are sometimes noted with herpes encephalitis, owing to the hemorrhagic nature of the lesions. The finding of a single granulocytic cell when the CSF is concentrated by a centrifuge, considered pathologic by many, should be considered normal if the total CSF white blood cell count is less than 5 cells/μL.[6] Bacterial meningitis is classically described as having CSF cell counts ranging from 100 to 10,000 cells/μL, with polymorphonuclear forms predominating early and lymphocytes appearing subsequently. The leukocyte esterase test can be used as a rapid, reasonably sensitive screening test for the determination of CSF polymorphonuclear leukocytes at concentrations of more than 10 cells/μL; its use, however, does not obviate the need for performance of the standard cell count and differential.[7]

Viral meningitis characteristically manifests a CSF lymphocytosis with cell counts on the order of 10 to 1000 cells/μL. There may be a marked predominance of neutrophils in the earliest stages of infection. Mononuclear cells usually predominate in cases of tuberculous and fungal meningitis, as well as in other causes of the aseptic meningitis syndrome. In the acute stages of viral encephalitis, a mild-to-moderate rise in mononuclear lymphocytes (e.g., 10 to 250 cells) is noted, with higher cell counts suggestive of concomitant meningeal involvement.

There is considerable overlap in the CSF findings of bacterial meningitis, the aseptic meningitis syndrome, and encephalitis. It has been reported that as many as 10% of patients with bacterial meningitis initially demonstrate a CSF lymphocytosis.[1,17] Moreover, both tuberculous and fungal meningitis may initially manifest CSF neutrophilia, and neutrophils may predominate throughout the course of illness. Patients with viral meningitis occasionally demonstrate CSF leukocytosis of greater than 1,000 cells/μL with more than 75% neutrophils, particularly early in their illness, but a second sample obtained within 8 to 24 hours generally shows a significant decrease in the proportion of neutrophils.

Several ancillary CSF tests are available to aid in the differentiation of bacterial from nonbacterial meningitis. The most helpful for use in the emergency setting are those that detect bacterial antigens (by counterimmunoelectrophoresis, latex agglutination, or enzyme-linked immunosorbent assay). These tests should be used without delaying critical antibiotic therapy. CSF lactic acid levels are usually normal in viral meningitis and elevated (greater than 3.5 mEq/L) in bacterial, fungal, and tuberculous meningitis.[14] Elevated CSF lactic acid, coupled with other CSF findings and the history and physical examination, may also be of diagnostic utility in partially treated meningitides.[11]

CSF obtained very early in the course of bacterial meningitis may be totally devoid of cells and organisms and may demonstrate no glucose or protein abnormalities. Occasionally, even in immunologically competent individuals, the CSF in fulminant meningitis (especially pneumococcal) demonstrates no cells but is teeming with bacteria. Although no single CSF laboratory value can, of itself, make the diagnosis of meningitis when the Gram stain is negative, certain patterns are more closely related to certain etiologic agents. A pattern of CSF neutrophilia, very low glucose (5 to 20 mg/dL), and elevated protein (100 mg/dL) strongly suggests bacterial meningitis. The CSF in tuberculous meningitis generally contains mononuclear cells, normal-to-decreased glucose, and elevated protein. In viral meningitis, there is a predominance of mononuclear cells (except for early in the illness, when polymorphonuclear cells may predominate), a normal glucose concentration, and a slightly to moderately increased protein level.

Cultures

The CSF should be cultured in all cases of suspected meningitis. The diagnosis is made only from the culture in almost 20% of cases, and, in all cases, definitive antimicrobial therapy is guided by these results.[2,8] Cultures take on even more importance in fungal and tuberculous meningitis, in which the India ink or acid-fast preparations are negative in 50% or more of cases.[1,22] Cultures for suspected fungal or tuberculous meningitis require large volumes of CSF, because the number of organisms per unit volume is small.

In individuals suspected of having partially treated meningitis, the CSF should be cultured for at least 7 days. The agent responsible for viral encephalitis or meningitis may sometimes be identified by polymerase chain reaction or viral isolation from CSF or brain; its identity can also be inferred from a fourfold or greater increase in viral antibody titers between acute and convalescent sera or by isolation of the virus from the throat or stool.

EMERGENCY DEPARTMENT MANAGEMENT

The patient who presents to the emergency department with headache and fever, with or without nuchal rigidity and with or without neurologic abnormalities, should be considered to have meningitis until proven otherwise. An altered sensorium accompanied by fever and headache should prompt consideration of encephalitis. A rapid but thorough physical examination should be carried out, intravenous access obtained, and appropriate laboratory testing ordered.

If there is concern about a possible mass lesion or increased intracranial pressure, intravenous antibiotics should be promptly administered and a computed tomographic scan obtained. If there are no contraindications, a lumbar puncture is done. In the severely ill patient, antimicrobial therapy should never be withheld pending lumbar puncture or laboratory confirmation of the clinical impression. Antibiotic administration is unlikely to alter CSF parameters within the first few hours.

Because the vast majority of patients with bacterial meningitis are infected with pneumococci or meningococci, empiric therapy should be directed against these organisms, but coverage for *H. influenzae* should be provided as well. Antibiotic therapy can be subsequently tailored to the results of the CSF Gram stain (Tables 183.1 and 183.2). If the examination suggests the possibility of herpes encephalitis, intravenous acyclovir is instituted at 10 mg/kg over 1 hour, every 8 hours for 10 days. The identification of nonviral agents of encephalitis (e.g., syphilis, toxoplasmosis, tuberculosis) will guide specific therapy.

Once the diagnosis of bacterial meningitis or encephalitis has been established, the patient's private physician or an infectious disease specialist should be contacted to assume responsibility for continuing management. Arrangements should be made for admission to a critical care unit. The emergency physician must insist on timely consultation in these potentially devastating illnesses. An infectious disease consultation should be considered for patients with suspected tuberculous or fungal meningitis.

TABLE 183.1. Empiric Parenteral Antibiotic Therapy for Meningitis

Ceftriaxone or cefotaxime (2 g)
If significant Streptococcus pneumoniae resistance in the community, trauma, recent surgery, or shunt, add vancomycin 2 g
If penicillin/cephalosporin allergic, vancomycin 2 g and chloramphenicol 25 mg/kg
If concomitant steroid use, ceftriaxone 2 g and rifampin 300 mg
If suspicion of Listeria, add ampicillin (2 g) + gentamicin (if allergic, trimethoprim-sulfamethoxazole)

TABLE 183.2. Gram Stain-Guided Parenteral Antibiotic Therapy for Meningitis

Organism	First-line Antibiotic	Alternative
Gram-positive cocci	Ceftriaxone Cefotaxime	Vancomycin
Gram-negative cocci	Penicillin Ampicillin Ceftriaxone Cefotaxime	Chloramphenicol Rifampin
Gram-positive bacilli	Ampicillin + aminoglycoside Penicillin + aminoglycoside	Trimethoprim-sulfamethoxazole
Gram-negative bacilli	Ceftriaxone + aminoglycoside Cefotaxime + aminoglycoside	Chloramphenicol Aztreonam

Patients with clinical evaluation suggestive of viral meningitis, but whose CSF demonstrates a predominant neutrophilia, should have a second lumbar puncture done in 8 to 24 hours, because more than 85% will then show a significant decrease in the proportion of neutrophils. The decision of whether to begin antibiotic coverage before the results of the second lumbar puncture are available must be made by the emergency physician on the basis of the patient's clinical picture, the presence of associated risk factors, and the availability of appropriate staff and facilities to monitor the patient's status closely.

Cases of uncomplicated viral meningitis (except those caused by herpes simplex virus) can be discharged from the hospital when the diagnosis is definite. Therapy consists of antipyretic analgesics to alleviate the headache and fever, as well as supportive care and arrangements for appropriate follow-up.

Chemoprophylaxis

Although no hard and fast rules exist for ascertaining who should receive chemoprophylaxis after exposure to individuals with bacterial meningitis, certain guidelines may be useful. Close contacts (e.g., families, roommates, daycare contacts) of patients with meningococcal and *H. influenzae* meningitis have an increased risk (200- to 1,000-fold) of contracting the disease.[21] Clearly, such individuals deserve the benefit of chemoprophylaxis. Paramedics and hospital personnel who have had close contact with the patient (e.g., mouth-to-mouth resuscitation) should also receive chemoprophylaxis. Others, including schoolmates, do not require prophylaxis.

Rifampin, 600 mg orally every 12 hours for a total of four doses, is the approved regimen for both *H. influenzae* and meningococcal meningitis. Ciprofloxacin (500-mg single dose) is an alternative regimen for meningococcal prophylaxis.[24] Pregnant individuals exposed to *N. meningitidis* should receive an intramuscular dose of ceftriaxone (250 mg) or a single oral dose of azithromycin (500 mg).[12] Individuals at risk for pneumococcal meningitis (e.g., postsplenectomy) should receive oral penicillin, 500 mg every 6 hours for 7 days.[13] Emergency physicians should use their broad public exposure to promote the use of preventative vaccines where appropriate.

COMMON PITFALLS

- Relying on classic signs and symptoms alone, which results in some cases of meningitis being missed because of atypical presentations
- Failure to appreciate occasional overlap in CSF findings between aseptic and bacterial meningitis
- Delay in starting antibiotic therapy when there is a reasonable suspicion of meningitis. Prior antibiotic administration will not materially affect CSF findings
- Failure to provide prophylaxis to significant contacts of patients with meningococcal or *H. influenzae* meningitis
- Failure to realize that organisms remain detectable on CSF Gram stain in 60% of persons with bacterial meningitis despite antibiotic administration

References

1. Benson CA, Harris AA. Acute neurologic infections. *Med Clin North Am* 1986;70:987.
2. Bohr V, Paulson CB, Rasmussen N. Pneumococcal meningitis: late neurological sequelae and features of prognostic impact. *Arch Neurol* 1984;41:1045.
3. Bolan G, Barza M. Acute bacterial meningitis in children and adults: a perspective. *Med Clin North Am* 1985;69:231.
4. Carpenter RR, Petersdorf RG. The clinical spectrum of meningitis. *Am J Med* 1962;33:262.
5. Centers for Disease Control. Summary of notifiable diseases, United States, 1991. *MMWR* 1992;40:1.
6. Conley JM, Ronald AR. Cerebrospinal fluid as a diagnostic body fluid. *Am J Med* 1983;76:102.
7. DeLozier JA, Auerback PS. The leukocyte esterase test for detection of cerebrospinal fluid leukocytosis and bacterial meningitis. *Ann Emerg Med* 1989;19:1191.
8. Dougherty JM, Jones J. Cerebrospinal fluid cultures and analysis. *Ann Emerg Med* 1986;15:317.
9. Dunn JD. Study reveals high-risk areas of emergency medical practice. *St. Paul Fire and Marine Insurance Company Malpractice Digest* 1987 (Spring).
10. Eng RHK, Seligman SJ. Lumbar puncture–induced meningitis. *JAMA* 1981;145:1456.
11. Genton B, Berger JP: Cerebrospinal fluid lactate in 78 cases of adult meningitis. *Intensive Care Med* 1990;16:196.
12. Girgis N, Sultan Y, Frenck RW Jr, et al. Azithromycin compared with rifampin for eradication of nasopharyngeal colonization by *Neisseria* meningitides. *Pediatr Infect Dis J* 1998;17:816.
13. Henry K, Crossley K. Meningitis: principles of diagnosis, advances in treatment. *Postgrad Med* 1986;80:59.
14. Lindquist L, Linne T, Hansson LO, et al. Value of cerebrospinal fluid analysis in the differential diagnosis of meningitis: a study in 710 patients with suspected central nervous system infection. *Eur J Microbiol Infect Dis* 1988;7:374.
15. Mancebo J, Domingo P, Blanch L, et al. The predictive value of petechiae in adults with bacterial meningitis. *JAMA* 1986;156:2820.
16. Odugbemi T, Jatto SA, Afolabi K. *Bacteroides fragilis* meningitis. *J Clin Microbiol* 1985;21:282.
17. Powers WJ. Cerebrospinal fluid lymphocytosis in acute bacterial meningitis. *Am J Med* 1985;19:216.
18. Ratzan KR. Viral meningitis. *Med Clin North Am* 1985;69:399.
19. Schuchat A, Robinson K, Wenger JD, et al. Bacterial meningitis is the United States in 1995. *N Engl J Med* 1997;337:970.
20. Seligman S. The rapid differential diagnosis of meningitis. *Med Clin North Am* 1973;57:1417.
21. Shapiro ED. Prophylaxis for bacterial meningitis. *Med Clin North Am* 1985;69:269.
22. Stockstill MT, Kauffman CA. Comparison of cryptococcal and tuberculous meningitis. *Arch Neurol* 1983;40:81.
23. Teele DW, Dashefsky B, Robinson T, et al. Meningitis after lumbar puncture in children with bacteremia. *N Engl J Med* 1981;305:1079.
24. Visakorpi R. Ciprofloxacin in meningococcal carriers. *Scand J Infect Dis Suppl* 1989;60:108.
25. Wilfert CM, Lehrman SN, Kaz SL. Enteroviruses and meningitis. *Pediatr Infect Dis* 1983;2:335.

CHAPTER 184

Central Nervous System Abscess

Ralph J. Riviello and
Douglas A. Rund

Intracranial suppurative infections include brain abscess, cranial subdural empyema, and cranial epidural abscess. Although uncommon, they can produce serious morbidity and mortality if their diagnosis is delayed. The emergency physician must consider these conditions when evaluating patients who present with headache, fever, alteration of consciousness, or new neurologic deficits. Early identification and immediate neurosurgical consultation can result in an improved outcome.

BRAIN ABSCESS

Brain abscesses can range from microscopic collections of inflammatory cells to necrosis of an entire hemisphere. Brain abscess is the most common intracranial focal suppurative process but only occurs about 2% as commonly as brain tumors. It accounts for four to ten cases per year on a busy neurosurgical service, or for approximately one in 10,000 hospital admissions.[4,12] The incidence had been declining due to improved therapy for otic and sinus infections; however, an increase in its incidence may be seen due to enhanced use of neurosurgical procedures, improved imaging techniques, and increased population of immunosuppressed patients.[4]

There is a 2 to 3:1 male-to-female predominance. The age distribution relates to the predisposing condition. Abscess from an otic origin usually occurs in those less than 20 years old or more than 40 years old. With a paranasal sinus focus, most patients are 10 to 30 years of age. Approximately 25% of cases occur in children less than 15 years old and are most commonly due to cyanotic congenital heart disease or otic sources. Abscess rarely occurs in those less than 2 years of age, but when it does, it is often secondary to gram-negative bacillary meningitis.[4,12]

Brain abscesses arise from either contiguous or hematogenous spread of a suppurative infection. Contiguous spread from craniofacial sites (middle ear, sinuses, dental) account for 19% to 40% of all cases.[8,11,12] Otitis media (chronic) and mastoiditis classically spread to the temporal lobe (50% to 75% of cases) and the cerebellum (one-third of cases). Approximately 85% to 99% of cerebellar abscesses are from an otic source. Frontal and ethmoidal sinusitis spread to the frontal lobe. Dental sources also tend to affect the frontal lobe.[4,12] Posttraumatic (penetrating) and postneurosurgical procedure abscesses now account for up to 24% of cases.[11] These contiguous infections can lead to abscess formation by two mechanisms: by direct extension through infected bone or by retrograde thrombophlebitis from emissary and diploic veins.[4,8,12]

About 25% of cases arise from hematogenous spread from a cardiac or pulmonary source, including lung abscess, bronchiectasis, cyanotic congenital heart disease (tetralogy of Fallot), and bacterial endocarditis. Hematogenously spread abscesses tend to be multiple and lie in the distribution of the middle cerebral artery at the gray-white junction where microcirculatory flow is poorest. Other causes include hereditary hemorrhagic telangiectasia (Osler-Weber-Rendu disease), dental extractions, abdominal or pelvic infections, and following esophageal stricture dilation and endoscopic sclerosis of esophageal varices.[4,12] In the remaining 10% to 15% of cases, there is no clearly identifiable cause.[12]

Improved microbiologic culture techniques have yielded a better understanding of the microbiology of brain abscesses. The microbiology is location dependent, and over 50% of abscesses involve mixed flora.[5,10,12] Anaerobes play a large role, with their being isolated in 40% to 60% of cases.[4] The most commonly isolated anaerobes are *Bacteroides* species (from ear or sinus infection) and anaerobic streptococci (from dental and chronic pulmonary infections). Aerobic and microaerophilic streptococci (*Streptococcus milleri, S. viridans*) are the most common bacteria isolated, being found in up to 70% of abscesses.[4] *Staphylococcus aureus* and *S. epidermis* are frequently isolated from posttraumatic or postsurgical abscesses. Gram-negative bacilli, found in 23% to 33% of cases, are associated with chronic otitis, postoperative infections, and abdominopelvic infection.[4,12]

The acquired immunodeficiency syndrome (AIDS) epidemic and the increasing use of immunosuppressive drug therapy have lead to more atypical, fungal, and protozoal brain abscesses, such as *Nocardia, Listeria, Cryptococcus, Mycobacterium, Aspergillus,* and *Candida. Toxoplasmosis gondii* is the most common cause of brain abscess in patients with AIDS.[3,4,7]

CLINICAL PRESENTATION

The triad of fever, headache, and focal neurologic deficit is present in less than half of patients who present with a brain abscess.[4] There are no other pathognomonic signs; therefore, history and a high clinical suspicion are important features to proper diagnosis.

Headache, the earliest presenting symptom, is present in 70% of patients and is oftentimes severe, hemicranial, and persistent. Fever is absent in more than 50% of patients. Alterations in consciousness, ranging from drowsiness to coma, occur in 50% of cases, as do nausea and vomiting. A focal neurologic deficit is seen in 50% to 75% of patients, and can include aphasia, hemiparesis, visual fields deficits, nystagmus, or ataxia. These physical findings may be helpful in localizing the abscess. Focal or generalized seizures occur in 30% of cases. Unfortunately, papilledema is a late and often absent finding.[4,9,12,14] The patient with a brain abscess is at risk for three major complications, producing sudden deterioration: uncal or tonsillar herniation, hemorrhage into an abscess, or rupture of abscess into the ventricular or subarachnoid space.[4,10,15]

DIFFERENTIAL DIAGNOSIS

Primary or metastatic brain tumor can mimic cerebral abscess on a computed tomography (CT) scan. History and CT appearance easily differentiate other infectious diseases, such as viral encephalitis, subdural empyema, epidural abscess, and meningitis. Subarachnoid hemorrhage, cerebral infarction, central nervous system (CNS) vasculitis, and migraines can mimic abscesses.[4,5,14,15]

AIDS patients account for a large proportion of patients presenting to the emergency department (ED) with intracranial mass lesions. Because of the wide variety of pathologic process involving the CNS of AIDS patients, brain biopsy is often needed for definitive diagnosis and treatment. *T. gondii* is the most commonly found organism and is often targeted when selecting empiric therapy. Other considerations include *Cryptococcus, Candida,* lymphoma, Kaposi's sarcoma, and progressive multifocal leukoencephalopathy.[3,7]

EMERGENCY DEPARTMENT EVALUATION

The history and physical examination should focus on sites of potential infection and the possibility of life-threatening complications. Routine laboratory evaluation is rarely helpful. Leukocytosis may be present, but approximately 30% to 40% of patients will have a normal white blood cell count. An elevated erythrocyte sedimentation rate is seen in 40% of cases; however, the C-reactive protein may help to distinguish abscess from tumor. Blood cultures are positive in about 10% of cases, but should be obtained even if the patient is afebrile. Although lumbar puncture is contraindicated in patients with brain abscess, if performed, the results will be normal or nonspecific (elevated opening pressure, mildly elevated protein and cell count). Cerebrospinal fluid (CSF) cultures rarely identify the causative organism.[4,5,9] Chest films may reveal a pulmonic source of infection; sinus or mastoid films may identify infection in these areas.

A CT scan of the brain, with and without contrast, should be obtained. CT has a reported sensitivity of 95% to 99%.[4] CT helps to localize the abscess and stage its evolution. During the "early cerebritis" stage (first 3 days), a CT scan reveals an irregular area of low density. This area does not enhance with contrast and represents the necrotic center of the abscess. In the late cerebritis stage, patchy enhancement is present. As the abscess evolves, a homogenous central area of low density is seen, and a thick, diffuse, ringlike pattern of enhancement is present. This enhancement correlates with formation of the collagen capsule. The ring becomes thinner as the capsular development progresses, and it is narrower on the ventricular surface of the abscess.[2] Features that help to identify the mass as an abscess include gas within the center of the mass, a thinner rim (less than 5 mm), and ependymal enhancement. Patients given corticosteroids may have diminished enhancement of the abscess ring.[4]

Magnetic resonance imaging (MRI) with gadolinium has become the diagnostic procedure of choice. MRI may not be readily available in most departments and not accessible to critically ill patients; therefore, a CT scan remains a very good alternative. MRI has better sensitivity and specificity than contrast CT. MRI better detects mass effect, edema, petechial hemorrhage, smaller lesions, and multifocal involvement. If clinical suspicion is high and a CT scan is negative, an MRI should be performed.

EMERGENCY DEPARTMENT MANAGEMENT

Initial management of the patient with a suspected brain abscess includes airway control, intravenous access, and maintenance of adequate ventilation and circulation. If signs of elevated intracranial pressure and/or impending herniation are present, one must act rapidly to reduce the pressure. These are, however, only temporizing measures and include intubating and hyperventilating the patient, elevating the head of the bed 30 degrees, and instituting pharmacologic therapy with mannitol and dexamethasone. Immediate neurosurgical consultation is required.

Definitive management includes antibiotic therapy and surgical decompression. Immediate surgical decompression is indicated if there is a deteriorating level of consciousness, increasing neurologic deficit, or signs of increasing intracranial pressure.[5] Surgical options include drainage, aspiration, or excision of the abscess.[9] Intravenous antibiotics should be initiated in the ED and should be selected to treat likely pathogens. Table 184.1 outlines the choice of empiric antibiotics based on the suspected source of the abscess and pathogens involved.[4,8,12] Pending culture and sensitivity results, one standard regimen includes a third-generation cephalosporin plus metronidazole (400 to 600 mg intravenously every 6 hours). In postsurgical or posttraumatic abscesses, vancomycin or an antistaphylococcal penicillin should be used to cover *Staphylococcus.* If *Pseudomonas* is thought to be a causative organism, ceftazidime plus an aminoglycoside should be used.[14]

Corticosteroids are used to reduce cerebral edema and help control intracranial pressure. The standard regimen is dexamethasone 10 to 12 mg intravenously, followed by 4 mg every 6 hours. Because corticosteroids may reduce antibiotic penetration into the abscess cavity and may delay encapsulation, they are indicated only when there is evidence of a significant mass effect, with progressive neurologic deficit or changing level of consciousness.[4,5,12]

DISPOSITION

All patients diagnosed with a brain abscess in the ED require admission to the hospital. Immediate neurosurgical consultation should be made. If a neurosurgeon is not available, arrange-

TABLE 184.1. Treatments for Brain Abscess Based on Pathogen and Site of Abscess

Predisposing Condition	Site	Isolate	Treatment
Otitis media/mastoiditis	Temporal lobe or cerebellum	Streptococci (aerobic or anaerobic), *Bacteroides fragilis*, Enterobacteriaceae	Third-generation cephalosporin + metronidazole
Sinusitis	Frontal or temporal lobe	Streptococci, Bacteroides spp., *S. aureus, Haemophilus* spp., Enterobacteriaceae	Third-generation cephalosporin + metronidazole + vancomycin
Dental	Frontal lobe	Mixed *Fusobacterium, Bacteroides, Streptococcus* spp.	Penicillin + metronidazole
Penetrating trauma or postsurgical	Related to wound	*S. aureus* and *Streptococcus* spp., Enterobacteriaceae, *Clostridium* spp.	Third-generation cephalosporin + vancomycin, *or* antistaphylococcal PCN
Congenital heart disease	MCA distribution	*Streptococcus* spp., *Haemophilus* spp.	Penicillin or ampicillin ± third-generation cephalosporin
Lung disease (empyema or abscess)	MCA distribution	*Fusobacterium, Actinomyces, Bacteroides, Streptococcus* spp., *Nocardia*	Penicillin + metronidazole + TMP/SMZ, or third-generation cephalosporin
Bacterial endocarditis	MCA distribution	Viridans streptococci, *S. aureus, Enterococcus* spp., *Haemophilus*	Antistaphylococcal PCN, ampicillin, *or* vancomycin ± aminoglycoside
GI source	MCA distribution	Enterobacteriaceae	Third-generation cephalosporin

PCN, penicillin; MCA, middle cerebral artery; TMP/SMZ, trimethoprim-sulfamethoxazole; GI, gastrointestinal.

ments should be made for transfer to a neurosurgical center after stabilization. Young persons, those without underlying disease, and those without neurologic deterioration or mental status changes have a better prognosis. With early diagnosis, advanced neuroradiologic imaging, and rapid treatment, mortality is less than 30%, but in patients presenting with signs of herniation, mortality is greater than 50%.[4,10,12] Persistent neurologic deficits, including seizure, intellectual or behavioral impairment, and motor deficits, are seen in 30% to 55% of patients.[4]

CRANIAL EPIDURAL AND SUBDURAL SPACE INFECTIONS

Subdural empyema and cranial epidural abscess are rare, but life-threatening, causes of intracranial suppurative infections. Subdural empyema accounts for 15% to 25% of focal intracranial infections, while cranial epidural abscess is much less common. Subdural empyema is a disease of teen-agers and young adults, with most cases occurring in the 10- to 40-year age group. On the other hand, epidural abscess rarely occurs in young children and has been reported in patients from ages 12 to 68. Both conditions exhibit a 3:1 male-to-female predominance.[4]

Subdural empyema forms between the dura mater and arachnoid mater, while cranial epidural abscess forms outside the dura mater. Both entities share a similar pathogenesis and etiology, and the two infections can coexist. The infections are thought to occur through direct extension or by hematogenous spread through the emissary veins.[4,12] Paranasal sinus disease, especially frontal and ethmoidal sinusitis, accounts for 60% to 70% of cases. Other causes include cranial osteomyelitis, mastoiditis, otitis media, head trauma, cranial surgery, ventriculoperitoneal shunt, halo traction pins, orbital infections, and chronic subdural hematoma.[4,6,8] In children, bacterial meningitis is the most common predisposing condition.[12]

The microbiology of these infections can be predicted by the primary source of infection. Aerobic, anaerobic, and microaerophilic streptococci are isolated in the majority of cases due to otorhinogenic origin. *S. aureus* and coagulase-negative staphylococci are found in sinus, otic, postoperative, and posttraumatic cases. Gram-negative bacilli can usually be seen in otic and posttraumatic sources. Polymicrobial infections are common, and a sterile culture may found in 20% to 30% of cases. In children, the most common causative agents are those responsible for the underlying meningitis (*H. influenzae, S. pneumoniae*).[4,6,12]

CLINICAL PRESENTATION

The clinical presentation of subdural empyema is fever, headache, and nuchal rigidity. The nonspecific symptoms of a sinus or ear infection, fever and malaise, rapidly progress to severe headache and meningismus. A classic presentation is a young male with frontal sinusitis, who develops progressive obtundation and hemiparesis.[8] Headache, present in 90% of cases, is focal but then becomes more generalized. Nausea and vomiting are common. Varying degrees of encephalopathy can be seen, ranging from mild confusion to coma. Focal neurologic signs (including hemiparesis, third and sixth cranial nerve palsies, and focal or generalized seizures) are seen in 75% of patients.[4,12] Postoperative and posttraumatic subdural empyema has a very indolent course due to the slow accumulation of fluid. Headache is often absent, and the disease course is more benign.[1,4]

The presentation of epidural abscess is more insidious. Symptoms can take weeks to months to develop. Patients often present with a long history of nonspecific symptoms, without focal signs or mental status changes. Once the fluid mass reaches critical size, nausea, vomiting, headache, drowsiness, and lethargy occur. Focal neurologic signs, seizure, and coma do not occur unless the infection spreads to the subdural space or cerebral herniation occurs. A patient with an epidural abscess involving the petrous bone may present with unilateral facial pain and fifth and sixth cranial nerve palsies, leading to lateral rectus weakness (Gradenigo syndrome).[1,4,6]

DIFFERENTIAL DIAGNOSIS

The initial presentation of subdural empyema and epidural abscess is similar to that of other intracranial processes. Meningitis, brain abscess, subdural hematoma, subarachnoid hemorrhage, herpes encephalitis, venous sinus thrombosis, and tumor should be considered.[1,4] CT scanning and the more sensitive MRI allow definitive diagnosis in most cases.

EMERGENCY DEPARTMENT EVALUATION

History and physical examination should focus on finding potential sources of infection. A detailed neurologic examination should be performed. Routine laboratory evaluation is of limited value. The white blood cell count may be only mildly elevated and oftentimes is normal. The sedimentation rate may be elevated if osteomyelitis is present.[6] CSF analysis is usually not helpful and is actually contraindicated, due to the risk of herniation.[1,4]

CT scanning with intravenous contrast remains the mainstay of ED diagnosis for both subdural empyema and cranial epidural abscess. Subdural empyema reveals a crescent-shaped, hypodense fluid collection in the subdural space, with displacement of the arachnoid. A mass effect is common, and an enhancing rim may be seen. Epidural abscess appears as a poorly defined, lentiform, extraaxial area of low or intermediate density. A hypointense, medial enhancing rim, representing inflamed dura, helps to differentiate it from a subdural collection.[13] Cranial osteomyelitis may be detected.[4,12]

MRI with gadolinium is more sensitive in detecting these processes, but may not be readily available in most EDs. MRI advantages include increased delineation between bone, CSF, and brain parenchyma; better ability to localize fluid to the epidural or subdural space; ability to characterize fluid type (blood, pus, or sterile effusion) in the collection; and ready detection of subtle edema and parenchymal abnormalities.[4,13] MRI should be used when CT scanning is negative in the face of high clinical suspicion.

EMERGENCY DEPARTMENT MANAGEMENT

Once the diagnosis is made, immediate neurosurgical consultation is required. If signs of impending herniation are present, temporizing measures must be employed.

Antibiotic coverage should begin in the ED. The choice of antibiotic should be tailored to the suspected source until culture results are available. A scheme for antibiotic selection is outlined in Table 184.1. If an otogenic source is suspected, a third-generation cephalosporin with metronidazole should be used. In postsurgical or posttraumatic abscesses, nafcillin or vancomycin should be used with a third-generation cephalosporin.[4,12]

DISPOSITION

All patients require admission. If neurosurgical services are not available, the patient, once stabilized, should be transferred to an appropriate center. Patients with an isolated cranial epidural abscess have an excellent prognosis. Most recover, with good neurologic outcome.

The mortality for subdural empyema ranges from 6% to 20%. Of those that survive, 15% to 44% have a persistent neurologic deficit (seizure disorder, hemiparesis, aphasia). Outcome is directly related to advanced patient age, degree of encephalopathy present, and delay to appropriate therapy.

COMMON PITFALLS

- Failure to order MRI after negative CT scan in patients suspected of having a subdural empyema or cranial epidural abscess
- Inappropriate antibiotic selection because the likely origin of the infection was not considered
- Delay in reducing intracranial pressure and neurosurgical consultation

References

1. Brock DG, Bleck TP. Extra-axial suppurations of the central nervous system. *Semin Neurol* 1992;12:263.
2. Enzmann DR, Britt DH, Placone R. Staging of human brain abscesses by computed tomography. *Radiology* 1983;146:703.
3. Hall WA. Neurosurgical infections in the compromised host. *Neurosurg Clin North Am* 1992;3:435.
4. Heilpern KL, Lorber B. Focal intracranial infections. *Infect Dis Clin North Am* 1996;4:879.
5. Kaplan K. Brain abscess. *Med Clin North Am* 1985;59:345.
6. Krauss WE, McCormick PC. Infections of the dural spaces. *Neurosurg Clin North Am* 1992;3:4.
7. Levy RM, Berger JR. Neurosurgical aspects of human immunodeficiency virus infection. *Neurosurg Clin North Am* 1992;3:443.
8. Luby JP. Southwestern Internal Medicine Conference: infections of the central nervous system. *Am J Med Sci* 1992;6:379.
9. Mampalam TJ, Rosenblum ML. Trends in the management of bacterial brain abscess: a review of 102 cases over 17 years. *Neurosurgery* 1988;23:451.
10. Osenbach RK, Loftus CM. Diagnosis and management of brain abscess. *Neurosurg Clin North Am* 1992;3:403.
11. Pruitt AA. Infections of the nervous system. *Neurosurg Clin North Am* 1998;2:419.
12. Townsend GC, Scheld WM. Infections of the central nervous sytem. *Adv Intern Med* 1998;43:403.
13. Weingarten K, Zimmerman RD, Becker RD, et al. Subdural and epidural empyemas: MR imaging. *AJR* 1989;152:615.
14. Wispelwey B, Scheld WM. Brain abscess. *Semin Neurol* 1992;12:273.
15. Yoshikawa T, Quinn W. The aching head: intracranial suppuration due to head and neck infections. *Infect Dis Clin North Am* 1988;2:265.

CHAPTER 185
Gonorrhea

Rodney Smith

Gonorrhea (GC) is a sexually transmitted disease caused by the small gram-negative diplococcus *Neisseria gonorrhoeae*. It is the second most frequently reported communicable disease after chlamydia. In 1997, approximately 325,000 cases were reported in the United States, and this figure represents only about half of the estimated number of cases treated.[4,5] The current epidemic of GC in the United States began in 1960, had a rapid rise in the number of annually reported cases, and peaked in 1975. Overall, there has been a gradual decrease in the annual incidence of GC since 1975, but the incidence has been stable or rising among adolescents.[22] There has also been a significant increase in antibiotic-resistant strains of *N. gonorrhoeae* since 1985. Thus, it is likely that gonococcal infections will continue to be a major public health problem.

GC is slightly more common in males, but the highest incidence is in females in the 15- to 19-year-old age group.[4,21] There is increased prevalence in non-Whites, in urban populations, in patients with lower socioeconomic status, in patients with multiple sex partners, among male homosexuals, and in patients with illicit drug use.[15] There is a seasonal variation, with more cases reported during the summer.[4]

Complications of GC, including pelvic inflammatory disease (PID), epididymitis and/or orchitis, prostatitis, ophthalmitis, septic arthritis, endocarditis, meningitis, and perihepatitis, are not reported separately, and their true incidence is unknown. Chronic sequelae such as infertility, ectopic pregnancy, blindness, urethral strictures, and abdominal adhesions represent a significant cause of morbidity.

Patients presenting to the emergency department with gonococcal disease usually fall into one of three categories: (1) those with symptoms due to localized infection; (2) those with symptoms attributable to disseminated disease; and (3) those who are asymptomatic contacts of partners known to be infected. The role of the emergency physician is to make the diagnosis, obtain suitable specimens for culture, institute appropriate antibiotic therapy, and arrange for timely follow-up.

CLINICAL PRESENTATION

The clinical manifestations of localized disease depend on the sex of the patient, the site of the infection, and the strain of gonococcus causing the infection. In heterosexual men, acute urethritis is the most common presentation. Symptoms begin within 1 to 14 days of exposure and consist of dysuria and a penile discharge. Physical examination reveals meatal erythema and, either spontaneously or with urethral stripping, a purulent urethral exudate. Asymptomatic gonococcal urethritis (GU) is not uncommon in sexually active men. It is estimated that 3% to 10% of newly acquired cases of GC in men may be asymptomatic and that the proportion of asymptomatic disease may approach 60% in some populations.[14] Because these men may not seek medical attention, they can constitute an important reservoir of disease in the community.

Primary GC in women is usually asymptomatic, and, when symptoms do occur, they are usually mild and nonspecific. Women with GC present to the emergency department with complaints of vaginal discharge, abnormal vaginal bleeding, urinary tract symptoms, and abdominal or pelvic pain.[2,13] Up to 20% of women with GC develop PID, and 33% to 81% of women with PID have GC.[20] Other local complications of GC include Bartholin abscess and perihepatitis (Fitz-Hugh-Curtis syndrome).

In patients with GC at any site, the pharynx has been found to be colonized in 3% to 7% of heterosexual men, 5% to 20% of women, 10% to 25% of homosexual men, and 39% to 96% of pregnant women.[8] Oropharyngeal GC is usually asymptomatic but can present as an acute exudative tonsillitis, a sore throat with minimal objective findings, or an acute ulcerative gingivostomatitis.

Anorectal involvement is common in both heterosexual women and homosexual men. Of women with GC, 26% to 63% may have positive rectal cultures, and most are due to autoinoculation of the rectum from vaginal infections.[2,15,22] Up to 6% of women have GC of the rectum in the absence of infection at another site.[22] In homosexual men, the rate of GC infection is as high as 55%, and half of these have no other site of infection.[1,22] Anorectal GC is often asymptomatic. When symptoms do occur, they are usually mild and consist of various combinations of pruritus ani, rectal discomfort, tenesmus, dyspareunia, hematochezia, and purulent or mucoid rectal discharge.[1,22]

Disseminated gonococcal infection (DGI) may complicate the course in 1% to 3% of patients, with the majority of cases occurring in patients with an asymptomatic primary infection.[6] About 80% of DGI cases occur in women, and about two-thirds of these occur within the first week after the onset of menses.[6] Pregnant or puerperal women and homosexual men are also at risk for developing DGI. The most common presentations of DGI are the arthritis–dermatitis syndrome, which occurs in approximately 60% of patients with DGI, and acute gonococcal arthritis. These probably represent different stages of a similar process, with a bacteremia leading to the arthritis–dermatitis syndrome, followed by frank suppurative arthritis.[5] Rare complications of DGI include pericarditis, endocarditis, perihepatitis, pyomyositis, osteomyelitis, and meningitis.[5]

Clinically, the arthritis–dermatitis syndrome presents with fever, chills, polyarticular arthritis or arthralgias, a characteristic rash, and tenosynovitis. The arthritis is migratory and occurs in only 30% to 40% of cases. The most frequently involved joints are the wrists, followed in frequency by the knees, hands, ankles, and elbows.[5,11] Although painful, the joints are usually not red or warm, and the effusion, if present, is small and usually sterile. The characteristic rash begins as petechiae or painful red papules involving the digits or distal extremities. These lesions either resolve spontaneously or evolve through vesicular and pustular stages to develop gray necrotic centers, often on hemorrhagic bases. There are usually fewer than 20 lesions per patient, and it is generally accepted that they represent septic emboli to small blood vessels during episodes of gonococcemia.[11] Skin lesions are seen in 50% to 75% of cases. Tenosynovitis occurs in up to 65% of cases and generally involves the extensor tendons of the hands, the wrists, or the tendons about the ankles.[11]

Gonococcal arthritis presents as an acute monoarticular or pauciarticular septic arthritis. The joint is red and warm and has an easily demonstrable effusion. The degree of systemic toxicity depends chiefly on the number and size of the joints involved.[11]

Patients with DGI should have cultures obtained from mucosal sites, as there is a high rate of recovery of GC from these sites.[5] For example, GC is cultured from the cervix in 90% of women and from the urethra in 50% to 75% of men. Pharyngeal cultures are positive in 20%, and rectal cultures in 15%. On the other hand, cultures of synovial fluid are positive for GC in only 50% of patients with frank arthritis, and in 25% to 30% of all patients with DGI. Blood cultures are positive in only 20% to 30%, and skin lesions in less than 5%.[5]

DIFFERENTIAL DIAGNOSIS

In men with urethritis, the major distinction to be made is between GU and nongonococcal (*Chlamydia trachomatis*) urethritis (NGU). Patients with GU are more likely to be Black, young, and of lower socioeconomic status than are patients with NGU.[12] Symptoms of GU are usually much more acute, and patients are more likely to complain of urethral discharge than are patients with NGU. The discharge in GU is usually purulent, whereas, in NGU, it is more often mucoid and scanty. Diagnosis is based on Gram stain of the urethral discharge. Other causes of NGU include *Ureaplasma urealyticum* (20% to 40%), *Trichomonas vaginalis* (25%), and, occasionally, herpes simplex virus.[4]

In women with symptoms attributable to GC, the differential diagnosis depends on the presenting symptoms. GC should always be considered in women presenting with a vaginal discharge. In studies of women with uncomplicated GC, no physical finding, including the character of the cervical discharge, reliably distinguishes between patients with GC and those whose symptoms are due to other pathogens.[2] Moreover, the finding of other pathogens on microscopy does not rule out coexistent GC. In one study, 35% of emergency department patients with GC also had trichomoniasis, and 19% had vaginal candidiasis.[2] Similarly, the results of urinalysis do not differentiate patients with GC from those whose urinary tract symptoms are due to other pathogens. GC should be considered in patients presenting with abnormal vaginal bleeding when another cause is not readily apparent, and it should always be a diagnostic consideration in sexually active women with complaints of abdominal or pelvic pain.

Gonococcal proctitis should be suspected in homosexual men presenting with rectal symptoms, but no symptoms are specific for anorectal GC. In studies of homosexual men presenting with rectal symptoms to venereal disease screening clinics, only 20% to 30% were found to have GC. Other causes of proctitis, including syphilis, herpes simplex, *Chlamydia*, *Entamoeba histolytica*, *Campylobacter*, anal fissure, anal fistula, and perianal abscess, should also be sought.

The differential diagnosis of patients presenting with signs and symptoms of DGI depends on the clinical manifestations of the process. In patients presenting with the classic arthritis–dermatitis syndrome, the major differential diagnosis is between disseminated *N. gonorrhoeae* and disseminated *N. meningitidis*. Clinical findings suggestive of meningococcemia include a larger number of skin lesions (greater than 100) and leukocytosis.[16] Other diagnostic considerations include acute rheumatic fever and Reiter syndrome. The fever and migratory polyarthralgias of DGI may suggest acute rheumatic fever, but high temperature (greater than 103°F [39.4°C]) is unusual in DGI, and skin lesions, if present, are distinctive. Features of DGI that distinguish it from Reiter syndrome are the more acute onset, increased frequency of migratory polyarthralgias, upper limb predominance, female predominance, and rarity of ocular involvement in DGI.[11] In men presenting with urethritis and arthritis, a Gram stain of the urethral discharge may be helpful.

The major differential diagnosis in patients presenting with acute monoarticular or pauciarticular septic arthritis is between gonococcal arthritis and other infectious arthritides. Gonococcal arthritis is the most frequent cause of septic arthritis in young, sexually active patients.[4] It predominantly affects the wrists and small joints of previously healthy women in the 15- to 35-year-old age group. Other types of infectious arthritis are uncommon in this population, predominantly involve the larger joints of the lower extremities, and affect men with underlying medical problems who are either preadolescent or more than 40 years old. Definitive diagnosis is based on culture and Gram stain.

EMERGENCY DEPARTMENT EVALUATION AND MANAGEMENT

In addition to the history and physical examination, the laboratory plays an important role in diagnosing GC. In symptomatic males, the Gram stain of urethral discharge approaches 100% sensitivity and specificity. In females and asymptomatic males, however, the Gram stain is less useful, with sensitivity as low as 45%. Culture for GC is considered the "gold standard," but proper collection and handling of the specimen is required to ensure accurate results. The specimen should be plated immediately and incubated in 3% to 5% CO_2 at 35°C to 37°C for 48 hours. More recently, nucleic acid amplification tests have been developed with high sensitivity and specificity for GC, and, in many sites, have replaced routine culture for the diagnosis of GC.[10] In addition to standard cervical and urethral specimens, these tests have been able to detect GC in first-voided urine samples, which allows a noninvasive method of screening patients for the disease.[18,19] In addition, testing for chlamydia can be performed on the same sample. Finally, GC has been detected by polymerase chain reaction in synovial fluid of patients with DGI, even when the culture is negative.[6]

The diagnosis and treatment of men presenting with acute urethritis are based on the results of a Gram stain of the urethral discharge. If a discharge cannot be expressed spontaneously or with urethral stripping, material for Gram stain may be obtained by inserting a calcium alginate swab about 2 cm into the distal urethra and rotating it gently. Patients with a positive Gram stain (polymorphonuclear leukocytes [PMNs] with intracellular gram-negative diplococci) or with a suggestive but nondiagnostic Gram stain (PMNs with extracellular gram-negative diplococci of typical *N. gonorrhoeae* morphology) should be treated for GC as will be outlined later. Patients with negative Gram stains (PMNs with either no organisms or bacteria not morphologically similar to gonococci) should be treated for NGU. If Gram stain is not available, a specimen should be obtained for culture or nucleic acid tests, and the patient treated for GC and *Chlamydia*.

The evaluation of women presenting with vaginal discharge, dysuria, PID, vaginal bleeding, and abdominal pain is discussed elsewhere in this text. The possibility of GC should always be considered, and cultures should be obtained if clinically indicated. Because of the high incidence of GC among adolescents, a GC culture should be obtained routinely whenever pelvic examination is done for whatever reason in this age group. When obtaining cervical cultures for GC, disinfectants and lubricants should not be used on the speculum, because even trace amounts may inhibit the growth of gonococci.[17] Excess cervical mucus should be removed, and a sterile swab should be inserted into the cervical canal and allowed to remain for 15 to 30 seconds. The swab should then be plated immediately onto a selective medium that is at room temperature. Rectal cultures are recommended in all women suspected of having GC, because they increase the diagnostic yield by 4% to 5%.[2,15,17] Blind rectal cultures may be obtained by inserting an unlubricated cotton-tipped swab past the anal canal into the rectum (about 3 cm) and moving it from side to side to sample the crypts. It should be left in place for 15 to 30 seconds. If there is stool on the swab when it is removed, it should be discarded and a new specimen obtained.

Routine culturing for *N. gonorrhoeae* in patients with pharyngitis is not indicated. Pharyngeal cultures for GC should probably be obtained in high-risk groups: homosexual men and prostitutes with pharyngitis, patients with sore throats and concurrent signs or symptoms of urogenital GC, pregnant women in whom GC is suspected, and patients with a history of exposure to GC and historic or clinical evidence of oropharyngeal involvement.

Homosexual men presenting with anorectal symptoms should have a careful physical examination for perianal erythema, ulcers, vesicles, fissures, tears, fistula, abscess, hemorrhoids, and other causes of their symptoms. An anoscopic examination should be performed in search of mucosal lesions or any exudate (which should be Gram stained). Anoscopy-directed Gram stain has a sensitivity of 60% to 79% in detecting GC.[1,7] The presence of other diagnostic lesions does not rule out coinfection with GC, and all patients with a negative Gram stain should have rectal cultures for GC.[1–3] Patients with acute proctitis after recent anal-receptive intercourse should be treated with ceftriaxone and doxycycline if anal pus is identified or the Gram stain demonstrates PMNs.[4]

Patients with signs or symptoms of DGI often have an asymptomatic primary infection. A careful physical examination for signs of complications should be performed. Cultures of the pharynx, rectum, and urethra or cervix should be obtained before initiating antibiotic therapy. Blood cultures should be obtained, and any joint effusions should be aspirated and specimens sent for cell count, microscopy for crystals, Gram stain, and culture. Pathologic cardiac murmurs or rubs suggest the possibility of endocarditis or pericarditis, and if meningeal signs are present, a lumbar puncture is indicated. Electrocardiographic evidence of myocarditis or pericarditis should be sought if clinically indicated.

Asymptomatic sexual contacts of patients with known cases of GC should be examined, have samples cultured, and undergo empiric treatment.[4] To await culture results before initiating therapy unnecessarily exposes these patients to the risks of complications. Up to 7% of women with untreated asymptomatic GC may develop PID during the 24 to 72 hours required to obtain culture results and have the patient come back for treatment.[15]

Current Centers for Disease Control and Prevention (CDC) guidelines for the treatment of GC are outlined in Table 185.1. There has been extensive clinical experience with ceftriaxone

TABLE 185.1. Treatment of Gonococcal Infection

UNCOMPLICATED INFECTIONS		
Ceftriaxone, 125 mg i.m.[a] *or* Cefixime, 400 mg PO *or* Ciprofloxacin, 500 mg PO[a,c,d] *or* Ofloxacin 400 mg PO[c,d]	*plus*	Doxycycline, 100 mg PO[h] bid for 7 days *or* Azithromycin, 1 g PO[b] *or* Ofloxacin, 300 mg PO b.i.d. for 7 days[d] *or* Erythromycin base, 500 mg PO q.i.d. for 7 days *or* Erythromycin ethylsuccinate, 800 mg PO q.i.d. for 7 days
DISSEMINATED INFECTIONS[e]		
Ceftriaxone, 1 g i.m. or i.v. q24h *or* Cefotaxime, 1 g i.v. q8h *or* Ceftizoxime, 1 g i.v. q8h *or* Ciprofloxacin, 500 mg i.v. q12h *or* Ofloxacin, 400 mg i.v. q12h *or* Spectinomycin, 2 g i.m. q12h[f]	*followed by*[g]	Cefixime, 400 mg PO b.i.d. *or* Ciprofloxacin, 500 mg PO bid[d] *or* Oflaxacin, 400 mg PO b.i.d.

[a]Recommended for pharyngeal infections.
[b]Safety and efficacy for persons younger than 16 years old have not been established.
[c]Not effective against incubating syphilis.
[d]Contraindicated in pregnant or nursing patients, or patients younger than 18 years old.
[e]Treatment of disseminated gonococcal infection should also include appropriate treatment for *Chlamydia*.
[f]For patients allergic to cephalosporins.
[g]Initial treatment continues for 24 to 48 hours after improvement begins; oral agents continue for a total of 7 days of treatment.
[h]Contraindicated in pregnant or nursing patients, or patients younger than 8 years old.
Adapted from Centers for Disease Control and Prevention. 1998 Guidelines for treatment of sexually transmitted diseases. *MMWR* 1998:47(RR-1).

that documents its efficacy against anal, genital, and pharyngeal GC, and resistance has not been identified. Its disadvantages are the added pain and expense of injection and the unavailability of vials of less than 250 mg. Pain on injection may be minimized by using 1% lidocaine as the diluent. Quinolone-resistant GC has rarely been reported in the United States, but a cluster of GC with reduced sensitivity to quinolones has been reported in the Cleveland, Ohio, area.[3,9] Spectinomycin (2 g intramuscularly) may be used in patients unable to take cephalosporins or quinolones, but, like the quinolones, it is ineffective against incubating syphilis.[4]

All patients treated for GC should have blood samples drawn for syphilis serology. Patients with incubating syphilis are likely to be cured by ceftriaxone or any of the regimens that include a 7-day course of doxycycline or erythromycin.[4] Patients with positive serologies should be treated as discussed in the section on syphilis. Because of a reported high incidence of human immunodeficiency virus (HIV) infection in patients presenting with sexually transmitted disease, it is recommended that these patients also be offered serologic testing for HIV, as well as appropriate counseling.

DISPOSITION

Patients with uncomplicated GC may be managed as outpatients and do not require follow-up evaluation for test of cure. Patients treated for GC should be advised to refrain from sexual activities until they and their sex partner or partners have completed antibiotic therapy and are completely asymptomatic.[4] Patients who are symptomatic after treatment have usually been reinfected, but they should be carefully evaluated for other sexually transmitted diseases or other causes of their symptoms, and should have culture of mucosal sites to look for resistant strains of GC.

The control of GC is highly dependent on contact tracing. Patients should be strongly encouraged to refer sexual contacts for treatment or to provide health-care personnel with the identities of exposed partners. The CDC recommends evaluation and treatment of persons who have had sexual contact with symptomatic patients within 30 days preceding onset of symptoms. If the index case is asymptomatic, sexual contacts within the preceding 60 days should be treated.[4] If the contact was before these time periods, the most recent sex partner should be treated. Special effort should be made to identify contacts of women with PID, because 20% to 60% of the infected sexual partners of these women may be asymptomatic.[14] Emergency physicians should be aware of and comply with state and local health department sexually transmitted disease–reporting guidelines.

Although hospitalization is recommended for patients with DGI, several centers routinely and successfully manage individuals with uncomplicated arthritis–dermatitis syndrome as outpatients. Only reliable patients with a typical presentation and ready access to follow-up care should be considered for outpatient treatment. It is imperative that these patients understand that anything other than a prompt response to therapy (definite improvement within 24 to 48 hours and essentially complete remission of symptoms within 72 hours of the initiation of therapy) necessitates an immediate return for further evaluation and possible hospitalization. Failure to respond rapidly to one of the recommended treatment regimens suggests either an alternative diagnosis or, rarely, infection with an antibiotic-resistant strain of GC. Patients in whom the diagnosis is uncertain, who have purulent synovial effusions, or whose psychosocial situation may make compliance unlikely or follow-up difficult should probably not be considered candidates for outpatient therapy. Patients with meningitis or endocarditis should be treated with ceftriaxone (1 to 2 g intravenously every 12 hours),[4] and infectious disease consultation should be requested.

COMMON PITFALLS

- The most common error in the management of GC is failure to diagnose. A significant proportion of men with GC remain asymptomatic, and the mild, nonspecific symptoms of primary GC in women require a high index of suspicion on the part of the emergency physician. This is especially true of adolescents, who have increasing rates of infection and often lack access to health care.[21] A detailed sexual history should be obtained from all patients presenting with urogenital or rectal complaints, and there should be a low threshold for obtaining cultures and instituting antibiotic therapy.
- The absence of symptoms should never lead the clinician to withhold antibiotics in a patient with known exposure to GC.
- Although a positive urethral or cervical Gram stain is highly specific for GC, the sensitivity is low in asymptomatic patients. Thus, a negative Gram stain should never be used to justify withholding therapy if there is a suspicion of GC.

References

1. Baker RW, Peppercorn MA. Gastrointestinal ailments of homosexual men. *Medicine* 1982;61:390.
2. Barlow D, Phillips I. Gonorrhoea in women: diagnostic, clinical, and laboratory aspects. *Lancet* 1978;1:761.
3. Centers for Disease Control and Prevention. 1998 Guidelines for treatment of sexually transmitted diseases. *MMWR* 1998;47(RR1).
4. Centers for Disease Control and Prevention. Summary of notifiable disease, United States, 1997. *MMWR* 1998;46(54).
5. Cucurull E, Espinoza LR. Gonococcal arthritis. *Rheum Dis Clin North Am* 1998;24:305.
6. Eisenstein B, Masi AT. Disseminated gonococcal infection (DGI) and gonococcal arthritis (GGA): I. Bacteriology, epidemiology, host factors, pathogen factors, and pathology. *Semin Arthritis Rheum* 1981;10:155.
7. Hook E, Holmes K. Gonococcal infections. *Ann Intern Med* 1985;102:229.
8. Hutt DM, Judson F. Epidemiology and treatment of oropharyngeal gonorrhea. *Ann Intern Med* 1986;104:655.
9. Knapp JS, Fox KK, Trees DL, et al. Fluoroquinolone resistance in *Neisseria gonorrhoeae*. *Emerg Infect Dis* 1997;3:33.
10. Koumans EH, Johnson RE, Knapp SJ. Laboratory testing for *Neisseria gonorrhoeae* by recently introduced nonculture tests: a performance review with clinical and public health considerations. *Clin Infect Dis* 1998;27:1171.
11. Masi AT, Eisenberg B. Disseminated gonococcal infection (DGI) and gonococcal arthritis (GCA): II. Clinical manifestations, diagnosis, treatment, complications, and prevention. *Semin Arthritis Rheum* 1981;10:173.
12. McCutchan A. Epidemiology of venereal urethritis: comparison of gonorrhea and nongonococcal urethritis. *Rev Infect Dis* 1984;6:669.
13. McNeeley SG Jr. Gonococcal infections in women. *Obstet Gynecol Clin North Am* 1989;16:467.
14. Potterat J, King R. A new approach to gonorrhea control: the asymptomatic man and incidence reduction. *JAMA* 1981;245:578.
15. Romanowski B, Harris JRW, Wood H, et al. Improved diagnosis of gonorrhea in women. *Sex Transm Dis* 1986;13:93.
16. Rompalo AM, Hook EW, Roberts PL, et al. The acute arthritis–dermatitis syndrome: the changing importance of *Neisseria gonorrhoeae* and *Neisseria meningitidis*. *Arch Intern Med* 1987;147:281.
17. Schin J, Keith L. Problems in the culture diagnosis of gonorrhea. *J Reprod Med* 1985;30[Suppl]:244.
18. Shafer MA, Pantell RH, Schachter J. Is the routine pelvic examination needed with the advent of urine-based screening for sexually transmitted diseases? *Arch Pediatr Adolesc Med* 1999;153:119.
19. Smith KR, Ching S, Lee H, et al. Evaluation of ligase chain reaction for use with urine for identification of *Neisseria gonorrhoeae* in females attending a sexually transmitted disease clinic. *J Clin Microbiol* 1995;33:455.
20. Sweet R. Pelvic inflammatory disease. *Sex Transm Dis* 1986;13:192.
21. Webster LA, Berman SM, Greenspan JR. Surveillance for gonorrhea and primary and secondary syphilis among adolescents, United States: 1981–1991. *MMWR* 1993;42(SS3).
22. Wexner SD. Sexually transmitted diseases of the colon, rectum, and anus. *Dis Colon Rectum* 1990;33:1048.

CHAPTER 186
Syphilis

Richard Wolfe

Syphilis has been a public health problem since the fifteenth century, when thousands died in a European epidemic. Over the years, syphilis evolved into an indolent disease manifested primarily by neuropsychiatric sequelae (20% of the patients in U.S. mental institutions in the 1920s had tertiary syphilis). The incidence of the disease dropped dramatically in the 1940s with the development of serologic screening programs and the introduction of penicillin. Between 1985 and 1990, a syphilis epidemic, due to the practice of "sex for drugs," in crack cocaine users occurred throughout the United States.[1,2,11]

Since 1990, syphilis rates have declined each year. The incidence of syphilis is highest in large metropolitan areas with relatively large minority populations. It remains substantially more common among Blacks than among other ethnic groups and continues to be concentrated in the southern region of the United States. Because the emergency department is the only access to health care for many high-risk patients, emergency physicians have a unique opportunity to detect cases of syphilis and aid in the public health effort to control and eradicate this disease.[6]

Syphilis infection occurs when *Treponema pallidum*, a spirochete, is disseminated through the body via the bloodstream or lymphatics. The primary pathologic lesion of syphilis is a focal endarteritis. *T. pallidum* is transmitted, most often during sexual activity, by contact between infectious lesions and sites of minor trauma. The risk of transmission varies significantly with the stage of disease and occurs primarily from contact with the lesions of primary and secondary syphilis. Among sexual partners of patients with infectious syphilis, approximately one-third will acquire the disease. Transmission may also occur later in the course of the disease, notably when congenital syphilis occurs in infants born to women with latent disease.

CLINICAL PRESENTATION

Primary Syphilis

Primary skin lesions (chancres) typically begin as papules at the site of inoculation. They quickly erode to form a painless ulcer, which is usually indurated, with characteristic cartilaginous consistency on palpation of the margins and the base (Fig. 186.1). The chancre is found commonly on the penis, labia, fourchette, or cervix, and occasionally on extragenital sites such as the perianal area (especially in homosexual men), oropharynx, fingers, and nipples. The lesions are usually single, but may be multiple in up to one-third of cases. Untreated chancres usually heal within 3 to 6 weeks.

Primary syphilis is associated with painless unilateral lymphadenopathy. Regional lymph nodes appear within 1 week of the onset of the lesion and are typically mobile, rubbery, and minimally tender.

Secondary Syphilis

The secondary stage of syphilis begins 4 to 10 weeks after the appearance of the chancre in virtually all cases of untreated primary syphilis. This stage is characterized by a broad spectrum of physical findings resulting from the immunologic response to the dissemination of *T. pallidum* in the bloodstream and lymphatics. Flulike symptoms, including myalgias, arthralgia, and low-grade fever, are common. Generalized lymphadenopathy with moderately enlarged, nontender lymph nodes is often present.

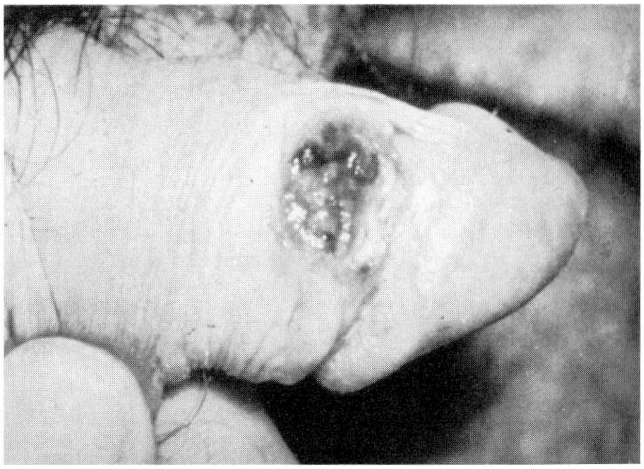

Figure 186.1. Syphilis: penile chancre.

The most prominent feature of secondary syphilis is the rash, which is present in more than 75% of cases. It is typically nonpruritic. The initial lesions are symmetrically distributed pink macules, typically 5 to 10 mm in diameter, over the trunk and proximal extremities. The lesions may evolve with time into a maculopapular rash, although papular papulosquamous and pustular lesions may occur. The widespread distribution involves the soles and the palms (Figs. 186.2 and 186.3). Skin findings may be subtle, and, in one-fourth of cases, patients fail to notice the rash.

Ten percent to 20% of patients with secondary syphilis develop large, pale, flat papules that coalesce to form broad-based, flat, or heaped-up fleshy lesions with a pearly gray appearance.

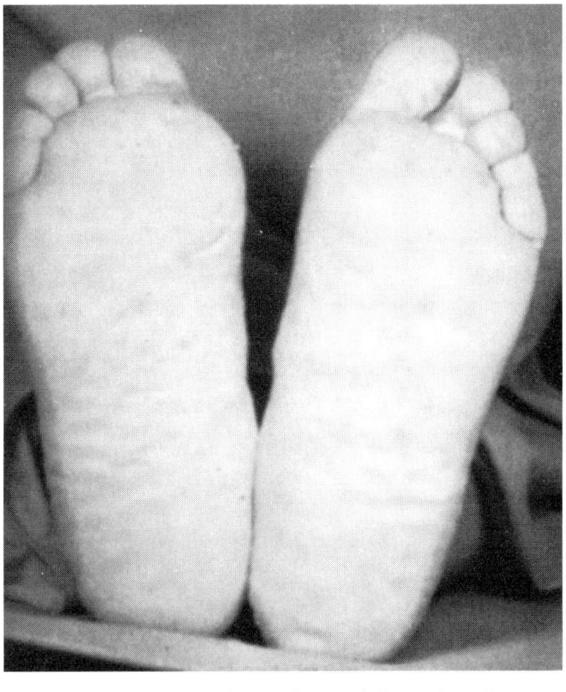

Figure 186.2. Lesions of secondary syphilis on the soles.

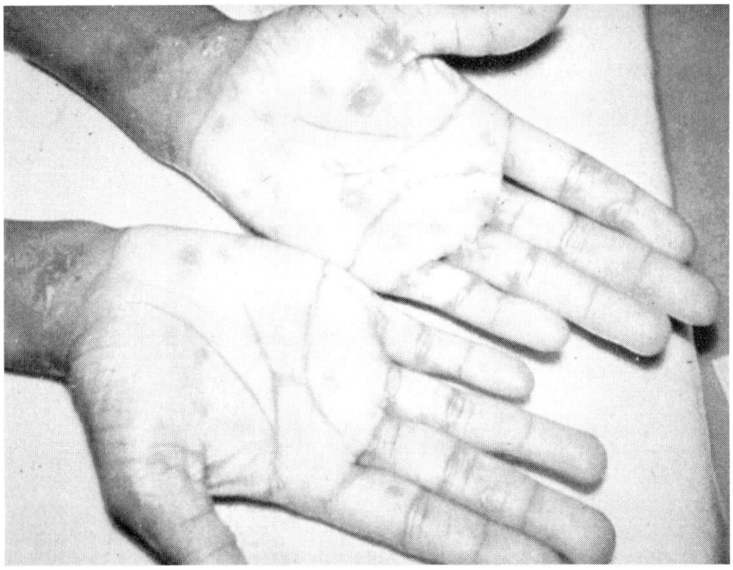

Figure 186.3. Lesions of secondary syphilis on the palms.

These highly infectious lesions are termed *condylomata lata* and are located in the warm, moist intertriginous areas, notably the anogenital regions (Fig. 186.4). They are particularly common during relapses, when they tend to be asymmetrically distributed and more infiltrated. Examination of the oral and genital mucosa may reveal painless, superficial lesions covered with a silver-gray membrane (mucous patches). Hair loss may occur in a diffuse spotty distribution (alopecia areata) affecting the scalp, eyebrows, and beard. The lesions of secondary syphilis heal within 2 to 6 weeks, and the infection becomes latent.

Gastrointestinal complaints are common in secondary syphilis and may be caused by hypertrophic gastritis, patchy proctitis, or an ulcerative lesion resembling a rectal neoplasm. Less common complications of secondary syphilis include hepatitis, nephropathy, arthritis, and periostitis. When symptomatic central nervous system (CNS) involvement occurs, ocular lesions (iritis, uveitis, retinitis, and optic neuritis) are the most common presentation. Patients with uveitis that has failed to respond to steroid therapy should thus be screened for syphilis.

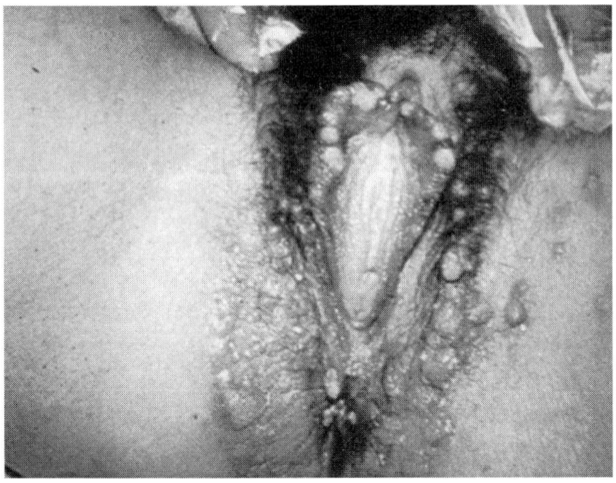

Figure 186.4. Condylomata lata.

Latent Syphilis

The latent period corresponds to the absence of clinical signs and symptoms but positive serologic test results (discussion follows). The World Health Organization arbitrarily divides latent syphilis into early latent (duration less than 1 year) and late (duration more than 1 year). However, because relapses of symptomatic syphilis can occur for up to 2 years and the risk of congenital syphilis continues to be high during this period, a 2-year cut-off (as used by the International Classification of Diseases) is more clinically accurate. Early latent syphilis is considered potentially infectious but requires a shorter course of treatment than late latent disease because *T. pallidum* is dividing more rapidly. Because the duration of infection cannot be established in many patients, however, it is safest to treat patients as if they had late latent syphilis but to manage their sexual contacts as if they had early latent disease.[7]

Tertiary Syphilis

Tertiary syphilis is rarely seen. It develops in only one-third of untreated patients, and, in the immunocompetent host, it occurs 4 to 30 years after the initial infection. Tertiary syphilis embraces a wide variety of manifestations: gummatous syphilis (approximately 15%), cardiovascular syphilis (10% to 26%), and neurosyphilis (8% to 10%).[4]

Gummas are circumscribed granulomas that develop on skin, mucous membranes, and subcutaneous tissue, predominantly at the site of trauma on the extremities, head, and neck. These lesions eventually become necrotic and develop central ulceration. Gummas also occur in the bone, most commonly the tibia.[8] Mass effects lead to the principal clinical manifestations: bony pain, obstructive jaundice, and perforation of the nasal septum.

Cardiovascular syphilis has become rare in the penicillin era. On the basis of postmortem data, it occurs in 25% of untreated patients. The most common lesions are aortic aneurysms (40%), aortic regurgitation (29%), and coronary ostial stenosis (26%). Cardiac hypertrophy, myocarditis, pulmonary arteritis, cardiac gummas, and coronary artery disease at sites other than the coronary ostia occur less often.

CNS involvement occurs at all stages of syphilis. It presents as one of many clinical syndromes or may remain asymptomatic, the diagnosis being based on the serologic testing of the cerebrospinal fluid (CSF). Patients with neurosyphilis commonly present with seizures or ocular findings.[5] Visual dysfunction, which may occur in both early and late syphilis, is often misdiagnosed in the active stages of the disease and underdiagnosed in the late stages.[10]

Syphilitic meningitis due to spirochetal spread tends to occur in the first 2 years after the initial infection. Patients with the disease may present with mild-to-moderate aseptic meningitis, with only a headache or with frank meningismus and associated cranial nerve abnormalities. Uveitis, retinitis, or optic neuritis may occur as isolated processes or in association with syphilitic meningitis.

In contrast, meningovascular syphilis occurs 5 to 10 years after infection and is due to involvement of small, medium, and large arteries. Patients present with a sudden cerebrovascular event occurring after months of a subacute encephalitic syndrome. For this reason, it is recommended that young patients presenting with stroke should have serologic testing to rule out syphilis.

The neurologic findings of tertiary syphilis are due to demyelination of the posterior columns, dorsal roots, dorsal root ganglia, and nerve trunks. Late neurosyphilis, once the most common form of CNS involvement, has also become very uncommon since the advent of penicillin. Tabes dorsalis and general paresis most often present from 10 to 20 years after infection. Tabes dorsalis is manifested by sudden episodes of pain predominantly in the lower extremities but occasionally in the larynx, rectum, vagina, and other organs. Physical findings include reflex changes, peripheral neuropathy, ataxia, urinary incontinence, and impotence. Ocular atrophy and an Argyll Robertson pupil (a poor reaction to direct light with a normal reaction to accommodation) are classically described. General paresis initially presents with mild personality changes; over time, memory loss, confusion, and, ultimately, organic psychosis develop.

DIFFERENTIAL DIAGNOSIS

Atypical lesions are common in primary syphilis, and, conversely, not all patients with "typical chancres" have syphilis. Other localized genital infections may occur in sexually active patients. Herpes simplex virus is a common cause of nonvesicular genital ulceration that can resemble a syphilitic chancre but is almost always painful.[3] Multiple ulcerations are usually found and present as grouped vesicles with a yellow-white membranous coating on an erythematous base. The associated lymphadenopathy is usually painful.

Chancroid, caused by infection with *Haemophilus ducreyi*, produces a painful soft ulcer with a necrotic base and undermined edges. Granuloma inguinale produces a painless, shallow, sharply demarcated ulcer with a beefy-red friable base. The characteristic Donovan bodies are found in scrapings from the ulcer base. In lymphogranuloma venereum, when ulceration occurs, the lesions often go unnoticed by the patient because they are small and painless. The associated lymph nodes are firm and painful, with overly dusky skin. Streptococcal, staphylococcal, and candidal infections may result in painful genital ulceration. Trauma, hypersensitivity to drugs, and neoplasm may present as a genital ulceration.

The diffuse symmetrical rash of secondary syphilis needs to be differentiated from other papulosquamous rashes, such as exanthems, drug eruptions, and pityriasis rosea. If the palms and soles are involved, the differential diagnosis may be limited to a few disorders, such as hand-foot-and-mouth disease and Rocky Mountain spotted fever. Clinically differentiating secondary syphilis from the acquired immunodeficiency syndrome (AIDS) may be extremely difficult, because both diseases share common risk factors and may coexist. AIDS may present as a diffuse macular, maculopapular, or pustular rash, and only laboratory studies will distinguish the eruption from syphilis.

Condylomata acuminata may be confused with genital warts in which the initial lesions may consolidate to form a large perianal cauliflower-like mass. However, genital warts are smaller and more sharply raised. Visceral involvement in secondary syphilis may suggest other causes of gastritis, hepatitis, or nephropathy.

Gastric syphilis may present as gastritis, peptic ulcer disease, or malignancy. Prolonged duration of symptoms and lack of improvement with H_2 blockers suggest the diagnosis. Findings at endoscopy are typically limited to the antral and pyloric regions, with the appearance of multiple erosions or shallow ulcers, nodularity, and hypertrophy of the rugae.[9]

Neurosyphilis should be differentiated from degenerative neurologic disorders, from granulomatous disease and other causes of aseptic meningitis, and from disorders involving the vasculature of the CNS. General paresis should be differentiated from other causes of organic brain syndrome.

EMERGENCY DEPARTMENT EVALUATION

A careful history and physical examination should suggest the possibility of syphilis in patients presenting with genital lesions or with a rash consistent with secondary syphilis. Laboratory testing is generally required to confirm the diagnosis.

Although *T. pallidum* cannot be cultured, dark-field microscopy can visualize spirochetes in exudates from chancres and condylomata lata, as well in lymph node aspirates in secondary syphilis. A concentration of treponemes of at least 104 is required to visualize the organism. The surface of the suspected lesion should be cleaned with saline solution and gauze without producing bleeding. Squeezing of the lesion may help produce serous fluid. Local cleansing with soap or application of topical antibiotics should be avoided before examinations.

Three negative examinations are required before a suspicious lesion is considered to be nonsyphilitic. When dark-field microscopy is unavailable, immunofluorescence may be utilized. Refinements in monoclonal antibody techniques have been shown to be just as accurate. Nonpathogenic treponemes are found in the mouth and gastrointestinal tract. Diagnosis of oral lesions should be made on the basis of clinical appearance, history, and serologic testing. Immunofluorescent microscopy is generally needed for biopsies of oral or rectal lesions.

The diagnosis of primary and secondary syphilis should be confirmed by serologic testing. The most common screening test, the Venereal Disease Research Laboratory (VDRL) and the rapid plasma reagin (RPR) tests are nontreponemal antibody tests. These are easier and less expensive but less specific than treponemal antibody tests such as the fluorescent treponemal antibody absorption (FTA-ABS) test or the microhemagglutination assay for antibody to *T. pallidum* [MHA-TP]. There are many causes of false-positive nontreponemal tests and a few for false-positive treponemal tests (Table 186.1).

The VDRL is positive in 60% to 80% of patients with primary syphilis. Serologic testing has the most utility shortly after the initial infection, but the highest titers are found during secondary syphilis and the early phase of latent syphilis. The VDRL is positive in 99% of patients with secondary syphilis. False-negatives occur in patients with such high titers of antibody that they are in antibody excess (prozone phenomenon). Dilution of the serum paradoxically results in conversion to a positive test in these cases.

TABLE 186.1. Common Causes of False-Positive Serologic Test Results for Syphilis

RPR/VDRL
Pneumococcal pneumonia
Bacterial endocarditis
Tuberculosis
Chancroid
Lymphogranuloma venereum
Malaria
Rickettsial disease
Mycoplasma pneumonia
Chickenpox
Human immunodeficiency virus infection
Measles
Infectious mononucleosis
Mumps
Viral hepatitis
Pregnancy
Connective tissue disease
Intravenous drug use
Multiple blood transfusions
Chronic liver disease
Multiple myeloma
Advanced cancer
Advanced age
TREPONEMAL TESTS
Lyme disease
Malaria
Infectious mononucleosis
Systemic lupus erythematosus

Because standard antibiotic therapy does not achieve treponemicidal levels in the CSF, a diagnosis of neurosyphilis implies the need for more intensive treatment. The diagnosis is based on a positive VDRL on the CSF and a reactive serum FTA-ABS test. It is generally agreed that a lumbar puncture should be done in all patients who demonstrate neurologic or neuropsychiatric findings and in certain high-risk individuals. These include those with syphilis of unknown duration, more than 1 year of untreated disease, or suspected treatment failure and all individuals who are positive for human immunodeficiency virus (HIV). Syphilis may progress more rapidly and present atypically in patients with HIV infection, and these individuals typically develop early neurosyphilis. False-negative serologic tests occur more commonly in these patients; a VDRL test should be performed on the CSF as well as the blood.

Although CSF findings suggestive of infection are rare in primary syphilis, CSF pleocytosis and elevated protein levels occur in more than 40% of patients with secondary or latent syphilis. Lumbar puncture is not useful in early syphilis in the absence of HIV infection. However, asymptomatic neurosyphilis occurs in later stages of the disease. Lumbar puncture should be performed if there is more than 1 year's duration of disease, when treatment failure has occurred, or when nonpenicillin therapy is planned. Lumbar puncture is mandatory in patients with cardiovascular syphilis, as 10% to 25% of these individuals have coexistent neurosyphilis.

EMERGENCY DEPARTMENT MANAGEMENT

Parenteral penicillin is the drug of choice for the treatment of all stages of syphilis. Primary, secondary, and early latent syphilis should be treated with a single intramuscular dose of 2.4 million U of benzathine penicillin. In penicillin-allergic patients, doxycycline (100 mg PO twice daily for 14 days) or erythromycin (500 mg four times a day for 14 days) may be used as an alternative. All sexual contacts within the previous 90 days should be identified and receive treatment for early syphilis. Importantly, the currently used treatment regimens for gonorrhea that include a β-lactam antibiotic appear to be effective against incubating syphilis.

Patients with late latent syphilis or cardiovascular syphilis should receive a similar dose of benzathine penicillin weekly for 3 weeks, or of oral doxycycline for 4 weeks.

Parenteral penicillin G is the only therapy with documented efficacy for neurosyphilis or for syphilis during pregnancy. Patients who report a penicillin allergy, including pregnant women with syphilis in any stage and patients with neurosyphilis, should be desensitized and treated with penicillin. Patients with neurosyphilis should be treated with either 2 million to 4 million U of penicillin G intravenously every 4 hours for 14 days, or with 2.4 million U of procaine penicillin G intramuscularly daily (with 500 mg of oral probenecid four times a day) for 14 days. Congenital syphilis is treated with penicillin G, 50,000 U/kg intravenously or intramuscularly every 8 hours for 14 days.

The Jarisch-Herxheimer reaction occurs in 50% of patients treated for primary syphilis, in 90% of patients with secondary syphilis, and in 25% of patients with early latent syphilis. The reaction, consisting of fever, myalgias, and headache, occurs within 2 hours of treatment and peaks within 7 hours of treatment. Vasodilatation, tachycardia, and mild hypotension may also be seen, and the lesions of secondary syphilis become more erythematous and edematous. These symptoms can almost always be managed with bedrest and aspirin, although rare cases of irreversible organ damage have occurred in some individuals with neurosyphilis or cardiovascular syphilis.

About 95% of patients with primary syphilis and about three-fourths of those with secondary or early latent syphilis revert to having a negative VDRL or RPR test within 2 years of appropriate treatment. These tests are thus used to monitor the effectiveness of treatment. Treponemal antibody titers are likely to remain positive indefinitely. They correlate poorly with disease activity and should not be used to assess treatment response.

DISPOSITION

All cases of syphilis must be reported to the state health department. Admission is indicated only for patients with neurosyphilis or congenital syphilis who require parenteral antibiotics. Some authorities have recommended that patients who are several months pregnant also be admitted to the hospital for treatment, basing their recommendation on the concern that a Jarisch-Herxheimer reaction may develop and that tocolytic therapy may be required. Patients should be warned that sexual partners require treatment, and all patients should be referred for follow-up to evaluate response to therapy.

COMMON PITFALLS

- Cleansing or applying topical antibiotics to chancres or other lesions, thereby possibly altering their appearance and reducing accuracy of dark-field examination of diagnostic specimens
- Failure to perform a lumbar puncture in high-risk patients, resulting in inadequate therapy
- Failure to order serologic testing for syphilis in the CSF of HIV-positive patients who undergo lumbar puncture
- Mistaking a febrile reaction 2 hours after the administration of penicillin for allergy to penicillin rather than a Jarisch-Herxheimer reaction

References

1. Centers for Disease Control. Primary and secondary syphilis—United States, 1997. *MMWR* 1998;47:493.
2. Centers for Disease Control. Guidelines for treatment of sexually transmitted diseases. *MMWR* 1998;47:1.
3. Chapel TA, Brown WJ, Jeffries C, et al. How reliable is the morphologic diagnosis of penile ulcerations. *Sex Transm Dis* 1977;4:150.
4. Clark EG, Danbolt N. The Oslo study of the natural course of untreated syphilis: an epidemiologic investigation based on a re-study of the Boeck-Bruusgaard material. *Med Clin North Am* 1964;22:1725.
5. Hira SK, Patel JS, Bhat SG, et al. Clinical manifestations of secondary syphilis. *Int J Dermatol* 1987;26:103.
6. Hook EW, Marra CM. Acquired syphilis in adults. *N Engl J Med* 1992;326:1060.
7. Hutchinson CM, Hook EW. Syphilis in adults. *Med Clin North Am* 1990;74:1389.
8. Kampmeir RM. The late manifestations of syphilis: skeletal, visceral, and cardiovascular. *Med Clin North Am* 1964;48:667.
9. Kolb JC, Woodward LA. Gastric syphilis. *Am J Emerg Med* 1997;15:164.
10. Spoor TC, Wynn P, Hartel WC, et al. Ocular syphilis: acute and chronic. *J Clin Neuroophthalmol* 1983;3:197.
11. Van Voorst Vader PC. Syphilis: management and treatment. *Dermatol Clin* 1998;16:699.

CHAPTER 187
Lyme Disease

Edward B. Bolgiano and Robert A. Barish

Lyme disease (LD), a tick-borne illness caused by the spirochete *Borrelia burgdorferi,* is the most common vector-borne disease in the United States.[8] *Ixodes scapularis* (the deer tick, formerly named *I. dammini*) and related tick species are the primary vectors in the transmission of the disease to humans. LD occurs worldwide and has been reported on every continent except Antarctica. The three major epidemiologic foci in the United States are the northeastern coastal states, from Massachusetts to Maryland; Wisconsin and Minnesota; and Northern California and Oregon.[5] Most human infections with *B. burgdorferi* occur during the months of May through August, when *I. scapularis* nymphal-stage activity and human outdoor activity are both at their peak. Early diagnosis and treatment are important to prevent morbidity (and, rarely, mortality) associated with later stages of the illness.

CLINICAL PRESENTATION

LD is a complex multisystem disorder with three clinical stages, each having a range of clinical manifestations and often overlapping with other stages (Table 187.1). Virtually any clinical feature may occur alone or recur at intervals, and late symptoms may occur without any preceding early symptoms.

The most recently recognized of the seven human spirochetal diseases, LD shares many features with them: (1) the skin or mucous membrane as a portal of entry; (2) spirochetemia early in the course of the disease, with wide dissemination; and (3) periods of latency followed by multisystemic involvement.

LD usually begins with localized infection of the skin, manifested by a lesion termed *erythema migrans* (EM), and its associated nonspecific constitutional symptoms. The lesion is followed by dissemination of the spirochete to other organs. Neurologic or cardiac symptoms may occur days to weeks later, and chronic arthritic and neurologic abnormalities may occur weeks to months later.

Early Localized Infection (Stage I)

LD begins with the inoculation of *B. burgdorferi* by the nymphal form of the tick vector during feeding, generally about 2 days after attachment.[15] The onset of symptoms is usually about 1 week (range, 3 to 32 days) after the tick bite.

EM, the most characteristic clinical manifestation of LD, is nevertheless absent in about 20% of patients. It usually (but not always) occurs at the site of a tick bite, beginning as red macules that expand centrifugally. There are two general forms: (1) an expanding red patch with varying intensities of redness within the patch (Fig. 187.1A) and (2) a central red patch surrounded by normal-appearing skin, that is, in turn, surrounded by an expanding red band, resembling a target or a ring-within-a-ring configuration (see Fig. 187.1B).

Most lesions are smooth, although scaling may be present, and the involved area is warmer than the surrounding normal-appearing skin. The centers of some lesions may become red and indurated, crusted, or vesicular and necrotic; partial or complete central clearing may occur. Most EM lesions are annular, but triangular and elongated patches may occur. Most demonstrate gradual enlargement, but others expand rapidly, forming a large patch in a relatively short period. Although a rash diameter of at least 5 cm is necessary to satisfy the Centers for Disease Control surveillance criteria, individual patients with LD may not have lesions this size. In patients seen 1 to 7 days after the appearance of lesions, the average size is 8 × 10 cm (ranges from 2 × 3 cm to 25 × 25 cm). Although most lesions are asymp-

TABLE 187.1. Clinical Stages of Lyme Disease

Stage	Time	Manifestations
Early localized infection	7–14 days; range, 3–30 days	Erythema migrans With or without nonspecific constitutional symptoms (fever, malaise, fatigue, headache, myalgia, and arthralgia) Asymptomatic
Early disseminated infection	Days to weeks	Multiple or secondary erythema migrans lesions Nervous system Musculoskeletal system Heart
Late disseminated disease	Weeks to months	Arthritis Chronic neurologic manifestations

A

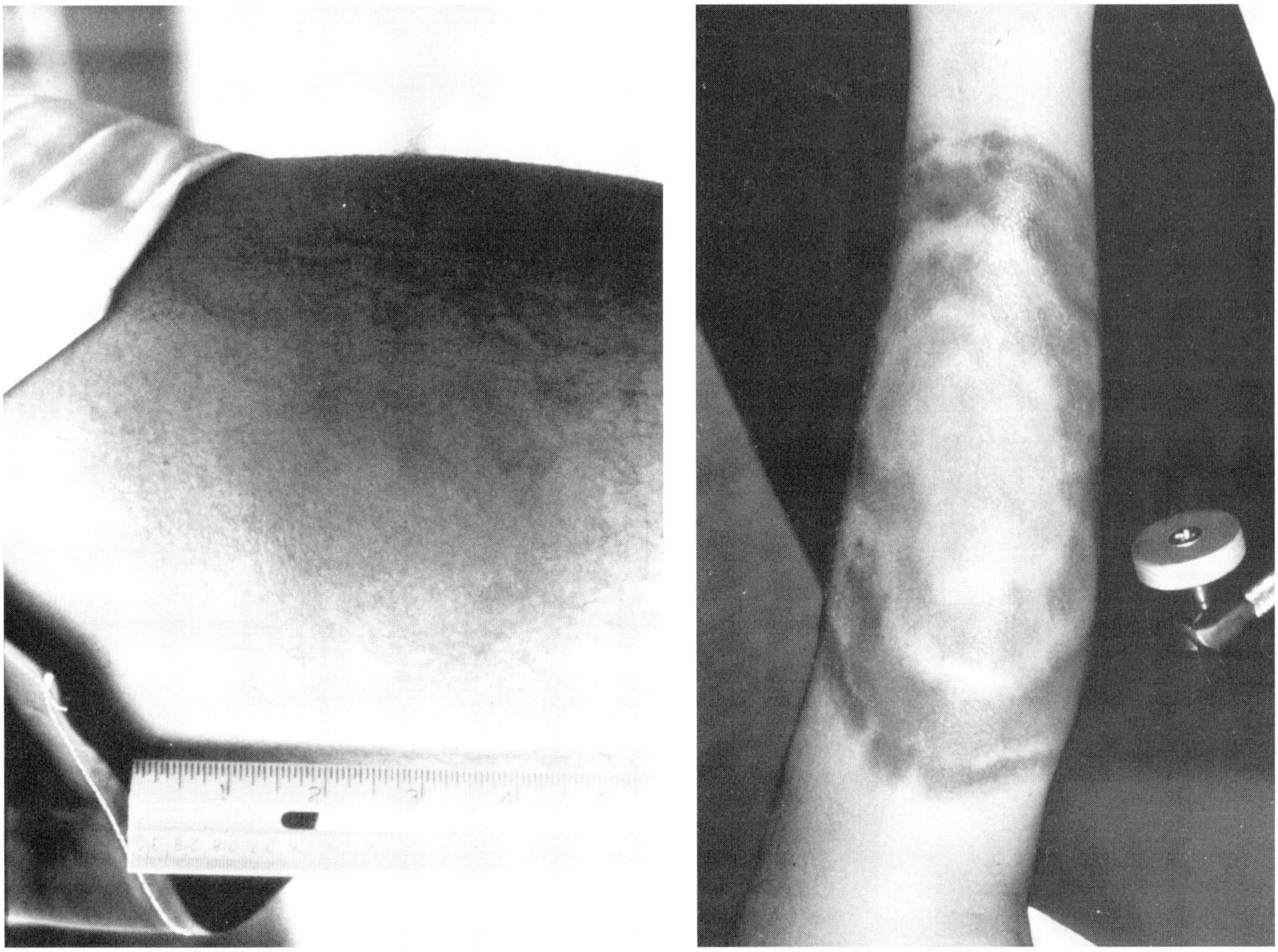

B

Figure 187.1. Two general forms of erythema migrans. (**A**) Expanding red patch. (**B**) Target configuration. (Courtesy of the Centers for Disease Control and Prevention.)

tomatic, some patients describe burning, itching, or, rarely, a painful sensation.[12]

The EM rash usually fades within several days of antibiotic therapy. Without treatment, primary and secondary lesions generally persist for about 28 days (range, 1 week to 14 months). Recurrent lesions may develop in patients who do not receive antibiotics. Untreated, the rash resolves over several weeks.

Minor constitutional symptoms commonly occur in stage I LD.[11,14] Malaise, fatigue, and lethargy are most common (approximately 80% of patients). Fever is typically low grade and intermittent. Regional lymphadenopathy in the distribution of the rash often accompanies EM. General lymphadenopathy and splenomegaly may occur. Musculoskeletal symptoms such as arthralgias and myalgias are common and characterized by a migratory, asymmetric, and evanescent pattern. Often, symptoms last only hours in one location and reappear later in another location. Frank arthritis with joint effusion may occur at this stage, but it is rare.

Upper respiratory symptoms such as sore throat occur less commonly. Signs and symptoms of hepatitis, including anorexia, nausea, vomiting, and abdominal pain, may be noted. Headache is a common complaint and may be accompanied by photophobia, nausea, vomiting, and stiff neck, but Kernig and Brudzinski signs are usually absent. At this stage, the neurologic examination and cerebrospinal fluid (CSF) both yield normal findings.

In the absence of the characteristic rash or a history of a tick bite, the nonspecific nature of the early signs and symptoms can easily result in misdiagnosis of stage I LD as a viral illness or collagen vascular disorder. Stage I symptoms usually last for several weeks in untreated patients but may persist for months.

Early Disseminated Infection (Stage II)

After a variable latent period, early disseminated symptoms usually occur from days to weeks after the initial infection, but there can be an overlap with other manifestations. The skin, nervous system, heart, and eyes are the main targets in early disseminated disease.

Within several days to several weeks, 20% to 50% of patients develop multiple annular secondary skin lesions, which are smaller than the initial ones. Usually asymptomatic, they typically spare the palms, soles, and mucous membranes.

Neurologic involvement occurs in approximately 15% of untreated patients. The most common neurologic manifestation is a fluctuating meningoencephalitis. Symptoms of cranial neuropathy, peripheral neuropathy, or radiculopathy may be superimposed, or may each occur alone.[9] Headache is usually present, and there may be nausea, vomiting, lethargy, or irritability. As in stage I, Kernig and Brudzinski signs are absent, and results of computed tomography are normal.[15,16] By contrast with stage I findings, however, CSF examination in stage II may reveal a lymphocytic pleocytosis and elevated protein level; glucose levels are normal.

Cranial neuropathy is seen in about 50% of patients with Lyme meningitis, most commonly, a unilateral peripheral seventh-nerve palsy (it may be bilateral in about a third of patients). Peripheral nervous system manifestations may include mononeuritis and motor or sensory radicular involvement or brachial plexitis.

Estimates of the incidence of cardiac involvement in untreated patients with LD range from 4% to 8%. Lyme carditis usually presents as transient myocarditis associated with varying degrees of atrioventricular block.[7] The average time from the initial illness to the development of carditis is about 5 weeks (range, 4 days to 7 months).[11] Common presenting symptoms of Lyme carditis are nonspecific, but include syncope, lightheadedness, dyspnea, palpitations, and chest pain. Atrioventricular block of some degree occurs in almost 90% of patients.[11] More than half of them have either high-grade or complete block, yet almost all are symptomatic. Left ventricular dysfunction has been documented by two-dimensional echocardiography and radionuclide studies; in most reported cases, it has been mild and transient. Pericarditis is uncommon, and the heart valves are spared.

A variety of ocular manifestations of LD have also been reported. They include conjunctivitis, keratitis, choroiditis, retinal detachment, optic neuritis, and blindness. Papilledema, with or without increased CSF pressure, is associated with Lyme encephalitis.

Late Disseminated Infection (Stage III)

The chronic phase of LD typically occurs months to years after the initial infection and is characterized by arthritic and, less commonly, neurologic symptoms. As is the case with syphilis, chronic manifestations follow a variable latent period.

Before antibiotic therapy for LD became standard, approximately 50% of untreated patients developed arthritis characterized by intermittent attacks of joint swelling and pain developing several weeks to several years after the onset of the illness.[16] The typical pattern of joint involvement is a monoarticular or asymmetric oligoarticular arthritis of the large joints. The knee is most often affected, with large, sometimes relatively asymptomatic joint effusions. The shoulder, elbow, temporomandibular joint, ankle, wrist, hip, and small joints of the hands and feet are involved less commonly. Episodes of arthritis are typically brief (weeks to months), separated by variable periods of complete remission.

Exacerbations and remissions often occur over a period of several years, with a gradual tendency toward less frequent and less severe occurrences. In untreated patients, there is a spontaneous long-term remission rate of 10% to 20% per year, but 10% of untreated patients develop chronic synovitis. An autoimmune response that persists after the pathogen has been eradicated may explain the unresponsiveness of some patients with chronic arthritis to antibiotic therapy. Chronic arthritis is much less common now, because most patients with early Lyme symptoms are recognized and treated.

Neurologic manifestations of late disease include a wide variety of abnormalities of the central and peripheral nervous systems, as well as fatigue syndromes.[9] The diagnosis is difficult because the symptoms may mimic those of a number of other neurologic conditions and because late neurologic symptoms may be the first symptoms of the disease.[14] Subtle encephalopathy with disturbances in mood, memory, or sleep may occur. Cases of cognitive dysfunction ranging from a mild "confusional" state to slowly progressive dementia have also been reported.[2,9] Incapacitating fatigue is a widely described late feature.

Late disease may also involve the cranial nerves, spinal roots, plexuses, or peripheral nerves. The neurologic symptoms of late disease commonly manifest as a subtle polyneuropathy, with spinal or radical pain or numbness and tingling in the hands and feet. A demyelinating condition with multiple sclerosis–like exacerbations and remissions has been described.[14]

Acrodermatitis chronica atrophicans is a late cutaneous manifestation of LD that occurs in approximately 10% of European patients but has rarely been reported in North America. It is characterized initially by an edematous infiltration that progresses to an atrophic lesion resembling that of localized scleroderma.

DIFFERENTIAL DIAGNOSIS

Although LD presents in many ways, each stage has characteristic clinical findings that are helpful in narrowing a differential diagnosis that may, at first, seem rather broad.

Stage I disease may easily be confused with a variety of other diseases, especially if the rash is absent. Even in endemic areas, most patients who present with "flulike" symptoms during the summer months do not have LD. The principal diagnostic distinction to be made is between LD and the enteroviral diseases and other causes of aseptic meningitis. The enteroviral diseases are frequently accompanied by diarrhea, which is not a feature of LD. Abdominal pain, anorexia, and nausea may suggest hepatitis. Sore throat, adenopathy, and fatigue, as seen in mononucleosis, may occur. When myalgias and arthralgias are the predominant symptoms, connective tissue disease may be considered. A distinctive feature of early LD, however, is that musculoskeletal pain is typically migratory and evanescent, and often occurs in brief attacks in one or a few locations at a time.

The characteristic initial skin lesion, EM, in its classic form is virtually pathognomonic for LD. Secondary skin lesions may, however, be confused with the target lesions of erythema multiforme. The lesions of erythema multiforme are generally smaller and nonexpanding and also involve the mucous membranes and palms and soles; EM does not. Hypersensitivity reactions to insect bites or spider bites may mimic EM, but these reactions usually occur within several hours of exposure, rather than 3 or more days after the exposure. Erythema nodosum has a predilection for the extensor surfaces of the legs and generally causes more painful induration than does EM.

Erythema marginatum secondary to acute rheumatic fever may mimic EM, but the lesions of EM are generally fewer, larger, and less evanescent, and they migrate more slowly. Other common cutaneous entities to be considered in the differential diagnosis of EM include cellulitis and fixed drug-related eruptions. A useful rule is that LD must be considered in a patient with an atypical rash that is accompanied by a flulike or meningitis-like illness during the months of peak incidence.

The cardiac manifestations of LD may suggest coronary artery disease, viral myocarditis, or acute rheumatic fever. As noted previously, varying degrees of heart block are characteristic. As with rheumatic fever, carditis in LD may follow pharyngitis and migratory polyarthritis. Although the clinical aspects of the Jones criteria may be satisfied by some patients with LD, several features serve to distinguish the two illnesses:

1. EM usually precedes the carditis in LD, whereas, in rheumatic fever, skin lesions usually occur with the onset of arthritis.
2. Evidence of a preceding streptococcal infection (elevated antistreptolysin-O titer) is lacking in patients with LD.
3. Valvular involvement is not a feature of Lyme carditis.

The differential diagnosis of the neurologic manifestations of LD is wide and includes aseptic meningitis, herpes simplex encephalitis, Bell's palsy, multiple sclerosis, Guillain-Barré syndrome, dementia, primary psychosis, cerebral vasculitis, and brain tumor. Lyme encephalopathy is usually associated with CSF abnormalities such as lymphocytosis, elevated protein, and the presence of antibody to the spirochete. Chronic fatigue syndrome and fibromyalgia are frequently misdiagnosed as LD.[18]

In contrast to patients with rheumatoid arthritis, those with Lyme arthritis rarely have symmetric polyarthritis, morning stiffness, positive rheumatoid factor, or subcutaneous nodules. LD is commonly mistaken for seronegative rheumatoid arthritis, but it is most similar to the rheumatoid variants, particularly Reiter syndrome. The absence of the extraarticular features of Reiter syndrome (conjunctivitis, urethritis or cervicitis, balanitis, keratodermia blennorrhagica) at the time of the arthritis helps distinguish LD from Reiter syndrome. In children, LD may mimic juvenile rheumatoid arthritis.

EMERGENCY DEPARTMENT EVALUATION

The diagnosis of LD is primarily clinical, based on the presence of EM and other specific manifestations, as well as a history of exposure in an endemic area. Diagnosis is difficult, however, especially in the early stages. A history of tick bite is present in only about one-third of cases. EM is present in most patients, but isolated late symptoms may appear months after the initial infection, and the patient might not recall having had a rash.

Routine laboratory studies are nonspecific and generally are not helpful in diagnosing LD. Culture of blood, tissue, and bodily fluids for *B. burgdorferi* are generally not clinically useful. Specialized laboratory studies must be cautiously interpreted within the clinical context and should be regarded as only adjuncts in the diagnosis.

Serologic testing for *B. burgdorferi* infection is the most practical and useful means of confirming clinical diagnosis of LD, but problems with the performance and interpretation of the tests often result in diagnostic confusion. The assays have not been standardized, and there is a significant interlaboratory and even intralaboratory variability. False-negative and especially false-positive results are common.

The antibody response to *B. burgdorferi* develops slowly. The peak of immunoglobulin M (IgM) titers appears between 3 and 6 weeks after the onset of illness, so assays for IgM are often negative during the first several weeks of infection. Moreover, IgM returns to nondiagnostic levels 4 to 6 weeks after peak. IgG antibody may be detectable 2 months after exposure and peaks approximately 12 months into the illness. Early antibiotic therapy may blunt or even abolish the antibody response. Patients with late disease usually have positive IgG antibody titer results. Nevertheless, a true-positive serologic result merely indicates previous exposure; the symptoms under evaluation need not be related to active LD. Long-term seropositivity may also result from previously treated LD.

Serologic cross-reactivity between *B. burgdorferi* and other spirochetes, most notably *Treponema pallidum*, can cause false-positive test results. Other illnesses known to be associated with false-positive serologic results include infectious mononucleosis, rheumatoid arthritis, and systemic lupus erythematosus.

Testing with the enzyme-linked immunosorbent assay (ELISA) is the cornerstone of the laboratory diagnosis of LD. Although ELISA alone has a sensitivity of 89% and a specificity of 72%, a positive result in patients with a pretest probability of LD of less than 0.20 is more likely to be a false positive than a true positive.[2] In patients with a positive or equivocal ELISA, a confirmatory Western blot should be ordered.[4] Polymerase chain reaction (PCR) has been used to amplify the genomic DNA of *B. burgdorferi* in skin, blood, CSF, and synovial fluid, but PCR has not been standardized for routine diagnostic use.[3]

In cases of suspected neurologic involvement, CSF should be examined for evidence of meningitis.[9] CSF serologic testing is generally not necessary, because almost all patients with neuroborreliosis have positive results on serum serologic testing.[2]

EMERGENCY DEPARTMENT MANAGEMENT

The emergency management of patients with suspected LD should be focused on recognizing the illness, obtaining appropriate diagnostic studies, delivering supportive care when necessary, and arranging appropriate follow-up.

Active *B. burgdorferi* infection is usually amenable to antibiotic therapy, and treatment can be begun in the emergency department. In making treatment decisions, however, the clinical findings and the meaning and the reliability of laboratory results must be closely analyzed on an individual basis. For this reason, decisions regarding antibiotic therapy (which are almost invariably nonurgent) are often made in consultation with the patient's primary physician. Table 187.2 is a summary of recommended antibiotic regimens. Treatment recommendations have been developed on the basis of disease stage and clinical manifestations.

Prompt treatment of early disease shortens the duration of symptoms and, more important, prevents progression to later stages in most patients. The decision of whom to treat is often difficult. As noted, early LD is diagnosed by clinical presentation alone, without the luxury of serologic confirmation. Patients are often seronegative at presentation, and curative antibiotic therapy may abort the development of a mature immune response and prevent seroconversion after treatment. Treatment is clearly indicated for a patient who has the characteristic skin lesion and a history of tick bite; there is no reason to wait for a positive antibody assay before beginning therapy. Patients in endemic areas who have a rash that is consistent with EM should be treated for LD without serologic testing.

Oral therapy with doxycycline is recommended for early LD (see Table 187.2).[1] Amoxicillin is an alternative for pregnant or lactating women and for children younger than 8 years old.[11] Jarisch-Herxheimer–like reactions (fever, chills, myalgias, headache, tachycardia, increased respiratory rate, and leukocytosis) may occur in the first 24 hours of treatment. Cefuroxime axetil appears to be as effective as doxycycline,[1] but cephalexin is ineffective in LD. Erythromycin is less effective than first-line antibiotics. Azithromycin was less effective than amoxicillin in one controlled trial.[10]

The duration of antibiotic therapy should be individualized according to the severity of illness and the rapidity of clinical response. EM and associated constitutional symptoms generally respond within days. Treatment failures or relapses despite recommended courses of antibiotics have been reported.

Neurologic Disease

Facial nerve palsy may occur within the first month of illness (mean time from the onset of EM is 20 days). For patients with Bell's palsy alone, oral therapy with doxycycline or amoxicillin can be used in the same dosage as for early disease (see Table 187.2), but the duration of therapy should be extended to 30 days. Corticosteroids have no identified role.

The decision to treat a patient who presents with facial palsy should be based on epidemiologic factors. Some authorities recommend lumbar puncture for all patients with LD-related Bell's

TABLE 187.2. Recommended Antibiotic Regimens

	Drug	Adult Dosage	Pediatric Dosage[a]
EARLY LYME DISEASE			
	Doxycycline[b]	100 mg PO b.i.d. for 14–21 days	
	or		
	Amoxicillin	250–500 mg PO t.i.d. for 21 days	25–50 mg/kg/d divided t.i.d.
Alternative	Cefuroxime axetil	500 mg PO b.i.d. for 21 days	250 mg b.i.d.
	or		
	Erythromycin (less effective than doxycycline or amoxicillin)	250 mg PO q.i.d. for 21 days	
NEUROLOGIC DISEASE			
Facial nerve paralysis	As an isolated finding, oral regimens for early disease, used for at least 30 days, may suffice.		
	As a finding associated with other neurologic manifestations, intravenous therapy is recommended.		
Lyme meningitis[c]	Ceftriaxone	2 g i.v. by single dose for 14–28 days	75–100 mg/kg/d i.v.
	Penicillin G	20 million U daily in divided doses for 14–28 days	300,000 U/kg/d i.v.
Alternative	Chloramphenicol	1 g i.v. q6h for 10–21 days	
CARDIAC DISEASE			
Mild[d]	Doxycycline[b]	100 mg PO b.i.d. for 21 days	
	or		
	Amoxicillin	250 mg–500 mg PO t.i.d.[a] for 21 days	25–50 mg/kg/d divided t.i.d.
More severe	Ceftriaxone	2 g i.v. daily by single dose for 14–21 days	75–100 mg/kg/d i.v.
	or		
	Penicillin G	20 million U daily in divided doses for 14–21 days	300,000 U/kg i.v.
ARTHRITIS			
Oral	Doxycycline[b]	100 mg PO b.i.d. for 30 days	
	or		
	Amoxicillin	500 mg PO t.i.d. for 30 days	50 mg/kg/d divided t.i.d.
Parenteral	Ceftriaxone	2 g i.v. by single dose for 14–28 days	75–100 mg/kg/d i.v.
	or		
	Penicillin G	20 million U daily in divided doses for 14–28 days	300,000 U/kg/d i.v.

[a]Pediatric dosage should not exceed adult dosage.
[b]Tetracycline 250–500 mg PO q.i.d. may be substituted for doxycycline. Neither doxycycline nor any other tetracycline should be used for children under 8 years old or for pregnant or lactating women.
[c]Regimens for radiculoneuropathy, peripheral neuropathy, and encephalitis are the same as those for meningitis.
[d]Oral regimens are reserved for mild cardiac involvement (see text).
Adapted from references 1 and 20.

palsy, and treatment with intravenous antibiotics if a pleocytosis is present. The implication of asymptomatic CSF pleocytosis is unknown, however.

For patients with more serious complications, such as meningitis, other cranial or peripheral neuropathies, cognitive deficits, or encephalitis, parenteral antibiotic therapy is required.

Cardiac Disease

Recommended antibiotic therapy for patients with cardiac involvement depends on the degree of heart block noted (see Table 187.2). Patients with minor cardiac involvement (first-degree atrioventricular block but a PR interval less than 0.30 second) can usually be treated orally, whereas those with more severe cardiac involvement (high-degree atrioventricular block) require intravenous antibiotics. Temporary cardiac pacing may be necessary in the latter group. Heart block generally resolves completely with antibiotic therapy.

Arthritis

Lyme arthritis usually responds to a 1-month course of oral doxycycline or amoxicillin (see Table 187.2). The response may be delayed for several weeks or months, however, regardless of antibiotic choice or route of administration. Oral regimens appear to be as effective as parenteral penicillin or ceftriaxone.

The diagnosis of LD should be confirmed by serologic testing of synovial fluid when possible. Chronic arthritis may not be responsive to antibiotic therapy (either oral or intravenous) in certain genetically susceptible individuals. Antiinflammatory agents may be useful in the treatment of this presumably immune-mediated syndrome.

Prophylaxis

Antibiotic treatment of asymptomatic patients who have been bitten by a tick is usually not recommended,[4] because the likelihood of acquiring LD is low, even in endemic areas. Infection is very unlikely unless the tick has remained attached beyond 72 hours.[12] The approximate duration of attachment can be assessed by inspecting of the tick for degree of engorgement. Early tick detection and removal limits the risk of disease transmission. Patients should still be counseled about the symptoms of early LD, however, and selective administration of antibiotics on an individualized basis (e.g., to pregnant women or those with engorged ticks) may be appropriate.

Vaccination

A LD vaccine (LYMErix) directed against the outer-surface protein A of *B. burgdorferi* is available. LYMErix is administered by injection of 0.5 mL (30 μg) into the deltoid muscle. Three doses are required for optimal protection. The first dose is followed by a second dose 1 month later, and a third dose administered 12 months after the first dose. In a randomized, controlled clinical trial involving over 10,000 subjects, the vaccine's efficacy in protecting against "definite" LD was 76% (95% CI = 58% to 86%).[17]

Vaccination will cause a positive ELISA result but a negative Western blot. LD vaccination should be considered for persons who reside, work, or enjoy recreation in areas of high or moderate risk and who engage in activities that result in frequent or prolonged tick exposure.[6]

DISPOSITION

Decisions regarding the disposition of patients with documented or suspected LD are made on the basis of disease stage and severity of clinical manifestations.

Almost all patients with early disease can be appropriately managed as outpatients. Many patients with the chronic neurologic and arthritic manifestations of late disease remain fully ambulatory and can be treated on an outpatient basis, although admission may be necessary for selected patients requiring intravenous antibiotics. Follow-up care by a primary care physician, rheumatologist, or infectious disease specialist should be arranged for patients who are discharged from the emergency department.

Hospital admission for cardiac monitoring is required for patients with Lyme carditis and any manifestation more severe than mild PR prolongation. Patients with prominent neurologic symptoms usually must be treated with intravenous antibiotics and often require a degree of supportive care that warrants hospital admission.

COMMON PITFALLS

- Late symptoms of LD may occur without any preceding early symptoms. Because late symptoms usually occur months after the initial tick exposure, there is no constant seasonal incidence suggestive of a tick-borne illness. The diagnosis of LD might therefore not be considered, for example, in a patient who presents during February with an isolated knee effusion.
- Disorders such as chronic fatigue syndrome and fibromyalgia are commonly misdiagnosed as LD, resulting in inappropriate treatment with antibiotics. Despite LD's variable presentations and the limitations that remain in serologic testing, in most cases, it is possible to distinguish between *B. burgdorferi* infection and these disorders.
- Antibiotic treatment for patients with a tick bite who have signs or symptoms of LD is usually not recommended, even in endemic areas.
- Specific diagnostic laboratory tests should not be used in screening, but rather to confirm the clinical diagnosis of LD. Even in endemic areas, most patients with "summer flu" do not have LD. Indiscriminate serologic testing of these patients results in a high rate of false-positive tests.

References

1. Abramowitz M, ed. Treatment of Lyme disease. *Med Lett* 1997;39(1000):47.
2. American College of Physicians. Guidelines for laboratory evaluation in the diagnosis of Lyme disease. *Ann Intern Med* 1997;127:1106–1108.
3. Brettschneider S, Bruckbauer H, Klugbauer N, et al. Diagnostic value of PCR for detection of *Borrelia burgdorferi* in skin biopsy and urine samples from patients with skin borreliosis. *J Clin Microbiol* 1998;36:2658–2665.
4. Centers for Disease Control. Notice to readers: recommendations for test performance and interpretation from the Second National Conference on Serologic Diagnosis of Lyme Disease. *MMWR* 1995;44:590–591.
5. Centers for Disease Control. Lyme disease—United States, 1996. *MMWR* 1997;46:531–535.
6. Centers for Disease Control and Prevention. Recommendations for the use of Lyme disease vaccine: recommendations of the Advisory Committee on Immunization Practices (ACIP). *MMWR* 1999;48(RR07):1–17.
7. Evans J. Lyme carditis. In: Rahn D, Evans J, eds. *Lyme disease*. Philadelphia: American College of Physicians, 1998:77–88.
8. Falagas ME, Gorback SL. *Infect Dis Clin Pract* 1996;5:217.
9. Logigian E. Neurologic manifestations of Lyme disease. In: Rahn D, Evans J, eds. *Lyme disease*. Philadelphia: American College of Physicians, 1998:89–106.
10. Luft BJ, Dattwyler RJ, Johnson RC, et al. Azithromycin compared with amoxicillin in the treatment of erythema migrans: a double-blind, randomized, controlled trial. *Ann Intern Med* 1996;124:785.
11. Nadelman RB, Wormser GP. Lyme borreliosis. *Lancet* 1998;352:557–565.
12. Nadelman R, Wormser G. Management of tick bites in early Lyme disease. In: Rahn D, Evans J, eds. *Lyme disease*. Philadelphia: American College of Physicians, 1998:49–76.
13. Pacher AR. *Borrelia burgdorferais* in the nervous system: the new "great imitator." *Ann NY Acad Sci* 1998;539:5b.
14. Rahn DW. Natural history of Lyme disease. In: Rahn D, Evans J, eds. *Lyme disease*. Philadelphia: American College of Physicians, 1998:35–48.
15. Sood SK, Salzman MB, Johnson BJ, et al. Duration of tick attachment as a predictor of the risk of Lyme disease in an area in which Lyme disease is endemic. *J Infect Dis* 1997;175:996–999.
16. Steere AC, Schoen RT, Taylor E. The clinical evolution of Lyme arthritis. *Ann Intern Med* 1987;107:725–731.
17. Steere AC, Sikand VK, Meurice F, et al. Vaccination against Lyme disease with recombinant *Borrelia burgdorferi* outer-surface lipoprotein A with adjuvant: Lyme Disease Vaccination Study Group. *N Engl J Med* 1998;339:209–215.
18. Steere AC, Taylor E, McHugh G, et al. The overdiagnosis of Lyme disease. *JAMA* 1993;269:1812–1816.

CHAPTER 188
Rocky Mountain Spotted Fever

Michael A. Gibbs

Rocky Mountain spotted fever (RMSF) is the most common tick-borne illness in the United States, and one of the most serious systemic infections seen in clinical practice. Emergency physicians must maintain a high index of suspicion for RMSF and consider early empiric therapy in the patient at risk.

Despite significant advances in diagnosis and therapy, the case-fatality rate of RMSF remains between 5% and 10%. The disease continues to confound physicians because of its sporadic occurrence and nonspecific clinical presentation. Difficulties in making the diagnosis are especially relevant, because the prognosis is directly related to the timeliness of appropriate treatment.

In one study, 90% of patients were seen by a physician within

5 days of the onset of symptoms, yet less than half received treatment before day 6. Patients who received antirickettsial therapy within 5 days were significantly less likely to die than were those who received treatment later (6.5% vs. 22.9%). Three independent predictors of a failure to initiate therapy on first presentation to a physician were absence of a rash, presentation between August 1 and April 30, and presentation within the first 3 days of illness.[3]

EPIDEMIOLOGY

RMSF is caused by *Rickettsia rickettsii,* an obligate intracellular bacterium. It is transmitted by several species of ticks that also serve as the reservoir or natural host. In the Eastern states, the wood tick, *Dermacentor andersoni,* is the major vector; the dog tick, *Dermacentor variabilis,* is the predominant vector in Western states. More than 95% of cases occur between April 1 and August 31, the incidence corresponding to the seasonal life cycle of the tick.

RMSF has been reported throughout the continental United States, Canada, and Mexico. The disease tends to be focally endemic, with clustering of cases within larger endemic areas. Although first described in Idaho and Montana, the disease is now infrequent in the Western states. There has been a steady increase in the number of cases in the Southeastern states, particularly North Carolina, Tennessee, and South Carolina.

Centers for Disease Control (CDC) surveillance data from 1981 to 1990 indicate that RMSF is most common among children 5 to 9 years of age and least common among people 10 to 29 years of age. The case fatality rate is highest for people 40 years of age or older (8.2%), compared with 2.3% for those less than 40 years old. The case-fatality rate is also higher for people whose treatment is begun more than 3 days after the onset of symptoms (6.2%) than for those treated within the first 3 days (1.3%). RMSF is more common in men than in women, reflecting a greater potential exposure to the tick vector. Despite the fact that RMSF is more common in Whites than in African Americans, the case-fatality rate is significantly higher in the latter group (16% vs. 3%),[5] a fact most likely related to the difficulty of detecting the characteristic rash on dark skin.

TABLE 188.1. Clinical Manifestations of Rocky Mountain Spotted Fever

	Any Time(%)	First 3 Days (%)
SIGN OR SYMPTOMS		
Fever (100°F–102°F)	99	73
Fever (>102°F)	90	63
Fever + rash + tick bite	67	3
DERMATOLOGIC		
Any rash	88	49
Rash, maculopapular	82	46
Rash, petechial or hemorrhagic	49	13
Rash on palms and soles	74	28
Edema	18	3
Conjunctivitis	30	13
NEUROLOGIC		
Headache, mild/moderate	91	71
Headache, severe	57	40
Altered mental status	26	6
Meningeal irritation	18	5
Decreased hearing	7	1
Seizures	8	2
CARDIOPULMONARY		
Pneumonitis	12	2
Dysrhythmias	7	1
Myocarditis	5	0
GASTROINTESTINAL		
Abdominal pain	52	30
Nausea/vomiting	60	38
Diarrhea	19	9
Jaundice	9	2
MUSCULOSKELETAL		
Myalgias, mild/moderate	83	57
Myalgias, severe	47	25

From Helmick CG, et al. Rocky Mountain spotted fever: clinical, laboratory, and epidemiological features of 262 cases. *J Infect Dis* 1984;150:480.

CLINICAL PRESENTATION

RMSF is a systemic vasculitis that may affect any organ system. For this reason, signs and symptoms are varied and nonspecific. A history of tick bite or presence of a tick is elicited in just over half of patients. The onset of illness is usually acute, with fever, headache, nausea, vomiting, abdominal pain, and myalgia, a presentation that is easily confused with a clinically benign viral illness. The clinical findings and their prevalence are summarized in Table 188.1.

A *rash* of one type or another is seen the majority of patients with RMSF, but "Rocky Mountain spotless fever" has been reported in 5% to 15% of cases.[6] When patients present at symptom onset, the rash is typically absent, which is one reason that diagnosis is difficult. Likewise, the rash may be unappreciated in patients with dark skin. This group is at especially high risk for delays in diagnosis and therapy, and thus increased morbidity.[5]

The rash usually appears on the third day of illness and is first seen on the palms, soles, wrists, and ankles and progresses centripetally, but the rash may begin on the trunk (approximately 10%) or have a diffuse onset (approximately 10%). Lesions are initially macular and later evolve to become petechial and maculopapular in 50% of cases. Application of a tourniquet or blood pressure cuff causes the appearance of additional lesions distally (Rumpel-Leede sign). In severe case, there may be extensive purpura, skin sloughing, ulceration, and gangrene. Rarely, an eschar may be seen at the site of the tick bite.[7]

The *central nervous system* is perhaps the most crucial target "organ" of RMSF. Varying degrees of meningeal inflammation and cerebral vasculitis cause a wide range of neurologic signs and symptoms. Rickettsial encephalitis, which is manifested by severe headache, confusion, stupor, coma, and seizures, carries a particularly grave prognosis.[8] Focal neurologic deficits, deafness, sensory neuropathy, tardive dyskinesia, and Guillain-Barré syndrome have all been described in patients with RMSF.[9,10]

Neuroimaging with computed tomography (CT) or magnetic resonance imaging (MRI) may reveal a variety of subtle nonspecific abnormalities, including infarcts, cerebral edema, meningeal enhancement, and increased signal of the perivascular spaces.[11] There is some evidence that the presence of these radiographic findings may be associated with a less favorable clinical outcome. In patients with central nervous system involvement, the cerebrospinal fluid is almost always abnormal (discussion follows).

The *cardiovascular* effects of RMSF are the result of myocarditis and myocardial vasculitis.[12] Clinical manifestations include varying degrees of atrioventricular (AV) block, dysrhythmias (atrial and ventricular tachycardia, atrial fibrillation), and left ventricular dysfunction. It has been hypothesized that cardiac involvement may play an important role in the cases of fatal RMSF.

Rickettsial *pneumonitis* results from microvascular injury and leakage of fluid into the interstitial tissues and alveolar airspaces. This potentially life-threatening complication occurs in 2% to 17% of patients. Signs and symptoms include cough, dyspnea, pleuritic chest pain, and hypoxemia. Chest radiography typically reveals diffuse patchy infiltrates.

Up to 80% of patients with RMSF have prominent *gastrointestinal* complaints early in the course of disease, including abdominal pain, nausea, vomiting, and diarrhea. This symptom complex may lead the clinician to incorrectly diagnose acute gastroenteritis, or even an acute surgical abdomen. Not surprisingly, patients with RMSF have undergone exploratory laparotomy for suspected appendicitis, cholecystitis, and perforated diverticulitis.[13] Acute hepatitis and clinical jaundice have been described in severe cases.[14]

Approximately 10% to 15% of patients with RMSF develop significant *renal* dysfunction, the result of systemic hypovolemia and prerenal azotemia, as well as direct injury to the glomerulus. Renal biopsy in these patients demonstrates acute glomerulonephritis with subendothelial immune deposits.

Ocular abnormalities are not uncommon in patients with RMSF. Conjunctivitis occurs in 15% to 60% of patients. Less common findings include anterior uveitis, retinal vasculitis and hemorrhage, papilledema, arterial occlusion, and iris nodules.

DIFFERENTIAL DIAGNOSIS

The clinical diagnosis of RMSF can be difficult despite a careful history and physical examination and appropriate screening laboratory studies. Depending on the constellation of signs and symptoms present, the individual patient with RMSF may be misdiagnosed as having a viral illness (e.g., measles, infectious mononucleosis, or nonspecific viral syndrome), meningococcemia, gastroenteritis, acute surgical abdomen, pneumonia, toxic shock syndrome, ehrlichiosis, or encephalitis. RMSF may also mimic noninfectious entities, including idiopathic thrombocytopenic purpura, thrombotic thrombocytopenic purpura, drug reaction, and immune-complex vasculitis.

As with RMSF, diagnosis must be made quickly and accurately in acute meningococcemia. Both diseases may present with headache, fever, nausea, vomiting, and upper respiratory symptoms. Meningococcemia is typically more abrupt in onset. In contrast to RMSF, the meningococcemic rash appears within 24 hours of symptom onset, is petechial at onset, and lacks a characteristic pattern. Gram stain of cerebrospinal fluid is diagnostic, and the causative organism can also be detected using latex agglutination and counterimmunoelectrophoresis. If either diagnosis is in question, immediate therapy for both RMSF and meningococcemia is mandatory.

Toxic shock syndrome is an acute febrile illness characterized by the appearance of a diffuse desquamating erythroderma. Mucous membrane involvement and conjunctivitis are typical. Headache, myalgias, nausea, vomiting, and diarrhea are often present. Criteria for toxic shock syndrome include (1) fever greater than 38.9°C, (2) the typical rash, (3) hypotension, and (4) involvement of at least three organ systems.

Distinguishing RMSF from an enteroviral infection can also be quite difficult. Fever, headache, aseptic meningitis, and a maculopapular rash are common to both presentations. The rash of enteroviral infections usually starts centrally, but may also involve the palms and soles. Petechial lesions are not uncommon.

Measles (rubeola) occurs most often in unimmunized children during the winter and early spring. A prominent respiratory prodrome (cough, coryza, conjunctivitis), and the presence of Koplik's spots are important distinguishing features. The rash of measles typically begins on the face and upper trunk and spreads to the extremities and downward.

Infectious mononucleosis is characterized by fever, fatigue, malaise, sore throat, and prominent lymphadenopathy. A maculopapular rash involving the trunk and extremities is often present, and it may become more prominent if the patient is inadvertently treated with ampicillin. The diagnosis is confirmed by a positive Monospot test, or by detection of antibodies against the Epstein-Barr virus.

EMERGENCY DEPARTMENT EVALUATION

Laboratory studies typically available in the emergency department offer little help in the diagnosis of RMSF. While routine studies may provide subtle clues, these are inconsistent and nonspecific. It must be emphasized that treatment must be based on clinical findings alone, and should never be withheld while waiting for specific serologic confirmation of the disease.

Hematologic findings seen in RMSF include a normal or decreased white blood cell count, anemia, thrombocytopenia, and a high peripheral band count. It has been suggested that the observation of an increased percentage of immature white cells in the absence of leukocytosis can help distinguish RMSF from meningococcemia. Anemia and thrombocytopenia are seen in 30% and in 30% to 50% of patients, respectively. Hyponatremia is seen in roughly one-fourth of cases. Elevation of serum transaminases and bilirubin may be noted in patients with hepatic involvement.

A lumbar puncture is mandatory in all patients with severe headache, fever, or signs of meningeal irritation. Elevated cerebrospinal fluid protein and pleocytosis are the typical finding in RMSF. Differential cell counts may reveal either lymphocytic or polymorphonuclear cell predominance. Of note, a cerebrospinal fluid white blood cell count more than 100 cells/μL is uncommon, occurring in only 11% of cases.[15]

Serologic tests are of value in the retrospective confirmation of RMSF, but are not helpful in the acute setting, as results are not reliably positive for 6 to 10 days after the onset of clinical illness. Currently, the most widely used tests, all of which rely on the presence of antibodies to *R. rickettsii* antigens, are the indirect immunofluorescent antibody assay (IFA), indirect hemagglutination assay (IHA), latex agglutination, and polymerase chain reaction (PCR).[16] These serologic tests may not be routinely available in all hospital settings, but they can usually be obtained through state health department laboratories. The Weil-Felix test, once a widely used assay for RMSF, lacks sensitivity and specificity and has fallen out of favor.

Identification of *R. rickettsii* in skin biopsy specimens is the best diagnostic test for RMSF in the acute setting. This technique can be used only when the rash is present. A punch biopsy should be obtained at the center of a well-defined lesion. Immunofluorescent staining of frozen-section samples demonstrates the organism in about 70% of cases.

EMERGENCY DEPARTMENT MANAGEMENT

For the majority of the conditions seen in emergency medicine, a diligent search for the cause is undertaken, and specific therapy is initiated based on the findings. This management paradigm is not realistic or acceptable in RMSF for several important reasons: (1) Clinical signs and symptoms are typically nonspecific; (2) the results of specific diagnostic tests are unavailable in a timely fashion; and (3) outcome is directly affected by delays in initiating therapy.

The most important factor contributing to the persistent case-fatality rate of 5% is delayed administration of specific therapy.[3] In one series, all patients treated within 5 days of symptom onset survived, whereas the mortality of those treated after the sixth day was 60%. It is not only appropriate, but essential for the clinician practicing in an endemic area to initiate antibiotic therapy in the patient with clinical findings suggestive of, but not necessarily diagnostic of, RMSF without the aid of serologic testing.

The tetracyclines and chloramphenicol are both effective in the treatment of RMSF and are considered the drugs of choice for therapy.[17] There are no randomized, controlled trials comparing the efficacy of these two agents. The fluoroquinolones have also been demonstrated to possess antirickettsial activity.[18] The penicillins, cephalosporins, erythromycin, sulfonamides, clindamycin, and aminoglycosides are ineffective against RMSF. Both the tetracyclines and chloramphenicol have significant adverse side effects; therefore, agent selection should be guided by the characteristics of the individual patient.

Because of a significant risk of thrombophlebitis and hepatotoxicity with the use of intravenous tetracycline, intravenous chloramphenicol is the preferred agent in the severely ill patient who cannot tolerate oral therapy. Chloramphenicol has also been advocated for treatment of RMSF during pregnancy. The recommended dosage is 50 to 100 mg/kg/d. Side effects associated with chloramphenicol include bone marrow depression, hemolytic anemia in patients with the Mediterranean form of glucose-6-phosphate dehydrogenase deficiency, "gray baby" syndrome in premature infants and neonates, and (rarely) aplastic anemia. Because chloramphenicol is metabolized by the liver, drug interactions may occur in patients taking either inhibitors or inducers of hepatic enzymes.

The tetracyclines are considered the drugs of choice for oral therapy in adults. The recommended dosages for tetracycline hydrochloride and doxycycline are 500 mg four times a day, and 100 mg twice a day, respectively. Doxycycline is the most favorable agent for the treatment of RMSF in children less than 9 years of age because of its documented effectiveness, broader margin of safety, and convenient dosing schedule. The recommended dosage is 4.4 mg/kg in divided doses every 12 hours for the first day of therapy, followed by a daily dose of 2.2 mg/kg.

Prior recommendations discouraged administration of doxycycline to children because of concerns about staining of the teeth. More recent evidence suggests that up to five short courses of doxycycline may be administered with minimal risk of dental staining.[19] Adverse effects associated with the use of tetracyclines include hepatitis, diarrhea, rash, thrombophlebitis, and impaired fetal bone formation.

Regardless of the agent selected, patients should be treated for at least 7 to 10 days, and therapy should be continued as necessary until the patient is afebrile and clinically improved for 24 to 48 hours.[20]

Successful treatment of the critically ill patient with RMSF requires meticulous attention to fluid and electrolyte balance. Widespread systemic vasculitis and resultant fluid shifts may cause hypotension, oliguric renal failure, disseminated intravascular coagulation, adult respiratory distress syndrome, and shock. In the treatment of these complications, the clinician must maintain a delicate balance between adequate restoration of intravascular volume and overresuscitation with precipitation of pulmonary edema. Isotonic saline should be given in small serial boluses. Vasopressors may be required in patients with impaired tissue perfusion that is unresponsive to fluid therapy. Hemodynamic monitoring with a pulmonary artery catheter may provide the treating physician with an extra margin of safety, and is recommended in the unstable patient.

Prevention

Emergency physicians play an important role in educating the public about disease prevention. People who reside or work in tick-infested areas should be informed about tick-borne diseases and their prevention. The optimal method for preventing RMSF is avoidance of tick-infested areas. People entering these areas should wear protective clothing and use tick repellent. Exposed areas of the body should be examined for tick attachment. Remove ticks by grasping them with fine tweezers at the point of attachment and pulling slowly and steadily.

DISPOSITION

When an otherwise healthy, clinically stable patient presents with one or several clinical findings suggestive of RMSF, it is appropriate to initiate empiric therapy without confirmatory diagnostic testing and discharge the patient with appropriate follow-up. In endemic areas, patients presenting with a flulike illness during the spring or summer months are frequently discharged home on doxycycline. In this situation, contact with a primary care provider, or a return visit to the emergency department in 24 to 72 hours, is a sensible part of the discharge plan.

Patients presenting with more severe disease should be admitted to the hospital. This group includes those with significantly abnormal vital signs, dehydration, or end-organ dysfunction. Patients with severe organ dysfunction (e.g., cerebritis, pneumonitis, myocarditis) or hemodynamic instability should be admitted to an intensive care unit. Prompt administration of antibiotics and early consultation with an intensivist and an infectious disease specialist are also appropriate.

COMMON PITFALLS

- Failure to consider the diagnosis of RMSF in the patient with fever and a "viral syndrome" during the peak season (April 1 to September 30) in an endemic area
- Failure to recognize that roughly 15% patients with RMSF present without a rash ("Rocky Mountain spotless fever"). Among ultimately fatal cases, a rash is absent at the time of first presentation to a physician in more than 80%.
- Failure to appreciate the often prominent gastrointestinal features of RMSF, resulting in an incorrect diagnosis of gastroenteritis
- Failure to initiate appropriate antirickettsial therapy in a timely fashion
- Overreliance on laboratory testing, which offers little in the acute phase of RMSF, or withholding of indicated therapy while waiting for definitive serologic confirmation of the disease

References

1. Bonawitz C, et al. Comparison of CT and MR features with clinical outcome in patients with Rocky Mountain spotted fever. *Am J Neuroradiol* 1997;18:459.
2. Cale DF, et al. Treatment of Rocky Mountain spotted fever in children. *Ann Pharmacother* 1997;31:492.
3. Centers for Disease Control. Current trends in Rocky Mountain spotted fever—United States, 1990. *MMWR* 1991;40:451.
4. Dalton MJ, et al. National surveillance for Rocky Mountain spotted fever,

1981–1992: epidemiologic summary and evaluation of risk factors for fatal outcome. *Am J Trop Med Hyg* 1995;52:405.
5. Faham RH, et al. Rocky Mountain spotted (and spotless) fever. *Compr Ther* 1992;18:18.
6. Hall GW, et al. White blood cell count and differential in Rocky Mountain spotted fever. *North Carolina Med J* 1979;40:212.
7. Helmick CG, et al. Rocky Mountain spotted fever: clinical, laboratory, and epidemiological features of 262 cases. *J Infect Dis* 1984;150:480.
8. Horney LF, et al. Meningoencephalitis as a major manifestation of Rocky Mountain spotted fever. *South Med J* 1988;81:915.
9. Kirk JL, et al. Rocky Mountain spotted fever: a clinical review based on 48 confirmed cases: 1943–1986. *Medicine* 1990;69:35.
10. Kirkland KM, et al. Therapeutic delay and mortality in cases of Rocky Mountain spotted fever. *Clin Infect Dis* 1995;20:1118.
11. Lochary ME, et al. Doxycycline and staining of permanent teeth. *Pediatr Infect Dis J* 1998;17:429.
12. Marin-Garcia J, et al. Myocardial function in Rocky Mountain spotted fever: echocardiographic assessment. *Am J Cardiol* 1983;51:341m.
13. Sexton DJ, et al. Rocky Mountain "spotless" and "almost spotless" fever: a world in sheep's clothing. *Clin Infect Dis* 1992;15:439.
14. Shaked Y. Rickettsial infection of the central nervous system: the role of prompt antimicrobial therapy. *Q J Med* 1991;79:301.
15. Trianabos T, et al. Detection of *Rickettsia rickettsii* DNA in clinical specimens by using polymerase chain reaction technology. *J Clin Microbiol* 1989;27:2866.
16. Voggli VL, et al. Pulmonary pathology of Rocky Mountain spotted fever (RMSF)in children. *Pediatr Pathol Lab Med* 1980;104:171.
17. Weber DJ, et al. Rocky Mountain spotted fever. *Infect Dis Clin North Am* 1991;5:19.
18. Wei TY, et al. Acute disseminated encephalomyelitis after Rocky Mountain spotted fever. *Pediatr Neurol* 1999;21:503.
19. Westerman EL. Rocky Mountain spotless fever: a dilemma for the clinician. *Arch Intern Med* 1982;142:1106.
20. Woodard TE, et al. Prompt confirmation of Rocky Mountain spotted fever: identification of rickettsiae in skin tissues. *J Infect Dis* 1976;134:297.

CHAPTER 189
Tuberculosis

Gregory J. Moran and David A. Talan

Tuberculosis (TB) causes more deaths worldwide than any other single infectious disease.[5] An estimated 30% to 60% of adults in developing countries are infected with *Mycobacterium tuberculosis*. Approximately 8 million new cases of active disease develop annually, resulting in as many as 3 million deaths worldwide. An estimated 10 to 15 million persons in the United States (4% to 6% of the population) are infected with *M. tuberculosis*.

The incidence of TB in the United States had been decreasing since the 1950s due to the introduction of better public health measures and effective anti-TB drugs. In the mid-1980s, however, that trend reversed itself and an increase in TB cases was noted. The resurgence of TB has disproportionately affected the poor, ethnic minorities, and immigrants, as well as prison and homeless populations. Multidrug-resistant strains of *M. tuberculosis* have also been found in increasing numbers, especially among immigrants and patients with the acquired immunodeficiency syndrome (AIDS). Increased efforts to control the disease in the United States have led to a decrease in TB cases in recent years.

M. tuberculosis is a slow-growing bacterium transmitted between persons by droplet nuclei produced from coughing and sneezing. The small size of the droplets allows them to remain suspended in the air for long periods of time. Infection may occur if contaminated droplets are inhaled and reach the alveoli. The risk of infection is a function of the level of contamination of the air and the length of time the air is breathed. Small, enclosed areas with poor ventilation are more likely to promote the spread of TB.

The small size of airborne droplet nuclei containing infectious organisms allows them to enter the alveoli of the lung. *M. tuberculosis* infection usually begins in the alveoli, where bacilli are able to multiply. Infection may spread through the lymphatics to regional lymph nodes, and subsequently to the bloodstream. In most persons, cell-mediated immunity will develop over 2 to 10 weeks and is adequate to contain the infection. The TB skin test usually becomes positive during this period. In this situation, in which the immune system prevents further spread, the person is said to have *M. tuberculosis* infection without disease. These people have no clinical symptoms of TB and cannot infect others.

M. tuberculosis survives within macrophages as a facultative intracellular parasite, and thus may remain dormant in the body for many years. Active TB develops within 2 years in about 5% of patients, and another 5% will develop reactivation disease at some later point over the course of a lifetime. Reactivation is more likely to occur in people with impaired cell-mediated immunity, such as those with diabetes, renal failure, immunosuppressive therapy, and malnutrition.

AIDS patients lack the ability to mount an effective cell-mediated immune response and are thus much more likely to progress to active disease. The incidence of TB in AIDS patients is almost 500 times that in the general population. The risk of developing active TB in human immunodeficiency virus (HIV)–infected persons with a positive tuberculin skin test is estimated to be 5% to 10% per year, compared with the 5% to 10% lifetime risk for people not infected with HIV.

Multidrug-resistant TB (MDR-TB) is defined as that due to an organism with resistance to two or more primary anti-TB drugs (currently, isoniazid [INH], rifampin, pyrazinamide [PZA], ethambutol, and streptomycin). Factors associated with the presence of MDR-TB include previous treatment (especially patients who were given an inadequate regimen or were not fully compliant), exposure to a known case of MDR-TB, birth or residence in an area of high MDR-TB incidence (e.g., Asia, South and Central America, and Africa), and living in environments such as homeless shelters and prisons, where there may be a high risk of MDR-TB transmission. HIV-infected patients who are exposed to MDR-TB are at especially high risk of developing disease.

Several factors contribute to the development and spread of MDR-TB. One of the most important is incomplete compliance with medications. Failure to take medication as prescribed may allow drug-resistant organisms to develop. The prescribed regimen must contain at least two drugs to which the organism is susceptible. Because susceptibility testing takes several weeks to complete, some patients receive inadequate treatment regimens while susceptibility results are pending. With ineffective therapy, the patient remains infectious and can spread the resistant organism to others.

Because patients on inadequate therapy are infectious for longer periods of time, MDR-TB may have a selective advantage over susceptible strains, which may lead to an increasing frequency of MDR-TB. Until more effective therapies or vaccines are available, the best weapon against TB is an aggressive infection control program focusing on early diagnosis, isolation, and directly observed therapy for TB patients.

CLINICAL PRESENTATION

The symptoms of TB vary dramatically, depending on the site and stage of infection as well as the overall health and immune status of the host. Some patients have mild symptoms that go unnoticed; some may be truly asymptomatic. Such patients may be identified only through exposure history, an abnormal chest radiograph, a positive TB skin test, or a positive TB culture.

Early pulmonary TB often causes no symptoms. As the disease progresses, patients may develop insidious constitutional symptoms such as fatigue, anorexia, weight loss, fevers, and night sweats. Cough may progress slowly over weeks to months, becoming productive of mucopurulent sputum. TB must be considered in any patient at risk who has a cough of more than 2 to 3 weeks' duration. Hemoptysis due to endobronchial erosion may be present, usually indicating more advanced disease. Some patients present with a more acute onset of fever, chills, cough, and myalgias, similar to an episode of acute bronchitis or pneumonia. Chest findings of rales or consolidation may be present. Patients may have a dull ache or tightness in the chest, or they may have pleuritic pain related to tuberculous pleuritis. Signs of pleural effusion may indicate a tuberculous empyema.

Most cases of disseminated TB have a subacute presentation with systemic symptoms. However, some patients with hematogenous dissemination of TB may present with an acute illness of fever, dyspnea, and cyanosis, mimicking bacterial sepsis. Physical findings may include hepatosplenomegaly, lymphadenopathy, erythema nodosum, and tuberculous lesions visible on examination of the optic fundi. Elderly patients are particularly prone to presenting with unexplained fever and hematologic abnormalities such as pancytopenia or leukemoid reaction.

TB may involve virtually any structure in the body and produce symptoms and signs related to the affected organs as well as systemic symptoms. In about 15% of TB cases, major involvement is seen at an extrapulmonary site. Granulomatous lymphadenitis is usually caused by *M. tuberculosis* in adults, but nontuberculous mycobacteria are a more common cause in children. The cervical and supraclavicular nodes are the most common sites of infection, but any nodes may be involved. Genitourinary TB may present as recurrent urinary tract infections without the growth of the usual bacterial pathogens, pyuria without bacteriuria, or simply recurrent fever. Skeletal tuberculosis is most common in the spine (Pott disease) and weight-bearing joints and usually presents as fever and localized pain.

Tuberculous meningitis is more common in small children as a complication of initial infection, but it can occur in any age group. TB meningitis typically has a subacute onset and may present as headache, altered mental status, or seizures. Cranial nerve signs attributable to involvement of the basilar meninges may be present. Some patients may have new psychiatric symptoms. The cerebrospinal fluid characteristically shows a moderate lymphocytic pleocytosis (usually 100 to 500 cells/mm^2), elevated protein, and low glucose.

HIV-infected patients are especially prone to having atypical presentations of TB. TB usually causes disease at an earlier stage of HIV infection than opportunistic pathogens such as *Pneumocystis carinii*, presumably because TB is more virulent than these other pathogens. Extrapulmonary involvement is much more common in HIV-infected patients with TB, occurring in 40% to 75% of cases, usually with concomitant pulmonary disease. In patients with advanced HIV infection, cavitary lung disease and localized extrapulmonary disease are relatively less common; diffuse interstitial pneumonia (mimicking *P. carinii* pneumonia) and disseminated infection are more typical.

DIFFERENTIAL DIAGNOSIS

Pulmonary TB can potentially mimic many other diseases, including pneumoconiosis, bacterial pneumonia, bronchiectasis, sarcoidosis, lung abscess, neoplasm, and fungal infections such as coccidioidomycosis or histoplasmosis or *P. carinii*. Factors that may be helpful in identifying TB as a cause of illness include history of exposure to TB; characteristic radiographic findings, such as cavitation or apical infiltrates; presence of acid-fast bacilli (AFB) on sputum smear; and results of skin testing. The diagnosis of TB ultimately rests on the culture of *M. tuberculosis*, but culture may take several weeks.

Difficulty may arise in distinguishing disease due to *M. tuberculosis* from disease due to other mycobacterial species. A number of mycobacterial species other than *M. tuberculosis* have been identified. Many are ubiquitous in the environment and are usually contaminants when isolated, but some have been found to be human pathogens. *Mycobacterium avium* complex (MAC, also known as *Mycobacterium avium-intracellulare* [MAI]), *M. kansasii*, and other mycobacteria are rare causes of pulmonary disease; most other mycobacterial species are associated with skin, soft-tissue, and lymph node infections. AFB identified in sputum smears may represent colonization by nonpathogenic mycobacteria, but until they can be definitively identified as such by culture they should be considered to represent *M. tuberculosis* in a patient with a clinical picture consistent with TB.

MAC is the most common mycobacterial species isolated from persons with AIDS in the United States. Infection typically occurs as a systemic febrile illness in end-stage AIDS patients, rather than as a pulmonary infection in earlier stage AIDS patients, as with *M. tuberculosis*.[19] A chest radiograph usually does not suggest mycobacterial disease, and pleuritis is uncommon. Acid-fast smears of stool are commonly positive, but acid-fast smears of sputum are often negative, suggesting that the gastrointestinal tract, rather than the lungs, is the portal of entry.

MAC infections in AIDS patients are often difficult to treat effectively, but they may respond to regimens containing clarithromycin or azithromycin, ethambutol, rifabutin, clofazimine, or ciprofloxacin.[9] HIV-infected patients with suspected pulmonary mycobacterial disease should generally be given empiric therapy against *M. tuberculosis* initially. Therapy can be adjusted later if MAC or other nontuberculous mycobacteria are cultured.

EMERGENCY DEPARTMENT EVALUATION

The most important test in the initial evaluation of patients with suspected pulmonary TB is the chest radiograph. Findings strongly suggestive of pulmonary TB include nodular densities, with or without cavities, that are commonly seen in the apical and posterior segments of the upper lobes or in the superior segments of the lower lobes (Fig. 189.1).

In disseminated TB, the chest radiograph often reveals a miliary pattern, but it may be normal in the early stages. TB may have many different radiographic appearances, ranging from lobar consolidation to a diffuse interstitial pattern. Patients with AIDS are especially likely to have TB without the typical radiographic pattern, and they are more likely to have lymphadenopathy on a chest x-ray.[15] A diffuse interstitial pattern that is easily misdiagnosed as *P. carinii* pneumonia may be seen in patients with AIDS (Fig. 189.2).

If pulmonary TB is suspected, sputum samples should be obtained for AFB smear and culture. Collection of sputum can put health-care workers and other patients at risk for exposure to TB, and should be performed only in an isolation room adequately equipped with outside ventilation and filters or ultraviolet light. Emergency departments may consider having the patient step outside to provide a specimen if these facilities are not available. Ideally, three successive early-morning sputum sam-

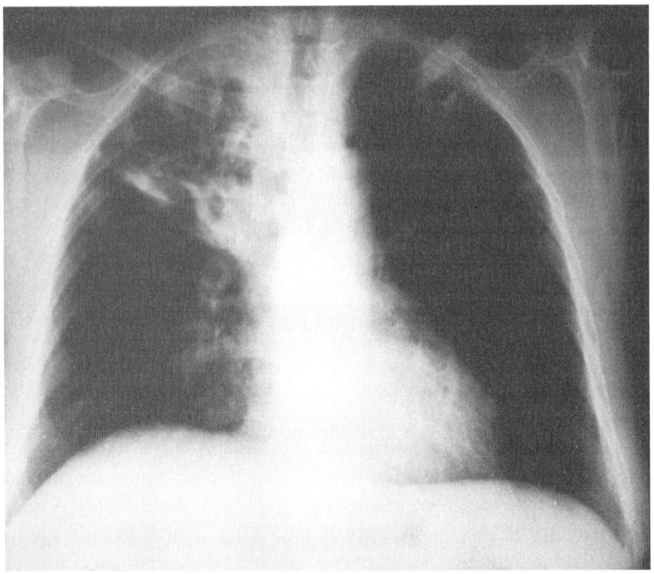

Figure 189.1. Chest radiograph demonstrating apical infiltrate with cavitation, typical of pulmonary tuberculosis.

ples should be obtained. In certain cases, they can be obtained on an outpatient basis.

A positive AFB smear supports a presumptive diagnosis of TB. A positive smear does not necessarily indicate infection with *M. tuberculosis,* however, because other mycobacteria (e.g., MAC) are also acid-fast. Patients with positive smears are potentially the most infectious, because they are usually coughing up large numbers of organisms. Because culture is more sensitive than AFB smear for the diagnosis of TB, the sample should be sent for culture even if the smear is negative.

AFB smear results are usually not available within the time frame of an emergency department visit. If there is a high likelihood of TB, the patient may be started on empiric therapy, with further AFB specimens obtained over the next couple of days. Empiric therapy will not significantly affect the diagnostic yield of specimens obtained over the next 1 to 2 days. Delays in diagnosis are a problem with current techniques, because culture usually takes 3 to 6 weeks, and susceptibility tests may take 8 weeks. Newer radiometric methods can provide results in as little as 10 to 15 days, but may not be available in many facilities. Nucleic acid amplification tests, such as polymerase chain reaction (PCR), can be used to rapidly verify *M. tuberculosis* in AFB smear–positive specimens.[12]

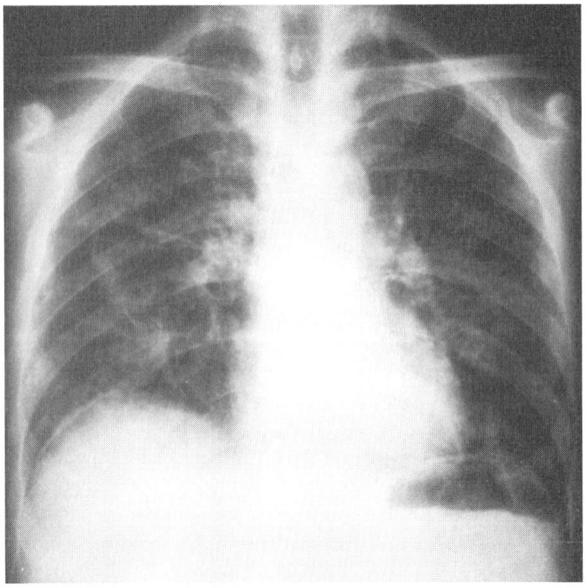

Figure 189.2. Chest radiograph of HIV-infected patient with tuberculosis, demonstrating hilar adenopathy and scattered interstitial infiltrates. This patient was initially misdiagnosed with *Pneumocystis carinii* pneumonia.

Intradermal tuberculin skin testing is the standard method for identifying persons infected with *M. tuberculosis.* The Mantoux test is performed by injecting 5 U (0.1 mL) of purified protein derivative (PPD) intradermally. The arm is then examined for 48 to 72 hours for induration at the site. Persons for whom TB skin testing is recommended are listed in Table 189.1, and interpretation of the test is summarized in Table 189.2.

A negative TB skin test does not rule out TB, because 60% of AIDS patients and up to 30% of those without HIV infection have a reaction of less than 5 mm even when they are infected. A skin test should nonetheless be performed in patients with AIDS, however, because it produces a positive reaction in up to 40% of those infected. False-positive reactions may be caused by cross-reaction with other mycobacteria, such as MAC.

A history of bacille Calmette-Guérin (BCG) vaccination generally does not alter the guidelines for interpretation of the skin test. BCG vaccination usually does not cause a reaction of more than 10 mm, and the extent of the reaction decreases with time. Because the vaccine is generally given only in areas with a high incidence of TB, a reaction greater than or equal to 10 mm should still be considered positive in these patients.[2]

The Centers for Disease Control and Prevention (CDC) recommend that facilities serving persons at high risk for HIV infection, TB infection, or both should provide screening for TB and encourage HIV testing. Facilities such as drug treatment centers, sexually transmitted disease clinics, correctional facilities, and homeless shelters have been suggested as important places for TB screening, and it has been recommended that TB case finding should be part of the regular health care provided to all homeless people.[8] Many persons at risk for TB and HIV come into contact with the health-care system only for episodic care in emergency departments.

Emergency department–based screening for TB could potentially identify many patients who require treatment.[16] However, the cost and time commitment necessary for an effective TB screening program may preclude the development of such a program in many emergency departments. If a TB screening program cannot be established in the emergency department, then patients at risk for TB should at least be referred to local public health clinics for testing. It is essential that all persons

TABLE 189.1. People in Whom PPD Skin Testing Is Indicated

People with signs, symptoms, or chest x-ray suggestive of active TB
Recent contacts of people known to have, or suspected of having, active TB
People with HIV infection
People with an abnormal chest x-ray compatible with past TB
People with other medical conditions that increase the risk of TB (e.g., intravenous drug use, diabetes, immunosuppressive therapy, renal failure, rapid weight loss)
Groups at high risk of recent infection with TB, such as immigrants from Asia, Africa, Latin America, and Oceania; medically underserved populations (e.g., homeless); personnel and residents in long-term care facilities and correctional institutions

TABLE 189.2. Criteria for Interpretation of PPD Skin Tests as Positive

INDURATION ≥ 5 MM
Close contact with someone with active TB Abnormal chest radiograph HIV infection
INDURATION ≥ 10 MM
Immigrants from an area with a high incidence of TB At risk because of low socioeconomic status—e.g., homeless, inner-city minority Intravenous drug users Residents or employees of long-term care facilities Demographic groups identified locally as being at risk for TB
INDURATION ≥ 15 MM
All others

with suspected active TB be reported to local public health authorities.[1]

EMERGENCY DEPARTMENT MANAGEMENT

Treatment of Active Tuberculosis

Rapid initiation of an effective drug regimen is important to prevent the spread of TB. Presumptive therapy can begin in the emergency department on the basis of clinical grounds alone if the patient is at risk for TB and has signs, symptoms, and radiographic findings suggestive of TB. Specimens should still be sent for AFB smear, culture, and sensitivity for subsequent management. If cultures are negative or yield only nontuberculous mycobacteria, treatment can be stopped or adjusted accordingly. It is crucial that patients can be followed up adequately, to ensure that treatment is appropriate and is being tolerated.

Active TB should always be treated with at least two drugs to which the organism is susceptible. Administration of a single drug can lead to the development of a bacterial population resistant to that drug. When two or more drugs are used simultaneously, each helps to prevent the emergence of TB resistant to the other. Because of concern about MDR-TB, the CDC recommends that initial therapy for TB include four drugs. The preferred initial regimen consists of daily INH, rifampin, PZA, and ethambutol or streptomycin.[6] Doses of these drugs can be found in Table 189.3. If four drugs are used in the initial regimen, it is very likely that the organism will not be sensitive to at least two of these drugs. The initial regimen is continued for 2 months, at which time the number of drugs and frequency of dosing can be reduced, depending in part on the results of susceptibility testing.

TABLE 189.3. Dosage Recommendation for the Initial Treatment of Tuberculosis

Drugs	Children ≤ 12	Adults
Isoniazid	10–20 mg/kg Maximum 300 mg	5 mg/kg Maximum 300 mg
Rifampin	10–20 mg/kg Maximum 600 mg	10 mg/kg Maximum 600 mg
Pyrazinamide	15–30 mg/kg Maximum 2 g	15–30 mg/kg Maximum 2 g
Ethambutol	15–25 mg/kg Maximum 2.5 g	5–25 mg/kg Maximum 2.5 g
Streptomycin	20–30 mg/kg Maximum 1 g	15 mg/kg Maximum 1 g

Adapted from Center for Disease Control. Initial therapy for tuberculosis in the era of multidrug resistance. Recommendations of the Advisory Council for the Elimination of Tuberculosis. *MMWR* 1993;42(RR7):3.

Immunocompetent patients usually cease to be infectious within 2 to 4 weeks of starting therapy, assuming the infecting organism is susceptible to the drugs being used and the patient is compliant. Expert advice should be sought if a patient is suspected of having MDR-TB. Alternative regimens may be recommended for these patients, including drugs such as cycloserine, ethionamide, amikacin, or quinolones.

Because rifampin interacts with protease inhibitors and nonnucleoside reverse transcriptase inhibitors, HIV-infected patients on these medications are treated with regimens that do not contain rifampin.[13] Rifabutin may be substituted in some cases, but is also contraindicated with some antiretroviral drugs. Expert consultation should be sought before initiating TB treatment for individuals taking antiretroviral drugs.

Certain low-risk patients in areas with a very low incidence of drug-resistant TB may be started initially on a three-drug regimen of INH, rifampin, and PZA. All others should be started on a four-drug regimen until sensitivity results are known. Those who are at especially high risk for MDR-TB include anyone with HIV infection, those with known exposure to MDR-TB, and persons from a geographic area or demographic group with a high incidence of MDR-TB. A five-drug regimen may be recommended for some very high risk patients. Treatment should be continued for at least 6 months in immunocompetent persons. HIV-infected patients who are unable to take rifampin or rifabutin may require 9 months of treatment.

Recommendations for treatment of extrapulmonary TB are generally the same as for pulmonary TB. However, children with miliary TB, bone or joint TB, or TB meningitis should receive a minimum of 12 months' treatment.[4]

Common side effects of these medications include hepatitis (INH, rifampin), peripheral neuropathy (INH), optic neuritis (ethambutol), and, rarely, purpura (rifampin). Adults should have baseline measurements of hepatic enzymes, bilirubin, serum creatinine or blood urea nitrogen, complete blood count, and platelet count. Serum uric acid should be measured if PZA is used, and a baseline examination of visual acuity should be obtained for patients to be treated with ethambutol. For this reason, unless resistance to other drugs is strongly suspected, ethambutol is not generally used for children younger than 6 years of age, in whom visual acuity cannot be assessed well.

Patients should be instructed to report any symptoms suggestive of hepatitis or thrombocytopenia. Pyridoxine (10 to 50 mg/d) may be given with INH to persons with conditions in which neuropathy is common, such as diabetes, alcoholism, or malnutrition. The rate of adverse reactions to antituberculous agents increases with age, and also appears to be higher in HIV-infected patients.

Management of Tuberculosis Exposure

Management of persons exposed to others with active TB involves several considerations: (1) the likelihood that the exposed person has been newly infected with *M. tuberculosis;* (2) the likelihood that the infecting strain is drug-resistant; and (3) the estimated likelihood that the newly infected contact will develop active TB. Contacts who are not immunosuppressed and do not have a history of a positive PPD skin test should receive a tuberculin skin test and, if indicated by symptoms, a chest radiograph and sputum examination. Those who have a PPD skin test reaction equal to 5 mm should be considered newly infected and should be considered for preventive therapy once active TB has been ruled out.

Persons with a high-risk exposure and a negative PPD should have a follow-up skin test 12 weeks after the exposure has ended; if the PPD test is still negative at that time, no further evaluation is necessary. Because the risk of developing TB is higher for young children, preventive therapy may be considered for all children younger than 5 years of age who are close contacts of TB cases until repeat skin testing is done at 12 weeks after exposure.

Persons who are known to be HIV-infected or otherwise immunosuppressed and who are close contacts of patients with infectious TB should be carefully evaluated for evidence of TB. If there are no findings suggestive of active TB, preventive therapy with INH may be recommended, even if PPD skin testing is negative.[4]

Management of Positive Tuberculosis Skin Tests

Persons with a positive TB skin test need to be evaluated for the presence of active TB with a chest radiograph. If the chest radiograph is abnormal or if symptoms suggest TB, an examination of sputum for AFB smear and culture is indicated. Those with no evidence of clinical disease should be referred for consideration of preventive therapy for TB. It is not necessary to initiate therapy urgently in this situation, but it is important that patients understand the importance of follow-up to obtain preventive therapy. It has been shown in numerous studies that preventive therapy substantially reduces the risk of latent infection's progressing to clinical disease. Immunocompetent persons who are not at risk for MDR-TB are generally treated with INH for 6 months.[4] HIV-infected persons who are not at risk for MDR-TB should receive preventive therapy with INH for a minimum of 9 months.[13] Alternatively, they may receive rifampin plus PZA daily for 2 months.

The effectiveness of preventive therapy for people exposed to MDR-TB strains has not been prospectively studied, and guidelines for management of such patients are less clear. If the infecting strain of TB is known to be less than 100% resistant to INH, then INH should be included in the preventive regimen; rifampin should be included for those with less than 100% resistance to rifampin. Those with exposure to strains resistant to both INH and rifampin who are at increased risk for developing active disease may be treated with regimens of PZA plus ethambutol or PZA plus a fluoroquinolone.[7]

Consultation with local infectious disease experts familiar with local patterns of resistance and current recommendations may be helpful in the management of such patients. Because the efficacy of drugs other than INH and rifampin for preventive therapy is unknown, persons on alternative therapies should have regular follow-up.

Recommendations for TB therapy are likely to continue to change because of shifting patterns of infection and drug resistance. The most current recommendations can be found in *Morbidity and Mortality Weekly Report* and the publications of the American Thoracic Society.

Preventing the Spread of Tuberculosis

The basic principles for preventing the transmission of TB include early identification of persons with active TB, early initiation of AFB isolation precautions in persons with suspected TB, and initiation of effective therapy to render the patient noninfectious. Lapses in infection control measures have led to nosocomial transmission of MDR-TB between patients and from patients to healthcare workers.[18]

The emergency department is potentially a high-risk area for the transmission of TB, because patients may be undiagnosed with TB when they present initially, and patients sometimes are crowded together for long periods of time, especially in busy inner-city emergency departments, which are likely to have a larger number of TB patients. There may be long delays in recognition and initiation of infection control measures for infectious TB patients in the emergency department, and HIV-infected patients appear to be even more likely to have delays in recognition, because they often have atypical presentations.[17]

Emergency departments should consider triage protocols to identify possible TB patients early. Those with possible TB should have an expedited chest radiograph, and can have a mask placed or wait outside while they are being evaluated for possible infectious TB.

Once a patient is suspected of having active TB, infection control measures should be initiated.[3,10] These measures are aimed at isolating the source from other patients and reducing the microbial contamination of indoor air. Recommendations include the use of a private room for the source patient, with negative pressure in relation to surrounding areas and a minimum of six air exchanges per hour. Air from the room should be exhausted directly to the outside. Use of ultraviolet lamps and/or high-efficiency particulate air filters to supplement ventilation may be considered.

Many emergency departments do not have the facilities to comply with these recommendations, and the costs associated with fitting a department with such facilities are substantial. If facilities that meet these standards are not available, it is important to at least designate an area for persons with possible TB that will keep them isolated from other patients and will minimize air exchange with other patient areas. Ordinary surgical masks may help reduce the amount of airborne droplets produced by patients who are coughing, but they are not truly effective for preventing the transmission of TB when worn either by TB patients or by those at risk for exposure. Masks used in the conventional manner are not designed to filter out particulates in the 1- to 5-μ range and can leak large amounts of air around the edges. The CDC recommends that health-care workers use masks capable of filtering out at least 95% of particles in the 1-μ range (commonly designated as N-95) for protection against TB. Individually fit-testing these masks may help ensure that they will provide adequate protection.[11]

DISPOSITION

Criteria for admission of patients with TB are similar to those for patients with other types of pneumonia. Patients who are not seriously ill and are not immunocompromised may safely be sent home with close follow-up, but precautions must be taken to avoid the spread of TB to others. Any patient who is discharged home with possible TB must be reported to local public health authorities. It may be assumed that household contacts have already been exposed, and will need to be tested.

Patients should be instructed to avoid crowded, enclosed, public areas and to wear a mask for at least the first 2 weeks of therapy to reduce the amount of airborne droplets produced by coughing. Other factors, such as homelessness, degree of compliance with medications, follow-up, and compliance with infection control measures should be considered when making decisions regarding admission. In the United States, laws vary among the states in regard to forced treatment and quarantine of patients who will not cooperate with therapy and are believed to be a public health hazard.[14]

COMMON PITFALLS

- Failure to consider the possibility of TB in a patient presenting with nonspecific systemic complaints
- Failure to rapidly initiate infection control measures for patients suspected of TB
- Risking the spread of TB in the emergency department by performing high-risk procedures such as sputum induction in infectious TB patients without proper isolation procedures
- Misdiagnosis of TB in AIDS patients as *P. carinii* or other infections
- Failure to refer patients at risk of TB for skin testing
- Failure to recognize and follow up patients whose cultures may become positive several weeks after an emergency department visit
- Failure to report persons with suspected TB to local public health authorities

References

1. American Thoracic Society. Control of tuberculosis in the United States. *Am Rev Respir Dis* 1992;146:1623–1633.
2. American Thoracic Society. Diagnostic standards and classification of tuberculosis. *Am Rev Respir Dis* 1990;142:725–735.
3. American Thoracic Society. Institutional control measures for tuberculosis in the era of multiple drug resistance. *Chest* 1995;108:1690–1710.
4. American Thoracic Society. Treatment of tuberculosis and tuberculosis infection in adults and children. *Am J Respir Crit Care Med* 1994;149:1359–1374.
5. Bloom BR, Murray CJ. Tuberculosis: commentary on a reemergent killer. *Science* 1992;257:1055–1064.
6. Center for Disease Control. Initial therapy for tuberculosis in the era of multidrug resistance. Recommendations of the Advisory Council for the Elimination of Tuberculosis. *MMWR* 1993;42(RR7):1–8.
7. Center for Disease Control. Management of persons exposed to multidrug-resistant tuberculosis. *MMWR* 1992;41(RR11):61–71.
8. Center for Disease Control. Prevention and control of tuberculosis among homeless persons. Recommendations of the Advisory Council for the Elimination of Tuberculosis. *MMWR* 1992;41(RR5):13–23.
9. Center for Disease Control. Recommendations on prophylaxis and therapy for disseminated *Mycobacterium avium* complex for adults and adolescents infected with human immunodeficiency virus. *MMWR* 1993;42(RR-9):17–20.
10. Centers for Disease Control and Prevention. Guidelines for preventing the transmission of *Mycobacterium tuberculosis* in health-care facilities, 1994. *Federal Register* 1994;58(208):54242–54303.
11. Centers for Disease Control and Prevention. Laboratory performance evaluation of N95 filtering facepiece respirators, 1996. *MMWR* 1998;47:1045–1049.
12. Centers for Disease Control and Prevention. Nucleic acid amplification tests for tuberculosis. *MMWR* 1996;45:950–952.
13. Centers for Disease Control and Prevention. Prevention and treatment of tuberculosis among patients infected with HIV: principles of therapy and revised recommendations. *MMWR* 1998;47(RR-20):1–58.
14. Gostin LO. Controlling the resurgent tuberculosis epidemic—a 50-state survey of TB statutes and proposals for reform. *JAMA* 1993;269:255–261.
15. Havlir DV, Barnes PF. Tuberculosis in patients with human immunodeficiency virus infection. *N Engl J Med* 1999;340:367–373.
16. Kirsch TD, Chanmugam A, Keyl P, et al. Feasibility of an emergency department-based tuberculosis counseling and screening program. *Acad Emerg Med* 1999;6:224–231.
17. Moran GJ, Talan DA, Morgan MT, et al. Lack of recognition and infection control for tuberculosis patients admitted through the emergency department. *Ann Emerg Med* 1993;22:936.
18. Pearson ML, Jereb JA, Frieden TR, et al. Nosocomial transmission of multidrug-resistant *Mycobacterium tuberculosis*. *Ann Intern Med* 1992;117:191–196.
19. Talan DA, Kennedy C. The management of HIV-related illness in the emergency department. *Ann Emerg Med* 1991;20:1355–1365.

CHAPTER 190
Infectious Mononucleosis

David Anthony Jerrard

Infectious mononucleosis is clinically defined by the triad of fever, lymphadenopathy, and pharyngitis, combined with the development of heterophil antibodies and atypical lymphocytosis. It is caused by the Epstein-Barr virus (EBV), which is also strongly implicated in the etiology of nasopharyngeal cancer and Burkitt's lymphoma. The most characteristic feature of the disease is its predilection for the young adult population, especially the 15- to 30-year age group. Early fall and spring are the two peak times of occurrence.[5]

Seroepidemiologic studies have shown that the presence of antibody to EBV (indicating exposure) correlates strongly with immunity and that its absence is highly indicative of susceptibility.[12] The age at which individuals develop the infection depends on socioeconomic factors as well as hygiene. Most children in developing countries have been exposed by the age of 3, whereas only 50% of those in economically advanced countries have antibodies by adolescence. Primary EBV infection during childhood is usually subclinical.[12] By adulthood, most individuals are seropositive.

Epidemiologic and laboratory evidence indicates that transmission occurs through the oropharyngeal route. EBV may be found in throat washings many months after clinical symptoms have abated, and may even be cultured from 10% to 20% of completely asymptomatic individuals. It is likely to be found in nearly 100% of patients with acquired immunodeficiency syndrome (AIDS).[12] Most transmission occurs from asymptomatic individuals to previously uninfected members of the population.

When EBV is transmitted by saliva, the initial site of replication is in the oropharynx. Both B lymphocytes and oropharyngeal epithelial cells have specific surface receptors for EBV, and replication takes place within these cells. Both humoral and cellular components are important in the immune response to EBV infection. The cellular response, consisting of the elaboration of T lymphocytes having very similar characteristics to suppressor-cytotoxic T lymphocytes,[12] is responsible for controlling B-cell proliferation.

CLINICAL PRESENTATION

The incubation period is 4 to 8 weeks. Nonspecific symptoms such as malaise, anorexia, fatigue, and chills often herald the illness and are followed by the development of fever, pharyngitis, and lymphadenopathy. Most patients seek medical care because of sore throat, but headache and myalgia are often complaints as well. Abdominal pain is rare in the absence of splenic rupture.

A pharyngeal exudate is present about one-third of the time,[12] and palatal petechiae may be observed. Anterior or posterior cervical lymphadenopathy is reported in about 90% of patients[10] and tends to be particularly impressive in these areas. Generalized adenopathy is often present; the nodes may be moderately tender or painless. Lymphadenopathy tends to be less prominent in patients older than the age of 40.[4]

Splenomegaly is noted in about 50% of patients, mostly in the second or third week of illness, and is usually not associated with pain. The presence of pain should alert the clinician to the possibility of impending or actual splenic rupture, an uncommon but well-documented complication of the disease that may be life-threatening if not identified and treated promptly.[1,2] Splenectomy is the most common treatment of choice. Splenic abscess has also been reported as a complication of infectious mononucleosis.[8]

Tonsillitis may occur during any stage of the illness, although it is usually most pronounced during the first 2 weeks of the postprodromal period. Tonsils hypertrophied to the point of "kissing" in the midline are not at all unusual and do not, in themselves, mandate hospital admission. The distinction between severe pharyngitis and airway compromise is necessary for obvious reasons, but tonsillar hypertrophy only rarely causes airway compromise.

Complications of infectious mononucleosis are rare, but the clinician must be alert for them. Autoimmune hemolytic anemia may appear within 1 to 2 months of initial symptoms; mild thrombocytopenia develops in about half of all cases. Both appear to be antibody mediated and are usually self-limited, lasting approximately 6 weeks. Glucocorticoids have been recommended for the treatment of both the thrombocytopenia and the hemolytic anemia, but there is little evidence to support their use.[12]

A number of neurologic complications of infectious mononucleosis have been described. Cranial nerve palsies (especially Bell's palsy) and various forms of encephalitis are the most common. Cerebellar dysfunction and episodes of Guillain-Barré syndrome have also been associated with infectious mononucleosis. Roughly 90% of patients with EBV-associated neurologic findings recover without sequelae.[12]

About 90% of patients with infectious mononucleosis have transient elevation of hepatic enzymes, although significant hepatic dysfunction is exceedingly unusual. Roughly half of the these patients have mild hepatic tenderness, but hepatomegaly is infrequent. Clinical jaundice may develop early in the illness, but resolution usually occurs within a few weeks. Subclinical illness that mimics mild viral hepatitis may in fact be due to infectious mononucleosis.

Although rare, airway obstruction secondary to extreme lymphoid hyperplasia is a potential complication. Airway compromise, as evidenced, for example, by stridor, requires active airway management.

DIFFERENTIAL DIAGNOSIS

The differential diagnosis of sore throat is lengthy (Table 190.1). Because several of the entities (e.g., foreign body, retropharyngeal abscess and hematoma, and, although less likely, adult epiglottitis) may be associated with airway compromise, it is vital to rule them out as possibilities. Compared with other causes of sore throat, infectious mononucleosis is likely to feature more prominent systemic complaints.

TABLE 190.1. Differential Diagnosis of Sore Throat

Retropharyngeal abscess
Epiglottitis
Esophageal candidiasis
Peritonsillar abscess
Foreign body
Uvulitis
Pharyngitis (bacterial or viral)[a]
Laryngitis
Cervical adenopathy

[a]Includes infectious mononucleosis.

Generalized lymphadenopathy prompts consideration of other viral illness, AIDS, leukemia, lymphoma, or tuberculosis.

The differential diagnosis of splenomegaly is broad as well. Infectious endocarditis, abscess, and disseminated tuberculosis are all possible infectious etiologies of splenic enlargement. Infiltrative processes such as lymphoma and leukemia must also be included for consideration.

EMERGENCY DEPARTMENT EVALUATION

If there is suspicion of adult epiglottitis or retropharyngeal abscess or hematoma, a soft-tissue lateral radiograph of the neck should be performed. In any patient presenting with the complaint of sore throat, indications of airway compromise should be sought.

The diagnosis of infectious mononucleosis is based on clinical, hematologic, and serologic criteria. In a patient strongly suspected of having infectious mononucleosis, certain laboratory features may aid in making a firm diagnosis.

A relative and absolute *lymphocytosis* is seen in 39% to 75% of patients with infectious mononucleosis.[7] The lymphocytosis is characterized by the presence of cells, roughly 10% of the total, that have atypical morphology. They are larger than mature lymphocytes and have large lobulated or indented nuclei and vacuolated or bluish cytoplasm. Lymphocytosis usually peaks in the second or third week of illness.

A significant number of patients with acute EBV infection, particularly those older than the age of 40,[4,7,11] do not fulfill the classic hematologic criteria for infectious mononucleosis, that is, lymphocytosis of at least 50%, with at least 10% atypical lymphocytes. Conversely, atypical lymphocytosis may be seen in other infections, such as toxoplasmosis, rubella, mumps, and hepatitis.[13] Complicating matters further, mononucleosis-like syndromes may be associated with cytomegalovirus infection, toxoplasmosis, and hepatitis A and B, and sometimes cannot be distinguished clinically from infectious mononucleosis due to EBV.

Because so many of the symptoms of infectious mononucleosis are nonspecific, serologic evidence may be required to make the diagnosis. *Heterophil antibodies* (defined as antibodies that react with antigens not responsible for their production) are characteristically produced in infectious mononucleosis.[3] The Monospot test is based on this tube dilution principle.

Heterophil agglutination is apparently almost never positive in persons of Japanese ancestry, for unknown reasons.[13] False-positive results have been known to occur in leukemia, lymphoma, malaria, rubella, hepatitis, pancreatic cancer, systemic lupus erythematosus, and hepatic abscess.[8,9,13] In addition, children younger than 4 years of age often fail to demonstrate heterophil antibody; likewise, the incidence of heterophil-negative infectious mononucleosis due to EBV increases with age.[4] The false-positive rate for heterophil antibody in adults is roughly 2%, and the false-negative rate is 5% to 7%. Only 70% of patients tested in the first week of the illness have a positive test, but 85% to 90% are positive by the third week. One study reported that positive titers were associated with four physical findings: palatal petechiae, posterior auricular adenopathy, axillary adenopathy, and inguinal adenopathy.[3]

More recently, latex agglutination tests have been developed for the detection of infectious mononucleosis–associated heterophil antibody.[6]

Because many individuals are heterophil antibody negative during the first week of illness, it seems reasonable to omit this test in patients with an illness of recent onset, unless the physical examination raises a high suspicion for mononucleosis. Patients should be instructed to return for testing if symptoms persist beyond 7 days.

Individuals with infectious mononucleosis also produce specific antibody directed against EBV antigens. Even though the development of detectable heterophil antibodies may be delayed, EBV antibody tests are rarely necessary, because 90% of cases are heterophil positive, and false-positive heterophil results are rare; more practically, illness is usually mild and self-limited.[6] Nevertheless, it should be noted that, as with heterophil antibodies, antibodies specific to EBV may sometimes not be detectable until several weeks after the onset of illness.

EMERGENCY DEPARTMENT MANAGEMENT

The treatment of infectious mononucleosis usually consists only of supportive care. Fever and pharyngeal pain may be ameliorated by acetaminophen. Aspirin should probably be avoided because of the risk of increasing any bleeding tendency due to thrombocytopenia. Adequate rest should be advised, although this does not seem to expedite recovery. Ampicillin, via an unknown mechanism, causes a rash in roughly 90% of those with infectious mononucleosis. When treating presumed streptococcal tonsillitis in patients with infectious mononucleosis, therefore, erythromycin or penicillin should be prescribed instead. Because of the small but real risk of splenic rupture, contact sports should be avoided for 6 to 8 weeks after the onset of illness. Some authors recommend that college and intramural athletics be avoided for 6 months.[10] Patients should be advised that feelings of malaise may linger, sometimes for months.

Severe pharyngitis may be treated with corticosteroids (prednisone, 40 to 60 mg/d, and tapered over 7 to 10 days). Impending airway obstruction or an inability to take oral medications may necessitate the use of dexamethasone. Symptoms of dysphagia and difficulty breathing are usually improved within 1 to 2 hours of administration of parenteral corticosteroids. As noted previously, active airway management is rarely necessary. Although corticosteroids do not decrease spleen size or reduce the likelihood of splenic rupture, some benefit may be obtained in decreasing neurologic, hematologic, and cardiac complications. Corticosteroid therapy is not generally recommended for uncomplicated infectious mononucleosis, however.

In patients presenting with abdominal pain, a computed tomography scan should be performed. Infectious mononucleosis may be the most common reason for splenic rupture.[1] Splenic rupture is unlikely to occur in the first 2 weeks of the illness, however; the capsular and trabecular changes that are necessary to permit rupture to occur do not develop for 2 to 4 weeks.

DISPOSITION

The vast majority of patients with infectious mononucleosis do quite well without any intervention whatsoever and can be discharged from the emergency department with instructions to return should abdominal pain develop and breathing or swallowing become difficult.

Consultation with appropriate specialists is indicated for neurologic or hematologic complications.

Patients who are unable to maintain oral intake because of difficulty in swallowing should be admitted and begun on parenteral corticosteroids. This also holds true if airway compromise becomes a concern.

In the unlikely event of splenic rupture, a surgical consult is imperative. Should either computed tomographic scanning or surgical backup not be available, immediate transfer to a center that does have these resources is crucial.

COMMON PITFALLS

- The differential diagnosis of sore throat includes more than simple viral or bacterial pharyngitis. Other infections localized to the throat can have disastrous consequences if they go undetected. These include retropharyngeal abscess and epiglottitis.
- Errors in management are usually the result of a failure to examine the patient thoroughly. This may result, for example, in a failure to diagnose splenic rupture (either spontaneous or posttraumatic), an uncommon but potentially dangerous complication. Patients should be strongly encouraged to refrain from contact sports for at least 6 months after their illness.
- Patients should be advised to seek medical attention promptly if they develop difficulty breathing or abdominal pain.
- Ampicillin should be avoided because of the high likelihood that a rash will develop.

References

1. Aldrete J. Spontaneous rupture of the spleen in patients with infectious mononucleosis. *Mayo Clin Proc* 1993;67:910.
2. Ali J. Spontaneous rupture of the spleen in patients with infectious mononucleosis. *Can J Surg* 1993;36(1):49.
3. Aronson M, Komaroff A, Puss T. Heterophil antibody in adults with sore throat. *Ann Intern Med* 1982;96:505.
4. Axelrod P, Finestone A. Infectious mononucleosis in older adults. *Am Fam Pract* 1990;42(6):1599.
5. Chatham M, Roberts K. Infectious mononucleosis in adolescents. *Pediatr Ann* 1991;20:208.
6. Dietrich W, Turner D, Vukich D. Use of the infectious disease laboratory in emergency medicine. *Emerg Med Clin North Am* 1991;9(2):263.
7. Fleisher G, Collins M, Fager S. Limitations of available tests for diagnosis of infectious mononucleosis. *J Clin Microbiol* 1983;17(4):619.
8. O'Dell K, Gordon R. Ruptured splenic abscess secondary to infectious mononucleosis. *Ann Emerg Med* 1992;21(9):1160.
9. Ridker P, Enders G, Lifton R. False positive mononucleosis screening test results associated with *Klebsiella* hepatic abscess. *Am J Clin Pathol* 1990;94:222.
10. Rutkow I. Rupture of the spleen in infectious mononucleosis. *Arch Surg* 1978;113:720.
11. Schmader K, Van der Horst C, Klotman M. Epstein-Barr virus and the elderly host. *Rev Infect Dis* 1989;2(1):64.
12. Schooley R. Epstein-Barr virus infections including infectious mononucleosis. In: Wilson J, Braunwald E, Isselbacher K, et al., eds. *Harrison's principles of internal medicine.* New York: McGraw-Hill, 1991:689.
13. Wallach J. Hematologic disease. In: Wallach J, ed. *Interpretation of diagnostic tests: a synopsis of laboratory medicine.* Boston: Little, Brown and Company, 1992:323.

CHAPTER 191
Influenza

Jonathan S. Olshaker

More people died in the 1918 influenza pandemic than in all of World War I.[18] Today, influenza remains a major killer and causes more morbidity and mortality than the acquired immunodeficiency syndrome (AIDS). In nonpandemic years, 20,000 to 40,000 persons die of influenza-related illness in the United States alone; in pandemic years, deaths can exceed 100,000.[8] Influenza infections account for several billion dollars in healthcare expenditures each year.[13]

Influenza is caused by large RNA viruses belonging to the myxovirus groups. Of the three immunologically distinct groups (A, B, and C), influenza A and B are encountered most frequently. Group A is responsible for the majority of the mortality and significant morbidity. It appears to cause more severe disease than type B, making secondary bacterial infection more likely, and is more common in older populations.[18] Not surprisingly, the vast majority of deaths occur in elderly individuals and in those with chronic medical conditions, particularly chronic obstructive pulmonary disease.[1]

CLINICAL PRESENTATION

Influenza is an extremely common respiratory illness, characterized by the abrupt onset of fever, sore throat, headache, myalgias, and nonproductive cough. The malaise is often much more extreme than that seen with most other common respiratory illnesses.[4] Symptoms last from a few days to a week in most patients. More severe illness can result if there is pulmonary involvement due to primary viral or secondary bacterial pneumonia, which is the most common cause of death. This occurs almost exclusively in the elderly, in the immunosuppressed, and in patients with chronic cardiovascular or pulmonary disease.

DIFFERENTIAL DIAGNOSIS

The differential diagnosis of influenza includes the myriad respiratory and infectious diseases seen in the emergency department. The clinician's major task should be to recognize serious illness that requires specific antibiotic treatment or other aggressive interventions.

Prominent severe headache, meningeal signs, or changes in mental status make it mandatory to rule out meningitis. Sore throat, often seen with influenza, may be due to peritonsillar abscess, epiglottitis, or streptococcal pharyngitis. Myalgia may be due to bacteremia or sepsis, particularly in the elderly. A finding of hypotension or marked orthostasis mandates evaluation for sepsis or toxic shock syndrome, particularly if there is evidence of multiple organ system involvement. Cough or difficulty breathing may be due to bacterial or viral pneumonia, acute bronchospasm, or cardiac processes such as congestive heart failure or myocardial ischemia.

Unfortunately, the differentiation of viral from bacterial pneumonia in the patient with influenza is difficult. Antibiotics should be instituted early if there is any suspicion of a bacterial process.

EMERGENCY DEPARTMENT EVALUATION

Initial management should focus on assessment of the airway, breathing, and circulation. Pulse oximetry is a simple, noninvasive test that may provide a quick indication of respiratory compromise. Physical examination should focus on the heart and lungs. A thorough examination of the skin should include a search for any cutaneous manifestations of infectious disease, such as purpura or petechiae.

Patients with significant cough, respiratory symptoms, or abnormalities on lung examination should have a chest radiograph. Lumbar puncture and urinalysis may be indicated if suggested by appropriate symptoms. A complete blood cell count, though nonspecific, may lend support to a diagnosis of superimposed bacterial infection. Tests to determine levels of electrolytes, blood urea nitrogen, creatinine, and blood glucose should be ordered in those patients with severe derangements of fluid balance or in those who have chronic medical problems or take medications, such as diuretics, that can affect electrolyte balance. Arterial blood gas analysis is appropriate when hypoxia or sepsis is suspected. Blood cultures should also be obtained if sepsis is a possibility.

Specific serologic testing for influenza cannot be carried out quickly enough to provide any benefit while the patient is in the emergency department.

EMERGENCY DEPARTMENT MANAGEMENT

Initial treatment for patients with suspected influenza is directed at ensuring adequate oxygenation and hemodynamic stability. Patients with viral or bacterial pneumonia, particularly the elderly or those with chronic obstructive pulmonary disease, can present *in extremis* with an immediate need for endotracheal intubation and mechanical ventilation. Supplemental oxygen should be given to patients with significant respiratory symptoms or low pulse oximeter readings.

Patients who are tachycardic, hypotensive, or orthostatic should have a large-bore intravenous line in place and receive initial fluid resuscitation with normal saline. Care should be taken to avoid overhydration, particularly in the elderly or in those with a history of congestive heart failure. Standard bronchodilator therapy is indicated for any accompanying reactive airway disease.

If the patient has a coexisting pneumonia, antibiotics should be instituted in the emergency department, because it is, as a rule, difficult to differentiate viral pneumonia from bacterial pneumonia. Antibiotics should provide adequate coverage against *Haemophilus influenzae* and group B *Streptococcus,* as well as *Staphylococcus aureus,* which is a relatively common bacterial pathogen associated with influenza outbreaks.[12]

The antiviral drugs rimantadine and amantadine are both effective in reducing the severity and duration of illness in high-risk individuals who have not been vaccinated or who have not received adequate protection by vaccination.[3,20] In addition, they can significantly reduce subsequent illness when given to nursing home residents exposed to an influenza outbreak. The most common adverse effects of these drugs relate to the central nervous system and the gastrointestinal tract. Rimantadine appears to cause fewer central nervous system side effects than amantadine and requires less dosage adjustment in patients with mild-to-moderate renal impairment. The normal adult dosage is 200 mg/d. Patients older than 65 should probably receive 100 mg/d because of the potential for side effects and renal toxicity.

Some evidence suggests that oral or aerosolized riboflavin can be of benefit in controlling influenza infections in high-risk individuals.[2] Also, zanamivir and other neuraminidase inhibitors are promising investigational antiviral agents that are just reaching clinical trials.[10] Remaining unresolved issues on these agents include prophylactic efficacy, cost efficiency, administration, and the emergence of resistance.

DISPOSITION

The majority of patients with influenza can be treated as outpatients. Close follow-up should be ensured, and the patient should be given specific instructions to return immediately if symptoms progress.

There should be a low threshold for admission for elderly patients, the immunocompromised, and those with chronic pulmonary or cardiac disease. These patients should be admitted if there is any evidence of pneumonia, which can often progress rapidly in these individuals. Admission to an intensive care unit should be considered for patients who are hypoxic or show any signs of significant respiratory difficulty.

PREVENTION/VACCINATION

Influenza vaccines have been shown in a number of studies to be effective in preventing clinical disease.[4,11] Each year, a different vaccine preparation is developed, using virus strains believed likely to appear in North America the following winter. As many as 90% of influenza cases can be prevented when there is a good match between vaccine and epidemic strains of the virus.[5] Influenza vaccine has also been extremely effective in reducing morbidity and mortality (by up to 80%) in vaccinated individuals who nevertheless develop clinical disease, particularly the elderly and the immunocompromised.[9] A number of studies have shown that vaccination reduces influenza-related hospitalizations and deaths in nursing home populations during epidemics.[6,7,9] Adverse effects of the vaccine itself have been minimal and should not deter its use in the high-risk patient.[15]

Despite the overwhelming evidence supporting the benefits and efficacy of influenza vaccines, many high-risk individuals go unvaccinated. Studies have shown poor vaccination rates in both the elderly and younger persons with high-risk medical conditions such as asthma.[20] One study also showed that only 60% of pediatric emergency physicians received an influenza vaccine with the past year.[14]

Emergency physicians can play a major role in educating patients and the general public about the need for vaccinations in high-risk groups. This should occur before the peak influenza season begins.[6,11] Target groups for vaccination programs are listed in Table 191.1. Vaccinations should be offered between late September and early November, depending on when regional influenza activity is expected to begin. Many emergency departments offer the vaccine on-site. This approach has been shown to be both needed and feasible,[17] even for most patients presenting with acute attacks of asthma requiring prednisone treatment.[16]

TABLE 191.1. Influenza Vaccination Target Groups

GROUPS AT RISK FOR INFLUENZA COMPLICATIONS
Adults and children with chronic respiratory or cardiovascular disorders
Healthy persons 65 years of age or older
Immunocompromised persons
GROUPS CAPABLE OF INFLUENZA TRANSMISSION
Residents of nursing homes and chronic care facilities
Physicians
Nurses
Hospital personnel who have close contact with high-risk patients
Home health-care or nursing home care providers

Emergency physicians are often in a position to recognize the outbreak of influenza in closed environments such as nursing homes. Rimantadine, 100 mg/d, should be administered prophylactically to residents of such an institution, whether or not they received influenza vaccine the previous fall.[19]

COMMON PITFALLS

- Failure to realize that the elderly, the immunosuppressed, and those with chronic cardiac or pulmonary disease are at high risk for complications from influenza or acute worsening of their baseline chronic disease
- Failure to realize that *Staphylococcus aureus* has a significant role as a pneumonia pathogen during influenza outbreaks
- Failure to use rimantadine in the high-risk patient with influenza. Dosage should be reduced to 100 mg/d in those older than 65.
- Failure to be on the alert for nursing home patients with influenza and to notify appropriate officials about potential outbreaks
- Failure to implement vaccination programs from late September through November

References

1. Barker WH, Mullooly JP. Pneumonia and influenza deaths during epidemics: implications for prevention. *Arch Intern Med* 1982;142:85.
2. Bernstein JM, Liss H, Erk SD. Comparison of oral and aerosol ribavirin regimens in the high risk elderly. *J Clin Pharmacol* 1989;29:128.
3. Centers for Disease Control. Control of influenza A outbreaks in nursing homes: amantadine as an adjunct to vaccine. *MMWR* 1991;13:841.
4. Centers for Disease Control. Prevention and control of influenza. *MMWR* 1992;15:1.
5. Douglas RG. Prophylaxis and treatment of influenza. *N Engl J Med* 1990;332:443.
6. Fattal-German M, Taillander J, Mathieu D, et al. Usefulness of influenza vaccination in the elderly. *Biomed Pharmacother* 1991;24:1.
7. Foster DA, Talsma A, Furumoto-Dawson A. Influenza vaccine effectiveness in preventing hospitalization for pneumonia in the elderly. *Am J Epidemiol* 1992;1:296.
8. Ghendon Y. Influenza—its impact and control. *World Health Stat Q* 1992;45:306.
9. Gross PA, Quinna GU, Rostein M. Association of influenza immunization with reduction in mortality in an elderly population: a prospective study. *Arch Intern Med* 1988;148:562.
10. Hayden FG. Antivirals for pandemic influenza. *J Infect Dis* 1997;176[Suppl 1]:556–561.
11. Hermogenes AW, Gross PA. Influenza vaccine: a need for emphasis. *Semin Respir Infect* 1992;7:54.
12. Jones A, MacFarlane J, Pugh S. Antibiotic therapy, clinical features and outcome of 36 adults presenting to hospital with proven influenza: do we follow guidelines? *Postgrad Med J* 1991;67:988.
13. Kennedy MM. Influenza viral infections: presentation, prevention, and treatment. *Nurse Pract* 1998;23(9):17–28.
14. Lane NE, Paul RI, Bratcher DF, et al. Pediatric emergency physicians and communicable diseases: can we be trusted to take care of ourselves? *Pediatr Emerg Care* 1997;13(5):308–311.
15. Margolis KL, Nichol KL, Poland GA, et al. Frequency of adverse reactions to influenza vaccine in the elderly. *JAMA* 1990;5:1139.
16. Pak CL, Frank AL, Sullivan M, et al. Influenza vaccination of children during acute asthma exacerbation and concurrent prednisone therapy. *Pediatrics* 1996;98(2 Pt 1):196–200.
17. Slobodkin D, Zielske PG, Kithas J, et al. Demonstration of feasibility of emergency department immunization against influenza and pneumococcus. *Ann Emerg Med* 1998;32(5):537–543.
18. Small PA. Influenza: pathogenesis and host defense. *Hosp Pract* 1990;25:51.
19. Wintermeyer SM, Nahata MC. Rimantadine: a clinical perspective. *Ann Pharmacother* 1995;29(3):299–310.
20. Zimmerman RK, Ruben FL, Ahwesh ER. Influenza, influenza vaccine, and amantadine/rimantadine. *J Fam Pract* 1997;45(2):107–122.

CHAPTER 192
Human Immunodeficiency Virus Infection and Related Disorders

Richard E. Rothman, Catherine A. Marco, and Gabor D. Kelen

Reports of Kaposi's sarcoma (KS) and *Pneumocystis carinii* pneumonia (PCP) in previously healthy homosexual males appeared in the literature beginning in 1981. These are now recognized to represent the earliest cases of the disease known as the acquired immunodeficiency syndrome (AIDS), which has since escalated to become a global public health issue. The medical, social, and economic impact of this disease is enormous and continues to grow.

As of June 1998, there have been more than 688,000 reported cases of AIDS in the United States.[4] Although true population-based seroprevalence surveys are difficult to conduct, current estimates indicate that well over 1.1 million persons are infected with the human immunodeficiency virus (HIV) (approximately one in every 250 Americans). New laws requiring mandatory reporting of HIV in over 20 states have resulted in the identification of a shift in the regional distribution of HIV and AIDS. While more than 50% of cases occurred in five large urban settings (New York, Newark, Miami, San Francisco, and Los Angeles) up until 1987, the majority of new HIV cases now occur outside of these centers, principally in smaller metropolitan areas.

EPIDEMIOLOGY

HIV infection results in a broad spectrum of clinical conditions, ranging from an asymptomatic seropositive state to severe immunocompromise. The most recent Centers for Disease Control and Prevention (CDC) definition of AIDS, published in 1993, is summarized in Table 192.1. The diagnosis of AIDS is usually made by laboratory evidence of HIV infection and the presence of one of more "indicator" conditions or laboratory evidence of severe immunosuppression (CD4 T-lymphocyte count of less than 200 cells/μL).

TABLE 192.1. Indicator Conditions for Case Definition of AIDS

Esophageal candidiasis
Cryptococcosis
Cryptosporidiosis
Cytomegalovirus retinitis
Herpes simplex virus
Kaposi's sarcoma
Brain lymphoma
Mycobacterium avium complex
P. carinii pneumonia
Progressive multifocal leukoencephalopathy
Brain toxoplasmosis
HIV encephalopathy
HIV wasting syndrome
Disseminated histoplasmosis
Isosporiasis
Disseminated *M. tuberculosis* disease
Recurrent *Salmonella* septicemia
ADDED IN 1993
CD4 cell count <200 cells/μL
Pulmonary tuberculosis
Recurrent bacterial pneumonia
Invasive cervical cancer

The majority of AIDS cases in the United States have occurred in men; 16% of cases are in women and less than 2% are in children. Approximately 87% of cases have occurred in individuals 20 to 49 years of age.[4] Risk factors associated with an increased likelihood of acquiring HIV infection include homosexuality or bisexuality, intravenous drug use, heterosexual exposure to a partner at risk, history of having received blood products before 1985, and horizontal maternal-to-neonatal transmission. Sexual partners of high-risk individuals and children of mothers engaging in high-risk behaviors are also at increased risk. A greater number of risk factors are associated with a greater likelihood of infection.[9]

The pattern of infection among high-risk individuals is changing. Worldwide, heterosexual transmission is the most common route of transmission of HIV infection, and heterosexual transmission accounts for the largest proportionate increase in HIV infection. In the United States, new infections among the homosexual population have significantly decreased in many areas, and in some regions are now rare. Meanwhile, the proportion of AIDS cases in women has increased rapidly, with the male-to-female ratio in certain populations approaching 1:1. During the past several years, the greatest increase in reported AIDS cases has occurred among women, minority populations, and children. Seroprevalence in one inner-city emergency department (ED) demonstrates these trends, with rates of HIV rising from 6% to 11% over a 4-year period.[13]

PATHOPHYSIOLOGY AND TRANSMISSION

HIV is a cytopathic retrovirus that kills infected cells. In humans, HIV appears to selectively attack cells within the immune system (primarily CD4 T-lymphocytes), a characteristic that accounts for much of the immunodeficiency it produces in affected individuals. Following infection of host cells, the viral genes, which are encoded by a single-stranded RNA molecule, are reverse-transcribed into DNA (using the enzyme reverse transcriptase), and then permanently integrated into the host's genome. Once integrated, retroviral DNA may lie dormant, or be actively transcribed and translated to produce virally encoded proteins and new HIV virions.

HIV protease converts viral protein precursors into functional enzymes required for virion infectivity. Antiretroviral therapy is directed at reducing levels of HIV RNA by interfering with the enzymes reverse transcriptase (nucleoside and nonnucleoside reverse transcriptase inhibitors) and HIV protease (protease inhibitors). Although the introduction of these agents has had a significant impact on disease progression, the emergence of mutant drug-resistant strains of HIV and the occurrence of drug toxicity have limited the ability to attain long-term and lasting inhibition of viral replication.

Proven modes of HIV transmission include via semen, vaginal secretions, blood or blood products, transplacental transmission *in utero*, and breast milk. There have been no documented cases of transmission by casual contact, although one report exists of possible transmission, by deep kissing, from an HIV-infected male with bleeding gums to a female partner.[7]

DISEASE PROGRESSION

The spectrum of HIV-induced disease ranges from asymptomatic to acute retroviral infection, to a wide variety of opportunistic infections, malignancies, and other symptoms directly attributable to HIV infection. Several weeks after exposure to the virus, an acute "flulike" illness is reported to occur in 50% to 90% of patients. During this stage of infection, high-level HIV RNA viremia occurs, along with a precipitous decline in CD4 cell counts. Symptoms, including fever, sore throat, fatigue, and myalgias, typically last for 2 weeks, after which there is a significant reduction in HIV RNA levels and moderate increases in CD4 counts.

Infectious disease experts suggest that it may be helpful to identify patients at this early stage, because it may be the optimal time to begin antiretroviral therapy. The best way to establish diagnosis during this acute stage is by quantitative plasma HIV RNA, because HIV antibody serology is usually negative until at least 4 weeks after infection. Median time from exposure to antibody detection has been estimated at 2.1 months, although delayed seroconversion of up to 11 months has been reported.

Disease progression varies among infected individuals. The average incubation time from initial infection to clinical AIDS has been estimated to be 8.23 years for adults, and 1.97 years for children under age 5. In the clinical setting, the laboratory variables that are most predictive of the stage of disease are CD4 cell counts and viral burden.

As the CD4 cell count drops below 500 cells/μL, patients present with a variety of conditions that may occur in the immunocompetent host, but are more common and more severe in the presence of HIV infection. Characteristic conditions that occur during "early symptomatic infection" include thrush, recurrent herpes zoster, persistent vulvovaginal candidiasis, and idiopathic thrombocytopenic purpura (ITP).

AIDS is defined by the appearance of any "indicator" condition (see Table 192.1) or a CD4 count of less than 200 cells/μL.[2] During this stage, a variety of opportunistic infections and malignancies are common. The average survival time after a diagnosis of AIDS has been estimated to be between 16 and 24 months.[25] Patients in this group should receive prophylaxis for opportunistic infections as well as antiretroviral therapy, as this has been shown to delay the time of onset of complications and death.[26] In patients with CD4 cell counts less than 50 cells/μL, median survival is 12 to 18 months, with common life-threatening complications, including disseminated *Mycobacterium avium* complex (MAC) and disseminated cytomegalovirus (CMV).

DIAGNOSIS OF HIV INFECTION

Diagnosing or testing for HIV directly in the ED as part of patient evaluation is rarely indicated, owing to difficulty in obtaining informed consent, appropriate counseling (particularly the time involved), maintaining confidentiality, and ensuring appropriate follow-up. Testing is appropriate in the ED for a few limited indications, such as when health-care providers are exposed to patients' blood.[8,9] For those patients with identified risk factors, or significant exposure to those with risk factors, emergency physicians play a critical role in referral for voluntary outpatient testing and counseling.[9,14]

The standard procedure for diagnosing HIV in the United States is viral antibody detection by the enzyme-linked immunoassay technique (EIA), followed by a confirming Western blot on EIA-positive specimens. EIA was initially developed to screen blood and blood products. There are several commercially available tests, each with a sensitivity and specificity greater than 98%. False-negative EIA tests can occur during acute disease before seroconversion or as a result of other factors, such as malignancy or long-term immunosuppressive therapy.

False-positive tests can also occur (among patients with severe liver disease, renal transplants, hematologic malignancies, and other disorders) and are most frequent in populations with a low seroprevalence for the disease. In children younger than 6 months of age, a positive test may be due to transplacentally acquired maternal antibodies and does not necessarily imply the presence of disease. Other false-positive results are due to cross-reacting antibodies, including anti–hepatitis A IgM, anti–hepatitis B core IgM, and antinuclear, anti–smooth muscle, antiparietal cell, and antimitochondrial antibodies.

When the EIA test indicates the presence of HIV antibodies, a second, more specific test, such as the Western blot test, is required before the diagnosis is established. The Western blot technique detects electrophoretically separated viral antigens in the patient's serum and is nearly 100% sensitive. In those cases in which the Western blot test is indeterminate (if bands are present that do not meet criteria for a truly positive test), it should be repeated; if it remains indeterminate, the entire testing sequence should be repeated in 3 to 6 months. An indeterminate test among those with risk factors usually indicates infection; however, among those without risk factors, true infection is rare.

Other less commonly used techniques for HIV testing include viral culture, p24 antigen assays, indirect immunofluorescence, monoclonal antibody detection, the production of reagent antigens by recombinant DNA techniques, and DNA amplification or polymerase chain reaction (PCR).

Measurement of the CD4 lymphocyte count is valuable in evaluating the clinical immunologic status of HIV-infected patients. When this test available, and in cases in which stage of disease is unknown, the total lymphocyte count (TLC) can be used to approximate the CD4 count. A TLC of less than 1,000 cells/μL is highly predictive of a CD4 count of less than 200 cells/μL.

EMERGENCY DEPARTMENT MANAGEMENT

It is reasonable to inquire about risk factors as part of the routine evaluation of all adult ED patients, especially in endemic areas, and particularly when patients present with atypical diseases or atypical presentations of common diseases. The infection rate may be surprisingly high, even in patients with presenting complaints not usually associated with HIV infection.[9] Furthermore, inquiries about risk factors help in the medical evaluation, remind physicians of the potential for occupational exposure to blood-borne infections, and afford the opportunity to offer counseling and referral for testing to those who engage in high-risk behaviors.

Patients with HIV infection may present with any number of symptoms and diseases, ranging from complaints unrelated to HIV infection to life-threatening complications. Virtually any organ system may be involved. The following focuses on some of the more common presentations that may be encountered in the ED.

Constitutional Symptoms and Fever

Systemic symptoms such as fever, malaise, and weight loss are common among patients with HIV infection.[11] For patients with newly acquired HIV, fever may occur in the course of primary infection, 8 to 12 weeks after exposure. When due to HIV infection alone, fever tends to occur in the afternoon or evening and is generally responsive to aspirin or acetaminophen. In patients with known HIV infection presenting with an acute febrile illness or a change in the patient's usual fever pattern, systemic infection and malignancy must be excluded. A thorough history and physical examination should be performed in an attempt to identify a site of infection and stage of disease.

Laboratory evaluation of fever may include blood cultures (aerobic, anaerobic, and fungal), blood tests for cryptococcal antigen and *Toxoplasma* and *Coccidioides* serologies, and chest radiography. Syphilis serology; viral hepatitis evaluation, purified protein derivative (PPD) with anergy panel; stool culture; stool examination for ova and parasites; urine culture for bacteria, fungus, and mycobacteria; and sputum smear and culture for fungus and mycobacteria may also be appropriate. If no other source of fever is identified and there are no contraindications, lumbar puncture should be performed, especially if there are neurologic signs or symptoms. Admission should be considered for patients with unexplained fever, particularly when oral intake and the patient's level of functioning have deteriorated.

Two of the more common infectious etiologies of fever to consider in patients with advanced disease are disseminated MAC and CMV infection. MAC is the most common opportunistic bacterial infection in AIDS patients, causing disseminated disease in up to 50% of patients at some time during their illness. It is usually associated with severe weight loss, diarrhea, and constitutional symptoms such as fever, malaise, and anorexia. Infection occurs most often in patients with CD4 counts of less than 100 cells/μL. The diagnosis may be made in one of several ways: A Ziehl-Neelsen (acid-fast) stain of stool or other body fluids is frequently positive, or the organism can also be cultured from blood.

Clarithromycin combined with ethambutol and rifabutin reduces bacteremia and improves symptoms, but is not curative. CMV is the most common cause of opportunistic viral infection in HIV-positive patients. Disseminated disease usually involves the pulmonary or gastrointestinal system, with definitive diagnosis often requiring biopsy, demonstrating intranuclear inclusion bodies. CMV retinitis (discussion follows) is the most important manifestation to recognize in the ED. Treatment is with foscarnet or ganciclovir.

A malignancy that frequently presents with fever is non-Hodgkin's lymphoma. New central nervous system (CNS) symptoms, particularly a change in mental status in the presence of fever, should be evaluated with neuroimaging. Definitive diagnosis requires biopsy. Effective treatment regimens include combined radiotherapy and chemotherapy.

Intravenous drug users (IDUs) who present with fever have been shown to be at increased risk for infective endocarditis (IE). The current standard of care is to admit all febrile IDUs, because there are no reliable clinical or laboratory predictors of this disease.[17] Inpatient evaluation for IE includes following blood culture results and findings on echocardiography. Recent studies suggest that a short ED-based evaluation for IE may be feasible, using echocardiography, culture, and new PCR-based technology as an alternative to blood culture.[21,22] Currently, however, inpatient hospitalization is advised due to the significant morbidity and mortality of missed IE and the difficulties associated with outpatient follow-up in this population.

Disposition of patients with fever depends on the patient's level of functioning and ability to maintain sufficient oral intake to prevent volume depletion, the availability of timely medical follow-up, and the physician's confidence that fever is due to a benign etiology that may be successfully managed on an outpatient basis.

Pulmonary Involvement

Pulmonary presentations are among the most frequent reasons for ED visits among patients with known HIV infection.[9,11] More than 80% of AIDS patients develop pulmonary disease. Presenting complaints may include cough, hemoptysis, shortness of breath, and chest pain. The differential diagnosis includes viral, bacterial, mycobacterial, fungal, and protozoal pneumonias, as well as malignancies. The more common etiologies are shown in Table 192.2. Although differentiation of these entities in the ED may be difficult, appreciation of the epidemiology and the common findings associated with various pathogens can assist the emergency physician in arriving at a working diagnosis and instituting appropriate treatment and disposition decisions.

The physical examination itself is not likely to aid in establishing a diagnosis. Patients with fever and productive cough are likely to have a bacterial pneumonia, whereas a nonproductive cough is more likely to accompany PCP, CMV pneumonia, fungal infection, or neoplasm. Hemoptysis is most often associated with pneumococcal pneumonia and tuberculosis (TB). Fulminant respiratory failure is most likely to be caused by PCP or CMV.

Evaluation of HIV-infected patients who present with pulmonary complaints should generally include pulse oximetry and chest radiograph; additional testing that may be helpful includes a complete blood cell count, electrolyte determination, arterial blood gas analysis, serum lactate dehydrogenase, sputum culture, Gram stain, and special stains (Gomori, Giemsa, acid-fast). Obtaining blood cultures may avoid delays in initiating antimicrobial therapy.

Findings of leukocytosis and focal infiltrates on plain chest radiography suggest bacterial pneumonia. A diffuse infiltrative process on chest radiography, especially in the absence of leukocytosis, is associated with PCP or CMV. PCP is suggested by an increased serum lactate dehydrogenase level and hypoxia more severe than expected from radiographic findings. Hilar adenopathy with diffuse pulmonary infiltrates suggests cryptococcosis, histoplasmosis, mycobacterial infection, or neoplasm. KS can present with cough, fever, and dyspnea; the chest radiograph may mimic that seen with PCP. PCP can be demonstrated by histologic techniques (Gomori, methenamine silver, or Giemsa stain) but cannot be cultured.

PCP is the most common opportunistic infection among AIDS patients. More than 70% of AIDS patients will acquire PCP at some time during their illness, and it is the initial opportunistic infection in 60% of cases. Although typically seen in HIV-infected adults with CD4 lymphocyte counts below 200/μL, pediatric cases may be seen with higher CD4 counts.

Classic presenting symptoms of PCP are an insidious cough (typically nonproductive), dyspnea, and fatigue. A determined

TABLE 192.2. Common Causes of Pulmonary Involvement in AIDS

INFECTION	
Viral	**Protozoa**
Cytomegalovirus	*Pneumocystis carinii*
Herpes simplex virus	*Toxoplasma gondii*
Adenovirus	**Bacteria**
Mycobacteria	*Streptococcus*
M. tuberculosis	*Staphylococcus aureus*
M. avium	*Haemophilus influenzae*
M. kansasii	*Legionella*
Fungi	*Nocardia*
Histoplasma	**MALIGNANCY**
Cryptococcus	Lymphoma
Coccidiodes	Kaposi's sarcoma
Candida	**PNEUMONITIS**
	Lymphoid interstitial pneumonitis

investigation of new or subtle symptoms may lead to an early diagnosis, which, in turn, may lead to a better outcome. Typical chest radiographic findings are diffuse interstitial infiltrates. Atypical x-ray findings are more common in patients with CD4 counts less than 100 cells/μL, and negative chest x-rays have been reported in up to 20% of patients with PCP.[6] Up to 10% of patients with PCP have been found to have pneumothoraces. In patients with PCP, arterial blood gas analysis may show hypoxemia and an increased alveolar–arterial oxygen gradient.

In the ED, a presumptive diagnosis of PCP is often made if there is hypoxia without any other explanation. Although bronchoscopy (bronchoalveolar lavage, brush biopsy, transbronchial biopsy) has been the mainstay of establishing the diagnosis, examination of induced sputum by indirect immunofluorescent staining using monoclonal antibodies has been shown to be a relatively easy and effective method of diagnosing PCP.

When PCP is suspected, treatment should be initiated without waiting to obtain a definitive diagnosis. Initial treatment is with 15 mg/kg/d of trimethoprim (TMP) and 75 mg/kg/d of sulfamethoxazole (SMZ), given either orally or intravenously in two to three daily divided doses for a total of 3 weeks. Intravenous pentamidine isethionate (4 mg/kg/d) is an alternative and equally efficacious initial choice for patients with adverse reactions (typically rash, fever, or neutropenia) to TMP/SMZ. Systemic corticosteroid treatment is recommended for patients with a PaO_2 less than 70 mm Hg, or an alveolar–arterial gradient of more than 35 mm Hg. Prednisone may be administered in a dose of 80 mg for 5 days, followed by 40 mg for 5 days, followed by 20 mg for an additional 11 days. Prophylactic therapy for PCP (with TMP/SMZ 1 DS PO qd) is recommended to prevent reinfection, and in all patients with CD4 cell counts less than 200 cells/μL.

The incidence of *M. tuberculosis* in HIV-infected patients is increasing, particularly in socioeconomically disadvantaged groups, including the homeless, immigrant, and intravenous drug–using populations. The incidence of TB in the AIDS population is estimated to be 200 to 500 times that of the general population.[19] Disease may occur from reactivation of prior infection or direct progression of disease from recently acquired infection. Because less immunosuppression is required to reactivate infection of this organism than that required to permit other opportunistic infections to become established, pulmonary TB may be the initial finding in HIV-infected patients, frequently occurring in patients with CD4 counts of 200 to 500 cells/μL.

Classic presenting symptoms of TB include cough (with hemoptysis), fever, nightsweats, and weight loss. In patients with severe immunosuppression, clinical manifestations are increasingly atypical, and extrapulmonary findings may occur. Frequent sites of dissemination include peripheral lymph nodes, bone marrow, and the genitourinary system. Typical pulmonary upper lobe lesions are less common in those with CD4 counts less than 200 cells/μL, and the chest radiograph may be indistinguishable from those due to a variety of other opportunistic infections.[6]

In the ED, physicians should maintain a high index of suspicion for TB among HIV-infected patients with pulmonary symptoms. For any patient in whom the diagnosis is being considered, immediate isolation should be instituted because of the high rate of person-to-person transmission.[20] Decisions for ongoing isolation and admission should be based on the results of chest x-ray and detailed historic and clinical information. Negative PPD tests are frequent among those infected. Attempts to diagnose TB by stain and culture of sputum may not be fruitful; bronchoscopy or biopsy of affected organs (e.g., lymph nodes, liver, brain) may be required. Patients with AIDS with TB should receive four-drug initial empiric therapy with isoniazid, rifampin, pyrazinamide, and streptomycin. All HIV-infected patients with a positive PPD should receive isoniazid or rifampin prophylaxis.

In HIV-infected patients, the most common pulmonary infections are nonopportunistic bacterial pneumonias, such as *Streptococcus pneumoniae, Mycobacterium pneumoniae,* and *Haemophilus influenzae*. In patients with severe immunosuppression, other pulmonary infections to consider include CMV infection, cryptococcosis, histoplasmosis, aspergillosis, and coccidioidomycosis. Malignancies, particularly KS and lymphoma, may also cause pulmonary involvement.

In patients with pulmonary symptoms who fall into high-risk groups but who do not carry a diagnosis of HIV infection, careful evaluation is nonetheless warranted. If initial ED tests (chest radiography, sputum examination, arterial blood gas analysis) are not helpful, the patient should be referred (or admitted, if warranted) for voluntary HIV testing, counseling, and follow-up. Disposition decisions for patients with pulmonary complaints are primarily dependent on respiratory status, oxygenation, and evidence of systemic toxicity.

Neurologic Involvement

CNS disease occurs in 90% of patients with AIDS, and 10% to 20% of AIDS patients initially present with CNS symptoms.[11,15] A wide variety of symptomatology may be seen, including altered mental status, coma, seizures, headache, and focal neurologic symptoms. Infection accounts for the vast majority of neurologic presentations and is often accompanied by fever. Noninfectious complications include HIV encephalopathy (AIDS dementia complex), lymphoma (primary and secondary), KS, intracerebral hemorrhage, subarachnoid hemorrhage, cerebral infarction, and cerebral edema.

A specific diagnosis may often be established with the aid of computed tomographic (CT) scanning, cerebrospinal fluid (CSF) studies, and, in some cases (e.g., lymphoma), biopsy. Patients with known HIV infection and those in high-risk groups who have a change in mental status, headache (new or different from previous pattern), seizure, or new neurologic finding should have a head CT performed on an emergent basis.[23] Lumbar puncture is also indicated unless there is a clinical contraindication. Specific CSF studies should include measurement of opening and closing pressures; cell count; glucose; protein; Gram stain; India ink stain; bacterial, viral, and fungal culture; and toxoplasmosis, cryptococcus, and coccidioidomycosis titers.

Toxoplasma gondii is the most common cause of focal encephalitis in patients with HIV infection. Typical manifestations include headache, confusion, lethargy, seizures, or other focal neurologic symptoms. Serologic testing is not useful because antibody to *T. gondii* is prevalent in the general population; the presence of *T. gondii* in the CSF is helpful, although there is a high rate of false negatives. Diagnosis is usually made by a contrast-enhanced head CT scan showing one or more ring-enhancing lesions associated with edema (Fig. 192.1).

A noncontrast CT scan can be used as an initial imaging study in the ED, because the addition of contrast has been shown to be of marginal value in patients with completely normal noncontrast CT scans. The typical appearance of toxoplasmosis on a noncontrast scan is multiple subcortical lesions, with a predilection for the basal ganglia. In cases in which the clinical suspicion for CNS pathology is high but the CT scan is equivocal or negative, contrast CT should be performed in the ED. The finding of multiple ring-enhancing lesions with surrounding edema is highly suggestive of toxoplasmosis.

Magnetic resonance imaging is slightly more sensitive than contrast CT but is usually not indicated in the ED. Patients with suspected toxoplasmosis should be admitted and treated with

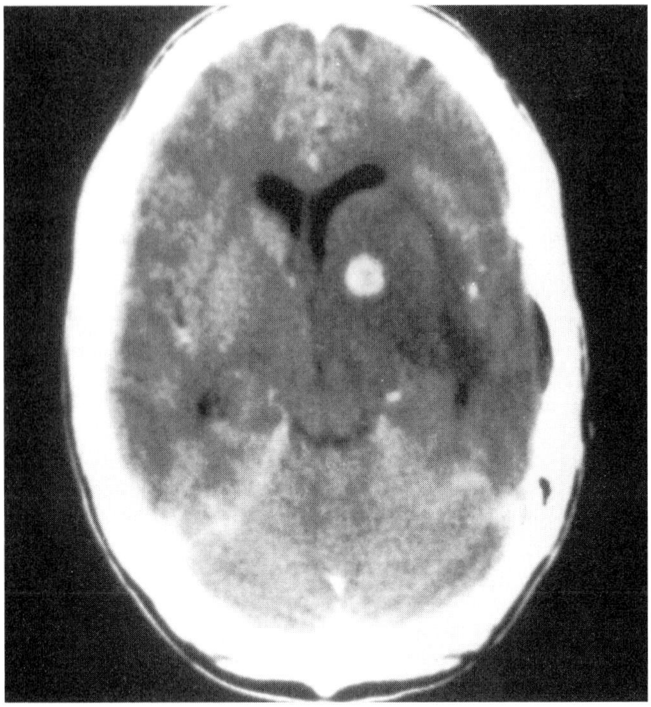

Figure 192.1. Contrast-enhanced CT scan with typical ring-enhancing lesions of cerebral toxoplasmosis.

sulfadiazine (4 to 8 g/d) and pyrimethamine (100 to 200 mg load, then 50 to 100 mg/d). Folinic acid may be added to blunt hematologic megaloblastic toxicity. Short courses of high-dose corticosteroids may also be used, particularly in cases in which significant edema or mass effect is noted. Presumptive treatment may be initiated before a definitive diagnosis is made. In cases in which the patient does not respond to therapy, alternative diagnoses should be considered.

Other focal lesions on CT that may be confused with toxoplasmosis include lymphoma, progressive multifocal leukoencephalopathy, and *Candida*. Definitive diagnosis may require biopsy. For those patients who respond to therapy, chronic suppressive treatment for toxoplasmosis is usually indicated because of the high likelihood of relapse.

Cryptococcus neoformans occurs in up to 10% of AIDS patients and may cause either focal cerebral lesions or diffuse meningoencephalitis. Presenting symptoms may be subtle (e.g., mild depression, headache, or dizziness without meningismus) but are often dramatic (e.g., cranial nerve palsies and seizures). The diagnosis depends on identifying organisms in the CSF by India ink preparation (60% to 80% sensitive), fungal culture (95% to 100% sensitive), or cryptococcal antigen (nearly 100% sensitive and specific). Serum cryptococcal antigen is also useful, but has a lower sensitivity (approximately 95%) than CSF cryptococcal antigen.[28]

Treatment of cryptococcal meningitis usually begins with intravenous amphotericin B (0.5 to 0.6 mg/kg/d), with or without 5-flucytosine, for 14 days. Fluconazole, 400 mg/d orally, or itraconazole may be considered as alternative therapies. The initial course of therapy should be followed by 8 to 10 weeks of oral fluconazole. Because of the high relapse rate (about 50%), chronic suppressive therapy is often continued after successful treatment. The major adverse effect of treatment for cryptococcal meningitis is marrow suppression.

Other infections, such as bacterial meningitis, TB meningitis, aseptic meningitis, brain abscess, CMV encephalitis, herpes simplex virus (HSV) encephalitis, aspergillosis, nocardial encephalitis, and neurosyphilis, may also be considered as possible causes of neurologic symptoms. Noninfectious CNS processes include CNS lymphoma, cerebrovascular accidents, metabolic encephalopathy, and AIDS dementia complex (HIV encephalopathy).

AIDS dementia is a common, progressive disorder characterized by impaired memory, lethargy, concentration difficulties, and other cognitive impairment. After other organic causes of neurologic symptoms are ruled out, the diagnosis of HIV encephalopathy may be made on the basis of neuropsychologic testing. CT scan typically shows atrophy and ventricular enlargement. HIV encephalopathy often responds to zidovudine therapy.

HIV-infected patients with new or changed CNS symptoms or signs should be considered for hospital admission, particularly if the ED evaluation is unrevealing. CT scan and lumbar puncture should usually be performed as part of the ED evaluation, although CSF culture and serologic results will not be available immediately. When CT and all CSF studies are unrevealing, magnetic resonance imaging may be helpful in identifying early CNS lesions.

Peripheral neuropathies are common in the HIV-infected population and may be caused by HSV, mononeuritis multiplex (possibly related to multifocal CMV), idiopathic sensory neuropathy, or drug reactions (specifically to dideoxyinosine and dideoxycytidine). In certain patients, symptomatic relief with pain-modifying agents such as amitriptyline or phenytoin may be helpful, although these agents should be used judiciously because of their potential for causing delirium in patients with concurrent HIV dementia. Narcotic analgesia may be indicated in severe cases.

Gastrointestinal Involvement

About one-half of all AIDS patients have symptoms due to infection of the gastrointestinal tract at some time during the course of their illness. The most common symptoms are abdominal pain, bleeding, and diarrhea. Table 192.3 contains a partial list of common etiologies of gastrointestinal infections.

Oropharynx

Oral candidiasis is the most common oral manifestation of HIV infection and affects more than 80% of AIDS patients. *Candida albicans* typically involves the tongue and buccal mucosa. It can be distinguished from hairy leukoplakia by its characteristic whitish, lacy plaques, which are easily scraped away from an erythematous base. Microscopic examination of the material on potassium hydroxide smear can confirm the diagnosis in the ED. Oral and esophageal involvement with *Candida* is considered predictive of a progressive course of HIV infection. Most oral lesions can be managed symptomatically on an outpatient basis, with topical treatment such as clotrimazole troches, 10 mg

TABLE 192.3. Common Gastrointestinal Infections in AIDS

BACTERIA	PARASITES
Salmonella	*Cryptosporidium*
Shigella	*Isospora belli*
Campylobacter	*Entamoeba histolytica*
Neisseria gonorrhoeae	*Giardia*
	Strongyloides
VIRUSES	**FUNGI**
Cytomegalovirus	*Candida*
Herpes simplex virus	
Adenovirus	

five times daily. Oral ketoconazole or fluconazole may be considered for refractory cases.

Painful oral and perioral ulcerations may be caused by HSV, which can be recognized by typical vesicular lesions and diagnosed in the ED by the identification of multinucleated giant cells in scrapings of the lesions. Oral HSV may be treated with acyclovir, 200 to 800 mg five times daily. Topical acyclovir is not effective.

Oral KS may appear as nontender, well-circumscribed, slightly raised, violaceous lesions anywhere in the oropharynx. Definitive diagnosis and therapy should be carried out by a consultant.

Hairy leukoplakia, thought to be caused by the Epstein-Barr virus, causes a benign epithelial thickening and typically involves the lateral borders of the tongue. The tongue may appear to have hairlike projections. Because it is usually asymptomatic and benign, no specific therapy is necessary.

Esophagus

Complaints of dysphagia or odynophagia are indicative of esophageal involvement. Candidal infection, HSV infection, and CMV infection may all cause painful esophagitis. Treatment of esophagitis in the ED is usually presumptive for *Candida*, which accounts for up to 70% of cases. Oral ketoconazole (100 to 200 mg/d) or fluconazole (200 to 400 mg/d) is equally efficacious. An air-contrast barium swallow may be obtained as part of the ED evaluation. An ulcerative pattern with plaques is characteristic of candidal esophagitis. HSV esophagitis typically produces easily seen punched-out ulcerations without associated heaped-up plaques. Endoscopy, fungal stains, viral cultures, and, occasionally, biopsy may be required to establish the definitive etiology.

Liver and Biliary Tract

Viral hepatitis occurs commonly among HIV-infected patients, and standard serologic testing and supportive care are indicated. Several opportunistic organisms, including CMV, *M. avium*, *M. tuberculosis*, and *Histoplasma*, can produce a hepatitis-like picture in patients with HIV infection. Most commonly, the patient presents with an elevation in the alkaline phosphatase level that is disproportionate to the levels of other liver enzymes.

Acalculous cholecystitis may be seen as a result of infection with CMV or *Cryptosporidium*.

Rectum

Anorectal disease is common in AIDS patients. Proctitis is characterized by painful defecation, rectal discharge, and tenesmus. Common causative organisms include *Neisseria gonorrhoeae*, *Chlamydia trachomatis*, syphilis, and HSV. Proctocolitis presents with the same symptoms but is accompanied by diarrhea. Typical causative organisms include those just listed, plus bacterial agents such as *Shigella*, *Salmonella*, *Campylobacter*, and *Entamoeba histolytica*. Diagnostic evaluation in the ED should include anoscopy with evaluation of stool or pus (or both) by Gram stain, culture, and testing for ova and parasites. A Thayer-Martin culture and chlamydial culture or immunoassay should be ordered. The diagnosis of rectal gonorrhea can be confirmed on a Gram stain of stool by the presence of leukocytes and intracellular organisms. HSV can be diagnosed by viral culture or by the identification of multinucleated giant cells on scrapings of anal lesions.

Diarrhea

Diarrhea is extremely common among AIDS patients, and may vary in severity from a few loose stools per day to massive fluid loss with prostration, fever, chills, and weight loss. ED evaluation should be directed toward stabilization, hydration, and laboratory studies, including cultures.

The differential diagnosis of diarrhea in the HIV-positive population is broad. Common identified etiologies include bacterial infections caused by *Salmonella*, *Shigella*, and *Campylobacter* species; viral infections, such as those from CMV, rotavirus, and Norwalk agent; fungal infections, such as histoplasmosis and candidiasis; and parasitic infections, such as *Giardia*, *Cryptosporidium*, and *Isospora belli*. Although a definitive diagnosis is usually not made in the ED, certain patterns may provide clues regarding the most likely etiology. Bacterial pathogens tend to follow an acute and fulminant course, while parasitic infections are more often indolent. Significant gastrointestinal bleeding has been associated with many pathogens, particularly CMV. *Cryptosporidium* and *Isospora* are associated with profuse, watery diarrhea. The most common agents in end-stage disease are CMV and *M. avium-intracellulare*.

The stool should be examined for leukocytosis, ova and parasites, and bacterial culture. When ordering stool cultures, it is important to specify which organisms are suspected, because not all are routinely cultured. The diagnosis of infection with mycobacteria, *Cryptosporidium*, and *Isospora* is made by acid-fast stain. Because of intermittent shedding, repeated examination of the stool for trophozoites, cysts, and larvae is often necessary to diagnose *Cryptosporidium* and *Isospora*, as well as amebiasis, giardiasis, and strongyloidiasis.

In general, patients who can tolerate oral intake and are not orthostatic may be discharged from the ED, with outpatient follow-up of test results. If bacterial infection is strongly suspected, empiric treatment with an antibiotic such as ciprofloxacin can be initiated. Patients who present with severe diarrhea may benefit from symptomatic therapy with agents such as attapulgite (Kaopectate), psyllium (Metamucil), and, if necessary, diphenoxylate hydrochloride with atropine (Lomotil).

Dermatologic Involvement

Skin disease may affect up to 90% of HIV-infected patients. Several cutaneous manifestations of AIDS are likely to be seen in the ED; cutaneous infection, dermatitis, and neoplasms are the most common. Viral infections may include HSV, herpes zoster, papillomavirus infection, and molluscum contagiosum.

HSVs are common in AIDS patients and can present as either a localized infection or systemic disease. Localized infections respond well to standard therapy with oral acyclovir (200 mg five times daily for 10 days). Intravenous therapy (15 to 30 mg/kg/d) may be required in cases of extensive disease. Reactivation of varicella zoster virus occurs more frequently in patients with HIV compared with the general population. The clinical course is prolonged, and complications are more common. In patients with single dermatomal involvement who are not significantly immunosuppressed, outpatient treatment with acyclovir (800 mg PO five times a day) or famciclovir (500 mg PO three times a day) for 7 days is usually sufficient. Patients with disseminated disease or ophthalmic zoster should be admitted to isolation beds for intravenous acyclovir.

Papillomavirus infection is manifested as warts, which may appear in various areas. Treatment may be initiated with topical salicylic acid, and referral to a dermatologist is generally indicated.

Molluscum contagiosum lesions are typically clusters of white umbilicated papules. Unless of cosmetic significance, molluscum lesions are considered benign, and treatment is not mandatory. If desired, referral to a dermatologist may be made for consideration of such therapy as cryosurgery or curettage.

Bacterial infections, such as staphylococcal infections (e.g., folliculitis, impetigo, cellulitis), are seen with increased frequency. Therapy involves standard antibiotic treatment, although the duration of treatment may need to be increased.

Several fungal infections are commonly seen. Dermatophyte infections, such as tinea corporis, tinea pedis, and tinea cruris, should be treated with topical antifungal agents such as miconazole or clotrimazole. Tinea versicolor should be treated with topical selenium sulfide. *C. albicans* infection may involve the oral, esophageal, nail, inguinal, and perianal areas with increased frequency. Treatment for mucosal infection is discussed in the section on gastrointestinal involvement; treatment for cutaneous infection may consist of topical antifungal agents such as clotrimazole or, in severe cases, oral ketoconazole, fluconazole, or intravenous amphotericin B.

Other types of dermatitis are also commonly seen. Seborrheic dermatitis manifests as erythematous scaly eruptions typically involving the nasolabial folds, cheeks, and chest, and is treated with a topical corticosteroid preparation. Diffuse xerosis (dry skin) and pruritus are common among HIV-infected patients. Treatment with topical emollients, oatmeal baths, and oral antihistamines such as diphenhydramine or hydroxyzine may be of benefit.

The most common cutaneous neoplasm is KS, which has involved approximately 25% of known AIDS cases, occurring most often in homosexual men. KS typically presents as raised, irregular, nonblanching, brown-black or purple macules or nodules. Cutaneous KS is generally not associated with significant morbidity or mortality; palliative therapy is indicated only for extensive, painful, or cosmetically disfiguring lesions. In addition to cutaneous involvement, KS may also involve the gastrointestinal tract, lungs, liver, spleen, and heart. Treatment may include antiretroviral therapy, radiation therapy, and chemotherapeutic agents.

Psychiatric Issues

HIV-infected patients may present with a variety of social and emotional issues, complicated by neuropsychiatric and cognitive components. Some of the common psychiatric conditions include depression, bipolar disease, suicidal ideation, anxiety, and adjustment disorder. Patients with depression tend to have lower CD4 counts, and they report more AIDS-related symptoms. All psychiatric symptoms should be evaluated with the goal of identifying treatable, reversible conditions, such as neurologic lesions or drug reactions.[16] Many patients will benefit from initiation of pharmacologic therapy in conjunction with social intervention and support. Suicidal potential should be taken seriously, particularly in patients who have limited social support; management at an inpatient facility is often required.

Ophthalmologic Manifestations

Eye complaints are common among patients with AIDS. Although a wide range of ophthalmic disease can occur, recognition of two is critical for the emergency physician.

CMV retinitis is the most serious ocular opportunistic infection and the leading cause of blindness in patients with AIDS, occurring in up to 40% of patients at some time during their illness. Presenting complaints are variable and may include changes in visual acuity, photophobia, scotoma, visual field cuts, eye redness, or pain. Funduscopic examination typically shows fluffy white perivascular lesions with areas of hemorrhage. These findings may be easily confused with retinal cotton wool spots, a benign lesion with no prognostic significance seen in patients with AIDS (indicative of retinal microvasculopathy). Because of the risk of blindness associated with CMV retinitis, any patient in whom there is suspicion of CMV retinitis requires immediate ophthalmologic consultation. Patients with CMV require immediate treatment to prevent progression of disease. The treatment regimen consists of induction therapy with intravenous ganciclovir (5 mg/kg every 8 hours for 14 to 21 days), followed by 6 mg/kg/d, oral or intravenous.

Herpes zoster ophthalmicus is another common cause of ocular damage in patients with HIV. The typical presentation is pain or paresthesia in the distribution of cranial nerve V_1, followed by the emergence of the vesicular zoster skin rash. Complications include conjunctivitis, episcleritis, iritis, keratitis, secondary glaucoma, and, rarely, retinitis. As with CMV, early recognition and treatment can prevent morbidity. Immunocompetent patients can be treated with acyclovir on an outpatient basis in consultation with ophthalmology; immunocompromised patients require admission for intravenous antibiotics.

Other Organ Systems

Several sexually transmitted diseases (STDs) are epidemiologically associated with HIV infection. Diseases causing genital ulcers are believed to provide vascular portals of entry for HIV. Increased STD surveillance in the ED has been recommended as a potential means to help control HIV transmission.[5,27]

Patients presenting with any symptoms suggestive of a possible STD should be evaluated for gonorrhea, chlamydia, and herpes. Serologic testing for syphilis with rapid plasma reagin (RPR) or Venereal Disease Research Laboratories (VDRL) tests should also be performed. Careful consideration should be given to identify patients with serologic false-negative results due to a lack of normal antibody response. In such cases, in which syphilis is clinically suspected, dark-field microscopy and direct fluorescent antibody staining from suspicious lesions may be undertaken. Empiric therapy may be instituted even without laboratory evidence of infection.

Primary (chancre) and secondary (rash, mucocutaneous lesions, adenopathy) syphilis should be treated with a single intramuscular dose of benzathine penicillin, 2.4 million U; latent syphilis, or secondary syphilis of unknown duration, requires three weekly injections. Patients with known or suspected syphilis should be evaluated for the presence of neurosyphilis, which has had a recent increase in incidence among HIV-infected individuals.

Renal complications of HIV include HIV-associated nephropathy, prerenal azotemia, vasculitis, drug reactions, and systemic infections. Renal involvement is often discovered incidentally on laboratory analysis, but initial ED presentations may include general malaise, edema, or oliguria. Because of the complexity of these disorders, management in consultation with a nephrologist or primary care provider is generally indicated.

Clinically significant cardiac involvement with HIV-related conditions is uncommon. Cardiac findings at autopsy in AIDS patients include cardiomyopathy, myocarditis, endocarditis, and pericardial effusion.

Antiretroviral Therapy

In 1996, the CDC reported a decline in the number of new AIDS cases and AIDS-related deaths for the first time since the beginning of the epidemic, attributed in large part to the use of antiretroviral therapy. Although not commonly instituted in the ED, antiretroviral therapy is an important aspect of management of HIV-infected patients.

Zidovudine (AZT) is a thymidine analog that inhibits the replication of HIV by interfering with the action of viral RNA-dependent DNA polymerase (reverse transcriptase). It is the first antiviral agent to have demonstrated clinical benefit, delaying progression to AIDS and decreasing mortality in patients with AIDS. Oral absorption is good, serum concentrations that inhibit viral replication are easily obtainable, and the drug is able to cross the blood–brain barrier to attack virus in the CNS. In several controlled trials, zidovudine has been shown to decrease the number and severity of opportunistic infections, as well as to improve general health and survival. Recent studies have shown that combination therapy, with two nucleoside reverse transcriptase inhibitors and a protease inhibitor, results in maximal clinical efficacy.[24] A large number of antiretroviral medications and combination regimens are currently prescribed.

Antiretroviral therapy is generally considered in patients with CD4 cell counts of less than 500 cells/μL, because the goal is to reduce viremia, bolster the CD4 cell count, and delay the onset of opportunistic infections. Treatment strategies are tailored to the individual patient, however, with attention to a variety of issues, including suppression of viral replication, preservation of immune function, drug side effects, drug interactions, and patient preference. Any decision regarding initiation and change in antiretroviral medications should be made in consultation with the patient's primary care provider or an infectious disease consultant.

TABLE 192.4. Considerations for Disposition Decisions for HIV-Infected Patients

Conditions Suggesting Admission	Conditions for Considering Discharge
New presentation of fever of unknown origin	Normal or baseline vital signs
Hypoxemia (worse than baseline) (PaO_2 <60)	Stable medical condition
Suspected PCP	Able to take PO/not orthostatic
Suspected tuberculosis	Follow-up and referral arranged
New CNS symptoms	Patient or caregiver understands instructions
Intractable diarrhea	Patient, caregiver, or hospice able to care for patient
Suicidality	
Suspected CMV retinitis	
Zoster ophthalmicus	
Cachexia/weakness	
Unable to care for self or receive adequate care	
Unable to assure appropriate follow-up	

Adverse Drug Reactions

Adverse drug reactions occur commonly among HIV-infected patients. These patients tend to be on multidrug therapy and, in addition, appear to have an increased risk of adverse effects. It is useful to be familiar with several of the most common adverse drug reactions in HIV-positive patients. TMP/SMZ reactions occur in up to 65% of AIDS patients, significantly more commonly than in the general population. Adverse effects generally become apparent after 7 to 14 days of therapy; the most common are nausea, vomiting, rash, fever, neutropenia, thrombocytopenia, hyponatremia, and hepatitis. Pentamidine can cause nausea, vomiting, diarrhea, neutropenia, hypoglycemia, hyperglycemia, renal impairment, hepatic toxicity, and orthostatic hypotension; about 50% of patients experience at least one adverse effect. AZT has been associated with several severe reactions, including anemia, neutropenia, headache, nausea, cardiomyopathy, and myopathy. Common etiologies of neurologic and psychiatric effects include therapy with acyclovir, amphotericin, corticosteroids, ganciclovir, pentamidine, TMP/SMZ, and zidovudine.

Drug reactions should be considered in the evaluation of all patients, and decisions to alter pharmacologic management should be made on an individual basis and in conjunction with the primary care provider. Review of current references and consultation with a hospital pharmacologist are indicated when drug reactions are suspected.

DISPOSITION

Disposition decisions for HIV-infected patients are based, as for any patient, on clinical condition, the availability of outpatient resources, and the ability to arrange adequate follow-up.

Patients who are known to be seropositive for HIV but who are not admitted to the hospital should be referred for follow-up, or for medical consultation and counseling if they do not have an established source of care. It has been found useful for each institution to have arranged appropriate mechanisms for these referrals. Patients who have symptoms or signs suggestive of HIV infection (e.g., weight loss, generalized adenopathy, chronic diarrhea, oral thrush) but who do not require admission should also receive similar referral.

Although the AIDS epidemic has raised grave concerns regarding the economic impact of the disease, financial considerations should not be a factor in determining management or disposition. General considerations related to discharge and admission decisions are listed in Table 192.4. When there is doubt about diagnostic or management options, consultation with an infectious disease specialist, neurologist, psychiatrist, AIDS specialist, or others is appropriate.

ETHICAL CONSIDERATIONS

Some experts contend that in the advanced stages of AIDS, major resuscitative measures are not appropriate because of the uniformly poor prognosis. Many patients may agree as they approach the terminal stages of their disease. However, decisions regarding the withholding of extraordinary resuscitation efforts are difficult to make in the ED, because the emergency physician is rarely in possession of sufficient information about individual patients, their wishes, the state of their disease, and the judgment and intentions of their physicians. In general, when confronted with a patient with AIDS, it is best to take the same actions that would otherwise be taken with any other patient, unless an advance directive is available, indicating that resuscitative efforts should be withheld.

Confidentiality is paramount in the care of patients with HIV-related diagnosis. Extra attention must be paid to this issue in the ED, where busy and crowded conditions make this aspect of patient care more challenging.

The management of patients with nonoccupational exposure to HIV (e.g., through sexual contact or injection drug use) may become a problem that will increasingly confront emergency physicians. Although clear guidelines exist regarding postexposure prophylaxis (PEP) following occupational exposure (discussion follows), the CDC has withheld making definite statements regarding PEP for nonoccupational exposure, owing to the lack of available data in this setting. PEP must, therefore, be considered on a case-by-case basis, and should generally be restricted to situations in which the risk of infection is high, the intervention can be initiated promptly (less than 36 hours), adherence to the regimen is likely, and the individual is most likely to maintain risk-reduction behavior over time. If the emergency physician is confronted with a case in which PEP is being considered, consultation should be sought with the patient's primary care provider (when available), an infectious disease specialist, or the CDC (via a 24-hour physician hotline: PEP Hotline, 1-888-448-4911).

PREVENTION/PRECAUTIONS

Health-care workers are often exposed to the blood and body secretions of AIDS patients or of other individuals who are at high risk of harboring the AIDS virus. Because there is no cure for AIDS at this time, the best strategy is to take proper precautions in handling potentially infectious body fluids. It should be noted, however, that the risk of acquiring HIV through occupational exposure appears to be very low. The rate of HIV infection after parenteral exposure has been calculated to be 0.32% (representing six infections in more than 2008 needlesticks involving HIV-infected blood).[18]

Several studies have shown that a substantial number of patients in the ED have unsuspected HIV infection and that HIV seroreactivity cannot be accurately predicted, even with the aid of risk factor assessment.[21] Because asymptomatic individuals who are HIV-antibody–positive can transmit the disease, *all* contacts with patients' blood or body secretions must be considered potentially infectious by ED personnel. Even if HIV is not suspected in a particular patient, the possibility of other bloodborne infections mandates the use of universal precautions with all patients when contact with body fluids is likely.[10,12]

HIV is a very labile virus. It is easily neutralized by heat and common disinfecting agents, such as 50% ethanol, 35% isopropyl alcohol, 0.3% hydrogen peroxide, Lysol, and a 1:10 solution of household bleach. Routine disinfection of surfaces that have come in contact with body fluids should be effective.

Although there is one unusual instance of HIV transmission from a dentist's practice to patients, evidence indicates that the risk of transmission of HIV infection to patients by health-care workers is extremely low, if present at all. Although still controversial, the debate concerning HIV-infected health-care workers, their ability to continue to work, and notification of patients possibly at risk has diminished, owing to the lack of further documented transmissions. Thus, routine screening of health-care personnel for HIV infection is not indicated. However, because HIV can potentially be transmitted to patients through contact with infected blood, body fluids, or secretions, the infected health-care worker should protect against exposing the patient to these sources of virus.

Guidelines for PEP of health-care workers following an occupational exposure have recently changed. The new policies are based on a recent case-control study of needlestick injures from an HIV-infected source, which found that AZT prophylaxis was associated with a 70% reduction in transmission.[1] PEP recommendations are based on exposure category, with the highest risk injuries associated with deep punctures and injuries caused by large-bore hollow needles.

Treatment regimens vary by type of exposure; all include AZT and 3TC.[3] Decisions should generally be made in consultation with an infectious disease specialist. Treatment should be initiated as quickly as possible, however, preferably within 1 to 2 hours. Antiretroviral therapy is not indicated in patients presenting more than 36 hours after exposure. Care of the exposed individual should include baseline testing, with follow-up testing at 6 weeks, 3 months, 6 months, and 1 year after the exposure. The exposed person should also be referred for counseling, which should include advice to practice safe sex. Documentation of the risk factors and HIV status of the source is also helpful.

Each hospital should have policies in place regarding testing of a source patient in cases of occupational exposure. When policies on HIV testing are developed, certain principles should be considered. There should be a mechanism for obtaining permission from the source patient. Special policies may be necessary for patients who are unable to give consent (e.g., unconscious patients). Provisions should be made for informing source patients of test results, and counseling should be made available. Confidentiality should be rigorously protected while still ensuring that the appropriate information is provided to the exposed individuals. Finally, the identification of a seropositive patient should not affect the delivery of appropriate health care.

COMMON PITFALLS

- Failure to recognize undiagnosed infection. Because patients often may not volunteer information regarding HIV risk factors, this information must be actively sought whenever a patient with possible opportunistic infection or other symptoms suggestive of HIV infection (e.g., weight loss, fever) is being treated.
- Failure to fully evaluate complaints of fever, headache, and shortness of breath in HIV-positive patients who appear well. Fever may indicate systemic infection; blood cultures should be obtained, even in patients who appear nontoxic. Chronic low-grade headache or headache different from a patient's usual pattern of headache may be suggestive of CNS infection or malignancy; a head CT and lumbar puncture are indicated in such patients. Subjective shortness of breath may be the only early sign of PCP.

References

1. Cardo DM, Culver DH, Ciesielski CA, et al. A case-control study of HIV seroconversion in health-care workers after percutaneous exposure. Centers for Disease Control and Prevention Needlestick Surveillance Group. *N Engl J Med* 1997;337:1485.
2. Centers for Disease Control and Prevention. 1993 revised classification system for HIV infection and expanded surveillance case definition for AIDS among adolescents and adults. *MMWR* 1993;41(RR-17):1.
3. Centers for Disease Control and Prevention. Update: Provisional Public Health Service recommendations for chemoprophylaxis after occupational exposure to HIV. *MMWR* 1996;45:468.
4. Centers for Disease Control and Prevention. Trends in the HIV and AIDS epidemic. CDC Web Site: www.cdc.gov/nchspt/od/trends.htm, 1999.
5. Ernst AA, Farley TA, Martin DH Screening and empiric treatment for syphilis in an inner-city emergency department. *Acad Emerg Med* 1995;2:765.
6. Huang L, Stanell JD. AIDS and the lung. *Med Clin North Am* 1996;80(4):775.
7. Katz MH, Gerberding JL. Postexposure treatment of people exposed to the human immunodeficiency virus through sexual contact or injection-drug use. *N Engl J Med* 1997;336:1097.
8. Kelen GD, Fritz S, Quaish B, et al. Unrecognized human immunodeficiency virus (HIV) infection in general emergency patients. *N Engl J Med* 1988;318:1645.
9. Kelen GD, Digiovanna T, Bisson K, et al. Human immunodeficiency virus infection in emergency department patients: epidemiology, clinical presentations and risk for health care workers: the Johns Hopkins experience. *JAMA* 1989;262:516.
10. Kelen GD. Human immunodeficiency virus and the emergency department: risks and risk protection for health care providers. *Ann Emerg Med* 1990;19:242.
11. Kelen GD, Johnson G, Digiovanna TA, et al. Profile of patients with human immunodeficiency virus infection presenting to an inner-city emergency department: preliminary report. *Ann Emerg Med* 1990;19:242.
12. Kelen GD, Hansen KN, Green GB, et al. Determinants of emergency department procedure- and condition-specific universal (barrier) precaution requirements for optimal provider protection. *Ann Emerg Med* 1995;25:743.
13. Kelen GD, Hexter DA, Hansen KN, et al. Trends in human immunodeficiency virus (HIV) infection. *Clin Infect Dis* 1995;21(4):867.
14. Kelen GD, Shahan SB, Quinn TC. Emergency department-based HIV screening and counseling: experience with rapid and standard serologic testing. *Ann Emerg Med* 1999;33(2):147.
15. Kieburtz K, Schiffer RB. Neurologic manifestations of human immunodeficiency virus infections. *Neurol Clin* 1989;7(3):447.
16. Lyketsos CG, Fishman M, Treisman G. Psychiatric issues and emergencies in HIV infection. *Emerg Med Clin North Am* 1995;13(1):163.
17. Marantz PR, Linzer M, Feiner CJ, et al. Inability to predict diagnosis in febrile intravenous drug addicts. *Ann Intern Med* 1987;106:823.
18. Marcus R, Cooperative Needlestick Surveillance Group. Surveillance of health care workers exposed to blood from patients infected with the human immunodeficiency virus. *N Engl J Med* 1988;319:1118.
19. Markowitz N, Hansen NI, Hopewell PC, et al. Incidence of tuberculosis in the United States among HIV-infected persons. *Ann Intern Med* 1997;126:123.

20. Moran GJ, McCabe F, Morgan TM, et al. Delayed recognition and infection control for tuberculosis in the emergency department. *Ann Emerg Med* 1995;26(3):290.
21. Rothman RE, Fein S, Quinn TC, et al. Rapid diagnosis of bacteremia using polymerase chain reaction in the emergency department (ED). *Acad Emerg Med* 1999;6(5):375.
22. Rothman RE, Londner M, Mehta, et al. Developing a 24-hour ED based diagnostic guidelines for 'ruling out' endocarditis in intravenous drug users (IDUs). *Acad Emerg Med* 1999;6(5):453.
23. Rothman RE, Keyl PM, McCarthur JC, et al. A decision guideline for emergency department utilization of noncontrast head computed tomography in HIV-infected patients. *Acad Emerg Med* 1999;6(10):1010.
24. Spooner KM, Lance C, Masur H. Antiretroviral therapy: reference guide to major clinical trails in patients infected with human immunodeficiency virus. *Clin Infect Dis* 1995;20:1145.
25. Vellq W, Chiesi A, Volpi A, et al. Differential survival of patients with AIDS according to the 1987 and 1993 CDC case definitions. *JAMA* 1994;271:1083.
26. Yarchoan R, Venzon DJ, Pluda JM, et al. CD4 count and the risk for death in patients infected with HIV receiving antiretroviral therapy. *Ann Intern Med* 1991;115(3):184.
27. Yearly DM, Greene TJ, Hobbs GD. Under recognition if cervical *Neisseria gonorrhoeae* and *Chlamydia trachomatis* infections in the emergency department. *Acad Emerg Med* 1997;4(10):962.
28. Zuger A, Louie E, Holzman RS, et al. Cryptococcal disease in patients with the acquired immunodeficiency syndrome. Diagnostic features and outcome of treatment. *Ann Intern Med* 1986;104(2):234.

CHAPTER 193
Spinal Infections

Ellen H. Taliaferro and Allan B. Wolfson

Vertebral osteomyelitis and epidural abscess are uncommon but devastating conditions that are easily overlooked in a busy emergency department. If undetected and untreated, they can result in vertebral collapse, cord compression, and paralysis.

The vertebral column is the most common site of hematogenous osteomyelitis in the adult, and most cases of vertebral osteomyelitis are blood-borne. Identifiable sites of antecedent infection include the genitourinary tract, soft tissues, the respiratory tract, infected vascular prostheses, and heart valves.[12] No source can be identified in approximately one-third of cases. Vertebral osteomyelitis can also occur by direct extension (e.g., from a retropharyngeal abscess) or by direct contamination (e.g., from trauma or after vertebral disc surgery).

Most patients with vertebral osteomyelitis fall into one of the following high-risk groups: patients older than the age of 50, intravenous drug users, and other immunocompromised individuals, including diabetics and alcoholics. Vertebral osteomyelitis is also reported occasionally in patients with sickle cell disease.[6] The incidence of spinal infection appears to be increasing in association with increases in intravenous drug use, iatrogenic immunosuppression, and the use of indwelling vascular and urinary catheters.

Pyogenic vertebral osteomyelitis in adults is most commonly caused by *Staphylococcus aureus* and *Escherichia coli*.[2–4,7,10,12] In intravenous drug users, the most common organisms are *Pseudomonas aeruginosa*, other gram-negative bacilli, *S. aureus*, and *Candida* species.[4] In the past, tuberculosis was a common cause of vertebral osteomyelitis (Pott disease), but the advent of effective antituberculous drugs has greatly reduced its role as a cause of this infection.

When osteomyelitis occurs by hematogenous spread, the richly vascularized flat bone adjacent to the disc cartilage is probably the first area involved (discitis).[4,8] Extension can occur longitudinally to other vertebrae or anteriorly to form a paraspinal abscess. When a disc and adjacent vertebral body have been destroyed, there may be vertebral collapse and kyphosis. Posterior extension can lead to meningitis or to epidural abscess and neurologic deficits such as paraplegia.

The introduction of antibiotics has changed the natural history of osteomyelitis. Early, aggressive treatment results in a high cure rate. With delayed or unsuccessful treatment, vertebral osteomyelitis may result in complications such as vertebral collapse, epidural abscess, cord compression, or vascular thrombosis.

CLINICAL PRESENTATION

Patients with vertebral osteomyelitis classically present with neck or back pain,[5,12,14] but early manifestations are often more subtle. Fever is commonly absent.[2,4,10,12] The onset of pain is often insidious; many patients have had back symptoms for months before seeking medical attention. Occasional patients present with an abrupt onset of the disease, however, and run an acute toxic course. Patients with Pott disease often present with nonspecific symptoms, such as fever, weight loss, nightsweats, and neck or back pain and stiffness.[15] Tuberculous osteomyelitis often runs a more indolent course than does pyogenic bacterial vertebral osteomyelitis.

Osteomyelitis most commonly affects the lumbar vertebrae (50% of cases); involvement of the thoracic spine is somewhat less frequent (35%).[12] Localized tenderness over the affected area of the spine is a major warning sign, and neck or back pain not relieved by rest is especially suggestive. Spasm of the paravertebral muscles is common but nonspecific. Some patients have limitation of back motion or a positive straight-leg raising sign.

Cord compression associated with osteomyelitis, reported in up to 40% of patients in some series, can result in irreversible deficits, especially when the compression is not treated surgically.[14] Abnormalities of bladder or bowel function or motor or sensory deficits of the lower extremities are clearly suggestive of spinal cord involvement.

The majority of patients with bacterial spinal epidural abscess also present with neck or back pain, which may have been present from 1 day to 2 months. Other symptoms include radicular pain, weakness of an extremity, sensory deficit, and cord symptoms.

DIFFERENTIAL DIAGNOSIS

Because back pain due to minor trauma or musculoskeletal strain is extremely common, back symptoms in emergency department patients are often attributed to these causes, especially when the symptoms are of relatively short duration. Spinal infection is suggested, however, by persistent pain and tenderness that localizes to one area of the midline, particularly in members of high-risk groups.

A sudden onset of neck or back pain, especially with neurologic signs, suggests a vascular event, such as spontaneous epidural hemorrhage. In sickle cell anemia, the difficulty of diagnosis may be compounded by the simultaneous presence of vasoocclusive complications.[6]

In the early stages, infection can be virtually indistinguishable from other septic conditions or may mimic malignancy. Moreover, it may be difficult to differentiate vertebral osteomyelitis from metastatic disease, severe degenerative changes, or postoperative changes on the basis of either plain films or radionuclide studies alone.

EMERGENCY DEPARTMENT EVALUATION

The emergency department evaluation begins, as always, with a careful history and thorough physical examination; a careful neurologic examination is critical. As noted earlier, localized vertebral tenderness, deformity, or neurologic signs are highly suggestive, particularly if they occur in a patient who is at risk.

Laboratory studies are of limited value. The white blood cell count is often elevated, but this finding is quite nonspecific. The erythrocyte sedimentation rate is nearly always elevated with vertebral osteomyelitis and epidural abscess, often above 100 mm/h. Blood cultures are positive in less than half of patients with vertebral osteomyelitis.[12,14]

Diagnostic imaging can often provide evidence for the diagnosis but tends to be less revealing in early cases. Plain radiography, often combined with tomography, is usually the initial imaging study ordered. The classic radiographic findings of osteomyelitis are lytic lesions, periosteal elevation, cortical irregularity, and demineralization. As the disease progresses, segments of devascularized and necrotic bone can separate and form sequestra; periosteal reaction and pathologic fracture may occur. In blood-borne vertebral osteomyelitis, the well-vascularized flat bone adjacent to the disc space tends to be involved earliest, and infection of the disc space (discitis) and the adjacent vertebral body follow. Radiographic findings usually do not appear, however, until at least 7 to 14 days after the onset of symptoms, and extensive destruction can occur before radiographic changes become evident.[9,11]

Computed tomographic scanning or radionuclide studies often reveal evidence of infection when plain radiographs are negative.[9–12] Technetium radionuclide scanning is sensitive but nonspecific; gallium scanning is more specific but less sensitive.[12]

Magnetic resonance imaging has superior sensitivity and specificity in detecting osteomyelitis.[10,11] It has the additional advantage of allowing direct visualization of the intervertebral discs, spinal cord, and soft tissues, making it extremely useful in detecting epidural pathology. Finally, it can differentiate infection from degenerative and neoplastic disease. When enhanced with gadolinium, magnetic resonance imaging readily detects actively inflamed tissues and appears to be the most useful diagnostic test for epidural abscess.[10,13]

The definitive diagnosis of osteomyelitis rests on the isolation of a pathogen from blood cultures or a bone lesion. Bone biopsy or aspiration is thus necessary for diagnosis if blood cultures are negative.[12,14] Sinus tracts, when present, should not be cultured, because the organisms that are identified from these sites bear little relation to the results of cultures obtained at surgery.[14]

EMERGENCY DEPARTMENT MANAGEMENT

Several factors have helped improve the outcome of vertebral osteomyelitis. They include greater awareness of the disease on the part of clinicians; the increasing availability of radionuclide imaging and magnetic resonance imaging; improved orthopedic techniques; and prophylactic antibiotic regimens for trauma, surgery, and invasive procedures.[14] The use of the newer antibiotics has improved outcomes in established infection as well. In most cases, osteomyelitis can be cured without surgical intervention.[12]

Treatment for osteomyelitis consists of 4 to 6 weeks of parenteral antibiotic therapy, sometimes followed by a prolonged course of oral antibiotics. Immobilization is also an accepted principle of treatment, at least during the initial phases.[1]

In view of the prolonged course of treatment that is generally required and the importance of eradicating the causative organism, the initiation of empiric antibiotic therapy in the emergency department is almost never appropriate. Definitive antibiotic therapy must be guided by culture results. In those few instances in which antibiotics might be started empirically before culture results are available, a combination of penicillinase-resistant penicillin and either a third-generation cephalosporin or an aminoglycoside would be a reasonable choice.

The more rapid the onset of symptoms and the more serious the manifestations, the more aggressive the clinician must be both in establishing the diagnosis and in obtaining specimens for culture. When cord compression or other neurologic complications occur, immediate surgical intervention is necessary to decompress the cord and stabilize the spine. Surgery is also indicated for abscess or significant bone necrosis.

DISPOSITION

Patients with suspected spinal infection require admission to the hospital for diagnostic evaluation and initiation of intravenous antibiotic therapy. Orthopedic or neurosurgical consultation is almost always mandatory. Patients with neurologic compromise should be transferred promptly to a tertiary care facility if rapid surgical intervention is not otherwise available.

COMMON PITFALLS

- An indolent spinal infection may be overlooked because of the paucity and nonspecific character of the patient's signs and symptoms. Although uncommon, the diagnosis must be considered in elderly or immunosuppressed individuals with persistent localized pain or tenderness in the neck or back, whether or not neurologic signs are present.
- Delays in treatment lead to a worse outcome.

References

1. Abramovitz JN, Batson RA, Yablon JS. Vertebral osteomyelitis: the surgical management of neurologic complications. *Spine* 1986;11:418.
2. Beltrani VP, Echols RM, Vedder DK. Vertebral osteomyelitis caused by *Haemophilus influenzae*. *J Infect Dis* 1987;156:391.
3. Carragee EJ. Pyogenic vertebral osteomyelitis. *J Bone Joint Surg* 1997;79A:874.
4. Case records of the Massachusetts General Hospital: case 16-1992. *N Engl J Med* 1992;326:1070.
5. Darouiche RO, Hamill RJ, Greenberg SB, et al. Bacterial spinal epidural abscess: review of 43 cases and literature survey. *Medicine* 1992;71:369.
6. Gardner RV. *Salmonella* vertebral osteomyelitis and epidural abscess in a child with sickle cell anemia. *Pediatr Emerg Care* 1985;1:87.
7. Gelfand MS, Miller JH. Pneumococcal vertebral osteomyelitis in an adult. *South Med J* 1987;80:534.
8. Honan M, White GW, Eisenberg GM. Spontaneous infectious discitis in adults. *Am J Med* 1996;100:85.
9. Jensen AG, Espersen F, Skinhoj P, et al. Bacteremic *Staphylococcus aureus* spondylitis. *Arch Intern Med* 1998;158:509.
10. Maslen DR, Jones SR, Crislip MA, et al. Spinal epidural abscess. *Arch Intern Med* 1993;153:1713.
11. Modic MT, Pflanze W, Feiglin DHI, et al. Magnetic resonance imaging of musculoskeletal infections. *Radiol Clin North Am* 1986;24:247.
12. Sapico FL, Montgomerie JZ. Vertebral osteomyelitis. *Infect Dis Clin North Am* 1990;4:539.
13. Teman AJ. Spinal epidural abscess: early detection with gadolinium magnetic resonance imaging. *Arch Neurol* 1992;49:743.
14. Waldvogel FA, Vasey H. Osteomyelitis: the past decade. *N Engl J Med* 1980;303:360.
15. Wurtz R, Quader Z, Simon D, et al. Cervical tuberculous vertebral osteomyelitis: case report and discussion of the literature. *Clin Infect Dis* 1993;16:806.

CHAPTER 194

Toxic Shock Syndromes

Frederick M. Schiavone

STAPHYLOCOCCAL TOXIC SHOCK SYNDROME

Toxic shock syndrome (TSS) associated with *Staphylococcus aureus* was originally described in 1978 and was found to be associated with tampon use in young women. The peak reported incidence, in 1980, has been followed by a marked and persistent decline.[4] Mortality from TSS has also declined—from 10% before 1980 to less than 5% in the early 1980s and to less than 1% in 1989.

Initial studies showed that this illness was associated with the use of new super-absorbent tampons during menses, and that vaginal colonization and infection by *S. aureus* played a major etiologic role. However, nonmenstrual cases of staphylococcal TSS were found in both sexes and in all age groups[11] and were associated with surgical procedures such as rhinoplasty, augmentation mammaplasty, liposuction, and burns. Nonmenstrual TSS has also been associated with influenza, sinusitis, tracheitis, intravenous drug use, human immunodeficiency virus (HIV) infection, cellulitis, burn wounds, gynecologic infections, and the postpartum period. The proportion of reported nonmenstrual cases has increased from 7% in 1980 to approximately 50% in recent years.[2]

A bacterial toxin, toxic shock syndrome toxin-1 (TSST-1), has been isolated in over 90% of menstruation-associated cases.[8] In contrast, TSST-1 has been detected in only half of the strains isolated in nonmenstrual TSS. Other toxins, such as staphylococcal enterotoxin B (SEB) and enterotoxins A (SEA) and C (SEC), are found in the remaining cases. The exotoxins are thought to be absorbed into the blood through inflamed or injured mucous membranes, leading to the production of cytokines, which produce widespread multisystem clinical effects such as fever, rash, emesis, hypotension, and shock.[8]

CLINICAL PRESENTATION AND DIFFERENTIAL DIAGNOSIS

Staphylococcal TSS often presents with flulike symptoms of malaise, myalgias, and chills, which progress over 2 to 3 days to a systemic shock–like syndrome. Some patients present with signs of hypovolemia due to diarrhea, generalized vasodilatation, or capillary leak. Others present with an abrupt onset of fever, tachycardia, tachypnea, and hypotension. A major feature of TSS is the erythematous rash, resembling a sunburn, which may be diffuse or patchy in distribution. The rash can be very subtle and may be misdiagnosed as a "fever flush." Desquamation of the skin occurs in 7 to 14 days at the sites of the previous rash, with full-thickness peeling of the skin involving the palms, soles, and fingers.

Criteria for the diagnosis of staphylococcal TSS are provided in Table 194.1.[10] TSS can involve every organ system and can produce a wide constellation of symptoms. Patients often complain of severe myalgias or edema of the face and eyelids, with hyperemia of the pharynx, tongue, and vaginal mucosa. Headache is common. There may be confusion, somnolence, lethargy, agitation, or combativeness, without focal neurologic signs. Gastrointestinal manifestations may include vomiting, diarrhea, abdominal pain, and hepatomegaly.

TABLE 194.1. Criteria for Staphylococcal Toxic Shock Syndrome

1. Fever of 102°F (38.9°C)
2. Presence of diffuse macular erythroderma ("sunburn" appearance)
3. Desquamation 1 to 2 wk after onset of illness, particularly of the palms and soles
4. Hypotension, defined as a systolic blood pressure of 90 mm Hg for adults and less than the fifth percentile for children younger than 16 years; an orthostatic decrease in diastolic blood pressure of 15 mm Hg with a position change from lying to sitting; orthostatic syncope; or orthostatic dizziness
5. Involvement of three or more of the following organ systems:
   - Gastrointestinal: history of vomiting or diarrhea at the onset of illness
   - Muscular: elevated creatine phosphokinase level or severe myalgia
   - Mucous membrane: nonpurulent conjunctivitis, oropharyngeal hyperemia, or vaginal hyperemia or discharge
   - Renal: abnormal results of renal function tests or urinalysis
   - Hepatic: elevated serum transaminase and bilirubin levels
   - Hematologic: thrombocytopenia
   - Central nervous system: disorientation or alteration in consciousness without focal neurologic signs and in the absence of hypotension or fever

   In addition, normal results of the following tests, if performed:
   - Blood, throat, cerebrospinal fluid cultures (blood culture may be positive for *Staphylococcus aureus*); antibody tests for Rocky Mountain spotted fever, ehrlichiosis, leptospirosis, and rubella

Toxic shock syndrome is "probable" when at least four of the five criteria are fulfilled.

Modified from American Academy of Pediatrics. Staphylococcal toxic shock syndrome. In: Peter G, ed. *1997 Red book: report of the Committee on Infectious Diseases*, 24th ed. Elk Grove Village, IL: American Academy of Pediatrics, 1997:481.

The differential diagnosis of TSS includes *streptococcal* toxic shock syndrome (discussion to follow), Kawasaki disease, staphylococcal scalded-skin syndrome, scarlet fever, Stevens-Johnson syndrome, Rocky Mountain spotted fever, ehrlichiosis, leptospirosis, meningococcemia, atypical measles, viral illness, anaphylaxis, heat stroke, gram-negative sepsis, and drug reactions.

EMERGENCY DEPARTMENT EVALUATION AND MANAGEMENT

The diagnosis of TSS must often be made on clinical grounds. Because the disorder is caused by toxins, blood cultures may be negative. Laboratory examination may demonstrate a marked thrombocytopenia (platelets less than 100,000), an elevated blood urea nitrogen and creatinine, and elevated liver function tests. The diagnosis is most often suggested by the characteristic blanching macular erythematous rash.

Initial treatment consists of intravenous fluid replacement. Large volumes of crystalloid or albumin are often required to maintain normal perfusion, and hemodynamic monitoring and vasopressors are sometimes necessary as well. Tampons, nasal packs, or other foreign bodies, if present, must be removed. Surgical wounds or areas of infection need to be incised and drained.

Antibiotics may not affect the clinical course, because the syndrome is caused by bacterial toxins rather than the bacterial infection *per se*. However, antibiotics may be beneficial if the patient is bacteremic or if there is a site of on-going infection. The drug of choice is a penicillinase-resistant synthetic penicillin or a first-generation cephalosporin. Vancomycin or clindamycin may be used as alternatives in penicillin-allergic patients.

Adjunctive treatments for TSS have included intravenous immunoglobulin, steroids, plasmapheresis, and monoclonal antibodies. At present, these therapies have not demonstrated a clear benefit. Some European studies have found corticosteroids to be effective in cases of severe TSS that are unresponsive to antibiotic therapy.

COMMON PITFALLS

- Failure to recognize staphylococcal TSS in young healthy patients with fever and an erythematous rash
- Failure to administer adequate fluid volumes to maintain tissue perfusion
- Failure to seek an occult source of staphylococcal colonization or infection

STREPTOCOCCAL TOXIC SHOCK SYNDROME

In the late 1980s, a disease similar to staphylococcal TSS, but caused by a strain of group A streptococci, was recognized.[13] This illness, characterized by hypotension and multiorgan failure, was termed *streptococcal toxic shock syndrome* (STSS). The Centers for Disease Control and Prevention case definition of this syndrome is shown in Table 194.2.[3]

Cases of STSS are often associated with minor nonpenetrating trauma or soft-tissue infection.[1,7] Viral infections, such as varicella[5] and influenza, are thought to provide a portal of entry in other cases, but, in many patients, no source of the organism can be identified. Bacterial toxins produced by group A streptococci (GAS), particularly streptococcal pyrogenic exotoxins (SPE), as well as host factors, are thought to play an important role in determining disease severity.[14] Blood cultures are generally positive. The young, the elderly, and the immunosuppressed are at greatest risk, but, significantly, a large proportion of patients with STSS are young, healthy adults.[6]

TABLE 194.2. Case Definition for the Streptococcal Toxic Shock Syndrome

1. Isolation of group A streptococci
   A. From a normally sterile site (e.g., blood, cerebrospinal fluid, peritoneal fluid, tissue biopsy, surgical wound)
   B. From a nonsterile site (e.g., throat, superficial skin lesion)
2. Clinical signs of severity
   A. Hypotension: systolic blood pressure 90 mm Hg in adults or less than fifth percentile for age in children, and
   B. Two or more of the following signs:
      Renal impairment: creatinine 2 mg/dL for adults or at least twice the upper limit of normal for age
      Coagulopathy: platelets less than 100,000/μL or disseminated intravascular coagulopathy
      Liver involvement: serum alanine aminotransferase (SGOT), aspartate aminotransferase (SGPT), or total bilirubin concentrations at least twice the upper limit of normal for age
      Adult respiratory distress syndrome
      A generalized erythematous macular rash that may desquamate
      Soft-tissue necrosis, including necrotizing fasciitis or myositis, or gangrene

An illness fulfilling criteria 1A and 2 (A and B) can be defined as a definite case.

An illness fulfilling criteria 1B and 2 (A and B) can be defined as a probable case if no other etiology for the illness is identified.

Modified from the Centers for Disease Control and Prevention. The Working Group on Severe Streptococcal Infection. Defining the group A streptococcal toxic shock syndrome: rationale and consensus definition. *JAMA* 1993;269:391.

CLINICAL PRESENTATION AND EMERGENCY DEPARTMENT EVALUATION

STSS often presents with a flulike syndrome of fever, malaise, myalgia, nausea, vomiting, and diarrhea. Hypotension is an essential part of the case definition of STSS. Half of patients have a normal blood pressure on admission but develop hypotension within a few hours of presentation. Hypotension may require aggressive fluid and vasopressor therapy. Organ system involvement also becomes evident. Renal dysfunction may be severe enough to require hemodialysis. Acute respiratory distress syndrome may require endotracheal intubation.

In distinction to staphylococcal TSS, a diffuse scarlatina-like rash is uncommon in STSS (less than 10%). A majority of patients have signs of a soft-tissue infection, such as localized swelling and erythema; of these, many progress to necrotizing fasciitis or myositis. Pain, out of proportion to physical findings, is usually severe and abrupt in onset, and occurs initially without associated tenderness. It may involve an extremity, the abdomen, the pelvis, or the chest. An ominous sign is the appearance of vesicles, which develop into violaceous or bluish bullae. These are an indication for emergent surgical exploration, both to establish the diagnosis of GAS infection and to debride nonviable tissue.

Despite prompt, aggressive medical and surgical management, the mortality rate of STSS is high, usually about 30%.

EMERGENCY DEPARTMENT MANAGEMENT

Early treatment with antibiotics is critical. Although *Streptococcus pyogenes* continues to be susceptible to beta-lactam antibiotics, including penicillin, several studies recommend treatment with both penicillin and clindamycin. However, because the differential diagnosis includes other infectious etiologies, initial broad-spectrum coverage is required. Prompt and aggressive surgical exploration and debridement of suspected deep-seated *S. pyogenes* infections are mandatory, however.

Massive quantities of intravenous fluids (up to 20 L/d) may be necessary. Vasopressors such as dopamine are frequently used, but outcome trials have not demonstrated their benefit. Cases of symmetrical gangrene of the digits have resulted with the use of vasopressors; however, it is difficult to determine whether this is due to pressors, infection, or both.

Case reports have described the successful use of intravenous gamma globulin infusions in a small number of patients with STSS.[9] Anecdotal reports of hyperbaric oxygen have been used in a handful of patients,[12] but it is unclear whether this treatment is useful.

COMMON PITFALLS

- Failure to consider the diagnosis of STSS early and to institute antibiotics promptly.
- Failure to debride soft-tissue infections aggressively. Areas of apparently minor, painful, erythematous swelling may represent the first sign of a serious GAS infection.

References

1. Bisno AL. Streptococcal infections of skin and soft tissues. *N Engl J Med* 1996;334:240.
2. Centers for Disease Control. Reduced incidence of menstrual toxic shock syndrome—United States 1980–1990. *MMWR* 1990;39:421.
3. Centers for Disease Control. The Working Group on Severe Streptococcal Infection. Defining the group A streptococcal toxic shock syndrome: rationale and consensus definition. *JAMA* 1993;269:391.
4. Centers for Disease Control. Epidemiologic notes and reports: toxic-shock syndrome—United States. *MMWR* 1997;46(22):492–495.
5. Doctor A, Harper MB, Fleisher GR. Group A B-hemolytic streptococcal bacteremia: historical overview, changing incidence, and recent association with varicella. *Pediatrics* 1995;96:428–433.
6. Hoge CW, Schwartz B, Talkington DF, et al. The changing epidemiology of invasive group A streptococcal infections and the emergence of toxic shock-like syndrome: a retrospective population-based study. *JAMA* 1993;269:384–389.
7. Kaul R, McGeer A, Low DE, et al. Population-based surveillance for group A streptococcal necrotizing fasciitis: clinical features, prognostic indicators, and microbiologic analysis of seventy-seven cases. *Am J Med* 1997;103:18–24.
8. Manders SM. Toxin-mediated streptococcal and staphylococcal disease. *Am Acad Dermatol* 1998;39:3.
9. Perez CM, Kubak BM, Cryer HG, et al. Adjunctive treatment of streptococcal toxic shock syndrome using intravenous immunoglobulin: case report and review. *Am J Med* 1997;102:111–113.
10. Peter G, ed. *1997 Red book: report of the Committee on Infectious Diseases,* 24th ed. Elk Grove Village, IL: American Academy of Pediatrics, 1997:481.
11. Reingold AL, et al. Nonmenstrual toxic shock syndrome: a review of 130 cases. *Ann Intern Med* 1982;96:871.
12. Riseman JA. Hyperbaric oxygen therapy for necrotizing fasciitis reduces mortality and the need for debridements. *Surgery* 1990;108:847.
13. Stevens DL, Tanner MH, Winship J, et al. Severe group A streptococcal infections associated with a toxic shock-like syndrome and scarlet fever toxin A. *N Engl J Med* 1989;321:1.
14. Stevens DL. Streptococcal toxic-shock syndromes: spectrum of diseases, pathogenesis, and new concepts in treatment. *EID* 1995;1:3.

CHAPTER 195

Bacteremia and Septic Shock

J. Stephan Stapczynski

Bacteremia is the presence of viable bacteria within the liquid component of blood.[3] Although bacteremia can be confirmed only by bacteriologic or immunologic tests, its potentially explosive course and high mortality rate mandate the institution of antibiotic therapy when its presence is suspected on clinical grounds, before the results of these tests are known.

Bacteremia can be *transient,* as is commonly seen after injury to mucosal surfaces (e.g., from tooth brushing, urethral catheterization, sigmoidoscopy, angiography), but intact host defenses usually neutralize the bacteria and their harmful products and prevent clinical infection. Bacteremia can be *primary* (without an identifiable focus of infection) or *secondary* to an extravascular or intravascular focal infection. Most bacteremias are secondary to an extravascular focus of infection.

A consensus conference of the American College of Chest Physicians and the Society of Critical Care Medicine, in August 1991, developed definitions for sepsis, severe sepsis, and septic shock to clarify the terminology and usage concerning these concepts[3] (Table 195.1). The conference first noted that physiologic alterations and organ dysfunction similar to those seen with bacterial infections can follow a wide variety of clinical insults. This clinical state was termed the *systemic inflammatory response* (SIRS) and was defined by changes in body temperature, heart rate, respiratory function, and peripheral leukocyte count. *Sepsis* was defined as the systemic host response to *infection,* the condition characterized by the presence of microorganisms or the invasion of normally sterile host tissue by those organisms. It should be noted that sepsis is defined by the host's reaction to infection and not only by the presence of microorganisms. The use of these recommendations is encouraged to avoid the confusion that has developed from the variety of bacteriologic, physiologic, and clinical meanings for the term *sepsis* and for the even less precise term *septicemia.*

TABLE 195.1. Definitions

Systemic Inflammatory Response Syndrome (SIRS): the physiologic response to a variety of severe clinical insults manifested by two or more of the following
- A. Temperature >38°C or <36°C
- B. Heart rate >90 beats/min
- C. Respiratory rate >20 breaths/min or a $PaCO_2$ <32 mm Hg
- D. White cell count (WBC) >12,000 cells/μL, <4,000 cells/μL, or >10% immature (band) forms

Sepsis: the systemic response to infection manifested by the presence of SIRS

Severe Sepsis: sepsis associated with organ dysfunction, hypoperfusion, or hypotension (systolic BP <90 mm Hg or a reduction of >40 mm Hg from baseline). Hypoperfusion and perfusion abnormalities may include, but are not limited to, lactic acidosis, oliguria, or an acute alteration in mental status.

Septic Shock: sepsis with hypotension, despite adequate fluid resuscitation, along with the presence of perfusion abnormalities that may include, but are not limited to, lactic acidosis, oliguria, or an acute alteration in mental status

Multiple Organ Dysfunction Syndrome (MODS): presence of altered organ function in an acutely ill patient such that homeostasis cannot be maintained without intervention

Adapted from American College of Chest Physicians, Society of Critical Care Medicine, Consensus Conference. Definitions of sepsis and organ failure and guidelines for the use of innovative therapies in sepsis. *Crit Care Med* 1992;20:864–874.

Septic shock was defined as sepsis with hypotension and evidence of inadequate tissue perfusion despite fluid resuscitation. In the case of bacterial infections leading to septic shock, circulatory insufficiency occurs when bacterial products interact with host cells and serum proteins to initiate a series of reactions leading to cell injury and death.[4] Not only are the bacterial products harmful, but the widespread and unregulated host response to these bacterial products also results in the elaboration of an extensive array of chemical mediators that lead to further cell damage.[22] The following systems and mediators are stimulated in septic shock: arachidonic acid metabolites (leukotrienes, prostaglandins, and thromboxanes), the complement system, coagulation cascade, the fibrinolytic system, catecholamines, glucocorticoids, prekallikrein, bradykinin, histamine, beta-endorphins, enkephalins, adrenocorticotropic hormone, circulating myocardial depressant factor(s), cachectin (tumor necrosis factor [TNF]), and interleukin-1 (IL-1).

Septic shock develops in fewer than half of patients with bacteremia; it occurs in about 40% of those with gram-negative aerobes such as *Escherichia coli, Klebsiella* species, *Pseudomonas aeruginosa,* and *Proteus* species, and in about 20% of those with gram-positive bacteremia with organisms such as *Staphylococcus aureus.* Multicenter studies of patients with septic shock have found that approximately 50% of patients have bacteremia, and another 30% have a documented bacterial infection without bacteremia.[4,6,14,18,19]

Septic shock is present in about a fourth of patients at the onset of sepsis syndrome.[18] While sepsis and septic shock are common events in hospitals, there are limited studies on the incidence or frequency of these syndromes. A multicenter study has identified a rate of approximately two cases per 100 hospital admissions for sepsis syndrome.[19] Of these cases, approximately half were diagnosed in the intensive care unit (ICU), 12% in the emergency department, and one-third in a non-ICU patient care unit.

With the development of advanced monitoring and cardiorespiratory support of patients with life-threatening illnesses, it has become increasingly clear that the major threat to survival is not the underlying disease or a specific complication, but a process of progressive failure of multiple independent organs. This process has been termed *multiple organ failure syndrome* and is the major cause of death in patients with severe sepsis and septic shock.[3–5,10]

CLINICAL PRESENTATION

Bacteremia is usually found in association with an acute illness and symptoms of fever, chills, and prostration—the so-called toxic state. Not all patients have such a classic presentation, particularly those at the extremes of age or in debilitated states. Bacteremia and septic shock are dynamic processes in which the observed clinical manifestations depend on when in the disease course the patient presents and on the ability of the patient's neurologic, cardiovascular, and pulmonary systems to respond to the various stimuli. For example, elderly patients may not manifest fever, but may present with hypothermia.

The mean age reported for SIRS and sepsis syndrome is 55 to 60 years old.[6,14,18,19] This is most likely because older patients have conditions (e.g., diabetes, surgical procedures, and cancer) that predispose them to bacterial infections. While there is no reason to suspect that the occurrence of sepsis and septic shock would vary according to the patient's age, two large-scale perspective studies of SIRS and sepsis syndrome have found a slightly higher percentage of men than women (55% to 60%).[18,19] This difference may reflect a higher rate of preceding surgical procedures in men as opposed to women.

The cardiovascular response in septic shock depends on the stage of disease. Initial hemodynamic measurements usually indicate the presence of vasodilation due to widespread arteriovenous shunting, a decrease in systemic vascular resistance, an increase in cardiac output, and an increase in oxygen consumption; this pattern is consistent with a distributive variety of shock.[4] Initially, blood pressure may not be altered much, and the abnormal hemodynamic parameters respond to volume infusion alone. Despite an increased cardiac output, there is impairment of myocardial function, with a decreased left ventricular ejection fraction and left ventricular dilatation.[12] As septic shock progresses, uncontrolled vasodilatation and capillary leakage of plasma lead to splanchnic pooling of circulating volume, decreased oxygen consumption, and a falling blood pressure. Typically, blood pressure falls 6 to 8 hours after the initial signs of bacteremia due to gram-negative organisms. Cardiac function may also be diminished by two other factors: inadequate coronary perfusion and the presence of humoral myocardial depressant factors.

Hemodynamic measurements in human bacteremia and septic shock are influenced by the administration of volume, inotropic, and vasoconstrictor agents. Persistently low systemic vascular resistance, regardless of cardiac output, is the major hemodynamic derangement in patients who die of septic shock. In advanced septic shock, depressed cardiac output and severe hypotension produce a vicious cycle of multiorgan failure that is usually unresponsive to volume and inotropic or vasoconstrictor therapy.

The initial pulmonary response to bacteremia and septic shock is hyperventilation with dyspnea and tachypnea.[4] The development of leaky pulmonary capillaries leads to noncardiogenic pulmonary edema, progressive hypoxemia, and ventilatory failure, termed the *adult respiratory distress syndrome* (ARDS). ARDS has been observed in 6% to 10% of patients with sepsis and in approximately 20% of those with septic shock.[18,19] Other significant complications from sepsis and septic shock include central nervous system (CNS) dysfunction, liver failure, acute renal failure, and disseminated intravascular coagulation (DIC).[4,8] The reported incidence of these complications from different studies for patients with sepsis is approximately 20% for CNS dysfunction, 12% for liver failure, 9% to 23% for acute renal failure, and 8% to 18% for DIC. In septic shock, DIC has been observed in approximately 40%, and acute renal failure in approximately 50%.

DIFFERENTIAL DIAGNOSIS

Acute infections due to viruses, rickettsiae, mycobacteria, fungi, and parasites may present as acute "sepsis," but severe infection due to these organisms is less common than that due to bacteria. Early diagnosis of these infections requires an awareness of specific predisposing host factors. Most affected patients have underlying depressed immunity. Specific antimicrobial therapy is often delayed, because diagnostic tests for nonbacterial infection are generally less routinely available and are more complicated to perform.

Hyperthermia and heat stroke may mimic many of the cardiopulmonary and neurologic manifestations of sepsis. Chills, however, are not expected with heat stroke.

Shock from other causes may also mimic sepsis; hemodynamic measurements are often helpful in narrowing the diagnostic possibilities. Septic shock should be suspected when hemodynamic measurements showing decreased vascular resistance and increased cardiac output are found.

The ultimate prognosis of gram-negative bacteremia is determined primarily by the presence of underlying host disease. Patients with rapidly fatal disease (such as acute leukemia and neutropenia) have a poor prognosis despite appropriate therapy, whereas patients with ultimately fatal disease (likely death within 5 years) and nonfatal disease (unlikely death within 5 years) do not.

The overall mortality in sepsis varies according to the degree of pathophysiologic derangement in the presence of a documented infection.[18] Mortality in SIRS has been reported to be about 8%, with mortality in sepsis syndrome of 16% to 20% and mortality from septic shock approximately 50%.[6,14,18,19] While there is a statistically significant trend for decreased mortality over the last 40 years in published studies, such reduction should be reviewed with caution, understanding the heterogeneity of the patients in question.[10]

EMERGENCY DEPARTMENT EVALUATION

Because sepsis may progress rapidly, the emergency department evaluation must be expeditious. Appropriate stabilization measures are often carried out simultaneously with assessment.

Vital signs must be reviewed. Unexplained tachycardia or tachypnea may be early clues to infection. Oral temperatures do not accurately reflect core temperature; rectal temperature measurement is recommended in any patient with suspected hypothermia or fever.

The physical examination should concentrate on potential sources for sepsis: The oral cavity, lungs, abdomen, urinary system, and skin are the most common locations. Violation of a mucosal or cutaneous barrier carries the risk of sepsis; all indwelling catheters and lines should be suspected as possible sources.

A wide variety of laboratory and ancillary tests are potentially useful in assessing the septic patient, but the following basic tests usually yield the most information: chest radiograph; serum electrolytes, glucose, blood urea nitrogen, and creatinine determinations; complete blood cell count, including white blood cell count and differential; urinalysis; blood cultures; and cultures of overt foci of infection. Initial antibiotic management is guided by the history and physical examination, not by the results of specific laboratory tests.

Most patients who present to the emergency department with fever and possible sepsis have localizing symptoms or signs, which identify a focal infection. More difficult to assess are those patients without localizing symptoms or signs. Mellors and coworkers found that five factors were useful in predicting the likelihood of bacteremia or occult focal bacterial infection in adults presenting to the emergency department with unexplained fever.[16] The risk of bacterial infection increased with the number of factors present (Table 195.2). Interestingly, the presence of high fever (greater than 103°F [39.4°C]) or a "toxic" appearance had no correlation with the presence of bacterial infection. These five factors have been further validated in hospitalized patients.

Other conclusions have been derived from studies of adults with unexplained fever:

1. Initially inapparent infections were most often due to common bacteria in common locations.
2. The incidence of diagnostic abnormalities on routine urinalysis and chest radiography was 13% to 16% and 3% to 4%, respectively.
3. Empiric use of urinalysis and chest radiography would have detected about half of the clinically occult infections.
4. About two-thirds of patients with "clinically occult" infections present with general findings that lead to hospital admission based on physician judgment, but among the one-third that are sent home, the incidence of bacterial infection is 20%.

Other studies have sought to develop prediction rules for the presence of bacteremia in different patient populations. A study of hospitalized patients found that shaking chills, a history of intravenous drug use, presence of an acute abdomen, major comorbidity, and a fatal or ultimately fatal underlying disease were all associated with an increased risk of bacteremia. These factors could be combined into a prediction rule, yielding estimates of the prevalence of bacteremia ranging from 1% to 2% for patients at the lowest risk to 15% for those at the highest risk.

TABLE 195.2. Presence of Bacteremia or Focal Bacterial Infection in Adults Presenting to the Emergency Department with Unexplained Fever

No. of Features Present	Bacteremia	Bacteremia and/or Focal Bacterial Infection
0	0/21 (0%)	1/21 (5%)
1	3/45 (7%)	15/45 (33%)
2	6/38 (16%)	15/38 (39%)
3–5	12/31 (39%)	17/31 (55%)

Features: age greater than 50; presence of diabetes mellitus; Wintrobe erythrocyte sedimentation rate greater than 30 mm/h; white blood cells greater than 15,000/μL; absolute neutrophil count greater than 1500/μL.

Adapted from Mellors JW, Horwitz RI, Harvey MR. A simple index to identify occult bacterial infection in adults with acute unexplained fever. *Arch Intern Med* 1987;147:666–670.

EMERGENCY DEPARTMENT MANAGEMENT

Stabilization often begins before assessment is complete. Adequate intravenous access should be ensured, supplemental oxygen should be administered, and cardiac monitoring instituted.

All patients with sepsis require supplemental fluids. The amount and rate of infusion are guided by an assessment of the patient's volume and cardiovascular status.[4,17] Because of vasodilatation and capillary leakage, large quantities of fluid may be required to support the peripheral circulation. Measurements of central venous pressure or pulmonary artery wedge pressure may provide confusing information about the inadequacy of intravascular volume. Volume administration is best guided by observing the response of the central venous pressure or pulmonary artery wedge pressure to aliquots of fluid given over a short period of time. A rise of more than 5 cm H_2O or 5 mm Hg after a volume infusion of several hundred milliliters indicates that the compliance of the vascular system is decreasing as further fluid is being given and that the intravascular space is most likely "full." Colloids (albumin, hetastarch) have no proven benefit over crystalloids (normal saline or Ringer's lactate) in the resuscitation of sepsis.[20]

Treatment beyond the supportive measures has four components: (1) parenteral antibiotics, often in combination; (2) removal or drainage of infected foci; (3) treatment of complications; and (4) pharmacologic interventions to prevent harmful host responses.[4,15]

Initial antibiotics should be administered in the emergency department. Selection of particular agents is empiric, based on assessment of the patient's underlying host defenses, potential sources of infection, and most likely responsible organisms.[4] Antibiotics must be "broad spectrum," covering both gram-positive and gram-negative bacteria, because both classes of organisms produce an identical clinical picture. Antibiotics must be given parenterally in doses adequate to achieve bactericidal serum levels; many studies have found that clinical improvement correlates with achievement of serum bactericidal levels rather than the number of antibiotics given.

Antistaphylococcal coverage is recommended for patients with a history of intravenous drug abuse or indwelling intravascular lines or devices. Coverage against anaerobes should be included for patients with intraabdominal or perineal infections. Antipseudomonal coverage is indicated in patients with neutropenia or burns. Immunocompetent patients can usually be treated with a single drug that has broad-spectrum coverage, for example, a third-generation cephalosporin such as cefotaxime, ceftriaxone, or cefuroxime. Monodrug therapy in the immunocompetent adult is also possible with either an antipseudomonal penicillin (ticarcillin or piperacillin) or a carbapenem (imipenem or meropenem). Alternatives would be ceftazidime plus either clindamycin or metronidazole; or a parenteral fluoroquinolone plus clindamycin.

Immunocompromised patients usually require coverage with two broad-spectrum antibiotics with overlapping coverage, such as an aminoglycoside plus either ticarcillin, piperacillin, or ceftazidime. Within these general guidelines, no one combination of antibiotics is clearly superior to another.

If the patient does not respond to several liters of isotonic crystalloid (usually 4 L or more) or there is evidence of volume overload, the depressed cardiovascular system can be stimulated by inotropic and vasoconstrictive agents.[4,17] Dopamine is the agent most commonly used for this purpose. Infusion should begin at a rate of 5 to 10 μg/kg/min intravenously and then adjusted according to the blood pressure and other hemodynamic parameters. Occasionally, patients may require higher doses of dopamine, in the range of 20 μg/kg/min. A pure vasoconstrictor, such as norepinephrine, can increase blood pressure, but the deleterious side effects on cardiac output and regional perfusion are significant. However, there are cases of survival when norepinephrine has been used to treat septic shock refractory to dopamine. Assessing response to the potent inotropes and vasoconstrictors by bedside observation is difficult in these very ill patients. Most patients require intravenous hemodynamic monitoring with arterial lines and pulmonary artery catheters.

While there is theoretical and experimental support for the use of large doses of corticosteroids in severe sepsis and septic shock, all randomized human studies (with the exception of one from 1976) have found that large doses of corticosteroids do not prevent the development of shock, reverse the shock state, or improve the 14-day mortality.[7,13] Thus, there is no support in the medical literature for the general use of high doses of corticosteroids in patients with sepsis or septic shock.

The insight that endotoxin, a lipid–polysaccharide compound found in the cell wall of gram-negative bacteria, plays a key role in initiating the cascades seen in septic shock has led to the hypothesis that neutralizing circulating endotoxin with intravenous administration of an antiendotoxin antibody might be beneficial. Several products have been developed and investigated in clinical trials. However, there has been no proven benefit with these agents to date.[15] Highlighting the uncertain benefits of antiendotoxin antibody therapy is the high cost, estimated to be at least $4,000 per course of treatment. Taurolidine, an antiendotoxin agent, has also not shown benefit in the treatment of sepsis syndrome.[21]

Serum levels of TNF and IL-1 are elevated in patients with septic shock.[22] Both cytokines produce hemodynamic effects that duplicate that found in sepsis. Many studies indicate that both mediators play a key role in sepsis and septic shock, and it is thought by some that TNF may be the central mediator in sepsis. Similar to the hypothesis concerning antiendotoxin antibodies, it is hypothesized that antibodies to TNF or IL-1 might be useful in septic shock. However, anti-TNF or anti–IL-1 antibodies have not been shown to improve the outcome in sepsis or septic shock in human trials.[1,2,9,15]

Agents such as naloxone, arachidonic acid inhibitors, prostaglandin E2, antihistamines, thyroid-releasing hormone, glucagon, and calcium channel inhibitors that antagonize humoral mediators elaborated in severe sepsis and septic shock have not proven beneficial in limited studies.[15]

DISPOSITION

The disposition from the emergency department of patients with a fever and no localizing signs of infection presents a dilemma. Otherwise healthy individuals in a stable clinical state and at low risk for occult bacterial infection can generally be discharged with instructions for fever control and a warning to return if symptoms persist or worsen. A "toxic" appearance itself is of little diagnostic value.[16]

Patients with underlying immunodeficiency or with disorders that predispose them to bacterial infection and bacteremia pose an additional dilemma. Careful consideration should be given to the decision whether to admit these patients or to discharge them with close follow-up. It is common practice to admit those patients with a reasonable risk for bacteremia (above 2% to 5%), even if they appear well, because of the difficulties in excluding potentially serious infections and predicting the clinical course. For example, it has been found clinically impossible to determine which febrile intravenous drug users have serious infections and which do not when they present to the emergency department.

The value of blood cultures in adults being discharged from the emergency department is controversial. The incidence of bacteremia in febrile adults presenting to an emergency department is 1% to 2%, and more than three-fourths of these patients are admitted to the hospital because of their clinical presentation. The use of outpatient blood cultures requires a reliable patient and an efficient call-back mechanism, but discharging these patients does entail a small but real risk of delay in treating a potentially explosive infection.

COMMON PITFALLS

- Failure to consider bacterial infection as a possibility in the assessment of subtle or confusing symptoms and signs
- Restriction of fluid resuscitation for fear of inducing pulmonary edema, even though large quantities of fluid may be required because of capillary leakage
- Delaying the administration of antibiotics until after all of the cultures are collected, the consultant is contacted, or the patient is admitted. All patients with suspected serious infections should receive antibiotics in the emergency department.
- Patients with an internal focus of infection often require surgical drainage or excision. Because many of these have serious or coexistent medical problems, surgery is often delayed to "get the patient into better shape." Experience teaches that such delays are usually not in the patient's best interest.

References

1. Abraham E, Glauser MP, Butler T, et al. p55 Tumor necrosis factor receptor fusion protein in the treatment of patients with severe sepsis and septic shock. A randomized controlled multicenter trial. *JAMA* 1997;277:1531–1538.
2. Abraham E, Wundernik R, Silverman H. Efficacy and safety of monoclonal antibody to human tumor necrosis factor alpha in patients with sepsis syndrome. A randomized, controlled, double-blind, multicenter clinical trial. *JAMA* 1995;273:934–941.
3. American College of Chest Physicians, Society of Critical Care Medicine, Consensus Conference. Definitions of sepsis and organ failure and guidelines for the use of innovative therapies in sepsis. *Crit Care Med* 1992;20:864–874.
4. Astiz ME, Rackow EL. Septic shock. *Lancet* 1998;351:1501–1505.
5. Beal AL, Cerra FB. Multiple organ failure syndrome in the 1990s. Systemic inflammatory response and organ dysfunction. *JAMA* 1994;271:226–233.
6. Brun-Buisson C, Doyon F, Carlet J. Incidence, risk factors, and outcome of severe sepsis and septic shock in adults. A multicenter prospective study in intensive care units. *JAMA* 1995;274:968–974.
7. Cronin L, Cook DJ, Carlet J. Corticosteroid treatment for sepsis: a critical appraisal and meta-analysis of the literature. *Crit Care Med* 1995;23:1430–1439.
8. Eidelman LA, Putterman D, Putterman C. The spectrum of septic encephalopathy. Definitions, etiologies, and mortalities. *JAMA* 1996;275:470–473.
9. Fisher CJ, Agosti JM, Opal SM, et al. Treatment of septic shock with tumor necrosis factor receptor: Fc fusion protein. *N Engl J Med* 1996;334:1697–1702.
10. Friedman G, Silva E, Vincent JL. Has the mortality of septic shock changed with time? *Crit Care Med* 1998;26:2078–2086.
11. Gattinni L, Brazzi L, Pelosi PA. A trail of goal-oriented hemodynamic therapy in critically ill patients. *N Engl J Med* 1995;333:1025–1032.
12. Guest TM, Ramanathan AV, Tuteur PG. Myocardial injury in critically ill patients. A frequently unrecognized complication. *JAMA* 1995;273:1945–1949.
13. Lefering R, Neugebauer EAM. Steroid controversy in sepsis and septic shock: a meta-analysis. *Crit Care Med* 1995;23:1294–1303.
14. Lundberg JS, Perl TM, Wiblin T. Septic shock: an analysis of outcomes for patients with onset on hospital wards versus intensive care units. *Crit Care Med* 1998;26:1020–1024.
15. Lynn WA, Cohen J. Adjunctive therapy for septic shock: a review of experimental approaches. *Clin Infect Dis* 1995;20:143–158.
16. Mellors JW, Horwitz RI, Harvey MR. A simple index to identify occult bacterial infection in adults with acute unexplained fever. *Arch Intern Med* 1987;147:666–670.

17. Rady MY, Rivers EP, Nowak RM. Resuscitation of the critically ill in the ED: responses of blood pressure, heart rate, shock index, central venous oxygen saturation, and lactate. *Am J Emerg Med* 1996;14:218–225.
18. Rangel-Frausto NS, Pittet D, Costigan M. The natural history of the systemic inflammatory response syndrome (SIRS). A prospective study. *JAMA* 1995;273:117–123.
19. Sands KE, Bates DW, Lanken PN. Epidemiology of sepsis syndrome in 8 academic medical centers. *JAMA* 1997;278:234–240.
20. Schierhout G, Roberts I. Fluid resuscitation with colloid or crystalloid solutions in critically ill patients: a systematic review of randomized trials. *BMJ* 1998;316:961–964.
21. Willatts SM, Radford S, Leitermann M. Effect of the anti-endotoxic agent, taurolidine, in the treatment of the sepsis syndrome: a placebo-controlled, double-blind trial. *Crit Care Med* 1995;23:1033–1039.
22. Wenzel RP, Pinsky MR, Ulevitch RJ. Current understanding of sepsis. *Clin Infect Dis* 1996;22:407–413.

CHAPTER 196
Infections in the Compromised Host

Judith C. Brillman and Sarah A. Stahmer

The aging of the population, the increasing frequency of transplants, advances in cancer chemotherapy, and the longer life spans of patients with chronic conditions have contributed to the increasing number of immunocompromised patients seen in emergency departments (EDs). The presence of an immunocompromised state alters ED evaluation and management by rendering patients more susceptible to infection, by altering or modifying the presenting signs and symptoms of disease, and by affecting management and disposition.

THE IMMUNE SYSTEM

The components of the immune system—nonspecific host defenses, antibodies, complement, granulocytes, and cell-mediated immunity—work synergistically to prevent infection.

NONSPECIFIC HOST DEFENSES

The skin and mucous membranes provide a physical barrier against microbes. The respiratory tract is protected by an aerodynamic filtration system and mucociliary transport away from the lungs. The defenses of the gastrointestinal tract include the acidic pH of the stomach, pancreatic enzymes, bile and intestinal secretions, peristalsis, epithelial cell turnover, and competition with normal bowel flora. The urinary tract resists microbial infection by frequent flushing, urinary pH and other antimicrobial constituents of urine, the hyperosmolarity of the kidney, and the length of the male urethra. The acid environment of the vagina is unfavorable to the growth of most pathogenic bacteria.

Patients in whom any of these host defenses are disrupted are at risk for infection. Iatrogenic breaching of physical barriers (e.g., by an indwelling urinary, intravenous catheter, or endotracheal tube) and alteration of protective indigenous flora by broad-spectrum antibiotics are important causes of infection.

Humoral Immunity

Antibody deficiency results in increased susceptibility to infection with encapsulated organisms such as *Streptococcus pneumoniae, Haemophilus influenzae, Mycoplasma, Staphylococcus aureus,* and *Neisseria meningitidis.* Sinopulmonary infections are most common. There is also an increased incidence of infections with gastrointestinal organisms such as *Salmonella, Shigella, Campylobacter,* and rotavirus.

There are several inherited disorders of humoral immunity, including X-linked common variable immunodeficiency and selective immunoglobulin A (IgA) deficiency. Acquired IgG deficiency is seen in malignancies such as multiple myeloma, Waldenström's macroglobulinemia, chronic lymphocytic leukemia, lymphoma, lymphosarcoma, and thymoma. In addition, immunoglobulins may be lost in protein-losing states such as severe burns, protein-losing enteropathies, and nephrotic syndrome. Immunoglobulin deficiency is also seen in human immunodeficiency virus (HIV) disease and after bone marrow transplantation.

Complement deficiency is usually inherited and results in susceptibility to infections such as pneumonia and meningitis with organisms such as *N. meningitidis, Neisseria gonorrhoeae, S. pneumoniae, H. influenzae,* and *S. aureus.* Acquired complement deficiency is most common in patients with autoimmune diseases, especially systemic lupus erythematosus (SLE) (5.9% of patients with SLE), discoid lupus, and glomerulonephritis.[14] Meningococcal disease is the most common infection in complement deficiency. Special attention should be paid to the risk for infection with encapsulated organisms, and blood cultures should be obtained. When stable, these patients should be referred for immunizations.

Multiple myeloma is associated with both decreased immunoglobulin production and impaired complement function. The degree of immunocompromise increases as the disease progresses, and, in advanced disease, cell-mediated immunity and granulocyte function are impaired as well. Pneumonia, urinary tract infection (UTI), and sepsis caused by *S. pneumoniae, H. influenzae,* and *Escherichia coli* are the most common infections.[6,13] The first 2 months of chemotherapy are a particularly high-risk period. With progressive disease and decreased granulocyte production, gram-negative and fungal bacteremia become more likely.

The spleen both produces antibody and clears bacteria from the blood. Splenectomized patients are at risk of infection from encapsulated organisms such as *S. pneumoniae, H. influenzae,* or *N. meningitidis.* Many patients have splenectomies during staging laparotomies for lymphoma or for treatment of leukemia or platelet dysfunction. Others are functionally asplenic because of sickle cell disease or other hemoglobinopathies, or are hyposplenic from a variety of systemic diseases. Patients who have splenectomy after trauma may have some residual splenic function because of seeding of the peritoneum by small splenic implants.

Overwhelming postsplenectomy infection (OPSI) occurs more commonly in children than in adults, but it must be considered in any postsplenectomy patient with a fever. Infections with *Babesia* (from tick bites) and *Capnocytophagia canimorsus* (from dog bites) are particularly severe and likely to result in sepsis. OPSI typically starts with a prodrome of fever, chills, sore throat, malaise, nausea, or vomiting in a relatively well-appearing patient. Rapid deterioration can occur, with hypotension, disseminated intravascular coagulation, respiratory failure, and coma developing over hours. Even with appropriate treatment, mortality is more than 50%.[15] OPSI can be associated with pneumonia, meningitis, or endocarditis. Vaccines against encapsulated organisms such as pneumococcus, *H. influenzae,* and *N. meningitidis* reduce the likelihood of OPSI, but do not eliminate it. Asplenic children may be taking prophylactic penicillin, or patients may have been given a supply of antibiotics to take when symptoms of infection appear.

Patients with defects in humoral immunity who present with symptoms of infection must be evaluated thoroughly. A complete history must include information about infectious exposures, immunizations, and prophylactic medications, if any. A chest x-ray, urinalysis and culture, and two sets of blood cultures are mandatory. If the bacterial load is high, a Gram stain of the buffy coat may demonstrate organisms. Patients should be closely observed in the hospital or observation unit for at least 24 hours after blood cultures are obtained. Empiric antibiotics appropriate for both the presumed infection site and encapsulated organisms should be started, especially in the ill-appearing patient.

Granulocytes

Neutrophils and macrophages are the granulocytes primarily responsible for phagocytosis of microbes and enzymatic destruction of their cell walls. Neutropenia is caused by cancer chemotherapy, a variety of drugs, bone marrow disease, or inherited conditions. Functional abnormalities of granulocytes can be caused by steroids, cancer chemotherapy, or irradiation.

The neutropenic patient is significantly immunosuppressed, and 50% to 60% of those with fevers have an infection.[7] Fever in this population is defined as a single oral temperature of greater than 38.3°C, or 38.0°C over at least 1 hour.[7] Neutropenia is defined as a neutrophil count less than 1,000/μL. The frequency and severity of infections is inversely proportional to the neutrophil count, so patients with neutrophil counts less than 500/μL are at even greater risk of infection. A rapid decline of the neutrophil count and a protracted duration further increase infection risk.[7] As with other patients, neutropenic patients may be infected but afebrile.

Neutropenic patients may have a blunted inflammatory response, resulting in vague or nonspecific clinical symptoms that do not indicate the location of the infection or its serious nature. History taking and physical examination must be careful and comprehensive. In the neutropenic cancer patient, infection is most likely to be found in the periodontium, pharynx, lower esophagus, lung, perineum and anus, skin, instrumentation sites, the ocular fundus, and the periungual area.[7] Patients with chronic hereditary neutropenia tend to have infections of the upper respiratory tract, periodontium, and skin. The most common bacterial causes of fever in neutropenic patients are *Staphylococcus* (*aureus, epidermidis,* and other coagulase-negatives), *Streptococcus* (*pneumoniae, pyogenes, viridans*), *Enterococcus faecalis/faecium, Corynebacterium* spp., *E. coli, Klebsiella* spp., and *Pseudomonas aeruginosa*.[7] Gram-positive organisms cause about 60% to 70% of infections.[7] Fungal infections are most common after courses of broad-spectrum antibiotics.

Neutropenic enterocolitis, also called typhlitis, is a fulminant necrotizing infection associated with severe neutropenia. Symptoms include nausea, vomiting, and abdominal pain. Bowel wall thickening or pneumatosis is a nonspecific but suspicious finding. Causative organisms are enteric and anaerobic bacteria, as well as *Candida* species. Both surgical and medical management have been successful, although mortality is more than 50%.

Laboratory evaluation must include a complete blood count (CBC); chest x-ray; and cultures of blood (peripheral and catheter), urine, lesions, and diarrheal stools. Liver function tests, electrolytes, creatinine, and blood urea nitrogen (BUN) are obtained to plan supportive care and to monitor for drug toxicity. Other tests are obtained as appropriate to the clinical presentation.

It is currently standard practice to administer high-dose in-

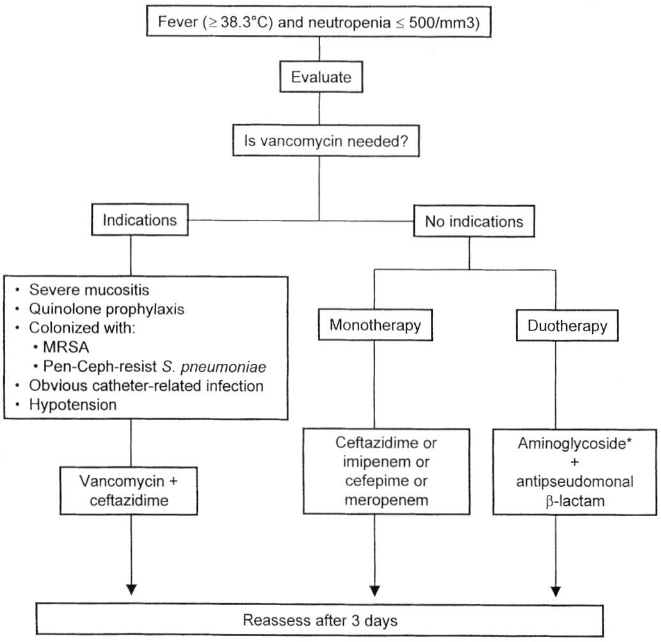

Figure 196.1. Guide to the initial management of the febrile neutropenic patient.
*Avoid if patient is also receiving nephrotoxic, ototoxic, or neuromuscular blocking agents; has renal or severe electrolyte dysfunction; or is suspected of having meningitis (poor CNS penetration). MRSA, methicillin-resistant *S. aureus;* Pen-Ceph-resist, penicillin–cephalosporin-resistant. (From Hughes WT, Armstrong D, Bodey GP, et al. 1997 Guidelines for the use of antimicrobial agents in neutropenic patients with unexplained fever. *Clin Infect Dis* 1997;25:551, with permission.)

travenous antibiotics (Fig. 196.1) to all patients with neutrophil counts less than 500, and in those with counts below 1000 in whom a further decrease is anticipated. More recent studies suggest that "low-risk" patients may be treated with oral amoxicillin–clavulanate plus ciprofloxacin.[4] High-risk factors include inpatient status when fever and neutropenia develop; a requirement for acute hospital care for problems in addition to the fever and neutropenia; uncontrolled cancer; allogenic bone marrow transplant; recent antibiotic use; renal failure; respiratory insufficiency; or evidence of specific infection.[4] Vascular access devices may often be left in place, even if infected, unless the infection is in the catheter tunnel or is causing septic emboli. Empiric antiviral or antifungal treatment is not routinely indicated.

Cell-Mediated Immunity

Impairment of cell-mediated immunity (CMI) results in infection with a wide variety of intracellular pathogens. These include certain bacteria (*Mycobacterium* spp., *Listeria monocytogenes, Legionella pneumophila, Salmonella* spp., *Nocardia* spp.), all viruses (particularly herpes simplex, varicella-zoster, cytomegalovirus, Epstein-Barr), and some fungi (*Candida, Cryptococcus, Mucor, Aspergillus, Histoplasma capsulatum, Coccoides immitis*) and protozoa (*Pneumocystis carinii, Toxoplasma gondii, Cryptosporidium, Strongyloides stercoralis*). Clinical infection with these organisms is rare in the normal host, except for tuberculosis, herpes, and varicella.

The classic example of a defect in CMI is the acquired immunodeficiency syndrome (AIDS) (see Chapter 192). Defects in CMI may be congenital and are often accompanied by defects in humoral immunity, because the systems are intertwined. In clinical practice, CMI usually results from drug or radiation therapy. Drugs used in organ transplants (cyclosporin and tacrolimus) and for autoimmune diseases, corticosteroids, antineoplastic agents, and total lymphoid irradiation (used for rejection in solid tumor transplants) are most commonly implicated. The likelihood of infection is related to the intensity and duration of immunosuppressive therapy. Defects of CMI also occur in malnutrition, aging, viral infections, lymphoma, lymphocytic leukemia, uremia, sarcoidosis, leprosy, trauma, and pregnancy.

Impairment of CMI may reduce the inflammatory response and mute the clinical presentation. The history and physical examination must be comprehensive and meticulous. Clues to infection must be aggressively pursued, and localizing signs must prompt attempts to identify a pathogen. The treatment threshold should be low.

Recommended antibiotic therapy for a number of common immunocompromised states is presented in Table 196.1.

TABLE 196.1. Antibiotic Choices in Immunodeficiency

Common Sites of Infection	Common Bacteria	Empiric Antibiotic Regimens
ASPLENIA		
Lungs	*S. pneumonia* *H. influenzae* *Mycoplasma* species	Cefotaxime Erythromycin + either ceftriaxone or cefotaxime
Heart	*S. aureus*	Vancomycin + either ceftriaxone or cefotaxime
Central nervous system	*N. meningitidis*	
COMPLEMENT DEFICIENCY		
As in asplenia		
DIABETES MELLITUS		
Skin/soft tissue	*S. pyogenes* *S. aureus* Enterobacteriaceae Anaerobes	Early/mild: first-generation cephalosporin Moderate: second- or third-generation cephalosporin + metronidazole; amoxicillin-clavulanate Severe: imipenem, meropenem
Urinary tract	Enterobacteriaceae *Candida* species Group B *Streptococcus*	Third-generation cephalosporin Trimethoprim-sulfamethoxazole Ciprofloxacin or other fluoroquinolone
Lungs	*S. pneumoniae* *S. aureus* *K. pneumoniae* Mouth anaerobes	Ticarcillin-clavulanate Third-generation cephalosporin
Malignant otitis externa	*Pseudomonas* species	Ciprofloxacin Ceftazidime Imipenem
ORGAN TRANSPLANTATION		
Blood	*S. aureus* *S. epidermidis* Enterobacteriaceae *P. aeruginosa* *L. monocytogenes* *Candida* species	Ceftazidime + ampicillin Piperacillin + tobramycin
Lungs	*S. aureus* Enterobacteriaceae *P. aeruginosa* *Nocardia* species Mycobacteria *Aspergillus* species *Pneumocystis carinii* Cytomegalovirus *Legionella*	Piperacillin + tobramycin Ceftazidime Trimethoprim-sulfamethoxazole + erythromycin
Central nervous system	*S. pneumoniae* *N. meningitidis* Enterobacteriaceae *P. aeruginosa* *L. monocytogenes* *C. neoformans*	Ampicillin + ceftazidime
Urinary tract	Enterobacteriaceae *P. aeruginosa* *Candida* species	Third-generation cephalosporin Ciprofloxacin
RENAL FAILURE		
Exit-site or tunnel infection	Coagulase-negative *Staphylococcus* *S. aureus* Streptococci "Skin flora"	Vancomycin
Peritonitis (nonseptic patient)	*S. aureus* *S. epidermidis* gram-negative	Vancomycin + gentamicin (intraperitoneal)
Urinary tract	Enterobacteriaceae *P. aeruginosa*	Fluoroquinolone Third-generation cephalosporin Trimethoprim-sulfamethoxazole

TABLE 196.1. *(Continued)*

Common Sites of Infection	Common Bacteria	Empiric Antibiotic Regimens
ELDERLY		
Bacteremia/sepsis (no obvious source) Nonimmunocompromised	Enterobacteriaceae Group A or D *Streptococcus* *S. pneumoniae* "Bacteroides" *E. coli* *S. aureus* Coagulase-negative *Staphylococcus* *Klebsiella* species	Ceftizoxime ± aminoglycoside Ampicillin + aminoglycoside + clindamycin Imipenem
Pneumonia		
Community-acquired	*S. pneumoniae* *H. influenzae* *Legionella pneumoniae* *Mycoplasma* Polymicrobial	Levofloxacin Macrolide ± second- or third-generation cephalosporin
Community-acquired; intensive care necessary	As above	Macrolide or Fluoroquinolone + either cefotaxime or ceftriaxone Beta-lactam/beta-lactamase inhibitor
Institutionalized (nosocomial)	*Klebsiella pneumoniae* *Pseudomonas* species *E. coli* *S. pneumoniae*	Ceftazidime Antipseudomonal PCN + aminoglycoside
Urinary Tract (not sepsis) Institutionalized, indwelling catheter, outlet obstruction, or upper tract symptoms	Consider MRSA *E. coli* *Proteus* species *Klebsiella* species *Pseudomonas* species *Enterococcus* *S. epidermidis* Often polymicrobial	± Vancomycin Ampicillin and gentamicin Piperacillin-tazobactam Imipenem
No modifying factors	*E. coli*	Fluoroquinolone Trimethoprim-sulfamethoxazole
Skin/Soft Tissue		
Cellulitis or erysipelas	Group A *Streptococcus* *S. aureus*	Dicloxacillin Nafcillin Cephalosporin
Pressure sore with systemic infection	Polymicrobial: anaerobic streptococci, Enterobacteriaceae, *Pseudomonas* species, *Bacteroides*	Amoxicillin-clavulanate Cefoxitin + aminoglycoside Imipenem Ampicillin-sulbactam
ALCOHOLISM		
Lungs	*S. pneumoniae* *S. aureus* *H. influenzae* *Klebsiella* "Atypicals" *M. tuberculosis*	Doxycycline and ciprofloxacin Third-generation cephalosporin or erythromycin + either piperacillin-tazobactam or ticarcillin-clavulanate
Lungs: aspiration	Anaerobes	Lexofloxacin or moxifloxacin or gatifoxacin + either clindamycin or metronidazole
Skin/soft tissue	*S. aureus* *S. pyogenes*	Cefazolin Cephalexin Dicloxacillin
Peritoneum	*S. pneumoniae* *S. pyogenes* *S. aureus* *S. faecalis* Enterobacteriaceae	Ampicillin + gentamicin Ticarcillin-clavulanate Piperacillin-tazobactam Cefotaxime
Blood	*S. aureus* *S. pneumoniae* Enterobacteriaceae	Aminoglycoside + third-generation cephalosporin Imipenem
CNS	*S. pneumoniae* *L. monocytogenes*	Ampicillin + either ceftriaxone or cefotaxime

TABLE 196.1. *(Continued)*

Common Sites of Infection	Common Bacteria	Empiric Antibiotic Regimens
INTRAVENOUS DRUG USE		
Skin/soft tissue	*S. aureus* *S. pyogenes* *C. tetani*	Cefazolin Cephalexin Dicloxacillin
Lungs	*S. pneumoniae* *S. aureus* Anaerobes *M. tuberculosis*	Erythromycin + second- or third-generation cephalosporin Consider vancomycin for MRSA Ticarcillin-clavulanate
Heart valves	*S. aureus* *P. aeruginosa* *Candida* species Viridans *Streptococcus* Enterococci	Vancomycin
Joints	*S. aureus* *S. pyogenes* *P. aeruginosa* *N. gonorrhoeae* Enterobacteriaceae	Vancomycin + either ceftriaxone, ceftazidime, or gentamicin
Endophthalmitis	*Bacillus cereus* *Candida* species	Intravitreal agent + either clindamycin or vancomycin

MRSA = Methacillin-resistant *S. aureus.*

SPECIFIC CLINICAL SITUATIONS

Transplantation

A host of factors predispose the transplant patient to infection. Chief among these are the immunosuppressive agents that are necessary to prevent transplant rejection. Cyclosporine and tacrolimus both affect T-lymphocyte function. Corticosteroids affect all aspects of immunity. Azathioprine is a cytotoxic agent that can lead to bone marrow suppression. Antilymphocyte and antithymocyte globulins decrease CMI.

Most transplant recipients are able to mount fevers in response to infection, despite their immunosuppressive therapy. Information about the type and amount of both immunosuppressive and antimicrobial prophylactic drugs should be obtained. A careful history and physical examination may demonstrate the source of the fever. Symptoms suggestive of a localized infection should be evaluated, even in the absence of a fever. Both the transplant and infectious disease services should be consulted early. If a parenchymal infection is located, efforts should be made to obtain samples for culture and smear.

These patients are hospitalized and started on antibiotics. Patients unable to go about their normal activities should also be hospitalized unless special arrangements can be made. A patient with a persistent fever greater than 38.5°C and an unknown source should be hospitalized for more intensive evaluation. The stable, well-appearing patient without an identified source may be observed without antibiotics. Noninfectious causes of fever, such as drug reaction or transplant rejection, should also be considered.

Diabetes Mellitus

Many mechanisms are responsible for immunosuppression for the diabetic patient. Chemotaxis, phagocytosis, bacterial killing, and T-lymphocyte response are impaired.[2,12] High tissue glucose levels enhance bacterial growth. Diabetic peripheral vascular disease results in ischemic tissue, which is more susceptible to infection. Autonomic and peripheral neuropathy predispose patients to repetitive injury of the lower extremities. Diabetic patients have a higher incidence of complications, such as septic shock, renal failure, and late superinfections.[2] A good rule of thumb is that a diabetic with any parenteral infection should be admitted for intravenous antibiotics, close follow-up for complications, and control of metabolic derangements (see Chapter 168).

The Elderly

Both cell-mediated and humoral immunity decrease with age. Increased skin fragility and decreased subcutaneous tissue also contribute to increased risk for skin infections and slower healing. A less vigorous cough and decreased mucociliary clearance may predispose to pneumonia. Impaired circulation, the presence of comorbid conditions, the use of immunosuppressive drugs, and the presence of foreign bodies (indwelling catheters and prostheses) all may predispose the elderly to infection.

The relative mortality of infections in the elderly is increased from three- to 15-fold over that of younger adults.[17] Respiratory, urinary tract, and soft-tissue infections (mnemonic: PUS, for *p*neumonia, *U*TI, and *s*oft tissue) are the predominant infections of the elderly and should be sought in every febrile older patient. Forty percent of all cases of bacteremia and sepsis occur in the elderly, and the elderly account for 60% of deaths from these conditions. More than 85% of elderly individuals have a medically supervised chronic disease[5] that may predispose to certain infections and increase morbidity. Those with chronic obstructive pulmonary disease (COPD) may get respiratory infections; those with an indwelling urinary catheter or prostatic hypertrophy may have UTIs; and those with degenerative or rheumatic heart disease, valvular prostheses, or pacemaker/defibrillators may develop endocarditis.

Nonspecific complaints—malaise, anorexia, nausea, vomiting, frequent falls, or a decline in functional or mental status—may be the only clue to the presence of a serious infection. Moreover, symptoms are often not referable to the infected area; for example, gastrointestinal symptoms are more common in urosepsis than are dysuria or urgency.

The physical examination can also be misleading. Fever is commonly absent in the elderly patient with an infection, although the presence of fever is significant. In one study of ambulatory patients, a bacterial infection was found 86.8% of the febrile elderly.[9] A tachycardic response can be limited by cardiovascular pathology or medications. Cellulitis or decubitus ulcers may be easily overlooked. New mental status changes may be attributed to chronic dementia.

Although test selection is guided by the history and physical, almost all elderly patients with fever need a chest x-ray and urinalysis. A CBC, blood cultures, and serum creatinine determination should be seriously considered. Elderly patients with a parenchymal infection, or infection of a system in which chronic disease is present, should be admitted for intravenous antibiotics. Those treated as outpatients should have close follow-up arranged.

Alcoholism

Chronic alcohol abuse or binge drinking is associated with an increased risk of infection. The infections that have been most closely linked to alcohol abuse are bacterial pneumonia, tuberculosis, and spontaneous bacterial peritonitis (SBP). Alcohol abuse has also been linked to an increased risk of acquiring hepatitis B and HIV infections, independent of the high-risk behaviors associated with alcohol abuse.[1,8,11]

The evaluation and disposition of these individuals is particularly challenging. The alcoholic presenting with an infectious disorder often has vague and nonspecific complaints of malaise, fever, tremulousness, or lethargy. Patients may be intoxicated or in withdrawal, often present without accompanying family or friends, and rarely have a close relationship with a single healthcare provider from whom one can obtain a medical history. The clinician should perform a meticulous examination and have a low threshold for ordering diagnostic tests such as radiographs and cultures, in order to avoid missing potentially life-threatening conditions. Alcoholics often minimize their complaints, and the fact that they are in the ED may be an important clue to the severity of their illness.

Initial management should focus on ensuring airway patency in the lethargic individual, optimizing hydration, assessing the serum glucose level, and observing for signs of withdrawal (tachycardia, tremor, seizures, or fever). Cough, pleuritic chest pain, and dyspnea suggest pneumonia, which may be due to a wide range of bacterial and atypical organisms. Chest radiographs, sputum, and blood cultures are helpful in identifying the causative agent, and patients should be covered broadly for *S. pneumoniae, H. influenzae, Klebsiella pneumoniae, Mycoplasma,* and *Legionella*. Individuals with suspected tuberculosis should be admitted for respiratory isolation and workup. Patients with seizures and/or persistent lethargy should be carefully assessed for meningitis after intracranial pathology and acute intoxication have been excluded. Fever is not always a feature of meningitis in these individuals. The cirrhotic patient with fever, abdominal pain, increasing abdominal distention, or acute hepatic insufficiency should be presumed to have SBP. Paracentesis is usually diagnostic, the fluid having a cloudy appearance and greater than 250 white blood cells (WBC)/μL. Broad-spectrum antibiotic coverage should be instituted. *E. coli* is identified in over half of positive peritoneal cultures.[10]

Disposition decisions should take into account the fact that these individuals may have inadequate social support, may be likely to drink immediately upon discharge, and may be poorly compliant with outpatient regimens. Alcoholic individuals with a disorder that has the potential for significant early morbidity or that requires compliance with treatment should be admitted to the hospital. For patients who are stable enough to be discharged, access to housing, food, prescriptions, and follow-up should be assessed and plans made for careful follow-up.

Injection Drug Use

Infectious complications are the most frequent reason for hospitalization and death among injection drug users, but immunosuppression directly related to intravenous drug injection plays a relatively minor role.

Infections in the injection drug use (IDU) patient are usually the direct result of the injection of substances into the skin and bloodstream. Injected drugs are typically unsterile and may be cut with any one of a large number of adulterants. Preparation of the drug for injection requires that it be dissolved, and the diluent is usually unsterile water or even saliva. Injection needles are frequently shared and are unlikely to be cleaned between uses.

Skin and soft-tissue infections of the extremities are thus common, but as peripheral injection sites are exhausted, almost any accessible part of the body is at risk. Infection introduced by needle into the bloodstream places the individual at risk for infections involving the vessels and heart, in addition to those organs secondarily infected by septic emboli, most notably the axial skeleton, brain, lungs, and kidneys.[3,16]

Smoking, promiscuous sexual behaviors, malnutrition, and concomitant alcohol and nonintravenous substance abuse are common in this group of patients, and place the individual at further risk for infection. HIV infection and its associated immune defects play an increasingly important role in determining the immunocompetence of the IDU patient and risk of infection, and must be taken into account when the HIV status of the individual is unknown.

The injection drug–using patient often presents to the ED with complaints that are vague and seemingly minor. They include localized skin infections, extremity pain, fatigue, malaise, fever, and back pain. Fever is often the only sign of serious illness. Up to 42% of intravenous drug users with fever have documented bacteremia, and 10% are eventually diagnosed with endocarditis. Moreover, it is difficult, if not impossible, in the ED for physicians to identify those individuals with fever who are bacteremic or have endocarditis. Furthermore, follow-up or compliance with outpatient treatment regimens is often unreliable. It is thus standard practice to admit these individuals to the hospital pending the results of blood culture and other ancillary studies.

Infections involving the skin are common and can be as simple as a superficial cellulitis or subcutaneous abscess, or as life-threatening as necrotizing fasciitis or gas gangrene. IDU patients with a painful skin condition should be asked about routes of injection and substances injected. They should also be examined carefully for evidence of muscle and/or compartment involvement or subcutaneous air. Patients with fever or a toxic appearance should have cultures taken of blood and wound and be admitted for intravenous antibiotics and definitive wound care.

Endocarditis is a particularly difficult diagnosis to make in the ED. It should be suspected in any IDU patient presenting with fever, even when there is a clear alternative source of infection, such cellulitis or pneumonia. Skin infections often lead to valvular infection; the lung, brain, axial skeleton, and kidney are common sites of infection secondary to endocarditis.[3,16] Patients in whom the diagnosis of endocarditis is suspected should have at least three peripheral blood cultures obtained before antibiotics are started. There is little value to routine screening of these patients with echocardiography prior to the finding of a positive culture. An exception is in individuals who have a partially treated infection, a new murmur or conduction delay, or hemodynamic instability.

Back pain, particularly when accompanied by fever, should always be considered a sign of serious underlying pathology among IDU patients. Although a common complaint in the ED, and usually benign in etiology, in this population, this complaint may indicate vertebral osteomyelitis or epidural space infection. Plain radiographs may be normal in the early stages, and laboratory studies, such as peripheral white count and erythrocyte sedimentation rate, even when elevated, are nonspecific markers of inflammation. Thus, the evaluation should include a diagnostic imaging study such as magnetic resonance imaging or bone scan.

References

1. Bagasra O, Kajdacsy-Balla A, Lischner HW, et al. Alcohol intake increases human immunodeficiency virus type I replication in human peripheral blood mononuclear cells. *J Infect Dis* 1993;176:789–797.
2. Carton JA, Maradon FJ, Nuno R, et al. Diabetes mellitus and bacteraemia: a comparative study between diabetic and non-diabetic patients. *Eur J Med* 1992;1:281–287.
3. Cherubin CE, Sapira JD. The medical complications of drug addiction and the medical assessment of the intravenous drug user: 25 years later. *Ann Intern Med* 1993;119(10):1017–1028.
4. Finberg RW, Talcott JA. Fever and neutropenia—how to use a new treatment strategy. *N Engl J Med* 1999;3341:362–363.
5. Garibaldi RA. Infections in the elderly. *Am J Med* 1986;81[Suppl A]:53–58.
6. Hargreaves RM, Lea JR, Griffiths H, et al. Immunological factors and risk of infection in plateau phase myeloma. *J Clin Pathol* 1995;48:260–266.
7. Hughes WT, Armstrong D, Bodey GP, et al. 1997 Guidelines for the use of antimicrobial agents in neutropenic patients with unexplained fever. *Clin Infect Dis* 1997;25:551–573.
8. Jacobson JM, Worner TM, Sacks HS, et al. Human immunodeficiency virus and hepatitis B virus infections in a New York City alcoholic population. *J Stud Alcohol* 1992;53(1):76–79.
9. Keating HJ, Klimek JJ, Levine DS, et al. Effect of aging on the clinical significance of fever in the ambulatory adult patient. *J Am Geriatr Soc* 1984;32:282–287.
10. Keou FM, Blochs F, Hoi AB, et al. Spontaneous peritonitis in cirrhotic hospital in-patients: retrospective analysis of 101 cases. *Q J Med* 1992;83(301):401–407.
11. MacGregor RR. Alcohol and infection. *Curr Clin Top Infect Dis* 1997;17:291–315.
12. Moutschen MP, Scheen AJ, Lefebvre PJ. Impaired immune responses in diabetes mellitus: analysis of the factors and mechanisms involved. Relevance to the increased susceptibility of diabetic patients to specific infections. *Diabetes Metab* 1992;18:187–201.
13. Oken MM, Pomeroy C, Weisdorf D, et al. Prophylactic antibiotics for the prevention of early infection in multiple myeloma. *Am J Med* 1996;100:624–628.
14. Ross SC, Densen P. Complement deficiency states and infection: epidemiology, pathogenesis and consequences of neisserial and other infections in an immune deficiency. *Medicine* 1984;63:243–273.
15. Styrt B. Infection associated with asplenia: risks, mechanisms, and prevention. *Am J Med* 1990;88:33–42.
16. Weisse AB, Heller DR, Schimenti RJ, et al. The febrile parenteral drug user: a prospective study in 121 patients. *Am J of Med* 1993;94:274–280.
17. Yoshikawa TT. Perspective: aging and infectious disease. *J Infect Dis* 1997;176:1053–1057.

CHAPTER 197
Parasitic Disease

Richard J. Ryan

Diagnosing parasitic disease in the emergency department is difficult: The physician must be aware of the many potential manifestations of infestation by parasites, a large group of organisms. Parasitic disease, however, can usually be diagnosed through methods available to most emergency physicians, and effective treatments are available that are generally minimally toxic to the human host.[3,9] A history of foreign travel or habitation in an endemic area, including certain regions of the United States, should alert the clinician to the possibility of parasitic infection.

Symptoms may not manifest themselves until well after the traveler has returned home. In addition, over the last two decades, the proportion of the United States population born abroad has increased steadily, with newer immigrants typically coming from Latin America and Asia.[19] The proper treatment of immigrants in the United States requires a familiarity with diseases common in the developing world, such as malaria, amebiasis, and neurocysticercosis.

Four major groups of organisms infest humans. *Protozoans* cause malaria, amebiasis, giardiasis, and many other diseases. Helminths or worms, including *nematodes* (roundworms), *cestodes* (tapeworms), and *trematodes* (flukes), are also responsible for a wide variety of human illnesses. A comprehensive review of parasitic diseases would encompass infections due to literally scores or organisms, so this chapter is limited to the parasitic diseases most common in emergency departments in the United States. (Trichomoniasis is excluded.) This chapter is divided into four discussions: systemic illnesses, predominantly gastrointestinal (GI) disease, predominantly central nervous system (CNS) disease, and ectoparasitic diseases.

SYSTEMIC ILLNESS

CLINICAL PRESENTATION

Fever in a patient with a history of recent travel or habitation in the tropics should suggest the diagnosis of malaria. Caused by four species of the protozoan *Plasmodium* (*P. vivax, P. ovale, P. falciparum*, and *P. malariae*), malaria is the most common parasitic disease in the world, accounting for an estimated 300 million cases and 1.5 to 2.7 million deaths annually.[12] Although malaria is no longer endemic in the United States, the increase in immigration from and travel to countries where the disease is common has made malaria a not infrequent presenting complaint at emergency departments in this country.[14] Patients with malaria are frequently misdiagnosed on their initial presentation to the emergency department, thus increasing their risk for serious morbidity and mortality.

Classic symptoms of malaria include fever, chills, and rigors. These symptoms last 4 to 10 hours, culminating in an episode of profuse diaphoresis followed by defervescence. This pattern may recur at 2- or 3-day intervals, depending on the species of *Plasmodium* involved. Other clinical signs and symptoms include general malaise, headache, and, occasionally, hypotension. Physical examination is not generally helpful. Splenomegaly and jaundice may be seen in established infections. Laboratory abnormalities include a mild anemia, neutropenia, thrombocytopenia, and increased prothrombin time. Clinical evidence of impaired hemostasis is rare, however.

The periodicity of the disease can be explained by examining the life cycle of the infecting organism. *Plasmodium* species may be injected into the human circulation following the bite of the *Anopheles* mosquito, after sharing needles or receiving a blood transfusion, and by congenital transmission. Immature sporozoites migrate to the liver, beginning the exoerythrocytic phase, the duration of which is species-dependent. Ultimately, mature parasites (merozoites) are released into the circulation and invade red blood cells, beginning the erythrocytic phase. Replication within red cells is followed 48 to 72 hours later by red cell lysis and release of further merozoites into the circulation, which again invade erythrocytes and repeat the cycle. The fever corresponds to episodes of red cell lysis.

The classic pattern of periodic fever is not always seen, however, particularly early in the course of the illness. The variability of the clinical course also depends on the infecting species and the host's immune status. People living in endemic areas often have partial "immunity" that results in much less severe manifestations and symptoms. It is presumed to be an acquired immunity caused by frequent exposure to the infecting organism. Months after leaving an endemic area, these persons may experience relapses that resemble the acute form of the disease, probably caused by a loss of immunity and the release of exoerythrocytic parasites from the liver. *P. vivax* and *P. ovale* can persist for long periods in the exoerythrocytic state. Even patients who have received adequate antimalarial therapy may experience relapses associated with the release of exoerythrocytic organisms.

P. falciparum causes the most severe type of malaria and is responsible for almost all complications and deaths related to malaria.[14] Falciparum malaria has two important features that account for differences in its presentation and in the severity of the disease it produces. First, this species causes widespread capillary obstruction, resulting in end-organ hypoxia and dysfunction, with severe complications that can include CNS dysfunction, hemolytic anemia, hypoglycemia, pulmonary edema, septicemia, renal failure, or splenic rupture. A second distinguishing feature of *P. falciparum* is that, unlike other malarial species that infect only the most mature red cells, it infects red cells of all ages, resulting in a greater degree of hemolysis and anemia and the potential for acute tubular necrosis.

EMERGENCY DEPARTMENT EVALUATION

The diagnosis of malaria is a difficult one to make because of the disease's nonspecific clinical features—fever, chills, headache, and malaise. Because approximately 90% of travelers who contract malaria do not become ill until returning home, the diagnosis should be entertained for anyone presenting to the emergency department with a febrile illness and a history of travel or habitation in an endemic area.[12] A high degree of suspicion is necessary for physicians who rarely encounter this disease. The most common incorrect diagnosis is a viral syndrome, but a history of recurrent fever generally distinguishes malaria from these disorders. Other disorders that cause fever and are endemic in foreign countries, such as viral hepatitis, dengue fever, typhoid fever, and amebiasis, should also be considered.

The standard way to make the diagnosis of malaria is through demonstration of intracellular forms of the parasite on a thin Giemsa-stained peripheral blood smear. If malaria is strongly suspected, negative blood films should be repeated every 12 hours for 2 days. Sometimes, it is necessary to use the thick-smear technique, which usually requires the expertise of a trained technician. Serologic tests may be helpful when there are very low levels of parasitemia, as in infection with *P. malariae*.[11]

EMERGENCY DEPARTMENT MANAGEMENT

Management of malaria in the emergency department is guided by the severity of the infection. Assessment of airway patency and respiratory, circulatory, and neurologic status should be performed in a timely fashion. The emergency physician should be prepared to treat potential complications such as anemia, coagulopathies, pulmonary edema, azotemia, hypoglycemia, metabolic acidosis, and hypotensive shock.[11]

Volume should be restored and fever controlled. Hypotension usually responds well to saline infusion. Fever usually responds to standard cooling measures; for temperatures less than 104°F, oral antipyretics are likely to be effective. Acetaminophen is recommended rather than aspirin because of the common occurrence of thrombocytopenia. For patients with high-density parasitemia, altered mental status, pulmonary edema, or renal failure, exchange transfusion may be helpful.[5]

Pharmacologic therapy of malaria is outlined in Table 197.1. Chloroquine remains the oral drug of choice for acute treatment of all infections except those due to chloroquine-resistant *P. falciparum* and *P. vivax*. For chloroquine-resistant *P. falciparum* infection or for severely ill patients with an unidentified malarial infection, quinine plus doxycycline or pyrimethamine and sulfadoxine or clindamycin is recommended.

In addition to acute therapy, patients infected with *P. vivax* or *P. ovale* require more prolonged treatment to prevent reactivation of exoerythrocyte forms. These patients should be treated with primaquine phosphate, 15 mg base/d for 14 days or 45 mg base/wk for 8 weeks. The pediatric dose is 0.3 mg base/kg/d for 14 days. Patients should be screened for G-6-PD deficiency before beginning primaquine therapy, and the drug is contraindicated during pregnancy.[5]

To prevent fatal outcomes in cases of falciparum malaria, the following are required: improved health information and preventive measures for travelers to malarious areas, improved recognition of infection by physicians, and prompt initiation of effective therapy.[12]

DISPOSITION

Hospital admission is indicated for patients with severe dehydration, significant underlying medical illness, inability to tolerate oral medications, or evidence of end-organ involvement such as stroke, renal failure, or pulmonary edema. Those whose ability to comply with an outpatient regimen is questionable should also be admitted. Suspected *P. falciparum* infection is commonly considered to require hospitalization because of the increasing prevalence of drug resistance and the potential for life-threatening complications. Severely ill patients or those with significant parasitemia (greater than 3% of red cells containing parasites) should be treated in an intensive care unit with intravenous medications.

Prophylaxis is the most important aspect of malaria control in the United States, given the frequency of foreign travel. Before going to an endemic area, travelers should consult an expert to determine whether chemical prophylaxis is indicated and whether chloroquine resistance has been reported in the area. Chloroquine is usually recommended for persons traveling to endemic areas but may not be necessary in all cases, particularly for a short trip to an urban area. The standard dose is 300 mg base (500 mg) orally once a week, beginning 1 week before and continuing for 4 weeks after exposure. Chloroquine is indicated even when traveling to chloroquine-resistant areas, because many strains are still sensitive in such areas. However, a second agent should be added if a febrile illness develops during travel. The particular medication chosen must depend on the pattern of resistance in the area. Mefloquine, 250 mg once a week, is the drug of choice for adults traveling to most chloroquine-resistant areas. Contraindications for the use of mefloquine include serious psychiatric illness, seizures, or serious cardiac arrhythmias.[6] Because no drug regimen guarantees protection against malaria, if fever develops within the first year

TABLE 197.1. Treatment of Malaria

Indication	Drug	Adult Dosage	Pediatric Dosage
MALARIA			
Oral drug of choice	Chloroquine phosphate	600 mg base (1 g), then 300 mg base (500 mg) 6 h later, then 300 mg base (500 mg)/d at 24 and 48 hours	10 mg base/kg (max 600 mg base), then 5 mg base/kg 6 h later, then 5 mg base/kg/d × 2 d
Parenteral drug of choice	Quinidine gluconate	10 mg/kg loading dose (max 600 mg) in normal saline slowly over 1–2 h, followed by continuous infusion of 0.02 mg/kg/min until oral therapy can be started	
	or Quinine dihydrochloride	20 mg/kg loading dose i.v. in 5% dextrose over 4 h, followed by 10 mg/kg over 2–4 h q8h (max 1,800 mg/d) until oral therapy can be started	Same as adult dose
Alternative	Artemether	3.2 mg/kg i.m., then 1.6 mg/kg/d	Same as adult dose
CHLOROQUINE-RESISTANT *P. FALCIPARUM* MALARIA			
Oral drugs of choice	Quinine sulfate plus	650 mg q8h × 3–7 d	25 mg/kg/d in 3 doses × 3–7 d
	doxycycline[a]	100 mg b.i.d. × 7 d	2 mg/kg/d × 7 d (>8 yr of age)
	or plus pyrimethamine–sulfadoxine	3 tablets at once on last day of quinine	<1 yr: one-fourth tablet 1–3 yr: one-half tablet 4–8 yr: 1 tablet 9–14 yr: 2 tablets
	or plus clindamycin[a]	900 mg t.i.d. × 5 d	20–40 mg/kg/d in 3 doses × 5 d
Alternatives	Mefloquine	750 mg followed in 12 h by 500 mg	25 mg/kg once (<45 kg)
	Halofantrine	500 mg q6h × 3 doses; repeat in 1 wk	8 mg/kg q6h × 3 doses (<40 kg); repeat in 1 wk
	Atovaquone[a]	1,000 mg qd × 3 d	11–20 kg: 250 mg 21–30 kg: 500 mg 31–40 kg: 750 mg
	plus proguanil	400 mg qd × 3 d	11–20 kg: 100 mg 21–30 kg: 200 mg 31–40 kg: 300 mg
	or plus doxycyclinea	100 mg b.i.d. × 3 d 4 mg/kg/d × 3 d	2 mg/kg/d × 3 d (>8 yr of age)
	Artesunate plus mefloquine	750 mg followed in 12 h by 500 mg	
CHLOROQUINE-RESISTANT *P. VIVAX* MALARIA			
Drug of choice	Quinine sulfate plus	650 mg q8h × 3–7 d	25 mg/kg/d in 3 doses × 3–7 d
	doxycycline[a]	100 mg b.i.d. × 7 d	2 mg/kg/d × 7 d (>8 yr of age)
	or plus pyrimethamine–sulfadoxine	3 tablets at once on last day of quinine	<1 yr: one-fourth tablet 1–3 yr: one-half tablet 4–8 yr: 1 tablet 9–14 yr: 2 tablets
	or Mefloquine	750 mg, followed in 12 h by 500 mg	25 mg/kg once (<45 kg)
PREVENTION OF RELAPSES (*P. VIVAX* AND *P. OVALE* ONLY)			
Drug of choice	Primaquine phosphate	15 mg base (26.3 mg)/d × 14 d or 45 mg base (79 mg)/wk × 8 wks	0.3 mg base/kg/d × 14 d

[a]An approved drug, but is considered investigational for this specific condition by the U.S. Food and Drug Administration.
Adapted from Drugs for parasitic infections. *Med Lett Drugs Ther* 1998;40:5.

after travel to a malarious area, travelers should be encouraged to seek medical attention.[5]

GASTROINTESTINAL DISEASE

The GI tract is commonly affected by parasites, because exposure occurs readily through fecal contamination of food and water. Protozoans and helminths are common causes of GI symptoms such as abdominal pain, malabsorption, obstruction, diarrhea, rectal prolapse, and pruritus ani. The protozoans that cause GI diseases *include Giardia lamblia, Entamoeba histolytica,* and *Cryptosporidium.*

G. lamblia, a flagellated protozoan, affects the small intestine. This infection may be transmitted through the ingestion of contaminated food or water, by person-to-person contact, or through male homosexual activity.[18] Most patients experience explosive, watery, foul-smelling diarrhea. Cramping epigastric pain is common; bloody diarrhea is unusual. Physical examination of the abdomen often reveals diffuse upper quadrant tenderness without evidence of peritoneal irritation. Malabsorption may be responsible for the substantial weight loss that may be associated with *Giardia* infestations.[18] Microscopic stool examination may demonstrate active trophozoites, but cysts are more commonly found. In homosexual men who have oral–anal contact, giardiasis may be associated with other bowel infections, particularly amebiasis and shigellosis. Diarrhea and other bowel symptoms occurring in this population, often with evidence of infection by several organisms, has been termed *gay bowel syndrome*. Because *Giardia* is most often transmitted by contaminated water or by the fecal–oral route, efforts at prevention should focus on these routes of transmission.

E. histolytica, upon invasion of the colonic mucosa, can cause amebic dysentery with abdominal pain, tenesmus, and bloody stools.[16] It may result in severe dehydration. The large bowel is typically most affected. Transmission of amebiasis is linked directly to hygiene and sanitation; risk factors for amebiasis include recent travel and institutionalization. The spectrum of clinical disease ranges from mild diarrhea to fulminant rectocolitis. Massive GI bleeding may occur when amebic trophozoites invade large areas of colonic mucosa and cause ulceration; toxic megacolon, perforation, and peritonitis are other severe complications of amebic dysentery. Extraintestinal infection, most commonly amebic liver abscess,[19] may occur with invasion of the trophozoites through the colonic mucosa. The diagnosis of amebic dysentery is made by stool examination for cysts and trophozoites or in biopsy specimens obtained by sigmoidoscopy or colonoscopy.[16]

Cryptosporidium may affect any part of the GI tract. Immunocompetent patients frequently experience a clinical syndrome similar to that of giardiasis, whereas immunodeficient ones typically develop more serious disease and may die of dehydration and electrolyte abnormalities. In addition to water sources, such as drinking water, pools, lakes, and water parks, there have been three food-borne outbreaks of cryptosporidiosis in the United States since 1993.[7,13] Diagnosis is based on the identification of fecal oocysts. The disease is typically self-limited.[5] Paromomycin has been used to treat cryptosporidiosis in several cases, but there is currently no effective therapy.

Infection by the helminths *Ascaris lumbricoides* and *Strongyloides stercoralis* and the hookworms *Necator americanus* and *Ancylostoma duodenale* causes cramping upper abdominal pain when associated with large worm burdens. Patients presenting from tropical climates, particularly Central America, South America, and Southeast Asia, may be infested with more than one of these GI parasites. Hookworms are also endemic in the southeastern United States.

Infection with *A. lumbricoides* and *S. stercoralis* may present with nonspecific abdominal pain and diarrhea. *Ascaris,* a roundworm, can migrate into the biliary system through the ampulla of Vater and induce inflammation and fibrosis of the biliary ducts through chemical irritation. They may also cause partial or intermittent obstruction of the bile ducts.[15] Midepigastric and right upper quadrant pain may also mimic peptic ulcer disease. *Ascaris* has also been reported to cause bowel obstruction, especially in children.[20] Upper respiratory symptoms can develop due to pulmonary migration of larvae (Loeffler syndrome). *S. stercoralis* larvae may mature within the GI tract, as the gravid adult female releases rhabditiform larvae that rapidly evolve into the invasive filariform larval form. The filariform larvae can penetrate the GI tract or perianal skin, causing the hyperinfection syndrome characteristic of strongyloidiasis;[9] this is particularly likely to appear in the immunocompromised patient. Both *Necator* and *Ancylostoma* penetrate the mucosa of the small bowel in heavy acute infestations and cause cramping epigastric pain. In addition, GI blood loss at worm attachment sites may result in a profound hypochromic microcytic anemia.

The physical examination of patients with worm infestation is often unremarkable. Minimal diffuse upper abdominal tenderness may be present, but peritoneal signs are unusual when the worms are intraluminal. Presentation as an acute abdomen does occur, however, when there is complete biliary obstruction or small bowel obstruction secondary to a massive worm burden, as may be the case with acute *Ascaris* infestation. A "whirlpool" pattern of intraluminal worms may be seen with plain abdominal x-rays.[20] In ascariasis and hookworm disease, microscopic examination of the stool often reveals typical ova. Rhabditiform and filariform larvae of strongyloidiasis may be seen in stool samples and Papanicolaou-stained gastric aspirate or sputum smears. The larval forms of *S. stercoralis* are more likely than ova to be visible in the stool samples from these patients. Eosinophilia is common with all helminthic infections and should alert the clinician to this possibility.

Trichuris trichiura and *Enterobius vermicularis* often present as an annoyance rather than the cause of serious illness. Rectal prolapse may occur with massive infestation by *T. trichiura*, the whipworm, particularly in children.[3] Large worm burdens with *T. trichiura* may cause a clinical pancolitis and a mild chronic illness,[10] which is referred to as "trichuris dysentery syndrome": chronic diarrhea, anemia, and growth retardation.[10] In patients with rectal prolapse from trichuriasis, the adult worms are normally visible on the exposed rectal mucosa. Microscopic examination of stool samples demonstrates the typical barrel-shaped ova of *T. trichiura.*

Infestation with the pinworm *E. vermicularis* is the most common helminthic infection of humans, with the prevalence highest among children ages 5 to 10.[10] Pinworm infection causes severe perianal pruritus, especially at night, when female worms crawl out onto the perianal skin to lay eggs.[9] This is typically the live worm seen by patients in the perianal region. Examination of the perineum may reveal secondary bacterial infection of perianal excoriated skin. On occasion, dead parasites or eggs deposited in ectopic sites may lead to the formation of granulomas or abscesses.[1] For diagnosis, clear cellulose tape may be placed against the perianal skin, lifted off, and then applied, adhesive side down, to a glass slide and viewed under a microscope to identify the characteristic eggs. Family members and other close contacts should be examined and, if necessary, treated. Pharmacologic therapy of GI parasitic disease is outlined in Table 197.2.

CENTRAL NERVOUS SYSTEM DISEASE

Several common parasitic diseases are responsible for CNS pathology. They require the emergency physician to have a basic understanding of the life cycle of the organisms involved.

Protozoal infestations such as malaria may present with neurologic manifestations. Falciparum malaria can cause sludging of parasitized red cells in brain capillaries, resulting in severe CNS dysfunction that can progress to coma and death. Early recognition and treatment are essential to prevent this outcome.

Helminthic CNS disease is caused primarily by two tapeworms: *Taenia solium* (pork tapeworm) and *Echinococcus granulosus. T. solium,* an intestinal parasite in humans, can invade other tissues in its larval form, causing cysticercosis. Although 60% of reported cases of cysticercosis involve the brain, it is believed that muscular and subcutaneous encystment is more common.[21] Humans may acquire the infestation by eating cured or undercooked pork meat that has been infected with the larvae

TABLE 197.2. Treatment of Gastrointestinal Parasitic Infections

Infection	Drug	Adult Dosage	Pediatric Dosage
Amebiasis (*Entamoeba histolytica*)			
Asymptomatic			
Drugs of choice	Iodoquinol	650 mg t.i.d. × 20 d	30–40 mg/kg/d (max 2 g) in 3 doses × 20 d
	or Paromomycin	25–35 mg/kg/d in 3 doses × 7 d	25–35 mg/kg/d in 3 doses × 7 d
Alternative	Diloxanide furoate	500 mg t.i.d. × 10 d	20 mg/kg/d in 3 doses × 10 d
Mild-to-moderate intestinal disease[a]			
Drugs of choice	Metronidazole	500–750 mg t.i.d. × 10 d	35–50 mg/kg in 3 doses × 10 d
	or Tinidazole[b]	2 g/d × 3 d	50 mg/kg (max 2 g) qd × 3 d
Severe intestinal disease, hepatic abscess[a]			
Drugs of choice	Metronidazole	750 mg t.i.d. × 10 d	35–50 mg/kg/d in 3 doses × 10 d
	or Tinidazole[b]	600 mg b.i.d. or 800 mg t.i.d. × 5 d	50 mg/kg or 60 mg/kg (max 2 g) qd × 3 d
Ascariasis (*Ascaris lumbricoides, roundworm*)			
Drugs of choice	Mebendazole	100 mg b.i.d. × 3 d or 500 mg × 1 dose	100 mg b.i.d. × 3 d or 500 mg × 1 dose
	or Pyrantel pamoate[c]	11 mg/kg × 1 dose (max 1 g)	11 mg/kg × 1 dose (max 1 g)
	or Albendazole[c]	400 mg × 1 dose	400 mg × 1 dose
Cryptosporidiosis (*Cryptosporidium*)			
Drug of choice	Paromomycin[c]	25–35 mg/kg/d in 3 or 4 doses	
***Enterobiasis vermicularis* (pinworm)**			
Drug of choice	Pyrantel pamoate	11 mg/kg × 1 dose (max 1 g); repeat in 2 weeks	11 mg/kg × 1 dose (max 1 g); repeat in 2 weeks
	or Mebendazole	100 mg once; repeat in 2 weeks	100 mg once; repeat in 2 weeks
	or Albendazolec	400 mg once; repeat in 2 weeks	400 mg once; repeat in 2 weeks
Giardiasis (*Giardia lamblia*)			
Drug of choice	Metronidazole[c]	250 mg t.i.d. × 5 d	15 mg/kg/d in 3 doses × 5 d
Alternatives	Tinidazole[a,b]	2 g × 1 dose	50 mg/kg × 1 dose (max 2 g)
	Furazolidone	100 mg q.i.d. × 7–10 d	6 mg/kg/d in 4 doses × 7–10 d
	Paromomycin[c,d]	25–35 mg/kg/d in 3 doses × 7 d	
Hookworm infection (*Ancylostoma duodenale, Necator americanus*)			
Drugs of choice	Mebendazole	100 mg b.i.d. × 3 d or 500 mg × 1 dose	100 mg b.i.d. × 3 d or 500 mg × 1 dose
	or Pyrantel pamoatec	11 mg/kg (max 1 g) × 3 d	11 mg/kg (max 1 g) × 3 d
	or Albendazolec	400 mg × 1 dose	400 mg × 1 dose
Strongyloidiasis (*Strongyloides stercoralis*)			
Drug of choice	Ivermectin	200 μg/kg/d × 1–2 d	50 mg/kg/d in 2 doses (max 3 g/d) × 2 d
Alternative	Thiabendazole	50 mg/kg/d in 2 doses (max 3 g/d) × 2 d	
Trichuriasis (*Trichuris trichiura, whipworm*)			
Drug of choice	Mebendazole	100 mg b.i.d. × 3 d or 500 mg × 1 dose	100 mg b.i.d. × 3 d or 500 mg × 1 dose
Alternative	*or* Albendazole[c]	400 mg × 1 dose	400 mg × 1 dose

[a]Treatment should be followed by drugs used to treat asymptomatic amebiasis.
[b]Not marketed in the United States.
[c]An approved drug, but is considered investigational for this specific condition by the U.S. Food and Drug Administration.
[d]Not absorbed. May be useful to treat giardiasis in pregnancy.
Adapted from Drugs for parasitic infections. *Med Lett Drugs Ther* 1998;40:1.

of *T. solium*.[21] In addition, infection may be acquired through the fecal–oral route by consuming contaminated food, such as raw vegetables, or water.[8] Cysts formed in the brain (i.e., neurocysticercosis) can cause seizures or produce symptoms through mass effect.[9] Worldwide and in the United States, cysticercosis is the most common parasitic disease of the CNS.[8] Immigrants from endemic areas, such as Mexico and Central America, account for the vast majority of cases in the United States. Cysticercosis is most prevalent in communities where there is close contact between humans and pigs, and where hygiene is poor.[8] *E. granulosus* also forms cysts in the CNS that can mimic neoplastic disease by causing compression effects or seizures.

CLINICAL PRESENTATION AND DIFFERENTIAL DIAGNOSIS

Although *T. solium* is the most common parasitosis of the human CNS, it is symptomatic in only 50% of patients.[21] Patients with cysticercosis of the brain may present with focal neurologic findings or impaired sensorium. The clinical features depend primarily on the location of the cyst. The cyst may be located in the meninges, brain parenchyma, or ventricles. The common presenting features include seizures (most prevalent), focal neurologic deficits, increased intracranial pressure, obstructive hydrocephalus, and stroke.[8,21] Neurocysticercosis should be considered when these features are noted in patients with a history of living in an endemic area. Status epilepticus and mechanical hydrocephalus are the most frequent causes of death.

EMERGENCY DEPARTMENT EVALUATION AND MANAGEMENT

The information obtained from laboratory examination is often limited. A mild peripheral leukocytosis and eosinophilia may be seen. Cerebrospinal fluid (CSF) findings suggestive of cysticercal arachnoiditis include an elevated protein level, eosinophilia, and a predominantly lymphocytic pleocytosis. Several immunologic tests of the serum and CSF have been developed to aid in the diagnosis of cysticercosis.[8] Microscopic examination of stool preparations may reveal typical eggs, proglottids (gravid uterus segments), or scolices, which are the heads of the worm. Although the patient with neurocysticercosis may no

TABLE 197.3. Treatment of Ectoparasite Infections

Infection	Adult and Pediatric Dosage
LICE (*PEDICULUS HUMANUS, P. CAPITIS, PHTHIRUS PUBIS*)	
Drugs of choice	1% Permethrin, topically *or* 0.5% Malathion, topically
Alternatives	Pyrethrins with piperonyl butoxide, topically[a] Ivermectin 200 mg/kg oral × 1 dose (adult and pediatric)[b]
MITES (SEE SCABIES)	
SCABIES (SARCOPTES SCABIEI)	
Drug of choice	5% Permethrin, topically
Alternatives	Ivermectin 200 mg/kg oral × 1 dose (adult and pediatric)[b] 10% Crotamiton, topically

[a]A second application is recommended in 1 week to kill hatchlings.

[b]An approved drug, but is considered investigational for this specific condition by the U.S. Food and Drug Administration.

Adapted from Drugs for parasitic infections. *Med Lett Drugs Ther* 1998;40:1.

longer have a tapeworm at the time the diagnosis is made, stools of both the patient and family members should be examined for several days.[8] Serologic diagnosis is necessary to confirm *E. granulosus* infection.

Laboratory personnel should be consulted to determine the most appropriate procedures for collecting and handling specimens. The laboratory should be informed of the patient's clinical diagnosis to assist in sample analysis. Consultation with an infectious disease expert may be helpful if the clinician is unfamiliar with the potential manifestations of a particular disease.

Computed tomography (CT) scanning of the head may show both calcified and uncalcified cysts.[8,15] Contrast-enhanced CT scanning may demonstrate ring-enhancing lesions in both cysticercosis and echinococcal cyst disease. Magnetic resonance imaging (MRI) has been shown to be more sensitive than CT scan for the detection of active neurocysticercosis, due to the superior ability of MRI to image cysts in the brainstem, subarachnoid space, and ventricles. CT, however, is a better modality for imaging inactive, calcified cysts.[15]

Treatment of parasitic CNS disease may involve medical or surgical interventions and depends on the clinical signs and symptoms, the presence of active noncalcified or inactive calcified cysts, and the occurrence of complications. In addition to symptomatic treatment, options for the treatment of neurocysticercosis include anticysticercal drugs, corticosteroids, CSF shunting, and surgical cyst removal.[8] Most parasitic infections in the active phase with viable cysts are readily treated with safe and effective agents. Patients can commonly be treated as outpatients, with appropriate follow-up.

If active neurocysticercosis is suspected, praziquantel (50 mg/kg/d in three divided doses for 15 days) or albendazole (400 mg two times a day for 8 to 30 days) should be initiated.[5] Corticosteroids should be given for 2 to 3 days before and during drug therapy.[5] Albendazole (400 mg two times a day for 28 days) has been used to treat echinococcal cysts. Surgical removal of cysts remains the most effective treatment.[5]

Patients who present with inactive disease (e.g., seizures secondary to parasitic calcifications) are not candidates for treatment with antihelminthic agents. Seizures are treated no differently than seizures from other causes. Neurologic or neurosurgical consultation is appropriate for these patients.

ECTOPARASITES

Ectoparasites live on the surface of the body. Those commonly seen in the emergency department include scabies (*Sarcoptes scabiei*), chigger mites (*Eutrombicula alfreddugesi* and *E. splendens*), body lice (*Pediculus humanus*), head lice (*P. humanus capitis*), and pubic lice (*Phthirus pubis*). Except for the common cold, *P. humanus capitis* affects more school-age children than all other communicable diseases combined.[17]

CLINICAL PRESENTATION

Ectoparasites may cause a pruritic rash, with pruritus alone or as a visual nuisance. The location of the complaints aids in the differential diagnosis. *S. scabiei* burrows under the superficial layers of the epidermis, causing small vesicles to form. Scratching may result in spread of the parasite, bleeding, and secondary bacterial infection. The most common sites for infestation include the interdigital and popliteal folds and the groin. Chigger mites, in contrast, attach to the skin surface and feed on tissue fluids, causing an intense pruritus and dermatitis. These mites attach to areas where clothing may be tight, such as the ankles, waist, and armpits. The human body lice or head lice can be found wherever personal or general hygiene is at a low level. The pubic or crab louse is found most commonly on the hairs of the genital region, although it may be found in other areas, such as the axilla and eyebrows. Lice may cause considerable distress from itching, scalp irritation, and potential secondary infection.[2]

EMERGENCY DEPARTMENT EVALUATION AND MANAGEMENT

S. scabiei may be identified by looking at a potassium hydroxide (KOH) skin scraping preparation under low-power magnification. *P. humanus* eggs or nits appear glistening white when seen in the hair. Wood's light examination may aid in the diagnosis, because the nits fluoresce under ultraviolet light.

Ectoparasites are managed primarily with topical lotions, although oral ivermectin may also be used[4] (Table 197.3). Because transmission of ectoparasites occurs by direct contact with infested persons or with their bedding or clothing, contacts should be treated as needed, and clothing should be washed in hot water. Children should remain home from school until the infestation has resolved.[2]

COMMON PITFALLS

- Failure to consider parasitic disease as a potential etiology for a variety of systemic, GI, CNS, and skin complaints. Parasitic disease should be considered in any patient presenting from an endemic area or with a travel history to an endemic area.
- Failure to consult reference textbooks concerning the appropriate diagnosis and treatment for these diseases

References

1. Avolio L, Avoltini V, et al. Perianal granuloma caused by *Enterobius vermicularis:* report of a new observation and review of the literature. *J Pediatr* 1998;132:1055.
2. Bainbridge CV, Klein GL, et al. Comparative study of the clinical effectiveness of a pyrethrin-based pediculicide with combing versus a permethrin-based pediculocide with combing. *Clin Pediatr* 1998;37:17.
3. Beaver PC, Jung RC, Cupp EW. *Clinical parasitology.* Philadelphia: Lea & Febiger, 1984.
4. Burkhart CN, Arbogast J. Head lice therapy revisited. *Clin Pediatr* 1998;37:395.

5. Drugs for parasitic infections. *Med Lett Drugs Ther* 1998;40:1.
6. Drugs for parasitic infections. *Med Lett Drugs Ther* 1998;40:47.
7. Food-borne outbreak of cryptosporidiosis—Spokane, Washington, 1997. *JAMA* 1998;280:595.
8. Garg RK. Neurocysticercosis. *Postgrad Med J* 1998;74:321.
9. Gibler WB. Parasitology: the emergency presentation. In: Rosen P, Barkin R, Braen GR, eds. *Emergency medicine—concepts and clinical practice.* St. Louis, Mosby, 1988.
10. Grencis RK, Cooper ES. Enterobius, trichuris, capillaria, and hookworm including *Ancylostoma caninum*. *Gastroenterol Clin North Am* 1996;25:579.
11. Jotte RS, Scott J. Malaria: review of features pertinent to the emergency physician. *J Emerg Med* 1993;11:729.
12. Kain KC, Keystone JS. Malaria in travelers: epidemiology, disease, and prevention. *Infect Dis Clin North Am* 1998;12:267.
13. Kramer MH, Goldstein ST, et al. First reported outbreak in the United States of cryptosporidiosis associated with a recreational lake. *Clin Infect Dis* 1998;26:27.
14. Kyriacou DN, Spira AM, et al. Emergency department presentation and misdiagnosis of imported falciparum malaria. *Ann Emerg Med* 1996;27:696.
15. Lamont EB, Sayah A. An occult cause of persistent nausea and vomiting. *J Emerg Med* 1996;15:633.
16. Li E, Stanley SL. Protozoa: amebiasis. *Gastroenterol Clin North Am* 1996;25:471.
17. Nguyen V, Robert P. Treatment of head lice. *N Engl J Med* 1997;336:734.
18. Ortega YR, Adam RD. *Giardia:* overview and update. *Clin Infect Dis* 1998;25:545.
19. Shandera WX, Bollam P, et al. Hepatic amebiasis among patients in a public teaching hospital. *South Med J* 1998;91:829.
20. Villamazir E, Mizrahinn M. *Ascaris lumbricoides* infestation as a cause of intestinal obstruction in children: experience with 87 cases. *J Pediatr Surg* 1996;31:201.
21. Yamashita P, Kelsey J, et al. Subcutaneous cysticercosis. *J Emerg Med* 1997;16:583.

CHAPTER 198

Blood and Body Fluid Exposures in the Health-Care Worker

Peter E. Sokolove

Despite the introduction of a safe and effective vaccine in 1982, hepatitis B remains a major problem among health-care workers. Although only about 4% of the estimated 300,000 cases of hepatitis B virus (HBV) infections in the United States each year occur in workers in health-care–related fields, seroprevalence studies indicate that health-care workers who have frequent contact with blood have a threefold to sixfold increase in seropositivity over that of the general population (15% to 30% vs. 5%).[4,16] It is also apparent that the more frequent the blood contact, the higher the rate of seroconversion. In studies of emergency medical personnel, emergency physicians exhibited a 12% to 16% seroprevalence rate,[11,12] emergency medical services personnel a 16% to 25% rate,[14,17,22] and emergency department nurses a 30% rate.[9]

Although the acquired immunodeficiency syndrome (AIDS) accounts for a much smaller number of cases than does hepatitis B, it often causes more concern among health-care workers. As of June 1997, there were only 52 confirmed occupational human immunodeficiency virus (HIV) infections among health-care workers in the United States,[5] compared with a previous Centers for Disease Control and Prevention (CDC) estimate of 12,000 health-care worker infections and 250 deaths each year from HBV.[3]

Previously known as non-A non-B hepatitis, hepatitis C virus (HCV) is now the most common chronic blood-borne infection in the United States. About 3.9 million Americans are infected with this virus, with about 36,000 new infections each year. While the overall prevalence of HCV in health-care workers is similar to that of the general population (1% to 2%), emergency department personnel are at high risk of exposure.[7] In one study from an inner-city emergency department, the prevalence of HCV infection among patients was 18%, compared with 5% for HBV and 6% for HIV.[13]

CLINICAL PRESENTATION

Health-care workers frequently present to the emergency department after exposure to material potentially infected with HBV, HCV, or HIV. First, the exposure must be assessed. Although blood is the single most important source of infection, other fluids may also transmit disease. Semen or vaginal secretions; cerebrospinal, synovial, pleural, peritoneal, pericardial, or amniotic fluids; and tissue are capable of transmitting HIV, HBV, and probably HCV. Unless blood is visible in them, feces, nasal secretions, sputum, sweat, and tears have not been identified as vehicles of transmission for HBV, HCV, or HIV infection. Transmission occurs most effectively through direct percutaneous exposure (e.g., needlestick); although far less likely, exposure through mucous membranes or open skin lesions can also result in HBV, HCV, and HIV transmission. Casual contact, airborne, and fecal–oral transmission have not been documented.[5,7,10]

EMERGENCY DEPARTMENT EVALUATION

An initial evaluation should be made to assess the risk of disease transmission. Information about the injury should be gathered, including the infectious material, instrument, procedure performed, depth of penetration, and volume of blood transferred. The source person should be evaluated for HIV and hepatitis risk factors, clinical signs of disease, previous HIV therapy, and viral load or CD4 count, if known.

The health-care worker should be evaluated for his or her medical history and immunization status for hepatitis B and tetanus. The source blood should be tested for hepatitis B surface antigen (HBsAg), HCV, and HIV antibodies. If the source is found to be positive for HBsAg, the source should also then be tested for hepatitis B e antigen (HBeAg). The health-care worker should be tested for hepatitis B surface antibody (HBsAb), HCV, HIV, and pregnancy, as appropriate. Testing of sharp instruments is not recommended or reliable.[5]

EMERGENCY DEPARTMENT MANAGEMENT

Hepatitis B Virus Exposure

Two types of products are available for the management of the exposed health-care worker. Hepatitis B immune globulin (HBIG), derived from plasma containing high titers of antibody to HBsAg, confers passive immunity. Side effects are minimal, and there is no evidence of HBV or HIV transmission with this product. For postexposure prophylaxis, the dose is 0.06 mL/kg intramuscularly. It should be administered within 72 hours of exposure (preferably within 24 hours), and is probably not useful beyond 7 days.[4] The average wholesale cost (in 1998) is $652 per dose.[18]

Hepatitis B vaccine is available for active immunization. It is a recombinant vaccine that is very safe, even in pregnancy. For postexposure prophylaxis of nonvaccinated individuals, 1 mL of vaccine is administered intramuscularly in the deltoid within 7 days of exposure and repeated at 1 month and 6 months.[4] Because about 10% of adults will not initially achieve the recommended antibody titer following this series, antibody levels should be checked 4 to 6 weeks after the series is completed. Health-care workers who are smokers, obese, over the age of 50, or immunocompromised are less likely to respond to the initial vaccination series.[20,23] Nonresponders may require a fourth dose of vaccine or intradermal administration. For health-care workers who achieve a level of at least 10 mIU/mL, the vaccine is essentially 100% effective in preventing subsequent HBV infection. The average wholesale price of HBV immunization is $165 per course.[18]

Whether to administer HBIG, HBV vaccine, both, or neither is based on the HBsAg status of the source person and the vaccination status of the exposed health-care worker (Fig. 198.1).[3a] A source person can transmit HBV if HBsAg is present, but the degree of infectivity is best correlated with HBeAg positivity. The risk of seroconversion after a percutaneous exposure to HBsAg-positive blood ranges from 2% (HBeAg negative) to 40% (HBeAg positive).[10] Of those infected with HBV, about 25% develop acute hepatitis, and 6% to 10% develop chronic infection.[3] These patients are at increased risk of cirrhosis and hepatocellular carcinoma.

Hepatitis C Virus Exposure

There are currently no agents available for managing exposure of the health-care worker to HCV.[7] Immune globulin is not useful for postexposure prophylaxis of HCV[19] for a number of reasons. In contrast to HBsAb, HCV antibody is only a marker antibody, not a neutralizing antibody. Even if a neutralizing antibody did exist among the donor population, immune globulin is derived from plasma donors that are excluded from donation if they test positive for HCV. Finally, HCV mutates rapidly, and new variants may be unaffected by neutralizing antibodies.

There is currently no vaccine against HCV, as this virus demonstrates great genetic heterogeneity and a high mutation rate.[1] Alpha-interferon, sometimes in combination with ribavirin, has been used successfully to treat patients with chronic hepatitis due to HCV.[15] Unfortunately, there is currently no evidence to support a role for such agents in postexposure prophylaxis.

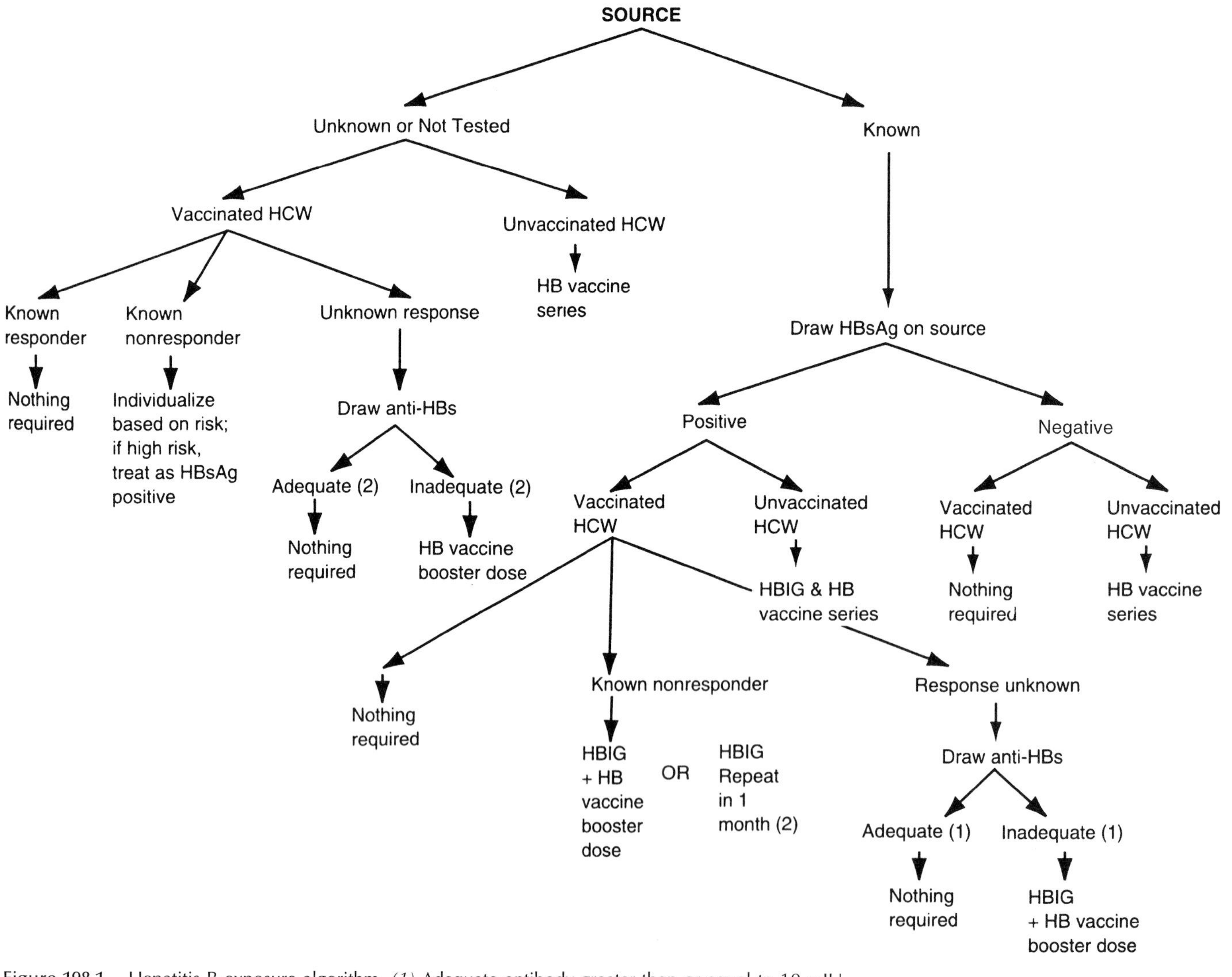

Figure 198.1. Hepatitis B exposure algorithm. *(1)* Adequate antibody greater than or equal to 10 mIU/mL. *(2)* Preferred for those who have failed to respond to at least four doses of vaccine. (Adapted from Centers for Disease Control. Immunization of health-care workers; recommendations of the Immunization Practices Advisory Committee (ACIP) and the Hospital Infection Control Practices Advisory Committee (HICPAC). *MMWR* 1997;46(RR-18):1.)

The average risk of acquiring HCV infection after percutaneous exposure is 1.8%, and ranges from 0% to 7%.[7] Of those who acquire HCV infection, approximately 75% to 85% develop chronic infection, of whom 60% to 70% have liver enzyme elevations.[6] Of patients with chronic HCV infection, about 10% to 20% develop cirrhosis, and about 1% to 5% develop hepatocellular carcinoma.[7]

Human Immunodeficiency Virus Exposure

Emergency department management of potential exposure to HIV materials consists of serologic testing of the exposed health-care worker and exposure source, counseling the health-care worker on the risk for infection, and consideration of postexposure prophylaxis. While previously the use of antiviral agents to prevent HIV seroconversion in exposed health-care workers was considered highly controversial, new evidence supports the use of certain drugs in many cases. The theoretical basis for postexposure prophylaxis is that there is a window of opportunity before HIV infection is established in the host. Antiviral agents may prevent or limit the replication of HIV in dendritic cells or regional lymph nodes, which appear to be the initial targets and route of spread of HIV.[5]

Many animal studies have demonstrated that the use of postexposure antiviral agents can prevent or delay HIV infection.[21] In human studies, when HIV-infected mothers were administered zidovudine (AZT) during pregnancy, perinatal transmission of HIV was decreased by 67%.[8] While transmission during pregnancy is different from percutaneous exposure, these data clearly demonstrate that antiviral agents can be used to prevent blood-borne infection in an HIV-negative individual. The most compelling evidence of postexposure prophylaxis efficacy, however, was a multinational case-control study, performed by the CDC.[2] In this study of health-care workers who had HIV exposures, mostly as a result of hollow-bore needlesticks, the risk for HIV infection was reduced by 81% if AZT was given following exposure. These new data prompted the Public Health Service to recommend postexposure prophylaxis for health-care workers exposed to HIV.[5]

AZT is a nucleoside reverse transcriptase inhibitor, and is administered in divided doses totaling 600 mg per day. Treatment should be continued for 4 weeks, but about one-third of health-care workers will discontinue therapy because of adverse symptoms. Short-term toxicity of AZT mostly consists of gastrointestinal (GI) discomfort and fatigue. Bone marrow suppression can be seen, but it is reversible and very rare in healthy individuals.

While AZT is the only drug shown to be beneficial for HIV postexposure prophylaxis in humans, multidrug regimens are often employed because of concerns about AZT-resistant strains of HIV, as well as a demonstrated synergistic effect of certain antiviral agents in the treatment of patients for AIDS. AZT resistance should be suspected if the source person is an HIV-positive patient who is not responding to AZT therapy. However, AZT-resistant strains can be found in HIV-positive patients who have never taken AZT.

Lamivudine (3TC) is another nucleoside reverse transcriptase inhibitor, and has been demonstrated to have synergistic antiviral activity when added to AZT to treat patients who have AIDS. The primary toxicity of 3TC is adverse GI symptoms, and pancreatitis is rare. 3TC is administered at a dose of 150 mg twice a day for 4 weeks. Because of the potential for increased efficacy without an increase in side effects, 3TC is usually added to the postexposure prophylaxis regimen whenever AZT is given.[5]

Protease inhibitors should be considered for use as a third agent in the postexposure prophylaxis regimen for certain high-risk exposures. These agents inhibit HIV aspartyl protease and are very potent antiviral agents. Unlike the nucleoside agents, protease inhibitors do not require phosphorylation to become active, providing the theoretical benefit of having an active agent present in the bloodstream very rapidly following exposure.

Indinavir or nelfinavir are generally the preferred agents for postexposure prophylaxis because of their rapid bioavailability and the fact that patients are able to start treatment at full dose. Indinavir is administered at a dose of 800 mg three times a day for 4 weeks. Its major side effects are GI discomfort, hyperbilirubinemia (10%), and renal stones (4%). Patients should be instructed to drink at least 1.5 L of fluid each day to help prevent stones. Nelfinavir is administered at a dose of 750 mg three times a day for 4 weeks.[5] This agent commonly results in diarrhea, so antimotility agents (e.g., loperamide) should be prescribed. All protease inhibitors may result in hyperglycemia. In rare cases, these agents may precipitate diabetic ketoacidosis, even in nondiabetic patients.

When determining whether to initiate postexposure prophylaxis, as well as which agents to choose, the physician must consider a number of factors. The type of exposure helps determine the risk of seroconversion, and thus the potential benefit of postexposure prophylaxis. As of this writing, there have been no reported cases of HIV seroconversion when blood has come in contact with intact skin. If the skin integrity is compromised, or if mucous membranes are exposed, transmission is unlikely but can occur.

The risk of transmission following a mucous membrane exposure to blood is about 0.1% (one in 1,000). The risk of transmission can be higher if a large volume of blood is involved or if prolonged contact occurs. The average risk for HIV transmission following percutaneous blood exposure is about 0.3% (one in 300) but depends on the severity of the exposure.[5] Table 198.1 lists the risk factors for HIV transmission after percutaneous blood exposure, as reported in the previously described CDC case-control study.[2]

The HIV status of the source person is also important when assessing the risk of transmission and choice of antiviral agents. If the source person is currently HIV-negative and has not had a recent retroviral-like illness (symptoms similar to those of acute mononucleosis), postexposure prophylaxis is not indicated. For HIV-positive source persons, the degree of infectivity is related to the patient's viral load. High viral loads are seen in patients with advanced AIDS or primary HIV infection. In 1998, the Public Health Service published a three-step algorithm for determining the need for and choice of HIV postexposure prophylaxis (Fig. 198.2).[5]

The timing of the initiation of postexposure prophylaxis is very important, as animal models have demonstrated an increased risk of infection with delays in AZT administration. It is best to initiate therapy promptly, preferably within 1 hour of ex-

TABLE 198.1. Risk Factors for HIV Transmission after Percutaneous Blood Exposure

Risk Factor	Odds Ratio	95% CI
Deep injury	15	6–41
Blood visible on device	6.2	2.2–21.0
Procedure with needle placed directly into artery or vein	4.3	1.7–12.0
Terminal AIDS in source patient	5.6	2–16
Postexposure zidovudine (AZT)	0.19	0.06–0.52

Adapted from Cardo DM, Culver DH, Ciesielski CA, et al. A case-control study of HIV seroconversion in health care workers after percutaneous exposure. *N Engl J Med* 1997;337:1487.

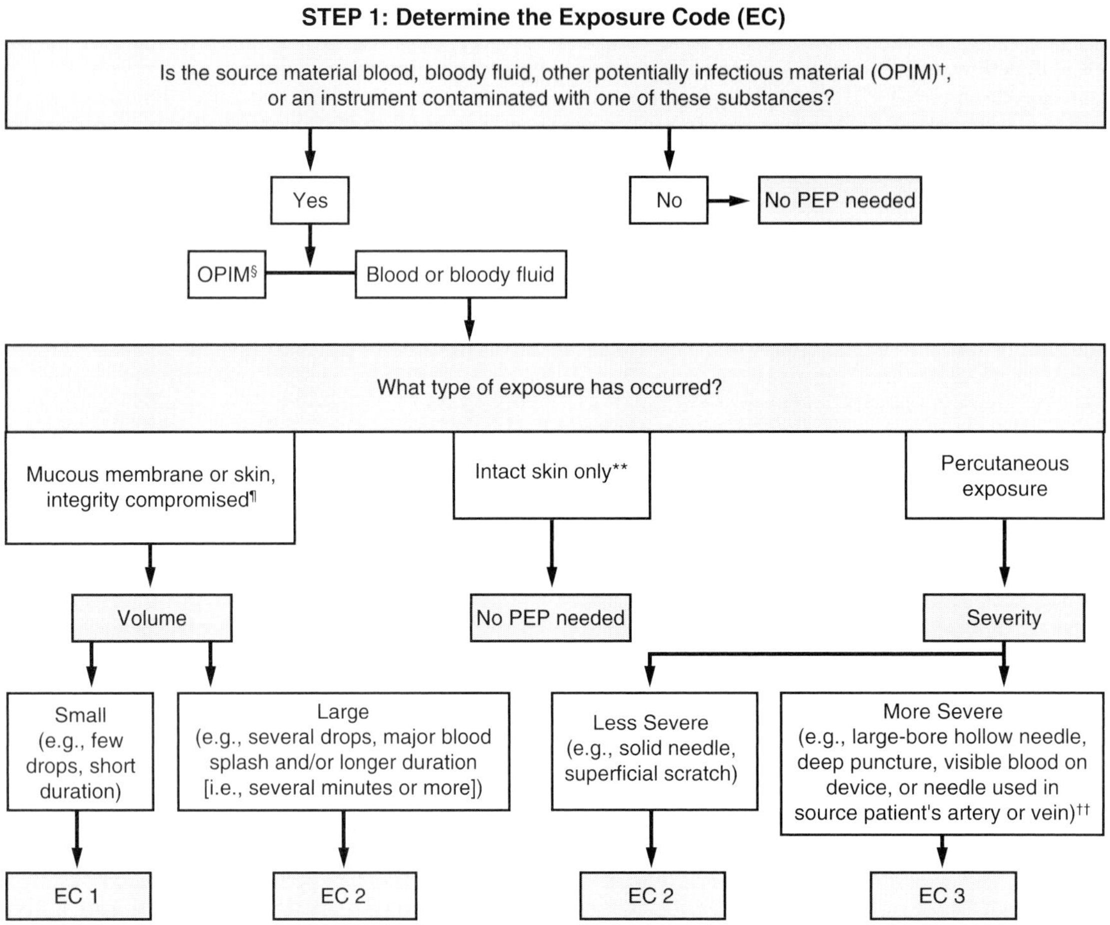

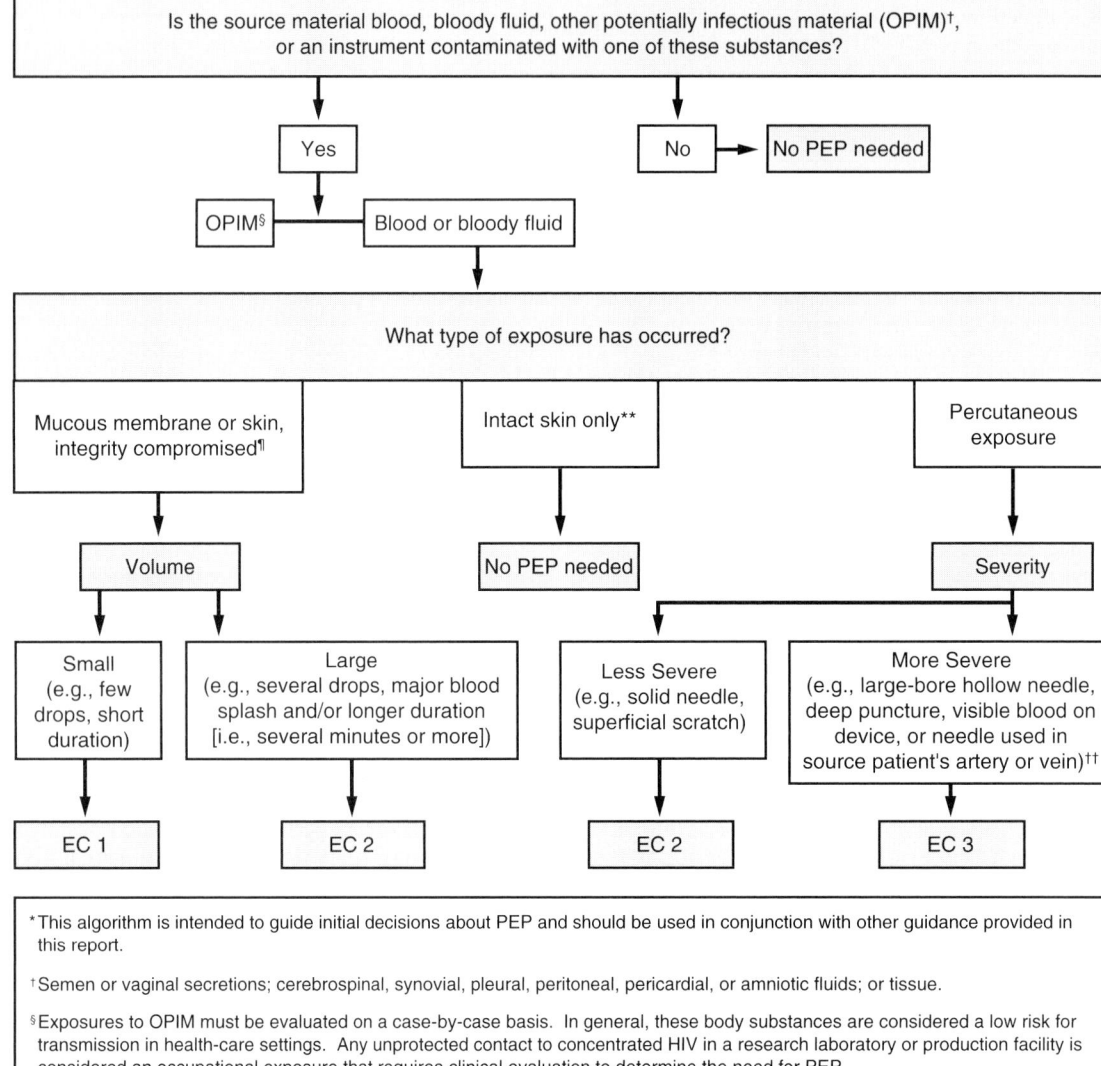

*This algorithm is intended to guide initial decisions about PEP and should be used in conjunction with other guidance provided in this report.

†Semen or vaginal secretions; cerebrospinal, synovial, pleural, peritoneal, pericardial, or amniotic fluids; or tissue.

§Exposures to OPIM must be evaluated on a case-by-case basis. In general, these body substances are considered a low risk for transmission in health-care settings. Any unprotected contact to concentrated HIV in a research laboratory or production facility is considered an occupational exposure that requires clinical evaluation to determine the need for PEP.

¶Skin integrity is considered compromised if there is evidence of chapped skin, dermatitis, abrasion, or open wound.

**Contact with intact skin is not normally considered a risk is for HIV transmission. However if the exposure was to blood, and the circumstance suggests a higher volume exposure (e.g., an extensive area of skin was exposed or there was prolonged contact with blood), the risk for HIV transmission should be considered.

††The combination of these severity factors (e.g., large-bore hollow needle and deep puncture) contribute to an elevated risk for transmission if the source person is HIV-positive.

Figure 198.2. Determining the need for HIV postexposure prophylaxis. (Adapted from Centers for Disease Control. Public Health Service guidelines for the management of health-care worker exposures to HIV and recommendations for postexposure prophylaxis. *MMWR* 1998;47(RR-7):14–15.)

posure. It is unclear how long following exposure treatment can be initiated and still be effective, but animal data suggest that some benefit may persist up to 36 hours.[21]

Summary of Acute Management

Acute management includes thorough washing of the exposed area with soap and warm water or flushing of mucous membranes. As with all wounds, the need for tetanus toxoid administration should be considered. HBIG or hepatitis B vaccine or both should be administered as indicated (see Fig. 198.1). HIV postexposure prophylaxis should be recommended based on the exposure type and the source HIV status (see Fig. 198.2). The health-care worker should be counseled regarding the risks of HBV, HCV, and HIV infection, as well as modifications of behavior (e.g., abstinence or condom use) to prevent secondary infection of others.

COMMON PITFALLS

A common error in the management of health-care worker exposures is to provide either unnecessary or inadequate treatment. Unnecessary treatment usually results from an overestimation of the infectious potential of an exposure, such as providing three-drug antiretroviral therapy for a blood splash onto intact skin. Undertreatment can occur if the treating physician is unaware of the benefit of postexposure prophylaxis, or if

STEP 2: Determine the HIV Status Code (HIV SC)

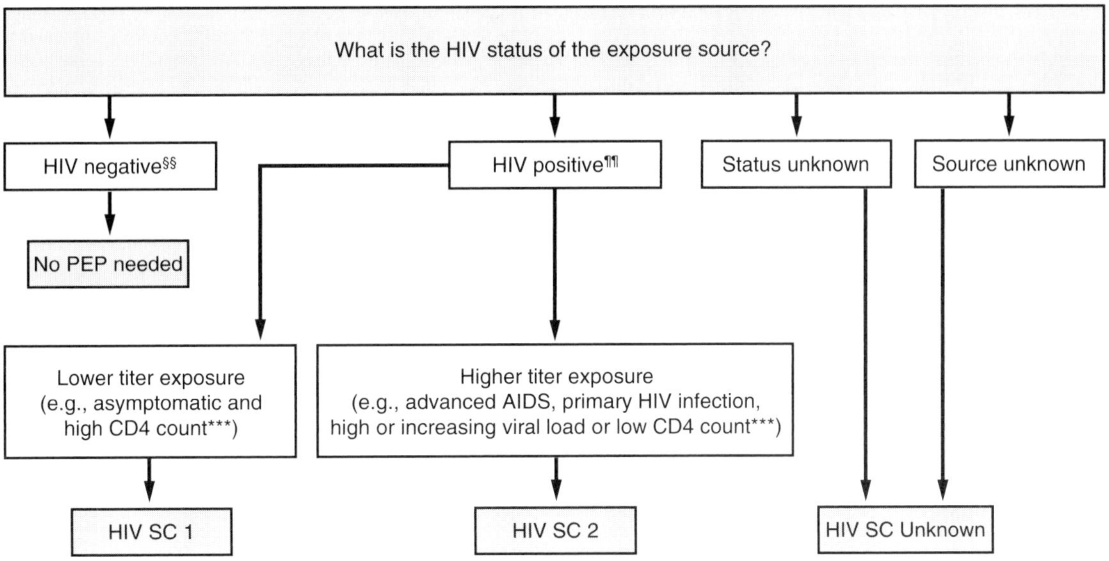

[§§]A source is considered negative for HIV infection if there is laboratory documentation of a negative HIV antibody, HIV polymerase chain reaction (PCR), or HIV p24 antigen test result from a specimen collected at or near the time of exposure and there is no clinical evidence of recent retroviral-like illness.

[¶¶]A source is considered infected with HIV (HIV positive) if there has been a positive laboratory result for HIV antibody, HIV PCR, or HIV p24 antigen or physician-diagnosed AIDS.

[***]Examples are used as surrogates to estimate the HIV titer in an exposure source for purposes of considering PEP regimens and do not reflect all clinical situations that may be observed. Although a high HIV titer (HIV SC 2) in an exposure source has been associated with an increased risk for transmission, the possibility of transmission from a source with a low HIV titer also must be considered.

STEP 3: Determine the PEP Recommendation

EC	HIV SC	PEP recommendation
1	1	**PEP may not be warranted.** Exposure type does not pose a known risk for HIV transmission. Whether the risk for drug toxicity outweighs the benefit of PEP should be decided by the exposed HCW and treating clinician.
1	2	**Consider basic regimen.**[†††] Exposure type poses a negligible risk for HIV transmission. A high HIV titer in the source may justify consideration of PEP. Whether the risk for drug toxicity outweighs the benefit of PEP should be decided by the exposed HCW and treating clinician.
2	2	**Recommend basic regimen.**[§§§] Exposure type represents an increased HIV transmission risk.
3	1 or 2	**Recommend expanded regimen.** Exposure type represents an increased HIV transmission risk.
Unknown		If the source or, in the case of an unknown source, the setting where the exposure occurred suggests a possible risk for HIV exposure and the EC is 2 or 3, consider PEP basic regimen.

[†††]Basic regimen is four weeks of zidovudine, 600 mg per day in two or three divided doses, and lamivudine, 150 mg twice daily.

[§§§]Expanded regimen is the basic regimen plus either indinavir, 800 mg every 8 hours, or nelfinavir, 750 mg three times a day.

Figure 198.2. *(Continued)*

treatment for HIV exposure is delayed. These pitfalls can be avoided by applying a standardized protocol, such as the algorithms presented here. In uncertain or complex cases, consultation with an employee health service or an infectious disease specialist is advised.

References

1. Bukh J, Miller RH, Purcell RH. Genetic heterogeneity of hepatitis C virus: quasi species and genotypes. *Semin Liver Dis* 1995;15:41.
2. Cardo DM, Culver DH, Ciesielski CA, et al. A case-control study of HIV seroconversion in health care workers after percutaneous exposure. *N Engl J Med* 1997;337:1485.
3. Centers for Disease Control. Guidelines for prevention of transmission of human immunodeficiency virus to health-care and public-safety workers. *MMWR* 1989;38(S-6):1.

3a. Centers for Disease Control. Immunization of health-care workers: recommendations of the Immunization Practices Committee (ACIP) and the Hospital Infection Control Practices Advisory Committe (HICPAC). *MMWR* 1997;46(RR-18):1.

4. Centers for Disease Control. Protection against viral hepatitis: recommendations of the Immunization Practices Advisory Committee (ACIP). *MMWR* 1990;39(RR-2):1.
5. Centers for Disease Control. Public Health Service guidelines for the management of health-care worker exposures to HIV and recommendations for postexposure prophylaxis. *MMWR* 1998; 47(RR-7):1.
6. Centers for Disease Control. Recommendations for follow-up of health-care workers after occupational exposure to hepatitis C virus. *MMWR* 1997;46:603.
7. Centers for Disease Control. Recommendations for prevention and control of hepatitis C virus (HCV) infection and HCV-related chronic disease. *MMWR* 1998;47 (RR-19):1.
8. Connor EM, Sperling RS, Gelber R, et al. Reduction of maternal-infant transmission of HIV type 1 with zidovudine treatment. *N Engl J Med* 1994;331:1173.

9. Dienstag JL, Ryan DM. Occupational exposure to hepatitis B virus in hospital personnel: infection or immunization? *Am J Epidemiol* 1982;115:26.
10. Gerberding JL. Drug therapy: management of occupational exposures to blood-borne viruses. *N Engl J Med* 1995;332:444.
11. Iserson KV, Criss EA, Barrett S, et al. The prevalence of hepatitis B serological markers in emergency physicians. *Am J Emerg Med* 1984;2:394.
12. Iserson KV, Criss EA. Hepatitis B prevalence in emergency physicians. *Ann Emerg Med* 1985;14:119.
13. Kelen GD, Green GB, Purcell RH, et al. Hepatitis B and hepatitis C in emergency department patients. *N Engl J Med* 1992;326:1399.
14. Kunches LM, Craven DE, Werner BG, et al. Hepatitis B exposure in emergency medical personnel. *Am J Med* 1983;75:269.
15. McHutchinson JG, Gordon SC, Schiff ER, et al. Interferon alpha-2b alone or in combination with ribavirin as initial treatment for chronic hepatitis C. *N Engl J Med* 1998;339:1485.
16. McQuillin GM, Fields HA, Polk BF. Seroepidemiology of hepatitis B virus infection in the United States. *Am J Med* 1989;87[Suppl 3A]:5S.
17. Pepe PE, Hollinger FB, Troisi CL, et al. Viral hepatitis risk in urban emergency medical services personnel. *Ann Emerg Med* 1986;15:454.
18. *Red book,* 1998 ed. Montvale, NJ: Medical Economics Company, 1998:296, 336.
19. Seeff LB, Zimmermann HJ, Wright EC, et al. A randomized, double blind controlled trial of the efficacy of immune serum globulin for the prevention of post-transfusion hepatitis. *Gastroenterology* 1977;72:111.
20. Shaw FE, Guess HA, Roets JM, et al. Effect of anatomic injection site, age and smoking on the immune response to hepatitis B vaccination. *Vaccine* 1989;7:425.
21. Shih CC, Kaneshima H, Rabin L, et al. Postexposure prophylaxis with zidovudine suppresses HIV type 1 infection in SCID-hu mice in a time-dependent manner. *J Infect Dis* 1991;163:625.
22. Valenzuela TD, Hook EW, Copass MK, et al. Occupational exposure to hepatitis B in paramedics. *Arch Intern Med* 1985;145:1976.
23. Wood RC, MacDonald KL, White KE, et al. Risk factors for lack of detectable antibody following hepatitis B vaccination of Minnesota health care workers. *JAMA* 1993;270:2935.

PART VI
Neurologic Disease

CHAPTER 199
Altered Mental Status and Coma

Gregory L. Henry

Coma is the most dramatic of the disorders of consciousness, but it is only the end point in a continuum of disease. Any disease process that can cause coma may initially present with mild alterations of mental status. It is often difficult or impossible to determine the direction and final outcome of a change in mental status until the most important test—the test of time—has been applied.

In severe nervous system disease, a change in mental status is often the first sign of a serious pathologic process.[14] It is generally recognized that the functional change is always greater and always precedes structural change in the brain and spinal cord. Of all the central nervous system functions, mental status is the most delicate and the most sensitive early indicator of advancing involvement of the nervous system.

Sophisticated evaluation of altered mental status always comes after the standard emergency medicine approach of initial stabilization, control of airway and breathing, and cardiovascular support.[19,20] When this has been achieved, the emergency physician should divide patients with severely altered mental status into two distinct groups: (1) those with diffuse metabolic or toxic causes of altered mental status and (2) those with focal disease that may require immediate surgical therapy. Although the differential diagnosis is exhaustive, the major job of the emergency physician is to differentiate between these two major groups. The management of toxic and metabolic disease is principally medical, and the management of focal disease is often surgical. To delay diagnosis may mean considerable harm to the patient.

When recording the patient's status, it is often better to describe in detail exactly which mental functions are present and which are not, rather than using potentially misleading nonspecific terms.[6] Such terms convey little information about the patient's neurologic functioning. The charting in the record of objective findings, such as the patient's ability to handle three-object retention and mathematic calculations, is much more effective than the use of terms such as *stuporous* or *lethargic*. *Consciousness* may be defined as an awareness of self and the environment. Disorders of consciousness can be divided according to levels of patient responsiveness.

CLINICAL PRESENTATION

Patients with altered mental status may present in multiple ways.[19] Sleep, a state of nonpathologic decreased mental status from which the patient can be easily aroused to full consciousness, may be a frequent finding in emergency departments. Although the sleepy patient experiences a transitory deterioration of mental status, the ability to return to normal function on arousal should separate sleep from pathologic conditions.

The term *lethargy* is, unfortunately, still part of medical jargon. *Lethargy* may best be defined as depressed mental status in which the patient may appear wakeful but has depressed awareness of self and environment globally and cannot be aroused to full function. However, the term is extremely vague and often causes as much confusion as enlightenment.

Stupor refers to an unresponsive condition from which the patient can be aroused with vigorous stimuli to purposeful activity. The stuporous patient, however, does not return to normal baseline awareness of self or environment.

Coma is the extreme end of the continuum of mental status change. A comatose patient is unresponsive and is not arousable by either verbal or physical stimuli to a level at which any purposeful or meaningful response can be made.

Like all aspects of emergency medicine, psychological factors are ever present. Psychogenic coma is a state of unresponsiveness, either voluntary or involuntary, from which the patient cannot be brought to reasonable cortical response by noxious, verbal, or physical stimuli, yet in which physiologic test results and electroencephalographic responses are normal.

Another major group of patients may appear awake but does not respond to stimuli. One group exhibits the abulic state, often referred to as akinetic mutism.[9,19] These patients are awake, with their eyes open, but are extremely slow in all mental processes and find it difficult to respond to questioning. Frontal lobe function is so depressed, from any number of processes, that they cannot respond meaningfully within a normal time frame. These patients often can process information, but because of the huge time delays in their ability to respond and answer, they are often misdiagnosed in the emergency department. They may take several minutes to respond to any problem or question posed.

A most unusual and dramatic form of seemingly awake but altered mental status is the locked-in syndrome. A patient with such a syndrome appears motionless, with eyes open. The lesion in the locked-in syndrome is the destruction of the ventral pontine motor tracts. The only function these patients maintain is vertical eye movement. Unresponsive patients who appear awake should be asked to look up. If a patient can look up but cannot move the eyes side to side in a horizontal plane, the diagnosis of locked-in syndrome is confirmed.[7–9]

TABLE 199.1. Toxic–Metabolic Disorders

Metabolic Disorders	Significant Differential Elements
Hyperglycemia/hypoglycemia	Diabetics at high risk, both insulin-dependent and users of oral hypoglycemics; also more prone to infectious disease and renal failure. Hypoglycemia may be seen in patients with certain tumors, chronic alcoholics.
Hepatic failure	Most common in long-standing alcohol abusers and/or hepatitis. May lead to rapid rises in serum ammonia. May be associated with hypoglycemia due to decreased glycogen storage.
Uremia	Affects intracellular cerebral water content.
Oxygen deprivation	All aspects of cardiopulmonary system may be involved. Severe anemia, decreased cardiac output due to poor myocardial contractility, and arrhythmias. Cerebral hypoperfusion secondary to medications. Rapid increases in CO_2 despite adequate O_2 will alter mental status.
Endocrine disorders	Rapid changes in serum sodium affect osmolality and cerebral water content. Hypothyroidism: gradual alteration of mental status. Hyperthyroidism: generally agitated and tremulous state; coma not seen until the patient is in extremely advanced disease.
Carcinoma	Remote effect of carcinoma and alteration of osmolality (i.e., syndrome of inappropriate secretion of antidiuretic hormone). Metabolic alkalosis with Cushing syndrome. Hyper- and hypocalcemic states may alter consciousness, but progressive multifocal leukoencephalopathies seen with lymphomas may present as depression of consciousness.
Poisons and toxins	Alcohol still most widely used and commonly seen metabolic poison, relatively short duration. Barbiturate comas may be of several weeks' duration.
Central nervous system infections	Meningitis (bacterial, viral, tuberculous, and fungal infections; acquired immunodeficiency syndrome: encephalopathy); mechanism poorly understood.

TABLE 199.2. Structural Disease

Structural Problem	Significant Differential Elements
Subdural empyema	Recent otolaryngologic surgery, particularly involving sinuses. Meningitis not associated with focal neurologic findings, but findings become localized when empyema forms. *Streptococcus* most common offending organism.
Subdural hematoma	Suspect in trauma, elderly patients, alcoholics, and patients on anticoagulants. Even if no focal neurologic findings, consider subdural hematoma in these groups. Bilateral subdural hematomas may compress structures diffusely, thus presenting much like a dementia or progressive encephalopathy. History of trauma, although helpful, is not necessary. In chronic subdural hematomas, symptoms can fluctuate mildly from day to day.[21]
Epidural hematoma	Almost always related to major trauma; bleeding usually rapid in onset and related to involvement of the middle meningeal artery due to fractures in the basilar skull. Rapid downhill course generally seen.[12]
Cerebrovascular accidents (CVAs)	Most thrombotic or embolic CVAs do not involve significant alteration of consciousness. Hemorrhagic CVAs commonly associated with unconsciousness. Bleeding associated with hypertension often does not disclose a discrete lesion.[1] Controlled reduction of blood pressure may be important in patients becoming progressively more obtunded.
Intraventricular hemorrhage	Associated with poor prognosis and increased intracranial pressure. Clinically difficult to differentiate intraventricular hemorrhage from pontine bleeding without CT scanning.
Cerebral neoplasms	Neoplasms (primary or more commonly metastatic) are rare causes of coma. More common for patient to present with a seizure and postictal depression that leads to the diagnosis of tumor during radiologic evaluation. Slow-growing superventricular tumors may produce mental status changes over time. Tumors in lateral and third ventricles may obstruct flow and cause acute pressure changes with rapidly deteriorating symptoms. In rare cases, the tumor infiltrates reticular activating formation, causing irreversible coma.
Infratentorial compressive syndromes	Infratentorial compressive causes of coma are lesions that do not usually originate within the brain stem itself and by their proximity may compress the brain.
Basilar artery occlusion	Basilar artery represents principal blood supply to the brainstem through the vertebrobasilar system. Supplies blood to the reticular activating formation, necessary for consciousness. Posterior circulation transient ischemic episodes may present as drop attacks.
Traumatic posterior fossa hemorrhage	Severe trauma may lead to hemorrhage without the destruction of the brainstem proper. Decreased mental status due to external compression of the brainstem represents a surgically correctable cause of coma. Requires timely diagnosis.
Acute cerebellar hemorrhage	Bleeding into the cerebellum usually is a result of an arteriovenous malformation. Head pain with sudden vertigo and conjugate deviation of the eyes to the opposite side of the cerebellar lesion strongly suggest acute bleeding. Most treatable of the intraparenchymal hemorrhages.[15]
Pontine hemorrhage	Devastating brainstem parenchymal lesion, difficult to initially separate from acute cerebellar hemorrhage or other forms of posterior fossa hemorrhage. Sudden decrease in consciousness, ataxia, irregular breathing, nonreactive pinpoint pupils, absent oculovestibular responses.
Brainstem tumors	Acute parenchymal lesions of brainstem (i.e., angiomas, gliomas, ependymomas) causing brainstem compression or destruction of actual pathways. Other posterior fossa tumors, including meningiomas and acoustic neuromas, generally present with cranial nerve findings before alteration of mental status.

Some patients appear awake but have psychogenic unresponsiveness (previously called the catatonic state). The level of unresponsiveness may vary; the patient may maintain normal motor posturing and neurologic testing but, for voluntary or involuntary reasons, cannot communicate with the examiner. Common psychiatric practice in the past was to use psychotropic medication to disinhibit such patients and to allow communication.

Patients may have altered mental status without actual depression of mentation. Acute confusional states exist in which the patient is alert and active but misinterprets external stimuli. The hallmark of such confusional states is global disorientation with an inability to appropriately process stimuli or an inability to make meaningful responses. Such findings are characteristic of toxic ingestions and metabolic encephalopathy and occasionally accompany central nervous system infections.

It is often a challenge to distinguish mental status changes caused by structural or chemical disease from those that are the result of psychological processes. The terms *encephalopathy* and *delirium* should be reserved for the former. In general, these organically based changes in mental status can be differentiated from psychological problems by certain characteristics.

An important difference has to do with *orientation*. In organic disease, orientation is virtually always lost in a predictable manner: Orientation to time is almost always lost before orientation to specific place, generic place, or person. When there is a loss of orientation that does not follow the expected order (i.e., time, specific place, generic place, and person), a psychological component should be suspected.

In contrast, abnormal *vital signs* should always raise suspicion of an organic process. Vital signs should be reassessed frequently as a usual part of patient evaluation. Be aware of the patient with altered vital signs who is diagnosed as having a "psychiatric condition."

Speech is perhaps the most sensitive indicator in differentiating between organic and psychiatric disease. Patients with an organic alteration of mental status generally have globally slowed speech patterns. There are often problems with articulation, particularly in toxic–metabolic encephalopathies. Speech that is rapid, well articulated, and well enunciated indicates that the vast majority of the nervous system is functioning normally. Even patients with severe psychiatric disorders often speak rapidly, clearly, and without any obvious hesitation.[6]

Thought content, as well as the way in which it is articulated, can also be extremely helpful. Patients with organic lesions rarely display bizarre or unusual ideation or associations and rarely have complex delusional systems. Patients with organic depression generally display a paucity of ideas or thought but no depressive content, morbid fears, or ideation.

Finally, the pattern of any *changes* in mental status provides important information. A progressive decline of alertness and slowing of mental activity are characteristic of organic neurologic disease. Similarly, many organic toxic–metabolic conditions (e.g., alcohol or drug intoxication) tend to improve progressively with time. Clouding of consciousness and a waxing and waning of alertness are also characteristic of delirium, however. In contrast, psychiatric patients often display moment-to-moment alterations in behavior that tend in different directions at different times. The psychiatrically unstable patient may be extremely active one minute and essentially catatonic the next. Thus, psychiatric disease must be a consideration if there are rapid up-and-down changes in alertness or behavior.

TABLE 199.3. Initial Evaluation and Management for Patients with Altered Mental Status

- Initial management
  - Airway established
  - Breathing checked (including auscultation to rule out pneumothorax)
  - Cardiac output assessed
  - Cervical spine immobilized
  - Obvious hemorrhage compressed
  - Intravenous line started
  - Vital signs (full set)
  - Thiamine, 100 mg i.v.
  - Glucose, 50 mL 50% i.v.
  - Naloxone, 2 ampules i.v. repeated if no response[11,16]
- The stable patient
  - Historic features obtained, including rate of onset, drugs, trauma, fever, prior episodes
- General physical examination
  - Signs of trauma: Battle sign, hemotympanum, scalp hematomas and lacerations, subcutaneous emphysema of the chest, etc.
  - Obvious lesions of the abdomen, lesions of the pelvis, and long-bone injuries
- Skin
  - Needle marks, cyanosis, pallor, rashes, dehydration
- Breath odors
  - Alcohol, acetone, fecal material, fetor hepaticus
- Cardiac examination
  - Rhythm, signs of decreased output, ausculation—endocarditis, valvular disease
- Abdominal findings
  - Organomegaly, ascites, bruits, flank ecchymoses (Grey Turner sign), rectal and pelvic examination as time permits
- Neurologic examination
  - Observation
  - Respiratory pattern[3,14,18]
    - Normal, Cheyne-Stokes, hyperventilation, apneustic breathing, ataxic breathing, agonal breathing
  - Automatisms
    - Yawning, coughing, hiccupping, vomiting
  - Mental status
    - Responds to voice, responds to touch, responds to noxious stimuli
  - Cranial nerves
    - Visual threat, inspection of fundi for papilledema and hemorrhages
  - Pupils
    - Size, reactions (direct and consensual)[4,8]
  - Extraocular movements[8]
    - Oculovestibular testing
    - Oculocephalic testing (if appropriate)
  - Corneal reflex
  - Facial asymmetry
  - Motor system
    - Posturing, ability of the limbs to move, stimuli[5]
  - Decerebration, decortication, or true abduction by high-level centers
  - Pathologic reflexes

DIFFERENTIAL DIAGNOSIS

There is a vast array of chemical agents and disease entities that can alter mental status. The emergency physician must have a basic framework in which to place all of these before considering the individual causes. From an operational standpoint, the neurologic examination and laboratory studies divide the causes of altered mental status into toxic–metabolic diseases and infratentorial lesions that affect the reticular activating formation (Tables 199.1 and 199.2).

EMERGENCY DEPARTMENT EVALUATION AND MANAGEMENT

Emergency department evaluation of the patient with severely depressed mental status or coma requires a systematic approach. The principles of management are to support the patient's airway, breathing, and circulation; treat most obvious

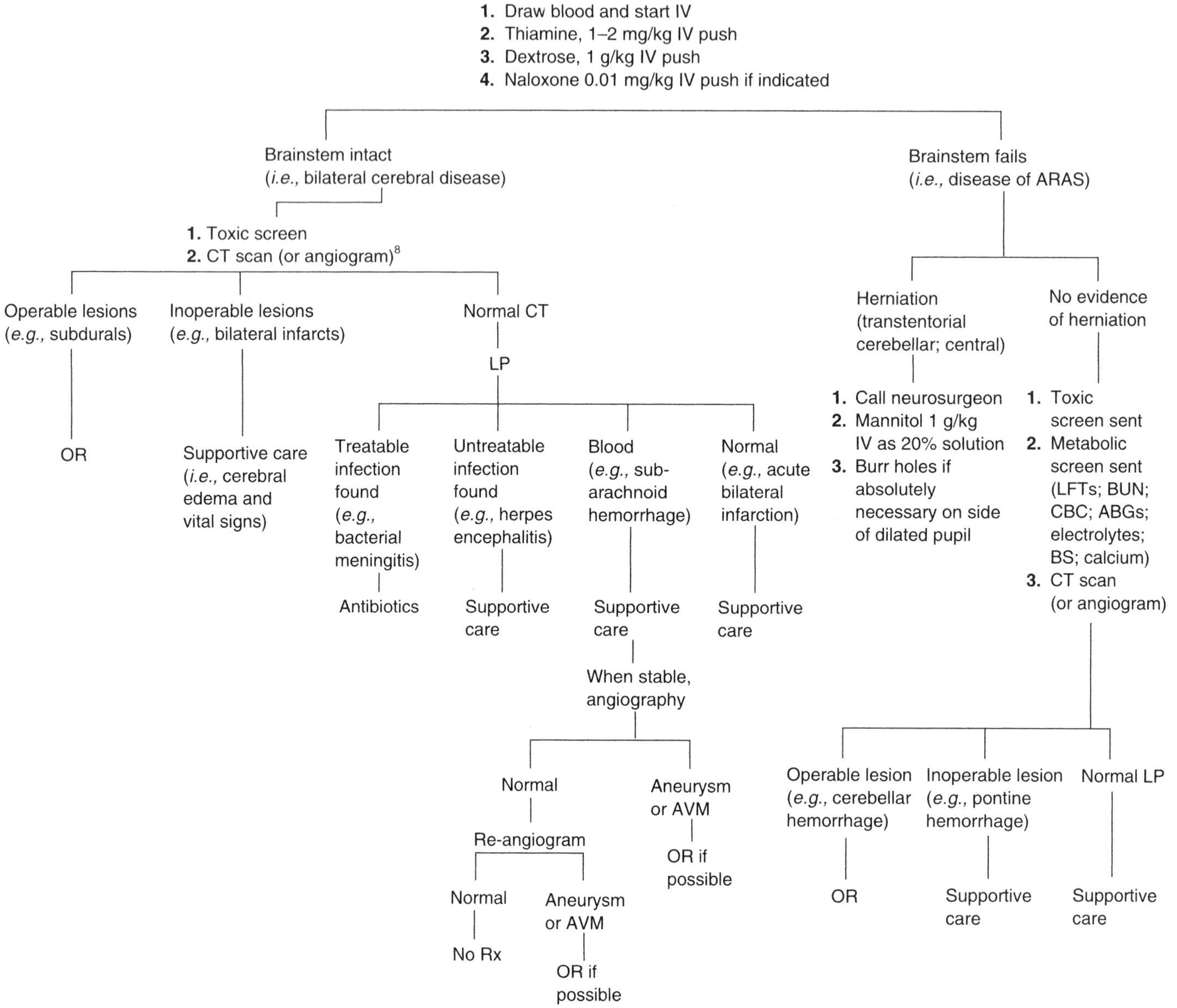

Figure 199.1. Diagnostic and treatment approach to coma.

causes first; perform a detailed examination; produce the specific diagnosis; and begin specific therapy. Table 199.3 lists initial management steps, both supportive and diagnostic measures, that should be performed on such patients.[10,11]

After initial supportive measures and examination, decisions on further examination must be made (Fig. 199.1).[17] The first step is to separate patients who have intact brainstem function from those who do not. As the algorithm of Fig. 199.1 shows, patients with acute brainstem failure can then be divided into those with obvious herniation syndromes or signs of transtentorial herniation and those without such findings. Patients without evidence of herniation require toxic–metabolic screens and a computed tomographic (CT) scan. Normothermic patients who have not received neurologically active drugs and have no brainstem reflexes are considered to have unsalvageable brain tissue.[2] Patients with evidence of focal herniation require immediate neurosurgical consultation; mannitol may be given if recommended by the neurosurgeon. In the patient who has developed the complete tentorial herniation syndrome, if an operating room is not immediately available, burr hole decompression on the side of the dilated pupil should be considered.

Similar decisions must be made about patients whose brainstem reflexes are intact. If CT scan results are normal, a lumbar puncture may be done. Bloody cerebrospinal fluid and a CT scan without a focal finding indicate subarachnoid hemorrhage. If the patient's condition is stable, angiography can be done; if a focal aneurysm or arterial venous malformation is found, surgery should be a serious consideration.

For patients with intact brainstem reflexes and initially positive CT scans, the neurosurgeon should decide whether the offending lesion is operable or inoperable.

In those patients who, after testing, are found to have toxic–metabolic conditions, appropriate medical therapy should be instituted without delay.

DISPOSITION

Consultation is immediately required on any potentially operable focal lesions, and immediate contact with a neurosurgeon is essential if the brain is to be saved. In patients in whom there is no surgically treatable disease, consultation with either a neurologist or internist for intensive care unit admission is indicated.

All patients with significantly altered mental status require admission after definitive diagnosis for continued evaluation and treatment.

When transferring comatose patients, it is important to provide basic support. Such patients generally require definitive airway control before transfer. Rapid transfer to a center with neurologic and neurosurgical diagnostic and treatment capabilities is essential in patients with potentially surgically treatable disease.

COMMON PITFALLS

- A major mistake is to wait for laboratory results when physical examination findings clearly point to a focal process requiring immediate surgical intervention. Many things in the evaluation of the comatose patient must be done simultaneously, and to wait for the sequential return of tests may doom the patient to permanent neurologic damage or death.
- Another common pitfall is failure to treat common causes first. Proper establishment of an airway, cardiovascular support, and provision of adequate oxygen and glucose are critical to proper care of the patient with severely altered mental status.[12,13]
- The most critical common pitfall in the evaluation of altered mental status is failure to reexamine the patient at intervals. Close attention to changes in level of consciousness, vital signs, speech patterns, and thought content is often helpful in separating organic from psychiatric conditions.

References

1. Adams RD. Aneurysmal subarachnoid hemorrhage. *Mod Concepts Cardiovasc Dis* 1981;50:49.
2. Bird TD, Plum F. Recovery from barbiturate overdose and with a prolonged isoelectric electroencephalogram. *Neurology* 1968;18:456.
3. Brown HW, Plum F. The neurologic basis of Cheyne-Stokes respiration. *Am J Med* 1961;30:849.
4. Byrnes D. Head injury and the dilated pupil. *Am Surg* 1979;45:139.
5. Davis RA, et al. Decerebrate rigidity in humans. *Neurosurgery* 1982;10:635.
6. Dziedzic L, et al. The use of the Mini-Mental status examination in the ED evaluation of the elderly. *Am J Emerg Med* 1998;16:686.
7. Feldman MH. Physiological observations in a chronic case of locked-in syndrome. *Neurology* 1971;21:459.
8. Fisher CM. Some neuro-ophthalmological observations. *J Neurol Neurosurg Psychiatry* 1967;30:383.
9. Fisher CM. The neurological examination of the comatose patient. *Acta Neurol Scand* 1969;45[Suppl 36]:1.
10. Gueye PN, et al. Empiric use of flumazenil in comatose patients: limited applicability of criteria to define low risk. *Ann Emerg Med* 1996;27(6):730.
11. Hoffman RS, et al. The poisoned patient with altered consciousness: controversies in the use of a "coma cocktail." *JAMA* 1995;274(7):562.
12. Jameson KG, Yelland JD. Extradural hematoma: report of 167 cases. *J Neurosurg* 1968;29:13.
13. Jefferson G. The tentorial pressure cone. *Arch Neurol Psychiatry* 1938;40:857.
14. Maragos GD. The unconscious child. *Pediatrics* 1978;8:142.
15. McKissock W, Richardson A, Walsh L. Spontaneous cerebellar hemorrhage: a study of 34 consecutive cases treated surgically. *Brain* 1960;83:1.
16. Moore RA, et al. Naloxone: underdosage after narcotic poisoning. *Am J Dis Child* 1980;134:156.
17. Plum F, Swenson AG. Central neurogenic hyperventilation in man. *Arch Neurol Psychiatry* 1959;81:535.
18. Plum F, Alvord EC. Apneustic breathing in man. *Arch Neurol* 1964;10:101.
19. Plum F, Posner J. *Diagnosis of stupor and coma,* 2nd ed. Philadelphia: FA Davis Co, 1972.
20. Shaffer MA. Limitation of the cross-table lateral view in detecting cervical spine injuries: a retrospective analysis. *Ann Emerg Med* 1981;10:508.
21. Vicario S, et al. Emergency presentation of subdural hematoma. *Ann Emerg Med* 1982;11:45.

CHAPTER 200
Organic Brain Syndrome

Sandra M. Schneider

Organic brain syndrome is a disorder of orientation, memory, intellect, judgment, and affect resulting from diffuse impairment of brain tissue.[5] This impairment leads to an altered mental status (either lethargy or excitement), confused thinking, and/or abnormal behavior. Organic brain syndrome may occur at any age. Although every intoxicated patient seen in the emergency department could be said to have "organic brain syndrome," the term is more commonly applied to older or debilitated patients in whom the etiology is less obvious.

CLINICAL PRESENTATION

Of the several types of organic brain syndrome, the two most important to emergency physicians are dementia and delirium. Tables 200.1 and 200.2 illustrate the important differences between dementia and delirium. The distinction is extremely important for diagnosis, prognosis, and determination of the need for hospitalization and treatment. Table 200.3 summarizes the clinical characteristics of delirium, dementia, and psychosis.

Dementia is the chronic insidious loss of intellectual function. Common causes are listed in Table 200.4. Correctable causes of dementia include thyroid dysfunction, vitamin deficiencies, and normal pressure hydrocephalus. Memory is impaired, along with other higher cerebral functions, such as abstract thinking, judgment, and personality. Although dementia is slow in onset and there may be fluctuations in mental function, complete return of normal function is rare. Patients are generally oriented and aware of their environment until quite late in the disease.[11] Some patients experience depression as they try to make sense of their impaired mental function and become fearful of their future dependence. This depression may then lead to additional alterations in affect.

Delirium, in contrast, is of acute onset and is transient, and recovery is common.[13] The majority of patients with delirium and no underlying dementia are able to return to independent living. Common causes are listed in Table 200.5. Delirium has been characterized as the loss of selective attention, that function that maintains coherent thought, orientation to surround-

TABLE 200.1. Diagnostic Criteria for Delirium (as defined by DSM-IV)

A. Disturbance of consciousness (i.e., reduced clarity of awareness of environment) with reduced ability to focus, sustain, or shift attention.
B. A change in cognition (such as memory deficit, disorientation, language disturbance) or the development of a perceptual disturbance that is not better accounted for by a preexisting, established, or evolving dementia.
C. The disturbance develops over a short period of time (usually hours to days) and tends to fluctuate during the course of the day.

From *Diagnostic and statistical manual of mental disorders*, 4th ed. Washington, DC: American Psychiatric Association, 1994.

TABLE 200.2. Diagnostic Criteria for Dementia (as defined by DSM-IV)

A. The development of multiple cognitive deficits manifested by both:
 1. memory impairment (impaired ability to learn new information or to recall previously learned information)
 2. one (or more) of the following cognitive disturbances:
  a. aphasia (language disturbance)
  b. apraxia (impaired ability to carry out motor activities despite intact motor function)
  c. agnosia (failure to recognize or identify objects despite intact sensory function)
  d. disturbance in executive functioning (i.e., planning, organizing, sequencing, abstracting)
B. The cognitive deficits in Criteria A1 and A2 each cause significant impairment in social or occupational functioning and represent a significant decline from a previous level of functioning.
C. The deficits do not occur exclusively during the course of a delirium.

From *Diagnostic and statistical manual of mental disorders*, 4th ed. Washington, DC: American Psychiatric Association, 1994.

ings, and organization of memory and perception.[9] Patients with delirium have a decreased ability to interact with the outside world. There is fluctuating level of consciousness, memory disturbance, decreased ability to shift or maintain attention, and, frequently, behavioral changes. Sleep–wake cycles become disturbed early.

Delirium is a common presenting complaint in the elderly. Approximately one in six elderly persons are delirious when admitted to the hospital,[12] and many (55%) develop acute confusion while hospitalized.[4] Dementia is also common, affecting one in 20 patients over the age of 65 and 20% of patients over the age of 80.[10] Delirium does occur in patients with dementia, presenting as an acute, often reversible worsening of the mental status. Mortality for patients with delirium is extremely high, two to five times higher than for age-matched controls, because of the severity of the underlying disease.[8]

It is often difficult in the emergency department to differentiate between acute delirium and the more chronic dementia.

TABLE 200.3. Clinical Characteristics of Delirium, Dementia, and Psychosis

Dellrium	Dementia	Psychosis
ONSET		
Rapid	Slow	Rapid
PATTERN		
Fluctuating	Fluctuating or stable	Stable
ORIENTED		
No	Yes	No
ATTENTION		
Disordered	Normal	Delusional
COGNITION		
Disordered impaired	Impaired	Selectively
SPEECH		
Incoherent	Perseveration	Rapid, pressured

TABLE 200.4. Common Causes of Dementia and Their Characteristics

ALZHEIMER DISEASE

Nonspecific dementia; insidiously worsening symptoms

PICK DISEASE

Generally more personality change than in Alzheimer's. Computed tomography often shows focal frontal and/or anterior temporal atrophy.

EXTRAPYRAMIDAL SYNDROMES WITH SUBCORTICAL DEMENTIA

Includes Parkinson disease, Wilson disease, and Huntington disease

MULTIPLE-INFARCT DEMENTIA

Highly variable presentation, often with stepwise deterioration and fluctuating course; may have history of previous cerebrovascular accidents or transient ischemic attacks. Focal neurologic deficits or pseudobulbar palsy may appear.

VIRUSES AND OTHER INFECTIOUS AGENTS

Includes progressive multifocal leukoencephalopathy (associated with human immunodeficiency virus), Jakob–Creutzfeldt disease, syphilitic general paresis, tuberculosis, fungi, and parasites

TOXIC AGENTS AND DEMENTIAS

Includes heavy metals, chronic drug abuse, industrial agents

METABOLIC DISORDERS

Includes dialysis dementia, hypothyroidism, hyperparathyroidism, porphyria, uremia, and hepatic encephalopathy

VITAMIN DEFICIENCIES

Vitamin B_{12}, folate, and niacin deficiencies

CENTRAL NERVOUS SYSTEM STRUCTURAL CHANGES

Hydrocephalus (obstructive and nonobstructive), head injury, neoplastic disorders, myelin disorders, and multiple sclerosis

PSYCHIATRIC DISORDERS

Depression, mania, schizophrenia, and hysteria

Patients with chronic dementia may develop acute delirium from very minor insults; the change may be discovered only after conversation with family or friends or after review of previous medical records.[14] The progressive cognitive deficiency of chronic mild dementia is often missed by examining physicians and denied or hidden by caring family members until a home crisis or acute delirium results in an emergency department visit.

DIFFERENTIAL DIAGNOSIS

Virtually every medical disease has been known to cause acute deterioration of mental status in a previously functional person, particularly in the elderly. Often, a minor event or illness can cause a functional elderly person to become disorganized and disoriented; there are several causes that, in combination, can lead to delirium.

Medications are, by far, the most common cause of acute delirium in patients without underlying dementia. Those drugs most commonly incriminated are the anticholinergic agents, especially those found in over-the-counter preparations. The elderly are particularly prone to confusion and hallucinations,

TABLE 200.5. Causes of Delirium

DRUG-INDUCED
Anticholinergics
Narcotic analgesics
Sedative hypnotics
Corticosterolds
Histamine blockers
Antibiotics
Cardiovascular drugs
INFECTION
Pneumonia
Urinary tract infection
Sepsis
FLUID AND ELECTROLYTE IMBALANCE
Dehydration
Hypoglycemia
Hyperglycemia
Hyponatremia
DRUG WITHDRAWAL
Alcohol
Narcotics
CENTRAL NERVOUS SYSTEM DISTURBANCES
Seizure activity
Cerebrovascular accident
PSYCHIATRIC DISEASE
Sensory deprivation
Depression
Mania
OTHER CAUSES
Vasculitis
Collagen vascular diseases
Encephalitis
Meningitis

even when taking therapeutic doses of anticholinergic medications. Other medications that have some anticholinergic side effects may cause similar symptoms. Meperidine, cimetidine, and ranitidine have anticholinergic properties, making them likely to cause delirium. Despite their sensitivity to anticholinergic medications, nearly 60% of nursing home residents and 23% of ambulatory elderly are prescribed drugs with anticholinergic properties.[3]

Nearly every drug can cause acute delirium in the elderly. In addition to anticholinergics, narcotics, nonnarcotic analgesics, sedative–hypnotics, corticosteroids, lithium, histamine blockers, antibiotics, and cardiovascular drugs, including antihypertensive agents, are commonly incriminated.[8,15]

Among younger individuals, trauma and medications, drug use, or poisonings are the leading causes of altered mental status; they often occur together. Infection is the second most common cause of delirium and is particularly common in patients with underlying dementia.[14] The infection need not be impressive or even physiologically apparent; fever and tachycardia are often absent. The urinary tract is the most common site,[14] and infection there is often asymptomatic in the elderly. Pneumonia is another common infection in the elderly, again often asymptomatic. Mental confusion may be the earliest sign of sepsis.[14]

Fluid and electrolyte imbalances can cause delirium and are found in patients with or without underlying dementia. Dehydration can arise from minor viral illnesses or diuretic therapy. Hyponatremia is particularly common after surgery, due to excessive use of hypotonic hydration.[2] Burns, trauma (major or minor), recent minor surgery, myocardial infarction, or steroid use may result in steroid (catecholamine) excess, hyperglycemia, and insulin resistance. Drug withdrawal, more commonly seen in younger individuals, causes delirium. Drugs and alcohol use are generally suspected or known by family members and friends, but in more socially isolated elderly, the use of illicit drugs or alcohol may go undiscovered. Patients may withhold information, fearing embarrassment; families may deny their suspicion of substance abuse.

Central nervous system (CNS) causes of acute alterations in mental status are relatively rare. The postictal state observed after grand mal seizure activity is rarely difficult to diagnose, but psychomotor seizures may be more subtle. Up to 20% of elderly patients with status epilepticus have nonconvulsive status.[8] Many patients, even elderly ones, have petit mal seizures.[8] Patients with cerebrovascular accidents can occasionally present with an acute organic brain syndrome in the absence of paralysis or other neurologic impairment.[8] Cerebrovascular accidents, particularly of the nondominant hemisphere in the area of the perisylvian cortex, can cause delirium without focality.[6]

Human immunodeficiency virus (HIV)–infected individuals are particularly prone to develop acute delirium. The differential diagnosis is quite different in these patients. Nearly 60% of patients with the acquired immunodeficiency syndrome (AIDS) develop neurologic deficits; up to 90% of patients have neuropathologic changes at autopsy. CNS infection is the most common cause of dementia and delirium and includes cryptococcal meningitis, toxoplasmosis, progressive multifocal leukoencephalopathy, cytomegalovirus, herpetic infections, and viral meningitis. CNS structural disease (including CNS lymphoma and AIDS dementia complex) leads to slow deterioration, but mental status changes may become acutely perceived by family or friends.

Psychiatric disease accounts for a small minority of the patients with acute organic brain syndrome. However, psychosocial factors may contribute significantly to the severity of confusion. Sensory impairment from poor vision or decreased hearing is common in the elderly. This may contribute to a patient's disorientation and confusion, making only minor confusion significantly worse.[8] Likewise, sensory deprivation caused by institutionalization or decreased mobility and social contact may contribute to cognitive impairment. "Sundowning," the onset of acute disorientation at night, is more common in patients with chronic mild dementia. This classic presentation in the hospitalized elderly is thought to be caused by a decrease in orienting stimuli at night and exacerbated by unfamiliar surroundings and disturbed sleep–wake cycles. Although sundowning is primarily associated with dementia, patients with acute delirium may also become more confused in new surroundings when orienting stimuli are diminished.

Finally, in up to 50% of patients with acute delirium, no cause can be identified.

EMERGENCY DEPARTMENT EVALUATION

A careful history should be obtained from the patient, family members, friends, neighbors, medical records, primary care physicians, or emergency medical services personnel. The goal of the history is to (1) establish the preexisting mental status; (2) establish the time pattern of the onset of the altered mental status; (3) establish rapport with the patient and with the family to avoid unnecessary restraints or sedating medications; and (4) identify current medical problems, medications (particularly over-the-counter medications), and stresses in the patient's life that may have predisposed to the alteration in mental status.

Some families may engage in denial about preexisting dementia symptoms or try to hide suspected drug or alcohol use. Access to alcohol, over-the-counter drugs, and prescription drugs, including narcotics, is an important clue to the diagnosis.

The physical examination should be directed at two items: establishing the existence and severity of delirium or dementia and identifying potential causes. Hypothermia or hyperthermia suggests sepsis or environmentally based disease. Some infections may be inapparent, and evidence for them should be sought (e.g., decubiti, dental caries, and perirectal disease). Even benign-looking decubiti should be examined thoroughly for underlying purulence. Fecal impaction may contribute to acute delirium, particularly in patients with underlying dementia. Rectal examination with disimpaction is appropriate in all patients.

The best way to assess the presence of an altered mental status is to use the Mini-Mental Status examination (Table 200.6).[7] This test has a high sensitivity (87%) and specificity (82%) when compared with a psychiatrist's opinion of the presence of delirium.[1] One of the earliest signs of acute delirium is the inability to recall three items after 3 minutes. Acute delirium can fluctuate rapidly; the patient who is currently lucid may be quite different 1 or 2 hours later.

The laboratory evaluation of patients with acute delirium should be directed at uncovering the cause or causes of the delirium. A tiered approach to laboratory ordering is perhaps best. The initial evaluation should include a complete blood cell count and differential; determination of levels of electrolytes and glucose; renal and liver function tests; and urinalysis (with culture when pyuria is present). When indicated, a chest radiograph, an electrocardiogram, and an arterial blood gas analysis should be performed. Patients with headache or a history of head trauma should have an urgent computed tomographic scan of the head. In debilitated, chronically ill, or malnourished individuals, knowledge of magnesium, calcium, and phosphorus levels may be helpful. Patients with no obvious cause of their mental status change should have computed tomography of the head, sedimentation rate determination, a serum and urine osmolality study (to screen for toxins such as methanol and ethylene glycol), and a toxicology screen, including levels of prescription drugs normally taken. Febrile patients warrant a more aggressive workup, often including a lumbar puncture if no other source of fever has been discovered or if there are signs of CNS infection or immunosuppression. HIV-positive individuals should have an early computed tomographic scan of the head and lumbar puncture. Finally, patients still without an obvious cause may require thyroid function tests, vitamin B_{12} and folate levels, and, if indicated, heavy-metal screens. The results of some of these tests will not be immediately available and are often best ordered in consultation with the primary physician. Electroencephalographic evaluation may be beneficial in selected patients to distinguish between fast activity (seen in drug-withdrawal states) and slow activity (seen with either toxic or other physiologic causes of acute delirium) and to detect the occasional patient with nonconvulsive status epilepticus.

TABLE 200.6. Mini-Mental Status Examination

	Maximum Points
ORIENTATION	
What is the year, date, day, month?	5
Where are we: state, country, town, hospital, floor?	5
REGISTRATION	
Recalling 3 objects immediately	3
ATTENTION	
Serial 7s or spell "world" backward	5
RECALL	
Renaming the above 3 objects after another exercise	3
LANGUAGE	
Name a pencil and a wristwatch	2
Repeat "no ifs, ands, or buts"	1
Follow 3 state commands (e.g., take a paper in your right hand, fold it in half, and put it on the floor)	3
Read and obey "close your eyes"	1
Write a sentence (not dictated)	1
Copy a design	1

EMERGENCY DEPARTMENT MANAGEMENT

Management should be directed toward three basic goals. As always, the first is to search for and correct potentially life-threatening causes (e.g., hypoxemia, temperature abnormalities, hypotension). The second goal is to discover and treat the underlying cause of delirium. All patients should have a bedside test to determine the serum glucose concentration or receive 50% dextrose. Naloxone should be given to any patient with a seriously depressed level of consciousness and possible narcotic exposure and to comatose patients for diagnostic purposes. In patients in whom the cause is obvious (e.g., infection, fluid or electrolyte imbalance), definitive treatment should eventually return the patient to a baseline state. Patients in whom the cause is less obvious may require a different approach. In these cases, it may be necessary to discontinue, or at least decrease, the dose of all medications with the potential to cause delirium. Patients identified as suffering from anticholinergic-induced delirium should be placed in a safe environment while the drug clears the body. Reversal of anticholinergic effects with physostigmine should be reserved for life-threatening arrhythmias and should not be used as a test for anticholinergic toxicity nor to reverse delirium. Administration of physostigmine can cause seizures and sudden death.

The final goal of management is to protect the patient while diagnostic evaluation and therapy proceed. Patients should be oriented to their new surroundings (the emergency department) to reduce anxiety. Patients should be kept in a well-lit room with as little extraneous noise as possible. Those who use hearing devices or glasses should be encouraged to wear them. Caregivers should be careful to introduce themselves and to explain their role and any planned procedures. Family and friends should be allowed to remain with the patient or to visit frequently.

Restraints may be necessary to control potentially dangerous behavior (e.g., wandering) and to prevent falls from bed. There are two types of restraints, physical and chemical, and the use of either should be reserved for patients who present a danger to themselves or whose behavior is extraordinarily disruptive. When physical restraints are used, there should be clear documentation on the chart stating their necessity. Explanation should be given to family members and visitors, as well as to other patients and visitors in close proximity to the patient. Mildly confused individuals can be reminded by soft restraints to stay in bed. More aggressive devices involving a netlike blanket or leather restraints can be used to control and protect more aggressive patients.

Chemical sedation is often preferable to physical restraints but may further add to the patient's confusion, and certainly will not aid in establishing the diagnosis. The ideal sedating drug would be one that calms the patient without worsening delirium, and it would have no anticholinergic or extrapyramidal side effects. The ideal drug could be given parenterally with no effect on blood pressure, the heart, or the respiratory system. Unfortunately, such ideal therapy does not exist. Haloperidol (5 to 10 mg intramuscularly) and droperidol (5 mg intramuscularly) are the agents most commonly used for acute sedation. Peak effect occurs at 30 minutes, and the dose can be repeated at that time. Major side effects include orthostatic hypotension, a decrease in seizure threshold, and, rarely, neuroleptic malignant syndrome. Other side effects of haloperidol or droperidol include dystonic reactions and akathisia. As an alternative, a benzodiazepine such as lorazepam (0.5 to 1.0 mg intramuscularly) can be given initially and repeated every hour. It can be used alone or as an adjunct to haloperidol. Several other psychotropic drugs, including chlorpromazine and thioridazine, have also been used for acute sedation.

DISPOSITION

Disposition is determined by the presence or suspicion of a serious underlying disease, the abruptness with which the organic brain syndrome has developed, and the ability of family and caretakers to provide a safe environment for the patient.

The following patients are likely to require admission:

Patients with identified infection, fluid or electrolyte imbalance, or CNS structural disease

Patients with acute confusion and no obvious underlying etiology, provided the confusion is significant or appropriate close follow-up is not available

Patients with a preexisting normal mental status who experience acute delirium, unless the delirium can be cleared while in the emergency department (e.g., as with hypoglycemia)

The chronically demented person who has not experienced an acute deterioration, but is often brought to the emergency department by exhausted caretakers looking for relief. The patient or family may have previously refused or been denied assistance through social services or long-term care placement.

In some hospitals, there are on-call teams to assist with the disposition of these individuals. However, without proper backup, many emergency physicians are forced to hospitalize such patients when caretakers are unable or unwilling to provide a safe environment for them.

COMMON PITFALLS

- Failure to appreciate the patient's true baseline mental status. It is often necessary to call neighbors and friends, rather than to rely on visiting, distant relatives.
- Failure to obtain a complete medication history, including the use of over-the-counter medications
- Failure to suspect substance abuse. Narcotics given for chronic pain relief may be abused or overused. Illicit drugs or alcohol may be used surreptitiously, often as self-treatment for depression.
- Failure to use appropriate restraints, leading to further injury of the patient within the emergency department. Soft restraints should be used on any confused patient who is not under direct observation by either staff or family at all times. More aggressive physical restraints, or chemical restraints, should be used as necessary to protect patients and others.
- Refusing admission to a patient in need
- Failure to recognize that patients with acute delirium are often able to return to baseline functional status
- Allowing admission decisions to become emotionally charged
- Failure to diagnose head trauma. Remote, seemingly minor injuries may lead to chronic subdural hematoma, leading to slow deterioration over a period of weeks to months, particularly in the elderly.

References

1. Anthony JC, LeResche L, Niaz U, et al. Limits of the "Mini-Mental State" as a screening test for dementia and delirium among hospital patients. *Psychol Med* 1982;12:397.
2. Arieff AL. Hyponatremia, convulsions, respiratory arrest, and permanent brain damage after elective surgery in healthy women. *N Engl J Med* 1986;314:1529.
3. Blazer DG, Federspiel CF, Ray WA, et al. The risk of anticholinergic toxicity in the elderly: a study of prescribing practices in two populations. *J Gerontol* 1983;38:31.
4. Chisholm SE, Deniston OL, Igvisan RM, et al. Prevalence of confusion in elderly hospitalized patients. *J Gerontol Nurs* 1982;8:87.
5. *Diagnostic and statistical manual of mental disorders,* 4th ed. Washington, DC: American Psychiatric Association, 1994.
6. Dunner JW, Leedman PG, Edis RH. Inobvious stroke: a cause of delirium and dementia. *Aust N Z J Med* 1986;16:771.
7. Folstein MF, Folstein SE, McHugh PR. "Mini-Mental State": a practical method for grading the cognitive state of patients for the clinician. *J Psychiatr Res* 1975;12:189.
8. Francis J, Kapoor WN. Delirium in hospitalized elderly. *J Gen Intern Med* 1990;5:65.
9. Geschwind N. Disorders of attention: a frontier in neuropsychology. *Philos Trans R Soc Lond B* 1982;298:1973.
10. Inneichen B. Measuring the rising tide: how many dementia cases will there be by 2001? *Br J Psychiatry* 1987;150:193.
11. Lipowski ZJ. Delirium (acute confusional states). *JAMA* 1987;258:1789.
12. Lipowski ZJ. Delirium in older adults. *Adv Psychosom Med* 1989;19:1.
13. Lipowski ZJ. Delirium in the elderly patient. *N Engl J Med* 1989;320:578.
14. Purdie FR, Homingman B, Rosen P. Acute organic brain syndrome: a review of 100 cases. *Ann Emerg Med* 1981;10:455.
15. Rodgers PT, Brengel GR. Famotidine-associated mental status changes. *Pharmacotherapy* 1998;18:404–407.

CHAPTER 201
Headache

E. John Gallagher and Adrienne J. Birnbaum

Head pain accounts for nearly 1 million emergency department (ED) visits annually in the United States. Fortunately, the vast majority of headaches presenting to the ED do not represent serious underlying disease. The goal in managing the patient with headache in the ED is to distinguish the small fraction of patients with serious illness who require immediate diagnosis and hospitalization from the great majority in whom the clinical focus is directed toward headache-specific, short-term pain management; prophylaxis against recurrence, as indicated; explanation; reassurance; and careful follow-up.

CLASSIFICATION OF HEAD PAIN

There are multiple axes along which headaches can be classified. The International Headache Society classifies head pain into 13 categories, which are further subdivided into a total of 129 di-

TABLE 201.1. International Headache Society Classification of Headache (Abridged)

1. Migraine
   a. With aura
   b. Without aura
2. Tension-type headache
   a. Episodic
   b. Chronic
3. Cluster headache
4. Head trauma
   a. Acute posttraumatic headache
   b. Chronic posttraumatic headache
5. Headache associated with vascular disorders
   a. Subarachnoid hemorrhage
   b. Intracranial hematoma
   c. Acute ischemic cerebrovascular disease
   d. Hypertension
6. Headache associated with nonvascular disorders
   a. Infection
   b. Neoplasm
   c. High cerebrospinal fluid pressure
   d. Low cerebrospinal fluid pressure
7. Headache associated with other cranial structures
   a. Neck
   b. Eyes
   c. Sinuses
   d. Temporomandibular joint
8. Cranial neuralgias
   a. Persistent pain
   b. Episodic (tic-like) pain
9. Headache associated with substances or their withdrawal
10. Headache associated with noncephalic infection
11. Headache associated with metabolic disorder
    a. Hypoxia/hypercapnia
    b. Hypoglycemia
    c. Dialysis
12. Miscellaneous, not associated with structural lesions
    a. Cold stimulus
    b. Cough
    c. Sexual activity
13. Headache unclassifiable

Adapted from the Headache Classification Committee of the International Headache Society. Classification and diagnostic criteria for headache disorders, cranial neuralgia, and facial pain. *Cephalalgia* 1988;8[Suppl 7]:1-96.

agnostic subcategories.[8] Although this classification offers a standardized and comprehensive taxonomy of headache, it is of limited clinical value to the emergency physician. It is presented for reference in an abbreviated form in Table 201.1.

Another means of categorizing headaches is to dichotomize them into primary headaches (e.g., migraine) versus secondary (or "organic") headaches that can be attributed to some underlying cause (e.g., subarachnoid hemorrhage [SAH]).

The pain-sensitive structures of the head include the blood vessels and all extracranial structures of the head and neck. The only intracranial structures sensitive to pain are the arteries at the base of the brain, their major branches, the periarterial dura mater, and the venous sinuses. The parenchyma of the brain itself and most of its meningeal coverings are not pain-sensitive.

For many years, traditional teaching held that there were three major mechanisms of head pain: vasodilatation within the cranial vasculature, causing a "vascular" headache; spasm of the neck and scalp muscles, causing a "muscle contraction" headache; and traction on blood vessels or inflammation around or within these and other pain-sensitive structures, causing a "traction–inflammatory" headache.

In light of more recent evidence, traditional concepts of the etiology of headache in general—and migraine in particular—have given way to more evidence-based explanations in which neuropeptides, most notably serotonin, and their many central nervous system (CNS) receptors play an important, though ill-defined, role. Experimental observations of the relationship between these neural transmitters and alterations in CNS vascular tone suggest that an exclusively neurogenic or vasogenic etiology is unlikely to provide a unifying theory of head pain.[7]

Perhaps the most useful categorization scheme for the emergency physician is to classify headache into one of four groups based on the temporal profile of the pain pattern: acute single headache; acute recurrent headache; subacute headache; and chronic headache (Table 201.2).[16]

Ten worrisome headache patterns are listed in Table 201.3. Only about 1% to 5% of headaches seen in the ED will fit any of these patterns, but they are among the most important headaches to diagnose.

TABLE 201.2. Differential Diagnosis of Headache

Acute Single Headache (presenting within hours of onset)	Acute Recurrent Headache (presenting within days to weeks of onset)	Subacute Headache (presenting within weeks to months of onset)	Chronic Headache (presenting within months to years of onset)
Bacterial meningitis	Migraine	Chronic subdural hematoma	Chronic tension-type headache
Subarachnoid hemorrhage	Cluster	Brain tumor	Transformational migraine
Cerebral ischemia	Episodic tension-type headache	Brain abscess	Analgesic abuse/rebound
Hypertension	Trigeminal neuralgia	Subacute/chronic sinusitis	Depression
Narrow-angle glaucoma	Postherpetic neuralgia	Temporomandibular joint syndrome	
Optic/retrobulbar neuritis	Coital headache	Chronic posttraumatic headache	
Acute sinusitis		Headache associated with low CSF pressure	
Spontaneous dissection of cranial arteries		Idiopathic intracranial hypertension	
Acute posttraumatic headache		Temporal arteritis	
Acute headache associated with metabolic disorder		Headache in HIV-positive patients	
Acute headache associated with substances or withdrawal			

TABLE 201.3. Ten Headaches to Worry About

1. Single acute headache, characterized as "first or worst" of the patient's life
2. Single acute or subacute headache with fever unexplained by other systemic illness
3. Single acute or subacute headache with vomiting unexplained by other systemic illness
4. Any headache associated with focal findings, unless focality known to be chronic and unchanged from baseline
5. Any headache associated with abnormal mental status, unless cognitive changes are known to be chronic and unaltered from baseline
6. Any headache associated with papilledema (specific, not sensitive for increased ICP)
7. Single acute headache with pain on neck flexion, but absent on rotation
8. Subacute headache, unremitting or progressively worsening
9. Acute or subacute headache in the elderly
10. Any headache in the immunocompromised host, especially if HIV-positive or with risk factors for HIV

DIFFERENTIAL DIAGNOSIS

Acute Single Headache

Bacterial Meningitis

Diffuse headache is a characteristic but not invariable feature of meningitis. Although only about two-thirds of community-acquired cases of bacterial meningitis have the triad of fever, nuchal rigidity, and altered mental status, all patients appear to demonstrate at least one of these features. Among these, fever (greater than or equal to 37.7°C or 100°F) is present in 95%, neck stiffness in nearly 90%, and altered mental status in about 80%.[5]

Subarachnoid Hemorrhage

Headache of SAH is the prototypic "first or worst" headache of the patient's life, presenting as a "thunderclap headache" of sudden onset, often associated with nausea, vomiting, neck stiffness, and a transient or prolonged alteration of consciousness. In patients with focal findings or sustained abnormalities of consciousness, the need for a neuroimaging study is apparent. However, in the many patients without neurologic findings, this entity may be clinically indistinguishable from a first attack of migraine, particularly in the case of SAH due to bleeding from an arteriovenous malformation, which may be considerably less dramatic than that of an aneurysm.

An especially difficult challenge for the emergency physician is identification of the "sentinel leak" that precedes major hemorrhage in more than one-third of patients. Detection of this premonitory bleed presents an opportunity to prevent a neurologic catastrophe.

Cerebral Ischemia

Although about 35% of stroke patients and about 25% of patients with transient ischemic attacks experience headache, the diagnosis is usually evident because the clinical picture is dominated by focal findings. It is difficult to distinguish hemorrhagic, thrombotic, and embolic causes of headache on clinical grounds alone.

Hypertension

Most headaches in hypertensive patients are either migrainous or tension-type, and only rarely are due to elevated blood pressure. In general, hypertensive headache requires an acute elevation of diastolic pressure by about 25% above baseline or sustained elevations in excess of 130 mm Hg.

Narrow-Angle Glaucoma

Ocular or periorbital pain distinguishes headache caused by narrow-angle glaucoma, along with diminished visual acuity, a pupil that is typically fixed in midposition, an edematous ("steamy") cornea, perilimbal injection, and increased intraocular pressure. Vomiting may be the dominant feature, especially in the elderly, who may also present with altered mentation.

Optic or Retrobulbar Neuritis

In optic or retrobulbar neuritis, the characteristic feature of this ocular–periorbital headache is the "deafferented" pupil, which paradoxically dilates when a bright light is moved from the contralateral to the involved eye. In optic neuritis, there is evidence of inflammation of the disc, but in retrobulbar neuritis, the fundus may appear normal. In contrast to acute papilledema, visual acuity is usually diminished in both optic and retrobulbar neuritis.

Acute Sinusitis

Although acute sinusitis can be a difficult clinical diagnosis, sinus inflammation that presents with local pain and tenderness over the involved sinuses is usually apparent.

Spontaneous Dissection of the Cranial Arteries

Spontaneous dissection of the cranial arteries is an uncommon syndrome, often associated with surprisingly minor trauma. It is marked by sudden onset of headache associated with neck pain and focal ischemic symptoms. The pain and its location are determined by the location of the dissection in the carotid or vertebrobasilar system. In the carotid system, the pain is anterior and often accompanied by monocular symptoms, Horner syndrome, and other focal findings. With dissection in the posterior circulation, the pain is occipital and brainstem findings predominate.

Acute Headache Associated with Metabolic Disorders

Most metabolic disorders produce acute single or acute recurrent headache. Of all patients presenting to the ED with headache, just over one-third have a systemic illness, usually associated with fever, causing their head pain. Other metabolic causes of headache include hypoglycemia, hypoxia, and hypercarbia.

Acute Headache Associated with Substances or Their Withdrawal

Among substance-related headaches, the single most important entity is carbon monoxide poisoning, which is the leading toxicologic cause of accidental death in the United States. Because the temporal profile of the headache associated with chemicals, drugs, and toxins depends on the pattern of exposure and withdrawal, substance-related head pain can fit any of the four categories of headache in Table 201.2.

Acute Recurrent Headache

The differential diagnosis of acute recurrent headache includes some of the serious entities discussed previously under "Acute Single Headache": SAH presenting as recurrent sentinel bleeds; repeated transient ischemic attacks; substance-related headache, varying as a function of exposure to toxins; and, rarely, severe hypertension, if the elevations are marked and episodic.

Tumors, brain abscesses, subdural hematomas, and idiopathic intracranial hypertension (pseudotumor cerebri) can present as acute recurrent headache, but these are more commonly subacute or chronic.

The differential diagnosis of acute recurrent headache centers around the two most common primary ("nonorganic") headache syndromes seen in emergency practice: migraine and episodic tension-type headache. However, this differential may represent a distinction without a meaningful clinical difference, because there is increasing evidence that tension-type headache may represent a migraine variant.[3]

Migraine

The definition of *migraine* has been broadened in recent years. Although migraine is classically defined as a throbbing, unilateral headache, neither the quality of the pain nor its location offers as much clinical discrimination between migraine and other causes of headache as do the associated symptoms and signs.[6] During the headache, most patients complain of photophobia, phonophobia, or gastrointestinal symptoms such as nausea (90%), anorexia (75%), vomiting (60%), and diarrhea (15%). *Constitutional symptoms* occur primarily during the prodrome (which precedes the aura) and the "postdrome." These include mood changes, fatigue, myalgias, food cravings, and irritability. *Neurologic symptoms* occur mainly during the migrainous aura (which occurs in a minority of patients), and include visual phenomena such as bright sparkling lights (scintillating scotomata), jagged lines (fortification spectra), and geometric figures. A unique characteristic of migrainous visual auras is their propensity to move across the visual field and to vary in color or intensity, sometimes shifting from positive to negative phenomena (scotomata). Less common migrainous auras include motor abnormalities (hemiparesis, ophthalmoplegia, aphasia), sensory dysesthesias, and brainstem disturbances (vertigo, ataxia).

Cluster Headache

In contrast to migraine, cluster headache is uncommon, affecting about 0.1% of the population, predominantly middle-aged men. Characteristic features are listed in Table 201.4. The first episode of cluster headache may be indistinguishable from SAH or from acute orbital, periorbital, or ocular disease. Usually, however, the short-lived, self-limited nature of the headache, accompanied by the findings in Table 201.4, clarify the diagnosis before further workup is necessary.

Episodic Tension-type Headache

Formerly known as muscle contraction headache, episodic tension-type headache may represent a migraine variant.[3,13] It is usually bilateral and dull, often bandlike, and occurs without nausea or vomiting. Tenderness of the pericranial musculature may be a feature of one form of this headache, although electromyographic studies have shown more muscle contraction with typical migraines than with tension-type headaches.[12]

Trigeminal Neuralgia

Trigeminal neuralgia is prototypic facial neuralgia characterized by repetitive, unilateral, lancinating pain in the distribution of one or more branches of the trigeminal nerve. Attacks may be triggered by some minor stimulus, such as a light touch on the face.

Postherpetic Neuralgia

The syndrome of postherpetic neuralgia results from a prior attack of herpes zoster. It is characterized by dermatomal hyperesthesia and pain that is often severe.

Coital Headache

Headache that occurs immediately before, during, or shortly after orgasm is termed *coital* or *orgasmic headache*. The pain is often severe and may persist for several hours. SAH must be excluded.[10]

Subacute Headache

A new and unremitting headache that is present for weeks warrants a complete neurologic investigation, particularly in patients who do not usually suffer from headache. There are only a few entities that conform to the temporal profile of subacute headache, but most of them are worrisome.

TABLE 201.4. Principal Distinguishing Features of Cluster and Migraine Headache

Feature	Cluster	Migraine
Location of pain	Always unilateral, periorbital	Unilateral (60%) or bilateral (40%)
Age at onset	20–50 yr	10–40 yr
Sex incidence	90% male	70% female
Occurrence of attacks	Daily for several weeks to several months with headache-free intervals	Intermittent
Time of day	Often nocturnal, same time each night	Anytime
Seasonal occurrence	More common in spring and fall	No variation
Duration of pain	10 min to 3 h	4–48 h
Aura	Absent	30% of cases
Nausea or vomiting	5%	90%
Lacrimation	Frequent, unilateral	Infrequent
Nasal congestion	70%, unilateral	Uncommon
Ptosis	30%	1% to 2%
Polyuria	2%	40%
Family history of vascular headaches	7%	90%
Miosis	50%	Absent
General appearance	Agitation, pacing	Lying immobile

Adapted from Diamond S, Dalessio DJ, eds. *The practicing physician's approach to headache*, 5th ed. Baltimore: William & Wilkins, 1992:90.

Chronic Subdural Hematoma

Chronic subdurals may be produced by minor trauma, especially in the elderly. As many as half the patients have no recollection of head trauma. Focal findings are often minimal and therefore go undetected about half the time. Alterations in mental status are often subtle and may require a knowledge of the patient's baseline level of cognition to be appreciated. In elderly patients with subdurals, a gradual deterioration in mental status may be misdiagnosed as dementia.

Brain Tumor

Headache is the presenting symptom of brain tumor in about 40% of cases. Like that of other space-occupying lesions, the headache is usually mild to moderate, diffuse, and often relieved by over-the-counter analgesics, at least initially. In about 90% of patients who can adequately describe their symptoms, the headache is intermittent, dull, rarely throbbing, and sometimes worse in the morning. Nausea and vomiting occur in about half the patients. In about 25%, the headache is worsened by Valsalva maneuvers (e.g., coughing or straining).

Brain Abscess

The headache of brain abscess is similar to that of brain tumor, but it is typically accompanied by fever and other evidence of infection. Often, it is associated with a chronic focus of infection in the ears or sinuses, a cerebrospinal fluid (CSF) leak from a basilar skull fracture, or an embolic cardiac or pulmonary source.

Subacute and Chronic Sinusitis

Subacute and chronic sinusitis may not present with headache or facial pain. Consequently, it can be extremely difficult to diagnose. Pain, if present, is usually dull and pressure-like, and may be associated with nasal congestion or rhinorrhea.

Temporomandibular Joint Syndrome

Temporomandibular joint syndrome is a poorly defined syndrome that may be caused by malocclusion, which produces masseter spasm. Features of tension-type headache and depression have also been reported.

Posttraumatic Headache

Although it may present acutely, posttraumatic headache is more commonly subacute. It is no longer classified as postconcussion syndrome because loss of consciousness is not a prerequisite for its development. Symptoms are usually present within the first 24 to 48 hours postinjury and are marked by a postural component to the head pain and associated postural dizziness. Typically, symptoms are improved by lying down. Transient neurocognitive impairment, depression, irritability, and emotional lability are common. The syndrome persists for more than 2 months in 60% of patients.

Headache Associated with Low Cerebrospinal Fluid Pressure

Headache after a lumbar puncture (LP) is thought to be due to low CSF pressure resulting from a post-LP CSF leak. It has some of the orthostatic features of the posttraumatic headache: worsening of pain, dizziness, and nausea when upright, and improvement on lying down. Usually, the history is diagnostic. If a repeat LP is performed to exclude arachnoiditis or infection, an opening CSF pressure of less than 30 mm H_2O strongly suggests this diagnosis.

Idiopathic Intracranial Hypertension (Pseudotumor Cerebri)

Headache in idiopathic intracranial hypertension is associated with high CSF pressures in the absence of intracranial structural disease. Pain is often postural and associated with pulsatile tinnitus, nausea, vomiting, and progressive visual loss. Papilledema is present in about 90% of patients. The diagnosis is confirmed by CSF pressures greater than 250 mm H_2O and no mass on computed tomography (CT).

Temporal (Cranial) Arteritis

Headache is the dominant complaint in this progressive, systemic, inflammatory disorder. It may occur anywhere in the scalp, and is localized to the temporal area in only half the cases. The syndrome tends to occur in patients over 50 years of age and is accompanied by constitutional symptoms such as anorexia and weight loss. The onset is gradual, with polymyalgia, proximal weakness, masseter claudication, and periocular discomfort developing over months to years. The diagnosis is suggested by a firm, tender, nonpulsatile cranial artery and an elevated erythrocyte sedimentation rate (greater than 50 mm/h), although about 25% of cases have only mild elevations of the sedimentation rate. Major complications include monocular blindness and stroke.

Headache in HIV-Positive and AIDS Patients

Headache in this group of patients is usually subacute, and is often associated with positive clinical findings. The list of possible opportunistic CNS infections includes mycobacteria (*Mycobacterium tuberculosis* and *Mycobacterium avium-intracellulare*), spirochetes (*Treponema pallidum*), viruses (herpes simplex, herpes zoster, cytomegalovirus, and HIV-1), fungi (*Cryptococcus*), protozoa (*Toxoplasma*), and actinomycetes (*Nocardia*). Noninfectious causes of headache include CNS lymphoma (primary and secondary) and Kaposi's sarcoma.

Chronic Headache

Patients presenting to the ED with chronic headache (i.e., headache that has been present for months to years) are part of what has been called the "last straw" syndrome.[6] Most of the serious entities included in this category have been discussed previously under subacute headache, and they usually conform to a similar temporal profile.

Chronic headaches can be divided clinically into several different groups, each requiring a different diagnostic and therapeutic strategy. These include patients with features of chronic tension-type headache, so-called transformational migraine (transformed from an episodic pattern to a chronic daily pattern), analgesic abuse, depression, and, rarely, tumor, subdural hematoma, idiopathic intracranial hypertension, and posttraumatic headache.

Most patients with chronic tension-type headache have mild-to-moderate pain, rarely see a doctor, and only occasionally come to the ED; fewer still see neurologists. Consequently, little is known about these patients other than the fact that, on the basis of anonymous prevalence surveys, they seem to exist in large numbers. One plausible speculation is that their headaches represent symptoms of depression.

The existence of transformational migraine supports the theory that migraine and many of the more severe tension-type headaches are related. Among a large cohort of migraineurs, 80% of whom had their first headache before the age of 26, 90% had developed chronic daily headache by age 45.[15] Many of these patients also suffered from superimposed periodic episodes of typical migraine.

Some patients with severe tension-type headache or frequent migraines overuse nonnarcotic analgesics or ergotamines, resulting in worsening of their headache. Gradual withdrawal provides relief, but it may require hospitalization for supervised detoxification.[1]

As noted previously, depression is a frequent concomitant of chronic headache of all varieties. This relationship may simply represent a response to living with constant pain, or it may reflect the central role of serotonin in both headache and depression.

Although chronic headache is rarely a presentation of a space-occupying lesion or increased intracranial pressure (ICP), most of these patients warrant a CT at some point in their management, especially if they do not respond to medical intervention.

EMERGENCY DEPARTMENT EVALUATION

A meticulous history is the key to headache diagnosis. Only in unusual circumstances does the neurologic examination, laboratory testing, or neuroimaging procedure reveal an abnormality that was completely unsuspected following a careful history.

Headache History

Temporal Profile

Because this is the primary axis along which headaches can be classified in the ED, this information should be obtained first in order to place the patient into one of the four groups shown in Table 201.2.

1. Single acute: Is this a "first and worst" headache of sudden onset?
2. Recurrent acute: What is the frequency, pattern, and duration of individual headache episodes?
3. Subacute: Is the headache progressively worsening?
4. Chronic: Has there been a pattern break or is this a "last straw" visit to the ED?

Associated Symptoms

In particular, look for transient loss of consciousness or imbalance at onset, nausea, vomiting, neck stiffness, unilateral lacrimation or rhinorrhea, photophobia, and phonophobia.

Circumstances of Onset

For single acute headaches, determine exactly what the patient was doing when the headache began. For recurrent headache, identify any usual precipitants.

Prodromes and Aura

Prodromes such as a shift in appetite or mood suggest migraine, and characteristic visual aura essentially define a subtype of migraine.

Location of Pain

Hemicranial, hemifacial, and unilateral ocular and periorbital pain have greater discriminating value than holocranial or bilateral pain.

Quality and Severity of Pain

This has limited value in identifying the type of headache, and correlates poorly with the seriousness of underlying disease.

Age at Onset

New-onset headache in the elderly is worrisome.

Recent Trauma

This is relevant to chronic subdural hematomas and posttraumatic headaches, although trauma may also precipitate a migraine or cluster headache.

Relief Measures

Headaches that are substantially relieved by lying down are usually posttraumatic or low CSF pressure (post-LP) headaches.

Family History

Migraine, depression, and, to a lesser extent, a predisposition to SAH are inherited.

Medical History

Ask about concurrent illnesses, medications (including oral contraceptives), hospitalizations, allergies, smoking, alcohol and drug use, and risk factors for HIV.

Occupational History

Note exposure to carbon monoxide, fumes, solvents, and other toxins.

Psychosocial History

Search especially for signs and symptoms of depression, anxiety, and marital or job-related stress.

Multiplicity

Many patients suffer from different kinds of headaches. To minimize confusion, it is important to determine this early and to obtain parallel but distinct histories of each headache type.

Physical Examination

General Examination

After obtaining vital signs, the remainder of the nonneurologic examination should be goal-directed, including the eyes, neck, face, and scalp. Visual acuity should be checked with a pinhole and the eye examined for ptosis, conjunctival injection (perilimbal vs. diffuse), corneal clouding, and pupillary size, reactivity, and equality. Any suggestion of acute glaucoma mandates measurement of intraocular pressure. The swinging flashlight test should be performed as described earlier to detect optic or retrobulbar neuritis.

A funduscopic examination is essential, looking specifically for signs of increased ICP, severe hypertension, optic neuritis, or subhyaloid hemorrhage (preretinal hemorrhages obscuring retinal vessels due to overlying blood in the subarachnoid space). Spontaneous venous pulsations (SVPs) are lost when the ICP exceeds about 200 mm H_2O. However, monitoring has shown enormous pressure fluctuations in patients with increased ICP, ranging from 50 to 500 mm over a 24-hour period. Thus, a patient with increased ICP might have SVPs if examined during a transient trough in intracranial pressure. In addition to the problem of false negatives (presence of SVPs in patients with increased ICP), there is the problem of false positives (absence of SVPs in patients with normal ICP), which is seen in about 20% of the normal population. Bilateral papilledema is a highly specific indicator of increased ICP, but, because it may lag behind acute elevations of ICP by several hours, this finding lacks sensitivity.

The neck should be examined for pain with flexion, which indicates meningeal irritation secondary to chemical or infectious meningitis. Tension-type headache also characteristically produces tightness in the paracervical muscles with discomfort on flexion. Unlike the nuchal rigidity of meningitis, tension-type headache causes pain with chin to shoulder rotation of the head. Because it may take several hours for subarachnoid blood to reach the cervical area of the meninges, and several more hours for it to produce a chemical meningitis, absence of nuchal rigidity early in the course of an SAH does not reliably exclude this entity.

The sinuses, temporomandibular joints, and scalp should be palpated for tenderness, paying special attention to the temporal arteries in older patients. In posttraumatic headache, hemotympanum, CSF otorrhea, infraorbital ecchymoses, posterior auricular ecchymoses, and CSF rhinorrhea indicate basilar skull fracture.

Neurologic Examination

Mental status assessment is a critically important feature of the neurologic examination that is commonly overlooked. Focality is detected most readily by pronator drift, asymmetry of cranial nerves II to VIII, and abnormalities of gait and station. In general, sensory examination (other than cranial nerve V), assessment of reflexes, and motor testing of individual muscle groups are not efficient use of the emergency physician's time in the evaluation of the patient with headache.

Laboratory Testing

As with the physical examination, laboratory tests are usually normal. In patients with a history strongly suggestive of a particular kind of headache (e.g., migraine), no laboratory tests are necessary. The erythrocyte sedimentation rate in patients suspected of having cranial arteritis is an exception to this rule. Other tests of occasional value include hemoglobin, leukocyte count, glucose, pulse oximetry, arterial blood gas, and carboxyhemoglobin level.

Imaging

When a diagnosis can be made on the basis of the history and clinical picture, no imaging is needed. Other patients with acute single or recurrent headache should probably have a CT or magnetic resonance imaging (MRI) at the time of their ED visit. Those with subacute and chronic headache may have an imaging procedure scheduled electively.

CT is preferred for the detection of acute intracranial bleeding, idiopathic intracranial hypertension, and hydrocephalus. Noncontrast CT, followed by a contrast CT, is useful in HIV-positive patients, in whom a ring-enhancing lesion suggests toxoplasmosis. Patients with suspected spontaneous SAH constitute a special case. State-of-the-art CT scans obtained within 12 hours of the onset of headache in suspected SAH have a sensitivity of 98% (95% CI, 94% to 100%), a specificity of 100% (95% CI, 94% to 100%), a negative likelihood ratio of 0.02 (95% CI, 0.005 to 0.06), and a positive likelihood ratio of at least 33 (95% CI, 11 to 316).[17]

Because a negative CT cannot completely exclude the diagnosis of SAH, the LP remains the criterion standard for this diagnosis. As shown by the likelihood ratios, a negative CT markedly reduces the probability of this entity by decreasing the odds of SAH by about 50-fold from the clinician's pretest estimates. Thus, the pretest probability of SAH would have to exceed 33% in order for the posttest probability of SAH to remain above 1% following a negative CT. The sensitivity of CT drops off as the time from headache onset increases. The sensitivity of MRI is inferior to that of CT during the first 24 hours, becomes slightly superior between 24 and 72 hours, and exceeds that of CT thereafter.[11]

The choice of CT versus MRI depends on the clinical picture, cost, and availability. In addition to late identification of SAH, MRI is preferred for imaging the posterior fossa (cerebellum and brainstem), detecting nonhemorrhagic strokes less than 2 days old, and visualizing transient ischemic attack, tumor, localized infection, or chronic subdural hematoma.

Finally, magnetic resonance angiography (MRA) promises to replace traditional angiography as the imaging modality of choice for aneurysms, arteriovenous malformations, and dissection of the cranial arteries.

Lumbar Puncture

There are two primary indications for an emergency LP in a patient with headache: suspicion of CNS infection (e.g., meningitis) or a substantial suspicion of SAH despite a normal CT. The other two circumstances in which an LP is the diagnostic standard is in headache due either to high (idiopathic intracranial hypertension) or low (post-LP) CSF pressure. In the first instance, the LP is clearly indicated and often therapeutic. In the case of a post-LP headache, another LP should be done only if the diagnosis is in serious doubt.

The risk of herniation after LP in patients with increased ICP or a mass lesion is low but unknown. Proponents of LP without prior CT argue that an association between herniation and LP has not been causally established. Proponents of CT prior to LP cite a small number of instances in which herniation has been temporally associated with LP. The difficulties inherent in studying this question suggest that the controversy will not soon be resolved. Because CT scanning is so widely and readily available, in the absence of definitive information supporting either position, many clinicians perform a CT prior to LP, provided that appropriate time-dependent emergency care (e.g., institution of antibiotics in suspected bacterial meningitis) is not delayed.

EMERGENCY DEPARTMENT MANAGEMENT AND DISPOSITION

Treatment of the following causes of headache is discussed in the corresponding chapters elsewhere in this text: bacterial meningitis, SAH, stroke, cranial artery dissection, hypertensive encephalopathy, acute glaucoma, optic neuritis, retrobulbar neuritis, sinusitis, temporomandibular joint syndrome, toxic–metabolic disorders, chronic subdural hematoma, brain tumor, and brain abscess.

Migraine

Table 201.5 lists some of the many therapies for management of acute migraine in the ED. Direct comparison of migraine abortive agents is confounded by a failure of clinical trials to target uniform end points, inconsistent documentation of adverse effects and recurrence rates, and variability in methods of pain measurement. Dihydroergotamine (DHE-45) is an effective abortive agent for the treatment of moderate-to-severe migraine. DHE and a dopamine antagonist provide the benefit of two effective abortive agents plus an antiemetic effect. Results of two randomized, placebo-controlled trials favor intravenous prochlorperazine over metoclopramide.[4,9]

Proposed doses of prochlorperazine range from 3.5 to 10 mg. When used in combination therapy with intravenous DHE, 3.5 mg may be nearly as effective as higher doses, but with fewer adverse effects, such as sedation and akathisia.[14] Intravenous diphenhydramine has recently been shown to be effective in preventing the akathisia associated with the use of prochlorperazine.[18] Sumatriptan is highly effective (70% of patients experience improvement within 1 hour of subcutaneous administration) and provides a more rapid onset of action than DHE. However, the drug is expensive, and a high proportion of patients (in one clinical trial, a majority,[2] and in another, 2.5 times that of DHE[20]) experience a recurrence of headache within 24 hours.

New triptans may be found to provide a longer duration of action and reduction in headache recurrence. At present, the oral, rectal, and nasal forms of sumatriptan have a limited role in the ED management of migraine. Prochlorperazine suppositories have been shown to be effective in the ED setting, but, like the alternative routes of administration for sumatriptan, do not work as rapidly as parenteral treatment. At the present time, for treatment of migraine, we recommend 10 mg of prochlorper-

TABLE 201.5. Emergency Management of Migraine and Related Headache

Drug	Indications	Dose	Route	Repeat Dose	Comments	Evidence[a] (Ref)
NSAID						
Ketorolac (Toradol)	Mild/moderate headache	60–90 mg	i.m.	30–45 mg i.m. in 6 h	Less effective than DHE + metoclopramide	Level I, Grade A
Indomethacin (Indocin)	Mild/moderate headache	50 mg	PO or PR	q6–8h	Prophylaxis against coital headache	Level I, Grade A
SEROTONIN AGONISTS						
Dihydroergotamine (DHE)	Moderate/severe migraine, cluster, status migrainosis, severe/intractable, tension-type headache	1 mg (0.25-mg test dose + 0.75 mg)	i.m./S.C. or i.v. over 30–60 min	0.5–1.0 mg i.m./s.c. or i.v. over 30–60 min (max 3 mg per attack)	Contraindicated in cardiovascular disease and pregnancy; D/C if chest pain, worsening headache or increased blood pressure	Level I, Grade A
Sumatriptan (Imitrex)	Moderate/severe migraine and cluster	6 mg	s.c.	6 mg s.c. in 1 h	More rapid action than DHE; 50% rebound within 24 h; higher cost	Level I, Grade A
DOPAMINE ANTAGONISTS						
Prochlorperazine (Compazine)	Moderate/severe migraine	10 mg	i.v. over 2 min	10 mg in 1 h	May cause dystonia (akathesia); PR less effective than i.v.	Level I, Grade A
Metoclopramide (Reglan)	Moderate/severe migraine	10–20 mg	i.v. in 50 mL D5W over 20 min	10 mg in 1 h	Enhances gastric emptying; may cause dystonia	Level I, Grade A
Chlorpromazine (Thorazine)	Moderate/severe migraine	12.5–25 mg	i.v. over 2 min	12.5 mg q20min × 2 (max 50 mg)	Give 500 mL saline, to offset orthostasis; drowsiness; may cause dystonia	Level I, Grade A
COMBINATION REGIMENS						
DHE + metoclopramide	Same as DHE	1 mg DHE + 10–20 mg metoclopramide	i.v. as above under individual agents	0.5 mg DHE + 10–20 mg metoclopramide in 1 h	Premedication with metoclopramide may reduce emesis from DHE	Level I, Grade A
DHE + prochlorperazine + diphenhydramine	Same as DHE	1 mg DHE + 10 mg prochlorperazine + 50 mg diphenhydramine	i.v. as above under individual agents; diphenhy-dramine may be i.v. push	0.5 mg DHE + 10 mg prochlorperazine in 1 h	Premedication with prochlorperazine may reduce emesis from DHE; diphenhydramine reduces dystonias	Level I, Grade A
CORTICOSTEROIDS						
	Status migrainosis, intractable episodic, cluster	10–20 mg dexamethasone	i.v.	60 mg prednisone tapering 5 mg/d	May decrease inflammation; interval medication until prophylactic agents take effect	Level II, Grade B
LOCAL ANESTHETICS						
Lidocaine	Moderate/severe migraine, cluster	0.5 mL (4% solution without epinephrine) in one nostril if unilateral, each nostril if bilateral	Intranasal	Repeat same dose after 2 min	Usefulness limited by high early relapse rate; may be useful while instituting other measures	Level I, Grade B
OPIOIDS						
	Last resort	75–125 mg meperidine + 25–50 mg hydroxyzine	i.m.	75–125 mg meperidine in 1–2 h	Most of above regimens provide superior pain relief in controlled trials	Level I, Grade A

[a]*Level of Evidence*
I: Evidence from at least one randomized controlled trial.
II: Evidence from well-designed controlled trials but without randomization; well-designed cohort or case-control studies; or dramatic results from uncontrolled experiments.
Class of recommendation
A: Good evidence to support procedure or treatment.
B: Fair evidence to support procedure or treatment.
Adapted, with modifications, from Ducharme J. Canadian Association of Emergency Physicians guidelines for the acute management of migraine headache. *J Emerg Med* 1998;17:137.

TABLE 201.6. Criteria for Hospitalization of Patients with Headache

1. Serious underlying disease
   a. CNS infection
      1) Bacterial meningitis
      2) Brain abscess
      3) Any evidence of infection in HIV-positive host
   b. CNS vascular disease
      1) Subarachnoid hemorrhage
      2) Cerebral ischemia
      3) Temporal arteritis
      4) Severe hypertension
      5) Spontaneous dissection of cranial arteries
   c. Space–occupying lesions
      1) Brain tumor
      2) Subdural hematoma
   d. Toxic–metabolic encephalopathy
   e. Acute sinusitis with evidence of spread or an ill-appearing patient
   f. Narrow–angle glaucoma
   g. Idiopathic intracranial hypertension, not responding to usual measures to reduce
   h. Headache associated with serious medical or surgical illness
2. Severe, intractable head or facial pain
   a. Status migrainosis
   b. Persistent cluster, unresponsive to usual measures
   c. Unremitting trigeminal or postherpetic neuralgia
3. Continuing vomiting, electrolyte imbalance, or inability to take PO (usually migraine or severe posttraumatic headache)
4. Analgesic abuse/rebound headache, requiring inpatient detoxification
5. Complex drug interactions and careful drug level monitoring required for headache management
6. Suicidal ideation associated with unremitting headache or severe depression
7. Social situation not conducive to outpatient management
8. Repeated ED visits

azine (10 mg of metoclopramide may be nearly equivalent),[4,9] 50 mg of diphenhydramine,[18] and 1 mg of DHE, all administered intravenously.[2,13,20]

Neurologic consultation is indicated in the ED if the diagnosis is in doubt, if the attack does not conform to the patient's typical migraine, or if intractable vomiting or unrelenting pain is encountered. Following successful treatment, patients should be referred to a neurologist or headache specialist. Indications for admission are summarized in Table 201.6.

Cluster

High-flow 100% oxygen should be administered as soon as the patient enters the ED. Because many patients with cluster are smokers, they should be observed for carbon dioxide retention while on oxygen. As indicated in Table 201.5, DHE and sumatriptan are effective in the ED management of cluster (sumatriptan has been shown to provide relief in about 10 minutes). However, concerns about coronary vasospasm limit the use of these drugs in patients with any cardiovascular risk factors. On discharge, patients with an exacerbation of cluster should receive a trial of prophylactic verapamil, starting at 80 mg t.i.d., if there are no contraindications. A tapering course of steroids should also be given until the verapamil can be increased to therapeutic levels (about 120 mg t.i.d.). Indications for admission are summarized in Table 201.6.

Episodic Tension-type Headache

In only a minority of cases do these patients require acute ED management. Those with severe symptoms may respond to a migraine regimen,[3] as indicated in Table 201.5. Most patients with mild episodic tension-type headaches can be managed with NSAIDs. Unless they have developed the syndrome of medication overuse, which requires inpatient detoxification,[1] these patients can usually be discharged with referral.

Trigeminal Neuralgia

This syndrome usually responds to carbamazepine, phenytoin, valproate, clonazepam, or baclofen. Superiority of one agent over another has not been established, and neurologic consultation may be helpful in choosing a drug. Some elderly patients with this syndrome become suicidal and require in-patient management, often beginning with intravenous or intramuscular fosphenytoin or intravenous phenytoin in the ED. Opioids may be necessary until other medications take effect. ED management of most patients is limited to referral for diagnostic confirmation and long-term care.

Postherpetic Neuralgia

Treatment with famciclovir prevents postherpetic neuralgia if given during an attack of zoster. Proposed treatments for postherpetic neuralgia include topical capsaicin cream (derived from hot peppers), amitriptyline, valproate, carbamazepine, and phenytoin. As with trigeminal neuralgia, neurologic consultation is helpful in choosing an appropriate regimen. Unless patients have unremitting pain, most can be discharged from the ED and referred for further management.

Coital Headache

Once an SAH has been excluded, these patients require explanation, reassurance, and referral. It is reasonable to offer the patient a therapeutic trial of indomethacin 50 mg PO, taken 1 to 2 hours before intercourse, if there is no contraindication.

Posttraumatic Headache (Acute and Chronic)

Once the diagnosis has been confirmed by a normal CT or MRI, these patients should be educated, reassured, and encouraged to spend as much time recumbent as possible. Confirmation that this is indeed "real," and that it will improve with time, is an important therapeutic intervention. Patients should be referred to a neurologist.

Headache Associated with Low Cerebrospinal Fluid Pressure

Traditional management of post-LP headache includes fluid replacement and bedrest. If the syndrome persists, 1 g of intravenous caffeine sodium benzoate, 500 mg over 15 minutes, followed by an additional 500 mg over 3 hours, may be administered. This increases CSF pressure by causing cerebral vasoconstriction, and should be considered only in young patients without cardiovascular risk factors or a history of arrhythmias. Continual monitoring is necessary. If caffeine is inadvisable or ineffective, an epidural blood patch may help. In most institutions, this requires anesthesia consultation. Unless individuals are incapacitated by the headache, they can be managed as outpatients.

Idiopathic Intracranial Hypertension

ED management requires neurologic consultation, ophthalmologic consultation, and administration of acetazolamide, often combined with furosemide. Repeated LP may be necessary to maintain reduced pressure. Steroids are used if these interventions fail. If this regimen does not reduce ICP, the headache can be treated with analgesics and migraine medications. However, control of pain does not treat the underlying threat to the patient's vision. If acuity worsens in spite of maximal medical management, an optic sheath decompression or ventricular shunt will be needed.

Temporal Arteritis

ED management requires ophthalmologic consultation for arterial biopsy and rheumatologic consultation for steroid management. Because 50% of untreated patients develop blindness, all patients with the working diagnosis of temporal arteritis should immediately receive steroids and then be admitted to the hospital for monitoring of symptoms and the sedimentation rate.

Headache in HIV-Positive and AIDS Patients

HIV-positive patients presenting with headache should be discharged only if they are afebrile, have an unaltered or baseline mental status (confirmed by a family member or caretaker), a negative contrast and noncontrast CT, and a negative LP. They should be followed by infectious disease or primary care physicians specializing in the management of AIDS.

Chronic Headache

Individuals with chronic headache are among the most challenging to manage in a busy ED. Within this heterogeneous group, one must try to identify treatable subsets and make the appropriate referrals. The only subgroup of chronic headache patients that may benefit from hospital admission are those with analgesic abuse. Individuals in this group require an inpatient washout and withdrawal protocol, utilizing DHE and a dopamine antagonist.[1]

In general, patients with chronic daily headache, including chronic tension-type headache, transformational migraine, analgesic abuse, and chronic headache as a depressive equivalent, are among those who can benefit most from the expertise of a headache specialist.

COMMON PITFALLS

- Failing to diagnose the sentinel leak of SAH until a major bleed occurs subsequently[19]
- Mistaking headache and other constitutional symptoms of carbon monoxide toxicity for a clustered outbreak of afebrile winter flu
- Misdiagnosing a chronic subdural hematoma in the elderly as progressive dementia because there is no history of head trauma
- Mistakenly attributing headache to hypertension, which is rarely the cause
- Failing to diagnose and treat migraine appropriately either because a large tension-type component is present or because the headache is not hemicranial. Nonthrobbing and bilateral pain occur in about 50% and 40%, respectively, of migraine patients during some episodes.[13]
- Presuming that response to certain medications necessarily defines the etiology of a headache. The headache of brain tumors, aneurysms, and SAH may respond to a migraine regimen.
- Missing a significant treatable component of depression associated with many headache disorders

References

1. Baumgartner CP, Wessely P, Bingol C, et al. Long-term prognosis of analgesic withdrawal in patients with drug-induced headaches. *Headache* 1989;29:510.
2. Cady RK, Dexter J, Sargent JD, et al. Efficacy of subcutaneous sumatriptan in repeated episodes of migraine. *Neurology* 1993;43:1363.
3. Cady RK, Gutterman D, Saiers JA, et al. Responsiveness of non-IHS migraine and tension-type headache to sumatriptan. *Cephalalgia* 1997;17:588.
4. Coppola M, Yealy DM, Leibold RA. Randomized, placebo controlled evaluation of prochlorperazine versus metoclopramide for emergency department treatment of migraine headache. *Ann Emerg Med* 1995;26:541.
5. Durand ML, Calderwood SB, Weber DJ, et al. Acute bacterial meningitis in adults: a review of 493 episodes. *N Engl J Med* 1993;328:21.
6. Edmeads J. Emergency management of headache. *Headache* 1988;28:675.
7. Edvinsson L. Neurogenic vs vascular mechanisms of sumatriptan and ergot alkaloids in migraine [Editorial]. *Cephalalgia* 1998;18:5.
8. Headache Classification Committee of the International Headache Society. Classification and diagnostic criteria for headache disorders, cranial neuralgia, and facial pain. *Cephalalgia* 1988;8[Suppl 7]:1.
9. Jones J, Pack S, Chun E. Intramuscular prochlorperazine versus metoclopramide as single-agent therapy for the treatment of acute migraine headache. *J Emerg Med* 1996;14:262.

9a. Luber AD, Flaherty JF. Famciclovir for treatment of herpes virus infections. *Ann Pharmacother* 1996;30:978.

10. Markus JS. A prospective follow up of thunderclap headache mimicking subarachnoid haemorrhage. *J Neurol Neurosurg Psychiatry* 1991;54:1117.
11. Ogawa T, Inugami A, Fujita H, et al. MR diagnosis of subacute and chronic subarachnoid hemorrhage: comparison with CT. *AJR* 1995;165:1257.
12. Olesen J. Clinical and pathophysiological observations in migraine and tension-type headache explained by integration of vascular supraspinal and myofascial inputs. *Pain* 1991;46:125.
13. Pryse-Phillips WE, Dodick DW, Edmeads JG, et al. Guidelines for the diagnosis and management of migraine in clinical practice. *Can Med Assoc J* 1997;156:1273.
14. Saadah HA. Abortive headache therapy in the office with intravenous dihydroergotamine plus prochlorperazine. *Headache* 1992;32:143.
15. Saper JR. Changing perspectives on chronic headache. *Clin J Pain* 1986;2:19.
16. Silberstein SD. Evaluation and emergency treatment of headache. *Headache* 1992;32:396.
17. Van der Wee N, Rinkel GJ, Hasan D, et al. Detection of subarachnoid haemorrhage on early CT: is lumbar puncture still needed after a negative scan? *J Neurol Neurosurg Psychiatry* 1995;58:357.
18. Vinson DR, Drotts DL. Diphenhydramine prevents akathisia induced by intravenous prochlorperazine. A randomized controlled trial. *Acad Emerg Med* 1999;6:533(abst).
19. Wasserberg J, Barlow P. Lesson of the week. Lumbar puncture still has an important role in diagnosing subarachnoid haemorrhage. *BMJ* 1997;315(7122):1598.
20. Winner P, Ricalde O, Le Force B, et al. A double-blind study of subcutaneous dihydroergotamine vs subcutaneous sumatriptan in the treatment of acute migraine. *Arch Neurol* 1996;53;180.

CHAPTER 202

Subarachnoid Hemorrhage

Phil Fontanarosa and Clifton Callaway

Spontaneous subarachnoid hemorrhage (SAH) is a relatively common yet devastating entity. Despite advances in resuscitation, critical care, cerebral pharmacotherapy, and microneurosurgical techniques, the overall mortality rate from SAH is 30% to 50%.[10,13] Of surviving patients, only half eventually have a good outcome, and less than one-third ever return to their premorbid functional status.[7,10,21]

SAH frequently affects healthy individuals in the most productive years of adult life and is responsible for half of all fatal strokes in patients younger than 45 years of age. The diagnosis of SAH is frequently delayed or missed entirely.[1] Because most patients with SAH initially seek medical attention in the emergency department, the emergency physician may be able to prevent death and limit disability from this potentially catastrophic disorder.

EPIDEMIOLOGY AND PATHOPHYSIOLOGY

In the United States, SAH accounts for approximately 10% of all acute cerebrovascular accidents and affects nearly 30,000 people each year, with an estimated annual incidence of five to ten cases per 100,000 persons.[13,21] Rupture of an intracranial aneurysm is responsible for most cases. The prevalence of asymptomatic intracranial aneurysms has been estimated from autopsy and neuroradiology studies at 0.5% or higher.[19]

The risk of rupture from these aneurysms is estimated to be 1% to 2% per year, and the risk of rupture increases with aneurysm size.[19] While few aneurysms less than 3 mm in diameter rupture, surgical clipping has been suggested for unruptured aneurysms of more than 5 to 7 mm in diameter.[15] Aneurysms are rare in children, but the incidence increases sharply in people after age 25 years and peaks at nearly 12% by age 60 years. Young and middle-aged Blacks have a substantially greater risk of aneurysmal SAH than do Whites of similar age.[6]

In contrast to most other cerebrovascular diseases, aneurysmal SAH is more common in women than in men. Factors leading to a state of relative estrogen deficiency, such as menopause and cigarette smoking, are associated with an increased risk. Among premenopausal women, the risk of hemorrhage appears greatest in the perimenstrual period and during pregnancy.[14] Smoking, hypertension, and a moderate-to-heavy alcohol consumption are risk factors for both men and women.[23]

Disorders that produce vascular wall defects, as well as certain connective tissue diseases, are associated with an increased likelihood of aneurysm formation. These include polycystic kidney disease, coarctation of the aorta, Marfan syndrome, Ehlers-Danlos syndrome, and fibromuscular hyperplasia. Consistent with and including these associations, genetic predisposition represents a nonmodifiable risk factor for SAH.[5]

Aneurysmal rupture typically is associated with sudden blood pressure surges, such as occur during strenuous physical activity, emotional stress, sexual intercourse, or during the Valsalva maneuver.[8] Other factors associated with increased risk of rupture include heavy alcohol consumption, cocaine or phencyclidine abuse, heavy cigarette smoking, and long-term use of aspirin or analgesics. Aneurysmal rupture may, however, be independent of any physical or environmental stress; SAH may occur during nonexertional, normal daily activity, or even during sleep.[1,8]

Nontraumatic SAH also may result from bleeding secondary to arteriovenous malformation (AVM), mycotic aneurysm, extension from parenchymatous hemorrhage, anticoagulant therapy, hemorrhagic encephalitis, or cerebral vasculitis. In approximately 20% of cases, an underlying cause cannot be determined.

CLINICAL PRESENTATION

Sudden, excruciating headache is the hallmark of SAH. The headache is typically severe, begins abruptly, peaks rapidly (within seconds to minutes), and differs from other headaches the patient has experienced. It may be described as "exploding," "bursting," or "the worst headache of my life," and is typically accompanied by nausea and vomiting. The pain is usually diffuse and poorly localized, but may be unilateral or confined to the frontal or occipital region. Headache is frequently accompanied by neck pain, and, on occasion, pain may radiate down the spine and to the legs.

Although the presentation of SAH is often dramatic, some patients present atypically, and the classic signs and symptoms may be absent or subtle. A sudden headache occurring days to weeks before the onset of SAH occurs in 30% to 50% of patients.[24] This "sentinel headache" has characteristics similar to those already discussed and may be accompanied by neurologic symptoms, vomiting, nuchal pain, dizziness, or drowsiness; it generally resolves in 2 to 3 days. The headache may be relatively mild and unimpressive, and its severity may be minimized by the patient. Such warning symptoms represent a premonitory "warning leak" that may reflect a minor initial hemorrhage (sentinel headache), enlargement or thrombosis of the aneurysm, isolated hemorrhage into the aneurysm wall, pressure exerted by an unruptured aneurysm, or local ischemia.

Syncope or coma is common, and most patients experience an alteration of consciousness of some degree at the onset of SAH.[12,15] Loss of consciousness may result from a sudden decrease in cerebral perfusion pressure as intracranial pressure (ICP) transiently approaches mean arterial pressure at the moment of aneurysmal rupture.

Seizures occur in as many as 25% of patients after SAH.[22] They are more common in younger patients and are not related to overall prognosis. Seizures occurring within 12 hours of SAH are thought to result primarily from increased ICP rather than from an irritative cerebral focus.

An alteration in mental status is common in patients with SAH, but focal neurologic findings are typically absent unless hemorrhage involves the brain substance or a large clot has produced a mass effect. Focal signs may also be caused by compression of cranial nerves or brain parenchyma by an unruptured but expanding intracranial aneurysm.[7] Nonfocal neurologic signs such as impaired memory, speech disorders, personality changes, and bilateral extensor plantar responses may be overlooked unless specifically sought or elicited. Patients may also complain of photophobia, dizziness, diplopia, or blurred vision.

Other physical findings may be present in the acute phase of SAH. Careful funduscopic examination may reveal preretinal or subhyaloid hemorrhages—small, smooth, round hemorrhages that usually occur near the optic nerve head. Although these hemorrhages are seen in only 10% to 20% of patients, they are pathognomonic for SAH when they occur with acute headache. Nuchal rigidity is common with SAH, but it may not develop for several hours after SAH and may be absent in patients with deep coma.

Systolic hypertension (greater than 200 mm Hg) occurs in up to 35% of patients with SAH. Acute blood pressure elevation may be due to increasing ICP (Cushing response) or may result from acute catecholamine release. Significant hypertension following SAH is associated with an increased incidence of cerebral vasospasm, an increased likelihood of hydrocephalus, and poor outcome. Hypotension is unusual immediately following SAH but is an ominous finding when present. Low-grade temperature elevation occurs in approximately 20% of patients with SAH and is thought to result from meningeal inflammation.

Cardiac dysrhythmias and ST-T wave abnormalities occur in most patients with SAH. Premature ventricular complexes, supraventricular tachycardia, and bradycardias are most common, but potentially life-threatening dysrhythmias (e.g., ventricular tachycardia, idioventricular rhythm, and complete heart block) have been documented in up to 40% of patients; they occur most frequently during the first 24 hours after SAH.[3] Acute ST-T wave changes similar to those associated with cardiac ischemia may also be noted.

Other characteristic electrocardiographic (ECG) changes associated with intracranial hemorrhage include peaked (deep, broad, symmetrically inverted) T waves, QRS complex prolongation, an increased QT interval, and large U waves. It is undetermined whether these ECG abnormalities are due to structural subendocardial myocardial damage associated with SAH or whether they result from alterations in autonomic input to the heart or increased levels of circulating catecholamines.[4]

Several clinical grading scales are used for patients with SAH (Table 202.1). These classification systems are useful for describing neurologic status and for timing surgical intervention.[12] In general, the poorer the clinical grade, the worse the prognosis. Thus, patients with severe neurologic impairment on presentation tend to have greater morbidity and mortality and usually require more intensive support.

Patients who are neurologically intact on admission require constant surveillance and prompt intervention to avoid the complications that can lead to neurologic deterioration. Major central nervous system (CNS) complications are common in patients who survive an initial SAH. They include rebleeding, vasospasm, and acute hydrocephalus.

Rebleeding is the most devastating CNS complication and is associated with mortality rates of greater than 50%.[4,25] The peak risk of rebleeding is during the first 48 hours after the initial SAH. Risk of rebleeding is about 4% of untreated patients during the first 24 hours, and 1% to 2% per day thereafter for the subsequent 4 weeks.[11]

Cerebral vasospasm, another major cause of delayed morbidity, accounts for 14% to 36% of poor outcomes in patients with SAH.[25] Vasospasm occurs in 20% to 30% of patients following SAH, with an onset 3 to 5 days after the initial bleed and maximal severity 5 to 10 days afterward.[15] Vasospasm can result in cerebral infarction or death. Cerebral vasospasm appears to be most common in patients in whom a large amount of blood is seen within the subarachnoid cisterns on initial computed tomography (CT) scan.

Hydrocephalus, which is also relatively frequent, is usually due to obstruction of the flow of cerebrospinal fluid (CSF) secondary to a clot blocking the basal cisterns and the foramen of the fourth ventricle. Depending on the location of the bleeding and the amount of blood in the subarachnoid space, acute hydrocephalus may develop as rapidly as a few hours after aneurysmal rupture; more typically, it occurs within the first few days. In the Cooperative Aneurysm Study, evidence of hydrocephalus was noted on the initial CT scan in approximately 16% of patients and was more common in patients who had severe neurologic impairment at the time of initial presentation.[2]

Patients with SAH are also subject to nonneurologic complications. Pulmonary complications, including aspiration pneumonia, hypoventilation due to decreased level of consciousness, and neurogenic pulmonary edema, may occur within the first hours or the first several days after SAH. Hyponatremia develops in up to 30% of patients after SAH; it may be due to inappropriate secretion of antidiuretic hormone or release of natriuretic peptides, and it contributes to cerebral edema, altered consciousness, and seizures.[4] Diabetes insipidus (with progressive hypernatremia) is most common in comatose patients with extensive SAH and elevated ICP. Late complications of SAH include systemic infections (e.g., sepsis), postoperative complications (e.g., meningitis), and venous thromboembolic disorders (e.g., pulmonary embolism).

DIFFERENTIAL DIAGNOSIS

The diagnosis of SAH is readily considered in the patient with an acute onset of severe headache accompanied by vomiting and loss of consciousness. SAH should be considered in the differential diagnosis of every patient with a clinical presentation that involves sudden-onset headache, with or without an altered level of consciousness (Table 202.2). Many patients, how-

TABLE 202.1. Clinical Grading Scales for Subarachnoid Hemorrhage

Grade	Description
HUNT–HESS SCALE	
I	Asymptomatic or mild headache
II	Moderate-to-severe headache, nuchal rigidity
III	Confusion, drowsiness, or mild focal signs
IV	Stupor or hemiparesis
V	Coma, moribund, and/or posturing
COOPERATIVE ANEURYSM SCALE	
I	Free of symptoms
II	Mildly ill—alert and responsive, headache
III	Moderately ill—lethargic, headache, no focal signs *or* alert, focal signs present
IV	Severely ill—stuporous, no focal signs *or* drowsy, focal signs
WORLD FEDERATION OF NEUROLOGICAL SURGEONS	
I	No headache or focal signs (GCS 15)
II	Headache, nuchal rigidity, no focal signs (GCS 15)
III	Headache, nuchal rigidity, no focal signs (GCS 13–14)
IV	Headache, nuchal rigidity *or* focal signs (GCS 13–14 or 9–12)
V	Headache, nuchal rigidity *or* focal signs (GCS 8 or less)

GCS, Glasgow Coma Scale.
From Award LA, Barnett GH. Acute, management of subarachnoid hemorrhage. In: Loftus CM ed. *Neurosurgical Experiences*, vol. I. Park Ridge, IL: American Association of Neurological Surgeons, 1994.

TABLE 202.2. Differential Diagnosis of Subarachnoid Hemorrhage

ACUTE HEADACHE
Migraine headache
Cluster headache
Muscle contraction headache
Meningitis
Encephalitis
Sinusitis
Temporal arteritis
Viral syndrome
Acute glaucoma
Carbon monoxide poisoning
Hypertensive crisis
ALTERED CONSCIOUSNESS/ABNORMAL NEUROLOGIC FINDINGS
Intracerebral hemorrhage
Cavernous sinus thrombosis
Cerebral infarction
Cerebral neoplasm
Cerebral metastasis
Lupus cerebritis
Seizure disorder
Head injury
Diabetic oculomotor nerve palsy
Alcohol/drug intoxication
Syncope
OTHER DISORDERS
Heat stroke
Acute myocardial infarction
Electrolyte imbalance
Cervical arthritis
Acute myositis

ever, present in a more benign fashion. The occurrence of an unusual headache, acute neck pain, a headache of sudden onset, or new unexplained headache should prompt consideration of SAH. Likewise, change in a chronic headache pattern, new-onset "migraine" headaches, or unexplained neurologic symptoms or signs should be strongly suspected as potential symptoms of SAH or cerebral aneurysm.

The differential diagnosis for acute headache in an awake patient includes new-onset migraine, muscle contraction headache, viral illness, encephalitis, meningitis, and musculoskeletal cervical pain. In patients with an altered level of consciousness, intracranial processes such as cerebral infarction may be confused with SAH. Because hypertension is common in the acute phase of SAH, hypertensive crisis may be an erroneous diagnostic consideration. Likewise, the ECG changes that frequently accompany SAH may be misinterpreted as representing acute cardiac ischemia.

Cranial CT scanning and, if necessary, lumbar puncture (LP) are performed to distinguish SAH from the more common causes of acute cephalgia. Although these tests exclude SAH in the vast majority of cases, the devastating consequences of failing to diagnose SAH in patients with unruptured aneurysms or warning leaks justifies the costs and risks of these procedures.

EMERGENCY DEPARTMENT EVALUATION

The goals of the emergency department evaluation are to establish the diagnosis of SAH, to identify associated complications, and to assist the neurosurgeon in determining the patient's fitness for angiography and surgery. In many cases, the clinical features are suggestive of the diagnosis, which can be confirmed simply and safely by cranial CT scanning and LP.

Unenhanced cranial CT scanning is the procedure of choice for diagnosing acute SAH, with a sensitivity estimated at between 80% and 90%, depending on the elapsed time between the onset of SAH and performance of the scan. Within 24 hours of SAH, CT demonstrates blood in the subarachnoid space or basal cisterns in 90% to 95% of cases of aneurysmal SAH (Fig. 202.1).[4,13] The sensitivity of CT declines with time after the initial hemorrhage and is lower in patients with relatively minor symptoms and normal neurologic examinations.

In the Cooperative Aneurysm Study, 8.2% of patients with SAH had normal CT scans; normal scans were significantly more frequent when obtained 3 or more days after SAH.[2] Even with later generation CT scanners, the overall sensitivity of CT scan alone for detecting SAH is greatest within 12 hours of symptom onset, and about 90% to 95% overall.[16,20] Thus, further testing is required after a normal CT scan in order to completely exclude SAH.

Besides establishing the diagnosis, CT provides important additional information. It reveals nonaneurysmal bleeding sources (e.g., hypertensive hemorrhages and AVMs), demonstrates acute complications that may require urgent intervention (particularly acute hydrocephalus or significant intraparenchymal hematoma), helps localize the probable site of aneurysmal rupture, helps determine the timing of surgical intervention, establishes a baseline for the diagnosis of complications (e.g., rebleeding, ischemia, or hydrocephalus), and serves as an important prognostic indicator for predicting ultimate neurologic outcome.

Magnetic resonance imaging (MRI) is less sensitive than CT scan for detecting SAH. Compared with CT scanning, MRI requires more time to perform, is often tolerated poorly by the patient, provides only limited emergency accessibility to the patient, and is available less frequently in some centers. Moreover, a positive MRI is usually no more likely than a positive CT to obviate the need for cerebral arteriography.[17] Although magnetic resonance angiography (MRA) can visualize some aneurysmal sources of SAH, the absence of rapid blood flow in the lumens of some aneurysms may render them less visible by MRA than by conventional angiography.

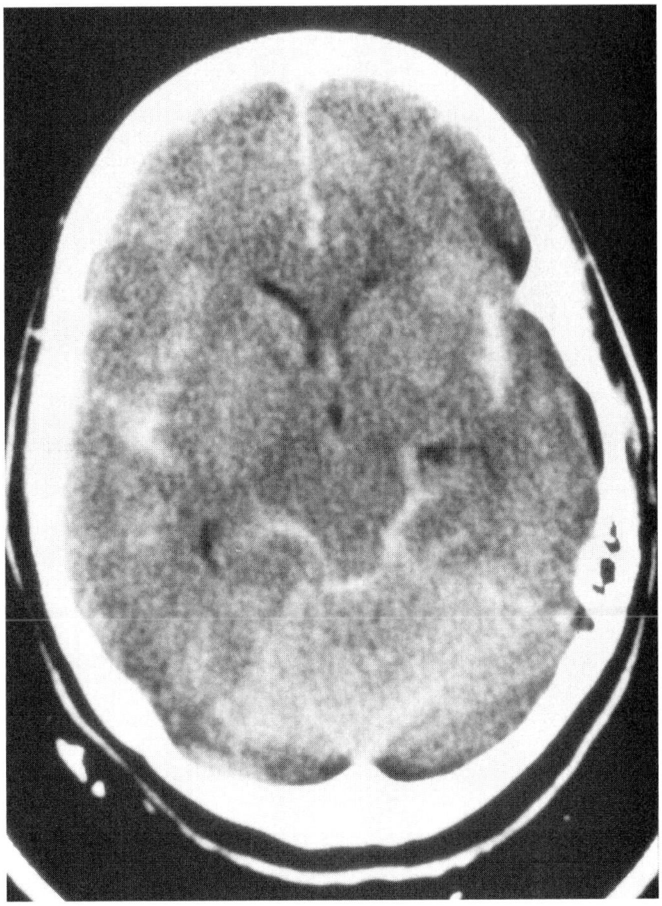

Figure 202.1. Cranial computed tomographic scan showing diffuse subarachnoid hemorrhage.

Although other diagnostic studies seldom aid directly in emergency management, they provide a baseline against which to assess subsequent complications. An ECG should be obtained, and continuous cardiac monitoring should be instituted. Chest radiographs, hematologic studies, and blood chemistry tests should also be ordered in the emergency department.

An LP is indicated in the symptomatic patient with suspected SAH if the CT scan is equivocal or negative. LP can identify subarachnoid blood missed on CT because of poor study quality, motion artifact, mixture of blood and CSF, severe anemia, or localized or subtle subarachnoid bleeding. However, it is generally recommended that CT be performed before the LP so that intracranial hematoma, mass effect, intracranial hypertension, and obstructive hydrocephalus may be ruled out. The risk of untoward neurologic events directly attributable to the performance of an LP in this situation is unknown.

The CSF is grossly bloody in acute SAH, usually containing from 100,000 to more than 1 million red blood cells (RBC)/μL. In rare cases, fewer than 100,000 RBC/μL are present, and greater than 1,000 RBC/μL has been used as a criterion for SAH in some studies.[16] Xanthochromia, the pink or yellow discoloration of the CSF supernatant caused by heme pigments released from the degradation of hemoglobin in CSF, is pathognomonic of SAH. Xanthochromia typically appears 4 to 6 hours after the initial hemorrhage, is present in virtually all patients 12 hours after aneurysmal SAH, and persists for up to 3 weeks in 70% of patients.

LP findings can be the cause of diagnostic confusion. Clinicians may have difficulty distinguishing blood in the CSF due to SAH from local bleeding into the CSF caused by the LP (traumatic tap). In SAH, comparable numbers of RBCs are present in the first and last (usually the fourth) specimen collection tube, whereas CSF samples taken after a traumatic tap usually yield decreasing number of RBCs in consecutively collected tubes. Patients whose presentation for care for SAH has been delayed may demonstrate decreasing numbers of RBCs in serially collected CSF specimen tubes, however, and the same number of RBCs may be seen in all specimens collected from some patients with traumatic taps.

The most accurate method for distinguishing subarachnoid bleeding from a traumatic tap is spectrophotometric examination of the CSF supernatant for the presence of xanthochromia. Xanthochromia is present in virtually all cases of SAH and is absent in most traumatic taps. Bedside visual inspection is insufficiently sensitive to rule out xanthochromia, however, so spectrophotometric analysis is required. Furthermore, because RBCs from a traumatic tap may lyse and discolor the supernatant if centrifugation and examination are delayed, analysis should be carried out on a freshly obtained specimen as soon as possible after collection.

Four-vessel cerebral angiography provides the definitive diagnostic information in patients with SAH or a sentinel headache. Angiography precisely defines the location of bleeding, delineates the cerebral anatomy, determines the degree of cerebral vasospasm, defines the extent and number of aneurysms, differentiates between aneurysm and AVMs, identifies unusual causes of SAH (e.g., tumors), and aids in decision making regarding surgical intervention. Angiography is not a routine part of the emergency department diagnostic evaluation in most centers, however. The admitting neurosurgeon generally determines the optimal timing of angiography in relation to plans for surgical intervention.

Although other diagnostic studies seldom aid directly in emergency management, they provide a baseline against which to assess subsequent complications. An ECG should be obtained, and continuous cardiac monitoring should be instituted. Chest radiographs, hematologic studies, and blood chemistry tests should also be ordered in the emergency department.

EMERGENCY DEPARTMENT MANAGEMENT

Emergency management of SAH involves the immediate stabilization of acute life-threatening conditions and the institution of appropriate supportive therapy. Once SAH is diagnosed, therapy is aimed at preventing complications such as seizures, rebleeding, and vasospasm, and preparations are made for angiography and possible surgical intervention.

The necessary supportive therapy depends on the patient's clinical status. Vital signs, cardiac rhythm, and oxygen saturation should be monitored, and an intravenous line should be established. A urinary catheter should be inserted in confused or obtunded patients. The head of the bed should be elevated 30 degrees from the horizontal to facilitate venous drainage and help reduce ICP. If possible, the patient should be kept in a quiet area, and visits by family or friends should be minimized.

Patients with respiratory compromise secondary to hypoventilation, obtundation, hypoxia, hypercarbia, loss of airway protective reflexes, or pulmonary edema require endotracheal intubation and assisted ventilation, as do those who require hyperventilation to reduce increased ICP. Controlled hyperventilation with target P_{CO_2} levels of 25 to 30 mm Hg is effective for acutely reducing elevated ICP. Adjunctive pharmacologic agents (e.g., lidocaine, sedatives, and neuromuscular blocking agents) may be necessary to ensure rapid, smooth, airway control and to minimize increases in ICP.

Adequate cerebral perfusion pressure must be maintained, and excessive increases or surges in mean arterial pressure must be avoided. Although hypertension at time of admission is associated with poor prognosis,[12] studies have failed to demonstrate a consistent benefit of antihypertensive treatment.[15] Thus, administration of antihypertensive agents should be performed in consultation with a neurosurgeon for most patients unless there is significant and sustained blood pressure elevation (diastolic greater than 120 to 130 mm Hg). For these patients, a titratable, short-acting agent, such as intravenous nitroprusside, should be employed. The drug should be titrated to reduce the diastolic pressure below 100 to 110 mm Hg diastolic over 20 to 30 minutes. Other agents, such as nifedipine or hydralazine, should be avoided, because they cannot be titrated and may cause excessive hypotension.

The administration of prophylactic anticonvulsant agents is a widespread practice. Anticonvulsants may prevent the seizures that can occur in as many as 25% of ruptured aneurysms.[22] Preventing seizures and the concomitant increases in ICP can reduce the risk of rebleeding. Phenytoin is typically used as a prophylactic anticonvulsant. Although studies have not demonstrated a consistent benefit from prophylactic anticonvulsant use, their short-term use in the interval after rupture and surgery has been recommended as a reasonable precaution.[15] Seizures should be aggressively managed if they occur. Diazepam or lorazepam may be used as first-line agents when seizures occur and should be followed by phenytoin loading. Phenobarbital loading is an effective alternative, but its sedating effects may interfere with subsequent neurologic assessment.

Antiemetics such as prochlorperazine or promethazine are indicated to control nausea and vomiting. Alert patients with significant headache or neck pain may require narcotic analgesics for pain control. Despite the lack of proven benefit of corticosteroids in decreasing cerebral edema associated with SAH, some neurosurgeons advocate their use to help reduce the irritative effects of blood in the subarachnoid space.

Treatment with a calcium channel blocker such as nimodipine (orally or via nasogastric tube) or nicardipine (intravenously) appears to be effective in reducing the risk and severity of cerebral vasospasm; patients who have a relatively good neurologic status after SAH derive the most benefit.[9,18]

Antifibrinolytic therapy (e.g., with aminocaproic acid) decreases the rate of rebleeding after SAH, but is associated with an increased risk of ischemic complications, including cerebral infarction, as well as hydrocephalus, pulmonary embolism, and deep venous thrombosis. Consequently, the use of antifibrinolytic agents has decreased with the trend toward earlier surgical intervention.

DISPOSITION

All patients with SAH require admission to the hospital for monitoring of neurologic status and evaluation for surgical intervention. A neurosurgeon should be consulted immediately once the diagnosis of SAH is established, and admission to a neurosurgical unit or critical care setting should be considered. The neurosurgeon evaluates the need to evacuate an acute intracerebral hematoma or to perform an intraventricular drainage procedure, and determines the pace of further evaluation, including angiography. The timing of definitive surgery for SAH secondary to ruptured cerebral aneurysm is somewhat controversial.

Early surgical intervention (i.e., within 24 to 48 hours after initial bleeding) appears to decrease the incidence of rebleeding and vasospasm and results in improved neurologic outcome, particularly for patients with good neurologic status after SAH. Prompt neurosurgical consultation is also indicated when there is evidence of increased ICP or progressive or lateralizing neurologic signs.

In hospitals without CT scanning or available neurosurgical expertise, the patient should be stabilized rapidly and transferred to a facility that has the necessary capabilities for treating patients with SAH.

COMMON PITFALLS

- Failure to consider the diagnosis and order the appropriate diagnostic studies. Although some patients with SAH may present with catastrophic hemorrhage, a significant proportion experiences less severe and relatively less impressive warning symptoms, most commonly consisting only of an unusual headache.
- Failure to perform an LP in a patient with suspected SAH in whom the head CT is negative. Conversely, performing an LP before obtaining a CT scan may result in substantial neurologic morbidity in the occasional patient who has a significant mass lesion or obstructive hydrocephalus.

References

1. Adams HP, Jergenson DD, Kassell NF, et al. Pitfalls in the recognition of subarachnoid hemorrhage. *JAMA* 1980;244:794.
2. Adams HP, Kassell NF, Torner JC, et al. CT and clinical correlations in recent aneurysmal subarachnoid hemorrhage: a preliminary report of the Cooperative Aneurysm Study. *Neurology* 1983;33:981.
3. Andreoli A, Pinelli G. Subarachnoid hemorrhage: frequency and severity of cardiac arrhythmias. *Stroke* 1987;18:558.
4. Awad IA, Barnett GH. Acute management of subarachnoid hemorrhage. In: Loftus CM, ed. *Neurosurgical emergencies,* vol I. Park Ridge, IL: American Association of Neurological Surgeons, 1994.
5. Bromberg JEC, Rinkel GJE, Algra A, et al. Subarachnoid hemorrhage in first and second degree relatives of patients with subarachnoid hemorrhage. *BMJ* 1995;311:288–289.
6. Broderick JP, Brott T, Tomsick T, et al. The risk of subarachnoid and intracerebral hemorrhage in blacks as compared with whites. *N Engl J Med* 1992;326:733.
7. Crowell RM. Management of subarachnoid hemorrhage. *Semin Neurol* 1989;9:210.
8. Fontanarosa PB. Recognition of subarachnoid hemorrhage. *Ann Emerg Med* 1989;18:1199.
9. Haley EC, Kassell NF, Torner JC. A randomized controlled trial of high dose intravenous nicardipine in aneurysmal subarachnoid hemorrhage: a report of the Cooperative Aneurysm Study. *J Neurosurg* 1993;78:537.
10. Inagawa T. Management outcome in the elderly patient following aneurysmal subarachnoid hemorrhage. *J Neurosurg* 1993;78:554.
11. Kassel NF, Torner JC. Aneurysmal rebleeding: a preliminary report from the cooperative aneurysm study. *Neurosurgery* 1983;13:479–481.
12. Kassel NF, Torner JC, Haley EC, et al. The international cooperative study on the timing of aneurysm surgery. Part I: overall management results. *J Neurosurg* 1990;73:18–36.
13. Longstreth WT, Nelson LM, Koepsell TD, et al. Clinical course of subarachnoid hemorrhage: a population based study in King County, Washington. *Neurology* 1993;43:712.
14. Longstreth WT, Nelson LM, Koepsell TD, et al. Subarachnoid hemorrhage and hormonal factors in women: a population based case control study. *Ann Intern Med* 1994;121:168.
15. Mayberg MR, Batjer HH, Dacey R, et al. Guidelines for the management of aneurysmal subarachnoid hemorrhage: a statement for healthcare professionals from a special writing group of the Stroke Council, American Heart Association. *Stroke* 1994;25:2315–2328.
16. Morgenstern LB, Luna-Gonzales H, Huber JC, et al. Worst headache and subarachnoid hemorrhage: prospective, modern computed tomography and spinal fluid analysis. *Ann Emerg Med* 1998;32:297–304.
17. Ogawa T, Inugami A, Shimosegawa E, et al. Subarachnoid hemorrhage: evaluation with MR imaging. *Radiology* 1993;186:345.
18. Pickard JD, Murray GD, Illingworth R, et al. Effect of oral nimodipine on cerebral infarction and outcome after subarachnoid hemorrhage: British aneurysm trial. *BMJ* 1989;298(6674):636.
19. Rosenon J, Eskesen V, Schmidt K. Unruptured intracranial aneurysms: an assessment of the annual risk of rupture based on epidemiological and clinical data. *Br J Neurosurg* 1988;2:369–377.
20. Sidman R, Connolly E, Lemke T. Subarachnoid hemorrhage diagnosis: lumbar puncture is still needed when the computed tomography scan is normal. *Acad Emerg Med* 1996;3:827–831.
21. Solomon RA, Fink ME. Current strategies for the management of aneurysmal subarachnoid hemorrhage. *Arch Neurol* 1987;44:769.
22. Sundaram MB, Chow F. Seizures associated with spontaneous subarachnoid hemorrhage. *Can J Neurol Sci* 1986;13:229–231.
23. Teunissen LL, Rinkel GJ, Algra A, et al. Risk factors for subarachnoid hemorrhage: a systematic review. *Stroke* 1996;27:544–549.
24. Verweij RD, Wijdicks EF, van Gijn J. Warning headache in aneurysmal subarachnoid hemorrhage—a case control study. *Arch Neurol* 1988;45:1019.
25. Whiting DM, Barnett GH, Little JR. Management of subarachnoid hemorrhage in the critical care unit. *Cleve Clin J Med* 1989;56:775.

CHAPTER 203
Cerebrovascular Disease

Phillip A. Scott and William G. Barsan

The term *stroke* refers to the sudden onset of a neurologic deficit of varying duration, caused by an acute vascular lesion of the brain that is either hemorrhagic, embolic, thrombotic, or aneurysmal in nature. *Cerebrovascular disease* is a broader term, encompassing stroke and other vascular causes of central nervous system dysfunction.

Stroke is the third leading cause of death in the United States, after heart disease and cancer. In 1995, there were over 700,000 new cases of stroke in the United States, with approximately 150,000 deaths and a cumulative total of 3 million stroke survivors, many requiring chronic care. The estimated annual cost of cerebrovascular disease in the United States exceeds $30 billion.

DIAGNOSTIC PROCEDURES IN CEREBROVASCULAR DISEASE

A knowledge of the common diagnostic procedures used to evaluate suspected cerebrovascular disease is essential for the emergency physician.

COMPUTED TOMOGRAPHY OF THE HEAD

Computed tomography (CT) has become the most commonly ordered examination in patients with symptoms of cerebrovascular disease. Image resolution can be optimized by the use of intravenous contrast material, which enhances the density of vascular structures and areas where the blood–brain barrier is breached.

Current scanners are capable of identifying hematomas of less than 1 cm in diameter and infarcts as small as 1.0 to 1.5 cm, provided the lesion is transected by a given slice and not lost in volume averaging. CT is less reliable in identifying lesions at the base of the brain and in the posterior fossa because of artifact from surrounding bony structures. In ischemic stroke, the infarct area becomes hypodense 6 to 72 hours after onset and by 10 days becomes isodense with the surrounding tissue. In hemorrhagic infarcts, the initially hyperdense area becomes isodense with surrounding tissue at 3 to 4 weeks. CT imaging identifies 95% of patients with subarachnoid hemorrhage (SAH) due to aneurysmal leak or rupture; lumbar puncture should be performed to rule out SAH in patients with a high index of suspicion and a normal CT scan.

MAGNETIC RESONANCE IMAGING

Magnetic resonance imaging (MRI) has several important advantages over CT in emergency care. First, MRI is superior in identifying lesions of the posterior fossa, brainstem, and skull base. Second, MRI accurately localizes gray and white matter pathology and is more sensitive than CT in the early detection of infarction. Third, major intracranial blood vessels can be visualized by MRI without the use of iodinated contrast media. This improved visualization makes MRI the preferred diagnostic study for suspected venous sinus thrombosis. Fourth, coronal and sagittal views are easily obtained with MRI, whereas reconstruction is required with CT. Finally, patients are not exposed to ionizing radiation with MRI.

Major limitations to the emergent use of MRI include its lack of availability, increased scanning time, and increased cost compared with CT. In addition, its sensitivity to motion artifact requires a high degree of patient cooperation in a tight, enclosed environment. There is limited access to the critically ill patient, and no ferromagnetic materials or monitors may be used while the patient is in the magnetic field.

DUPLEX SCANNING

Vascular duplex scanning combines high-resolution, brightness-modulated (B-mode) imaging of the vessel wall with pulsed-wave spectral analysis of the intravascular flow velocity. This combination of modalities improves the reliability of noninvasive carotid studies to greater than 90% for identifying significant carotid artery disease.

Indications for emergent duplex scanning of the carotid system include transient ischemic attacks (TIAs) and completed ischemic strokes in which vascular dissection is suspected. Duplex scanning is also useful in evaluating asymptomatic bruits and in identifying nonstenotic vascular lesions. It is a safe, noninvasive test to screen patients for extracranial carotid disease before angiography.

Duplex scanning has several limitations. It is unreliable for imaging high in the internal carotid and intracranial arterial systems, and its ability to evaluate the vertebrobasilar system is unproved. The accuracy of duplex scanning in distinguishing severe carotid stenosis from complete occlusion is controversial.

CEREBRAL ANGIOGRAPHY

There are several potential indications for emergent cerebral angiography: (1) evaluation of stenotic lesions seen on carotid duplex scanning in patients being considered for emergent endarterectomy; (2) detection of vertebrobasilar or carotid artery dissection in young adults presenting with a new ischemic stroke; and (3) localization of bleeding in patients presenting with acute SAH. Other indications for scheduled angiography include definitive evaluation of extracranial and intracranial arterial stenosis, arteriovenous malformations, aneurysms, and vasculitis.

Limitations of cerebral angiography include its lack of universal availability and its associated morbidity. There is a 0.1% to 1.0% risk of stroke from the procedure that is angiographer-dependent. There is also the possibility of hemorrhage from the femoral puncture site and the risk of anaphylactoid reactions and renal failure from the contrast media employed.

ISCHEMIC CEREBROVASCULAR DISEASE

Ischemic neurologic deficits are commonly categorized by their time course. Deficits persisting less than 24 hours are referred to as *transient ischemic attacks;* those persisting up to 6 weeks are termed *reversible ischemic neurologic deficits;* those with progressive symptoms are *strokes in evolution;* and stable deficits are classified as *completed strokes*. In the Dutch TIA study trial, a relevant infarct corresponding to a clinical deficit was found on CT scanning in 13% of patients with TIAs, 35% of patients with reversible ischemic neurologic deficits, and 49% of patients with "minor" strokes.[14] This suggests that these temporal classifications should be thought of as a continuum rather than as separate entities with specific causes, prognoses, and treatments. Nevertheless, this classification is useful for the emergency physician evaluating the patient at a single point early in the disease process. Other classification systems define stroke syndromes by probable cause or anatomic location.

RISK FACTORS

Not surprisingly, risk factors for ischemic cerebrovascular disease parallel those for atherosclerotic heart disease. Hypertension is the major risk factor for stroke and accounts for a fourfold increase in the incidence of atherothrombotic brain infarction as compared with normotensive subjects. The degree of risk corresponds to the level of elevation of either the systolic or diastolic pressure and may be reduced by appropriate antihypertensive therapy. The presence of coronary heart disease triples the risk of stroke. Left ventricular hypertrophy, atrial fibrillation, and acute myocardial infarction (AMI) are all independent risk factors for ischemic stroke. Patients with diabetes have a prevalence of stroke 2.5 to four times higher than persons with normal glucose levels.

There are significant associations of ischemic cerebrovascular disease with age, sex, and race. The incidence of all strokes increases with age, doubling with each decade of life. In 1990, 13% of the population in the United States was over 65 years of age, and this group accounted for more than 75% of all strokes. There is a slightly higher risk in men compared with women, and Black men and women have age-adjusted stroke incidence rates that are 1.5 to 2.3 times higher, respectively, than those in Whites.[9] The Japanese population shares this higher incidence of stroke relative to the White population of the United States. Cerebrovascular disease in both Blacks and Japanese is typically intracranial, rather than the extracranial disease more common in White males.

Other medical conditions predisposing to stroke include a history of migraine headaches, elevated fibrinogen levels or hematocrit (causing increased blood viscosity), and advanced age with elevated total serum cholesterol levels.

Environmental risk factors for ischemic cerebrovascular disease include smoking and heavy alcohol consumption. Women taking oral contraceptives, particularly high-estrogen formulations, are also at increased risk for stroke. This risk is more pronounced in women smokers older than 35 years of age and in those with other cardiovascular risk factors.

Finally, patients with a history of ischemic stroke represent a high-risk population, with 1- and 5-year recurrence rates among survivors of 10% and 20%, respectively.[16]

Transient Ischemic Attacks

Although TIA is arbitrarily defined as a deficit that resolves within 24 hours, the typical carotid TIA lasts less than 15 minutes. TIAs serve as a warning sign, though the exact number progressing to completed stroke is the subject of numerous studies and much debate. If untreated, TIAs carry a cumulative risk of 5% to 6% per year for completed stroke (30% to 35% over 5 years), but the risk may be as high as 20% in the first month. Other studies, however, indicate that 3% to 9% of patients with TIAs experience a stroke within 1 week and approximately 15% have additional TIAs over this period.

Classically, the majority of TIAs were believed to result from plaque ulceration or embolism of platelet aggregates from extracranial or intracranial atherosclerosis. After impeding local blood flow, these emboli break up, accounting for the transient nature of the episode. Other sources of emboli include prosthetic heart valves and infective or marantic vegetations on valve leaflets. However, one report indicates that small-vessel disease in penetrating cerebral arteries may actually be the most common cause of TIAs and that these "lacunar" TIAs may represent a subgroup with a better prognosis than TIAs with cortical symptoms.[12] Hypotension and mechanical kinking of the extracranial vessels are less common causes of TIAs. Cardiac dysrhythmias are also an important potential etiology.

CLINICAL PRESENTATION

Carotid artery syndrome results from transient disruption of the anterior circulation of one cerebral hemisphere or of the retina. Hemispheric ischemia results in an abrupt onset of contralateral monoparesis or hemiparesis, numbness, tingling, aphasia, or hemianopia. Occlusion of the ophthalmic branch of the internal carotid artery results in retinal ischemia, causing temporary monocular blindness (amaurosis fugax). The patient complains of a "fog," "mist," "cloud," or "shade being drawn" over the visual field of one eye. Funduscopic examination of the involved eye may reveal cholesterol crystals (Hollenhorst plaques) in the retinal vessels.

Transient ischemia involving the posterior circulation (the brainstem or occipital lobes) is termed *vertebrobasilar artery syndrome*. Interruption of brainstem circulation may result in symptoms of vertigo, dizziness, ataxia, nausea, and vomiting secondary to involvement of the vestibular nuclei. Dysarthria, dysphagia, and perioral numbness may also occur. Occipital lobe ischemia results in blurred or dim vision or total cortical blindness. Diplopia may result from loss of conjugate gaze.

Basilar artery TIAs may cause *drop attacks*, which are brief paretic spells resulting in the patient dropping to his or her knees. There is no loss of consciousness, distinguishing it from true syncope, and the patient attempts to rise immediately after falling.

Transient global amnesia is thought to be caused by ischemia of the temporal lobes or thalamic area supplied by the posterior cerebral arteries. These episodes affect men more frequently than women and are characterized by a rapid development of retrograde memory loss and confusion, with preservation of self-identity. The length of retrograde amnesia gradually shortens until only the period during the attack remains lost.

DIFFERENTIAL DIAGNOSIS

The differential diagnosis of TIAs includes (1) transient deficits secondary to mass lesions from either tumor or hemorrhage (these patients often have a residual neurologic deficit detectable on examination); (2) infection (as with focal abscess, septic emboli, meningitis, or encephalitis); (3) seizure with a subsequent Todd's paralysis; (4) complicated migraine; (5) exacerbation of multiple sclerosis; (6) hypoglycemia; and (7) syncope from any cause, particularly cardiac dysrhythmias.

EMERGENCY DEPARTMENT EVALUATION

Clinical investigation of TIA is directed toward identifying whether the deficit involves the anterior or posterior circulation, establishing the source of the TIA, and ruling out other causes of focal deficits. A detailed history often provides the most significant information. The patient may not be aware of any deficits, and the family should be questioned, if possible, along with the patient.

The onset and course of symptoms should be carefully elicited. Were there any prior episodes and, if so, how many; and were the events in the same or differing vascular distributions? "Crescendo" TIAs are defined as more than three events occurring in a 72-hour period, and these patients represent a high-risk group. A history of multiple events in differing territories points to a cardiac or other proximal source of emboli. Is there a history of intravenous drug use? Are there any medications predisposing the patient to decreases in blood pressure? Are there risk factors for cerebrovascular disease, or is there evidence of peripheral vascular disease?

Is there a history of claudication in an exercised arm occurring simultaneously with symptoms of vertebrobasilar insufficiency? With significant occlusion of the brachiocephalic or left subclavian artery, exercise of the ipsilateral extremity results in a reversal of blood flow through the vertebral arteries, shunting blood to the involved limb and causing posterior circulation symptoms (subclavian steal syndrome). Is there a history of significant arthritis predisposing the patient to formation of cervical osteophytes that could mechanically compress the extracranial vessels? This would indicate a need for radiologic evaluation of the cervical spine.

The neurologic examination in patients with TIAs is often unremarkable, but a complete assessment is essential. Orthostatic blood pressures should be measured in patients with vertebrobasilar TIAs, because symptoms are often related to postural changes. Auscultation for cervical and subclavian bruits should be performed, as well as evaluation for cardiac dysrhythmias, murmurs, and left ventricular dysfunction.

Laboratory evaluation of patients with suspected TIA include a complete blood cell count to assess hemoglobin and hematocrit (anemia or polycythemia), coagulation studies (prothrombin time and partial thromboplastin time), and a glucose determination. An erythrocyte sedimentation rate is useful for suspected vasculitis, and a serologic test for syphilis should also be obtained if clinically indicated. An electrocardiogram and cranial CT scan should be performed. Transthoracic and/or transesophageal echocardiography is indicated when cardiac emboli are suspected.

Patients with anterior circulation TIAs who have no obvious cardiac etiology and no contraindications for vascular surgery should be screened with duplex ultrasonography for significant carotid artery stenosis. These patients represent a subgroup of TIA patients known to have an improved outcome with carotid endarterectomy; they should be identified as early as possible.

EMERGENCY DEPARTMENT MANAGEMENT

All patients with a diagnosis of TIA should be placed on a cardiac monitor and have potentially correctable causes (e.g., hypoglycemia) immediately addressed. If infective endocarditis is suspected, serial blood cultures should be obtained and appropriate antibiotic therapy initiated. Extended cardiac monitoring is indicated for patients with suspected dysrhythmias.

Medical therapy is indicated for patients with posterior circulation TIAs, those with anterior circulation TIAs who have less than 50% stenosis on carotid duplex scanning, and patients who are not candidates for carotid endarterectomy. Medical treatment options are limited to antiplatelet therapy and anticoagulation.

Antiplatelet therapy with aspirin (30 to 1500 mg/d) reduces the incidence of nonfatal stroke, nonfatal myocardial infarction, and death from all vascular causes in patients with TIAs. Because the lower dosages require several days to achieve maximal platelet inhibition, therapy in the emergency department should be initiated with 300 to 325 mg/d. The ESPS-2 trial found dipyridamole (200 mg b.i.d.) to have an additive protective effect when used with low-dose (50 mg/d) aspirin, with a combined 37% reduction in recurrent stroke in patients with previous stroke or TIA.[7] This is the first study to report an independent effect of dipyridamole when used with aspirin.

Ticlopidine (Ticlid, 250 mg b.i.d.), an antiplatelet agent inhibiting adenosine diphosphate (ADP)–dependent platelet activation, is slightly more effective than aspirin alone in preventing recurrent TIAs. Because of concern over side effects (diarrhea, rash, neutropenia) and increased cost, its use should be reserved for patients who cannot tolerate aspirin or continue to have TIAs while on aspirin.[3,10] Clopidogrel (Plavix, 75 mg daily) is a newer ADP inhibitor and, though structurally similar to ticlopidine, does not cause neutropenia. Its role as a primary or secondary agent in the treatment of TIA is still unclear, given its cost and the small (0.5%) improvement it provides in reducing risk for stroke, AMI, and vascular death in patients with atherosclerotic vascular disease compared with aspirin alone.

Although heparin has traditionally been used in selected patients with TIA, no prospective randomized study of significant size has demonstrated a clear benefit. Its use is probably best reserved for "high-risk" patients. These are patients with crescendo TIAs, vertebrobasilar TIA, recurrent TIA while receiving maximum antiplatelet therapy, high-grade carotid stenosis, or a suspected cardiac source for emboli. Because the use of anticoagulants is controversial, neurologic consultation is advisable when initiating heparin therapy.

A subset of patients with TIAs have surgically correctable carotid stenosis and represent an important group for the emergency physician to identify. Those with greater than or equal to 50% carotid stenosis on duplex scanning are potential candidates for endarterectomy and should begin medical therapy in the emergency department pending a final decision. Carotid angiography is typically used to define the specific characteristics of these lesions before surgery and in cases in which duplex scanning is inadequate.

The North American Symptomatic Carotid Endarterectomy Trial (NASCET) found that symptomatic patients with high-grade (70% to 99%) stenosis randomized to carotid endarterectomy had a 17% reduction in the risk of ipsilateral stroke after 2 years, compared with the optimal medical treatment group. Carotid endarterectomy was usually performed within 2 days after the TIA, and no patients died or had a stroke during this interval. The data comparing surgical to medical therapy for patients with moderate (30% to 69%) stenosis found a smaller risk reduction (10.1%) at 5 years for those with 50% to 69% stenosis and no benefit from surgery for those with less than 50% stenosis.[2] The beneficial effect of endarterectomy for high-grade stenosis is further supported by the European Carotid Surgery Trial.[8]

DISPOSITION

Patients who have an anterior circulation TIA and who are potential surgical candidates should not be discharged without an evaluation of the carotid arteries. If duplex scanning is unavailable, the patient should be admitted (either to an inpatient setting or to an emergency department clinical decision unit) and started on antiplatelet therapy while undergoing frequent neurologic assessments. Carotid duplex scanning should be performed as soon as possible and vascular consultation requested for patients determined to have greater than or equal to 50% stenosis.

Patients with an anterior circulation TIA who are not "high risk" (as defined previously) and have less than 50% carotid stenosis on duplex scanning may be discharged home on antiplatelet therapy, with close follow-up. High-risk patients should be admitted and neurologic consultation obtained to address the issue of anticoagulation. Patients with suspected dysrhythmias require a monitored bed and evaluation for ischemic heart disease, as appropriate.

Standard protocols for patients with TIAs should be jointly developed with neurologic specialists in each institution. Active collaboration can ensure the provision of efficient and consistent patient care and facilitate future modifications as new treatments become available.

COMMON PITFALLS

- Failure to recognize a TIA when the symptoms are remote in time from the emergency department presentation. Establishing the diagnosis becomes more difficult when the patient is unable to recall the specific events surrounding the TIA.
- Discharging patients with anterior circulation TIAs before determining whether there is a potentially surgically correctable carotid lesion. This carries a high medicolegal risk.
- Failure to consider heparinization in high-risk patients: those with crescendo TIAs, vertebrobasilar TIA, recurrent TIA on maximal antiplatelet therapy, high-grade carotid artery stenosis, or presumed cardioembolic source

Ischemic Stroke

Ischemic strokes have traditionally been classified by clinical presentation, time course of onset, progression of deficits, accompanying symptoms, and risk factor profiles. The clinical description of the deficit identifies the extent and location of the stroke and allows accurate communication regarding patient status. The time course and progression of symptoms suggest certain etiologies; for example, prolonged, "stuttering" deficits indicate a thrombotic phenomenon, while an abrupt onset of the maximal deficit suggests an embolic event. Associated symptoms reveal other causes of neurologic deficits (e.g., a seizure preceding a Todd's paralysis or a migraine headache preceding an ischemic stroke of vascular origin). Consideration of cerebrovascular risk factors helps to classify the stroke as lacunar, embolic, thrombotic, extracranial, or intracranial.

Pathologically, ischemic strokes are divided into *bland* and *hemorrhagic* infarcts. A bland infarct is a pale region, caused by an occluding thrombus, with red blood cells found only at the periphery. Hemorrhagic infarcts are thought to occur after fragmentation of an occluding embolus and show large numbers of red blood cells in the infarcted area secondary to reperfusion of the injured arterial bed. This is consistent with data indicating a higher frequency of hemorrhagic transformation among cardioembolic strokes. The absolute level and rate of change of arterial blood pressure also plays an important role in this "hemorrhagic transformation." The timing of hemorrhagic transformation is variable, occurring hours to weeks after symptom onset. The clinical effects are also variable, ranging from asymptomatic to catastrophic. Hemorrhagic transformation should be considered in any patient who experiences an abrupt decrease in neurologic function after a stroke.

CLINICAL PRESENTATION

Anterior Cerebral Artery Syndrome

Patients with infarction in the territory of the anterior cerebral artery present with hemiparesis involving the leg more than the face or arm. Urinary incontinence and primitive reflexes (grasp and suck) are often present. The patient may perseverate with speech or motor movements and respond slowly to questions. If both anterior cerebral arteries originate from a common trunk, a bilateral parasagittal infarct may occur, with paraplegia and speechlessness (anarthria).

Middle Cerebral Artery Syndrome

Infarction in the distribution of the middle cerebral artery is the most common of the stroke syndromes. Patients with infarcts of the middle cerebral artery present with weakness of the face and arm greater than that of the leg, often with corresponding cortical sensory loss. The presence of aphasia localizes the lesion to the dominant hemisphere. Inattention, extinction on double simultaneous sensory or visual testing, neglect, or constructional or dressing apraxia indicates nondominant hemisphere involvement. Homonymous hemianopia and conjugate eye deviation toward the side of the infarct may also be found. All of these findings are present in the patient with a proximal trunk occlusion and variably present when branches of the middle cerebral artery are involved.

Posterior Cerebral Artery Syndrome

Infarcts in this territory present with homonymous hemianopia secondary to visual cortex involvement. The patient is often unaware of the deficit until formally tested. Motor involvement is minimal, but sensory loss, including both light touch and pinprick, may be severe. There is no aphasia or disruption of nondominant hemisphere functions. Small branches of the posterior cerebral artery anastomose with branches of the anterior and middle cerebral arteries in border zones between the arterial distributions. These areas are at risk for *watershed infarcts* during periods of decreased blood flow.

Vertebrobasilar Artery Syndrome

The classic sign of brainstem stroke is the presence of crossed symptoms: ipsilateral cranial nerve palsy and contralateral hemiplegia. One of the most common strokes in this region is due to occlusion of the vertebral or posterior inferior cerebellar artery, resulting in the *lateral medullary (Wallenberg) syndrome*. Patients may present with ipsilateral facial pain (described as a sharp or stabbing sensation to the face or eye), vertigo, headache, limb ataxia, Horner syndrome, and weakness of the soft palate, with dysphagia and dysphonia. Contralateral symptoms include loss of pinprick and temperature sensation in the arm and leg. Other brainstem syndromes may result in deafness, nausea, vomiting, vertigo, and diplopia.

Cerebellar Infarction

A subset of posterior circulation strokes are those that involve the cerebellum. The most common initial symptom is the sudden inability to walk or stand. This may be followed by complaints of headache, nausea, vomiting, central vertigo, and, possibly, a stiff neck. Cranial nerve findings may also be present. Although the initial CT scan is often unremarkable, one-third of patients develop significant posterior fossa edema. In this confined space, edema produces pressure on the brainstem, causing a decrease in the level of consciousness, typically after a stable period of 6 to 12 hours. Pathologic respiratory patterns and pupillary dilation are late findings, indicating impending herniation. Recognition of cerebellar infarction is critical, and frequent neurologic assessment imperative. Repeat CT scanning or MRI is indicated for patients with a declining level of consciousness. Surgical decompression or the use of diuretics and corticosteroids to prevent edema may be lifesaving.

Lacunar Syndromes

Lacunar infarcts cause several distinct stroke syndromes. Lacunes are found almost exclusively in the basal ganglia, internal capsule, thalamus, and brainstem and are associated with hypertensive arteriopathy. Approximately 20% of patients with lacunar infarctions have had a prior TIA, and the onset of symptoms is often surprisingly gradual (over 36 hours in up to 30% of patients). Deficits often improve with time, and treatment is aimed at control of hypertension after the acute episode resolves. An evaluation for embolic sources should also be undertaken. Lacunar strokes are classified by clinical presentation.

The most frequent lacunar syndrome, *pure motor stroke*, causes paresis or plegia of the face, arm, and leg. It is easily diagnosed when the deficit involves all three areas equally, but may also present as a partial deficit. The location of the lacune may be in the internal capsule or pons. Cortical sensory deficits are notably absent.

Pure sensory stroke is the result of infarction of the ventral posterior nuclei of the thalamus and results in sensory loss in the face, arm, and leg. The patient may also complain of paresthesias involving the affected side. There is no hemiplegia or other cortical signs.

Patients with *clumsy hand–dysarthria syndrome* present with slurred speech and weakness and ataxia of the upper limb. Facial weakness may also be present. The syndrome is most commonly associated with lesions of the anterior limb and genu of the internal capsule and typically has a good functional outcome.

DIFFERENTIAL DIAGNOSIS

Table 203.1 lists conditions that may mimic ischemic stoke and is divided into structural and nonstructural diseases. CT scanning is used initially to evaluate these possibilities and to rule out structural causes of neurologic deficits.

Diseases presenting with features similar to posterior circulation strokes can be difficult to distinguish from stroke. Wernicke's encephalopathy presents as the triad of ophthalmoplegia, ataxia, and confusion and is found typically in chronic alcoholics. Ménière disease, with its characteristic triad of vertigo, tinnitus, and deafness, occurs in patients between the ages of 30 and 60 and is paroxysmal in nature. Gross ataxia and cranial nerve deficits should be absent. Multiple sclerosis presents in the third to fourth decades of life and has variable symptoms, depending on the location of demyelination. Symptoms of phenytoin toxicity include sedation, nystagmus, vertigo, ataxia,

TABLE 203.1. Differential Diagnosis of Ischemic Stroke

Structural Causes	Nonstructural Causes
Intracerebral hemorrhage	Meningitis
Epidural hematoma	Encephalitis
Subdural hematoma	Hypertensive encephalopathy
Acute	Wernicke's encephalopathy
Chronic	Hypoglycemia
Intracranial tumor	Complicated (hemiplegic) migraine
Intracranial abscess	Todd's postictal paralysis
	Peripheral nerve palsy (Bell's palsy)
	Labyrinthitis
	Menière disease
	Demyelinating disease (multiple sclerosis)
	Drug toxicity (phenytoin, lithium)

and nausea. Central nervous system symptoms of acute lithium toxicity include confusion, hyperreflexia, tremors, and cranial nerve deficits; dysarthria also may be a prominent feature.

Special consideration should be given to stroke patients younger than 50 years of age or those who have preexisting heart disease, hematologic disorders, or vasculitis. These patients typically fall into the cardioembolic, other, or unknown subtype classifications and may have reversible etiologies or other contributing disease states that should be identified as rapidly as possible. Conditions associated with each of these groups are listed in Table 203.2. An extensive discussion of each of these entities is beyond the scope of this chapter.

EMERGENCY DEPARTMENT EVALUATION

Like myocardial infarction, stroke is an acute disease necessitating early identification and treatment. Patients with stroke symptoms should be advised to access 911, because studies indicate that a significant delay in obtaining medical care occurs among those contacting their personal physician initially.

Prehospital personnel should obtain information surrounding the onset of symptoms, particularly noting the time that deficits started. Patients found lying immobile for prolonged periods are at risk for decubitus ulcers, dehydration, hypothermia or hyperthermia, and rhabdomyolysis. Intravenous access should be obtained and a fingerstick glucose level determined when possible. In the prehospital phase, it is unusual for patients with ischemic stroke to have an altered level of consciousness; an altered sensorium suggests the presence of other etiologies. Glucose-containing solutions and routine administration of dextrose (D_{50}) should be avoided unless hypoglycemia is documented or strongly suspected. Narcan is generally not required unless there are historic features or pinpoint pupils, suggesting opiate ingestion.

On arrival in the emergency department, stroke patients re-

TABLE 203.2. Differential Diagnosis of Special Patient Groups with Ischemic Stroke

Condition	Comments
YOUNG ADULTS WITH STROKE	
Arterial dissection	Age between 15 and 50 Accounts for 20% of strokes in the young, often preceded by minor trauma
Cardioembolism	Mitral valve prolapse, patent foramen ovale with paradoxical emboli, rheumatic heart disease
Premature atherosclerosis	Hyperlipidemia
Migrainous stroke	Female predominance
Air embolism	Scuba diving, medical procedures
Substance abuse	Heroin, cocaine, amphetamines, LSD
PREEXISTING CARDIAC DISEASE	
Ischemic heart disease	Peripheral emboli from mural thrombus
Dysrhythmias	Atrial fibrillation, ventricular tachycardia, sick sinus syndrome, etc.
Valvular heart disease	Rheumatic heart disease, prosthetic valves
Dilated cardiomyopathies	Peripheral emboli from mural thrombus
Endocarditis	Associated fever and murmur
HEMATOLOGIC DISORDERS	
Hyperviscosity syndromes	Cancer, myeloproliferative diseases, dysproteinemia, thalassemia, sickle cell disease, polycythemia
Coagulopathies	Disseminated intravascular coagulation, protein C or S deficiencies, antithrombin III deficiency, antiphospholipid antibody syndrome
Thrombotic thrombocytopenic purpura	Rare disorder with fever, microangiopathic hemolytic anemia, thrombocytopenia, neurologic and renal impairment
VASCULAR DISORDERS	
Infectious vasculitis	Herpes zoster, human immunodeficiency virus infection, syphilis, tuberculosis, aspergillosis
Noninfectious vasculitis	
Necrotizing	Polyarteritis nodosa
Nonnecrotizing	Giant cell arteritis (patients >age 50; females > males), Takayasu's arteritis
Cerebral venous thrombosis	Presents with headache and papilledema; magnetic resonance imaging is diagnostic

quire a monitored bed and have a rapid assessment of airway, breathing, and circulatory status. Complete vital signs should be obtained, including a core temperature. A rapid general physical examination should be performed, including a search for evidence of head trauma. The neck should be examined for meningeal signs present with either infection or SAH. Auscultation for carotid bruits, particularly on the side opposite a clinical deficit, should be performed. The heart is examined for rate, regularity, and murmurs, searching for conditions predisposing to stroke, such as atrial fibrillation and mitral valvular disease. The extremities should be assessed for evidence of peripheral vascular disease or emboli, and the skin examined for needle tracks or evidence of petechiae or ecchymosis, suggesting endocarditis, sepsis, or coagulopathy.

A focused neurologic examination should follow. Initially, a brief mental status examination is performed, including assessment of level of consciousness, language, memory, and interpretation. A careful eye examination should follow, with testing of both visual acuity and visual fields. Pupillary size, reactivity, and extraocular movements provide information on brainstem function and cranial nerves III, IV, and VI. Asymmetry of the pupils suggests a third-nerve palsy due to tentorial herniation. Conjugate eye deviation toward the normal arm and leg suggests a hemispheric lesion, while deviation toward the paretic arm or leg suggests a brainstem lesion. Funduscopic examination of the retina may reveal papilledema, hypertensive changes, Hollenhorst plaques, diabetic changes, or Roth spots suggestive of endocarditis. Cranial nerves V and VII through XII may quickly be assessed by examining facial and corneal sensation; smiling symmetry, eyebrow raising, and forehead wrinkling; gross auditory acuity; gag reflex; shoulder shrug (trapezius strength); head rotation against resistance (sternocleidomastoid strength); and tongue protrusion, respectively.

Motor strength and tone should be assessed in both proximal and distal muscle groups. Pronator drift is a sensitive indicator of upper extremity weakness.

The sensory examination is the most subjective part of the neurologic examination and should be interpreted in view of the patient's ability to cooperate and the overall examination. Double simultaneous extinction is tested at this time, particularly if visual field deficits were identified. The ability of a patient to identify, by touch, common objects such as keys or pens (stereognosis) and to identify a number drawn on the skin surface (graphesthesia) is an easy test of sensory function done in the emergency department.

Cerebellar function can be assessed by finger-to-nose and heel-to-shin tests; these are particularly useful with the bedridden patient. Important reflex arcs to test routinely include the biceps (C-5, C-6), triceps (C-6, C-7, C-8), patellar (L-2, L-3, L-4), and Achilles (L-5, S-1), as well as pathologic reflexes. Asymmetry of deep tendon reflexes or a unilateral Babinski sign may indicate corticospinal tract lesions.

Assessment of station and gait is one of the most revealing parts of the neurologic examination and the part most frequently neglected. Subtle weakness, ataxia, rigidity, and sensory defects can be identified by observation of the gait, toe-walking, heel-walking, tandem walking, and Romberg tests.

Further diagnostic evaluation in the emergency department should include a 12-lead electrocardiogram, chest radiograph, complete blood cell count, electrolyte and glucose determinations, and renal function studies. A serum creatine phosphokinase determination should be considered (along with urine myoglobin) in patients with prolonged immobilization. Coagulation studies are often ordered to provide a baseline evaluation for patients who may require anticoagulation. Arterial blood gases, blood cultures, toxicologic screens, and other studies are ordered as necessary.

A nonenhanced CT scan of the head should be obtained in all patients to identify intracranial hemorrhage and to rule out other causes for neurologic deficits. An ischemic stroke does not become hypodense for 6 to 72 hours after vessel occlusion and is often not visible on initial CT evaluation. If CT scanning is unavailable, the patient should be stabilized and transferred as rapidly as possible to a facility with CT capability.

MRI, carotid ultrasonography, echocardiography, and angiography have limited roles in the acute evaluation of most patients with ischemic stroke and are utilized in selected cases after hospital admission. An exception is the patient with a possible vertebrobasilar or carotid artery dissection. These patients should be considered for emergent ultrasound, angiography, or MR angiogram (MRA), because dissection is commonly treated with anticoagulation.

Advances in the evaluation of acute ischemic stroke continue. As MRI becomes faster and more available, it may become the diagnostic test of choice, allowing earlier assessment of the size of infarction and measurement of tissue perfusion and metabolism. Xenon CT now allows identification of regional cerebral blood flow. Transcranial Doppler can noninvasively identify occlusion of the middle cerebral artery. These may prove useful in the future in selecting patients for thrombolytic therapy.

EMERGENCY DEPARTMENT MANAGEMENT

The goal of acute stroke management in appropriate patients who present within 3 hours of symptom onset is the reversal of clinical deficits by reestablishing cerebral blood flow with intravenous thrombolytic agents. In patients presenting beyond 3 hours, there is no intervention that has proven effective in reducing infarct size; the objective of treatment is to limit infarct progression and recurrence. Current approaches to preventing or minimizing infarct progression include maintenance of adequate cardiac output to preserve cerebral blood flow, regulation of core temperature, and control of the blood glucose level. Strategies to prevent infarct recurrence focus on anticoagulation and antiplatelet therapy.

Thrombolytic Therapy

Current recommendations by the American Heart Association and American Academy of Neurology support the use of recombinant tissue plasminogen activator (r-TPA) in carefully selected patients when the diagnosis has been established by physicians with expertise in stroke and the cranial CT has been interpreted by a qualified individual. These recommendations followed Food and Drug Administration approval for use of r-TPA in acute ischemic stroke and are based primarily on the results of the NIH/NINDS Stroke Study, Parts I and II. These trials found that stroke patients treated with r-TPA were at least 30% more likely to have minimal or no disability 3 months after the event, compared with those who received placebo (absolute increase in favorable outcome, 11% to 13%). Though treated patients had a symptomatic hemorrhage rate of 6.4% (vs. 0.6% for placebo), there was no significant difference in mortality at 3 months (17% r-TPA, 21% placebo).[17] Post-hoc analyses do not support withholding therapy from any patient on the basis of suspected stroke subtype, age, clinical deficit, or CT findings of early ischemic changes.

Concern has been raised regarding the fact that only the NINDS trials have shown benefit, while four other trials (ASK, MAST-E, MAST-I, and ECASS) found either no benefit or they found potential harm. It should be noted that there were many fundamental differences between the NINDS trials and the other studies, which make direct comparison problematic. These differences include thrombolytic agent used, dose, time-to-treatment, blood pressure management, and number of protocol violations. Two subsequent trials (ECASS II and ATLANTIS) specifically evaluated the use of intravenous r-TPA beyond 3 hours and found no benefit.

Other concerns address the reproducibility of the results in the community setting. Ten postapproval studies involving more than 500 r-TPA–treated patients have all found results similar to those of the NINDS trials. One of these studies involved patients treated by emergency physicians at hospitals using standardized treatment protocols.[21]

The development of treatment guidelines for stroke may improve patient selection and speed the delivery of thrombolytics to appropriate patients. The National Institutes of Health recommends that stroke patients undergo evaluation by a physician within 10 minutes of emergency department arrival, CT within 25 minutes, and CT interpretation by 45 minutes. Total "door-to-needle" time for patients meeting appropriate inclusion criteria, and no exclusion criteria, should not exceed 60 minutes.

Table 203.3 outlines inclusion and exclusion criteria for the use of r-TPA in acute stroke. Eligible patients should be treated with 0.9 mg/kg of r-TPA (maximum dose, 90 mg), with 10% given as a bolus over 1 to 2 minutes, and the remainder given over 60 minutes via infusion pump. Table 203.4 presents pre- and posttreatment blood pressure control guidelines. An algorithm for the management of suspected intracranial hemorrhage secondary to thrombolytic therapy is shown in Fig. 203.1.

TABLE 203.3. TPA in Ischemic Stroke: Inclusion and Exclusion Criteria[1,17,18,20]

Inclusion Criteria	**Yes**	**No**
1. Age 18 or older		
2. Clinical diagnosis of ischemic stroke causing a measurable neurologic deficit defined as impairment of language, motor function, cognition and/or gaze, vision, or neglect. (Ischemic stroke is defined as an event characterized by the sudden onset of an acute focal neurologic deficit presumed to be due to cerebral ischemia after CT excludes hemorrhage.)		
3. Time of onset well established to be less than 180 minutes before treatment would begin. *"Time of onset" of stroke is defined as that point at which a change in the baseline neurologic function occurred. If that time is not known (e.g., the patient awakens from sleep with new symptoms), the last time the patient was observed to be neurologically intact must be considered to be the time of onset.*		
Medical History Exclusions	**Yes**	**No**
1. [a]Current use of oral anticoagulants (e.g., warfarin sodium) AND a prothrombin time greater than 15 seconds or an INR greater than 1.7?		
2. [a]Use of heparin in the previous 48 hours AND a prolonged partial thromboplastin time?		
3. History of another stroke (any type) in previous 3 months?		
4. History of a serious head injury in the previous 3 months?		
5. History of major surgery or biopsy of a parenchymal organ within the preceding 14 days?		
6. History of any prior intracerebral hemorrhage (any type)?		
7. History of intracranial neoplasm, arteriovenous malformation, or aneurysm?		
8. History of seizure at the time of stroke onset?		
9. History of gastrointestinal or urinary bleeding within the preceding 21 days?		
10. History of myocardial infarction in the past 14 days?		
11. History of pregnancy or parturition within the previous 30 days?		
12. History of known hereditary or acquired abnormal hemostasis?		
13. History of recent (within 7 days) lumbar puncture?		
14. History of recent (within 30 days) arterial puncture at a noncompressible site?		
Clinical Examination Exclusions	**Yes**	**No**
1. Rapidly improving neurologic signs?		
2. Isolated, mild neurologic deficits, such as ataxia alone, sensory loss alone, dysarthria alone, or minimal weakness (NIH stroke scale less than 4 AND normal speech AND visual fields)?		
3. Clinical presentation that suggests SAH, even if initial CT scan is normal.		
4. Pretreatment hypertension: systolic blood pressure greater than 185 mm Hg OR diastolic blood pressure greater than 110 mm Hg prior to treatment? (Hypertension may be treated with nitroglycerine paste and/or 1 to 2 doses of intravenous labetalol and TPA initiated if reduction to above levels occurs. More aggressive treatment to reduce blood pressure excludes the patient from treatment with TPA).		
5. Presumed septic embolus as etiology of stroke (any stroke with a fever)?		
6. Glucose less than 50 mg/dL or greater than 400 mg/dL (hyperglycemia is a relative contraindication)?		
7. Platelet count less than 100,000/mm?		
8. Clinical presentation suggesting stroke secondary to aortic dissection extension?		
Cerebral CT Exclusions	**Yes**	**No**
1. High-density lesion consistent with hemorrhage or possible hemorrhage of any degree or type on CT?		

[a]In patients without recent use of oral anticoagulants or heparin, treatment with r-TPA can be initiated before the availability of coagulation study results, but should be discontinued if either the PT is greater than 15 seconds (INR greater than 1.7) or the PTT is elevated by local laboratory standards.

TABLE 203.4. Blood Pressure Management in Acute Stroke[18]

Pretreatment

A. Monitor blood pressure (BP) every 15 minutes.
B. If systolic BP is > 185 mm Hg or diastolic BP is > 110, the BP may be treated with one to two 10- to 20-mg doses of labetalol given i.v. push within 1 hour and/or nitroglycerin paste.
C. If these measures do not reduce the BP below 185/110 and keep it down, the patient should not be treated with TPA.

Posttreatment

A. If systolic BP is 180 to 230 mm Hg or if diastolic BP is 105 to 120 on two or more readings 5 to 10 minutes apart:
   1. Give labetalol 10 mg i.v. over 1 to 2 minutes. The dose may be repeated or doubled every 10 to 20 minutes, up to 150 mg.
   2. Monitor BP every 15 minutes during labetalol treatment and observe for development of hypotension.
B. If systolic BP is > 230 mm Hg or if diastolic BP is in the range of 121 to 140 mm Hg for two or more readings 5 to 10 minutes apart:
   1. Give labetalol 10 mg i.v. over 1 to 2 minutes. The dose may be repeated or doubled every 10 to 20 minutes, up to 150 mg.
   2. Monitor BP every 15 minutes during labetalol treatment and observe for development of hypotension.
   3. If unsatisfactory response, infuse sodium nitroprusside (0.5 to 10.0 μg/kg/min). Continuous arterial monitoring is advised if sodium nitroprusside is used.
C. If diastolic BP is > 140 mm Hg for two or more readings 5 to 10 minutes apart:
   1. Infuse sodium nitroprusside (0.5 to 10.0 μg/kg/min).
   2. Continuous arterial monitoring is advised if sodium nitroprusside is used.

The development of institution-specific evaluation and treatment guidelines is recommended to identify local responsibilities concerning thrombolytic delivery and posttreatment care and disposition. A multidisciplinary approach will deliver the highest level of care in a time-critical setting.

Hypertension Management

Acute elevations of blood pressure typically decline, without treatment, within a few days to prestroke levels. Because the benefit of blood pressure control is unproved, it is reasonable to avoid treating hypertension in the absence of specific indications such as thrombolytic therapy for acute stroke, AMI, hypertensive encephalopathy, arterial dissection, and hemorrhagic transformation.

In stroke patients requiring antihypertensive therapy (and not treated with r-TPA), the goal is a gradual reduction of blood pressure by 15%, with a systolic blood pressure of 170 to 220 mm Hg and a diastolic blood pressure of 90 to 120 mm Hg being acceptable targets. Although these are commonly used end points, no specific values have been supported by good clinical or experimental evidence.

The ideal antihypertensive agent in patients with ischemic stroke is also unclear. Nitroprusside remains a standard agent because of its rapid onset, ease of control, and short duration of action. Other useful agents include labetalol, hydralazine, and trimethaphan (Arfonad). Esmolol (Brevibloc) has been used to control hypertension postoperatively in patients undergoing intracranial surgery and, like nitroprusside, is easily titrated. It is probably best to avoid oral calcium channel blockers because of their potential for causing precipitous declines in blood pressure. The use of antihypertensive agents requires frequent neurologic checks so that treatment may be discontinued if neurologic deterioration occurs.

Volume Management

Maintenance of intravascular volume is important in optimizing cardiac output in stroke patients. These patients are often unable to maintain adequate oral intake, and up to one-third may be significantly hypovolemic. Volume deficits should be corrected as rapidly as possible and followed by maintenance fluids. Patients with underlying cardiac or renal disease may require invasive hemodynamic monitoring to guide fluid management. Aggressive hypervolemic therapy to increase cerebral blood flow should be avoided, because it does not improve outcome and may contribute to cerebral edema. Hemodilution has also not been proven to alter stroke outcome and cannot be recommended.

Temperature Regulation

Temperature regulation of the ischemic stroke patient is often neglected in the emergency department. Experimentally, hypothermia has a protective effect on ischemic neurons, whereas hyperthermia may worsen damage by increasing cellular metabolic demand. Fever is not uncommon in stroke patients and should be promptly treated.

Glucose Regulation

The ideal serum glucose level for stroke patients is unknown. Although Pulsinelli and colleagues[19] reported a worse neurologic outcome in stroke patients whose blood glucose exceeded 120 mg/dL, later studies have found no association.[15] Because the optimal glucose level is unknown, it is reasonable to treat excessive blood glucose levels with insulin and to avoid the overadministration of glucose-containing solutions.

Anticoagulation

Although anticoagulation has been used for more than 50 years, its role in the treatment of stoke is still controversial. In patients with completed thrombotic strokes, and particularly strokes involving large areas or accompanied by hypertension, anticoagulation has no proven benefit and carries the risk of hemorrhage into the infarcted area. Anticoagulation with heparin is often empirically started in patients with stuttering deficits to, presumably, prevent clot extension. These "progressing strokes," however, may not represent "progressing clot," but secondary neuronal injury. No well-controlled, randomized, clinical trial has demonstrated a benefit from anticoagulation in this setting.

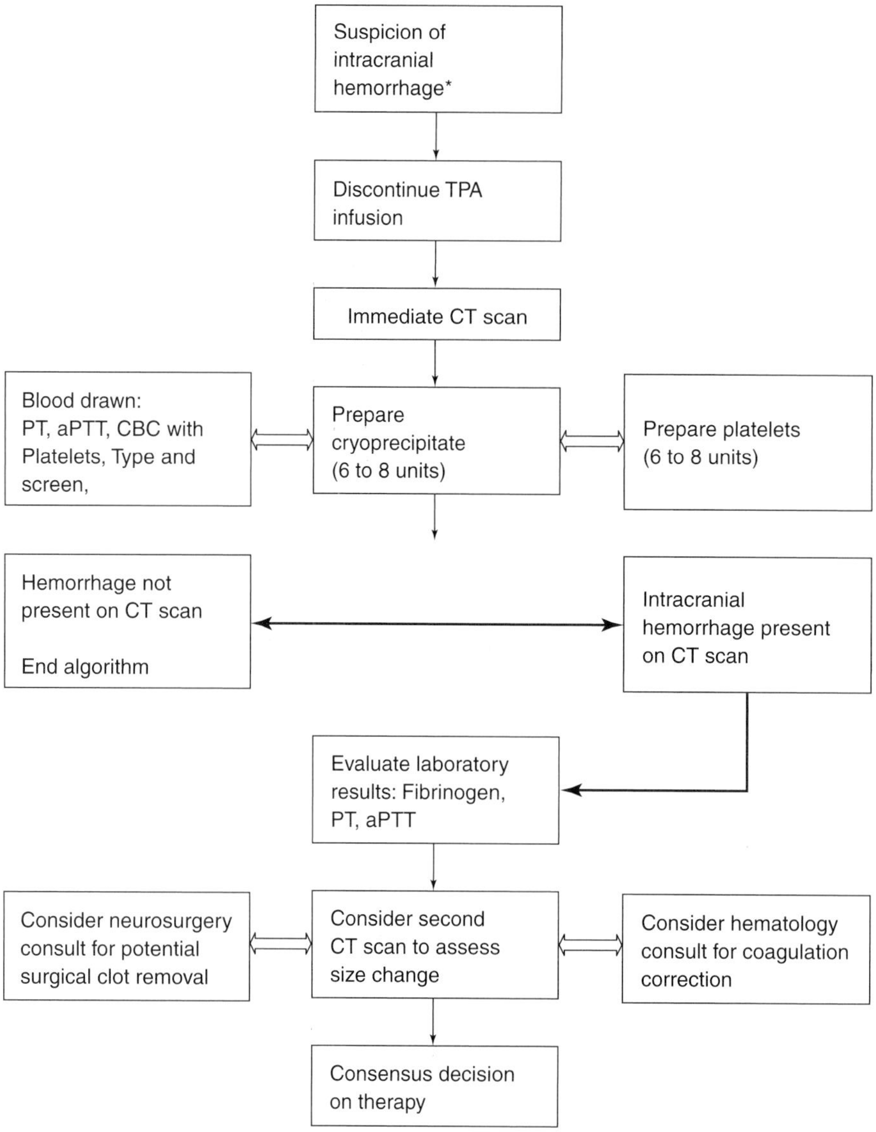

Figure 203.1. Management of suspected intracranial hemorrhage.
* Symptoms such as neurological deterioration, new headache, acute hypertension, nausea, vomiting.

Given the uncertainties regarding anticoagulation in the face of progressing clinical deficits, consultation is recommended prior to its initiation. All anticoagulants should be withheld for 24 hours following the use of r-TPA in acute stroke.

The role of anticoagulation is only slightly better defined in patients with cardioembolic stroke. It is estimated that 10% to 15% of these patients suffer a second embolic stroke within 3 weeks, and some series report an early recurrence rate as high as 21%.[5,6] The benefits of anticoagulation to prevent recurrence, however, must be weighed against the risk of intracerebral hemorrhage. Patients with embolic stroke are at increased risk for hemorrhagic transformation, particularly in the first 48 hours. This risk is increased in patients with large infarctions, uncontrolled hypertension, and advanced age. The Stroke Council of the American Heart Association states that no recommendations regarding the use of heparin can be made, because the data are considered insufficient and conflicting. The use of heparin, therefore, has been left to the preference of the treating physician. When initiated, an International Normalized Ratio (INR) between 2 and 3 is adequate.

Other potential emergency indications for anticoagulation include vertebrobasilar or carotid artery dissection, hypercoagulable states, and cerebral venous thrombosis.

Antiplatelet Therapy

Antiplatelet therapy is a cornerstone of stroke management and reflects the central role of platelet activation in clot formation. The use of aspirin in patients with a previous mild stroke or TIA results in a 20% reduction in stroke risk. In patients treated within 48 hours of stroke onset, with 300 mg of aspirin daily, there was a statistically significant reduction in recurrent ischemic stroke at 14 days, with no increase in risk of hemorrhagic stroke.[11] Initiation of aspirin therapy should begin in the emergency department with 300 to 325 mg in patients who are not treated with thrombolytic therapy or have aspirin sensitivities.

Ticlopidine (Ticlid) is slightly more effective than aspirin in preventing stroke recurrence and clopidogrel (Plavix) is slightly more effective than aspirin in preventing stroke, AMI, and vascular death. Studies have not evaluated their use in acute stroke, however, and ticlopidine requires serial complete blood counts to monitor for neutropenia. Their onset of action is delayed for several days, suggesting they should not be relied on acutely to inhibit platelet function. Given these limitations and their increased cost, the emergent use of these agents is best reserved for aspirin-intolerant patients or those failing aspirin therapy.

Future Therapies

Future treatment of ischemic stroke may involve neuroprotective agents, new antiplatelet strategies, and thrombolytic therapy with novel agents or delivery mechanisms. Neuronal protective agents are aimed at attenuating the biochemical cascade of events leading to cellular death after hypoxic insult. Drugs presently under investigation include excitatory neurotransmitter antagonists and inhibitors of local inflammatory responses. The use of a glycoprotein IIb/IIIa platelet inhibitor in acute stroke was found to be safe in a phase II dose escalation trial and may offer the potential for use alone or in combination with thrombolytic therapy. New thrombolytic agents with higher clot specificity are undergoing testing. A trial of the antifibrinolytic agent Ancrod recently reported positive outcomes when used in stroke patients treated within 3 hours.[8a,22] A trial on the delivery of intraarterial prourokinase also reported improved outcomes in patients with proximal middle cerebral artery occlusions in patients treated out to 6 hours.[8a]

DISPOSITION

Factors influencing disposition in the patient with ischemic stroke include infarct location, time of symptom onset, infarct size, stroke etiology, concurrent medical conditions, and social resources available to the patient. The vast majority of stroke patients are admitted to the hospital, often to a specialized unit or floor skilled in the care of patients with neurologic deficits. Cardiac monitoring should be arranged for those with potential dysrhythmias either as an etiology or as a consequence of the infarct.

Patients with minor, completed strokes are potential candidates for evaluation in an emergency department clinical decision unit. Predefined protocols for neurologic consultation, subsequent neurologic and vascular imaging, and initiation of therapy to prevent recurrent stroke in this setting speed patient care and reduce length of hospital stay.

Patients treated with r-TPA and those with impaired gag or swallowing reflexes or mental status changes should be admitted to the intensive care unit. Intensive care unit admission is also indicated for patients with cerebellar strokes and should be considered for patients with large hemispheric strokes who are at risk for the development of cerebral edema 24 to 48 hours after the event.

Stroke patients are often cared for in the inpatient setting without neurologic consultation. Neurologic consultation in the emergency department is indicated when the diagnosis is unclear or when further evaluation is required (e.g., arterial dissection, migrainous infarct, unusual hematologic conditions). Because anticoagulation is controversial, it is reasonable to consult a neurologist before initiating heparin, particularly in the patient with a progressing deficit. Patients with cerebellar infarction should have neurosurgical consultation, because decompressive craniectomy may be lifesaving in selected patients.

COMMON PITFALLS

- Failure to identify, evaluate, refer, and/or treat stroke patients who are eligible for thrombolytic therapy
- Failure to perform a complete history and physical examination, particularly in uncooperative elderly patients. The history and physical examination are the basis for determining the extent of a stroke and its etiology.
- Failure to consider unusual etiologies of stroke, such as arterial dissection and emboli in younger patients with new neurologic deficits
- Misdiagnosis of cerebellar stroke as alcohol or drug intoxication, labyrinthitis, benign positional vertigo, or severe gastroenteritis, and failure to obtain neurosurgical consultation
- Failure to optimize cardiac output and to treat temperature elevations in the emergency department
- Managing blood pressure too aggressively. Reduction of blood pressure may reduce cerebral blood flow and cause extension of an ischemic stroke.

HEMORRHAGIC CEREBROVASCULAR DISEASE

Intracerebral hemorrhage (ICH), defined as hemorrhage directly into the brain parenchyma, affects 10% to 15% of all stroke patients. Major risk factors for intracranial hemorrhage include advancing age, hypertension, and race. Blacks have a higher incidence of ICH than do Whites; Asians have an even higher incidence. Other risk factors include cigarette smoking and alcohol use.

The most common site for ICH is the putamen, which accounts for 35% to 50% of all hemorrhages. Next in frequency are the subcortical white matter (30%), the cerebellum (16%), the thalamus (10% to 15%), and the pons (5% to 12%).[13] Pathologically, these are areas of the brain supplied by small arteries that are 50 to 200 μm in size.

CLINICAL PRESENTATION

The onset of ICH is usually heralded by a sudden headache, vomiting, and neurologic deficit. The majority of patients exhibit a decreased level of consciousness due to elevated intracranial pressure (ICP). ICH often occurs during activity and only rarely has its onset during sleep. In one-third of cases, clinical deficits are maximal at onset. In the remaining two-thirds, the symptoms follow a steadily progressive course over the first 30 minutes. Coma is a poor prognostic sign and is associated with larger hemorrhages and ventricular extension. Headache and vomiting are typically absent in ischemic strokes and thus are of help in identifying patients with ICH. Early seizures are uncommon in ICH involving the putamen, thalamus, and pons but may be present in up to one-third of patients with subcortical white matter ("lobar") hemorrhages. Hypertension is noted in over 90% of patients with ICH.

The clinical deficits are related to the location and size of the hemorrhage. Putaminal hemorrhages cause a dense contralateral hemiplegia with sensory loss and homonymous hemianopia. The eyes show conjugate deviation away from the paralyzed side, which may be overcome with caloric testing or doll's-eye reflex testing. Thalamic hemorrhages cause similar motor and sensory findings but may also cause conjugate downward gaze with pinpoint, unresponsive pupils. Deficits from a lobar hemorrhage depend on the size and location of the hemorrhage. Pontine hemorrhage typically causes a severe occipital headache, followed rapidly by a decreased level of consciousness; coma is present in 80% of patients. Patients may become hyperthermic and may have severe neurologic deficits. These include quadriplegia, loss of corneal reflexes, and pinpoint pupils with absent horizontal eye movements on caloric or doll's-eye reflex testing. Cerebellar hemorrhage causes extremity and truncal ataxia and an inability to walk. These symptoms are commonly accompanied by vomiting, dysequilibrium, and headache. An ipsilateral gaze palsy may also be present.

Patients with cerebellar hemorrhage may initially appear stable but can deteriorate rapidly to coma and death.

DIFFERENTIAL DIAGNOSIS

The presence of intracerebral blood on head CT should not automatically be ascribed to a hypertensive hemorrhage. Various nonhypertensive causes of ICH include arteriovenous malformation, berry aneurysm, sympathomimetic drug use, intracranial tumor, anticoagulant and thrombolytic agent use, hematologic disorders (e.g., leukemia, thrombotic thrombocytopenic purpura, hemophilia), cerebral vasculitis, and mycotic aneurysm.

EMERGENCY DEPARTMENT EVALUATION

The evaluation of patients with suspected ICH is similar to that for ischemic stroke. However, patients with ICH may exhibit rapid neurologic deterioration and a decreased level of consciousness, necessitating acute airway intervention. Vital signs should be monitored closely, and frequent neurologic assessments are required. Laboratory data should be obtained to help identify possible contributing causes, such as coagulopathy, thrombocytopenia, or platelet dysfunction. Toxicologic screening is indicated for patients with atypical presentations and for younger patients without a history of hypertension. Cardiac monitoring is essential, because dysrhythmias are common from either increased sympathetic discharge or impending tonsillar or uncal herniation.

The CT scan typically shows high attenuation in the area of hemorrhage. There is usually a "ring" of low attenuation surrounding the hemorrhage because of edema of the adjacent tissue. Angiography and/or MRI/MRA should be considered when an aneurysm, arteriovenous malformation, or central nervous system tumor is strongly suspected.

EMERGENCY DEPARTMENT MANAGEMENT

The goals of emergency care for ICH are rapid diagnosis, management of the airway, control of ICP, and early neurosurgical consultation. Oxygen should be administered to all patients. Intubation is indicated for airway protection or hyperventilation to reduce ICP. Rapid-sequence intubation with paralytic agents may be necessary to obtain adequate CT images in a combative patient.

Management of hypertension in the patient with ICH is directed at managing the competing interests of decreasing ongoing hemorrhage against overreduction of cerebral perfusion pressure. Current recommendations[4] are to initiate treatment for systolic pressures greater than or equal to 180 mm Hg or diastolic pressures greater than or equal to 105 mm Hg and to maintain a mean arterial pressure below 130 mm Hg in persons with a history of hypertension. In patients with an ICP monitor, cerebral perfusion pressure (mean arterial pressure − ICP) should be kept above 70 mm Hg. Useful antihypertensive agents in the setting of ICH include nitroprusside, esmolol, and labetalol.

ICP control is important in the patient with ICH. Acute elevations in ICP, as manifested by decreasing level of consciousness and neurologic deterioration due to mass effect, are initially managed with elevation of the head (30 degrees), osmotherapy, and hyperventilation. Although there is no universally accepted standard therapy for the management of ICH, current recommendations support the use of a stepwise approach[4] beginning with mannitol (20% solution; 0.25 to 0.5 g/kg every 4 hours) in patients with progressively increasing ICP values or clinical deterioration. Furosemide (10 mg every 2 to 8 hours) may be administered simultaneously with osmotherapy.

Reduction of the pCO_2 to 30 to 35 mm Hg lowers ICP by 25% to 30% in most patients, though peak ICP reduction may be delayed up to 30 minutes after the pCO_2 is changed. Because hypocarbia causes cerebral vasoconstriction, overaggressive reduction in pCO_2 may reduce cerebral blood flow below critical values; this should thus be avoided.

In general, ICP monitoring is indicated in patients with a Glasgow Coma Scale score of less than 9 and in those whose condition is thought to be deteriorating due to increases in ICP. Other patients may warrant ICP monitors, however, particularly those with intraventricular hemorrhage.

Neurosurgical consultation should be obtained early, and, if unavailable, the patient should be stabilized and transferred. The indications for hematoma evacuation depend on many factors, including patient age, hemorrhage location, and surgical accessibility. Patients who present initially with coma or loss of brainstem function generally do not benefit from surgical evacuation, whereas those who experience progressive deterioration after a lobar hemorrhage are often operated on. In patients with cerebellar hemorrhage, surgery is recommended for all hematomas exceeding 3 cm in diameter. All patients with ICH should be admitted to a neurosurgical intensive care unit for close observation and monitoring.

COMMON PITFALLS

- Failure to diagnose cerebellar hemorrhage. Patients may be misdiagnosed with acute viral syndrome, labyrinthitis, or intoxication. Surgical intervention may be lifesaving.
- Delay in transport. Patients with ICH require early neurosurgical consultation and should be transported to an appropriate facility if immediate neurosurgical attention is not otherwise available.

References

1. Adams HP Jr, Brott TG, Furlan AJ, et al. Guidelines for thrombolytic therapy for acute stroke: a supplement to the guidelines for the management of patients with acute ischemic stroke. A statement for healthcare professionals from a special writing group of the Stroke Council, American Heart Association. *Circulation* 1996;94:1167–1174.
2. Barnett HJM, Taylor DW, Eliasziw M, et al., for the North American Symptomatic Carotid Endarterectomy Trial Collaborators. Benefit of carotid endarterectomy in patients with symptomatic moderate or severe stenosis. *N Engl J Med* 1998;339:1415–1425.
3. Bellavance A. Efficacy of ticlopidine and aspirin for prevention of reversible cerebrovascular ischemic events: the Ticlopidine Aspirin Stroke Study. *Stroke* 1993;24:1452.
4. Broderick JP, Adams HP, Barsan W, et al. Guidelines for the management of spontaneous intracerebral hemorrhage. A statement for healthcare professionals from a special writing group of the Stroke Council, American Heart Association. *Stroke* 1999;30:905–915.
5. Cerebral Embolism Task Force. Cardiogenic brain embolism. *Arch Neurol* 1986;43:71.
6. Cerebral Embolism Task Force. Cardiogenic brain embolism: the second report of the Cerebral Embolism Task Force. *Arch Neurol* 1989;46:727.
7. Diener HC, Cunha L, Forbes C, et al. European Stroke Prevention Study 2. Dipyridamole and acetylsalicylic acid in the secondary prevention of stroke. *J Neurol Sci* 1996;143:1–13.
8. European Carotid Surgery Trialists' Collaborative Group. MRC European Carotid Surgery Trial: interim results for symptomatic patients with severe (70%–99%) or with mild (0%–29%) carotid stenosis. *Lancet* 1991;337:1235.
8a. Furlan A, Higashida R, Wechsler L, et al. for the PROACT Investigators. Intra-arterial prourokinase for acute ischemic stroke. The PROACT II Study: A randomized controlled trial. *JAMA* 1999;282:2003.
9. Gillum RF. Stroke in blacks. *Stroke* 1988;19:1.
10. Hass WK, Easton JD, Adams HP Jr, et al. A randomized trial comparing ticlopidine hydrochloride with aspirin for the prevention of stroke in high-risk patients: Ticlopidine Aspirin Study Group. *N Engl J Med* 1989;321:501.
11. The International Stroke Trial Collaborative Group: The International Stroke Trial (IST): a randomized trial of aspirin, subcutaneous heparin, both, or neither among 19,435 patients with acute ischemic stroke. *Lancet* 1997;349: 1569–1581.

12. Kappelle LJ, van Latum JC, Koudstaal PJ, et al. Transient ischemic attacks and small-vessel disease. *Lancet* 1991;337:339.
13. Kase CS, Mohr JP, Caplan LR. Intracerebral hemorrhage. In: Barnett HJM, Mohr JP, Stein BM, et al., eds. *Stroke: pathophysiology, diagnosis and management*, 2nd ed. New York: Churchill Livingstone, 1992:561.
14. Koudstaal PJ, van Gijn J, Frenken CWGM, et al. TIA, RIND, minor stroke: a continuum, or different subgroups? *J Neurol Neurosurg Psychiatry* 1992;55:95.
15. Matchar DB, Divine GW, Heyman A, et al. The influence of hyperglycemia on outcome of cerebral infarction. *Ann Intern Med* 1992;117:449.
16. Matsumoto N, Whisnant JP, Jurland LT, et al. Natural history of stroke in Rochester, Minnesota, 1955 through 1969: an extension of a previous study, 1945 through 1954. *Stroke* 1973;4:20.
17. The National Institute of Neurological Disorders and Stroke (NINDS) rt-PA Stroke Study Group. Tissue plasminogen activator for acute ischemic stroke. *N Engl J Med* 1995;333:1581–1587.
18. The National Institute of Neurological Disorders and Stroke (NINDS) rt-PA Stroke Study Group: A Systems Approach to Immediate Evaluation and Management of Hyperacute Stroke—Experience at Eight Centers and Implications for Community Practice and Patient Care. Stroke 1997;28:1530-1540.
19. Pulsinelli WA, Levy DE, Sigsbee B, et al. Increased damage after ischemic stroke in patients with hyperglycemia with or without established diabetes mellitus. *Am J Med* 1983;74:540.
20. Report of the Quality Standards Subcommittee of the American Academy of Neurology. Practice advisory: thrombolytic therapy for acute ischemic stroke—summary statement. *Neurology* 1996;47:835–839.
21. Scott PA, Chudnofsky CR, Grant RJ, et al. Emergency physician administration of rt-PA in acute stroke: analysis of treatment and outcome. *Stroke* 1999;30:244(abst).
22. Sherman DG, Atkinson RP, Chippendale T, et al. for the STAT participants: Intravenous Ancrod for treatment of acute ischemic stroke. The STAT Study: A randomized controlled trial. *JAMA* 2000;283:2395.

CHAPTER 204

Peripheral Neuropathies

Phyllis A. Vallee and Kevin M. Reilly

Peripheral neuropathies are confusing entities for both neurologists and nonneurologists. The types and etiologies of peripheral neuropathy are numerous, and the pathophysiology is not well understood in many cases. Nevertheless, only 15% to 30% of patients undergoing intensive evaluation fail to have a diagnosis made.[2,5]

The peripheral nervous system begins within the spinal canal with the spinal nerve roots and extends outward to include all distal nerve tissue. When faced with disorders of this system, emergency physicians should examine the chronicity, pattern, and symmetry of symptoms to establish a working differential diagnosis.[1,2,5] In general, peripheral neuropathies can be divided into several basic categories: polyneuropathy, plexopathy, radiculopathy, and mononeuropathy.

POLYNEUROPATHY

Polyneuropathy results from the simultaneous dysfunction of multiple peripheral nerves. Symptoms include diffuse motor or sensory loss or both, with variable autonomic nervous system dysfunction.

Acute Polyneuropathy

CLINICAL PRESENTATION

Polyneuropathies that develop over several days to 2 weeks are considered acute. Of these, Guillain-Barré syndrome (GBS), also known as acute inflammatory demyelinating polyradiculoneuropathy, is the most common.[7,9,15,17] GBS is a worldwide, nonseasonal, acute polyneuropathy that affects all ages, with a yearly incidence of 0.6 to 2.4 cases per 100,000 population.[17] Men are affected slightly more than women by a ratio of 1.25 to 1.5:1.[7,9,15,17] The exact etiology is unclear, but pathologic examination reveals inflammation and segmental demyelination as the primary defect in 85% of cases, while primary axonal degeneration occurs in 15% of cases.[9]

Classically, patients experience a prodromal event such as upper respiratory tract infection, gastroenteritis (especially due to *Campylobacter jejuni,* which is the most commonly identified pathogen associated with GBS[9,10]), surgery, vaccination, or infection with agents such as *Mycoplasma,* the herpesviruses, and the human immunodeficiency virus (HIV). This is followed in 1 to 3 weeks by the onset of a symmetric ascending motor paralysis that progresses to its peak over 10 to 14 days. Motor weakness is both proximal and distal, with legs being involved prior to the arms and trunk. Additional findings include hyporeflexia or areflexia within 1 week of symptom onset, distal paresthesias and numbness, minimal sensory losses, cranial nerve palsies, and autonomic dysfunction. Bowel and bladder disturbances are uncommon (15%) and brief in duration.[1] Patients are afebrile and mental status is unaffected. It is not unusual for patients to present with low-back, hip, and thigh pain that is confused with disc disease or lumbar strain.

Several atypical presentations or variants of GBS are described. In pure motor GBS, there are no sensory losses or paresthesias.[9,18] Pure sensory GBS involves ascending sensory loss and areflexia without motor weakness.[15,18] The Miller Fisher variant of GBS consists of ophthalmoplegia, ataxia, and areflexia.[9,15,18] A regional variant, pharyngeal-cervical-brachial GBS, presents with motor weakness limited to the neck, pharynx, shoulders, upper arms, and diaphragm; in the paraparetic GBS variant, motor weakness is limited to the legs.[18] In the pure pandysautonomia variant, autonomic dysfunction and areflexia occur without motor or sensory loss.[15,18]

The various presentations and variants of GBS make diagnosis difficult. However, marked or persistent asymmetry of weakness, lack of facial and respiratory muscle weakness in a patient with generalized paralysis, prolonged incontinence, a sharp sensory level, or fever strongly suggests another diagnosis.[1,17]

DIFFERENTIAL DIAGNOSIS

Poliomyelitis

In the United States, nearly all cases of polio are related to the use of the live attenuated oral vaccine. Patients with polio first develop an acute viral illness with fever, headache, meningeal signs, and muscle pain and tenderness. These symptoms are present 1 to 2 days before weakness develops. Polio paralysis is more proximal than distal; legs are involved more than arms; and, classically, involvement is asymmetric. Sensory loss is extremely rare, and its presence should raise the suspicion of other diagnoses, especially GBS. The most serious complication of polio is respiratory muscle paralysis. Progression of paralysis abates when patients become afebrile.[12]

Tick Paralysis

Tick paralysis typically affects children in the spring and summer months. Symptoms, which are nearly identical to those of GBS, result from a toxin that is present in the saliva of ticks (usually *Dermacentor*) that have been attached to the human host for a period of 5 to 7 days. The diagnosis is made when the offending tick is located, and treatment consists of removal of the tick and supportive care. Symptoms begin to improve within hours of removal, and generally resolve completely within 2 to 3 days. One tick species found only in Australia, *Ixodes holocyclus*, is associated with paralysis that can progress despite tick removal. For this species, a hyperimmune serum has been developed.[8,12]

Botulism

Exposure to botulinum toxin, which inhibits the release of acetylcholine at neuromuscular junctions, results from the ingestion of improperly canned foods or raw honey or, rarely, from cutaneous infection with *Clostridium botulinum*. Initial symptoms begin hours to several days after exposure and include nausea, vomiting, and dry mouth in patients who have ingested the toxin. Neurologic symptoms begin with cranial nerve palsies with prominent ocular findings, followed by symmetric, descending motor weakness. Sensation and mental status are not affected. Fever is absent. Treatment consists of antitoxin therapy (available through the Centers for Disease Control [CDC]) and supportive care, including respiratory support as necessary.[12]

Acute Intermittent Porphyria

In this disorder, stimulation of an enzymatically deficient heme synthesis pathway results in the buildup of neurotoxic precursors. Acute attacks classically begin with severe abdominal pain, which is followed by tachycardia, hypertension, and mental status changes. Seizures may occur. A sensorimotor polyneuropathy that can be symmetric or asymmetric, and ascending or descending, may develop and can progress to respiratory failure and death. Treatment consists of intravenous glucose and hematin to shut down the defective pathway, beta blockers to control hypertension, and supportive care.[1,3,5]

Heavy Metals

Most neuropathies due to heavy-metal poisoning are subacute or chronic. Acute presentations are associated with thallium exposure and massive arsenic exposure. Thallium ingestion produces abdominal pain, vomiting, and diarrhea, followed by painful paresthesias and the rapid onset of diffuse motor weakness. Differentiation from GBS is often made 1 to 2 weeks after the onset of symptoms, when thallium-induced alopecia becomes apparent. Acute arsenic polyneuropathy, which is also clinically similar to GBS, begins 8 to 20 days after a large exposure and is associated with gastrointestinal symptoms, renal failure, hepatic failure, and mental status changes.[1]

Diphtheria

Diphtheria begins as a pharyngeal infection caused by an exotoxin-producing *Corynebacterium diphtheriae*. Subsequent toxicity, both cardiac and neurologic, correlates with the severity of the pharyngeal disease. Paralysis of local pharyngeal muscles, followed by cranial nerve palsies, occurs in the first or second week of infection. Cardiac toxicity begins 1 to 2 weeks after the onset of illness. The polyneuropathy, which is mainly motor, does not develop until 5 to 8 weeks after onset. Weakness may begin in all extremities simultaneously, or it may first appear in proximal muscles and then spread distally. Occasionally, the primary site of infection is a skin wound, in which case sensorimotor changes are first noted near the infected wound. Treatment of diphtheria involves use of antitoxin within the first 48 hours of infection. Treatment of the neuropathy consists of supportive care.[12]

Others

Acute polyneuropathy may also be a complication of collagen vascular disease, uremia and dialysis, malignancy, critical illness, nutritional deficiencies, infectious agents, or a host of toxins and drugs. Myasthenia gravis, transverse myelitis, lumbar disc disease, spinal cord compression, and acute myopathy are other neuromuscular disorders that can present with weakness that must be differentiated from GBS. Weakness produced by metabolic disorders such as acute hypophosphatemia, hypermagnesemia, hyperkalemia, hypokalemia, and periodic paralysis may mimic GBS. Finally, hysteria and malingering should also be considered.

EMERGENCY DEPARTMENT EVALUATION AND MANAGEMENT

Patients presenting with the acute onset of weakness warrant rapid assessment of airway, ventilatory capacity, and cardiovascular status. Following stabilization, history and physical examination, including a detailed neurologic examination, are the principal methods of emergency department diagnosis of GBS. The emergency physician should obtain a complete blood count, serum electrolytes, calcium, magnesium, phosphate, glucose, blood urea nitrogen, creatinine, erythrocyte sedimentation rate, chest radiograph, and electrocardiogram on all patients.

Additional studies may be needed to rule out other causes of acute weakness; they include antinuclear antibodies, rheumatoid factor, thyroid function tests, liver function tests, creatinine phosphokinase, serum and urine protein electrophoresis, cryoglobulins, vitamin B12, heavy-metal screens, urinary porphobilinogens, and serologic tests for HIV, Lyme disease, and Epstein-Barr virus (EBV).[1–5,13,15] Some of these studies might be obtained by the emergency physician if clinical evaluation raises the suspicion of a specific disease process. Otherwise, additional testing should be left to the consulting neurologist following characterization of the neuropathy by nerve conduction studies and electromyography.

Patients suspected of having GBS should undergo lumbar puncture, even though cerebrospinal fluid changes may be delayed 1 to 2 weeks after the onset of symptoms. The characteristic findings are normal pressure and albuminocytologic dissociation (elevated protein level with fewer than 10 mononuclear cells/μL). An increased cell count should raise the suspicion for HIV or Lyme disease as the precipitating event.[3,13,15,17]

Baseline measurements of pulmonary function are important, because 25% to 33% of patients with GBS eventually require mechanical ventilation.[10,15] Forced vital capacity (FVC) or inspiratory force (IF) should be tested in the emergency department. The hospital respiratory therapist may be able to provide the appropriate portable devices if they are not available in the department. A quick bedside test is to have the patient take a deep inspiration and then count as long as possible; the ability to count to 25 correlates with an FVC of 2 L, and a count to only 10 with an FVC of 1 L.[15] FVC of less than 12 to 15 mL/kg or an IF of less than 20 cm H_20 are indications of impending respiratory failure and the need to initiate mechanical ventilation.[3,7,15] Patients who remain in the emergency department for several hours should have serial pulmonary function testing. Bulbar muscle strength should also be followed, as intubation may be required to maintain a patent airway and prevent aspiration. Frequent vital signs and continuous cardiac monitoring are essential to identify autonomic dysfunction. Blood pressure fluctuations should be treated, as needed, with fluids and short-acting agents.

DISPOSITION

Every patient with an acute polyneuropathy should be evaluated by a neurologist. Admission to the hospital for further diagnostic studies and continued monitoring of vital signs and respiratory status is required. Whether an intensive care unit is necessary for all patients is controversial. Clearly, any patient with significant respiratory impairment (e.g., FVC less then 20 mL/kg,[7,17] IF less than 25 cm H_20,[7] difficulty swallowing, etc.) or autonomic instability should be admitted to an intensive care unit. For all others, the decision depends on the adequacy of monitoring in other settings. Patients with severe or rapidly progressive GBS benefit from early plasma exchange or immune globulin therapy; therefore, these patients should be transferred to a facility capable of providing such therapies.[1,7,17]

COMMON PITFALLS

- Mistaking the low back pain of GBS for disc disease or back strain
- Failing to admit patients with minimal, but suggestive, symptomatology
- Monitoring inadequately for respiratory and autonomic dysfunction
- Ascribing the symmetric weakness of GBS or other acute polyneuropathies to a psychiatric disorder
- Failure to recognize variant presentations of GBS

Subacute Polyneuropathy

Polyneuropathy that develops over a period of several weeks to months is said to be subacute; however, the distinction between subacute and acute polyneuropathy is not always clear. For example, while half of patients with GBS present with symptoms that develop over 10 to 14 days, in the other half, symptoms progress over 3 to 4 weeks.[3,5] Subacute polyneuropathies may be symmetric or asymmetric. Symmetric disease generally begins with distal sensorimotor losses and tends to produce marked sensory impairment. Asymmetric neuropathies are frequently the result of neuronal ischemia; nerves are randomly affected, producing patchy sensorimotor losses.

DIFFERENTIAL DIAGNOSIS

The differential diagnosis of *symmetric* subacute polyneuropathy includes GBS, chronic inflammatory demyelinating polyneuropathy, diabetes mellitus, collagen vascular and autoimmune diseases, nutritional deficiencies, uremia, amyloidosis, heavy-metal intoxication, industrial solvents (e.g., glue sniffing), a multitude of toxins and medications, Lyme disease, and HIV infection.

The etiologies of *asymmetric* disease include diabetes mellitus (e.g., diabetic amyotrophy), collagen vascular and other autoimmune diseases, peripheral vascular disease, sarcoidosis, neoplastic disease, paraproteinemia, leprosy, Lyme disease, HIV infection, and idiopathic disease.

Other diseases that produce subacute weakness and may be confused with subacute polyneuropathy are myasthenia gravis, amyotrophic lateral sclerosis, Parkinson disease, and depression.

EMERGENCY DEPARTMENT EVALUATION, MANAGEMENT, AND DISPOSITION

History and physical examination are the principal methods of evaluation. Key historic elements to elicit are a history of neuromuscular or systemic disease, medications (prescription and nonprescription), and potential infectious or toxic exposure. Laboratory studies should include complete blood count, serum electrolytes, calcium, magnesium, phosphate, glucose, blood urea nitrogen, creatinine, and a screening chest radiograph. As with acute neuropathies, further studies should be obtained only if a specific etiology is suspected following evaluation of the patient.[4]

Most patients with subacute polyneuropathy may be referred to their primary care physician for outpatient evaluation and referral to a neurologist. If a medication is suspected as the etiology, it should be discontinued or changed after consultation with the primary care physician. Short-term follow-up should be arranged.

COMMON PITFALL

Assuming that subacute polyneuropathy is secondary to a chronic medical condition, thus overlooking potentially treatable causes

Chronic Polyneuropathy

Chronic polyneuropathy develops over months to years. Patients generally have marked sensory changes, but motor losses are prominent as well. Muscle wasting and foot deformities are clinical clues to a chronic neuropathy. The differential diagnosis is vast; it includes both acquired conditions and numerous hereditary disorders. Adults presenting for primary evaluation of a peripheral neuropathy that, by history and examination, appears to be chronic should be referred to their primary care physicians.

Plexopathy and Radiculopathy

CLINICAL PRESENTATION

A plexopathy is a disorder that affects the brachial or lumbosacral plexus. Symptoms include pain and mixed motor and sensory deficits in a pattern that cannot be attributed to individual peripheral nerves or nerve roots.

Acute or subacute plexopathies are associated with local trauma (e.g., shoulder dislocation), compression (e.g., retroperitoneal hematoma or abdominal aortic aneurysm), vascular disease (usually due to diabetes or collagen vascular disease), or infection (e.g., Lyme disease), or they may be idiopathic.[16] Chronic plexopathy is associated with infections, vascular disease, collagen vascular disease, tumor, infiltrative processes, and radiation therapy.

Idiopathic lumbosacral plexopathy is rare,[5,16] but acute idiopathic brachial plexopathy is well described. It is seen most commonly in men in the third or fourth decade of life,[11] and there appears to be some association with recent viral illnesses and immunizations.[5,11] Symptoms begin with the sudden onset of severe shoulder pain that may extend into the neck and upper arm. Less commonly, the lower plexus cords may be affected, producing symptoms in the forearm and hand. Within days to weeks, motor weakness and sensory loss develop, usually coinciding with resolution of pain.[5,11,16] About 90% of patients recover good neurologic function by 3 years.[11]

In contrast to plexopathy, a radiculopathy affects spinal nerve roots. Symptoms include pain and sensorimotor deficits in a pattern consistent with the involved nerve root (e.g., lancinating pain along the L-5 nerve root dermatome). Frequently, several adjacent roots are affected, making differentiation from a plexopathy or multiple mononeuropathies clinically impossible. The etiologies of radiculopathy include all those of a plexopathy, as well as specific spinal canal or cord disorders such as herniated disc, spinal stenosis, and epidural tumor, abscess, hematoma, granuloma, and infection.[1,6]

DIFFERENTIAL DIAGNOSIS

The differential diagnosis of brachial plexopathy and lumbosacral plexopathy includes polyneuropathy, multiple mononeuropathies, and spinal cord and root disorders. Brachial plexopathy can easily be confused with C-5 root compression, and lumbosacral plexopathy with L-4 compression.[6] The pain of idiopathic brachial plexopathy tends to resolve as motor symptoms develop, unlike the persistent pain of C-5 root compression.[6] In addition, C-5 root pain increases with neck movement, coughing, and sneezing, while brachial plexopathy pain increases with shoulder movement.[5] Pain from both lumbosacral plexopathy and L-4 root compression is persistent. Iliopsoas weakness is common in lumbosacral plexopathy but is not seen with L-4 root lesions.

Thoracic outlet syndrome (TOS) can mimic brachial plexopathy by producing pain and weakness in the arm. Provocative maneuvers suggestive of TOS include loss of the radial pulse and onset of symptoms when the patient inhales deeply and the shoulder is hyperabducted and externally rotated with the head turned to the unaffected side (Wright's maneuver) or the neck is extended with the head rotated to the affected side (Adson's test).[14] Other local joint or tendon disorders, muscular disorders, and amyotrophic lateral sclerosis may also mimic plexopathy, but can usually be differentiated by their lack of sensory abnormalities.

EMERGENCY DEPARTMENT EVALUATION AND MANAGEMENT

The history and physical examination, including a detailed neurologic examination, are essential in management decisions. In patients with chronic symptoms, minimal immediate diagnostic workup is necessary. A chest and neck radiograph or lumbosacral films are reasonable screening tools for such patients.

Acute symptomatology, on the other hand, requires an aggressive approach. Patients with symptoms of *acute brachial plexopathy* should have cervical spine, chest, and shoulder radiographs.[5,11] Laboratory studies such as complete blood cell count, serum electrolytes, glucose, blood urea nitrogen, creatinine, and sedimentation rate may be considered if the history or physical examination suggests infection, diabetes, or collagen vascular disease.

Acute lumbosacral plexopathy generally occurs secondary to another disease process. A complete blood cell count, serum electrolytes, glucose, blood urea nitrogen, creatinine, erythrocyte sedimentation rate, and lumbosacral films are appropriate. An abdominal ultrasound or computed tomography is indicated if an aortic aneurysm or other retroperitoneal pathology (e.g., bleed, tumor) is suspected. A determination of postvoid residual urine volume will aid in defining the extent of the neurologic deficit.

The approach to an *acute radiculopathy* is dictated by the history and physical examination. An evaluation consistent with an acute herniated disc and no objective neurologic deficits may require only conservative management with analgesia, muscle relaxants, limited activity, and close follow-up. Most other etiologies require an aggressive evaluation, including blood testing, a determination of postvoid residual urine volume, and spinal imaging.

DISPOSITION

Acute symptoms resulting from plexopathies are often difficult to distinguish from root and spinal cord disorders.[5,6] Therefore, both generally require urgent neurosurgical consultation. Spinal computed tomography, magnetic resonance imaging, or myelography may be required to determine the correct diagnosis, and hospital admission to complete such testing is recommended. Outpatient follow-up is appropriate for patients with chronic symptoms.

COMMON PITFALLS

- Attribution of symptoms to mononeuropathy, and thereby failing to proceed with the appropriate diagnostic evaluation required for plexopathies and radiculopathies
- Failure to consider potentially catastrophic etiologies for acute plexopathies (e.g.,abdominal aneurysm)
- Failure to consider potentially catastrophic etiologies for acute radiculopathies (e.g., spinal epidural abscess or acute cord compression)

Mononeuropathy

CLINICAL PRESENTATION

Mononeuropathies produce variable symptoms of pain and sensorimotor loss in the distribution of a single peripheral nerve. The actual neuronal injury may be classified as neuropraxia (a "stunned" nerve with an intact, but nonconducting axon), axonotmesis (damaged axon in an intact nerve trunk), or neurotmesis (disrupted nerve trunk).[11,14] The speed and degree of neurologic recovery are related to the type of injury present.

Nerve compression and entrapment are the most frequently encountered etiologies for mononeuropathies in the emergency department. Entrapment syndromes (e.g., carpal tunnel syndrome) have been associated with pregnancy, rheumatoid arthritis, osteoarthritis, gout, hypothyroidism, acromegaly, amyloidosis, multiple myeloma, collagen vascular disease, local tumors, and repetitive activity.[1,5] Other causes of mononeuropathies are trauma (mechanical, electrical, or thermal), collagen vascular disease, diabetes mellitus, vascular disease, infection, granulomatous disease, infiltrative disorders, neoplasia, radiation therapy, and primary nerve tumors.

A unique form of mononeuropathy is mononeuritis multiplex. This entity involves the simultaneous or near-simultaneous dysfunction of two or more peripheral nerves. It may result from multiple pressure palsies, infections (e.g., leprosy, Lyme disease, HIV infection), infiltrative or neoplastic disease, vascular disease, or collagen vascular disease.[5] The abrupt onset of mononeuritis multiplex in patients with a collagen vascular disease or other vasculitis is of specific concern, as it generally indicates an acute necrotizing vasculitis that requires aggressive treatment.[1]

DIFFERENTIAL DIAGNOSIS

The differential diagnosis of a mononeuropathy includes radiculopathy, plexopathy, polyneuropathy, local joint or muscular disorders, hysteria, and malingering.

EMERGENCY DEPARTMENT EVALUATION AND MANAGEMENT

The evaluation of mononeuropathies should focus on identification of a specific etiology. Once the nature of the deficit and its mode of onset are reviewed, the history should elicit any traumatic injury, occupational factors (e.g., repetitive activity), or symptoms suggestive of diabetes or collagen vascular disease. The physical examination should include a detailed neurologic examination to determine whether the deficits fit the distribution of a single peripheral nerve. An excellent summary of peripheral nerve dermatomes can be found in Appendix A in *Disorders of Peripheral Nerves,* by Schaumburg et al.[19] Evidence of systemic disease, trauma, and possible entrapment sites should be sought.

Complete blood cell count, electrolytes, blood glucose, erythrocyte sedimentation rate, antinuclear antibody testing, thyroid function tests, and serum protein electrophoresis are indicated only if a systemic disorder is suspected. Radiographs may be helpful in cases associated with trauma or when bone abnormalities are a possible cause of entrapment.

DISPOSITION

Most patients with a mononeuropathy can be discharged, with a splint, to outpatient follow-up. Identified etiologies, such as diabetes or repetitive activities, should be addressed, and patients in whom the etiology is unclear should be referred to their primary care physician or a neurologist for further testing, which may include nerve conduction studies and electromyography. Posttraumatic mononeuropathy should be evaluated urgently by a plastic surgeon, orthopedic surgeon, or neurosurgeon, although expectant management is generally the preferred approach to care.

Admission to the hospital is indicated for acute mononeuropathy multiplex in patients with known or suspected collagen vascular disease or vasculitis. As previously mentioned, this disorder usually indicates an acute necrotizing vasculitis, which requires aggressive steroid and/or other immunosuppressive therapy.[1]

COMMON PITFALLS

- Failure to differentiate a mononeuropathy from a polyneuropathy, plexopathy, or radiculopathy
- Failure to detect systemic signs of collagen vascular disease or other vasculitis disorder in patients with mononeuropathy multiplex

References

1. Adams RD, Victor M, Ropper AH, eds. *Principles of neurology,* 6th ed. New York: McGraw-Hill, 1997.
2. Barohn RJ. Approach to peripheral neuropathy and neuronopathy. *Semin Neurol* 1998;18(1):7.
3. Bella I, Chad DA. Neuromuscular disorders and acute respiratory failure. *Neurosurg Clin North Am* 1998;16(2):391.
4. Dyck PJ, Dyck JB, Grant IA, et al. Ten steps in characterizing and diagnosing patients with peripheral neuropathy. *Neurology* 1996;47:10.
5. Dyck PJ, Thomas PK, eds. *Peripheral neuropathy,* 3rd ed. Philadelphia: WB Saunders, 1993.
6. Fager CA. Identification and management of radiculopathy. *Neurosurg Clin North Am* 1993;4(1):1.
7. Fulgham JR, Wijicks FM. Guillain-Barré syndrome. *Crit Care Clin* 1997;13(1):1.
8. Grattan-Smith PJ, Morris JG, Johnston HM, et al. Clinical and neurophysiological features of tick paralysis. *Brain* 1997;120:1975.
9. Hahn AF. Guillain-Barré syndrome. *Lancet* 1998;352:635.
10. Hughes RA, Rees JH. Clinical and epidemiologic features of Guillain-Barré syndrome. *J Infect Dis* 1997;176[Suppl 2]:S92.
11. Leffert RD. Neurological problems. In: Rockwood CA, Matsen FA, eds. *The shoulder.* Philadelphia: WB Saunders, 1990:750.
12. Mandell GL, Bennett JE, Dolin R, eds. *Mandell, Douglas and Bennett's principles and practice of infectious diseases,* 4th ed. New York: Churchill Livingstone, 1995.
13. McLeod JG. Investigation of peripheral neuropathy. *J Neurol Neurosurg Psychiatry* 1995;58(3):274.
14. Nuber GW, Assenmacher J, Bowen MK. Neurovascular problems in the forearm, wrist, and hand. *Clin Sports Med* 1998;17(3):585.
15. Pascuzzi RM, Fleck JD. Acute peripheral neuropathy in adults: Guillain-Barré syndrome and related disorders. *Neurol Clin* 1997;15(3):529.
16. Pryse-Phillips W, Murray TJ, eds. *Essential neurology,* 4th ed. New York: Elsevier Science, 1992.
17. Rees J. Guillain-Barré syndrome: clinical manifestations and directions for treatment. *Drugs* 1995;49(6):912.
18. Ropper AH, Wijdicks EFM, Traux BT. *Guillain-Barré syndrome.* Philadelphia: FA Davis Co, 1991.
19. Schaumburg HH, Berger AR, Thomas PK. *Disorders of peripheral nerves,* 2nd ed. Philadelphia: FA Davis Co, 1992.

CHAPTER 205

Myopathies and Disorders of Neuromuscular Transmission

James J. Walter

Weakness is a commonly encountered symptom in patients presenting for emergency medical care, but only rarely is it due to a primary disorder of muscle or neuromuscular transmission. These primary disorders are not only uncommon, but also often subtle and variable in presentation and, therefore, easy to misdiagnose. Because these disorders may be serious and potentially life-threatening, they should always be included in the differential diagnosis of true weakness.

Once considered, the most important way to diagnose these neuromuscular disorders is an appropriately focused history and physical examination. Emergency physicians must also be knowledgeable about the diagnostic tests commonly used to help identify these disorders.[11]

Many neuromuscular disorders can present as rapidly progressive, generalized weakness that has the potential to cause life-threatening ventilatory compromise. When faced with a severely weak patient, the emergency physician must know how to intervene safely and rapidly while simultaneously considering the differential diagnosis and possible acute precipitants.

MYOPATHIES

Primary muscle disease presents with muscular weakness as the predominant symptom. Weakness is generally proximal and symmetric in distribution. Deep tendon reflexes are preserved, and there are no sensory complaints, distinguishing the myopathies from acute inflammatory polyneuropathy (Guillain-Barré syndrome). Myopathic weakness is not marked by diurnal variation and usually spares the extraocular, facial, and bulbar muscles (distinguishing the myopathies from myasthenia gravis and other disorders of the neuromuscular junction). Pain may occasionally be present (e.g., tenderness in polymyositis, or the pain and swelling infrequently seen in acute rhabdomyolysis). Although myopathic disease characteristically is of gradual onset with a slow progression of symptoms, several disorders can present with rapidly progressive, generalized weakness, and are thus of particular concern to emergency physicians. An overview of the spectrum of myopathic disorders is given in Table 205.1.

The hereditary myopathies include the various forms of muscular dystrophy as well as the metabolic myopathies and periodic paralysis. The *muscular dystrophies* are characterized by the insidious onset of muscle weakness, with progressive deterioration over time. The types are differentiated by mode of inheritance, age at onset, rate of progression, and the selectivity of muscle involvement.[8] Diagnosis is made on the basis of family history, clinical features, and the results of creatine phosphokinase determination, electromyography, and muscle biopsy. The muscular dystrophies should be included in the differential diagnosis of chronic and subacute progressive weakness. It is also important to remember that the muscular dystrophies are associated with an increased frequency of cardiac failure, arrhythmias, pneumonia, and respiratory failure, as well as an increased susceptibility to anesthetic-induced malignant hyperthermia. Thus, the threshold for instituting close monitoring of cardiopulmonary function should be lower in patients with these disorders.

Metabolic myopathies are disorders of glucose or lipid utilization and energy production in skeletal muscle. The best known is muscle phosphorylase deficiency (McArdle disorder). Primarily affecting males, it occurs in the late teens and is characterized by painful muscle cramps, stiffness, and weakness after intense exercise, resulting from an enzymatic block in the glycolytic pathway and subsequent depletion of high-energy phosphate stores. Overexertion in these patients may lead to rhabdomyolysis and myoglobinuria. The disorder is diagnosed by a careful history and confirmed by a forearm ischemic exercise test and muscle biopsy. Treatment involves dietary measures and exercise limitation. This disorder should be considered in patients presenting with a history of intense postexercise muscle pain.

The several types of *periodic paralysis* (hypokalemic, thyrotoxic, hyperkalemic, and normokalemic) are caused by defects in muscle membrane permeability to sodium and potassium. Although rare, these are disorders that the emergency physician should be familiar with so that an appropriate history can be elicited, a diagnosis made, and correct therapy initiated. Although these episodic disorders usually spare the respiratory muscles, respiratory arrest has been reported and is always a danger in the profoundly weak patient.

In hypokalemic periodic paralysis, attacks characteristically begin in adolescence and recurrences are usually more than a month apart. Attacks last from hours to days and are triggered by sleep, exertion, high carbohydrate intake, cold, and stress. Symmetric weakness of the proximal limb muscles is noted. The diagnosis is based on patient history and serum potassium determination (usually 2.5 to 3.5 mEq/L during attacks). If attacks are infrequent, provocative testing with glucose and insulin infusion may be needed (performed in a controlled setting by a neurologist). Acute therapy is with potassium chloride (10 mEq/h intravenously or 40 to 60 mEq PO, repeated in 1 hour if needed). Acetazolamide prophylaxis and avoidance of high-carbohydrate meals are useful in chronic management.

Thyrotoxic periodic paralysis is a variant of hypokalemic periodic paralysis and occurs most frequently in young Asian and Hispanic males, often with only minimal clinical evidence of hyperthyroidism. The weakness can be mild to severe, primarily affects the lower extremities, and tends to occur at night or in the early morning. Therapy consists of the cautious administration of oral or intravenous potassium (rebound hyperkalemia is common) and control of the hyperthyroid state.[12,13]

In the less common, hyperkalemic form of period paralysis, attacks typically begin in the first decade of life, occur more frequently, and are of shorter duration (usually less than 2 hours). They may be precipitated by exercise, cold exposure, fasting, or potassium ingestion. During an attack, the serum potassium is usually greater than 5 mEq/L, although the level may remain normal (normokalemic periodic paralysis is a clinically indistinct variant of the hyperkalemic form). The brief attacks seldom require emergency treatment. If necessary, acute attacks may be treated with oral glucose, with inhalation of nebulized beta-adrenergic agents, or with glucose and insulin (1 ampule $D_{50}W$ with 5 U regular insulin). To prevent attacks, a thiazide diuretic may be used, along with avoidance of known precipitants.

Diagnosis is the challenge of these uncommon episodic illnesses for the emergency physician. Brief recurrent attacks of limb weakness should not be attributed to psychiatric causes without considering periodic paralysis. Similar previous episodes should be identified, and serum potassium and thyroxine levels should be measured. Other causes of hypokalemia and hyperkalemia should be considered as well.

Polymyositis, an inflammatory disorder of skeletal muscle, is the most common primary myopathy to affect adults but is nonetheless a rare disease (annual incidence of one per 100,000).[1] Muscle damage is caused by cell- and antibody-mediated autoimmune attack, but the ultimate etiology is unknown. Dermatomyositis, a common variant, is polymyositis with characteristic skin changes. Approximately 20% of patients with

TABLE 205.1. Classification of Myopathies

HEREDITARY
Muscular dystrophies
Metabolic myopathies
Periodic paralysis
INFLAMMATORY
Idiopathic (polymyositis, dermatomyositis)
Other connective tissue disorders
Infectious (toxoplasmosis, trichinosis, Lyme disease, viral infection)
ENDOCRINE/METABOLIC
Endocrine (thyroid, adrenal, parathyroid, pituitary)
Electrolyte abnormality (sodium, potassium, calcium, magnesium, phosphate)
DRUG INDUCED
Myopathy/myositis (alcohol, corticosteroids, chloroquine, clofibrate, lovastatin, colchicine, zidovudine, others)
Rhabdomyolysis (alcohol, opiates, barbiturates, cocaine, phencyclidine, amphetamines, others)
Malignant hyperthermia (general anesthetics, depolarizing muscle relaxants)
Neuroleptic malignant syndrome (neuroleptics)
OTHER
Trauma, ischemia, sepsis

polymyositis or dermatomyositis have an associated connective tissue disease such as scleroderma, lupus, or rheumatoid arthritis.

The disease begins with the gradual onset of symmetric weakness of the proximal extremities that progresses over weeks to months, classically ascending from the lower to the upper extremities and finally involving the neck and pharyngeal muscles. Rarely, the disease presents in a fulminant form with severe generalized weakness, respiratory insufficiency, and rhabdomyolysis.

Characteristically, the patient notes difficulty in performing everyday activities such as rising from a chair, climbing stairs, or reaching overhead. Muscle pain and tenderness are occasionally noted. The facial and extraocular muscles are not involved.

The diagnosis of inflammatory myositis may be made by a combination of proximal muscle weakness, elevated muscle enzymes (creatine phosphokinase and aldolase), characteristic electromyogram, magnetic resonance imaging, and muscle biopsy. Autoantibodies may be positive. The erythrocyte sedimentation rate is often normal or only mildly elevated and is not a reliable indicator of disease severity.[1]

Long-term treatment of polymyositis is with corticosteroids; a cytotoxic drug such as azathioprine is occasionally used as well. Although relapse can occur, most patients with idiopathic polymyositis or dermatomyositis improve with therapy, and up to 50% can eventually discontinue corticosteroid treatment. For severe weakness, high-dose intravenous immunoglobulin can be helpful.[6] Plasma exchange has not proven effective.

EMERGENCY DEPARTMENT EVALUATION AND DIFFERENTIAL DIAGNOSIS

After initial attention to ventilatory status, evaluation of the patient presenting with the acute or subacute development of muscular weakness should focus on the history: the time course of the illness, progression of symptoms (including whether the weakness is periodic, fluctuating, or progressive), precipitating factors, associated pain or stiffness, any sensory complaints, and whether there is any associated fever, rash, arthralgia, or other symptoms. Information should be elicited about family history, any underlying illnesses, medication use, and exposure to home-canned or other contaminated food.

On physical examination, the patient should be tested for the ability to perform simple tasks (e.g., lifting arms above head, ability to make a tight fist, rising from a chair, rising on the toes), and the distribution of muscle involvement should be determined (including whether the extraocular, facial, or bulbar musculature is involved). Pathologic fatigue of muscles may be elicited by having the patient sustain an upward gaze, count loudly, or hold the arms horizontally. The muscles should be inspected for size and irritability and palpated for tenderness. The neurologic examination must include an evaluation of pupillary size and reactivity, sensory function, and deep tendon reflexes. Evidence should be sought for any potential precipitating illness; when appropriate, an adherent tick should be carefully sought. Using the history and physical examination, it is generally possible to exclude upper and lower motor neuron disease, myelopathy, and peripheral neuropathy from the differential diagnosis.

Elements of the diagnostic evaluation may include a complete blood cell count; determination of glucose, electrolyte, blood urea nitrogen, creatinine, creatine phosphokinase, calcium, magnesium, and phosphorus levels; sedimentation rate; electrocardiogram; chest radiograph; arterial blood gas analysis; and bedside spirometry. Additional studies may be necessary in the course of evaluation after referral to an internist or neurologist.

The differential diagnosis of subacute or chronically progressive weakness includes polymyositis (progressive, proximal limb weakness; sparing of extraocular muscles; elevated creatine phosphokinase); the muscular dystrophies (distinguished by family history, progression of symptoms over years, and selective pattern of muscle involvement); myasthenia gravis (almost always presenting with early involvement of extraocular and facial muscles and confirmed by a response to a short-acting anticholinesterase and characteristic results on repetitive nerve stimulation testing); polymyalgia rheumatica (proximal muscle pain and stiffness without true weakness, elevated erythrocyte sedimentation rate); and drug-induced myopathy. Thyroid or other endocrine myopathy can also present as proximal muscle weakness, as can severe hypokalemia, hypophosphatemia, or hypermagnesemia. Chronic alcohol abuse can produce a syndrome of proximal muscle wasting and weakness, often with coexistent evidence of alcoholic peripheral neuropathy. Finally, infectious etiologies of myositis or myopathy should be sought.

The differential diagnosis of acutely developing weakness includes myasthenia gravis; inflammatory polyneuropathy (Guillain-Barré syndrome); neurotoxin exposure (e.g., botulism, tick paralysis, organophosphate poisoning); severe electrolyte abnormality; drug- and alcohol-induced myopathy; periodic paralysis; and (rarely) polymyositis.

EMERGENCY DEPARTMENT MANAGEMENT

In patients with neuromuscular disease presenting with *severe and rapidly progressing weakness,* the crisis is usually precipitated by an intercurrent illness, most commonly a respiratory tract infection. These patients often present with ventilatory compromise, ineffective cough, and difficulty handling secretions. Decompensation to respiratory failure can be rapid. Immediate attention should be directed to oxygenation and ventilatory status. Serial physical examination, arterial blood gas determination, and spirometry are essential, and endotracheal intubation should be performed at the earliest sign of difficulty. Normal levels of pCO_2 and pO_2 are often maintained nearly to the point of profound respiratory failure and respiratory arrest.

The need for intubation and mechanical ventilation is best guided by serial measurement of vital capacity. A declining vital capacity or a vital capacity less than 15 mL/kg is an indication for urgent intubation. Testing of maximum inspiratory (PI_{max}) and expiratory (PE_{max}) pressures is also helpful in quantitating respiratory muscle weakness (PI_{max} less than 20 cm H_2O and PE_{max} less than 40 cm H_2O are correlated with inadequate ventilation and ineffective cough, respectively). Patients with severe weakness should be ventilated, at least initially, in the controlled mode.

Attention to hemodynamic stability is the next priority, with continuous electrocardiographic monitoring and evaluation of fluid needs. Creatine phosphokinase determination and urinalysis are mandatory to identify acute rhabdomyolysis. Patients with severe weakness require admission to an intensive care setting for supportive care, monitoring of cardiorespiratory status, treatment of any underlying illness, and further diagnostic evaluation.

In patients with *slowly progressive neuromuscular weakness,* the first priority is, likewise, to ensure cardiorespiratory stability. After appropriate diagnostic testing, these patients may require hospital admission for clinical observation, identification and treatment of any underlying illness, and further evaluation. Admission is indicated if there is any concern about the patient's respiratory reserve, if the degree of pharyngeal muscle weakness suggests a risk of aspiration, if rhabdomyolysis is suggested by creatine phosphokinase determination and urinalysis, or if the patient cannot function satisfactorily at home. The decision to manage the problem on an outpatient basis must be made after consultation with the primary care physician, internist, or neurologist, and on the condition that follow-up can be reliably arranged.

DISORDERS OF NEUROMUSCULAR TRANSMISSION

Myasthenia Gravis

Understanding disorders of the neuromuscular junction (Table 205.2) is of special importance for emergency physicians, because patients with these disorders may present with critical neuromuscular dysfunction requiring rapid diagnostic evaluation and specific management. The emergency physician must also be aware of the commonly used medications that can cause precipitous worsening of muscle strength in these patients.

Myasthenia gravis, the most common disorder of the neuromuscular junction, is an autoimmune disorder in which antibodies are directed against the acetylcholine receptor, reducing the number of available receptors and impairing neuromuscular transmission.[7] In the majority of patients, the disease is associated with an abnormality of the thymus gland, either thymoma or thymitis. The thymus appears to be the site where B cells are sensitized to the acetylcholine receptor, initiating the disease process. The disease can occur at all ages but is most common in women in their mid-20s. The peak incidence for men is in the sixth or seventh decade.

The hallmark of myasthenia gravis is pathologic fatigue, owing to the loss of the generous physiologic reserve that normally supports transmission across the neuromuscular junction. Muscle weakness worsens with sustained activity and improves with rest; patients commonly report worsening of symptoms as the day progresses.

Myasthenia gravis is a disease of insidious onset, developing over a period of weeks to months. The muscle weakness occurs at first in transient attacks, at times precipitated by infection, stress, or pregnancy. The extraocular muscles are most commonly affected, and the most typical presentation is one of recurring episodes of diplopia and ptosis that are often noticed later in the day. There may also be weakness of eye closure, weakness of the muscles of facial expression, or difficulty chewing; transient dysarthria and dysphagia are common. Patients may also have involvement of the proximal limb and truncal and respiratory muscles and note difficulty climbing stairs or combing their hair.

The disease is extremely variable in its clinical presentation and may affect diverse muscle groups in an asymmetric, unpredictable manner, fluctuating in intensity over time. Spontaneous remissions and relapses are common, and the ultimate progression of the disease is highly variable. Respiratory crisis requiring mechanical ventilation occurs in up to 20% of patients.[9]

Immunosuppressive therapy for myasthenia, which is quite successful in controlling the disease, is responsible for a significant proportion of long-term morbidity and mortality. Fortunately, a large percentage of patients show marked improvement with treatment and can often be weaned off immunosuppressive agents. With proper management, mortality for the disease itself, previously as high as 30%, is now less than 5%.[7]

TABLE 205.2. Disorders of Neuromuscular Transmission
AUTOIMMUNE
Myasthenia gravis, Eaton-Lambert syndrome
TOXIN INDUCED
Botulism, tick paralysis, envenomation (coral snakes, black widow spiders), paralytic shellfish poisoning
DRUG INDUCED
Aminoglycosides, procainamide, penicillamine, phenytoin, chloroquine, psychotropic drugs, others
POISONING
Organophosphates, carbamates

EMERGENCY DEPARTMENT EVALUATION AND DIFFERENTIAL DIAGNOSIS

For the patient presenting with a history of episodic weakness and fatigue involving extraocular, facial, and/or bulbar musculature, the evaluation should focus on obtaining a careful history, ruling out an underlying precipitating illness, demonstrating pathologic fatigue on physical examination, and developing a differential diagnosis.

On physical examination, provocative maneuvers to demonstrate weakness after repetitive or sustained muscle activity can assist in suggesting the diagnosis of myasthenia (e.g., ptosis or diplopia provoked by prolonged upward gaze, dysarthria or dysphonia with loud counting, inability to hold a tongue blade tightly in clenched teeth, or fatigue on holding the arms abducted or with repeated deep knee bends). Physical examination should also carefully assess pupillary response, sensation, and deep tendon reflexes, which should all be normal in the patient with myasthenia gravis. Underlying or precipitating illness should be carefully sought. The examination should also focus on the status and reserve of the respiratory system, especially on the adequacy of the resting tidal volume and the ability to manage secretions.

Patients with localized or mild symptoms suggestive of myasthenia gravis are usually referred to a neurologist for confirmatory testing. Testing includes an anticholinesterase test, in which the short-acting agent edrophonium is given intravenously while observing the patient for resolution of weakness in an affected muscle group. A repetitive nerve stimulation test is more definitive and is recommended as the next step in diagnosis. In myasthenia, a decrement in the amplitude of the muscle action potential is noted when the motor nerve is repetitively stimulated at 3 cycles per second. Further evaluation includes an assay for circulating antiacetylcholine receptor antibodies (found in 90% of patients with generalized disease), computed tomography scanning of the thymus, thyroid function tests, and serologic screening for the presence of other autoimmune diseases.

The differential diagnosis includes drug-induced myasthenia, botulism, tick paralysis, organophosphate poisoning, Eaton-Lambert myasthenic syndrome, inflammatory polyneuropathy (Guillain-Barré syndrome), a primary or secondary myopathy, other causes of oculomotor palsy (diabetes, multiple sclerosis, aneurysm), and neurasthenia. History, physical examination, and simple laboratory data should enable the clinician to readily distinguish among these entities. However, myasthenia gravis (like periodic paralysis and multiple sclerosis) can easily be misdiagnosed as a psychiatric problem (depression, anxiety, or a somatoform disorder). One should be extremely wary of making a diagnosis of a psychiatric or functional illness in a patient complaining of weakness, without carefully considering the possibility of one of these diagnoses.

EMERGENCY DEPARTMENT MANAGEMENT

Unrecognized airway and ventilatory problems remain the greatest danger in myasthenia gravis. If there is any concern about progression of the disease from whatever cause, neurologic consultation and monitoring of the patient in an intensive care unit is warranted. Underlying respiratory tract infection or other precipitant should be identified and treated aggressively. Early antibiotic therapy is of utmost importance in the treatment of an associated infectious illness.

Management should focus on the patient's respiratory status and ability to handle secretions. The picture may be complicated by poor oral intake and, occasionally, by drug-induced muscarinic side effects such as bronchorrhea and bronchospasm. Arterial blood gas analysis and bedside spirometry should be performed. One should be aware that respiratory failure can develop insidiously and that it may occur despite normal arterial blood gases and apparently good peripheral motor strength. The deterioration to respiratory arrest can be precipitous. Endotracheal intubation should be performed at the earliest suggestion of respiratory compromise, which is best detected by serial measurements of vital capacity, inspiratory and expiratory force, and the patient's ability to clear secretions.

Respiratory infections are common precipitants of myasthenic crisis and must be diagnosed and treated aggressively. Electrolyte abnormalities that may be exacerbating the clinical picture should likewise be identified. Prominent muscarinic side effects from cholinergic overmedication (e.g., bradycardia, abdominal cramping, bronchorrhea) may be treated with atropine. All medications should be withdrawn, any underlying illness treated, and volume status and caloric intake normalized if possible. Improvement is often relatively rapid, and the patient is commonly restarted on anticholinesterase medication within 48 hours. For patients who do not respond to the aforementioned measures, plasmapheresis is, as a rule rapidly effective and has dramatically reduced morbidity from respiratory failure. Muscle strength typically recovers within 5 days after the initiation of plasmapheresis or plasma exchange.[5] Intravenous immunoglobulin has also proven useful and has the advantage of not requiring specialized equipment.[15] High-dose corticosteroids are also commonly administered to patients in crisis.

Long-term treatment of myasthenia gravis involves several different modalities. Anticholinesterase agents, which potentiate the action of acetylcholine at the postsynaptic membrane, are the drugs of first choice in treatment. Although they provide symptomatic relief, improvement is usually incomplete, and they do not influence the progression of the disease. Pyridostigmine, at an initial dose of 60 mg three times a day, is the agent most commonly chosen. An experienced neurologist should initiate and monitor anticholinesterase therapy in myasthenia gravis. The medication dose is adjusted cautiously while clinical signs are monitored; the edrophonium test may be repeated to help gauge therapy. Muscarinic side effects can be troublesome, but more serious is the development of a depolarizing neuromuscular block secondary to overmedication, the so-called cholinergic crisis.

Thymectomy leads to improvement in most patients and is increasingly recommended for patients with generalized myasthenia gravis and persistent symptoms.[19]

Corticosteroids produce favorable results in over 80% of patients but, because of side effects, are usually reserved for patients with inadequate response to anticholinesterase therapy and thymectomy. Corticosteroids reduce antiacetylcholine receptor antibody levels and probably have additional direct effects on the neuromuscular junction. They may initially aggravate muscle weakness, however, so it is generally recommended that therapy be initiated with low doses and inhospital observation. Azathioprine or cyclosporine can be used as supplemental agents or in patients unable to tolerate corticosteroid therapy.

A patient with known myasthenia gravis who presents with severe weakness may be suffering from either a rapid worsening of the disease ("myasthenic crisis") or a depolarizing neuromuscular block as a result of cholinergic overmedication ("cholinergic crisis"). Myasthenic crisis is the much more common of the two and may be precipitated by poor compliance with medication, drug interaction, underlying infection, or other stress.[2,17] The patient with cholinergic crisis is more likely to present with symptoms of cholinergic overactivity, including miosis, sweating, salivation, and gastrointestinal distress (muscarinic effects), as well as muscular cramps and fasciculations (nicotinic effects). However, the presentation of a patient with progressive weakness who has been treated with increasing doses of anticholinesterase medication may be confusing, even to the most experienced clinician. In practice, the distinction between myasthenic crisis and cholinergic crisis is of little clinical relevance to the emergency physician, because the management approach is the same. Attempting to distinguish myasthenic from cholinergic crisis with an edrophonium test in the severely weak patient is both unreliable and hazardous.

The emergency physician must be aware that a number of medications can impair neuromuscular transmission and exacerbate weakness in patients with myasthenic gravis (Table 205.3). These drugs include aminoglycoside antibiotics, certain cardiovascular drugs, phenothiazines, and anticonvulsants.[14,20] These drugs act either by preventing release of acetylcholine from the presynaptic membrane or by binding to the postsynaptic membrane, producing a curare-like effect. Benzodiazepines and potent analgesics such as morphine and meperidine can also aggravate weakness in myasthenics. All of these agents should be avoided whenever possible in the management of patients with myasthenia; when required, they must be used cautiously and with careful monitoring. Acute intercurrent medical and surgical problems in patients with myasthenia gravis should always be managed in consultation with a neurologist.

TABLE 205.3. Common Drugs Capable of Impairing Neuromuscular Transmission or Exacerbating Weakness in Patients with Myasthenia Gravis

ANTIBIOTICS	**HORMONAL AGENTS**
Aminoglycosides, tetracycline, fluoroquinolones, clindamycin, sulfonamides, erythromycin, ampicillin, chloroquine	Corticosteroids
	PSYCHOTROPICS
	Phenothiazines, lithium
ANTICONVULSANTS	**ANALGESICS/SEDATIVES**
Phenytoin, phenobarbital	Morphine, meperidine, benzodiazepines, antihistamines
CARDIOVASCULAR	
β-blockers, calcium-channel blockers, lidocaine, quinidine, procainamide, diuretics	

Other Disorders of Neuromuscular Transmission

Several other disorders of neuromuscular transmission should enter into the differential diagnosis of muscular weakness. The *Eaton-Lambert syndrome* is a very rare syndrome of weakness and fatigability caused by a defect in the release of acetylcholine from the presynaptic membrane of the neuromuscular junction. It is usually a paraneoplastic condition, associated particularly with small-cell carcinoma of the lung. Clinically, there is weakness of the proximal limb muscles, hyporeflexia, dry mouth, and impotence. The extraocular and facial muscles are usually spared. When the motor nerve is stimulated at high frequency during electromyographic testing, an incremental response of the muscle action potential is observed, the opposite of what occurs in myasthenia gravis. Treatment includes anticholinesterase agents, immunosuppressants, plasmapheresis, and therapy for the underlying tumor.[18]

Botulism is caused by a neurotoxin produced by the anaerobic organism *Clostridium botulinum*. Botulinum toxin, considered to be the most powerful poison known (0.1 μg of toxin A can be lethal in humans), binds irreversibly to the presynaptic membrane, blocking calcium-mediated release of acetylcholine, and thus interfering with neuromuscular and cholinergic autonomic transmission.[4] The principal source of the toxin is inadequately prepared food; home-canned products are most often incriminated. Infantile botulism is an insidious form of the disease in which viable bacilli are ingested and survive in the infant's intestine, where toxin is then elaborated. Infants with this disease are often seen by a physician several times before the diagnosis is considered.

Wound botulism is a rare entity (most recent cases occurring in injection drug abusers) in which the clostridial organisms grow and produce toxin in injured, devitalized tissue.[4] The responsible wound is often surprisingly benign in appearance.

Botulism may vary from a mild illness to a fulminant, fatal one. Prodromal symptoms of nausea, vomiting, diarrhea, and a dry, painful throat develop hours to days after ingestion of contaminated food. Neurologic symptoms are usually noted within 72 hours of ingestion and include anticholinergic effects (dry eyes, dry mouth, dilated pupils, ileus, and urinary retention) and fluctuating but rapidly progressive weakness, with early involvement of the extraocular and bulbar muscles (with ptosis, diplopia, dysphagia, and dysphonia as common early symptoms). The disease then progresses over several days to involve all the muscles of the trunk and extremities. Respiratory compromise can develop rapidly as the symmetric paralysis descends. There are usually no cognitive or sensory abnormalities; deep tendon reflexes are normal to decreased.[10,16]

The diagnosis of botulism must be made primarily on clinical evidence (acute onset of gastrointestinal, autonomic, and cranial nerve dysfunction), aided by epidemiologic, laboratory, and electrophysiologic findings. If the disease is suspected, state health authorities and the Centers for Disease Control and Prevention should be contacted for assistance in performing assays for the toxin, for release of botulinum antitoxin, and for the initiation of appropriate control measures. A blood sample should be sent for toxin assay, and specimens of food, gastric contents, and stool should be sent for toxin assay and culture. Wounds can also be cultured and assayed for toxin.

Because only one-third of patients with food-borne botulism have detectable toxin in the blood, confirmation, in most cases, depends on demonstration of botulinum toxin in stool or leftover food.[14] However, laboratory confirmation, even when successful, is often delayed. The edrophonium test is often helpful in distinguishing botulism from myasthenia gravis, but a positive test is occasionally seen with botulism. Findings on repetitive nerve stimulation are similar to those in patients with the Eaton-Lambert syndrome.

Treatment consists of efforts to eliminate the toxin, provision of respiratory and other supportive care, and early use of trivalent botulinum antitoxin. Precipitous respiratory failure is the primary cause of death, and serial measurements of vital capacity and inspiratory and expiratory force are thus essential. Approximately one-third of patients require mechanical ventilation, often for several weeks or more. The current mortality rate for food-borne botulism in the United States is about 10%.[16] Recovery is characteristically very slow, with weakness and autonomic symptoms often persisting for months. Infantile botulism, once diagnosed, is usually a self-limited disease that does not require antitoxin or antibiotics. In wound botulism, wound debridement and high-dose penicillin are indicated.

Tick paralysis is an ascending flaccid paralysis caused by a neurotoxin elaborated by an engorged tick that has been adherent to the human host for several days. The toxin blocks release of acetylcholine at the neuromuscular junction and also impairs conduction in peripheral motor nerves. In the United States, the disease occurs primarily in children during the late spring and summer in the Rocky Mountain and northwestern regions and is caused by a female wood tick (*Dermacentor andersoni*) or common dog tick (*Dermacentor variabilis*). The presenting symptom is an ascending, symmetric paralysis that progresses over 1 to 2 days to involve the extraocular and bulbar muscles. If the cause is unrecognized, respiratory paralysis can follow. Ataxia may be an early finding. Patients are alert and afebrile. Sensory changes are rarely noted, and deep tendon reflexes are markedly decreased.

The differential diagnosis of this acutely developing disorder includes Guillain-Barré syndrome, poliomyelitis, diphtheritic polyneuropathy, botulism, myasthenia gravis, and transverse myelitis. Any patient presenting with an afebrile ascending paralysis requires a careful physical examination to detect an adherent tick, often found on the scalp. After removal of the tick, neurologic recovery occurs within 24 to 48 hours. Unrecognized, the disease has proved fatal in 10% of patients.[3]

The venom of the *black widow spider* causes uncontrolled release, and eventually depletion, of acetylcholine from presynaptic terminals; that of the elapid and hydrophid *snakes* causes a nondepolarizing, postsynaptic, neuromuscular block; and the neurotoxin elaborated by dinoflagellates in *paralytic shellfish poisoning* decreases sodium-channel permeability in nerves, leading to weakness, paresthesias, and ataxia.

The same drugs that can exacerbate myasthenia gravis can also produce varying degrees of neuromuscular blockade and weakness in patients without underlying neurologic disease (see Table 205.3). Because there is normally ample reserve supporting neuromuscular transmission, a noticeable clinical effect is generally restricted to elderly patients, patients with associated electrolyte abnormalities, those with muscle weakness due to another condition, and those with high serum drug levels secondary to overdose or impaired elimination. These drugs act either presynaptically or postsynaptically and produce symptoms that resemble naturally occurring myasthenia gravis. Treatment includes discontinuing the offending agent and providing supportive care. Calcium gluconate or an anticholinesterase can be used acutely to reverse severe symptoms.

COMMON PITFALLS

- Attributing a history of episodic weakness to psychiatric disorder without considering the possibility of a neurologic disease (e.g., periodic paralysis, myasthenia gravis, or multiple sclerosis)

- Failure to take a careful, focused history in a patient presenting with a possible neurologic complaint. Misdiagnosis is common if historic information is overlooked.
- Failure to rule out electrolyte abnormalities in evaluating the weak patient
- Failure to perform a thorough search for an underlying precipitating illness in a patient with myopathy or myasthenia gravis who presents with an exacerbation
- Attempting an edrophonium test or other pharmacologic maneuvers in the acute management of myasthenic patients presenting in crisis. Acute treatment initially involves attention to airway and ventilatory status (with a low threshold for endotracheal intubation), treatment of any underlying illness, withdrawal of medications, and volume replacement. Management decisions should be made in consultation with a neurologist.
- Prescribing medications that may exacerbate weakness in myasthenia gravis. Emergency physicians must be aware of drugs that can impair neuromuscular function. Treatment decisions should be made in consultation with a neurologist.

References

1. Amato A, Barohn R. Idiopathic inflammatory myopathies. *Neurol Clin* 1997;15:615.
2. Berrouschot J, Baumann I, Kalischewski P, et al. Therapy of myasthenic crisis. *Crit Care Med* 1997;25:1228.
3. Centers for Disease Control and Prevention. Tick paralysis? Washington, 1995. *JAMA* 1996;275:1470.
4. Cherington M. Clinical spectrum of botulism. *Muscle Nerve* 1998;21:701.
5. Clark W, Rock G, Buskard N, et al. Therapeutic plasma exchange: an update from the Canadian Apheresis Group. *Ann Intern Med* 1999;131:453.
6. Dalakas M. Intravenous immune globulin therapy for neurologic diseases. *Ann Intern Med* 1997;126:721.
7. Drachman D. Myasthenia gravis. *N Engl J Med* 1994;330:1797.
8. Emery A. The muscular dystrophies. *BMJ* 1998;317:991.
9. Evoli A, Batocchi A, Tonali P. A practical guide to the recognition and management of myasthenia gravis. *Drugs* 1996;52:662.
10. Hayes M, Soto O, Ruoff K. Weekly clinicopathologic exercises: case 22-1997: a 58 year old woman with multiple cranial neuropathies. *N Engl J Med* 1997;337:184.
11. LoVecchio F, Jacobson S. Approach to generalized weakness and peripheral neuromuscular disease. *Emerg Med Clin North Am* 1997;15:605.
12. Manoukian M, Foote J, Crapo L. Clinical and metabolic features of thyrotoxic periodic paralysis in 24 episodes. *Arch Intern Med* 1999;159:601.
13. Miller JD, Quillian W, Cleveland W. Nonfamilial hypokalemic periodic paralysis and thyrotoxicosis in a 16 year old male. *Pediatrics* 1997;100:412.
14. Pascuzzi R. Drugs and toxins associated with myopathies. *Curr Opin Rheumatol* 1998;10:511.
15. Qureshi A, Choudhry M, Akbar M, et al. Plasma exchange versus intravenous immunoglobulin treatment in myasthenic crisis. *Neurology* 1999;52:629.
16. Shapiro R, Hatheway C, Swerdlow D. Botulism in the United States: a clinical and epidemiologic review. *Ann Intern Med* 1998;129:221.
17. Thomas C, Mayer S, Gungor Y, et al. Myasthenic crisis: clinical features, mortality, complications, and risk factors for prolonged intubation. *Neurology* 1997;48:1253.
18. Weinberg D. Case records of the Massachusetts General Hospital: Lambert-Eaton myasthenic syndrome. *N Engl J Med* 1994;331:528.
19. Wilkins K, Bulkley G. Thymectomy in the integrated management of myasthenia gravis. *Adv Surg* 1999;32:105.
20. Wittbrodt E. Drugs and myasthenia gravis: an update. *Arch Intern Med* 1997;157:399.

CHAPTER 206
Seizures

Andy Jagoda and Silvana Riggio

Seizures account for an estimated 1% to 2% of emergency department visits. Two to 4 million Americans have epilepsy, a condition of recurrent unprovoked seizures. A much larger number of people have seizures provoked by an underlying pathologic process.

Seizures result from any of a variety of pathologic processes that provoke excessive and disorderly neuronal discharge in the cerebral cortex. The manifestations of a seizure reflect the area of the brain in which neurons are discharging. Seizure discharges may be focal or may be generalized throughout the cerebral cortex. Consequently, the clinical spectrum of seizures includes focal or generalized motor activity, altered mental status, sensory or psychic experiences, or autonomic disturbances.

Ictus refers to the period during which a seizure occurs. An aura, or "warning," represents the beginning of a partial seizure, which can remain focal or can spread into a generalized event; a corollary is that patients with a primary generalized seizure disorder do not have an aura. The period after a seizure but before the patient returns to baseline is called the postictal period.

Status epilepticus is the condition in which seizures last more than 30 minutes or in which there are recurrent seizures without a return to baseline mental status between events. There are a projected 126,000 to 195,000 cases of status epilepticus each year in the United States, with an overall mortality of 22%. There is a bimodal distribution of cases, with the highest incidence occurring in the first year of life and after the age of 60. Over one-half of patients presenting to the emergency department in status epilepticus have no prior seizure history.

The classification of seizures (Table 206.1) is based on the behavioral and electrophysiologic features of the event rather than on specific pathophysiologic mechanisms or anatomic localiza-

TABLE 206.1. Classification of Seizures

I. PARTIAL SEIZURES
A. Simple Partial
1. Motor
2. Somatosensory
3. Autonomic
4. Psychic
B. Complex Partial
C. Secondary Generalized
II. GENERALIZED SEIZURES
A. Nonconvulsive (absence)
B. Convulsive
1. Tonic–clonic
2. Clonic
3. Tonic
4. Myoclonic
5. Atonic
III. STATUS EPILEPTICUS
A. Convulsive generalized
B. Convulsive focal
C. Nonconvulsive

tion. Seizures can be broadly divided into primary generalized seizures and partial seizures (also called focal seizures). *Primary generalized seizures* do not have an inciting focus, but begin bilaterally in both hemispheres of the cerebral cortex. *Partial seizures* begin in a localized area of the brain; they may remain focal but can also spread to incorporate both hemispheres, in which case, the seizure is termed *secondary generalized.*

Primary generalized seizures are broadly classified further as convulsive or nonconvulsive. All primary generalized seizures, except myoclonic seizures, are associated with an altered level of consciousness. Thus, it is not possible to have a bilateral tonic–clonic event with preservation of mental status, and this criterion can be helpful at times in distinguishing neurogenic seizures from psychogenic seizures

Absence seizures are primary generalized events characterized by an alteration in mental status without significant motor activity. They are more frequent in the young, usually beginning between the ages of 5 and 10 years, and are infrequent after the mid-teens. The average duration is 10 seconds, and there is rarely a postictal period.

Partial seizures are subdivided according to associated impairment of consciousness. Simple partial seizures have no impairment of consciousness and are categorized according to clinical presentation (see Table 206.1). Partial seizures that are associated with an impairment of consciousness are termed *complex partial seizures.*

Aside from the seizure activity itself, seizures may have harmful secondary consequences. A transient impairment of consciousness may result in a fall or a motor vehicle accident. The convulsive movements of a seizure may result in injury from direct trauma to head, trunk, or limbs. There are also metabolic consequences. There is typically a period of transient apnea and hypoxia, the duration of which varies with the duration of seizure activity. There is an increase in blood pressure, serum lactate and serum glucose levels, and white blood cell (WBC) count (but with no increase in bands). Body temperature is frequently elevated.[14] Acidosis due to elevated lactate occurs within 60 seconds of a convulsive event and normalizes within 1 hour after ictus.[12] A transient cerebrospinal fluid pleocytosis of up to 20 WBC/μL has been reported to occur in 2% to 23% of seizure patients (Table 206.2).

If the seizure lasts more than 30 minutes, the body's homeostatic regulating mechanisms begin to deteriorate; blood pressure begins to decrease, and the blood pH and lactate level can normalize if the patient's respiratory status is not compromised. It is hypothesized that even if systemic factors such as acidosis and hypoxia are controlled, prolonged status epilepticus results in neuronal damage secondary to the release of neurotoxic excitatory amino acids and influx of calcium into cells.

TABLE 206.2. Physiologic and Systemic Consequences of Convulsive Seizures

PHYSIOLOGIC
Hyperthermia
Acidosis
Hypoglycemia/hyperglycemia
Hypoxia
Acidosis
Leukocytosis
Cerebrospinal fluid pleocytosis
SYSTEMIC
Central nervous system edema
Pulmonary edema
Hypertension followed by hypotension
Dysrhythmias
Rhabdomyolysis
Disseminated intravascular coagulation
Fractures/dislocations

CLINICAL PRESENTATION AND DIFFERENTIAL DIAGNOSIS

A number of conditions can be confused with seizure disorders, among them syncope, arrhythmia, migraine, vertigo, sleep disorders, decerebrate posturing, drug reactions, tetanus, strychnine poisoning, and psychogenic events. A detailed history and physical can usually differentiate among these.

Syncope can be associated with occasional twitching movements that can be misdiagnosed as a seizure. Tonic–clonic movements, tongue biting, and postictal amnesia have not been commonly described in convulsive syncope. When put in the context of when and where the event occurred, length of event, and type of movements, convulsive syncope can usually be fairly reliably differentiated from seizure.

Migraine with an aura can be confused with nonconvulsive seizures. This is compounded by the finding that many migraine patients have abnormal electroencephalograms (EEGs). Basilar migraine can result in loss of consciousness, making the differentiation even more difficult.

Other entities that have been confused with seizures include narcolepsy, hyperventilation syndrome, hypoglycemia, and dystonic reactions. Of note, tonic, clonic, and tonic–clonic seizures are associated with altered consciousness, while dystonic reactions are not.

Psychogenic seizures, also referred to as pseudoseizures, are functional events with a clinical presentation mimicking neurogenic seizures, yet with no corresponding alteration in EEG activity. These events are often conversion reactions and not under the patient's conscious control. It is estimated that 20% of patients followed in epilepsy clinics are misdiagnosed and actually have psychogenic seizures.[6]

Psychogenic seizures often last longer than neurogenic events, frequently for more than 5 minutes. There usually is not a postictal period; patients can often recall events during the seizure, have not been incontinent, and do not incur physical injury. However, it must be stressed that exceptions to all of the aforementioned are commonly found, including incontinence and prolonged postictal periods. Psychogenic seizures are classically manifested by forward-thrusting pelvic movements and head-turning from side to side.[6]

Several maneuvers and tests are useful in diagnosing psychogenic seizures. These patients often avoid or resist noxious stimuli. They may display gaze aversion and look away from an examiner, regardless of position. On laboratory testing, psychogenic seizure patients do not have a metabolic acidosis, which is nearly universal with generalized convulsive seizures, and there is not a postictal increase in serum prolactin levels.

Seizures may be the result of acute or progressive neurologic insults or systemic stressors, and the evaluation of the patient with seizures must always look for these potentially reversible or treatable causes (Table 206.3). The two most commonly identified etiologic antecedents to seizures are neurologic injury from birth (8%) and cerebrovascular disease (11%).[7] Other identified etiologies of secondary seizures include trauma (5.5%), neoplasm (4%), degenerative disease (3.5%), and infection (2.5%).

Metabolic and toxin-related etiologies must always be considered in the differential diagnosis. Hypoglycemia is the most common metabolic cause of seizures; hyponatremia, hypocalcemia, and hypomagnesemia are much less common.[18] Interestingly, the metabolic encephalopathies, such as non-

TABLE 206.3. Etiology of Seizures

I. IDIOPATHIC	
II. STRUCTURAL	
	A. Degenerative disease (e.g., multiple sclerosis, tuberous sclerosis)
	B. Neoplasm
	C. Scar from birth trauma, other trauma, anoxic damage
III. INFECTION: BACTERIAL, VIRAL, PARASITIC, SYPHILITIC	
	A. Meningitis
	B. Encephalitis
	C. Abscess
IV. METABOLIC	
	A. Hypoglycemia
	B. Hyperosmolar states
	C. Hyponatremia
	D. Hypocalcemia
	E. Hypomagnesemia
	F. Hypoxia
	G. Uremia
	H. Thyroid disease
	I. Nutritional deficiency
V. TOXIN	
	A. Drug withdrawal
	B. Drug overdose
VI. VASCULAR	
	A. Subdural hematoma
	B. Epidural hematoma
	C. Intraparenchymal hemorrhage
	D. Stroke
	E. Subarachnoid hemorrhage
	F. Arteriovenous malformation
VII. ECLAMPSIA	

ketotic hyperglycemia and uremia, can cause both focal and generalized seizures. Alcohol is the toxin most commonly associated with seizures, followed by tricyclic antidepressants, cocaine, amphetamines, antihistamines, theophylline, and isoniazid. Drug withdrawal, including noncompliance with anticonvulsant medications in patients with a known seizure disorder, is a leading cause of recurrent seizures.[14]

Acute central nervous system (CNS) infections are responsible for 4% to 12% of acute isolated seizures and up to 28% of cases of refractory status epilepticus.

A number of physiologic and psychological stressors can activate seizure disorders. These stressors include fatigue, sleep deprivation, hyperventilation, photic stimulation, emotional stress, and menstruation. In rare cases, seizures can be triggered by colors, objects, music, and voices. Pregnancy can also result in the onset of a seizure disorder, separate from eclamptic seizures.

EMERGENCY DEPARTMENT EVALUATION

The evaluation of the patient who has had a seizure should begin with a careful history that includes a description of the event and an indication of the frequency, pattern, and duration of recent or previous seizures. A history of incontinence, loss of consciousness, and self-injury during the event should be elicited. It should be determined whether there was an aura or a postictal period. Every attempt should be made to interview observers and to obtain a clear description of the seizure to avoid misdiagnosing nonseizure events.

The circumstances preceding a seizure must be elucidated. Inciting factors such as medication noncompliance, infection, pregnancy, sleep deprivation, alcohol use, or other drug or medication use should be identified. A history of head trauma, headaches, diabetes, cancer, cerebrovascular disease, electrolyte imbalances, or infections can prove vital to making a diagnosis.

The physical examination begins with the vital signs, which can provide important red flags of underlying pathology. Signs of trauma should be sought, and a careful neurologic examination performed. Both unilateral and bilateral pupillary dilatation as a result of seizure has been reported. A focal deficit can represent a metabolic derangement such as hypoglycemia, an old lesion, new intracranial pathology, or a Todd paralysis secondary to the seizure. Todd paralysis can be manifested as either a motor or a sensory deficit. Although it typically resolves within hours of seizure, neuroimaging is usually necessary to differentiate a Todd paralysis from other causes of acute focal neurologic dysfunction.

Note should be made of the patient's mental status before and after a seizure. Postictal confusion is common, but almost always resolves over a few hours. Other causes of altered mental status must be strongly considered in patients whose mental status remains impaired, or when family or friends note an abnormally long postictal phase or unusual behavior manifestations. It is estimated that approximately 15% of patients treated for convulsive status epilepticus continue to be in nonconvulsive status after their motor activity is controlled; this unrecognized status may be a factor in the high mortality associated with status epilepticus and suggests the need for EEG monitoring in the "postictal" period.[6] Causes of altered mental status in patients who have had a seizure are listed in Table 206.4.

Patients are often brought to the emergency department after having had an episode of loss of consciousness of unknown cause. The differential diagnosis in these difficult cases includes seizures, and there are clues that can suggest that a seizure occurred. Postictal patients often have hyperreflexia, upgoing toes, evidence of incontinence, or a tongue laceration. Laboratory testing in postictal patients often demonstrates a metabolic acidosis or an elevated serum creatine phosphokinase level. These findings can be helpful and should be sought, but, unfortunately, they are time and patient dependent and their absence does not rule out the possibility that a seizure occurred.

The details of the history and physical examination should dictate the urgency and course of any further emergency department evaluation. Of all laboratory tests, serum glucose determination followed by a serum sodium determination has been found to be the most valuable in diagnosing an unsuspected etiology of seizure.[1,15] The decision to measure other electrolytes, creatinine, blood urea nitrogen, calcium, and magnesium is based on the individual patient assessment; generally, these tests are of limited value in patients with no underlying medical problems who have returned to baseline. An arterial blood gas analysis is indicated when hypoxia or an underlying acidosis is suspected. A pregnancy test should be obtained in all

TABLE 206.4. Causes of Altered Mental Status in Patients Who Have Had a Seizure

Postictal state
Persistent nonconvulsive seizures
Metabolic abnormality
Hyperosmolar state
Central nervous system infection
Central nervous system vascular event
Drug effect
Psychiatric dysfunction

TABLE 206.5. Drugs Used in the Treatment of Epilepsy

Drug	Trade Name	Route	Seizure Type	Loading Dose (mg/kg)	Daily Dose for Adults (mg)	Therapeutic Range (μg/mL)
Phenytoin	Dilantin	PO, i.v.	P, GC	20	300–400	10–20
Fosphenytoin	Cerebex	i.v., i.m.	P, GC	20	—	10–20
Carbamazepine[a]	Tegretol	PO	P, GC	—	800–1,600	6–12
Valproate[b]	Depakene	PO	All	—	1,000–3,000	50–120
Divalproex sodium	Depakote	PO	All	—	1,000–4,800	50–120
	Depacon	i.v.	All	10–20	—	50–120
Phenobarbital		PO, i.v., i.m.	P, GC	10–20	90–150	15–35
Primidone	Mysoline	PO	P, GC	—	750–1,250	6–12
Clonazepam	Klonopin	PO	A, M	—	1.5–20.0	0.02–0.08
Ethosuximide[c]	Zarontin	PO	A	—	750–1,250	40–100
Lamotrigine	Lamictal	PO	All	—	200–600	—
Felbamate[d]	Felbatol	PO	P, GC	—	1,800–4,800	—
Gabapentin[e]	Neurontin	PO	P, GC	—	1,200–4,800	—
Topiramate	Topamax	PO	P, GC	—	200–600	—
Tiagabine		PO	P, GC	—	32–48	—
Diazepam[f]	Diastat	Rectal	All	0.2–0.5	—	—

PO, orally; i.v., intravenous; P, partial seizure; GC, generalized seizure; i.m., intramuscular; A, absence seizure; M, myoclonic seizure.
[a] Drug of choice for partial seizures, with or without secondary generalization.
[b] Drug of choice for primary generalized tonic–clonic seizures.
[c] Drug of choice for absence seizures.
[d] Associated with aplastic anemia in one in 5,000 patients; hepatic failure in one in 30,000.
[e] Only anticonvulsant that is renally metabolized; recommended in patients with multiple medical problems.
[f] Used primarily in children to control clusters of breakthrough seizures.

women of childbearing age.[1] Serum anticonvulsant levels should be checked in patients with epilepsy who have had a seizure and in patients for whom a history cannot be obtained (Table 206.5).

Alcohol is by far the most common drug of abuse associated with seizures, followed by cocaine. Serum alcohol and theophylline levels and urine drug-screening tests should be ordered based on clinical suspicion. It is worth remembering that patients with epilepsy can have other medical problems (e.g., depression), so other possibilities (e.g., tricyclic overdose) should not be overlooked.

Patients who have had a seizure but who are not immunocompromised and who do not have an abnormal mental status, fever, or meningeal signs do not require a lumbar puncture as part of their emergency department evaluation.[5] However, seizures, especially status epilepticus seizures, are associated with hyperthermia, leukocytosis, and altered mental status, thus often forcing consideration of meningitis. It is also important to note that, as mentioned previously, seizures can cause cerebrospinal fluid pleocytosis, further confusing the issue occasionally. Antibiotics, once started, must be continued until cerebrospinal fluid culture results are available.

Computed tomographic (CT) scanning of the head should be performed in the emergency department when an acute intracranial event, such as subdural or subarachnoid hemorrhage, is suspected. Patients with a history of acute trauma or malignancy, or with an abnormal neurologic examination, are most likely to have an abnormal imaging study.

All patients who have had a first-time seizure need an imaging study, but not necessarily an emergent CT scan obtained in the emergency department. If the patient has a normal mental status and neurologic examination and is judged to be reliable for follow-up, it is reasonable, after consultation with a neurologist, to arrange for outpatient magnetic resonance imaging (MRI). MRI is superior to CT scanning in identifying structural epileptogenic abnormalities.[2]

EEG monitoring is not a standard practice in the emergency department, yet there are clear indications for its use on an emergent basis. Any patient with altered mental status in whom nonconvulsive status epilepticus is suspected requires an emergent EEG. An emergent EEG is also indicated in patients with refractory status epilepticus who have been managed with paralysis or barbiturate coma.

Additional laboratory and radiographic testing may be indicated to identify underlying complicating factors, such as cardiac dysrhythmia, urinary tract infection, sepsis, or pulmonary disease.

EMERGENCY DEPARTMENT MANAGEMENT

Most seizures are self-limited and do not require immediate intervention. If the patient is seen during the seizure, the focus should be on protecting the patient from injury. Airway patency should be ensured, but objects should not be inserted into the patient's mouth. Patients who have experienced a seizure once are at risk for recurrent seizure episodes, so proper precautions should be taken to keep the guard rails on stretchers up and to prevent the patient from ambulating unaccompanied.

First-Time Seizures

Patients who have had a single, unprovoked seizure have about a 35% risk of recurrence within the next 5 years; the risk of recurrences increases to approximately 75% after two or three seizures.[11] When a cause of the seizure is identified, management is based on the underlying pathology. When no cause can be identified, a risk–benefit analysis regarding initiation of antiepileptic therapy must be performed. There are significant psychosocial consequences of a diagnosis of epilepsy, as well as potential dangers from the chronic use of antiepileptic medications. Thus, one must be cautious when labeling patients as epileptic and instituting treatment from the emergency department.

Intravenous phenytoin or fosphenytoin loading, 20 mg/kg, can be accomplished quickly and leads to therapeutic blood levels within 1 hour of the infusion's completion. Intravenous phenytoin loading can be associated with local infusion site irritation, hypotension, confusion, and ataxia; consequently, infusions should not be run faster than 50 mg/min in adults.

Fosphenytoin is a water-soluble disodium phosphate ester of phenytoin, which does not need a propylene glycol vehicle and has a more physiologic pH than does phenytoin. It has fewer side effects than phenytoin, though rapid infusion can still cause hypotension, ataxia, and confusion. Fosphenytoin can be given safely by the intramuscular route, with 100% bioavailability and therapeutic serum levels within 1 hour of a loading dose.[7] Oral phenytoin loading is another option; it results in unpredictable absorption, however, with only 60% of patients being therapeutic at 12 hours after a 1-g dose. A daily maintenance dose of 300 mg can be given at bedtime, although, in some patients, divided dosing can provide better seizure control by minimizing variations in the blood level.

Recurrence of Seizures in Patients with Known Seizure Disorder

Noncompliance with anticonvulsant medication is, by far, the most common cause of seizure recurrence in a patient with a known seizure disorder. A patient who has been on phenytoin, but has a subtherapeutic level, should be given supplemental intravenous phenytoin or fosphenytoin to reestablish serum levels in the therapeutic range. Intramuscular fosphenytoin is another option and eliminates the need for infusion pumps and cardiac monitoring. The patient can then be discharged with instructions to resume oral dosing within 12 hours. Likewise, patients with subtherapeutic valproic acid levels can be supplemented with intravenous valproic acid administered over 1 hour at a rate no faster than 20 mg/min, and discharged on their oral regimen.

Patients managed on carbamazepine who have a seizure due to noncompliance present more of a management problem, because this drug cannot be loaded orally or intravenously. In these cases, if the patient can tolerate phenytoin, consideration should be given to loading the patient with phenytoin and continuing on this drug until therapeutic levels of carbamazepine are achieved.

Patients who have seizures despite therapeutic anticonvulsant levels must be evaluated carefully for precipitating factors such as infection, new anatomic lesions, or new medications. Decisions to increase the drug dose should be made only after communication with the patient's primary care physician. A second anticonvulsant should be added to the patient's regimen only when seizures are refractory to monotherapy and there are clinical signs of toxicity.

The evaluation of pregnant patients with new-onset seizures should follow the same principle as in other patients. However, if no etiology is identified, anticonvulsants should be withheld and the patient referred for close follow-up. Eclampsia is an additional consideration in patients at more than 20 weeks' gestation.

Noncompliance and sleep deprivation are the two most common causes of seizure recurrence in pregnant patients with epilepsy.[4] Active seizures should be treated pharmacologically just as in the nonpregnant patient, because the risks to the fetus of hypoxia and acidosis are greater than the potential teratogenicity of anticonvulsant medications. Phenytoin and phenobarbital have similar teratogenetic profiles; carbamazepine is probably the safest of the anticonvulsants to use in pregnancy. Beyond 24 weeks' gestation, fetal monitoring should be provided during and after a seizure.

Alcohol-Related Seizures

Alcohol-related seizures deserve special mention, because alcohol use is frequently involved in patients presenting to emergency departments with seizures. Alcohol-withdrawal seizures classically occur 6 to 48 hours after a significant reduction in the serum alcohol level, but they have also been associated with *rising* blood ethanol levels in some patients.

Alcohol-related seizures are temporally associated with alcohol use but are not necessarily solely the result of the alcohol. Alcoholics are susceptible to cerebrovascular insults, trauma, metabolic disorders, and infections, and are thus at increased risk for seizures.

Management of the alcoholic who has had a seizure focuses on determining whether the event was a withdrawal seizure or due to another etiology. Patients with a first-time alcohol-related seizure should be evaluated fully in the same manner as any other patient.

The diagnosis of alcohol-withdrawal seizures is based on the history, and the clinician must always consider the possibility that another etiology is responsible. Benzodiazepines alone are sufficient to prevent successive withdrawal seizures in the acute setting, but there is no good evidence to support the use of phenytoin either acutely or chronically in the management of alcohol-withdrawal seizures. Patients who have had one alcohol-withdrawal seizure and have been observed to remain seizure-free and at baseline mental status for 6 hours, with no evidence of withdrawal, can be discharged if a suitable environment is available.[3]

Psychogenic Seizures

Psychogenic seizures should be suspected in patients who are refractory to anticonvulsants and whose clinical presentation is atypical. The diagnosis is suspected particularly when a convulsing patient does not have a metabolic acidosis, and it can be confirmed, when possible, by demonstrating that the clinical convulsion is not accompanied by an abnormal EEG. Management of psychogenic seizures is dependent on making the correct diagnosis; although this sounds obvious, the anxiety associated with evaluating a convulsing patient often leads to the initiation of pharmacologic interventions before an adequate assessment can be performed.[8] The key to management is avoiding iatrogenic harm by aggressive pharmacologic interventions or supportive measures such as intubation. Long-term management usually involves a comprehensive evaluation in an epilepsy monitoring unit, with a coordinated approach involving both an epileptologist and a psychiatrist.

Status Epilepticus

The management of convulsive status epilepticus involves simultaneous maintenance of the patient's airway, breathing, and circulation; diagnostic testing; and pharmacologic intervention (Fig. 206.1). Status epilepticus tends to occur more frequently in patients with an underlying neurologic insult, either old or new, and refractory status epilepticus almost always indicates the presence of an underlying CNS disorder. Morbidity and mortality in status epilepticus is related to the etiology, duration, and systemic consequences of the event.

Airway support should be aggressive, and continuous pulse oximetry should be employed. Patients should be intubated at any sign of hypoxia or loss of protective gag reflex. Intravenous access should be secured using a non–dextrose-containing solution, because phenytoin precipitates if it is inadvertently administered with dextrose (dextrose will not precipitate fosphenytoin); fluids should be run at keep-open rates unless the patient is hypotensive, because status epilepticus can be associated with both cerebral and pulmonary edema.[19]

The blood glucose level should be checked immediately by bedside testing. Consideration should be given to sending blood for determination of electrolytes, magnesium, phosphate, cal-

Patient in Convulsive Status Epilepticus

Stabilization

1. Airway: Intubate early
2. Breathing: Use pulse oximetry to monitor oxygenation.
3. Circulation: Watch for hypotension or hypertension.
4. ECG/Monitor: Watch for dysrhythmias and/or indicators of toxic or metabolic insult.
5. Foley catheter.
6. Nasogastric tube.
7. EEG: Especially for patients who are paralyzed, in barbiturate coma, or in whom nonconvulsive status is suspected.
8. Periodically recheck IV access to ensure proper function and drug delivery.

Diagnostic Investigation

1. Send blood for:
   Electrolytes, BUN, Cr, Mg, Ca, PO_4
   Liver functions, PT, PTT
   Alcohol Level
   Toxicology Screen
   CBC with WBC differential
   Anticonvulsant drug levels
2. Check for hypoglycemia initially and periodically throughout the resuscitation.
3. Urinalysis
4. Pregnancy testing in all women of childbreaing age.
5. Consider lumbar puncture.
6. Consider head CT.
7. Rectal temperature initially and monitor throughout the resuscitation.

Pharmacologic Intervention

1. A. Dextrose to patients with hypoglycemia.
   B. Antibiotics if infection is suspected.
   C. Thiamine 100 mg IV and magnesium 1–2 g to all alcoholic and/or malnourished patients.
   D. Lorazepam 2 mg/min IV up to 10 mg.
   E. Phenytoin 20 mg/kg at 50 mg/min. If patient is on phenytoin, give 10 mg/kg or fosphenytoin 20 mg/kg at 150 mg/min.
2. If seizures continue, give phenobarbital 10-20 mg/kg at 100 mg/kg <u>OR</u> consider second phenytoin infusion of 10 mg/kg.
3. If seizures continue:
   A. Initiate pentobarbital anesthesia 5 mg/kg at 25 mg/min followed by 2.5 mg/kg/hr <u>OR</u>
   B. Midazolam 0.2 mg/kg i.v. followed by 0.75–10 mg/kg/min
   C. Lidocaine 100 mg bolus IV
   D. Propofol 1–2 mg/kg followed by 2–10 mg/kg/hr.

Figure 206.1. Approach to patient in status epilepticus. (Modified from Jagoda A, Riggio S. Refractory convulsive status epilepticus. *Ann Emerg Med* 1993;22:1343.)

cium, liver and renal function, hematocrit, WBC count, platelet count, anticonvulsant levels, and drug screen, including alcohol. The urine should be checked for evidence of rhabdomyolysis, and a pregnancy test should be sent on all women of childbearing age.

Patients in status epilepticus should be placed on a cardiac monitor, and an electrocardiogram should be done. A nasogastric tube should be placed to prevent gastric distention, and a Foley catheter should be placed to help monitor volume status. A head CT scan should be done at some point in all patients. Consideration should be given to performing a lumbar puncture.

The pharmacologic management of status epilepticus begins while the patient is being stabilized and diagnostic testing performed. Hypoglycemia is treated immediately with thiamine and dextrose. Antibiotics should be given very early in the management of any patient in whom meningitis or sepsis is suspected.

The benzodiazepines diazepam and lorazepam are considered the first-line drugs in the management of status epilepticus. Lorazepam (2 mg/min, up to 10 mg) or diazepam (5 mg/min, up to 20 mg) will stop seizures in the majority of cases. Both drugs are efficacious, but lorazepam is preferred because its anticonvulsant action lasts up to 12 hours, compared with 20 minutes for diazepam. Consequently, if lorazepam terminates the seizure activity, no additional anticonvulsant needs to be immediately given; a long-lasting anticonvulsant such as phenytoin must be added when diazepam is used, because, otherwise, the patient is at high risk of seizure recurrence.[13]

When seizures persist despite a full loading dose of a benzodiazepine, phenytoin or fosphenytoin is added at a rate of 50 mg/min or 150 mg/min, respectively. Status epilepticus that does not terminate at this point is usually the result of some significant underlying CNS lesion. If seizures persist, the current recommendation is to give additional phenytoin, up to a total dose of 30 mg/kg.[13]

If seizures persist after the phenytoin infusion, phenobarbital (20 mg/kg) should be given intravenously at a rate of 100 mg/min. Because respiratory depression is all but inevitable at that point, intubation is likely to be necessary, if it has not already been performed.

Patients who continue to seize despite the aforementioned interventions should be put into pentobarbital coma by giving 5 mg/kg at 25 mg/min, followed by 2.5 mg/kg/h as an infusion. Besides requiring ventilatory support, these patients are at significant risk for hypotension, and therefore require hemodynamic monitoring. Hypotension should be treated with fluids and vasopressors as needed. EEG monitoring should be instituted to evaluate for continued seizure activity.[13]

Many other drugs have been tried in the management of refractory status epilepticus, but no controlled trials support their use.[9] These include continuous infusions of benzodiazepines, propofol, intravenous lidocaine, and rectal chloral hydrate.[13,15]

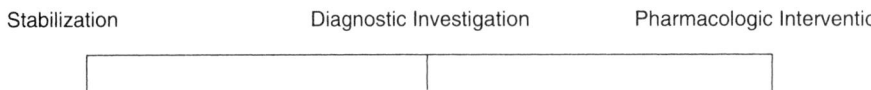

Current recommendations would support use of these drugs only if it is not possible to administer pentobarbital anesthesia.

Nonconvulsive Status Epilepticus

Nonconvulsive status epilepticus presents as altered mental status ranging from a mild behavioral alteration noticeable only to family or friends to frank coma.[10,16] Other manifestations may include speech arrest, cognitive deficits, delusions, paranoia, hallucinations, or psychosis. Because, by definition, there is rarely a significant motor component, the diagnosis is often missed, and there are many case reports of these patients initially being diagnosed with a psychiatric illness. Nonconvulsive status epilepticus has been reported in every age group, can be the initial presentation of a seizure disorder, and has been reported to last as long as 8 weeks.

The diagnosis should be suspected in patients with a seizure history who present with a prolonged postictal period or an unusual behavior pattern. It should also be considered in patients without a seizure history who present with altered mental status of undetermined etiology. The diagnosis is made by electroencephalography. Treatment is the same as for convulsive status epilepticus, beginning with lorazepam, 2 mg/min, until the EEG normalizes or a total of 10 mg is administered. This should be followed by phenytoin loading, although it is questionable whether phenytoin is effective in absence status.[17]

DISPOSITION

The disposition of patients who have had a seizure depends on the etiology of the event and, often, on the socioeconomic environment to which the patient will return. Of prime importance is communication with the primary care provider who will be responsible for following up on the patient's diagnostic tests and medications.

Hospital admission should be considered when the cause of a seizure is unclear, when seizure recurrence has not been controlled, when the seizure is secondary to a treatable underlying illness, or when there is concern that the patient will not receive timely outpatient evaluation. All patients who have been in status epilepticus should be admitted, usually to an intensive care setting.

COMMON PITFALLS

- Failure to maintain and protect the airway during the management of status epilepticus
- Failure to check a Dextrostick in patients with seizures or refractory status epilepticus
- Infusion of phenytoin with a dextrose solution
- Failure to perform a complete secondary survey in postictal patients
- Assumption that altered mental status is due to a postictal state and failure to consider other possible etiologies
- Confusion of decerebrate posturing for a tonic seizure
- Failure to obtain a pregnancy test in women of childbearing age
- Failure to make a reasonable effort to obtain witnesses' accounts of a seizure
- Failure to recognize a psychogenic seizure as a nonneurologic event
- Failure to advise a patient who has had a seizure not to drive or operate dangerous equipment
- Increasing a patient's anticonvulsant medication dose without obtaining a proper history for precipitating stressors or medication compliance
- Failure to communicate with the primary care provider

References

1. American College of Emergency Physicians. Clinical policy for the initial approach to patients presenting with a chief complaint of seizure, who are not in status epilepticus. *Ann Emerg Med* 1997;29:706.
2. American College of Emergency Physicians, American Academy of Neurology, American Association of Neurological Surgeons, American Society of Neuroradiology. Practice parameter: neuroimaging in the emergency patient presenting with seizure [Summary Statement]. *Ann Emerg Med* 1996;27:113.
3. Chance J. Emergency department treatment of alcohol withdrawal seizures with phenytoin. *Ann Emerg Med* 1991;20:520.
4. Delgado-Escueta A, Janz D. Consensus guidelines: preconception counseling, management, and care of the pregnant woman with epilepsy. *Neurology* 1992;42[Suppl 5]:149.
5. Engel J. Diagnostic evaluation. In: Engle J, ed. *Seizures and epilepsy.* Philadelphia: FA Davis Co, 1989:312.
6. Gates J, Ramini V, Whalen S. Ictal characteristics of pseudoseizures. *Epilepsia* 1983;24:246.
7. Hauser W, Anneger J, Kurland L. Incidence of epilepsy and unprovoked seizures in Rochester, Minnesota: 1935–1984. *Epilepsia* 1993;34:453.
8. Howell S, Owen L, Chadwick D. Pseudostatus epilepticus. *Q J Med* 1989;71:507.
9. Jagoda A, Riggio S. Refractory status epilepticus in adults. *Ann Emerg Med* 1993;22:1337.
10. Lee S. Nonconvulsive status epilepticus: ictal confusion in later life. *Arch Neurol* 1985;42:778.
11. Lowenstein D, Alldredge B. Status epilepticus. *N Engl J Med* 1998;338:970.
12. Orringer C, Eustace J, Wunsch C, et al. Natural history of lactic acidosis after grand-mal seizure. *N Engl J Med* 1977;297:796.
13. Osorio I, Reed R. Treatment of refractory generalized tonic clonic status epilepticus with pentobarbital anesthesia after high dose phenytoin. *Epilepsia* 1989;30:464.
14. Simon R. Physiologic consequences of status epilepticus. *Epilepsia* 1985; 26[Suppl 1]:58.
15. Tardy B, LaFond P, Convers P, et al. Adult first generalized seizure: etiology, biological tests, EEG, CT scan, in an ED. *Am J Emerg Med* 1995;13:1.
16. Tomson T, Lindbom U, Nilsson B. Nonconvulsive status epilepticus in adults: thirty-two consecutive patients from a general hospital population. *Epilepsia* 1992;33:829.
17. Treiman D, Meyers P, Walton N, et al. A comparison of four treatments for generalized convulsive status epilepticus. *N Engl J Med* 1998;339:792.
18. Turnbull T, Vanden Hoed T, Howes D, et al. Utility of laboratory studies in the emergency department patient with a new-onset seizure. *Ann Emerg Med* 1990;19:373.
19. Working Group on Status Epilepticus. Treatment of convulsive status epilepticus: recommendations of the Epilepsy Foundation of America's working group on status epilepticus. *JAMA* 1993;270:854.

CHAPTER 207
Demyelinating Disease

Adrienne J. Birnbaum

Multiple sclerosis (MS) is a disease of the central nervous system (CNS) in which the myelin sheath that surrounds axons is damaged as a result of an inflammatory process. The scattered areas of demyelination in the brain and spinal cord are known as plaques. Axons are relatively spared, although there is recent evidence that substantial axonal damage can occur, especially in the later phases of the disease. MS is believed to be immunologically mediated and to occur in genetically susceptible individuals.

Clinically, MS is characterized by neurologic symptoms and signs that are attributable to lesions in the different locations and that appear at different times over the patient's course. It is primarily a disease of young adults, the majority of patients reporting their first symptoms between 20 and 45 years of age. The incidence is approximately two to ten cases per 100,000 people per year.[6] Women are affected 1.8 times as often as men, and Whites twice as often as Blacks. Apart from trauma, MS is the most significant cause of neurologic disability afflicting young adults,[18] with major consequences for patients, families, and society.

The course of MS is variable and relatively unpredictable. It is characterized by exacerbations of acute or subacute onset that last for days to months. Exacerbations are more commonly manifested by the reappearance of previous signs and symptoms than by the development of new ones. Recovery between exacerbations may be incomplete, however. *Relapsing, remitting disease* refers to a situation in which the clinical course between exacerbations is stable. In general, a pattern of intermittent exacerbations is more frequent in the earlier stages of the disease, while progressive deterioration, with or without superimposed exacerbations, is more common in the later stages (secondary progressive course). A small percentage of patients experience disease progression from the onset, with or without superimposed exacerbations (progressive relapsing and primary progressive disease).[11]

CLINICAL PRESENTATION

New Patient with Acute Focal Neurologic Deficit

The diagnosis of MS neither can nor should be definitively made in the emergency department (ED). First, most diagnostic frameworks incorporate elements of a clinical picture that changes over time; this is unavailable to the emergency physician seeing the patient at only one point in time. Second, diagnostic test results that enhance the confidence of a clinical diagnosis of MS are often not immediately available in the ED. Third, the diagnosis of MS imposes a significant psychological burden on the patient and should not be made without a substantial degree of certainty.

Symptoms of MS generally develop over hours or days, but may sometimes occur with the suddenness usually characteristic of strokes. Negative signs or symptoms (e.g., loss of vision, strength, or sensation) are due to slowed or blocked conduction in axons that undergo demyelination. The demyelinating process can also result in the generation of ectopic impulses, as well as abnormal transmission of impulses between neighboring nerve fibers. These phenomena are the basis for the generation of "positive" symptoms, such as Lhermitte's sign, an electric shock–like, tingling, or vibrating sensation in the torso or extremities that is produced by flexion of the neck. Despite the fact that demyelination can occur anywhere within the CNS, MS lesions have a predilection for certain sites, resulting in a relatively limited distribution of initial symptoms.[15]

The possible clinical manifestations of MS are extremely varied and may take the form of virtually any neurologic symptom. While no symptoms or neurologic findings are pathognomonic, some are characteristic and may heighten the clinician's diagnostic suspicions (Table 207.1). The majority of patients present with one or more of these signs and symptoms.

Decreased visual acuity and symptoms related to oculomotor dysfunction (e.g., diplopia) are among the most common initial presenting symptoms of MS. Optic neuritis characteristically presents with monocular blurred vision (bilateral in 30%), and, often, retroorbital pain or headache and alteration of color vision.[15] The optic disc may appear normal or swollen, blurred or hyperemic. An afferent pupillary defect (Marcus Gunn pupil), consisting of diminished response to a direct light stimulus and a normal consensual response to a light stimulus in the opposite eye, may be noted. Optic nerve involvement may remain as an isolated manifestation, but roughly half of these patients are diagnosed with MS within 15 to 20 years.[16,17] Neuromyelitis optica or Devic disease, an uncommon disorder, consists of optic neuritis and transverse myelitis.

TABLE 207.1. Common Initial Symptoms of Multiple Sclerosis

Optic neuritis
Diplopia and oculomotor dysfunction
Weakness: monoparesis, paraparesis
Paresthesias and numbness
Incoordination, unsteady gait, abnormal balance
Vertigo
Bladder, bowel dysfunction
Tremor

Nystagmus and diplopia occur commonly in patients with MS. The finding of internuclear ophthalmoplegia, especially in a young adult, is very suggestive. This form of dysconjugate gaze, referable to the medial longitudinal fasciculus of the brainstem, involves limited adduction of one eye and nystagmus in the abducting eye on lateral gaze.

Paresthesias and dysesthesias are characteristically bilateral and ascending but may affect both hands or one side of the body. Motor weakness may occur as paraparesis, hemiparesis, or monoparesis and is generally accompanied by signs of upper motor neuron dysfunction (e.g., hyperreflexia and positive Babinski sign). Transverse myelitis can be the initial neurologic event; symptoms include ascending weakness and numbness below the level of the lesion.

Transient attacks of paroxysmal dysarthria and ataxia are also suggestive of demyelinating disease when they occur in a young person without vascular risk factors.

Patients with Known Multiple Sclerosis

In most cases, the natural history of MS is characterized by episodes of neurologic dysfunction alternating with periods of stabilization or remission of symptoms. Common signs and symptoms of chronic disease are listed in Table 207.2. Patients with known MS may present to the ED because of an exacerbation of previous deficits, because of the development of new deficits, or because of medical complications of the disease.

Factors that have been cited as having an association with the occurrence of MS exacerbations are infection (including minor respiratory infections), emotional stress, spinal anesthesia, heat exposure, and the postpartum period. Pregnancy itself has not been associated with an increase in the frequency of attacks.[10]

Common secondary complications in patients with MS are pneumonia, infections of the urinary tract, septicemia, respiratory failure, pulmonary embolism, bladder and renal calculi, and pressure ulcers of the skin.[15] Elevated body temperature, occurring as a result of infection or because of exposure to heat, can be associated with a transient increase in neurologic symptoms. Fever-related exacerbations that include dysphagia can result in aspiration pneumonia.

Fatigue is a common complaint of patients with MS. It typically increases with exercise, heat exposure, or as the day progresses. This pattern of fatigue is distinct from that associated with depression, which is more likely to be present earlier in the day or to be constant.[12] Spasticity, a manifestation of upper motor neuron disease, is characterized by increased muscle tone, hyperreflexia, decreased mobility, painful muscle spasms, and

TABLE 207.2. Common Chronic Problems of Multiple Sclerosis

Problem	Drugs Used in Treatment[15,19]
Weakness: monoparesis, paraparesis, hemiparesis, quadriparesis	Corticosteroids, potassium channel blockers (i.e., 4-aminopyridine, 3,4-diaminopyridine)
Spasticity	Baclofen (oral or intrathecal), benzodiazepines, dantrolene, tizanidine
Paresthesias	Amitriptyline, carbamazepine, gabapentin, corticosteroids if disabling
Bladder dysfunction	Depends on type of impairment
Optic atrophy, blurred vision, central scotomata	Intravenous methylprednisolone for acute optic neuritis
Internuclear ophthalmoplegia, diplopia	Corticosteroids
Loss of balance, incoordination, ataxia, tremor	Clonazepam for tremor; corticosteroids for balance
Cognitive changes	Serotonin reuptake inhibitors
Depression	
Sexual dysfunction	
Fatigue	Amantadine, CNS stimulants, fluoxetine
Vertigo	Meclizine, promethazine, diazepam, metoclopramide
Paroxysmal symptoms: itching, burning, twitching, Lhermitte's sign	Carbamazepine, phenytoin, tricyclic antidepressants, low-dose antipsychotics, gabapentin
Pseudobulbar palsy	Amitriptyline, levodopa, bromocriptine

weakness. There is conflicting evidence as to whether seizures occur more frequently in MS patients than in the general population. When seizures occur, they should not be attributed to MS until other causes have been ruled out. Similarly, aphasia and dementia should prompt a search for alternate causes.

DIFFERENTIAL DIAGNOSIS

The differential diagnosis of an acute focal neurologic deficit is broad and includes the intracranial and spinal cord processes listed in Table 207.3. Some of the more common diseases capable of causing multifocal CNS lesions disseminated over time are systemic lupus erythematosus, Lyme disease, sarcoidosis, and CNS vasculitis. Because MS is a disease that is confined to the CNS, patients generally lack the rheumatologic and constitutional symptoms and laboratory abnormalities that are present in many of these other disease states. Spinal cord compression by mass lesions or hematomas must be considered in the patient who presents with symptoms referable to the spinal cord. The differential diagnosis of transverse myelitis includes both infectious (e.g., herpes simplex) and postinfectious causes.

EMERGENCY DEPARTMENT EVALUATION

When faced with a patient with one or more focal neurologic deficits in whom MS is suspected, one of the emergency physician's major tasks is the exclusion of other more treatable disease entities. The definitive diagnosis of MS is most appropriately left to the neurologist in the non-ED setting. MS remains primarily a clinical diagnosis, requiring the demonstration of focal neurologic signs and symptoms scattered over time and space. Just as no neurologic findings are pathognomonic for MS, no laboratory test is universally diagnostic. Imaging studies of the brain and spinal cord, cerebrospinal fluid (CSF) examination, and evoked potentials are the major adjuncts used to increase one's confidence in the clinically suspected diagnosis.

Magnetic resonance imaging (MRI) is superior in sensitivity to contrast-enhanced computed tomography (CT) for evaluation of the lesions of MS. A negative MRI does not, however, have sufficient sensitivity or negative predictive value to rule out the diagnosis.[14] MRI is well suited for the diagnostic workup of patients suspected of having MS and for monitoring the course of the disease and its response to therapy. The number, size, and distinctive location of areas of increased signal found

TABLE 207.3. Differential Diagnosis of Acute Focal Neurologic Deficit

BLEEDING (SPONTANEOUS OR TRAUMATIC)
Subdural hematoma
Intraparenchymal hemorrhage
Epidural hematoma
Subarachnoid hemorrhage
INFECTION
Abscess
Brain
Epidural
Subdural
Meningitis/encephalitis
NEOPLASM
Primary
Metastatic
VASCULAR
Thrombosis
Embolism
METABOLIC
Hypoglycemia
Hyperosmolar hyperglycemia
B_{12} deficiency (spinal cord)
MISCELLANEOUS
Postictal
Migraine
Bell's palsy
Psychogenic (diagnosis of exclusion)

on MRI help distinguish MS from other neurologic diseases. Multiple white matter and periventricular lesions are characteristic, and lesions are commonly seen in the brainstem and cerebellum as well. Signal enhancement with gadolinium is characteristic of the disruption of the blood–brain barrier that occurs with active inflammatory lesions.

Newer and faster MRI techniques show promise of achieving even greater sensitivity for the lesions of MS. Findings on MRI are common in patients with optic neuritis, even when there is no other clinical evidence of MS, and MRI has been demonstrated to have prognostic value in predicting conversion from isolated syndromes, such as optic neuritis, myelitis, and internuclear ophthalmoplegia, to MS.[2,4,15] MRI is also useful in identifying alternate diagnoses, such as intracranial neoplasm, vascular abnormalities, and spinal cord lesions.

Examination of the CSF can help to confirm the diagnosis. Useful findings are the presence of myelin basic protein (indicative of rapid myelin degradation); an elevated level of immunoglobulin G (IgG), out of proportion to that in serum; and the presence of oligoclonal immunoglobulin bands on protein electrophoresis. Other common CSF findings include elevated total protein and a modestly increased mononuclear cell count (less than 50 cells/μL). In addition, CSF analysis permits the exclusion of infection as the cause of symptoms.

Evoked potentials (EPs) are electrodiagnostic studies that measure the electrical potentials (voltages) that are evoked in response to the application of brief sensory stimuli. Demyelination causes abnormal axonal conduction that can be picked up on EP testing as abnormal potentials. This modality falls into the domain of the neurologist and is not part of the ED evaluation.

EMERGENCY DEPARTMENT MANAGEMENT

Treatment of acute exacerbations of MS is most appropriately undertaken in consultation with a neurologist. Immunosuppression with corticotropin (ACTH) or corticosteroids, traditionally a mainstay of therapy for relapses in patients with known disease, is predicated on the presumed immune basis for the disease. High-dose intravenous bolus methylprednisolone is superior to placebo in decreasing the recovery time with MS relapses.[5,13] Critical analysis of the benefit of corticosteroids in shortening the duration of relapse, preventing relapse, and modifying long-term disease progression is ongoing.[6]

Preliminary studies comparing different steroid regimens (e.g., intravenous vs. oral) have failed to demonstrate a clear advantage of one over the other.[1] An exception is the use of corticosteroids in the treatment of optic neuritis. A reduction in the rate of development of MS has been demonstrated at 2 years for short-term treatment with intravenous methylprednisolone followed by prednisone, but not for prednisone alone.[2] Intravenous methylprednisolone has also shown short-term benefit in improving visual acuity, but this benefit diminishes over time. Prednisone has not demonstrated this same benefit and is actually associated with an increased risk of new episodes of optic neuritis compared with placebo.[3] New modalities for the treatment of relapses, based on the known pathophysiology of the myelin plaque, are currently in clinical trials.

Prevention of the exacerbations associated with MS and alteration of the progression of neurologic disability are currently the focus of extensive research. Therapeutic interventions aimed at limiting demyelination, enhancing remyelination, and improving conduction in demyelinated fibers are being investigated. Interferon beta-1b, interferon beta-1a, and copolymer 1 have shown significant promise and are the first drugs to have been demonstrated to alter the course of relapsing disease. Beta-interferons have been shown to decrease clinical relapse rate and the severity of exacerbations, and to result in a lower lesion burden on MRI.[7,8] Copolymer 1 has been shown to reduce relapse rate and improve disability status.[9] Administration of these drugs falls under the domain of the neurologist.

In the patient with known disease who presents with fever, sources of infection should be sought and treated aggressively. Patients with bladder dysfunction are particularly susceptible to urinary tract infection; decubitus ulcers and pneumonia are other common sources of infection that should be considered. In any event, antipyretics should be administered. An elevated temperature that is related solely to heat exposure should be treated by active cooling measures.

DISPOSITION

The new patient with clinically suspected MS may warrant hospital admission to complete the diagnostic workup, to exclude other causes of signs and symptoms, and to undergo aggressive treatment of debilitating symptoms. For the patient with known MS, determination of the need for hospitalization depends on the general medical condition as well as the neurologic status. Patients may also require hospitalization for medical complications of MS (e.g., infection), for the administration of aggressive treatment of neurologic symptoms, and for the supportive care necessary because of disability during disease exacerbations.

COMMON PITFALLS

- Failure to identify and treat other disease entities in the patient with known or suspected MS
- Failure to consider the possibility of intercurrent medical illnesses, especially those that commonly affect the chronically ill neurologic patient (e.g., urinary tract infection, pneumonia, decubitus ulcers)
- Failure to consider MS in the young patient presenting with focal neurologic signs and symptoms. The presenting symptoms of MS can be vague and transient, and can seem bizarre. A psychogenic etiology remains a diagnosis of exclusion.
- Failure to realize that rheumatologic or constitutional symptoms or abnormal laboratory values should call the diagnosis of MS into question

References

1. Barnes D, Hughes RA, Morris RW, et al. Randomised trial of oral and intravenous methylprednisolone in acute relapses of multiple sclerosis. *Lancet* 1997;349:902.
2. Beck RW, Cleary PA, Trobe JD, et al. The effect of corticosteroids for acute optic neuritis on the subsequent development of multiple sclerosis. *N Engl J Med* 1993;329:1764.
3. Beck RW, Cleary PA, Anderson MM, et al. A randomized controlled trial of corticosteroids in the treatment of acute optic neuritis. *N Engl J Med* 1992;326:581.
4. Beck RW, Arrington J, Murtagh FR, et al. Brain magnetic resonance imaging in acute optic neuritis—experience of the optic neuritis study group. *Arch Neurol* 1993;50:841.
5. Durelli L, Cocito D, Riccio A, et al. High dose intravenous methylprednisolone in the treatment of multiple sclerosis: clinical-immunologic correlations. *Neurology* 1986;36:238.
6. Filippini G, Brusaferri L, Sibley WA, et al. Corticosteroids or ACTH for acute exacerbations in multiple sclerosis (Cochrane Review). In: The Cochrane Library, 1, 1999. Oxford.
7. The IFNB multiple sclerosis study group. Interferon beta-1b is effective in relapsing remitting multiple sclerosis. *Neurology* 1993;43:655.
8. Jacobs LD, Cookfair DL, Rudick RA, et al., and the Multiple Sclerosis Collaborative Research Group (MSCRG). Intramuscular interferon beta-1a for disease progression in relapsing multiple sclerosis. *Ann Neurol* 1996;39:285.
9. Johnson KP, Brooks BR, Cohen JA, et al., and the Copolymer 1 Multiple Sclerosis Study Group. Copolymer 1 reduces relapse rate and improves disability in relapsing remitting multiple sclerosis: results of a phase III multicenter double-blind, placebo-controlled trial. *Neurology* 1995;45:1268.

10. Lynch SG, Rose JW. Multiple sclerosis. *Dis Monogr* 1996;11:10.
11. Lublin FD, Reingold SC, et al. Defining the clinical course of multiple sclerosis: results of an international survey. *Neurology* 1996;46:907.
12. Minden SL, Moes E. A psychiatric perspective. In: Rao SM, ed. *Neurobehavioral aspects of multiple sclerosis*. New York: Oxford University Press, 1990.
13. Milligan NM, Newcombe R, Compston DAS. A double-blind controlled trial of high dose methylprednisolone in patients with multiple sclerosis. *J Neurol Neurosurg Psychiatry* 1987;50:511.
14. Mushlin AI, Detsky AS, Phelps CE, et al. The accuracy of magnetic resonance imaging in patients with suspected multiple sclerosis. *JAMA* 1993;269:3146.
15. Raine CS, McFarland HF, Toutellotte WW, eds. *Multiple sclerosis: clinical and pathogenetic basis*. London: Chapman & Hall, 1997.
16. Rizzo JF, Lessell S. Risk of developing multiple sclerosis after uncomplicated optic neuritis: a long-term prospective study. *Neurology* 1988;38:185.
17. Rodriguez M, Siva A, Cross SA, et al. Optic neuritis: a population-based study in Olmsted County, Minnesota. *Neurology* 1995;45:244.
18. Solari A, Uitdehaag B, Giuliani G, et al. Aminopyridines for symptomatic treatment in multiple sclerosis (Cochrane Review). In: The Cochrane Library. 1, 1999. Oxford: Update software.
19. van Oosten BW, Truyen L, Barkof F, et al. Multiple sclerosis therapy: a practical guide. *Drugs* 1995;49(2):200.

CHAPTER 208
Parkinsonism

Brendan R. Furlong

Parkinsonism, or Parkinson syndrome, is a group of progressive degenerative central nervous system disorders characterized by cardinal motor signs of bradydyskinesia, tremor, rigidity, and postural instability. Idiopathic Parkinson disease (PD) is the most common cause of parkinsonism and accounts for 80% of cases. Secondary parkinsonism, from a host of disparate causes, constitutes the remaining 20% (Table 208.1).

The incidence of parkinsonism and PD is approximately 20 per 100,000 and increases with age.[8,10] There does not appear to be a genetic predisposition for PD when the disease begins after age 50, although there may be one for early-onset disease.[10] There is no gender difference, but PD appears to be more common in Whites than in other groups.[11] The survival rate for appropriately treated PD approximates that of the general population, whereas that of secondary parkinsonism is markedly less and the clinical course more complicated.[6]

Although the precise cause and pathophysiology of PD is not known, profound localized depletion of the neurotransmitter dopamine in the substantia nigra is the biochemical marker for the disease.[2,9] The mainstay of therapy for PD is neurotransmitter replacement in the form of levodopa. Infections (von Economo's pandemic of encephalitis lethargica), toxins (the designer drug methylphenyl tetrahydropyridine [MPTP]), and medications (phenothiazines) are known causes of secondary parkinsonism (see Table 208.1).

In practice, the diagnosis of parkinsonism and PD is made on clinical grounds, but the ultimate diagnosis still rests with neuropathologic confirmation at autopsy.[3] The various secondary parkinsonian syndromes show etiology-specific pathologic changes in the extrapyramidal system and the cortex of the brain. PD has distinct cellular degeneration of the substantia nigra with characteristic Lewy bodies.[4] Precisely how the neurochemical and pathologic changes in parkinsonism result in dysfunction of the regulation of tone and motor activity is not completely understood.[6]

TABLE 208.1. Causes of Parkinsonism

Parkinson disease (PD)
Neurodegenerative processes
Multiple system atrophy (MSA)
Progressive supranuclear palsy (PSP)
Corticobasal degeneration (CBD)
Drugs—phenothiazines, butyrophenones, anticonvulsants
Toxins—Methylphenyl tetrahydropyridine (MPTP), carbon monoxide, manganese
Trauma
Malignancy—lymphoma, glioma
Arteriosclerotic parkinsonism
Infections—epidemic encephalitis, von Economo's encephalitis

CLINICAL PRESENTATION

Patients can present to the emergency department (ED) with complaints referable to undiagnosed parkinsonism or with complications of previously diagnosed illness. Although emergent interventions are rarely needed for the disease itself, because effective symptomatic treatment is available and there is the possibility of preventing disease progression, it is desirable to make the diagnosis as early as possible.

The clinical manifestations of parkinsonism develop insidiously and gradually. Motor deficiencies are usually asymmetric. Rigidity may be present on flexion and extension of the extremities and neck, and "cogwheel" rigidity on passive extension of the elbow or circumduction of the wrist may be noted. Early on, ambulation is generally slow; short or shuffling steps (*march à petits pas*), instability, and falls occur later. The classic tremor of PD is a 3- to 6-Hz distal resting tremor that increases in periods of anxiety and disappears during sleep or voluntary motor activity. Monotonous speech and decreased speech volume are other early features, and there is eventual development of drooling, dysphagia, and masked facies. Sensory findings are generally absent. The Mini-Mental State Examination is usually normal early in the disease. Depression may occur. The presence of early dementia and psychosis (unrelated to medicines), autonomic dysfunction (orthostasis), cerebellar findings, and supranuclear gaze palsy suggest one of the secondary causes of parkinsonism.[3,6]

In patients with known PD, complications of therapy or a worsening of symptoms while on therapy is often the reason for presentation to the ED. The so-called on–off phenomenon, sudden wide fluctuations in motor function, ranging in severity from dyskinesia to freezing, can be particularly troubling to patients. "Wearing off," or loss of therapeutic effect, should prompt a reassessment of the medication regime and also confirmation that secondary parkinsonism has not been erroneously diagnosed as PD. Orthostasis, nausea, vomiting, and acute psychosis can be caused by various dopaminergic and anticholinergic agents. Differentiating disease progression from medication inadequacy or excess can be difficult, but is an important part of ED management.

Other complications related to general motor disability (e.g., traumatic injuries due to falls) are significant reasons for ED presentation. In addition, many older patients, the cohort most affected by parkinsonism, have multiple medical conditions that can be more difficult to manage in the setting of progressive parkinsonism.

DIFFERENTIAL DIAGNOSIS

The primary entities in the differential diagnosis of parkinsonism are idiopathic PD and secondary parkinsonism. To help distinguish PD from other causes of parkinsonism on a clinical basis, Gelb et al.[3] have suggested specific diagnostic criteria for PD: bradykinesia, rigidity, and the asymmetric onset of resting tremor, all of which must have a substantial and sustained response to levodopa or dopamine agonist therapy. The presence of postural instability, freezing phenomena, hallucinations, dementia, severe dysautonomia, or supranuclear gaze palsy within the first 3 years of disease presentation suggests a secondary form of parkinsonism.[3] PD has a gradually progressive course; rapid progression strongly suggests another form of parkinsonism.[3]

EMERGENCY DEPARTMENT EVALUATION

The ED evaluation of a patient with clinical symptoms suggestive of parkinsonism consists primarily of a history and physical examination. For patients with new symptoms, clinical assessment is aimed at identifying parkinsonism and then differentiating between the secondary parkinsonian syndromes and PD.

For patients previously diagnosed with parkinsonism, evaluation should focus on progression of disease, complications of medical treatment, and concomitant medical conditions.

EMERGENCY DEPARTMENT MANAGEMENT

Strategies for the management of parkinsonism in the ED should be coordinated with the physician who will treat the patient for the long term.

For patients who are *newly diagnosed* with PD, treatment includes agents to alleviate disabling symptoms, as well as agents that are potentially neuroprotective. Table 208.2 outlines treatment options. The centrally acting dopamine agonist levodopa is the mainstay of symptomatic treatment. It is desirable to use the minimum amount of levodopa necessary to control symptoms, because the metabolism of levodopa is thought to contribute to an excess of oxyradicals in the substantia nigra, leading to further cell degeneration. Levodopa's peripheral side effects (nausea, vomiting, and orthostasis) are thus limited as well.[9] Carbidopa blocks the peripheral metabolism of levodopa, allowing lower doses of levodopa to be effective centrally. For this reason, the levodopa–carbidopa combination drug, Sinemet, has become a mainstay of treatment. The dopamine agonists bromocriptine and pergolide are often used as adjuvant therapy and help reduce the dose of levodopa required while themselves serving as neuroprotective agents. The monoamine oxidase (MAO) B inhibitor selegiline is utilized primarily as a neuroprotective agent, but may also have some symptomatic benefit. The anticholinergic drug benztropine is prescribed selectively for patients with tremor predominance. Surgical options are generally used only in those with severe disease refractory to medical management.

For patients with *known* PD, ED management is directed at recognizing the inadequacy or excess of the medication regimen and adjusting dosages accordingly. The "on–off" phenomenon is thought to be due to fluctuations in drug concentrations. Changing doses and/or dosing intervals and adding other antiparkinsonism agents may be necessary. A sustained-release levodopa–carbidopa combination appears to reduce the total levodopa requirement, as well as variations in drug concentration.[1] Medication excess may cause acute psychiatric and cognitive side effects, such as psychosis, hallucinations, delusions, agitation, and confusion. This may require a decrease in dopaminergic and anticholinergic medications and the initiation of clozapine.[9] The peripheral side effects of excessive dopamine (nausea, vomiting, and orthostasis) are treated by reducing levodopa doses. Optimizing the balance of various

TABLE 208.2. Management of Parkinson Disease

MEDICAL
Dopamine Precursor
Levodopa: precursor of the pathologically deficient dopamine, which is able to cross the blood-brain barrier; improves symptoms; most often used in combination with carbidopa
Side effects: dyskinesia, anorexia, nausea vomiting, postural hypotension
Peripheral Dopa-decarboxylase Inhibitor
Carbidopa: peripheral dopa-decarboxylase inhibitor; decreases peripheral breakdown of levodopa, allowing lower dose therapy
Side effects: may exacerbate central dopaminergic side effects when levodopa dose not reduced sufficiently
Dopamine Agonist
Bromocriptine: dopamine agonist used as adjuvant to levodopa; decreases the dopamine requirement, thus allowing lower dose levodopa therapy[7]; also appears to decrease dyskinesias and "on-off" side effects
Side effects: hypotension, nausea, vomiting, constipation, fatigue, hallucinations
Pergolide: dopamine agonist used as adjuvant to levodopa; also used by some as monotherapy, particularly early in young-onset PD
Side effects: hypotension, nausea, vomiting, constipation, confusion, hallucinations, dyskinesias, dystonias
MAO-B Inhibitor
Selegiline: MAO-B inhibitor thought to reduce the peroxide produced as MAO-B metabolizes dopamine[9]; may also have some therapeutic effect
Side effects: sleep disturbances, psychosis, agitation, confusion, dyskinesias
Anticholinergic Drugs
Benztropine: striatal muscarinic blocker; useful in treating the tremor of PD
Side effects: typical anticholinergic symptoms and signs
SURGICAL
Electrical deep-brain stimulation
Posteroventral pallidotomy
Neural cell transplantation

agents can be difficult and should be coordinated with the patient's primary physician.

The management of the parkinsonian syndromes other than PD is generally less effective. Parkinsonism due to prescription medications may improve with cessation of the implicated agent, but parkinsonism associated with prior MPTP use is not reversible. Symptoms of neurodegenerative parkinsonism can be managed with the same agents as used for those of PD, but there tends not to be a sustained response to therapy.

For all parkinsonian syndromes, injuries from falls, infections (e.g., aspiration pneumonia), and concomitant medial conditions should be evaluated and managed as with other patients, keeping in mind the limitations imposed by the patient's chronic level of functioning.

DISPOSITION

Whether the diagnosis of parkinsonism is made in the ED or the patient is being seen for complications of therapy or progression of symptoms, the patient's primary care physician or neurologist should be consulted. This assures continuity of care, which is essential to optimize the management of this chronic condition. Rarely is admission to the hospital or transfer to a tertiary care center indicated for parkinsonism itself. Complications such as sepsis or injuries from falls are more likely to be indications for inpatient management.

COMMON PITFALLS

- The diagnosis of parkinsonism may be missed in patients with vague complaints of dizziness, unsteadiness, or inability to walk, unless the signs are specifically sought on careful neurologic examination
- The complex medical regimens for PD require precise modifications to maximize clinical benefit while minimizing side effects

References

1. Capildeo R. Implications of the 5-year CR FIRST trial. *Neurology* 1998;50:[Suppl 6]:S15.
2. Duvoisin RC. A brief history of parkinsonism. *Neurol Clin* 1992;10:301.
3. Gelb DJ, et al. Diagnostic criteria for Parkinson disease. *Arch Neurol* 1999;56:33.
4. Gibb WRG. Neuropathology of Parkinson's disease and related syndromes. *Neurol Clin* 1992;10:361.
5. Little NE. Parkinson disease. In: Harwood-Nuss AL, Linden CH, Luten RC, et al., eds. *The clinical practice of emergency medicine,* 2nd ed. Philadelphia: Lippincott–Raven Publishers, 1996:897.
6. Litvan I. Parkinsonian features: when are they Parkinson disease? *JAMA* 1998;280:1654.
7. Olanow CW, Koller WC, eds. An algorithm (decision tree) for the management of Parkinson's disease: treatment guidelines. *Neurology* 1998;50[Suppl 3]:S1.
8. Rajput AH, et al. Epidemiology of parkinsonism: incidence, classification, and mortality. *Ann Neurol* 1984;16:278.
9. Stern MB. Contemporary approaches to the pharmacotherapeutic management of Parkinson's disease: an overview. *Neurology* 1997;49[Suppl 1]:S2.
10. Tanner CM, et al. Parkinson disease in twins: an etiologic study. *JAMA* 1999;281:341.
11. Tanner CM. Epidemiology of Parkinson's disease. *Neurol Clin* 1992;10:317.

CHAPTER 209
Drug-Induced Hyperthermic Syndromes

Sandra M. Schneider

Neuroleptic malignant syndrome (NMS), malignant hyperthermia (MH), and serotonin syndrome (SS) all have similar clinical presentations, but they differ in their pathophysiology. (See Chapter 370.) As a group, they have been termed *drug-induced hyperthermic syndromes*. All three are rarely encountered in the emergency department but are important to identify and treat promptly.

NMS is a rare idiosyncratic reaction to neuroleptic medication that occurs in only 0.5% to 2.4% of patients taking neuroleptics.[3] It is more common in patients on longer-acting (depo) medications and those with strong D2-receptor antagonism. It also occurs during drug "holidays," when levodopa therapy has been withdrawn. NMS is thought to result from dopamine depletion in the brain, possibly in combination with increased anticholinergic activity.[5,14,16] There is an increased risk in patients of Japanese heritage, and in those with dehydration, malnutrition, physical exhaustion, or organic brain disease.[11]

NMS is also reported in patients taking lithium. Although it is most often seen with initiation of new medication or a dosage adjustment, it can occur without dose or medication alteration. Reexposure to the medication causes a recurrence of NMS in only 50% of cases.[15] While an intensive search for a genetic link has been undertaken, no association with chromosomal or enzymatic abnormality has been discovered.

MH is a rare, genetically determined reaction to anesthetics and other agents (Table 209.1).[4,6,7] For unknown reasons, nearly half of cases occur in children under 15 years of age. [13] Males are twice as commonly affected as females and have a higher mortality. In affected patients, anesthetic exposure triggers the release of calcium by the sarcoplasmic reticulum, resulting in increased muscle contraction and oxygen consumption. Depolarizing muscle relaxants are more likely to cause MH than are inhaled anesthetic gases. It is most commonly seen after exposure to halothane or succinylcholine. Other risk factors are listed in Table 209.2.

SS, first described in 1955,[10] is a reaction to serotonin-active agents. It most commonly occurs after an increase in dosage of a

TABLE 209.1. Agents in Malignant Hyperthermia

Agents Potentially Causing MH	Agents Probably Safe in MH
Halothane	Nitrous oxide
Succinylcholine	Barbiturates
Enflurane	Local anesthetics
Isoflurane	Narcotics
Desflurane	
Sevoflurane	
Decamethonium	
Suxamethonium	

TABLE 209.2. Risk Factors Associated with Potential for Malignant Hyperthermia

History of MH during surgery
First-degree relative with MH
Family member with multiple episodes of MH
History of neuromuscular disease
High creatine phosphokinase
History of NMS or heatstroke

drug, or with the addition of a new drug to another serotonin-active agent. The combination of a monoamine oxidase (MAO) inhibitor and a serotonin reuptake inhibitor can cause effects within minutes. The severity of SS is related to the degree of serotonin elevation and its duration.

Common serotonin receptor agonists and their approximate half-lives are listed in Table 209.3. Serotonin reuptake inhibitors are used in a variety of disorders, including appetite reduction, bulimia, depression, obsessive–compulsive disorder, diabetic neuropathy, and panic disorder. Several of the serotonin-active drugs are metabolized by the P450 system, and about 8% of Caucasians are poor metabolizers of drugs degraded by this cytochrome.[2] These individuals may show increased sensitivity to serotonin-active drugs and an increased incidence of SS.

While MH occurs by a peripheral reaction, NMS and SS are centrally mediated. Although the complex role of neurotransmitters in heat regulation is not clearly understood, dopamine is involved. The extrapyramidal system, which maintains equilibrium and muscle tone, involves the activity of a number of neurotransmitters, including dopamine, serotonin, acetylcholine, and GABA.

TABLE 209.3. Drugs That May Cause Serotonin Syndrome and Their Relative Half-Lives

Selective inhibitors of serotonin uptake	
Fluoxetine (Prozac)[a]	Long
Paroxetine (Paxil)[a]	Short
Sertraline (Zoloft)	Short
Trazodone	
Meperidine	
Dextromethorphan[a]	
Fluvoxamine (Luvox)	Short
Specific serotonin agonists	
Buspirone	Short
LSD	Short
Mescaline	
Nonspecific serotonin agonists	
Bromocriptine	Short
Bupropion	
Phenytoin	
Tryptophan	
Levodopa	Short
Lithium	Short
Other drugs	
Chlorpheniramine[a]	Long
Brompheniramine[a]	Long
Ginseng	
St. John's wort	
Tramadol[a]	Short
Nonspecific inhibitors of serotonin reuptake	
Clomipramine (Anafranil)[a]	Long
Venlafaxine (Effexor)[a]	Short
Nefazodone (Serzone)	
Agents that increase serotonin release	
Amphetamine	
MDMA (Ecstasy)	
Cocaine	
Codeine	
Reserpine	
Monoamine oxidase inhibitors	
Pargyline (Eutonyl)	Long
Phenelzine (Nardil)	Long
Selegiline (Eldepryl)	Long
Isocarboxazid (Marplan)	Long
Procarbazine (Malulane)	
Trancypromine (Parnate)	Long
Isoniazid	Long
Moclobemide	Short

Half-lives: short, <24 h; medium, 24–72 h; long, >72 h.
[a] Metabolized by CYP4502D6.

CLINICAL PRESENTATION

NMS presents with altered mental status, autonomic instability, hyperpyrexia, and muscular rigidity, which develop rapidly over 1 to 3 days. Not every patient presents with all signs, although hyperpyrexia and altered mental status are nearly always present. Diagnostic criteria for NMS are presented in Table 209.4. Temperature in excess of 41°C has been reported. Muscular rigidity of the thorax may impair breathing. Autonomic dysfunction may cause severe variations of both blood pressure and pulse. Some patients may develop seizures, trismus, opisthotonos, and positive Babinski's signs.

MH can occur at any interval after initiation of anesthetics. Masseter muscle spasm is generally noted initially, and then generalized muscle rigidity leads rapidly to hyperpyrexia. Some patients develop recurrent symptoms 48 hours after the initial episode.

SS was first described in 1955 but, most notably, was likely the cause of death in the Libby Zion case.[1] It involves an alteration in mental status, autonomic dysfunction, and increased neuromuscular activity, the latter causing a rise in temperature. Diagnostic criteria for SS are presented in Table 209.5. Mental status changes may be manifested as agitation, confusion, drowsiness, coma, and/or seizures. Autonomic dysfunction may produce nausea, salivation, tachycardia, diaphoresis, diarrhea, hyperthermia, hypertension, and mydriasis.

Reported neuromuscular findings can include ankle clonus, hyperreflexia, rigidity, tremor, ataxia, head twitching, mutism, bilateral Babinski's, and myoclonus. Many of the findings are similar to those of NMS, but mydriasis is seen with SS and lead-pipe rigidity with NMS. Symptoms can be seen within 15 minutes and can last for up to 6 hours. The duration of symptoms in other cases is dependent on drug half-life, but, in severe cases, symptoms can persist for up to 6 weeks.

Because all three syndromes share similar presentations, with severe muscle contraction and hyperpyrexia, they share common complications of rhabdomyolysis, myoglobinemia, and intravascular hemolysis. Patients may also develop pulmonary embolism, cardiovascular collapse, myocardial infarc-

TABLE 209.4. Diagnostic Criteria for Neuroleptic Malignant Syndrome

Patient taking neuroleptic with
Fever
Muscle rigidity
↑ CPK
Or two of the above, plus four of the following:
Tachycardia
Abnormal blood pressure
Tachypnea
Altered mental status
Diaphoresis
Leukocytosis

TABLE 209.5. Diagnostic Criteria for Serotonin Syndrome

The addition or increase in dosage of a serotonergic agent
Plus three of the following:
- Agitation
- Mental status changes
- Diaphoresis
- Diarrhea
- Myoclonus
- Fever
- Tremor
- Hyperreflexia
- Incoordination

No neuroleptic has been involved.

TABLE 209.6. Treatment of Malignant Hyperthermia

Discontinue precipitating agent.
Administer dantrolene 2 mg/kg i.v., up to 10 mg/kg/d.
Infuse saline with sodium bicarbonate to maintain urinary output.
 Monitor systemic pH to prevent alkalosis.
Cool patient with cooling blanket, ice packs, or evaporation.
Monitor for electrolyte imbalance and cardiac dysrhythmias.
 Avoid the use of calcium antagonists or digoxin.

tion, and acute respiratory failure. The brain is particularly sensitive to heat. Temperatures above 42°C cause central nervous system (CNS) damage, initially to the more sensitive cerebellum and eventually to the cerebral cortex, brainstem, and spinal cord.

DIFFERENTIAL DIAGNOSIS

Infectious etiologies, particularly meningitis, are generally the primary consideration in the differential diagnosis. Many authors suggest initial empiric CNS coverage in all patients suspected of having NMS.

In fever, the hypothalamic "set point" is altered so that the body seeks to stay at an elevated temperature. Fever appears to be mediated by prostaglandins and can be reduced by the use of prostaglandin inhibitors. Such medications have no effect on environmental hyperthermia or drug-induced hyperthermia.

Drugs may increase basal heat production by increasing metabolism, stimulating beta receptors, impairing sweating, or uncoupling oxidative phosphorylation (e.g., salicylates). All three syndromes increase metabolism. In addition, neuroleptic medications may impede sweating through anticholinergic mechanisms.

Lethal catatonia is a disorder similar to these syndromes, and occurs in patients with psychiatric disorders (primarily schizophrenia) who are not taking antipsychotic medications. The pathogenesis is unknown, although dopamine antagonism or depletion appears to underlie the disorder.[8] Patients initially develop mood swings, anorexia, and insomnia, followed by muscular rigidity, severe agitation, and psychosis. Autonomic instability (labile blood pressure and pulse and severe hyperthermia) is also seen.

Finally, patients can develop catatonia with profound muscular rigidity and continued hyperthermia. Patients with lethal catatonia are at risk for similar complications, including acute renal failure, rhabdomyolysis, acute respiratory failure, and disseminated intravascular coagulation. Management is directed at reducing temperature and preventing renal failure and rhabdomyolysis. Bromocriptine, amantadine, and dantrolene have been used, but with variable response. Benzodiazepines have also been useful. Electroconvulsive therapy given early in the course of lethal catatonia is reported to be particularly effective.[12]

EMERGENCY DEPARTMENT EVALUATION AND MANAGEMENT

As in all patients, attention to the ABCs takes priority. All should receive high-flow oxygen and have at least two intravenous (i.v.) sites established. Rapid cooling should be initiated by the use of fans and cool-water spray.

Renal failure may be prevented or lessened by saline diuresis (up to 150 mL/h) accompanied by an osmotic agent (e.g., mannitol) or a diuretic (e.g., furosemide). Rhabdomyolysis can be prevented or lessened by sodium bicarbonate by increasing urinary pH. In theory, sodium bicarbonate will inhibit the formation of ferrihemate, a nephrotoxin. Hyperkalemia may accompany extensive rhabdomyolysis and can be treated by calcium gluconate, insulin and glucose, or exchange resins.

Monitoring of cardiac rhythm and core temperature is essential. Electrolyte abnormalities, including hypocalcemia, hyperkalemia, and hyperphosphatemia, are common, as is leukocytosis, with or without a left shift. Liver damage from hyperthermia is reflected in elevated transaminases and alkaline phosphatase. A computed tomography scan should be performed to rule out a cerebral bleed, and a lumbar puncture may need to be performed to rule out bacterial meningitis.

With the increasing emergency department use of succinylcholine for rapid-sequence intubation, emergency physicians need to be aware of the early signs of MH. Masseter muscle contraction or any developing muscular rigidity should lead to immediate treatment, which is outlined in Table 209.6. Agents safe for use in patients with MH include vecuronium, pancuronium, etomidate, propofol, opiates, barbiturates, benzodiazepines, and ester-based local anesthetics such as lidocaine. Dantrolene, the mainstay of treatment, is a muscle relaxant that decreases the release of calcium by the sarcoplasmic reticulum. The dosage is 0.8 to 3.0 mg/kg i.v. q6h, up to a maximum of 10 mg/kg/d.

Specific treatment for NMS is not well established. Neuroleptic agents should be discontinued. Dantrolene appears to be most useful in patients with prominent muscle contraction. Bromocriptine mesylate, a dopamine agonist, is widely used alone or in combination with dantrolene; the dosage is 2.5 to 7.5 mg orally q8h. Bromocriptine is most useful when hyperthermia is not accompanied by dramatic muscle rigidity. Amantadine, another dopamine agonist, also has been used with some success. Levodopa and carbidopa–levodopa are useful in many patients, particularly those in whom NMS is associated with the recent withdrawal of these medications.

Treatment of SS consists of discontinuing the offending medication and providing supportive care. Benzodiazepines have been useful in decreasing hyperactivity, as has chlorpromazine, though with somewhat variable efficacy. Cyproheptadine (4 mg/h) or methysergide (2 mg b.i.d.) has been reported to decrease the symptoms of SS.[9]

DISPOSITION

All patients with these syndromes require inpatient treatment, generally in the intensive care unit, with consultation with a psychiatrist (for NMS, SS) or anesthesiologist (for MH). Mortality has fallen dramatically in all three syndromes with increased recognition and early aggressive treatment.

COMMON PITFALLS

- Very high temperatures (in excess of 42°C) are rarely due to bacterial or viral infection; thus, more unusual causes of hyperthermia should be considered. Nonetheless, patients with NMS, SS, or MH should undergo evaluation for infection, generally including lumbar puncture.
- Patients receiving succinylcholine as a component of rapid-sequence intubation are at potential risk of MH. Periodic evaluation for masseter spasm may alert the physician to developing MH.
- Patients with severe hyperthermia (greater than 41°C) require immediate cooling, regardless of the underlying etiology. Antipyretics are not effective for environmental hyperthermia or in drug-induced syndromes such as MH, SS, or NMS. Hyperthermic individuals should be monitored for signs of rhabdomyolysis, renal failure, or other end-organ damage.
- Patients receiving serotonin agonists should not receive other serotonin-active drugs, including such commonly prescribed medications as meperidine and dextromethorphan.

References

1. Asch DA, Parker RM. The Libby Zion case; one step forward or two steps backward? *N Engl J Med* 1988;318:771–775.
2. Brosen K, Neilsen DN, Brusgeard K, et al. CYP2D6 genotype determination in the Danish population. *Eur J Clin Pharmacol* 1994;47:221–225.
3. Delay J, Pichot P, Lemperior MT, et al. Un neuroleptique majeur nonphenothiazineque et non reserpinique, l'halidol, dans le traitment des psychoses. *Ann Med Psychol* 1960;118:145.
4. Denborough MA, Lovell RRH. Anaesthetic deaths in a family. *Lancet* 1960;2:45.
5. Jauss M, Krack P, Franz M, et al. Imagine of dopamine receptors with ^{123}I Iodobenzamide single-photon emission-computed tomography in neuroleptic malignant syndrome. *Mov Disord* 1996;11:726–728.
6. Johnson C, Edleman KJ. Malignant hyperthermia: a review. *J Perinatol* 1992;12:61.
7. Lazarus A, Mann SC, Caroff SN. *The neuroleptic malignant syndrome and related conditions*. Washington: American Psychiatric Press, 1989.
8. Mann SC, Caroff SN, Bleir HR, et al. Lethal catatonia. *Am J Psychiat* 1986; 143:1374–1381
9. Martin TG. Serotonin syndrome. *Ann Emerg Med* 1996;28:520–526.
10. Mitchell RS. Fatal toxic encephalitis occurring during iproniazid therapy in pulmonary tuberculous. *Ann Intern Med* 1955;42:417.
11. Na Ganuma H, Fuji I. Incidence and risk factors in neuroleptic malignant syndrome. *Acta Psychiatr Scand* 1994;90:424–426.
12. Philbrick KL, Rummans TA. Malignant catatonia. *J Clin Psychiat Neurosci* 1994;6:1–13.
13. Stazis KP, Fox AW. Malignant hyperthermia: a review of published cases. *Anesth Analg* 1993;77:297.
14. Tanii H, Taniguchi N, Niigawa H, et al. Development of an animal model for neuroleptic malignant syndrome: heat exposed rabbits with haloperidol and atropine administration exhibit increased muscle activity, hyperthermia and high serum creatine phosphokinase level. *Brain Res* 1996;743:263–270.
15. Wells AJ, Sommi RW, Crismon MC. Neuroleptic rechallenge after neuroleptic malignant syndrome: case report and literature review. *Drug Intell Clin Pharmacol* 1988;22:475–480.
16. Yamawaki S, Lai H, Horita A. Dopaminergic and serotonergic mechanisms of thermal regulation; mediation of thermal effects of apomorphine and dopamine. *Pharmacol Exp Ther* 1983;227:383.

PART VII

Hematology/Oncology

CHAPTER 210
Bleeding Disorders

Kathleen C. Hubbell

Emergency physicians encounter bleeding on a daily basis: Bleeding lacerations, epistaxis, bruising, hematuria, gastrointestinal (GI) bleeding, and blunt and penetrating trauma are common complaints in the emergency department. Most of these patients have normal clotting function and are bleeding because of a local lesion. Their bleeding can be controlled by pressure, packing, suturing, or other local therapy aimed at the specific lesion, and bleeding does not recur if the lesion is properly treated.

On the other hand, a patient with a bleeding disorder may bleed spontaneously as well as after trauma, and treatment of the local lesion may not control the bleeding or prevent its recurrence. The disorder may be congenital or acquired, and may involve one or more components of the body's complex coagulation system.

PATHOPHYSIOLOGY

Hemostasis is normally maintained by the balanced functioning of four elements: the blood vessel wall, the platelets, the clotting factors (Table 210.1) and inhibitors, and the fibrinolytic system. Altered function of any of these components may lead to bleeding or thrombosis.

Normally, the *vascular endothelium* provides a barrier between the fluid blood and the adhesive proteins collagen, von Willebrand factor (vWF), and fibronectin, which are synthesized in the endothelial cells and secreted into the extracellular matrix. It also prevents coagulation through the action of thrombin inhibitors, such as thrombomodulin, that are bound to the endothelial cell membranes. When the endothelium is disrupted by trauma, immune complexes, proteolytic enzymes, bacterial endotoxin, viruses, or other stimuli, the adhesive molecules are exposed.

Platelets adhere to these proteins through their glycoprotein (GP) 1b/IX complexes. Adherence stimulates pseudopod formation and release of various substances involved in the coagulation process from the alpha and dense granules of the platelets. During the release, granule cell membranes merge with the platelet cell membranes, exposing other glycoproteins that serve as binding sites for coagulation factors. The release induces a change in the GP IIb/IIIa complexes that allows them to bind fibrinogen and link one platelet to another (aggregation). Products released from the injured endothelium and from the platelets, in addition to the presence of binding sites and cofactors for coagulation on the platelet membrane, encourage the initiation of the *clotting factor* cascade, which terminates in the formation of the fibrin clot.

The cascade has two initially separate pathways that join to form the common pathway (Fig. 210.1). The intrinsic pathway uses components normally found in plasma; the extrinsic pathway requires initial activation by tissue factor, previously known as thromboplastin. This classic version of the cascade has been supplemented by information from new studies, which shows additional interactions between the two pathways and a predominant role for the extrinsic pathway in the initiation of factor activation. The tissue factor (of the extrinsic pathway) released from the injured endothelial cells forms a complex with factor VII that activates not only factor X, as previously known, but also factor IX. Activated factor IX can then proceed through the last step of the intrinsic pathway to activate additional factor X, which, in turn, contributes to the formation of thrombin. Thrombin can activate factor XI, reinforcing the activation of the factors of the intrinsic pathway. As the extrinsic pathway initiates the cascade, an inhibitor called "tissue factor pathway inhibitor" is formed and prevents further activation of factors IX and X through the extrinsic arm of the cascade, leaving the intrinsic pathway as the main route to the activation of thrombin. These newly discovered coagulation mechanisms explain such previous observations as the lack of bleeding diathesis in patients with factor XII and prekallikrein deficiency, as contrasted to the severe disease seen in patients with low levels of factors VIII and IX. Several steps in the pathways require the presence

TABLE 210.1. Concentration of Blood Clotting Factors Needed for Normal Hemostasis

Factor	Common Name	Concentration Required
I	Fibrinogen	100 mg/dL
II	Prothrombin	30%–40%
III	Tissue thromboplastin	—
IV	Calcium	—
V	Labile factor, proaccelerin	30%–40%
VII	Proconvertin	30%–40%
VIII	Antihemophilic globulin	30%–40%
IX	Christmas factor	30%–40%
X	Stuart–Prower factor	30%–40%
XI	Plasma thromboplastin antecedent	20%
XII	Hageman factor	None
XIII	Fibrin-stabilizing factor	1%
Prekallikrein	Fletcher factor	None
High-molecular-weight kininogen	Williams–Fitzgerald–Fleaujeac factor	None

Adapted from White GC, Marder VJ, Colman RW, et al. Approach to the bleeding patient. In: Colman RW, Hirsh J, Marder VJ, et al., (eds). *Hemostasis and thrombosis, basic principles and clinical practice*, 2nd: ed. Philadelphia: JB Lippincott Co. 1987.

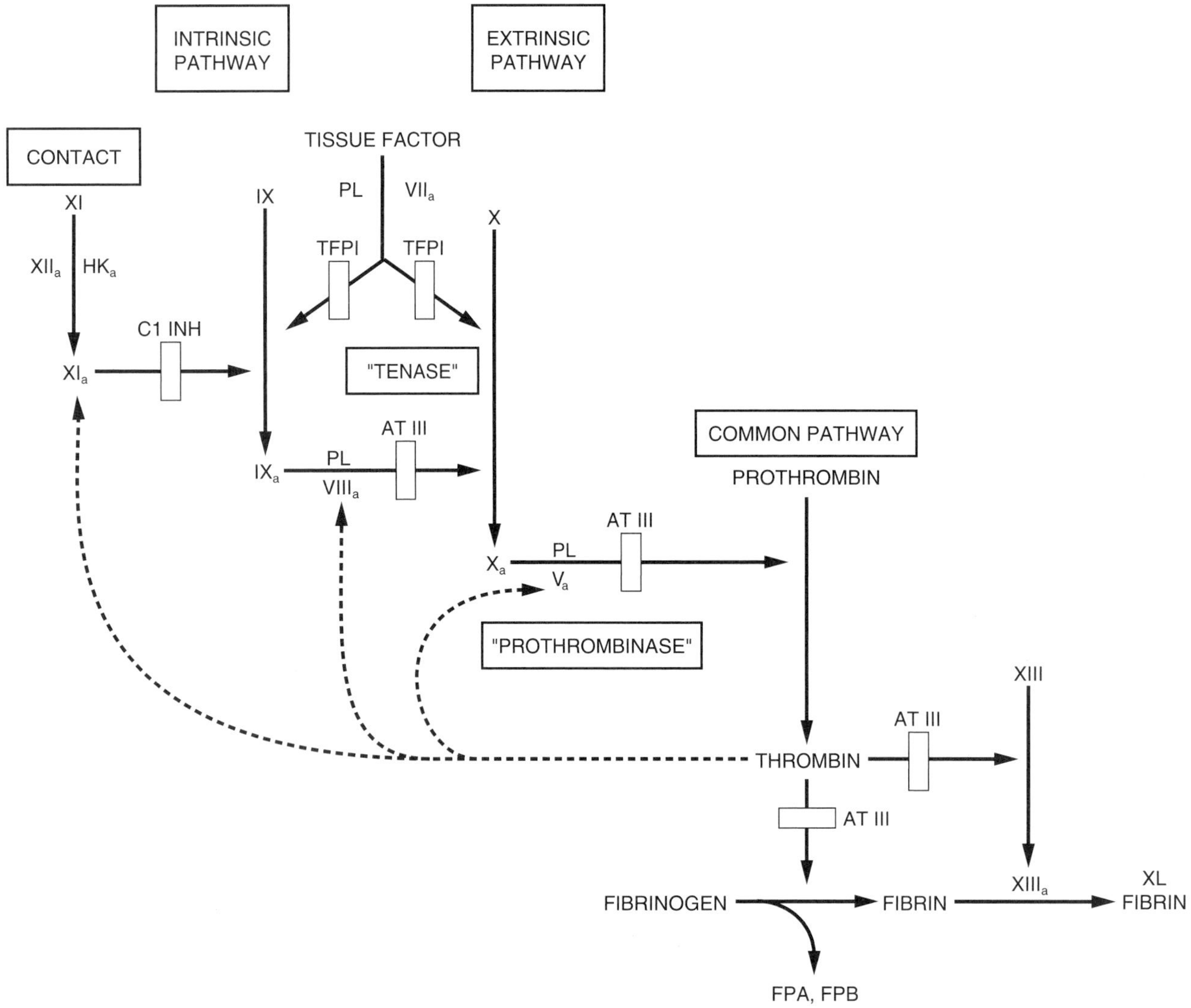

Figure 210.1. The clotting cascade. The central precipitating event is considered to involve tissue factor *(TF),* which, under physiologic conditions, is not exposed to the blood. With vascular or endothelial cell injury, TF acts in concert with activated factor VIIa and phospholipid *(PL)* to convert factor IX to IXa and factor X to Xa. The "intrinsic pathway" includes "contact" activation of factor XI by the XIIIa/activated high-molecular-weight kininogen *(HKa)* complex. Factor XIa also converts factor IX to IXa, and factor IXa, in turn, converts factor X to Xa, in concert with factors VIIIa and PL (the "tenase" complex). However factor Xa is formed, it is the active catalytic ingredient of the "prothrombinase" complex, which includes factor Va and PL and converts prothrombin to thrombin. Thrombin cleaves fibrinopeptides *(FPA, FPB)* from fibrinogen, allowing the resultant fibrin monomers to polymerize, and converts factor XIII to XIIIA, which cross-links *(XL)* the fibrin clot. Thrombin accelerates the process *(interrupted lines)* by its potential to activate factors V and VIII, but continued proteolytic action also dampens the process by activating protein C, which degrades factors Va and VIIIa. Thrombin activation of factor XI to XIa is a proposed but not yet proven pathway. Natural plasma inhibitors retard clotting: C1-inhibitor *(C1 INH)* neutralizes factor XIIa, TF pathway inhibitor *(TFPI)* blocks factor VIIa/TF, and antithrombin III *(ATIII)* blocks factors IXa, Xa and thrombin. *Arrows,* active enzymes; *open rectangles,* sites of inhibitor action; *dashed lines,* feedback reactions.

of calcium and a platelet phospholipid surface. Platelets thus are necessary not only to fill the endothelial defect initially, but also to provide elements needed for the operation of the clotting cascade, which serves to localize thrombus generation to the area of endothelial injury.[2,12,18]

Clotting *factor inhibitors,* such as antithrombin III (AT III) and protein C, provide a negative-feedback effect to limit the formation of clot.[2,12]

The *fibrinolytic system* is activated by many of the same substances that activate the clotting cascade. Active plasmin cleaves fibrin to lyse the clot. Activation of plasminogen by substances found in the clot localizes fibrinolysis to the clot.[2,12]

When all systems operate in a normal, balanced fashion, there is neither unchecked hemorrhage nor thrombosis in the vascular tree. However, when an inherited or acquired disorder produces an abnormality in one or more components of the system, bleeding may occur. The abnormality may be in the structure of the vascular tree; in the number of platelets; in the platelets' functional ability to adhere, aggregate, and release their dense-granule contents; in the activity of clotting factors; or in the activity of the fibrinolytic system. The emergency physician must use information from the clinical and laboratory evaluation to identify the abnormal component and treat the patient correctly.

EMERGENCY DEPARTMENT EVALUATION

When taking the history in a bleeding patient, the physician should try to establish whether the bleeding is part of a systemic disorder and what the etiology of the disorder might be (i.e., congenital vs. acquired, vascular vs. platelet vs. coagulation factor disorder).

A *systemic* disorder is suggested by bleeding from multiple sites, either at the time of presentation or in the past; spontaneous bleeding from sites in the absence of trauma or a known lesion; or unusually severe bleeding.[22] If a systemic disorder is suspected, further information regarding etiology is sought. Because of the large number of identified congenital bleeding disorders, the personal and family histories are closely scrutinized for clues to an inherited condition. Such patients often have had symptoms of bleeding since infancy (e.g., from the umbilical cord or after circumcision), have had unusual amounts of bleeding from previous trauma or surgery, and have a family history of bleeding.

Although these clues are helpful, mild forms of inherited bleeding disorders may be associated with significant bleeding only after severe trauma, and thus may not yet have caused any symptoms in the patient's life. The absence of a family history also does not rule out an "inherited" bleeding disorder: Up to 20% of cases of hemophilia A result from spontaneous mutation.[22]

If the patient has a family history of unusual bleeding, the pattern of inheritance may help identify the disorder. Sex-linked recessive disorders, such as hemophilia A and B and the Wiskott-Aldrich platelet disorder, are seen in multiple generations of a family in males only. Autosomal recessive conditions, such as deficiencies of factors II, V, VII, X, and XII, prekallikrein, and high-molecular-weight kininogen, are seen in both sexes and are manifested only in the proband's generation, because the parents are heterozygous and therefore asymptomatic. Autosomal dominant inheritance is seen in von Willebrand disease (vWD) and Osler-Weber-Rendu disease (hereditary telangiectasia); both sexes of multiple generations are affected.[22]

Patients with acquired bleeding disorders are more likely to be adults who have an underlying illness that affects platelet number or function or clotting factor levels (e.g., hepatic or renal disorder, disseminated intravascular coagulation [DIC], cancer, or an immunologic process). The development of acquired inhibitors to individual clotting factors is rare in nonhemophiliac patients but is associated with severe, often fatal, bleeding.[13,20,21] Factor VIII inhibitors are, by far, the most common. Patients are usually previously healthy individuals, often older, and often with a history of recent injury or surgery. Eighteen percent have an autoimmune disease; 5% note recent penicillin, sulfa, or other drug use. Some postpartum cases have been reported.[13]

Acquired bleeding disorders are often linked to the use of medications that interfere with normal coagulation (e.g., coumadin, heparin, aspirin, and nonsteroidal antiinflammatory drugs [NSAIDs]).[1] The effects of aspirin on platelet function are irreversible, lasting the 7- to 10-day lifespan of the platelet[16]; those of NSAIDs last about three to five drug half-lives, after which platelets again participate normally in clot formation (Tables 210.2 and 210.3).

Further information as to the probable etiology of a bleeding disorder can be obtained by asking about the characteristics of the bleeding. Vascular and platelet abnormalities produce one pattern of bleeding, coagulation factor deficiencies another.[1,22] Patients with vascular disorders, thrombocytopenia, and platelet function disorders complain of easy bruising, epistaxis, gingival bleeding, prolonged bleeding after dental extraction, hematuria, excessive menstrual flow, and GI bleeding. Bleeding may be either spontaneous or secondary to trauma. It may continue for hours, but, once stopped, does not recur.

Coagulation factor deficiencies, in contrast, typically cause

TABLE 210.2. Acquired Hemostatic Defects Associated with Selected Underlying Clinical Conditions

Underlying Clinical Condition	Type of Hemostatic Defect	Cause
Liver disease	Factor deficiency	Decreased synthesis
	Fibrinolysis	Decreased clearance of activators
	Hypercoagulable state	Antithrombin III and protein C deficiency, decreased clearance of activated clotting factors
	Thrombocytopenia	Splenic sequestration
Renal disease	Thrombocytopenia	Decreased marrow production
	Platelet defect	Retained metabolites in the blood
Malabsorption	Multiple factor deficiency	Vitamin K malabsorption
Acute leukemia (especially promyelocytic)	Thrombocytopenia	Decreased megakaryocytopoiesis
	DIC	Increased cellular procoagulant activity
Myeloproliferative disease	Platelet defect	Abnormal thrombopoiesis
	Thrombocythemia/thrombocytopenia	Hyperplastic or replaced (fibrotic) marrow, splenic sequestration
Lymphoma/chronic lymphocytic leukemia	Decreased von Willebrand factor	Adsorption onto tumor, autoantibody
	Low factor VIII	Autoantibody
	Thrombocytopenia	Marrow replacement, splenic sequestration
Dysproteinemia	Thrombocytopenia	Decreased marrow production
	Prolonged thrombin time	Inhibition of fibrin monomer polymerization
Amyloidosis	Factor X deficiency	Adsorption by amyloid
	Capillary fragility	Amyloid vascular infiltration
Systemic lupus	Lupus inhibitor[a]	Antibody to acidic phospholipids
	Factor deficiency	Autoantibodies to coagulation proteins
	Thrombocytopenia/thrombocytopathia	Autoantibodies to platelet glycoproteins

[a]Although the lupus inhibitor produces prolongation of clotting assay results and may exist coincidentally in patients with thrombocytopenia or clotting factor deficiency that predisposes to bleeding, the lupus inhibitor itself is characterized by a thrombotic rather than a hemorrhagic tendency.

Adapted from White GC, Marder VJ, Colman RW, et al. Acquired disorders of hemostasis. In: Colman RW, Hirsh J, Marder VJ, et al., eds. *Hemostasis and thrombosis, basic principles and clinical practice*, 3rd ed. Philadelphia: JB Lippincott Co., 1994.

TABLE 210.3. Acquired Disorders of Hemostasis Associated with Drugs

PLATELET FUNCTION DEFECTS
Aspirin
Nonsteroidal antiinflammatory agents
Heparin
Dipyridamole
Theophylline
Penicillins
Cephalosporins
Tricyclic antidepressants
Phenothiazines
Clofibrate
Antihistamines
Ethanol
Dextrans
THROMBOCYTOPENIA
Immune Destruction
Quinidine
Quinine
H_2 antagonists
Heparin
Phenytoin
Antibiotics
Methyldopa
Decreased Production
Ethanol
Thiazides
Chemotherapeutic agents
COAGULATION FACTOR DEFICIENCIES
Coumadin
Penicillins
Cephalosporins

deep intramuscular hematomas, retroperitoneal bleeding, or hemarthrosis. Bleeding may not start until hours after trauma and may recur at a later time. This occurs because, although initial hemostasis is normal (due to properly functioning platelets), an adequate fibrin clot is not formed. Normal fibrinolysis then results in delayed bleeding.

Intracranial hemorrhage is the leading cause of death in hemophiliacs, accounting for 33% of deaths. Only about half of hemophiliacs with intracranial hemorrhage have a history of recognized head trauma; even in patients with known trauma, neurologic manifestations may be delayed 1 to 6 days.[3] Therefore, hemophiliacs with any neurologic symptom or sign should receive a computed tomography (CT) scan, even in the absence of trauma. The same approach should be followed in patients with significant factor depletion due to an acquired disorder (e.g., coumadin therapy).

Several articles in the literature suggest that hemophiliac and anticoagulated patients who have no history of loss of consciousness or posttraumatic amnesia, and who have a normal mental status and neurologic examination, may not need a CT scan of the head. These studies have shown either no CT abnormalities or no clinical findings of neurologic injury on follow-up if CT not done.[4,7,9,17] However, these studies are retrospective and involve small numbers of patients. The physician should consider the patient's past as well as recent history, social circumstances, and the availability of follow-up care, and err on the side of obtaining a CT if there is even the slightest suspicion of intracranial injury or any problem with follow-up.

Some bleeding disorders combine features of both platelet and clotting factor deficiencies. Examples include DIC, liver disease, and severe vWD. vWD results from a deficiency in the complex of two proteins, factor VIII and vWF, that circulate together in plasma. vWF promotes adhesion of platelets to the subendothelium of damaged vessels and induces platelets to bind fibrinogen, which facilitates the platelet interactions essential for formation of the hemostatic plug. Factor VIII plays its part in the clotting factor cascade in the activation of factor X. Most patients with vWD have bleeding typical of a platelet disorder, but those with severe disease display both mucosal and deep bleeding.

The physical examination is directed toward identifying all bleeding sites and recognizing signs of underlying illness. Jaundice, organomegaly, adenopathy, and abnormal masses are sought.[22]

Laboratory Tests

When intelligently combined with a careful history and physical examination, a few basic laboratory tests are sufficient for the emergency evaluation of bleeding disorders: the activated partial thromboplastin time (aPTT), the prothrombin time (PT), and the platelet count. Other tests can pinpoint specific factor deficiencies or functional platelet disorders, but these assays are unavailable on an emergency basis and are unnecessary for emergency treatment.

The aPTT detects abnormalities of the intrinsic and common pathways and is prolonged by deficiencies of high-molecular-weight kininogen; prekallikrein; factors XII, XI, IX, VIII, X, V, and II; and fibrinogen. The aPTT is also prolonged in the presence of antiphospholipid antibody (formerly termed the *lupus anticoagulant*) and by heparin, coumadin, and fibrin degradation products. The test is performed by exposing plasma to an activating surface such as kaolin and adding calcium and the necessary phospholipid (partial thromboplastin). The time required for clotting in this test is usually 25 to 40 seconds.[12,22]

The PT reflects the activity of the factors of the intrinsic and common pathways. It is prolonged by deficiencies of factors VII, X, V, and II and fibrinogen; by coumadin; and by heparin in high concentrations. The test is performed by adding thromboplastin (a phospholipid-protein extract of lung, brain, or placental tissue) and calcium to the plasma. The time required for clotting is normally 10 to 14 seconds, shorter than the aPTT because the initial time-consuming steps of the intrinsic pathway have been bypassed with the direct activation of factor X by thromboplastin-activated factor VII. The PT is more affected by reduced levels of factors VII, V, and X than by decreases in factor II and fibrinogen.[12,22]

When the PT is used to monitor coumadin therapy, the PT ratio (the ratio of the patient's PT to a control's PT) has been superseded by the international normalized ratio (INR):[10]

$$\text{INR} = (\text{PT ratio})^{\text{ISI}}$$

The ISI is the international sensitivity index, which relates the thromboplastin's activity to that of a single batch of human brain thromboplastin, designated as the first international reference preparation by the World Health Organization in 1977. Using the ISI to standardize the PT ratio removes the variability in the determination of the PT caused by the use of thromboplastins manufactured from different organ sources and by different extraction techniques. The INR can be interpreted by the clinician as a reflection of the patient's degree of anticoagulation, whereas the PT ratio may reflect only the reactivity of the thromboplastin used to perform the test.

The thromboplastins now used in the United States are much less responsive to reductions in vitamin K–dependent clotting factors than those used from the 1940s through the 1960s. Hence, in the 1970s and 1980s, higher doses of coumadin were required to produce the desired PT prolongation; clinicians prescribed higher doses of coumadin to achieve the same laboratory value, but they were actually overanticoagulating their patients. The use of the INR has made it possible to avoid this error.

Another result of this change has been a reevaluation of the research that formed the basis for anticoagulant dosage recommendations. Revised recommendations published in 1989 use INR values and endorse lower PT ratios as the basis for safe and appropriate anticoagulation.[10] Ratios of 1.3 to 1.5 are now recommended for most conditions. Less intense anticoagulation is effective for the prevention and treatment of venous thrombosis and pulmonary embolism and for use in patients with tissue heart valves, atrial fibrillation, myocardial infarction, and valvular heart disease; more intense anticoagulation is appropriate for patients with mechanical prosthetic valves and recurrent systemic embolism (Table 210.4).

Patients with factor VIII and IX deficiencies (hemophilia A, B, and vWD) have a prolonged aPTT and a normal PT. Patients with a normal aPTT and a prolonged PT have a factor VII deficiency, because that is the only factor of the extrinsic pathway not involved in the common pathway. Isolated factor VII deficiency occurs as a congenital abnormality and is seen in the acquired form in mild liver disease and in the initial stages of oral anticoagulation or vitamin K deficiency. Although the aPTT, as well as the PT, are prolonged in the fully coumadinized patient, the PT is used for monitoring because of its simplicity. Both the PT and the aPTT are prolonged in moderate-to-severe liver disease, vitamin K deficiency, heparin and coumadin use, afibrinogenemia, and consumptive coagulopathies such as DIC.[12,22]

Specific factor assays can be done to confirm the diagnosis suspected from the history or from abnormalities of the screening PT and aPTT and to provide exact activity levels. However, these assays are rarely available on an emergency basis, and emergency treatment must be initiated without the benefit of such tests.

The platelet count is the first step in the evaluation of possible platelet disorders. Patients with counts less than 100,000/μL are considered thrombocytopenic; if platelet function is normal, the bleeding time increases in direct proportion to the decrease of the count below 100,000/μL. Patients with platelet counts below 5,000 to 10,000/μL are at risk for spontaneous bleeding. Platelet counts above 50,000 to 60,000/μL are usually sufficient to control bleeding caused by trauma or local pathology. However, the platelet count should never be the only criterion considered when assessing a patient's risk of hemorrhage. The underlying condition leading to thrombocytopenia must be sought, and platelet function must also be considered.[19]

No tests are available on an emergency basis that specifically screen for platelet function, as opposed to platelet number. A thorough history and physical examination, however, may suggest that the patient is at risk for a functional platelet disorder (e.g., alcohol or aspirin use). The bleeding time, a laboratory test that evaluates both platelet number and function, is determined by measuring the time required for bleeding to stop after a standard incision 1 to 2 mm deep and 5 mm long is made on the patient's forearm while an inflated blood pressure cuff on the upper arm maintains venous pressure at 40 mm Hg. The normal bleeding time is 4 to 7 minutes. If the platelet count is normal, a prolonged bleeding time suggests a functional platelet disorder.[22]

A few bleeding disorders produce no abnormalities in the available screening tests. Patients with vascular disorders, simple and senile purpura, factor XIII deficiency, and mild forms of other factor deficiencies (factor levels greater than 20% to 25% of normal) have normal aPTTs, PTs, and platelet counts.[12,22]

TABLE 210.4. Recommended Values for Anticoagulant Therapy Monitoring

Indication	INR	PT Ratio (ISI = 2.4)
Prophylaxis of venous thrombosis Treatment of venous thrombosis Treatment of pulmonary embolism Prevention of systemic embolism Tissue heart valves Acute myocardial infarction Valvular heart disease Atrial fibrillation	2.0–3.0	1.3–1.5
Mechanical prosthetic valves Recurrent systemic embolism	3.0–4.5	1.5–2.0

Adapted from Hirsh J, Poller L, Deykin D, et al. Optimal therapeutic range for oral anticoagulants. *Chest* 1989;95:7S.

EMERGENCY DEPARTMENT MANAGEMENT

Appropriate treatment of bleeding disorders depends on the physician's success in determining the most likely etiology of the bleeding.

The initial management of the bleeding patient includes airway control, if necessary, and adequate ventilation and oxygenation. If bleeding has led to hypovolemia, crystalloid resuscitation is started, and packed red blood cells given as needed. Local measures to control bleeding (e.g., pressure, packing, suturing, immobilization, gastric lavage) are used. As these basic measures are instituted, information from the history, physical examination, and laboratory tests can be combined to assess the probability that a platelet, coagulation factor, or mixed disorder is present.

If there is active bleeding typical of that caused by a platelet disorder and the platelet count is below 50,000/μL, platelet transfusions are given.[19] Active bleeding with a platelet count above 50,000/μL should prompt a search for another cause of bleeding, such as a functional platelet disorder or a coagulation factor deficiency. Controversy continues regarding the platelet count below which prophylactic transfusion to prevent spontaneous hemorrhage should be given. It is thought that platelets play an essential role in the maintenance of vascular endothelial integrity and that a minimum number are required to fulfill that function. Below this threshold, thinning and fenestration of the endothelium may lead to spontaneous bleeding. Studies suggest that 5,000 to 10,000 platelets/μL can maintain vascular integrity and that prophylactic transfusion should be given for values below that to prevent intracranial and other hemorrhage. However, factors such as fever, presence of an anatomic bleeding risk (e.g., a known GI lesion), rate of decrease of platelet count, presence of coexisting coagulation defects, and etiology of the thrombocytopenia affect the likelihood of bleeding and must be considered in the decision to transfuse. For these reasons, some experts recommend a higher level of 15,000/μL.[19]

There are several benefits to decreasing unnecessary prophylactic platelet transfusions, including reduced cost and disease transmission. More importantly, avoidance of alloimmunization decreases the incidence of unresponsiveness to subsequent transfusions and may enhance the success of bone marrow transplantation, which may be a lifesaving procedure in some patients.

Patients who need prophylactic transfusion or who are actively bleeding because of thrombocytopenia should receive 10 bags of pooled random-donor platelets (RDPs) or a single-donor platelet (SDP) unit, which is equivalent to six to eight RDPs. One RDP unit raises the platelet count by 5,000 to 6,000/μL in healthy adults, and probably less in ill, bleeding patients and those with platelet-destructive or -consumptive disorders. A posttransfusion platelet count should be obtained to guide further transfusion.[11,19]

Although immune destruction or consumption of transfused platelets may occur in patients with certain disorders, the temporary effect of the transfusion may be lifesaving in the actively bleeding patient; thus, platelets should be given while attempts are made to treat the underlying disorder. Two conditions are exceptions to this recommendation. In thrombotic thrombocytopenia purpura and in heparin-induced thrombocytopenia, platelet transfusions are considered to be harmful, because they can lead to increased microangiopathic thrombosis.[19]

Hemostatic defects in uremia are multifactorial, but are primarily related to defects in platelet function defects. Only in the severely nephrotic patient should significant coagulation factor deficiencies be suspected. Platelet counts are somewhat decreased, but rarely below 100,000/μL. The functional platelet defect is due to toxic retained metabolites, which can quickly reduce the effectiveness of newly transfused platelets. Dialysis at least partially reverses this toxic effect but may not be immediately available for the bleeding patient. Two pharmacologic adjuncts can help.[11] DDAVP can shorten the bleeding time within 2 hours in uremia. The effect lasts only 12 hours and decreases with repeated doses. The mechanism of action is not known. Conjugated estrogens decrease the bleeding time within 6 hours, and a 5-day course will maintain the effect for 2 weeks. Along with the administration of platelets, these should be considered primary therapy of bleeding in the uremic patient. If they fail, cryoprecipitate can be given. Its efficacy is controversial, and its mechanism of action unclear.

Maintaining a hematocrit greater than 25% also appears to decrease bleeding time in uremia. It has been proposed that an adequate number of red cells distribute the platelets closer to vessel walls, where they can fulfill their function.[11]

If the clinical evaluation suggests a congenital single-factor deficiency (e.g., hemophilia A or B), the location of the bleeding determines the therapeutic approach. Bleeding into the central nervous system (CNS), neck, or retroperitoneal spaces is life-threatening. All hemophiliacs with suspected bleeding in these high-risk sites should receive immediate factor replacement therapy with 50 U/kg of the appropriate factor, without waiting for the results of the aPTT, factor levels, or head CT or other scans. If the bleeding is in the joint space, oral cavity, GI tract, soft tissues, or muscles, 20 U/kg of factor VIII or 15 U/kg of factor IX is recommended. The half-life of factor VIII is 12 hours, so maintenance therapy should be infused every 12 hours or given as a continuous infusion. (Factor IX maintenance therapy is given every 24 hours.) Factor administration should be continued for 14 days if bleeding is located in the CNS, neck, or retroperitoneum.[4,8,14] Admission for observation should be strongly considered in those patients with injury or suspected bleeding in the high-risk sites.

Recognition of the role of pooled plasma products in the transmission of hepatitis, the human immunodeficiency virus (HIV), and other viral diseases to a majority of severe hemophiliacs spurred the development of the safer and more highly purified products available today. The emergency physician should be knowledgeable about selecting the appropriate product for each patient. No HIV, hepatitis B, or hepatitis C seroconversion has been reported in previously unexposed hemophiliacs since 1987. However, there have been outbreaks of thermoresistant and non–lipid-enveloped hepatitis A and parvovirus B19 infection associated with virucidally treated factor VIII preparations.[15]

Another problem associated with factor concentrates is the large amount of non–factor VIII plasma proteins included in the preparations. Repeated exposure to these contaminants has been associated with significant and progressive alterations in immune function (e.g., lowering of CD4 counts and development of anergy) in HIV-infected hemophiliacs. A purification method called "immunoaffinity," which uses monoclonal antibodies against factor VIII or vWF to separate the factor from the other proteins, produces an extremely pure product that should be used in the HIV-positive hemophiliac.[14,15]

Recombinant factor VIII (produced in hamsters) has been shown to have full hemostatic function and a normal half-life in humans. Although there has been concern that the recombinant factor may be more likely to induce the production of inhibitors than plasma-derived factor, these effects have generally been no greater than with any other factor VIII preparation.[14] Recombinant factor VIII products are usually more expensive than the other products.

The choice of appropriate factor VIII product for each hemophilic patient is one that should be made in concert with the patient's hematologist, if possible. All currently marketed factor VIII products are considered safe from the standpoint of HIV and hepatitis B and C transmission. High-purity products are those from which non–factor VIII protein contaminants have been removed. Intermediate-purity products contain plasma protein, but not viral contaminants.

Another approach to the treatment of non–life-threatening bleeding in patients with mild or moderate hemophilia A or with type I vWD is the use of DDAVP. The intravenous dose is 0.3 μg/kg, and the intranasal dose is 1 spray in children and 1 spray in each nostril in adults. A two- to threefold increase in factor VIII and vWF is seen, peaking about 30 to 60 minutes after the dose.[14]

Patients with types II and III vWD who have abnormal or absent vWF do not benefit from DDAVP, which simply stimulates factor release from the endothelial cells. A factor VIII preparation that also contains significant vWF, such as Humate P, must be used for these individuals.[14]

Antibodies against factor VIII, termed *inhibitors*, develop in 15% to 35% of hemophiliacs,[21] usually early in life and after relatively few factor VIII transfusions. These inhibitors render the patient unresponsive to factor VIII given to treat bleeding episodes. In patients with low inhibitor titers, regular or high doses of factor VIII usually continue to be effective. Patients with high titers of inhibitors often require use of porcine factor VIII at starting doses of 50 to 100 U/kg. Another approach is administration of activated prothrombin complex concentrates (aPCCs) (Autoplex T, FEIBA VH), which "bypass" factor VIII and are usually effective in stopping bleeding. However, repeated use is associated with thrombotic complications, and factor levels cannot be monitored to assess therapy.[14] Most recently, recombinant factor VII has become available and has been shown to be safe and effective in patients with inhibitors.[6]

Inhibitors also occur *de novo* in nonhemophiliac patients, those directed against factor VIII being the most common. Treatment of life-threatening bleeding is similar to that described previously, which uses high doses of human factor VIII, porcine factor VIII, aPCCs, and recombinant factor VII. To arrest synthesis of the inhibitor, steroids and immunosuppressants, such as azathioprine or cyclophosphamide, are given. Spontaneous remission is thought to be fairly common.[13,20,21]

Patients with complex conditions such as liver disease or DIC usually have deficiencies of multiple coagulation factors and, often, of platelets as well. If laboratory tests confirm these abnormalities and the patient is actively bleeding, fresh-frozen plasma and platelets are given to replace the needed components.

When heparin or coumadin is implicated as a cause of bleeding, a knowledge of the mechanisms by which it anticoagulates the blood helps the physician to treat the bleeding logically.[16]

Heparin acts immediately on administration by accelerating 1,000-fold the reaction by which factor II (thrombin) combines with the plasma protease inhibitor antithrombin III (AT III). The complex is inactive, and the AT III–bound thrombin cannot activate fibrinogen. Heparin is not consumed in the reaction and is available for further activity. Fortunately, the half-life of heparin is short, about 1 hour at usual doses and longer at higher doses. Therefore, when bleeding occurs in the heparinized patient, discontinuation of the drug leads to a rapid fall in the plasma heparin concentration. For severe bleeding, it may be necessary to administer protamine sulfate, a specific heparin antidote that combines with heparin to form a stable complex with no anticoagulant activity. One milligram of protamine neutralizes 100 U of heparin. The physician should estimate the amount of heparin remaining in the plasma and give the protamine at a rate no faster than 50 mg over 10 minutes.

The mechanism of action of coumadin is quite different. It interferes with the carboxylation of the vitamin K–dependent clotting factors II, VII, IX, and X in the liver. Factor synthesis is decreased 30% to 50 %, and biologic activity is decreased to 10% to 40% of normal because of inadequate carboxylation.[16] The onset of anticoagulant activity is delayed 8 to 12 hours because it depends on the gradual decrease in factor levels that is a consequence of the decreased rate of their synthesis, although their normal rate of degradation is unchanged. Factor VII has the shortest half-life (about 6 hours),[12] and some anticoagulant effect is noted as factor VII levels drop. However, the longest-lived of the four factors, factor II, has a half-life of 60 hours, so that 2 to 3 days are required before the full anticoagulant effect of coumadin can be expected.

The effects of coumadin cannot be reversed rapidly by discontinuing it, because time is required for synthesis of the factors. If severe hemorrhage occurs in a patient on coumadin, fresh-frozen plasma must be given to provide the needed coagulation factors immediately.

Because of the large volume and, possibly, repeated doses of fresh-frozen plasma needed to reverse an intensely anticoagulated patient, some authors recommend the use of aPCCs, which specifically contain the vitamin K–dependent coagulation factors.[11] There is a small risk of thrombosis associated with the use of this product because of the presence of activated factors. The risk is greatest in patients with liver disease or previous thrombotic events. Vitamin K, 5 to 10 mg by slow intravenous injection, should also be given to promote factor synthesis. One should always maintain an awareness of the risk of thrombotic complications occurring as a result of the reversal of anticoagulation, and careful judgment should be exercised.[5]

Because so many bleeding disorders are associated with underlying diseases, attention should always be directed to the potential associated condition while immediate lifesaving transfusions of blood components are provided.

DISPOSITION

An acutely bleeding patient should be transferred to another facility only if a service unavailable at the initial hospital can be provided at the second facility. For example, a child with a head injury and hemophilia would benefit from transfer to a hospital where neurosurgical services are available, despite the risk of transport. The ABCs must always be attended to and the hematologic parameters normalized as much as possible by transfusion of the appropriate components before transfer.

COMMON PITFALLS

- Bleeding is a common occurrence in the emergency department, and most patients have no bleeding disorder. In most cases, the history and a physical examination directed toward the identification of a congenital or acquired bleeding disorder constitute adequate screening. Such information should be recorded on the medical record of every patient with bleeding or injury.
- Delayed bleeding is characteristic of coagulation factor deficiencies. Because the initial stage of hemostasis is normal, these patients may appear to have their bleeding well controlled in the emergency department and may be discharged, only to experience life-threatening hemorrhage a few hours later. Factor transfusion should be given immediately in the emergency department to patients with potential bleeding in high-risk sites such as the CNS, neck, and retroperitoneal space without waiting for results of coagulation or imaging studies. Admission for observation should be considered in these patients.
- The emergency physician must use judgment in deciding whether to perform invasive procedures in patients with bleeding disorders. When possible, such procedures should be delayed until appropriate treatment has normalized clotting parameters.

References

1. Bick RL. Acquired platelet function defects. *Hematol Oncol Clin North Am* 1992;6:1203.
2. Colman RW, Marder VJ, Salzman EW, et al. Overview of hemostasis. In: *Hemostasis and thrombosis: basic principles and clinical practice,* 3rd ed. Philadelphia: JB Lippincott Co, 1994:3.
3. DeBehnke DJ, Angelos MG. Intracranial hemorrhage and hemophilia: case report and management guidelines. *J Emerg Med* 1985;8:423.
4. Dietrich AM, James CD, King DR, et al. Head trauma in children with congenital coagulation disorders. *J Pediatr Surg* 1994;29:28.
5. Ferrera PC, Bartfield JM. Outcomes of anticoagulated trauma patients. *Am J Emerg Med* 1999;17:54.
6. Gallistl S, Cvirn G, Muntean W. Recombinant factor VIIa does not induce hypercoagulability in vitro. *Thromb Haemost* 1999;81:245.
7. Garra G, Nashed AH, Capobianco L. Minor head trauma in anticoagulated patients. *Acad Emerg Med* 1999;6:121.
8. Gill JC. Therapy of factor VIII deficiency. *Semin Thromb Hemost* 1993;19:1.
9. Hennes H, Losek JD, Sty JR, et al. Computerized tomography in hemophiliacs with head trauma. *Pediatr Emerg Care* 1987;3:147.
10. Hirsh J, Poller L, Deykin D, et al. Optimal therapeutic range for oral anticoagulants. *Chest* 1989;95:5S.
11. Humphries JE. Transfusion therapy in acquired coagulopathies. *Hematol Oncol Clin North Am* 1994;8:1181.
12. Kottke-Marchant K. Laboratory diagnosis of hemorrhagic and thrombotic disorders. *Hematol Oncol Clin North Am* 1994;8:809.
13. Kunkel LA. Acquired circulating anticoagulants. *Hematol Oncol Clin North Am* 1992;6:1341.
14. Lusher JM. Transfusion therapy in congenital coagulopathies. *Hematol Oncol Clin North Am* 1994;8:1167.
15. Mannucci PM. Modern treatment of hemophilia: from the shadows toward the light. *Thromb Haemost* 1993;70:17.
16. Majerus PW, Broze GJ, Miletich JP, et al. Anticoagulant, thrombolytic, and antiplatelet drugs. In: Hardman JG, Limbird LE, eds. *Goodman and Gilman's the pharmacological basis of therapeutics,* 9th ed. New York: McGraw-Hill, 1996:1341.
17. Morgan LM, Kissoon N, deVebber BL. Experience with the hemophiliac child in the pediatric emergency department. *J Emerg Med* 1993;11:519.
18. Nemerson Y. The tissue factor pathway of blood coagulation. In: Colman RW, Hirsh J, Marder VJ, et al., eds. *Hemostasis and thrombosis: basic principles and clinical practice,* 3rd ed. Philadelphia: JB Lippincott Co, 1994:81.
19. Rintels PB, Kenney RM, Crowley JP. Therapeutic support of the patient with thrombocytopenia. *Hematol Oncol Clin North Am* 1994;8:1131.
20. Scott-Timperley LJ, Haire WD. Autoimmune coagulation disorders. *Rheum Dis Clin North Am* 1997;23:411.
21. Sohngen D, Specker C, Bach D, et al. Acquired factor VIII inhibitors in non-hemophiliac patients. *Ann Hematol* 1997;74:89.
22. White GC, Marder VJ, Colman RW, et al. Approach to the bleeding patient. In: Colman RW, Hirsh J, Marder VJ, et al., eds. *Hemostasis and thrombosis: basic principles and clinical practice,* 3rd ed. Philadelphia: JB Lippincott Co, 1994:1134.

CHAPTER 211
Disseminated Intravascular Coagulation, Thrombotic Thrombocytopenic Purpura, and Hemolytic–Uremic Syndrome

Kathleen C. Hubbell

A number of disease processes initiate tissue and vessel wall damage that leads to activation of the coagulation cascade and intravascular deposition of an obstructive mesh of fibrin strands. Red cells passing through these vessels are physically damaged, and the result is what is referred to as microangiopathic hemolytic anemia. Platelets and clotting factors are consumed to varying degrees, and may be responsible for thrombotic and bleeding complications that are usually more significant clinically than the associated hemolysis. With diffuse vascular involvement, these disorders often affect multiple body systems.

Disseminated intravascular coagulation (DIC), thrombotic thrombocytopenia purpura (TTP), and the hemolytic–uremic syndrome (HUS) are characterized by the combination of microangiopathic hemolytic anemia, thrombocytopenia, multisystem involvement, and varying degrees of coagulation factor depletion.

The presence of schistocytes on the peripheral blood smear should always alert the examiner to the presence of microangiopathic hemolytic anemia. The diagnosis is further supported by findings of decreased hematocrit, increased indirect bilirubin, decreased haptoglobin, and increased reticulocyte count. Thrombocytopenia is seen in DIC, TTP, and HUS; prolonged prothrombin time (PT) and partial thromboplastin time (PTT), decreased fibrinogen, and elevated fibrin degradation products are seen predominantly in DIC alone.

Microangiopathic hemolytic anemia can also be seen in malignant hypertension, eclampsia, collagen vascular disease, rejection of a renal allograft, disseminated carcinomatosis, and hemangiomas. In these conditions, anemia usually resolves with treatment of the specific disease.

DISSEMINATED INTRAVASCULAR COAGULATION

DIC is a condition of deranged and unbalanced activity of the clot-forming and clot-dissolving systems that normally function to maintain unimpeded blood flow through the body. DIC occurs only in conjunction with a variety of well-recognized conditions that have in common the release of procoagulant substances into the circulation. These conditions include sepsis; malignancy; trauma, including burns, crush injuries, and head injuries; obstetric conditions, such as abruptio placenta and retained fetus; and intravascular hemolysis, as seen with transfusion reactions[3,18] (Tables 211.1 and 211.2).

TABLE 211.1. Frequency of Conditions Associated with DIC

Condition	% of Total
Infection	26–29
Malignancy	18–24
Surgery	18–20
Liver disease	8–10
Obstetric	4–6
Trauma	2–5
Other	18–23

The procoagulant substances released activate the coagulation cascade through the tissue factor pathway, leading to the formation of thrombin. Thrombin plays its normal pivotal role in coagulation, cleaving fibrinogen to form fibrin, activating factor XI of the intrinsic pathway, and activating platelets. Thrombin is also involved in the body's normal method of terminating the clotting process, by inhibiting coagulation through a number of mechanisms. As the procoagulant substances are continuously released into the circulation as part of the patient's illness, they drive the coagulation cascade and the coactive inhibitory mechanisms, yielding both fibrin clots throughout the vascular system and large amounts of inactivated factors. The fibrin mesh of the clots traps platelets as they flow past. An eventual depletion of factors, inhibitors, and platelets occurs, causing hemorrhage.

Further contributing to this clotting disorder is activation of the fibrinolytic system. Plasmin attacks fibrinogen and fibrin, producing fibrin degradation products (FDPs). FDPs interfere with the polymerization of fibrin, which is necessary to create functional clots, and they cause a severe functional platelet defect.

In most patients, fibrinolysis does not keep pace with the intravascular coagulation, so the microvasculature fills with occlusive thrombi. The resultant tissue ischemia and necrosis manifest as severe organ dysfunction, which is the usual cause of death in DIC. Although bleeding can be dramatic and many physicians think of DIC as a hemorrhagic disorder, it is essential to realize that it is a thrombohemorrhagic condition. Interventions to arrest the clotting process must be a part of the therapy.[3,5,13,29]

These procoagulant substances that initiate the thrombohemorrhagic processes vary according to the underlying illness with which the DIC is associated. In sepsis, bacterial endotoxin and cytokines induce the production and surface expression of tissue factor by circulating monocytes and endothelial cells.[5,7,29] Many tumor cells also make tissue factor in large amounts. Severe trauma, intravascular hemolysis, and obstetric conditions such as abruptio placenta all release large quantities of tissue factor into the general circulation from damaged cells.

CLINICAL PRESENTATION AND DIFFERENTIAL DIAGNOSIS

DIC occurs in an acute, fulminant form and in a low-grade, chronic form. The acute form usually is associated with sepsis, trauma, transfusion reactions, and acute obstetric events. The incidence of DIC in severe sepsis is 18% and in septic shock, 38%.[29] Bleeding in these clinical settings should cause suspicion of DIC. Bleeding may occur from surgical or traumatic wounds despite local treatment and from venipuncture and arterial puncture sites. Petechiae, purpura, hemorrhagic bullae, and subcutaneous hematomas can be seen. Gastrointestinal, urinary

TABLE 211.2. Conditions Associated with DIC

INFECTIONS	MALIGNANCIES	SURGERY, TRAUMA
Bacterial	**Carcinomas**	Extracorporeal circulation
Gram-negative sepsis (very common)	Lung	Extensive surgery
Neisseria meningitidis	Colon	Severe burns
Neisseria gonorrhoeae	Stomach	Head trauma
Klebsiella	Pancreas	Trauma with shock, acidosis
Serratia	Breast	**OBSTETRIC**
Proteus mirabilis	Gallbladder	Abruptio placenta
Pseudomonas aeruginosa	Esophagus	Amniotic fluid embolism
Escherichia coli	Kidney	Saline or septic abortion
Salmonella	Melanoma	Missed abortion
Gram-positive sepsis (less common)	Prostate	Eclampsia
Streptococcus pneumoniae	**Leukemias**	**MISCELLANEOUS**
Staphylococcus aureus	Acute promyelocytic	Collagen vascular diseases
Staphylococcus albus	Acute myelocytic	Major transfusion reactions
Legionnaires' disease	Chronic myelocytic	Snake bites
Bacteroides	Eosinophilic	Heat stroke
Haemophilus meningitis	Hairy cell	Cardiac arrest
Typhoid fever	**Other**	Conditions of anoxia, acidosis
Shigella	Pheochromocytoma	Giant hemangiomas
Clostridium welchii	Neuroblastoma	Aortic aneurysms
Mycoplasmal	Sarcomas	
Mycoplasma pneumonia	Histiocytosis X	
Rickettsial	Polycythemia vera	
Rocky Mountain spotted fever		
Viral		
Varicella, disseminated		
Measles pneumonia		
Dengue fever		
Herpes simplex		
Influenza		
Yellow fever		
Rubella, congenital		
Chlamydial		
Psittacosis		
Fungal		
Aspergillosis		
Candidiasis		
Histoplasmosis		
Mycobacterial		
Tuberculosis		
Protozoal		
Malaria (*P. falciparum*)		

tract, and pulmonary bleeding are common. Typical patients with DIC bleed from at least three sites. They are often febrile and hypotensive. Signs of thromboses may be more subtle and manifest as abnormal mental status, dyspnea, abdominal pain, acral cyanosis, and gangrene.[3]

Patients with the chronic form of DIC usually have malignancy, liver disease, collagen vascular disease, or an obstetric condition such as retained fetus. Bleeding is rarely severe; instead, thrombotic disorders such as thrombophlebitis, pulmonary embolism, and nonbacterial thrombotic endocarditis predominate. Diagnosis of a thrombotic event, followed by recognition of typical laboratory abnormalities of DIC, may lead to the diagnosis of an occult malignancy.[3,18]

EMERGENCY DEPARTMENT EVALUATION

An appropriate clinical setting with a typical physical examination is highly suggestive of DIC and should spur the physician to seek laboratory evidence of the diagnosis. To support a diagnosis of DIC, results should show abnormalities in four areas: (1) depletion of coagulation factors; (2) depletion of coagulation inhibitors; (3) activation of the fibrinolytic system; and (4) evidence of end-organ damage.[3] The tests that are most sensitive and specific for detecting abnormalities in these areas may not be available on an emergency basis. Those that are available may not be sensitive or specific and must be used with an understanding of their limitations.

Examination of the peripheral blood smear will show schistocytes in 50% of patients with fulminant DIC.[3] Thrombocytopenia is usually evident on the smear, and large platelet forms (young platelets) are commonly seen because of increased platelet turnover.

Readily available laboratory tests that confirm depletion of coagulation factors include the PT and PTT and the fibrinogen level.[3] The PT and PTT are prolonged in only about 50% of cases of DIC, because activated factors and degradation products may interfere with these tests. Therefore, normal PT or PTT values do not rule out DIC. The fibrinogen level is less than 150 mg/dL in only 70% of cases, probably because it is an acute-phase reactant and its baseline level can be increased in acute illness. Other, more reliable tests exist but are not generally available in the emergency department.

The consumption of coagulation inhibitors can be measured directly by checking the antithrombin III (AT III) level, which is decreased in 89% of patients with DIC, but will rarely be available to the emergency physician.

Activation of the fibrinolytic system is best demonstrated by elevation of the D-dimer level, which is seen in 93% of patients with DIC and has an 80% specificity.[3,5] D-dimer is produced by the action of plasmin on cross-linked fibrin. FDPs, which are increased in 75% to 100% of patients with DIC, are not as specific for DIC as the D-dimer level.

Laboratory tests reflecting end-organ damage are lactic dehydrogenase (LDH), serum creatinine, and arterial blood gases. Other useful tests are hemoglobin and platelet count, urinalysis, pregnancy test, and imaging studies as guided by history and examination to search for the inciting illness. Platelet counts range from 2,000 to 100,000/μL, averaging about 60,000/μL.[3]

Thus, of the laboratory analyses available to the emergency physician for the diagnosis of DIC, the most sensitive is D-dimer. The PT, PTT, fibrinogen, and FDP should be ordered, but may be normal in patients with early DIC. Similarly, in cases of mild or chronic low-grade DIC, the PT, PTT, fibrinogen level, and platelet count may all be normal, because the bone marrow and liver can increase the synthesis and release of the clotting components. FDPs and D-dimer are elevated, however, and the peripheral smear is abnormal.

Appropriate coagulation studies should be drawn early in patients with sepsis, trauma, and other conditions with high risk for DIC. Laboratory abnormalities are usually present before severe hemorrhage occurs.

EMERGENCY DEPARTMENT MANAGEMENT

Treatment of DIC is an area lacking consensus and clarity. The heterogenicity of underlying causes has made it difficult to perform prospective clinical trials with results applicable to the individual patient. Treatment must be individualized and based on a current understanding of the pathologic basis of the condition underlying the DIC. An expanding choice of agents is becoming available as knowledge of hemostasis grows.

There is one area of universal agreement in DIC treatment. The underlying illness must be aggressively attacked with surgery, antibiotics, chemotherapy, or other appropriate therapy so as to stop the continuous release of the procoagulant factor and persistent activation of the coagulation cascade.[3,5,7,19] For example, in abruptio placenta, DIC terminates immediately upon evacuation of the uterus. Correction of hypovolemia, hypotension, acidosis, and hypoxia should also begin in the emergency department, and disease-specific interventions should be initiated promptly whenever possible.

If the patient is bleeding, transfusion with packed red blood cells and platelets to correct anemia and thrombocytopenia is indicated. A platelet count less than 50,000/μL should prompt transfusion in the bleeding patient, and the additional contribution of functional platelet disorders to the bleeding tendency should be remembered.[5] Although some clinicians fear "fueling the fire" of coagulation by giving fresh-frozen plasma (FFP) or cryoprecipitate to patients with DIC, this event has not been shown to occur in most cases, especially if concurrent therapy to arrest the consumption of coagulation factors is under way.[3,5,7,19] Six units of cryoprecipitate will raise fibrinogen by about 50 mg/dL. A level of at least 100 mg/dL is desired.

Other specific treatments for DIC are generally initiated after admission. A number of agents, including heparin, AT III, antifibrinolytics, protein C, hirudin, tissue factor pathway inhibitor (TFPI), thrombomodulin, and tissue plasminogen activator (TPA), have been investigated. None so far has been shown to decrease mortality in humans, although several are associated with improvement in coagulation abnormalities, lung function, and duration of symptoms.

Heparin has shown neither significant benefit nor harm in acute DIC. Some recommend it in conditions such as purpura fulminans, in which devastating thrombi are obvious. Many specifically recommend against its use in cases in which potential central nervous system (CNS) bleeding is of concern (e.g., head trauma).[3,7,19]

AT III appears promising. It has been shown to decrease duration of symptoms, improve coagulation parameters, improve oxygenation, and decrease intensive care unit (ICU) and ventilator days and the need for dialysis in patients with sepsis and trauma. It also has been associated with a trend toward decreased mortality. Most agree that it should be given in doses that achieve very high serum levels.[3,5,7,12,18]

Fibrinolytic inhibitors such as epsilon amino caproic acid (EACA) or tranexamic acid are usually contraindicated in DIC because the thrombotic aspects of the condition are those most associated with morbidity.[3,5,7,19]

DISPOSITION

The primary role of the emergency physician in the management of DIC is to be aware of its association with severe illness and injury, to perform the appropriate physical examination and laboratory screening tests to identify its presence, and to initiate immediate stabilization of airway, breathing, and circulation. The importance of immediate specialty consultation once DIC is suspected cannot be overemphasized, owing to the importance of treating the underlying cause. Antibiotics and replacement blood component therapy (as well as preparation of the patient for surgery, if needed) should be initiated in the emergency department.

The prognosis in patients with DIC is poor, even with proper treatment, which is not surprising, because the appearance of DIC signifies severe illness or injury and extensive tissue damage. In trauma patients, mortality rises from 14% in those without DIC to 59% in those with it. Mortality quadruples from 10% to 40% in meningococcal sepsis in children when DIC supervenes.[15]

Patients with acute DIC are very ill and should not be transferred from an institution that has facilities to care for them. However, because treatment of the underlying condition is so essential to the termination of the coagulation abnormalities, transfer should be arranged after initial stabilization if the hospital does not offer the required surgical, obstetric, or intensive care services. If transfer is anticipated, the emergency physician must ensure adequate airway, breathing, and circulation and should initiate appropriate blood component replacement. Other modalities, such as antibiotic therapy, should also be started prior to transfer, preferably after consultation with the accepting physician.

COMMON PITFALLS

- Failing to consider DIC in the appropriate clinical setting. Because of its association with severe illness or injury and its effect on mortality, signs of DIC should be sought in all patients at risk. The identification of such signs should prompt the physician to order the appropriate laboratory tests to confirm the diagnosis.
- Allowing the bleeding associated with DIC to distract the physician from the search for and treatment of the underlying causative illness. Any therapeutic plan that fails to include measures directed against the underlying cause is likely to be unsuccessful.

THROMBOTIC THROMBOCYTOPENIC PURPURA AND HEMOLYTIC–UREMIC SYNDROME

TTP and adult HUS appear to be closely related disorders that each present with some of the elements of the classic pentad of microangiopathic hemolytic anemia, thrombocytopenia, neurologic abnormalities, fever, and renal dysfunction. In TTP, neurologic abnormalities predominate, and renal dysfunction is seen less often; the opposite is characteristic of HUS. These syndromes occur twice as often in women and peak in the fourth and fifth decades of life.[17] U.S. mortality data from the years 1968 through 1991 seem to suggest that the incidence of TTP is increasing.[27]

There is an epidemiologically distinct form of HUS seen in children 6 months to 4 years of age, with an equal distribution between the sexes. This childhood illness is often preceded by febrile, diarrheal, or respiratory symptoms and has been linked to infection with cytotoxin-producing strains of *Escherichia coli* and *Shigella* that damage the renal vascular endothelium. About 90% of cases of pediatric HUS are associated with *E. coli* enterocolitis.[2]

The etiology of adult TTP-HUS is unknown. It occurs in association with other conditions, such as pregnancy; autoimmune diseases; cancer; bacterial and viral infections, including the human immunodeficiency virus (HIV) and HTLV-1; and in conjunction with the use of various medications, including ticlopidine, and chemotherapeutic agents, mitomycin-C and 5-fluorouracil in particular.[4,14,17,25] However, most cases occur in otherwise healthy patients, and no etiologic link has been convincingly drawn among the various associated conditions and TTP-HUS.

There is, however, a uniformity of pathologic findings in TTP-HUS. The characteristic lesion is the platelet thrombus found in the capillaries and arterioles of involved organs without evidence of vessel wall pathology or perivascular inflammation. The clot consists of platelets held together by von Willebrand factor (vWF) with very little fibrin deposition. This symptom corresponds to the laboratory findings of TTP, which include thrombocytopenia but no depletion of coagulation factors, as manifested by normal PT, PTT, and fibrinogen in 80% to 90% of patients. Focal necrosis and hemorrhage caused by ischemia are seen in the areas of occluded vessels.[17]

The pathophysiologic basis of the platelet thrombus is thought to be related to unusually large vWF (ULvWF) multimers seen in patients with TTP-HUS.[17] These multimers are produced and stored in the endothelial cells and platelets in all people, but once released into the plasma, they are reduced in size by a cleaving protease enzyme. It has been shown that some patients with TTP have congenital absence of this enzyme and others have an inhibitor to the enzyme.[8,16] The ULvWF multimers are more active in inducing platelet aggregation than are normal-sized multimers, so larger and more numerous platelet thrombi are formed. Both the platelet count and levels of ULvWF drop simultaneously during a TTP episode, suggesting that both are consumed in the clotting process. Patients in whom ULvWF is detectable after a clinical recovery from TTP are those who go on to have recurrent episodes of the disease.[17]

Two-thirds of patients have a single episode of TTP. One-third have intermittent, irregularly recurring episodes. A very small number has chronic relapsing TTP with frequent episodes that occur at regular intervals.[17]

CLINICAL PRESENTATION AND DIFFERENTIAL DIAGNOSIS

Although the pentad of symptoms and laboratory findings is considered classic in these diseases, it is important to realize that only about 40% of patients manifest all five criteria. In those with a diagnosis of TTP, 50% to 70% have neurologic dysfunction and 50% to 75% have renal involvement. Less than 15% have severe renal dysfunction with creatinine greater than 5 mg/dL.[14,17] Only about one-third of HUS patients have neurologic dysfunction. Fever has been reported in 60% to 100% of patients.[26]

The most frequent initial neurologic abnormality is altered mental status, which may be manifested by subtle personality change, lethargy, agitation, or confusion. Seizures, hemiplegia, aphasia, paresthesias, and visual disturbances occur in somewhat less than half of patients and more often in the later stages of the disease. Visual symptoms may be caused by thromboses in the CNS or in the retinal vessels.

Although 20% of patients may complain of gross hematuria, renal dysfunction is usually discovered only on laboratory studies. Bleeding (e.g., epistaxis, hematuria, gastrointestinal or vaginal hemorrhage) is seen in about 30% to 40% at initial presentation. Abdominal pain, usually without an identifiable source, may be part of the presentation in 30% to 40%.

This type of multisystem symptomatology requires the emergency physician to entertain a broad differential diagnosis that includes DIC, CNS infection, collagen vascular disease, bacterial endocarditis, and malignant hypertension, among others. History and physical examination directed to the identification of salient characteristics of each condition may narrow the differential. Laboratory studies can be very helpful in confirming the diagnosis of TTP-HUS, as the laboratory abnormalities of the pentad are more consistently present than the clinical symptoms.

EMERGENCY DEPARTMENT EVALUATION

Laboratory studies directed toward the etiology of fever, bleeding, and neurologic and renal abnormalities should be ordered. Complete blood count, platelet count, PT, PTT, fibrinogen, fibrin degradation products, D-dimer, and examination of the peripheral blood smear often suggest the diagnosis. All patients with TTP-HUS are anemic; 90% have hemoglobin less than 10 g/dL, and 40% have less than 6 g/dL. The peripheral smear reveals schistocytes and a decreased number of platelets; 50% of patients have a platelet count less than 20,000/μL. The PT and PTT are normal in 90%, and fibrinogen is less than 100 mg/dL in only 5% of TTP-HUS patients. In DIC, by contrast, tests reflective of coagulation factor consumption are usually abnormal.[17]

The LDH, blood urea nitrogen (BUN), creatinine, electrolytes, blood cultures, and computed tomography (CT) scan of the head can provide further important diagnostic information. Lumbar puncture should be considered, but severe thrombocytopenia may lead the clinician to defer this procedure. Serum LDH is uniformly and greatly elevated in TTP-HUS patients; median levels are often six times normal. This is a much larger elevation than is seen in other hemolytic anemias, suggesting tissue sources in addition to red blood cell lysis. LDH measurements show LDH5 from liver and skeletal muscle to be the isoenzyme most elevated.[6] It has been suggested that because LDH is greatly elevated in most cases and decreases rapidly in response to therapy, it should be considered a sensitive marker of TTP-HUS.[26] The combination of a greatly elevated LDH, microangiopathic hemolytic anemia, and thrombocytopenia is often considered sufficient to make a diagnosis of TTP-HUS, even in the absence of fever and renal or neurologic abnormalities.

Abnormalities of BUN and creatinine are universal in patients in whom HUS is diagnosed, and are seen in 40% to 50% of patients with TTP.

EMERGENCY DEPARTMENT MANAGEMENT

As always, airway, breathing, and circulation should receive primary attention. In febrile patients in whom infection is suspected, antibiotic therapy should be initiated after obtaining appropriate cultures in the emergency department. When the diagnosis of TTP-HUS is suspected on clinical and laboratory grounds, a hematologist should be consulted. The emergency physician should be aware that despite significant thrombocytopenia and clinical bleeding, platelet transfusions are contraindicated in TTP.[17] Several case reports note clinical deterioration following platelet administration, and it is assumed that more thrombi are formed in the tissues when additional platelets are supplied. Platelet transfusions are sometimes given as a stopgap measure in patients with intracranial bleeding demonstrated on CT.

The mainstay of current therapy for TTP is plasma exchange.[14,20] The specific mechanism of efficacy is unknown, but it is postulated that the enzyme needed to cleave vWF multimers is provided or an inhibitor removed by the exchange.[8] An infusion of approximately 10 U of FFP per 24-hour period should be started, and arrangements made for plasmapheresis if there is not prompt improvement. An exchange of one plasma volume per day is recommended initially, with an increase or decrease according to the patient's response. Seriously ill patients with coma, cardiac failure, or renal dysfunction should have plasmapheresis as soon as possible.[17]

The benefits of plasma exchange using FFP are clear. In a study comparing plasma exchange with plasma infusion, 47% of those receiving exchange had an increased platelet count after the first treatment cycle, compared with 26% of those receiving infusion. The death rate was four times greater in the infusion group.[20] Another study noted an 81% reduction in the risk of development of end-stage renal disease in patients who received plasma exchange, compared with those who did not.[11] Red cell transfusions are rarely needed, but should be considered if the patient is symptomatic from severe anemia.

Prednisone in doses of 1 mg/kg/d or greater is often given on the basis of historic precedent. Thirty of 100 patients were noted to have complete resolution of symptoms and laboratory abnormalities after receiving prednisone only, without plasma therapy.[3] Inhibitors of platelet function, such as aspirin, dipyridamole, sulfinpyrazone, and prostacyclin, are often given, despite conflicting reports of their efficacy.[17]

Therapies under investigation include aurin tricarboxylic acid, which prevents binding of ULvWF to platelets, and exposure of plasma from TTP patients to immunoadsorbent substances to bind antibodies or immune complexes.[9,17]

PEDIATRIC HEMOLYTIC–UREMIC SYNDROME

E. coli O157:H7 is now recognized as the leading cause of HUS in the United States, Canada, and Europe,[2] although cases associated with HIV infection, chemotherapeutic agents, and radiation therapy continue to be reported. The organism attaches to colonic cells and produces a so-called Shiga toxin that enters the circulation and destroys or damages endothelial cells, especially in the kidney and brain, where a specific glycosphingolipid receptor is found.[22,24] This cellular damage may lead to the release of the ULvWF multimers that are thought to cause platelet aggregation, which leads to vessel obstruction by thrombi.[17,22]

E. coli O157:H7 is transmitted by contaminated food and water. In the United States, the largest outbreak was associated with undercooked, contaminated hamburger meat. More recently, there have been outbreaks related to unpasteurized apple juice, lettuce, and alfalfa sprouts in the United States and to radish sprouts in Japan. Well water contaminated with run-off from cattle pastures led to infection of more than 100 people in New York in 1999. Person-to-person spread is also reported in institutions, childcare centers, and within families.[2]

Five percent to 14% of children with *E. coli* O157:H7 infection develop HUS with microangiopathic hemolytic anemia, thrombocytopenia, and renal dysfunction. Most laboratory abnormalities resolve within 2 weeks. Twenty-five percent of patients will have severe HUS with more than 7 days of anuria, more than 14 days of oliguria, or stroke. Five percent die, usually from thrombotic CNS involvement, which occurs in about 30% of pediatric HUS cases. Thirty-five percent to 50% of survivors have chronic kidney damage; 3% have end-stage disease.[2,24]

A number of studies agree that use of antibiotics to treat the diarrheal illness does not prevent HUS.[2] However, most are retrospective analyses and involve a wide variety of antibiotics administered by intravenous and oral routes. It has been suggested that the use of oral fluoroquinolones to treat the diarrheal illness is associated with a lower incidence of HUS, absence of Shiga toxin in the gut, and eradication of *E. coli* O157:H7 from the gut.[10,23] An orally administered Shiga toxin–binding resin is under study but, so far, has shown no efficacy in preventing HUS.[2,24,28]

The general management of pediatric diarrhea-associated HUS is supportive, with careful management of fluids and electrolytes and dialysis when needed.[28] Plasma exchange is generally reserved for those more severe cases that resemble TTP with CNS involvement.[21,24]

DISPOSITION

Patients with TTP-HUS require high levels of nursing care and blood bank support, and should be admitted to an ICU. If plasmapheresis is not available, transfer to another institution should be arranged while plasma infusion therapy is begun.

Response to plasma therapy generally follows a predictable pattern. Neurologic abnormalities are the first to resolve, usually within 3 days. LDH levels normalize in about 5 days, and platelet counts in 10 days. Renal function is the last to normalize, typically requiring about 2 weeks to return to baseline. It usually takes about nine plasmapheresis treatments to produce sustained improvement.[26]

Other treatments that may be used by the admitting physician, if there is rapid deterioration or no response to plasmapheresis, include immunosuppressive agents such as vincristine and splenectomy.[17,26] In one series of 44 patients, about 30% underwent splenectomy.

Relapse is fairly common. Most relapses (84%) occur within the first month after diagnosis, and 97% within 2 months. A small percentage of relapses occurs years after the initial episode.[1]

Since the advent of plasma therapy, overall survival in patients with TTP-HUS has been about 80% to 90%. Recovery from neurologic, hematologic, and renal abnormalities is usually complete.

COMMON PITFALLS

- Only about a third of patients have all five criteria of the classic diagnostic pentad of TTP-HUS at the time of presentation. The clinical components of the syndrome are variable in their appearance, and may be subtle or absent.

- The multisystem abnormalities seen in cases of TTP-HUS suggest a wide variety of possible diagnoses. Despite its rarity, TTP-HUS should always be considered in patients with neurologic, renal, or hemostatic abnormalities.
- No specific laboratory abnormality is diagnostic of TTP-HUS. However, the combination of microangiopathic hemolytic anemia, thrombocytopenia, an extremely high LDH, and normal PT and PTT is characteristic of the syndrome and distinguishes it from DIC.
- Administration of platelets is associated with deterioration in TTP-HUS.

References

1. Bell BP, Griffin PM, Lozano P, et al. Predictors of hemolytic uremic syndrome in children during a large outbreak of *Escherichia coli* O157:H7 infections. *Pediatrics* 1997;100:E12.
2. Besser RE, Griffin PM, Slutsker L. *Escherichia coli* O157:H7 gastroenteritis and the hemolytic uremic syndrome: an emerging infectious disease. *Annu Rev Med* 1999;50:355.
3. Bick RL. Disseminated intravascular coagulation: objective clinical and laboratory diagnosis, treatment, and assessment of therapeutic response. *Semin Thromb Hemost* 1996;22:69.
4. Brailey LL, Brecher ME, Bandarenko N. Apheresis and the thrombotic thrombocytopenic purpura syndrome: current advances in diagnosis, pathophysiology, and management. *Ther Apher* 1999;3:20.
5. Carey MJ, Rodgers GM. Disseminated intravascular coagulation: clinical and laboratory aspects. *Am J Hematol* 1998;59:65.
6. Cohen JA, Brecher ME, Bandarenko N. Cellular source of serum lactate dehydrogenase elevation in patients with thrombotic thrombocytopenic purpura. *J Clin Apheresis* 1998;13:16.
7. de Jonge E, Levi M, Stoutenbeek CP, et al. Current drug treatment strategies for disseminated intravascular coagulation. *Drugs* 1998;55:767.
8. Furlan M, Robles R, Morselli B, et al. Recovery and half-life of von Willebrand factor-cleaving protease after plasma therapy in patients with thrombotic thrombocytopenic purpura. *Thromb Haemost* 1999;81:8.
9. Gaddis TG, Guthrie TH Jr, Drew MJ, et al. Treatment of plasma-refractory thrombotic thrombocytopenic purpura with protein A immunoabsorption. *Am J Hematol* 1997;55:55.
10. Higami S, Nishimoto K, Kawamura T, et al. Retrospective analysis of the relationship between HUS incidence and antibiotics among patients with *Escherichia coli* O157 enterocolitis in the Sakai outbreak. *Kansenshogaku Zasshi* 1998;72:266.
11. Hollenbeck M, Kutkuhn B, Aul C, et al. Haemolytic-uraemic syndrome and thrombotic-thrombocytopenic purpura in adults: clinical findings and prognostic factors for death and end-stage renal disease. *Nephrol Dial Transplant* 1998;13:76.
12. Inthorn D, Hoffman JN, Hartl WH, et al. Antithrombin III supplementation in severe sepsis: beneficial effects on organ dysfunction. *Shock* 1997;8:328.
13. Mammen EF. Antithrombin: its physiological importance and role in DIC. *Semin Thromb Hemost* 1998;24:19.
14. Martinez FA, Pereira A, Ordinas A. Thrombotic thrombocytopenic purpura and hemolytic uremic syndrome (TTP/HUS). Description of a series of 35 patients. *Med Clin (Barc)* 1997;109:49.
15. Mertens R, Peschgens T, Granzen B, et al. Diagnosis and stage-related treatment of disseminated intravascular coagulation in meningococcal infections. *Klin Paediatr* 1999;211:65.
16. Moake JL, Chow TW. Thrombotic thrombocytopenic purpura: understanding a disease no longer rare. *Am J Med Sci* 1998;316:105.
17. Moake JL, Eisenstaedt RS. Thrombotic thrombocytopenic purpura and the hemolytic uremic syndrome. In: Colman RW, Hirsh J, Marder VJ, et al., eds. *Hemostasis and thrombosis: basic principles and clinical practice,* 3rd ed. Philadelphia: JB Lippincott Co, 1994.
18. Penner JA. Disseminated intravascular coagulation in patients with multiple organ failure of non-septic origin. *Semin Thromb Hemost* 1998;24:45.
19. Riewald M, Riess H. Treatment options for clinically recognized disseminated intravascular coagulation. *Semin Thromb Hemost* 1998;24:53.
20. Rock GA, Shumak KH, Buskard NA, et al. Comparison of plasma exchange with plasma infusion in the treatment of thrombotic thrombocytopenic purpura. Canadian apheresis study group. *N Engl J Med* 1991;325:393.
21. Ruggenenti P, Remuzzi G. Pathophysiology and management of thrombotic microangiopathies. *J Nephrol* 1998;11:300.
22. Sassetti B, Vizcargüénaga MI, Zanaro NL, et al. Hemolytic uremic syndrome in children: platelet aggregation and membrane glycoproteins. *J Pediatr Hematol Oncol* 1999;21:123.
23. Shiomi M, Togawa M, Fujita K, et al. Effect of early oral fluoroquinolones in hemorrhagic colitis due to *Escherichia coli* O157:H7. *Pediatr Int* 1999;41:228.
24. Siegler RL. Hemolytic uremic syndrome in children. *Curr Opin Pediatr* 1995;7:159.
25. Sutor GC, Schmidt RE, Albrecht H. Thrombotic microangiopathies and HIV infection: report of two typical cases, features of HUS and TTP, and review of the literature. *Infection* 1999;27:12.
26. Thompson CE, Damon LE, Ries CA, et al. Thrombotic microangiopathies in the 1980s: clinical features, response to treatment, and the impact of the human immunodeficiency virus epidemic. *Blood* 1992;80:1890.
27. Török TJ, Holman RC, Chorba TL. Increasing mortality from thrombotic thrombocytopenic purpura in the United States—analysis of national mortality data, 1968–1991. *Am J Hematol* 1995;50:84.
28. Trachtman H, Christen E. Pathogenesis, treatment, and therapeutic trials in hemolytic uremic syndrome. *Curr Opin Pediatr* 1999;11:162.
29. Vervloet MG, Thijs LG, Hack CE. Derangements of coagulation and fibrinolysis in critically ill patients with sepsis and septic shock. *Semin Thromb Hemost* 1998;24:33.

CHAPTER 212
Sickle Cell Disease

Donald M. Yealy and Larry D. Weiss

Sickle cell disease is a hereditary disorder of hemoglobin structure and function. Hemoglobin S (for "sickle") differs from the normal hemoglobin A, in that valine is substituted for glutamic acid in position 6 of the globin beta-chain. Both hemoglobins function similarly in the oxygenated state, but deoxygenated hemoglobin S tends to polymerize and gelate, leading to red cell sickling. Erythrocytes with less total hemoglobin or less hemoglobin S are more resistant to sickling, as are younger and smaller cells.

Individuals who are homozygous for the sickle cell gene (SS) are said to have *sickle cell disease.* Their erythrocytes contain at least 90% hemoglobin S. Patients who are heterozygous for the sickle cell gene (SA) are said to have *sickle cell trait.* Their erythrocytes contain both hemoglobin A (50% to 60%) and hemoglobin S (30% to 40%). Common sickle variants include *SC disease* (in which patients are heterozygous for both hemoglobin S and hemoglobin C) and *sickle-thalassemia.* These variants display lower red blood cell (RBC) levels of hemoglobin S and are associated with less morbidity than sickle cell disease.

An estimated 8% to 10% of Black Americans carry the sickle cell gene, and about one in 400 to 600 manifests sickle cell disease. The sickle variant diseases are less common and are regarded as less severe disorders compared with homozygous disease.[15,16] Most patients with sickle trait or variants have a normal lifespan and rare crises, although there is an increased risk of sudden death during exertion.

The anemia of sickle cell disease is due to both chronic and acute hemolysis. The red cell membranes are damaged with repeated episodes of sickling, leading to increased fluid and electrolyte permeability and fragility. RBCs have an average lifespan of about 10 to 20 days in SS disease, compared with 120 days in normal subjects.

During an acute painful crisis, the involved red cells undergo sickling. Initially, this is a reversible process, but after repeated episodes, the RBCs become irreversibly sickled and are destroyed. The microvascular circulation is slowed or obstructed because of the sickling, increased viscosity, and increased endothelial adherence of RBCs. Local tissue ischemia and acidosis lead to further sickling, and organ damage results because of tissue ischemia and infarction.

The clinical severity of sickle cell disease is variable. Some patients follow a mild clinical course with infrequent pain crises, but others are more severely affected. An increased frequency of painful crises, particularly chest crises (discussion follows), is associated with a shorter life expectancy.[15,16] Most homozygous patients develop painful crises before the age of 1 year, and by 5 years nearly all sickle cell disease patients have experienced a crisis.

Neonates and infants are often spared from crisis symptoms because of the protective effects of fetal hemoglobin (HbF), which persists in significant amounts during the first 6 to 12 months of life. Patients with sickle trait may develop painful crises when they undergo physiologic stress or spend time at higher elevations.

Infection is a leading cause of mortality in patients with sickle cell disease. The life expectancy of these patients is increasing because of aggressive medical therapy, particularly treatment of infection. Currently, most sickle cell patients survive into middle adulthood.[15,16] Patients with sickle trait, SC, and sickle-thalassemia all have near-normal life expectancies and suffer far fewer symptoms.

CLINICAL PRESENTATION AND DIFFERENTIAL DIAGNOSIS

Painful vasoocclusive crisis is the most common presenting problem for sickle cell patients in the emergency department. Although a proximate inciting event is not always discovered, several triggers have been identified. These include infection, systemic acidosis, dehydration, hypoxia, cold exposure, pregnancy, and physical or emotional stress. Identifying one or more of these factors helps guide therapy and may prevent sequelae. Episodes of painful sickle crises commonly last 48 hours to several days.

Bony pain is very common during acute vasoocclusive crises. In young children, pain and swelling often occur in the metacarpal and metatarsal areas, whereas older children and adults usually complain of back and proximal extremity pain. When evaluating a patient with suspected bony vasoocclusive pain, other causes, such as trauma or infection, must be considered.

The association between sickle cell anemia and *Salmonella* osteomyelitis is well described, yet staphylococci remain the most common pathogen causing osteomyelitis. Repeated episodes of bony ischemia can lead to aseptic necrosis, particularly in the femoral head[12] and carpal navicular areas, causing persistent pain that is frequently mistaken for acute vasoocclusion.

Abdominal pain, nausea, and vomiting are common with episodes of vasoocclusion. Local ischemia is thought to be the cause of these symptoms. However, a careful evaluation to rule out other causes of abdominal pain is mandatory. Because of persistent hemolysis, sickle cell patients develop calcium bilirubinate gallstones and symptomatic cholelithiasis. In addition, other causes of acute abdominal pain, including pancreatitis, appendicitis, renal colic, and peptic ulcer disease, should be considered before concluding that a vasoocclusive crisis is the sole cause.

The presence of active bowel sounds and a lack of high fever or signs of peritonitis favor a nonsurgical etiology. The risk of infectious hepatitis is higher in sickle cell patients because of previous transfusion therapy and an increased incidence of drug abuse. Jaundice does not necessarily indicate liver disease, because it is commonly due to chronic hemolysis.

The pregnant sickle cell patient with abdominal pain poses a diagnostic and therapeutic challenge. Identifying appendicitis or cholecystitis is more difficult because of the anatomic changes associated with pregnancy. Preterm labor, placental ischemia and abruption, and spontaneous abortion are also more common in sickle cell patients than in the general population.

Low-grade fever during a vasoocclusive episode is not uncommon. If the temperature exceeds 38°C, an infectious source should be sought. Viruses probably account for most infections, but because of functional asplenia, these patients are at risk for bacteremia, especially with encapsulated organisms such as *Streptococcus pneumoniae* and *Haemophilus influenza*. The functional asplenia of sickle disease is due to autoinfarction of the spleen, which is usually completed by school age in those with homozygous disease. Patients with sickle trait or sickle cell variants generally have normal splenic function and immunity.

Chest pain is also common in vasoocclusive crises.[1,13,15–17] Pleuritic pain is often due to vasoocclusion (with or without pulmonary infarction), although distinguishing it from an infectious etiology is difficult. Low-grade fever, hypoxemia, and leukocytosis are common in both vasoocclusive crisis and pneumonia. The radiographic diagnosis of an infiltrate is difficult because chronic interstitial changes are present in many patients and some new opacities represent atelectasis or infarction (the latter termed *sickle chest syndrome*). A productive cough, high fever, elevated total and immature neutrophil count, or Gram stain evidence of infection supports the diagnosis of pneumonia. The best clinical indicator of infarction is the absence of these infectious clues and the presence of occlusive symptoms in another area. *S. pneumoniae* and *H. influenzae* are the most frequent causes of pneumonia in sickle cell patients.[17] In adults, chest pain can also result from myocardial ischemia.

Focal or generalized neurologic signs and symptoms (including seizures) can follow vasoocclusion in the cerebral circulation, with both small and large vessels affected. Acute retinal ischemia with visual loss and "floaters" from vitreous hemorrhages secondary to vessel disruption are also reported in sickle cell patients.

Priapism is a manifestation of local sequestration and vasoocclusion and may present in all age groups. It often responds to vigorous medical therapy, including hydration, analgesia, local ice packs, or exchange transfusions. In refractory cases, surgical decompression is indicated. Testicular or ovarian ischemia can also result from vasoocclusion, presenting with pain in the affected area. Another complication of vasoocclusion is rhabdomyolysis, which requires aggressive fluid therapy to diminish the risk of acute renal failure.

Most patients with sickle cell disease and many with sickle trait or variants are at increased risk for dehydration because of a renal concentrating defect. Chronic renal failure (from repeated infarction and papillary necrosis) is common in sickle disease and may be associated with hypertension.

Besides painful vasoocclusive crisis, the patient with sickle cell disease is subject to other less common, episodic hematologic crises. These are categorized as sequestration, hemolytic, megaloblastic, or aplastic crises. In *sequestration crisis*, acute anemia, hypotension, and even shock occur because of sequestration of RBCs in the spleen. This often follows a viral illness and usually occurs in younger children with SS disease before autoinfarction, or in older patients with sickle cell variants. *Hemolytic crisis* can occur during a fulminant vasoocclusive episode, when large numbers of irreversibly sickled cells are lost. Severe anemia, with increased reticulocytosis and jaundice, is found. Marrow failure, resulting from either *megaloblastic crisis* (often from folate deficiency) or *aplastic crisis*, presents with a falling hematocrit and deficient reticulocytosis.

In addition to the organ ischemia induced by RBC sickling, sickle cell disease is frequently associated with enhanced coagulation, leading to arterial and venous thrombotic events. This is due to a variety of procoagulant syndromes seen more often in these patients, including protein C and S deficiencies and circulating antiphospholipid antibodies.[24]

EMERGENCY DEPARTMENT EVALUATION

The rapid evaluation and treatment of the sickle cell patient with acute pain is a formidable challenge. Vasoocclusive crises are common and may mask other serious pathology, while other types of sickle crises are less frequent and easily overlooked.

The diagnosis of uncomplicated vasoocclusive crisis is one of exclusion. A common but dangerous error is to attribute all pain in sickle cell patients to this cause. The initial investigation should seek evidence of an acute infection or other precipitating event. Chest pain can result from pneumonia, pulmonary embolism, pulmonary infarction, or myocardial ischemia; abdominal pain may reflect a surgical emergency. By the third decade of life, many sickle cell patients have undergone cholecystectomy and appendectomy, either because of demonstrable pathology or because abdominal pain during a previous vasoocclusive crisis suggested an acute abdominal emergency.

A focused history and examination are the cornerstones of the evaluation of sickle cell patients. A knowledge of the frequency and severity of past crises and complications, the medication history, and baseline laboratory values are helpful in the initial evaluation and treatment of patients with acute pain. Especially ominous are any new neurologic signs or symptoms, which require computed tomographic (CT) scanning, transcranial ultrasound, or (rarely) lumbar puncture.

Based primarily on unquestioned dogma, a complete blood and reticulocyte count (CBC and RC) are commonly ordered in sickle cell patients presenting for emergency department care. These can help screen for marrow failure (from sickle disease or hydroxyurea therapy), sequestration crisis, or infection. In a clinically uncomplicated vasoocclusive crisis that is similar to previous episodes in patients not treated with hydroxyurea, these tests add little to the clinical management. In other patients, especially those with suspected infection or nonocclusive crisis, the CBC and RC should be obtained.

When interpreting a blood count, a few points must be kept in mind. Most sickle cell patients have a persistent mild leukocytosis and a moderate anemia (hematocrit of 20% to 30%, although lower values are seen in some individuals). The total leukocyte count should be adjusted for nucleated RBCs to avoid factitious elevation. Because of ongoing hemolysis and anemia, the reticulocyte count is elevated (usually to 8% or greater) compared with normal subjects. An abrupt drop in the hematocrit suggests a sequestration or hemolytic crisis, while an abnormally low reticulocyte count suggests marrow failure. The erythrocyte sedimentation rate (ESR) is low in most patients with SS disease and is not helpful unless it is extremely elevated.[10]

The urine should be screened for evidence of infection or infarction, especially in patients with pelvic or back pain. If symptoms of urinary tract infection are present, with pyuria or bacteriuria, a urine culture should be obtained to help guide follow-up therapy.

Some authors believe that all sickle cell patients with acute pain deserve routine chest radiography to screen for occult infection,[17] but data validating this as a routine practice in low-risk patients are lacking. Clearly, fever, chills, or any pulmonary symptoms or signs suggesting a new abnormality mandate chest radiography, because the difference between sickle chest syndrome and pneumonia can be difficult to assess from clinical history and examination alone.[13,17] Because of the risk of bacteremia and sepsis, blood cultures should be obtained when there is evidence of pneumonia or pyelonephritis, or when high fever or leukocytosis occurs without an apparent source.

Other tests may have a role, depending on the clinical presentation. An electrocardiogram is indicated with chest pain or other symptoms suggestive of myocardial ischemia. Serum electrolytes, blood urea nitrogen, and creatinine determinations are sometimes helpful to assess hydration and renal function, but they are not mandatory in clinically uncomplicated mild-to-moderate crises. In cases of unexplained abdominal pain, a serum amylase, liver enzymes, abdominal x-rays, gallbladder ultrasound, or CT scan may be indicated.[21] In previously undiagnosed cases, a sickle prep and hemoglobin electrophoresis will confirm the diagnosis.

Although quantifying fetal hemoglobin levels may aid in assessing long-term prognosis, electrophoresis for this or other reasons is not helpful in the acute management of painful crisis. In patients with stroke, myocardial ischemia, or other arterial or venous thrombotic signs or symptoms, a hypercoagulable workup may be helpful, beginning with measurement of prothrombin and partial thromboplastin times.

An assessment of oxygen saturation is important, especially if there are any pulmonary or chest symptoms or abnormal physical findings. The pulse oximeter is minimally affected by sickle cell disease.[14] Arterial blood gas analysis is indicated when an acid–base abnormality is suspected or when oximetry signals are inadequate or otherwise unreliable.

EMERGENCY DEPARTMENT MANAGEMENT

In unstable patients, airway stabilization and circulatory assistance are the primary concerns. Otherwise, routine emergency department management can proceed while an appropriate diagnostic workup is begun. Treatment is usually supportive, because definitive treatment of crisis based on the underlying pathophysiology is still lacking. Often, the best treatment is rehydration and analgesia, with oral regimens preferred whenever possible.[1,4,23]

The choice of fluids is controversial. Patients with orthostasis or hypotension should receive isotonic saline initially. However, in the absence of significant volume depletion, hypotonic fluids have theoretical benefits. Experimentally induced hyponatremia decreases the mean corpuscular hemoglobin concentration and interferes with gelation of hemoglobin S. In one trial, desmopressin (DDAVP) combined with a diuretic and a low-sodium diet induced hyponatremia and decreased the frequency and duration of painful crises.[19] Despite these investigations, there are no clinical data to support the routine use of parenteral hypotonic solutions in vasoocclusive crisis. Outside of the United States, oral regimens are often used successfully. Irrespective of the fluid chosen, the physician must pay attention to the total volume administered to avoid iatrogenic pulmonary edema.[9]

Traditionally, all sickle cell patients received supplemental oxygen during painful crises. Although oxygen reverses some sickling *in vitro,* it has never been shown to affect the incidence, duration, or severity of clinical vasoocclusive crises. Oxygen can depress erythropoietin levels and reticulocytosis, potentially interfering with a natural compensatory response and paradoxically increasing the number of irreversibly sickled cells.[3]

Currently, there are no clinical data supporting or refuting the routine use of oxygen, although pragmatism suggests that those with clinically important hypoxemia are most likely to benefit. The latter has not been defined rigorously, although an oxygen saturation of less than 85% or a drop of greater than 5% from a known baseline is often used as a threshold at which to initiate therapy.

Achieving adequate pain control in vasoocclusive crisis is challenging.[11] By late adolescence, many patients with sickle cell disease require opioid analgesics in high doses to gain relief. Complicating the management of these patients are physician and nursing fears of drug abuse and secondary gain. Subjectively reported pain is generally the only tool available to measure discomfort; it is not possible to reliably identify "feigned" pain on clinical grounds. Optimal treatment of vasoocclusive pain is based on multifaceted, inexpensive regimens that offer the best chance of timely relief with a minimum of complications.

In addition, caregivers must encourage patients to participate actively in the process of pain relief, rather than reinforcing a passive "lie there and we'll take care of it" approach. This means a frank discussion about the goals of therapy (pain relief, albeit not always extinction, without harm) and the need for nonpharmacologic adjuncts, including counseling and behavior modification. The goals of pain management in sickle cell disease and metastatic cancer are analogous, because both are incurable diseases.[2] Analgesia must be titrated to need rather than to arbitrary ceiling doses, using regimens that rapidly achieve and sustain effective drug levels.

Oral analgesics are the mainstays for most patients with mild-to-moderate pain, with parenteral regimens reserved for those who cannot tolerate oral agents or are in severe pain. Aside from young children, most older patients presenting for care in the United States receive opioids in addition to hydration and acetaminophen. Because the pain of vasoocclusion is caused by ischemia, the analgesic effects of nonsteroidal antiinflammatory drugs (NSAIDs) are less prominent than in other syndromes in which prostaglandin excess is the major biochemical trigger (e.g., inflammatory or postoperative pain).[26] Additionally, the risk of renal failure may be higher than in non–sickle cell patients due to the renal arterial ischemia frequently present.[8] Given these considerations, NSAIDs are best avoided in these patients.[20]

Hydrocodone, oxycodone, morphine, and hydromorphone are good choices of an opioid for patients with refractory or more intense pain who can tolerate oral therapy. Other agents that have been found useful in the management of other chronic pain syndromes (e.g., antidepressants or phenothiazines) have been suggested for sickle cell pain, but their effectiveness is not supported by controlled trials.

For those who require parenteral therapy, there is no ideal opioid. The key is choosing an adequate dose and dosing regimen based on individual patient response; the ceiling dose is whatever relieves pain or causes side effects. Intravenous regimens (by either repeated injections, continuous infusion, or patient-controlled administration) offer ease of titration, rapid analgesia, and less risk of side effects.[6] Intramuscular injections should be reserved for selected cases when oral therapy is impractical and venous access unobtainable.

Meperidine is commonly used for sickle crisis but has some disadvantages, primarily related to its short duration of action and the accumulation of toxic metabolites, which can cause seizures. Morphine is inexpensive, but it is short-acting and frequently causes nausea, requiring the use of antiemetic agents. In patients who are not on outpatient opioid therapy, a mixed or partial opioid agonist (e.g., butorphanol, pentazocine, nalbuphine, or buprenorphine) offers analgesia with less euphoria and a ceiling on respiratory depression. For others, a longer acting opioid agonist (e.g., hydromorphone) may be an ideal choice.

A minority of sickle cell patients are deliberate opioid abusers. This has led some centers to initiate "contracts" with their patients in an effort to limit abuse while ensuring prompt and humane treatment when a painful crisis occurs. Often, the patient agrees in writing to take oral opioids only for severe pain and to contact a designated physician or emergency department during a crisis. The patient also agrees to not seek alternate opioid sources. This provides adequate care while limiting the total amount of opioid prescribed over a specified period.

For documented or suspected bacterial infections, a broad-spectrum antibiotic should be administered early while awaiting culture results. Sickle cell patients should take folic acid supplements daily to avoid megaloblastic crisis.

Transfusion therapy is indicated in selected sickle syndromes. In patients with priapism or aplastic, sequestration, or hemolytic crisis, exchange transfusion is preferable to simple transfusion because it avoids the risk of iron overload and is generally more effective. With central nervous system (CNS) vasoocclusion, exchange transfusion can reverse some neurologic symptoms and lower the incidence of recurrence.[7] Prophylactic transfusion is best reserved for patients requiring immediate surgery and for those in impending or active labor. Anemia alone is not an indication for emergency transfusion, in the absence of signs or symptoms of deficient oxygen delivery to the heart or brain.

Several new approaches to the treatment of SS disease are currently under evaluation. Hydroxyurea disrupts RBC endothelial adhesion and enhances hemoglobin F production and can diminish the frequency and severity of crises.[18,22] The long-term safety of this treatment is still not well defined, with marrow failure a limiting side effect. Other methods of altering hemoglobin production, through gene manipulation, bone marrow transplantation, or a combination of hydroxyurea and recombinant erythropoietin, show promise in reducing the frequency of clinical vasoocclusive crises.[18]

High-dose corticosteroids (dexamethasone 0.3 mg/kg every 12 hours for three doses) may augment inpatient analgesic regimens in children and adolescents with sickle crisis, especially the sickle chest syndrome.[1a,5] The mechanism and true effect of steroids are debated, and there are currently no data confirming their utility in the treatment in acute sickle crisis. Similarly, inhaled nitric oxide may provide pain relief when used together with standard therapies, especially with chest syndromes, but it remains under investigation.

DISPOSITION

Patients with uncomplicated painful crises who are adequately hydrated and obtain sufficient pain relief in the emergency department can be discharged with close follow-up. There is no absolute rule to determine how long an "adequate" analgesia and hydration trial in the emergency department should be, because individual patients, physicians, and local resources vary. If pain relief is obtained in an uncomplicated vasoocclusive crisis, oral analgesics should be prescribed for 3 to 5 days, because crises commonly last this long. Each patient should be encouraged to obtain further care from the same institution or a single physician (or group) to ensure continuity.

The inability to control pain is the most common indication for admission in adults. Patients with proven or suspected sequestration, aplastic, or hemolytic crisis require admission. The presence of any new neurologic sign or symptom, priapism, or an acute abdomen also mandates hospitalization.

In general, bacterial infection mandates admission, because it is largely through the aggressive treatment of infections that the life expectancy for SS patients has been increased. Two groups of patients may be discharged home if close outpatient follow-up within 24 hours can be arranged: adults with a minor respiratory tract infection and non–toxic-appearing children (age 6 months to 12 years) with fever less than 40°C, no clinical evidence of pneumonia or pyelonephritis, and a leukocyte count between 5,000 and 30,000.[25] In the latter group, blood cultures should be obtained to screen for bacteremia, and ceftriaxone (50 mg/kg i.m.) should be given before discharge. In addition to these specific instances, admission is indicated for patients with fever, unexplained leukocytosis (especially with immature forms), or uncertain compliance with follow-up schedules.

Because continuity of care is especially important in sickle cell disease, the patient's primary physician should be contacted during the emergency department visit. Consultation with the internal medicine or hematology service is advisable for routine admissions, with other subspecialty consultation obtained as needed.

Finally, patients should be counseled to avoid any sympathomimetic drugs (including over-the-counter decongestants and illicit cocaine) and alcohol (which may suppress a stressed marrow). Pneumococcal and influenza vaccines can be offered or made available in follow-up, along with potential long-term oral penicillin prophylaxis for those with frequent bacterial infections .

COMMON PITFALLS

- Do not assume that abdominal pain is due to a vasoocclusive crisis without considering other causes, especially surgical pathology.
- It is easy to overdiagnose pneumonia in sickle cell patients, but underdiagnosis can be fatal. Because an acute infiltrate often represents an infarct rather than infection, other signs and symptoms of pneumonia should be sought. If the diagnosis is not clear, it is prudent to err on the side of caution and begin antibiotic therapy.
- Some complications of sickle disease are mistaken for crisis pain (e.g., osteomyelitis, aseptic necrosis of bone).
- Although transfusions are ordered too frequently and unnecessarily, exchange transfusion therapy is often not started early enough in the setting of neurologic changes or priapism.
- Humane and adequate analgesia should be provided to each patient, with precautions to avoid abuse. Many patients benefit by entering into a written treatment contract with their primary care providers and emergency department staff.
- Patients should be educated about avoiding triggers, maintaining hydration, and initiating self-titrated analgesia early to limit the need for recurrent emergency department visits.

References

1. Athanasou NA, Hatton C, McGee JO, et al. Vascular occlusion and infarction in sickle cell crisis and the sickle chest syndrome. *J Clin Pathol* 1985;138:659.

1a. Bernini JC, Rogers ZR, Sandler ES, et al. Beneficial effect of intravenous dexamethasone in children with mild to moderate severe acute chest syndrome complicating sickle cell disease. *Blood* 1998;92:3082.

2. Brookoff D, Polomano R. Treating sickle cell pain like cancer pain. *Ann Intern Med* 1992;116:364.
3. Embury SH, Garcia JF, Mohandas N, et al. Effects of oxygen inhalation on endogenous erythropoietin kinetics, erythropoiesis, and properties of blood cells in sickle cell anemia. *N Engl J Med* 1984;311:291.
4. Friedman EW, Webber AB, Osborn HH, et al. Oral analgesia for treatment of painful crisis in sickle cell anemia. *Ann Emerg Med* 1986;15:787.
5. Griffin TC, McIntire D, Buchanan GR. High-dose intravenous methylprednisolone therapy for pain in children and adolescents with sickle cell disease. *N Engl J Med* 1994;330:733.
6. Gonzalez ER, Bahal N, Hansen LA, et al. Intermittent injection vs patient-controlled analgesia for sickle cell crisis pain. Comparison of patients in the emergency department. *Arch Intern Med* 1991;151:1373.
7. Haruda F, Friedman JH, Ganti SR, et al. Rapid resolution of organic mental syndrome in sickle cell anemia in response to exchange transfusion. *Neurology* 1981;31:1015.
8. Hardwick WE, Givens TG, Monroe KW, et al. Effect of ketorolac in pediatric sickle vaso-occlusive pain crisis. *Pediatr Emerg Care* 1999;15:179.
9. Haynes J, Allison RC. Pulmonary edema: complication in the management of sickle cell pain crisis. *Am J Med* 1986;80:833.
10. Lawrence C, Fabry ME. Erythrocyte sedimentation rate during steady state and painful crisis in sickle cell anemia. *Am J Med* 1986;81:801.
11. Maxwell K, Streetly A, Bevan D. Experiences of hospital care and treatment seeking for pain from sickle cell disease: a qualitative study. *BMJ* 1999;318:1585.
12. Milner PF, Kraus AP, Sebes JI, et al. Sickle cell disease as a cause of osteonecrosis of the femoral head. *N Engl J Med* 1991;325:1476.
13. Morris C, Vichinsky E, Styles L. Clinician assessment for acute chest syndrome in febrile patients with sickle cell disease: is it accurate enough? *Ann Emerg Med* 1999;34:64.
14. Ortiz FO, Aldrich TK, Nagel RL, et al. Accuracy of pulse oximetry in sickle cell disease. *Am J Respir Crit Care Med* 1999;159:447.
15. Platt OS, Brambilla DJ, Rosse WF, et al. Mortality in sickle cell disease. Life expectancy and risk factors for early death. *N Engl J Med* 1994;330:1639.
16. Platt OS, Thorington BD, Brambilla DJ, et al. Pain in sickle cell disease. Rates and risk factors. *N Engl J Med* 1991;325:11.
17. Pollack CV, Jorden RC, Kolb JC. Usefulness of empiric chest radiography and urinalysis testing in adults with acute sickle cell pain crisis. *Ann Emerg Med* 1991;20:1210.
18. Rodgers GP, Dover GJ, Uyesaka N, et al. Augmentation by erythropoietin of the fetal-hemoglobin response to hydroxyurea in sickle cell disease. *N Engl J Med* 1993;328:73.
19. Rosa RM, Bierer BE, Thomas R et al. A study of induced hyponatremia in the prevention and treatment of sickle cell crisis. *N Engl J Med* 1980;303:1138.
20. Schaller S, Kaplan BS. Acute nonoliguric renal failure in children associated with nonsteroidal antiinflammatory agents. *Pediatr Emerg Care* 1998;14:416.
21. Serafini AN, Spolianski G, Skafianakis GN, et al. Diagnostic studies in patients with sickle cell anemia and acute abdominal pain. *Arch Intern Med* 1987;147:1061.
22. Steinberg MH. Management of sickle cell disease. *N Engl J Med* 1999;340:1021.
23. Ware MA, Hambleton I, Ochaya I, et al. Day-care management of sickle cell painful crisis in Jamaica: a model applicable elsewhere? *Br J Haematol* 1999;104:93.
24. Westerman MP, Green D, Gilman-Sachs A, et al. Antiphospholipid antibodies, protein C and S, and coagulation changes in sickle cell disease. *J Lab Clin Med* 1999;134:352.
25. Williams JA, Flynn PM, Harris S, et al. A randomized study of outpatient treatment with ceftriaxone for selected febrile children with sickle cell disease. *N Engl J Med* 1993;329:472.
26. Wright SW, Norris RL, Mitchell TR. Ketorolac for sickle cell vaso-occlusive crisis pain in the emergency department: lack of a narcotic sparing effect. *Ann Emerg Med* 1992;21:925.

CHAPTER 213
Anemia

Louis S. Binder

Anemia is defined as a decrease in the number of circulating red blood cells, with a concomitant decrease in the capacity of the blood to carry oxygen to tissues. Anemia is a manifestation of disease rather than a diagnostic entity in and of itself.

Anemia can be classified into disorders of decreased red cell production, disorders of increased red cell destruction, and anemia resulting from blood loss.[8,12] Each of these diagnostic groups has its own clinical presentation and differential diagnosis (Table 213.1) and, in general, requires its own approach to emergency department evaluation and management.

Anemia of any cause may present acutely or chronically, and the aggressiveness of intervention and management depends on the acuteness of onset and on the severity of the clinical presentation. For example, anemia secondary to acute gastrointestinal blood loss may require vigorous fluid resuscitation, transfusion therapy, and intensive care management; anemia secondary to chronic occult gastrointestinal bleeding leads to a well-compensated iron deficiency anemia that can be evaluated and treated on an outpatient basis.[1,11,14]

Defective red blood cell production may be due to interruption in the availability or synthesis of any of the three moieties of the hemoglobin molecule: iron, heme, and globin. Hence, anemia may result from iron deficiency, from toxins or enzymatic deficits that interfere with heme synthesis, or from genetic defects in globin synthesis.[12,14] Disorders and deficiencies that affect the proliferation of erythroid stem cells in the bone marrow may also result in anemia from decreased red cell production.[3,7,15]

Red cell destruction may result from either intrinsic or extrinsic causes. Intrinsic abnormalities of hemoglobin, enzymes, or red cell membranes may result in hemolytic anemia.[18] Extrinsic destruction may be due to immunologic, mechanical, or environmental causes, or to hypersequestration (hypersplenism).[6,16,18]

Blood loss resulting in anemia may be acute or chronic and may originate from intraperitoneal, retroperitoneal, pelvic, pleural, gynecologic, or gastrointestinal sources.[8,11]

CLINICAL PRESENTATION

Patients with anemia secondary to acute blood loss present with hypovolemia. A source of blood loss may be readily identifiable on clinical evaluation; menstrual blood loss and losses from the gastrointestinal tract are the most common sources for occult bleeding if the locus is unclear.[8,11] A history of underlying disease (e.g., cirrhosis, bleeding diathesis, malignancy, or infection) or of medication use (e.g., use of salicylates, nonsteroidal antiinflammatory drugs, or anticoagulants) may be useful in guiding initial evaluation and management. Hypovolemia may be relatively well tolerated in the young patient without underlying disease, but can be a significant stress to elderly or chronically ill individuals whose compensatory mechanisms may be overwhelmed and whose tissue perfusion may be marginal at baseline.[13]

Patients with anemia secondary to chronic blood loss or to decreased red cell production often present with progressive fatigue, malaise, and a "washed-out" feeling. Dizziness, dyspnea on exertion, decreased exercise tolerance, or exacerbation of congestive heart failure may also be prominent symptoms. Gastrointestinal symptoms such as anorexia or nausea may reflect compensatory hypoperfusion of the splanchnic bed. Patients with asymptomatic underlying atherosclerotic vascular disease may present with angina pectoris, claudication, syncope, or focal neurologic deficits when decreased oxygen-carrying capacity is superimposed on local ischemia from vascular lesions. Other important historic information includes ethnicity and family history (predisposition to certain hemoglobinopathies and pernicious anemia), drug use, dietary history, use of ethanol, recent hospitalization (anemia of chronic disease is common in hospitalized patients), and history of underlying disease (renal, hepatic, thyroid, collagen vascular, or neoplastic disease; previous anemia; or recurrent jaundice).[4,5,12,13,17,18]

Pallor of the skin or mucous membranes is the cardinal sign of anemia, although it may be difficult to ascertain in some patients. Jaundice is suggestive of a hemolytic process. Tachycardia with a wide pulse pressure and hyperdynamic precordium (reflecting increased cardiac output) and a systolic ejection murmur may be present.[8,13]

Petechia and purpura may indicate a concomitant thrombocytopenia. Signs of chronic disease (rheumatologic, endocrine, hepatic, or neoplastic disease) manifest as lymphadenopathy, rash, thyromegaly, myxedema, or the stigmata of liver failure.[4,17] Hepatosplenomegaly may suggest underlying disease or extramedullary hematopoiesis.[12]

Other signs may suggest specific causes of anemia. Vitamin B_{12} deficiency affects exfoliating cell populations and demyelination of the dorsal columns, resulting in atrophy and tenderness of mucous membranes (particularly glossitis) and stocking–glove anesthesia of the distal lower extremities with impaired position and vibratory sense.[2,5]

The symptoms, signs, and laboratory findings of anemia may be the initial presenting manifestations of pancytopenia.[3,7,15] The etiology of pancytopenia is multifactorial. Pancytopenia is most commonly idiopathic (50%), but may result from chemical and physical agents, autoimmunity, or vitamin B_{12} or folic acid deficiency. Pancytopenia may follow viral illness, including upper respiratory infection, hepatitis, Epstein-Barr infection, and human immunodeficiency virus infection.[15] It may also be associated with hypersplenism, myelodysplasia, bone marrow failure, or marrow replacement.[15] Clinically, pancytopenia may present as a viral illness, preceding the symptomatic presentation of anemia over several weeks, or as an insidious presentation of anemia with clinical evidence of thrombocytopenia (petechia, purpura, or mucous membrane bleeding).[3,7,15]

Patients with anemia secondary to acute hemolysis are likely to present with signs and symptoms similar to those seen with mild chronic anemia. In more severe presentations, there may be jaundice and dark urine. Fever, prostration, abdominal and back pain, and hemoglobinuria suggest acute intravascular hemolysis, similar to that associated with transfusion reaction.[8,12] A family history of anemia suggests an intrinsic cause of hemolysis, whereas exposure to drugs or toxins suggests an extrinsic cause.[18] Immunologic destruction of red blood cells may be due to autoantibodies.[18] Mechanical destruction is seen in some patients with prosthetic heart valves.[6,16,18] Disseminated intravascular coagulation leading to microangiopathic hemolytic anemia is suggested by diffuse bleeding.[6,16] A finding of hepatosplenomegaly may suggest either sequestration or an autoimmune process.[18]

DIFFERENTIAL DIAGNOSIS

A complete differential diagnosis is presented in Table 213.1.

EMERGENCY DEPARTMENT EVALUATION AND MANAGEMENT

After anemia is identified by a complete blood count or hematocrit determination in the emergency department, further laboratory evaluation includes the measurement of red blood cell indices and reticulocyte count. Examination of a peripheral smear may show heterogeneity of cells, evidence of hemolysis, basophilic stippling, ringed sideroblasts, or hypersegmented leukocytes.[8,12] Additional diagnostic tests are normally neither necessary nor available in the emergency department. However, serum iron, total iron-binding capacity (TIBC), and serum ferritin determinations should be considered in hypochromic, microcytic anemia; folate and vitamin B_{12} levels, liver function tests, and thyroid function tests in macrocytic anemia; and direct and indirect Coombs' tests, fractionated serum bilirubin count, and plasma and urine tests for free hemoglobin in hemolytic anemia.[1,5,8,12,14,18] Inpatient evaluation may include further laboratory evaluation for specific disease and a bone marrow biopsy for evaluation of any unexplained anemia or pancytopenia.[3,7,8,12,15]

Potential diagnostic errors of importance include the following:

1. Not suspecting acute blood loss and impending hypovolemic shock with any unexplained normocytic normochromic anemia
2. Confusing anemia with other entities that also cause constitutional symptoms (e.g., uremia, collagen vascular disease, fluid and electrolyte imbalance, infections, drug effects)
3. Confusing iron deficiency anemia, which presents with low iron, increased TIBC, and low ferritin, with anemia of chronic disease, which presents with low iron, low TIBC, and normal ferritin associated with a chronic disease or recent hospitalization[1,4,14,17]
4. Confusing hemolytic anemia with other entities that also cause acute jaundice (particularly acute hepatitis)

TABLE 213.1. Differential Diagnosis of Anemia

ANEMIA SECONDARY TO BLOOD LOSS (ACUTE OR CHRONIC)
Intraperitoneal
Retroperitoneal
Pelvic
Urinary tract
Gastrointestinal tract
Gynecologic (vaginal bleeding, placenta previa, abruption)
Epistaxis
Hemoptysis
External bleeding
Drug-related (coumadin, heparin)
Traumatic
ANEMIA SECONDARY TO DECREASED RBC PRODUCTION (Insidious-Onset, Decreased Reticulocyte Count)
Hypochromic/Microcytic
Iron deficiency
Thalassemia
Sideroblastic (including lead)
Chronic disease (infection, chronic inflammation, neoplasm, diabetes, liver failure, uremia, thyroid disease)
Macrocytic
Hypothyroidism
Folic acid deficiency
Chemotherapy, radiotherapy, immunosuppressive therapy
Liver disease
Vitamin B_{12} deficiency
Scurvy
Normocytic
Primary bone marrow disorder (aplastic anemia, myeloid metaplasia, myelofibrosis, myelophthistic anemia)
Secondary bone marrow disease (endocrinopathy, uremia, chronic inflammation, liver disease, ethanol ingestion)
ANEMIA SECONDARY TO INCREASED RBC DESTRUCTION (Increased Reticulocyte Count, Free Hemoglobin, RBC Fragmentation)
Intrinsic
Enzyme defect (G6PD, pyruvate kinase)
Membrane abnormality (spherocytosis, elliptocytosis, spur cell, paroxysmal nocturnal hemoglobinuria)
Hemoglobin abnormality (hemoglobinopathy, thalassemia)
Extrinsic
Immunologic (alloantibody, autoantibody, cold agglutinins, e.g., mononucleosis)
Neoplastic (especially leukemia, lymphoma)
Collagen vascular (lupus, rheumatoid arthritis, periarteritis nodosa)
Infections (mycoplasma, syphilis, malaria, bartonella, viral)
Other (thyroid disease, ulcerative colitis)
Mechanical (microangiopathic hemolytic anemia, prosthetic valve)
Abnormal sequestration (hypersplenism)
Environmental (drugs, toxins, hyperthermia, drowning)

Modified from Hamilton GC, Braen GR, Anemia and white blood cell disorders. In: Rosen P, Barkin RM, Braen GR, et al., eds. *Emergency medicine: concepts and clinical practice*. 3rd ed. St. Louis: Mosby, 1992:1673.

5. Overlooking pancytopenia by focusing on a clinical picture of anemia and low hemoglobin, while neglecting findings of leukopenia and thrombocytopenia

The need for rapid intervention in both prehospital and emergency department patients is limited to identifying and treating hypovolemic shock. For certain anemic patients, treatment is best begun in the emergency department without waiting for definitive outpatient evaluation. Anemia of pregnancy is treated with prenatal vitamins (one daily) and iron replacement (ferrous sulfate 325 mg three times per day), and hypochromic microcytic anemia associated with an identified source of blood loss (presumed to be due to iron deficiency anemia) is treated similarly, with iron replacement therapy.[1,14]

These patients should be reevaluated after 4 to 6 weeks to assess the adequacy of the therapeutic response.[1,5,14] A reticulocyte count may be checked after a few days of therapy if more immediate confirmation of a therapeutic response is desired.[8–10,12] In megaloblastic anemia presumed to be due to folic acid or vitamin B_{12} deficiency, treatment may be initiated with 1 mg/d of oral folic acid or with 100 μg/d of cobalamin parenterally for 1 week, after specimens for serum vitamin B_{12} and folic acid levels are drawn and follow-up is arranged.[5,8,12,13] In mild or asymptomatic anemia of chronic disease, therapy is generally directed to control the underlying disease.[4,17] For severe or symptomatic anemia, however, consultation and, usually, hospital admission are advisable.

In many cases of newly identified anemia, drug therapy and other interventions are frequently not indicated in the emergency department setting, and patients are referred to a consultant for further evaluation and management.

DISPOSITION

Consultation or referral for follow-up, in most cases, is to the patient's primary care physician. Most anemic patients have iron deficiency anemia, vitamin B_{12} or folic acid deficiency anemia, or anemia of pregnancy; these cases can be treated and followed up on an outpatient basis.

Urgent consultation and hospital admission should be sought for the following indications[8,12,13]:

1. Hypovolemia or ongoing bleeding
2. Need for urgent transfusion, generally because of a hemoglobin level less than 9 g/dL in a bleeding or symptomatic patient[11]
3. Severe symptoms (e.g., chest pain, dyspnea, syncope) that impair the patient's ability to function at home
4. Pancytopenia requiring diagnostic evaluation[3,7,15]
5. Anticipated need for extensive diagnostic or therapeutic intervention

Unless active bleeding is present or the patient is hemodynamically unstable, there is usually no contraindication to routine transfer for specialized evaluation.

COMMON PITFALLS

- Failure to suspect and identify bleeding and hypovolemia
- Failure to appreciate the possibility of anemia from the clinical presentation, and, hence, not ordering a hemoglobin or hematocrit determination. This is especially likely in hemolytic anemia or when chest pain, dyspnea, dizziness, or claudication is the presenting complaint.
- Failure to ensure referral or appropriate follow-up for evaluation of therapeutic response or the need for additional diagnostic testing

References

1. Baynes RD, Bothwell TH. Iron deficiency. *Annu Rev Nutr* 1990;10:133.
2. Beck WS. Neuropsychiatric consequences of cobalamine deficiency. *Adv Intern Med* 1991;36:33.
3. Besa EC. Myelodysplastic syndromes (refractory anemia): a perspective of the biologic, clinical, and therapeutic issues. *Med Clin North Am* 1992;76:599.
4. Cash JM, Sears DA. The anemia of chronic disease: spectrum of associated disease in a series of unselected hospitalized patients. *Am J Med* 1989;87:638.
5. Chanarin I. How to diagnose (and not misdiagnose) pernicious anemia. *Blood Rev* 1987;1:280.

6. Colon-Ortero G, Menke D, Hock CC. A practical approach to the differential diagnosis and evaluation of the adult patient with microangiopathic anemia. *Med Clin North Am* 1992;76:581.
7. Glader BS. Red blood cell aplasia in children. *Pediatr Ann* 1990;19:168.
8. Hamilton GC, Braen GR. Anemia and white blood cell disorders. In: Rosen P, Barkin RM, Braen GR, et al., eds. *Emergency medicine: concepts and clinical practice*, 3rd ed. St. Louis: Mosby, 1992:1673.
9. Henry DH. Changing patterns of care in the management of anemia. *Semin Oncol* 1992;19[Suppl 8]:3.
10. Humphries JE. Anemia of renal failure: use of erythropoietin. *Med Clin North Am* 1992;76:711.
11. Jain R. Use of blood transfusion in the management of anemia. *Med Clin North Am* 1992;76:727.
12. Kellermeyer RW. General principles of the evaluation and therapy of anemia. *Med Clin North Am* 1984;68:533.
13. Mansuri A, Lipschitz DA. Anemia in the elderly patient. *Med Clin North Am* 1992;76:619.
14. Massey AC. Microcytic anemia: differential diagnosis and management of iron deficiency anemia. *Med Clin North Am* 1992;76:549.
15. Rappeport JM, Bunn HF. Bone marrow failure: aplastic anemia and other primary bone marrow disorders. In: Wilson JD, Braunwald E, Isselbacher KJ, et al., eds. *Principles of internal medicine*, 12th ed. New York: McGraw-Hill, 1991:1567.
16. Rosse WF. Microangiopathic hemolytic anemia. In: Williams WJ, Beutler E, Erslev AJ, et al., eds. *Hematology*, 3rd ed. New York: McGraw-Hill, 1983.
17. Sears DA. Anemia of chronic disease. *Med Clin North Am* 1992;76:567.
18. Tabbara IA. Hemolytic anemia: diagnosis and management. *Med Clin North Am* 1992;76:649.

CHAPTER 214

Transfusion Reactions and Complications

Gregory W. Hendey

Each year, over 23 million units of blood components, including 11.4 million packed red blood cell (PRBC) units, are transfused to patients in the United States.[1,8] The incidence of transfusion reactions is estimated to be only 1%, and the majority of reactions are simple febrile or minor allergic reactions.[16] The exceptionally low rate of serious transfusion reactions is mainly due to strict adherence to blood-banking techniques, careful transfusion practices, and extensive testing of donated units.

Life-threatening reactions occur rarely, but it is critical that physicians recognize them quickly and respond appropriately in order to avert a disastrous outcome. Transfusion reactions may be categorized in many ways, but it seems most useful clinically to divide them by severity and time of onset (Table 214.1).

TABLE 214.1. Blood Transfusion Reactions and Complications

ACUTE, SEVERE REACTIONS
Acute hemolysis
Anaphylaxis
Septic
Transfusion-related acute lung injury
Congestive heart failure
ACUTE, MINOR REACTIONS
Simple febrile
Allergic
DELAYED REACTIONS
Delayed hemolysis
Graft-versus-host disease
Hepatitis
HIV
CMV
Other infections: Epstein-Barr virus, cytomegalovirus, syphilis, trypanosomiasis, babesiosis, malaria, toxoplasmosis, brucellosis
MASSIVE TRANSFUSION
Coagulopathy
Hypothermia
Citrate toxicity (hypocalcemia)
Hyperkalemia
Lactic acidosis

CLINICAL PRESENTATION

Acute, Severe Reactions

Acute Hemolysis

One of the most serious (and most preventable) blood transfusion reactions is acute hemolysis caused by incompatibility between recipient and donor ABO blood groups. The incidence is between one in 250,000 and one in 1 million PRBC units transfused.[8] The resulting IgM–antigen complex fixes complement, leading to rapid intravascular hemolysis, with massive release of hemoglobin, acute renal failure, disseminated intravascular coagulopathy (DIC), and cardiovascular collapse.

The most common cause is simple clerical error—the wrong unit is given to the wrong patient. For that reason, painstaking efforts must be taken to double-check every step in the identification process prior to a transfusion.

The clinical signs of an acute hemolytic reaction are usually not subtle in the awake patient but may be difficult to recognize quickly in the unconscious, intubated patient. Unfortunately, the latter is just the type of patient that emergency physicians often need to transfuse. In an acute reaction, patients experience a rapid onset of fever, chills, back pain, vomiting, tachycardia, and hypotension.

The most important aspect of care is early recognition and discontinuation of the transfusion, because the severity of the reaction is related to the volume of blood transfused. For this reason, a physician or nurse should be at the bedside during the first 5 minutes of transfusion. Although there is no specific remedy, treatment of acute hemolysis centers around aggressive supportive care to minimize shock and maximize renal perfusion (Fig. 214.1). In hemodynamically unstable patients, early use of invasive monitoring is warranted, along with vasopressors and forced diuresis with crystalloids and loop diuretics (e.g., furosemide). Dopamine may be added—in "renal" doses (2 to 3 $\mu g/kg/min$)—for its potential benefit in increasing renal blood flow. Other treatments, such as steroids, mannitol, or heparin for DIC, are more controversial.

Anaphylaxis

Anaphylaxis is, fortunately, rare during a blood transfusion, but when it does occur, it is most often in IgA-deficient individuals who react to the IgA present in the transfused unit. The incidence has been estimated to be between one in 20,000 and one in 150,000 transfusions.[14,16] Unfortunately, these reactions cannot be reliably predicted, even by testing for the presence of IgA antibody in the patient's serum.[14]

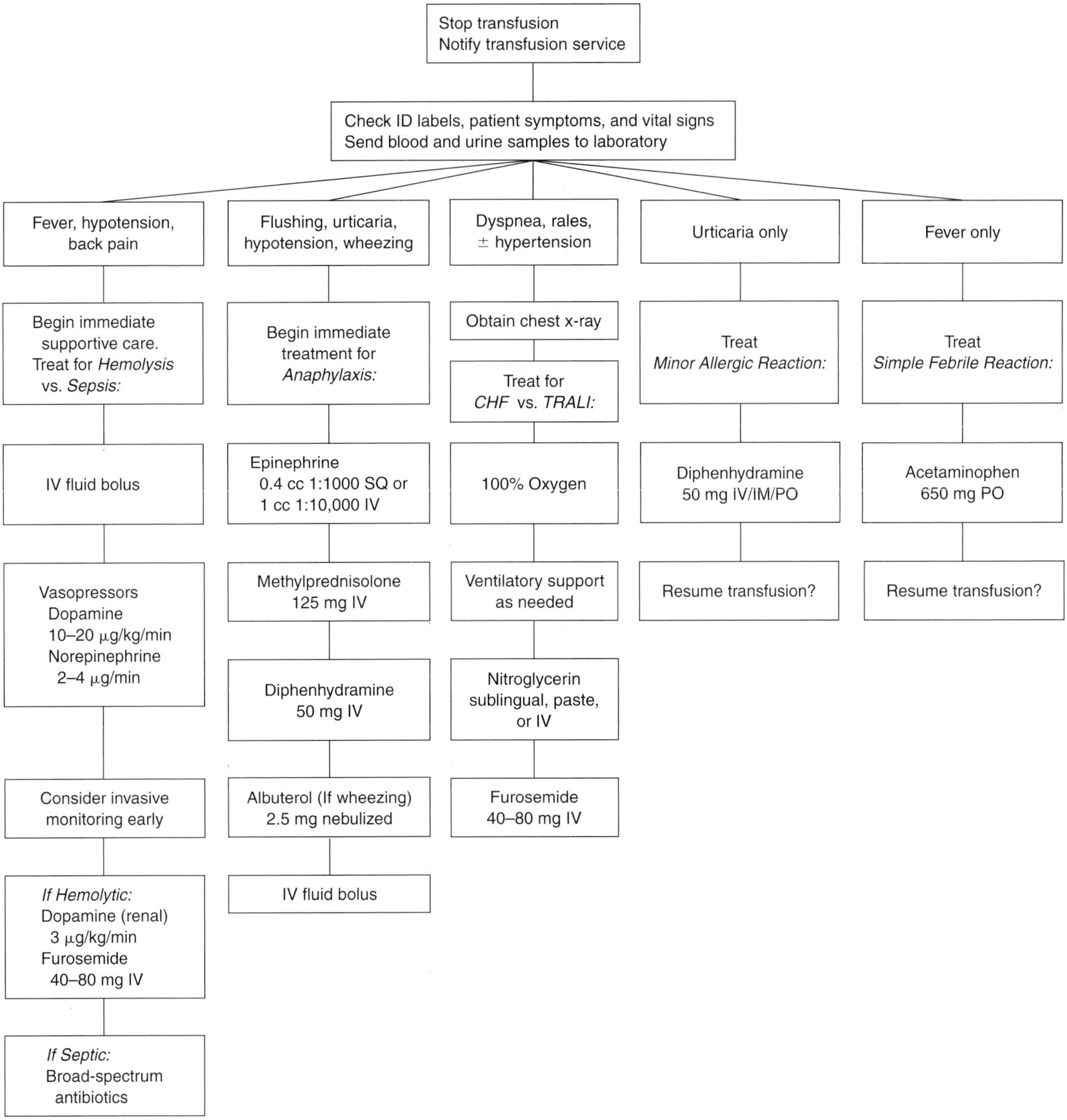

Figure 214.1. Clinical algorithm for suspected transfusion reaction. Many hospitals have developed policies and guidelines for actions to be taken in case of a transfusion reaction. Physicians should be informed regarding local hospital policy. TRALI = transfusion-related acute lung injury.

The onset is generally within the first minutes of transfusion and may present as sudden flushing, pruritus, laryngospasm, bronchospasm, and hypotension.

Treatment must be rapid and consists of epinephrine (intravenous [i.v.] or subcutaneous), steroids (methylprednisolone 125 mg i.v.), diphenhydramine (50 mg i.v.), and nebulized albuterol if wheezing is present. Intravenous crystalloid boluses and vasopressors may be necessary to treat hypotension.

Patients with a history of serious allergic reactions to blood products may be given washed RBCs or frozen–deglycerolized RBCs in an effort to prevent allergic reactions. IgA-deficient donors are often available when the transfusion can be planned in advance.

Hypotensive reactions to platelet transfusions have also been reported. These are not thought to be allergic in origin but may initially lead the clinician to suspect anaphylaxis. These reactions appear to be uncommon and resolve quickly with cessation of the platelet transfusion.[9]

Sepsis

Another potentially fatal transfusion reaction occurs when a contaminated blood product is transfused. This is a rare event with PRBC, with a risk between one in 500,000 and one in 2.5 million.[4,8,16] The risk is much higher, however, in platelet transfusions (between one in 1600 and one in 12,000) because they are stored at room temperature to maintain platelet activity.[4,8] Single-donor apheresis platelet units carry a lower risk for bacterial contamination than do random-donor pooled platelets, as do fresher units with less storage time.[4,16] Many bacteria have been implicated in platelet transfusions, including *Staphylococcus aureus, Klebsiella pneumoniae, Serratia marcescens,* and *Staphylococcus epidermidis,* and the mortality has been reported at 26%.[8] The most common agent in PRBC units, however, is *Yersinia enterocolitica,* which grows well under refrigerated conditions.[2,4,8]

When the contaminated unit is transfused, it may produce the acute onset of a sepsis syndrome, with fever, chills, and hypotension. A septic reaction, especially when caused by a gram-negative organism, could easily be confused with the early stages of hemolytic or anaphylactic reactions in the early stages.

Treatment should consist of stopping the transfusion, sending cultures of the patient's blood, and immediately returning the donor unit to the laboratory for Gram staining, cultures, and hemolysis workup. The Gram stain is positive in most cases of bacterial contamination, but if the suspicion of a septic reaction is high, broad-spectrum antibiotics should be administered without waiting for these results. Antibiotic coverage for a contaminated platelet transfusion should include an antistaphylococcal agent as well as a third-generation cephalosporin. Coverage for a contaminated PRBC transfusion must include a third-generation cephalosporin or quinolone to cover *Yersinia.* Intravenous fluids and vasopressor support may also be necessary.

Transfusion-Related Acute Lung Injury

Transfusion-related acute lung injury (TRALI) is a noncardiogenic pulmonary edema occurring unpredictably in one in 5,000 to one in 10,000 units of PRBC transfused.[8,16] It is probably caused by antileukocyte antibodies in the donor unit reacting with the patient's white blood cells (WBCs). This reaction leads to increased pulmonary capillary permeability and produces an adult respiratory distress syndrome (ARDS) during or just following transfusion. It should be differentiated from acute congestive heart failure (CHF) by the patient's history and the typical chest x-ray finding of diffuse interstitial edema without cardiomegaly.

Treatment is supportive and consists of oxygenation, ventilatory support, and intensive care unit (ICU) care. Diuresis and steroids are generally not effective. Such reactions should be reported to the laboratory so that donors found to have antileukocyte antibodies can be excluded from future donations.

Congestive Heart Failure

The cardiovascular systems of most patients can easily accommodate the rapid change in intravascular volume that a blood transfusion provides. Elderly patients, however, and those with preexisting cardiomyopathy or diastolic dysfunction may have difficulty handling an acute change in volume and preload, and the result is pulmonary edema. Transfusions are often necessary or even lifesaving in these patients, but they must be carried out with extra care and attention.

These patients must not be rapidly transfused and discharged home. In those with a low-to-medium risk for CHF, it may be sufficient to transfuse slowly (over 3 to 4 hours) and allow a period of time between each subsequent unit transfused. Administration of a loop diuretic (e.g., furosemide) between units may also be helpful. Vigilant observation and monitoring is the key. In high-risk patients, invasive monitoring of right or left ventricular filling pressures (or both) in the ICU may be necessary.

If a patient receiving a transfusion develops pulmonary edema, it should first be determined whether the patient has CHF or noncardiogenic pulmonary edema. The patient history and chest x-ray will be helpful in this determination. CHF should be treated as usual, with nitrates (i.v., sublingual, paste, etc.), diuretics (furosemide), oxygen, close monitoring, and ventilatory support, as needed.

Acute, Minor Reactions

Simple Febrile Reaction

This is the most common transfusion reaction, with an incidence of 1%. It is thought to be due to antileukocyte and antiplatelet antibodies, or to transfused pyrogenic cytokines that accumulate in stored blood as leukocytes break down. Patients who receive frequent transfusions or who have a history of febrile reactions may be given leukocyte-reduced units of blood to reduce the likelihood of this reaction. It is most important to carefully differentiate this benign reaction from the potentially lethal acute intravascular hemolytic reaction discussed earlier.

The simple febrile reaction should be treated with oral acetaminophen. There is controversy about whether the transfusion may be carefully resumed after clinical observation and appropriate laboratory testing have ruled out a hemolytic reaction.

Allergic Reaction

Minor allergic reactions occur largely in response to transfused plasma proteins. The incidence is estimated to be 0.1%, but it may be underreported.[16] The reaction is more common with platelet or plasma transfusions, but PRBC units also carry some residual plasma. The patient develops urticaria or flushing and pruritus, without any dyspnea or hypotension. As with other reactions, the transfusion should be stopped while the patient is assessed to be certain that the more dangerous anaphylaxis is not present. Diphenhydramine should be administered, and the transfusion may be carefully resumed with close monitoring for any sign of recurrence.

Delayed Reactions

Adverse transfusion reactions may occur days to months after the transfusion. These include delayed hemolysis, graft-versus-host disease (GVHD), and a number of infections. Many infectious diseases may be transmitted by blood transfusion, including the human immunodeficiency virus (HIV), hepatitis, syphilis, malaria, cytomegalovirus (CMV), Epstein-Barr virus (EBV), trypanosomiasis, toxoplasmosis, babesiosis, and brucellosis.[4,7,17] The most clinically significant in the United States are hepatitis, HIV, and CMV.

Delayed Hemolysis

Delayed hemolysis is unusual, but may occur 5 to 7 days post-transfusion. The incidence is between one in 1,000 and one in 2,500 units transfused.[4,7,17] It is most commonly caused by reactivation of antibodies to the minor RBC antigen systems such as Rh, Kell, Kidd, and Duffy. It presents in a less severe and dramatic way than the acute hemolytic reaction, though progression to renal failure is still a concern. In contrast to acute hemolysis, there is usually less free hemoglobin circulating at any given time, and thus the renal insult tends to be less severe.[16] Worsening anemia is the most common clinical problem that must be evaluated.

Laboratory studies should reveal signs of recent hemolysis (anemia, indirect hyperbilirubinemia, and a positive direct Coombs' test), and one or more new antibodies may be identified. However, the haptoglobin may be normal, and the serum and urine lack the pink discoloration of acute hemolysis. If further transfusion is required, units lacking the problematic antigen must be used.

Graft-Versus-Host Disease

GVHD occurs when lymphocytes from a donated unit of blood attack an immunocompromised host who is unable to combat the foreign cells, or when lymphocytes from an immunologically similar donor are not recognized as foreign by the host. Signs and symptoms may include fever, rash, nausea, and vomiting, as well as elevation of transaminases and pancytopenia. This is a particular danger in neonates and bone marrow transplant recipients.

Although there is no specific treatment beyond supportive care, preventive measures exist. Irradiation of PRBC and platelet units suppresses any white cells that may be transfused along with the desired component. This is the only effective means of preventing GVHD in these high-risk patient groups.

Hepatitis

Transfusion-associated hepatitis was a major problem in the 1970s and 1980s. It has been estimated that during the early 1970s, transfusion-associated hepatitis occurred in up to 33% of transfusions.[11] Since then, aggressive screening of donors and the development of specific assays for hepatitis B and C have greatly reduced the risk.

Donahue reported a decrease in the risk of posttransfusion hepatitis C from approximately one in 200 during 1985 to one in 3,300 in 1991, after hepatitis C testing became available.[3] With further advances in testing, the current estimated risk of transfusion-transmitted hepatitis B is one in 63,000, and of hepatitis C is one in 103,000.[15] Although the hepatitis C test successfully eliminated the majority of non-A, non-B hepatitis, the small risk of non-A, non-B, non-C hepatitis remains.

Human Immunodeficiency Virus

Although it is now exceedingly rare, the transfusion complication that has received the most public attention is HIV infection. It has been estimated that the risk of HIV transmission in some metropolitan areas was as high as one in 100 units transfused in 1983, before HIV testing was available to blood banks in March of 1985.[8] Now, thanks to aggressive predonation screening, along with HIV-1 antibody and p24 antigen testing, the current risk is estimated to be between one in 450,000 and one in 660,000.[4] Donated blood is also screened for HIV-2, although this strain is rare in the United States.

The use of concentrated pooled plasma products resulted in a majority of hemophiliacs in the 1980s contracting the acquired immunodeficiency syndrome or hepatitis. Highly purified, lyophilized factor VIII concentrate and recombinant products have eliminated these tragic complications of therapy.

Cytomegalovirus

Although CMV is generally not a significant pathogen in immunocompetent individuals, the immunosuppressed, especially premature neonates, HIV patients, and bone marrow and organ transplant recipients, are especially susceptible to CMV infection transmitted by blood transfusion. The risk may be greatly reduced through the use of blood collected from CMV-negative donors, or by using either leukocyte-reduced or frozen–deglycerolized units of blood.[3]

Massive Transfusion

Several alterations are present in stored blood that are insignificant in small transfusions but may become clinically relevant in the setting of massive transfusion. *Massive* is usually defined as transfusion of the equivalent of one blood volume, or 10 to 12 units of PRBC, within 24 hours. Fortunately, it is rare that the emergency physician would be faced with this situation, but it may occur in the setting of major trauma or gastrointestinal (GI) bleeding when definitive care is delayed for whatever reason.

Hyperkalemia and lactic acidosis may result from the transfusion of multiple units of older stored blood, but the effects tend to be relatively mild and transient. Citrate toxicity may result in hypocalcemia in the setting of massive transfusion, which caused substantial problems in the past when it was common to transfuse whole blood units. However, in the era of component therapy, whole blood is rarely (if ever) available or indicated, and units of PRBC contain far less citrate. Hypothermia may cause or make patients more prone to becoming coagulopathic. Blood warmers lessen this problem, but they also slow the rate of transfusion, which is problematic in the hypotensive, hemorrhaging patient. Methods of mixing PRBC units with heated crystalloids, making the transfusion both faster and warmer, have been described.[5,10]

The coagulopathy associated with massive transfusion is multifactorial and difficult to predict prospectively. Clotting factors and platelets decrease, at least in part, because of dilutional effects after multiple units of PRBC are transfused, because these units contain negligible amounts of clotting factors and platelets. Coagulation times may rise beyond 1.5 times control, and clinically relevant bleeding occurs in some patients. Trauma patients who receive more than 10 units in 24 hours are more likely to develop serious coagulopathy in the presence of hypothermia, acidosis, or hypotension. Among severely injured patients who receive massive transfusion, virtually all become coagulopathic when all of the noted risk factors are present.[6] Although platelet counts fall during massive transfusion, the decrease is much less than would be predicted from dilution alone.[13] This is thought to be due to release of platelets into the circulation from storage in the spleen or from the bone marrow. Platelet counts usually remain above 50,000 until 20 units of PRBC are transfused, but coagulation times exceed 1.5 times control in patients receiving more than 12 units.[12]

Routine prophylactic administration of fresh-frozen plasma (FFP) and platelets is not usually recommended for patients receiving massive transfusion, because there is substantial variability in the number of units it takes to make a patient coagulopathic or thrombocytopenic. There is even more variability in whether the patient has only a laboratory abnormality or clinically significant bleeding. Physicians must, however, be vigilant for the development of coagulopathic bleeding and be prepared to treat it quickly.

In general, patients who are bleeding and have platelet counts of less than 50,000 should receive platelet transfusion, and those with prothrombin times or partial thromboplastin times greater than 1.5 times control should receive FFP.[17] Cryoprecipitate may be used to replenish fibrinogen if it becomes depleted. One should consider the *prophylactic* administration of FFP after massive transfusion when there are other complicating factors, such as hypothermia, acidosis, or hypotension, because individuals with these conditions are at greater risk for developing significant coagulopathy.[6]

DIFFERENTIAL DIAGNOSIS

The patient who develops any adverse symptoms early in a blood transfusion must be carefully evaluated for the possibility of one of the acute, severe reactions. However, many patients who receive emergent transfusions have underlying disease that may have symptoms in common with transfusion reactions. For example, when trauma patients or those with GI bleeding become hypotensive during a transfusion, the hypotension may represent either increasing hemorrhage or an acute, severe transfusion reaction. Sepsis and some drug overdoses may also present with symptoms that are similar to those of a transfusion reaction.

Although many of the signs and symptoms of transfusion reactions are nonspecific and can be confused with many disease processes, most transfusion reactions occur during or soon after a transfusion. A delayed hemolytic reaction must be differentiated from other causes of jaundice and anemia, but the indirect hyperbilirubinemia should cue the physician that hemolysis has occurred.

EMERGENCY DEPARTMENT EVALUATION

In the patient with an acute reaction, the clinician must rapidly decide whether the signs and symptoms are consistent with one of the severe reactions or one of the more benign febrile or allergic reactions (see Fig. 214.1). Differentiation may sometimes be done clinically by evaluating the constellation of findings, without extensive testing. One may also employ quick, simple testing, such as observing the serum (after centrifugation of a blood sample) or the urine for pink discoloration during a hemolytic reaction.

The evaluation should also involve immediate reporting to the laboratory and sending blood samples for testing. Based on the clinical setting, the laboratory will often confirm the ABO types of the patient and donor unit, perform a direct Coombs' test, and search for evidence of hemolysis (an elevated indirect bilirubin, decreased haptoglobin, schistocytes on a peripheral smear, or hemoglobinuria). Testing may also include Gram staining and cultures, especially after platelet transfusions, if bacterial contamination is suggested.

The transfusion should be stopped during this evaluation in case the patient is in the early stages of a severe reaction. In some cases of minor reactions, especially allergic ones, the clinician may choose to treat the symptoms and restart the transfusion after determining that a severe reaction is not present, although this procedure is controversial. One should quickly involve the laboratory and transfusion service for consultation when a reaction occurs. Most institutions have policies or guidelines to help the clinician in evaluating and reporting transfusion reactions.

EMERGENCY DEPARTMENT MANAGEMENT

Treatment, of course, depends on which type of reaction has occurred (see Fig. 214.1). The first step is always to stop the transfusion and carefully evaluate the patient to determine whether a transfusion reaction is occurring and, if so, which type. The treatment of acute hemolysis is largely supportive, with special attention to maintaining renal perfusion. Anaphylaxis should be treated with epinephrine, steroids, diphenhydramine, and i.v. fluids, regardless of the cause. Sepsis from bacterial contamination requires aggressive supportive care, including i.v. fluids, vasopressors, and broad-spectrum antibiotics. TRALI and CHF are treated with ventilatory support, as well as nitrates and diuresis for CHF. Simple febrile and allergic reactions are treated with acetaminophen and diphenhydramine, respectively.

DISPOSITION

Most patients receiving blood transfusions in the emergency department are ultimately admitted to the hospital, whether or not they have a transfusion reaction. However, acute, severe reactions usually necessitate ICU admission, regardless of the patient's original disposition. Simple febrile or allergic reactions do not necessarily require a change in the patient's treatment plan.

COMMON PITFALLS

- Failing to carefully identify patients when drawing pretransfusion blood samples, and failing to carefully match identities of blood components, their paperwork, and the recipient. This is the most frequent cause of fatal hemolytic reactions.
- Failing to adequately evaluate a patient who develops symptoms during a blood transfusion. The large majority are simple febrile or allergic reactions, but the few dangerous reactions must be discovered and treated immediately.
- Failing to recognize a severe reaction in an intubated patient. Because the patient cannot complain of symptoms, it is more difficult to differentiate a transfusion reaction from underlying disease. An acute, severe reaction may initially appear as isolated hypotension or a change in urine color.
- Rapidly transfusing an elderly patient who is inadequately observed. Congestive failure can be avoided by slow, intermittent transfusion and diuresis.
- Failing to transfuse an appropriate patient because of the misconception that complications of transfusion are more common than they actually are. Blood transfusion is safer now than it ever has been, and it remains a lifesaving intervention.

References

1. American Association of Blood Banks. http://www.aabb.org/docs/facts.html
2. Center for Disease Control, BaCon Study web site: http://www.cdc.gov/ncidod/hip/bacon/bacon.htm
3. Donahue J, Munoz A, Ness P, et al. The declining risk of post-transfusion hepatitis C virus infection. *N Engl J Med* 1992;327:369–373.
4. Chamberland M, Khabbaz R. Emerging issues in blood safety. *Infect Dis Clin North Am* 1998;12:217–229.
5. Cohn S, Stack G. In vitro comparison of heated saline-blood admixture with a heat exchanger for rapid warming of red blood cells. *J Trauma* 1993;35:688–690.
6. Cosgriff M, Moore M, Sauaia M, et al. Predicting life-threatening coagulopathy in the massively transfused trauma patient: hypothermia and acidoses revisited. *J Trauma* 1997;42:857–862.
7. Dobroszycki J, Herwaldt B, Boctor F, et al. A cluster of transfusion-associated cases traced to a single asymptomatic donor. *JAMA* 1999;281:927–930.
8. Goodnough L, Brecher M, Kanter M, et al. Transfusion medicine. First of two parts. Blood transfusion. *N Engl J Med* 1999;340:438–447.
9. Hume H, Popovsky M, Benson K, et al. Hypotensive reactions: a previously uncharacterized complication of platelet transfusion? *Transfusion* 1996; 36:904–909.
10. Iserson K, Knauf M, Anhalt D. Rapid admixture blood warming: technical advances. *Crit Care Med* 1990;18:1138–1141.
11. Labadie L. Transfusion therapy in the emergency department. *Emerg Med Clin North Am* 1993;11:379–406.
12. Leslie S, Toy P. Laboratory hemostatic abnormalities in massively transfused patients given red blood cells and crystalloid. *Am J Clin Pathol* 1991;96:770–773.
13. Reed R, Ciavarella D, Heimbach D, et al. Prophylactic platelet administration during massive transfusion. *Ann Surg* 1986;203:40–47.
14. Sandler S, Mallory D, Malamut D, et al. IgA Anaphylactic transfusion reactions. *Transfus Med Rev* 1995;9:1–8.

15. Schreiber G, Busch M, Kleinman S, et al. The risk of transfusion-transmitted viral infections. The Retrovirus Epidemiology Donor Study. *N Engl J Med* 1996;334:1685–1690.
16. Sloop G, Friedberg R. Complications of blood transfusion. how to recognize and respond to noninfectious reactions. *Postgrad Med* 1995;98:159–162.
17. Storer D. Blood and blood component therapy. In: Rosen P, Barkin R, eds. *Emergency medicine, concepts and clinical practice*, 4th edition. St. Louis: Mosby, 1998:129–134.

CHAPTER 215
Hematologic Malignancies

Daniel Brookoff

ACUTE LEUKEMIA

Acute leukemia is rarely overlooked or misdiagnosed.[3] Most patients with acute leukemia present with complaints of fatigue, weight loss, or bleeding and are found on physical examination to have petechiae, lymphadenopathy, splenomegaly, or sternal tenderness.

A complete blood count with examination of the blood smear is usually sufficient to make a provisional diagnosis. In acute leukemia, the white blood cell count may be increased (in 50% of patients), normal, or decreased (in up to 33% of patients), but blast cells usually make up more than 5% of circulating white cells. The definitive diagnosis is made on examination of the bone marrow with the finding of more than 30% blast cells.

The most common complications of leukemia that precipitate emergency department visits are infection (responsible for 70% of deaths from acute leukemia) and bleeding.

Infection

In patients with acute leukemia, neutropenia is caused by replacement of normal marrow by leukemic cells or is the result of cytotoxic chemotherapy. In addition, most patients have qualitative defects of the circulating neutrophils. With prolonged neutropenia (less than 1,000 neutrophils per microliter), the mucous membranes and skin lose their effectiveness as barriers to infection. Infections in leukemic patients, therefore, tend to be due to bowel or skin flora. These include *Pseudomonas aeruginosa, Escherichia coli, Proteus* species, and *Staphylococcus aureus*. In patients with indwelling catheters, *Staphylococcus epidermidis* and *Streptococcus viridans* have become major causes of infection. Leukemia does not interfere with the ability to mount a fever and is rarely the primary cause of fever.

Any patient with known or suspected leukemia who presents with intermittent or sustained fever greater than 100.5°F should be assumed to be septic and promptly treated with broad-spectrum antibiotics after blood is drawn for cultures. In patients without an obvious source of infection, a combination of an antipseudomonal penicillin or cephalosporin and an aminoglycoside is commonly used. For patients with a history of allergy to penicillin or cephalosporin, broad-spectrum quinolone antibiotics (e.g., ciprofloxacin) or imipenem may be substituted.

Hemorrhage

Until platelet transfusions came into widespread use, hemorrhage was almost as important as infection as cause of death among leukemic patients. Even now, hemorrhage due to thrombocytopenia continues to account for more than 15% of deaths from leukemia. Most patients with thrombocytopenia present with petechiae and microscopic hematuria. With platelet counts below 20,000/mL, there is a high risk of intracranial hemorrhage.[2]

Transfusion of random-donor platelets is usually sufficient to prevent hemorrhage due to thrombocytopenia. The usual goal is to raise the platelet count above 50,000/mL. In nonimmunized patients, 1 U of platelets can be expected to raise the count by between 5,000 and 10,000, but the patient who has had repeated platelet transfusions may have become immunized to platelet-borne tissue antigens and may require human leukocyte antigen–matched platelets. The blood bank is usually aware of these individuals because of their previous transfusions.

Leukoagglutinin reactions, usually manifested by body aches, fever, rigors, or shortness of breath, are common in patients receiving pooled platelets, because pooled platelets contain a high concentration of viable leukocytes. Symptoms can usually be prevented by using a Leukapor filter and by administering acetaminophen 650 mg by mouth and diphenhydramine 50 mg intravenously 10 to 20 minutes before the transfusion.

A less common cause of hemorrhage is disseminated intravascular coagulation (DIC), which is seen most often in patients with acute promyelocytic leukemia or acute monocytic leukemia. DIC should be considered in leukemic patients who present with ecchymosis rather than petechiae. DIC causes prolongation of both the prothrombin and partial thromboplastin times. The diagnosis is confirmed by finding depressed levels of fibrinogen and high concentrations of fibrinogen degradation products. Patients with acute leukemia and DIC often require emergent replacement of plasma coagulation factors and platelets before being treated with cytotoxic drugs. Heparin is often administered to interfere with uncontrolled coagulation, but its usefulness is controversial and there is no compelling reason to administer it in the emergency department.

Hyperleukocytotic Syndromes

A small proportion of patients with myelogenous leukemia (5% of acute leukemias and 15% of patients with chronic leukemia) present with hyperleukocytotic syndromes. In these conditions, the high concentration of leukemic cells interferes with circulation to the brain, eye, lung, ear, or penis. Clinical features include tachypnea, dyspnea, pulmonary infiltrates, retinal hemorrhages, dizziness, stupor, visual blurring, and priapism. Intracranial hemorrhages are a rare but catastrophic manifestation. These problems usually occur when the white cell count is greater than 75,000/mL in acute leukemia or is greater than 250,000/mL in chronic myelogenous leukemia. Patients with chronic lymphocytic leukemia generally do not develop problems related to leukostasis until the peripheral white cell count exceeds 1 million per milliliter.

Patients with hyperleukocytotic syndromes can be treated with emergent leukapheresis. If this modality is not available in a timely fashion, cytotoxic drugs can be used to reduce the peripheral white blood cell count. Cytotoxic therapy, however, carries the risk of "tumor lysis syndrome," manifested by the rapid onset of hyperuricemia, hyperphosphatemia, hyperkalemia, and lactic acidosis. A commonly used cytotoxic agent that is easy to administer is hydroxyurea, an oral medication given in doses of 500 to 2,000 mg four times per day. Patients with hyperleukocytosis who will be treated with hydroxyurea should be given allopurinol at least 3 to 6 hours before the first dose; the serum electrolytes and blood counts must also be monitored closely. Tumor lysis syndrome is also associated with rapidly growing lymphomas.

Other Complications of Hematologic Malignancies

Patients with hematologic malignancy can present with signs and symptoms referable to anemia. Infiltration of leukemic or lymphoma cells into various organs can also be a feature of the initial presentation and is often associated with relapse after treatment. Patients with Burkitt lymphoma often present with an abdominal mass, and sometimes with obstructive symptoms due to mesenteric infiltration by cancer cells. More than 75% of patients with acute leukemia have enlargement of lymph nodes, liver, and spleen.

In the patient who gives a history of cured leukemia or leukemia in remission, relapse of the disease must always be considered. A common site of relapse is the central nervous system; symptoms can include headache, cranial nerve dysfunction, or signs of meningeal irritation and carcinomatous meningitis. Meningeal leukemia is most often seen in children and in leukemia of lymphoid origin. It usually presents with signs of increased intracranial pressure. A computed tomography scan of the head is usually normal in these patients, and examination of the cerebrospinal fluid reveals a pleocytosis, often with identifiable leukemic cells. Patients with meningeal leukemia require emergent hospital admission and intrathecal chemotherapy.

LYMPHOMA

Certain lymphomas are associated with medical emergencies. Patients with multiple myelomas often have extensive bone lesions, and bone pain is a presenting feature in 70% of patients. The emergency physician must maintain a high suspicion for fracture, even when presented with a story of pain that is gradual in onset or waxing and waning. Vertebral metastases are common in myeloma, and many patients report having already noticed a loss of height before the diagnosis of myeloma is made. Myeloma is a common cause of spinal cord compression.

More than 60% of patients with myeloma develop hypercalcemia during the course of their disease.[1] Symptoms such as anorexia, nausea, vomiting, polyuria, and constipation can develop rapidly, and patients may progress to develop lethargy and coma. Rarely, profound hypercalcemia may not be accompanied by these symptoms because circulating myeloma proteins are binding the calcium. It is thus useful to measure the free ionized calcium level before beginning therapy.[6] Patients with hypercalcemia are usually volume-depleted, and initial therapy almost always includes saline infusion. Diuretics can be used if volume overload is a concern, but they should be avoided as initial therapy unless volume overload is present initially.

Another emergency related to lymphoid malignancies is hyperviscosity syndrome, which has an incidence ranging from 2% in patients with myeloma to 50% in patients with macroglobulinemia. The common manifestations are bleeding disorders (e.g., epistaxis, purpura, or gastrointestinal bleeding), visual impairment, and a broad range of neurologic symptoms.[8] Serum viscosity is easily measured in the laboratory. The normal range of relative serum viscosity is 1.4 to 1.8. Symptoms usually appear at values greater than 4, and a relative viscosity of 6 or greater is associated with severe manifestations.[7] Patients with severe hyperviscosity syndrome (e.g., central nervous system findings or hemorrhage) require emergent plasmapheresis.

POLYCYTHEMIA AND THROMBOCYTHEMIA

Overproduction of erythrocytes or platelets may also precipitate medical emergencies. A hemoglobin level greater than 17 g/dL or a hematocrit greater than 55% may signal polycythemia vera, an uncontrolled clonal overproduction of erythrocytes. Other conditions that should be considered in patients presenting with a high hematocrit include volume depletion, hypoxia, and polycythemia due to cigarette smoking or exposure to high altitudes. Patients with polycythemia vera are usually middle-aged and generally have a normal arterial oxygen saturation (greater than 92%) and splenomegaly. They often have leukocytosis (greater than 12,000 white blood cells/mL) as well as thrombocytosis (greater than 400,000 platelets/mL).

Emergencies due to polycythemia are related to hypervolemia and hyperviscosity. Patients may present with headache, vertigo, angina pectoris, or claudication. Thirty percent of patients with polycythemia vera suffer thrombotic episodes, and stroke is a common complication and cause of death. Elevated hematocrit findings can also interfere with platelet function; thus, some patients with uncontrolled polycythemia suffer hemorrhagic complications, most commonly in the gastrointestinal tract. Many patients with polycythemia also have thrombocythemia (platelet counts greater than 600,000/mL), a finding that is also associated with abnormal bleeding.

Polycythemic patients with signs or symptoms of hyperviscosity or thrombotic complications should have their blood volume and hemoglobin concentration reduced to normal as quickly as possible.

Even without symptoms, a hemoglobin level of 18 g/dL or a hematocrit reading of 60% or higher is also an indication for emergent phlebotomy or cytapheresis. Patients who are otherwise healthy can usually tolerate a rapid phlebotomy of 500 mL, although more gradual treatment may be required in the elderly or in those with known coronary artery disease. With the attainment of a normal hematocrit, the platelet defect that gives rise to thrombosis and bleeding is eventually corrected, but this can take weeks to occur. Elective surgery and dental procedures in polycythemic patients should thus be delayed until the red cell mass and platelet count have been normalized for at least 2 months. Polycythemic patients in need of emergency surgery require emergent phlebotomy or cytapheresis.[4]

Primary thrombocythemia is a myeloproliferative disorder characterized by platelet counts of more than 600,000/mL and a clinical course marked by hemorrhagic and thrombotic episodes. The disease may be associated with polycythemia vera. Other causes of thrombocytosis include chronic inflammatory disorders (e.g., rheumatoid arthritis, ulcerative colitis), iron deficiency, carcinoma, or recent administration of epinephrine. A thromboembolic event often brings the patient initially to medical attention. Neurologic symptoms are common and usually include headache, dizziness, paresthesia, or transient ischemic attacks. More than half of patients with primary thrombocythemia experience arterial thrombosis, most commonly in the legs, coronary arteries, and renal arteries. In addition, many suffer gastrointestinal hemorrhage.

Individuals with platelet counts greater than 1 million per milliliter and either thrombosis or hemorrhage require rapid plateletpheresis to reduce the platelet count to less than 500,000/mL. If plateletpheresis is not available, cytotoxic drugs can be used; nitrogen mustard, uracil mustard, and hydroxyurea are the agents of choice. The use of antiplatelet agents is controversial because of the increased risk of hemorrhage. Asymptomatic patients with platelet counts of less than 2 million per microliter should have prompt evaluation and treatment, but do not require emergent therapy.[5]

References

1. Bergsagel DE, Griffith KM, Haut A. The treatment of plasma cell myeloma. *Adv Cancer Res* 1967;10:311.
2. Glover DJ, Glick JH. Oncologic emergencies and special complications. In: Carbone P, Schein P, Rosenberg S, eds. *Medical oncology*. New York: Macmillan, 1987.
3. Henderson E. Acute leukemias: general considerations. In: Williams WJ, Beutler E, Erslev AJ, et al., eds. *Hematology*, 4th ed. New York: McGraw-Hill, 1990.
4. Hoffman R, Boswell HS. Polycythemia vera. In: Hoffman R, Benz EJ, Shattil SJ, et al., eds. *Hematology: basic principles and practice*. New York: Churchill Livingstone, 1991.
5. Hoffman R, Silverstein MN. Primary thrombocythemia. In: Hoffman R, Benz EJ, Shattil SJ, et al., eds. *Hematology: basic principles and practice*. New York: Churchill Livingstone, 1991.
6. Jaffe JP, Mosher DF. Calcium binding by a myeloma protein. *Am J Med* 1979;67:343.
7. McGrath MA, Penny R. Paraproteinemia: blood hyperviscosity and clinical manifestations. *J Clin Invest* 1976;58:1155.
8. Somer T. Hyperviscosity syndrome in plasma cell dyscrasias. *Adv Microcirc* 1975;6:1.

CHAPTER 216

The Cancer Patient in the Emergency Department

Daniel Brookoff

Patients who have been diagnosed with cancer have usually been warned by their oncologists that certain symptoms, such as fever while on chemotherapy, require emergent evaluation. When other symptoms appear, patients and their families are, as a rule, quite concerned about how the new problem may be related to the cancer or its treatment. These patients commonly suffer from chronic anxiety and uncertainty about their disease, its treatment, and its prognosis, and they pose a significant challenge to the emergency physician.

Cancer patients nevertheless deserve special attention for even apparently minor problems, because catastrophic oncologic emergencies often present with subtle complaints and findings. For example, mild radicular low back pain with a positive "straight leg-raising sign" may be the first sign of impending spinal cord compression in a patient with a history of lung cancer. Likewise, a vague complaint of dyspnea or malaise in a patient with a history of breast cancer may be due to a pericardial effusion that has progressed nearly to the point of frank tamponade.

Similarly, apparently minor aches and pains may herald the appearance of new metastases. Thus, a heightened sense of suspicion is always appropriate when treating a patient with a history of cancer. All cancers are not the same, however; for effective assessment, the emergency physician must determine the type of cancer involved and must have some familiarity with its natural history. The pattern of any metastasis or previous complications should be established, as well as specific details about therapy (e.g., which drugs have been administered, which sites have been irradiated, and when).

In the emergency department, it is important to set reasonable treatment goals that are consistent with the long-term treatment plan formulated by the patient's oncologist. They can range from immediate pain relief to complex treatments designed to restore functional status.[7] As with all patients, the treatment should be tailored to the patient's physical and psychological state and prognosis. Is the patient responding to treatment? Is there hope for cure or sustained palliation, or is the patient terminally ill? Thus, early consultation with the oncologist is usually appropriate to ensure consistency and continuity of care.

What follows is a discussion of common oncologic emergencies, organized by the usual presenting complaint. These are often complaints that the emergency physician evaluates every day, but when any of them is coupled with a history of cancer, the malignancy must figure prominently on the list of potential etiologies. Some of the many complications of cancer therapy that can prompt visits to the emergency department are also addressed.

SHORTNESS OF BREATH

The emergency physician's first priority in dealing with shortness of breath is to assess the airway, seeking evidence of obstruction. Upper airway obstruction is seen with far-advanced hypopharyngeal and laryngeal cancers. Superior vena cava obstruction due to lymphoma or lung cancer can cause pharyngeal edema, but this symptom is very rare.[1]

Usually, the patient with a malignant upper airway obstruction has a history of chronic, gradually worsening dyspnea that has progressed over weeks or months, and that is worsened by exertion. The patient may also have noted increasing hoarseness over the prior few weeks or months. Assessment can be carried out with laryngoscopy and soft-tissue radiographs of the neck. Treatment may involve surgery, radiation, or chemotherapy. It is also safe to administer a dose of steroids emergently and, if there is significant obstruction, to administer oxygen–helium mixtures to improve gas flow.

An exception to the pattern of gradually developing airway compromise is rapid obstruction due to fast-growing neck tumors, such as anaplastic thyroid cancers or Burkitt's lymphoma. In addition, partial upper airway obstruction from a laryngeal tumor may be exacerbated by infection, hemorrhage, or retained secretions and may present as a critical obstruction. In the critical situation, one must be prepared to establish a surgical airway, although there is usually time to use suction, to administer nebulized racemic epinephrine, and, if necessary, to attempt endotracheal intubation so that definitive intervention can be performed on a nonemergent basis.

In addition to obstructing the upper airway, tumors (usually lung, esophageal, or thyroid carcinomas) can also impinge directly on the trachea. The trachea is rarely the site of primary or metastatic tumor, however. Tracheal obstruction is usually due to complications of treatment, such as tracheomalacia following prolonged intubation or edema secondary to radiation therapy. Tracheostomy is often necessary in these patients, as endotracheal intubation is likely to be unsuccessful and the obstruction is below the level of the cricothyroid membrane. Attempts at bronchoscopy may worsen tracheal edema.

Bronchial obstructions are usually due to primary lung carcinoma or, rarely, endobronchial metastases from other primaries (notably breast, colon, and renal cancer). As with upper airway obstruction, bronchial obstruction is usually asymptomatic until there is greater than 75% obstruction. The usual presentation includes cough, hemoptysis, wheezing, or palpable rhonchi. Patients with a history of breast cancer who present with new-onset asthma and a nonspecific chest radiograph may have widespread endobronchial metastases that can respond to hormone therapy or chemotherapy; these patients should thus not simply be treated with bronchodilators without investigating this possibility.

Another cause of dyspnea in the cancer patient, especially the patient with a history of lymphoma or lung, breast, or ovarian cancer, is pleural effusion. Pleural effusions usually occur because of metastases that infiltrate the pleura and cause exudation of fluid and increased capillary permeability. These collections of tumor can also erode into blood vessels and block lymphatic outflow. Overall, about 30% of patients with cancer develop malignant pleural effusion.[13] In a large series of patients with metastatic breast cancer, about half developed pleural effusion during the course of their disease, and half of these required specific treatment.

Malignant pleural effusion usually presents with dyspnea that worsens with exertion or when supine, and commonly with a dry cough. Chest examination typically reveals dullness to percussion, a pleural friction rub, and decreased breath sounds on the affected side. Radiographs of the chest confirm the diagnosis. An effusion that is visible on an upright radiograph has a volume of more than 300 mL; the threshold of detection on decubitus films is 100 mL. In the case of new pleural effusions, thoracentesis is both diagnostic and therapeutic. Pleural fluid samples should be sent for cytology, culture, cell count, and protein and lactate dehydrogenase determinations. The oncologist should be consulted for consideration of more definitive treatment modalities, such as sclerosis, pleurectomy, or chemotherapy.

Pericardial effusion also often presents with dyspnea and carries with it the danger of cardiac tamponade. Pericardial effusions are not uncommon in advanced cancer; they are usually found in the setting of lung or breast cancer but can occur in patients with lymphoma, leukemia, melanoma, sarcoma, or gastrointestinal tumors.[6] Fewer than 30% of patients with malignant pericardial effusions have symptoms of pericarditis.[7] As with the other malignant processes mentioned, pericardial effusions leading to tamponade are usually the result of long-standing processes that may evolve into critical clinical problems over the course of a few hours. The severity of tamponade is related to the rapidity with which fluid accumulates, because the pericardium can usually stretch a great deal to accommodate a slow-growing effusion. If the pericardium is thickened by fibrosis, as is often the case in patients who have received radiation therapy to the mediastinum, a small effusion can cause significant compression. Thus, a small heart on chest radiograph does not exclude cardiac tamponade.

Although a nonconstricting pericardial effusion usually does not cause specific symptoms, as the pericardium distends and compression worsens, patients develop dyspnea, chest pain relieved by leaning forward, cyanosis, or even dysphagia. Some patients with impending tamponade complain of hoarseness, epigastric discomfort, or hiccups. They often look like patients with congestive heart failure. On physical examination, the patient is typically anxious and diaphoretic, with tachycardia and decreased systolic pressure and pulse pressure. The lungs are clear; the neck veins are often engorged, and the heart sounds may be muffled. An increased pulsus paradoxus and Kussmaul's sign (inspiratory swelling of the neck veins) may be noted. With chronic pericardial constriction, the patient may develop peripheral edema, hepatojugular reflux, hepatomegaly, and, eventually, ascites.

On chest radiograph, most of these patients have increased heart size, an irregular heart border, or a globular cardiac silhouette. The electrocardiogram (ECG) typically shows sinus tachycardia and may show low-voltage QRS complexes or global ST elevation. Electrical alternans is pathognomonic of significant pericardial effusion, but this finding can disappear as compression worsens. The diagnosis of tamponade can be made definitively by echocardiography or by right heart catheterization showing equalization of diastolic pressures. Vigorous administration of intravenous fluids to maintain filling pressure can usually buy enough time to get the patient to surgery for a pericardial stripping procedure. The indications for emergent pericardiocentesis include shock, cyanosis, decreased level of consciousness, or a pulsus paradoxus greater than 50% of the pulse pressure.[20]

Superior vena caval obstruction also usually presents with a chief complaint of dyspnea, which is due to edema of the lower airway. The superior vena cava syndrome is not rare—it develops in 5% to 15% of lung cancer patients during the course of their disease. The manifestations of venous distention and facial swelling are well known, but most patients with superior vena cava syndrome do not have these signs. Superior vena cava syndrome can also cause hoarseness, dysphagia, headache, and chest pain. The symptoms are usually worsened by positional change, such as bending forward, stooping, or lying down. There is generally enough time to do diagnostic procedures if the identity of the primary tumor is unknown.

The indications for emergent therapy include decreased cardiac function, upper airway edema, or cerebral dysfunction secondary to brain edema, all of which are, fortunately, rare on presentation.[1] Nearly all patients with superior vena cava syndrome have evidence of a mass on chest radiograph (usually in the right hilum, but 20% have their lesions on the left). Superior vena cava obstruction can also cause pleural effusion (usually right-sided).[4] The most common causes of superior vena cava syndrome are bronchogenic carcinoma (predominantly small cell cancer) and lymphoma, but it can also be caused by metastases from breast and testicular cancer. In patients without a lung mass, superior vena cava syndrome may be due to mediastinal fibrosis, goiter, tuberculosis, or thrombosis around indwelling venous catheters or pacemaker leads. Computed tomography (CT) scanning of the chest is a reliable diagnostic tool.

Because patients with cancer are generally at increased risk for thrombosis, pulmonary embolism must always be considered as a potential cause of dyspnea. One issue that may arise in the treatment of cancer patients with presumed pulmonary embolism is whether the presence of brain metastases precludes the emergent use of anticoagulants. Because of the greater dangers of pulmonary embolism, these patients are generally treated with anticoagulants.

Another diagnosis that should be considered in the cancer patient presenting with shortness of breath is pulmonary fibrosis, especially among patients who have received bleomycin, high-dose cyclophosphamide, or radiation therapy to the chest. Other reasons for dyspnea include pneumonia, sepsis, or metabolic acidosis, particularly in those who are immunocompromised because of their primary tumor (especially those with a history of leukemia and lymphoma) or because of immunosuppressive therapy with cytotoxic drugs, steroids, or radiation.

HEADACHE OR LETHARGY

When evaluating the cancer patient complaining of headache or lethargy, one of the first considerations is brain metastasis. The most common tumors that spread to the brain are lung, breast, and genitourinary cancers and melanoma. As the primary treatments for these diseases improve and prolong lifespan, emergency physicians can expect to see an increasing incidence of brain metastasis. For example, 10% to 30% of patients with metastatic breast cancer develop clinically significant brain metastases during the course of their disease. The symptoms often develop over weeks, and signs depend on the location of the metastases.

Because over 90% of brain metastases are located in the cerebrum, patients often present with a history of progressive lethargy, memory loss, aphasia, paresis, or sensory disturbance.[18] Cerebellar metastases, which account for 8% of clinically important brain metastases, usually cause dysmetria or gait disturbance. A common complaint in all patients with brain metastases is headache, which is typically worse on awakening and may resolve during the course of the morning. Fewer than 25% of patients with clinically significant brain metastases have papilledema on presentation; about 15% present with new seizures.

Brain metastasis is easily diagnosed by CT scanning or magnetic resonance imaging (MRI) of the brain. Corticosteroids reduce headache and improve function in 60% to 75% of patients with brain metastasis. Dexamethasone is the drug of choice because of its high central nervous system (CNS) penetration; the usual starting dose is 4 to 10 mg intravenously. Steroid treatment should be initiated promptly. If there are physical or radiographic signs of increased intracranial pressure, an intravenous bolus of 50 g of mannitol should be given and the radiation therapist consulted emergently.

In the patient who presents with a history of seizure, anticonvulsant therapy should be begun, but it is important to keep in mind that dexamethasone reduces the serum half-life of phenytoin. Whether to begin anticonvulsant therapy in patients who have brain metastases but who have not had a seizure is a decision often left to the oncologist. However, because these patients are at increased risk for seizure, they should be warned against driving or operating machinery.

Carcinomatous meningitis can also present with headache or lethargy. It most commonly complicates breast, lung, or genitourinary tumors; leukemia; or lymphoma. Carcinomatous meningitis is especially insidious because it can develop in the face of a systemic remission. Symptoms are usually subtle and tend to develop gradually over weeks or months before the diagnosis is made. They may include headache, nausea, photophobia, back pain, memory loss, and nonspecific mental status, memory, or personality changes. Only 40% of patients with carcinomatous meningitis show evidence of cranial nerve dysfunction on presentation, usually diplopia, hearing loss, or facial numbness.

When confronted with vague CNS symptoms in a patient with a predisposing cancer, one should always include carcinomatous meningitis in the differential diagnosis, and, after ascertaining that there are no brain masses, a spinal tap should be performed. Carcinomatous meningitis should continue to be suspected even if the cerebrospinal fluid (CSF) is negative for malignant cells, because only 45% of patients with carcinomatous meningitis have the diagnosis made on the first tap; 30% of patients have the diagnosis made on the second tap, and 10% only on the third tap.[8] An opening pressure greater than 160 mm, CSF leukocytosis, increased CSF protein concentration, and decreased CSF glucose should reinforce suspicions about the presence of meningitis, although these findings are not specific for a malignant cause.

Patients with impaired cellular immunity (e.g., a history of leukemia or lymphoma or recent steroid use) can present with lethargy or subtle changes in mental status due to meningitis caused by *Cryptococcus neoformans* or *Listeria monocytogenes*. These individuals are generally not neutropenic. In cryptococcal meningitis, examination of the CSF reveals mononuclear pleocytosis and a mildly decreased glucose. The India ink stain for fungus is positive in only 50% of patients, and serologic tests for cryptococcal antigen in the serum and CSF are often needed to make the diagnosis.

Patients with *Listeria* meningitis often present with a sustained course of low-grade fevers, personality changes, and, sometimes, headache. The CSF white cell count is usually 5,000 to 15,000/μL and can consist predominantly of either neutrophils or monocytes. The CSF protein concentration is usually increased (100 to 300 mg/dL). The CSF glucose is often only mildly decreased, and organisms (gram-positive rods) are often not identified on initial examination of the CSF smear. The organism is generally sensitive to penicillin or ampicillin and is resistant to third-generation cephalosporins.[17]

Other infections that can cause a change in mental status or lethargy in cancer patients include herpes simplex and varicella zoster encephalitis. The CSF may show a mild pleocytosis and the protein is usually elevated, but CSF glucose is usually normal. CT and MRI scans often show no specific findings. Treatment is usually started on the basis of clinical suspicion. Bacterial brain abscess can also present with headache or lethargy and is usually related to contiguous bacterial infections (e.g., sinusitis, otitis, or dental abscess). These are usually apparent on CT images, as are other CNS infections that can present with a subacute or chronic history, including toxoplasmosis, nocardiosis, aspergillosis, candidiasis, and mucormycosis.

Metabolic disturbances related to cancer and its treatment are often the cause of lethargy or a change in mental status.[2] Hypercalcemia is common, especially in patients with breast, lung, renal, head and neck, esophageal, or thyroid cancers or multiple myeloma.[12] Between 10% and 20% of cancer patients develop hypercalcemia during the course of their illness; a serum calcium level greater than 13 mg/dL is a medical emergency. These patients generally respond well to saline infusion; they will often also require magnesium and potassium repletion. Loop diuretics such as furosemide are reserved for patients who cannot easily handle the volume load, and should be administered only after rehydration with saline.[15] If saline diuresis is not effective in lowering the serum calcium, other agents, such as calcitonin, mithramycin, steroids, or bisphosphates, can be used. In addition to saline diuresis, a common initial treatment for hypercalcemia is pamidronate 90 mg, given intravenously over 4 hours, and hydrocortisone 250 to 500 mg intravenously every 6 hours.

Hyponatremia, another metabolic disturbance that presents with lethargy, is usually due to ectopic secretion of antidiuretic hormone in patients with oat cell, prostate, adrenal, pancreatic, or esophageal tumors; brain metastases; or recent treatment with vincristine or cyclophosphamide.[3] Hypoglycemia should be suspected in lethargic patients, especially those with a history of insulinoma, islet cell tumors, sarcoma, hepatoma, or gastrointestinal or adrenal tumors.

Tumor lysis syndrome is a rare metabolic disorder that is associated with rapid necrosis of tumor, usually following treatment. It is most commonly seen in patients with lymphoma, acute lymphocytic leukemia, and myelogenous leukemia, but has also been reported in cases of small cell lung cancer and breast cancer. Widespread necrosis of tumor can cause severe hyperuricemia, hyperkalemia, and hyperphosphatemia, precipitating renal failure due to urate nephropathy. Metastatic calcification can exacerbate renal dysfunction and lead to cardiac dysrhythmias as well. The serum calcium may be low because of precipitation of calcium phosphate salts in soft tissues. Aggressive hydration and diuresis are the usual treatments. Urine alkalinization can help enhance uric acid execration, but in the presence of high phosphate levels, it can lead to calcium phosphate precipitation in the renal tubules. Patients with tumor lysis syndrome and severe electrolyte abnormalities or volume overload may require emergent dialysis.

MUSCULOSKELETAL PAIN

Musculoskeletal pain, a common complaint among patients in the emergency department, takes on special importance in the cancer patient. The sudden onset of pain, commonly in the upper arm, leg, or pelvis, may mean a pathologic fracture, especially in the patient with a history of prostate, breast, or lung cancer or myeloma. These fractures often occur within the sites of previous radiation therapy portals. A recent negative bone scan can be misleading in this regard, especially in cancers with purely lytic lesions, as occurs in most cases of myeloma and up to 10% of prostate cancers. The diagnosis is easily made with plain radiographs. Patients with pathologic fractures or with lytic lesions involving more than 25% of the cortex of a weight-bearing bone require immediate therapy, which calls for emergent consultation with an orthopedist and radiation therapist. Fractures often require internal fixation, because poor results are obtained with casting or bracing of these fractures.

Back pain of recent onset in the cancer patient should alert the emergency physician to the possibility of vertebral metastases, epidural metastases, and the potential for spinal cord compression. Ninety percent of cancer patients with spinal cord compression have back pain as a presenting symptom. The majority have back pain for weeks or months before neurologic signs become apparent. Patients with spinal cord compression face irreversible neurologic damage unless the diagnosis is made rapidly and therapy is initiated without delay. Most lesions causing spinal cord compression arise from tumor metastatic to the vertebral bodies; 70% of compressing lesions are in the thoracic spine, 20% are in the lumbosacral spine (especially metastatic colon cancer), and 10% occur in the cervical spine.[5]

Spinal cord compression develops in 1% to 5% of all cancer patients during the course of their disease. Patients with malignant spinal cord compression typically have a history of 1 to 6 months of back pain, which may have the features of radiculopathy and which may be made worse by the patient's lying down, bearing weight, coughing, or sneezing. The pain may radiate to the abdomen.

These patients can have many of the features of musculoskeletal back pain (e.g., paresthesias, positive straight leg-raising sign). The earliest specific sign of cord compression is motor dysfunction, usually manifested by lower extremity weakness. Subtle leg weakness cannot be assessed with the patient lying down. All patients with back pain must have their gait and the ability to walk on the toes and on the heels assessed.

On initial presentation, about half of patients with cord compression show some loss of light touch or temperature sensation. Loss of pain sensation and bowel or bladder dysfunction are usually late signs of cord compression. Patients with cauda equina syndrome typically exhibit saddle anesthesia, with sensory disturbances in the urethral, vaginal, and perianal regions. Deep tendon reflexes may be present, and even brisk, in the face of cord compression. They are usually diminished with nerve root compression.

More than 70% of patients with malignant spinal cord compression have positive spine radiographs, although those of patients with lymphoma or retroperitoneal sarcomas are generally negative. Epidural metastases are usually detectable before the onset of cord injury.[19] Suspicion that epidural metastasis are causing cord compression should prompt the immediate involvement of the neurologist and neurosurgeon. Steroids should be started and a diagnostic procedure emergently arranged.

MRI scanning is very useful for assessing the spinal cord and is usually adequate for evaluation, but myelography (plain or CT scanning) is the most precise means of assessing the extent of compression and dural involvement. Suspicion of malignant cord compression is certainly an indication for an emergent MRI scan.

In the face of a positive study, treatment (usually radiation or laminectomy) must be initiated emergently, because compression by the tumor and surrounding edema can progress rapidly to cause irreversible paraplegia or bowel or bladder dysfunction. Lest the physician become nihilistic in treating impending cord compression, one study showed that more than half of the cancer patients referred for rehabilitative treatment after malignant spinal cord compression lived for more than 1 year after the initial injury.[16]

Pain is a feature of cancer in nearly all patients, but is almost always amenable to treatment. Mild-to-moderate pain is often relieved by nonsteroidal antiinflammatory drugs or acetaminophen; more severe pain requires opioids. Pain medication must be given in adequate doses and with adequate frequency. A patient who is still in pain 1 hour after a dose of parenteral narcotics is not at high risk of developing respiratory depression from an additional dose. Various drugs are available, but no opioid is more effective than morphine. Physicians should be familiar with the equianalgesic doses and different dosing regimens of oral and parenteral opioid preparations.[10] Morphine allergy is rare (less than 1%); nausea and pruritus (secondary to the direct histamine-releasing effects of narcotic analgesics) are much more common, but can be avoided or managed with the use of antihistamines and antiemetics. Synthetic opioids, such as hydromorphone (Dilaudid), are as effective as morphine and generally have fewer side effects.

COMPLICATIONS OF CANCER TREATMENT

Nearly all cancer patients receive some sort of specific anticancer therapy, and many of these regimens can lead to complications requiring emergency treatment. The complications of cancer surgery, such as intestinal obstruction, form one broad category. The side effects of radiation therapy, another important category, depend on the site of treatment and the dose administered. A common complaint of the patient receiving mediastinal radiation is severe dysphagia. This may be mild enough to be treated with oral viscous lidocaine, or it may be severe enough to cause significant dehydration and require parenteral fluids and opioid analgesics. In general, it is reasonable to consult the radiation therapist or oncologist about complaints that relate to a site that was recently irradiated.

Patients with chronic lymphedema after cancer surgery or radiation therapy commonly present with complaints of increased swelling, pain, or redness in the involved extremity. Because of the very high risk of infection due to impaired lymphatic drainage, such individuals should be considered to have cellulitis of the limb until proven otherwise. Venipuncture, intravenous lines, and even blood pressure measurement should be avoided in the affected extremity, and antibiotics effective against staphylococci and streptococci should be started immediately.

Cytotoxic chemotherapy is fraught with side effects, some of which can be life-threatening. Because different chemotherapeutic agents have different side effects, it is useful to have some familiarity with the different agents and their side effects. The most common and serious side effect of chemotherapy is delayed-onset neutropenia. The fact that many of the drugs used in cancer treatment can also mask the clinical signs of infection helps to make acute bacterial infection the most common cause of death for patients under treatment for cancer.[11]

TABLE 216.1. Regimens for Initial Intravenous Therapy of Neutropenic Sepsis

SINGLE-DRUG REGIMENS	
Use of these antibiotics covers gram-negative organisms well and avoids the risk of nephrotoxicity. None of these covers coagulase-negative staphylococci, methicillin-resistant *Staphylococcus aureus*, enterococci, and viridans streptococci. Ceftazidime has poor anaerobic coverage.	
Ceftazidime (Fortaz, Tazidime)	2 g q8h
Cefepime (Maxipime)	2 g q8h
Imipenem-cilastin (Primaxin)	500 mg q6h
Meropenem (Merrem, Meronem)	1 g q8h
TWO-DRUG REGIMENS	
These usually include an aminoglycoside (gentamicin, tobramycin, amikacin) and an antipseudomonal beta-lactam antibiotic.	
Aminoglycosides	
Gentamicin-tobramycin	2-mg/kg loading dose, then 1.5 mg/kg q8h
Amikacin (Amikin)	8-mg/kg loading dose, then 7.5 mg/kg q8h
Antipseudomonal Beta-lactams	
Ticarcillin (Ticar)	2 g q6h
Ticarcillin and clavulanate (Timentin)	3.1 g q6h
Piperacillin (Pipracil)	3 g q4h
Piperacillin and tazobactam (Zosyn)	4 g q8h
Mezlocillin (Mezlin)	4 g q6h
Ceftazidime (Fortaz, Tazidime)	2 g q8h
Cefoperazone (Cefobid)	3 g q12h

Adapted from Pazdur R, Coia LR, Hoskins WJ, et al. Cancer management: a multidisciplinary approach. PRR: Melville NY: 1999.

NEUTROPENIC FEVER

Any patient with a recent history of chemotherapy and even a minimal fever (greater than 100.5°F) should be assumed to be neutropenic (and septic) until proven otherwise. Patients with fever and an absolute neutrophil count less than 1,000/μL should be hospitalized. Treatment should not be delayed; in neutropenic patients who die of gram-negative sepsis, death usually occurs within 48 hours of the development of fever.[11] Antibiotics should be started immediately after blood is drawn for counts and cultures. Because most lethal infections are caused by gram-negative bacilli, the febrile patient without an obvious source should receive antibiotic coverage for a broad spectrum of organisms that include *Escherichia coli, Enterobacter,* and *Pseudomonas* species. Initial treatment should include a combination of antibiotics with good gram-negative coverage.[17] Table 216.1 lists several alternative regimens for the initial empiric therapy of cancer patients with fever and neutropenia. The choice of initial antibiotic therapy must take into account the patient's allergies and hepatic and renal function.

In recent years, gram-positive infections have become more prominent with the increasing use of long-term indwelling intravenous catheters. Such infections have led to the frequent use of vancomycin in the emergency department, and antibiotics started on admission tend to be continued in the hospital until bacterial susceptibilities are available. The Centers for Disease Control has advised against the empiric use of vancomycin unless the patient has specific indications (Table 216.2). In patients who have been on prolonged courses of broad-spectrum antimicrobial therapy or on steroids, fungal infections must also be considered.

CHEMOTHERAPY-INDUCED EMESIS

Another common side effect of cancer therapy is severe nausea and vomiting that may not be amenable to treatment with the antiemetics usually used in the emergency department. The medications that most commonly cause delayed nausea (usually occurring 1 to 3 days after treatment) are intravenous cyclophosphamide, ifosfamide, and platinum. Ondansetron, high-dose intravenous metoclopramide, or parenteral benzodiazepines (e.g., lorazepam) are effective in treating the patient who is suffering from severe chemotherapy-induced nausea.[9] Chlorpromazine and haloperidol are also very effective treatments for chemotherapy-induced nausea and emesis.

CARDIOPULMONARY RESUSCITATION IN CANCER PATIENTS

A cancer patient who has significant therapeutic options should have vigorous resuscitative measures applied, just as would any other patient without the diagnosis of cancer.[14] Rates of successful resuscitation and hospital discharge for cancer patients who suffer sudden death are similar to those of patients without cancer.[21] In fact, cancer is rarely a cause of sudden, unexpected death.[22] Thus, in the absence of well-documented advanced refractory disease, an attempt at resuscitation should be undertaken. Conversely, patients who are known to have refractory advanced disease are not appropriate candidates for resuscitation, should sudden death occur.[14]

TABLE 216.2. Indications for Vancomycin for Initial Therapy of Neutropenic Sepsis

- Patients with clinically obvious catheter-related infections
- Patients with severe mucositis (especially those who have recently been treated with high-dose cytarabine [Ara-C], which increases the risk of viridans streptococci)
- Patients who had been receiving prophylactic treatment with quinolone antibiotics before the onset of fever
- Patients who are known to have been colonized with resistant pneumococci or methicillin-resistant *Staphylococcus aureus*
- Patients with hypotension or other evidence of cardiovascular instability

COMMON PITFALLS

- Failing to begin antibiotics promptly in febrile patients who are neutropenic
- Failing to treat pain aggressively. Severe pain is an emergency that requires timely treatment.
- In the cancer patient who presents with shortness of breath and a normal chest radiograph, failing to consider pulmonary embolism or cardiac tamponade
- Failing to evaluate patients with altered mental status or personality changes for treatable causes, such as hypercalcemia, hyponatremia, medication effects, carcinomatous meningitis, or subacute bacterial meningitis
- Failing to suspect spinal cord compression in a patient with cancer who presents with back pain, with or without associated neurologic complaints. Strong consideration of this entity and aggressive evaluation are imperative. The physician must keep in mind that, in patients with cord compression who have findings referable to the lumbosacral spine, the compressing lesion may be in the thoracic cord. It is therefore imperative that emergent MRI scans in these patients include the thoracic cord.
- Adopting a nihilistic attitude. Many patients with cancer have reversible illness and may have months or years of productive life ahead of them.

References

1. Ahmann F. A reassessment of the clinical implications of the superior vena cava syndrome. *J Clin Oncol* 1984;2:961.
2. Cohen LF, Balow JE, Magrath IT, et al. Acute tumor lysis syndrome. *Am J Med* 1980;68:486.
3. Ebie N, Ryan W, Harris J. Metabolic emergencies in cancer medicine. *Med Clin North Am* 1986;70:1151.
4. Escalante CP. Management of superior vena cava syndrome. *Oncology* 1993;7:61–68.
5. Gezelius C, Erikson A. Neoplastic disease in medicolegal autopsy material. *Z Rechstmed* 1988;101:115.
6. Gilkey S, Reyes CV. Cardiac tamponade in lung cancer. *J Surg Oncol* 1985;28:301.
7. Glick JH, Glover D. Oncologic emergencies. In: *American Cancer Society textbook of clinical oncology*. Atlanta: American Cancer Society, 1995.
8. Gonzalez-Vitale JC, Garcia-Bunuel R. Meningeal carcinomatosis. *Cancer* 1976;37:2906.
9. Gralla RJ, Tyson LB, Kris MG, et al. The management of chemotherapy-induced nausea and vomiting. *Med Clin North Am* 1987;71:289.
10. Jacox A, Carr DB, Payne R, et al. Management of cancer pain. Washington: U.S. Department of Health and Human Services, AHCPR Publication No. 94-0592, 1994.
11. Hughes WT, Armstrong D, Brodey GP. 1997 Guidelines for the use of antimicrobial agents in neutropenic patients with unexplained fever. *Clin Infect Dis* 1997;25:551–573.
12. Theriault RL. Hypercalcemia of malignancy: pathophysiology and implications for treatment. *Oncology* 1993;7:47–50.
13. Memon A, Zawadzki ZA. Malignant effusions, diagnostic evaluation and therapeutic strategy. *Curr Probl Cancer* 1981;5:3.
14. Morris JC, Holland JF. Oncologic emergencies In: Holland JF, Frei E, Bast RC, et al., eds. *Cancer medicine*. Philadelphia: Lea and Febiger, 1993.
15. Mundy GR, Guise TA. Hypercalcemia of malignancy. *Am J Med* 1997;103:134–145.
16. Murray PK. Functional outcome and survival in spinal cord injury secondary to neoplasia. *Cancer* 1985;55:197.
17. Pizzo PA, Meyers J, Freifeld AG, et al. Infections in cancer patients. In: DeVita VT, Hellman S, Rosenberg SA, eds. *Cancer, principles and practice of oncology*, 5th ed. Philadelphia: JB Lippincott Co, 1996.
18. Posner JB. Neurologic complications of systemic cancer. *Med Clin North Am* 1979;63:783.
19. Rodichok LD, Harper GR, Ruckdeschel JC, et al. Early diagnosis of spinal epidural metastases. *Am J Med* 1981;70:1181.
20. Theologides A. Neoplastic cardiac tamponade. *Semin Oncol* 1978;5:181.
21. Vitelli CE, Cooper K, Rogatko A, et al. Cardiopulmonary resuscitation and the patient with cancer. *J Clin Oncol* 1991;9:111.
22. Wachter RM, Luce JM, Hearst N, et al. Decisions about resuscitation: inequities among patients with different diseases but similar prognoses. *Ann Intern Med* 1989;111:525.

PART VIII

Allergy and Immunology

CHAPTER 217

Anaphylaxis

David N. Zull

Anaphylaxis is an acute, life-threatening condition; immediate recognition and treatment are critical. Its manifestations may range from minor symptoms such as rash or lip swelling to sudden, life-threatening upper airway obstruction or shock. Even the patient who presents with urticaria alone can subsequently develop hypotension, bronchospasm, or laryngeal edema and should thus be treated with the same urgency as the patient with the full-blown anaphylactic syndrome.

The constellation of anaphylactic symptoms results from massive release of chemical mediators from mast cells and basophils throughout the body. For anaphylaxis to occur, there must have been previous sensitization to a foreign substance, against which immunoglobulin E (IgE) was made by antibody-producing B lymphocytes. IgE binds to mast cells and basophils. On reexposure to the foreign substance, antigen binds to the IgE, and chemical mediators are released from these cells. The term *anaphylactoid reaction* denotes a clinical syndrome that is identical to anaphylaxis but is distinguished by the fact that mast cell mediator release results from an IgE-independent mechanism.[20]

Mediators released from activated mast cells include histamine, leukotrienes, prostaglandins, platelet activating factor, and cytokines. These mediators cause capillary leakage and vasodilation, thereby resulting in hypotension, urticaria, and angioedema of the skin, upper airway, and gastrointestinal tract. Leukotrienes are potent bronchoconstrictors as well.

Penicillin is the most feared cause of life-threatening anaphylaxis: More than 1% of the population is sensitive to penicillin. Reactions generally are manifested by urticaria alone, but an estimated 25 of 100,000 patients treated with penicillin experience a severe anaphylactic reaction; one will die.[10] There is cross-reactivity among all penicillin derivatives, as well as imipenem, but not with aztreonam. Cephalosporin cross-reactivity in penicillin-allergic patients appears to be less than 2% overall, and is rare with second- and third-generation agents; however, caution is still advised in patients with a history of anaphylaxis to pencillin.[1,10]

The reaction rate to bee stings is 0.4% to 5.0%, with at least 40 anaphylactic deaths per year.[20] The administration of iodinated contrast media (as in CT scanning with IV contrast) results in anaphylactoid reactions in 1% to 2% of patients, with one to ten fatalities per 100,000 patients, accounting for 40 to 50 deaths per year in the United States.[8] Foods are an increasingly recognized cause of fatal or near-fatal anaphylaxis,[15] and now appear to be the most common cause of anaphylaxis, accounting for one-third of cases overall and for more than one-half of episodes in children. Peanuts, other nuts, and shellfish are most commonly implicated, with highly allergic individuals reacting to the mere touch or smell of the food.[9,13,16] Nonsteroidal antiinflammatory agents are the most common medications causing anaphylaxis, often unrecognized due to over-the-counter availability.[14] Exercise, especially in combination with food or drug ingestion, can cause or aggravate anaphylaxis.[22]

Table 217.1 summarizes etiologic factors in anaphylaxis.

Repeated intermittent exposure to a substance or drug increases the risk of sensitization; the more direct the route to the systemic circulation, the greater the likelihood and severity of a reaction. The possible routes of exposure, in descending order of severity of potential reactions, are intravenous, intramuscular, subcutaneous, intradermal, oral, through other mucous membranes, and topical.

The onset of symptoms of anaphylaxis usually occurs less than 30 minutes after exposure, but is often immediate. Antigens given orally may have a 2-hour delay before symp-

TABLE 217.1. Etiologic Agents in Anaphylaxis

IgE MEDIATED—PROTEINS
Venoms: Hymenoptera (e.g., yellow jacket, honey bee), fire ant, kissing bug, rattlesnake, jellyfish[17,20]
Foods: peanuts, nuts, shellfish, grains, milk, eggs
Allergy extracts: pollens, danders
Enzymes: streptokinase, chymopapain
Human proteins: insulin, ACTH, seminal fluid
Equine antisera: botulinum toxin, snake antivenom
Vaccines: influenza, MMR, yellow fever (egg), tetanus
Miscellaneous: latex, protamine
IgE MEDIATED—HAPTENS
Antibiotics: penicillins, caphalosporins, sulfonamides, fluoroquinolones, tetracyclines[1,10]
PROSTAGLANDIN INHIBITION
NSAIDs: aspirin (excluding nonacetylated salicylates), indomethacin, ibuprofen, naproxen, etc.[14]
COMPLEMENT ACTIVATION
Blood products: gamma globulin, plasma, whole blood
Dialysis related
DIRECT MAST CELL DEGRANULATION
Drugs: opiates, vancomycin, curare, thiopental
Vitamins: thiamine, vitamin K
Polysaccharides: dextrans
Radiocontrast media: ionic >> nonionic
PHYSICAL FACTORS
Exercise-induced anaphylaxis[22]
Food- or NSAID-related anaphylaxis unmasked by exercise
Cold-induced urticaria and anaphylaxis
IDIOPATHIC[18]

toms occur. In general, the more immediate the reaction, the more life-threatening it is. Symptoms may last only a few minutes, even without therapy, but, on the average, persist for 2 to 4 hours, with the exception of angioedema, which often persists up to 24 hours, regardless of the location. Rarely, the whole anaphylactic syndrome persists beyond 24 hours,[3,7,9] and in about 3% of patients there is a biphasic course, with recurrent anaphylaxis within 24 hours, despite earlier complete resolution.[4]

CLINICAL PRESENTATION

Anaphylaxis is often heralded by premonitory symptoms (Table 217.2). Pruritus of the palms and soles, tingling about the mouth and tongue, generalized warmth, tightness in the chest, and a lump in the throat are commonly described. Dizziness or syncope secondary to hypotension may also be presenting manifestations of anaphylaxis in the absence of any other signs or symptoms of allergic reaction.

More than 90% of patients have urticaria or angioedema. Urticaria (edema of the upper dermis) appears as raised erythematous wheals in evanescent pruritic patches. Angioedema represents edema of the deep dermis and appears as puffy, nonpitting areas of skin or mucous membrane. Angioedema is generally painless and nonpruritic; patients note only tingling and swelling in the affected areas. It tends to be most prominent about the face and lips, and less so on the hands and arms.[3,7,25]

Laryngeal edema resulting in acute upper airway obstruction is the principal cause of death from anaphylaxis. The onset can be dramatic, and may be mistaken for a sudden dysrhythmic death or an apparent "café coronary." Angioedema of the lips, uvula, tongue, and oropharynx is less likely to obstruct the airway but must be treated aggressively because of the likelihood of concomitant edema of the larynx. Uvular edema, in particular, is a helpful marker for potential laryngeal involvement. Frequently, however, the patient complains of hoarseness and a lump in the throat, and the examination of the oropharynx is completely normal. Indirect laryngoscopy may reveal supraglottic or laryngeal edema, but this examination should not delay the prompt administration of epinephrine in a patient with these complaints.

TABLE 217.2. Symptoms and Signs of Anaphylaxis

Reaction	Symptom	Sign
Urticaria	Itching	Raised wheals diffusely, wandering, evanescent
Angioedema	Nonpruritic tingling	Swelling of lips, eyes, hands, uvula, tongue
Laryngeal edema	Hoarseness Dysphagia Lump in throat Airway obstruction Sudden death	Inspiratory stridor Intercostal and clavicular retractions Cyanosis
Bronchospasm	Cough, dyspnea, chest tightness	Wheezing, tachypnea, retractions
Hypotension	Dizziness Syncope Confusion	Hypotension (mild to severe) Tachycardia Oliguria
Rhinitis	Nasal congestion Itching and fluid	Mucosal edema
Conjunctivitis	Tearing Itching	Lid edema, injection, chemosis
Gastroenteritis	Cramping Diarrhea Vomiting	Normal examination

Rhinitis and conjunctivitis are other common manifestations of mucous membrane involvement, but they are not life-threatening.[3,8]

Bronchospasm is common in the anaphylactic syndrome, but it tends to be mild unless the patient has a preexisting history of asthma. Pulmonary edema, although reported in anaphylaxis, is generally considered a rare terminal event and not part of the syndrome.

Refractory hypotension is second only to laryngeal edema as a cause of death from anaphylaxis. A drop in blood pressure of 20 to 30 mm Hg is typical, but there is great variability. When sudden in onset, syncope or sudden death may occur.

Although it is usually overshadowed by other symptoms, abdominal cramping is common in anaphylaxis. Angioedema of the gut lining causes this colic as well as vomiting, diarrhea, and, rarely, hematochezia.

Myocardial infarction and ventricular tachycardia have been reported, and nonspecific ST-T wave changes are commonly seen on the electrocardiogram in patients suffering from anaphylaxis. These cardiac manifestations are generally attributed to hypotension, hypoxia, and overzealous epinephrine therapy, although histamine itself may induce coronary vasospasm and cardiac dysrhythmias.[23]

DIFFERENTIAL DIAGNOSIS

The diagnosis of anaphylaxis is often obvious when antigen exposure is rapidly followed by urticaria, angioedema, bronchospasm, upper airway edema, and hypotension. Confusion in the diagnosis may occur when a delay in the development of symptoms obscures a cause-and-effect relation or when the syndrome is only partially expressed. Anaphylaxis often presents as the acute development of only one component of the syndrome. Differentiating acute, severe urticaria, for example, from anaphylaxis is a moot point. The greatest confusion may arise when anaphylaxis presents as isolated hypotension; it should therefore be considered in the differential diagnosis of syncope and vascular collapse.

The acute development of isolated angioedema of the skin and upper airway is a common presentation of anaphylaxis, but it may also be due to hereditary angioedema. This rare disease is characterized by the absence of a functional C1′ esterase inhibitor, allowing free activation of the complement cascade. Hereditary angioedema is characterized by repeated episodes of angioedema of the skin, upper airway, and gut. Episodes generally date from adolescence and are often provoked by minor trauma. Gastrointestinal involvement is usually very prominent, often mimicking an acute abdomen. Both urticaria and hypotension are absent in hereditary angioedema, and the administration of epinephrine, antihistamines, and steroids is ineffective. A reduction in the C4 level is diagnostic. Fresh-frozen plasma, C1 esterase inhibitor concentrate, or epsilon aminocaproic acid are options in the treatment of an acute attack.[6]

Rapid development of edema of the upper airway may also result from viral or bacterial infection. However, pain, fever, and findings of erythema and exudate are not present in anaphylaxis.

Angiotensin converting enzyme inhibitors produce life-threatening tongue and palatal angioedema in 0.1% to 0.2% of patients. Although the appearance is indistinguishable from anaphylactic swelling, its development is more gradual and other features of anaphylaxis are absent.[21]

Rarely, patients may experience stridor and obstructive airway symptoms secondary to vocal cord dysfunction or as a manifestation of hysteria; indirect laryngoscopy is the only means to verify these suspicions.

Scombroid fish poisoning may mimic anaphylaxis, presenting with acute, severe urticaria, nausea and vomiting, headache, and dysphagia. This syndrome occurs shortly after eating fish with a high histidine content (such as tuna or mahi-mahi) that has spoiled slightly, so that the histidine has been broken down to histamine.

The flushing seen in monosodium glutamate reactions may be confused with anaphylaxis, but the prominence of headache and burning chest discomfort distinguishes it from an allergic reaction.

Systemic mastocytosis and the carcinoid syndrome may present with intense flushing and hypotension, mimicking anaphylaxis; prominent gastrointestinal symptoms, hepatomegaly, and provocation by alcohol help distinguish these entities.[8]

The systemic capillary leak syndrome is a rare disorder characterized by life-threatening episodes of hypovolemic shock, often accompanied by facial and extremity swelling. Transient polycythemia and hypoalbuminemia during attacks are pathognomonic; the presence of a monoclonal gammopathy may provide a clue to the diagnosis between attacks.[19]

EMERGENCY DEPARTMENT EVALUATION AND MANAGEMENT

Evaluation of the upper airway and careful blood pressure monitoring are the immediate priorities in the care of the patient with possible anaphylaxis. Angioedema of the lips, tongue, uvula, and soft palate, as well as symptoms of hoarseness, stridor, dysphagia, or lump in the throat, should alert the physician to progressive airway compromise. Such patients are treated immediately with epinephrine 0.3 mL (1:1000 dilution) subcutaneously before attempting any further evaluation. Beta-adrenergic stimulation promotes the synthesis of cyclic AMP in mast cells, which blocks further release of chemical mediators. Epinephrine also exerts a therapeutic benefit by its alpha-adrenergic effect, causing vasoconstriction with resulting improvement in blood pressure and decreased swelling of edematous tissues.[2,3,7]

The patient is placed on a cardiac monitor and given oxygen by cannula, and an intravenous line of normal saline is established. If hypotension is profound and unresponsive to saline loading, or if airway obstruction appears imminent (as evidenced by drooling and audible stridor), intravenous epinephrine is considered. The most common error made in this situation is to give too much epinephrine too fast, precipitating cardiac dysrhythmias. The recommended dose is 1.0 mL of 1:10,000 epinephrine diluted in 10 mL of normal saline, and given as a slow intravenous push over 3 to 5 minutes. If life-threatening symptoms persist, the intravenous dose may be repeated as clinically indicated.[2,5,18] In this dire situation, a cricothyroidotomy may have to be performed if air exchange is further compromised. Aerosolized epinephrine may decrease supraglottic and laryngeal edema for a few minutes, thereby buying time while preparations are made to establish an airway and parenteral epinephrine is given. If symptoms are resolving, epinephrine can be continued in a dose of 0.3 mL subcutaneously at 20-minute intervals, or an epinephrine drip can be considered (1 to 10 μg/min intravenously).[2]

Hypotension generally responds to saline infusion, with most adults requiring 1 to 2 L over the first hour. Epinephrine is an important component of therapy and can be given intramuscularly or subcutaneously if perfusion is adequate, reserving the intravenous route for use only if shock ensues. If intravenous access is unavailable, sublingual or intraosseous injection or endotracheal administration of epinephrine is considered. Other possibly helpful interventions include placing the patient in the Trendelenburg position and applying the MAST suit.[3,12] Cimetidine, 300 mg intravenously, may be useful if hypotension is refractory to standard measures.[3,5]

Most patients with anaphylaxis do not require such intensive therapy, however. In general, one or two doses of epinephrine subcutaneously at 15- to 20-minute intervals (based on symptom response) and 1 L of saline intravenously are adequate. Patients with acute, severe urticaria alone may benefit from a single dose of epinephrine, yet it is usually not necessary, because there is no life threat. Bronchospasm in anaphylaxis is responsive to epinephrine alone, but in patients with preexisting asthma, repeated albuterol nebulizations may be necessary.[3]

Corticosteroids are recommended in all patients with anaphylaxis. Although there is no immediate benefit to their administration, steroids speed the resolution of angioedema and urticaria, and are thought to prevent a biphasic course in anaphylaxis.[3,4] Dosage recommendations are similar to those for status asthmaticus: methylprednisolone (Solu-Medrol), 125-mg intravenous push, repeated every 4 to 6 hours in patients whose symptoms persist despite standard therapy.[3,7,8]

All patients with anaphylaxis should receive an antihistamine such as diphenhydramine (Benadryl), 25 to 50 mg, to a maximum of 100 mg, in more severe reactions. The route of administration depends on the severity of the reaction. An H_2 blocker such as cimetidine may be preferable to diphenhydramine if sedation is undesirable[12] or if hypotension is a prominent feature of the reaction. The combination of H_1 and H_2 blockers appears superior to either agent alone, especially in severe anaphylaxis.[3,10,12] The use of intravenous famotidine 20 mg or ranitidine 50 mg is anecdotal, but the drugs are probably equivalent to cimetidine in effect. Antihistamines alone, however, are usually inadequate in the treatment of acute anaphylaxis and should not be relied on as the sole treatment.

Preventing further exposure to the antigen is critical; for instance, a tourniquet can be placed above an injection site, the stinger of a honey bee can be removed, and any offending chemicals can be washed off.

Throughout therapy, the vital signs are reassessed frequently and the airway is checked for edema of the uvula or oropharynx. The patient is asked about symptoms of laryngeal edema or bronchospasm and examined for signs of stridor, retractions, or wheezing. These assessments are made at 1- or 2-minute intervals at first, with the intervals lengthened as the patient stabilizes.

With patients over age 50 or those with a cardiac history, saline is given cautiously for hypotension, while monitoring closely for volume overload. Epinephrine should not be withheld in patients with potential upper airway obstruction or in those with hypotension unresponsive to volume loading. A test dose of epinephrine, 0.15 mL (1:1000) subcutaneously or intramuscularly, can generally be given safely. If no chest pain or cardiac dysrhythmias develop, another test dose or a full dose is then given. However, intravenous epinephrine should be avoided in these patients unless death appears imminent without its use.[2]

Another special situation arises when anaphylaxis occurs in a patient who is taking a beta-adrenergic blocker, in which case, epinephrine therapy may have a net alpha-adrenergic effect only, thereby limiting its efficacy. In this situation glucagon, 1 to 2 mg given intravenously over 5 minutes may be of great benefit. Terbutaline, 0.25 mg subcutaneously or an isoproterenol drip, may also be considered.[3,5,7,12]

Table 217.3 summarizes treatment guidelines for anaphylaxis.

TABLE 217.3. Treatment of Anaphylaxis

1. Remove antigen, delay absorption.
2. Maintain an adequate airway.
3. Epinephrine
   0.3 ml SC 1:1000; repeat at 5- to 20-min intervals.
   If severe (hypotension, stridor) give IM and may increase dose to 0.5 mL.
   If shock or incipient airway obstruction, give 1 mL of 1:10,000 dilution IV over 5 min, repeating as indicated by clinical response.
   If protracted severe symptoms, start a drip: 1 mg in 250 mL DSW, 1–10 μg/min.
   If patient is >50 yr old or has a cardiac history and life-threatening symptoms exist, give a test dose of 0.1–0.15 mL SC or IM (1:1000). If shock resistant to other measures or immlnent airway closure, consider a drip as above.
4. Volume expansion with saline or lactated Ringer's
   Shock: 1 L over 15 min, then reassess.
5. Antihistamines
   Diphenhydramine:
   25–50 mg IM or IV push. May repeat within 15 min to a maximum of 100 mg, then smaller doses q2–4h as needed.
   Cimetidine:
   300 mg IV, repeated at 6-h intervals as needed; given as an adjunct to diphenhydramine if refractory to treatment or if sedation is a problem.
6. Methylprednisolone
   125 mg IV push; may repeat q4h if persistent symptoms.
7. If resistant hypotension:
   Trendelenburg position
   Dopamine infusion (5–20 μg/kg/min)
   Cimetidine 300 mg IV
   MAST suit
8. If imminent airway obstruction (stridor, drooling, hoarseness):
   Nebulized racemic epinephrine (0.5 mL of 2.25% in 2.5 mL normal saline) or epinephrine (5 mL of 1:1000 dilution)
   Prepare for intubation or cricothyrotomy
   Consider IV epinephrine
9. If resistant bronchospasm (usually preexistent asthma):
   Albuterol by nebulization (3–6 mL of 0.083% solution); repeat as needed.
10. If beta blocker–accentuated anaphylaxis:
    Glucagon 1 mg IV push over 4–5 min; repeat as needed for hypotension and wheezing.
    Isoproterenol drip
    Terbutaline 0.25 mg SC
11. Outpatient regimen if stable for discharge:
    Diphenhydramine 25 mg q4–6h as needed for 3 d.
    Prednisone 40–60 mg/d for 3 d.
    Prescribe EpiPen and refer to allergist if idiopathic or high risk of recurrence (food, bee sting).

DISPOSITION

Indications for Admission

If all symptoms of anaphylaxis resolve rapidly and completely with initial therapy, the patient can be observed in the emergency department without further treatment. If symptoms do not recur in the next 2 to 3 hours, the patient may safely be discharged and should continue on a 3-day course of prednisone (40 mg/d) and diphenhydramine (25 mg every 4 hours as needed) or cimetidine (400 mg every 8 hours as needed). Discharge instructions should caution the patient to avoid any suspected inciting cause, such as medications, foods, chemicals, or even exercise. The patient should be instructed to return to the emergency department immediately if hoarseness, dysphagia, wheezing, dyspnea, dizziness, or worsening rash and swelling develop. Follow-up with an allergist should be recommended, particularly if no obvious etiology has been identified in the emergency department.[18]

Patients who had a life-threatening manifestation on presentation (shock or upper airway obstruction), even if it resolved with acute therapy, should be admitted. Those who had a slow or incomplete response to therapy or any worsening of symptoms during emergency department evaluation and treatment also require admission, as do elderly or debilitated patients or those with serious underlying cardiac disease.

Transfer Considerations

Because anaphylaxis can progress in such a fulminant manner, transfer to another institution is not recommended unless prolonged observation in the emergency department has shown the patient to be stable.

COMMON PITFALLS

- Giving dangerously large doses or inappropriate concentrations of epinephrine intravenously[2]
- Withholding epinephrine therapy in the elderly or cardiac patient with imminent airway obstruction or refractory shock
- Not recognizing the possibility of recrudescence of symptoms 4 to 8 hours after an initial complete response to therapy[16]
- Not identifying common etiologies of anaphylaxis, such as antiinflammatory drugs (especially over-the-counter preparations), foods (shellfish, nuts), antibiotics (despite the lack of previous reactions and regardless of duration of therapy), antihypertensive drugs (beta blockers, angiotensin converting enzyme inhibitors), and exercise
- Not treating upper airway symptoms, such as hoarseness and dysphagia, with appropriate aggressiveness
- Not recognizing uvular and pharyngeal angioedema as warning signs of laryngeal involvement
- Misdiagnosing anaphylaxis as the flushing of a monosodium glutamate reaction or as scombroid fish poisoning
- Failing to recognize that anaphylaxis can present with shock or acute airway obstruction alone, without any other manifestations of the classic anaphylactic syndrome
- Failing to prescribe EpiPen and to provide allergy referral to patients with idiopathic anaphylaxis and those at high risk for recurrent episodes

References

1. Anne S, Reisman RE. Risk of administering cephalosporin antibiotics to patients with histories of penicillin allergy. *Ann Allergy Asthma Immunol* 1995;74:167.
2. Barach EM, Nowack RM. Epinephrine for treatment of anaphylactic shock. *JAMA* 1984;25:2118.
3. Bochner BS, Lichtenstein LM. Anaphylaxis. *N Engl J Med* 1991;324:1785.
4. Brady WJ Jr, Luber S, Carter CT, et al. Multiphasic anaphylaxis: an uncommon event in the emergency department. *Acad Emerg Med* 1997;4(3):193.
5. Brown AF. Anaphylactic shock: mechanisms and treatment. *J Accid Emerg Med* 1995;12:89.
6. Elnicki DM. Hereditary angioedema. *South Med J* 1992;85:1084.
7. Freeman TM. Anaphylaxis: diagnosis and treatment. *Prim Care* 1998;25:809.
8. Horan RF, Pennoyer DS, Sheffer AL. Management of anaphylaxis. *Immunol Allergy Clin North Am* 1991;2(1):117.
9. Kemp SF, Lockey RF, Wolf BL, et al. Anaphylaxis. A review of 266 cases. *Arch Intern Med* 1995;155:1749.
10. Lin RY. A perspective on penicillin allergy. *Arch Intern Med* 1992;152:930.
11. Moscati RM, Moore GP. Comparison of cimetidine and diphenhydramine in the treatment of acute urticaria. *Ann Emerg Med* 1990;19:12.
12. Perkin RM, Anas NG. Mechanisms and management of anaphylactic shock not responding to traditional therapy. *Ann Allergy* 1985;54:202.
13. Novembre E, Cianferoni A, Bernardini R, et al. Anaphylaxis in children: clinical and allergologic features. *Pediatrics* 1998;101:E8.

14. Quiralte J, Blanco C, Castillo R, et al. Anaphylactoid reactions due to nonsteroidal anti-inflammatory drugs: clinical and cross-reactivity studies. *Ann Allergy Asthma Immunol* 1997;78:293.
15. Sampson HA, Mendelson L, Rosen JP. Fatal and near-fatal anaphylactic reactions to food in children and adolescents. *N Engl J Med* 1992;327:380.
16. Stark BJ, Sullivan TJ. Biphasic and protracted anaphylaxis. *J Allergy Clin Immunol* 1986;78:76.
17. Stafford CT. Hypersensitivity to fire ant venom. *Ann Allergy Asthma Immunol* 1996;77:87.
18. Stoloff R, Adams SL, Orfan N, et al. Emergency medical recognition and management of idiopathic anaphylaxis. *J Emerg Med* 1992;10:693.
19. Tahirkheli NK, Greipp PR. Treatment of the systemic capillary leak syndrome with terbutaline and theophylline, a case series. *Ann Intern Med* 1999;130(11):905.
20. Valentine MD. Anaphylaxis and stinging insect hypersensitivity. *JAMA* 1992;268:2830.
21. Vleeming W, van Amsterdam JG, Sticker BH, et al. ACE inhibitor-induced angioedema: incidence, prevention and management. *Drug Saf* 1998;18:171.
22. Volcheck GW, Li JT. Exercise-induced urticaria and anaphylaxis. *Mayo Clin Proc* 1997;72:140.
23. Yunginger JW. Anaphylaxis. *Ann Allergy* 1992;69:87.

CHAPTER 218
Angioedema

Joyce M. Mitchell-Savinsky

Angioedema, characterized by areas of cutaneous and visceral swelling, has a predilection for the face, oral areas, distal extremities, and genitalia; it may also involve the larynx, gastrointestinal tract, and central nervous system. The swelling is deep rather than superficial. Unlike urticaria, the cutaneous lesions of angioedema are not usually pruritic.[7]

There are two main forms of angioedema: acquired and hereditary. The acquired form is more common, often occurring in association with urticaria, and is usually the result of a reaction to certain stimuli, such as food, drugs, infections, inhalants, insect bites, blood products, and physical factors (e.g., cold, heat, vibration, exercise), or systemic illness (e.g., collagen vascular disease).[1,9,10,12]

Angiotensin converting enzyme (ACE) inhibitors have been recognized as a common cause of this disorder. Angioedema can first occur months or even years after the ACE inhibitor was first taken, and patients sometimes report having had previous episodes that subsided spontaneously while they continued taking the drug.[2] Acquired angioedema usually lasts for hours to days. A chronic form (by definition, persisting more than 6 weeks) is more common in middle-aged adults; often, no inciting factor can be identified.[7]

Hereditary angioedema (HAE), an inherited deficiency of the inhibitor of the activated first component of complement (C1 INH), is manifested by recurrent attacks of angioedema not associated with urticaria. Compromise of the airway occurs in up to two-thirds of these patients at some time and is the cause of death in many patients with the disease.[5,14] A rare acquired form of C1′ esterase INH deficiency is seen in association with hematologic and other malignancies.[4]

Histologically, both forms of angioedema show vascular dilatation and increased permeability with interstitial edema. These changes occur in the deep dermis and subcutaneous tissues, unlike those of urticaria, which are seen in the upper dermis.[7]

CLINICAL PRESENTATION

The clinical presentation depends on the sites or organ systems affected. Most commonly, there is localized swelling that develops acutely, typically on the face or upper lip, especially with ACE inhibitor–associated disease. Some patients complain of pruritus due to associated urticaria and tightness or burning in the angioedematous areas.[7] Involvement of the gastrointestinal tract, seen more commonly in HAE, can cause abdominal pain, nausea, vomiting, and diarrhea. The pain is usually diffuse and colicky and may be associated with peritoneal signs, mimicking an acute surgical abdomen but without fever or leukocytosis. Radiologic findings suggestive of bowel wall edema may be seen.[8] Neurologic involvement is rare but, when it occurs, may be associated with altered consciousness, headache, seizures, and focal deficits. These typically resolve without permanent sequelae.[11]

The most emergent presentation of angioedema is life-threatening upper airway obstruction with dysphagia, a "tightness" in the throat, dyspnea, cough, hoarseness, and stridor. Airway involvement is unusual in acquired angioedema, it but can progress rapidly.[9] Fatal airway obstruction has been reported with the use of ACE inhibitors.[1,10] In HAE, airway edema can progress over several hours, with increasing hoarseness, difficulty swallowing, and aphonia prior to complete airway obstruction.[13]

DIFFERENTIAL DIAGNOSIS

Other entities that can cause swelling must be considered, including cellulitis and erysipelas, congestive heart failure, lymphedema, renal disease, and venous obstruction.

EMERGENCY DEPARTMENT EVALUATION

Evaluation in the emergency department is directed at identifying inciting agents, assessing the severity of illness, and considering the possibility of HAE or other underlying disorder.[7] The crucial aspect of the physical examination is assessment of airway status. A common pitfall is to underestimate airway involvement and the potential for obstruction. Laboratory studies are seldom useful in acute episodes, except to eliminate other causes of edema.

EMERGENCY DEPARTMENT MANAGEMENT

For patients with upper respiratory involvement, the most important aspect of emergency care is maintenance of a patent airway. These patients should receive subcutaneous epinephrine (0.3 mL of 1:1000) and a parenteral H_1-blocker antihistamine. There is no reported added benefit of administering epinephrine intravenously. Continuous monitoring of airway status is critical. The decision to establish an airway is sometimes difficult. When in doubt, however, aggressive intervention should be undertaken, using orotracheal or nasotracheal intubation or cricothyrotomy.

The mainstays of drug treatment of acute acquired angioedema are epinephrine and H_1-blocker antihistamines such as diphenhydramine, hydroxyzine, and cyproheptadine.[7,10] In chronic angioedema, corticosteroids have been used, with varying success, in conjunction with H_2 blockers.[4,8–10] Patients presenting with uncomplicated cutaneous swelling should be treated with oral or intramuscular diphenhydramine (25 to 50 mg) or hydroxyzine (25 to 50 mg).[7] If there is gastrointestinal involvement, additional symptomatic and supportive therapy should be provided. Patients taking ACE inhibitors should stop doing so and henceforth avoid taking that class of drugs.

Epinephrine, antihistamines, and corticosteroids have not been reported consistently to be useful in the treatment of acute attacks of HAE.[13] Androgen derivatives (e.g., danazol) and antifibrinolytic agents (e.g., ϵ-aminocaproic acid and tranexamic acid) can decrease the frequency of attacks, but they do not arrest acute episodes.[3,4,13] Significant improvement has been seen with infusion of C1 INH concentrates.[3,6,13] No therapy is required for simple cutaneous episodes, and isolated gastrointestinal attacks likewise require only symptomatic and supportive care. With impending airway obstruction, maintenance of airway patency is the prime consideration. Infusion of C1 INH concentrate (or, less preferably, fresh-frozen plasma when the concentrate is unavailable) may be beneficial.[4,6,13] Patients with acquired C1 INH deficiency may require much higher doses than those with the hereditary form.[4]

DISPOSITION

In patients with previously diagnosed HAE, management should be discussed with the patient's primary care physician.

In both acute and hereditary forms of angioedema, patients with simple cutaneous swellings who have shown no progression of symptoms during several hours of observation in the emergency department can often be discharged, with follow-up scheduled in 1 to 2 days. Because airway compromise occasionally develops unpredictably many hours after the episode of angioedema, some clinicians admit all such patients to the hospital for observation, particularly if there is any doubt as to the reliability of follow-up. Patients who are reliable and safe to be discharged, however, should be instructed to return immediately if airway symptoms develop. Patients who have been taking ACE inhibitors should consult their primary care physician for initiation of a different antihypertensive medication.

Patients with airway compromise or worsening symptoms despite therapy require immediate hospital admission. These patients and those with severe neurologic symptoms should be placed in a critical care setting.

If the patient must be transferred to a facility offering a higher level of care, the airway must be secured before transport. The patient should be transferred by the most expeditious route and by personnel who are skilled in airway management.

COMMON PITFALLS

- The worst error made in the management of patients with angioedema is failure to establish airway control.
- Failure to recognize an ACE inhibitor as the underlying cause of angioedema may result in repeated episodes if the drug is not discontinued.
- The diagnosis of angioedema can be missed when the patient presents with gastrointestinal and neurologic complaints. Careful attention to associated cutaneous lesions or to a history of previous episodes should alert the physician to the diagnosis of angioedema.
- In acute attacks of HAE, epinephrine and antihistamines have not been proven to be beneficial, and their use may lead to a false sense of security.

References

1. Agah R. Angioedema: the role of ACE inhibitors and factors associated with poor clinical outcome. *Intensive Care Med* 1997;23:793–796.
2. Brown N. Recurrent angiotensin-converting enzyme inhibitor-associated angioedema. *JAMA* 1997;278:232.
3. Cicardi M. Pathogenetic and clinical aspects of C1 inhibitor deficiency. *Immunobiology* 1998;199:366.
4. Heymann W. Acquired angioedema. *J Am Acad Dermatol* 1997;36(4):611.
5. Kulp-Shorten C. Urticaria, angioedema, and rheumatiologic disease. *Rheum Dis Clin North Am* 1996;22(1):95.
6. Kunschak M. A randomized, controlled trial to study the efficacy and safety of C1 inhibitor concentrate in treating hereditary angioedema. *Transfusion* 1998;38:540.
7. Kwong K. Urticaria and angioedema: pathophysiology, diagnosis, and treatment. *Pediatr Ann* 1998;27(11):719.
8. Mullins R. Visceral angioedema related to treatment with an ACE inhibitor. *Med J Aust* 1996:165:319.
9. Pillans P. Angiooedema and urticaria with angiotensin converting enzyme inhibitors. *Eur J Clin Pharmacol* 1996;51:123.
10. Sabroe R. Angiotensin-converting enzyme (ACE) inhibitors and angiooedema. *Br J Dermatol* 1997;136:153.
11. Sunder T. Neurological manifestations of angioedema. *JAMA* 1982;247(14):2005.
12. Van Rijnsoever E. Angioneurotic edema attributed to the use of losartan. *Arch Intern Med* 1998;158:2063.
13. Visentin D. C1-esterase inhibitor transfusions in patients with hereditary angioedema. *Ann Allergy Asthma Immunol* 1998;80:457.
14. Winnewisser J. Type I hereditary angio-oedema. Variable of clinical presentation and course within two large kindreds. *J Intern Med* 1997; 241(1):39.

CHAPTER 219
Drug Allergy and Other Drug Reactions

Donna Kinser

Adverse drug effects occur in up to 15% of drug regimens and are said to be the basis of the majority of iatrogenic illness. Patients with acute symptoms are likely to present to the emergency physician for diagnosis and care.

Adverse drug reactions are predictable (80%) or unpredictable (20%). Predictable reactions are those related to known pharmacologic activity; they include side effects of immediate expression, side effects of delayed expression (carcinogenicity, teratogenicity), effects of overdosage or toxicity, secondary or indirect effects, and drug interactions. Unpredictable reactions are those related to individual immunologic response or genetic difference; they include drug intolerance, drug idiosyncrasy, allergic reaction and pseudoallergic reaction, plus psychophysiologic reaction (vasovagal, hyperventilation).

DRUG ALLERGY

Drug allergy or hypersensitivity accounts for 5% to 10% of adverse drug reactions. Characteristically, allergic drug reactions occur in a minority of patients receiving a particular drug. There is typically a history of prior uneventful use of the drug, although allergic reactions can occur during the first course of therapy if continuing for more than about a week. There may be rapid reaction on reexposure to a small dose of the same or a related drug. Reactions typically conform to a characteristic pattern.

Risk factors for drug allergy include the degree of host reactivity, the characteristics of the drug, the degree of exposure, and the route of administration (topical and parenteral administration is associated with greater risk than oral administration.) Some drugs are complete antigens (e.g., insulin, streptokinase, and heterologous antisera), but most are low-molecular-weight incomplete antigens that must form a stable bond with tissue or plasma proteins to become immunogenic. Usually, it is one or more of the drug's metabolites that form the union. Because the metabolites of most drugs are not well identified (the notable exception being penicillin), tests to confirm specific drug sensitivity and to elucidate the mechanism of reactivity are limited.

Immunologic or allergic adverse drug reactions can be categorized according to the classification system of Gell and Coombs.

Type I: IgE-Mediated Immediate Hypersensitivity

Type I reactions are mediated by preformed drug-specific IgE antibodies attached to the surface of tissue mast cells and circulating basophils. Bridging of the IgE antibodies by the drug in antigenic form results in mediator release and clinical sequelae such as urticaria, angioedema, laryngeal edema, bronchospasm, and hypotension. Maculopapular rashes may also be type I reactions.

Type II: Cytotoxic Antibody Reactions

Cytotoxic reactions result when IgG or IgM antibodies interact with cell-bound drug and mediate cell injury through complement activation or mononuclear cell activation. Almost all type II reactions involve injury to formed elements of the blood, for example, manifesting as immune hemolytic anemia or thrombocytopenia.

Type III: Immune Complex–Complement Reactions

In type III reactions, circulating immune complexes (consisting of drug plus IgG or drug plus IgM) fix complement and lodge in tissue, where tissue injury ensues. Clinically, the reaction is characterized by fever, rash (ranging from urticaria to palpable purpura), arthralgia, and lymphadenopathy. Serum sickness is the prototype of the type III reaction; penicillins and foreign antisera are among the recognized causes. Other examples of type III reactions are drug-induced, lupus-like syndromes and infiltrative lung disease secondary to inhaled drug allergens.

Type IV: Cell-Mediated Delayed Hypersensitivity

Type IV reactions are mediated by sensitized lymphocytes that recognize a particular drug antigen and recruit other lymphocytes and mononuclear cells to the site of that antigen. Type IV reactions primarily occur as contact dermatitis.

Other Reactions

A number of drug reactions do not strictly fit the Gell and Coombs classification but are presumed to be immunologic. They include Stevens-Johnson syndrome, exfoliative dermatitis, toxic epidermal necrolysis, drug-induced fever, the anticonvulsant hypersensitivity syndrome, and certain cases of pulmonary, hepatic, and renal hypersensitivity. They also include vasculitis syndromes such as hypersensitivity angiitis and leukocytoclastic vasculitis.

A set of reactions that resembles type I IgE-mediated hypersensitivity reactions, but do not involve IgE, are termed *pseudoallergic reactions*. They are clinically indistinguishable from true allergic reactions because comparable mediators produce comparable target-organ sequelae. When life-threatening, they are termed *anaphylactoid*. Commonly used agents that can cause nonspecific mast cell and basophil release of preformed and generated mediators include iodinated radiocontrast media (RCM), opiates, and dextrans. Drugs such as succinylcholine, vancomycin, and ciprofloxacin can cause either IgE-mediated or non–IgE-mediated systemic reactions. The "red man syndrome" is a dose-dependent reaction to vancomycin caused by direct stimulation of mast cells to release histamine; it may be attenuated by reducing the infusion rate. Aspirin and nonsteroidal antiinflammatory agents are hypothesized to cause pseudoallergic respiratory reactions through their effects on the cyclooxygenase pathway. Angiotensin converting enzyme (ACE) inhibitors are hypothesized to cause pseudoallergic reactions through their effects on the kallikrein system.

Diagnosis

The diagnosis of adverse drug reactions hinges on the history of drug exposure. Improvement of symptoms after withdrawal of the suspected drug is suggestive information. Confirmatory tests are generally unavailable. Skin testing to detect immediate hypersensitivity has only a limited role for some high-molecular-weight compounds and for penicillin. Patch testing may be performed for drug-induced contact dermatitis. *In vitro* radioallergosorbent or enzyme-linked immunosorbent tests are applicable in special circumstances. The indirect Coombs' test is a diagnostic aid in immune hemolytic anemia. Direct challenge is potentially hazardous and rarely indicated, but it occasionally has a role in evaluating local anesthetic reactions.

Management

The standard management of adverse drug reactions includes prompt discontinuation of the medication and provision of supportive care that is specific to the type and severity of manifestations. Mild pruritis, flushing, and rash may be treated with antihistamines. Corticosteroids are usually administered only for more severe systemic reactions. Early epinephrine is the mainstay of treatment for anaphylactic reactions. Oxygen and airway support, inhaled beta agonists, intravenous fluids, and pressors also may be required.

Certain steps can be taken to prevent or minimize drug reactions. Medications should be prescribed only when necessary; in one study of anaphylactic deaths, 40% of the cases involved drugs for which there was no clear indication. The oral route should be used when possible. Preparations that are less sensitizing (e.g., human insulin rather than pork insulin) are preferred when available. Drug history should be carefully elicited. Frequently, information that can prevent an adverse drug reaction is available from the patient, the patient's relatives, or previous medical records. Documentation in the medical record of any apparent reaction may help avert a similar or worse reaction. Finally, when potentially immunogenic parenteral agents are given in the emergency department, patients should be observed for at least 20 minutes after administration. Discharge instruction should include cautions regarding possible reaction.

PENICILLIN ALLERGY

Penicillin and its derivatives are among the most widely prescribed antibiotics and are the most common cause of drug-induced allergic reactions. Penicillin may be responsible for any of the four main types of reactions: IgE-mediated urticaria, angioedema, anaphylaxis (type I); cytotoxic hemolytic anemia, thrombocytopenia (type II); immune complex serum sickness (type III); or cell-mediated contact dermatitis (type IV). Penicillin may also cause other reactions, such as interstitial nephritis, exfoliative dermatitis, and drug fever.

The overall incidence of adverse reactions to penicillins is estimated to be 2% (range, 0.7% to 10%), and the incidence of anaphylaxis is thought to be 0.015% to 0.04% of treatment courses. Approximately 10% of anaphylactic episodes are fatal, accounting for more than 400 deaths annually in the United States and making penicillins the leading cause of anaphylactic death. Anaphylaxis is usually an immediate reaction (occurring within 30 minutes of administration), but, in approximately 10% of cases, symptoms begin more than 1 hour after administration.

IgG and IgM antibodies to penicillin–protein complexes are produced on first exposure to penicillins in virtually all individuals, whereas IgE antibodies develop in only a small subset. Sensitization may occur through medical use or through occult food, environmental, or medication exposure. There seems to be a genetic predisposition to formation of IgE antibodies, but atopy is not a risk factor. IgE production usually occurs within 1 to 3 weeks of exposure. Depending on the individual, the half-life varies from days to years.

Early reactions consistent with a generalized systemic response (e.g., generalized urticaria angioedema, bronchospasm, or hypotension) are usually categorized as anaphylactic, even if they are mild, and these should be treated promptly. Therapy should be tailored to the severity of the reaction, and, after epinephrine, may include antihistamines, corticosteroids, intravenous fluids, and pressors. Penicillin and penicillin derivatives should thereafter be avoided in these patients. Regarding risk of future use of the other beta-lactam antibiotics, cross-reactivity is high with the carbapenems (e.g., imipenem), less with the cephalosporins, and minimal with the monobactams (e.g., aztreonam). If there is not an acceptable or effective alternative to penicillin (e.g., for central nervous system syphilis or gestational syphilis), the patient should be considered for penicillin skin testing and inhospital desensitization.

When a patient develops a maculopapular rash after receiving penicillin, it may represent an allergic reaction, mediated by either IgE, IgG, or IgM. Alternatively, the rash may be an unrelated manifestation of the underlying disease. In some cases, the disease plus the penicillin drug result in the adverse reaction. For example, patients with infectious mononucleosis are likely to develop a morbilliform rash 3 to 8 days after commencing ampicillin or amoxicillin therapy. A similar rash may develop in patients with cytomegalovirus infection, hyperuricemia, or lymphocytic leukemia.

When a maculopapular rash attributable to penicillin allergy occurs, the antibiotic should be discontinued. Additionally, the patient should be instructed to avoid all penicillins. Even if the reaction were actually due to allergy to the specific side chain of a penicillin derivative (e.g., amoxicillin) and not the group common to penicillin drugs, this cannot be distinguished clinically (hence, the need to advise avoidance of all). Whether to use a cephalosporin antibiotic for future infections requires consideration of the risks and benefits in the clinical circumstances. The baseline risk of reaction to a cephalosporin is felt to be approximately 2%. The previously accepted estimate—an increase to 8% to 10% risk of reaction when first- or second-generation cephalosporins are used in patients with history of penicillin allergy—is being questioned. Recent information and analysis suggest that the incidence is much lower than this, and, for third-generation cephalosporins, it is not above the baseline incidence for the general population.

LOCAL ANESTHETIC REACTIONS

Local anesthetics are among the most frequently administered drugs in emergency medicine. They can be divided into two main chemical groups: the esters and the amides (Table 219.1).

TABLE 219.1. Local Anesthetic Chemical Groups

GROUP I: ESTERS (MAY CROSS-REACT)
Benzocaine (Americaine)
Procaine (Novocain)
Proparacaine (Alcaine, Ophthaine)
Tetracaine (Pontocaine)
GROUP II: AMIDES (UNLIKELY TO CROSS-REACT)
Bupivacaine (Marcaine, Sensorcaine)
Lidocaine (Xylocaine)
Mepivacaine (Carbocaine)
Prilocaine (Citanest)
OTHERS: FOR MUCOUS MEMBRANES
Dibucaine (Nupercainal)
Dyclonine (Dyclone)
Pramoxine (Tronothane)

The amides have a longer half-life in tissues and are favored for local anesthesia. Although true allergic reactions are rare, many patients report "allergy to 'caines," because a variety of nonallergic reactions are associated with the administration of local anesthesia. The differential diagnosis includes hyperventilation, vasovagal reaction, sympathetic stimulation, and toxic drug levels.

The approach to the patient who reports allergy to local anesthesia depends on the analysis of the available information. When the history supports prior nonallergic reaction to local anesthesia, any of the standard anesthetic agents may be used. When the suspected drug can be identified, an agent from a structurally unrelated group is preferred. Hypersensitivity and intragroup cross-reactivity occur more prominently with ester anesthetics.

When all local anesthetic agents seem contraindicated, local anesthesia may be provided by the use of diphenhydramine. Diphenhydramine 1% (1.5 to 5.0 mL intradermally) provides effective anesthesia for repair of minor lacerations. Pain during initial administration is greater than with lidocaine, but pain during the procedure is equally well controlled. Sleepiness occasionally occurs after anesthesia with 1% diphenhydramine. Lower concentrations (e.g., 0.5%) seem less effective for anesthesia, and higher concentrations (2% to 5%) have been associated with local irritation, burning, erythema, vesicle formation, skin sloughing, and prolonged anesthesia or paresthesias.

Patients for whom local anesthetics will be needed in the future, but which cannot be ascertained as safe by history, should be referred for allergy testing. There are protocols for testing serial dilutions of the agent in question. Experience has shown that true-positive reactions are rare (less than 1%) and that the sensitivity does not seem to correlate with the presence of paraben or methylparaben preservatives. Although serial testing could be conducted in the emergency department, time constraints usually make it impractical.

RADIOCONTRAST MEDIA REACTIONS

More than 10 million radiographic evaluations using RCM are performed each year in the United States. Diatrizoates and iothalamates are the ionic contrast agents that have been most widely used. They are referred to as high-osmolality contrast media because their osmolality is several-fold higher than that of plasma.

In the 1970s, low-osmolality agents were introduced. Their osmolality is only approximately twice that of plasma; most of them are also nonionic (Table 219.2). Compared with their fore-

TABLE 219.2. Radiocontrast Media Categories

	Approximate Osmolality (mOsmol/kg water)	Ionic
HIGH OSMOLALITY		
Diatrizoate sodium	1,500	Yes
Diatrizoate sodium (8%) and meglumine (52%)	1,500	Yes
Iothalamate meglumine (60%)	1,400	Yes
LOW OSMOLALITY		
Iohexol	300–800	No
Iopamidol	600	No
Ioversol	700	No
Ioxaglate sodium (19.6%) and meglumine (39.3%)	600	Yes

runners, these low-osmolality agents seem to provide comparable quality of opacification and to carry a lower overall risk of complications. They have not fully supplanted the high-osmolality agents, however, because of their expense.

Immediate adverse effects from contrast media can be subdivided into two broad categories. The first consists of those reactions that are related to the physicochemical properties of the media, particularly hyperosmolality. Physiologic effects that correlate with high osmolality include vasodilation, hemodilution, erythrocyte deformity, disturbance of the blood–brain barrier, and alteration of left ventricular end-diastolic pressure and arterial pressure. Reduction in the incidence of cardiovascular side effects, heat sensation, and local pain have been demonstrated when low-osmolality (nonionic) agents are used in place of high-osmolality (ionic) agents. Overall rates of immediate adverse reactions attributable to physicochemical properties are estimated to be 1% to 3% for the former and 4% to 12% for the latter.

The other broad category of immediate adverse reactions is anaphylactoid reactions. They typically follow intravascular injection of RCM but, in rare instances, may occur after contrast is introduced into extravascular structures. The anaphylactoid reactions tend to be more severe and less dose- and concentration-dependent than the physicochemical reactions. Bronchospasm, laryngeal edema, widespread urticaria or angioedema, hypotension, and/or arrhythmias manifest within 30 minutes of the infusion. Although the initiating pathophysiology does not seem to be that of an IgE-mediated allergic reaction, there is comparable release of histamine and other mediators from mast cells. Therefore, the treatment is the same as for true anaphylaxis. Estimated rates of incidence are 0.22% for the high-osmolality (ionic) contrast agents versus 0.04% for low-osmolality (nonionic) contrast agents. Deaths have been reported with the use of each type of agent. Patients with allergic diathesis, asthma, or cardiac disease are at increased risk for these anaphylactoid reactions. Patients with a history of contrast reaction have more than five times the incidence of a subsequent reaction in comparison with previous nonreactors.

The most significant late-occurring adverse reaction is that of nephrotoxicity. The mechanism is not completely understood, but the clinical picture is that of an increase in the serum creatinine level that begins within 24 hours of exposure to the agent. Risk factors for nephrotoxicity include advanced age, dehydration, preexisting renal insufficiency, diabetes mellitus, diuretic therapy, hepatic insufficiency, multiple myeloma, recent large dose of RCM, and sickle cell anemia. Although the degree of protective benefit is not uniform or certain, low osmolality (nonionic) agents are recommended for patients with one or more of the risk factors for nephrotoxicity.

Fever, chills, rash, arthralgias, diarrhea, nausea, vomiting, headache, and other nonspecific symptoms may occur as a delayed reaction 30 minutes to 3 days after contrast media injection in 4% to 8% of patients. Fever typically abates within 8 hours and is speculated to represent a hypothalamic response to RCM injection. Patients who have recently received interleukin-2 seem to have an increased frequency and severity of delayed reactions. Treatment of delayed reactions is supportive.

The risk-to-benefit ratio of a contrast study should be considered before it is ordered and performed, especially in patients with a history of anaphylactoid reaction. In some situations, a study that does not require contrast (e.g., ultrasound or magnetic resonance imaging) can be substituted. In others, the radiocontrast test can be delayed for 12 to 36 hours, during which time the patient can be pretreated with corticosteroids and antihistamines to decrease the likelihood of recurrent anaphylactoid reaction. One established protocol is to administer methylprednisolone, 32 mg by mouth, 12 hours and 2 hours before contrast administration, and diphenhydramine, 50 mg by mouth or intramuscularly, 1 hour before contrast administration. Pretreatment can be expected to reduce the incidence of reactions to high-osmolality agents by approximately one-third. Simply using low-osmolality agents alone may reduce risk to a similar level. Combining pretreatment and low-osmolality agents may provide extra protection but extends the time until the test can be performed.

ANGIOTENSIN CONVERTING ENZYME INHIBITOR REACTIONS

The propensity of the ACE inhibitors to cause cough and angioedema has been increasingly recognized and studied in recent years. These reactions are not allergic in nature and appear to involve the kinin system.

Cough is the more frequent but less serious of the two adverse reactions and occurs in 5% to 20% of patients treated with ACE inhibitors. It occurs more often in females and may be dependent on dose. The onset of cough is typically within 1 week of initiation of therapy, but it may develop up to 6 months later. There is no associated alteration in pulmonary function. The diagnosis is a clinical one. In most cases, management consists simply of withdrawal of the ACE inhibitor, and the diagnosis is confirmed by resolution of the cough within a week. Subsequent challenge with the same agent or another ACE inhibitor almost always results in recurrence of cough.

Angioedema, typically of the face, neck, or upper airway, occurs in 0.1% to 0.2% of patients treated with ACE inhibitors (and also has been reported in patients treated with angiotensin II receptor antagonists). The reaction can progress rapidly to airway obstruction and death. The risk is highest in the first few hours to first week of treatment but can also occur in patients who have been taking the drug uneventfully for months to years. The risk abates within hours of stopping the drug.

When angioedema secondary to an ACE inhibitor occurs, administration of the standard allergic anaphylaxis treatment of subcutaneous epinephrine, diphenhydramine, and corticosteroids cannot be relied on to reverse the process. Furthermore, the progression of the edema is unpredictable, and there may be rebound. Early airway control is therefore recommended, because massive edema of the tongue and pharynx can make orotracheal and nasotracheal intubation difficult, and neck edema may make creation of a surgical airway difficult as well.

Bibliography

Asaverreaza EE. Penicillin allergy: a review. *Tex Med* 1989;85:37.

Cohan RH, Leder RA, Ellis JH. Treatment of adverse reactions to radiographic contrast media in adults. *Radiol Clin North Am* 1996;84:1055.

deShazo RD, Kemp SF. Allergic reactions to drugs and biologic agents. *JAMA* 1997;278:1895.

deShazo RD, Nelson HS. An approach to the patient with a history of local anesthetic hypersensitivity: experience with 90 patients. *J Allergy Clin Immunol* 1979;63:87.

DeSwarte RD. Drug allergy—problems and strategies. *J Allergy Clin Immunol* 1984;74:209.

Ernst AA, Anand P, Nick T. Lidocaine versus diphenhydramine for anesthesia in the repair of minor lacerations. *J Trauma* 1993;34:354.

Greenberger PA, Patterson R. The prevention of immediate generalized reactions to radiocontrast media in high-risk patients. *J Allergy Clin Immunol* 1991;4:867.

Israili ZH, Hall WD. Cough and angioneurotic edema associated with angiotensin-converting enzyme inhibitor therapy. *Ann Intern Med* 1992;117:234.

Kim K, Evans R III, Mahr TA. Drug allergy. *Allergy Proc* 1990;11:299.

King BF, Hartman GW, Williamson B. Low-osmolality contrast media: a current perspective. *Mayo Clin Proc* 1989;6:976.

Lin RY. A perspective on penicillin allergy. *Arch Intern Med* 1992;152:930.

Suresh A, Reisman RE. Risk of administering cephalosporin antibiotics to patients with histories of penicillin allergy. *Ann Allergy Asthma Immunol* 1995;74:167.

Westhoff-Bleck M, Bleck JS, Jost S. The adverse effects of angiographic radiocontrast media. *Drug Saf* 1991;6:28.

PART IX

Rheumatology

CHAPTER 220

Monoarticular Arthritis

Alan C. Heffner and Stephen A. Coluciello

Monoarticular arthritis is a common emergency condition, the outcome of which depends on rapid diagnosis and treatment.[1] In the case of septic arthritis, delay or misdiagnosis may lead to joint destruction or even death.

Gout and disseminated gonococcal infection are the most common causes of monoarticular arthritis; infections due to *Staphylococcus aureus* and other bacteria are the most serious. Monoarticular arthritis may also be the initial presentation of a systemic polyarticular disease.

CLINICAL PRESENTATION

Gonococcal Arthritis

Gonococcal arthritis may be monoarticular, migratory, or polyarticular, and usually involves the wrist, knee, or ankle. At least half of patients exhibit a rash that consists of scattered hemorrhagic pustules on an erythematous base, usually on the extremities. Maculopapular and petechial lesions may also occur. Tenosynovitis frequently involves the extensor tendons of the hand and wrist and tends to be fleeting and migratory. The degree of toxicity varies greatly, and fever and leukocytosis may be absent.

Nongonococcal Septic Arthritis

Nongonococcal septic arthritis involves, in descending order of frequency, the knee, hip, shoulder, ankle, elbow, hand, or wrist. Patients with a history of intravenous drug use can present with involvement of unusual joints such as the sternoclavicular, sacroiliac, or manubriosternal joints. Septic arthritis may develop in a fulminant fashion, with marked toxicity, fever, and confusion, or may be subacute and insidious, with malaise, anorexia, and little or no fever. In the elderly or those with rheumatoid arthritis, the onset is often gradual, and multiple joint involvement occurs in up to 9% of patients.[5,13] This combination of rheumatoid arthritis and septic arthritis is deadly; the mortality rate is reported to be as high as 19%.[4]

Crystal-Induced Monoarthritis

Most cases of acute gout affect a single joint, but the attack may be polyarticular in up to 40% of cases.[10] Pseudogout, or calcium pyrophosphate deposition disease (CPPD), usually develops after the age of 50; attacks may be mono- or polyarticular, often affecting the knees, wrists, ankles, and elbows. In both disorders, patients may demonstrate systemic symptoms such as fever or confusion.[11]

DIFFERENTIAL DIAGNOSIS

Monoarticular arthritis may be due to hemorrhagic, mechanical, neoplastic, ischemic, inflammatory, or infectious causes (Table 220.1). In patients with hemophilia or those who take anticoagulants, hemorrhage may occur spontaneously or in association with mild trauma. Patients without coagulopathy who develop acute traumatic hemarthrosis usually have significant injury to bone, joint, or ligament.

The most common causes of crystal-related arthritis are monosodium urate (gout) and calcium pyrophosphate dihydrate (pseudogout). On occasion, a variety of other crystals, including apatites and calcium oxalate, may produce inflammatory joint changes. Gout develops when sodium urate crystals

TABLE 220.1. Differential Diagnosis of Acute Monoarticular Arthritis

Infectious	Bacterial
	Gonococcal
	Nongonococcal
	Mycobacterial (tuberculosis and atypical)
	Spirochete (Lyme, syphilis)
	Fungal
	Viral (HIV, hepatitis B, rubella, others)
	Postinfectious
Crystal-induced	Gout (monosodium urate)
	Pseudogout (CPPD)
	Calcium apatite
Traumatic	Fracture
	Ligamentous injury
	Overuse injury
Ischemic	Avascular necrosis
	Sickle cell vasoocclusive crisis
	Decompression illness
	Spontaneous osteonecrosis
Hemorrhagic	Posttraumatic
	Hemophilia
	Systemic anticoagulation
Neoplastic	Metastasis
	Osteochondroma
	Osteoid osteoma
	Pigmented villonodular synovitis
Systemic disease	Remote infection, infectious endocarditis
	Rheumatic fever
	Seronegative spondyloarthropathies (ankylosing spondylitis, inflammatory bowel disease, psoriatic, reactive)
	Reiter syndrome, Behçet disease
	Rheumatoid arthritis, SLE
	Sarcoidosis, amyloidosis

precipitate in joints and initiate an inflammatory reaction. Although chronic hyperuricemia is necessary for gout to develop, during an acute attack the serum uric acid may be normal, high, or low. Ninety percent of primary, or idiopathic, gout is due to underexcretion of uric acid; attacks are precipitated by excessive purine intake, joint trauma, or alcohol use. Secondary gout is associated with systemic disease, such as malignancy or diabetes, or with alcoholism or use of certain medications. Diuretics are frequent offenders. Gout occurs far more frequently in men than in women. It may occasionally develop in early adulthood, but males usually experience their first attack in their 40s, and women rarely contract the disease until well after menopause. Pseudogout is caused by disposition of calcium pyrophosphate dihydrate crystals, and is associated with osteoarthritis and diseases such as hyperparathyroidism, hemochromatosis, and acromegaly.[17]

A wide variety of inflammatory states, including rheumatoid arthritis and the seronegative arthropathies, although usually polyarticular, may affect a single joint. The seronegative arthritides, characterized by the absence of rheumatoid factor, include ankylosing spondylitis, psoriatic arthritis, enteropathic arthritis (associated with inflammatory bowel disease), and reactive arthritis (such as Reiter syndrome). Rheumatoid arthritis, gout, pseudogout, and the seronegative spondyloarthropathies may all display similar clinical pictures.

Trauma, foreign bodies, or osteochondral fragments in a joint lead to mechanical arthritis. Neoplasms may develop within the capsule (e.g., pigmented villonodular synovitis), or they may occur in juxtaarticular bone (e.g., osteoid osteoma or metastatic cancer). Ischemic arthritis, including that due to decompression illness, is rare. Systemic corticosteroids can lead to aseptic necrosis of the hip, shoulder, or knee.

Of all joint disease, infectious arthritis is of the greatest concern to the emergency physician. It can be due to bacteria, mycobacteria, fungi, and viruses, although bacterial processes are, by far, the most common and the most serious. The degree of inflammation varies among pathogens. Staphylococcal infections are the most destructive; gonococcal arthritides are usually much less devastating.

Disseminated gonococcal infection (DGI) is responsible for most cases of monoarticular arthritis in sexually active adults. Conversely, 3% of patients with gonorrhea may present with this syndrome.[2] Although the classic triad of DGI consists of dermatitis, tenosynovitis, and migratory polyarthritis, many patients have only monoarticular arthritis. Most cases of DGI are seen in young adults, but the syndrome occurs in sexually active octogenarians as well.

Women are more frequently affected, possibly because longer asymptomatic colonization increases the chance of dissemination; they are especially affected during the perimenstrual period and pregnancy. Gonococcal arthritis begins as an immune complex disorder that produces an inflammatory but sterile joint effusion. If left untreated at this stage, subsequent bacterial invasion may produce an infected joint.

Nongonococcal bacterial arthritis usually occurs in patients who have underlying medical problems such as diabetes, alcoholism, and malignancy. Rheumatoid arthritis, collagen vascular disease, and immunosuppressed states increase susceptibility, and patients who are elderly, malnourished, or being treated with corticosteroids are also predisposed to develop a septic joint. Prior joint abnormality, whether secondary to trauma, noninfectious arthritis, or a prosthetic joint, significantly increases the risk of septic arthritis, especially in the presence of bacteremia. Bacterial seeding may occur by direct inoculation from a puncture wound or skin ulcer overlying the joint, or it may result from hematogenous spread associated with a remote infection such as pneumonia, urinary tract infection, endocarditis, or cellulitis.

Contiguous osteomyelitis may erupt into a joint space. *S. aureus* is responsible for up to 75% of cases of nongonococcal bacterial arthritis, and other gram-positive organisms, such as *Streptococcus*, play a significant role.[5,13] Gram-negative and anaerobic bacteria may be found in up to 20% of patients, particularly the elderly or immunocompromised. Rarely, *Salmonella* arthritis develops in patients with sickle cell anemia or systemic lupus erythematosus. Acute HIV infection, as well as other viral infections, may produce monoarticular viral arthritis, and fungal and tubercular arthritides occur occasionally, almost always in an immunosuppressed host. Spirochetal disease, such as syphilis or Lyme disease, must also be included in the differential diagnosis of infectious arthritis.

Monoarticular arthritis must be distinguished from periarticular conditions such as cellulitis, tendinitis, and bursitis. A significant proportion of patients with apparent monoarticular arthritis actually have a soft-tissue process, usually bursitis. Bursitis is characterized by pain over bony prominences, and little or no pain on range of motion. Trochanteric bursitis may masquerade as a septic hip, while rotator cuff injuries, subacromial bursitis, and adhesive capsulitis are common mimics of the septic shoulder joint. Olecranon bursitis must be differentiated from arthritis of the elbow.

The acute worsening of a patient with a prior joint abnormality presents a diagnostic challenge. A flare of rheumatoid arthritis may be clinically indistinguishable from acute joint infection, and it is very difficult to separate mechanical loosening of a prosthesis from an indolent septic process.[7]

EMERGENCY DEPARTMENT EVALUATION

The diagnosis of acute monoarticular arthritis is greatly assisted by history, physical examination, and, above all, arthrocentesis. The emergency physician must recognize the infected joint during the first visit in order to prevent joint destruction and possible death. In contrast, most other monoarticular arthritides pose significantly less risk of acute or chronic morbidity and may be treated symptomatically pending definitive diagnosis.

The patient should be questioned regarding recent or remote joint trauma, a history of dysuria or urethral discharge (in men), or the presence of lower abdominal pain or vaginal discharge (in women). Fever, chills, or systemic symptoms suggest infection but are nonspecific. A history of inflammatory bowel disease, nephrolithiasis, psoriasis, lupus, or hemophilia implicates the associated types of monoarticular arthritis. The patient must be assessed for the presence of immunosuppression, alcohol abuse, diabetes, intravenous drug use, and human immunodeficiency virus (HIV) risk factors. The use of medications such as corticosteroids, immunosuppressive agents, and diuretics provides additional diagnostic clues. Recent antibiotic use raises the possibility of a partially treated septic arthritis in which cultures of joint fluid may be negative. In endemic areas, the history of a tick bite or the typical rash of erythema migrans suggests Lyme disease. Recent medical or dental procedures predispose to endocarditis and subsequent septic arthritis.

Rheumatoid arthritis is one of the most common predisposing factors for septic arthritis. In patients with rheumatoid arthritis, it should be determined whether intraarticular steroids have been administered within the last 3 to 6 months; as many as one in 2000 of such injections results in late septic arthritis.[14] A history of other attacks of joint pain, recent joint instrumentation, or the presence of a prosthetic joint is also significant. The diagnosis of gout can be made on clinical grounds alone in patients who present with acute podagra and a history of gout. A family history of gout may be helpful.

The physical examination should not focus solely on the affected joint. A search for remote sites of infection may reveal pneumonia, endocarditis, urinary tract infection, or osteomyelitis, any of which may be associated with a septic arthritis. Tophi may be aspirated and examined under the microscope for sodium urate crystals. The skin lesions of psoriasis, erythema migrans (Lyme disease), erythema marginatum (rheumatic fever), and erythema nodosum (systemic lupus erythematosus, sarcoid, vasculitis) can provide strong clues to etiology.

Other informative rashes include the scattered pustules of DGI on the distal extremities and the characteristic eruptions of Reiter syndrome (keratoderma blennorrhagicum on the soles of the feet and circinate balanitis around the glans penis). Stigmata of parenteral drug use (e.g., needle tracks or skin-popping ulcers) suggest infection as the cause of arthritis, as do signs of bacterial endocarditis such as splinter hemorrhages, Osler's nodes, and Janeway lesions. Discharge or other evidence suggestive of infection should be sought on genital or pelvic examination.

The involved joint should first be examined to distinguish arthritis from periarticular inflammation. Pain on motion, whether active or passive, is the hallmark of joint inflammation. If the patient can move the joint through the full range of motion with minimal pain, acute arthritis is unlikely. One should also look for periarticular puncture wounds or ulcerations and for joint effusions. The presence of lymphangitis or nodes proximal to the involved area argues more for cellulitis than arthritis. The Patrick test or FABER test (pain on forced *f*lexion, *ab*duction, and *e*xternal *r*otation of the hip) identifies involvement of the sacroiliac joint.

Radiography is of variable utility in the evaluation of acute monoarticular arthritis. Plain films detect fractures or effusions, show foreign bodies or loose bone chips within the joint, and can demonstrate subchondral bone erosion, joint space narrowing, and, occasionally, intraarticular gas. Osteomyelitis, bone tumors, Paget disease, and osteochondritis dissecans are also visible. Calcification of the cartilage (chondrocalcinosis) may accompany pseudogout, but is not diagnostic of this condition. Advanced gout produces a characteristic pattern of punched-out bony erosions, juxtaarticular or periarticular soft-tissue swelling, and joint space narrowing.

A computed tomography (CT) scan may be useful in certain situations, such as juxtaarticular osteomyelitis, bony tumors, or periarticular abscesses, and can help to distinguish articular from periarticular processes.[1] Magnetic resonance imaging accurately detects ligamentous and cartilage damage, soft-tissue inflammation, and intramedullary osteomyelitis, but has little utility in the emergency setting. Radionuclide scans highlight joint inflammation, but are rarely necessary for acute evaluation, except in the case of a suspected prosthetic joint infection.

The evaluation of a painful *prosthetic joint* may require a variety of imaging studies. Plain films can detect fractures or loosening of the prosthesis, whereas a radionuclide scan can help to distinguish infectious from noninfectious etiologies of joint pain.

The emergency physician must recognize the limitations of the laboratory in the evaluation of acute arthritis. Blood tests cannot conclusively determine the etiology of monoarticular arthritis, nor can they distinguish articular from periarticular inflammation. The white blood cell (WBC) count is increased in fewer than 60% of cases of infection.[13] The erythrocyte sedimentation rate (ESR) is elevated in 90% or more of cases; a normal sedimentation rate makes bacterial arthritis less likely, *but does not rule out the possibility*. Furthermore, elevated white counts and sedimentation rates are not specific for infectious arthritis, occurring commonly in crystal-induced arthritis and other inflammatory conditions. Likewise, the serum uric acid level is not helpful and, in fact, may be misleading in the emergency setting, because 40% of patients with acute gout have normal or low levels,[12] while many patients *without* gout have high levels.

When DGI is a consideration, urethral or cervical culture should be obtained, even if the patient denies a discharge. Gonorrhea is far more likely to be isolated from the genital tract than from joint cultures. Up to 80% of DGIs can be detected by genital cultures, whereas only 30% of patients have culture-positive joint fluid. Even asymptomatic individuals should have genital cultures obtained, because nearly half of patients with DGI have no genitourinary complaints. Culturing of the rectum and the pharynx can be expected to increase the yield further.

Serologic tests for syphilis, Lyme disease, and HIV may occasionally be useful in establishing a diagnosis, but rarely affect emergency management. Lyme titers in particular can be misleading.

Synovial fluid analysis is the single most important test in the emergency evaluation of acute monoarticular arthritis. Arthrocentesis should be attempted in all cases of monoarticular arthritis, with the possible exception of classic recurrent gout. Most joints can be readily aspirated by the emergency physician, but for certain joints, such as the hip and sacroiliac joints, specialty consultation is generally required and aspiration is performed under fluoroscopic, CT, or ultrasonographic guidance. In the case of a dry tap, nonbacteriostatic saline may be injected into the joint and reaspirated for Gram staining and culture. When aspiration of the first metatarsal joint is attempted and no fluid is obtained, sodium urate crystals can sometimes be expressed from the needle bore onto a glass slide.

Synovial fluid analysis requires only 1 to 2 mL of fluid, but if only a drop is obtained, it should be sent for culture. Laboratory analysis should include cell count and differential, Gram stain, culture, and examination for crystals. Synovial fluid chemistries such as lactate dehydrogenase, glucose, and protein are traditionally recommended, but they provide little useful information and are often misleading or redundant.[18] Arthrocentesis remains an accurate method of detecting infection in a *prosthetic* joint, but it should probably be performed only after orthopedic consultation.

The synovial fluid white cell count can be used to categorize effusions as (1) noninflammatory (less than 2000 WBC/μL), (2) inflammatory (2,000 to 50,000 WBC/μL), and (3) infectious (greater than 50,000 WBC/μL).[13] In general, there is a broad overlap of the WBC count in inflammatory and infectious conditions. A significant percentage of patients with septic arthritis have synovial WBC counts of less than 50,000/μL, and patients with gout may have WBC counts of greater than 100,000/μL.

Gram stain and culture of the fluid are also critical components of the evaluation. The Gram stain is positive in 50% to 75% of nongonococcal septic arthritis, but in less than 25% of cases of gonococcal arthritis.[2] Culture yields similar percentages. In immunosuppressed patients, both aerobic and anaerobic cultures should be requested and the laboratory should be alerted if fungal, mycobacterial, or viral etiologies are suspected.

Polarized light microscopy is extremely helpful in the diagnosis of crystal-related arthropathies.[15] Monosodium urate crystals appear as strongly negatively birefringent needles that may be either intra- or extracellular. Calcium pyrophosphate dihydrate crystals are more rod-shaped and have weak positive birefringence. Apatite crystals shine in nonbirefringent clumps and can be further demonstrated using special stains.

EMERGENCY DEPARTMENT MANAGEMENT AND DISPOSITION

Gonococcal Arthritis

Because of antibiotic resistance, third-generation cephalosporins are preferred over penicillin in the management of gonococcal arthritis (Table 220.2). Ceftriaxone, 1 g parenterally every 24 hours, is the treatment of choice. Other Centers for Disease Control–approved regimens include cefotaxime 1 g intravenously (i.v.) every 8 hours, or ceftizoxime 1 g i.v. every 8 hours. Spectinomycin 2 g intramuscularly (i.m.) every 12 hours, or ciprofloxacin 500 mg i.v. every 12 hours, may be given to persons who are allergic to beta-lactam drugs. After the patient demonstrates clinical improvement with parenteral treatment, an approved oral regimen may be started (e.g., cefixime 400 mg orally twice a day, or ciprofloxacin 500 mg orally twice a day). Traditionally, patients with gonococcal arthritis have been treated as inpatients. However, compliant, nontoxic patients with involvement of a non–weight-bearing joint may be discharged after initial parenteral antibiotic loading with instructions to return for daily ceftriaxone therapy. Patients who are toxic-appearing or immunocompromised must be admitted for intravenous therapy.

In any event, clinical improvement should occur within 48 hours. Patients should be treated for a total of 7 days, but oral therapy may be substituted once symptoms have resolved. All patients with presumed gonococcal arthritis should also be tested for concurrent chlamydial infection and syphilis and treated with doxycycline or tetracycline. All patients with a sexually transmitted disease should be counseled regarding the use of condoms and referred for HIV testing.

Patient comfort may be increased by immobilizing involved patients in the position of function, but passive range of motion exercises should be instituted as early as possible to avoid the development of adhesive capsulitis. Arthrocentesis is usually performed daily until the joint is no longer tense.

Nongonococcal Bacterial Arthritis

Nongonococcal septic arthritis represents a true emergency. Antibiotics should be started in the emergency department. Antibiotic selection depends on the findings on Gram stain of the synovial fluid, or on the organism that is suspected to be responsible based on such factors as a history of parenteral drug use, the patient's age, the presence of a prosthetic joint, and the history of a puncture wound. After blood cultures and joint cultures are obtained, empiric antibiotic therapy is most safely begun with a penicillin-resistant synthetic penicillin (e.g., nafcillin) and a third-generation cephalosporin. Vancomycin plus either an intravenous fluoroquinolone or an antipseudomonal aminoglycoside is appropriate therapy for patients who are suspected of having infection with methicillin-resistant *S. aureus* (MRSA), such as those with prosthetic joints. Rifampin may provide synergistic benefit.

All patients with nongonococcal arthritis must be admitted to the hospital. Orthopedic consultation is highly advisable, because certain joints, such as the shoulder and hip, may require arthrotomy and open drainage. While joints such as the knee and wrist are often treated with daily aspiration, formal arthrotomy or arthroscopic drainage may provide better results in certain circumstances.[9] Intraarticular antibiotics may cause a chemical synovitis and should not be given.[16] Infected prosthetic joints require orthopedic consultation for possible removal of the prosthesis.

Crystal-Induced Arthritis

Colchicine has been used for acute gout for decades. It complexes with microtubules to inhibit leukocyte function, blunting the intraarticular inflammatory response. The therapeutic effect of colchicine is reasonably specific for gout and pseudogout, but it may also work in sarcoid arthropathy. It is most effective when administered early in an attack. The usual dose is 0.5 to 0.6 mg orally every 30 to 60 minutes until joint pain resolves or gastrointestinal (GI) side effects supervene, but no more than 4 to 6 mg should be given in a 24-hour period. Side effects include abdominal pain, nausea, vomiting, and diarrhea, and occur in up to 80% of patients who receive the full therapeutic dose.[20]

GI side effects are minimized with intravenous administration, which often yields very dramatic results, aborting painful attacks within 20 to 30 minutes, with minimal GI side effects. A single intravenous dose of 1 to 2 mg can be given over 10 minutes in a free-flowing intravenous line to prevent chemical thrombophlebitis. There have been several deaths secondary to inappropriately large doses of intravenous colchicine in compromised patients, but it remains a safe and effective drug when

TABLE 220.2. Treatment of Monoarticular Arthritis

Type	Treatment	Alternative
Infectious		
Empiric and nongonococcal (all ages)	PCN-ase-resistant synthetic PCN* and third generation cephalosporin (*nafcillin is the preferred choice) Ciprofloxacin or an aminoglycoside	Vancomycin
Isolated gonococcal	Ceftriaxone 1 g i.v. q24h Cefotaxime 1 g i.v. q8h Ceftizoxime 1 g i.v. q8h Treat also for concurrent chlamydia	Spectinomycin 2 g i.v. q12h Ciprofloxacin 500 mg i.v. q12h
Crystal-induced	Indomethacin 50 mg PO t.i.d. × 3 d, followed by taper over 4–6 days	Colchicine 0.6 mg PO q1h until relief, GI upset, or 8 mg max (or comparable NSAID) 1–2 mg i.v. over 30 min Corticosteroids Prednisone 30–50 mg PO qd for 3 d and taper over 5 days 5–60 mg intraarticular methylprednisolon acetate
Traumatic	Joint aspiration for tense effusion Rest, ice, compression, elevation Orthopedic follow-up as needed	
Hemorrhagic	Correct coagulopathy Rest, ice, compression, elevation	
Inflammatory	Indomethacin 50 mg PO t.i.d. with taper (or other comparable NSAID) High-dose ASA for RA	

used as directed. Colchicine should not be given to patients with leukopenia or to those with underlying liver or kidney disease. Patients who receive a full loading dose of colchicine (either intravenous or oral) in the emergency department should not take any additional colchicine for the next 7 days.

Nonsteroidal antiinflammatory drugs (NSAIDs) have substantially replaced colchicine as the primary treatment of acute gout.[3] Side effects include GI irritation and azotemia and, occasionally, central nervous system (CNS) side effects such as confusion or lethargy, particularly in the elderly. Relative contraindications include peptic ulcer disease, gastritis, and renal insufficiency. Indomethacin is the most widely used agent to treat acute gout, but other nonsteroidal drugs may be equally effective.

Corticosteroids (parenteral, oral, or intraarticular) are useful in patients who are not candidates for NSAIDs or colchicine, or in those who fail to respond to other drugs. Oral prednisone is often given in a dose of 40 mg/d for 5 days, with a subsequent taper. Before using intraarticular corticosteroids, the emergency physician must be extremely confident that the patient does not have an infectious arthritis.

Patients with an acute gouty attack should not receive the uricosuric agent probenecid or the xanthine oxidase inhibitor allopurinol, as these drugs can exacerbate the attack. They may be started 10 to 14 days later, after the acute attack has subsided.

Like gout, pseudogout may be managed with NSAIDs, colchicine, or intraarticular steroids. Most patients with crystal-induced arthritis can be treated at home with oral agents, but if the patient appears toxic or the synovial fluid white count is very high, admission is advisable. Although rare, septic arthritis can coexist with crystal-induced arthropathy, particularly pseudogout. Patients with inflammatory arthritis benefit from elevation and short-term splinting, and should follow up with their caregiver within several days. They must be instructed to return to the emergency department immediately for any worsening of symptoms.

COMMON PITFALLS

- Failing to obtain synovial fluid for analysis
- Believing that a normal complete blood count and the absence of fever rule out septic arthritis Assuming that acute symptoms in the setting of chronic arthritis are due to a rheumatic flare or gout rather than infection
- Forgetting that any sexually active person can develop gonococcal arthritis
- Ordering a serum uric acid level in the emergency department to confirm or exclude gout
- Prescribing additional colchicine in the first week following maximal colchicine loading in the emergency department
- Prescribing allopurinol or probenecid for a patient with an acute gouty attack

References

1. Baker DG, Schumacher HR. Acute monarthritis. *N Engl J Med* 1993;329:1013.
2. Cucurull E, Espinaoza LR. Gonococcal arthritis. *Rheum Dis Clin North Am* 1998;24:305–323.
3. Emmerson BT. The management of gout. *N Engl J Med* 1996;334:445–451.
4. Goldenberg DL. Infectious arthritis complicating rheumatoid arthritis and other chronic rheumatic disorders. *Arthritis Rheum* 1989;32:496.
5. Goldenberg DL. Septic arthritis. *Lancet* 1998;351:197–202.
6. Gristina AG, Kolkin J. Total joint replacement and sepsis. *J Bone Joint Surg* 1983;65:128–134.
7. Lane JG, Falahee MH, Wojtys EM, et al. Pyarthrosis of the knee: treatment considerations. *Clin Orthop* 1990;252:198.
8. Lawry GV, Fan PT, Bluestone R. Polyarticular vs. monoarticular gout: a prospective comparative analysis of clinical features. *Medicine* 1988;67:335.
9. Masuda I, Ishikawa K. Clinical features of pseudogout attack: a survey of 50 cases. *Clin Orthop* 1988;229:173.
10. McCarty DJ. Gout without hyperuricemia. *JAMA* 1994;271:302.
11. McCutchan HJ, Fisher RC. Synovial leukocytosis in infectious arthritis. *Clin Orthop* 1990;257:226.
12. Ostensson A, Geborek P. Septic arthritis as a non-surgical complication in rheumatoid arthritis: relation to disease severity and therapy. *Br J Rheumatol* 1991;30:35.
13. Pioro MH, Mandell BF. Septic arthritis. *Rheum Dis Clin North Am* 1997;23:239–258.
14. Reginato AJ, ed. *Atlas of synovial fluid in crystal identification*. Philadelphia: Lea & Febiger, 1991:121.
15. Renner JB, Agee MW. Treatment of suppurative arthritis by percutaneous catheter drainage. *Am J Rheum* 1990;154:135.
16. Schumacher HR, Reginato AJ. Calcium pyrophosphate dihydrate crystal deposition. In: Schumacher HR Jr, ed. *Primer on the rheumatic diseases*, 11th ed. Atlanta: Arthritis Foundation, 1997.
17. Shmerling RH, Tosteson AN, Trentham DE. Synovial fluid test: what should be ordered? *JAMA* 1990;264:1009.
18. Wallace SL, Singer JZ. Review of systemic toxicity associated with the intravenous administration of colchicine: guidelines for use. *J Rheumatol* 1988;15:495.

CHAPTER 221
Polyarticular Arthritis

Harold A. Thomas, Jr. and Richard S. Hartoch

The emergency physician encounters polyarthritis in two contexts: the patient with joint pain that is as yet undiagnosed and the patient with complications of a known rheumatologic disease, most commonly rheumatoid arthritis (RA).

Many polyarthritis syndromes have a gradual onset and sometimes defy precise diagnosis, despite months of sophisticated workup (Table 221.1). Many symptoms of systemic lupus erythematosus (SLE), RA, and other collagen–vascular diseases are overlapping, and laboratory test results are often equivocal. Thus, a definitive diagnosis is not usually made on any single emergency department visit. This discussion focuses on those polyarthritides that typically have an acute presentation (Table 221.2).

TABLE 221.1. Polyarthritic Syndromes

Rheumatoid arthritis	Symmetric, additive involvement initially of small joints; morning stiffness, positive rheumatoid factor 75%
Systemic lupus erythematosus	Multiple organ system involvement; symmetric evanescent involvement of any joint; serologic autoreactivity (e.g., anti-DNA)
Osteoarthritis	Lower extremity involvement; Heberden nodes; lack of inflammatory signs
Ankylosing spondylitis	Insidious involvement of spine (occasionally hips and shoulders); uveitis in 25%, HLA-B27 positive 90%
Colitic arthritis	Large joints; parallels course of ulcerative colitis or regional enteritis
Psoriatic arthritis	Distal interphalangeal joint involvement; symmetric or asymmetric; skin disease begins first; 80% have pitting of nails

TABLE 221.2. Acute Polyarticular Arthritis: Clinical Features

Acute rheumatic fever	Migratory polyarthritis; carditis; erythema marginatum; subcutaneous nodules; chorea
Gonococcal arthritis	Early tenosynovitis and diffuse arthralgias; common wrist involvement; characteristic rash
Lyme disease	Brief, recurrent; involves knees; preceded by characteristic rash (erythema chronicum migrans); cardiac and neurologic involvement
Reiter syndrome	Asymmetric involvement of lower extremities; urethritis; conjunctivitis; skin lesions
Viral arthritis	Symmetric involvement of fingers, wrists, and knees
Serum sickness	Migratory involvement of large and small joints; associated rash

EMERGENCY DEPARTMENT EVALUATION

In an undiagnosed patient, sudden onset of joint pain (developing over several hours, rather than days) strongly suggests gout (almost always monoarticular) or infection. The most important joint disorder to diagnose accurately and early is infectious arthritis.

Symmetric joint involvement is seen in RA or SLE; asymmetric joint involvement is seen in the seronegative arthritides (e.g., Reiter syndrome). Migratory involvement (leaving one joint before involving another) is typical of acute rheumatic fever (ARF). A family history of arthritis supports a diagnosis of RA or one of the seronegative spondyloarthropathies. Thiazides are known to increase the serum uric acid level and may precipitate gout. Hydralazine, procainamide, isoniazid, and phenytoin can induce a lupus-like reaction.

Inflammation in the periarticular soft tissues (tendons, bursae) can cause swelling and limitation of motion, simulating joint disease. Arthritis usually limits both active and passive motion equally, whereas acute tendinitis or bursitis usually limits active motion significantly more than passive motion. Synovitis is indicative of joint inflammation, but usually results from chronic disease and does not necessarily indicate an acute flare of activity. A diagnosis of polyarthritis demands objective evidence of inflammation in at least two joints.

To assess the pattern of involvement and chronicity, all joints should be examined, not just those that are symptomatic. Several acute polyarthritides are associated with a characteristic rash. Subcutaneous nodules are seen in 35% of patients with RA (2% to 3% of those with ARF). Psoriatic arthritis is usually associated with characteristic pitting of the nails, as well as the typical papulosquamous rash. A general physical examination may note such important findings as a pleural effusion in SLE or RA, or clinical signs of liver inflammation in the arthritis associated with hepatitis. A pelvic examination should be performed on all women with unexplained arthritis to rule out *Neisseria gonorrhoeae*. Generalized lymphadenopathy or oral thrush may suggest the human immunodeficiency virus (HIV).

For either the previously undiagnosed patient or the patient with diagnosed disease and a new acute complaint, the most important laboratory test is examination of the joint fluid. Specific diagnostic tests (e.g., antinuclear antibody, rheumatoid factor, HIV, hepatitis screen) are seldom available on an emergency basis. They should be ordered, however, in appropriate patients for use in subsequent evaluation. The erythrocyte sedimentation rate (ESR) can be elevated in any inflammatory condition and is of little help in the differential diagnosis, but it may be useful to monitor the activity of a chronic arthritis.

Radiographs help little in evaluating the patient with nontraumatic joint pain. Radiographically visible inflammatory changes (such as symmetric erosions of the wrist and metacarpophalangeal joints in RA) occur late in the course of disease, and a normal radiograph does not rule out a diagnosis of arthritis. The main use of radiographs in the emergency department is to exclude complications in patients with chronic arthritis.

Rheumatoid Arthritis

The most commonly encountered etiology of chronic polyarthritis is RA, characterized by symmetric joint inflammation, constitutional symptoms, and, in some cases, extraarticular organ involvement. The disorder ranges in severity from a mild nonprogressive arthritis to a fulminant, sometimes fatal illness, with destruction of joints and serious systemic and organ system involvement.

The onset of RA may be acute or insidious. Inflammation in multiple joints in almost any combination may be present, although symmetric involvement of the hands, wrists, and feet is most common. RA virtually never affects the thoracic or lumbar spine. Systemic manifestations include malaise, anorexia, fever, myalgia, weight loss, and Raynaud phenomenon. In some patients, especially those with high titers of rheumatoid factor and more severe joint disease, there is specific organ involvement, most commonly of the lungs and heart.

The diagnosis of RA is based largely on observation of the clinical course over a period of months to years. Rheumatoid factor, although not a specific marker for RA, is present in the serum of 75% to 80% of patients. Clinical criteria for review include morning stiffness, patterns of joint involvement, and rheumatoid nodules.

Acute Rheumatic Fever

Although the incidence of ARF has dramatically declined over the past 40 years, recent reports have described episodic outbreaks. The diagnosis of ARF requires fulfillment of the modified Jones criteria (Table 221.3).

Arthritis, the most common finding in ARF, is seen in more than 75% of first attacks. It is typically migratory and most often affects the large joints of the lower extremities, but rarely the hips, hands, or feet.

Carditis, seen in 40% to 50% of acute cases, is the most serious finding. The diagnosis of carditis requires one of the following: new organic heart murmur (usually mitral regurgitation), cardiomegaly, pericarditis, or congestive heart failure. A recent report found echocardiographic evidence of mitral regurgitation in many patients with no clinical evidence of carditis.

TABLE 221.3. Modified Jones Criteria for Diagnosis of Acute Rheumatic Fever

Major Criteria	Minor Criteria
Carditis	History of acute rheumatic fever
Polyarthritis	Fever
Chorea	Arthralgia
Erythema marginatum	Elevated sedimentation rate
Subcutaneous nodules	Prolonged PR interval

The diagnosis of acute rheumatic fever requires two of the major criteria and one of the minor criteria, or one of the major criteria and two of the minor criteria plus evidence of recent group A streptococcal pharyngitis (positive culture or increased ASO titer).

Chorea occurs in 5% of cases. It develops several months after streptococcal infection and is characterized by involuntary movements that cease with sleep.

Erythema marginatum (5% of cases) begins as a macule that extends outward, with central clearing. It may resemble erythema chronicum migrans, the rash of Lyme disease (LD). It is not painful or pruritic. It usually fades within hours but may recur.

Subcutaneous nodules, seen in less than 10% of patients, are firm, painless, and of variable size (2 to 10 mm). They are most commonly seen over the extensor joint surfaces.

The diagnosis of ARF requires laboratory confirmation of recent group A streptococcal pharyngitis. An elevated antistreptolysin-O (ASO) titer is seen in most patients.

Gonococcal Arthritis

Gonococcal arthritis (GA) is the most common bacterial arthritis among healthy young people. Disseminated gonococcal infection (DGI) is characterized by a clinical triad: dermatitis, tenosynovitis, and migratory polyarthritis. Joint involvement is predominantly asymmetric, often affecting the knee, elbow, wrist, and ankle. HIV patients are infected in unusual joints (hip and sternoclavicular) and may present with a more aggressive course.

A painless, nonpruritic skin rash is seen in roughly 50% of patients. *N. gonorrhoeae* is cultured in only half of affected joints. One is significantly more likely to obtain a positive culture from the mucosal surface of initial infectious contact (throat, cervix, urethra, or rectum). Polymerase chain reaction (PCR) may be useful in identifying gonococcal infection from a joint that is culture-negative.

Lyme Disease

LD is caused by the spirochete *Borrelia burgdorferi,* which is transmitted by the bite of the deer tick *Ixodes*. A characteristic rash, erythema chronicum migrans, develops in 60% of patients. It starts as a single red macule that expands to form a large annular lesion with a red outer border and central clearing. Two weeks to 2 years after the initial skin lesion, 60% of patients develop an acute arthritis, typically asymmetric and oligo- or monoarticular, involving large joints, most commonly the knee. About 10% of patients develop cardiac abnormalities, most often atrioventricular (AV) block. Although cardiac involvement is transient, some patients require temporary pacemakers. About 10% of patients develop significant neurologic abnormalities, including meningitis, encephalitis, and cranial neuropathies.

Reiter Syndrome

Reiter syndrome may occur as a reactive arthritis in young, often human leukocyte antigen (HLA) B-27–positive men. It classically presents as a triad: nongonococcal urethritis, asymmetric polyarthritis, and conjunctivitis. The arthritis is usually acute in onset, involving the large joints of the lower extremities, particularly the knees and ankles. Urethritis usually precedes the development of arthritis, although it is commonly asymptomatic; it may be suggested only by the finding of white blood cells on microscopic examination of a first-voided, morning urine. Conjunctivitis occurs in 30% of patients, and iritis in 10%. Two distinctive skin lesions are occasionally seen. Keratoderma blennorrhagica (15% of patients), scaling lesions on the palms and soles that begin as erythematous macules, may progress to lesions indistinguishable from those of psoriasis. Circinate balanitis (25% of patients) produces painless superficial ulcers of the glans penis. Reiter syndrome is usually associated with a fever and may be confused with GA. The synovial fluid is inflammatory but sterile, although chlamydial antigen has been detected in joint fluid in some cases.

Viral Arthritis/Postinfection Arthritis

Transient arthritis has been associated with viral infection, the two best documented being hepatitis B and rubella. The arthritis of hepatitis B is believed to be due to the deposition of circulating immune complexes in affected joints. It typically occurs during the prodrome of the illness, before the appearance of clinical jaundice. Liver enzymes are usually elevated, and HBsAg or anti-HBc may be positive. The most common presentation is that of a migratory symmetric arthritis potentially involving the small joints of the hand, wrist, elbow, and ankle. It can be painful, with prominent morning stiffness, but seldom lasts more than 3 weeks.

Both natural and vaccine-induced rubella are associated with an asymmetric polyarthritis involving the large joints (knees, elbows, and ankles). It typically appears after the rash, is characterized as painful, with significant morning stiffness, and lasts 5 to 10 days.

Polyarthritis syndromes have also been described in association with enteric infections (*Yersinia, Shigella, Salmonella, Clostridium difficile*) and respiratory infection (mycoplasma).

Serum Sickness

Serum sickness, typically occurring 6 to 10 days after an antigenic stimulus, presents with the abrupt onset of fever, lymphadenopathy, and migratory arthralgia. Urticaria or angioedema may also develop. Less frequently, it is accompanied by glomerulonephritis, carditis, aseptic meningitis, or peripheral neuropathy. A more severe reaction tends to result after subsequent exposure to the same antigen. Penicillin is, by far, the most commonly implicated causal agent, but many other drugs have been implicated as well.

AIDS Arthritis

Several polyarthritic syndromes have been described in association with HIV infection. A painful, asymmetric, oligoarticular arthritis affecting the knees and ankles has been widely reported. Also seen are seronegative spondyloarthritis (particularly Reiter syndrome and psoriatic arthritis) and lupus-like syndromes. These polyarthritides may occur at any stage of HIV infection and have been reported to develop months or years before the actual diagnosis of HIV. Etretinate has been used to treat AIDS-related Reiter disease.

EMERGENCY DEPARTMENT MANAGEMENT

The mainstay of treatment for polyarthritis is nonsteroidal anti-inflammatory drugs (NSAIDs). These agents control both pain and inflammation. A common mistake is to prematurely conclude that a drug is ineffective or to advance too rapidly to more potent agents, such as corticosteroids. Even if one NSAID fails to control symptoms, another in a different class may work well.

Recent research into the etiology of the inflammatory process has revealed that two enzymes, cyclooxygenase 1 and 2 (COX-1, COX-2), are fundamental. Aside from being a mediator of inflammation, COX-1 plays a cytoprotective role in the gastrointestinal (GI) tract. Typical NSAIDs inhibit COX-1 and thus place the GI tract at risk for erosive damage. COX-2 is also instrumental in the inflammatory process but has not been demonstrated to be cytoprotective to the GI tract. Recently developed COX-2 blocking agents thus appear to have a lower likelihood of causing gastric erosions while inhibiting the inflammatory process.

Several disorders, however, require more specific treatment. Patients with a first attack of ARF should be hospitalized and closely monitored for worsening carditis and arrhythmias, the most common of which is first-degree AV block. High-dose salicylates are used for arthritis. Steroids are reserved for patients with significant carditis. A course of penicillin is recommended to eradicate any remaining streptococci, and the patient should be kept on low-dose penicillin prophylaxis indefinitely thereafter.

Most patients with gonococcal arthritis should be hospitalized. Therapy is initiated with a parenteral third-generation cephalosporin, or spectinomycin if there is a history of a major allergic reaction to penicillin. Repeated joint aspirations may be required. In most cases, dramatic clinical improvement is noted in 2 to 4 days, and oral antibiotics may then be substituted for a total of 7 days of therapy. Most patients should be treated at the same time for chlamydia with doxycycline or azithromycin, or with erythromycin if the patient is pregnant.

LD is generally treated with doxycycline. Advanced cases may require treatment with ceftriaxone. Reiter syndrome, once diagnosed, is incurable, but treatment of the initial urethritis may prevent development of the full-blown disease. Arthritic inflammation is treated symptomatically.

RA that does not respond satisfactorily to NSAIDs may be treated with "disease-modifying agents," which include antimalarials, gold salts, penicillamine, methotrexate, cytotoxic agents, and prednisone.

Complications of Rheumatoid Arthritis

RA, the most common and most serious of the chronic polyarthritides, may be associated with a number of emergent complications (Table 221.4). In addition to suffering direct complications of the disease, patients are also subject to the potential toxic effects of treatment. The emergency physician must be aware of the potential for acute problems in patients with well-established RA.

Radiographic abnormalities of the cervical spine are common, especially with subluxation of C-1 on C-2. Usually, these abnormalities are asymptomatic, but the appearance of neurologic symptoms or signs necessitates immediate neurosurgical consultation. Patients may note a peculiar slipping sensation with neck movements that is associated with either exacerbation or relief of symptoms. Flexion and extension views of the cervical spine aid in the diagnosis. A patient with RA who sustains even minor cervical trauma should have careful examination of the neck; similarly, the potential for cervical spine instability should be considered when intubating a patient with chronic RA.

TABLE 221.4. Complications of Rheumatoid Arthritis

Organ	Manifestations
Neurologic	Subluxation C-1, C-2 (cord compression); entrapment neuropathy (carpal tunnel); peripheral neuropathy; myositis; necrotizing vasculitis (central nervous system)
Musculoskeletal	Septic arthritis; tendon rupture; synovial cyst knee (pseudophlebitis); rheumatoid nodules
Larynx	Cricoarytenoid arthritis (airway)
Lung	Pleurisy; effusion; fibrosis
Cardiac	Pericarditis; tamponade; conduction defects; valvular (nodules); myocardial infarction (coronary arteritis)
Hematologic	Anemia; leukopenia; hyperviscosity; Felty syndrome (splenomegaly, neutropenia)
Ocular	Sjögren syndrome; episcleritis; scleritis
Blood vessels	Vasculitis (usually dermal, can be widespread)

Various entrapment neuropathies occur in RA; carpal tunnel syndrome is the most common. Patients initially complain of sensory changes over the distribution of the median nerve and a "toothache-like" pain at the wrist. Tinel sign, the induction of a tingling sensation in the same distribution upon tapping over the median nerve with a reflex hammer, is a useful physical finding. The diagnosis is confirmed with electromyography and nerve conduction studies. Treatment consists of splinting the wrist and arranging consultation with a rheumatologist or orthopedist. Local corticosteroid injection is occasionally performed; surgical release of median nerve entrapment is sometimes necessary. Generalized muscle wasting, weakness, and peripheral neuropathy in RA patients may also be manifestations of systemic vasculitis.

Rupture of the extensor tendons of the hand is not uncommon in advanced RA. Once one tendon ruptures, the increased strain on the remaining tendons may lead to rupture of others. Patients cannot extend the fingers actively at the metacarpophalangeal joints, but passive extension is still possible. The treatment is elective surgical repair.

The development of a synovial cyst behind the knee is common in RA. Synovial inflammation may result in large knee effusions, and high pressure generated during flexion of the knee may cause cyst formation in the popliteal fossa. These cysts may rupture, dissecting into the calf, or may obstruct venous return. Because the resulting calf pain, swelling, and redness may be confused with thrombophlebitis, venography is usually required to rule out deep vein thrombosis. A careful history may reveal that the patient noted a fullness in the popliteal area that diminished a few days before the development of calf symptoms. The diagnosis is confirmed by an arthrogram of the knee joint. Ultrasonography may be helpful, but is less accurate. Treatment involves joint aspiration and local corticosteroid injection.

The cricoarytenoid joint is a synovial articulation and can be involved in RA. Patients may present with stridor and significant airway obstruction or, with less severe involvement, with dyspnea, dysphagia, painful speech, foreign-body sensation, or hoarseness. There may be tenderness over the thyroid cartilage. Indirect laryngoscopy reveals redness and edema over the arytenoids and abnormal bowing of the vocal cords during inspiration. Intubation may be difficult, and cricothyrotomy or tracheostomy is often necessary to secure the airway. Local or systemic corticosteroids and cool humidification are useful for milder cases. Extubation has been associated with acute airway obstruction.

The most common type of vasculitis associated with RA involves small dermal vessels, causing relatively benign infarctions in the periungual areas of the fingers. Occasionally, patients develop a necrotizing vasculitis, which can follow a fulminant course; the presenting manifestations may be large ulcerations, digital gangrene, neuropathies, mesenteric ischemia, or coronary arteritis. Patients with systemic vasculitis usually have fever, leukocytosis, high titers of rheumatoid factor, an elevated ESR, and antinuclear antibodies. They should be admitted to the hospital for initiation of high-dose corticosteroids. At times, cytotoxic agents or apheresis is useful. The prognosis in patients with extensive vasculitic involvement is poor.

Sjögren syndrome (keratoconjunctivitis sicca), which is not uncommonly associated with RA, is characterized by dry eyes and dry mouth and is caused by decreased lacrimal and salivary gland function. Patients complain of grittiness in the eyes and thick mucus beneath the eyelids. The diagnosis is made by the Schirmer test, which measures tear production, or by noting filamentous keratitis on slit-lamp examination. Treatment consists of the use of artificial tears, humidified air, and eye goggles to minimize tear evaporation.

Episcleritis, also associated with RA, is usually benign, but should be followed by an ophthalmologist because it can lead to scleritis. A brief course of topical corticosteroids, prescribed by an ophthalmologist, is usually beneficial.

With scleritis, which is a more diffuse process that can lead to uveitis, glaucoma, and rupture of the globe, patients complain of a deep aching sensation and have tenderness on gentle palpation of the globe. Slit-lamp examination reveals a cellular exudate in the anterior chamber. Prompt ophthalmologic consultation is indicated.

Hematologic problems, including anemia, leukopenia, and hyperviscosity occur in RA. Felty syndrome (the triad of RA, splenomegaly, and neutropenia) is associated with severe disease. These patients are prone to recurrent infections and usually have hepatic dysfunction and recurring cutaneous ulcers; splenectomy is occasionally beneficial.

Pleurisy and pleural effusions are common in RA but are not usually life-threatening. Pericarditis is also common, but only rarely does pericardial tamponade or constrictive pericarditis occur. Rheumatoid nodules may affect the heart valves or cardiac conduction system. Myocardial infarction secondary to vasculitis involving the coronary arteries has been reported.

COMMON PITFALLS

- Failure to analyze synovial fluid in a patient with undiagnosed arthritis or in one with new joint tenderness, warmth, and swelling
- Failure to recognize an acute septic joint in a patient with underlying polyarthritis
- Failure to recognize rheumatic fever and initiate appropriate therapy to prevent cardiac damage
- Failure to recognize symptoms due to therapy rather than to underlying disease
- Failure to appreciate extraarticular manifestations of chronic polyarthritis
- Failure to consider underlying HIV infection in a person with a newly diagnosed, seronegative spondyloarthropathy or lupus-like syndrome

Bibliography

Cucurull E., Espinoza JLR. Gonococcal arthritis. 1998;24(2):305.
Cuellar M. HIV infection associated inflammatory musculoskeletal disorders. *Rheum Dis Clin North Am* 1998;24(2):403.
Firestein, G. Rheumatic arthritis. *Sci Am* 1998;3:15 II.
Golbus J. Rheumatic disease and AIDS. *Postgrad Med* 1992;92(4):1233.
Kaye B. Rheumatologic manifestations of infection with human immunodeficiency virus. *Ann Intern Med* 1989;111:158.
Leicht Ng, Harrington TM, David DE, et al. Cricoarytenoid arthritis: a cause of laryngeal obstruction. *Ann Emerg Med* 1987;16:885.
Masferrer JL, Isakson PC, Seibert K. NSAIDs, eicosanoids and the gastroenteric tract. *Gastroenterol Clin* 1996;25(2):363.
Massell BF, Chute CG, Walker AM, et al. Penicillin and the marked decrease in morbidity and mortality from rheumatic fever in the United States. *N Engl J Med* 1988;318:280.
Rose CD, Eppes SC. Infection related arthritis. *Rheum Dis Clin North Am* 1997;23,3:677.
Sigal LH. Pitfalls in the diagnosis and management of Lyme disease. *Arthritis Rheum* 1998;41(2):195.
Snyderman R, Haynes BF. The Medical Clinics of North America. *Adv Rheumatol* 1997;81(1):57.
Stanley KL, Weaver JE. Pharmacologic management of pain and inflammation in athletes. *Clin Sports Med* 1998;17(2):375.
Veasy GL, et al. Persistence of acute rheumatic fever in the intermountain area of the United States. *J Pediatr* 1994;24:9.
Weiner SR. Emergencies in rheumatoid arthritis. *Am Fam Physician* 1984;29:127.
Williams H. Etretinate and AIDS-related Reiter's disease. *Br J Dermatol* 1991;124:389.
Winchester R. The co-occurrence of Reiter's syndrome and acquired immunodeficiency. *Ann Intern Med* 1987;106:19.

CHAPTER 222
Multisystem Autoimmune Disease

Laurie Vande Krol and Theodore I. Benzer

Patients with multisystem autoimmune disorders may present for initial medical evaluation with a bewildering array of symptoms or complaints. Many of the tests needed to diagnose these "rheumatic disorders" cannot be performed during an emergency department visit. However, the emergency physician must recognize that an autoimmune disorder may be responsible for the patient's clinical picture and must decide which patients require admission and which can safely undergo an outpatient evaluation. Likewise, when a patient with known multisystem autoimmune disease presents to the emergency department with new symptoms, the physician must determine whether they represent an exacerbation of known disease, a manifestation of an unrelated disorder, or a complication of therapy.

Evolving therapies and variations in individual response to treatments make rheumatologic consultation appropriate in many cases. Although the ultimate cause of the autoimmune disorders remains a mystery, it is increasingly clear that specific autoantibodies directed against cellular components are markers for, and probable causes of, many of the manifestations. Positive tests for these antibodies not only correlate with current symptoms, but are also predictive of the patient's course. The use of these specific disease markers can improve accuracy in diagnosis and can guide therapy directed at specific pathologic entities.

Despite the fact that definitive therapies for most autoimmune disorders are lacking, there is often much that can be done to alleviate symptoms and prevent progression of tissue damage. Nevertheless, every pharmacologic treatment has a potential for toxicity that must be balanced against the potential benefit it may provide to the patient.

SYSTEMIC LUPUS ERYTHEMATOSUS

Systemic lupus erythematosus (SLE) is the prototypical autoimmune disease. Its prevalence is one in 2,000, with a 10:1 predominance of women over men and a predilection for non-Whites. The prevalence is one in 750 for Black women between the ages of 20 and 64.[6]

The cause of SLE remains unknown; hormonal, metabolic, genetic, environmental, and infectious factors have all been proposed as etiologic agents. The pathophysiology of SLE involves the production of autoantibodies initiated by an unknown stimulus. These antibodies react with cell constituents and initiate an inflammatory response that results in the fixing of complement and the elaboration of chemotactic factors and other inflammatory mediators. Antibody-dependent cytotoxic leukocytes are also activated.

Antinuclear antibodies (ANAs) are almost invariably detected in patients with SLE. Although ANAs are found in low titers in many other autoimmune and nonrheumatologic disorders, high titers are more specific for SLE; high titers of antibodies to double-stranded DNA are seen only in patients with SLE.[16] Antibodies to the Smith antigen are also specific for SLE, as well as being associated with more severe symptoms. During active SLE, complement levels are depressed and may be helpful in following the course of disease.[6]

CLINICAL PRESENTATION

SLE can affect any tissue or organ and, in fact, has been said to have replaced syphilis as "the great imitator" of other diseases.[6] Patients often make multiple visits to physicians before SLE is initially recognized. Some of the more common manifestations are listed in Table 222.1.

The most typical initial complaints are fatigue and arthralgias, but fever, anemia, anorexia, and a malar rash are other common presenting symptoms. The arthralgias are commonly fleeting and migratory, typically appearing in the proximal interphalangeal and metacarpophalangeal joints, the wrists, and the knees, but they may also be due to frank synovial inflammation.

The rash of SLE varies from a slight blush to a well-demarcated and somewhat edematous maculopapular erythematous eruption covering both cheeks and the bridge of the nose. It tends to spare the nasolabial folds, but can cause scarring and atrophy of skin structures. It is characteristically exacerbated by sun exposure and may often cause a patient to seek medical attention before any other symptoms of SLE have developed.

Although the kidneys are commonly affected in SLE, nephrotic syndrome and peripheral edema are rarely seen before other manifestations of disease have led to the diagnosis of SLE.[12] Patients with SLE frequently present with acute, potentially life-threatening problems. Complaints of chest pain, abdominal pain, and neurologic dysfunction can indicate an acute flare of disease or a serious complication of therapy. Patients with acute chest pain, with or without fever, may have pleuritis, pericarditis, or pneumonitis. Abdominal pain may indicate an acute flare of polyserositis.

Table 222.1. Systemic Lupus Erythematosus: Characteristic Features and Suggestive Signs and Symptoms

System	Presentation
Constitutional	Fever, fatigue, malaise, weight loss
Vascular	Raynaud's phenomenon, arterial occlusion, extremity ulcers
Dermatologic	Diffuse alopecia, malar rash, discoid rash, photosensitivity
Hematologic	Hemolytic anemia, leukopenia, thrombocytopenia, thrombosis
Immunologic	False-positive serologic test for syphillis
Gastrointestinal	Nausea, vomiting, oral ulcers
Cardiac	Pericarditis, myocarditis
Pulmonary	Diffuse interstitial pneumonitis, pleuritis, pleural effusion
Musculoskeletal	Nonerosive arthritis
Renal	Glomerulonephritis, nephrotic syndrome
Reproductive	Spontaneous abortion, preeclampsia
Neurologic	Psychosis, depression, mania, seizures, headache, organic brain syndrome, aseptic meningitis, peripheral neuropathy

Neurologic problems of virtually any type may be seen in SLE. Most common are central disorders ranging from mood disorders to frank psychosis. Seizures are also common, especially in younger patients. SLE should be in the differential diagnosis of new-onset seizures, especially in young women.

The lupus anticoagulant, also called the anticardiolipin antibody or antiphospholipid antibody, is an antibody that produces an artifactually prolonged partial thromboplastin time *in vitro*, but a "paradoxical" procoagulant effect *in vivo*. Although antiphospholipid antibodies are associated with SLE, they may occur as a part of a distinct pathologic entity referred to as the antiphospholipid syndrome.[1,8] Both conditions can lead to deep venous thrombi, pulmonary emboli, stroke, chronic ulcers of the extremities, and thrombocytopenia.[1,8] Patients with recurrent or unusual thrombosis should be evaluated for antiphospholipid autoantibody and SLE.[13]

Patients with *known* SLE may present to the emergency department with either exacerbations of their disease or complications of therapy.

DIFFERENTIAL DIAGNOSIS AND EMERGENCY DEPARTMENT EVALUATION

Given the variety of possible presentations, the differential diagnosis of SLE is exceedingly broad. A thorough history and physical examination are required to identify multisystem involvement and recurrent symptoms. The differentiation of SLE from the other autoimmune syndromes may require repeated rheumatologic evaluation and specific autoantibody testing.

Tan and associates[20] have published a list of 11 criteria diagnostic for SLE (Table 222.2); the diagnosis is established if four or more of these findings are present serially or simultaneously. A medication history must be elicited to rule out drug-induced lupus. Attention to detail in evaluating the patient with nonspecific symptoms may lead one to suspect the diagnosis of SLE. The diagnosis should be particularly entertained in women of childbearing age who have recurrent or vague symptoms that do not clearly point to a discrete disease entity.

Drug-induced SLE is a distinct entity that has been associated with many medications, including procainamide, hydralazine, anticonvulsants, chlorpromazine, isoniazid, methyldopa, penicillamine, quinidine, propylthiouracil, and sulfasalazine. Drug-induced SLE has a milder course than idiopathic SLE and does not cause renal and central nervous system involvement.[18] Specialized ANA testing panels reveal only histone-binding ANAs rather than the multiple varieties characteristic of SLE.[6]

The evaluation of patients with established SLE should focus on the presenting complaint. However, attention should also be given to signs and symptoms of the potentially life-threatening complications of SLE, such as thrombotic disease, pleural and pericardial effusions, and infections secondary to immunosuppressive therapy.

Patients presenting with new-onset monoarthritis or oligoarthritis generally require diagnostic arthrocentesis to rule out infection or crystal-induced arthritis. Fluid should be sent for Gram stain, culture, cell count and differential, and examination for crystals. The synovial fluid in autoimmune arthritis is typically inflammatory, with an elevated white cell count (20,000 to 80,000/μL mixed polymorphonuclear cells and lymphocytes), a negative Gram stain, and no crystals.

The specific organs affected by SLE and the severity of the disease vary widely between individuals and over time in any given individual. Not only does the variability of the disease make diagnosis difficult but, with the exception of the charac-

TABLE 222.2. Diagnostic Criteria for Systemic Lupus Erythematosus[a]

1. Malar rash	Fixed erythema, flat or raised, over the malar eminences
2. Discoid rash	Erythematous raised patches with adherent keratotic plugging; atrophic scarring may occur
3. Photosensitivity	
4. Oral ulcers	Incudes oral and nasopharyngeal, observed by physician
5. Arthritis	Nonerosive arthritis involving two or more peripheral joints, characterized by tenderness, swelling, or effusion
6. Serositis	Pleuritis or pericarditis documented by electrocardiogram or rub or evidence of pericardial effusion
7. Renal disorder	Proteinuria greater that 0.5 g/d or greater than 3+, or cellular casts
8. Neurologic disorder	Seizures without other cause, or psychosis without other cause
9. Hematologic disorder	Hemolytic anemia or leukopenia (less than 4,000/μL) or lymphopenia (less than 1,500/μL) or thrombocytopenia (less than 100,000/μL) in the absence of offending drugs
10. Immunologic disorder	Positive lupus erythematosus cell preparation or anti-dsDNA or anti-Sm antibodies or false-positive VDRL
11. Antinuclear antibodies	An abnormal titer of ANAs by immunofluorescence or an equivalent assay at any point in time in the absence of drugs known to induce ANAs

[a] If four of these criteria are present at any time during the course of disease, a diagnosis of SLE can be made with 98% specificity and 97% sensitivity.

teristic rash, each of the manifestations of lupus may occur from other causes. Although a presentation of one of these conditions alone would not prompt consideration for autoimmune disease, recurrent symptoms or the sequential development of multiple conditions associated with lupus warrants referral for ANA testing.

EMERGENCY DEPARTMENT MANAGEMENT AND DISPOSITION

The specific clinical presentation dictates the management indicated in the emergency department. Patients presenting with mild symptoms may require nothing more than screening for renal and hematologic involvement with a urinalysis and complete blood cell count. More severe symptoms are managed as in any other disease. For example, a large pleural effusion should be tapped, and heparin should be given for thromboembolic disease.

ST elevations and PR depressions seen on the electrocardiogram that are associated with a pericardial friction rub indicate pericarditis. If pericarditis is suspected, a careful evaluation should be made for signs of pericardial tamponade. Elevated neck veins, elevated pulsus paradoxus, or hypotension should prompt an urgent echocardiogram to rule out tamponade. Infectious complications should be considered in patients with established disease who are taking chronic immunosuppressive medications.

Patients with significant pleural or pericardial effusion, or any thrombotic complication, require hospital admission and rheumatologic consultation. Immunosuppressed patients with documented infection require admission for parenteral antibiotics.

Neuropsychiatric complications are frequent in SLE. Cerebritis, aseptic meningitis, seizures, ischemic strokes, peripheral neuropathy, and acute psychosis are all recognized manifestations of SLE. In addition, corticosteroid treatment and other immunosuppressive agents predispose to infectious meningitis and corticosteroid-induced psychosis.

The acute presentation of an SLE patient with a neuropsychiatric complaint is always a challenge. The diagnosis of lupus flare should be made only after infectious etiologies have been ruled out. Patients presenting with severe disease are often treated with "stress" doses of corticosteroids (hydrocortisone, 100 mg intravenously; or methylprednisolone, 125 mg intravenously) and often receive empiric broad-spectrum antibiotic coverage after samples of blood, urine, and sputum are obtained for culture.

Patients with established disease who present with a flare of symptoms may require the initiation of corticosteroids or an increase in the dose. When more than 5 to 10 mg of prednisone a day is required, many rheumatologists prescribe combination therapy in an effort to limit adverse effects. Medications commonly used include nonsteroidal antiinflammatory drugs (NSAIDs), antimalarial agents, azathioprine, and cyclophosphamide. Because every therapeutic agent has adverse effects, the risks of medication must be weighed against the morbidity of the clinical presentation. The aggressiveness and urgency of treatment depends on the presence of major organ involvement. Changes in a patient's usual medication regimen are best carried out in conjunction with the patient's rheumatologist.

Patients with suspected or newly diagnosed SLE may be managed as outpatients if the manifestations are mild and a life-threatening pathologic process is absent. An ANA panel should be ordered. Rheumatologic consultation can be obtained by telephone concerning any further studies, initiation of corticosteroid therapy, and appropriate follow-up. Newly diagnosed patients with SLE should be educated about the importance of adequate sleep and avoidance of ultraviolet light. Ibuprofen and estrogens may exacerbate disease and should be avoided.[12] Hypertension should be controlled rigorously because it appears to have a synergistic effect in exacerbating renal disease. In drug-induced lupus, after the medication is discontinued, symptoms usually resolve within days to weeks.[9,18]

COMMON PITFALLS

- Failure to recognize vague, atypical complaints as a presentation of SLE or other autoimmune disease
- Failure to include SLE in the differential diagnosis of patients with pericarditis, pleuritis, renal dysfunction, neurologic symptoms, or recurrent venous thrombosis
- Failure to differentiate disease exacerbation from an adverse effect of therapy
- Failure to suspect infection in an immunocompromised patient

RHEUMATOID ARTHRITIS

Rheumatoid arthritis (RA) is a chronic autoimmune disorder characterized by widespread synovial inflammation and, often, progressive destruction of joints. It affects women three times as often as men; its prevalence increases with age and is approximately 1%.

The pathophysiology of RA involves the production of immunoglobulins against native IgG; these are referred to as rheumatoid factor. Helper T cells are also activated and produce lymphokines that promote cellular proliferation.[15] Activation of the inflammatory response leads to the elaboration of vasoactive substances, chemotactic factors, and complement in synovial tissues. Mononuclear cells infiltrate the subsynovial stroma, and polymorphonuclear cells appear in the synovial fluid. A "pannus" of inflamed, thickened, redundant synovium invades and replaces cartilage and periarticular bone and tendon. Polymorphonuclear cells in the synovial fluid release lysozymes, which break down hyaluronic acid polymers in the synovial fluid and articular cartilage.[6] Although the symptoms and signs are primarily related to the joints, RA is a multisystem autoimmune disease that frequently involves the heart, lungs, and blood.

CLINICAL PRESENTATION

RA typically presents initially as constitutional symptoms such as low-grade fever, weight loss, fatigue, and lymphadenopathy. Stiffness in the morning or after periods of inactivity may also be a complaint.

Articular symptoms initially involve any number or size of joints. Either arthralgia (pain) or arthritis (inflammation) may be present in an unpredictable pattern. Later, in established disease, the typical symmetric pattern of arthritis develops.

The most commonly affected joints are the metacarpophalangeal and proximal interphalangeal joints, wrists, knees, and upper spine. Although some cases of RA remain mild or even resolve, the typical course is one of unpredictable exacerbations and remissions, with progressive deformity and disability.

As tissue damage progresses, typical ulnar deviation of the carpometacarpal joints and valgus deformity of the knees develop. Baker cysts may develop in the popliteal fossa. Of prime importance for the emergency physician is the development of instability of the atlantoaxial joint, with laxity and even rupture of the transverse ligament. The result is an unstable cervical spine, which may lead to spinal cord compression following even apparently trivial injury.[13]

RA, however, is a systemic disease. Over time, subcutaneous nodules over the elbows, occiput, and sacrum, thought to be vasculitic in origin, develop in 20% to 25% of patients. Pericarditis, pleuritis, pulmonary fibrosis, scleritis, Sjögren syndrome, nerve entrapment, and vasculitis may also occur. Felty syndrome, consisting of splenomegaly, anemia, thrombocytopenia, and granulocytopenia, sometimes complicates RA.

DIFFERENTIAL DIAGNOSIS AND EMERGENCY DEPARTMENT EVALUATION

RA is rarely misdiagnosed when it reaches the stage of symmetric polyarthritis in characteristic joints. At earlier stages, or with milder involvement, the clinical picture may be suggestive of inflammatory or infectious joint disease or other autoimmune diseases. When joint manifestations become apparent, infectious and crystalline synovitis must be considered.

In practice, most patients presenting to the emergency department with oligoarthropathy should have joint aspiration to rule out infection or crystal-induced arthritis. Although RA or another autoimmune disorder may be suspected, the definitive diagnosis is made at follow-up, when further data, such as final culture results, rheumatoid factor tests, and response to antiinflammatory therapy, are available.

Table 222.3. Criteria for the Diagnosis of Rheumatoid Arthritis

1. Morning stiffness[a]
2. Arthritis of three or more joints[a]
3. Swelling of proximal interphalangeal, metacarpophalangeal, or wrist joint[a]
4. Symmetric arthritis[a]
5. Rheumatoid nodules
6. Presence of rheumatoid factor
7. Erosions or periarticular osteopenia in radiographs of hands or wrists

[a] Duration of at least 6 weeks required.

The American Rheumatism Association has developed a set of seven criteria, four of which must be present to establish the diagnosis (Table 222.3).[2] In practice, most such patients presenting to the emergency department must have other significant disease ruled out (e.g., infectious arthritis, SLE); and although there may be a suspicion of RA, the definitive diagnosis is usually made on further evaluation at follow-up.

Patients with known RA who present with an exacerbation of joint inflammation require evaluation for possible secondary infections or crystalline arthropathy. Others may present with new systemic symptoms. Although the problem may be related to RA, this should not be assumed to be the case until other serious causes have been excluded. Evaluation based on presentation should be pursued as in any patient without RA. Special consideration should be given to complications of therapy; for example, pulmonary interstitial disease may be a result of either RA or treatment.

If a diagnosis of RA is considered, a rheumatoid factor titer should be ordered. If other autoimmune disorders are considered possible, other autoantibody titers, complement levels, and an erythrocyte sedimentation rate (ESR) may be indicated. Monoarticular or oligoarticular arthritis should cause one to consider crystalline and infectious arthritis. Joint aspiration is indicated, as well as oropharyngeal and genital cultures for *Neisseria gonorrhoeae*.

Few laboratory tests results are abnormal in RA, and, in general, the results tend to be nonspecific. The ESR is elevated and parallels disease activity. There may be a mild normocytic anemia. A test for mixed cryoglobulins, reflecting large amounts of circulating immune complexes, may be positive, but complement levels are usually normal. Arthrocentesis of involved joints typically yields sterile fluid with hallmarks of inflammation: decreased mucin clot formation and 20,000 to 80,000 white blood cells per microliter, of which 50% to 70% are polymorphonuclear cells.[3] The classic laboratory finding of a positive serum rheumatoid factor is found in 80% of patients, but a positive rheumatoid factor can also be found in 1% to 5% of persons without RA (e.g., patients with other rheumatic disorders, leprosy, tuberculosis, liver disease, or bacterial endocarditis).

EMERGENCY DEPARTMENT MANAGEMENT AND DISPOSITION

NSAIDs are the mainstay of chronic treatment of RA. Patients experiencing a flare of known disease often require second-line therapy in addition to NSAIDs. These include heat modalities, antimalarial agents, sulfasalazine, gold salts, D-penicillamine, azathioprine, cyclophosphamide, chlorambucil, methotrexate, and surgical replacement of joints.

Corticosteroids are usually reserved for the treatment of extraarticular manifestations. Each of the therapeutic agents has associated adverse effects. Sulfasalazine may cause leukopenia. Gold salts and D-penicillamine have renal and myeloid toxicity. Gold may also cause a pruritic rash and mouth ulcers. The antineoplastic agents can all cause myelosuppression and a host of other adverse effects.[5] Second-line agents should be initiated only after discussion with a rheumatologist who will be observing the patient.

Appropriate disposition depends on the severity of the presenting symptoms. Outpatient treatment is appropriate in individuals who do not appear toxic, even those with a new diagnosis of RA. These patients should be started on a standard dose of an NSAID and have rheumatologic follow-up arranged. Patients who appear ill require hospital admission for more intensive evaluation, particularly to rule out infectious disorders, and rheumatologic consultation. Hospitalization may be required for social reasons or if disability prevents adequate functioning at home.

COMMON PITFALLS

- Prescribing corticosteroids as a first-line therapy for RA
- Failure to recognize nonspecific complaints as a manifestation of autoimmune disease
- Failure to recognize a monoarticular flare of RA as a possible septic joint
- Failure to consider the possible severity of cervical spine trauma in an RA patient
- Failure to consider possible C1-C2 instability when intubating an RA patient

SCLERODERMA

Scleroderma (or systemic sclerosis) is an autoimmune disorder characterized by abnormal collagen production that results in pathologic fibrosis of the skin and internal organs. It occurs equally in all races and geographic areas, but it is four times more common in women than in men. In most cases, the onset is during the third decade of life.[17] The course is typically progressive over decades, but it may be fulminant and fatal. Collagen accumulation and endothelial cell proliferation in the vascular intima lead to severe narrowing of the arterial lumen.

Scleroderma can be classified according to its predominant manifestations. The CREST syndrome consists of subcutaneous *c*alcinosis, *R*aynaud's phenomenon, *e*sophageal dysmotility, *s*clerodactyly, and *t*elangiectasia and is associated with a specific antibody.[14,19] "Diffuse scleroderma" denotes the full systemic disease. A third subset is mixed connective-tissue disease or undifferentiated connective-tissue disorder, which combines features of SLE, scleroderma, and polymyositis.[4] Clinical criteria have been developed for the diagnosis of systemic sclerosis (Table 222.4).

CLINICAL PRESENTATION

Patients with scleroderma most commonly present to the emergency department because of painful fingers due to Raynaud's phenomenon, dyspnea due to restrictive lung disease, or dysphagia due to esophageal dysfunction. Malignant hypertension due to scleroderma renal disease is a true emergency.

Raynaud's phenomenon is present in virtually all cases of scleroderma and is the initial manifestation in 70% of cases. Skin involvement is usually first manifested as edema of the fingers. As the disease progresses, the skin becomes shiny and taut, with loss of the normal skin folds. Joints become immobilized from tight encasement in thickened skin, as well as from contractures of muscles, tendons, and palmar fascia.

DIFFERENTIAL DIAGNOSIS AND EMERGENCY DEPARTMENT EVALUATION

Established scleroderma causes a characteristic taut, smooth appearance of the hands and face. This sign should be apparent to the physician, although the patient may not have noticed the gradual changes.

Early disease may be difficult to recognize, however. The most common early symptom is painful fingers due to Raynaud's phenomenon, but this is a nonspecific feature of many autoimmune disorders that may also be due to occlusive arterial disease, repetitive trauma to the fingers, cryoglobulinemia, neurogenic lesions, or vasospastic drugs. In fact, Raynaud's phenomenon unassociated with scleroderma is extremely com-

TABLE 222.4. Clinical Criteria for the Diagnosis of Systemic Sclerosis

MAJOR CRITERION	
Proximal scleroderma	Typical sclerodermatous skin changes involving areas proximal to the metacarpophalangeal or metatarsophalangeal joints, affecting other parts of the extremities, face, neck, or trunk; usually bilateral, symmetric, and almost always including similar changes in the digits
MINOR CRITERIA	
Sclerodactyly	Sclerodermatous skin changes limited to the digits
Digital pitting, scars, or loss of substance from the finger pad	Depressed areas at the tips of digits or loss of digital pad substance from the finger pad tissue as a result of digital ischemia rather than trauma or exogenous causes
Bibasilar pulmonary fibrosis	Bilateral reticular pattern of linear or lineonodular densities that are most pronounced in basilar portions of the lungs on standard chest roentgenogram; may assume appearance of diffuse mottling or "honeycombing lung," and should not be attributable to primary lung disease

Classification as definite systemic sclerosis requires the presence of (1) the major criterion or (2) two or three of the minor criteria.[21]

mon in women. Specific autoantibody testing may distinguish early cases of scleroderma from other causes of Raynaud's phenomenon. Radiography of the hand may also be helpful. Subcutaneous calcinosis and resorption of the tufts of the distal phalanges are pathognomonic findings. More than 90% of patients with scleroderma have a positive ANA test.

An awareness of the systemic manifestations of disease is important in the evaluation of the patient with known scleroderma. Systemic collagen deposition may result in cardiac conduction abnormalities or cardiomyopathy, restrictive lung disease and pulmonary hypertension, gastrointestinal dysmotility and malabsorption, and renal arteriolar necrosis leading to malignant hypertension. Recognition of these manifestations in patients with advanced illness is critical.

EMERGENCY DEPARTMENT MANAGEMENT AND DISPOSITION

The majority of patients with Raynaud's syndrome do not have symptoms requiring treatment in an emergency department. Patients with persistent vasospasm may, however, respond to simple interventions, such as warming of the hands or oral administration of nifedipine. Only rarely are more invasive maneuvers, such as interarterial or local phenoxybenzamine or prazosin, required.

Systemic manifestations may require evaluation for dysfunction caused by scarring in many organ systems. Intestinal hypomotility may be treated with metoclopramide. Esophageal reflux should be treated with antireflux maneuvers and medications, as necessary. Patients with increased blood pressure, renal failure, and internal organ involvement are frequently treated with angiotensin converting enzyme inhibitors.

Most patients with scleroderma do not require hospitalization, but admission may be necessary for dehydration due to gastrointestinal dysfunction or for pulmonary compromise. Patients with hypertensive emergency due to renal crisis should be placed on nitroprusside and admitted to an intensive care unit.

Only those women with severe Raynaud's phenomenon and those men without a history of trauma to the hands require periodic monitoring for the development of scleroderma. Patients should be instructed in the importance of keeping the hands warm and avoiding nicotine and caffeine. Suppressive pharmacologic therapy may be necessary if attacks are frequent.

Patients with signs and symptoms beyond Raynaud's phenomenon should be referred for diagnostic autoantibody testing, occupational therapy, or orthopedics.

COMMON PITFALLS

- Failure to consider the systemic manifestations of scleroderma
- Failure to recognize scleroderma as the cause of a hypertensive emergency

GIANT-CELL ARTERITIS

Giant-cell arteritis is characterized by inflammation of branches of the carotid artery (temporal arteritis) or the aortic arch (Takayasu's arteritis), and can present with emergent manifestations.

CLINICAL PRESENTATION

Temporal arteritis usually occurs in women over 50 years of age. Symptoms may be nonspecific: fever, headache, myalgias, and fatigue. Patients may have the syndrome of polymyalgia rheumatica, manifested by chronic stiffness and aching of the neck, shoulder, and hip girdle. However, chronic or subacute headache is often the presenting complaint.

The temporal artery may be tender and nodular,[7] and there may be jaw claudication. The chief complication of temporal arteritis is monocular visual loss due to ischemic optic neuritis. Visual loss or impairment generally occurs 3 or 4 months after onset of initial symptoms.[10]

Takayasu's arteritis has a predilection for involvement of branches of the aortic arch. It is a rare disease. Patients are usually young women who present with nonspecific symptoms of fever, nightsweats, fatigue, myalgias, and weakness. Signs of large vessel occlusion with decreased peripheral pulses, cerebrovascular accidents, or myocardial ischemia occur only months to years after initial presentation.[11]

DIFFERENTIAL DIAGNOSIS AND EMERGENCY DEPARTMENT EVALUATION

The differential diagnosis of patients with temporal arteritis is wide because of the nonspecific symptoms. Mild anemia is typical. A markedly elevated ESR in a patient over 50, with headache and nonspecific symptoms, particularly polymyalgia rheumatica, should prompt further evaluation.

Takayasu's arteritis, although rare, should be considered in any young female patient with signs of large vessel ischemia (e.g., cerebrovascular accident, upper extremity ischemia, cardiac ischemia).

EMERGENCY DEPARTMENT MANAGEMENT AND DISPOSITION

Patients with suspected temporal arteritis rarely need admission to the hospital. However, prompt diagnosis and treatment is essential in order to prevent visual impairment. In the emergency department, patients should be started on 40 to 60 mg of prednisone daily. Arrangements should be made for definite follow-up and semiurgent temporal artery biopsy. Response to corticosteroid treatment is usually dramatic, with relief of systemic symptoms and headaches within days. Treatment is generally continued for 1 to 2 years.

The diagnosis of Takayasu's arteritis is not usually made in the emergency department. The diagnosis should be entertained in young women who need admission for large vessel occlusive disease. Angiography of the affected vessels shows narrowing or occlusion of large vessels, with well-developed collateral circulation.[21] No treatment has been proven effective, but corticosteroids and cyclophosphamide have been used.

COMMON PITFALLS

Failure to initiate corticosteroid therapy in the emergency department in a patient suspected of having temporal arteritis

DERMATOMYOSITIS AND POLYMYOSITIS

Dermatomyositis and polymyositis are inflammatory disorders of skeletal muscle, characterized by weakness in the muscles of the pharynx, neck, shoulder, and hip. Women are affected twice as often as men. There is a bimodal peak of incidence: in the early teen years and around age 50. Infection with toxoplasmosis and coxsackievirus has been implicated. Ten percent of cases of polymyositis and 15% of those of dermatomyositis are associated with malignant tumors, most commonly of the breast, lung, ovary, and stomach.

CLINICAL PRESENTATION

An insidious onset of muscular weakness may bring patients to the emergency department. Careful questioning for specific dysfunction typically reveals a history of proximal muscle weakness. Patients complain of difficulty getting out of a chair, climbing stairs, combing the hair, and raising their heads from the pillow.

Dermatomyositis presents as a characteristic rash consisting of heliotrope (violet) plaques over the eyelids and knuckles. Muscle wasting becomes evident later in the course, and dysphagia and dysarthria may develop. Interstitial lung disease may develop as an associated manifestation.

DIFFERENTIAL DIAGNOSIS AND EMERGENCY EVALUATION

The differential diagnosis includes many causes of muscular weakness: polymyalgia rheumatica, fibrositis, muscular dystrophy, myasthenia gravis, thyroid disease, metabolic defects, and corticosteroid myopathy.

Evaluation centers on differentiating the type of muscle process involved. Patients with polymyositis have elevated levels of creatine phosphokinase, myoglobin, and transaminases, whereas enzyme levels are normal in polymyalgia rheumatica and fibrositis. The ESR may be elevated but does not correlate with clinical disease severity. Autoantibodies are detectable in 90% of patients; tests for ANA and extractable nuclear antigen should be ordered. Although there is an association of these disorders with malignancy, the search for a tumor is rarely productive. Unless the clinical evaluation discloses signs and symptoms of a specific tumor, further evaluation in the emergency department is not necessary.

A referral for electromyography may reveal characteristic changes. A muscle biopsy in an area with abnormal electromyographic activity confirms the diagnosis.

EMERGENCY DEPARTMENT MANAGEMENT AND DISPOSITION

The treatment of choice for polymyositis unrelated to malignancy is corticosteroids. Prednisone, 60 to 100 mg/d, is used initially. The dose is tapered when the enzyme levels have returned to normal. Azathioprine is used as a second-line agent. Because this drug has severe immunosuppressive, gastrointestinal, and neoplastic adverse effects, it should be given only under the direction of the rheumatologist who will be observing the patient. If an associated tumor is found, symptoms of polymyositis often resolve after resection.

Patients able to carry out activities of daily living can usually be managed as outpatients. Patients with an unstable gait or who are unable to navigate stairs in their homes require hospital admission.

COMMON PITFALLS

- Considering weakness a normal senile change
- Considering only endocrine and electrolyte imbalances as causes of weakness
- Confusing disease exacerbation with corticosteroid myopathy

References

1. Alarçon-Segovia D. Clinical manifestations of the antiphospholipid syndrome. *J Rheumatol* 1992;19:1778.
2. Arnett FC, Edworthy SM, Block DA, et al. The American Rheumatism Association 1987 revised criteria for the classification of rheumatoid arthritis. *Arthritis Rheum* 1988;31:315.
3. Benzer TI, Leonard K, Raymond F. Evaluating bodily fluids. In: Flomenbaum N, et al., eds. *Emergency diagnostic testing,* 2nd ed. St. Louis: Mosby, 1995:291–328.
4. Black C, Isenberg DA. Mixed connective tissue disease—goodbye to all that. *Br J Rheumatol* 1992;31:695.
5. Brooks PM. Clinical management of rheumatoid arthritis. *Lancet* 1993;341:286.
6. Condemi JJ. The autoimmune diseases. *JAMA* 1992;268:2882.
7. Fauci AS, Haynes BF, Katz P. The spectrum of vasculitis: clinical, pathologies, immunologic, and therapeutic considerations. *Ann Intern Med* 1978;89:660.
8. Feinstein DI, Francis RB. The lupus anticoagulant and anticardiolipin antibodies. In: Wallace DJ, Hahn BH, eds. *Dubois' lupus erythematous,* 4th ed. Philadelphia: Lea & Febiger, 1993:246–253.
9. Fritzler MG, Rubin RL. Drug induced Lupus. In: Wallace DJ, Hahn BH, eds. *Dubois' lupus erythematous,* 4th ed. Philadelphia: Lea & Febiger, 1993:442–443.
10. Goodman BW. Temporal arteritis. *Am J Med* 1979;67:839.
11. Hall S, et al. Takayasu's arteritis. A study of 32 North American patients. *Medicine (Baltimore)* 1985;64:89.
12. Kotzin BL, O'Dell JR. Systemic lupus erythematous. In: Frank MM, et al., eds. *Sammter's immunologic diseases,* 5th ed. Boston: Little, Brown and Company, 1995:667–697.
13. Kramer J, Jolesz F, Kleefiend J. Rheumatoid arthritis of the cervical spine. *Rheum Dis Clin North Am* 1991;17:757.
14. LeRoy EC, et al. Scleroderma (systemic sclerosis): classification, subsets, and pathogenesis. *J Rheumatol* 1988;15:202.
15. Panayi GS. The immunopathogenesis of rheumatoid arthritis in the thorax. *J Thorac Imaging* 1992;7:19.
16. Pisetsley DS. Antinuclear antibodies. *Rheum Dis Clin North Am* 1992;18:1.
17. Silman AJ. Epidemiology of scleroderma. *Ann Rheum Dis* 1991;50:846.
18. Skaer TL. Medication-induced systemic lupus erythematosus. *Clin Ther* 1992;14:496.
19. Sturgess A. Recently characterized autoantibodies and their clinical significance. *Aust N Z J Med* 1992;22:279.
20. Tan EM, Cohen AS, Fries JF, et al. The 1982 revised criteria for the classification of systemic lupus erythematosus. *Arthritis Rheum* 1982;25:1271.
21. Yamato M, et al. Takayasu's arteritis: radiographic findings in 59 patients. *Radiology* 1986;161:329.

PART X

Dermatology

CHAPTER 223

Papulosquamous Eruptions

John J. Kelly and William H. Spivey

Papulosquamous lesions are characterized by papules and scaly desquamation of the skin. The lesions may also be macular and erythematous. Diseases in this group include psoriasis, seborrheic dermatitis, pityriasis rosea, lichen planus, and secondary syphilis. Other diseases that may be part of the differential diagnosis include tinea, discoid lupus erythematosus, mixed connective-tissue diseases, and scabies. Papulosquamous eruptions are the most common cutaneous manifestations of human immunodeficiency virus (HIV) infection, and their appearance may be the first clue of HIV infection in an otherwise asymptomatic host.[1] In addition, a large number of drugs are known to cause papulosquamous eruptions.

When evaluating a papulosquamous eruption in the emergency department, the physician should look for clues to help differentiate the possible etiologies. Is the rash disseminated or localized? Does it appear on specific areas of the body, such as the elbows, knees, scalp, palms, soles, web spaces, or sun-exposed areas? Is it a well-marginated, ring-shaped, or isolated lesion (herald patch)? Are the papules pruritic or purple? Answering these basic questions and using the algorithm in Fig. 223.1, most papulosquamous diseases are diagnosed without dermatologic consultation.

PSORIASIS

Psoriasis, the most common papulosquamous dermatosis, is found in 1% to 2% of the general population.[5] It is equally distributed between males and females, but is more common in Whites than in Blacks. Although it is more common during the second and third decades, it may manifest itself at any age. The etiology of psoriasis is not known, although genetic predisposition appears to play an important role.[11] There is a family history of psoriasis in one-third of those affected. Psoriasis may also have a neuroimmunologic etiology.[4] Three factors that are implicated as disease triggers are psychological stress, skin injury and infection.[6]

CLINICAL PRESENTATION

Psoriatic lesions are characterized by well-delineated, salmon-colored papules that are soon covered by silvery-white scales (Fig. 223.2). They involve both the dermis and epidermis; the depth of involvement depends on their age and location. As the lesions age, the epidermal layer thins, exposing underlying capillary beds. These capillary beds may bleed when the overlying keratotic epidermis is sheared away by mechanical force. This phenomenon, known as the Auspitz sign, is diagnostic of psoriasis. Common sites for psoriasis are the scalp, extensor surfaces of the extremities, presacral region, palms, soles, and nails. Arthritis is seen in 5% to 7% of patients with psoriasis, and nail abnormalities are seen in up to 50% of patients.[6] The nails are commonly pitted and show a brownish or whitish discoloration and an accumulation of scale on the nail bed.

Pustular psoriasis is characterized by erythematous areas covered with pustules. It may be localized or general, and may affect the hands and feet in addition to the trunk and extremities. Generalized pustular psoriasis has an acute onset associated with malaise, pyrexia, and leukocytosis, and it is potentially fatal if untreated. Factors known to induce generalized pustular psoriasis include a tapering of the dose of systemic corticosteroids, withdrawal of potent topical steroids, nonsteroidal antiinflammatory agents, pregnancy, viral upper respiratory tract infections, and beta-hemolytic streptococcal infections.[6]

Guttate psoriasis usually follows streptococcal infections; lesions appear on the trunk and extremities.

DIFFERENTIAL DIAGNOSIS

The differential diagnosis of psoriasis includes tinea cruris, candidiasis, secondary syphilis, pityriasis rosea, cutaneous lupus erythematosus, and seborrheic dermatitis,[5] as well as intertrigo when the eruption occurs in the intertriginous areas. Seborrheic dermatitis may resemble psoriasis of the scalp, but usually has finer and more widespread yellow scaling. A helpful clue in differentiating psoriasis from other conditions is the presence of psoriatic nail changes: pitting of the nails and separation of the nail from the underlying nail bed.[5] Guttate psoriasis on the trunk is easily confused with pityriasis rosea.

EMERGENCY DEPARTMENT MANAGEMENT

Psoriasis is a chronic disease that waxes and wanes, often for no apparent reason. Minor cases may respond to lubricants and emollients, exposure to sunlight, and avoidance of stress. More

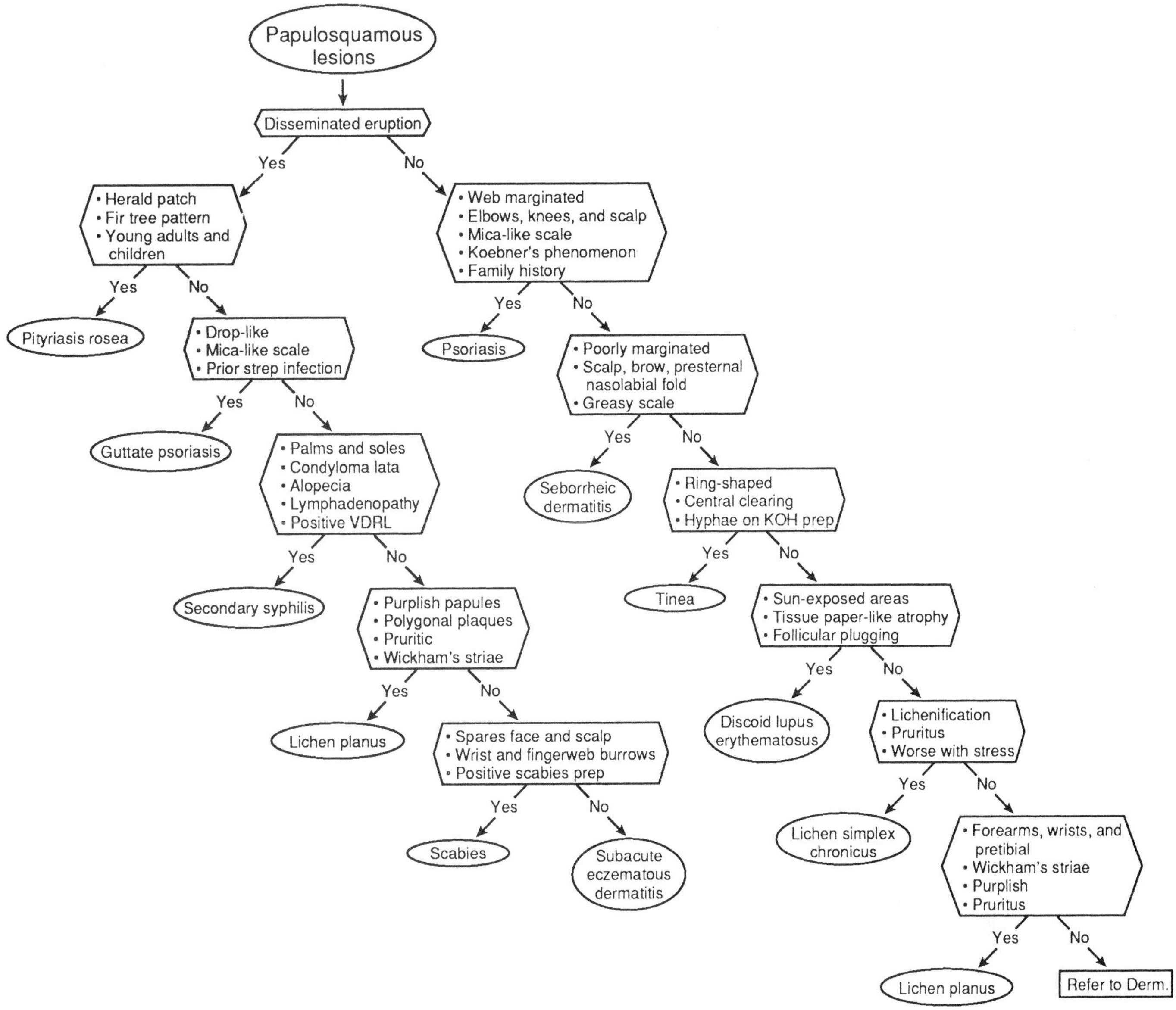

Figure 223.1. Algorithm for papulosquamous diseases. (From Flowers FP, Krusinski PA. *Dermatology in ambulatory and emergency medicine.* Chicago, Year Book Medical, 1984.)

commonly, crude tar 2% and tar paints such as Zetar, which are added to bath water, are needed. Ultraviolet light exposure, in conjunction with topical tar application, is often effective, even in severe cases.

Large, thick lesions on the trunk and extremities may be treated with a fluorinated corticosteroid ointment. Hydrocortisone 1% is not strong enough to treat these lesions, but it may be used to treat lesions in the intertriginous areas, where striae and atrophy occur, with stronger preparations.[18] Newer treatments include calcipotriene ointment, anthralin ointment, and tazarotene gel.[5] Methotrexate has been used in severe cases of psoriasis, but up to a third of patients develop liver toxicity. In PUVA therapy, psoralen (P) is combined with long-wavelength ultraviolet light (UVA) to interfere with the DNA synthesis of psoriatic lesions. This treatment should be performed only in a hospital or physician's office. Immunotherapeutic agents (e.g., cyclosporine) and drugs approved for other indications, such as zidovudine, may also be initiated by a dermatologist.[8] Pustular psoriasis requires systemic antibiotics (e.g., penicillin 500 mg four times a day for 10 days) and a topical antibiotic steroid ointment. Often, pustular psoriasis is difficult to treat, and methotrexate, retinoids, hydroxyurea, and other antimetabolites may be required for severe cases.[6] Guttate psoriasis is usually self-limited but may be helped by coal tar or steroid preparations.

DISPOSITION

Psoriasis is rarely dangerous or life-threatening and is usually best cared for by a dermatologist who can follow the patient over time. Topical steroids or coal tar may be initiated in the emergency department, but treatment with UVA or methotrexate should be performed under the direction of a dermatologist, usually in the hospital. The patient who appears toxic should be admitted for intravenous antibiotics.

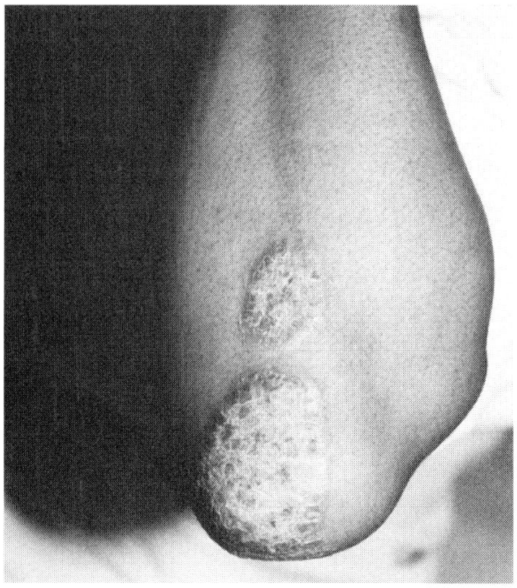

Figure 223.2. Well-defined erythematous, scaling plaques on the extensor surface of the arm in a patient with psoriasis.

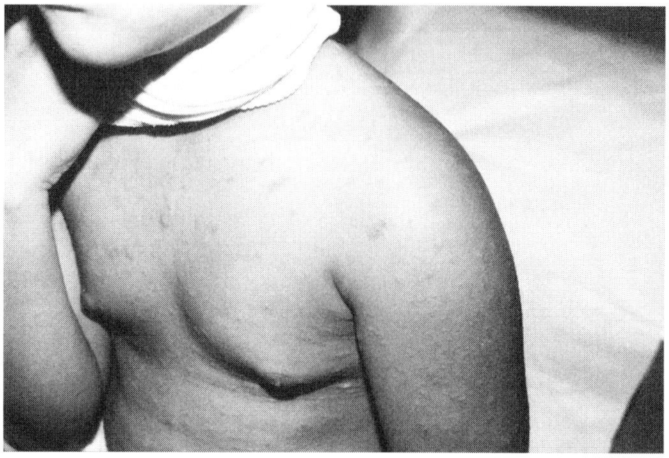

Figure 223.3. Circular and ovoid papules and plaques with scaling on the trunk and proximal extremities in a patient with pityriasis rosea.

COMMON PITFALLS

- Psoriasis of the trunk and extremities is rarely confused with other diseases, but in the intertriginous areas, it may be confused with tinea cruris, candidiasis, or intertrigo. Close examination with a Wood's light and potassium hydroxide (KOH) preparation should help differentiate these diseases.
- If steroids are used to treat psoriasis, systemic steroids should be avoided. They are very effective but can cause long-term side effects, and the disease often rebounds when steroids are stopped.
- New cases of psoriasis; sudden, severe exacerbations; or cases recalcitrant to treatment should alert the clinician to the possibility of HIV infection.[1]

PITYRIASIS ROSEA

Pityriasis rosea is an acute, self-limited, inflammatory dermatosis seen most commonly in children and young adults, although it can appear at any age.[7] It affects both sexes equally and accounts for about 1% of patients seen by dermatologists.[12] The incidence is lowest during the summer.[7] The etiology is unknown, although it is presumed to be related to a viral infection.[6]

CLINICAL PRESENTATION

Pityriasis rosea is characterized by oval, salmon-colored, pruritic, scaling patches on the neck and trunk that follow skin cleavage lines (Fig. 223.3). On the back, this produces a so-called Christmas tree pattern. The rash is rarely found on the palms and soles,[16] and it may involve the oral mucosa and gingiva.[17] Characteristically, this generalized eruption is preceded by a 2- to 5-cm herald patch, but it is absent in 10% to 15% of patients. Within 7 to 14 days, other lesions appear, which, in young children, may involve the face, scalp, and distal extremities.[9] An atypical presentation (inverse pityriasis rosea) spares the trunk, only affecting the face and extremities.[6] The rash usually lasts 4 to 7 weeks.

The most common complaints associated with pityriasis rosea are pruritus and mild constitutional symptoms such as malaise, fever, and lymphadenopathy. It poses no risk to the fetus if it occurs in pregnant women. It does not appear to be contagious.

DIFFERENTIAL DIAGNOSIS

The differential diagnosis includes tinea corporis when there are a few lesions, and secondary lues when there are many (although luetic lesions tend to be less pruritic). The herald patch is commonly misdiagnosed as ringworm. A KOH preparation of scrapings from the lesions is negative, however. Examination of tinea corporis with a Wood's light produces a bright green fluorescence, but no fluorescence is seen with pityriasis rosea. Guttate psoriasis, which is distributed mainly on the trunk, has thicker, more silvery scales than does pityriasis rosea. Lichen planus may have a similar appearance, but the lesions are purple, not salmon-colored. Eruptions resembling pityriasis rosea may be caused by gold, bismuth, methopromazine, metronidazole, captopril, barbiturates, nonsteroidal antiinflammatories, and clonidine.[7] Because the skin eruption of secondary syphilis may mimic that of pityriasis, a VDRL or rapid plasma reagin (RPR) should be drawn.

EMERGENCY DEPARTMENT MANAGEMENT AND DISPOSITION

Pityriasis is a benign, self-limited disease that does not require therapy. Symptomatic treatment for pruritus may include antihistamines and intermediate-strength topical steroids. UVA may accelerate resolution of the lesions.

If the diagnosis is made with certainty, consultation with a dermatologist is unnecessary. The patient may be discharged to follow-up with the family physician. If the diagnosis is in question, the patient should be referred to a dermatologist.

COMMON PITFALLS

- Pityriasis rosea is often misdiagnosed. The herald patch can resemble tinea corporis and may be incorrectly treated with antifungal medication until the generalized rash appears. Later, the generalized rash may be mistaken for lichen planus or a drug eruption. A careful history and physical examination decrease the likelihood of these errors. The wise clinician draws a VDRL or RPR to rule out "the great masquerader."

TABLE 223.1. Drugs Causing Lichenoid Drug Reactions

Beta blockers	Captopril
Methyldopa	Thiazides
Furosemide	Gold
Antimalarials	Quinidine
Oral hypoglycemic agents	Phenytoin
Carbamazepine	Antituberculous agents
Antihistamines	Phenylbutazone
Antipsychotics	Bismuth
p-Aminosalicylic acid	Lithium

LICHEN PLANUS

Lichen planus is a relatively uncommon inflammatory dermatitis characterized by violaceous, flat-topped papules. The disease is most common between ages 30 and 60 and is seen with equal frequency in men and women. It is responsible for about 1% of visits to dermatologists.[7] Viral and bacterial agents, as well as genetic predisposition,[15] have been suggested as causes. Drugs have also been implicated in causing a lichen planus–like eruption (Table 223.1).[2]

CLINICAL PRESENTATION

The lesions of lichen planus are flat-topped, slightly scaly, polygonal, and purple, with a fine reticular pattern of white dots and lines on their surface (Fig. 223.4). They are commonly found on the wrist, volar surface of the forearms, and pretibial areas, but may also appear on the palms, soles, lips, and penis. On the palms and soles, they are commonly yellowish and nonpruritic. The lesions commonly develop at sites of trauma (Koebner phenomenon). For this reason, they are often found in a linear pattern, presumably due to scratching. Over half of patients with cutaneous lichen planus have oral mucosal lesions as well. These are whitish plaques with a lacy, whitish, reticular pattern (Wickham striae).

DIFFERENTIAL DIAGNOSIS

The differential diagnosis of lichen planus includes psoriasis, fungal infection, secondary syphilis, pityriasis rosea, and discoid lupus erythematosus. When the mucous membranes are involved, leukoplakia and candidiasis are considerations.

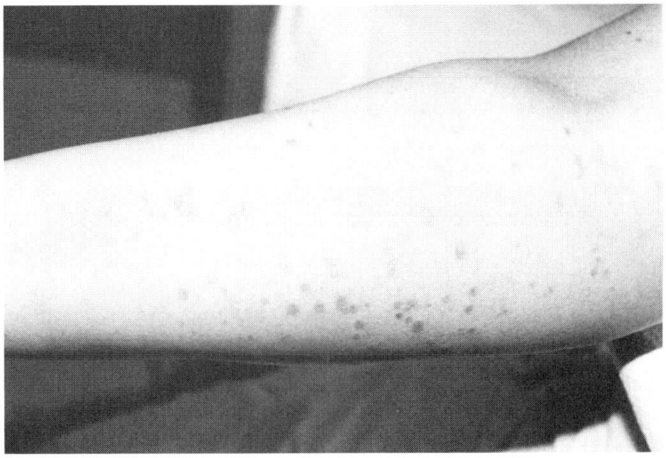

Figure 223.4. Gray to violaceous flat-topped papules (some with Wickham striae) on the flexural surface of the forearm in a patient with lichen planus.

EMERGENCY DEPARTMENT MANAGEMENT AND DISPOSITION

Lichen planus is a self-limited disease that may last weeks to years. Most patients experience a spontaneous resolution within a year. A few cases of squamous cell carcinoma have been reported in association with oral lichen planus. Treatment includes antihistamines for pruritus and topical steroids for inflammatory lesions. Occasionally, with widespread lesions, systemic steroids may be used. Patients with lichen planus should be referred to a dermatologist for long-term follow-up, although treatment may be initiated in the emergency department.

COMMON PITFALLS

- Lichen planus frequently involves the oral mucosa; in fact, 15% to 25% of patients with oral lichen planus never develop skin lesions. It is also one of the few rashes that may affect the palms and soles. A close physical examination, not only of the obvious lesions on the arms and trunk, but also of the mouth, palms, and soles, is important in making the correct diagnosis.

SEBORRHEIC DERMATITIS

Seborrheic dermatitis is a chronic, superficial, inflammatory process affecting regions of the body with increased sebaceous gland activity. It is more common in males, and occurs in infants under 12 months, among adolescents, and in elderly persons. It is more severe in winter. It is particularly common in patients with HIV infection. The etiology is unclear, but it may be caused by dysfunctional sebaceous gland activity[7] or a reaction to the common skin yeasts *Malassezia ovalis*[14] and *Pityrosporum ovale*.[3]

CLINICAL PRESENTATION

The lesions of "oily" seborrheic dermatitis are characterized by poorly defined margins, mild erythema, and greasy yellow scales. "Dry" seborrheic dermatitis exhibits small, dry, powdery scales and little or no erythema.[3] Secondary lesions due to scratching may be seen around the primary lesions. Areas commonly affected include the scalp, face (especially the eyebrows and nasolabial folds), axilla, groin, buttocks, and inframammary folds. In infants, the scalp is frequently affected and is known as cradle cap. When the scalp is affected in adults, it is called dandruff.

DIFFERENTIAL DIAGNOSIS

The differential diagnosis includes psoriasis, tinea, and atopic dermatitis in children. Lesions affecting the scalp, axilla, and groin may be difficult to differentiate from psoriasis.[12] Involvement of the knees, elbows, and nails favors psoriasis. Persistent pruritic lesions that do not respond to therapy may be tinea. In infants, seborrheic dermatitis is commonly seen on the scalp, axilla, and diaper area. Lesions on the forearms and shins favor atopic dermatitis.

EMERGENCY DEPARTMENT MANAGEMENT AND DISPOSITION

Antiseborrheic shampoos containing sulfur, salicylic acid, coal tar, or selenium sulfide provide adequate therapy for most patients. They should be used daily and rubbed into the scalp, with a 5- to 10-minute wait before rinsing. Involvement of the face or intertriginous regions may be treated topically with hydrocortisone 1% to 2% or another nonfluorinated corticosteroid twice daily. The use of 2% ketoconazole cream has been reported to provide satisfactory relief of this chronic dermatitis.[10] Patients with seborrheic dermatitis may be treated on an outpatient basis by the emergency physician, and then referred to a dermatologist or the patient's family physician. The possibility of HIV infection should be considered.

COMMON PITFALLS

- Seborrheic dermatitis is often misdiagnosed. It occurs in infancy as cradle cap and usually does not appear again until puberty. It is associated with an oily complexion and is often precipitated by fatigue or stress.

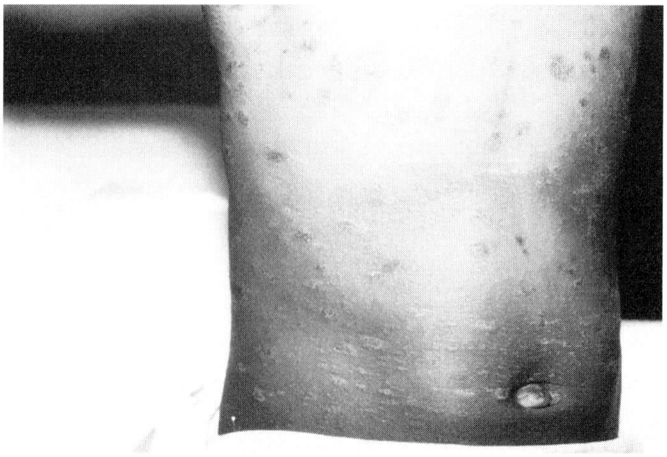

Figure 223.5. Diffuse erythematous papules and plaques with scaling in a patient with the rash of secondary syphilis.

SECONDARY SYPHILIS

Syphilis is a sexually transmitted infectious disease caused by *Treponema pallidum*. The rash of secondary syphilis appears 9 to 90 days after the onset of the chancre; the average is 3 weeks.[13] Most individuals contract the disease from sexual activity with a person in the early stages of syphilis. The risk of transmission ranges from 10% to 60%, and approximately one-third of individuals with a single exposure to early syphilis become infected.[13]

CLINICAL PRESENTATION

The rash of secondary syphilis is generalized, painless, and nonpruritic. It involves the skin as well as the mucous membranes in 30% to 50% of the cases.[13] On the skin, it tends to follow the lines of cleavage, especially on the trunk. It has a special predilection for the palms and soles. The lesions are scaling, red-brown papules and plaques that are discrete and sharply demarcated rather than confluent (Fig. 223.5). Annular plaques on the mouth, nose, and lip areas are virtually diagnostic.[16] The patient's presenting complaint may be an apparently unrelated other symptom, such as headache, sore throat, malaise, and generalized arthralgia.

DIFFERENTIAL DIAGNOSIS

The differential diagnosis of secondary syphilis includes pityriasis rosea, Rocky Mountain spotted fever, meningococcemia, drug reaction, and lichen planus. Palmar lesions that mimic secondary syphilis may be secondary to drug eruption.[16]

EMERGENCY DEPARTMENT MANAGEMENT AND DISPOSITION

Diagnostic studies such as VDRL or RPR should be ordered. Dark-field examination of scrapings from lesions may also be performed. If either test is positive, the patient is treated in the emergency department with either benzathine penicillin G (2.4 million units intramuscularly) or aqueous procaine penicillin G (600,000 units intramuscularly daily for 8 days). Patients allergic to penicillin may be treated with tetracycline or doxycycline for 2 weeks.

If the diagnosis of secondary syphilis cannot be made in the emergency department, the patient should be referred to a private physician or clinic pending the results of VDRL or RPR testing. Hospital admission is unnecessary for secondary syphilis, but the patient should be instructed to abstain from sexual contact until the diagnosis is clear and any necessary treatment has been administered, and to refer all sexual partners to testing and treatment, as indicated.

COMMON PITFALLS

- Failing to elicit a history of a primary lesion preceding the rash. This history and an adequate sexual history are helpful in the initial diagnosis.
- Failing to appreciate the typical erythematous, hyperpigmented, scaly papules on the palms and soles may lead to an inappropriate diagnosis
- Because of the strong association of HIV and syphilis, patients newly diagnosed with syphilis should be referred for HIV testing.[13]

ACKNOWLEDGMENT

The authors thank Howard Goldman, DO, Associate Professor of Dermatology at Philadelphia College of Osteopathic Medicine, for contributing the photographs used in this chapter.

References

1. Aftergut K, Cockerell CJ. Update on the cutaneous manifestations of HIV infection. Clinical and pathologic features. *Dermatol Clin* 1999;17:445–471, vii.
2. Crowson AN, Magro CM. Recent advances in the pathology of cutaneous drug eruptions. *Dermatol Clin* 1999;17:537–560, viii.
3. Faergemann J. Pityrosporum infections. *J Am Acad Dermatol* 1994;31:S18–20.
4. Farber EM, Raychaudhuri SP. Is psoriasis a neuroimmunologic disease? *Int J Dermatol* 1999;38:12–15.
5. Feldman SR, Clark AR. Psoriasis. *Med Clin North Am* 1998;82:1135–1144, vi.
6. Ferrera PC, Dupree ML, Verdile VP. Dermatologic problems encountered in the emergency department. *Am J Emerg Med* 1996;14:588–601.
7. Fox BJ, Odom RB. Papulosquamous diseases: a review. *J Am Acad Dermatol* 1985;12:597–624.
8. Guzzo C. Recent advances in the treatment of psoriasis. *Dermatol Clin* 1997;15:59–68.
9. Hartley AH. Pityriasis rosea. *Pediatr Rev* 1999;20:266–269.
10. Hay RJ, Graham-Brown RA. Dandruff and seborrheic dermatitis: causes and management. *Clin Exp Dermatol* 1997;22:3–6.
11. Henseler T. The genetics of psoriasis. *J Am Acad Dermatol* 1997;37:S1–11.
12. Lookingbill DP, Marks JG. Scaling papules, plaques and patches. In: Lookingbill DP, Marks JG, eds. *Principles of dermatology*. Philadelphia: WB Saunders, 1993.
13. Rosen T, Brown TJ. Cutaneous manifestations of sexually transmitted diseases. *Med Clin North Am* 1998;82:1081–1104, vi.

14. Schmidt A. Malassezia furfur: a fungus belonging to the physiological skin flora and its relevance in skin disorders. *Cutis* 1997;59:21–24.
15. Scully C, Beyli M, Ferreiro MC, et al. Update on oral lichen planus: etiopathogenesis and management. *Crit Rev Oral Biol Med* 1998;9:86–122.
16. Tonecki KJ, Dijkstra JWE. Treponemes, rickettsia, and mycobacteria. In: Sams WM, Lynch PJ, eds. *Principles and practice of dermatology*. New York: Churchill Livingstone, 1996.
17. Vidimos AT, Camisa C. Tongue and cheek: oral lesions in pityriasis rosea. *Cutis* 1992;50:276–280.
18. Yoder F. Papulosquamous diseases. In: Flowers FP, Krussinsky PA, eds. *Dermatology in ambulatory and emergency medicine*. Chicago: Yearbook Medical, 1984.

CHAPTER 224
Blistering Disorders

M. Andrew Levitt

Vesicular lesions are commonly seen in the emergency department. Like other dermatologic lesions, vesicles can present a challenge in determining their etiology, contagiousness, and proper treatment.[3–6]

Vesicles are circumscribed epidermal elevations 1 to 4 mm in diameter that usually contain clear fluid. Several characteristics help distinguish the lesion from other vesicular disorders, including the nature of the contained fluid (seropurulent, serosanguineous), the shape of the lesion's apex (rounded, acuminate, umbilicated), the pattern of the eruption (discrete, irregularly scattered, grouped, linear), and the distribution over the body and associated mucous membrane involvement.

In this discussion, there are two types of vesicular disorders: those appearing in groups and those that are individual or disseminated. Algorithms for each appear in Figs. 224.1 and 224.2.

GROUPED LESIONS

Herpes Simplex

The lesions of herpes simplex are typically tightly clustered on an erythematous base and evolve into pustules and erosions over 5 to 7 days. Grouped, crusted erosions are the typical presentation. Associated symptoms may include fever, local pain, regional lymphadenopathy, fatigue, and malaise. Urinary retention occasionally occurs with genital lesions and generally requires hospital admission.

Primary lesions usually are not tightly clustered, but are more widespread with a bilateral distribution. Recurrent lesions more typically are tightly clustered, are unilateral, and occur in the same location as previous episodes of infection. Approximately 50% of patients with recurrent lesions have a 24-hour prodrome of local itching, burning, tingling, and stinging. Precipitating factors for recurrence appear to include upper respiratory infections, fever, sunburn, menstruation, trauma, or other stress.

Primary lesions usually resolve in 2 to 3 weeks, but the duration may be longer in immunocompromised patients. Typical sites of involvement are the oral, genital, and periorbital areas and the fingertips (herpetic whitlow). With periorbital lesions, fluorescein staining of the cornea is necessary to rule out herpetic keratitis. These patients should be referred to an ophthalmologist. A Tzanck smear or viral culture may be helpful in the diagnosis.

With the increasing incidence of the acquired immunodeficiency syndrome and the growing use of bone marrow and solid organ transplantation, more severe manifestations of herpes infections are being seen.[8] Acyclovir is the most widely used antiviral agent in clinical use. Treatment with 200 mg of oral acyclovir five times per day for 10 days is indicated for primary genital herpes. However, the duration of symptoms is decreased only minimally with this therapy and only if started within 24 hours after onset of the rash. Time to crusting decreases from 2.7 days to 2.2 days. In immunocompromised patients, a dose of 400 mg is recommended. Other medications that are effective and available for treating herpetic infections are famciclovir, valacyclovir, and topical penciclovir 1% cream. The latter can minimally reduce average time to healing of recurrent orolabial herpes simplex virus infections by 0.7 days and the duration of pain by 0.6 days.[10] Intravenous therapy (5 mg/kg every 8 hours) should be considered for patients with urinary retention, compromised immunity, or disseminated infection, which might be life-threatening. Topical viscous lidocaine preparations may be useful for short-term pain control of oral or genital lesions. All three oral agents have been shown to reduce the frequency of symptomatic recurrences of genital herpes. Recommended doses are acyclovir 400 mg b.i.d., famciclovir 250 mg b.i.d., and valacyclovir 500 mg b.i.d.[11] Importantly, patients receiving suppressive antiviral medication should be counseled that they may still transmit herpes simplex virus to their sexual partners.

Herpes Zoster

Herpes zoster (shingles) occurs in individuals with a history of chickenpox when varicella-zoster virus that is dormant in dorsal root ganglia is reactivated. Patients are most often older, with a peak age of 50 to 70 years. Thoracic and trigeminal nerve dermatomes are the most common sites of involvement, with tightly clustered lesions on an erythematous base present in a linear fashion distributed along one or two adjacent dermatomes. A prodrome of painful hyperesthesia is often described in the same dermatomes 5 to 7 days before the lesions appear. Resolution generally occurs within 3 weeks. The pain associated with herpes zoster is the principal reason that patients seek medical care. Traditionally, pain that is present while the rash persists or in the first 30 days from onset has been termed *acute pain*. Pain that is present after this period is generally termed *postherpetic neuralgia* and may persist for more than 6 months. The incidence of postherpetic neuralgia increases sharply with increasing age. Nearly half of patients older than 60 years have this complication. Postherpetic neuralgia is also more severe and persists longer in older patients than in younger individuals.

A metaanalysis found that acyclovir reduces pain duration and prevalence, especially in patients 50 years of age or older.[15] The treatment generally recommended is acyclovir 800 mg five times a day for 7 days. It is unclear whether treating longer with acyclovir or adding prednisolone is of added benefit.[13,14] Famciclovir 750 mg or valacyclovir 1,000 mg t.i.d. for 7 days has also been shown to decrease the median duration of postherpetic neuralgia.[2,12] Symptomatic treatment with Burow solution–soaked compresses three times a day is often helpful as well. Ophthalmologic consultation is indicated if the ophthalmic division of the trigeminal nerve is involved. Dissemination beyond the original dermatomes should raise the suspicion of immunodeficiency.

Hospital employees who are exposed to patients with herpes zoster should be tested for antibody to the varicella-zoster virus.

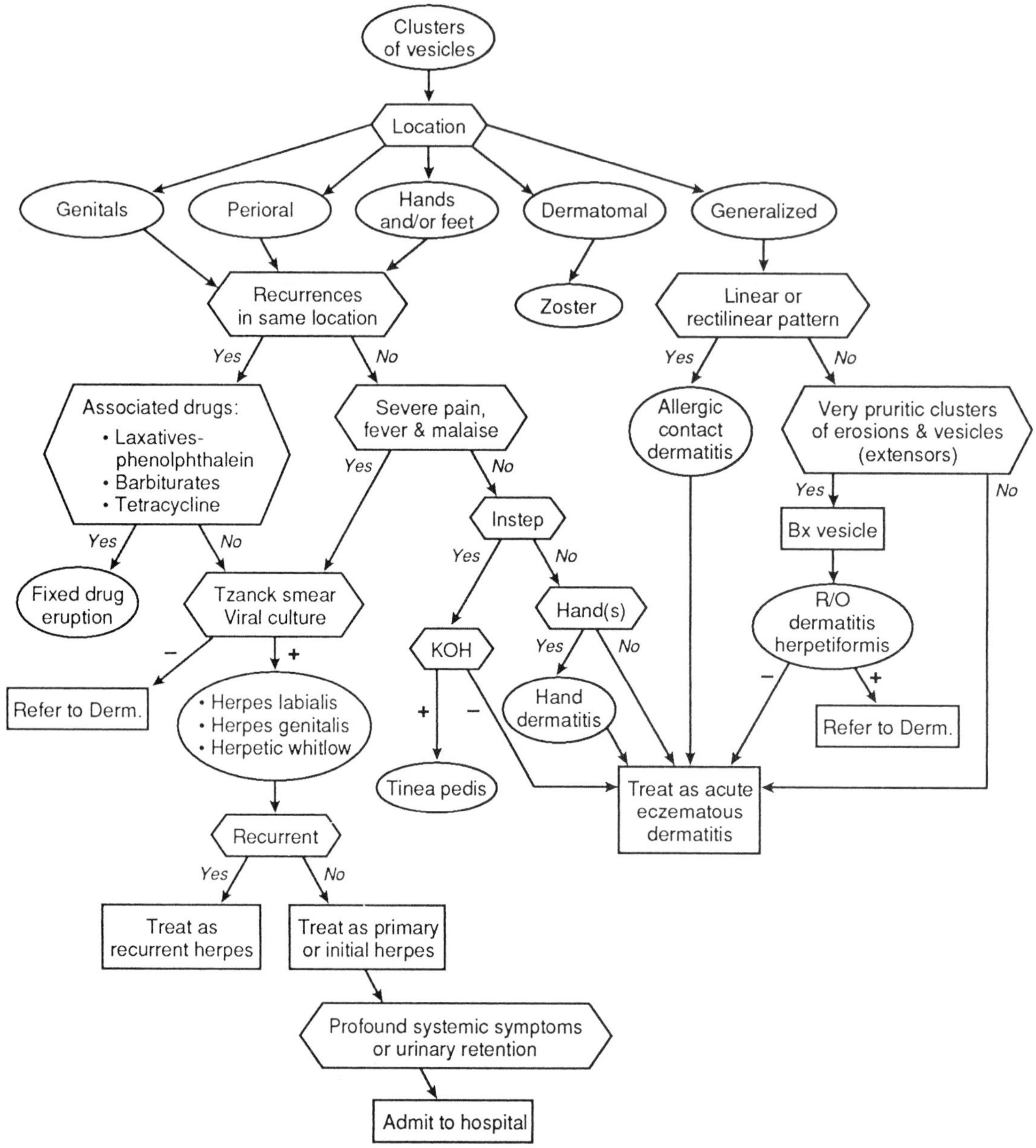

Figure 224.1. Algorithm for vesiculobullous diseases. (From Flowers FP, Krusinski PA. *Dermatology in ambulatory and emergency medicine*. Chicago: Year Book Medical, 1984, with permission.)

Isolation for 8 to 21 days after exposure is recommended when antibody is not detected. If antibody is present, isolation is unnecessary.[9]

Allergic Contact Dermatitis

Because allergic contact dermatitis is a result of delayed hypersensitivity, skin lesions may appear hours to days after exposure to the offending antigen, and it is often difficult to identify that antigen. Commonly identified etiologic agents include poison ivy, oak, and sumac; soaps; detergents; and perfumes. Pruritus is the initial symptom, which is quickly followed by erythema and vesiculation. Areas with a thin stratum corneum (such as eyelids and genitalia) may swell severely. Without treatment, symptoms may persist for 2 to 3 weeks.

Mild contact dermatitis may be treated with topical corticosteroids. For severe cases, oral prednisone (40 to 60 mg/d for 7 days) accelerates resolution of symptoms (usually within 24 to 48 hours) and poses minimal risks of adverse effects.

Fixed Drug Eruption

Like herpes simplex, fixed drug eruption causes recurrent episodes of skin lesions in one location. Unlike herpes simplex, however, fixed drug eruption generally leaves persistent slate-gray to brown hyperpigmentation after the attack resolves. The most commonly implicated drugs include phenolphthalein (e.g., Ex-Lax, Feen-a-Mint), tetracycline, sulfa, and barbiturates. Symptoms usually arise 1 to 2 days after ingestion. Pruritus generally occurs first, followed by the appearance of clusters of vesicles or bullae in a hyperpigmented macule. The process resolves in 2 to 3 weeks, after discontinuation of the offending agents.

Other Causes of Vesicular Eruptions

Dyshidrotic eczema (pompholyx) usually occurs on the medial and lateral aspects of the fingers and sometimes on the palms and soles. It is intensely pruritic and responds to topical corticosteroids. If severe, oral steroids can be used.

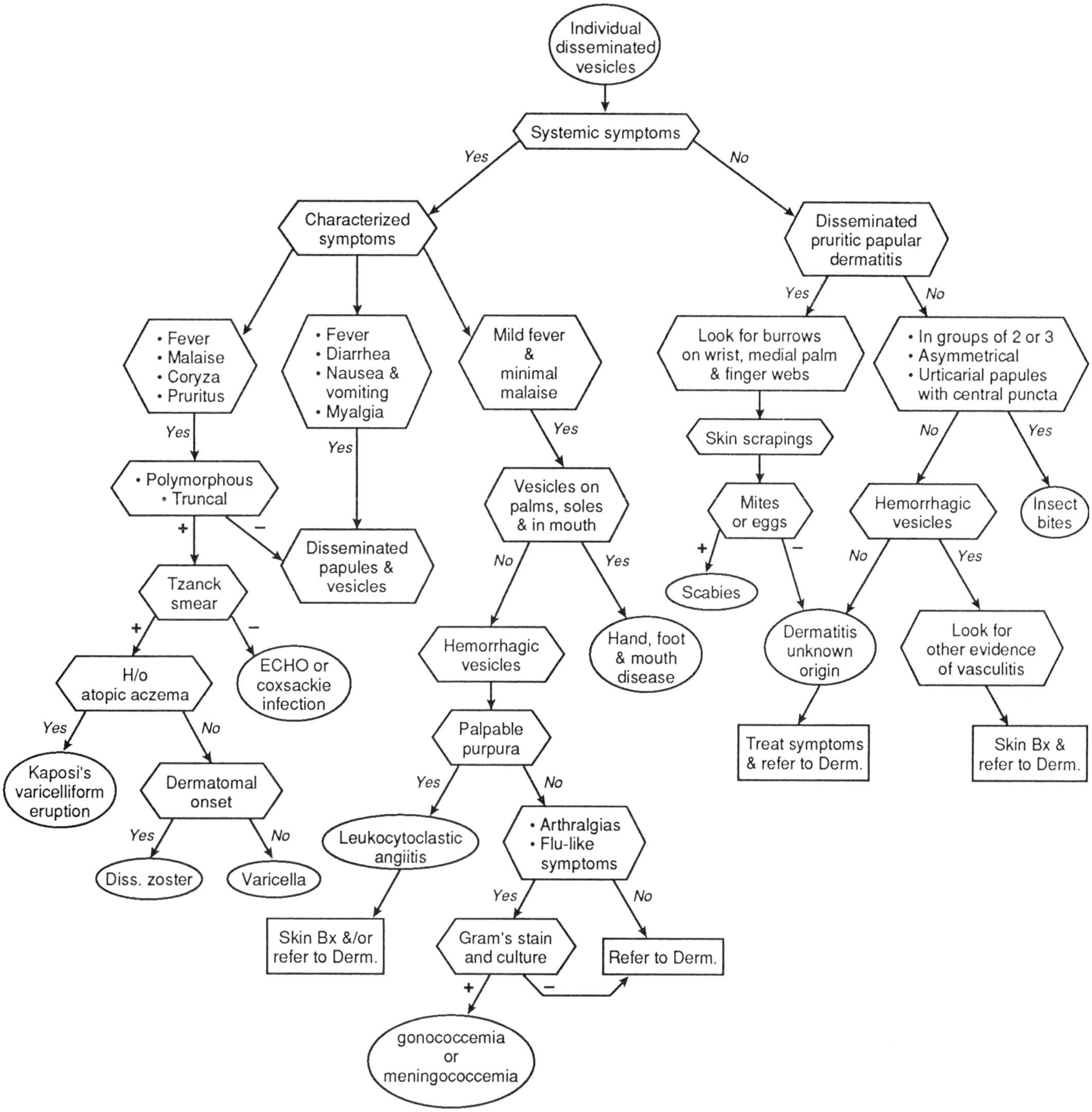

Figure 224.2. Algorithm for vesicular dermatoses. (From Flowers FP, Krusinski PA. *Dermatology in ambulatory and emergency medicine.* Chicago: Year Book Medical, 1984, with permission.)

The vesicular eruption of tinea pedis may usually be diagnosed clinically by potassium hydroxide staining of vesicle fluid. Treatment is with a topical antifungal agent such as clotrimazole. Accompanying involvement of the hands is often an eczematous reaction.

Atopic dermatitis is generally accompanied by a personal or family history of eczema, allergic rhinitis, asthma, or urticaria. Nonetheless, the eruption is usually precipitated by physical irritation (wool gloves, soap and water) or emotional stress. Treatment with topical steroids is effective.

Dermatitis herpetiformis (unrelated to the herpes viruses) may be confused with scabies or neurotic excoriations. It generally presents with broken, excoriated vesicles on an erythematous base. It usually begins on extensor surfaces and is pruritic. Treatment is with dapsone and oral antihistamines.

INDIVIDUAL OR DISSEMINATED VESICLES

Varicella

Varicella (chickenpox) is not uncommon in adults. It presents with a polymorphic rash, predominantly on the trunk, consisting of vesicles, umbilicated pustules, and hemorrhagic crusts, which heal to leave atrophic scars. A key diagnostic feature is the simultaneous presence of lesions in all stages of development. It is often accompanied by a prodrome of fever, malaise, myalgia, and coryza, and there may be a clear history of exposure 10 to 14 days before the rash. Pruritus may be severe, and excoriations may be evident. The patient is considered contagious until all of the lesions have crusted over, generally 5 to 6 days after the first appearance of the eruption.

A Tzanck smear and viral culture may aid in making the diagnosis. Pneumonia and encephalitis are uncommon and rarely life-threatening complications. Patients who have pneumonia but no respiratory distress or significant comorbid disease can probably be safely treated as outpatients.[1] Treatment is symptomatic, with oral antihistamines and tepid compresses.

Coxsackievirus and Echovirus Infections

Coxsackievirus and echovirus infections may cause papulovesicular lesions that are evenly spread across the face and torso. Associated symptoms may include fatigue, malaise, fever, vomiting, and diarrhea. Resolution occurs spontaneously in 10 to 14 days, and treatment is symptomatic.

Hand–foot–mouth disease caused by coxsackieviruses presents with tender, flat-topped, whitish vesicles 3 to 4 mm in diameter on the palms and soles and in the mouth. It is commonly associated with mild systemic complaints. The duration is generally 4 to 5 days, and no treatment is necessary.

Scabies

Scabies, an infestation by *Sarcoptes scabiei,* causes pruritus and a mild, disseminated, papulovesicular dermatitis that develops insidiously over several weeks. The pruritus typically worsens at night. Vesicles typically appear on the volar aspects of the wrists, the medial palms, and the interdigital web spaces, but they also may be seen on the areolae, glans penis, elbows, and axillary folds. The face and scalp are not affected in adults. Skin scrapings from the lesions may demonstrate mites, eggs, or feces. Burrows may be identified by applying ink to suspected areas and then wiping clean with alcohol; the burrows retain the color of the ink.

Treatment of scabies has two components. First, lindane (Kwell) solution is applied after bathing, allowed to remain on the skin for 8 to 12 hours, and then washed off. The patient is rendered noninfective 24 hours after treatment, but this procedure should be repeated after 1 week. Recurrence implies reinfection or, possibly, resistance to lindane. Because the incubation period may be 1 to 2 months, asymptomatic contacts and family members should be treated. Pregnant women should be treated with crotamiton (Eurax) twice a day for 2 to 3 weeks. The anthelminthic agent ivermectin, 200 μg/kg, has been found to be effective in treating scabies in both healthy and human immunodeficiency virus–positive individuals.[7]

The second component of treatment is laundering of all clothes and bedding. Items that cannot be washed can be used safely after being set aside for 3 days, because the female mite dies after 2 to 3 days without human contact.

Insect Bites

Vesiculobullous skin lesions may occur as hypersensitivity reactions to insect bites, commonly those of fleas, bedbugs, and mites. A clue to the diagnosis is a linear or grouped pattern of lesions; some may have central puncta. Treatment is with topical corticosteroids and oral antihistamines, and avoidance of further contact with the insect.

COMMON PITFALLS

- Failure to instruct patients with contagious disorders, such as herpes simplex virus, about measures to prevent transmission to others
- Failure to admit patients with herpes who are immunocompromised or have urinary retention or disseminated infection
- Failure to consult an ophthalmologist if there is periorbital herpetic infection

References

1. Baren JM, Henneman PL, Lewis RJ. Primary varicella in adults: pneumonia, pregnancy and hospital admission. *Ann Emerg Med* 1996;28:165–169.
2. Beutner KR, Friedman DJ, Forszpaniak C, et al. Valaciclovir compared with acyclovir for improved therapy for herpes zoster in immunocompetent adults. *Antimicrob Agents Chemother* 1995;39:1546–1553.
3. Dahl M. The blistering diseases. In: Dahl M. *Common office dermatology.* New York: Grune & Stratton, 1983.
4. Domonkos AN, Arnold HL, Odom RB. *Andrews disease of the skin.* Philadelphia: WB Saunders, 1982.
5. Flowers FP, Krusinski PA. *Dermatology in ambulatory and emergency medicine.* Chicago: Year Book Medical, 1984.
6. Furey N. Blistering disorders. In: Roenigk H, ed. *Office dermatology.* Baltimore: Williams & Wilkins, 1981.
7. Meinking TL, Taplin D, Hermida JL, et al. The treatment of scabies with ivermectin. *N Engl J Med* 1995;333:26–30.
8. Sasadeusz JJ, Sacks SL. Systemic antivirals in herpes virus infections. *Dermatol Clin* 1993;11:171.
9. Sayre MR, Lucid EJ. Management of varicella-zoster-virus exposed hospital employees. *Ann Emerg Med* 1987;16(4):421.
10. Spruance SL, Rea TL, Thoming C, et al. Penciclovir cream for the treatment of herpes simplex labialis. A randomized, multicenter, double-bind, placebo-controlled trial. *JAMA* 1997;277:1374–1379.
11. *The Medical Letter* 1997;39:69.
12. Tyring S, Barbarash RA, Nahlik JE, et al. Famciclovir for the treatment of acute herpes zoster: effects on acute disease and postherpetic neuralgia—a randomized, double-blind, placebo-controlled trial. *Ann Intern Med* 1995;123:89–95.
13. Whitley RJ, Weiss H, Gnann JW, et al. Acyclovir with and without prednisolone for the treatment of herpes zoster—a randomized, placebo-controlled trial. *Ann Intern Med* 1996;125:376–383.
14. Wood MJ, Johnson RW, McKendrick MW, et al. A randomized trial of acyclovir for 7 days or 21 days with and without prednisolone for treatment of acute herpes zoster. *N Engl J Med* 1994;330:896–900.
15. Wood MJ, Kay R, Dworkin RH, et al. Oral acyclovir therapy accelerates pain resolution in patients with herpes zoster: a meta-analysis of placebo-controlled trials. *Clin Infect Dis* 1996;22:341–347.

CHAPTER 225
Purpuric Eruptions

Steven M. Joyce and Stephen C. Hartsell

The term *purpura* (Latin, meaning "purple") refers to any skin or mucous membrane eruption caused by bleeding into the skin. Purpura is a sign of underlying disease, usually a disorder of platelets or small vessels and only rarely of clotting factors. The cause of purpura varies, ranging from the trivial (e.g., actinic purpura in the elderly) to the life-threatening (e.g., thrombotic thrombocytopenic purpura) (Table 225.1).

The lesions of purpura vary in size, consistency, and distribution. Lesions smaller than 3 mm are called *petechiae* and usually result from platelet or vascular abnormalities, whereas larger lesions are termed *ecchymoses* and generally are secondary to trauma or clotting disorders.[7] Lesions vary from red to purple and do not blanch with pressure, because the lesions represent extravasated blood in the dermis rather than erythema due to dilated vessels. Lesions may be flat and nonpalpable when inflammation is absent (as in thrombocytopenic purpura) or palpable papules or macules when inflammation is present (as in septic embolic disease or vasculitis).[8] Purpura

TABLE 225.1. Disorders Causing Purpura

EXTRAVASCULAR (nonpalpable)—loss of dermal vascular connective tissue
Actinic disorders (senile purpura)
Scurvy
Corticosteroid therapy
Amyloidosis
Hereditary connective tissue disorders (Ehlers-Danlos syndrome, Marfan syndrome)
VASCULAR—damage to vessel walls
Mechanical (nonpalpable)—vessel walls normal
Increased intravascular pressure (vomiting, cough, straining at childbirth, Valsalva maneuver)
Suction to skin ("love bites," suction cups, depilatory waxing)
Trauma (bruise)
Factitial (self-induced by various methods)
Stasis purpura (increased hydrostatic pressure)
Anoxic (nonpalpable)—microvascular obstruction
Consumptive coagulopathies (DIC, TTP, HUS, purpura fulminans)
Fat emboli
Thrombocytosis, polycythemia, myeloproliferative disorders
Dysgammaglobulinemias
Inflammatory Vasculitis (palpable)
Drug-induced (see Table 225.2)
Hypersensitivity vasculitis—Henoch-Schönlein and other allergic purpuras, collagen–vascular disorders, certain infections, dysgammaglobulinemias, malignant neoplasms, cryoglobulinemia, serum sickness
Granulomatous vasculitis—Wegener, giant cell
Infectious vasculitis (embolic or dermal Shwartzman reaction)—meningococcus, streptococcus, gonococcus, measles, mumps, smallpox, Rocky Mountain spotted fever
INTRAVASCULAR/HEMATOLOGIC (nonpalpable)
Thrombocytopenia
Decreased platelet production (bone marrow disorders)—radiation, chemicals, chemotherapeutic agents and other drugs (see Table 225.2), bone marrow failure or neoplasm
Increased platelet destruction—immune-mediated (ITP, SLE, CLL, HIV, drugs [see Table 225.2], posttransfusion, neonatal), nonimmune (artificial surfaces, snake venoms, consumptive coagulopathies (DIC, TTP, HUS, purpura fulminans)
Platelet sequestration—hypersplenism, hypothermia
Infections (by above listed mechanisms and others)
Viral, rickettsial, bacterial, mycotic, protozoal
Functional Platelet Disorders
Drug-induced (see Table 225.2)
von Willebrand
Storage pool disorders (rare, inherited)
Other—diabetes, hemachromatosis, liver disease, myeloma, myeloproliferative syndrome, uremia
Coagulopathies
Hemophilias
von Willebrand
Consumptive coagulopathies (DIC, TTP, HUS, purpura fulminans)

Many disorders may cause purpura by several different mechanisms. See references 1, 4–6, 10–12, 14.

DIC, disseminated intravascular coagulation; *TTP*, thrombotic thrombocytopenic purpura; *HUS*, hemolytic–uremic syndrome; *ITP*, idiopathic thrombocytopenic purpura; *SLE*, systemic lupus erythematosus; *CLL*, chronic lymphocytic leukemia; *HIV*, human immunodeficiency virus.

TABLE 225.2. Common Drugs That May Cause Purpura

ANALGESICS
- Acetylsalicylic acid
- Acetaminophen
- Nonsteroidal antinflammatory drugs (NSAIDs)
- Codeine

ANTIBIOTICS
- Antituberculous agents
- Penicillins
- Sulfonamides
- Chloramphenicol
- Nitrofurantoin
- Tetracyclines
- Erythromycin
- Cephalosporins
- Aminoglycosides
- Streptomycin

ANTICONVULSANTS
- Barbiturates
- Carbamazepine
- Diphenylhydantoin
- Primldone
- Valproate sodium

ANTIHYPERTENSIVES
- Methyldopa
- Reserpine

ANTICOAGULANTS
- Coumarin
- Heparin

CARDIOVASCULAR AGENTS
- Atropine
- Quinidine
- Digitalis
- Nitroglycerin
- Propranolol

ANTIRHEUMATICS
- NSAIDs
- Gold
- Prednisone

DIURETICS
- Thiazides
- Furosemide
- Spironolactone

HYPOGLYCEMICS
- Tolbutamide
- Chlorpropamide

SEDATIVES, HYPNOTICS
- Meprobamate
- Phenobarbital
- Chlordiazepoxide

ANTIPSYCHOTICS, ANTIDEPRESSANTS
- Tricyclics
- Phenothiazines

MISCELLANEOUS
- Antimetabolites, chemotherapeutic agents
- Alcohol
- Allopurinol
- Serum
- Estrogens, oral contraceptives
- Heroin
- Quinine
- Benadryl
- Clofibrate
- Chlorpheniramine
- Arsenicals
- Cimetidine
- Griseofulvin
- Iodides
- Dextroamphetamine
- Bismuth
- Organic hair dyes
- Menthol
- Insecticides
- Benzene
- Metal compounds

Mechanisms include direct or immune-mediated thrombocytopenia, vascular injury, platelet inhibition, and coagulopathies. Many drugs may cause purpura by several of these mechanisms.[13]

may appear with a variety of other lesions, again depending on the underlying cause (e.g., immune-mediated vasculitis may progress from areas of urticaria to necrotic, confluent ecchymoses). The skin and mucous membrane lesions are the outward signs of a systemic process in most cases, and the effects of visceral bleeding, infection, and inflammation must be considered.

Purpura may occur in any age group, may be rapidly or slowly progressive, and may be accompanied by either few or many systemic manifestations.

In addition to various medical conditions, purpura may be caused by a variety of drugs, which can cause small vessel or platelet disorders by direct toxicity, inhibition of function, or immune-mediated mechanisms. Almost every class of drug has been implicated as a cause of purpura (Table 225.2).

CLINICAL PRESENTATION

Patients with purpura present to the emergency department for a variety of reasons. Some patients may simply be concerned about the rash itself, whereas others present because of manifestations accompanying the rash (e.g., abnormal bleeding, easy bruising, or constitutional symptoms such as fever, malaise, and arthralgias). Less commonly, severe manifestations of the underlying illness, such as spontaneous bleeding or mental status changes due to intracranial hemorrhage or meningococcal meningitis, are the reason the patient presents to the emergency department.

Regardless of the appearance of the rash or associated symptoms and signs, the presence of spontaneous bleeding ("wet" purpura) is a grave diagnostic sign requiring immediate intervention.[2] Bleeding gums, epistaxis, intraocular hemorrhage, guaiac-positive stool, menorrhagia, or hematuria are all included in this category. The cause is usually thrombocytopenia.

The immediate threat to life is intracranial hemorrhage. Severe anemia and shock from blood loss are possible but not common. Patients without spontaneous bleeding ("dry" purpura) may have extensive petechiae or ecchymoses on the skin and mucous membranes, but are in less immediate danger. Spontaneous bleeding may develop at any time, so rapid determination of the cause is indicated.

Any patient presenting with purpura and mental status changes requires immediate evaluation for intracranial hemorrhage or central nervous system (CNS) infection. Empiric treatment (e.g., platelet transfusion or intravenous antibiotics) based on the presumptive diagnosis and preliminary laboratory results (complete blood count [CBC] with platelets, prothrombin time, partial thromboplastin time [PTT]) may be instituted during such evaluation.

DIFFERENTIAL DIAGNOSIS

The lesions of purpura are characteristic and difficult to mistake for other disorders. Some lesions appear purpuric but do not reflect an underlying illness. Normal bruising resulting from trauma is technically a form of ecchymosis. Purpuric lesions may be created by pressure or suction in normal skin. Examples include facial and conjunctival petechiae due to increased venous pressure (as with protracted vomiting or sneezing) or isolated ecchymosis from suction applied to the skin (as with "love bites" or electrocardiographic suction cups). These lesions are classified as mechanical or factitial purpura.[5,6] Other erythematous rashes, such as viral exanthems and urticaria, can be differentiated from purpura by their light red color and in that they blanch with pressure (because they represent hyperemia rather than extravasation of blood). Similarly, telangiectases and hemangiomata are discrete collections of abnormally dilated blood vessels that appear bright red and usually blanch with pressure. Diascopy, the use of a glass slide to apply pressure over a lesion, is a simple visual method to differentiate lesions due to vascular dilation (which blanch with pressure) from those due to purpura (which do not).

The lesions of Kaposi's sarcoma begin as reddish macules and evolve in 1 to 2 weeks into purple or brown rounded lesions measuring from several millimeters to centimeters in size.[3]

EMERGENCY DEPARTMENT EVALUATION

The history and physical examination should be directed toward identifying the underlying cause of the purpura. The history should include recent infections, recent drug ingestion, radiation or chemical exposure, and systemic symptoms. A personal or family history of purpura or abnormal bleeding after surgical or dental procedures or trauma, as well as hepatic, renal, rheumatologic, or hematologic disease or malignancy, should also be elicited.

A complete list of medications and allergies should be obtained. Except for hereditary coagulation disorders, which rarely present as purpura, and rare hereditary thrombocytopenias, the family history is usually unremarkable. The social history should include questions regarding alcohol and drug use and risk factors for human immunodeficiency virus (HIV) infection. Patients may report easy bruising, prolonged bleeding after surgical or dental procedures, or spontaneous bleeding such as epistaxis, menorrhagia, or melena.

The physical examination should allow rapid differentiation between trivial and serious causes of purpura. The distribution of the rash may be an indicator of the cause of the purpura. Senile or actinic purpura occurs on sun-exposed areas, usually the forearms, of elderly patients. Vasculitic purpura is usually symmetric and predominates in the lower extremities (e.g., Henoch-Schönlein purpura) (Fig. 225.1). A more generalized distribution of discrete petechiae may be noted when purpura is associated with bacterial illness such as meningococcemia or subacute bacterial endocarditis. Purpuric lesions in thrombocytopenia tend to occur in areas of minor trauma or areas of pressure, such as the belt line or over bony prominences.[7] The purpura of scurvy classically appears as perifollicular petechiae, whereas that of Rocky Mountain spotted fever begins over the distal joints and spreads centrally. The lesions of purpura fulminans are large, symmetric ecchymoses of the lower extremities and buttocks, often with infarcted areas or bullae.

The morphology of purpuric lesions may likewise suggest their cause. Raised or "palpable" purpura signifies dermal inflammation, usually caused by a vasculitis, whether infectious or immune-mediated (see Table 225.1). Flat, nonpalpable petechiae or ecchymoses usually indicate thrombocytopenia or coagulation defects. When bacterial infections cause purpura, the lesions may have a central purulent papule (e.g., disseminated gonococcemia). Immune-mediated vasculitides often have lesions of erythema, bullae, or urticaria in association with purpura. Coumarin-associated vasculopathy results in necrotizing ecchymoses.

The physical examination may further reveal specific abnormalities in certain causes of purpura. In thrombocytopenia, the

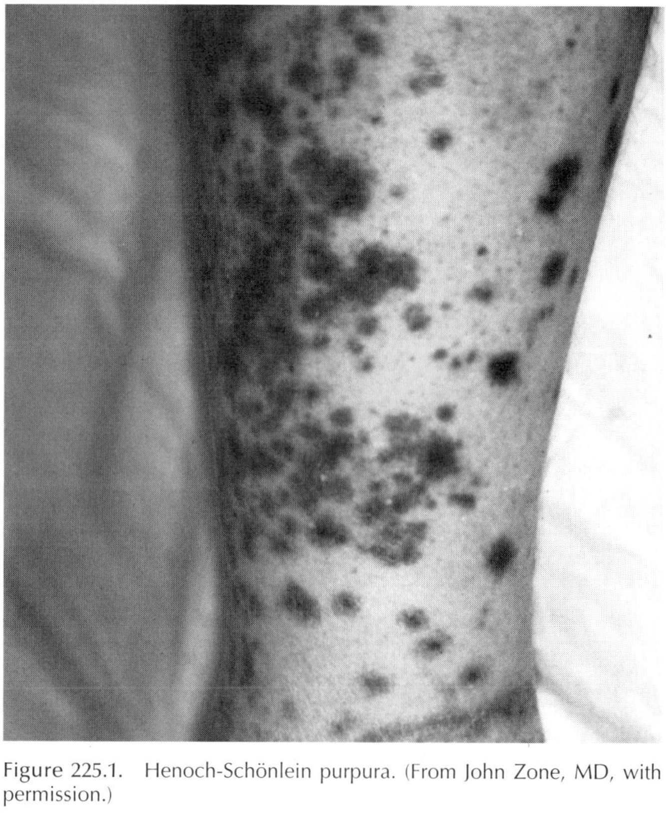

Figure 225.1. Henoch-Schönlein purpura. (From John Zone, MD, with permission.)

optic fundi and mucous membranes may show petechiae. Painful joint effusions may accompany various types of immune-mediated purpura, disseminated gonococcemia, and coagulation disorders. Lymphadenopathy or lesions characteristic of Kaposi's sarcoma may be indicators of HIV seropositivity, which may present with purpura in up to 9% of cases.[9] Lymphadenopathy may also be found in patients with lymphoma, infectious mononucleosis, and leukemia. Splenomegaly, as well as other forms of hypersplenism, may also be noted in these same illnesses, but is absent in most other types of thrombocytopenic purpura and coagulation defects.[7]

All but the trivial causes of purpura (e.g., actinic, mechanical) require laboratory studies to elucidate the underlying cause. Initial emergency department studies should include a CBC with differential (to screen for anemias, bone marrow disorders, various malignancies, infection, or hemolysis), platelet count (to screen for thrombocytopenia, although purpura and spontaneous bleeding rarely occur until the platelet count drops below 50,000/μL), and prothrombin times and PTTs (to screen for coagulation or mixed platelet and/or coagulation disorders).[10,14]

Determination of bleeding time may be of limited use in the emergency department in confirming platelet dysfunction or vascular disorders. The fibrinogen level, along with fibrin–fibrinogen degradation products (FDP, D-dimer), may also be useful.[10] Because therapy with blood products is often necessary, and their use may confound subsequent diagnosis, extra tubes for type and screen and for other platelet and coagulation assays should be obtained before treatment.

On subsequent (usually as an inpatient) evaluation, the following tests may be indicated, depending on the suspected etiology: bone marrow aspiration (almost always necessary in suspected anemia or thrombocytopenia), skin biopsy, bleeding time, autoimmune disease screening tests, clotting factor assays, and platelet function tests.[14]

EMERGENCY DEPARTMENT MANAGEMENT

First, life-threatening complications of spontaneous bleeding should be stabilized, and efforts should be made to ascertain the cause of purpura. As described, the history, physical examination, and laboratory studies should allow rapid determination of the category of illness causing the purpura and associated symptoms.

When thrombocytopenia is the cause of purpura, platelet transfusion should be considered only when there has been abnormal bleeding. Generally, each unit of platelets may be expected to raise the platelet count by about 5,000 to 10,000/μL.[12] Spontaneous mucous membrane or CNS bleeding can usually be controlled when the platelet count is restored to more than 20,000/μL. Platelet transfusion is relatively contraindicated in disorders caused by intravascular thrombosis (such as disseminated intravascular coagulation [DIC]), because platelets may contribute to further thrombosis.

When immune-mediated thrombocytopenia is likely, as in idiopathic thrombocytopenic purpura or posttransfusion purpura, the half-life of transfused platelets is short (in hours) compared with that for other disorders (in days).[2] In these cases, alternative inpatient therapy, such as splenectomy or plasmapheresis, may eventually be indicated.

If purpura is thought to be due to a drug, regardless of the suspected mechanism, that drug should be discontinued. Anticoagulants or platelet inhibitors (in proper dosages) may be reinstituted, if indicated, when the disorder is controlled.

Specific therapy directed to underlying disorders should be initiated once those etiologic factors have been defined.

DISPOSITION

Because purpura may reflect hematologic, rheumatologic, or infectious disorders, once trivial causes of purpura have been ruled out, consultation is obtained from appropriate specialists. When the diagnosis is unclear, a dermatology consultation can be helpful.

Because the underlying disorders that are responsible for purpura often have the potential for progressing to life-threatening emergencies, patients with purpura are often admitted to the hospital for confirmation of the diagnosis and definitive treatment. For example, patients with thrombocytopenia usually require a bone marrow biopsy or aspirate to confirm the exact cause of illness. If vasculitis secondary to penicillin is suspected, however, and signs and laboratory abnormalities are mild, the drug may be withdrawn and outpatient follow-up provided. In general, however, the consultant should choose between inpatient and outpatient treatment. Patients presenting with spontaneous bleeding or life-threatening complications, such as septic shock or CNS hemorrhage, require immediate hospital admission, usually to an intensive care unit.

Emergency transfer of patients with life-threatening complications of purpuric illness is indicated when the needed blood products, specialty consultation, or level of care is not available. Stabilization with intravenous fluids and emergently indicated blood products (when available) should be accomplished before transfer, after consultation with the accepting physician. Patients whose illness may progress rapidly (e.g., meningococcemia, DIC) should be considered for air ambulance transfer when ground transport times would be prolonged.

COMMON PITFALLS

- Failure to recognize the trivial causes of purpura may result in unnecessary time and expense spent in pursuing a diagnostic workup.
- Drugs are a common cause of purpura and, unless an adequate history of drug exposure is obtained, the causal agent may initially be missed.
- When spontaneous bleeding is noted, consultation should be obtained immediately and platelet transfusion (when indicated) should be initiated to minimize the chance of CNS hemorrhage.
- Premature administration of drugs or blood products may delay laboratory diagnosis and, in some cases, may worsen the disease process causing purpura.

References

1. Bick RL. Alterations of hemostasis associated with surgery, cardiopulmonary bypass, and prosthetic devices. In: Ratnoff OD, Forbes CD, eds. *Disorders of hemostasis*. Orlando, FL: Grune & Stratton, 1984:319.
2. Crosby WH. Wet purpura, dry purpura. *JAMA* 1975;232(7):744.
3. Friedman-Kien AE, Laurenstein LJ, Rubinstein P, et al. Disseminated Kaposi's sarcoma in homosexual men. *Ann Intern Med* 1982;96:693–700.
4. Gibson LE, Danielson WP. Cutaneous vasculitis. *Rheum Dis Clin North Am* 1995;21:1097–1113.
5. Koblenzer CS. Cutaneous manifestations of psychiatric disease that commonly present to the dermatologist—diagnosis and treatment. *Int J Psychiatry Med* 1992;22:47–63.
6. Lyell A. Cutaneous artifactual disease. *J Am Dermatol* 1979;1:391–407.
7. Masaione AS. An approach to purpura. *Cutis* 1973;12:41.
8. Pierre WW. Hematologic diseases. In: Freideberg IM, Eisen AZ, Wolff K, et al., eds. *Dermatology in general medicine,* 5th ed. New York: McGraw-Hill, 1999:1867.
9. Ratner L. Human immunodeficiency virus–associated autoimmune thrombocytopenic purpura: a review. *Am J Med* 1989;86:194.
10. Rogers GM, Bithell TC. The diagnostic approach to the bleeding disorders. In: Lee GR, Foerster J, Lukens J, et al., eds. *Wintrobe's clinical hematology,* 10th ed. Baltimore: Williams & Wilkins, 1999:1557.
11. Sauer GC. Vascular dermatoses. In: Hall JC, Saver GC, (eds.) *Saver's Manual of skin diseases,* 8th ed. Philadelphia: JB Lippincott Williams & Wilkins, 2000.

12. Schafer AI. Acquired disorders of platelet function. In: Loscalzo J, Schafer A, eds. *Thrombosis and hemorrhage,* 2nd ed. Baltimore: Williams & Wilkins, 1998:707.
13. Swinyer LJ. Drug eruptions in an emergency department setting. *Emerg Med Clin North Am* 1985;3(4):717.
14. Taylor RE, Blatt PM. Clinical evaluation of the patient with bruising and bleeding. *J Am Acad Dermatol* 1981;4:348–368.

CHAPTER 226
Urticaria

Theodore A. Christopher and Joseph D. Kim

Urticarial rash may be the most common skin lesion seen in emergency medicine. Making the diagnosis is not nearly as challenging to the emergency physician as defining the etiology, which very often remains elusive.

Urticaria, or "hives," is a vascular reaction of skin, resulting in wheals, raised white or red welts that itch and sting. It can occur in any age group, but young adults are most commonly afflicted. An estimated 20% of the population experiences at least one attack of urticaria in a lifetime.

Acute urticaria is characterized by symptomatic attacks lasting 6 weeks or less. It occurs with equal frequency in men and women and is often associated with an atopic history or an allergic etiology. *Chronic* urticaria is more common in middle-aged women and is characterized by attacks that last longer than 6 weeks; the attacks tend to be less frequent and less severe than acute attacks. Half of the patients with chronic urticaria have the disease for 5 years, and 25% have it for 20 years. In 90% of cases, no specific etiology can be identified.

Histologically, the fact that urticaria involves the superficial dermis only distinguishes it from angioedema, which involves the deeper dermis. Perivascular lymphocytic and mast cell infiltration are also features. Mast cell degranulation, with release of mediators such as histamine, acetylcholine, serotonin, neuropeptides, cytokines, prostaglandins, anaphylatoxins, leukotrienes, eosinophilic chemotactic factor, platelet activating factor, and bradykinin, appears to be responsible for the pathogenesis of urticaria.[9,12] Degranulation is initiated by immunologic (type I, type III) and nonimmunologic (chemicals, foods, drugs) mechanisms, but numerous modulating factors also undoubtedly play significant roles.

CLINICAL PRESENTATION

Urticaria presents as pruritic, edematous, slightly erythematous, raised wheals or papules that persist for less than 24 hours on unexposed areas of skin. Urticaria can be circumscribed, annular, or serpiginous; central clearing may or may not be present. The lesions commonly blanch with pressure, reflecting local vasodilatation.

Table 226.1 summarizes types and causes of urticaria. Foods and drugs are probably the most common causes of both acute and chronic urticaria. Among foods, nuts, berries, shellfish, chocolate, fish, tomatoes, and eggs are frequent offenders in acute urticaria. In chronic urticaria, milk, cereals, beef, pork, cheese, garlic, onions, and spices may be responsible. Food additives, both natural and synthetic, also appear to be important etiologic factors. Acute reactions occur within minutes of ingestion, whereas delayed symptoms may develop several hours later, presumably when a reactive antigen is formed by the digestive actions of proteolytic enzymes.

TABLE 226.1. Classification of Urticaria

IMMUNOLOGIC URTICARIAS
Atopic disease history
Physical
Cholinergic
Dermatographism
Pressure
Cold
Solar
Vibratory
Aquagenic
Heat
Adrenergic
Contact
Food
Insects
Inhalants
Drugs
NONIMMUNOLOGIC URTICARIAS
Drugs
Aspirin/NSAIDs
Opiates
Antibiotics
Antihypertensives
Curare
Radiocontrast media
Food additives
IDIOPATHIC
CHRONIC
Systemic vasculitis/collagen vascular disease/malignancy
Infections
Genetic

Penicillin heads a lengthy list of drugs that cause urticaria; both immunologic and nonimmunologic mechanisms are thought to be active.

Aspirin intolerance has been identified in 20% to 50% of patients with urticaria and is thought to act by a nonimmunologic mechanism.[2] Increased prostaglandin levels have been found in affected patients. Urticaria may occur 15 minutes to 20 hours after aspirin ingestion and is often accompanied by wheezing, increased bronchial secretions, rhinorrhea, and flushing. Many other drugs cause urticaria by inducing histamine release, most notably morphine, codeine, *d*-tubocurarine, and many oral and topical antibiotics.

Another class of urticaria is physical urticaria, in which wheals and itching develop at sites of a physical stimulus.[8] *Dermatographism* is defined as a whealing reaction of skin within 10 minutes of receiving a moderate stroke stimulus of less than 36 g/mm^2.[3] Clinically, dermatographism typically occurs within seconds after stimulation and usually fades within 30 minutes. It is often due to contact with seatbelts, garters, or brassieres. In contrast to dermatographism, pressure urticaria occurs when more sustained physical pressure applied to the skin produces itchy, often painful wheals. These lesions can present as early as 30 minutes after application of pressure, but typically present in 6 hours and often last up to 72 hours.[3] Common causes are tight-fitting garments and prolonged walking (feet) or sitting (buttocks).

Cholinergic urticaria is characterized by pruritic 1- to 4-mm wheals surrounded by a red flare and produced within 15 minutes of any stimulus that causes an increase in core temperature.[3] Exercise, hot baths, and emotional stress can precipitate episodes of cholinergic urticaria, which usually begins on the upper thorax and neck before spreading to the entire body, usually sparing the palms and soles. The exact pathophysiology is unclear, but appears to involve the release of acetylcholine and degranulation of histamine from mast cells.[14] Clinically, patients can present with varied symptoms, including lacrimation, salivation, diarrhea, abdominal pain, weakness, flushing, and headache. Rarely, severe, life-threatening symptoms (e.g., angioedema, bronchospasm, vascular collapse, and hypotension) can occur.[14]

Solar urticarias present as a whealing response within 10 minutes in skin exposed to ultraviolet or visible radiation from any source.[3] In addition to hives, symptoms may include wheezing, dizziness, and (rarely) hypotension; all resolve within 1 to 3 hours after the light stimulus is removed. Both histamine and prostaglandins have been implicated.[1]

Cold urticaria occurs on exposed areas, such as the face and hands, and is commonly induced by swimming. It occurs within minutes of exposure, usually during rewarming, and can be elicited by placing an ice cube on the skin, holding cold objects in the hand, or drinking cold fluids (leading to lip swelling). It also may be associated with other symptoms, including syncope and shock.[15]

Other physical urticarias include generalized aquagenic urticaria, which is induced by contact with water of any temperature; vibratory urticaria, in which localized swelling occurs within minutes of local vibration; and adrenergic urticaria, a variant of stress-related urticaria, characterized by increased blood levels of norepinephrine and epinephrine.[10]

The third major class of urticaria consists of those associated with infection (bacterial, fungal, viral, and parasitic). In most cases, urticaria does not appear to be related to hypersensitivity to the infectious agent.

Insect bites can cause widespread urticarial lesions that are distinct from the common local erythematous and vesicular reaction. Wasps, hornets, fleas, gnats, mites, mosquitoes, and bedbugs are common offenders.

Contact urticaria is whealing of the skin due to exposure to certain substances in susceptible patients. A diverse range of agents has been implicated, including food, metals (nickel, platinum, rhodium), and hair-care products.[16] Of particular concern to health-care workers is the emergence of natural rubber latex allergy, which presents as a local or generalized urticaria but can rapidly progress to angioedema and anaphylaxis.

Finally, several underlying systemic diseases may be responsible for unexplained chronic urticaria. Malignancies (leukemia, lymphoma), collagen vascular disease, serum sickness, and C1 esterase inhibitor deficiency are all recognized causes. Hepatitis B and C, Lyme disease, and chronic tinea pedis have also been associated with urticaria.[4]

DIFFERENTIAL DIAGNOSIS

Urticaria must be differentiated from angioedema, which involves the deeper dermis and mucous membranes, is often associated with abdominal symptoms, and is more often life-threatening. The two most common causes of angioedema are angiotensin converting enzyme inhibitors and hereditary angioedema.[5] Cutaneous vasculitis causes lesions that may be clinically indistinguishable from urticaria, but they last 24 to 72 hours and are generally nonpruritic; secondary pigmentation and scaling are common, as are systemic symptoms. Serum sickness usually begins 7 to 14 days after antigenic exposure and is associated with fever, arthralgia, and lymphadenopathy. Finally, urticaria must be distinguished from other cutaneous lesions, such as erythema multiforme, bullous pemphigoid, dermatitis herpetiformis, and urticaria pigmentosa.

EMERGENCY DEPARTMENT EVALUATION

The evaluation of urticaria in the emergency department consists of a detailed history to identify any of the previously mentioned inciting factors, paying particular attention to medications, exposures, contacts, underlying illness, allergies, diet, and family history. A general physical examination follows. The patient is undressed and the skin examined thoroughly to localize characteristic lesions. All urticarial lesions are described in detail as to size, shape, number, pattern, color, and temperature. Evidence of systemic illness is sought. If deep cutaneous edema is noted, the physician must ensure that the airway is patent and uninvolved.

In 75% of cases, an underlying cause of urticaria cannot be identified.[11] Thus, beyond a good history and physical examination, extensive evaluation in the emergency department is not indicated. However, simple maneuvers, such as placing an ice cube on the forearm (cold urticaria), immersing a hand in warm water (cholinergic urticaria), or "writing" on the skin (dermatographism), may be performed in an attempt to elicit symptoms if the clinical history is suggestive.

EMERGENCY DEPARTMENT MANAGEMENT

Treatment of urticaria depends on the severity and extent of the reaction. All identifiable offending agents and exposures should be eliminated, especially because reexposure often results in a more severe reaction. Nonspecific vasodilators (alcohol, aspirin, heat, exertion, stress) should also be avoided, although broad elimination diets are seldom helpful. Opiates are also another commonly prescribed class of drugs that exacerbate urticaria.

First-generation H_1 antagonists such as diphenhydramine (Benadryl, 25 to 50 mg), chlorpheniramine (Chlor-Trimeton, 4 mg), and hydroxyzine (Atarax, 10 to 25 mg) are commonly prescribed to relieve intense pruritus when sedation is desired; they may also be given in liquid or parenteral formulations when necessary.[7] Patients should be instructed to repeat the dose whenever hives return, or after 30 minutes if hives are not relieved.

Second-generation H_1 antagonists such as cetirizine (Zyrtec, 10 mg/d) and loratadine (Claritin, 10 mg/d) are now the first line of treatment in urticaria. These antihistamines have only minor sedative and anticholinergic side effects and have longer half-lives, permitting once-a-day dosing. Astemizole (Hismanal) should not be prescribed if a patient is taking macrolide antibiotics, imidazole antifungal agents, or quinine, because of the risk of inducing torsade de pointes.[13] First- and second-generation antihistamines may be prescribed together, with a first-generation antihistamine given at bedtime and a second-generation agent during the day.

The H_2 antagonists cimetidine (300 mg) and ranitidine (150 mg) alone are ineffective in urticaria and may actually increase the incidence of hives. In refractory cases, however, when combined with an H_1 antihistamine, they may suppress urticarial reactions more completely.[9]

Other agents used for treatment of urticaria include calcium channel blockers such as nifedipine. In combination with antihistamines, dosages from 10 mg twice a day to 20 mg three times a day have been shown to be effective in some cases,[13] but the routine use of such a regimen is not recommended. Doxepin is a tricyclic antidepressant with both H_1 and H_2 activity, and at dosages of 10 mg three times a day, it has been shown to be efficacious in treatment. Because of it side effects, however, it is best taken only at night.[4]

Severe pruritus unresponsive to antihistamine therapy may be managed by adding antipruritic lotions (phenol or menthol preparations), colloidal oatmeal baths, and cool showers or baths. Sympathomimetics such as ephedrine, metaproterenol, and terbutaline (commonly in combination with a barbiturate to control tremor) have been most successful when used in combination with an H_1 antagonist.[12]

Corticosteroids have a role in the treatment of acute urticaria. A course of prednisone 40 to 60 mg a day for 5 days can relieve symptoms of severe urticaria. Steroid therapy is not typically recommended for patients with chronic urticaria, but short-term therapy is effective in controlling an acute exacerbation. Prednisone at dosages of 20 to 30 mg/d for less than 5 days is recommended. Exacerbations of urticaria can occur after treatment if steroids are given to patients with chronic urticaria for more than 5 days.[13]

Life-threatening urticaria accompanied by laryngeal edema, hypotension, or wheezing requires the administration of intravenous fluids and epinephrine (1 to 2 mL of 1:10,000 solution intravenously over several minutes, repeated cautiously as necessary or followed by a drip of 2 μg/min). In less extreme circumstances, epinephrine can be given subcutaneously or intramuscularly (0.2 to 0.5 mL of 1:1000 solution every 15 to 20 minutes for a maximum of three doses). Antihistamines and corticosteroids should also be given. Some urticarial syndromes respond well to specific agents and modalities.[6]

DISPOSITION

Most acute urticaria begins to respond to treatment within 2 hours. Patients should generally be observed for at least this period of time, or until definitive improvement is documented, but discharge is the rule. Only patients with airway compromise (i.e., laryngeal spasm, bronchospasm) or hemodynamic instability (hypotension) require admission. Antihistamines and steroids, if necessary, should be continued on an outpatient basis.

COMMON PITFALLS

- Urticaria is commonly undertreated with H_1-blocker antihistamines, often resulting in poor control of symptoms and another visit to the emergency department. Patients who respond to antihistamine therapy in the emergency department should be given an adequate supply on discharge. Those who do not respond require the addition of another antihistamine; the administration of steroids should be strongly considered.
- Expensive laboratory workups in the emergency department should be discouraged. A thorough history and physical examination are more likely to identify an etiology.
- Urticarial skin lesions may be the first manifestation of infection, infestation, or systemic diseases such as systemic lupus erythematosus, pemphigoid, dermatitis herpetiformis, vasculitis, and occult malignancy, particularly lymphoma.

References

1. Armstrong RB. Solar urticaria. *Dermatol Clin* 1986;4:253.
2. Asad SI, Kermeny DM, Youlten LJF, et al. Effect of aspirin in "aspirin sensitive" patients. *BMJ (Clin Res)* 1984;288:745.
3. Black AK, Lawlor F, Greaves MW. Consensus meeting on the definition of physical urticarias and urticarial vasculitis. *Clin Exp Dermatol* 1996;21:424.
4. Charlesworth EN. Urticaria and angioedema: a clinical spectrum. *Ann Allergy Asthma Immunol* 1996;76:484.
5. Condemi, JJ. Update in allergy and immunology. *Ann Intern Med* 1996;125(9):744–750.
6. Duc J, Pécoud A. Successful treatment of idiopathic cold urticaria with the association of H_1 and H_2 antagonists: a case report. *Ann Allergy* 1986;56:355.
7. Goldsmith P, Dowd PM. The new H_1 antihistamines: treatment of urticaria and other clinical problems. *Dermatol Clin* 1993;11:87.
8. Greaves MW, Sabroe RA. ABC of allergies: allergy and the skin. I: Urticaria. *BMJ* 1998;316(7138):1147–1150.
9. Juhlin L, Landor M. Drug therapy for chronic urticaria. *Clin Rev Allergy* 1992;76:805.
10. Kaplan AP. Urticaria and angioedema. In: Meddleton E Jr, Reed CE, Ellis EE, et al., eds. *Allergies: principles and practice,* 3rd ed. St. Louis: Mosby, 1988:1377.
11. Leung DY, Diaz LA, DeLeo V, et al. Allergic and immunologic skin disorders. *JAMA* 1997;278(22):1914–1923.
12. Soter NA. Urticaria: current therapy. *J Allergy Clin Immunol* 1990;86:1009.
13. Tharp MD. Chronic urticaria: pathophysiology and treatment approaches. *J Allergy Clin Immunol* 1996;98(6 Part 3):325–330.
14. Volcheck GW, Li JT. Exercise-induced urticaria and anaphylaxis. *Mayo Clin Proc* 1997;72(2):140–147.
15. Wanderer AA, Grandel KE, Wasserman SI, et al. Clinical characteristics of cold-induced systemic reactions in acquired cold urticaria syndromes. *J Allergy Clin Immunol* 1986;78:417.
16. Warner MR, Taylor JS, Leow YH. Agents causing contact urticaria. *Clin Dermatol* 1997;15:623.

CHAPTER 227
Life-Threatening Dermatoses

Alan T. Forstater and Kenneth J. Neuberger

Cutaneous lesions are often the first clinical sign of serious systemic disease. In this chapter, the focus is on the recognition and acute management of the common life-threatening dermatoses listed in Table 227.1. These disorders can be conveniently grouped into diffuse red rashes, vesiculobullous eruptions, localized or discrete lesions, and purpuric or hemorrhagic lesions.

Several entities are not discussed in detail here but deserve brief mention. Palpable purpura is a skin manifestation of vasculitis; it is not a manifestation of thrombocytopenia or clotting disorder. Involvement may be limited to the skin or may be systemic. Treatment is for the underlying vasculitic disorder.

Generalized exfoliative erythroderma (formerly called exfoliative dermatitis) is a diffuse, widespread dermatitis that covers most of the body surface. This condition not only causes pruritus and pain, but also may be complicated by hypothermia; fluid, electrolyte, and protein loss; invasion of bacteria and opportunistic organisms through the skin; and high-output congestive heart failure secondary to severe vasodilatation. The causes of exfoliative erythroderma include previously existing skin diseases (e.g., psoriasis, atopic eczema, contact dermatitis) (50%); drug eruptions (10%); lymphoproliferative disorders (e.g., Hodgkin disease, leukemia, Sézary syndrome) (15%); and idiopathic (25% to 40%). Mortality is less than 5%.

Other potentially life-threatening entities, such as angioedema and disseminated herpetic infection, are discussed in other chapters.

DIFFUSE RED RASHES

Staphylococcal scalded skin syndrome (SSSS) (Fig. 227.1) occurs in children and, rarely, adults, and is caused by an exotoxin

TABLE 227.1. Life-Threatening Dermatoses

DIFFUSE RED RASHES	VESICULOBULLOUS DISEASES
Urticaria with anaphylaxis	Pemphigus[a]
Toxic shock syndrome[a]	Pemphigoid[a]
Kawasaki disease	Stevens-Johnson syndrome[a]
Toxic epidermal necrolysis[a]	Toxic epidermal necrolysis[a]
Staphylococcal scalded skin syndrome[a]	Disseminated zoster
Generalized exfoliative erythroderma[a]	Disseminated herpes simplex
Pustular psoriasis	
Cutaneous T-cell lymphoma	
Systemic lupus erythematosus	
LOCALIZED OR DISCRETE LESIONS	**PURPURIC OR HEMORRHAGIC**
Erysipelas and cellulitis[a]	Meningococcemia[a]
Gonococcemia[a]	Gonococcemia[a]
Ecthyma gangrenosum[a]	Disseminated intravascular coagulation
Brown recluse spider bite	Palpable purpura[a]
Behçet syndrome	Brown recluse spider bite
Malignant melanoma	Rocky Mountain spotted fever[a]
Kaposi sarcoma and AIDS	Miscellaneous hematologic disorders

[a] Discussed in chapter.

From Krusinski PA, Flowers, FP, life-threatening dermatoses. In: Flowers FP, Krusinski PA. *Dermatology in ambulatory and emergency medicine, a clinical guide with algorithums*. Chicago: Year Book Medical, 1984.

from an infecting strain of coagulase-positive *Staphylococcus aureus*. The disease may present as a prodrome of fever, irritability, malaise, and exquisite skin tenderness; in other cases, the child presents with the sudden onset of generalized erythema. The skin is red, warm, and very tender. Flaccid bullae that are ill

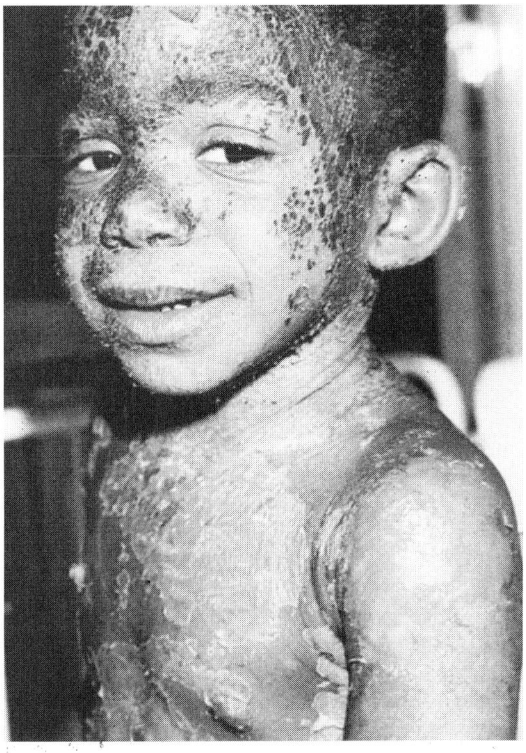

Figure 227.1. Staphylococcal scalded skin syndrome. The skin becomes raw and eroded. The similarity to impetigo is clear. The condition responds rapidly to antibiotics. (From du Vivier A. *Atlas of clinical dermatology*. London: Gower Medical Publishing, 1986, with permission.)

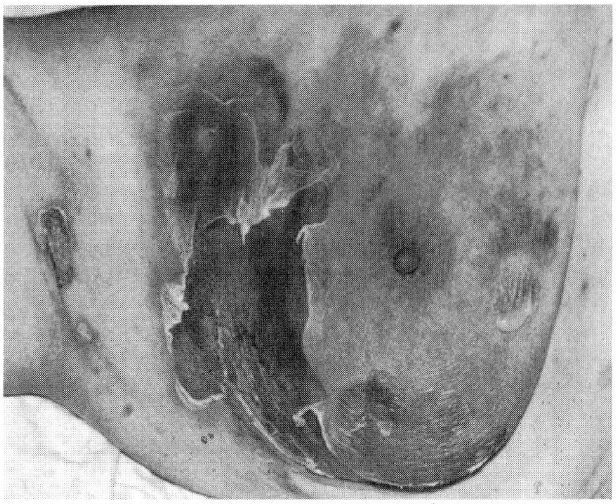

Figure 227.2. Toxic epidermal necrolysis. There is "sheeting" of the skin, leaving a raw, denuded area. This was secondary to a barbiturate. (From du Vivier A. *Atlas of clinical dermatology*. London: Gower Medical Publishing, 1986, with permission.)

defined and hard to see then desquamate in large sheets. Gentle lateral stroking of the skin causes the epidermis to separate (Nikolsky sign).

Therapy consists of systemic antibiotics effective against penicillinase-producing *Staphylococcus*. Children older than 1 year and with mild symptoms may be treated as outpatients. Children who appear toxic and infants should be admitted. Despite proper treatment, most of the superficial body surface will desquamate; but because the site of blister cleavage is in the superficial layer of the dermis, healing occurs rapidly over 10 to 14 days.

Toxic epidermal necrolysis (TEN) (Fig. 227.2) is a disease of adults in which the skin also sloughs in large sheets. Although it is very similar in appearance to SSSS, it is quite different. It may actually represent the most severe form of erythema multiforme and begins, like erythema multiforme, with constitutional symptoms of fever, malaise, and myalgia. The skin is initially diffusely painful, hot, and red. Within 24 hours, blisters and large areas of denuded skin develop; erosive, sloughing lesions of the oral mucosa are common. The Nikolsky sign is positive.[6]

The differences between TEN and SSSS are noteworthy. SSSS almost always occurs in children and is secondary to staphylococcal infection. TEN almost always occurs in adults and is precipitated by drugs such as phenytoin, sulfas, penicillins, and some nonsteroidal antiinflammatory agents[17] or by graft-versus-host reactions (e.g., after bone marrow transplantation) or blood product transfusions. Mucous membrane involvement in SSSS is rare and limited to the lips, but, in TEN, erosive oral lesions are common. Although SSSS sloughs only the superficial layers of epidermis, TEN desquamates the entire thickness of the epidermis, accounting for the high associated mortality rate: The mortality rate in SSSS is very low, while that of TEN is more than 50%.[7]

The diagnosis of TEN is made by clinical presentation and confirmed by biopsy. Treatment is removal of the precipitating agent, if possible, and, as in burn patients, judicious fluid and electrolyte therapy and prevention of infection. Early transfer to a burn center is associated with significantly decreased bacteremia and mortality.[22] Corticosteroid treatment is controversial because it may not speed recovery, yet may predispose the patient to infectious complications.[18,19]

Toxic shock syndrome (TSS) is an acute, febrile illness associated with localized infection by strains of *S. aureus* that produce an exotoxin (TSST-1) believed to be the cause of the clinical signs and symptoms. Characteristic signs and symptoms include an early macular rash, hypotension, abnormalities in multiple organ systems, and acral desquamation occurring 1 to 2 weeks after the onset of the illness. About 90% of the *S. aureus* isolates from patients with TSS produce the exotoxin. Eighty-five percent to 90% of cases are reported in menstruating women.[12] In fact, the disease was originally described in association with the use of highly absorbent vaginal tampons that could be kept in place for many hours before being discarded. Other cases are associated with localized infection in men, children, and nonmenstruating women.[4]

The early cutaneous rash is scarlatiniform and blanches with pressure; it can be difficult to appreciate because it is often quite pale. Coincident with the rash, there is often erythema of the mucous membranes of the oropharynx, conjunctivae, and vagina. Desquamation of the skin of the distal extremities occurs 1 to 2 weeks after the onset. Hair and nail loss follows 1 to 2 months later.[1]

Strict criteria for the diagnosis of TSS are fever, hypotension or orthostasis, an erythematous macular rash, involvement of at least three organ systems (Table 227.2), and the presence of an *S. aureus* infection. Most patients have facial and extremity edema. Hypoalbuminemia and hypocalcemia not accounted for by the decreased albumin level have been described.[13] The illness can proceed rapidly. Hypotension may appear early; most patients present to the hospital with at least orthostasis.

The differential diagnosis of TSS includes Rocky Mountain spotted fever (RMSF), scarlet fever, sepsis, Kawasaki disease (rare in those older than 8 years), leptospirosis, Colorado tick fever (in which photophobia is common), and other viral infections. Supportive treatment for dehydration and hypotension includes fluid replacement and the use of pressors, if necessary.

TABLE 227.2. Revised Case Definition of Staphylococcal Toxic Shock Syndrome

Fever: temperature ≥38.9°C (102°F)
Rash: diffuse macular erythroderma
Desquamation: 1 to 2 weeks after onset of illness, particularly of palms and soles
Hypotension: systolic blood pressure ≤90 mm Hg for adults or below fifth percentile by age for children below 16 years of age, orthostatic drop in diastolic blood pressure ≥15 mm Hg from lying to sitting, orthostatic syncope, or orthostatic dizziness
Multisystem involvement—three or more of the following:
- GI: vomiting or diarrhea at onset of illness
- Muscular: severe myalgia or creatine phosphokinase level at least twice the upper limit of normal for laboratory
- Mucous membrane: vaginal, oropharyngeal, or conjunctival hyperemia
- Renal: blood urea nitrogen or creatinine at least twice the upper limit of normal for laboratory or urinary sediment with pyuria (≥5 leukocytes per high-power field) in the absence of urinary tract infection
- Hepatic: total bilirubin, SGOT,* SGPT† at least twice the upper limit of normal for laboratory
- Hematologic: platelets ≤100,000/µL
- CNS: disorientation or alterations in consciousness without focal neurologic signs when fever and hypotension are absent

Negative results on the following tests, if obtained:
- Blood, throat, or cerebrospinal fluid cultures (blood culture may be positive for *Staphylococcus aureus*)
- Rise in titer to Rocky Mountain spotted fever, leptospirosis, or rubeola

* SGOT denotes serum aspartate transaminase.
† SGPT denotes serum alanine transaminase.
Reproduced with permission from Reingold AL, et al. Toxic shock surveillance in the United States 1980–1981. *Ann Intern Med* 1982; 96(Pt 2):875–880.

TABLE 227.3. Proposed Case Definition for the Streptococcal Toxic Shock Syndrome[a]

I. Isolation of group A streptococci (*Streptococcus pyogenes*)
  A. From a normally sterile site (e.g., blood, cerebrospinal, pleural or peritoneal fluid, tissue biopsy, surgical wound)
  B. From a nonsterile site (e.g., throat, sputum, vagina, superficial skin lesion)
II. Clinical signs of severity
  A. Hypotension: systolic blood pressure ≤90 mm Hg in adults or <5th percentile for age in children
  and
  B. ≥2 of the following signs
    1. Renal impairment: creatinine ≥177 µmol/L (≥2 mg/dL) for adults or ≥2 times the upper limit of normal for age. In patients with preexisting renal disease, a ≥2-fold elevation over the baseline level
    2. Coagulopathy: platelets ≤100 × 10^9/L (≤100,000/µL) or disseminated intravascular coagulation defined by prolonged clotting time, low fibrinogen level, and the presence of fibrin degradation products
    3. Liver involvement: alanine aminotransferase (SGOT), aspartate aminotransferase (SGPT), or total bilirubin levels ≥2 times the upper limit of normal for age. In patients with preexisting liver disease, a ≥2-fold elevation over the baseline level
    4. Adult respiratory distress syndrome defined by acute onset of diffuse pulmonary infiltrates and hypoxemia in the absence of cardiac failure, or evidence of diffuse capillary leak manifested by acute onset of generalized edema, or pleural or peritoneal effusions with hypoalbuminemia
    5. A generalized erythematous macular rash that may desquamate
    6. Soft-tissue necrosis, including necrotizing fasciitis or myositis, or gangrene

[a] An illness fulfilling criteria IA and II (A and B) can be defined as a *definite* case. An illness fulfilling criteria IB and II (A and B) can be defined as a *probable* case if no other etiology for the illness is identified.
From The Working Group on Severe Streptococcal Infections. Defining the group A streptococcal toxic shock syndrome: rationale and consensus definition. *JAMA* 1993;269:391.

The adult respiratory distress syndrome is common in serious cases.

Although it has not been proved that antibiotics are always necessary for recovery, provided the site of located staphylococcal infection is drained (e.g., removal of tampons or incision of abscesses), treatment with a penicillinase-resistant penicillin or a first-generation cephalosporin is considered mandatory if the diagnosis cannot be excluded. In the penicillin-allergic patient, vancomycin or clindamycin is an appropriate alternative. Because TSS recurs in a large proportion of women with tampon-associated TSS who continue to use tampons, it is recommended that these women forego their use. All symptomatic patients suspected of having TSS require admission to the hospital for vigorous supportive treatment.

The hallmark of streptococcal TSS, first described in the mid 1980s, is a relatively early onset of shock and multiorgan failure. The currently proposed criteria for streptococcal TSS are isolation of group A streptococci from a sterile or nonsterile site, hypotension, and at least two of the following: renal impairment, coagulopathy, liver function test abnormalities, adult respiratory distress syndrome, soft-tissue necrosis, and rash (which may be generalized macular or possibly scarlatiniform and may desquamate) (Table 227.3).[20] Treatment is with high-dose penicillin (20 to 24 million units/d); cephalosporins, clindamycin, erythromycin, vancomycin, and penicillinase-resistant penicillins are also effective. Aggressive supportive care is mandatory, as is surgical drainage or debridement for abscess, pyonecrosis, or necrotizing fasciitis. Even with prompt treatment, mortality is reported to be between 20% and 30%.[21]

VESICOBULLOUS DISEASES

The spectrum of acute, self-limited immunologic reactions causing vesicles includes bullous erythema multiforme, Stevens-Johnson syndrome, and TEN. The causes are the same as those listed in the previous discussion of TEN, although erythema multiforme is often related to herpes simplex, and Stevens-Johnson syndrome is usually related to drugs. The classic lesion of erythema multiforme is the target lesion, a central gray wheal or bulla surrounded by concentric rings of erythema and normal skin. As the name implies, however, many types of lesions may be present simultaneously: macules, papules, urticaria (though nonpruritic), and bullae. The extremities are involved more than the trunk; the palms and soles are often affected. The rash appears abruptly and may be accompanied by fever, malaise, and pruritus.

Further along the spectrum is Stevens-Johnson syndrome: bullous erythema multiforme accompanied by constitutional symptoms and involving at least two mucous membranes.[6] A prodrome of fever, malaise, and myalgia is followed by the explosive appearance of blisters on mucous membranes and skin. Symmetric blistering begins on the dorsa of the hands and feet and on extensor surfaces. Erosive lesions begin on oral mucosa, lips, and bulbar conjunctiva and can extend to the pharynx, larynx, esophagus, and genital mucosa (Fig. 227.3). Ocular lesions can result in corneal ulceration, panophthalmitis, and even blindness, requiring early recognition and treatment. The prognosis of Stevens-Johnson syndrome is usually excellent.[16] However, the disorder may progress to an illness clinically indistinguishable from TEN, with large confluent bullae and sloughing of epidermis in sheets.

Milder cases of Stevens-Johnson syndrome can be treated with oral antihistamines and topical corticosteroids; more severe cases require hospital admission. The use of systemic corticosteroid therapy is controversial.[17,18]

Pemphigus vulgaris, a rare disease, occurs mostly in adults 40 to 60 years old and is distinguished from other blistering diseases by its fulminant course. Early identification and aggressive treatment may avert a poor outcome. Initially, blisters may be localized to small areas of the mucous membranes or skin; lesions may be present for months before the blistering becomes generalized. The lesions are typically painful flaccid bullae that may rupture easily or painful erosions where bullae have ruptured. The Nikolsky sign is positive. Half of patients present initially with oral lesions; 90% have oral lesions at some time during the course of the illness. These painful erosions or collapsed bullae can persist despite successful treatment of skin lesions.[6]

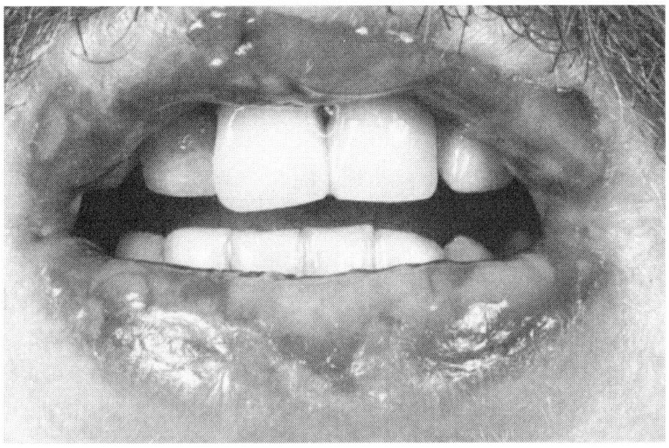

Figure 227.3. Stevens-Johnson syndrome. Severe blistering and ulceration of the mucous membranes occur. Ulceration is present on the lips and in the mouth. (From du Vivier A. *Atlas of clinical dermatology*. London: Gower Medical Publishing, 1986, with permission.)

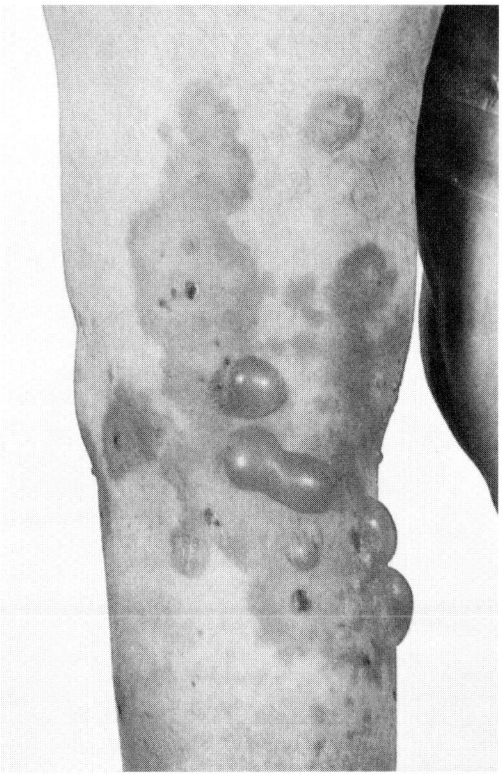

Figure 227.4. Bullous pemphigoid. Large, tense blisters are characteristic, in contrast to the flaccid blisters of pemphigus. (From du Vivier A. *Atlas of clinical dermatology*. London: Gower Medical Publishing, 1986, with permission.)

The diagnosis of pemphigus is made by biopsy of intact skin adjacent to a bulla. Direct immunofluorescent staining for antiepithelial antibodies localized to the epidermal cell membrane are confirmatory. Indirect immunofluorescence of the patient's serum or blister fluid detects a pemphigus antibody that reacts with epithelial cell membranes of most species. Therapy is with corticosteroids and immunosuppressive agents.

Bullous pemphigoid is an autoimmune blistering disease occurring mostly in the elderly. The bullae of bullous pemphigoid, unlike those of pemphigus vulgaris, are tense rather than flaccid, and oral lesions are less common (Fig. 227.4). The Nikolsky sign is positive. Bullous pemphigoid is characterized by spontaneous remissions and exacerbations and a low mortality rate; most patients experience complete remission.[6] As with pemphigus vulgaris, the diagnosis is made by biopsy of the skin adjacent to a blister. Direct immunofluorescence studies reveal antibodies bound to the basement membrane; these antibodies can often be found in the serum as well. Mild cases are treated with erythromycin, topical corticosteroids, or intralesional injections; severe cases require systemic corticosteroids with or without immunosuppressive agents.[7]

LOCALIZED OR DISCRETE LESIONS

Patients with gram-negative sepsis may manifest the skin lesions known as ecthyma gangrenosum (Fig. 227.5). Originally described in *Pseudomonas* septicemia, they may also occur with bacteremia due to *Escherichia coli* or *Klebsiella* and have been reported in the absence of disseminated infection.[19] Because the lesions of ecthyma gangrenosum are manifestations of life-threatening illness, the diagnosis must be made early. Ecthyma gangrenosum is a true dermatologic emergency; patients with it are critically ill and usually immunocompromised (e.g., with leukemia or lymphoma).

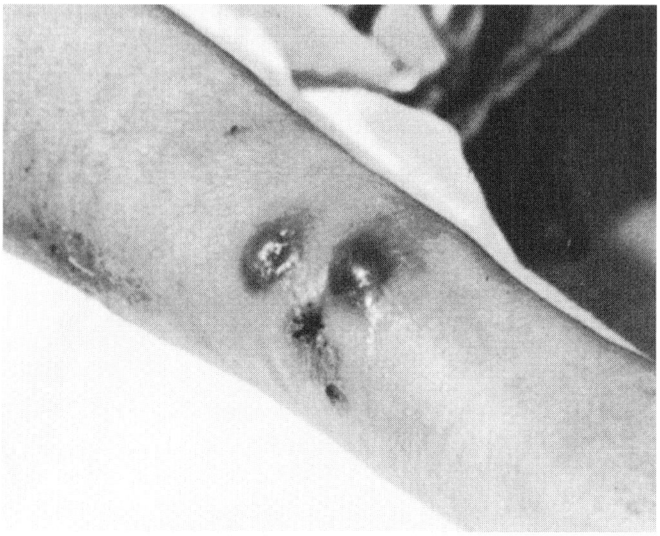

Figure 227.5. Ecthyma gangrenosum. Deep-seated hemorrhagic necrotic nodules on forearm. (From Greene S, et al. Ecthyma gangrenosum: report of clinical histopathologic and bacteriologic aspects of eight cases. *J Am Acad Dermatol* 1984;11:781, with permission.)

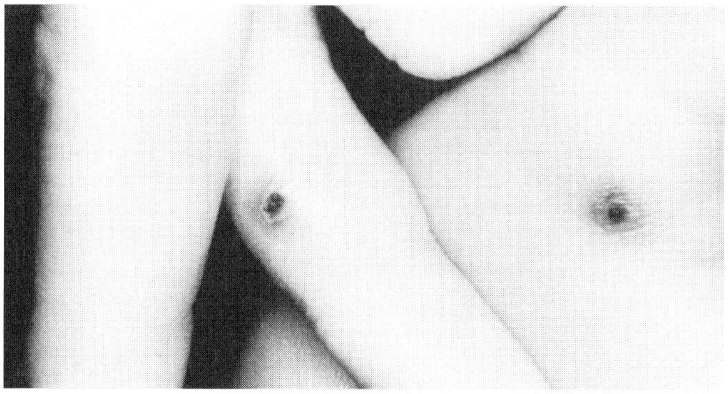

Figure 227.6. Gonococcemia. The lesions are hemorrhagic pustules on an erythematous base. The extremities, particularly the hands, are affected. (From du Vivier A. *Atlas of clinical dermatology*. London: Gower Medical Publishing, 1986, with permission.)

The appearance of the lesion can vary, depending on the stage of the illness at presentation. Beginning as a painless macule or vesicle, it indurates and assumes the appearance of a pustule or bulla on a blue or red base. The lesion then sloughs, leaving a gangrenous ulcer. These solitary or multiple lesions usually occur on the arms, hands, and feet or in the perineal region.

Disseminated gonococcal infection (DGI) usually occurs in individuals with asymptomatic infection of the pharynx, rectum, or genitalia. The patient commonly presents with fever, skin lesions, arthritis, periarthritis, tenosynovitis, or any combination of these signs. DGI occurs most commonly in women during menstruation or pregnancy, but it can occur in any patient with gonococcal infection.

The skin lesions are pustules or vesicles on an erythematous base about 5 mm in diameter, but they may also be petechial, bullous, papular, or hemorrhagic. There are usually relatively few (fewer than ten to as many as 30), and they typically appear on the extremities and resolve rapidly (usually in less than a week). The periarthritis of DGI presents with joint swelling and tenderness, which are often transient and migratory. Septic arthritis occurs most commonly in the larger joints (knees, hands, ankles, and elbows, in descending order of occurrence). Complications such as endocarditis, meningitis, and sepsis are rare.

The diagnosis of gonococcemia (Fig. 227.6) is a clinical one. Any sexually active person with polyarthritis, tenosynovitis, and typical skin lesions can be given a presumptive diagnosis of gonococcemia with little doubt as to its accuracy. Gonococcal cultures should be performed on specimens obtained from all mucous membrane surfaces, as well as blood and (when appropriate) joint fluid. The diagnosis can also be made on the basis of a response to empiric treatment; DGI responds quite promptly to antibiotic treatment (see Chapter 185).

The differential diagnosis should include Reiter syndrome (a syndrome of urethritis, conjunctivitis, and arthritis that usually occurs after a diarrheal illness, has dissimilar skin lesions, and does not respond to antibiotics), meningococcemia (which has more numerous petechial lesions), immune complex diseases (which may have joint manifestations but a different type of skin lesion), and rheumatic fever.

Admission is probably required only for patients with severe systemic signs and symptoms or severe joint involvement (especially of weight-bearing joints) and those who cannot be followed closely as outpatients.

Erysipelas is a superficial cellulitis that progresses rapidly in extent and involves the associated lymphatic channels. The classically described offending organism is the group A streptococcus, but groups C and D streptococci and *S. aureus* have also been isolated.[14] The infection is most common in infants and children and in the elderly. The source, in most cases, is probably an inapparent wound. Erysipelas may range from a self-limited process that resolves spontaneously, even without antibiotics, to a rapidly progressive and severe infection leading to bacteremia. Admission is indicated for patients with extensive facial or neck involvement or for patients with fever and a toxic appearance.

The involved skin is erythematous, warm, and tender to palpation and has an advancing margin that is slightly elevated. Fever is common. The diagnosis is usually clinical, because local aspiration is rarely positive. Punch biopsy may be useful, but it is usually not readily available. The differential diagnosis includes cellulitis, maxillary or frontal sinus infections (if localized to the face), and erysipeloid (if located to the hands).

Treatment with penicillin is rapidly effective if erysipelas is due to streptococci, but, because it is rarely easy to identify the causative organism, either a first-generation cephalosporin or a penicillinase-resistant penicillin should be used to cover *Staphylococcus*. Clindamycin or vancomycin may be used in the penicillin-allergic patient. Hospital admission is based on the patient's clinical status. Some affected individuals may be treated as outpatients with close follow-up, and admitted if there is no response or any worsening after 1 to 2 days of oral antibiotic therapy.

Cellulitis, an acute, spreading inflammation of the skin and subcutaneous tissue, appears as a warm, tender, erythematous area with indistinct margins. Its differentiation from erysipelas is based on the appearance of the advancing edge of the infection: In cellulitis, the edge is not raised. In practice, the clinical management of patients with erysipelas and with cellulitis is similar. Erysipelas is more likely, however, to require prompt initiation of antibiotic therapy because it can progress so rapidly.

PURPURIC OR HEMORRHAGIC LESIONS

Neisseria meningitidis colonizes the nasal mucosa in humans (5% to 15%) but may invade the bloodstream and cause disease. Most cases occur in children and adolescents, although any age group may be affected.[11] The mortality of meningococcemia is higher than that of meningococcal meningitis.

Meningococcemia usually follows an upper respiratory tract infection with flulike symptoms of headache, myalgias, nausea, and vomiting. The severity of the disease can range from an indolent, slowly evolving infection to a fulminating illness causing prostration within a few hours after the onset of symptoms. The classic skin lesions can be petechial, macular, or maculopapular with pale gray vesicular centers. All are a few millimeters in size but may progress to a confluent hemorrhagic rash.[2] They are most commonly localized to the extremities and trunk but may appear on any part of the body. Meningitis presents with the usual symptoms of meningeal irritation—neck soreness, photophobia, headache—while, in meningococcemia, meningeal signs are typically absent.

Gram stain and culture of scrapings of the skin lesions are positive in only about half of cases.[11] The diagnosis must often rest on clinical findings and is confirmed by positive cultures of blood or cerebrospinal fluid.

One should entertain the diagnosis of meningococcemia in any patient who presents with fever, malaise, and a petechial or maculopapular rash, and include it in the differential diagnosis of other bacteremias (e.g., *H. influenzae, S. pneumoniae, S. aureus*), subacute bacterial endocarditis, gonococcemia (few distal papular, hemorrhagic lesions), vasculitis (usually distal purpuric lesions), enteroviral exanthems, and RMSF.

The treatment of choice for meningococcemia is high-dose intravenous antibiotics. Penicillin G (2 million units every 2 hours), ampicillin (2 g every 6 hours), chloramphenicol (4 g/d), and ceftriaxone (up to 4 g/d [100 mg/kg] in children) have all been shown to be effective. Complications such as shock, disseminated intravascular coagulation, adult respiratory distress syndrome, or metabolic acidosis require aggressive supportive care. Prophylaxis is recommended for close school and household contacts. Rifampin, 600 mg (10 mg/kg for children, 5 mg/kg for infants younger than 1 month old), is given orally twice daily for 2 days.

A related syndrome, chronic meningococcemia, presents as periodic fever, localized rash, myalgia, and arthralgias lasting for several days. The number of skin lesions is small. Episodes may recur over a period of weeks to months. The diagnosis is established by positive cultures (especially of blood) during the febrile episodes. A fair percentage of patients proceed, if untreated, to an acute phase of disease. The differential diagnosis includes subacute bacterial endocarditis, rheumatic fever, gonococcemia, and Henoch-Schönlein purpura.

Treatment is the same as for acute meningococcal disease, except that lower doses of intravenous antibiotics are generally considered sufficient to eradicate the infection. All patients suspected of having meningococcal disease should be admitted to the hospital for evaluation and treatment, regardless of clinical appearance.

RMSF is an acute infectious disease caused by *Rickettsia rickettsii* and transmitted by the bites of several species of ticks (*Dermacentor andersoni* in the western United States, *Dermacentor variabilis* in the eastern United States, and *Amblyomma americanum* in some southwestern areas). It is not limited to the Rocky Mountain area; in fact, the areas of highest incidence are in the south-Atlantic region and western south-central states.[15] The organisms can be introduced directly into the skin by a tick bite or may enter broken skin with the tick's feces. Once the infection is established, the organisms invade vascular endothelial cells, causing localized thrombosis and necrosis. The disease is manifested clinically by fever, rash, myalgia, and headache. It ranges in severity from a mild, self-limited illness to severe, life-threatening disease.[10]

RMSF is seen most commonly in the late spring and early summer. The incubation period ranges from 3 to 12 days. There is an abrupt onset of fever, chills, arthralgia, and headache and sometimes nausea, vomiting, and photophobia. The rash appears between the second and sixth days of the illness, beginning peripherally on the wrists, ankles, and forearms as a macular erythematous rash and extending to the palms, soles, and torso. The lesions become maculopapular in a few days in most cases and become petechial shortly thereafter (2 to 4 days after the start of the rash). The rash may be absent in 12% to 17% of cases and may be difficult to appreciate in dark-skinned individuals.[15] Areas of decreased circulation, such as the distal extremities, nose, and ear lobes, may develop areas of infarction; finding such lesions on the scrotum or vaginal area can be an additional clue to the diagnosis.

In severe cases, multiple organ systems are involved. Manifestations of central nervous system involvement can range from headache to coma and seizures. The cerebrospinal fluid may show a mildly increased protein level and a pleocytosis, but these findings are nonspecific. Disseminated intravascular coagulation can occur. Due to the early capillary invasion, capillary permeability is increased; there may be third-spacing of fluids and concomitant edema, hypoalbuminemia, and hypovolemia. Hyponatremia due to the syndrome of inappropriate secretion of antidiuretic hormone is noted in 20% of cases but occurs most commonly in those who are critically ill.[10] The white blood cell count is usually normal.

The diagnosis of RMSF is a clinical one based on the findings of fever, headache, rash, and other associated symptoms and signs. However, it is critical to keep in mind that only about 70% of patients with the disease give a history of tick exposure.[15] Although serologic testing can confirm the diagnosis, seroconversion is not apparent early in the disease. (The indirect fluorescent antibody titer has a sensitivity of 94%, and indirect hemagglutination has a sensitivity of 96%. The Weil-Felix, latex agglutination, and complement fixation tests are considerably less sensitive.[9]) Another promising diagnostic modality (particularly for rapid diagnosis) is immunofluorescent staining of skin biopsy specimens.[15]

The differential diagnosis of RMSF includes TSS, meningococcal meningitis, Kawasaki disease, measles, leptospirosis, Colorado tick fever, enteroviral infections, any cause of disseminated intravascular coagulation and vasculitis, mononucleosis, rat-bite fever, atypical measles, and other rickettsial diseases. Among the latter are murine typhus and epidemic typhus, which both have rashes that usually begin on the trunk rather than on the distal extremities.

The treatment of choice for RMSF is tetracycline (25 to 50 mg/kg in divided doses four times daily, not to exceed 2 g/d) or doxycycline (100 mg every 12 hours) for 7 to 10 days. Because of concern over dental effects of tetracycline, chloramphenicol (50 to 100 mg/kg/d in four divided doses) may be used to treat children. Tetracycline usually does not affect enamel formation in the incisors, canines, and bicuspids after age 7.[8] Moreover, in children younger than 5 years old, it is unlikely to result in any apparent change in tooth color when fewer than five courses of therapy are given in the usual oral dosage.[8]

Most patients require inpatient care due to the severity of the illness, but some patients with mild disease have been treated as outpatients on oral medication and with close follow-up.[16] Most patients improve after a few days of treatment; antibiotics should be continued for 2 to 4 days after fever abates. Lifelong immunity appears to develop after infection.

COMMON PITFALLS

- TEN can easily be confused with SSSS. TEN requires the removal of any possible precipitating agent, most commonly a drug; SSSS must be treated with appropriate antibiotics. The prognosis of the two diseases is markedly different.

- The rash of TSS may be indistinct. The diagnosis should be considered in any patient with fever and signs of volume depletion, even in the absence of a history of tampon use. The disease can occur in men and children.
- Bullous pemphigoid can easily be confused with pemphigus vulgaris. Early consultation with a dermatologist may be necessary to avoid misdiagnosis and inappropriate treatment.
- In a febrile, seriously ill patient, skin lesions may be a manifestation of sepsis. The lesions should be opened and their contents Gram stained and cultured.
- Rapid identification and treatment are crucial in ecthyma gangrenosum. The underlying septic process can be fatal if not treated promptly.
- The diagnosis of gonococcemia is often overlooked in persons presenting with tendinitis without any history of injury.
- The early rash of meningococcemia may be macular or maculopapular as well as petechial, as classically described.
- In RMSF, the rash is absent in a significant proportion of cases. An increased index of suspicion is necessary for any patient presenting with a viral-like illness in the late spring or early summer.

References

1. Bach MC. Dermatologic signs in toxic shock syndrome: clues to diagnosis. *J Am Acad Dermatol* 1983;8:3.
2. Baxter P, Priestly B. Meningococcal rash. *Lancet* 1988;2:1166.
3. Dahl M. The blistering diseases. In: Dahl M. *Common office dermatology*. New York: Grune & Stratton, 1983.
4. Davis JP, et al. Toxic shock syndrome: epidemiologic features, recurrence, risk factors and prevention. *N Engl J Med* 1980;303:1429.
5. Domonkos AN, Arnold HL, Odom RB. *Andrews' diseases of the skin*. Philadelphia: WB Saunders, 1982:311.
6. Fergie J, Patrick C, Lott L. *Pseudomonas aeruginosa* cellulitis and ecthyma gangrenosum in immunocompromised children. *Pediatr Infect Dis J* 1991;10:496.
7. Flowers FP, Krusinski PA. *Dermatology in ambulatory and emergency medicine*. Chicago: Year Book Medical, 1984:813.
8. Fury N. Blistering disorders. In: Roenigk H. ed. *Office dermatology*. Baltimore: Williams & Wilkins, 1981:171.
9. Grossman ER, et al. Tetracyclines and permanent teeth. *Pediatrics* 1971;47:567.
10. Hoge CW, Schwartz B, Talkington DF, et al. The changing epidemiology of invasive group A streptococcal infections and the emergence of streptococcal toxic shock-like syndrome. *JAMA* 1993;269(3):384.
11. Kaplan JE, Schonberger LB. The sensitivity of various serologic tests in the diagnosis of Rocky Mountain spotted fever. *Am J Trop Med Hyg* 1986;35:840.
12. McGee T, Munster A. Toxic epidermal necrolysis syndrome: mortality rate reduced with early referral to a regional burn center. *Plast Reconstr Surg* 1998;102(4):1018–1022.
13. Peters W, Zaidi J, Douglas L. Toxic epidermal necrolysis: a burn center challenge. *Can Med Assoc J* 1991;144:1477.
14. Petri WR. Tick-borne diseases. *Am Fam Physician* 1988;37:95.
15. Raman GV. Meningococcal septicaemia and meningitis: a rising tide. *BMJ* 1988;296:1141.
16. Reingold AL, et al. Toxic shock surveillance in the United States, 1980–1981. *Ann Intern Med* 1982;96:875.
17. Schopf E, et al. Toxic epidermal necrolysis and Stevens-Johnson syndrome. *Arch Dermatol* 1991;127:839.
18. Shands KN. Toxic shock syndrome in menstruating women. *N Engl J Med* 1980;303:1436.
19. Swartz MN, Weinberg AN. Infections due to gram-positive bacteria. In: Fitzpatrick TB, Eisen EZ, Wolff K, et al., eds. *Dermatology in general medicine*, 3rd ed. New York: McGraw-Hill, 1987:2100.
20. Taylor J, et al. Toxic epidermal necrolysis: a comprehensive approach. *Clin Pediatr* 1989;28:404.
21. The Working Group on Severe Streptococcal Infections. Defining the group A streptococcal toxic shock syndrome: rationale and consensus definition. *JAMA* 1993;269:390.
22. Wright S. North American tick-borne diseases. *Ann Emerg Med* 1988;17:964.

CHAPTER 228

Pigmented Lesions and Skin Tumors

Thomas P. Graham and George W. Go

PIGMENTED LESIONS

Pigmentation of the human skin is influenced by a variety of factors, most importantly, the relative quantity and depth of the pigment melanin. The production of melanin, a protein-bound polymer derived from tyrosine, is influenced by genetic and environmental factors as well as intrinsic regulators. Other factors contributing to skin pigmentation include the thickness of the horny layer, the degree of vascularity, and the oxygen saturation of blood hemoglobin.[12]

Patients do not commonly present to the emergency department with the chief complaint of hyperpigmented or hypopigmented skin lesions. However, such lesions are frequently encountered by emergency physicians during a physical examination or are mentioned by patients while a history is being taken. It is therefore important for emergency physicians to be familiar with the differential diagnosis of such lesions, particularly those that are malignant or have malignant potential.

Hypopigmented Lesions

Skin hypopigmentation may result from a defect in one of several pathways in the synthesis, transport, and deposition of melanin.[12] Such lesions may be secondary to an intrinsic dysfunction in one of these pathways or, occasionally, may be manifestations of an otherwise occult systemic disorder.

CLINICAL PRESENTATION

Although patients with hypopigmented lesions may complain of "white spots," they may have presenting complaints unrelated to their skin lesions. The patient may therefore not relate the presence of lesions to the emergency physician. Fortunately, they are usually recognized easily on physical examination, prompting a careful search to delineate their extent and to discover other skin findings.

DIFFERENTIAL DIAGNOSIS

Tinea versicolor, or pityriasis versicolor, is a common fungal infection of the skin. Lesions begin as small, well-circumscribed circular macules that may be white, pink, or even hyperpigmented. Most commonly encountered on the trunk, they are rarely found on the face. The color is uniform in each individual. Although they may be pruritic, lesions are usually asymptomatic. Potassium hydroxide preparation reveals hyphae and yeast forms, with Wood's light examination revealing pale yellow to white fluorescence.[7]

Pityriasis alba is an idiopathic, usually asymptomatic disorder characterized by round or oval, white or pink scaly patches.

The most commonly affected areas are the face, upper trunk, shoulders, and arms. Lesions may become more obvious in summer months, as they fail to tan after sun exposure. Young children, particularly atopic individuals, are commonly affected.[15]

Vitiligo is an idiopathic, possibly multifactorial, disorder characterized by progressively enlarging, circumscribed, hypopigmented macules. Melanocytes are absent from the affected areas. Lesion distribution is variable, but frequently affected areas include bony prominences, perioral and periorbital regions of the face, the dorsum of the hands, and body folds such as the axillae and genitalia. The macules have a well-defined border, which may be rimmed with hyperpigmentation or a red halo.[7] Often familial, vitiligo can be associated with a host of systemic diseases, including adrenal insufficiency, hypothyroidism, diabetes mellitus, and pernicious anemia. Spontaneous repigmentation occurs in up to 25% of cases.

Albinism is characterized by congenital absence of pigment in the skin, hair, and eyes (oculocutaneous albinism) or in the eyes alone (ocular albinism). The skin is a milky pinkish-white, and scalp hair is pale yellow with a fine texture. The eyes are striking because of red pupils and bluish or pink irides. Photophobia and nystagmus may be present. These patients suffer from the constant threat of sunburn and are prone to basal cell and squamous cell carcinomas.[7]

Piebaldism is a congenital disorder characterized by patches of hypopigmentation (similar to vitiligo) most commonly located the chest, abdomen, and midregion of the upper and lower extremities. The characteristic feature of piebaldism is the striking white forelock present on the frontal scalp or forehead. Islands of hyperpigmented macules may frequently be found within hypopigmented areas as well as on normal skin.[7]

Tuberous sclerosis is an autosomal dominant disease characterized by hypopigmented, oval or "ash-leaf" shaped macules in association with early onset seizures, mental retardation, facial angiofibromas, periungual fibrosis, and the so-called shagreen patch. The shagreen patch is a soft, yellow or lightly colored plaque with an irregular surface that has been likened to pigskin, occurring most commonly in the lumbosacral region. Shagreen patches represent the earliest sign of tuberous sclerosis.[15]

EMERGENCY DEPARTMENT MANAGEMENT AND DISPOSITION

For tinea versicolor, treatment should be directed at the underlying infection, with the use of topical antifungal agents such as clotrimazole or miconazole, or selenium sulfide (2.5%) lotion or shampoo.[2] Systemic therapy is generally not recommended. Although weak topical steroids and tar solutions have been used to treat pityriasis alba, the hypopigmentation is self-limited and gradually improves after puberty. Therefore, no therapy other than skin lubrication is needed.

Patients with newly diagnosed vitiligo should be referred to a dermatologist. Therapeutic options include cosmetic cover-up, photochemotherapy, and repigmentation. Before disposition, an underlying systemic cause for the lesions should be considered. Albinotic and other patients with severe hypopigmentation have a least a partial melanin deficiency, and therefore lack the protection that melanin normally provides from the sun's ultraviolet radiation. These patients are exquisitely sensitive to sunlight and are at risk for severe sunburn as well as skin tumors.[15] Proper skin shielding (and eye protection for albinotic patients) is essential, and these patients should be under the care of a dermatologist.

COMMON PITFALLS

- Whether the skin lesions are the presenting complaint or an incidental finding, the possibility of an underlying systemic illness in these patients should be considered.
- Hypopigmentation can dramatically affect the patient's lifestyle, especially when lesions are located on visible areas. Such patients should be referred to a dermatologist.

Hyperpigmented Lesions

Skin hyperpigmentation results from disorders of melanin production, whether from augmented synthesis or transport, or from an increase in the size of melanosomes. A variety of skin lesions may result.[15]

While maintaining a high degree of suspicion for malignancy, emergency physicians should be able to diagnose many benign dermatoses, thereby allaying patient anxiety and avoiding inappropriate dermatologic referral. This section deals with hyperpigmented lesions, excluding skin tumors, which are discussed in the next section.

CLINICAL PRESENTATION

As with most other dermatoses, patients frequently mention hyperpigmented lesions as a secondary complaint while in the emergency department, or they may be unaware of lesions detected during physical examination. However, it is not uncommon for patients to present to the emergency department, expressing concern about such a lesion being malignant.

DIFFERENTIAL DIAGNOSIS

When skin tumors are excluded, the differential diagnosis of hyperpigmented lesions is not extensive. Ephelides, or freckles, are irregularly shaped tan macules that form on sun-exposed areas, most notably the nose, cheeks, hands, and upper trunk. Typically less than 5 mm in diameter, they occur in genetically predisposed persons who are susceptible to sunburn. Freckles are benign lesions, and therefore require no treatment.[7]

Senile or solar lentigos, also known as "liver spots," are discrete, irregularly shaped macules occurring on sun-exposed skin. Common sites of involvement include the forehead and dorsum of the hands. Sparing of the knuckles and phalanges is characteristic. They are of cosmetic significance only and require no treatment.[7]

Juvenile lentigos, or lentigo simplex, are sharply defined brown or black macules that appear anywhere on the skin or mucosa, and are clinically indistinguishable from junctional (*vide infra*) nevi. There is no predilection *for* sun-exposed skin. They may appear in patients of any age but often arise in childhood. Because there is no tendency for neoplastic change, no therapy is indicated.[8]

Peutz-Jeghers syndrome is an autosomal dominant disorder characterized by brown-to-black macules from 1 to 5 mm in diameter, involving the oral mucosa, lips, and perioral area. The sacral region may also be involved. Lesions are associated with gastrointestinal polyps.[3] The color and size of the macules in Peutz-Jeghers syndrome are not affected by sunlight, as they are in freckles.

Mongolian spots are bluish-gray macules or patches that vary from 2 to 8 cm in diameter. Lesions occur in Asian, African-American, Native-American, and southern European patients.

Although multiple lesions may occur in a widespread distribution, they are typically solitary and located in the sacral region of newborns. Mongolian spots usually disappear during childhood.

Café-au-lait spots are uniformly hyperpigmented pale-brown macules with sharply circumscribed borders. They may be present at birth, and occur in up to 20% of normal children. They range in size from a few millimeters to 20 cm, and increase in number and size with age.[15] The presence of six or more spots greater than 1.5 cm in diameter is presumptive evidence of neurofibromatosis (von Recklinghausen disease), although most people with café-au-lait spots do not have this disorder. Macules that mimic café-au-lait spots but are darker and have a more irregular border are seen in Albright syndrome in association with fibrous dysplasia of the long bones and precocious puberty in girls.[12,15]

Melasma, also known as the "mask of pregnancy," is an irregular, brown, macular hyperpigmentation usually noted on the back and neck. It occurs during the second or third trimester of pregnancy, fades after delivery, and darkens with subsequent pregnancy. Melasma worsens with sun exposure and is therefore more obvious in the summer. Melasma may also occur in women taking oral contraceptives.[12]

Acanthosis nigricans is characterized by symmetric brown or "velvety" hyperpigmentation located most commonly along skin folds, including the axillae and groin, as well as the flexural area of the neck. The skin may become thickened and develop leathery or warty patches. Commonly idiopathic, acanthosis nigricans may be associated with endocrinopathies and gastrointestinal malignancies.[7]

EMERGENCY DEPARTMENT MANAGEMENT AND DISPOSITION

Although often not part of the presenting complaint, pigmented skin lesions should always prompt a careful search to delineate their extent and the extent of other skin findings, as well as to detect the presence of underlying illness. If the lesion is benign and systemic illness is not suggested, patients can be discharged with follow-up as needed only.

Some benign pigmented lesions can mimic malignant melanoma. Although emergency physicians should be familiar with the lesions discussed here, it is frequently not possible to completely exclude malignant or premalignant lesions from the differential diagnosis. If the nature of a pigmented lesion is questionable, dermatology referral is indicated.

COMMON PITFALLS

- Despite their nonemergent nature, potentially malignant skin lesions should never be ignored. Dermatologic referral is indicated when any uncertainty exists.
- As with other dermatoses, the possibility of an associated underlying disease should be considered.

SKIN TUMORS

The incidence of skin cancer continues to rise annually, accounting for over 500,000 cases each year in the United States. Melanoma of the skin accounts for over 7,000 deaths each year in the United States, and affects young as well as older individuals. It is projected that, within the next few years, one in 90 people will develop melanoma (an increase from a one in 123 risk in 1987).[3] A number of factors, including depletion of the ozone layer (with resultant increase in radiation exposure), increased longevity, and increased recreational sun exposure, have been implicated.[4,13]

Historically, primary care physicians have had difficulty making the diagnosis of skin cancer clinically. Furthermore, access to specialists may be restricted by the widening influence of managed care, and has always been difficult to obtain for indigent patients. Nevertheless, even highly malignant skin tumors may be curable if detected early. The emergency physician is in an excellent position to prevent serious morbidity and mortality by considering the presence of, and diligently searching for, suspicious lesions.[5]

CLINICAL PRESENTATION

Unlike many problems encountered in the emergency department, skin tumors are generally asymptomatic and may be an incidental finding on physical examination. As such, the emergency department physical examination provides an opportunity to screen for suspicious lesions. Bleeding, ulceration, or pain is sometimes associated with malignancy, generally in the later stages, and may be a presenting complaint.

Most skin tumors are easily recognized as benign lesions and present no diagnostic dilemma, but some are concerning to the patient and challenging for the emergency physician. Early tumors can often be treated successfully, whereas more advanced ones (particularly in the case of melanoma) can be devastating.

DIFFERENTIAL DIAGNOSIS

The most important distinction to make is the one between benign and malignant lesions. A familiarity with several of the more commonly encountered tumors and their characteristics is thus essential.

Benign Tumors

Nevi, commonly known as "moles," are the most common benign tumors of the skin. They vary in size, shape, and color, but each nevus tends to remain uniform in surface characteristics. Although various shades may be present in a single lesion, the colors are distributed over the surface uniformly. Lesions are typically round or oval, with regular borders. They may be macular (intraepidermal or junctional nevi) or raised (dermal or compound nevi). They may be present at birth and tend to increase in number during childhood, reaching a peak at puberty. There is a strong correlation between sun exposure and the number of nevi. Except for certain types of nevi, such as dysplastic nevus and large congenital nevus, most nevi have little malignant potential unless encountered in large numbers.[6,9]

Several types of vascular tumors occur on the skin, including hemangiomas, nevus flammeus, Kaposi's sarcoma, and pyogenic granulomas. Kaposi's sarcoma is discussed in the section, "Nonmelanoma Malignant Tumors."

Hemangiomas represent a broad category of vascular lesions caused by proliferation of vascular endothelium in the dermis. They usually develop during the neonatal period, and their appearance and growth rate vary. Ulceration is the most common complication, although profuse bleeding is rare. Hemangiomas often resolve with minimal scarring.[2]

Nevus flammeus (port-wine stain) is a vascular malformation, usually unilateral, that frequently occurs on the face. The lesion appears as an irregular red-to-purple patch. It may be a component of neurocutaneous syndromes, such as Sturge-Weber syndrome (encephalotrigeminal angiomatosis), in association with mental retardation, epilepsy, visual impairment, and angioma of the meninges. Salmon patches (stork bite, angel's kiss) are variants of nevus flammeus. They are red irregular patches most commonly located on the nape of the neck.

Pyogenic granulomas are rapidly growing, yellow-to-bright red, dome-shaped lesions that are thought to result from trauma. Most often seen on the extremities, especially the fingers, they have a fragile surface that bleeds easily.

Telangiectases are permanently dilated vessels consisting of arterioles, capillaries, or venules. They accompany a wide variety of diseases.

Hereditary hemorrhagic telangiectasia (Rendu-Osler-Weber disease) is an autosomal dominant disease characterized by telangiectases involving the lips, tongue, nasal mucosa, and gastrointestinal tract. Recurrent bleeding represents the most serious complication.

Nevus araneus, or spider angiomas, are prominent arterioles (spider's body) that radiate capillaries (spider's legs). Though sometimes seen in normal individuals, they are more common and may increase in number during pregnancy and in patients with liver disease.[8]

Seborrheic keratoses are oval or round plaques of variable color with sharply circumscribed borders. They vary from a few millimeters to more than 3 cm in diameter. Lesions are usually seen on the head, trunk, and extremities of patients older than 40 years.[12] Sometimes rough in texture, seborrheic keratoses often appear "stuck on" the skin surface. They originate in the dermis, are of unknown origin, and have no malignant potential. Lesions can occasionally become darkly pigmented and irregular, thereby resembling melanoma. In addition, their sudden appearance or an increase in their number or size has been reported as a marker for internal malignancy (Leser-Trélat sign).[9]

Lipomas are fatty tumors that are usually solitary and tend to occur more in women. They usually appear during the fourth or fifth decade of life and commonly affect the posterior neck, trunk, abdomen, forearms, buttocks, and thighs. Most are soft, mobile, subcutaneous masses 2.5 to 5.0 cm in diameter. The tumor is encapsulated and composed of adipose tissue, which has the same appearance as normal subcutaneous fat.[8]

Acrochordons, or "skin tags," are papules or pedunculated lesions that range in color from the patient's skin tone to hyperpigmented. They are of no significance, other than cosmetic.

Dermatofibromas are benign, sometimes slightly pruritic, pink–brown hyperpigmented papules. They are characteristically firm and will dimple when lateral compression is applied. Lesions most commonly occur on the anterior surface of the legs.[2]

Injury or surgery can cause abnormally prominent scarring in some individuals. Keloids, to which African Americans are more susceptible, extend beyond the wound margins and do not regress. Hypertrophic scars are abnormally large but remain confined to the wound site and regress over time.

Milia are 1- to 2-mm white cysts usually found on the face of middle-aged patients, especially around the eyes. Epidermal cysts, also called sebaceous cysts, are similar to milia in that epidermal tissue is trapped within the dermis. The cyst wall is lined with stratified squamous epithelium, which produces keratin. However, epidermal cysts are larger and deeper, and frequently prompt visits to the emergency department when they become inflamed or infected. They occur primarily on the face, posterior neck, chest, and back. Pilar cysts are similar to epidermal cysts except that they occur on the scalp. Syringomas are small papules, yellow or matching the patient's skin, that occur primarily on the lower eyelids. They are benign sweat duct tumors that appear during the third and fourth decades.

Keratoacanthoma is a benign epithelial tumor, possibly of viral origin, that occurs in the elderly. It appears as a smooth, dome-shaped red papule resembling molluscum contagiosum, which then develops a central keratin-filled crater that is frequently covered with crust. It frequently regresses over a period of 2 to 12 months and heals with scarring. Most common locations are sun-exposed areas, such as the back, face, and dorsum of the hands. Clinical differentiation from squamous cell carcinoma may be difficult.[8]

Tumors with Malignant Potential

Dysplastic nevus was initially identified in families with a high incidence of melanoma as a cutaneous marker for increased malignancy risk. It may also occur in patients without a family history of skin cancer. The presence of ten or more dysplastic nevi is associated with a 12-fold increase in the risk of developing melanoma.[18] Dysplastic nevi are larger than common moles. The surface has a mixture of colors, with an irregular, indistinct border that fades into the surrounding skin. A characteristic presentation is an irregular pigmented papule surrounded by an irregular macular collar of pigmentation, giving a "fried egg" appearance. The lesions, not present at birth, begin to appear during childhood as common moles. However, their appearance changes at puberty and newer lesions continue to appear throughout life. Dysplastic nevi occur not only in sun-exposed areas, as do common moles, but also at unusual sites, such as the scalp, buttocks, and breast. They are most commonly seen on the back.

Congenital nevus is present at birth and may vary in size from a few millimeters to several centimeters in diameter. It may cover wide areas of the face, an extremity, or the trunk. It may contain hair (congenital hairy nevus). Very large lesions have potential for malignant transformation.[9]

The most common premalignant skin tumor is actinic keratosis, also known as solar keratosis or senile keratosis. It is a hyperpigmented, well-circumscribed, and usually scaly macular lesion occurring in middle-aged or older patients and especially in light-complected individuals.[8,12]

Malignant Melanoma

Malignant melanoma is one of the most frequently encountered cancers among many age groups, and the incidence is increasing. Although melanoma represents less than 2% of all skin cancers, it accounts for over 60% of all skin cancer deaths.[1,8,10,14] The incidence of melanoma continues to rise, possibly due to an increase in recreational exposure to the sun's ultraviolet radiation. People who experience acute episodic exposures may be at greater risk than those with constant exposure.

Melanoma arises from the pigment-producing melanocytes of the basal layer, from melanocytes in dysplastic nevi, and from malignant transformation of large congenital nevi. It can metastasize widely. Because there is a high cure rate when melanoma is detected early, it is important for the primary care physicians to screen for the disease and for patients to perform self-examination.

The "ABCD" method recommended by the American Academy of Dermatology (Table 228.1) is a commonly used guide for the early identification of malignant melanoma. Melanomas tend to have *a*symmetry, irregular *b*orders, variegated *c*olor, and greater *d*iameter than benign lesions. Patients with lesions that meet any of these criteria should be given

TABLE 228.1. "ABCD" Method as a Guide for Early Detection of Malignant Melanoma

Asymmetry	Two halves of lesion do not appear identical
Border	Uneven, notched, scalloped, or rugged
Color	Different shades of black/brown/red/white/blue
Diameter	Greater than 6 mm in diameter or changing in size

follow-up for dermatologic evaluation and possible biopsy.[11] Other characteristics that should raise suspicion are the development of bleeding, tenderness, and pruritus. Although clinical suspicion depends primarily on direct visual inspection of a lesion without much regard for its evolution, certain traits are known to place individuals at higher risk for melanoma. These include fair complexion, red or blonde hair, excessive sun exposure, a positive family history, previous melanoma, and the presence of a large congenital nevus or dysplastic nevus syndrome.[1,7]

Nonmelanoma Malignant Tumors

By far, the most common cutaneous malignancy is basal cell carcinoma. It arises from the epidermis and consists of histologically normal-appearing basal cells. Typical lesions are hyperpigmented, smooth or waxy nodules, often with irregular borders and uneven pigmentation. They are classically described as pink pearly papules with prominent telangiectatic vessels. There may be central ulceration. However, there are a variety of forms, and lesions may be indistinguishable from Bowen disease, psoriasis, or even eczema. About 90% of basal cell carcinomas occur on sun-exposed areas of the neck and face, particularly the nose. Metastasis is rare, although local extension of the tumor into cartilage, bone, nerve, and other tissues may produce complications.[13]

Squamous cell carcinoma accounts for about 20% of all cases of skin cancer.[14] Like basal cell carcinoma, it arises from the epidermis and is common on sun-exposed areas. However, it grows more rapidly and can occur at any anatomic site. Although there is no classic lesion, many are firm, scaly papules with ulcerations or crusting.[13] Lesions may mimic a patch of psoriasis. Squamous cell carcinoma may arise on skin that has been chronically damaged by sun exposure (actinic keratosis) or chronic inflammation (Marjolin ulcer). Several strains of human papillomavirus are associated with squamous cell carcinoma and may lead to increased risk of developing a malignancy.[14]

Kaposi's sarcoma is a vascular neoplasm with several different forms. It is described in genetically predisposed individuals of European or African descent, as well as in immunocompromised patients (particularly patients with acquired immune deficiency syndrome [AIDS]). Usually beginning on the feet as red, bluish, or purple macules and papules, lesions may occur in a variety of forms and locations, particularly in AIDS patients.

Marjolin ulcer refers to squamous cell carcinoma that arises from malignant changes in chronic ulcers of the skin or sinuses, or in previous burn scars. A majority occur on the extremities. These tumors are typically more aggressive than those that develop from actinic keratosis or Bowen disease.

Bowen disease is also referred to as squamous cell carcinoma *in situ*. It occurs more frequently in light-complected individuals, but lesions are equally distributed between sun-exposed and nonexposed skin. Lesions are characteristically red, scaly plaques with well-defined borders. Erythroplasia of Queyrat of the penis resembles Bowen disease and is thought to be the same entity, although metastases may occur more frequently than from lesions at other sites. It appears under the foreskin of the uncircumcised penis. Vulvar lesions are described but are rare.[14]

Verrucous carcinoma, a variant of squamous cell carcinoma, is a slow-growing, exophytic, fungating tumor that rarely metastasizes. In the early stages, it is often mistaken for a common wart.

Paget disease of the breast results from invasion of the epidermis of the nipple and surrounding skin by malignant cells originating from a ductal carcinoma. The process begins insidiously with a small area on the nipple that may drain and form a cyst. The inflammation initially may be attributed to trauma, and partial healing may support this false impression. The appearance may be similar to eczema, but Paget disease of the breast is a unilateral disease, whereas eczematous inflammation of the nipple is nearly always bilateral.[8]

Mycosis fungoides, a form of cutaneous T-cell lymphoma (CTCL), can present with skin lesions that initially may be confused with eczema, contact dermatitis, or psoriasis. Visceral involvement occurs much later in the course. Other forms of CTCL include Sézary syndrome and lymphoma cutis.

Finally, metastases to skin may develop in 1% to 2% of patients with underlying malignancy.[17]

EMERGENCY DEPARTMENT MANAGEMENT AND DISPOSITION

The emergency physician should carefully inspect any questionable skin lesion, delineate the number and extent of coexisting lesions, and question the patient regarding their development and any associated conditions.

Nevi are generally easily diagnosed and require no special follow-up, but may rarely be found in association with melanoma. Therefore, any nevus undergoing suspicious changes or arising for the first time in patients more than 20 years old, should be referred for biopsy.

Patients should be reassured that most hemangiomas resolve spontaneously without therapy, whereas therapeutic interventions often produce scarring.[16] However, referral is warranted in order to follow the lesion. Treatment for pyogenic granuloma consists of curettage and electrodesiccation.[2]

Except for cosmetic considerations, lipomas, acrochordons, and dermatofibromas require no treatment or referral. Keloids can be treated with cryotherapy or intralesional steroid injections. Surgical excision may lead to keloids that recur and are larger than the original lesion. For milia and syringoma, the cyst may be opened and contents expressed for cosmetic reasons. Epidermal cysts may be opened and drained, although in order to achieve long-term results, the cyst wall must be excised as well.[16]

None of these entities requires urgent treatment in the emergency department. However, if malignancy is suspected, the patient should be promptly referred for biopsy. Therapeutic options for the various malignant tumors include excision, curettage and electrodesiccation, radiation therapy, systemic or topical chemotherapy, micrographic surgery, and cryosurgery.[13]

COMMON PITFALLS

- Patients with skin lesions suspicious for malignancy require prompt specialty referral for further care. A "watch and wait" attitude in these cases can be disastrous.
- Pigmented lesions that are asymmetric, painful, pruritic, increasing in size, irregularly colored, or otherwise atypical should be considered malignant until proven otherwise by biopsy.

References

1. Buzaid AC, Bolognia JL, Poo W, et al. Management of cutaneous melanoma. *Resid Staff Physician* 1993;39(6):19.
2. Fitzpatrick TB, Johnson RA, Wolff K, et al., eds. *Color atlas and synopsis of clinical dermatology,* 3rd ed. New York: McGraw-Hill, 1997:730.
3. Friedman RJ, Rigel DS, Silverman MK, et al. Malignant melanoma in the 90's: the continued importance of early detection and the role of physician examination and self-examination of the skin. *CA Cancer J Clin* 1991;41(4):201.
4. Goldstein AM, Tucker MA. Etiology, epidemiology, risk factors, and public health issues of melanoma. *Curr Opin Oncol* 1993;5:358.
5. Grant-Kels JM, Bason ET, Grin CM. The misdiagnosis of malignant melanoma. *J Am Acad Dermatol* 1999;40(4):539.
6. Higgins E, du Vivier A. Malignant melanoma—a review: early diagnosis is the key. *Br J Clin Pract* 1991;45(2):109.
7. Kang S, Sober AJ. Disturbances of melanin pigmentation. In: Moschella SL, Hurley HJ, eds. *Dermatology,* 3rd ed. Philadelphia: WB Saunders, 1992:1442.
8. Koh HK, Bhawan J. Tumors of the skin. In: Moschella SL, Hurley HJ, eds. *Dermatology,* 3rd ed. Philadelphia: WB Saunders, 1992:1721.
9. Langley RGB, Sober AJ. Clinical recognition of melanoma and its precursors. *Hematol Oncol Clin North Am* 1998;12(4):699.
10. Lee JA. Trends in melanoma: incidence and mortality. *Clin Dermatol* 1992;10:9.
11. Lefkovits AM. The practitioner's approach to the atypical mole. *Mt Sinai J Med* 1992;59(3):203.
12. Maize JC, Ackerman AB. *Pigmented lesions of the skin.* Philadelphia: Lea & Febiger, 1987.
13. Mora RG. Non-melanoma skin cancer. *Prim Care* 1989;16(3):665.
14. Rose LC. Recognizing neoplastic skin lesions: a photo guide. *Am Fam Physician* 1998;58(4):873.
15. Saur GC, Hall JC, eds. *A manual of skin diseases,* 7th ed. Philadelphia: Lippincott–Raven Publishers, 1996.
16. Scott MA. Benign cutaneous neoplasms. *Prim Care* 1989;16(3):645.
17. Sober AJ, Kang S, Barnhill RL. Discerning individuals at elevated risk for cutaneous melanoma. *Clin Dermatol* 1992;10:15.
18. Tucker MA, Halpern A, Holly EA, et al. Clinically recognized dysplastic nevi. A central risk factor for cutaneous melanoma. *JAMA* 1997;227:1439.

PART XI
Psychiatry

CHAPTER 229

Medical Clearance: Distinguishing Medical and Psychiatric Causes of Disturbed Behavior

Phillipph I. Bialecki, Douglas A. Rund, and William R. Dubin

Patients with psychiatric conditions often present with various somatic complaints; conversely, some patients with medical conditions present with abnormal thought or behavior that resembles psychiatric complaints. Treatment depends on differentiating between predominant psychiatric illness and predominant medical illness in patients who present in these various ways. The prevalence of physical illness among psychiatric patients in one review was 50% overall.[12] The patient's physical condition was considered to be the cause of the psychiatric disorder in 8% of cases and to be an exacerbating factor in 22%.[11] Almost 60% of the physical illness had not previously been diagnosed. Another study, specifically reviewing emergency department practice, found that 80% of patients in whom medical disease should have been identified in the emergency department were instead documented as "medically clear."[21]

There is a lack of standardized nomenclature in this area. The terms *organic disease* and *functional disease* are, perhaps, most frequently used. Organic disease denotes nonpsychiatric causes, and functional disease indicates a psychiatric cause. To call one mental disorder organic, however, implies that a nonorganic or functional mental disorder is unrelated to physical or biologic factors or processes.[12] In fact, many chemical neurophysiologic and genetic factors have been documented to be related to psychiatric disease.

The Diagnostic and Statistical Manual of Mental Disorders, Fourth Edition (DSM-IV) eliminates the terms *organic* and *functional* and distinguishes "mental disorders that are due to a general medical condition" from "primary mental disorders."[1] An example of a mental disorder due to a medical condition is delirium, a clinical condition seen often in emergency department patients.

CLINICAL PRESENTATION

Delirium, or acute confusional state, is a reversible condition, the essential feature of which is a disturbance of consciousness accompanied by a change in cognition or a perceptual disturbance.[1,13–15] It develops over a short period, usually hours to days, and has a fluctuating course during any one day. Reduced awareness of the environment is manifested by an impaired ability to focus, sustain, or shift attention. During the clinical interview, patients have problems focusing on any given question and may shift from topic to topic or perseverate on one question. They are distracted easily by irrelevant stimuli, and their thought process may seem disjointed or incoherent.

Cognitive changes include memory impairment, disorientation, or language disturbances. Recent memory is most commonly affected.[1] Disorientation, especially to time and place, may be the first sign of mild delirium; disorientation to self is uncommon. Speech that is rambling, pressured, or incoherent may lead the clinician to mistakenly diagnose a primary mental disorder such as mania or a psychosis-related disorder. When gathering information from the patient is difficult or impossible, it is important to talk with family or friends, who often can provide critical information about time course and related symptoms, as well as relevant medical history.

Patients with delirium may experience delusions, hallucinations, and illusions that are often mistaken for those occurring with primary mental disorders.[2] Such a patient may be referred prematurely to psychiatric care before medical conditions are investigated. Paranoia about hospital staff may exist and may involve elaborate schemes that integrate hallucinations. The patient may misinterpret the sound of a dropped stethoscope as a gunshot and act accordingly. Hallucinations are usually visual, but may take any form.

Patients commonly display both restlessness and excitement. The sleep–wake cycle is often affected, causing the patient to appear stuporous during the day and hyperalert at night. Symptoms follow a varied time course; patients often may be coherent during the afternoon and symptomatic by evening. Rapid and unpredictable shifts in emotion are common. Displays of fear, anxiety, sadness, anger, euphoria, and apathy are not unusual, but are not necessarily present. Some patients display aggressive or violent behavior.

Children are susceptible to delirium when affected by a febrile illness and when given certain medications (e.g., anticholinergics).[17] Patients aged 65 years old and older are the most vulnerable. In these patients, approximately 10% exhibit delirium on admission, and 10% to 15% may become delirious while in the hospital.[1,7] Postoperative and severely burned patients are also notably prone to confusional states.

The time course of delirium is usually one of hours to days, with symptoms typically having an acute onset. The duration depends on the etiologic factors. The more promptly the underlying medical condition is diagnosed and treatment initiated, the shorter the time course. Acuteness of onset is an important factor differentiating delirium from dementia or primary mental disorders: Onset is more likely to be recent and rapid in delirium.

DIFFERENTIAL DIAGNOSIS

The differential diagnosis of delirium is so extensive that there may be a tendency to avoid searching for the cause. For example, an elderly delirious patient may have pulmonary insufficiency, cardiac failure, and preexisting brain damage and may be taking multiple medications.[23] In such a patient, each problem is a possible contributor to delirium and must be pursued and evaluated independently.

The differential diagnosis can be divided into two categories: emergent and urgent. Life-threatening emergent conditions that require immediate intervention include meningitis and encephalitis, hypoglycemia, hypertensive encephalopathy, diminished cerebral oxygenation, anticholinergic delirium, intracranial hemorrhage (spontaneous or traumatic), and Wernicke encephalopathy. Most other causes, although not emergencies, may be urgent enough to require treatment in the emergency department (Table 229.1).

Delirium that manifests with hallucinations, delusions, language disturbances, and agitation must be differentiated from primary mental disorders, including brief psychotic disorder, schizophrenia, and mood disorder with psychotic features, among others. Psychotic symptoms that fluctuate, are fragmented, and are not particularly systematized are likely to be secondary to delirium. Memory impairment, disorientation, and reduced ability to maintain and shift attention are not usually present in primary mental disorders.[10]

TABLE 229.1. Treatable Causes of Acute Mental Disorders Due to a General Medical Condition

CARDIAC	**ELECTROLYTE IMBALANCE**
Arrhythmias Congestive heart failure Myocardial infarction	Hyponatremia Hypernatremia Hypercalcemia
PULMONARY	**VITAMIN DEFICIENCIES**
Chronic obstructive pulmonary disease Pulmonary emboli	Thiamine Niacin Riboflavin Folate Ascorbic acid Vitamin A Vitamin B_{12}
HEPATIC	
Cirrhosis Hepatitis Wilson disease	
	DRUG-INDUCED
RENAL	Alcohol Tranquilizers Over-the-counter preparations Any drug used to treat medical illness (e.g., phenytoin, aminophylline, digitalis, steroids)
Worsening of mild nephritis by urinary tract infection Dehydration with elevation of BUN >50 mg/dL	
VASCULAR	
Subdural hematoma Cerebrovascular accident	**EXOGENOUS TOXINS**
INFECTION	Carbon monoxide Bromide Mercury Lead
ENDOCRINE DISEASE	
Thyroid disease Cushing disease Diabetes Addison disease Hypoglycemia	**TUMORS**
	NONCONVULSIVE STATUS EPILEPTICUS
	NORMAL PRESSURE HYDROCEPHALUS
	DEPRESSION

EMERGENCY DEPARTMENT EVALUATION

Emergency physicians are often called on to medically clear patients judged to have primary mental disorders before their psychiatric care begins. As discussed, the physician's judgment that a patient has been medically cleared is often inaccurate. In one study, 33% of patients bearing this label did not even have vital signs recorded on the chart, and almost half had no mental status examination recorded.[19] No physical examination at all was noted in 8% of patients, and at least one standard portion of the physical examination was missing in 80% of patients. Only 8% of patients had a complete neurologic examination.

A thorough evaluation must include a complete history and physical examination, with special attention to the neurologic and mental status examinations. The entire workup should be well documented on the patient's chart in the place of the phrase "medically clear." Laboratory data also should be well documented.

Useful laboratory studies include a complete blood count, serum glucose evaluation, electrolytes study, blood urea nitrogen, and creatinine. In some cases, blood alcohol level, toxicology screen, chest radiograph, electrocardiogram, and arterial blood gas measurement will be appropriate. Patients who present with an acute change of behavior and clouded consciousness that is not explained by this laboratory evaluation may require computed tomography, followed by a lumbar puncture and, in some cases, an electroencephalogram (EEG).

The EEG is helpful in making the diagnosis of delirium, as certain EEG changes are typical of delirium, including generalized slowing.[6,16] Also, the EEG can occasionally unexpectedly reveal that the patient's altered mental status is due to nonconvulsive status epilepticus.

EMERGENCY DEPARTMENT MANAGEMENT

Extreme agitation is often part of the syndrome of delirium and can significantly interfere with evaluation. Rapid tranquilization (RT) is a safe and effective method for controlling agitated, potentially assaultive, or overtly violent delirious patients.[5] RT is accomplished by administering a standard dose of a high-potency antipsychotic medication, such as haloperidol or droperidol, in 30- to 60-minute intervals. Research indicates that the combination of antipsychotic medication with lorazepam is more effective than either medication alone, though the synergistic effects may cause excessive sedation.[8]

Table 229.2 outlines suggested doses. Most patients respond after one to three doses, each dose being double the previous dosage until an effective dose is reached. No ceiling dose has ever been established for RT; even in severely ill medical patients, high doses of antipsychotic medication alone or in combination with lorazepam are safe and well tolerated.[4]

The most common side effects of RT are dystonic reactions or akathisia. These are effectively treated with benztropine (Cogentin) 2 mg, intramuscularly or intravenously, or diphenhydramine (Benadryl) 50 mg, propranolol 20 to 40 mg or lorazepam 1 to 2 mg.

DISPOSITION

The treatment of delirium is based on detection of the underlying cause. Hospital admission is necessary if the patient's be-

TABLE 229.2. Recommended Doses for Rapid Tranquilization[a]

Medication is given in 30–60-minute intervals, up to 6 doses/24 h
Haloperidol (Haldol) 5 mg i.m. or 10 mg concentrate
Droperidol (Inapsine) 2.5–5.0 mg i.v. or i.m.
Thiothixene (Navane) 10 mg i.m. or 20 mg concentrate
Loxapine (Loxitane) 10 mg i.m. or 25 mg concentrate
OR
Lorazepam (Ativan) 2–4 mg i.m. combined with haloperidol (Haldol) 5 mg i.m. or thiothixene (Navane) 10 mg i.m.

[a] With older or debilitated patients, the recommended doses should be reduced by 50%.
i.m., intramuscularly; i.v., intravenously.

havior jeopardizes further medical evaluation or care. If no specific cause can be found while in the emergency department, the patient should be admitted for further workup, with psychiatric consultation as needed. A patient should be discharged only after a cause has been identified, treatment has been initiated, and adequate follow-up has been ensured.

The fluctuating time course of delirium must be considered, because a patient may initially improve only to have symptoms recur when inadequate resources are available.

Identified illnesses associated with a risk of morbidity or mortality also warrant hospital admission.[23]

COMMON PITFALLS

- Delirious patients who present to the emergency department are often inappropriately referred to a psychiatrist. This is especially true for those who present with bizarre and agitated behavior. There are several reasons for misdiagnosis and premature psychiatric referral.
- Psychiatric patients who behave in a bizarre, disruptive manner may not be approached with the same sense of urgency or seriousness as are patients with cardiovascular disease or trauma. Often, such decisions are based on a single symptom or item of history, or on a previous diagnosis. Out of a sense of discomfort and an urgency to get to the "really sick" patients, the physician may decide that the patient is "medically clear" without conducting a complete and thorough evaluation.
- A common misunderstanding is that delusions, hallucinations, and disorganized thoughts are diagnostic of primary mental disorders. On the contrary, such symptoms, like fever or pain, are nonspecific and occur in both primary mental disorders and mental disorders caused by a medical condition, as well as in certain personality disorders.
- There is a tendency to refer violent patients prematurely to a psychiatrist. Yet, like disordered perception, violence is etiologically nonspecific. A significant proportion of violence that occurs in psychiatric settings results from underlying medical illness or drug intoxication.[20] Thus, the evaluation of the violent patient must include a search for these conditions.
- The least tolerated patients are those who are believed to create their own disease (e.g., alcoholic patients, drug abusers, and suicidal patients).[22] Thus, a patient who overdoses on tricyclic antidepressants and is fully alert and clinically stable may be treated with an inappropriate lack of urgency. Similarly, Wernicke encephalopathy is rarely given consideration in confused, belligerent patients who present with chronic alcoholism.[18]
- Finally, clinicians often fail to take seriously the complaints of elderly patients, commonly attributing their symptoms to "old age."[9] This attitude is particularly unfortunate when the patient is demented, because 60% of all dementias are treatable or reversible.[3] For many clinicians, dementia implies a chronic, progressive, irreversible deterioration of higher intellectual functions. Dementia is not etiologically specific, however, and does not imply irreversibility. Premature labeling tends to preclude the exhaustive physical, neurologic, and laboratory evaluation necessary to identify potentially reversible causes of dementia or delirium.

References

1. American Psychiatric Association. *Diagnostic and statistical manual of mental disorders*, 4th ed. Washington, DC: American Psychiatric Press, 1994.
2. Carlson RJ, Nayar N, Sur M. Physical disorders among emergency psychiatric patients. *Can J Psychiatry* 1981;26:65.
3. Dubin WR. Assessment and management of psychiatric manifestations of organic brain disease. In: Dubin WR, Hanke N, Nickens HW, eds. *Clinics in emergency medicine: psychiatric emergencies*. New York: Churchill Livingstone, 1984.
4. Dubin WR. Rapid tranquilization: antipsychotics of benzodiazepines. *J Clin Psychiatry* 1988;49[Suppl]:5.
5. Dubin WR, Weiss KJ, Dorn JM. Pharmacotherapy of psychiatric emergencies. *J Clin Psychopharmacol* 1986;6:210.
6. Engel GL, Romano J. Delirium, a syndrome of cerebral insufficiency. *J Chron Dis* 1959;9:260.
7. Flint FJ, Richards SM. Organic basis of confusional states in the elderly. *BMJ* 1956;2:1537.
8. Garza-Trevino ES, Hollister LE, Overall JE, et al. Efficacy of combination of intramuscular antipsychotics and sedative-hypnotics for control of psychotic agitation. *Am J Psychiatry* 1989;146:1588.
9. Goodstein RK. Common clinical problems in the elderly, camouflaged by ageism and atypical presentation. *Psychiatr Ann* 1985;15:299.
10. Hall RCW, Popkin MK, Devaul RA, et al. Physical illness presenting as psychiatric disease. *Arch Gen Psychiatry* 1978;35:1315.
11. Koranyi EK. Morbidity and rate of undiagnosed physical illness in a psychiatric clinic population. *Arch Gen Psychiatry* 1979;36:414.
12. Koranyi EK, et al. Physical illnesses underlying psychiatric symptoms. *Psychother Psychosom* 1992;58(3-4):155.
13. Lipowski ZJ. Delirium, clouding of consciousness and confusion. *J Nerv Ment Dis* 1967;145:22.
14. Lipowski ZJ. Delirium updated. *Compr Psychiatry* 1980;21:190.
15. Lipowski ZJ. Transient cognitive disorders. *Am J Psychiatry* 1983;140:1426.
16. Pro JD, Wells CE. The use of the electroencephalogram in the diagnosis of delirium. *Dis Nerv Syst* 1977;38:804.
17. Rabins PV, Folstein MF. Delirium and dementia: diagnostic criteria and fatality rates. *Br J Psychiatry* 1987;140:149.
18. Reuler JB, Girard DE, Cooney TG. Wernicke's encephalopathy. *N Engl J Med* 1985;16:1035.
19. Riba M, Hale M. Medical clearance: fact or fiction in the hospital emergency room. *Psychosomatics* 1990;31(4):400.
20. Tardiff K, Sweillam A. Assault, suicide, and mental illness. *Arch Gen Psychiatry* 1980;37:164.
21. Tintinalli JE, Peacock FW, Wright MA. Emergency medical evaluation of psychiatric patients. *Ann Emerg Med* 1994;23:859.
22. Weissberg MP. Emergency room medical clearance: an educational problem. *Am J Psychiatry* 1979;136:787.
23. Wise MG. Delirium. In: Hales RE, ed. *Textbook of neuropsychiatry*. Washington, DC: American Psychiatric Press, 1987.

CHAPTER 230
Depression and Suicide

Robert S. Hockberger and Roger Yang

Depression is the most common psychological disturbance affecting humankind. Its prevalence is 10% to 20% in the general population and 20% to 50% in patients seen by physicians in general practice settings.[1] Suicide, the most notable sequela of depression, is the eighth most common cause of death in the United States, accounting for approximately 30,000 deaths annually.[1,2] The overall incidence of suicide nationwide does not appear to be increasing; however, recent epidemiologic studies have shown an increase among certain groups, including the young (particularly adolescents), inner-city minorities, and patients with acquired immune deficiency syndrome (AIDS).[1,2]

Patients frequently seek nonpsychiatric medical care shortly before committing suicide. It is sometimes difficult for physicians without formal psychiatric training to recognize and evaluate depression and suicide potential in their patients, because many of these patients do not specifically complain of depression or readily admit their suicidal ideation or intentions unless specifically questioned.[12,13] Emergency physicians are further hampered by the hectic environment of an emergency department, constantly changing priorities that limit one's ability to spend significant time with individual patients, and the difficulty in obtaining after-hours psychiatric consultation. Nevertheless, the emergency physician's ability to make these assessments and to decide when to seek urgent psychiatric referral or hospitalization for potentially suicidal patients is a vital link in the effective management of a highly disabling and often fatal affliction.

CLINICAL PRESENTATION

Depressed patients commonly complain of multiple vague, ill-defined somatic symptoms such as weakness, malaise, weight loss, headache, and back pain; however, a thorough medical evaluation should be made before attributing such physical complaints to a psychological cause. Depressed people frequently admit to a diminished sense of self-esteem and general physical and mental well-being; loss of interest in or lack of enjoyment of pleasurable activities; loss of energy; poor appetite; sleep disturbances, including insomnia or hypersomnia; decreased attention span and ability to concentrate; decreased effectiveness or productivity at school, work, or home; episodes of tearfulness or crying; irritability or excessive anger; a pessimistic attitude toward the future; and recurrent thoughts of death.[12]

The potential for suicide should be considered in the following groups of patients, among others:

- Patients who have made a recent suicide attempt or have experienced recent suicidal ideation. While most completed suicides involve firearms, drug overdose accounts for 70% to 90% of all suicide attempts.[2] Major and minor tranquilizers and antidepressants have replaced barbiturates and other sedatives as the major agents involved in intentional overdose.
- Patients who state that they are depressed or who complain of symptoms of depression
- Patients who present with problems related to chronic alcoholism, drug withdrawal, or any psychiatric disorder (particularly affective disorders, psychosis, and panic attacks)
- Patients who present with apparently unintentional overdoses or self-inflicted gunshot wounds, lacerated wrists, falls from heights, or motor vehicle accidents of unclear cause, particularly when only one vehicle and one victim are involved

DIFFERENTIAL DIAGNOSIS

A number of psychiatric and medical disorders may present with symptoms of depression. Approximately 80% of people suffering bereavement have one or more symptoms of depression for 1 year or more following the death of a loved one.[2] Persons suffering from an adjustment disorder may develop similar symptoms within several months of the onset of psychosocial stresses (e.g., economic loss, physical illness, or trouble with interpersonal relationships) with which they are unable to cope. The diagnosis of organic affective syndrome is made when symptoms of depression are found to accompany organic neurologic disease such as organic brain syndrome, stroke, tumor, or trauma. Symptoms of depression may be exacerbated or even caused by medications, including antihypertensive drugs (beta blockers, clonidine, methyldopa, and reserpine), antidepressants, antihistamines, neuroleptic agents, sedative–hypnotic drugs, cimetidine, and alcohol.[10]

When these diagnostic possibilities have been eliminated in a patient exhibiting symptoms of depression, a final diagnosis of dysthymic disorder (depressive neurosis, or minor depression) or major affective syndrome (major depression) should be considered. The difference is one of degree, and establishment of the final diagnosis is best left to a psychiatrist.

EMERGENCY DEPARTMENT EVALUATION AND MANAGEMENT

The clinical assessment of depression and suicide potential is an art as well as a science. Patients feel at ease to talk about difficult personal issues when health professionals exhibit a friendly, nonjudgmental, supportive attitude and convey their willingness to listen to problems and understand feelings. Several studies have shown that this is frequently not the case, however, particularly among emergency department staff. Reasons cited for these lapses include inadequate time and staffing, patient behavior that is perceived as either abusive or manipulative, value conflicts, and staff frustration regarding ineffective disposition and follow-up options.[6,8] Expression of a negative or hostile attitude by a respected authority figure, such as a physician or nurse, reinforces a depressed patient's feeling of diminished self-worth and may actually increase the likelihood of another suicide attempt.

Patients who are not overtly depressed or suicidal but who exhibit one or more high-risk presentations should be assessed in a sympathetic but direct manner. First, the presenting complaint should be addressed by asking general questions about the patient's home, work, and social situation. This can be followed with specific questions regarding the signs and symptoms of depression. Finally, the physician should ask direct questions regarding suicide, such as, "Have you ever felt so bad that you thought about killing yourself?" or "Do you have thoughts of harming yourself now?" and "What plans have you made to do this?" Physicians are occasionally reluctant to ask patients directly about suicidal thoughts, fearing that this type of questioning will surface subconscious thoughts and result in suicidal acts. There is no evidence to support this concern; to the contrary, most depressed patients are relieved at the opportunity to discuss their problems openly when the clinician demonstrates an interest and a willingness to listen.

Patients who are judged to be markedly depressed or who present a potential immediate suicide risk should be relieved of medications or weapons and placed in a quiet area of the emergency department that is free of potentially dangerous objects, and where they can be kept under observation by a staff member at all times. No potentially suicidal patient should be allowed to leave the emergency department before an evaluation is completed; all states have statutes permitting detention by physicians of individuals deemed to be dangerous to themselves or others. Mechanical restraints should be used only if they are necessary to protect the patient or health-care providers. Chemical restraints may inhibit psychiatric evaluation and should be avoided, if possible.

Following the medical management of a patient's overdose,

TABLE 230.1. SAD PERSONS Score

	Description	Points
S = Sex	Male	1
A = Age	<19 or >45 years old	1
D = Depression or hopelessness	Admits to depression or decreased concentration, appetite, sleep, libido	2
P = Previous attempts or psychiatric care	Previous attempt, or previous inpatient or outpatient psychiatric care	1
E = Excessive alcohol or drug use	Stigmata of chronic addiction or recent frequent use	1
R = Rational thinking loss	Organic brain syndrome or psychosis	2
S = Separated, divorced, or widowed	Recent or on anniversary	1
O = Organized or serious attempt	Well-thought-out plan or life-threatening presentation	2
N = No social supports	No close family, friends, job, or active religious affiliation	1
S = Stated future intent	Determined to repeat attempt, or ambivalent	2
		SCORE

Score	Risk
<6	Low
6–8	Intermediate
>8	High

injury, or associated medical problems, the patient's degree of depression and potential for suicide should be assessed. Many studies have attempted to identify patients likely to engage in self-destructive behavior. Although no combination of clinical characteristics has been found that accurately identifies all patients likely to manifest suicidal behavior, a number of high-risk characteristics have been isolated. For example, a young woman who takes a few aspirin after fighting with her boyfriend is usually at low risk for actually committing suicide; an elderly man who takes the same action on the anniversary of his wife's death is another matter. Most patients fall somewhere between these two extremes, and estimating any particular patient's risk for self-harm is often difficult.[11]

Several high-risk characteristics have been incorporated into the mnemonic SAD PERSONS, which can help the clinician assess potentially suicidal patients (Table 230.1).[3,7] In a nonintoxicated patient whose history can be corroborated by family or friends, the numerical SAD PERSONS score appears to be correlated closely with the need for hospitalization as determined by a psychiatrist after an in-depth evaluation. In one study, hospitalization was deemed necessary in almost all patients with a high SAD PERSONS score (greater than 8), in approximately half of patients with intermediate scores (6 to 8), and in almost none of the patients with low scores (less than 6).[3] While the SAD PERSONS score is a convenient tool to help organize, document, and communicate the assessment of a patient's suicide potential, a low score should not preclude emergent psychiatric consultation when the physician is uncomfortable with his or her assessment or when the patient requests to see a psychiatrist.

DISPOSITION

Potentially suicidal patients generally require admission to an inpatient psychiatric unit. Discharge from the emergency department should not be considered unless the following conditions have been met:

- The patient's injuries or associated medical problems do not necessitate hospitalization.
- The patient states that he or she is no longer suicidal, and is not intoxicated, demented, or psychotic.
- The acute precipitant of the crisis has been identified and, in some way, addressed.
- The patient has cooperated with an evaluation and is deemed to be at low risk for suicide. In general, nonpsychotic younger patients whose attempts involve low risk, high likelihood of rescue, and high manipulative intent can be discharged safely.
- Psychiatric consultation has been obtained (at least by telephone) and hospitalization has been judged unnecessary or inadvisable.
- Short-term outpatient follow-up (within 1 to 2 days) has been arranged. The reliability of such patients in scheduling and keeping follow-up appointments is poor. When emergency department personnel demonstrate a positive, supportive attitude and when the patient is given a scheduled outpatient follow-up appointment at the time of emergency department discharge, patient compliance with follow-up improves markedly.[4,5,9]
- The patient agrees to return to the emergency department immediately if further self-destructive urges arise.
- A positive, supportive environment with family or friends is available into which the patient can be released. Arrangements should be made to remove all pills, poisons, and weapons from the patient's home.

A potentially suicidal patient should not be transferred to another medical facility or to a psychiatrist's office unless accompanied by medical personnel or family members who have agreed to deliver the patient to the stated destination and to maintain close observation of the patient during transport.

COMMON PITFALLS

- "Accidental" trauma may be a manifestation of self-destructive behavior. When the stated mechanism of injury is questionable or inconsistent with the injury seen, a more in-depth evaluation of the patient's mental state and motives is warranted.
- The information obtained from a potentially suicidal patient must be corroborated with family or friends. Patients who vehemently deny suicidality, give abrupt answers to questions, or appear anxious to leave the emergency department may be committed to finishing the act they began.
- Anxiolytics, antidepressants, or any other potentially lethal medication should not be prescribed to patients who are depressed or potentially suicidal. More than half of patients who die by intentional overdose use a single prescription drug.

References

1. Cooper-Patrick L, Krum RM, Ford DE. Identifying suicidal ideation in general medical patients. *JAMA* 1994;272:1757.
2. Hirschfeld RM, Russell JM. Assessment and treatment of suicidal patients. *N Engl J Med* 1997;337:911.
3. Hockberger RS, Rothstein RJ. Assessment of suicide potential by non psychiatrists using the "SAD PERSONS" score. *J Emerg Med* 1988;6:99.
4. Jellinek M. Referrals from a psychiatric emergency room: relationship of compliance to demographic and interview variables. *Am J Psychiatry* 1978;135:209.
5. Knesper DJ. A study of referral failures for potentially suicidal patients: a method of medical care evaluation. *Hosp Commun Psychiatry* 1982;33:49.
6. Pallikkathayil L, Morgan SA. Emergency department nurses' encounters with suicide attempters: a qualitative investigation. *Scholar Inquiry Nurs Pract* 1988;237:2.
7. Patterson WM, Dohn HH, Brid J, et al. Evaluation of suicidal patients: the SAD PERSONS scale. *Psychosomatics* 1983;24:343.
8. Soukas J, Lonnquist J. Work stress has negative effects on the attitudes of emergency personnel towards patients who attempt suicide. *Acta Psychiatr Scand* 1989;474:79.
9. Spirito A. Emergency department assessment of adolescent suicide attempters: factors related to short-term follow-up outcome. *Pediatr Emerg Care* 1994;10:6.
10. Thienhaus OJ. Assessment of suicide risk. *Psychiatr Serv* 1997;48:293.
11. Tueth NJ. Predicting suicide in the emergency department. *Am J Emerg Med* 1996;14:434.
12. Verdick BM, Homes CB, Waln RF. Recognition of suicide signs by physicians in different areas of specialization. *J Med Educ* 1983;58:716.
13. Weissberg M. The meagerness of physicians' training in emergency psychiatric intervention. *Acad Med* 1990;65:747.

CHAPTER 231
Acute Psychiatric Illness in the Emergency Department

Douglas A. Rund and Philliph I. Bialecki

The prevalence of psychiatric illness in a typical emergency department population is significant. In some cases, the psychiatric illness is the basis of the primary complaint; in others, it is an associated condition. The major goals of the emergency physician's evaluation are immediate stabilization and patient restraint, as necessary; diagnosis of life-threatening medical conditions that present as abnormal thought and behavior; and determination of a disposition that effectively addresses the patient's medical and psychiatric needs.

ANXIETY DISORDERS

Anxiety is a prominent complaint in 10% to 15% of all medical outpatient visits. It is subjectively experienced as a terrible sense of apprehension, worry, and nervousness and is often accompanied by physical symptoms that reflect intense sympathetic activity (e.g., palpitations, dry mouth, dizziness, paresthesia, faintness, and exhaustion). Anxiety is a pathologic condition when the patient's physical and emotional responses surpass the normal response to a perceived threat, and can interfere with optimal functioning. Anxiety may be triggered by a specific source and thus may be expected when that source is present (i.e., cued anxiety). Sometimes, however, anxiety is free-floating; in such cases, anxiety attacks may be unexpected and occur without a recognizable cue (i.e., uncued anxiety).[2]

Most medical conditions are associated with some degree of anxiety, but certain conditions can present with anxiety as a predominant feature. Examples include hypoglycemia, pulmonary embolism, myocardial infarction, hypoxia, drug intoxication or withdrawal, caffeine toxicity, mitral valve prolapse, paroxysmal atrial tachycardia, thyrotoxicosis, pheochromocytoma, and carcinoid syndrome.[8] In addition, anxiety itself may cause comorbidity because its associated symptomatic responses create demands on previously impaired organ systems. Ruling out a primary or comorbid medical disorder is an important aspect of the initial and ongoing assessment. A focused history and physical examination initiate the assessment when medical illness or comorbidity is suspected. Screening laboratory tests typically include complete blood count, urinalysis, renal and hepatic studies, thyroid function tests, serum calcium and phosphorus tests, pulse oximetry, and a standard 12-lead electrocardiogram. Other tests can then be ordered, based on the findings of the initial evaluation.

DIFFERENTIAL DIAGNOSIS AND EMERGENCY DEPARTMENT EVALUATION

Anxiety that is not associated with general medical illness or substance abuse may be due to any of a number of reasonably well-defined disorders. The emergency physician should have a general understanding of the varying diagnostic criteria for these disorders, the generally used chronic treatment modalities, and the emergency department assessment and management of acute presentations.

Panic Attack

A panic attack is a sudden or "out of the blue" discrete period of intense fear or discomfort, in which at least four of the following symptoms develop abruptly and reach a peak within 10 minutes: (1) palpitations, pounding heart, or accelerated heart rate; (2) sweating; (3) trembling or shaking; (4) sensations of shortness of breath or smothering; (5) a feeling of choking; (6) chest pain or discomfort; (7) nausea or abdominal distress; (8) feeling dizzy, unsteady, light-headed, or faint; (9) derealization (a feeling of unreality) or depersonalization (being detached from oneself); (10) fear of losing control or going crazy; (11) fear of dying; (12) paresthesia; and (13) chills or hot flashes. Panic attacks can also be seen in association with any of the medical conditions previously discussed. These attacks are an extremely common psychiatric cause for presentation to the emergency department, with patients typically feeling unable to breathe or having atypical chest pain.

Panic attacks are the predominant feature of panic disorder, but also may be seen in depression, social phobia, simple phobia, and posttraumatic stress disorder (PTSD). Panic attacks associated with panic disorder and depression may occur without an associated trigger, the so-called unexpected or uncued panic attacks. Situational-bound or cued panic attacks occur immediately after exposure to, or in anticipation of, the specific situational trigger and are characteristic of social and specific phobias. A third type of panic attack is called situational-predisposed, which is most likely to occur when the patient is exposed to the situational trigger (cue) but is not invariably associated with the cue. In addition, it does not necessarily occur immediately after the exposure. Situational-predisposed attacks are most frequently seen in patients with panic disorder, but may, at times, occur in association with a specific or social phobia.

Panic Disorder

Panic disorder is characterized by four panic attacks per month, or recurrent, unexpected panic attacks that are followed by 1 month (or more) of persistent concern about having additional attacks, worry about the implications of the attacks or their consequences, or a significant change in behavior related to the attacks. The disorder may be associated with agoraphobia, which is an anxiety about being in places or situations from which escape might be difficult or embarrassing, or in which help may not be available if an unexpected or situational predisposed panic attack occurs. Agoraphobic fears typically involve characteristic clusters of situations that include being outside the home, being in a crowd or standing in a line, being on a bridge, and traveling in a bus, train, or car. The frequency and severity of the attacks vary, but the illness is generally chronic. Rates of suicide attempts among individuals with panic disorder have been found to be more than twice as high as those among patients with other psychiatric disorders, and 18 times higher than that occurring in a nonpsychiatric population.[14] Such comorbidity must be considered when treating such patients in the emergency department and deciding on their disposition.

Specific Phobia

Specific phobia is a marked and persistent fear that is excessive or unreasonable, cued by the presence of a specific object or situation (e.g., flying, heights, animals, receiving an injection, seeing blood). Exposure to the stimulus almost invariably provokes an immediate anxiety response, which may take the form of a situationally predisposed panic attack. In this disorder, the patient recognizes that the fear is excessive, but feels powerless to prevent it, except by avoiding the trigger. This "phobic avoidance" then significantly interferes with normal, routine occupational, social, or relationship functioning.

Social Phobia

Social phobia is similar to specific phobia, except that the cue or trigger involves a marked or persistent fear of one or more social or performance situations. Patients fear that they will act in a humiliating or embarrassing manner. The anxiety generated by this fear may lead to a situationally bound or predisposed panic attack.

Obsessive Compulsive Disorder

Patients with obsessive compulsive disorder suffer from obsessions or compulsions (most commonly, both). They usually recognize that their behavior is excessive or unreasonable and are distressed because their behavior causes marked impairment in everyday function. Obsessions are recurrent or persistent thoughts, impulses, or images that are experienced as intrusive and inappropriate and cause severe anxiety. These are not excessive worries about real-life problems, and the patient attempts to ignore, suppress, or neutralize them with other thoughts or actions. Patients recognize that the obsessional thoughts, impulses, or images are products of their own mind. Compulsions are repetitive behaviors (e.g., repetitive hand washing, ordering, or checking) or mental acts (e.g., repetitively praying or counting, or repeating words silently) that the patient feels driven to perform in response to an obsession, or according to rules that must be rigidly applied. This behavior significantly impairs normal functioning.

Posttraumatic Stress Disorder

Patients with PTSD have usually experienced or witnessed an event that involves actual or threatened serious personal injury, death, or a threat to the physical integrity of self or others. The response to such an event involves intense fear, helplessness, or horror. The traumatic event is typically reexperienced by either recurrent and intrusive recollections of the event or distressing dreams of the event. The patient may act or feel as if the event were recurring, or may experience intense psychological distress at exposure to internal or external cues that resemble some aspect of the event. Such feelings are then acted out by persistent avoidance of stimuli associated with the trauma and a general numbing of responsiveness to any event, related or not. Such patients manifest symptoms of increased arousal, with difficulty falling or staying asleep, irritability or outbursts of anger, difficulty concentrating, hypervigilance, or an exaggerated startle response. The diagnosis is made only if the disturbance has persisted for more than 1 month and has caused significant social or occupational dysfunction.

Acute Stress Disorder

Acute stress disorder is similar to PTSD, except that there is a closer temporal association between the traumatic event and the onset of symptoms, typically a period of less than 4 weeks. Patients experience dissociative symptoms during or immediately following the event. Symptoms may include a subjective numbing, detachment, or absence of emotional responsiveness; a reduction in awareness of the surrounding environment, such as "being in a daze"; feelings of derealization or depersonalization; and dissociative amnesia.

Generalized Anxiety Disorder

Patients presenting with generalized anxiety disorder display excessive anxiety and worry that occur on most days for at least 6 months. Patients have difficulty controlling the worry and have associated symptoms of restlessness or feeling on edge, fatigability, difficulty concentrating, irritability, muscle tension, or sleep disturbances. To classify the anxiety as a disorder, the symptom should significantly impair everyday functioning.

EMERGENCY DEPARTMENT MANAGEMENT AND DISPOSITION

Reassurance is the first-line intervention in patients with anxiety disorder. Patients should be assured that they are safe and that they are going to receive help. A firm, direct approach in a quiet, comfortable environment helps the patient feel secure and in better control. If a supportive interview does not work, pharmacologic intervention should be considered.

The benzodiazepines have long been considered the drugs of choice in the treatment of acute anxiety.[1] As a group, benzodiazepines are similar in their clinical effect, although they differ in pharmacokinetic properties. Short-acting benzodiazepines (half-life, 5 to 20 hours) include lorazepam (Ativan) and alprazolam (Xanax). The long-acting benzodiazepines (half-life, 20 to 200 hours) include diazepam (Valium), chlordiazepoxide (Librium), and clonazepam (Klonopin). These medications are usually effective for anxiety disorders.

When used chronically, however, benzodiazepines can cause physical dependence. Furthermore, when used acutely in the emergency department, administration of the medication can reinforce the belief that the only way to control anxiety is by the use of a chemical substance. The patient may subsequently turn to alcohol and nonprescription drugs when the prescription medication expires or no longer provides the needed relief. Patients may also begin to medicate themselves in anticipation of anxiety. This is often the beginning of a cycle of dependency.

For this reason, a new emphasis has been placed on the use of interpersonal psychotherapies, neurolinguistics, biofeedback, and behavior modification in the chronic management of such conditions.[14] Although not all forms of anxiety are successfully treated by such techniques, there is a growing attitude that they should be tried, because they often bring partial, if not total, relief of symptoms.

Propranolol and other beta blockers have been used to control the autonomic symptoms of anxiety, such as tremor, tachycardia, and palpitations. If such symptoms can be relieved, the anxiety itself often abates. Propranolol is the treatment of choice in mitral valve prolapse–associated panic attacks and in the prevention of performance anxiety or stage fright.

Selective serotonin reuptake inhibitors (SSRIs) are now commonly used for many anxiety disorders, such as generalized anxiety disorder and panic disorder, even in the absence of depression. This is generally a safe and effective alternative to benzodiazepine use. They require approximately 1 month to take effect, however, so the more rapidly acting benzodiazepines may be needed concurrently in the short term.

The high rate of suicide attempts among patients with panic disorders must be considered, especially because approximately half of those who attempt suicide by overdose do so by using medication prescribed within the week prior to the attempt. If benzodiazepines are prescribed, only a small quantity should be prescribed, and close follow-up and subsequent psychiatric evaluation should be arranged. More importantly, the patient should first be assessed for suicidal potential.

Administration of intravenous benzodiazepines is appropriate in two particular anxiety states. The first is the patient who is so anxious that a threat is posed to self or others, especially if there is a history of poor impulse control. The second indication involves nonpathologic anxiety states, such as in a patient ready to undergo a potentially painful emergency department procedure.[8] For such indications, lorazepam (Ativan), a short-acting benzodiazepine, can be given in doses of 0.5 mg every 20 minutes.

COMMON PITFALLS

- Assuming that an acutely anxious patient who is known to suffer from an anxiety disorder has no medical problem. Patients presenting with anxiety must be presumed to have a medical condition as the cause until it is ruled out by an appropriate emergency evaluation.
- Discharging the patient with anxiety disorder before suicidal and violence potential has been assessed. Patients who are actively suicidal, violent, or significantly disabled by their anxiety should be admitted to the hospital. Likewise, when the cause of acute anxiety is unclear, short-term admission for further medical and psychiatric evaluation should be considered.

SCHIZOPHRENIA AND OTHER PSYCHOTIC DISORDERS

Psychosis is the predominant clinical feature of schizophrenia and the other psychotic disorders. The central clinical feature of psychosis involves an impaired perception of reality. The psychotic patient incorrectly interprets internal and external stimuli, even when there is evidence to the contrary. Characteristic features of schizophrenia and similar disorders include delusions, hallucinations, disorganized speech, grossly disorganized (or catatonic) behavior, and abnormal affect.[3] Schizophrenic patients who have come to the emergency department may be actively hallucinating, delusional, or agitated. Such behavior is likely to have attracted the attention of family, friends, bystanders, bartenders, police, or a social worker who has brought the patient to the emergency department for evaluation.

Delusions are ideas that are fixed, false beliefs. The delusions of schizophrenia and related disorders are typically bizarre, patently false, and seem strange to others.[12] Persecutory and paranoid delusions may involve beliefs that the patient is being followed, watched, or controlled by machines or "outside forces." Patients may have somatic delusions ("my body is rotting away") or delusions of reference ("the television is talking about me"). Hallucinations are typically auditory and well organized. A voice may keep up an ongoing commentary on the person's behavior or thoughts, or voices may converse with one another. Such voices sometimes insult the patient about sexual topics or may instruct the patient to act in bizarre or even dangerous ways. The schizophrenic patient's speech can be incoherent or rambling and typically displays shifting of ideas without any apparent association (looseness of association). Behavior may be disorganized and may be manifested, among other ways, by a disheveled appearance. In schizophrenia, apparent emotion (affect) is impaired. *Flattened affect* refers to an apathetic or unemotional tone. Lack of volition or apparent thought (alogia) may also be present.

DIFFERENTIAL DIAGNOSIS AND EMERGENCY DEPARTMENT EVALUATION

There are several subtypes of schizophrenia, including paranoid, disorganized, catatonic, undifferentiated, and residual. Related psychotic disorders have been termed *schizophreniform disorder, schizoaffective disorder, delusional disorder,* and *brief psychotic disorder*. Detailed psychiatric evaluation is typically required to differentiate among these disorders.

The primary focus of emergency department evaluation is the differentiation of psychiatric illness from life-threatening medical conditions. Such conditions include meningitis, encephalitis, central nervous system hemorrhage, hypoglycemia, hypoxia, shock, hypertensive encephalopathy, poisoning (e.g., anticholinergic), and Wernicke encephalopathy. Other common medical conditions causing abnormal thought or behavior include drug intoxication or withdrawal, alcohol syndromes, liver or kidney failure, seizure, and ictal or postictal states. The suggested evaluation strategy for such entities is detailed in Chapter 229.

The psychiatric evaluation includes a brief interview consisting initially of open-ended or undirected questions about the patient's chief complaint or reason for being in the emergency department. The physician should be understanding, calm, and nonjudgmental. The patient's speech and behavior are observed for signs of disorganization, delusions, or hallucinations. The second phase of the interview involves some questioning about medical history, the onset of illness, previous psychoactive medications, psychiatric hospitalizations, and other psychiatric care. The mental status should be assessed as part of the evaluation for acute medical illness. This should include, at a minimum, an assessment of general appearance, level of consciousness, spontaneous speech, and orientation to time and place. Additional testing for memory, calculation, and judgment should also be performed, if possible. The third phase of the psychiatric interview involves a brief summary by the physician and a statement of the plan for subsequent management, for example, telling the patient that a psychiatrist will be called in to help with additional evaluation. Answers to the patient's questions should be clear, concise, and straightforward.

EMERGENCY DEPARTMENT MANAGEMENT AND DISPOSITION

The acutely psychotic patient needs psychiatric evaluation and, probably, hospitalization if the potential for violence or self-harm is suspected. The psychotic patient who expresses suicidal or self-harming thoughts or who has attempted suicide is at risk because he or she can exhibit unpredictable behavior in the immediate future.

New psychiatric symptoms (not caused by medical illness) or worsening symptoms (suggesting some kind of crisis or management failure) should ideally be managed in the emergency department by a psychiatrist.

Patients with chronic, stable psychiatric illness that is apparently under good control can probably be referred for outpatient management as circumstances dictate, but telephone consultation with the patient's psychiatrist may facilitate evaluation and help ensure adequate follow-up.

COMMON PITFALLS

- Missing a life-threatening medical condition that presents as abnormal thought and behavior
- Neglecting to consider suicidal potential. Patients with certain psychiatric illness have a much higher suicide rate than those without such illnesses. Psychiatric conditions that place a patient at risk for suicide include major depressive disorder, bipolar disorder, alcoholism, panic disorder, borderline personality disorder, and schizophrenia.
- Neglecting to consider the potential for violence. The psychotic patient can suddenly and unexpectedly become explosively violent.

ACUTELY AGITATED OR VIOLENT PATIENT

A patient presenting to the emergency department who manifests violent or potentially violent behavior represents a threat to the safety of other patients and staff members. Measures to bring such a situation under control must be instituted immediately and usually involve summoning security personnel or police. A "show of force" may quiet the agitated patient and may be sufficient to bring the situation under control. If this is not successful, physical restraint, involving the minimum force needed to control the patient, becomes necessary.

DIFFERENTIAL DIAGNOSIS AND EMERGENCY DEPARTMENT EVALUATION

The evaluation of the violent patient involves the differentiation of psychiatric from medical causes (Table 231.1) and, specifically, an assessment for potentially life-threatening medical illness. Vital signs, general appearance, and mental status examination are among the most helpful aspects of such an evaluation. The differentiation of psychiatric from medical disorders is discussed in Chapter 229.

Psychiatric illnesses associated with violent behavior include schizophrenia, affective disorder, personality disorders, adjustment disorders, and intermittent explosive disorder.

Schizophrenic Disorders

In psychotic episodes associated with the schizophrenic disorders, patients may react to stimuli unseen or unheard by the medical staff members. Violent outbursts may, therefore, be unexpected. Those with paranoid delusions may be attempting to protect themselves from others who are perceived as enemies. Mute and catatonic patients can be unpredictable and should be approached with caution.

TABLE 231.1. Diagnostic Considerations in the Evaluation of the Violent Patient

MEDICAL DISORDERS
Intoxication
Alcohol
Anticholinergics
Amphetamines
Barbiturates
Cocaine
Hallucinogens
Phencyclidine
Other drugs
Withdrawal
Alcohol
Barbiturates
Other drugs
Adverse Reaction to Prescribed Medication
Corticosteroids
Others
Metabolic Disorders
Hypoglycemia
Hyperthyroidism
Electrolyte imbalance
Anorexia
Infection
Sepsis
Meningitis
Encephalitis
Head Injury and CNS Hemorrhage
Seizure Disorders
PSYCHIATRIC DISORDERS
Schizophrenia
Affective Disorders
Mania
Personality Disorders
Antisocial
Borderline
Adjustment Disorders
Intermittent Explosive Disorder

Mania, Depression

Both mania and depression can be associated with hostile or violent behavior, but manic patients are more likely to present with agitated, hyperactive behavior. Such patients may become hostile if they feel their plans are being thwarted or they are not being taken seriously (e.g., being kept in the hospital away from things they need or want to do). Such persons may experience psychosis and may become visibly hostile. A show of force is often sufficient to suppress physical violence in these situations.

Antisocial Personality

Antisocial personality is often the diagnosis in those who have a history of lying, stealing, cheating, defying authority, pyromania, truancy, childhood aggression, excessive drinking, and substance abuse. It is not surprising, therefore, that such persons often are in prison or have a prison record. By definition, such patients feel little or no remorse for their actions, and so are among the most dangerous of hostile patients. They can be extremely difficult to manage because they often make promises to the staff but quickly break the agreement. Talking therapy is typically unsuccessful.

Adjustment Disorder

The essential feature of adjustment disorder is an emotional or behavioral response to a known psychosocial stressor. The response may include the symptom of anxiety, depression, or a disturbance in conduct, or some combination of these three. Disturbances in conduct result in a violation of the rights of others or of major age-appropriate societal norms and rules. Adjustment disorder is common, occurring in all age groups and in either gender equally. Talking with patients about the stressors in their lives and the options available to deal with them may help to avoid violent behavior.

Intermittent Explosive Disorder

Intermittent explosive disorder is a rare condition characterized by episodes of failure to resist aggressive impulses, resulting in serious assaultive acts or destruction of property. It is more common in men than in women. The degree of aggressiveness is out of proportion to any precipitating psychosocial stressor. The patient often feels remorseful or embarrassed by the violent outburst. The behavior usually causes significant impairment in both personal and work environments.

EMERGENCY DEPARTMENT EVALUATION AND PRECAUTIONS

Providing a safe physical setting minimizes the chance of harm by violent patients. This can be achieved only if the patient is quickly dispatched to an appropriate treatment area. Security personnel, the physician, and the head nurse should be notified. The use of a separate, isolated, quiet room tends to decrease the patient's agitation. The room should allow constant monitoring, either via shatterproof glass or a television camera. The room should be empty of any medical equipment and be sparsely furnished. Anything that could possibly be used by patients to harm themselves or others should be removed.

Both the history of the illness and the medical history are vital to accurate diagnosis. Other than the patient, who is often uncooperative, important sources of information include the patient's family and friends, paramedics, police, and possibly a mental health worker who knows the patient. Topics of particular relevance include the onset and course of agitated or violent symptoms, a history of previous threats or violence, a history of psychiatric illness, history of present drug or alcohol abuse, recent stressors, work-related problems, a family history of violence, or any childhood problems.

As in any life-threatening disease, the vital signs are among the most important parameters to assess. A brief, focused physical examination is helpful, when possible. On neurologic examination, any lateralizing signs may indicate an intracranial pathologic condition. Changes in pupil size or reactivity may indicate toxic ingestion. A brief mental status examination that assesses general appearance, affect, attention, language, orientation, and the presence of paranoid delusions, hallucinations, or other frankly psychotic symptoms is similarly helpful.

Any patient who requires an examination may need to be restrained first. The emergency department staff should be cautious, especially because physical contact is the most threatening form of interaction for an agitated patient. Considerable verbal reassurance may be required before an unrestrained patient submits to physical examination.

In addition to overtly violent behavior, indicators of possible violent actions by the patient include hostile behavior, verbal aggressiveness, statements about violent intent, or violent behavior immediately before arrival at the emergency department.

EMERGENCY DEPARTMENT MANAGEMENT

A presence of security officers conveys the message that aggressive behavior is not tolerated. Security staff members should be properly trained in their role, and they should not behave aggressively.

All staff members should be trained in the use of physical and chemical restraint before a crisis arises. The use of a code word to alert security, nursing, and physicians may be helpful. For example, calling for "Dr. Armstrong" when staff members feel that a patient is imminently dangerous can provide the same cohesive response provided by a trauma code in the appropriate setting.[11]

A threatening patient evokes many emotions, including fear, anger, disgust, and pity, among emergency department staff members. Their actions or attitudes may be perceived by the patient as a threat to an already fragile ego. The patient's personal space and boundaries should be respected initially. A reasonable amount of space between patient and staff members helps to protect the staff and does not threaten the patient unnecessarily. Space can be reduced as the patient deescalates and develops some trust that the staff is there to help and not to harm, threaten, or demean. Assuming a nonconfrontational physical posture and moving and speaking slowly help to create an atmosphere of safety. Direct eye contact should be avoided as much as possible. Active listening, especially in the beginning, allows the patient to vent and ultimately feel that the staff members are concerned.[9]

Active listening refers to a technique in which patients are allowed to talk, and their words are then fed back by the interviewer in a slightly different way. This allows patients to feel heard and provides the opportunity for them to hear their thoughts expressed in a more objective way. Using a patient's own language creates a feeling of empathy. A confident style of active listening helps to put the patient more at ease. The staff members provide safety by letting the patient know, through their own behavior, that they will maintain control and will not tolerate certain behaviors.

Patients who are most likely to require physical restraint include the intoxicated, the actively psychotic (especially those with paranoid delusions), the antisocial personalities, those who are manic, and those with nonpsychiatric causes of their behavior. The most common pitfall in the use of physical restraint is in hesitating to act after it becomes evident that restraint is needed. The use of physical restraint is humane, safe, legal, and ethically appropriate for patients who pose a threat to themselves or others. Physical restraint should be carried out in the same coordinated manner as a trauma or cardiac arrest code. A team of at least five staff members must act together under the direction of one experienced team leader. Each team member is responsible for control of one limb, preferably at the major joint, and the team leader is in control of the head.

In a coordinated effort, the team leader directs the staff while letting the patient know exactly what is happening. The less hesitation exhibited by the staff, the more safely restraint can be accomplished. Such coordination can be accomplished only when staff members are trained and practiced. A predesigned flowsheet aids in coordinating the team's actions and is an important source of documentation. Many patients feel calmer after being restrained, when uncontrollable impulses are diminished. Restraints are applied with the minimum amount of force necessary. The patient should be secured on his or her side if there is a danger of aspiration. A weapons search should immediately follow restraint, if one has not already been performed.

Physical restraint is often made unnecessary by effective chemical restraint, if it can be administered without risk to the patient or staff members. If physical restraint is the only option initially, once accomplished, it should be followed immediately by appropriate pharmacologic intervention.

The butyrophenones are the most widely used neuroleptic agents in the emergency department. Haloperidol (Haldol) has higher potency, is less sedating, and has a lower incidence of hypotension and cardiotoxic side effects than other neuroleptic agents.[5] A typical dose for chemical restraint or rapid treatment of psychosis is 5 mg intramuscularly every 30 to 60 minutes, up to a total of six doses in 24 hours. Most patients respond to one to three doses. Haloperidol is a Food and Drug Administration class C drug and, as such, is not recommended for use in pregnant or lactating women. The primary side effects are extrapyramidal syndrome (EPS), usually presenting as an acute dystonia that can be treated with benztropine (Cogentin) 1–2 mg IM or diphenhydramine 50 mg IM or IV. Some clinicians administer benztropine prophylactically with the first dose of halperidol. Neuroleptic malignant syndrome is a rare complication.

Benzodiazepines have been especially effective in manic patients and those with alcohol and drug intoxication. Lorazepam (Ativan), 2 mg intramuscularly, has gained favor in recent years. Using haloperidol 5 mg in combination with lorazepam 2 mg provides effective control of most acute symptoms in most situations.[6] The two can be mixed in the same syringe and be given as a single intramuscular injection.

Droperidol (Inapsine), given intramuscularly or intravenously, can also be used for chemical restraint. It works within minutes but has a shorter duration of activity than haloperidol (half-life, 2.2 hours vs. 10 to 19 hours). Droperidol is more sedating than haloperidol, and its major side effect is hypotension, which is usually transient but can be treated with the Trendelenburg position or intravenous fluids.[13] An often-missed side effect of both agents is akathisia, an intense sense of restlessness or inability to sit still. If determined to be present, it is best treated with a benzodiazepine or a beta blocker, both of which are preferred to an anticholinergic agent.

DISPOSITION

Any patient who is a threat to self or others may be involuntarily detained. The amount of time a patient may be detained without court intervention varies from state to state; all emergency physicians should be aware of the provisions of their state's laws. Heroic measures often lead to harm to patient and staff, and should be avoided. The patient should be allowed to leave if no organized restraint is immediately available. If a suicidal or homicidal patient does leave the emergency department, the physician is under an ethical and legal obligation to notify the police and any persons specifically threatened.

Most patients who require physical or chemical restraint require psychiatric consultation and admission to the hospital, usually through a psychiatrist, after nonpsychiatric illness has been excluded. The one common exception is the alcohol- or drug-intoxicated patient who, after being restrained, "sleeps off" the intoxication and is no longer violent or agitated.

The emergency physician is often under pressure from staff members, police, and family to make a quick disposition. Careful and conservative management is the best course to take with potentially violent patients. Even psychiatrists have been shown to be not particularly good at predicting future violence.[7] All patients who pose a threat to self or others, who are under the influence of alcohol or drugs, or who are actively psychotic should be detained until expert consultation directs otherwise.

COMMON PITFALLS

- Waiting for the agitated patient to become violent before intervening with physical or chemical restraint. The agitated patient who has not yet become violent is considerably easier to sedate than the actively violent patient.
- Assuming that agitation is due solely to a psychiatric condition. The use of physical or chemical restraint necessitates a more careful evaluation for the presence of a medical condition that may be responsible for abnormal behavior.

References

1. Abramowicz M. Drugs for psychiatric disorders. *Med Lett Drugs Ther* 1991;33:43.
2. American Psychiatric Association. *Diagnostic and statistical manual of mental disorders,* 4th ed. Washington, DC: American Psychiatric Press, 1994.
3. Bellack AS. *Schizophrenia—treatment, management, and rehabilitation.* New York: Grune & Stratton, 1984.
4. Bick PA, Hannah AL. Intramuscular lorazepam to restrain violent patients [Letter]. *Lancet* 1986;1:206.
5. Clinton JE, Sterner S, Stelmachers Z, et al. Haloperidol for sedation of disruptive emergency patients. *Ann Emerg Med* 1987;16:319.
6. Dubin WR. Rapid tranquilization: antipsychotics or benzodiazepines? *J Clin Psychiatry* 1988;49[Suppl]:12.
7. Dubin WR, Wilson SJ, Mercer C. Assaults against psychiatrists in outpatient settings. *J Clin Psychiatry* 1988;49:339.
8. Kercher E. Anxiety. Psychiatric aspects of emergency medicine. *Emerg Med Clin North Am* 1991;9:161.
9. Kercher E. Crisis intervention in the emergency department. Psychiatric aspects of emergency medicine. *Emerg Med Clin North Am* 1991;9:219.
10. Konikoff F, Kuritzky A, Jerushalmi Y, et al. Neuroleptic malignant syndrome induced by a single injection of haloperidol. *BMJ* 1984;289:1228.
11. Rice M, Moore G. Management of the violent patient. Psychiatric aspects of emergency medicine. *Emerg Med Clin North Am* 1991;9:13.
12. Rund DA, Hutzler J. *Emergency psychiatry.* Chicago: Mosby, 1983.
13. Thomas H, Schwartz E, Petrilli R. Droperidol versus haloperidol for chemical restraint of agitated and combative patients. *Ann Emerg Med* 1992;21:407.
14. Weissman MM. Suicidal ideation and suicide attempts in panic disorder and attacks. *N Engl J Med* 1989;321:18.
15. Goldberg RJ. *Practical guide to the care of the psychiatric patient,* 2nd edition, St. Louis, Mosby, 1998.

CHAPTER 232

Factitious Illness, Malingering, and Conversion Disorder

Jeffrey Dubin and Mark Smith

Factitious illness, malingering, and conversion disorder constitute a spectrum of medical conditions in which the patient's symptoms are false, pretended, or grossly exaggerated. The patient's symptoms may be voluntary (malingering and factitious illness) or may be an involuntary expression of an underlying psychological conflict (conversion disorder).[2] Distinguishing the physiologic conditions from the functional while addressing the patient's psychological issues is a test of the emergency physician's diagnostic acumen and therapeutic skill.

FACTITIOUS ILLNESS

CLINICAL PRESENTATION

Factitious illness is classified by the American Psychiatric Association according to whether the patient's presenting symptoms are psychological or physical.[2] In the syndrome of factitious illness with psychological symptoms, which is not discussed here, the patient presents with pretended psychological complaints, such as hallucinations, suicidal ideation, memory loss, or dissociative feelings.

The syndrome of factitious illness with physical symptoms is better known as Munchausen syndrome, named by Asher[3] after the character in a book who had a penchant for telling fabricated stories, based on an actual eighteenth-century, retired German cavalry officer. In the novel by Rudolf Raspe, the baron enjoyed a series of fanciful, fantastic, and fabricated adventures. Like the baron, the patient with Munchausen syndrome is often a peregrinating impostor, that is, a wanderer and a liar.

Munchausen patients are impostors who invent bizarre and often fantastic stories and accept painful and potentially dangerous procedures (e.g., cardiac catheterization, exploratory laparotomy) to reach their presumed goal: to become a patient admitted to the hospital. There seems to be no other secondary gain, thus distinguishing the Munchausen patient from the malingerer.

Munchausen patients typically present to the emergency department in a dramatic fashion, with a constellation of physical symptoms, plausibly suggesting the presence of substantial pathologic illness that is not present. Munchausen patients may simulate signs of disease (e.g., mixing a drop of their own blood into their urine sample) or actually induce a disease state in themselves (e.g., injecting exogenous material in themselves to produce fever and infection). They are typically young or middle-aged men (although the age range spans the pediatric to the geriatric), have a history of extensive travel, and report a medical history of previous hospitalizations and operations that have usually been performed in other cities. They are knowledgeable about hospital routines, but are often vague or inconsistent about medical details. Although Munchausen patients are clever, realistic, and facile in their simulation of clinical reality, the extent and severity of symptoms are often out of proportion to physical findings and demeanor, and may seem almost too classical in their constellation. Even about subjects other than their illness, Munchausen patients often exhibit pathologic lying (pseudologia fantastica).

Munchausen patients have been characterized as hostile, dependent persons with poor impulse control and a history of self-destructive behavior. They tend to be socially isolated, rarely are accompanied to the emergency department by friends or family, and, once admitted to the hospital, usually have no visitors. When confronted, they usually become hostile and querulous, deny the allegation of factitious illness, and sign out of the hospital against medical advice.

Munchausen patients simulate the broad spectrum of illnesses with varying degrees of authenticity. They may offer a history of advanced human immunodeficiency virus but have a normal physical appearance, or simulate life-threatening gastrointestinal hemorrhage or placenta previa.[4,5,13] The different and often fantastic clinical presentations of the Munchausen patient have been described as laparotomaphilia migrans, cardiopathic fantastica, neurologica diabolica, hyperpyrexia figmentatica, lithiasis nephrologica, dermatitis autogenica, and hemorrhagica histrionica.[3,9,10]

When parents falsify illness in their children, the disorder is termed *factitious disorder by proxy* (FDBP) or *Munchausen syndrome by proxy* (MBP). MBP describes abuse in which the perpetrator (most often the mother) is motivated by the desire to assume the sick role by proxy or to seek attention from the hospital staff. Whenever this diagnosis is considered, it is important to define the specific abuse to the child. FDBP refers to the context of the abuse and the disorder of the parent. FDBP is child abuse and should be treated as such.[11] FDBP often presents with apnea, cyanosis, and seizures (from smothering and poisonings) in infants, whereas older children frequently present with toxin-induced diarrhea and vomiting. Child protective services need to be involved in these cases, and inpatient admission may be warranted. Children may suffer permanent disability or death.[6]

Less likely to present to the emergency department is the patient, usually a young woman, and often a nurse, with a distinctive subtype of chronic factitious illness. In contrast to the typical Munchausen patient, these patients tend to have persistent unexplained symptoms accompanied by documented self-induced physical abnormalities. These patients often have stable social and professional lives, and they usually develop strong attachments to individual physicians as their "illnesses" persist over time. Their medical problems include self-induced infections, nonhealing wounds, fevers, endocrine disorders (e.g., from self-administration of insulin or thyroxine), water intoxication, anemia, and bleeding disorders (e.g., from self-administration of anticoagulants).[1] Admission to the hospital is sometimes required to observe the patient in a controlled environment.

DIFFERENTIAL DIAGNOSIS

Munchausen syndrome must be distinguished from organic disease and malingering, and from three conditions in which the production of nonorganically based symptoms is not voluntary: conversion disorder, somatization disorder, and hypochondriasis.

In the absence of explicit evidence to the contrary, the clinician should presume that there is an organic basis for the patient's complaints. When the patient fits the pattern of presentation for Munchausen syndrome, however, evidence should be sought to confirm or disprove that suspicion.

An accurate delineation of the patient's medical history is generally the most useful information for making the diagnosis. The patient commonly relates a history of previous hospitalizations and physician contacts, all of which need to be either confirmed or identified as false. This activity may require a dogged devotion to tracking down medical records at other hospitals and contacting the patient's previous physicians, many of whose names are misrepresented.

In contrast to the Munchausen patient, the malingerer has a clearly understandable external incentive and goal other than wanting to be a patient (e.g., to receive room and board, to receive drugs, to avoid work). Once that goal is met, the feigned illness resolves. Malingering may overlap with Munchausen syndrome in that a component of drug-seeking behavior exists in both; a substantial percentage of Munchausen patients want, as a secondary goal, to acquire narcotic analgesics.[12]

In the three somatoform disorders (conversion disorder, somatization disorder, and hypochondriasis), the patient's symptoms are neither consciously willed nor voluntary. Conversion disorder is discussed in subsequent paragraphs. The patient with somatization disorder has a chronic history of multiple symptoms involving different organ systems in a fluctuating and recurrent pattern that is not adequately explained by a physical disorder. The hypochondriacal patient presents with fear and concern about the presence of disease and, despite reassurance, misinterprets normal bodily sensations and physical signs as pathologic conditions.

EMERGENCY DEPARTMENT MANAGEMENT

Until a diagnosis of Munchausen syndrome is confirmed, the patient should be treated as if an organically based disease is present. The usual diagnostic and therapeutic procedures should be followed.

If Munchausen syndrome is suspected but not confirmed, the physician may treat the patient in a modified manner (e.g., withhold large doses of morphine in patients with persistent chest pain and a normal electrocardiogram).

When Munchausen syndrome is confirmed, the patient should be managed with the goal of ameliorating symptoms. The physician may elect to confront the patient in a supportive and nonthreatening manner, although the establishment of a therapeutic alliance between patient and physician is unlikely.

Patients who are labeled with Munchausen syndrome can still become organically ill. Procedures that have been performed because of their imposture may predispose them to real illness (e.g., a small bowel obstruction may occur as a result of adhesions from a previous exploratory laparotomy for abdominal pain). Other patients may need medical treatment for self-induced physical ailments. The physician must not neglect to care for these patients because of their underlying psychopathologic condition.

DISPOSITION

If any doubt exists about the diagnosis of Munchausen syndrome and if the purported illness warrants admission, the patient should be admitted to the hospital for further evaluation. If the diagnosis of Munchausen syndrome is certain, however, the patient should be denied admission to the hospital for the presenting complaint. The refusal can be couched in medical terms (e.g., stating that the chest pain is noncardiac in nature), or the physician may confront the patient gently with the fact that there is a history of imposture. The physician may offer the option of psychiatric care, although it is likely to be refused.

MALINGERING

CLINICAL PRESENTATION

Malingering is the voluntary and conscious presentation of false and exaggerated physical or psychological symptoms in pursuit of a recognizable goal. Such goals typically include avoiding work or other unpleasant obligations, obtaining shelter, obtaining controlled substances, or obtaining financial compensation through litigation. Malingerers may either exaggerate or invent symptoms.

In contrast to factitious illness, in malingering, the goal is clear and understandable, the behavior is conscious and situationally appropriate, and the symptoms abate once the goal is attained.

Malingerers present to the emergency department with a variety of demands or complaints. Some patients who complain of migraine headache, renal colic, or sickle cell crisis are seeking narcotic analgesics. The evaluation of renal colic may be impeded by an inability of the patient to void under direct observation or by a volunteered history of allergy to intravenous contrast media. Other individuals may present to the emergency department after missing several days or even weeks of work and request a retroactive "sick slip" because of a medical problem, the presence of which is difficult to document definitively. Patients who have been in minor motor vehicle accidents may present with exaggerated symptoms of cervical or lumbar strain in an effort to document damages and collect financial compensation.

Patients with underlying psychiatric disorders may feign exacerbations of mood and thought disorders in order to be hospitalized for secondary gain. As many as one-fourth of emergency department psychiatric visits may represent malingering. These patients can be difficult to evaluate; often, they are admitted to the psychiatric service with a comorbid psychiatric diagnosis, with malingering strongly suspected.[18]

DIFFERENTIAL DIAGNOSIS

Malingering is suggested if the patient overdramatizes complaints, symptoms, or physical signs; overreacts during the physical examination; is uncooperative during the diagnostic evaluation; declines to appear when scheduled for diagnostic testing; or is reluctant to accept a favorable prognosis. The history, physical examination, and laboratory data may not support the severity of the patient's complaints, particularly those that lack objective correlates for diagnosis (e.g., migraine headache). During their evaluation, some patients may reveal their true objectives (e.g., a prescription for narcotic analgesics or a medical excuse from work).

Patients apparently suffering an acute neuromuscular syndrome may complain of symptoms that do not fit an anatomically consistent pattern or may exhibit weakness during testing that is belied by their ability to carry out other activities when they are not being examined. Patients complaining of low back strain may demonstrate a large disparity between the "straight leg-raise" test performed in a sitting versus supine position, and, while in the supine position, the patient may not make an appropriate effort at raising the affected leg (detectable by placing a hand under the contralateral heel and feeling for the expected downward pressure associated with true effort).

If drug-seeking behavior is suspected, telephone contact with other emergency departments or a review of past medical records may reveal that the patient has exhibited a suspicious pattern of similar behavior.

EMERGENCY DEPARTMENT MANAGEMENT

Because the malingering patient may become defensive, angry, and hostile when confronted with the suspicion that the symptoms are false or exaggerated, the physician is often tempted to comply with the patient's demands rather than risk a confrontation. Furthermore, the diagnosis of malingering can rarely be made with complete certainty. Because each patient reacts to illness or injury differently, the degree of volition or willfulness that underlies the patient's exaggeration of symptoms is not always clear.

Perhaps the most prudent way to deal with a suspected malingerer is to give the patient a minimal amount of gratification and to invoke general rules or established policies that prevent the physician from filling the patient's demands completely. It is worthwhile to record on the patient's chart suspicions or questions about the patient so that the next treating physician is aware of the concerns. In flagrant cases, neighboring emergency departments should be contacted.

DISPOSITION

The usual criteria for admission to the hospital should apply, depending on the patient's complaint. If the physician is convinced that the patient is malingering, a firm stand should be taken against admission, despite the patient's wishes, although there are times when, in order to avoid a disruptive confrontation, it may be more prudent to admit the patient to the hospital and allow the details to be sorted out later.

CONVERSION DISORDER

CLINICAL PRESENTATION

Patients with conversion disorder present with physical symptoms that are not under voluntary control, that cannot be explained as a manifestation of a physical disorder or on the basis of a pathophysiologic mechanism, and that are unconscious expressions of underlying psychological conflict. Often, these symptoms are immediately preceded by an acute psychological stress, and that precipitant should be sought. Conversion disorder was previously called "hysterical neurosis, conversion type."

The most typical conversion symptoms involve loss of neurologic function: blindness, aphonia, pseudoseizures, paralysis, anesthesia, tunnel vision, gait abnormality, unresponsiveness, and amnesia.[14] The conversion disorder symptom usually has a sudden onset. *La belle indifférence,* an attitude of relative unconcern despite the seriousness of the symptom, may be present, but its diagnostic importance is minimal. Patients with conversion disorder may also present with vomiting or symptoms of pregnancy (pseudocyesis).

The diagnosis of conversion disorder depends on demonstrating that the patient's symptoms are not due to organically based malfunction. With most neurologic presentations of conversion disorder, this is not difficult, because the patient's deficits usually do not make neuroanatomic sense. The physician's knowledge of neuroanatomy is usually better than the patient's; moreover, the patient is not consciously trying to fool the physician.

Typical "mistakes" made by the conversion disorder patient with neurologic symptoms include the following:

Acute onset of sensory loss in a sharp stocking-glove pattern (although this may be mimicked by the peripheral neuropathies of diabetes or alcoholism, and vascular lesions such as aortic dissection or subclavian vein thrombosis)

Complete paralysis and sensory loss of one leg, with preservation of deep tendon reflexes and antigravity muscle activity

Hemianesthesia without contralateral pain–temperature loss or with nonanatomic midline splits in vibratory sensation

Complete loss of motor function on one side of the body, with inability to turn the head to the side of paralysis (indicating contralateral sternocleidomastoid muscle dysfunction)

Pseudoseizures: seizure-type movements unaccompanied by characteristic electroencephalographic (EEG) patterns. Patients with a true seizure disorder may also experience pseudoseizures. Features suggestive of pseudoseizures include the presence of fluttering eyelids, thrashing of extremities or side-to-side head movement, dramatic vocalizations, and evidence of responsiveness to environmental stimuli during an apparent grand mal seizure. In addition, there is typically absence of tongue biting, incontinence, physical injury, or postictal depression. Differentiating a pseudoseizure from a true seizure can be difficult; for example, a complex partial seizure, with its seemingly purposeful behavior, may be mistakenly identified as a pseudoseizure.[8]

Cogwheel response on manual muscle testing[6,17]

Slowness of motion. Patients with nonorganic muscle weakness may exhibit a general slowing of motor movements, not realizing that certain tests require more strength when performed slowly (e.g., deep knee squat).[16]

Inconsistencies in physical signs during unresponsiveness. The patient with nonorganic unresponsiveness often does not permit an upraised and suspended arm to strike the face when released, but rather allows it to glide harmlessly over the face (note that substantial injury can occur to the nose and mouth if the arm does drop directly onto them). Such a patient often vigorously resists manual eye opening by the physician; if opened, the eyes may be closed actively, in contrast to the smooth, effortless glide seen in the organically unresponsive patient.[16]

Nonorganically unresponsive patients always demonstrate both the fast and slow components of nystagmus on oculovestibular stimulation (cold calorics). Patients with a cortical lesion but an intact brainstem show only tonic deviation of the eyes; patients without either cortical or brainstem function show no deviation of the eyes whatsoever.

Inconsistencies in blindness. The patient for whom blindness is a conversion symptom demonstrates a remarkable ability to avoid injury and misstep. For patients complaining of tunnel vision, the visual field extending into space may be described as cylindrical rather than cone-shaped.

Nonneurologic presentations of conversion disorder are uncommon. Persistent unexplained vomiting may be a manifestation of revulsion and disgust; a psychological conflict that triggered the symptom should be sought. False pregnancy can be confirmed with a negative pregnancy test; the task is then to assess the patient's underlying psychiatric diagnosis.

DIFFERENTIAL DIAGNOSIS

Conversion disorder must be distinguished from organic illness, malingering, and Munchausen syndrome, as well as from somatization disorder and hypochondriasis.

The tendency should be strongly resisted to diagnose conversion disorder in any patient with vague symptoms. Up to 30% of patients who, at some time, have been given a diagnosis of conversion disorder are eventually found to have organic disease that could explain these symptoms.[7] Illnesses such as systemic lupus erythematosus, multiple sclerosis, and hyperthyroidism may present in the emergency department as subtle perturbations of physical functions; hypoglycemia can present in myriad different guises.

The diagnosis of conversion disorder should not be made solely on the basis of a negative organic workup; the precipitating emotional stress and the unconscious conflict that the symptoms are designed to solve must be identified.[9]

Patients with conversion disorder lack the characteristic features of the Munchausen patient: There is no tendency to submit to multiple procedures, and there is a lack of sophistication with respect to medical terminology. Unlike the malingering patient, there is no conscious fabrication of illness or disability.

EMERGENCY DEPARTMENT MANAGEMENT

Patients with conversion disorder must be handled delicately, deftly, and with respect. It is unacceptable to confront the patient with an assertion or proof that the illness is faked or not real. The patient should be told that, although the symptoms are bothersome, they do not appear to be manifestations of a serious illness. Symptoms can sometimes be relieved by planting the suggestion that they will improve over the next several hours. Patients with aphonia can be told that they will be able to whisper; patients with paralysis can be told that they will begin to experience movement in their toes.

Simultaneously, the physician can probe for underlying psychosocial conflicts that might have led to the appearance of the symptom. Hypnosis may aid in identifying the underlying emotional conflict. An amobarbital interview may be useful in the management of the psychogenically unresponsive patient and in certain types of discrete conversion disorder.[15]

DISPOSITION

The neurologic consultant may assist the physician in differentiating organic from nonorganic illness. If the diagnosis of conversion disorder is secure and the patient's symptoms persist and prevent the patient from carrying out the activities of ordinary living, a psychiatric consultant may assist in the process of symptom resolution in the emergency department, using talk therapy, hypnosis, or amobarbital.

Many patients with conversion disorder experience resolution of their physical symptoms during their emergency department stay, but some require admission to the hospital. If the diagnosis of conversion disorder is uncertain and if the presenting symptom could signify dangerous illness, hospital admission is warranted. Even when the diagnosis of conversion disorder is clear, patients whose manifestations persist and who cannot manage on their own (e.g., psychogenic unresponsiveness or paralysis) require inpatient care.

COMMON PITFALLS

- Failing to appreciate that the patient has an unusual presentation of an organic illness
- Permitting unpleasant aspects of the patient's personality to result in dismissal of the patient's problem as "psychogenic"
- Inadequately distinguishing among malingering, conversion disorder, and Munchausen syndrome
- Classifying all patients with symptoms having no discernible anatomic cause as "crocks"
- Losing interest in caring for the patient once it has been determined that the patient's symptoms are not organically based

References

1. Aduan RP, Fauci AS, Dale DC, et al. Factitious fever and self-induced infection. *Ann Intern Med* 1979;90:230.
2. American Psychiatric Association. *Diagnostic and statistical manual of mental disorders,* 4th ed. Washington, DC: American Psychiatric Press, 1994.
3. Asher R. Munchausen's syndrome. *Lancet* 1951;1:339.
4. Byard RW, Beal SM. Munchausen syndrome by proxy: repetitive infantile apnoea and homicide. *J Paediatr Child Health* 1993;29:77.
5. Dickson H, Cole A, Engel S, et al. Conversion reaction presenting as acute spinal cord injury. *Med J Aust* 1984;141:428.
6. Duffy TP. The Red Baron. *N Engl J Med* 1992;327:408.
7. Ifudu O, Kolanski SI, Friedman EA. Brief report: kidney-related Munchausen's syndrome. *N Engl J Med* 1992;327:388.
8. Kounis NG. Munchausen syndrome with cardiac symptoms, cardiopathia fantastica. *Br J Clin Pract* 1979;33:67.
9. Lazare A. Conversion symptoms. *N Engl J Med* 1981;305:745.
10. Manolis AS, Sanjana VM. Cardiopathia fantastica and arteritis factitia as manifestations of Munchausen syndrome. *Crit Care Med* 1987;15:526.
11. Meadow R. Fictitious epilepsy. *Lancet* 1984;2:25.
12. Mendel JG. Munchausen's syndrome: a syndrome of drug abuse. *Compr Psychiatry* 1974;15:69.
13. Perry JC, Jacobs D. Overview: clinical applications of the Amytal interview in psychiatric emergency settings. *Am J Psychiatry* 1982;139:552.
14. Samuels MP, Southall DP. Munchausen syndrome by proxy. *Br J Hosp Med* 1992;47:759.
15. Swartz MS, McCracken J. Emergency room management of conversion disorders. *Hosp Commun Psychiatry* 1986;37:828.
16. Trimble MR. Pseudoseizures. *Neurol Clin North Am* 1986;4:531.
17. Warden RE, Johnson EW, Burk RD. Diagnosis of hysterical paralysis. *Arch Phys Med* 1961;4:122.
18. Watson CG, Buranen C. The frequency and identification of false-positive conversion reactions. *J Nerv Ment Dis* 1979;167:243.
19. Weintraub MI. Hysteria, a clinical guide to diagnosis. *Clin Symp* 1977;29.
20. Zuger A, O'Dowd MA. The Baron has AIDS: a case of factitious human immunodeficiency virus infection and review. *Clin Infect Dis* 1992;12:211.

SECTION V

Section Editor: Phyllis Hendry Stenklyft

Pediatrics

PART I
Resuscitation

CHAPTER 233
Newborn Resuscitation

Brian P. Gilligan

Approximately 5% to 10% of all newborns require resuscitation following birth to establish spontaneous respirations.[1,6] However, newborns delivered in or transported to the emergency department are considered high risk, and nearly 40% receive some form of resuscitation.[7] Fortunately, the majority of these infants will respond to simple maneuvers such as drying, suctioning, oxygen, and gentle stimulation. Occasionally, more invasive resuscitation efforts are required. The key to successful neonatal resuscitation in the emergency department is to anticipate the special needs of the newborn, organize equipment, and prepare personnel to deliver appropriate, timely care.

PATHOPHYSIOLOGY

The goal of newborn resuscitation is to facilitate the transition from fetal to extrauterine life. Prior to delivery, fetal lungs are fluid-filled, gas exchange occurs through the placenta, and intra- and extra-cardiac circulation shunts blood through the foramen ovale and ductus arteriosis, largely bypassing the left side of the heart and lungs. After clamping the umbilical cord and the newborn's first breath, physiologic changes occur to allow survival in the extrauterine environment.

During the first initial respirations, fetal lung fluid is displaced, functional residual capacity is established, and pulmonary vascular resistance decreases. Clamping of the umbilical cord leads to increased systemic vascular resistance, resulting in closure of the foramen ovale and ductus arteriosis. The combination of these events leads to increased pulmonary blood flow and the establishment of normal extrauterine circulation. This normally smooth transition can be precluded by antepartum events that cause asphyxia.[1]

There are many factors associated with neonatal asphyxia, but all asphyxiated newborns undergo a well-defined sequence of events. Initial deprivation of oxygen leads to a period of rapid breathing, followed by progressive bradycardia, decreased neuromuscular tone, and, finally, primary apnea.[2,7] Oxygen and stimulation will induce spontaneous respirations in most newborns at this stage. If asphyxia continues, however, irregular gasping respirations occur with profound bradycardia, hypotension, and flaccidity until the infant takes his or her last gasp and enters into secondary apnea. Once secondary apnea occurs, death is imminent unless resuscitation with assisted ventilation and oxygen is initiated. From a practical standpoint, it is difficult to distinguish primary from secondary apnea; therefore, all apneic newborns are assumed to be in secondary apnea and are treated with ventilatory assistance.

EMERGENCY DEPARTMENT EVALUATION AND MANAGEMENT

Resuscitation of the newborn follows an orderly approach based on heart rate (HR), respiratory effort, and color. Though most newborns do not require invasive resuscitation, all should receive certain interventions (drying, warming, positioning, suctioning, and stimulation). Of those who require more advanced resuscitation, the majority will respond to supplemental oxygen or bag-valve-mask (BVM) ventilation. Very few infants require chest compressions, endotracheal intubation, or drugs for successful resuscitation.[4] It is helpful to remember the inverted pyramid concept when encountering a newborn resuscitation (Fig. 233.1). Following this stepwise approach, excessive morbidity can be prevented by avoiding unnecessary procedures.

Although most emergency department resuscitations occur without notice, adequate preparations can be made, specifically in the areas of equipment and personnel assignments that can facilitate the resuscitation process. It cannot be overemphasized that due to the abrupt, unexpected nature of emergency department resuscitations, unless equipment is meticulously organized and readily available, even the most sophisticated personnel will be unable to perform successful newborn resuscitations.

Preparation

Preparation for newborn resuscitation can be divided into two phases: (1) the remote phase (prior to notification of an impending birth) and (2) the immediate phase (after such notification).

Remote Preparation

Table 233.1 outlines equipment that should be maintained in every emergency department and readily accessible at all times. It is convenient to organize certain items in a newborn resuscitation tray. Equipment and drug cards containing correct equipment sizes and drug doses for different-sized newborns (full-term, premature) are also helpful. A radiant warmer should be kept on at all times, and personnel skilled in newborn resuscitation should be available. The American Heart Association and the American Academy of Pediatrics sponsor a neonatal resuscitation course, and the Pediatric Advanced Life Support course includes a newborn lecture and skill station.

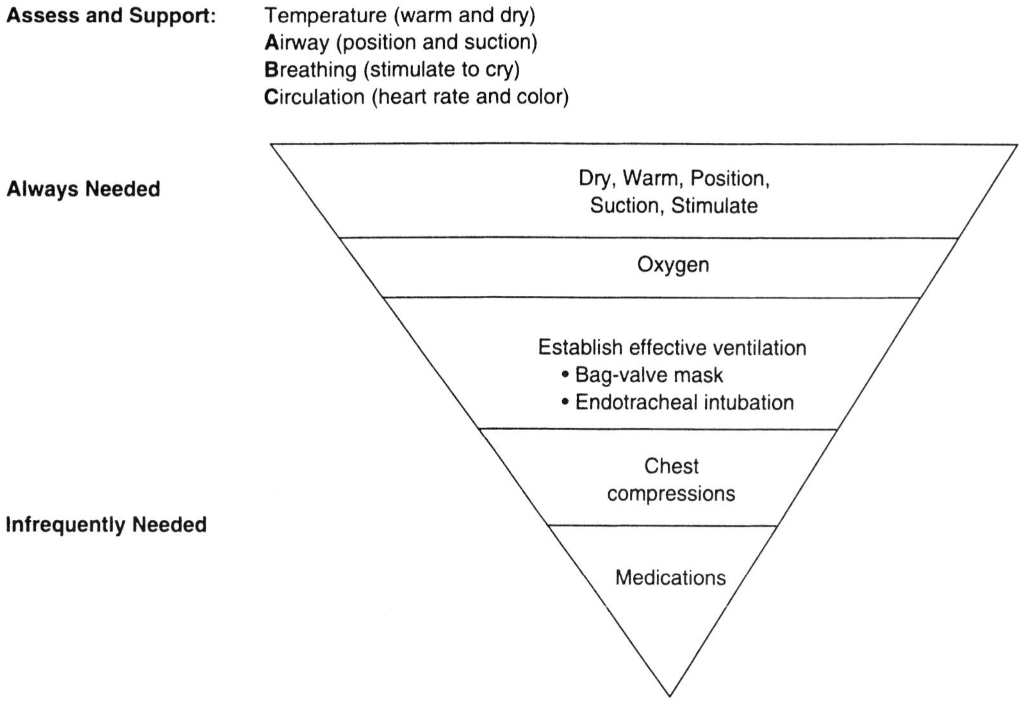

Figure 233.1. The reverse pyramid graphically represents the relative frequency that various modalities are needed to successfully resuscitate a newborn. Note that very few infants actually require the most invasive intervention, and most infants respond to noninvasive procedures. (Adapted from American Heart Association, American Academy of Pediatrics. Neonatal resuscitation. In: *Textbook of pediatric advanced life support*. Dallas: American Heart Association, 1997.)

Immediate Preparation

The resuscitation of a severely depressed and asphyxiated newborn requires at least two people: one to ventilate (and intubate) and the other to monitor HR (and perform chest compressions). If a prolonged resuscitation is required, the assistance of a third person, to insert intravascular catheters and administer medications, is highly desirable. Assignments must be made quickly, and personnel must adhere to their assigned duties.

Although there is little time for an in-depth history, specific information is useful in preparing for resuscitation. Questions should be addressed concerning multiple gestations, gestational age, and the presence of meconium. A history of maternal drug use and vaginal bleeding may also be helpful. This information will alert personnel to the specific needs of the newborn and allow time for additional preparation, if necessary (Table 233.2).

TABLE 233.1. Neonatal Resuscitation Equipment

Radiant warmer, warm blankets, gowns, infant caps
Suction, suction catheters (5F, 8F, 10F)
Resuscitation bags (250 mL for premature only, 450 mL, 750 mL)
Face masks (premature, newborn, infant sizes)
Laryngoscope with Miller (straight) blades (no. 0 and 1)
Medications (epinephrine, naloxone, dextrose, bicarbonate)
Volume expanders (normal saline, Ringer's lactate, O^- blood)
Gowns, gloves, masks, eye protection (universal precautions)
The following can be organized into a specific newborn tray:
Bulb syringe, tape, scissors
Endotracheal tubes with stylet (2.5, 3.0, and 3.5 mm)
Umbilical catheter with insertion kit (3.5F and 5.0F)
Three-way stopcock, syringes (10 cc)
Obstetric kit/umbilical cord cutting materials
Meconium aspirator

Assessment

Immediately following birth, all newborn infants should undergo the same initial assessment and basic resuscitation. It should be emphasized that several interventions may occur simultaneously and not in isolated, consecutive steps. For newborns delivered out of hospital who present vigorous and crying, the same initial assessment should be followed. When newborns deliver out of hospital but present intubated or with cardiorespiratory depression, airway management is the immediate priority, followed by the remaining steps of newborn resuscitation.

The initial phase of newborn resuscitation involves preventing heat loss, opening the airway, and evaluating the infant in terms of respiratory effort, HR, and color.[2] These steps must be done quickly, so that more advanced resuscitation efforts can be performed if required.

Initial Resuscitation

On delivery, the umbilical cord is clamped and cut, and the newborn is placed under a radiant warmer. Unless meconium is present, the newborn is thoroughly dried with warm blankets to prevent heat loss and stimulate spontaneous respirations. Wet blankets should be removed immediately. The infant is positioned supine, with a rolled towel under the shoulders, and head midline. This will facilitate optimal opening of the airway in the slightly extended neck position. Suctioning of the mouth, then the nose can be accomplished with a bulb syringe or mechanical suction device. If mechanical suction is used, negative pressure should not exceed 100 mm Hg, and is used for only 3 to 5 seconds to prevent vagally mediated apnea and bradycardia. If further stimulation is required, gently rubbing the back or flicking the soles of the feet can be effective. Following this process, evaluation of respiratory effort, HR, and color are performed.

TABLE 233.2. Significant Maternal History

History	Newborn Significance
1. Prematurity	Most require intubation
2. Multiple gestations	Multiple resuscitation set-ups; more personnel are needed.
3. Meconium	Suction hypopharynx/trachea before stimulation
4. Maternal drug (opiate) abuse	Avoid naloxone; it may precipitate withdrawal signs (seizures).
5. Maternal opiate administration	Consider naloxone for respiratory depression.
6. Maternal bleeding	May require fluid resuscitation

Spontaneous *respiratory effort* is adequate if the infant is able to improve color and maintain HR above 100 beats/min.[6] Following delivery, most infants respond to the tactile stimulation of the extrauterine environment by crying and gradually become pink. Some infants, however, require additional brief stimulation and 100% blow-by oxygen. Infants who are outright apneic or have gasping respirations require BVM ventilation with 100% oxygen. Institution of BVM ventilation should not be delayed by providing prolonged stimulation and blow-by oxygen. Once the respiratory effort has been evaluated and appropriately managed, HR can be assessed.

HR is determined by ausculting the chest, feeling the brachial pulse, or, most conveniently, palpating the base of the umbilical cord. In the uncompromised infant, the HR should remain greater than 100 beats/min. HR less than 100 needs to be closely monitored and BVM ventilation initiated (or continued). If the HR remains less than 60 to 100, further interventions with chest compressions or medications may be required.

The *color* of a healthy newborn will remain pink without supplemental oxygen. Acrocyanosis, or peripheral cyanosis, is not an unusual finding at birth. It is thought to occur secondary to cold stress and initially sluggish circulation, not to hypoxemia.[2] True cyanosis, or central cyanosis, is determined by examining central structures and mucous membranes. Infants with central cyanosis, regardless of HR and respiratory effort, require supplemental oxygen and, generally, BVM ventilation and endotracheal intubation.

The Distressed Newborn

Following the initial assessment and resuscitation, there are two general outcomes that occur. The newborn is either vigorous and requires no further intervention other than close observation and postresuscitation care, or the newborn is distressed, mandating further resuscitative efforts. One situation that precludes normal resuscitation is that of the infant born with meconium in the amniotic fluid.

Meconium staining of the amniotic fluid generally implies fetal distress. It is found in 8% to 20% of all deliveries, predominantly in small for gestational age (SGA) and postterm stressed newborns.[1] The clinical concern is to avoid meconium aspiration, with the resultant complications of meconium aspiration syndrome (hypoxemia, acidosis, and persistent fetal circulation). Interventions are aimed at depressed newborns and those born with thick, particulate meconium. Controversy exists over whether a vigorous baby with meconium-stained fluid requires tracheal suctioning.[5,6]

Clearing meconium from the airway begins with the delivery of the head, at which time a 10F or greater catheter is used to suction the mouth, pharynx, and nose. Following delivery, the infant is placed on the radiant warmer and care taken to avoid stimulation. The hypopharynx is suctioned under direct visualization on all infants exposed to meconium who are depressed and in any infant passing thick, particulate meconium. The trachea is then intubated and meconium suctioned from the lower airway. Repeat intubation and suctioning can be performed until meconium is no longer recovered, provided the infant's HR remains above 60 beats/min.[6] Unless vigorous, most infants will remain intubated, requiring positive-pressure ventilation (PPV). Following tracheal suctioning, the infant should be dried, warmed, and stimulated like other infants.

Distressed newborns require ongoing resuscitation. Following the initial evaluation, any infant who has apnea, gasping respirations, HR less than 100, or persistent central cyanosis requires BVM ventilation with 100% oxygen at 40 to 60 breaths per minute. Initial breaths may require 30 to 40 cm H_2O pressure to establish adequate lung volumes, but all subsequent breaths should be delivered at the lowest possible pressure. Good chest rise should be observed; if not, reposition the infant's head and attempt ventilation again. It is important to ensure a good seal between the mask and the infant's face. Placement of an orogastric tube, to prevent gastric distension, will be necessary if more than 2 minutes of BVM ventilation is required. After 30 seconds of PPV, the HR should be evaluated.

The HR is an internal monitor of ventilation adequacy. If the HR is greater than 100, observe for spontaneous, effective respirations and discontinue PPV. If the HR is 60 to 100 and increasing, continue PPV and reassess the HR in 2 to 3 minutes. A HR that is 60 to 80 and not increasing requires continued PPV and chest compressions. When the HR is less than 60 after the initial 30 seconds of PPV, or if, at any time, the HR is absent, chest compressions should accompany PPV with 100% oxygen.[2]

There are two acceptable techniques for neonatal chest compressions. Both thumbs may be placed on the lower third of the infant's sternum, just below the nipple line, with hands encircling the infant's chest. Alternatively, the sternum may be compressed, using two fingers (ring and middle or index and middle fingers) at the same location.[9,10] The sternum should be compressed to a depth of one-half to three-fourths inch and accompanied by PPV at a rate of one ventilation for every three compressions, delivering 120 events per minute (90 chest compressions + 30 ventilations).[8] Chest compressions should be smooth, with the fingers or thumbs not leaving the infant's sternum between compressions. Care should be taken to avoid applying pressure to the xiphoid process, as this may injure abdominal organs. Compressions may be discontinued if the infant's spontaneous HR exceeds 80 beats/min.

Endotracheal intubation is necessary whenever BVM ventilation is ineffective, prolonged PPV is required, or tracheal suctioning is necessary (e.g., meconium aspiration). It is also recommended when a diaphragmatic hernia is suspected to avoid gastric distension associated with BVM ventilation. Equipment size for intubation can be selected based on the infant's estimated weight and gestational age (Table 233.3). In general, premature newborns require a 2.5-mm endotracheal tube (ETT), while term newborns need a 3.0- to 3.5-mm ETT. A laryngoscope with a straight (Miller) blade is preferred (size 0 to premature, size 1 to term infants) to visualize the newborn's glottis and vocal cords. If a stylet is used, care must be taken to prevent

TABLE 233.3. Equipment Size Based on Estimated Age and Weight

Age (wk)	Weight (kg)	ETT (mm)	Insertion Depth (cm)	Blade
<28	<1	2.5	7	0
28–34	1–2	3.0	8	0
34–38	2–3	3.5	9	0–1
>38	>3	3.5–4.0	10	1

the tip from protruding beyond the end of the ETT and injuring the airway. After intubation, proper ETT placement should be determined by careful physical examination and chest radiograph. Lack of chest rise, asymmetry of chest movement, and the lack of improvement in HR and/or color are signs of inappropriate ETT placement.[6]

Medications

Medications are rarely indicated during a newborn resuscitation and are reserved for specific situations.[3] Epinephrine is recommended for asystole and bradycardia (HR less than 60 to 80) despite PPV with 100% oxygen and chest compressions for 30 seconds. Volume expansion with 10 mL/kg of crystalloid (normal saline, lactated Ringer's) or colloid (O^- blood, 5% albumin) is indicated when acute blood loss is suspected and signs of hypovolemia are present (pallor, poor perfusion, weak pulse). Naloxone is useful when there is severe respiratory depression and a history of maternal narcotic administration within 4 hours of delivery. Naloxone should not delay other resuscitation efforts, such as airway management, and should never be used if chronic maternal narcotic drug use is suspected, as it can precipitate withdrawal signs in the newborn. The use of sodium bicarbonate remains controversial. It is only indicated during a prolonged arrest that does not respond to other therapy after adequate ventilation is established. Glucose should be administered for documented hypoglycemia (less than 30 mg/dL in preterm, less than 40 mg/dL in term infants). A dopamine infusion should be considered when signs of shock continue despite volume expansion. Table 233.4 outlines the recommended doses and routes of administration of resuscitation medications. High-dose epinephrine is not recommended in neonatal resuscitations.

The administration of medications can occur via several routes. In general, the quickest route to give epinephrine and naloxone is down the ETT. Medications given down an ETT should be two to three times the intravenous dose, flushed with 1 to 2 mL of normal saline and followed by BVM ventilation. Although intravenous access can be established in newborns, the umbilical vein may be the most rapidly accessible route to give all resuscitation medications, including volume expanders. The use of intraosseous lines in newborn resuscitation is not common because of the fragility of small bones, the small intraosseous space in premature infants, and the easily accessible umbilical vein.[6] However, when other means of vascular access are not available, the intraosseous route may be attempted.

Vascular Access

When vascular access is needed, the umbilical vein is the most accessible site. Using sterile technique, a tie is placed around the base of the umbilical stump to control bleeding, and a scalpel is used to cut the cord 1.0 cm above the skin. The umbilical vein is easily distinguished from the two smaller arteries, which are usually constricted (Fig. 233.2). Flush a sterile 3.5F (premature) or 5.0F (term) umbilical venous catheter with normal saline and attach it to a three-way stopcock. The catheter is advanced into the umbilical vein until good blood return is obtained (5 to 8 cm). Wedged hepatic positions are recognized by subsequent failure of free blood return after introduction. If this occurs, the catheter should be withdrawn to a position where blood can be easily aspirated. Secure the umbilical venous catheter to the skin with tape.

Special Situations

Congenital Airway Obstruction

Newborns with choanal atresia present with cyanosis at rest but become pink with crying. This occurs secondary to membranous or bony obstruction of the nasal passages and is confirmed by the inability to pass a 5F catheter through the nares. An oral airway is useful, but endotracheal intubation may be required for adequate airway management. Infants with large tongues and a small hypopharynx may benefit from an oral airway and prone positioning.

Congenital Diaphragmatic Hernia

Infants suspected of having a diaphragmatic hernia present in respiratory distress immediately after birth, with a scaphoid abdomen and displaced cardiac impulse. Ventilation by BVM

TABLE 233.4. Medications

Medication	Concentration	Dose	Route
Epinephrine	1:10,000	0.1–0.3 mL/kg	i.v., ETT*
Volume expanders	Normal saline Ringer's lactate O^- blood, 5% albumin	10 mL/kg	i.v.
Naloxone	1.0 mg/mL	0.1 mL/kg	i.v., ETT i.m., SQ
Sodium bicarbonate	4.2% solution (0.5 mEq/mL)	2–4 mL/kg	i.v. (1–2 mEq/kg)
Glucose	$D_{10}W$	2–4 mL/kg	i.v.
Dopamine	$\frac{\text{wt (kg)} \times 6 \times \mu\text{g/kg/min}}{\text{mL/h}} = \text{mg in 100 mL fluid}$ For example, if kg × 6 × 5, then 1 mL/h = 5 μg/kg/min Continuous i.v. infusion at 5–20 μg/kg/min		

*ETT = endotracheal tube

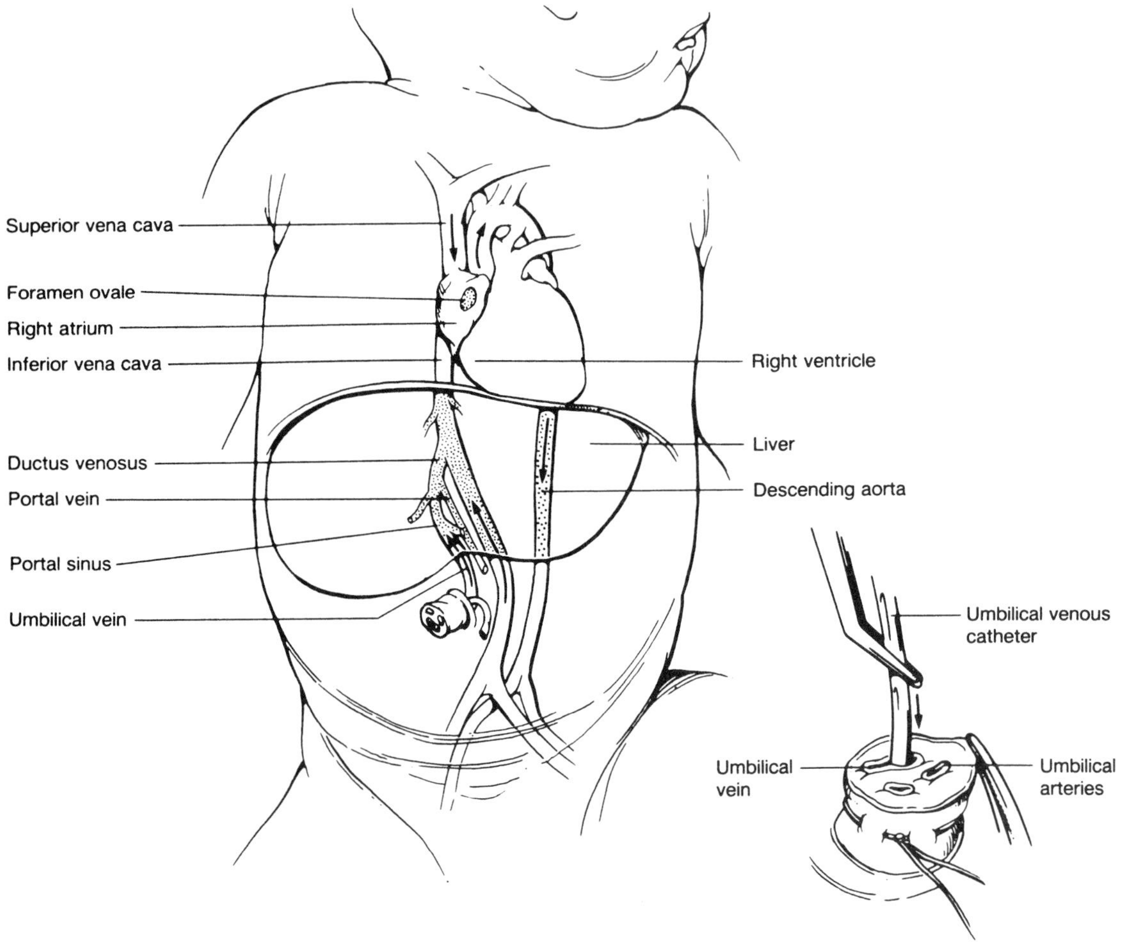

Figure 233.2. Insertion of the umbilical venous catheter.

should be avoided, because it increases gastric distension and further compromises lung expansion. Infants may require endotracheal intubation and gastric decompression.

Congenital Heart Disease

Infants who remain cyanotic despite adequate resuscitation efforts may have congenital heart disease or persistent fetal circulation. Referral to a pediatric cardiologist for echocardiography is required. Prostaglandin E_1 may be necessary to maintain patency of the ductus arteriosis.

Maternofetal Hemorrhage

Vaginal bleeding may be a sign of placenta previa or abruptio placenta. Infants are at increased risk for hypovolemia and may require volume replacement before they will respond to other forms of resuscitation. Infants placed on the mother's abdomen prior to cord clamping are at risk for hypovolemia as well.

Multiple Births

Additional equipment and personnel will be required to manage multiple births. Resuscitation is frequently required secondary to mechanical complications of delivery and compromised cord blood flow.

Pneumonia/Sepsis

Newborns occasionally present with respiratory distress and signs of sepsis. Common bacterial causes include group B *Streptococcus, Escherichia coli,* and *Listeria monocytogenes*. After appropriate cultures and stabilization, treatment with ampicillin and gentamicin (or cefotaxime) is indicated.

Pneumothorax

Pneumothorax is not uncommon in the newborn who receives aggressive resuscitation. Symptomatic pneumothoraces are relieved with needle decompression at the second intercostal space, midclavicular line, or the anterior axillary line at the level of the nipples. Chest tube placement can occur after stabilization.

Prematurity

Premature newborns are prone to respiratory distress secondary to immature lungs and surfactant deficiency. Most will require intubation. They are also at increased risk for hypoglycemia, heat loss, and intraventricular hemorrhage during resuscitation.[6] Expeditious transfer to a neonatal intensive care unit (NICU) is recommended.

DISPOSITION

All newborns require admission to the hospital nursery or an NICU following resuscitation. Consultation with a pediatrician or neonatologist is necessary at the earliest possible time to facilitate ongoing care and transfer, if necessary. If the newborn requires transfer to another hospital, an advanced cardiac life-support unit should be requested. Often, the accepting hospital will have a neonatal or pediatric transport team available.

Newborns remaining in the emergency department for an extended time will need ongoing postresuscitation care.

Postresuscitation Care

Following stabilization of the newborn, special care should be taken to maintain temperature, avoid hypoglycemia, and monitor HR, blood pressure, and oxygen saturation. Infants remaining in the emergency department for any prolonged time should have labs sent, including CBC, arterial blood gas (ABG), and glucose level. A chest x-ray to assess ETT placement and rule out a pneumothorax is recommended. The infant can be ventilated at a rate of 40 to 60 breaths per minute until the ABG results are obtained. Maintenance intravenous fluids can be started with $D_{10}W$ at 80 cc/kg/d, as electrolytes are generally not required in the first 24 hours of life. Lorazepam 0.1 mg/kg is effective to sedate the intubated newborn.

Some emergency departments receive infants who have already been resuscitated. In rural areas, for instance, many children are born at home or in transit, and present to the emergency department after resuscitation. Even in the successfully resuscitated infant, one should assume an airway complication until proven otherwise. It is very easy for an ETT to become dislodged or plugged and for a pneumothorax to be produced by overzealous ventilation. These newborns must be assessed immediately on arrival to the emergency department. Once stabilized, they should be transferred to the NICU as soon as possible.

The Apgar score (Table 233.5) is assigned at 1 and 5 minutes to all infants born in the delivery room and is helpful in documenting their transition to extrauterine life. It serves as a shorthand notation of an infant's condition and change in status, as well as a general prediction of outcome, although it has limitations. Application of the score to the extremely preterm infant is not standardized, and scoring in the presence of resuscitative interventions is not uniform. The Apgar score, although of prognostic value, should not be used as a guide to resuscitation of the depressed newborn in the emergency department. HR, respiratory effort, and color should serve as the guides to successive steps of resuscitation.

SUMMARY

For most newborns, the asphyxial stress of birth is mild and brief and there is no need for sophisticated intervention. When the stress is excessive or the neonate's ability to compensate is decreased, resuscitation may be necessary.

Because newborn resuscitation rarely occurs in the emergency department, skilled emergency physicians and staff accustomed to adult resuscitation may find themselves unprepared or anxious. For this reason, it is important to assign roles in advance and to have appropriate equipment ready and available at all times. It is helpful to have the newborn inverted pyramid posted near or attached to the newborn equipment or tray (see Fig. 233.1).

After a successful resuscitation, transfer to the newborn nursery or to the NICU should be expedited. In the interim, particular attention should be paid to postresuscitation needs, such as temperature control and airway maintenance.

TABLE 233.5. Apgar Score

Sign	0	1	2
Heart rate	Absent	Slow (<100)	>100
Respirations	Absent	Slow, irregular	Good; crying
Muscle tone	Limp	Some flexion	Active motion
Reflex irritability	No response	Grimace	Vigorous
Color	Blue, pale	Acrocyanosis	Pink

COMMON PITFALLS

- Failure to have specific neonatal resuscitation equipment set up and readily accessible, including a radiant warmer
- Lack of familiarity with newborn resuscitations in the emergency department; ongoing practice with mock codes is helpful
- Failure to initiate basic resuscitation techniques (dry, warm, position, suction, and stimulate) before invasive procedures
- Failure to adequately clear meconium from the hypopharynx and trachea before stimulating
- Failure to obtain a basic maternal history: twins, gestational age, meconium

ACKNOWLEDGMENT

The author gratefully acknowledges the contribution of Ann K. Leahy and Robert C. Luten, who wrote the previous edition of this chapter.

References

1. Bloom R. Delivery room resuscitation of the newborn. In: Fanaroff A, Martin R, eds. *Neonatal-perinatal medicine, diseases of the fetus and infant*. St. Louis: Mosby, 1997:376–401.
2. Bloom R, Cropley C, for the AHA/AAP Neonatal Resuscitation Program Steering Committee. *Textbook of neonatal resuscitation*. Dallas: American Heart Association, 1994.
3. Burchfield D, Berkowitz I, et al. Medications in neonatal resuscitation. *Ann Emerg Med* 1993;22:435–439.
4. Chameides L, Hazinski M, for the AHA/AAP. Neonatal resuscitation. In: *AHA, AAP textbook of pediatric life support*. Dallas: American Heart Association, 1997.
5. Cleary G, Wiswell T. Meconium-stained amniotic fluid and the meconium aspiration syndrome: an update. *Pediatr Clin North Am* 1998;45(3):511–529.
6. Kattwinkel J, Niermeyer S, et al. Resuscitation of the newly born infant. An advisory statement from the Pediatric Working Group of the International Liaison Committee on Resuscitation. *Circulation* 1999;99:1927–1938.
7. Khan N, Luten R. Neonatal resuscitation. *Emerg Med Clin North Am* 1994; 12:239–256.
8. Orlowski J. Optimum position for external cardiac compression in infants and young children. *Ann Emerg Med* 1986;15:667–663.
9. Standards and guidelines for cardiopulmonary resuscitation (CPR) and emergency cardiac care (ECC). *JAMA* 1992;268:2776.
10. Slywka B, Whitelaw C, Goldsmith L. Comparison of the two finger vs the two thumb compression. *Acad Emerg Med* 1998;5:398(*abst*).

CHAPTER 234
Pediatric Resuscitation

John A. Brennan and Neena Gupta

Resuscitation of an infant or child can be one of the most challenging and anxiety-producing experiences any physician will encounter in the emergency department (ED). The ability to recognize and treat life-threatening conditions requires prior preparation, experience, a substantial knowledge base, adequate airway and vascular access skills, and appropriate use of all resources.

The events just before, during, and after a pediatric resuscitation are all critical components to the successful resuscitation of an infant or child. The physician must be able to treat the family, as well as the patient, during and after the resuscitation. He or she must help the parents have some sense of understanding and control as their child is taken to a pediatric intensive care unit or help the parents begin the grieving process if the resuscitation efforts have been unsuccessful.

Annually there are 12.7 to 19.7[14] pediatric arrests in the United States per every 100,000 children.[13] Approximately half of the arrests are in children less than 1 year old.[14] The survival rate of a child with cardiopulmonary arrest is between 0% and 13%. The most common initial rhythm is asystole.

Because most EDs have very few true pediatric emergencies, preparedness and education are crucial aspects of pediatric resuscitation. Less than 5% to 7% of pediatric ED visits are considered critical, and in less than 1% is cardiac or respiratory resuscitation required.

The pathophysiology of cardiopulmonary arrest and shock in children differs from that of adults in many aspects. Most pediatric cardiopulmonary arrests are caused by progressive deterioration in respiration or circulation due to traumatic or medical illness. Children have a remarkable physiologic compensation mechanism and maximize it just before the cardiopulmonary arrest. For this reason, there is significant intracellular hypoxemia and acidosis that decrease the cardiovascular system's ability to respond to medications and defibrillation.

CLINICAL PRESENTATION

Children who present in emergency conditions usually follow one of two pathways to cardiopulmonary arrest. The most common path leading to cardiopulmonary collapse involves respiratory failure (i.e., inadequate oxygenation–ventilation).

Causes of respiratory arrest can be divided into two categories. First, there is upper airway pathology, which includes anatomic abnormalities, infectious disease, inflammatory reactions, and foreign bodies. The second category is lower airway pathology, which includes interstitial disease, alveolar disease, and bronchus or bronchiole disease.

Shock (inadequate cellular energy supply) is the next most common pathway predisposing the child to cardiopulmonary arrest. Shock has many different etiologies, the most common of which is hypovolemia, either from dehydration or bleeding. Distributive shock is secondary to anaphylaxis, spinal cord injuries, or sepsis. Cardiogenic shock is secondary to an arrhythmia or mechanical abnormality, whether structural or infectious (i.e., myocarditis). Obstructive shock, secondary to cardiac tamponade or tension pneumothorax, and dissociative shock, secondary to hemoglobin abnormalities (carbon monoxide poisoning or methemoglobinemia), complete the list.

Thus, assessment of cardiopulmonary stability is of paramount importance. A rapid survey assessment (known as the Pediatric Assessment Triangle[9]) allows rapid evaluation of the child's appearance, breathing, and circulation status. This assessment can be completed during the first 15 to 30 seconds of the child's initial presentation.

Specifically, the parameters involved include the rapid assessment of the child's airway, breathing, and cardiac status; general appearance,[9] skin color, and capillary refill; and a general neurologic assessment of the child that includes the child's mental status and best verbal, motor, and eye responses.

Throughout this chapter, fundamental differences, similarities, and intragroup differences related to size and age are highlighted as they affect resuscitation. Management goals of pediatric resuscitation are to correct hypoxemia and ventilation abnormalities, correct metabolic abnormalities (e.g., acidemia), and improve coronary, renal, and cerebral perfusion. A successful outcome depends on adequate alveolar oxygenation and carbon dioxide exchange, maintaining vascular perfusion, and correcting the underlying cause of the cardiopulmonary arrest.

EMERGENCY DEPARTMENT MANAGEMENT

Cardiopulmonary Resuscitation Overview

Single-rescuer cardiopulmonary resuscitation (CPR) should activate EMS after 1 minute of rescue breathing and compressions if the patient is less than 8 years old (more likely respiratory than cardiac).[5] Infants and children should have a compression rate of 100 per minute and 20 ventilations per minute (5:1). The resuscitator's hand should be on the lower half of the sternum and a depth of one-third to one-half the depth of the chest. Foreign-body maneuvers include back blows and chest thrusts for infants and the Heimlich maneuver for children. There are many investigational alternative methods for CPR, but none has been shown to have better outcomes than those described in the American Heart Association (AHA) guidelines for CPR.

Airway

The foundation of all pediatric resuscitative attempts is appropriate airway management. Because the airway in childhood is in dynamic growth, the clinician must deal with variables such as its anatomic location, caliber, and length. Consideration must also be given to variability in head size (occipital prominence), tongue, and mandible size.[5]

As the child grows, the larynx descends from its relatively superior and anterior position in infancy to the adult location, which it reaches by about age 10 years (range, 8 to 12 years). The narrowest portion of the extrathoracic airway in a child younger than 8 years is the cricoid ring, while in older children and adults it is the glottic opening. Head size, equal to or larger than chest circumference in the neonate, grows to adult proportions by adolescence.

Positioning the infant requires careful attention to the tendency of the prominent occiput to cause neck flexion and resultant airway occlusion. Mild extension of the head (nontraumatic arrest) to achieve the "sniffing" position will provide airway patency in the child with adequate mandibular muscle tone. Overextension may cause airway obstruction by compressing the compliant trachea.

The large tongue may still occlude the airway, even with proper head–neck position. When hypotonia occurs, the mandible will no longer be maintained in a stable open position by the child, so the tongue will fall against the posterior pharyngeal wall, obstructing the airway. Appropriate maneuvers, such as a chin lift or jaw thrust, will move this block of tissue anteriorly and will open the airway. Airway devices, such as nasopharyngeal tubes for conscious children or oropharyngeal airways in unconscious patients, may be helpful once the airway has been opened manually. When the airway cannot be maintained using these maneuvers, or when other indications exist, an endotracheal tube (ETT) may need to be inserted.

There are many physiologic and anatomic differences between adult and pediatric airways. The previous section mentioned many of the anatomic differences in normal children. The physician taking care of children must also be prepared to treat patients with congenital malformations such as webs, tracheolaryngeal malacia, hemangiomas, cranial facial disorders, subglottic stenosis, and extrinsic and intrinsic foreign bodies. Physiologic differences between adults and children include the higher metabolic and oxygen consumption of children (which causes them to become hypoxic sooner), the smaller functional reserve capacity of children, their exaggerated vagal responses, and the higher airway resistance of children.

If the child has inadequate oxygenation or ventilation unresponsive to basic airway treatment, intubation is indicated. Preparations for this procedure should be started while the child is being properly positioned and oxygenated. A bag-valve-mask device with supplemental oxygen and oxygen reservoir can provide a 90% inspired concentration of oxygen, and the child can be ventilated until intubation preparations are complete.

Endotracheal intubation offers the following advantages:

It protects the airway from aspiration.
It provides a conduit for suctioning of secretions and debris.
It permits alveolar ventilation and corrects respiratory acidosis without compromising chest compressions.
It permits 100% oxygen instillation to the trachea with the possibility of applying positive end-expiratory pressure.

Full preparation includes an adequate large-bore suction device for clearing the oral and hypopharynx, a range of ETT sizes, smaller suction catheters for the ETT following insertion, and a laryngoscope with the proper size and shape of blade.

In general, a straight blade is preferable in children 4 years of age and younger. The curved blade should be used for older children. The straight blade is better in the younger child because the epiglottis and larynx are more cephalad and anterior. This anatomic configuration allows the straight blade to be placed in proper position easier than the curved blade. The curved blade must be placed in the vallecula for ideal use, whereas the straight blade is placed posterior to the epiglottis and does not require strict anatomic matching to the curvature of the tongue. The child's anterior and superior anatomy may preclude visualization of the entire anteroposterior dimensions of the glottic opening, even with sufficient help, lighting, positioning, and preparation. In fact, the clinician may be able to visualize only the posterior one-third of that opening.

A rapidly available supply of tubes in a wide range of sizes is needed to accommodate the size- and age-related differences of childhood. In most instances, ETTs without cuffs should be used in children younger than 7 or 8 years of age because the cricoid ring is small enough to produce an air seal. Controversy exists regarding the use of tubes with cuffs in children younger than 8 when a child has ingested a poison, because gastric lavage may potentially lead to aspiration. Theoretically, a cuff could provide better airway protection than could an uncuffed tube. As with any cuffed ETT, cuff pressure must be monitored and maintained at 20 cm H_2O or less to minimize the risk of mucosal ischemia and necrosis. This complication can also be avoided by using an uncuffed tube small enough to allow a minimal leak audible on positive-pressure ventilation.

The appropriate-sized ETT can be found by using a table of approximate sizes. These tables, however, require an accurate age or weight estimation for access of appropriate-sized equipment. Length has been shown to be the most accurate predictor of correct ETT size in children.[11] The Broselow Pediatric Emergency Tape (a length-based resuscitation tape) provides accurate equipment selection as well as resuscitation drug doses with a single length measurement. Two additional tubes should be available, one-half size smaller and one-half size larger. The child's small finger can serve as an approximation of his or her tracheal diameter, and an infant's length corresponds to the ETT size.

Because ETTs for children are short and easily dislodged from the trachea, one must be wary of tube movement and carefully secure the tube in position. Holding the tube and the corner of the mouth together until the tube is taped or otherwise held in position usually maintains this security. Once the ETT has passed between the vocal cords, proper position must be determined by auscultating the lung fields in both axillas. An endotracheal vapor cloud may be seen, and apparent breath sounds may be heard, even with esophageal intubation. The latter is especially common in small infants. The *sine qua non* of proper ETT placement is a patient whose vital signs improve, whose chest rises, and whose tissue perfusion improves. If the patient does not improve or if doubt exists, tube position may be checked by direct visualization using a laryngoscope. Alternate airway methods and personnel must be available for the difficult airway that cannot be ventilated or intubated.

Breathing

Once the airway is secured, attention should focus on breathing. The physiologic goals of oxygenation and ventilation require patency of airway and alveoli, normal alveolar capillary membranes, and matching of perfusion with ventilation. Patients with patent airways who require ventilatory support with bag-valve-mask devices must have the proper "bagging" technique employed to avoid complications.

Proper bag-valve-mask use demands a good mask–face seal with an appropriate-sized mask and the use of a bag that allows the provider to supply the necessary tidal volume. The mask must fit over the nose and mouth without compressing the eyes (compression of the eyes may lead to vagal-induced bradycardia) and without extending beyond the chin. A properly sized mask minimizes artificial airway dead space. A self-inflating bag is most commonly used. Overventilation may lead to unilateral or bilateral pneumothoraces; underventilation will lead to carbon dioxide retention and respiratory acidosis.

Whether using a mask or ETT, the clinician should provide a tidal volume that causes the chest to rise. A pop-off valve, if present, allows for a preset maximum inspiratory pressure. Additional tidal volume can be delivered at higher pressures by holding a finger on the valve while delivering the breath with the self-expanding bag. Ideally, an in-line manometer should be used to monitor peak inspiratory pressure.

Resting tidal volume in children and adults is 5 to 7 mL/kg, while ventilatory supported tidal volume may be 10 to 15 mL/kg. Rather than calculating a value, attention should be paid to lung and chest wall compliance while bagging, and the volume should be varied according to chest rise. Resuscitation bags for premature neonates should have a 250-mL capacity; 500-mL bags should be used for term newborns, infants, and small children. Adolescents require 750-mL bags.

Circulation

Adequacy of circulation is a clinical determination based on physical examination. The primary indication for assisting circulation with chest compressions is pulselessness. In neonates, chest compressions are also indicated when the heart rate remains below 60 beats/min despite effective maneuvers to oxygenate and ventilate the patient, or when the heart rate is between 60 and 80 beats/min and not increasing.

Access to the vascular space of infants and small children is required when there is an immediate need to restore circulating blood volume or to infuse medications that can be given by no other route. The most common cause of cardiopulmonary failure in children older than 1 year of age is trauma; most of these children are large enough to allow for rapid intravenous cannulation. Nontraumatic arrests in children younger than 1 year old are most often secondary to respiratory failure.

Consequently, appropriate airway management may preclude full arrest, and if cardiac arrest does ensue, the endotracheal cannula provides a route for administration of certain necessary medications.

The most common sites for intravenous cannulation are dorsal hand veins, superficial veins on the dorsum of the foot, antecubital veins of the forearm, superficial scalp veins, the external jugular veins, and the femoral vein in the inguinal canal. Once the airway is patent and maintained, any one or more of these sites may be used. Standard cleansing and cannulation techniques should be used.

Both the external jugular vein and the femoral vein may provide passage to the central venous circulation through guidewire and long-line insertion. These procedures should not be first-line attempts; rather, short, reasonably large-bore cannulas should be placed first. When the patient is stable, these lines can be replaced under more controlled conditions.

An alternate site for access to the vascular space is the bone marrow. Infusion of blood, fluids, and medications into the circulation using the bone marrow has been done for over 50 years.[10] Intraosseous (IO) cannulation can be accomplished using either the distal femur (proximal to the physis) or the proximal tibia (distal to the physis).

The bone marrow can be used to facilitate infusion of all resuscitation drugs and for volume resuscitation with fluids or blood.[2] These sites are used in the patient in full cardiopulmonary arrest who needs intravenous medications when intravenous access is not obtainable within 90 to 120 seconds.

Pediatric disposable IO infusion needles are available in various sizes for infants and children younger than 7 years of age but can be used in older children. Standard aseptic technique should be used. The IO needle can be removed once one or more intravenous catheters have been placed and are stabilized.

For most resuscitation medications, the intravenous doses are well recognized and standardized. For optimum action, these drugs should be given as close as possible to the heart. In the absence of specific pediatric recommendations, accepted intravenous dosage schedules should be used. Drugs given through the ETT should be delivered well down into the bronchial system for optimum mucosal absorption via a feeding tube (two to three times the dosage for lidocaine, atropine, and naloxone, and ten times the intravenous epinephrine dose). Drugs given through the bone marrow have dosages identical to the intravenous dosage and should be followed with a 2- to 5-mL saline flush to aid delivery to the central circulation. Some authorities also recommend a 2- to 5-mL saline flush after bolus intravenous medication administration.

Equipment selection, medication, and defibrillation dosing errors can be minimized by using standardized charts, forms, tables, and the Broselow Pediatric Emergency Tape. All information should be displayed in large type in an easy-to-read format and be prominently located for reference during critical situations. The AHA publishes resuscitation algorithms and drug dosages in the pocket-sized *Handbook of Emergency Cardiovascular Care for Healthcare Providers.*

Resuscitation Medications

All of the drugs used during adult CPR can be used for children. For the most part, they function through the same molecular mechanisms. Thus, alpha- and beta-adrenergic receptors must be stimulated by exogenous agonists, as must the dopaminergic receptors. However, children may have fewer available receptors because of underlying maximal endogenous stimulation or incomplete development. The concerns after restoration of cardiovascular function include prolonged tachycardia and potential hypertension.

Oxygen, the mainstay of any resuscitation attempt, is the most important "drug" used during pediatric resuscitation. It has no contraindications, and airway management must be the first therapeutic modality instituted.

Fluids such as normal saline or Ringer's lactate should be used in the hypotensive infant or child. The initial fluid bolus is 20 cc/kg, which may be repeated up to three times, depending on the clinical condition. Packed red blood cells are dosed at 10 cc/kg.

Epinephrine, with both alpha- and beta-receptor action, is a potent medication to help reverse cardiac collapse, treat lethal arrhythmias, treat symptomatic bradyarrhythmias, and treat hypotension not related to hypovolemia. The cardiac beta-receptor action may improve output when heart rate is slow. Thus, epinephrine is often used in neonates and young infants to accelerate heart rate.

The alpha-adrenergic receptor activity that predominates in the doses used for cardiopulmonary arrest has many effects. It increases coronary and cerebral perfusion pressures; increases intravascular resistance of the skin, muscles, and splanchnic vessels; prevents arterial collapse of intrathoracic arteries; increases heart rate, myocardial contractility, and cardiac automaticity; and increases myocardial oxygen demand. All neonatal dosages are 0.01 mg/kg. Higher doses are not used because of the increased incidence of intracranial bleeding in this age group.

The initial intravenous/IO dose of epinephrine for patients outside the neonatal range in pulseless arrest is 0.01 mg/kg (0.1 mL/kg) of the 1:10,000 solution. All endotracheal doses[2] and subsequent intravenous doses are 0.1 mg (0.1 mL/kg) of the 1:1,000 solution for pulseless arrest. Note that the first dose of epinephrine, subsequent doses of epinephrine, as well as endotracheal epinephrine doses have the same amount of milliliters; only the concentration of the drug changes. These doses may be administered every 3 to 5 minutes during arrest. There is no evidence-based literature to support the use of high-dose epinephrine. High-dose epinephrine may increase return of spontaneous circulation (ROSC) but it does not improve survival to hospital discharge.[4,8] In addition to increasing myocardial oxygen demand, epinephrine postresuscitation may cause prolonged hypertension and tachycardia after ROSC. For bradycardia, epinephrine may be given intravenously or IO at 0.01 mg/kg of the 1:10,000 solution, or 0.1 mg/kg of the 1:1,000 solution per ETT.

Atropine is a parasympatholytic drug used in cardiorespiratory arrest. It accelerates sinus and atrial pacemakers, reduces cardiac vagal tone, and increases atrioventricular conduction. Atropine increases heart rate and therefore improves cardiac output. In children, an improvement in cardiac output generally relies much more on heart rate than on an increase in stroke volume. Atropine is indicated for symptomatic bradycardia after oxygenation–ventilation and epinephrine have been given. It also attenuates vagolytic effects of infants and children during intubation.

The recommended dose of atropine is 0.02 mg/kg, with a minimum dose of 0.1 mg and a maximum single dose for a child of 0.5 mg and for an adolescent of 1.0 mg. The initial dose may be repeated once. The total of the two doses should not exceed 1.0 mg for the child or 2.0 mg for the adolescent. The endotracheal dosage of atropine is unknown but is generally given at higher than the intravenous dose (two to three times the intravenous dose). Side effects of atropine include paradoxical bradycardia and tachycardia, and increased myocardial oxygen demand.

Glucose is a medication uncommonly used during adult cardiorespiratory arrest. In infants and small children, the small reserve of endogenous glucose in the form of hepatic glycogen is readily exhausted during stress. Rapid bedside glucose testing, with easily usable equipment that provides accurate results, is mandatory in any location that resuscitation of a child may occur. Serum glucose and its anaerobic end product lactate can be monitored during the resuscitation process. If needed, glucose can be given intravenously or intraosseously in a dose of 2 to 4 mL/kg of 25% dextrose in water. Because dextrose concentrations over 12.5% may cause loss of integrity of small peripheral veins, it should be given in as large a vein as possible. The 10% solution should be used in neonates.

Naloxone is a narcotic antagonist and is used for potential narcotic overdose. The dosage is 0.1 mg/kg up to 20 kg, and 2 mg for anyone over 20 kg. There are no adverse side effects, but it does have a short half-life. It needs to be monitored, especially if the child has taken a long-acting narcotic.

Recommended indications for *calcium* are calcium channel blocker toxicity, hypocalcemia, hyperkalemia, and hypermagnesemia. If given, calcium chloride should be used in a dose of 20 mg/kg (0.2 mL/kg).

Respiratory and lactic acidosis are secondary to hypoventilation and hypoperfusion. Correction of acidemia is primarily by ventilation–oxygenation and restoration of circulation. *Sodium bicarbonate* is indicated for acidemia after a prolonged arrest when adequate ventilation–oxygen and cardiac compressions are being performed. During CPR, sodium bicarbonate should be given intravenously or intraosseously. The dose of sodium bicarbonate is 1 mEq/kg of the 8.4% solution. In the neonate, the dose is the same, but the solution should be 4.2%. The 8.4% solution can be converted to 4.2% by diluting it 1 : 1 with sterile water (not sterile saline). Side effects include hypernatremia, hyperosmolarity, alkalemia, and paradoxical cerebrospinal fluid and intracellular acidosis.

Dopamine is used to enhance urine output and treat hypotension not related to hypovolemia. Renal dosages are 2 to 5 μg/kg/min; beta-adrenergic effects, 2 to 10 μg/kg/min; and alpha-adrenergic effects, 15 to 20 μg/kg/min.

Lidocaine is used in ventricular tachycardia (VT) and ventricular fibrillation (VF) or symptomatic ventricular arrhythmias. The initial dosage is a 1-mg/kg bolus, followed by a 20- to 50-μg/kg/min drip.

Electrical Treatment of Rhythm Disturbances

Electrical dysfunction of cardiac muscle in childhood is most often secondary to respiratory failure and/or congenital heart disease. The most common rhythm disturbance after asystole is sinus bradycardia. It will respond to adequate ventilation and oxygenation, if provided early enough, and rarely requires medication. Sinus tachycardia is also seen and may present as the earliest sign of impending cardiopulmonary arrest. Both of these rhythms must be interpreted in light of possible causes, and the underlying cause should be treated. The ventricular arrhythmias in pediatrics are more difficult to treat, because children have a prolonged compensatory stage and therefore are much more acidotic and hypoxic than an adult who has a sudden collapse secondary to a ventricular arrhythmia. Electricity is the immediate treatment for pulseless VT or VF.

Electrical conversion energy levels for supraventricular tachycardia are 0.25 to 1.0 J/kg, while delivered energy for VF or pulseless VT starts at 2 J/kg. Figure 234.1 illus-

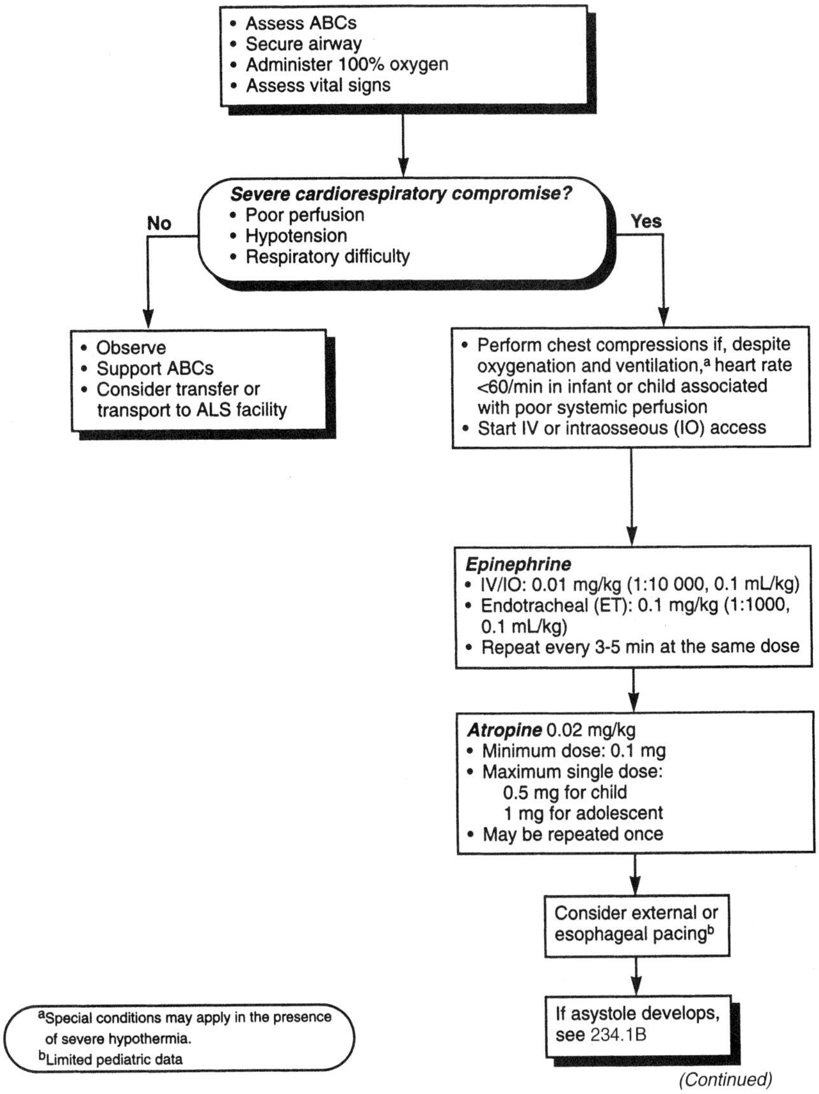

A

Figure 234.1. Treatment algorithms for pediatric advanced life support. **(A)** Bradycardia algorithm. **(B)** Asystole and pulseless arrest algorithm. **(C)** Tachycardia with poor perfusion algorithm. (From American Heart Association. *Textbook of pediatric advanced life support.* Dallas: American Heart Association, 1997.)

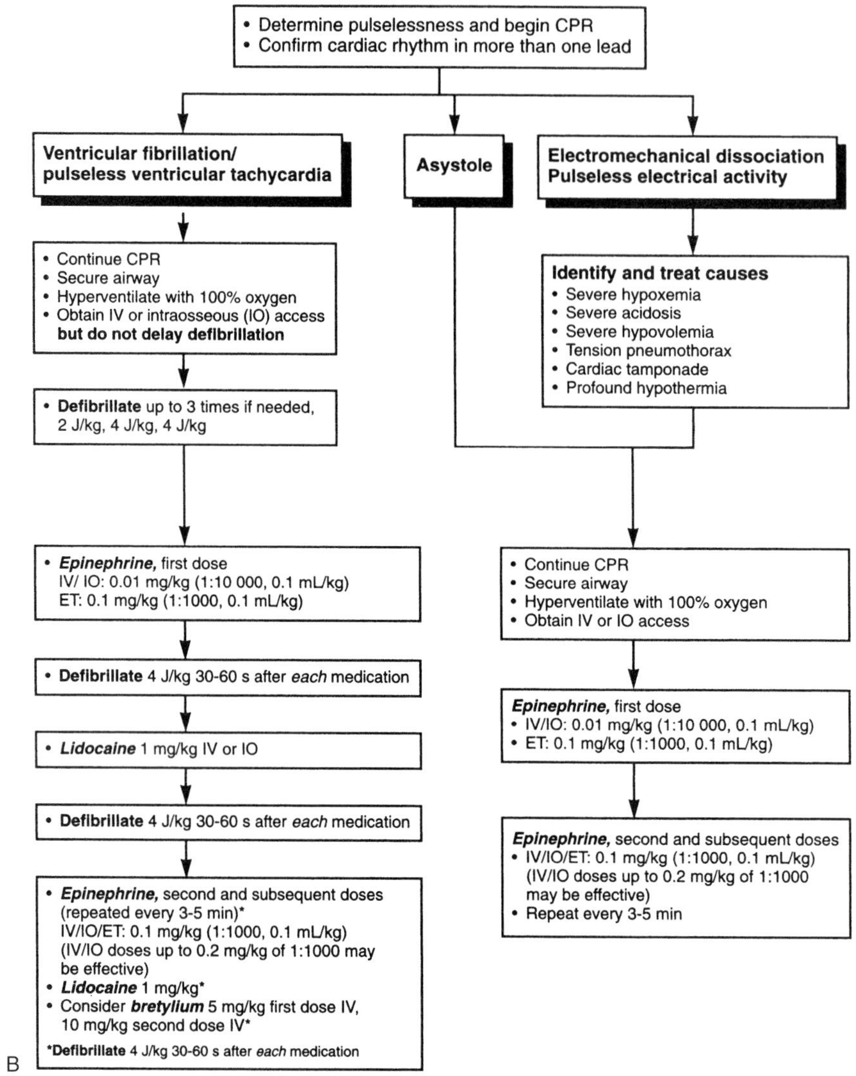

Figure 234.1. *(Continued)*

trates current treatment algorithms for potentially lethal arrhythmias.

When electricity is being used to convert an unstable rhythm, appropriate-sized paddles must be placed in an appropriate position. The recommended paddle size for small children (less than 10 kg) is 4.5 cm in diameter, and up to 8 cm in diameter in larger children and adolescents. If only large paddles are available, they should be placed in the anteroposterior position. Regardless of position, a proper conducting medium must be used with full paddle contact on the chest wall.

Paying attention to the underlying ionic, metabolic, or mechanical causes of the unstable rhythm in a child is the mainstay of therapy. The child should be assessed for hypothermia or hyperthermia, hypoglycemia or hyperglycemia, and alterations in oxygen, potassium, calcium, sodium, and magnesium. Acid–base alterations must be corrected. Mechanical causes of pulseless electrical activity (PEA), such as hypovolemia due to dehydration, cardiac tamponade, tension pneumothorax, and ETT obstruction or misplacement should be rapidly addressed.

Implementing Resuscitation Principles

Successful resuscitation requires applying the principles of resuscitation, practicing psychomotor skills, and using proper equipment and drugs. One barrier to optimal results can be the difficulties caused by variations in the size of pediatric patients: It is not uncommon for valuable resuscitation time to be lost calculating drug doses or selecting appropriately sized equipment. This is compounded by the provider's anxiety and the potential for error inherent in this process.[12] In adults, this problem is virtually nonexistent, because size variations and, therefore, drug and equipment needs do not change significantly from one patient to another. See Table 234.1 for a list of recommended ED equipment and supplies.

A system based on length has been introduced. The Broselow Pediatric Emergency Tape relates the patient's length to his or her weight and, therefore, to the appropriate drug dosage and also to appropriate equipment sizes. The tape provides immediate access to the correct drug dosage, as well as equipment selection, based on a single measurement. It is not enough to have the knowledge and the skills to resuscitate; any barriers to implementation of that knowledge must also be eliminated. Appropriate personnel, training, equipment and medications, and preparedness are the keys to a successful resuscitation.

Postresuscitation Stabilization

Avoiding secondary injury and frequent assessment of the ABCs, neurologic status, urine output, fluid administration, monitors, laboratory results, and vital signs are mandatory for

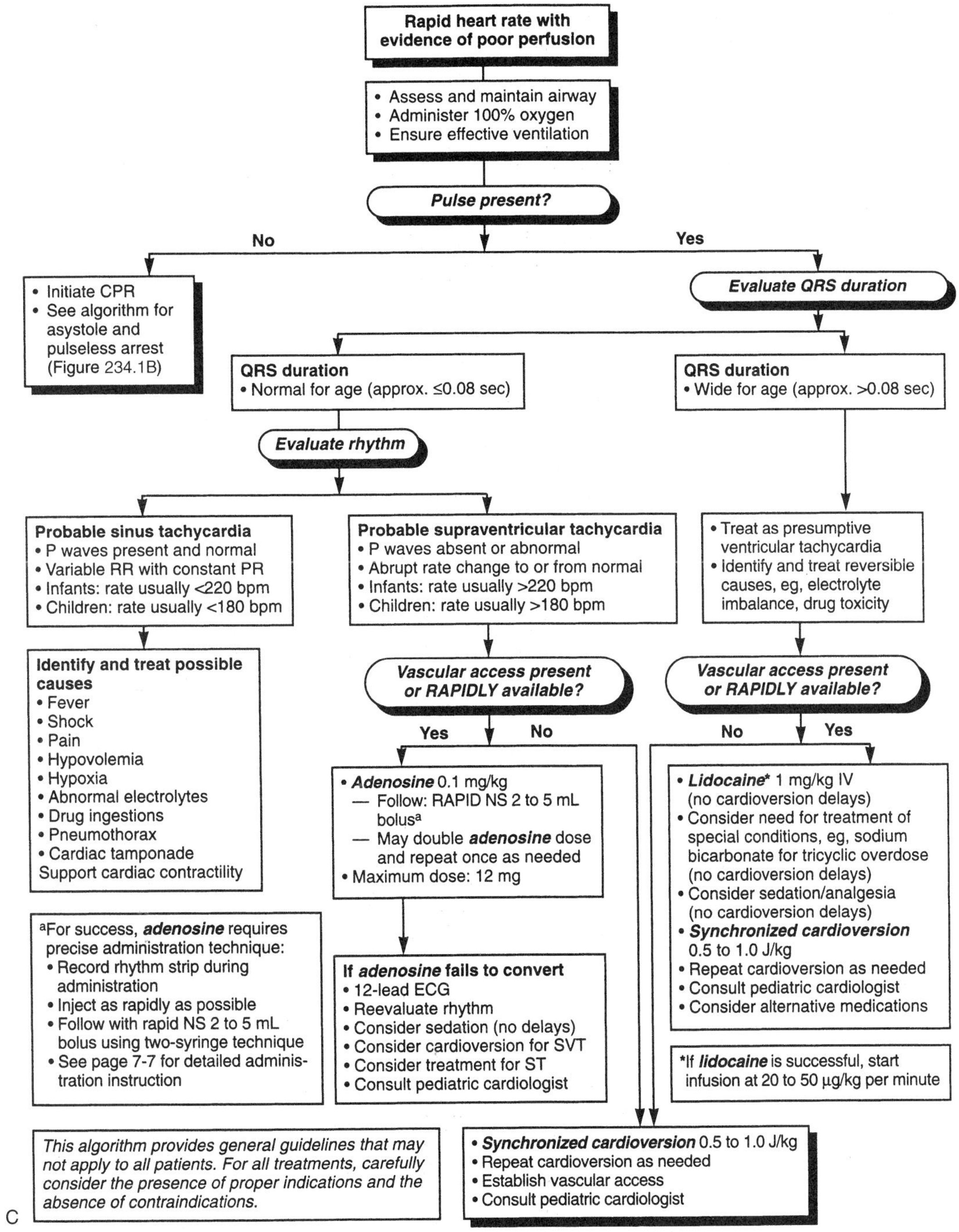

Figure 234.1. *(Continued)*

successful postresuscitation stabilization. Sedation and pain management must also be appropriately addressed and monitored. Family members and friends must be continuously updated on the status of the patient.

Outcome Predictors

Respiratory arrests without cardiac arrests have a much higher survival rate. Patients in whom return of spontaneous circulation has occurred with less than 5 minutes of CPR and with fewer than two doses of epinephrine (vs. multiple doses) have a better chance of survival. Those patients who arrested because of VF and are treated rapidly have better outcomes than all other causes of cardiopulmonary arrest. Patients who arrest secondary to sepsis have the lowest rate of survival. Those patients who arrest and have a family member begin CPR have higher survival rates than patients who do not get immediate CPR.[13]

Family Members' Involvement with Pediatric Resuscitation

Parent surveys have indicated that most parents find being at their child's bedside during a code helps them begin the grieving process if the resuscitation is unsuccessful. Prewritten protocols and a health-care professional who can be with the family and answer questions as the code proceeds are a must for successful implementation.[1] These health-care providers can help explain procedures and recognize potential problems parents may encounter during the resuscitative effort.

TABLE 234.1. Guidelines for Minimum Equipment and Supplies for Care of Pediatric Patients in Emergency Departments

MONITORING
Cardiorespiratory monitor with strip recorder
Defibrillator (0- to 400-J capability) with pediatric and adult paddles (4.5 cm and 8.0 cm)
Pediatric and adult monitor electrodes
Pulse oximeter with sensor sizes for newborn through adult
Thermometer/rectal probe[a]
Sphygmomanometer
Doppler blood pressure device
Blood pressure cuffs (neonatal, infant, child, adult, and thigh sizes)
Method to monitor endotracheal tube and placement[b]
VASCULAR ACCESS
Butterfly needles (19- to 25-gauge)
Catheter-over-needle devices (14- to 24-gauge)
Infusion device[c]
Tubing for the above
Intraosseous needles (16- and 18-gauge)[d]
Arm boards (infant, child, and adult sizes)
Intravenous fluid/blood warmers
Umbilical vein catheters (sizes 3.5F and 5F)[e]
Seldinger technique vascular access kit (with pediatric sizes 3F, 4F, 5F catheters)
AIRWAY MANAGEMENT
Clear oxygen masks (preterm, infant, child, and adult sizes)
Non-rebreather masks (infant, child, and adult sizes)
Oral airways (sizes 00–5)
Nasopharyngeal airways (12F–30F)
Bag-valve-mask resuscitator, self-inflating (450- and 1,000-mL sizes)
Nasal cannulae (infant, child, and adult sizes)
Endotracheal tubes: uncuffed (sizes 2.5 to 8.5) and cuffed (sizes 5.5 to 9.0)
Stylets (pediatric and adult)
Laryngoscope handle (pediatric and adult)
Laryngoscope blades, curved (sizes 2 and 3) and straight (sizes 0 to 3)
Magill forceps (pediatric and adult)
Nasogastric tubes (sizes 6F–14F)
Suction catheters: flexible (sizes 5F–16F) and Yankauer suction tip
Chest tubes (sizes 8F–40F)
Tracheotomy tubes (sizes 00 to 6)[f]

[a] Suitable for hypothermic and hyperthermic measurements with temperature capability from 25°C to 44°C.
[b] May be satisfied by a disposable ET_{CO_2} detector, bulb, or feeding tube methods for endotracheal tube placement.
[c] To regulate rate and volume.
[d] May be satisfied by standard bone marrow aspiration needles, 13- or 15-gauge.
[e] Available within the hospital.
[f] Ensure availability of pediatric sizes within the hospital.
From the Committee on Pediatric Equipment and Supplies for Emergency Departments, National Emergency Medical Service for Children Resource Alliance. Guidelines for pediatric equipment and supplies for emergency departments. *Ann Emerg Med* 1998;31:56.

Terminating an Unsuccessful Cardiopulmonary Arrest and Informing the Parents

Patients in cardiopulmonary arrests continuing longer than 30 minutes, unless they are hypothermic, have very little chance of survival. Informing the parents of a child's death is a skill in which very few physicians have any formal training. Most training focuses on interactions with the dying patient, not the bereaved family. Some general guidelines include telling both parents together, knowing the name of the deceased, telling the parents their child has *died* (not that their child is *dead*), looking professional, preparing the patient before the family enters the room, having counselors available, having a private grieving room, and making sure the staff has an adequate debriefing.[6]

PEDIATRIC RESUSCITATION PEARLS

Preparation and competent personnel are mandatory to adequately resuscitate children. Team approaches, with clear identification of individual roles, helps prevent confusion and potential chaos during a pediatric code. Resuscitation rooms in the ED, which are designed to facilitate pediatric resuscitations, help lower the stress of a very stressful situation. They have the appropriate equipment, medications, and room to facilitate the resuscitative efforts. Carts, which are color coded by length, have helped decrease medication errors during these resuscitative efforts.

Neonatal patients are usually not given atropine for bradycardia. The second dose of epinephrine for neonates in VF or pulseless VT is not increased as it is with all other VF and pulseless VT arrests. If the neonatal patient requires sodium bicarbonate, it is given at half strength. The umbilical vein is an excellent vascular access site in neonates. Suction pressure should not exceed 100 mm Hg in neonates and should not last greater than 2 to 3 seconds in any pediatric patient.

All medications given by intravenous, IO, or ETT routes should be followed by a small normal saline bolus. All children in cardiopulmonary arrest should have their glucose immediately checked. A bedside warmer should be used during all pediatric resuscitations. Pediatric patients should be kept in a slight Trendelenburg position during resuscitation efforts, to help prevent aspiration. Airway equipment and alternative airway equipment must be checked every shift to make sure it is always in working condition. The most important medication for any pediatric patient is oxygen.

Appropriate airway management and ventilation of an arrested child can be the difference between a successful and an unsuccessful resuscitation. The rhythm strip should be carefully examined in any pediatric arrest. Cardiopulmonary arrest secondary to sepsis has a very high mortality rate. Always consider child abuse or neglect if there are any inconsistencies in the caregivers' history or the physician's physical examination. Finally, be prepared to help a family begin their grieving process if the resuscitative efforts are unsuccessful.

COMMON PITFALLS

- Failure to have an organized system for stocking appropriate pediatric equipment and supplies
- Failure to perform routine mock codes and assessments of pediatric preparedness in the ED
- All staff should be aware of the anatomic and physiologic differences between pediatric and adult airway management.
- All staff should be knowledgeable about neonatal resuscitations and medications.

References

1. Adams S, Whitlock M, Baskett PJF, et al. Should relatives be allowed to watch resuscitation? *BMJ* 1994;308:1687.
2. American Academy of Pediatrics: Committee on Drugs. Alternative routes of drug administration: advantages and disadvantages (subject review). *Pediatrics* 1997;100:143.
3. Appleton GO, Cummins RO, Larson MP, et al. CPR and the single rescuer: at what ages should you "call first" rather than "call fast?" *Ann Emerg Med* 1995;25:492.
4. Carpenter TC, Stenmark KR. High-dose epinephrine is not superior to standard-dose epinephrine in pediatric in-hospital cardiopulmonary arrest. *Pediatrics* 1997;99:403.
5. Chameides L, Hazinski MF, eds. Pediatric airway management. In: *Textbook of pediatric advanced life support*. Dallas: American Heart Association, 1997.
6. Committee on Pediatric Emergency Medicine. Death of a child in the emergency department. *Pediatrics* 1994;93:861.
7. Committee on Pediatric Equipment and Supplies for the Emergency Department, National Emergency Medical Service for Children Resource Alliance. Guidelines for pediatric equipment and supplies for emergency departments. *Ann Emerg Med* 1998;31:56.
8. Dieckmann RA, Vardis R. High-dose epinephrine in pediatric out-of-hospital cardiopulmonary arrest. *Pediatrics* 1995;95:901.
9. Gausche M, ed. The pediatric emergency medicine course: instructor manual, 3rd ed. Dallas: American College of Emergency Physicians and Elk Grove Village, IL: American Academy of Pediatrics, 1998.
10. Hodge D. Intraosseous infusions: a review. *Pediatr Emerg Care* 1985;1:215.
11. Luten RC, Wears RL, Broselow J, et al. Length-based endotracheal tube sizing for pediatric resuscitation. *Ann Emerg Med* 1992;21:900.
12. Oakley P. Inaccuracy and delay in decision making in pediatric resuscitation and a proposed reference chart to reduce errors. *BMJ* 1988;297:817.
13. Sirbaugh PE, Pepe PE, Shook JE, et al. A prospective population-based study of the demographics, epidemiology, management, and outcome of out-of-hospital pediatric cardiopulmonary arrest. *Ann Emerg Med* 1993;33(2):174.
14. Young KD, Seidel JS. Pediatric cardiopulmonary resuscitation: a collective review. *Ann Emerg Med* 1999;33:195.

CHAPTER 235
Rapid-Sequence Induction in Children

Robert C. Luten and Phyllis Hendry Stenklyft

Because all patients requiring emergent intubation, for whatever reason, must be assumed to have a full stomach, they are at risk for aspiration, and intubation must be done with all precautions taken to prevent this complication. Also, manipulating the airway can cause hemodynamic changes, including increases in intracranial pressure (ICP), which, in the head-injured patient, may lead to further central nervous system insult. Using rapid-sequence induction (RSI) with the aid of potent induction agents, muscle relaxants, and cricoid pressure to prevent passive regurgitation, patients can be quickly rendered fully unconscious, facilitating intubation and preventing the side effects of airway manipulation, especially iatrogenic ICP increases. The exposure time to the risk of aspiration can also be reduced. RSI helps facilitate endotracheal intubation in the combative or seizing patient, or in other patients in whom inadequate muscle relaxation prevents endotracheal intubation. The decision to employ the technique of RSI for emergent intubation should be based on a structured assessment of patient stability and the perceived difficulty of obtaining successful endotracheal intubation with the standard oral laryngoscopic technique.[1,2] Figure 235.1 demonstrates the Universal Emergency Airway Algorithm adapted from the *National Emergency Airway Management Course*.[12] Defined plans or algorithms for crash, difficult, and failed airways must be part of the armamentarium of any practitioner who utilizes RSI, and patients must be selected accordingly. Details of this process are beyond the scope of this chapter, which will focus on standard RSI.

The steps of RSI are

1. Preparation
2. Preoxygenation
3. Premedication
4. Induction and paralysis
5. Cricoid pressure
6. Intubation

Figure 235.2 presents a timed flowchart of the procedure. Tables 235.1, 235.2, and 235.3 outline the medications used in the scheme.

PREPARATION

Without adequate preparation, no amount of skill or expertise can ensure successful intubation. Lack of preparation also increases the likelihood of complications. *Advance preparation* includes equipment, medications, and team function, education, and orientation. *Immediate preparation* includes selecting appropriate equipment, selecting and preparing appropriate medications, and assigning team roles.

Advance Preparation

Table 235.4 lists the equipment needed to perform RSI in children. Most pediatric equipment is age- or size-appropriate. Because the child's age and weight are usually not known in

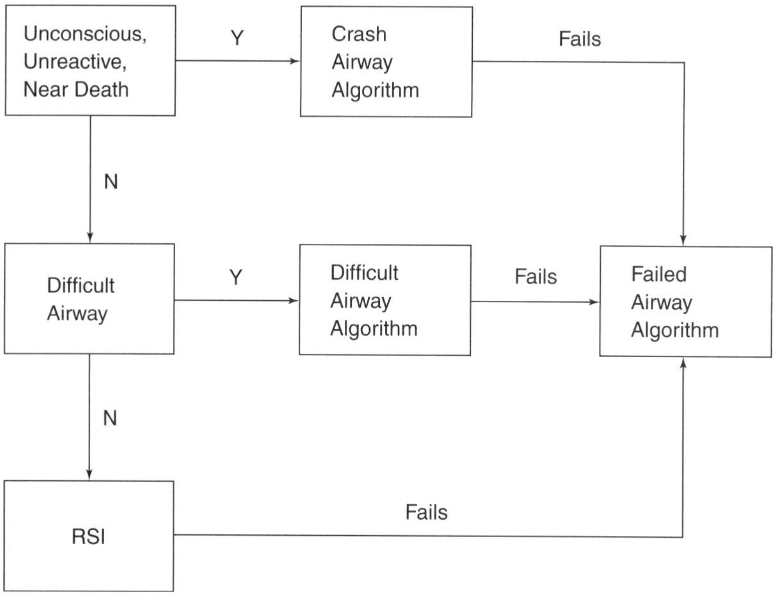

Figure 235.1. The Universal Emergency Airway Algorithm, adapted from the *National Emergency Airway Management Course*.

emergencies, using a length measurement such as the Broselow Pediatric Emergency Tape allows for correct selection of equipment and drug dosages.

Adequate training for team participants is critical. Physicians must be skilled in advanced airway management and RSI, and nursing personnel also need practice with the mechanics of the procedure (e.g., cricoid pressure, the logistics of medication preparation). The Advanced Pediatric Life Support course includes a chapter and skill station on RSI, and there are now several national advanced airway courses available for training. Mock codes and practice sessions help prepare the team and ensure that resources are available.

Immediate Preparation

Early, prehospital length measurement permits timely equipment selection and drug dosage preparation. Team roles (e.g., leader, cricoid pressure designee) are immediately assigned, and the timing of the procedure is monitored by the team leader.

PREOXYGENATION

During RSI, the patient sustains a variable period of complete apnea. To prevent hypoxia by extending the time of adequately saturated blood, the patient must be preoxygenated. The purpose of preoxygenation is to produce nitrogen washout by having the patient breathe 100% oxygen, creating an oxygen reservoir.

In the patient who is spontaneously breathing, 2 to 5 minutes of 100% oxygen delivery by a non-rebreather mask should allow 2 to 4 minutes of apnea without hypoxia. In the apneic or inadequately ventilated patient, preoxygenation with a bag-valve-mask for 1 to 2 minutes should produce the same result. Cricoid pressure is applied during bag-valve-mask ventilation to prevent gastric insufflation.

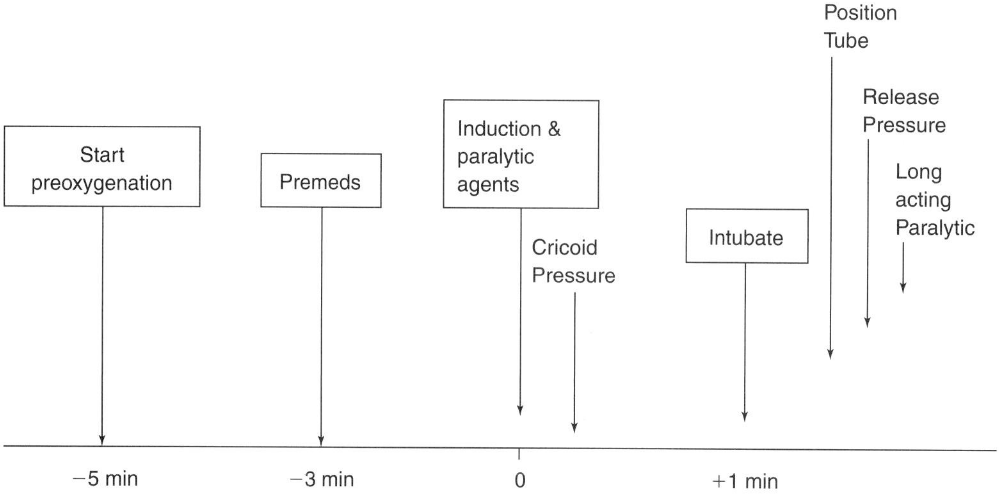

Figure 235.2. Rapid-sequence induction. This chart reflects details of timed activity of the procedure in the stable patient. All time intervals may be abbreviated by the clinician, if deemed necessary, because of less than optimal or deteriorating clinical status.

TABLE 235.1. Common Premedications in Rapid-Sequence Induction

Drug	Dose (i.v.)	Action
Lidocaine	1.5 mg/kg	Lowers ICP
Atropine	0.02 mg/kg	Prevents bradycardia associated with airway manipulation and succinylcholine
Pancuronium/ vecuronium (defasciculating dose)	0.02 mg/kg	Prevents fasciculations and ICP elevations from succinylcholine in patients >5 years of age
Fentanyl (optional)	1–3 μg/kg	Attenuates sympathetic discharge and resultant elevations in ICP. Use with caution. May cause respiratory depression or blunt compensatory sympathetic tone

TABLE 235.2. Common Agents for Induction of Unconsciousness in RSI

Drug	Dose (i.v.)	Onset	Duration
Thiopental	3–5 mg/kg	10–30 s	10–30 min
Ketamine	1–2 mg/kg	1–2 min	15–30 min
Midazolam	0.2 mg/kg (maximum 5 mg)	1–2 min	30–60 min
Etomidate	0.2–0.4 mg/kg	1 min	30–60 min
Propofol	1.0–2.0 mg/kg	30–60 s	10–15 min

TABLE 235.4. Equipment Required for Rapid-Sequence Induction

Oxygen source
Bag-valve masks
Face masks (100% nonrebreather)
Oral airways
Laryngoscope handles
Laryngoscope blades
Suction system
Endotracheal tubes
Stylet
Cardiac monitor
Pulse oximeter
Cricothyroidotomy supplies
End-tidal CO_2 detector

TABLE 235.5. Medications Required for Rapid-Sequence Induction

PREMEDICATIONS
Atropine
Lidocaine
Defasciculating agent
SEDATION
Ketamine
Thiopental
Midazolam
Propofol
Etomidate
MUSCLE RELAXANTS
Succinylcholine
Vecuronium
Pancuronium
Rocuronium

PREMEDICATION

Certain medications used as adjuncts to RSI are given before the muscle relaxant (Table 235.5). *Lidocaine* 1.5 mg/kg is of benefit in lowering ICP. *Atropine* 0.2 mg/kg dries secretions and prevents reflex vagal tone and bradycardia due to airway manipulation and succinylcholine administration. It is recommended for all children below 5 years or 20 kg, and any child receiving succinylcholine as the muscle relaxant. An alternative is to give atropine as a premedication to all children, regardless of age or paralyzing agent used. It is a relatively benign drug and can help maintain heart rate—and therefore perfusion—in the face of potential hypoxia- or drug-induced bradycardia.

If succinylcholine is used as a muscle relaxant, a pretreatment dose of a nondepolarizing agent is given to prevent muscle fasciculations and ICP elevations secondary to the succinylcholine. For children less than 5 years old or 20 kg (less muscle mass than older children and adolescents), this additional step is unnecessary. For the sake of simplicity, all premedications can be given 3 minutes prior to the administration of the induction and paralytic agent.

SEDATION/INDUCTION

The choice of induction agent depends on two variables: clinical condition and perfusion status. Advantages and disadvantages of the commonly used sedatives are listed in Table 235.6. Table 235.7 gives examples of the use of thiopental, midazolam, and ketamine, based on the patient's perfusion status and clinical condition.[4,7] Other agents frequently used include propofol, etomidate, and diazepam, and all have advantages and disadvantages.

Of the agents mentioned, etomidate is an agent that can be

TABLE 235.3. Common Agents for Muscle Relaxation in RSI

Drug	Dose (i.v.)	Onset	Duration
Succinylcholine	1.0–1.5 mg/kg (>10 kg)	30–60 s	4–10 min
	1.5–2.0 mg/kg (<10 kg)		
Vecuronium	0.2–0.25 mg/kg (RSI)	60–90 s	90 min
	0.1 mg/kg (standard dose)	2–3 min	25–40 min
	0.01 mg/kg (defasciculating dose)		
Pancuronium	0.1 mg/kg	2–5 min	45–90 min
	0.01 mg/kg (defasciculating dose)		
Rocuronium	1.0–1.2 mg/kg	30–60 s	25–60 min

TABLE 235.6. Advantages/Disadvantages of Common Sedation/Induction Agents

Drug	Advantages	Disadvantages
Thiopental	Rapid onset and duration Cerebroprotective effect Decreases ICP	Causes hypotension Histamine release → bronchospasm
Ketamine	Rapid onset Increases BP Bronchodilator	Increases ICP Emergence reactions
Diazepam	Antiepileptic	Long duration
Midazolam	Antiepileptic Short duration	
Fentanyl	Reversible Analgesic effect Attenuates hemodynamic parameters	Possible ICP elevation Chest wall rigidity Variable dose response
Etomidate	Cerebroprotective effect Minimal hemodynamic effect	Cortisol suppression—not usually a problem in acute one-time use. Myoclonic jerks
Propofol	Cerebroprotective effect	Causes hypotension

used in almost any clinical situation, and it and has one of the best cardiovascular profiles. It is the agent of choice in RSI for many emergency department physicians.[2]

CRICOID PRESSURE: THE SELLICK MANEUVER

The Sellick maneuver consists of digital cricoid pressure to occlude the esophagus and prevent passive regurgitation. The anatomic structure of the cricoid cartilage—a complete ring—prevents collapse of the airway while occluding the esophagus. If the patient vomits, cricoid pressure is immediately released to avoid esophageal rupture. Pressure is initiated as soon as the patient becomes sedated and is not released until the position of the endotracheal tube is verified. Cricoid pressure is always applied when using a bag-valve-mask to ventilate an apneic patient.

PARALYSIS

Paralytic agents are used to provide total muscle relaxation for optimal intubating conditions. There are two categories of muscle relaxants: the depolarizing agents (succinylcholine is the principal agent) and nondepolarizing agents (e.g., vecuronium, pancuronium, atracurium, and the newer, shorter acting agent rocuronium). The ideal agent acts quickly, thereby reducing the time to intubation. It should have a short duration of action, because if the patient cannot be intubated, he or she will require bag-valve-mask ventilation until the paralysis wears off. The agent should have minimal side effects.[6,9]

The ideal drug for RSI is succinylcholine. Although it has many side effects, in the acute situation, they are rarely of practical concern. Pretreatment with a defasciculating dose of a nondepolarizing agent prevents rises in ICP. As noted, this is necessary only in the muscular patient (more than 5 years and 20 kg). Atropine pretreatment prevents the bradycardia associated with succinylcholine; such bradycardia is especially common if a second dose of succinylcholine is needed to achieve or prolong paralysis.

Nondepolarizing agents such as vecuronium or rocuronium can also be used as the paralyzing agent and require no pretreatment with defasciculating doses. However, the time to intubation is prolonged with the nondepolarizing agents. They also have a longer duration of action.[11] Newer nondepolarizing agents, such as rocuronium, offer the advantage of short onset of action without the potential side effects of succinylcholine or the need for a defasciculating dose for the older child.

INTUBATION

The intubation procedure during RSI is no different from the procedure in other situations. Patience is needed to await complete paralysis (approximately 45 seconds). A stylet is recommended for better control of the endotracheal tube. Tube position should be verified by auscultating the chest and colorimetric CO_2 detection before releasing cricoid pressure. After succinylcholine administration, a nondepolarizing agent should be given to continue paralysis.

SUMMARY

Table 235.8 summarizes the medications used in the pediatric patient undergoing RSI. The scheme is one approach only and can be modified using alternative induction agents and paralytics if preferred.

COMMON PITFALLS

- Failing to have a system in place for RSI that includes all participants (i.e., medical specialists and nursing personnel)

TABLE 235.7. Examples of Induction Agent Choices Considering Perfusion and Clinical Condition[a]

Clinical Condition:	*Head Trauma*		*Hemorrhage*		*Asthma*	
Perfusion Status	Normal	Decreased	Normal	Decreased	Normal	Decreased
AGENT						
	Thiopental	Low-dose thiopental or midazolam	Midazolam	Ketamine	Ketamine or midazolam	Ketamine
RATIONALE						
	Cerebroprotective	Myocardial depressant effect, less at reduced dose		Elevates BP	Ketamine is bronchodilator	Ketamine bronchodilates and elevates BP

[a] Etomidate can be used in any of these clinical conditions.

TABLE 235.8. Summary of Medications Used in Rapid-Sequence Induction

0–5 min	Start preoxygenation
0–3 min	Atropine[a]
0	Etomidate + succinylcholine[b]
0 + 45 s	Intubate

[a] For elevated ICP, add lidocaine and a defasciculating agent (if >20 kg). Fentanyl may be considered, but caution must be used because of the respiratory-depressant sympathetic blockade effect in the compromised patient.
[b] Substitute rocuronium for patients at risk for hyperkalemia.

- Lack of preparation of equipment and drugs before initiating the procedure
- Failing to preoxygenate
- Using bag-valve-mask ventilation in the spontaneously breathing patient
- Failing to perform the Sellick maneuver; failing to relax cricoid pressure if active regurgitation occurs
- Attempting intubation before muscle relaxation
- Failing to secure the endotracheal tube adequately after intubation
- Confusing a defasciculating dose with a paralyzing dose of a nondepolarizing agent before using succinylcholine
- Failing to follow succinylcholine with a nondepolarizing agent in patients requiring prolonged mechanical ventilation
- Failing to verify endotracheal tube position both clinically and with an end-tidal CO_2 detector

References

1. American College of Emergency Physicians, American Academy of Pediatrics. *APLS: the Pediatric Emergency Medicine Course.* Dallas: American College of Emergency Physicians, and Elk Grove Village, IL: American Academy of Pediatrics, 1998.
2. Bergen JM, Smith DC. A review of etomidate for rapid sequence intubation in the emergency department. *J Emerg Med* 1997;15(2)221.
3. Berry FA, Yemen TA. Pediatric airway in health and disease. *Pediatr Clin North Am* 1994;41:153.
4. Gerardi MJ, Sacchetti AD, Cantor RM, et al. Rapid sequence intubation of the pediatric patient. *Ann Emerg Med* 1996;28(1):55.
5. Gnauck K, Lungo JB, Scalzo A, et al. Emergency intubation of the pediatric medical patient: use of anesthetic agents in the emergency department. *Ann Emerg Med* 1994;23:1242.
6. Gronert BJ, Brandom BW. Neuromuscular blocking drugs in infants and children. *Pediatr Clin North Am* 1994;41(1):73.
7. L'Hommedieu CS, Arens JJ. The use of ketamine for the emergency intubation of patients with status asthmaticus. *Ann Emerg Med* 1987;16:568.
8. Nakayama DK, Gardner MJ, Rowe MI. Emergency endotracheal intubation in pediatric trauma. *Ann Surg* 1990;211:218.
9. Nugent SK, Lavarvuso R, Rogers MC. Pharmacology and use of muscle relaxants in infants and children. *J Pediatr* 1979;94:481.
10. Perkin R, Van Stralen D, Mellick LB. Managing pediatric airway emergencies: anatomic considerations, alternative airway and ventilation techniques, and current treatment options. *Pediatr Emerg Med Rep* 1996;1:1–12.
11. Tullock WC, Diana P, Cook DR, Wilks DH, et al. Neuromuscular and cardiovascular effects of high-dose vecuronium. *Anesth Analg* 1990;70:86.
12. Walls RM, Luten RC, Murphy, et al. *National Emergency Airway Management Course manual,* 3rd ed. Wellesley, MA: Airway Management Education Center, 1999.
13. Walls RM. Rapid sequence intubation in head trauma. *Ann Emerg Med* 1993;22:1008.
14. Yamamoto LG, Yim GK, Britten AG. Rapid sequence anesthesia induction for emergency intubation. *Pediatr Emerg Care* 1990;6:200.

CHAPTER 236
Shock

Lucian K. DeNicola and James H. McCrory

Shock is a complex syndrome resulting from insufficient substrate and oxygen delivery (DO_2) to meet tissue metabolic demands (VO_2) (i.e., DO_2 less than VO_2). Untreated, it leads to metabolic acidosis, organ dysfunction, and death. Recognition, diagnosis, and treatment prior to irreversible organ failure can substantially reduce morbidity and mortality.[3,6,7]

DO_2 is a direct function of cardiac output (CO) and arterial oxygen content (CaO_2); that is,

$$DO_2 = CO \times CaO_2$$

CO = heart rate (HR) × stroke volume (SV). SV is the difference between the end diastolic volume (EDV) and the end systolic volume (ESV) and is influenced by preload, afterload, and contractility. CaO_2 is a function of the hemoglobin concentration (Hgb), arterial oxygen saturation (SaO_2) and arterial oxygen tension (PaO_2) (i.e., $CaO_2 = (Hgb \times 1.39 \times SaO_2) + 0.003 \times PaO_2$). Thus, DO_2 can be increased by increasing heart rate, preload, hemoglobin concentration, or arterial oxygenation and by improving the metabolic milieu or, occasionally, by decreasing afterload within certain parameters (Fig. 236.1).

The pathophysiology of shock is far more complex than simple hemodynamics. Decreased DO_2 leads to cellular hypoxia and subsequent alterations in cytochrome oxidation. Reactive oxygen species (oxygen radicals) increase, causing further damage to tissue and initiating inflammatory pathways that lead to release of tumor necrosis factor, interleukin-1, arachidonic acid, complement, and myocardial depressant factors.[4] In septic shock, endotoxin and lipopolysaccharide also stimulate these highly reactive substances.[5] Although much has been accomplished in identifying and understanding these complex interrelationships, and specific treatments have been devised to block deleterious pathways,[2] the successful treatment of shock continues to be based on early hemodynamic improvement to prevent a vicious cycle of cellular destruction.

CLINICAL PRESENTATION

The early diagnosis of shock requires a high index of suspicion based on an understanding of conditions that predispose children to shock. The diagnosis is made by a thorough physical examination that focuses on the adequacy of tissue perfusion, because hypotension is a late and premorbid sign in children due to their ability to sustain pressure by increasing systemic vascular resistance (Fig. 236.2).

The organ systems that are observable include the following:

Neurologic: Fluctuating mental status is a hallmark of poor cerebral perfusion, beginning with lethargy, agitation, and combativeness and progressing to unresponsiveness—even to painful procedures and coma. In infants, in the absence of meningitis, the anterior fontanelle may be sunken.

Skin and Extremities: In order to maintain vital organ perfusion, circulation to the skin and extremities will be diverted. The skin and mucous membranes may be cool, with pallor, cyanosis, and mottling. Rashes may be consistent with classic bacterial, viral, or rickettsial infections. Capillary refill at the

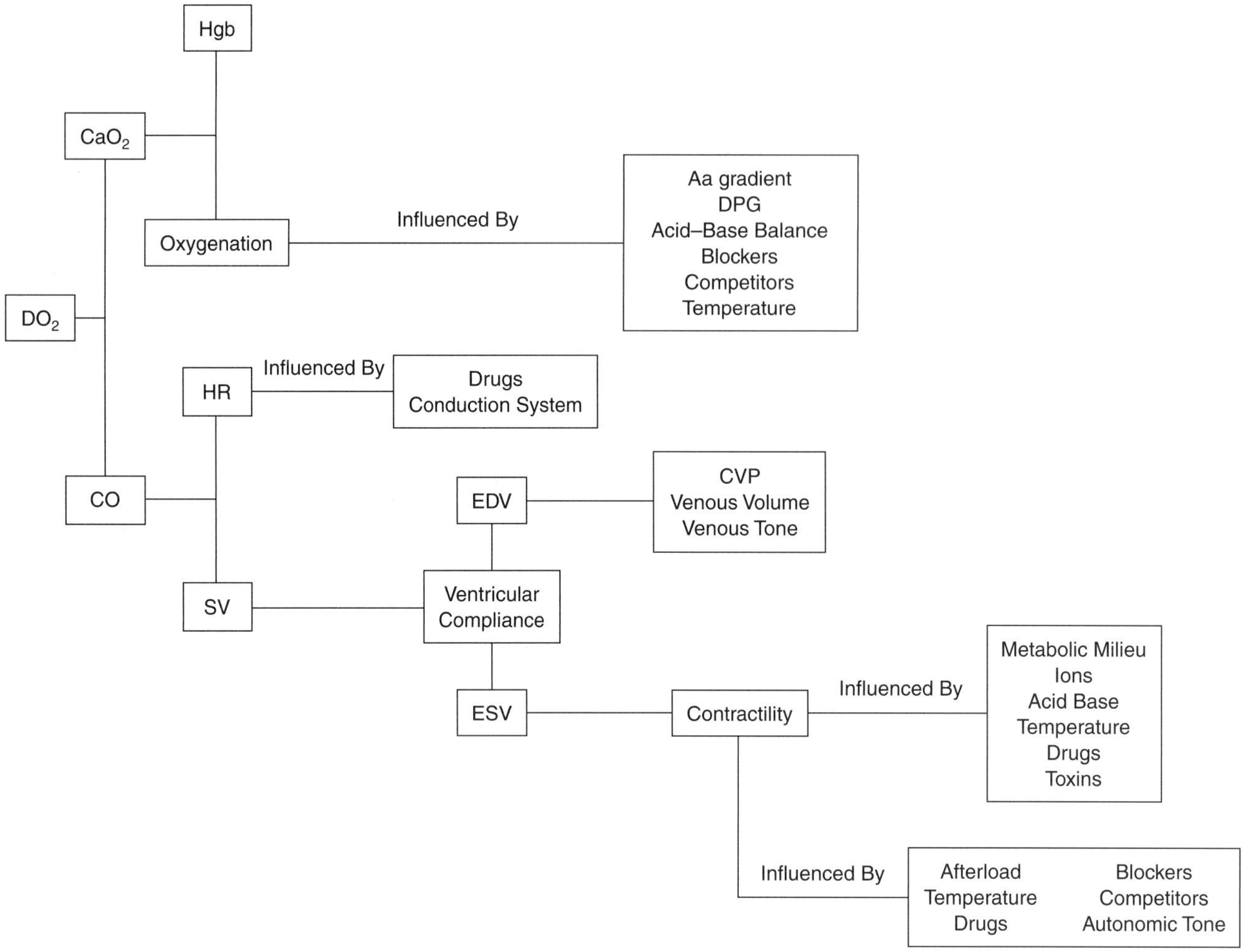

Figure 236.1. Factors affecting oxygen delivery.

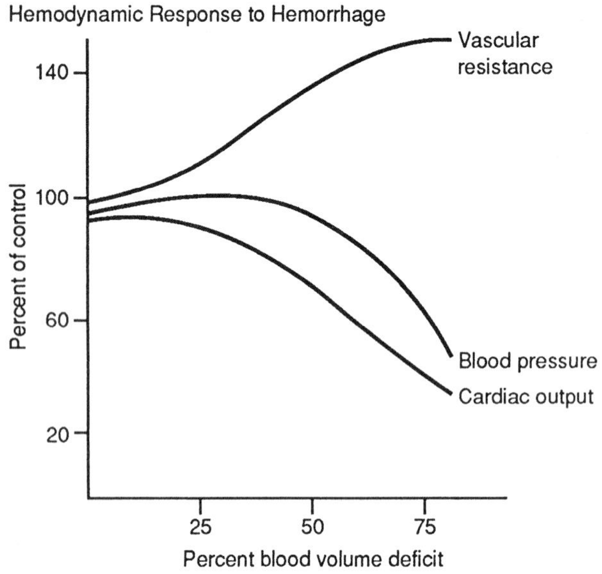

Figure 236.2. Cardiovascular response to hypovolemia from hemorrhage in puppies (based on normative data). (From Schwaitzberg SD, Bergman KS, Harris BH. A pediatric trauma model of continuous hemorrhage. *J Pediatr Surg* 1988;23:605.)

nail beds will be greater than 2 seconds, and peripheral pulses at the wrist and ankles may be weak or absent. Poor muscle tone reflects decreased muscle perfusion and, coupled with central nervous system dysfunction, leads to prostration.

Cardiopulmonary: Hyperpnea and tachycardia may be the only cardiopulmonary signs in early, compensated shock, as increases in HR compensate for decreased SV, and hyperpnea compensates for metabolic acidosis. Auscultation of the chest is often normal unless the source of the shock is pulmonary edema or infection, supraventricular tachycardia, pneumothorax, cardiac tamponade, or undiagnosed congenital heart disease.

Renal: As organ perfusion diminishes, so does glomerular filtration rate. The first compensation for decreased perfusion is urinary concentration, followed by decreased-to-absent urine output. This decrease will not be readily apparent by examination but may be elicited by history or bladder intubation.

DIFFERENTIAL DIAGNOSIS

Although there are many classifications of shock (Table 236.1), it is important to recognize that precise identification may be arduous and require prolonged laboratory examination. Time is critical, and treatment cannot wait for precise classification. Lacking immediate physical signs that indicate precise etiology,

TABLE 236.1. Etiologic Classification of Shock States

HYPOVOLEMIC SHOCK
Hemorrhage
Internal
External
Serum/plasma loss
Burn
Third-spacing (i.e., nephrosis, bowel ischemia)
Septic
Diabetes insipidus and mellitus
Gastrointestinal loss
Drugs (i.e., diuretics, laxatives)
CARDIOGENIC SHOCK
Myocardial
Ischemia
Infectious/septic
Toxic/drugs (i.e., hypocalcemia, beta blockers, etc.)
Dysrhythmia
Congenital
Usually ductus arteriosus-dependent lesion (i.e., coarctation, hypoplastic left heart, critical aortic stenosis)
DISTRIBUTIVE SHOCK
Anaphylactic
Neurogenic
Increased intracranial pressure
Spinal cord injury
Septic
OBSTRUCTIVE SHOCK
Pneumothorax
Pericardial tamponade
Dissecting aortic aneurysm
METABOLIC/TOXIC SHOCK
Heat
CO, cyanide
Endocrine
Thyroid
Adrenal
Parathyroid

the history and, occasionally, the laboratory findings are needed to differentiate the causes of shock.

Physiologically, with the exception of some forms of cardiogenic shock, absolute or relative hypovolemia is usually present, causing decreased preload and decreased SV. With the exception of pericardial tamponade, the size of the cardiac shadow on chest radiogram reflects the intracardiac volume and can be used as a determinate of the need for volume replacement (Fig. 236.3). Even cardiogenic shock, without pulmonary edema, may improve with judicious volume replacement.[1]

EMERGENCY DEPARTMENT EVALUATION

The diagnosis of shock should be made by a primary and secondary survey. Initially, airway patency is assessed and, in the absence of cervical instability, can be corrected by positioning or provision of an artificial airway. Assessment of breathing may be difficult. Hypoventilation in the face of shock signals central nervous system dysfunction and requires immediate attention. Hypoxia also requires immediate attention. Hyperventilation may be compensatory for metabolic acidosis or may be a response to obstructive shock or fever.

The adequacy of peripheral circulation is observed by inspection of cutaneous vasoconstriction, mottling, cool extremities, and prolonged capillary refill greater than 2 seconds. Palpation of the peripheral pulse correlates better with tissue blood flow than does the blood pressure, which may be preserved by intense vasoconstriction until just prior to cardiac arrest.

Once the primary survey is completed and resuscitation measures instituted, a secondary survey may be undertaken to investigate the etiology and extent of the shock state. There should be a complete physical examination, with emphasis placed on the primary shock organs, including the neuroaxis, pulmonary, and cardiac systems and a careful abdominal examination. A complete blood count; determination of serum electrolytes, glucose, blood urea nitrogen, and creatinine; and acid–base determination are usually necessary. The patient's history guides the remainder of the laboratory examination and

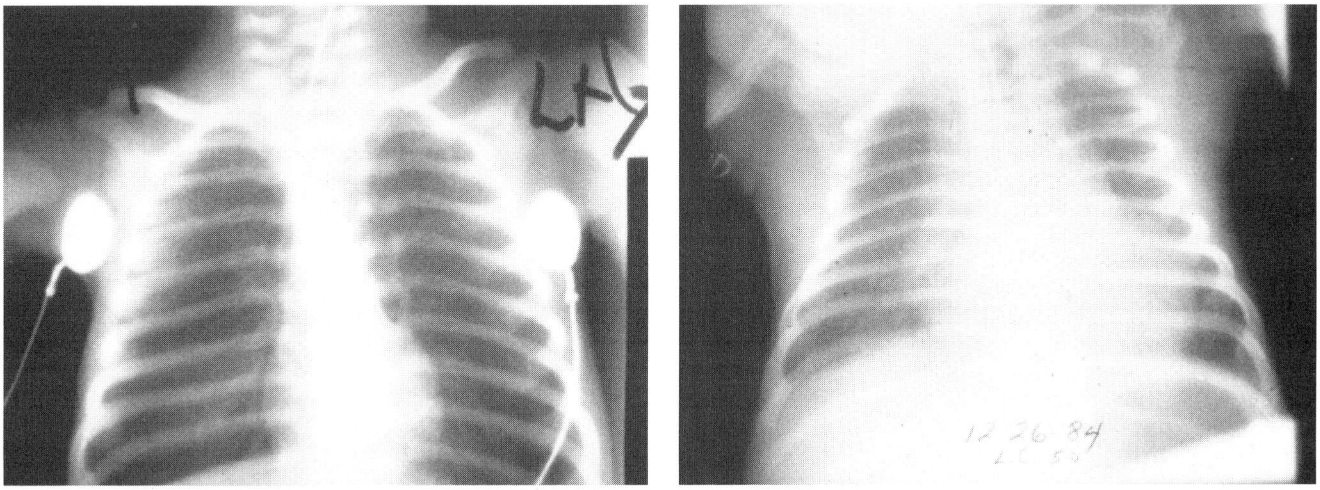

A B

Figure 236.3. **(A)** Chest x-ray from a 6-week-old premature infant showing small heart shadow in hypovolemic shock secondary to gastroenteritis. **(B)** Chest x-ray from a 3-day-old term infant showing large heart shadow in cardiogenic shock secondary to an inborn error of metabolism. The size of the cardiac shadow is directly proportional to the intravascular volume and can be used to distinguish cardiogenic shock from those etiologies that produce an absolute or relative hypovolemia. (From American Heart Association. *Pediatric Advanced Life Support Course.*)

may include a reticulocyte count, determination of serum protein and albumin, liver or cardiac enzymes, drug screens, or cultures. Arrhythmias require sequential electrocardiograms, and when congenital heart disease is considered, a pediatric echocardiogram is imperative.

A plain film of the chest has both diagnostic and therapeutic significance. In addition to revealing heart or lung disease, including pneumothorax, the size of the heart can be used as an indicator of volume status. The size of the cardiac silhouette on serial x-rays may be used to guide the degree of volume replacement.

EMERGENCY DEPARTMENT MANAGEMENT

All children in shock should be maintained at physiologic temperatures and provided with sufficient oxygen to maintain their oxygen saturation above 90% to 92% by pulse oximetry. Heart rate and rhythm should be continuously monitored, and blood pressure, temperature, fluid intake, and fluid output must be assessed frequently. A calm and reassuring manner may reduce pain and anxiety, thus decreasing wasted oxygen consumption without resorting to the use of analgesics or sedatives that might impede physiologic compensation.

Endotracheal intubation is indicated for any patient with a compromised or unstable airway. Provision of positive-pressure ventilation is indicated for respiratory arrest, persistent apnea, hypoventilation, presumed intracranial hypertension, and acute hypercapnea, or when deep anesthesia is required for definitive therapeutic interventions. When absolute indications are lacking, mechanical ventilation should be postponed until adequate preload is established, because positive-pressure ventilation may impede right heart return. Establishment of adequate vascular access is essential and is addressed in the following chapter. When the etiology of the shock is clearly discernible (i.e., anaphylaxis, chest trauma, known hypoparathyroidism, known steroid dependency) and definitive treatment is quickly available, early attempts should then be made for primary correction (i.e., removal of antigen, insertion of chest tube, correction of profound hypocalcemia, administration of steroids). In most cases, however, a general approach to the treatment of shock is required.

Volume Expansion

Volume resuscitation is the mainstay of all forms of shock therapy and is oriented toward restoring intravascular volume relative to the vascular space and optimizing ventricular preload. Even in shock due to myocardial failure, judiciously optimizing left ventricular preload (using aliquots of 5 cc/kg of 0.9% saline) can improve stroke volume. Initially, the resuscitation fluids of choice are either normal saline (0.9% NaCl) or lactated Ringer's solution. Except for shock due to myocardial failure, aliquots of 10 to 20 mL/kg are given rapidly over 2 to 10 minutes. The end point of volume resuscitation is clinical improvement in perfusion as assessed by a decrease in HR and compensatory hyperventilation, an increase in blood pressure, capillary refill, muscle tone and strength of peripheral pulses, and improvement in affect and skin color. These improvements may require from 60 to 100 mL/kg in fluid replacement. If no improvement is seen after 40 to 60 mL/kg of resuscitation fluid has been given, consider ongoing fluid losses or alternative causes of shock, such as adrenal insufficiency, intestinal ischemia, pericardial effusion, or pneumothorax. A chest radiogram may be useful to visualize heart size as a measure of the adequacy of volume resuscitation. When central venous access is obtainable, determination of central venous pressure may be useful in guiding further volume therapy. Early determination of serum glucose, electrolytes, calcium, acid–base status, and hemoglobin concentration will help guide the choice of solutions for definitive therapy.

Cardiotonic Infusions

Lack of unusual fluid losses by history, preexisting heart disease, hepatomegaly, rales, cardiomegaly, and failure to improve perfusion with provision of adequate oxygenation, ventilation, HR, and volume expansion should suggest a cardiogenic or distributive component to the patient's shock state. Cardiotonic and vasoactive drug infusions can further improve cardiac output and tissue perfusion by inotropy, chronotropy, or altering blood flow distribution.

Prior to the administration of cardiotonic–vasoactive drugs, the goals of therapy and the criteria for monitoring the end point must be established. Although a variety of agents are available, only a few drugs are appropriate for the acute resuscitation period in pediatric patients (Table 236.2) The child's outcome is dependent on both the expeditious reversal of the shock state and the definitive treatment of the underlying cause. Administration of antibiotics, antihistamines, hormones, antidotes or surgical intervention may preclude the need for prolonged cardiotonic treatment.

DISPOSITION

Specific subspecialty referral is dependent on the etiology of the child's shock. In all cases, these children will require admission to an inpatient facility with the trained staff and facilities to care

TABLE 236.2. Suggested Drugs, Dosages, and End Points for Cardioactive Drugs for Pediatric Shock

Drug	Dose	Effect	End Point
Epinephrine	0.05–0.15 μg/kg/min	Increases heart rate, improves contractility and increases systemic vascular resistance	Tachycardia, increased blood pressure
Dopamine	2–20 μg/kg/min Dopaminergic effects at low dose, beta-1 effects at medium dose, alpha effects at high dose	Increases renal and splanchnic blood flow, increases cardiac contractility, and, at high doses, will increase heart rate and vascular resistance	Improved perfusion and urine output; may improve blood pressure
Dobutamine	1–15 μg/kg/min	Increases contractility and may reduce systemic resistance	Improved perfusion; may slightly lower blood pressure
Prostaglandin E-1	0.05–0.1 μg/kg/min	Maintains patency of ductus arteriosus for neonates with cardiac lesions that are duct dependent	Improved perfusion

for a critically ill child. The child in shock should be transported by appropriate transport personnel that have pediatric experience and necessary equipment and medications.

COMMON PITFALLS

- The most common pitfall is failure to recognize pediatric shock, either due to the child's ability to maintain blood pressure by increasing HR and systemic resistance or due to early hyperdynamic septic shock where perfusion is maintained. To avoid this pitfall, the physician must have a high index of suspicion and perform a complete physical examination, with emphasis on the shock organs.
- Another common diagnostic error is to assume that all "shocky" children are septic when the true diagnosis may be a neurologic or cardiologic problem or an abdominal vascular crisis (i.e., volvulus or intussusception).
- A major treatment pitfall is inability to obtain adequate vascular access when a child is in shock. If peripheral access cannot be obtained within 3 minutes, alternate routes (intraosseus, central line) should be attempted.
- Another treatment pitfall is failing to rapidly administer the appropriate amount of volume expansion. Children have a higher blood volume relative to weight than do adults, and thus may require substantial volumes of resuscitation fluid. Determining the end point of volume expansion is based on clinical improvement and aided by serial chest radiographs to evaluate heart size. If central access was obtained, a simple beside central venous pressure can be done by lowering a free-running intravenous line to observe the distance above the heart that backflow occurs. Conversely, excessive volume administration to a child with myocardial failure may lead to overwhelming pulmonary edema and possibly acute respiratory distress syndrome. When an infant less than 1 week of age presents in shock, be sure to consider congenital heart disease as well as sepsis. An initial chest radiograph showing cardiomegaly should preclude overly vigorous volume resuscitation and evoke an immediate pediatric cardiology consultation.
- Shock that is unresponsive to volume resuscitation and cardiotonic administration requires a broadened differential diagnosis that should include adrenal crisis, hypoglycemia, and hypocalcemia, as well as obstructive shock and abdominal crisis. Fingerstick glucose levels can be checked, and prospective treatment with cortisone and calcium is not contraindicated.

References

1. Bengur AR, Meliones JN. Cardiogenic shock. *New Horiz* 1998;6:139–149.
2. Christman JW, Holden EP, Blackwell TS. Strategies for blocking the systemic effects of cytokines in the sepsis syndrome. *Crit Care Med* 1995;23:955–963.
3. Crone RK. Acute circulatory failure in children. *Pediatr Clin North Am* 1980;27:525–538.
4. Flowers F, Zimmerman JJ. Reactive oxygen species in the cellular pathophysiology of shock. *New Horiz* 1998;6:169–180.
5. Murphy K, Haudek SB, Thompson M, et al. Molecular biology of septic shock. *New Horiz* 1998;6:181–193.
6. Perkin RM, Levin DL. Shock in the pediatric patient. Parts I and II. *J Pediatr* 1982;101:163–169, 319–332.
7. Perkin RM, Levin DL. Shock in the pediatric patient. Part II. J *Pediatr* 1982;101:319.

CHAPTER 237
Vascular Access in Children

Talaat A. Abdelmoneim and Lucian K. DeNicola

It is well known that establishing intravenous access in an infant or young child is challenging even under normal circumstances. In an acute setting, intravenous access is needed for the delivery of resuscitative medications, antibiotics, administration of volume expanders, correction of electrolyte abnormalities, and blood sampling for diagnostic tests. In the less emergent scenario, intravenous access allows provision of maintenance fluids for patients unable to maintain adequate oral hydration. Peripheral venous cannulation is the easiest and safest method of access and should be attempted before attempting more invasive methods.

The method selected for intravenous access is determined by the child's age, developmental level, and acuity status. In newborn resuscitation, the umbilical vessels may be used for vascular access. In children younger than 6 years of age who are critically ill or injured, the intraosseous (IO) route is an excellent alternative for intravenous access. Percutaneous central venous access may be attempted in a child of any age in an emergency. Another alternative that is less commonly used in pediatric emergencies is peripheral venous cutdown. Utilizing nonvascular methods for drug administration includes endotracheal, intragastric, intramuscular, subcutaneous, rectal, and inhalation routes. Arterial cannulation provides a direct means of continuously measuring blood pressure and sampling.

This chapter reviews various methods of vascular access and briefly addresses nonvascular routes used for emergency administration of some medications. The role of ultrasonography as an aid in the localization and cannulation of vessels is addressed.

PERIPHERAL INTRAVENOUS LINES

When emergent administration of fluid or medication is indicated, an intravenous catheter must be placed rapidly. The vein that appears easiest to cannulate should be attempted first. The child's developmental level is helpful in determining the best site to be accessed:

Infants: median antecubital basilic, median cephalic veins, scalp veins, and the dorsal veins of the hand
Toddlers: dorsal veins of the hand or foot, antecubital veins
Children greater than 2 years old: hand, forearm, and antecubital veins

The greater saphenous vein is often selected in pediatric patients because of its large size and consistent anatomy, and it may be cannulated successfully without palpation or visualization.[12]

Another useful access site in infants is the external jugular vein, although the infant must often be immobilized and placed in a dependent posture for safe insertion at the site. Unfortunately, external jugular catheters are difficult to stabilize and are easily dislodged.

The use of an arm board to immobilize the site, tourniquets, heat lamps, and transillumination devices can be helpful. It is extremely important to have adequate assistance in immobilizing the site and handling vascular supplies. Caretakers will usually become very emotional or angry if their child requires multiple intravenous sticks secondary to movement or unskilled health-care providers. The skin should be cleansed with alcohol or iodophor before the skin is punctured. A tourniquet should be placed proximal to the intended site of cannulation. A T-connector is often attached from the hub of the catheter to the intravenous tubing to avoid putting tension on the catheter. Sterile dextrose water or saline is then flushed through the catheter to ensure that it infuses freely into the vein.[4] The catheter is taped securely to the skin, and the extremity is immobilized with a padded arm board. One or both hands may need to be immobilized or "mittened" to prevent the small child from pulling out the intravenous catheter.

PERIPHERALLY INSERTED CENTRAL CATHETER LINES

Peripherally inserted central catheter (PICC) lines are long-term intravenous access devices for peripheral insertion. They can be placed peripherally or advanced into the central circulation. Because the silicone PICCs are especially soft and pliable, they must be inserted with a through-the-needle technique either with or without a guidewire or forceps. Venipuncture is performed in the antecubital fossa. Before insertion, the basilic, median cubital, and cephalic veins need to be thoroughly assessed. A chest x-ray will confirm that the tip is correctly placed.[10] Complications that may result from peripheral intravenous catheterization include hematoma formation, cellulitis, thrombosis, phlebitis, pulmonary embolism, and air embolism.

CENTRAL VENOUS CATHETERS

The central venous catheter is one of the most commonly used invasive tools in the management of critically ill children. Indications vary from routine access to emergent situations (Table 237.1).

A central venous catheter should not be inserted in a site where skin is infected or burned or in an extremity that has vascular insufficiency, hematoma, thrombus, or abscess.[7] Percutaneous central venous catheter kits are available in various sizes. A 3.0F or 4.0F catheter should be used in infants younger than 1 year, while 4.0F to 5.5F catheters can be used in children 1 to 12 years of age. Catheters may be inserted percutaneously into the subclavian, femoral, or internal jugular veins using the Seldinger technique.[13]

The femoral vein is the easiest and safest central vein to cannulate in emergencies because of its anatomic landmarks and large size, and it can be accessed without interfering with resuscitation.[8] The leg is abducted and externally rotated. The groin is prepped with iodophor and draped. The femoral vein is located medial to the femoral artery, which can be palpated as a guide.

TABLE 237.1. Indications for Central Venous Access

Inability to establish peripheral venous access and the patient is hemodynamically unstable
Administration of large volumes of potentially caustic or incompatible medications
Delivery of parenteral nutrition
Hemodynamic monitoring in patients not responsive to resuscitative efforts

The area below the inguinal ligament, medial to the femoral artery is infiltrated with 1% lidocaine; be careful not to inject any intravenously or intraarterially. The introducer needle (with syringe attached) is then directed at a 30- to 45-degree angle to the skin, starting about 1 cm below the inguinal ligament and aiming toward the contralateral shoulder. Traction is applied to the plunger of the syringe once the needle has broken the skin. When blood return is noted, the syringe is disconnected from the needle; be careful not to change the angle of the needle in the process. The hub of the needle is covered with a thumb to prevent air embolism during a spontaneous breath.

A guidewire is then threaded through the needle, starting with the J-tip, until at least one-fourth of the wire is in the vein. The needle is removed, leaving the wire in place, and the scalpel is used to enlarge the skin entry site. A dilator is then threaded over the wire and advanced, with a twisting motion, through the skin. The tip of the wire is held in place to prevent its migration into the patient. The dilator is removed, and the catheter (which has been previously flushed with saline) is threaded over the wire through the skin entry site and into the vein. The catheter is not advanced past the skin until it is possible to grasp the tip of the wire at the external end of the catheter. This may require pulling out some of the wire that was previously placed. The catheter then may be inserted to the proper location, determined at the beginning of the procedure. The wire is removed, and a syringe of heparin flush is used to confirm good blood return and to flush the line to prevent clotting. The catheter is sutured in place, and a radiograph is performed to confirm proper position of the catheter.[1]

Internal jugular and subclavian venous approaches also can be performed by experienced personnel, but these procedures carry the additional risks of pneumothorax and hemothorax.[11]

INTRAOSSEOUS ACCESS

The IO route is probably the most useful and versatile of the emergency nonperipheral vascular access sites and should be considered in all children younger than 6 years when emergent access is crucial and attempts at peripheral vascular sites are unsuccessful. In extreme circumstances, the IO technique can be used in older children and adults when other vascular attempts are unsuccessful. The marrow cavity is much smaller in older children. Any drug or fluid that can be administered intravenously can be infused through the IO route. The IO route also provides a means for rapid and effective volume resuscitation using crystalloids, colloids, or blood products.[9] The bone marrow can also be a source of laboratory studies for diagnostic as well as therapeutic interventions.[5,14] The preferred site for IO infusion is the flat, anteromedial surface of the proximal tibia 1 cm inferior to and 1 cm medial to the tibial tubercle (Fig. 237.1). Other sites include the distal femur, the distal tibia proximal to the medial or lateral malleoli, and the iliac crests. There are several styles of commercially available IO infusion needles, and Jamshidi-type bone marrow aspiration needles can be used.

The skin over the anterior tibia should be sterilized with iodophor and a towel roll or intravenous fluid bag placed under the knee to stabilize the lower leg. Starting 1 to 3 cm below the tibial tuberosity (to avoid damaging the growth plate), the needle is directed at a 90-degree angle to the medial surface of the tibia. When the needle passes through the cortex of the bone, a decrease in resistance will be apparent. Several signs help to confirm that the needle is in the marrow cavity:

- The needle will stand upright without support.
- When a syringe is attached to the needle, marrow can be aspirated (in approximately 50% of cases).
- Fluid infuses freely without signs of subcutaneous infiltration.

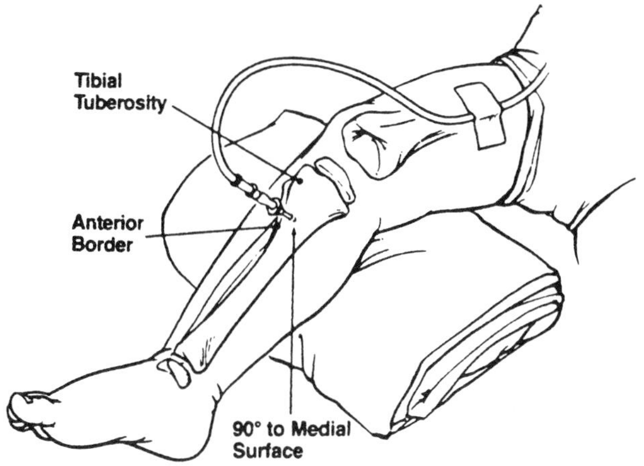

Figure 237.1. Intraosseus cannulation technique. (From American Heart Association. *Textbook of pediatric advanced life support.* Dallas: American Heart Association, 1997, with permission.)

Complications of IO infusions are rare but include osteomyelitis, compartment syndrome, tibial fracture, and skin necrosis.[1,5,14]

VASCULAR CUTDOWN

Surgical venous cutdown has decreased in popularity since the resurgence of the IO technique, but remains useful in emergency situations when attempts at percutaneous access and IO have failed or cannot be performed. The long saphenous vein that courses anterior to the medial malleolus at the ankle is the preferred site for cutdown.

The lower extremity is immobilized, with the foot turned laterally, exposing the saphenous vein anterior to the medial malleolus. A sterile field is prepared, and 1% lidocaine is injected subcutaneously over the vein. An incision perpendicular to the vein is made, and the vein is gently isolated by blunt dissection with a curved hemostat. Two silk sutures are looped around the vein; the distal one may be used to ligate the vein. With tension applied to the proximal suture loop, a venotomy is made with a no. 11 blade inserted into the lateral wall of the vessel and drawn upward. This avoids complete transection of the vessel. Finally, the cannula is inserted into the vein, advanced, and secured in place by tying a proximal suture loop. The wound is then closed with simple nylon sutures and dressed.

Percutaneously placed peripheral catheters are limited by short-term access, moderate infusion volumes, and solutions that are of low osmolarity. The most important complication in the use of peripheral vascular catheters is their potential to become partially dislodged or occluded, thereby resulting in leakage of nonphysiologic fluids into the extravascular tissue.[2]

UMBILICAL VASCULAR ACCESS

In neonates, the umbilical vessels may be directly accessed during the first several days of life directly or by intraumbilical cutdown. Both the umbilical vein (UV) and the umbilical artery (UA) may be used for blood sampling and fluid or drug infusion. The UA and the UV may be used for blood pressure and central venous pressure monitoring, respectively. Normally, two UAs and one UV exist. At skin level, the UV is usually in the 12 o'clock position and has a thinner wall and wider lumen than does the UA. The infant must be supine and restrained; maintenance of temperature and sterile technique is mandatory. The umbilicus is scrubbed with a bactericidal solution and draped, and a silk suture is looped around the base of the umbilicus stump. The distal end of the stump is cut off, and the vessels are occluded to prevent blood loss.

A 3.5F to 5.0F catheter is flushed with saline and inserted into the lumen of the desired vessel. Advancement of a UA catheter should place the tip above the celiac axis but below the ductus arteriosis. The UV catheter tip should lie a few centimeters into the UV or inferior vena cava (4 to 5 cm). Plain radiographs should be taken to confirm placement.[3] Complications of umbilical catheters include hemorrhage, infection, air embolism, and perforation of a blood vessel.[8]

ARTERIAL ACCESS

Arterial cannulation for continuous blood pressure and arterial blood gas monitoring is often necessary in critically ill infants and children. Sites available for arterial access include the radial, axillary, femoral, posterior tibial, and dorsalis pedis arteries. Most commonly, the radial artery is used. It lies between the distal radius laterally and the flexor carpi radialis tendon medially. It is important to assess the adequacy of collateral flow to the hand before radial artery cannulation, using a modified Allen test or Doppler flow evaluation.[1]

The hand is secured on an arm board, with slight extension of the wrist to avoid excessive median nerve stretching. The fingertips should be left exposed when the hand is taped down so that any peripheral ischemic changes can be observed. Palpate the artery for maximal pulsation and introduce the cannula (22- or 24-gauge catheter) at an angle of 30 degrees. Making a nick into the skin at the point of entry with a larger needle facilitates introduction of the cannula. Blood is aspirated to confirm the intraarterial position of the cannula. Radial arterial cannulation can also be accomplished by the Seldinger technique or cutdown, these techniques being similar to that described for venous access. Similar techniques are used for cannulation of other arteries.[3]

The most common complications of arterial catheterization include minor skin lesions, localized hematoma, arterial bleeding, and arterial thrombosis with distal ischemia. The catheter should be removed immediately if any evidence of tissue ischemia develops.

ACCESSING PERMANENT INDWELLING CENTRAL VENOUS CATHETERS

Indwelling central catheters are placed in patients who require long-term chemotherapy, parenteral nutrition, antibiotics, and deferoxamine chelation therapy in patients with sickle cell disease. A variety of catheters (e.g., Hickman, Broviac) and implantable venous devices, or "ports" (e.g., Infus-a-port, MediPort), are used in pediatric patients. Familiarity with the technique of accessing indwelling catheters in a child who has one inserted can save multiple painful attempts at venous and arterial punctures, which are not without complication. The most common complications of chronic central catheters are infection, formation of thrombi, and breakage of the catheter.

THE ROLE OF ULTRASONOGRAPHY

In some situations, such as marked hypotension, pulses may not be easily palpable, making arterial catheterization extremely difficult and standard intravenous access difficult or impossible. The use of Doppler ultrasonography has been advocated to aid in the localization and cannulation of both arteries and veins.

A recently introduced device incorporates a disposable ultrasound transducer within the lumen of a thin-wall vascular needle (P.D. Access, Advanced Medical Inc., Philadelphia). This allows detection of both arterial and venous sounds, and the intended vessel can be selected for access while avoiding trauma to other structures. The absence of a vessel can also be verified to potentially eliminate further trauma. Another device uses a Doppler transducer with a central orifice that allows passage of the needle through the transducer, once the vessel has been located, using B-mode ultrasonography (Site Rite II, Dymax Corp., Pittsburgh).

EMERGENCY ALTERNATIVES TO INTRAVENOUS ACCESS

A number of other procedures have been used in the past as alternatives to intravenous access when access could not be readily achieved. These included intradermal clysis, rectal clysis, intraperitoneal infusion, sublingual injection, and intracardiac injection.

In the past, intradermal clysis was usually performed with a needle inserted subcutaneously on the back between the scapulae. Clysis was used for volume replacement in dehydration states, but when perfusion is compromised because of hypovolemia or shock, clysis is unreliable and not sufficiently rapid. Rectal clysis involves the infusion of fluid into the rectum for volume replacement. It is also unreliable and erratic and risks rectal perforation, septicemia, and increased volume loss from rectal stimulation and diarrhea.

Intraperitoneal infusion has also been used for volume replacement and, although more effective than clysis, it is clearly not as effective as IO or intravenous fluid administration and risks viscus perforation, injury to other abdominal organs, and the introduction of infection and peritonitis.

Sublingual injection cannot be used for volume infusion, but the sublingual area is a route for the administration, in an emergency, of drugs such as epinephrine, atropine, or lidocaine. Sublingual injection is based on the preferential maintenance of perfusion to the face and brain, even in states of hypovolemia or shock. There is a rich vascular plexus on the underside of the tongue. Unfortunately, studies have demonstrated that the sublingual and intralingual injection of drugs is not very effective in shock or arrest states.

Intracardiac injection was widely practiced in the 1950s and 1960s as a means of administering emergency drugs when an intravenous route was not available, and also of directly administering drugs to the heart when intravenous administration was ineffective. The intracardiac injection of drugs was abandoned by the American Heart Association in the late 1970s, when studies demonstrated that the risks of intracardiac injection exceeded the benefits.[1]

References

1. American Heart Association. Vascular access. In: Chameides L, Hazinski, MF, eds. *Pediatric advanced life support.* Dallas: 1997:5-1.
2. Clark VL, Kruse JA. Arterial catheterization. *Crit Care Clin* 1992;4(8):687–696.
3. Dyer BJ, Weiman MG, Ludwing S. Central venous catheters in the emergency department—access, utilization and problem solving. *Pediatr Emerg Care.* 1995;11:112–117.
4. Engle WA, Rescorla FJ. Vascular access and blood sampling techniques in infants and children. In: Roberts JR, Hedges JR, eds. *Clinical procedures in emergency medicine,* 2nd ed. Philadelphia: WB Saunders, 1991:268–287.
5. Fiallos M, Kissoon N, Abdelmoneim T, et al. Fat embolism with the use of intraosseous infusion during cardiopulmonary resuscitation. *Am J Med Sci* 1997;314(2):73–79.
6. French J. *Pediatric emergency skills.* St. Louis: Mosby, 1995.
7. Gauderer MW. Vascular access techniques and devices in the pediatric patient. *Surg Clin North Am* 1992;72:1267–1284.
8. King D, Conway EE. Vascular access. *Pediatr Ann* 1996;25(12):693–698.
9. Kissoon N, Rosenberg H, Gloon J, et al. Comparison of the acid-base status of blood obtained from intraosseous and central venous sites during steady-and-low flow states. *Crit Care Med* 1993;21:1765–1769.
10. Meares C. P.I.C.C. and M.L.C. lines—options worth exploring. *Nursing* 1992;22(10):52–55.
11. Orlowski JP. Emergency alternatives to intravenous access. *Pediatr Clin North Am* 1994;41(6):1183–1199.
12. Stovroff M, Teague WG. Intravenous access in infants and children. *Pediatr Clin North Am* 1998;45(6):1373–1393.
13. Strauss RH. Pediatric vascular access. In: Fuhrman BP, Zimmerman JJ, eds. *Pediatric critical care.* St. Louis: Mosby, 1998:126–139.
14. Vidal R, Kissoon N, Gayle M. Compartment syndrome following intraosseous infusion. *J Pediatr* 1993;91:1201–1202.

PART II
Signs and Symptoms

CHAPTER 238
Abdominal Pain

Javier I. Escobar II and Steven A. Godwin

Abdominal pain is a common complaint in children presenting to emergency departments (EDs). It is estimated that abdominal pain alone accounts for approximately 5% of ED visits,[3] and that abdominal pain accompanied by vomiting and diarrhea account for nearly 20 % of general and pediatric ED visits.[10]

Abdominal pain in children is caused by a variety of disorders, and, in each stage of childhood, the common causes of abdominal pain differ. The emergency physician must be able to recognize causes of abdominal pain in children of all ages, from neonatal surgical emergencies to the more typical adult problems of the teen-ager.

Although most etiologies of abdominal pain are benign, it is imperative to identify those that are true emergencies. Prompt recognition of abdominal emergencies, with rapid institution of treatment, can significantly reduce morbidity and mortality in pediatric patients. Unfortunately, early recognition of serious abdominal disorders is often difficult. As an example, one study showed that 28% of pediatric appendicitis cases were initially misdiagnosed.[12] Accurate diagnosis is further complicated by the atypical presentation of abdominal emergencies. It has been reported that the classic triad for intussusception—currant jelly stool, colicky abdominal pain, and vomiting—is noted in as few as 10% to 40% of patients.[5]

A useful method for facilitating the evaluation of children complaining of abdominal pain involves separating the various disorders on an age-related basis (Table 238.1).

CLINICAL PRESENTATION

The most common condition of infancy, presenting with apparent abdominal pain, is colic.[6] The predominant symptom is prolonged, continuous crying. The infant may have mild abdominal distention and may pull the knees up against the abdomen, giving the parents the impression that the infant is experiencing abdominal pain. The infant may be inconsolable, although rocking, swinging, or a car ride may calm the baby. The pattern of the pain is predictable, coming on suddenly in the late afternoon or evening. Feeding irregularities, such as excessive air swallowing and gulping, inadequate burping, or bottle propping by the caregiver, may be historic clues.

The physical examination, except for the infant's crying, is often unremarkable. In contrast to the colicky baby, an infant with a serious abdominal disorder often has signs of intestinal obstruction with vomiting and distention. Of particular mention is the infant with bilious vomiting, which should prompt the emergency physician to suspect a mechanical obstruction proximal to the ligament of Treitz. This suspicion should be greatly increased in the absence of rhinitis, sneezing, fever, diarrhea, and other symptoms associated with a systemic viral illness.[13] Nonsurgical causes of bilious vomiting include sepsis, urinary tract infection, and inborn errors of metabolism. Surgical causes include intussusception and malrotation complicated by midgut volvulus.

Intussusception is the most common cause of intestinal obstruction in children less than 2 years of age, and can be defined as a telescoping of a proximal section of bowel into a more distal segment. It typically has a dramatic, acute onset in a previously thriving baby with an otherwise uncomplicated gastroenteritis. The pain appears to come in waves, with the infant relatively normal between attacks. There may be similarly intermittent waves of extreme pallor and diaphoresis. The triad for intussusception includes abdominal pain, emesis, and the hallmark currant jelly stool that is typically a late finding. Additionally, patients may present with profound lethargy and miosis, presumably from an intussusception-induced endogenous opioid secretion.[15] Naloxone has been successful in the reversal of these symptoms.

Malrotation complicated by midgut volvulus is a surgical emergency. Malrotation is a congenital anomaly in bowel migration and mesentery fixation, which predisposes the bowel to twist on itself, resulting in a volvulus. Bowel injury in patients with malrotation develops rapidly, with bowel necrosis occurring in 1 to 2 hours. These infants often present with an acute onset of pain followed, by distention, obstipation, and, frequently, bilious emesis.

Appendicitis in the infant will present as peritonitis in over 90% of cases.[11,14] Irritability, crying, refusal of feeding, and vomiting, in conjunction with fever, distention, and shallow, grunting respirations, constitute the clinical presentation. In advanced cases, the infant may present in shock. The physical examination may reveal an indurated and erythematous abdominal wall in these delayed presentations. Older children present with more classic symptoms of appendicitis, such as low-grade fevers, anorexia, and periumbilical pain that localizes to the right lower quadrant. On physical examination, McBurney's point tenderness, Rovsing's sign, and peritonitis may be noted. The diagnosis of appendicitis should be made in a timely manner. This urgency is highlighted by the increased risk of appendiceal perforation with time, as the majority of cases will perforate within 48 hours of symptom onset.[2]

TABLE 238.1. Differential Diagnosis of Abdominal Pain in Children

Infants	Toddlers	School-Aged	Teenager
Colic	Acute gastroenteritis	Idiopathic	Appendicitis
Intussusception	Urinary tract infection	Appendicitis	Pelvic inflammatory disease
Malrotation	Constipation	Acute gastroenteritis	Peptic ulcer disease
Volvulus	Referred pain	Constipation	Ectopic pregnancy
Hirschsprung disease	Appendicitis	Urinary tract infection	Mittelschmerz
Necrotizing enterocolitis		Peptic ulcer disease	
Incarcerated hernia			

Gastroesophageal reflux may present with only a vague suggestion of abdominal pain but a perplexing array of symptoms. They include failure to thrive, respiratory disturbances (obstructive apnea, stridor, pneumonia, bronchospasm), or neurobehavioral aberrations (seizure-like episodes, Sandifer syndrome).[9]

Chronic idiopathic constipation, or Hirschsprung disease, may present with crampy, recurrent abdominal pain. A previously unrecognized case of Hirschsprung disease may be complicated by toxic megacolon in 9% to 12% of cases.[8] Patients with Hirschsprung disease will appear ill and have signs of peritonitis and obstruction.

Carbohydrate intolerance typically presents with cramps, gas, bloating, and diarrhea and is commonly due to lactose intolerance following infectious gastroenteritis.[4] Other carbohydrates, however, may be involved and hidden in the diet (e.g., sorbitol in fruit juice, candy, or medication).

Recurrent abdominal pain is the most common somatic complaint of school-age children and is usually psychophysiologic in origin.[7] Subjective pain with associated pallor, sweaty palms, and anxiety may be present during examination. The child is more likely to be female (2:1), with periumbilical or epigastric pain that lasts less than 3 hours and does not awaken the child from sleep.

Recurrent abdominal pain associated with fever, diarrhea, and growth or sexual maturational arrest may indicate the presence of inflammatory bowel disease.

Cholecystitis may occur as right upper quadrant pain and is uncommon in the younger child unless associated with a chronic hemolytic anemia (sickle cell disease, thalassemia, spherocytosis) or Kawasaki disease.[1] As the teen years approach, cholelithiasis and cholecystitis become more common. They are often associated with female gender, obesity, pregnancy, and previous ileal surgery.

Abdominal pain following trauma may be the chief and only complaint with blunt abdominal contusion. Signs of hemodynamic instability suggest spleen or liver injury. Peritoneal signs suggest a hollow viscus injury or free peritoneal blood. Delayed presentation with recurrent emesis may indicate a mural duodenal hematoma. Handlebar injuries may result in traumatic pancreatitis.

A postpubertal female presenting with abdominal pain should be carefully examined for evidence of reproductive tract sources, such as ectopic pregnancy, pelvic inflammatory disease, tuboovarian abscess, and corpus luteal cyst.

The presentation of abdominal pain and fever in the child with immunodeficiency, nephrotic syndrome, or ascites suggests primary peritonitis.

Sexual abuse may also manifest itself as a vague abdominal complaint in some children. A high degree of suspicion is therefore required by the emergency physician to include this diagnosis as part of the differential that must be thoroughly investigated. Once sexual abuse is suspected, prompt involvement by the appropriate local and state authorities is required.

DIFFERENTIAL DIAGNOSIS

Abdominal pain in children may indicate a primary abdominal process or a condition far removed. Evaluation by the emergency physician should establish first whether there is a surgical emergency (ischemia, obstruction, or peritonitis). Ischemic pain is often of sudden onset and associated with torsion or volvulus. Obstruction is most commonly associated with incarcerated hernia, intussusception, malrotation, Hirschsprung disease, and adhesions from previous surgery. If the evaluation suggests peritonitis, the most frequent etiologies are appendicitis, ruptured viscus from trauma or foreign body, and a complication of bowel obstruction. Nonabdominal conditions such as pyelonephritis or sickle cell disease must also be considered as the underlying cause of peritonitis in some patients.

EMERGENCY DEPARTMENT MANAGEMENT

A detailed history is essential for diagnosis and management of infants and children presenting to the ED with abdominal pain. The history should be obtained from the caregiver most familiar with the child's illness and from the verbal child. Due respect should be given to a parent's intuitive feeling for the child's illness: Such information is essential but difficult to articulate.

The emergency physician should approach the physical examination in a friendly, deliberate manner, with younger children remaining in the parent's lap. Close inspection for distention, asymmetry, or abdominal wall erythema is followed by auscultation with a warm stethoscope. Palpation should then proceed with a soft, warm hand on the abdomen, palpating very slowly for tenderness or masses, initially in the area of the abdomen away from the suspected pathology. The groin should always be examined for hernia or torsion. The anus should be inspected carefully, but rectal examination should be performed only if there is a specific indication (e.g., to rule out impaction or appendicitis or to check for blood in the stool). Percussion of the back evaluates for renal tenderness. The rest of the examination follows, with delay of potentially painful procedures, such as otoscopy, for last. The pelvic examination is reserved for the sexually active or postmenarchal patient.

Laboratory investigations should be tailored by clinical suspicion and may include complete blood count, electrolytes, blood urea nitrogen, glucose, liver enzymes, bilirubin, amylase, blood cultures, urinalysis with culture, and, for the postmenarchal patient, a pregnancy test. In selected cases, the stool may be examined for blood, polymorphonuclear leukocytes, culture, and parasites. Radiographic studies are obtained primarily to rule out an intestinal obstruction or perforation. An occult lower lobe pneumonia causing abdominal pain should not be overlooked and may also be evaluated with chest films. Ultrasound may be helpful in the evaluation of appendicitis, cholecystitis, free peritoneal blood, masses, or the urinary tract. Computed tomographic scanning may be necessary in the trauma patient or to evaluate suspected masses.

If there are signs of hemodynamic instability, vascular access should be obtained promptly. Nasogastric decompression should be performed if there are signs of intestinal obstruction. Prompt pediatric surgical, general pediatric, or urologic consultation is in order whenever obstruction, peritonitis, bleeding, or testicular torsion is suspected. Midgut volvulus is an extreme emergency; rapid detorsion of the mesenteric vessels is necessary to prevent devastating bowel gangrene.

DISPOSITION

Role of the Consultant

If volvulus, intraabdominal bleeding, or torsion is suspected, immediate surgical consultation and attention are mandatory, and a prompt response to the ED should be expected. If there are signs of septic shock or respiratory compromise, pediatric critical care consultation should be obtained.

Indications for Admission

All children with intestinal obstruction, intraabdominal trauma or bleeding, peritonitis, or cardiorespiratory instability should be admitted promptly. Emergency conditions such as volvulus, torsion, or bleeding should be triaged directly to the operating room. In unclear cases, patients should be admitted for observation until the suspected abdominal emergency can be excluded. Parental exhaustion or inability to deal with a fussy child is a legitimate reason to admit a child.

Transfer Considerations

Surgical emergencies in infants require a surgeon with specific expertise; if one is unavailable, the patient may need to be transferred to a pediatric facility.

COMMON PITFALLS

- Beware of a history of previous abdominal surgery; it may predispose the patient to various emergent conditions (obstruction, cholecystitis, intussusception).
- Intussusception is common and easily missed. Early diagnosis requires a high index of suspicion, given the fleeting and intermittent nature of intussusception as a complication of acute gastroenteritis.
- Always err on the conservative side with children in whom the diagnosis is unclear. Admission for observation or recheck in 8 to 12 hours should be the rule.

ACKNOWLEDGMENT

The authors gratefully acknowledge the contribution of Dr. Lowell Clark, who wrote the previous version of this chapter.

References

1. Bailey PV, et al. Changing spectrum of cholelithiasis and cholecystitis in infants and children. *Am J Surg* 1990;158:585.
2. Braveman P, Schaff VM, Egerter S, et al. Insurance related differences in the risk of ruptured appendix. *N Engl J Med* 1994;331:444–449.
3. Brewer RJ, Golden GT, et al. Abdominal pain: an analysis of 1000 consecutive cases in a university hospital emergency room. *Am J Surg* 1976;131:219–223.
4. Hyams J. A simple explanation for chronic abdominal distress. *Contemp Pediatr* 1991;8:88.
5. McLario D, Rothrock SG. Understanding the varied presentation and management of children with acute abdominal disorders. *Pediatr Emerg Med Rep* 1997;2(11).
6. Miller A, Barr R. Infantile colic: Is it a gut issue? *Pediatr Clin North Am* 1991;38:1407.
7. Oberlander T, Rappaport L. Recurrent abdominal pain during childhood. *Pediatr Rev* 1993;14:313.
8. Orenstein JB. Hirschprung disease. In: Barkin RM. *Pediatric emergency medicine,* 2nd ed. St. Louis: Mosby–Year Book, 1997:850
9. Orenstein SR. Gastroesophageal reflux. *Pediatr Rev* 1992;13:174.
10. Rothrock SG, Green SM, et al. Plain abdominal radiography in the detection of acute medical and surgical disease in children: a retrospective analysis. *Pediatr Emerg Care* 1991;7:280–285.
11. Rothrock SG, Skeock G, et al. Clinical features of misdiagnosed appendicitis in children. *Ann Emerg Med* 1991;20:45.
12. Samuels GA. Appendicitis in children. *West Indian Med J* 1971;20:105.
13. Seashore JH, Touloukian RJ. Midgut volvulus: an ever-present threat. *Arch Pediatr Adolesc Med* 1994;148:43–46.
14. Stevenson R, Ziegler M. Abdominal pain unrelated to trauma. *Pediatr Rev* 1993;14:302.
15. Tenebien M, Wiseman NE. Early coma in intussusception: endogenous opioid induced? *Pediatr Emerg Care* 1987;3:22–23.

CHAPTER 239
Altered Mental Status

Lindsey Alan Johnson

A prioritized, disciplined approach to the child with altered mental status (AMS) is critical in order to maximize outcome. The greatest priority is for the physician to ensure that the ABCs of basic and advanced life support are attended to first, before being drawn into lengthy diagnostic considerations. During the initial evaluation, the astute practitioner will often be led to the diagnosis and etiology of the patient's condition by careful observation and the ongoing collection of clinical data.

Because the status of the cervical spine in a child with AMS may be unknown, the possibility of a traumatic injury must be entertained early in the evaluation process. Thus, cervical spine immobilization must be maintained until clinically or radiologically cleared. The airway of the child with AMS may be vulnerable due to the potential loss of laryngospastic and cough reflexes, thus predisposing to aspiration and asphyxiation. Endotracheal intubation may be necessary to continue adequate oxygenation and ventilation, to protect the airway from aspiration, and to decrease elevation of intracranial pressures (ICPs). Supplemental oxygen should be given until adequate oxygenation is verified by pulse oximetry and arterial blood gases. Once hemoglobin dysfunction has been excluded, as in carbon monoxide poisoning and methemoglobinemia, oxygenation may be followed by pulse oximetry. Ventilation can be assessed by venous or capillary blood gas pCO_2 values, or by end-tidal CO_2 monitoring in intubated patients. The status of the circulatory system should be evaluated in terms of cardiac rhythm, pulse rate, blood pressure, and perfusion, with intravenous or intraosseous access obtained to allow for interventions.

Grading the pediatric patient's level of consciousness can be done in a variety of ways.[9,11,12] However, it is essential that, whichever method one employs, frequent and serial neurologic status examinations continue in order to assess for changes that may dictate modifications in therapy. In the older child and adolescent, the Glasgow Coma Scale may be used. In the infant and

TABLE 239.1. Modified Glasgow Coma Scale

EYES OPENING			
	>1 Year	*<1 Year*	
4	Spontaneously	Spontaneously	
3	To verbal command	To shout	
2	To pain	To pain	
1	No response	No response	
BEST MOTOR RESPONSE			
	>1 Year	*<1 Year*	
6	Obeys	Spontaneous	
5	Localizes pain	Localizes pain	
4	Flexion-withdrawal	Flexion-withdrawal	
3	Flexion-abnormal (decorticate rigidity)	Flexion-abnormal (decerebrate rigidity)	
2	Extension (decerebrate rigidity)	Extension (decorticate rigidity)	
1	No response	No response	
BEST VERBAL RESPONSE			
	>5 Years	*2–5 Years*	*0–23 Months*
5	Oriented and converses	Appropriate words and phrases	Smiles, coos appropriately
4	Disoriented and converses	Inappropriate words	Cries, consolable
3	Inappropriate words	Persistent cries and/or screams	Persistent, inappropriate crying and/or screaming
2	Incomprehensible sounds	Grunts	Grunts, agitated/restless
1	No response	No response	No response
Total: 3–15			

nonverbal small child, a modified Glasgow Coma Scale is employed (Table 239.1). Other methods of assessment include applying standard verbal and painful stimuli and then accurately observing and documenting the child's motor, eye, and verbal responses. Deterioration in a child's neurologic examination at any time should prompt an immediate investigation as to the cause of the decline in status.

DIFFERENTIAL DIAGNOSIS

The acronym AEIOU-TIPS (Table 239.2) can help remind the physician of key diagnostic considerations.

AMS is often multifactorial, and even though a primary cause may be discovered, it does not exclude the possibility of other contributory factors. As examples, an adolescent who has suffered a closed head injury and cerebral contusion may also have indulged in one or more recreational drugs or alcohol prior to the motor vehicle accident that caused head injury. A dehydrated infant may also be hypoglycemic, hypothermic, septic, or a victim of child abuse. The time course of events leading to the onset of AMS is paramount to making the diagnosis.

TABLE 239.2. Key Diagnostic Considerations

A—Alcohol
E—Encephalitis/meningitis
I—Insulin
O—Overdose
U—Uremia/metabolic encephalopathy
T—Trauma, tumor
I—Infarction, intracranial hemorrhage
P—Psychiatric
S—Seizures
O—Other

A—Alcohol

Alcohol use must be entertained in adolescents, and may be confirmed by assessing breath odor and serum ethanol levels. Alcohol intoxication also may occur in a toddler who has access to alcoholic beverages left out by adults.

E—Encephalitis

There are different types of encephalitis to consider:

1. Encephalitis with positive cerebrospinal fluid (CSF) findings
2. Parainfectious encephalitis: similar in presentation to encephalitis, but the virus (Epstein-Barr) cannot be cultured from the CSF
3. Parainfectious encephalopathy: distinguished from the first two by acellular CSF. Parainfectious encephalopathy may occur with or without increased ICP. When the ICP is increased, Reye syndrome, herpes, or mycoplasma encephalopathy are considerations. Infectious encephalopathy without brain swelling is toxin mediated. The *Shigella* toxin is the most common and should be suspected if there is a history of diarrhea in the patient or contacts or if a rectal examination documents blood or mucus.[3] Endotoxin has also been incriminated as a cause of parainfectious encephalopathy.
4. Postinfectious encephalomyelitis: Varicella and other childhood exanthems are the most common causes. A history of preceding rash is helpful in suggesting this diagnosis.
5. Meningitis
6. Brain abscess

The lumbar puncture is key to many of the diagnoses in the encephalitis category. However, several of these diagnoses are complicated by increased ICP, which is a relative contraindication to a lumbar puncture. Therefore, caution should be exercised regarding the timing and performance of a lumbar puncture in a child with AMS. If possible, computed tomography (CT) should be quickly obtained to rule out a severe increase in ICP before a lumbar puncture. Alternatively, a lumbar puncture should be carried out with a small-gauge needle, to withdraw a minimal amount of fluid, and with an intravenous line in place and a bag-mask-valve unit on hand to institute hyperventilation in the event of sudden deterioration.

I—Insulin

Insulin, either too much or too little, represents diagnosis that is easily ruled out with a Chemstrip, quantitative glucose testing, and blood gas analysis. In particular, it is unacceptable to delay the diagnosis of hypoglycemia by relying on a quantitative glucose when a Chemstrip could make or strongly suggest the diagnosis within 2 minutes. If a quick bedside glucose test cannot be performed or is equivocal, a trial dose of 25% dextrose in water, 2 mL/kg, can be given.

O—Overdose

Overdose, a possibility at any age, occurs most commonly in toddlers (accidental) and adolescents (nonaccidental). Table 239.3 is a partial list of substances associated with AMS when taken in overdose by toddlers or adolescents. Those substances for which emergency treatment may be indicated, beyond general support of vital functions, are listed with a superscripted, italic "a," along with physical and laboratory findings that might lead the physician to the correct diagnosis. Worthy of special mention are the use of a trial dose of naloxone to diagnose narcotic overdose and the routine performance of a 12-lead electrocardiogram to screen for the possibility of tricyclic antidepressant overdose. In most cases, a careful history of specific drug and toxin availability plus rapid comprehensive drug screening of urine and blood will be the keys to diagnosis. Flumazenil is generally reserved for cases of known benzodiazepine ingestion, and is avoided in patients with known seizure disorder, because the reversal of benzodiazepine effect in these patients may induce seizure activity.

U—Uremia/Metabolic Encephalopathies

Uremia is one of many metabolic encephalopathies that may result in AMS. Most of these can be remembered by considering various organ system failures (Table 239.4). Additional considerations include status after anoxia, electrolyte disturbances, hypothermia and hyperthermia, and inborn errors of metabolism. Although this category includes a large number of possibilities, a careful physical examination and a few routine laboratory studies will diagnose most of these conditions. A reasonable initial laboratory evaluation would include electrolytes, with calcium, blood urea nitrogen, and creatinine; arterial blood gas analysis, with carboxyhemoglobin level (and methemoglobin level if the blood appears brown); and liver function studies, including a serum ammonia level. Simple dehydration without frank shock is an entity that may, occasionally, have a deceivingly subtle clinical appearance and a normal or near-normal laboratory evaluation. If there is a history of fluid loss or even minimal clinical evidence of dehydration with no evidence of increased ICP, a fluid challenge should be considered.

TABLE 239.3. Substances Associated with Altered Mental Status

Alcohols[a]—osmolar gap
Antihistamines
Barbiturates
Carbon monoxide[a]—carboxyhemoglobin
Narcotics[a]—miosis, response to a naloxone trial dose
Salicylates[a]—hyperpnea, overcompensated metabolic acidosis
Phenothiazines
Tricyclic antidepressants[a]—atropinic signs, widened QRS complex
Atropinics
Anticonvulsants
Organophosphate insecticides[a]—increased respiratory secretions, miosis
PCP
Heavy metals (Pb)[a]—basophilic stippling, lead lines, paint chips on kidney-ureter-bladder x-ray, elevated CSF protein

[a] Substances with additional emergency treatments or antidotes beyond the general support of vital functions.

TABLE 239.4. Metabolic Encephalopathies (According to System) That May Cause Altered Mental Status

Lung—hypoxia, hyperpnea
Cardiovascular—shock
Kidney—uremia, hypertensive encephalopathy
Liver—hepatic encephalopathy
Thyroid—hyperthyroidism, hypothyroidism
Adrenal—addisonian crisis

T—Trauma/Tumor

Trauma (head trauma with cerebral edema or hemorrhage) and tumors are most expeditiously diagnosed by prompt CT scanning. The absence of any external signs of trauma in no way eliminates trauma as a possibility. For example, in the shaken-baby syndrome, the only physical finding, other than AMS, may be retinal hemorrhages. A tumor presenting as acute AMS is unusual; when this does occur, acute hemorrhage into the tumor is the likely explanation.[8]

I—Infarction/Intracranial Hemorrhage

Infarction and intracranial hemorrhage not secondary to trauma include several unusual diagnoses:[7]

Acute hemiplegia of childhood
Embolism (usually secondary to congenital heart disease)
Intraoral trauma to the carotid artery
Arteriovenous malformation[3]
Hemorrhage secondary to a bleeding diathesis
Venous thrombosis secondary to severe dehydration
Arterial thrombosis secondary to sickle cell disease

The last of these diagnoses is the most common and demands that any Black child presenting with AMS be promptly screened for sickle cell disease if the sickle cell status is unknown. Most of the remaining diagnoses in this category can be ruled out by contrast medium–enhanced CT scanning and a nontraumatic lumbar puncture, looking for red blood cells in the CSF. This category should also remind the clinician to screen for clotting disorders with a prothrombin time, partial thromboplastin time, and platelet count.

P—Psychiatric

Psychiatric causes of AMS primarily include conversion reaction and hysterical coma. Appropriate challenge tests, used discreetly and with respect for the patient's obvious emotional disturbance, will readily diagnose hysterical coma. Such challenge tests include eye blinking in response to the examiner's hand moving suddenly toward the patient's opened eye, smelling salts, and a calm bedside discussion with the nursing staff regarding the possible need for an nasogastric tube or Foley catheter. A true coma conversion reaction is more difficult to diagnose; fortunately, in the pediatric age group, this diagnosis is exceedingly rare. It is, to a large extent, a diagnosis of exclusion aided by a patient history or a family history of psychiatric disturbance.

S—Seizures

Seizures may be subtle in infants. Typical tonic–clonic movements are often not present. Careful examination of the eyes for rhythmic movements or tonic deviation will often be the only suggestion of seizure activity. Pupillary dilatation, if not caused by medication or ingestion, may also suggest seizure activity. Unequal muscle tone or increased muscle tone greater than that expected for the child's level of consciousness is another clue. Occasionally, a stat electroencephalogram or a cautious trial of an anticonvulsant such as lorazepam will be needed to diagnose seizure activity.

Even more difficult than the diagnosis of subtle seizure activity is the diagnosis of a postictal state in a child who has experienced an unwitnessed seizure. Once again, this becomes a diagnosis of exclusion aided by the finding of steady recovery of mental status. A partial paralysis (Todd paralysis) may also be evidence of a postictal state. However, one must be careful not to ascribe a paralysis too quickly to a postictal state before ruling out head trauma and other central nervous system catastrophes, as described earlier.

O—Other

"Other" is a category that must be included in every diagnostic acronym. In the case of coma in childhood, "other" represents at least three diagnoses: intussusception, hydrocephalus, and vasculitis. Of these, intussusception is the most common and most difficult to diagnose. At least 10% of infants with intussusception will present solely with a depressed level of consciousness. They will not have had the typical prodrome of rhythmic irritability, hematochezia, and vomiting. An abdominal mass may provide a clue to this diagnosis in some infants. However, the key to this diagnosis is the routine performance of a barium or air-contrast enema in any patient between 6 months and 3 years of age with a depressed level of consciousness that remains unexplained after a reasonable workup for other causes.

Hydrocephalus, either spontaneously developing (e.g., after a recent episode of meningitis) or as a result of a blocked shunt, is easily diagnosed by a CT scan of the head.

Vasculitis presenting as a primary alteration in level of consciousness is extremely rare in the pediatric age group. An elevated erythrocyte sedimentation rate in an adolescent girl without other obvious cause for the alteration in level of consciousness should prompt consideration of this diagnosis.

EMERGENCY DEPARTMENT MANAGEMENT

After managing the ABCs, the emergency department focus should be to quickly diagnose and treat those entities discussed earlier that require prompt recognition for successful treatment.

Laboratory and radiographic results will lead to an ongoing revision of the working diagnosis. Often, the patient is admitted or transferred before the definite diagnosis is determined. The patient should be continually reassessed for improvements or deteriorations in the ABCs and mental status.

DISPOSITION

Disposition depends on both specific diagnosis and degree of alteration of level of consciousness. Any persistent alteration in level of consciousness requires admission. Any profound alteration in level of consciousness requires admission to an intensive care unit. If an artificial airway is required, the unit chosen must be experienced in dealing with children. Until admission, the child with an altered level of consciousness requires both continuous electronic monitoring and continuous nursing monitoring. In particular, the child with an altered level of consciousness should not be sent to the radiology department without both forms of monitoring.

COMMON PITFALLS

- Failure to address the ABCs first
- Failure to consider certain diagnoses that uncommonly present as AMS: infectious encephalopathy without CSF pleocytosis, selected poisonings, selected metabolic encephalopathies, cerebral infarction with a negative CT scan, hysterical coma, seizures without tonic–clonic activity, and intussusception
- Failure to prioritize the evaluation of the child with AMS in a fashion that considers both the relative emergent nature of various diagnoses and the potential for iatrogenic complications: lumbar puncture causing cerebral herniation; intubation or uncontrolled fluid therapy, resulting in an exacerbation of increased ICP; positioning for CT scan resulting in exacerbation of an unstable cervical spine injury

Bibliography

Cheatham ML, Block EF, Nelson LD. Evaluation of acute mental status change in the nonhead injured trauma patient. *Am Surg* 1998;64(9):900–905.

Giannoni C, Sulek M, Friedman EM. Intracranial complications of sinusitis: a pediatric series. *Am J Rhinol* 1998;12(3):173–178.

Khan WA, Dhar U, Salam MA, et al. Central nervous system manifestations of childhood shigellosis: prevalence, risk factors, and outcome. *Pediatrics* 1999;103(2):E18.

Maggi G, Aliberti F, Petrone G, et al. Extradural hematomas in children. *J Neurosurg Sci* 1998;42(2):95–99.

Perry HE, Wright RO, Shannon MW, et al. Baclofen overdose: drug experimentation in a group of adolescents. *Pediatrics* 1998;101(6):1045–1048.

Rothrock SG, Green SM, Wren J, et al. Pediatric bacterial meningitis: is prior antibiotic therapy associated with an altered clinical presentation? *Ann Emerg Med* 1992;21(2):146–152.

Singer JL. Erroneous diagnosis within the cranial vault. *Pediatr Emerg Care* 1992;8(5):297–299.

Snyder H, Robinson K, Shah D, et al. Signs and symptoms of patients with brain tumors presenting to the emergency department. *J Emerg Med* 1993;11(3):253–258.

Tatman A, Warren A, Williams A, et al. Development of a modified pediatric coma scale in intensive care clinical practice [published erratum appears in *Arch Dis Child* 1998;78(3):289]. *Arch Dis Child* 1997;77(6):519–521.

Weinbroum AA, Flaishon R, Sorkine P, et al. A risk-benefit assessment of flumazenil in the management of benzodiazepine overdose. *Drug Saf* 1997;17(3):181–196.

Westbrook A. The use of a pediatric coma scale for monitoring infants and young children with head injuries. *Nurs Crit Care* 1997;2(2):72–75.

Wilson JT, Pettigrew LE, Teasdale GM. Structured interviews for the Glasgow Outcome Scale: guidelines for their use. *J Neurotrauma*, 1998;15(8):573–585.

CHAPTER 240
Apnea

Ghazala Q. Sharieff

Apnea, one of the many different types of breathing problems presenting to the emergency department, is seen predominantly in the neonate and young infant. In 1987, the Consensus Statement of the National Institutes of Health Consensus Development Conference on Infantile Apnea and Home Monitoring was published in an effort to serve as a guide for future research.[2] The definitions published in the consensus statement will be used in this chapter (Table 240.1). The focus of this chapter is on the evaluation, differential diagnosis, and management of the neonate and young infant with apnea and briefly mentions other causes of apnea in older children.

EPIDEMIOLOGY

Sudden infant death syndrome (SIDS) occurs in about two per 1,000 live births in the United States. The National Institute of Child Health and Development Cooperative Epidemiological Study of SIDS found that only 2% to 4% of cases had a hospital record of apnea of prematurity, and less than 7% had a history of an acute life-threatening event (ALTE). ALTEs have been reported to occur in up to 3% of all children.[1] The mortality of patients with apnea of infancy varies in the literature from 2% to 6%. Infants presenting with apnea during sleep may have up to 10% mortality, with the risk of death tripling with two or more recurrences. In over 50% of ALTEs, no definitive cause can be found.

TABLE 240.1. Definitions of Apnea

Apnea—Cessation of respiratory airflow. The respiratory pause may be central or diaphragmatic (i.e., no respiratory effort), obstructive (usually due to upper airway obstruction), or mixed. Short (<15 s) central apnea can be normal at all ages.
Pathologic Apnea—A respiratory pause is abnormal if it is prolonged (>20 s) or associated with cyanosis; abrupt, marked pallor or hypotonia; or bradycardia.
Periodic Breathing—A breathing pattern in which there are three or more respiratory pauses of greater than 3 seconds' duration with less than 20 seconds of respiration between pauses. Periodic breathing can be normal.
Apnea of Prematurity—Periodic breathing with pathologic apnea in a premature infant. Apnea of prematurity usually ceases by 37 weeks' gestation (menstrual dating) but occasionally persists for several weeks past term.
Apparent Life-Threatening Event (ALTE)—An episode that is frightening to the observer and that is characterized by some combination of apnea (central or occasionally obstructive), color change (usually cyanotic or pallid but occasionally erythematous or plethoric), marked change in muscle tone (usually marked limpness), choking, or gagging. In some cases, the observer fears the infant has died.
Apnea of Infancy—An unexplained episode of cessation of breathing for 20 seconds or longer, or a shorter respiratory pause associated with bradycardia, cyanosis, pallor, or marked hypotonia. The term *apnea of infancy* generally refers to infants who are greater than 37 weeks' gestational age at onset of pathologic apnea. Apnea of infancy should be reserved for those infants for whom no specific cause of an ALTE can be identified. In other words, these are infants whose ALTEs were idiopathic and believed to be related to apnea.

From Consensus Statement. National Institute of Health Consensus Development Conference on Infantile Apnea and Home Monitoring. *Pediatrics* 1987;79:293.

PATHOPHYSIOLOGY

In general, apnea is the final common pathway of many pathophysiologic processes, especially in the neonate and young infant. Respiratory function is a complex, precise system regulated in the pons and medulla, which receive afferent stimuli from numerous receptors. These vary from chemoreceptors to stretch receptors found in the bronchioalveolar tree. The efferent impulses from respiratory centers are mainly found in the vagus, phrenic, and intercostal nerves. The neonate has more nerve endings and smooth muscle surrounding the walls of small airways and a thinner pulmonary arterial wall, contributing to the decreased vascular resistance.

These changes, coupled with the immaturity of all the systems, may translate into sudden changes in both pulmonary vascular and distal airway resistance, causing ventilatory–perfusion disturbances, with possible intrapulmonary shunting and hypoxemia. Also, gastroesophageal reflux has been associated with central, obstructive, or mixed apnea due to reflex hypoxemic episodes.

CLINICAL PRESENTATION

There is no typical clinical setting or presentation of a child with apnea. Most children are brought to the emergency department in stable condition by the parents, who say the child "stopped breathing." The child may present, however, in cardiopulmonary arrest or in respiratory distress with an unstable airway (Fig. 240.1). It is important to determine the child's position, activity, and exact sequence of events before and during the apneic episode.[8] The child may have a spontaneous inspiratory effort or require stimulation after an apneic episode. The child may also experience a change in color, usually cyanosis, but the color may vary from pallid to erythematous. Associated change in muscle tone can be seen before or during the apneic event. This change in tone may vary from arching or extension of the extremities to marked hypotonia and limpness after the apneic spell.[10] An understanding of the sequence may help guide the diagnosis; for instance, arching with apnea after feeding, with or without formula in the oronasal passages, can be seen in gastroesophageal reflux.[4]

In general, there are two clinical types of apnea: obstructive and central. An absence of respiratory airflow with effort in respiration and chest wall movement suggests obstructive apnea. The absence of respiratory effort, chest wall movement, and respiratory airflow is consistent with central apnea.

The parents are usually extremely frightened by what they have seen, and frequently believe that their child is dying. In most cases, parents administer some form of cardiopulmonary resuscitation (CPR) or stimulation. A thorough history is vital in order to determine whether the CPR was actually clinically indicated.

DIFFERENTIAL DIAGNOSIS

The differential diagnosis of obstructive, central, and mixed apnea in neonates, infants, and older children is shown in Tables 240.2 through 240.4. The most common diagnoses to consider in neonates and infants include sepsis, hypoglycemia, seizures, gastroesophageal reflux, anemia, and electrolyte and acid–base

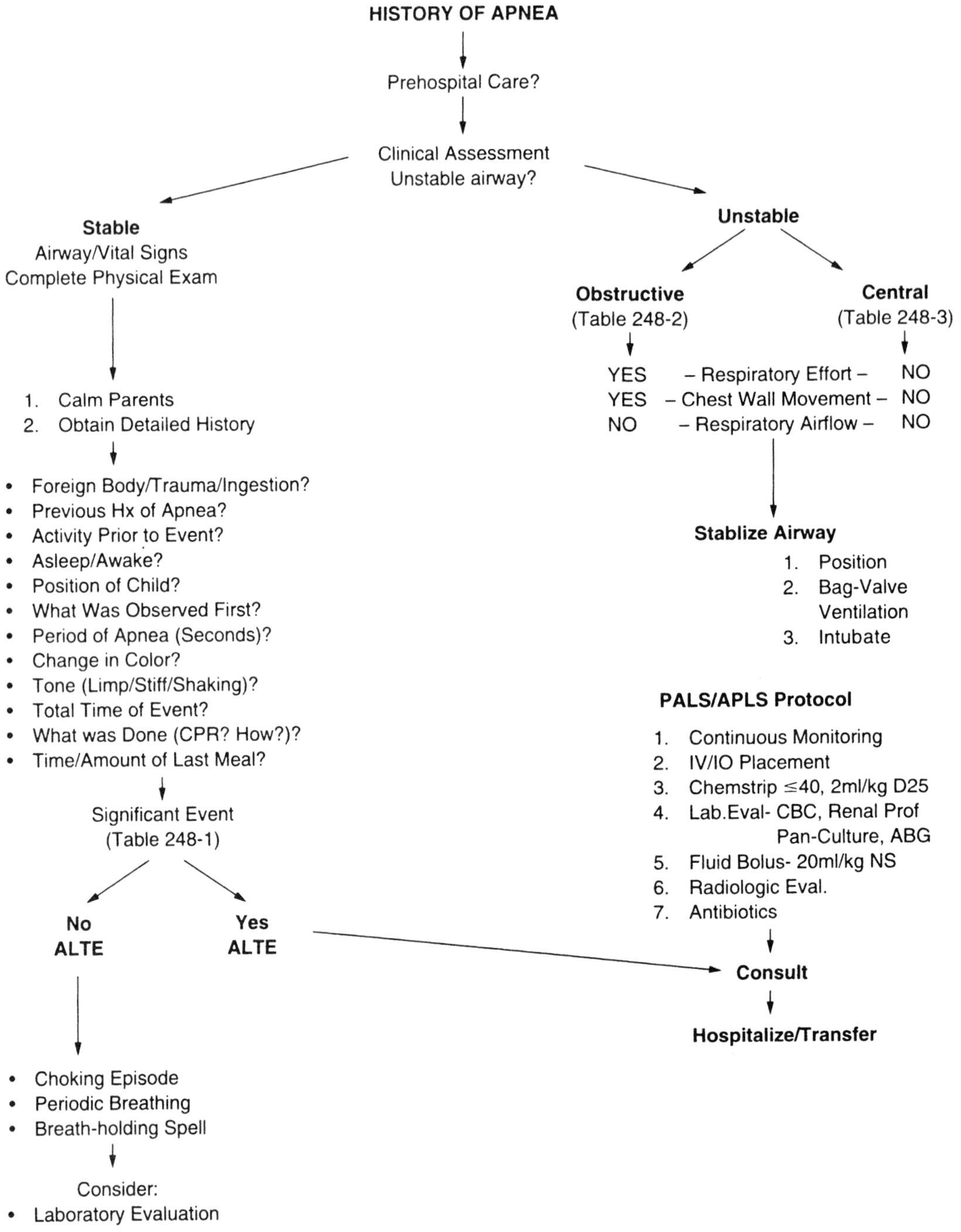

Figure 240.1. Algorithm for emergency department management and evaluation of apnea in an infant/young child.

disturbances. In a septic child, there may be associated hypothermia or hyperthermia, thready pulses, prolonged capillary refill, or mottled skin. Apnea may be the only manifestation of a seizure, or a seizure may be precipitated by a hypoxic event. In the toddler and young child, foreign-body ingestion and poisoning should also be considered.

The clinician must differentiate between a breath-holding spell and an ALTE: A breath-holding spell is an involuntary event that occurs during an awake state in a healthy toddler or young child during expiration. The most common type is the cyanotic or classic spell, which begins with crying, usually after a known precipitating event. The child then stops breathing in end expiration, with resultant cyanosis and loss of consciousness. The spell usually resolves spontaneously, with resumption of breathing and gradual recovery to the patient's baseline state. There may be associated body jerks and urinary incontinence.[3] The clinical sequence and definition of a breath-holding spell does not apply to spells occurring during sleep. The pallid breath-holding spell involves a sudden painful incident, with resultant vagally mediated bradycardia or asystole. The patient turns pale and limp and may experience tonic–clonic seizure activity, but then ultimately resumes normal behavior.

Child abuse should be considered if retinal hemorrhages or signs of increased intracranial pressure are present. Cyanotic congenital heart disease usually presents in the first few weeks of life. The cause of the cyanosis is the right-to-left shunt, and it can vary in degree, depending on the pulmonary blood flow (i.e., the lower the pulmonary blood flow, the greater the degree

TABLE 240.2. Differential Diagnosis of Obstructive Apnea

Neonate/Infant	Both	Toddler/ Young Child
STRIDOR		
Vascular ring	Vocal cord paralysis Foreign body Croup/epiglottitis	
PREMATURITY		
	Positional Laryngomalacia Tracheomalacia	Laryngeal web Tracheostomy plug Subglottic stenosis Bronchopulmonary dysplasia
ABNORMAL AIRWAY		
Choanal atresia/ stenosis Tracheoeophageal fistula	Craniofacial abnormalities	Large tonsils/ adenoids
OTHER		
	Gastroesophageal reflux Hemangioma/ lymphangioma Pharyngeal/ retropharyngeal mass	

of cyanosis). These children tend to have difficulty feeding, with associated diaphoresis and poor weight gain. The administration of 100% oxygen can clinically differentiate pulmonary from cardiac causes of cyanosis. The oxygen saturation measurement and PaO_2 increase when the cyanosis is secondary to a pulmonary cause, and they fail to due so in the cardiac patient.

Many infants with known apnea who are on home monitors are brought to the emergency department for "frequent alarms." False alarms account for greater than 90% of monitor alarm events[7] and typically are due to shallow breathing or loose lead placement.[9] A thorough history usually helps to differentiate between a true apneic event and a false alarm. However, if there is any doubt, the child should be admitted for further evaluation.

TABLE 240.3. Differential Diagnosis of Central Apnea

Neonate/ Infant	Both	Toddler/ Young Child
CENTRAL NERVOUS SYSTEM		
CNS immaturity Aberrant thermo-regulation	Seizures Brainstem tumor Chiari type I malformation Increased intracranial pressure Vascular malformation/ hemorrhage Congenital central hypoventilation syndrome	Apneustic breathing (achondroplasia)

TABLE 240.4. Differential Diagnosis of Mixed Apnea

Neonate/Infant	Both	Toddler/ Young Child
CARDIOVASCULAR		
	Shock Dysrhythmias Congenital heart disease Q-T prolongation	
INFECTIOUS DISEASES		
Infant botulism Respiratory syncytial virus	Sepsis Pertussis Meningitis Encephalitis Pneumonia	
OTHER		
	Anemia Trauma Poisoning Neuromuscular disorders Child abuse/ Munchausen syndrome by proxy Metabolic disorders	

EMERGENCY DEPARTMENT EVALUATION AND MANAGEMENT

Most infants who present to the emergency department with a history of apnea are in stable condition and have a normal physical examination. The clinician must ensure a stable airway, because positioning (i.e., excessive neck flexion or extension) may predispose to upper airway obstruction, especially in patients with anatomic anomalies. A thorough physical examination, correlating the vital signs with chest wall movements, respiratory effort, and airflow, helps to differentiate between obstructive and central apnea. All patients presenting with apnea should be placed on a pulse oximeter and cardiac monitor, and an intravenous line should be placed.

The questions in Fig. 240.1 can be used to determine high-risk groups, such as those that meet the criteria for an ALTE, patients with previous events, occurrence during sleep, and events requiring either vigorous stimulation or any form of CPR.[6] In addition, these questions may help differentiate events that appear similar, such as a breath-holding spell.

After taking a methodical history and performing a complete physical examination, the physician should be able to conclude whether the child has had an ALTE and whether the apneic event was obstructive, central, or mixed (see Tables 240.2 through 240.4). If there is a significant event consistent with ALTE, a consultant should be notified for further inpatient evaluation and management.

If the patient has an unstable airway, positioning, oxygen, and bag-valve ventilation may be the only necessary immediate support to stabilize the child. If there is no improvement, endotracheal intubation is necessary to secure the airway. Continuous monitoring and intravenous access are necessary.

A common error is failing to obtain an immediate bedside glucose level; hypoglycemia, commonly seen in sepsis, can be treated with 2 to 4 mL/kg of D_{25} intravenously or intraosseously. Neonates should be treated with 4 to 6 mL/kg of

D_{10}, because higher glucose concentrations can cause sclerosis. The laboratory evaluation consists of a complete blood count, renal profile, and pan-cultures. Testing for respiratory syncytial virus should be done in infants who were premature and in patients with congenital heart disease; this virus is associated with an increased risk of apnea in these populations.[5]

A lumbar puncture should be strongly considered in patients less than 2 months of age, regardless of whether they are febrile, to rule out meningitis–encephalitis. Pertussis and chlamydia cultures should be obtained if these diseases are clinically suspected. The radiographic evaluation consists of a chest radiograph and, if upper airway obstruction is suspected, anteroposterior and lateral soft-tissue radiographs of the neck. Many patients are on caffeine or aminophylline; therefore, a theophylline level should be checked, with a therapeutic range of 8 to 12 μg/mL.[7]

An electrocardiogram should be obtained to rule out arrhythmias and prolonged QT syndrome. Head computed tomography should be obtained in patients with an altered level of consciousness, abnormal muscle tone, focal neurologic findings, or retinal hemorrhages. Further inpatient evaluation may include an electroencephalogram, swallowing studies, esophageal pH probe, and polysomnography.[1]

DISPOSITION

Any child who meets the criteria for an ALTE, despite a normal workup and physical examination, should have the appropriate consultation and be admitted for further evaluation, observation, and parental education. The stable child can be admitted to a general pediatric ward with an apnea–bradycardia monitor to help determine the frequency and length of the apneic episodes and any associated bradydysrhythmia. Children who required any type of resuscitative measures in the prehospital course or in the emergency department should be monitored in a pediatric step-down or pediatric intensive care unit, depending on the severity of the event.

Indications for transfer depend on whether the facility has a pediatric intensive care unit or is capable of the necessary workup. The transfer should be done by personnel trained in pediatric advanced life support.

COMMON PITFALLS

- Failing to believe the caretaker about the event, particularly when the child is happy and alert or if the parents are young
- Failing to obtain an immediate bedside glucose level. It should be repeated within 5 minutes after giving the dextrose bolus. Sepsis can present with respiratory instability, and hypoglycemia must be treated.

ACKNOWLEDGMENT

The author gratefully acknowledges the contribution of Manuel Carmona Jr., who wrote the previous version of this chapter.

References

1. Brooks JG. Apparent life-threatening events. *Pediatr Rev* 1996;17:257.
2. Consensus Statement. National Institutes of Health Consensus Development Conference on Infantile Apnea and Home Monitoring. *Pediatrics* 1987;79:292.
3. Evans OB. Breath-holding spells. *Pediatr Ann* 1998;26:410.
4. Halstead LA. Role of gastroesophageal reflux in pediatric upper airway disorders. *Otolaryngol Head Neck Surg* 1999;120:208.
5. Kneyber MC, Brandenburg AH, de Groot R, et al. Risk factors for respiratory syncytial virus associated apnoea. *Eur J Pediatr* 1998;157:331.
6. Palfrey S. Overcoming ALTEphobia: a rational approach to "spells" in infants. *Contemp Pediatr* 1999;16:132.
7. Palfrey S. When and how to manage infants who have "spells." Part 2. *Contemp Pediatr* 1999;16:79.
8. Ponsonby Al, Dwyer T, Couper D. Sleeping position, infant apnea and cyanosis: a population based study. *Pediatrics* 1997;99:E3.
9. Rosenbaum RA, Levine BJ, Sweeney TA. Another false alarm? Apnea monitor activation in a neonatal intensive care unit graduate. *J Emerg Med* 1997;15:855.
10. Steinschneider A, Richmond C, Ramaswamy V, et al. Clinical characteristics of an apparent life-threatening event (ALTE) and the subsequent occurrence of prolonged apnea or prolonged bradycardia. *Clin Pediatr* 1998;37:223.

CHAPTER 241
Chest Pain

Edward J. Bayne and Carissa J. Kostecki*

Chest pain is an increasingly common presenting complaint in school-aged children and adolescents. This is particularly the case because there is increasing public awareness of this symptom as a warning sign of myocardial infarction. Cardiac disease, particularly coronary artery disease, is the most important differential consideration in the adult patient with chest pain. In a child who presents with this symptom, however, a systemic approach should be taken. There are many causes of chest pain in a child, most of which are noncardiac.[4] The clinician should avoid relying on routine laboratory tests for cardiac disease, unless they are specifically indicated by either history or physical examination.

PATHOPHYSIOLOGY

Superficial chest wall pain arises from sensory neurons of the intercostal nerve plexus and travels to the dorsal root ganglia along spinal afferents to the brain.[7] This type of superficial pain is frequently reproducible on physical examination. Pain also may arise in the dorsal root ganglion (from spinal cord irritation or compression) and may travel along the intercostal neurons.

Visceral pain is less well localized and is usually not reproducible.[7] The chest wall is covered by dermatomes T1 to T8. Pain presenting in the T1 to T4 distribution may arise from the esophagus, mediastinum, pericardium, aorta, pulmonary arteries, or myocardium. This pain is experienced maximally in the retrosternal or precordial areas. Abdominal organs (the gallbladder, pancreas, stomach, duodenum, liver, or peritoneal surfaces) may produce chest pain in the T5 to T8 distribution, maximal in the xiphoid region with frequent radiation to the back. Diaphragmatic pain may be experienced in the lower chest, the neck, or the shoulder because of more complex innervation. Cardiac pain may also be experienced as deep, visceral pain or as sharp, superficial pain due to crossed innervation.

Hyperventilation is common, either as a primary disorder or accompanying and intensifying other types of chest pain.[11] Hyperventilation probably causes pain by producing aerophagia with resultant gastric distention. Hypocapnic alkalosis may produce temporary coronary artery constriction and diaphragmatic muscle spasm, which may also be a part of this mechanism for chest pain.[3]

TABLE 241.1. Differential Diagnosis for Pediatric Chest Pain (Using the Mnemonic CHEST PAINS)

C	Cardiac (mitral valve prolapse, aortic stenosis, cardiomyopathy, arrhythmias, vasodepressor syncope, myocardial infarction[18])
H	Hematologic/oncologic (sickle cell anemia, acute chest syndrome,[15,22] tumor); hyperventilation
E	Esophagitis and other gastrointestinal etiologies; endocrine (breast enlargement)
S	Skeletal/muscular (costochondritis, chest wall syndrome[5])
T	Trauma; toxins (cocaine,[10,12] marijuana, tobacco)
P	Psychogenic; pneumonia; "precordial catch"[19]; pulmonary embolism; pneumothorax
A	Asthma (exercise-induced asthma)[16,23]
I	Idiopathic; infectious (pericarditis, pneumonia)
N	Neurologic (scoliosis, radiculopathy, autonomic dysfunction)
S	Sports (with undiagnosed cardiac lesions such as HCM, AS)[6]; syndromes (Marfan)[8]

AS, aortic stenosis; HCM, hypertrophic cardiomyopathy.

DIFFERENTIAL DIAGNOSIS

Causes for chest pain in children and adolescents are listed in Table 241.1, using the mnemonic CHEST PAINS. The differential diagnosis can usually be accomplished through careful history and physical examination. Laboratory testing should not be dictated by strict adherence to established protocol. Although cardiac causes are included in this discussion, noncardiac causes should be considered more frequently in children.

History of recent trauma, or of recent respiratory infection with excessive coughing, should suggest a musculoskeletal cause, particularly costochondritis. Such chest pain may be intensified by change in position and occurs more commonly on the left side. Costochondritis is usually reproducible on examination.[5]

Psychogenic chest pain is common, particularly in older school-aged children and adolescents. Depressive affect or recent history of chest pain in an older relative should suggest this diagnosis. Psychogenic chest pain is frequently recurrent and may be accompanied by additional history of headache or abdominal pain.[1]

History of pleuritic chest pain, dyspnea, fever, and cough should prompt a search for an infectious cause, particularly pneumonia or bronchitis. Constant substernal pain with fever and friction rub should suggest the possibility of pericarditis. Increasingly, bronchial hypersensitivity, especially exercise-induced asthma, is found to be a cause of chest pain. Diagnostic testing and treatment of these entities may be beneficial.[9,15]

Esophagitis may mimic cardiac chest pain, as in the older patient. There may be an increase in chest pain with change in position or with consumption of certain foods. Atypical peptic ulcer disease also should be considered.

Cardiac causes, although uncommon in children, deserve careful consideration. Chest pain accompanied by a soft systolic ejection murmur on physical examination should not automatically suggest a cardiac cause, because the majority of such murmurs are innocent or functional.

A history of palpitations or of atypical, sharp chest pain in a thin individual with a systolic click on examination should suggest mitral valve prolapse (MVP).[3,11] MVP is almost always congenital but may not be recognized until adolescence. MVP is more common in females and is frequently associated with Marfan syndrome, straight-back syndrome, pectus excavatum, and scoliosis. Although an electrocardiogram (ECG) is usually normal, it may reveal biphasic T-waves. An echocardiogram is diagnostic.[11]

Any patient with Marfan syndrome who presents with chest pain or palpitations should be specifically evaluated for MVP. This defect is present in 80% to 100% of Marfan syndrome patients and is the most common cause of morbidity. Aortic root dilation, aortic dissection, and aortic aneurysm are uncommon in the adolescent with Marfan's, but this possibility must be considered, particularly with severe pain and radiation to the back.[8] Marfanoid patients are more prone to spontaneous pneumothorax, which may present with sharp chest pain. A chest x-ray should be obtained in any patient who presents with chest pain and has marfanoid features on physical examination.[8] Pneumothorax should be considered in any patient with cough and sudden onset of sharp chest pain, although this is seldom a life-threatening disorder.

Aortic stenosis (AS) accounts for approximately 5% of cardiac malformations in childhood. Rarely, an older child with previously undiagnosed aortic stenosis may present with angina, fatigue, dizziness, or syncope secondary to severe obstruction to left ventricular outflow. Physical findings include an early systolic ejection click, the second heart sound may be split paradoxically (wider upon expiration), and a fourth heart sound may be heard. Typically, the murmur is heard at the upper right sternal border and radiates to the neck and down the left sternal border. There is usually a thrill in the sternal notch, and an apical thrust with an enlarged left ventricle. The ECG is usually within normal limits, although there may be evidence of left ventricular hypertrophy and strain, with inverted T-waves in the precordial leads. These patients may present following strenuous physical activity and should be kept away from competitive sports pending a complete workup.[6,14]

Cardiomyopathies, although uncommon in children, may also manifest with insidious onset of congestive heart failure, chest pain, dyspnea, arrhythmia, or sudden death.

Hypertrophic cardiomyopathy (HCM) has been shown to be a frequent cause of sudden death in adolescents and young adults. Symptoms prior to sudden death may be exertional chest pain, particularly with dizziness or loss of consciousness.

Physical examination reveals a brisk pulse, a systolic ejection murmur along the left sternal border and apex, left ventricular lift, and a double apical impulse. The murmur may increase with exercise and decrease with Valsalva or assuming an erect position. The ECG reveals left ventricular hypertrophy and may or may not show ST-segment depression and T-wave inversion. Any suspicion of cardiomyopathy should warn against the administration of digitalis, diuretics, or inotropic agents, all of which could exacerbate this condition.[14]

Chest pain occurring on exertion and relieved by rest (angina) is unusual in childhood but should suggest a significant cardiac cause, particularly if accompanied by a loud (grade III-IV/VI) murmur.

Chest pain in children and adolescents rarely indicates a life-threatening emergency.[6,13] Coronary insufficiency or myocardial infarction must be ruled out if there is a strong suspicion of cocaine abuse.[10] Significant arrhythmias can occur with abuse of this substance, and such patients deserve careful observation and monitoring.

EMERGENCY DEPARTMENT EVALUATION AND MANAGEMENT

A careful history and physical examination, including careful palpation and auscultation of the chest, should suggest the appropriate diagnosis in most cases. Chest radiographs are not routinely indicated in the evaluation of pediatric chest pain but are helpful to rule out intrapulmonary or cardiac disorders if suggested by history or physical examination, or both. An ECG is indicated if there is a history of palpitation, angina, or syncope with chest pain. ECGs should not be routinely ordered, because there may often be confusion in the interpretation of ST-T segments in adolescents, particularly in Black patients. Cardiac enzymes and echocardiograms are seldom helpful in the evaluation of pediatric chest pain, unless directed by specific concerns from history or examination.

Routine reliance on cardiac diagnostic studies may intensify the child's or parent's concerns about the possibility of cardiac disease. Once the unlikely possibility of a significant cardiac problem has been ruled out by history and examination, reassurance is most helpful in the management of pediatric chest pain.

Nonsteroidal antiinflammatory agents such as ibuprofen are helpful for the management of musculoskeletal or inflammatory chest pain. After appropriate reassurance, the patient with idiopathic or psychogenic chest pain should be referred to an appropriate primary caretaker (pediatrician or family physician), because many of these cases may be recurrent.[9,20]

COMMON PITFALLS

- The emergency physician can relieve anxiety in the patient and family by not routinely obtaining a battery of studies to rule out heart disease. A thorough history and physical examination are the most important diagnostic tools in the evaluation of pediatric chest pain.[21]
- The emergency physician should not assume that pediatric chest pain is either cardiac or musculoskeletal. The extended differential diagnosis is often not remembered.
- Chest pain during or after exercise, especially with dizziness or loss of consciousness, merits careful evaluation to rule out a cardiac etiology.
- Acute chest syndrome should be actively considered in all sickle cell anemia patients presenting with fever and chest discomfort.
- Childhood chest pain, particularly in the adolescent with psychogenic pain, can often be a recurrent problem.[17] It is imperative to arrange appropriate follow-up with a primary physician for such patients.
- ECGs may reveal ST-segment and T-wave "abnormalities" that can often be considered as normal variants (e.g., ST elevation from early repolarization).[2] Close clinical correlation, especially with the medical history, is recommended before accepting computerized electrocardiographic readings.
- Chest pain in the child or adolescent with underlying congenital heart disease is an unusual symptom, and additional causes should be considered before attributing the pain to a cardiac disorder in such patients.
- Drugs, especially cocaine, should be considered as an important cause for true angina in an otherwise healthy adolescent. Cocaine abuse has been associated with coronary insufficiency, myocardial infarction, and sudden death during adolescence.[12]
- Hyperventilation is often an important primary etiology or secondary exacerbating element in pediatric chest pain.

References

1. Asnes RS, Santulli R, Bemporad JR. Psychogenic chest pain in children. *Clin Pediatr* 1981;20:788.
2. Brady WJ, Chan TC. Electrocardiographic manifestations: benign early repolarization. *J Emerg Med* 1999;17:473.
3. Brenner JI, Ringel RE, Berman MA. Chest pain in children: identifying a source. *Md Med J* 1985;34:481.
4. Brenner JI, Ringel RE, Berman MA. Cardiologic perspectives of chest pain in childhood: a referral problem? to whom? *Pediatr Clin North Am* 1984;31:1241.
5. Brown RT. Costochondritis in adolescents. *J Adolesc Health Care* 1981;1:198.
6. Cantwell JD. Preparticipation physical evaluation: getting to the heart of the matter. *Med Sci Sports Exerc* 1998;30:S341.
7. Coleman WL. Recurrent chest pain in children. *Pediatr Clin North Am* 1984;31:1007.
8. Dowd MD, Tarantino C, Borders J. Case 02-1994: a tall, thin 15-year-old male with chest pain. *Pediatr Emerg Care* 1994;10:117.
9. Driscoll DJ, Glicklich LB, Gallen WJ. Chest pain in children: a prospective study. *Pediatrics* 1976; 57:648.
10. Gordon NM, Thompson PD. Cardiac complications of recreational cocaine use. *Cardiovasc Rev Rep* 1987; 8:29.
11. Greenwood RD. Mitral valve prolapse in children. *Postgrad Med* 1986;80:257.
12. Hoffman RS, Hollander JE. Evaluation of patients with chest pain after cocaine use. *Crit Care Clin* 1997;13:809.
13. Izumi N, Haneda N, Mori C. Methacholine inhalation challenge in children with idiopathic chest pain. *Acta Paediatr Jpn* 1992;34:441.
14. Luckstead EF. Cardiovascular evaluation of the young athlete. *Adolesc Med* 1998;9:441.
15. Morris C, Vichinsky E, Styles L. Clinical assessment for acute chest syndrome in febrile patients with sickle cell disease: is it accurate? *Ann Emerg Med* 1999;34:64.
16. Nudel DB, Diamant S, Brady T, et al. Chest pain, dyspnea on exertion, and exercise-induced asthma in children and adolescents. *Clin Pediatr* 1987;26:388.
17. Panteil RH, Goodman BW Jr. Adolescent chest pain: a prospective study. *Pediatrics* 1983;71:881.
18. Perry RF, Garlisi AP, Allison EJ, et al. Acute myocardial infarction in a 16-year-old boy with no predisposing factors. *Pediatr Emerg Care* 1997;13:413.
19. Pickering D. Precordial catch syndrome. *Arch Dis Child* 1981;56:401.
20. Rowland TW, Richards MM. The natural history of idiopathic chest pain in children. *Clin Pediatr* 1986;25:612.
21. Selbst SM. Consultation with the specialist. Chest pain in children. *Pediatr Rev* 1997;18:169.
22. Sprinkle RH, Cole T, Smith S, et al. Acute chest syndrome in children with sickle-cell disease. *Am J Pediatr Hematol Oncol* 1986;8:105.
23. Weins L, Sabath R, Ewin L, et al. Chest pain in otherwise healthy children and adolescents is frequently caused by exercise-induced asthma. *Pediatrics* 1992;90:350.

CHAPTER 242
Constipation

Elisa Alter Zenni

Although there are relatively few situations in which disorders of bowel control are truly emergent, concerns about constipation frequently result in emergency room visits. The emergency physician should be able to discern abnormal situations as well as advise concerned parents about the developmental process of bowel control, including normal stooling patterns and normal makeup of stool.

There is a wide variation in "normal" stool patterns. The normal newborn passes a meconium stool in the first 48 hours of life and then passes a mean of four stools per day during the first week, with a range of zero to 12.[5] Meconium stools are sticky, greenish-black, and odorless. Transitional stools, which are passed within 3 to 5 days, are thinner, greenish-brown, and commonly mixed with milk curds if the newborn is bottle-fed. The stools of breast-fed infants are pale yellow, occasionally slightly green, and are homogeneously mushy. Breast-fed newborns often pass a small stool after each feeding, which may be as frequent as eight to 15 times daily, although an occasional infant may not have a bowel movement for 7 to 10 days.[7] In contrast, bottle-fed infants tend to have firm, formed, yellow, putty-like stools one to four times daily. Many infants strain, grunt, and turn red in the face during bowel movements, and parents often erroneously interpret this behavior as signaling constipation. When infants are 3 to 4 months of age, stool frequency decreases, with the occasional bottle-fed infant passing only one stool every other day. For children beyond infancy, the normal frequency ranges from passing one stool every other day to passing three daily. Most children develop the adult pattern of having a mean of 1.2 stools per day by age 4 years.[5]

During the first year of life, defecation is a reflex act.[4] Maturational voluntary control of the external anal sphincter occurs in the second year, and bowel continence then becomes physiologically possible. Between the ages of 2 and 3 years, most American parents begin to toilet train their children, although the techniques and timing vary between cultural and socioeconomic groups. An important pathophysiologic concept relative to bowel control is that of stool retention.[7] Stool retention usually occurs in boy toddlers, with the common starting point being simple constipation, which leads to painful passage of stool. Parents may describe their children as spending long periods of time straining and trying to have a bowel movement, when, in reality, the children are trying not to have a bowel movement. The association of pain with defecation leads to the cycle of pain, retention to avoid painful defecation, increasing fecal mass, and further retention to avoid pain. Anal fissures are common and may start the process because of their associated pain or may exacerbate the problem by causing pain with the passage of each large stool. The rectum and sigmoid become dilated, the anal canal shortened, and the normal stretch-defecation reflexes blunted. Eventually, the fecal mass may become impacted, and unformed liquid stool leaks around the impaction, resulting in soiled pants. The process becomes established and may continue into the child's school years, at which time, hectic schedules and unsuitable school toilet facilities tend to worsen the situation. Because such fecal soilage occurs beyond the normal training period, the child's emotional or psychological constitution is invariably questioned. If emotional problems are found, they are as likely to be the result of this form of encopresis as the cause. There is also an association between stool retention and recurrent urinary tract infections, enuresis, and urinary incontinence.[1]

A single definition of *constipation* has not been agreed on. Although many parents focus on the length of time between bowel movements, any determination of *normal* should encompass stool consistency and the ease with which the stool is passed. A child who defecates twice daily but painfully passes only small, dry pellets is constipated, whereas a child who produces a large, soft stool every other day is probably normal. It is simplest to define *constipation* as the difficult passage of large or hard stools, irrespective of frequency. The epidemiology and clinical scenarios commonly associated with constipation vary with age.[5] In infants and toddlers, constipation occurs equally in boys and girls. In older, prepubertal children, constipation is more common in boys, with a male-to-female ratio of 3:1. This ratio reverses during adolescence, with constipation being three times more common in postpubertal girls.

CLINICAL PRESENTATION

A newborn infant discharged before 48 hours of age will occasionally present to the emergency department with a history of constipation, progressive abdominal distention, and vomiting, which may become bilious. In relation to constipation, this may be caused by imperforate anus, anal stenosis, meconium plug syndrome, meconium ileus, or Hirschsprung disease.

Constipation in the older infant or child is far less likely to be a serious or life-threatening process, yet is a source of great anxiety and frustration for some parents. Onset of constipation is commonly related to changes in diet, especially from breast milk to prepared formula or baby foods. Inadequate fluid intake is a common predisposing factor, as is any illness that may produce dehydration and inactivity. Constipation may arise with overly zealous efforts at toilet training. The school-aged child may present with constipation simply from reluctance to use the school bathroom.

The child with rectal retention and encopresis has fecal soiling of the underpants and may paradoxically complain of diarrhea. A lower abdominal mass may be found by palpation, and a shortened anal canal with huge fecal impaction may be found on rectal examination.

Older children may present with a clinical picture of acute abdomen.

DIFFERENTIAL DIAGNOSIS

Although there are many primary pediatric diseases with constipation as a symptom, most constipation does not suggest serious underlying disease. Anatomic malformations and congenital intestinal disorders are more likely to present in infancy than at a later age, but nonorganic causes of constipation predominate at all ages.[5] The more common serious causes of constipation in the newborn are imperforate anus, anal stenosis, meconium plug syndrome, meconium ileus, Hirschsprung disease, volvulus, hypothyroidism, and any of the numerous causes of newborn bowel obstruction. Imperforate anus is easily diagnosed by inspection, which reveals no anal opening. In anal stenosis, the anus appears small, with a central black dot of meconium. In meconium plug syndrome or meconium ileus, there is scanty or no meconium and progressive signs of intestinal obstruction. Meconium plug syndrome is strongly related to Hirschsprung disease. Gentle digital examination produces passage of a dry, hard plug of meconium. Hirschsprung disease is suggested by an empty rectal vault and a long, sleevelike anal canal around the examining finger. It may be complicated by enterocolitis with paradoxical diarrhea, abdominal distention, and shock. In meconium ileus, there is delayed or no passage of meconium, with progressive intestinal obstruction and, often, serious complications (e.g., volvulus or perforation). Meconium ileus is strongly associated with cystic fibrosis; however, the respiratory symptoms of cystic fibrosis are usually absent in the newborn, and the clinical picture is dominated by the bowel obstruction. In an infant presenting with constipation, inadequate fluid intake should always be considered.

When the infant is beyond the immediate newborn period, constipation tends to be less emergent in nature, with most cases having either an idiopathic or dietary cause.[6] The more common identifiable causes of constipation include excessive cow's milk intake, lack of dietary roughage, anal fissure, cerebral palsy, anterior displacement of the anus, and dehydration. Less common causes include Hirschsprung disease, drug intake (e.g., phenytoin, methylphenidate, imipramine, codeine), spinal cord lesions, chronic intestinal pseudoobstruction, infant botulism, prune-belly syndrome, presacral teratoma and other tumors, hypocalcemia, hypercalcemia, and hypothyroidism.

Hirschsprung disease is considered whenever there is significant constipation in the pediatric patient. It is caused by the congenital absence of submucosal and myenteric ganglion cells in a segment or all of the colon. It is more common in boys and is occasionally associated with Down syndrome. The cardinal sign is failure to pass meconium within the first 48 hours of life, followed by ongoing constipation and small-diameter (ribbonlike) stools in infants. Hirschsprung disease is the cause of 20% to 25% of neonatal intestinal obstruction. Necrotizing enterocolitis (toxic megacolon) is a complication that may develop in infants. Newborns who are not diagnosed may present later in childhood with chronic constipation, abdominal distention, and, often, failure to thrive.

A rectal examination of a child should be performed gently and deliberately. The physical examination may reveal well-formed fecal masses suprapubically or in either lower quadrant. Pertinent findings may include an anteriorly displaced anus (anal ectopy), a tight and stenotic anus (anal stenosis), anal fissure, or a sleevelike anal canal with empty ampulla (Hirschsprung disease). The signs of hypothyroidism (coarse facial features, umbilical hernia, macroglossia) should raise suspicion of that diagnosis.

EMERGENCY DEPARTMENT EVALUATION AND MANAGEMENT

Evaluation of the constipated patient should include careful history and physical examination, which often provide the diagnosis without requiring further studies in the emergency department. Dietary habits, changes in diet, fluid intake, stooling habits, and associated urinary tract abnormalities should be considered. Physical examination should include abdominal palpation for masses, especially fecal masses in the left lower quadrant; inspection of the anus for fissure, anterior displacement, or stenosis; and inspection of the sacrum for signs of myelodysplasia. Gentle rectal examination with a well-lubricated little finger should be attempted but not forced on an unwilling child. If the history is chronic, a urine culture should be taken to avoid missing the occult urinary tract infection. Exhaustive laboratory and radiographic investigation is not appropriate in the emergency department.

Dietary management of simple constipation includes increasing fluid intake, adding bulk to the diet, and adding fruits such as prunes or plums to the diet. Maltsupex (barley malt extract) or Karo syrup can be safely recommended for infants in a dosage of 1 to 2 teaspoons two to four times daily, added to formula, juice, or food. Cathartics, suppositories (other than small glycerin suppositories), and, especially, enemas should generally be avoided in infants. Hypertonic phosphate enemas have been associated with severe, acute hypocalcemia and cardiac arrest in infants.[8] Tap water enemas have been associated with acute hyponatremia, seizures, and death.[9] In the older infant and toddler, milk of magnesia 1 to 3 mL/kg/d, mineral oil 1 to 4 mL/kg/d (contraindicated in children at risk for aspiration), or lactulose 1 to 2 mL/kg/d, all given once or twice per day, can be used. Docusate (Colace) 5 to 10 mg/kg/d or senna extract (Senokot) 5 to 10 mL daily can be safely used in older children.

If an anal fissure is discovered, management includes frequent, gentle, thorough cleansing of the anus and liberal lubrication with petroleum jelly. A stool softener must be used, and a topical anesthetic ointment such as dibucaine may be necessary.[3] Aggressive care of the simple fissure is necessary to prevent the pain-retention cycle from becoming established.

DISPOSITION

Role of the Consultant

Consultation for simple constipation is unnecessary. Infants with suspected Hirschsprung disease or bowel obstruction should be expeditiously referred to a pediatrician or pediatric surgeon, and prompt response to the emergency department should be expected, because such conditions may constitute a surgical emergency. Older children with chronic constipation with or without encopresis should be referred to a pediatrician for long-term management. Older children with suspected Hirschsprung disease should be referred to a pediatric gastroenterologist or pediatric surgeon.

Indications for Admission

The following are indications for admission: failure to pass meconium, bowel obstruction, and toxic megacolon complicating Hirschsprung disease. Occasionally, the need for complicated disimpaction and initiation of a therapeutic regimen for chronic constipation with encopresis may require admission, but this is quite rare in the current era of cost containment and emphasis on ambulatory care.

Transfer Considerations

Bowel obstruction or toxic megacolon in the newborn requires specific pediatric expertise on an emergent basis, and transfer to a pediatric facility may be necessary. Before transfer, venous access should be secure, gastric suction and decompression begun, and antibiotics considered. Hypothermia should be vigorously avoided.

COMMON PITFALLS

- The newborn or young infant who presents with constipation should be seriously considered so that Hirschsprung disease is not missed, only to occur later with necrotizing enterocolitis.
- Enemas, especially hypertonic phosphate enemas, should be avoided in infants.

References

1. Dohil R, Roberts E, Jones KV, et al. Constipation and reversible urinary tract abnormalities. *Arch Dis Child* 1994;70:56.
2. Fitzgerald JF. Constipation in children. *Pediatr Rev* 1987;8:10
3. Felt B, Wise CG, et al. Guideline for the management of pediatric idiopathic constipation and soiling. *Arch Pediatr Adolesc Med* 1999;153:380.
4. Green M. *Constipation in pediatric diagnosis.* Philadelphia: WB Saunders, 1986:234.
5. Lewis LG, Rudolph CD. Practical approach to defecation disorders in children. *Pediatr Ann* 1997;26:260.
6. Loening-Baucke V. Chronic constipation in children. *Gastroenterology* 1993; 105:1557.
7. Rappaport L, Levine M. The prevention of constipation and encopresis: a developmental model and approach. *Pediatr Clin North Am* 1986;33:859.
8. Reedy J, Zwiren J. Enema-induced hypocalcemia and hyperphosphatemia leading to cardiac arrest during induction of anesthesia in an outpatient surgery center. *Anesthesiology* 1983;59:578.
9. Ziskind A, Gellis SS. Water intoxication following tap water enemas. *Am J Dis Child* 1958;96:699.

CHAPTER 243

Crying, Fussy Infant

Naghma S. Khan and Agoritsa G. Baka

Crying is one of the most important forms of communication between infants and their caretakers.[2] Few studies exist on normal infant crying patterns during the first year of life, but they tend to agree that crying follows a circadian rhythm.[8] Crying is generally considered to signal an unmet need or distress, and, as such, evokes significant apprehension in both the parents and health-care providers. Persistent infant crying, though, can be an important source of family disruption and has been shown to play a role in child abuse.[3] Parental temperament and experience greatly determine the crying limit at which medical help is sought. An emergency department encounter is likely to be precipitated by prolonged, inconsolable, and recurrent episodes of crying that are usually two or three times longer than normal controls,[8] or if a single act of crying is abnormally high-pitched or associated with a look of pain or anxiety. Repeated, unpredictable, paroxysmal attacks of screaming provoke anxiety in parents and physicians. Emergency physicians must be able to distinguish between normal crying, colic, and the occasional acute illnesses, some of which may be life-threatening.

CLINICAL PRESENTATION

Parents tend to seek assistance from health-care providers when they cannot identify the cause of their infant's crying or cannot console the infant, or when crying continues for longer than usual. Most commonly, the presentation is in the late evening or the middle of the night. A febrile infant with extreme irritability and fussiness does not pose as much of a diagnostic dilemma as does an afebrile child with the same symptoms.

DIFFERENTIAL DIAGNOSIS

It is important to differentiate recurrent benign crying syndromes such as colic from the single episode of excessive crying that may be a harbinger of some life-threatening pathologic process. The presence of fever with acute-onset, high-pitched, inconsolable crying may suggest meningitis or infection, although fever is not always present in young infants with serious bacterial infection.

Occult urinary tract infections may present as recurrent crying or as a single episode of excessive crying and should be ruled out in almost every case.

Excessive, persistent crying (greater than 3 hours) is a well-documented side effect of the diphtheria-pertussis-tetanus (DPT) vaccination and is probably related to an extremely painful local reaction at the site of inoculation.[1]

With the use of disposable diapers, an open diaper pin is seldom a cause for excessive crying, but this should be ruled out in infants wearing cloth diapers.

A strangulated finger, toe, penis, or clitoris, usually with an encircling hair or a sock fiber, and insect bites, especially brown recluse spider bites, may go unrecognized by parents, as may burns, particularly scald burns on the buccal mucosa or tongue (from milk bottles heated in the microwave oven).

Infants appear to demonstrate a relative corneal anesthesia; thus, they may not exhibit all the symptoms and signs of corneal abrasions or foreign body in the eye, and yet may show extreme irritability related to the injury and complete resolution of symptoms when the cause is treated.[4] The ears are difficult to examine in an infant, particularly a neonate, because of the narrow canal and the horizontal positioning of the tympanic membrane. Assistance may be required to immobilize the infant so that the examiner can see the membrane to rule out otitis.

Hyperpnea may point to metabolic acidosis or salicylate poisoning. Supraventricular tachycardia may present with irritability as the sole manifestation.

Head trauma, fractures, and other signs of child abuse and neglect should be sought carefully, lest these potentially life-threatening entities be missed.

A high degree of suspicion is needed to rule out intussusception, anal fissures, testicular torsion, and incarcerated hernias.

Cocaine exposure (including passive inhalation) and drug withdrawal should be considered as part of the differential diagnosis.

Finally, "infantile colic" is arbitrarily defined by the rule of threes: an otherwise healthy, thriving infant crying for more than 3 hours a day, more than 3 days in a week, for more than 3 weeks.[9] The typical colic episode is described as paroxysmal crying that develops into a piercing scream, with legs drawn up, abdominal distention, and passage of flatus. The infant appears to be in severe abdominal pain.[6,9] Normal infant crying peaks in the afternoon and evening hours from 1 to 3 months of age and is reported to last a mean of 2.0 to 2.5 hours a day. Cow's milk allergy, infant temperament, and overstimulation have been implicated in the cause of "colic," while others regard it as the extreme end of normal crying.[5] It is obvious from the foregoing that the cause of infantile colic is unknown, but we do know that it subsides spontaneously by 4 to 5 months of age.

Table 243.1 lists conditions associated with abrupt onset of inconsolable crying in young infants.

EMERGENCY DEPARTMENT EVALUATION

An orderly approach to the evaluation of the crying infant yields the most information with the least morbidity to the parents and the infant (Fig. 243.1). The importance of a careful history, documenting the onset, frequency, duration, and associated events (vaccinations, particularly pertussis), cannot be overemphasized. A thorough physical examination of a completely undressed infant (including the diaper) yields vital information in nearly 54% of patients,[7] circumventing the need for invasive procedures. The initial history and physical examination must focus on ruling out potentially life-threatening causes of crying, such as meningitis, shaken-baby syndrome and other forms of child abuse, acute abdominal catastrophes (e.g., intussusception), incarcerated hernias, metabolic disorders, and intoxications; the less critical causes are collectively more common. A review of the vital signs is essential to rule out cardiac dysrhythmias and respiratory problems. A catheterized or suprapubic urine specimen should be obtained in all infants when the cause is not obvious.

Fluorescein staining and ultraviolet light eye examination is essential to rule out corneal abrasions. Eversion of the eyelids may be needed to visualize a foreign body in the eye. A funduscopic examination should be attempted; if visualization is difficult and the index of suspicion is high for shaken-baby syndrome, this examination should be repeated after dilating the pupils. A careful otoscopic examination may show an unsuspected otitis media.

The head should be examined for any signs of trauma and for a bulging fontanel. The extremities and joints (especially the hips) should be carefully palpated and maneuvered to rule out fractures, osteomyelitis, and septic joint.

An abdominal examination is difficult to perform in a crying infant. It is important to examine the abdomen and chest and listen to the heart before attempting any invasive or painful procedures; if possible, this should be done while the infant is in the mother's lap and sucking on a bottle or pacifier. Flexing the legs at the hip may help relax the abdominal muscles enough to allow a good abdominal examination. Before attempting a rectal examination, the physician should check the anal area for signs of trauma or anal fissures.

If a careful history and physical examination do not reveal or suggest a cause for crying, further studies are indicated. Skeletal roentgenography and cranial computed tomography scanning are indicated in suspected child abuse. If an abnormal cardiac rhythm is auscultated, initial cardiac monitoring and a subsequent 12-lead electrocardiogram may reveal the diagnosis. Suspected gastrointestinal problems should be confirmed with appropriate studies, such as a barium enema or an esophagram. A sepsis workup is indicated if there is any suspicion of an infectious etiology. An elevated anion gap or abnormal urinalysis

TABLE 243.1. Causes of Excessive Crying in Afebrile Infants

HEAD AND NECK

Head
Head trauma (intracranial hemorrhage, shaken-baby syndrome)
Meningitis
Encephalitis
Pseudotumor cerebri

Eye
Corneal abrasions
Ocular foreign body

Ear
Otitis media

Throat
Oral mucosal burns
Teething
Herpangina
Herpes stomatitis
Foreign body in oropharynx
Oral thrush

CHEST

Cardiac
Supraventricular tachycardia
Congestive heart failure
Coarctation of the aorta
Anomalous left coronary artery

Respiratory
Pneumonia
Rib fractures

ABDOMEN

Intussusception, volvulus
Appendicitis
Gastroenteritis
Constipation
Gastroesophageal reflux

GENITOURINARY

Urinary tract infection
Incarcerated hernia
Strangulated penis, clitoris (hair tourniquet syndrome)
Torsion testis

EXTREMITIES

Fractures
Strangulated digit (hair tourniquet syndrome)
Osteomyelitis
Septic arthritis
Open pin in diaper
Pain at vaccination site (especially after DPT)
Insect bites (brown recluse)

METABOLIC

Inborn errors of metabolism
Metabolic acidosis
Aspirin overdose

MISCELLANEOUS

Colic
Night terrors
Overstimulation
Maternal depression
Environmental deprivation (starvation, neglect)
Idiopathic

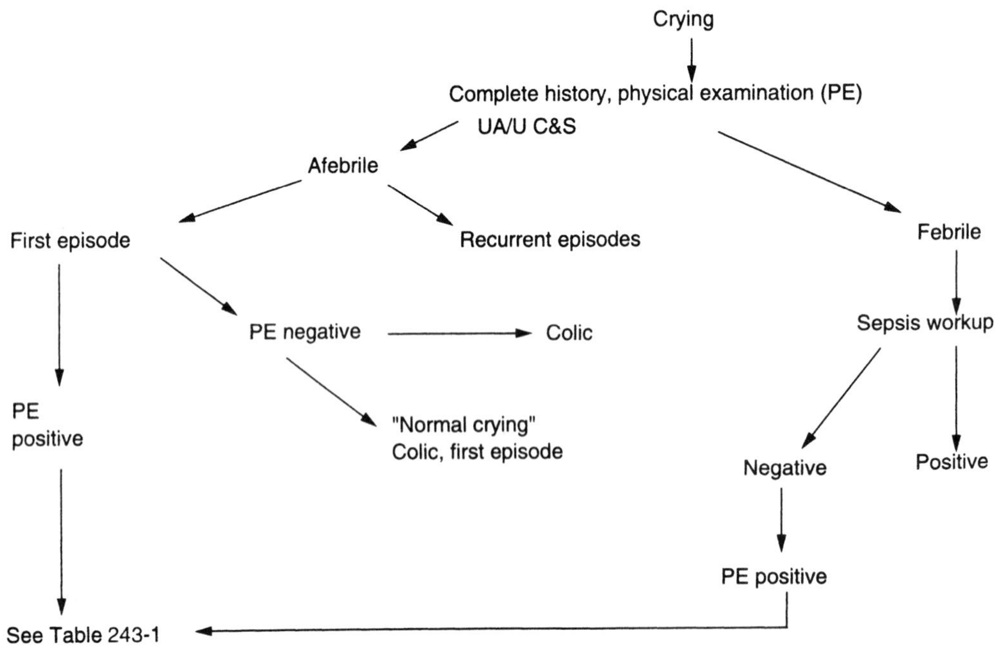

Figure 243.1. Evaluation of the crying infant.

and electrolyte levels may point toward an inborn error of metabolism or endocrinopathy.

EMERGENCY DEPARTMENT MANAGEMENT

Most infants have a completely normal examination and workup. If the history and physical examination are compatible, a diagnosis of colic should be entertained. Parents who present to the emergency department with a crying infant usually do not readily accept the diagnosis and the inability to treat the cause with medications. Multiple studies have shown the danger of using alcohol-based preparations and Dramamine–Donnatal combinations.[10] About 4% of infants may benefit from changing to a protein hydrolysate formula due to cow's milk allergy.[5] It is important to empathize with the parents and to take time to counsel them on methods to console the child early; possible intervention techniques include rocking slowly in a quiet room, warm compresses to the abdomen, feeding, frequent burping, and diaper changing.

Other etiologies of crying should be managed as outlined in the appropriate chapters of this book.

DISPOSITION

All children who present to the emergency department with crying need appropriate follow-up to ensure an adequate weight gain and no progression of symptoms, especially if the diagnosis is "colic." Consultation with subspecialists and admission are determined by the diagnosis.

COMMON PITFALLS

- A hurried and superficial history and physical examination on this group of infants will lead to misdiagnosis and inadequate care. On the other hand, doing complete sepsis workups in all infants with crying would subject a large population of colicky infants to unnecessary tests with extremely low yield. A rational approach is to tailor the workup based on a reliable history and physical examination.
- Corneal abrasions are difficult to diagnose without fluorescein staining. Similarly, retinal hemorrhages may not be noted on a cursory ophthalmoscopic examination in a crying, uncooperative patient unless the pupils are dilated.
- Careful attention should be paid to the vital signs, lest the physician miss fever, tachypnea, and supraventricular tachycardia.
- Listen to the parents. Do not underestimate their distress and ability to determine the degree of illness in their infant.
- Avoid terms and diagnoses such as "difficult infant."[8]
- If neglect can be safely ruled out, reassure the parents about their parenting skills.

References

1. Blumberg DA, Lewis K, Mink CM, et al. Severe reactions associated with DPT vaccine: detailed study of children with seizures, hypotonic-hyporesponsive episodes, high fevers, and persistent crying. *Pediatrics* 1993;91:1158.
2. Brazelton TB. Crying in infancy. *Pediatrics* 1962;29:579.
3. Frodi A. When empathy fails: aversive infant crying and child abuse. In: BM Lester, CFK Boukydis, eds. *Infant crying: theoretical and research perspectives.* New York: Plenum Publishing, 1985.
4. Harkness MJ. Corneal abrasion in infancy as a cause of inconsolable crying. *Pediatr Emerg Care* 1989;5(4):242.
5. Lucassen PLBJ, Assendelft WJJ, et al. Effectiveness of treatments for infantile colic: systematic review. *BMJ* 1998;316:1563–1569.
6. Miller AR, Barr RG. Infantile colic: is it a gut issue? *Pediatr Clin North Am* 1991;38:1407.
7. Poole SR. The infant with acute, unexplained, excessive crying. *Pediatrics* 1991;88:448.
8. St. James-Roberts I, Halil T. Infant crying patterns in the first year: normal community and clinical findings. *J Child Psychol Psychiatry* 1991;32:951.
9. Wessell MA, Cobb SC, Jackson EB, et al. Paroxysmal fussing in infancy sometimes called "colic." *Pediatrics* 1954;14:421.
10. Williams J, Watkin-Jones R. Dicyclomine: worrying symptoms associated with its use in some small babies. *BMJ* 1984;288:901.

CHAPTER 244
Dehydration

Naghma S. Khan

Young infants are especially vulnerable to dehydration because 8% to 10% of their body water is turned over on a daily basis. This turnover represents fluid deficits from the extracellular (mostly intravascular) compartment through insensible losses, urinary losses, and gastrointestinal losses. (Adults, by comparison, turn over less than 5% of body water daily.) It is easy to see, therefore, how hydration, a dynamic state, can be affected through illness. Decreased intake through fasting and vomiting, increased losses through diarrhea, or an increase in insensible losses secondary to fever or respiratory distress can easily upset this balance and leave the infant deficient in total body water. For this reason, any infant who presents with fever, vomiting, diarrhea, or respiratory distress, regardless of etiology, must be assessed for potential dehydration. In addition, dehydration is the single most common initial diagnosis among both children and adults in the early-return and return-admission population in the emergency department.[1]

CLINICAL PRESENTATION

History

The physician must obtain an accurate history of the volume and composition of oral intake; the frequency, consistency, and volume of diarrhea; the presence or absence of fever and vomiting; recent body weight; and frequency of urination.

Fulminant diarrhea can rapidly progress to cause dehydration, particularly when associated with vomiting, fever, and decreased intake. The potential for dehydration in this situation is inversely proportional to the child's age. Total body water and the percentage of daily fluid turnover is highest in infants less than 6 months old. In these infants, fulminant rotaviral gastroenteritis, shigellosis, or salmonellosis can easily cause dehydration in minutes to hours. Therefore, even if the infant does not appear clinically dehydrated at the time of examination, continued close observation is necessary to prevent progression.

Physical Evaluation

The diagnosis of dehydration is based on clinical criteria, not on laboratory values.[2,4,9] However, a low serum bicarbonate (less than or equal to 13 mEq/L) appears to correlate with more severe dehydration and an inability to tolerate oral fluids.[5,10] Signs and symptoms of dehydration are listed in Table 244.1. Multiple

TABLE 244.1. Clinical Assessment of Hydration Status and Percentage Dehydration

	Mild, (5%–8%)	Moderate (9%–12%)	Severe (>12%)
Mucous membranes	Sl. dry	Dry	Parched
Skin turgor	Normal	Decreased	Tenting
Skin	Normal	Cool	Mottled/blue
Fontanel	Normal	Sunken	Markedly sunken
Eyes	Normal	Sunken	Markedly sunken
Mental status	Normal	Normal	Depressed
Pulse rate	Full, normal	Rapid	Weak, rapid
Systolic BP	Normal	Low normal	Shock
Urine output	Decreased	Decreased	Anuria

classification schemes exist, none of which has been well validated.[2] The degree of dehydration is expressed as a percentage of the pre-illness body weight. Less than 5% dehydration is clinically inapparent, but an infant that is more than 15% dehydrated is moribund, cold and clammy, and near death from hypovolemic shock. The physical examination helps to define mild, moderate, and severe dehydration. The diagnosis of dehydration does not require the use of laboratory values; these are only confirmatory in nature. Treatment should never be delayed while awaiting the results of laboratory tests.

Infants that are 5% to 8% dehydrated typically exhibit an alert and hypoactive affect. They follow the caregiver around with their eyes but appear quiet and listless in bed. With severe dehydration, they exhibit hypotonia, lethargy, mottling, cool skin, and irritability. Before initiating fluid therapy, it is important to feel the liver to assess its size. Cardiogenic shock, although rare, is frequently misdiagnosed as hypovolemic shock. The patient must be reevaluated after every bolus, because it is easy to overshoot and cause congestive cardiac failure with only a few hundred milliliters of extra fluid.

In hypernatremic dehydration, redistribution of fluid out of the intracellular compartment into the extracellular compartment masks the signs of dehydration, even in the face of significant weight loss. The skin consistency is doughy.

In hyponatremic dehydration, the intravascular volume is severely compromised as fluid translocates into the intracellular compartment to maintain osmotic equilibrium. Infants with hyponatremic dehydration exhibit signs of shock in the face of minimal weight loss.

EMERGENCY DEPARTMENT MANAGEMENT

Although most dehydration cases are urgencies, poor management can escalate the problem and lead to shock and a true emergency.

Minimal dehydration (less than 5%) can be managed with an oral fluid challenge (5 to 10 mL/kg every hour).[7] Frozen oral hydration solutions (Revital-Ice, Pedialyte popsicles) have proven to be particularly effective in the initial management of mild-to-moderate dehydration.[8] Refusal of oral fluids or failure to tolerate the oral fluids should prompt initiation of intravenous hydration. If dehydration is estimated to be severe, it is prudent to achieve intravenous access and to give a fluid bolus and replacement fluids for a few hours before attempting oral rehydration.[3,6] If the child is in shock (as evidenced by signs of extreme dehydration, thready pulse, poor end-organ perfusion, capillary refill greater than 3 seconds), vascular access is obtained immediately, and successive fluid boluses of 20 mL/kg of an isotonic solution (lactated Ringer's or normal saline) are given until clinical improvement is noted. After three boluses

TABLE 244.2. Type of Dehydration Based on Serum Sodium Concentration

Hypotonic (hyponatremic) dehydration: <130 mEq/L
Isotonic (isonatremic) dehydration: 130–150 mEq/L
Hypertonic (hypernatremic) dehydration: >150 mEq/L

with crystalloid solution (60 mL/kg), the use of colloids may be appropriate, because only 25% of a bolus of crystalloid remains in the intravascular compartment after equilibration. If the child is not in shock but is clinically dehydrated, the 20-mL/kg fluid bolus may be given more slowly (i.e., over a period of 30 minutes to 1 hour). If two or three attempts at intravenous access fail, obtain intraosseous access.

Blood should be drawn for laboratory studies, which should include electrolyte levels, a bedside screening to rule out hypoglycemia, and venous gas measurements.

Subsequent management consists of calculating the deficit of fluids and evaluating the acid–base and electrolyte disturbances, but this kind of management is not necessarily the responsibility of the emergency physician.

In the consolidation phase, the total volume of fluid needed is determined by calculating deficit fluids, maintenance fluids, and ongoing losses.

To calculate deficit fluids:

1. Determine the patient's admission weight. If the weight is unavailable, the weight in kilograms can be estimated by using a length-based system (Broselow Resuscitation Tape) or by doubling the patient's age in years and adding 10.
2. Calculate the free water deficit. The deficit in milliliters equals 100 divided by the percentage dehydration × weight in kilograms × 10.
3. Calculate the sodium and potassium deficits. First determine whether the dehydration is hypotonic, isotonic, or hypertonic, based on the criteria in Table 244.2. Then determine the electrolyte deficits, based on Table 244.3.
4. Calculate the rate of deficit replacement. For isotonic and hypotonic dehydration, the first half of the deficit is replaced in 8 hours, and the second half in 16 hours. For hypertonic dehydration, the total deficit is replaced over 30 to 36 hours. The rate of decline in serum sodium should not exceed 0.5 mEq/L/h.

To calculate maintenance fluids:

1. Free water needs are 100 mL/kg/d for the first 10 kg of body weight, or 4 mL/kg/h; 50 mL/kg for the second 10 kg, or 2 mL/kg/h; and 20 mL/kg for more than 20 kg of body weight, or 1 cc/kg/h.
2. Sodium requirements are 2 to 3 mEq/kg/d.
3. Potassium requirements are 1 to 2 mEq/kg/d.

An alternate method to is to refer to the appropriate kilogram section of the Broselow Resuscitation Tape for maintenance or bolus intravenous therapy.

To calculate ongoing losses, fluid losses from vomiting and diarrhea can be replaced milliliter for milliliter with normal

TABLE 244.3. Free Water and Electrolyte Deficits in Dehydration

	Water (mL/kg)	Sodlum (mEq/kg)	Potassium (mEq/kg)
Isotonic	100–120	8–10	8–10
Hypertonic	100–120	2–4	0–4
Hypotonic	100–120	10–12	8–10

saline every 4 to 6 hours, unless these losses are severe; if so, more frequent replacement may be required. Usually, however, once parenteral fluids are initiated, these losses diminish rapidly to an insignificant level and do not need to be taken into consideration.

Management of Acidosis

Acidosis rarely needs to be corrected by intravenous administration of sodium bicarbonate, because repletion of the intravascular compartment usually corrects this problem. However, if the pH is below 7.20, sodium bicarbonate administration is needed (1 mEq/kg over 30 minutes).

Management of Hyponatremic Seizures

Hyponatremia is a serum sodium level of less than 130 mEq/L. Usually, a rapid fall in serum sodium to less than 120 mEq/L within 24 hours results in nausea, vomiting, muscle twitching, seizures, and coma. Symptoms related to acute hyponatremia are relieved when the serum sodium is raised to 125 mEq/L. The amount of 3% hypertonic saline (513 mEq/L) needed for the correction can be calculated by subtracting the present level of serum sodium from the desired level and multiplying that figure by 0.6 and by the patient's weight in kilograms. Three percent NaCl contains 0.5 mEq NaCl/mL; therefore, the desired increase in mEq/L must be multiplied by a factor of 2 to obtain the milliliters of 3% NaCl needed.

Management of Hypoglycemia

Hypoglycemia can be addressed early by obtaining a bedside measurement and giving intravenous dextrose. The bedside test may then be confirmed by a laboratory serum glucose measurement. The 25% dextrose needed is given at a 2- to 4-mL/kg slow intravenous push.

Vascular Access

Vascular access can be a problem, especially in the dehydrated infant. Chapter 237 discusses the intraosseous infusion procedure that can be effective in hypovolemic shock secondary to dehydration. Otherwise, most infants can be resuscitated effectively with peripheral intravenous cannulation and fluid boluses.

DISPOSITION

In many centers, the clinical diagnosis of dehydration mandates intravenous therapy and, therefore, admission. This is the more classical and accepted management, but some centers advocate intravenous rehydration for selected infants in the emergency department over a period of 3 to 4 hours; the physician then determines the need for admission. Infants requiring more than one fluid bolus of 20 mL/kg or those with acidosis, ongoing losses, electrolyte abnormalities, intolerance to oral fluids, or social needs should be admitted.

Oral rehydration with specifically designed oral solutions has been tried in certain situations, especially in Third World countries, but is of little use in the routine emergency department management of dehydrated infants. This mode of therapy should be reserved for infants with ongoing losses who present with less than 5% dehydration and have reliable parents and adequate follow-up. Pedialyte is a maintenance fluid and is not adequate replacement therapy for losses secondary to vomiting and diarrhea; Rehydralyte is a more appropriate replacement fluid. Clear liquids should not be continued for longer than 24 hours, and if losses continue, the patient should return for evaluation.

COMMON PITFALLS

- Failing to appreciate the acuity of the ongoing process
- Failing to recognize and treat shock secondary to dehydration. This includes failing to give boluses of 20 mL/kg until end-organ perfusion is improved, or the use of nonisotonic fluids to accomplish this task.
- Failing to monitor ongoing therapy, which may result in overhydration or underhydration
- Failing to address associated abnormalities of electrolyte and acid–base balance
- Failing to address the underlying cause of dehydration (e.g., pyloric stenosis, diabetic ketoacidosis, child abuse or neglect)
- Misdiagnosing cardiogenic shock as hypovolemic shock

References

1. Gordon JA, Lawrence CA, Hayward RA, et al. Initial emergency department diagnosis and return visits: risk versus perception. *Ann Emerg Med* 1998;32(5):569–573.
2. Gorelick MH, Shaw KN, Murphy KO. Validity and reliability of clinical signs in the diagnosis of dehydration in children. *Pediatrics* 1997;99(5):E6.
3. Kallen RJ. The management of diarrheal dehydration in infants using parenteral fluids. *Pediatr Clin North Am* 1990;37:2.
4. Narchi H. Serum bicarbonate and dehydration severity in gastroenteritis. *Arch Dis Child* 1998;78:70–71.
5. Reid SR, Bonadio WA. Outpatient rapid intravenous rehydration to correct dehydration and resolve vomiting in children with acute gastroenteritis. *Ann Emerg Med* 1996;28(3):318–323.
6. Rosenstein BJ, Baker MD. Pediatric outpatient intravenous rehydration. *Am J Emerg Med* 1987;5:183.
7. Santosham M, Daum RS, Dillman L, et al. Oral rehydration in infantile diarrhea. *N Engl J Med* 1982;306:1070.
8. Santucci KA, Anderson AC, Lewander WJ. Frozen oral hydration as an alternative to conventional enteral fluids. *Arch Pediatr Adolesc Med* 1998;152: 142–146.
9. Teach SJ, Yates EW, Feld LG. Laboratory predictors of fluid deficit in acutely dehydrated children. *Clin Pediatr* 1997;36(7):395–400.
10. Vega RM, Avner JR. A prospective study of the usefulness of clinical and laboratory parameters for predicting percentage of dehydration in children. *Pediatr Emerg Care* 1997;13(3):179–182.

CHAPTER 245
Diarrhea

Ghazala Q. Sharieff

Diarrheal illness continues to be a significant cause of pediatric morbidity and mortality. In the United States, approximately 200,000 children less than 5 years of age are hospitalized annually for acute gastroenteritis, which accounts for more than 875,000 inpatient hospital days.[2] Dehydration secondary to diarrhea is responsible for 300 to 500 pediatric deaths per year. The incidence of diarrhea in children less than 3 years of age is estimated to be 1.3 to 2.5 episodes per child per year, with higher rates in children enrolled in daycare.[6]

Pathophysiologically, the insult most often leading to diarrhea is infectious. Enteroinvasive pathogens cause osmotic diarrhea by invading and destroying enterocytes of the villous tip, resulting in failure of water and electrolyte absorption and damage to the brush border disaccharidase enzymes. Unabsorbed carbohydrates are fermented to organic acids, which impart an acid reaction to the stool (pH less than 5.5), and undigested carbohydrates may appear as reducing substances. In addition, the organic acids increase the osmotic load and result in increased water loss into the stool. In contrast, enterotoxigenic pathogens generally result in secretory diarrhea, in which enterotoxins affect cAMP and cGMP pumps. Secretion of chloride and sodium, followed by water and potassium, results in large-volume diarrhea, usually without acid reaction or reducing substances. Invasion of the mucosa by bacterial pathogens may produce a leukocytic reaction in the stool, demonstrable by staining with methylene blue.

CLINICAL PRESENTATION

The most common presenting condition of children with diarrhea is infectious gastroenteritis, with viral agents accounting for 75% of cases. Acute diarrhea typically lasts less than 2 weeks, and the history is one of a distinct change in stool frequency, volume, and color. The stools may be less well formed and yellowish, loose and green, or watery and voluminous. The presence of bloody, mucoid stools increases the possibility of a bacterial cause. Vomiting is common, especially with viral disorders. However, bilious vomiting demands close attention and raises the possibility of intestinal obstruction. Intussusception may complicate an otherwise mild gastroenteritis. Low-grade fever is common, but if it exceeds 40°C, a bacterial etiology is more likely.

Important history to obtain from the caretaker includes the use of antibiotics; recent travel or other exposures, such as day care; pets; or unsanitary water supply. The patient's prior weight, duration of illness, and associated signs and symptoms, such as fever, abdominal pain, vomiting, rash, seizures, and activity level can aid in determining the degree and severity of dehydration. A vital component of the history is the type of oral intake given to the child. The use of hyperosmolar fluids, such as carbonated soft drinks, apple juice, or excess sodium due to improper formula preparation, can result in hypernatremia, while hypotonic fluid replacement can result in hyponatremia.

Of foremost clinical importance on presentation is the presence of signs of dehydration. Infants may become critically dehydrated over a period of only a few hours and may present with sepsis. The signs and symptoms of progressive dehydration are listed in Table 245.1. As the vascular space contracts, the extremities become cool with decreased distal pulses, and alterations in mental status occur. Gorelick et al.[5] discovered that the findings of three or fewer of the clinical signs of dehydration correlated with a 5% fluid deficit, three to five signs correlated with 5% to 9% dehydration, and more than six signs, with a fluid deficit of 10% or greater.

Rotaviral gastroenteritis accounts for 30% to 60% of acute diarrheal disease, with a peak incidence in children between the ages of 4 and 23 months.[10] However, up to 25% of severe cases occur in patients over 2 years of age. Rotavirus is responsible for at least 50% of the hospitalizations for gastroenteritis during the peak season of October to May.[3] Transmission occurs by the fecal–oral route and by person-to-person transmission. The illness presents with fever and vomiting prior to the onset of diarrhea; bloody stools are uncommon. The patient may have concomitant respiratory disease. A new vaccine has been developed to prevent rotaviral illness and has shown efficacy in preventing severe disease.

Norwalk virus is responsible for up to 40% of gastroenteritis cases in older children. Transmission is via airborne droplets, person-to-person contact, contaminated food, and contaminated water. The incubation period is 12 to 48 hours, with symptoms consisting of nonbloody diarrhea, vomiting, fever, headache, myalgias, and abdominal cramping. Other viruses associated with enteritis include adenovirus, astrovirus, calicivirus and torovirus.[12]

Campylobacter gastroenteritis is the leading cause of bacterial gastroenteritis in the United States. The organism's reservoirs are newborn puppies, chicken, and turkey, with person-to-person transmittal. The incubation period is 2 to 5 days, with symptoms consisting of fever, abdominal pain, bloody stools, vomiting, myalgias, and headache.

Salmonella gastroenteritis is transmitted by the fecal–oral route, and has an incubation period ranging from 6 to 72 hours. The minimum infective dose is 10 million organisms. The highest attack rate involves those less than 1 year of age. Complications such as pneumonia, bacteremia, septic arthritis, osteomyelitis, meningitis, endocarditis, and urinary tract infections may be seen. *Salmonella typhi* presents with fever, headache, myalgias, organomegaly, and rose spots. Infection with this agent causes a prolonged gastroenteritis.

Shigella gastroenteritis is extremely virulent in that the minimum infective dose in only 100 organisms, with an incubation period of 1 to 5 days. Typical presenting symptoms include fever, malaise, febrile seizures, and tenesmus, with possible resultant rectal prolapse.

Yersinia gastroenteritis presents with fever, vomiting, headache, and pharyngitis and may mimic appendicitis, with severe right lower quadrant pain. Erythema multiforme and a reactive arthritis may also be present.

Diarrhea associated with *Escherichia coli* 0157:H7 may result in hemolytic–uremic syndrome.[1] The organism has a bovine reservoir and is transmitted by undercooked meat, contaminated water, unpasteurized milk, or person-to-person contact. The illness usually begins as nonbloody diarrhea and may progress to grossly bloody stools. Severe abdominal pain is common, at times mimicking an acute surgical condition. After

TABLE 245.1. Signs and Symptoms of Dehydration

Clinical Findings	Mild (≤5%)	Moderate (10%)	Severe (≥15%)
Mental status	Alert	Irritable	Lethargic
Tears	Present	Decreased	Absent
Mucous membranes	Moist	Dry	Very dry
Urine output	Normal	Oliguric	Anuric
Systolic blood pressure	Normal	Normal	Decreased
Heart rate	Normal	Normal-rapid	Rapid
Fontanelle	Normal	Flat	Sunken
Eyes	Normal	Sunken	Glassy
Capillary refill	<2 s	2–3 s	>3 s

the gastroenteritic phase of the disease seems to have resolved, the patient may develop irritability, pallor, and oliguria. Laboratory examination reveals anemia with schistocytes and helmet cells, thrombocytopenia, and azotemia. Peritoneal dialysis may be required.

Profuse sudden-onset diarrhea, especially when associated with vomiting and abdominal cramps but no fever, raises the possibility of bacterial toxin food contamination, such as that caused by *Staphylococcus aureus* or *Clostridium perfringens*. Such illnesses tend to be explosive in onset but brief in duration. Acute-onset diarrhea associated with cranial nerve weaknesses suggests botulism.

Noninfectious diarrhea is less likely to have a febrile and dehydrating onset. Food intolerance as to sorbitol in candy and gum, hyperosmolar juices (pineapple), or, occasionally, even simply overfeeding may precipitate a brief bout of diarrhea. Allergic diarrhea presents, sometimes explosively, soon after exposure to the offending food and may be part of a larger picture of anaphylaxis. Breast milk colitis, caused by sensitivity to maternally ingested proteins, occurs in breast-fed infants and presents as bloody diarrhea with negative microbial studies in an otherwise thriving infant.

A key observation in the child with chronic diarrhea is the presence of failure to thrive, as determined by anthropometric measurements. Such children often lose calories in the stool by malabsorption and do not grow normally. Usually, the malabsorption is accompanied by bulky, malodorous stools that may be oily on close inspection. Disorders with such a presentation include chronic giardiasis, cystic fibrosis, pancreatic diseases, celiac disease, and immunodeficiency disorders, including acquired immunodeficiency syndrome.

The presence of chronic diarrhea without failure to thrive suggests irritable bowel syndrome. These children tend to have frequent, large, occasionally explosive stools early in the day but otherwise appear well. Questioning often reveals a history of colic as an infant and a family history of irritable bowel syndrome.

Acquired disaccharide intolerance is common and presents with flatulence, bloating, cramps, and watery diarrhea. The history often reveals a preceding bowel insult, most commonly infectious. Disaccharide intolerance may also complicate cystic fibrosis, celiac disease, or postoperative states.

In children, especially infants, diarrhea may accompany almost any acute or chronic illness, especially if antibiotics are given. Although fulminant pseudomembranous enterocolitis is uncommon, milder antibiotic-associated diarrhea is often seen. The most frequent drugs that can result in pseudomembranous colitis are clindamycin, third-generation cephalosporins, and anticancer drugs.

TABLE 245.2. Common Causes of Acute Diarrheal Illness

BACTERIAL	PARASITIC
Campylobacter	*Giardia lamblia*
Salmonella	*Cryptosporidium*
Shigella	*Entamoeba histolytica*
Yersinia	**OTHER**
Escherichia coli	Medication-induced
Clostridium perfringens	Parenteral: otitis media, upper respiratory infection, urinary tract infection
Clostridium botulinum	Food intolerance
Clostridium difficile	Psychogenic: anxiety
Cholera	Necrotizing enterocolitis
Staphylococcus aureus	Cystic fibrosis
Aeromonas	Adrenal insufficiency
VIRAL	Organophosphates
Rotavirus	Heavy metals (iron)
Norwalk virus	Hirschsprung disease
Adenovirus	Intussusception
Calicivirus	
Astrovirus	
Torovirus	

DIFFERENTIAL DIAGNOSIS

The differential diagnosis is broad: Diarrhea may accompany almost any pediatric illness at any given point in its course. The differential diagnosis may be categorized as acute or chronic. There may be important diagnostic clues based on age, character of the stool, associated symptoms, and effect on the child's general health.

The most common causes of acute diarrheal disease are listed in Table 245.2. The differential diagnosis of chronic diarrhea includes postinfectious disaccharide intolerance, irritable bowel syndrome, milk or soy protein intolerance, giardiasis, maternal deprivation syndrome, cystic fibrosis, celiac disease, immunodeficiency disorders, short bowel syndrome (postoperative), and, uncommonly, inflammatory bowel disease, tumors (neuroblastoma, carcinoid), stagnant loop syndrome, and acrodermatitis enteropathica.[14] The presence or absence of blood, leukocytes, reducing substances, an acid reaction, or fat in the stool can be helpful in the differential diagnosis. Blood and white cells suggest bacterial gastroenteritis or inflammatory bowel disease. Reducing substances and an acid pH suggest disaccharide intolerance. Fat on Sudan stain suggests malabsorption, most commonly cystic fibrosis, celiac disease, or chronic giardiasis.

EMERGENCY DEPARTMENT EVALUATION AND MANAGEMENT

The goals of diarrhea management include prevention of dehydration by early fluid administration, treatment of dehydration with an oral rehydration solution (ORS), continued feeding during the diarrhea, and selective use of antibiotics and avoidance of antidiarrheal medications.[4,11]

A thorough history should determine acute or chronic status. Preliminary studies that may be indicated for chronic diarrhea include a stool examination for blood, parasites, culture, Sudan fat stain, and alpha-1-antitrypsin. If there is significant failure to thrive or dehydration, the child should be admitted; otherwise, the patient should be referred to a pediatrician for further evaluation.

If the diarrhea is acute, the primary concern is the existence of dehydration, acidosis, electrolyte disturbances, shock, or associated sepsis. The physical examination determines dehydration according to the signs previously described. If dehydration is not present, laboratory studies may be unnecessary. However, the presence of significant dehydration calls for the measurement of electrolytes, blood urea nitrogen, and glucose.[7] Other than a guaiac test or culture, stool studies such as fecal leukocytes, Rotazyme, pH, reducing substances, and ova and parasites are usually not helpful in the emergency setting. A complete blood count may aid in diagnosis, as patients with *Shigella* typically have a white blood cell count less than 10,000 with a marked left shift. If the ratio of bands to total polymorphonuclear leukocytes (PMNs) is greater than 0.10, a bacterial etiology such as *Shigella, Salmonella,* or *Campylobacter* should be suspected.

Dehydration exceeding 5% to 10% or significant electrolyte disturbances are considerations for admission, with rehydration beginning in the emergency department. In patients who are

TABLE 245.3. Contents of Commercial Oral Rehydration Solutions

Solution	Na (mEq/L)	K (mEq/L)	Other (mEq/L)	Cl (mEq/L)	Base (mEq/L)	Carbohydrate (g/L)
Pedialyte	45	20		35	30	25
Rehydralyte	75	20		65	30	25
Infalyte	50	25		45	34	30
Resol	50	20	8	50	34	20
WHO solution	90	20		80	30	20

mildly to moderately dehydrated and are refusing oral intake, a nasogastric tube can be placed to initiate replacement therapy. In severely dehydrated children, intravenous fluids should be initiated. Normal saline boluses of 20 cc/kg should be initiated, with repeat boluses, as needed, to restore intravascular volume. It is not uncommon to administer 60 to 100 cc/kg in the initial phase of fluid resuscitation. Close monitoring of the pulmonary status is important in children with underlying cardiac or pulmonary conditions, to avoid iatrogenic pulmonary edema. Once intravascular volume has been restored, dextrose-containing maintenance fluid should be initiated, avoiding potassium replacement until the patient is spontaneously voiding and is known to have normal renal function.

In mild dehydration and in selected cases of moderate dehydration, outpatient oral rehydration therapy should begin with a commercially available ORS.[8,9] Homemade solutions and electrolyte–glucose beverages for athletes should be avoided; in the former, serious errors may be made in preparation, and the latter contain too little sodium, too much sugar, and almost no potassium. Each liter of a commercial ORS contains about 45 to 75 mEq sodium, 20 to 25 mEq potassium, 2% glucose, and a mixture of chloride and base as anions (Table 245.3). This ratio of electrolytes and glucose promotes the coupled mucosal transport of sodium and glucose, with water absorption following.

If oral rehydration is chosen, it is best started during an extended period of monitored therapy in the emergency department, and it may be implemented in any child who can drink and is not in shock. A safe program for 5% or less infant rehydration is listed in Table 245.4. After successful oral rehydration, a prompt return to age-appropriate diet is indicated. It should be stressed to parents that the objective is to "feed through" the diarrhea, and that loose stools will persist for a few days but should decrease in volume and frequency. In general, smaller but more frequent feedings should be given so that the total daily intake approaches normal.[4]

Subsequent diet depends on the child's dietary status before the illness. If formula was the primary nutrition, a return to half-strength formula for 12 to 24 hours, followed by full-strength formula, is advised. If there is impressive return of diarrhea following refeeding of a standard cow's milk–based formula (Enfamil or Similac), a lactose-free formula (Lactofree, ProSobee, or Isomil) may be tried, again gradually advancing through half- to full-strength formulas. Continued diarrhea on these preparations may require an elemental formula such as Alimentum or Pregestimil. For older children on a mixed diet, a bland diet of rice or rice cereal, bananas, potatoes, noodles, crackers, and toast should be offered in increasing quantities and then advanced to a balanced intake over 24 to 48 hours. Although lactose in milk may cause an osmotic diarrhea, fermented milk products such as yogurt are generally well tolerated. The breast-fed infant with diarrhea generally has a milder illness for which evaluation and reassurance alone may suffice. If significant dehydration exists, oral rehydration should proceed using the previously mentioned guidelines with no or minimal interruption of breast-feeding.

Most episodes of diarrhea do not require antimicrobial therapy. Bloody diarrhea with PMNs probably represents bacterial gastroenteritis, and antibiotic therapy should be considered. Antibiotic selection should be made and adjusted based on stool culture and sensitivity results. For *Shigella,* the episode may be treated with trimethoprim–sulfamethoxazole (TMP/SMX) (TMP 8 mg/kg/d divided b.i.d.) or erythromycin (40 mg/kg/d q.i.d.) for 5 to 7 days. *Campylobacter* enteritis has been shown to be resistant to TMP/SMX, and should be treated with erythromycin for 5 to 7 days. Antibiotics should be avoided in *Salmonella* gastroenteritis, because they prolong the carrier state. Exceptions include certain populations prone to *Salmonella* bacteremia, such as infants less than 4 months old and patients with immunodeficiency or sickle cell disease. These high-risk patients should be admitted and given intravenous antibiotics. If *Giardia* is demonstrated by stool testing, furazolidone (6 mg/kg/d divided q.i.d. for 7 days) or metronidazole (15 mg/kg/d divided t.i.d. for 7 days) is indicated. If *C. difficile* cytotoxin is found in the stool, oral vancomycin (50 mg/kg/d divided q.i.d. for 7 days) or metronidazole is usually effective.

The American Academy of Pediatrics does not recommend the use of antiemetic, antisecretory, or antiperistaltic drugs.[11] The use of narcotic-based agents are specifically contraindicated in bacterial gastroenteritis, because they may induce bowel stasis and promote more aggressive bacterial invasion.

Parents should be instructed on hygienic precautions for diaper handling and good hand-washing practices. The child should be excluded from the daycare center if there is diarrhea not contained by diaper or toilet use, if stools contain mucus or blood, or if there is associated fever.

TABLE 245.4. Emergency Department Management of Acute Diarrhea with Mild Dehydration

- Estimate daily fluid requirements and degree of dehydration.
- Maintenance: 100 mL/kg for first 10 kg body weight, 50 mL/kg for each additional kg over 11–20 kg, and 20 mL/kg for each kg over 20 kg
- Deficit requirement for 5% dehydration is 50 mL/kg
- While patient is being monitored in the ED, give 50 mL/kg ORS over 4 h. ORS is best tolerated as small, frequent volumes rather than larger boluses. If vomiting occurs, give the solution 1–2 teaspoons every 5–10 min.
- Replace ongoing losses with 10 mL/kg ORS for each diarrheal stool.
- If stable and retaining fluids, the child may be discharged after deficit fluid is replaced, with phone contact 4–6 h later.
- The remainder of calculated fluids (deficit plus maintenance) should be given at home as maintenance ORS, such as Pedialyte, Infalyte, or Resol. Any fluid intake desired by the child beyond calculated should be provided as water or dilute juice.
- Infants should be offered breast milk or half-strength formula in increasing amounts. Older infants and children should be offered rice cereal, rice, potatoes, toast, bananas, and noodles, and rapidly advanced to full caloric intake.

DISPOSITION

Role of the Consultant

If more than 5% dehydration is present, a pediatrician should be consulted for probable admission, with rehydration efforts beginning in the emergency department. With chronic diarrhea, consultation with a pediatrician or pediatric gastroenterologist is in order. Diarrhea may paradoxically complicate surgical conditions (e.g., Hirschsprung disease), in which case, a pediatric surgeon should be consulted.

Indications for Admission

Patients with the following should be admitted: greater than 5% dehydration, significant electrolyte disturbances, suspected sepsis, intractable vomiting, bilious vomiting, or complicated chronic diarrhea with failure to thrive. Sepsis and serious illness in infants less than 1 month old may be clinically subtle or occult. Even mild dehydration in young infants deserves careful consideration for admission. Poor social situation, parental noncompliance or inability to follow prescribed therapy, and suspected deprivation or neglect are other reasons for admission.

Transfer Considerations

Simple diarrhea with dehydration requires only judicious oral or intravenous rehydration and rarely requires transfer unless there are no inpatient pediatric services. Complicated cases of dehydration (e.g., hypernatremic) or those of chronic duration usually require specific pediatric expertise.

COMMON PITFALLS

- The young infant with diarrhea may initially appear well but develop serious dehydration over a short period.
- Because of renal immaturity, infants less than 3 months old may continue to pass urine even when dehydrated.
- Not relying on the caregiver's history of lack of urine output, lethargy, and the patient's inability to tolerate fluids may lead to inappropriate management and disposition.
- Underestimating the degree of hypovolemia and missing the subtle signs of shock
- Antidiarrheal agents should be avoided. The narcotic-based antidiarrheals may cause apnea in infants or predispose to systemic invasion of certain bacterial pathogens.

ACKNOWLEDGMENT

The authors gratefully acknowledge the contribution of Lowell Clark, who wrote the previous version of this chapter.

References

1. Bolton FJ, Aird H. Verocytotoxin producing *Escherichia Coli* 0157: public health and microbiological significance. *Br J Biomed Sci* 1998;55:127–135.
2. Cicirello HG, Glass RI. Current concepts of the epidemiology of diarrheal diseases. *Semin Pediatr Infect Dis* 1994;5:162–167.
3. Committee on Infectious Diseases, American Academy of Pediatrics. Prevention of rotavirus disease: guidelines for use of rotavirus vaccine. *Pediatrics* 1998;1484–1489.
4. Gastanaduy AS, Begue RE. Acute gastroenteritis. *Clin Pediatr* 1999;38:1–12.
5. Gorelick MH, Shaw KN, Murphy K. Validity and reliability of clinical significance in the diagnosis of dehydration in children. *Pediatrics* 1997;99:5.
6. Kilgore PR, Holman RC, Clark MJ, et al. Trends of diarrheal disease associated mortality in US Children, 1968–1991. *JAMA* 1995;27:1143–1148.
7. Liebelt EL. Clinical and laboratory evaluation and management of children with vomiting, diarrhea, and dehydration. *Curr Opin Pediatr* 1998;10:461–469.
8. Lifschitz CH. Treatment of acute diarrhea in children. *Curr Opin Pediatr* 1997;9:498–501.
9. Merrick N, Davidson B, Fox S. treatment of acute gastroenteritis: too much and too little care. *Clin Pediatr* 1996;35:429–435.
10. Parashar UD, Holman RC, Bresee JS, et al. Epidemiology of diarrheal disease among children enrolled in four West Coast health maintenance organizations. Vaccine Safety Datalink Team. *Pediatr Infect Dis J* 1998;17:605–611.
11. Provisional Committee on Quality Improvement, Subcommittee on Acute Gastroenteritis, American Academy of Pediatrics Practice parameter. The management of acute gastroenteritis in young children. *Pediatrics* 1996;97: 424.
12. Sherman PM, Petric M, Cohen M. Infectious gastroenterocolitides in children. An update on emerging pathogens. *Pediatr Clin North Am* 1996;43:391–405.
13. Sullivan PB. Nutritional management of acute diarrhea. *Nutrition* 1998; 14:758–762.
14. Vanderhoof JA. Chronic diarrhea. *Pediatr Rev* 1998;19:418–422.

CHAPTER 246
Failure to Thrive

Marc Linares and Bruce J. Quinn

The concept of failure to thrive is commonly used in the pediatric literature but lacks a clear definition.[8] *Failure to thrive* is frequently defined as a failure to gain weight (weight less than the third percentile for age, or weight for height below the fifth percentile); however, the definition should be more global and should include any decrease of growth velocity leading to a decline of two major percentiles, using the National Center for Health Statistics growth charts. The term *failure to thrive* is used less and less by some experts; terms such as *undernutrition* or *malnutrition* are preferred.[3] Measurements of weight, height, and head circumference are necessary to define and classify growth failure. Failure to thrive is common in inner-city emergency departments, with rates from 15% to 30% reported.[4]

DIAGNOSIS

Except for familial short stature and constitutional growth delay, the etiology of failure to thrive is malnutrition.

Failure to thrive can be arbitrarily classified into three groups (Table 246.1). The most common form is secondary to caloric insufficiency. The child presents with a markedly decreased weight compared with height and head circumference. Decreased caloric intake is usually secondary to parental poverty, maternal disorganization, or neglect. Social history and envi-

TABLE 246.1. Classification of Failure to Thrive

GROUP I
Most common type. Normal head circumference; weight reduced out of proportion to height. In most cases of failure to thrive, malnutrition is present as a result of either deficient caloric intake or malabsorption.
GROUP II
Normal or enlarged head circumference for age; weight only moderately reduced, usually in proportion to height; structural dystrophies, constitutional dwarfism, endocrinopathies.
GROUP III
Subnormal head circumference; weight reduced in proportion to height; primary CNS deficit; intrauterine growth retardation.

From Kempe CH, Silver HK, O'Brien D, eds. *Current pediatric diagnosis and treatment*, 6th ed. Los Altos, CA: Lange, 1980:624.

ronmental circumstances are important keys to the diagnosis. Less commonly, caloric intake can be impaired by diseases causing regurgitation (e.g., severe gastroesophageal reflux, pyloric stenosis, rumination syndrome) or malabsorption (e.g., cystic fibrosis, lactase deficiency, renal tubular acidosis). To the fortunate emergency physician, a history of chronic disease may explain the malnutrition.

The second group of children presents with weight and height equally affected. The head circumference is normal or enlarged. Most of these patients have a metabolic disorder (e.g., hypothyroidism, growth hormone deficiency, galactosemia, renal tubular acidosis).

The third group consists of children whose weight, height, and head circumference are all reduced. This category includes patients with genetic disorders (e.g., Turner syndrome, structural dystrophies) or congenital problems (e.g., fetal alcohol syndrome, small for gestational age).

Often a child does not clearly fit into any one particular group, making the differential diagnosis of growth deficiency difficult. Even after hospitalization and a thorough evaluation, 24% of patients will not have a definite etiology for their failure to thrive.[7]

The major challenge for the emergency physician is to recognize growth deficiency. This is more difficult to do when caretakers use the emergency department as their primary care center. When a child is brought to the emergency department with an acute illness, it is not uncommon for both parents and physicians to fail to recognize the insidious and potentially more serious problem of growth failure. Weight measurement should be part of the initial evaluation of any child seen in the emergency department, and it should be routinely charted in the growth chart. When the diagnosis of failure to thrive is suspected, a thorough history, physical examination, and growth pattern evaluation must be done.

EMERGENCY DEPARTMENT MANAGEMENT

The emergency physician's responsibility is to diagnose the condition, *not* to determine its cause. Environmental factors are the leading cause of failure to thrive, principally maternal deprivation. If child abuse or neglect is suspected, proper referral to child protective services should be made. Laboratory tests are of limited value in most cases of failure to thrive, but they can help diagnose some serious conditions that require immediate attention. Tests commonly performed in the emergency department are a complete blood count with differential, a urinalysis with culture, and routine chemistries. More specific tests should be individualized.

DISPOSITION

Traditionally, patients with failure to thrive were admitted and evaluated in the hospital, but over the past few years, outpatient treatment has been advocated.[5,6] When failure to thrive is mild, with no obvious organic cause, outpatient management is encouraged if private physician follow-up is possible.[2] A multidisciplinary team approach, involving a social worker, psychiatrist, and nutritionist, is more likely to be successful than the private doctor alone in both inpatient and outpatient treatment. A recent randomized, controlled trial showed that the use of a health visitor significantly improved the growth rate of children, compared with conventional management.[9] Inpatient evaluation and treatment are reserved for cases in which outpatient management has failed. Also, severe cases of failure to thrive, the presence of an organic etiology, young age, or concerns that the child is at risk for abuse should prompt inpatient management.[1] In all cases of failure to thrive, communication between the emergency physician and the primary physician helps in decision making.

COMMON PITFALLS

- Failing to consider the diagnosis by addressing only the acute illness of presentation
- Failing to look for signs and symptoms of neglect
- Failing to screen for serious disease
- Failing to provide adequate follow-up

References

1. Bithoney W, Dubowitz H, Egan H. Failure to thrive/growth deficiency. *Pediatr Rev* 1992;13(12):453.
2. Bithoney W, McJunkin J, Michalek J, et al. Prospective evaluation of weight gain in both nonorganic and organic failure-to-thrive children: an outpatient trial of a multidisciplinary team intervention strategy. *J Dev Behav Pediatr* 1989;10(1):27.
3. Cahagan S, Holmes R. A stepwise approach to evaluation of undernutrition and failure to thrive. *Pediatr Clin North Am* 1998;1:169–187.
4. Frank D, Zeisel S. Failure to thrive. *Pediatr Clin North Am* 1988;35:1187.
5. Kirkland R. Failure to thrive. In: Oski F, DeAngelis C, Feigin R, et al., eds. *Principles and practice of pediatrics*. Philadelphia: JB Lippincott Co, 1990:969.
6. Schmitt B, Mauro R. Nonorganic failure to thrive: an outpatient approach. *Child Abuse Negl* 1989;13:235.
7. Sills R. Failure to thrive—the role of clinical and laboratory evaluation. *Am J Dis Child* 1978;132:967.
8. Wilcox W, Nieburg P, Miller D. Failure to thrive: a continuing problem of definition. *Clin Pediatr* 1989;28(9):391.
9. Wright CM, Callum J, Birks E, et al. Effect of community based management in failure to thrive: randomized controlled trial. *BMJ* 1998;317:571–574.

CHAPTER 247
Fever and Petechiae

R. Kemp Crockett and Elizabeth Rincon

The combination of fever and petechiae is a common finding in infants and children. Approximately 2 % of febrile children evaluated in an emergency department have a petechial rash.[10] The majority of such children have benign, self-limited illnesses. A rare patient, however, will have a life-threatening infection such as meningococcemia or Rocky Mountain spotted fever. Unfortunately, no controlled trials comparing strategies for evaluation and management of children with fever and petechiae have been conducted. In fact, there are only two relatively small, prospective studies of fever and petechiae in children from which conclusions may be drawn.[3,10]

Petechiae are defined as minute (less than 2 mm in diameter), nonblanching, macular hemorrhagic spots. They result from bleeding into the skin secondary to thrombocytopenia, vasculitis, or abnormal platelet function. In addition, petechiae often develop from purely mechanical causes.

From the limited evidence available, it appears that the child with a benign illness can be differentiated from the child with a life-threatening illness by a careful history and physical examination emphasizing toxicity, distribution of the petechiae, and the presence or absence of purpura. Laboratory tests may also be helpful in certain situations.

CLINICAL PRESENTATION

The typical child with a benign cause of fever and petechiae is 3 to 36 months of age, well-appearing, and smiling, with good tone, color, and eye contact. Onset is usually acute, and the height of the fever is from 38°C to 42°C. Purpura is absent. The findings most helpful in ruling out serious disease are the distribution of the petechiae and the absence of toxicity. In the two prospective studies of fever and petechiae in children, none of the children with petechiae isolated solely above the nipple line had serious disease. Baker et al.[3] found no serious invasive disease in children with petechiae above the nipple line, even in the absence of a mechanical explanation for the petechiae. Ill appearance was also found to be 100 % sensitive for serious illness in the largest study to date.[10]

Less frequently, one encounters a child with a life-threatening illness as the cause of fever and petechiae. Such children are ill-appearing, typically with acute onset of fever, irritability, tachycardia, lethargy, and signs of meningeal irritation or shock. The petechiae may be tender and lack a characteristic distribution. The petechiae of meningococcemia are usually on the extremities and trunk and may appear in "crops."[16] The presence of purpura in combination with petechiae is an extremely worrisome finding and mandates aggressive evaluation.[10]

DIFFERENTIAL DIAGNOSIS

Approximately 40% of children have a clear mechanical explanation for their petechiae.[10] Such petechiae typically develop on the face and upper chest immediately following coughing, vomiting, or vigorous crying. Petechiae that develop in this manner are usually distributed above the nipple line (including the upper arms) and are presumably due to increased intravascular pressure in the superior vena cava. A similar mechanism explains petechiae that develop distal to tourniquets or blood pressure cuffs. Contrary to the common wisdom that mechanically induced petechiae are *limited* to the skin above the nipple line, many patients will also be found to have some petechiae below the nipple line.[10]

In another 40% of patients, a benign viral or bacterial illness explains their petechiae.[3,12] Streptococcal pharyngitis,[5,10] respiratory syncytial virus,[5] and otitis media are common identifiable causes. Streptococcal pharyngitis is particularly common in children older than 18 months, accounting for 26% of such cases in one study.[10]

Brucellosis, dengue, endocarditis, gonococcemia, ehrlichiosis, and illness due to adenovirus, enterovirus,[3] and Epstein-Barr virus can all cause fever with a petechial rash. Clues to the diagnosis include contact with farm animals or ingestion of raw milk (brucellosis), recent travel to Central or South America (dengue), history of heart disease (endocarditis), urethritis and polyarthritis (gonococcemia), or onset during the summer or fall (enterovirus).[3]

Finally, a small number of children with fever and petechiae have a potentially serious disease, such as sepsis (usually meningococcal sepsis), leukemia, or idiopathic thrombocytopenic purpura (ITP). In endemic areas, Rocky Mountain spotted fever also should be considered.[2,6,8,14] Because meningococcemia is, by far, the most common serious disease causing fever and petechiae in children, it is described in depth in the following section.

MENINGOCOCCEMIA

Meningococcemia is an infectious disease emergency. The disease spectrum ranges from transient bacteremia to fulminant septic shock and death within hours, despite appropriate therapy.[1,4,5,7,13] Peak incidence occurs in the late winter and early spring; infants younger than age 2 represent 90% of cases.

CLINICAL PRESENTATION

The onset of meningococcemia is usually abrupt, with high fever, petechiae, lethargy, and headache. The rash, when present, may be petechial, urticarial, or maculopapular.[1] Maculopapular lesions are often tender. Lesions are sparse and generalized. Purpuric lesions have been described in 60% to 100% of cases and indicate fulminating disease with a high incidence of shock and disseminated intravascular coagulation.[1,15] Other signs and symptoms include evidence of an upper respiratory tract infection, myalgias, and joint pains. Meningitis occurs in about half of the patients with meningococcemia.[15]

Approximately 25% of children with meningococcal bacteremia will have neither a petechial rash nor a toxic appearance. They may be initially evaluated in an office or emergency department and sent home.[5,9] Such children with "occult meningococcemia" have, on average, a higher band count than other febrile children. However, because of the rarity of this disease, the predictive value of the band count is almost useless.

EMERGENCY DEPARTMENT EVALUATION

Children with unexplained fever and petechiae should be triaged as urgent or emergent and rapidly assessed. It is useful to divide children into three groups: well-appearing children with a mechanical cause for their petechiae, well-appearing children *without* a clear mechanical cause, and toxic- or ill-appearing children. The evaluation and management of the first and last groups is straightforward, while the evaluation of the middle group is less clear.

In the well-appearing child with a readily apparent mechanical cause, it is reasonable to forego laboratory investigation. A platelet count may be done to rule out thrombocytopenia, although this is extremely unlikely in the child with a typical history and physical examination for mechanical petechiae.

At the opposite end of the spectrum is the septic or toxic–appearing child. Laboratory evaluation should include a chest radiograph; complete blood count (CBC) with differential and platelet cell count; prothrombin time (PT); partial thromboplastin time (PTT); determination of electrolyte levels, including glucose and calcium; blood culture; and urinalysis with urine culture.

A lumbar puncture should be performed in all patients stable enough to tolerate the procedure. Tests to determine the presence of meningococcal antigens in cerebrospinal fluid may be helpful, especially in cases in which prior antibiotic therapy has been given, making culture results unreliable.[1] In contrast, a positive antigen detection test in urine is not helpful, as the sensitivity and specificity in urine are less than 50%.[1]

Unfortunately, there is no consensus as to the appropriate management of the child whose petechiae are not clearly mechanical in origin.[11] In the absence of purpura or toxicity, the vast majority of these children will have either a benign viral illness or streptococcal pharyngitis.[3,10] Mandl et al.[10] found that none of 357 "well-appearing" children with fever and petechiae had invasive illness.[10] However, other studies have not found clinical judgment to be as sensitive.[3,9] Unfortunately, these studies were not designed to look specifically at clinical criteria, as was Mandl's.

The data on using the peripheral white blood cell (WBC) count as a screen for meningococcemia are discouraging. At present, it seems that the WBC is too nonspecific to be useful.[3,9,10] Its sensitivity in meningococcemia is also unclear. Mandl et al. found an abnormal WBC count (defined as either greater than 15,000 or less than 5,000) in all patients with invasive bacteremia. All of these children were also assessed as clinically "ill." Thus, it is not clear whether the WBC count adds anything to the sensitivity of clinical assessment in the subgroup of well-appearing children with fever and petechiae.

The patient's age, degree of fever, and identification of a fever source should also be considered. Many emergency department physicians still commonly order a "screening CBC and platelet count" and a blood culture on well-appearing children with fever and petechiae. This is often done for medical–legal reasons.

Perhaps most important in the evaluation of the well-appearing child lacking a mechanical cause for petechiae are careful serial examinations. One should look specifically for the appearance of additional petechiae (showers or crops of petechiae, an acral distribution, or tender petechiae), the appearance of purpura, abnormalities of vital signs (tachycardia, hypotension), or subtle changes in perfusion, mental status, or appearance. Any other workup should be directed toward specific signs and symptoms (throat culture for streptococcal disease, PT/PTT for purpura, etc.).

EMERGENCY DEPARTMENT MANAGEMENT AND DISPOSITION

In the well-appearing child with a readily apparent mechanical cause for the petechiae, no specific laboratory evaluation is necessary. These children may be discharged home.

The toxic-appearing child with fever and petechiae should be assumed to have meningococcemia, and a complete septic workup should be performed. Children at risk for meningococcemia should receive continuous cardiovascular monitoring and frequent examinations, looking for subtle signs of shock. Management includes prompt institution of antibiotics, treatment of coagulopathy if present, and volume expansion and inotropic support for signs of inadequate tissue perfusion. Antibiotics should be administered promptly, even in the child in which lumbar puncture cannot be performed. If you are unable to obtain intravenous access, antibiotics may be administered intramuscularly.

Because hypotension is a late manifestation of shock in children, repeated evaluations of mental status, skin perfusion, urine output, and pulse quality are important. Evidence of inadequate tissue perfusion should initially be treated with volume expansion. Myocardial dysfunction is common in meningococcemia and inotropic agents may be required.[4]

Rapid deterioration is well documented in meningococcemia. Sudden deterioration within minutes of antibiotic administration has been noted. This phenomenon is likely due to massive endotoxin release from the destruction of organisms, and thus monitoring should be particularly vigilant immediately after the administration of the first dose of antibiotics.

If bacterial meningitis is confirmed, dexamethasone 0.6 mg/kg/d in four divided doses, should be considered in infants and children older than 2 months to reduce hearing loss and/or other neurologic sequelae.[1] Efficacy is currently established only for bacterial meningitis due to *Haemophilus influenzae* type b. If used, it is most effective if administered at the time of or slightly before antibiotics are given. In cases in which there is a strong suspicion of bacterial meningitis (signs of meningitis and cloudy spinal fluid on lumbar puncture), it is reasonable to administer dexamethasone, followed by antibiotics, immediately after obtaining a lumbar puncture.

All patients with suspected meningococcemia should be admitted to a facility able to handle children in severe septic shock, usually one in which a pediatric intensivist is available and that has a pediatric intensive care unit. The potential for rapid deterioration during transport should be anticipated. Rapid transport should be done by personnel trained in advanced cardiac life support, preferably a pediatric critical care transport team. Inotropes should be mixed in advance, and infusion rates established. Intubation before transport should be strongly considered in patients in shock. Two secure intravenous lines are desirable.

Antibiotic prophylaxis and careful observation are recommended for all close contacts of persons with invasive meningococcal disease. What constitutes a *close contact* has been meticulously described in the American Academy of Pediatrics *1997 Red Book*,[1] and include household contacts and childcare or nursery school contacts in the previous 7 days.

In addition, persons who have had direct exposure to the patient's oral secretions (including kissing, sharing of toothbrushes or eating utensils, mouth-to-mouth resuscitation, unprotected intubation, or suctioning before antibiotic therapy was begun) should receive prophylaxis. The recommended prophylactic regimen is rifampin 10 mg/kg per dose (maximum dose, 600 mg), given every 12 hours for a total of four doses over 2 days. Alternatives include ceftriaxone or ciprofloxacin. Chemoprophylaxis should be done in consultation with local public health authorities.

The most difficult decision is in the management of the well-appearing child with petechiae lacking a clear mechanical cause. Most of these patients do not have serious illnesses. A period of careful observation in the emergency department, although unstudied, is a common approach. The child should be observed for progression of petechiae (looking for showers of new petechiae), development of purpura, and signs or symptoms of meningitis or altered perfusion. Patients who remain stable, smile, have good tone and color, develop no further petechiae, and have no purpura can safely be discharged home with close follow-up by a primary care physician. Well-appearing, febrile children with petechiae, no fever source, and a WBC count greater than 15,000 are often given ceftriaxone intramuscularly or intravenously pending blood culture results.

COMMON PITFALLS

- Failure to detect petechiae in a febrile child often occurs because the patient is not totally undressed.
- Delay in antibiotic administration in a child with meningitis, either due to lack of intravenous access or due to a delay in performing a lumbar puncture, is a frequent but risky occurrence. Remember: Antibiotics may be given intramuscularly if intravenous access is unavailable.
- Failure to diagnose shock in infants and children is common. Once recognized, inadequate fluid resuscitation may occur. Children in septic shock can require massive amounts of volume and potent inotropic agents.
- Mechanically induced petechiae are a common finding in infants and children with or without fever. Although they do not seem to be a risk factor for meningococcemia, neither do they "immunize" a child against serious disease. The literature is clear that meningococcemia is clinically occult in approximately 25% of children on initial presentation.[9] Thus, meningococcemia and mechanical petechiae may occur simultaneously simply due to chance. All infants with fever, with or without mechanical petechiae, need careful evaluation and close follow-up.

References

1. American Academy of Pediatrics. Peter G, Hall CB, Halsey NA, et al., eds. *1997 Red book: report of the Committee on Infectious Diseases,* 24th ed. Elk Grove Village, IL: American Academy of Pediatrics, 1997:357–362.
2. Anonymous. Rocky Mountain spotted fever and human ehrlichiosis—United States, 1989. *MMWR* 1990;39:281–284.
3. Baker RC, Seguin JH, Leslie N, et al. Fever and petechiae in children [see comments]. *Pediatrics* 1989;84(6):1051–1055.
4. Bausher JC, Baker RC. Early prognostic indicators in acute meningococcemia: implications for management. *Pediatr Emerg Care* 1986;2:176–179.
5. Dashefsky B, Teele DW, Klein JO. Unsuspected meningococcemia. *J Pediatr* 1983;102:69–72.
6. Fishbein DB, Kaplan JE, Bernard KW. Surveillance of Rocky Mountain spotted fever in the United States, 1981–1983. *South Med J* 1984;150:609–611.
7. Friedman AD, Fleisher GR. Unsuspected meningococcemia treated with orally administered amoxicillin. *Pediatr Infect Dis J* 1982;1:38.
8. Helmick CG, Bernard KW, D'Angelo LJ. Rocky Mountain spotted fever: clinical, laboratory, and epidemiological features of 262 cases. *J Infect Dis* 1984;150:480–488.
9. Kupperman N, Malley R, Inkelis SH, et al. Clinical and hematologic features do not reliability identify children with unsuspected meningococcal disease. *Pediatrics* 1999;103:E20.
10. Mandl KD, Stack AM, Fleisher GR. Incidence of bacteremia in infants and children with fever and petechiae. *J Pediatr* 1997;131:398–404.
11. Nelson DG, Leake J, Bradley J, et al. Evaluation of febrile children with petechial rashes: is there consensus among pediatricians? *Pediatr Infect Dis J* 1998;17:1135–1140.
12. Nguyen QV, Nguyen EA, Weiner LB. Incidence of invasive bacterial disease in children with fever and petechiae. *Pediatrics* 1984;74:77–80.
13. Sullivan TD, LaScolea LJ. *Neisseria meningitides* bacteremia in children: quantitation of bacteremia and spontaneous clinical recovery without antibiotic therapy. *Pediatrics* 1987;80:63–67.
14. Tanaka R. Rocky Mountain spotted fever—United States, 1986. *MMWR* 1987;36(20):314–315.
15. Toews WH, Bass JW. Skin manifestations of meningococcal infection. *Am J Dis Child* 1974;127:173–176.
16. Weiner LB. Management of young children with fever and rash. *Pediatr Infect Dis J* 1991;10:416–417.

CHAPTER 248
Fever of Acute Onset

Maureen D. McCollough and David A. Talan

Fever is present in 25% of infants and children brought to the emergency department (ED), either as the sole complaint or in conjunction with other symptoms. Fever produces tremendous parental anxiety, often reinforced by health-care personnel. Fever, in and of itself, is usually not harmful, but it may be an early sign of an emergency condition, such as meningitis or other bacterial infections.[21]

The ED evaluation of fever focuses first on identifying life-threatening sepsis syndromes. A source of infection is also sought through a careful history and physical examination. The extent of laboratory testing (to confirm a suspected focus of infection or evaluate the likelihood of occult infection) and the decision to initiate empirical antimicrobial therapy depend on several variables. The patient's age, degree of fever, illness severity, and presence or absence of a clinically suspected source of infection are most important to determine the need for further diagnostic testing. Other factors that must be considered include the patient's history of underlying medical conditions, the examiner's skill, the child's course during a period of observation, laboratory resources, and availability of follow-up.

Both the likelihood and consequences of serious infections are increased in febrile children with immunocompromising diseases, such as sickle cell anemia and leukemia.

Signs of serious illness, such as meningitis, can be subtle. When the examiner's experience is limited, greater laboratory evaluation may be justified. For example, most experts recommend a lumbar puncture for febrile infants less than 1 month old. The ability to determine signs of meningitis in older infants depends on the physician's experience in interpreting infant behavior and clinical examination findings.

Assessing behavior in young children can be difficult, even for experienced examiners. Observation of trends in behavior over time, including alertness, consolability, social interactions, and feeding, is perhaps the most sensitive means to discern the presence or absence of a serious infection in a child with an initially equivocal presentation. Expectant antibiotic therapy for young children with fever without source and presumed occult bacteremia may be justified when a hospital's laboratory requires 48 hours to identify and report on a positive blood culture. But in a hospital that uses radioisotope techniques to identify positive cultures in 12 hours, the justification for empiric antibiotic therapy is less.

AVAILABILITY OF FOLLOW-UP

When follow-up is uncertain, extensive evaluation and cautious disposition are justified. For example, a 3-year-old nontoxic, toilet-trained girl with reliable follow-up might be discharged to return with a voided urine specimen for urinalysis and culture in 12 hours. But if follow-up is uncertain, it might be appropriate to catheterize the child during the ED visit. Children at risk for unreliable follow-up include those with parents who are young, who have no access to transportation, or who believe their child is not ill.[25]

DEFINITION, MEASUREMENT, AND INTERPRETATION OF FEVER

Traditionally, a rectal temperature (for neonates and young children) or oral temperature (older children and adolescents) at or above 38°C (100.4°F) has been defined as fever. Note that temperature varies diurnally 0.5°C or 1.0°F, and a temperature of 37.0°C (98.6°F) in the early morning hours (e.g., 4 a.m.) may represent a low-grade fever.[19,29] Rectal temperatures are generally about 0.3°C or 0.5°F higher and less variable than oral temperatures.[13] Bundling of a nonfebrile child should not cause a fever when the temperature is taken rectally.[17] Axillary temperatures have been shown to be unreliable.[22] Although previously not advocated, tympanic thermometers, when used after proper training, may be more reliable than previously thought.[28]

Recent antipyretic use could interfere with fever identification, although, typically, fever is not eliminated and the antipyretic effect dissipates approximately 2 hours after the last dose.[30] It should be noted that the degree of fever response to antipyretic therapy bears no relation to the likelihood of bacterial infection, and thus is irrelevant in clinical decision making.[4,8] Elevated body temperature is not generally harmful unless the temperature rises above approximately 106.5°F.[21]

INITIAL EVALUATION

All children who are evaluated for fever should receive a thorough physical examination. The initial examination should start with an evaluation of the child's ABCs. Signs of respiratory distress, hypoperfusion, or shock should be treated immediately.

TABLE 248.1. Key Historic and Physical Findings Relevant to the Evaluation of the Acutely Febrile Infant or Child

HISTORY
Behavior: activity level, consolability, irritability when moved (may be sign of meningitis), lethargy
Hydration status: fluid intake, urine output
Respiratory symptoms: cough, difficulty breathing
Gastrointestinal symptoms: vomiting, diarrhea (with blood), travel
Renal symptoms: abdominal pain, dysuria, frequency, urgency, hematuria
Other: focal pain (e.g., limp, sore throat, earache, abdominal pain, rash)
Medical history: immunization status, chronic medical conditions, ill contacts
PHYSICAL EXAMINATION
General appearance: activity, eye contact, muscle tone, color, consolability
Hydration status: mucous membranes, fontanelle, capillary refill, skin color, mottling
Respiratory: respiratory rate, grunting, nasal flaring, rales, bronchial breath sounds (may be only finding in child with pneumonia), retractions
HEENT: adenopathy, meningismus (may not be present in meningitic infants <1 yr old), pharyngitis, otitis media (bulging, decreased mobility; redness as the only sign is insufficient to diagnose otitis)
Cardiovascular: heart rate, murmur
Abdomen: tenderness, guarding, organomegaly, CVA* tenderness
Skin: rash (including viral, Kawasaki disease, measles, Coxsackie virus, scarlet fever, roseola, Henoch-Schönlein purpura, varicella)
Musculoskeletal: bone or joint tenderness, swelling, erythema, ability to ambulate

*CVA = costovertebral cortex.

The child's mental status and interaction with the environment are especially important to evaluate. A happy and playful infant with a fever of 40.0°C is less concerning than a lethargic child with no eye contact with a fever of 38.5°C. Febrile children should be undressed to look for skin infections and rashes, including petechiae (e.g., meningococcemia) and vesicles (e.g., *coxsackie* or *varicella* virus infection). Walking an ambulating child will help evaluate for occult joint infections. Table 248.1 lists other key symptoms and signs that should be pursued as part of the emergency evaluation of febrile infants and children.

DIFFERENTIAL DIAGNOSIS AND EMERGENCY DEPARTMENT MANAGEMENT BY AGE

Tables 248.2 and 248.3 list noninfectious and infectious causes of fever, respectively, along with the clinical features that should trigger their consideration. Table 248.4 presents an approach to the evaluation of the acutely febrile infant or child. This protocol assumes the absence of underlying chronic medical conditions and the presence of a skilled examiner and laboratory, as well as reliable follow-up. A few of the more common fever syndromes by age and clinical findings are discussed next.

Fever in the Neonate (0 to 28 Days)

Neonates, once infected with a bacterial process in one area, such as the urinary tract, are at risk for seeding of the bacteria into other areas, such as the meninges. Because bacterial sepsis and meningitis can have such subtle presentations in this age group (e.g., change in sleep or feeding pattern, diarrhea, jaundice), a complete septic workup, including lumbar puncture, and hospital admission are generally recommended.[10,23] In most circumstances, neonates should be treated with intravenous antibiotics until the culture results are known. Ampicillin (200 mg/kg/d) and cefotaxime (150 mg/kg/d) are recommended as initial empirical therapy (and continued therapy for confirmed meningitis), with gentamicin (7.5 mg/kg/d, or 5 mg/kg/d if less than 1 week postterm age) later substituted for cefotaxime if the cerebrospinal fluid (CSF) is negative. These combinations will provide adequate coverage for the most common bacterial pathogens in this age group, including group B *Streptococcus, Listeria monocytogenes,* and *Escherichia coli.* Studies suggest that some febrile, well-appearing neonates with negative initial septic workups can be successfully managed with admission and observation without empiric antibiotic treatment, or even discharged.[3] Currently, however, this is not considered a standard approach.

TABLE 248.2. Noninfectious Causes of Acute Fever in Infancy and Childhood

ENVIRONMENTAL
Overbundling (may raise skin temperature but not rectal temperature[17])
Heat stroke
COLLAGEN-VASCULAR
Rheumatic fever (prolonged fever, recent sore throat, rash, arthralgia)
Juvenile rheumatoid arthritis (prolonged fever, rash, arthritis)
POISONING
Atropine or other anticholinergics (dry mucous membranes, flushed)
Salicylates (tinnitus, hyperventilation)
Amphetamines (pupillary dilation, agitation, tremor, hypertension, tachycardia, hyperreflexia)
Antidepressants
OTHER
Kawasaki disease (prolonged fever, conjunctivitis, rash, adenopathy, erythematous mucous membranes)
Drug reaction
Prolonged seizures
Hemolysis

Fever in the Young Infant (1 to 3 Months)

Infants 1 to 3 months of age also may have subtle manifestations of serious infection, and, until just a few years ago, febrile infants as old as 12 weeks were routinely admitted to the hospital after a complete septic workup. Several studies now support use of specific guidelines in order to stratify the risk of serious bacterial infection in children 1 to 3 months of age. The Rochester criteria (Table 248.5) are a well-validated set of clinical and laboratory criteria that, if met, place a young infant at low risk for a bacterial infection, such that he or she can be managed as an outpatient.[6,7] Based on these criteria, the estimated risk of bacteremia and meningitis is 1.1% and 0.5%, respectively. For children meeting Rochester criteria, urine and blood cultures are recommended, and routine lumbar puncture and empirical antimicrobials are considered optional.[2,12] If an empiric antibiotic is to be used, intramuscular ceftriaxone (50 mg/kg) is recommended. Because of difficulty in clinically evaluating meningitis in this age group, and the concern for undiagnosed partially treated meningitis, it is recommended that lumbar puncture be performed if antimicrobials are to be administered. Discharged infants should be followed up in 24 hours. Standard manage-

TABLE 248.3. Common Infectious Processes Causing Fever in Children*

CNS	
	Meningitis
	Encephalitis
HEENT	
	Pharyngitis/tonsillitis
	Gingivostomatitis
	Common cold/influenza
	Sinusitis
	Parotitis (viral or suppurative)
	Tonsillar/pharyngeal abscess (uncommon)
	Peritonsillar cellulitis/abscess (uncommon)
RESPIRATORY	
	Pneumonia
	Croup
	Epiglottitis (uncommon)
	Bronchliolitis
	Bronchitis
CARDIOVASCULAR	
	Myocarditis (uncommon)
	Endocarditis (uncommon)
GI	
	Acute gastroenteritis
	Appendicitis
GU	
	Urinary tract infection
	Acute salpingitis (fever generally not the primary symptom)
	Epididymitis (fever generally not the primary symptom)
CELLULITIS/SUPPURATIVE ADENITIS	
	Periorbital cellulitis
	Facial cellulitis
	Cervical adenitis
	Inguinal adenitis
MUSCULOSKELETAL	
	Osteomyelitis
	Septic arthritis
SYSTEMIC	
	Bacterial sepsis/bacteremia
	Viremia
	Rocky Mountain spotted fever
	Toxic shock syndrome

*Boldface indicates common emergency conditions.

ment is to administer a second dose of ceftriaxone until the cultures are finalized as negative.

Fever in Infants and Children Older Than 3 Months by Clinical Findings

In children older than 3 months of age, signs such as mentation and behavior are more reliably present when serious bacterial infections are present. Young infants with meningitis may have a bulging fontanel, and infants older than 12 to 18 months usually have meningeal signs. Careful, repeated assessments of the patients' general appearance, especially just before discharge from the ED, are the key to reasonably excluding meningitis in children 3 to 36 months of age. If the febrile child becomes lethargic or is persistently irritable or inconsolable, then a lumbar puncture is recommended, regardless of other physical findings or laboratory parameters.

Fever and Rash

Vesicles or ulcers isolated to the oropharynx are possibly herpes simplex or Coxsackie virus. If vesicles are also present on the hands or feet, then hand-foot-mouth disease is likely. Diffuse vesicular lesions on an erythematous base suggest the presence of varicella.

A febrile, ill-appearing child with an acute onset of a petechial or purpuric rash should be considered to be meningococcemic until proven otherwise. Petechiae may develop on the face or neck area due to severe coughing or vomiting. It is recommended that any child with fever and petechiae not thought to be due to vomiting or coughing should undergo a complete septic workup. If the child remains well-appearing after a period of observation, no new petechiae have developed, and the child has a negative septic workup, then it may be possible to discharge the child with close follow-up.[20] Henoch-Schönlein purpura (HSP), a multisystem vasculitis, is suggested by subacute onset of a petechial or purpuric rash of the lower extremities, associated with painful swollen joints and abdominal pain in a slightly older child. As opposed to meningococcemia, these children rarely appear acutely ill. If HSP is suspected, stool for occult blood and urine for hematuria should be evaluated.

The pink maculopapular rash of roseola infantum will develop after a high fever has defervesced in an otherwise well-appearing infant. The maculopapular rash of measles will usually be associated with an ill-appearing young child with fever, cough, coryza, conjunctivitis, and Koplik's spots in the mouth. Kawasaki disease is uncommon but has the potential for serious morbidity. Kawasaki disease usually presents in a young child with a several-day history of high fever that progresses to a macular–papular diffuse rash, conjunctivitis, erythematous or fissured lips, strawberry tongue, cervical lymphadenopathy, and edema or desquamation of hands or feet. Children with Kawasaki disease are at risk for developing aneurysms of the coronary arteries. The treatment includes high-dose aspirin, immunoglobulin therapy, and serial echocardiograms.

Fever and a Red Tympanic Membrane

Acute otitis media remains one of the most common discharge diagnoses for young children with fever. Because an erythematous tympanic membrane can result from the fever alone or from crying, this finding alone is not sufficient to diagnose acute otitis media. A bulging membrane or immobility during insufflation is necessary for this diagnosis to be reasonably considered.

Fever and Pharyngitis

Group A beta-hemolytic *Streptococcus* remains a concern as a cause of pharyngitis and fever in children generally older than 5 years of age. This infection is often associated with prominent gastrointestinal symptoms in children. Scarlet fever is likely when a fine, "sandpapery," raised maculopapular rash is also present. A rapid streptococcal antigen test is a relatively specific aid to diagnosis. If it is negative, however, a throat culture is necessary to exclude this diagnosis. Adolescents with exudative pharyngitis accompanied by prominent cervical adenopathy and splenomegaly may have mononucleosis; atypical lymphocytes on a blood smear or a Monospot test help to confirm this diagnosis.

TABLE 248.4. Evaluating the Acutely Febrile Child[a]

Age	
<28 d[b,c]	Septic workup,[d] empirical antimicrobials, supportive care and monitoring, and hospital admission
1–3 mo[b]	Septic workup[d] Ill appearing infants or those with positive septic workup or not meeting Rochester criteria (see Table 248.5) should receive empirical antimicrobials, supportive care and monitoring, and hospital admission. If nontoxic with a negative septic workup (i.e., meeting Rochester criteria), discharge home with close follow-up with or without intramuscular antibiotics[d]
3–36 mo	Ill-appearing infants and young children should receive empirical antimicrobials, supportive care and monitoring, and hospital admission. If non-toxic-appearing, temperature > 39.0°C to 39.5°C,[e] and no source on examination[f]: UA and UC for girls <2 to 3 years old and for uncircumcised boys <6 to 12 months old Chest x-ray if signs of lower respiratory tract disease Additional laboratory workup and management considerations in this age group are dependent on general appearance and change over time or specific physical findings, such as meningismus or bulging fontanelle (e.g., lumbar puncture), painful swollen joint (e.g., arthrocentesis), and petechial rash (e.g., possible meningococcemia requiring parenteral antimicrobials and hospital admission). If no infectious source is identified, various approaches include discharging home, with close follow-up; blood cultures and empirical antimicrobial therapy for all febrile children, or for those with peripheral WBC >15,000/μL or ANC >10,000/μL, or for those with special risk (i.e., temperature >40.0°C to 41.0°C, lack of complete HIB vaccination, sickle cell disease, unreliable follow-up).
>36 mo	History and physical examination are usually reliable to identify presence of serious (e.g., meningitis or septic shock) or localized infection, and will dictate the extent of laboratory workup and management. UA and UC should be considered for girls if no source found on examination, or if vomiting, abdominal pain, or tenderness exists.

[a] Simplified approach to evaluation of fever; many variables must be taken into account, including prematurity, past medical conditions, ability to follow up.
[b] Fever defined as 38.0°C in this age group.
[c] Age is defined as postterm age; body weight and past medical conditions should be considered when determining category for workup.
[d] CBC, blood culture, urinalysis (UA), urine culture (UC), stool for WBCs and culture if diarrhea, chest x-ray if symptoms or signs of lower respiratory infection are present. Lumbar puncture and CSF analysis recommended <1 month of age; 1 to 3 months of age optional if no signs of CNS infection, but recommended if antimicrobials are to be prescribed.
[e] The risk of bacterial infection as a cause for the fever increases with the level of the fever.
[f] Otitis media, upper respiratory infections and gastroenteritis are not necessarily considered reliable sources of fever, such that other diagnoses can be excluded.

Fever and Cough, Wheezing, or Tachypnea

Upper respiratory symptoms associated with fever in the winter and early spring are often due to respiratory syncytial virus (RSV) bronchiolitis and can range in severity from mild cough and wheezing to severe respiratory distress with tachypnea, retractions, grunting, and nasal flaring. The chest x-ray typically shows hyperinflation with peribronchial cuffing. A nasal wash for rapid RSV antigen testing can quickly be obtained. If the child clinically appears to have bronchiolitis and the RSV antigen test is positive, the yield from blood cultures and urine cultures looking for other sources of fever is low.[1]

TABLE 248.5. The Rochester Criteria for Evaluating Young Infants

Previously healthy, non-toxic-appearing[a] term infant
No previous antimicrobial use
No focal infection on examination
WBC count 5,000–15,000/μL
Band count < 1,500/μL
Stool WBC count ≤5 WBC/HPF when diarrhea present
≤10 WBCs/HPF in spun urine

[a] Includes activity, alertness, color, strength of cry, consolability, irritability, eye contact, social responsiveness, and respiratory effort

Pneumonia in pre–school-age children is most often due to viral infection; *Mycoplasma* pneumonia is more common in older children and adolescents. Toxic-appearing, febrile children of any age may have pneumonia due to pyogenic bacteria such as *Streptococcus pneumoniae*. The signs of pneumonia in young children that are indications to consider a chest radiograph include tachypnea, retractions, nasal flaring, grunting, abnormal auscultatory findings, and a pulse oximeter reading of less than 92%.[11]

Fever and Vomiting, Diarrhea, or Abdominal Pain

Fever presenting with vomiting, diarrhea, or abdominal pain has a variety of causes, depending on the child's age. Gastrointestinal causes are the most likely source of the fever and associated symptoms. Acute gastroenteritis is a very common cause of fever with vomiting or diarrhea in young children and can have a viral or bacterial etiology. The most common cause of gastroenteritis in young children is *Rotavirus*. The vomiting frequently precedes the diarrhea by 24 hours. Rehydration is the cornerstone in treating the vomiting and diarrhea. If oral rehydration appears as an option, encourage the parents to try small amounts of fluids (e.g., 5 cc or 1 teaspoon every 2 to 3 minutes for young children). The child's diet should be advanced to a regular diet as soon as possible.

Bacterial causes of enteritis include *Shigella, Salmonella, Campylobacter*, and enterotoxic *E. coli*. Laboratory evaluation of children with fever, hematochezia, and abdominal pain may include a stool culture. A child found to have a bacterial pathogen as the cause of the diarrhea, with the exception of *Salmonella*, should be treated with the appropriate antimicrobial. Treating *Salmonella* may lead to a chronic carrier state and is recommended only for infants less than 3 months of age, patients with immunosuppressive illness, and toxic patients. The fluoroquinolones are relatively contraindicated in young children, due to the potential risk to growth.

Appendicitis also remains a serious cause of fever and abdominal pain in young children. Young children have higher perforation rates compared with older children, due in part to the difficulty in making the diagnosis. Children with appendicitis are often discharged home with diagnoses of gastroenteritis or urinary tract infection (UTI) before the final diagnosis of appendicitis is made. The omentum in young children is less capable of walling off focal areas of infection, such as appendicitis. Peritonitis with diffuse abdominal tenderness is therefore more common. Ultrasound and computed tomography (CT) scan are two modalities that are now used more commonly to diagnose appendicitis in young children.

Streptococcal pharyngitis in older children may present with fever, abdominal pain, and associated dysphagia. Lower lobe pneumonia can sometimes present with abdominal pain and fever. Adolescent girls with fever and abdominal pain should be questioned regarding sexual activity and possibly evaluated for pelvic inflammatory disease. UTIs are also a common cause in girls with fever and abdominal pain. In young children, UTIs may present with fever and vomiting, often without abdominal pain. UTI should be considered in febrile girls less than 2 years old and in uncircumcised boys less than 1 year old.

Fever and vomiting without diarrhea can be a sign of a neurologic process. Meningitis, particularly bacterial meningitis, is the most serious cause. Children with a central nervous system (CNS) ventricular shunt should be evaluated for the possibility of obstruction and meningitis. This evaluation may include a head CT scan and lumbar puncture or shunt tap for CSF evaluation. Finally, acute otitis media can also present with fever and diarrhea in young children.

Fever and Swollen Joint or Limp

Febrile children who are nonambulatory, walk with a limp, or have local joint symptoms should be evaluated for a joint infection. Toxic synovitis, a benign condition related to coincident viral infection, must be differentiated from septic arthritis, which can rapidly be destructive. Joint effusions should be aspirated and analyzed for cell counts, Gram stain, and culture. If the hip joint is suspected, ultrasound appears to be a reliable test to evaluate the presence of an effusion, and can then be used to guide joint aspiration. Sexually active adolescents may have arthritis or tenosynovitis due to disseminated gonococcal infection.

Fever without Source in Young Children (3 to 36 Months)

After a thorough physical examination, often no identifiable infection source for the fever is found in infants and children younger than 36 months of age. The presence of some clinical diagnoses can reasonably explain fever, including Coxsackie pharyngitis (and hand-foot-mouth disease) and chickenpox. The presence of acute otitis media does not necessarily exclude other diagnoses as the cause of fever.

Fever may be the only indication of a UTI in a young child. Up to 7% of febrile young children without a source found on physical examination have a UTI as a cause of their fever.[26] In one study, up to 4% of young febrile children less than 2 years old, with either acute otitis media or gastroenteritis as a source for the fever, also had a UTI.[27] A urinalysis and culture are recommended as part of the workup of girls less than 2 years old and of uncircumcised boys less than 12 months old. Urinalysis is insufficiently accurate to be used alone to evaluate the presence of UTI in young children.[18] Therefore, a urine culture should be sent in addition to the urinalysis. Enhanced urinalysis, using Gram stain or hemocytometer, has been shown to improve the capabilities of the urinalysis.[18] Bag urine specimens are also more likely to produce contaminant flora, compared with catheterized specimens. Pneumonia is rarely present without signs of disease (see previous discussion).[14]

When no source is found on physical examination, and pneumonia and UTI have been ruled out by either physical examination or laboratory tests, the potential for occult bacteremia should be considered. Previous studies have shown that 3% to 5% of children with no focus of infection and with temperatures above 39.5°C are bacteremic with *S. pneumoniae, Haemophilus influenzae*, or *Neisseria meningitidis*.[5] Previously, up to 25% of these bacteremic children would have seeding of other areas, causing other serious bacterial infections, such as meningitis or septic arthritis.[5] Due to *H. influenzae* type b vaccine, this virulent bacteria is now almost nonexistent as a cause of occult bacteremia, with *S. pneumoniae* accounting for over 90% of cases. The risk of pneumococcal bacteremia causing meningitis is much lower, at less than 3%.[24] Although occult pneumococcal bacteremia ultimately spontaneously resolves in the vast majority of children, both oral and parenteral antimicrobial agents may reduce the risk of focal bacterial infections and possible meningitis in children with occult bacteremia.

The relative benefit of possible averted infectious sequelae, and the risk and cost of unnecessary blood cultures (and consequences of contaminants, etc.) and antimicrobials, compared with careful follow-up alone, is not clear.[16] Currently, no consensus exists as to the need or means to identify and empirically treat children who may be bacteremic among all those with fever without source.

Approaches include blood cultures and empirical antimicrobials for all nontoxic children 3 to 36 months of age with fever without source; for only those at high risk (e.g., temperature greater than 41.0°C, under- or nonimmunized against *H. influenzae*, or a combination of temperature greater than 39.0°C and absolute neutrophil count [ANC] greater than 10,000/μL); and close follow-up without testing or treatment.[16] If empiric antibiotics are to be utilized, intramuscular ceftriaxone (50 mg/kg) is appropriate, especially for the child who is not fully immunized against *H. influenzae*. For other children, oral amoxicillin (60 to 90 mg/kg/d) is a reasonable alternative. A new protein-conjugate pneumococcal vaccine for young children was recently approved and appears to be 80% to 100% effective in preventing bacteremia and meningitis.[9] Soon, the justification for empiric antimicrobial therapy for presumed occult bacteremia will be significantly less in fully vaccinated children.

EMERGENCY DEPARTMENT DISPOSITION AND INSTRUCTIONS TO PARENTS

Fever control with acetaminophen (15 mg/kg every 4 to 6 hours) or ibuprofen (10 mg/kg every 4 to 6 hours); cool, clear liquids; and light dressing are advised. Sponging may be used but is of questionable value. Body temperature is determined

TABLE 248.6. Indications for Reevaluation[a]

AGE OR TREATMENT
Any child less than 3 mo old Any child given antibiotics for fever without a source
BEHAVIOR
Persistent lethargy or irritability
HYDRATION STATUS
Signs of dehydration (decreased urine output, decreased tears)
RESPIRATORY
Worsening cough Difficulty breathing
GASTROINTESTINAL
Persistent vomiting Bilious vomiting Worsening diarrhea
OTHER
New rash Pain

[a] Telephone contact my be sufficient in some cases.

by the temperature regulatory center in the hypothalamus. Acetaminophen resets the regulatory center, but sponging has no effect on it and a minimal effect on lowering the temperature for any significant period of time. Sponging usually results in an irritated, agitated child.[15]

Although experimental evidence suggests that fever may be adaptive and stimulate the immune system, fever reduction has not proven to be deleterious, and does lead to increased patient comfort and decreased metabolic demands and fluid loss. Therefore, fever control is recommended.

The second component of discharge instructions consists of the indications for urgent return for reevaluation (Table 248.6). The most important indications for urgent reevaluation are lethargy and persistent irritability. Even with continued fever, if the child's behavior and disposition improve, urgent reevaluation is not necessary. A child less than 3 months old or a child given empiric antibiotics should generally be followed up in 12 to 24 hours by a primary care physician or clinic. That follow-up may consist of a telephone call to the caretaker or, if there is reason for additional concern, a repeat examination.

COMMON PITFALLS

- Do not forget to consider noninfectious disease processes as a cause for the fever.
- Remember to account for an infant's age in determining the extent of the fever evaluation.
- Do not forget to carefully evaluate and document the child's general appearance.
- Do not overrely on acute-phase reactants such as the white blood cell or ANC.

References

1. Antonow JA, Hansen K, McKinstry CA, et al. Sepsis evaluations in hospitalized infants with bronchiolitis. *Pediatr Infect Dis J* 1998;17(3):231–236.
2. Baker MD, Bell LM, Avner JR. Outpatient management without antibiotics of fever in selected infants. *N Engl J Med* 1993;329(20):1437–1441.
3. Baker MD, et al. The applicability of an established outpatient management protocol for febrile 0–1 month old infants. SAEM 1997 Annual Meeting. *Acad Emerg Med* 1997;427(abst 258).
4. Baker MD, Fosarelli PD, Carpenter RO. Childhood fever: correlation of diagnosis with temperature response to acetaminophen. *Pediatrics* 1987;80(3):315–318.
5. Baraff LJ, Bass JW, Fleisher GR, et al. Practice guideline for the management of infants and children 0 to 36 months of age with fever without a source. Agency for Health Care Policy and Research. *Ann Emerg Med* 1993;22(7):1198–1210.
6. Baskin MN, Fleisher GR, O'Rourke EJ. Outpatient management of febrile infants 28 to 90 days of age with intramuscular ceftriaxone. *Am J Dis Child* 1988;142:391(abst).
7. Baskin MN, O'Rourke EJ, Fleisher GR. Outpatient treatment of febrile infants 28 to 89 days of age with intramuscular administration of ceftriaxone. *J Pediatr* 1992;120(1):22–27.
8. Berkowitz CD, Schiff D, Black JL, et al. Effect of acetaminophen on clinical assessment of febrile infants. *Am J Dis Child* 1988;142:393(abst).
9. Black S, Shinefield H, Ray P, et al. Efficacy of heptavalent conjugate pneumococcal vaccine in 37,000 infants and children: results of the Northern California Kaiser Permanente Efficacy Trial (abst LB-9). 1998 Interscience Conference on Antimicrobial Agents and Chemotherapy, San Diego, California, September 1998.
10. Bonadio WA. Incidence of serious infections in afebrile neonates with a history of fever. *Pediatr Infect Dis J* 1987;6(10):911–914.
11. Bramson RT, Meyer TL, Silbiger ML, et al. The futility of the chest radiograph in the febrile infant without respiratory symptoms. *Pediatrics* 1993;92(4):524–526.
12. Brik R, Hamissah R, Shehada N, et al. Evaluation of febrile infants under 3 months of age: is routine lumbar puncture warranted? *Isr J Med Sci* 1997;33(2):93–97.
13. Chamberlain JM, Grandner J, Rubinoff JL. Comparison of a tympanic thermometer to rectal and oral thermometers in a pediatric emergency department. *Clin Pediatr* 1991;30[Suppl 4]:24–29; discussion, 34–35.
14. Crain EF, Bulas D, Bijur PE, et al. Is a chest radiograph necessary in the evaluation of every febrile infant less than 8 weeks of age? *Pediatrics* 1991;88(4):821–824.
15. Friedman AD, Barton LL. Efficacy of sponging vs acetaminophen for reduction of fever. Sponging Study Group. *Pediatr Emerg Care* 1990;6(1):6–7.
16. Green SM, Rothrock SG. Evaluation styles for well-appearing febrile children: are you a "risk-minimizer" or a "test-minimizer"? *Ann Emerg Med* 1999;33(2):311–214.
17. Grover G, Berkowitz CD, Lewis RJ, et al. The effects of bundling on infant temperature. *Pediatrics* 1994;94(5):669–673.
18. Hoberman A, Wald ER, Penchansky L, et al. Enhanced urinalysis as a screening test for urinary tract infection. *Pediatrics* 1993;91(6):1196–1199.
19. Mackowiak PA, Wasserman SS, Levine MM. A critical appraisal of 98.6 degrees F, the upper limit of the normal body temperature, and other legacies of Carl Reinhold August Wunderlich. *JAMA* 1992;268(12):1578–1580.
20. Mandl KD, Stack AM, Fleisher GR. Incidence of bacteremia in infants and children with fever and petechiae. *J Pediatr* 1997;131(3):398–404.
21. May A, Bauchner H. Fever phobia: the pediatrician's contribution. *Pediatrics* 1992;90(6):851–854.
22. Morley CJ, Hewson PH, Thornton AJ. Axillary and rectal temperature measurements in infants. *Arch Dis Child* 1992;67(1):122–125.
23. Roberts KB, Borzy MS. Fever in the first eight weeks of life. *Johns Hopkins Med J* 1977;141(1):9–13.
24. Rothrock SG, Harper MB, Green SM, et al. Do oral antibiotics prevent meningitis and serious bacterial infections in children with *Streptococcus pneumoniae* occult bacteremia? A meta-analysis. *Pediatrics* 1997;99(3):438–444.
25. Scarfone RJ. Compliance with scheduled visits to a pediatric emergency department. *Acad Emerg Med* 1994;1: (abst 41).
26. Shaw K. Predicting urinary tract infections in febrile young children in the emergency department. SAEM 1997 Annual Meeting. *Acad Emerg Med* 1997;427(abst 257).
27. Shaw K, Gorelick M, McGowan K, et al. Prevalence of urinary tract infections in febrile young children in the emergency department. *Pediatrics* 1998;102:E16.
28. Terndrup TE, Rajk J. Impact of operator technique and device on infrared emission detection tympanic thermometry. *J Emerg Med* 1992;10(6): 683–687.
29. van der Bogert. *J Pediatr* 1937;10:795.
30. Vauzelle-Kervroedan F, d'Athis P, Pariente-Khayat A, et al. Equivalent antipyretic activity of ibuprofen and paracetamol in febrile children. *J Pediatr* 1997;131:683–687.

CHAPTER 249
Gastrointestinal Bleeding

Michael O. Gayle and Niranjan Kissoon

The causes of bleeding from the gastrointestinal (GI) tract vary with the child's age. The site of bleeding is also important in diagnosis and therapy, and can often be determined by the presenting symptoms. Hematemesis is the vomiting of blood and implies a source proximal to the ligament of Treitz. Vomited blood may have the appearance of coffee grounds or may be bright red, implying ongoing bleeding. Blood from the upper GI tract or proximal small bowel, when passed per rectum, is typically black or tarry, is sticky, has a characteristic aroma, and is called *melena.* Bright red blood per rectum or maroon stools (hematochezia) implies a more distal GI source. Upper GI bleeding, however, may present as gross blood rectally (hematochezia), if the hemorrhage is large and transit time is short.

Tables 249.1 and 249.2 outline the causes of GI bleeding in children and illustrate the wide, age-related differential diagnosis.

CLINICAL PRESENTATION

Bleeding from anal fissures and bleeding from the upper GI tract are the most common reasons children with GI bleeding visit the emergency department. Life-threatening hemorrhage is a rare presentation to the emergency department. More commonly, GI bleeding in the child presents as anemia from chronic upper GI bleeding (typically microcytic) or occult bleeding in the stool (e.g., cow's milk protein sensitivity).[6] Acute bleeding can be classified as occult, overt, or massive. Massive bleeding (e.g., variceal bleeding) is the most dramatic presentation and is usually accompanied by compromised cardiac output or tissue oxygenation.

DIFFERENTIAL DIAGNOSIS

Reaching the exact diagnosis in a child with GI bleeding is usually unnecessary in the emergency department, because most patients are stable and the differential diagnosis is large (see Tables 249.1 and 249.2). A thorough history and clinical examination can usually make the diagnosis. For the emergency physician, it is most important to determine whether the source of bleeding is in the upper or the lower GI tract. The easiest method is to atraumatically pass a small, soft, nasogastric tube and perform a gastric lavage with tap water or normal saline at room temperature. Water appears to be as efficacious as saline, and there does not appear to be any benefit of cold versus room-temperature solution.[12] If blood is not evident on lavage, it is unlikely that the bleeding is above the ligament of Treitz (i.e., bleeding from the nose, esophagus, and stomach).

Measuring the ratio of blood urea nitrogen to creatinine (BUN/Cr), as described by Felber and colleagues,[4] may also provide supportive evidence of upper GI bleeding. A ratio exceeding 30 suggests bleeding from the upper GI tract; less than 30 might be consistent with either an upper or a lower GI bleeding site. This ratio also provides a useful means of assessing the amount of blood loss and predicting when a significant bleed has ceased.[19]

Newborn (0 to 1 Month)

Most causes of bleeding in neonates are never identified, as most bleeding usually stops between 24 and 48 hours of life. Significant upper GI bleeding may result from stress ulcers or hemorrhagic gastritis in the neonate with sepsis, an intracranial lesion, or other major illness. Hematemesis in the neonate may also result from hemorrhagic disease of the newborn (vitamin K deficiency) or congenital bleeding disorders such as hemophilia. The swallowing of a mixture of amniotic fluid and maternal blood is a frequent cause of hematemesis but may also present as dark red rectal bleeding. Swallowed maternal blood (adult hemoglobin) can be easily differentiated from upper GI bleeding in the fetus (fetal hemoglobin) by adding sodium hydroxide to a blood sample. This test is known as the alum precipitated toxoid test, or the Apt. Fetal hemoglobin resists alkaline degradation and remains pink; adult hemoglobin gives a brownish color.

Anal fissure and local trauma are the most common causes of rectal bleeding in the first month of life. However, both necrotizing enterocolitis and enterocolitis due to Hirschsprung disease may present with occult or overt rectal bleeding. Necrotizing enterocolitis is more common in the preterm infant but is also seen in the stressed term infant. Bilious vomiting, abdominal distention, and rectal bleeding are the most common clinical features and may also be due to surgical emergencies such as midgut volvulus. Finding air in the bowel wall (pneumatosis intestinalis) on an abdominal radiograph is pathognomonic for necrotizing enterocolitis.

Infant (1 Month to 2 Years)

Upper GI bleeding is frequently caused by esophagitis, gastritis, or stress ulcers. However, congenital malformations such as

TABLE 249.1. Differential Diagnosis of Lower GI Bleeding

Newborn (0–1 mo)	Infant (1 mo–2 yr)	Preschool (2–5 yr)	School Age (>5 yr)
Anal fissure	Anal fissure	Anal fissure	Anal fissure
Local trauma	Hirschsprung disease	Juvenile polyp	Juvenile polyp
Swallowed maternal blood	Allergic colitis	Infectious colitis	Infectious colitis
Upper GI bleeding	Intussusception	Meckel's diverticulum	Hemorrhoids
Necrotizing enterocolitis	Infectious colitis	Hemolytic–uremic syndrome	Inflammatory bowel disease
Malrotation with volvulus	Meckel's diverticulum	Henoch-Schönlein purpura	Pseudomembranous colitis
Infectious colitis	Intestinal duplication	Inflammatory bowel disease	Lymphonodular hyperplasia
Hirschsprung disease	Lymphonodular hyperplasia	Intussusception	Hemolytic–uremic syndrome
Allergic colitis	Pseudomembranous colitis	Pseudomembranous colitis	
Coagulopathy		Lymphonodular hyperplasia	

TABLE 249.2. Differential Diagnosis of Upper GI Bleeding

Newborn (0–1 mo)	Infant (1 mo–2 yr)	Preschool (2–5 yr)	School Age (>5 yr)
Idiopathic	Esophagitis	Esophagitis	Esophagitis
Swallowed maternal blood	Gastritis	Gastritis	Gastritis
Esophagitis	Stress ulcer	Peptic ulcer	Peptic ulcer
Stress ulcer	Mallory-Weiss tear	Varices (esophageal, gastric)	Varices (esophageal, gastric)
Vitamin K deficiency	Vascular anomalies	Mallory-Weiss tear	Mallory-Weiss tear
Blood dyscrasia	Foreign body	Foreign body	Inflammatory bowel disease
Vascular anomalies	Duplication	Blood dyscrasia	
		Vascular anomalies	

duodenal web, although more likely to present in the newborn period, can present after 1 month of life.[14]

Lower GI bleeding is most commonly due to anal fissure, but other anorectal lesions, such as juvenile polyps, should also be considered. Intussusception, which classically presents with currant jelly stools, is most common in infants 7 to 12 months old. Infectious colitis is usually secondary to species of *Salmonella* and *Shigella* and to *Campylobacter jejuni, Yersinia enterocolitica,* and both enterohemorrhagic and enteroinvasive *Escherichia coli*. Other organisms that should be considered include *Aeromonas hydrophila* and *Entamoeba histolytica*. With the increasing number of children with the acquired immunodeficiency syndrome, cases of GI bleeding secondary to opportunistic infections such as cytomegalovirus will be seen with increased frequency.[3]

Preschool (2 to 5 Years)

Varices in both the upper and the lower GI tracts can lead to massive, life-threatening hemorrhage in this age group. Two-thirds of patients with portal hypertension sustain bleeds before 5 years of age, and 85% do so by age 10 years. On physical examination, other signs of portal hypertension or liver disease are found, such as splenomegaly, hepatomegaly, and dilated abdominal veins.[1] Foreign-body ingestion, although uncommon, should also be considered as a cause of upper GI bleeding.

Anal fissure and juvenile polyps are the most frequent cause of lower GI bleeding. Polyps are usually solitary and nonmalignant and can be felt on rectal examination. Massive GI bleeding from Meckel's diverticulum is sometimes seen in preschool children. Infectious enterocolitis from infectious agents similar to those described for the infant may also present with bloody stools. Multisystem diseases such as hemolytic–uremic syndrome and Henoch-Schönlein purpura are less common causes of bloody stools.

School Age (Over 5 Years)

Esophagitis, gastritis, and peptic ulcer disease account for most cases of upper GI bleeding. Erosions of the gastric mucosa may occur acutely after any major stress, such as trauma, shock, burns, or sepsis. Peptic ulcer disease may be either primary or secondary to other conditions, such as cystic fibrosis medications (e.g., corticosteroids and nonsteroidal antiinflammatory agents).

Anal fissure and juvenile polyps account for most cases of lower GI bleeding. Intestinal lymphonodular hyperplasia of childhood has a peak incidence between 6 and 10 years; inflammatory bowel diseases (e.g., Crohn disease and ulcerative colitis) have a peak incidence in children over 5 years.[8] With the increased prevalence of cocaine use, drug intoxication should be considered in cases of unexplained shock and hemorrhagic diarrhea in this age group.[13]

EMERGENCY DEPARTMENT EVALUATION

The emergency physician's initial step is to determine the site and magnitude of bleeding and whether it is ongoing at the time of evaluation. If the patient presents with signs and symptoms of cardiovascular compromise, immediate attention to restoring intravascular volume is necessary. Usually, however, the evaluation can be done in a leisurely manner, beginning with a thorough history and physical examination.

Important elements of the history and physical examination are outlined in Table 249.3. A nasogastric tube should be inserted and fluid aspirated, unless a distal source is obvious. A positive aspirate for blood almost certainly indicates that the site of bleeding is proximal to the ligament of Treitz. However, a negative aspirate does not exclude an upper GI bleeding site beyond the pylorus.

In most cases, the cause of bleeding is evident, but sometimes, before beginning an expensive and possibly invasive workup, it may be necessary to confirm that the patient is actually passing blood. Many foods and medications (e.g., tomato or cranberry juice, flavored gelatin, Kool-Aid, red licorice, ampicillin, rifampin, iron, and bismuth preparations [Pepto-Bismol]) can give stools a bloody appearance or test positive for blood. In most hospitals, guaiac benzidine or benzidine derivative test pads (Hemoccult or Hematest) are used to detect blood. These tests use a hydrogen peroxide developer and are based on the peroxidase activity of hemoglobin and its derivatives. In the presence of hydrogen peroxide, these substances catalytically oxidize substrates such as guaiac or benzidine. The oxidation produces a color change in the substrate, indicating a positive test. However, false-negative results can be obtained if the patient has ingested large doses of ascorbic acid or if intestinal bacteria have degraded the hemoglobin to porphyrin. False-positive results can be seen if the patient has eaten rare red meat or peroxidase-containing fruits and vegetables such as broccoli, radishes, cauliflower, cantaloupe, or turnips. A new test, HemoQuant, appears to be more sensitive.[6,7] Laboratory studies

TABLE 249.3. History and Physical Examination for GI Bleeding

HISTORY	PHYSICAL EXAMINATION
Characteristic bleeding (duration, quantity, color, rectal vs. oral)	Vital signs
Associated pain	Site of bleeding (nose, mouth, outside GI tract)
Vomiting/diarrhea	Acuity or chronicity
Medication history (e.g., aspirin, alcohol)	Anthropometric data
Illicit drugs (e.g., cocaine)	Cutaneous signs (e.g., spider nevi)
Systemic diseases	Abdominal tenderness/mass
Family history	Hepatomegaly
Social history	Splenomegaly
	Anorectal examination

TABLE 249.4. Laboratory Studies

Blood count: CBC with reticulocyte count
Coagulation profile: platelet count, prothrombin time, partial thromboplastin time, fibrinogen
Hepatic profile: bilirubin, SGPT, SGOT
Renal profile: BUN/Cr
Blood bank: type and crossmatch
Stools: leukocytes, aerobic and anaerobic stool cultures, microscopy for ova and parasites

(Table 249.4) should include a complete blood count with platelet and reticulocyte counts and a coagulation profile. If bleeding is severe, blood should also be sent for a crossmatch. The BUN/Cr ratio is useful in localizing the source of bleeding to the upper GI tract and may provide an estimate of the severity of blood loss from the upper GI tract. Also, an elevated BUN level is more likely to be associated with an upper than a lower GI bleed.[19] Hepatic and renal function tests (to assess liver function and to obtain the BUN/Cr index) should be obtained. If an infective cause is thought likely, stool should be examined promptly for fecal leukocytes, aerobic and anaerobic cultures, and microscopy for ova and parasites.[14]

Plain radiography and sonography are noninvasive and minimally distressing for a child and may give definitive information, such as a classic appearance of multiple short fluid levels in the abdomen in a neonate with volvulus, or the appearance of an intraluminal mass on sonography, in a case of intussusception.

If the source of bleeding is not obvious after these investigations, more detailed testing, including endoscopy and complex radiographic procedures, is necessary. However, most of these will not be conducted as part of the emergency department workup. In children with a positive nasogastric aspirate, endoscopy within the first 24 hours can determine the source of upper GI bleeding in 90% of cases. Fiberoptic endoscopy in children has shown that the most common causes of bleeding are gastritis, esophagitis, duodenal ulcers, and esophageal varices.[9] Endoscopy is especially recommended in children with a history of esophageal varices, because the source of bleeding may be from other lesions. Upper GI barium studies are less accurate than endoscopy and may interfere with subsequent endoscopic examination.

Both endoscopy and barium studies fail to determine the source of bleeding in patients with massive bleeding (greater than 0.5 mL/min, making endoscopic examination impossible). In these patients, arteriographic examination of the superior and mesenteric arteries and the celiac axis may reveal some common causes of bleeding, as well as some unusual causes, such as hepatic artery aneurysms, traumatic hematobilia, or malformations (e.g., arteriovenous lesions and hemangiomas). Nuclear medicine scans have fewer complications and are preferred by some clinicians.[15]

If the nasogastric aspirate is negative, a rectal examination and proctosigmoidoscopy can identify the source of rectal bleeding in 80% of cases. Additional studies are needed to identify the other 20%. Dark blood mixed with stool, in the absence of abdominal pain or diarrhea, may indicate Meckel's diverticulum, intestinal duplication, or right-sided colonic polyps. A bleeding Meckel's diverticulum is the cause in 80% of cases and can often be diagnosed by a nuclear medicine scan. Colonoscopy and, ultimately, an air-contrast barium enema should be performed if the scan is inconclusive.

EMERGENCY DEPARTMENT MANAGEMENT

Management depends on the child's clinical status and the severity and site of bleeding (Fig. 249.1).

Assessment of Cardiovascular Status

Initial management is based on the child's condition, including factors such as age; source, rate, and amount of bleeding; and associated medical illnesses. Assessment of cardiopulmonary status and prompt attention to any derangements are always necessary. Oxygen administration and venous access, followed by fluid boluses of crystalloids (20 mL/kg lactated Ringer's or normal saline), are mandatory, particularly if the patient has signs of volume compromise (anxiety, tachycardia, weak pulses, delayed capillary refill, hypotension, tachypnea). Additional fluid boluses are given as indicated by frequent reevaluations. A nasogastric tube is then placed in the stomach, and lavage with tap water or saline begins.

Occult Bleeding

In the stable child with occult bleeding, management is geared toward making the diagnosis and excluding more serious conditions. Investigations are dictated by the history and physical examination, but most tests, including cultures, radiologic and nuclear medicine scans, and endoscopy, can be performed on an outpatient basis. The cause of occult upper GI bleeding in children is often not from the GI tract. Although anal fissures account for most cases of occult blood in stools, the physician should always consider the possibility of a less benign cause (e.g., necrotizing enterocolitis or intussusception in the ill-looking neonate or infant). Occult bleeding may also presage other serious events, such as Meckel's diverticulum.

Overt Bleeding

Administration of crystalloids (normal saline or Ringer's lactate) to restore intravascular volume is the management priority. Blood is sent for urgent type and crossmatch, or O-negative blood is made immediately available. The child who has lost 10% to 20% of his or her blood volume does not necessarily require blood replacement, provided the bleeding has stopped. If, after 20% of the blood volume has been replaced by crystalloid, the child still has orthostatic hypotension, blood should be given. The child's age and physical condition also dictate the need for blood; for example, children with heart and chronic lung disease may require earlier transfusion. Platelets, fresh-frozen plasma, or vitamin K (1 mg per year of age, up to 10 mg) is given as necessary to correct an identified coagulopathy. In the neonate suspected of vitamin K deficiency, vitamin K (1 mg) is given intramuscularly. Antacid therapy, H_2 blockers, and sucralfate have proven to be efficacious in minimizing or preventing bleeding in patients with stress or peptic ulcer from trauma, shock, or sepsis, if gastric pH levels are kept above 4. H_2 blockers are best given intravenously by continuous infusion. The recommended intravenous dosage is 20 to 30 mg/kg/d for cimetidine or 7.5 mg/kg/d for ranitidine.

Massive Bleeding

Although the incidence of massive GI bleeding in children is low, the emergency physician must be prepared to treat these patients aggressively. Aggressive fluid resuscitation and administration of blood components usually suffice. However, in some cases, endotracheal intubation, to secure the airway and to decrease the work of breathing, is needed in a patient with low cardiac output. Endotracheal intubation allows adequate sedation without the risk of hypoventilation or aspiration, and it also facilitates endoscopy. Continuous monitoring of vital signs, urine output with a Foley catheter, and oxygen saturation with pulse oximetry is essential. Central venous catheter placement,

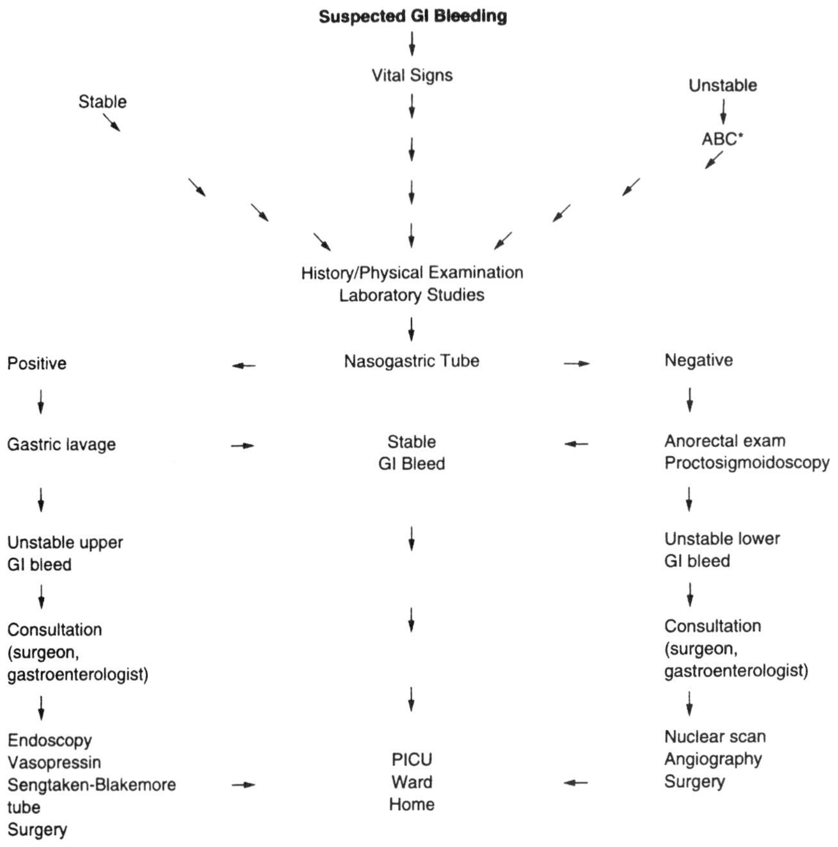

Figure 249.1. Flow diagram of suggested management of GI bleeding in the emergency department. ABC (*) includes attention to respiratory status (may include endotracheal intubation) and cardiovascular support (including vascular access, crystalloid and blood infusions).

although not mandatory, may be helpful in monitoring the volume status.

Management of the child with massive variceal bleeding from portal hypertension may include intravenous vasopressin (0.1 to 0.4 U/min), variceal injection, or ligation using endoscopy.[1]

Massive bleeding can also occur in children with Meckel's diverticulum; these patients also require aggressive resuscitation initially. Following cardiovascular stabilization, the site of bleeding can be confirmed by a nuclear medicine scan or by arteriography.

If massive bleeding precludes stabilization, immediate laparotomy may be required.

DISPOSITION

Role of the Consultant

Conditions that require urgent surgical evaluation include volvulus, vascular malformations, and necrotizing enterocolitis in the neonate. Some cases of GI bleeding from stress ulcers, variceal bleeding, or intussusception require urgent surgical evaluation. The emergency physician should always be in direct communication with physicians who will assume inpatient care of the child. Consultation with a pediatric gastroenterologist, pediatric surgeon, and/or pediatric intensivist may be necessary early in management. Panendoscopy to establish a specific diagnosis and to assess the rapidity of bleeding, the risk of rebleeding, and, possibly, the administration of definitive therapy may be required.

Transfer Considerations

In the prehospital setting or during interhospital transfer of the child with GI bleeding, attention must be paid to the airway, breathing, and circulation. Oxygenation and vascular access with the administration of crystalloid are priorities if there is evidence of vascular compromise. Continuous monitoring to ensure an adequate airway and stable vital signs is mandatory. Although personnel skilled in advanced pediatric life support should accompany the child, attention to stabilization before transport should minimize the need for interventions during transport.

COMMON PITFALLS

- Assuming the colored material is blood. Many foods and medicines can give secretions or stools a bloody appearance.
- Failing to perform an Apt test on a neonate's stool to rule out swallowed maternal blood.
- Using the wrong-sized nasogastric tube. Smaller bore tubes may be adequate for assessing bleeding, but not for removing clots.
- If the nasogastric aspirate does not sample duodenal contents, or if bleeding is intermittent, a false-negative aspirate may result.
- A carelessly placed nasogastric tube may yield a false-positive aspirate and cause distress to the patient. Iodine, supplemental iron, and ingestion of red meat may cause false-positive results.
- A normal hemoglobin level does not exclude significant, rapid GI bleeding.

- A normal or increased blood pressure in children does not exclude hypovolemia.
- Assuming the blood is from the GI tract
- Performing a barium study before endoscopy
- Not considering sexual abuse as a cause of anal fissures
- Failing to consider nonorganic causes (e.g., Munchausen syndrome by proxy) of GI bleeding

References

1. Alvarez F. Long-term treatment of bleeding caused by portal hypertension in children. *J Pediatr* 1997;131:798.
2. Chaibou M, Tucci M, Dugas MA, et al. Clinically significant upper gastrointestinal bleeding acquired in a pediatric intensive care unit: a prospective study. *Pediatrics* 1998;102:933.
3. Dolgin SE, Larsen JG, Shah KD, et al. CMV enteritis causing hemorrhage and obstruction in an infant with AIDS. *J Pediatr Surg* 1990;25:696.
4. Felber S, Rosenthal P, Henton D. The BUN/creatinine ratio in localizing GI bleeding in pediatric patients. *J Pediatr Gastroenterol Nutr* 1988;7:685.
5. Fonkalsrud EW. Treatment of variceal hemorrhage in children. *Surg Clin North Am* 1990;70:475.
6. Fuchs G, Dewier M, Hutchinson S, et al. GI blood loss in older infants: impact of cow milk vs. formula. *J Pediatr Gastroenterol Nutr* 1993;16:4.
7. Gopalswamy N, Stelling HP, Markert RJ, et al. A comparative study of eight fecal occult blood tests and HemoQuant in patients in whom colonoscopy is indicated. *Arch Fam Med* 1994;12:1043.
8. Grand RJ, Ramakrishna J, Calenda KA. Inflammatory bowel disease in the pediatric patient. *Gastroenterol Clin North Am* 1995;24:613.
9. Kay MH, Wyllie R. Alcohol isn't for kids: endoscopic hemostasis of bleeding peptic ulcers in pediatric patients. *J Pediatr* 1998;133:802.
10. McRury JM, Barry RC. A modified Apt test: a new look at an old test. *Pediatr Emerg Care* 1994;10:189.
11. Pearl RH, Irish MS, Caty MG, et al. The approach to common abdominal diagnoses in infants and children. Part II. *Pediatr Clin North Am* 1998;45:1287.
12. Ponsky JL, Hoffman M, Swayngim DS. Saline irrigation in gastric hemorrhage: the effect of temperature. *J Surg Res* 1980;28:204.
13. Riggs D, Weibley RE. Acute hemorrhagic diarrhea and cardiovascular collapse in a young child owing to environmentally acquired cocaine. *Pediatr Emerg Care* 1991;7:154.
14. Sarda AK, Cannan R. Massive lower GI hemorrhage due to ascariasis. *Am J Gastroenterol* 1992;87:1233.
15. Szeasi IJ, Morrison RT, Lyster DM. Technetium^{99}m-labeled red blood cell scanning to diagnose occult GI bleeding. *Can J Surg* 1985;28:512.
16. Teach SJ, Fleisher GR. Rectal bleeding in the pediatric emergency department. *Ann Emerg Med* 1994;32:1252.
17. Thompson EC, Brown MF, Bowen EC, et al. Causes of gastrointestinal hemorrhage in neonates and children. *South Med J* 1996;89:370.
18. Treem WR. Gastrointestinal bleeding in children. *Gastrointest Endosc Clin N Am* 1994;4:75.
19. Urashima N, Toyoda S, Nakano T, et al. BUN/creatinine ratio as an index of GI bleeding mass in children. *J Pediatr Gastroenterol Nutr* 1992;15:89.
20. Vinton NE. Gastrointestinal bleeding in infancy and childhood. *Gastroenterol Clin North Am* 1994; 23:93.

CHAPTER 250
Headache

Laurie Jeanne Burton and Harold K. Simon

Headaches, a common complaint among children presenting to the emergency department, are often associated with other systemic signs and symptoms that can help determine their etiology. Headaches can be acute or chronic, recurrent or of new onset, and often vary in how they progress or resolve. The child's description of the duration, specific location, and intensity is often difficult to elicit and makes classification and treatment a challenge for the physician in the emergency department.

While often a diagnostic and management problem for physicians, headaches in children are equally frustrating and concerning for families. Families confronted with a child who complains of headache are often concerned with severe, life-threatening possibilities such as meningitis or intracranial lesions. For this reason, many families bring their childre to an emergency center for evaluation. In addition, for those with chronic headaches, lack of symptomatic relief is a major precipitating factor in bringing a child for evaluation.

Even though most children with acute or chronic headaches do not have life-threatening etiologies or intracranial lesions, these must be of foremost concern for the emergency department physician and must be ruled out by a careful and detailed history and physical examination.[1,5,6] An in-depth knowledge of the mechanisms and presentations of the various forms of headaches is therefore paramount for the emergency department physician.

Most children presenting to the emergency department are found to have headaches related to minor febrile illnesses, sinusitis, stress, or migraines. Serious neurologic conditions are found in approximately 7% of cases, many of these being viral meningitis.[1] Even so, one cannot be lulled into thinking that all children with the complaint of headache have relatively benign, non–life-threatening concerns.

CLINICAL PRESENTATION AND DIFFERENTIAL DIAGNOSIS

Headache is often a chief complaint, but it is more often part of a series of concerns. The complaint can be acute or chronic, intermittent or persistent, localized or focal, and mild to extremely intense. The severity of the presentation is related to the general appearance of the child, historic and physical findings, as well as associated signs and symptoms. Most commonly, the concern of headache is associated with viral or self-limited illnesses. Emotional problems and new types of stress (school or home) should be identified.

Certain historic and physical findings raise the suspicion for significant medical conditions. These include historic findings of sudden onset of headache, visual disturbances, weight loss, morning vomiting, neck pain, significant changes in behavior, and persistent and unremitting headache. Physical findings on presentation that would point toward more worrisome conditions include ill appearance of the child, change in mental status, focality on neurologic examination, papilledema, retinal hemorrhages, cranial bruits, nuchal rigidity, fever with petechiae or purpura, café-au-lait spots, hypertension, or signs of nonaccidental trauma.[5]

The two most commonly seen primary headache disorders in the pediatric population are migraine (vascular) and tension (functional) headaches. It may be difficult to distinguish the two types in some pediatric patients, but it is important to do so, because the treatments are somewhat different. Children with migraine headaches usually have a positive family history. Migraines are more commonly unilateral but may present as bilateral throbbing or pulsatile pain located in the regions of the eye, forehead, and temple. The headache may last anywhere from hours to days. It is often associated with nausea and vomiting, and it may be preceded by an aura.

Light, noise, and movement usually aggravate the pain. Motion sickness is prominent in about 45% of children with migraine headaches. Tension headaches, on the other hand, are usually bandlike and nonpulsatile in quality; lack the nausea, vomiting, photophobia, and phonophobia components; and do not have an aura.[3] Environmental triggers, anxiety, and depression are often associated with tension headaches.

The differential diagnosis of pediatric headache is outlined in Fig. 250.1.

EMERGENCY DEPARTMENT EVALUATION

A complete history often points the clinician toward the correct diagnosis and helps identify concerns for an underlying serious neurologic condition, including central nervous system (CNS) infection or structural pathology. All patients seen in the emergency department with a complaint of headache must have a complete set of vital signs, including measurement of temperature and blood pressure. A complete physical examination is useful diagnostically, and there are several highlights to mention.

The best assessment of CNS "well-being," or perfusion and oxygenation, is the level of consciousness. In the HEENT examination, any signs of trauma, minor infections such as pharyngitis, otitis media, or sinus tenderness could be diagnostic. Given that the frontal sinuses become pneumatized between the ages of 6 to 10 years, there is potential for frontal sinus infection in children aged 6 and older. The patient with frontal sinusitis may have tenderness in the forehead above the inner canthus of the eye. The teeth and gums should be checked carefully for signs of dental caries or abscesses.

Auscultation for a cranial bruit, a very rare finding, can be attempted. The neck should be examined carefully for signs of meningismus, especially for Brudzinski's and Kernig's signs. In the infant, the fontanelle should be checked for bulging, indicative of increased intracranial pressure from such causes as CNS infection or structural pathology. Funduscopy should be attempted on every patient with headache. Although papilledema may not be present early in the patient with increased intracranial pressure, the presence of venous pulsations would effectively rule it out. Retinal hemorrhages are indicative of child abuse until proven otherwise. Performing a complete neurologic examination is fundamental in the evaluation of patients with headache.

Laboratory evaluation is clinically guided and may include a rapid streptococcal throat screen or culture, sinus radiographs, lumbar puncture, toxicology assays in patients with altered consciousness or carbon monoxide exposure, and pregnancy testing. Radiographic evidence of sinusitis includes air–fluid levels, mucosal thickening of greater than 4 to 5 mm, or complete opacification. Indications for a lumbar puncture include any patient with fever and meningismus, bulging fontanelle, or suspicion of subarachnoid hemorrhage.

In the child who has abnormal neurologic findings, controversy exists over whether to perform a lumbar puncture prior to or after a computed tomography (CT) scan. A CT scan confirms there are no signs of increased intracranial pressure that could precipitate herniation. If a lumbar puncture is undertaken prior to CT scan, the risks can best be minimized with the use of a small-bore needle. Obtaining an opening pressure is critical if there is suspicion of intracranial hypertension.

Indications for a CT scan of the head include abnormal neurologic findings without a clear etiology. More specific indications include recurrent morning headaches, persistent emesis without clear etiology, paroxysmal onset of excruciating headache, lethargy, papilledema, retinal hemorrhages, or head trauma with severe headache. The clinician should have a low threshold for obtaining a head CT scan in the following types of pediatric patients: the infant with persistent irritability of unclear etiology, the child under 5 years of age with severe headache, the sickle cell or bleeding diathesis patient with headache, and the ventriculoperitoneal (VP) shunt patient with headache. For the patient with a VP shunt and headache, a shunt series should also be obtained to ensure that there is no shunt disconnection or migration. Lastly, the pediatric patient 6 years of age or older with frontal sinus tenderness and severe persistent headache could have contiguous CNS spread from the sinuses best diagnosed by CT.

In the patient with a migraine headache associated with neurologic deficits, or a "complicated migraine," CNS imaging is recommended. The preferred imaging test, if available, is a magnetic resonance imaging with angiogram. Otherwise, a head CT, with and without contrast, will suffice.

EMERGENCY DEPARTMENT MANAGEMENT

Treatment should be based on the presumptive diagnosis. Most tension headaches or headaches due to minor illnesses can be treated successfully in the pediatric population simply with analgesics such as acetaminophen or ibuprofen (in patients over 6 months of age). Migraines deserve special mention. Currently, there are no specific practice guidelines for migraine headaches in the pediatric population. Several classes of drugs are used to treat the acute migraine, including various analgesics, vasoconstrictors, serotonin agonists, and antiemetic sedatives. If the patient suffers from chronic migraines, the best approach might be to ask what medications have successfully aborted attacks in the past. Milder migraine pain often responds to acetaminophen; ibuprofen; a dark, quiet room; and rest. More moderate pain often responds to intravenous ketorolac 1 mg/kg (maximum, 60 mg).

Management of a child over 12 years of age is similar to that of an adult, and a serotonin agonist such as sumatriptan can be given to the nonpregnant patient intranasally or orally at a dose of 25 mg.[2,3] When using these agents, it is important to make a correct diagnosis of migraine, because the serotonin agonists do not work in the patient with tension or other types of headache. Care should be taken not to mix the serotonin agonists with the ergotamines, because side effects can be potentiated. A frequently used ergotamine in the migraine patient aged 12 years and older is dihydroergotamine (DHE) at a dose of 0.5 mg/kg intravenously. For severe pain, opioids such as morphine can be used, as long as serious etiologies of the headache have been carefully excluded. Regarding the younger child, analgesics such as acetaminophen and ibuprofen are first-line therapy. Anecdotally, sumatriptan is effective even in children as young as 6 years of age.[4] In younger children with more severe migraine pain, inducing sleep is a common therapeutic approach. Antiemetics–sedatives are employed for this purpose, such as Phenergan 0.25 to 0.5 mg/kg per dose PO, PR, intramuscularly or intravenously.

DISPOSITION

There are several scenarios involving the pediatric patient with headache wherein consultation is indicated. Neurosurgical consultation should be sought for any patient with CNS hemorrhage or midline shift. If the etiology of the bleed is from trauma, and no neurosurgical support is available at the site of care, stabilization and transfer should be expedited. Consultation with a neurologist should be considered for a patient with focal neurologic findings or unexplained altered mental status, as well as for patients with papilledema, severe migraine unresponsive to medical management, and a head CT showing a mass lesion that is not felt to be a CNS bleed.

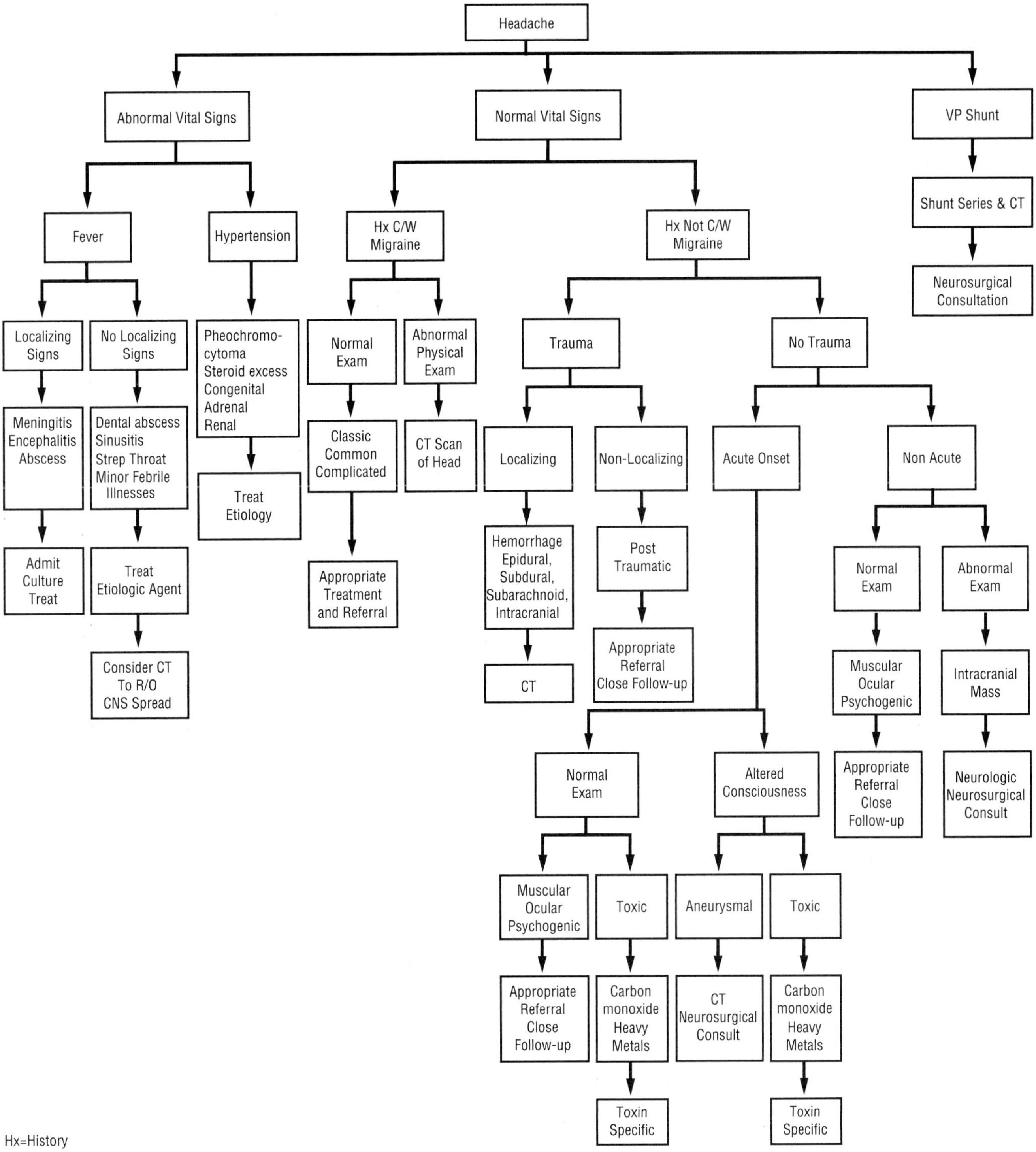

Figure 250.1. Differential diagnosis of headache in the pediatric patient.

Complicated migraines also warrant consultation with a neurologist. Such migraines, by definition, are associated with abnormal neurologic findings. Examples include migraine with hemiplegia, ataxia, transient blindness or visual field defect, acute confusional state, Alice-in-Wonderland syndrome (visual hallucinations wherein objects appear distorted in size), and olfactory or gustatory hallucinations.[5] Toxicology consultation with the local poison center should be considered in high-risk populations, such as the adolescent with altered mental status.

Indications for hospital admission include pain control that cannot be maintained in an outpatient setting, altered mental status or focal neurologic findings, suspected increased intracranial pressure, possible bacterial meningitis or encephalitis, severe headache after head trauma, complicated frontal sinusitis, and any CNS pathology.

Patients discharged from the emergency department should be instructed to seek medical attention if the headache worsens, changes, or persists for more than 2 to 3 days. They should also be encouraged to see their primary care provider to ensure proper follow-up and to avoid delays in diagnosis of inapparent or undeclared structural lesions.

COMMON PITFALLS

- All children with headache should have a screening blood pressure. The normal value for the systolic blood pressure in children can be approximated by the formula 2 × patient's age (in years) + 90 mm Hg. Diastolic blood pressure is approximately two-thirds of that value.
- In the setting of head trauma, do not forget about the possibility of occult neck injury.
- Always perform an opening pressure on the patient with headache who is undergoing a lumbar puncture. Many pediatric lumbar puncture kits do not come with manometers. One should be secured in advance, ideally before the first drop of cerebrospinal fluid is obtained.
- Have a low threshold for obtaining a head CT in children with frontal sinusitis and severe, persistent headache. Frontal sinusitis spreading to CNS involvement is not uncommon, particularly in the adolescent population.
- Always palpate the anterior fontanelle in infants under 1 year of age. It may be "full," especially if the infant is crying, but it should not bulge over the dimensions of the scalp. Life-threatening causes of a bulging fontanelle include not only CNS infection, but also CNS hemorrhage or edema, possibly from abuse.
- In the ambulatory child, the presence of up-going toes is indicative of CNS pathology, whereas the preambulatory child has a Babinski reflex normally.
- Subtle signs of altered mental status can be easy to miss in the "sleepy" patient presenting to the emergency department during the overnight hours. In this scenario, one should have a lower threshold to obtain ancillary testing such as head CT and toxicology screening.
- Meningismus can be a sign not only of CNS infection, but also of occult cervical spine injury or subarachnoid hemorrhage, the latter seen in the pediatric population almost exclusively in the perinatal period.
- CT scanning of the head without contrast more than 7 days posttrauma may miss an intracranial bleed, because the breakdown of blood often causes it to be isodense with surrounding tissue. The use of contrast may be warranted.

ACKNOWLEDGMENT

The authors gratefully acknowledge the chapter authors of the previous edition, Raymond Gyarmathy and Khal Aboudan.

References

1. Burton L, Quinn B, Pratt-Chaney J, et al. Headache etiology in the pediatric emergency department. *Pediatr Emerg Care* 1997;13:1–4.
2. Diener HC, Kaube H, Limmroth V. A practical guide to the management and prevention of migraine. *Drugs* 1998;56(5):811–824.
3. Lanzi G, et al. Guidelines and recommendations for the treatment of migraine in paediatric and adolescent patients. *Funct Neurol* 1996;11(5):269–275.
4. MacDonald JT. Treatment of juvenile migraine with subcutaneous sumatriptan. *Headache* 1994;34:581–582.
5. Molofsky WJ. Headaches in children. *Pediatr Ann* 1998;27:614–621.
6. Rosenberg NW, Cruz NM, Schor J, et al. The emergency department headaches conundrum. *Pediatr Emerg Care* 1997;13:437–440.

CHAPTER 251
Heart Murmurs

Edward J. Bayne

Heart murmurs are heard frequently in children, particularly in toddlers and school-age children. The incidence of significant congenital heart disease is about 1% (eight per 1,000 live births), but with careful auscultation, heart murmurs can be found in an estimated 40% to 60% of children. Most of these sounds are "normal," "functional," or "innocent," and do not require extensive evaluation, consultation, or diagnostic testing.[5–8] As Fyler and Nadas[4] wrote, "The most cost-effective tool for cardiac diagnosis is the stethoscope."

Murmurs arise from the heart and circulatory system for various reasons. Pathologic murmurs may arise because of valvular stenosis or insufficiency or because of an abnormal communication between chambers or vessels (e.g., ventricular septal defect). The high incidence of normal murmurs in infants and children can be explained by several factors, including

- The relatively thin chest wall in many children, and close proximity between the heart and the stethoscope
- Vigorous circulation through relatively small vessels[9]
- Conditions under which the child is examined, such as anxiety or fever, both of which increase the intensity of sound

In recent years, echocardiography and Doppler echocardiography have been used to better define the origins of pathologic murmurs and normal murmurs.[9]

CLINICAL PRESENTATION

Cardiac murmurs can be heard in infants and children at any age. Most cases of symptomatic congenital heart disease manifest before 6 months of age. The infant with a large ventricular septal defect with left-to-right shunt and symptoms and signs of congestive heart failure typically presents at 4 to 8 weeks of age with a loud, long, and harsh systolic murmur at the lower left sternal border, usually with an associated diastolic murmur or gallop and hyperdynamic circulation. The infant with tetralogy of Fallot (ventricular septal defect plus right ventricular or pulmonary artery obstruction) presents with a loud, harsh systolic murmur heard over the precordium and over the anterior and posterior chest. Such an infant shows signs of cyanosis and tachypnea but not of congestive heart failure.

The emergency physician may be the first person to hear a murmur in an older infant or child. High fever and anxiety increase the chances of hearing a cardiac murmur, and, in the absence of symptoms or signs of cardiorespiratory distress, it is unlikely that such a murmur is associated with significant pathology. When children with recognized congenital cardiac pathology are examined in the emergency or acute care setting, factors increasing cardiac output (such as fever) will increase the intensity of heart murmurs, and that increased intensity of sound may not necessarily correlate with worsening condition. Hearing a heart murmur in a child presenting with chest pain should not automatically implicate a cardiac etiology for the source of the pain.

Fever in the child with known congenital heart disease may alert the examiner to the possibility of infectious endocarditis. In such patients, a new or different murmur (e.g., appearance of the high-pitched diastolic murmur of aortic insufficiency in a patient with known aortic stenosis) makes the diagnosis of endocarditis more likely.

DIFFERENTIAL DIAGNOSIS

Table 251.1 lists five common innocent murmurs, along with their differential characteristics.[1] The second heart sound should split normally with inspiration, although appreciation of normal versus abnormal splitting takes considerable practice. Using the commonly accepted scale of I to VI, innocent murmurs are almost never greater than grade III/VI in intensity, even under conditions of fever. Loud murmurs, especially if associated with high-frequency thrills felt over the chest wall, should raise the index of suspicion for a significant cardiac lesion.

Diastolic murmurs (with the exception of the venous hum) are more likely to be pathologic. Except for "physiologic" peripheral pulmonary artery stenosis in young infants, it is unusual to hear normal or innocent murmurs radiating to the back. Significant findings, such as failure to thrive, respiratory distress, or cyanosis, make cardiovascular pathology more likely.

EMERGENCY DEPARTMENT MANAGEMENT

Figure 251.1 presents a management scheme for cardiac murmurs. Patients presenting with cardiorespiratory distress require prompt stabilization. Once symptomatic measures have been instituted to relieve respiratory distress or cyanosis, evaluation proceeds with a chest x-ray and electrocardiogram, and consultation is sought.

If the examiner discovers a new murmur in an otherwise asymptomatic child, further diagnostic evaluation at the time of the emergency visit is generally inappropriate, and, in most cases, the patient and family can be reassured.[10]

The source of fever should be sought for the child with known structural congenital heart disease. If a definite source of fever is identified and the patient is well compensated, he or she is managed like any other patient. If no definite source of fever is identified, blood cultures are obtained, along with other diagnostic studies (e.g., a complete blood count and differential white blood cell count), before starting antibiotics. Close follow-up should be arranged.[2,3]

TABLE 251.1. "Normal" Murmurs in Infants and Children

Murmur	Characteristics
Still's	Vibratory, musical quality at LLSB to apex: louder in supine position; disappears with Valsalva
Pulmonary flow	Raspy quality at ULSB; normal S_2; not heard in back
Venous hum	Loudest in seated position; disappears when supine; continuous (systolic-diastolic)
Carotid bruits	Short ejection murmurs over one or both clavicles to carotids
"Physiologic" PPS	Short ejection murmur with quality of breath sounds; heard in axillae and back; age <6 months

LLSB, lower left sternal border; PPS, peripheral pulmonic stenosis; S_2, second heart sound; ULSB, upper left sternal border.

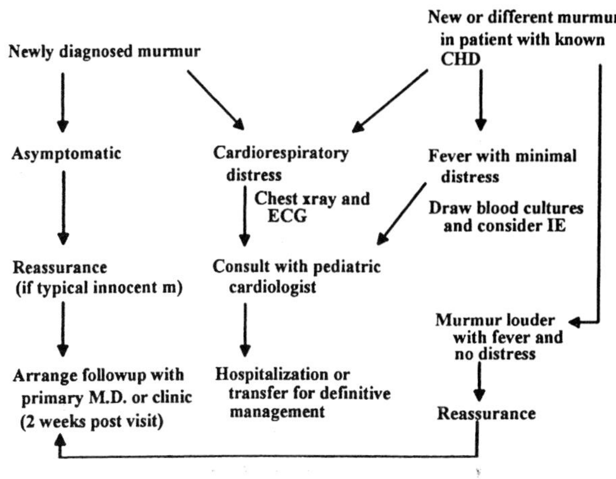

Figure 251.1. Scheme for the emergency department evaluation and management of cardiac murmurs in infants and children. CHD, congenital heart disease; ECG, electrocardiogram; IE, infective endocarditis; m, murmur.

DISPOSITION

Emergent consultation is sought for the infant with murmur and cardiorespiratory distress or cyanosis. Young infants with cardiorespiratory distress or cyanosis and murmur generally require hospitalization in a tertiary center with full pediatric cardiovascular services. Prompt communication with specialists at the referral center should include instructions for appropriate stabilization and transport.

For the asymptomatic child with a newly discovered murmur, follow-up with the primary physician or clinic should be arranged. A primary referral to the pediatric cardiology subspecialist is usually not indicated, because, with the resolution of fever, many loud murmurs are considerably less impressive on reexamination. Likewise, it is usually better to delay more involved diagnostic studies, such as echocardiography, until the child can be reexamined at a later time.

COMMON PITFALLS

- Heart murmurs are more commonly identified in infants and children than in adults. The presence of a murmur in an asymptomatic child does not usually imply significant pathology. Other symptoms, such as fever, can greatly exaggerate the intensity of a cardiac murmur.
- Most infants with significant structural congenital heart disease will present with a heart murmur. However, the absence of a murmur in an infant with cardiorespiratory distress or cyanosis should not rule out cardiovascular pathology. Some of the sickest infants with advanced congestive failure or with cyanosis may not present with murmurs.
- Increased intensity of a murmur in a child with known congenital heart disease and fever does not necessarily imply worsening condition.
- Chest pain is a common presenting complaint in the emergency department. Cardiac murmurs are also common findings, and the presence of a murmur in a child with chest pain does not necessarily imply a cardiac etiology.
- On palpation of the chest, transmitted bronchial congestion is often misinterpreted as a cardiac thrill, particularly in infants. A thrill is a well-localized, high-frequency vibration or buzz.

References

1. Bayne EJ. Etiology, diagnosis, and management of congenital cardiac disorders. *Compr Ther* 1988;14(8):31.
2. Brook MM. Pediatric bacterial endocarditis. Treatment and prophylaxis. *Pediatr Clin North Am* 1999;46:275.
3. Dajani AS, Taubert KA, Wilson W, et al. Prevention of bacterial endocarditis. Recommendations by the American Heart Association. *JAMA* 1997;277:1794.
4. Fyler DC, Nadas AS. History, physical examination, and laboratory tests. In: Fyler DC, ed. *Nadas' pediatric cardiology*. Philadelphia: Hanley & Belfus, 1992:101.
5. McCrindle BW, Shaffer KM, Kan JS, et al. Cardinal clinical signs in the differentiation of heart murmurs in children. *Arch Pediatr Adolesc Med* 1996;150:169.
6. Pelech AN. Evaluation of the pediatric patient with a cardiac murmur. *Pediatr Clin North Am* 1999;46:167.
7. Rajakumar K, Weisse M, Rosas A, et al. Comparative study of clinical evaluation of heart murmurs by general pediatricians and pediatric cardiologists. *Clin Pediatr (Phila)* 1999;38:511.
8. Rosenthal A. How to distinguish between innocent and pathologic murmurs in childhood. *Pediatr Clin North Am* 1984;31:1229.
9. Schwartz ML, Goldberg SJ, Wilson N, et al. Relation of Still's murmur, small aortic diameter and high aortic velocity. *Am J Cardiol* 1986;57:1344.
10. Swenson JM, Fischer DR, Miller SA, et al. Are chest radiographs and electrocardiograms still valuable in evaluating new pediatric patients with heart murmurs or chest pain? *Pediatrics* 1997;99:1.

CHAPTER 252
Hematuria

Lina Abujamra and Madeline Matar Joseph

Hematuria is the presence of blood in the urine, which usually alarms the patient, the parents, and the physician. It can be macroscopic (visible to the naked eye) or microscopic. Microscopic hematuria represents one of the most frequently encountered genitourinary abnormalities in children, occurring in 0.5% to 6.0% of school-age children undergoing routine screening.[10] Currently, the American Academy of Pediatrics recommends performance of a screening urinalysis at school entry (ages 4 to 5 years) and one time during adolescence. The prevalence of hematuria is 0.5% for boys and 1.0% for girls, with an annual new case incidence of 0.4% for both sexes. In the absence of gross hematuria, the primary tool for hematuria screening is a urine dipstick. Greater than 1+ blood is considered positive. The dipsticks used for detection of blood in the urine are very sensitive in detecting red blood cells (RBCs) as well as minute amounts of free hemoglobin and myoglobin. All positive dipstick screens should be confirmed by a microscopic examination of the urine to confirm the presence of RBCs and exclude false-positive and -negative dipstick results. Causes of false-positive dipstick reactions include myoglobinuria (rhabdomyolysis); hemoglobinuria (seen in conditions causing hemolysis); oxidizing contaminants, such as bacterial peroxidases from a urinary tract infection (UTI); delay in reading the dipstick; and interfering compounds, such as beets or aniline dyes. A false-negative dipstick result can occur in urine with high specific gravity and in urine containing large amounts of a reducing agent, such as ascorbic acid.

The definition of *hematuria* is somewhat arbitrary. The presence of five to ten erythrocytes by high power field (HPF) in a centrifuged urine is considered significant by a number of authors.[11] Hematuria can originate from any part of the urinary tract. Localizing the source of the bleeding to the kidney or the lower urinary tract can facilitate the workup and assist the emergency physician in developing the most efficient diagnostic plan. A good approach is to classify the origin of hematuria anatomically from the glomeruli, renal tubules–interstitium, or urinary tract. In children, the cause is more often glomerular in origin. Glomerulonephritis is usually accompanied by proteinuria and RBC casts in the urine. This etiology is discussed elsewhere in this text. The nonglomerular causes of hematuria can be further subdivided into renal parenchymal disease and extrarenal disease (Table 252.1).[11]

CLINICAL PRESENTATION

Once the presence of hematuria is confirmed by microscopic urinalysis, further information regarding the presentation will help guide the investigation. Children with glomerular bleeding will present with cola-colored urine, red cell casts (pathognomonic), renal insufficiency, and proteinuria, whereas lower tract bleeding colors the urine red or pink. Passing blood clots in the urine usually points to the bladder or urethra as the source of bleeding.[11] A recent upper respiratory tract infection is often seen with immunoglobulin-A (IgA) nephropathy (Berger disease). Poststreptococcal glomerulonephritis is generally preceded by a sore throat or impetiginous lesion by 7 to 21 days. Dysuria, frequency, or abdominal pain suggests a UTI.

A history of recent trauma, strenuous exercise, menstruation, or bladder catherization may account for transient hematuria and exclude the need for further workup. An adolescent's history should include certain habits, such as masturbation, excessive bicycle riding, or urethral foreign-body insertions. A recent or earlier history of renal colic or passage of a stone in the urine, as well as a family history of hypercalciuria and renal stones, should be elicited, because hypercalciuria is one of the most common causes of hematuria in children.

Certain medical conditions are commonly associated with hematuria. Children with hemoglobinopathies (sickle cell trait) and coagulopathies should be carefully evaluated. The use of drugs such as furosemide for congenital heart disease can lead to hypercalciuria and, subsequently, hematuria. Antibiotics and over-the-counter medications may cause interstitial nephritis. Chemotherapy and radiation for malignancies can explain isolated hematuria in children. In the neonatal period, hematuria can be caused by thrombosis of the renal vein or artery after use of umbilical catheters. A history of tuberculosis exposure is important to identify children with genitourinary tuberculosis, a rare but reported cause of hematuria.[3]

A family history can be extremely critical in elucidating the cause of hematuria in the presenting child. Alport syndrome is frequently seen in family members with hearing deficits and renal failure. Other diseases that carry a genetic origin include systemic lupus erythematosus (SLE), sickle cell anemia, hemophilia, and other coagulation factor deficiencies. Nephrolithiasis and IgA nephropathy also have a familial association. The thin basement membrane of the glomerulus is a common cause of benign familial hematuria in children. Family members may not be aware that they have microscopic hematuria and should be screened with a microscopic urinalysis.

The physical examination of the patient with hematuria is not specific, but several elements deserve attention. An accurate blood pressure is essential, because the presence of elevated blood pressure should alert the emergency physician to the possibility of a more severe underlying condition. The height and weight of the child should be plotted carefully to detect failure to thrive associated with long-standing acidosis or chronic renal insufficiency. A funduscopic examination of the retina, looking for evidence of long-standing hypertension or lenticonus as seen

TABLE 252.1. Causes of Hematuria

GLOMERULAR	NONGLOMERULAR
Primary Glomerulonephritis	**Renal Parenchymal**
Poststreptococcal glomerulonephritis	Anatomic: hydronephrosis
IgA nephropathy (Berger disease)	Ureteropelvic junction obstruction
Membranoproliferative glomerulonephritis	Polycystic kidney disease
Focal glomerulosclerosis	**Vascular Malformation**
Secondary Glomerulonephritis	Renal vein thrombosis
Systemic lupus erythematosus	Arteriovenous fistula
Henoch-Schönlein purpura	Sickle cell disease
Hemolytic–uremic syndrome	**Metabolic**
Familial	Hypercalciuria
Alport syndrome	Hyperuricosuria
Thin basement membrane disease	**Infectious**
	Urinary tract infection, pyelonephritis
	Tuberculosis
	Foreign Body to Urethra or Bladder
EXTRARENAL	
Tumors: Wilms', tuberous sclerosis	
Other	
Drugs and toxins	
Trauma and exercise	
Coagulopathy	
Dehydration	
Other: menstruation, masturbation, fever	

in Alport syndrome, should be performed. Periorbital edema is frequently the first site of edema in children. The chest should be examined for signs of fluid overload. Costovertebral angle tenderness may indicate a UTI. Recent trauma can be detected by findings of flank bruises and pain. Examining the abdomen for masses is critical for the identification of malignancies (Wilms' tumor), polycystic kidneys or hydronephrosis. Ascites suggests nephrosis. The examination of the skin can give evidence of pallor or rashes. This may be significant in diseases such as hemoglobinopathies, leukemia, HSP (Henoch-Schönlein purpura; petechial or purpuric lesions on the lower extremities), and SLE (malar rash). The genital examination should be included to identify abuse or trauma, discharge, and meatal stenosis, all of which can cause hematuria.

DIFFERENTIAL DIAGNOSIS

The causes of hematuria are numerous. A careful history and physical examination are essential in guiding the investigation for the correct etiology. It is important to first determine the site of bleeding in the presenting child. In infants, blood on the diaper can originate from the vagina or rectum and be confused with hematuria. In the menstruating girl, vaginal bleeding can be confused with urinary blood (obtain a catheterized urine specimen). The "red diaper syndrome" in infants has two causes: One is a group of healthy infants whose soiled diapers develop a red color after 24 to 36 hours, which is attributed to *Serratia marcescens;* the second is due to urate crystals. The former is rarely seen, due to the popularity of disposable diapers.

The differential diagnosis for childhood hematuria can be remembered by using the alphabetic sequence A through I[8]:

*A*natomy/vascular (renal cysts, arteriovenous malformations, obstruction with hydronephrosis)
*B*oulders (renal stones, hypercalciuria and hyperuricosuria)
*C*ancer (Wilms' tumor or adenocarcinoma and infiltration of the kidney by leukemia or solid tumors)
*D*rugs (over-the-counter or illicit drugs, methicillin, cyclophosphamide, anticoagulants)
*E*xercise
*F*oreign body, familial (Alport's) or factitious
*G*lomerulonephritis
*H*ematology (hemoglobinopathy, coagulopathy)
*I*nfection (cystitis caused by adenovirus, tuberculosis, schistosomiasis in patients with recent travel to the Middle East or Africa)

EMERGENCY DEPARTMENT EVALUATION

The diagnosis of hematuria requires an organized and systematic approach. Figure 252.1 suggests an approach to emergency department evaluation. If the history and physical examination fail to disclose the diagnosis of hematuria, a stepwise laboratory evaluation is necessary. If the initial urine dipstick tests positive for blood, two tests are absolutely required: a test for proteinuria and a microscopic examination of the urine for RBCs and RBC casts. Proteinuria should not exceed 2+ if the only source of protein is from the blood. If the child has 2+ protein, or more than 500 mg per 24 hours, both in the supine and standing positions, the investigation is directed toward glomerulonephritis and nephrotic syndrome. This evaluation should include a complete blood count (hemolytic–uremic syndrome), throat culture, streptozyme panel, and serum C3 concentration (acute poststreptococcal glomerulonephritis), and serum creatinine and potassium concentrations (looking for renal insufficiency). The same is true if RBC casts are noted on microscopic urinalysis. RBC morphology by phase contrast microscopy can be helpful in localization of hematuria. Dysmorphic cells indicate glomerular bleeding. However, this is thought to be a costly test, offering little additional information to the evaluation of microscopic hematuria in children.[10] A urine culture should be sent because a third of UTIs are associated with hematuria. Also, UTIs are the most common cause of macroscopic hematuria.[11] The urine culture is especially important in the child with white blood cells on microscopic urinalysis. Urinalysis testing in family members may be needed, in some cases, to identify familial causes of hematuria.

Another notable cause of hematuria is hypercalciuria, seen in 28% to 35% of children referred for evaluation of hematuria. This condition precedes overt urolithiasis by 1 to 6 years. A spot urine calcium–creatinine (Ca/Cr) ratio can easily rule out hypercalciuria as an etiology (normal is less than 0.21). Another method to identify hypercalciuria is by measuring a urinary calcium excretion of greater than 4 mg/kg/d. The normal values for Ca/Cr are age related and are much higher in infants than in older children and adults. A serum C3 level may be helpful in the advanced evaluation of hematuria. The complement C3 level is low in acute poststreptococcal glomerulonephritis, membranoproliferative glomerulonephritis, and SLE.

Patients who are at risk for sickle cell disease should be screened for it. Finally, the initial evaluation should include a renal ultrasound to rule out polycystic kidney disease, Wilms' tumor, renal stones, and obstruction as possible causes of hematuria. The renal ultrasound is capable of detecting gross lesions as effectively as can intravenous urography, and has replaced the latter as the diagnostic study of choice. There is rarely a reason for performing cystoscopy or retrograde urography. Children thought to need further diagnostic imaging should be referred to a nephrologist.

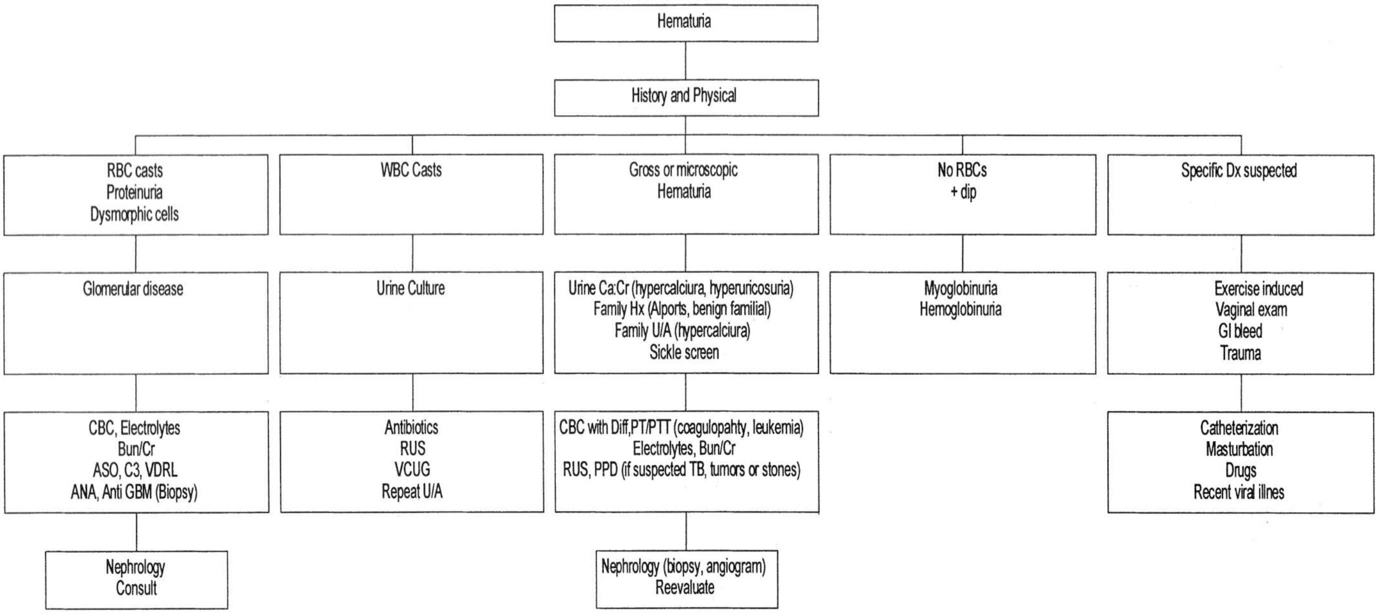

Figure 252.1. Approach to the diagnosis of hematuria in children.

The remainder of the evaluation should be based on the history and the results of the previous tests. This part of the workup should not be performed in the emergency department. Less common causes of hematuria in children are sought, such as coagulation problems and some anatomic and vascular abnormalities.[11] Most of the conditions requiring advanced workup (Table 252.2) should be referred to a pediatric nephrologist.

A renal biopsy is usually performed on children who have significant hematuria and proteinuria but who do not have a diagnosis of poststreptococcal glomerulonephritis. The pediatric nephrologist can perform a renal biopsy on those patients who have hematuria and significant proteinuria that do not have laboratory or clinical findings consistent with poststreptococcal glomerulonephritis. A renal biopsy should be considered only if treatable, progressive, or hereditary glomerular disease is suspected.

EMERGENCY DEPARTMENT MANAGEMENT

The patient with hematuria should be managed according to the etiology of the disease condition. Asymptomatic hematuria does not need acute management in the emergency department. An exception to this rule includes evaluation for UTIs. Younger infants and dehydrated or ill-appearing patients with UTI warrant hospitalization and intravenous antibiotics. A recent study recommended treating UTI in children aged 1 to 24 months with oral cefixime for 14 days.[6] Older patients can be treated with oral trimethoprim–sulfamethoxazole for 3 to 10 days.

Children with suspected hypercalciuria should increase water intake to attempt to decrease the concentration of calcium in the urine. A low-calcium diet and hydrochlorothiazide therapy have been shown to decrease urinary calcium excretion; a short course can result in the disappearance of microscopic hematuria. A child with a suspected renal calculus should have a urologic consultation in the emergency department.

When there are no indications for immediate medical intervention, the parents can be reassured that a life-threatening condition does not exist and that most cases of isolated hematuria do not require treatment.

DISPOSITION

Referral to a pediatric nephrologist should take place if the child has gross hematuria, a coexistent significant proteinuria, hypertension, abnormal kidney function tests, persistent hypocomplementemia, or findings suggesting a systemic disease; or if there is a family history of glomerulonephritis, nerve deafness, chronic renal failure, end-stage renal disease, or familial hema-

TABLE 252.2. Evaluation of the Child with Hematuria

INITIAL EVALUATION OF CHILD WITH HEMATURIA
History
Physical examination
Family history
Initial laboratory evaluation
Urinalysis with microscopy, protein measurement
Red blood cell morphology
Urine culture
Calcium–creatinine ratio
Sickle cell screen, if applicable
Complete blood count, creatinine and blood urea nitrogen levels
Urine of first-degree relatives
Renal ultrasound
ADVANCED EVALUATION OF CHILD WITH HEMATURIA
Complement level
Membranoproliferative glomerulonephritis
SLE, postinfectious glomerulonephritis
Antistreptolysin-O and anti-DNAase B
Acute poststreptococcal glomerulonephritis
Antinuclear antibody
SLE
Audiogram
Alport syndrome
Anti-glomerular basement membrane antibodies
Antineutrophil cytoplasmic antibodies
Active crescenteric glomerulonephritis
Tuberculosis testing
Renal biopsy

turia. If parental anxiety is high, referral to a pediatric nephrologist may help alleviate compounding fears and serve as additional reassurance to the family that dangerous and treatable conditions have been ruled out by the primary physician.

Rarely does a patient with hematuria need to be hospitalized. Patients with newly diagnosed renal disease should be admitted with pediatric nephrologist consultation. A toxic-appearing child with a UTI is admitted for intravenous antibiotics.

For the patient with persistent microscopic hematuria who does not have hypertension, proteinuria, or RBC casts, follow-up urinalysis should be performed every 2 to 4 months for 1 year. This should be done by the primary care or subspecialty physician. Blood pressure and a dipstick test for proteinuria should also be checked periodically. If proteinuria or gross hematuria develops during this follow-up period, the patient should be referred to a nephrologist.

It is important to remember that the most common causes of microscopic hematuria without casts or proteinuria are benign and untreatable. The prognosis for these children is very good. A poor prognosis is associated with proteinuria at presentation, persistent hematuria, and hypertension.

COMMON PITFALLS

- Failure to perform a urine dipstick and urinalysis to confirm the presence of blood in the "red urine" can lead to unnecessary performance of numerous laboratory tests.
- Failure to obtain relevant information in the history (recent pharyngitis, trauma, or a family history of renal stones) can make the determination of the cause of hematuria more cumbersome.
- Although most children with microscopic hematuria have an excellent prognosis, failure to detect proteinuria, hypertension, and the subtle signs of fluid overload can be detrimental to the prognosis of such patients.

References

1. Ahmed Z, Lee J. Asymptomatic urinary abnormalities. Med Clin North Am 1997;81(3):641–651.
2. Benbassat J, Gergawi M, et al. Variability in management of symptomless microhaematuria in schoolchildren. *Postgrad Med J* 1998;74:161–164.
3. Chattopadhyay A, Bhatnagar V, et al. Genitourinary tuberculosis in pediatric surgical practice. *J Pediatr Surg* 1997;32(9):1283–1286.
4. Feld LG, Waz WR, et al. Hematuria. *Pediatr Clin North Am* 1997; 44(5):1191–1209.
5. Fitzwater DS, Wyatt RJ. Hematuria. *Pediatr Rev* 1994;15(3):102–108.
6. Hoberman A, Wald ER, et al. Oral versus initial intravenous therapy for urinary tract infections in young febrile children. *Pediatrics* 1999;104(1):79–86.
7. Levy FL, Kemp RD, et al. Macroscopic hematuria secondary to hypercalciuria and hyperuricosuria. *Am J Kidney Dis* 1994;24(3):515–518.
8. Neiberger RE. The ABC's of evaluating children with hematuria. *Am Fam Physician* 1994;49(3):623–628.
9. Perrone HC, Stapleton FB, et al. Hematuria due to hyperuricosuria in children: 36-month follow-up. *Clin Nephrol* 1997;48(5):288–291.
10. Ward JF, Kaplan GW, et al. Refined microscopic urinalysis for red blood cell morphology in the evaluation of asymptomatic microscopic hematuria in pediatric population. *J Urol* 1998;160:1492–1495.
11. Yadin O. Hematuria in children. *Pediatr Ann* 1994;23(9):474–485.

CHAPTER 253
Intoxications

Jay L. Schauben and Dawn Ruskosky-Sollee

The 1997 annual report of the American Association of Poison Control Centers analyzed 2,192,088 human exposures reported to 66 centers.[14] As in the past, the victim's age was one of the major prognostic factors. Of the reported exposures, 52.5% occurred in children under age 6 years, in contrast to the 7.0% and 7.3% that occurred in children ages 6 to 12 years and 13 to 19 years, respectively. Eighty-six percent of the exposures were termed *accidental,* 86.2% involved exposure to a single substance, and the product was orally ingested in 74% of the cases. About 7.5% of the total exposures were suicide attempts. Symptoms related to the exposure developed in only 22.1% of the cases, and almost 74.9% were treated at the site of exposure (home). In short, most of these toxic exposures appear in children, and most of the patients do not develop symptoms.

Management of the poisoned or overdosed patient revolves around certain basic principles: initial stabilization, assessment of history, documentation of findings on physical examination and correlating these symptoms with known toxidromes, institution of techniques aimed at preventing further absorption, use of antidotal and supportive therapies, and modalities to enhance elimination. Age-related factors may warrant modification in some of these techniques. Also, recent changes in some of these procedures have been recommended in the literature and have left us with a seemingly more rational approach to management.

Errors in judgment may occur when the diagnostic, prognostic, and therapeutic management guidelines for adults are directly translated to childhood intoxications. The presence of age-dependent pharmacokinetic variations, the unpredictability and variability in handling of toxins, and differences in sensitivity to the effects of toxic exposures dictate a modified approach to the management of the poisoned child. For example, transit time through the gastrointestinal (GI) tract is shorter and much more variable in the infant, approaching adult values after about 2 to 3 years of age. The importance of this factor is evident, because it may affect the time course of an overdose, especially because GI exposure appears to be the most common route of poisoning in children.[11]

Decisions on the initiation of therapeutic maneuvers in children should be based on knowledge of the exposure (e.g., what, how, when, where, how much), the potential of the ingested substance(s) to cause toxicity, the prognostic factors relating to the toxin, the risk–benefit ratio when considering the use of invasive therapeutic and diagnostic maneuvers, and patient presentation.

The incidence and etiologic factors behind pediatric exposures differ from those of adult intoxications. History may be more accurate with accidental ingestions in children because they often occur under observation. This is usually not true of ingestions in adolescents and adults, wherein drug abuse, drug experimentation, and suicide come into play. The clinician should be suspicious when assessing the history, as it may be misleading, confusing, or unreliable. The specific product container in question should be produced, if possible. Toxic and nontoxic products may share the same phonetic name, product formulations may be changed over time by the manufacturer, and certain product lines have numerous varieties of the same product with small changes in their ingredients. Prescription bottles should be emptied and the contents counted, specifically identified, then compared with the label information. Patients sometimes use medication bottles to store different, and often multiple, types of medication.

Adult and adolescent suicide attempts often involve polydrug ingestions, and the history obtained is unreliable. In contrast, most accidental ingestions in children involve only a single substance. The accidental ingestion of a bad-tasting household product often results in only one swallow (5 mL) in the child, whereas the suicidal adolescent may ingest much larger quantities. Medications mistaken for candy by children, or those intentionally flavored for pediatric use, are often ingested in multiple quantities.

The following information is obtained to allow accurate assessment of whether the victim is in immediate danger, potential danger, or no danger at all:

- Source of the exposure
- Severity of the symptomatology present
- Nature of the toxin as assessed by the labeled ingredients; place and date purchased; name of the company or person who purchased, obtained, or used the product; and the color, odor, and intended use of the product
- Other medications or products available in the environment
- Time of exposure
- Approximate amount involved
- Actions taken before emergency department presentation
- Reliability of the informant
- Assessment of intent: accidental, therapeutic overdose, or suicide attempt

Accidental ingestions, whether toxic or nontoxic, may warrant investigation into the home situation if

- The ingestion occurs in a child over age 5 years. This usually signals a cry for help.
- More than one episode of "accidental" ingestion occurs. This may signal inadequate parental concern, inadequate poison prevention education, or, possibly, neglect.
- The "accidental" ingestion occurs in a child under 1 year of age. Infants this young often do not possess the physical or mental capabilities required to self-administer a toxin.

The importance of history and an assessment of toxin availability is crucial to the awareness of what type of poisoning, if any, has occurred. GI decontamination may be considered when a potentially toxic amount of a substance has been ingested within a specified period of time.

EMERGENCY DEPARTMENT EVALUATION

Stabilization

Stabilizing vital functions should always precede definitive poison management procedures. The airway is evaluated, as well as ventilatory function, heart rate and rhythm, temperature, and blood pressure, with adequate caution for the cervical spine. Trauma and overdose are not mutually exclusive. Any patient presenting with severe central nervous system (CNS) or respiratory depression is intubated with an endotracheal tube (cuffed in a patient over age 9 years to protect against aspiration). If the patient will not tolerate placement of the endotracheal tube, chances are that he or she does not need it.

If hypotension fails to improve after establishment of adequate ventilation and oxygenation, the patient is placed in the Trendelenburg position to aid venous return. A fluid challenge should be used and will improve the circulatory function if hypovolemia is the problem. If the child does not respond to adequate fluid challenges (20 mL/kg), more invasive critical care monitoring is considered (e.g., central venous pressure, pulmonary capillary wedge pressure measurements) to further guide fluid administration and prevent overload. Cautious use of fluid resuscitation may also be prudent in light of the many drugs and toxins that can alter the permeability of the alveolar capillary beds, increasing the risk for development of pulmonary edema and adult respiratory distress syndrome. Vasopressors or inotropic agents may be required if myocardial depression or vasodilatation is present. The appropriate choice of vasopressor or inotropic agent may depend on the mechanism behind the toxicologic derangement.

The comatose patient should receive the following, either during or soon after the vital functions are stabilized:

1. Oxygen
2. Rapid bedside glucose evaluation or, if unavailable, 0.5 g/kg glucose as 10% to 25% dextrose in water (after a blood specimen for glucose determination is obtained)
3. Naloxone 0.1 mg/kg (up to 2 mg in a child), every 3 to 5 minutes for two doses, unless partial response or high suspicion of opiate intoxication exists, when dosing may proceed up to a total of 10 mg. Given naloxone's short half-life, a naloxone infusion may be considered if adequate response is obtained with bolus dosing. The appropriate dose is calculated as two-thirds of the cumulative initial reversal dose given per hour. Nalmefene is a newer, longer-acting option for opiate antagonism. It may substitute for naloxone infusions using the adult dosing regimen of 0.5 mg/70 kg intravenously.
4. Thiamine (50 to 100 mg intramuscularly or intravenously) may be considered in adolescents and adults if the patient is malnourished or a chronic alcoholic.
5. Flumazenil, a specific benzodiazepine antagonist, can be safely utilized in the pediatric population as long as the signs and symptoms of cyclic antidepressant intoxication are absent. Caution should be exercised in children on benzodiazepines chronically, because a withdrawal reaction may be precipitated. The adult dosing regimen, often used in pediatric overdose, is 0.2 mg administered intravenously over 30 seconds. If no effect is seen within 30 seconds of administration, an additional 0.3 mg is administered; then 0.5 mg. This dose can be readministered until a total of 3 mg has been given. If a partial response has been obtained, dosing in 0.5-mg increments is continued until a total of 5 mg has been administered. Resedation is very common in overdose. Vital sign instability may require an infusion (1 to 5 mg/h) to maintain an adequate reversal.
6. Assessment (if warranted and guided by toxidrome recognition) of arterial blood gases, blood urea nitrogen, creatinine, liver enzyme tests, blood ammonia and electrolytes, blood culture, osmolality, toxicology screen, and an additional tube of blood held in reserve.

Physical Examination

Repeated examinations and clinical assessments, with continuous monitoring of vital signs, are mandatory, because the patient's condition may change with dramatic rapidity. Recognition of a specific toxic syndrome (toxidrome) may help to direct diagnostic, therapeutic, and analytic techniques. The neurologic survey, noting the degree and progression of altered mental status, is particularly important. In children, their behavior and interaction with parents and the examiner are noted. Pupil size, reactivity to bright and dim light, accommodation, shape, equality, presence of nystagmus, irregularities in ocular movements, and presence of funduscopic changes are also useful in recognizing a toxidrome. Abnormal motor system function and reflexes and the presence of focal neurologic findings are noted. One of the most important diagnostic considerations is the differentiation of a structural CNS disorder, which requires advanced radiologic evaluation (computed tomography scan) and neurosurgical consultation, from a toxic–metabolic or systemic disorder, which requires meticulous supportive and possibly antidotal therapy.

EMERGENCY DEPARTMENT MANAGEMENT

The first priorities are the management and maintenance of vital functions. Next comes an attempt to diagnose the intoxication, although the agent's identity may be unknown. Most ingestions in young children involve nontoxic products or those that cause only minor toxicity.[14] A common error is to treat all ingestions aggressively, even when such treatment is unnecessary.

Ocular and Dermal Exposures

Ocular exposures warrant immediate attention by irrigation with copious water or saline. Wrapping the child in a sheet or blanket, papoose-style, may help control the writhing infant. The parent or guardian may help calm the child and make him or her more amenable to treatment. Dermal exposure requires removal of clothes, followed by complete soap-and-water washing (including the hair, fingernails, and navel) in an attempt to limit further percutaneous absorption. Again, enlisting the parent's help is suggested and may limit the child's fear.

Caustic or Corrosive Exposures

In caustic or corrosive ingestions, dilution with milk or water is warranted. Contraindications include an inability to swallow and signs of upper airway obstruction, esophageal perforation, or shock. Administering more than 15 mL/kg in a child (to a maximum of 250 mL) may result in vomiting, an event to be avoided. Dilutional therapy as a general overdose management procedure has other drawbacks. Ingesting a large volume of water may enhance GI absorption of certain toxins by increasing the solubilization of the product.[7,8] The use of specific neutralization techniques with caustic or corrosive ingestions is controversial and requires further study. It was believed that neutralization created an exothermic reaction resulting in the release of thermal energy and gas formation, leading to distention. However, several recent studies in animals have questioned this belief.[12]

Gastrointestinal Decontamination

Ipecac

Syrup of ipecac contains two alkaloids that cause local stimulation in addition to central stimulation of the vomiting center in the brain. The administration of ipecac decreased dramatically over the 1990s (10.1 % of exposures in 1987 to 1.5 % in 1997).[14] After review of the available clinical studies, insufficient data were found to support or exclude the administration of ipecac to poisoned patients.[3] No evidence was found that demonstrates that this GI decontamination modality improves patient outcome.[3] Syrup of ipecac, in the health-care setting, has been found to delay the administration of the more effective decontamination method, activated charcoal, and should therefore be avoided in the emergency department.[3,11]

Syrup of ipecac may be used in the home setting if an asymptomatic patient has ingested a potentially harmful amount of a toxin, but it must be within 1 hour of the ingestion.[3] Because emesis carries its own dangers, the unnecessary and routine administration of ipecac should be avoided. The following are contraindications to the use of ipecac[3]:

1. Relative contraindications
   a. The ingestion of a high-viscosity petroleum distillate, a very low viscosity hydrocarbon, and certain other hydrocarbons in small quantities
   b. The ingestion of an agent likely to produce rapid depression of consciousness or to induce convulsions
   c. A child under 6 months of age, who may have immature protective airway reflexes
   d. The ingestion of a foreign body; emesis is usually ineffective in removing the object and increases the risk of creating or worsening airway obstruction.
2. Absolute contraindications
   a. The ingestion of a caustic or corrosive product
   b. A comatose or seizing patient
   c. The presence of hematemesis
   d. Lack of or depression of upper airway protective reflexes

Some clinicians argue that ipecac is safe to administer at home in children aged 6 months or older.[11] The appropriate dose should be based on the child's age: less than 1 year old, 5 to 10 mL; 1 to 12 years old, 15 mL; 12 years old to adult, 30 mL.[3] This dose of ipecac may be repeated once if the child does not vomit within 15 to 20 minutes. Water (120 mL in infants and small children, 240 mL in older children) should accompany the ipecac.[3] Expiration of the ipecac should not preclude its administration.

Although normal ipecac doses pose little threat of toxicity, ipecac has reportedly produced mild adverse effects, with the most common being protracted vomiting, diarrhea, and lethargy. Symptoms, if noted, should not be mistaken for part of a toxic syndrome.

Gastric Lavage

The use of gastric lavage as a decontamination method has decreased from 3.4% to 2.4% of exposures reported to the American Association of Poison Control Centers during the past 4 years.[14] Lavage is indicated if a patient has ingested a life-threatening amount and presents to the emergency department within 1 hour of the ingestion.[2] However, gastric lavage has not been shown to improve patient outcome and, in fact, may increase morbidity by increasing the chance of aspiration.[2,17] Complications can be minimized by respecting these contraindications[2]:

- Caustic or corrosive ingestions without previous assessment of esophageal damage
- Absence of protective upper airway reflexes without previous insertion of an endotracheal tube
- Ingestion of certain petroleum distillates or hydrocarbons

The best results are obtained from gastric lavage when the largest bore tube that can be reasonably and safely inserted is used. Although many argue that children cannot tolerate large orogastric tubes, others say that a 36F orogastric hose can be safely passed in children as young as 1 year of age. Most commonly, a 24F to 28F orogastric tube is utilized after lubrication. Once the tube is placed, aspiration of gastric contents is followed by positive identification of tube placement, which precedes instillation of any lavage fluid.

If the child is to be endotracheally intubated before lavage, a cuffed endotracheal tube should not be used in a child less than 9 years old for fear of tracheal damage. If a cuffed tube is used in the older child, it is deflated immediately after lavage.[7]

Without elective endotracheal intubation, the patient is placed in the left lateral decubitus position, with the head 15 to

20 cm lower than the hips (Trendelenburg position). This will help to prevent aspiration if vomiting does occur without physical airway protection.[15]

Although the standard lavage fluid in adults is either water or saline, children should be lavaged with normal saline.[15] The use of an alternative fluid composition in children may lead to hyponatremia or other severe electrolyte imbalances.[2] Although adults may tolerate up to 250 to 350 mL, only 10 to 15 mL/kg should be used in children.[2] If this volume is exceeded, the stomach contents may be forced through the pylorus into the intestine, or vomiting may result. Lavage is continued until there is a consistently clear fluid return. Activated charcoal is given after the lavage procedure is completed.

Concretions

The physician should remember that specific ingestants are known to cause gastric concretions (e.g., ferrous sulfate, meprobamate, glutethimide, and salicylates), as do large amounts of dry tablets. A concretion may require prolonged, forceful, whole bowel irrigation to dissolve, break up, or otherwise remove the bolus of material. This may be an indication for the use of multiple-dose activated charcoal in combination with whole bowel irrigation. As a last resort, endoscopic or surgical removal may be required. Clues to the presence of concretions include failure to respond to appropriate treatment, continued deterioration despite therapy, or measured blood concentrations that do not decrease with adequate GI decontamination.

Activated Charcoal

Despite previous practices, activated charcoal should no longer be administered to every overdose patient presenting to the emergency department.[4] With few exceptions, administration of activated charcoal should be considered in patients who ingest a potentially toxic amount of a substance less than 1 hour prior to their arrival in the emergency department.[4] Insufficient data are available to support or exclude the use of activated charcoal more than 1 hour postingestion.[4]

Activated charcoal, with its ultrasmall particle size and very large surface area, is known to adsorb a number of chemical agents. The standard-grade activated charcoals commonly used have a surface area of over 1,000 to 1,500 square meters per gram. Even though activated charcoal has been shown to produce a mean decrease in bioavailability of approximately 69% if given within 1 hour of the ingestion, it has not been proven to improve patient outcome.[4] Charcoal should not be given with ingestions involving a caustic or corrosive product because it does not effectively adsorb these compounds, may cause vomiting, and will most probably hinder any endoscopic attempts to evaluate the esophageal or gastric mucosa.

Activated charcoal cannot adsorb all known toxins. It has limited usefulness with boric acid, caustics, corrosives, cyanide, ethylene glycol, iron, iodides, lithium, and other elemental metal ingestions.[18] Certain pesticides and other poorly water-soluble compounds also may not be effectively captured by the charcoal complex. The alcohols may be adsorbed to a limited extent by charcoal, but this appears to have little clinical significance because the systemic absorption of the alcohols is so rapid.

The dose of standard-grade activated charcoal is usually 1 to 2 g/kg in children. The charcoal is given as a slurry in at least 100 mL of water solution, and is given orally or through a gastric tube.

Charcoal administration in children is more easily discussed than performed. Using a firm approach will make the child more likely to comply. The charcoal slurry is placed in an opaque container with a fitted lid to mask its color. The suspension is sipped through one or two straws, alternating with sips of a clear fluid such as water. If attempts to get the child to drink this antidote within 15 to 20 minutes have failed, a nasogastric tube is placed and the charcoal slurry administered through it.[4] Activated charcoal may be used in smaller and more frequent doses, making administration easier in the child by virtue of the absolute volume given per dose. In fact, this may be more efficacious in small children, because it is more likely that the slurry will be retained when smaller volumes are given.

The role of multiple doses of activated charcoal, given every 2 to 6 hours to enhance elimination, is not very clear, despite its common usage. Multiple-dose therapy appears useful in cases of long-acting or sustained-release agents, preparations resulting in concretions, and agents undergoing enterohepatic or enterogastric recirculation. Activated charcoal can produce a "gastric dialysis" in addition to serving as a stool marker, indicating that no further compound is available for absorption.[6,13] This dialysis concept has proven useful for agents administered both orally and parenterally, for such ingestions as phenobarbital, salicylate, theophylline, digoxin, cyclic antidepressants, phenytoin, and carbamazepine.[6,13] The efficacy of this procedure is reportedly due to the creation of a concentration gradient out of the systemic circulation, with the charcoal acting as an adsorbent sink. This enhances the rate of back-diffusion from the central compartment into the GI tract.

Nonetheless, multiple-dose charcoal should not be given indiscriminately without evaluating the risks, the clinical symptomatology, and its reported usefulness for a particular compound. Multiple doses of charcoal should not be given to a patient who has absent bowel sounds or any evidence of ileus.

For multiple dosing in children, give 0.5 to 1.0 g/kg of activated charcoal every 2 to 4 hours with water.

Cathartics

Cathartics are used to shorten the transit time of the toxin or toxin–charcoal mixture through the GI tract and prevent the formation of "charcoal briquets" in the GI tract when multiple-dose activated charcoal is administered. Despite their previously common use in the management of poisoning, there is no scientific or clinical proof to support the efficacy of cathartics when administered alone.[1,15] Likewise, there are no data to support the use of cathartics with single doses of activated charcoal, because constipation has not been seen after a single dose.[1] Adverse effects of cathartic administration, such as fluid loss and moderate-to-severe electrolyte imbalances, appear to be more common in children. Fleet's Phospho-Soda should never be used in children, due to the risk of severe electrolyte complications.

Sorbitol is used most commonly because it improves the palatability of charcoal and is a better cathartic than magnesium or sodium salts. The use of sorbitol in children is not without concern, because it may induce significant diarrhea and electrolyte imbalances.[9] For this reason, prepared charcoal–sorbitol mixtures should not be used, especially in multiple-dose therapy. Children should receive no more than a 35% concentration and must be monitored carefully for dehydration and electrolyte disturbances.[1] Sorbitol is not recommended for children under 1 year of age and should be used cautiously in those under 3 years of age.

Sorbitol can be given in doses of 1 to 2 g/kg of no greater than a 35% solution, once every 12 hours.[18] With multiple-dose regimens, standard commercially prepared charcoal–sorbitol slurries should not be used, because they lock the clinician into giving sorbitol every 2 to 4 hours, which is far too often. It is safer and more rational to stock the aqueous charcoal slurry and to add a specific dose of sorbitol when, and if, necessary.

Whole Bowel Irrigation

Although whole bowel irrigation has been shown to decrease

the bioavailability of ingested substances, it has not yet been shown to improve patient outcome.[5] Whole bowel irrigation may be considered for ingestions of iron, lithium, and other toxins not effectively bound by charcoal, as well as ingestion of massive quantities and sustained-release products, and ingestions of illicit drugs by body packers and stuffers.[5,20] This procedure may pose a significant risk of fluid and electrolyte imbalance in children unless a balanced solution (polyethylene glycol–electrolyte) is used.[20]

A nasogastric tube is placed and secured in the patient, who is seated on a commode. The room-temperature polyethylene glycol–electrolyte solution is given by gravity into the stomach at a rate of 25 mL/kg/h up to a maximum of 500 mL/h in toddlers and preschoolers.[20] Adolescents and adults will tolerate up to 2 L/h. If vomiting occurs, the rate should be slowed and then gradually increased back to full rate.[20] The end of the procedure comes with clear return from the rectum.

Whole bowel irrigation is contraindicated if an ileus, bowel obstruction or perforation, unprotected airway, or persistent vomiting is present.[5]

Enhancing Elimination

Other methods of enhancing the elimination of certain toxins, besides multiple doses of activated charcoal, include ion trapping to enhance the renal clearance of certain compounds and the use of extracorporeal methods of removal.

Alkalinizing the urine, by virtue of its ability to produce an ion-trapping effect, can significantly increase the elimination of phenobarbital, barbital, and salicylates. However, a volunteer study found that multiple-dose activated charcoal was superior to urinary alkalinization to enhance the elimination of phenobarbital.[10] Urinary alkalinization is accomplished by raising the urine pH to 7.5 to 8.0, without allowing the blood pH to go beyond 7.55. This goal is attained by giving intravenous sodium bicarbonate (1- to 2-mEq/kg bolus, followed by an infusion); this, in itself, requires close monitoring of the urinary and plasma pH. This procedure may also place the patient at risk for hypokalemia or hypocalcemia.

The use of forced diuresis, where fluid and possibly a diuretic is given to stimulate urine flow three to six times that of normal, has been abandoned due to the associated risks. The use of fluid administration to induce a high urine flow rate may result in cerebral edema, pulmonary edema, disturbances in acid–base and electrolyte balance, and drug-induced SIADH (e.g., barbiturates, opioids, salicylates, cyclic antidepressants, sulfonylureas, biguanides, carbamazepine), placing the patient at a higher risk for morbidity.[16] This is especially true in children, in which administration of large fluid loads and sodium bicarbonate presents a more pronounced problem than in adults. This problem is compounded when, by virtue of the specific toxicologic action, certain exposures actually produce cerebral or pulmonary edema or renal failure. Likewise, acid diuresis accomplished with the use of intravenous ammonium chloride has been abandoned in amphetamine, quinine, strychnine, and phencyclidine poisoning, because it may cause severe metabolic acidosis, precipitation of myoglobin in the renal tubules, and severe electrolyte shifts.[16]

Although fairly useful with certain adult poisonings, extracorporeal means of removing toxic substances may have limited utility in children and small infants, depending on the patient's age and the clinical characteristics of the exposure. These modalities are rarely first-line choices; they are reserved for severe, life-threatening poisonings that are amenable to dialysis or hemoperfusion. These measures are also useful if maintenance of appropriate acid–base balance becomes difficult or refractory, severe electrolyte imbalances arise, overhydration due to acute renal failure is evident, or the patient develops uremia and its related syndromes. Consultation with the nephrologist should be sought when

- Progressive deterioration occurs despite intensive supportive care
- Severe intoxication results in refractory hypoventilation, hypothermia, or hypotension
- Complications arise that depict catastrophic deterioration
- Impairment of normal drug excretory pathways is evident

Even though peritoneal dialysis is reportedly only one-twentieth as effective as hemodialysis, it is easier and less hazardous to perform. It is particularly useful in small children, whose blood vessel size and small blood volume make hemodialysis difficult.[16] Peritoneal dialysis has been successful in ingestions of barbiturate, bromide, phenytoin, ethanol, ethchlorvynol, ethylene glycol, inorganic mercury, isopropyl alcohol, lithium, methyprylon, quinidine, salicylate, and theophylline.[16] Peritoneal dialysis is contraindicated if the patient has had recent abdominal surgery or if there is evidence of an intraabdominal infection.

Exchange transfusions, primarily used in young infants and children, are effective with highly protein-bound drugs exhibiting a low volume of distribution. They have limited use in older children.

Antidotal Therapy

Table 253.1 summarizes the indications, dosages, and considerations for the use of specific antidotes.[19]

DISPOSITION

If adequate facilities are available, emergency department observation for 4 to 8 hours, depending on the toxic potential, is usually long enough to unmask most of the delayed-onset toxic reactions. Children under 1 year of age are at a higher risk for toxicity. Because children often do not show the classic adult symptomatology, caution should be used in their early discharge.

Appropriate indications for admission, other than a patient who is already manifesting signs and symptoms, include exposure to an agent known to be highly toxic, a dose or exposure to a toxin sufficient to anticipate the development of toxicity, or a history of an intentional ingestion. The adequacy of the home environment is assessed before discharge. Older children with suicidal ideation are evaluated before release.

Prevention

Treatment is incomplete until the existing problem is addressed, whether it is inadequate poison-proofing in the home, undersupervision of the child, a cry for help, or even child abuse. If warranted, the proper social service authorities should be contacted. If it was truly an accidental ingestion, poison prevention should be emphasized to avoid a repeat of the episode. This important modality is often overlooked. Each training session should be tailored to the patient and family situation.

1. Safety packaging has contributed significantly to the decline in pediatric accidental ingestions. Urge members of households with children to use these packages.
2. Instruct parents to keep products in their original containers and to discard containers safely.
3. Medicine should never be called "candy" and should never be taken in front of children, who are great imitators.

TABLE 253.1. Pediatric Dosages of Selected Antidotes

Antidote	Indications	Pediatric Dose
N-Acetylcysteine	Acetaminophen toxicity	Loading: 140 mg/kg orally or i.v. (not FDA approved by this route) Maintenance: 70 mg/kg q 4 h × 17 doses orally or 12 doses i.v. as a 5% solution
Atropine	Organophosphates/carbamates and other severe cholinergic poisonings	0.05 mg/kg (2 mg max) i.v. every 2–5 min until cessation of symptoms (e.g., pulmonary secretions)
Calcium	Calcium channel blocker toxicity or black widow spider enveromation	10% calcium gluconate 0.2–0.3 mL/kg or 10% calcium chloride 0.1–0.2 mL/kg slow i.v.
Cyanide kit	Cyanide poisoning	See below

Hemoglobin	Sodium Nitrite 3% (initial dose: max 10 mL)	Sodium Thiosulfate (Initial dose: 12.5 g max)
8 g	0.22 mL/kg (6.6 mg/kg)	1.10 mL/kg
10 g	0.27 mL/kg (8.7 mg/kg)	1.35 mL/kg
12 g*	0.33 mL/kg (10 mg/kg)	1.65 mL/kg
14 g	0.39 mL/kg) (11.6 mg/kg)	1.95 mL/kg

*If hemoglobin unknown, use this dose.

Antidote	Indications	Pediatric Dose
Deferoxamine	Iron intoxication	Therapeutic dose: slow Intravenous infusion up to 15 mg/kg/h
Diazepam	Seizures resulting from intoxication	0.1–0.3 mg/kg up to 10 mg i.v. slowly over 2 min
Dimercaprol (BAL)	Intoxications from lead, arsenic, gold, mercury, copper, nickel, antimony	IM use only: 3–5 mg/kg initially, followed by 2.5 mg/kg q4h for 2 days, then q 6–12h Note: Dosage and duration vary with specific intoxicant and severity; see recommendations for each poisoning. Caution: in peanut oil
Diphenhydramine	Dystonic reactions from phenothiazine and related compounds	1–2 mg/kg IM or i.v. over 2 min
Ethanol	Methanol, ethylene glycol toxicity	Loading: 7.6–10 mL/kg of a 10% solution in D_5W over 30 min i.v.: or 0.8–1.0 mL/kg 95% ETOH diluted to a 20%–30% solution for oral administration Maintenance: 1.4 mL/kg/h of a 10% ETOH solution i.v. (0.15 mL/kg/h PO 95%); add 91 mL/h if patient on dialysis
Fomepizol (Antizol)	Ethylene glycol, methanol toxicity	Loading: 15 mg/kg i.v. over 30 min Maintenance: 10 mg/kg q12h for 4 doses then 15 mg/kg q12h Note: Dosage needs to be adjusted during hemodialysis.
Glucagon	Beta-blocker or calcium channel blocker intoxication	50–150 µg/kg i.v. over 1 min followed by infusion of 1–5 mg/h tapered over 5–12 h Note: Do not use supplied diluent in older formulations (contains phenol).
Methylene blue	Methemoglobinemia	0.1–0.2 mL/kg of a 1% solution (1–2 mg/kg) i.v. over 5 min
Naloxone	Opioid toxicity	0.1 mg/kg i.v. if no response to initial dose Note: Many clinicians use normal adult doses in children; maintenance infusion is the initial reversal dose used, per hour.
Physostigmine	Severe anticholinergic poisoning	0.5 mg i.v. over 2 min repeated to a max dose of 2 mg if required Note: reserved for severe, life-threatening toxicity when conventional therapy has failed
Pralidoxime (2-PAM)	Organophosphate poisoning	25–50 mg/kg i.v. over 2 min or i.m. repeat every 8–12 h if needed; or infusion of 5–10 mg/kg/h
Succimer (Chemet)	Lead poisoning	10 mg/kg q8h for 5 days, followed by 10 mg/kg q12h for 14 days

From Schauben JL, Mofenson HC, Caraccio TR. Problems in the management of intoxications. In: Luten RC, ed. *Problems in pediatric emergency medicine*. New York: Churchill Livingstone, 1988:245.

4. Old and out-of-date medications and those no longer used should be discarded.
5. Medications and household products should be kept out of reach of children.
6. Children must be taught never to eat anything without checking with a parent or caretaker.
7. Stress the appropriate storage and use of ipecac syrup, and provide information about the poison control center.

COMMON PITFALLS

- Failing to appreciate a difference in historic factors may lead to a misinterpretation of the event's actual toxic potential. This may lead to underly or overly aggressive management.
- The variation in pharmacokinetic handling of a toxin in children should always be considered. If not, a serious error may be incurred when predicting the time course and toxic potential of an exposure.
- Directly translating poisoning management procedures for adults to children, without regard to the differences between adult and pediatric protocols, may be harmful.
- Assuming that all overdose patients require GI decontamination. This may place the patient at risk for unnecessary complications.

References

1. American Academy of Clinical Toxicology and European Association of Poisons Centres and Clinical Toxicologists Joint Position Statement. Cathartics. *J Toxicol Clin Toxicol* 1997;35:743–752.

2. American Academy of Clinical Toxicology and European Association of Poisons Centres and Clinical Toxicologists Joint Position Statement. Gastric lavage. *J Toxicol Clin Toxicol* 1997;35:711–720.
3. American Academy of Clinical Toxicology and European Association of Poisons Centres and Clinical Toxicologists Joint Position Statement. Ipecac syrup. *J Toxicol Clin Toxicol* 1997;35:699–710.
4. American Academy of Clinical Toxicology and European Association of Poisons Centres and Clinical Toxicologists Joint Position Statement. Single-dose activated charcoal. *J Toxicol Clin Toxicol* 1997;35:721–742.
5. American Academy of Clinical Toxicology and European Association of Poisons Centres and Clinical Toxicologists Joint Position Statement. Whole bowel irrigation. *J Toxicol Clin Toxicol* 1997;35:753–762.
6. Bradberry SM, Vale JA. Multiple-dose activated charcoal: a review of relevant clinical studies. *J Toxicol Clin Toxicol* 1995;33:407–416.
7. Chin L. GI dilution of poisons with water: an irrational and potentially harmful procedure. *Am J Hosp Pharm* 1971;28:712.
8. Cuprit GC, Temple AR. GI decontamination in the management of the poisoned patient. *Emerg Med Clin North Am* 1984;2:15.
9. Farley TA. Severe hypernatremic dehydration after use of an activated charcoal-sorbitol suspension. *J Pediatr* 1986;109:719.
10. Frenia ML, Schauben JL, Wears JL, et al. Multiple-dose activated charcoal compared to urinary alkalinization for the enhancement of phenobarbital elimination. *J Toxicol Clin Toxicol* 1996;34:169–175.
11. Gaudreault P, McCormick MA, Lacouture PG, et al. Poisoning exposures and use of ipecac in children less than 1 year old. *Ann Emerg Med* 1986;15:808.
12. Homan CS, Singer AJ, Thomajan C, et al. Thermal characteristics of neutralization therapy and water dilution for strong acid ingestion: an in-vivo canine model. *Acad Emerg Med* 1998;5:286–292.
13. Levy G. GI clearance of drugs with activated charcoal. *N Engl J Med* 1982;307:676.
14. Litovitz TL, Klein-Schwartz W, Dyer KS, et al. 1997 Annual report of the American Association of Poison Control Centers toxic exposure surveillance system. *Am J Emerg Med* 1998;16:443.
15. Perry H, Shannon M. Emergency department gastrointestinal decontamination. *Pediatr Ann* 1996;25:19–26.
16. Pond SM. Diuresis, dialysis, hemoperfusion—indications and benefits. *Emerg Med Clin North Am* 1984;2:29.
17. Pond SM, Lewis-Driver DJ, Williams GM, et al. Gastric emptying in acute overdose: a prospective randomised controlled trial. *Med J Aust* 1995; 163:345–349.
18. Rumack BH, Toll LL, Gerlman CR, eds. General or unknown (management/treatment protocol). In: *POISONDEX ® system*. Englewood, CO: Micromedex, Inc. (edition expired August 8, 1999).
19. Schauben JL, Mofenson HC, Caraccio TR. Problems in the management of intoxications. In: Luten RC. ed. *Problems in pediatric emergency medicine*. New York: Churchill Livingstone, 1988:245.
20. Tenenbein M. Whole bowel irrigation as a GI decontamination procedure after acute poisoning. *Med Toxicol* 1988;3:77.

CHAPTER 254
Limp

Jonathan I. Singer

Locomotion is accomplished by a graceful succession from a stance phase to a swing phase. The stance phase is initiated by the heel striking the ground and terminates with toeing-off. The swing phase begins with flexion of the knee and hip, followed by extension of the knee, and ends with dorsiflexion of the foot, which permits heel contact. Altered locomotion and gait disturbance are generic terms for any deviation from this rhythmic movement. Paralysis implies loss or impairment of neuromuscular mechanisms. Pseudoparalysis is a physiologically intact neuromuscular apparatus but with a refusal to walk or an inability to support weight.[4,20] A child who limps has faulted cadence of the swing and stance phase. When pain is the cause of acute loss of rhythm, the gait is described as antalgic.[18]

When a previously healthy child has either an acute or insidious onset of gait disturbance, it may benefit the emergency physician to consider anatomic units that may be functionally deranged. Lesions of the central nervous system, spine, peripheral nervous system, intraabdominal contents, hip, knee, ankle joints, feet, or any of the weight-bearing long bones can lead to distinct patterns of altered locomotion. By organizing the characteristic history and demonstrating the accompanying physical findings, the emergency physician may readily establish the affected organ system.[17]

Unfortunately, because of the close proximity of these structures, many disease states that alter locomotion are likely to involve a combination of them. This fact may make it more difficult to draw a prompt conclusion as to the pathogenesis of the altered gait, but, often, historic, physical, and adjunctive laboratory features may help in characterizing its probable origin.[16]

CLINICAL PRESENTATION

Take the history in a setting comfortable for both the parent and the child. The physician should attempt to remain as inconspicuous as possible, and the historian should be encouraged to distract the child's attention from the physician. The physician should inquire about the length of time the child has been symptomatic. With gait disturbance, symptoms may be acute, constant, of a brief duration, or insidious with inconstant manifestations.

Are there temporal relationships or patterns related to physical activity? Ask the parent what part of the body appears to be the source of the child's problem. Determine whether there is pain associated with the gait disturbance. Attempt to identify the site, if pain is present. Focus on posture during sleep and rest, avoidance of a particular position, and discomfort with handling a specific body part.

Seek the history of an acute traumatic event, such as a fall, a twisting injury, a direct blow, or penetration by a foreign body. Inquire about the presence of fever, which may accompany an inflammatory or infectious problem. Is there exposure to contagion? Is there an antecedent infectious process? Is the child currently being treated with antibiotics for an intercurrent infection? The review of symptoms should emphasize cutaneous lesions such as a scarlatiniform erythroderma, erythema marginatum, erythema migrans, erythema nodosum, urticaria, or purpura. Make inquiry regarding weight loss, morning stiffness, decreased motor strength and agility, a change in bladder or bowel control, altered mental status, headache, rhinorrhea, cough, anorexia, nausea, vomiting, and abdominal pain. Exclude exposures to animals, ticks, and potential intoxicants, such as heavy metals, insecticides, alcohol, or various medications, such as hydantoin, isoniazid, antimetabolites, and steroids.

Determine whether there have been recent intramuscular injections, including immunizations. Is there a history of previous joint disease, prior lumbar puncture, or underlying disease state, such as endocrinopathy, sickle hemoglobinopathy, diabetes mellitus, or immunocompromised state? Is there a family history of inflammatory bowel or joint disease? Is there any suggestion of physical abuse, sexual assault, or psychosocial disturbances that would predispose to a conversion reaction? Has there been acquisition of any new footwear?[6,18]

In the preschool-aged child, first carry out the physical examination with the child on a parent's lap. Begin with inspection. Observe the position of the patient at rest, and look at the child's passive movements. Focus on the skin, looking for evidence of hemorrhagic diathesis, occult trauma, and penetrating wounds. Look for soft-tissue swelling and skin changes that suggest pyoderma, varicella, cellulitis, or a deeper plane infection. Look for asymmetry of gluteal, thigh, and popliteal creases.

Determine whether there is effusion or distension of the joint capsules of the hip, knee, or ankle.

Only after inspection should the physician palpate for localized induration, warmth, or tenderness over the bones, particularly metaphyseal regions of long bones. Gently examine the joints for motion, avoiding the probable area of pathology until last. Handle the limb systematically and delicately, providing anxiolytic, distracting speech. Determine the degree of restriction of flexion, extension, abduction, and rotation. Palpate the spine in the midline, looking for paraspinal muscle spasm or scoliosis. Determine whether there is any sensory disturbance, asymmetry of deep tendon reflexes, loss of motor strength, cranial nerve abnormalities, or nuchal rigidity. Finally, examine the feet and footwear for embedded foreign objects.

Transfer the patient onto an examining table. Readdress positive physical findings. With the patient recumbent, look for abdominal guarding or palpable mass in the iliac fossa. Perform a pelvic rock. With a rectal examination, exclude a mass in the pelvic floor. Perform a Valsalva maneuver, heel strike, and straight leg raise.[10,18] Remove the patient from the examining table, and place him or her on the floor in a sitting position. Observe the method chosen to achieve the erect position. If the child refuses to arise, stand the child on the floor at a distance from the parent. Determine whether the child refuses to bear weight on one of the limbs or simply walks with an antalgic gait.

DIFFERENTIAL DIAGNOSIS

A wide variety of problems have a presenting complaint of limp. The ones most common in the emergency department are listed in Table 254.1. Because of their frequency, overt or occult trauma and infectious diseases should be part of the differential diagnosis for any child with an acute gait disturbance.[4,17]

Trauma to the lower extremities is the principal cause of gait disturbance, especially in early childhood. In children less than 5 years old, multiple obstacles may impede this diagnosis. A fracture of the tibia or fibula should be considered the probable diagnosis in an afebrile child less than 5 years old who suddenly refuses to walk or place any weight on a single lower extremity. The absence of direct trauma should not rule out the diagnosis, because these fractures may occur as the result of trivial, indirect injury associated with the child's daily activity.[19]

Older children may limp from stress fractures of the femoral head, tibial tubercle, and tibial or fibular shaft. They also may limp from avulsion of the ischial apophysis, lesser trochanter, or navicular tuberosity, or from lacerations and compression of cartilage plates, fracture of the epiphyseal ossification centers, shaft fractures, and infractions at various levels of the long-bone metaphyses. These traumatic lesions may present singly or in various combinations. They may appear acutely or insidiously, caused by repeated injury during sports. Trauma and repeated stress may be important factors in the genesis of slipped capital femoral epiphysis, transient synovitis, and Legg-Calvé-Perthes disease, three of the most common hip afflictions associated with antalgic gait.[8,9]

TABLE 254.1. Principal Causes for Altered Childhood Locomotion

Overt and occult trauma
Cellulitis
Osteomyelitis
Pyarthrosis
Sickle cell, vasoocclusive crisis
Drug intoxication
Transient synovitis
Legg-Perthes disease
Appendicitis
Juvenile rheumatoid arthritis

Modified and reproduced with permission from Singer J. The cause of gait disturbance in 425 pediatric patients. In: Ludwig S, Fleisher G, eds. *Pediatric emergency care*, vol 1. Baltimore: Wiliams & Wilkins, 1985:7.

Among the nontraumatic conditions that can cause altered locomotion, potentially serious infectious diseases predominate. A history of an antecedent infectious process with or without fever in the preceding 2 weeks should heighten concern for a serious infectious disease in the child with a gait disturbance. Similarly, current treatment with antibiotics for a recognized infection, especially of the skin or respiratory tract, in a child with gait disturbance should raise suspicion for a more serious infection.

The most common infectious conditions associated with gait disturbance are focal cellulitis of the lower extremity, unifocal pyarthrosis of a weight-bearing joint, and osteomyelitis of the femoral or tibial metaphyses. On clinical grounds alone, it may be difficult to differentiate these three conditions. The final diagnosis rests with isolation of an offending organism from either the skin and soft tissues, synovial fluid, or subperiosteal space.[16]

Patients with sickle hemoglobinopathy may present acutely with a gait disturbance from dactylitis, stasis of blood in tendons and periarticular and synovial tissues, bone infarction, osteomyelitis of the long bones, and avascular necrosis of a femoral head.[16]

Dose-dependent toxic reactions from alcohol or diphenylhydantoin and prolonged exposure to heavy metals, insecticides, and toluene-containing compounds may produce clumsiness, incoordination, and unsteady gait with overt ataxia or inability to walk. This diagnosis depends on the medication history and potential exposure to toxins.[16]

In acute synovitis, there is a transient, unilateral inflammatory reaction in the hip. There may be antecedent minor trauma or recent upper respiratory tract symptoms, possibly associated with low-grade fever. An affected child presents with either acute or progressive discomfort in the hip, anteromedial thigh, or ipsilateral knee, eventually leading to an antalgic gait. Clinically, this condition is indistinguishable from Legg-Calvé-Perthes disease. In both cases, children do not appear systemically ill. They will choose a position with the thigh flexed, abducted, and externally rotated. They guard the hip during examination and have pain with internal rotation of the hip and, to a lesser extent, with hip extension.[9]

Patients with uncomplicated appendicitis, or a perforated or abscessed appendix, exhibit a gait disturbance manifested by a cautious, slow gait, often accompanied by flexion of the trunk. An outright right-sided limp is seen occasionally. The gait resembles that seen with cervicitis or any pelvic inflammatory disease.[16]

The clinical manifestations of juvenile rheumatoid arthritis are so varied that it may be difficult to distinguish this disease when first encountering a patient. The mode of onset varies considerably, from involvement of a single joint with no constitutional reactions, to a more widespread polyarthritis of varying severity, to a generalized systemic onset with extraarticular manifestations.[16]

Major Emergency Entities

An early presumptive diagnosis for the cause of gait disturbance must be established for a few conditions (Table 254.2). Failing to consider these conditions at the initial encounter may lead to deformity, functional disability, or death.[16]

Pain associated with osteomyelitis of the long bones is primarily located over the affected metaphysis. Direct pressure

TABLE 254.2. Disease States Associated with Limp That Require Prompt Recognition

Osteomyelitis
  Long bone, spine, pelvis
Pyarthrosis
  Hip, knee, ankle
Sacroiliac infection
Psoas abscess
Deep-plane infection
Epidural abscess
Slipped capital femoral epiphysis
Cord tumor
Guillain-Barré syndrome
Tick paralysis
Meningitis
Encephalitis
Cerebral abscess
Appendicitis

Modified and reproduced with permission from Singer J. Evaluation of acute and insidious gait disturbance in children less than 5 years of age. In: Barness LA, et al., eds. *Advances in padiatrics*, vol 26. Chicago: Year Book, 1979.

over the affected metaphysis produces extreme discomfort. Swelling is limited to the immediate metaphyseal area initially, but it can spread rapidly to involve an entire extremity or adjacent periarticular tissue. Joints adjacent to the infected metaphysis may have some limitation of motion caused by voluntary guarding or sympathetic effusion. If the joints are handled gently, slowly, and persistently, motion is not as restricted as in septic arthritis, and full range may be possible. Neck pain, back pain, and refusal to walk may signal the presence of osteomyelitis of the spine. Fever associated with back, buttock, or hip pain with gait disturbance may be the initial expression of osteomyelitis of the pelvis. [16]

Patients with pyarthrosis are readily diagnosed because of the protective posturing imposed by joint capsule distention. When there is hip involvement, children assume a position of comfort, with the thigh on the affected side in moderate flexion, abduction, and external rotation. Children place the affected limb on the ground in the same position as when it is supine, and often hold the foot in plantar flexion.[12] If the knee or ankle is involved, it is erythematous, warm, swollen, and painful to palpate, with limited range of motion. Minimal active motion, extreme muscle spasm, and pain with passive movement are distinguishing features of pyarthrosis in weight-bearing regions.[16]

Suppuration may be limited to the sacroiliac joint and causes gait disturbance in rare cases. Patients have pain in the buttocks and lower back that radiates to the hip, lateral thigh, lower leg, or abdomen. They may hold a single hip guarded, abducted, and externally rotated, but flexion, abduction, external rotation, and hip extension are permitted. Another differentiating feature is pain caused by direct compression of the sacroiliac joint or pain in the sacroiliac joint during rectal examination or from compression of the ileal wings. Often, the straight leg-raising test is positive.[5]

Hip, groin, abdomen, lower back, buttock, or upper thigh pain associated with fever and limping may occur with a psoas abscess. Like patients with septic arthritis of the hip, those with psoas abscess may assume the position of hip flexion, abduction, and external rotation. Hip extension and internal rotation that stretches the iliopsoas muscle may cause increased pain. Rotation of the fully flexed hip is typically pain-free. When they attempt to walk, patients keep the affected extremity advanced in relation to the unaffected side, with the trunk deviated toward the affected side, the pelvis tilted down, and the knee and hip flexed slightly. Several findings may differentiate psoas abscess from septic arthritis or osteomyelitis: the presence of abdominal guarding with tenderness in both lower quadrants, or a palpable mass in the iliac fossa or pelvic floor that may be detectable by rectal examination. Patients also may have bulging of the flank with or without cutaneous edema, scoliosis, immobility of the spine with spasm of the paravertebral muscles, or decreased excursions of the diaphragm.[14]

Deep-plane infection refers to suppuration that extends to the depth of fascia or muscle. In necrotizing fasciitis, fat and fascia are destroyed. Muscle is typically uninvolved, and skin, on occasion, may be spared.[7] In bacterial myositis, the striated muscle is involved, and there may be localized abscess formation within the muscle (pyomyositis).[3]

Clinical features of fasciitis and myositis overlap. Neither is common in immunologically intact children. Predisposing conditions including diabetes mellitus, chronic cardiac or pulmonary disease, collagen vascular disease, varicella complicated by pyoderma, and antecedent blunt trauma. There is a predilection for involvement of the lower extremities, especially the groin and thigh. Symptoms are often insidious, starting with poorly localized extremity pain that impairs gait. Fever may be absent or only of low grade. Pain that is out of proportion to the degree of physical findings may be the only clue to the correct diagnosis at the initial encounter.[1]

With varicella, a violaceous hue about a cluster of pox lesions may be the clue to deep-plane infection. In those without varicella, rapidly developing skin changes suggest the diagnosis. These include a localized soft-tissue swelling, erythema, and either darker discoloration of the skin (pyomyositis) or bullae formation, and spontaneous sloughing (necrotizing fasciitis). If misdiagnosed at the time there is painful gait without skin changes, children may return in extremis within 24 to 48 hours in septic shock.[1,3]

Hip pain and limp may be the presenting complaints with epidural abscess, but most patients seek medical attention because of unremitting back pain. At the onset, most patients exhibit fever, headache, malaise, and aching midline back pain. Patients may have tenderness on palpation of the spinous processes at the level of the subjective back pain. Neck stiffness is present in more than one-third of patients, and when altered sensorium is an accompanying feature, the disease may mimic meningitis. Overt cord involvement may be heralded by weakness of voluntary muscles and bowel and bladder sphincters, or by sensory abnormalities, most often characterized as ascending anesthesia.[14]

Deep groin pain and hip, distal medial thigh, or knee pain may be of sudden onset or progressive over weeks as result of acute or chronic slipped capital femoral epiphysis. Classically, pain is vague, dull at rest, and exacerbated by ambulation. Children seek comfort by externally rotating the leg when walking. They limp, and there is often a truncal shift with ambulation to accommodate hip abductor weakness. Examination demonstrates a partially flexed, irritable hip maintained in external rotation. Maximal hip flexion is restricted, and complete internal rotation is not possible. Delay in recognition of an acute slip may result in further displacement or may increase the risk for avascular necrosis.[6]

A diagnosis of cord tumor must be considered in any child with a gait disturbance who also has a recent history of altered bowel pattern or an insidious onset of motor weakness of the lower extremities, subjective sensory disturbance (including leg and neck pain), or back pain that is usually progressive. The back pain associated with a cord tumor is classically increased in the supine position and increased in intensity by the Valsalva maneuver. Physical examination may reveal weakness of the lower extremities, paraspinal or hamstring muscle spasm, nuchal rigidity, scoliosis, back stiffness, spine tenderness, relaxed sphincter tone, and absence of fever. Even when cord tumors present precipitously, the absence of systemic manifestations helps to discriminate them from acute epidural abscess.[16]

Alterations in gait seen with Guillain-Barré syndrome can be secondary to subjective complaints of foot or leg pain, impairment of position sense, or profound leg weakness with loss of voluntary movement. The clinical hallmark of Guillain-Barré syndrome is rapidly progressive, relatively symmetric motor impairment. The motor deficit may range from isolated lower limb weakness to total paralysis of the muscles of all four extremities and the trunk. Mild sensory symptoms or signs strongly support the diagnosis. Severe sensory dysfunction with pain as a dominant expression is a clinical variant. Such patients may experience bilateral pain in the large proximal muscles, including the lower back, buttocks, and anterior and posterior aspects of the thighs. Such sensory disturbances can precede the onset of clinically demonstrable weakness.[16]

The prognosis for full functional recovery from tick paralysis depends on establishment of the diagnosis. After a brief period with nonspecific symptoms, patients experience a progressive weakness of the lower extremities, usually without pain or paresthesias. The weakness or attendant ataxia can lead to inability to walk, and the patient may seek medical attention before the development of a generalized flaccid paresis.[16]

Children may be reluctant to assume an upright position or to walk because of cephalalgia, myalgia, electrolyte imbalance, compromised circulatory status, and altered sensorium from encephalitis or meningitis. The cardinal symptoms of cerebral abscess include severe and intractable headache, altered sensorium, vomiting, fever, and neurologic abnormalities that include seizure, paresthesias, incoordination, unsteady gait, or hemiparesis.[16] Early recognition of these intracranial infections can prevent significant morbidity and mortality.

EMERGENCY DEPARTMENT EVALUATION

Among the benign and potentially life- or limb-threatening causes of gait disturbance, several have a classic profile. By recognizing the characteristic history and subsequently demonstrating the accompanying physical findings, the physician may establish a diagnosis. Where the pathogenesis is clear, no diagnostic investigation is an option. When the provisional diagnosis is elusive, ancillary tests from phlebotomy or imaging may be helpful.

A complete blood count may facilitate the diagnosis of systemic infection, hemoglobinopathy, or blood dyscrasia. The erythrocyte sedimentation rate (ESR) correctly identifies over 75% of all patients with limb pain who have an inflammatory or infectious disease.[11] About 70% of patients with an ESR of more than 30 mm/h have arthralgia or arthritis of infectious or inflammatory origin. Those with an ESR of 40 mm/h or more have bacterial infections as the cause of their refusal to walk.[4]

When the area of pain has been localized, radiographs limited to the area of interest have proven diagnostic efficacy. Plain radiographs may aid in the diagnosis of periostitides, osteochondroses, benign and malignant tumors, mechanical disturbances, metabolic derangements, and infectious diseases. Films that appear negative should never hinder therapeutic strategies. Several noteworthy conditions that present with gait disturbance, such as tibial fracture in the toddler, septic hip in the child over 1 year old, osteomyelitis of the long bone or pelvis, sacroiliac joint infection, and intervertebral disk infection, may be associated with normal radiographs. Radiographs are often insensitive and unreliable, especially in the early course of these disorders.[2,13]

Ultrasonography may be helpful in the investigation of hip irritability. Sonography may demonstrate intraarticular effusion when plain films are normal.

Radionuclide scans rarely establish an unexpected diagnosis, but they do provide important positive and negative information central to inpatient management. A positive technetium scan reflects any condition that results in increased bone formation or blood flow. A negative technetium scan does not rule out an infectious process and should be followed by a gallium scan. Gallium accumulates in leukocytes independent of blood supply. A positive gallium scan supports a provisional diagnosis of infection, and negative technetium and gallium scans refute it. The diagnostic accuracy of these procedures is augmented only when both scans are performed sequentially.

Computed tomography (CT) scanning is useful for the study of tumors and inflammatory and infectious problems of the musculoskeletal system in children. Magnetic resonance imaging (MRI) is superior to both plain films and CT scans for soft-tissue detail. MRI may be the most sensitive means of establishing an early diagnosis of Legg-Calvé-Perthes disease, differentiating bone infarction from osteomyelitis in the sickle cell patient and benign from malignant bone tumors. MRI may be useful in certain anatomic regions that are difficult to evaluate with plain films (e.g., region of the sacroiliac joint, vertebral bodies, and intervertebral disks).[12] All of these imaging modalities, however, are of limited assistance to the emergency physician, who must make a prompt diagnosis.[15–17]

EMERGENCY DEPARTMENT MANAGEMENT

The intensity of the emergency department management of patients with gait disturbances rests with the physiologic derangement at the time of presentation. Rarely, a patient with limp, pseudoparalysis, or paresis requires establishment of an airway or ventilatory support. Cardiovascular instability, which can occur with a few of the infectious diseases (notably deep-plane infection, meningitis, and appendiceal abscess), requires fluid resuscitation. Neurologic deficits may be rapidly progressive in a few conditions associated with gait disturbance. Continuous monitoring of neurologic status is warranted for patients suspected of having Guillain-Barré syndrome, poliomyelitis, acute transverse myelitis, tick paralysis, brain abscess, meningitis, and cerebral vascular accident. A few conditions associated with gait disturbance require specific emergency department treatment to forestall functional disability. Various therapeutic modalities include splinting of fractures, antibiotic administration, arthrocentesis to reduce intraarticular pressure, and removal of a tick to definitively treat tick paralysis.

DISPOSITION

When presented with a child who has a gait disturbance, the physician has a major responsibility to distinguish between those children who require emergency department intervention and immediate hospitalization and those who have self-limited conditions. The following features, when present, may be helpful in characterizing patients who require greater scrutiny. Be more cautious when the gait disturbance is more likely to be from illness rather than from injury. In nontraumatic states, have a heightened awareness for adverse outcome when a gait disturbance is associated with a rapid progression of signs and symptoms or when there is an indolent illness with sudden change.

Admission is warranted for children with gait disturbance in certain circumstances. Admit all patients who appear to have a serious bacterial infection. History and physical examination are more likely to uncover serious bacterial infection than are ancillary laboratory investigations. Maintain a high index of suspicion for serious bacterial diseases in those patients who have recently been febrile or are currently being treated with antibiotics for benign intercurrent illness.

Certain clinical findings suggest that serious bacterial illness is present. They include fever, even if of low grade; nuchal rigidity; limitation of joint motion; lower limb direct metaphyseal pain; compression tenderness over a spinal process; pain in the sacroiliac joint, with pelvic rock; and back pain enhanced with Valsalva movement, heel strike, or straight leg raising. Additional features that suggest serious bacterial infection include pain that is disproportionate to physical findings or neurologic abnormalities. In the context of a likely infectious disease, do not be dissuaded by a normal white blood cell count or normal ESR. Conversely, do not admit a child who has no historic or clinical findings to suggest serious bacterial infection when there is an isolated finding of leukocytosis or elevated sedimentation rate.

Admission is warranted for all patients with neurologic abnormalities, such as altered consciousness, cranial nerve involvement, subjective or objective sensory disturbance, ataxia, alteration of sphincter tone, urinary retention, altered deep tendon reflexes, or loss of voluntary movement. Admit patients with gait disturbance who might have been physically abused.

COMMON PITFALLS

- Think of trauma when there is an abrupt onset of gait disturbance without prodromal events in a previously healthy child.
- Deemphasize the history of trauma, even if witnessed, when there is an antecedent or current infectious process; this scenario suggests serious bacterial infection.
- Fever, leukocytosis, and elevated ESR may not uniformly accompany infectious diseases associated with gait disturbance.

References

1. Barton LL, Jeck DT. Necrotizing fasciitis in children: report of two cases and review of literature. *Arch Pediatr Adolesc Med* 1996;150:105.
2. Blatt SD, Rosenthal BM, Barnhart DC. Diagnostic utility of lower extremity radiography of young children with gait disturbance. *Pediatrics* 1991;87:138.
3. Boyle MF, Singer J. Necrotizing myositis and toxic strep syndrome in a pediatric patient. *J Emerg Med* 1992;10:577.
4. Callahan DL. Causes of refusal to walk in childhood. *South Med J* 1982;75:20.
5. Carlson SA, Jones JS. Pyogenic sacroiliitis. *Am J Emerg Med* 1994;12:639.
6. Clark MC, Iwiniski HJ. The limping child: meeting the challenges of an accurate assessment and diagnosis. *Pediatr Emerg Med Rep* 1997; 2:123–133.
7. Halsey NA, Abramson JS, Chesney PG, et al. Severe invasive group A streptococcal infections: a subject review. *Pediatrics* 1998; 101:136–140.
8. Illingworth CM. One hundred twenty-eight limping children with no fracture, sprain or obvious cause. *Clin Pediatr* 1987;17:139.
9. Koop S, Quambecke B. Three common causes of childhood hip pain. *Pediatr Clin North Am* 1996;43:1053.
10. Lawrence LL. The limping child. *Pediatr Clin North Am* 1998;16:911.
11. McCarthy PL, Wasserman D, Spiesel SZ, et al. Evaluation of arthritis and arthralgia in the pediatric patients. *Clin Pediatr* 1980;19:183.
12. McLario DJ, Burton LJ, Bruce RW, et al. Pseudoparalysis of the lower extremity in an infant. *Pediatr Emerg Care* 1998;14:277.
13. Myers MT, Thompson GH. Imaging of the child with a limp. *Pediatr Clin North Am* 1997;44:637.
14. Peterson JA, Paris P, Williams AC. Acute epidural abscess. *Am J Emerg Med* 1987;5:287.
15. Schwaitzberg SD, Pokorny WJ, Thurston RS, et al. Psoas abscess in children. *J Pediatr Surg* 1985;20:339.
16. Singer J. Evaluation of acute and insidious gait disturbance in children less than 5 years of age. *Adv Pediatr* 1979;26:209.
17. Singer J. The cause of gait disturbance in 425 pediatric patients. *Pediatr Emerg Care* 1985;1:7.
18. Singer J. Altered locomotion: an approach to the assessment of the child with a limp. In: Barkin RM, ed. *The emergently ill child.* Rockville, MD: Aspen, 1987.
19. Singer J, Tobin R. Occult fractures in the production of gait disturbance in childhood. *Pediatrics* 1979;64:192.
20. Singer J. Neonatal psoas pyomyositis simulating pyarthrosis of the hip. *Pediatr Emerg Care* 1993;9:87.

CHAPTER 255
Respiratory Distress

Bruce Quinn and Marc Linares

Respiratory distress is a compensatory state in response to impaired oxygen delivery to the tissues, with or without decreased carbon dioxide elimination. When the patient's capacity for compensation is overwhelmed, respiratory failure occurs.

The respiratory system can be divided into two anatomic categories: the lungs, or gas-exchange portion; and the "respiratory pump," consisting of the nervous system, respiratory muscles, and thorax.[12] Pathology involving any of these areas can potentially lead to the signs and symptoms of respiratory distress. Depending on the etiology of the respiratory compromise and the time until presentation in the emergency department, these signs and symptoms may be subtle.

A number of differences exist between the pediatric and the adult patient that place the child at greater risk for respiratory compromise. Infants and young children have a subglottic airway that is smaller and has less supporting cartilage than that found in adults, therefore making it easier for obstruction to occur secondary to edema, secretions, constriction, or compression.[4] The smaller the airway, the greater the resistance for a given decrease in lumenal diameter. Dynamic collapse of a partially obstructed airway, as can be seen in croup during inspiratory, is a direct consequence of the high compliance of the pediatric airway.[4] Children less than 1 to 2 years of age may not have the anatomic pathways or "collateral ventilation" that allow aeration distal to an obstructed airway, thereby increasing the risk of atelectasis and ventilation–perfusion mismatching.[12] Due to the increased chest wall compliance of the pediatric patients, some of the diaphragmatic contractions force is wasted distorting the rib cage rather than expanding the lungs.[12] The younger the child, the greater the pliability of the chest wall, placing the neonate at greatest risk for fatigue, respiratory failure, and cardiopulmonary arrest.

In addition to anatomic differences, the higher metabolic rate in children, compared with that in adults, places them at a further disadvantage by increasing their oxygen demand. With the onset of hypoventilation, hypoxemia will occur more rapidly in the child.[4]

CLINICAL PRESENTATION

The presentation of a child in respiratory distress varies, depending on a number of factors, including the specific etiology, duration of illness, age, underlying medical conditions, and interventions prior to arrival in the emergency department. Any degree of respiratory compromise needs to be quickly detected and appropriate therapy instituted, in order to avoid potential deterioration to respiratory failure and cardiopulmonary arrest.

Signs of respiratory distress can be separated into two categories: visual and audible (Table 255.1). Initially, simply looking at a child and listening, avoiding prolonged eye contact and use of a stethoscope, can provide a great deal of information with minimal, if any, anxiety being produced in the patient.

Visual inspection begins with the child's behavior. Normal behavior in a child does not rule out underlying pathology, but it does inform the clinician that the child is comfortable and in no need of urgent intervention. However, a quiet, serious child, who prefers sitting upright in a sniffing position, is a cause for concern and requires immediate assessment. Behavior changes such as restlessness or irritability can be subtle clues of hypoxemia. Any alteration in mental status can represent either generalized central nervous system (CNS) disease or hypercarbia, with or without hypoxemia.

The presence of either tachypnea or bradypnea is taken as evidence of respiratory compromise. It is important, therefore, to be aware of the normal range of respiratory rates in the pediatric population. Hooker et al.[14] found normal respiratory rates to be higher than in previously published studies with a wide range of "normal." In addition, fever, pain, and anxiety increase the respiratory rate in the absence of pulmonary disease. In Hooker's study, patients younger than 1 year of age had a mean respiratory rate of 39 ± 11 with a minimum of 22 breaths per minute to a maximum of 65.[14] Patients 2 to 3 years of age had a mean rate of 28 ± 4, with rates at 8 years of age falling into the adult range (20 ± 4).[14]

Rather than an absolute respiratory rate, a better marker of respiratory distress may be a change in the respiratory rate for a particular child, as well as an assessment of the depth of respirations. Shallow respirations are often seen in diseases causing lower airway obstruction, while deep respirations are often associated with diseases causing metabolic acidosis and represent a central compensatory mechanism.[22] The presence of chest retractions indicates respiratory distress. They begin subcostally with mild disease, and progress upward as the disease process worsens.[34] Nasal flaring can be a subtle sign, more commonly present in the infant and younger child, and is usually associated with lower tract disease. Head bobbing with each breath and "see-saw" or "rocky" respirations, in which the chest pulls in while the abdomen thrusts out, are signs of severe distress; the latter is an inefficient means of ventilation that can quickly lead to respiratory failure.[4] Cyanosis is not apparent until at least 5 g of desaturated hemoglobin per deciliter of capillary blood is present; this usually correlates with a PO_2 below 40 and an arterial oxyhemoglobin saturation of 85% or less.[5,20] Because anemic patients can be acyanotic and profoundly hypoxic, cyanosis should not be considered a dependable or an early indicator of hypoxemia.[4]

Certain indicators of respiratory distress can be heard without the use of a stethoscope. Persistent, forceful, nonproductive coughing may indicate a foreign body lodged in the upper airway, with the potential for complete obstruction. Stridor is a harsh, crowing sound, occurring during inspiration[28] and commonly seen in the pediatric population. It signifies upper airway pathology being produced by rapid, turbulent air flow through a narrowed area.[34] Wheezing represents expiratory obstruction of the lower airways.[22] If heard without chest auscultation, it clearly indicates serious disease and the need for urgent intervention. Grunting, an end-expiratory sound, is produced by glottic closure during exhalation in an attempt to provide physiologic positive end-expiratory pressure (PEEP).[22] When detected, it indicates a disease process causing alveolar and/or interstitial fluid.[22] An abnormal voice or cry, particularly if muffled in quality, should alert the clinician to possible upper airway disease and the need for prompt, nonthreatening evaluation.

In the absence of visual and audible signs of respiratory distress, the likelihood of an infant or child having serious respiratory pathology requiring emergent intervention is small.

DIFFERENTIAL DIAGNOSIS

Determining the precise etiology of respiratory distress in the pediatric patient can be challenging; the differential diagnosis is substantial (Table 255.2.). The clinician needs to recognize the signs and symptoms of respiratory distress in a child and determine the degree of severity. In moderate-to-severe degrees of distress, a rapid assessment of the likely etiology is needed so that proper therapy can be initiated.

The presence of stridor indicates some degree of upper airway obstruction and, when associated with fever, one should suspect an infectious etiology. Croup classically presents between 6 months and 3 years of age, with a history of a low-grade fever and upper respiratory infection (URI) symptoms for a few days, followed by the sudden onset of a barking cough, hoarseness, and stridor, with or without chest retractions.

In any child thought to have croup, the diagnosis of epiglottitis must be considered and ruled out. Although the incidence of epiglottitis has declined dramatically since the introduction of the *Haemophilus influenzae* type b conjugate vaccine,[13,35] the physician must remain vigilant for this potentially life-threatening disease. Epiglottitis usually occurs between 3 and 8 years of

TABLE 255.1. Indicators of Actual or Possible Respiratory Compromise

VISUAL	AUDIBLE
Chest retractions	Cough
Abnormal behavior	Stridor
Altered mental status	Wheezing
Tachypnea/bradypnea	Grunting
Shallow/deep respirations	Abnormal voice or cry
Nasal flaring	
Head bobbing	
"See-saw" respirations	
Cyanosis	

TABLE 255.2. Etiologies of Respiratory Distress

INFECTIOUS	TRAUMA/MECHANICAL
Respiratory Tract	Hemothorax
Upper	Pneumothorax
Croup	Pulmonary contusion
Epiglottitis	Flail chest
URI	Spinal cord injury
Bacterial tracheitis	Intracranial hemorrhage
Peritonsillar abscess	Abdominal distension
Retropharyngeal abscess	**ENVIRONMENTAL**
Lower	Foreign body
Pneumonia	Smoke inhalation
Bronchiolitis	Near drowning
Central Nervous System	Ingestions
Meningitis	**OTHER**
Encephalitis	Seizures
Brain abscess	Cardiac failure
HYPERACTIVE AIRWAY	Cystic fibrosis
Asthma	Metabolic acidosis
Anaphylaxis	Vocal cord dysfunction
	Congenital anomalies
	Hypocalcemia

age, although it can be seen as early as 6 months and as late as adulthood.[33] Sudden onset of high fever is often the earliest manifestation.[5] Losek et al.[21] reported that among children with epiglottitis, 95% of those aged 2 years and older had a history of sore throat, and that 92% of all children had a change in voice or cry. At physical examination, the most common signs of epiglottitis were found to be stridor (88%), retractions (81%), and temperature 38°C or higher (85%); drooling (66%) and a preference for sitting (58%) were less common.[21] The time course from first clinical sign to respiratory distress can be rapid, usually occurring within 12 hours.[5]

In distinguishing between epiglottitis and croup in a child presenting with fever, stridor, and retractions, the importance of the history cannot be overemphasized. Drooling in the absence of spontaneous cough is the most specific indicator of acute epiglottitis.[24] It is important to note, though, that cough can be seen in epiglottitis, and that its presence in no way eliminates it from the differential diagnosis.[5,21]

Not infrequently, a URI alone will cause signs of mild-to-moderate respiratory distress in the very young infant. Simply suctioning the nares, using several drops of normal saline and a bulb syringe, is usually all that is required.

Other, less common etiologies to consider in a child with fever and stridor include bacterial tracheitis and peritonsillar or retropharyngeal abscesses. Patients with bacterial tracheitis typically have symptoms of croup initially and then go on to develop high fever, toxicity, and purulent tracheal secretions, resulting in airway compromise.[5] Peritonsillar abscesses are most common in older adolescents and young adults in their early 20s.[11] There is sudden elevation of temperature, toxicity, and unilateral throat pain following an earlier tonsillitis.[5] The patient complains of trismus and has drooling, difficulty speaking, and a muffled voice.[7] Examination may reveal bilateral tonsillar hypertrophy, but one tonsil will be more enlarged and possibly cause deviation of the uvula.[7] Unlike peritonsillar abscesses, retropharyngeal abscesses usually present in young children, from infancy to 3 years of age.[5] The clinical picture is similar to that seen with epiglottitis, but with a less sudden onset.[7] If the child is stable, a diagnostic lateral neck x-ray should be done.

Infectious etiologies of the lower respiratory tract that may cause respiratory distress include bronchiolitis and pneumonia. Bronchiolitis is any wheezing-associated illness in the first years of life that is preceded by a URI.[39] Differentiation from acute attacks of asthma, often triggered by viral infections, may be difficult.

In those patients presenting in respiratory distress not obviously associated with infection, the history and physical examination should quickly solve the mystery. Most commonly, a diagnosis of asthma will be made. An important etiology to include in the differential diagnosis is anaphylaxis, a multisystem syndrome involving the cutaneous, respiratory, cardiovascular, and gastrointestinal systems; involvement of two or more systems is required for the diagnosis.[6] Both the upper and lower airways can be involved, leading to hoarseness, stridor, wheezing, and cough. Early diagnosis and distinction of anaphylaxis from more benign conditions is essential, as these patients can progress rapidly to anaphylactic shock.[6]

Environmental causes of respiratory distress, such as smoke inhalation and near drowning, will usually be evident from the history. Others, particularly foreign-body aspirations, may be difficult to determine. An infant or young child found in the midst of peanuts or similar sized objects, who subsequently develops a persistent cough with stridor, should obviously be evaluated for foreign-body aspiration. Often, however, the history of a foreign-body aspiration is less apparent, with the parents reporting only that their previously well child suddenly "began coughing out of the blue." Stridor or wheezing not responsive to appropriate therapy requires further evaluation, beginning with lateral and anteroposterior x-rays of the neck and chest.

Etiologies of respiratory distress associated with trauma should be evident from clinical examination. Tension pneumothorax and hemothorax need to be rapidly diagnosed and treated. Respiratory depression in the trauma patient without obvious respiratory tract pathology should raise the possibility of injury to the CNS.

Other important causes of respiratory compromise in the child include seizures, congestive heart failure, cystic fibrosis, and metabolic acidosis due to sepsis, diabetic ketoacidosis, renal disease, and certain ingestions (e.g., salicylate, methanol). Neuromuscular diseases, including Guillain-Barré, botulism, and myasthenia gravis, also need to be considered. Vocal cord dysfunction, believed to represent a conversion disorder, results in either inspiratory or expiratory stridor that may be confused with wheezing.[36] Congenital anomalies should be considered in infants less than 6 months old who present with stridor; such anomalies include vascular rings, laryngeal webs, vocal cord paralysis, and laryngomalacia.[20] Hypocalcemia, in addition to having neurologic, cardiovascular, and psychiatric manifestations, can also result in apnea, laryngeal spasm, bronchospasm, or biphasic respiratory noises and needs to be included in the differential diagnosis of any patient with respiratory distress.[1]

EMERGENCY DEPARTMENT EVALUATION

The goals of the emergency department evaluation are to reach a diagnosis quickly, with minimal stress on the patient, and to promptly begin appropriate therapy and monitoring. Assessing the degree of respiratory distress is important, but mild distress must not be underestimated, as some diseases or conditions can progress rapidly (e.g., epiglottitis). The initial evaluation begins when the physician enters the room, noting any visual and audible indicators of actual or possible respiratory compromise. The child in respiratory distress must be approached in a gentle, reassuring manner and allowed to find the most comfortable position, whether it be on the examining table or on a parent's lap. In the child who is alert and behaving normally, the evaluation can proceed with the history and physical examination. However, any child who has an altered mental status, or one who is irritable or restless, with other signs of distress, needs to have an immediate assessment of airway, breathing pattern, and circulatory status, the ABCs of resuscitation. Further assessment or therapeutic intervention follows this initial evaluation.

Important historic points include underlying medical problems (e.g., asthma, cystic fibrosis, or seizure disorder), the onset and type of current symptoms, and the possibility of a foreign-body aspiration or ingestion or poisoning. If epiglottitis is suspected, forced visualization of the pharynx should be avoided in the emergency department.[33] Although such attempts by Mauro and colleagues[24] in six patients did not lead to complications, forced visualization may result in a vasovagal response, causing cardiopulmonary collapse, respiratory obstruction, and death.[8] We recommend the traditional approach of taking the child with suspected epiglottitis to the operating room for direct visualization of the airway in the presence of personnel skilled in establishing the airway.

After the history and physical examination, the etiology of the respiratory distress is usually clear. Noninvasive monitoring can be used to help with clinical assessment. Pulse oximetry provides a continuous, generally valid measure of the arterial hemoglobin oxygenation status and arterial pulse. Obtaining blood gas measurements stress an already distressed child, and should therefore generally be avoided early in the evaluation.

Sometimes, the diagnosis may not be obvious from the history and examination, and further evaluation may be needed. In situations in which aspiration of a foreign body is suspected, lateral and anteroposterior neck and/or chest x-rays should be obtained; if normal, either an assisted expiratory film, bilateral decubitus x-rays, or fluoroscopy should be done.[3] If the distinction between croup and epiglottitis is not obvious, and the child is stable and only mildly ill, a lateral neck radiograph with close monitoring has been traditionally viewed as appropriate. However, Ragosta and colleagues[30] found lateral neck films to be of limited value in the initial evaluation of suspected epiglottitis and recommend against their use.

Repeated evaluations at regular intervals, as well as noninvasive monitoring, are essential in any child presenting to the emergency department in respiratory distress. Once the diagnosis is determined and appropriate therapy instituted, the response to therapy must be constantly reassessed. Often, the best way to determine whether an adult or older child is improving is simply to ask, "Are you feeling better?" In the nonverbal or frightened child, however, the response to therapy must be assessed by using changes in clinical parameters. Repeated examinations, although difficult in busy emergency departments, can be lifesaving for the child in respiratory distress.

EMERGENCY DEPARTMENT MANAGEMENT

The importance of a gentle, nonthreatening approach cannot be overemphasized. Interventions of any sort are usually poorly tolerated by young children and, at least temporarily, may result in a worsening of their condition. The benefit of any intervention must always be weighed against its potential for adversely affecting the child.

Management of the child in respiratory distress generally involves two goals: keeping the patient as calm and comfortable as possible, and providing appropriate therapy. Therapy begins with humidified oxygen. Infants and some children often do not tolerate masks well, and depending on their oxygen requirement, may best be served with blow-by oxygen administered by the parent. In addition to the physical examination, pulse oximetry is useful in following the oxygenation status. Normal pulse oximetry readings have been reported as 91.5% to 100% in awake infants 6 months and younger,[25] and 96% to 100% (median, 99.5%) in asleep children 2 to 16 years of age.[27] If the anxiety produced by the administration of oxygen to children in mild distress worsens their condition, then the oxygen is clearly doing more harm than good and should be avoided. However, the anxiety elicited by the administration of oxygen is usually transient. An attempt at oxygen delivery should be made for all children in respiratory distress, except, perhaps, for the rare patient with chronic obstructive pulmonary disease (COPD). For severely distressed or cyanotic patients, 100% humidified oxygen must be provided quickly, irrespective of their acceptance.

The next step in management is to provide disease-specific therapy. Common diagnoses that respond to specific medical therapy include croup, asthma, and bronchiolitis. Children presenting with croup and stridor at rest can be provided a trial of humidified air. However, a beneficial effect of mist therapy on the upper airway edema found with croup has not been established.[9,23] Steroids, given orally, parenterally, or via nebulizer, have been shown to be effective in the management of croup.[9,23] A single oral dose of dexamethasone (0.15 mg/kg) significantly reduced the need for follow-up in children discharged from an emergency department with mild croup; 16.7% of the placebo group required additional medical care versus 0% of the steroid group.[10] In patients with moderately severe croup, parenteral dexamethasone and, to a lesser extent, nebulized budesonide were shown to provide clinical improvement; both significantly reduced hospital admissions.[15] For severe croup, nebulized epinephrine can rapidly relieve distress, but its effect lasts only 1 to 3 hours.[32] Either racemic epinephrine or L-epinephrine can be used, the latter having been shown to be as safe and effective as the more commonly prescribed racemic form.[38] Although nebulized epinephrine's activity is short lived, studies indicate that when it is used with steroids (e.g., dexamethasone, 0.6 mg/kg, intramuscularly or orally), patients can be safely discharged home after 2 to 4 hours if clinically well (e.g., without retractions and stridor at rest).[16,18,19,29,32] Caution should be used when employing nebulized epinephrine if epiglottitis is suspected, as it may precipitate airway obstruction.[17]

The mainstays of therapy for acute asthma are inhaled beta-adrenergic bronchodilators and corticosteroids, either orally or parenterally.[37] Anticholinergic agents, widely recognized as important therapy for chronic asthma and COPD, have been shown to be effective for asthma exacerbations as well.[2] Combining a nebulized anticholinergic agent with a beta-adrenergic agent appears to provide better bronchodilation than either drug alone.[26]

Although the effectiveness of inhaled bronchodilators in the management of bronchiolitis is controversial, an initial trial of inhaled beta-adrenergic agents is recommended.[37,39] In addition, Reijonen and colleagues[31] found nebulized racemic epinephrine to be safe and useful.

DISPOSITION

The disposition of the child in moderate-to-severe distress depends on the hospital's capacity to accommodate the patient's needs. Often, an inpatient pediatric floor or a pediatric intensive care unit (PICU) is required.

For the stable child in moderate distress, admission to an inpatient pediatric floor is appropriate. When there is a concern that the patient may deteriorate due to the particular disease process (e.g., anaphylaxis) or medical history (e.g., an asthmatic previously requiring intubation), admission to a PICU should be considered. If necessary, transfer to the nearest hospital having a PICU should be arranged in accordance with federal guidelines. The transfer should done by personnel skilled in airway management (i.e., an advanced cardiac life-support unit or the pediatric transfer team of the receiving hospital). Ground transport is adequate for the stable child in only moderate distress.

Any child in severe distress should be admitted to a PICU. If transfer is necessary, consideration should be given to intubating and stabilizing the airway before departure, rather than risk deterioration and the need for a potentially difficult intubation en route. Transfer by ground units with personnel skilled in airway management is adequate for most patients in severe distress. However, the need for ground versus air transport must always be individualized.

COMMON PITFALLS

- Taking a blood pressure before giving therapy to the well-perfused patient
- Starting an intravenous line not needed for initial therapy[22]
- Forcing oxygen on the child in mild distress who will not tolerate it
- Obtaining blood for blood gas analysis in a severely distressed patient before providing therapy
- Doing a detailed history and physical examination before intervening in the severely distressed child[22]

- Not allowing the patient to assume a comfortable poistion[22]
- Misinterpreting decompensation for improvement
- During pulse oximetry monitoring, determining a sleeping infant to be hypoxic without further evaluating him or her in an awake state

References

1. Abrunzo TJ. An infant fatality associated with inspiratory and expiratory wheezing: another wheeze that wasn't asthma. *Pediatr Emerg Care* 1995;11:48.
2. Beakes DE. The use of anticholinergics in asthma. *J Asthma* 1997;34:357.
3. Brownstein DR. Foreign bodies of the gastrointestinal tract and airway. In: Barkin RM, ed. *Pediatric emergency medicine concepts and clinical practice,* 2nd ed. St. Louis: Mosby–Year Book, 1997:371.
4. Chameides L, Hazinski MF, eds. *Pediatric advanced life support.* Dallas: American Heart Association, American Academy of Pediatrics, 1997.
5. Davis HW, Gartner JC, Galvis AG, et al. Acute upper airway obstruction: croup and epiglottitis. *Pediatr Clin North Am* 1981;28:859.
6. Edwards KH, Johnston C. Allergic and immunologic disorders In: Barkin RM, ed. *Pediatric emergency medicine concepts and clinical practice,* 2nd ed. St. Louis: Mosby–Year Book, 1997:619.
7. Fleisher GR. Infectious disease emergencies. In: Fleischer GR, Ludwig S, eds. *Textbook of pediatric emergency medicine,* 3rd ed. Baltimore: William & Wilkins, 1993:613.
8. Fulginiti VA. Acute supraglottitis (epiglottitis): to look or not? *Am J Dis Child* 1988;142:597.
9. Geelhoed GC. Croup. *Pediatr Pulmonol* 1997;23:370.
10. Geelhoed GC, Turner J, MacDonald WBG. Efficacy of a small single dose of oral dexamethasone for outpatient croup: a double blind placebo controlled clinical trial. *BMJ* 1996;313:140.
11. Hammerschlag PE, Hammerschlag MR. Peritonsillar, retropharyngeal, and parapharyngeal abscesses. In: Feigin RD, Cherry JD, eds. *Textbook of pediatric infectious diseases,* vol 1, 4th ed. Philadelphia: WB Saunders, 1998:164.
12. Helfaer MA, Nichols DG , Rogers MC. Developmental physiology of the respiratory system. In: Rogers MC, ed. *Textbook of pediatric intensive care,* 3rd ed. Baltimore: Williams & Wilkins, 1996:98.
13. Hickerson SL, Kirby RS, Wheeler JG, et al. Epiglottis: a 9-year case review. *South Med J* 1996;89:487.
14. Hooker EA, Danzl DF, Brueggmeyer M, et al. Respiratory rates in pediatric emergency patients. *J Emerg Med* 1992;10:407.
15. Jonson DW, Jacobson S, Edney PC, et al. A comparison of nebulized budesonide, intramuscular dexamethasone, and placebo for moderately severe croup. *N Engl J Med* 1998;339:498.
16. Kelly PB, Simon JE. Racemic epinephrine use in croup and disposition. *Am J Emerg Med* 1992;10:181.
17. Kissoon N, Mitchel I. Adverse effects of racemic epinephrine in epiglottitis. *Pediatr Emerg Care* 1985;1:143.
18. Kunkel NC, Baker MD. Use of racemic epinephrine, dexamethasone, and mist in the outpatient management of croup. Pediatr Emerg Care 1996;12:156.
19. Ledwith CA, Shea LM, Mauro RD. Safety and efficacy of nebulized racemic epinephrine in conjunction with oral dexamethasone and mist in the outpatient treatment of croup. *Ann Emerg Med* 1995;25:331.
20. Letourneau MA, Schuh S, Gausche M. Respiratory disorders. In: Barkin RM, ed. *Pediatric emergency medicine concepts and clinical practice,* 2nd ed. St. Louis: Mosby–Year Book, 1997:1056.
21. Losek JD, Dewitz-Zink BA, Melzer-Lange M, et al. Epiglottitis: comparison of signs and symptoms in children less than 2 years old and older. *Ann Emerg Med* 1990;19:55–58.
22. Luten R. Respiratory distress. In: Harwood-Nuss A, Linden C, Shepherd S, et al., eds. *The clinical practice of emergency medicine.* Philadelphia: JB Lippincott Co, 1991:681.
23. MacDonald WBG, Geelhoed GC. Management of childhood croup. *Thorax* 1997;52:757.
24. Mauro RD, Poole SR, Lockhart CH. Differentiation of epiglottitis from laryngotracheitis in the child with stridor. *Am J Dis Child* 1988;142:679.
25. Mok JYQ, McLaughlin J, Pintar M, et al. Transcutaneous monitoring of oxygenation: what is normal? *J Pediatr* 1986;108:365.
26. Nichols DG. Emergency management of status asthmaticus in children. *Pediatr Ann* 1996;25:394.
27. Poets CF, Stebbens VA, Samuels MP, et al. Oxygen saturation and breathing patterns in children. *Pediatrics* 1993;92:686.
28. Poole SR, Mauro RD, Fan LL, et al. The child with simultaneous stridor and wheezing. *Pediatr Emerg Care* 1990;6:33.
29. Prendergast M, Jones JS, Hartman D. Racemic epinephrine in the treatment of laryngotracheitis: can we identify children for outpatient therapy? *Am J Emerg Med* 1994;12:613.
30. Ragosta KG, Orr R, Detweiler MJ. Revisiting epiglottis: a protocol—the value of lateral neck radiographs. *J Am Osteopath Assoc* 1997;97:227.
31. Reijonen T, Korppi M, Pitkäkangas S, et al. The clinical efficacy of nebulized racemic epinephrine and albuterol in acute bronchiolitis. *Arch Pediatr Adolesc Med* 1995;149:686.
32. Rizos JD, DiGravio BE, Sehl MJ, et al. The disposition of children with croup treated with racemic epinephrine and dexamethasone in the emergency department. *J Emerg Med* 1998;16:535.
33. Ruddy RM. Respiratory distress in a child in the office. *Pediatr Emerg Care* 1990;6:314.
34. Saipe C. Respiratory emergencies in children. *Pediatr Ann* 1990;19:637
35. Schroeder LL, Knapp JF. Recognition and emergency management of infectious causes of upper airway obstruction in children. *Semin Respir Infect* 1995;10:21.
36. Snyder HS, Weiss E. Hysterical stridor: a benign cause of upper airway obstruction. *Ann Emerg Med* 1989;18:1991.
37. Stempel DA, Redding G. Management of acute asthma. *Pediatr Clin North Am* 1992;39:1311.
38. Waisman Y, Klein BL, Boenning DA, et al. Prospective randomized double-blind study comparing L-epinephrine and racemic epinephrine aerosols in the treatment of laryngotracheitis (croup). *Pediatrics* 1992;89:302.
39. Welliver JR, Welliver RC. Bronchiolitis. *Pediatr Rev* 1993;14:134.

CHAPTER 256
Seizures

Christopher S. Kennedy

A seizure in a child can be a dramatic event, provoking fear and panic in parents and caregivers. The majority of parents will bring their child to the emergency department (ED) for evaluation, even if the child has seemed to fully recover. The initial step in this process requires determining whether the seizure has stopped and whether the child has returned to his or her prior neurologic baseline. If the child is continuing to have seizure activity on arrival to the ED, stopping the seizure is the first priority.

A seizure is a series of excessive, abnormal electrical discharges from cerebral neurons that produce transient involuntary alterations in functioning, including consciousness, motor activity, behavior, and/or autonomic regulation. Affecting 4% to 6% of children by age 16, seizures are the most common childhood neurologic disorder. The incidence is highest in newborns, and higher in childhood than in later life.

During seizure activity, consumption of oxygen and glucose is increased in cerebral tissues. Early physiologic changes include hypertension, hyperglycemia, and hypoxemia. With subsequent or prolonged seizure activity, progressive lactic acidosis, rhabdomyolysis, hyperkalemia, hyperthermia, and hypoglycemia may develop, leading to possible permanent neurologic damage.

Most childhood seizures are brief and isolated, and they have a good outcome. In some children, seizures are prolonged and recurrent. *Status epilepticus,* defined as recurrent or continuous seizure activity that lasts longer than 30 minutes without recovery of baseline mental functioning, is one of the most common neurologic emergencies encountered in children. Because seizures are one of the more common pediatric symptoms that lead to an ED visit, and stopping the seizure and its complications is time dependent to prevent sequelae, the ED physician should be familiar with all aspects of seizure management. These aspects include initial stabilization, primary investigation of cause, acute management, and disposition.

CLINICAL PRESENTATION

The single most important clinical finding when a child presents with a seizure is whether there is ongoing seizure activity. Seizures are classified as either generalized or partial. Generalized seizures may be convulsive or nonconvulsive and may manifest with an altered level of consciousness and with or without bilateral motor activity. Partial seizures may be simple, without affecting consciousness; or complex, with impaired mental status. In the ED, ongoing seizures may manifest with a wide array of clinical presentations, from tonic, clonic, tonic–clonic, or myoclonic activity; or by clouding of, or loss of, consciousness; eye deviations; repetitive, stereotyped movements; or by isolated behavioral changes, such as continuous crying or bicycling movements seen in infants. Whether the child responds to a caregiver's presence or voice can also be a useful clinical clue.

If the seizure has already stopped, additional related clinical findings include presence of a postictal phase, loss of bowel and/or bladder control, or focal neurologic deficit. A hemiparesis or other focal neurologic deficit (without signs of increased intracranial pressure [ICP]), also called a Todd's paralysis, is an important localizing sign and suggests that the seizure had a focal onset. If it is new and persists, a structural cause for the seizure should be sought. Fever is the most common cause of seizures in childhood; discussion of febrile seizures follows in a subsequent section. Clinical signs of neurologic disease or remote neurologic events that predispose a child to seizures include skin findings associated with neurocutaneous disorders (such as ash leaf spots or adenoma sebaceum, suggesting tuberous sclerosis; café-au-lait spots, suggesting neurofibromatosis; or port-wine staining of the face, suggesting Sturge-Weber syndrome), microcephaly, dysmorphic features, spasticity, hemiplegia, or quadriplegia. Stroke, increased ICP, or meningitis may be associated with acute clinical findings such as hemiparesis, papilledema and bulging fontanelle, or stiff neck. Unexplained superficial bruising should raise the suspicion of a bleeding disorder or child abuse.

TABLE 256.1. Acute Causes of Seizures by Age

NEONATAL
Birth injury and congenital abnormalities
Metabolic disorders (e.g., hypoglycemia, hyponatremia)
Inborn error of metabolism
Infections
Epilepsy (e.g., infantile spasms)
Pyridoxine deficiency
EARLY CHILDHOOD
Past birth-related injury
Febrile convulsions (6 mo to 6 yr)
Infections
Metabolic disorders
Neurocutaneous syndromes
Cerebral degenerative disorders
Tumors
Head trauma (shaking or direct injury)
Epilepsy
CHILDREN AND ADOLESCENTS
Head trauma
Infection
Epilepsy (± medication noncompliance)
Cerebral degenerative disorders
Tumors
Idiopathic
ANY AGE GROUP
Ventriculoperitoneal shunt malfunction or infection
Toxins
Pesticides, phenothiazines, phencyclidine
Lidocaine, lindane, lithium
Alcohol, amphetamines, antihistamines, antidepressants, anticholinergics
Salicylates
Theophylline
Insulin, isoniazid, Inderal
Camphor, caffeine, carbon monoxide, cocaine

DIFFERENTIAL DIAGNOSIS

A seizure is not a diagnosis but a clinical symptom of an underlying disease or process with many potential causes, which vary with age (Table 256.1). Other entities that may be confused with seizures include underlying neurologic disease, such as spasticity, and acute dystonic reactions, neither of which has associated loss of consciousness. A detailed history of the seizure event from a witness is the single most important feature for accurate diagnosis. It is important to determine whether the child has actually had a seizure, because many childhood conditions can easily be mistaken for a seizure. These disorders can be classified by one of three presentations: sudden loss of consciousness, paroxysmal movements, or sudden change in behavior.

Disorders with sudden loss of consciousness include breath-holding spells, syncope, cardiac dysrhythmias, and complicated migraines, and each is differentiated from a seizure because a postictal state is rare. Breath-holding spells occur in two forms, cyanotic and pallid, usually in children between 6 months and 4 years of age. Cyanotic spells begin with vigorous crying, followed by apnea, cyanosis, and, occasionally, myoclonus. Pallid spells begin with a painful stimulus (even fear), followed by pallor and loss of consciousness. Vasovagal syncope, the most common cause of syncope in childhood, may be preceded by light-headedness and dizziness, followed by loss of consciousness. The loss of consciousness is brief, and recovery is rapid. Syncopal events from cardiac dysrhythmias are usually associated with a positive family history; they are characterized by a brief loss of consciousness, with myoclonic movements, and rapid recovery. Electrocardiographic (ECG) or Holter monitoring as an outpatient may be needed for confirmation. With complicated migraines, loss of consciousness may be associated with or preceded by blurred vision, blindness, dizziness, or loss of postural tone.

Disorders with paroxysmal movements include tics, shuddering attacks, benign sleep myoclonus, and pseudoseizures. These are differentiated from seizures because a loss of consciousness is rare. Tics are brief, stereotyped, nonrhythmic movements that may be precipitated by stress; usually, some voluntary control is exhibited. Shuddering attacks are characterized by rapid tremors of the entire body, which may occur up to 100 times a day. They are usually inherited, are self-limited, may be precipitated by stress, and may require an electroencephalogram (EEG) (which is normal) to convince the family that they are seizures. Benign sleep myoclonus usually presents in infancy with benign, self-limited, sudden, jerky movements of one or more extremity. Although more common when the child is falling asleep, they may occur throughout sleep. Pseudoseizures may be difficult to distinguish from seizures in the ED and may require video EEG monitoring for diagnosis. They present with paroxysmal movements, lack of coordination, and moaning or talking during the episode, and can even be seen in patients with a seizure disorder.

Disorders with sudden behavioral changes include night terrors. These are differentiated from seizures by their characteristic findings. Night terrors, a form of parasomnia, occurs in preschoolers, with sudden awakening from sleep with fits of crying, sweating, and rapid breathing, and there may be associated stereotyped movements.

EMERGENCY DEPARTMENT EVALUATION

History and physical examination are the most useful tools in ED evaluation. History should focus on a detailed description of the seizure and finding an acute cause of it, such as trauma, infection, recent immunization, or intoxication, and history of seizures and anticonvulsant use. Physical examination should search for signs of trauma, increased ICP, and meningeal irritation. Laboratory testing should be guided by the history and examination. Useful studies may include a rapid bedside glucose, serum electrolytes, calcium, magnesium and ammonia, a complete blood count (CBC), and a urine toxicology screen.

A lumbar puncture is not indicated for the nonfebrile child with a seizure, but should be considered in a neonate. Magnetic resonance imaging has become the imaging modality of choice for new-onset seizure in children, but it usually is not required on an emergent basis. Brain imaging studies for the ED patient at most institutions consist of a cranial computed tomography (CT) scan. Indications for CT in the ED include a focal deficit on neurologic examination, signs of increased ICP, an infant less than 12 months old (possible child abuse), patients with ventriculoperitoneal shunts, and suspected head trauma. EEG monitoring is rarely used emergently, except for refractory status or if a diagnosis of nonconvulsive status is considered (EEG may be the only way to accurately diagnose this disorder).

EMERGENCY DEPARTMENT MANAGEMENT

Seizure activity in the ED should be considered status epilepticus until further history can be obtained, and the main priorities should be resuscitation of the child and stopping the seizure. A brief history should focus on finding an acute cause of the seizure, such as trauma, infection, or intoxication, and history of seizures and anticonvulsant use. A rapid physical examination should search for signs of trauma, increased ICP, and meningeal irritation. If meningitis is a concern, appropriate antibiotics should be given.

Management of Status Epilepticus

The following protocol is suggested to manage status epilepticus.

0 to 5 minutes
- Maintain airway, give oxygen, support ventilation, and consider cervical spine immobilization for trauma patients.
- Obtain intravenous access, check bedside glucose, and send blood samples for electrolytes, CBC, glucose, and anticonvulsant levels.
- Monitor vital signs, pulse oximetry, and ECG.
- Consider intravenous glucose 2 mL/kg of D_{25}, and/or pyridoxine 100 mg for neonates (or isoniazid overdose).

At 5 to 15 minutes, if seizure continues
- Lorazepam 0.05 to 0.1 mg/kg intravenously, or diazepam 0.2 to 0.4 mg/kg intravenously; if no intravenous access, consider diazepam 0.5 to 1.0 mg/kg PR, or midazolam 0.2 mg/kg intramuscularly.
- Repeat up to two times every 5 minutes.

At 15 to 30 minutes, if seizure continues
- Fosphenytoin 15 to 20 mg phenytoin equivalents (PE)/kg intravenously or intramuscularly, not to exceed 150 mg PE/min; or phenytoin 15 to 20 mg/kg intravenously, not to exceed 1 mg/kg/min.
- Consider phenobarbital 15 to 20 mg/kg intravenously.
- Reevaluate airway and consider need for intubation.
- Check electrolyte results; consider need for intravenous hypertonic saline.

At beyond 30 minutes, if seizure continues
- Consider additional fosphenytoin 5 mg PE/kg or phenytoin.
- Consider consultation with neurologist. Discuss need for EEG monitoring.
- Contact pediatric intensivist to arrange transport and need for pentobarbital, midazolam, or propofol coma. Consider general anesthesia in consultation with an anesthesiologist.

At beyond 60 minutes, if seizure continues
- Begin alternative (coma) regimen and consider transfer to appropriate facility or location.

Brief Overview of Pharmacotherapy

First-line drugs for the management of status include benzodiazepines, fosphenytoin or phenytoin, and phenobarbital. Benzodiazepines are the current drugs of choice for initial management of status epilepticus, and should be used only in patients with active seizures. Lorazepam, diazepam, and midazolam may be used to manage status. Lorazepam is preferred for its longer half-life (24 hours). If diazepam is used initially, consideration should be given to an additional longer acting agent, such as fosphenytoin or phenytoin. Benzodiazepines cause respiratory depression and, in higher doses, may cause hypotension. Diazepam can be given rectally if intravenous access is not available. The rectal dose is 0.5 mg/kg, to a maximum dose of 20 mg, and is given via a short no. 8 feeding tube or a needleless 1-mL Tb syringe. Recently developed Diastat, a viscous solution for rectal administration, is available in prefilled, rectal-tipped syringes in a variety of doses.

Fosphenytoin or phenytoin is utilized if a seizure continues after benzodiazepine use. Fosphenytoin, a newly developed prodrug of phenytoin, is often preferred for use in children because it causes fewer side effects, such as respiratory depression and cardiac and tissue necrosis. Fosphenytoin can also be given intramuscularly if vascular access has not been established.

Phenobarbital is the drug of choice for neonatal seizures and for complex febrile seizures that are unresponsive to benzodiazepines. Noteworthy is the increased risk of respiratory depression when phenobarbital is given concomitantly with benzodiazepines.

DISPOSITION

Children with first-time seizure can be followed as outpatients if they appear well, the parents are comfortable with outpatient management, and follow-up can be assured. These children frequently do not require maintenance anticonvulsant therapy, but the decision to start therapy, and which agent to use, should be done in consultation with a pediatric neurologist and the primary care physician. Hospital admission is reserved for children with a prolonged seizure or status epilepticus, even if successfully treated in the ED. Children requiring intubation and ventilatory support or those with prolonged refractory status should be transported to a tertiary care facility with pediatric subspecialists.

FEBRILE SEIZURES

Febrile convulsions are the most common form of seizures in childhood, occurring in 2% to 5% of children. Generally, febrile seizures are defined by a seizure in association with a febrile illness, without central nervous system infection or electrolyte imbalance. They usually occur between the ages of 6 months and 6 years; peak incidence is approximately 18 months of age. Febrile seizures are classified as simple or complex. A febrile seizure is complex if it is focal, prolonged more than 15 minutes, or multiple (more than one seizure during the febrile illness). The majority of febrile seizures are simple febrile seizures that are brief, isolated, and generalized. Although the pathophysiology of febrile seizures remains unclear, it appears that the absolute peak temperature plays a key role. Mortality is extremely rare, and there are no differences in cognitive abilities after a febrile seizure, even when prolonged.

EVALUATION, MANAGEMENT AND DISPOSITION

To diagnose a febrile seizure, meningitis, encephalitis, electrolyte imbalances, and other acute neurologic disease must be ruled out. Most of these can be eliminated by a careful history or physical examination. In 1996, the American Academy of Pediatrics issued guidelines for the evaluation of children with simple febrile seizures who are between the ages of 6 months and 5 years. According to these guidelines, a lumbar puncture should strongly be considered in all infants less than 12 months of age, should be carefully considered in all children between 12 and 18 months, and should not be considered necessary in well-appearing children over 18 months, without symptoms of meningitis. Neuroimaging of any kind is not routinely required, and additional routine blood studies are of limited value. If the child arrives in the ED in apparent status from a febrile seizure, it should be treated as such. Benzodiazepines are the drugs of choice, but the most studied agent is diazepam, as discussed.

Other than evaluation and treatment of the underlying cause of the fever, the majority of cases will require only reassurance and education of parents about febrile seizures. Anticonvulsant prophylaxis is not routinely recommended.

COMMON PITFALLS

- Failure to address airway, breathing, and circulation as the first priority in status epilepticus management
- Failure to recognize and treat the underlying disease causing the seizure
- Failure to consider shaking or child abuse in young children
- Failure to diagnose meningitis in infants with a febrile seizure

Bibliography

American Academy of Pediatrics. Committee on Quality Improvement. Practice parameter: the neurodiagnostic evaluation of the child with a simple febrile seizure. *Pediatrics* 1996;97:769.

Dunn DW. Status epilepticus in infancy and childhood. *Neurol Clin North Am* 1990;8:647–658.

Liu Z, Yang Y, Silviera DC, et al. Consequences of recurrent seizures during early brain development. *Neuroscience* 1999;92(4):1443–1454.

Maytal J, Shinnar S. Status epilepticus in children. *Pediatr Adolesc Med* 1995;6:111.

Morton LD, Rizkallah E, Pellock JM. New drug therapy for acute seizure management. *Semin Pediatr Neurol* 1997;4:51.

Pellock JM. Status epilepticus. In: Swaiman KF, Ashwal S, eds. *Pediatric neurology: principles and practice,* 3rd ed. St. Louis: Mosby, 1999:683–691.

Shinnar S, Pellock JM, Berg AT, et al. An inception cohort of children with febrile status epilepticus: cohort characteristics and early outcomes. *Epilepsia* 1995;36[Suppl 4]:31.

CHAPTER 257
Vomiting

Anthony P. Pohlgeers

Vomiting is a common nonspecific complaint of children presenting to the emergency department. It can be a presenting finding in a variety of medical and surgical diagnoses. In determining a cause, a complete history and physical examination may be all that is required. Laboratory and radiologic studies may become useful to confirm a suspected diagnosis.

Vomiting in children is usually associated with a transient illness and has little clinical significance. However, it may also be a response to a serious or potentially life-threatening illness.[1] Initial treatment is usually directed at stabilization while the diagnosis is being made.

EMERGENCY DEPARTMENT EVALUATION AND DIFFERENTIAL DIAGNOSIS

Factors important in evaluating the patient with vomiting are age, appearance at presentation, and presence of associated symptoms. The majority of cases of vomiting are due to self-limiting infectious illness and can be diagnosed based on associated symptoms and physical findings. The patient's age is important when considering the differential diagnoses (see Table 257.1).

Birth to Three Months

In infants, the history should focus on the time of onset, the duration of vomiting, the description of the emesis, and any associated gastrointestinal or other complaints. Most commonly, gastroesophageal reflux (GER) presents during this time. Excess vomiting secondary to GER is a common cause of failure to thrive.[5] A majority of these infants present with regurgitation of formula or breast milk after feeds, clinically are in no distress, and are well appearing. As a result, they can be managed conservatively with cereal-thickened feedings and antireflux precautions.

This condition must be distinguished from hypertrophic pyloric stenosis (HPS). HPS usually presents with projectile vomiting of formula shortly after feeding and is typically well described by the parents (see Chapter 289) The classic presentation of the 3- to 6-week-old infant presenting with hypochloremic metabolic alkalosis and severe dehydration is no longer common. Earlier diagnosis with ultrasound results in earlier surgical repair and decreased morbidity.[3]

Other obstructive lesions to consider include duodenal and jejunal atresia as well as malrotation with midgut volvulus. These entities were typically seen in the newborn nursery but now are seen in the emergency department secondary to early hospital discharge. Infants with these conditions are typically ill appearing, have bilious vomiting, and have abdominal tenderness and various degrees of abdominal distention.[2] Plain radiographs may reveal a gasless abdomen. Rapid stabilization and surgical intervention are required.

Medical illness and metabolic disorders may also present with vomiting as an associated finding. Infectious illness such as pneumonia, sepsis, meningitis, and inborn errors of metabolism are examples. These diagnoses are usually suspected because of other associated symptoms and are confirmed with laboratory and radiologic evaluation.

TABLE 257.1. Life-Threatening Causes of Vomiting

NEWBORN (BIRTH TO 2 WK)
Anatomic anomalies—esophageal stenosis/atresia, intestinal obstructions (T.49.1.E), especially malrotation and volvulus, Hirschsprung's disease
Other GI causes (necrotizing enterocolitis, peritonitis)
Neurologic—kernicterus, mass lesions, hydrocephalus
Renal—obstructive anomalies, uremia
Infectious—sepsis, meningitis
Metabolism—inborn errors, especially congenital adrenal hyperplasia
OLDER INFANT (2 WK TO 12 MO)
Gastroesophageal reflux, severe
Esophageal disorders
Rumination
Intestinal obstruction (T. 49.1, II.E), especially pyloric stenosis, intussusception, incarcerated hernia
Other GI causes, especially gastroenteritis (with dehydration)
Neurologic—mass lesions, hydrocephalus
Renal—obstruction, uremia
Infectious—sepsis, meningitis, pertussis
Metabolic—inborn errors
Drugs—aspirin, theophylline, digoxin
OLDER CHILD (> 12 MO)
GI obstruction, especially intussusception (T49.1, III.A)
Other GI causes, especially appendicitis, peptic ulcer disease
Neurologic—mass lesions
Renal—uremia
Infectious—meningitis
Metabolic—diabetic ketoacidosis, Reye syndrome, adrenal insufficiency
Toxins, drugs—aspirin, ipecac, theophylline, digoxin, iron, lead
OLDER CHILD AND ADOLESCENT
Gastroenteritis
Appendicitis/peritonitis; pancreatitis
Reflex vomiting due to stimuli from GU tract; pyelonephritis; calculi
Labyrinthine disorders (e.g., motion sickness)
Metabolic disorders
Intracranial lesions
Migraine
Drugs and alcohol
Pregnancy
Ulcers
Functional or self-induced
CAUSES COMMON TO ALL AGE GROUPS
Head trauma
Intracranial infections or space-occupying lesions
Drug overdose
Chemotherapeutic agents and radiation
Intestinal obstruction
Food poisoning

Henntig FM, Vomiting. In: Fleisher G, Ludwig S eds. *Textbook of pediatric emergency medicine*. Baltimore: Williams & Wilkins, 1988:331.

Three Months to Two Years

The most common cause of vomiting in children 3 months to 2 years old is infectious gastroenteritis, most commonly of viral etiology. Fever and diarrhea typically accompany the vomiting. Presentation can vary from a well-appearing child (early) to a severely dehydrated one (late). Laboratory evaluation may direct therapy, especially when hyponatremia, hypernatremia, or hypoglycemia is present. Other medical conditions to consider, especially in the absence of diarrhea, include pneumonia, meningitis, and increased intracranial pressure.

Surgical causes in this age group include intussusception, incarcerated hernia, and volvulus. Intussusception is the most common surgical condition in this age group. This typically involves the child less than 1 year of age with paroxysmal, cramping abdominal pain, followed by vomiting and periods of lethargy. The classic triad of vomiting, currant jelly stools, and right-sided mass may be present in only 20% of cases. Physical examination may reveal a right sided mass (85%) and various degrees of distention.[2] Plain films may be nonspecific and, early in the illness, may be normal.[6] Because of this, a high index of suspicion, not laboratory findings or plain radiography, should direct the management. A contrast enema or air is commonly both diagnostic and therapeutic. Once the intussusception is reduced, admission for observation is indicated.

Older Child and Adolescent

The most common cause of vomiting in this age group is infectious gastroenteritis. A viral etiology is the most common of these cases. Fever and diarrhea typically accompany the vomiting. Dehydration as a complication of acute viral gastroenteritis is far less common in the older child and adolescent and, if present, should alert the physician to consider other diagnoses.

The most common surgical etiology of vomiting is acute appendicitis. Associated symptoms include migrating pain to the right lower quadrant, associated anorexia, and low-grade fever. In addition, diarrhea has been noted to be present in 16% of patients.[4] However, especially in the child less than 6 years old, the typical findings are not always present and the physical examination is often difficult. Consequently, the diagnosis is often missed in the child less than 6 years of age.[4] The physical examination may prove more reliable in the older child. A high index of suspicion is based on the history and physical examination. Laboratory or radiographic evidence may be used to support the diagnosis, but normal studies are common. Surgical consultation is indicated with positive physical findings.

Other causes of vomiting in the adolescent include pregnancy, pelvic inflammatory disease, undiagnosed diabetic ketoacidosis, and self-induced vomiting (bulimia). These entities can usually be confirmed with history, examination, and supportive laboratory evaluation.

EMERGENCY DEPARTMENT MANAGEMENT

Regardless of the etiology of the vomiting, the initial management of the patient should include a rapid cardiopulmonary assessment and a determination of the stability of the patient. The management is then guided by these findings. The unstable patient may require fluid resuscitation while a diagnostic evaluation is being completed. Certain rapid diagnostic tests may be indicated, based on suspicion of illness. For example, in a lethargic vomiting child less than 3 months of age, a rapid determination of serum glucose is indicated. In a child with moderate-to-severe dehydration, an infusion of 20 mL/kg of crystalloid solution is given and the patient is reassessed. Dextrose-containing fluids should not be used in the initial fluid resuscitation. If hypoglycemia is present, a separate infusion of dextrose should be administered. If the patient's clinical appearance and physical examination are suspicious for an obstructive lesion, surgical consultation should proceed prior to return of laboratory values or radiologic studies.

Antiemetics are contraindicated, except when used for predictable, limited causes (e.g., chemotherapy, motion sickness). Most antiemetics have variable, unpredictable side effects, and, more importantly, the cessation of vomiting may lead to a delay in diagnosis of a life-threatening condition (e.g., meningitis).

DISPOSITION

Admission to the hospital should be considered for children with vomiting and dehydration who require intravenous fluid boluses and for children with suspected but unproven surgical etiologies. Patients admitted for observation should be made NPO if a surgical diagnosis is being ruled out. Children that are discharged home should have explicit instructions regarding when to return for reevaluation.

COMMON PITFALLS

- Vomiting in the infant may be due to overfeeding.
- Plain radiographs of the abdomen may be normal in early intussusception.
- Diarrhea can be present with acute appendicitis.
- Antiemetics should be used with caution, especially in young children.

References

1. Crain EF, Gershel JC, Gallagher EH. *Clinical manual of emergency pediatrics*. New York: McGraw-Hill, 1992.
2. Irish MS, Pearl RH, Caty MG, et al. The approach to common abdominal diagnoses in infants and children. *Pediatr Clin North Am* 1998; 45:729.
3. Papadakis K, Chen EA, Luks FI, et al. The changing presentation of pyloric stenosis. *Am J Emerg Med* 1999;17:67–69.
4. Rothrock SG. When appendicitis isn't classic. *Emerg Med* 1996;00:108–124.
5. Rowe MI, O'Neill JA, Grosfeld JL, et al., eds. *Essentials of pediatric surgery*. St. Louis, Mosby–Year Book, 1995.
6. Swischuk LE. *Emergency imaging of the acutely ill or injured child,* 3rd ed. Baltimore: Williams & Wilkins, 1994.

PART III

Specific Diseases

CHAPTER 258

Abuse: Sexual

J. M. Whitworth

Until recent years, sexual abuse in children was considered an uncommon problem. It is now clear that sexual abuse or sexual molestation affects at least one in four girls and one in seven boys before age 18.[7] The short- and long-term physical and psychological effects of sexual abuse depend on many factors, including the severity of the abuse, the length of time of involvement, the relationship of the abuser to the child, and the sensitivity of intervening professionals and family members after the problem has come to light.

The needs of sexually abused children differ from the needs of sexually assaulted adults. Although children are sometimes raped, the usual case is characterized by a long-term process perpetrated by an older person who is well known to the child, and results in totally different evidentiary, evaluation, and treatment approaches. The "child sexual abuse accommodation syndrome" describes characteristics seen in these children and points out the challenges in approaching child victimization, as compared with adults. Children are gradually entrapped in a secret arrangement with a trusted adult or adolescent and feel helpless. They accommodate to the abuse and often display delayed and conflicting disclosure, followed by retraction of the allegation.[25] A specially trained professional interviewer is needed to begin addressing these specific issues often seen in children.

The emergency department response to sexual abuse of children must address the child's medical needs and must be equally considerate of his or her psychological needs. The emergency department visit can serve as the first step in a therapeutic process. The forensic examination is a small part of a multidisciplinary effort to evaluate and protect the child; the examiner must have the time, effort, and skill to minimize the traumatic aspects of the encounter. If such a commitment cannot be ensured, the emergency department should consider referring cases to another facility for evaluation.

CLINICAL PRESENTATION

A few child sexual abuse cases present to the emergency department as a medical emergency, usually with a history of genital bleeding or clinical suggestions of acute abdominal trauma or peritoneal irritation. In these cases, matters of evidence collection, forensic evaluation, and reporting are secondary to the need for immediate intervention to stabilize the child's condition. Resuscitation takes precedence.

More typically, patients present in one of two ways. First, the child may present with a chief complaint of sexual abuse by personal report or because of a caretaker's suspicion. Second, the child may present with a seemingly unrelated chief complaint, and the examiner suspects sexual abuse because of findings in the history or physical examination.

The approach to these presentations may be different, but the examiner's immediate reaction should always be the same. After an assessment to determine whether there are immediate medical needs, a team of professionals must become involved to obtain a detailed interview, to recommend and perform necessary interventions, and to ensure the child's safety. Psychosocial assessment and treatment plans must be addressed early in case development. This requires the involvement of the local child protection agency, law enforcement, and, ideally, a multidisciplinary child protection team in the community.[2,3]

Whenever sexual abuse is suspected, the health-care professional must make a report to child protective services or to a law enforcement agency in the community.[23] Local and state laws determine the physician's responsibility for reporting.

EMERGENCY DEPARTMENT EVALUATION

History

In the sexually abused child, the medical history is separate from the detailed interview. The medical history focuses on the information necessary to make a diagnosis, determine assessment needs, determine public health issues, and plan treatment. Taking a medical history should not be seen as an opportunity to do a detailed interview, unless there is no other resource available in the community.

The exact history and source of the information should be clearly recorded in the chart. If possible, the history should come from the child to ensure greatest reliability. It should be taken in the least threatening environment possible; adequate time must be taken to develop rapport with the child. Generally, the child should be interviewed alone. The examiner must spend enough time with the child to ascertain his or her names for body parts and bodily functions. If the child volunteers specific information, it is recorded as direct quotes. Information gathered from others is considered hearsay. Questions must be presented in a format that does not lead the child; if a question can be answered "yes" or "no," it is probably leading. If the child says nothing, this fact should be recorded in the chart, documenting that the child was asked to give information about the case.

The history should also include an assessment of evidence for other kinds of abuse, family violence, and any other significant medical problems.

The decision as to the type and extent of medical intervention should be made by a health-care professional. It should not be based on the supposed needs of the legal system or a child protection agency. This medical responsibility for protecting the child cannot be abrogated to others who may not understand the potential trauma of a forensic examination in a child.

Physical Examination

Before the examination, the child should be told what to expect, and he or she should receive constant reassurance during the procedure.

The examination of the genitalia of a sexually abused child should always be done in the context of a complete standard pediatric physical examination. This approach is necessary to ensure that other significant problems are documented and addressed, and it is also necessary to reassure the child that he or she has been completely examined by a health professional and is intact. Abused children generally perceive themselves as "damaged goods."

Abnormal findings should never be reported in the child's presence. Likewise, assurances by the physician that the child is not at fault and is believed are remembered by the child long after the minor trauma of the examination has faded. The physician should approach the child in a warm, friendly, age-appropriate manner and should not engage in extensive play or subterfuge to accomplish the examination, because playing games and subterfuges are often approaches used by an abuser.

If the child will not or cannot cooperate, the examination can be done at another time or in another place. With adequate preparation and patience, examination under anesthesia or with sedation is rarely necessary.

In a busy emergency department, an examination for sexual abuse of a child may have unanticipated negative effects. Other patients and the procedures performed on them may frighten the child. The examination should be done in a quiet environment. A support figure—never the suspected abuser—should be present and should be selected by the child. Blood samples, if necessary, can be obtained shortly after the examination.

The examination of the genitalia of a prepubertal child is primarily a process of description and observation based on a knowledge of normal structures and deviations from normal. A child's genitalia differ in appearance from adult structures, so review of a standard pediatric gynecology reference is essential.[24]

Proper positioning of the child for a genital examination varies depending on the child's age, comfort, and degree of cooperation. An adequate examination can be performed with a small child on the mother's lap. Preferable positions, from the examiner's viewpoint, are the knee–chest and frog-leg positions. In the frog-leg position, direct inspection and moderate downward and outward pressure on the labia majora allow adequate visualization of all structures germane to the examination. In the knee–chest position, structures can usually be visualized directly without pressure or traction on the labia, but this position is often difficult to accomplish because it makes the child feel more vulnerable.

There are significant differences in the appearance of normal anatomic structures in different positions, as well as with different degrees of relaxation in the same child. For this reason, only findings that clearly indicate scarring from trauma, consistent changes in reflex response, or active infection should be considered definitive.

Invasion with a speculum or digit is seldom necessary or helpful, except in much older children or children who are sexually active. Cultures or specimen collection should be done with the smallest swab available. Inspection of the labia and introitus should include attention to evidence of old or new lacerations or abrasions.

Hymenal configuration should be noted and may be described as annular, crescentic, cribriform, septate, or imperforate.[13] Congenital absence of the hymen does not occur.[15] Thickness of the membrane should be described, along with any scarring located, and recorded as related to the face of a clock. The hymenal opening diameter in lateral and anteroposterior aspects is carefully measured and recorded. In the past, the lateral hymenal diameter was considered extremely important in making the diagnosis of sexual abuse or molestation, but currently, this measurement seems less important than evidence of chronic scarring or acute injury.

If the vaginal canal can be visualized, a description of general appearance, rugous folds, and any scars may be important.

Abnormalities in the prepubertal child fall into several categories[1,6,13,14,18–21]:

1. Findings diagnostic of sexual abuse
   a. Presence of sperm or semen in a prepubertal child
   b. Presence of a sexually transmitted disease with no reasonable possibility of nonsexual transmission (i.e., gonorrhea, syphilis)
   c. Witnessed or photographically documented sexual abuse with or without physical findings
2. Findings diagnostic of penetration and consistent with a history of sexual abuse
   a. Healed or fresh vaginal tear
   b. Healed or fresh hymenal tear
   c. Missing section(s) of hymen in the posterior half
   d. Fresh or healed rectal tears
   e. Immediate reflex anal dilatation (greater than 20 mm) in the absence of stool in the ampulla
3. Findings diagnostic of genital trauma (insult) and consistent with a history of sexual abuse
   a. Microlacerations of the posterior fourchette
   b. Abrasions of the fossa navicularis or perihymenal tissues
   c. Bruises of genital tissues
   d. Presence of other sexually transmitted diseases (a disease not exclusively sexually transmitted, such as chlamydia or herpes)
   e. Rectal fissures
4. Findings that neither support nor negate an allegation of sexual abuse
   a. Redness or irritation of the genital area
   b. Agglutination of the labia minora
   c. Variations in the vascular pattern seen without attendant scars
   d. Enlargement of the hymenal opening
   e. Attenuated hymen without scarring
   f. Vaginitis (other than sexually transmitted diseases)

In cases of documented sexual abuse, definite physical findings are present in only about 50% to 60%; this is also true in many cases of known penetration.[22] The physical examination, therefore, can never be used to negate an allegation of sexual abuse.

Findings should be recorded, for future reference, on a standard anatomic chart. Color photography is strongly recommended but is not always readily available in the emergency department.

When reaching a conclusion, external pressures always suggest that a definitive "yes" or "no" answer is necessary. This is not always possible, and the examiner should not be tempted to make definitive statements if the history and physical examination are not definitive. The physician may conclude that the examination is diagnostic of sexual abuse, consistent with sexual abuse, or neither confirms nor negates a history of sexual abuse. The examiner will probably be asked to support his or her conclusions at a later date.

Laboratory Evaluation

Useful forensic evidence is almost never found beyond 72 hours after an assault. If forensic evidence collection is needed, an evidence collection packet must be sought from local law enforcement sources, and the physician must be knowledgeable about the use of the kit before doing the examination. Thorough training in maintaining the chain of evidence and evidence collection techniques is mandatory and varies from jurisdiction to jurisdiction. Training is available from adult sexual assault centers or from police departments.

Sexual abuse victims must always be assessed for sexually transmitted diseases, but the extent of the search is a matter of clinical judgment. Cultures for *Neisseria gonorrhoeae* should be obtained from all prepubertal patients from the vagina, rectum, and throat, assuming a reasonable history or finding that suggests potential transmission. Cultures for *Chlamydia trachomatis* are useful if facilities are available. The use of screening or presumptive tests for chlamydia or gonorrhea is not recommended.[12]

Wet mounts are done with anogenital discharges, and darkfield examinations are done on genital ulcers. Viral cultures for herpes simplex are indicated with vesicular lesions, and routine bacteriologic cultures should be done in all patients with a demonstrable discharge. The utility of cultures for herpes and human papillomavirus in determining sexual transmission is limited. Routine serologic tests for syphilis should not be done unless there are clinical indications.

Human immunodeficiency virus transmission can occur with sexual abuse but is uncommon. Routine testing is not recommended but should be available for any patient with high-risk exposure, or on request.[9] There are compelling clinical reasons for testing only in a setting where adequate preparation and follow-up with counseling services are provided.

EMERGENCY DEPARTMENT MANAGEMENT

The first priority is to alleviate any urgent or life-threatening medical needs. Subsequent treatment should be responsive to time-sensitive evidence collection and the treatment of sexually transmitted diseases. Presumptive treatment is never advisable; treatment should be undertaken only after definitive culture evidence exists or when there are life-threatening infectious disease issues.

In selecting treatment choices, the physician should always seek a history of drug sensitivity and should be familiar with the expected sensitivity of organisms in the community. Treatment recommendations are shown in Table 258.1.[5,8,10]

TABLE 258.1. Treatment Recommendations for Children Who Have Contracted a Sexually Transmitted Disease through Sexual Abuse

Agent	Drug	Dosage
Neisseria gonorrhoeae	Ceftriaxone	125 mg i.m.
	or	
	Azithromycin	1 g PO if ≥45 kg
Herpes genitalis	Acyclovir	400 mg PO t.i.d. for 7–10 d
Chlamydia trachomatis	Erythromycin ethylsuccinate	50 mg/kg/d for 10 d
	or	
	Azithromycin	1 g PO if ≥45 kg
Treponema pallidum	Benzathine penicillin G	50,000 U/kg i.m. (max, 2.4 million units)
Trichomonas vaginalis	Metronidazole	15 mg/kg/d divided t.i.d. for 7 d, or 40 mg/kg (max, 2 g) as a single dose

Data from Barone[5] and Committee on Infectious Diseases, American Academy of Pediatrics.[8]

COMMON PITFALLS

- The examiner should not become confused when a child recants a history of sexual abuse. This phenomenon is common and often results from fear, parental coaching, the observed response of authority figures, or the realization that intervention may result in jail for a family member or family separation. Recantation is so common that it does not necessarily interfere with prosecution or with therapy for the patient. Documentation of the emergency department visit assumes greater importance in these cases.
- Investigators may think that the absence of physical findings means that sexual abuse did not occur or that a case cannot be prosecuted. This is contrary to current knowledge and experience with sexually abused children and can actually lead to further victimization. Because a child's disclosure of sexual abuse is generally accurate, and because serious sexual abuse can occur without physical findings, the history is the critical piece of evidence. The absence of physical findings does not hinder the ability to obtain a conviction.[9,16,22]
- The examiner must record all data, because he or she may need to recall the information in detail months or years later in a courtroom. Meticulous attention to detail in the examination and in the recording of the history and examination findings is essential to minimize this problem.

References

1. Adams JA, Harper K, Knudsen S. A proposed system for the classification of anogenital findings in children with suspected sexual abuse. *Adolesc Pediatr Gynecol* 1992;5:73.
2. American Academy of Pediatrics Committee on Child Abuse and Neglect. Guidelines for the evaluation of sexual abuse of children. *Pediatrics* 1991;87:254.
3. *AMA guidelines for the evaluation of child sexual abuse*. Chicago: American Medical Association, 1992.
4. Atabaki S, Paradise JE. The medical evaluation of the sexually abused child: lessons from a decade of research. *Pediatrics* 1999;104:178.
5. Barone MA, ed. *The Harriet Lane handbook,* 14th ed. St. Louis: Mosby–Year Book, 1996.
6. Berenson A, Heger A, Hayes J, et al. Appearance of the hymen in prepubertal girls. *Pediatrics* 1992;89:387.
7. Berkowitz CD. Child sexual abuse. *Pediatr Rev* 1992;13:443.
8. Committee on Infectious Diseases, American Academy of Pediatrics. *Report of the Committee on Infectious Diseases (red book),* 24th ed. Elk Grove Village, IL: American Academy of Pediatrics, 1997.
9. DeJong A, Rose M. Legal proof of child sexual abuse in the absence of physical evidence. *Pediatrics* 1991;88:506.
10. Gellert G, Durfee M, Berkowitz C, et al. Situational and sociodemographic characteristics of children infected with HIV from pediatric sexual abuse. *Pediatrics* 1993;91:39.
11. Hammerschlag M. Sexually transmitted diseases in sexually abused children. *Adv Pediatr Infect Dis* 1988;3:1.
12. Hammerschlag MR, Rettig PJ, Shields ME. False-positive results with the use of chlamydial antigen detection tests in the evaluation of suspected sexual abuse in children. *Pediatr Infect Dis J* 1988;7:11.
13. Heger A, Emans S. *Evaluation of the sexually abused child.* New York: Oxford University Press, 1993.
14. Hobbs C, Wynne J. Sexual abuse of English boys and girls: the importance of anal examination. *Child Abuse Negl* 1989;13:195.
15. Jenny C, Kuhns MLD, Arakawa F. Hymens in newborn female infants. *Pediatrics* 1987;80:399.
16. Jones D, McGraw J. Reliable and fictitious accounts of sexual abuse to children. *J Interpers Viol* 1987;2(1):27.
17. Kini N, Brady WJ, Lazoritz S. Evaluating child sexual abuse in the emergency department: clinical and behavioral indicators. *Acad Emerg Med* 1996;3:966.
18. McCann J, Voris J. Perianal injuries resulting from sexual abuse: a longitudinal study. *Pediatrics* 1993;91:390.

19. McCann J, Voris J, Simon M. Genital injuries resulting from sexual abuse: a longitudinal study. *Pediatrics* 1992;89:307.
20. McCann J, Voris J, Simon M, Wells R. Perianal findings in prepubertal children selected for nonabuse: a descriptive study. *Child Abuse Negl* 1989;13:179.
21. McCann J, Wells R, Simon M, Voris J. Genital findings in prepubescent girls selected for nonabuse: a descriptive study. *Pediatrics* 1990;86:428.
22. Muram D. Child sexual abuse: relationship between sexual acts and genital findings. *Child Abuse Negl* 1989;13:211.
23. Ricci LR. Child sexual abuse: the emergency department response. *Ann Emerg Med* 1986;7:711.
24. San Philippo JS. *Pediatric and adolescent gynecology*. Philadelphia: WB Saunders, 1994.
25. Summit R. The child sexual abuse accommodation syndrome. *Child Abuse Negl* 1983;7:177.

CHAPTER 259

Abuse and Neglect: Physical

J. M. Whitworth

An awareness of child abuse and neglect is of particular importance in the emergency department setting. Any visit by a child may afford the health-care professional an opportunity to protect a child from further harm. The visit may also provide a rare window into a family that may desperately need intervention and supportive services.

The problem of child abuse affects about 2 million children yearly in the United States and results in the deaths of 2,000 to 5,000 children. Because many of these children receive only episodic medical care or care at a time of medical crisis, the emergency department or acute care clinic plays a special role in identification and reporting of child abuse and neglect. Although the physician is legally required to report suspected child abuse and is protected from liability for making a report in all states, the more important responsibility of the physician is to protect the child from further harm, and, therefore, cause an investigation to be done by the appropriate agency.[2] More detailed information as to state reporting requirements and procedures should be sought from local law enforcement or child protection agencies.

PHYSICAL ABUSE

Physical abuse occurs in all cultural, ethnic, socioeconomic, and racial groups. There are some geographic and regional differences in the prevalence of given types of abuse, but not in overall incidence. The incidence of abuse in a socioeconomic subgroup is most closely related to the presence of significant stresses in that population (i.e., joblessness, homelessness, drug and alcohol abuse). In any parent dyad, the parent with caretaking responsibilities is more likely to abuse a child. Abusive parents are usually not psychotic and generally respond to their children in a pattern similar to that experienced in their own childhood. They fairly consistently have unrealistic expectations of their children, with limited knowledge of developmental norms, and are unable to cope with the failure of the child to meet expectations. Triggering behaviors in the child, such as excessive crying or colic, are frequently seen.

EMERGENCY DEPARTMENT EVALUATION

Presentation

The history from an abused child or an abusive parent remains the most important evaluative tool for the physician. The veracity of a child's history must be assumed until there is good reason to assume otherwise. If children lie, they usually do so to hide the abuse rather than to bring it to light. The history from an abusive parent usually reflects a significant delay in seeking medical attention, and if a primary physician exists, parents have usually not sought his or her advice. There is almost always a history disparate from the severity or type of injury. If repeated questions are used to elicit the history, there is usually considerable variation in detail. Injury may be attributed to a sibling or to someone not present to verify the occurrences. Parents often simply cannot relate any explanation for the injuries sustained. A brief interview of witnesses to trauma can often quickly obviate a need for investigation of a case.

Physical Assessment

The initial physical assessment of the child may show findings that are strong indicators that further evaluation for abuse is necessary:

1. Bruises in unusual locations or where an accidental etiology is implausible due to the age or developmental status of the child (e.g., nonambulatory infant with multiple bruises)
2. Bruises that have a characteristic pattern, suggesting an object used to inflict the injury (e.g., hand print, belt mark)
3. Second-degree burns without bullae that show a characteristic pattern (e.g., the sole plate of an iron)
4. Second-degree burns with bullae and no evidence of splash marks and an unusually sharp line of demarcation (e.g., glove or stocking burns of an extremity)
5. Burns limited to the perineum
6. Swelling of any part of the body out of proportion to the severity of described injury (e.g., may indicate underlying fracture)
7. Unexplained or implausibly explained sudden changes in neurologic status
8. Retinal hemorrhages
9. Failure to thrive without a history suggestive of chronic or debilitating disease

The physical finding most commonly present in abused children is a bruise. Bruises are also the most commonly found accidental injury in children. Accidental bruises are located in areas most frequently exposed to injury in play or other normal childhood activities. These areas include the elbows, knees, and skin over the anterior tibia. The occasional bruise in less usual locations is of little concern and generally occurs over a bony prominence. The only commonly occurring lesion that may be mistaken for a bruise is the Mongolian spot. Mongolian spots are most common in darker skinned infants and are characteristically shiny and blue-black and limited to the back.

Bruises that occur in clusters and in unusual locations, such as on the abdomen, the back, or buttocks, and that show unusual severity or varying stages of resolution should cause concern, because they are rarely accidental. Resolution of bruises takes place in a sequence related to the severity and location of the injury. While there are findings that indicate an acute injury, such as swelling and tenderness, the color of a bruise cannot be used to date the injury accurately. A bruise has usually resolved after about 2 to 4 weeks.[12] Much more specific sequencing can be accomplished by experience in observing many bruises. Photographic documentation of these findings may become critically important to those pursuing the investigation of abuse, and this must be anticipated in completing the medical record.

Children who have been injured in falls from a height often present challenges in assessment for abuse versus an accidental cause. Although there have been poorly designed papers in the literature that would suggest otherwise, a significant head injury requires a fall from a distance of 4 feet or higher. Falls from a bed or sofa never result in serious injury beyond an uncomplicated fracture or bruise.[4]

Laboratory Evaluation

Laboratory evaluation in suspected physical abuse cases should include bleeding and clotting studies when bruises are present and when there is any suggestion of easy bruisability. At a minimum, these studies should include a prothrombin time, partial thromboplastin time, and platelet count. In addition, a photographic record of any finding is always preferable to a written or schematic description alone. Radiographic studies are indicated when evidence of trauma is noted and in children for which abuse is identified by some other means. These studies should include the chest, skull, and long bones in addition to the area of suspected injury. Films should be reviewed for fractures as well as evidence of osteopenia, increased trabeculation, and presence of excessive numbers of wormian bones in the skull. These findings, along with an appropriate family history, might suggest the presence of osteogenesis imperfecta. If fractures are seen, they should be related to the history of the type of injury. For example, spiral fractures occur in response to a torsional force, and chip fractures of the metaphysis occur with traction of the extremity or with a shearing force across the end of the bone. Metaphyseal chip fractures are rarely accidental.[8]

In addition, it is often necessary to estimate the age of fractures in comparison to the history. Fractures of differing ages without good evidence of multiple accidental trauma are virtually diagnostic of physical abuse. Healing of a fracture takes place in a predictable sequence. Periosteal new bone is formed as early as 4 to 10 days after the fracture, and soft callus formation may be seen as early as 10 to 14 days. Hard callus formation may occur as early as 14 days, and remodeling may begin by 3 months after the acute fracture.[9]

Computed axial tomography of the head is indicated in those children with retinal hemorrhages or evidence of acute neurologic deterioration. The presence of intracranial hemorrhage with or without skull fracture and in the absence of a history of major trauma is diagnostic of child abuse until proven otherwise.[6] Magnetic resonance imaging is a useful tool in identifying small areas of bleeding and to more carefully determine areas of bleeding that have occurred at different times.[1] The use of bone scans is usually not indicated, except under special circumstances in which abuse is clearly a likely possibility and in which fractures may be suspected that are not yet visible on routine films.

With abdominal trauma, one might expect to see evidence of acute anemia associated with intraabdominal bleeding or an elevated amylase with trauma to the pancreas. Hematuria is not an uncommon occurrence with paddling or spanking, in which one or more blows has strayed cephalad.

ASSOCIATED SYNDROMES

Shaken-Baby Syndrome (Acceleration–Deceleration Injury)

Shaken infants rarely present with a history of shaking. The most common presentation is that of respiratory difficulty, apnea, or unexplained seizures. The basic insult is the presence of intracranial bleeding, which may be characterized as subdural, epidural, interhemispheric, or intraparenchymal. Symptoms are usually a result of increased intracranial pressure. Retinal hemorrhages are the single most common physical finding and, outside the newborn period, provide presumptive evidence of intracranial bleeding due to trauma. Although retinal hemorrhages may be seen with other head trauma, they should be considered the hallmark of the shaken-baby syndrome until another plausible explanation is found. The hemorrhages seen are usually superficial and diffuse, as compared with the deeper flame-type hemorrhages seen in hypertension. The diagnosis is made by a careful history after documentation of intracranial bleeding by computed tomography or magnetic resonance imaging. The mechanism of injury was once believed to be totally due to rotational and shear forces created by the to-and-fro motion of the head in shaking. Later studies strongly suggest that similar lesions can be caused by significant increased venous pressure transmitted from squeezing of the chest as part of shaking or in any type of injury in which significant increases in intraabdominal or intrathoracic pressure are sustained.[6] The latest studies suggest that impact of the head is necessary to produce the full clinical picture and that acceleration–deceleration forces are important.[5]

As might be expected, other skeletal injuries can be seen with shaking. The child is commonly held by the thorax or the extremities with enough force to cause fractures at those sites. The combination of intracranial bleeding, as described here, and metaphyseal chip fractures of the distal tibias is indicative of the child being held by the feet and cracked like a whip. The clinical outcome in this syndrome is dismal, in that approximately 65% of children will die or have significant neurologic sequelae as a result. Milder forms of this syndrome undoubtedly exist with milder neurologic sequelae but are yet to be carefully documented. This syndrome is frequently missed or misdiagnosed in the clinical setting.

Failure to Thrive

Failure to thrive is often categorized as organic and nonorganic, although there are often some elements of both types in most individual cases. The child presents with the weight being greater than two standard deviations below the mean expected for age, and there may be associated growth failure as well. In most cases of organic failure to thrive, a strong suggestion of the underlying etiology will be evident from the history or physical examination. Suggestions of a nonorganic etiology may be evident in observing the interactions between the mother and child. The mother and child often show little interaction, and nonnurturing behavior is evident on the part of the mother. The child often shows little eye contact and is generally withdrawn from the environment.[3] Most commonly, nonorganic failure to thrive requires a period of observation in a hospital setting for accurate diagnosis.

Munchausen Syndrome by Proxy

This unusual type of child abuse occurs when a caretaker describes or produces factitious illness in a child as a response to their own psychiatric pathology. This is a diagnosis of which the emergency physician should be aware but is not a diagnosis to be made in the emergency department. This diagnosis requires intense record review and, usually, inpatient evaluation.[10]

EMERGENCY DEPARTMENT MANAGEMENT

After a decision to report has been made, the next dilemma is to decide whether to tell the parents about the report. Under most circumstances, the physician should calmly inform the parents that a report is being made because he or she is required to do so by state law and therefore has no choice in the matter. It is generally good to relieve some of the mystery of what will happen after the report is made by informing the parents about the steps in the investigation process. The circumstance when it is better not to inform the parents is one in which the physician feels the parents are likely to flee with the child and further endanger the child's health and welfare.

Meticulous attention to the chart is essential in all abuse cases. The examiner is often called on to recall the encounter with the patient and parents in great detail months or years later. The use of direct quotes from the child is helpful in avoiding questions of hearsay information. The use of detailed body charts to delineate injuries and findings, including careful measurements, is important. Even better is the inclusion of photographs of findings as part of the medical record.

The emergency department physician should be aware of community agencies that provide investigative and intervention services to abusive families and abused children, so that he or she has immediate access to information and consultation on individual cases. If the services of a multidisciplinary team are available, participation in the activities of the team is often very valuable in receiving feedback as to case outcome and progress.

COMMON PITFALLS

The most common pitfall in the diagnosis of child abuse is the failure of the physician to seriously consider this etiology in the differential diagnosis of trauma to children. The presence of documented findings of trauma with an implausible history should provide more than adequate impetus for further evaluation and careful documentation.

References

1. Alexander RC, Schor DP, Smith WL. Magnetic resonance imaging of intracranial injuries from child abuse. *J Pediatr* 1986;109:975.
2. American Medical Association. *Guidelines for the management of physical abuse of children*. Chicago: American Medical Association, 1992.
3. Bithoney WG, Dubowitz H, Egan H. Failure to thrive/growth deficiency. *Pediatr Rev* 1992;13:453.
4. Chadwick D, Chin S, Salerno C, et al. Deaths from falls in children: how far is fatal? *J Trauma* 1993;31:1353.
5. Duhaime AC, Alario AJ, Lewander WJ, et al. Head injury in very young children: injury types and ophthalmologic findings in 100 hospitalized patients younger than 2 years of age. *Pediatrics* 1992;90:179.
6. Dykes LJ. The whiplash shaken infant syndrome: what has been learned? *Child Abuse Negl* 1986;10:211.
7. Jenny C, Hymel K, Ritzen A, et al. Analysis of missed cases of abusive head trauma. *JAMA* 1999;281:621.
8. Leventhal JM, Thomas SA, Rosenfield NS, et al. Fractures in young children: distinguishing child abuse from unintentional injuries. *Am J Dis Child* 1993;147:87.
9. O'Conner JF, Cohen J. Dating fractures. In: Kleinman PK, ed. *Diagnostic imaging of child abuse*. Baltimore: Williams & Wilkins, 1987.
10. Rosenberg DA. Web of deceit: a literature review of Munchausen syndrome by proxy. *Child Abuse Negl* 1987;11:547.
11. Schimdt BD. The child with nonaccidental trauma. In: Helfer ME, ed. *The battered child*, 3rd ed. Chicago: University of Chicago Press, 1983.
12. Schwartz A, Ricci L. How accurately can bruises be aged in abused children? *Pediatrics* 1996;97:254.

CHAPTER 260
Appendicitis

Maureen D. McCollough

Appendicitis is the most common surgical emergency in childhood, with an estimated 80,000 children affected annually.[2] Despite the decline in mortality since the introduction of antibiotics, morbidity has remained unchanged over the past 40 years, due primarily to perforation because of delays in diagnosis. Perforation rates are higher in children, occurring in 50% to 70% of preschoolers with appendicitis, versus 10% to 20% in an adult population.[10,14] This highlights the importance of early diagnosis and treatment in the prevention of significant morbidity.

Obstruction of the appendiceal lumen, caused most commonly by a fecalith (calcified fecal material), is the primary cause of appendicitis. Other less common causes of obstruction include inflamed lymphoid tissue; vegetable and fruit seeds; intestinal worms (especially Ascaridae); bacterial infection with *Yersinia, Salmonella,* or *Shigella;* and, rarely, retained barium from previous radiographic studies, or anomalies of mucus-secreting glands, as in cystic fibrosis.[13,20]

Luminal obstruction of the appendix causes distention and increased intraluminal pressure, resulting in obstruction of the blood supply. Bacterial invasion occurs, and, ultimately, the ischemic appendix becomes gangrenous and perforates. Bacteriologic cultures of perforated appendices have revealed polymicrobial organisms, including *Escherichia coli, Bacteroides fragilis,* and enteric streptococci.[8]

The progression from appendiceal obstruction to perforation is more rapid in children. What starts as vague abdominal complaints can quickly progress to ileus, nausea, vomiting, fever, tachycardia, localized pain, and, finally, peritonitis. The inability of omentum in young children to wall-off localized infections contributes to the development of diffuse peritonitis. Therefore, appendicitis must be recognized early and proper management instituted without delay.[14]

CLINICAL PRESENTATION

The symptoms of acute appendicitis correlate with the pathophysiology of the disease. Obstruction and distention of the appendix stimulates stretch receptors, relaying pain through visceral nerve fibers to the tenth thoracic ganglion, resulting in the perception of periumbilical pain. Bacterial invasion and inflammation then lead to fever, nausea, or vomiting in up to 80% of children. As the inflammation extends to surrounding tissues, localized pain depends on the location of the appendix. Up to one-third of appendices are located in areas other than the usual intraperitoneal location. This results in up to 30% of children with appendicitis having localized pain in areas other than the right lower quadrant. A retrocecal location of the appendix may cause back or flank pain, a pelvic appendix may cause suprapubic pain, and a retroileal location may cause referred pain to the testicle.

If appendicitis is allowed to progress without surgical intervention, appendiceal rupture will occur. The diagnosis of perforation is easier to make. The child is usually ill appearing, toxic, and dehydrated. Particularly in younger children, the incompletely developed greater omentum is incapable of walling off the inflammatory process. Therefore, the abdominal pain is more diffuse and may decrease in intensity just after perforation, becoming much more severe as peritonitis develops.

Examining a young child with abdominal pain is often fraught with difficulty. Because young children are often frightened of doctors and "white coats," observing the child from the doorway or across the room can be revealing. A young child who is ambulating easily around the room, interested in his or her surroundings, is less concerning than a child who is ill appearing and lying very quietly. A slight limp in the child's gait, hesitation to climb onto the examination table, and inability to stretch the right leg may suggest appendicitis even before the full evaluation. The child usually prefers to lie still in the supine position with the thighs, particularly the right, drawn up, because any motion increases pain. Vital signs are essentially normal, but a child with simple appendicitis may show a mild temperature elevation. Tachycardia may be present if the child is dehydrated, febrile, or in pain.

Examination of the abdomen for bowel sounds and tenderness can often frighten young children. Distraction of the young child, using a hand puppet or other toy, may help achieve a better examination. Bowel sounds are usually normal in early appendicitis. Advanced inflammation, perforation, or both, usually result in an ileus and a quiet abdomen.

Abdominal palpation should start away from the painful area. Muscular resistance to palpation of the abdomen parallels the severity of the inflammatory process. Early in the disease process, resistance, if present, consists of voluntary guarding. With the progression of peritoneal irritation, muscle spasm increases and becomes involuntary. The classic physical finding is point tenderness at McBurney's point (3 to 5 cm from the anterior–superior iliac spine on a straight line drawn from that process to the umbilicus).[20]

Physical signs usually associated with acute appendicitis are as follows:[24]

1. Rovsing's sign. This may be found if local peritoneal inflammation is present. By testing for tenderness in the left lower quadrant, referred tenderness can be elicited in the right lower quadrant.
2. Psoas sign. The child lies on the left side, then stretches the psoas muscle by slowly extending the right thigh. Alternatively, the child lies supine and flexes the right hip against a hand placed just above the knee. Pain elicited by either maneuver can indicate an irritating focus in proximity to the psoas muscle.
3. Obturator sign. A positive obturator sign occurs when passive internal rotation of the flexed thigh with the patient supine produces right-sided abdominal pain. This sign indicates irritation around the obturator internus muscle.

A positive psoas or obturator sign suggests retrocecal or retrocolic inflammation. Although these signs (Rovsing, psoas, and obturator) are often quoted as associated with appendicitis, there have been few studies published evaluating the accuracy of the clinical examination for appendicitis.[24] A metaanalysis regarding the clinical signs most likely to identify patients (both children and adults) at increased likelihood for appendicitis was published. The clinical signs with the highest positive likelihood ratios were right lower quadrant pain, rigidity, and migration of initial periumbilical pain to the right lower quadrant. Clinical signs with the highest negative likelihood ratios for ruling out appendicitis were absence of right lower quadrant pain and presence of similar previous pain.[24] The diagnostic value of the rectal examination in children is limited; rectal tenderness is present in 50% of all children with or without appendicitis.[3]

DIFFERENTIAL DIAGNOSIS

The differential diagnosis in children depends on three major factors: the anatomic location of the inflamed appendix, the stage of the process (simple or ruptured), and the age and sex of the patient. The five main groups of differential diagnoses are as follows:[13,19,20,23]

1. Intestinal diseases: mesenteric adenitis, viral and bacterial enteritis, Meckel's diverticulitis, intussusception, enteric duplication
2. Uterine or tuboovarian pathology: ovarian or testicular torsion, acute epididymitis, pelvic inflammatory disease, ectopic pregnancy, endometriosis, mittelschmerz
3. Urinary tract pathology: acute pyelonephritis, cystitis, renal stones
4. Respiratory and systemic diseases: basal pneumonia, Henoch-Schönlein purpura, sickle cell crisis, diabetic ketoacidosis
5. Trauma: accidental or nonaccidental injury

Acute Mesenteric Lymphadenitis

Mesenteric adenitis is most often confused with acute appendicitis in children. A careful history almost invariably reveals the presence of upper respiratory symptoms in these patients. Laboratory procedures are usually of limited value in differentiation, although a relative lymphocytosis may suggest mesenteric adenitis or a generalized viral syndrome. The abdominal pain is usually more diffuse and less severe, and generalized lymphadenopathy may be noted on physical examination.

Pelvic Inflammatory Disease

A history of vaginal discharge in a sexually active adolescent can often be elicited. Interviewing adolescents alone, without parental presence, may offer a more revealing and true history regarding sexual activity. Pain is most often bilateral and lower in location. Physical examination reveals Chandelier's sign (pain with motion of the cervix).

Acute Gastroenteritis

Acute gastroenteritis usually can be differentiated from appendicitis. Often, there is a history of other ill contacts. These patients have nausea, vomiting, watery diarrhea, and intermittent, crampy abdominal pain. Often, the vomiting precedes the diarrhea by 24 hours. Localizing signs on the abdominal examination are usually absent.

Meckel's Diverticulitis

Preoperative differentiation is unnecessary, because the signs and symptoms of Meckel's diverticulitis are similar to those of acute appendicitis, and surgical treatment is indicated for both.

Intussusception

Differentiating between intussusception and acute appendicitis is important and relatively straightforward. Appendicitis is rare in children younger than 2 years of age, whereas nearly all intussusceptions occur in children younger than age 2 years. Intussusception typically occurs suddenly in an otherwise healthy infant. The infant "doubles up" with apparent colicky pain, but is usually without pain between attacks. A bloody mucoid stool is usually passed several hours after the onset of pain. Physical examination may reveal a sausage-shaped mass in the right lower quadrant. Occasionally, infants with intussusception present with an altered mental status. Treatment of intussusception is reduction by barium or air enema (see Chapter 277).

Henoch-Schönlein Purpura

Henoch-Schönlein purpura, a diffuse vasculitis, classically presents with joint pain and swelling and purpura. Abdominal pain may also be a prominent symptom. Rectal examination should be performed for occult blood. Urinalysis to evaluate for hematuria due to nephritis should also be performed.

Mittelschmerz

These patients are at the midpoint of their menstrual cycle. The pain of mittelschmerz is usually sudden in nature and may be localized to one side of the lower abdomen, or diffuse in nature.

Ovarian or Testicular Torsion

A number of nonspecific symptoms may exist, including anorexia, nausea, and vomiting. The correct diagnosis can be made by always including the genitalia in the physical examination, which usually reveals the subtle findings of asymmetry in gonadal size or position. A normal examination of the ovarian or testicular size or position does not completely rule out the diagnosis of torsion, however.

Urinary Tract Infection

Bacteria or white blood cells may be present in the urine specimen of approximately 17% of children with acute appendicitis.[1] This occurs if the appendix lies near the ureter or bladder. With the exception of an elevated specific gravity due to dehydration, the urinalysis is normal in more than 80% of children with acute appendicitis.

EMERGENCY DEPARTMENT EVALUATION

The most important steps in making a correct diagnosis of appendicitis are eliciting a complete history and performing a complete physical examination, including examining the external genitalia in boys and performing an internal pelvic examination in adolescent girls. However, because the sensitivity of the clinical examination has been reported to be as low as 63%, other modalities have been utilized to improve diagnostic capabilities.[7]

Indicated laboratory studies include a complete blood count with differential and urinalysis. Moderate leukocytosis (10,000 to 18,000 white blood cells/mL) with a predominance of polymorphonuclear cells is classically seen but does not necessarily correlate with the severity of the disease.[4] A left shift in the differential may precede a total leukocytosis in children. It must be noted that a normal white blood cell count does not rule out the diagnosis of appendicitis.

Abdominal radiographs are not particularly helpful, as the presence of a fecalith is shown in only 10% to 20% of children with appendicitis.[13] Nonspecific findings on plain abdominal films include isolated distended loops of bowel in the right lower quadrant and obliteration of the psoas shadow. Because lesions that irritate nerves at the T10 to T12 level may simulate the referred pain distribution of appendicitis, a chest film may be required to rule out right lower lobe pneumonia, especially if signs or symptoms of lower respiratory tract disease exist.

Other noninvasive imaging studies, such as ultrasonography or computed tomography, may help make the diagnosis and have gained popularity. Ultrasound in children has been shown to have a sensitivity and specificity of 90% and 97%, respectively, with an overall accuracy of 96%.[11] The classic finding of appendicitis, when viewed by ultrasound, is a thickened, noncompressible, nonperistaltic appendix. Ultrasonography in adolescent girls is especially useful to differentiate appendicitis from tuboovarian disease (e.g., a tuboovarian abscess or ovarian cyst). A normal appendix should be visualized to rule out the diagnosis of appendicitis.[11,17,21] Computed tomography of the abdomen, with rectal contrast, has been shown to have sensitivity and specificity of 94% and negative predictive value of 97%.[6] Computed tomography also has been shown to reduce the number of inpatient prediagnosis observation days, operations, and negative laparotomies.[7]

It has been shown that 20% to 40% of children with acute appendicitis are given the wrong diagnosis on the first visit to a physician.[7,14,18] The most common erroneous preoperative diagnoses, in descending order of frequency, are acute mesenteric lymphadenitis, no organic pathologic condition, acute pelvic inflammatory disease, ovarian cyst, mittelschmerz, and acute gastroenteritis. These account for more than 75% of all missed diagnoses. A thorough history and physical examination should result in a higher degree of accuracy.[19]

There is a higher incidence of perforation in younger children and in children with a history of prolonged symptoms. Symptoms suggestive of perforation are as follows:[23]

- Duration of symptoms more than 36 hours
- Temperature greater than 102°F
- White blood cell count of more than 15,000/mL
- Physical findings of peritonitis

The surgical consultant should be contacted as soon as the diagnosis of acute appendicitis is entertained, to avoid the complication of late diagnosis and perforation. Perforated appendicitis has a mortality rate of 5% and a morbidity rate of up to 46% in some series, compared with a mortality rate of 0.1% for nonperforated appendicitis.[5,12,19]

EMERGENCY DEPARTMENT MANAGEMENT

Appendicitis is a surgical emergency. All children thought to have an abdominal surgical emergency should be seen by a surgeon as soon as possible. The initial emergency department management of simple and perforated appendicitis is essentially the same. Once the diagnosis is made, the child must be fluid-resuscitated intravenously and kept NPO. In a child who has been vomiting, obtaining serum electrolyte levels should be considered while intravenous fluid therapy is begun. Those children who have clinical signs or symptoms of dehydration should receive 0.9 NaCl or Ringer's lactate boluses at 10 to 20 mL/kg to maintain urine output at 1 to 2 mL/kg/h. Once the child is considered fluid-resuscitated, dextrose 5% in 0.45 or 0.225 normal saline and 20 mEq/L KCl at 1.5 times maintenance should be given, as long as the child is not oliguric. If the patient has eaten or vomited within a few hours of the operation, insertion of a nasogastric tube to empty the stomach may be requested by the surgeon. If the child is febrile, an acetaminophen suppository may be given.

The use of routine antibiotic coverage in children with uncomplicated appendicitis continues to be debated. It appears that short-term perioperative antibiotic prophylaxis in children with acute nonperforated appendicitis may decrease the rate of postoperative infectious complications.[22] Absolute indications for extended therapy and a broader spectrum of antibiotic coverage are systemic signs of toxicity, sepsis, suspected perforation, and the presence of underlying conditions that predispose the patient to complications of bacteremia (i.e., infants younger than 6 months of age and children with congenital or acquired cardiac anomalies, sickle cell disease, diabetes mellitus, chronic renal failure, or other states of immune suppression).[19] One commonly used regimen includes ampicillin (100 mg/kg/24 h in four doses), gentamicin (5 mg/kg/24 h in three doses), and clindamycin (40 mg/kg/24 h in four doses). This particular regimen ensures coverage of aminoglycoside-resistant enterococci, gram-negative bacilli, and anaerobes, respectively.[5,16] Other antibiotic combinations or single-drug therapy can be used as long as the same microbial coverage is obtained in the setting of acute noncomplicated disease.

DISPOSITION

All children with appendicitis should be admitted to the hospital for surgical exploration. In certain cases of appendiceal abscess, a surgeon may opt for admission to the hospital for intravenous antibiotics or percutaneous drainage, with an interval appendectomy several weeks later.[15]

If there is doubt about the correct diagnosis, but the suspicion for appendicitis is still high, the child should be admitted to the hospital for serial physical examinations. If the suspicion is low but still a consideration, the child may be discharged with clear instructions to return in 6 to 8 hours for a reexamination of the abdomen. If there is any doubt about the ability of the child to return for a revisit, the child should be admitted to the hospital for serial physical examinations.

The child may require transfer to another facility if appropriate surgical staff is unavailable at the initial hospital. This should be done expediently after resuscitation has been started.

COMMON PITFALLS

- Immediate diagnosis of acute appendicitis in children is essential. Rapid progression of disease in this age group necessitates early suspicion, diagnosis, and operation if perforation is to be avoided. Late diagnosis results in significantly higher morbidity and mortality.
- The evaluating physician must be thorough in obtaining the history and performing the physical examination. In some cases, children or adolescents have been admitted to the hospital for observation with a diagnosis of "rule out appendicitis," when the actual, unrecognized diagnosis was testicular torsion or pelvic inflammatory disease, which could have been recognized if a complete physical examination had been performed.

ACKNOWLEDGMENT

The author gratefully acknowledges the contribution of Bonnie Beaver, who wrote the previous version of this chapter.

References

1. Arnbjornsson E. Bacteriuria in appendicitis. *Am J Surg* 1988;155:356.
2. Ballantine TVN. Appendicitis. *Surg Clin North Am* 1981;6:117.
3. Bower RJ, Bell MJ, Ternberg JL, et al. Controversial aspects of appendicitis management in children. *Arch Surg* 1981;116:885.
4. Coleman C, Thompson JE Jr, Bennon RS, et al. White blood cell count is a poor predictor of severity of disease in the diagnosis of appendicitis. *Am Surg* 1998;64:983.
5. Douville C, Birinyi L, Stevenson RJ. Complicated appendicitis in children. *Hosp Physician* 1986;22:33.
6. Garcia Pena BM, Mandl KD, Kraus SJ, et al. Ultrasonography and limited computed tomography in the diagnosis and management of appendicitis in children. *JAMA* 1999;282:1041.
7. Garcia Pena BM, Taylor GA, Lund DP. Effect of computed tomography on patient management and costs in children with suspected appendicitis. *Pediatrics* 1999;104:440.
8. Gilbert SR, Emmens RW, Putnam TC. Appendicitis in children. *Surg Gynecol Obstet* 1985;161:261.
9. Gilchrist BF, Lobe TE, Schropp KP, et al. Is there a role for laparoscopic appendectomy in pediatric surgery? *J Pediatr Surg* 1992;27:209.
10. Graham JJ, Pokorny WJ, Harberg FJ, et al. Acute appendicitis in preschool age children. *Am J Surg* 1980;139:247.
11. Hahn HB, Hoepner FU, Kalle T, et al. Sonography of acute appendicitis in children: 7 years experience. *Pediatr Radiol* 1998;28:147.
12. Karp MP, Caldarola VA, Cooney DR, et al. The avoidable excesses in the management of perforated appendicitis in children. *J Pediatr Surg* 1986;21:506.
13. Kottmeier PK. Appendicitis. In: Welch KJ, Randolph JG, Ravitch MM, et al., eds. *Pediatric surgery*, 3rd ed. Chicago: Year Book, 1986:989.
14. Linz DN, Hrabovsky EE, Franceschi D, et al. Does the current health care environment contribute to increased morbidity and mortality of acute appendicitis in children? *J Pediatr Surg* 1993;28:321.
15. Mazziotti MV, Marley EF, Winthrop AL, et al. Histopathologic analysis of interval appendectomy specimens: support for the role of interval appendectomy. *J Pediatr Surg* 1997;32:806.
16. Neilson IR, Laberge JM, Nguyen LT, et al. Appendicitis in children: current therapeutic recommendations. *J Pediatr Surg* 1990;25:1113.
17. Rubin SZ, Martin DJ. Ultrasonography in the management of possible appendicitis in childhood. *J Pediatr Surg* 1990;25:737.
18. Savrin RA, Clatworthy HW. Appendiceal rupture: a continuing diagnostic problem. *Pediatrics* 1979;63:37.
19. Scherer LR. Acute appendicitis. In: Cameron JL, ed. *Current surgical therapy*, 4th ed. St. Louis: Mosby–Year Book, 1992:217.
20. Schwartz SI. Appendix. In: Schwartz SI, ed. *Principles of surgery*, 6th ed. New York: McGraw-Hill, 1994:1307.
21. Siegel MJ, Carel C, Surratt S. Ultrasonography of acute abdominal pain in children. *JAMA* 1991;266:1987.
22. Soderquist-Elinder C, Hirsch K, Bergdahl S, et al. Prophylactic antibiotics in uncomplicated appendicitis during childhood—a prospective randomised study. *Eur J Pediatr Surg* 1995;5:282.
23. Stone HH, Sanders SC, Martin JD. Perforated appendicitis in children. *Surgery* 1971;69:673.
24. Wagner JM, McKinney WP, Carpenter JL. Does this patient have appendicitis? *JAMA* 1996;276:1589.

CHAPTER 261
Asthma

Jeffrey F. Linzer

Asthma is the most prevalent chronic disease in children.[1] In 1995, it accounted for almost 3% of all children's visits to the emergency department (ED) in the United States. Visit rates were almost four times higher among Black children than among White children (2.8 and 0.7 visits, respectively, per 100 children).[7]

Asthma can simply be defined as recurrent reversible bronchospasm due to a trigger (Table 261.1). There are underlying inflammatory and neural mechanisms that make the airways

TABLE 261.1. Triggers of Asthma Symptoms in Various Age Groups

	Infancy	Early Childhood	Late Childhood	Adolescence
Viral infections	++++	+++	±	+++
Exercise	+	++	+++	+++
Irritants	+	++	+++	+++
Foods	++	+	()	()
Indoor inhalants	±	+++	+++	+++
Pollens	()	++	+++	++
Emotions	()	+	+	+

Adapted from Pearlman DS, Lemanske RF Jr. Asthma (bronchial asthma): principals of diagnosis and treatment. In: Bierman CW, Pearlman DS, Shapiro GG, et al., eds. *Allergy, asthma and immunology from infancy to adulthood.* Philadelphia: WB Saunders, 1996:492.

TABLE 261.2. Classification of Severity of Asthma Exacerbation

	Mild	Moderate	Severe	Respiratory Arrest Imminent
SYMPTOMS				
Breathlessness	While walking	While talking (infant softer, shorter cry; difficulty feeding)	While at rest (infant stops feeding)	
	Can lie down	Prefers sitting	Sits upright	
Talks in	Sentences	Phrases	Words	
Alertness	May be agitated	Usually agitated	Usually agitated	Drowsy or confused
SIGNS				
Respiratory rate	Increased	Increased	Often >30/min	
Guide to normal rates of breathing in awake children:				
Age	*Normal rate*			
<2 mo	<60/min			
2–12 mo	<50/min			
1–5 yr	<40/min			
6–8 yr	<30/min			
Use of accessory muscles; suprasternal retractions	Usually not	Commonly	Usually	Paradoxical thoracoabdominal movement
Wheeze	Moderate, often only end expiratory	Loud; throughout exhalation	Usually loud; throughout inhalation and exhalation	Absence of wheeze
Pulse/minute	<100	100–120	>120	Bradycardia
Guide to normal pulse rates in children:				
Age	*Normal rate*			
2–12 mo	<160/min			
1–2 yr	<120/min			
2–8 yr	<110/min			
Pulsus paradoxus	Absent (<10 mm Hg)	May be present (10–25 mm Hg)	Often present (20–40 mm Hg)	Absence suggests respiratory muscle fatigue
FUNCTIONAL ASSESSMENT				
PEF				
% predicted or % personal best	>80%	Approx. 50%–80% or response lasts <2 h	<50% predicted or personal best	
PaO_2 (on air)	Normal (test not usually necessary)	>60 mm Hg (test not usually necessary)	<60 mm Hg: possible cyanosis	
and/or				
PCO_2	<42 mm Hg (test not usually necessary)	<42 mm Hg (test not usually necessary)	≥42 mm Hg; possible respiratory failure	
SaO_2 % (on air) at sea level	>95% (test not usually necessary)	91%–95%	<91%	
Hypercapnia (hypoventilation) develops more readily in young children than in adults and adolescents.				

Adapted from National Heart, Lung, and Blood Institute, National Institutes of Health. *Expert panel report 2: guidelines for the diagnosis and management of asthma.* NIH Publication No. 97-4051, Bethesda, MD, 1997.

more sensitive to the triggers and result in bronchial hyperresponsiveness. A number of preformed and generated mediators cause the airway epithelium to become fragile and denuded and the epithelial subbasement membranes to thicken. Also, mucus production and consistency increase, and endothelial leakage results in mucosal edema.[3] Mediator-induced abnormalities in the parasympathetic and nonadrenergic noncholinergic nervous systems may also lead to increased bronchial hyperresponsiveness.

CLINICAL PRESENTATION

Acute asthma exacerbations vary in severity and duration. They can resolve without any intervention. The patient or family may not even have realized there was a problem. An asthma attack can be divided into two phases: early and late asthmatic responses. The early asthmatic response (EAR) occurs soon after trigger exposure, producing bronchospasm, and usually lasts 1 to 2 hours. About 50% of patients go on to develop a late asthmatic response (LAR), with reoccurrence of bronchospasm about 4 hours after the initial trigger exposure. The LAR episode usually lasts 12 to 24 hours but may persist up to several days in some children.

Clinical events such as symptoms, spirometry, and ventilation–perfusion measurements poorly correlate with each other.[10] Spirometry tends to reflect the degree of bronchoconstriction in large and medium airways. Ventilation–perfusion mismatch is more related to obstructive changes in the peripheral airways. Patients who are admitted to a hospital tend to have more severe airway obstruction.[5]

Classically, with an acute asthma attack, the child presents with wheezing and respiratory distress. Bronchospasm, however, can also present as cough, chest pain, shortness of breath, and fatigue with exertion. This can make the diagnosis and appropriate management more difficult. Acute asthma attacks can be divided into mild, moderate, severe, and impending respiratory failure[12] (Table 261.2).

With a mild attack, the child usually has been symptomatic for a short period of time and may still be in the EAR. There may be some increase in the respiratory rate, with a tight, hacking cough or end-expiratory wheezing. There is good air exchange, with minimal breathlessness and no accessory muscle use. Room air oxygen saturation (SaO_2) is greater than 95%, and peak expiratory flow rate (PEFR) or forced expiratory volume in one second (FEV_1) greater than 80% predicted or personal best.

In a more moderate attack, symptoms may have been ongoing for several hours to days, indicating LAR. There is an increase in the work of breathing, with tachypnea and accessory muscle use. Expiratory wheezing may be audible on entering the examination room, and inspiratory–expiratory wheezing may be present. The child may become breathless while talking and be somewhat agitated. An infant may have a less vigorous but more irritable cry and pull away from an offered bottle. Oxygen saturation will be in the low normal range, and PEFR/FEV_1 less than 80% predicted or personal best.

Severe attacks are similar to moderate in their time of onset and duration. There is marked respiratory distress, work of breathing, and tachypnea. Accessory muscle use is associated with intercostal and tracheosternal retractions and nasal flaring. Breath sounds can range from inspiratory–expiratory wheezing to a somewhat quiet chest. The child will be breathless at rest. Neurologically, the child may range from anxious and agitated to somnolent and difficult to arouse. Infants will range from very agitated to unusually quiet and will refuse to take a bottle. Hypoxia is present, and the $PaCO_2$ may rise above 40 mm Hg. PEFR/FEV_1 will be less than 50% predicted or personal best.

While type I respiratory failure (hypoxia without CO_2 retention) can develop with a moderate-to-severe asthma attack, type II failure (hypoxia with CO_2 retention) develops as the child becomes fatigued from the increased work of breathing. Respiratory efforts are labored to the point of paradoxical respiratory movement. The chest may be quiet because of the inability to move any air. The level of consciousness will be depressed. Bradycardia may develop because of hypoxia. Oxygenation may remain significantly low (SaO_2 less than 92% and PaO_2 less than 60 mm Hg) despite adequate supplementation (greater than or equal to 40% O_2).

It is important to remember that a child may present with symptoms from any and all of the mentioned categories, and symptoms thus do not always lend themselves to easy classification.

DIFFERENTIAL DIAGNOSIS

The clinician's careful history and physical examination can help locate from which part of the respiratory tract the symptoms originate. It is important to note that the term *reactive airways disease* refers to a group of conditions that affect the lower airways. Generally, the diagnosis of asthma can be made after documentation of three or more episodes of bronchodilator responsive bronchospasm.[19]

Cough or rattling chest sounds that could mimic asthma are most commonly heard with upper airway pathology. These sounds can occur in children with an upper respiratory infection and in older children and adolescents with allergic rhinitis and sinusitis. These conditions also can contribute to an asthma exacerbation. Similar sounds can be produced in infants with choanal atresia and in children with hypertrophy of the tonsils or adenoids. The examiner should especially be aware of the potential of foreign bodies in toddlers and young children.

Middle-airway pathology can not only cause cough, but also result in wheezing and chest sensations that a young or preverbal child may indicate to be chest pain. Stridor, which is an inspiratory sound, should not be confused with wheezing. Examples of conditions that produce stridor include croup, epiglottitis, and pharyngeal foreign bodies. Fortunately, epiglottitis in the post-*Haemophilus influenzae* vaccination era has become rare in children. Unfortunately, laryngotracheobronchitis ("wheezy croup") and tracheal foreign bodies can produce wheezing.

In infants, anatomic conditions that can cause cough and wheeze include laryngomalacia, tracheomalacia, tracheoesophageal fistula, and hemangiomas. Laryngeal webs, vascular rings, and slings are seen in older infants and toddlers. Vocal cord dysfunction is rare and usually seen in older children and adolescents. In all of these conditions, there is minimal, if any, improvement in symptoms with asthma therapy.

The lower airway causes of asthma-like symptoms are more difficult to differentiate from asthma. Cystic fibrosis can present with symptoms that initially respond well to asthma therapy. Children with cystic fibrosis can go on to develop digital clubbing, which is rarely seen with asthma. Now less common due to surfactant therapy, bronchopulmonary dysplasia can occur in ex-premature infants who required prolonged ventilatory support. Chronic aspiration and gastroesophageal reflux, which can exacerbate underlying asthma, can produce cough and wheezing on their own. Inhalation of chemical and toxic substances and foreign bodies must also be considered.

Viral bronchiolitis is a common cause of wheezing in children under 2 years of age, although viral infections can trigger wheezing in any age group. Bronchitis should be considered an adult or adolescent disease. *Chlamydia trachomatis* (infants under 3 months), pertussis (especially in infants under 6 months of age), pneumonia, and chronic *Chlamydia pneumoniae* in asthmatics can present like or worsen asthma.

Rare lower airway conditions to consider include complications of congenital cardiac conditions, alpha$_1$-antitrypsin deficiency, pulmonary hemosiderosis, and pulmonary eosinophilia (Löffler syndrome).

EMERGENCY DEPARTMENT EVALUATION

Determination of the severity of the attack is based on a rapid initial assessment that includes a brief history, directed physical examination, and baseline SaO_2 measurement, which should be done in a calm and reassuring manner. PEFR or FEV_1 should be obtained in all children 6 years of age and older (Fig. 261.1).

The presentation and duration of symptoms and response to any therapy prior to arrival in the ED help determine whether the child is in LAR. Identifying contributing factors (e.g., fever, choking) assists in determining the need for ancillary tests or other therapy. The number and timing of similar episodes, prior ED visits and hospitalization (including intensive care unit admissions and the need for bilevel positive airway pressure [BiPAP] nasal mask ventilation and/or intubation), and medication history (including last exposure to systemic steroids) will reveal the severity and risk of the child's disease.

The physical examination should rapidly determine the child's work of breathing by evaluating the degree of breathlessness, use of accessory muscles and nasal flaring, and listening to breath sounds. Neurologic status is reflected by the degree of irritability and interaction with the examiner. Measurement of PEFR or FEV_1 allows objective monitoring of lung function. It should be expressed as a percentage of a predicted value based on height, age, and sex from any of several available tables. A better comparison is the child's own personal best value that was obtained during a symptom-free period.

Routine radiographs are not needed for the straightforward asthma attack that improves with ED treatment. Plain chest films should be considered if there is a fever or suspicion of pneumothorax or pneumomediastinum. Care should be taken not to "overread" the x-ray. Hilar prominence and patchy atelectasis are common findings and sometimes misinterpreted as pneumonic infiltrates. Inspiratory–expiratory (or left and right lateral decubitus in infants and toddlers) chest views showing unilateral hyperinflation are useful in evaluation for possible inhaled foreign bodies. Portable chest films are appropriate for any child who has a worsening of symptoms in the ED or is in impending respiratory failure. Children with chronic reoccurring exacerbations may benefit from sinus films to determine the presence of sinusitis. An untreated or undertreated sinusitis may be causing the reoccurrences. Upper airway radiographs should be obtained if middle airway pathology is suspected.

The use of pulse oximetry and noninvasive end-tidal CO_2 monitors has diminished the need for arterial and capillary blood gases. Blood gases are indicated for patients who have persistent hypoxia on greater than 40% O_2, elevated end-tidal CO_2 trends, or impending respiratory failure or arrest. A serum level should be obtained for all patients taking theophylline. Routine complete blood counts or electrolyte determinations generally do not provide useful information in uncomplicated asthma attacks.

Clinical asthma scores (CAS) are an additional method of monitoring the child's progress in the ED. Many CAS have been developed over the years and are variations and improvements of the Wood-Downes-Lecks respiratory failure score.[20] An ED can develop and validate a simple scoring system based on the current National Heart, Lung, and Blood Institute (NHLBI) guidelines.

EMERGENCY DEPARTMENT MANAGEMENT

Beta-Agonists

Inhaled, intermediate-acting beta-agonists (albuterol, terbutaline, biosterol, pirbuterol) are the mainstay of acute asthma therapy. The inhaled medications are preferred because they have been shown to be more effective and have fewer side effects than their oral or parenteral counterparts.[2,11,15] Children respond better to aggressive high-dose albuterol therapy than do adults. There is a significant relationship between albuterol dosing and improvement in pulmonary function.[13] Higher and more frequent administration also leads to greater bronchodilatation.[18]

The initial dosage of albuterol is 0.15 mg/kg (2.5 mg minimum) by oxygen-powered nebulizer. This dose may be repeated at 20-minute intervals during the first hour, as indicated by the patient's response. Subsequent doses at 0.15 to 0.3 mg/kg (10 mg maximum) may be given every 1 to 4 hours, depending on the child's response. Children with moderate-to-severe exacerbations may benefit from continuously nebulized albuterol.[14] The dosage is 0.5 mg/kg/h (7.5 mg minimum) or the equivalent of three intermittent treatments over 1 hour. This may be repeated in severe attacks or impending respiratory failure.

A metered-dose inhaler (MDI) with spacer has been shown to be equivalent to nebulized albuterol in mild-to-moderate exacerbations.[9] Four to eight puffs (each puff taken at 30- to 60-second intervals) of albuterol, pirbuterol, or biosterol are taken every 20 minutes, as needed, in the first hour. The dose may then be repeated every 1 to 4 hours, as needed, while the patient is in the ED.

Subcutaneous injections of epinephrine or terbutaline have no advantage over the inhaled beta-agonists. Their use should be limited to those patients with very poor air exchange. The dose for terbutaline (1 mg/mL) and epinephrine (1:1000 solution) is the same: 0.01 mL/kg (0.1 mL minimum, 0.3 mL maximum). This may be repeated at 15- to 20-minute intervals to a maximum of three doses.

There is no intravenous beta-agonist approved in the United States. The injectable preparation of terbutaline has been used for children with impending respiratory failure.[8] A loading dose of 10 μg/kg is given over 10 minutes, followed by a maintenance infusion of 0.4 μg/kg/min. The dose is titrated in increments of 0.2 μg/kg/min until desired respiratory effects are achieved or unacceptable tachycardia occurs. The usual effective dose is 3 to 6 μg/kg/min. The most common side effects of beta-agonists, tremors and tachycardia, are dose related.

Ipratropium

Ipratropium bromide is a quaternary ammonium derivative of atropine. This greatly diminishes its systemic absorption and side effects. By itself, ipratropium has a relatively long onset but a prolonged duration of action when compared with the beta-agonists. Its anticholinergic activity does provide an additional mechanism of bronchodilation. When given with albuterol, there appears to be greater improvement in pulmonary function than when the same medications are given individually.[16] This appears to be especially true for children with moderate-to-severe attacks.[17] Also, because cough is more a large-airway (rich in cholinergic innervation) function, this medication may be of benefit when there is a significant cough component.

The dose for ipratropium is 0.25 mg for infants and 0.5 mg for older children and adolescents. It may be repeated at 20-minute intervals during the first hour and is mixed in the same nebulizer with the albuterol. Repeated doses are given every 2 to 4 hours. Add 0.5 to 1.0 mg to any continuous albuterol treatment.

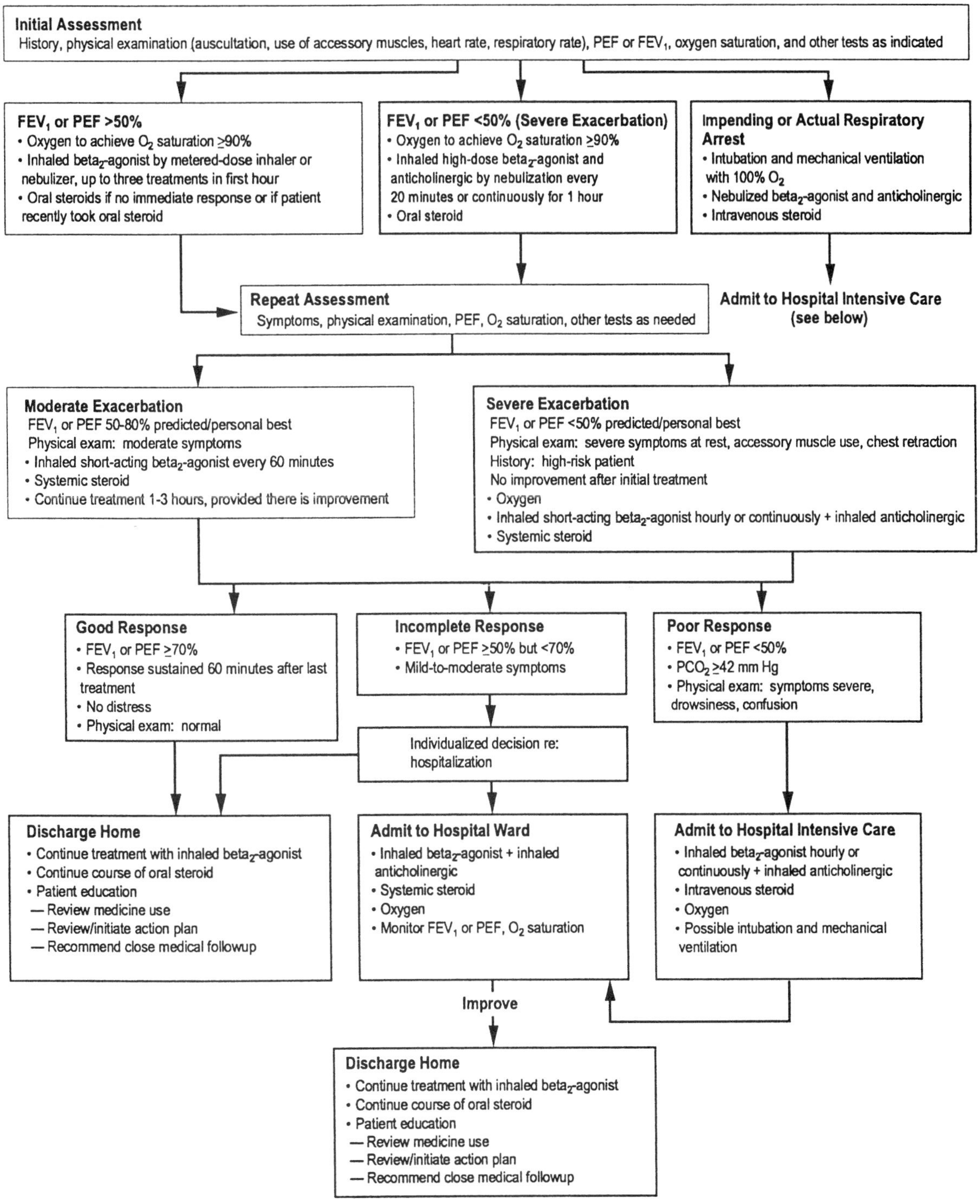

Figure 261.1. NHLBI ED/Hospital Care management algorithm. (Modified from National Heart, Lung, and Blood Institute, National Institutes of Health. *Expert panel report 2: guidelines for the diagnosis and management of asthma.* NIH Publication No. 97-4051, Bethesda, MD, 1997:112.)

Corticosteroids

Systemic corticosteroids are important in controlling LAR. They also decrease the relapse rate during the first week after an asthma exacerbation. Oral and parenteral forms appear equally effective. The onset of antiinflammatory activity is approximately 4 to 8 hours;[16a] however, corticosteroids appear to up-regulate the beta receptors in about 1 hour.[4]

Oral prednisone, prednisolone, or methylprednisolone, 1 to 2 mg/kg (60 mg maximum), should be given within the first hour of ED arrival to children with moderate-to-severe attacks. If the child is unable to tolerate oral medications, then 1 to 2 mg/kg (120 mg maximum) of methylprednisolone intravenously, or 0.15 to 0.6 mg/kg (30 mg maximum) of dexamethasone intramuscularly, may be given. There may be no benefit in using corticosteroids in children with EAR. The oral and intravenous doses may be repeated every 6 hours, up to 48 hours. The higher dose of intramuscular dexamethasone will provide 2 to 3 days of corticosteroid coverage.

GREEN ZONE: Doing Well

- No cough, wheeze, chest tightness, or shortness of breath during the day or night
- Can do usual activities

And, if a peak flow meter is used,
Peak flow: more than ________________
(80% or more of my best peak flow)

My best peak flow is:________________

Take These Long-Term-Control Medicines Each Day (include an anti-inflammatory)

Before exercise ❑ ____________________ ❑ 2 or ❑ 4 puffs 5 to 60 minutes before exercise

YELLOW ZONE: Asthma Is Getting Worse

- Cough, wheeze, chest tightness, or shortness of breath, or
- Waking at night due to asthma, or
- Can do some, but not all, usual activities

-Or-

Peak flow: _____ to _____
(50% - 80% of my best peak flow)

FIRST **Add: Quick-Relief Medicine – and keep taking your GREEN ZONE medicine**

____________________ (short-acting $beta_2$-agonist) ❑ 2 or ❑ 4 puffs, every 20 minutes for up to 1 hour ❑ Nebulizer, once

SECOND **If your symptoms (and peak flow, if used) *return to GREEN ZONE* after 1 hour of above treatment:**
❑ Take the quick-relief medicine every 4 hours for 1 to 2 days.
❑ Double the dose of your inhaled steroid for __________ (7-10) days.

-Or-

If your symptoms (and peak flow, if used) *do not return to GREEN ZONE* after 1 hour of above treatment:
❑ Take: ____________________ (short-acting $beta_2$-agonist) ❑ 2 or ❑ 4 puffs or ❑ Nebulizer
❑ Add: ____________________ (oral steroid) ________ mg. per day For _______ (3-10) days
❑ Call the doctor ❑ before/ ❑ within __________ hours after taking the oral steroid.

RED ZONE: Medical Alert!

- Very short of breath, or
- Quick-relief medicines have not helped, or
- Cannot do usual activities, or
- Symptoms are same or get worse after 24 hours in Yellow Zone

-Or-

Peak flow: less than______
(50% of my best peak flow)

Take this medicine:

❑ ____________________ (short-acting $beta_2$-agonist) ❑ 4 or ❑ 6 puffs or ❑ Nebulizer
❑ ____________________ (oral steroid) ________ mg.

Then call your doctor NOW. Go to the hospital or call for an ambulance if:
- You are still in the red zone after 15 minutes AND
- You have not reached your doctor.

DANGER SIGNS

- **Trouble walking and talking due to shortness of breath**
- **Lips or fingernails are blue**

- **Take ❑ 4 or ❑ 6 puffs of your quick-relief medicine *AND***
- **Go to the hospital or call for an ambulance (____________________) *NOW!***

Figure 261.2. NHLBI ED/Hospital Care asthma action plan form. (Modified from National Heart, Lung, and Blood Institute, National Institutes of Health. *Practical guide for the diagnosis and management of asthma*. NIH Publication No. 97-4053, Bethesda, MD, 1997:45.)

Oxygen

Any child with significant respiratory distress will benefit from oxygen, even with a normal SaO_2. Low-flow oxygen (1 to 2 L/m) by nasal cannula is usually sufficient. Warm, humidified oxygen is preferable because dry oxygen can irritate the respiratory tree. High-flow oxygen should be administered via a nonrebreather mask whenever the child is hypoxic.

Alternative Therapies

For the child with a severe asthma attack or impending respiratory failure who is not responding to conventional treatment, there are limited alternatives. BiPAP has been shown to be of benefit in children with moderate hypoxia as an alternative to intubation.[6] The use of Heliox, Ketamine (1 mg/kg IV loading dose and a maintenance drip at 0.5–.75 mg/kg/hr.), and magnesium sulfate (25 mg/kg intravenously; max, 2 g) remains controversial. There are some subgroups of patients who may benefit from these alternatives. Theophylline is no longer considered first-line therapy for an acute asthma attack.

Antibiotics

There is no benefit to the routine use of antibiotics in the management of an acute asthma attack. They should be used when findings are consistent with pneumonia or other clinical bacterial infection. Therapy is directed to the most likely organism (see Chapter 288).

DISPOSITION

Patient disposition depends on the severity of the attack, response to treatment, and contributing risk factors. It is important that the patient be reassessed after initial therapy and observed for an appropriate period of time for relapse while in the ED.

A child who has had a mild attack, required no more than one or two albuterol treatments, and whose PEFR or FEV_1 was not less than 70% may be sent home after a short (30-minute) observation period. All other patients should be observed for at least 1 hour for signs of relapse. Patients with an incomplete or poor response to therapy should be considered for admission. The decision to watch a patient in an observation unit or an inpatient ward is dependent on local policy and capabilities. Children presenting in impending or actual respiratory failure or who have deteriorated in the ED should be admitted to a pediatric intensive care unit.

Discharged children should be sent home with inhaled beta-agonists (albuterol, pirbuterol, biosterol) if they do not already have the medication. Normal oxygen saturation and a respiratory assessment should be documented at time of discharge. An MDI and appropriate spacer (with or without a mask) can be used in children as young as 1 month of age. Older children and adolescents can use an MDI with autoactuator or dry powder inhaler. The initial MDI dose is two to six puffs (separated by 1 minute) every 3 to 4 hours for the first 24 to 48 hours following ED treatment. For patients with a home nebulizer, the dose is 2.5 mg per treatment. The patient should be weaned as rapidly as possible to four times a day, with rescue use up to every 3 to 4 hours, as needed. A good rule of thumb is to use this intensive course of beta-agonist for as long as the patient is taking corticosteroids (3 to 14 days).

Children respond well to short courses ("bursts") of corticosteroids and generally do not need to be "weaned" from the systemic steroid effects. The dose of prednisone, prednisolone, or methylprednisolone is 1 to 2 mg/kg (60 mg maximum) in one or two divided doses. The length of treatment is a 3- to 7-day course, depending on patient's severity and rapidity of response. Use a tapering dose if the child has taken systemic corticosteroids in the previous 30 to 60 days, has had three bursts in the past 6 months, or has had four bursts in the past 12 months. The taper should be over 7 to 14 days. Because of the potential risk of disseminated disease and death, the risks of using systemic (not inhaled) steroids in children with active varicella must be carefully weighed against the benefits. In some cases, it is appropriate to start preventative therapy with inhaled corticosteroids on discharge from the ED.

Children should be sent home with an asthma plan that details what treatment the patient received and how they should manage continuing problems at home. Children 6 years old and older should be sent home with a PEFR meter. The PEFR is done two to four times a day, and the results used to trigger part of the action plan (Fig. 261.2).

All children who have an ED visit for asthma exacerbation should be referred back to their primary care physician or specialist for follow-up. At a minimum, the parent should make phone contact within 24 hours of discharge to advise the physician of the child's progress.

COMMON PITFALLS

- Failure to provide early, aggressive treatment can lead to unnecessarily prolonged ED care or hospitalization.
- Failure to educate parents and children about potential triggers and how to avoid them. Smoking is a significant environmental trigger and is potentially harmful to the child, even if the parent "smokes outside."
- Do not use the term *reactive airway disease* or *bronchitis* if the child has asthma. They are different entities. If the child has not been diagnosed with asthma, then use symptom- and complaint-based terminology (e.g., wheezing, shortness of breath, respiratory distress).
- Asthma is an inflammatory disease. Viral infections are an important trigger. There is no need to routinely use antibiotics unless there is a bacterial focus of infection.
- Corticosteroids are like any other medication with appropriate and inappropriate uses. Not every child who comes to the ED with an asthma attack needs corticosteroids.
- Send the patient home with a written action plan. It can provide guidance and help avoid an unnecessary ED visit.

References

1. Benson V, Marano MA. Current estimates from National Health Interview Survey, 1995. National Center for Health Statistics. *Vital Health Stat* 1998;10(199):78.
2. Ben-Ziv Z, Lam C, Hoffman J, et al. An evaluation of the initial treatment of acute asthma. *Pediatrics* 1982;70:348.
3. Bradding P, Freezer NJ, Sheffer AL, et al. Asthma. In: Frank MM, Austen KF, Claman HN, et al., eds. *Samter's immunologic diseases,* 5th ed. Boston: Little, Brown and Company, 1995:1293–1327.
4. Ellul-Micallef R, French FF. Effect of intravenous prednisolone in patients with diminished adrenergic responsiveness. *Lancet* 1975;2:1269.
5. Ferrer A, Roca J, Wagner PD, et al. Airway obstruction and ventilation-perfusion relationships in acute severe asthma. *Am Rev Respir Dis* 1993;147:579.
6. Fortenberry JD, Del Toro J, Jefferson LS, et al. Management of pediatric acute hypoxemic respiratory insufficiency with bilevel positive pressure (BiPAP) nasal mask ventilation. *Chest* 1995;108:1059.
7. Freid VM, Makuc DM, Rooks RN. Ambulatory health care visits by children: principal diagnosis and place of visit. National Center for Health Statistics. *Vital Health Stat* 1998;13(137):60.
8. Fuglsang G, Pederson S, Borgstrom L. Dose-response relationships of intravenously administered terbutaline in children with asthma. *J Pediatr* 1989;114:315.
9. Kerem E, Levison H, Schuh S, et al. Efficacy of albuterol administered by nebulizer versus spacer device in children with acute asthma. *J Pediatr* 1993;123:313.

10. Lagerstrand L, Bylin G, Hedenstierna G, et al. Relationships among gas exchange, spirometry and symptoms in asthma. *Eur J Med* 1992;1:145.
11. Louridas G, Kakoura M, Galanis N, et al. Bronchodilatory effect of inhaled versus oral salbutamol in bronchial asthma. *Respiration* 1983;44(6):439.
12. National Heart, Lung, and Blood Institute, National Institutes of Health. *Expert panel report 2: guidelines for the diagnosis and management of asthma*. NIH Publication No. 97-4051, Bethesda, MD, 1997.
13. Nelson HS, Spector SL, Whitsett TL, et al. The bronchodilator response to inhalation of increasing doses of aerosolized albuterol. *J Allergy Clin Immunol* 1983;72:371.
14. Papo MC, Frank J, Thompson AE. A prospective, randomized study of continuous versus intermittent nebulized albuterol for severe status asthmaticus in children. *Crit Care Med* 1993;21:1479.
15. Pierce RJ, Payne CR, Williams SJ, et al. Comparison of intravenous and inhaled terbutaline in the treatment of asthma. *Chest* 1981;79:506.
16. Reisman J, Galdes-Sebalt M, Kazim F, et al. Frequent administration by inhalation of salbutamol and ipratropium bromide in the initial management of severe acute asthma in children. *J Allergy Clin Immunol* 1988;81:16.
16a. Scarfore RJ, Fuchs SM, Nager AL, Shane SA. Controlled trial of oral prednisone in the emergency department treatment of children with acute asthma. *Pediatrics* 1993;92:513.
17. Schuh S, Johnson DW, Callahan S, et al. Efficacy of frequent nebulized ipratropium bromide added to frequent high-dose albuterol therapy in severe childhood asthma. *J Pediatr* 1995;126:639.
18. Schuh S, Parkin P, Rajan A, et al. High- versus low-dose, frequently administered, nebulized albuterol in children with severe, acute asthma. *Pediatrics* 1989;83:513.
19. Skoner DS. Asthma. In: Fireman P, Slavin RG, eds. *Atlas of allergies*. Philadelphia: JB Lippincott Co, 1991.
20. Wood DW, Downes JJ, Lecks MS. A clinical scoring system for the diagnosis of respiratory failure. *Am J Dis Child* 1972;123:227.

CHAPTER 262

Bleeding Disorders

James L. Harper and Paul A. Pitel

Bleeding disorders in children arise from defects in either the cellular (platelet) or humoral components of the coagulation system. These defects, congenital or acquired, may be either qualitative or quantitative in nature. The most common bleeding disorders in children are immune thrombocytopenic purpura, von Willebrand disease, and the hemophilias.

IMMUNE THROMBOCYTOPENIC PURPURA

Immune thrombocytopenic purpura (ITP) is an acquired syndrome characterized by thrombocytopenia, without abnormality in other cell lines, caused by the immune-mediated destruction of circulating platelets, primarily in the spleen. About 85% of cases in children are acute, lasting less than 9 months; the rest are chronic, lasting variable periods. Patients with ITP soon exhibit rapid clearance of circulating platelets, resulting in severe thrombocytopenia, despite increased platelet production in the bone marrow.

ITP may occur at any age, but the typical child is 2 to 6 years old. Prepubertal children are more likely to have the acute form than are postpubertal children.

CLINICAL PRESENTATION

The classic presentation is that of an otherwise healthy child with a recent viral syndrome noted to have an acute onset of petechiae and ecchymoses. Apart from the bleeding diathesis, the history and physical examination are normal; in particular, there is no history of significant fever, weight loss, bone or joint pain, or anorexia. The physical examination reveals no significant adenopathy, hepatosplenomegaly, or masses. Bruising can range from rare scattered petechiae to severe, diffuse ecchymoses. Bleeding in the oral mucosa and other mucous membranes is also seen.

Occasionally, gastrointestinal (GI) or renal bleeding or, rarely, intracranial bleeding is seen. The key element in the laboratory evaluation of ITP is the lack of any hematologic abnormality other than severe thrombocytopenia. Anemia secondary to bleeding (e.g., GI or renal) is occasionally seen.

DIFFERENTIAL DIAGNOSIS

The differential diagnosis of a child who, on a physical examination, is normal, except for the presence of petechiae and ecchymoses, should include child abuse; bone marrow failure (aplastic anemia); bone marrow replacement, as in acute lymphoblastic leukemia or metastatic neuroblastoma; sepsis; and disseminated intravascular coagulation. Children with organomegaly or involvement of more than one hematologic cell line must be more extensively evaluated.

EMERGENCY DEPARTMENT EVALUATION

Evaluation should include a thorough physical examination, with close attention to detecting hepatosplenomegaly, significant lymphadenopathy, or soft-tissue or intraarticular bleeding. Any of these findings warrants a complete hematologic evaluation. Laboratory evaluation should include a complete blood count with manual differential, platelet count, reticulocyte count, and careful morphologic review of the Wright-stained smear. Most children with ITP have profoundly low platelet counts (usually less than 20,000/μL). Large (young) platelets are often observed on the peripheral smear. Any evidence of abnormality in another hematologic cell line (red or white cell) without obvious explanation necessitates a hematologic consultation.

The optimal evaluation of the child with ITP remains controversial. Anything in the history, physical examination, or laboratory studies inconsistent with ITP necessitates a full evaluation, including bone marrow aspiration or biopsy. Many hematologists perform these tests on all patients to confirm the diagnosis and to allay fears of a misdiagnosis.

EMERGENCY DEPARTMENT MANAGEMENT

ITP may be treated expectantly or with intravenous gamma globulin (IVIG), prednisone, or, in rare refractory cases (life-threatening emergencies), splenectomy. Because most children do not experience severe or life-threatening bleeding despite nearly undetectable platelet counts, a growing number of hematologists are treating these children expectantly. Most hematologists recommend treatment with immunosuppression, either IVIG or corticosteroids, for children with platelet counts below 10,000/μL, associated with moderate-to-severe bruising.

IVIG has the advantage of rapid onset, relatively few side effects, and minimal effect on other hematologic cell lines. The major disadvantage of IVIG is its expense. It may be given as a single dose (1 g/kg intravenously over 4 to 6 hours) or given over several days (250 mg/kg/dose intravenously over 4 to 6 hours daily for 4 days).[1,2,7,9] IVIG is preferred if the bone marrow cannot be examined before beginning therapy.

Corticosteroids (prednisone, methylprednisolone) are also effective in producing a prompt rise in the platelet count. They should be avoided if a definitive diagnosis has not been made. Patients with acute lymphoblastic leukemia may be placed in a temporary remission with prednisone alone. A typical course of prednisone is 2 to 4 mg/kg/d orally, in two or three divided doses for 4 days, followed by 1 to 2 mg/kg/d, in divided doses, to complete a 14-day course.

Intraoral bleeding is usually not a significant problem in children with ITP, but in the case of a child with thrombocytopenia and gingival hemorrhage, the use of topical collagen (INSTAT) is reportedly an effective means of control.[8,10] Splenectomy is reserved for refractory chronic ITP and rare life-threatening bleeding, particularly intracranial hemorrhages. Clamping the splenic pedicle is associated with an almost immediate increase in the platelet count.

DISPOSITION

Role of the Consultant

In the initial management of the child with suspected ITP, the physician's role is to rule out other etiologies, such as marrow failure or replacement. A pediatric hematologist should promptly evaluate any child with abnormalities of the history, physical examination, or laboratory studies inconsistent with a diagnosis of ITP.

Indications for Admission

Once a diagnosis is established, the patient may be managed by the primary care physician and hematologist in either a clinic or an inpatient setting. Most patients can be managed primarily on an outpatient basis. Admission is indicated if there are clinical features suspicious for child abuse or suggestive of another hematologic disorder. Admission is also indicated if there is evidence of severe bleeding, or if reliable outpatient follow-up is problematic. In general, these patients may be managed on general pediatric floors.

Transfer Considerations

The rare patient with severe bleeding may require more intensive monitoring. The patient should be transferred if the initial center does not have pediatric hematology support. The skill level of the transport should be dictated by the severity of the bleeding, which is usually minor.

VON WILLEBRAND DISEASE

Von Willebrand disease (vWD) is a relatively common (1% of population) congenital coagulation defect. Inherited, most commonly, in an autosomal dominant fashion, it is caused by deficient, defective, or absent von Willebrand factor (vWF). vWF is a high-molecular-weight multimeric coagulation factor with a primary role in platelet adhesion to vascular surfaces.

There are several variants of vWD. Type I vWD, the most common form, is caused by deficient production of normal vWF. Type 2 vWD is associated with production of an abnormal vWF, resulting in impaired function. Type 2A is associated with an abnormal isotype that has decreased platelet adhesion. Type 2B is associated with an abnormal vWF that tightly binds to platelets and may produce thrombocytopenia. Type 2N (type 2 Normandy) is a rare form of vWD in which the binding site for factor VIII is dysfunctional, with a resulting phenotype similar to classical hemophilia. Type 3 vWD is the complete absence of circulating vWF in a patient with homozygous disease (from two affected parents), and is clinically most severe.

CLINICAL PRESENTATION

vWD causes an abnormality of platelet adhesion to vessel walls, producing a delay in the formation of the hemostatic platelet plug. The clinical presentation is prolonged mucocutaneous bleeding (e.g., nosebleeds, excessive bleeding from sites of dental extractions, prolonged menstrual bleeding, petechiae, excessive bruising). vWF also stabilizes the factor VIII molecule; therefore, a severe (homozygous) deficiency of circulating vWF may result in a deficiency of factor VIII procoagulant, producing soft-tissue and joint bleeding similar to that seen in hemophilia. Symptoms of this disease are variable in any given patient.

DIFFERENTIAL DIAGNOSIS

The differential diagnosis includes platelet defects, either qualitative or quantitative in nature, and abnormalities of the humoral coagulation system, such as hemophilia. A history of a variable bleeding tendency suggests vWD. Because the inheritance of vWD is autosomal dominant, women are also clinically affected.

EMERGENCY DEPARTMENT EVALUATION

The initial evaluation of a patient with known vWD who is actively bleeding should focus on determining, from the patient or records, the type of vWD present in order to plan appropriate therapy. Laboratory evaluation of a newly diagnosed patient would include a platelet count, prothrombin time (PT) and partial thromboplastin time (PTT), factor VIII level, factor VIII–related antigen ([FVIII Rag, von Willebrand antigen] the antigenic measure of the vWF), and a ristocetin cofactor ([RcoF] a measure of vWF activity). Studies of vWF multimers may be needed to further classify the type of vWD, and will almost certainly necessitate consultation with a hematologist.

EMERGENCY DEPARTMENT MANAGEMENT

The management of the bleeding patient with vWD centers on raising the circulating level of vWF to hemostatic levels. Depending on the type and severity of the patient's vWD, several options are useful. For patients with mild-to-moderate type I vWD, DDAVP (0.3 μg/kg) infused over 30 minutes is often effective in controlling bleeding. Intranasal DDAVP (Stimate) may be used to treat minor bleeding in those patients known to respond to this preparation. For patients with severe type I, type 2B, or type 3, DDAVP should be avoided, and factor replacement using cryoprecipitate (0.2 U/kg) or intermediate purity FVIII concentrates (such as Humate-P or Koate-HP) should be pursued. These factor concentrates are dosed according to guidelines for hemophilia A (Table 262.1). If the type of vWD is unknown, the patient should be managed using factor replacement therapy. If the diagnosis of the factor deficiency is uncertain, consultation with a hematologist is indicated for proper planning of factor replacement.

TABLE 262.1. Emergency Factor Dosages for Bleeding Episodes in Hemophiliacs

Site	Factor VIII (U/kg)	Factor IX (U/kg)
EXTREMITY		
Muscle	20–30	30
Joint	30	30
ABDOMEN		
Iliopsoas	30	30-40
Intraabdominal	40	50
CHEST		
Chest wall	30	30
Intrathoracic	50	50–70
HEAD/NECK		
Intracranial	50	50–70
Airway	50	50–70
Mouth/face	30	30

Note: Subsequent therapy should be coordinated with the patient's hematologist. Bleeding in soft tissues that encroaches on a major neuromuscular structure or the airway should be treated with 50 U/kg of the appropriate factor.

DISPOSITION

The role of the emergency physician in the treatment of acute bleeding in patients with vWD is principally limited to ongoing therapy and the treatment of patients who develop soft-tissue or joint bleeding. Patients who develop such a bleed should be referred to an experienced center for follow-up. Patients with type 2B vWD may develop thrombocytopenia if given DDAVP. These patients have a more complicated course and should be referred to an experienced hematologist.

HEMOPHILIA

Hemophilia A (factor VIII) and hemophilia B (factor IX) are X-linked recessive congenital deficiencies of circulating coagulant factors. The incidence of factor VIII deficiency is one in 100,000 White males and accounts for 85% of hemophilia cases; factor IX deficiency accounts for most of the rest. Factor VIII deficiency has a high incidence of spontaneous mutation, with about 30% of cases arising *de novo*. Both diseases are classified into three severity groupings according to the circulating level of factor. Severe disease is defined as less than 1% of normal activity (normal range, 50% to 150%); moderate disease, 1% to 5%; and mild disease, 5% to 30%.

CLINICAL PRESENTATION

The clinical presentation varies with the severity of the deficiency. Severe hemophilia may be diagnosed soon after birth, with intracranial bleeding associated with difficult labor or excessive bleeding from circumcision or other bleeding sites.

After the neonatal period, the typical patient is spared significant bleeding problems until toddler age, when the child begins walking (and falling). Even at this age, the diagnosis may not be obvious. Patients with a severe deficiency of either factor are prone to spontaneous bleeding in muscles and joints, body cavities, and the head and neck. Moderate hemophiliacs may experience excessive bleeding due to trauma or surgery, but they experience spontaneous bleeding episodes less frequently.[3,5,10] Mild hemophiliacs may often go undiagnosed until they require surgery or suffer major trauma, at which time they will have excessive bleeding.

EMERGENCY DEPARTMENT MANAGEMENT

The two principal goals are stabilization and protection of normal function, and prompt hemostasis. A patient with a life-threatening bleed is treated promptly with factor concentrates to restore normal hemostasis.

Bleeding may occur at any site, but some sites are of greater concern. Bleeding in the head and neck area is emergent if it encroaches on either the intracranial space or the airway. Intracranial bleeding is most often manifested by headache and vomiting, and it occurs spontaneously in 60% of cases. Intracranial bleeding is most common in children, with 50% of all bleeding episodes occurring in boys less than 10 years old, and 75% in boys less than 20 years old. The mortality rate may reach 30%, depending of the site of bleeding.[12] Human immunodeficiency virus (HIV) infection should not be blamed for any mental status changes seen in an HIV-infected hemophiliac until a hematoma or other space-occupying lesion has been ruled out.[1]

Other areas of the head and neck region may be the site of an emergent bleed, especially if the bleed may encroach on the airway. Areas of particular concern are the posterior half of the oropharynx, the tongue, the soft tissues of the anterior triangle of the neck, and the retropharyngeal space. Any bleeding or mass in these areas must be considered as potentially life-threatening and treated aggressively. After initial treatment with factor VIII or IX at 50 U/kg, to achieve levels approaching 100% activity, and the patient is stabilized, he should be transferred to a center experienced in the care of hemophilia.

Less emergent sites of bleeding in the head and neck include lip lacerations and dental extraction sites. Usually, these are successfully treated with 20 to 30 U/kg of clotting factor, with additional antifibrinolytic therapy to combat the fibrinolytic effect of saliva and to stabilize the clot. Tranexamic acid (4.8% aqueous solution) may be used as a mouth rinse. Epsilon-aminocaproic acid (Amicar) is also useful (100 U/kg orally every 6 hours for 7 days). These bleeding episodes generally resolve without incident, but close follow-up should be arranged, as blood may dissect between soft-tissue planes to cause compartment compression if bleeding is not well controlled.

Abdominal bleeding usually presents as vague abdominal discomfort, although if presentation is delayed, a palpable mass may be noted. Bleeding in the abdomen requires a high level of factor replacement and is generally treated with 40 U/kg of factor VIII replacement product or 50 U/kg of factor IX replacement product. Factor replacement is required for several days, and subsequent therapy should be coordinated with the patient's hematologist. Occasionally, patients develop painless hematuria not related to trauma, inflammation of the kidney, or renal calculus. Once other causes are ruled out, hydration and observation are generally sufficient treatment.[9]

Bleeding in the retroperitoneum is most commonly located in the iliopsoas muscle. The classic clinical presentation is a combination of severe acute back pain and the inability to extend the hip on the affected side due to pressure on the muscle body from the evolving hematoma. This is generally treated with 30 U/kg of either factor VIII or IX. Unlike other sites of bleeding in the musculoskeletal system, these bleeding episodes frequently require several days of factor replacement, as well as narcotic analgesia.

Bleeding into the joints (hemarthrosis) is the most common bleeding problem seen in hemophilia. Early treatment with clotting factor and local measures, such as ice packs, rest, and immobilization, typically result in resolution within a couple of days. Delay in factor replacement results in more bleeding into the joint space and the potential development of a so-called target joint. Leukocytes produce greater damage to the synovium, resulting in synovial hypertrophy. The resulting spongy synovium is more prone to additional bleeding. Hemophiliacs may thus develop target joints that bleed more frequently than others. The clinical presentation of a hemarthrosis is warm, painful swelling of the joint, with limited range of motion. Erythema may accompany the swelling if considerable inflammation is present, although erythema is generally not prominent. These bleeding episodes are treated with 20 U/kg of factor VIII (same dose for factor IX). Subsequent factor replacement may be needed to control severe bleeds. Factor VIII is usually given at 20 U/kg every 12 hours for 2 to 3 days, and factor IX at 20 U/kg daily for 2 or 3 days. Ice, compression, elevation, and rest are also important in treatment.

Intramuscular bleeding is the second leading cause of long-term disability, after hemarthrosis. Delayed or insufficient replacement therapy may result in a hematoma with compartment compression and subsequent injury. The usual clinical presentation is swelling and pain over a muscle body. These bleeds are most common in the large muscles of the extremities, but they may occur in any muscle. They are treated with 30 U/kg of either factor VIII or IX. Subsequent therapy should be coordinated by a hemophilia center, and, generally, several days of factor replacement is required. Following hemarthrosis and hematoma formation, an aggressive physical therapy program should be encouraged, once the bleeding has resolved.

In patients with a mild deficiency of factor VIII, DDAVP (0.3 μg/kg intravenously over 30 minutes) is effective in controlling minor bleeds. It should not be used for life- or limb-threatening bleeding. Another contraindication is a bleed likely to require more than 3 days to resolve. The response to DDAVP diminishes over time. By 48 to 72 hours, many patients develop significant tachyphylaxis.[12] Intranasal DDAVP has also been found to be effective in patients with mild factor VIII deficiency.

Severe hemophiliacs have little or no circulating factor, and thus fail to develop immune tolerance to the factor in which they are deficient. About 15% of patients with severe hemophilia A develop an antibody to infused factor VIII, an inhibitor that negates the function of subsequently infused factor VIII. Inhibitors vary in titer and in affinity. Clinically, they may complicate therapy for bleeding episodes by neutralizing the replacement factor before hemostasis can be achieved. Patients with a previously undiagnosed inhibitor often present with a bleed unresponsive to the usual therapy. The diagnosis is made by measuring the titer of the inhibitor. Therapy for these patients, particularly those with high-titer inhibitors, is complex and requires an experienced center.[4]

COMMON PITFALLS

Bleeding disorders in children are a relatively uncommon problem in the emergency department. Failing to recognize some of the nuances of these diseases can lead to misdiagnosis and mistreatment. Knowledge of the following facts can help avoid errors.

- Children with significant adenopathy, organomegaly, or other abnormalities apart from their bleeding diathesis probably do not have ITP.
- ITP produces isolated thrombocytopenia; an unexplained abnormality of another cell line is inconsistent with the diagnosis of ITP.
- Half of all children with acute lymphoblastic leukemia have normal white cell counts, indistinguishable from a child with ITP.
- ITP produces a systemic decrease in platelet numbers. Bruises and petechiae occur in a widespread, symmetric, and random fashion. Child abuse usually results in bruises that are asymmetric and nonrandom and may form patterns, such as a belt mark.
- vWD patients often have a variable coagulopathy and may have an episodic bleeding history.
- Sixty percent of all intracranial hemorrhages in hemophilic boys occur spontaneously. Headache and vomiting are the most common symptoms.
- HIV infection may complicate bleeding in hemophilia due to HIV-induced thrombocytopenia.
- Mild hemophilia commonly is asymptomatic until excessive bleeding from an injury occurs. It should be considered in any boy who develops excessive or prolonged bleeding after an injury. Hemophiliacs with potentially life- or limb-threatening bleeds should receive factor concentrates before any imaging studies are done.
- Recombinant human factor VIII concentrates should be used preferentially in boys with hemophilia A, and ultrapure factor IX concentrates in boys with hemophilia B.
- If the specific factor deficiency is not known, fresh-frozen plasma (10 mL/kg, if tolerated) is the product of choice for factor replacement. Fresh-frozen plasma is also the product of choice for the treatment of rare clotting-factor deficiencies.
- DDAVP (0.3 μg/kg) is effective for the treatment of mild hemophilia A and mild type I vWD. It is not useful in severe deficiencies or in factor IX deficiency.
- DDAVP may be helpful in controlling excessive bleeding in patients with uremia and qualitative platelet disorders, but it is not helpful in treating bleeding due to thrombocytopenia.
- Intranasal DDAVP (Stimate) may be useful in controlling minor bleeding in suitable patients, but it should not be relied on for treatment of patients that have not been shown to respond to it previously, as the response rates differ for intravenous versus intranasal DDAVP.

References

1. Bale JF, Contant CF, Garg B, et al. Neurologic history and examination results and their relationship to HIV type I serostatus in hemophilic subjects. *Pediatrics* 1993;91:736.
2. Blanchette VS, Kirby MA, Turner C. Role of intravenous immunoglobulin G in autoimmune hematologic disorders. *Semin Hematol* 1992;29[3, Suppl 2]:722.
3. Bloom AL. Progress in the clinical management of haemophilia. *Thromb Haemost* 1991;66(1):166.
4. Bloom AL. Management of factor VIII inhibitors: evolution and current status. *Haemostasis* 1992;22:268.
5. DiMichele D, Neufeld EJ. Hemophilia, a new approach to an old disease. *Hematol Oncol Clin North Am* 1998;12(6):1315.
6. Fleming P. Dental management of the pediatric oncology patient. *Curr Opin Dent* 1991;1:577.
7. George JN, Woolf SH, Raskob GE. Idiopathic thrombocytopenic purpura: a practice guideline developed by explicit methods for the American Society of Hematology. *Blood* 1996;88(1):3–40.
8. Green JG, Durham TM. Application of INSTAT hemostat in the control of gingival hemorrhage in the patient with thrombocytopenia. *Oral Surg Oral Med Oral Pathol* 1991;71(1):27.
9. Imbach P. Immune thrombocytopenic purpura and intravenous immunoglobulin. *Cancer* 1991;68[6, Suppl]:1422.
10. Logan LJ. Treatment of von Willebrand's disease. *Hematol Oncol Clin North Am* 1992;6:1079.
11. Lusher JM, Warrier I. Hemophilia A. *Hematol Oncol Clin North Am* 1992;6:1021.
12. Mannucci PM, Cattaneo M. Desmopressin: a nontransfusional treatment of hemophilia and von Willebrand disease. *Haemostasis* 1992;22:276.

13. Mannucci PM, Bettega D, Cattaneo M. Patterns of development of tachyphylaxis in patients with haemophilia and von Willebrand disease after repeated doses of desmopressin (DDAVP). *Br J Haematol* 1992;82:87.
14. de Tezanos Pinto M, Fernandez J, Perez Bianco PR. Update of 156 episodes of CNS bleeding in hemophiliacs. *Haemostasis* 1992;22:259.

CHAPTER 263
Bronchiolitis

Kathy N. Shaw

Each epidemic season, the emergency physician is faced with evaluating and treating infants and young children with bronchiolitis and determining their disposition. Unlike children with reactive airway disease, their lower respiratory tract symptoms are caused by inflammation of the bronchiolar epithelium by an acute infection. The resultant necrosis of epithelium and plugging of the 75- to 300-μm airways by cellular debris may result in air trapping or atelectasis distal to the obstruction.[1] This lower airway pathology may manifest as tachypnea, wheezing, rales, increased work of breathing, and/or hypoxemia.

Respiratory syncytial virus (RSV) is probably the most important respiratory pathogen among young children and may cause serious morbidity and mortality. Over 50% of infants will acquire RSV infection during the first epidemic that they experience, and 40% will progress from upper to lower respiratory tract illness. One in ten infants will require hospitalization. The peak incidence of lower airway disease occurs in infants 2 to 5 months of age.[8,9,13] Two major subtypes of the virus, strains A and B, circulate concomitantly, with one predominating during a given season. Subtype A is more commonly associated with more severe disease.[16] Children in the first few months of life, those with a history of prematurity, children with congenital heart disease (CHD), especially uncorrected pulmonary hypertension, and those who are immunosuppressed or have chronic lung disease are most at risk for severe disease and death.[6,11,15,22] Although RSV is the most common pathogen, other viruses, such as parainfluenza, influenza, adenovirus, and rhinoviruses, may cause bronchiolitis.[9,13]

CLINICAL PRESENTATION

The presentation of the infant or young child with bronchiolitis ranges from the smiling, interactive child with mild tachypnea and end-expiratory wheezing to the child who presents with severe respiratory distress or failure. Typically, there is a several-day history of upper respiratory tract symptoms of coryza and congestion before the onset of lower respiratory tract symptoms. The parent may have noted that the child started with a cold and now is not as active, is breathing faster, and has difficulty feeding. Although most have tachypnea, cough, wheezing, and increased work of breathing, the young infant may present with lethargy or irritability, apnea or tachypnea, and have few lower respiratory findings.[10,22] Fever is often present early in the course of illness, but may be absent or low grade at the time that lower respiratory tract symptoms manifest. Once lower respiratory tract involvement occurs, it usually progresses and peaks within 3 to 5 days. However, resolution of symptoms, including cough, wheezing, and some degree of hypoxemia, may take days to weeks.

DIFFERENTIAL DIAGNOSIS

Because bronchiolitis is so endemic during the winter months, the emergency physician must remember to consider other causes of acute onset of lower respiratory tract distress in infants. Congestive heart failure in the infant is often thought initially to be bronchiolitis during epidemics, as the infant may present with a history of poor feeding and tachypnea, rales, and wheezing on examination. Congenital lesions compromising the airway, such as vascular rings, slings, or teratomas, may appear to have acute onset. Aspiration from gastroesophageal reflux or tracheoesophageal "H-type" fistulas should cause symptoms around feeding. Congenital infections such as chlamydia pneumonia are prevalent throughout the year. Community-acquired bacterial pneumonia should also be considered in children of all ages. Foreign-body aspiration should also be suspected in young children.

In older infants and children, it is often difficult to distinguish bronchiolitis from asthma or reactive airway disease. The first episode of wheezing with upper respiratory tract symptoms in the young child should be considered bronchiolitis. Children with prior episodes of wheezing responsive to bronchodilator therapy, atopy, and a family history of asthma may have reactive airway disease. Repeat episodes of bronchiolitis are not uncommon, even with RSV. Additionally, infants who have had RSV bronchiolitis may be more prone to have repeated episodes of wheezing.[23] Whether the viral infection causes pulmonary damage or immunologic changes or the child who develops lower respiratory tract illness has a predisposition to reactive airway disease is the subject of debate.

EMERGENCY DEPARTMENT EVALUATION

No single fact or finding during emergency department (ED) evaluation is sensitive enough to predict which child will develop severe disease.[18,22] A combination of historic, physical examination, and laboratory measures must be considered when determining risk for significant morbidity and mortality (Table 263.1). In taking a history, it is important to determine the gestational age at birth and whether there were any perinatal complications, such as bronchopulmonary dysplasia (BPD). Underlying diseases or anomalies such as congenital heart disease, cystic fibrosis, or immunodeficiencies may put the infant at increased risk. It is also important to determine whether the child is in the first few days of illness, in which the disease will continue to progress, or beyond the 3- to 5-day peak of illness. Social issues, such as the mother's ability to care for a sick infant or return if the disease progresses, are also important to evaluate.

The overall appearance of the child is a sensitive indicator of disease severity. The child's respiratory rate, accessory muscle use for breathing, and air exchange are important to evaluate at presentation and after therapeutic trials. The infant's oxygen saturation, as determined by pulse oximetry, is the single most objective predictor of more severe disease and should be measured on all infants and children presenting to the ED with bronchiolitis.[22] Assessment of the child's hydration status by physical examination (moistness of mucous membranes, capillary refill at the fingertip, presence or absence of tears) should also be done, as many have a history of poor oral intake.

Radiographs are indicated in infants or young children with their first episode of wheezing or in children with high fever or

TABLE 263.1. Risk Factors Associated with More Severe Disease

Moderate Risk	High Risk
HISTORIC FACTORS	
Prematurity 34–37 wk	Prematurity <34 wk
Age <3 mo	History of cyanosis or apnea
First 3 d of illness	Underlying condition
	Pulmonary disease
	Congenital heart disease
	Immunodeficiency
PHYSICAL EXAMINATION FINDINGS	
General appearance: ill, not toxic	General appearance: toxic
Moderate accessory muscle use	Marked accessory muscle use
Respiratory rate: 60–70/min	Respiratory rate: >70/min
TESTING	
Oxygen saturation: 95%–96%	Oxygen saturation: <95%
Atelectasis on chest radiograph	
RSV infection, subtype A	

Data from Eriksson et al.,[6] Green et al.,[8] Hall et al.,[10,11] McConnochie et al.,[16] Opavsky et al.,[18] and Shaw et al.[22]

severe disease. The majority of radiographs will show some degree of hyperaeration (flattening of the diaphragms on lateral view or increased radiolucency with small heart size on the anterior view) or peribronchial thickening. Atelectasis or infiltrates occur in less than 10% of children presenting for outpatient evaluation.[22] Most areas of opacity represent atelectasis, but pneumonia cannot be excluded as a cause.

Evaluation of fever in infants less than 2 or 3 months of age should be done as per usual practice. For infants over 2 months of age with classic bronchiolitis, fever is unlikely to indicate serious bacterial illness and more likely to indicate early viral illness, pneumonia, or otitis media.[3,14] Therefore, routine culture of the blood or urine may be unnecessary. Complete blood cell counts are rarely useful. Microbiologic testing to determine viral etiology is indicated only for those with or at great risk for severe disease (BPD, CHD) or for cohorting purposes for hospital admission.

EMERGENCY DEPARTMENT MANAGEMENT

Children with moderate or severe respiratory distress should be allowed to assume a position of comfort, and 100% oxygen should be delivered. Suctioning of copious nasopharyngeal secretions may relieve some distress caused by airway obstruction. A trial of bronchodilators and/or racemic epinephrine should be delivered. Intubation is required for the child with severe respiratory distress not responding to these measures.

Table 263.2 lists current treatment options for children with bronchiolitis. Most children presenting to the ED with bronchiolitis have mild or moderate severity of illness. Those with very mild disease require supportive therapy only. The use and effectiveness of bronchodilators such as nebulized albuterol is controversial.[5,12,17,21] A trial of two nebulized treatments of albuterol (0.15 mg/kg per dose) given 20 to 30 minutes apart is usually given to infants and young children with moderate-to-severe symptoms. Assessment for objective improvement in oxygen saturation, lowering of the respiratory rate, or improved aeration indicates response. For those without improvement, there is no need or benefit to continue further treatments.[5] Nebulized racemic epinephrine has been more effective than β_2 agonists in several clinical trials and may be tried for those who do not respond and will require hospitalization.[17,21] Cromolyn sodium and immunoglobulin therapies are used for preventive care and have no role in the ED.[2,20] Ribavirin, an expensive antiviral agent, is probably not effective and also has no role in the ED.[19] Steroids, either inhaled or oral, have not been proven to be effective.[4] They should be reserved for children who have reactive airway disease. Antibiotics are indicated only when a specific bacterial infection has been diagnosed or for neonates with fever.[7] Many children with bronchiolitis have or develop bacterial ear infections.[3]

DISPOSITION

Indications for Admission

Most infants and children with bronchiolitis do not require admission. Clearly, those in respiratory distress or with hypoxia require intervention and admission. Among those with mild or moderate disease, no single factor can predict necessity for admission.[18,22] Children at high risk for developing more severe

TABLE 263.2. Treatment Options

Therapy	Indications	Effectiveness
Supportive (suctioning, mist)	Mainstay of therapy for mild or moderate bronchiolitis; suctioning prior to feeding helps infant to feed better.	Moistening of inspired air may be as beneficial as β_2 agonists in treatment.[5,21]
Oxygen	Oxygen saturation: <94%	Protects against hypoxia
Antibiotics	Not indicated empirically or for treatment of bronchiolitis	Use only for specific diagnosed bacterial infections, such as otitis media or pneumonia.[3,7,14]
Steroids (oral or inhaled)	Not indicated for bronchiolitis	Not proven to be helpful[4]
Bronchodilators (β_2 agonists, anticholinergics)	Poor air exchange Respiratory rate >50/min Marked work of breathing Oxygen saturation: <97%	Undetermined: probably helps some children; for infants <6 mo, less than half respond[5,12]
Racemic epinephrine	No response to trial of β_2 agonists and persistent severe symptoms requiring admission	Multiple clinical trials have shown effectiveness for moderate-to-severe disease.[17,21]
Cromolyn sodium	To prevent or limit future episodes of wheezing	Undetermined; not indicated at this time[20]
Ribavirin	Not useful in the ED	Probably not effective, even for those hospitalized for severe disease[19]
Immunotherapy (RSV-IGIV or palivizumab)	For prevention only	Proven to be beneficial in reducing hospitalization and severity of disease for infants who were premature or have bronchopulmonary dysplasia; not indicated for congenital heart disease[2]

disease (see Table 263.1) should be considered for admission or close outpatient observation. Any child who is early in the course of the illness or has moderate severity of illness, not requiring admission, should have follow-up arranged in 24 hours.

Role of the Consultant

Children with underlying medical conditions should have their subspecialist physicians consulted about treatment and indications for admission. For example, the pediatric cardiologist can determine whether the child with congenital heart disease has significant uncorrected pathology putting them at higher risk. If the diagnosis of bronchiolitis is not clear, a pediatrician may offer further help with the differential diagnosis or workup.

Transfer Considerations

Children with respiratory failure requiring intubation should be transferred to a facility with a pediatric intensive care unit. Children with underlying medical conditions or at high risk for severe disease or mortality should also be transferred to a facility with pediatric subspecialists and a pediatric intensive care unit.

COMMON PITFALLS

- Failure to identify that the child is in the first few days of illness and may get progressively worse. These children who appear to have mild illness may progress over the next hours or days and require close outpatient follow-up. The caregiver should be given specific instructions of what to look for and when to return.
- Failure to identify that the child has an underlying condition or history of prematurity. It is important to ask and document whether the child has risk factors that put him or her at high risk for morbidity and mortality.
- Persistence in using bronchodilators despite no evidence of response. Less than half of infants with bronchiolitis will respond to bronchodilators. If they have mild disease, they should be sent home with symptomatic care instructions and follow-up arrangements.
- Failure to use pulse oximetry to identify children with hypoxemia. This is the most specific and objective indicator of more severe disease. Cyanosis detectable on physical examination does not occur until the oxygen saturation is less than 85%!
- Use of routine laboratory tests or radiographs. Evaluation of infants and young children with bronchiolitis should be tailored to the individual patient.

References

1. Aherne W, Bird T, Court SD, et al. Pathological changes in virus infections of the lower respiratory tract in children. *J Clin Pathol* 1970;23:7.
2. American Academy of Pediatrics. Committee on Infectious Diseases and Committee on Fetus and Newborn. Prevention of respiratory syncytial virus infections: indications for the use of palivizumab and update on the use of RSV-IGIV. *Pediatrics* 1998;102(5):1211.
3. Andrade MA, Hoberman A, Glustein J, et al. Acute otitis media in children with bronchiolitis. *Pediatrics* 1998;101:617.
4. De Boeck K, Van der As N, Van Lierde S, et al. Respiratory syncytial virus bronchiolitis: A double blind dexamethasone efficacy study. *J Pediatr* 1997;131:919.
5. Dobson JV, Stephens-Groff SM, McMahon SR, et al. The use of albuterol in hospitalized infants with bronchiolitis. *Pediatrics* 1998;101:361.
6. Eriksson M, Forsgren M, Sjoberg S, et al. Respiratory syncytial virus infection in young hospitalized children: identification of risk patients and prevention of nosocomial spread by rapid diagnosis. *Acta Paediatr Scand* 1983;72:47.
7. Field CMB, Connolly JH, Murtagh G, et al. Antibiotic treatment of epidemic bronchiolitis—a double-blind trial. *BMJ* 1966;1:83.
8. Green M, Brayer A, Schenkman KA, et al. Duration of hospitalization in previously well infants with RSV infection. *Pediatr Infect Dis J* 1989;8:601.
9. Glezen WP, Denny FW. Epidemiology of acute lower respiratory disease in children. *N Engl J Med* 1973;288:498.
10. Hall CB, Kopelman AE, Douglas RG, et al. Neonatal respiratory syncytial virus infection. *N Engl J Med* 1979;300:393.
11. Hall CB, Powell KR, MacDonald WE, et al. RSV infection in children with compromised immune function. *N Engl J Med* 1986;315:77.
12. Kellner JD, Ohlsson A, Gadomski AM, et al. Efficacy of bronchodilator therapy in bronchiolitis. a meta-analysis. *Arch Pediatr Adolesc Med* 1996;150(11):1166.
13. Kim HW, Arrobio JO, Brandt CD, et al. Epidemiology of respiratory syncytial virus in Washington, DC. Importance in different respiratory tract disease syndromes and temporal distribution. *Am J Epidemiol* 1973;98:216.
14. Kuppermann N, Bank DE, Walton EA, et al. Risks for bacteremia and UTI in young febrile children with bronchiolitis. *Arch Pediatr Adolesc Med* 1997;151:1207.
15. MacDonald NE, Hall CB, Suffin SC, et al. Respiratory syncytial viral infection in infants with congenital heart disease. *N Engl J Med* 1982;307:397.
16. McConnochie KM, Hall CB, Walsh EE, et al. Variation in severity of respiratory syncytial virus with subtype. *J Pediatr* 1990;117:52.
17. Menon K, Sutcliffe T, Klassen TP. A randomized trial comparing the efficacy of epinephrine with salbutamol in the treatment of acute bronchiolitis. *J Pediatr* 1995;126:1004.
18. Opavsky MA, Stephens D, Wang EEL. Testing models predicting severity of respiratory syncytial virus infection on the PICNIC RSV database. *Arch Pediatr Adolesc Med* 1995;149:1217.
19. Randolph AG, Wang EEL. Ribavirin for respiratory syncytial virus lower respiratory tract infection. *Arch Pediatr Adolesc Med* 1996;150:942.
20. Reijonen T, Korppi M, Kuikka L, et al. Anti-inflammatory therapy reduces wheezing after bronchiolitis. *Arch Pediatr Adolesc Med* 1996;150(5):512.
21. Reijonen T, Korppi M, Pitkakangas S, et al. The clinical efficacy of nebulized racemic epinephrine and albuterol in acute bronchiolitis. *Arch Pediatr Adolesc Med* 1995;149(6):686.
22. Shaw KN, Bell LM, Sherman NH. Outpatient assessment of infants with bronchiolitis. *Am J Dis Child* 1991;145:151.
23. Sigurs N, Bjarnason R, Sigurbergsson F, et al. Asthma and immunoglobulin E antibodies after respiratory syncytial virus bronchiolitis: a prospective cohort study with matched controls. *Pediatrics* 1995;95(4):500.

CHAPTER 264
Cellulitis

Christopher S. Kennedy and Madhumita Sinha

Cellulitis is an acute inflammation of the skin and subcutaneous soft tissue that is commonly caused by bacterial infection. The age of the child, the history, and the location of the infection serve as important determinants of the most likely bacterial agent. Cellulitis may occur by local tissue invasion following minor skin breaks, by puncture wounds by an object or tooth, or from hematogenous dissemination of a pathogenic organism. More common in the pediatric population, periorbital and facial cellulitis occurs in children less than 5 years of age, and may be accompanied by fever and ill appearance. Unique to the newborn period is neonatal omphalitis (infection of the umbilicus and surrounding tissues).

In most instances, children with cellulitis recover uneventfully. However, the recent resurgence of invasive group A β-hemolytic *Streptococcus* (GABHS) infection, characterized by necrotizing fasciitis, bacteremia, and toxic shock, reminds us that the potential for serious complications exists, and emphasizes the need for accurate diagnosis and appropriate management.

EPIDEMIOLOGY

During the course of normal play, children incur minor injuries with breaks of the skin. Any injury or skin opening that disrupts the protective barrier of the skin can serve as portal of entry for pathogens, most commonly GABHS or *Staphylococcus aureus*. Puncture wounds by a contaminated object such as a cat claw or a nail penetrating a tennis shoe may predispose to other causative pathogens, such as *Pasteurella* sp. and *Pseudomonas* sp., respectively. Likewise, animal and human bites result in an increased likelihood of *Pasteurella multocida* and *Eikenella corrodens* infections.

Omphalitis, or infection of the umbilicus, with accompanying erythema of the abdomen, is a diagnosis unique to the newborn period, usually occurring in the first few weeks of life. The cord stump may serve as a portal of bacterial entry for *S. aureus*, GABHS, group B streptococci, and gram-negative enterics.

The epidemiology of childhood facial cellulitis has changed dramatically since the introduction of *Haemophilus influenzae* type B (HIB) vaccine. HIB had been the cause of more than 50% of cases of facial cellulitis, but, in the postvaccine era, it has become a rare agent. Now, common organisms include GABHS, *S. aureus*, and *Streptococcus pneumoniae*. Facial and periorbital infections caused by HIB and *S. pneumoniae* usually spread by a hematogenous route, and hence can be isolated by blood culture.

Primary dental infection may lead to bacterial seeding of adjacent facial soft tissues by a variety of aerobic and anaerobic bacteria, such as *Bacteroides* and *Fusobacterium*.

Important preexisting conditions that may predispose to infections include other traumatic injuries, particularly crush injuries, preexisting vascular or lymphatic compromise, chronic cutaneous conditions such as eczema, and immunocompromised states. More recently, case reports of necrotizing fasciitis due to GABHS infection have indicated a predisposition for severe varicella infection.

CLINICAL PRESENTATION

The most reliable way to diagnose cellulitis is to recognize the characteristic clinical features: localized erythema, warmth, edema, and pain. Most often, cellulitis involves the extremities, usually the lower extremities in children. Demarcation between involved and adjacent normal skin may be indistinct. There may be associated lymphangitis, appearing as red streaks radiating from the margin of the lesion, and also enlargement and tenderness of regional lymph nodes. The white blood cell (WBC) count is usually normal. Children with cellulitis of an extremity may exhibit limitation of movement of the affected limb due to pain from the infection. In 10% to 20% of cases, cellulitis may be associated with fever and other systemic symptoms, such as chills, myalgias, malaise, and even emesis. When fever is present, a concomitant bacteremia should be presumed and leukocytosis expected.

Distinct clinical entities include erysipelas, periorbital cellulitis, omphalitis, and necrotizing fasciitis. Erysipelas, a more superficial cellulitis most often associated with GABHS infection, typically has very sharp, elevated margins that rapidly spread outward, with central clearing and tenderness to palpation.

Periorbital cellulitis, a form of facial cellulitis usually seen in children less than 5 years old, presents with swelling of the eyelids, erythema of a violaceous hue, normal eye movements, and absence of proptosis. Bacteremia and leukocytosis may be associated particularly with infection by *H. influenzae* or *S. pneumoniae* in as many as 90% of cases.

Omphalitis presents in the newborn as purulent, foul-smelling discharge from the umbilical stump and erythema of the abdominal wall. Associated fever, hypothermia, lethargy, and irritability may be seen late in the course. Laboratory studies such as a WBC count will be normal in early localized infections. The diagnosis of omphalitis can be challenging, because drainage and small areas of erythema may be present without true infection, and there are no definitive criteria. Suggestive findings include anterior abdominal erythema and circumferential erythema of the umbilicus. Infection is clearly indicated when induration and erythema of the anterior abdominal wall are present.

Deeper infections of the skin and soft tissues may include fasciitis, myonecrosis, and gas gangrene. Necrotizing fasciitis initially presents as a cellulitis, but the subsequent development of purpura, blistering, necrosis (manifested clinically by pain out of proportion to the cutaneous findings), and severe systemic toxicity with tachycardia, and even hypotension, suggest a more serious infection. The child may be lethargic, disoriented, and in profound shock.

DIFFERENTIAL DIAGNOSIS

Any tender, erythematous swelling of the skin and subcutaneous soft tissue may resemble cellulitis. Trauma, insect bites or stings, localized urticarial eruptions, swelling overlying a sprain or fracture, or a joint with septic arthritis may be mistaken for cellulitis. Mosquito bites may induce significant lymphedema surrounding the bite site, which develops over hours. The bites are usually described as itching rather than painful. Bee stings and spider bites may also cause significant lymphedema, warmth, and even tenderness, and they may be more difficult to distinguish from cellulitis.

"Popsicle panniculitis" can also mimic facial cellulitis. Thought to be a cold-induced histamine response from eating water ice, typically the skin involvement begins at the labial crease and spreads outward with a warm, mildly tender cheek. Insect bites and stings, panniculitis, and contusions all lack fever, a relatively common symptom of cellulitis. Localized, specific soft-tissue infections, such as folliculitis (infection of a pilosebaceous follicle), furuncles and carbuncles (deep follicular abscess, either solitary or multiple), impetigo (vesiculopustular lesion), ecthyma (ulcerated impetigo), and others, should be differentiated from cellulitis by their characteristic clinical appearances.

Extremity cellulitis, as mentioned earlier, may cause limitation of movement of the affected limb; for that reason, it may be difficult to distinguish from deeper tissue infection such as osteomyelitis or septic arthritis.

EMERGENCY DEPARTMENT EVALUATION

In most situations, diagnosis of cellulitis is made on clinical grounds. Blood culture and WBC count should be reserved for patients presenting with fever or associated systemic toxicity or for those who are immunocompromised. Certain clinical features are specific enough to make a reasonable etiologic assumption. Erysipelas, with its characteristic rapidly advancing, raised, sharply demarcated margin, is usually caused by GABHS. A bluish or violaceous discoloration of the area involved by cellulitis suggests infection by *H. influenzae* or *S. pneumoniae*.

With the reemergence of suppurative GABHS infections, it is important to distinguish early streptococcal necrotizing fasciitis from cellulitis, as fasciitis may require surgical debridement. Necrotizing fasciitis is characterized by diffuse swelling with extreme tenderness at the local site, followed by bulla formation with rapid purplish discoloration and extension into deeper fascial planes. Streptococcal toxic shock syndrome may be associated with necrotizing fasciitis in as many as 50% of cases.[1]

Cellulitis in the buccal or perineal area that develops after a human or animal bite, or cellulitis in an area involving devitalized or necrotic tissue, should raise the concern for the anaerobic organisms *Bacteroides, Fusobacterium,* and *Clostridium.* Cellulitis caused by pet bites is often associated with *Pasteurella.* Cellulitis due to water-contaminated wounds is often caused by *Aeromonas* and *Vibrio* species. Severe systemic symptoms in any patients with cellulitis should suggest the possibility of concurrent bacteremia. Presence of immunocompromised states should alert the clinician to the possibility of atypical infectious agents as the etiologic agents of cellulitis.

In any patient with periorbital cellulitis, it is particularly important to rule out orbital cellulitis, a much more severe infection that may need surgical intervention. In a patient with orbital cellulitis, unlike periorbital cellulitis, the ocular movements are restricted and painful, and proptosis is usually present.

Although the combination of clinical features and epidemiologic considerations may suggest the etiology of cellulitis, definitive bacteriologic diagnosis requires isolation of the causative organism. In the past, because of the high prevalence of bacteremia with *H. influenzae,* blood cultures were routinely done in children with cellulitis. In the post-HIB vaccine era, however, the association of bacteremia with cellulitis in children has reduced dramatically, and recent studies indicate that the practice of obtaining blood cultures routinely may not be cost effective.[5,6] Of note, positive blood cultures are most commonly associated with younger age, active varicella, and soft-tissue infections such as osteomyelitis or septic arthritis.

Needle aspiration of the cutaneous inflammatory lesion, accompanied by prompt Gram stain and culture, is a rapid and specific tool to establish a bacteriologic diagnosis. Aspiration is performed by inserting a 22-gauge needle attached to a 1-cc syringe into the advancing edge of the cellulitis. If no material is aspirated, 0.1 mL of normal saline may be injected in to the area, followed by immediate aspiration. The yield of needle aspiration, however, is modest; a positive aspiration rate in different studies varies from 5% to 50%.[4]

If underlying deeper trauma or infection is suspected, appropriate imaging should be done. In a patient with severe periorbital cellulitis, a computed tomography scan is recommended if orbital involvement is suspected or cannot be excluded by examination of the eye, and if inflammation progresses despite optimal antibiotic treatment.[3]

EMERGENCY DEPARTMENT MANAGEMENT

Application of warm compresses to the affected area, elevation of the affected limb, and bed rest are often useful. Analgesics may be needed for control of pain. Antibiotic therapy, in most cases, except in the mildest form of cellulitis, is warranted. Given the low yield of microbiologic workup, in most situations antibiotic therapy is empirical but should be based on sound clinical judgment.

Hospital admission and parenteral antibiotic therapy should be strongly considered in any febrile child with cellulitis. All neonates with suspected omphalitis should be promptly admitted and started on parenteral antibiotics. In infants less than 3 months of age, cellulitis is commonly caused by group B streptococcus and should be treated with parenteral penicillin along with an aminoglycoside and hospital admission. Between 3 months and 3 years of age, *H. influenzae* and *S. pneumoniae* are the likely organisms, and third-generation cephalosporins (ceftriaxone or cefotaxime) should be administered. Some 10% to 40% of *H. influenzae* isolates are resistant to ampicillin, which should not be used alone. Ampicillin with a beta-lactamase inhibitor such as clavulanic acid may be used instead.

Erythromycin also is not appropriate for treatment of cellulitis. Beyond age 3 years, patients with well-localized cellulitis and without fever or systemic toxicity may be treated on an outpatient basis with an antistaphylococcal oral antibiotic, including penicillinase-resistant penicillin or newer cephalosporins such as cefuroxime. Ceftriaxone, with its once-a-day intramuscular dosing, may also be used in appropriate patients.

Any patient with cellulitis who shows severe systemic toxicity or does not improve within 48 hours of oral antibiotic therapy should receive high-dose intravenous broad-spectrum antibiotic therapy covering both streptococci and staphylococci. Patients suspected of a severe infection with GABHS, such as fasciitis, may need parenteral clindamycin in addition to penicillin, a surgical consultation, and close monitoring for signs of shock.

Patients who respond promptly to parenteral antibiotics may be changed over to oral antibiotics, but, in most cases of cellulitis, total duration of therapy should be at least 7 days. Patients with immunosuppressed conditions often develop cellulitis caused by atypical organisms, *Corynebacterium, Pseudomonas,* atypical mycobacteria, and even fungi. A microbiologic diagnosis should be vigorously pursued in these patients, particularly when initial empirical therapy fails to show any response.

Complications of cellulitis usually develop from extension of infection to deeper underlying tissue, often resulting in osteomyelitis or arthritis. Septicemia may develop in patients with severe, suboptimally treated infections, and meningitis, arthritis, endocarditis, or other metastatic complications may develop. Immunocompromised patients and younger patients are at the greatest risk for such complications. Patients with cellulitis involving the dangerous area of the face are susceptible to the complication of cavernous sinus thrombosis.

DISPOSITION

All infants younger than 6 months old who have cellulitis should be admitted, as should patients who appear to be toxic and have severe systemic symptoms and those who are immunosuppressed. Patients with facial cellulitis and a fever of more than 38.5°C and patients with extremity cellulitis and a fever of more than 38.5°C and a WBC count of more than 15,000/mL should be admitted. All other patients with cellulitis may be started on antibiotics on an outpatient basis, with follow-up arranged at 48-hour intervals. The recommendations for hospital admission are essentially based on the risk of bacteremia associated with cellulitis and the consequent need for intravenous antibiotics. However, with the decreasing incidence of *H. influenzae* cellulitis and associated bacteremia and the availability of potent oral antibiotics, more and more patients with cellulitis will probably be managed as outpatients in this age of managed care and cost containment.

COMMON PITFALLS

- With the recent increase in invasive GABHS infections, early recognition is important, as it may drastically change management.
- Orbital cellulitis should always be considered in the differential diagnosis of periorbital cellulitis.
- In immunocompromised patients with cellulitis, atypical and opportunistic infections are common, and microbiologic diagnosis should be actively pursued.

- Patients with cellulitis who are treated as outpatients should have follow-up within 48 hours.

References

1. Bisno A, Stevens DL. Streptococcal infections of skin and soft tissues. *N Engl J Med* 1996;334:240.
2. Doctor A, Harper MB, Fleisher GR. Group A β hemolytic streptococcal bacteremia: historical overview, changing incidence, and recent association with varicella. *Pediatrics* 1995;96:428.
3. Goldberg F, Berne AS, Oski FA. Differentiation of orbital cellulitis from preseptal cellulitis by computed tomography. *Pediatrics* 1978;52:1000.
4. Sachs MK. Cutaneous cellulitis. *Arch Dermatol* 1991;127:493.
5. Sadow KB, Chamberlain JM. Blood cultures in the evaluation of cellulitis. *Pediatrics* 1998;101:E4.
6. Schwartz GR, Wright SW. Changing bacteriology of periorbital cellulitis. *Ann Emerg Med* 1996;28:617.

TABLE 265.1. Etiology and Pathophysiology of Low Cardiac Output

LEFT-SIDED OBSTRUCTION
Aortic stenosis
Hypoplastic left heart
Coarctation of the aorta
Interrupted aortic arch
POOR MYOCARDIAL FUNCTION
Cardiomyopathy
Myocarditis
Glycogen storage diseases
Coronary artery anomaly
POOR VENTRICULAR FILLING
Congenital mitral stenosis
Tachyarrhythmias
Pulmonary venous obstruction

CHAPTER 265

Congenital Heart Disease, Congestive Heart Failure, and Other Cardiac Presentations

Randall M. Bryant

Emergency care required by the child with cardiac disease may be quite variable, with symptoms from a variety of etiologies (congenital heart defects, arrhythmias, cardiomyopathies). This potentially broad range of presentations makes definitive diagnosis and treatment a complex topic.[4] In general, the symptomatic child or infant with heart disease will present with low cardiac output, congestive heart failure, or cyanosis. Unfortunately, the diagnostic tools available to the emergency physician are often limited to the chest radiograph, the electrocardiogram (ECG), and, of course, the physical examination. Appropriate management of the cardiac patient requires a timely response by the emergency physician, coordinated with the primary care physician and the pediatric cardiologist or cardiovascular surgeon. Herein, we discuss the clinical presentation, initial evaluation, and management of these patients in the emergency department.

LOW CARDIAC OUTPUT

The discerning emergency physician should easily recognize the child with low cardiac output. These children usually present with tachypnea with or without distress, pallor or mottling of the extremities, peripheral cyanosis, diminished or asymmetric pulses, and oliguria and/or acidosis.[9] Because of decreased peripheral perfusion, venous or arterial access may be difficult to obtain, although necessary for resuscitation. They may present with hemodynamic instability or may initially appear stable hemodynamically and then quickly deteriorate. Depending on the degree of distress at presentation, a specific congenital heart defect may not be characterized until the patient's postmortem study.

The pathophysiology of low cardiac output in the pediatric cardiology patient generally falls into three categories: left-sided obstructive lesions, poor myocardial function, and poor ventricular filling (Table 265.1).

Left-Sided Obstructive Lesions

The timing of presentation of a left-sided obstructive lesion is variable and is dependent on the degree of obstruction. The most common lesions that present in the emergency setting are aortic valve stenosis, hypoplastic left heart syndrome (HLHS), coarctation of the aorta and interrupted aortic arch (IAA). The patient with mild aortic stenosis due to a bicuspid aortic valve may present in late childhood when a murmur is noted during an otherwise normal physical examination. The patient with severe aortic stenosis may present in early infancy and have very little murmur due to the small orifice of a unicuspid aortic valve and associated diminished cardiac output. These patients may appear cyanotic due to right-to-left shunting across a patent ductus arteriosus (PDA), their main source of systemic blood flow. Alternatively, they may present obtunded with severe acidosis following spontaneous ductal closure. Likewise, infants with HLHS and IAA may present in an obtunded state following ductal closure. Patients with coarctation of the aorta may have a progressive course, depending on the degree of obstruction. Symptomatic infants generally present at 2 weeks of age due to progressive ductal closure, while older children with less severe coarctations may present with hypertension and multiple collateral vessels. Unlike patients with aortic stenosis and HLHS, who present with diminished pulses throughout, patients with coarctation of the aorta and IAA have asymmetric upper and lower extremity pulses.

The radiographic findings in patients with left-sided obstructive lesions may vary, depending on the lesion. With chronic aortic stenosis, there may be evidence of cardiomegaly with poststenotic dilatation of the ascending aorta. However, infants with HLHS may, surprisingly, have normal radiographic findings. Infants with coarctation of the aorta who present in failure may have cardiac dilatation; however, older children may have a normal heart size with visible indentation at the coarctation site and evidence for collateral blood vessels, characterized by rib notching. Infants with IAA in general have cardiac dilatation and pulmonary congestion at the time of presentation. A narrowed mediastinum on chest radiograph suggests the absence of a thymus. This finding, along with hypocalcemia, suggests the presence of DiGeorge syndrome.

Electrocardiographic findings vary considerably. In most of these lesions, the ECG may be normal. As the patient develops evidence of ventricular failure, evidence of LV hypertrophy and lateral T-wave inversion may arise. Patients with coarctation often have evidence of right ventricular hypertrophy, characterized by a Q wave in the anterior precordial leads. The hypocalcemia accompanying IAA with DiGeorge syndrome can result in QTc prolongation.

If cyanotic, a patient with low cardiac output due to left-sided obstruction will increase their PaO_2 greater than 20 mm Hg when challenged with oxygen.

The appropriate treatment of low cardiac output in a child depends on the etiology. If there is concern regarding a *left-sided obstructive lesion,* initiation of prostaglandin E_1 (PGE_1) with inotropic support is indicated to maintain systemic blood flow via a PDA. In some congenital heart defects (e.g., HLHS), it is acceptable to decrease the F_iO_2 less than 21% to increase pulmonary vascular resistance and promote systemic blood flow across the PDA. A prompt referral to a pediatric cardiologist or pediatric cardiovascular surgeon is indicated for evaluation and treatment.

Poor Myocardial Function

Clinical signs of diminished cardiac output may occur in patients with poor myocardial function due to a cardiomyopathy or myocarditis. A cardiomyopathy may occur as a result of ischemia due to a coronary anomaly, a glycogen storage disease, a previous viral infection, a muscular dystrophy, or an inherited or idiopathic myopathy. The degree of symptomatology is usually related to the degree of cardiac dysfunction. The patient with mild dysfunction may present with only mild cardiomegaly on a routine chest radiograph, while the patient with an end-stage cardiomyopathy may present in florid congestive heart failure requiring emergent resuscitation. Likewise, the child with acute myocarditis may present with severe cardiac dysfunction and an associated tachyarrhythmia (e.g., polymorphic ventricular tachycardia) or bradyarrhythmia (e.g., complete atrioventricular [AV] block).

The radiographic findings in these patients are cardiomegaly and, frequently, pulmonary edema. Depending on the etiology, the cardiomegaly is usually LV in origin.

Patients with a "dilated," poorly functioning hypertrophic cardiomyopathy may have evidence of increased voltages throughout the precordium, with evidence of ST-segment or T-wave changes. Children with glycogen storage diseases, such as Pompe disease, may have evidence of a short PR interval with very large precordial QRS voltages. Decreased amplitudes, manifested as a *low-voltage QRS* (less than 5 mm total in each frontal lead), suggest the presence of myocarditis. Patients with an anomalous left coronary arising from the pulmonary artery will have evidence of an LV infarct with an abnormal Q wave in leads aVL and I, as well as T-wave and ST-segment changes laterally.[5]

If cyanotic, a patient with low cardiac output due to poor ventricular function will increase the PaO_2 greater than 20 mmHg when challenged with oxygen.

If the etiology of the low cardiac output appears to be due to poor myocardial function, then oxygen is indicated with inotropic support, including afterload reduction. These measures are used to reduce cardiac work in an attempt to improve cardiac output. The use of steroids in myocarditis is controversial.

Poor Ventricular Filling

Diminished cardiac output may occur in children with poor ventricular filling as a result of congenital or rheumatic mitral valve stenosis, pulmonary venous obstruction, and tachyarrhythmias. These children may not only present with evidence of poor systemic blood flow, but also, in the most severe cases, often have evidence of pulmonary edema and right heart failure, manifested by hepatomegaly and peripheral edema.

Radiographically, these patients will have electrocardiographic evidence of cardiac enlargement and pulmonary edema. Patients with mitral stenosis have the classic radiographic findings of left atrial enlargement, with pulmonary edema and dilation of the pulmonary vasculature. In patients with pulmonary venous obstruction, the left atrium is usually small, with pulmonary edema and right heart enlargement. In particular, the pulmonary blood vessels may be massively dilated due to chronic pulmonary hypertension. Patients with sustained tachyarrhythmias usually have cardiac enlargement as a result of LV failure and, as such, demonstrate LV enlargement on the chest radiograph.

Patients with congenital mitral stenosis have electrocardiographic evidence of left atrial enlargement and LV voltages, while patients with tachyarrhythmias tend to have retrograde P waves while in supraventricular tachycardia (SVT) or V-A dissociation if in ventricular tachycardia.

If cyanotic, a patient with low cardiac output due to poor ventricular filling will increase their PaO_2 greater than 20 mmHg when challenged with oxygen.

In patients with poor ventricular filling as their etiology of poor cardiac output, oxygen administration and diuresis are usually indicated. If symptomatic, many patients may also require correction of a severe metabolic acidosis. If obstruction is significant, these patients can become severely ill in a short period of time. Although administration of PGE_1, in some cases, can promote systemic blood flow via a patent ductus, prompt referral to a pediatric cardiovascular surgeon is required for surgical repair or palliation.

If the patient has a tachyarrhythmia, conversion either by adenosine (0.1 to 0.3 mg/kg per dose) or, if hemodynamically compromised, DC cardioversion (0.5 to 2.0 J/kg) is indicated.[8] Calcium channel blockers in children, particularly in infants, are contraindicated. They are negative inotropes as well as a peripheral vasodilators and, as such, can produce dramatic hemodynamic compromise and, in some cases, cardiac arrest.

CONGESTIVE HEART FAILURE

Children with congestive heart failure generally present with symptoms similar to adults: tachypnea, tachycardia, and diaphoresis.[1] Because the majority of work performed by infants and small children occurs during feeding, many of these children will also have feeding intolerance and failure to thrive. Uncommonly, they may have peripheral edema. Most infants with a significant left-to-right shunt will present at 6 to 8 weeks of life as their pulmonary vascular resistance naturally drops to permit pulmonary overcirculation.

The pathophysiology of congestive heart failure in these children is increased pulmonary blood flow, pulmonary interstitial edema, and volume overload. The congenital heart defects most commonly associated with congestive heart failure are those that result in pulmonary recirculation via a large left-to-right shunt. They include ventricular septal defects, AV canal, PDA, atrial septal defects, aortopulmonary windows, and truncus arteriosus (Table 265.2).

The clinical findings of "stiff, wet lungs" and a large heart correlate with the radiographic findings. Typically, there is car-

TABLE 265.2. Etiology and Pathophysiology of Congestive Heart Failure[a]

PATHOPHYSIOLOGY
Increased pulmonary blood flow
Pulmonary interstitial edema
Volume overload (dilation)
CONGENITAL DEFECTS
Ventricular septal defects
Atrioventricular canal
Patent ductus arteriosus
Atrial septal defects
Aortopulmonary window
Truncus arteriosus

[a] Stiff lungs, large heart, and increased pulmonary vascular markings.

diac enlargement and increased pulmonary vascular markings, with pulmonary edema.

The electrocardiographic findings may be nonspecific, depending on the level of the shunt; however, a QRS axis of –30 degrees to –120 degrees in an infant, particularly one with trisomy 21, is consistent with an AV canal.

If cyanotic, these children will increase their PaO_2 by greater than 20 mm Hg in response to oxygen.

The treatment, in general, is respiratory support and inotropic support. Afterload reduction and intravenous diuretics are often indicated; however, those patients who have feeding intolerance may present with dehydration, in which case initiation of intravenous diuretics should be withheld until the patient is appropriately rehydrated.

CYANOSIS

The cyanotic child is usually diagnosed in infancy; however, due to multiple factors, including (1) the ratio of fetal-to-adult hemoglobin, (2) the concentration of deoxyhemoglobin, and (3) the total hemoglobin, cyanosis may go undetected. Also, it is not uncommon for a child to have unrecognized cyanosis while at rest, only to become hypercyanotic when agitated. Interestingly, as these patients become more cyanotic, their murmur gets softer as blood is shunted right to left, away from the area of obstruction. In general, pediatric patients with cyanosis have one of three presentations: (1) a normal heart size with decreased pulmonary vascular markings (2) a small heart with pulmonary edema, and (3) a large heart with increased pulmonary vascular markings (Table 265.3).

TABLE 265.3. Etiology of Cyanosis Based on Radiographic and Clinical Findings

NORMAL/LARGE HEART WITH DECREASED PVMS
Tetralogy of Fallot
Double-outlet right ventricle with pulmonary stenosis
Pulmonary atresia, severe pulmonary stenosis
Transposition of great arteries with VSD and PS
Tricuspid atresia
Ebstein's anomaly of the tricuspid valve
SMALL HEART WITH PULMONARY EDEMA
Total anomalous pulmonary venous return with obstruction, often below the diaphragm to the portal system
LARGE HEART WITH INCREASED PVMS
Transposition of the great arteries
Total anomalous pulmonary venous return
Truncus arteriosus
Double-outlet right ventricle
Single ventricle

PVMs, pulmonary vascular markings; PS, pulmonary stenosis; VSD ventricular septal defect.

Normal or Large Heart with Decreased Pulmonary Vascular Markings

Patients with a normal or large heart size with decreased pulmonary vascular markings typically have some degree of obstruction of pulmonary blood flow. Because of an atrial or ventricular right-to-left shunt, they have mixing of desaturated blood with systemic blood, resulting in cyanosis. Their degree of cyanosis is variable, depending on the degree of obstruction and the degree of shunt at the time of presentation. The congenital heart defect most associated with these symptoms is tetralogy of Fallot but may also include double-outlet right ventricle with pulmonary stenosis, pulmonary atresia or severe pulmonary stenosis, transposition of the great arteries with a ventricular septal defect and pulmonary stenosis, tricuspid atresia, and Ebstein's anomaly of the tricuspid valve.

These patients typically present with central cyanosis but may also have a history of hypercyanotic spells. At the time of cyanosis, they are often hyperpneic. Occasionally, they may present with acidosis due to a low cardiac output as a result of closure of a ductus arteriosus.

Radiographically, these patients may present with an increased heart size. Classically, Ebstein's anomaly is the congenital heart defect with a "wall-to-wall heart." Also, transposition of the great arteries and tricuspid atresia may demonstrate cardiac enlargement on chest radiograph. If there is a narrowed mediastinum with an "egg on a string" appearance, transposition of the great arteries should be considered. Patients with tetralogy of Fallot and a right aortic arch or patients with pulmonary atresia may have an absent pulmonary artery segment, thereby giving the heart a "boot-shaped" appearance.

Electrocardiographically, these patients may have right ventricular hypertrophy (tetralogy of Fallot, double-outlet right ventricle, pulmonary stenosis, transposition of the great arteries, or Ebstein's anomaly) or decreased right ventricular forces (tricuspid atresia and pulmonary atresia). If the QRS axis is negative with right atrial enlargement, then tricuspid atresia should be considered.

Because these patients have an obligatory shunt or a fixed obstruction to pulmonary blood flow, then their PaO_2 would increase less than 20 mm Hg in response to oxygen. Because oxygen can be an effective pulmonary vasodilator, in some cases, a decrease in pulmonary vascular resistance may diminish right-to-left shunting, resulting in a significant increase in PaO_2 in response to oxygen, In patients with hypercyanosis, the treatment of choice includes oxygen and sedation. Often, the mother is allowed to hold the child, and all attempts at intravenous access are withheld until the patient is adequately sedated with low-dose morphine (0.05 to 0.1 mg/kg intravenously or intramuscularly) or, in some cases, ketamine (1 mg/kg intravenously or 2 mg/kg intramuscularly). In addition, maneuvers such as "knee-to-chest" positioning and volume administration are performed to increase systemic vascular resistance. In refractory cases, alpha agonists (e.g., phenylephrine) should be considered to increase systemic vascular resistance and promote pulmonary blood flow by diminishing the right-to-left shunt. Referral to a pediatric cardiologist or pediatric cardiovascular surgeon is indicated for balloon palliation or surgical palliation or repair.

Small Heart with Pulmonary Edema

These patients may present in severe distress, with tachypnea, metabolic acidosis, low cardiac output, and central cyanosis. The pathophysiology of these findings is obstruction of pulmonary venous return. Typically, this is due to a total anomalous pulmonary venous return (TAPVR) with obstruction. Often, this occurs below the diaphragm at the portal but may also occur supradiaphragmatically.

The chest radiograph generally demonstrates a heart that is either normal or small in appearance, with pulmonary edema. Patients with supracardiac TAPVR may demonstrate a "snowman sign," due to the ascending vertical vein. These patients are much less commonly obstructed.

Electrocardiographic findings may be normal or demonstrate right ventricular hypertrophy.

The response to oxygen may be variable. In general, the PaO_2 increases less than 20 mm Hg when challenged with oxygen; however, in the presence of a PDA that shunts right to left and secondary pulmonary hypertension, oxygen may result in improved PaO_2.

Treatment generally requires aggressive inotropic support and immediate intervention, which may include balloon atrial septostomy, balloon dilation at the site of obstruction, or surgical repair or palliation.

Large Heart with Increased Pulmonary Vascular Markings

The pathophysiology of cyanosis in children with a large heart and increased pulmonary vascular markings includes pulmonary recirculation and "stiff lungs." These congenital heart defects include transposition of the great arteries, TAPVR (unobstructed), truncus arteriosus, double-outlet right ventricle, and single ventricle. In general, these patients present with central cyanosis, tachypnea, tachycardia, feeding intolerance, failure to thrive, and, occasionally, acidosis.

Radiographic findings may demonstrate a narrowed mediastinum in patients with transposition of the great arteries and, occasionally, double-outlet right ventricle ("egg on a string"), or "snowman sign" in those patients with supracardiac TAPVR. Electrocardiographically, there may be right ventricular or LV hypertrophy.

Response to oxygen depends on the congenital heart defect. Patients with transposition of the great arteries and TAPVR increase their PaO_2 less than 20 mm Hg. Patients with truncus arteriosus, double-outlet right ventricle, and single ventricle may increase their PaO_2 by greater than 20 mm Hg.

Treating these patients may or may not include oxygen therapy, depending on the congenital heart defect. In general, however, oxygen is not detrimental, as many of these patients are not dependent on the PDA as their means of systemic blood flow. Diuretics are indicated with inotropic support and, occasionally, afterload reduction. Balloon atrial septostomy or surgical palliation or repair is indicated.

SUPRAVENTRICULAR TACHYCARDIA

SVT may present in an emergency department setting at almost any age.[2] Typically, SVT is diagnosed between 2 and 4 months of age. These patients may demonstrate symptoms of tachypnea and feeding intolerance. If SVT is sustained for several hours, the patient may present with decreased cardiac output and metabolic acidosis. In general, however, SVT is well tolerated.

The majority of SVTs are reentrant and therefore respond to intravenous adenosine.[8] The initial recommended dose for adenosine is 0.1 mg/kg as a rapid bolus, followed by a rapid push of 5 to 10 mL of normal saline. Following adenosine therapy, the patient may have a short break in tachycardia, with early recurrence requiring additional doses. The infant may require up to 0.3 mg/kg by intravenous push in a peripheral intravenous line. Usually, the adenosine dose required is lower if central venous access is obtained. In general, calcium channel blockers are contraindicated in infants and children.[6] An ECG should be obtained prior to and at the time of conversion to document the underlying rhythm. If preexcitation is present, digoxin and calcium channel blockers are contraindicated for chronic therapy. Additionally, intravenous beta blockers are almost never required in infants and children for conversion from a reentrant arrhythmia. In all cases, chronic therapy in an infant should be decided after consultation with a pediatric cardiologist.

Although reentrant SVT is often well tolerated, without evidence of clinical compromise, certain "chronic" tachycardias may present with evidence of a tachycardia-induced cardiomyopathy. These patients may have evidence of severe metabolic acidosis and diminished cardiac output requiring resuscitation. In general, these "chronic" tachycardias are automatic in nature, such as atrial ectopic tachycardia (AET) or junctional ectopic tachycardia. However, an incessant reentrant arrhythmia, such as a permanent junctional form of reciprocating tachycardia (PJRT), may also present with this clinical scenario.

In automatic tachycardias, the arrhythmia is due to an abnormal focus located in the atrial, AV nodal, or ventricular myocardium. AET (Fig. 265.1) is, by far, the more common of these arrhythmias. Administration of adenosine will only block the AV node but will not terminate the tachycardia. In this case, you will see P waves continue to march through at their tachycardia rate until AV nodal conduction returns, at which time, SVT will resume. In general, this tachycardia is not as rapid as a reentrant arrhythmia; however, due to its chronic nature, it may result in a cardiomyopathy. Usually, support of the circulation is beneficial until appropriate referral to a pediatric cardiologist is obtained. Administration of intravenous sympathomimetic agents to improve cardiac output may only exacerbate the tachyarrhythmia, resulting in further clinical compromise. In these patients, administration of intravenous digoxin in the emergency setting may result in either reduction in the tachycardia rate or decreased AV nodal conduction. Occasionally, a calcium channel blocker or a beta blocker is required in the treatment of this arrhythmia; however, given their negative inotropic effects, they are less desirable. Intravenous amiodarone or procainamide is usually better tolerated and more effective in the treatment of this arrhythmia acutely. The therapy of choice in the older child is radiofrequency ablation.

PJRT is a special type of reentrant tachycardia that is usually incessant in nature, thereby resulting in a cardiomyopathy. Like AET, the heart rate is generally less than 200 beats per minute, even in the smallest infants. Unlike AET, PJRT can be terminated with adenosine; however, it is not uncommon that there is

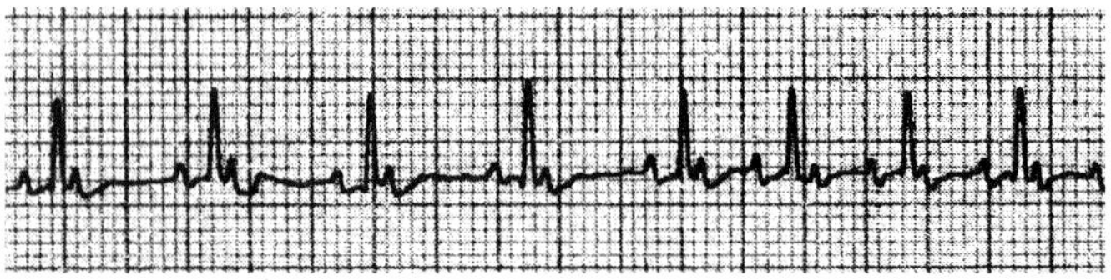

Figure 265.1. Atrial ectopic tachycardia. P waves with abnormal morphology and variable AV conduction in a 1-month-old that presented with feeding intolerance, tachypnea, and poor peripheral perfusion. This infant required amiodarone infusion before his tachycardia converted to normal sinus rhythm.

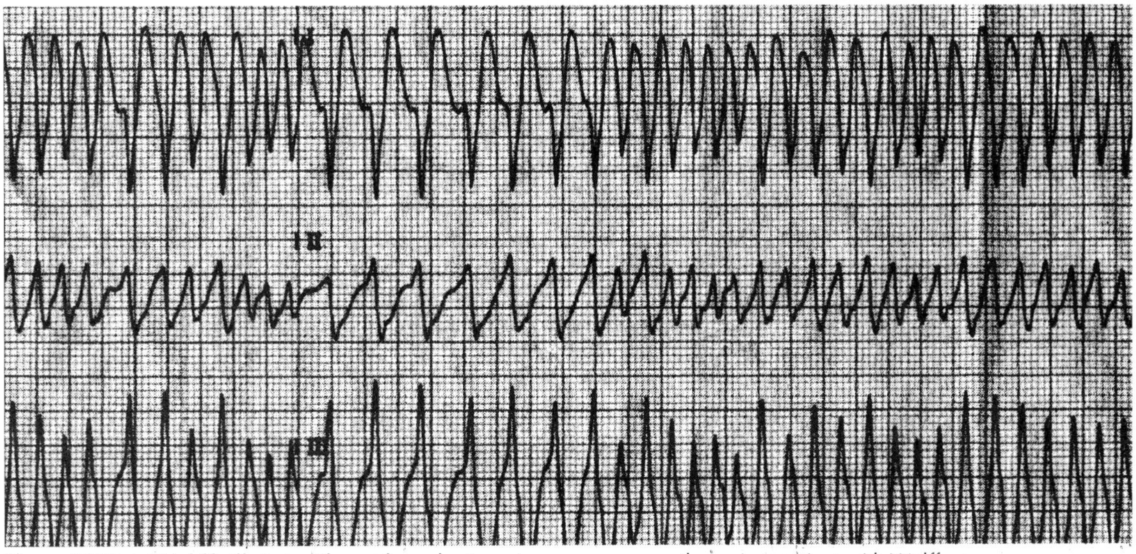

Figure 265.2. Atrial fibrillation with rapid conduction via an accessory pathway in a patient with Wolff-Parkinson-White syndrome. This patient presented without hemodynamic compromise. There was no response to adenosine.

immediate recurrence once adenosine is metabolized. Furthermore, the hypotension that can accompany adenosine often results in a release of endogenous catecholamines that may increase the tachycardia rate. Like patients with AET, these patients may be treated with intravenous antiarrhythmics (e.g., digoxin, amiodarone, or procainamide) or nodal blocking agents. However, the treatment of choice for both PJRT and AET is radiofrequency ablation.

Although uncommon, hemodynamically unstable arrhythmias require immediate and aggressive therapy. The two most common arrhythmias of this type include ventricular tachycardia and rapid conduction of atrial fibrillation in a patient with Wolff-Parkinson-White syndrome. Patients with ventricular tachycardia who are hemodynamically compromised require immediate DC cardioversion. Electrolyte abnormalities should be considered in patients who are refractory to cardioversion. Patients with a history of intoxication (e.g., with cocaine) may require pharmacologic therapy in addition to cardioversion, such as with lidocaine or beta blockers. In patients with a history of digoxin toxicity, DC cardioversion should be avoided, and treatment with digoxin-specific Fab fragments initiated. These patients require cardiopulmonary resuscitation while managing their malignant arrhythmia in order to avoid permanent central nervous system injury.

In patients with atrial fibrillation and Wolff-Parkinson-White syndrome, there may be rapid conduction to the ventricles.[3] Electrocardiographically, this may mimic rapid ventricular tachycardia (Fig. 265.2). However, these patients may be surprisingly hemodynamically stable initially and then deteriorate rapidly if they remain in this arrhythmia. Again, DC cardioversion is the treatment of choice; however, if the patient appears stable, infusion with intravenous procainamide or ibutilide may be tolerated. In general, treatment with adenosine will not result in any arrhythmia change. Because digoxin and calcium channel blockers may increase accessory pathway conduction, resulting in ventricular fibrillation, these medications are contraindicated whenever this arrhythmia is suspected.

SYNCOPE

The evaluation of the child with syncope in the emergency department can be difficult.[7,10] Most of these children will have normal findings indicative of a neurocardiogenic mechanism. The confounding factor is that most children who die of sudden cardiac death have a history of syncope. Therefore, the child who presents with syncope cannot be taken lightly. It is important to obtain a good clinical and family history, as well as perform a thorough physical examination. The family history should ensure that there is no familial sudden death, arrhythmia, or early cardiac disease. The clinical history should ensure that syncope is not exercise- or catecholamine-induced, which is suggestive of an arrhythmic etiology or coronary anomaly. An ECG should be performed in all children with their first syncopal episode or nonfebrile seizure to ensure that there is a normal corrected QT interval. If the ECG is normal, along with the physical examination and clinical and family histories, the patient can be safely discharged from the emergency department, with appropriate follow-up by their primary care physician or pediatric cardiologist.

COMMON PITFALLS

- Infants with cardiogenic shock and septic shock can present similarly with cardiomegaly and metabolic acidosis. However, it is an important distinction to make, because septic shock requires fluid resuscitation and cardiogenic shock often requires diuresis.
- All "first-time wheezers" require a chest x-ray to rule out cardiomegaly. Hyperinflation from bronchiolitis should result in a normal or small cardiac silhouette. Cardiomegaly in a child with wheezing suggests "cardiac asthma" due to myocarditis, anomalous left coronary from the pulmonary artery, or other cardiac etiologies.
- All patients should undergo electrocardiography after an initial syncopal episode or nonfebrile seizure to rule out an arrhythmic cause (e.g., long QT syndrome).
- Intravenous calcium channel blockers are almost always contraindicated in infants and small children.

References

1. Barkin RM. Congestive heart failure in children. *J Emerg Med* 1986;4(5):379–382.
2. Binder LS, Boeche R, Atkinson D. Evaluation and management of supraventricular tachycardia in children. *Ann Emerg Med* 1991;20(1):51–54.

3. Bromberg BI, Lindsay BD, Cain ME, et al. Impact of clinical history and electrophysiologic characterization of accessory pathways on management strategies to reduce sudden death among children with Wolff-Parkinson-White syndrome. *J Am Coll Cardiol* 1996;27(3):690–695.
4. Burton DA, Cabalka AK. Cardiac evaluation of infants. The first year of life. *Pediatr Clin North Am* 1994;41(5):991–1015.
5. Daliento L, Fasoli G, Mazzucco A. Anomalous origin of the left coronary artery from the anterior aortic sinus: role of echocardiography. *Int J Cardiol* 1993;38(1):89–91.
6. Epstein ML, Kiel EA, Victorica BE. Cardiac decompensation following verapamil therapy in infants with supraventricular tachycardia. *Pediatrics* 1985;75(4):737–740.
7. Gutgesell HP, Barst RJ, Humes RA, et al. Common cardiovascular problems in the young. Part I. Murmurs, chest pain, syncope and irregular rhythms. *Am Fam Physician* 1997;56(7):1825–1830.
8. Losek JD, Endom E, Dietrich A, et al. Adenosine and pediatric supraventricular tachycardia in the emergency department: multicenter study and review. *Ann Emerg Med* 1999;33(2):185–191.
9. Prasodo AM. Management of congenital heart disease. *Paediatr Indones* 1989;29(3–4):78–90.
10. Wolff GS. Unexplained syncope: clinical management. *Pacing Clin Electrophysiol* 1997;20(8 Pt 2):2043–2047.

CHAPTER 266
Croup and Epiglottitis

Timothy G. Givens

Croup is a clinical syndrome characterized by a barklike cough, hoarseness, inspiratory stridor, and respiratory distress of variable severity. The two most common forms are viral (laryngotracheobronchitis [LTB]) and spasmodic croup. The former is due to infection with parainfluenza viruses types 1, 2, and 3; respiratory syncytial virus; influenza virus type A; or adenovirus.[7,9] The virus causes inflammation of the subglottic tissues and sometimes of the tracheal mucosa. The supraglottic structures are normal.

Spasmodic croup is of uncertain etiology, although seen more commonly in patients with a family history of asthma, allergies, or recurrent episodes of croup. The peak incidence of LTB is during late fall and early winter. It can occur in all age groups but is most often seen during the second year of life. There is a 2:1 male-to-female ratio, with a recurrence rate of 5%.[7] Most cases of croup are mild to moderate in severity and are self-limited.

Epiglottitis, in contrast, is an acute bacterial process that is life-threatening. While the epiglottis and the aryepiglottic folds become inflamed and swollen, the glottis and subglottis remain normal. Epiglottitis is usually caused by *Haemophilus influenzae* type B (HIB).[7,9,18] Its incidence has fallen dramatically since the introduction of HIB vaccination.[1,6,17,21] Epiglottitis occurs throughout the year. It traditionally afflicts preschool children (2 to 6 years old) but can present in almost any age group, including adults. Because of widespread HIB vaccination, cases are now more often seen in older children and adolescents. Epiglottitis does not recur after the first infection.[7] The onset of epiglottitis is usually rapid, with a fulminant course that leads to respiratory arrest from either complete airway obstruction or fatigue associated with a partial airway obstruction. If properly managed, the signs and symptoms of the acute infection resolve within 24 to 72 hours.

CLINICAL PRESENTATION

Inspiratory stridor, a barking cough, and hoarse voice with mild-to-moderate respiratory distress are the common presenting symptoms of LTB. One to 2 days of coryza with a low-grade fever is the usual prodrome. The symptoms peak by 2 to 3 days, with improvement and resolution noted by 5 to 7 days.[7,9] Respiratory distress worsens when the patient cries or becomes agitated. Some patients may present with wheezing, tachypnea, and stridor. These patients have a combined illness of bronchiolitis and croup. A clinical scoring system may assist the physician in assessing the degree and progression of respiratory distress.[3] In spasmodic croup, the same barking cough, stridor, and labored breathing are observed, but the patient is afebrile and does not have the upper respiratory symptoms that precede LTB. Patients with spasmodic croup are usually responsive to cool, humidified air and often improve by time they reach the emergency department.

Patients with epiglottitis usually have the abrupt onset of sore throat, high fever, and one or more of the four D's: dysphagia, dysphonia, drooling, and distress. Inspiratory stridor may be audible, but there is usually no cough. Secretions, laryngospasm, and fatigue can further compromise breathing.[7] Classically, patients assume a tripod sitting position, with the mandible extended forward in an effort to maintain airway patency. Patients appear very apprehensive and often toxic because of sepsis.[18]

DIFFERENTIAL DIAGNOSIS

With a typical presentation of croup, the diagnosis is clinical, and laboratory and radiographic studies are unnecessary.[9] Atypical clinical features should prompt other considerations. Occasionally, a child with LTB caused by parainfluenza or influenza virus will present with stridor and wheezing and is diagnosed as having bronchiolitis. Epiglottitis is differentiated by its more acute and fulminant presentation (Table 266.1). A history of HIB vaccination does not rule out epiglottitis. Ludwig's angina (a rapidly spreading inflammation of the sublingual, submandibular, and submaxillary spaces) and retropharyngeal

TABLE 266.1. Comparison between Epiglottitis and Laryngotracheobronchitis

Characteristic	LTB	Supraglottitis
Age	6 mo–3 yr	2–6 yr
Onset	Gradual	Rapid
Etiology	Viral	Bacterial
Swelling site	Subglottic	Supraglottic
Symptoms		
Cough-voice	Hoarse cough	No cough Muffled voice
Posture	Any position	Sitting
Mouth	Closed; nasal flaring	Open-chin forward, drooling
Fever	Absent to high	High
Appearance	Often not acutely ill	Anxious, acutely ill
Radiograph	Narrow subglottic area	Swollen epiglottis and supraglottic structures
Palpation larynx	Nontender	Tender
Recurrence	May recur	Rarely recurs
Seasonal incidence	Winter	None

From Backofen JE, Rogers MC. Upper airway disease. In: Rogers MC, ed. *Textbook of pediatric intensive care*, vol 1. Baltimore: Williams & Wilkins, 1987.

and peritonsillar abscesses are suspected based on inspection of the oral cavity. If membranes are noted in the oropharynx, diphtheria and infectious mononucleosis must also be considered. Bacterial tracheitis may be suspected when there is no response to the standard management for LTB, or when the patient's symptoms worsen. If the patient is afebrile or has a history of choking, the possibility of aspiration of a foreign object should be investigated, using noninvasive techniques such as inspiratory and expiratory chest radiographs, fluoroscopy, or computed tomography scanning. Direct visualization by laryngobronchoscopy may be required.[7,18] For recurrent or persistent stridor or a clinical presentation of LTB during an atypical time of year, the following also should be considered: congenital airway anomalies, acquired tracheal stenosis secondary to previous intubations, congenital heart disease with associated vascular anomalies, tracheal hemangiomas, or recurrent angioneurotic edema.[7]

EMERGENCY DEPARTMENT EVALUATION

The child in respiratory distress should not be separated from parental comfort unless respiratory arrest is imminent.[7,9] Minimal manipulation is necessary so as not to increase the child's work of breathing and worsen the respiratory distress. The physical examination consists of inspection and observation at a comfortable distance from the patient. Oxygen can be delivered in a manner tolerable to the child. Venipuncture should be deferred to avoid distressing the patient. When epiglottitis is highly suspected, immediate arrangements must be made to transport the patient to an operating room in order to secure placement of an artificial airway. Further evaluation of the airway by direct visualization can then be done with the patient anesthetized. A physician experienced in airway management must accompany the child during transport to the operating room.

If the history and physical examination suggest LTB, the physician may apply a clinical scoring system to assess the patient's degree of compromise (Table 266.2).[3] Sequential scoring is done after each intervention. If the diagnosis is in doubt and the child is stable, an inspiratory soft-tissue lateral neck radiograph and chest radiograph may be helpful (see Figs. 266.1 through 266.3).[7] Classic radiographic signs of epiglottitis include the thumb sign (enlarged epiglottis), swelling of the aryepiglottic folds, blunting of the vallecula, and obliteration of the piriform sinuses. In LTB, the steeple sign (a gradual narrowing at the subglottic area) may be observed, but all supraglottic structures should appear normal. Radiographic widening of the soft tissue between the air column and cervical vertebrae points to retropharyngeal abscess or cellulitis.

EMERGENCY DEPARTMENT MANAGEMENT

Maintenance or provision of an adequate airway is the first priority in any illness in which airway obstruction is possible. Each institution must establish an epiglottitis protocol that can be rapidly activated.[7] Once the diagnosis of suspected epiglottitis is made, appropriate personnel must be mobilized. The patient must be taken to the operating room immediately, where inhalation anesthesia is given with the patient in a sitting position. The hypopharynx is then visualized, and rapid intubation is performed with an endotracheal tube 0.5 to 1.0 mm smaller in diameter than that predicted for the patient's age and weight. A surgeon skilled in pediatric tracheostomy should be prepared to perform an emergency tracheostomy, if necessary. Intravenous access and laboratory studies are obtained at the discretion of the anesthesiologist, usually after induction of anesthesia.

Patients with LTB who have a clinical score of 7 or greater and who do not respond quickly to initial therapeutic maneuvers may also be candidates for endotracheal intubation. Continuous pulse oximetry monitoring will reveal any deterioration in the patient's oxygenation status in a noninvasive fashion.[19] Ventilatory failure should be suspected if the patient loses head control or becomes lethargic. Because of airway narrowing, an endotracheal tube size smaller in diameter than that predicted for the child's age and weight should be used if intubation becomes a necessity.

For patients who present to the emergency department with impending or complete respiratory arrest, the airway must be addressed immediately. Bag-valve-mask ventilation with 100% oxygen should be initiated. Higher positive pressures are sometimes necessary, requiring a two-handed technique to obtain an adequate chest rise. If these measures are unsuccessful within 15 to 30 seconds, a rapid oral intubation should be attempted. Tips for intubating children with epiglottitis include using a smaller size endotracheal tube, using a stylet, and looking for an air bubble at the glottic opening while someone compresses the chest.

If intubation is impossible, emergency cricothyrotomy must be done. A large-bore (14-gauge) angiocatheter is inserted through the cricothyroid membrane at a caudad angle and attached to a 3.0 endotracheal tube. This maneuver may provide a temporary open airway for bag ventilation or direct connection to a pressurized continuous-flow oxygen source.[18] A pediatric surgeon or otolaryngologist should be consulted for emergency tracheostomy. Complications associated with the disease, as well as the artificial airway placement, include pulmonary edema, tension pneumothorax, subcutaneous emphysema, pneumomediastinum, bleeding, endotracheal tube plugging, accidental extubation, and bronchospasm.[7,18]

In LTB, therapy is provided commensurate with the patient's level of respiratory distress. In mild cases (croup score less than

TABLE 266.2. Clinical Croup Score

	0	1	2
Inspiratory breath sounds	Normal	Harsh with rhonchi	Delayed
Stridor	None	Inspiratory	Inspiratory and expiratory
Cough	None	Hoarse cry	Barking cough
Retractions/flaring	None	Flaring, suprasternal retractions	As in 1 plus subcostal/intercostal retractions
Cyanosis *or*	None	In room air	In 40% O_2
PaO_2 (mm Hg)	70–100	<70	<70
CNS function	Normal	Depressed/agitated	Coma

Modified from Downes JJ, Raphaely R. Pediatric intensive care. *Anesthesiology* 1975;43:242.

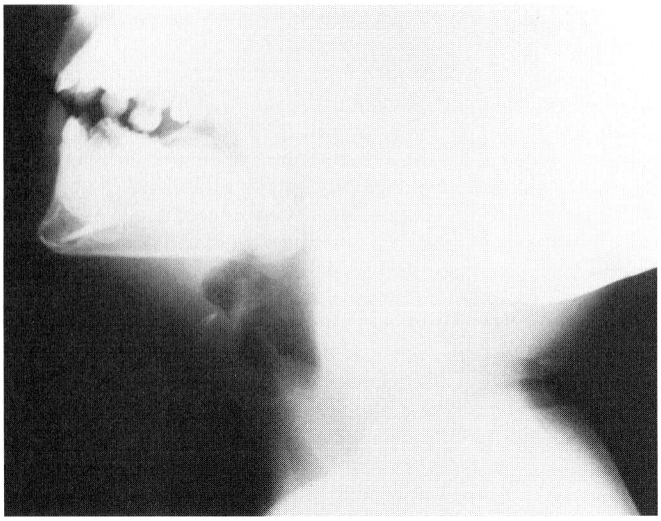

Figure 266.1. Normal inspiratory soft-tissue lateral neck radiograph.

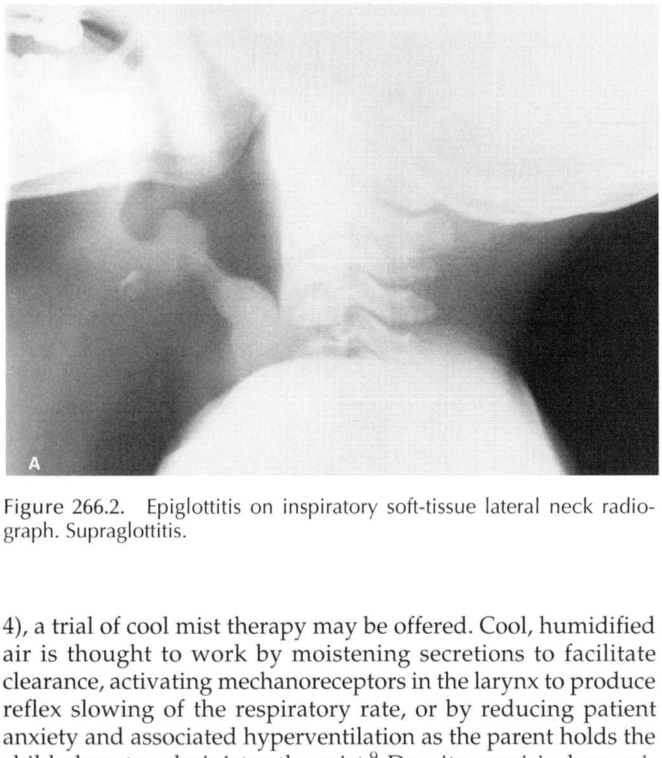

Figure 266.2. Epiglottitis on inspiratory soft-tissue lateral neck radiograph. Supraglottitis.

4), a trial of cool mist therapy may be offered. Cool, humidified air is thought to work by moistening secretions to facilitate clearance, activating mechanoreceptors in the larynx to produce reflex slowing of the respiratory rate, or by reducing patient anxiety and associated hyperventilation as the parent holds the child close to administer the mist.[9] Despite empirical experience, no significant benefit to cool mist therapy has ever been proven. Because croup tents may actually interfere with observation of the patient or increase anxiety, their use to administer mist therapy has become passé.[9]

Patients with LTB who have a clinical score of 4 or greater or inspiratory stridor at rest should receive oxygen and nebulized epinephrine (0.05 mL/kg per dose [max dose, 0.5 mL] of a 2.25% solution diluted in 3 mL of saline, repeated as necessary).[7,9,15,18] Equivalent doses of either racemic epinephrine or L-epinephrine, which is more readily available and less expensive, have been shown to be equally efficacious.[23] There should be almost immediate clinical improvement due to reduction of the edema and vasoconstriction of the inflamed mucosa through the stimulation of the α-adrenergic receptors. Parents should be encouraged to deliver the nebulized treatment in a nonthreatening manner. Heart rate should be monitored during treatment with nebulized sympathomimetics. The treatment should be stopped

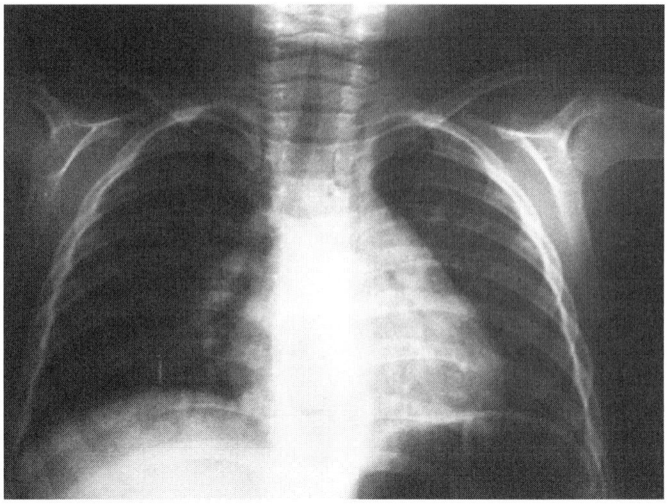

Figure 266.3. Croup. Steeple sign on a soft-tissue neck radiograph.

when the heart rate exceeds 200 beats per minute or if dysrhythmias occur.

Previously, all patients who received nebulized epinephrine were admitted to the hospital because of a possible rebound effect, a clinical worsening due to vasodilation, and increased mucosal edema as the adrenergic effects abate. This phenomenon usually occurs within 2 to 4 hours after epinephrine treatment.[7] Recently, the need for hospitalization has been reassessed. Several studies suggest that discharge from the emergency department is safe following epinephrine therapy if, after 3 to 4 hours of observation, the patient has no stridor at rest and has normal air entry, normal color, and normal level of consciousness.[9,13,14,16]

There is now ample evidence to suggest that corticosteroids are of benefit to patients with croup. Steroids promote resolution of laryngeal edema through antiinflammatory activity. Dexamethasone (Decadron), 0.3 to 0.6 mg/kg, administered either orally or as a single intramuscular injection, has been shown to reduce the severity of symptoms,[2,4,10,20] rate of hospital admissions,[4] need for subsequent nebulized epinephrine treatments,[20] and duration of hospital stay or observation in the emergency department.[4,5] Dexamethasone has a half-life of 54 hours, so one dose is sufficient. A smaller 0.15-mg/kg oral dose of dexamethasone, compared with placebo, has been shown to reduce the number of return visits to the emergency department in children with mild croup that were discharged home.[5] Both oral and intramuscular routes have been shown to be effective compared with placebo, but to date there have been no data directly comparing the two routes.[9] As effects from corticosteroid treatment take 6 hours, early use is most beneficial.[22] All patients who require epinephrine therapy should also receive steroids. Inhaled corticosteroids (budesonide) have a rapid onset (within 2 to 4 hours) and are effective in mild-to-moderate croup.[3,8,11,12] More studies are needed, however, before steroids can be recommended routinely.

Antibiotics are unnecessary for patients with LTB. Patients with epiglottitis should receive intravenous antibiotics beginning in the operating room. Options include ceftriaxone (100 mg/kg/d at 12-hour intervals), cefuroxime (150 mg/kg/d at 8-hour intervals), cefotaxime (150 mg/kg/d at 8-hour intervals), or chloramphenicol (100 mg/kg/d at 6-hour intervals). Bronchospasm secondary to secretions can be treated with β_2-agonist nebulization (e.g., albuterol) and suctioning. Additional supportive treatment includes antipyretics and intravenous fluids for patients with compromised oral intake.

DISPOSITION

Intubated patients (including all epiglottitis patients) must be admitted to a pediatric intensive care unit, accompanied by personnel skilled in pediatric airway placement. LTB patients with a clinical score of 4 or greater (significant respiratory distress), those with persistent stridor at rest, and those with minimal to no response to nebulized adrenergic treatment should be admitted. Instructions to parents whose children are sent home include monitoring the child's work of breathing (respiratory rate, retractions, and agitation), implementing a method of rapid and easy communication access between physician and family, placing a humidifier at the child's bedside, and ensuring minimal stimulation.

COMMON PITFALLS

- Separating children from parents during initial assessment or during administration of nebulized medications or oxygen
- Underestimating the degree of respiratory distress
- Increasing agitation and respiratory distress by performing medical procedures (vital signs, laboratory and x-ray studies)
- Obtaining radiographic studies when the diagnosis by history and clinical presentation is clear
- Delaying the establishment of an artificial airway or not having the appropriate equipment readily available
- Failure to have a physician skilled in establishing artificial airways accompany the child during transport
- Using too large an endotracheal tube during intubation

ACKNOWLEDGMENT

The author gratefully acknowledges the contribution of Jose S. Martinez and James H. McCrory, who wrote the previous version of this chapter.

References

1. Alho O-P, Jokinen K, Pirila T, et al. Acute epiglottitis and infant conjugate *Haemophilus influenzae* type b vaccination in northern Finland. *Arch Otolaryngol Head Neck Surg* 1995;121:898.
2. Cruz MN, Stewart G, Rosenberg N. Use of dexamethasone in the outpatient management of croup. *Pediatrics* 1995;96:220.
3. Downes JJ, Raphaely R. Pediatric intensive care. *Anesthesiology* 1975;43:242.
4. Geelhoed GC. Sixteen years of croup in a Western Australian teaching hospital: effects of routine steroid treatment. *Ann Emerg Med* 1996;28:621.
5. Geelhoed GC, Macdonald WBG. Oral dexamethasone in the treatment of croup: 0.15 mg/kg vs. 0.3 mg/kg vs. 0.6 mg/kg. *Pediatr Pulmonol* 1995;20:362.
6. Gorelick MH, Baker MD. Epiglottitis in children, 1970–1992. Effects of *Haemophilus influenzae* type b immunization. *Arch Pediatr Adolesc Med* 1994;148:47.
7. Hen J Jr. Current management of upper airway obstruction. *Pediatr Ann* 1986;15(4):274.
8. Husby S, Agertoft L, Mortensen S, et al. Treatment of croup with nebulised steroid (budesonide): a double blind, placebo controlled study. *Arch Dis Child* 1993;68:3:352.
9. Kaditis AG, Wald ER. Viral croup: current diagnosis and treatment. *Pediatr Infect Dis J* 1998;17:827–834.
10. Kairys SW, Olmstead EM, O'Connor GT. Steroid treatment of laryngotracheitis: a meta-analysis of the evidence from randomized trials. *Pediatrics* 1989;83:683.
11. Klassen TP, Feldman ME, Watters LK, et al. Nebulized budesonide for children with mild-to-moderate croup. *N Engl J Med* 1994;331:285.
12. Klassen TP, Watters LK, Feldman ME, et al. The efficacy of nebulized budesonide in dexamethasone-treated outpatients with croup. *Pediatrics* 1996;97:463.
13. Kunkel NC, Baker MD. Use of racemic epinephrine, dexamethasone, and mist in the outpatient management of croup. *Pediatr Emerg Care* 1996;12:156.
14. Ledwith CA, Shea LM, Mauro RD. Safety and efficacy of nebulized racemic epinephrine in conjunction with oral dexamethasone and mist in the outpatient management of croup. *Ann Emerg Med* 1995;25:331.
15. McDonogh AJ. The use of steroids and nebulized adrenaline in the treatment of viral croup over a seven year period at a district hospital. *Anaesth Intensive Care* 1994;22(2):175.
16. Prendergast M, Jones JS, Hartman D. Racemic epinephrine in the treatment of laryngotracheitis: can we identify children for outpatient therapy? *Am J Emerg Med* 1994;12:613.
17. Progress toward eliminating *Haemophilus influenzae* type b disease among infants and children—United States, 1987–1997. *MMWR* 1998;47(46):993.
18. Rogers MC. *Textbook of pediatric intensive care,* vol 3. Baltimore: Williams & Wilkins, 1996.
19. Stoney PJ, Chakrabarti MK. Experience of pulse oximetry in children with croup. *J Laryngol Otol* 1991;105:295.
20. Super DM, Cartelli NA, Brooks LJ, et al. A prospective randomized double-blind study to evaluate the effect of dexamethasone in acute laryngotracheitis. *J Pediatr* 1989;115:323.
21. Takala AK, Peltola H, Eskola J. Disappearance of epiglottitis during large-scale vaccination with *Haemophilus influenzae* type b conjugate vaccine among children in Finland. *Laryngoscope* 1994;104:731.
22. Tibballs J, Shann TA, Landau LI. Placebo-controlled trial of prednisolone in children intubated for croup. *Lancet* 1994;340:745.
23. Waisman Y, Klein BL, Boenning DA, et al. Prospective randomized double-blind study comparing *l*-epinephrine and racemic epinephrine aerosols in the treatment of laryngotracheitis (croup). *Pediatrics* 1992;89:302.

CHAPTER 267
Diabetic Ketoacidosis

Timothy G. Givens

Diabetic ketoacidosis (DKA) is caused by either an absolute or a relative insulin deficiency accompanied by increased action of four counterregulatory hormones: glucagon, epinephrine, cortisol, and growth hormone.[14,16,20] Counterregulatory hormone activity increases the patient's insulin resistance, thus compounding the effects of insulin deficiency. The results of this imbalance are hyperglycemia, dehydration, ketosis, and acidosis.

Precipitating events for this cascade include acute infection, inflammatory reactions, trauma, psychological stress, or medical noncompliance in patients known to have insulin-dependent diabetes mellitus (IDDM). Recurrent DKA is almost always due to insulin omission.[6,7] Approximately 30% of cases of new-onset IDDM present as DKA;[16] a high index of suspicion is required to make the diagnosis in infants and children. Mortality in DKA is primarily due to the development of cerebral edema.[17]

CLINICAL PRESENTATION

Children with DKA have a variable clinical picture, and the diagnosis may be difficult, particularly in patients not known to have IDDM. Acutely, the child may appear moderately dehydrated and be misdiagnosed as having viral gastroenteritis or a urinary tract infection. Presenting symptoms include nausea, vomiting, abdominal pain, hyperpnea, fruity breath odor, dehydration, and lethargy or coma. Polyuria, polydipsia, and polyphagia—three classic features of diabetes—as well as weight loss, should signal the physician to consider DKA.

DIFFERENTIAL DIAGNOSIS

Because new-onset IDDM presenting as DKA may be mistaken for gastroenteritis or a urinary tract infection, a history of polyuria and polydipsia should be sought in every case of a child who is vomiting, particularly in very young children. Occasionally, dehydrated children with gastroenteritis will have hyperglycemia and glucosuria due to stress and do not have IDDM;[2] they are usually nonketotic.

It is unclear whether patients with stress-induced hyperglycemia are at risk for future development of IDDM.[19,21] If the history is obscure or unavailable in a child who presents with altered mental status, the differential diagnosis widens to include intoxication, inborn errors of metabolism, Reye syndrome, sepsis, meningoencephalitis, nonketotic hyperglycemic coma, or hypoglycemic coma.[16] In children with known IDDM, the differential diagnosis includes precipitants for the development of DKA, such as bacterial infections, viral gastroenteritis, appendicitis, pancreatitis, or other acute intraabdominal disorders.

EMERGENCY DEPARTMENT EVALUATION

The initial evaluation of a child who presents as described previously consists of

1. Establishing the diagnosis of DKA
2. Assessing and correcting dehydration and electrolyte imbalance
3. Providing adequate insulin to restore normal metabolism
4. Searching for the precipitating event for DKA
5. Avoiding complications of therapy (cerebral edema, hypoglycemia, hypokalemia)

Hyperglycemia (serum glucose greater than 200 mg/dL), ketonuria, and metabolic acidosis (venous pH less than 7.3 or serum bicarbonate less than 15 mEq/L) confirm the diagnosis of DKA.[16,18]

The physical examination should focus, as always, on the ABCs first. Next, attention is directed toward establishing the degree of dehydration, as well as identifying processes that may have precipitated DKA. Because the extracellular fluid of children with DKA is hyperosmolar, the percentage of dehydration is commonly underestimated when relying on physical signs that correlate with extracellular volume (e.g., hydration of mucous membranes, skin turgor, and temperature). In general, one should assume at least 10% dehydration in all patients with DKA.[13,18]

Measurement of serum electrolyte levels may assist in assessment but must be interpreted in light of the physiologic derangements that accompany DKA. The measured sodium level is often low because of the dilutional effects of water flowing into the vascular compartment to compensate for hyperosmolarity generated by high plasma glucose levels. Treatment of this "pseudohyponatremia" with administration of excessive sodium is not required, as the sodium level should rise as the glucose level falls with treatment for DKA. Serum potassium is usually elevated—despite the fact that the patient's total body potassium stores are depleted—because intracellular potassium ions are exchanged for extracellular hydrogen ions in the presence of acidosis. Low-normal potassium levels in DKA indicate extreme total-body potassium depletion. Continuous electrocardiographic monitoring for evidence of cardiac dysrhythmias is necessary in DKA, particularly in patients with alterations in their serum potassium concentrations.

EMERGENCY DEPARTMENT MANAGEMENT

Fluid replacement and correction of dehydration should begin as soon as possible. Volume expansion with isotonic fluid such as normal saline, 20 mL/kg, is given during the first 1 to 2 hours. Unless the patient is in shock, initial fluid boluses beyond 20 mL/kg should be avoided because of the risk of cerebral edema. Lactated Ringer's solution is less commonly used, owing to a theoretical risk of hyperchloremic acidosis.[6]

After the first hour, fluids are adjusted to correct the remainder of the patient's water deficit (10% dehydrated = 100 mL/kg) over the next 48 hours. As a general principle, slow correction of hyperosmolarity is desirable. Maintenance fluids are calculated in the usual manner (100 mL/kg for the first 10 kg, 50 mL/kg for the second 10 kg, and 20 mL/kg for every additional kg) and added to estimates of ongoing losses and rehydration fluids to calculate an infusion rate. This calculation can be accomplished with a solution of 0.45% sodium chloride (which closely approximates the fluid lost in DKA), with the addition of 40 mEq/L of potassium as the chloride and/or phosphate salt. The use of higher sodium concentrations may prevent the development of cerebral edema during the treatment of DKA,[10] although this theory has not been proved.[17] Dextrose is added to fluids when the plasma glucose level approaches 300 mg/dL; the desired goal is maintenance of a glucose level between 200 and 300 mg/dL.

Hypophosphatemia and deficiency of 2,3-diphosphoglycerate are well-known features of DKA. They occur because of osmotic diuresis and phosphate competition with glucose for reabsorption at the renal tubules. Potassium phosphate has thus been proposed as an alternative to potassium replacement with the chloride salt; correction of phosphate homeostasis, however, has not been shown to clinically benefit children with DKA.[1,12,16] Its use should be limited to those patients with extremely low serum phosphate concentrations (less than 1 mg/dL) or when potassium concentrations in the intravenous fluid greater than 40 mEq/L are needed.

Once hyperglycemia and ketosis confirm the diagnosis of DKA, a continuous infusion of intravenous insulin at a rate of 0.1 U/kg/h should be begun. While insulin administration has been effective using intramuscular or subcutaneous routes, continuous low-dose intravenous infusion allows for slower, more even correction of hyperglycemia and fewer episodes of hypoglycemia than do other forms of insulin administration,[3,4,16] and is preferable in children. Although some sources recommend an initial bolus of 0.1 U/kg prior to the continuous infusion, there is no evidence that it is helpful.[16] When mixing the insulin for infusion, the concentration of insulin should be at least 0.5 U/mL, and the infusion line should be primed to overcome insulin binding to the intravenous infusion equipment.[11]

The use of bicarbonate is highly controversial in the treatment of DKA, largely because its reported benefits and risks have been unproven.[8,13,14,18] The potential advantages of bicarbonate are improved myocardial function; reduction of potential for dysrhythmias; decreased insulin resistance; and through avoidance of hypochloremia, a more rapid correction of acidosis. Major disadvantages of bicarbonate use are its potential for generation of paradoxical central nervous system acidosis, due to increased diffusion of carbon dioxide across the blood–brain barrier; increased hemoglobin affinity for oxygen (increased tissue hypoxia, due to reduced off-loading); and promotion of hypokalemia. If bicarbonate is used, it should be given as a slow infusion over several hours, not as a bolus. Rapid infusion may produce hypokalemia and exacerbate the degree of hyperosmolarity.

Plasma glucose levels should be monitored hourly. Serum electrolyte concentrations and venous blood gases should be monitored every 2 to 4 hours, and calcium and phosphate concentrations should be checked every 8 hours. The rate of decrease in glucose should be no faster than 50 to 100 mg/dL/h.[13,16]

In spite of improvements in DKA management, mortality due to cerebral edema has not changed.[9,16] Data suggest that a large percentage of patients in DKA have subclinical cerebral edema on computed tomography scans;[15] however, clinically significant cerebral edema is present in less than 1% of cases of DKA.[5,10,17] Typically, signs of increased intracranial pressure present several hours into therapy, as the patient experiences a sudden decline in sensorium, headache, sluggish pupillary reflexes, or change in vital signs despite an apparent improvement in metabolic and other clinical parameters.

Thus, cerebral edema is thought to be the result of (overly vigorous) treatment for DKA.[5,9,10,13,16,17] Specific mechanisms remain elusive but are thought to relate to overly rapid hydration, with a concomitant precipitous drop in effective serum osmolarity, leading to intracerebral fluid shifts and intracellular swelling. Once clinically apparent, cerebral edema leads to mortality in 60% to 80% of cases, with long-term neurologic morbidity in most of the remaining patients. There are few reliable predictors of risk for significant cerebral edema, although children less than 5 years of age with new-onset IDDM and a prolonged period of untreated DKA are at increased risk.[16]

If evidence of cerebral edema develops, the patient should receive rapid, aggressive intervention with intravenous mannitol (1 g/kg).[17] Intubation and hyperventilation should be considered. Because of the devastating outcomes in patients who develop this complication, the need for frequent neurologic reassessment and early intervention must be underscored.

DISPOSITION

Children in moderate-to-severe DKA should be admitted to a pediatric intensive or intermediate care unit because of the frequency and extent of monitoring that is required. Patients with new-onset IDDM should be admitted to a facility where age-appropriate diabetes education can be given.

Patients who can retain oral intake without vomiting and who are not significantly dehydrated or acidotic (pH greater than 7.25) may be discharged home from the emergency department if appropriate follow-up care can be arranged. Follow-up includes frequent telephone contact over the ensuing 24 hours with an individual knowledgeable in diabetes management.

COMMON PITFALLS

- Failure to administer adequate insulin, which may result from errors in insulin dilution or infusion. Concerns about therapy-related hypoglycemia are addressed by adding dextrose to the fluid replacement, not by slowing or stopping the insulin infusion.
- Failure to treat the precipitating process. Patients with refractory DKA should be thoroughly reexamined for a source of infection or intraabdominal disorder, such as pancreatitis or appendicitis.
- Inadequate volume expansion from failure to monitor the patient's fluid input and output
- Too-rapid correction of the hyperosmolarity may lead to cerebral edema and brainstem herniation.
- Inadequate potassium replacement during correction of acidosis, which leads to a shift of potassium into the cells and resultant hypokalemia

ACKNOWLEDGMENT

The author gratefully acknowledges the contribution of Robert P. Hoffman, who wrote the previous version of this chapter.

References

1. Becker DJ, Brown DR, Steranka BH, et al. Phosphate replacement during treatment of diabetic ketosis. *Am J Dis Child* 1983;137:241.
2. Boulware SD, Tumborlane WV. Not all severe hyperglycemia is diabetes. *Pediatrics* 1992;89:330.
3. Butkiewicz EK, Leibson CL, O'Brien PC, et al. Insulin therapy for diabetic ketoacidosis. *Diabetes Care* 1995;18:1187.
4. Drop SLS, Duval Arnold BJM, Sober AE, et al. Low-dose insulin infusion versus subcutaneous insulin injection: a controlled comparative study of diabetic ketoacidosis. *Pediatrics* 1977;59:733.
5. Duck SC, Wyatt DT. Factors associated with brain herniation in the treatment of diabetic ketoacidosis. *J Pediatr* 1988;113:10.
6. Glasgow AM, Weissberg-Benchell J, Tynan WD, et al. Readmissions of children with diabetes mellitus to a children's hospital. *Pediatrics* 1991;88:98.
7. Golden MP, Herrold AJ, Orr DP. An approach to prevention of recurrent diabetes ketoacidosis in the pediatric population. *J Pediatr* 1985;107:195.
8. Green SM, Rothrock SG, Ho JD, et al. Failure of adjunctive bicarbonate to improve outcome in severe pediatric diabetic ketoacidosis. *Ann Emerg Med* 1998;31:41.
9. Harris GD, Fiordalisi I. Physiologic management of diabetic ketoacidemia: a 5-year prospective pediatric experience in 231 episodes. *Arch Pediatr Adolesc Med* 1994;148:1046.
10. Harris SD, Fiordalisi I, Harris WL, et al. Minimizing the risk of brain herniation during treatment of diabetic ketoacidemia: a retrospective and prospective study. *J Pediatr* 1991;117:221.
11. Hersch JI, Fratkin MJ, Wood JH, et al. Clinical significance of insulin absorption by polyvinyl chloride infusion systems. *Am J Hosp Pharm* 1977;34:583.
12. Keller U, Berger W. Prevention of hypophosphatemia by phosphate infusion during treatment of diabetic ketoacidosis and hyperosmolar coma. *Diabetes* 1980;29:87.
13. Klekamp J, Churchwell KB. Diabetic ketoacidosis in children: initial clinical assessment and treatment. *Pediatr Ann* 1996;25:387.
14. Krane EJ. Diabetic ketoacidosis: biochemistry, physiology, treatment and prevention. *Pediatr Clin North* Am 1987;34:935.
15. Krane EJ, Rockoff MA, Wallman JK, et al. Subclinical brain swelling in children during treatment of diabetic ketoacidosis. *N Engl J Med* 1985;312:1147.
16. Rogers MC. *Textbook of pediatric intensive care,* vol 3. Baltimore: Williams & Wilkins, 1996:1261.
17. Rosenbloom AL. Intracerebral crises during treatment of diabetic ketoacidosis. *Diabetes Care* 1990;13:22.
18. Rosenbloom AL, Schatz DA. Diabetic ketoacidosis in childhood. *Pediatr Ann* 1994;23:284.
19. Schatz DA, Kowa H, Winter WE, et al. Natural history of incidental hyperglycemia and glycosuria of childhood. *J Pediatr* 1989;115:676.
20. Schatz DA, Rosenbloom AL. Diabetic ketoacidosis: management tactics in young patients: correcting metabolic derangements to prevent DKA-related deaths. *J Crit Illness* 1988;3:31.
21. Vandi P, Sheharde N, Etzioni A, et al. Stress hyperglycemia in childhood: a very high risk group for the development of type 1 diabetes. *J Pediatr* 1990;117:75.

CHAPTER 268
Diaper Rash

Lindsey Alan Johnson

Diaper rash is a nonspecific term used to describe a variety of dermatologic conditions that occur in the diaper area of the infant. Diaper rashes are the most common dermatologic problem seen in infants and children from birth to 24 months old, with a peak incidence at 7 to 9 months of age.[5,7–9]

The cause of diaper dermatitis can be complex. In simplest terms, it is caused by irritation, infection, or an underlying skin condition, but factors such as friction and increased permeability of skin, as well as how often the baby's diaper is changed, may contribute to the development or severity of the rash. The role of urine and feces in the pathophysiology of diaper rash has been the subject of much debate.[2,3,6,7,9,10]

The practice of using disposable diapers has become commonplace, and use of the traditional cloth diaper has become relatively uncommon in the United States. The disposable diaper, with its exterior plastic film, maintains humidity and heat between the skin and the diaper, predisposing to the growth of *Candida albicans* and bacteria. Injuries to the epidermis from prolonged exposure to urine and feces result in areas easily infected.

Alterations in gastrointestinal flora due to viral infections or antibiotic use contribute in particular to the development of candidal dermatitis with satellite lesions. The most frequently seen diaper rash is that which arises after the onset of diarrhea caused by a viral gastroenteritis or diarrhea associated with antibiotic therapy. The usual sequence of skin changes following the onset of diarrhea is an initial hyperemia to the skin covered by the diaper, with development of candidal colonization within 72 hours.

As the diarrhea continues, the initial candidal colonization may progress to the development of satellite *C. albicans* lesions. When the diaper area is then cleansed during diaper changes, the infant may experience pain due to the irritation of cleaning solutions or commercially prepared wipes, or the skin may become excoriated and secondarily infected with bacteria.

The infant is usually brought for medical attention because the diaper rash has been prolonged or unresponsive to over-the-counter preparations or is worsening in severity and extent.

DIFFERENTIAL DIAGNOSIS

Diaper rash due to irritation is common and may be divided into causes such as mechanical, intertrigo, miliaria, and contact irritation. Mechanical irritation is caused by constant friction of the wet, excessively hydrated skin of the diaper area against both the diaper and skin folds. It is aggravated by frequent overvigorous cleansing. The infant's diaper area appears chafed, with shiny, erythematous patches that tend to wax and wane in severity. Any diaper dermatitis induced by other factors can be aggravated by mechanical irritation.

Intertrigo occurs in areas where skin surfaces are apposed, such as the groin or intergluteal cleft. It is produced when heat, moisture, and sweat retention combine to cause maceration and irritation. Intertrigo is characterized by red denuded areas in the skin folds.

Miliaria, or prickly heat, is the result of contact of the hot, moist diaper with the infant's skin. It is characterized by small, clear superficial vesicles that are nonerythematous in the newborn, or by small erythematous papules and pustules in the older infant.

There are two types of contact irritation: allergic and primary irritant. Allergic contact diaper dermatitis is caused by the development of a sensitivity to detergents, chemicals in the diaper, or creams and medications used in the diaper area. The rash of contact dermatitis usually begins with tiny erythematous vesicles that rupture and adopt an eczematous appearance. The distribution of the rash is characteristic and involves skin surfaces in contact with the diaper, such as the convexities of the buttocks, the medial thighs, and scrotum, while the skin folds are spared.

Primary irritant contact dermatitis is thought to be caused by the effect of noxious components of urine and feces on skin that is already sensitive or irritated from other causes.[1] Primary irritant dermatitis is most often described as a parchment-like erythema, resembling a scald, that involves the convex surfaces. In boys, inflammation of the urethral meatus is common.

Infectious causes of diaper rash are yeast, bacterial, viral, and fungal. *C. albicans* is commonly found in the gastrointestinal tract of infants and is frequently implicated as a cause of diaper rash.[6] The rash consists of small, beefy-red papules that may be coalesced centrally but appear to spread outward as small satellite lesions. Usually, the perianal area and skin folds are spared. Examination of the mouth may show the characteristic lesions of thrush, the finding of which will help support the diagnosis.

Staphylococcus aureus can cause bullous impetigo in the diaper area. The bullae are large and flaccid and tend to rupture very quickly. Very often, only the red, moist, denuded base with peeling edges will be apparent on presentation. *S. aureus* is also the cause of folliculitis.[10] The distribution is usually over the buttocks, thighs, and lower abdomen. The lesions are small red follicular papules or pustules. Folliculitis is most prevalent in the summer and occurs as a complication in infants with chronic miliaria.

Although uncommon as a cause of diaper rash, several viruses may produce vesicular eruptions in the diaper area. Among these are herpes simplex, herpes zoster, coxsackievirus, and varicella. Herpes simplex infection is usually either congenitally acquired or caused by sexual abuse.[10] The lesions are small singular, coalescing, or grouped vesicles that rupture to form small crusted ulcers on an erythematous base. Herpes zoster is recognized by the dermatomal distribution of the vesicular eruption. Hand-foot-and-mouth disease, caused by coxsackievirus A16, and chickenpox are distinguished by the involvement of other skin surfaces.

Dermatophytosis of the diaper area has been described by several authors and may be more common than traditionally thought.[4,8,10] The most common fungi responsible are *Trichophyton rubrum*, *Epidermophyton floccosum*, and *Microsporum audouini*, the same fungi responsible for tinea cruris in adults. Patients present because of a diaper rash that has been unresponsive to conventional therapy. The rash consists of slightly raised erythematous patches with scaly margins. If topical corticosteroids have been applied to the area, the rash may be atypical and difficult to recognize.

Underlying skin conditions that cause rashes in the diaper area vary. Seborrheic dermatitis is common in infancy and appears at 3 or 4 weeks of age. Most cases subside spontaneously by 3 to 4 months of age. Seborrheic dermatitis is characterized by a sharply demarcated zone of erythema that commonly starts in the skin folds and spreads out over convex skin areas. It may be accompanied by small papules that are similar in appearance to the satellite lesions of *C. albicans*. Seborrheic dermatitis can be distinguished from intertrigo by the involvement of other areas of the body, such as the axilla, face, and scalp.

Atopic dermatitis usually does not occur in warm, moist environments such as the diaper area.[10] When it does present in the diaper area, the lesions are red and scaly, similar to seborrheic dermatitis. The primary differentiating points are that atopic dermatitis generally has its onset later in life, at about 2 months of age, and is intensely pruritic.[6] Atopic dermatitis also has the tendency to become eroded, with the development of crusting, oozing, eczematous-appearing lesions. At this point, the infant runs the risk of secondary infection of the involved areas.

Other less common causes of diaper rash should be considered when clinical presentation varies or response to therapy is not adequate. These include syphilis, Letterer-Siwe disease, psoriasis, granuloma gluteale infantum, nutritional disorders, and other bullous eruptions.

EMERGENCY DEPARTMENT EVALUATION

The diagnosis can usually be established on the basis of history and physical examination. The history for the rash should include age at onset; laundering and diapering practices; frequency of bathing; use of creams and medications, especially antibiotics that may alter gastrointestinal flora; any recent gastroenteritis with accompanying diarrhea; response to previous therapy; and family history. The physical examination should note the morphology, color, and distribution of the rash. Diagnostic errors occur because of failure to do a full physical examination to rule out underlying conditions that may present as a diaper rash.

Diaper rash is common and usually easily diagnosed and treated. Because more serious clinical entities may initially present as a diaper rash, however, several clinical caveats are in order:

- Seborrheic dermatitis in an infant younger than 6 months of age that does not respond to conventional therapy should alert the physician to the possibility of Letterer-Siwe disease.
- Many conditions may be secondarily infected with yeast or bacteria and should be treated accordingly.
- Sexually transmitted diseases are a cause of diaper rash. The possibility of congenital infection or sexual abuse must be entertained.
- Dermatophytosis is uncommon but occurs in the diaper area.
- Psoriasis presents after the resolution of another primary skin condition and may lack the typical thick, silvery scale.

EMERGENCY DEPARTMENT MANAGEMENT

The management of diaper rash begins with a discussion of the pathophysiology of the rash in terms the parents can understand. The emergency department physician must explain the effects that infrequent diaper changes, prolonged exposure of the skin to urine and stool, diarrhea, and antibiotic use have on the production of the diaper rashes.

For mild irritant dermatitis or seborrheic dermatitis, a 1% hydrocortisone cream is usually effective. For more severe dermatitis, such as atopic dermatitis, or psoriasis, a more potent fluorinated corticosteroid, such as 0.1% betamethasone valerate, is used twice daily initially. As inflammation subsides, 1% hydrocortisone is used. Infection with *C. albicans* is common and may be treated with 1% hydrocortisone cream and a topical imidazole or nystatin cream twice daily, or after each diaper change, if the area is cleaned. If thrush is a consideration, oral nystatin suspension, 1 mL three times a day for 5 to 7 days, is prescribed.

Dermatophytes are treated with topical antifungal agents, such as miconazole nitrate 2% applied twice daily for 2 to 4 weeks. Bullous impetigo or folliculitis is treated with systemic antibiotics, such as cephalexin 40 to 60 mg/kg/d, divided into three to four doses, or other antibiotics with good activity against *S. aureus,* such as mupirocin 2% ointment topically, three times a day.

Zinc oxide ointment can be used to protect the area once the primary rash has resolved, but one must remember that creams are generally preferred to ointment bases, because ointments tend to be occlusive and cause sweat retention. Potent corticosteroids are used only for short periods of time to avoid local and systemic side effects.

DISPOSITION

Consultation or admission is rarely needed for the treatment of a diaper rash. Exceptions are cases refractory to therapy, those in which an underlying systemic disorder is suspected, or those in which parental neglect or inability to properly care for the child is suspected.

COMMON PITFALLS

- Failure to do a full history and physical examination
- Neglecting attention to simple general care
- Not providing the parents with specific, written instructions
- Failure to recognize secondary infection and treat it accordingly
- Overuse of potent corticosteroids
- Failure to recognize more serious underlying disorders or infections, especially when they present as a chronic or refractory problem

ACKNOWLEDGEMENT

The author gratefully acknowledges the contribution of Jane Knapp, who wrote the previous version of this chapter.

References

1. Anderson PH, Bucher AP, Saeed I, et al. Faecal enzymes: in vivo human skin irritation. *Contact Dermatitis* 1994;30(3):152–158.
2. Berg RW, Milligan MC, Sarbaugh FC. Association of skin wetness and pH with diaper dermatitis. *Pediatr Dermatol* 1994;11(1):18–20.
3. Boiko S. Treatment of diaper dermatitis. *Dermatol Clin* 1999;17(1):235–240.
4. Higuchi R, Mizukoshi M, Koyama H, et al. Intractable diaper dermatitis as an early sign of biotin deficiency. *Acta Paediatr* 1998;87(2):228–229.
5. Holden C. Infant napkin dermatitis. *J Wound Care* 1998;7(8):417–418.
6. Hoppe JE. Treatment of oropharyngeal candidiasis and candidal diaper dermatitis in neonates and infants: review and reappraisal. *Pediatr Infect Dis J* 1997;16(9):885–894.
7. Philipp R, Hughes A, Golding J. Getting to the bottom of nappy rash. ALSPAC Survey Team. Avon Longitudinal Study of Pregnancy and Childhood. *Br Hosp Gen Pract* 1997; 47.
8. Roul S, Ducombs G, Leaute-Labreze C, et al. "Lucky Luke" contact dermatitis due to rubber components of diapers. *Contact Dermatitis* 1998;38(6):363–364.
9. Singalavanija S, Frieden IJ. Diaper dermatitis. *Pediatr Rev* 1995;16(4):142–147.
10. Sires UI, Mallory SB. Diaper dermatitis. How to treat and prevent. *Postgrad Med* 1995;98(6):79–84, 86.

CHAPTER 269
Exanthems

Mary A. Hegenbarth

The sudden onset of a rash, particularly with fever, is a frequent cause of emergency department (ED) visits. Definitive diagnosis may not be possible in the ED. Most patients have a nonspecific, self-limited viral illness rather than a classic disease such as measles. The physician should focus on identifying diseases that require specific therapy (e.g., scarlet fever) or have public health implications, and should exclude life-threatening illnesses with rash (see Chapter 247).

Patient history should establish the initial location, spread, duration, and changes in appearance of the rash. Any fever or other associated symptoms, such as sore throat, cough, vomiting, headache, and neck pain, should be characterized. A history of recent exposure to a highly contagious disease, such as varicella or measles, is often helpful. Recent medication use may suggest a drug reaction. If either the patient or a household contact is a neonate, pregnant, or immunocompromised, the management of an otherwise benign illness may be altered.

Physical examination should focus on assessing the general severity of illness (e.g., irritability, state of hydration) and should thoroughly characterize skin and mucous membrane lesions. Complications such as otitis media, cellulitis, pneumonia, and encephalitis should be sought.

DISEASES WITH MACULOPAPULAR ERUPTIONS

Nonspecific viral eruptions commonly have maculopapular lesions, often resembling the classic childhood diseases. Differentiating features of illnesses with characteristic maculopapular eruptions are shown in Table 269.1.

EPIDEMIOLOGY AND CLINICAL PRESENTATION OF SPECIFIC DISEASES

Measles

Measles (rubeola) is caused by a paramyxovirus. The incidence of measles has declined greatly since widespread vaccination began, but outbreaks still occur. Recent outbreaks that occured between 1989 and 1991 involved primarily unvaccinated preschool-aged children in urban areas, but cases may also be seen in older children and young adults, particularly those receiving only a single dose of vaccine. Many recent measles cases in the United States have been due to importation from endemic areas.[7] The diagnosis of measles has important public health implications, as prompt recognition of a local outbreak helps control spread. Health-care facilities, including EDs, may serve as sites of significant exposure risk to patients and staff.[8,13]

Measles has a characteristic 3- to 4-day prodrome, characterized by fever, malaise, and the "3 C's"—cough, coryza, and conjunctivitis. A pathognomonic enanthem known as Koplik's spots precedes the rash and consists of small red patches capped

TABLE 269.1. Differentiating Features of Selected Diseases with Maculopapular Eruptions

Disease	Ages Most Affected	Typical Seasons	Type/Distribution of Skin and Oral Lesions	Common Associated Symptoms/Signs	Complications
Measles	Children, young adults	Winter, spring	Skin—purple-red maculopapules spreading from the hairline downward, confluent on face and neck Oral mucosa—Koplik's spots	Prodrome of high fever, coryza, cough, conjunctivitis	Common: otitis media, pneumonia Rare: encephalitis, severe laryngotracheitis
Rubella	Children, young adults	Winter, spring	Skin—discrete, pink-red maculopapules spreading from face downward Soft palate—Forchheimer's spots	Children—lymphadenopathy, minimal fever Adolescent/adult—febrile prodrome, joint pains	Common: arthritis in older patients Very rare: encephalitis, purpura Prenatal exposure: congenital rubella syndrome
Roseola infantum	6 mo to 3 yr	Spring, fall, summer	Discrete, small rose-pink macules spreading from trunk to rest of body	High fever for 3–4 days before rash, mild pharyngitis, otitis, and adenopathy	Common: febrile seizures Very rare: encephalitis
Erythema infectiosum	2 to 12 yr	Late winter, spring	1st stage—"slapped-cheek" malar rash 2nd stage—truncal/extremity, rash, fading in lacelike pattern 3rd stage—recurrence of rash with stimuli	Asymptomatic or mild fever	Rare: arthritis (especially in adults), hemolytic anemia, encephalitis, fetal loss
Scarlet fever	3 to 12 yr	Winter, spring	Skin—face flushed with circumoral pallor, trunk/extremities with "sandpapery," blanching pinpoint red rash most prominent in creases, Pastia lines Mucosa—pharyngitis/tonsillitis, palatal petechiae, strawberry tongue	Fever, sore throat, vomiting, abdominal pain, tender anterior cervical nodes	Early: otitis media, peritonsillitis, cervical adenitis Late: rheumatic fever, glomerulonephritis

by bluish-white specks (resembling sprinkles of salt), seen first on the buccal mucosa opposite the molars, with subsequent spread and coalescence within the mouth. Koplik's spots resolve by the second or third day of rash and have often disappeared by the time the patient is seen. The rash appears on the third or fourth day of illness, and consists of purplish-red maculopapules that begin at the hairline and spread downward, tending to be confluent on the face and neck.

A comparison of the progression of skin findings in measles, rubella, and scarlet fever is shown in Fig. 269.1. The child with full-blown measles appears miserable ("measly"), with high fever, impressive conjunctivitis, marked cough, and rhinorrhea. The severity of symptoms peaks on the second day of the rash, with subsequent rapid recovery in uncomplicated cases. Measles is highly contagious, with infectivity from about 2 days before onset of illness to 4 days after the rash appears. The incubation period is 8 to 12 days from exposure to onset of illness.

Otitis media, diarrhea, dehydration, pneumonia, and croup are common complications of measles. Severe laryngotracheobronchitis has been a frequent complication among recently hospitalized infants and young children; endotracheal intubation may be required to relieve airway obstruction.[9,16] Encephalitis is a rare complication. Although measles is seldom fatal in the United States, approximately 1 million deaths per year occur worldwide.[7] Vitamin A deficiency is associated with increased morbidity and mortality from measles; treatment with vitamin A appears to reduce measles complications in developing countries.[2] Significant numbers of children with measles in the United States have been found to have low levels of vitamin A; supplementation may be indicated in selected patients (see Emergency Department Management).[1,2]

Rubella

Rubella (German measles) is a mild disease caused by *Rubivirus.* Its major significance is its ability to cause severe illness and birth defects in prenatally infected infants. Since vaccination began, the incidence of rubella and congenital rubella syndrome has greatly decreased; however, approximately 10% of young adults remain susceptible.[1]

Rash is usually the first symptom of rubella, beginning with discrete pink-red maculopapules on the face that rapidly spread downward (see Fig. 269.1). A nonspecific enanthem of small reddish dots on the soft palate (Forchheimer's spots) may be seen. The rash often coalesces on the trunk and usually fades within 3 days. Generalized lymphadenopathy, particularly postauricular and suboccipital, is typical. Adolescents and adults tend to have a febrile prodrome and commonly develop arthralgias or arthritis. Serious complications, such as encephalitis or purpura, are extremely rare. First-trimester prenatal infection may cause severe anomalies and illness in the fetus, including congenital heart disease, deafness, cataracts, microcephaly or mental retardation, hepatosplenomegaly, and purpura.

Roseola

Roseola infantum (exanthem subitum) is a commonly recognized clinical syndrome in young children. Human herpesvirus 6 (HHV-6) is the primary etiologic agent, although human herpesvirus 7 (HHV-7) appears to cause a similar illness.[17] HHV-6 is a very common cause of acute febrile illness in young children seen in the ED, peaking at 6 to 9 months of age.[10] However, only about 15% to 20% of HHV-6 infections present as typical roseola.[10,11] Almost all children acquire HHV-6 by 2 years of age.

Classic roseola has a characteristic history of abrupt onset of high fever for 3 to 4 days, followed by sudden defervescence that coincides with the onset of rash. The skin lesions are small, discrete, rose-pink macules or maculopapules that appear first on the trunk before spreading to the rest of the body. The rash resolves within 1 to 2 days. When seen during the febrile phase, the child may be irritable but often appears otherwise well. Diarrhea and cough are common associated symptoms. Physical findings may include a bulging fontanelle, periorbital edema, erythematous papules on the soft palate and base of the uvula (Nagayama's spots), inflamed tympanic membranes, and cervical adenopathy.[6,11] Febrile seizures are common. Serious complications such as encephalitis are rare.

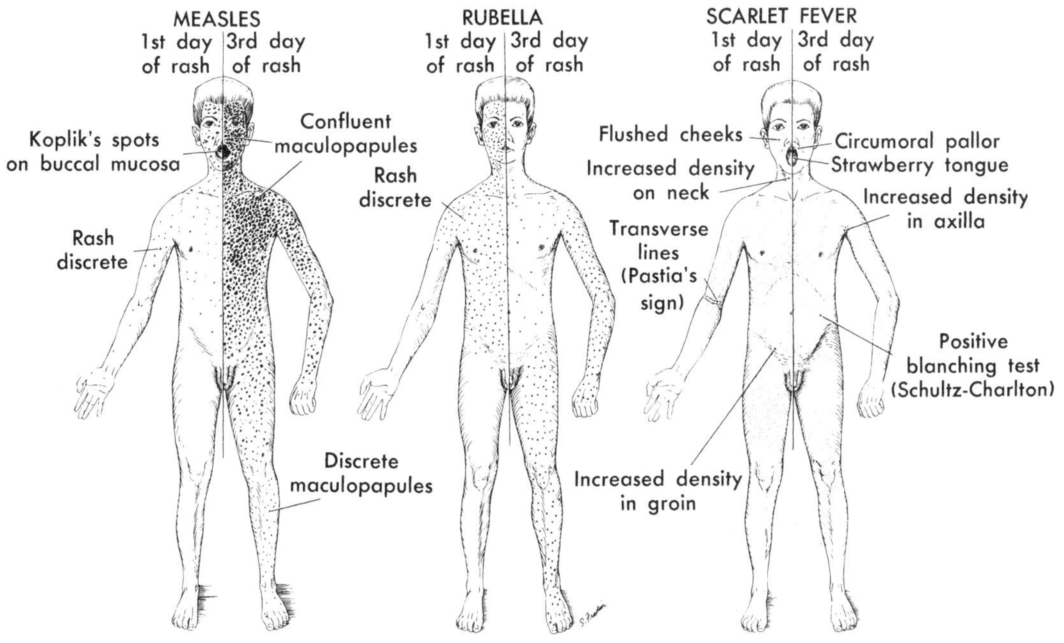

Figure 269.1. Differences in appearance and progression of rashes in measles, rubella, and scarlet fever. (From Krugman S, et al. *Infectious diseases of children,* 8th ed. St. Louis: CV Mosby, 1985, with permission.)

Erythema Infectiosum

Erythema infectiosum, or "fifth disease," is caused by human parvovirus B19. Parvovirus B19 is also responsible for other illnesses, including nonspecific febrile illnesses and rashes, aplastic crises in patients with chronic hemolytic anemia (e.g., sickle cell anemia), chronic anemia in immunocompromised persons, and arthritis. Maternal infection, particularly in the first half of pregnancy, may result in fetal anemia, hydrops, and fetal death.

Erythema infectiosum typically affects school-aged children in epidemics. A viremic phase occurs approximately 1 week before the onset of rash; some children have a nonspecific febrile illness during this time, but many are asymptomatic. The skin findings appear in three stages. A bright red, raised macular rash on the cheeks that spares the nasal bridge and mouth appears first, giving the child a distinctive "slapped-cheek" appearance. The second stage begins about 1 day later with a symmetric maculopapular rash on the extremities and trunk (appearing first on the arms and extensor surfaces), which becomes lacy-appearing as confluent areas clear. During the third stage, lasting weeks to months, the rash may reappear with various stimuli, such as bathing, temperature extremes, or local irritation.

Occasional complications in children include arthralgias and arthritis; symmetric polyarthritis is common in women. Patients with fifth disease are not contagious once they have a rash; however, patients with aplastic crisis are highly infectious. The risk of fetal death in proven infection in the first half of pregnancy is under 10%, and less in the second half.[1] The overall risk of an adverse fetal outcome when a pregnant woman is exposed to parvovirus B19 is only 1% to 2%; at least 50% of women have had previous unrecognized infection and are immune.[1,12]

Scarlet Fever

Scarlet fever (scarlatina) is a rash seen in association with group A beta-hemolytic streptococcal (GABHS) infections caused by strains producing an erythrogenic toxin. A similar clinical picture may be caused by other organisms, including *Staphylococcus aureus* and *Arcanobacterium haemolyticum.* Scarlet fever is most common in school-age children in the winter and spring and is more prevalent in temperate or colder climates. The clinical symptoms are usually those of streptococcal pharyngitis, although other types of GABHS infections, such as pyoderma, may occasionally present with scarlatina. The rash appears within 1 to 2 days, beginning on the trunk and spreading rapidly. The skin is red, blanches, and has fine punctate bumps that feel like sandpaper. The face is flushed and has circumoral pallor. The rash is prominent in skin folds, and Pastia lines (areas of hyperpigmentation and petechiae) may be seen in joint creases such as the antecubital fossae (see Fig. 269.1). Desquamation after resolution of symptoms is characteristic. The complications of scarlet fever are the same as those of streptococcal pharyngitis (rheumatic fever, glomerulonephritis).

Other Agents

Many other agents cause nonspecific maculopapular eruptions. A rash that is usually maculopapular but may be urticarial, vesicular, hemorrhagic, or similar to erythema multiforme occasionally accompanies infectious mononucleosis. Rashes are seen commonly in patients with mononucleosis who have received ampicillin. *Mycoplasma pneumoniae* infections have a wide variety of associated rashes, including maculopapular and vesicular types. Enteroviruses are a common cause of nonspecific febrile exanthems as well as more distinctive vesicular eruptions.

DIFFERENTIAL DIAGNOSIS

The presumptive diagnosis of a specific disease or nonspecific "viral exanthem" is usually made clinically, because definitive diagnosis requires methods such as viral culture or titer tests that are generally not useful in the ED. Many other conditions are associated with maculopapular skin lesions, including drug reactions, rheumatic diseases, and Kawasaki disease. Scarlatiniform rashes are commonly seen in streptococcal and staphylococcal toxic shock syndromes. Other life-threatening infections, such as meningococcemia and Rocky Mountain spotted fever, occasionally present with a benign-appearing rash. These possibilities should be considered in the child with severe or unusual symptoms.

EMERGENCY DEPARTMENT EVALUATION

The child's overall degree of illness is the most important assessment, as laboratory tests are rarely helpful or indicated in the child who is only mildly ill. A throat culture or rapid strep test (with confirmatory culture if negative) should be obtained if the child has a sore throat or suspected scarlet fever. Antibody titers may be useful for confirming suspected cases of measles, rubella, and parvovirus B19 exposure (pregnant contacts). White blood cell counts and blood cultures are helpful in evaluating the ill-appearing child who is suspected of having complications or a more serious disease. Further workup should be aimed at confirming clinically suspected complications such as pneumonia or encephalitis.

EMERGENCY DEPARTMENT MANAGEMENT

A child with an uncomplicated, presumably viral illness should be treated symptomatically with acetaminophen or ibuprofen and oral fluids; antibiotics should be reserved for secondary bacterial infection. Scarlet fever requires treatment with penicillin or an alternative.

Children with suspected measles or rubella should be isolated within the ED and reported to the health department. Treatment with vitamin A may be indicated for selected children with measles, such as infants 6 months to 2 years of age hospitalized with complications, and children with immunodeficiency, impaired intestinal absorption, malnutrition, or recent immigration from areas with high measles mortality rates.[1,2]

Attempts at prevention or amelioration of measles may be indicated for susceptible household contacts, particularly infants younger than 1 year, pregnant females, and immunocompromised persons. Intramuscular immune globulin, given within 6 days of exposure, is the primary mode of prevention in such cases. Measles vaccine may be used for susceptible household contacts (unless pregnant or immunocompromised) if given within 72 hours of exposure; however, this is seldom possible, because the diagnostic findings of measles are not present until the third or fourth day of illness.[1]

DISPOSITION

A pediatrician or infectious disease specialist should be consulted if the child appears to have a serious complication, is a neonate, or is immunosuppressed, or if a potentially serious disease is under consideration. Indications for hospitalization include dehydration, pneumonia, measles croup, encephalitis, and clinical toxicity.

Obstetric follow-up should be arranged for pregnant patients who may have been exposed to rubella or parvovirus B19; antibody titer tests may be indicated. Children with erythema infectiosum need not be isolated or restricted from school or daycare attendance, because they have already passed their period of infectivity.

Patients discharged home should follow up with their private physician or the ED if their illness worsens or does not resolve within the expected time course. Occasionally, the physician or parent may be uncomfortable with a diagnosis of "nonspecific viral exanthem." If the child is not acutely ill, outpatient consultation is appropriate.

Transfer to a tertiary pediatric facility should be considered if the child needs a level of care or expertise (e.g., intensive care or subspecialists) that is not available at the treating facility.

COMMON PITFALLS

- Children with benign, nonspecific febrile exanthems do not need lengthy diagnostic evaluation unless they are ill-appearing.
- Early scarlet fever may be subtle and easily overlooked, especially in children with minimal pharyngitis.

DISEASES WITH VESICULAR OR PUSTULAR LESIONS

Viral vesicular rashes and enanthems are frequently distinctive, allowing a presumptive diagnosis in many cases. The basic approach to the history and physical examination is described earlier in this chapter.

EPIDEMIOLOGY AND CLINICAL PRESENTATION OF SPECIFIC DISEASES

Varicella

Varicella (chickenpox) is a common contagious childhood disease caused by the varicella-zoster virus. Most cases occur in children, but adolescents and adults tend to have a severe course, with more frequent complications. Chickenpox is most common in late winter and spring. The frequency of varicella is likely to decrease as the vaccine becomes more widely used.

Signs and symptoms of varicella in healthy children include mild systemic symptoms, fever, and rash following an incubation period of 10 to 21 days. The skin lesions appear in crops, beginning as macules that rapidly progress to papules, then vesicles that eventually rupture and crust. The classic early vesicle is small and surrounded by erythema, resembling a dewdrop on a rose petal. The first lesions often develop on the face and scalp.

As the rash spreads, lesions of all stages (papules, vesicles, crusts) are characteristically present within a single affected area. Shallow ulcers often occur in the mouth but may also be seen on other mucous membranes. The number of skin lesions generally correlates with the height of fever and severity of symptoms. Pruritis is common, and scarring may result if the lesions are traumatized by severe scratching or become infected. The patient is contagious from 1 day before onset of the rash until all of the lesions are crusted, or until 6 days from the onset of rash.

Serious complications are unusual in normal children. Secondary bacterial skin infections, manifested by impetigo, cellulitis, or local abscess, are the most common complications seen in young children. Recently, there have been increased reports of invasive group A beta-hemolytic streptococcal (GABHS) infections associated with chickenpox, including necrotizing fasciitis and streptococcal toxic shock syndrome.[3,18] GABHS infection should be suspected in children with varicella who develop localized skin swelling, warmth, redness, or pain, and in those with fever persisting beyond the fourth day of illness or who have recurrence of fever after becoming afebrile.[3] Pain out of proportion to the degree of clinical findings is common.

Other serious complications seen occasionally in children include neurologic problems such as acute cerebellar ataxia, encephalitis, and Reye syndrome. Varicella pneumonia is relatively common in adolescent and adult patients but is rare in children. Unusual complications include hepatitis, eye involvement (keratoconjunctivitis or uveitis), coagulopathy, arthritis, orchitis, nephritis, and other invasive bacterial infections (e.g., osteomyelitis).

Patients with altered cell-mediated immunity, such as leukemic children receiving chemotherapy, are susceptible to disseminated varicella with hemorrhagic lesions, pneumonitis, and encephalitis. Fetal infection during the first or early second trimester of pregnancy may result in the congenital varicella syndrome. Newborns exposed to perinatal maternal varicella are at risk for severe illness. Children recently treated with corticosteroids (particularly systemic, high doses) may be at increased risk of severe varicella, although this is controversial. A case-control study found little increased risk in otherwise normal children.[15]

Herpes Zoster

Herpes zoster (shingles) is caused by reactivation of latent varicella-zoster virus in sensory ganglia. Children are less commonly affected than are adults, and younger patients tend to have a less painful course and little postherpetic neuralgia. The characteristic findings include grouped, vesicular lesions in a dermatomal distribution, accompanied by pain and tenderness along the pathway of the nerves involved. Fever and local lymphadenopathy are common. The presence of lesions on the tip of the nose signals possible eye involvement.

Herpes Simplex

Primary infection with herpes simplex viruses (usually HSV-1) in childhood is extremely common and often asymptomatic. The most common form seen in the ED is acute herpetic gingivostomatitis, primarily affecting children aged 1 to 4 years. Symptoms include high fever, irritability, and reluctance to eat or drink. The child looks uncomfortable, drools, and has marked gingival redness, swelling, and friability. Ulcerations or plaques may be seen on the tongue, buccal mucosa, palate, and pharynx. Vesicles may be present on the lips, and there is tender cervical adenopathy. Lesions can occasionally be seen on the fingers or genitalia from autoinoculation. Dehydration is not uncommon. Symptoms may last 1 to 2 weeks.

Other primary and recurrent herpes infections, including herpes labialis, herpetic whitlow, and herpes keratoconjunctivitis, may be seen in children. Children with atopic dermatitis may develop extensive herpes simplex infection on eczematized areas (eczema herpeticum, also called Kaposi's varicelliform eruption). Although herpetic vulvovaginitis can be a rare manifestation of innocently acquired primary herpes simplex infection in young children, the possibility of sexual abuse must be strongly considered.

Enteroviruses

Nonpolio enteroviruses are a frequent cause of febrile illnesses and exanthems. Pathogens include group A and B coxsackieviruses, echoviruses, and enteroviruses. Epidemics occur during the summer and fall, affecting primarily 1- to 4-year-old children. The vesicular exanthems and enanthems are often distinctive and easily recognized. Occasional complications include dehydration and aseptic meningitis.

Hand-foot-and-mouth disease is a distinctive clinical syndrome. Children have fever and lesions on the oral mucosa and tongue that progress from small red macules to vesicles on an erythematous base to discrete ulcers. The skin lesions are oval or linear vesicles (about 3 to 7 mm) surrounded by erythema. They occur on the dorsum of the hands and feet, the interdigital areas, and the palms and soles. Some patients have mild diarrhea or cervical adenopathy. Serious complications, such as meningitis, myocarditis, and pneumonia, are unusual.

Herpangina presents with fever, sore throat, and dysphagia. Examination discloses small vesicles or punched-out ulcers involving the tonsillar pillars, tonsils, pharynx, and soft palate. The illness resolves in 5 to 6 days.

DIFFERENTIAL DIAGNOSIS

Classic varicella is usually easily recognized, although early cases may require a meticulous search to find the first vesicles. Herpes zoster and herpes simplex infections can overlap in presentation, and viral vesiculopustular lesions are sometimes confused with impetigo. Herpetic gingivostomatitis may be confused with herpangina, Vincent's angina, or aphthous stomatitis. Herpetic whitlow is often misdiagnosed as a paronychia. Many other disorders may present with vesicular lesions.

A definitive diagnosis of herpes simplex or varicella-zoster virus infection may be needed in immunocompromised or severely ill patients. There are numerous testing methods available (e.g., enzyme immunoassay, latex agglutination, indirect fluorescent antibody, fluorescent antibody-to-membrane antigen); the practitioner should consult with the laboratory and pertinent specialists, if necessary (i.e., infectious diseases), to determine the best available methods. Immunofluorescent staining of vesicle scrapings, using monoclonal antibodies, can distinguish between herpes simplex virus and varicella-zoster virus.

Herpes simplex is easily cultured; polymerase chain reaction (PCR) testing for herpes simplex virus is sensitive, but false positives occur. Less accurate but helpful when more sophisticated tests are unavailable is the Tzanck preparation, which demonstrates multinucleated giant cells in both varicella-zoster and herpes simplex infections.

Virus isolation or PCR testing (e.g., from throat, stool, cerebrospinal fluid) may be helpful in the diagnosis of enterovirus infections, although isolation from stool is of uncertain clinical significance.

EMERGENCY DEPARTMENT EVALUATION AND MANAGEMENT

ED evaluation includes assessment of the child's degree of clinical toxicity, state of hydration, and ability to take oral fluids. Laboratory evaluation is indicated for suspected complications or in high-risk patients in whom definitive diagnosis is necessary.

Symptomatic therapy for chickenpox includes acetaminophen and measures to decrease itching and discomfort. Children with chickenpox should not receive aspirin because of its association with Reye syndrome. Recently, there has been concern that ibuprofen use may be associated with an increased risk of necrotizing fasciitis in children with chickenpox.[18] Although causal evidence is lacking, some authors caution against the use of ibuprofen and other nonsteroidal antiinflammatory drugs in patients with varicella. Topical measures, such as cool baths, calamine lotion, and colloidal oatmeal baths, may help alleviate pruritis. Oral antihistamines (diphenhydramine or hydroxyzine) may be helpful for severe itching; topical antihistamines are less desirable because of the risks of sensitization and excessive systemic absorption through nonintact skin.

Oral acyclovir started within 24 hours of rash onset in normal children with chickenpox has shown modest benefit in reducing the number of lesions, duration of fever, and severity of constitutional symptoms.[4] However, most authorities do not recommend the routine use of acyclovir in healthy children who are likely to have an uncomplicated course. Acyclovir treatment (20 mg/kg four times a day for 5 days; maximum single dose, 800 mg) beginning within 24 hours of rash onset may be advisable for children with varicella who appear to be at risk of moderate-to-severe disease. Such patients include adolescents (over age 12), children older than 12 months of age with chronic skin or pulmonary disorders, children on chronic salicylate therapy, and patients recently treated with short, intermittent, or aerosolized courses of corticosteroids.[1] Although acyclovir and related drugs are commonly used to treat adults with shingles, normal children seldom have severe symptoms or develop postherpetic neuralgia, and treatment is not routinely recommended. Significantly immunocompromised patients with varicella-zoster infections should be hospitalized and treated with intravenous rather than oral acyclovir.

Acyclovir and related drugs are commonly used to treat adults with severe or recurrent herpes simplex infections, but there is little pediatric data. One study found that oral acyclovir (15 mg/kg five times a day for 7 days) started within 72 hours of the onset of herpes gingivostomatitis reduced symptoms and duration of illness.[5] Although some authors recommend routine use of acyclovir for children with gingivostomatitis and other herpes simplex infections,[14] the optimal dose has not been established, and routine use remains controversial. There seems to be more agreement that children with severe illness requiring hospitalization should be treated; immunocompromised patients (including neonates) should receive intravenous acyclovir.

Children with oral vesicles and ulcers, especially those with herpetic gingivostomatitis, may refuse to drink. Cold substances such as Popsicles, ice cream, and nonirritating fluids are often accepted. Acetaminophen or ibuprofen usually suffices for symptomatic relief in mild cases. However, children with severe mouth pain may require narcotic analgesia. Oral anesthetics (e.g., viscous lidocaine) are seldom helpful in children with widespread stomatitis and should be used sparingly to avoid toxicity. Intravenous hydration may be required. Antibiotics should be given only for secondary bacterial infections.

Patients with varicella should be isolated in the ED. Passive immunization with varicella-zoster immune globulin may be indicated within 96 hours of exposure of a susceptible, high-risk patient.[1]

DISPOSITION

Children with chickenpox who have significant or rapidly progressing cellulitis should be hospitalized for intravenous antibiotics and carefully observed for the development of necrotizing fasciitis. Neonates or immunocompromised patients with suspected varicella-zoster or herpes simplex infection should be referred to a specialist (e.g., for infectious disease, oncology, neonatology, pediatrics). These patients usually require hospitalization for intravenous acyclovir. An ophthalmologist should be consulted when herpes keratoconjunctivitis is suspected.

Children with uncomplicated viral stomatitis or rash are discharged on symptomatic therapy, with outpatient follow-up scheduled if further symptoms develop or the child does not improve within a few days.

Transfer to a tertiary pediatric facility should be considered if the child is seriously ill or needs intensive care, or when subspecialty consultation is indicated.

COMMON PITFALLS

- Children with vesicular skin infections or stomatitis are often uncomfortable, and their parents are frequently frustrated. Give reassurance and careful explanations about the expected course, communicability, and self-limited nature of the disease.
- If the term *herpes infection* is used, explain to the parents the innocent acquisition of most childhood infections, to avoid confusion and anxiety.
- Avoid potentially toxic preparations such as oral viscous lidocaine or topical diphenhydramine.
- Antibiotics should be prescribed only for the infrequent bacterial superinfection.
- Acyclovir is not indicated for healthy children presenting more than 24 hours after the onset of chickenpox lesions.

References

1. American Academy of Pediatrics. *1997 Red book: report of the Committee on Infectious Diseases,* 24th ed. Elk Grove Village, IL: American Academy of Pediatrics, 2000.
2. American Academy of Pediatrics, Committee on Infectious Diseases. Vitamin A treatment of measles. *Pediatrics* 1993;91:1014–1015.
3. American Academy of Pediatrics, Committee on Infectious Diseases. Severe invasive group A streptococcal infections: a subject review. *Pediatrics* 1998;101:136–140.
4. American Academy of Pediatrics, Committee on Infectious Diseases. The use of oral acyclovir in otherwise healthy children with varicella. *Pediatrics* 1993;91:674–676.
5. Amir J, Harel L, Smetana Z, et al. Treatment of herpes simplex gingivostomatitis with aciclovir in children: a randomised double blind placebo controlled study. *BMJ* 1997;314:1800–1803.
6. Asano Y, Yoshikawa T, Suga S, et al. Clinical features of infants with primary human herpesvirus 6 infection (exanthem subitum, roseola infantum). *Pediatrics* 1994;93:104–108.
7. Centers for Disease Control and Prevention. Advances in global measles control and elimination: summary of the 1997 international meeting. *MMWR* 1998;47(RR-11).
8. Farizo KM, Stehr-Green PA, Simpson DM, et al. Pediatric emergency room visits: a risk factor for acquiring measles. *Pediatrics* 1991;87:74–79.
9. Fortenberry JD, Mariscalco M, Louis PT, et al. Severe laryngotracheobronchitis complicating measles. *Am J Dis Child* 1992;146:1040–1043.
10. Hall CB, Long CE, Schnabel KC, et al. Human herpesvirus-6 infection in children: a prospective study of complications and reactivation. *N Engl J Med* 1994;331:432–438.
11. Katz SL, Gershon AA, Hotez PJ. *Krugman's infectious diseases of children,* 10th ed. St. Louis: Mosby–Year Book, 1998.
12. Markenson GR, Yancey MK. Parvovirus B19 infections in pregnancy. *Semin Perinatol* 1998;22(4):309–317.
13. Mason WH, Ross LA, Lanson J, et al. Epidemic measles in the postvaccine era: evaluation of epidemiology, clinical presentation and complications during an urban outbreak. *Pediatr Infect Dis J* 1993;12:42–48.
14. Murph JR, Grose C. Routine acyclovir therapy: isn't it time? *Contemp Pediatr* 1999;16(4):79–99.
15. Patel H, Macarthur C, Johnson D. Recent corticosteroid use and the risk of complicated varicella in otherwise immunocompetent children. *Arch Pediatr Adolesc Med* 1996;150:409–414.
16. Ross LA, Mason WH, Lanson J, et al. Laryngotracheobronchitis as a complication of measles during an urban epidemic. *J Pediatr* 1992;121:511–515.
17. Suga S, Yoshikawa T, Nagai T, et al. Clinical features and virologic findings in children with primary human herpesvirus 7 infection. *Pediatrics* 1997;99:E4.
18. Zerr DM, Alexander ER, Duchin JS, et al. A case-control study of necrotizing fasciitis during primary varicella. *Pediatrics* 1999;103:783–790.

CHAPTER 270
Eye Disorders

Janet G. Alteveer and Kathryn McCans

A complete pediatric eye examination includes inspection of the eyelids, conjunctivae, pupil, and iris; evaluation of the extraocular muscles; funduscopy; and testing of visual acuity. This examination is an essential part of the evaluation in any child presenting with primarily ophthalmologic conditions such as conjunctivitis, periorbital edema, visual change or loss, trauma, or neurologic complaints.

Inspection of the eyelids and conjunctivae should document the presence of erythema, ecchymosis, edema, proptosis, or masses. The cornea should be evaluated for normal contour and clarity. A bulging or hazy cornea in a neonate may indicate congenital glaucoma. The cornea should be stained, using topical anesthetic drops and fluorescein test strips, after the rest of the examination is completed so as not to interfere with visual acuity testing. Shining a Wood's light on the cornea in a darkened room will reveal stain adherent to corneal defects caused by an abrasion, herpetic infection, or ulcer. The pupil should be assessed for contour, bilateral symmetry and reactivity to light. An abnormally shaped or reactive pupil may indicate defects in the iris or disruption of the afferent or efferent nerve pathways to the eye.

Extraocular muscle testing can be accomplished by 4 months of age. By this age, a normal, full-term infant should be able to fixate on and follow a small, brightly colored toy held 6 to 12 in. from the baby's face. By 5 to 6 months, the infant should fixate and follow an object through the full range of motion. By 2 to 3 years of age, most children, with gentle encouragement, will follow a light or finger.[2]

Evaluation of the posterior chamber via direct ophthalmoscopy is dependent on the child's age and cognitive development, becoming easier as cooperation increases. The use of a short-acting topical parasympatholytic such as tropicamide (Mydriacyl 0.5%), will facilitate the examination of the retina. To encourage the child to look beyond the examiner and away from the direct light, use a brightly colored toy or have the parent wave at the child from directly behind the examiner. The minimal examination in an infant is the documentation of a normal red reflex. The presence of an abnormal red reflex (leukocoria), which could indicate a cataract or intraocular tumor, mandates formal consultation with a pediatric ophthalmologist.

The corneal light reflex, or Hirschberg test, is useful in detecting strabismus or an ocular muscle palsy. It is conducted by shining a penlight, held 3 ft (1 m) away, centrally onto the child's face. In a normal child, the light will reflect centrally on both pupils when the child is fixated on the light or a small toy held in front of the face. If the light reflex is eccentric on one eye, a strabismus or palsy is present.[2]

Visual acuity testing is an extremely important aspect of the complete eye examination. The manner of testing is dependent on the age and cognitive ability of the child. Visual acuity also varies by age (Table 270.1). To assess an infant, have the baby fixate (on a bright toy or light) and cover one eye gently with your thumb. If the uncovered eye has normal vision, the child will continue to fixate on the object. If the uncovered eye has

TABLE 270.1. Visual Acuity by Age

Age	Visual Acuity
6 mo	20/60 to 20/100
3 yr	20/25 to 20/30
5–7 yr	20/20 to 20/25
By 8 yr	20/20

poor vision, the child may lose interest, push the covering thumb away, or protest.[6]

By 3 years of age, depending on developmental and cognitive ability, more objective visual testing can be achieved. The Allen chart, HOTV matching test, or "Tumbling E" game can be used. By 5 years of age, most cognitively normal children can use the Snellen chart. Testing with the Snellen, Tumbling E, or HOTV chart should be performed at a distance of 20 ft (6 m). The Allen test can be performed at 10 ft (3 m).[2]

In all of these charts, letters or objects are presented as a group. Children with poor vision have increased difficulty identifying objects when presented as a group (the crowding phenomenon) and will perform better when objects are presented singly.[2]

THE RED EYE

Children frequently present to the emergency department (ED) with a complaint of one or both eyes being reddened. The most common diagnosis will be conjunctivitis due to bacterial or viral infection, chemical, or allergic exposure. The etiologies of infectious conjunctivitis after the neonatal period are nontypable *H. influenzae, Streptococcus pneumoniae, Moraxella catarrhalis,* herpesvirus, and adenovirus.[26] Uncommonly, gonococcal conjunctivitis may occur after the neonatal period and in the prepubescent child, who is not sexually active. Sexual abuse must be excluded; however, cases of transmission from an infected caregiver who is not abusing the child have been reported.[1]

The syndrome of conjunctivitis–otitis was first described in 1982 by Boder. Nontypable *H. influenzae* will commonly cause concomitant otitis and conjunctivitis. Additionally, as many as 60% of children presenting with conjunctivitis without clinical findings or symptoms of otitis will develop an otitis within 2 weeks.[24]

Herpesviruses can cause ocular involvement during primary or recurrent infections. Herpes simplex virus (HSV) is ubiquitous and is transmitted from person to person during primary and recurrent infections that may or may not be symptomatic. Periocular inoculation can occur from the HSV-1 perioral infections so common in children. Herpes zoster represents a reactivation of latent varicella-zoster virus. When it occurs in the dermatomal distribution of the trigeminal nerve, it can cause a keratitis with conjunctivitis.[1]

Adenoviral conjunctivitis may be associated with two distinct clinical syndromes: pharyngoconjunctival fever and epidemic keratoconjunctivitis. Pharyngoconjunctival fever is caused by adenovirus types 3 and 7. It is most commonly spread by person-to-person contact, but has also been reported to be spread through swimming; thus, the infection may be referred to as "swimming pool" conjunctivitis. Adenovirus types 8, 19, and 37 cause epidemic keratoconjunctivitis. This entity is transmitted by direct contact with infected people or contaminated instruments and is often iatrogenic. Attention to frequent hand washing prevents transmission.[26]

Infectious neonatal conjunctivitis is caused by *Neisseria gonorrhoeae, Chlamydia trachomatis,* and, less commonly, HSV. The infant is infected at birth during passage through the birth canal. The incubation period for gonococcal conjunctivitis (ophthalmia neonatorum) is 2 to 7 days. Neonatal prophylaxis for ophthalmia neonatorum with a 1% silver nitrate solution, 0.5% erythromycin ophthalmic ointment, or 1% tetracycline ophthalmic ointment is recommended universally in the United States. Only silver nitrate solution is effective in prevention of infection by a penicillinase-producing gonococcus. Neonatal chlamydial conjunctivitis develops a few days to several weeks after birth. Fifty percent of infants born to infected women acquire *C. trachomatis,* and, of those, 25% to 50% develop conjunctivitis. Neonatal ophthalmic prophylaxis is not effective in the prevention of chlamydial conjunctivitis. Neonatal HSV infection occurs in one per 3,000 to one per 20,000 live births. The infant is most at risk if the mother has a primary infection at the time of delivery. The risk to an infant born to a mother with a recurrent infection is much lower. Neonatal infections are of three types: generalized infection, localized central nervous system (CNS) infection, or disease localized to the skin, eye, and mouth (SEM).[1]

The most common cause of allergic conjunctivitis in children is seasonal rhinoconjunctivitis. The symptoms are caused by a localized IgE-mediated hypersensitivity reaction to airborne allergens, with resultant release of histamine and other products from mast cells. Pollens and grasses are the most common allergens. In up to 25% of children, ocular findings may be the sole manifestation. The findings are caused by the release of products from mast cells, predominantly histamine.[4,21]

Chemical conjunctivitis is most often caused by ocular medications. Neomycin has the greatest incidence of contact sensitivity. Silver nitrate is a common cause in the neonate. Accidental environmental exposure to a toxin, such as cleaning agents, is also common.

CLINICAL PRESENTATION

The clinical presentation, while not completely specific, may help the clinician determine the etiology of conjunctivitis. Bacterial conjunctivitis is more often unilateral and occurs predominantly in infants and preschool-aged children. There is usually a mucopurulent exudate, and the palpebral and bulbar conjunctivae are erythematous but not hemorrhagic. Eyelid erythema and swelling may be present, and the child may be febrile. A neonate with ophthalmia neonatorum may appear toxic, with a copious purulent discharge. *C. trachomatis* infection causes a beefy red conjunctiva.[1]

Viral conjunctivitis, on the other hand, is often bilateral and occurs in school-aged children. A mucopurulent discharge may be present, but the presence of a conjunctival inflammatory membrane is diagnostic. The discharge is often copious and clear. Marked periorbital edema can be present, leading to a false diagnosis of periorbital cellulitis.[20] Pharyngoconjunctival fever is manifested by pharyngitis, fever to 40°C (104°F), and conjunctivitis. Conjunctival findings may persist from 4 days to 2 weeks. Epidemic keratoconjunctivitis lacks upper respiratory symptoms and fever. Corneal involvement predominates, with an early keratitis that causes photophobia and a foreign-body sensation. Subepithelial opacities develop 7 to 10 days after onset, which may cause a temporary mild decrease in visual acuity. These opacities resolve without scarring of the cornea.[26]

HSV infection of the eye is of the SEM type; however, skin and mouth lesions may not be present at the time of presentation. The conjunctiva is erythematous, and keratitis may be present. Characteristic dendritic keratitis may be seen with fluorescein staining for both varicella-zoster virus and herpes simplex virus. Varicella-zoster infection of the first division of the trigeminal nerve affects the eye. There may be characteristic vesicular lesions on the forehead and eyelid. The conjunctivae are usually injected. Herpes zoster is a unilateral infection, and, often, periorbital pain precedes the appearance of the vesicles.[1]

Allergic conjunctivitis is bilateral, with variable conjunctival injection and watery eye discharge. Other allergic symptoms, such as boggy nasal turbinates, watery nasal discharge, and allergic shiners (dark circles around the eye), may or may not be present.

Chemical conjunctivitis presents with conjunctival injection and, often, a burning sensation.

DIFFERENTIAL DIAGNOSIS

The differential diagnosis of the red eye includes conjunctivitis, periorbital cellulitis, corneal abrasion, uveitis, iritis, Kawasaki syndrome, glaucoma, dry-eye syndromes, blepharitis, dacryocystitis and Parinaud oculoglandular syndrome (a syndrome of cat scratch disease involving the conjunctiva and ipsilateral preauricular lymph node).

EMERGENCY DEPARTMENT EVALUATION

The ED evaluation of the red eye begins with a detailed history and physical, including a complete age-appropriate eye examination. A slit-lamp examination in an older child who is cooperative is helpful. Outside of the neonatal period, conjunctival cultures are rarely obtained. Fluorescein staining should be considered, especially with severe photophobia or corneal changes.

All young infants in whom the diagnosis of ophthalmia neonatorum or SEM secondary to HSV is being considered require a full evaluation for disseminated disease. In addition to blood and cerebrospinal fluid (CSF) studies (complete blood count, chemistries, blood culture, CSF culture for bacteria and viruses, glucose, protein, Gram stain), conjunctival cultures for bacteria and viruses should be obtained. In suspected gonococcal infection, a Gram stain of the eye is helpful in early confirmation of the diagnosis.[26] A Tzanck preparation may be helpful in herpetic infections. A conjunctival scraping is more sensitive than swab cultures.[26] When a chlamydial infection is suspected, cultures or specimens for rapid antigen testing of the conjunctiva and nasopharynx should be obtained.[1] A chemical conjunctivitis is suggested when a history of ocular exposure to a toxin or ophthalmic medication is elucidated in the presence of conjunctival injection.

EMERGENCY DEPARTMENT MANAGEMENT

The management of conjunctivitis is dependent on the suspected etiology and the age of the child. Treatment ranges from supportive care to hospital admission for parenteral antibiotics. Bacterial conjunctivitis is most frequently treated with topical ophthalmic antibiotics. Trimethoprim–polymyxin B, gentamicin sulfate, and sodium sulfacetamide all have high rates of cure.[25] Trimethoprim–polymyxin B eradicates *H. influenzae* most effectively.[24] The topical agent is administered every 4 hours, while the patient is awake, for 5 to 7 days.

In the instance of conjunctivitis–otitis syndrome, oral therapy with an appropriate antibiotic to treat *H. influenzae,* such as amoxicillin–clavulanate, will cure both the otitis and the conjunctivitis. Oral therapy for conjunctivitis without otitis has been shown to decrease the occurrence of otitis in the ensuing 2 weeks.[24] Further data are needed to substantiate the efficacy of oral treatment of conjunctivitis.

Table 270.2 lists the etiologies of neonatal conjunctivitis with the indicated treatment.

Localized herpesvirus infections involving the eye should be treated with intravenous acyclovir 30 mg/kg/d in three divided doses for children less than 1 year of age, and, for older children, 1500 $mg/m^2/d$ in three divided doses for 7 to 10 days. Higher dosing is used for disseminated or CNS disease.[1]

Adenoviral conjunctivitis is treated with supportive therapy. To prevent the spread of infection to other family members, the family should be counseled to wash hands frequently and to avoid sharing wash cloths. The infected child should be kept away from immunocompromised persons and neonates, because this group is at increased risk for severe disease.

The treatment of allergic conjunctivitis is avoidance of the allergen and topical therapy with antihistamines, vasoconstrictors, or nonsteroidal antiinflammatory agents.[21] Cool compresses may be soothing.

DISPOSITION

Bacterial conjunctivitis outside of the neonatal period is an outpatient disease. Follow-up with a primary care provider should be recommended.

If large corneal defects or defects involving the visual axis are detected, emergent ophthalmologic evaluation by a provider skilled in pediatric ophthalmology is necessary. All cases of suspected ophthalmia neonatorum, HSV, and varicella-zoster ophthalmic infection should be referred to a pediatric ophthalmologist emergently. The risk for ocular damage and permanent visual loss is high.

Neonatal and herpetic conjunctivitis requires inpatient therapy at a facility well versed in pediatric care and with pediatric ophthalmologic resources. When chlamydial infection is suspected, consultation with a pediatrician is helpful.

TABLE 270.2. Etiology of Neonatal Conjunctivitis and Therapy

Organism	Medications	Other Therapy
N. gonorrhea	Ceftriaxone 25–50 mg/kg i.v. or i.m., not to exceed 125 mg; given once *or* Cefotaxime 100 mg/kg i.v. or i.m.	Frequent eye irrigation with saline
C. trachomatis	Erythromycin 50 mg/kg/d divided q.i.d. PO for 14 d	
Herpes simplex virus	Acyclovir 30–60 mg/kg/d i.v. divided q8h Duration: 14 to 21 d *and* 1% to 2% trifluridine, 1% iododeoxyuridine, or 3% vidarabine, applied topically	Ophthalmologic consultation

Data from American Academy of Pediatrics.[1]

COMMON PITFALLS

- Failure to recognize herpetic infection of the eye. Delay in treatment can often lead to visual loss, CNS disease, or systemic disease.
- Failure to treat bacterial conjunctivitis results in delayed cure and progression of disease.
- Failure to recognize otitis in association with conjunctivitis

THE SWOLLEN EYE

Children with a swollen, red eye represent a relatively common problem in the ED. Most children with periorbital (PO) or orbital cellulitis (OC) are under the age of 5, with very few older than 10 years of age. The pathogenesis of PO/OC may occur via three different routes. The skin barrier near the eye may be broken by local trauma, an insect sting, or the lesions of varicella or herpes zoster, with local spread of infected material to the periorbital tissues. There may be contiguous spread to the orbital tissues from infected frontal, ethmoidal, or maxillary sinuses. Alternatively, there may be seeding of periorbital tissues from bacteremia.[18]

A bacterial pathogen is identified in only up to 30% of cases, with most of these, in the past, identified by blood culture. Prior to the introduction of the *H. influenzae* vaccine (HIB), 50% of the cultures were positive for *H. influenzae*. Widespread usage of the vaccine has resulted in a 90% decrease in the incidence of *H. influenzae*-related PO/OC.[3,8] The most common organisms, currently, are *S. aureus*, group A *Streptococcus* species, and *S. pneumoniae*. *S. aureus* and group A *Streptococcus* are more likely to be involved when there is a history of local trauma or a wound. *S. pneumoniae* is more likely in the younger child with a history of an upper respiratory infection and sinusitis. Anaerobic bacteria and *M. catarrhalis* should be considered in the older child with documented sinusitis.[8] *H. influenzae* should still be considered in the child who has not received, or not completed, the primary series of HIB vaccination (2, 4, 6 months).[22]

Periorbital cellulitis is defined as an inflammatory or infectious process superficial to the orbital septum. If untreated, it has the potential to spread via blood vessels to the CNS or to penetrate the orbital septum and result in OC. *Orbital cellulitis* is thus defined as inflammation or infection deep to the orbital septum. OC may involve the ocular structures, causing abscess formation and loss of vision. It may also spread to the CNS via the cavernous sinus, causing cavernous sinus thrombosis or meningitis.

CLINICAL PRESENTATION

The thin skin and loose connective tissue of the eyelid allow for easy and rapid accumulation of fluid. A child with PO/OC may often present within hours of onset with a red and swollen eyelid. Ninety-five percent of cases are unilateral, with the actual color of the lid described as violaceous or purple. Seventy-five percent of children are febrile. Two-thirds will have an upper respiratory infection; one-third, a history of minor trauma; one-fourth, an acute otitis media; and one-fifth, an associated conjunctivitis.[18] In PO, palpation of the periorbital tissues will elicit tenderness, but the eye itself should move freely and painlessly. In advanced OC, the eye may be proptotic and extremely painful to voluntary movement of the extraocular muscles, and visual acuity may be reduced. There may be diplopia on upward gaze. The child may appear "toxic" or irritable, with early meningeal signs.

DIFFERENTIAL DIAGNOSIS

The most common differential diagnoses to consider are local allergic reactions, blunt trauma, swelling secondary to an underlying sinusitis, and bulbar or retrobulbar neoplasms. The history of an insect bite, the presence of loose swelling and itching, and the absence of systemic symptoms should aid in the diagnosis of a local allergic reaction. Likewise, the history of recent trauma to the area surrounding the eye, the presence of a "shiner," or the dissection of hematoma downward from a frontal contusion should be obtainable on careful questioning of the parent and child. Sinusitis is thought to cause swelling by obstruction of venous drainage from the overlying skin. The swelling is usually painless and not erythematous, but it sometimes may be difficult to distinguish from true PO. The time course for neoplasms of the lids and orbit is usually much more insidious. While retrobulbar tumors may cause proptosis and decreased vision, the lid swelling and periorbital cellulitis are usually not present.

EMERGENCY DEPARTMENT EVALUATION

The ED evaluation begins with a careful history and physical. The rapidity of onset; the history of trauma, insect bite, or skin lesions; the presence of an upper respiratory infection or sinusitis; and immunization status, particularly HIB, must be ascertained. The examination of the eye must include not only gentle palpation of the periorbital area, but also an assessment of whether the globe is proptotic, the function of the extraocular muscles, and whether there is any pain with movement of the eye. Visual acuity must be assessed, if necessary, with the use of lid retractors.

Laboratory studies are of limited value, although a white blood cell count greater than 15,000 may suggest bacteremia. Cultures of any wounds near the eye should be obtained; however. conjunctival or nasopharyngeal swabs are generally not helpful.[18] Blood cultures have been reported positive in up to 30% of children; however 70% to 80% of these were *H. influenzae* in the prevaccine era.[3,8,22] It seems likely that blood cultures will identify fewer and fewer organisms. In the pre-HIB era, lumbar puncture (LP) was considered almost mandatory in the young child because of the invasive and virulent character of *H. influenzae* bacteremia. Currently, most authors reserve LP for children under 1 year of age (increased risk of *S. pneumoniae* bacteremia),[10] those who are "toxic" or irritable, or those who have not yet received or completed the HIB vaccination series.

Computerized tomography (CT) of the orbit may be useful in delineating sinusitis, orbital involvement, proptosis, abscess, or foreign body. It should be reserved for the child who presents with proptosis, pain on extraocular movement, decreased visual acuity, or inability to conduct a full eye examination.[10]

EMERGENCY DEPARTMENT MANAGEMENT

After appropriate cultures have been obtained, an intravenous line should be started and antimicrobial therapy initiated with a third-generation cephalosporin:

Ceftriaxone 50 to 75 mg/kg intramuscularly or intravenously q24h, *or*
Cefotaxime 50 mg/kg per dose intravenously q6h

plus Clindamycin 10 mg/kg per dose q8h, or nafcillin 100 to 200 mg/kg/d q6 h.[18]

DISPOSITION

Immediate consultation with an ophthalmologist should be undertaken if there are any physical findings suggestive of orbital involvement (proptosis, pain on eye movement, or decreased visual acuity), if there is difficulty obtaining an adequate eye examination, or if there has been failure to respond to parenteral antimicrobial therapy. Some of these children may be found to have an abscess that will require emergent surgical evacuation.

All children with OC and most children with PO should be admitted to the hospital. The inpatient unit should have the capability to care for children and have an ophthalmologist available for urgent consultation. Recently, certain selected children with PO have been managed on an outpatient basis. There are several criteria that need to be met before the child can be discharged: There must be *no* orbital involvement (proptosis, opthalmoplegia, decreased visual acuity), the child should be well-appearing, and there should be no purulent wound near the eye. Furthermore, the support system should be such that, not only are the parents willing and able to take the child home, but also willing and able to return the child immediately should there be a worsening in the child's condition. If *all* of these criteria are met and appropriate cultures are taken, an initial dose of ceftriaxone 50 mg/kg intramuscularly or intravenously (not to exceed 1 g) is given, followed by ampicillin–clavulanate 45 mg/kg/d in two divided doses orally for 7 to 10 days.[8] In the penicillin-allergic child, give azithromycin 12 mg/kg (max, 500 mg/d) once a day for 5 days.[13] The choice of outpatient antibiotics should reflect *S. pneumoniae* and group A *Streptococcus* resistance within the community. The child should be brought back for daily examinations to document and follow resolution, until blood cultures are negative (usually 48 hours).[18,22]

COMMON PITFALLS

- Failure to conduct a thorough eye examination, thus missing signs of orbital involvement
- Failure to perform an LP in a child under 12 months of age or in a child with early meningeal signs or irritability, thereby missing CNS involvement
- Failure to consult an ophthalmologist early in cases of orbital involvement, which could result in a poor outcome, possible visual impairment, or loss of the eye
- Discharging a child who does not meet all of the criteria for outpatient management, resulting in a poor outcome from OC or abscess or spread to the CNS

ABNORMAL VISION

Children with complaints related to vision rarely present to the ED. When they do, the visit is prompted by their own complaints of abnormal vision or complaints from their parents, teachers, or school nurses. Occasionally, the ED physician, during the course of an examination, discovers a particular finding that necessitates urgent ophthalmologic referral. The complaints and etiologies for visual loss can vary greatly with the age of the child.

Cataracts, glaucoma, intraocular tumors, optic nerve problems, and nystagmus may all present in infancy. The incidence of congenital cataracts is one to four of 10,000 live births in industrialized countries and five to 15 of 10,000 births in the developing world. Cataracts usually present in the newborn nursery.[11] However, with home births and the easy movement of populations between developing countries and the industrialized world, it is conceivable that the first presentation may be in the ED. Cataracts are strongly associated with several chromosomal abnormalities (trisomy 13, 18, 21), perinatal infections (rubella, toxoplasmosis, or varicella-zoster), and inborn errors of metabolism.[11] Infantile glaucoma has an incidence of less than one in 10,000 live births. The sclera of an infant is more elastic than that of an older child. Increased intraocular pressure results in a gradual expansion of the globe. While the predisposition is congenital, the term *infantile* is used to express the variability in the time of onset from birth to clinically apparent disease.[16]

Retinoblastoma is the most common intraocular malignancy. The average age of presentation is 18 months, with most occurring prior to 3 years of age. One-third of tumors are bilateral and present earlier than unilateral tumors. The underlying genetic defect is felt to be associated with changes to one of the genes on chromosome 13.[23]

Nystagmus in childhood may be congenital or acquired. The etiologies of congenital nystagmus are essentially the same as those that cause visual impairment in infancy. Nystagmus that develops in the older child is usually either drug-induced or associated with severe visual loss or intracranial neoplasm.[19]

By far, the most common complaint in the toddler and preschool-age child that is seen in the primary care office is strabismus, or ocular malalignment. The prevention of amblyopia (abnormal vision in an anatomically normal eye) is the major visual concern in this age group. If not detected and treated appropriately, the child may be left with a functionally blind eye.[12,16]

Visual loss in childhood may result from compression of the optic nerve by tumor, inflammation of the optic nerve, and heredodegenerative conditions. Ten percent of rhabdomyosarcomas occur in the eye, arising from the intraocular muscles. The peak incidence is at age 8, with 75% occurring before age 10.[16] Optic neuritis in the child is felt to be a postviral autoimmune phenomenon. The most common preceding infections are measles, mumps, varicella, pertussis, mononucleosis, and postimmunization. Unlike in young adults, there is not a strong association with multiple sclerosis.[19]

Optic gliomas and craniopharyngiomas are the two most common tumors that compress the optic nerve. Optic gliomas are intrinsic tumors of the optic nerve. They usually occur between 4 and 8 years of age. There is a strong association with neurofibromatosis. Craniopharyngiomas are the third most common brain tumor of childhood, representing 10% of all tumors in childhood. They arise from the embryonic rests of Rathke's pouch near the sella turcica. Craniopharyngiomas affect visual acuity by compressing the optic chiasm or the optic nerve.[19]

CLINICAL PRESENTATION

The clinical presentation of visual loss varies with age and ability to express oneself. The infant may be brought to the ED because the parents have noted unilateral swelling of the globe or haziness of the cornea. The parents may complain that the 2- to 3-month-old infant does not seem able to fix on and follow objects. There may be no complaints at all, and the physician may discover one of these findings or note an abnormal red reflex or the presence of nystagmus.

The parents of a preverbal child may bring him or her to the ED because of perceived strabismus or a persistent head tilt. Intraocular tumors may present as decreasing visual acuity, leukocoria (absent red reflex), strabismus, or gradually increasing proptosis and corneal edema.[12] Rhabdomyosarcoma may present explosively, with rapid development of proptosis and decreased visual acuity.[23] Craniopharyngiomas may present with advanced visual defects, with or without headache, and sometimes with an unusual vertical "see-saw" nystagmus.[19] By contrast, optic neuritis presents with sudden, severe visual loss, often bilateral. There may be a history of an antecedent viral infection.

On examination, there is reduced vision, nonreactive pupils, and swollen optic nerves. Hemorrhages and exudates may be seen on the optic disc.[19] For a general differential diagnosis, refer to Table 270.3.

EMERGENCY DEPARTMENT EVALUATION

A complete history is very important to help narrow the differential diagnosis. The second most important step is a methodic and complete, age-appropriate eye examination. When a tumor is suspected, neuroimaging, beginning with a CT scan, is imperative. Particularly, any finding of proptosis, with or without decreased vision, necessitates an urgent CT scan. The evaluation of optic neuritis includes magnetic resonance imaging and an LP. The LP usually reveals a monoclonal pleocytosis and mild protein elevation.[19]

EMERGENCY DEPARTMENT MANAGEMENT

The emphasis in management, in the majority of these conditions, should be on recognition of the potential severity of the problem; timely neuroimaging, when applicable; and prompt, sometimes emergent, referral.

Therapy for optic neuritis is based on randomized clinical trials conducted in adults. However, because the use of high-dose steroids is felt to be associated with more rapid visual improvement, most ophthalmologists also offer this treatment to children. Treatment is begun with methylprednisolone 15 to 30 mg/kg/d for 10 to 14 days.[5] This is followed by a slow prednisone taper over 1 to 2 months. Too rapid a taper has been associated with a recurrence of optic neuritis and compounded visual loss.[19]

DISPOSITION

Tumors, glaucoma, cataracts, and optic neuritis often involve urgent admission to the hospital. The facility, as well as the consultant, should be experienced in pediatric eye disorders. Because the growth of some tumors, such as rhabdomyosarcoma, can be explosive, consultation with an experienced ophthalmologist is emergent.

The presence, in an infant, of leukocoria or a swollen anterior chamber requires urgent referral to an ophthalmologist comfortable with the treatment of pediatric cataracts, tumors, or glaucoma. The treatment of these conditions is largely surgical. Because infancy represents a critical period in normal visual maturation, failure to remove the obstruction to clear vision could result in a functionally blind eye.

TABLE 270.3. Differential Diagnosis of Abnormal Vision[a]

Physical Finding	Age	Differential Diagnosis
Leukocoria	Infant	Cataract
	Older child	Retinoblastoma
		Other tumor
Tearing	Neonate	Congenital nasal lacrimal duct obstruction
		Glaucoma
Failure to fix or follow	2–3 mo	Abnormal visual development
		Any cause of decreased vision
		Strabismus
Nystagmus	Infant	Benign
	Older child	Any cause of decreased vision
		Tumor
		Amblyopia
		Drug-induced
Decreased visual acuity (monocular)	Infant	Cataract
		Glaucoma
		Tumor
		Refractive errors
	Child	Amblyopia
		Refractive errors
		Tumor
		Orbital cellulitis
	Older child	Optic neuritis
	Adolescent	Tumor
		Trauma
		Refractive errors
Decreased visual acuity (binocular)	Variable ages	Glaucoma
		Retinoblastoma
		Optic neuritis
		Refractive errors
Proptosis	All ages	Rhabdomyosarcoma
		Other tumor
		Retrobulbar infiltrative process
Strabismus	All ages	Amblyopia
		Muscle palsy
		Large unilateral refractive error

[a] This table is intended as a guide to the more common diagnoses and is not comprehensive.

Because nystagmus can represent a structural lesion as well as amblyopia, referral on a semiurgent basis to an ophthalmologist should be done.

The finding of strabismus in the preverbal or preschool child mandates outpatient referral to an ophthalmologist.

COMMON PITFALLS

- Failure to perform an age-appropriate, complete eye examination
- Failure to refer a time-dependent process urgently to an appropriate ophthalmologist

CORNEAL ABRASION IN INFANTS

Corneal abrasion occurs in infants as a result of known or occult trauma. Infants under 1 year of age are more likely to present without a history of trauma and without any physical findings that point to the eye.[17]

CLINICAL PRESENTATION

Infants may present, as with older children, with eye pain, tearing, photophobia, blepharospasm, conjunctival injection, eye-rubbing, and lid edema. On the other hand, they may present with only excessive crying or irritability. The infant may present only with grunting respirations, without any evidence of respiratory compromise.[17]

DIFFERENTIAL DIAGNOSIS

In the infant who presents with injection, tearing, and blepharospasm, the differential diagnosis includes other etiologies of the "red eye." In the infant who presents with crying, irritability, or grunting, the differential needs to include systemic causes, such as respiratory insufficiency, sepsis, and meningitis.

EMERGENCY DEPARTMENT EVALUATION

A history and full eye examination should be done in infants with physical findings pointing to the eye. A corneal abrasion is diagnosed by staining the cornea with fluorescein-impregnated strips and shining a Wood light on the surface of the eye. An abrasion will stand out as a stained defect on the surface of the cornea. Both eyelids should be everted to search for a retained foreign body.

In the infant who presents with excessive crying, irritability, or grunting, a drop of topical anesthetic may be diagnostic as well as therapeutic.[17] The infant may calm down almost immediately.

EMERGENCY DEPARTMENT MANAGEMENT

Treatment of corneal abrasions includes the use of a lubricating antibiotic ointment, such as erythromycin, bacitracin, or Polysporin. Cyclopentolate 1% drops may be used if significant pain or ciliary spasm is present. Patching the affected eye may also be comforting to the infant. Any contact lenses should be removed.

DISPOSITION

Immediate consultation with an ophthalmologist should be sought if penetration past the superficial layers of the cornea is suspected. The abrasion should be followed daily until resolution of symptoms. This can be accomplished by the ED physician or primary care physician. If the abrasion is large or central (involving the visual axis), the infant should be referred to an ophthalmologist for examination within 24 hours.

COMMON PITFALLS

- Failure to recognize a deep abrasion or corneal ulcer, which could result in corneal scarring or deep infection of the eye
- Failure to consider corneal abrasion in the infant with otherwise unexplained crying or irritability

CONGENITAL NASOLACRIMAL DUCT OBSTRUCTION AND DACRYOCYSTITIS

Congenital nasolacrimal duct obstruction (CNLDO) is a common problem of infancy, with 20% of children exhibiting some symptoms within the first year of life.[16] Canalization of the nasolacrimal duct may not be complete at birth. In most of these children, a membranous obstruction is the etiologic factor; however, a nasolacrimal duct cyst may also result in obstruction.[14] Ninety-six percent of infants with CNLDO show spontaneous resolution of the obstruction by the first birthday.[16]

Dacryocystitis, or infection of the nasolacrimal duct, may be acute or chronic. It may occur as a complication of CNLDO or of acquired nasolacrimal duct obstruction (ANLDO). In the neonatal period, dacryocystitis is rare, occurring in less than 2% of infants with CNLDO. However, if a duct cyst is the etiology of the obstruction, the risk of dacryocystitis is greater, with earlier presentation, usually by 2 weeks of age.[14] The causative organisms are most often *S. aureus, S. epidermidis,* and alpha-hemolytic streptococci. *Corynebacterium* diphtheria and Epstein-Barr virus have also been reported.[7] The risk of bacteremia is higher in the neonatal period than in the older infant or child. ANLDO may occur as the result of ethmoidal sinusitis or maxillary fracture through the wall of the nasolacrimal duct.[7]

CLINICAL PRESENTATION

Symptoms of CNLDO may be present at birth or may be delayed for several weeks, until normal tear production develops. Signs include excessive tear lake, tear overflow, or a mucoid discharge that is produced by the lacrimal sac. There may be crusting or stickiness of the eye; however, the conjunctivae are clear, the eye is neither red nor swollen, and fever should not be present. The tearing is often distressing to the parent.[16]

Dacryocystitis is characterized by erythematous and swollen skin over the lacrimal sac and purulent drainage from the punctum. Fever may be present, and periorbital or orbital cellulitis may develop as a complication of dacryocystitis.[7]

DIFFERENTIAL DIAGNOSIS

The differential diagnosis includes corneal abrasion, conjunctivitis of various etiologies, local insect bite, or local trauma with resultant infection.

EMERGENCY DEPARTMENT EVALUATION

A careful history and physical should differentiate CNLDO from dacryocystitis. In the latter case, cultures of any purulent drainage, as well as blood cultures, need to be obtained. A complete blood count may be helpful, a high white blood cell count indicating a higher risk of bacteremia. In the infant who is 1 month old or younger, a full sepsis workup, including LP, should be done.

EMERGENCY DEPARTMENT MANAGEMENT

In dacryocystitis, antibiotics to cover *Staphylococcus* and *Streptococcus* species should be started immediately after cultures are obtained. The choice of particular antibiotics should reflect *Staphylococcus* and *Streptococcus* resistance within each community.

Suggested choices include the following:

Nafcillin 150 mg/kg/d intravenously in four divided doses
Cefuroxime 150 mg/kg/d intravenously in three divided doses

In the penicillin-allergic infant or child, vancomycin can be used.

DISPOSITION

All patients with acute dacryocystitis should be admitted to the hospital, on the service of a pediatrician capable of dealing with the potential complications of sepsis and/or meningitis. Immediate consultation with an ophthalmologist is needed, because early nasolacrimal duct probing is important to the successful treatment of acute dacryocystitis. Because neonatal dacryocystitis is often associated with a nasolacrimal duct cyst, a complete intranasal examination at the time of surgery and marsupialization of any cyst are imperative to prevent recurrence.[14]

The treatment of chronic or "low-grade" dacryocystitis is primarily surgical, with duct probing within several weeks. Systemic antibiotics are not necessary, although some consultants recommend a topical antibiotic ointment such as polymixin B.[7]

Dacryocystitis after facial fracture or sinusitis requires referral to the appropriate specialist; ophthalmology; ear, nose, and throat; or plastics.[7]

Conservative management of CNLDO includes warm-water compresses (to remove the mucoid discharge) and nasolacrimal duct massage. The latter is performed by occluding the common canaliculus with the index finger and then stroking firmly downward. This maneuver increases the hydrostatic pressure in the nasolacrimal sac, with the ultimate goal of overcoming the membranous obstruction. The massage should be repeated five to ten times, four to six times a day. Erythromycin ophthalmic ointment applied four times a day is recommended; however, its efficacy in speeding recovery has not been proved. Referral to an ophthalmologist is recommended for those cases that do not resolve with conservative management. Probing will cure 90% of these infants.[7]

COMMON PITFALLS

- Failure to consider bacteremia, sepsis, or meningitis in the neonate or young infant
- Failure to consult an ophthalmologist early in cases of acute dacryocystitis

PARASITIC INFESTATION OF THE EYELASHES

Lice infestation of the eyelashes is caused by the genus *Phthirus*, otherwise known as the crab or pubic louse. Transmission may occur via the hand from infestation in the genital area, but it may also occur from contaminated towels and bedding. Infants may become infected as a result of close contact with an infested caretaker.

The adult lice feed on the host's blood, depositing their excrement at the base of the lashes. The females lay eggs (nits), which are firmly cemented in groups to the lashes. Exposure to the lice saliva and feces results in a dermal hypersensitivity reaction, causing severe pruritus. The intense desire to scratch often results in excoriations of the eyelids and, often, secondary bacterial infections.

CLINICAL PRESENTATION

Patients present with a history of itching and irritation of the eyes and eyelids, often of several weeks' duration. The lids may appear reddened, with a brownish crust at the base of the lashes. Close observation may reveal adult lice as well as clusters of nits on the upper and lower lashes. The nits appear as small, pearly, oval structures cemented to the base of the lashes. The palpebral conjunctiva may be red and inflamed. The cornea is rarely involved. There may be preauricular node swelling, reflecting secondary bacterial involvement.[9]

DIFFERENTIAL DIAGNOSIS

Bacterial, viral, or allergic conjunctivitis represents the main differential diagnoses. Identification of adult lice and nits should effectively rule these out.

EMERGENCY DEPARTMENT EVALUATION

Slit-lamp examination should reveal, in addition to adult lice and nits, a brownish granular crust at the bases of the lashes (lice feces). Blue spots (maculae ceruleae) on the lid margins are characteristic of lice infestation and represent bite marks. A full eye examination, including fluorescein staining of the cornea to rule out concomitant corneal abrasion, should be done.

EMERGENCY DEPARTMENT MANAGEMENT

Eliminating lice infestation involves several management issues: killing adult lice, removing existing nits, and preventing reinfestation. In the cooperative patient, mechanical removal can be accomplished by using a slit-lamp, cotton swabs, and fine-toothed forceps. This needs to be followed by medical treatment aimed at killing the lice when they hatch. Several ophthalmic preparations have been endorsed over the years. The only clearly nontoxic preparation is petroleum jelly, applied to the eyelashes several times a day for 8 days, in order to suffocate the organisms.[9] Yellow mercuric oxide ointment is pediculicidal, but a case of mercury poisoning has been reported in a 4-month-old infant. Physostigmine ointment likewise kills the lice, but it may cause such unwanted side effects as miosis and ciliary spasm. The argon laser has been used to kill lice and nits, but its use requires a cooperative patient as well as a skilled operator.

DISPOSITION

The patient needs to be evaluated for infestation of other body sites, and appropriate therapy instituted. If genital infestation is found, the possibility of sexually transmitted diseases needs to be addressed and treated. In order to prevent reinfestation, the caretaker needs to be educated on the sterilization of bedding, towels, and clothing, as well as the discarding of any cosmetic products used about the eye. Evaluation of potential infestation in the parent, especially in the case of an infant, should also be done.[9]

COMMON PITFALLS

- Failure to entertain the diagnosis of louse infestation in the eyelashes
- Failure to educate the caretaker on the necessary measures needed to prevent reinfestation

SUPERGLUE IN THE EYE

Superglue (cyanoacrylate glue) in the eye usually occurs as the result of an accidental "squirt" while using the glue to repair an object, or by mistaking the bottle for an ophthalmic preparation and directly instilling glue in the eye. Cyanoacrylates form strong bonds between opposing surfaces within seconds. In the eye, they may form a layer covering the conjunctival and corneal surfaces, or they may tightly seal the lids and lashes together. They may also cause corneal abrasions, eyelid skin excoriation, and loss of eyelashes.[15]

CLINICAL PRESENTATION

The clinical presentation is usually that of eyelids firmly glued together. If the cyanoacrylate has seeped into the eye, there may be pain, photophobia, tearing, and decreased vision. A film of glue may be adherent to the corneal surface of the eye, or there may be fragments under the lids.

DIFFERENTIAL DIAGNOSIS

Corneal abrasions present with similar symptoms, and may result from glue in the eye.

EMERGENCY DEPARTMENT EVALUATION

When the eyelids are firmly sealed together, the condition of the underlying eye needs to be inferred indirectly from complaints of pain, foreign-body sensation, tearing, and ability to move the globe without pain. As complete an examination as possible should be carried out.

EMERGENCY DEPARTMENT MANAGEMENT

Eyelids that are firmly bonded together are generally allowed to separate on their own, which will occur in 1 to 4 days. Trimming the involved eyelashes may facilitate separation of the lids. If the lashes are not pulled out, they should grow back normally. In the case of glue that is adherent to the cornea, the treatment is the same as for a corneal abrasion, with antibiotic preparations, mydriatic agents, and possible eye patching. Pain medication should be administered as needed.

DISPOSITION

Reexamination in 24 hours is recommended to evaluate for any signs of infection. The appearance of purulent drainage necessitates ophthalmologic consultation and surgical separation of the lids in order to evaluate fully the cornea and the globe. In the case of glue that is adherent to the cornea, follow-up evaluation often reveals spontaneous separation of the glue from the cornea, with a resultant epithelial defect. This corneal abrasion is usually superficial and requires continued therapy with antibiotic drops and mydriatics.[15]

COMMON PITFALLS

- Unnecessary, early surgical separation of the lids, with pulling and subsequent loss of eyelashes
- Application of "home remedies" or chemicals that are potentially harmful to the eye, in an effort to "unbond" the lids

References

1. American Academy of Pediatrics. Chlamydial infections, gonococcal infections, herpes simplex, and varicella zoster. In: Peter G, ed. *1997 Red book: report of the Committee on Infectious Diseases,* 24th ed. Elk Grove Village, IL: American Academy of Pediatrics; 1997:170–174, 212–219, 266–276, 573–585.
2. Bacal DA, Rousta ST, Hertle RW. Why early vision screening matters. *Contemp Pediatr* 1999;16(2):155–156,159–163, 167.
3. Barone SR, Aiuto LT. Periorbital and orbital cellulitis in the *Haemophilus influenzae* vaccine era. *J Pediatr Ophthalmol Strabismus* 1997;34(5):293–236.
4. Bielory L, Wagner RS. Allergic and immunologic pediatric disorders of the eye. *J Investig Allergol Clin Immunol* 1995;5(6):309–317.
5. Brady KM, Brar AS, Lee AG, et al. Optic neuritis in children: clinical features and visual outcome. *J Aapos* 1999;3(2):98–103
6. Broderick P. Pediatric vision screening for the family physician. *Am Fam Physician* 1998;58(3):691–700, 703–704.
7. Campolattaro BN, Lueder GT, Tychsen L. Spectrum of pediatric dacryocystitis: medical and surgical management of 54 cases. *J Pediatr Ophthalmol Strabismus* 1997;34(3):143–153.
8. Donohue SP, Schwartz G. Preseptal and orbital cellulitis in childhood: a changing microbiologic spectrum. *Ophthalmology* 1998;105(10):1902–1906.
9. Dornic DI Ectoparasitic infestation of the eyelashes. *J Am Optom Assoc* 1985;56(9):716–719.
10. Dudin A, Othman A. Acute periorbital swelling: evaluation of management protocol. *Pediatr Emerg Care* 1996;12(1):16–20.
11. Foster A, Gilberr C, Rahi J. Epidemiology of cataract in childhood: a global perspective. *J Cataract Refract Surg* 1997;23[Suppl 1]:601–604.
12. King RA. Common ocular signs and symptoms in childhood. *Pediatr Clin North Am* 1993;40(4):753–766.
13. Langtry HD, Balfour JA. Azithromycin: a review of its use in paediatric infectious diseases. *Drugs* 1998;56(2):273–297.
14. Leuder GT. Neonatal dacryocystitis associated with nasolacrimal duct cysts. *J Pediatr Ophthalmol Strabismus* 1995;32(2):102–106.
15. Maitra AK. Management of complications of cyanoacrylate adhesives. *Br J Clin Pract* 1984;38:284–286.
16. Olitsky SE, Nelson LB. Common ophthalmologic concerns in infants and children. *Pediatr Clin North Am* 1998;45(4):993–1012.
17. Poole SR. Corneal abrasion in infants. *Pediatr Emerg Care* 1995;11(1):25–26.
18. Powell KR. Orbital and periorbital cellulitis. *Pediatr Rev* 1995;16(5):163–167.
19. Repka MX. Common pediatric neuro-ophthalmologic conditions. *Pediatr Clin North Am* 1993;40(4):777–788.
20. Ruttum MS, Ogawa G. Adenovirus conjunctivitis mimics preseptal and orbital cellulitis in young children. *Pediatr Infect Dis J* 1996;15(3):266–267.
21. Sabbah A, Marzetto M. Azelastine eye drops in the treatment of seasonal allergic conjunctivitis or rhino conjunctivitis in young children. *Curr Med Res Opin* 1998;14(3):161–170.
22. Schwartz GR, Wright SW. Changing bacteriology of periorbital cellulitis. *Ann Emerg Med* 1996;28(6):617–620.
23. Shields JA, Shields CL. Ocular tumors in childhood. *Pediatr Clin North Am* 1993;40(4):805–826.
24. Wald ER. Conjunctivitis in infants and children. *Pediatr Infect Dis J* 1997;16[2 Suppl]:S17–S20.
25. Wallace DK, Steinkuller PG. Ocular medications in children. *Clin Pediatr (Phila)* 1998;37(11):645–652.
26. Weiss A. Acute conjunctivitis in childhood. *Curr Probl Pediatr* 1994;24(1):4–11.

CHAPTER 271
Foreign-Body Ingestion

Linda L. Settle

Infants enjoy using their mouths to help them assess new objects. They continue this into the toddler years, when they are mobile and therefore have greater opportunities to find small objects. It is not surprising, then, that the peak years for foreign-body ingestions are the toddler ones.[6] Of the more than 94,023 foreign-body ingestions reported to 66 poison control centers in 1997, 72% occurred in children younger than 6 years of age.[17]

CLINICAL PRESENTATION

When children present with a history of foreign-body ingestion, a choking or gagging episode has usually been witnessed by an adult or has been reported to the parent by an older child. Many of these children are asymptomatic on presentation. The greater diagnostic challenge is the symptomatic child who presents without a positive history. Diagnosis in this case requires awareness of the range of presenting symptoms. In one review of 125 children with foreign-body ingestions, the most frequent complaints were gagging or vomiting, choking, neck and throat pain, foreign-body sensation, and dyspnea.[6] In a review of esophageal foreign bodies, the most common presenting symptoms of the 343 children studied were refusal to eat, salivation, pain and discomfort on swallowing, and vomiting.[19]

In addition to the more common presentations, children with esophageal foreign bodies may present with symptoms referable to the respiratory tract (i.e., stridor, persistent cough, wheezing, and chronic pneumonia).

DIFFERENTIAL DIAGNOSIS

When there is a positive history for ingestion, localizing the foreign body within the gastrointestinal tract is important, even if the child is asymptomatic.[2] One study showed that 17% of asymptomatic children with a history of coin ingestion were found to have coins in the esophagus.[14] Delay in removal of esophageal foreign bodies may result in obstruction, because an inflammatory reaction and edema develop, with the resultant possibility of aspiration; perforation or erosion through the esophagus; or formation of a tracheoesophageal fistula or tracheoaortic fistula.

Esophageal foreign bodies may present very much like airway foreign bodies. Again, it is important to remember that stridor, cough, or wheezing may represent an esophageal foreign body.[3,22]

EMERGENCY DEPARTMENT EVALUATION

When there is a clinical suspicion of ingested foreign body, radiographic evaluation should include a lateral soft-tissue view of the neck in addition to an anteroposterior view, as well as films of the chest and abdomen. Foreign bodies are often missed when only an anteroposterior view is ordered. Lateral views are also necessary to demonstrate multiple coins in rouleau. Nonradiopaque items can usually be demonstrated with contrast.

There is some controversy about obtaining x-rays on asymptomatic children with a history of coin ingestion, even though there are reports of esophageal placement in asymptomatic children, as previously noted. With a clear history for coin or similar object ingestion, an alternative way to locate the coin is with a metal detector.[10] If it can be located clearly below the diaphragm, an x-ray could be deferred. If it can be located low in the chest, where it is most likely at the lower esophageal sphincter, an observation period and repeat metal detector scan would be indicated, as objects at this location are likely to pass into the stomach. If the metal detector places the coin or other round object high in the chest, an x-ray is indicated.[1,24]

EMERGENCY DEPARTMENT MANAGEMENT

Most foreign bodies pass through the digestive tract without problems. Although most objects lodged in the esophagus require immediate removal because of the reasons listed earlier, a brief observation period (12 to 24 hours) has been recommended by some clinicians for asymptomatic patients with coins in the esophagus, particularly at the lower esophageal sphincter.[9,20] Once objects have been demonstrated to have passed beyond the esophagus, however, they rarely represent a hazard to the patient: 95% pass without incident.[12] Objects can enter a Meckel's diverticulum or appendix and cause obstruction; therefore, a repeat x-ray should be done in a week if the object has not passed. Instructions are given to the parents to return the child for repeat x-ray if any abdominal symptoms are noted. Sharp objects pose an increased risk for perforation, and elongated objects sometimes cannot traverse the C loop of the duodenum. For such objects, closer follow-up is needed to monitor development of signs of potential obstruction or peritonitis. A repeat x-ray is mandatory if the object has not passed in a few days.

Endoscopic removal is indicated for objects retained in the stomach or rectum. Operative removal is indicated if the object remains at the same site in the duodenum or small intestine longer than 7 days or if symptoms develop. Enemas are usually successful at dislodging retained colonic foreign bodies.[12]

The amount of time it takes for a foreign body to pass through the entire gastrointestinal tract varies widely. In one study, 85% had passed within 72 hours and 99.9% within 7 days.[17]

Removal of esophageal foreign bodies traditionally has been done by using a rigid endoscope. Recently, use of the flexible scope has been reported and may be an alternative for select patients when done by those skilled in its use with children.[4] In the 1960s, reports described removal of blunt objects by using a Foley catheter under fluoroscopy.[5,23] This method avoids the use of general anesthesia, which is necessary for rigid endoscopy. The largest report of experience with this method in children describes successful removal of foreign bodies in 322 of 337 patients, without complications.[13] This procedure should be done only by someone skilled in management of the pediatric airway and with the necessary equipment available. Some recommend that an individual be present who can use the rigid endoscope, if that becomes necessary.[15] This method should be used only with recent ingestions of blunt, nonorganic radiopaque objects and in patients with a normal esophagus. At some centers, esophageal bougienage is used for coin ingestions, with low complication rates, when strict selection criteria are used.[8,11] With both Foley catheter removal and esophageal bougienage advancement into stomach, there is no direct visualization of the esophagus. Therefore, there are the risks of missing a second radiolucent object and intrinsic disease.

Disk batteries lodged in the esophagus pose a high risk for

serious injury to the patient. However, a review of 2,382 battery ingestions, including 2,320 button cells and 62 cylindrical cells, showed that most cases follow a benign course.[16] There were no deaths, and only two cases demonstrated a major effect (both of these represented lodgement in the esophagus). All patients with a history of battery ingestion should have a radiograph done to determine the battery's location. If it is lodged in the esophagus, immediate removal is indicated. Burns have occurred at 4 hours and perforation at 6 hours after ingestion of a battery.[7,21,25] If the battery is not in the esophagus and is less than 15 mm in diameter, stools should be checked, and radiography considered at 1 week if the battery does not pass. Earlier evaluation would be indicated by abdominal pain with tenderness or hematochezia.

If the battery is greater than 15 mm in diameter (3% of cases), radiography in 48 hours is recommended because of delayed transit through the stomach for this size battery in children younger than 6 years old. Endoscopic removal is recommended if the battery is still present in the stomach at 48 hours.

Mercuric oxide batteries (usually 15.6 mm) have a greater likelihood of splitting. Mercury (blood or urine) levels should be obtained only if splitting or radiopaque droplets are noted. Elevated mercury levels and mercury poisoning are rare.

Ipecac is contraindicated with battery ingestions. One study suggests that cimetidine and metoclopramide may have a protective effect against tissue injury when there is gastric retention of batteries.[15]

For objects with possible lead content, such as bullets, shot, fishing sinkers, and curtain weights, a baseline lead level and close follow-up are indicated. A rising level indicates the need for medical and surgical treatment.[18]

DISPOSITION

Children with retained esophageal foreign bodies should be referred to a physician that is skilled in the removal of foreign bodies in children. Foreign bodies beyond the gastroesophageal junction may be observed on an outpatient basis, with follow-up to include x-ray if the object is elongated, sharp, or a disk battery. Forty-eight-hour follow-up radiographs are recommended for disk batteries lodged in the stomach that are greater than 15 mm in diameter.[13]

COMMON PITFALLS

- Failure to recognize the child with an esophageal foreign body who presents with *respiratory* symptoms
- Failure to obtain lateral radiographic views, which may result in failure to visualize opaque foreign bodies

References

1. Arena L. Use of a metal detector to identify ingested metallic foreign bodies. *AJR* 1990;155:803.
2. Bailey P. Pediatric esophageal foreign body with minimal symptomatology. *Ann Emerg Med* 1983;12:452.
3. Beer S, Avidan G, Vivre E, et al. A foreign body in the oesophagus as a cause of respiratory distress. *Pediatr Radiol* 1982;12:41.
4. Bendig DW. Removal of blunt esophageal foreign bodies by flexible endoscopy without general anesthesia. *Am J Dis Child* 1986;140:789.
5. Bigler FC. The use of a Foley catheter for removal of blunt foreign bodies from the esophagus. *J Thorac Cardiovasc Surg* 1966;51:751.
6. Binder L, Anderson WA. Pediatric gastrointestinal foreign body ingestions. *Ann Emerg Med* 1984;13:112.
7. Blatnik BS, Toohill RJ, Lehman RH. Fatal complications from an alkaline battery foreign body in the esophagus. *Ann Otol Rhinol Laryngol* 1977;86:611.
8. Caravati EM, Bennett DL, McElwee NE. Pediatric coin ingestion: a prospective study on the utility of routine roentgenograms. *Am J Dis Child* 1989;143:549.
9. Cohen SR. Unusual presentations and problems created by mismanagement of foreign bodies in the aerodigestive tract of the pediatric patient. *Ann Otol Rhinol Laryngol* 1981;90:316.
10. Conners GP, Chamberlain JM, Weiner PR. Pediatric coin ingestion: a home-based survey. *Am J Emerg Med* 1995;13:638.
11. Emslander HC. Efficacy of esophageal bougienage by emergency physicians in pediatric coin ingestion. *Ann Emerg Med* 1996;27:726.
12. Graff DB. Foreign bodies and bezoars. In: Welch KJ, Randolph JG, Ravitch MM, et al., eds. *Pediatric surgery*, 4th ed. Chicago: Year Book Medical, 1986.
13. Harned RK, Strain JD, Hay TC, et al. Esophageal foreign bodies: safety and efficacy of Foley catheter extraction of coins. *AJR* 1997;168:443.
14. Hodge D, Tecklenburg F, Fleisher G. Coin ingestion: does every child need a radiograph? *Ann Emerg Med* 1985;14:443.
15. Korock M. No-confidence vote on catheter removal of foreign bodies. *JAMA* 1982;247:3304.
16. Litovitz TL, Schmitz BF. Ingestions of cylindrical and button batteries: an analysis of 2382 cases. *Pediatrics* 1992;89:747.
17. Litovitz TL, et al. 1997 Annual report of the American Association of Poison Control Centers' Toxic Exposure Surveillance System. *Am J Emerg Med* 1998;Sept:443.
18. Mowad E. Management of lead poisoning from ingested fishing sinkers. *Arch Pediatr Adolesc Med* 1998;152:485.
19. Nandy P, Ong GB. Foreign body in the oesophagus: review of 2394 cases. *Br J Surg* 1978;65:5.
20. Schunk JE, Corneli H, Bolte R. Pediatric coin ingestion: a prospective study of coin location and symptoms. *Am J Dis Child* 1989;143:546.
21. Shabino CL, Feinberg AN. Esophageal perforation secondary to alkaline battery ingestion. *J Am Coll Emerg Phys* 1979;8:360.
22. Smith PC, Swischuk LE, Fagan CJ. An elusive and often unsuspected cause of stridor or pneumonia (the esophageal foreign body). *AJR* 1974;122:80.
23. Symbas PN. Indirect method of extraction of foreign body from the esophagus. *Ann Surg* 1968;167:78.
24. Tidey B. The use of a metal detector to locate ingested metallic foreign bodies in children. *J Accid Emerg Med* 1996;13:341.
25. Votteler TP, Nash JC, Rutledge JC. The hazard of ingested alkaline disk batteries in children. *JAMA* 1983;249:2504.

CHAPTER 272
Glomerulonephritis and the Nephrotic Syndrome

Asad Tolaymat and Anne Schaefer

ACUTE GLOMERULONEPHRITIS

Glomerulonephritis is a term that is generally reserved for a variety of renal diseases in which proliferation and inflammation of the glomerulus occurs. Poststreptococcal acute glomerulonephritis (PSAGN) is the most common form of glomerulonephritis seen in children in the United States.[8] It is rare in children younger than 3 years of age; the mean age at onset is 6 to 7 years. The true incidence is unknown, because many cases are subclinical.

PSAGN is known to follow infections of the skin or upper respiratory tract with certain nephrogenic strains of group A β-hemolytic streptococci. PSAGN is associated with pharyngitis more often during the winter months and with pyoderma more often during the summer. Pyoderma-related AGN is typically seen more in the southern regions of the United States and may account for as many as 60% to 70% of the cases.[15] Characteristically, there is a latent period between the onset of the streptococcal infection and the onset of nephritis (8 to 14 days for pharyngitis and 14 to 21 days for skin infection).[3] PSAGN can occur as sporadic cases or in well-recognized epidemics.

Most AGN is immunologically mediated. In PSAGN, evidence suggests that immune complexes formed with streptococcal antigens localize on the glomerular capillary wall, activate the complement system, then initiate a proliferative and inflammatory response.[18]

CLINICAL PRESENTATION

The intensity of the disease varies, as does the clinical presentation, but many patients are not markedly ill. Hematuria and edema are the most common complaints. Gross hematuria (tea-colored urine) has been reported in 70% of hospitalized patients, and microscopic hematuria is present in virtually all children with the disease.[18] Characteristically, the edema in PSAGN is dependent, and therefore shifting in nature. The initiating streptococcal infection usually has resolved by the time of the illness presentation, although impetigo may still be present. Table 272.1 lists the clinical manifestations in patients with PSAGN in order of frequency.[10] A variety of laboratory and radiographic abnormalities are observed in these patients.[8] Table 272.2 summarizes some of these abnormalities.

DIFFERENTIAL DIAGNOSIS

Entities that may mimic the presentation of postinfectious glomerulonephritis are listed in Table 272.3, with some differentiating features. It is impossible to make a final causal diagnosis in the emergency department. It is important, however, to recognize that the patient has nephritis and to be aware of possible life-threatening complications, such as hypertension and hyperkalemia.

EMERGENCY DEPARTMENT EVALUATION

Many patients have no symptoms, and their disease is discovered only by examination of the urine. At the other extreme is the child with severe disease manifested by edema, hypertension, oliguria, and azotemia. The history should include questions about previous illnesses and medications. It is important to obtain a full set of vital signs. The unstable patient should be placed on a cardiac monitor. The glomerular filtration rate is usually reduced, and physical examination may reveal signs of circulatory overload. Periorbital edema is a common finding. Laboratory abnormalities vary with the severity of the disease.

Hematuria is the most consistent urinary abnormality, but the urinalysis can be normal.[15] The sediment reveals red blood cell casts. Pyuria and hyaline granular casts are common. Proteinuria may be present but is usually less than 2 g/m^2/24 h.

In a small number of patients, there is profound azotemia with elevations of blood urea nitrogen (BUN), serum creatinine, and even serum inorganic phosphate, the latter signifying a reduction of approximately 80% in glomerular filtration. Hyponatremia, hyperkalemia, and metabolic acidosis also can occur. The complete blood cell count may show a dilutional anemia. Rising antistreptolysin-O titers suggest previous streptococcal infection; however, anti-DNase B is more apt to be increased following streptococcal pyoderma. Early antibiotic use may interfere with rising antibody titers. The C3 component of complement is decreased in most patients.[16] Cultures from the throat and skin should be sent for analysis in an effort to isolate a nephrogenic strain of *Streptococcus*.

Consistent findings on chest radiography include cardiomegaly, pulmonary edema, pleural effusion, and edema of the soft tissues.[4]

TABLE 272.1. Clinical Findings in Acute Poststreptococcal Glomerulonephritis

MOST FREQUENT PRESENTING MANIFESTATIONS
Edema (periorbital-anasarca)
Hematuria (microscopic-gross)
Hypertension (mild-moderate)
Oliguria
Nonspecific systemic symptoms
Anorexia, nausea, fever, malaise, abdominal pain
Pallor
LESS FREQUENT ASSOCIATED FINDINGS
Urinary tract syndrome
Flank-loin pain, dysuria, frequency
Circulatory congestion
Mild symptoms of congestive heart failure
Frank pulmonary edema
Hypertensive encephalopathy
Headaches, vomiting, confusion, somnolence, visual disturbances, aphasia, convulsions

TABLE 272.2. Laboratory Investigations

URINE	
Sediment	
Hematuria, red blood cell casts ± hyaline granular casts, proteinuria	
BLOOD	
Biochemistry	
BUN: ↑	
Creatinine: N or ↑	
Sodium: N or ↓	
Potassium: N or ↑	
Chloride: N or ↑	
Albumin: N or ↓	
Serology	
Antistreptolysin-O: ↑ (with pharyngitis)	
Anti-DNase: B ↑	(with impetigo)
Antihyaluronidase: ↑	(with impetigo)
Complement components	
Hemolytic complement activity: ↓	
C3: ↓	
Clq, C4: N or rarely minimally ↓	
Hematology	
Hgb and Hct: N or ↑	
Platelets: N	
CULTURES	
Throat	
Skin	
RADIOGRAPHIC STUDIES	
Chest	
± Cardiomegaly	
± Pulmonary congestion	
± Pleural effusion	
Abdomen	
± Ascites	

TABLE 272.3. Differential Diagnosis of Acute Poststreptococcal Glomerulonephritis

Disease	Distinguishing Features
Acute exacerbation of chronic glomerulonephritis	Absence of latent period Significant azotemia and anemia History of known renal disease
Idiopathic hematuria (focal nephritis, benign hematuria, IgG/IgA nephropathy)	Usually hematuria without edema, hypertension, or azotemia Coincides with infection or exercise History of preceding upper respiratory tract infection
Nephritis of Henoch-Schönlein purpura	Abdominal pain, purpuric rash, arthralgia C3 usually normal
Lupus nephritis	Rash, arthralgia, lupus serology (antinuclear, antibody, anti-DNA) Prolonged hypocomplementemia, hemolytic anemia common
Membranoproliferative glomerulonephritis (MPGN)	Most likely if C3 still decreased after 6–8 wk and glomerular filtration rate still decreased after 3 wk Rising antistreptolysin-O titers favors poststreptococcal glomerulonephritis, but 25% of patients with MPGN have preceding streptococcal infection.
Nephritis secondary to toxins (e.g., lead, mercury, hydrocarbons)	Suggested by history and other clinical findings of suspected toxin

EMERGENCY DEPARTMENT MANAGEMENT

In most cases of acute poststreptococcal glomerulonephritis, there is no specific therapy that influences healing of the glomerular lesions. Antibiotics do not alter the course of the disease but may decrease the spread of nephrogenic strains of *Streptococcus* in patients with positive cultures.[13]

Appropriate therapy, as listed in Table 272.4, should be instituted promptly for the child who presents with acute renal failure, hypertension, or hyperkalemia. Symptoms suggestive of hypertensive encephalopathy consist of headache, nausea, vomiting, seizures, and transient cortical blindness. Although there is an armament of medication to treat hypertensive emergencies in children,[6,11] experience with PSAGN hypertension is limited to the medications listed in Table 272.4.

DISPOSITION

When a child with AGN presents to the emergency department, a pediatrician or nephrologist should be consulted for admission or follow-up care. Because of the possible complications, such as hypertension, hyperkalemia, and acute renal failure, most consultants choose either to admit all children with AGN or to ensure close follow-up. The decision to discharge a patient with possible AGN should never be made without consulting the primary care physician.

COMMON PITFALLS

- Hematuria is the most common urinary abnormality, but the presence of polymorphonuclear leukocytes and renal epithelial cells may be the only abnormalities early in the disease. Thus, the patient may be mistakenly diagnosed as having a urinary tract infection.
- It is extremely important to differentiate between AGN and the nephrotic syndrome, because the management may be entirely different. Patients with nephritis may have signs of fluid overload and should be fluid restricted. Diuretics should be used in the management of circulatory congestion. Those with the nephrotic syndrome may also present with edema despite being intravascularly volume depleted. The use of diuretics, here, however should be done with great care, because it may lead to severe hypovolemia.
- It is important to remember that too rapid a correction of the elevated blood pressure can be dangerous, and it is therefore essential that the patient be monitored closely during treatment.[6]

NEPHROTIC SYNDROME

The nephrotic syndrome is a clinical entity characterized by proteinuria, hypoalbuminemia, hypercholesterolemia, and edema.[16] Hypertension, hematuria, and reduced glomerular filtration rate are not usually observed in idiopathic nephrotic syndrome of childhood, although a small number of patients may have these features. The primary abnormality is increased permeability of the glomerular capillary wall to plasma proteins, resulting in excessive urinary loss of protein, principally albumin.[12]

The nephrotic syndrome is categorized into primary and secondary forms, as listed in Table 272.5. Minimal-change nephrotic syndrome, or "nil" disease, is the most common primary form seen in children, accounting for 80% to 85% of cases.[9] In these patients, renal biopsy reveals minimal glomerular abnormalities. Ninety-two percent of such patients will respond to a course of corticosteroid therapy with complete cessation of proteinuria, unlike other forms of nephrotic syndrome, which carry a worse prognosis.[19] Nephrotic syndrome can occur at any age, but 70% of children with minimal-change nephrotic syndrome have the onset of their disease between ages 2 and 7 years, with a male-to-female ratio of 2:1. The incidence and prevalence of this condition in children younger than 16 years of age are about 1.6 and 13 per 100,000, respectively.[2]

TABLE 272.4. Emergency Department Management of Complications of Acute Glomerulonephritis

A. Acute Renal Insufficiency
   1. Fluid restriction
      a. Insensible water loss (300 mL/m^2/24 h) + urine output − planned weight loss
   2. Diet
      a. Low sodium (1–2 g NaCl/m^2/24 h)
      b. Low protein: 0.5 g/kg/24 h (if BUN is >75)
   3. Correction of metabolic acidosis (serum bicarbonate <12)
      a. 0.6 × weight × (desired − observed HCO^3) given i.v. over 4–6 h[a]
B. Hypertension
   1. Encephalopathy
      a. Oxygen
      b. Diazoxide 2–5 mg/kg i.v. (maximum dose of 150 mg)
      c. Furosemide 1 mg/kg per dose i.v.
   2. No encephalopathy
      a. Nifedipine 0.10–0.50 mg/kg per dose PO or SL; may repeat in 4–6 h[b]
      b. Hydralazine 0.1–0.2 mg/kg i.v.
C. Hyperkalemia
   If serum K >6.5 mEq/L with ECG changes:
   1. Calcium: 10–15 mg/kg of elemental calcium i.v. over 15–30 min with continuous ECG monitoring
   2. Bicarbonate: 1–3 mEq/kg (short-term effect)
   3. Glucose and insulin: 1 mL/kg D_{50} with 0.2 U insulin per gram of glucose given
   4. Kayexalate: 1 g/kg with dextrose and water (enema) or with sorbitol (oral)
   5. Dialysis if above measures are unsuccessful
D. Hyponatremia
   1. Fluid restriction
E. Congestive Cardiac Failure
   1. Oxygen
   2. Fluid restriction
   3. Correct hypertension
   4. Diuretics (i.e., furosemide)
   5. Dialysis

[a] May exacerbate hypertension.
[b] Causes profound hypotension in adults.

TABLE 272.5. Etiology of Nephrotic Syndrome

PRIMARY OR MINIMAL CHANGE

Congenital
Steroid-responsive
Steroid-resistant

SECONDARY

Associated with Systemic Disease
Systemic lupus erythematosus
Henoch-Schönlein purpura
Sickle cell disease
Diabetes mellitus
Lymphoma
Berger disease (IgA nephropathy)
Postinfectious glomerulonephritis
  Syphilis
  Malaria
  Hepatitis
  Schistosomiasis
  Toxoplasmosis
  Cytomegalovirus
  HIV
Amyloidosis

Associated with Medications
Nonsteroidal antiinflammatory drugs
Penicillin
Gold salts
Tridione
Heroin

Associated with Toxins or Allergens
Bee sting
Poison oak
Vaccination
Food allergy

CLINICAL PRESENTATION

Regardless of the histopathologic abnormalities, edema is the most prominent clinical manifestation of the nephrotic syndrome in most children. The classic explanation for edema formation in the nephrotic syndrome is that hypoalbuminemia leads to decreased intravascular oncotic pressure, allowing water to extravasate into the interstitial space. The resulting contraction of intravascular volume stimulates renin release and provides an osmotic stimulus for the release of antidiuretic hormone, with activation of the renin–angiotensin–aldosterone sequence. The result is small volumes of concentrated urine containing little sodium. When plasma volume is measured in patients with the nephrotic syndrome, however, it is not uniformly decreased. This latter observation suggests that sodium retention in the nephrotic syndrome is due to intrarenal factors.

Other symptoms, such as anorexia, abdominal pain, diarrhea, and vomiting, also can be present and may be related to the severity of the edema. With anasarca and abdominal distention, respiratory distress, umbilical and inguinal hernias, and rectal prolapse may be seen. Family members may notice that the child has puffy eyes (periorbital edema) or has gained weight recently. Some children have proteinuria for 1 to 2 months before the edema becomes apparent.

The initial episode and subsequent relapses may follow a viral upper respiratory tract infection. Microscopic hematuria occurs in approximately 20% of children with minimal-change nephrotic syndrome and in 50% of those with membranoproliferative glomerulonephritis. Thus, hematuria is not a common presenting symptom in most cases of prednisone-responsive childhood nephrotic syndrome.

Blood pressure is usually normal in minimal-change nephrotic syndrome, but in 6% to 13% of patients, hypertension (above the 98th percentile for age) has been reported. Persistent hypertension is uncommon and should suggest a histologic lesion other than minimal-change nephrotic syndrome.

Laboratory findings diagnostic of the nephrotic syndrome include the following:

1. Proteinuria
   a. Greater than 3 g/1.73 m^2 of body surface area/24 h, or 50 mg/kg/24 h or 40 mg/h/m^2 of body surface area.[9] (This is usually compatible with a 4+ reading on the urinary dipstick.)
   b. Spot urine protein-to-creatinine ratio greater than 2
2. Hypoproteinemia: serum albumin value less than 2.5 g/dL
3. Hyperlipidemia: Elevation of serum levels of triglycerides, cholesterol, and total lipids is a constant feature of minimal-change nephrotic syndrome.
4. Serum creatinine is usually normal.
5. Serum BUN is normal or sometimes slightly increased secondary to hypovolemia.
6. Increased hemoglobin is frequently observed secondary to hemoconcentration.

DIFFERENTIAL DIAGNOSIS

The differential diagnosis includes the various causes of the nephrotic syndrome (see Table 272.5). Although nephrosis may be the presenting manifestation in the secondary forms, there is usually other clinical evidence of the underlying disorder.

Minimal-change disease carries a better prognosis, with a relatively good response to corticosteroid therapy. Disorders in which gross hematuria occurs in association with the nephrotic syndrome are listed in Table 272.6.

EMERGENCY DEPARTMENT EVALUATION

Many children with nephrotic syndrome are apparently healthy and have edema as their only obvious presenting abnormality. The emergency physician should perform a thorough physical examination, however, paying particular attention to the cardiovascular and respiratory systems, because respiratory difficulties secondary to ascites and pleural effusions can occur. The presence of edema can be deceptive, giving the impression of fluid overload, when, in fact, many patients are intravascularly volume-depleted secondary to their hypoproteinemia. The child with tachycardia and hypotension may require prompt fluid resuscitation.

Children with the nephrotic syndrome are prone to serious infections, and fever in such a child warrants careful evaluation. Coagulation abnormalities and thrombotic tendencies are infrequently observed. Common sites for thrombosis include cerebral veins, renal veins, pulmonary arteries, femoral arteries, and cerebral arteries.

Initial laboratory investigations fall into two categories: those necessary to establish the diagnosis and those that may elucidate its cause. Initial diagnostic tests should include a complete blood cell count, serum electrolytes, calcium, phosphorus, BUN, creatinine, total protein, albumin, globulin, cholesterol, triglycerides, complement (C_3 and C_4), urinalysis, and a spot urine protein-to-creatinine ratio. It is also important to consider testing for the human immunodeficiency virus.

Depending on the clinical findings, other laboratory studies may be performed, such as antinuclear antibodies, antistreptolysin-O titer, syphilis serology, and hepatitis B surface antigen.

TABLE 272.6. Disorders in Which Gross Hematuria Can Occur with the Nephrotic Syndrome

Urinary tract infection
Acute postinfectious glomerulonephritis
Sickle cell hemoglobinopathies
Renal vein thrombosis
Membranoproliferative glomerulonephritis
Systemic disease (e.g., systemic lupus erythematosus, syphilis, vasculitides)
Congenital or inherited renal diseases (e.g., Alport syndrome, Finnish type)
IgA nephropathy

The chest radiograph may be helpful in differentiating the nephrotic syndrome from glomerulonephritis. In the nephrotic syndrome, the heart may be normal to small in size; the lungs are relatively clear, and there is usually a much greater accumulation of pleural fluid than is seen in glomerulonephritis.[4]

EMERGENCY DEPARTMENT MANAGEMENT

Specific treatment of the nephrotic syndrome is not an emergency. Most consultants will admit all newly diagnosed patients to the hospital; admission provides an opportunity to make a specific diagnosis and initiate treatment. During this time, the family can be educated about the disease, its natural course, and its long-term management, such as diet modification. They also can be given instructions regarding the serious complications of this disease, how to recognize complications, and when to seek emergency care. It is in the management of these complications that the emergency physician plays an important role.

General measures to treat nephrotic syndrome include salt restriction (no-added-salt diet) and bed rest.[9] The initial treatment of minimal-change nephrotic syndrome of childhood consists of oral prednisone, 2 mg/kg/d (not to exceed 80 mg daily) divided into three doses[10] or given as one dose. Ninety-two percent of patients with this form of the disease will respond by becoming proteinuria-free.[19] This dose is continued for 1 week beyond this point. The dose is then doubled and given every other day; it is then gradually tapered until the patient is weaned off of prednisone at about 8 to 10 weeks after initiation of therapy. Parents can be taught to use the urinary dipstick and should be advised to return should relapse occur.

Relapses are common, and these patients may present to the emergency department. Patients who are otherwise stable do not necessarily need admission to the hospital. The treatment of relapses is not usually emergent, and the emergency physician can contact the patient's primary care pediatrician or nephrologist to ensure follow-up within the next few days.

Many complications of the nephrotic syndrome can be life-threatening and require prompt treatment.[1,20] A number of these complications are related to the edema. The patient may present in respiratory distress, with pleural effusions or massive ascites that further impairs respiration. Such patients will require diuretic therapy, but extreme care must be taken when using diuretics. The intravascular volume may be low in these patients, and giving potent diuretics may lead to hypotension and shock. The patients should be placed on a cardiac monitor, and the physician should pay close attention to the heart rate and blood pressure. Serum electrolyte levels should also be monitored.

Furosemide (Lasix) is the diuretic of choice for nephrotic patients with severe discomfort due to fluid retention. It is given orally or intravenously in a dose of 1 to 2 mg/kg and is usually given in combination with an infusion of salt-poor albumin. A useful regimen is to give furosemide intravenously, then 1 g/kg of 25% salt-poor albumin solution intravenously over 2 hours, followed by a second dose of furosemide at the end of the infusion. Again, the patient should be observed closely for hypotension or hypertension.

Some patients will require thoracentesis for relief of their respiratory distress. Paracentesis should only be performed for ascites that impairs respiration, because there is a risk of causing peritonitis with this procedure.

It is not uncommon for the nephrotic patient to present to the emergency department in hypovolemic shock. Clinically, this can be a difficult diagnosis, because the patient is edematous. Treatment here consists of prompt fluid resuscitation and hospital admission. Albumin, when available, is the preferred fluid for intravascular resuscitation.

Infections and related complications account for up to 70% of deaths in patients with childhood nephrotic syndrome. This is because of their altered immune systems. There is a high incidence of invasive infections, such as septicemia, pneumonia, cellulitis, and peritonitis caused by *Streptococcus pneumoniae*. These patients are also susceptible to gram-negative organisms such as *Escherichia coli, Pseudomonas,* and *Haemophilus influenzae*. Because the pneumococcal vaccine incorporates antigen from a limited number of strains of *S. pneumoniae,* immunization with this vaccine does not guarantee protection against these organisms. Any child with nephrotic syndrome and fever should be evaluated thoroughly and admitted to the hospital with broad-spectrum antibiotic coverage, taking into account the emergence of penicillin-resistant *S. pneumoniae* in some regions.[7] Because their immune systems are compromised, children with the nephrotic syndrome are particularly at risk for severe varicella infections. Treatment with acyclovir and or varicella-zoster immune globulin may be indicated in these patients. Consultation with a pediatric infectious disease specialist should be obtained in this circumstance.[14]

Total serum calcium is decreased in patients with the nephrotic syndrome. Hypoalbuminemia leads to a decrease in protein-bound calcium, but ionized calcium levels can also be decreased because of excessive loss of vitamin D–binding protein in the urine, leading to decreased absorption of calcium. Symptomatic hypocalcemia is rare, although bone demineralization and osteomalacia may occur.

Occasionally, a patient will present to the emergency department with tetany or muscle cramps. Such a patient should be placed on a cardiac monitor and given an initial dose of 0.5 to 1.0 mL/kg of a 10% solution of calcium gluconate intravenously over 3 to 5 minutes. Calcium gluconate is preferable to calcium chloride because it is less sclerosing to the patient's veins. When symptoms are relieved, calcium gluconate may be added to the intravenous solution at a dose of 100 mg elemental calcium/kg/24 h, or calcium may be administered orally (10% calcium gluconate contains 9 mg elemental calcium/100 mg of the salt).

Another serious complication of the nephrotic syndrome is the increased risk of vascular thromboses.[5] Thromboses have been demonstrated in all the major arteries and veins and may occur more commonly in children than is recognized by clinical symptoms and signs. Renal vein thrombosis should be suspected in a patient with acute flank pain, renal enlargement, hematuria, unexplained deterioration in renal function, oliguria, and renal failure. Many reasons for this susceptibility to thromboses have been proposed. Nephrotic patients have increased levels of plasma fibrinogen and coagulation factors V and VIII. A decrease in the circulating level of antithrombin III has been observed, and the platelets of some patients show an increase in spontaneous aggregation. Hyperviscosity of the plasma resulting from hyperfibrinogenemia and volume depletion may increase the likelihood of vascular thromboses; thus, diuretics should be used with caution. The value of routine anticoagulant and antiplatelet therapy has not been adequately assessed. An existing thrombotic lesion should be managed as for a nonnephrotic patient.

DISPOSITION

Children who are newly diagnosed as having the nephrotic syndrome should probably be admitted to the hospital for evaluation, initiation of therapy, and education of family members about the disease. Patients who were in remission and present to the emergency department with a relapse do not necessarily need to be hospitalized. The primary care pediatrician or nephrologist should be contacted, and, if follow-up can be arranged within a few days, treatment may be postponed until then. If timely follow-up is impossible, the emergency physician, usually in consultation with the primary care pediatrician, may restart prednisone therapy. Patients with life-threatening complications, such as respiratory distress, infection, hypovolemia, and thromboses, should be admitted to the hospital.

COMMON PITFALLS

- Children with the nephrotic syndrome have an increased risk of life-threatening infections; those on corticosteroid medications are even more immunocompromised. It may be safer to isolate these children in the emergency department, where they are in danger of contracting a serious infection from other patients.
- Patients presenting with periorbital edema as the only obvious manifestation of their disease may be mistakenly diagnosed as having an allergy. It is advisable to perform a urinary dipstick test on these patients to check for the presence of proteinuria.
- Emergency physicians should resist the temptation to treat the edema of the nephrotic patient in the absence of respiratory compromise or significant discomfort because of the risk of profound hypotension.

References

1. Adhikari M, Coovadia HM. Abdominal complications in black and Indian children with nephrotic syndrome. *S Afr Med J* 1993;83:253.
2. Barratt TM, Clark G. Minimal change nephrotic syndrome and focal segmental glomerulosclerosis. In: Holliday MA, Barratt T, Avner ED, eds. *Pediatric nephrology,* 3rd ed. Baltimore: Williams & Wilkins, 1994:767.
3. Boineau F, Levy J. Glomerulonephritis associated with infection. In: Massry SG, Glassock RJ, eds. *Textbook of nephrology,* vol 1. Baltimore: Williams & Wilkins, 1989.
4. Caffey J. Acute glomerulonephritis. In: Silverman FN, ed. *Caffey's pediatric x-ray diagnosis: an integrated imaging approach,* 9th ed. Chicago: Year Book Medical, 1993.
5. De Mattia D, Penza R, Giordano P, et al. Thromboembolic risk in children with nephrotic syndrome. *Haemostasis* 1991;21:300.
6. Fivush B, Neu A, Furth S. Acute hypertensive crises in children: emergencies and urgencies. *Curr Opin Pediatr* 1997;9:233–236.
7. Ilyas M, et al. Serious infections due to penicillin resistant *Streptococcus pneumoniae* in two children with the nephrotic syndrome. *Pediatr Nephrol* 1996;10:639–641.
8. Jordan SC, Lemire JM. Acute glomerulonephritis, diagnosis and treatment. *Pediatr Clin North Am* 1982;29:857.
9. Makker S. Nephrotic syndrome in children. *Curr Probl Pediatr* 1988;18:199.
10. McEnery P, Strife C. Nephrotic syndrome in childhood: management and treatment in patients with minimal change disease, mesangial proliferation, or focal glomerulosclerosis. *Pediatr Clin North Am* 1982;29:875.
11. Michael J, Groshong T, Tobias JD. Nicardipine for hypertensive emergencies in children with renal disease. *Pediatr Nephrol* 1998;12:40–42.
12. Nash MA, Edelmann CM Jr, Burnstein J, et al. The nephrotic syndrome. In: Edelmann CM Jr, ed. *Pediatric kidney disease,* 2nd ed. Boston: Little, Brown and Company, 1992:1247.

13. Pelayo JC. Acute streptococcal glomerulonephritis. In: Ichikawa I, ed. *Pediatric textbook of fluids and electrolytes*. Baltimore: Williams & Wilkins, 1990:308.
14. *Red book report of the Committee of Infectious Disease 1997,* 24th ed. Dallas: American Academy of Pediatrics, 1997:573–585.
15. Sanjad S, Tolaymat A, Whitworth J, et al. Acute glomerulonephritis in children: a review of 153 cases. *South Med J* 1977;70:1202.
16. Schnaper HW. Primary nephrotic syndrome of childhood. *Curr Opin Pediatr* 1996;8:141–147.
17. Shroff KJ, Ravichandran R, Acharya VN. ASO titre and serum complement (C3) in post-streptococcal glomerulonephritis. *J Postgrad Med* 1984;30:27.
18. Travis LB. Acute postinfectious glomerulonephritis. In: Rudolph AM (ed): Pediatrics, 20th ed. Norwalk, CT: Appleton & Lange, 1996:1352.
19. Travis LB. The nephrotic syndrome. In: Rudolph AM, ed. *Pediatrics,* 20th ed. Norwalk, CT: Appleton & Lange, 1996:1366.
20. Tsau YK, Chen CH, Tsai WS, et al. Complications of nephrotic syndrome in children. *J Formos Med Assoc* 1991;90:555.

CHAPTER 273
Human Immunodeficiency Virus (HIV)

Ronald M. Ferdman and Jeffrey F. Linzer

In the early 1980s, a novel immunodeficiency was first seen in children. Its clinical presentation was similar to that of severe combined immunodeficiency (SCID), but included distinct clinical and pathologic findings. In 1982, these first cases of pediatric acquired immunodeficiency syndrome (PAIDS) were reported. By 1983, the causative agent of AIDS was identified as human immunodeficiency virus (HIV), and, in 1985, a commercial assay to detect HIV became available.

HIV is an RNA retrovirus that attacks primarily CD4+ T-lymphocytes (T-helper), though other cells, including monocytes and macrophages, are at risk as well. The chemokine receptors CXCR4 and CCR5 have been recently identified as necessary coreceptors. Viral RNA is transcribed by reverse transcriptase to DNA. A provirus is formed that can remain "latent" for a prolonged period (up to several years). New virus copies are produced after activation of the host cell. This activation can lead to direct cellular cytotoxicity and the spread of virus to cause eventual depletion, and through a variety of mechanisms, dysregulation of the immune system. T-helper cells become depleted and the ratio of T-helper to T-suppressor cells becomes reversed.

The most serious clinical consequence of HIV infection—AIDS—is defined in children according to certain immunologic (Table 273.1) and clinical parameters (Tables 273.2 and 273.3), as defined by the Centers for Disease Control and Prevention (CDC). Between 1982 and 1998, over 8,000 cases of PAIDS were reported to the CDC. Many more children are HIV infected, but do not meet the criteria for AIDS.

Of the reported cases with PAIDS, 78% occurred in children under 5 years and 90% in children born to HIV-infected mothers. Currently, vertical transmission accounts for all but a few isolated cases of new pediatric HIV infections. Children born to untreated HIV-infected mothers have approximately a 20% to 30% chance of being infected. With recent recommendations for universal HIV screening of pregnant women and effective prenatal and postnatal prophylaxis, transmission can be reduced to below 5%, and it is expected that the number of new cases of PAIDS will dramatically decline.

CLINICAL PRESENTATION

The presentation of an HIV-infected child may vary, depending on whether the diagnosis of HIV infection had been previously known. The child with HIV may be outwardly growing well and have no more than the usual number of routine childhood infections. Therefore, it is not uncommon for previously undiagnosed HIV-infected children to present through the emergency department (ED) with the first clinical manifestations of HIV disease, and an index of suspicion must be kept for HIV, even in relatively healthy older children. Suspicion for HIV should be raised in children with unexplained poor growth and developmental delay, with recurrent or chronic infections. Recurrent infections do not need to be severe or debilitating. The most common infections seen are frequent otitis media, sinusitis, pneumonia, adenitis, and diarrhea. Certainly, any opportunistic infection (OI) should immediately suggest an underlying immunodeficiency. Probably the most common physical finding is diffuse lymphadenopathy (LAD), especially with axillary or subclavicular involvement and hepatic or splenic enlargement. Parotid enlargement is a common finding. The presence of persistent or chronic oral candidiasis, especially in a child over 1 year of age should suggest immune dysfunction. Common hematologic findings include anemia, leukopenia, and especially thrombocytopenia. Nonspecific liver enzyme elevation is often seen, as is hypoalbuminemia and hyperproteinemia, with a resultant increased globulin fraction. Sedimentation rate, though nonspecific, is often markedly elevated.

TABLE 273.1 CDC Classification System for HIV Infection in Children Less Than 13 Years of Age: Immune Categories Based on Age-Specific CD4+ T-Lymphocyte and Percentage

	Age of Child		
	<12 mo	1–5 yr	6–12 yr
Immunologic Category	cells/cc (%)	cells/cc (%)	cells/cc (%)
1: No suppression	>1,500 (>25)	>1,000 (>25)	>500 (>25)
2: Moderate suppression	750–1,500 (15–24)	500–999 (15–24)	200–499 (15–24)
3: Severe suppression	<750 (<15)	<500 (<15)	<200 (<15)

Modified from Centers for Disease Control and Prevention. 1994 Revised classification system for human immunodeficiency virus infection in children less than 13 years of age. *MMWR* 1994;43(RR-12):1–10.

TABLE 273.2. Clinical Categories for Children with Human Immunodeficiency Virus Infection

N: NOT SYMPTOMATIC
Children who have no signs or symptoms considered to be the result of HIV infection or who have only one of the conditions listed in category A
CATEGORY A: MILDLY SYMPTOMATIC
Children with *two* or more of the following conditions but none of the conditions listed in categories B and C:
Lymphadenopathy ($\geq$0.5 cm at more than two sites; bilateral = one site)
Hepatomegaly
Splenomegaly
Dermatitis
Parotitis
Recurrent or persistent upper respiratory infection, sinusitis, or otitis media
CATEGORY B: MODERATELY SYMPTOMATIC
Children who have symptomatic conditions other than those listed for category A or category C that are attributed to HIV infection. Examples of conditions in clinical category B include, but are not limited to, the following:
Anemia ($<$8 g/dL), neutropenia ($<$1,000/μL), or thrombocytopenia ($<$100,000/μL) persisting $\geq$30 days
Bacterial meningitis, pneumonia, or sepsis (single episode)
Candidiasis, oropharyngeal (i.e., thrush) persisting for $>$2 months in children aged $>$6 months
Cardiomyopathy
Cytomegalovirus infection with onset before age 1 month
Diarrhea, recurrent or chronic
Hepatitis
Herpes simplex virus (HSV) stomatitis, recurrent (i.e., more than two episodes within 1 year)
HSV bronchitis, pneumonitis, or esophagitis with onset before age 1 month
Herpes zoster (i.e., shingles) involving at least two distinct episodes or more than one dermatome
Leiomyosarcoma
Lymphoid interstitial pneumonia (LIP) or pulmonary lymphoid hyperplasia complex
Nephropathy
Nocardiosis
Fever lasting $>$1 month
Toxoplasmosis with onset before age 1 month
Varicella, disseminated (i.e., complicated chickenpox)
CATEGORY C: SEVERELY SYMPTOMATIC
Children who have any condition listed in the 1987 surveillance case definition for acquired immunodeficiency syndrome, with the exception of LIP (which is a category B condition)

Modified from Centers for Disease Control and Prevention. 1994 Revised classification system for human immunodeficiency virus infection in children less than 13 years of age. *MMWR* 1994;43(RR-12):1–10. Erratum *MMWR* 1998;47(15):316.

Sudden presentation with an OI is not an uncommon manner in which a child with undiagnosed HIV may present to the ED. *Pneumocystis carinii* pneumonia (PCP) remains the most common presenting OI in undiagnosed children. Although it can occur at any age, it typically presents at under a year of age. Symptoms include dyspnea, tachypnea, cough, and fever, with relatively clear lung sounds and disproportionate hypoxemia. Severity of symptoms may range from mild upper respiratory symptoms to severe respiratory distress. A chest radiograph shows a diffuse interstitial pattern. Lymphoid interstitial pneumonitis (LIP) and pulmonary lymphoid hyperplasia (PLH) are common causes of respiratory symptoms and may mimic respiratory infections. Children with LIP/PLH often have radiographic findings out of proportion to their respiratory symptoms; they usually have LAD and hepatosplenomegaly (HSM) and can have digital clubbing. The most common organisms causing respiratory infections in HIV-infected children remain the typical pediatric respiratory pathogens, such as *Streptococcus pneumoniae* and *Haemophilus influenzae.*

Mycobacterium avium-intracellulare (MAI), seen in children with advanced disease, can present with prolonged fevers and nightsweats, chronic diarrhea, abdominal pain, and weight loss. Oral thrush is common, and esophageal candidiasis should be suspected in a child with oral thrush accompanied by fever, refusal to eat, irritability, and weight loss. Diarrhea is common and is most often due to *Salmonella* sp., *Shigella* sp., and *Campylobacter* sp. Infections with *Clostridium difficile, Escherichia coli, Yersinia* sp., and *Vibrio cholerae* are also seen with increased prevalence. Parasitic infection, specifically with *Giardia* and *Cryptosporidium,* is also prevalent. Cytomegalovirus (CMV) and herpes simplex virus (HSV) can cause especially severe enteritis.

Other OIs, such as toxoplasmosis, histoplasmosis, and cryptococcosis, can be seen in children but are rare; these occur primarily in adults. Herpesvirus infections (HSV, varicella-zoster virus [VZV], CMV) can be particularly severe and can present as disseminated disease. CMV retinitis, a common cause of acute blindness in adults, is very uncommon in children, but it can occur with advanced disease. Malignancies, especially lymphomas, occur at an increased rate, and may be primary central nervous system (CNS) or disseminated. Kaposi's sarcoma, common in immunocompromised adults, is rare in children. Acute cardiac and renal manifestations are uncommon, but myocardi-

TABLE 273.3. Conditions Included in Clinical Category C for Children Infected with Human Immunodeficiency Virus

Serious bacterial infections, multiple or recurrent (i.e., any combination of at least two culture-confirmed infections within a 2-year period), of the following types: septicemia, pneumonia, meningitis, bone or joint infection, or abscess of an internal organ or body cavity (excluding otitis media, superficial skin or mucosal abscesses, and indwelling catheter-related infections)
Candidiasis, esophageal or pulmonary (bronchi, trachea, lungs)
Coccidioidomycosis, disseminated (at site other than or in addition to lungs or cervical or hilar lymph nodes)
Cryptococcosis, extrapulmonary
Cryptosporidiosis or isosporiasis with diarrhea persisting >1 month
Cytomegalovirus disease with onset of symptoms at age >1 month (at a site other than liver, spleen, or lymph nodes)
Encephalopathy (at least one of the following progressive findings present for at least 2 months in the absence of a concurrent illness other than HIV infection that could explain the findings): (a) failure to attain or loss of developmental milestones or loss of intellectual ability, verified by standard developmental scale or neuropsychological tests; (b) impaired brain growth or acquired microcephaly demonstrated by head circumference measurements or brain atrophy demonstrated by computerized tomography or magnetic resonance imaging (serial imaging is required for children <2 years of age); (c) acquired symmetric motor deficit manifested by two or more of the following: paresis, pathologic reflexes, ataxia, or gait disturbance
Herpes simplex virus infection causing a mucocutaneous ulcer that persists for >1 month; or bronchitis, pneumonitis, or esophagitis for any duration affecting a child >1 month of age
Histoplasmosis, disseminated (at a site other than or in addition to lungs or cervical or hilar lymph nodes)
Kaposi's sarcoma
Lymphoma, primary, in brain
Lymphoma, small, noncleaved cell (Burkitt's), or immunoblastic or large-cell lymphoma of B-cell or unknown immunologic phenotype
Mycobacterium tuberculosis, disseminated or extrapulmonary
Mycobacterium, other species or unidentified species, disseminated (at a site other than or in addition to lungs, skin, or cervical or hilar lymph nodes)
Mycobacterium avium complex or Mycobacterium kansasii, disseminated (at site other than or in addition to lungs, skin, or cervical or hilar lymph nodes)
Pneumocystis carinii pneumonia
Progressive multifocal leukoencephalopathy
Salmonella (nontyphoid) septicemia, recurrent
Toxoplasmosis of the brain with onset at >1 month of age
Wasting syndrome in the absence of a concurrent illness other than HIV infection that could explain the following findings: (a) persistent weight loss >10% of baseline *or* (b) downward crossing of at least two of the following percentile lines on the weight-for-age chart (e.g., 95th, 75th, 50th, 25th, 5th) in a child ≥1 year of age, *or* (c) <5th percentile on weight-for-height chart on two consecutive measurements, ≥30 days apart *plus* (a) chronic diarrhea (i.e., at least two loose stools per day for ≥30 days) *or* (b) documented fever (for ≥30 days, intermittent or constant)

From Centers for Disease Control and Prevention. 1994 Revised classification system for human immunodeficiency virus infection in children less than 13 years of age. *MMWR* 1994;43(RR-12):1–10.

tis with congestive heart failure and acute renal failure have been described. Although chronic HIV-associated encephalopathy and developmental delay are common, acute CNS manifestations are not, and etiologies such as infection, space-occupying lesions, and thromboembolic events should be investigated. Infected children are at increased risk for sepsis and meningitis with the usual pediatric pathogens.

Less acute symptoms commonly seen in the ED include skin rashes, such as molluscum, warts, and drug eruptions. The child with PAIDS is at greater risk for cutaneous herpesvirus infections, and can have recurrent or chronic chickenpox, zoster, or mucocutaneous HSV. Oral aphthous ulcers are common and present with shallow oropharyngeal ulcers, which can be quite painful and result in decreased oral intake and dehydration. Aphthous ulcers need to be differentiated from oral HSV infections, as corticosteroids are often needed to resolve the aphthous ulcer.

Children previously diagnosed with HIV may present differently. In patients on appropriate drug regimens who are compliant with recommended therapy, most OIs, especially PCP and MAI, are much more rare. If the child is on effective antiretroviral therapy, in general, infections should be less common and less severe, though he or she remains at risk for all of the previously listed conditions.

Common presentations for HIV-infected children under treatment often involve adverse effects from their medications. Acute pancreatitis can be seen with several of the antiretroviral agents and can be quite severe and life-threatening. Drug eruptions, ranging from mild nonspecific erythroderma and urticaria to overwhelming Stevens-Johnson syndrome, can be seen with many of the agents used to treat HIV. Nausea, vomiting, diarrhea, and hepatitis are common adverse effects. Drug-induced hematologic abnormalities that may be seen in the ED include bleeding from thrombocytopenia, congestive heart failure from anemia, and secondary infections from granulocytopenia.

DIFFERENTIAL DIAGNOSIS

Because HIV can cause such a wide and varied pattern of symptoms, its differential diagnosis is extensive, and there are a number of conditions that can cause a child to present to the ED with manifestations similar to those of HIV infection. The symptoms of primary immunodeficiencies can be virtually identical to those of HIV.

PAIDS most resembles the T-cell deficiencies, the most common being severe SCIDS and DiGeorge syndrome. There are many variants of SCIDS, and they can be either autosomal recessive or X-linked. Children with SCIDS usually present with overwhelming infections within the first few months of life and rarely live more than 1 or 2 years without treatment. Patients with DiGeorge syndrome can have similar infections, but often also have severe hypocalcemia, cardiac, and other anatomic and morphologic abnormalities. Other T-cell disorders have similar presentation but are much rarer. Of the B-cell disorders, the most common are X-linked agammaglobulinemia and common variable immune deficiency. Both result in immunoglobulin deficiency and typically present with recurrent encapsulated bacterial infections, mostly of the respiratory tract. *Giardia* and enteroviral disease are also commonly seen.

In the newborn and young infant, other congenital infections, such as CMV, rubella, syphilis, toxoplasmosis, HSV, and Epstein-Barr virus (EBV), can present with developmental delay, failure to thrive, HSM, and LAD. Lymphoma, leukemia, and other malignancies can present with weight loss, HSM, LAD, fevers, cytopenias, and OI. Recurrent pneumonias and sinus disease, along with chronic diarrhea and poor weight gain, are common presenting symptoms for cystic fibrosis. Certain autoimmune diseases, such as lupus or systemic juvenile rheumatoid arthritis, as well as metabolic and mitochondrial diseases may have similar initial presentations. Many chronic conditions can cause secondary immunodeficiencies with presenting symptoms similar to those of HIV. Examples of secondary immunodeficiencies include protein calorie malnutrition or specific nutrient (i.e., zinc) deficiencies, nephrotic syndrome, inflammatory bowel diseases, and protein-losing enteropathies, among many others.

EMERGENCY DEPARTMENT EVALUATION

The ED evaluation depends on whether the child has known HIV infection or is presenting for the first time with a suspected but undiagnosed immunodeficiency. A careful physical examination and history should be taken, especially for parental HIV risk factors. However, absence of risk factors should not override clinical suspicion of HIV. In a well-appearing child with suspicious history, physical, or laboratory findings, a referral for in-depth testing and evaluation may be more appropriate than testing in the ED. A child with significantly abnormal physical findings, laboratory values, or illness should be admitted for a full immunologic evaluation.

For the child with known HIV infection, ED evaluation should be based on the presenting problem (e.g., fever, diarrhea, respiratory distress), taken in conjunction with immunologic status. The risk of significant bacterial infections and OI is related to the degree of the child's immunocompetency as well as to the medication regimen.

In general, children who are in the CDC clinical category N (no signs/symptoms) or A (mild signs/symptoms) or in immunologic category 1 (no evidence of immune suppression) can receive the same evaluation as would a noninfected child with similar clinical symptoms. Children in more advanced categories are at higher risk for serious illness and require proportionately more intensive evaluations.

Because the range of possible presenting symptoms is wide, it is impossible to list all evaluations that should be done in every case. Oftentimes, an HIV-infected child will have so many chronic problems that evaluation in any system will yield abnormal results. Therefore, evaluations should be acute symptom–specific.

A source of fever should always be sought. Febrile children should have a complete blood count (CBC) and routine blood culture. Children with severe immunosuppression should have blood cultures sent for acid-fast bacilli, viral (especially CMV), and fungus as well. Chest radiographs and pulse oximetry (blood gases, if severe) are indicated in patients with cough, wheeze, or respiratory distress. Elevated lactose dehydrogenase (LDH) is suggestive of PCP, although it can be elevated with other pneumonias. Sputum culture should be obtained in older children.

With any acute diarrheal illness, stool cultures for routine bacteria, ova and parasite, and rotavirus, as well as fecal leukocytes, are indicated. Specific evaluation for *Giardia* and *C. difficile* should be considered, and in children with advanced disease, cultures for *Cryptosporidium,* acid-fast bacilli, and other viruses (CMV, adenovirus) can be included. In patients with chronic or severe acute diarrhea, electrolyte abnormalities are common, and levels of electrolytes, including calcium and magnesium, should be monitored.

For acute abdominal pain, serum amylase and lipase, especially if the patient is on antiretrovirals, and tests of liver function should be ordered. Abdominal imaging may be indicated for severe or chronic pain. For acute skin rashes, a history of recent changes in medication within the past few weeks should be obtained. When possible, cultures should be taken of any infectious-appearing skin lesion of unknown etiology. Children with acute CNS symptoms should have appropriate CNS imaging studies, as well as consideration for lumbar puncture, if deemed safe.

The diagnosis of HIV in adults and children over 2 years old is relatively straightforward, and is made by demonstrating the presence of HIV antibodies in the blood. In young children, the diagnosis is more difficult. All children born to HIV-infected mothers will have transplacentally acquired HIV antibodies, which may persist until 18 to 24 months. Therefore, although HIV antibody testing identifies a child at risk, definitive diagnosis in children under 2 years requires demonstration of the presence of the virus itself, not only antibody to the virus. The preferred method of testing is via polymerase chain reaction (PCR) against proviral DNA. Serial testing is often necessary to prove infection, but PCR is highly reliable, with over 90% accuracy with one test alone. Because results of testing are rarely available during the ED stay, the decision to test patients in the ED should be done only when appropriate counseling and follow-up are available. As the HIV-infected child is often the index case, the implications of testing a child or the parents and other siblings must be taken into account.

EMERGENCY DEPARTMENT MANAGEMENT

The presenting illness in the HIV-infected child in CDC immune category 1 or clinical categories N or A can generally be managed similarly to that of any noninfected child. For other categories, the stage of the underlying disease needs to be taken into consideration to determine appropriate ED management. Consultation with the child's primary care physician or infectious disease specialist is indicated to help determine appropriate management. Often, ED-determined abnormalities are well known to the primary service and may, in fact, be chronic changes. Other times, the primary service is aware of factors unique to the patient that need to be incorporated into the management plan.

It is important to remember that HIV is not spread by casual contact; as with all patients, however, take universal precautions when dealing with body fluids.

The principles of empiric antibiotic treatment in a child with HIV are similar to those in ill-appearing, non-HIV infected children. Obviously, children with advanced HIV disease require more aggressive treatment, both in terms of threshold to begin treatment as well as in antibiotic choice. Empiric antibiotic therapy is based on source of infection and likely organisms. For the febrile child in whom bacteremia is suspected but who does not appear septic, ceftriaxone (50 to 75 mg/kg) parenterally could be considered in a child to be sent home from the ED. Ceftriaxone, followed by a course of an oral antibiotic effective against beta-lactamase–positive agents, is also a good choice for community-acquired pneumonia or a chronic otitis media or sinusitis. Children with relatively good immune function or with mild infections can often be treated with oral antibiotics alone.

Broader spectrum antibiotics are indicated if the child has failed previous antibiotics or is on chronic antibiotic prophylaxis. Occasionally, quinolone antibiotics are the only oral antibiotics available, but they should be started only after consultation with the child's primary service and should be restricted to patients with documented *Pseudomonas* infections or failure of conventional antibiotics. If the patient's clinical condition warrants hospital admission, then broad-spectrum intravenous antibiotic coverage should be started. The presence of a central venous catheter should suggest the use of an agent effective against gram-negative and coagulase-negative *Staphylococcus* organisms, especially if the child appears septic.

A high index of suspicion should be kept for unusual organisms and OI. The presentation of PCP is varied, and any child at risk (Table 273.4) who presents with respiratory symptoms and hypoxemia, especially with characteristic radiographic and laboratory findings, should be suspected of having PCP. Children with early or mild PCP often have only minimal changes on chest radiograph, and their only symptoms may be tachypnea, and dyspnea and hypoxemia on exertion. Even children with mild PCP, although often treatable with oral antibiotics alone, should be admitted for definitive diagnosis with bronchioalveolar lavage (BAL) and to ensure nonprogression of respiratory symptoms. Empiric treatment with trimethoprim-sulfamethoxazole (TMP/SMX) should be started immediately, as BAL will detect *P. carinii*, even several days after initiation of treatment. Administration of corticosteroids is definitely indicated in any child with moderate-to-severe PCP, and is typically given even in mild cases.

The differentiation of community-acquired pneumonia from other respiratory conditions can be a challenge for the ED clinician. While the radiographic findings in LIP/PLH may mimic respiratory infections, they rarely cause acute respiratory symptoms. Acute exacerbations are usually due to a superimposed viral infection and may manifest with fever, cough, wheezing, and dyspnea. If it is possible to obtain previous radiographs, they can be useful to differentiate old from new findings. For acute exacerbations, symptomatic treatment with bronchodilators and oral corticosteroids is often effective. Antibiotics should be reserved for patients with suspected secondary infections or with new radiographic changes. Short courses of oral glucocorticoids, such that might be used for LIP/PLH, acute asthma attacks, or a severe allergic reaction, are rarely absolutely contraindicated in HIV-infected children. The rare exceptions include patients with an active viral infection, such as herpesviruses, and those with severe underlying immune dysfunction. Nevertheless, it is always appropriate to contact the patient's primary service before beginning home systemic glucocorticoids.

Diarrhea is treated as in non–HIV-infected children, and dietary changes are often all that is necessary to control symptoms. Dehydration can be treated with oral or intravenous rehydration, depending on the severity.

Specific therapy should be withheld pending culture results, but, in certain cases, empiric antibiotics can be started. Children with fever and more than 5 white blood cells per high-power field may benefit from empiric TMP/SMX treatment. Infectious diarrheas often become chronic (such as with *Giardia, C. difficile,* and *Cryptosporidium*), and empiric therapy is based on past response to medications.

It is generally not appropriate to institute or make major changes in antiretroviral therapy, prophylactic therapy, or other chronic medications in the ED. Changes should be made only after discussion with the child's primary service, and they are best left to the outpatient clinic setting.

TABLE 273.4. Risk for PCP in HIV-Infected Children

Age	Risk for PCP
<4 wk	Low
4 wk–12 mo	Any infected infant
1–5 yr	CD4 <500 cells/cc or <15%
6–12 yr	CD4 <200 cells/cc or <15%
Any age	If history of previous PCP
	If CD4 (count or %) rapidly decreasing or class C disease present

Modified from Centers for Disease Control and Prevention. 1995 Revised guidelines for prophylaxis against *Pneumocystis carinii* pneumonia for children infected with or perinatally exposed to human immunodeficiency virus. *MMWR* 1995;44(RR-4):1–11.

Chemoprophylaxis after Suspected Exposure to HIV

Children may present to the ED after exposures that put them at risk for HIV infection. Such exposures include accidental puncture wounds they might incur by playing with discarded needles found outside or inside the house, or from sexual abuse.

Determination must first be made as to the risk of HIV transmission. If the source is known to be HIV-infected, then recommendations for chemoprophylaxis are based on type of exposure (percutaneous, mucous membrane, or skin) and source material (blood, other infectious body fluids, such as semen and vaginal secretions). Larger volume or area of exposure, higher HIV titer, and prolonged contact all increase the risk of transmission. Most often, the HIV status of the previous needle user or sexual contact is not known. In such an instance, recommendations for chemoprophylaxis should be made, case by case, on the basis of the exposure risk and likelihood of HIV infection of the source. Chemoprophylaxis should be recommended for children with high-risk exposure. Prophylaxis should be offered to children with low but nonnegligible exposures, balancing the lower risk versus the use of drugs of uncertain efficacy and toxicity. For exposures with negligible risk (i.e., exposure to urine, normal household contacts, etc.), chemoprophylaxis should not be offered.

There is no drug regimen that has proven superiority, and certainly there are many cases of chemoprophylaxis failure. Drug regimens should be based on the profile of antiretroviral drug resistance of the source case, local availability of drugs, the patient's preexisting medical condition and drug therapy, and drug toxicity.

In general, triple-drug combination therapy is recommended. In most cases, the combination should include zidovudine combined with another reverse transcriptase inhibitor and a protease inhibitor. Recent CDC guidelines suggest zidovudine, lamivudine, and indinavir as empiric therapy. When possible, these drugs should be started after consultation with specialists having expertise in antiretroviral therapy. Postexposure prophylaxis should be initiated as soon as possible after exposure, preferably within 1 to 2 hours.

Although animal studies suggest that prophylaxis is not effective when started more than 36 hours after exposure, the interval after which there is no benefit in humans is not known. Some sources recommend initiating therapy as long as 1 to 2 weeks after a very high risk exposure, so that even if infection is not prevented, early treatment of HIV infection may be of benefit. The optimal duration of postexposure prophylaxis is unknown, but the regimen should be administered for at least 4 weeks if tolerated, or until the source is proven HIV-negative. The child should be tested for HIV at initiation of chemoprophylaxis to confirm the absence of preexisting HIV infection. Chemoprophylaxis should be offered in conjunction with appropriate counseling as the to risks and benefits of antiretroviral therapy and the risk of the exposure. Arrangements should be made for ongoing counseling and follow-up testing.

DISPOSITION

As with any chronic disease, children who are suspected of having HIV infection need to be followed by a primary service experienced in their management. Children who are suspected of having undiagnosed HIV and who do not have significant clinical findings should be referred to an appropriate consultant in infectious disease or immunology. Discussion with the consultant prior to discharge from the ED can help to determine whether the child may be safely evaluated as an outpatient, and to arrange for a definitive appointment. Known HIV-infected children with mild disease can be managed at home and should have follow-up arranged with their primary service.

Children requiring hospitalization should be carefully evaluated to determine whether admission to an intensive care or step-down unit is required. For most infectious processes, consultation with an infectious disease specialist is indicated. If BAL is required, a pediatric pulmonologist should be contacted. If the hospital is not equipped to manage seriously ill, HIV-infected children, or if the necessary specialist consultations are not available, the patient should be transported to an appropriate center by qualified transport personnel.

COMMON PITFALLS

- Not all parents will volunteer that their child is HIV-infected, and may deny their own risk factors. Every attempt should be made to elicit appropriate historic information, but decisions on whether to suspect a child is HIV-infected may need to be based on strong clinical suspicion.
- In any suspected immunodeficient patient under a year of age, the presence of tachypnea and hypoxemia should suggest PCP, and empiric therapy should not be withheld while waiting for definitive diagnosis. Although breakthroughs are rare, even children on prescribed PCP prophylactic medications may develop PCP.
- Any child over a year old with persistent or recurrent oral thrush should be considered immunodeficient until proven otherwise.
- Because of the risk of more serious disease, significantly immunosuppressed children should receive more intensive evaluation and treatment than might be done in an otherwise normal child. When in doubt, it is better to err on the side of caution when deciding to treat or admit.
- If a child's HIV status is unknown, but there is risk for HIV, either by history or suggestive clinical findings, he or she should be assumed to be infected and treated accordingly.
- As much as possible, a source for any fever should be sought, and all appropriate cultures should be obtained.
- As with any immunodeficient patient, all live virus vaccines should be avoided in the ED, and all blood products should be irradiated and CMV-free.
- Reasonable efforts should be made to contact the HIV-infected child's primary service before final evaluation and disposition. Effective follow-up is key to successful management and minimization of future ED visits.

Bibliography

Centers for Disease Control and Prevention. 1994 revised classification system for human immunodeficiency virus infection in children less than 13 years of age. *MMWR* 1994;43(RR-12):1–10.

Centers for Disease Control and Prevention. 1995 revised guidelines for prophylaxis against *Pneumocystis carinii* pneumonia for children infected with or perinatally exposed to human immunodeficiency virus. *MMWR* 1995;44(RR-4):1–11.

Centers for Disease Control and Prevention. *HIV/AIDS surveillance report.* 1998;10:1.

Centers for Disease Control and Prevention. Public health service recommendations for the management of health-care worker exposures to HIV and recommendations for post-exposure prophylaxis. *MMWR* 1998;47:1–28.

Centers for Disease Control and Prevention. USPHS/IDSA guidelines for the prevention of opportunistic infections in persons infected with human immunodeficiency virus: a summary. *MMWR* 1999;48:1.

Frank MM, Austen KF, Claman HN, et al. *Samter's immunologic diseases,* 5th ed. New York: Little, Brown and Company, 1995.

Moore JP. Co-receptors: implications for HIV pathogenesis and therapy. *Science* 1997;276:51–52.

Pizzo PA, Wilfert CM. *Pediatric aids: the challenge of HIV infection in infants, children, and adolescents,* 3rd ed. Baltimore: Williams & Wilkins, 1999.

Working Group on Antiretroviral Therapy and Medical Management of HIV-Infected Children. Guidelines for the use of antiretroviral agents in pediatric HIV infection. http://hivatis.org/guidelines/Pediatric/text/ped_12.pdf/. The HIV/AIDS Treatment Information Service (ATIS). Rockville, MD, Jan. 2000.

CHAPTER 274
Immunizations

Mary A. Hegenbarth and Hisham A. Omran

Although the vast majority of routine immunizations are administered by private physicians and health departments, an emergency department (ED) visit by an underimmunized child can be viewed as an opportunity for vaccination, and some authors promote the administration of missed vaccines in the ED.[11]

Table 274.1 summarizes recent recommendations from the American Academy of Pediatrics (AAP), the Centers for Disease Control and Prevention (CDC), and the American Academy of Family Physicians (AAFP) for routine childhood immunizations. Immunization practices are rapidly changing; many new vaccines and changes in the vaccine schedule are expected. Updated information on vaccines, adverse events, and schedules can be found on AAP websites (http://www. aap.org), AAFP (http://www.aafp.org), the National Immunization Program of the CDC (http://www.pcdc.gov/ nip), or in the American Academy of Pediatrics *Red Book.*[1]

Serious complications from currently used vaccines are rare; minor febrile and local reactions are common. In addition to specific vaccine reactions, the general complications associated with intramuscular injections (e.g., sterile and infected abscesses, nerve or vascular injuries) are sometimes seen.

TABLE 274.1. Routine Childhood Immunization Schedule United States, June 2000

Vaccine	Age: Birth	1 mo	2 mos	4 mos	6 mos	12 mos	15 mos	18 mos	24 mos	4–6 yrs	11–12 yrs	14–16 yrs
Hepatitis B		←Hep B→										
			←Hep B→			←Hep B→						
Diphtheria, Tetanus, Pertussis			DTaP	DTaP	DTaP		←DTaP→			DTaP	←Td→	
H. influenzae type b			Hib	Hib	Hib	←Hib→						
Polio			IPV	IPV		←IPV→				IPV		
Measles, Mumps, Rubella						←MMR→				MMR		
Varicella							←Var→					
Hepatitis A									Hep A-in selected areas			
Pneumococcal (PCV7)			PCV7	PCV7	PCV7	←PCV7→						

Adapted from recommendations of the Advisory Committee on Immunization Practices (ACIP), the American Academy of Pediatrics (AAP), and the American Academy of Family Physicians (AAFP).

Recent controversy over rare vaccine complications, particularly encephalopathy and other possible neurologic sequelae, has heightened parental anxiety toward immunization reactions.[6] The Institute of Medicine has extensively analyzed suspected vaccine complications and categorized adverse effects into five categories that favor or reject a causal relationship for the vaccine involved. For many suspected vaccine complications, there is insufficient evidence to accept or reject a causal relationship, and further study is needed.[7,9,10,12]

CLINICAL PRESENTATION: VACCINE COMPLICATIONS

Diptheria, Tetanus, and Pertussis

Diphtheria, tetanus, and pertussis combination vaccines contain diphtheria and tetanus toxoids and either whole-cell pertussis (DTP/DTwP) or acellular pertussis antigens (DTaP). Acellular pertussis vaccines are now recommended for the initial series, as they are highly effective and cause fewer local and systemic reactions, such as fever, seizures, and constitutional symptoms, than whole-cell vaccine.[1,2]

Common adverse reactions to DTwP vaccine are seen in more than half of recipients and usually occur within 48 hours. They include local redness, swelling, pain, fussiness, and moderate fever (less than 40.5°C). Giving acetaminophen at the time of administration and 4 to 8 hours later reduces the incidence of febrile and local reactions.[1] The occurrence of immediate anaphylaxis or encephalopathy within 7 days of administration contraindicates further doses of any pertussis vaccine. The following findings (less common after DTaP than dTwP) are considered "precautions," which should be considered before further doses of either pertussis vaccine are administered[1,7]:

1. Seizures within 3 days
2. Persistent, inconsolable screaming or crying for more than 3 hours within 48 hours
3. Collapse or shocklike state (hypotonic–hyporesponsive episode) within 48 hours
4. Unexplained fever over 40.5°C within 48 hours

Recent estimates of the risk of acute encephalopathy after whole-cell pertussis vaccine are from zero to 10.5 episodes per million immunizations.[7] The American Academy of Pediatrics has concluded that pertussis vaccine has not been proven to be a cause of brain damage.[1,3] It should be stressed that neurologic complications occur with much higher frequency in natural pertussis disease.

Haemophilus influenzae Type B

There are four *Haemophilus influenzae* type b conjugate vaccines (HbCV) licensed for use in the United States: PRP-OMP (PedvaxHIB), HbOC (HibTITER), PRP-T (ActHIB/OmniHIB), and PRP-D (ProHIBiT). The vaccines differ in their carrier proteins, polysaccharide molecular size, and method of conjugation; as a result, they differ in immunogenicity.

The primary series begins at 2 months of age (two doses for PRP-OMP, three doses for HbOC or PRP-T), with a later booster dose of any of the vaccines. A dramatic decrease in the incidence of invasive *H. influenzae* disease has occurred since the introduction of these vaccines, with a 99% decline in invasive disease in children less than 5 years of age.[8] All of the vaccines are well tolerated, with about 25% of children having mild local reactions. HbCV vaccines are also available in combination with other vaccines (see later section, Combination Vaccines).

Hepatitis B

Universal immunization with hepatitis B vaccine, beginning at birth, is now recommended. Currently used recombinant vaccines may occasionally cause local soreness or fever but are otherwise well tolerated.

Measles, Mumps, Rubella

The live measles, mumps, and rubella (MMR) vaccine is generally well tolerated; occasionally, children develop fever or rash

7 to 12 days after immunization. Thrombocytopenia may occur within 2 months of administration; it is usually transient and benign. The risk of thrombocytopenia appears to be increased in children with a history of prior thrombocytopenia or thrombocytopenic purpura. Acute arthralgia or arthritis may be seen, particularly in postpubertal girls. Allergy to egg is no longer considered a contraindication to MMR administration; rare anaphylactic reactions to MMR are thought to be due to traces of gelatin, neomycin, or other substances in the vaccine.[1]

Polio

Oral polio vaccination programs have resulted in the eradication of wild polio in the Americas, and progress continues to be made toward worldwide eradication. There is an extremely small risk of vaccine-associated paralytic polio in live oral polio vaccine (OPV) recipients and their contacts; this low risk is now felt to be unacceptable in the United States. Therefore, inactivated polio vaccines (IPVs), which do not carry a risk of paralysis, are now recommended for the entire series of vaccinations in the United States. Allergic reactions are rare after polio vaccines, which contain trace amounts of neomycin and other antibiotics.

Pneumococcus

Heptavalent pneumococcal conjugate vaccine (PCV7, PREVNAR™) has recently been recommended for universal use in children less than or equal to 23 months of age and for selected older children.[5] The vaccine contains seven pneumococcal antigens conjugated to a nontoxic diphtheria protein. The most common adverse effects seen after pneumococcal vaccine (usually given simultaneously with other routine immunizations) include local reactions, fever, irritability, drowsiness, and decreased appetite.

Varicella

Live-attenuated varicella vaccine is generally well tolerated; adverse effects include local pain and redness, occasional fever, and rash at the injection site or elsewhere (up to a month after vaccination). Vaccine-induced immunity appears to be long lasting, with no increased incidence of zoster.[1] Varicella may occur in vaccinated children but is usually mild.

Combination Vaccines

Many new combination vaccines are being marketed or are under investigation. They aim to limit the number of injections and health-care visits, thereby limiting discomfort and increasing compliance with the extensive schedule of recommended immunizations. Current combination vaccines include DTP plus *H. influenzae* (Tetramune), and hepatitis B plus *H. influenzae* (Comvax). When *H. influenzae* vaccine is administered simultaneously with DTP, there is no change in the expected rate of systemic or local reactions from that expected with DTP alone.

DIFFERENTIAL DIAGNOSIS

The cause of neurologic problems that appear temporally related to vaccination is often difficult to determine, because infants are in an age group in which neurologic disorders and seizures commonly first occur. Most seizures seen shortly after immunization are simple febrile seizures. The child with fever after vaccination may have an infection (e.g., otitis media) as the cause.

EMERGENCY DEPARTMENT EVALUATION AND MANAGEMENT

Mild febrile or local reactions require only reassurance and symptomatic treatment. Children with suspected serious neurologic complications often require further evaluation, such as lumbar puncture or neuroradiologic imaging.

Passage of the National Childhood Vaccine Injury Act of 1986 instituted strict legal requirements for administering immunizations. There is now a National Vaccine Injury Compensation Program, which is a no-fault system for compensating persons experiencing severe or fatal vaccine complications. Detailed written information about risks and benefits, using official Vaccine Information Statements (VISs), must be provided before giving vaccines with pertussis, measles, mumps, rubella, polio, or tetanus–diphtheria toxoids, and the provision of such materials and informed consent should be documented. VISs will likely be required for other routine vaccinations in the future.

When a vaccine is administered, the following information must be recorded: (1) date; (2) vaccine type; (3) manufacturer; (4) lot number and expiration date; (5) site and route of administration; and (6) name, address, and title of the person administering the vaccine. Serious events suspected to be related to vaccine administration, including anaphylaxis, encephalopathy, brachial neuritis (tetanus toxoid), paralytic polio, chronic arthritis (rubella), thrombocytopenic purpura (measles), and early onset HIB disease (within 7 days of vaccination), must be reported the United States Department of Health and Human Services Vaccine Adverse Event Reporting System (VAERS), telephone 1-800-822-7967 or website (http://www.cdc.gov/nip/vaers.htm.)

DISPOSITION

Consultation with a pediatrician, infectious disease specialist, or neurologist should be obtained when a severe immunization reaction is suspected. Children with significant neurologic symptoms, anaphylaxis, or other serious vaccine complications should be hospitalized. Serious vaccine complications must be reported (see VAERS information in preceding section). The child's physician should provide follow-up care for discharged patients and be notified of the suspicion of an immunization reaction. Transfer to a tertiary pediatric facility should be considered if further subspecialty consultation or intensive care is needed.

COMMON PITFALLS

- Do not automatically attribute fever occurring after immunization to vaccination; thoroughly examine the child for a treatable focus of infection.
- Typical local and febrile reactions are not a contraindication to further doses of the vaccine.
- Routine immunizations are not contraindicated in children with minor febrile illnesses.

References

1. American Academy of Pediatrics. *2000 Red book: report of the Committee on Infectious Diseases,* 25th ed. Elk Grove Village, IL: American Academy of Pediatrics, 2000.
2. American Academy of Pediatrics, Committee on Infectious Diseases. Acellular pertussis vaccine: recommendations for use as the initial series in infants and children. *Pediatrics* 1997;99:282–288.
3. American Academy of Pediatrics, Committee on Infectious Diseases. The relationship between pertussis vaccine and central nervous system sequelae: continuing assessment. *Pediatrics* 1996;97:279–281.

4. American Academy of Pediatrics, Committee on Infectious Diseases. Poliomyelitis prevention: revised recommendations for use of inactivated and live oral poliovirus vaccine. *Pediatrics* 1999;103:171–172.
5. American Academy of Pediatrics, Committee on Infectious Diseases. Recommendations for the prevention of pneumococcal infections, including the use of pneumococcal conjugate vaccine (Prevnar), pneumococcal polysaccharide vaccine, and antibiotic prophylaxis. AAP website, www.aap.org, June 2000.
6. Ball LK, Evans G, Bostrom A. Risky business: challenges in vaccine risk communication. *Pediatrics* 1998;101:453–458.
7. Centers for Disease Control and Prevention. Update: vaccine side effects, adverse reactions, contraindications, and precautions—recommendations of the Advisory Committee on Immunization Practices (ACIP). *MMWR* 1996;45(RR-12):1–35.
8. Centers for Disease Control and Prevention. Progress toward eliminating *Haemophilus influenzae* type B disease among infants and children—United States, 1987–1997. *MMWR* 1998;47:993–998.
9. Institute of Medicine, Howson CP, Howe CJ, Fineberg HV, eds. *Adverse effects of pertussis and rubella vaccines*. Washington, DC: National Academy Press, 1991.
10. Institute of Medicine, Stratton KR, Howe CJ, Johnston RB, eds. *Adverse effects associated with childhood vaccines: evidence bearing on causality*. Washington, DC: National Academy Press, 1994.
11. Robinson PF, Gausche M, Gerardi MJ, et al. Immunization of the pediatric patient in the emergency department. *Ann Emerg Med* 1996;28:334–341.
12. Stratton KR, Howe CJ, Johnston RB. Adverse events associated with childhood vaccines other than pertussis and rubella: summary of a report from the Institute of Medicine. *JAMA* 1994;271:1602–1605.

CHAPTER 275
Impetigo

Jeffrey G. Michael and Jane F. Knapp

Impetigo is the most common infection of the skin in children.[7,8,12] It is more prevalent during warm, humid summer months in temperate climates, but year round in more tropical climates. Impetigo affects the entire pediatric population, with a mean patient age of 5 years.[8]

Impetigo is caused by either *Staphylococcus aureus* or group A beta-hemolytic streptococci (usually *S. pyogenes*), or both. Within the past decade, penicillin-resistant *S. aureus* has emerged as the predominant pathogen causing impetigo.[4,5,7,9,10]

Generally, bacterial invasion occurs through a break in the skin traumatized by a scratch, abrasion, or insect bite. Two distinct clinical forms have been described. Classic or nonbullous impetigo may be either staphylococcal or streptococcal or a mixed infection. Bullous impetigo is generally agreed to be due to *S. aureus* alone. In nonbullous impetigo, the lesion begins as a papule or vesicle that erodes and forms a thick, honey-colored crust. The lesions are initially discrete but may coalesce with progression of infection. When the crust is removed, a cloudy serous fluid exudes from a moist erythematous base. The lesions of bullous impetigo are flaccid bullae filled with a cloudy fluid. The bullae are often ruptured before presentation, leaving a shiny, lacquered, erythematous base with peeling edges.

The lesions of both forms of impetigo are usually not painful. Impetigo is most commonly encountered on the extremities, face, or buttocks. Fever and systemic involvement are rare, although nonbullous impetigo frequently is accompanied by lymphadenopathy. When treated, impetigo heals completely without scarring.

CLINICAL PRESENTATION

The patient with nonbullous impetigo generally seeks treatment because the infection is spreading or has been unresponsive to topical antibiotics. The child with bullous impetigo is usually brought for medical attention soon after infection because of parental alarm at the appearance of the bullae. The neonate with bullous impetigo is at risk for systemic involvement. The source of infection is often the nursery where the baby was born. When the possibility of bullous impetigo secondary to *S. aureus* occurs in a neonate in the period 2 weeks post discharge from the nursery, the emergency department should alert the newborn nursery of the possibility of an *S. aureus* epidemic.

The major complication of impetigo, acute poststreptococcal glomerulonephritis, has an incidence of 1% to 5%, with higher occurrences during epidemic infections.[7,12] Treatment with antibiotics does not prevent the development of acute glomerulonephritis. The nephritis most commonly affects patients between 3 and 7 years of age and has a latent period averaging 18 to 21 days. Anti-DNAase B titers are elevated when the source of infection is the skin, with antistreptolysin-O titers rising minimally to none at all. Rheumatic fever has not been established as a sequel of impetigo.[7,8]

Other rare but possible complications of impetigo include cellulitis, regional adenitis, osteomyelitis, and sepsis.

DIFFERENTIAL DIAGNOSIS

The diagnosis of impetigo is commonly made on the basis of the typical appearance of the lesions. The differential diagnosis includes other vesicular or crusted dermatologic conditions or thermal burns. On occasion, impetigo may be mistaken for burns, especially cigarette burns, but cigarette burns are usually deeper, more punched-out-appearing lesions and do not have the distribution characteristic of bullous impetigo. Bullous impetigo on the buttocks has been difficult to differentiate from suspected child abuse due to submersion scald burns.[11] Chickenpox is distinguished by the appearance of a macular, papular erythematous rash, which then turns into vesicles. The rash and vesicles start centrally and progress peripherally, appear in crops, may be present on mucous membranes, and are often accompanied by systemic symptoms of illness.

Herpes zoster is distinguished by its characteristic dermatomal distribution. Herpes simplex should be suspected when the vesicles have a grouped or tightly coalesced appearance. The child may complain of itching, burning, or pain, and there may be a history of previous occurrences at the same site. Hand-foot-and-mouth disease is usually caused by a coxsackievirus infection. The vesicles are individual, firm, and oval and are most often located on the palms and soles and in the mouth. Scabies is frequently vesicular or pustular in children. Helpful points in differentiation of scabies are its characteristic distribution on the wrists and in the web spaces of the fingers and toes, complaints of intense pruritus, and presence of similar lesions in other family members.

Contact dermatitis such as poison ivy can be vesicular or crusted. There is usually a history of exposure, and the lesions are pruritic and grouped in streaks. Occasionally, tinea corporis may be mistaken for impetigo when the lesions are crusted.

EMERGENCY DEPARTMENT EVALUATION

Impetigo can usually be identified by the characteristic appearance of its lesions, and cultures are not typically needed. Many skin conditions in children become impetiginized. Common examples are chickenpox, scabies, and atopic dermatitis. Patients with atopic dermatitis have been noted to have an increasing incidence of streptococcal impetigo in addition to increased colonization of *S. aureus*.[1] All patients with impetiginized skin conditions need to be treated with antibiotics.

EMERGENCY DEPARTMENT MANAGEMENT

Impetigo is treated with systemic antibiotics, although mupirocin 2% (Bactroban) has been studied extensively and has been found to be as effective as systemic antibiotics when used alone for limited infections, which are generally described as a few lesions to one area of the body.[2,3] Penicillin is no longer recommended as a therapy option due to resistance issues.[8] The oral antibiotics chosen should have good *S. aureus* coverage. Infants with bullous impetigo may need admission and intravenous therapy if they have systemic signs of illness. Appropriate oral therapy includes the macrolides, clindamycin, cloxacillin, and cephalexin. The dosage of cloxacillin is 50 to 100 mg/kg/d, divided in four equal doses. Erythromycin estolate can be given as 40 mg/kg/d, divided in two or four equal doses. The dosage for erythromycin ethylsuccinate is 40 to 50 mg/kg/d, divided in three or four equal doses. The maximum dosage for each is 1 g/kg/d, not to exceed 250 mg four times per day.

In 1994, clarithromycin was approved for uncomplicated skin infections in children at a dosage of 15 mg/kg/d, divided two times per day. This medication has been shown to have fewer gastrointestinal side effects, and the dosing schedule suggests improved compliance, perhaps offsetting the increased cost.[7] Cephalexin can be given as 40 to 50 mg/kg/d, divided three to four times per day. The dosage of clindamycin is 15 mg/kg/d, divided three or four times per day. Concern for increased association of the development of *Clostridium difficile* toxin–associated diarrhea has been reported with clindamycin. Thus, tempered with the fact that any antibiotic can change the normal intestinal flora, leading to overgrowth of *C. difficile* and the risk of toxin-mediated diarrhea, clindamycin is a less desirable choice. All oral therapy is recommended for 7 to 10 days.

Currently, the rate of erythromycin resistance to *S. aureus* in children reported from studies in the United States is 10% to 20%. Israel and Australia have reported rates in the range of 30% to 50%. Treatment failure rates with erythromycin are higher in areas of known ethyromycin-resistant strains than in areas with erythromycin-sensitive strains. The treating physician's knowledge of regional sensitivity of erythromycin against *S. aureus* is helpful when making a decision to use this medication.[6,7,9]

DISPOSITION

Consultation with a dermatologist or infectious disease specialist is generally not required. Rarely does a child need to be admitted to the hospital, except in cases of extensive disease, immunocompromised states, or infants with bullous impetigo with systemic involvement. Unfortunately, some cases of impetigo may be unresponsive to therapy due to parental inability to effectively provide the medication, and thus these children may warrant admission for compliance issues. In most cases, follow-up is not indicated unless a satisfactory clinical response is not achieved in 7 days, at which point, a culture of the site is recommended to evaluate for resistance.[7]

COMMON PITFALLS

- Treatment failures due to error in diagnosis, poor compliance with medication, or medication resistance
- Difficulty differentiating impetigo from burns due to child abuse
- Recognition that bullous impetigo in neonates may be related to nursery epidemics

References

1. Adachi J, et al. Increasing incidence of streptococcal impetigo in atopic dermatitis. *J Dermatol Sci* 1998;17:45.
2. Bass JW, et al. Comparison of oral cephalexin, topical mupirocin and topical bacitracin for treatment of impetigo. *Pediatr Infect Dis J* 1997;16:708.
3. Booth JH, Benrimoj SI. Mupirocin in the treatment of impetigo. *Int J Dermatol* 1992;31:1.
4. Bisno AL, Stevens DL. Streptococcal infections of skin and soft tissues. *N Engl J Med* 1996;334:240.
5. Brook I, Frazier EH, Yeager JK. Microbiology of nonbullous impetigo. *Pediatr Dermatol* 1997;14:192.
6. Darmstadt GL. Antibiotics in the management of pediatric skin disease. *Dermatol Clin* 1998;16:509.
7. Darmstadt GL, Lane AT. Impetigo: an overview. *Pediatr Dermatol* 1994;11:293.
8. Melish ME, Bertuch AA. Bacterial skin infection. In: Feigin RD, Cherry JD, eds. *Textbook of pediatric infectious diseases*, 4th ed, vol 1. Philadelphia: WB Saunders, 1998:741.
9. Misko ML, Terracina JR, Diven DG. The frequency of erythromycin-resistant *Staphylococcus aureus* in impetiginized dermatoses. *Pediatr Dermatol* 1995;12:12.
10. Sadick SS. Current aspects of bacterial infections of the skin. *Dermatol Clin* 1997;15:341.
11. Scales JW, et al. Bullous impetigo. *Arch Pediatr Adolesc Med* 1997;151:1168.
12. Shriner DL, Schwartz RA, Janniger CK. Impetigo. *Cutis* 1995;56:30.

CHAPTER 276

Infestations: Scabies, Lice, and Pinworms

R. Wayne Wolfram, Kevin R. Kowaleski, Eugene Izsak, and Amy S. Spangler

SCABIES

Scabies (from the Latin *scabere*, meaning "to scratch") is a highly contagious, pruritic skin rash caused by the mite *Sarcoptes scabiei*. The female mite, 0.3 mm in length, burrows beneath the skin while laying two to three eggs per day. Eggs hatch after 3 to 4 days, and the larvae migrate toward the surface of the skin, where they mature from the nymph stage into adults in 2 weeks. After mating, the adult female migrates more deeply into the skin, continuing the mite's life cycle (which totals 30 days).

Transmission usually occurs via close personal contact. Other varieties of scabies (dog, cat, bird, horse) may transiently infest humans, but this is a self-limited infestation, as these mites cannot reproduce in humans. Scabies is most commonly seen during the winter. Live mites have been recovered from floors, furniture, and clothing, but transmission from fomites is thought to be unusual. The incubation period is 10 to 30 days. However, the rash is a delayed type IV hypersensitivity, so a recurrent infestation may produce symptoms within 24 hours.

Prevalence has increased in the United States over the past several years. The highest incidence is in the pediatric age group.

CLINICAL PRESENTATION

Patients usually present with persistent generalized pruritus. Itching is typically worse at night, and it may precede the actual rash. The rash may consist of papules (often crusted), vesicles, pustules, or nodules. The classic lesion (not seen in the majority of patients) is a 2- to 10-mm-long, threadlike, raised serpiginous burrow with a terminal papule or vesicle. The mite may be visible as a black dot at the leading end. More commonly, lesions consist of multiple, small, erythematous papules, often excoriated. Lesions have a predilection for the hands and feet (particularly the web spaces), axilla, flexor aspects of the wrists or forearms, buttocks crease, genitalia, female breasts and nipples, and umbilicus or belt line. The face and scalp are generally spared, except in young children.

Chronic lesions tend to be more nodular and reddish brown. They are most likely to be seen on the genitalia or in the axillae. Mites may not be found in these lesions.

Neonatal scabies is uncommon but tends to be more generalized, with pustules and eczematoid changes. Such an infant may manifest irritability due to pruritus.

Norwegian scabies presents with gross scaling, especially of the hands, feet, scalp, and pressure-bearing areas. Pruritus is variable and may be minimal. This form is more likely to be seen in the immunocompromised or debilitated patient. Norwegian scabies is extremely contagious: An affected individual may harbor millions of mites (versus the usual dozen or so that are present in a typical infestation).

Secondary bacterial infection of lesions is not uncommon, and scabies may also complicate other dermatoses. Treatment with topical steroids may alter the inflammatory component of the rash and decrease pruritus.

DIFFERENTIAL DIAGNOSIS

Atopic dermatitis is commonly confused with scabies, but it tends not to involve the web spaces, axilla, or wrists. Hand-foot-mouth disease is usually seen with fever and mucosal lesions. Dyshidrotic eczema may manifest as vesicles on the sides of the fingers. Papular urticaria may cause confusion with scabies, but these lesions are self-limited and do not spread over time. Acropustulosis of infancy consists of recurring crops of pruritic papules, vesicles, and pustules. Other considerations in the differential diagnosis include contact dermatitis, dermatitis herpetiformis, syphilis, folliculitis, pityriasis rosea, impetigo, seborrhea, nodular lymphoma, psoriasis, lichen planus, fiberglass exposure, histiocytosis X, and keratosis follicularis.

EMERGENCY DEPARTMENT EVALUATION

Microscopic examination of a skin scraping for mites, eggs, or feces is 90% to 95% sensitive when done properly (many emergency departments are not equipped to do this test). To perform this test, choose a nonexcoriated burrow or papule. Place a drop of mineral oil on the lesion, then scrape it with a no. 15 blade deeply enough to produce no more than a speck of blood. Transfer the scraping to a glass slide and examine it under 40× magnification.

Detection of burrows may be facilitated by applying topical tetracycline, wiping it away, then using a Wood lamp (burrows retain the tetracycline and fluoresce). Alternatively, rub a suspected site with a washable felt-tip marker and wipe it away with alcohol (the burrow retains the ink).

EMERGENCY DEPARTMENT MANAGEMENT

Permethrin 5% (Elimite) has replaced lindane (Kwell) as the treatment of choice for scabies. In randomized studies, permethrin has proved more efficacious than lindane and is also less absorbed through the skin (less than 2% vs. 10%), with lower potential for toxicity. Permethrin is neurotoxic to mites, causing paralysis.

Permethrin should be applied from the neck or hairline to the toes and washed off in 10 to 12 hours. Many authorities advise a second application in 1 week. The only contraindication to its use is known hypersensitivity to permethrin (or formaldehyde, one of its ingredients). It has been classified as category B for pregnant patients (usually safe, but benefits must outweigh risks). The patient may experience mild stinging or burning. Children, adolescents, and adults should apply cream over the entire body below the head. Permethrin may be safely used in children past 2 months of age. With infants and toddlers, the cream should be applied over the head, neck, and body (avoiding the eyes), with special attention to postauricular areas, hands, and feet, and should be washed off after 10 to 12 hours.

Alternative therapies, which should be needed rarely, include lindane (Kwell , Scabine), crotamiton (Eurax) cream or lotion, sulfur in petrolatum, and Ivermectin (0.2 mg/kg orally for one dose). Lindane is contraindicated in infants less than 6 months of age and in pregnant women, and it is applied as the permethrin cream. Lindane should not be applied after a warm bath, because absorption may be enhanced. It should be removed in 8 to 12 hours, with a repeat application in 1 week. Crotamiton is applied to the whole body once a day for 2 days followed by a bath 48 hours after the last application. Retreatment with crotamiton in 2 weeks is suggested. Sulfur ointment 6% to 8% is an old treatment that is less effective, smelly, and causes stains.

Response to treatment is not dependent on the number of lesions present. The patient should be advised that symptoms may not resolve for 2 to 4 weeks; the nodular form may persist for many weeks after treatment. Therefore, it is prudent to prescribe antipruritic therapy: diphenhydramine, hydroxyzine, or a judicious use of topical steroids. Usually, patients are no longer infectious 24 hours after treatment.

All clothing, bedding, and towels contacted within the 2 days prior to treatment should be either washed in hot water, dry cleaned, or stored for 1 week. It is best to treat every person in the household simultaneously (even asymptomatic individuals), as the prolonged incubation period makes it difficult to know with certainty who is infested. Secondarily infected lesions should be treated with appropriate antimicrobial medication.

DISPOSITION

Follow-up in 2 weeks with the patient's primary care physician should suffice in most cases. Dermatology consultation may be prudent in severe cases or in immunocompromised patients.

COMMON PITFALLS

- Consider scabies in any patient with pruritus, even if skin findings are minimal. Be alert to the varying manifestations.
- Treat all family and household contacts simultaneously, whether symptomatic or not.
- Consider other sexually transmitted diseases in those who have contracted scabies through sexual contact.
- Do not prescribe repeated courses of Lindane, due to its cumulative neurotoxicity.

- Do not fail to treat secondary bacterial infection with appropriate antimicrobials.
- Provide families with adequate anticipatory guidance regarding the use of medications. Inform patients that even successful treatment may result in little improvement for several weeks afterward.
- Inadequate anticipatory guidance related to environmental measures: At the time of treatment, all clothing and linens should be dry-cleaned or washed with hot water and put in a hot dryer for 20 minutes. Items unable to be washed or dry-cleaned should be placed in a sealed plastic container for at least 7 days (until eggs hatch).
- Inadequate anticipatory guidance related to personal care: Avoid overbathing, as it may cause further irritation of the skin.

LICE

Lice are blood-sucking, wingless ectoparasites. Three species commonly infest humans: *Pediculus humanus capitis* (head louse), *Pediculus humanus corporis* (body louse), and *Phthirus pubis* (pubic louse or crab). *Pediculus* species can interbreed. The pubic louse is morphologically distinct from the other two and primarily infests the pubic and anogenital areas, but it may infest the eyelashes, brows, beard, axilla, and, rarely, the scalp.

P. capitis has worldwide distribution. In the United States, it is the louse that most commonly produces infestation. Most infestations involve between 10 and 20 lice. Hair length and cleanliness are not significant factors in infestation. The louse is spread by close physical contact and by shared fomites, such as combs, brushes, hats, or bedding. School-age children have the highest prevalence—an estimated 10% to 40% in U.S. schools. Incidence is greatest in late summer and autumn. African Americans in the United States have a lower rate of infestation than do other racial or ethnic groups. Head lice are not known vectors for other diseases.

P. corporis has a life cycle similar to that of the head louse, except that it lives in clothing and inhabits the host's skin only to feed. It is generally found on those with poor hygiene and living in overcrowded conditions. Unlike the head louse, the body louse is a known vector of rickettsial diseases.

P. pubis is commonly transmitted via sexual contact. Infested individuals have a 30% to 40% risk of another sexually transmitted disease, and should therefore be investigated for such infections. If found on children, sexual abuse should be suspected. *P. pubis* can inhabit any hair-bearing area, but it is usually found in the pubic and perineal regions. It is the only louse known to infest eyelashes and eyebrows.

CLINICAL PRESENTATION

Pruritis is the most common symptom. Careful inspection may reveal nits cemented in place at the base of the hair shaft. Detection is aided by the use of a Wood lamp to reveal the fluorescent nits. Nits greater than 10 mm from the scalp are either hatched or nonviable. Body lice lay nits in the seams of the clothing, not on the host directly. Head lice most commonly inhabit the hair line near the ears and the nape of the neck.

DIFFERENTIAL DIAGNOSIS

Any condition with itching and scalp or skin irritation should be considered:

Tinea capitis
Contact dermatitis
Seborrheic dermatitis
Atopic dermatitis
Superficial skin infections
Scabies
Eczema

EMERGENCY DEPARTMENT EVALUATION

A history of exposure and/or intense pruritis should prompt a careful search for nits or adult lice, using a Wood lamp to help find the nits. Excoriations, secondary infections, and local lymphadenopathy may be present.

EMERGENCY DEPARTMENT MANAGEMENT

Pediculicides

Body lice do not require medications if infested clothing can be removed and destroyed (or disinfected).

For head lice, 1% permethrin (available over the counter under the brand name Nix) is effective in over 90% of cases. It is a topical cream rinse, applied after the hair is washed with an over-the-counter shampoo. In addition to killing adult lice, it also has ovicidal activity. Hair should not be rewashed for 24 hours after application.

Pyrethrins, which contain piperonyl butoxide (A-200, Rid) is another class of agents for treatment. These medications are contraindicated in patients with ragweed allergy. Pyrethrin is not ovicidal, so retreatment is necessary in 7 to 10 days to kill newly hatched nymphs.

Lindane (1%) shampoo (Kwell) is also available but has been associated with seizures. Therefore, lindane is usually recommended for patients who fail to respond to permethrin or pyrethrin. Lindane is contraindicated in infants and pregnancy. The lindane shampoo is applied as a cream rinse after washing the hair with a nonmedicated shampoo. Allow the medication to remain in place for no more than 4 minutes and then rinse thoroughly. For body lice, apply it as a cream or lotion, leave it on for 8 to 12 hours, and then rinse. For pubic lice, apply it as a shampoo for 10 minutes, then rinse, and apply it again in 2 weeks.

Malathion lotion (0.5% and 1.0%) is an alternative therapy that binds to the hair shaft for 4 weeks. However, it is flammable and must be used with caution. Its potential for toxicity is still being investigated. This medication is no longer available in the United States. In other countries, the recommended use is for the 1% shampoo. It is to be utilized in two 10-minute applications approximately 7 days apart.

New on the market is the oral antihelmintic, ivermectin. A single dose of 0.2 mg/kg is highly effective, with virtually no side effects. Retreatment is often recommended in 7 days to kill any residual surviving adults and nits.

An infestation of the eyelashes can be treated with petroleum ointment (Vaseline) applied to coat the lashes two to three times a day for 8 to 14 days. Using a small beard or mustache comb to mechanically remove nits on eyelashes is a necessary adjunct to petroleum ointment.

Nit Removal

An important adjunct to the use of pediculicides is the use a fine-tooth comb to remove nits in treated individuals. Most U.S. schools have a "no-nit" policy to prevent the classroom spread of lice infestations. Therefore, it is important to instruct patients and families on the differentiation between nits and benign hair casts. This will prevent reinfection as well as unnecessary retreatment, which can be a toxic hazard.

A proper comb and correct technique in combing the hair are essential for adequate nit removal. Most pediculicides include a nit-removal comb. A minimum of 20 minutes should be spent combing damp hair—divided into 1-in. sections—working from the crown of the head downward. Special attention should be given to the postauricular and nape areas, because head lice preferentially seek these regions of the scalp.

The cement used to attach the nit to the hair shaft can be loosened using a 50:50 rinse solution of vinegar and water. The solution should be applied to the hair, covered with a warm, moist towel for 30 minutes, and then the hair combed as described previously. A commercial product (Step 2) containing 8% formic acid may also aid in nit removal. When infestation is heavy, a haircut may be preferable to tedious nit removal.

Environmental Measures

Environmental measures are necessary for adequate treatment and prevention of reinfestation. Machine washing in hot water and hot-cycle drying of all clothing, headgear, bedding, and linen kills adult lice and nits. Combs, brushes, and hair accessories should be soaked in hot water (128.3°F), with or without a pediculicide shampoo, for 15 minutes, followed by a hot-water rinse. Items unable to be washed (stuffed animals, etc.) should be either dry cleaned or placed in a well-sealed plastic bag for 10 days to kill both adults and nits.

Family members, friends, school or daycare contacts, and other contacts should be examined for asymptomatic infestation.

DISPOSITION

Simultaneous treatment of all family members is recommended to prevent intrafamily reinfestation. In addition , children found to be infested with *P. pubis* should be evaluated for other sexually transmitted diseases and possible sexual abuse.

COMMON PITFALLS

- Failure to reassure patients and families that lice infestation is not a social disease
- Inadequate evaluation and treatment of close contacts
- Failure to adequately educate patients and families regarding procedures to fully remove nits and nit differentiation
- Failure to educate patients and families on the necessity to retreat in 7 days
- Failure of the health-care provider to suspect sexually transmitted diseases and sexual abuse in children infested with *P. pubis*
- Failure to treat secondary infection with appropriate antimicrobial agents
- Inadequate anticipatory guidance to patients and/or parents regarding adequate procedures to remove nits and adult lice from fomites and the environment
- Failure to remember that pyrethrins are contraindicated in patients with ragweed allergy

ENTEROBIASIS (PINWORMS)

Enterobius vermicularis, a small nematode, is a common cause of helminthic infestation in the United States. All socioeconomic levels are affected, and infestation often occurs in family clusters. Infestation does not equate with poor home sanitary measures. Prevalence is greatest in 5- to 9 year-old children, but all ages can be affected. One widely quoted source (Pomeranz and Fairley, 1998) estimates a prevalence of 5% to 15% in the general population, with this rate declining in recent years.

E. vermicularis is an obligate parasite, with humans as the only natural host. Both males and females are affected. Fecal–oral contamination via fomites (toys, clothes) is a common method of infestation. After ingestion, eggs usually hatch in the duodenum within 6 hours. Worms mature in as little as 2 weeks. Adult worms normally inhabit the terminal ileum, cecum, vermiform appendix, and proximal ascending colon. The worms live free in the intestinal lumen, and little evidence exists to support invasion of healthy tissue under normal conditions. The female worm migrates to the rectum after copulation. If not expelled during defecation, she migrates to the perineum (often at night), where she releases an average of 11,000 eggs and then dies. Eggs can survive in the environment for up to 3 weeks under optimum conditions.

CLINICAL PRESENTATION

Pruritus ani and pruritus vulvae are common presenting complaints. One study (Hogan et al., 1991), however, failed to find an increase of these symptoms in infested children, compared with matched controls. Occasionally, the gravid female may migrate aberrantly into the human female genitalia and produce vaginitis. Association with small and large intestine ulcerations, appendicitis, perianal abscesses, intestinal pain, transient synovitis, or enuresis is not causal.

DIFFERENTIAL DIAGNOSIS

Other diagnoses to consider include appendicitis (more severe abdominal discomfort), cervicitis (localized tenderness and inflammation of the cervix), dermatitis, contact dermatitis, giardiasis, inflammatory bowel disease (mucoid or bloody stools), roundworm or tapeworm infestation (eosinophilia), and vulvovaginitis.

EMERGENCY DEPARTMENT EVALUATION

Patients often have excoriation or erythema of the perineum and/or vulvae, but infestation can occur without these signs. Visual sighting of a worm by a reliable source (i.e., a parent) is usually accepted as evidence of infestation and grounds for treatment. Worms are commonly found among stools or on the patient's perineum at night. Without a visual report, diagnosis can be confirmed by using the knowledge that eggs are normally deposited in great quantities on the perineum of a host at night. Wide (2-in.) transparent tape pressed against the perineum in the morning before the patient washes will capture eggs. Diagnosis is made by identifying eggs under the low-power lens of the microscope, using a slide to which dilute sodium hydroxide or toluene is added.

EMERGENCY DEPARTMENT MANAGEMENT

Treatment of pinworms is via family education and medications administered as an outpatient. Fear and guilt are common parental reactions to parasitic worm infestation. Many families come to the emergency department with misconceptions about pinworms. It is helpful to inform them that infestation occurs in spite of proper child and household hygiene. Families also should be counseled to avoid overreaction through aggressive sanitary measures.

DISPOSITION

Pyrantel pamoate (11 mg/kg; maximum, 1,000 mg) with a repeat treatment in 2 weeks is effective. An alternative is mebendazole (100 mg, regardless of weight), also repeated in 2 weeks. Because asymptomatic infestation of other members in a household is frequent, it may be reasonable to treat all household members simultaneously. Families should be informed that repeat infestations are common. If reinfestation occurs, it is treated in the same fashion as an initial infestation.

Symptomatic relief of pruritus can be obtained by applying topical antipruritic ointments or creams (1% hydrocortisone) to the perianal region.

COMMON PITFALLS

- Failure to assure patients and families that pinworm infestation is not a social disease, and is a self-limited disease with frequent reinfections
- Failure to consider that families may need to be treated as a group
- Failure to instruct patients and families that no special hygienic measures are necessary. However, reassurance can be provided that using simple, prudent measures, such as clipping fingernails (a favorite repository for eggs), washing hands frequently, showering daily in the morning, and normal laundering of linen weekly, are activities that can help prevent recurrence.

Bibliography

Scabies

Amer M, El-Gharib I. Permethrin versus crotamiton and lindane in the treatment of scabies. *Int J Dermatol* 1992;31:357–358.

Hogan DJ, Schachner L, Tanglertsampan C. Diagnosis and treatment of childhood scabies and pediculosis. *Pediatr Clin North Am* 1991;38:41–57.

Molinaro MJ, Schwartz RA, Janniger CK. Scabies. *Cutis* 1995;56:317–321.

Peterson CM, Eichenfield LF. Scabies. *Pediatr Ann* 1996;25:97–100.

Pomeranz AJ, Fairley JA. The systematic evaluation of the skin in children. *Pediatr Clin North Am* 1998;45:49–63.

Schult MW, et al. Comparative study of 5% permethrin cream and 1% lindane lotion for the treatment of scabies. *Arch Dermatol* 1990;126:167–170.

Sciammarella J. Scabies. In: Plantz S, ed. *Emergency medicine online reference text* (http://www.emedicine.com/emerg) 1999.

Lice

American Academy of Pediatrics. Pediculosis. In: American Academy of Pediatrics. *Report of the committee on infectious diseases,* 24th ed. Elk Grove Village, IL: American Academy of Pediatrics, 1997:387–390.

Bradenburg K, et al. 1% permethrin cream rinse vs. 1% lindane shampoo in treating pediculosis capitis. *Am J Dis Child* 1986;140:894–896.

Colven RM, Prose NS. Parasitic infestations of the skin. *Pediatr Ann* 1994;23:436–442.

Hogan DJ, et al. Diagnosis and treatment of childhood scabies and pediculosis. *Pediatr Clin North Am* 1991;38:941–957.

Drugs for head lice *Med Lett* January 17, 1997.

Drugs for parasitic infections. *Med Lett* January 2, 1998.

Wolfram RW. Lice. In: Plantz S, ed. *Emergency medicine online reference text* (http://www.emedicine.com/emerg) 1999.

Pinworms

American Academy of Pediatrics. *Enterobius vermicularis.* In: American Academy of Pediatrics. *Report of the committee on infectious diseases,* 24th ed. Elk Grove Village, IL: American Academy of Pediatrics, 1997:407–408.

Symmers W St C. Pathology of oxyuriasis. *Arch Pathol* 1950;50:475.

Weller TH, Sorenson CW. Enterobiasis: its incidence and symptomatology in a group of 505 children. *N Engl J Med* 1941;224:143.

Wolfram RW. Pinworms. In: Plantz S, ed. *Emergency medicine online reference text* (http://www.emedicine.com/emerg) 1999.

CHAPTER 277
Intussusception

Jonathan I. Singer

Intussusception, an invagination of a proximal portion of the intestine into a distal adjacent part, is a common cause of intestinal obstruction. Classically, it occurs in well-nourished children, most often boys. Approximately two-thirds of cases are seen prior to age 2, with most of those occurring between the fifth and ninth month.[14] Intussusceptions that occur beyond age 2 tend to cluster around the third year, but intussusceptions have been reported throughout the age spectrum, including adulthood.[11]

In all age groups, ileocolic intussusceptions predominate (75% to 95%), and greater than 90% are idiopathic.[1] Abnormal lead points include Meckel's diverticulum, polyps, duplication cysts, hemangioma, and tumors.[3] Irrespective of cause, early diagnosis is essential; the duration of intussusception before treatment bears a close relationship to its morbidity and mortality.[5,14]

CLINICAL PRESENTATION

The cardinal symptoms of intussusception are abdominal pain, vomiting, and rectal bleeding. In a typical case, there is a sudden onset of severe abdominal pain that may last several minutes. After an asymptomatic interval, repeated paroxysms will cause the child to cry out again. The child may be impossible to console or may seem comfortable only in a knee–chest position in the arms of an attendant. Vomiting may occur either with the initial painful episode or soon after. Concurrent with vomiting, the child usually has one or more bowel movements, which vary from thin liquid to formed stools. Within 12 to 24 hours, mucus, blood, or both may be passed per rectum.[20]

This classic triad of paroxysmal pain, vomiting, and rectal bleeding is found in less than one-third of all patients.[1,5] Only 85% manifest colicky abdominal pain. Approximately 75% of patients experience vomiting. Nonbilious vomiting may become bilious as bowel obstruction progresses. Rectal bleeding is a less constant historic feature and may be found in as little as 40% of patients.[11] Frank blood, or blood-streaked stools, may be present within a few hours of the first painful episode. "Currant jelly" stools, which are bloody, maroon, and mucus-laden, account for a minority of bloody stools and are typically seen after prolonged symptomatology.[2,20]

Recognition of the stereotypic history facilitates the diagnosis. When there is historic aberrancy, a less than classic presentation contributes to diagnostic uncertainty.[10] Among the factors that contribute to misdiagnosis, several predominate. Altered mental status contributes most to delayed diagnosis. Apathy or listlessness may occasionally be the dominant concern of the parent. This altered sensorium with intussusception may be seen in the context of prolonged symptomatology or as the initial complaint.[12,15] Intussusception may not be considered when it occurs later in childhood.[11] A painless event may occur in 15% of cases and reduces diagnostic accuracy.[2] Sometimes, blood never passes per rectum. Stool from the rectal examination early in the course may be normal-appearing, and guaiac may be negative.

The physical appearance of an affected child may be variable.[5] Most children will be alert and hydrated. Those with advanced disease complicated by either fluid or electrolyte imbalance or blood loss may appear less responsive.[7] Not uncommonly, a child with a very brief history of enteric manifestations may be obtunded at presentation.[6] Other findings are limited to the abdominal examination.

On inspection, the abdomen may appear scaphoid. The right lower quadrant may seem empty (Dances sign).[9] A sausage-shaped, sometimes ill-defined, and variably tender mass is present in 25% to 89% of patients. The mass will be subhepatic early in the course of ileocolic intussusception. Abdominal guarding and distention are infrequent. A mass may be palpable on rectal examination. On rare occasions, even with a short history, the advancing mass prolapses through the anus.

DIFFERENTIAL DIAGNOSIS

Intussusception is readily diagnosed in the 10% to 17% of young children who present with the constellation of abdominal pain, vomiting, rectal bleeding, and abdominal mass.[5,16] When the picture is less complete, other diagnoses that may be entertained include intestinal obstruction from other causes, such as malrotation with midgut volvulus or incarcerated hernia. Other considerations include pseudomembranous or infectious enterocolitis, acute gastroenteritis, Hirschsprung disease, appendicitis, appendicial abscess, and peritonitis.[1,2] Metabolic derangement, endocrinopathy, intoxication, occult cranial trauma, sepsis, and meningitis may be considered in those patients with intussusception who present with altered mental status.[6,8]

EMERGENCY DEPARTMENT EVALUATION

Several laboratory investigations may guide the medical decision making in patients with a provisional diagnosis of intussusception.[7,14] A stool examination for occult blood has a high benefit-to-cost ratio. A negative guaiac should not be used to exclude the diagnosis, yet a positive stool guaiac should reduce the threshold for further evaluative and management decisions. When symptoms are brief and the child appears nontoxic and well hydrated, blood chemistries and a hemogram are not warranted. However, a complete blood count, serum electrolytes, blood urea nitrogen, creatinine, and urinalysis may facilitate decision making concerning a child who appears to be volume depleted. A blood sugar is required for the child with altered mental status. Further, the child who appears septic should have cultures of blood, urine, stool, and cerebrospinal fluid.[15]

A variety of imaging procedures can be utilized for a provisional diagnosis of intussusception.[17,18] When there is a high index of suspicion, supine and upright or supine and left lateral decubitus radiographs of the abdomen should be obtained.[6,9] Depending on the time course at presentation, age of the patient, and presence of a lead point, films may be normal or reveal nonspecific findings such as localized air–fluid levels or reduced intestinal air. The presence of a mass or obliteration of usual gas shadows of the colon is suggestive of intussusception. The presumed diagnosis can be confirmed only by plain film findings if the head of the intussusception is clearly visible in the bowel lumen. Those with nonspecific or suggestive findings should have either a barium or an air contrast enema.[19] Those patients with radiographic evidence of complete bowel obstruction, intraperitoneal air, ascites, or pneumatoses intestinalis should not be subjected to contrast enema.

When there is a lower index of suspicion for intussusception, ultrasonography may be useful.[8] Suggestive findings are created by the edematous head of the intussusception.[2] Findings include a "target" or "donut" sign on transverse section and a "pseudokidney" sign viewed on longitudinal section.[9]

EMERGENCY DEPARTMENT MANAGEMENT

Unless there is ischemic bowel with peritonitis, sepsis, massive volume loss, coagulopathy, or respiratory distress from massive pneumoperitoneum, the patient with intussusception should not require airway intervention, respiratory support, or volume resuscitation. Monitoring should be initiated that is appropriate for the degree of patient instability. Those who evidence mild-to-moderate dehydration should be given a normal saline bolus, followed by polyionic intravenous fluids pending serum electrolytes. Although not universally performed, pending imaging procedures, a nasogastric tube is recommended. All patients should be placed NPO.

If imaging is to be carried out beyond the emergency department, provide information to the radiologist and surgeon. A decision must be made concerning whether there are contraindications to nonoperative attempts at reduction of the intussusception. For patients without contraindication, the surgeon and radiologist can determine whether air inflation or barium should be employed. Attempts at reduction should never be done without the consent of the surgeon, who must accept the responsibility of operating if the reduction is unsuccessful or if the patient sustains a perforation. If either hydrostatic pressure or pneumatic reduction techniques fail to reduce the intussusception, sedation of the patient, with repeated efforts at nonoperative reduction or operative interventions, is an option.[3,9]

DISPOSITION

Whether under ultrasonographic or fluoroscopic guidance, both air and barium reductions have success rates ranging from 65% to 90%.[3,13] Recurrence of a successfully reduced intussusception within 1 to 3 days following reduction may occur in approximately 10% of patients.[3,13] It is not possible to establish which patients are likely to have recurrent intussusception based on presenting signs and symptoms, age, or sex. Therefore, admission for a 24-hour period may be customary at many institutions but considered unnecessary at others. If the child is discharged home, the emergency physician must ascertain that parents know the indications that warrant a return for further medical attention.

COMMON PITFALLS

- Obstacles to accurate diagnosis include failure to recognize the typical history, failure to perform a rectal examination, reluctance to accept the diagnosis in a well-appearing child with a prolonged history, and failure to consider the disease in older children.
- Marked variation from the classic picture may lead to misdiagnosis. The absence of pain, lack of a mass, the presence of bright red rectal bleeding, or neurologic aberrations should not dissuade one from the diagnosis.[4,11,12]
- A normal plain abdominal radiograph should not deter performance of the reduction techniques.[14]
- An inopportune hour of the patient encounter should not prevent recruitment of the radiologist or the surgeon.

References

1. Bergdahl S, Hugosson C, Lauren T, et al. Atypical intussusception. *J Pediatr Surg* 1972;7:700.

2. Buchert GS. Abdominal pain in children: an emergency practitioners guide. *Emerg Med Clin North Am* 1989;7:497.
3. Champoux AN, Del Beccaroma, Nazar-Stewart V. Recurrent intussusception: risks and features. *Arch Pediatr Adolesc Med* 1994;148:174.
4. Eins S, Stephens C. Intussusception: 354 cases in 10 years. *J Pediatr Surg* 1971;6:16.
5. Fanconi S, Berger D, Rickham P. Acute intussusception: a classic clinical picture? *Helv Paediatr Acta* 1982;37:345.
6. Felter RA. Nontraumatic surgical emergencies in children. *Emerg Med Clin North Am* 1991;9:589.
7. Gierup J, Jorulf H, Livaditis A. Management of intussusception in infants and children: a survey based on 288 consecutive cases. *Pediatrics* 1972;50:535.
8. Harrington L, Connolly B, Hu X, et al. Ultrasonographic and clinical predictors of intussusception. *J Pediatr* 1998;132:836.
9. Irish MS, Pearl RH, Katy MG, et al. The approach to common abdominal diagnoses in infants and children. *Pediatr Clin North Am* 1998;45:729.
10. Losek JD. Intussusception: don't miss the diagnosis! *Pediatr Emerg Care* 1993;9:46.
11. Luks FI, Yazbeck S, Perreault G, et al. Changes in the presentation of intussusception. *Am J Emerg Med* 1992;10:574.
12. McCabe J, Singer J, Love T, et al. Intussusception: a supplement to the mnemonic for coma. *Pediatr Emerg Care* 1987;3:118.
13. McLario D, Rothrock SG. Understanding the varied presentation and management of children with acute abdominal disorders. *Pediatr Emerg Med Rep* 1997;Nov:111–122.
14. Ravitch M. Considerations of errors in the diagnosis of intussusception. *Am J Dis Child* 1952;84:17.
15. Singer J. Altered consciousness as an early manifestation of intussusception. *Pediatrics* 1979;64:93.
16. Singer J. Acute abdominal conditions that may require surgical intervention. In: Strange G, ed. *A comprehensive study guide in pediatric emergency medicine.* New York: McGraw-Hill 1998:313–319.
17. Smith DS, Bonadio WA, Losek JD, et al. The role of abdominal x-rays in the diagnosis and management of intussusception. *Pediatr Emerg Care* 1992;8:325.
18. Swischuk L. Acute vomiting and abdominal pain in an infant. *Pediatr Emerg Care* 1986;2:201.
19. Tamanaha K, Winbish K, Talwalker Y, et al. Air reduction of intussusception in infants and children. *J Pediatr* 1987;111:733.
20. Yamamoto LG, Morita SY, Boychuk RB, et al. Stool appearance in intussusception: assessing the value of the term "currant jelly." *Am J Emerg Med* 1997;15:293.

CHAPTER 278

Kawasaki Disease

James A. Wilde

Kawasaki disease (KD), also known as mucocutaneous lymph node syndrome, was first described in Japan in 1967[4] and reported in the United States literature in 1974.[5] Although initially thought to be a new disease, KD was soon recognized to be clinically indistinguishable from infantile periarteritis nodosa.[6] The disease is primarily a vasculitis that affects the coronary arteries most significantly, but it can also produce pathology in the central nervous system, liver, gallbladder, lungs, and digits.

There are 2,000 estimated cases of KD in the United States annually, most commonly in children less than 5 years of age (80%), although it has also been reported in young adults.[11,12] Peak incidence is the second year of life. Intense efforts to identify the causative agent have failed to yield an etiology, although certain clinical and epidemiologic features favor an infectious cause.

There is no diagnostic assay that can definitively identify a case of KD, so cases must be presumptively diagnosed based on characteristic clinical features and laboratory findings. Adding to the difficulty in identifying cases of the disease is that some children have been described with an incomplete form of KD that does not fit the classic case definition.[1,3,7] These children are also at risk for development of significant cardiac sequelae. Twenty-five percent to 30% of KD patients will develop coronary artery aneurysms without therapy, while only 5% to 8% do so with the current recommended regimen of intravenous immune globulin (IVIG) and aspirin.[9] The overall mortality rate is 1% to 3% in untreated KD,[8] but, with recommended therapy, may be as low as 0.08%.[15]

CLINICAL PRESENTATION

Classic KD is diagnosed by clinical criteria as originally described by Dr. Kawasaki, with only slight modifications. These criteria include fever of at least 5 days' duration, at least four of five physical findings, and no other explanation for the illness (Table 278.1). A diagnosis of KD can be made in a patient with less than 5 days' fever if all the remaining clinical criteria are met.[10] The fever is generally over 39°C, spiking, remittent, and prolonged in untreated patients, with some children remaining febrile for 2 to 4 weeks.

The conjunctivitis is primarily bulbar, spares the area around the limbus, and is not associated with an exudate. Changes in the lips may include erythema, bleeding, dryness, and fissuring. The oral mucosa may show erythema with a strawberry tongue, but exudates and oral ulcerations are not found. Hands and feet may show edema, erythema, or both, primarily on the palms and soles, with characteristic desquamation 1 to 2 weeks after the onset of the illness. The rash can be quite variable, but it is most commonly diffuse, maculopapular, and erythematous.

Cervical lymphadenopathy is usually unilateral, is nonfluctuant, and is defined by a node diameter of at least 1.5 cm. Each of the clinical criteria is found in approximately 90% of cases, with the exception of the cervical lymphadenopathy, which occurs in only 50% to 75% of cases. An additional, commonly reported finding is extreme irritability in excess of that seen in other childhood febrile illnesses.[10]

Multiple organ system involvement has been reported, including pericarditis, myocarditis, arthritis, cerebrospinal fluid pleocytosis,[2] peripheral extremity gangrene,[13] pulmonary infiltrates, and hydrops of the gallbladder.[10] A desquamated, erythematous, perineal rash in the first 3 to 4 days is an early finding that is helpful in making a diagnosis.[14]

Approximately 1 to 2 weeks after the onset of the acute symptoms, resolution of the fever, rash, and lymphadenopathy can be expected, although the conjunctival injection often persists. It is during this subacute stage that desquamation of the digits occurs. This is also the stage at which coronary artery aneurysms develop and the risk of sudden death is at its highest.

Incomplete KD, or atypical Kawasaki disease (AKD), was first described in a number of case reports and case series in the early 1980s.[1] Most of these patients were under 6 months of age,

TABLE 278.1. Diagnostic Criteria for Kawasaki Disease

Fever of at least 5 days' duration
Presence of four out of five physical findings:
Bilateral, nonpurulent conjunctival injection
Inflammatory changes of the lips and oral mucosa
Erythema or swelling of the hands or feet
Nonvesicular rash, primarily truncal
Cervical lymphadenopathy, usually unilateral
Illness not explained by other known disease

but cases in older children have also been reported.[7] AKD is a febrile illness that does not meet the case definition for KD but that can result in similar cardiac sequelae. In most cases reported to date, one to three of the physical findings typical of KD have been present, but several cases of AKD have been manifested solely by fever. Indeed, one investigator has suggested that AKD be considered in any child with prolonged fever of unknown etiology.[7]

DIFFERENTIAL DIAGNOSIS

There are several diseases that can mimic KD, but careful attention to the clinical criteria, as outlined, can help to avoid misdiagnosis. Among these diseases are scarlet fever, measles, toxic shock syndrome, Stevens-Johnson syndrome, leptospirosis, and Rocky Mountain spotted fever. Tonsillar exudates help to differentiate KD from an illness caused by group A streptococci, such as scarlet fever, as does the characteristic scarlet fever rash. Prominent respiratory symptoms, particularly cough, should suggest measles. Many of the symptoms of toxic shock are similar to those of KD, but hypotension is an uncommon finding in KD unless heart failure secondary to severe carditis is present.

Recent exposure to inciting drugs, the presence of oral lesions, an exudative conjunctivitis, and the typical "target lesion" rash can serve as a clues to the diagnosis of Stevens-Johnson syndrome. The centripetal spread of a petechial rash that begins on the hands or feet, severe myalgias, and seasonal and epidemiologic clues might point to Rocky Mountain spotted fever. Chills, myalgia, and abdominal pain may lead to the diagnosis of leptospirosis. Serologic tests are of limited value in the acute stage of any of these illnesses, but they can be helpful during the recovery phase for retrospective diagnoses.

In the emergency department, the diagnosis of KD is usually one of exclusion and is often not considered until a child has presented to a clinic or emergency setting multiple times.

EMERGENCY DEPARTMENT EVALUATION

Immediate workup of a suspected case of KD should include a complete blood count and differential, platelet count, blood cultures, erythrocyte sedimentation rate (ESR), and a chemistry panel including serum transaminases, total protein, and albumin. White blood cell counts are usually elevated, with polymorphonuclear cell predominance; leukopenia is uncommon. Platelet counts are usually normal in the acute stage, but after a week increase markedly, often rising to above 1 million per microliter. The ESR is virtually always elevated during the acute stage.[10]

Serum transaminases are often two to three times the normal value. Marked rises in serum immunoglobulin levels in the acute stage may result in an elevation in the serum protein level. Lumbar puncture may reveal aseptic meningitis,[2] and urinalysis may reveal a sterile pyuria.

Further workup should include a baseline electrocardiogram to search for evidence of myocarditis or pericarditis. A baseline echocardiogram should also be obtained but should not delay therapeutic interventions.

EMERGENCY DEPARTMENT MANAGEMENT

Uncomplicated presentations require no more than supportive management in the emergency department: an antipyretic for fever and intravenous fluids for rehydration and maintenance. Cardiovascular decompensation must be treated as appropriate, and may require inotropic support.

DISPOSITION

Children with a presumptive diagnosis of Kawasaki disease should ideally be admitted to a tertiary care pediatric center with pediatric cardiologists and infectious disease consultants available. Therapy to be instituted in the hospital includes high-dose IVIG at 2 g/kg over a 10-hour period. IVIG has been shown to substantially reduce the incidence of serious cardiac sequelae, particularly coronary artery aneurysms, if administered early in the course of the disease.[9,11] High-dose aspirin therapy at 100 mg/kg is also begun on admission and is continued until the acute phase has resolved. Transfer to a pediatric intensive care unit should be considered for patients with signs of cardiac decompensation.

COMMON PITFALLS

- Failure to consider KD in the differential diagnosis of prolonged fever in young children
- Failure to consider AKD in prolonged fever in children
- Failure to monitor for or identify cardiac decompensation
- Failure to use certain laboratory screening tests, such as ESR, to help differentiate KD from common childhood viral exanthems
- Failure to obtain early input from an experienced pediatric cardiologist
- Failure to recognize the importance of early admission and institution of therapeutic interventions such as IVIG and aspirin

References

1. Burns JC, Wiggins JW, Toews WH, et al. Clinical spectrum of Kawasaki disease in infants younger than 6 months of age. *J Pediatr* 1986;109:759–763.
2. Dengler LD, et al. Cerebrospinal fluid profile in patients with acute Kawasaki disease. *Pediatr Infect Dis J* 1998;17(6):478–481.
3. Fukushige J, Takahashi N, Ueda Y, et al. Incidence and clinical features of incomplete Kawasaki disease. *Acta Paediatr* 1994;83:1057–1060.
4. Kawasaki T. Acute febrile mucocutaneous lymph node syndrome: clinical observation of 50 cases. *Jpn J Allergy* 1967;16:178.
5. Kawasaki T, Kosaki F, Okawa S, et al. A new infantile acute febrile mucocutaneous lymph node syndrome (MLNS) prevailing in Japan. *Pediatrics* 1974;54(3):271–276.
6. Landing BH, Larson EJ. Are infantile periarteritis with coronary artery involvement and fatal MLNS the same: comparison of 20 patients from North America with patients from Hawaii and Japan. *Pediatrics* 1977;59:651–662.
7. Levy M, Koren G. Atypical Kawasaki disease: analysis of clinical presentation and diagnostic clues. *Pediatr Infect Dis J* 1990;9:122–126.
8. Morens DM, Anderson LJ, Hurwitz ES. National surveillance of Kawasaki disease. *Pediatrics* 1980;65:21–25.
9. Newburger JW, Takahashi M, Beiser AS, et al. Single infusion of intravenous gamma globulin compared to four daily doses in the treatment of acute Kawasaki syndrome. *N Engl J Med* 1991;324:1633–1639.
10. Rowley AH, Shulman ST. Kawasaki syndrome. *Pediatr Cardiol* 1999;46(2):313–329.
11. Rowley A, Taubert K, et al. (Barron KS, Shulman ST, co-eds). Report of the National Institutes of Health workshop on Kawasaki disease. *J Rheumatol* 1999;26:170–190.
12. Taubert KA. Epidemiology of Kawasaki disease in the United States and worldwide. *Prog Pediatr Cardiol* 1997;6:181–185.
13. Tomita S, Chung K, et al. Peripheral gangrene associated with Kawasaki disease. *Clin Infect Dis* 1992;14:121–126.
14. Urbach AH, McGregor RS, Malatack JJ, et al. Kawasaki disease and perineal rash. *Am J Dis Child* 1988;142:1174.
15. Yanagawa H, Nakamura Y, Yashiro M, et al. Update of the epidemiology of Kawasaki disease in Japan: from the results of the 1993–1994 nationwide survey. *J Epidemiol* 1996;6:148–157.

CHAPTER 279
Lymphadenitis

Nizar F. Maraqa and Mobeen H. Rathore

Lymph nodes are commonly palpated in children's necks. Cervical nodes greater than 10 mm are considered abnormal and are often referred to as lymphadenopathy.[5] Lymphadenitis is one type of lymphadenopathy. Although some define *lymphadenitis* as broadly as an "inflammation of a lymph node," others restrict the definition to include only bacterial infections of the lymph gland.[5,18]

After invading regional tissues, microorganisms enter the lymphatic system, where they are trapped and destroyed by phagocytes. This, in conjunction with the lymphocytic proliferation and transformation that occurs, results in swelling of the node. Abscess formation ensues when neutrophils accumulate.[5,7]

Group A β-hemolytic streptococci and *Staphylococcus aureus* are the most frequent pathogens of bacterial lymphadenitis. Children with staphylococcal infections generally have a longer history of symptoms and an increased incidence of fluctuance, compared with those with streptococcal infections.[5,7,15]

CLINICAL PRESENTATION

Cervical lymphadenitis presents most commonly in children between 1 and 4 years of age, and there is no significant difference in incidence between genders. It is helpful to determine whether the cervical lymphadenitis developed in an acute, subacute, or chronic manner. The acute bacterial nodal enlargement usually develops acutely and unilaterally. These nodes are typically very tender and sometimes feel fluctuant. Erythema of the overlying skin is occasionally noted. Affected children often experience malaise and irritability and may be febrile. Frequently, a concurrent pharyngitis, otitis media, upper respiratory tract infection, dental abscess, or adjacent skin infection can be detected, or a recent history of infection can be elicited. Subacute or chronic lymphadenitis develops over 2 to 3 weeks and tends to be relatively painless. It may be caused by cat-scratch disease, atypical mycobacteria, or tuberculosis.

There are rarely significant sequelae when adenitis is managed appropriately. Of particular concern is the possibility of misdiagnosing and consequently mismanaging another more serious problem.[2]

DIFFERENTIAL DIAGNOSIS

Obtaining a careful history and performing a complete examination can often differentiate the disorders most commonly confused with adenitis.[2]

Viral Lymphadenopathy

Viral illnesses, especially those that produce viremia, are common causes of lymphadenopathy that subsides within a few days to 2 weeks. Often bilateral, causative agents include respiratory viruses such as adenovirus, Epstein-Barr virus (EBV), cytomegalovirus (CMV), human herpesvirus 6, coxsackievirus, rubella, rubeola, and varicella.[5,7]

Bacterial Lymphadenitis

The presence of erythema, warmth, and tenderness overlying a node typically indicates the acute inflammatory response of pyogenic bacterial lymphadenitis. Most acutely infected nodes in children are rubbery or firm in consistency and are freely mobile. Left untreated, these nodes, often unilateral, tend to suppurate and may rupture onto the skin or, less commonly, dissect into the underlying soft tissues.[5,7,15]

Infectious Mononucleosis

EBV causes infectious mononucleosis. It often presents as acute or subacute cervical lymphadenopathy. These nodes tend to be posterior cervical, bilateral, and moderately painful.[7] Associated findings include malaise, fever, tonsillopharyngitis, hepatosplenomegaly, and generalized lymph node enlargement. A positive heterophil test (Monospot) confirms the diagnosis, except in children less than 4 years of age, for whom specific EBV titers should be done. Treatment is supportive. The patient should be instructed to avoid contact sports for several months after the illness.

Cat-Scratch Disease

Most cases of cat-scratch disease are caused by *Bartonella henselae*. In approximately 50% of cases, there is a primary lesion at the site of a 7- to 14-day-old scratch or bite by a cat. This lesion begins as an indurated erythematous papule and later may become vesicular or pustular. It resolves within 10 to 20 days. Cat-scratch disease usually presents subacutely. Several days to weeks later, the lymph nodes draining this area become progressively enlarged. These nodes are typically only moderately tender, but, occasionally, they will suppurate. Sometimes, patients are febrile and may experience headache, myalgia, or malaise. Other complications, such as encephalitis, hepatosplenic abscesses, and osteolytic lesions, are uncommon. Although the diagnosis is usually made on clinical grounds, it should be confirmed serologically. Antibiotics are of no proven value, and the adenopathy generally resolves in 6 to 8 weeks, with supportive treatment only. Fluctuant nodes often need surgical intervention.[5,8,9,16]

Atypical Mycobacterial Lymphadenitis

Atypical mycobacterial cervical lymphadenitis usually presents as subacute or chronic unilaterally enlarged lymph nodes that do not respond to antibiotics.[5,10] Nontuberculous mycobacterial lymphadenitis generally occurs in early childhood. Infected nodes tend to be relatively painless but are sometimes tender and may even suppurate and drain. Systemic symptomatology is uncommon. Tuberculin skin testing is unreliable. Antituberculous drugs are not recommended, and the treatment of choice is excisional biopsy.[11]

Kawasaki Disease

Also known as mucocutaneous lymph node syndrome, Kawasaki disease is diagnosed in the presence of fever, plus four of the five diagnostic criteria (cervical lymphadenopathy, rash, oral exanthem, conjunctival injection, and swelling and redness of palms and soles) and exclusion of other illnesses. Cervical lymphadenopathy is found in only 50% of cases. Nodes are usually unilateral and confined to the anterior triangle, moderately tender, nonfluctuant, and firm, with or without overlying erythema. The early diagnosis of Kawasaki disease is critical, because treatment with salicylates and intravenous immunoglobulin can prevent the most serious complication, namely, coronary aneurysm.[16]

Tuberculous Lymphadenitis

Tuberculous lymphadenitis is rarely seen.[6,16,17] Diseased nodes are similar to those of nontuberculous mycobacterial adenitis. To exclude the diagnosis, the family should be questioned about exposure to tuberculosis, a tuberculin skin test should be done, and a chest radiograph should be ordered. Tuberculous lymph nodes should never be aspirated, because this could lead to sinus development. Antituberculous drugs are effective in treating this condition. Infection should be reported to public health authorities.

Group B Streptococcal Cellulitis–Adenitis Syndrome

The group B streptococcal cellulitis–adenitis syndrome occurs in neonates.[14] The neonate presents with the abrupt onset of fever and facial or submandibular erythema and swelling. An affected infant is irritable, feeds poorly, and appears toxic. About 80% have an ipsilateral otitis media. Meningitis may accompany lymphadenitis. The organism can be isolated from blood and from aspirates of the lymph node or the cellulitis. A complete sepsis workup should be performed, and the infant must be admitted to the hospital for intravenous antibiotic therapy.[1,14,16]

Toxoplasmosis

Acquired toxoplasmosis sometimes presents as a single, enlarged, posterior cervical node that may or may not be tender.[5,12,19] These nodes tend to vary in size but do not suppurate. The diagnosis can be made by performing serial toxoplasma titers. Pharmacologic therapy should be withheld unless fever or a complication such as pneumonitis, myocarditis, meningitis, or encephalitis ensues.

Neoplasms

Neoplasms are rare in children, occurring in 1.4% of patients younger than 17 years of age with a superficial lump on any part of the body. Cancerous nodes may be single or multiple. They are classically painless and are often immobile and indiscrete. Careful follow-up of all lymphadenopathy is mandatory, especially if it is associated with fever or weight loss or if it fails to resolve.[4,5,9]

Other causes of cervical lymphadenopathy are even more uncommon and include *Pasteurella multocida, Yersinia pestis,* histoplasmosis, and CMV.

A few other entities may be confused with adenopathy or adenitis. These include dermoid cysts, thyroglossal duct cysts, benign neoplasms, branchial cleft defects, cystic hygromas, and hematomas.[4]

EMERGENCY DEPARTMENT EVALUATION

Many of the aforementioned diagnoses can be made simply by taking a complete history and performing a thorough examination. The following points should be addressed when questioning the family: duration of adenopathy, history of an adjacent skin lesion, earache, upper respiratory tract infection, sore throat, or dental problem; presence of fever or weight loss; exposure to tuberculosis; contact with cats; and travel.[5,7] The size, consistency, mobility, and tenderness of each affected node must be noted.[5,15] Marking the dimensions with ink and recording them in the emergency department record can be helpful to the next physician who evaluates the patient. The head, ears, eyes, nose, oropharynx, and neck are examined, and the child is evaluated for hepatomegaly, splenomegaly, and other adenopathy.[5]

Useful studies include a complete blood cell count, erythrocyte sedimentation rate, a Monospot or EBV serology, a throat culture for group A *Streptococcus,* and a tuberculin skin test. It is, however, unnecessary to order all of these tests on every patient. They prove most helpful when the cause of the adenopathy is unknown. A blood culture should be obtained if the patient appears particularly ill. Older children with cervical adenitis are rarely bacteremic, but neonates often are and must be evaluated for possible sepsis.[1] Additional studies may be needed in the older child, depending on the history and physical examination (e.g., serology for cat-scratch disease or EBV might be drawn). Sometimes, a definitive diagnosis is not made until a biopsy is performed and results evaluated.

Needle aspiration is useful both diagnostically and therapeutically, and any fluctuant node should be aspirated if tuberculous lymphadenitis can be excluded. An ultrasound can help determine whether a node is cystic or solid, if necessary.[13] The largest, most fluctuant node is selected, the overlying skin is cleansed, a 20-gauge needle attached to a 20-mL syringe is inserted into the fluctuant region, and aspiration is done. If pus is not obtained, 1 to 2 mL of sterile, nonbacteriostatic saline is injected into the node, which is reaspirated. The aspirate is sent for Gram stain and cultures for aerobic and anaerobic bacteria, mycobacteria, and fungi.[5,7,15]

EMERGENCY DEPARTMENT MANAGEMENT

In addition to percutaneous needle aspiration of fluctuant nodes, if bacterial cervical lymphadenitis is suspected, it should be treated with antibiotics effective against the principal bacterial pathogens, group A β-hemolytic *Streptococcus* and *S. aureus.* Analgesics and warm compresses may also be helpful.[5]

Outpatient therapy is as follows:[3,5,12]

Cephalexin: 50 mg/kg/d, divided q6h PO
Clindamycin : 20 mg/kg/d, divided q6h PO
Dicloxacillin: 25 mg/kg/d, divided q6h PO

Failure to respond to oral antibiotics does not necessarily mean that the cause of adenitis is not bacterial; parenteral antibiotics may be required. For inpatients, the following agents can be used:[3,5,12]

Cefazolin: 100 mg/kg/d, divided q8h i.v.
Cephalothin: 125 mg/kg/d, divided q4h–6h i.v.
Oxacillin: 125 mg/kg/d, divided q6h i.v.

If the lymphadenitis is associated with dental disease, anaerobic infection needs to be considered, and the following agents are recommended:[3,5]

Clindamycin: 20 mg/kg/d, divided q6h PO; 40 mg/kg/d, divided q6h–8h i.v.
Amoxicillin–clavulanate (Augmentin): 45 mg/kg/d, divided q12h PO

Treatment should last at least 10 days.[5,12] After a good response to parenteral antibiotics is observed, oral agents can be substituted.[5]

DISPOSITION

Most children can be managed successfully as outpatients. They should be reevaluated, to monitor their progress, within 2 to 3 days of the emergency department visit. Follow-up is very important and is done best by the patient's primary care physician, who should reexamine the child serially until the node regresses.

Admission for intravenous antibiotics is warranted if the child appears to be toxic, if the adenitis is severe (e.g., node diameter greater than 3 to 4 cm, or high fever), if the adenitis fails to respond to oral medications, or if the patient is a neonate or cannot tolerate oral antibiotics.[12] Admission for further evaluation is recommended if there is mediastinal adenopathy on the chest radiograph or if the child has lost weight or been febrile for more than 1 week, or if Kawasaki disease is suspected.[9]

Biopsy is indicated if the node increases in size or does not decrease in 4 to 6 weeks or return to normal in 8 to 12 weeks.[9] Particularly worrisome findings are weight loss, persistent fever, or fixation to adjacent tissues or overlying skin.[4,5,7]

COMMON PITFALLS

- Treating patients with severe adenitis orally and delaying an inevitable admission for intravenous antibiotics
- Failure to consider atypical mycobacterial lymphadenitis, Kawasaki disease, and cat-scratch disease in the differential diagnosis

References

1. Albanyan EA, Baker CJ. Is lumbar puncture necessary to exclude meningitis in neonates and young infants: lessons from the group B streptococcus cellulitis-adenitis syndrome. *Pediatrics* 1998;102:984.
2. Armstrong WB, Giglio MF. Is this lump in the neck anything to worry about? *Postgrad Med* 1998;104:63.
3. Barone MA, ed. *The Harriet Lane handbook.* St. Louis: Mosby–Year Book, 1996.
4. Brown RL, Azizkhan RG. Pediatric head and neck lesions. *Pediatr Clin North Am* 1998;45:889.
5. Chesney PJ. Cervical adenopathy. *Pediatr Rev* 1994;15:277.
6. Kanlikama M, Gokalp A. Management of mycobacterial cervical lymphadenitis. *World J Surg* 1997;21:516.
7. Kelly CS, Kelly RE. Lymphadenopathy in children. *Pediatr Clin North Am* 1998;45:875.
8. Klein JD. Cat scratch disease. *Pediatr Rev* 1994;15:349.
9. Knight PJ, Mulne AF, Vassy LE. When is lymph node biopsy indicated in children with enlarged peripheral nodes? *Pediatrics* 1982;69:391.
10. Losurdo G, et al. Cervical lymphadenitis caused by nontuberculous mycobacteria in immunocompetent children: clinical and therapeutic experience. *Head Neck* 1998;20:245.
11. Makhani S, et al. Atypical cervicofacial mycobacterial infections in childhood. *Br J Oral Maxillofac Surg* 1998;36:119.
12. Marcy SM. Cervical adenitis. *Pediatr Infect Dis* 1985;4[Suppl 3]:523.
13. Na DG, et al. Differential diagnosis of cervical lymphadenopathy: usefulness of color Doppler sonography. *AJR* 1997;168:1311.
14. Rathore MH. Group B streptococcal cellulitis and adenitis associated with meningitis. *Clin Pediatr* 1989;28:411.
15. Rathore MH, Barton LL. Cervical adenitis. In: Koplan SL, ed. *Current therapy in pediatric infectious diseases.* St. Louis: Mosby–Year Book, 1993:20–21.
16. *Red book: report of the Committee on Infectious Diseases,* 24th ed. 1997; American Academy of Pediatrics, Elkgrae, IL.
17. Smith MHD, Marquis JR. Tuberculosis and other mycobacterial infections. In: Feigin RD, Cherry JD, eds. *Textbook of pediatric infectious diseases.* Philadelphia: WB Saunders, 1987:1342.
18. *Stedman's medical dictionary,* 24th ed. Baltimore: Williams & Wilkins, 1982.
19. Wilson CB, Remington JS. Toxoplasmosis. In: Feigin RD, Cherry JD, eds. *Textbook of pediatric infectious diseases.* Philadelphia: WB Saunders, 1987:2067.

CHAPTER 280
Meningitis and Encephalitis

James A. Wilde

Central nervous system (CNS) infections are a source of significant morbidity and mortality, and are often included in the differential diagnosis of a febrile child. Bacterial meningitis and viral disease presenting as meningitis, encephalitis, or meningoencephalitis are the most common forms of CNS infection in children. They present a formidable challenge to the emergency physician, both diagnostically and therapeutically, because of their relative rarity, often subtle presenting signs and symptoms, and, sometimes, fulminant course.

The organism that causes bacterial meningitis bears a relationship to the age of the patient. Among neonates, group B *Streptococcus* (GBS) is, by far, the most commonly isolated bacterium. Other less common but significant organisms include *Listeria monocytogenes* and gram-negative enteric bacilli such as *Escherichia coli, Klebsiella* and *Enterobacter* spp., *Citrobacter diversus,* and *Salmonella* spp. GBS and *L. monocytogenes* typically present as "late-onset" meningitis at 1 to 12 weeks of life, while meningitis due to the gram-negative enteric bacteria often presents during the first 2 weeks. Beyond the age of 3 months, *Streptococcus pneumoniae* and *Neisseria meningitidis* are the major pathogens, with *S. pneumoniae* predominating from 1 to 23 months and *N. meningitidis* predominating from 2 to 18 years.[39] Meningitis due to *Haemophilus influenzae* type B (HIB) is now rare because vaccines have improved.

The leading pathogens caused an estimated 2,800 cases of bacterial meningitis in U.S. children under 18 years in 1995.[39] This represents a dramatic decline, resulting from the near disappearance of HIB meningitis over the preceding decade. While two-thirds of patients with bacterial meningitis in 1986 were between 1 month and 5 years of age, by 1995 meningitis in this age group had dropped by 87%, and the median age of bacterial meningitis cases rose from 15 months to 25 years.

Bacterial meningitis is almost always preceded by a hematogenous spread of bacteria. The mechanism whereby bacteria gain access to the intravascular space is unclear, although some data indicate that a breach of the normal mucosal barriers may be caused by viral upper respiratory infections.[31] It is also unclear how bacteria gain access to the CNS from the bloodstream.

One point that is clear is that most instances of bacteremia do not progress to invasion of the CNS.[11] Once in the CNS, bacteria can initially multiply relatively unimpeded because of poor immunologic defenses in normal cerebrospinal fluid (CSF).[27] It is only after local release of bacteria-associated chemotactic factors that a significant defense is mounted in the CNS. The resulting inflammation, edema, and CNS dysfunction are manifested as severe headache, nuchal rigidity, photophobia, or seizures (i.e., classic symptoms of meningitis). A patient with fever can be anywhere on this continuum, but in the absence of CSF for evaluation, it is impossible to state definitively that the child has reached the meningitic stage. Bacterial meningitis can also result from direct invasion of the CNS after trauma or erosion through an infected sinus, but this is a much less common mechanism.

Several infectious or noninfectious agents can cause aseptic meningitis, that is, meningitis without evidence of a bacterial pathogen detectable in CSF. Among the most common infectious etiologies are the enteroviruses (ECHO and coxsackievirus) and mumps virus.

Encephalitis is an inflammation of the brain that can occur as the primary pathologic event, as in arbovirus encephalitis, or as a simultaneous event with a primary meningitis. The latter is more correctly termed *meningoencephalitis,* and is common in bacterial meningitis. Among the many infectious causes of encephalitis are the enteroviruses, arboviruses (La Crosse strain of the California encephalitis virus [CEV], St. Louis encephalitis), herpes simplex virus (HSV), varicella virus, and mumps virus.[42] The enteroviruses and the arboviruses occur during the warmer months, with the latter paralleling mosquito activity. Infection by CEV is typically seen in young boys exposed to hardwood forests or small pools of stagnant water, where mosquitoes breed.[14] HSV encephalitis can occur at any age, including a neonatal form that presents during the second to third week of life.

CLINICAL PRESENTATION

Due to the protean clinical manifestations of bacterial meningitis in infants and young children, physicians must maintain a high index of suspicion for meningitis. Inflammation of the meninges can be manifested by headache, nausea and vomiting, fever, photophobia, mental confusion and lethargy, or excessive irritability in children. Clinical findings indicative of CNS dysfunction, such as seizures, focal neurologic signs (hemiparesis, quadriparesis, cranial nerve palsies, visual field defects), and ataxia suggest meningitis, but no single sign is pathognomonic. The symptoms and signs of meningitis vary and depend, in part, on the patient's age, the duration of illness, and the host's response to the infection,[19] especially in neonates and young infants, in whom the clinical findings may be subtle and may include only such nonspecific manifestations as disinterest in feeding, lethargy, respiratory distress, or jaundice. Fever is commonly not present in neonates with bacterial meningitis.[6]

A change in the child's affect or state of alertness is one of the most important signs of bacterial meningitis. In one study, 36% to 60% of children with this diagnosis were described as toxic or moribund, and 73% to 100% lethargic or comatose, depending on the age of the patient.[45] These findings were generally not present in infants younger than 3 months in this study. *Lethargy* refers to a decreased level of consciousness and interaction with the environment, bordering on unconsciousness. True lethargy is an ominous finding and warrants further investigation. A febrile child who is playful, smiling, or interactive is unlikely to have bacterial meningitis in the absence of other signs or symptoms suggestive of the disease.

Seizures are found at presentation in 20% to 30% of children with bacterial meningitis.[37] However, seizures are rarely the sole manifestation of meningitis in febrile children; most children with seizures secondary to bacterial meningitis will have a significant, prolonged alteration in their level of consciousness or focal findings on physical examination.[21] This is in marked contrast to children with simple febrile seizures, who, after a short postictal period, usually return quickly to their baseline mental status and have no neurologic deficits on examination.

Bacterial meningitis in infants and children can present either insidiously over several days or acutely in a fulminant fashion. The prognosis may be worse for the second group,[23] a group that is generally not difficult to recognize at presentation. Delays are common in diagnosing those with an insidious presentation, despite the best efforts of physicians. It is unclear whether these delays contribute to the subsequent morbidity or mortality.[9,18,22,36] Enteroviral infection is typically insidious in onset and may have a biphasic presentation. The patient does not usually appear seriously ill unless the infection occurs during the neonatal period.[13]

Differentiating HSV infection of the CNS from bacterial meningitis may be difficult because the nonspecific symptoms just described are found in both. Helpful clues include the absence of bacteria on CSF Gram stain, negative cultures of blood and CSF, the presence of focal seizures, and difficult-to-control seizures. Cutaneous vesicles are found at presentation in only 30% to 50% of infants with neonatal HSV, and are uncommon at any stage of HSV encephalitis in older children. St. Louis encephalitis and La Crosse encephalitis can present either in a mild form, consisting of a 2- to 3-day prodrome of low-grade fever, headache, malaise, and vomiting with subsequent development of higher fever, lethargy, and meningeal signs, or a severe form, characterized by the abrupt onset of fever and headache, followed rapidly by generalized or focal seizures, focal neurologic signs, and coma.[42] HSV encephalitis in the older child may be similar to this severe form of arboviral encephalitis.

An altered state of consciousness is apparent in most children with encephalitis due to the brain parenchymal involvement. This may be manifested by only lethargy or delirium, but in severe cases, the lethargy may progress to a stuporous state or frank coma.

DIFFERENTIAL DIAGNOSIS

Although not always apparent at presentation, nuchal rigidity is probably the one clinical sign that physicians most consistently associate with meningitis. However, nuchal rigidity may be associated with a variety of illnesses:[43]

- Infections: meningitis, encephalitis, brain abscess, epidural abscess, Guillain-Barré syndrome, transverse myelitis, acute cerebellar ataxia, poliomyelitis, tetanus, cervical adenitis, retropharyngeal abscess, vertebral body osteomyelitis, discitis, epiglottitis, trichinosis, tonsillitis, otitis media, pyelonephritis, mumps, hepatitis, shigellosis, malaria, typhoid fever
- Vascular abnormalities: subarachnoid hemorrhage, intracranial venous thrombosis
- Neoplasms: meningeal leukemia, intracranial and brainstem tumors, tumors of the cervical vertebrae (osteoid osteoma, eosinophilic granuloma)
- Metabolic disorders: infantile Gaucher disease, maple syrup urine disease, kernicterus
- Toxins: phenothiazines, strychnine, lead
- Bony or muscular disorders: vertebral anomalies; subluxations, dislocations, and fractures of the cervical spine; myositis; fibromyositis; congenital torticollis
- Miscellaneous causes: juvenile rheumatoid arthritis, black widow spider bite, effects of lumbar puncture (LP), Arnold-Chiari malformation.

Viral infections such as influenza, dehydration, and lethargy due to gastroenteritis, and other febrile illnesses often mimic meningitis. Children often look toxic one minute and then become alert and playful an hour later, when their fever decreases.

EMERGENCY DEPARTMENT EVALUATION

History

A careful history can help to differentiate a child with a serious systemic bacterial infection such as sepsis or meningitis from one with a self-limited viral infection. It is important to remember that the overwhelming majority of children with fever do not have bacterial meningitis; if each child under 2 years of age had only one febrile illness per year of life, the expected rate of bacterial meningitis in this age group in the United States would be approximately one case per 4,000 febrile episodes. Most children in this age group have more than one febrile illness per year, so the actual rate is much less than one case per 4,000 febrile episodes. Information gathered from the history and physical examination can help to determine who requires LP for further evaluation (Table 280.1).

Bacterial meningitis leads to inflammation of the brain and meninges, which causes symptoms such as extreme irritability, photophobia, vomiting, headache, lethargy, and seizures. In infants, excessive sleep or poor feeding may result. The emergency department physician should initially focus on these historic items when assessing a febrile child. Their absence does not rule out meningitis but does make it less likely. Conversely, their presence should heighten suspicions of meningitis.

In addition, questions should be directed toward establishing a source for the fever. Are there any ill contacts with fever? Are there signs or symptoms that are temporally related to the fever and that together constitute a self-limited viral illness? Prior or current antibiotic administration is another important historic item to ascertain.

In evaluating a neonate with fever, ask the mother about infections during pregnancy or at delivery. The physician should ask about pruritic or burning vaginal lesions, antibiotic use during pregnancy, ingestion of raw dairy products during pregnancy (listeriosis), parental history of or exposure to HSV, perinatal complications in the mother or child, prolonged care in the nursery after delivery, the mother's GBS status at the time of delivery, and any antibiotic use in the child since birth.

In all febrile children, a history of exposure to someone with tuberculosis, HIB or *N. meningitidis* should be sought. Travel history and animal contact are important factors to consider when dealing with the less common causes of CNS infections. Mosquito bites may suggest an arbovirus infection.

TABLE 280.1. Indications for Lumbar Puncture and/or Immediate Empiric Treatment for Meningitis

Recommended	Strongly Consider
Unexplained fever and:	**Unexplained fever and:**
Lethargy	Seizure in child under 18 mo or over 5 yr of age
Coma	Severe headache
Shock	No obvious source for fever, child under 3 mo of age
Extreme irritability in infant	Poor feeding in infant
Age <1 mo	Increased sleep in infant
New neurologic deficit	Petechial or purpuric rash
Nuchal rigidity	**Any afebrile, toxic-appearing child with symptoms from either column**
Photophobia	
Uncontrolled seizure	
Seizure in child under 6 mo of age	
New-onset focal seizure	

A history of lethargy should be cause for concern. However, parents tend to use the word *lethargic* to describe their children when, in fact, true lethargy is not present. A less playful or a sleepier child is not necessarily a lethargic child. These symptoms are almost universally present in young children with febrile illnesses. Questions should be directed toward establishing the presence or absence of true lethargy.

Physical Examination

A complete physical examination is critical in the evaluation of a febrile child to detect a CNS infection or to establish a reasonable alternative explanation for the fever. An abnormal blood pressure or prolonged capillary refill time in the absence of dehydration suggests a potentially life-threatening bacterial infection. Does the child have symptoms of an acute upper respiratory infection? Does the child have an obvious pharyngitis, or oral lesions consistent with herpangina or herpetic gingivostomatitis? Is there a rash consistent with a clear etiology, such as varicella or the sandpaper rash of scarlet fever? Does the child have conjunctivitis or otitis?

Examine the chest, abdomen, and extremities to rule out other foci of involvement, including pneumonia, myopericarditis, hepatitis, arthritis, and osteomyelitis. Look for the presence of a bulging anterior fontanelle in infants in the seated position, an indication of increased intracranial pressure (ICP). Although the funduscopic examination is usually normal in acute CNS infections, the presence of papilledema should raise concern for a brain abscess, subdural empyema, or venous sinus thrombosis. A complete neurologic examination is required to determine the presence and severity of a CNS insult and to document a baseline against which the response to therapy can be gauged.

In all patients with suspected CNS infection, signs of meningeal irritation are sought by examining for nuchal rigidity and Kernig and Brudzinski signs. Especially in a very young child who is frightened by the emergency department setting, forceful flexion of the neck can be misleading, because the child's natural tendency is to resist the examiner. A toy or flashlight placed at the sitting child's umbilicus usually causes the child to flex the neck spontaneously, and may be more helpful in excluding nuchal rigidity. Kernig's sign is positive when pain is elicited with the knee extended from its initial flexed position, with the patient supine and the leg flexed at the hip. The Brudzinski sign consists of spontaneous flexion of the lower extremities after passive flexion of the neck. Meningeal signs are almost invariably present at the time of diagnosis in children older than 13 months with bacterial meningitis, but are only rarely present in children younger than 6 months.[45]

Careful attention to the child's affect or state of alertness is critical, to distinguish those who should undergo LP for further evaluation from the vast majority who need no further invasive tests. The emergency physician should carefully document the general appearance of the child.

Laboratory Evaluation

The definitive diagnosis of meningitis requires CSF analysis, generally after performance of an LP. This procedure should include an opening pressure, if available, cellular analysis, glucose (including simultaneous serum glucose) and protein determinations, Gram-stained smear, and appropriate cultures. Viral, mycobacterial, and fungal cultures should be reserved for special circumstances, and are not considered routine in otherwise healthy children.

LP should be delayed in the presence of cardiopulmonary instability, signs of significantly increased ICP, evidence of bacterial infection in or around the LP site, coma, focal seizures, and new focal neurologic deficits, or if there are signs or a history of a bleeding disorder. These situations may warrant immediate therapeutic interventions aimed at saving the child's life, or radiologic procedures to assess for increased ICP.

If the LP is to be delayed, blood cultures are obtained and empiric antibiotics administered immediately; lifesaving therapy takes priority over diagnostic procedures. The laboratory diagnosis of bacterial meningitis rests on demonstration of bacteria or inflammation in the CSF. While early antibiotics may prevent the isolation of bacteria in subsequent CSF culture, obvious laboratory markers of inflammation persist for days to weeks in most cases.[7] In addition, bacteria can be isolated from blood culture in up to 80% of patients with bacterial meningitis.[8] The various rapid antigen diagnostic tests, including countercurrent immunoelectrophoresis, latex particle agglutination, and enzyme-linked immunosorbent assay, also may be helpful in establishing the etiologic agent if antibiotics have already sterilized the CSF.

A head computed tomography (CT) scan is not necessary before performance of LP[26,28] if the clinical scenario is consistent with uncomplicated meningitis or encephalitis. However, if the patient has focal neurologic findings, has signs of a severe increase in ICP, or is comatose (making neurologic examination unreliable), a brain imaging study such as a contrast-enhanced CT would be prudent to determine the advisability of performing an LP.

Results of CSF analysis can give important clues to the etiology of the CNS infection (Table 280.2). However, in approximately 1% of cases of bacterial meningitis, CSF cell counts, glucose, and protein are normal, and there are no organisms on Gram stain.[41] A "normal" CSF profile does not rule out the possibility of bacterial meningitis, but it does render this diagnosis very unlikely. Viral infections of the CNS are typically associated with a lymphocyte pleocytosis of less than 500/μL, with relatively normal glucose and protein concentrations initially. However, the first CSF examination in a child with enterovirus meningitis may have a predominance of polymorphonuclear leukocytes, and the cell count may rarely exceed 1,000/μL.

Interpreting a traumatic tap is difficult, and previous recommendations for estimating the number of white cells based on the ratio of white to red cells in peripheral blood may be inaccurate.[10]

In addition to blood culture and CSF analysis, the minimum laboratory evaluation should also include a complete blood count with differential and platelet count, coagulation studies if thrombocytopenia is present, serum electrolytes, urine sodium concentration, urinalysis, and, in some cases, a chest radiograph.

In suspected cases of encephalitis, helpful studies include viral cultures of CSF and mucosal surfaces, specific viral detection in CSF by polymerase chain reaction, electroencephalogram, and brain imaging studies.[29,38]

EMERGENCY DEPARTMENT MANAGEMENT

Supportive care and stabilization are of the utmost importance with CNS infections. Among the initial complications encountered are septic shock with its associated metabolic derangements, coagulopathy, intracranial hypertension, seizures, and hyponatremia resulting from the syndrome of inappropriate antidiuretic hormone (SIADH) secretion. The emergency department physician must be prepared to support the patient with acute meningitis and manage complications until transfer to an intensive care unit (ICU) setting can be arranged for definitive care.

Septic Shock

Simultaneous shock and cerebral edema present a theoretic therapeutic dilemma, because the treatment of one may adversely affect the other. However, correcting systemic hypotension must take priority, and fluid resuscitation is an integral part of the management of septic shock. Massive amounts of crystalloid or colloid may be required, but if there is no response after 40 mL/kg, pharmacologic support should be instituted with pressor agents such as dopamine. Patients who require this level of intervention should ideally be managed in an ICU setting, with a central venous pressure line, Foley catheter, and cardiorespiratory monitors.

Previous recommendations for the fluid management of children with meningitis have stressed fluid restriction to avoid cerebral edema resulting from SIADH.[12] New data, however, have led to the hypothesis that an elevated ADH and the concomitant increase in extracellular water may be part of a compensatory mechanism to overcome elevated ICP and maintain adequate cerebral blood flow.[34,40] A study in children with acute bacterial meningitis demonstrated poorer survival among those who received restricted fluids.[40] Further studies are required to determine optimal fluid management in these patients,[17] but restriction of fluids should no longer be considered standard.[46] If the patient is not dehydrated and the cardiovascular system is stable, maintenance fluids can be initiated, using a solution containing one-fourth to one-half normal saline in 5% dextrose.

Increased Intracranial Pressure

The upper limit of normal for ICP is about 50 mm H_2O in neonates and 85 mm H_2O in older infants and children, but it can be much higher in CNS infections.[18–20] In patients with suspected intracranial hypertension, the head of the bed is elevated 15 to 30 degrees.[47] Although the practice is somewhat controversial, some physicians use mannitol (0.25 to 1.0 g/kg infused over 10 minutes), with or without diuretics, to treat intracranial hypertension. Hyperventilation is another effective means of

TABLE 280.2. Typical Cerebrospinal Fluid in Infants and Children[a]

Component	Normal Children	Normal Newborn	Bacterial Meningitis	Viral Meningitis	Herpes Meningitis
Leukocytes/μL	0–6	0–30	>1,000	100–500	10–1,000
Neutrophils (%)	0	2–3	>50	<40	<50
Glucose (mg/dL)	40–80	32–121	<30	>30	>30
Protein (mg/dL)	20–30	19–149	>100	50–100	>75
Erythrocytes/μL	0–2	0–2	1–10	0–2	10–500

[a] The values shown should be used only as a guide to diagnosis, because there is considerable overlap in CSF values for the different etiologic categories.

Modified from Wubbel L, McCracken GH. Management of bacterial meningitis 1998. *Pediatr Rev* 1998; 19:78–84.

decreasing ICP in the severely affected patient. If hyperventilation is utilized, the $PaCO_2$ should be kept at 25 to 30 mm Hg.[16] ICP should be monitored continuously in patients requiring hyperventilation and mannitol infusions.

Several clinical trials have advocated the use of adjunctive dexamethasone therapy for bacterial meningitis, particularly in disease due to HIB.[25,33] However, a recent large multicenter study failed to demonstrate any improvement in neurologic or developmental outcome in children who received steroids for bacterial meningitis.[44] Other authors have pointed out that, in light of the low incidence of side effects and the potential benefits, administration of steroids is appropriate,[30] particularly if CSF Gram stain or epidemiologic clues point to a likely case of HIB meningitis. The AAP Committee on Infectious Diseases has suggested the use of dexamethasone in suspected bacterial meningitis but has stopped short of recommending it as routine therapy, unless disease is due to HIB.[2] If dexamethasone is used, it should be given only to children over age 6 weeks with suspected bacterial meningitis, at a dose of 0.15 mg/kg intravenously just before the first parenteral dose of antibiotic.

Seizures

Early seizure activity occurs in 20% to 30% of patients with bacterial meningitis. Effective anticonvulsants include diazepam or lorazepam acutely, and phenobarbital or phenytoin as maintenance. Seizures associated with hyponatremia require infusion of hypertonic sodium solutions. Generally 4 cc/kg of 3% NaCl is infused over 10 minutes; repeat doses may be necessary.[35]

Disseminated Intravascular Coagulation

Treating the underlying disease process and correcting the shock and metabolic derangements constitute the best approach to reversing disseminated intravascular coagulation (DIC). If the patient is actively bleeding from peripheral sites or from the gastrointestinal or urinary tract, treatment options include platelet transfusions to raise the count above 50,000/μL, vitamin K to correct a prolonged prothrombin time, and infusions of fresh-frozen plasma to correct a prolonged activated partial thromboplastin time. In the setting of DIC and thrombotic manifestations, heparin therapy may be considered, although its use in this setting is controversial.

Antimicrobial Therapy

Table 280.3 lists the antibiotics and dosages suggested for the initial therapy of suspected bacterial meningitis.[19,35] Because penicillin- and cephalosporin-resistant pneumococci have been reported throughout the United States, vancomycin should be added to the regimen any time infection due to *S. pneumoniae* is suspected.[24] Previous concerns about reduced penetration of vancomycin into the CNS after administration of dexamethasone appear to be unwarranted.[1] If HSV encephalitis is strongly suspected, acyclovir therapy is instituted at 10 mg/kg every 8 hours.

DISPOSITION

Role of the Consultant

Pediatric infectious disease consultation is suggested for the management of CNS infections in children. Neurosurgical consultation for placement of an ICP monitoring device may also be required.

TABLE 280.3. Initial Antimicrobial Therapy for Suspected Bacterial Meningitis

Age	Drug	Dosage (mg/kg)
Newborn–30 d	Ampicillin	50–75
	and	
	Gentamicin	2.5
	or	
	Cefotaxime	50
30 d–3 mo	Ampicillin	50–75
	and	
	3rd-generation cephalosporin	
	• Ceftriaxone	80–100
	• Cefotaxime	50–75
>3 mo	Ceftriaxone or cefotaxime	
	and	
	Vancomycin	15

Indications for Admission

All patients with potential bacterial meningitis or HSV encephalitis require immediate hospitalization with intensive monitoring. CNS infections of probable enteroviral or arboviral origin may require hospitalization for diagnostic purposes or for supportive care. Sometimes, the results of the initial CSF examination do not distinguish between a bacterial and a viral process. If patients have been pretreated with antibiotics, are younger than 6 months, or are clinically unstable, they should initially be managed as if bacterial meningitis were present.

If clinical signs and symptoms and laboratory analysis of CSF suggests viral meningitis, outpatient management may be appropriate. Some authors suggest observation for 4 to 8 hours and repeat LP for suspected viral meningitis cases.[46] Lymphocyte predominance, no significant worsening of pleocytosis, normal glucose and protein, and continued absence of bacteria on CSF Gram stain would be expected on the second LP in the setting of viral meningitis.

Transfer Considerations

According to the report of the Task Force on Diagnosis and Management of Meningitis, "It is advisable to manage infants and children with meningitis in a hospital that has specialized equipment and staff with expertise in caring for infants and children who are critically ill. The staff should include physicians who are capable of managing the complications of meningitis."[19] Therefore, transport to a pediatric referral center should be strongly considered for any child with meningitis. If LP has been performed, an aliquot of the CSF should be sent with the patient, along with documentation of clinical management up to the point of transfer.

PREVENTION

If meningitis is due to *N. meningitidis* or HIB, rifampin chemoprophylaxis should be considered for the child's household contacts.[3,4] The dosage regimen is 10 mg/kg (maximum dose, 600 mg) every 12 hours for four doses, and 20 mg/kg (maximum dose, 600 mg) once daily for 4 days, respectively. With HIB, chemoprophylaxis is given only if there is at least one unvaccinated household contact younger than 48 months. Rifampin should not be given to a pregnant patient. Medical personnel exposed to a case of meningococcal infection need chemoprophylaxis only if that exposure was intimate (e.g., mouth-to-mouth resuscitation). The use of appropriate isolation precautions (mask and gown, hand-washing) for suspected cases of bacterial meningitis eliminates any need for prophylaxis in most situations.

RISK MANAGEMENT

Failure to diagnose meningitis is one of the leading causes of malpractice litigation among physicians who care for children.[15] While failing to diagnose and treat meningitis in a child with a fulminant presentation probably does constitute a breach of the standard of care, failing to recognize meningitis in a child with an insidious presentation may not. Consider a 10-month-old child who presents to Doctor "A" on day 2 of a febrile illness. If the child is not toxic-appearing, has no nuchal rigidity or photophobia, is alert, has good state variation (cries when examined but is easily consolable when left with the mother), and has symptoms consistent with a viral illness, few (if any) physicians would perform an LP.

If the child is then diagnosed with bacterial meningitis 2 days later, a reasonable explanation is that the child had not yet seeded the meninges when seen by the first physician. However, that physician may still find him- or herself the defendant in a lawsuit. The physician can do substantial harm to the case by failing to fully document the aforementioned findings, particularly the general appearance of the patient. After good medical care, good documentation is the best defense against malpractice litigation. Finally, careful follow-up instructions, including specific symptoms or circumstances that should prompt the parent to seek immediate care, are a part of good medical practice and also serve to protect the physician who may be a target in malpractice litigation.

COMMON PITFALLS

- Consider bacterial meningitis and perform an LP in lethargic, irritable infants, even in the absence of classic signs of meningitis.
- Consider meningitis in infants with fever without a source.
- Consider CNS infection in febrile or afebrile, vomiting children, with or without diarrhea.
- Do not discount the diagnosis of bacterial meningitis in the presence of strong clinical clues simply because the CSF white cell count is normal or the Gram-stained smear is negative for bacteria.
- Always obtain a Gram-stained smear of the CSF if bacterial meningitis is in the differential.
- Consider repeat LP if the clinical setting suggests meningitis, even if a CSF culture obtained hours or days earlier was negative.
- Always reassess a child with a positive blood culture. LP should be considered if the febrile illness persists or if any suggestions of meningitis are present.
- Consider the possibility of a CNS infection in a child who has had a simple febrile seizure. Although LP is not mandatory, it should be considered in a child less than 18 months of age, especially if the child has not returned to the baseline mental status.
- Always obtain a blood culture before instituting antibiotic therapy for suspected bacterial meningitis.
- Document the physical examination thoroughly, particularly the general appearance of the child.
- Always provide adequate discharge instructions, especially reasons for immediate return to the emergency department.

ACKNOWLEDGMENT

The author gratefully acknowledges the contribution of William J. Barson, who wrote the previous version of this chapter.

References

1. Ahmed A. A critical evaluation of vancomycin for treatment of bacterial meningitis. *Pediatr Infect Dis J* 1997;16:895–903.
2. American Academy of Pediatrics. Dexamethasone therapy for bacterial meningitis in infants and children. In: Peter G, ed. *1997 Red book: report of the Committee on Infectious Diseases,* 24th ed. Elk Grove Village, IL: American Academy of Pediatrics, 1997:620–623.
3. American Academy of Pediatrics. *Haemophilus influenzae* infections. In: Peter G, ed. *1997 Red book: report of the Committee on Infectious Diseases,* 24th ed. Elk Grove Village, IL: American Academy of Pediatrics, 1997:220–231.
4. American Academy of Pediatrics. Meningococcal infections. In: Peter G, ed. *1997 Red book: report of the Committee on Infectious Diseases,* 24th ed. Elk Grove Village, IL: American Academy of Pediatrics, 1997:357–362.
5. Archer BD. Computed tomography before lumbar puncture in acute meningitis: a review of the risks and benefits. *Can Med Assoc J* 1993;148(6):961–965.
6. Bell AH, Brown D, Halliday HL, et al. Meningitis in the newborn—a 14 year review. *Arch Dis Child* 1989;64:873–874.
7. Blazer S, Berant M, Alon U. Bacterial meningitis: effect of antibiotic treatment on CSF. *Am J Clin Pathol* 1983;80:386.
8. Bohr V, Rasmussen N, Hansen B, et al. Eight hundred seventy-five cases of bacterial meningitis: diagnostic procedures and the impact of preadmission antibiotic therapy. *J Infect* 1983;7:193–202.
9. Bonadio WA. Medical-legal considerations related to symptom duration and patient outcome after bacterial meningitis. *Am J Emerg Med* 1997;15(4):420–423.
10. Bonadio WA, Smith DS, Goddard S, et al. Distinguishing CSF abnormalities in children with bacterial meningitis and traumatic LP. *J Infect Dis* 1990;162:251.
11. Bratton L, Teele DW, Klein JO. Outcome of unsuspected pneumococcemia in children not initially admitted to the hospital. *J Pediatr* 1977;90:703–706.
12. Brown LW, Feigin RD. Bacterial meningitis: fluid balance and therapy. *Pediatr Ann* 1994;23(2):93–98.
13. Cherry JD. Enteroviruses. In: Feigin RD, Cherry JD, eds. *Textbook of pediatric infectious diseases*. Philadelphia: WB Saunders, 1992:1705–1753.
14. Cherry JD, Shields WD. Encephalitis and meningoencephalitis. In: Feigin RD, Cherry JD, eds. *Textbook of pediatric infectious diseases*. Philadelphia: WB Saunders, 1992:445–454.
15. Committee on Medical Liability. Liability issues in diagnosing meningitis. In: Robertson WO, Lockhart JD, eds. *Medical liability for pediatricians.* Elk Grove Village, IL: American Academy of Pediatrics, 1995:99–103.
16. Dacey RD. Monitoring and treating increased ICP. *Pediatr Infect Dis J* 1987;6:1161.
17. Duke T. Fluid management of bacterial meningitis in developing countries. *Arch Dis Child* 1998;79:181–185.
18. Feigin RD, Kaplan SL. Commentary. *Pediatr Infect Dis J* 1992;11(9):698–699.
19. Feigin RD, McCracken GH, Klein JO. Diagnosis and management of meningitis. *Pediatr Infect Dis J* 1992;11:785–814.
20. Goitein KJ, Tamir I. Cerebral perfusion pressure in central nervous system infections of infancy and childhood. *J Pediatr* 1983;103:40–43.
21. Green SM, Rothrock SG, Clem KJ, et al. Can seizures be the sole manifestation of meningitis in febrile children? *Pediatrics* 1993;92(4):527–534.
22. Kallio MJT, Kilpi T, Anttila M, et al. The effect of a recent previous visit to a physician on outcome after childhood bacterial meningitis. *JAMA* 1994;272:787–791.
23. Kilpi T, Anttila M, Kallio M, et al. Severity of childhood bacterial meningitis and duration of illness before diagnosis. *Lancet* 1991;338:406–409.
24. Klugman KP, Friedland IR, Bradley JS. Bactericidal activity against cephalosporin resistant *Streptococcus pneumoniae* in cerebrospinal fluid of children with acute bacterial meningitis. *Antimicrob Agents Chemother* 1995;39(9):1988–1992.
25. Lebel MH, Freij BJ, Syrogiannopoulos GA, et al. Dexamethasone therapy for bacterial meningitis. Results of two double-blind, placebo-controlled trials. *N Engl J Med* 1988;319:964.
26. Lipton JD, Schafermeyer RW. Pediatric meningitis [Letter]. *Ann Emerg Med* 1994;24(1):118
27. Lipton JD, Schafermeyer RW. Evolving concepts in pediatric bacterial meningitis. Part I: pathophysiology and diagnosis. *Ann Emerg Med* 1993;22:1602–1615.
28. Lipton JD, Schafermeyer RW. Evolving concepts in pediatric bacterial meningitis. Part II: current management and therapeutic research. *Ann Emerg Med* 1993;22:1616–1629.
29. Lukeman FD, Whitley RJ, National Institute of Allergy and Infectious Diseases Collaborative Antiviral Study Group. Diagnosis of herpes simplex encephalitis: application of polymerase chain reaction to cerebrospinal fluid from brain-biopsied patients and correlation with disease. *J Infect Dis* 1995;171:857.
30. McIntyre PB, Berkey CS, King SM, et al. Dexamethasone as adjunctive therapy in bacterial meningitis. *JAMA* 1997;278:925–931.
31. Michaels RH, Myerowitz RL. Viral enhancement of nasal colonization with *Haemophilus influenzae* type b in the infant rat. *Pediatr Res* 1983;17:472–473.
32. Nichols DG, Yaster M, Lappe DG, et al., eds. Shock and fluid resuscitation. In: *Golden hour, the handbook of advanced pediatric life support*. St. Louis: Mosby–Year Book, 1991:88.
33. Odio CM, Faingezicht I, Paris M, et al. The beneficial effects of early dexamethasone administration in infants and children with bacterial meningitis. *N Engl J Med* 1991;324:1525.
34. Powell KR, Sugarman LI, Eskenazi AE, et al. Normalization of plasma arginine vasopressin concentrations when children with meningitis are given maintenance plus replacement fluid therapy. *J Pediatr* 1990;117(4):515–522.
35. Quagliarello VJ, Scheld WM. Treatment of bacterial meningitis. *N Engl J Med* 1997;336:708–716.
36. Radetsky M. Duration of symptoms and outcome in bacterial meningitis: an analysis of causation and the implications of a delay in diagnosis. *Pediatr Infect Dis J* 1992;11:694–698.

37. Rosman NP, Peterson DB, Kaye EM, et al. Seizures in bacterial meningitis: prevalence, patterns, pathogenesis, and prognosis. *Pediatr Neurol* 1985;1:278–285.
38. Schroth G, Gawehn J, Thron A, et al. Early diagnosis of *Herpes simplex* encephalitis by MRI. *Neurology* 1987;37:179.
39. Schuchat A, Robinson D, Wenger JD, et al. Bacterial meningitis in the United States in 1995. *N Engl J Med* 1997;337:970–976.
40. Singhi SC, Singhi PD, Srinivas B, et al. Fluid restriction does not improve the outcome of acute meningitis. *Pediatr Infect Dis J* 1995;14:495–503.
41. Sivakmaran M. Meningococcal meningitis revisited: normocellular CSF. *Clin Pediatr* 1997; 36:258–262.
42. Tsai TF. Arboviral diseases of North America. In: Feigin RD, Cherry JD, eds. *Textbook of pediatric infectious diseases.* Philadelphia: WB Saunders, 1992:1390–1423.
43. Tunnessen WW. Nuchal rigidity. In: Tunnessen WW, ed. *Signs and symptoms in pediatrics.* Philadelphia: JB Lippincott Co, 1988:259.
44. Wald ER, Kaplan SL, Mason EO, et al. Dexamethasone therapy for children with bacterial meningitis. *Pediatrics* 1995;95:21.
45. Walsh-Kelly C, Nelson DB, Smith DS, et al. Clinical predictors of bacterial versus aseptic meningitis in childhood. *Ann Emerg Med* 1992;21:910–914.
46. Wubbel L, McCracken GH. Management of bacterial meningitis 1998. *Pediatr Rev* 1998;19:78.
47. Yatsiv I. Central nervous system support techniques. In: Holbrook PR, ed. *Textbook of pediatric critical care.* Philadelphia: WB Saunders, 1993.

CHAPTER 281
Newborn Problems

Michael O. Gayle and Niranjan Kissoon

Neonates present to the emergency department (ED) with a wide range of minor to life-threatening problems. Their assessment is more difficult than that of older children or adults because the history is often incomplete and unclear, or it is based on a care provider's opinion of the problem. In addition, signs are usually subtle and, even when recognized, may not be helpful in pinpointing the exact diagnosis. For example, respiratory distress may be due to respiratory or cardiac disease, sepsis, intraabdominal pathology, or metabolic derangements, or it may be factitious. Evaluation of the neonate is time consuming, requiring knowledge of the infant's postconceptual age as well as requiring special skills in approaching both the infant and the parents. Many visits to the ED are triggered by parental concerns regarding breathing, feeding, weight gain, and the consistency, color, or frequency of stools. Physicians caring for neonates in the ED, therefore, should be aware of the patterns of normal vegetative functions of the neonate.

PHYSIOLOGY AND PATHOPHYSIOLOGY

Significant physiologic changes occur in the newborn to allow the transition from intrauterine to extrauterine life. Some of these changes occur in the first few days of life, but others occur in the weeks following birth. The fetus depends on uteroplacental blood flow while in the uterus and pulmonary blood flow and alveolar gas exchange following delivery. *In utero,* the pulmonary vascular resistance is high, which leads to significant shunting across the foramen ovale and ductus arteriosus. At birth, systemic vascular resistance is increased, with a subsequent decrease in pulmonary vascular resistance, leading to a substantial reduction in the right-to-left shunt across the foramen ovale and ductus arteriosus. In addition, pulmonary blood flow increases, improving oxygenation, allowing increases in left atrial pressure, which eventually reduces the shunt across the foramen ovale. This adult circulatory pattern can revert to the neonatal pattern within the first 2 weeks of life (longer in premature infants). This occurs when the neonate is exposed to stress (e.g., hypoxemia, acidosis, shock, hypothermia, hypercarbia and hypovolemia).

In the neonate, maturation of the cardiovascular system is incomplete. Contractile elements, such as mitochondria and myofibrils in myocardial muscle mass, are not well organized in the neonate. There is a reduction in the muscle mass in neonates, with 30% of muscle mass composed of contractile mass compared with 60% in adults. This is partly responsible for the neonate's cardiac output being heart rate dependent.

The neonate has a respiratory system that is efficient for growth but inefficient for gas exchange. In the upper airway of the neonate, the large head, small face, short neck, small external nares, small mandible, relatively large tongue for mouth size, high larynx, long and floppy epiglottis, and small cricoid ring in the subglottic area make the maintenance of a patent airway in the unconscious neonate difficult. This configuration makes it easier for the neonate to protect the airway during swallowing, but it increases the chance of aspiration in cases in which conscious level is decreased. The development of lung tissue is not complete until 7 years of age, with immaturity of the alveoli leading to high closing volumes. There is a deficiency in elasticity of the lungs, which leads to an increased tendency to atelectasis. This decrease in total lung volume in the neonate makes the neonate less tolerant to hypoxia.

Neonates are at risk for hypothermia because of a large surface area in relation to their mass; lack of subcutaneous tissue for insulation; a large scalp, which has a large blood flow; and lastly, their inability to alter surroundings to prevent heat losses. A sick or unconscious neonate will be unable to increase heat generation and, because of limited mass, will cool rapidly. Hypothermia in the neonate is a significant stress, as the neonate will try to maintain body temperature by increasing oxygen consumption and cardiac output. These can be the final decompensating events in the sick neonate.

The neonate is at much greater risk from dehydration, in view of the increased fluid losses related to body surface area, and during illnesses, when water losses are high (e.g., fever or diarrhea) or when water intake is restricted (e.g., coma, vomiting, etc). For growth and development, the neonate requires a high caloric expenditure, and hence high oxygen consumption. In addition, neonates have high glucose needs and low glycogen stores. As a result, during periods of stress and high-energy requirements, the infant may become hypoglycemic.

NORMAL VEGETATIVE FUNCTIONS OF THE NEONATE

Respiratory Patterns

Respiratory patterns vary widely in the first month of life. During sleep, the normal full-term infant may have episodes of "central apnea." Central apnea is an absence of drive from the central nervous system (CNS) respiratory control center. When central apnea occurs in a regular repeating pattern (three or more episodes of apnea of less than 20 seconds each), with short bursts of breathing in between, it is referred to as periodic breathing. Normal infants may exhibit apnea of 25 to 30 seconds without apparent adverse effects. Recent studies suggest that some apnea associated with hypoxemia is normal in young infants.

Feeding

Most normal newborns dictate their own feeding pattern by the first month of life. Breast-fed infants may require feeding every 2 to 4 hours, whereas bottle-fed infants usually require six to nine feedings every 24 hours. Most term infants rapidly increase their intake from 30 mL to 90 mL every 3 to 4 hours at 4 to 5 days of life. Infants have wide variation in their intake and parents require frequent reassurance that their infant is obtaining adequate nutrition. Adequate nutritional intake should be judged by factors other than frequency of feeding, such as weight gain.

Weight Gain

In the bottle-fed infant, caloric intake can be determined accurately, but this is rarely necessary. In the breast-fed neonate, estimation of intake is difficult. Consistent and appropriate weight gain in an infant who is content between feedings indicates adequate intake. Intake is deemed satisfactory if the neonate is back to its birth weight by 5 to 7 days and gains 10 to 30 g/d by 12 to 14 days of age.

Stool Characteristics

The normal bowel patterns in neonates vary widely. The number, color, and consistency of bowel movements vary greatly in the same infant and between infants, regardless of diet or environment. Breast-fed infants tend to have more frequent stools, but frequency ranges from one every few days to six to ten per day. Infrequent bowel movements do not necessarily mean constipation; both bottle- and breast-fed infants may go 5 to 7 days without a bowel movement. The presence of blood in the stool is the most significant color change and should prompt an examination for benign lesions, such as fissures, or for significant pathologic conditions, such as bleeding diathesis or enterocolitis.

CLINICAL PRESENTATION

Table 281.1 lists the presenting signs and symptoms of the neonate in the ED. These complaints should be more accurately described as "symptom complexes" because they are nonspecific and indicative of the diverse diseases seen in the neonate.

TABLE 281.1. The Neonate in the Emergency Department: Presenting Signs and Symptoms

Crying/irritability/lethargy
See Table 281.2 for differential diagnosis
Cardiorespiratory symptoms and signs
Tachypnea (see Table 281.3)
Cough and nasal congestion
Noisy breathing and stridor
Apnea and periodic breathing
Blue spells and cyanosis
Other organ systems
Neurologic
Seizures
Intracranial bleed
Encephalitis, meningitis
Gastrointestinal tract symptoms and signs
Feeding problems
Regurgitation
Vomiting
Diarrhea
Constipaton
Abdominal distention
Jaundice
Eye discharge/redness
Diaper rash and oral thrush
Fever/sepsis
Sudden infant death syndrome

DIFFERENTIAL DIAGNOSIS, EVALUATION, AND MANAGEMENT

An astute emergency physician is alert to the possibility of either an acquired or congenital disorder to account for the symptom complexes listed in Table 281.1.

The neonate who is crying, irritable, or lethargic is difficult to treat, even when there is an identifiable cause. Most neonates cry at times during a 24-hour period. The infant who exhibits acute inconsolable crying, however, should be assessed for an underlying cause (Table 281.2).

TABLE 281.2. Differential Diagnosis of Neonate with Uncontrollable Crying/Irritability/Lethargy

Improper feeding practices
Intestinal colic
Infections
Otitis media
Meningitis
Generalized sepsis
Urinary tract infection
Gastroenteritis
Septic arthritis
Surgical
Incarcerated hernia
Testicular torsion
Pyloric stenosis
Anal fissure
Metabolic Disorders
Hypoglycemia
Hypocalcemia
Trauma
Child abuse (eg, burns, fractures)
Accidental injuries, skull or extremity fractures
Strangulation of finger or penis
Abrasion of cornea, foreign body in eye

Improper Feeding Practices

An inexperienced parent may engage in improper feeding practices, such as overfeeding, with inadequate burping during feeds. The infant swallows large amounts of air, with progressive bowel distention and, occasionally, respiratory distress. Improper feeding with bowel distention may result in an irritable infant with periods of inconsolable crying. A thorough history and physical examination usually provide clues to the diagnosis. Instructing the parent in proper feeding techniques alleviates the problem.

Intestinal Colic

One of the most common causes of repeated crying episodes in neonates is intestinal colic. The incidence of colic is higher in premature infants. Colic usually occurs in healthy, thriving babies in the second or third week of life and persists until 3 months of age. Episodes commonly occur in the late afternoon or evening. The infants scream, draw up their knees as if in pain, and often pass flatus. Although intestinal colic does not have any grave clinical significance or long-term effects, it may be complicated by gastroesophageal reflux. Treatment of colic should begin with a careful history, physical examination, and appropriate laboratory investigations. This approach is important in the ED to exclude the more serious conditions listed in Table 281.2. If the physician is in doubt as to the diagnosis, the infant should be admitted for observation. In many cases, parents have already seen several physicians and are angry, frustrated, exhausted, or dissatisfied with the advice or care given.

Colic cannot be cured in the ED, but the physician can assist by recommending some calming techniques, such as swaddling the infant; using slow, smooth motions; holding the infant in a flexed position; and rocking and holding the infant. Other suggestions include changing the environment (e.g., changing background noise, taking a car ride, or trying a feeding change). Changes in diet are helpful if the infant has other manifestations, such as visible peristalsis, persistent regurgitation, or symptoms following ingestion of cow's milk protein. Removal of cow's milk from the diet of a mother who is breast feeding may also be attempted. However, the discontinuation of breast feeding or the routine switching of formula is not recommended. The use of medications, such as sedatives or antispasmodics, especially in premature babies, should be discouraged. A sympathetic and supportive ED physician who emphasizes the normalcy of the infant and parents may be the best therapy.

Metabolic Disorders

One of the common causes of lethargy and subsequent collapse in the neonate is hypoglycemia. Hypoglycemia may be secondary to multiple causes, but in the first few days of life, it is often seen in infants of diabetic mothers. The physician should be aware of other causes, such as sepsis or inborn errors of metabolism. Hypoglycemia accompanied by lethargy, jitteriness, and seizures requires urgent treatment. Hypoglycemia can be rapidly diagnosed by a bedside test using a drop of blood and a reagent strip. Intravenous glucose at a dose of 1 to 2 mL/kg of 10% dextrose is required, followed by an infusion of $D_{10}W$ at a rate of 100 mL/kg/d or 4 mL/kg/h. Rebound hypoglycemia frequently occurs, and it is therefore important that a continuous glucose infusion follows the bolus.

The neonate is particularly susceptible to hypocalcemia due to hypoparathyroidism, abnormal vitamin D metabolism, a low calcium intake, or a high phosphate intake. Infants of diabetic mothers as well as critically ill neonates are also often hypocalcemic. In symptomatic neonates, irritability, muscular twitching, jitteriness, and tremors are common clinical manifestations. However, apnea and seizures may occur. A serum calcium concentration below 7 mg/dL establishes the diagnosis. Serum phosphate as well as an electrocardiogram should be performed. In the symptomatic neonate, treatment consists of intravenous injection of 2 mL/kg of a 10% solution of calcium gluconate.

Infections

Infections in the neonate may be of varied etiology and nonspecific symptomatology. The infected neonate presents with a variety of symptoms and signs, such as feeding difficulties, fever, jaundice, or respiratory distress. The classic signs, such as stiff neck and the Kernig or Brudzinski sign, are usually absent in the presence of meningitis. The septic neonate may present with a normal temperature, fever, or hypothermia. The documented temperature at home should be considered in decision making. Infants who are bundled and have borderline fever should be unbundled, and their temperatures should be documented again in 10 to 20 minutes. Urinary tract infections in neonates may manifest as irritability, diarrhea, or poor feeding. The diagnosis is established by urine culture, preferably obtained by suprapubic puncture.

Opinions differ regarding the management of the febrile infant younger than 28 days of age. There is general consensus, however, that all neonates with possible sepsis should be hospitalized and given broad-spectrum antibiotics after initiation of a full sepsis workup (complete blood count, blood and urine cultures, urinalysis, chest radiograph, and cerebrospinal fluid examination).

In the neonate, herpes simplex virus (HSV) infection can manifest as (1) generalized, systemic infection involving the liver and other organs, including the CNS ; (2) localized CNS disease; or (3) disease localized to the skin, eyes, and mouth. HSV infection in the neonate should be considered when there is any history of a sexually transmitted disease in the mother. If HSV infection is considered in the differential diagnosis, the antiviral agent acyclovir should be added to the broad-spectrum antibiotics.

Surgical Lesions

Surgical lesions such as incarcerated hernia (umbilical or inguinal), pyloric stenosis, and testicular torsion may present with nonspecific signs in the infant. The more common symptoms and signs include irritability, crying, poor feeding, vomiting, constipation, and abdominal distention. Projectile vomiting in a baby 2 to 3 weeks of age, especially if the infant is a first-born male, should suggest a diagnosis of pyloric stenosis. In the infant with a testicular torsion or an incarcerated hernia, physical examination may reveal a red, edematous, tender lump at the site of a hernia or testicular torsion. Examination of the infant with possible pyloric stenosis should be done with the infant relaxed and the stomach empty. Prominent gastric waves may be seen going from left to right, and a firm olive-sized mass may be felt by palpating under the liver edge. Malnutrition and dehydration may be evident if symptoms are prolonged. Hospitalization is required for rehydration and surgical consultation. Anal fissures may also present at this age. If the anal fissure is not obvious during the physical examination, it may be diagnosed by inserting a small test tube into the anal verge and inspecting the area through the bottom glass surface.

Trauma

Trauma is not common in the neonate. However, the infant is at risk for both accidental and nonaccidental (child abuse) trauma. A careful history, looking for inconsistent or implausible explanations, should be obtained in every case of neonatal trauma. The diagnosis of child abuse can often be based on the history alone, although physical examination may provide further support by revealing unexplained injuries. Injuries may include multiple bruises or bruises of varying ages, burns, extremity fractures, and skull fractures. Neonates who are shaken are at risk for "whiplash" or "shaken-baby syndrome," which may present with subtle, nonspecific signs; seizures; coma; or respiratory insufficiency. A thorough funduscopic examination is important in these patients, because the presence of retinal hemorrhage, especially in the absence of external signs of trauma, is a common finding.

The examination of the eye is also useful to rule out an eyelash in the eye or a corneal abrasion as a reason for an infant's irritability and crying. Although rare, congenital glaucoma may also present with irritability and crying. Other uncommon reasons for distress in the neonate include piercing of the skin with an open diaper pin and strangulation of integuments with hair.

Cardiorespiratory Symptoms and Signs

The anatomic and physiologic characteristics of the neonatal respiratory system predisposes the child to frequent respiratory problems. Unfavorable anatomic factors include small nares, a relatively large tongue relative to the size of the mandible, smaller upper and lower airway diameters, flattened diaphragm, limited movement of diaphragm by abdominal compression, and barrel-shaped chest. In addition, the higher closing volumes and high compliance of the chest wall, low compliance of the lung, and less fatigue-resistant fibers in the diaphragm and intercostal muscles contribute to diminished respiratory reserve.

The cardiorespiratory symptoms listed in Table 281.1 are nonspecific and may be due to primary organ failure (cardiovascular or respiratory) or secondary to a variety of systemic diseases, such as sepsis, metabolic acidosis, abdominal pathology, and severe meningitis. Regardless of the cause, the first priority is assessment and stabilization of airway, breathing, and circulation. Establishment of the diagnosis is a secondary concern.

Tachypnea

Tachypnea can be due to a life-threatening illness (e.g., sepsis) or to a minor problem (e.g., abdominal distention due to swallowed air) (Table 281.3). A neonate who is grunting or breathing rapidly should be considered to have a serious pathologic illness. Hospital admission for investigations, monitoring, and therapy should be considered in all cases. If a cause for tachypnea cannot be identified on initial presentation, a full sepsis workup is warranted, and broad-spectrum antibiotic therapy should be instituted.

Pneumonia. Pneumonia, whether bacterial or viral, may present with irritability, nasal congestion, and poor appetite, followed by either low- or high-grade fever, nasal flaring, grunting, retractions, tachypnea, and tachycardia (see Table 281.3). Bacterial pneumonias are usually caused by *Streptococcus pneumoniae* (pneumococcus), *Haemophilus influenzae, Staphylococcus aureus,* or other *Streptococcus* species. Viral pneumonias caused by respiratory syncytial virus (RSV) and parainfluenza, however, are more common. *Chlamydia* pneumonia usually occurs after 3 weeks of age and is accompanied by conjunctivitis in more than 50% of cases. The infants are usually afebrile and have tachypnea and a prominent cough. Chest examination reveals rales but few wheezes. A chest radiograph shows hyperinflation with diffuse patchy infiltrates. Aspiration pneumonia is more likely to occur in debilitated infants and in those with tracheoesophageal fistula or swallowing dysfunction. Aspiration of gastric contents may result in cough, tachypnea, and wheezing. Neonates with pneumonia should be admitted to the hospital for monitoring and institution of antibacterial therapy. Immunocompromised infants, such as the children infected with the human immunodeficiency virus (HIV), should be suspected of having an infection with *Pneumocystis carinii.*

TABLE 281.3. Causes of Tachypnea in the Neonate

Pneumonia
Bacterial
Viral
Chlamydial
Aspiration
Bronchiolitis
Bronchopulmonary dysplasia
Nonpulmonary symptoms
Septicemia
Gastrointestinal tract—abdominal distention, gastroenteritis
Metabolic acidosis
Cardiac—supraventricular tachycardia
Congenital disorders
Respiratory
Tracheal stenosis, web
Tracheoesophageal fistula
Tracheomalacia
Delayed presentation of diaphragmatic hernia
Lobar emphysema
Cardiac
Cardiac failure (e.g., critical aortic coarctation of aorta, aortic stenosis, hypoplastic left heart, patent ductus arteriosus)
Cyanotic disease (e.g., transposition of great arteries)
Vascular ring
Neuromuscular disease (e.g., myopathy)

Bronchiolitis. Acute bronchiolitis usually presents in infancy as a serous nasal discharge accompanied by sneezing. These symptoms are followed by fever (38.5°C to 39°C), diminished appetite, cough, dyspnea, irritability, and, commonly, periods of apnea. Apnea is more common in infants less than 3 months of age and usually presents in the first 3 days of the illness. On examination, the infant usually has tachypnea (respiratory rate greater than 60 breaths per minute), is cyanotic, has intercostal and subcostal retractions, and has a palpable liver and spleen due to hyperinflation of the lungs. Expiration is prolonged, and wheezes and fine rales are present. Chest radiographs usually reveal hyperinflation with atelectasis. A trial of a β_2-agonist, such as albuterol, is warranted in all cases, because it is difficult to differentiate infants with pure reactive airway disease. All infants with a history of apnea should be admitted to the hospital for monitoring; infants who are moderately ill should be considered for admission as well. All high-risk infants should be admitted, and antiviral therapy should be considered. Infants with a history of severe prematurity, chronic lung disease, congenital heart disease, and immune deficiency are at high risk for respiratory failure, and should all be admitted.

Bronchopulmonary Dysplasia. Bronchopulmonary dysplasia (BPD) is the chronic pulmonary disease of infancy that usually follows ventilator and oxygen therapy for neonatal respiratory distress syndrome. Although new therapies, such as exogenous surfactant administration, high-frequency ventilation, and administration of steroids (prenatal and postnatal), and other changes in patient care may have altered the severity of BPD, chronic lung disease remains a major clinical problem. With continued improvement in survival of extremely preterm newborns, BPD is one of the most significant sequelae of neonatal intensive care; therefore, these surviving infants will be increasingly seen in EDs. Chronic abnormalities in lung function and gas exchange, as well as cardiovascular problems, such as pulmonary and systemic hypertension and cardiac hypertrophy, are among the long-term complications. Other clinical problems include growth, nutrition, metabolic, neurologic, and developmental issues.

The underlying pulmonary disease results in limited reserve and in visits to the ED with respiratory tract infections. RSV is the most frequent cause of respiratory distress in these patients during winter and early spring months. Other viral infections, such as influenza and parainfluenza, are also implicated. Bacterial organisms may also be likely pathogens. Infections in the infant with BPD can rapidly progress to severe respiratory failure, especially if treatment is delayed. Respiratory distress is generally due to severe airflow obstruction, which may be alleviated by bronchodilator therapy. Early hospitalization of the patient with BPD should be considered in an infant with even mild-to-moderate distress.

Congenital Disorders

Respiratory Disease. Although rare, H-type tracheoesophageal fistula may present in the first month of life or later, with recurrent pneumonia, respiratory distress after feeds, or difficulty handling mucus and secretions. Congenital stenosis of the trachea may initially present with noisy breathing, high-pitched cry, or respiratory distress, especially when associated with mild upper respiratory infection. Tracheomalacia, weakness of the cartilaginous rings of the trachea, may present in the neonate with cough, stridor, dyspnea, and cyanosis. This is often a diagnosis of exclusion, and management is usually conservative therapy.

Cardiac Disease. Neonates with congenital heart disease may present with rapid breathing, but this is usually not associated with significant retractions or use of accessory muscles. Congenital heart disease should be considered in the neonate with unexplained tachypnea and cyanosis. Neonates may present in congestive heart failure due to transposition of the great arteries, with a ventricular septal defect, critical coarctation of the aorta, or supraventricular tachycardia. Signs of heart failure may be subtle but are life-threatening and require emergent referral. Clinical examination may reveal dyspnea, cyanosis, weak peripheral pulses, cardiomegaly, and hepatomegaly.

Neuromuscular Disease. Muscle weakness from any cause, including myopathies, may be associated with shallow breathing and an increase in respiratory rate as a compensatory mechanism.

Cough/Nasal Congestion

Coughing may be a primary symptom of many respiratory illnesses as well as cardiac disease. It may also be the initial presentation of a variety of congenital anomalies, including cleft palate, laryngotracheomalacia, laryngotracheal cleft, tracheal webs, tracheoesophageal fistula, tracheal hemangiomas, and vascular rings. Cough and nasal congestion in the neonate may be a result of congenital malformations, but, in most instances, cough is due to a viral upper respiratory infection. Treatment of the underlying condition is the treatment of choice in the coughing neonate. Cough suppressants should be avoided in neonates because there is a possibility of respiratory depression. Nasal congestion is best treated with instillation of saline drops and suctioning with a bulb syringe.

Noisy Breathing/Stridor

In the neonate, noisy breathing is a common presenting complaint and is usually benign. Stridor is usually due to congenital anomalies (webs, cysts, atresia, stenosis, clefts, hemangiomas) extending anywhere from the nose to the tracheobronchial area. Infants requiring prolonged intubation in the neonatal period are prone to develop subglottic stenosis. Infection (croup, epiglottitis, retropharyngeal abscess) as a cause of stridor is rare in the neonate. Stridor, which worsens with crying, is suggestive of laryngomalacia or subglottic hemangioma; stridor and feeding difficulties are suggestive of vascular ring, laryngeal cleft, or tracheoesophageal fistula; stridor with hoarseness is suggestive of vocal cord paralysis. Laryngomalacia is the most common cause of stridor in the neonate and is characterized by noisy, crowing inspiratory sounds. The first upper respiratory infection usually accentuates these noisy sounds. This condition usually improves in the first year of life.

Periodic Breathing and Central Apnea

Normal neonates may have episodes of *periodic breathing,* defined as absence of breathing for less than 20 seconds, which is not usually accompanied by bradycardia or color changes. This pattern of breathing is different from apnea, which is usually associated with adverse effects such as bradycardia or cyanosis. Periodic breathing may precede apnea, however, and both may occur in the same patient. Apnea in a neonate usually signifies critical illness and warrants prompt investigation and hospital admission. Central apnea may be precipitated by any of the causes of rapid breathing listed in Table 281.3. Because there is a deficiency in fatigue-resistant respiratory muscle fibers in the neonate, apnea may indicate respiratory muscle fatigue and impending respiratory arrest. After the apneic infant is stabilized, that is, after airway support and ventilation are provided, a thorough search for the inciting condition should be undertaken. If an obvious cause is not found, the neonate should be presumed to be septic, and the appropriate cultures obtained. Broad-spectrum antibiotics should then be started. Antibiotic therapy should not be delayed, however, if there is difficulty in obtaining all cultures.

Blue Spells and Cyanosis

Blue spells or cyanosis in infants may be caused by a variety of disorders. If breathing is rapid but not labored, the most likely cause is cyanotic congenital heart disease with right-to-left shunting. Although rare, methemoglobinemia may present with similar findings. Sepsis, meningitis, cerebral edema, or intracranial hemorrhage may be associated with irregular or shallow breathing and cyanosis. Labored breathing (grunting, indrawing) is most likely due to pulmonary disease (pneumonia, bronchiolitis). Infants with cyanosis should be admitted to the hospital for monitoring and further investigation.

Other Organ Systems

Illness involving other organ systems, such as generalized sepsis, meningitis, gastroenteritis, or metabolic acidosis, may cause tachypnea in the newborn. Disease outside of the lung should always be suspected in the infant with respiratory distress as the predominant symptom.

Neurological Symptoms and Signs

Neonatal seizures are fairly common. Arriving at the diagnosis of seizure in the neonate may be difficult, as seizures manifest in a variety of nonspecific symptoms due to immaturity of the nervous system. Seizures may be either generalized, tonic–clonic, absence, focal or associated with subtle motor activities such as ocular changes, oral–buccal–lingual movements, cycling–swimming limb movements, or apnea. There are several possible etiologies for seizure-like activity in the neonate. These include metabolic causes (e.g., hypoglycemia), infections, intracranial hemorrhage, and cerebral malformations. The first step in management of these infants is to ensure stability of vital functions, such as airway, breathing, and circulation. Evaluation should include a blood count, bedside glucose determination, serum glucose, a serum calcium, lumbar puncture, and, possibly, a brain imaging study such as computed tomography or magnetic resonance imaging. The usual first choice of anticonvulsant in a neonate is phenobarbital, although some physicians favor a benzodiazepine such as lorazepam or diazepam. For adequate blood levels (20 to 40 mg/mL), a full 18- to 20-mg/kg phenobarbital load must be given. Thereafter, additional 5- to 10-mg/kg boluses may be given until a serum level of 40 mg/mL is reached. When considering the differential diagnosis of CNS infections in the neonate, in addition to broad-spectrum antibiotics to cover gram-positive and gram-negative organisms, strong consideration should be given to the initiation of intravenous acyclovir for the possibility of HSV encephalitis.

Gastrointestinal Tract Symptoms and Signs

Neonates presenting with gastrointestinal symptoms may either have no significant problems or be seriously ill.

Feeding Difficulties. Feeding difficulties could arise from parental misconceptions or improper feeding, anatomic abnormalities (e.g., cleft palate), obstruction to the esophagus, or localized or systemic infection.

Regurgitation. Regurgitation of small amounts is common in the neonate, due to reduced lower esophageal sphincter pressure and relatively increased intragastric pressure. Rare causes, such as compression of the esophagus or, occasionally, compression of the trachea, however, may also cause regurgitation. Dysphagia, irritability, anemia due to chronic blood loss, and malnutrition are sequelae of chronic regurgitation with esophagitis, but this condition is rare. If the neonate has a history of significant regurgitation, as evidenced by weight loss, pulmonary infiltrates, and irritability, consultation with a pediatrician or a pediatric gastroenterologist should be arranged as an in- or outpatient depending on patient stability. In most instances, reassurance and referral are all that is necessary from the ED physician. Specific investigations and therapy in the ED are rarely required.

Vomiting. Vomiting during the first few weeks of life is uncommon and often is confused with regurgitation. The neonate who vomits from birth is likely to have an anatomic abnormality, such as tracheoesophageal fistula, upper gastrointestinal obstruction, or midgut rotation. Acute-onset vomiting, however, is more commonly part of the symptom complex of some other disease, such as infection, raised intracranial pressure, or hepatobiliary disease. Projectile vomiting usually indicates pyloric stenosis, especially in male neonates. Inborn errors of metabolism should also be considered as a cause of vomiting in this age group. The physical examination of the neonate with vomiting should include assessment of hydration status, level of consciousness, and nonspecific signs such as jaundice. Laboratory evaluation should include electrolytes, glucose, and acid–base status. Infants less than 2 months of age who are vomiting should be admitted to the hospital for evaluation and therapy.

Diarrhea. The complaint of diarrhea often reflects ignorance of the normal variation in neonatal stool frequency and consistency. Diarrhea may be associated with systemic diseases, however, such as generalized sepsis or localized infections of the ear or bladder. Nonspecific diarrhea that neither contains blood or mucus nor is associated with other illnesses is termed *parenteral diarrhea.*

Diarrhea may be secondary to infectious causes and is usually associated with fever. The most common cause is a viral infection, with rotavirus and enteroviruses being the most common. Bacterial causes include *E. coli, Salmonella,* and *Shigella.* Parasitic causes include *Entamoeba histolytica* and are rare in immunocompetent neonates. Diarrhea may be one of the presenting features of HIV infection in infants. Causes of bloody diarrhea in the neonate include necrotizing enterocolitis, bacterial enteritis, antibiotic-associated diarrhea, milk allergy, and, rarely, intussusception. The neonate with diarrhea should be assessed for signs of dehydration. Close attention should be paid to the nutritional status as well as to fluid and electrolyte balance. Infants who are moderately or severely dehydrated should be admitted to the hospital for treatment, whereas infants with mild dehydration can be followed closely as outpatients if periodic reassessment can be arranged.

Necrotizing enterocolitis occurs more commonly in the premature neonate than in the older infant. It may occur in the full-term neonate, however, and usually presents with other signs of sepsis (jaundice, lethargy, poor feeding, poor perfusion). Abdominal radiography may demonstrate pneumatosis intestinalis. True milk allergy presents with abdominal distention, explosive bloody diarrhea, and, in severe cases, shock. Intussusception usually occurs in the older infant and toddler but can also occur in the neonate. It may present with abdominal distention, feeding difficulties, and a mass in the right upper quadrant.

Constipation. True constipation in the neonate may suggest meconium ileus or plug, Hirschsprung disease, hypothyroidism, intestinal stenosis, or atresia. Hirschsprung disease should be suspected in the constipated neonate when there is absence of feces on rectal examination and an abrupt change in bowel luminal size on barium enema. The diagnosis is confirmed by the absence of ganglion cells on a rectal biopsy. In a neonate with constipation, feeding problems, a weak and hoarse cry, hypothermia, hypotonia, and peripheral edema, a diagnosis of hypothyroidism should be entertained.

Abdominal Distention. Abdominal distention in the neonate is common and is usually due to lax abdominal musculature, relatively large intraabdominal organs, and frequent swallowing of air. If the neonate is feeding well and has a soft abdomen, there should be no concern. Generalized sepsis, gastroenteritis, or constipation, however, may also result in an ileus and abdominal distention. Organomegaly from congenital or acquired hepatomegaly, splenomegaly, or renal enlargement may also present as abdominal distention.

Jaundice. Jaundice is a yellowish green or yellowish orange pigmentation of the skin and sclera due to excess bilirubin (Table 281.4). It may appear at various times during the neonatal period but usually appears on the second or third day of life and resolves in 7 to 10 days in the term infant. If jaundice persists for more than 10 days, however, a complete diagnostic evaluation is warranted. Jaundice during the first 24 hours rarely presents to the ED. The most common cause of jaundice seen in the ED is physiologic, which is usually benign, and treatment is rarely necessary. Other common causes seen in the ED include jaundice secondary to sepsis, breast milk jaundice, and, occasionally, hemolysis due to other immune congenital causes.

Physiologic jaundice is due to the breakdown of fetal red blood cells, with bilirubin rising at a rate of less than 5 mg/dL/24 h, with a peak of 5 to 6 mg/dL during the second to fourth day of life, returning to less than 2 mg/dL by 5 to 7 days. The infant with sepsis and hyperbilirubinemia has other features of sepsis, such as vomiting, abdominal distention, respiratory distress, and poor feeding. Like physiologic jaundice, breast milk jaundice is associated with prolonged unconjugated hyperbilirubinemia, which may start as early as the third to fourth day of life and reach a peak of 10 to 27/mg/dL by week 3. Discontinuation of breast feeding causes a rapid decline of the bilirubin in 2 to 3 days. This is thought to be due to the presence of substances that inhibit glucuronyl transferase in breast milk.

A complete history and physical examination often provide a clue to the cause of jaundice in the newborn. The well-looking infant who is gaining weight and feeding well is unlikely to be septic. Laboratory evaluation should include a full blood count for anemia, a smear for hemolysis, direct and total bilirubin evaluation, a reticulocyte count, and a Coombs' test. For the neonate who looks unwell and has any of the symptoms or signs listed in Table 281.4, appropriate cultures should be drawn, broad-spectrum antibiotics should be instituted, and the patient

TABLE 281.4. Common Causes of Jaundice in Neonates

FIRST DAY OF LIFE
Erythroblastosis fetalis
Sepsis
Congenital infections (rubella, toxoplasmosis, cytomegalovirus)
Hematoma
2 TO 3 DAYS
Physiologic
Sepsis
Intrauterine infections
3 DAYS TO 1 WEEK
Breast milk jaundice
Sepsis, atresia of bile ducts
Viral hepatitis
Congenital hemolytic anemias (spherocytosis, sickle cell anemia)
Hemolytic anemia due to drugs (e.g., in glucose-6-phosphate dehydrogenase deficiency)
Hypothyroidism
Rubella
Galactosemia

should be admitted to the hospital. In all cases, arrangements should be made to monitor bilirubin and hemoglobin levels. Most well infants can be monitored out of the hospital, but infants who are anemic or have bilirubin levels approaching exchange transfusion levels (approximately 20 mg/dL) should be admitted for phototherapy and close observation.

Eye Discharge and Redness

The most common cause of red eye in the neonate is conjunctivitis, and although the most common cause of neonatal conjunctivitis is chemical, due to silver nitrate administration, this rarely presents to the ED. The most common causes of conjunctivitis during the first 2 weeks of life are infection with *Chlamydia, Neisseria gonorrhoeae,* and gram-negative bacilli (*E. coli* and *Pseudomonas*). Neonates older than 2 weeks of age may also have conjunctivitis secondary to infections with such organisms as herpesvirus and *Staphylococcus* and *Streptococcus* species.

Gonococcal conjunctivitis begins after an incubation period of 2 to 5 days with a mild inflammation accompanied by a serosanguineous discharge that becomes purulent within 24 hours. *Chlamydia trachomatis* has an incubation period of 5 to 14 days and is associated with a thick, purulent discharge in an afebrile and alert infant. It may also accompany pneumonia in the neonate older than 3 weeks of age. After obtaining appropriate cultures, infectious causes should be treated. A neonate with a red eye and irritability may also be suffering from a corneal irritation or abrasion that is usually due to an eyelash or fingernail scratch. Acute glaucoma is rare and presents as a red, teary eye. In these instances, the cornea may be stained or cloudy, the anterior chamber shallow, and intraocular pressure increased. Prompt ophthalmologic consultation should be obtained in all cases of suspected glaucoma.

Diaper Rash and Oral Thrush

Diaper dermatitis is fairly common in the neonate. *Candida albicans* is the most common cause of diaper dermatitis and presents as an erythematous plaque with a scalloped border and a sharply demarcated edge studded by satellite lesions. It usually occurs in the moist, occluded diaper area and intertriginous zones and results from the action of organisms harbored in the gastrointestinal tract. Treatment consists of applying an anticandidal agent with each diaper change, or four times daily. Protection of the area with zinc oxide paste overlying the cream prevents friction. In severe cases, an oral course of treatment is warranted to prevent colonization of the gut.

Oral lesions are white, flaky plaques covering the tongue, lips, and gingival and mucous membranes. These lesions are common in debilitated infants, especially those with immunodeficiency disorders and those neonates on antibiotic therapy. A neonate with oral lesions may have decreased intake because of the pain and discomfort associated with these lesions. Treatment consists of administration of a topical antifungal agent and an anesthetic gel before feeding. Cool liquids may prevent discomfort and pain. Infants with significantly decreased intake or who exhibit evidence of dehydration should be admitted for further management.

Fever and Sepsis

Fever in the neonate is most commonly due to infectious causes. Infections occurring in the first 5 days of life are usually acquired by vertical transmission from the mother. Bacterial infections are usually caused by streptococci (30%), *E. coli* (30% to 40%), other gram-negative enteric organisms (15% to 20%), and gram-positive cocci (10%). Viral infections are common, however, and are most likely due to enteroviruses (coxsackievirus and echovirus) acquired at the time of delivery or to RSV acquired postnatally. All toxic-appearing infants and all febrile infants younger than 28 days of age should be hospitalized for parenteral antibiotic therapy after a full sepsis workup (Tables 281.5 and 281.6).

Listeria monocytogenes is an uncommon but potentially lethal cause of sepsis and meningitis in neonates. Like group B *Streptococcus,* it tends to occur in an early and a late form, and the signs and symptoms are similar to those seen with group B *Streptococcus* infection. The differential diagnosis should also include the possibility of HSV infection. In addition to broad-spectrum antibiotics, the antiviral agent acyclovir should be added if there is a clinical suspicion of an HSV infection.

Apparent Life-Threatening Events

Apparent life-threatening events (ALTEs) should be considered a chief complaint rather than a specific diagnosis. *ALTE* is defined as "an episode that is frightening to the observer and is characterized by some combination of apnea, color change, marked change in muscle tone, choking or gagging. In some cases the observer fears that the infant has died." There has been previously used terminology such as *aborted crib death* or *near-miss SIDS*. These terms should be abandoned because they imply a possibly misleading, close association between this type of event and SIDS (sudden infant death syndrome). Although SIDS should be considered in these cases, catastrophic deterioration is more likely to be due to infectious causes (septicemia,

TABLE 281.5. Signs and Symptoms of Neonatal Sepsis

Temperature instability
Fever, hypothermia
Central nervous system dysfunction
Lethargy, irritability, seizures
Respiratory distress
Apnea, tachypnea, grunting
Feeding intolerance
Vomiting, poor feeding, gastric distention, diarrhea
Jaundice
Itching, rash

TABLE 281.6. Antibiotic Therapy for Infections[a]

Indications	Drugs
Bacterial pneumonia Generalized sepsis Necrotizing enterocolitis Bacterial meningitis Gonococcal infections	Ampicillin (100 mg/kg/d q6h); and gentamicin (7.5 mg/kg/d q8h) or cefotaxime (200 mg/kg/d q8h)
Urinary tract infections	Length of therapy depends on infection being treated.
Bronchiolitis (respiratory synctial virus)	Ribavirin (nebulized) 20 mg/mL water for 12–18 h/d for 3–5 days
Conjunctivitis (bacterial)	Sodium sulamyd 10% or topical erythromycin 2 drops to each eye, q4h for 5–7 days or erythromycin 40 mg/kg/d q6h for 14 days
Pneumonia (chlamydial)	Erythromycin 40 mg/kg/d q6h for 14 days
Oral thrush	Oral nystatin suspension 100,000 U q4–6h after feeds for 7–14 days
Candida dermatitis	Nystatin or amphotericin cream to affected area q4–6h for 7–14 days
Herpesvirus infection	Acyclovir 30 mg/kg/d q8h

[a] Antibiotic dosages as well as type may change. Consultation with the most recent *Report of the Committee on Infectious Diseases* (*Red Book*) is recommended.

meningitis), trauma (intracranial bleed, child abuse), inborn errors of metabolism (medium-chain acyl dehydrogenase deficiency), gastroesophageal reflux, seizures, cardiac dysrhythmia, or Munchausen syndrome by proxy. In most cases of SIDS, cardiopulmonary resuscitation is unsuccessful because the myocardium has suffered severe hypoxic ischemic damage. If the infant appears hemodynamically stable at the time of presentation, a very careful history and physical examination should be performed. Most infants, who present acutely after an ALTE, require hospitalization. If the infant presents with a history of apnea, following stabilization of airway support and ventilation, a thorough search for the inciting condition should be undertaken. If an obvious cause is not found, the neonate should be presumed to be septic, and the appropriate cultures (blood, urine, and cerebrospinal fluid) should be obtained. Broad-spectrum antibiotics, and possibly antiviral therapy with acyclovir, should then be started. However, antibiotic therapy should not be delayed if there is difficulty in obtaining all cultures. In true cases of SIDS, the cause of death is unknown; therefore, appropriate samples (blood, urine, skin biopsy) and a complete autopsy should be obtained.

DISPOSITION

Role of the Consultant

The emergency physician should be aware of the conditions that require urgent medical or surgical subspecialty evaluation. These include the cyanotic infant with possible congenital heart disease, requiring a pediatric cardiology consultation, or the neonate with an acute abdomen, requiring pediatric surgical evaluation.

Transportation

Transporting the neonate either in the prehospital setting or during interhospital transport requires attention to the airway, breathing, and circulation. Because of their increased heat loss, neonates also need maintenance of temperature. Continuous monitoring to ensure adequate oxygenation, temperature, and other vital signs is necessary. Transport personnel should be able to provide advanced pediatric life support in case the neonate becomes unstable during transport. Appropriate-sized resuscitation equipment and medications should be readily available during transport. Consideration should always be given to the risk–benefit of any transport action.

COMMON PITFALLS

- Unfamiliarity with the patterns of normal vegetative functions in the neonate
- Failure to recognize the extent of volume loss in the critically ill neonate
- Missing the signs of child abuse
- Excluding congenital causes in the differential diagnosis
- Not obtaining appropriate samples to exclude a metabolic disorder in a child dying of SIDS
- Failure to recognize signs and symptoms of impending respiratory failure
- Failure to provide parental reassurance and support

Bibliography

American Academy of Pediatrics. *Report of the Committee on Infectious Diseases*. Elk Grove Village, IL: American Academy of Pediatrics, 1997.

Baraff LJ, Bass JW, Fleisher GR, et al. Practice guidelines for the management of infants and children 0 to 36 months of age with fever without source. *Pediatrics* 1993;92:1.

Behrman RE, Kliegman RM, Arvin AM. *Nelson textbook of pediatrics*, 15th ed. Philadelphia: WB Saunders, 1996.

Burton BK. Inborn errors of metabolism in infancy: a guide to diagnosis. *Pediatrics* 1998;102:E69.

Chameides L, Hazinski MF, eds. *Pediatric advanced life support*. Dallas: American Heart Association, 1997:9-1–9-10.

Committee on Drugs, 1996 to 1997, Liaison Representatives, and AAP Section Liaisons. Drugs for pediatric emergencies. *Pediatrics* 1998;101:E13.

Dillon PW, Cilley RE. Newborn surgical emergencies: gastrointestinal anomalies, abdominal wall defects. *Pediatr Clin North Am* 1993;40:1289.

Gayle MO, Kissoon N, Hered R, et al. Retinal hemorrhage in the young child. A review of etiology, predisposed conditions and clinical implications. *J Emerg Med* 1995;13:233.

McIntosh N. Pain in the newborn, a possible new starting point. *Eur J Pediatr* 1997;156:173.

Stafstrom CE. Neonatal seizures. *Pediatr Rev* 1995;16:248.

Trocinski DR, Pearigen PD. The crying infant. *Emerg Med Clin North Am* 1998;16:895.

CHAPTER 282
Nursemaid's Elbow

Julide Ayse Ozan

Subluxation of the radial head (nursemaid's elbow or pulled elbow) is a common injury in the preschool-aged child.[4] The synonymous terms *supermarket elbow* and *temper tantrum elbow* lend further causal description to this injury. It often occurs in grocery stores, on stairways, or in other situations, when the parent or guardian is in a hurry or the child is misbehaving. The injury is caused by sudden traction of the hand, with the elbow extended and the forearm pronated. There may be a history of pulling a child as he or she stumbles to prevent a fall, lifting a child by the hand, or pulling the hand through the sleeve of a garment. Occasionally, it may be attributed to a fall on the arm.

The peak incidence occurs in children aged 1 to 4 years. It is rare after age 5 and has been reported in 6- to 12-month-old infants.[2] It occurs more often in boys, and the left elbow is involved more often than the right.

The pathophysiology is partly explained by the anatomic features of the region. The annular ligament is thinly attached to the periosteum of the radial neck in children younger than 5 years of age, whereas this attachment is stronger in the older child. Traction exerted on the upper extremity when it is in a pronated, extended position causes a transverse tear in the distal attachment of the annular ligament to the periosteum of the radial head. The head of the radius then moves distally. When traction is released, the ligament is carried up and becomes impacted between the radius and the capitellum (Fig. 282.1). Because the shape of the radial head is not completely regular, the ligament can be replaced by slight flexion and supination—thus, the method of treatment.

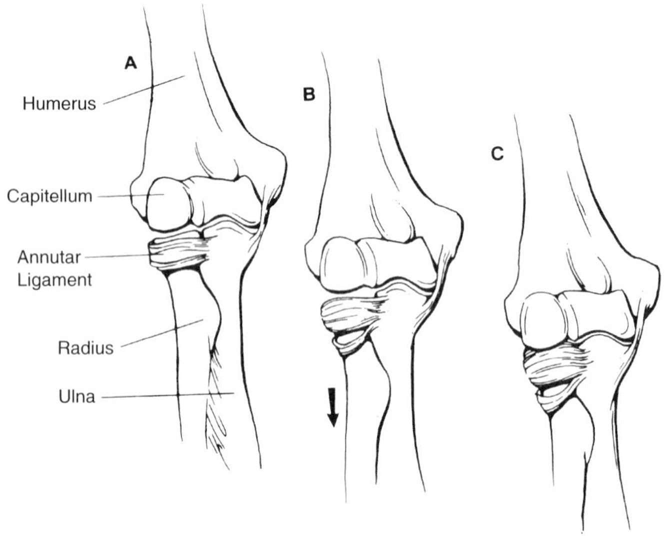

Figure 282.1. Pathology of pulled elbow. **(A)** Normal annular ligament that attaches the radius to the ulna. **(B)** Traction on the radius, causing a tear in the attachment of the annular ligament. **(C)** When traction is released, fibers of the ligament are caught between the radial head and the capitellum.

CLINICAL PRESENTATION AND EMERGENCY DEPARTMENT EVALUATION

The diagnosis of subluxation of the radial head is made by the typical clinical findings. Immediately after injury, the child cries in pain and refuses to use the affected arm. The child holds the elbow slightly flexed and the forearm pronated. Local tenderness may be palpated over the anterolateral aspect of the radial head. There is no restriction to flexion and extension of the elbow, but supination of the forearm is markedly limited and voluntarily resisted. The diagnosis may be missed if supination of the forearm is not tested. A clear history should be obtained before examining the toddler in the parent's arms. Gentle manipulation of the contralateral arm first may make examination of the injured arm easier.

Radiographic findings are minimal and generally not helpful. It is a soft-tissue injury, and although subluxation of the radial head does occur, it is minimal and usually not demonstrable radiographically.[1,5] A radiograph to rule out fracture may be made, however. This may prove therapeutic rather than diagnostic, because reduction is often accomplished when the arm is positioned by the technician.

DIFFERENTIAL DIAGNOSIS

Other causes of pain and limited motion should be kept in mind. Shoulder dislocations, brachial plexus injuries, fractures, and wrist sprains can present in a similar manner, as can infectious processes (i.e., osteomyelitis and septic arthritis).

EMERGENCY DEPARTMENT MANAGEMENT AND DISPOSITION

Reduction of the subluxation is usually effected readily in the emergency department. A parent or assistant restrains the child in the sitting position. The palm of the child's hand is grasped as if to shake it. The elbow is encircled with the other hand, with the thumb over the annular ligament of the radius. Then the palm of the hand is gently supinated, and, with a continuous motion, the elbow is flexed to the shoulder. During the flexion maneuver, the physician may feel a "click" with the thumb that lies over the radial head. This maneuver results in instantaneous relief of pain and reuse of the arm within 30 minutes in 90% of patients.[2,4]

Recent studies have shown that hyperpronation of the wrist of the affected arm may provide an alternative method of reducing the subluxation if the supination maneuver is initially unsuccessful.[2] Also, the supination maneuver may be repeated several times during the initial visit. The child should be seen again in 24 hours for repeated manipulation if he or she is still not using the arm normally. At the second visit, if the child does not use the arm within 30 minutes, he or she should be completely reevaluated. Septic arthritis, osteomyelitis, and fractures above and below the elbow, including the clavicle and humerus, should be considered.

Immobilization is unnecessary if it is the first time subluxation has occurred. A sling may be applied if the child does not use the arm, to prevent anyone pulling on the elbow. If treatment is delayed for more than 12 hours, some clinicians immobilize the upper arm in a long-arm posterior splint with the elbow in 90-degree flexion and the forearm in full supination for 10 days.

Recurrence of subluxation as a result of a subsequent pull on the hand occurs in about 25% of cases.[6] After manipulative reduction of a recurrent case, it is best to immobilize the upper limb in a long-arm cast for at least 2 or 3 weeks.

In a small number of children, the subluxated radial head is irreducible by closed manipulation and requires open reduction by an orthopedic surgeon.

COMMON PITFALLS

- With nursemaid's elbow, there is usually no swelling, bruising, or other evidence of injury. If these are present, another diagnosis should be considered.
- Before discharge, the mechanism of injury should be explained to the parents. This might help prevent a recurrence.

ACKNOWLEDGMENT

The author gratefully acknowledges the contribution of Ann K. Leahy, who wrote the previous version of this chapter.

References

1. Bretland PM. Pulled elbow in childhood. *Br J Radiol* 1994;67:1176.
2. Marcias CG, Bothner J, Wiebe R. A comparison of supination/flexion to hyperpronation in the reduction of radial head subluxations. *Pediatrics* 1998;102:E10.
3. Sachetti A, Ramoska EE, Glascow C. Nonclassic history in children with radial head subluxations. *J Emerg Med* 1990;8:151–153.
4. Schutzman SA, Teach S. Upper-extremity impairment in young children. *Ann Emerg Med* 1995;26:474.
5. Snyder HS. Radiographic changes with radial head subluxation in children. *J Emerg Med* 1990;8:265.
6. Teach SJ, Schutzman SA. Prospective study of recurrent radial head subluxation. *Arch Pediatr Adolesc Med* 1996;150:164.

CHAPTER 283
Osgood-Schlatter Disease

Todd Wylie

In 1903, Osgood and Schlatter each described, in separate papers, a disturbance of the tibial tuberosity in adolescents, which came to be known as Osgood-Schlatter disease.[6,9] The condition is thought to be a traction apophysitis of the tibial tubercle resulting from repeated normal stresses or overuse.[7] Generally, the pathology is considered to be a result of partial avulsion of developing ossification centers and overlying cartilage from the anterior surface of the tibial apophysis.[5] Radiologic studies have demonstrated changes in the patellar tendon at the insertion on the tibial tuberosity, suggesting that patellar tendinitis may be a significant source of the clinical symptoms seen in patients with Osgood-Schlatter disease.[8]

Patients are usually between 10 to 15 years of age at onset of Osgood-Schlatter disease.[5] Boys are affected more often than girls. The condition is usually unilateral, but it may be bilateral in 35% to 56% of boys and approximately 18% of girls.[3,4] It is usually a self-limiting condition but should be distinguished from a fracture, tumor, or infection.

CLINICAL PRESENTATION

Osgood-Schlatter disease rarely presents as an acute complaint. The pain may have been present intermittently for a period of time before the patient seeks medical attention. Common complaints include knee pain that is exacerbated by running, kneeling, squatting, and climbing or descending stairs.[7] Children almost always point specifically to the tibial tubercle as the site of discomfort. There may also be a history of relief of pain with rest or cessation of strenuous activities.

Physical findings include localized swelling and tenderness over the tibial tuberosity at the site of patellar tendon insertion. Effusion and other abnormalities of the joint should be absent. The pain is reproducible by extending the knee against resistance.

EMERGENCY DEPARTMENT EVALUATION

A reasonably certain diagnosis can be made from the history and physical examination. If Osgood-Schlatter disease is suspected from the history, the diagnosis usually can be confirmed by having the patient sit on the edge of the examination table, hang his or her legs off the table, and point to the site of greatest tenderness. If the patient points to the tibial tubercle, the diagnosis is reasonably certain.

Radiographs are not necessary in all cases of Osgood-Schlatter disease. Radiographs may help confirm the diagnosis but are more helpful in ruling out other disorders, such as fractures and occult bone tumors. Anteroposterior knee radiographs usually appear normal. A lateral knee radiograph is best for demonstrating abnormalities, which may include areas of calcification in the tibial tubercle region, separate ossicles from the anterior border of the tubercle, and prominence of the tubercle.[7]

EMERGENCY DEPARTMENT MANAGEMENT

Treatment of Osgood-Schlatter disease is usually symptomatic. Restriction of vigorous activities for 2 to 4 months is recommended, based on the severity of symptoms. Total restriction from all athletic activities is generally not necessary. Stretching exercises for the quadriceps and hamstrings are advisable. Icing after sporting activities and use of nonsteroidal antiinflammatory agents may be helpful. Corticosteroid injections are not recommended and may actually cause complications.[10,11] In severe or persistent cases, a knee immobilizer is recommended for 3 to 6 weeks. In rare cases, immobilization in a cylinder cast may be necessary.

DISPOSITION

Patients with Osgood-Schlatter disease should be referred to their primary care physicians for follow-up care. Orthopedic referral may be indicated in persistent or severe cases. Symptoms usually resolve with conservative treatment. In almost all cases, resolution of symptoms is final at skeletal maturity, when the apophysis of the tibial tubercle fuses to the metaphysis of the tibia. Occasional patients develop chronic pain, associated with a discrete ossicle in the patellar tendon. Surgical excision provides predictable relief in these rare cases.[1]

COMMON PITFALLS

- Radiographs may be incorrectly interpreted as an acute fracture.
- Do not forget to stress the importance of activity restriction to the patient, parents, and school.

ACKNOWLEDGMENT

The author gratefully acknowledges the contribution of Daniel Cavallaro and Jeffrey B. Neustadt, who wrote the previous version of this chapter.

References

1. Binazzi R. Surgical treatment of unresolved Osgood-Schlatter lesion. *Clin Orthop Rel Res* 1993;289:202.
2. Dunn JF. Osgood-Schlatter disease. *Am Fam Physician* 1990;41:173.
3. Ehrenborg G. The Osgood-Schlatter lesion. A clinical and experimental study. *Acta Chir Scand (Suppl)* 1962;288:1.
4. Kujala UM, Kvist M, Heinonen O. Osgood-Schlatter's disease in adolescent athletes. Retrospective study of incidence and duration. *Am J Sports Med* 1985;13:236.
5. Morrissy RT, ed. *Lovell and Winter's pediatric orthopaedics,* 4th ed. Philadelphia: Lippincott–Raven Publishers, 1996.
6. Osgood RB. Lesions of the tibial tubercle occurring during adolescence. *Boston Med Surg J* 1903;148:114.
7. Rockwood CA, ed. *Fractures in children,* 4th ed. Philadelphia: Lippincott–Raven Publishers, 1996.
8. Rosenberg ZS, et al. Osgood-Schlatter lesion: fracture or tendinitis? Scintigraphic, CT, and MR imaging features. *Radiology* 1992;185:853.
9. Schlatter C. Veletzungen des schnabelfermigen Fertsatzeo der oberon Tibiaepiphyse. *Bruns Beitr Klin Chir* 1903;38:874.
10. Smith JB. Knee problems in children. *Pediatr Clin North Am* 1986;33:1439.
11. Wojtys EM. Sports injuries in the immature athlete. *Orthop Clin North Am* 1987;18:689.

CHAPTER 284
Otitis Externa

Katalin I. Koranyi

External otitis is an inflammatory condition of the auricle, the ear canal, or the outer surface of the tympanic membrane. It is caused by infection, inflammatory dermatitis, or local trauma to the skin. Acute diffuse external otitis (swimmer's ear) is the most common infection of the external ear in children. Perspiration and hearing aids contribute to the retention of moisture in the car canal.[4] It must be differentiated from acute *localized* external otitis (impetigo, folliculitis, herpes simplex) and from chronic external otitis (infection secondary to a coexisting drainage from the middle ear) or as secondary to seborrhea.

CLINICAL PRESENTATION

This bacterial (occasionally fungal) infection usually affects persons after prolonged and frequent swimming, particularly when the weather is hot and humid. As water is retained in the external ear canal, the normal resident flora of the area are altered, with an increase in the proportion of gram-negative organisms. The normally acid pH of the ear canal becomes more alkaline, and this wet and alkaline debris is a good culture medium. The infection causes edema and pain, which may be severe. The presenting symptoms are itching and ear pain. The pain is worse on touching the ear and on swallowing. Most cases are caused by *Pseudomonas,* gram-negative organisms, and *Staphylococcus aureus.*[3] Anaerobic bacteria or a polymicrobial etiology is also possible.[2] Fungal external otitis (*Aspergillus, Candida*) is rare in the United States.

DIFFERENTIAL DIAGNOSIS

Ear pain may be due to infection *outside* the ear (mastoiditis, parotitis, periauricular adenitis, tonsillitis, temporomandibular joint dysfunction). If the pain originates *in the ear,* foreign body, impacted cerumen, and otitis media must be differentiated from external otitis. Differentiation from otitis media may be, at times, difficult or impossible, because both conditions may coexist, and also, the tympanic membrane may not be visualized due to edema of the ear canal. Acute otitis media is more common in the spring and winter, fever may be present, and, on examination, the tympanic membrane appears red, bulging, or retracted and has decreased mobility. External otitis, in contrast, is more common in the summer, and the tympanic membrane appears normal on examination, or it may be covered by whitish debris. In cases of uncertainty, physicians may have to treat for both otitis media and external otitis.

Another differential diagnosis of swimmer's ear is necrotizing "malignant" external otitis. Although it occurs mainly in the elderly, the diabetic, and the immunocompromised adult, it may occasionally occur in children.[1] The patient is febrile and appears ill. The infection (usually *Pseudomonas*) often spreads to deeper tissues. Patients with malignant external otitis require hospital admission and parenteral antimicrobial therapy.

EMERGENCY DEPARTMENT MANAGEMENT

The most important step in the management of external otitis is the careful cleaning of all debris and the drying of the ear canal. In the very mild case of external otitis, dry-mopping with a small tuft of cotton attached to a wire applicator is sufficient. In the more severe cases, in which the ear canal is occluded by secretions, gentle suction can be used in the external ear canal. This is followed by irrigation with a warm solution (at body temperature). The irrigant solutions include 3% saline, acetic acid 2% in Burow solution (Otic Domeboro solution), or a solution of rubbing alcohol and acetic acid in equal parts. After irrigation, drying can be accomplished by suctioning, compressed air, or use of a hair dryer. When the tympanic membrane is perforated or a perforation is suspected, solutions containing acid or rubbing alcohol should be avoided (because they produce a stinging sensation); 3% saline solution is used in these situations. Home rinsing with Otic Domeboro or a solution of rubbing alcohol and vinegar is often useful and prescribed.

The infection usually can be treated with 2% acetic acid ear drops (Otic Domeboro or propylene glycol Vō Sol, Vō Sol HC otic drops). Otic preparations containing antibiotics are more expensive but are not more effective in treating the infection. However, in the presence of a perforated tympanic membrane, the antibiotic preparations are better tolerated. Polymyxin–neomycin–hydrocortisone (Cortisporin otic suspension) four times a day can be prescribed. Cortisporin otic solution is more irritating. Ciprofloxacin (Cipro HC Otic) solution or ofloxacin (Floxin Otic) solution is appropriate for *Pseudomonas* infection. For fungal external otitis (otomycosis), the therapy is the same as for bacterial infections. If this treatment fails, 25% M-cresyl acetate (Cresylate), given three times a day, or tolnaftate (Tinactin) may be prescribed.[5] For external otitis secondary to seborrhea, control of seborrhea with regular use of dandruff shampoo is a helpful additional measure to the use of antibiotic ear drops.

In the treatment of external otitis, instructions need to be given regarding the proper application of ear drops. The child should lie on his or her side, with the affected ear up. The ear drops are instilled, with the child remaining is this position for 1 to 2 minutes. A piece of cotton can be applied to occlude the ear canal. If there is significant edema of the ear canal, a wick can be placed and left in for 24 hours, with periodic soaking with the ear drops. The treatment is continued with administration of ear drops directly into the ear canal four times a day thereafter, usually for 7 to 10 days. For the treatment of pain, oral analgesics such as acetaminophen alone or in combination with codeine are prescribed. Swimming is not allowed during the course of treatment. If there is therapeutic failure in 48 hours, the patient should be reexamined and a deeper infection, such as an abscess or cellulitis, should be sought. For prophylaxis of the patient with frequent episodes of swimmer's ear, ear drops containing 2% acetic acid (Otic Domeboro solution, VōSol) or a solution of rubbing alcohol and acetic acid in equal parts soon after swimming can be prescribed.

DISPOSITION

Patients with cellulitis extending beyond the external ear canal require admission to the hospital and parenteral antibiotic therapy. When necrotizing malignant external otitis is suspected, consultation with an otolaryngologist needs to be sought and the patient admitted for intensive parenteral antimicrobial therapy.

COMMON PITFALLS

- Diagnosis of swimmer's ear when the problem is really pus in the ear canal draining from a perforated tympanic membrane or through ventilation tubes. In this case, local therapy should be complemented with administration of systemic antibiotics. Improper application of the ear drops into an edematous ear canal may be the cause of "therapeutic failure" (the ear drops do not penetrate completely, or they do not penetrate at all). A cotton wick needs to be left in the ear canal for 24 hours and soaked periodically with the medication.
- Diagnosis of swimmer's ear in the child who has a different dermatosis (seborrheic dermatitis, folliculitis, or herpetic eruption)

References

1. Bergstrom L. Diseases of the external ear. In: Bluestone CD, Stool SE, eds. *Pediatric otolaryngology,* 2nd ed, vol 1. Philadelphia: WB Saunders, 1990:311.
2. Brook I, Frazier EH, Thompson DH. Aerobic and anaerobic microbiology of external otitis. *Clin Infect Dis* 1992;15:955.
3. Marcy SM. External otitis due to infection. *Pediatr Infect Dis* 1985;14:S27.
4. Mirzan N. Otitis externa. Management in the primary care office. *Postgrad Med* 1996;99:153.
5. Pelton SI, Klein JO. The draining ear: otitis media and externa. *Infect Dis Clin North Am* 1988;12:117.

CHAPTER 285
Otitis Media and Mastoiditis

Katalin I. Koranyi

OTITIS MEDIA

Acute otitis media is one of the most common infectious conditions for which children visit a physician.[7] It is the most common indication for the prescription of an antimicrobial agent in childhood. By 3 years of age, 80% of children have had at least one episode of otitis media.[6] The peak occurs between 6 and 24 months of age and during the periods of high incidence of viral upper respiratory tract infections in winter and spring.

The most important factor in the pathogenesis of otitis media appears to be eustachian tube dysfunction.[2] The increased incidence of otitis media in young children is due to the fact that their eustachian tubes are shorter and lie more horizontally than in the older child and adult. Dysfunction of the eustachian tube prevents middle ear secretions from draining into the nasopharynx, and the negative pressure created in the middle ear allows the aspiration of nasopharyngeal secretions into the middle ear. Other important factors include infection, immunologic status, allergy, passive smoking, breast feeding, and socioeconomic status.

CLINICAL PRESENTATION

The usual presentation is that of a child who, having had several days of symptoms of an upper respiratory tract infection, suddenly develops ear pain, fever, decreased hearing, or ear drainage. In infancy, irritability, crying, and difficulty sleeping can be the presenting features. Some children have minimal symptoms or none at all, and otitis media is diagnosed during a routine physical examination. Tugging at the ears may be a sign of otitis media, but often a misleading one, because children may tug or pull at their ears for other reasons.

Thus, the diagnosis of otitis media is based on the appearance and the mobility of the tympanic membrane rather than on symptomatology. The tympanic membrane is red or yellow, dull, and bulging; it has decreased or absent mobility when examined with a pneumatic otoscope. Bulging is best interpreted by the absence of the normal bony landmarks, which, in an early case, may be limited to the pars flaccida.

Some of the difficulties in diagnosing otitis media include the presence of wax in the ear canal, which obscures the visualization of the tympanic membrane, and a crying or febrile child in whom a hyperemic tympanic membrane could be falsely interpreted as early otitis media. Bullous myringitis is a form of acute otitis media in which bullae form between the outer and middle layers of the tympanic membrane. Children with bullous myringitis usually present very acutely with severe otalgia. Purulent otorrhea constitutes a reliable sign for an otitis media with perforation. Hearing loss may be a presenting sign of otitis media, but it will not be the complaint in the young child and it can also easily be missed by parents.

The diagnosis of otitis media in the newborn and very young infant is even more difficult, because their tympanic membranes may be naturally gray and dull. In these infants, the diminished or absent mobility may be the only physical findings for otitis media. If tympanocentesis is performed, a purulent middle ear aspirate is usually obtained. Although not an emergency department procedure, tympanometry usually reveals an effusion pattern.

The microbiology of otitis media from middle ear aspirates demonstrates that the three most common pathogens are *Streptococcus pneumoniae, Haemophilus influenzae,* and *Moraxella catarrhalis. Streptococcus pyogenes* group A, *Staphylococcus aureus, Mycoplasma pneumoniae,* and viruses have also been isolated from the middle ear. The microbiology of acute otitis media in the newborn (i.e., a child in the first 4 weeks of life) is different from that in later life. *S. aureus* and gram-negative enteric organisms should be considered in addition to the other organisms that cause otitis media in the older child.[2] *Chlamydia trachomatis* also may cause acute otitis media in the first few months of life.[2]

DIFFERENTIAL DIAGNOSIS

Earache could be caused by pain referred from sore throat, toothache, external otitis, parotitis, a foreign body in the ear canal, or impacted ear cerumen. Injected blood vessels at the periphery of the tympanic membrane and along the malleus can be seen with fever or crying.

COMPLICATIONS

Acute otitis media may resolve without treatment, but spontaneous rupture of the tympanic membrane and otorrhea may occur. Complications such as ossicle necrosis, retraction pockets, cholesteatoma, mastoiditis, meningitis, cerebral thrombophlebitis, hearing loss, and speech delay are rare but may occur. The introduction of antimicrobial therapy has produced a decline in the frequency of these complications.

EMERGENCY DEPARTMENT MANAGEMENT

Most children who present with symptomatology of otitis media or fever can be easily diagnosed by examining the tympanic membranes and pneumatoscopy. If obscured by cerumen, the ear canals should be cleaned, remembering that irrigation of the ear canal could cause a temporary injection of the blood vessels in the tympanic membrane. Newborns with fever or irritability and otitis media are often hospitalized for a sepsis evaluation and parenteral antibiotic treatment pending culture results.

Systemic Antibiotics

Many episodes of acute otitis media resolve spontaneously. Antimicrobial therapy is directed against the major pathogens: *S. pneumoniae, H. influenzae,* and *M. catarrhalis.* Drug resistance is now common in otitis media. Surveillance data from 1998 demonstrate that up to 34% of all clinical isolates of pneumococci are no longer susceptible to penicillin, and many of these strains are also resistant to other classes of antimicrobials.[9] In the United States, the incidence of β-lactamase–producing *H. influenzae* varies but can be as high as 20% to 25% (for *M. catarrhalis,* up to 70%). *M. catarrhalis* and *H. influenzae* tend to clear spontaneously and have few suppurative complications.

For most physicians, amoxicillin is the drug of choice. Amoxicillin is inexpensive and has only a few side effects (diarrhea, rash). Physicians now favor the higher dosing range of amoxicillin to treat the intermediates and some of the highly resistant *S. pneumoniae.*[7] In the very ill appearing and febrile child (particularly the young infant or the child already on amoxicillin), or for therapeutic failures, an alternative drug should be used.

Second-line therapy includes amoxicillin–clavulanate or cefuroxime axetil.[7] The reformulated amoxicillin–clavulanate (7:1) has fewer gastrointestinal side effects than the old formulation (4:1). Safety and tolerability of a new formulation (90 mg/kg/d, divided every 12 hours) of amoxicillin–clavulanate (14:1) was recently reported.[3] Many of the 13 other Food and Drug Administration–approved otitis media drugs are not very effective against drug-resistant pneumococcus.[4] (For dosages, see Table 285.1.)

If the physician shortens the previously recommended course of therapy from 10 days to 7 days in the child over 24 months, and to 5 days in the child under 24 months of age, the patient is less likely to develop antibiotic resistance and more likely to comply with the regimen. Ceftriaxone as a single daily dose for 1 to 3 days is reserved for the child who is vomiting or unlikely to take oral antibiotics.[5]

Amoxicillin and trimethoprim-sulfamethoxazole are the least expensive drugs. Trimethoprim-sulfamethoxazole does not reliably treat *S. pyogenes* group A. Cefixime has increased activity against *H. influenzae* but decreased activity against *S. pneumoniae.*

Symptomatic relief should occur within 48 to 72 hours after the initiation of therapy. The patient and the parents should be advised to seek medical attention if symptomatology continues beyond that time. If, at this point, the child still has very red and bulging tympanic membranes, a change to a broader spectrum antimicrobial (a β-lactamase–resistant one) should be considered.

In the child who clinically responds well to therapy, a reexamination must be performed by the child's physician in 2 to 3 weeks, in a search for resolutions of acute signs of otitis media. At this checkup, about half of the children still have evidence of serous effusion of the middle ear.

Antibiotic Ear Drops

In the child with considerable purulent drainage from the ear, ear drops can occasionally be prescribed. Gentle cleansing with normal saline solution or diluted sterile vinegar may be followed for a few days by use of an antibiotic–corticosteroid ear drop suspension. Chronic otorrhea may be caused by *Pseudomonas* species, *S. aureus,* or fungal pathogens.

Also, careful evaluation as to possible complications of the acute otitis media or to a coexisting condition (meningitis, brain abscess, or mastoiditis) should be done. In addition, the emergency physician needs to advise the parents to seek prompt medical attention if, during the course of treatment, symptoms of lethargy, irritability, vomiting, or relapse of the fever develop.

TABLE 285.1. Antimicrobial Therapy for Otitis Media

Drug	Dosage
Amoxicillin	80–90 mg/kg/d PO q8h or q12h
Amoxicillin-clavulanate	45 mg/kg/d PO q12h
Azithromycin	10 mg/kg/d loading dose, then 5 mg/kg/d PO q24h
Cefixime	8 mg/kg/d PO q12-24h
Cefpodoxime proxetil	10 mg/kg/d PO q12h
Ceftibuten	9 mg/kg/d PO q24h
Ceftriaxone	50 mg/kg/d i.m. or i.v. q24h
Cefuroxime axetil	30 mg/kg/d PO q12h
Clarithomycin	15 mg/kg/d PO q12h
Trimethoprim-sulfamethoxazole	8–12 mg/kg/d of trimethoprim component PO q12h

Analgesics and Antipyretics

The child with severe earache may need acetaminophen or even codeine during the first 2 or 3 days of treatment. The use of an oral decongestant is ineffective in the treatment of otitis media; it should be prescribed only for relief of symptoms of concomitant upper respiratory tract infection.

DISPOSITION

The vast majority of children with acute otitis media can be discharged with subsequent follow-up by their physicians in about 2 weeks. In older children, follow-up may be arranged in 6 weeks. Most infants in the first 6 weeks of life, those older children who appear toxic and severely ill, or those with immunodeficiency must be evaluated for a coexisting, more serious infection, such as sepsis or meningitis. Some of these children will require hospital admission. Children who have mastoiditis complicating otitis media need otolaryngologic consultation and possible hospital admission.

COMMON PITFALLS

- Overdiagnosis of otitis media in a febrile or crying child who has only hyperemic (injected) tympanic membranes on otoscopic examination
- Failure to consider other diagnoses and neglecting to consider a more serious and even life-threatening disease, such as meningitis, sepsis, or pneumonia, coexisting with acute otitis media

MASTOIDITIS

Mastoiditis is an infection of the mastoid air cells of the temporal bone. Due to the anatomic contiguity of the middle ear, cleft, and the mastoid air cells, mastoiditis is actually part of the otitis media.[1] It becomes clinically relevant when the inflammation of the mastoid air cells progresses, causing invasion of the bony structures of the mastoid. At this stage, the signs and symptoms of mastoiditis are distinguishable from those of acute otitis media.

The incidence of mastoiditis has greatly decreased since the advent of antimicrobial agents, but it still occurs, causing significant morbidity and, rarely, life-threatening conditions. The clinical significance of the mastoid air cells is their proximity to contiguous structures such as the posterior cranial fossa, the semicircular canals, the facial nerve, and the petrous tip of the temporal bone.

According to the pathologic stage, acute mastoiditis is subdivided into acute mastoiditis, acute mastoiditis with periostitis, and acute mastoid osteitis with or without subperiosteal abscess.[1]

Acute mastoiditis is caused by the same organisms responsible for acute otitis media, namely *S. pneumoniae,* group A *Streptococcus, S. aureus,* and *H. influenzae* (rare). Chronic mastoiditis is caused by gram-negative enteric bacteria such as *Escherichia coli, Proteus, Pseudomonas,* and *S. aureus.*

CLINICAL PRESENTATION

Due to the communication of the middle ear (antrum) with the mastoid air cells through the aditus ad antrum, inflammation of the mastoid air cells is a natural extension of acute otitis media. At this stage, the signs and symptoms are those of acute otitis media, and they are not specific for mastoiditis. These signs and symptoms include otalgia, decreased hearing, and fever. On examination, the signs are those of acute otitis media. Radiographically, the mastoids are hazy or cloudy, and the bony structures are intact. Therapy for *acute mastoiditis* is the same as for acute otitis media. Most cases resolve spontaneously or respond to antimicrobial therapy. Surgery is not indicated. If resolution does not occur, acute mastoiditis may progress, causing a more severe involvement of the mastoid air cells.

In *acute mastoiditis with periostitis,* the infection spreads, involving the periosteum covering the mastoid process and causing periostitis. This condition may or may not be accompanied by subperiosteal abscess. There is no radiologic evidence for osteitis, and, clinically, it is difficult to differentiate from acute mastoiditis.

Acute mastoid osteitis (also known as acute coalescent mastoiditis or acute surgical mastoiditis) may be accompanied by subperiosteal abscess. At this stage, the infection within the mastoid air cells has progressed, causing destruction (i.e., "coalescence") of the bony trabeculae that separate the mastoid cells. Physical examination reveals mastoid empyema. The clinical findings include swelling, tenderness to touch, and erythema of the mastoid bone. The pinna is displaced outward and downward. A fluctuant subperiosteal abscess of the mastoid area may be evident, occasionally accompanied by a draining fistula.

On examination of the external ear canal, swelling of the posterior and superior ear canal wall can be found. A purulent drainage through the perforated tympanic membrane is present. In most acute cases, the patient appears febrile and toxic. Pus from acute mastoid osteitis may spread to the middle ear through aditus ad antrum with resolution of this process. It also may spread to the soft tissue below the pinna or behind the sternocleidomastoid muscle of the neck (Bezold abscess). When it spreads to the petrous air cells, it causes petrositis. If the extension is to the calvarium, it may cause osteomyelitis. At times, the acute middle ear effusion drains through the eustachian tube with resolution of the otitis media, but the obstruction due to swelling of aditus ad antrum causes infection of the mastoid air cells with development of osteitis.

In the case of a normal-appearing tympanic membrane, and especially when there are no external signs such as subperiosteal abscess, computed tomography of the mastoid is necessary to demonstrate mastoiditis. Radiographs show haziness and destruction of the septa between the mastoid air cells (i.e., coalescent mastoiditis).

Chronic mastoiditis is always associated with chronic suppurative otitis media. It can be treated medically, but it is most often managed surgically (mastoidectomy) by the otolaryngologic specialist.

DIFFERENTIAL DIAGNOSIS

A displaced pinna with swelling around it due to mastoiditis can be confused with parotitis (mumps or bacterial parotitis). In the case of parotid involvement, the swelling is behind, below, and anterior to the pinna, causing the displacement of the ear lobe out and upward. In addition, the tympanic membrane and the external ear canal are normal on examination. Lymphadenitis of occipital and suboccipital nodes could mimic mastoid swelling, but the ear examination is normal. Severe external otitis with spread of the cellulitis to the surrounding tissue could be confused with mastoiditis, but radiographs of the mastoid air cells are normal in this case.

EMERGENCY DEPARTMENT MANAGEMENT

A diagnosis of acute mastoiditis calls for consultation with an otolaryngologist. In the case of subperiosteal abscess, the child should be admitted. Treatment should include analgesia, administration of parenteral antimicrobial agents, and evacuation of the pus by tympanocentesis or myringotomy. The material obtained should be sent for Gram stain and culture.

The initial antimicrobial therapy is a penicillinase-resistant penicillin such as nafcillin at 150 mg/kg/d, or a cephalosporin such as cefuroxime, 100 to 150 mg/kg/d for 10 days.[6] Once the culture and susceptibility tests return, the antimicrobial agent may need to be changed accordingly. Parenteral therapy can be switched to oral therapy once adequate drainage has been accomplished and the child has been afebrile for 36 to 48 hours. Surgery should be done only after the culture has been obtained, antibiotic therapy has been initiated, and the child is stable. The type of surgery will depend on the stage of infection. For chronic *Pseudomonas* mastoiditis, in preparation for surgery, intravenous mezlocillin or ticarcillin, 200 to 300 mg/kg/d, given intravenously and divided every 4 to 6 hours for 7 days, is recommended.[6] Daily cleansing of the ear canal is also important.

DISPOSITION

The child should be admitted to the hospital, and consultation with an otolaryngologist obtained. If it is necessary to transfer the child to another medical center, do so after initial stabilization and initiation of antibiotic therapy.

COMMON PITFALLS

- Failure to be aware of the clinical presentation of mastoiditis because of its infrequent occurrence, which may lead to nonaggressive management of this serious condition
- Failure to consider other coexisting or complicating conditions, such as meningitis or brain abscess

References

1. Bluestone CD, Klein JO. Intratemporal complications and sequelae of otitis media. Mastoiditis. In: Bluestone CD, Stool SE, eds. *Pediatric otolaryngology,* 3rd ed, vol 1. Philadelphia: WB Saunders, 1996:618.
2. Bluestone CD, Klein JO. Otitis media, atelectasis, and eustachian tube dysfunction. In Bluestone CD, Stool SE. *Pediatric otolaryngology,* 3rd ed, vol 1. Philadelphia: WB Saunders, 1996:388.
3. Bottenfield GW, Burch DJ, Hendrick JA, et al. Safety and tolerability of a new formulation (90mg/kg/day divided every 12h) of amoxicillin/clavulanate (Augmentin™) in the empiric treatment of pediatric acute otitis media caused by drug-resistant *Streptococcus pneumoniae. Pediatr Infect Dis J* 1998;17:963.
4. Dowell SF, Butler JC, Giebink GS, et al. Acute otitis media: management and surveillance in an era of pneumococcal resistance—a report from the drug-resistant *Streptococcus pneumoniae* therapeutic working group. *Pediatr Infect Dis J* 1999;18:1.
5. Green SM, Rothrock SG. Single-dose intramuscular ceftriaxone for acute otitis media in children. *Pediatrics* 1993;91:23.
6. Nelson JD. *Pocket book of pediatric antimicrobial therapy,* 13th ed. Baltimore: Williams & Wilkins, 1998–1999:22.
7. Pool MD. Implications of drug-resistant *Streptococcus pneumoniae* for otitis media. *Pediatric Infect Dis J* 1998;17:953.
8. Schappert SM. Office visits for otitis media: United States, 1975–90. Advance data from vital and health statistics of the Centers for Disease Control/National Center for Health Statistics NII214. Hyattsville, MD: Public Health Service 1992;214:1–20.
9. Schwartz B. Surveillance data presented at the Centers for Disease Control Therapeutic Working Group on Drug-Resistant *Streptococcus pneumoniae* in Otitis Media, Atlanta, March 20–21, 1997.

CHAPTER 286
Pertussis

Samir Midani and Hanif Kamal

Pertussis is a common respiratory illness that occurs worldwide in all age groups, but it is recognized primarily in young, unprotected infants and children. The source of infection is usually an infected older sibling or adult who has mild or asymptomatic infection.[3,8] The risk of the disease is highest in children less than 5 years of age. Mortality and hospitalization rates are highest in unimmunized infants younger than 6 months of age.[4] Neonatal pertussis is particularly severe with maternal peripartum pertussis as the usual source. Premature infants are more likely to have severe presentations.

The etiologic agent is *Bordetella pertussis,* a gram-negative, pleomorphic bacillus. Less frequently, the disease can be caused by *Bordetella parapertussis.* The descriptive name of the disease, "whooping cough," is derived from the characteristic sound of the inspiratory effort that follows the paroxysmal coughing. Transmission is by respiratory droplets, with extremely high attack rates (70% to 100%) for susceptible hosts. The incubation period is 6 to 20 days, with a mean of 7 to 10 days.[2]

The incidence of pertussis has decreased markedly since the institution of the pertussis vaccine. Although immunization reduces the incidence and mortality of pertussis, it is neither complete nor permanent. There is no evidence of a causal relationship between pertussis vaccine and brain damage.[1] Natural immunity to pertussis could be lifelong, whereas 12 years after vaccination, 95% of the vaccinees are susceptible to pertussis.[6] Susceptible hospital staff can acquire the infection easily, and although most of these infections are mild, on occasion, the infection can be incapacitating.

CLINICAL PRESENTATION

The clinical manifestation of pertussis depends on age and previous immunization or infection. The classic illness, which lasts for 6 to 10 weeks, occurs as a primary infection in unimmunized children and is generally divided into three stages: the catarrhal stage, the paroxysmal stage, and the convalescent stage. The course of the disease may not always be typical in adults or in infants.[7]

The catarrhal stage is characterized by rhinorrhea, lacrimation and mild cough, and low-grade or no fever. This stage lasts 1 to 2 weeks, and the diagnosis is usually not suspected, yet patients are more contagious in this stage than during any other.

In the paroxysmal stage, episodes of coughing increase in severity and number. A characteristic repetitive series of six to 12 forceful coughs during a single expiration is followed by a sudden, massive inspiratory effort that produces the classic whoop as air is inhaled forcefully against a narrow glottis. Cyanosis, bulging eyes, protrusion of the tongue, salivation, lacrimation, and distention of the neck veins may occur during these episodes of coughing. The paroxysms are frequently precipitated by a variety of events, such as feeding, crying, or even hearing another person cough.

Physical examination during this stage may reveal conjunctival hemorrhages and petechiae over the neck and head. Some patients can have diffuse rhonchi and rales on auscultation. In very young infants, the paroxysm and whoop are often absent.

Infants usually present with choking spells, apnea, bradycardia, cyanosis, and unresponsiveness. Seventy percent of fatal cases occur in infancy, and it is estimated that 18% of infants who were victims of sudden infant death syndrome had positive tests for *B. pertussis*.

In the convalescent stage, which usually lasts 1 to 2 weeks, symptoms gradually abate, but the cough may persist for several months.

Complications of pertussis include otitis, seizures, pneumonia, encephalopathy (risk, 1:12,000), and death. Pneumonia can be due to *B. pertussis* or to secondary bacterial infection. Other complications include interstitial or subcutaneous emphysema, atelectasis, ulcer of the tongue frenulum, epistaxis, melena, subdural hematoma, rectal prolapse, syndrome of inappropriate antidiuretic hormone secretion, and nutritional disturbances. The case fatality rate is 1.3% in children younger than 1 month and 0.3% in infants 2 to 11 months of age. Premature infants are especially at increased risk for severe disease, with the major cause of death being secondary bacterial infection.

DIFFERENTIAL DIAGNOSIS

In classic disease, the clinical diagnosis of pertussis should be made without difficulty. Other infectious agents that cause similar illness include *Mycoplasma pneumoniae, Chlamydia trachomatis, Chlamydia pneumoniae,* adenoviruses, and other respiratory viruses. *B. parapertussis* and *B. bronchiseptica* occasionally produce a pertussis-like syndrome.

Spasmodic attacks of coughing may be observed in infants and children with bronchiolitis, bacterial pneumonia, cystic fibrosis, tuberculosis, an airway foreign body, and other diseases that cause lymphadenopathy and extrinsic compression of the trachea and bronchi. These attacks also can occasionally be seen with sinusitis.

Difficulty in recognizing pertussis occurs in the catarrhal stage, in mild illness, and in adults or very young infants. Pertussis should be included in the differential diagnosis of all infants presenting with choking or apneic episodes and in children who present with a history of severe, spasmodic coughing or posttussive emesis

EMERGENCY DEPARTMENT EVALUATION

A child or infant suspected to have pertussis should be observed for signs and symptoms of respiratory distress. Paroxysmal coughing episodes should be documented. These attacks may be triggered by eating, drinking, yawning, sneezing, or other physical activities. Between attacks, patients may appear normal and are usually in no distress. It is important to remember that young infants require hospitalization and close observation, in spite of looking well in between paroxysms.

Evaluation of the white blood cell count may be helpful. Leukocytosis of 20,000 to 60,000 cells/mL with an absolute lymphocytosis is characteristic in severe disease. Nasopharyngeal secretion culture remains the gold standard for diagnosis. Dacron or calcium alginate swabs are used to collect the specimen. A selective medium such as Bordet-Gengou should be rapidly inoculated (within 1 to 2 hours) for optimal isolation of the organism. Recovery of *B. pertussis* from nasopharyngeal secretions is highest during the catarrhal stage. Direct immunofluorescent assay of nasopharyngeal secretions has a low sensitivity and a variable specificity, and is not reliable for laboratory confirmation.[2,5] Chest radiograph findings are nonspecific and may include perihilar infiltrate, atelectasis, or emphysema.

EMERGENCY DEPARTMENT MANAGEMENT

Treatment is mostly supportive and can be managed at home for older children and for mild forms of the disease. Young infants or children with severe disease require hospitalization, and perhaps admission to an intensive care unit, for close observation.

In the emergency department, if the patients are unable to handle the mucoid secretions, they should be placed in a head-down position (45 to 60 degrees) to take advantage of gravity. Suction of the oropharynx with a catheter large enough to permit flow of tenacious secretions is required during paroxysms. In a severely ill child, oxygen may be needed. Hydration must be monitored and maintained, as well as caloric intake. Apneic infants may require active airway and ventilation management. Children less than 6 months of age are more likely to be hospitalized, tend to have longer hospitalization, and are more likely to require intensive care monitoring.

The paroxysmal coughing episodes may prove to be exhausting, and avoidance of factors that provoke such attacks may be helpful. Patients with severe paroxysms should be monitored to ensure early recognition of hypoxia or bradycardia. Corticosteroids and albuterol may reduce the frequency and severity of symptoms, but before they can be recommended, further evaluation is required to establish their safety and efficacy. Maintenance of hydration and nutritional status is of utmost importance for optimal recovery, especially in infants with severe disease and in children with posttussive vomiting.

Antimicrobial agents, if given early during the course of illness, may ameliorate the symptoms. However, once paroxysmal coughing is established, antibiotics have no discernible effect on the course of illness, but they are recommended to limit the spread of the organism to other susceptible individuals.

The first choice for treatment is oral erythromycin. The dosage for children is 40 to 50 mg/kg/d, given every 6 hours (maximum, 2 g/d) for 14 days. Other macrolides, such as clarithromycin 15 mg/kg/d in two divided doses (maximum, 1 g/d), are likely to be effective and are thus alternatives for patients who cannot tolerate erythromycin. Trimethoprim-sulfamethoxazole (8 to 40 mg/kg/d orally in two divided doses) is another alternative, but its efficacy is unproved.

In addition to standard precautions, droplet precautions are recommended for 5 days after initiation of effective antimicrobial therapy. Chemoprophylaxis with erythromycin, 40 to 50 mg/kg/d, given every 6 hours (maximum, 2 g/d) for 14 days, is recommended for all household contacts, irrespective of age and immunization status.[4]

DISPOSITION

Patients with severe disease and those younger than 6 months of age with clinical evidence of pertussis should be hospitalized because of the high rate of complications in this age group. Older children and those with milder forms of illness may be discharged home after appropriate evaluation and initiation of antimicrobials.

COMMON PITFALLS

- Failure to recognize and diagnose pertussis, especially when presenting in an atypical fashion
- To assume that infants younger than 6 months of age will have a benign illness
- Failure to administer chemoprophylaxis to contacts
- Incorrect specimen collection and delay in plating secretions on appropriate media

- Failure to diagnosis pertussis in adolescents who present with an aura of suffocation followed by coughing episodes
- Failure to know that there is no effective transplacental immunity

References

1. American Academy of Pediatrics. Committee on Infectious Diseases. The relationship between pertussis vaccine and brain damage. *Pediatrics* 1991;88:397–400.
2. American Academy of Pediatrics. Pertussis. In: Peter G, ed. *1997 Red book: report of the Committee on Infectious Diseases,* 24th ed. Elk Grove Village, IL: American Academy of Pediatrics, 1997:394–407.
3. Beiter A, Lewis K, et al. Unrecognized maternal peripartum pertussis with subsequent fatal neonatal pertussis. *Obstet Gynecol* 1993;82(4):691–693.
4. Cherry JD, Heininger U. Pertussis and other *Bordetella* infections. In: Fegin RD, Cherry JD, eds. *Textbook of pediatric infectious disease.* Philadelphia: WB Saunders, 1997:1423–1435.
5. Friedman RL. Pertussis: the disease and new diagnostic methods. *Clin Microbiol Rev* 1998;1:365–376.
6. Lambert HJ. Epidemiology of small pertussis outbreak in Kent County, Michigan. *Publ Health Rep* 1992S;80:365–339.
7. Nelson JD. The changing epidemiology of pertussis in young infants. *Am J Dis Child* 1978;132:371–373.
8. Robertson PW, Goldberg M, Jarvie BM, et al. *Bordetella* pertussis infection: a cause of persistent cough in adults. *Med J Aust* 1987;147:522–523.

CHAPTER 287
Acute Pharyngitis

Karen Camasso-Richardson
and Martha S. Wright

Sore throats often bring pediatric patients to the emergency department. Most of these children have acute pharyngitis. Many infectious agents cause acute inflammation of the tonsils and pharynx, including Epstein-Barr virus (EBV), adenovirus, parainfluenza virus, group A and other β-hemolytic streptococci, and *Mycoplasma pneumoniae.*[1,8] Nonbacterial agents are the cause of pharyngitis in 70% to 80% of patients, especially in adolescents and in children less than 2 years of age. The most important agent for diagnostic, treatment, and public health considerations remains group A β-hemolytic *Streptococcus* (GABHS).[1,2]

If inadequately treated, infection with this organism can lead to suppurative complications, including peritonsillar and retropharyngeal abscess, mastoiditis, and cervical adenitis, as well as the nonsuppurative complication of acute rheumatic fever (ARF).

CLINICAL PRESENTATION

Most children with pharyngitis present with one or more subjective complaints of sore throat, rhinitis, cough, headache, abdominal pain, or vomiting.[5] The parent may report that younger children will not drink. On physical examination, these children have fever, pharyngeal inflammation with or without tonsillar exudate, and tender cervical adenopathy. Children with GABHS infection may have characteristic features, such as a fine, diffusely papular erythroderma ("sandpaper" or scarlatiniform rash) or palatal petechiae.[14] Numerous studies have demonstrated that clinicians can differentiate GABHS from non-GABHS pharyngitis with only 50% to 75% accuracy.[6,17] Although patients infected with GABHS often have more pharyngeal inflammation and tender lymphadenopathy, these findings are not reliably predictive.[7,15] Greater than 70% of GABHS cultures will be positive in school-age children (5 to 15 years) with fever and pharyngitis and an absence of upper respiratory symptoms (conjunctivitis, rhinorrhea, or cough).[17]

DIFFERENTIAL DIAGNOSIS

Acute pharyngitis may be accompanied by more serious infectious entities, such as peritonsillar and retropharyngeal abscesses and peritonsillar cellulitis. All three require more aggressive treatment and possible hospitalization. Marked pharyngeal erythema, leukocytosis, and fever characterize peritonsillar cellulitis. This may progress to abscess formation in either the parapharyngeal or the tonsillar space. Clinically, patients with tonsillar and peritonsillar abscesses present with fever, trismus, a muffled ("hot potato") voice, and swelling of the affected tonsil with deviation of the uvula. Sore throat may not be a primary complaint. Younger children with acute pharyngitis may develop lymphadenitis of retropharyngeal lymph nodes, which may become retropharyngeal abscesses. This should be considered in a toxic-appearing child with dysphagia, drooling, airway obstruction, and neck stiffness.

Many organisms are known to cause pharyngitis. The majority of the time, a self-resolving virus is the causative organism. *Mycoplasma* often presents with a history of prolonged cough. EBV may present with a prolonged cough, extreme fatigue, a highly exudative pharynx, or an enlarged spleen. Gonococcal pharyngitis should be considered in both the sexually active adolescent and in the younger child in whom sexual abuse is suspected.

EMERGENCY DEPARTMENT EVALUATION AND MANAGEMENT

When evaluating the pediatric patient with pharyngitis, it is necessary to assess for airway patency and hydration status. Edematous tonsils can cause upper airway obstruction, resulting in stridor and accessory muscle use. A nasopharyngeal airway may be necessary to ensure airway patency. Often, children refuse to drink and can become significantly dehydrated. Intravenous fluid resuscitation and pain treatment may be necessary. The patient should be evaluated for suppurative complications, such as peritonsillar abscess, by palpating edematous regions to check for fluctuance. A soft-tissue x-ray or computed tomography scan of the neck may be necessary if abscess is suspected.

The primary goal for evaluation of uncomplicated pharyngitis is to determine whether GABHS is the causative agent. Rapid antigen detection tests (RADTs) provide highly specific (95% to 99%) identification of the GABHS antigen, but lack sensitivity (75% to 85%).[1,7,15] It is recommended that two throat swabs be done for both a rapid antigen test and culture in those patients with a higher risk of GABHS. If the rapid antigen test is negative, a confirmatory throat culture should be sent. For those patients less likely to have GABHS, a throat culture alone is recommended, to decrease the cost of evaluation.[12] The swabs should be obtained from the posterior pharynx and tonsillar pillars.[1] RADTs have been shown to increase appropriate care of GABHS in the emergency department.[10]

If GABHS is the responsible organism, antibiotic therapy is indicated. Penicillin, an inexpensive drug with a narrow spectrum of activity and proven efficacy and safety, remains the drug of choice for GABHS initial therapy.[1,9] Oral penicillin V is recommended at 400,000 U (250 mg) two to four times daily for 10 days, or, in those that may not complete a 10-day course, benzathine penicillin G, 600,000 U intramuscularly in children less than 27 kg (60 lb) and 1.2 million U in larger children.[9] In penicillin-allergic patients, erythromycin ethylsuccinate (40 mg/kg/d) or erythromycin estolate (20 to 40 mg/kg/d) in two to four divided doses for 10 days is recommended.[4] A more recent treatment alternative is daily azithromycin for 5 days. Although there is evidence that cephalosporins may have a potentially lower failure rate of GABHS eradication and may allow a shorter course of therapy, comprehensive studies are not yet available.[11,13] Empiric therapy is not recommended. Therapy can be postponed up to 9 days from initial symptoms and still safely prevent both suppurative and nonsuppurative sequelae, such as ARF.[2,3] Symptomatic relief for patients with pharyngitis can be provided with topical and systemic analgesics. The adjunctive use of steroids for pain relief is not recommended, as their role has not been adequately studied in children.

Follow-up throat cultures and RADTs are not indicated in patients who are asymptomatic and have completed a full course of antibiotics. A positive culture or RADT in most properly treated individuals would indicate the carrier state. Follow-up testing is indicated in these exceptions: outbreaks of ARF and poststreptococcal glomerular nephritis, outbreaks in closed or semiclosed communities, and when a "ping-pong" spread is occurring in a family.[1] Treatment of the carrier state should be reserved for the exceptions just noted and in individuals living with someone with ARF or in health-care workers.[16]

DISPOSITION

Most children with pharyngitis can be evaluated and managed as outpatients. An otolaryngologist should evaluate suspected cellulitis or abscess for possible surgical intervention. Often, admission is needed for surgical treatment and intravenous antibiotics. Admission should be considered in the dehydrated patient or in the child with evidence of airway obstruction. Any airway compromise should be evaluated by an otolaryngologist, and the patient should be admitted to a monitored bed for close observation.

COMMON PITFALLS

- Avoid treatment of nonbacterial pharyngitis with antibiotics.
- The missed diagnosis of GABHS may be secondary to improper culture technique or a negative RADT not confirmed with throat culture.
- Always look closely for peritonsillar, tonsillar, or retropharyngeal abscesses.
- Do not forget to evaluate and document the airway examination.

References

1. Bisno AL, Gerber MA, Gwaltney JM, et al. Diagnosis and management of group A streptococcal pharyngitis: a practice guideline. *Clin Infect Dis* 1997;25:574.
2. Bronze MS, Dale JB. The reemergence of serious group A streptococcal infections and acute rheumatic fever. *Am J Med Sci* 1996;311:41.
3. Catanzaro FJ, Stetson CA, Morris AJ, et al. The role of the streptococcus in the pathogenesis of rheumatic fever. *Am J Med* 1954;17:749.
4. Dajani AS. Current therapy of group A streptococcal pharyngitis. *Pediatr Ann* 1998;27:277–280.
5. Denny FW Jr. Tonsillopharyngitis 1994. *Pediatr Rev* 1994;15:185.
6. Dobbs F. A scoring system for predicting group A streptococcal throat infection. *Br J Gen Pract* 1996;46:461.
7. Gerber MA. Diagnosis of group A streptococcal pharyngitis. *Pediatr Ann* 1998;27:269–273.
8. Glezen WP, Clyde WA, Senior RJ, et al. Group A streptococci, mycoplasmas and viruses associated with acute pharyngitis. *JAMA* 1976;202:119.
9. Klein JO. Management of streptococcal pharyngitis. *Pediatr Infect Dis J* 1994;13:572–575.
10. Lieu TA, Fleisher GR, Schwartz JS. Clinical evaluation of a latex agglutination test for streptococcal pharyngitis: performance and impact on treatment rates. *Pediatr Infect Dis J* 1988;7:847.
11. Pichichero ME. Streptococcal pharyngitis: is penicillin still the right choice? *Compr Ther* 1996;22:782–787.
12. Pitetti RD, Wald ER. Strep throat: weighing the diagnostic options. *Contemp Pediatr* 1998;15:68.
13. Scaglione F, Demartini G, Arcidiacono MM, et al. Optimum treatment of streptococcal pharyngitis. *Drugs* 1997;53:86–97.
14. Schartz RH. Pharyngeal findings of group A streptococcal pharyngitis. *Arch Pediatr Adolesc Med* 1998;152:927–928.
15. Schulman ST. Streptococcal pharyngitis: diagnostic considerations. *Pediatr Infect Dis J* 1994;13:567.
16. Tanz RR, Schulman ST. Streptococcal pharyngitis: the carrier state, definition, and management. *Pediatr Ann* 1998;27:281–285.
17. Wald ER, Green MD, Schwartz B, et al. A streptococcal score card revisited. *Pediatr Emerg Care* 1998;14:109.

CHAPTER 288
Pneumonia

David A. Schaeffer

Pneumonia—inflammation of the lungs—typically refers to an inflammatory process of the parenchymal component of the lung that results from infection, although there are also noninfectious etiologies. Acute respiratory tract infections are a major cause of morbidity at any age, and young children characteristically develop six to eight upper respiratory infections per year, even more for children in daycare settings. The attack rates for lower respiratory tract infections (e.g., croup, tracheobronchitis, bronchiolitis, pneumonia) are highest in children ages 6 to 12 months and decline thereafter.[9] Attack rates for pneumonia showed an average of 40 episodes for every 1000 children ages 6 months to 5 years, 22 of 1000 for children ages 5 to 9 years, 11 of 1000 for children ages 9 to 12 years, and 7 of 1000 for children ages 12 to 15 years.

Poor socioeconomic status, number of siblings, parental smoking, and prematurity may all be associated with an increased risk of pneumonia in children. There is seasonal variation in the prevalence of certain pathogens. For example, respiratory viruses cause winter epidemics of bronchiolitis and pneumonia, and every few years there are epidemics of pneumonia due to *Mycoplasma pneumoniae*.

PATHOGENESIS AND ETIOLOGY

Respiratory viruses are transmitted primarily by direct contact with infected secretions from objects or hands of one person to the hands of another. The conjunctival or nasal mucosa is then inoculated with contaminated secretions. The inoculated virus attacks the airway, and viral replication occurs. This causes sloughing of the ciliated epithelial layer of the respiratory tract mucosa, leading to loss of ciliary activity and increased colonization of the airway with bacteria. Suppression of alveolar macrophage function is thought to be the primary mechanism allowing bacterial infection of the lungs.

The causes of acute infectious pneumonia in children may be divided into bacterial and nonbacterial agents (i.e., viruses, fungi, or parasites). *Mycoplasma* infections are usually considered separately from other bacterial infections, because the clinical course and treatment differ from that of other bacterial infections. Pneumonia is also described as typical or atypical in its presentation. Typical pneumonia is characterized by sudden onset of fever, chills, pleuritic chest pain, and productive cough. Typical pneumonia is usually caused by bacteria, most commonly *Pneumococcus*. Atypical pneumonia has a gradual onset over days to weeks and is associated with low-grade fever, malaise, nonproductive cough, and, often, headache and sore throat. Atypical pneumonia may be due to viruses, *Mycoplasma*, or *Chlamydia*. In infants, an afebrile pneumonia syndrome may be caused by *Chlamydia trachomatis*, viruses, *Ureaplasma urealyticum*, or *Pneumocystis carinii*. *Bordetella pertussis* may also cause atypical pneumonia in infants and young children. *Mycobacterium tuberculosis* may cause pneumonia in healthy or immunocompromised children, and the clinical onset resembles bacterial pneumonia. Pneumonia in the immunocompromised child with immunodeficiency or immunosuppression secondary to cancer chemotherapy or human immunodeficiency virus (HIV) infection may be caused by the usual viral and bacterial pathogens as well as *Legionella* species, herpesviruses, mycobacteria, fungi, and protozoa.

Noninfectious causes of pneumonia include foreign-body aspiration (often with secondary infection), chronic aspiration of oral secretions, gastroesophageal reflux with aspiration, congenital heart disease with bronchial compression from enlarged pulmonary arteries or chamber enlargement, smoke inhalation, hypersensitivity pneumonitis, pulmonary edema, pulmonary hemosiderosis, leukemia or lymphoma, metastatic tumor, and idiopathic interstitial pneumonitis. Pneumonia may be mistakenly diagnosed when there is atelectasis secondary to mucous plugging or migratory recurrent atelectasis in children with asthma.

Bacteria are the major cause of pneumonia in newborns. Beyond 1 month of age, viruses, *Mycoplasma*, and *Chlamydia* cause most pneumonias. The diagnosis of bacterial pneumonia can be made by a positive blood culture, although blood cultures are positive in less than 10% of cases of pneumonia.[21] Direct lung puncture and needle aspiration may be positive for a bacterial pathogen in up to 62% of children with pneumonia, but this technique is seldom used.[5] Recent studies using bacterial antigen and antibody testing showed that bacterial causes of pneumonia are more common than previously reported. Serologic evidence of pneumococcal infection was found in 5% to 11% of children between 3 months and 14 years as a single infection and in 15% to 25% of children who had mixed infections with more than one etiologic agent. The highest incidence of pneumococcal infections was found in children of ages 3 months to 4 years.[13] As shown in Table 288.1, an etiologic diagnosis for pneumonia can be established in about half the cases, and a bacterial cause can be identified in about one-fourth of children.[13,15,20,21,27]

The causes of pneumonia in children vary with age, and knowing the likely causative agents for a given age range allows the physician to select the appropriate diagnostic methods and most effective antibiotic therapy. In the first month of life, pneumonia is commonly due to group B streptococci and gram-negative bacilli (*Escherichia coli, Klebsiella pneumoniae, Listeria monocytogenes*) acquired during or before delivery. Between 1 and 3 months of age, infants may develop an afebrile pneumonia syndrome with a staccato cough caused by infection with *C. trachomatis*, viruses, *U. urealyticum*, or *P. carinii*.[25] Viral infections are the most common causes of pneumonia in children ages 1 month to 5 years (Table 288.2). Respiratory syncytial virus (RSV) causes up to 70% of all viral pneumonias in children. Other viruses causing pneumonia and characteristics of the pneumonia syndromes are listed in Table 288.3. Bacterial pneumonia in children of ages 1 month to 5 years is most commonly due to *Streptococcus pneumoniae*. *Haemophilus influenzae* is unlikely in children who have received the HIB vaccination. Staphylococcal pneumonia is now uncommon.

Historically, in children 6 years and older, *Mycoplasma pneumoniae* is the most common etiologic agent, accounting for up to 21% of cases of pneumonia.[3] *S. pneumoniae* has been the next most common bacterial pathogen in older children. Viral pneumonia from influenza, parainfluenza, or adenovirus is also frequently seen in this age group.

Pneumonia in the immunocompromised host is often caused by the usual viral and bacterial pathogens, and also by oppor-

TABLE 288.1. Common Causes of Pneumonia in Children (in Percentages)[13] (n = 201)

Bacterial	41
S. pneumoniae	28
H. influenzae	6
Other bacteria	0
Chlamydia	14
Mycoplasma	22
Viruses	15
Mixed viral and bacterial	10
No etiology	34

TABLE 288.2. Relative Causes of Pneumonia in Children by Age

	<3 mo	4 mo–5 yr	≥6 yr
Bacterial	+	++	+
Mycoplasmal	−	++	+++
Chlamydia pneumonia	−	++	++
Viral	+++	+++	++
Afebrile pneumonia syndrome	++	−	−

+++, most frequent; ++, frequent; +, occasional; −, rare.

TABLE 288.3. Viral Causes of Pneumonia in Children

Virus	Age	Season	Syndrome
Respiratory syncytial virus	Infants and preschool	Winter	Bronchiolitis Pneumonia
Parainfluenza viruses	Infants and preschool	Fall and spring	Bronchiolitis Croup Pneumonia
Influenza viruses	Preschool and school-aged	Winter	Pneumonia
Adenoviruses	All ages	Year-round	Bronchiolitis Pneumonia

tunistic agents that do not usually cause infections, except in patients with altered immune status. Children with agamma- or hypogammaglobulinemia are susceptible to repeated bacterial pneumonias and may develop bronchiectasis. They may also develop pneumonia from *Aspergillus* or *P. carinii*. *Legionella* species may cause a severe bacterial pneumonia in any immunocompromised child. Children with cancer and chemotherapy-induced neutropenia or anergy and decreased T-cell lymphocyte function are susceptible to viral pneumonias such as cytomegalovirus (CMV), herpesvirus, and varicella-zoster virus.[24] Fungal infections with *Candida* may also occur. Children with lymphomas may develop infection with *Toxoplasma gondii* and *Cryptococcus neoformans*. *P. carinii* pneumonia is uncommon in patients receiving trimethoprim–sulfamethoxazole prophylaxis. In children with the acquired immunodeficiency syndrome (AIDS), major causes of pneumonia include bacterial pneumonias, *P. carinii*, CMV, and mycobacteria.[18]

CLINICAL PRESENTATION

Symptoms and signs of pneumonia in children vary with age and may be nonspecific in the youngest patients. Infants under 2 months of age may present with fever and tachypnea and no signs of pulmonary consolidation. Most children have 1 or 2 days of prodromal symptoms, including rhinitis, low-grade fever, decreased appetite, and decreased activity. Common symptoms and signs are listed in Table 288.4.

Pneumonia is characterized by evidence of lung consolidation on the physical examination or chest x-ray. Typical physical findings include decreased breath sounds, dullness to percussion, or crackles on lung auscultation. On the chest x-ray, different patterns of pulmonary infection may be seen: (1) diffuse peribronchial thickening, often with hyperinflation of the lungs from air-trapping (indicated by flattening of the diaphragm); (2) a diffuse, patchy interstitial pattern; and (3) focal lobar consolidation. Diffuse, patchy infiltrates, often with shaggy peribronchial infiltrates in the perihilar regions, are commonly seen with viral infections, although bacterial infections may also show a similar pattern. Lobar consolidation may be difficult to distinguish from atelectasis secondary to mucous plugging, although signs of volume loss with a shift of the trachea and unaffected lung to the atelectatic side are usually evident. Focal lobar consolidation may sometimes present as a "round" pneumonia and be mistaken for a chest mass. Expiratory chest x-rays may be misinterpreted as pneumonia, because normal vascular and airway markings will be accentuated if the lungs are underinflated when the film is taken at the end of expiration.

Pneumonia may be complicated by pleural effusion, which may occur as a parapneumonic exudative effusion, empyema, pneumatocele, or abscess formation. A small pleural effusion is occasionally seen with viral pneumonia. About 20% of patients with mycoplasmal pneumonia develop a pleural effusion. Complicated pneumonias are now most commonly caused by *S. pneumoniae*.[12] Pleural effusions were reported in 29% of a recent series of 257 episodes of pneumococcal pneumonia, with 14% of patients having pleural fluid characteristics of an empyema.[25] Pneumonia due to *Staphylococcus aureus* is uncommon but unusually severe and is characterized by 80% of cases occurring in children less than 1 year of age. Staphylococcal pulmonary pneumatoceles present early in the course, pleural effusions are common in up to 70% of cases, and pneumothorax occurs in up to 41% of cases. The combination of pneumothorax and empyema or pyopneumothorax is very suggestive of staphylococcal pneumonia.

Primary tuberculosis (TB) pneumonia is more common in urban or lower socioeconomic areas, in recent immigrants to the United States, and in children exposed to contacts with TB or HIV. Usual findings of pneumonia are common, with lobar consolidation, frequently hilar adenopathy and, less frequently, cavitary lesions or pleural effusion.

TABLE 288.4. Symptoms and Signs of Pneumonia in Children

INFANTS < 6 MONTHS OF AGE
Fever
Cough
Poor feeding
Irritability
Tachypnea (RR >60/min)
Retractions
Apnea
Toxic appearance
Abdominal distention
CHILDREN
Fever
Cough
Chills
Chest or abdominal pain
Respiratory distress
Nasal flaring, grunting
Retractions
Decreased breath sounds
Rhonchi, crackles, wheezing
Tachypnea (RR >50/min, 6–12 mo; >40/min, 1–3 yr; >25/min, >3 yr)

RR, respiratory rate.

DIFFERENTIAL DIAGNOSIS

The physician must try to determine which children have bacterial infections so that appropriate antibiotic therapy can be started. Although the clinical features of viral versus bacterial versus mycoplasmal pneumonia do not guarantee a correct diagnosis, it is helpful to seek the typical features of the different etiologies. Unfortunately, there are no clear radiographic patterns or laboratory studies (white blood cell [WBC] and neutrophil counts, C-reactive protein, or erythrocyte sedimentation rate) to differentiate the various causes of pneumonia (Table 288.5).

The possibility of coexistent bacterial and viral infections should also be considered. In a report of 136 infants and children ages 1 month to 6 years admitted for bronchiolitis and pneumonia, half were given antibiotics and half were not.[10] A viral infection was diagnosed in about half of the patients, predominately RSV. There were no significant differences in the course of acute disease, frequency of fever relapse, or pulmonary complications between the children not given antibiotics and those treated with antibiotics. In another report of the risk of secondary bacterial infection in infants hospitalized with RSV, the frequency of a secondary bacterial pneumonia was increased to 2.7% in infants treated with parenteral antibiotics, compared with 0.6% in those who received no antibiotics. Children with serious, mixed respiratory viral and bacterial infections usually demonstrate an atypical course of bronchiolitis or pneumonia characterized by persistent fever and respiratory distress.[26] Atypical bacterial infections, such as *Mycoplasma* or *Chlamydia*, may also coexist with viral infections or with typical bacteria, such as *Pneumococcus*.[11,13] Although other studies report the incidence of mixed respiratory viral and bacterial infections to be

TABLE 288.5. Typical Features of Acute Pneumonia in Children by Etiologic Agent

Variable	Bacterial	Viral	Mycoplasmal
Age	Any	Any	Over 5 yr
Fever	>39°C	<39°C	<39°C
Onset	Abrupt	Gradual	Gradual
Others ill at home or school	No	Yes, at same time	Yes, weeks apart
Other symptoms	Otitis media	Myalgia, rash, conjunctivitis, pharyngitis, diarrhea, otitis media	Headache, sore throat, myalgia, rash, conjunctivitis, otitis media
Cough	Productive	Nonproductive	Hacking, paroxysmal
Pleuritic chest pain	Yes	No	No
Toxicity	Marked	Moderate	Mild
Auscultation	Localized crackles, dullness	Diffuse crackles, wheezing	Unilateral crackles, wheezing
Chest x-ray	Segmental or lobar infiltrate	Hyperinflation, interstitial, perihilar, diffuse infiltrate	Patchy infiltrate in single or adjacent to lower lobe
Pleural fluid	Large, exudate or empyema	Minimal	Small in 20%
WBC count	>15,000/mm^3, increased PMNs	<15,000/mm^3, increased lymphocytes	Normal to <15,000/mm^3

as high as 39%, the clinical significance of these mixed infections is unclear.[14,17]

Other diseases that may be mistaken for pneumonia should also be considered. Asthma occurs in about 10% of children, and acute episodes are commonly triggered by viral respiratory infections associated with pulmonary infiltrates caused by atelectasis from mucous plugging. Children with asthma may experience recurrent febrile episodes with migratory atelectasis, which may be misdiagnosed as recurrent or persistent pneumonia. Often, the typical history of asthma with chronic cough and wheezing associated with common triggers of airway hyperreactivity goes unrecognized.[22] Many children with clinically diagnosed pneumonia, who have wheezing and are treated with antibiotics and bronchodilators, actually have underdiagnosed asthma.

Foreign-body aspiration may also cause pneumonia due to bronchial obstruction and may be missed if the initial aspiration episode is not recognized. Thus, questions should be asked about an acute choking episode in all children presenting with suspected pneumonia. Foreign-body aspiration is most common between ages 6 months and 3 years, and food is responsible for 80% of the objects aspirated (specifically peanuts in half of the cases). Many episodes of foreign-body aspiration present more than 1 week after the aspiration episode.

Children with congenital heart disease have a greater incidence of respiratory infections, especially those with large left-to-right shunts, as in patent ductus arteriosus or atrial or ventricular septal defect. Enlarged pulmonary arteries or cardiac chamber enlargement may cause bronchial compression, resulting in atelectasis or pneumonia. Pulmonary edema may also be mistaken for pneumonia. Cystic fibrosis should be considered in the child with recurrent pneumonia associated with chronic diarrhea and failure to thrive, although 20% of children with cystic fibrosis initially present only with respiratory problems.

EMERGENCY DEPARTMENT EVALUATION

The diagnosis of pneumonia is most often suspected after clinical presentation with fever, cough, tachypnea, crackles on lung auscultation, and chest x-ray evidence of consolidation. The precise etiology may not be readily apparent without further investigation. There is general agreement that routine chest x-rays are not needed for children with acute episodes of fever in the absence of specific respiratory findings (see Table 288.4). However, a recent report shows that "occult" pneumonias were found in 26% of children with leukocytosis (WBC count greater than 20,000/mm^3) and triage temperature in the emergency department of greater than or equal to 39.0°C and no clinical evidence of pneumonia as judged by absence of specific respiratory findings.[1]

A complete blood count and differential do not reliably differentiate the etiology of pneumonia. In general, higher white cell counts, with a greater number of polymorphonuclear forms, are seen with bacterial infection. Eosinophilia may be seen in the afebrile pneumonia syndrome in infants. Blood cultures should be considered in all febrile patients suspected of having bacterial pneumonia, but they are positive in only less than 10% of patients with bacterial infection. Mantoux PPD tuberculin skin tests should be considered for high-risk children. Thoracentesis should be performed for analysis and culture of pleural fluid in children who are moderately ill and present with a significant pleural effusion. Analysis of pleural fluid characteristics can differentiate uncomplicated parapneumonic effusion from pleural empyema and help guide initial therapy and decision to place a chest tube for drainage.

Bacterial antigen detection by latex agglutination from samples of serum, urine, and pleural fluid is available for group B streptococci, *S. pneumoniae,* and *H. influenzae*. Bacterial antigens may still be detected in patients already treated with antibiotics. Problems with bacterial antigen detection tests include poor sensitivity, as evidenced by reports of inability to detect pneumococcal antigen in serum or urine from children with blood cultures positive for *S. pneumoniae*.[15] The specificity has also been questioned by reports of *S. pneumoniae* and *H. influenzae* antigenuria in 4% of healthy children and 16% of children with otitis media without pneumonia, and also false-positive tests for *H. influenzae* in children with pneumonia as well as in controls.[15,21]

Rapid diagnostic tests are available to detect viral and chlamydial antigen by fluorescent antibody tests performed by ELISA. Samples are obtained from nasal washings and scrapings, and test results are available quickly. Rapid diagnosis of RSV, influenza, parainfluenza, and adenovirus is readily available. The sensitivity of rapid antigen detection for viruses is as high as 90% but is less than 50% for the detection of chlamydia. Viral cultures are specific but take several days to be completed. Rapid diagnostic tests are currently being developed (but not widely available) using polymerase chain reaction (PCR) assay for antigen detection for *Mycoplasma* and *Chlamydia pneumoniae*. *Legionella* pneumonia antigen detection by immunofluorescence staining in urine is currently available for rapid diagnosis.

Antibody assays may diagnose bacterial or viral infections by demonstrating a fourfold increase in specific antibody titers over a 2- to 4-week period, but they usually are clinically impractical due to the lack of immediate results. Specific IgM antibody by complement fixation against *Mycoplasma* or an IgG titer greater than 1:128 is consistent with *Mycoplasma* infection. A positive serum cold agglutinin reaction as a bedside test is helpful to diagnose *Mycoplasma* infection, although serum cold agglutinins may also be present with viral infections. Approximately 30% to 75% of patients with *Mycoplasma* pneumonia will be positive for cold agglutinins in a titer greater than 1:32. A "bedside" cold agglutinin test can be performed by adding 0.4 mL of blood to a standard blue- or purple-top tube, then placing the tube on wet ice for several minutes. A positive test shows agglutination or clumping, which disappears when the tube is warmed.

EMERGENCY DEPARTMENT MANAGEMENT AND DISPOSITION

Optimal treatment of pneumonia requires the following:

1. Knowing the most likely causative agents for a given age range
2. Judicious use of available diagnostic methods
3. Selecting the most appropriate antibiotic therapy when necessary
4. Supportive therapy, such as hospitalization, oxygen, or intravenous fluids

Optimal treatment focuses on determining whether the child needs to be hospitalized and considering the most likely cause of pneumonia for the child's age to determine whether antibiotic therapy is required. About 20% to 30% of children require hospitalization for treatment of pneumonia. Most infants under the age of 3 months should be hospitalized, as should older children who appear toxic, have significant respiratory distress, are hypoxemic, or have a complicated pneumonia. Other indications for hospitalization include apnea or poor feeding in infants, a family that cannot care for the child at home, persistent fever for greater than 2 to 3 days, poor response to outpatient treatment, dehydration, vomiting, and underlying conditions that would increase the risk for complications. Underlying conditions include young age, prematurity, congenital heart disease, bronchopulmonary dysplasia, immunodeficiency, cancer, AIDS, multiple congenital anomalies, and neurologic or metabolic disease.

If a diagnosis of viral pneumonia is made, supportive treatment is indicated and antibiotics are unnecessary, unless an atypical course is observed with toxicity and persistent fever. A high index of suspicion for secondary bacterial pneumonia is needed in children with measles, varicella, or pneumonia due to influenza. Specific antiviral therapy with ribavirin is available but ineffective for RSV in ventilated infants and of uncertain clinical efficacy in nonventilated infants.[4] The antiviral agents amantadine and rimantadine may be considered for treatment of influenza A infection to reduce the severity and duration of illness, although efficacy studies in children are limited.

If hospitalization is necessary, supportive treatment includes oxygen to prevent hypoxemia, intravenous fluids to maintain adequate hydration, and intravenous antibiotics for suspected bacterial infection. Close observation and monitoring for increased respiratory distress and oxygen saturation monitoring using pulse oximetry are indicated for children with severe pneumonia. Arterial or capillary blood gas measurements should be obtained for children with worsening respiratory distress or impending respiratory failure.

Suggested initial therapy for suspected bacterial pneumonia is listed in Table 288.6.[5,6,15,16,18,19,23] Most febrile infants under the age of 3 months should be admitted and treated with intravenous antibiotics for suspected sepsis. Infants aged 1 to 3 months with suspected afebrile pneumonia syndrome may be treated as outpatients if they are not significantly ill, but initial treatment in the hospital with oral erythromycin, clarithromycin, or azithromycin may be preferable. For children over age 3 months and treated as outpatients, antibiotics should be selected to cover *S. pneumoniae, M. pneumoniae,* and *C. pneumoniae*. Erythromycin, clarithromycin, or azithromycin are again suggested.[2] When a lobar pneumonia is present and atypical pneumonia is not a consideration, amoxicillin, a second- or third-generation cephalosporin, amoxicillin–clavulanate, and trimethoprim–sulfamethoxazole are alternatives to cover adequately for *S. pneumoniae*.

For children over age 3 months and treated as inpatients for suspected bacterial pneumonia, intravenous cefuroxime, cefotaxime, or ceftriaxone is indicated to treat probable *S. pneumoniae*. Nafcillin or clindamycin should be added when staphylococcal disease is suspected. Clindamycin is also indicated for suspected aspiration pneumonia or a lung abscess. An oral or intravenous macrolide antibiotic may be added if an atypical pneumonia is suspected. In a recent series of children with *S. pneumoniae,* there were no differences in clinical course or outcome between patients with penicillin-resistant versus -sensitive isolates, and only three of 16 with penicillin-resistant isolates were treated with vancomycin.[25] Vancomycin should be considered in patients who have a high level of resistance to penicillin or are critically ill. Identification of a specific bacteria may guide further treatment by the antibiotic sensitivity pattern.

Most children with uncomplicated bacterial pneumonia can be treated with oral antibiotics. Some physicians routinely treat children initially with an intramuscular antibiotic, often ceftriaxone, followed by oral antibiotics. Dagan et al.[6] concluded that 1 or 2 days of intramuscular ceftriaxone 50 mg/kg/d, followed by a second-generation oral cephalosporin, was safe and effective. No difference has been found between intramuscular penicillin versus oral amoxicillin in treating outpatient pediatric pneumonia. There are no strict criteria or definitive controlled studies to recommend inpatient versus outpatient treatment or oral versus parenteral treatment.

Intravenous antibiotics for children hospitalized with pneumonia should be continued until the fever defervesces and the child improves clinically. Treatment failure or the development of a complicated pneumonia should be suspected if fever persists for more than 72 hours. Oral antibiotic therapy can then be continued to complete 10 days of treatment. Children with complicated pneumonias should be treated with intravenous antibiotics for 1 to 2 weeks and then with oral antibiotics to complete a 2- to 3-week course.

Children with pneumonia should be reevaluated after 2 to 3 weeks, and a follow-up chest x-ray should be obtained at that

TABLE 288.6. Treatment of Bacterial Pneumonia in Children

<3 mo	1–3 mo (Afebrile Pneumonia Syndrome)	>3 mo
OUTPATIENT		
If febrile, admit	PO erythromycin, clarithromycin, or azithromycin	Atypical: PO erythromycin, clarithromycin, or azithromycin Lobar: as above or amoxicillin, or PO second- or third-generation cephalosporin,[a] or amoxicillin clavulanate, or TMP/SMX For selected cases of lobar pneumonia, i.m. ceftriaxone every day × 1–2 days, followed by above[b]
INPATIENT		
i.v. ampicillin + cefotaxime or aminoglycoside	PO/i.v. erythromycin or PO clarithromycin or azithromycin	i.v. cefuroxime or cefotaxime or ceftriaxone, plus consider PO/i.v. erythromycin or PO PO/i.v. erythromycin or PO clarithromycin or azithromycin, clarithromycin or azithromycin

PO, oral; i.m., intramuscular; i.v., intravenous; TMP/SMX, trimethoprim-sulfamethoxazole.
[a] Second- or third-generation cephalosporins: cefuroxime, cefprozil, cefixime.
[b] Consider as alternative to hospitalization only in children >6 months who are not severely toxic, are able to take oral fluids, do not require oxygen, and who will be compliant with follow-up for a recheck in 24 hours. Might also consider for failure of previous oral antibiotic therapy. Follow parenteral treatment with oral antibiotics to complete 10 days of therapy.

time for a severe or complicated pneumonia. For the child with an uncomplicated course, a follow-up chest x-ray may be done at 6 to 8 weeks to look for unsuspected atelectasis or persistent infiltrate, which may indicate a retained foreign body, congenital malformation of the lung, or undiagnosed chronic lung disease such as cystic fibrosis.[28] If a foreign body is suspected, bronchoscopy is indicated. Rigid bronchoscopy is preferred for foreign-body removal.

COMMON PITFALLS

- Do not forget to consider congestive heart failure in the young infant or newborn with a x-ray diagnosis of pneumonia.
- Consider underlying disease, either pulmonary disease or general immunodeficiency syndrome (e.g., cystic fibrosis, AIDS), in patients with recurrent pneumonia.
- Consider foreign-body aspiration in the patient with recurrent or persistent pneumonia.
- Provide close follow-up for the patient with suspected bacterial pneumonia.
- Suspect asthma in a child diagnosed with recurrent or persistent migratory infiltrates and wheezing.

References

1. Bachur R, Perry H, Harper MB. Occult pneumonia: empiric chest radiographs in febrile children with leukocytosis. *Ann Emerg Med* 1999;33:166.
2. Block Stan, Hedrick James, et al. *Mycoplasma pneumoniae* and *Chlamydia* pneumonia in pediatric community-acquired pneumonia: comparative efficacy and safety of clarithromycin vs. erythromycin ethylsuccinate. *Pediatr Infect Dis J* 1995;14:471–477.
3. Broughton RA. Infections due to *Mycoplasma pneumoniae* in childhood. *Pediatr Infect Dis J* 1986;5:71.
4. Committee on Infectious Diseases. Use of ribavirin on the treatment of respiratory syncytial virus infection. *Pediatrics* 1993;92:501.
5. Dagan R. Antibiotic treatment of pediatric community-acquired lower respiratory tract infections: challenges and possible solutions. *Respiration* 1993; 60:38.
6. Dagan R, Syrogiannopoulos G, Ashkenazi S. Parenteral–oral switch in the management of paediatric pneumonia. *Drugs* 1994;47[Suppl 3]:43.
7. Davies HD, Matlow A, et al. Brief reports: prospective comparative study of viral, bacterial, and atypical organisms identified in pneumonia and bronchiolitis in hospitalized Canadian infants. *Pediatr Infect Dis J* 1996;15:371–375.
8. Demuri GP. Community-acquired respiratory infections in children: afebrile pneumonia in infants. *Prim Care* 1996;23(4):849–860.
9. Denny FW, Clyde WA Jr. Acute lower respiratory tract infections in nonhospitalized children. *J Pediatr* 1986;108:635.
10. Friis G, Andersen P, Brenoe E, et al. Antibiotic treatment of pneumonia and bronchiolitis. *Arch Dis Child* 1984;59:1038.
11. Hall CB, Powell KR, Schnabel KC, et al. Risk of secondary bacterial infection in infants hospitalized with respiratory syncytial viral infection. *J Pediatr* 1988;113:266.
12. Hardie WD, Roberts NE, Reising SF, et al. Complicated parapneumonic effusions in children caused by penicillin-nonsusceptible *Streptococcus pneumoniae*. *Pediatrics* 1998;101:388.
13. Heiskanen-Kosma T, Korppi M, et al. Etiology of childhood pneumonia: serologic results of a prospective, population-based study. *Pediatr Infect Dis J* 1998;17:986–991.
14. Hietala J, Uhari M, Tuokko H, et al. Mixed bacterial and viral infections are common in children. *Pediatr Infect Dis J* 1989;8:683.
15. Isaacs D. Problems in determining the etiology of community-acquired childhood pneumonia. *Pediatr Infect Dis J* 1989;8:143.
16. Jadavji T, Law B, et al. A practical guide for the diagnosis and treatment of pediatric pneumonia. *Can Med Assoc J* 1997;156(5):5703–5711.
17. Korppi M, Leinonen M, Koskela M, et al. Bacterial coinfection in children hospitalized with respiratory syncytial virus infections. *Pediatr Infect Dis J* 1989;8:687.
18. Krasinski K, Borkowsky W, Bonk S, et al. Bacterial infections in HIV-infected children. *Pediatr Infect Dis J* 1988;7:323.
19. Leibovitz E, Tabachnik E, Fliedel O, et al. Once-daily intramuscular ceftriaxone in the outpatient treatment of severe community-acquired pneumonia in children. *Clin Pediatr* 1990;29:634.
20. Nohynek H, Eskola J, Laine E, et al. The causes of hospital-treated acute lower respiratory tract infection in children. *Am J Dis Child* 1991;145:618.
21. Ramsey BW, Marcuse EK, Foy HM, et al. Use of bacterial antigen detection in the diagnosis of pediatric lower respiratory tract infections. *Pediatrics* 1986;78:1.
22. Schaeffer DA. Chronic cough in children. *Am J Asthma Allerg Pediatr* 1988; 1:201.
23. Schutze GE, Jacobs RF. Management of community-acquired bacterial pneumonia in hospitalized children. *Pediatr Infect Dis J* 1992;11:160.
24. Shaw NJ, Elton R, Eden OB. Pneumonia and pneumonitis in childhood malignancy. *Acta Paediatr* 1992;81:222.
25. Tan TQ, Mason EO, Barson WJ, et al. Clinical characteristics and outcome of children with pneumonia attributable to penicillin-susceptible and penicillin-nonsusceptible *Streptococcus pneumoniae*. *Pediatrics* 1998;102:1369.
26. Tristram DA, Miller RW, McMillan JA, et al. Simultaneous infection with respiratory syncytial virus and other respiratory pathogens. *Am J Dis Child* 1988;142:834.
27. Turner RB, Lande AE, Chase P, et al. Pneumonia in pediatric outpatients: cause and clinical manifestations. *J Pediatr* 1987;111:194.
28. Wald ER. Recurrent and nonresolving pneumonia in children. *Semin Respir Infect* 1993;8:46.

CHAPTER 289
Pyloric Stenosis

Maureen Campbell and Lisa Horton

Hypertrophic pyloric stenosis is the most common cause of obstruction in the pediatric age group; consequently, the emergency physician should be able to recognize the clinical manifestations and treat the patient appropriately.

The incidence of pyloric stenosis is estimated at three per 1,000, affecting five times as many boys as girls. Heredity plays some role, as the incidence of pyloric stenosis in the children of affected parents rises to 6.9%.[2,9]

The etiology of pyloric stenosis remains unclear. Infants with pyloric stenosis have significantly higher levels of prostaglandin E2, a potent smooth muscle contractor, and prostaglandin F2 than their normal counterparts, leading investigators to speculate a causative role of prostaglandins in pyloric stenosis.[8] The pathology is characterized by diffuse hypertrophy and hyperplasia of antral smooth muscle cells. This results in elongation and thickening of the pylorus and antrum. The stomach then becomes dilated and uniformly hypertrophied.

CLINICAL PRESENTATION

Hypertrophic pyloric stenosis typically presents in the third week of life, although symptoms have been reported as early as the first week and as late as the fourth month of life.[5] The initial symptom is occasional vomiting, which then becomes more forceful and frequent over time, until it is projectile in nature, occurring shortly after every feeding. The emesis is nonbilious and is occasionally blood tinged; in severe cases, "coffee ground" emesis is seen. The stools are small and infrequent, and the infants characteristically fail to gain weight appropriately, in the absence of anorexia. In advanced cases, infants may present with severe dehydration and electrolyte abnormalities. Electrolyte loss due to repetitive vomiting can result in a characteristic hypokalemic, hypochloremic, metabolic alkalosis. Jaundice occurs in 2% to 9% of affected infants. Currently, patients with hypertrophic pyloric stenosis present less frequently with the clinical hallmarks of the disease. The use of imaging studies to establish the diagnosis has become common practice. The result has been the diagnosis of hypertrophic pyloric stenosis before alkalosis has developed, a shorter clinical course, less morbidity, and a shorter postoperative hospital stay.[11,12]

DIFFERENTIAL DIAGNOSIS

The differential diagnosis for projectile nonbilious vomiting in an infant includes overfeeding, gastroenteritis, gastroesophageal reflux, pyelonephritis, sepsis, drug withdrawal, gastric or duodenal web, adrenal insufficiency, formula intolerance, pylorospasm, poor maternal infant interaction, and intracranial hypertension. Most of these entities are easily differentiated from pyloric stenosis by history, physical examination, laboratory values, and simple observation of the child when feeding. However, it is sometimes difficult to rule out gastroesophageal reflux and gastrointestinal malformations without radiologic studies.

EMERGENCY DEPARTMENT EVALUATION

The history of present illness should be obtained to determine duration of symptoms, urine output, and the infant's level of activity, so as to assess the severity of dehydration. A history of the presence of fever, diarrhea, prior surgery, or trauma is important to exclude other diagnostic entities. The physical examination reveals varying degrees of dehydration, depending on the duration of symptoms. Examination may reveal slightly dry mucous membranes in infants with mild dehydration or, in severe cases, listlessness, prolonged capillary refill, and a sunken anterior fontanelle. Skin turgor is decreased in most infants as a result of decreased caloric and fluid intake. Inspection of the abdomen often reveals peristaltic waves of the hypertrophied stomach moving from the left upper quadrant to the right upper quadrant just after a feeding. The waves are most readily visualized beneath a strong light directed tangentially to the abdomen. The peristaltic wave can sometimes be elicited by gently tapping the epigastric area. The wave begins as a ball-like prominence in the left upper quadrant, preceded by an area of depression that moves across the abdomen. Palpation of the hypertrophied pylorus, or "olive," is pathognomonic for hypertrophic pyloric stenosis. It is said to be palpable in 70% to 90% of affected infants. Palpation of the olive is best accomplished by using the left hand and standing on the right side of the infant, while using the right hand to gently lift the feet and relax the abdominal wall. Palpation of the infant's epigastrium then should reveal a firm olive-sized mass ballottable just above and to the right of the umbilicus.[5] The mass is the consistency of the tip of the nose and is very mobile. Decompression of the stomach, by placement of a 12F to 14F orogastric tube, further facilitates examination. Aspiration of more than 3 oz of formula from the stomach of a vomiting infant is strong evidence of the presence of pyloric stenosis, because these infants characteristically have large residual volumes. Once the olive is felt, the diagnosis is made, and further diagnostic work-up is unnecessary. If, after several minutes, an olive cannot be palpated, further evaluation is warranted. Electrolytes, glucose, blood urea nitrogen, pH, pCO_2, and urinalysis should be obtained, as well as a complete blood count. Once other diagnostic possibilities, such as pyelonephritis and sepsis, have been ruled out, one may proceed to radiologic studies.

EMERGENCY DEPARTMENT MANAGEMENT

After completing the history and physical examination, intravenous access should be obtained. If the infant is markedly dehydrated, a bolus of 20 mL/kg of an isotonic fluid should be initiated immediately. If the infant's hydration status is adequate, maintenance intravenous fluids should be started at a rate of 100 to 150 mL/kg/d. As soon as the infant voids, potassium should be added to the infusion. The blood chemistry values typically reveal a hypochloremic metabolic alkalosis due to the large loss of hydrochloric acid through vomiting. The serum CO_2 can be as high as 35 to 40 mEq/L. The alkalosis leads to an intracellular exchange of potassium for hydrogen ion. Also, the decrease in intravascular volume stimulates aldosterone secretion, which promotes sodium and water reuptake in the kidney at the expense of potassium loss. As the serum potassium level drops, the kidney preferentially exchanges hydrogen ion for sodium instead of potassium, resulting in characteristic acid urine in the presence of a serum alkalosis and a total body deficit of potassium.[13] The complete blood count may reveal a high hematocrit due to hemoconcentration, as well as a marked leukocytosis due to stress.

In centers where sonographers are experienced in imaging the pylorus, ultrasound is the study of choice. Ultrasound avoids the radiation exposure of fluoroscopy and the risk of a reaction to contrast. In experienced hands, the differing echogenicities of the various layers of the pylorus afford clear delineation of the area. It is generally agreed that a pyloric muscularis layer of greater than 4 mm, a pyloric diameter of greater than 15 mm, and a pyloric length of greater than 18 mm are indicative of pyloric stenosis.[1,6] A transverse section of the hypertrophic area can be seen as a "doughnut" or "bull's eye."[9] Ultrasound currently can diagnose pyloric stenosis in over 70% of affected infants.[10] If the ultrasound is negative or not available, an abdominal flat plate and upper gastrointestinal (GI) contrast series may be obtained. It is strongly recommended that the upper GI be used only when careful physical examination and/or ultrasonography is inconclusive.[5] On flat plate, the dilated stomach can be seen, with the gastric air bubble found as low as L2 to L3. An upper GI series characteristically demonstrates the "string sign," a narrow stream of barium passing through the thickened pyloric canal. Once a barium study is obtained, the barium should be quickly removed from the stomach. This eliminates the possibility of the infant vomiting and subsequently aspirating the barium, as well as avoids possible leakage of barium into the peritoneum should the pyloric mucosa be entered accidentally during surgery.

DISPOSITION

Once the diagnosis is made, either by physical examination or radiologic studies, pediatric surgery consultation and admission is the appropriate disposition, even if this requires transfer of the patient to a tertiary care center. In experienced hands, the mortality rate of pyloromyotomy is 0.3%, and the average hospital stay is 2 days or less. Pending admission or transfer to the operating room, the emergency department physician should continue to provide gastric decompression and rehydration, and follow vital signs and urine output.

COMMON PITFALLS

- Early in the course of pyloric stenosis, the diagnosis is difficult to differentiate from gastroesophageal reflux, and a high degree of suspicion is required in these cases. Examination of the infant's abdomen after feeding may be helpful. If a mass is palpated, further workup is unnecessary. If a pediatric surgeon is readily accessible, it may be more appropriate not to proceed with radiologic studies prior to surgical consultation, because physical examination by an experienced surgeon can obviate the need for further studies in the many affected infants.
- Failure of the physician to adequately rehydrate the dehydrated infant
- Failure to decompress the infant's stomach prior to sending the child to surgery

References

1. Bowen A. The vomiting infant's recent advances and unsettled issues in imaging. *Radiol Clin North Am* 1988;26:377.
2. Carter CO, Evans KA. Inheritance of congenital pyloric stenosis. *J Med Genet* 1969;6:233.
3. Chen E., Luks F, Gilchrist B, et al. Pyloric stenosis in the age of ultrasonography: fading skills, better patients? *J Pediatr Surg* 1996;31(6):829.
4. Cohen H, Zinn H, Haller J, et al. Ultrasonography of pylorospasm: findings may simulate hypertrophic pyloric stenosis. *J Ultrasound Med* 1998;17:705.
5. Garcia VF, Randolph JG. Pyloric stenosis: diagnosis and management. *Pediatr Rev* 1990;11:292.
6. Haller JO, Dohen HL. Hypertrophic pyloric stenosis: diagnosis using ultrasound. *Radiology* 1986;161:335.
7. Hulka F, Campbell T, Campbell J, et al. Evolution in the recognition of infantile hypertropic pyloric stenosis. *Pediatrics* 1997;100:E9.
8. LaFerla G, Watson J, Fyfe A, et al. The role of prostaglandins E2 and F2 alpha in infantile hypertrophic pyloric stenosis. *J Pediatr Surg* 1986;21:410.
9. McKeown T, MacMahon B. Infantile hypertrophic pyloric stenosis in parent and child. *Arch Dis Child* 1955;30:497.
10. Mollitt DL, Golladay ES, Williamson S, et al. Ultrasonography in the diagnosis of pyloric stenosis. *South Med J* 1987;80:47.
11. Papadakis K, Chen E, Luks F, et al. The changing presentation of pyloric stenosis. *Am J Emerg Med* 1999;17:67.
12. Poon T, Zhang A, Cartmill T, et al. Changing patterns of diagnosis and treatment of infantile hypertrophic pyloric stenosis: a clinical audit of 303 patients. *J Pediatr Surg* 1996;31(12):1611.
13. Stevenson RJ. Non neonatal intestinal obstruction in children. *Surg Clin North Am* 1985;65:1217.

CHAPTER 290
Rheumatic Fever

Robert D. Schremmer and Jane F. Knapp

Although Guillaume de Baillou first differentiated arthritis from gout in the sixteenth century, it was not until 1889 that acute rheumatic fever (ARF), as it is known today, was described by Walter Cheadle.[3] With the early 1930s came the discovery of an association between rheumatic fever and group A *Streptococcus*, which was not proven until years later.[14] T. Duckett Jones' landmark article in 1944[7] standardized the diagnosis of ARF. By specifying major and minor criteria, Dr. Jones hoped to improve accuracy of diagnosis. A poorly understood, sudden decrease in the incidence of ARF occurred in the postwar years,[3,14] lasting into the 1980s.[10,15,16] During the past decade, regional outbreaks of strongly rheumatogenic strains of group A *Streptococcus* were noted.[15,16] Even with these resurgences, the incidence of ARF has remained well below that of pre–World War II.

Rheumatic fever is an inflammatory disorder involving multiple organ systems. Peak incidence is between 5 and 18 years, with equal affinity for both sexes throughout the world.[14] Sydenham's chorea, a manifestation of ARF, mainly affects postpubertal girls.[11] Disease prevalence is highest in developing countries,[10] probably secondary to malnutrition,[18] crowding, and inadequate access to medical care.

It seems that several factors are involved in the host–pathogen relationship for ARF to occur. First, the strain of *streptococcus* must be rheumatogenic. These highly contagious strains preferentially cause pharyngitis and do not infect the skin.[15] The M protein, a component of the cell wall, appears to be one primary factor determining a strain's rheumatogenicity.[2] Second, the host must be susceptible. There are common antigens between certain human tissues (i.e., heart valves and synovium) and the streptococcal cell wall. Discovery of this "molecular mimicry" has led to a better understanding of the pathophysiology of ARF. The shared epitopes confuse the immune system's ability to differentiate self and nonself, inducing an autoimmune reaction.[14] Despite this knowledge, many aspects of the pathogenesis of ARF are not understood.

CLINICAL PRESENTATION

Signs and symptoms of ARF are variable in intensity. A symptom-free period follows an episode of pharyngitis. It is notable, however, that the majority of patients from the local outbreaks in the 1980s did not recall sore throat.[3] The silent period is followed by an acute onset of symptoms, such as fever, malaise, and pallor not representative of the degree of anemia.[14]

To establish the diagnosis of ARF, the Jones criteria must be fulfilled (Table 290.1). Although these criteria have undergone revision four times since their original publication, the general structure remains intact. The major manifestations are considered such because of their specificity and frequency of occurrence.[14] On the other hand, the minor criteria are much less specific, but are frequently seen with the disease. Only three exceptions to the Jones criteria are noted in the 1992 revision. A patient who presents late in the disease course may manifest only chorea or indolent carditis. Furthermore, a patient with the presumed diagnosis of recurrent rheumatic fever may be difficult to diagnose if there is a history of rheumatic heart disease. Evidence of streptococcal infection is still required, but the diagnosis in such a patient otherwise only requires the presence of one major or several minor criteria.

Arthritis is the most common of the major manifestations, occurring in 70% to 80% of patients.[6,14] This arthritis is typically migratory and involves larger joints, such as knees, ankles, and wrists. Erythema, warmth, swelling, and severe pain are often present, as is decreased range of motion. Untreated, the arthritis typically lasts about 4 weeks and resolves without deformity.[1] Characteristic of rheumatic arthritis is its exquisite responsiveness to salicylate therapy. If no response has been seen after the first 2 days of therapy, other diagnoses should be considered.

Carditis is the second most commonly seen manifestation, with up to 50% to 60% of patients affected.[6] Pancarditis is classic, but patients also commonly present with symptoms of valvular disease. Mitral regurgitation is the most frequently encountered lesion, followed by aortic regurgitation.[17] A new or changing murmur is the usual finding, although tachycardia, friction rubs, cardiomegaly, and, rarely, heart failure may be seen. Morphologically, valvulitis is manifested as a later finding by focal nodular thickening of the leaflets.[17] The role of echocardiography in diagnosis is controversial, but it may be used to confirm the presence of valvular disease in a patient with a new or changing murmur.

TABLE 290.1. Rheumatic Fever Manifestations

MAJOR
Carditis
Arthritis
Chorea
Subcutaneous nodules
Erythema marginatum
MINOR
Clinical Findings
Arthralgia
Fever
Laboratory Findings
Elevated acute-phase reactants
Erythrocyte sedimentation rate
C-reactive protein
Prolonged PR interval
Supporting evidence of antecedent group A streptococcal infections
Positive throat culture or rapid streptococcal antibody titer
Elevated or rising streptococcal antibody titer

Adapted from Jones TD. The diagnosis of rheumatic fever. *JAMA* 1944;126:431. modified in *JAMA* 1992;268:2069.

The other major manifestations include Sydenham's chorea, subcutaneous nodules, and the erythema marginatum rash. Chorea, named for Thomas Sydenham, who first described it in 1686, is present in only 10% to 20% of rheumatic fever patients.[11] A disorder of the central nervous system, it is characterized by sudden, involuntary, and purposeless movements, usually of the upper extremities and face. Often, psychological or psychiatric symptoms may be present as well. Chorea is diagnosed by clinical signs alone, but can be easily missed if emotional lability is the only sign.[8] Often, chorea is a late manifestation. Subcutaneous nodules, often seen in patients with carditis, are firm, small, and nontender, and they are often found on extensor surfaces, tendons, bony prominences, and the occipital region. Rarely seen, these nodules are present only a few days. Erythema marginatum is also rarely seen. A rash with a serpiginous reddish pink border, it is nonpruritic and blanches with pressure. It is usually present on areas of the body hidden by clothing and also disappears in a few days.

The minor criteria are divided into clinical and laboratory findings. Fever, a common sign in many disorders, must be at least 39°C to be considered for the diagnosis. Arthralgia, joint pain with no evidence of inflammation, should not be regarded as a minor manifestation if arthritis is also present. Laboratory findings include elevated acute-phase reactants and prolonged PR interval on electrocardiography. Erythrocyte sedimentation rate and C-reactive protein are the commonly used acute-phase reactants.

Signs and symptoms associated with, but not specific for, ARF include epistaxis, serositis, and lung, kidney, and eye involvement. Tachypnea, cough that may be nonproductive or productive of blood-streaked sputum, and chest pain are characteristic of pulmonary disease.[4] Scleritis, uveitis, and glaucoma have been reported in a patient with ARF.[12] Hematuria may occur in 5% of patients,[14] but renal failure is rare.

DIFFERENTIAL DIAGNOSIS

The differential diagnosis of ARF is extensive. Each of the three types of juvenile rheumatoid arthritis (JRA) may resemble ARF. Systemic JRA is characterized by high fevers with chills, hepatosplenomegaly, generalized lymphadenopathy, and rash. Rheumatoid rash shares a common typical distribution with erythema marginatum, but may occur anywhere on the body and is composed of small red-pink macules that may coalesce. Many patients may also develop pleuritis or pericarditis and pleural or pericardial effusion. The arthritis may be initially overlooked, given the patient's ill appearance. Polyarticular JRA will involve five or more joints, often in the hand. A small fraction of patients may be rheumatoid factor positive, but most are negative. Girls are more commonly affected than boys. Systemic symptoms may include low-grade fever, anorexia, malaise, slight hepatosplenomegaly and lymphadenopathy, and mild anemia. Patients with pauciarticular JRA will manifest arthritis in four or fewer joints. The involved joints are often large and symmetric. Affected girls will more often have a positive antinuclear antibody, and boys will more likely show a positive HLA B27. Rheumatoid factor is generally negative in both genders. Girls show an increased risk for iridocyclitis, and boys are at an increased risk for developing ankylosing spondylitis. Systemic symptoms are similar to that of polyarticular JRA. In all forms of JRA, the joint pain tends to be less severe than that of ARF, but it lasts much longer.

Several infections can manifest joint symptoms. Septic arthritis is usually accompanied with fever and will involve a single joint. Aspiration of synovial fluid for examination and culture will confirm the diagnosis. Systemic infections that may have an associated arthritis include infectious mononucleosis, hepatitis, influenza, Lyme disease, fifth disease (erythema infectiosum), varicella, tuberculosis, gonorrhea, and brucellosis. These infections are often easily ruled out by their associated signs and symptoms.

Leukemia and sickle cell anemia patients may also demonstrate severe joint pain; both disorders may be diagnosed by a complete blood count and peripheral smear. Inflammatory bowel disease also initially presents with arthritis, but will soon be associated with gastrointestinal symptoms. Legg-Calvé-Perthes disease, slipped capital femoral epiphysis, and toxic synovitis should be considered in any child complaining of hip pain. Although systemic lupus erythematosus can fulfill many of the Jones criteria, other aspects of the illness will differentiate it from ARF. Similarly, other collagen vascular diseases can be distinguished by other manifestations. Kawasaki disease has diagnostic criteria that may partially overlap the Jones criteria, but the clinical appearances are dissimilar. Henoch-Schönlein purpura is recognized by the characteristic rash on the lower extremities. Subacute bacterial endocarditis should be considered in any child with a new or changing murmur and fever. Finally, poststreptococcal reactive arthritis has alternatively been considered a separate disorder and an atypical presentation of ARF.

EMERGENCY DEPARTMENT EVALUATION

To establish an accurate diagnosis, the revised Jones criteria are used. The presence of two major manifestations or of one major and two minor manifestations coupled with evidence of a preceding streptococcal infection indicates a high probability of ARF.[1] The 1992 revision recognizes that the criteria are only useful during the initial attack and not during recurrences.

Only laboratory evidence of recent streptococcal pharyngitis is acceptable and may include positive throat culture or rapid antigen assay, antistreptolysin-O titer, anti-DNase B, and antihyaluronidase. A complete blood count and blood culture may be useful to rule out other diseases. Chest x-ray may be indicated if cardiomegaly, pericardial, or pleural effusion is suspected. Echocardiography can be used to confirm valvulitis, but is not indicated without auscultatory findings, unless Sydenham's chorea is present. Finally, an electrocardiogram can be obtained to determine PR interval prolongation.

EMERGENCY DEPARTMENT MANAGEMENT

Treatment is focused on prevention of ARF through early identification and treatment of streptococcal pharyngitis. This strategy terminates the ongoing exposure of streptococcal antigen to the host immune system.[14] Nonsteroidal antiinflammatory drugs (NSAIDs) are extremely useful in treating rheumatic arthritis and may also be used for mild carditis. Moderate-to-severe rheumatic carditis, however, requires oral corticosteroids. Prednisone 1 to 2 mg/kg/d for 10 to 15 days, followed by a slow taper over at least a month, will ensure adequate treatment. NSAIDs are unnecessary if corticosteroids are used.[14] Treatment of Sydenham's chorea may require haloperidol, valproic acid, or carbamazepine.[11]

DISPOSITION

Traditionally, patients with ARF have required hospitalization. Recently, however, over 50% of cases have been managed on an outpatient basis, with the severity of carditis or the presence of arthritis determining inpatient necessity.[9] Follow-up should be with the child's primary care physician. Pediatric cardiology or neurology consultations should be considered if symptomatology warrants.

COMMON PITFALLS

- Do not fail to perform a thorough joint examination.
- Do not focus exclusively on the joint examination in a patient with obvious joint disease.
- The diagnosis of ARF is easily overlooked in the patient with vague complaints of joint pain. A new or changing murmur may be the only apparent indication of carditis.
- Chorea must be considered in the differential diagnosis of emotional lability.

References

1. American Heart Association. Guidelines for the diagnosis of rheumatic fever. Jones criteria, 1992 update. *JAMA* 1992;268(15):2069–2073.
2. Bessen DE, et al. Serologic evidence for a class I group A streptococcal infection among rheumatic fever patients. *J Infect Dis* 1995;172:1608–1611.
3. Bronze MS, Dale JB. The reemergence of serious group A streptococcal infections and acute rheumatic fever. *Am J Med Sci* 1996;311(1):41–54.
4. Burgert SJ, et al. Rheumatic pneumonia: reappearance of a previously recognized complication of acute rheumatic fever. *Clin Infect Dis* 1995;21:1020–1022.
5. Feder HM, et al. Once-daily therapy for streptococcal pharyngitis with amoxicillin. *Pediatrics* 1999;103(1):47–52.
6. Hoey J. The disease that "bites the heart and licks the joints." *Can Med Assoc J* 1998;158(10):1335.
7. Jones TD. The diagnosis of rheumatic fever. *JAMA* 1944;126:481–484.
8. Kanabar DJ, et al. An emotional 13-year old girl. *Lancet* 1996;348:1000.
9. Loeffler AM, et al. Identification of cases of acute rheumatic fever managed on an outpatient basis. *Pediatr Infect Dis J* 1995;14(11):975–978.
10. Markowitz M. Rheumatic fever—a half-century perspective. *Pediatrics* 1998;102(1):272–274.
11. Marques-Dias MJ, et al. Sydenham's chorea. *Psychiatr Clin North Am* 1997; 20(4):809–820.
12. Ortiz JM, et al. Scleritis, uveitis, and glaucoma in a patient with rheumatic fever. *Am J Ophthalmol* 1995;120(4):538–539.
13. Outlaw KK, O'Leary JP. Wolfgang Amadeus Mozart 1756–1791: a mysterious death. *Am Surg* 1995;61:1025–1027.
14. da Silva NA, Pereira BA. Acute rheumatic fever. Still a challenge. *Rheum Dis Clin North Am* 1997;23(3):545–568.
15. Stollerman GH. Rheumatic fever. *Lancet* 1997;349:935–942.
16. Taubert KA, et al. Seven-year national survey of Kawasaki disease and acute rheumatic fever. *Pediatr Infect Dis J* 1994;12(8):704–708.
17. Vasan RS, et al. Echocardiographic evaluation of patients with acute rheumatic fever and rheumatic carditis. *Circulation* 1996;94(1):73–82.
18. Zaman MM, et al. Association of rheumatic fever with serum albumin concentration and body iron stores in Bangladeshi children: case-control study. *BMJ* 1998;317:1287–1288.

CHAPTER 291
Sickling Syndromes

Paul A. Pitel and James L. Harper

Sickle cell anemia is an autosomal recessive hemoglobinopathy characterized by hemolytic anemia, recurrent vasoocclusion, and end-organ dysfunction. The heterozygous state (AS), sickle cell trait, is found in 8% to 10% of American Blacks. The homozygous state (SS), sickle cell anemia, occurs in one in 400 to

600 Black newborns. The disease is seen less commonly in the Hispanic, southern European, and Middle Eastern populations.

The molecular basis of the disease is the substitution of glutamine for valine at the sixth position of the globin beta chain. This permits the crystallization of the hemoglobin molecules in conditions of relative hypoxemia. The cell becomes irreversibly sickled, leading to premature cell destruction (hemolysis) and blood vessel obstruction.

Hemoglobin electrophoresis permits the accurate diagnosis of sickle cell anemia, sickle cell trait, hemoglobin sickle cell disease, and other sickle variants as early as the newborn period. The sickle cell prep (Sickledex) is inaccurate before age 4 to 6 months. In the older infant or child with sickle cell anemia, the hemoglobin averages 8 g/dl, the hematocrit 24%, and the reticulocyte count 10%, with an elevated platelet count and a white count of 13,000 to 17,000.

Unexplained anemia in a Black child should raise the issue of a hemoglobinopathy. The presence of any sickle forms on a peripheral blood smear is presumptive evidence of sickle cell anemia. Children with sickle cell trait have normal hematologic values.

The emergency department evaluation depends on the presentation or type of crisis of the current illness. Clinical symptoms may begin as early as 3 to 4 months of age, when significant amounts of hemoglobin S become present. Referral for ongoing treatment and parent education, preferably through a sickle cell center, is vital.

DACTYLITIS (HAND–FOOT SYNDROME)

The hand–foot syndrome is the most common presentation of the child with sickle cell anemia from age 6 to 24 months. Painful swelling of the hands or feet, or both, results from symmetric infarction of the metacarpals and metatarsals. Low-grade fever (less than 101.5°F) is common, and no significant changes in hematologic values are noted. Radiographs initially show only soft-tissue swelling, but osteolytic and periosteal changes are seen 2 to 3 weeks after the onset of symptoms. The presentation is often classic but must be differentiated from osteomyelitis (either unifocal or multifocal) and trauma. Therapy consists of hydration at 150% to 200% maintenance (oral or intravenous fluids) and analgesia. Pain and swelling commonly require 2 to 5 days to resolve. Recurrence is not rare, but the syndrome generally ends by age 2 as the vascular supply to these bones collateralizes.

INFECTION

Bacterial infection is the most common cause of serious morbidity and mortality in children with sickle cell anemia.[6] The primary pathogens are the encapsulated organisms *Streptococcus pneumoniae* and *Haemophilus influenzae,* but *Salmonella* osteomyelitis and severe *Mycoplasma pneumoniae* infections are also seen. The primary cause is functional asplenia secondary to autoinfarction, which may occur as early as 5 months of age but is routine by age 5 years. Defects in complement and opsonization are also noted in sickle cell patients.

Bacterial meningitis and septicemia are more than 600 times more common in sicklers than in normal children.[17] Bacterial pneumonia is 100 times more common in sicklers. Pneumococcal sepsis in sicklers carries a 14% mortality, often within hours of presentation, even when recognized and treated. Pneumococcal disease is most common before age 6 and is particularly common in the first 2 to 3 years of life.[14]

Prophylactic daily penicillin should be started at age 3 to 4 months and continued at least until age 5 years at a dose of 125 mg orally twice daily.[4] A dose of 250 mg orally twice daily is given from ages 3 to 5 years. Also, *H. influenzae* type B (HIB) and pneumococcal (Pneumovax) vaccines are given routinely. Educating the family is critical.

Despite optimal treatment, children with sickle cell anemia may present with fever and potential bacterial infections. Initial evaluation should include

- A careful history of the present illness. Bacteremia is more likely to be of only several hours' duration and associated with a fever above 103°F.
- A careful review of the medical history, including penicillin prophylaxis and possible missed doses
- A careful physical examination. Focal sites of infection can coexist with bacteremia.
- For fever above 101.5°F, a complete blood count with differential, a reticulocyte count, and a blood culture are probably minimal requirements. Marked leukocytosis (above the baseline 13,000 to 17,000) or a left shift is usually seen. Lumbar puncture and chest radiographs may be indicated. The erythrocyte sedimentation rate and C-reactive protein assessment are unreliable.

Children less than age 1 year with fever are routinely admitted for appropriate intravenous antibiotics. In selected cases, older children with a fever below 103°F and no focal source of infection may be discharged home after obtaining appropriate cultures and giving ceftriaxone 75 mg/kg intramuscularly.[15] Reliable follow-up must be assured. A repeat dose of ceftriaxone should be administered 24 hours later. With a focal source, blood cultures and ceftriaxone should be followed up with appropriate oral antibiotics. Children with fevers above 103°F should routinely be admitted and observed on appropriate antibiotic coverage. Antibiotic choice should depend on local patterns of bacterial sensitivity; however, coverage of both *H. influenzae* and *S. pneumoniae* is necessary in the young child. The emergence of resistant or partially resistant *S. pneumoniae* must be considered. Children older than 8 or 9 years can often be managed with penicillin alone.

VASOOCCLUSIVE EPISODES

The hallmark of sickle cell anemia is the painful "crisis" caused by arterial occlusion by irreversibly sickled cells. Vasoocclusion may be precipitated by dehydration, hypoxia, acidosis, or infection, but it often occurs without ready explanation. Symptoms vary according to the location of vascular obstruction, but pain secondary to tissue hypoxemia is common. Pain episodes commonly involve the extremities or abdomen, but head pain (calvarial) or chest wall pain (rib, sternal) is common in older children. Low-grade fever is often noted.

Therapy consists of aggressive hydration (twice maintenance) and analgesics. For mild pain, ibuprofen or acetaminophen may be adequate. For moderate pain, intravenous or intramuscular morphine sulfate or meperidine may be appropriate, followed by hydration and transfer to oral agents such as acetaminophen with codeine.[1,18] Severe pain requires intravenous morphine sulfate, fluids, and hospitalization.[12] The use of multiple doses of meperidine should be avoided because of the drug's short duration of action and because its metabolic by-product normeperidine lowers the seizure threshold.[11]

CEREBROVASCULAR ACCIDENT

About 7% of sickle cell patients suffer a central nervous system event, often a stroke. In the younger child, the event is usually thrombotic; in the adolescent or adult, it may be hemorrhagic.[10] These events are unpredictable. They routinely involve major cerebral arteries and can be devastating. In the emergency department, any untoward neurologic event in a sickle cell patient is considered a cerebrovascular accident until proven otherwise.

Initial evaluation should include a careful history for precipitating events, a formal neurologic examination, insertion of an intravenous line, and measurement of baseline laboratory values. Computed tomography scanning without contrast is needed routinely. Neurology and hematology consultations are obtained. Arteriography is usually not needed and can precipitate further sickling in the untransfused patient.

Acute therapy usually includes intravenous hydration and exchange transfusion to decrease the percentage of hemoglobin S to below 30%. Prompt recognition and treatment in an intensive care setting usually results in a gratifying outcome.[7] Long-term treatment necessitates hypertransfusion for several years to reduce the 66% chance of a recurrent cerebrovascular accident.[9,13,16]

ACUTE SPLENIC SEQUESTRATION

Splenic sequestration is a life-threatening condition seen in young children before the onset of autoinfarction of the spleen. Over a period of hours, a significant portion of the circulating blood volume is sequestered in the spleen because of vasoocclusion in the splenic vein. Thus, the patient develops hypovolemia, pallor, massive splenomegaly, and, occasionally, shock and death. Families should be educated in splenic palpation. Evaluation demonstrates splenomegaly (often massive), anemia, and reticulocytosis.

Treatment is aimed at sustaining blood volume until the condition spontaneously reverses, releasing the sequestered blood. Careful monitoring and, often, a transfusion of 10 mL/kg of packed red blood cells may be required.[8] Overtransfusion should be avoided, as the condition will reverse.

APLASTIC CRISIS

The term *aplastic crisis* refers to acute anemia that may be superimposed on sickle cell patients by episodes of marrow hypoplasia. The severely decreased red cell survival in these patients necessitates a marked reticulocytosis (greater than 10%) to maintain baseline hemoglobin levels. Episodes of erythroid hypoplasia, manifested by progressive anemia with reticulocytopenia (less than 1%), occur both sporadically and epidemically in association with the human parvovirus B19.[5] Packed red blood cell transfusion may be necessary until erythroid production returns, usually within a few weeks. Patients with aplastic crisis require close monitoring because their hemoglobin may fall to 4 g% or lower within a few days.

ACUTE CHEST SYNDROME

Episodes of cough, chest pain, fever, and pulmonary infiltrates are common. In younger children, the cause is usually infection, and in older children and adolescents, infarction. A syndrome of progressive infection and infarction may develop, with diffuse lung involvement. *M. pneumoniae* can produce severe and unusual patterns of infection in these patients. Treatment focuses on appropriate antibiotic coverage. Oxygen supplementation, transfusion, or both, may be indicated.

PRIAPISM

Priapism is painful, involuntary penile erection. Sickling within the penile cavernous sinuses is most common in adolescents and young adults. Any episode lasting more than 3 hours is unlikely to resolve spontaneously and requires intravenous hydration and narcotic analgesia. Hematologic consultation regarding transfusion or exchange transfusion should be considered. Episodes persisting more than 24 hours require surgical intervention. Physiologic sexual impotence commonly occurs from chronic scarring of the erectile tissue.[2]

DISPOSITION

Most children with sickle cell disease are followed by a pediatric hematologist and a primary care physician.[3] It is essential that these physicians be advised of the patient's emergency visit and consulted regarding the discharge plan.

COMMON PITFALLS

- Failing to recognize that any sickled cell on peripheral smear is presumptive evidence of sickle cell anemia
- Failing to appreciate the immune status of the sickle cell patient. The febrile sickle cell child requires careful evaluation and often hospitalization and intravenous antibiotics.
- Failing to recognize that sickle cell anemia can be diagnosed in the newborn; symptoms may begin by age 3 to 4 months. Many states have mandatory newborn screening programs.
- Failing to recognize that the sickle prep is inaccurate before 4 to 6 months of age
- Failing to consider a cerebrovascular accident when evaluating any untoward neurologic event in a sickle cell patient
- Failing to consider aplastic crisis and acute splenic sequestration in the acutely anemic sickle cell patient

References

1. American Academy of Pediatrics, Committee on Genetics. Health supervision for children with sickle cell diseases and their families. *Pediatrics* 1996;98:467.
2. Emond A, Holman R, Hayes R, et al. Priapism and impotence in homozygous sickle cell disease. *Arch Intern Med* 1980;140:1434.
3. Frush K, Ware RE, Kinney T. Emergency department visits by children with sickle hemoglobinopathies: factors associated with hospital admission. *Pediatr Emerg Care* 1995;11:9.
4. Gaston M, Verter J, Woods G, et al. Prophylaxis with oral penicillin in children with sickle cell anemia. *N Engl J Med* 1986;314:1593.
5. Kelleher J, Luban N, Cohen B, et al. Human serum parvovirus as the cause of aplastic crisis in sickle cell disease. *Am J Dis Child* 1984;138:401.
6. Platt OS, Dover GJ. *Hematology of infancy and childhood*. Philadelphia: WB Saunders/Harcourt Brace Jovanovich, 1993:732.
7. Platt OS, Thorington BD, Brambilla DJ, et al. Pain in sickle cell disease: rates and risk factor. *N Engl J Med* 1991;325:11.
8. Porter JBV, Heuhns ER. Transfusion and exchange in sickle cell anemia, with particular reference to iron metabolism. *Acta Haematol* 1987;78:198.
9. Rao S, Gooden S. Splenic sequestration in sickle cell disease; role of transfusion therapy. *Am Pediatr Hematol Oncol* 1985;127:298.
10. Russell M, Goldberg H, Hodson A, et al. Effect of transfusion therapy on arteriographic abnormalities and on recurrence of stroke in sickle cell disease. *Blood* 1984;63:162.
11. Serjeant GR. *Sickle cell disease*. Oxford: Oxford University Press, 1985:326.
12. Shapiro BS. The management of pain in sickle cell disease. *Pediatr Clin North Am* 1989;36:1029.

13. Tang R, Shimomura S, Rotblatt M. Meperidine-induced seizures in sickle cell patients. *Hosp Formul* 1980;15:764.
14. Wayne AS, et al. Transfusion management of sickle cell disease. *Blood* 1993;81:1109.
15. Wilimas JA, Flynn P, Harris S, et al. A randomized study of outpatient treatment with ceftriaxone for selected febrile children with sickle cell disease. *N Engl J Med* 1993;329:472.
16. Williams J, Goff J, Anderson H, et al. Efficacy of transfusion therapy for 1 to 2 years in patients with sickle cell and cerebrovascular accidents. *J Pediatr* 1980;96:205.
17. Zarkowsky H, Gallager D, Sill F, et al. Bacteremia in sickle hemoglobinopathies. *J Pediatr* 1986;109:579.
18. Zimmerman SA, Ware RE, Kinney TR. Gaining ground in the fight against sickle cell disease. *Contemp Pediatr* 1997;14:154.

CHAPTER 292
Sinusitis

Elizabeth A. Wedemeyer
and Vinay M. Nadkarni

Sinusitis is an infection or inflammation of the paranasal sinuses: the maxillary, ethmoid, frontal, and sphenoid sinuses. The sinuses develop during gestation as outpouchings of the nasal mucosae. The maxillary and ethmoid sinuses are pneumatized at birth and can potentially harbor infection in infancy. In contrast, the frontal and sphenoid sinuses are only rudimentary at birth. The frontal sinuses expand from the middle meatus of the frontal bone and do not assume their characteristic supraorbital location until about 6 years of age.[4] The sphenoid sinuses do not pneumatize until 2 to 3 years of age, and they do not become clinically important until the second decade of life.

Acute sinusitis is usually preceded by an upper respiratory infection. The mucosal lining of the sinuses is contiguous with that of the nasopharynx. With an upper respiratory infection, this lining becomes hyperemic and edematous, causing obstruction of the sinus ostia. This obstruction, which may also result from anatomic or allergic causes, results in the development of negative pressure within the sinus. When the obstruction is relieved, this negative pressure predisposes the normally sterile sinus to bacterial invasion and infection.[8]

In most cases of childhood sinusitis, the maxillary sinus is the primary site of involvement. The location of its ostium (high on the medial wall of the sinus) hinders gravity drainage of the sinus.[12] In addition to maxillary involvement, the ethmoid sinus is readily obstructed by mucosal swelling. After the age of 10 years, the frontal sinuses are an increasingly common site of sinus infection. In children with chronic sinusitis, predisposing conditions need to be considered; these include sinus ostia obstruction from allergic rhinitis, chronic indwelling nasoenteral feedings tubes, or impaired mucociliary clearance in children with cystic fibrosis or ciliary dyskinesia syndromes.

CLINICAL PRESENTATION

Sinusitis can present as an acute or chronic infection, characterized by different but overlapping groups of symptoms. Acute sinusitis is estimated to complicate between 5% and 10% of upper respiratory infections.[2,13] A child with sinusitis may not present with the typical symptoms seen in an adult (i.e., facial pain, headache, fever).[14] Instead, the parent may describe a persistent cold (more than 10 days) that is more severe than usual, with copious nasal discharge (clear to purulent) and associated cough that is present during the day but may worsen at night. Parents commonly note that their preschool child has fetid breath without evidence of pharyngitis.[12,14] A less common but severe presentation of acute sinusitis is high fever (greater than 39.0°C), purulent nasal discharge, headache, and, occasionally, periorbital swelling.[5,12] Subacute or chronic sinusitis (which may be infectious, allergic, or related to chronic nasal ostia obstruction) can present as a persistent cold with prolonged nasal congestion, causing nasal obstruction, cough of more than 30 days without improvement, and sore throat due to mouth breathing. On physical examination, there is mucopurulent discharge in the nose or pharynx, with erythematous nasal mucosa. Usually, there is not impressive cervical adenopathy. In more severe cases, there can be periorbital swelling or facial tenderness.

Major complications of sinusitis include periorbital cellulitis, orbital cellulitis or abscess, meningitis, osteomyelitis, epidural abscess, subdural empyema, cavernous sinus thrombosis, and cerebral abscess.[1,2,7,12,16]

DIFFERENTIAL DIAGNOSIS

Sinusitis is predominately a clinical diagnosis based on history and clinical examination and, occasionally, on supportive radiographic studies and cultures. Standard radiographic projections of the cranium include an anteroposterior (Caldwell) view for the frontal and ethmoidal sinuses, lateral and submentovertex views for the sphenoid sinus, and occipitomental (Waters) view for the maxillary sinuses. The findings most diagnostic of bacterial sinusitis include air–fluid levels or complete opacification of the sinuses. However, children less than 5 years of age with biopsy-proven sinusitis do not always show air–fluid levels or opacification, and the amount of sinus mucosal thickening that is diagnostic of bacterial sinusitis is not agreed on (most authors suggest that mucosal thickening of greater than 4 mm is diagnostic).[2,14]

Complete opacification and air–fluid levels of the maxillary sinuses on plain radiography correlates well with computed tomography (CT).[8] When clinical signs and symptoms suggesting acute sinusitis are accompanied by abnormal maxillary sinus radiographs, bacteria will be present in the sinus aspirate more than 75% of the time.[15] However, a normal radiograph does not rule out bacterial sinusitis.[6] Radiographic evaluation is recommended only if the child has been seriously ill, has had recurrent episodes, has chronic symptoms, or has a suspected suppurative complication.[1,13,14,16] When the diagnosis is obvious on clinical grounds, radiologic evaluation may not be necessary.

Transillumination of the sinuses is not reliable, and ultrasound evaluation has not been used enough in children to recommend universally.[12,13] CT scans may be helpful in evaluating sinus involvement but are reserved for patients with severe disease, or those with orbital involvement usually undergoing CT for other reasons. Although useful in defining the soft-tissue structures surrounding the sinuses, magnetic resonance imaging (MRI) does not image the bone well; hence, MRI is useful in delineating the spread of a nasal tumor, but CT scan remains the modality of choice in evaluating sinus disease.[11]

The "gold standard" for clinical diagnosis is sinus aspiration or functional endoscopic sinus surgery (biopsy is more sensitive as a research tool).[5] These techniques are usually reserved for those with severe pain unresponsive to medical therapy, those who are seriously ill, those with immunologic deficiencies, or those presenting with suppurative complications of sinusitis.[1,10,12,14] In a study of 79 aspirates from 50 children with acute maxillary sinusitis, 28% grew *Streptococcus pneumoniae*, 19% grew *Moraxella catarrhalis*, 19% grew *Haemophilus influenzae*, 7% grew *Streptococcus* spp., *Eikenella corrodens*, *Peptostreptococcus*, and other *Moraxella* spp., and 34% were culture negative.[5] Surface cultures of the nasopharynx, nose, or throat are not at all predictive of the causative organism.[15] Directed cultures of the middle meatus, however, correlate with chronic maxillary or ethmoid sinusitis organisms.[9]

The complications of sinusitis are secondary to the contiguous spread or hematogenous spread of infection and include periorbital (preseptal) and orbital cellulitis, blindness, meningitis, epidural abscess, subdural empyema, venous sinus thrombosis, cerebral abscess, and cranial osteomyelitis.

EMERGENCY DEPARTMENT EVALUATION

All patients presenting to the emergency department with signs or symptoms of sinusitis require a thorough history and physical examination to rule out serious sequelae. Only those children with severe illness, recurrent symptomatology, or suspected suppurative complication deserve radiographs. Referral to an otorhinolaryngologist for further evaluation and management should be considered in cases of systemic toxicity, severe pain unresponsive to medical outpatient therapy, failure of medical therapy, suppurative complications or immune compromise.[1,10]

EMERGENCY DEPARTMENT MANAGEMENT

Medical therapy with an antimicrobial agent is recommended in children diagnosed with acute sinusitis. Treatment should be directed toward *S. pneumoniae, H. influenzae*, and *M. catarrhalis*.[3] In areas where the prevalence of beta-lactamase–positive, ampicillin-resistant *H. influenzae* and *M. catarrhalis* is relatively low, amoxicillin is the drug of choice. In areas of prevalent ampicillin resistance or in treatment failures, alternative therapies include amoxicillin–clavulanate or cefaclor. For patients allergic to penicillin, alternatives include trimethoprim–sulfamethoxazole or the combination of erythromycin–sulfisoxazole. In older children, cefuroxime axetil may be used. The trimethoprim-sulfamethoxazole combination may be ineffective in patients with concomitant group A beta-hemolytic streptococcal infections. Cefixime, which is less active against *S. pneumoniae*, is a less optimal choice.[2,10,12]

Clinical improvement should be rapid, with resolution of the fever and reduced nasal discharge and cough within 48 to 72 hours. The duration of recommended therapy is 10 to 14 days (after 1 week in an adult study, 20% of sinus aspirate cultures still grew pathogenic bacteria). If the patient is improved but not completely recovered, continuation of antibiotic therapy for another week is recommended.

Chronic infectious sinusitis should be treated with antibiotics. In addition, in children with chronic sinusitis and asthma, in whom underlying allergic rhinitis is suspected, a course of topically applied corticosteroids (beclomethasone or flunisolide) may be useful.[10]

DISPOSITION

Emergent consultation with an otorhinolaryngologist, neurologist, or ophthalmologist may be indicated if the sequelae of sinusitis are apparent on presentation. The otorhinolaryngologist may be asked to evaluate and aspirate sinus fluid in patients who are severely ill, are recurrently or persistently infected, are immunocompromised, or have suppurative complications. These patients also warrant admission. All patients should be followed up at the completion of therapy, and those with persistent nasal discharge treated with an additional 7 days of antibiotics. Patients should be advised to return if symptoms of fever, headache, facial swelling or pain, cough, and purulent nasal drainage worsen or do not improve within 72 hours of initiation of therapy.

COMMON PITFALLS

- Because pneumatization of the sinuses is variable in children, radiographs may be misleading.
- Typically, children with sinusitis do *not* exhibit the classic triad of adult symptoms: fever, headache, and facial pain.
- Complete a thorough neurologic examination to reduce the chance of missing associated intracranial or suppurative sequelae.

References

1. Fairbanks DN, Milmoe GF. Sinusitis: complications and sequelae: an otolaryngologist's perspective. *Pediatr Infect Dis J* 1984;4:S75.
2. Fireman P. Diagnosis of sinusitis in children—emphasis on the history and physical examination. *J Allergy Clin Immunol* 1992;90:433.
3. Hopp R, Cooperstock M. Medical management of sinusitis in pediatric patients. *Curr Probl Pediatr* 1997;27:178.
4. Isaacson G. Sinusitis in childhood. *Pediatr Clin North Am* 1996;43:1297.
5. Kennedy DW. Overview. *Otolaryngol Head Neck Surg* 1990;103:847.
6. Lazar R, Younis R, Parvey L. Comparison of plain radiographs, coronal CT, and intraoperative findings in children with chronic sinusitis. *Otolaryngol Head Neck Surg* 1992;107:29.
7. Lusk R, ed. *Pediatric sinusitis*. New York: Raven Press, 1992.
8. Lusk R, Lazar R, Muntz H. The diagnosis and treatment of recurrent and chronic sinusitis in children. *Pediatr Clin North Am* 1989;36:1411.
9. Orobello P, Park R, Blecher L, et al. Microbiology of chronic sinusitis in children. *Arch Otolaryngol Head Neck Surg* 1991;117:980.
10. Ott NL, O'Connell EJ, Hoffman AD, et al. Childhood sinusitis. *Mayo Clin Proc* 1991;66:1238.
11. Rai VM, El-Noveam KI. Sinonasal imaging: anatomy and pathology. *Radiol Clin North Am* 1998;36:921.
12. Wald ER. Acute sinusitis in children. *Pediatr Ann* 1998;27:811.
13. Wald ER, Guerra N, Byers C. Upper respiratory infections of young children: duration and frequency of complications. *Pediatrics* 1991;87:129.
14. Wald ER, Milmoe GJ, Bowen A, et al. Acute maxillary sinusitis in children. *N Engl J Med* 1981;304:749.
15. Wald ER, Pang D, Milmoe GJ, et al. Sinusitis and its complications in the pediatric patient. *Pediatr Clin North Am* 1981;28:777.
16. Wehrle PF, Hawkins DB. Sinusitis: complications and sequelae: a pediatrician's perspective. *Pediatr Infect Dis J* 1985;4:S73.

CHAPTER 293
Submersion Injuries

Madeleine Matar Joseph and Lisa Santer

Submersion injuries are the result of a person's being submerged in a liquid, with at least a temporary loss of consciousness. Traditionally, they are divided into drownings (fatal submersion injuries) and near-drownings (survival for at least 24 hours after submersion injury). Although the number of deaths due to unintentional drowning had declined from 5,700 in 1986 to 3,959 in 1996, drowning rates have barely declined among children. In fact, the mortality rate has increased among children younger than 1 year.[8]

An even greater number of lives are affected by nonfatal submersion injuries. For every child who drowns, four children are hospitalized for near-drowning. One-third of those who are comatose on admission and survive suffer significant neurologic impairment.[2] Submersion injuries have a bimodal age distribution, with peaks in toddlers and adolescents.

The availability of bodies of water and the climate, geography, and socioeconomics of a community determine its most likely site of submersion injury. Databases from state surveillance systems have identified for each age category both the location of drowning and the activity performed. Children less than 1 year of age most frequently drown in bathtubs and buckets; children aged from 1 to 4 years most often drown in swimming pools. Children and adolescents aged from 5 to 19 years most frequently drown in lakes, ponds, rivers, and pools.[2] Lack of adult supervision is a factor in most pediatric submersion injuries.[9] Alcohol is a factor in many adult and adolescent submersion injuries.[3,7]

Predisposing conditions of the victim include seizures, alcohol ingestion, and trauma (unintentional and intentional child abuse and homicide). The possibility of child abuse must be considered in home submersion injuries, such as in bathtubs or buckets.[5] Morbidity and mortality are related more to the promptness and quality of field care than to hospital care.

PATHOPHYSIOLOGY

The injury of submersion is global hypoxia. The events of a submersion injury follow a predictable pattern. Initially, the victim struggles to reach the surface. During this struggle, the victim consciously controls the urge to breathe. Eventually, asphyxia forces the submerged person to inspire. Liquid enters the larynx and causes laryngospasm, which temporarily prevents liquid from entering the lungs. Because the mouth is full of water, the swallowing mechanism tries to clear the oral cavity, and fills the stomach with water. As asphyxia worsens, the laryngospasm relaxes and the diaphragm contracts, pulling water into the lungs in about 85% of cases. This aspiration causes surfactant washout or inactivation (fresh and salt water, respectively), with subsequent atelectasis. Aspiration can also cause transient electrolyte changes, particularly with fresh-water submersion.

The pulmonary response to hypoxia is reflex-mediated pulmonary hypertension with intrapulmonary shunting. Aspiration-induced atelectasis worsens ventilation–perfusion mismatch and produces further hypoxia. Aspiration of pulmonary irritants such as emesis or caustic substances also contributes to pulmonary injury. Myocardial hypoxia results in cardiac arrest within minutes of the submersion. In addition, hypothermia can cause decreased myocardial contractility and dysrhythmias. Prompt, effective resuscitation can minimize these effects.

In the patient who has been severely asphyxiated, the delayed responses of vital end organs to hypoxia and resulting acidosis include acute tubular necrosis and sloughing of bowel mucosa, resulting in profuse, bloody diarrhea. Cerebral edema results from generalized neuronal death and develops within hours (cytotoxic cerebral edema). Cerebral edema leads to increased intracranial pressure, which decreases the cerebral perfusion pressure and cerebral blood flow, causing further ischemic injury. Central nervous system (CNS) injury is the most common cause of death after successful cardiac resuscitation, and the most common cause of permanent sequelae.

Acute respiratory distress syndrome, which also begins within hours of the injury, is present in 5% to 15% of submersion victims ill enough to require intensive care. The delayed immersion syndrome is an uncommon, delayed pulmonary response to hypoxia, occurring up to 24 hours after submersion in victims who initially looked well. Myocardial failure due to hypoxia occurs within hours of submersion. Although uncommon, coagulopathies or renal failure may develop after hypoxia and hypothermia. Myoglobinuria or hemoglobinuria may also precipitate renal failure. Despite transient electrolyte changes due to aspiration and absorption of fresh and salt water, electrolytes are almost always normal by the time the patient arrives in the emergency department. There are, however, reports of a correlation between an elevated initial blood glucose level and poor outcome.[1,4]

The outcome of submersion victims is generally bimodal: intact survival or death. The duration of submersion and resuscitation are the most common predictors of outcome, but no set of parameters is absolutely predictive for bad outcome in all cases. Criteria predicting death or survival with severe neurologic sequelae are submersion for more than 10 minutes and a resuscitation that lasts more than 25 minutes.[7] The most reliable predictors for poor outcome (death or survival with severe neurologic sequelae) include cardiac arrest requiring more than 25 minutes of advanced cardiac life support, ongoing cardiopulmonary resuscitation in the emergency department, and a submersion duration of more than 25 minutes.[9]

Criteria predicting good outcome are the presence of sinus rhythm, reactive pupils, and neurologic responsiveness.[7] Among comatose children, unfavorable outcome (vegetative state and death) was predicted by a combination of absent pupillary light reflex, increased initial blood glucose concentration, and male sex.[4]

EMERGENCY DEPARTMENT EVALUATION

As always, the ABCs are primary: the *a*irway is cleared of vomitus or other foreign material, adequate *b*reathing efforts are ensured, and *c*irculation is assessed by monitoring heart rate, rhythm, pulse pressure, and capillary refill time. The cause of the submersion injury is noted. Initial signs and symptoms usually reflect cardiopulmonary and cerebral hypoxic injury. However, because occult injury to the head, cervical spine, or other areas may be present, the cervical spine must be immobilized if trauma is suspected. Hypothermia may not be recognized unless a rectal temperature is obtained along with other vital signs. The temperature is taken with a thermometer that can register low temperatures.

Altered mental status, if present, is probably due to cerebral hypoxia, but other possibilities, such as drug ingestion, intracranial injury, hypothermia, or a postictal state, should be considered. A blood alcohol and drug screen is recommended on all but the youngest children. A baseline hematocrit level, electrolyte measurements, and a chest x-ray are obtained. A blood gas measurement should be obtained in patients with respiratory or CNS symptoms.

EMERGENCY DEPARTMENT MANAGEMENT

The goal of therapy is to reverse hypoxia. Appropriate, aggressive airway management in the field is essential. Many apneic, unresponsive victims respond to positive-pressure ventilation alone by breathing and waking. Intensive care protocols have failed to improve outcome. The patient in cardiac arrest is resuscitated in the usual manner. If hypothermia (less than 34°C) is present, death should not be pronounced before the asystolic victim is rewarmed.

Arterial oxygen levels are kept at normal levels or above by increasing positive end-expiratory pressure, F_iO_2, and other parameters as needed. Borderline oxygenation or ventilation is unacceptable in a brain-injured patient. Positive end-expiratory pressure is helpful when there is evidence of intrapulmonary shunt on the arterial blood gas. Avoid high positive end-expiratory pressure, which can compromise the cardiac output. The patient is hyperventilated ($PaCO_2$ of 25 to 30 mm Hg) to decrease intracranial pressure.

If the patient is in shock and not responding to respiratory therapy, fluid boluses and inotropes can be given. The physician should consider myocardial infarction secondary to asphyxia, even in young children. Unless hypovolemia is present, the rate of intravenous fluids can be restricted to minimize intracranial pressure. Cerebral perfusion pressure should be maximized. Fluid shifts and electrolyte changes are not significant clinical problems for submersion victims.[9] Glucose levels are often high in severely asphyxiated patients, so glucose-containing intravenous fluids should be used only if hypoglycemia occurs.

Gastric aspiration is avoided by placing a nasogastric tube, as the stomach is usually full of swallowed liquid.

DISPOSITION

Alert Patients with Spontaneous Respirations

Patients with a history of at least temporary loss of consciousness should be observed for 12 to 24 hours for organ failure, especially of the lungs. The observation should be done in a setting that can recognize deteriorating pulmonary function and provide appropriate intensive care or transport.

If a child has had a momentary period of asphyxia, admission to a local hospital may still be appropriate. If the child was submerged longer than 5 minutes or did not waken at the scene, observation close to a pediatric intensive care unit is suggested.

Patients without Spontaneous Respirations

The decision to transfer a patient who has been treated aggressively in an emergency department but does not have spontaneous respirations is problematic. The patient who has only a return of heartbeat has little, if any, chance of intact survival. The prognosis should be communicated to the family at an appropriate time. Too often, the family feels that if the patient has a heartbeat on arrival at the intensive care unit, his or her condition will markedly improve.

Patients with causes of decreased mental status other than hypoxia and no spontaneous respirations may have a better outcome. They should be admitted to an intensive care unit. Victims who are potential organ donors also merit consideration of intensive care unit admission.

PREVENTION

It is much easier to prevent a submersion injury than to treat one. Emergency physicians can support groups such as the American Red Cross, American Heart Association, and Safe Kids, which educate lay people, legislators, and professionals about water safety.

COMMON PITFALLS

- Failure to place a nasogastric or orogastric tube may result in vomiting and aspiration.
- Inadequate oxygenation may worsen the hypoxic insult that occurred as a result of submersion.
- Inadequate fluid resuscitation and the use of inotropes in a hypovolemic patient can worsen the ischemic insult.
- The asymptomatic patient with a history of significant submersion may be at risk for respiratory deterioration.
- Many bathtub near-drowning victims suffer from abuse or neglect. Therefore, medical evaluation should include social services consultation and a search for other accompanying injuries.

References

1. Ashwal S, Schneider S, Tomasi L. Prognostic implications of hyperglycemia and reduced cerebral blood flow in childhood near-drowning. *Neurology* 1990;40:820.
2. Committee on Injury and Poison Prevention, 1993 to 1994. Drowning in infants, children, and adolescents. *Pediatrics* 1993;92(2):292–294.
3. Cummings P, Quan L. Trends in unintentional drowning, the role of alcohol and medical care. *JAMA* 1999;281(23):2198–2202.
4. Graf WD, Cummings P, Quan L, et al. Predicting outcome in pediatric submersion victims. *Ann Emerg Med* 1995;26(3):312–319.
5. Lavelle J, Shaw K, Seidl T, et al. Ten-year review of pediatric bathtub near-drownings: evaluation of child abuse and neglect. *Ann Emerg Med* 1995; 25(3):344–348.
6. Orlowski JP. Drowning and near-drowning and ice water submersions. *Pediatr Clin North Am* 1987;34:75.
7. Quan L, Kinder D. Pediatric submersions: prehospital predictors of outcome. *Pediatrics* 1992;90:909.
8. Smith G, Howland J. Declines in drowning, exploring the epidemiology of favorable trends. *JAMA* 1999;281(23):2245–2246.
9. Wintemute GJ. Childhood drowning and near-drowning in the United States. *Am J Dis Child* 1990;144:663.

CHAPTER 294
Torticollis

Gregory G. Gaar

The word *torticollis* is derived from the Latin words *tortus*, meaning "twisted," and *collum*, meaning "neck." Medically, *torticollis* is defined as "a contraction, often spasmodic, of the muscles of the neck, chiefly those supplied by the spinal accessory nerve; the head is drawn to one side and usually rotated so that the chin points to the other side."[12] It is a manifestation of illness, not a disease in itself, which means the etiology and pathophysiology can be very wide-ranging. As many as 80 different etiologies have been documented in the medical literature.[11]

CLINICAL PRESENTATION

The clinical presentation of torticollis in the newborn is often a firm, nontender, unilateral enlargement in the sternocleidomastoid muscle, which is noticed shortly after birth.[5] Older children and adults present with the head rotated on the neck, tilted to the affected side, with the chin pointed to the opposite direction.

DIFFERENTIAL DIAGNOSIS

The most commonly accepted categories of torticollis are congenital and acquired, depending on the etiology and time of onset and recognition.

Congenital Torticollis

The congenital causes can be subdivided into those caused by malformations and those caused by deformations. Malformations are due to a defect during morphogenesis, whereas deformations occur secondary to intrauterine postures and crowding.

Malformations can develop in the cervical spine, the cervical musculature, or the central nervous system. Rare cervical spine anomalies cause torticollis: odontoid hypoplasia, cervical spine fusions (Klippel-Feil syndrome), hemivertebrae, spina bifida, or congenital scoliosis.[1,13] Hypertrophy or absence of the cervical musculature is one etiology.[13] An arteriovenous fistula at the craniocervical junction has been reported.[2]

Pseudotumor of infancy and congenital muscular torticollis are reported with an incidence of 0.4% to 1.3%, respectively.[6] The condition results from a unilateral fibrous contraction of the sternocleidomastoid muscle.[1,4,6] It usually appears at ages younger than 1 month and resolves by the age of 6 months.[4] Physical examination often reveals a firm, nontender, immobile mass in the sternocleidomastoid muscle.[5] The exact etiology is unknown. There is a higher prevalence in breech and difficult deliveries assisted by forceps. Although most cases resolve spontaneously, some 10% to 20% of the cases will develop progressive torticollis.[4]

Congenital ocular disturbances can be a cause of torticollis that presents later in life. In one series, 4% of the total number of children with torticollis had ocular abnormalities. These were usually a fourth nerve palsy with resultant strabismus.[1]

Deformations of the spine leading to torticollis can happen in the presence of uterine tumors, oligohydramnios, and multiple fetuses.[13] These cases of torticollis secondary to intrauterine postures are usually transient and resolve within a few months.

Brachial plexus palsies due to birth trauma can also cause torticollis.[1]

Acquired Torticollis

The causes of acquired torticollis are extremely varied. Often, the cause is associated with involvement of the cervical spine. Trauma to the cervical spine, resulting in subluxations or fracture and dislocations, is one cause. This trauma can be relatively minor, such as the hyperflexion or hyperextension of a "whiplash" injury. Onset of symptoms can be delayed by several months.[13] The most common areas affected are the atlantoaxial area and C-2 on C-3.[13] Ligamentous laxity in the atlantoaxial region is commonly a cause of subluxation, which can present as torticollis. These cases are often associated with underlying disorders, such a trisomy 21 (Down syndrome), mucopolysaccharidosis, and invasive erosion from surrounding soft-tissue infections.[1,10] Infections of the cervical spine, such as osteomyelitis and discitis, can present as torticollis,[13] as can metastatic or primary osteomas.[10]

Other causes of torticollis do not involve the cervical spine. Clavicle fractures, with resultant splinting of that area because of pain, has been recognized as a cause.[1,10] Infections of the surrounding soft tissues, such as nasopharyngeal abscesses, retropharyngeal abscesses, cervical adenitis, tonsillitis, mastoiditis, and sinusitis, have been reported in the literature as etiologic agents.[1,13] The twisting of the neck found on physical examination in these cases is felt to be due to pain from underlying cervical muscle spasms and not from an underlying spinous abnormality. If the infection is extensive, erosion of paraspinous ligaments has been reported, with subsequent rotatory subluxation in the atlantoaxial region.[13]

Torticollis appearing later in childhood can be due to compensation for underlying strabismus or diplopia.[1,10]

Paroxysmal torticollis of infancy is due to vestibular dysfunction. It typically presents between the ages of 2 and 8 months.[8] This episodic torticollis often is associated with vomiting, pallor, ataxia, or irritability.[9] It is usually a self-limiting disease that resolves by age 2 to 3 years.[3]

Dystonic reactions to medication can present as torticollis. These are most commonly due to phenothiazine ingestions. Differentiation, in these instances, is usually made by the presence of ocular symptoms suggestive of oculogyric crisis.

The nuchal rigidity of bacterial meningitis can be confused with torticollis in younger patients. The mental status, behavioral, and physiologic changes that accompany meningitis are the key to differentiation.

EMERGENCY DEPARTMENT EVALUATION

Careful historic questioning concerning the location, severity, and onset of pain and abnormal posture of the neck is important. Patients should be asked about radiation of any pain. In classic cases of torticollis, there is unilateral neck pain. The pain may radiate to the ipsilateral shoulder but no further. Historic information about fever and constitutional signs and symptoms is important in determining infectious or inflammatory causes of torticollis. The possibility of phenothiazine exposure should be explored.

In older children and adults, acute torticollis often presents after trauma. Even with seemingly mild trauma, careful evaluation of the cervical spine, including appropriate radiographs, is necessary to rule out cervical spine fractures. In the absence of such fractures, a thorough examination of the head, eyes, ears, nose, and throat should be performed to search for inflammatory causes. Careful physical examination should distinguish torticollis from the nuchal rigidity of bacterial meningitis. Palpation of the clavicles is necessary to isolate bony pain or crepitus. On neurologic examination, there should be no motor or sensory deficit in congenital muscular torticollis or that due to muscle spasm.

In infants, especially those less than 1 month of age, historic data concerning the birth should be collected. Information concerning birth presentation and the use of forceps may be found only by review of the birth medical records. Careful physical examination in these cases is likely to find the mass in the sternocleidomastoid, which helps to make the diagnosis of pseudotumor of infancy. Signs consistent with brachial plexus palsy are diagnostic of torticollis due to that etiology.

The evaluation of chronic torticollis differs if it is episodic or static in nature. For patients with recurring episodes, the emergency physician should perform a careful history of drug usage and a careful neurologic examination. Torticollis that is constant requires careful ophthalmologic and neurologic examination for strabismus and subtle cerebellar or other neurologic signs, which might be indicative of central nervous system lesions.

EMERGENCY DEPARTMENT MANAGEMENT

Patients who are younger than 1 month and present with a physical examination consistent with pseudotumor of infancy or brachial plexus palsy from a birth injury can be referred to their pediatricians for further workup and follow-up. Similarly, those whose history and examination are consistent with an intrauterine deformity due to multiple births, uterine tumor, or oligohydramnios can be referred for follow-up.

All other patients who present with an acute onset of torticollis that is not chronic and paroxysmal in nature, and those who present to be evaluated for the first time with a history of static torticollis, should have radiographs of their cervical spines after proper immobilization. This is necessary to rule out fracture or subluxation. It must be remembered that ligamentous instability from a congenital cause can often present as the result of a minor injury received several months prior to the emergency department visit.

When no radiographic fracture or subluxation is identified, further history and physical examination will help to uncover the underlying etiology of the torticollis. The management then follows based on the etiology and pathophysiology. If there are any abnormalities on neurologic examination, computerized tomography of the brain or magnetic resonance imaging is indicated. If there are signs and symptoms of an infection or inflammatory process, appropriate diagnostic studies should be obtained prior to institution of antibiotic therapy. If the torticollis is felt to be related to phenothiazine use, diphenhydramine or benztropine in appropriate dosages can be given to counteract the dystonic reaction.

Depending on the etiology, consultation with neurosurgery, neurology, or radiology colleagues should be considered.

DISPOSITION

Neurosurgical consultation and admission should be obtained for all patients with evidence of cervical spine fractures, subluxation, or dislocation. Ambulatory follow-up by the primary care pediatrician is sufficient in those infants with pseudotumor or congenital muscular torticollis. In some cases, conservative therapy in the form of manual stretching is all that is necessary.[7] Some children eventually require surgical treatment.[7]

Appropriate treatment for the underlying cause of the torticollis is the mainstay of good therapy.

COMMON PITFALLS

- Failure to consider the myriad nonmuscular causes of torticollis
- Failure to immobilize the neck
- Failure to obtain cervical spine films to rule out a fracture or subluxation in the patient with potential traumatic etiology
- Failure to consider phenothiazine side effects, even when used in an appropriate therapeutic dosage

References

1. Ballock RT, Song KM. The prevalence of nonmuscular causes of torticollis in children. *J Pediatr Orthop* 1996;16:500.
2. Bayraker B, Aysun S, Firat M. Arteriovenous fistula: a cause of torticollis. *Pediatr Neurol* 1999;20:146.
3. Bratt HD, Menelaus MB. Benign paroxysmal torticollis of infancy. *J Bone Joint Surg Am* 1992;74:449.
4. Bredenkamp JK, Hoover LA, Berke GS. Congenital muscular torticollis: a spectrum of disease. *Arch Otolaryngol Head Neck Surg* 1990;116:212.
5. Chandler FA, Altenberg A. "Congenital" muscular torticollis. *JAMA* 1944;125:476.
6. Cheng JCY, Au AW. Infantile torticollis: a review of 624 cases. *J Pediatr Orthop* 1994;14:802.
7. Cheng JCY, Tang SP, Chen TMK. Sternocleidomastoid pseudotumor and congenital muscular torticollis in infants: a prospective study of 510 cases. *J Pediatr* 1999;134:712.
8. Deonna T, Martin D. Benign paroxysmal torticollis in infancy. *Arch Dis Child* 1981;56:956.
9. Hanukoglu A, Somekh E, Fried D. Benign paroxysmal torticollis in infancy. *Clin Pediatr* 1984;23:272.
10. Kahn ML, Davidson R, Drummond DS. Acquired torticollis in children. *Orthop Rev* 1991;20:667.
11. Kiwak KJ. Establishing an etiology for torticollis. *Postgrad Med* 1984;75:126.
12. Spraycar M, ed. *Stedman's medical dictionary*, 26th ed. Baltimore: Williams & Wilkins, 1995.
13. Suchowersky O, Caine DB. Non-dystonic causes of torticollis. *Adv Neurol* 1988;50:501.

CHAPTER 295
Urinary Tract Infections

Thomas G. McLoughlin, Jr.

Urinary tract infections (UTIs) in children pose particular problems in diagnosis and management. A high index of suspicion is necessary to diagnose UTI in infants because they present with nonspecific symptoms. Diagnosis and management depend on the age and sex of the child. Accurate diagnosis and prompt therapy are important in infants and young children because they are at higher risk for vesicoureteral reflux (VUR) and renal scarring.

The cumulative risk for a primary symptomatic UTI to occur in a child from age 1 to 11 years is 1.1% for a boy and 3% for a girl, with the highest risk occurring during infancy and decreasing with increasing age.[19] Among febrile children 2 months to 2 years of age with no apparent source of fever, the prevalence of UTI is 5%. Girls are at higher risk, with a 2:1 predominance in the first year of life and a 4:1 predominance in the second year of life. In circumcised boys, the prevalence is very low, 0.2% to 0.5%. Recurrence rates are higher in girls, reaching 40%.[19]

Evidence suggests that most infections in children under 5 years involve the renal parenchyma.[19] The incidence and severity of VUR are highest among the youngest infants. Delay in treatment and recurrent UTIs increase the risk of renal scarring, emphasizing the importance of early diagnosis and treatment. The long-term consequences of childhood UTIs may include hypertension, impaired renal function, and end-stage renal disease. These adverse effects are more common in children with intrauterine renal damage.[5]

CLINICAL PRESENTATION

The clinical presentation of patients with UTI varies with age. Children younger than age 2 usually present with fever alone or other nonspecific symptoms. Other symptoms include vomiting, diarrhea, failure to thrive, and irritability. A rash or jaundice may be present. In evaluating febrile children, the likelihood that a UTI is the source varies by the presence of associated illnesses as well as the patient's age and sex. Patients with bronchiolitis have been shown to have a relatively decreased risk of UTI.[13] The presence of otitis media does not affect the risk of UTI.[17]

Clinical presentation does not reliably differentiate cystitis from pyelonephritis nor predict those with associated bacteremia. The large majority of young children with UTIs have renal parenchymal involvement seen by technetium 99m dimercaptosuccinic acid (DMSA) renal scan.[19] In this age group, all UTIs should be presumed to be pyelonephritis. The overall risk of bacteremia in children less than 5 years old with UTI is 5%, with the highest prevalence in those less than 6 months of age (8%).[2] Routine blood cultures are appropriate in those less than 6 months and those who appear toxic.

Preschool children may present with traditional symptoms of suprapubic pain, urgency, dysuria, and frequency. At this age, they still have symptoms not localized to the urinary tract, such as fever, generalized abdominal pain, and diarrhea. Enuresis that has recurred in a previously continent child is also an indicator of possible infection.

In the school-age child with a UTI, symptoms referable to the urinary tract are usually present. Fever is frequently present, and although it suggests upper tract disease, it is seen with cystitis as well. Fever may be absent in a patient with significant renal involvement. In this age group, the overwhelming majority of patients are girls, with a higher risk among white girls.

DIFFERENTIAL DIAGNOSIS

In infants, UTI should be included in the differential diagnoses of fever, irritability, gastroenteritis, failure to thrive, and sepsis. Although the infant will present with nonspecific symptoms, such as those listed previously, careful questioning may uncover additional symptoms that would direct attention to the urinary tract. Signs such as dribbling, poor stream, frequency, and malodorous urine may be present, although not the presenting complaint (Table 296.1).

When the preschool-age and older child present with urgency, dysuria, or frequency, the differential diagnosis for this complex of symptoms should include urethritis, pinworms, vaginitis, and child abuse. Children with constipation are at increased risk of UTIs, and the diagnosis should also be considered in these patients.

EMERGENCY DEPARTMENT EVALUATION

Screening tests for UTIs include the reagant tests nitrite and leukocyte esterase (LE) and microscopy for leukocytes and bacteria. In a recently published practice guideline, the American Academy of Pediatrics reviewed the literature on these tests, and estimated their sensitivities and specificities as seen in Table 296.2.[1]

Several considerations are important. The large range in specificity and sensitivity for the microscopy tests reflects the inconsistency in technique and quality in various laboratories. The white cell count is an unstandardized test. There is no agreement between studies of what constitutes significant pyuria on spun specimens. Most clinicians consider greater than 5 white blood cells (WBCs) to be significant. An "enhanced urinalysis" has been proposed that consists of an unspun urine sample using a standardized hemocytometer (Neubauer) and a Gram stain using a standardized amount of urine. The enhanced urinalysis (UA) was found to have a sensitivity of 85%, compared with 65% for the standard spun UA and microscopy.[9] Presence of pyuria is a nonspecific test, because children with other febrile illnesses, dehydration, appendicitis, or inflammatory processes also may have this finding. Spun samples reduce the specificity of microscopy, probably by releasing cellular fragments that appear similar to bacteria.[14] Sensitivity of the reagent tests may be reduced up to 35% by a 3-hour delay in processing.[12] Also note that when urine is collected and promptly analyzed, the combination of LE, nitrite, or bacteria on microscopy is sensitive but not specific. Although samples for these screening tests can be collected by the most convenient means, they do not replace the need for appropriately collected specimens for culture.

Interpretation of culture results depends on the collection technique. In incontinent children, urine for culture should be collected by catheter or bladder tap. Bag samples have no practical value because the contamination rate is so high. In continent children, the clean-catch technique is quite sensitive, but the specificity depends on interpretation of the quantitative results.

Bacteria may be introduced into a specimen when it is obtained with a catheter. With growth of 100,000 colony-forming units (CFU)/mL from such a specimen, there is a 95% likelihood of infection; with 10,000 CFU/mL, there is a 50% likelihood of infection.[3] Many authors consider $> 10^4$ CFU/ml of a single organism or a catheterized sample to be diagnostic of UTI.[19] Any bacteria seen on examination per high-power field, or growth on culture from a specimen obtained by suprapubic aspiration, probably represents infection.[16]

Various strategies have been proposed for evaluating children with UTIs. Clinical judgment and circumstances will play an important role. Regardless of the particular strategy, remember to always obtain an appropriate sample of urine for culture prior to starting antibiotic therapy. The following approach is recommended. In children less than 2 months of age with fever (greater than 100.4°F), a UA and culture should be obtained routinely as part of the "sepsis workup." The sample should be collected by bladder catheterization or suprapubic bladder aspiration. UA and culture should also be strongly considered in any child less than 3 years of age with fever without an identified source. In incontinent children, catheterization is recommended, while continent children can provide a sample from a clean-catch, midstream void. A negative UA in circumcised boys older than 1 year may be sufficient to rule out UTI, but a culture should be sent for younger boys, girls, and uncircumcised boys, even when the UA is negative. Additionally, when there are clinical signs and symptoms of UTI in older infants and children, UA and culture should be collected.

Many tests have been proposed to aid in localization of infection within the urinary tract, including urinary lactate dehydrogenase, antibody-coated bacteria, and serum antibodies. Results have been conflicting, and none has been shown to be reliable in children. The presence of WBC casts indicates origin of an inflammatory process in the kidney but does not necessarily indicate infection. Failure to maximally concentrate the urine is an indicator of renal involvement and is usually a transient finding with acute pyelonephritis.[18] Elevated C-reactive protein and erythrocyte sedimentation rate are seen with pyelonephritis, but absence of elevation does not rule out upper tract infection.[4]

TABLE 296.1. Indications for Obtaining Urine Specimens for Analysis and Culture

ABSOLUTE

All febrile infants younger than 2 months
Temp: 39°C without a source and male younger than 6 months
Temp: 39°C without a source and female younger than 2 years
Enuresis in previously continent child
Symptomatology of urinary tract infection
Failure to thrive

CONSIDER

Child with abdominal pain
Infants with vomiting, diarrhea, poor feeding, and irritability

TABLE 296.2 Screening Tests for UTI

Test	Sensitivity %	Specificity %
LE	67–94 ~83	64–92 ~78
Nitrite	15–82 ~53	90–100 ~98
LE or nitrite	90–100 ~93	58–91 ~72
WBCs (>5)	32–100 ~73	45–98 ~81
Bacteria	16–99 ~81	11–100 ~83
LE, nitrite, or WBCs	99–100 ~99.8	60–92 ~70

Renal cortical scintigraphy (99m DMSA scan) can reliably diagnose pyelonephritis in children,[15] but its role in the acute evaluation of UTI is not well established. In short, localization of UTIs in children is unreliable and generally unnecessary for acute management. UTIs should be considered pyelonephritis until proven otherwise in children under 5 years of age.

EMERGENCY DEPARTMENT MANAGEMENT

Management of patients with suspected UTIs in the emergency department includes making a presumptive diagnosis, appropriate collection of urine samples for culture, and initiation of antibiotic therapy. Collection of blood for complete blood count, blood culture, electrolytes, blood urea nitrogen, and creatinine should be considered in those less than 3 years of age and should be routinely collected in those less than age 6 months. For patients with equivocal clinical and negative laboratory findings, treatment may be postponed until culture results are available.

Treatment is indicated if there is any growth from a specimen obtained by suprapubic aspiration. Growth of more than 150,000 CFU/mL of a single organism from a catheterized specimen or from a voided specimen represents infection and should be treated. For patients who are febrile or otherwise highly symptomatic, treatment before availability of culture results may be indicated. In less symptomatic children, results of the UA and microscopy can be used to determine the likelihood of infection and the need to start treatment empirically. The presence of pyuria, urinary nitrites, or bacteriuria suggests infection, and empiric therapy while awaiting culture results may be appropriate.

Antibiotic coverage depends on the age of the child. For febrile infants younger than 2 months of age, broad-spectrum antibiotic coverage with ampicillin and gentamicin or ampicillin and a third-generation cephalosporin is appropriate until culture results are available.

Treatment options for children greater than 2 months of age depend on the patient's clinical state. All children who appear toxic, are vomiting, and are unlikely to tolerate PO medicines, or those who may be noncompliant, should be admitted for intravenous antibiotics until they are afebrile, culture results are available, and indicated imaging studies are completed. In addition, most clinicians recommend hospitalization and intravenous antibiotic therapy for all children less than 1 year of age. Initial parenteral antibiotic therapy should be with ceftriaxone (75 mg/kg/d divided q24h), cefotaxime (150 mg/kg/d divided q6h), gentamicin (7.5 mg/kg/d divided q8h). One should keep in mind the ototoxicity and nephrotoxicity of aminoglycosides. The change to an appropriate oral drug may be made after clinical response, and is based on culture sensitivity and resistance.

A recent study evaluated outpatient management of children greater than 1 month of age, using oral cefixime (16 mg/kg administered in the emergency department, followed by 8 mg/kg/d for 13 additional days), and found outcomes similar to a 3-day course of intravenous cefotaxime followed by oral cefixime.[7] While this study suggests an increasing role for outpatient management of pyelonephritis in children, routine application is not appropriate. Only patients who are nontoxic, are tolerating PO administration, and are likely to be compliant can be considered for outpatient management.

Older children with cystitis can be treated as outpatients. Antimicrobials for outpatient treatment include trimethoprim–sulfamethoxazole, amoxicillin–clavulanate, and second- or third-generation cephalosporins. Community resistance patterns of *Escherichia coli* to trimethoprim–sulfamethoxazole are important and may be higher than 15% in some areas.[8]

Recommendations on the duration of therapy vary. Because short-course and single-dose therapies have been successful with women, short-course regimens may be acceptable for uncomplicated cystitis in adolescent girls. Because studies of short-course therapy in children have yielded conflicting results, a 7- to 10-day course of antibiotics is recommended in prepubertal children. In addition, the difficulty with accurately identifying all cases of upper tract disease in children makes short-course therapy less acceptable in children.

DISPOSITION

Hospital admission is indicated for all infants younger than age 2 months and should be strongly considered in those less than 1 year of age. As noted previously, clinical judgment may be used for those infants who do not appear ill, who are more than 2 months old, and who will comply with oral antibiotics and recommended follow-up in 24 hours. In any patient managed as an outpatient, an initial oral dose of antibiotics or an i.m. or i.v. dose of ceftriaxone should be given in the emergency department. All admitted infants need evaluation by ultrasonography or intravenous pyelography (IVP), for possible obstruction and renal involvement. All children less than 5 years of age with UTI and fever should have a renal ultrasound and voiding cystourethrogram (VCUG) as soon as possible. For those patients who are treated as outpatients, it is essential to establish follow-up for radiographic evaluation of the urinary tract, if indicated, and repeat cultures.

Radiographic assessment of the urinary tract generally includes a renal ultrasound and either a VCUG or radionuclide cystography (RNC). Although these studies are not performed in the emergency department, an understanding of their role in the management of UTIs is important when determining a patient's disposition. The ultrasound evaluates renal and bladder anatomy. It is effective in revealing renal anomalies, hydronephrosis, ureteral dilatation, ureteroceles, calculi, and bladder wall thickening. It does not diagnose VUR and is not sensitive for renal scarring. The VCUG is obtained after the acute inflammation has subsided and details the anatomy of the urethra, bladder, and renal fossa. It demonstrates the presence of reflux and posterior urethral valves quite well. The RNC also demonstrates reflux but does not evaluate the urethra, and is thus unreliable in ruling out posterior urethral valves. Males of any age and girls less than age 5 should have an ultrasound (or IVP) as soon as possible to detect any obstructive process or renal disease. In those with a poor response to antibiotic therapy, the ultrasound should be performed in 48 to 72 hours.[1] A VCUG for evaluation of reflux may be delayed until after the infection has cleared, because infection predisposes to reflux.

In the past, radiographic evaluation of girls older than 1 year of age was reserved for those with pyelonephritis or those with recurrent lower tract infections. As many as 40% of UTIs have been found to be inadvertently diagnosed as respiratory or gastrointestinal infections, making history regarding previous infections unreliable.[6] Also, because younger children are most likely to have renal injury with UTIs, most experts now recommend radiographic evaluation for all symptomatic children younger than 5 years of age with their first UTI.[3,6] One study found fever to be indicative of a treatable urologic problem in 42% of girls younger than 5 years of age with UTIs.[11]

COMMON PITFALLS

- Failure to consider UTI as a source of fever in otherwise asymptomatic children leads to missed or incorrect diagnoses.

- Failure to obtain appropriate specimens before administering antibiotics in the septic infant may lead to delay in diagnosis of obstructive lesions of the urinary tract.
- Mild respiratory and gastrointestinal symptoms do not preclude UTI as the source of fever in the young child.
- Failure to arrange adequate follow-up for radiographic studies and repeat cultures may result in failure to find treatable causes of renal disease.

ACKNOWLEDGMENT

The author gratefully acknowledges the contribution of Linda Settle, who wrote the previous version of this chapter.

References

1. American Academy of Pediatrics. Practice parameter: the diagnosis, treatment, and evaluation of the initial urinary tract infection in febrile infants and young children: American Academy of Pediatrics, Committee on Quality Improvement, Subcommittee on Urinary Tract Infection. *Pediatrics* 1999; 103:686–693.
2. Bachur R, Caputo GL. Bacteremia and meningitis among infants with urinary tract infections. *Pediatr Emerg Care* 1995;11:280–284.
3. Carvajal HF, Travis LB. Infections of the urinary tract. In: Rudolph AM, Hoffman J, eds. *Pediatrics,* 18th ed. Norwalk, CT: Appleton & Lange, 1987.
4. Durbin WA, Peter G. Management of urinary tract infections in infants and children. *Pediatr Infect Dis* 1984;3:564.
5. Hellerstein S. The long-term consequences of urinary tract infections: a historic and contemporary perspective. *Pediatr Ann* 1999;28:69.
6. Hellerstein S, Wald ER, Winberg J, et al. Consensus: roentgenographic evaluation of children with urinary tract infections. *Pediatr Infect Dis* 1984;3:291.
7. Hoberman A, Wald E, Hickey RW, et al. Oral versus initial intravenous therapy for urinary tract infections in young febrile children. *Pediatrics* 1999;104:79–86.
8. Hoberman A, Wald ER. Treatment of urinary tract infections. *Pediatr Ann* 1999;28:688–692.
9. Hoberman A, Wald ER. UTI in young children: new light on old questions. *Contemp Pediatr* 1997;14:140–156.
10. Johnson CE. New advances in childhood urinary tract infections. *Pediatr Rev* 1999;20:335–343.
11. Johnson CE, Shrum PA, Marchant CD, et al. Identification of children requiring radiologic evaluation for urinary infection. *Pediatr Infect Dis* 1985;4:656.
12. Kierkegaard H, Feldt-Rasmussen U, Horder M, et al. Falsely negative urinary leucocyte counts due to delayed examination. *Scand J Clin Lab Invest* 1980;40:259–261.
13. Kupperman N, Bank DE, Walton EA, et al. Risks for bacteremia and urinary tract infections in young febrile children with bronchiolitis. *Arch Pediatr Adolesc Med* 1997;151:1207–1214.
14. Littlewood J, Jacobs S, Ramsden C. Comparison between microscopical examination of unstained deposits of urine and quantitative culture. *Arch Dis Child* 1977;52:894–896.
15. Pennington DJ, Zerin M. Imaging of the urinary tract in children. *Pediatr Ann* 1999;28:678–686.
16. Pryles CV, Lustik B. Laboratory diagnosis of urinary tract infection. *Pediatr Clin North Am* 1971;18:233.
17. Roberts KB, Channey E, Eseren RJ, et al. Urinary tract infections in infants with unexplained fever: a collaborative study. *J Pediatr* 1983;103:864.
18. Rubin MI, Baliah T. Urinalysis and its clinical interpretation. *Pediatr Clin North Am* 1971;18:245.
19. Shaw KN, Gorelick MH. Urinary tract infection in the pediatric patient. *Ped Clin North Am* 1999;46(6):1111.
20. Winberg J, Anderson HJ, Bergstom T, et al. Epidemiology of symptomatic urinary tract infection in childhood. *Acta Paediatr Scand* 1974;252[Suppl]:1.

CHAPTER 296
Ventricular Shunt Problems

Naghma S. Khan and Geoffrey Jackman

There is an increasing population of children with ventricular shunts placed for obstructive hydrocephalus. Emergency physicians must familiarize themselves with the different types of cerebrospinal fluid (CSF) shunts that are commonly used in their area of practice and be able to evaluate shunt function, dysfunction, and infection.[11] Early diagnosis and management of ventricular shunt problems are important to prevent the sequelae of increased intracranial pressure (ICP) (e.g., death, blindness, and cerebral white matter destruction).

Children are shunted for a variety of congenital and acquired conditions. These include congenital aqueductal stenosis, myelomeningocele and Arnold-Chiari malformation, Dandy-Walker cyst, brain tumor, postinfectious or posttraumatic scarring, and growths related to tuberous sclerosis or neurofibromatosis. There is an increasing number of children born prematurely who were shunted after intraventricular hemorrhage.

Ventricular shunts are one-way calibrated systems made of silicone rubber, a material biologically well tolerated by the body. They consist of a ventricular catheter, a reservoir, and a distal catheter. The ventricular catheter allows CSF drainage through perforations along its length. Valve mechanisms in the tubing allow only unidirectional flow of CSF away from the ventricles; they are calibrated to open when a certain pressure differential is reached.[6] A pumping chamber enables easy assessment of shunt function. When compressed, CSF should empty distally without resistance; when released, CSF should refill the chamber without delay. Distal tubing consists of silicone rubber. Most shunts end in the peritoneal cavity. Another site of CSF drainage is the atrium, and, rarely, the pleura, gallbladder, or urethra may be the distal site of drainage. A reservoir is placed proximal to the valve apparatus. CSF can be removed for sampling, or antibiotics and dyes can be instilled after manually occluding the system downstream from the reservoir.

An antisiphon device may be added to the shunt system to alleviate symptoms associated with excessive CSF runoff related to the creation of a negative intraventricular pressure on standing or with respirations. This device runs a serious risk of CSF underdrainage, leading to increased ICP. On–off devices are added distal to the valve mechanism to shut off the shunt so that alternative means of fluid drainage can be tested and the patient can gradually be weaned off the shunt. These devices drain automatically under high pressure, in case they are turned off for long periods of time.

Shunt problems include infection, mechanical dysfunction, and miscellaneous complications, depending on the terminal site of the shunt.[3,12]

Infection is the main complication in shunted patients, but a majority of shunt revisions occur for malfunction rather than infection of the shunt.[12] Some important risk factors for infection are age younger than 6 months, duration of surgery, reinsertion after previous infection, and postsurgery wound infection. Five percent to 15% of ventricular shunts become infected, 70% within the first month of surgery and 90% within 6 months of surgery.[4] A single preoperative dose of ceftriaxone may be a safe and effective way of preventing shunt infections.[1]

Common mechanical problems of ventricular shunts include proximal obstruction, distal obstruction, and "slit ventricle syndrome."

Miscellaneous, less common complications are related to the site of distal tubing insertion. In the peritoneum, migration of the tubing out of the peritoneal cavity into a hollow or solid organ, kinking or plugging of the distal end, volvulus, intestinal obstruction, and pseudocyst formation may occur. In the atrium, complications include endocarditis leading to shunt nephritis, pulmonary embolism, cardiac tamponade, and pulmonary hypertension. Gallbladder complications include atony, cholecystitis, obstructive jaundice, and fistula formation. Hydrothorax, pneumocranium, and pneumothorax occur in the pleura.

CLINICAL PRESENTATION

Shunted children may present with problems ranging from fever or headache to impending herniation related to ICP.

In most cases, the symptoms of shunt dysfunction are nonspecific but suggestive of increased ICP. These include fussiness, irritability, poor feeding, poor suck, altered sleep pattern, paradoxical crying, mental status changes, bulging fontanelle, seizures, apnea, bradycardia, and vomiting. Seizures occurring in children with therapeutic anticonvulsant levels should be suspected to be secondary to shunt malfunction. In a child old enough to talk, the most common presenting symptom associated with a shunt malfunction is headache. The problem with this complaint is that most individuals with shunts have headaches regularly. Headaches that are associated with shunt malfunction, however, are relentlessly progressive and are not ameliorated by lying down. Irritability and lethargy follow, as do personality change, lack of interest, and poor school performance.[14] Other presenting symptoms include blurred vision, neck pain, back pain, puffiness around the eyes, gait disturbances, urinary incontinence, and subtle behavior change.[9,13] When a patient is shunt dependent, the time between the onset of shunt obstruction and coma may be only a few hours.[14]

Children with ventriculitis may present with an insidious onset of symptoms of increased ICP, meningismus, abdominal pain (with ventriculoperitoneal shunts), and fever. Infection with *Staphylococcus epidermidis* accounts for more than 50% of shunt infections and usually presents with low-grade fever and an illness of insidious onset. *Staphylococcus aureus* and gram-negative infections may present as fulminating, life-threatening situations.

Patients with slit ventricle syndrome present with signs and symptoms of increased ICP, but a computed tomography (CT) scan shows either normal or slitlike collapsed ventricles and may sometimes show calvarial thickening and premature synostosis.[2] Some of the factors contributing to slit ventricle syndrome include low pressure from overdrainage of CSF; normal pressure and shunt function, but development of secondary high pressure waves from sudden vasodilation; periods of high pressure from intermittent proximal catheter obstruction; and intermittent high pressure despite normal catheter function.

DIFFERENTIAL DIAGNOSIS

The symptoms and signs of ventricular shunt problems are nonspecific. As such, they may mimic myriad common pediatric emergencies, ranging from viral infections, ear infections, and gastroenteritis to sepsis and shock. The prompt diagnosis and treatment of shunt malfunction and its discrimination from routine childhood illnesses such as gastroenteritis are critical to the well-being of the child.[14] It is important to avoid treating all the presenting complaints as shunt related, thereby failing to investigate all other diagnostic possibilities. As with nonshunted children, other causes of fever and increased ICP must be included in the differential diagnosis.

Migraine headaches are a difficult diagnostic dilemma. Children with migraine headaches may present with headache, vomiting, and altered sensorium. If the ventricles are small on CT scan, adequate shunt function can be documented by physical examination and shunt series; if family history is positive, the diagnosis of migraines can be entertained and unnecessary surgery avoided.[7]

EMERGENCY DEPARTMENT EVALUATION

A detailed history should document the number of shunts in place, underlying cause for placement, time of initial placement, number of revisions, types of infections, and other complications.

The site and type of shunt, number of craniotomy scars, and skull defects should be evaluated. Signs of increased ICP include a bulging fontanelle, bulging craniotomy site, distended scalp veins, widely split sutures, and sun-setting eyes. Older children present with headaches, vomiting, and photophobia. Cushing's triad is a late finding of impending herniation. If the fontanelle or craniotomy site is sunken, overdrainage of CSF and decreased ICP should be suspected. A mobile reservoir or fluid-filled swelling over the shunt site suggests a disconnection or perforation. The presence of cellulitis, frank pus, or skin breakdown is associated with a high incidence of ventriculitis and shunt malfunction. The tubing should be palpated all the way down to the abdomen. Swelling, kinking, or disruption of continuity should be sought. Shunt breakages tend to occur most commonly 2 to 4 cm above the neck incision in ventriculoatrial shunts and just cephalad to the clavicle in ventriculoperitoneal shunts.[8]

Manual Testing

Once the pumping chamber is identified, the system can be tested by compressing the pump. Effortless emptying on compression suggests distal patency of the tubing, whereas difficulty on compression suggests distal obstruction rather than loculated CSF. If there is immediate refill on release of the pumping chamber, the tubing is probably patent proximally. If there is delayed refill or no refill, partial or complete proximal obstruction should be suspected. A click on compression may be felt with a malfunctioning valve. The sensitivity of the shunt pumping test is only 18% to 20%, and the predictive value of a negative pumping test, indicating shunt patency, is only 65% to 81%.[13]

A patient who is unstable at presentation, with or without signs of increased ICP, should be monitored with telemetry as well as a pulse oximeter and should never be transported for further radiologic evaluation without establishing a stable airway, undertaking measures to control ICP, and obtaining vascular access.

Radiologic Testing

A shunt series and neuroimaging[5] are essential for further evaluation. Shunt series include anteroposterior and lateral skull and neck films, anteroposterior chest film, and right and left decubitus films of the abdomen. The latter are obtained to note the change in position of the abdominal end of the shunt tubing to determine whether the tip is free-floating. Tube migration, a fixed or stuck distal catheter, and curling within the abdominal wall or in pseudocysts can all be shown on plain film. Fusiform swelling of the distal end of the catheter suggests distal end obstruction. Abdominal ultrasound is a useful adjunct to plain films in detection of abdominal complications.

Initial evaluation requires head CT without contrast. The most important point in evaluating cranial CT scans is to have the last CT scan available for comparison of ventricular size. Normal or minimally enlarged ventricles may be related to increased ICP if the previous film showed small ventricles. The CT scan may also be helpful in delineating proximal shunt migration outside the ventricles. The most common malfunction is that of occlusion of the ventricular catheter by choroid plexus or glial tissue that has grown into the lumen of the catheter. Diagnosis can only be inferred from static imaging studies and plain x-rays that show enlarged lateral ventricles despite a well-placed ventriculostomy tube and intact connections of the shunt system.[2]

Pressure measurements, CSF assay, and radionuclide clearance are studies used to assess shunt function and infection. Using sterile technique, the clinician accesses the reservoir or pumping chamber with a 23-gauge butterfly needle, and the opening pressure, drip interval, and closing pressure are measured.[15] Fluid is obtained for analysis and, if indicated, for decompression of the ventricles. A "shuntogram" may be obtained by injecting technetium Tc 99m (to check for patency and clearance of CSF) through the system when the symptoms are vague and clinical testing and CT scan are equivocal. Fifty percent of radionuclide activity should clear in 5 minutes, and scout films at 15, 30, and 45 minutes should show steady clearance of dye into the abdominal cavity. Flow studies (using Tc 99m) may be falsely normal in one-third of cases with shunt disconnection, because the dye may be transported in a fibrous band of tissue surrounding the disconnected shunt tubing, even when there is increased ICP secondary to shunt malfunction.

A pressure of more than 15 cm H_2O or reflux of dye into ventricles without spontaneous clearance suggests distal obstruction, whereas difficulty in obtaining CSF suggests proximal obstruction. Extravasation of dye into the surrounding soft tissue occurs with disruption of tubing continuity. An abnormal cell count, culture, or Gram stain suggests ventriculitis. Normal function is determined if ICP is less than 20 cm H_2O, 50% of technetium is cleared in 5 minutes, there is good dissemination in the abdominal cavity, and fluid is easily obtained for laboratory analysis.

EMERGENCY DEPARTMENT MANAGEMENT

History, physical examination, and laboratory and radiologic evaluation enable the emergency physician to determine whether the patient's presenting complaint is related to a shunt problem and whether the cause is mechanical dysfunction or infection, or both. In either case, in the presence of increased ICP, the initial emergency department management is the same.

Mildly elevated ICP may be managed with osmotic agents or diuretic agents alone, whereas extremely elevated pressures would require rapid-sequence intubation, hyperventilation, osmotic diuretics, and, sometimes, manual decompression of the ventricles through a butterfly needle.

Emergency department management of ventriculitis consists of obtaining the appropriate laboratory data and early institution of broad-spectrum intravenous antibiotics. Blood cultures are rarely positive unless the shunt terminates in the circulation (e.g., ventriculoatrial shunts), so CSF cultures must be obtained before starting antibiotics. If CSF cannot be obtained from the shunt, a lumbar puncture should be considered after ruling out increased ICP. Initial therapy consists of antibiotic coverage for gram-positive and gram-negative organisms. Vancomycin 10 mg/kg and ceftazidime 50 mg/kg offer optimal initial antibiotic coverage. Oral rifampin 10 mg/kg may be added for synergy. Operative and antibiotic management of ventriculitis is controversial, especially regarding intraventricular antibiotic therapy. A high degree of success has been documented with intravenous antibiotic therapy, externalization of the distal catheter, and subsequent revision of the shunt, once the infection is under control.[10]

Slit ventricle syndrome is managed surgically by placement of an antisiphon device.

DISPOSITION

Role of the Consultant

Neurosurgical consultation is necessary for all patients diagnosed with shunt malfunction, ventriculitis, or any other shunt-related problems. Most neurosurgeons prefer to tap the shunt themselves; therefore, the ED physician should consult the neurosurgeon before attempting to tap a ventricular shunt. Most shunt malfunctions and some shunt infections require shunt revision or externalization.

Indications for Admission

If there are any signs of increased ICP, the patient should be admitted to the intensive care unit for close monitoring with telemetry and pulse oximetry. All patients with shunt-related infections should be admitted for antibiotic therapy.

Transfer Considerations

For patients with shunt-related problems who are being transferred to a tertiary care center, ensure an adequate airway, adequate control of ICP, and intravenous access. The patient's status and the transferring physician's concerns should be discussed in depth with the accepting agency's physician. Only Advance Cardiac Life-Support units should be used, and, in the case of an unstable patient, air transport should be used.

COMMON PITFALLS

- The most common pitfalls in assessing children with shunts are the tendency to attribute all presenting complaints to shunt-related problems and failure to pursue other possible diagnoses. On the other hand, failing to assess for shunt-related problems, even when the child presents with an upper respiratory infection, can be potentially fatal.
- All patients with ventricular shunts do not necessarily require a shunt series and a CT scan at every emergency department presentation, but they do require clear documentation of an infectious focus, if they present with fever, and a thorough assessment of the central nervous system and shunt and tubing sites. If there is any doubt that the symptomatology is related to shunt malfunction, a neurosurgical consultation and isotope clearance studies are necessary.
- Lack of availability of comparison films can pose a problem. If the CT scan shows no signs of hydrocephalus, then there is no issue. However, in the face of dilated ventricles, one is left with the dilemma of determining the clinical significance when comparison views are not available. In most cases, the neurosurgeon will opt to observe the patient if symptoms suggestive of increased ICP present.

References

1. Arnaboldi L. Antimicrobial prophylaxis with ceftriaxone in neurosurgical procedures. A prospective study of 100 patients undergoing shunt operations. *Chemotherapy* 1996;42(5):384–390.
2. Barkovich J, Edwards MSB. Applications of neuroimaging in hydrocephalus. *Pediatr Neurosurg* 1992;18:65.
3. Casey AT, Kimmings EJ, Kleinlugtebeld AD, et al. The long-term outlook for hydrocephalus in childhood. A ten-year cohort study of 155 patients. *Pediatr Neurosurg* 1997;27(2):63–70.
4. Choux M, Genitori L, Lang D, et al. Shunt implantation: reducing the incidence of shunt infection. *J Neurosurg* 1992;77(6):875.
5. Goeser CD, McLeary MS, Young LW. Diagnostic imaging of ventricular–peritoneal shunt malfunctions and complications [Review]. *Radiographics* 1998;18(3):635–651.
6. Hirsch JF, Hoppe-Hirsch E. Shunts and shunt problems in childhood. *Adv Tech Stand Neurosurg* 1988;16:177.
7. James HE, Nowak TP. Clinical course and diagnosis of migraine headaches in hydrocephalic children. *Pediatr Neurosurg* 1991–1992;17:310.
8. Langmoen IA, Lundar T, Vatne K, et al. Occurrence and management of fractured peripheral catheters in CSF shunts. *Childs Nerv Syst* 1992;8(4):222.
9. Lee TT, Uribe J, Ragheb J, et al. Unique clinical presentations of pediatric shunt malfunction. *Pediatr Neurosurg* 1999;30(3):122–126.
10. Morissette I, Gourdeau M, Francoeur J. CSF shunt infections: a fifteen-year experience with emphasis on management and outcome. *Can J Neurol Sci* 1993;20:118.
11. Naradzay JF, Browne BJ, Rolnick MA, et al. Cerebral ventricular shunts [Review]. *J Emerg Med* 1999;17(2):311–322.
12. Odio C, McCracken GH, Nelson JD. CSF shunt infections in pediatrics. *Am J Dis Child* 1984;138:1103–1108.
13. Piatt JH. Physical examination of patients with cerebrospinal fluid shunts: is there useful information in pumping the shunt? *Pediatrics* 1992;89(3):470.
14. Rekate HL. Shunt revision: complications and their prevention. *Pediatr Neurosurg* 1991–1992;17:155.
15. Sood S, Kim S, Ham SD, et al. Useful components of the shunt tap test for evaluation of shunt malfunction. *Childs Nerv Syst* 1993;9:157.

PART IV

Pediatric Trauma

CHAPTER 297

Multiple Trauma

Thom A. Mayer

Nearly 22 million children are injured each year in the United States—almost one out of every three children.[3] Trauma is the leading cause of death in children aged 1 to 15 years and is responsible for over one-third of all deaths in children younger than 1 year of age. More than 20,000 children (birth to 19 years) die of injuries from trauma each year.[23]

Although injuries from trauma are a common cause of death and disability in children, these injuries are spread over such a wide geographic area that it is uncommon for any single emergency department or emergency physician to have extensive experience in the care of pediatric trauma victims. One reason for this is that the majority of ill and injured children are initially taken care of in the community emergency department setting.

It is extremely important to recognize that any well-trained emergency physician should have the diagnostic and therapeutic skills required to care for the pediatric multiple trauma victim. The numerous significant differences between adult and pediatric trauma victims preclude a totally unified approach to all multiple trauma patients. A protocol-oriented approach to the care of pediatric victims with multiple trauma, accentuating differences between adults and children, is presented in this chapter.

Most important to the care of the pediatric multiple trauma victim is *preparation* of the entire emergency department and surgical backup teams to care for pediatric patients with acute injuries. There is a thin margin for error in caring for severely injured children: The physician and nurse must be familiar with the appropriate elements of evaluation and resuscitation, including normal baseline parameters in children. Although caring for seriously injured children can be among the most demanding of emotional and psychological experiences, the appropriate preparations can result in a well-organized resuscitation with excellent outcomes. A general emergency department seeing 20,000 undifferentiated patients per year may see only four or five seriously injured children per year, but the time and effort necessary to prepare for such events are well worthwhile. In this respect, pediatric multiple trauma is a low-frequency but extremely high-yield event.

The major causes of pediatric trauma include motor vehicle accidents, automobile–pedestrian collisions, burns and smoke inhalation, falls, poisonings, and child abuse. Data from the National Pediatric Trauma Registry indicate that about 90% of childhood injuries are due to blunt trauma.[20] The remaining 10% of injuries are penetrating and tend to occur in urban settings or are due to farm-related accidents or hunting injuries. Mechanisms of injury vary considerably by age. Most infants or toddlers suffer trauma as a result of falls, vehicular accidents as a passenger, or child abuse.[13] As the child approaches the preschool and grade-school age group, automobile–pedestrian accidents become increasingly common as a source of injury for the child. However, passengers in motor vehicles also account for a large percentage of injuries in this age group. In the adolescent years, motor vehicle accidents (with or without the influence of drugs and alcohol) become the most common cause of pediatric trauma.

ANATOMIC AND PHYSIOLOGIC DIFFERENCES

One of the most common statements in pediatric training programs is, "Children are not simply small adults." This is true, and it is important to review the differences between adults and children that result in differences in therapy and evaluation.

Because children are smaller, the amount of medication or fluids given to injured children varies according to a child's lean body mass. The most accurate way of calculating fluid or medication dosages is by using lean body mass calculations, but, in the emergency department setting, this is impractical at best and futile at worst.[12] Instead, fluid and medication dosages can be calculated on the basis of the child's overall weight. At the time of evaluation, the child's weight is not often known; more important, when a child is severely injured and requires resuscitative efforts, there is no time to weigh the child or check with the parents regarding the last known weight. Because of this, it is important to establish general guidelines for predicting the child's weight by age or length.

First, many pediatric critical care centers publish charts and tables that can be placed on the wall of the resuscitation area. These include weight as related to age and indicate the appropriate-sized tubes and drug calculations for resuscitation. Second, Luten and Broselow have developed a resuscitation tape that can be used to measure the child's length; from this measurement, the child is placed in a color zone that lists specific fluid and drug dosages, as well as resuscitative equipment.[12] Third, the child's weight can generally be predicted, with a fair degree of accuracy, based on age. The Broselow Resuscitation Tape or some other length-based system is the method of choice in estimating the child's weight.

There are important anatomic differences between adults and children. The child's head occupies a larger total body surface area and weight than in the adult. Head injuries occur in approximately 75% of all seriously injured pediatric patients but in only about 50% of adult patients.[13] Because the head is the major organ for heat loss, a greater percentage of loss, and therefore temperature instability, may occur in children. The occiput is more prominent in children, which affects airway positioning. The child's cranial sutures are open at birth and gradually fuse by the age of 12 to 18 months. Because of this, palpating the anterior and posterior fontanelles can be an important source of information in children with increased intracranial pressure. The child's brain also has a higher percentage of white matter versus gray matter, resulting in a greater overall "plasticity" and the ability to withstand deceleration injuries.

The child's neck is considerably shorter and has more subcutaneous tissue than in an adult. In addition, the cervical spine is more cartilaginous and is far less commonly fractured than an adult's. Nonetheless, cervical cord injuries are not uncommon in children, although fully two-thirds of such injuries result in spinal cord injuries without radiographic abnormalities (SCIWORA) present to the cervical spine (see Chapter 300). Because the young child has a shorter neck, with more subcutaneous tissue, evaluating the midline position of the trachea and neck veins can be considerably more difficult.

The larynx is located in a more cephalad and anterior position in children, which makes intubation considerably more difficult. The epiglottis sits at nearly a 45-degree angle and is far more cartilaginous in children. The narrowest portion of the pediatric airway is not at the glottis, as in the adult; rather, the level of the cricoid cartilage is the narrowest portion until about age 10.[13] In addition, the cricoid cartilage is also the site of very loose, abundant areolar columnar epithelium, which reacts easily to either infectious processes or pressure necrosis.

The chest in children is more compliant, less bony, and more cartilaginous than in an adult. There is far less overlying muscle and fat in the child, so that forces applied to the chest can easily be transmitted to underlying tissues. The mediastinum is not well fixed in children, so pneumothorax easily progresses to tension pneumothorax in children. Children's diaphragms are much more distensible than adults', and they insert at a more horizontal angle. As a result, gastric distention may easily cause pulmonary compromise by pushing the diaphragm superiorly.

As with the chest, the child's abdomen is less protected by overlying muscle and fat, so that mild forces applied to the abdominal wall can injure the abdominal structures. Children are diaphragmatic, or "belly," breathers, which means they require full diaphragmatic excursion to produce normal respirations. They are far less able to recruit the intercostal muscles to assist in respiration than are adults. For this reason, the restriction of movement of the diaphragm from irritation secondary to blood may cause respiratory compromise. The bladder is well protected by the overlying pubic bone in adults, whereas this organ is an intraperitoneal structure in young children and is far more prone to injury from blunt trauma.[11]

The long bones of children accommodate growth through the epiphyses or growth plates. The epiphyseal–metaphyseal junction is the weakest portion of the child's joint, so that ligamentous structures are actually stronger than the growth plate junction. For this reason, epiphyseal fractures are common in children.

THE PRIMARY AND SECONDARY SURVEYS

Because of the numerous differences between adults and children, the emergency physician must clearly understand a protocol approach to evaluating such patients in a rapid but thorough fashion. By far, the easiest way of attaining this is to integrate the child's care with the adult's to whatever extent possible. The simplest way of doing this is to use the primary survey–secondary survey format initially described by the American College of Surgeons Committee on Trauma in the *Advanced Trauma Life Support* (ATLS) course.[3] The primary survey is an initial assessment of the patient's airway, oxygenation, ventilation, circulation, perfusion, and overall level of consciousness. It is a physiologic survey that assesses the overall compromise to the patient's vital systems.

TABLE 297.1. Primary Survey Approach to the Pediatric Trauma Patient

A	—Airway (with cervical spine immobilization)
B	—Breathing
C	—Circulation
D^2	—Disability
	Diagnosis and treatment of shock
E^2	—Expose
	Environment

Adapted from American College of Surgeons Committee on Trauma. *Textbook of advanced trauma life support.* Chicago: American College of Surgeons, 1997.

Differences between adults and children require modification of the primary survey (Table 297.1). This modification simply recognizes the important differences in the diagnosis and treatment of shock in children, as well as the importance of maintaining a normal homeostatic thermoregulatory environment for infants and young children. The essential tenets of the primary survey are similar, however.

Because it is common to encounter serious physiologic derangements in children, it may be necessary to interrupt the primary survey to provide life-saving resuscitative measures. Using such a protocol approach allows the emergency physician to give this care and then to return immediately to a structured evaluation.

The primary survey resuscitative phase should take only a few minutes to perform, but it gives the emergency physician an accurate baseline assessment of the child's overall physiologic status. By using a protocol approach to the patient, the emergency physician can be assured that potential threats to life and limb are identified in sequential yet complete fashion. One must remember the important differences between adults and children in provision of an airway; maintenance of cervical spine immobilization; use of appropriate ventilation; recognition of circulatory stability and shock; provision of vascular access; role of oxygenation, ventilation, and perfusion in pediatric head injury; and maintenance of a normal homeostatic regulatory environment.

During the primary survey, the patient is fully undressed for a detailed secondary survey, which is a timely, directed evaluation of each body area, usually performed in head-to-toe fashion. The secondary survey assesses the type and severity of injury, as well as the body system's potential contribution to physiologic instability. The examination should not delay evaluation or treatment of life-threatening injuries. In addition to identifying specific injuries in each body region and their overall severity, it is also important to begin to assess the appropriate definitive care for the injury, as well as the priority of therapy as compared with others identified in the secondary survey.

AIRWAY

The highest priority in caring for either adult or pediatric patients with multiple trauma is providing a patent airway with adequate ventilation and oxygenation. However, significant differences in the pediatric airway require an approach different from that for an adult.

Although cervical spine injuries are less common in children than in adults, it is extremely important to protect the cervical spine throughout all airway manipulations in injured children. As mentioned, fully two-thirds of all children with spinal cord injuries have no radiographic abnormalities apparent on initial or follow-up radiographs. Most of these children have symptoms of transient paresthesias or numbness that occur at the time of the impact injury.[13] In particular, extreme caution must be used in caring for children who are at extremely high risk for the development of cervical spine injuries (e.g., unrestrained infants in motor vehicle deceleration injuries, children struck by automobiles, or any patient who has fallen from a height greater than 10 ft). In these children, even if the initial lateral cervical spine radiograph is normal, cervical spine integrity must be protected.

By far, the most underrated mechanism of protecting the cervical spine in children is in-line cervical immobilization. Because of the child's smaller size, providing such immobilization is more often effective in children than in adults, although it often requires a two-rescuer approach in the struggling child. One rescuer holds the cervical position while maintaining the airway, while the other ensures that the distal portions of the body are also immobilized until more permanent means can be obtained. All emergency medical services providers should have rigid pediatric cervical spine collars available for field use. Children injured in infant seats should usually be left in the infant seat and transported after appropriate padding has been placed to prevent movement during transport.

If the patient's cervical spine has not been immobilized in the field, the emergency physician should immediately provide in-line cervical immobilization while a rigid cervical collar, sandbags, and tape are applied. It is often possible to use both a rigid cervical collar and sandbags with tape to immobilize a child's cervical spine without compromising the airway. The anterior portion of the rigid collar can be removed once sandbags and tapes are present, so that the airway can be evaluated.

Concurrently with stabilizing the cervical spine, the airway should be evaluated and positioned. Although many common errors are made in the evaluation and maintenance of the pediatric airway, by far the most frequent and obvious is failure to position the airway properly. Because the larynx is both more anterior and more cephalad in a child, positioning the airway similar to the adult trauma patient will not result in effective airway positioning. In addition, in severely injured children, the tongue and other muscular tissue attached to the mandible often fall posteriorly. This "mandibular block" of tissue can cause significant respiratory compromise. Figure 297.1 summarizes the significant differences in the child's airway.

To ensure that the airway is patent in a child, the child is placed in the "sniffing position" (with the neck slightly flexed on the spinal axis and the head slightly extended on the neck). It is called the sniffing position because it approximates the position a child's airway would be in if he or she were sniffing a flower. In practical terms, this position can be obtained by placing either the rescuer's hand or a small towel under the occiput of the head. Because the occiput is more prominent, only slight elevation is usually required. In addition, a jaw thrust or chin lift maneuver should be provided to ensure that the mandibular block of tissue does not fall posteriorly and obstruct the airway, and also to provide appropriate extension of the head on the neck. The jaw thrust maneuver is far more practical in the child and is also easily obtainable because of the child's smaller size.

Unless the airway is appropriately positioned as described here, it is often difficult to provide appropriate oxygenation or ventilation, even in the presence of otherwise acceptable bag-valve-mask ventilation or endotracheal (ET) intubation. Proper airway positioning in the child must be practiced in advance, both on mannequins during appropriate training and also in evaluating non–critically ill children in the emergency department. *It is the emergency physician's responsibility to ensure that prehospital care providers and emergency department staff are fully aware of these factors and can provide appropriate airway positioning in the child.*

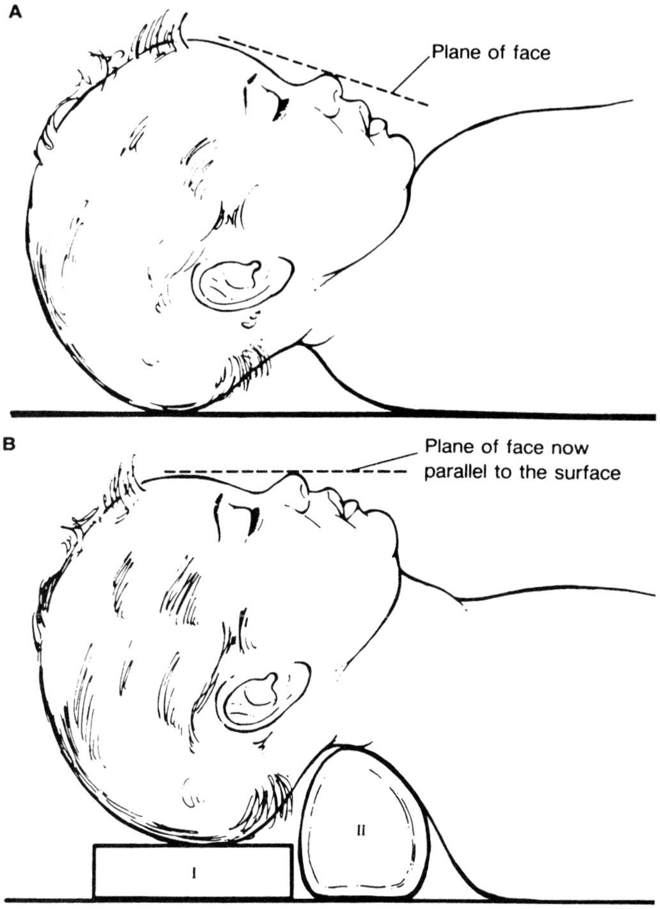

Figure 297.1. **(A)** Airway at high risk for occlusion. Flexion of the neck on the thorax is caused by a prominent occiput. **(B)** Sniffing position, which gives maximum possibility for a patent airway. Note the mild extension of the head. Flexion is now corrected by elevation of the head *(I)* and/or posterior neck support *(II)*.

Once the airway has been appropriately positioned, a rapid assessment should be made for airway patency and adequacy of ventilation. If airway obstruction exists, manual clearing or suction with a rigid tonsillar suction should be provided, after which the airway should be repositioned. In addition, the respiratory effort should be at the appropriate rate and should provide adequate bilateral chest wall rise. The presence or absence of cyanosis should also be noted. Supplemental oxygen should be provided to all pediatric multiple trauma victims until the airway can be completely evaluated. Up to about age 4 to 6 months, children are obligate nasal breathers, so nasal obstruction must be quickly and effectively relieved to allow spontaneous ventilation.

A second common error in the evaluation of the pediatric patient is failure to recognize the presence or absence of adequate ventilation. Because children have small tidal volumes, the chest wall rise that is usually present may be subtle. For this reason, it is important to observe normal ventilation in children who present to the emergency department who are *not* in respiratory distress. Both the rate and depth of ventilation should be assessed rapidly but effectively. Table 297.2 indicates the appro-

TABLE 297.2. Ranges for Pediatric Vital Signs[a]

	Pulse/min		Respiratory Rate/min		Systolic Blood Pressure (mm Hg)	
Age	Min	Max	Min	Max	Min	Max
0–1 mo	100	160	30	60	60 (term) 50 (premature)	80
1 mo–1 yr	100	140	20	40	70	100
1–2 yr	90	130	20	30	70+ 2 × age (yr)	105
2–6 yr	75	120	20	30	70+ 2 × age (yr)	105–110
6–14 yr	60	110	15	25	70+ 2 × age (yr)	115–130

Min, 2nd percentile, minimal acceptable value (calm, sleeping); Max, 98th percentile, maximal acceptable value (agitated, crying).
[a] Vital signs must be correlated with clinical picture.

priate ventilation ranges for children by age. To assess the adequacy of air movement, it is often helpful for the examiner to moisten his or her cheek and place it close to the child's nose and mouth to feel whether air is being exchanged. Placement of the cheek close to the child's mouth also allows simultaneous assessment of rise of the chest wall.

Although this assessment may seem relatively simple, it is often neglected by even the best emergency physicians and trauma surgeons in the early care of the pediatric multiple trauma patient. It cannot be overstated that *the positioning and initial assessment of the child's airway are critical to appropriate care.*

Oral and Nasal Airways

In unconscious adult trauma patients, oral or nasal airways are often used to assist in ensuring airway patency. However, such airways are less commonly useful in children for several reasons. First, in the conscious child, oral or nasal airways can produce significant vomiting or laryngospasm. For that reason, their use should be strictly limited to unconscious patients. Second, the posterior pharynx of a child is the site of highly vascular adenoidal tissue, which is almost always traumatized by the insertion of a nasal tube. The significant amount of bleeding that can be produced from such tubes may interfere with further efforts to secure the airway. Third, and most important, there is a tendency to assume that the placement of an oral or nasal airway helps ensure that the child's airway is in a proper position. This is certainly not the case in children, as the mandibular block of tissue can easily obstruct the portion of the airway just above the glottis, even in the presence of either a nasal or oral airway. For all of the these reasons, airways have a much more limited role in pediatric patients.[13]

Bag-and-Mask Ventilation

In pediatric multiple trauma patients with a compromised airway, there is a natural tendency to rush toward ET intubation. This is an extremely common but potentially fatal mistake. Most children can be initially ventilated in an adequate fashion by bag-and-mask ventilation, assuming the physician remembers several factors.

First, giving bag-and-mask ventilation to children is much easier than in adults because of the child's smaller size: It is much easier to generate appropriate tidal volumes and airway pressures in children than in adults.

Second, providing an adequate seal by face mask is usually much easier in children than in adults. In the adult, there are often significant air leaks around the mask, but in a child it is usually easy to provide an adequate seal between the face and the mask (assuming that the appropriate size is used) by pressing firmly with one hand on the mask and with the other either under the child's head or neck. In small children or infants, the thumb can be placed on the mask and the fingers underneath the head. The appropriate-sized mask can be selected by choosing one that easily fits from the bridge of the nose to the bony portion of the symphysis of the mandible. A full range of sizes of pediatric ventilation masks should be available in all emergency departments, as well as to all prehospital care providers. The bag-and-mask technique should be taught to all emergency services personnel in both the prehospital and in-hospital settings.

One of the most frequent criticisms of bag-and-mask ventilation versus ET intubation is protection of the airway from aspiration. However, the judicious use of Sellick's maneuver precludes the possibility of aspiration if applied appropriately. This maneuver consists of placing pressure on the cricoid cartilage posteriorly, which occludes the esophagus against the spinal column, thereby preventing regurgitation. Although care should be taken not to occlude the carotid arteries, this maneuver can be performed easily and ensures that vomiting and subsequent aspiration will not occur.

The adequacy of assisted ventilation should be assessed by ensuring that there is equal bilateral chest wall rise at appropriate rates. Listening to the child's chest with a stethoscope may be of some benefit, but it is important to recognize that children's chests transmit sound easily. This results in inaccurate estimations of presence or absence of pneumothoraces, right main stem bronchus intubation, and so forth. By far, the best single guide to adequacy of ventilation is the presence of bilateral chest wall rise.

Nasogastric Tube Placement

Whenever assisted ventilation is provided to the pediatric multiple trauma victim, a nasogastric tube should be placed. Aerophagia and gastric distention are common in the pediatric multiple trauma victim and may result in distention of the left hemidiaphragm, compromising ventilation. Placement of an appropriate nasogastric tube should empty both air and some particulate matter from the patient's stomach.

Assessment of appropriate nasogastric tube position should not be done by injecting air into the stomach. In addition to further filling and distending the stomach, the pediatric patient's gastroesophageal junction is far less patent than in the adult. It is common to hear air bubbling over the stomach, even when the nasogastric tube is in the esophagus. More importantly, the purpose of the nasogastric tube is to empty the stomach. It is possible that the tube may be in the stomach but positioned anteriorly, and therefore not emptying the stomach. Therefore, the best means to assess appropriate positioning of the nasogastric tube is to place 15 mL of normal saline through the tube and ensure that a like quantity can be aspirated easily.

Endotracheal Intubation

As indicated previously, most children can be adequately ventilated initially by bag-and-mask ventilation, but there are three general indications for ET intubation in the pediatric multiple trauma patient[18]:

1. Inability to adequately ventilate the child by bag-and-mask methods
2. The need for prolonged control of the airway, including prevention of aspiration
3. The need for controlled hyperventilation in patients with serious head injury

When any of these indications are present, adequate bag-and-mask ventilation with 100% oxygen is continued until appropriate preparations can be made for ET intubation. A length-based system can be used to select the appropriate-sized ET tube and intubation equipment.[12]

Other preparations necessary before ET intubation include adequate preoxygenation of the patient by bag-and-mask ventilation with 100% oxygen. In most cases, a stylet should be placed in the ET tube to prevent deflection of the tube away from the vocal cords. However, it is important to ensure that the stylet does not advance past the level of the ET tube, because tracheal perforation has been reported in such instances. The child should be suctioned adequately to allow optimal visualization of the cords.

In general, a straight laryngoscope blade is more helpful in children. A curved blade that is adequately lodged in the vallecula may not allow adequate visualization of the vocal cords, because the larynx is both more anterior, more cephalad, and obscured by the floppy epiglottis that sits at a nearly 45-degree angle. For this reason, a straight laryngoscope blade is usually better able to allow visualization of the cords in the child. In any cases in which there is a chance of cervical spine injury, in-line cervical immobilization during ET intubation should be maintained.

Airway positioning is critical during ET intubation. The child is placed in the sniffing position, and a Sellick maneuver is used to prevent vomiting and aspiration. Pulse oximetry readings should be monitored to assess oxygenation. If oxygen saturation drops, the intubation attempt should be stopped and 100% oxygen should be administered prior to further attempts.

Once the tube has been placed within the trachea, the best way to ensure proper position is to watch for bilateral, symmetric chest wall rise commensurate with the rescuer's efforts of using bag ventilation on the child. Listening to the chest in the child is much less helpful than in the adult, because the chest transmits sound very easily in children. It is not uncommon for the rescuer to hear relatively clear breath sounds on both sides in the child, even though the tube is either in the esophagus or in the right main stem bronchus. The presence of bilateral, symmetric chest wall rise and improvement in the child's overall color and condition should confirm placement of the tube. Colorimetric or quantitative end-tidal CO_2 detectors are also recommended for confirmation. If there is any question, one can try to revisualize that the tube is between the vocal cords. A chest radiograph can be obtained to ensure that the tube is in the proper position in the trachea.

The tube is secured to the upper lip with benzoin and taped to ensure that it is not dislodged during further resuscitative efforts.

Oral Versus Nasotracheal Intubation

In adult trauma patients in whom ET intubation is required and in whom the cervical spine has not been adequately cleared, blind nasotracheal (NT) intubation is sometimes utilized, assuming that in-line cervical immobilization is carefully maintained. Should blind or visualized NT intubation be used in the pediatric patient? Several facts argue against the *routine* use of this procedure in children.

First, as indicated previously, although cervical spine injuries are less common in children than in adults, they still occur with sufficient frequency to require careful maintenance of cervical spine protection in children at risk for injury.

Second, numerous anatomic differences between the adult and the child make it much more difficult to perform either blind or visualized NT intubation in the child. First among these differences is the fact that the larynx sits farther forward and more cephalad and is protected by the nearly 45-degree angle of the epiglottis. For this reason, blind NT intubation in a child requires the tube to take a sharp anterior angle after clearing the level of the nasopharynx. This can sometimes be obviated by firm rearward cricoid pressure (Sellick maneuver), but this does not always produce sufficient posterior displacement.

In addition, the child's nasopharynx is the site of highly vascular adenoidal tissue, which is often traumatized by the passage of the NT tube. Once such bleeding is present, it is extremely difficult to stop and may complicate efforts at oral intubation.

The rapid sequence induction (RSI) technique for emergency intubation has gradually become the standard for intubating most critically injured trauma patients. This technique is described in detail in Chapter 235. Most patients will have a suspected cervical spine injury or will require intubation before adequate radiographs and definitive examination. Appropriate measures must be taken to stabilize the cervical spine, and a neurologic examination must be done before RSI. The RSI technique in a trauma patient requires one person to stabilize the cervical spine, one to hold cricoid pressure, and a third to intubate and supervise the airway. In those exceedingly rare cases in which direct laryngeal injury is present and precludes ET intubation, needle cricothyroidotomy should be performed.

Needle cricothyroidotomy should be used only in rare circumstances in children.[13,18] It is largely a means to avoid surgical cricothyroidotomy, which is difficult in the child. Because the child can almost always be ventilated by bag-and-mask techniques, even with severe laryngeal injury, needle cricothyroidotomy and surgical cricothyroidotomy are rare in children. Although surgical cricothyroidotomy has been performed successfully in numerous adult series of patients, the cricoid is the narrowest portion of the pediatric airway, and significant bleeding often occurs during this technique. Several series in pediatric trauma patients have indicated that this technique should not be used in children, except in the extremely experienced hands of pediatric surgeons or pediatric otolaryngologists.[9,13,18]

In those rare circumstances in which an airway is needed immediately because of massive facial or laryngeal trauma in the child, needle cricothyroidotomy is an alternate technique. In this technique, a 14- to 16-gauge catheter is placed in the midline through the cricoid cartilage and is advanced distally (Fig. 297.2).

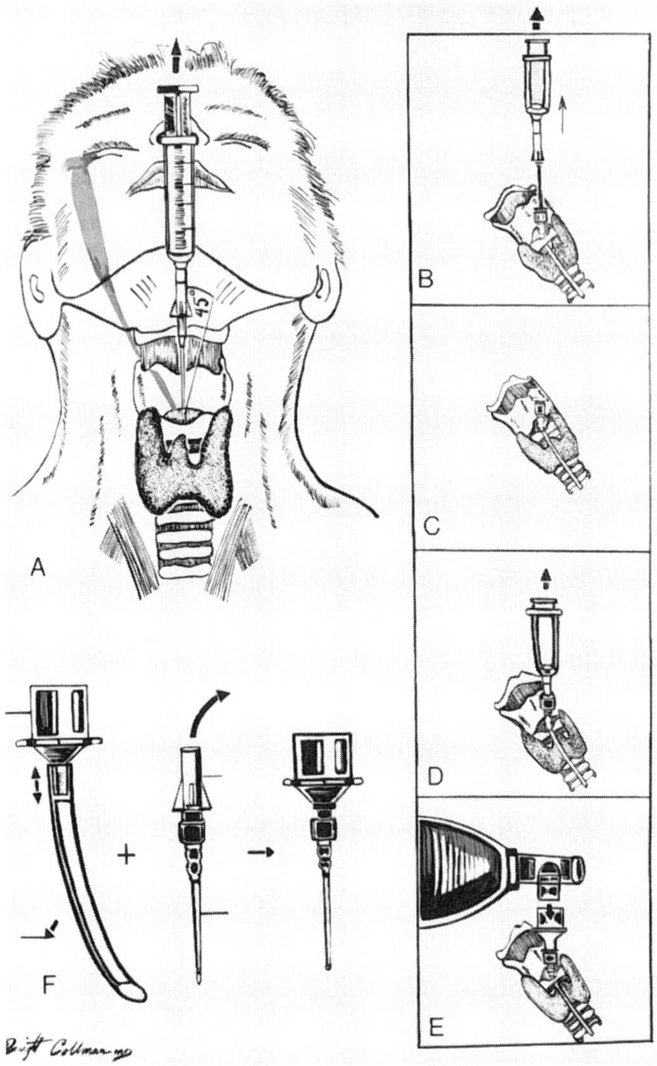

Figure 297.2. Needle cricothyroidotomy. **(A)** The cricothyroid cartilage is palpated in the midline, between the thyroid and cricoid cartilage, and is punctured at a 45-degree angle with a 5- or 10-mL syringe attached to a 14-gauge catheter. **(B)** As the catheter is advanced, the syringe should be aspirated, with free and rapid entry of air into the syringe indicating position in the trachea. **(C)** After initial entry into the trachea, the catheter is carefully advanced distally. **(D)** After the catheter is advanced, tracheal position should be carefully rechecked by again aspirating the syringe. **(E)** Ventilation is provided either by bag and mask (as shown) or by jet ventilation. **(F)** A 3.5-mm pediatric endotracheal tube adapter fits easily into the hub of the catheter, allowing ventilation. (From Mayer T, ed. *Emergency management of pediatric trauma*. Philadelphia: WB Saunders, 1985.)

Summary: Airway

Evaluating and managing the pediatric airway is the most critical aspect of the care of the pediatric trauma victim. In most cases, bag-and-mask ventilation can be used to maintain adequate oxygenation and ventilation during the initial evaluation. When the airway must be secured on a more definitive basis, the emergency physician should be skilled at performing RSI. Cervical spine immobilization should be maintained during all types of airway manipulations.

CIRCULATION

Once the airway has been secured and adequate ventilation and oxygenation are provided, attention is turned to the patient's circulation. The major goals are to assess overall circulatory status, including pulse and perfusion, while obtaining reliable venous access with the fewest possible complications and controlling any internal or external hemorrhage. Assessing and treating the circulatory system correspond closely to an accurate assessment of the presence and degree of shock in the pediatric patient.

The initial assessment of the overall circulatory status of pediatric multiple trauma patients involves determining the patient's *pulse* and *perfusion*. Palpating the carotid, femoral, brachial, or radial pulse may be done during proper airway positioning. The initial circulatory assessment should include palpating the pulse for quality (strong, normal, thready), rate, and regularity.

Although tachycardia is a normal response to hypovolemia in both adult and pediatric patients, the tachycardic response to blood loss is much more profound in children than in adults. Therefore, the earliest sign of altered circulation in impending shock in children is tachycardia. In general, any child with tachycardia (as defined by rates exceeding those in Table 297.2) should have a venous access line in place and appropriate fluid bolus.

Assessing the patient's overall tissue perfusion lies at the heart of the early diagnosis and recognition of shock and is discussed more fully in *Chapter 236*. Basic measures of peripheral perfusion include assessment of capillary refill and pallor of the mucous membranes. However, children's total peripheral resistance rises rapidly in response to initial blood loss, so they tend to "clamp down" in their peripheral circulation rapidly. For this reason, capillary refill is an early sign of shock. Pallor of the mucous membranes usually takes somewhat longer to occur but should be assessed.

Indicators of central perfusion include more sensitive measures of total peripheral resistance (diastolic blood pressure or pulse pressure), maintenance of central nervous system perfusion, and decreases in renal blood flow (decreased urine output). Because head injury occurs in up to 80% of patients with serious multiple trauma, following the status of the central nervous system may be difficult as a measure of central perfusion. Measuring urine output, essential in the care of the shock patient, requires at least 30 minutes to 1 hour to ensure accuracy, because it is a dynamic rather than a static measurement. For this reason, the emergency physician must be able to follow the pulse rate, pulse pressure, and diastolic blood pressure as indirect measurements of the central perfusion of the child in shock.

Venous Access

Rapid, efficient venous access is one of the most challenging problems facing the emergency physician responsible for caring for pediatric multiple trauma victims. The alternatives include percutaneous peripheral venous cannulation, intraosseous infusion, peripheral venous cutdown, and percutaneous central venous access. One should select the route that is the most rapid and yet involves the fewest possible complications for the child. In addition, the vascular access site and technique should allow for the most rapid means of replenishing vascular volume.

In most cases, the pediatric patient will be well served by initial placement of a percutaneous peripheral venous catheter whenever possible. When this fails in a child younger than age 6, intraosseous infusion should be used immediately. Following this, or in cases in which an intraosseous line cannot be placed, one must decide whether to pursue central venous cannulation or peripheral venous cutdown. Whichever technique is used, the emergency team should have prepared in advance for such eventualities and should plan carefully which vascular access technique is to be used. Appropriate equipment for either procedure should be available in most emergency departments.

See *Chapter 237* for a detailed review of vascular access techniques.

HEAD INJURY

Because the primary survey is a resuscitative survey of the critically injured patient, the assessment of the level of head injury is an important yet secondary one in the pediatric multiple trauma patient. As mentioned previously, head injuries are present in nearly 80% of all severely injured multiple trauma patients. However, maintaining a patent airway with adequate ventilation and ensuring adequate central and peripheral perfusion are extremely important in treating the head-injured child. Providing the "ABCs" is critical to the survival of head-injured children.

During the primary survey, the goal is simply to assess the general level of injury, and the best way to assess the overall central nervous system injury is the patient's level of consciousness. The Glasgow Coma Scale (GCS) is the best way to assess level of consciousness in a definitive fashion, but during the primary survey, it is only important to get a general assessment of the patient's overall level of consciousness. For this reason, the ATLS course recommends the AVPU mnemonic[3]:

A: Alert
V: Responsive to verbal stimuli
P: Responsive to painful stimuli
U: Unresponsive

By using this brief, simple assessment, the emergency physician can gain a sense of whether any neurologic injury is present. In general, a patient who responds only to painful stimuli or does not respond at all should be assumed to have a major head injury until a GCS score can be assessed. Although children with severe head injuries (GCS less than 8) were often hyperventilated (pCO_2 28 to 32) in the past, more recent studies clearly indicate that children should receive only minimal hyperventilation (pCO_2 35 to 40) unless intracranial pressure cannot be controlled by other means.[1]

In addition to assessing the overall level of consciousness, the examiner should quickly check for the size and reactivity of the pupils and the presence of any posturing or lateralizing findings. A more detailed neurologic examination can be done in the secondary survey.

SHOCK

To recognize the early stages of hypovolemic shock in children, the emergency physician must have an astute eye and a clear understanding of the differences between adults and children. *The earliest finding in pediatric patients in shock is tachycardia.*[9,14,18] Table 297.2 lists pulse values by age. Any child who has undergone major trauma and has a pulse rate above these values should be assumed to be in shock until proven otherwise, particularly if other findings of shock are present. A vascular access line is established rapidly, and at least 20 mL/kg of a crystalloid solution (usually lactated Ringer's) is given. Strict attention is paid to preinfusion and postinfusion parameters to assess the patient's response to fluid therapy. See *Chapter 236* for more details on shock.

SECONDARY SURVEY

After an overall survey of the patient's cardiorespiratory, neurologic, and shock status, the patient is undressed fully for an adequate secondary survey. Although it is important to ensure the child is undressed rapidly and appropriately, infants and small children, up until the age of about 2 years, may require warming lights or blankets to maintain their temperature at a normal level. Even in older children, particularly in the development of hypovolemic shock, the child should be covered when the secondary survey is not being performed. Children's homeostatic thermoregulatory responses are not nearly as well developed as those of adults. Undressing a small child in an air-conditioned emergency department, infusing relatively cold intravenous fluids, and placing alcohol or povidone–iodine solutions on the skin all serve to make the child hypothermic.

Two additional points are important before proceeding to the secondary survey. First, because the condition of pediatric patients may deteriorate rapidly and because these patients often present with subtle signs and symptoms, the elements of the primary survey must continually be reassessed over the course of the patient's initial emergency department resuscitation. The examiner must keep updated on the status of the airway, breathing, circulation, response to shock therapy, neurologic disability, and core body temperature. If there are signs of sudden deterioration, one can quickly run through a mental checklist of possible causes of deterioration (Table 297.3).

Second, if a nasogastric tube and indwelling bladder catheter have not been placed, the examiner should assess whether they are necessary. A nasogastric tube should be placed in any child receiving assisted ventilation, even bag-and-mask ventilation, and in patients in which there is suspicion of intraabdominal trauma or when aerophagia or crying is causing appreciable abdominal distention. An indwelling bladder catheter is placed in all patients who have signs or symptoms of shock or who may develop shock. The amount of fluid in the bladder at the time of catheterization is noted and saved in a separate container. One must not routinely place a bladder catheter in extremely young children or in those with evidence of urethral injury.

The secondary survey is usually performed in a head-to-toe fashion, which allows for an easily followed protocol approach. One must not neglect the cardiorespiratory system during the head-to-toe evaluation: The major threats to life in the *early* evaluation of the pediatric multiple trauma patient come from the cardiorespiratory system.[9] Although head injury is the most common cause of death in pediatric multiple trauma victims, providing oxygenation and ventilation, as well as central perfusion, addresses the earliest threats to life.

TABLE 297.3. Checklist for Sudden Deterioration

AIRWAY
Adequate airway position?
Adequate tidal volume?
Adequate rate?
Pneumothorax?
Tension pneumothorax?
ENDOTRACHEAL TUBE
Dislodged?
Plugged?
Right main stem bronchus?
INTRAVENOUS ACCESS
Functional?
Adequate size?
Medications infusing?
UNRECOGNIZED BLEEDING
Pelvis
Chest
Abdomen
Thighs
Retroperitoneum
UNRECOGNIZED INJURIES

Finding one severe injury during the evaluation should not cause the physician to cease evaluation, except to treat life-threatening injuries. Multiple systems injuries are common in pediatric patients, and a detailed evaluation of each body system is necessary.

Early in the secondary survey, an appropriate history is taken from the patient, the family, or the paramedics who brought the patient to the emergency department. The history should include all events leading up to the accident, the mechanism of injury, the biomechanics of injury, time of injury, initial status at the scene of injury, and clinical course during transportation. Additional details on chronic illnesses or injuries, allergies, medications, and the time of the last meal should be taken. The ATLS course of the American College of Surgeons Committee on Trauma uses the AMPLE mnemonic:

A: Allergies
M: Medications
P: Past illnesses or injuries
L: Last meal eaten before injury
E: Events preceding the injury

Physical Examination

Head

The secondary survey should begin with an in-depth evaluation of the child's head and neck, including the soft tissues, bones, ears, eyes, and neck. Any signs of obvious trauma are noted. Bleeding is stopped with pressure dressings. Mucous membranes are examined for paleness and overall hydrational status. The eyes are examined for random eye motions, pupil size and reactivity, and foreign bodies. A funduscopic examination should be performed. When direct ocular trauma is suspected, the presence or absence of hyphema must be documented. The bones and soft tissues of the midface are examined for evidence of instability or direct trauma. "Raccoon eyes" or the Battle sign may indicate anterior or posterior basal or skull fractures, respectively. The patient's upper airway, including the nasopharynx and oropharynx, is reexamined. If blood or clear fluid is present in the nares, it should be tested for cerebrospinal fluid rhinorrhea. The ears, including the tympanic membranes, should be examined for perforation, infection, or hemotympanum. In children younger than age 2, one should carefully examine the fontanelles, because they may reveal important information regarding intracranial pressure.

A detailed neurologic examination is performed during the secondary survey but is usually delayed until after the rest of the survey, unless the patient has a rapidly declining level of consciousness.

Neck

Children have shorter, more cartilaginous necks with a great deal of subcutaneous tissue, making this area more difficult to evaluate. Any evidence of cervical spine injury should be noted, including detailed information regarding the mechanism of injury and history of the accident. Pediatric patients in motor vehicle accidents occurring at over 45 mi/h, in motor vehicle accidents in which the occupant is unrestrained, in automobile–pedestrian collisions, in falls from greater than 10 ft, and with direct trauma to the posterior neck are all at higher risk for cervical spine injury. Muscular spasm is much less common in young children than it is in adults and older children, and, until proven otherwise, one should assume that a cervical spine injury is present whenever muscular splinting does occur. Because up to two-thirds of children with spinal cord injuries have no radiographic abnormality, whenever either focal muscular splinting or neurologic findings are present or if the history strongly suggests a cervical spine injury, the neck should remain immobilized, even if the cross-table lateral cervical spine film is normal.

Tracheal deviation and shifting of the midline position of the trachea are more difficult to determine in children because of their inherent anatomic differences, but both should be carefully assessed. Distended neck veins may be a sign of tension pneumothorax or cardiac tamponade, and tracheal deviation is often seen in cases of tension pneumothorax.

Chest

Examination of both the chest and the abdomen should follow the "look, listen, and feel" rule. One of the most neglected aspects of the chest examination in children is looking at the patient's spontaneous respirations and chest wall movements. Emergency physicians should be adept at noticing the normal pattern of respiration in children and how it differs from that of adults. Bilateral, symmetric chest wall rise should be present unless there is some element of chest injury. Decreased chest wall rise may be due to chest wall contusion, splinting, pneumothorax, hemothorax, or inadvertent ET intubation of the right main stem bronchus. When splinting is present, that side of the hemithorax is evaluated for any additional signs of trauma. Any signs of abrasions, lacerations, contusions, or ecchymosis may be associated with underlying pulmonary or cardiac injury.

Because the chest wall in children has less muscle and fat, it is not uncommon for forces applied to the external thorax to be transmitted to the underlying pulmonary parenchyma. The presence of retractions is a significant finding and indicates significant respiratory difficulty. Whenever such external signs of trauma are seen, a chest film is obtained to ensure that there is no underlying pulmonary contusion or hemopneumothorax.

After one looks carefully at the chest, then both sides of the thorax should be listened to in all lung fields, including both anteriorly and posteriorly. As mentioned previously, breath sounds are easily transmitted across the child's small, resilient thorax, so the value of the presence or absence of lung sounds is less important in children than in adults. Nonetheless, the chest should still be carefully auscultated, because the soft crackling sounds of subcutaneous emphysema may occasionally be heard in patients with pneumothorax or penetrating chest injury.

Finally, all aspects of the thorax should be carefully felt for tenderness or other signs of injury. Conscious patients should be asked where they hurt, and palpation should be begun away from that site.

Abdomen

Examining the abdomen of the pediatric trauma patient can yield a great deal of information regarding the presence or absence of abdominal injury. The abdominal examination requires extensive expertise in evaluation of children, but this does not necessarily mean that only the surgeon or pediatric surgeon has the skills to do it. Indeed, most emergency physicians should have a wealth of experience in examining the normal pediatric abdomen, because up to 25% of all patients presenting to the emergency department are children. Only by doing a careful, detailed examination on each pediatric patient presenting to the emergency department can this expertise be gained.

The examination is begun by carefully looking at the child's abdomen for evidence of splinting, contusions, abrasions, ecchymosis, or distention. Both the front and back of the abdomen are examined for these signs of trauma. Listening to the abdomen for bowel sounds is probably the least helpful of the aspects of the physical examination, because the presence or absence of bowel sounds neither indicates nor precludes the presence of abdominal injury in children.

The most helpful aspect of the pediatric abdominal examination is palpation. Conscious patients should be asked where they hurt, and the examination is then begun as far away from that site as possible. The patient needs to be reassured as much as possible, and the examination should be done gently. It may help to have the patient place a hand on top of the examiner's hand to reassure the patient that no undue pain or pressure will be exerted. Rebound tenderness should always be evaluated last, because it is difficult to obtain information from palpation after this potentially painful procedure. Attention must be paid to examining the suprapubic area, because the bladder is an intraperitoneal organ in the child.

Repeat examinations of the abdomen are necessary in the child. The child will initially be frightened and will cry during the examination, which may make abdominal examination difficult. Repeated examinations commonly reveal significant findings that would have been missed with a single examination. In cases in which potential abdominal injury is present, a soft nasogastric tube is placed to prevent abdominal distention and to empty the stomach to whatever degree possible. The abdominal girth is measured and marked on the child's skin with a pen so that any difference may be noted on reexamination. In children, abdominal distention may be an early finding of abdominal injury.

A rectal examination must be performed on all children, gently and with a well-lubricated, gloved finger. Most children can be talked through this examination quite easily, and the entire pelvic rim can be palpated for signs of injury.

Pelvis

After the abdomen is examined, the bony pelvis and the perineum are inspected. The entire bony pelvis is palpated for instability or tenderness. The patient is asked to gently flex and abduct the hip, because this may detect subtle pelvic fractures. Assessment is done for urethral meatal blood and evidence of scrotal hematoma or swelling.

Musculoskeletal Evaluation

The examiner should palpate carefully over the entire bony skeleton for tenderness or swelling. All bony areas are examined visually for deformity, abrasion, contusion, or hematoma. An obvious deformity is splinted and compared with the opposite side; appropriate radiographs should be taken. In particular, any asymmetric motions of the extremities should be noted, because this may be an early sign of a fracture. In general, one should assume a fracture exists, until proven otherwise, in any extremity that the child is not moving normally. The examiner should evaluate and document the pulse and neurologic status of the extremities.

Neurologic Examination

In completing the secondary survey, a neurologic examination is done. Correlation of the history is critical in determining whether a neurologic injury is present, as well as the extent of the injury. The mechanism of injury and any potential injury transfer are carefully assessed, as well as the progression of neurologic findings since the time of injury. The paramedics are critical in obtaining this information and should be spoken to directly when they present to the emergency department with a pediatric multiple trauma patient.

By far, the most critical aspect in evaluating the potentially head-injured patient is the overall level of consciousness. The best way to accomplish this is with the GCS.[5,15] The GCS assesses patients with regard to eye opening, verbal stimuli, and motor responses. This scale has been tested on thousands of adult and pediatric patients and has been found to correlate extremely well with outcome. In children in the preverbal age group (younger than 2 to 3 years old), the score is modified by giving any child who cries a full verbal score; this reflects the fact that comatose children do not cry.[15] In testing motor response, the response is recorded on both the right and left sides, although the best response is considered the GCS score. A pediatric GCS has been proposed but is not widely used (Table 297.4).

Patients with a GCS score of 10 or less are considered to have a potentially serious head injury, and neurosurgical consultation is obtained after ensuring ventilation, oxygenation, and perfusion. The GCS is also extremely accurate in evaluating changes in the level of consciousness. A loss of two points in the score indicates severe neurologic deterioration, while a three-point decline usually is an indication for immediate neurosurgi-

TABLE 297.4. Pediatric Glasgow Coma Score

Glasgow Coma Score	Pediatric Modification	
Eye opening	**Eye opening**	
≥ 1 year	*0–1 year*	
4 Spontaneously	Spontaneously	
3 To verbal command	To shout	
2 To pain	To pain	
1 No response	No response	
Best motor response	**Best motor response**	
≥ 1 year	*0–1 year*	
6 Obeys command	Normal spontaneous movements	
5 Localizes pain	Withdraws to touch	
4 Flexion withdrawal	Flexion withdrawal	
3 Flexion abnormal (decorticate)	Flexion abnormal (decorticate)	
2 Extension (decerebrate)	Extension (decerebrate)	
1 No response	No response	
Best verbal response	**Best verbal response**	
> 5 years	*2–5 years*	*0–2 years*
5 Oriented and converses	Appropriate words and phrases	Cries appropriately, smiles, and coos
4 Disoriented and converses	Inappropriate words	Cries
3 Inappropriate words	Cries/screams	Inappropriate crying/screaming
2 Incomprehensible sounds	Grunts	Grunts
1 No response	No response	No response

cal intervention. The overall level of consciousness, and thus the GCS score, can be affected by hypoxia, hypotension, the presence of intoxicants, or a postictal state, but one must assume that the patient has a head injury until proven otherwise. See *Chapter 299* for a detailed discussion of pediatric head trauma.

After the level of consciousness is assessed, the patient's vital signs are reassessed to ensure adequate oxygenation, ventilation, and perfusion. The pupils are examined for size and reactivity, as well as the presence of random eye movements. Movement of the extremities, including lateralizing findings, are evaluated. The plantar responses, deep tendon reflexes, and presence of oculovestibular reflexes are tested. Oculocephalic reflexes ("doll's eyes" reflexes) should not be assessed until it is absolutely certain that the cervical spine is uninjured.

Laboratory Studies and Radiologic Evaluation

In any patient in which the primary and secondary surveys have identified possible or documented evidence of shock, altered level of consciousness, or evidence of either single- or multisystem injury, a complete set of trauma laboratory studies should be ordered. This should consist of the following: blood cell count; determination of electrolyte, glucose, blood urea nitrogen, and amylase levels; urinalysis; type and screen or crossmatch for one-half to one-fourth the total blood volume; prothrombin time; partial thromboplastin time; and platelet count. In patients with respiratory compromise or on whom artificial ventilation is being performed, an arterial blood gas analysis is obtained. The nasogastric and rectal contents for occult blood are examined. In older children, alcohol or other intoxicants may contribute to the patient's response to injury, so appropriate toxicologic studies are ordered. The need for additional laboratory studies should be guided by the patient's physical findings and clinical course.

Radiography has a limited role in the initial management of the pediatric trauma victim. Certainly, the cervical spine may need radiographic evaluation, although its limitations have been pointed out earlier. The physical examination is the clinician's first resource in caring for all injured pediatric patients; radiographic studies should simply confirm or verify suspicions. In evaluating the pediatric multiple trauma victim, chest and cervical spine radiographs have the highest priority, while abdominal, pelvis, and extremity films are less urgently needed. Additional radiographic studies, such as computed tomography of the head, chest, and abdomen; ultrasonography; and contrast studies, should be guided by the patient's physical findings, the clinical course, and the availability of such resources.[6,8,10,11] The emergency physician, trauma surgeon, and radiology department should agree in advance on the appropriate protocols for pediatric multiple trauma victims. Controversies regarding radiologic studies should be settled in advance whenever possible.

DEFINITIVE CARE

Consultation

Whether the pediatric multiple trauma victim is resuscitated in a general hospital emergency department or a pediatric trauma center, the best available resources for the child's care should be implemented at the earliest possible time. *Immediate surgical consultation is required for any pediatric multiple trauma victim with either single-system or multisystem injury or in whom there has been an altered level of consciousness or documented shock.* Although an increasing number of pediatric multiple trauma victims can be managed without surgery, this in no way implies that the evaluation and care of such patients can be handled by nonsurgeons. Indeed, the decision whether to operate requires considerable surgical expertise.[4]

Because 80% of children have head injuries in association with multiple trauma, appropriate neurosurgical consultants should be readily available. One must use caution in assuming that children have isolated head injuries: Although up to 50% of patients with severe head trauma have relatively minor additional injuries, each child requires a detailed evaluation to ensure that no occult injuries are present. In such cases, consultation with both the neurosurgeon and the appropriate pediatric or trauma surgeon should be obtained.

Indications for Transfer

The decision to transfer a pediatric multiple trauma patient to a definitive care facility depends largely on the patient's stability and on the availability of resources of a nearby pediatric trauma center. In some cases, severe intraabdominal bleeding may require immediate operative intervention to obtain appropriate hemostasis. However, these cases represent a small minority of pediatric trauma cases. For that reason, it is important to consult in advance with the appropriate pediatric trauma centers within each emergency department's geographic area to ensure that the initial resuscitation reflects the standards of the nearby center. Whenever possible, the initial resuscitative and management approach in the emergency department should reflect standards similar to those of the tertiary pediatric critical care center to which the patient may be transferred. Most centers are extremely active in outreach education and appreciate the opportunity to work with outlying hospital emergency departments in continuing medical education and quality assurance programs. *The overall outcome of the pediatric patient depends less on how long it takes the child to reach the pediatric critical care center than it does on ensuring that the regional center's expertise is applied as early as possible in the referring hospital.*[4]

Indications for Admission

Obviously, a child with a GCS score of 8 and major cardiovascular instability needs to be admitted to the intensive care unit, but determining the criteria for admission for the "gray area" patients is much more difficult. In general, any pediatric patient who has lost consciousness (however briefly) or in whom single-system or multisystem injury has required the placement of an intravenous line should be observed in the hospital for at least 24 hours. This is to ensure that continued and complete observation of the patient results in a clear delineation of the extent and severity of injuries. Furthermore, the numerous differences between adults and children require a careful approach to childrens' injuries and a complete evaluation.

OUTCOME FROM PEDIATRIC MULTIPLE TRAUMA

The single most important determinant of outcome in pediatric multiple trauma patients is the presence or absence of severe head injury.[5,7,8,15,16,21] Numerous outcome studies have documented that patients with severe head injuries have a poorer outcome than those without such injuries. However, the outcome from head injury in pediatric patients is much better than in adults.[5] Even in patients with GCS scores of 3 or 4, a good recovery can be expected in fully 30%. For that reason, virtually all pediatric multiple trauma patients should be resuscitated aggressively. In general, the overall mortality from severe pediatric trauma (in which two or more body systems are injured to a severe degree) is still only 10% to 15%. Recent data from numerous pediatric trauma centers indicate that these mortality figures may be decreasing with the advent of a systems management approach to such patients.

Pediatric Trauma Scoring

As with any medical or surgical disease, the only way to appropriately study a subject is to be able to quantify it. Because detailed studies on pediatric trauma have been relatively recent, specific efforts to quantify pediatric trauma have also been limited to several recent studies. Mayer and colleagues developed the Modified Injury Severity Scale (MISS) score to reflect differences in pediatric versus adult trauma victims.[15,16] This scale focused on neurologic injuries and used elements of the GCS score to quantify the nature of head injury in pediatric patients. This score was later modified to include the presence or absence of a mass lesion, as well as other details on the severity of initial impact, to allow for more accurate scoring of pediatric trauma victims. This scale was used in retrospective studies primarily, and it was well recognized that a prehospital score was needed to help classify injury severity in pediatric patients.

Accordingly, Tepas and Ramenofsky developed the Pediatric Trauma Score (PTS) in an attempt to further recognize the importance of the unique needs of the pediatric trauma with regard to prehospital and emergency department classification.[17,18,20] This score (Fig. 297.3) allows easy classification of the pediatric trauma victim in either the prehospital or emergency department setting. Studies on over 6,000 pediatric patients indicate that the PTS has a high validity as a predictor of injury severity in both settings.

Nonetheless, some studies indicate that comparison of adults and children in utilizing the Trauma Score (TS) and Revised Trauma Score (RTS) shows fewer differences between adults and children than have been predicted in the past.[7,8] Most pediatric surgeons and pediatric emergency physicians use the PTS to calculate injury severity in the prehospital setting.

COMMON PITFALLS

- Failure to complete the primary survey before starting the secondary assessment may lead to missed opportunities to provide treatment of life-threatening injuries.
- Lack of advance preparation and organization of equipment, medications, resources, and personnel will result in a disorganized resuscitation phase with the potential for poor outcomes.

Component	+2	+1	−1
Size	>20 kg	10–20 kg	<10 kg
Airway	Normal	Maintainable	Unmaintainable
CNS	Awake	Obtunded	Coma
Systolic BP	>90 mm Hg	90–50 mm Hg	<50 mm Hg
Open Wound	None	Minor	Major
Skeletal	None	Closed Fx	Open/Mult Fx's
		TOTAL (PTS)	____________

Figure 297.3. Pediatric trauma score.

References

1. American Association of Neurological Surgeons. *Guidelines for the management of severe head injury.* New York: Gitken Neuroscience Center, 1997 (212-772-0608).
2. American College of Emergency Physicians—Trauma Committee. Guidelines for trauma care systems. *Ann Emerg Med* 1993;22:1079.
3. American College of Surgeons—Committee on Trauma. *Advanced trauma life support course.* Chicago: American College of Surgeons, 1997.
4. American College of Surgeons—Committee on Trauma. *Pediatric trauma care. Resources for the optimal care of the injured patient: 1999.* Chicago: American College of Surgeons, 1998.
5. Bruce DA, Schut L, Bruno LA, et al. Outcome following severe head injuries in children. *J Neurosurg* 1978;48:679.
6. Cooney DR. Splenic and hepatic trauma in children. *Surg Clin North Am* 1981;61:1165.
7. Eichelberger MR, Champion HR, Sacco WJ, et al. Pediatric coefficients for TRSS analysis. *J Trauma* 1993;34:319.
8. Eichelberger MR, Mangubat EA, Sacco WJ, et al. Outcome analysis of blunt injury in children. *J Trauma* 1988;4:1109.
9. Eichelberger MR, Randolph JG. Pediatric Trauma: an algorithm for diagnosis and therapy. *J Trauma* 1983;23:91.
10. Ein SH, Shandling B, Simpson JS, et al. Non-operative management of the traumatized spleen in children: how and why. *J Pediatr Surg* 1978;13:117.
11. Karp MP, Cooney DR, Pros GA, et al. The non-operative management of pediatric hepatic trauma. *J Pediatr Surg* 1983;19:512.
12. Lubitz DS, Seidel JS, Chameides L, et al. A rapid method for estimating weight and resuscitation drug dosages from length in the pediatric age group. *Ann Emerg Med* 1988;17:576.
13. Mayer T. Initial evaluation and management of the injured child. In: Mayer T. ed. *Emergency management of pediatric trauma.* Philadelphia: WB Saunders, 1985.
14. Mayer TA. Pediatric multiple trauma. In: Howell JM, ed. *Emergency medicine.* Philadelphia: WB Saunders, 1998:1091–1100.
15. Mayer T, Clark P, Walker ML. Further experience with the Modified Injury Severity Scale. *J Trauma* 1984;24:31.
16. Mayer T, Walker ML, Matlak ME. Causes of morbidity and mortality in severe pediatric trauma. *JAMA* 1981;245:719.
17. Ramenofsky ML, Ramenofsky MB, Jurkovich IJ, et al. The predictive validity of the Pediatric Trauma Score. *J Trauma* 1988;4:1038.
18. Ramenofsky ML, Morese TS. Standards of care for the critically injured pediatric patient. *J Trauma* 1982;22:921.
19. Taylor GA, Fallat ME, Potter BM, et al. The role of computed tomography in blunt abdominal trauma in children. *J Trauma* 1988;4:660.
20. Tepas JJ, Ramenofsky ML, Mollitt DL, et al. The Pediatric Trauma Score as a predictor of injury severity: an objective assessment. *J Trauma* 1988;4:425.
21. Wesson DE, Williams JI, Salmi LR, et al. Evaluating a pediatric trauma program. *J Trauma* 1988;4:1226.
22. Rhodes M, Smith S, Boorse D. Pediatric trauma patients in an "adult" trauma center. *J Trauma* 1993;35:384.
23. Widone MD, ed. *Injury prevention and control for children and youth.* Elk Grove, IL: American Academy of Pediatrics, 1997.

CHAPTER 298
Hemorrhagic Shock

Thom A. Mayer

Perhaps one of the most overused words in the English language is *shock.* What is surprising is that even physicians and other health-care professionals use the word imprecisely and incorrectly. Many physicians may think about shock the way Supreme Court Justice John Potter Stewart described pornography: "I may not be able to define it, but I know what it is when I see it." Because of the imprecision of definition and recognition of shock, especially in children, the central goal of this chapter is to give a working definition of *hemorrhagic shock,* to tell how to recognize it immediately in children, and to provide an effective treatment plan for patients who present in shock.

The simplest definition of *shock* is that it is a generalized state of inadequate tissue perfusion that results in impaired cellular respiration.[11] Although maintaining adequate tissue perfusion involves a number of extremely complicated cardiovascular, neurohumoral, and other factors, perhaps the best and most simple analogy is a mechanical one: Maintaining adequate tissue perfusion requires a properly functioning pump (the heart) that can deliver an adequate type and volume of fluid (blood) through appropriate vessels (arteries, veins, and capillaries) without obstruction. Failure to perfuse the tissues adequately may result from defects of the pump, fluid, or vessels or from an obstruction to flow.

During the immediate phase of care of the pediatric trauma victim, shock is nearly always due to hypovolemia, usually caused by external or internal hemorrhage.[7] In the vast majority of pediatric trauma victims presenting in shock, the shock is caused by hemorrhagic factors. An exception would be patients suffering from major burns, in which plasma is the major volume constituent lost; virtually all other pediatric trauma victims have at least some element of hemorrhagic shock.

PATHOPHYSIOLOGY

Development of shock is a dynamic process, involving many systems that progressively produce well-defined signs and symptoms of the disease. The problem is that the symptoms produced are clear only to the clinician who recognizes the overall pathophysiology of the disease. Although some aspects of the pathophysiology of hemorrhagic shock in adults and children are similar, there are also important differences.

In both the adult and pediatric patient, the patient's earliest response to either major or minor blood loss consists of local factors, including spasm of local blood vessels and activation of the clotting cascade. This is followed immediately by a rapid outpouring of catecholamines, which have both local and systemic effects. One of the major differences between adults and children is that the child's cardiovascular system is particularly capable of increasing vasomotor tone in response to this catecholamine surge.[7,11] This increase in vasomotor tone is particularly noticeable in the large venous beds and in the skin. Because the child's skin is thinner and lacks the more stratified epithelium of the adult, the effects of increased vasomotor tone are more visible in the child than in the adult. This accounts for the extremely mottled skin appearance that is a classic finding in children, even in early stages of hemorrhagic shock. Because up to 60% of the total circulating blood volume may reside in large venous beds and in the circulation to the skin and extremities, the profound "autotransfusion" effect seen in children allows them to compensate extremely well for even relatively large and acute blood losses.

In addition to the catecholamine effect on vascular resistance and stroke volume, children are also sensitive to the inotropic effects of the norepinephrine output. Thus, the child's earliest response to either minor or major hemorrhage is to produce increased vascular resistance and tachycardia. The increased vascular resistance becomes apparent to the clinician as an increase in the pulse pressure or as a prolonged capillary refill time, because perfusion to the extremities is both decreased and more noticeable.

As blood loss increases or continues, extracellular fluid from the interstitial space is mobilized into the vascular space. As further losses continue, decreased organ perfusion results in anaerobic metabolism. If hemorrhage either continues or ongoing losses are not replaced, the cell's sodium–potassium pump begins to fail, and structural damage, acidosis, and functional damage ensue (Fig. 298.1).

EMERGENCY DEPARTMENT EVALUATION

Because the child's response to the early catecholamine output is more profound than an adult's, recognizing shock in children (Table 298.1) requires a complete understanding of this difference, as well as astute clinical skills. Until the child loses about 15% of total blood volume, the only signs of shock will be local swelling and bleeding and an increased heart rate. For this reason, *tachycardia out of proportion to that seen in adults is often the only finding early in the course of hemorrhagic shock in the pediatric patient.*[4,7] However, children's pulse rates vary widely according to age. While there are charts that summarize the maximum pulse rate in children, it is easiest to remember that the pulse should be less than 140 in newborns, less than 120 in ages 1 month to 2 years, less than 100 in ages 2 to 10 years, and less than 75 in children 10 years and older.[6] *Any child with a heart rate above these levels should be assumed to be in shock until proven otherwise.*

Physicians too often assume that tachycardia is due to either anxiety, fright, pain, or reaction to parental stimulation. This is a dangerous precedent: Many such children are in the earliest stages of shock and require immediate fluid resuscitation. The patient's vital signs should always be noted carefully, paying particular attention to the pulse rate. During the initial evaluation, the pulse rate should be retaken, because the patient's initial anxiety and pain should have abated somewhat. If tachycardia persists, one should assume that the patient is in shock and administer appropriate treatment.

In addition to changes in the normal pulse rate, children also have a different normal circulating blood volume and blood

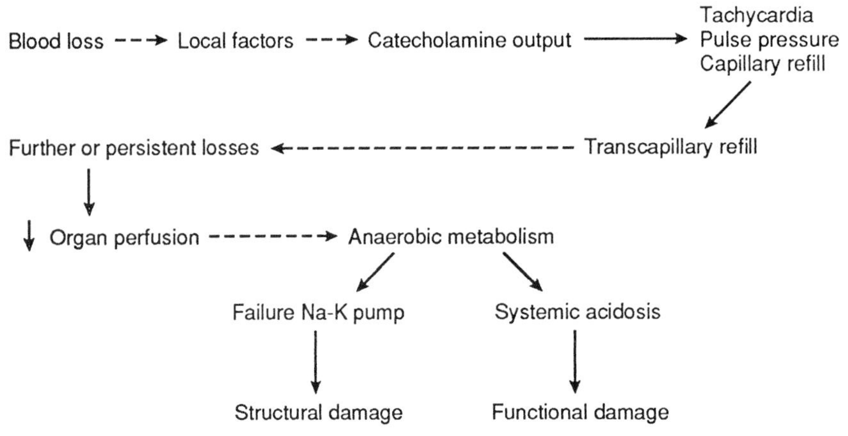

Figure 298.1. Pathophysiology of pediatric hemorrhagic shock.

TABLE 298.1. Clinical Signs of Acute Hemorrhagic Shock

% Blood Loss	Clinical Signs
≤15	Slightly increased heart rate Local swelling, bleeding
15–25	Increased heart rate Increased diastolic blood pressure Prolonged capillary refill
25–50	Above findings plus: Hypotension Confusion Acidosis Decreased urine output
>50	Refractory hypotension Refractory acidosis

pressure than do adults.[9,11] Children have larger total blood volumes, about 8.5% of body weight; the average blood volume of a man is about 7% of body weight, and it is about 7.5% in women. The best general estimate for general circulating blood volume in children is 85 mL/kg.

Children's blood pressure also varies according to age. Again, tables and charts are available to indicate a child's appropriate blood pressure, but the following simple formula gives a *minimal* systolic blood pressure:

Newborn: 60 mm Hg
Infant: 70 mm Hg
Child: 70 + (2 × age in years)

The diastolic blood pressure in a child should be about two-thirds of the systolic blood pressure.[1] Both the systolic and diastolic blood pressures should be assessed in every pediatric patient. Because an increase in the total peripheral resistance causes an early rise in the diastolic pressure (and therefore a fall in the pulse pressure), diastolic blood pressure should be assessed routinely in all children. All emergency departments should have a wide range of pediatric blood pressure cuffs. A correctly sized cuff should cover two-thirds of the distance between the point of the child's shoulder and the olecranon process.

When the child has lost about 15% of total blood volume, the sole sign of shock may be a slight increase in pulse rate. When 15% to 25% of blood volume has been lost, additional factors come into play. Adrenergic stimulation is maximal, venous beds are fully contracted, and peripheral resistance is elevated, resulting in increased diastolic blood pressure (or decreased pulse pressure). In addition, prolonged capillary refill time and further increases in heart rate may be seen. Although increased respiratory rate, anxiety, and thirst are often present in adults with shock at this level, these criteria are more difficult to evaluate in the child.

Although up to 25% of the child's total blood volume may have been lost, shock can be detected only by looking carefully at the heart rate, the diastolic blood pressure, and the capillary refill time. *Not until blood loss reaches 25% to 30% of total blood volume are hypotension, confusion, decreased urine output, and acidosis evident.*

The accentuated response to adrenergic stimulation is the primary reason that hypotension develops so late in the child with hemorrhagic shock.[6,7,11] Waiting for hypotension to develop before recognizing shock threatens the child's life. A complete set of vital signs should be obtained, including an accurate pulse rate and systolic and diastolic blood pressures, on each patient who presents with even minor trauma. Paying careful attention to such details in all pediatric patients helps the clinician develop the clinical judgment necessary to recognize pediatric patients in early stages of shock.

If blood loss continues or progresses, decreased urine output, altered mental status, and the development of systemic acidosis occur. However, using any of these factors to recognize shock has severe limitations. Up to 80% of all pediatric multiple trauma victims have some element of head injury, making it difficult to follow mental status as a primary indicator of central perfusion. In addition, it can be difficult to assess mental status in young children.

Urine output is an excellent indicator of overall central perfusion in the ongoing management of the pediatric and adult shock victim, because it accurately reflects renal blood flow (in the absence of postrenal obstruction). One of the body's earliest responses to hypovolemia is to decrease blood flow to the renal bed, which, under normal conditions, receives 20% of the cardiac output. However, although urine output is an excellent ongoing measure of central perfusion, it is difficult to assess within the first 15 to 30 minutes of trauma resuscitation, because it is a dynamic rather than a static value. If children are delayed in the emergency department for an hour or more, the normal urine output in a child is at least 1 mL/kg/h. In any patient with signs or symptoms of shock, a catheter should be placed and the amount of urine present in the bladder at the time of trauma should be noted. This urine should be placed in a separate container, because it does not reflect ongoing urine output after the development of shock.

EMERGENCY DEPARTMENT MANAGEMENT

There are three primary goals of shock therapy: (1) to restore effective circulatory volume, (2) to maximize oxygen delivery, and (3) to decrease ongoing blood loss.

Restoring Effective Circulatory Volume

Any increase in blood flow will result in an increase in overall cardiac output and tissue perfusion. The central tenet in shock therapy in pediatric patients is to immediately restore the effective circulatory volume. Any child with any signs of shock, including persistent tachycardia, should receive an intravenous line and an appropriate fluid bolus.

All emergency physicians should be skilled in placing percutaneous peripheral intravenous lines in children, as well as alternative means of obtaining vascular access in children (percutaneous central venous cannulation, intraosseous infusion, or, rarely, peripheral venous cutdown).[3,10] Although peripheral venous cutdown and percutaneous central venous cannulation require a moderate level of skill, placement of a needle into bone marrow can be mastered with minimal training.[8]

Regardless of the site of infusion, children require an immediate and appropriate fluid bolus of 20 mL/kg. The bolus is given as quickly as possible, over no more than 5 to 10 minutes. In many cases, this initial fluid bolus therapy occurs over 20 to 30 minutes, during which time the child continues to bleed internally.

The prevailing wisdom in both adult and pediatric trauma patients is that the initial fluid infusion should be a crystalloid solution, even though some pediatric authorities claim that colloids are better in the resuscitation of the pediatric patient. Colloids play virtually no role in the emergency department, and crystalloids should be used in the initial treatment of the pediatric patient presenting in shock.[2,4,6,7] The initial fluid bolus therapy is usually lactated Ringer's solution. Normal saline can also be used, but large fluid infusions with 0.9% sodium chloride can result in hyperchloremic acidosis.

Children who present with hypotension in addition to tachycardia and a decreased pulse pressure have lost at least 25% to 30% of their total circulating blood volume and are in extreme danger of rapid decompensation. Under such circumstances, immediate infusion of an initial fluid bolus of 40 mL/kg is done. Weight can be estimated by a length-based system such as the Broselow Resuscitation Tape.[5]

One of the most common problems in pediatric trauma resuscitation is the physician's reluctance to infuse the appropriate fluid volume to a child with signs and symptoms of shock. For example, if a 4-year-old boy presents after a motor vehicle accident, with a pulse rate of 130 beats per minute and a blood pressure of 90/75 mm Hg, some clinicians may not recognize the presence of shock. This preschooler's heart rate is above 120 beats per minute, while the systolic blood pressure is adequate and the diastolic blood pressure is elevated. This child has therefore lost at least 15% to 25% of his total blood volume and requires immediate infusion of 20 mL/kg for effective therapy. If this child's weight is an estimated 20 kg, he should immediately receive about 400 mL of lactated Ringer's solution.

The single most important determinant of the adequacy of ongoing fluid resuscitation is the child's response to the fluid infusion. For this reason, one must make a mental note of the initial pulse, respirations, blood pressure, and diastolic blood pressure at the time the initial fluid infusion is begun. Furthermore, the nurse responsible for charting should also note carefully the time that the infusion is begun. After infusion of the appropriate fluid bolus, the shock parameters are reassessed to determine whether the patient's condition is improving, staying the same, or deteriorating.

The second aspect of restoring effective circulatory volume is transfusion. In the pediatric patient, packed red blood cells are infused if the patient fails to respond to a total of 40 to 60 mL/kg of crystalloid infusion. Based on the extent of physical findings, rapid infusion of 5 to 10 mL/kg of packed red blood cells is warranted, through a blood warmer if possible. Rapidly infusing cold blood into a child can cause major problems with hypothermia, which may make the child resistant to the usual resuscitative measures.

If the child's cardiovascular parameters respond to the initial fluid bolus of 20 mL/kg, one should monitor the child closely. If the cardiovascular parameters remain stable, the total fluid infusion should be according to the principles in Table 298.2. If the child has lost less than 25% of total blood volume, the total amount of blood lost should be replaced with 3 mL of lactated Ringer's solution for each estimated milliliter of blood lost. (This formula accounts for the phenomenon of transcapillary refill, in which interstitial fluid is mobilized into the vascular space by the body's normal physiologic response.) If the patient has lost more than 25% of total blood volume, half of the loss is corrected with lactated Ringer's solution on the basis of 3 mL of lactated Ringer's solution per milliliter of blood loss. The rest of the child's lost blood volume is corrected on a milliliter-per-milliliter basis with packed red blood cells. All patients who require transfusion to maintain their cardiovascular parameters should be observed closely, because major hemorrhage has occurred.

TABLE 298.2. Total Fluid Infusion in Pediatric Hemorrhagic Shock

% Blood Loss	Replacement
<25	3 ml LR per mL blood loss
25–50	1/2 volume = 3 mL LR per mL blood
	1/2 volume = 1 mL PRBC per mL blood loss
>50	Type specific or O negative or O positive
	Amount titrated to ongoing urine output

LR, lactated Ringer's solution; PRBC, packed red blood cells.

One additional means of potentially restoring effective circulatory volume is by using pneumatic antishock garments, also known as military antishock trousers (MAST). It was initially thought that antishock trousers could result in large "autotransfusions" of blood to the body, but studies in adults indicated this was not so. MAST have not been effective in the treatment of hemorrhagic shock in major pediatric trauma, with the occasional exception of pelvic fractures, and may cause complications such as compartment syndrome and ischemia. Because of the child's dramatic increase in vasomotor tone to adrenergic output, it is highly unlikely that antishock trousers result in any significant autotransfusion in the child.[1]

Maximizing Oxygen Delivery

The second goal of shock therapy is to maximize oxygen delivery. By far, the most important aspect in doing so is to ensure an adequate airway. A stable airway is critical in the pediatric multiple trauma victim, particularly one in hemorrhagic shock. In addition, adequate oxygen should be supplied. Virtually all multiple trauma patients should receive 100% humidified and warmed oxygen in both the prehospital and emergency department phases of care.

Other potential means of maximizing oxygen delivery is by transfusing packed red blood cells to increase oxygen-carrying capacity and by improving myocardial contractility in patients in whom this factor is depressed. Decreasing oxygen demand is also of potential benefit but is usually more pertinent to the intensive care unit phase of care.

Decreasing Blood Loss

The time-honored principles of decreasing blood loss in the shock victim have remained largely unchanged. Pressure is placed on any external bleeding points, which are then elevated. The head of pediatric trauma patients with external hemorrhage should be elevated, but pressure dressings must always be put on the head before elevating it; in the event of a dural sinus tear, an air embolism could be produced by elevating the head without an appropriate dressing. In general, the only bleeding sites that should be controlled with hemostats are ones that are extremely superficial and those on the head. On the extremities, the vascular and neurologic bundles travel in close proximity, and nerves may be inadvertently clamped unless extreme caution is used. Patients who continue to hemorrhage, either externally or internally, may need surgery. Finally, transfusion with either platelets, fresh-frozen plasma, or cryoprecipitate may be necessary in selected patients with specific bleeding disorders. Such transfusions are limited only to patients with documented bleeding abnormalities.

DISPOSITION

Role of the Consultant

The immediate resuscitation of the pediatric trauma victim with hemorrhagic shock is the emergency physician's responsibility. Emergency physicians should be trained in evaluating and resuscitating pediatric trauma victims, including those with hemorrhagic shock. They should be capable of recognizing the manifestations of shock, placing an appropriate intravascular line, and beginning initial fluid resuscitation. However, in virtually all patients who require intravenous fluid therapy, either a pediatric surgeon or a general surgeon skilled in the care of the pediatric trauma patient should be consulted for final disposition. Patients who receive intravenous lines and fluid bolus therapy and those whose shock parameters do not immediately return to normal should be observed for at least 24 hours to rule out unrecognized ongoing bleeding.

In most cases in which ongoing fluid therapy is required, the skills of a radiologic imaging specialist should be obtained to determine which studies will be required. Additional expertise in the field of pediatric neurosurgery, pediatric intensive care, and other surgical subspecialties may be necessary, depending on the type and extent of the patient's injuries.

As with any emergency, the patient is best served by a prospective approach. Emergency departments can provide better care for injured children by discussing in advance the appropriate treatment and diagnostic therapy protocols. Emergency physicians should consult with trauma surgeons, pediatric surgeons, and radiologists to develop a consensus approach to all phases of pediatric trauma care.

Indications for Admission

Any patient who manifests any signs or symptoms of hemorrhagic shock should be admitted for observation. Exceptions are patients who present with relatively minor trauma and signs of tachycardia who respond immediately to initial fluid bolus therapy and are not found to have any significant injuries, but even these patients need to be observed in the emergency department for several hours before discharge.

Transfer Considerations

Each emergency department caring for pediatric patients should have appropriate transfer arrangements with a pediatric critical care center or pediatric trauma center in the area. Although 75% to 85% of all pediatric trauma victims can be cared for locally, the remainder who require the resources of a regional pediatric trauma center must be transferred rapidly, so that the center's resources can be used as early as possible. Consultation with the center is done ahead of time, so that the protocols for patient care can be used at the referring hospital as well.

For children with hemorrhagic shock who are transferred to a regional pediatric trauma center, one must ensure there is a functioning intravenous line before the transfer. It is better to take the extra time to ensure a functioning line than to risk having no intravenous access during the transfer. Providing an adequate airway with appropriate oxygenation and ventilation, in most cases, will require placing an endotracheal tube in patients with serious illnesses or injuries. Patients in mild phases of hemorrhagic shock may not require endotracheal intubation.

In most cases, an indwelling bladder catheter will be required to allow ongoing monitoring of urine output during the transfer. Because 80% of pediatric trauma victims have head injuries, appropriate care should be given to management of head injury during the transfer.

COMMON PITFALLS

- Lack of attention to detail while evaluating the patient. The only way to recognize the sometimes subtle signs and symptoms that present in early pediatric hemorrhagic shock is to become familiar with normal physical findings and their variance in the wealth of pediatric patients seen in the emergency department.
- Failure to recognize that tachycardia is the earliest and most consistent sign of shock in the pediatric patient
- The tendency to attribute tachycardia to factors such as anxiety or pain rather than to shock. Because tachycardia's role in the early development of shock often goes unrecognized, many physicians fail to place an intravenous line in such patients and give an appropriate fluid bolus.
- The tendency to underinfuse with an appropriate intravenous fluid. Some physicians fail to give at least 20 mL/kg. Some patients still are given nonisotonic crystalloid solutions.
- Failure to follow the ongoing shock parameters in the pediatric multiple trauma victim, even after appropriate fluid bolus therapy

References

1. American Heart Association and American Academy of Pediatrics. *Textbook of pediatric advanced live support*. Dallas: American Heart Association, 1997.
2. Carcillo JA, Davis AL, Zaritsky A. Role of early fluid resuscitation in pediatric septic shock. *JAMA* 1991;266:1242.
3. Hodge D, Fleisher G. Pediatric catheter flow rates. *Am J Emerg Med* 1985;3:403.
4. Kallen RJ, Lonergan JM. Fluid resuscitation of acute hypovolemic hypoperfusion in pediatrics. *Pediatr Clin North Am* 1990;37:287
5. Lubitz DS, Seidel JS, Chameides L, et al. A rapid method for estimating weight and resuscitation drug dosages from length in the pediatric age group. *Ann Emerg Med* 1988;17:576.
6. Mayer T. Initial evaluation and management of the injured child. In: Mayer T, ed. *Emergency management of pediatric trauma*. Philadelphia: WB Saunders, 1985.
7. Mayer T. Management of hypovolemic shock. In: Mayer T, ed. *Emergency management of pediatric trauma*. Philadelphia: WB Saunders, 1985.
8. Parrish GA. Intraosseous infusion in the emergency department. *Am J Emerg Med* 1986;4:59.
9. Perkin S, Levin L. Shock in the pediatric patient: I and II. *J Pediatr*1 982;101:163.
10. Rowe MI, O'Neill JA Jr, Grosfeld JL, et al. *Vascular access: essentials of pediatric surgery*. Philadelphia: Mosby, 1995:138.
11. Tobin JR, Wetzel RC. Shock and multisystem organ dysfunction. In: Rogers MC, ed. *Textbook of pediatric intensive care*. Baltimore: Williams & Wilkins, 1996.

CHAPTER 299
Head Trauma

Dee Hodge III and Kimberly S. Quayle

Trauma is the leading cause of death in children older than 1 year in the United States; 75% or more of these deaths are associated with significant central nervous system (CNS) injury.[17] Approximately 150,000 to 300,000 children are hospitalized each year as a result of head injury.[2,10] Falls are the leading cause of head injuries in children, especially in those younger than 5 years of age.

Motor vehicle collisions with bicyclists and pedestrians become more significant in school-age children, while motor vehicle occupant injuries, assaults, and sports injuries are more common in the adolescent age group. Motor vehicle collisions are the leading cause of severe and fatal head injuries for all pediatric age groups, except for infants, for whom nonaccidental trauma is the most common cause of serious injury.[1,22]

ORGAN SYSTEMS

Anatomy

Figure 299.1 shows the cross-sectional anatomy of the head and associated CNS injuries.[18] The types of injury can be grouped by location.

Injuries to the scalp are the most common complication of head injury. These injuries include swelling, contusions, and lacerations. Causes of swelling of the scalp must be differentiated. Subgaleal hematomas are common in children. In neonates, subgaleal hematomas present with diffuse swelling that does not transilluminate. This presentation differs from that of the cephalohematoma, which is focal swelling. Porencephalic or leptomeningeal cysts also present as focal swelling, but these have increased transillumination.

The presence of skull fractures means that significant force has been applied to the cranium, but the presence of fractures does not guarantee intracranial hemorrhage. Likewise, intracranial hemorrhage is seen in the absence of skull fracture. Seventy-five percent of skull fractures are linear fractures. Basilar skull fractures involve the frontal, ethmoid, sphenoid, temporal, and occipital bones. Signs of basilar skull fracture include "raccoon eyes," the Battle sign, cerebrospinal fluid (CSF) otorrhea or rhinorrhea, and hematotympanum. Compound fractures, those with laceration of the scalp, carry a risk of complicating infection of the CNS.

Depressed skull fractures are seen when force is applied over a small surface area. A depressed fracture greater than a few millimeters needs surgical elevation. Diastatic fractures are unique to children and are seen in the first 4 years of life. These fractures represent separation of the sutures. "Growing" fractures are caused by the formation of porencephalic or leptomeningeal cysts in the site of linear or diastatic fractures. These cysts occur during the first 6 months after injury and are most often seen in children younger than 3 years of age.

Traumatic intracranial hemorrhage includes subdural, epidural, and subarachnoid hemorrhages. Subdural hemorrhages occur five to ten times as often as epidural hemorrhages. There is a relatively slow onset of symptoms because these are usually venous in origin. Signs and symptoms of the hemorrhage are secondary to increased intracranial pressure. In infants, these hemorrhages may present with seizures. Although rare in children, the mortality rate of 10% to 20% associated with epidural hematomas makes their early recognition essential. The usual presentation is one of rapid and focal neurologic deterioration. The classic triad is of concussion with an intervening lucent phase, followed by deterioration. These hemorrhages usually represent a tear in the middle meningeal artery. In the child, hemorrhages from the meningeal and diploic veins are also seen. Although these hemorrhages are always associated with fractures in adults, this association is observed in only 50% of the pediatric patients. Subarachnoid hemorrhages are a common computed tomographic (CT) finding in severe pediatric head trauma.

Penetrating head injuries are less common in children. Puncture wounds are seen with lawn darts, other missile-type projectiles, and dog-bite wounds in young children. These injuries are often associated with lacerations of the brain.

Contusions and lacerations of the cerebral cortex are often adjacent to sites of significant focal impact or at locations that predispose the brain to accelerative forces. Coup injuries represent contusions directly beneath the site of impact, while contrecoup injury occurs against the skull surface opposite the site of impact. The signs are often focal and are associated with local swelling on a CT scan. These injuries are not necessarily the cause of unconsciousness.

Concussions are a functional injury. Mild concussions are associated with brief impairment of consciousness. Associated symptoms include anorexia, vomiting, pallor, or abnormal behavior lasting up to several hours. Severe concussions may present with signs ranging from lethargy to coma. All grades have

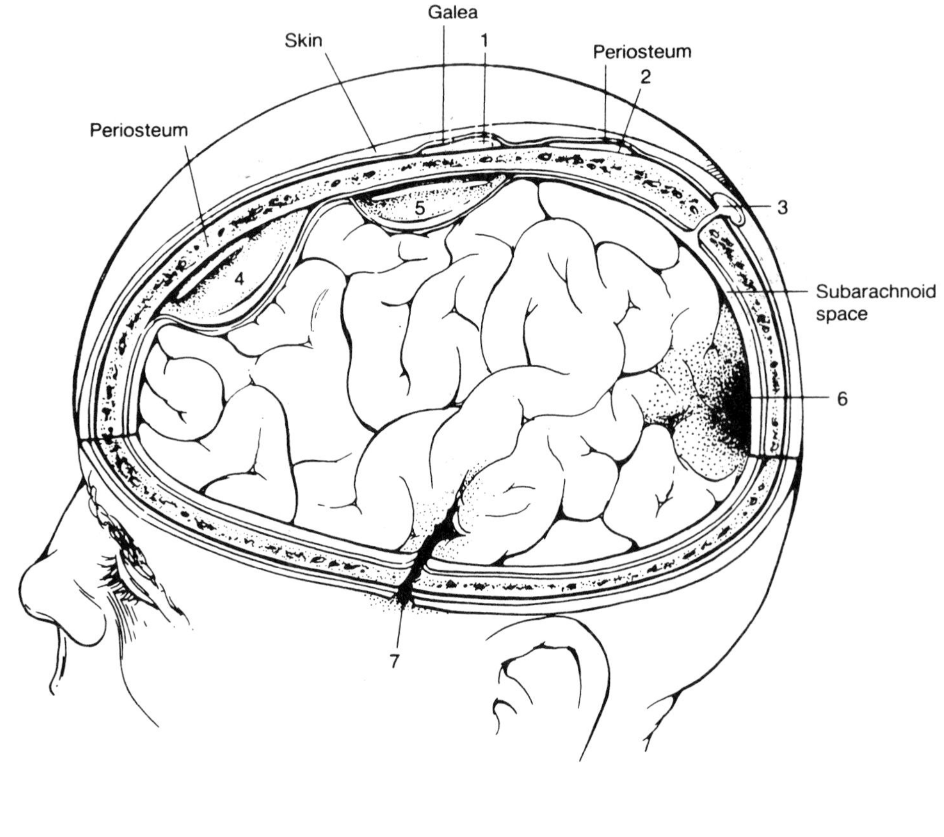

Figure 299.1. Cross-sectional anatomy of the head and associated central nervous system injuries. *1,* Subgaleal hematoma; *2,* cephalohematoma; *3,* porencephalic cyst; *4,* epidural hematoma; *5,* subdural hematoma; *6,* cerebral contusion; *7,* cerebral laceration. (Modified from Rosman NP, Oppenheimer EY, O'Conner JF. Emergency management of pediatric head injuries. *Emerg Med Clin North Am* 1983;1:141.)

an associated amnesia either retrograde, permanent retrograde, or temporary posttraumatic antegrade. Alternative presentations in infants and younger children include lethargy, irritability, and vomiting not associated with loss of consciousness. These symptoms usually subside within 48 hours.

Pathophysiology

The types of injuries can also be classified as primary and secondary. Primary injuries occur at the time of impact and cannot be prevented. These include fractures, concussions, contusions, lacerations, and neuronal or vascular injury on impact. Secondary injuries occur after the initial impact and include cerebral hyperemia, vascular autoregulatory dysfunction, cerebral edema, hemorrhagic lesions, and seizures. These CNS reactive lesions are either preventable or may be minimized by good medical management. If untreated, these lesions lead to mechanical distortion, ischemia, and hypoxic injury.

Cerebral edema and increased intracranial pressure account for a large degree of the morbidity in the pediatric head trauma patient. Injury occurs because the volume of the cranium is fixed. The relationship is expressed by the following formula:

$$\text{Volume CSF} + \text{volume blood} + \text{volume brain} + \text{volume other} = \text{constant}$$

An increase in the volume of one means a reduction in the size of the others. A buffering capacity is important in the early stages of increasing pressure. With an increase in brain volume or a mass lesion, CSF is displaced, followed by a decrease in blood flow. Once the intracranial volume increases beyond the buffering capacity, the intracranial pressure increases and the brain subsequently herniates.[7]

Differences in the growth and maturation of head structures account for the different injuries seen in children and adults. The prevalence of head trauma in children is partly because the young child's proportionally larger head size and weight give a higher center of gravity. The cranial vault is more pliable and less dense in young infants. The open fontanelle and sutures in the younger child, along with the larger subarachnoid space and cisterns, offer a greater extracellular space. This allows better tolerance of expanding mass lesions, up to a point. The dura mater's tight adherence to the skull accounts for the lower incidence of mass hemorrhages in children (less than 30%, compared with 40% to 50% in adults) and the variable and occasional subacute presentation of epidural hemorrhage. Because myelination continues for the first 6 months of life, subcortical white matter tears are often present in this age group, as opposed to the contusions and hemorrhages seen in toddlers. Finally, cerebral edema and increased intracranial pressure as a result of severe head injury occur in 80% of pediatric cases, as opposed to 40% to 50% of the cases in adults.[1,11,16]

EMERGENCY DEPARTMENT EVALUATION

As with most emergencies, evaluation, assessment, and management is a multifaceted, ongoing process until the patient is stabilized and appropriate disposition is made. Although the classic systematic approach of history, physical examination, radiographic evaluation, and management are presented here, these often occur simultaneously.

The history is often obtained from an adult caretaker who may or may not have been present at the time of injury. One must elicit and document details of the accident, including the height of any falls and the type of surface struck, and include a history of loss of consciousness, memory loss, disorientation, and visual disturbance. A brief seizure at the time of impact may be part of the history but may have no diagnostic or prognostic significance, in contrast to seizures that occur after injury. Vomiting is another useful symptom, especially when it is protracted or occurs more than 6 hours after injury.

The physical examination should not be limited to the head; significant physical findings may be found elsewhere. The initial respiratory rate and pattern are noted, and pulse and blood pressure are measured. The examiner should quickly evaluate the level of consciousness using the mnemonic AVPU (*a*lert, responds to *v*oice, responds to *p*ainful stimuli, *u*nconscious). The Glasgow Coma Scale, a fast, objective, and reproducible scoring system, evaluates the best eye opening, verbal, and motor response of the patient (Table 299.1) and has been modified for the preverbal child (Table 299.2).[13] Ocular signs, including pupil

TABLE 299.1. Glasgow Coma Scale

EYE OPENING	
Spontaneous	4
To voice	3
To pain	2
None	1
VERBAL RESPONSE	
Oriented	5
Confused	4
Inappropriate words	3
Incomprehensible words	2
None	1
MOTOR RESPONSE	
Obeys command	6
Localizes pain	5
Withdrawal	4
Abnormal flexion	3
Extensor response	2
None	1

E + V + M = 3 to 15

From Raimondi AJ, Hirschauer J. Head injury in the infant and toddler. *Childs Brain* 1984;11:12.

TABLE 299.2. Glasgow Coma Scale Modified for the Preverbal Child

EYE OPENING	
Spontaneous	4
To voice	3
To pain	2
None	1
VERBAL RESPONSE	
Coos, babbles	5
Irritable cries	4
Cries to pain	3
Moans to pain	2
None	1
MOTOR RESPONSE	
Spontaneous movements	6
Withdraws to touch	5
Withdraws to pain	4
Abnormal flexion	3
Extensor response	2
None	1

E + V + M = 3 to 15

From Raimondi AJ, Hirschauer J. Head injury in the infant and toddler. *Childs Brain* 1984;11:12.

size and response and extraocular movement, should be checked, and an early funduscopic examination, looking for retinal hemorrhages and papilledema, should be done. The head is examined for signs of trauma, including scalp lacerations and abrasions, hematomas, hematotympanum, the Battle sign, raccoon eyes, and CSF leaks from the ears or nose. A complete neurologic examination should be part of the secondary survey. This should also include a search for signs of injury at other sites.[16]

Recommendations for imaging remain somewhat controversial; however, most experts do not advocate routine skull radiographs in the evaluation of head-injured children. Although the risk for intracranial injury is increased with the presence of a skull fracture, as many as 50% of intracranial injuries occur without skull fractures.[4,9,12,15] Head CT has become the imaging modality of choice for the evaluation of possible intracranial injury, including epidural and subdural hematomas, and parenchymal contusions and edema. The head CT can also delineate facial, orbital, and sinus injuries, as well as linear and depressed skull fractures.

Clinical features, such as depressed level of consciousness, focal neurologic deficits, palpable skull depressions, seizures, and signs of a basilar skull fracture, indicate children at higher risk for intracranial injuries.[4,13,15] These children should undergo head CT imaging. However intracranial injury also occurs in the absence of these findings in 3% to 7% of symptomatic children who appear neurologically normal.[4,9,15,19] Head CT imaging should be considered in symptomatic children who are neurologically normal; however, careful observation by a reliable caretaker may be another option.

The presentation of intracranial injury in infants may be very subtle, often occurring without symptoms.[6,8,15] Unlike older children, the great majority of intracranial injuries in infants occur in association with a skull fracture. Moreover, most skull fractures in infants are associated with scalp hematomas or contusions.[5,20] In asymptomatic infants with scalp hematomas, skull radiographs may serve as a screen for serious head injury. If a skull fracture is present, these infants should undergo head CT imaging. Any symptomatic infant should also undergo head CT imaging.

EMERGENCY DEPARTMENT MANAGEMENT

Major Head Trauma

Patients with major head trauma are at the highest risk for intracranial injury. They may have findings of depressed level of consciousness, focal neurologic signs, decreasing level of consciousness, penetrating injury or palpable depressed skull fracture, or a combination of these problems.

Airway and cervical spine control are critical in these patients. Airway patency is assessed and any obstructions are removed. Once the airway has been opened, ventilatory effort is assessed and assisted with bag-valve-mask ventilation in an attempt to keep the PaO_2 above 100 mm Hg. Good cerebral oxygenation is necessary for the prevention of secondary injury. Cricoid pressure is useful to avoid regurgitation and aspiration. A secure airway must be maintained. Endotracheal intubation should be considered in children with a Glasgow Coma Scale score less than 8; rapid-sequence intubation is the method of choice in this situation. With an assistant providing cricoid pressure and oxygenation, atropine sulfate 0.02 mg/kg is given intravenously to reduce secretions and for vagolytic effect; then a sedative and amnestic agent (diazepam, midazolam, thiopental, or etomidate) should be administered. Etomidate is preferred in the hypotensive patient. Confirmation that the patient can be ventilated manually is followed by the administration of succinylcholine, rocuronium, vecuronium, or pancuronium, for muscle relaxation (see *Chapter 235*, "Rapid Sequence Induction and Emergency Airway Management").

Circulation is maintained within normal physiologic limits. Shock may be explained by large scalp lacerations in older children or epidural hemorrhage in infants, but, more commonly, the source of blood loss is elsewhere. Shock is treated with crystalloid boluses. Once normal blood pressure is established, fluids are given at one-half to two-thirds of the maintenance rates.

The goal of treatment of increased intracranial pressure is to prevent displacement (herniation) of the brain. Elevating the patient's head to 30 degrees promotes venous drainage. Controlled hyperventilation reduces cerebral blood flow by reducing arteriolar diameter. Some studies have promoted the use of moderate hyperventilation. $PaCO_2$ is maintained in the 30 mm Hg range.[14,21] Diuretic therapy is used in an attempt to shift water from the brain into the vascular compartment, but these agents should be used with caution in the hypovolemic patient. Intravenous mannitol at 0.25 g/kg is generally recommended. Intracranial pressure increases initially after mannitol administration as a result of an increase in cerebral blood flow secondary to expansion of the vascular volume and increased cardiac output. Intravenous furosemide (Lasix) 0.5 to 1.0 mg/kg is useful in cases of diffuse cerebral edema.

Patients with major head trauma require emergency CT scanning as soon as they are stable enough to tolerate the procedure. Neurosurgical consultation is obtained as soon as possible.[7]

Minor Head Trauma

Children with altered mental status, focal neurologic deficit, signs of a basilar skull fracture, palpable skull depression, or seizure should undergo head CT imaging. Head CT imaging should be considered for neurologically normal children who are symptomatic with a history of vomiting, headache, amnesia, loss of consciousness, drowsiness, or irritability. Careful observation of these children at home by a reliable caretaker may be an alternative strategy. Children with progressive or persistent symptoms should return for reevaluation and head CT imaging. Children who have a normal head CT scan after minor head injury will very rarely develop delayed intracranial sequelae.[3] They can be safely discharged home for further observation. Neurologically normal children without symptoms may also be discharged home without imaging studies.

Skull radiographs are recommended only for evaluation of nonaccidental trauma and for asymptomatic infants with scalp hematomas or contusions. Infants with skull fractures should have head CT imaging to exclude intracranial injury. Infants younger than 12 months who develop symptoms following head trauma should also undergo head CT imaging.

DISPOSITION

Neurosurgical consultation should be sought for patients with major head trauma, including those with abnormal head CT scans, altered mental status, focal neurologic deficit, penetrating injury, or depressed skull fracture. A patient with major head trauma should be stabilized and transported to a facility with a pediatric intensive care unit. The patient should be transported by personnel experienced in caring for critically ill and injured children. Vital signs and neurologic status must be followed closely. The patient's head should be elevated at 30 degrees, and adequate ventilation should be maintained in intubated patients. An intravenous infusion of dextrose 5% in an isotonic solution should be given at one-half to two-thirds of maintenance rates.

Children with minor head trauma should be hospitalized for intracranial injuries identified on the head CT and for persistent neurologic abnormality despite a normal head CT. Children with suspected child abuse and children without a reliable caretaker should also be admitted for observation. Discharge instructions for home observation following head trauma should include indications to return for persistent vomiting, weakness, worsening headache, pupillary asymmetry, lethargy, or difficulty with gait or balance. Symptomatic children and children with isolated skull fractures should be seen by their physician 24 hours after discharge from the emergency department.

COMMON PITFALLS

- Failure to recognize the protean manifestations of head injury in children. Because the open fontanelle and sutures in the younger child, along with the larger subarachnoid space and cisterns, offer a greater extracellular space, a better tolerance of expanding mass lesions is allowed, up to a point.
- Failure to take an adequate history, perform a complete examination, and recognize signs of retinal hemorrhage and increased intracranial pressure. This can lead to a delay in diagnosis and treatment.
- Failure to suspect child abuse, especially shaken-baby syndrome
- Failure to consider other causes of altered mental status, such as CNS infections, metabolic disorders such as hypoglycemia, and toxins, when there are no obvious signs of trauma.

References

1. Adelson PD, Kochanek PM. Head injury in children. *J Child Neurol* 1998;13:2–15.
2. Bruce DA. Head injuries in the pediatric population. *Curr Probl Pediatr* 1990;20:61–107.
3. Davis RL, Hughes M, Gubler KD, et al. The use of cranial CT scans in the triage of pediatric patients with mild head injury. *Pediatrics* 1995;95:345–349.
4. Dietrich AM, Bowman MJ, Ginn-Pease ME, et al. Pediatric head injuries: can clinical factors reliably predict an abnormality on computed tomography? *Ann Emerg Med* 1993;22:1535–1540.
5. Greenes DS, Schutzman SA. Infants with isolated skull fractures: What are their clinical characteristics, and do they require hospitalization? *Ann Emerg Med* 1997;30:253–259.
6. Greenes DS, Schutzman SA. Occult intracranial injury in infants. *Ann Emerg Med* 1998;32:680–686.
7. Griffith JE, Brasfield JC. Increased intracranial pressure. *Pediatr Rev* 1981;2:269.
8. Gruskin KD, Schutzman SA. Head trauma in children younger than 2 years. Are there predictors for complications? *Arch Pediatr Adolesc Med* 1999;153:15–20.
9. Hahn YS, McLone DG. Risk factors in the outcome of children with minor head injury. *Pediatr Neurosurg* 1993;19:135–142.
10. Kraus JF, Rock A, Hemyari P. Brain injuries among infants, children, adolescents, and young adults. *Am J Dis Child* 1990;144:684–691.
11. Lillehei KO, Hoff JT. Advances in the management of closed head injury. *Ann Emerg Med* 1985;14:789.
12. Lloyd DA, Carty H, Patterson M, et al. Predictive value of skull radiography for intracranial injury in children with blunt head injury. *Lancet* 1997;349:821–824.
13. Masters SJ, McClean PM, Arcarese JS, et al. Skull x-ray examinations after head trauma. Recommendations by a multidisciplinary panel and validation study. *N Engl J Med* 1987;316:84–91.
14. Muizelaar JP, Marmarou A, Ward JD, et al. Adverse effects of prolonged hyperventilation in patients with severe head injury: a randomized clinical trial. *J Neurosurg* 1991;75:731–739.
15. Quayle KS, Jaffe DM, Kupperman N, et al. Diagnostic testing for acute head injury in children: when are head computed tomography and skull radiographs indicated? *Pediatrics* 1997;99:1–8.
16. Raimondi AJ, Hirschauer J. Head injury in the infant and toddler. *Childs Brain* 1984;11:12.
17. Rivara FP. Pediatric injury control in 1999: where do we go from here? *Pediatrics* 1999;103:883–888.
18. Rosman NP, Oppenheimer EY, O'Conner JF. Emergency management of pediatric head injuries. *Emerg Med Clin North Am* 1983;1:141.
19. Schunk JE, Rodgerson JD, Woodward GA. The utility of head computed tomographic scanning in pediatric patients with normal neurologic examination in the emergency department. *Pediatr Emerg Care* 1996;12:160–165.
20. Shane SA, Fuchs SM. Skull fractures in infants and predictors of associated intracranial injury. *Pediatr Emerg Care* 1997;13:198–203.
21. Stringer A, Hasso AN, Thompson JR, et al. Hyperventilation induced cerebral ischemia in patients with acute brain lesions: demonstration by xenon-enhanced CT. *Am J Neurosurg Res* 1993;14:475–484.
22. Zuckerman GB, Conway EE. Accidental head injury. *Pediatr Ann* 1997;26:621–632.

CHAPTER 300

Evaluation of the Cervical Spine

David M. Cosentino and Francis M. Fesmire

Unlike the adult cervical spine, the developing pediatric cervical spine has unfused synchondroses, incomplete ossification centers, and epiphyseal growth plates. To understand the nuances of radiographic interpretation, the emergency physician must have an understanding of developmental anatomy. Because of the dynamic changes that occur with bone and ligament development in the pediatric cervical spine, distribution patterns of fractures and dislocations within the cervical spine itself differ from the distribution of injuries in the adult spine. Furthermore, a significant percentage of pediatric spinal cord injuries occur in the absence of radiographically identifiable fractures and dislocations.

DEVELOPMENTAL ANATOMY

The first cervical vertebra (atlas) develops from three primary ossification centers: the body and two neural arches (Fig. 300.1). The neural arches ossify *in utero* and fuse posteriorly at approximately the third year of life. The body of C1 is not ossified at birth and does not become visible until approximately 1 year of age. The synchondroses between the body and neural arches (neurocentral synchondroses) fuse at approximately the seventh year of life.[3,8,22]

The second cervical vertebra (axis) is the most difficult to interpret radiographically because of its four primary ossification centers: the odontoid, body, and two neural arches (Fig. 300.2). All four ossification centers are visible at birth. A secondary ossification center appears at the apex of the odontoid (summit ossification center) at approximately 3 to 6 years and fuses with the odontoid by the twelfth year of life. The synchondroses of the posterior neural arches fuse at approximately the third year. The synchondrosis between the odontoid–body of C2 and the neural arches fuses at approximately the third to sixth year. Before fusion, these synchondroses may be confused with fracture lines. The fusion line of the synchondrosis between the odontoid and the body of C2 commonly remains visible until age 11, and one-third of individuals have a visible fusion line throughout life.

In the remaining C3 to C7 cervical vertebrae, there are three major ossification centers—the body and two neural arches—all of which are visible at birth (Fig. 300.3). The posterior synchondroses of the neural arches fuse at approximately the third year

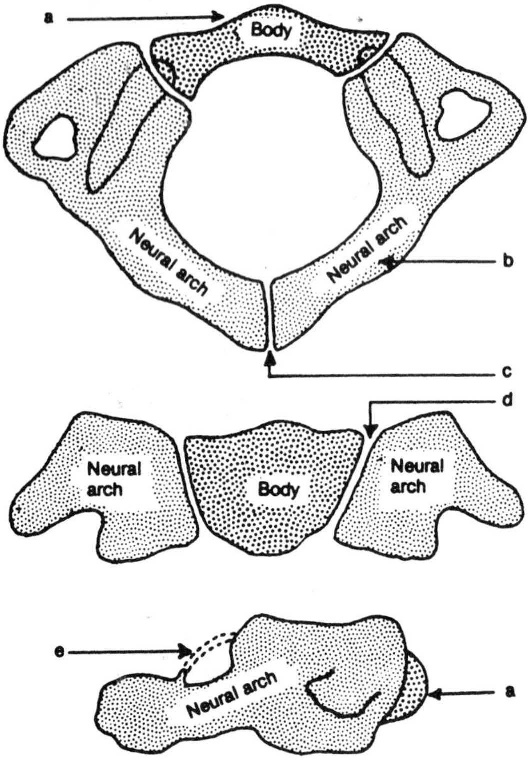

Figure 300.1. The first cervical vertebra (atlas). *(a)* Body: ossification center becomes visible during first year of life. *(b)* Neural arches: ossification center appears *in utero* at approximately the seventh fetal week. *(c)* Synchondrosis of spinal process: fuses at approximately the third year of life. *(d)* Synchondrosis about the body (neurocentral synchondrosis: fuses at approximately the seventh year of life. *(e)* Ligament surrounding the superior vertebral notch: may ossify later in life. (From Fielding JW. Cervical spine injuries in children. In: The Cervical Spine Research Society, eds. *The cervical spine.* Philadelphia: JB Lippincott Co, 1983:268–281, with permission.)

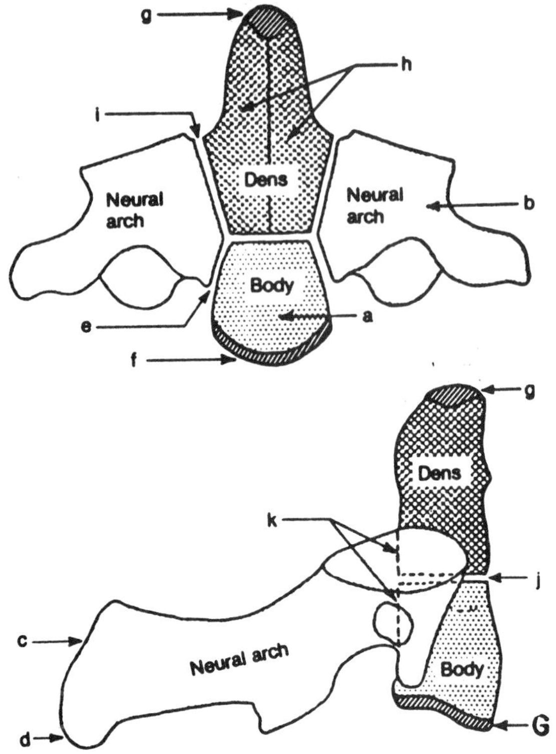

Figure 300.2. The second cervical vertebra (axis). *(a)* Body: ossification center appears by the fifth fetal month. *(b)* Neural arches: appear by the seventh fetal month. *(c)* Synchondrosis of spinous process: fuses by the third to sixth year of life. *(d, e)* Neurocentral synchondrosis: fuses by the third to sixth year. *(f, G)* Inferior epiphyseal ring: appears at puberty and fuses to body at approximately 25 years of life. *(g)* Summit ossification center for odontoid: appears at approximately the third to the sixth year and fuses with the odontoid by the twelfth year of life. *(h)* Odontoid: develops from two ossification centers that fuse by the seventh fetal month. *(j)* Synchondrosis between the odontoid and body: fuses at approximately the third to sixth year of life. (From Fielding JW. Cervical spine injuries in children. In: The Cervical Spine Research Society, eds. *The cervical spine.* Philadelphia: JB Lippincott Co, 1983:268–281, with permission.)

of life. The neurocentral synchondroses fuse at approximately the third to sixth year of life. Secondary ossification centers appear at puberty along the superior and inferior aspects of the cervical bodies (superior and inferior epiphyseal rings) and at the tips of the spinous processes. Before fusion, these ossification centers may be mistaken for chip fractures of the cervical bodies and clay shoveler's fractures of the spinous processes, respectively. These secondary ossification centers fuse with the main body by age 25 years. Table 300.1 summarizes the major radiographic changes seen in the development of the pediatric cervical spine.

NORMAL VARIANTS AND CONGENITAL ANOMALIES

Because of the laxity of the ligaments in the pediatric cervical spine, absent lordosis is a frequent finding on the lateral radiograph. In adults, this finding may signify ligamentous injury. In one study, lordosis was absent in 14% of 160 healthy children aged 16 years and younger.[6]

During the ossification process of the immature cervical bodies, an appearance of anterior wedging is produced. The finding of anterior wedging in several adjacent vertebrae suggests that it is a developmental finding and not a compression fracture (Fig. 300.4).

The extreme laxity of ligaments creates a pseudosubluxation of adjacent vertebrae in 46% of children younger than 8 years old.[6] This finding is most pronounced at the level of C2 to C3 (see Fig. 300.4). To distinguish pseudosubluxation from true subluxation, Swischuk[21,23] has developed the concept of the posterior cervical line (Fig. 300.5). This line is drawn by connecting the anterior aspects of the spinous processes of C1 and C3. If the anterior aspect of the spinous process of C2 misses this line by 2 mm or more (1.5 mm is borderline), this finding is suggestive of a true subluxation or a hangman's fracture of the neural arches of C2. This posterior cervical line can be applied only in children demonstrating subluxation or pseudosubluxation of C2 on C3. If no subluxation or pseudosubluxation exists, the anterior aspect of the spinous process of C2 commonly misses the posterior cervical line by more than 2 mm.

In adults, widening of the predental space frequently signifies a rupture of the transverse ligament or subluxation of C1 on C2. Twenty percent of children younger than 8 years old demonstrate a predental space of 3 mm or more, and distances up to 5 mm may be seen in nonpathologic instances (see Fig. 300.4).[6,10] Distances greater than 3.5 mm should be considered abnormal, however, until proven otherwise.

Widening of the prevertebral soft tissue due to hemorrhage and edema is an important adult radiographic finding. In children, suggested norms have included soft-tissue space less than 7 mm anterior to C2 or less than three-fourths of the adjacent vertebral body's width.[2] The younger the child, however, the

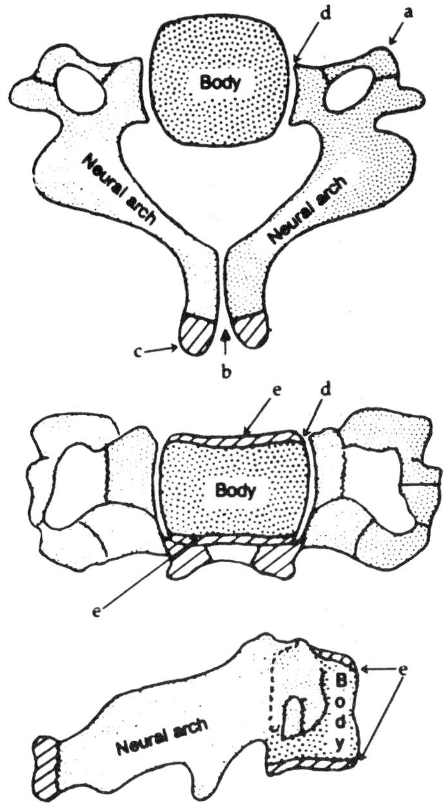

Figure 300.3. Typical cervical vertebrae (C3-C7). *(a)* Anterior portion of transverse process: may develop from a separate ossification center that fuses by the sixth year. *(b)* Synchondrosis between the spinous processes: fuse by third year. *(c)* Secondary centers for bifid spinous processes: appear at puberty and fuse by 25 years of life. *(d)* Neurocentral synchondrosis: fuses at approximately third to sixth year of life. *(e)* Superior and inferior epiphyseal rings: appear at puberty and fuse with body by 25 years of life. (From Fielding JW. Cervical spine injuries in children. In: The Cervical Spine Research Society, eds. *The cervical spine.* Philadelphia: JB Lippincott Co, 1983:268–281, with permission.)

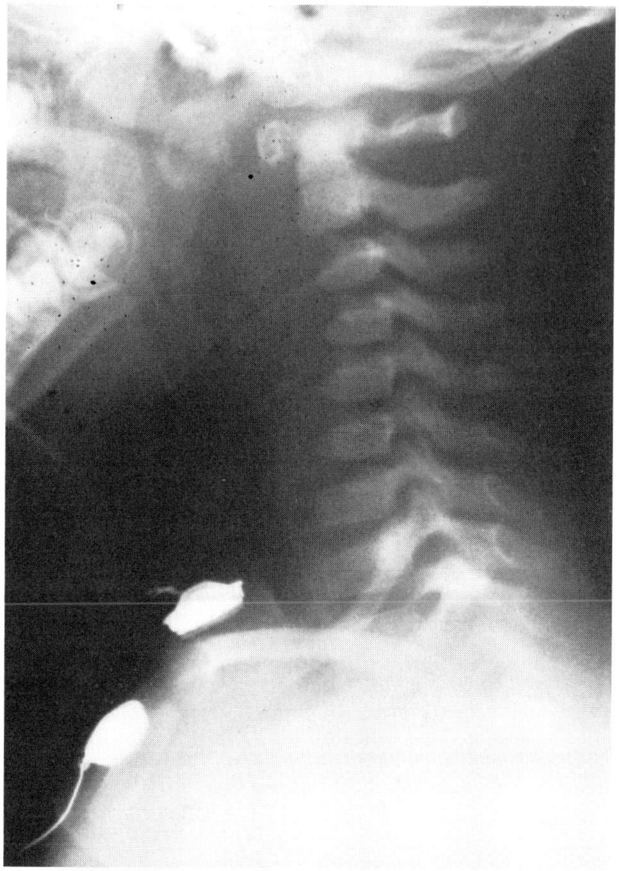

Figure 300.4. Three-year-old with a 4-mm anterior pseudosubluxation of C2 on C3 and a nonpathologic, widened predental space of 4 mm. Note that the anterior aspect of the spinous processes of C1 through C3 lies on a straight line. This line would be broken in a true subluxation. The synchondrosis between the dens and body of C2 is unfused. Also note the normal anterior wedging of the vertebral bodies, as well as the increased soft-tissue space anterior to the cervical spine. (From Fesmire FM, Luten RC. The pediatric cervical spine: developmental anatomy and clinical aspects. *J Emerg Med* 1989;7:133–142, with permission.)

more unreliable these norms, because dramatic increases in soft-tissue density occur during expiration or when the neck is held in mild flexion (see Fig. 300.4).

Excluding major congenital malformations, os odontoideum and ossiculum terminale are two congenital malformations that occasionally occur.[9,25] Os odontoideum is a failure of the odontoid to fuse with the body of C2. The odontoid is separated from the body of C2 by a thin layer of hyaline cartilage, and fairly insignificant trauma can result in odontoid subluxation, resulting in death or quadriplegia. Os odontoideum can also occur secondarily from the failure of an odontoid fracture to heal. Ossiculum terminale is a failure of the apical segment of the odontoid (summit ossification center) to fuse with the main body of the odontoid. This is generally a benign condition, but one case of this anomaly has led to progressive atlantoaxial dislocation, resulting in quadriplegia and death.[20]

TABLE 300.1. Radiographic Development of the Pediatric Cervical Spine

Age	Developmental Change
6 mo	Body of C1 not visible; all synchondroses open
1 yr	Body of C1 visible
3 yr	Synchondroses of posteriorly located spinous processes fuse
3–6 yr	Neurocentral syncondroses fuse; synchondrosis between odontoid and body of C2 fuses; summit ossification center appears at superior aspect of odontoid; anterior wedging of vertebral bodies resolves
8 yr	Pseudosubluxation and widening of predental space resolve; spine assumes a more lordotic appearance
Puberty	Secondary ossification centers appear at the tips of the spinous processes; superior and inferior epiphyseal rings appear; summit ossification center of odontoid fuses
25 yr	Secondary ossification centers at tips of spinous processes fuse; superior and inferior epiphyseal rings fuse to the main body

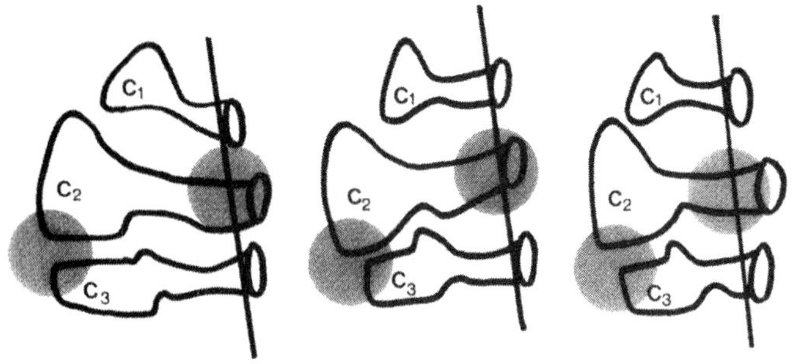

Figure 300.5. The posterior cervical line (PCL) is drawn by connecting the anterior aspect of the spinous processes of C1 and C3. The concept of the PCL can be applied only if subluxation or pseudosubluxation is present. **(A)** Pseudosubluxation is absent: The anterior aspect of the spinous process of C2 will commonly miss the PCL by 2 mm—*Normal or Abnormal* (PCL cannot be applied). **(B)** Pseudosubluxation is present: The anterior aspect of the spinous process of C2 lies on the PCL—*Normal*. **(C)** Subluxation is present: The anterior aspect of the spinous process of C2 misses the PCL by 2 mm. This finding is suggestive of a hangman's fracture of the neural arches of C2—*Abnormal*. (From Fesmire FM, Luten RC. The pediatric cervical spine: developmental anatomy and clinical aspects. *J Emerg Med* 1989;7:133–142, with permission.)

CLINICAL ASPECTS

Radiographically apparent cervical spine injury is rare in the pediatric age group. Approximately 2% of all cervical spine fractures and dislocations occur in children younger than 16 years old, and only approximately 1.2% of all pediatric cervical spine radiographs reveal an abnormality.[11,19]

The incidence of cervical spine fractures and dislocations increases with age. Radiographically apparent cervical spine injury, excluding birth trauma, is virtually nonexistent in children younger than 16 months of age.[2,7,11,13,19] The cause of cervical spine fractures and dislocations is broad, but motor vehicle accidents account for approximately 35% to 50%; diving injuries and falls, approximately 30% to 35%; and sports injuries, approximately 20% to 25%.[2,7,11,13,19]

Types of pediatric cervical spine injuries can be divided into those of the upper cervical spine (C1 to C2) and those of the lower cervical spine (C3 to C7). Injuries most commonly seen in the upper cervical spine are fracture or synchondral separation of the odontoid, with atlantoaxial dislocation and hangman's fracture of the neural arches of C2. Abnormalities most frequently encountered in the lower cervical spine are anterior subluxation or dislocation, compression fractures, teardrop fractures, and spinous process fractures.

Children younger than 8 years old have a high preponderance of upper cervical spine fractures and dislocations, whereas children older than 12 years have a distribution of injuries resembling that of adults, with a preponderance of low cervical lesions (Table 300.2).[2,7,11,13] Children aged 8 to 12 years are in a transition state between the two. The preponderance of high cervical injuries in children younger than 8 years of age relates to the relatively heavy head of the child, coupled with the laxity of ligaments and nearly horizontal facet joints. This combination results in high torques and shear forces being applied to the C1 to C2 regions.

The incidence of pediatric spinal cord injuries ranges from less than 1% to 9.4% of all spinal cord injuries.[5,16] The incidence of spinal cord deficits resulting from cervical spine fractures and dislocations is approximately 30%.[2,11,13] Of those children with a spinal deficit, approximately 12% are rendered quadriplegic. The incidence of neurologic deficit with cervical spine fractures and dislocations increases with age, with neurologic deficit occurring in 20% of children younger than 8 years of age and in approximately 40% of children aged 8 to 16 years.[2,11,13]

Pediatric cervical injuries related to the use of front-passenger airbags have been increasingly described in the literature. Airbag deployment has produced a pattern of cervical injuries in older children traveling in front seats and crush injury to the skull of infants in rear-facing safety seats.[17] Currently, the National Highway Traffic Safety Administration recommends placing infants in rear-facing child safety seats in the back seat and that children under 12 should ride seat-belted in a rear seat at all times.

The reported incidence of spinal cord injury without radiographic abnormality (SCIWORA) ranges from 4% to 67% of all pediatric spinal injuries.[1,16,18] An extensive epidemiologic analysis of 16 California counties found an incidence of 20% of all pediatric spinal injuries that probably most accurately reflects true incidence of this syndrome.[16]

The pathophysiology of SCIWORA is thought to result from a combination of a diverse multitude of mechanisms, all resulting in a disruption of microvascular blood supply. Mechanisms proposed include hyperextension with inward bulging of the interlaminar ligaments, reversible disc prolapse, flexion compression of the cord, longitudinal distraction of the cord, and vertebral artery spasm.

A detailed study of SCIWORA in 24 children revealed that 83% of these lesions involved the cervical spinal cord.[17] There were seven cases of complete cord transection, all of which occurred in patients younger than 8 years old. In this study, 54% of the children had a delayed onset of neurologic deficit (range, 30 minutes to 4 days; mean, 1.2 days). More than half of the children in the delayed-onset group later recalled transient paresthesias at the time of the injury.

TABLE 300.2. Correlation of Level of Cervical Fractures/Dislocations with Age[a]

Level of Fracture	Age	Henrys[11]	Hill[13]	Apple[2]	Dietrich[7]	Total	C1-C2 (%)
C1-C2	<8 yr	7	6	4	11	28	
C3-C7	<8 yr	1	0	0	6	7	80
C1-C2	8–12 yr	4	6	5	6	21	
C3-C7	8–12 yr	0	6	2	4	12	64
C1-C2	>12 yr	2	13	4	7	26	
C3-C7	>12 yr	2	41	13	18	74	26

[a] Excluding birth trauma.

EMERGENCY DEPARTMENT MANAGEMENT

All children with potential cervical spine injury should have their necks immobilized. Prehospital cervical spine immobilization is best accomplished using a rigid plastic cervical collar and a backboard, combined with tape, sandbags, or a commercially available head-immobilization device.[14] The disproportionate head size of young children causes cervical flexion to occur in children younger than 7 years old when they are immobilized on a standard flat backboard.[12] This flexion can be prevented either by placing padding underneath the back to raise the level of the thoracic spine or by using a spinal backboard with a recess for the occiput. The cervical spine is properly positioned when a line drawn through the external auditory meatus and the anterior aspect of the shoulder is parallel to the backboard. When an alert child vigorously resists attempts at immobilization, however, these attempts could potentially worsen an injury. As a general rule, children rarely ingest central nervous system depressants such as ethanol and, if alert, will not move a significantly injured portion of the body. Thus, it is acceptable to not immobilize the cervical spine of a young alert child with no obvious injuries who is vigorously resisting all attempts.

All children who arrive at the emergency department with a new neurologic deficit consistent with a spinal cord injury and a history of trauma or suspected trauma should undergo treatment with high-dose methylprednisolone as soon as possible.[4] Recommended dosing consists of a loading dose of 30 mg/kg over 15 minutes, followed by a maintenance infusion of 5.4 mg/kg/h for 23 hours. Due to the existence of SCIWORA, workup should not delay the initiation of high-dose methylprednisolone in patients with spinal cord injury.

The management of the threatened airway in a child can be an urgent dilemma.[24] Ventilation can frequently be accomplished with a chin lift alone (which elevates the tongue off the hypopharynx) or in combination with bag-valve-mask ventilation. Oral intubation, which is preferred in younger children, is best performed using manual in-line traction to maintain cervical immobilization. Young children require little, if any, extension to visualize the glottis. Nasotracheal intubation should be attempted only in older children with spontaneous respirations.

Jaffe and coworkers[15] retrospectively analyzed 206 children with suspected cervical spine injury and developed a clinical algorithm for identifying patients at high risk for cervical spine injury. They found that the clinical criteria of any one of the following—history of direct neck trauma; neck pain; neck tenderness; limitation of mobility; abnormality in flexion, strength, or sensation; or decreased mental status—had a sensitivity of 98% and a specificity of 54% for detecting cervical spine injuries. They also found that the standard lateral roentgenogram detected 95% of the injuries, and 100% of the injuries when combined with the anteroposterior view. Until further studies are performed, however, attempts should still be made to also obtain an open-mouth odontoid view, although, in our experience, this radiograph is frequently impossible to obtain in young children. Figure 300.6 demonstrates an approach to children with no history of direct neck trauma who arrive at the emergency department with the cervical spine immobilized by rescue personnel.

Due to the potential of SCIWORAs developing despite normal radiographs, all children with potential spinal injury should be questioned specifically concerning transient paresthesias at the time of the injury. Such children should be assumed to have a spinal injury until a neurosurgical consultation establishes otherwise. The diagnosis of SCIWORA should be a diagnosis of exclusion and should not be made until occult bony, ligamentous, or disc injuries are ruled out by fluoroscopically guided flexion and extension radiographs, computed tomography scanning, magnetic resonance imaging, or myelography.

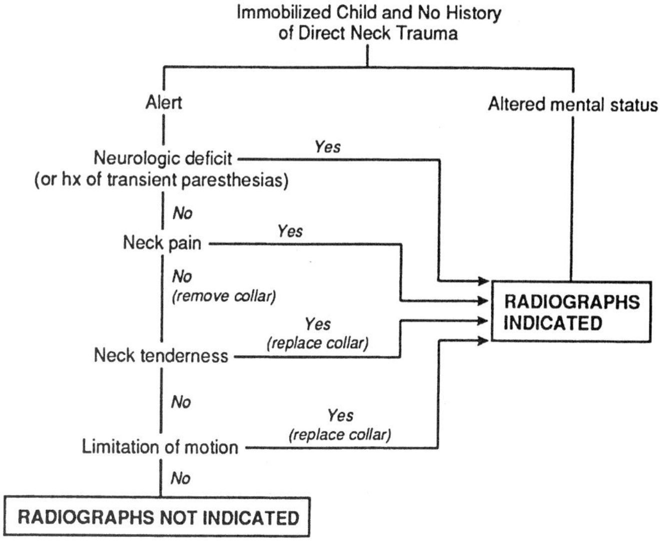

Figure 300.6. Protocol for deciding which pediatric patients arriving immobilized in the emergency department need radiographs. (Modified from Wales LR, Knopp RK, Morishima MS. Recommendations for evaluation of the acutely injured cervical spine: a clinical radiologic algorithm. *Ann Emerg Med* 1980;9:422, with permission.)

Pending further studies concerning the nature of cervical spine fractures and dislocations, as well as the nature of SCIWORA, it seems prudent to conservatively admit to the hospital all children with suspected cervical spine injury.

COMMON PITFALLS

- Physicians may confuse open synchondrosis and secondary ossification centers with fractures.
- Physicians may not realize that absent lordosis, anterior wedging of cervical bodies, pseudosubluxation of C2 on C3, increased prevertebral soft-tissue density, and widening of the predental space can be normal.
- A normal radiograph does not rule out cervical spinal cord injury in the pediatric age group, because spinal cord injuries frequently occur in the absence of radiographically detectable injuries. All children with suspected neck injury should be questioned specifically for transient paresthesias at the time of the injury, because approximately one-half of all patients with delayed onset of SCIWORA have this finding.

References

1. Anderson JM, Schutt AH. Spinal injury in children: a review of 156 cases seen from 1950–1978. *Mayo Clin Proc* 1980;55:499.
2. Apple JS, Kirks DR, Merten DF, et al. Cervical spine fractures and dislocations in children. *Pediatr Radiol* 1987;17:45.
3. Bailey DK. The normal cervical spine in infants and children. *Radiology* 1952;59:712.
4. Bracken MB, Shepard MJ, Collins WF, et al. A randomized, controlled trial of methylprednisolone or naloxone in the treatment of acute spinal-cord injury: results of the Second National Acute Spinal Cord Injury Study. *N Engl J Med* 1990;322:1405.
5. Burke D. Spinal cord trauma in children. *Paraplegia* 1971;9:1.
6. Cattell HS, Filtzer DK. Pseudosubluxation and other normal variations in the cervical spine in children. *J Bone Joint Surg* 1965;47A:1295.
7. Dietrich AM, Ginn-Pease ME, Bartkowski HM, et al. Pediatric cervical spine fractures: predominately subtle presentation. *J Pediatr Surg* 1991;26:995.

8. Fesmire FM, Luten RC. The pediatric cervical spine: developmental anatomy and clinical aspects. *J Emerg Med* 1989;7:133.
9. Garber JN. Abnormalities of the atlas and axis vertebrae: congenital and traumatic. *J Bone Joint Surg* 1964;46A:1782.
10. Gerlock AJ, Kirchner SG, Heller RM, et al. *The cervical spine in trauma.* Philadelphia: WB Saunders, 1978:13.
11. Henrys P, Lyne ED, Lifton C, et al. Clinical review of cervical spine injuries in children. *Clin Orthop* 1977;129:172.
12. Herzenberg JE, Hensinger RN, Dedrick DK, et al. Emergency transport and positioning of young children who have an injury of the cervical spine: the standard backboard may be hazardous. *J Bone Joint Surg* 1989;71:15.
13. Hill SA, Miller CA, Kosnik EJ, et al. Pediatric neck injuries: a clinical study. *J Neurosurg* 1984;60:700.
14. Huertta C, Griffith R, Joyce SM. Cervical spine stabilization in pediatric patients: evaluation of current techniques. *Ann Emerg Med* 1987;16:1121.
15. Jaffe DM, Binns H, Radowski NA, et al. Developing a clinical algorithm for early management of cervical spine injury in child trauma victims. *Ann Emerg Med* 1987;16:270.
16. Kewalramani LS, Orth MS, Kraus JF, et al. Acute spinal cord lesions in pediatric population: epidemiological and clinical features. *Paraplegia* 1980;18:206.
17. Marshall KW, Koch BL, Egelhoff JC. Air bag-related deaths and serious injuries in children: injury patterns and imaging findings. *Am J Neuroradiol* 1998;19(9):1599–1607.
18. Pang D, Wilberger JE. Spinal cord injury without radiographic abnormalities in children. *J Neurosurg* 1982;57:114.
19. Rachesky I, Boyce WT, Duncan B, et al. Clinical prediction of cervical spine injuries in children. *Am J Dis Child* 1987;141:199.
20. Sherk H, Nicholson J. Rotary atlanto-axial dislocation associated with ossiculum terminale and mongolism. *J Bone Joint Surg* 1969;51A:957.
21. Swischuk LE. Anterior displacement of C2 in children—physiologic or pathologic. *Radiology* 1977;122:759.
22. Swischuk LE. *Radiology of the newborn and young infant,* 2nd ed. Baltimore: Williams & Wilkins, 1980:834.
23. Swischuk LE. *Emergency imaging of the acutely ill or injured child,* 3rd ed. Baltimore: Williams & Wilkins, 1994:653.
24. Tecklenburg F. Problems in managing cervical spine injuries. In: Luten RC, ed. *Problems in pediatric emergency medicine.* New York: Churchill Livingstone, 1988:110.
25. Truex RC, Johnson CH. Congenital anomalies of the upper cervical spine. *Orthop Clin North Am* 1978;9:891.

CHAPTER 301

Abdominal Trauma

Khaled Mutabagani and Donna A. Caniano

EPIDEMIOLOGY

Data from the National Pediatric Trauma Registry (NPTR) indicate that the incidence of abdominal injuries in children is 8%. Multiple injuries are twice as common as isolated abdominal injuries and twice as lethal. Abdominal injuries are present in up to 30% of children admitted to the hospital because of trauma, and 2% of all trauma-related deaths are secondary to abdominal organ injury. The mortality of serious abdominal organ injury is 15%.[6,7]

Over 85% of abdominal injuries in children are due to blunt trauma.[7] Motor vehicle-related accidents (passenger, pedestrian, motorcycle, bicycle, and other motor vehicles) are, by far, the most frequent mechanism of injury in children, followed by falls, sport-related injuries, and assault.[6,7] Penetrating abdominal injuries in children are uncommon; however, with the increase in urban violence in recent years, the number of children with gunshot or stab wounds to the abdomen is increasing.[12,16]

Abdominal trauma from child abuse is uncommon,[10,16] but it should be suspected if any of the following apply: history of accidents, vague or unclear accident history, history of injury incompatible with the child's developmental stage or the type of trauma, admission by the child that he or she has been abused, delay in seeking medical attention, unstable family situation, or unusually withdrawn or compliant behavior on the part of the child.

CLINICAL PRESENTATION

Children with abdominal trauma can present with a variety of complaints, from the rare child who is completely asymptomatic to the patient *in extremis*. Most children with abdominal injury complain of abdominal pain, nausea, or vomiting. From a management perspective, children with abdominal trauma can present in one of two ways.

The first and most common presentation is that of a hemodynamically stable patient transported to the emergency department (ED) minutes to hours after the injury. Prehospital personnel have usually instituted initial resuscitative measures, such as administration of supplemental oxygen and intravenous fluids and application of a cervical immobilization collar. The evaluation of a hemodynamically stable patient in the ED can then proceed in a calm and unhurried fashion. The second type of presentation is that of a hemodynamically unstable child, usually transported from the scene, where the immediate diagnostic and therapeutic maneuvers of trauma physicians are necessary for the patient's survival.

EMERGENCY DEPARTMENT EVALUATION

Children with abdominal trauma, either blunt or penetrating, can have one or more organs injured. The management of these injuries can vary from bed rest and observation (e.g., a splenic laceration) to abdominal exploration (e.g., a small-bowel perforation).[6] Although clinical assessment is very helpful in reaching the correct diagnosis, a diagnostic test, usually radiologic, is essential in many patients to identify the specific injury.[2,4,5,11,14] The primary focus of the evaluation performed in the ED is to determine the organ injured and the severity of the injury, in order to initiate appropriate management.

Advanced Trauma Life Support (ATLS) guidelines must be followed in the evaluation of all trauma patients.[2] First, the primary survey is performed to identify and treat any life-threatening injury. This is followed by the secondary survey, in which a head-to-toe examination of the patient is completed. The abdomen is evaluated during the secondary survey.[2,10]

Because the ED evaluation and management differ according to the hemodynamic status of the patient, they are discussed separately.

The Hemodynamically Unstable Patient

After thoracic and central nervous system (CNS) causes of hemodynamic instability are excluded, the evaluation of a hemodynamically unstable child is directed toward the immediate identification of the source of bleeding. Although a small amount of pericardial blood can cause hypotension (ascertained by pericardiocentesis or echocardiography), there are only a few areas of the body in which exsanguinating hemorrhage can accumulate: the pleural space (quickly identified by clinical assessment, a chest radiograph, or placement of chest tubes), the thigh (diagnosed clinically), the pelvis or retroperitoneum (determined with ultrasound or computed tomography [CT]), and, most commonly, the peritoneal cavity.[2] Diagnostic peritoneal lavage (DPL) or ultrasound, especially focused abdominal sonography for trauma (FAST), are the two best modalities to quickly and reliably diagnose exsanguinating intraperitoneal hemorrhage.[14] Differentiation between intraperitoneal hemorrhage and other sources of bleeding is important, because bleeding from a pelvic fracture is managed optimally by pelvic stabilization and angiographic control rather than by laparotomy.

The hemoglobin, hematocrit, and blood type and crossmatch are the most important laboratory values in hemodynamically unstable patients. Chest and pelvis radiographs can provide very helpful information. In cases in which immediate surgical intervention to control bleeding is indicated, x-rays should not be obtained if to do so would cause any delay in exploration.

The Hemodynamically Stable Patient

In the hemodynamically stable child, a thorough clinical assessment can provide very useful information and help guide further diagnostic tests. The likelihood of preexisting medical conditions in children is low, but pertinent information regarding the patient's medical history should be obtained in addition to the information related to the accident. Abdominal examination focuses on the presence of any sign of significant injury, including abdominal distension, rigidity, tenderness, especially diffuse abdominal tenderness, abrasions, ecchymoses, and the "seat belt" sign.[17] Abdominal examination includes inspection and palpation of both flanks, the back, genitalia, perineum, and a rectal digital examination.[5,10]

Laboratory values useful for decision making or therapeutic intervention in blunt abdominal trauma include hemoglobin and hematocrit to assess bleeding, serum transaminase (AST and ALT) levels (60% of patients with levels over 100 to 200 IU have identifiable hepatic injuries), amylase (for suspected pancreatic injuries), and urinalysis.[1,11] A blood type and screen should be obtained if it is anticipated that blood products will be used later in the hospital course.

Plain x-rays are of little help in most cases of blunt trauma to the abdomen. The vast majority of abdominal films only show nonspecific findings that do not add information helpful to management decisions. One exception is in children with intestinal perforation, in which the demonstration of free intraperitoneal air on a plain film necessitates proceeding to the operating room for laparotomy.

Plain films will show bony abnormalities and should be performed in cases of suspected spine or pelvic fractures. Plain x-rays of the abdomen and chest should be obtained in patients with penetrating injuries. Two views, with entrance and exit skin markers at the site of the projectile, can yield very helpful information on the type of projectile, trajectory, fragmentation, and location of fragments.

Chest radiographs can provide useful information in patients with an abdominal injury. They may show lower-rib fractures (ribs 6 to 12), hemothoraces, or abnormal diaphragmatic contour, all of which may be associated with an abdominal organ injury or a diaphragmatic tear. Also, trauma patients often have injuries to more than one anatomic area, especially in motor vehicle accidents (MVAs). These radiographs may demonstrate thoracic injuries that are not suspected from clinical assessment.

Currently, CT is the preferred radiologic test for the evaluation of children with suspected intraabdominal injuries who are hemodynamically stable.[4,11,14] Helical or spiral CTs, with intravenous contrast, can be performed rapidly (in minutes), with a sensitivity and specificity greater than 90%. CT is noninvasive; can evaluate intraabdominal, retroperitoneal, and lower thoracic structures; is not operator dependent; and is widely available. Some of the drawbacks of CT include expense, having to transport the patient to the scanner's location, radiation exposure, and the possibility of a side effect from intravenous contrast. Although its sensitivity in identifying intestinal perforations is only about 50%, it still is the most sensitive radiologic test for these injuries.[14]

Ultrasonography, both the complete abdominal sonographic examination and FAST, are emerging as useful radiologic tests in the evaluation of children with suspected abdominal injuries. Ultrasound is noninvasive and portable, requires no intravenous contrast, and poses no radiation risks. In addition, FAST can be performed in minutes by members of the trauma team during the resuscitation phase. A complete abdominal ultrasonogram is more time consuming and is similar to CT in cost. Both tests, however, are operator-dependent and less sensitive than CT. FAST is used primarily as a screening test, while complete abdominal ultrasound examinations are performed instead of CT in a few trauma centers.[14]

DPL is a quick, inexpensive, and extremely sensitive test for the presence of free intraperitoneal blood (98%); however, it is also nonspecific and invasive, it does not evaluate the retroperitoneum, and it is associated with a 1% to 2% risk of intestinal or vascular injuries.[2,5] Because the vast majority of children with abdominal trauma have blunt injuries, are hemodynamically stable, and are now managed nonoperatively, the mere presence of blood in the peritoneal cavity (detected by DPL) does not provide information useful in the management plan.[9,16] The more sensitive and specific CT has now replaced DPL as the preferred test for the evaluation of blunt abdominal trauma in children. DPL is used mainly to determine the need for immediate laparotomy in the hemodynamically unstable child who suffered blunt injury.[5,10,16]

Penetrating Injuries

In children (as in adult trauma patients) with penetrating injuries, the velocity and trajectory of the projectile, in addition to clinical findings, determines the necessary diagnostic tests and the need for laparotomy. Most (greater than 85%) high-velocity penetrating injuries that violate the peritoneum cause enough organ damage that surgical repair is necessary.[8] A smaller percentage of low-velocity injuries cause significant organ damage, but surgical intervention depends on the projectile trajectory, clinical findings, and results of laboratory tests and x-rays.[8,12] Patients with stab wounds require surgical repair in only one-third of cases and can therefore be managed selectively with exploration reserved for patients with worsening clinical findings.[8]

EMERGENCY DEPARTMENT MANAGEMENT

The Hemodynamically Unstable Patient

All hemodynamically unstable patients should undergo resuscitation concurrent with the primary and secondary survey, as per ATLS protocols. Ringer's lactate (preferably) or normal saline should be administered via intravenous or intraosseous access, with at least one site above the diaphragm.[2,10,16] Resuscitative fluids must be infused as rapidly as needed to maintain vital organ perfusion. Many children with abdominal injuries have an associated head injury. In these patients, avoiding hypotension and maintaining adequate cerebral perfusion are important to minimize any secondary brain injury.

Nasogastric tubes (NGTs) should be inserted unless a contraindication is identified. Contraindications include visible blood or cerebrospinal fluid in the nose, significant facial injury, or a basilar skull fracture. Urinary drainage catheters should also be placed, unless a contraindication is found. These include blood at the urethral meatus, a perineal or scrotal hematoma, or a high-riding prostate.

After excluding an intrathoracic or CNS cause for the hemodynamic instability, abdominal sources of bleeding are then sought in an orderly fashion. DPL or FAST is performed to determine the presence of intraperitoneal blood, which would justify immediate laparotomy. Blood samples are obtained for type and crossmatch and hemoglobin and hematocrit measurement, and intravenous antibiotics are administered. Analgesics and tetanus prophylaxis are administered, as indicated.

The Hemodynamically Stable Patient

For the hemodynamically stable patient, management depends on the injuries identified and investigations planned. Laboratory values and radiographic studies are performed with specific indications. In most pediatric cases, a hemoglobin and hematocrit, AST/ALT, urinalysis, and a blood type and crossmatch are done. NGTs and Foley catheters should be placed for specific indications, not routinely. NGTs are indicated for nausea, vomiting, or suspected gastric distension, and Foley catheters are placed to decompress the bladder or if urine output measurement is important. As mentioned, Foley catheters should not be placed routinely in children. In addition to the psychological trauma of their placement, they can cause significant urethral injury in boys, especially if they are younger than 5 years of age.

Most blunt solid-organ (liver, spleen, kidney, and pancreas) injury in children can be successfully managed nonoperatively. Surgical intervention is needed for intestinal perforations, intraperitoneal bladder rupture, and most high-velocity penetrating traumas. A selective approach can be safely followed in children with abdominal stab wounds. Therefore, once the patient's workup is completed, he or she is promptly admitted to the surgical service.

SPECIFIC INJURIES

Spleen and Liver

The spleen and liver are the most commonly injured abdominal organs in children. Splenic injury should be suspected in children with a history of left-sided trauma, complaints of left upper quadrant or left shoulder pain, and anemia. Hepatic injuries are associated with a higher morbidity and mortality. Stable children with hepatic injury usually complain of right upper quadrant pain and have an elevation in hepatic enzymes.

The majority of hepatic and splenic injuries can be successfully managed nonoperatively. Nonoperative management consists of strict bed rest for 5 to 7 days, followed by a gradual return to full activities. Monitoring of hemodynamic parameters and measurement of serial hemoglobin and hematocrit values are required for the first few days after injury. Requirements for nonoperative therapy include hemodynamic stability, operating capabilities on a 24-hour basis, and blood transfusion requirements less than 40 cc/kg (one-half blood volume).[4]

Intestinal Perforation

Intestinal perforations are unusual in children and often have a nonspecific presentation. Intestinal injuries are usually diagnosed on clinical grounds within the first 24 hours after injury, occasionally with radiologic investigations. Surgical intervention is always required.[9]

Kidney, Bladder, and Urethra

Minor trauma can unmask asymptomatic renal anomalies. Between 5% and 10% of children with congenital anomalies of the genitourinary (GU) system are first diagnosed because of renal trauma.[1] Similar to splenic and hepatic injuries, renal trauma is usually due to a blunt mechanism and can be managed nonoperatively in over 90% of patients, even with urinary extravasation. Usually, a CT scan is performed to evaluate microscopic hematuria, regardless of the hemodynamic status of the patient. Bladder perforation can be diagnosed with cystography or CT scan and usually requires surgical repair.

Urethral injury in girls is rare; however, in boys, it should be suspected in those with a pelvic fracture, blood at the meatus, scrotal hematoma, a high-riding prostate, and inability to void or pass a Foley catheter. A retrograde urethrogram must be performed in these patients to evaluate the urethra and guide surgical repair.[13]

Pancreas

Because of the location of the pancreas in the retroperitoneum, pancreatic injuries are uncommon. The identification of injuries to this organ, however, remains difficult, and delays in diagnosis are common. Serum amylase level, lipase level, and abdominal CT are the most useful tests, but they still have a low sensitivity when performed during the initial evaluation. Most types of pancreatic injuries can be managed successfully nonoperatively, although this subject remains controversial.[11]

Diaphragm

Diaphragmatic injuries are rare in children and are usually due to penetrating trauma.[7] Irregular contour of the hemidiaphragm on radiologic examinations can suggest the diagnosis, although this finding is present in less than 50% of patients. Laparoscopy and DPL have been suggested as diagnostic tools, and surgical repair remains the standard of care for these injuries.[5]

Musculoskeletal

Pelvic fractures are uncommon in children, occurring in only 2% to 3% of all trauma admissions. Pedestrian injury poses the biggest risk. A pelvic x-ray quickly establishes the diagnosis and guides management. Pubic rami fractures are the most common, followed by those of the ilium or pelvic rim and, finally, the sacrum.[3] DPL can be performed in children with pelvic fractures, with specific modifications in the technique and a recognized higher false-positive rate. Open supraumbilical placement is recommended.

Angiographic intervention, for diagnosis and treatment, should be considered in hemodynamically unstable children without other sources of bleeding. The presence of multiple fractures of the pelvic rim is a predictor of associated abdominal or GU injury.[3] Lumbosacral spine fractures are unusual but should be suspected in patients with the "seat belt" sign or tenderness on palpation. A Chance fracture consists of a transverse lumbar fracture due to hyperflexion over the fulcrum of the seat belt.

"Seat Belt Syndrome"

Seat belt use has been clearly shown to decrease MVA-related deaths.[15] It is associated, however, with a specific pattern of injuries to the small intestine and lumbar spine from compression, burst, or shearing. A seat belt sign across the lower abdomen should be investigated, preferably, with a CT scan, and the patient should be admitted for observation because of the increased risk of small-bowel perforation.[17]

DISPOSITION

Role of the Consultant

All children suspected of having intraabdominal organ injury must be evaluated by a surgeon familiar with pediatric trauma. Clinical assessment, including history of significant injury, radiologic findings, and laboratory results, should be considered when deciding on the need for surgical consultation. Surgical consultation is especially indicated in any one of the following conditions:

Hemodynamic instability
Seat belt sign
Penetrating trauma
Abdominal tenderness (localized or diffuse)
Elevated AST/ALT, decreased hemoglobin and hematocrit, or hematuria
Pelvic fracture

Indications for Admission

All children with abdominal tenderness on clinical evaluation, laboratory abnormalities, or radiologic evidence of an intra-abdominal organ injury must be admitted for monitoring. Children who appear well but are unable to tolerate liquids should also be admitted. The determination of which hospital unit is most appropriate for the care of these children depends on the severity of the injury and the type of monitoring provided in each unit. Patients with a major solid-organ injury (e.g., grade IV splenic laceration) should be admitted to the intensive care unit and monitored closely. Children with suspected pancreatic or renal injury based on elevated amylase or hematuria, but without radiologic abnormalities, may be admitted to the general ward. A small group of children who appear well, have minimal abdominal discomfort, or near-normal workup can even be observed in the ED for a few hours, reexamined, and then discharged home from the ED if their symptoms resolve.

Transfer Considerations

The reasons for transferring a patient to a higher-level trauma unit depend on the patient's clinical status and the medical facilities and expertise available. Transfer indications related specifically to abdominal injury include blunt abdominal trauma, with either hemodynamic instability or signs of intestinal perforation, or penetrating abdominal injury. These represent the patients with the highest possibility for requiring surgical intervention.

COMMON PITFALLS

- Inability to promptly recognize hemodynamic instability in children
- Failure to quickly identify patients with exsanguinating intraabdominal or retroperitoneal bleeding
- Inadequate volume resuscitation (crystalloid and blood products) in patients with significant bleeding
- Failure to recognize clues of child abuse

References

1. Abou-Jaoude WA, Sugarman JM, Fallat ME, et al. Indicators of genitourinary tract injury or anomaly in cases of pediatric blunt trauma. *J Pediatr Surg* 1996;31:86.
2. American College of Surgeons. In: *Advanced trauma life support (ATLS) for doctors student course manual,* 6th ed. Chicago: American College of Surgeons, 1997.
3. Bond JB, Gotschall CS, Eichelberger MR. Predictors of abdominal injury in children with pelvic fracture. *J Trauma* 1991;31:1169.
4. Bond SJ, Eichelberger MR, Gotschall CS, et al. Nonoperative management of blunt hepatic and splenic injury in children. *Ann Surg* 1996;223:286.
5. Boulanger BR, McLellan BA. Blunt abdominal trauma. *Emerg Med Clinic North Am* 1996;14:151.
6. Colombani P, Buck J, Dudgeon D, et al. One-year experience in a regional pediatric trauma center. *J Pediatr Surg* 1985;20:8.
7. Cooper A, Barlow B, DiScala C, et al. Mortality and truncal injury: the pediatric perspective. *J Pediatr Surg* 1994;29:33.
8. Demetriades D, Rabinowitz B. Indications for operation in abdominal stab wounds. *Ann Surg* 1987;205:129.
9. Jerby BL, Attori JR, Morton D. Blunt intestinal injury in children: the role of the physical examination. *J Pediatr Surg* 1997;32:580.
10. Kapklein MJ, Mahadeo R. Pediatric trauma. *Mt Sinai J Med* 1997;64:302.
11. Keller MS, Stafford PW, Vane DW. Conservative management of pancreatic trauma in children. *J Trauma* 1997;42:1097–1100.
12. Laraque D, Barlow B, Durkin M, et al. Children who are shot: a 30-year experience. *J Pediatr Surg* 1995;30:1072.
13. McAleer IM, Kaplan GW, Scherz HC, et al. Genitourinary trauma in the pediatric patient. *Urology* 1993;42:563.
14. Mutabagani KH, Coley BD, Zumberge DW, et al. Preliminary experience with focused abdominal sonography for trauma (FAST) in children: is it useful? *J Pediatr Surg* 1999;34:48.
15. Newman KD, Bowman LM, Eichelberger MR, et al. The lap belt complex: intestinal and lumbar spine injury in children. *J Trauma* 1990;30:1133.
16. Spitalnic SJ, Berns SD. Big trauma, little patients: emergent approach to blunt trauma in pediatric patients. *Hosp Physician* 1998;17.
17. Tso EL, Beaver BL, Haller JA. Abdominal injuries in restrained pediatric passengers. *J Pediatr Surg* 1993;28:915.

CHAPTER 302
Burns

Donna A. Caniano and Marc Downing

Annually, burns result in 10,000 severe disabilities and in 2,000 deaths among children, a significant cause of morbidity and mortality. Burns represent the third leading cause of traumatic death in children, surpassed only by motor vehicle collisions and drownings. Most children with minor burns are treated at home without the aid of a physician, while the majority of patients treated in the emergency department are managed on an outpatient basis. Thus, it is important that emergency department physicians are skilled in the up-to-date care of acute and complicated pediatric burn injury.

The majority of children admitted to the hospital have total body surface area (TBSA) burns of less than 20%. The most common burn injury in children is a scald before age 4, typically involving the head, chest, and arms. Seventy percent of pediatric burns are scalds from hot liquids associated with cooking or bathing, and nearly 20% of these involve abuse, particularly tap water immersion. The remaining 30% are the result of flame, contact burns, chemical injury, high-voltage electrical burns, or tar injuries.[9]

CLINICAL PRESENTATION

The severity of thermal trauma is most closely related to the depth and extent of injury, but may also be related to inhalation injury or specific locations of the burn injury, such as joints, face, or genitalia. Other factors that contribute to the severity of the injury include the causative factors, age of the patient, toxic exposures, and concomitant traumatic injuries. The depth of injury depends on the source type, the source temperature, and the length of exposure. A scald injury usually results in partial-thickness burns, while a flame injury typically results in full-thickness burns. Infants and young children have a much thinner dermal layer of skin (compared with adults), which has a greater propensity for deep burns. Certain causative agents, such as grease, chemicals, and electricity, have the potential to cause a deeper, more severe injury because of their higher temperature, greater heat-transferring ability, sustained effect, and internal effect.

Depth of burn trauma refers to the level of destruction of the epidermis, a thin layer of epithelial cells, and the dermis, which is composed of fibrous connective tissue, blood vessels, nerves, hair follicles, and sebaceous and sweat glands (Fig. 302.1). A *first-degree* burn involves only the epidermis and presents as intact erythematous skin; this type of burn is not included in calculations of TBSA. A *second-degree* burn involves the dermis and is characterized by blistering and pain. *Third-degree* burns destroy the epidermis and dermis down to the subcutaneous fat, and if the subcutaneous fat is completely involved, the burn injury can be described as *fourth degree* (Fig. 302.1).

Another nomenclature describes burns as *superficial partial-thickness* burns that extend into the upper dermis and present with erythema, tenderness, and blistering. The pain associated with these injuries reflects the intact nerve endings in the dermis. These burns heal completely within 21 days without scarring because of epidermal cell migration from appendages remaining in the dermis. *Deep partial-thickness* burns involve more of the dermis, with fewer remaining epidermal appendages. These deeper burns can heal without grafting over prolonged periods of time, but the functional result is often improved with grafting. Superficial partial-thickness burns tend to have more exudative moisture and be hypersensitive compared with deep partial-thickness injuries, which are pale and sensitive only to deep pressure. Pain is related to the depth of injury but is not reliable for determining the depth of injured dermis, because receptors may not function in the acute phase of injury.

Full-thickness burns destroy the entire epidermis and dermis. As a result, these wounds are insensate and generally appear dry and leathery, with a pale-to-brown color. These injuries will not heal spontaneously unless the injury is very small (2 to 3 cm), because repair results from epithelial cell migration from the wound edges. Differentiating between deep partial-thickness and full-thickness burns in infants and children may be difficult or impossible in the emergency department because of the relative thinness of children's skin and overlapping clinical presentations.

The extent of burn injury can be mathematically described in terms of TBSA involvement. An accurate assessment is essential for calculating fluid requirements and determining the severity of injury. Children have relatively larger heads and smaller lower extremities than do adults, making the "rule of nines" inaccurate for patients younger than 10 years of age. By the pediatric rule of nines, the head is calculated as 18% of the TBSA and the legs as 14% each of the TBSA. A modification of the Lund and Browder chart considers these unique anatomic factors in children (Fig. 302.2). Another useful method for smaller burns is estimating the area of the burn using the patient's hand. The palm of the hand is approximately equal to 0.5% of the TBSA, and the entire palmar surface is 1% of the TBSA. Calculating the extent of the injury requires complete examination of the undressed patient and should be performed only after initial stabilization.

Electrical Burns

Electrical burns may present with small, unimpressive external wounds that obscure extensive deep-tissue destruction. The electrical current passes along neurovascular bundles, causing thrombosis of blood vessels and damage to adjacent muscle and bone. Patients with extensive muscle damage may develop myoglobinuria and may require intravenous fluids to prevent acute renal failure.

Myocardial injury from the electrical current can result in infarction and arrhythmias. An electrocardiogram should be obtained along with determination of cardiac isoenzyme values and continuous cardiac monitoring. An injury peculiar to children is the burn to the lip and commissure of the mouth caused by chewing an electrical cord. These patients should be admitted and observed for delayed hemorrhage of the labial artery and oral splinting.

Chemical Burns

Household cleaners often cause chemical burns in children. Ingestion should be suspected in any young child with a chemical burn. The burn should be copiously irrigated with warm water or normal saline for 20 minutes after removal of the child's clothing. Then the extent and depth of the burn can be assessed and treated with appropriate topical agents.

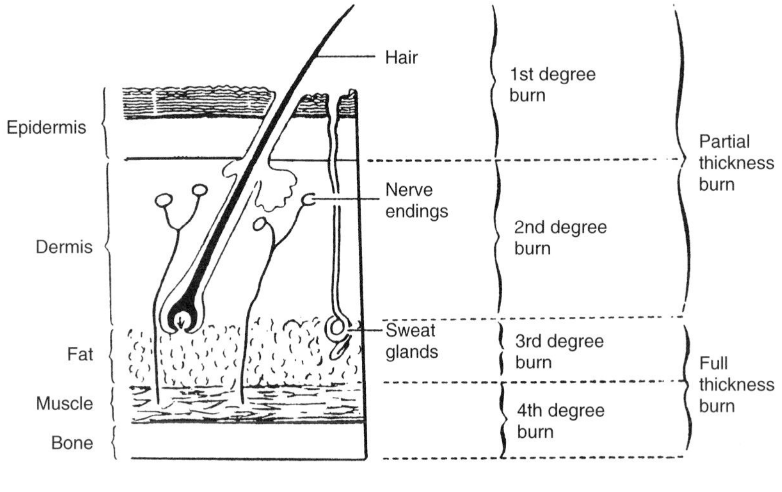

Figure 302.1. Cross-section of skin demonstrates various depths of burn

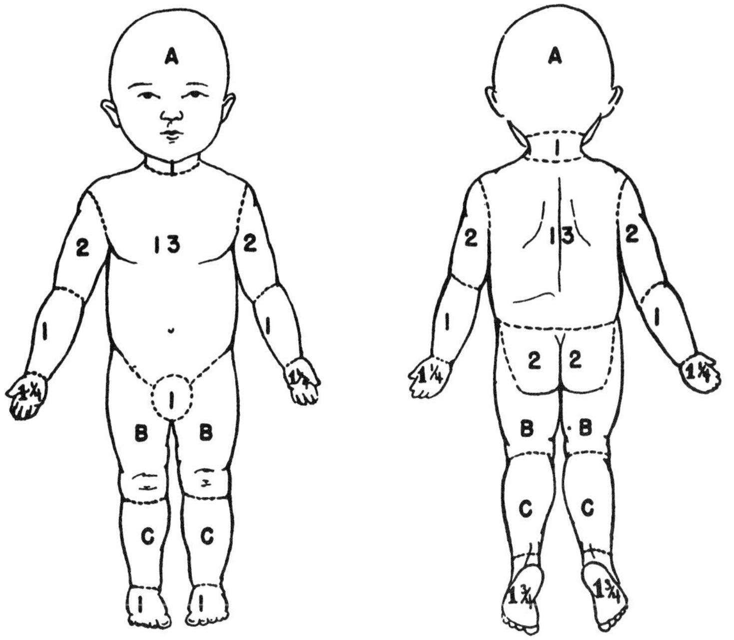

RELATIVE PERCENTAGES OF AREAS AFFECTED BY GROWTH

Area	Age 0	1	5
A = ½ of Head	9½	8½	6½
B = ½ of One Thigh	2¾	3¼	4
C = ½ of One Leg	2½	2½	2¾

% BURN BY AREAS

Probable 3rd° Burn { Head_____ Neck_____ Body_____ Up. Arm_____ Forearm_____ Hands_____ Genitals_____ Buttocks_____ Thighs_____ Legs_____ Feet_____

Total Burn { Head_____ Neck_____ Body_____ Up. Arm_____ Forearm_____ Hands_____ Genitals_____ Buttocks_____ Thighs_____ Legs_____ Feet_____

Sum of All Areas________ **Probably 3rd°** ________ **Total Burn**________

Figure 302.2. Modified Lund and Browder chart for estimation of body surface area burn involvement in infants and children.

DIFFERENTIAL DIAGNOSIS

Children sometimes present to the emergency department with apparent burn injuries but no witnessed burn event. Although such a presentation is often the result of a self-inflicted injury denied by the child or can be indicative of a nonaccidental injury, other medical conditions should be considered before a burn wound is conclusively diagnosed. *Toxic epidermal necrosis* produces diffuse epidermal sloughing related to drug usage. Severe presentations involving the mucosa and conjunctiva are known as *Stevens-Johnson syndrome,* and oropharyngeal involvement may require intubation. Clinically, it is difficult to distinguish from staphylococcal scalded skin syndrome, and a biopsy is necessary for final confirmation. Topical antibiotics are used to prevent superinfection and desiccation, and grafting may be necessary in large affected areas.

Purpura fulminans can present with extensive blistering of the skin as a complication of meningococcal sepsis. Treatment is initially directed toward resolution of the septicemia but may include excision and grafting of wounds. *Scalded skin syndrome* is associated with staphylococcal exotoxin that causes separation of the epidermal granular layer. Mucosal surfaces and conjunctiva are never involved, and the wounds heal spontaneously, provided infection and desiccation are avoided.

EMERGENCY DEPARTMENT EVALUATION

Airway

Inhalation injuries are relatively uncommon, with only 15% of admitted patients having such complications, but the high correlation with mortality emphasizes the need for careful initial evaluation of the patency and adequacy of the airway of any child with a burn injury. Airway injuries result from mucosal exposure to heat or toxins, and cause edema to the epithelial lining of the larynx, trachea, and bronchus. Clinical or historic evidence of inhalation injury demands prophylactic intubation in children, because the smaller overall size of the airway creates more flow resistance with even minimal edema, as well as the inherent difficulties associated with pediatric intubation.[4]

Physical findings consistent with inhalation injury include tachypnea, stridor, wheezing, cough, hoarseness, dysphonia, head and neck burns, oronasopharyngeal soot, swallowing difficulties, loss of consciousness, or altered mental status. Historic information that suggests the need for intubation includes a fire in a closed space and exposure to superheated gas vapor. Carbon monoxide and oxygen levels, as well as pulmonary function tests, are not helpful in determining the need for intubation. Chest radiographs and bronchoscopy are likewise not useful, and lateral cervical radiographs are not sensitive for identifying airway edema.[8]

Breathing

All burn patients should be treated with 100% oxygen during the initial evaluation period. Absolute indications for endotracheal intubation of the burned infant or child include upper airway obstruction, confirmed inhalation injury, respiratory depression, nasolabial full-thickness bums, and circumferential neck burns. Circumferential burns of the chest or abdomen may also lead to respiratory compromise that requires intubation. The choice of nasotracheal or orotracheal intubation depends on the patient's clinical condition and physician's technical skill. Of paramount importance is careful stabilization of the endotracheal tube with adhesive tape, if possible, or by other means if the face is burned, because reintubation of a patient with edema of the neck or posterior pharynx may be difficult or impossible.

Circulation

Circulation can be initially evaluated by the presence of peripheral pulses, and the character of the pulse is a clue to the overall volume status. If pulses cannot be evaluated because of overlying burns or poor overall perfusion, capillary refill can provide evidence of adequate circulation. Circulation distal to circumferential burns should be evaluated frequently to identify compromised distal perfusion. The absence of circulation should first be addressed with adequate fluid resuscitation, followed by emergent escharotomy if circulation remains poor after adequate volume resuscitation.

Secondary Survey

Although the tendency is strong to focus on the obvious burn injury, a disciplined, systematic approach to the patient is critical, particularly if other mechanisms of potential injury are reported, such as an explosion, vehicle collision, or abuse. With these mechanisms, altered mental status may reflect a head injury rather than the effects of narcotics or respiratory insufficiency, and a computed tomography (CT) scan of the head must be considered. The potential of a head injury necessitates evaluation of the cervical spine with a lateral radiograph and a cervical collar until assessment is complete.

A chest radiograph should be performed as part of the initial evaluation for any significant burn injury, and attention should also be directed toward traumatic injuries such as pneumothorax, skeletal fractures, and mediastinal injuries. Suspicion of abdominal injury should prompt careful observation, laboratory evaluation of hepatocellular enzymes and amylase, and possibly a CT of the abdomen. The remainder of the examination should evaluate the extremities and back for skeletal and soft-tissue injuries distinct from the burn injuries. A baseline neurologic examination will provide important information for future comparison, because the initial examination will be least complicated by the sequelae of the burn injury.

Abuse

As many as 20% of all hospitalized burn patients incur their injuries as a result of child abuse[7]; thus, the physician must consider the possibility that each pediatric burn injury represents a nonaccidental injury. Circumstances suggestive of intentional burn injury include a history of "accidents," a history inconsistent with the injuries, conflicting stories from the caregivers and child, or a history incompatible with the child's developmental stage. Over one-half of children with intentional burn injuries have previous injuries or abuse, and almost the same percentage have delays in their presentation.[7]

Findings consistent with abuse include a contact burn with a recognizable or symmetric pattern, coexistent musculoskeletal or soft-tissue trauma, and well-demarcated, bilateral, or circumferential burns of buttocks, perineum, or extremities. Scald burns represent the majority of intentional burns and commonly result from immersion into hot water. Typically, these injuries have an absence of splash marks and a sparing of flexion creases. Victims of abuse are more likely to have an unstable family situation, a single-parent home, and lower socioeconomic status.

EMERGENCY DEPARTMENT MANAGEMENT

Fluid Resuscitation

Once the depth and extent of the burn injury are determined, the injury can be categorized according to the system in Table 302.1. Children with burns of greater than 20% TBSA require intravenous fluid resuscitation due to the systemic impact of burns of this extent. Patients with lesser burns who have suspected inhalation injury should be treated cautiously with intravenous fluids in order to minimize contributions to airway edema. Two intravenous catheters of the largest possible size in an unburned area are preferable.

If peripheral intravenous access cannot be established, intraosseous access can be established at the tibia, femur, or sternum, especially in children less than 6 years of age. Other intravenous options include a saphenous vein cutdown at the medial ankle and central venous access via the jugular, subclavian, or femoral routes. Due to the higher BSA-to-weight ratio in children, fluid losses are increased relative to body weight. As a result, the classic burn resuscitation formula has been modified for children.

The modified Parkland formula administers lactated Ringer's solution over the first 24 hours from the time of injury, using the following calculation: 4 mL/kg/%TBSA plus maintenance volume. One-half of the burn resuscitation fluid is given over the first 8 hours, and the remainder over the subsequent 16 hours. For example, a child weighing 20 kg with a 40% burn should receive 3,200 mL of resuscitation fluid in the first 24 hours plus 60 mL of maintenance fluid hourly. If the child arrives 1 hour after the injury with an intravenous line at 100 mL/h, the new rate would be 283 mL/h ((1,600 − 40)/7 = 223 + 60 = 283) for the next 7 hours and 160 mL/h (1,600/16 + 60)

TABLE 302.1. Burn Classification

Minor burn injury	<15% TBSA burn <10% TBSA burn in children <10 yr old <2% TBSA full-thickness burn
Moderate burn injury	15%-25% TBSA burn 10%-20% TBSA burn in children <10 yr old <10% TBSA full-thickness burn involving the face, eye, ear, hand, foot, or perineum
Major burn injury	>25% TBSA burn >20% TBSA burn in children <10 yr old >10% TBSA full-thickness burn Injury involving the face, eye, ear, hand, foot, or perineum, with likely functional and/or cosmetic disability High-voltage electrical burn injury All burn injuries with concomitant inhalation injury or major trauma

for the subsequent 16 hours. This formula provides only a guideline and should be adjusted according to urine output, which should be greater than 1 mL/kg/h for children less than 14 years of age, and greater than 2 mL/kg/h for those less than 3 years of age.

The insertion of a Foley catheter is essential for following the adequacy of the resuscitation. Additional parameters that are useful for assessing response to intravenous fluids are pulse quality, heart rate, and peripheral perfusion.

Initial laboratory tests should include a complete blood cell count, electrolytes, type and screen, urinalysis, and arterial blood gas analysis. A carboxyhemoglobin level should be obtained, and a cyanide level considered, on patients with suspected inhalation injury or a history of fire in a closed space. The urine should be screened for free hemoglobin or myoglobin in significant burns. A nasogastric tube is necessary in all patients with burns greater than 20% TBSA, due to anticipated intestinal ileus.

Escharotomy

Full-thickness burns create a leathery coagulum of necrotic tissues known as the eschar. If the full-thickness burn is circumferential in an extremity, the inflexible eschar and progressive edema beneath the eschar can lead to increased compartment pressures that impede venous return initially and arterial inflow ultimately. If this circumferential burn involves the chest and upper abdomen, the restriction of chest expansion and diaphragm excursion can result in respiratory embarrassment. Either of these circumstances may warrant an escharotomy. If a surgeon is not available or is delayed, emergent escharotomy may be necessary to preserve a limb or a life in the case of thoracic circumferential burns. Skeletal trauma and electrical burns may necessitate a fasciotomy, which should be accomplished in the operating room.

An incision through the burn eschar to the underlying subcutaneous fat can be accomplished by using a scalpel or electrocautery. Because the eschar and underlying tissue are insensate, analgesia is not required, but sedation should be considered. Bleeding should be minimal and can be treated effectively with gentle pressure. Release of the eschar is accomplished with medial and lateral incisions of the arms and legs, including involved joints, with care to avoid superficial blood vessels and nerves.

Escharotomy is indicated in limbs with distal cyanosis, decreased capillary refill, decreased pulses, or progressive neurologic change. Serial Doppler flow measurements of vessels distal to the burn are useful in deciding whether an escharotomy is adequate. Impending respiratory failure should prompt intubation and bilateral escharotomy of the chest along the anterior axillary line. If ventilation remains impaired, the chest escharotomy can be extended with one or two horizontal incisions connecting the lateral escharotomies at their superior or inferior extents.

Hands and fingers with circumferential burns are important areas to assess because of the potential disability that can result from delay in diagnosis of ischemia or from injury related to attempted escharotomy. Doppler signals of the radial and ulnar arteries do not adequately predict hand perfusion; thus, flow in the superficial palmar or digital arteries must be confirmed to ensure adequate hand circulation.

Other clinical indications for escharotomy in the hand or fingers include pain, inability to passively straighten the fingers, loss of nailbed capillary refill, and tenseness of the tissue on palpation. Escharotomy of the fingers requires only one incision axially on the ulnar surface between the neurovascular bundle and the extensor apparatus. The thumb can be approached similarly, with an incision along the radial aspect. The dorsum of the hand can be released with one or more incisions between the metacarpals. The wrist can be released medially and laterally, avoiding the superficial radial and ulnar nerves.

Outpatient Care of the Burn Wound

The care of burn wounds in the emergency department can be complicated and time consuming. Keys to success include adequate pain relief and thorough cleansing of the burn wound. Analgesia in the form of narcotics and sedation in the form of benzodiazepines should be used liberally for the initial phase. Moist saline dressings provide some pain relief and may limit the ultimate depth of burn injury, but they should be employed only with small wounds, due to the risk of hypothermia. Thirty minutes after the administration of narcotics and cool towels, the wound should be cleansed thoroughly, using mild antiseptic soap, and loose tissue should be debrided. Intact blisters that are not over mobile areas can be left intact, although large blisters should be unroofed.

Following cleansing and debridement, burns can be covered with a 3- to 5-mm layer of silver sulfadiazine (Silvadene 1%), which provides broad-spectrum bacterial coverage. The topical agent can then be covered with a nonstick, porous gauze and wrapped in a bulky occlusive dressing. For wounds that require further debridement, the nonstick gauze can be omitted; thus, the dressing removes loose tissue when it is taken off. This dressing will need to be changed twice daily, with all topical agents completely removed. Caregivers should be informed that the yellow color in the dressing is not indicative of infection.

Mafenide (Sulfamylon 8.5%) has properties similar to those of silver sulfadiazine but has little role in the outpatient care of burns because of the pain experienced with application. Povidone–iodine 1% ointment can be used in areas prone to maceration, because this ointment has a drying effect. For children with sulfa allergies or burns of the ears, gentamicin cream can be applied twice daily. This agent should not be considered a first-line agent, because it does not cover gram-positive organisms, and it should not be used on large burns because of the risk of ototoxicity and nephrotoxicity. Bacitracin ointment can be applied four times daily for minor neck and facial burns, because silver sulfadiazine is irritating to the eyes.

Tetanus toxoid (0.5 mL intramuscularly) should be given to any child who has not had a booster within 5 years or whose last immunization date is unknown. If the child has had no immunizations, 250 U of intramuscular tetanus human immune globulin should be given, along with the first of a series of active immunizations with tetanus toxoid.

The goals of outpatient care are to prevent infection and maintain mobility of involved joints. Education of the caregiver becomes the most critical aspect of the patient's care. Oral pain relief in the form of codeine (often with acetaminophen) is essential. The patient should also be given a prescription for diphenhydramine for pruritus. The child's caretaker needs to be carefully instructed in dressing care and given prescriptions for necessary supplies and topical medications. Caregivers should be instructed to immediately initiate mobilization at least five times daily, with gentle stretching, to prevent loss of function. All patients should be reevaluated in 24 to 48 hours in the emergency department or with a primary physician.

Hospitalization for Burn Wound Care

Once the decision to admit a patient with burns has been made (Table 302.2) and the patient is physiologically stable, transport should be expedited so that debridement and dressings can be initiated. No topical treatments should be applied prior to trans-

TABLE 302.2. Admission Criteria

Greater than 10% second-degree burns	Other major medical problems
Greater than 2% third-degree burns	Oral pain management insufficient
Burn of hand, foot, face, perineum, or genitalia	Family cannot perform dressing changes
Inhalation injury	Inadequate social support
Significant electrical or chemical burn	Suspicion of child abuse or neglect
	Follow-up compliance dubious

fer, as they will interfere with initial inspection of the wound and may preclude the use of some types of burn wound coverings.

Transfer to Burn Care Centers

Patients with major burns should be transferred to burn centers, where an integrated team approach can decrease mortality by 30% and morbidity by 40%.[2] Because sepsis resulting from burn wound infections is the major source of mortality in extensive burns (greater than 15%), some consideration should be given to prevention of burn wound contamination during the initial evaluation. Dry and clean dressings allow adequate dissipation of wound heat without contributing to hypothermia and protect the wound from further contamination. A "sterile" approach to the burn patient is both unrealistic and unnecessary; at the same time, gloves and masks should be worn by health care providers, and sterile sheets should cover the patient.

Meticulous attention must be paid to stabilizing the patient before transport, including two peripheral intravenous lines, a nasogastric tube, and Foley catheter. The patient's airway must be secured; if there is any question about a child's respiratory status, intubation should be performed before transport. Appropriate intravenous fluid resuscitation should be initiated, and monitoring should be employed throughout transport. Analgesics should not be administered intramuscularly in major burns, because absorption may be unpredictable.

COMMON PITFALLS

- Intubation is often delayed because inhalation injury is unrecognized or unappreciated.
- Inappropriate discharge can result from underestimation of the depth and extent of the burn.
- The severity of electrical injury is easily underestimated, resulting in delayed transfer to a burn center.
- Child abuse cannot be recognized if it is not suspected.
- Too narrow an approach to the patient can result in failure to identify associated injuries.
- At discharge, do not forget to explain dressing care to caretakers, to provide adequate pain control, to arrange appropriate follow-up, and to provide or give a prescription for necessary wound-care supplies.

References

1. American College of Surgeons Committee on Trauma. *Advanced trauma life support for doctors.* Chicago: American College of Surgeons, 1997.
2. Demling RH. The advantage of the burn team approach. *J Burn Care Rehabil* 1995;16: 569–572.
3. Hansbrough JF, Hansbrough W. Pediatric burns. *Pediatr Rev* 1999;20:117–1124.
4. Hantson P, Butera R, Clemessy JL, et al. Early complications and value of initial clinical and paraclinical observations in victims of smoke inhalation without burns. *Chest* 1997;111:671–675.
5. Hermans MHE. Results of a survey on the use of different treatment options for partial and full thickness burns. *Burns* 1998;24:539–551.
6. Herndon DN, ed. *Total burn care.* Philadelphia: WB Saunders, 1996.
7. Hultman CS, Priolo D, Cairns BA, et al. Return to jeopardy: the fate of pediatric burn patients who are victims of abuse and neglect. *J Burn Care Rehabil* 1998;19:367–376.
8. Muehlberger T, Kunar D, Munster A, et al. Efficacy of fiberoptic laryngoscopy in the diagnosis of inhalation injuries. Arch Otolaryngol Head Neck Surg 1998;124:1003–1007.
9. Sheridan RL. The seriously burned child: resuscitation through reintegration. *Curr Probl Pediatr* 1998;28:105–127, 139–167.
10. Silverman SH, Purdue GF, Hunt JL, et al. Cyanide toxicity in burned patients. *J Trauma* 1988;28:171–176.
11. Smith MA, Munster AM, Spence RJ. Burns of the hand and upper limb—a review. *Burns* 1998;24:493–505.

CHAPTER 303

Fractures and Sports Injuries

Christopher S. Kennedy

Fractures account for up to 10% to 15% of emergency department (ED) visits of children, owing to their high activity level, youthful fearlessness, poor judgment, and underdeveloped motor coordination. High-energy trauma has become more significant, although the incidence may decrease with stricter car seat and seat belt laws and enforcement. Also, over the past decade, as participation in organized youth sports programs has increased, so has the spectrum of injuries sustained by children.

Children's fractures are not smaller versions of adult fractures. Because children's bones are actively growing, children have a distinct bony architecture different from that of adults, and active growth may make different growth areas more susceptible at different stages. Actively growing bones are described by three areas: the epiphysis, metaphysis, and diaphysis.

Generally, children's bones are more porous, more pliable, and overall have less strength than those of adults. Likewise, because ligamentous attachments are stronger than their bony attachments, fractures (e.g., avulsions) are more common than sprains, strains, or dislocations. Children's fractures have a high rate of healing and potential for deformity correction through remodeling. Pediatric fracture healing is complicated by problems such as plastic deformation, growth arrest, and progressive angulation.

A thorough examination is necessary, not only of the fracture site, but also to rule out any associated or occult injury. This can be challenging with a frightened, uncooperative patient who is in pain, and with concerned parents hovering nearby. After taking a history and performing a searching physical examination, further diagnostic studies, usually plain radiographs, are obtained. Laboratory evaluation has minimal utility in most fracture decision making. If an isolated extremity injury is the presumptive diagnosis, adequate pain control should be strongly considered and may be started before plain films are performed. Occasionally, pelvic fractures and multiple long-bone fractures may cause enough blood loss to result in hemodynamic compromise. Barring suspicion of these injuries, hemodynamic instability merits a careful examination to seek others sources of blood loss.

Treatment is based on the complete diagnosis and should include pain control. Options include definitive treatment by the emergency physician, splinting and referral, or immediate consultation with orthopedic or other specialists.

EMERGENCY DEPARTMENT EVALUATION

Accurate, complete diagnosis is of paramount importance. Common fracture patterns and associations are easily recognized if the treating physician is familiar with them. Management, based on some knowledge of the natural history, is usually straightforward if the diagnosis is correct and complete. An incorrect or delayed diagnosis can result in complications. Although the rapid healing of children's fractures is generally beneficial, it can decrease the time frame in which interventions are possible, usually to about a week or so.

History

It is tempting to take a quick history, believing that the x-rays will show everything, but it is important to establish the circumstances and mechanism of injury. The time spent obtaining the history also allows the physician time to establish rapport with the parent and to calm and gain the trust of the child.

When the nature of the injury seems implausible, child abuse must be considered. If high-energy trauma was involved, occult intraabdominal or intracranial injury must be sought. If the cause of the fracture is a mystery to the child, the physician must consider the possibility of seizures, leading to a fall.

The mechanism of injury provides clues as well. The common fall on an outstretched arm can produce wrist, forearm, or elbow fractures, or a combination of these. Falls from a height may result in calcaneus fractures associated with lumbar spine fractures. A dashboard injury can fracture the patella and can cause a hip fracture or dislocation.

Physical Examination

It is difficult to overemphasize the importance of the physical examination. The uninjured extremities and the spine are examined first; the physician should reassure the child that he or she will not cause pain unexpectedly. This may reveal occult injuries while the child is most cooperative and least upset.

When examining the injured extremity, the examiner should start at the end farthest from the painful area. Careful, thorough palpation of the entire limb is important. Any significantly tender areas should be x-rayed.

When possible, joints should be taken through a range of motion to assess for possible dislocation, particularly in the older child. This is most important for the shoulder, elbow (including pronation and supination), and hip. The joints should be palpated as well; radial head and proximal fibula fractures are frequently missed.

The skin should be thoroughly assessed, including the part hidden by splints applied as first aid. A laceration over a joint requires exploration to rule out an arthrotomy, a condition requiring urgent management. A break in the skin associated with a fracture is usually an open fracture, particularly if it has a continuous, slow oozing of dark blood, characteristically associated with fat droplets. This requires emergent intervention as well.

Neurologic and vascular examinations must not be omitted. Frequently, the child will cooperate with at least a sensory examination for light touch. More encouragement may be rewarded with a limited motor examination. A wiggle is better than nothing.

Compartment syndrome must not be overlooked. It is most common in the forearm and lower leg as a result of either fracture or crushing injuries, leading to bleeding and swelling within inelastic fascial compartments. Elevated pressures lead to ischemia at the capillary level and, untreated, can threaten the entire limb from muscle and nerve necrosis. The hallmarks are pain out of proportion to the degree of injury, and extreme pain with passive range of motion of the fingers or toes. Paresthesias, pulselessness, and pallor are all late manifestations. A compartment syndrome is a true orthopedic emergency, and early consultation with an orthopedist is warranted. Definitive diagnosis should be in concert with an orthopedist to measure compartment pressure. Emergent fasciotomy is required to preserve limb function.

Unfortunately, a fracture during childhood may be a manifestation of child abuse in up to 5% to 18% of cases. Suspicion for child abuse should be high when an infant (less than 1 year old) has a fracture, there are inconsistencies between the history and the fracture type or developmental abilities of the child, there are multiple fractures in different stages of healing, or there are multiple complex or depressed fractures. Certain fracture types are associated with child abuse. Especially noteworthy would be a spiral fracture of the femur or tibia in a nonambulating child, spiral fracture of the humerus, an avulsion of the clavicle or acromion process, or a metaphyseal chip fracture. Any suspicious finding constitutes grounds for reporting to local social service officials and consultation with the nearest center providing comprehensive care for the abused child.

Radiographic Evaluation

Obtaining high-quality radiographs is nearly as important as the physical examination. Performing an inadequate examination and accepting poor radiographs can mean missing a fracture. Long bone fractures should be splinted, preferably with plaster, before taking x-rays. Unstable joint injuries also may be splinted, although this sometimes obscures crucial detail.

X-rays should be made at 90 degrees (orthogonal) to each other. With diaphyseal fractures, radiographs should be taken of the joint above and below, particularly if there is any tenderness or if the physical examination is limited. The wrist and elbow cannot be adequately evaluated with regular forearm films. Foregoing additional radiographs and missing an associated fracture is, obviously, a false economy.

Comparison views can be helpful. An anteroposterior view of the pelvis, with a lateral view of the affected hip, should be routinely ordered, rather than an anteroposterior and lateral view of the hip. Elbows can be difficult to evaluate without a contralateral control, even for the subspecialist. Comparison views are also frequently indicated for ankle fractures or shoulder injuries. Oblique x-rays can aid in diagnosis as well, particularly in the knee, ankle, and elbow.

Some injuries have a high rate of missed associated fractures. Cervical spine and pelvic radiographs should be part of the protocol for high-energy trauma. Chest x-rays should be evaluated for bony injuries. A calcaneus fracture due to a fall should prompt lumbar spine films. Suspected child abuse should be routinely pursued with a skeletal survey.

Poor-quality films must not be accepted. The child may be uncomfortable and the radiologic technician may shy away from getting good films, but the duty of diagnosis ultimately rests with the physician, who should insist on films with good anteroposterior views and truly lateral laterals. Excessive obliquity easily obscures subtle fractures. After the failure to perform an adequate physical examination, the most common cause of overlooked injuries is probably poor-quality films.

Additional imaging techniques are sometimes helpful. Stress views are commonly used to evaluate acromioclavicular joint injuries and occult knee-joint growth plate or ligament injuries. Computed tomography (CT) scanning is frequently used for spine injuries and has replaced tomography in most areas. More intensive techniques, such as arthrography, arteriography, bone scanning, and magnetic resonance imaging are of great benefit when indicated, but are typically considered to be the domain of the consultant.

DESCRIPTION OF FRACTURES

Proper use of fracture nomenclature can do much to elevate the status of the emergency physician in the eyes of the consultant. Simplicity is the key, avoiding unfamiliar eponyms and references to bony landmarks.

The description should begin by naming the injured bone. In the hand, use of the terms *thumb, index finger, long finger, ring finger,* and *small finger* is preferable to numeric description, due to confusion as to whether the thumb is counted or if the count starts medially or laterally.

Fractures are classified by where they are on the bone. Shaft fractures are diaphyseal. The flare is the metaphysis. The radiolucent growth plate is the physis, and the epiphysis is the secondary ossification center. "Proximal" or "distal" is the best way to distinguish one end of the bone from the other.

Displacement is relative to the width of the shaft. Nondisplaced fractures show only a hairline fracture. Displacement of only 5% to 10% of the shaft width is termed *minimally displaced*. Further displacement is described by percentage.

Angulation is described separately from displacement, by both degrees of angulation and direction, with the apex as the reference direction. For example, the common Colles' fracture is volar angulation, even though the hand is deformed in a dorsal direction.

Various fracture configurations are described below (Fig. 303.1).

Growth plate injuries are classified by the Salter-Harris scheme (Fig. 303.2), with the risk of growth problems increasing with grade. Salter III and IV are further complicated by the potential for intraarticular displacement. Salter V fractures are often diagnosed only in retrospect.

It is important to describe any associated injuries, particularly the nature of the injury (i.e., open or closed) and the child's neurovascular status, as these can alter crucial treatment decisions.

EMERGENCY DEPARTMENT MANAGEMENT

The treatment options are to treat the fracture definitively in the ED, to splint and provide temporary treatment with later referral to a specialist, or to seek immediate consultation.

Some simple fractures with low risk of problems and uniformly good outcomes may be cared for completely in the ED. Factors in this decision include the physician's degree of confidence in fracture management, ease of providing follow-up care, and acceptance by the parents of the treatment plan.

Temporary splinting with later referral is more common. Common indications are nondisplaced or minimally displaced fractures and fractures with a low risk of short-term complications such as neurovascular compromise or compartment syndrome.

Immediate consultation should be sought for all open fractures, arthrotomies, and unreduced dislocations. Open fractures should be regarded as orthopedic emergencies. They should be treated with prophylactic intravenous antibiotics (e.g., broad-spectrum cephalosporins), tetanus prophylaxis, and orthopedic consultation. Neurovascular injury and compartment syndrome require emergent surgical intervention. Consultation is also indicated when there is a high index of suspicion but adequate evaluation has failed to establish a diagnosis. Triage of displaced fractures that require reduction depends on the relationship between the emergency physician and the orthopedist. Many orthopedists prefer to see the child initially and perform

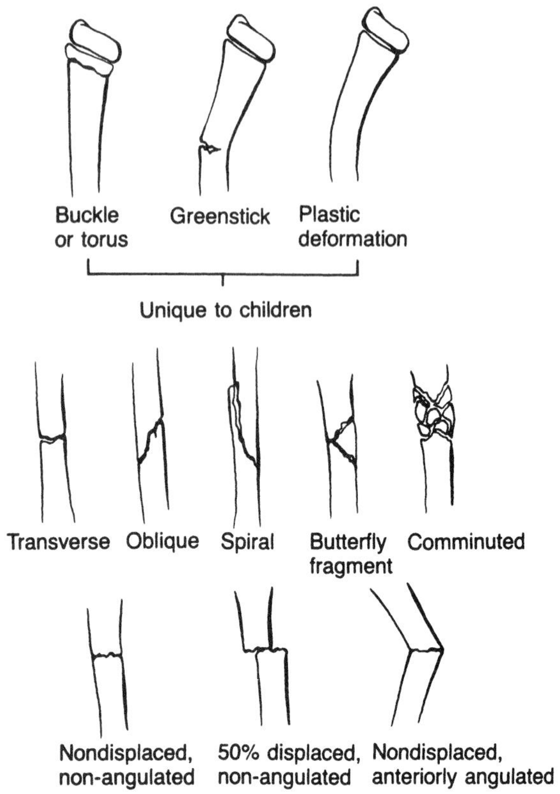

Figure 303.1. Descriptive terminology for pediatric fractures.

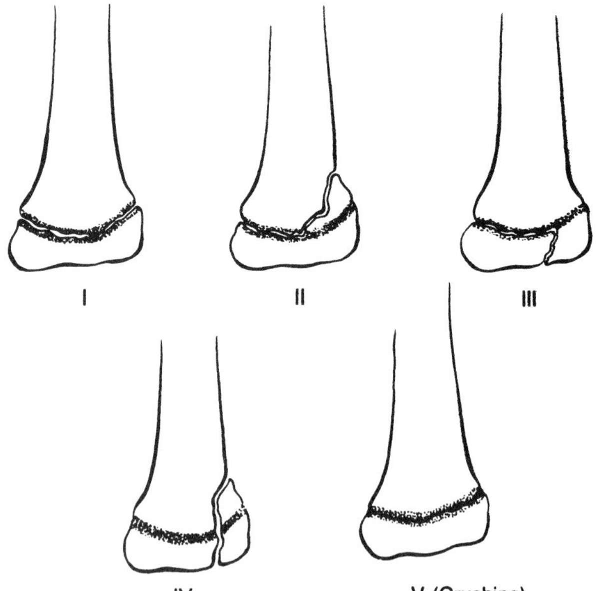

Figure 303.2. Salter-Harris nomenclature of representative fractures involving the growth plate in children.

the reduction in the ED, where there is appropriate equipment and support personnel.

Immobilization

Immobilization decreases the discomfort in the injured limb. It also can maintain the fracture in a reduced position and prevent further injury by jagged fracture fragments.

Choices for immobilization are varied. Splints are the most popular, and plaster of Paris is best, owing to its ease of molding, although prepadded, fiberglass splint material is being used in many areas. A good plaster splint requires adequate padding, with particular attention to bony prominences. The splint should hold the joint above and below the fracture. Too long is better than too short. Fifteen layers of plaster is the standard. It should be applied and overwrapped while wet for a good mold. Movement while hardening greatly weakens the splint. Commercial splints are much less desirable due to the difficulty of proper fitting and the resulting poor immobilization. Inflatable splints may exert external pressure on already traumatized tissue.

Casts are less commonly used by emergency physicians due to problems associated with swelling inside a rigid cast. This difficulty may be alleviated to some degree by splitting the cast. Ice and elevation are critically important in managing swelling in all fractures. Proper cast application requires skill and practice to achieve the proper balance between being tight enough to maintain the immobilization and loose enough to avoid problems with swelling. Overall, a splint is more easily applied and is superior to a poorly fitting cast. Neurovascular status distal to the affected limb should be evaluated and documented both before and after splinting.

If the child is being transferred or referred for later treatment, the fracture fragments must not be left in a position that tents the skin. Skin necrosis can result in conversion to an open fracture in only a few hours.

Operative Treatment

Detailed discussion is beyond the scope of this chapter. Operative intervention is usually indicated for fractures with a high degree of instability, such as supracondylar humerus fractures; a high risk of problems from displacement, such as intraarticular fractures or severe growth plate injuries; and open fractures, to remove contaminated, necrotic tissue and to reduce the risk of infection. Internal fixation is also used to make overall management easier in head-injured and multiply injured children.

Complications

Neurovascular injury and compartment syndrome, discussed previously, may result in loss of function or even loss of the limb. Angular deformity is common, but many deformities remodel if sufficient growth remains and the deformity is in the plane of joint motion. A general rule is that remodeling will be adequate if the child's deformed bone fits within the outline of the adult bone. No remodeling is to be expected in rotational deformity, nor in displaced Salter III and IV fractures.

The child's growth potential can lead to problems with physeal fractures. Partial or complete growth arrest leads to progressive angular malalignment or limb-length discrepancy, respectively, and requires surgery for correction, often with compromised results.

Discharge Instructions

The parents should be taught routine care of the cast or splint, the importance of frequent neurovascular checks, and that adequate pain medication should be provided, and the importance of ice and elevation must be stressed. The parents must understand the need for follow-up care and the risk of complications if this is neglected.

Treatment of Specific Fractures

Shoulder

The clavicle is the most commonly fractured bone in childhood. Usually resulting from a fall in children less than 10 years old, the majority can be managed without orthopedic referral. Clavicular fractures in children less than 2 years of age should raise concern for intentional injury. Fractures of the clavicle can usually be treated with a figure-of-eight strap or a sling for comfort. Minimally displaced proximal or diaphyseal humerus fractures can be splinted. A shoulder injury requires either an axillary or a good "Y" scapular lateral view to rule out dislocation. The hallmark of posterior dislocation is loss of external rotation.

Elbow

Pediatric elbow fractures have high rates of complications, even in the hands of experts. In order to confirm the diagnosis, a true lateral film of the elbow is required. Radiographic evidence of a torus fracture may be subtle, and a nondisplaced fracture may be difficult to diagnose. Radiographs must be carefully inspected for the presence of abnormal fat pads, especially the presence of a posterior fat pad. Also important is the alignment of the radial head with the capitellum. To evaluate this alignment, a line drawn through the central axis of the radius should pass through the center of the capitellum. Comparison views of the unaffected extremity may prove helpful if the diagnosis is not clear. Isolated abnormalities in the fat pads should be considered signs of occult fracture; immobilization and prompt follow-up should be arranged in consultation with an orthopedist. In general, any displaced distal humerus fracture requires pinning. Supracondylar fractures have a high incidence of neurovascular injury and compartment syndrome. Late deformity results from less-than-anatomic reduction. Medial epicondyle fractures in younger children have a high association with elbow dislocation. Minimally displaced radial head fractures are usually treated with early motion.

Forearm

Forearm fractures are common fractures of childhood. Good results are the norm, even with growth plate injury. Isolated distal ulna torus fractures usually have an associated distal radius physeal fracture. True buckle fractures require only 3 to 4 weeks of immobilization.

Hand

Children's hand fractures, unless the injury is severe, are generally free of the stiffness problems that plague adults. Phalangeal fractures involving the growth plate or through the joint should be followed up by an orthopedist, but can be splinted in the ED. Before splinting, each phalangeal injury should be examined for the presence of rotational or malrotation deformity, which may be missed if the digit is examined only in extension. To examine for rotational deformity, the fingers should be flexed to make sure all fingers point in the same direction. Overlapping of the digits occurs if rotational deformity is present and reduction is needed. A nailbed injury with the nail pulled out proximally and overlying the eponychial fold is generally associated with a

Salter fracture of the distal phalanx. This is an easily overlooked open fracture. Nailbed injuries require precise repair.

Hip

A slipped capital femoral epiphysis is easily missed. The child usually presents with no or minimal trauma, groin aching, or simply medial thigh and knee pain. Hallmarks on physical examination are mandatory abduction and external rotation when the hip is brought into flexion. Delay in diagnosis is associated with progressive slipping. Radiographic findings can be subtle, especially in early cases; therefore, good lateral radiographs are required.

Knee

Knee pain can be referred from the hip. Strong consideration should be given to the routine use of anteroposterior pelvic and lateral hip x-rays when evaluating knee pain. Ligament injuries are less common in children's knees than are occult growth plate injuries. Stress views can establish the diagnosis only if the child is relaxed and cooperative. A dislocated patella may be reduced simply by bringing the knee into extension. Tibia fractures may be a common cause of compartment syndrome.

Leg

The term *toddler fracture* refers to an oblique nondisplaced fracture of the distal tibia, usually occurring in children under 4 years of age. These children may present to the ED with complaints of a limp and a history of a minor accident, and physical findings may be subtle. Pain with gentle twisting of the leg may be the only localizing physical finding. Because they may poorly localize, complete radiographs of both lower extremities are needed. Immobilization usually provides relief of symptoms, and at least telephone consultation with a pediatric orthopedist is advisable.

Ankle

The fracture pattern varies with age. An example of this age variation is the distal tibia fracture called a "Tillaux fracture," which is unique to adolescents. As skeletal maturity is achieved and growth plates are beginning to close, the medial distal tibial epiphysis closes prior to the lateral. This creates a fulcrum through which a Salter-Harris III fracture may occur, just lateral to the point of fusion. Due to growth plate involvement and a potential need for open fixation, a prompt orthopedic consultation is indicated. Intraarticular injury is common. Widening of the mortise may require surgery. CT scans are useful in evaluating complex fracture patterns. Comparison views may help in difficult cases.

Foot

Lawn mower injuries are a common cause of open fractures. Severe contamination and degree of injury may require operative debridement. Athletes are subject to metatarsal stress fractures, particularly in adolescence. Fractures at the very base of the fifth metatarsal require only minimal treatment, but proximal metaphyseal fractures outside the articular area (Jones fractures) need cast immobilization and a period of nonweightbearing. Malalignment at the base of the metatarsals, particularly the second, suggests a Lisfranc dislocation, which has a high risk of associated complications.

Sports Injuries

Over the past decade, larger numbers of children began to participate in organized youth sports programs. This has led to an increase in sports-related injuries. Common among these injuries, other than various acute fractures, are overuse injuries, avulsion fractures, stress fractures, and ligamentous injuries. The following are specific examples.

Peripheral Nerve Injuries: The Stinger

A "stinger" is a peripheral nerve injury that involves an upper limb unilaterally. This nerve injury is most commonly caused by a compressive overload of the head and neck, such as caused by tackling in football. The athlete experiences a burning pain in the affected limb, which may last from seconds to hours, and there may be associated weakness. More than single-limb involvement should raise concern for possible cervical spine injury. The athlete should be immobilized on the field and transported to the ED. Most athletes transported to the ED with cervical immobilization for a tackling injury require cervical spine radiographs before removing the cervical collar. Cervical spine fracture is a rare diagnosis. Most patients should be advised in the ED to discontinue play until cleared by a follow-up visit with their primary care, sports medicine, or orthopedic specialist, and some will require aggressive physical therapy.

Overuse Injuries

Stress Fractures. Stress fractures are becoming more common in children. Risk factors include a high-"volume" or repetitive activity and improper training or overtraining. The most common sites of injury in children are the tibia, fibula, and the pars interarticularis segment of the vertebra (i.e., spondylolysis). Each of these stress fractures may cause localized tenderness; most require more than plain films, and so are not usually diagnosed in the ED. One exception may be spondylolysis, the most common cause of back pain in a child to yield an anatomic diagnosis. The thin segment of bone between facet joints is subject to high forces, especially with marked lordosis, or heavy lifting. Most commonly seen in the early teen years, the frequency may reach 20% of those athletes competing in wrestling, gymnastics, or weight lifting. While pain will be exacerbated by straight leg raising, radiation of pain into the legs is rare. Plain film radiography may reveal the diagnosis and is best visualized on oblique views. The most frequent location is at L5, followed by L4. Management is conservative, and the athlete should be discouraged from sports participation if activity is painful. Outpatient follow-up with a bone scan may be needed.

Little League Elbow. Little League elbow is an overuse injury seen in young pitchers. The usual presentation is elbow pain and a subtle flexion contracture, most commonly caused by valgus strain during the acceleration phase of throwing. Plain films of the elbow are normal. Treatment should include rest from play until the child is cleared by a qualified physician. No immobilization is needed.

Iliac Crest Apophysitis. Iliac crest apophysitis is an overuse injury commonly seen in runners and hockey, soccer, or football players. The main symptom is pain over the affected iliac crest that is worsened with running. Plain radiographs are normal. Treatment is conservative.

Patellofemoral Stress Syndrome. Patellofemoral stress syndrome is the most common complaint in young female athletes. The common presentation is of aching knees, with pain increased by jumping or climbing. Physical findings usually include pain on compression of the patellar region; joint effusion and swelling are rare. Plain films are normal. Treatment includes relative rest and physical therapy.

Sever Disease. Sever disease, or calcaneal apophysitis, is a common complaint of adolescent boys. The chief complaint is pain in the heel that is worsened by running. No swelling or deformity is noted on physical examination; only tenderness is noted with lateral and medial compression of the calcaneus. Radiographs are not helpful. Treatment includes plantar flexibility exercises. The disease is usually self-limited.

Avulsion Fractures

Avulsion fractures may occur at virtually any muscular insertion point. Two noteworthy examples in children include avulsions about the pelvis and avulsions about the tibial spine or intercondylar eminence. Avulsion fractures of the hip may occur at a muscular attachment typically pulled off during strong, active resistance. Pain is localized but may be significant with weight bearing. Often, the diagnosis can be made by plain film radiographs. Treatment is conservative, with partial or no weight bearing for 4 to 6 weeks.

Intercondylar eminence or tibial spine fracture occurs from anterior cruciate ligament injury resulting from either noncontact or collision trauma. Typically, this happens with abrupt decelerating or direction changes, with or without an audible "pop." Gross swelling about the knee joint is a prominent physical finding, as is intense pain. Plain film radiographs may reveal the fragment as nondisplaced (type I), minimally displaced (type II), or with rotation or significant displacement (type III). This injury should prompt consultation with an orthopedist, and treatment may include drainage of the associated effusion or open reduction and pinning.

COMMON PITFALLS

- Most pediatric fractures heal very well, but proper treatment is essential.
- Misdiagnosis is avoided by taking a history, performing a searching and thorough physical examination, and obtaining acceptable radiographs. Based on the diagnosis, proper treatment can be initiated and appropriate referral or consultation made.
- Complications are minimized by early recognition and, while uncommon, have significant long-term consequences.
- Child abuse should be considered when there are inconsistencies between the history of injury, developmental stage, and the fracture type.
- Children with fractures need adequate outpatient pain control.

ACKNOWLEDGMENT

The author gratefully acknowledges the contribution of John Churchill, who wrote the previous version of this chapter.

Bibliography

Cramer KE. Orthopedic aspects of child abuse. *Pediatr Clin North Am* 1996; 43(5):1035–1051.
England SP, Sundberg S. Management of common pediatric fractures. Pediatr Clin North Am 1996;43(5):991–1012.
Green NE, Swiontkowski MF, eds. *Skeletal trauma in children*. Philadelphia: WB Saunders, 1994.
Outerbridge AR, Micheli LJ. Overuse injuries in the young athlete. *Sport Med Clin North Am* 1995;14(3):503–516.
Rockwood CA, Wilkins KE, King RD, eds. *Fractures in children*, 3rd ed. Philadelphia: JB Lippincott Co, 1991.

CHAPTER 304
Facial Trauma

Barry Steinberg

Pediatric facial trauma is a relatively common occurrence. Fractures of facial bones in children under the age of 12, however, constitute less than 5% of all maxillofacial skeletal injuries.[7] Under age 5 years, this percentage falls to 1% or less. The low incidence of facial fractures in young children is due to significant plasticity of the facial bones and the prominence of the calvarium. Essentially, the forehead and cranium "protect" the upper midface from impact injury.

Additionally, the fact that the sinuses are poorly pneumatized in the young child further decreases the likelihood of upper facial fractures. Maxillofacial injuries can be caused by a variety of mechanisms. Posnick et al.[8] reported that 50% of pediatric facial fractures were caused by motor vehicle accidents and 25% by falls, and 15% were sports-related.

The mandible is the site of 75% to 90% of all pediatric facial fractures.[4,5,10] Fractures of the mandible in the young child, however, are a relatively rare phenomenon because of the resiliency and small size of the lower jaw.[6] The nasal bones also account for a significant portion of skeletal–facial injuries in the pediatric population, and injuries to them may be the most difficult to diagnose. Other associated injuries are common and of greatest significance to the emergency physician. Gussack et al.[3] found that other systemic injuries are associated with pediatric facial trauma in 73% of presentations.

The care of a child with maxillofacial injuries is not unlike that of the adult. There are, however, some special considerations when caring for the child. For example, blood loss from facial injuries is rarely life-threatening in the adult but can be a concern in the younger child. As in the adult patient, reconstruction and achievement of a good esthetic repair are important. The effects of trauma on future facial growth and development, however, are a concern unique to the pediatric population. Discussions with the child's family about these issues are probably best managed by the surgeon, who will be primarily responsible for definitive care.

CLINICAL PRESENTATION

Obtaining a complete history of the traumatic event and clinical evaluation can be quite difficult in the pediatric patient. For example, examination of extraocular muscles to determine the extent of orbital injuries requires that the child be able to follow commands. Dentoalveolar, mandibular, and lower maxillary fractures may alter the dental occlusion. Changes may be so slight that only the patient can feel the mild change in the way the teeth come together. Getting the child to relay this information following a traumatic incident is often impossible.

The child with the isolated dental injury usually presents in a stable condition. There may be some mild bleeding from the gingiva and pain. If a tooth has been completely avulsed, there can be bleeding from the socket and possibly associated lacerations. As the severity of the maxillofacial injuries increases, so does the risk to hemodynamic stability. For example, a simple scalp laceration with blood losses of 200 cc that does not cause blood pressure instability in the adult may account for a significant loss of blood volume in the small child. There also may be significant loss of blood from skeletal fractures posterior to the oropharynx that go unnoticed.

Airway compromise is always a potential issue in oral and maxillofacial injuries. The lost single tooth can be aspirated and should be accounted for. Bleeding, swelling, and displaced fractures can contribute to the loss of an airway.

DIFFERENTIAL DIAGNOSIS

The diagnosis of simple dental and dentoalveolar injury is easily made. Injury will be missed only if associated with more significant facial or systemic injuries. Tumors and infections can cause oral and facial swelling. Usually, the general appearance and a brief history will lead to the appropriate differential diagnosis of traumatic facial injury in the child.

EMERGENCY DEPARTMENT MANAGEMENT

The initial assessment of the pediatric patient with facial trauma is the same as that for the adult. The risk of airway compromise is clear. Loose tissues, malpositioned facial bones, dental segments, edema, and foreign debris can easily occlude the airway and should be dealt with early in the emergency department (ED) presentation. Blood in the airway should be suctioned, and loose debris, bone fragments, and avulsed teeth, loose teeth, or dental prosthesis (from orthodontic treatment) are to be removed. The specialist who will definitively treat the child can address replacement.

Certain types of fractures (i.e., bilateral subcondylar fracture of the mandible and retrodisplaced maxillary fractures) can compromise the airway; temporary reduction (traction) may restore adequate breathing. Interestingly, Siegel et al.[9] found the association between mandibular fractures and airway compromise to be very low. The airway can often be protected by intubation, although nasal intubation should be avoided when there are injuries to the nasoethmoidal region.

Obtaining a surgical airway in the emergency setting is rarely indicated and is reserved for massive midface and mandibular fractures. A formal tracheotomy, if required, can be done under more controlled circumstances when the patient is brought to the operating room for definitive management of the injuries.

Blood loss from maxillofacial injuries can cause hypovolemic shock in children. Control, using direct pressure, is the first line of therapy and may include packing of the lacerations or the placement of intranasal packs to control bleeding from nasal and maxillary fractures. On rare occasions, repositioning of displaced fractures will control the bleeding; this is most likely to be effective with maxillary fractures but is generally ineffective with mandibular and dentoalveolar injuries.

Initial evaluation of the alert child with maxillofacial injury requires patience and compassion. Often, the patient and family's apprehension may exceed that normally associated with similar adult injuries. This apprehension and the effects of the injuries themselves can increase the difficulty or make impossible a complete clinical examination. Sedation, in those cases in which neurologic injuries are not suspected, may help in examination and treatment of the injured child.

After the ABCs, the clinical examination proceeds in an orderly manner. The general appearance of the head and face is reviewed for obvious deformity.

Facial Soft-Tissue Injuries

It is important to consider that lacerations can cause injury to the facial nerve. When possible, function of the nerve should be tested. In children who will follow instructions, facial nerve function can be grossly evaluated by having the child purse the lips as if he or she is going to whistle, raise the eyebrows, and wrinkle the nose. The examiner may help the process by demonstrating these movements to the child. Of note, edema from the injury may temporarily decrease facial nerve function, even with intact nerve fibers. Lacerations can also transect the parotid duct. If transection is suspected, the duct may cannulated intraorally and the wound checked for duct integrity.

Management

Soft-tissue injuries to the face should be vigorously irrigated and debris removed. Simple wounds can be closed in the ED; sedation may be necessary. Ketamine has been found useful, particularly in the younger population. Shallow, simple wounds can be closed with tissue glue.

The long-term outcome of facial laceration repair is highly dependent on the techniques used in closure. Wide scars are due to lack of or inadequate approximation of deep tissues. Depressed scars result from improper repair of underlying muscles or extensive loss of subcutaneous tissue. Therefore, after local anesthesia has been obtained, more complex wounds are closed in layers, using 5.0 Vicryl deep sutures.

The skin may be closed with a 6.0 nonresorbable suture. In young children, in whom removal may be difficult, fast-absorbing gut suture can be used. Minimal tissue should be removed initially, although very ragged edges and devitalized tissue can be trimmed to enhance the esthetic outcome.

Take great care when attempting to close lacerations that cross over the vermilion border of the lip and those involving the eyebrows. The first skin suture should precisely line up the borders, because any discrepancy leads to a visually obvious deformity. Do not shave the eyebrow prior to closure, as this structure aids in wound-edge alignment. Lacerations to the eyelids and to structures with underlying cartilage (nose and ear) require special care and should be referred to a specialist in otolaryngology, plastic surgery, or maxillofacial surgery. All skin closures should be well everted to diminish scar width. Eversion may be accomplished with the aid of mattress suturing techniques.

Annually, there are over 1 million dog bites; 70% of those in the pediatric population occur in the face and neck.[2] Treatment includes tetanus prophylaxis and, possibly, management for potential rabies. Antibiotics should be given and, particularly in the case of dog bites, cover *Pasteurella multocida*. Augmentin is often prescribed in these cases, although penicillin can cover most of the potential organisms transferred with the bite. Copious irrigation is very important prior to closure.

Intraoral Soft-Tissue Injuries

Intraoral examination is the next stage of the evaluation. Any remaining debris or loose fragments are dealt with at this time. As with lacerations of the scalp and face, all of these must be examined for underlying skeletal injury. Mucosal ecchymosis often represents loss of underlying periosteal integrity, indicating potential associated skeletal injury.

Management

Treat lacerations of the oral mucosa by closing them with a resorbable suture such as Vicryl or chromic gut (3.0 to 4.0). Scarring is not a major concern. Tongue lacerations may not always need closure. If they are not very deep and there is little or no bleeding, they can be left untreated. Severe, uncontrollable bleeding from the tongue may be managed by passing a large suture through the midline from dorsal to ventral surface (near the base of the tongue) and tying it laterally on the side that is bleeding. This "tourniquet" suture is left in place until the source of the bleeding is found and definitely controlled.

Skeletal Injuries: Skull and Upper Face

Use palpation and gentle manipulation to search for skeletal injury. Examine the scalp for depressions or "rough" edges that would indicate underlying skull fractures. Palpate the forehead for depression, crepitus, and tenderness, which might indicate fractures of frontal bone or the frontal sinus. Examine the orbital rims for step-off or depressions, which might indicate orbital fractures.

Adjunctive examination would include visual acuity and extraocular muscle function. For example, limitation of upward gaze and binocular diplopia is suggestive of orbital floor fracture with entrapment, which limits the eye movement in the upward direction. A decrease in the sensation of the infraorbital nerve (checked grossly by brushing the skin from just beneath the orbit to the top of the upper lip) is suggestive of an orbital or zygomaticomaxillary complex fracture. The presence of the latter fracture would be supported by depression of the malar eminence (a flattening of the cheeks).

Standing behind the seated, partially reclined patient (bird's-eye view) might help in observing the depressed and rotated zygomaticomaxillary segment. However, these changes may not be readily obvious when swelling is significant.

Placing the thumb and forefinger on the bridge of the nose and gently moving from side to side and up and down will help test for upper maxillary fractures (LeFort II and III) and nasoethmoidal injuries. Widening of the space between the medial canthi (telecanthus) suggests nasoethmoidal fractures with disruption of the canthal attachments.

The "bowstring" test would support the presence of such an injury. This test is accomplished by placing a finger beneath the medial attachment and pulling laterally on the lower eyelid. A rounding out of the medial corner of the eye indicates loss of canthal attachment. If the corner of the eye remains sharp, there probably is no disruption of the medial canthal ligaments.

Determination of isolated nasal injuries is more difficult; diagnosis may require knowledge of the traumatic event as well as what the nose looked like before the event. Generally, there is pain on palpation, and there may be deviation of the tip of the nose. A depression of the nasal dorsum or of the lateral nasal bones indicates the presence of treatable fractures.

Computed tomography (CT) scans are the standard for suspected fractures in this region. On occasion, a thin-section coronal CT series is useful for evaluation of orbital floor injuries.

Management

Only significant depression of the skull fractures may require treatment. Basilar skull fractures may cause otorrhea or rhinorrhea, which may need to be addressed. Often, only conservative follow-up is needed, and antibiotic coverage is controversial. Neurosurgical intervention may be needed in cases that do not resolve spontaneously, or with reduction of associated fractures.

Fractures of the frontal sinus may need to be treated. Generally, if the depression of the outer table is equal to the thickness of the bone of the outer table, open reduction is required to prevent deformity. Additionally, the sinus lining should be removed and the sinus obliterated with bone, fat, or fascia to prevent remucosalization and the potential for mucopyocele formation. Fractures involving the posterior wall of the frontal sinus may require removal of the posterior wall (cranialization) of the sinus. Fractures in this region in the very young child are rare, because the sinus may not be fully formed.

Initial ED management of potential orbital injury centers on ruling out direct injury to the globe and retrobulbar hematoma. Both of these injuries require emergent care. Ophthalmologic consultation is required for globe injury, and lateral canthotomy is the choice of emergent care for retrobulbar hematoma. A sharp scissors is placed in the corner of the eye between the lateral attachments of the upper and lower lids. A full-thickness cut is made, ensuring that the lateral canthal attachments (particularly the inferior limb) are fully transected and released from the bone. This incision should allow decompression of the hematoma and prevent further injury to the eye. Treatment of orbital floor fractures follows when the patient is stable.

Persistent diplopia and entrapment lasting for more than 1 to 2 weeks are indications for exploration. Other indications include CT evidence of a large orbital defect, early enophthalmos, or associated fractures of the rim.[6] Unfortunately, diplopia in younger children (0 to 9 years of age) has been found to take much longer to resolve (10 to 18 months) than diplopia in an older population.[1]

No management in the ED is necessary for zygomaticomaxillary complex fractures. Reduction during definitive therapy usually results in an acceptable aesthetic outcome.

If nasal injury is suspected, careful examination of the internal nose, to rule out the presence of septal hematoma, is of primary importance. The presence of such an injury requires early drainage and nasal packing to prevent the loss of septal cartilage.

Midface Fractures (LeFort I)

Asking the patient whether the occlusion feels like it did before the injury is the first step in the examination for maxillary and mandibular fractures. If the patient feels that the bite is "off," the suspicion for fracture increases. The presence of an anterior open bite that was not present before the traumatic event also is suggestive of skeletal injury. The examiner should place the forefinger on the inner surface and the thumb on outer surface of the upper teeth (if still present) or alveolar ridge and test for mobility. Placing the thumb and forefinger of the other hand on the nasal bridge may help in the detection of movement, which is indicative of maxillary injury. There can be confusion with an alveolar fracture, which can also show mobility in this area. Crepitus is suggestive of violation of the maxillary sinus, which occurs in LeFort fractures as well as in isolated anterior wall fractures of the maxilla. A CT scan helps to determine the extent of the injuries.

Management

The severely impacted, retrodisplaced maxillary fracture can impinge on the airway. Therefore, the initial care provided in the ED should be to ensure patency of the airway. If there is evidence of airway compromise secondary to the maxillary injury, then grasping the anterior maxilla and pulling down and forward may alleviate the problem.

On occasion, this maneuver requires the use of special disimpaction forceps, which is best accomplished in the operating room and with an established airway (intubation or tracheostomy). There also can be bleeding from maxillary fractures, which is stopped by reduction of the segments. There remains some controversy as to the effects on growth due to maxillary injuries. Some authors suggest that these injuries, particularly those associated with the nasomaxillary complex, can interfere with normal facial development.[6]

Mandibular Fractures

Checking for changes in occlusion (using wear facets and patient feedback) helps in the determination of mandibular fractures. There may be deviation on opening in the presence of condyle injury. The lower jaw will shift to the contralateral side if the condyle is dislocated anterior to the fossa; a unilateral condylar fracture causes deviation to the ipsilateral side on opening. A patient with bilateral condylar injuries may present with an anterior open bite that was not obvious prior to the trauma. The examiner should be aware that the presence of a fracture in the anterior mandible (parasymphysis) could be associated with a contralateral subcondylar injury (contrecoup).

Evaluation of the mandible includes bimanual palpation both intra- and extraorally to look for mobile, fractured segments. As mentioned previously, the presence of lacerations or ecchymosis can be suggestive of an underlying fracture. CT studies of the mandible should be ordered for the severely traumatized patient who cannot have plain studies performed. When possible, a panoramic film of the mandible, a Towne's view for the condyles, and lateral oblique mandibular films should be obtained. Careful review of these studies is important, because nondisplaced fractures of the mandible in young children can be difficult to see on radiographs due to the presence of numerous tooth buds.

Management

Severely displaced mandible fractures can cause airway compromise that must be addressed early in the ED management. In grossly mobile segments, a 23- or 24-gauge stainless steel wire can be wrapped around the teeth on either side of the fracture to gain temporary stabilization and make the patient more comfortable. On occasion, the specialist may not come to the ED, but will ask that the stable child with an isolated mandibular injury be discharged for follow-up and treatment. Pain medication should be prescribed, as well as antibiotics (penicillin or clindamycin) for open fractures. Of note, all fractures that pass through segments of the mandible containing teeth are considered open, whether or not there is an obvious laceration. Closed fractures of the condyle and ramus do not require antibiotic therapy. The lack of erupted teeth, the presence of primary teeth only, and underlying tooth buds make the definitive care of mandibular fractures in children more of a challenge when compared with that of the adult. The use of splints and resorbable bone plates to treat fractures is more commonplace in the pediatric population.

Dentoalveolar Injuries

Evaluation

The intraoral examination, in addition to checking for fractures, should look for injury to teeth and supporting alveolar bone. The empty tooth socket with associated bleeding is suggestive of an avulsed tooth. It is important to ascertain that the tooth was lost during the traumatic incident rather than as part of normal development. If the tooth cannot be accounted for, a chest film to rule out aspiration might be indicated. Loose teeth, particularly permanent teeth, and loose alveolar segments are managed by the specialist.

Management

Primary teeth are not to be reimplanted. Permanent teeth that have been completely avulsed need to be handled with care. The best technique is to replace the tooth into the socket after minimal manipulation. If replacement is not feasible, then the tooth should be placed in saliva, balanced salt solution, or milk. A dental specialist should be immediately notified, because the chance of successful reimplantation of the tooth is critically dependent on timing of treatment. The greatest success rate occurs if reimplantation takes place within 30 minutes. The dental specialist, generally with splinting of various methods, manages loose teeth and alveolar fractures.

DISPOSITION

The type of institution and the level of trauma care it can provide determine the timing and the role of the maxillofacial specialist. In level-one trauma centers, the physicians in the ED or the trauma surgeons initially manage the patient. They will establish the airway as needed. Hemorrhage may be controlled by the primary service; however, on occasion, the maxillofacial specialist may be required to obtain hemostasis because of their specialized skills. Early consultation with the specialist is recommended regardless of the level of trauma care provided by the institution.

Indications for Admission

Clearly, the young patient with multiple system injuries should be admitted. Admission is indicated for a potential closed head injury associated with facial injuries. Patients with isolated maxillofacial injuries require admission if these injuries involve possible airway compromise or uncontrollable bleeding. Severely mobile fractures are uncomfortable and are treated quickly; therefore, patients with these injuries are admitted. The threshold for admission of children with facial injuries is much lower than that of the adult. Transfer to another facility is essentially dependent on whether a maxillofacial specialist is on staff. Many smaller hospitals do not have such expertise; therefore, transfer is recommended.

COMMON PITFALLS

- Do not forget to account for all missing teeth, to ensure that a tooth is not aspirated.
- Do a complete assessment, because facial injuries are often associated with other systemic trauma.
- Do not forget that intracranial injuries are more common in pediatric maxillofacial trauma than they are in that of adults.
- Mandibular fractures in the pediatric population can be associated with child abuse.

References

1. Cope MR, Moos KF, Speculand B. Does diplopia persist after blow-out fractures of the orbital floor in children? *Br J Oral Maxillofac Surg* 1997;35:46.
2. Farrior RT, Clark DA. Soft tissue trauma in children. In: Smith JD, Bumsted R, eds. *Pediatric facial plastic and reconstructive surgery.* New York: Raven Press, 1993:263.
3. Gussack GS, Luterman A, Rogers A, et al. Pediatric maxillofacial trauma: unique features in diagnosis and treatment. *Laryngoscope* 1987;97:925.
4. Iizuka T, Hanna T, Annino DJ, et al. Midfacial fractures in pediatric patients. *Arch Otolaryngol Head Neck Surg* 1995;121:1366.
5. Khan AA. A retrospective study of injuries to the maxillofacial skeleton in Harare, Zimbabwe. *Br J Oral Maxillofac Surg* 1988;26:435.

6. Koltai PJ. Maxillofacial injuries in children. In: Smith JP, Bumstead R, eds. *Pediatric facial plastic and reconstructive surgery.* New York: Raven Press, 1993:283.
7. McGraw BL, Pediatric maxillofacial trauma. *Arch Otolaryngol Head Neck Surg* 1990;116:41.
8. Posnick JC, Wells M, Pron GE. Pediatric facial fractures: evolving patterns of treatment. *J Oral Maxillofac Surg* 1993;51:836.
9. Siegel MB, Wetmore RF, Potsic WP, et al. Mandibular fractures in the pediatric patient. *Arch Otolaryngol Head Neck Surg* 1991;117:533.
10. Zachariades N, Papavassiliou D, Koumoura F. Fractures of the facial skeleton in children. *J Craniomaxillofac Surg* 1990;18:151.

PART V

Administrative and Clinical Issues

CHAPTER 305

Sedation and Pain Management

William F. Coombs

Appropriate relief of pain and anxiety should always be a priority in the overall management of the acutely sick or injured child. Historically, the medical profession has done a poor job of alleviating such symptoms, preferring to focus on the diagnostic evaluation.[16] This attitude has been especially prevalent in the care of children.[15]

Dramatic advances in procedural sedation techniques, along with a greater understanding of the pharmacodynamics of available sedatives and analgesics, have led to safer, more effective sedation and analgesia in children.[14] The Agency for Health Care Policy and Research, noting the widespread inadequacy of pain management, has stated in its guidelines that it is the physician's "ethical obligation to manage pain and relieve the patient's suffering" and that such pain management should be at the core of every health-care professional's commitment.[1]

GUIDELINES FOR PEDIATRIC SEDATION AND ANALGESIA

The first attempts at developing uniform guidelines for children requiring sedation or analgesia for diagnostic or therapeutic procedures occurred in 1985, when the National Institutes of Health (NIH) and the American Academy of Pediatrics (AAP) published consensus documents on procedural sedation.[3] Subsequent revisions have attempted to accurately define the various states of sedation encountered in the management of these patients. In 1996, the American Society of Anesthesiologists (ASA) Task Force on Sedation and Analgesia by Non-Anesthesiologists published their own guidelines, which were, in essence, a compromise of those proposed by the various subspecialty societies.[4] The ASA rejected the term *conscious sedation* and offered the following definitions, stressing that these states represent different points on a continuum and that movement along this continuum can occur in any direction at any time:

Analgesia: Relief of perception of pain without intentional production of a sedated state.

Sedation–analgesia: Medically induced state of depressed consciousness, during which there is a margin of safety wide enough to have a reasonable expectation that the patient

a. will be easily aroused
b. will maintain intact protective reflexes
c. will maintain patent airway independently
d. will have appropriate responses to stimulation, commands

Deep sedation: Medically induced state of depressed consciousness, during which it is reasonable to expect that the patient

a. may not be easily aroused
b. may develop partial or complete loss of protective reflexes
c. may lose ability to maintain independent airway
d. may be unable to respond appropriately to physical stimulation or verbal commands

General anesthesia: Medically induced state of unconsciousness, during which the patient has

a. complete loss of protective reflexes
b. inability to maintain independent airway
c. inability to respond to any stimulation or command

The nature of procedures performed in the emergency room often necessitates deep sedation to ensure an appropriate level of analgesia and cooperation. Besides attempting to define the various states of sedation, these guidelines also discuss the preparation that should be undertaken prior to the start of a procedure. It is important to note that these are not absolute rules but rather recommendations that may be adopted, modified, exceeded, or rejected according to clinical needs and constraints.[7] The Joint Commission on Accreditation of Hospital Organizations (JCAHO) does not recommend a specific set of guidelines, but mandates that hospitals develop institution-specific policies and procedures regarding procedural sedation that ensure all patients receive "one standard of care," regardless of what area of the hospital it occurs in.[7] This mandate should not be misinterpreted as requiring *identical* care in all areas of the hospital.

PATIENT SELECTION AND MONITORING

Administration of sedatives–analgesics should occur in a facility suitable for appropriate evaluation and monitoring of the patient and for the performance of emergency resuscitative measures if needed. Monitoring and emergency equipment suitable for children of all ages and sizes must be available (Table 305.1). It should include a positive-pressure oxygen delivery system, suction apparatus, blood pressure monitor, pulse oximeter, and

TABLE 305.1. Equipment

Positive-pressure oxygen delivery system
Suction apparatus
Blood pressure and CR monitor
Pulse oximeter
Emergency crash cart

an emergency crash cart. Reversal agents should be readily available. The practitioner responsible for administering the sedative and monitoring the patient must be someone other than the one performing the diagnostic or therapeutic procedure, and should be appropriately trained and certified.

A full evaluation of the patient's health and medical history should be performed, with consideration given to the physiologic reserve of the patient's major organ systems, as defined by the ASA physical status classification (Table 305.2). Patients who are ASA class I or II are usually considered appropriate candidates for sedation–analgesia or deep sedation. Patients in ASA class III or IV present special problems that require additional and individual considerations.[4]

Evaluation of the patient's recent food and fluid intake must also occur. Standard NPO guidelines are as follows:

1. Infants less than 6 months: no milk or solids for 4 hours prior to procedure
2. Infants greater than 6 months: no milk or solids for 6 hours prior to procedure

All patients, regardless of age, are allowed to ingest clear liquids until 2 hours prior to the procedure. In emergent circumstances, in which NPO guidelines cannot be followed, sound clinical judgment should be exercised and the risks of aspiration versus the benefits of the procedure should be weighed very carefully.

Most guidelines dictate that the following parameters be monitored carefully: oxygenation, ventilation, airway, and level of consciousness. Proper documentation calls for the person who administers sedation to obtain appropriate informed consent from the parents and to record the patient's vital signs, oxygen saturation, medications given, and any remarkable or unexpected events (Table 305.3). The frequency of documentation varies with the level of sedation. It is recommended that the heart rate, respiratory rate, blood pressure, and oxygen saturation be recorded prior to the sedation, every 15 minutes during sedation–analgesia, every 5 minutes for deep sedation, and once again prior to discharge. After the procedure is terminated and sedation is no longer desired, monitoring and recording should be continued until the patient has recovered sufficiently to meet the following discharge criteria:

1. Cardiovascular function and airway patency are satisfactory and stable.
2. The patient can be easily aroused, and protective reflexes are intact.
3. The patient can talk and sit up (age-appropriate).
4. Hydration is adequate.

For the very young or special-needs child who is incapable of the usual expected responses, the presedation level of responsiveness or a level as close as possible to the child's baseline should be achieved. Appropriate discharge instructions include anticipatory guidance regarding sleep, diet, and activity, as well as specific instructions on how to access care in the event of untoward effects or unexpected complications.

TABLE 305.2. American Society of Anesthesiologists Physical Status Classification

Class I	A healthy patient
Class II	A patient with mild systemic disease
Class III	A patient with severe systemic disease
Class IV	A patient with severe systemic disease that is a constant threat to life
Class V	An ill patient not expected to survive without an operation

TABLE 305. 3. Documentation

Monitor	Document
Oxygenation	Consent
Ventilation	Vital signs
Airway	Oxygen saturation
Level of consciousness	Medications
	Untoward events
	Recovery

PHARMACOLOGIC THERAPY

The ideal drug for sedation or pain control would be painless to administer and easily titratable by virtue of its fast and predictable rate of absorption, onset, and duration of action. It would also be reversible and inexpensive and would have no side effects or contraindications. Unfortunately, such a drug does not exist.

There are, however, many drugs available that, when used alone or in combination for the right indications, are very effective and relatively safe (Table 305.4). In selecting an agent, the physician must consider the effects desired, the risks and benefits, and the logistics of administration for each situation (Table 305.5). When pure sedation is the desired end point, agents such as benzodiazepines and barbiturates are excellent choices. These agents, however, do not inhibit perceptions of pain and should never be used as the sole agent for pain management.

Purely sedative agents can be used for painful procedures in conjunction with other agents to provide sedation as an adjunct to analgesia. Sedative analgesics such as narcotics, on the other hand, are excellent choices for painful procedures. Although they have varying degrees of sedation, they should rarely be used as a single agent for providing control for a painless diagnostic study. Combining different classes of agents is a way to produce an effect not present in either agent alone. Such combinations must be used with caution, because they enhance not only desired responses, but also adverse effects.

Pure Analgesics (Nonnarcotics)

Indications: Relief of mild-to-moderate pain
Complications: Gastritis, peptic ulcer disease

Specific Agents

Acetaminophen: Pure analgesic agent with antipyretic properties. Standard dose is 15 mg/kg every 4 hours, can be given orally or rectally, and can be combined with narcotics such as oxycodone and hydrocodone.

Ibuprofen: Nonsteroidal antiinflammatory agent with analgesic and antipyretic properties. Standard dose is 10 mg/kg by mouth every 6 hours.

Ketorolac: Nonsteroidal antiinflammatory agent best suited for relief of biliary and renal colic. Standard dose is 0.4 to 1.0 mg/kg intravenously (i.v.) or intramuscularly (i.m.).

TABLE 305.4. Pharmacologic Therapy

	Sedatives			
	Midazolam	Pentobarbital	Thiopental	Methohexital
Class	Benzodiazepine	Short-acting barbiturate	Ultrashort-acting barbiturate	Short-acting barbiturate
Peds dose	0.1–0.2 mg/kg i.v. 0.5–0.7 mg/kg PO	2–6 mg/kg i.v.	4–6 mg/kg i.v.	1 mg/kg i.v.
Adult dose	0.025–0.05 mg/kg	—	0.5–1.0 mg/kg	—
Onset	0.5–5.0 min i.v. 5–20 min PO	1–5 min	30 s	1–5 min
Duration	15–80 min	30–60 min	3–5 min	3–10 min
Effects	Hypotension Apnea Skeletal muscle relaxation Anticonvulsant	Hypoxia Apnea Hypotension Decreased ICP	Hypotension Apnea Decreased ICP Bronchospasm	Fewer cardiorespiratory effects than thiopental

Note: Reversal Agents: *Naloxone (Narcan)*. Dose: 0.01–0.1 mg/kg; how supplied: 1-mg/mL, 0.4-mg/mL, 0.02-mg/mL vials. *Flumazenil (Mazicon)*. Dose: 0.3 mg repeat q1min to maximum of 3 mg; how supplied: 0.1 mg/mL in 5- and 10-mL vials.

TABLE 305.5. Clinical Applications

Desired Effect	Age	Options
Moderate-to-severe painful condition	Infant, child, and adolescent	Morphine 0.1–0.2 mg/kg i.v.
Painless diagnostic study	Infant	Pentobarbital 2–6 mg/kg i.v.
	Child and adolescent	Midazolam 0.1 mg/kg i.v. or 0.5 mg–0.7 mg/kg PO
Sedation-Analgesia	Infant and child	Ketamine 3–5 mg/kg i.m. or 1–2 mg/kg i.v.
	Child and adolescent	Fentanyl 1–2 μg/kg and midazolam 0.1 mg/kg i.v. (titrate to effect), or Nitrous oxide inhalation

Pure Sedative

Indications: Sedation for nonpainful diagnostic or therapeutic procedures

Complications: Dose-dependent respiratory depression, hypotension, "paradoxical" (disinhibitory) effects

Specific Agents

Benzodiazepines

Midazolam: Potent sedative with amnesic and anxiolytic properties, a rapid onset, and short duration of action. Standard dose is 0.02 to 0.1 mg/kg i.v., 0.5 to 0.7 mg/kg orally, and 0.3 mg/kg intranasally. When titrating intravenously, remember that onset of sedation may take 2 to 5 minutes. Children younger than 5 years of age often will become excited and agitated when given midazolam.[18] Whether this represents a paradoxical or disinhibitory effect and whether higher doses would eliminate the effect are not known. For this reason, the use of midazolam as a single agent for sedation in this age group should be reconsidered.

Barbiturates

Pentobarbital: Sedative agent best used intravenously for nonpainful diagnostic studies. Onset of action is within 1 to 2 minutes, with duration of 30 to 60 minutes. Standard dose is 2 to 6 mg/kg i.v. It is recommended to start with an initial dose of 2 mg/kg and titrate to effect with subsequent doses of 1 to 2 mg/kg every 30 seconds as needed.

Thiopental: Ultrashort-acting agent that can cause profound respiratory depression and hypotension. Standard dose is 3 to 5 mg/kg i.v. or 25 mg/kg rectally.

Methohexital: Ultrashort-acting agent with dose-dependent respiratory depression and apnea but minimal associated cardiovascular side effects. Standard dose is 1 mg/kg i.v.

Others

Etomidate: Ultrashort-acting sedative hypnotic with onset of action less than 1 minute and duration of 3 to 5 minutes; it has minimal cardiorespiratory effects. Standard dose is 0.1 to 0.3 mg/kg i.v. There is minimal experience with this drug for pediatric sedation.

Propofol: Ultrashort-acting sedative hypnotic with onset of action within one circulation time following i.v. administration. Patients are usually awake within 5 to 10 minutes of infusion termination.[11] It has potent, dose-dependent respiratory depressant effects and can produce significant hypotension with rapid bolus injection. Standard initial dose is 1 to 3 mg/kg, followed by either repeated boluses or a constant infusion at 25 to 130 μg/kg/min.

Choral Hydrate: Sedative hypnotic with a long history of safety in pediatrics. Onset of sedation is unpredictable and can be as long as 40 to 60 minutes. Recovery time is also prolonged and highly variable, limiting its use in the emergency setting. Standard dose is 25 to 100 mg/kg orally or rectally.

Sedative Analgesics

Indications: Moderate-to-severe pain management, painful procedures

Complications: Respiratory depression, nausea, vomiting

Specific Agents

Narcotics

Morphine: The "gold standard" against which all other narcotics are compared. Standard dose is 0.1 to 0.2 mg/kg i.v.

TABLE 305.4. Pharmacologic Therapy (Continued)

	Sedatives		*Sedative-Analgesics*	
	Etomidate	Propofol	Fentanyl	Ketamine
Class	Nonbarbiturate hypnotic	Nonbarbiturate hypnotic	Synthetic opiate	Dissociative anesthetic
Peds dose	0.3–0.4 mg/kg i.v.	1.5–3.0 mg/kg i.v.	1–2 μg/kg i.v. 10 mg/kg PO	1–2 mg/kg i.v. 3–5 mg/kg i.m.
Adult dose	0.1–0.3 mg/kg	0.5–1.0 mg/kg	0.5–1.0 μg/kg	0.5–1.0 mg/kg
Onset	30 s	30 s	30 s	30 s
Duration	5–10 min	5–10 min	30–60 min	5–15 min i.v. 20–40 min i.m.
Effects	Relative cardiovascular and respiratory stability Myoclonus Adrenal suppression	Hypotension Apnea Myoclonus Anaphylaxis with soy and egg allergy	Bradycardia Apnea Antiemetic Hypotension (less than morphine) Chest wall rigidity	Increased heart rate and blood pressure Airway reflexes intact Bronchodilation Increased IOP & ICP Emergence reaction

Fentanyl: The most potent of the commonly used narcotics, it has a rapid onset of action (1 to 10 minutes) and a relatively brief duration of 30 to 60 minutes. It has fewer respiratory and cardiovascular depressive effects than other narcotics but can cause severe respiratory depression and apnea when combined with benzodiazepines. Standard dose is 1 to 2 μg/kg i.v. administered slowly.[5] Rapid boluses have been associated with chest wall rigidity and should be avoided.[14] Although available in transmucosal form as a lollipop, the high incidence of nausea and vomiting has limited its acceptability.[6]

DPT cocktail: The most widely used "cocktail" for sedation in the pediatric patient has been the combination of Demerol, Phenergan, and Thorazine. Its popularity stems from extensive past experience, reliability, and ease of administration by a single intramuscular injection. Reports questioning the safety of such combinations, along with their unpredictable onset and significantly prolonged duration of action, make them poor choices for procedural sedation in the emergency setting.[3]

Nonnarcotics

Ketamine: Ketamine is unique among the sedative analgesics in that it produces a dissociative state between the thalamus and limbic systems, which is characterized by four features: sedation, analgesia, amnesia, and catalepsis. It possesses positive inotropic and bronchodilatory effects, with preservation of spontaneous respirations and protective airway reflexes. These qualities make it an ideal choice for outpatient procedures, with an excellent safety and efficacy record documented in over 11,000 children.[8,9] Standard dosages are 1 to 2 mg/kg i.v., 3 to 5 mg/kg i.m., and 10 mg/kg PO.[10] The clinical state produced by ketamine differs from that of other sedatives in that the patient's eyes often remain open but with a disconnected stare and marked nystagmus. This "lights on, nobody home" look can be disconcerting to parents, and they should be forewarned prior to administration of the drug. Potential side effects of ketamine include increased salivary and tracheobronchial secretions and emergence reactions.[9] Secretions can be ameliorated by adding atropine (0.01 mg/kg) or glycopyrrolate (0.005 mg/kg; max, 0.25 mg). Emergence reactions are uncommon in children under 8 years of age and can be reduced by premedication with a benzodiazepine (midazolam 0.05 mg/kg mixed in with the ketamine and antisialagogue of choice). Laryngospasm following administration of ketamine has been documented in small infants (less than 3 months) with respiratory tract infections, and use of ketamine is therefore contraindicated in this patient population.[3]

Inhalation Agents

Nitrous Oxide: This is the only inhalation agent in common use, usually in concentrations of 30% to 70% N_2O. It is a safe, effective sedative–analgesic with a rapid onset and short duration of action upon withdrawal. Nitrous oxide is inexpensive and easy to administer by experienced hands. It is very operator-dependent, with a substantial learning curve. As with hypnosis, suggestion is very important, and the patient must be well prepared in regard to expectations. This method of sedation is best used in older children and adolescents who are more likely to cooperate.

Reversal Agents

These are available for narcotics and benzodiazepines:

Naloxone (Narcan): Narcotic antagonist; dose: 0.01 mg/kg to 0.1 mg/kg i.v. or i.m.

Flumazenil (Mazicon): Benzodiazepine antagonist; dose: 0.3 mg i.v., repeat q1min to maximum of 3 mg.

NONPHARMACOLOGIC THERAPY

The involvement of child life specialists in the management of pain and anxiety in the pediatric patient can be invaluable. By providing the patient with age-appropriate information regarding the procedures to be undertaken and teaching appropriate coping strategies, these specialists often succeed in lessening the child's fear and anxiety, thereby reducing and occasionally eliminating the need for pharmacologic intervention. Distraction techniques such as listening to music with headsets, singing, or imagery can also be powerful coping strategies. Finally, parental support at the bedside can play a significant role in reducing the child's distress.[2]

COMMON PITFALLS

- Inappropriate monitoring during and after a painful procedure
- Selecting a sedative agent without analgesia for a painful procedure
- Not giving enough medication because of time factors or fears about side effects, especially respiratory depression
- Selecting an agent that titrates too slowly and fails to produce the desired state
- Not having reversal agents readily available
- Not anticipating disinhibitory effects with the use of benzodiazepines in small children
- Not preparing the parents for the nystagmus and catalepsy seen with ketamine

References

1. Agency for Health Care Policy and Research. Clinical practice guideline: acute pain management: operative or medical procedures and trauma. U.S. Department of Health and Human Services, AHCPR Pub. No. 92-0032, Rockville, MD, 1992.
2. Algren JJ. Sedation and analgesia for minor pediatric procedures. *Pediatr Emerg Care* 1996;12(6):435–440.
3. American Academy of Pediatrics, Committee on Drugs. Guidelines for monitoring and management of pediatric patients during and after sedation for diagnostic and therapeutic procedures. *Pediatrics* 1992;89:1110–1115.
4. American Society of Anesthesiologists. Practice guidelines for sedation and analgesia by non-anesthesiologist. *Anesthesia* 1996;84(2):459–470.
5. Chudnofsky CR, Wright SW, Dronen SC, et al. The safety of fentanyl use in the emergency department. *Ann Emerg Med* 1989;18:635–639.
6. Cote CJ. Sedation for the pediatric patient—a review. *Pediatr Clin North Am* 1994;41:31–59.
7. Green SM, Whittaker WA. Meeting the guidelines and standards for pediatric sedation and analgesia. *Emerg Med Rep* 1997;2(7):67–78.
8. Green SM, Nakamura R, Johnson NE. Ketamine sedation for pediatric procedures. Part 1: a prospective series. *Ann Emerg Med* 1990;19:1024–1032.
9. Green SM, Johnson NE. Ketamine sedation for pediatric procedures. Part 2: review and implications. *Ann Emerg Med* 1990;19:1033–1046.
10. Green SM, Hummel CB, et al. What is the optimal dose of intramuscular ketamine for pediatric sedation. *Acad Emerg Med* 1999;6:21–26.
11. Hertzog JH, Campbell JK, et al. Propofol anesthesia for invasive procedures in ambulatory and hospitalized children. *Pediatrics* 1999; 103:3.
12. Krauss BS, Shannon M, et al. Guidelines for pediatric sedation. *Am Coll Emerg Physicians* 1995.
13. Qureshi FA, Mellis PJ. Efficacy of oral ketamine for providing sedation and analgesia to children requiring laceration repair. *Pediatr Emerg Care* 1995;11(2):93–97.
14. Sachetti A, Schafermeyer R, et al. Pediatric analgesia and sedation. *Ann Emerg Med* 1994;23:237–250.
15. Selbst SM, Clark M. Analgesic use in the emergency department. *Ann Emerg Med* 1990;12:1010.
16. Wilson JE, Pendelton JM. Oligoanalgesia in the emergency department. *Am J Emerg Med* 1989;7:620–623.
17. Wright SW, Chudnofsky CR, Dronen CR, et al. Midazolam use in the emergency department. *Am J Emerg Med* 1990;8:97–100.
18. Vander Bijl P, Roelofse JA. Disinhibitory reactions to benzodiazepines—a review. *J Oral Maxillofac Surg* 1991;49:519–523.

CHAPTER 306

Emergency Medical Services for Children

Deborah Mulligan-Smith

The term *emergency medical services for children* (EMSC) originated in the 1980s, when landmark legislation provided for a federal EMSC grant program based in the Maternal and Child Health Bureau (MCHB) of the U.S. Department of Health and Human Services. The name has come to encompass a wide spectrum of efforts underway to ensure that all children in the United States have access to the same quality of emergency care as adults. Although the term *emergency medical services* (EMS) is generally used to mean prehospital care, the scope of EMS has expanded to include public education, injury prevention, access to public emergency services, emergency department care, inpatient and critical care services, and rehabilitation of the acutely ill and injured patient. The goal of EMSC is not to create a segregated EMS system for children, but to integrate comprehensive pediatric emergency care into existing systems and services and to increase awareness of pediatric issues in all aspects of EMS. The federal EMSC program has provided individual state grants to address all of the issues special to children who experience an emergency illness or trauma.

Despite significant progress, a 1993 study by the National Academy of Science's Institute of Medicine (IOM) documented many remaining gaps and deficiencies in pediatric EMS. In 1995, a panel of expert advisers joined MCHB and the National Highway Traffic Safety Administration (NHTSA) staff to convert the IOM's recommendations into a 5-year plan for EMSC. The achievement of proposed activities led to a data base from which to revise the objectives and restate them in a way that is measurable. As stated in the introduction to the plan, it can be fully implemented only with the assistance and involvement of a variety of groups and organizations, each addressing the aspect of EMSC relevant to its particular area of expertise and work. In addition, the plan's objectives can be met only if there is communication and collaboration among these organizations.

Thus, an interorganizational consortium is needed to further the goals for the program by addressing specific objectives of the plan and by ensuring ongoing communication and collaboration. Contracts were developed with 14 professional associations, with each contract including activities, related tasks, and objectives in the 5-year plan. A new document, EMSC *5 Year Plan: Midcourse Review 1995–2000*, provides the nation with an updated overview of the plan. As of 1998, EMSC grants had helped all 50 states, the District of Columbia, Puerto Rico, and three territories to make significant progress toward optimum emergency care for all children.

This chapter focuses on prehospital EMSC issues. Emergency department–based caregivers will find that they face many of these issues; in fact, emergency department practitioners have much in common with their partners in the field.

EPIDEMIOLOGY

Children from the newborn to those 12 years of age make up only 3% to 7% of all EMS calls in the United States. This figure increases to 10% when 13- to 18-year-olds are included. About half of all pediatric calls are for trauma; vehicular trauma and falls are the most common mechanisms of injury. Respiratory difficulty, seizures, ingestions, near-drowning, and altered mental status are among the most common medical complaints. Medical complaints predominate in children under age 3 and increase again among adolescents. Traumatic complaints occur at all ages but are more prevalent in school-aged children and adolescents.

The National EMSC Data Analysis Resource Center (NEDARC) provides technical support to the EMSC community in linking various data sets to improve understanding about the unique needs of children and awareness of areas requiring additional system development. Epidemiologic studies suggest that prehospital services are simultaneously over- and underused by children. Only one out of every three to five children transported by EMS has a serious or critical illness or injury. However, this does not mean that all pediatric EMS patients are not sick: Children arriving at an emergency department via EMS are five to eight times more likely to be admitted than those arriving by nonmedical transport. Studies also show that most seriously ill children arrive at the emergency department by private transport. The most important factor in this perceived underuse of EMS may be the relative ease with which a sick small child can be carried from place to place.

In summary, paramedics and emergency medical technicians (EMTs) encounter children on only 3% to 10% of their calls. About half of those children are trauma victims. About a third of pediatric EMS patients require simple or complex advanced life-support (ALS) procedures by field personnel. Private vehicle or other public transport takes many children who might benefit from advanced prehospital care directly to the emergency department.

EMS PREPAREDNESS FOR PEDIATRIC PATIENTS

While the majority of trained prehospital EMS personnel are volunteers, they cover only 20% of the population. Until recently, personal experience has been the primary instructor for EMTs and paramedics. But considering that only three to ten out of every 100 calls involve children, and that only one to three of those patients are significantly ill, personal experience can not adequately suffice. Standard curricula for basic training in the recent past required that EMTs receive only 2 hours of neonatal and pediatric training out of a 100- to 200-hour course. Paramedics were required to cover an additional 6 to 12 hours of pediatrics in a 450- to 1,100-hour course. Curricula have included basic skills such as airway management and assessment of pediatric vital signs, but they have also focused on diagnoses such as meningitis, epiglottis, and Reye syndrome rather than the assessment of general patient status and common clinical syndromes. Although pediatric clinical experiences are available with varying frequency throughout the country, many training programs have not required their inclusion in basic curricula.

The EMSC movement has helped to produce a positive change in basic and continuing pediatric EMS education. A cornerstone of this movement lies in the training provided to EMTs, who deliver the bulk of the prehospital emergency care in the United States. The new EMT-Basic curriculum is assessment-based, has an expanded pediatric section, and integrates pediatrics through the entire course. EMSC advocates are campaigning for similar changes in the paramedic curriculum. Teaching hospitals and EMS training programs are offering courses in pediatric emergency care, such as the Pediatric Advanced Life Support (PALS) course or Pediatric Education for Prehospital Providers (PEPP). Some of these courses have been modified to suit the special needs of prehospital care providers. Instructor resource manuals and provider assessment-based courses have been developed to help bridge the knowledge gap that still exists in the specialized field of prehospital pediatric care. Pediatric workshops and lectures are increasingly available at regional and national EMS meetings, and several texts and videotapes are available for reference. Many of the available educational programs are products of the federal EMSC grant program.

Recognizing that their basic training and experience may not be enough, many EMTs and paramedics are taking advantage of the new accessibility of pediatric education. As a result, they are gaining not only skills and knowledge, but confidence as well.

EMS systems must also prepare for pediatric patients. Another product of the EMSC movement is the increased participation of pediatricians and other physician advocates in medical control issues. Pediatric ALS and basic life-support (BLS) protocols and procedures for EMS are now widely available. Several consensus documents have been published that provide guidelines for minimum EMS pediatric and neonatal equipment, procedures, and assessment-based protocols. Pediatricians have become more active in local, state, and national EMS advisory and oversight organizations. EMSC issues are now addressed in most EMS texts. Base-station physicians, nurses, and other direct medical control personnel are also being encouraged to keep pace with their prehospital colleagues' advancing pediatric capabilities and knowledge.

SPECIAL CHALLENGES

Differing Anatomy and Physiology

EMS providers practice in a system that traditionally emphasizes their role in the recognition and treatment of cardiovascular insufficiency, the leading killer of adults. The pediatric patient demands a different focus. Problems with airway and breathing are the most common causes of acute deterioration in children; cardiovascular compromise usually occurs secondary to hypoxia or trauma. For this reason, the basic ABC approach is even more important for children than for adults. The ability to recognize, categorize, and anticipate respiratory dysfunction is key in pediatric management. These assessment skills are best learned and reinforced through guided patient contact and immediate feedback from receiving hospital personnel. Unfortunately, few prehospital providers have access to such pediatric educational experiences.

Treatment priorities must change to conform to assessment priorities. When faced with a very sick child, the reflex of many emergency care providers is to rush to start an intravenous line, but, in reality, few field intravenous lines are truly "lifelines" for children. The real lifelines for the pediatric patient are an intact airway and adequate oxygenation and ventilation. Routine attempts to insert intravenous lines in children may even be counterproductive, as they can increase the patient's oxygen demands (because of pain and anxiety), delay transport to definitive care, and distract the medic from more important tasks, such as monitoring the ventilatory status.

Pediatric anatomy influences both injury patterns and emergency intervention. When assessing both the scene and the patient, the EMT must remember that the child's large head, increased body surface area, relatively poorly protected abdominal cavity, and general soft-tissue and bony elasticity may contribute to or protect against various injuries. Spinal immobilization procedures must be modified to compensate for the large head and narrow body. Airway maneuvers are slightly different because of the large tongue and tonsils, as well as the position and conformation of the larynx. Gastric decompression becomes more important because of the predominance of diaphragmatic breathing. Temperature regulation is a priority because of the increased risk of hypothermia in children. All of these factors must be rapidly assessed and integrated into the EMT's plan of action.

Probably the most important difference between adult and pediatric field management is the emphasis on BLS skills. About two-thirds of all pediatric EMS patients can be managed effectively with only BLS interventions. Even patients for whom endotracheal intubation is the optimal airway can often be treated adequately with a scrupulous bag-valve-mask technique if necessary. Children respond well to simple interventions. Invasive procedures should be performed only if the benefits clearly outweigh the risks; if they are needed, invasive procedures can and should be performed by properly trained paramedics. A good pediatric paramedic needs confidence, strong assessment and BLS skills, patience, and a high degree of comfort with a "low-tech, high-touch" approach.

All of these anatomic and physiologic principles influence practice by both prehospital and emergency department personnel. They present a special challenge, however, to the field provider. Emergency department personnel have the luxury of resources such as advanced diagnostic equipment, reference materials, consultants, and time. EMTs have less experience and training, far fewer specialized resources, and much less time in which to integrate these principles into a focused patient assessment and treatment plan that will form the foundation of the care that will be delivered in the emergency department.

Skills Performance and Maintenance

Table 306.1 lists pediatric ALS skills and procedures performed by paramedics in the United States. Several of the skills in general use for adults may be restricted by local medical directors for use in children. Rectal and aerosolized drug administration and intraosseous line placement are relatively new to the prehospital setting. They are not yet universally performed but are quickly gaining acceptance. Some jurisdictions have been slow to allow their medics to intubate children; this attitude is also changing. Other procedures may be limited because of equipment expense or relative risk. The third column of the table lists procedures used in adults but considered of limited utility for children due to safety considerations or lack of proven efficacy.

Because of the infrequent need for pediatric ALS interventions in the field, and because of their relative lack of basic pediatric clinical training, paramedics often feel uncomfortable performing such procedures on children. Fortunately, the actual procedural steps vary little from those needed for adults. Continuing education through agency in-service programs or formal courses can help medics gain confidence in their abilities to give the same level of care to children as they give to adults. Hands-on practice with real children in a supervised setting is difficult to arrange, but many pediatric emergency departments welcome paramedics as observers. Even this kind of patient contact can be a valuable educational opportunity.

Triage and Transport Decisions

EMS providers face an additional challenge when formulating a care plan for a child in the field. Not all emergency departments can provide the full spectrum of acute pediatric care, especially trauma, critical care, and subspecialty services. Transport destinations for children are more limited than for adults. EMS personnel must be familiar with the pediatric care capabilities of facilities in their area, and must sometimes be prepared to bypass the closest facility in favor of one better qualified to care for their patient. Formal EMS triage and transport guidelines for children should be established for every service area.

EMTs must also factor resource management and social and medicolegal issues into their triage and transport decisions. Could EMS services to an area be compromised if a unit transports a patient out of its territory to the closest pediatric facility? Should the patient be taken instead to a closer, but less capable, facility? Should an EMS unit transport a child and family members to an emergency department just because the parents are too shaken to drive or have no transportation? Should injured adult and child family members be taken to the same facility, even though the quality of care might be affected? How does the system handle unaccompanied minors with nonemergent complaints or parental service refusals when the child obviously is at increased risk for significant morbidity or mortality? These decisions must all be supported by standing policies that address these pediatric-specific issues, or by knowledgeable on-line medical control assistance. Medics must also be allowed the freedom to use their own judgment to adapt triage and transport guidelines to the case at hand.

Emotional Aspects

An axiom among pediatricians is that the hardest part of pediatrics is not the patients, it is the parents. The medical team

TABLE 306.1. Pediatric ALS Procedures Performed by Paramedics

General Practice	Subject to Local Variation	Limited Use in Pediatrics
Bag-valve-mask ventilation	Orotracheal intubation	Nasotracheal intubation
Peripheral venous access	Retrograde endotracheal intubation	Needle cricothyrotomy
Subcutaneous drug administration	Needle thoracostomy	Surgical cricothyrotomy
Intravenous administration of resuscitation and anticonvulsant drugs	Rectal drug administration	Transcutaneous pacing
	Aerosolized drug administration	Automatic external defibrillation
Synchronized cardioversion	Naso- or orogastric intubation	Pneumatic antishock garment application
Defibrillation	Intraosseous line placement	
	Central line placement	
	Chest tube insertion	
	Pulse oximetry	
	End-tidal CO_2 monitoring[a]	

[a] Used mostly by aeromedical and interfacility transport teams.

works best when family members and other caregivers assist in a child's care. Parents and caretakers must fulfill two important roles during an actual emergency. First and foremost, adults must know how to access and activate their local EMS network. In most communities, that means dialing 911. In a poisoning emergency, however, this may mean calling the nearest poison center. Adults should provide needed first aid to the injured child. This can range from covering the child with a blanket to providing lifesaving procedures such as cardiopulmonary resuscitation. The emotional stress surrounding an ill or injured child sometimes impairs the caregivers' ability to function as a part of the team. Young children take their cues primarily from the adult caregivers they know best. Parents may feel guilt, fear, or helplessness in aiding their child. Depending on the developmental stage, a child's response and understanding of the situation at hand may be affected by curiosity, need for autonomy, desires for modesty and privacy, fears of death or mutilation, guilt, or misinterpretation of overheard discussions. EMS providers must be sensitive to these reactions and prepared to support the caregivers through applied psychology and good communication skills, while simultaneously providing medical care to the patient. In essence, the family members may become patients as well, requiring supportive therapy to restore their normal psychological and emotional function. This must always be a second priority, after medical support of the child, but it is an important aspect of pediatric emergency care. Such sensitivity improves the perception of EMS care by the family and helps to prepare the caregivers to take an active role in the child's treatment and recovery.

Emergency care providers also have strong emotional reactions to ill and injured children. Many have children of their own and cannot help seeing their child in place of the patient. EMTs are almost universally protective of children and may have significant feelings of anger when faced with a child injured in a preventable accident or one who has been abused or neglected. Likewise, they may suffer from feelings of guilt and self-doubt when a child has a poor outcome. Pediatric calls are common triggers for formal critical incident stress debriefing. Because their emotional instincts and reactions are so similar when it comes to children, it may be helpful to bring together the entire emergency health-care team (prehospital and emergency department staff) for such debriefings.

EMS PROVIDERS AS AN EXTENSION OF THE EMERGENCY DEPARTMENT TEAM

Prehospital care providers are essential members of the emergency care team. They extend the services of the emergency department into the homes and streets of the community. They act as the eyes, ears, and hands that gather necessary information and initiate patient and family care. This information-gathering function is more important for many children than it is for adults. EMTs observe and elicit scene details that help clarify mechanisms of injury, thereby adjusting the index of suspicion for occult injuries through an analysis of the forces applied to children of varying body sizes and maturity. They may also report environmental signs of neglect, or detect incongruities between the scene and the alleged mechanism of injury. EMTs may notice environmental hazards such as chemicals or pill bottles that might explain a puzzling patient presentation. Prehospital providers are often the only medical team members with direct knowledge and access to questions and answers about the scene.

EMTs can, and should, share a voice with their emergency department counterparts. Emergency care providers have long led efforts toward public education and illness and injury prevention. EMTs have the advantages of public trust and respect and the ability to take information to the people who need it most. Every EMS agency should participate in public education programs as a routine part of their mission in the community.

ROLE OF EMERGENCY PHYSICIANS IN EMSC

Encouragement

The pediatric aspects of EMS and the impact of children on EMS providers have long been downplayed or ignored. As a result, the patients may suffer from suboptimal care, and the providers may suffer from a lack of self-confidence and fulfillment. EMTs must be encouraged to develop greater self-assurance and a more positive attitude toward their pediatric patients. Emergency department staff members can assist by reinforcing such attitudes, providing positive feedback to EMTs for tasks well done and constructive input for those that might have been done better. Patient follow-ups provide EMS crews with not only an educational opportunity, but also gratification and emotional closure. Whenever possible, EMTs should be encouraged to spend time with children in the emergency department setting; likewise, emergency department staff will benefit from spending time with EMS crews in the field.

Education

Education begins with each EMS response. Every pediatric EMS patient is a teaching opportunity. Emergency physicians should make an effort to try to answer questions the EMS crew might have about their pediatric patient. They should point out the objective findings that support their immediate clinical impression of "sick" or "not sick." The crew should be encouraged to observe therapeutic or diagnostic procedures and alerted to other interesting cases in the department. EMS crews do not always have time to stay and watch or ask questions, but they truly appreciate the opportunity when they can take advantage of it.

Emergency physicians should alert EMS agencies to formal pediatric education programs sponsored by their facilities. Perhaps the administration could open grand rounds, trauma conferences, and so forth, to EMS personnel. The PALS course, the Neonatal Resuscitation Program, and other standardized pediatric courses should be available to local paramedics. Emergency department staff members with pediatric experience and expertise should be encouraged to share their knowledge with local EMS providers. EMS-oriented pediatric emergency care lectures or skill labs could be assigned as projects for residents and fellows. The Pediatric Education for Prehospital Professionals (PEPP) is complementary to PALS. Ideally, individuals would take both courses to strengthen the skills needed for caring for ill and injured children.

Advocacy and Involvement

The EMSC movement needs the support of all emergency care providers. Emergency physicians provide a significant amount of both acute and primary pediatric care as a part of their duties every day. In doing so, they must recognize the importance of providing every child with access to the same quality of care given to adults. Advocacy for EMSC projects and legislation means advocacy for an integrated, comprehensive system of pediatric and family care that spans the continuum from public education to prehospital care to the emergency department and beyond.

TABLE 306.2. Resources for EMSC Information

LOCAL
Local pediatric or emergency medicine residency program Local pediatric emergency medicine fellowship program Local pediatric emergency department Local trauma center Local pediatric or medical society Local EMS agencies
STATE
State EMS office State Chapter of the American Academy of Pediatrics State Chapter of the American College of Emergency Physicians
NATIONAL
American Academy of Pediatrics Committee on Pediatric Emergency Medicine Section of Pediatric Emergency Medicine 141 Northwest Point Blvd. PO Box 927 Elk Grove Village, IL 60009-0927 (800) 433-9016
American College of Emergency Physicians Pediatric and Emergency Medical Services Sections PO Box 619911 Dallas, TX 75261-9911 (800) 798-1822
NATIONAL RESOURCE CENTERS
EMSC Clearinghouse 2070 Chain Bridge Road, Suite 450 Vienna, VA 22182 (703) 902-1203
EMSC National Resource Center (NRC) Children's National Medical Center 111 Michigan Avenue, NW Washington, DC 20010 (202) 884-4927 www.ems-c.org
National EMSC Data Analysis Resource Center (NEDARC) 410 Chipeta Way, Suite 222 Salt Lake City, UT 84108-1226 (801) 581-6410
FEDERAL AGENCIES
Centers for Disease Control and Prevention National Center for Injury Prevention and Control 1600 Clifton Road, NE, Mailstop F-36 Atlanta, GA 30333 (404) 639-3311
Federal Interagency Committee on EMS U.S. Fire Administration Federal Emergency Management Agency 16825 S. Seton Avenue Emmitsburg, MD 21727 (301) 447-1080
U.S. Department of Health and Human Services Maternal and Child Health Bureau 5600 Fishers Lane, Room 18A-38 Rockville, MD 20857 (301) 443-2250
U.S. Department of Transportation National Highway Traffic Safety Administration 400 Seventh Street, SW Washington, DC 20590-0001 (202) 366-5440

Emergency physicians can become personally involved in EMSC projects by participating in formal EMSC grant-supported programs, or through local pediatric and EMS programs and organizations. Pediatric courses need instructors; EMS agencies need guidance in preparing and supervising pediatric protocols, quality improvement, and educational programs. Emergency physicians also can help educate primary care practitioners about the EMS system, helping them better understand its functions as well as teach their patients and families how to use the system properly.

CONCLUSION

Because EMS providers encounter so few children during their everyday interventions, they have fewer opportunities to develop and practice their skills in pediatric care. Until recently, a correspondingly small percentage of time, money, and effort was allocated toward optimizing pediatric care in a primarily adult-oriented system. The EMSC movement works to integrate a comprehensive pediatric care plan into the EMS systems that already exist. EMSC programs affect all emergency care providers and strive to strengthen the EMS team.

This chapter discussed just a few of the EMSC issues challenging prehospital and hospital-based emergency care providers. The EMSC program has undertaken initiatives over the last few years in addition to the ones described in this chapter. Examples include the national EMSC Resource Alliance, national consensus documents developed on pediatric equipment for transport vehicles and on pediatric equipment for hospital emergency departments; children and disasters; children with special health-care needs; cultural competence; injury prevention; family-centered care in emergencies; and data collection and analysis. For more information on EMSC principles and projects, the reader may contact any of the resources listed in Table 306.2 or consult the references in the Bibliography.

ACKNOWLEDGMENT

The author gratefully acknowledges the contribution of Lou E. Romig, who wrote the previous version of this chapter.

Bibliography

American Academy of Pediatrics, Committee on Pediatric Emergency Medicine. The emergency physician and the office-based pediatrician. *Pediatrics* 1998;101:936.

Allen K, Ball J, Helfer B. Preventing and managing childhood emergencies in schools. *J Sch Nurs* 1998;14:20.

Athey JL, Henderson DH, O'Malley P, et al. Emergency medical services for children: beyond lights and sirens. *Prof Psychol Res Pract* 1998;28:464.

Athey JL. *Emergency medical services for children. Health and welfare for the families in the 21st century*. Boston: Jones and Bartlett, 1999.

Cook RT Jr. The Institute of Medicine report on emergency medical services for children: thoughts for emergency medical technicians, paramedics, and emergency physicians. *Pediatrics* 1996; [1 Pt 2]:199.

Cooper A, Barlow B. The surgeon and emergency medical services for children. *Pediatrics* 1996;[1 Pt 2]:184.

Dieckmann R, Schafermeyer R. EMS for children. In: Roush W, ed. *Principles of EMS systems*, 2nd ed. American College of Emergency Physicians, 1994.

Dieckmann R, ed. *Pediatric emergency care systems: planning and management*. Baltimore: Williams & Wilkins, 1992.

Durch J, Lohr K, eds. *Emergency medical services for children*. Washington DC: Institute of Medicine/National Academy Press, 1993.

EMSC National Task Force. EMS for children: recommendations for coordinating care for children with special health care needs. *Ann Emerg Med* 1997;30:274.

Foltin G, Cooper A. Pediatric issues. In: Kuehl A, ed. *Prehospital systems and medical oversight*, 2nd ed. St. Louis: Mosby Lifeline, 1994.

Foltin G, Romig L. Prehospital/emergency medical services. In: Surpure J, ed. *Synopsis of pediatric emergency care*. Boston: Andover Medical, 1993.

Gausche M. A prospective randomized study of the effect of out-of-hospital pediatric intubation on patient outcome. *Acad Emerg Med* 1998;5:878.

Gausche M, Henderson D, Brownstein D, et al. Education of out-of-hospital emergency medical personnel in pediatrics: report of a national task force. *Ann Emerg Med* 1998;31:74.
Gonsalves D. Historical background of emergency medical services in the U.S. *Emerg Care Q* 1989;4:73.
Hirschfeld J. Emergency medical services for children in rural and frontier America: diverse and changing environments. *Pediatrics* 1996;[1 Pt 2]:179.
Mulligan-Smith DA, Puranik S, Coffman S. Parental perception of injury prevention practices in a multicultural metropolitan area. *Pediatr Emerg Care* 1998;14:10.
National Academy of Science, Division of Medical Science. *Accidental death and disability: the neglected disease of modern society*. Washington, DC: National Academy of Science/National Research Council, 1996.
Seidel JS. et al. Priorities for research in emergency medical services for children: results of a consensus conference. *Ann Emerg Med* 1999;33:206.
U.S. Department of Health and Human Services, Health Resources and Services Administration Maternal and Child Health Bureau. *5 year plan: midcourse review: emergency medical services for children, 1995–2000*. Washington DC: EMSC National Resource Center, 1997.

CHAPTER 307

Dealing with Death or Catastrophic Illness

Phyllis Hendry Stenklyft

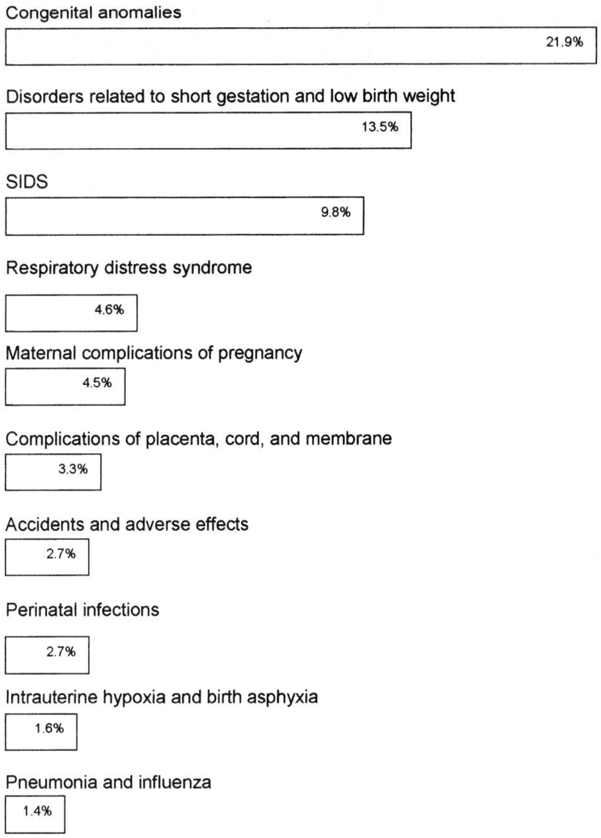

Figure 307.1. Top ten causes of infant mortality in the United States. (Adapted from Guyer B, MacDorman MF, Martin JA, et al. Annual summary of vital statistics—1997. *Pediatrics* 1998;102:1333.)

Emergency physicians and prehospital care providers often face the task of telling a family that their child has died or has a catastrophic illness. Dealing with death in the emergency department is difficult for many reasons. The hectic surroundings and the lack of acquaintance with the family or patient make a difficult situation even worse. Deaths in infants or children differ from those in adults in etiology and in the emotions they create in family and staff members.

EPIDEMIOLOGY OF INFANT AND PEDIATRIC DEATH

The common causes of death in infants (less than 1 year of age) are congenital anomalies, sudden infant death syndrome (SIDS), disorders related to prematurity, and respiratory distress syndrome (Fig. 307.1). Infant mortality in the United States has declined by 40% since 1980. Many infant deaths occur in the neonatal period, often before the infant goes home from the hospital. Birth weight is one of the most important predictors of infant mortality.[8]

Death due to suspected SIDS is commonly encountered by the emergency physician. SIDS deaths are particularly tragic: A family puts a happy, well baby down for a nap and faces unanticipated death hours later. The emergency physician should be knowledgeable about the epidemiology and differential diagnosis of SIDS. Many states have death review teams for unexplained infant deaths. Deaths due to carbon monoxide poisoning, asphyxia in mechanically unsafe sleeping environments, and overlying (smothering) are often initially labeled as possible SIDS. Fortunately, after slow declines during the 1980s, SIDS rates have fallen by 42% since 1992, when the American Academy of Pediatrics issued a recommendation to reduce the risk of SIDS by placing infants on their backs or sides to sleep.[2,3,5,11]

The physical examination of infants who present with sudden, unexplained death or arrest should include a search for signs of abuse, metabolic disorders, and congenital syndromes. Child abuse can be a great imitator of medical and traumatic disease. About 2,000 children die each year of abuse or neglect; 50% of these victims are less than 1 year old.[5,11]

After the infant year, the death rate of children decreases. Injury (usually from motor vehicle accidents) is the most common cause of death in children older than 1 year. Pedestrian accidents, falls, bicycle injuries, and house fires are other common causes of lethal injury. In adolescents, an adult pattern is seen, with death caused by motor vehicle accidents, firearm injuries, and suicide. In some western and southern states, drowning is the leading cause of death in children over age 1 year.[8,9]

Most pediatric deaths are sudden and unexpected. Malignancy, asthma, congenital heart disease, acquired immunodeficiency syndrome, and seizures are the more common preexisting disorders seen in pediatric sudden deaths. In 1997, mortality due to human immunodeficiency virus infection declined by 47%.[8]

GRIEF REACTIONS

In general, society reacts to pediatric death or terminal illness with disbelief, helplessness, and, often, anger. Children are expected to remain healthy and reach adulthood. The high infant mortality rates of past decades are no longer accepted. Parents and family members will usually express guilt feelings, especially when the death was a result of accidental injury. If the death was associated with inadequate parental supervision, family members may blame one another. Hostility among family members may be increased in cases of divorced or separated parents.[4]

Infants and children have often had a recent primary care visit before a sudden death occurs, and parents commonly express anger at the last physician who treated the child. An example is a SIDS death in an infant who recently received immunization shots. Parents may ask the emergency physician why their regular physician failed to see that something was wrong with the child.

SUPPORT AND COUNSELING

Interventions for helping survivors cope with grief are reviewed in Chapter 409. Parental guilt must be addressed soon after the news of death or illness is given to the family. Assure parents that guilt feelings are an expected reaction, and praise them for the positive things they did for their child. Avoid statements such as, "At least you have other children," after a pediatric or neonatal death or a miscarriage. When SIDS is suspected, inform the family that SIDS is a diagnosis of exclusion and that other investigation is required.

Emergency departments should have advance directives, a plan addressing notification of family, burial arrangements, organ donation, autopsy requests, and family support. The support team may include physicians, nursing staff, social workers, chaplains, the primary care physician, and other local support groups. An example of an emergency department death protocol is shown in Fig. 307.2.[1,4,6,10,15]

Encourage, but do not force, family members to view the body or spend time saying goodbye to the child. This experience can be enhanced by providing a quiet room, privacy, blankets, or a rocking chair. Many emergency departments provide foot- or handprints, a lock of hair, or photographs. This is especially applicable in neonatal or infant deaths, when no pictures of the child have been taken before death.

A follow-up support plan should be in place when the parents leave the emergency department. Often, support services will not be accepted for days or weeks after the death. National support organizations are listed in Table 307.1.

TABLE 307.1. National Support Organizations

The Compassionate Friends
P.O. Box 3696
Oakbrook, IL 60522-3696
(630) 990-0010
Support for bereaved parents, siblings, and grandparents; chapters in all states.

American SIDS Institute
6065 Rosewell Road, #876
Atlanta, GA 30328
(800) 232-SIDS

SIDS Alliance
1314 Bedford Avenue, Suite 210
Baltimore, MD 21208
(800) 221-SIDS

Pregnancy and Infant Loss Center
1421 East Wayzata Blvd., Suite 30
Wayzata, MN 55391
(612) 473-9372

SIBLING AND CHILDHOOD BEREAVEMENT

The emergency physician should also be knowledgeable about the grieving process in surviving children. The American Academy of Pediatrics recommends addressing the following questions:

1. What is death?
2. What made the person die?
3. Where is the person?
4. Can it happen to me?
5. Who will take care of me?

Table 307.2 lists manifestations of grief in children by age and developmental level. The child's pediatrician or primary care physician should be involved in monitoring the grief process.[1]

AUTOPSY

The emergency department staff should be aware of state and local requirements for reporting deaths and for organ donation. Postmortem examinations by state medical examiners are often

TABLE 307.2. Manifestations of Grief in Children

Young Children (<3 yr of age)	Preschool Children	School-age Children	Adolescents
Regression	Increased activity	Deterioration of school performance caused by loss of concentration, disinterest, lack of motivation, failure to complete assignments, and day dreaming in class	Depression
Sadness	Constipation	Resistance to attending school	Somatic complaints
Fearfulness	Encopresis	Crying spells	Delinquent behavior
Anorexia	Enuresis	Lying	Promiscuity
Failure to thrive	Anger and temper tantrums	Stealing	Suicide attempts
Sleep disturbance	"Out-of-control" behavior	Nervousness	Dropping out of school
Social withdrawal	Nightmares	Abdominal pain	
Developmental delay	Crying spells	Headaches	
Irritability		Listlessness	
Excessive crying		Fatigue	
Increased dependency			
Loss of speech			

Adapted from American Academy of Pediatrics. The pediatrician and childhood bereavement. Committee on Psychosocial Aspects of Child and Family Health. *Pediatrics* 1992;89:516.

PROCEDURE: Pediatric Death In The ED
Support For Survivors

Physician Responsibilities

1. Notify chaplain early, as soon as death appears inevitable. Ask clerk or nurse to page chaplain via operator
2. Talk with family (listen!)
   - Intervene early and report progress
   - Answer specific questions to the best of your ability
   - Assure the family that medical care was complete
   - Allay parental guilt
   - Take PA/Nursing staff with you
   - *Remember:* Doing nothing is doing something! Some people just cannot be consoled or reached acutely
3. Allow family to view or hold their child.

Nursing Responsibilities

1. Assign consistent nurse to the family
2. Facilitate ED phase
3. Accompany physician and chaplain
4. Provide a quiet room and rocking chair
5. Complete ED checklist
6. Personally ensure paperwork forwarded to ED Nurse Manager's office
7. Attach letter requesting medical examiner's report to Notice of Death worksheet

Follow-Up Phase

1. Chaplain phone call to parents 1-2 weeks after death to coordinate support group participation
2. Patient relations to coordinate physician/survivor meeting to review autopsy findings or answer questions

Checklist for Pediatric Deaths

Patient name________ Unit #________ Date________

Relative name________ Address________

Phone #________ Account #________

Initial Emergency Department Phase

____ Staff person assigned to family members, who?
____ Ask family if patient has had a primary physican or medical clinic
____ If so, who?
____ Medical examiner notifed
____ Family notification of death and tentative cause (essential family members present in emergency department)
____ Family permitted to see baby/tangible evidence of death offered (eg, lock of hair), special requests honored, if so, what? ________
____ Family allowed to express grief; respond to individual needs
____ Family members understand how they may receive autopsy report
____ Family informed of follow-up procedures and given a phone number to call if they have questions
____ ED chart completed (including ED form)
____ Copy of chart enclosed
____ Organ donation

EMS Office Phase

Family physician/clinic notified of death on________ Phone #________ by________

Copy of checklist retained in EMS office? _____ Yes _____ No

Comments________

Chaplain's Phase

Phone call to family (3–5 days after death) on________ by________

Comments________

Phone call to family (2–3 weeks after death) on________ by________

Comments________

Support group offered on________ by________

Comments________

Patient Relations Phase

Autopsy results requested on________ by________

Appointment made for follow-up with physician on________ by________

Appointment date________ Physician________

Comments________

Physician/EMS office Phase

Physician's comments after meeting________

____

Checklist/chart returned to Chaplain's office by EMS office on________ by________

Chaplain's Phase

Call made to family (6 months following death) on________ by________

Comments________

Checklist/chart returned to EMS office for final filing on________ by________

Comments________

Figure 307.2. Example of emergency department death protocol.

required in all sudden deaths of patients in apparently good health. The jurisdiction of medical examiners varies among states but usually includes death as a result of accident, homicide, suicide, or suspected SIDS. Autopsies in infant deaths are strongly encouraged, to find evidence of familial genetic disease, infection, public health threats, or child abuse and neglect.

This subject is difficult to approach. Advise parents that an autopsy allows them and their physician to understand why the child died and how other or future children might be affected. Autopsy results should be made available to the parents in lay terms.

Pediatric autopsies require expertise in pediatrics, pathology, child abuse, and forensic pathology. The fact that many jurisdictions do not have such experts may lead to underreporting, misclassification, and mismanagement of pediatric deaths.

EMERGENCY DEPARTMENT STAFF CONCERNS

A review by Schmidt and Tolle[13] found that emergency physicians responded to a mean of 17 patient deaths per year and were exposed to a much higher death rate than were other specialties. Pediatric deaths usually make up a very low proportion of these deaths, but the exposure to death varies, depending on the patient population, the number of shifts worked, and other factors. Most emergency physicians feel uncomfortable dealing with death and giving bad news to families, and they receive little training in this area.

Pediatric deaths are particularly stressful for staff members; staff should be observed for signs of depression, hostility, burnout, or substance abuse. A crisis intervention team should be considered if an unusual number of pediatric deaths occur or if a mass-casualty incident exposes the staff to many deaths at one time. Death policies and crisis counseling skills should be part of the orientation program for new emergency department staff members.[7,12–14,16]

COMMON PITFALLS

- Do not assume that unexplained infant deaths are due to SIDS without looking for signs of abuse, congenital disorders, or sepsis.
- Do not handle deaths on a haphazard, day-to-day basis; have an organized plan or protocol.
- Do not ignore the grieving of the emergency department staff.
- Do not ignore grief reactions in siblings.
- Remember to contact the primary care physician.

References

1. American Academy of Pediatrics. The pediatrician and childhood bereavement. Committee on Psychosocial Aspects of Child and Family Health. *Pediatrics* 1992;89:516.
2. American Academy of Pediatrics. Distinguishing SIDS from child abuse fatalities. Committee on Child Abuse and Neglect. *Pediatrics* 1994;94:124.
3. Corey TS, McCloud LC, Nichols GR, et al. Infant deaths due to unintentional injury. *Am J Dis Child* 1992;146:968.
4. Edlich RF, Kübler-Ross E. On death and dying in the emergency department. *J Emerg Med* 1992;10:225.
5. Emery JL. Child abuse, SIDS, and unexpected infant death. *Am J Dis Child* 1993;147:1097.
6. Greenberg LW, Ochsenschlager D, Cohen GJ, et al. Counseling parents of a child dead on arrival: a survey of emergency departments. *Am J Emerg Med* 1993;11:225.
7. Greenberg LW, Ochsenschlager D, O'Donnell R, et al. Communicating bad news: a pediatric department's evaluation of a simulated intervention. *Pediatrics* 1999;103;1210.
8. Guyer B, MacDorman MF, Martin JA, et al. Annual summary of vital statistics—1997. *Pediatrics* 1998;102:1333.
9. Keeling JW, Knowles SA. Sudden death in childhood and adolescence. *J Pathol* 1989;159:221.
10. Krahn GL, Hallum A, Kime C. Are there good ways to give bad news? *Pediatrics* 1993;91:578.
11. Reece RM. Fatal child abuse and SIDS: a critical diagnostic decision. *Pediatrics* 1993;91:423.
12. Schmidt TA, Norton RL, Tolle SW. Sudden death in the ED: educating residents to compassionately inform families. *J Emerg Med* 1992;110:643.
13. Schmidt TA, Tolle SW. Emergency physicians' responses to families following patient death. *Ann Emerg Med* 1990;19:125.
14. Smith TL, Walz BJ, Smith RL. A death education curriculum for emergency physicians, paramedics, and other emergency personnel. *Prehosp Emerg Care* 1999;3:37.
15. Walsh-Kelly CM, Lang KR, Cheevako EL, et al. Advance directives in a pediatric emergency department. *Pediatrics* 1999;1103:826.
16. Wolfram RW, Timmel DJ, Doyle CR, et al. Incorporation of a "coping with the death of a child" module into the pediatric advanced life support (PALS) curriculum. *Acad Emerg Med* 1998;5:242.

CHAPTER 308
Optimal Pediatric Care in a Nonpediatric Emergency Department

John P. Santamaria

More than 31 million children receive emergency department care in the United States each year, accounting for approximately one-third of the 91 million emergency department visits. The annual rate for visits to the emergency department by people under 21 years of age is 41.2 per 100 persons, compared with 36.1 for the general population. A child or adolescent comes to the emergency department on the average of once every second. Thirty percent of all pediatric visits are for children under 3 years of age, and 50% of pediatric resuscitations occur in infants. Most children are seen in emergency departments of general hospitals, not children's hospitals. Children have special needs in these settings, and general hospital emergency departments should be capable of accommodating the pediatric patient.

The care of children in the emergency department of the general hospital can be separated or integrated, depending on the situation and the pediatric volume. Resources can be shared among different subsections of the emergency department. This chapter discusses emergency department design, staffing, and personnel use, as well as equipment and resources. The differences and complexities of each emergency department necessitate unique solutions, and, if optimally planned, no two emergency departments should be exactly the same.

The realistic pediatric emergency department is a balance of institutional resources and patient care needs. The concept of providing for the needs of a specific patient group is not unique to pediatrics. Women with pelvic disease require specialized beds for their examinations; ear, nose, and throat patients often require a specialized chair. The special needs of children are more diverse than these simplistic adult analogies, but the concept is the same.

OPTIONS: SEPARATE VERSUS INTEGRATED FACILITIES

1. *Separate facility.* An annual volume of at least 15,000 pediatric visits is usually required to justify a separate pediatric emergency department with separate staff. A separate emergency facility for the care of children in a general hospital may have drawbacks. In a separate facility, the staffing patterns, equipment, and support services are less efficient and more expensive than when they are integrated into a general emergency department. Some emergency departments open and staff a separate pediatric facility only during peak hours.
2. *Dedicated space and staff.* Fiscal responsibility usually dictates that pediatric emergency services share facilities with the rest of the emergency department. Needs and resources must be carefully examined so that the proper balance of resource sharing and services is achieved. Such a balance allows the greatest degree of flexibility while allowing hospitals to provide excellent pediatric care.
3. *Complete integration.* Complete integration of pediatric patients into the general emergency department maximizes use of space and staff but has a negative impact on the "pediatric experience." This option should not be seriously considered, because it precludes the delivery of optimal pediatric care.

EMERGENCY DEPARTMENT DESIGN

Emergency department configuration is dictated by financial and structural limitations. A newly designed facility is preferable to a renovated structure. The entrance to the pediatric emergency department should be easily identified at all levels. Curbside assistance and convenient short-term parking should be available. Parents may feel uncomfortable if they cannot accompany their children into the hospital as care is initiated.

Optimally, entry into the emergency department is by a path completely separate from the regular entrance, to minimize the exposure of the child to frightening sights and sounds. It is preferable that ambulatory and ambulance patients enter by different paths. A warm, welcoming environment in the receiving area allays some of the anxiety patients feel upon entering the emergency department. Friendly, courteous staff contribute to a patient's positive first impression. It is important that the patient and family perceive from the outset that the department is oriented to the child and family unit.

Play areas, telephones, and access to food and educational materials ease the stress of the waiting period. Optimal facility planning allows family participation in the child's care when possible. Traffic through the emergency department is minimized by use of alternate hallways that circumvent patient care areas.

Bedside registration, although more staff-intensive, allows the parent to be with the child at all times. Although not always possible, bedside registration should be available if the patient's condition makes central registration impractical. Initial care of the acutely ill patient should not be delayed for the sake of collecting demographic information.

A centrally located nursing station provides optimal patient observation. An effective emergency department design centralizes staff services, minimizes circulation distances, and reduces staffing requirements. If design constraints preclude creation of a centralized station, satellite nursing stations provide a similar reasonable observation point.

The function of each patient care area should be carefully evaluated. Safety issues should be considered, including child access to choking hazards (small parts), electrical outlets, and needle containers. Provision should be made for the isolation of infectious patients. Visual and acoustic isolation is also an important consideration.

A designated pediatric procedure room gives the older patient a sense of security, because painful procedures such as phlebotomy and intravenous line placement only occur in a designated space. If space is limited, an acute care room, which may otherwise be underused, fulfills this purpose and allows centralized stocking of equipment. Allowing children to master their anxiety about procedures by "playing out the event" with an appropriately trained staff member helps reduce anxiety and addresses emotional and developmental needs.

A dedicated resuscitation room is optimal for management of critically ill children. Visual and acoustic isolation helps reduce the anxiety of other patients and families. It is particularly important that equipment in this area be well organized so that it is easily accessible for use during a true emergency.

STAFFING

Medical care is ideally rendered by staff with specific interest, training, and experience in pediatric emergency medicine. Patient volume may not support full-time, dedicated pediatric coverage; a review of patient flow studies may determine appropriate times for such coverage.

Nurses with specific experience in emergency medicine and pediatrics are important resources for the orientation and continuing education of other staff. Cross-training in adult and pediatric emergency medicine maximizes efficiency. Nurse extenders and emergency department technicians allow nurses to function at the highest level possible, minimizing nonnursing functions and clerical duties. All personnel should have a pediatric orientation. Staff should be encouraged to take courses in pediatric advanced life support.

The collection of blood from infants and small children can be emotionally taxing and technically difficult. Unless staffing allows for blood collection by nurses or physicians, it is imperative that phlebotomists be experienced in pediatrics. Phlebotomy is often the most memorable event of the emergency department visit and a frequent focus of patient complaints; it must be performed with compassion and technical competence.

Airway management is crucial to optimal pediatric emergency care. If respiratory therapists are not dedicated to pediatrics, then specific pediatric training and experience should be a minimum requirement.

Radiology technicians with pediatric experience can best cone down views to the smallest appropriate field, are familiar with appropriate restraining and sedation techniques, and can judge exposure requirements in a wide range of patient sizes.

Medical and psychiatric social workers, as well as child life specialists, can be of great help to the patient and family in the emergency setting.

EQUIPMENT

A dedicated pediatric resuscitation cart should be well organized and contain equipment appropriate for the smallest neonate and the largest adolescent. In an emergency setting, the child's weight is often unknown. A Broselow Resuscitation Tape is recommended for determining equipment sizes and medication dosages on a length-based system. Equipment must be restocked after each use. A low-dose defibrillator is an integral part of the resuscitation equipment. Monitoring capability must be consistent with the level of care provided.

Appropriate sizes of all equipment, such as intravenous catheters, endotracheal tubes, orthopedic supplies, and blood sample containers, should be stocked in the pediatric area. The Committee on Pediatric Equipment and Supplies for Emergency Departments, National Emergency Medical Services for Children Resource Alliance, has published a list of recommended pediatric equipment for emergency departments (Table 308.1).

QUALITY IMPROVEMENT

Quality improvement is the responsibility of all who serve the emergency department. Even in the busiest emergency department, the presentation of a critically ill or injured child may not be a daily event. It is imperative that the pediatric team be constantly challenged. Coordination of personnel is the key; mock scenarios help clarify team members' roles.

In addition to its role in patient care, the pediatric emergency staff should be involved in continuing education of prehospital and other hospital personnel. National courses, such as Pediatric Advanced Life Support and Advanced Pediatric Life

TABLE 308.1. Guidelines for Minimum Equipment and Supplies for Care of Pediatric Patients in Emergency Departments

MONITORING

Cardiorespiratory monitor with strip recorder
Defibrillator (0- to 400-J capability) with pediatric and adult paddles (4.5 cm and 8.0 cm)
Pediatric and adult monitor electrodes
Pulse oximeter with sensors (sizes newborn through adult)
Thermometer/rectal probe[a]
Sphygmomanometer
Doppler blood pressure device
Blood pressure cuffs (neonatal, infant, child, adult, and thigh sizes)
Method to monitor endotracheal tube placement[b]

VASCULAR ACCESS

Butterfly needles (19- to 25-gauge)
Catheter over-needle devices (14- to 24-gauge)
Infusion device[c]
Tubing for above
Intraosseous needles (16- and 18-gauge)[d]
Arm board (infant, child, and adult sizes)
Intravenous fluid/blood warmers
Umbilical vein catheters (sizes 3.5F and 5.0F)[e]
Seldinger technique vascular access kit (with pediatric sizes 3F, 4F, 5F catheters)

AIRWAY MANAGEMENT

Clear oxygen masks (preterm, infant, child, and adult sizes)
Non-rebreathing masks (infant, child, and adult sizes)
Oral airways (sizes 00–5)
Nasopharyngeal airways (12F–30F)
Bag-valve-mask resuscitator, self-inflating (450- and 1,000-mL sizes)
Nasal cannulae (infant, child, and adult sizes)
Endotracheal tubes: uncuffed (sizes 2.5–8.5) and cuffed (sizes 5.5–9.0)
Stylets (pediatric and adult sizes)
Laryngoscope blades: curved (sizes 2 and 3) and straight (sizes 0–3)
Magill forceps (pediatric and adult)
Nasogastric tubes (sizes 6F–14F)
Suction catheters: flexible (sizes 5F–16F) and Yankauer suction tip
Chest tubes (sizes 8F–40F)
Tracheostomy tubes (sizes 00 to 8)[f]

RESUSCITATION MEDICATIONS

Medication chart, tape, or other system to ensure ready access to information on proper per-kilogram doses for resuscitation drugs and equipment sizes[g]

MISCELLANEOUS

Infant and standard scales
Infant formula and oral rehydrating solutions
Heating source[h]
Towel rolls/blanket rolls or equivalent
Pediatric restraining devices
Resuscitation board
Sterile linen[i]

SPECIALIZED PEDIATRIC TRAYS

Tube thoracotomy with water seal drainage capability
Lumbar puncture (spinal needle sizes 20-, 22-, and 25-gauge)
Urinary catheterization with pediatric Foley catheters (sizes 5F–16F)
Obstetric pack
Newborn kit
—Umbilical vessel cannulation supplies
—Meconium aspirator
Venous cutdown
Surgical airway kit[j]

FRACTURE MANAGEMENT

Cervical immobilization equipment (sizes child to adult)[k]
Extremity splints
Femur splints (child and adult sizes)

DESIRABLE EQUIPMENT AND SUPPLIES

Medical photography capability

[a] Suitable for hypothermic and hyperthermic measurements, with temperature capability from 25°C–44°C.
[b] May be satisfied by a disposable, end-tital CO_2 or $ETCO_2$ detector, bulb, or feeding tube methods for endotracheal tube placement.
[c] To regulate rate and volume.
[d] May be satisfied by standard bone marrow aspiration needles, 13- or 15-gauge.
[e] Available within the hospital.
[f] Ensure availability of pediatric sizes within the hospital.
[g] System for estimating medication doses and supplies may use the length-based method with color codes or other predetermined weight (kilogram)/dose method.
[h] May be met by infrared lamps or overhead warmer.
[i] Available within hospital for burn care.
[j] May include any of the following items: tracheostomy tray, cricothyrotomy tray, ET JV tray (needle jet).
[k] Many types of cervical immobilization devices are available. These include wedges and collars. The type of device chosen depends on local preference and policies and procedures. Whatever device is chosen should be stocked in sizes to fit infants, children, adolescents, and adults. The use of sandbags to meet this requirement is discouraged because sandbags may cause injury if the patient has to be turned.

From Committee on Pediatric Equipment and Supplies for Emergency Departments, National Emergency Medical Services for Children Resource Alliance. Guidelines for pediatric equipment and supplies for emergency departments. *Ann Emerg Med* 1998;31(1):56, with permission.

Support, are generally well received and can be included in the education program. It is also beneficial to offer pediatric classes to the general public and first responders. They can be taught that a critically ill child is often more appropriately transported to the emergency department by trained prehospital care providers than by well-intentioned family members or friends. In addition to enhancing prehospital pediatric care, such training courses raise public awareness of the emergency department's pediatric preparedness.

SUMMARY

Emergency department design, staffing, equipment, and quality improvement greatly affect the quality of pediatric care delivered in the emergency department setting. A less tangible factor is the overall pediatric "orientation" of the department. This child-friendly atmosphere is best witnessed by the way staff approaches and interacts with patients and families. The optimal approach to the ill or injured child is greatly dependent on the severity of illness and on the patient's age and developmental stage. Attention to parental concerns enhances the parent–physician relationship, thereby enhancing the overall satisfaction of all involved.

In preparing an emergency department to care for sick children, limitations should also be recognized. In many instances, institutional limitations and the availability of other excellent pediatric emergency care minimize the need for elaborate pediatric resources in all emergency departments. In such cases, coordination of care within a region and cooperative referral patterns best serve the needs of children.

Bibliography

American Academy of Pediatrics, American College of Emergency Physicians. *Preparedness for pediatric emergencies in the general hospital emergency department. APLS: the Pediatric Emergency Medicine Course*. Dallas: American College of Emergency Physicians, and Elk Grove, IL: American Academy of Pediatrics, 1998.

Committee on Pediatric Equipment and Supplies for Emergency Departments, National Emergency Medical Services for Children Resource Alliance. Guidelines for pediatric equipment and supplies for emergency departments. *Ann Emerg Med* 1998;31:54–57.

Santamaria JP. Design considerations in pediatric emergency care. In: Riggs L. ed. *Emergency department design*. Dallas: American College of Emergency Physicians, 1993.

Weiss HB, Mathers LJ, Forjuoh SN, et al. *Child and adolescent emergency department visit databook*. Pittsburgh: Center for Violence and Injury Control, Allegheny University of the Health Sciences, 1997.

SECTION VI

Section Editor: Christopher H. Linden

Toxicology

CHAPTER 309
Approach to the Poisoned Patient

William A. Watson and Christopher H. Linden

The principal objectives in the evaluation and treatment of the poisoned or potentially poisoned patient are listed in Table 309.1. Appropriate treatment is determined by both existing and predicted toxicity. The former is relatively easy to assess by the physical examination and routine ancillary studies. The latter requires information that may not always be available: an accurate history and knowledge of the mechanism of action, biologic disposition (pharmacokinetics), and effects of a given dose of a drug or chemical (pharmacodynamics) and of potential interactions between them.

The mechanism of action (intrinsic toxicity) of a substance determines the location and nature of toxicity. Effects limited to the site of exposure are usually due to nonspecific chemical reactions such as desiccation, oxidation, protein denaturation, and solvent activity. In contrast, systemic effects usually result from selective interactions between a substance (or its metabolite) and specific target sites (e.g., membrane receptors or enzymes of a particular tissue or organ).

Pharmacokinetic parameters include absorption, protein binding, distribution, and elimination (i.e., metabolism, excretion, or secretion). Pharmacodynamic equations define dose–response and concentration–response relations. A general understanding of these variables as they relate to overdoses is essential for predicting the course of a potential poisoning.

Absorption and distribution and, in some cases, biotransformation are required before systemic toxicity is seen. Pulmonary and intravenous administration produces the most rapid absorption. With toxic doses, the rate of oral absorption is often erratic. More rapid absorption may occur with substances in solution, because most drugs have first-order absorption (i.e., the rate is proportional to the concentration). Solid dosage forms require disintegration and dissolution before absorption can occur. The ingestion of toxic doses can result in slower absorption when these processes are impaired or when the solubility of the compound in gastrointestinal (GI) fluids is exceeded.[19] With toxic doses, the rate of tissue distribution, also a first-order process, usually remains unchanged, but the extent may be increased. This may be due to the presence of more free drug (i.e., the binding capacity of plasma proteins is exceeded) or changes in pH that increase the amount of un-ionized drug available to diffuse across cell membranes.

TABLE 309.1. Goals of Patient Evaluation and Management in Poisoning

Evaluation	Management
Recognition of poisoning	Provision of supportive care
Identification of the poison	Prevention of poison absorption
Prediction of toxicity	Administration of antidotes
Assessment of severity	Enhancement of poison elimination
	Prevention of reexposure

The severity of systemic effects is determined by the target tissue concentration of a substance: The larger the dose, the greater the tissue concentration, and hence the effect. However, blood concentrations accurately correlate with those in tissue only if distribution (or redistribution) occurs faster than absorption (or elimination). Because these conditions are not always met, blood levels may be higher than tissue levels during absorption and distribution and lower than tissue levels during elimination and redistribution. Hence, the phase of disposition should always be considered when interpreting blood levels.

Elimination is usually accomplished by metabolic (mainly hepatic) inactivation and renal excretion. The rate and route vary from chemical to chemical. Regardless of whether elimination is constant (zero-order), concentration-dependent (first-order), or saturable (Michaelis-Menten equation), it takes longer to reach nontoxic concentrations as the dose increases. Hence, the duration of effects also depends on the dose. When the rate of elimination is constant or becomes constant (i.e., saturable), increasing the dose results in a proportionately greater (i.e., nonlinear) increase in blood levels, time for elimination, and duration of effects.

The response to a substance depends on biologic variables (e.g., the structure, activity, and integrity of external and internal membrane barriers to chemical translocation; body water, fat, and muscle content, which depend on age, sex, and habitus; serum protein levels and organ function, which reflect the current state of health; genetic influences; and prior chemical exposures) and the physical characteristics (e.g., molecular size and charge, and lipid and water solubility) and dose of the substance. Hence, pharmacokinetic and pharmacodynamic relations are distributed within the population according to a normal (gaussian) curve, and the disposition of a substance or the response to a given dose in a particular person cannot be precisely predicted from mean values (those reported in the literature).

CLINICAL PRESENTATION

Poisoning is most frequently reported and encountered by physicians after ingestion, but other routes of exposure include dermal, inhalational, ophthalmic, envenomation (bites and stings), and parenteral injection. Rare exposures may occur by rectal, vaginal, urethral, or other routes. Acute exposures (those that occur over a short period of time) are more common than chronic ones (those that occur repeatedly or over a prolonged period).

Unintentional poisoning may result from misidentification of a substance (the label may be misread or not read at all, or the label is absent), its misuse or abuse, therapeutic misadventures, or true accidents, such as unforeseen exposures in adults or children. Misuse can apply to either accidental exposure (due to carelessness or ignorance) or intentional exposure (excessive self-dosing to achieve a greater or faster response). Abuse is the intentional use of a substance for its psychotropic effects. Therapeutic misadventures may result from dosing errors or may simply be an adverse reaction to an appropriate dose. Intentional poisoning usually implies attempted (or successful) suicide with a chemical agent. It may also refer to the use of substances to harm another person (e.g., attempted murder, child abuse, chemical warfare).

The agents most frequently involved in reported exposures are pharmaceuticals (particularly analgesics and cough or cold preparations), cleaning products, cosmetics, plants, and hydrocarbons. Ingestion of substances available in the home by children under age 6 is, by far, the most common scenario. Serious or fatal poisoning usually occurs in suicidal adults but is increasingly reported in teenagers and the elderly. Agents commonly implicated in poisoning fatalities include carbon monoxide, antidepressants, cardiovascular drugs, sedative–hypnotics, inorganic chemicals, alcohols, glycols, and iron.

Poisoned patients may present with a wide variety of signs and symptoms. Subjective complaints may occur without objective findings. The severity of poisoning may range from minor to life-threatening. Manifestations may be local (confined to the surface of exposure), systemic, or both.

Chemicals that cause local effects may be classified as weak irritants, strong irritants, or corrosives, depending on whether exposure results, respectively, in mucosal irritation only, mucosal and skin irritation, or severe burns, potentially resulting in permanent tissue damage or death. Systemic effects may be behavioral, biochemical, cognitive, or physiologic. Substances that produce systemic effects may be categorized as extremely toxic, highly toxic, moderately toxic, slightly toxic, practically nontoxic, or relatively harmless, based on a corresponding oral LD_{50} (median lethal dose) of less than 1 mg/kg, 1 to 50 mg/kg, 50 to 500 mg/kg, 0.5 to 5.0 g/kg, 5 to 15 g/kg, or more than 15 g/kg. Products with the three most potent toxicity ratings may be labeled with the words "Danger," "Warning," or "Caution," respectively.

Patients who eventually become severely poisoned may be relatively asymptomatic on presentation. Substances with toxicity, which is characteristically delayed, include acetaminophen, antitumor agents, antimetabolites, carbon tetrachloride, colchicine, digoxin, ethylene glycol, heavy metals, methanol, mushrooms, opioids (especially diphenoxylate), salicylates, and slow- or sustained-release medications (e.g., carbamazepine, enteric-coated tablets, lithium, phenytoin, theophylline).

A history of exposure may be absent when the victim is confused, comatose, unaware of an exposure or its relation to harmful effects (e.g., victims of animosity, chronic or insidious exposures, and therapeutic misadventures), or unable or unwilling to admit to an exposure (e.g., infants and toddlers, victims of attempted abortion or suicide, drug addicts, these attempting to conceal or smuggle illicit drugs in body cavities, recreational users of illicit drugs, and patients with Munchausen syndrome). Because the signs and symptoms of poisoning are usually nonspecific, the diagnosis may be missed unless it is included in virtually every differential diagnosis.

Poisoning should always be suspected in patients with a sudden or unexplained illness or injury; those with a history of psychiatric problems or a recent change in behavior, health, economic status, or social relations; those who use chemicals at work or for hobbies; and those who become ill soon after arriving from a foreign country or being arrested or incarcerated for criminal activity (suspect illicit drugs concealed in a body cavity), or after ingesting food, drink (especially ethanol), or medications.

DIFFERENTIAL DIAGNOSIS

The vital signs and mental status are the most useful physical findings for determining the cause of poisoning by an unknown substance.[15] The overall clinical picture usually suggests either generalized physiologic stimulation or generalized physiologic depression. Increased blood pressure, pulse and respiratory rates, and temperature and central nervous system (CNS) excitation indicate the former; decreased vital signs and CNS activity are manifestations of the latter.

Physiologic stimulation (Table 309.2) is usually caused by one of four mechanisms of action: sympathetic nervous system stimulation, cholinergic inhibition, central hallucinogenic activity, or drug withdrawal (i.e., sympathetic hypersensitivity). Similarly, physiologic depression (Table 309.3) usually results from one of four mechanisms: sympathetic inhibition, cholinergic stimulation, opioid receptor stimulation, or sedative–hypnotic activity. Agents that commonly cause physiologic stimulation or depression are listed according to mechanism of action in Table 309.4.

Less commonly, discordance among or between vital signs and CNS activity may be seen. This usually results from metabolic and membrane effects, multiple mechanisms of action, or selective action leading to compensatory or opposing autonomic responses (refer to Table 309.4). In addition, extreme (preterminal) physiologic stimulation may result in coma and cardiovascular collapse as a consequence of anaerobic metabolism or depletion of neurotransmitters. Analogously, severe poisoning by physiologic depressants (except for sedatives) may result in seizures and tachyarrhythmias as a consequence of shock, hypoxia, stimulation of specific (e.g., opioid) receptors, or membrane destabilization. In most of these cases, however, the overall physiologic picture usually suggests a predominance of either stimulation or depression.

And finally, the vital signs and mental status may be normal. In this situation, care must be taken to exclude exposure to "toxic time bombs" (agents with delayed onset of action; see Table 309.4) before diagnosing a nontoxic ingestion or psychogenic illness After the physiologic status has been characterized, an attempt should be made to narrow the diagnosis to a specific syndrome, corresponding to one of the mechanisms of action previously noted, or to a particular causative agent.

Eye, skin, and neuromuscular findings can be helpful in the differential diagnosis. Although mydriasis may be caused by any physiologic stimulant, and miosis by any depressant, markedly dilated pupils that are minimally responsive to light and accommodation are typical of anticholinergic poisoning.

TABLE 309.2. Manifestations of Stimulant Poisoning

Severity	Signs and Symptoms
Grade 1	Diaphoresis, hyperreflexia, irritability, mydriasis, tremors
Grade 2	Confusion, fever, hyperactivity, hypertension, tachycardia, tachypnea
Grade 3	Delirium, mania, hyperpyrexia, tachyarrhythmias
Grade 4	Coma, convulsions, cardiovascular collapse

Adapted from Espelin DE, Done AK. Amphetemine poisoning: effectiveness of chlorpromazine. *N Engl J Med* 1968;278:1361.

TABLE 309.3. Manifestations of Depressant Poisoning

Severity	Signs and Symptoms
Grade 1	Lethargic; able to answer questions and follow commands
Grade 2	Comatose; responsive to pain; brainstem and deep tendon reflexes intact
Grade 3	Comatose; unresponsive to pain; most reflexes absent; respiratory depression
Grade 4	Comatose; unresponsive to pain; all reflexes absent; cardiovascular and respiratory depression

Adapted from Reed CE, Driggs MF, Foste CC. Acute barbituate poisoning: a study of 300 cases based an a physiological system of classification of the severity of intoxication. *Ann Intern Med* 1952;37:290.

TABLE 309.4. Differential Diagnosis of Poisoning Based on Vital Signs and Mental Status

PHYSIOLOGIC STIMULATION	PHYSIOLOGIC DEPRESSION	MIXED PHYSIOLOGIC EFFECTS	ABSENT PHYSIOLOGIC EFFECTS
Sympathomimetics	**Sympatholytics**	**Asphyxiants**	**Agents with Slow Absorption**
Amphetamines	Adrenergic blockers	Carbon monoxide	Carbamazepine
Beta-adrenergic agonists	Antiarrhythmics	Cyanide	Digitalis preparation
Caffeine/theophylline	ACE inhibitors	Hydrogen sulfide	Dilantin Kapseals
Cocaine	Calcium channel blockers	Inert gases	Enteric-coated pills
Decongestants (oral)	Clonidine	Inhaled irritants	Lomotil
Ergot alkaloids	Cyclic antidepressants (late)	Methemoglobinemia	Salicylates
MAO inhibitors	Digitalis	Nitrophenol herbicides	Sustained-release preparations
Thyroid hormones	Imidazoline decongestants	**CNS syndromes**	**Agents with Slow Distribution**
Anticholinergics	Neuroleptics	Disulfiram	Digitalis preparations
Antihistamines	**Cholinergics**	Extrapyramidal reactions	Heavy metals
Belladonna alkaloids	Bethanecol	Isoniazid	Lithium
Cyclic antidepressants (early)	Carbamate insecticides	Neuroleptic malignant syndrome	Salicylates
Cyclobenzaprine	Drugs for myasthenia gravis	Serotonin syndrome	**Agents That Are Activated Metabolically**
Drugs for Parkinson disease	Edrophonium	Strychnine	Acetaminophen
GI/GU antispasmodics	Organophosphate insecticides	Volatile hydrocarbons	Chloramphenicol
Mydriatics (topical)	Physostigmine	**Membrane-Active Agents**	Chlorinated hydrocarbons
Orphenadrine	Pilocarpine	Amantadine	Ethylene glycol
Phenothiazines	Nicotine	Antiarrhythmic agents	L-thyroxine
Plants/mushrooms	**Opioids**	Antimalarial agents	Methanol
Hallucinogens	Analgesics	β-Adrenergic blockers	Paraquat
LSD and its analogues	Antidiarrheal agents	Cyclic antidepressants (late)	Some methemoglobin inducers
Marijuana	Heroin	Fluorides	Some organophosphates
Mescaline and its analogues	**Sedative–hypnotics**	Heavy metals	Thyroxine
Phencyclidine	Alcohols	Lithium	**Inhibitors of Metabolic Pathways**
Psilocybin mushrooms	Anticonvulsants	Local anesthetics	Disulfiram
Drug Withdrawal	Barbiturates	Meperidine	Fluoride
Antidepressants	Benzodiazepines	Neuroleptic agents	Inhibitors of thyroid hormone synthesis
Beta blockers	Bromide	Propoxyphene	MAO inhibitors
Clonidine	Ethchlorvynol	**Metabolic Acidosis (Low Lactate; High Anion Gap)**	Salicylates
Ethanol	Hydrocarbons	Alcoholic ketoacidosis	**Inhibitors of Nucleic Acid Synthesis**
Opioids	Gamma-hydroxybutyrate (GHB)	Ethylene glycol	Anticancer agents
Sedative–hypnotics	Glutethimide	Methanol	Antiviral agents
	Methyprylon	Formaldehyde/paraldehyde	Immunosuppressive drugs
	Muscle relaxants	Salicylate	Mushrooms (amatoxins)
		Sulfur/sulfate	Podophylline
		Toluene	**Nontoxic Exposure**
		Valproic acid	**Psychogenic Illness**

Pinpoint pupils suggest opioid poisoning. The alpha-adrenergic blocking effects of phenothiazines may also cause pronounced miosis. Similarly, horizontal nystagmus and disconjugate gaze may be due to any sedative–hypnotic agent, but vertical or rotatory nystagmus suggests lithium or phencyclidine poisoning.

Hot, dry, flushed skin is characteristic of anticholinergic poisoning. Flushing may also be due to boric acid, monosodium glutamate, rifampin, or scombroid poisoning or to a disulfiram–ethanol or niacin reaction. Diaphoresis and pallor suggest either sympathetic stimulation (sympathomimetic, hallucinogenic, or hypoglycemic agent poisoning, or drug withdrawal) or cholinergic hyperactivity. Brown, gray, or purple cyanosis that is unresponsive to oxygen suggests methemoglobinemia. Amiodarone may cause a blue discoloration of the skin that can be mistaken for cyanosis. External contamination of the skin or nails with blue dye may also be confused with cyanosis; wiping the affected area with acetone or isopropyl alcohol will reveal the true cause. Hair loss, nail growth abnormalities, and mucosal pigmentation suggest chronic heavy-metal poisoning.

Tremors may result from poisoning by lithium or physiologic stimulants. Fasciculations are typically seen with cholinergic insecticide poisoning, but they may also be a manifestation of sympathetic hyperactivity. Muscle rigidity may be due to severe sympathomimetic poisoning, the neuroleptic malignant syndrome, or the serotonin syndrome. Dystonic posturing suggests a neuroleptic reaction or strychnine poisoning. Myoclonus and choreoathetoid movements are usually manifestations of excessive anticholinergic activity. Weakness and muscle wasting suggest chronic alcohol, heavy-metal, or solvent poisoning.

Seizures may be caused by physiologic stimulants, cholinergic agents, some opioids (e.g., propoxyphene), membrane-active physiologic depressants (e.g., antiarrhythmics, antimalarials, beta blockers, cyclic antidepressants), and agents with metabolic or mixed effects. Except for theophylline and hypoglycemic agents, seizures caused by poisoning are almost always generalized. Hence, the presence of focal neurologic findings should suggest these agents or another cause (e.g., a structural CNS lesion).

Routine laboratory findings may also suggest the cause of poisoning by an unknown agent. The anion gap, acid–base status, and osmolal gap can be useful, because abnormalities suggest poisoning by agents that require early, specific therapy to prevent progressive toxicity and irreversible tissue damage (Fig. 309.1)[1] The anion gap—the difference between the serum sodium concentration and the sum of the chloride and bicarbonate concentrations (sodium − [chloride + bicarbonate])—is normally 13 (±4) mEq/L, and the osmolal gap—the difference between the serum osmolality measured by freezing point depression (but not the vapor pressure or head space method) and that calculated from the serum sodium, glucose, and blood urea nitrogen (BUN) ([2 × sodium] + [glucose/18] + [BUN/3])—is normally 5 (±7).

An increased anion gap metabolic acidosis due to lactic acid may occur in any poisoning accompanied by hypoxemia, cellular hypoxia, hypotension, or seizures. In the absence of these complications (and diabetic ketoacidosis or uremia), methanol, ethylene glycol, and salicylate poisoning and alcoholic ketoacidosis are the leading suspects. Concomitant visual symptoms point to methanol; back pain suggests ethylene glycol; tinnitus or hearing loss implicates salicylate. Similarly, the presence of crystalluria and hypocalcemia suggests ethylene glycol, and a mixed acid–base disorder suggests salicylate. Ketosis may be seen in salicylate as well as ethanol poisoning. An increased osmolal gap with an increased anion gap acidosis supports a diagnosis of either methanol or ethylene glycol poisoning. However, the absence of either or both does not necessarily rule out their presence, because the sensitivity of these findings is low.

The osmolal gap may also be increased by other low-molecular-weight substances, including "unmeasured" sugars or electrolytes, and the magnitude of this gap can be used to estimate the amount (Table 309.5). The presence of an oxygen saturation gap (the difference between the oxygen saturation calculated from the PO_2 and that measured directly by co-oximetry) indicates the presence of an abnormal hemoglobin, such as carboxyhemoglobin or methemoglobin.

Hypokalemia may be due to beta-adrenergic stimulation (e.g., acute poisoning by beta agonists, caffeine, or theophylline), acute barium poisoning, chronic diuretic or laxative use, or toluene abuse. Hyperkalemia may result from alpha-adrenergic stimulation (e.g., by sympathomimetics), beta-adrenergic blockade, and digitalis, fluoride, or lithium poisoning. Hypoglycemia may be a manifestation of poisoning with alcohol, a beta-adrenergic blocker, a hypoglycemic agent, quinine, or salicylate; hyperglycemia may be seen with acetone, beta agonist, calcium channel blocker, iron, or theophylline intoxication.

An elevated serum creatinine with a normal BUN suggests acetone or isopropyl alcohol poisoning, because acetone, a metabolite, or isopropyl alcohol interferes with the colorimetric assay for creatinine. Crystalluria may be seen with primidone as well as ethylene glycol poisoning. Heme (orthotoluidine)-positive urine in the absence of red cells on microscopic examination suggests hemoglobinuria or myoglobinuria due to hemolysis or rhabdomyolysis, respectively. Clear serum with a decreased hematocrit, increased unconjugated bilirubin level, and abnormal red cell morphology is seen in the former; pink serum with increased creatine kinase, aldolase, and lactate dehydrogenase levels is present in the latter.

Agents that cause hemolysis include arsine gas, antibiotics (in patients with glucose-6-phosphate dehydrogenase deficiency), and oxidizing compounds (which also cause methemoglobinemia). Rhabdomyolysis may result from grade 3 or 4 and occasionally grade 2 physiologic stimulation or depression (see Tables 309.2 and 309.3) of any cause. Acute renal failure may result from dehydration, shock, or nephrotoxins such as acetaminophen, cancer chemotherapeutics, carbon tetrachloride, ethylene glycol, heavy metals, immunosuppressants, and

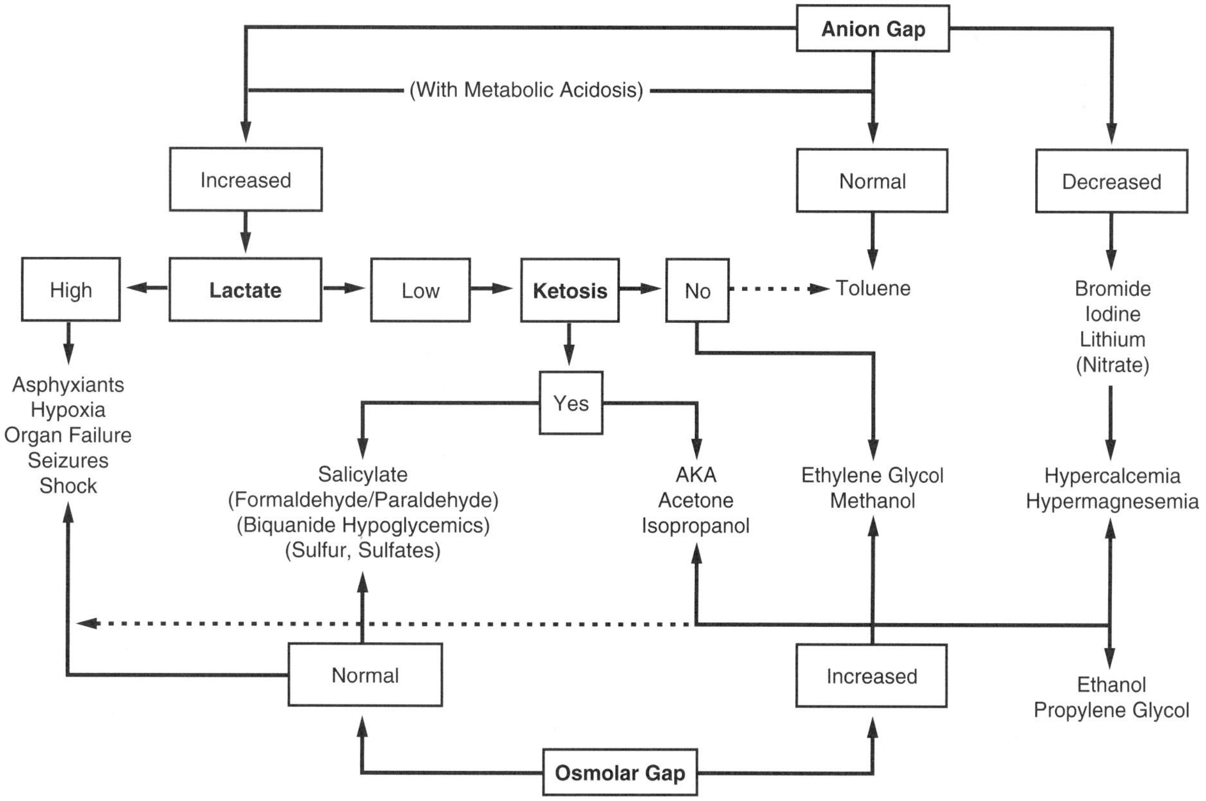

Figure 309.1. Use of routine laboratory findings and calculated gaps in the differential diagnosis of poisoning.

TABLE 309.5. Amount of Solute That Increases Serum Osmolality by 1 mOsmol/kg

Solute	Serum Concentration (mg/dL)[a]
Alcohols, glycols, and ketones	
Acetone	5.8
Ethanol	4.6
Ethylene glycol	5.2
Isopropanol	6.0
Methanol	2.6
Propylene glycol	7.6
Electrolytes	
Calcium	4
Magnesium	2.4
Sugars	
Mannitol	18
Sorbitol	18

[a] Equivalent to 2 mmol/L of electrolyte and 1 mmol/L of other solutes.

nonsteroidal antiinflammatory agents. In most cases, however, the BUN and creatinine levels and the urinalysis are normal at presentation.

The electrocardiogram (ECG) may also provide clues to the diagnosis. Sinus tachycardia or bradycardia with a concomitant increase or decrease in blood pressure may be caused by any physiologic stimulant or depressant, respectively. Tachycardia may also be a reflex response to hypovolemia or vasodilatation. In such cases, the blood pressure is usually low, but it may be normal or even increased. The combination of tachycardia and hypotension may be seen in poisoning by agents such as beta agonists, caffeine, theophylline, carbon monoxide, cyanide, and various antihypertensive drugs (e.g., alpha-adrenergic blockers, nitrates, direct-acting vasodilators). Similarly, bradycardia may be a homeostatic response to hypertension. This combination usually results from alpha-adrenergic stimulation caused by agents such as phenylpropanolamine or imidazoline (e.g., clonidine, guanabenz, and tetrahydrozoline) poisoning.

Ventricular tachyarrhythmias may be due to anticholinergics, chloral hydrate, digitalis, solvents (particularly chlorinated hydrocarbons), sympathomimetics, and agents that cause QRS and Q-T interval prolongation as a result of depressant effects on cardiac membrane activity. Membrane-active agents include amantadine, cardiac drugs (e.g., antiarrhythmics, beta blockers), fluoride (due to its ability to cause hypocalcemia), heavy metals (e.g., arsenic, thallium), magnesium, potassium, organophosphate insecticides, quinine, and psychotherapeutic agents (e.g., antipsychotics, cyclic antidepressants, lithium). Torsades de pointes (polymorphous ventricular tachycardia) suggests a prolonged Q-T interval as the underlying cause.

Atrioventricular block and bradyarrhythmias may be caused by potent alpha agonists (most notably phenylpropanolamine), antiarrhythmics, beta blockers, calcium channel blockers, digitalis, cholinergic agents, and psychotherapeutic medications. In patients with any type of rhythm disturbance, hypoxia, hypoglycemia, hypothermia, hyperthermia, hypovolemia, and acid–base and electrolyte (including calcium and magnesium) abnormalities should be considered as causative or contributing factors.

Radiographs are occasionally useful in the differential diagnosis. An abdominal film that reveals radiopaque densities in the GI tract suggests the presence of calcium salts, chloral hydrate, chlorinated hydrocarbons, enteric-coated tablets, heavy metals, magnesium, phenothiazines, or salicylate. A "double bubble," representing an air–fluid or fluid–fluid interface, may be seen with hydrocarbon ingestion, because this fluid is less dense than water and thus layers on top of the gastric contents. Ingested drug packages may be visible all along the GI tract as uniform oval or round, marble-sized densities.

A chest film that reveals pulmonary edema without cardiomegaly (acute respiratory distress syndrome) may be seen in patients with carbon monoxide, cyanide, opioid, paraquat, sedative–hypnotic, or salicylate poisoning. This picture may also be noted in patients with irritant gas inhalation (e.g., acid fumes, chlorine, mercury vapor, metal or polymer fumes, or nitrogen dioxide) and hydrocarbon aspiration. Pulmonary edema and aspiration pneumonitis are common but nonspecific findings in patients with coma, seizures, or prolonged shock of any cause.

EMERGENCY DEPARTMENT EVALUATION

The history in patients with a known exposure should include the time, route, dose, location (e.g., home or work), surrounding circumstances, and intent. The specific name and amount (weight, volume, concentration, or duration of contact) of all substances involved should be determined. The time of onset, nature, and severity of symptoms; the type of first aid undertaken; and the victim's medical and psychiatric history should also be noted.

If the history is vague or of questionable reliability, an attempt should be made to obtain or verify as much information as possible from paramedics, police, family, and friends. Communicating with the patient's employer, pharmacist, or physician may also be valuable. A search of the patient's clothes, home, or place of discovery may reveal a suicide note, pill bottle, or chemical container. All available chemicals or other evidence of exposure or intent should be brought to the hospital for identification.

If the exposure involves a chemical or product whose ingredients are unknown, consultation with a regional poison control center, reference text, or poison information system may provide the desired data. Drugs can be identified by the pill or tablet imprint code (now required by law) or by their street slang names. The composition of a brand-name product may also be determined from reference sources or by calling the manufacturer. The odor or use of an unknown chemical may also suggest its identity. Local nurseries, horticultural and mycologic societies, botany departments of academic institutions, and field guides may help to identify an unknown plant. Similarly, pet stores, zoos, veterinarians, entomologists, herpetologists, and zoologists may help to identify unknown insects, reptiles, snakes, and other potentially poisonous animals.

A complete physical examination is necessary in all patients. It should begin with vital signs and initially be directed toward assessment of cardiovascular stability, respiratory function, and neurologic status. The accurate measurement of all vital signs, including the respiratory rate (measured over a full minute) and core (rectal) temperature, is essential to detect subtle abnormalities. The neurologic examination should include evaluation of the mental status.

Evidence of underlying illness and coexisting trauma, especially head injury, also should be sought. When the history suggests the possibility of illicit drug concealment, all orifices and body cavities should be visually or digitally examined for the presence of drug packages. The odor of the breath and any vomitus, the urine color, eye findings (e.g., nystagmus, papilledema, pupil size and reactivity), bowel and bladder activity (e.g., bowel sounds, distention, incontinence), and the condition of the skin and mucosa (e.g., color, warmth, moisture, burns, bullae, pressure sores, puncture marks) should be noted.

The vital signs and physical examination must be repeated frequently. Poisoned patients can suddenly and precipitously deteriorate with little or no warning signs.

The need for routine ancillary studies is primarily determined by the clinical presentation. Laboratory studies in symptomatic patients, particularly those with unreliable histories, should include a complete blood count, determination of electrolyte, BUN, creatinine, and glucose levels, and a urinalysis. In asymptomatic patients, blood and urine samples should be obtained on presentation and saved for later (baseline) analysis in the event of subsequent deterioration.

Depending on the history and physical examination, measurement of serum osmolality and ketone levels and arterial blood gas analysis may also be helpful. Patients with respiratory complaints or grade 2 or greater physiologic dysfunction should have a chest radiograph as well as arterial blood gas analysis. The methemoglobin level should be measured in patients with cyanosis despite a normal PO_2. The evaluation of patients with grade 3 or 4 stimulation or depression should include measurement of serum amylase, calcium, magnesium, and creatine phosphokinase levels and liver function tests. Anion, osmolal, and oxygen saturation gaps should be calculated whenever their determinants are available.

Unless the exposure is clearly trivial, evaluation of the cardiac rhythm by continuous monitoring is prudent. Symptomatic patients, those exposed to agents with cardiovascular toxicity, and those with an abnormal rhythm strip should have a 12-lead ECG.

Toxicology screening—the qualitative analysis of urine, blood, and, sometimes, gastric contents, or a sample of the chemical itself—may confirm or rule out a suspected diagnosis.[9,13] Comprehensive screening is expensive and generally requires 2 to 6 hours to perform. It is of greatest value in patients with severe and unexplained findings, such as acid–base disturbances, cardiovascular instability, coma, multiple-organ dysfunction, nonsinus cardiac rhythms, respiratory depression, and seizures. In these patients, the results may prompt a significant change in treatment but usually not in disposition. Depending on the clinical findings, selective ordering of a stimulant, hallucinogen, depressant (coma), or drugs of abuse screen may increase the speed and utility of qualitative testing. In contrast, routine screening is neither clinically useful nor cost effective in patients who are asymptomatic or have clinical findings consistent with the reported history. Despite increased diagnostic certainty and specificity, only rarely do the results lead to a change in treatment or disposition, particularly in mildly poisoned patients. Because of their ready availability, delayed onset of toxicity, and need for specific therapy, acetaminophen and salicylate are exceptions, and levels of these drugs should generally be measured in all patients with intentional overdose.

Optimal use of the toxicology laboratory requires knowledge of which tests (e.g., thin-layer, gas–liquid, high-performance liquid chromatography; colorimetric, fluorometric, and enzyme-multiplied assays and radioimmunoassays; gas chromatography; mass spectrometry) are used for screening and subsequent confirmation of any chemicals that are detected, and the sensitivity (i.e., limit of detection) and specificity of each test. Personal communication with laboratory personnel is recommended in all cases; it is essential when laboratory results do not agree with clinical findings.

A negative screen should never be interpreted as excluding a diagnosis of poisoning: It may indicate only that the suspected agent cannot be detected by the test used, that a chemical is present but cannot be positively identified, or that its concentration is too low for detection in the specimen submitted.

In many cases, it is more appropriate to obtain a quantitative serum level of a specific chemical than a toxicology screen. The results of quantitative analyses are often available within 1 hour. Acetaminophen, acetone, alcohols (ethylene glycol as well as ethanol, isopropanol, and methanol), antiarrhythmics, antiepileptics, barbiturates, carbon monoxide, digoxin, electrolytes, heavy metals, lithium, salicylate, and theophylline are agents whose quantitative measurement is necessary for optimal patient management.

Antidotes may be used for diagnostic purposes. Prompt resolution of mental status and vital sign abnormalities after the intravenous administration of dextrose, naloxone, or flumazenil is virtually diagnostic of hypoglycemia, opioid poisoning, or benzodiazepine intoxication, respectively. Rapid reversal of an acute dystonic (extrapyramidal) reaction after the intravenous administration of diphenhydramine (or another anticholinergic) indicates a drug etiology. A change in urine color after deferoxamine can be used to confirm but not exclude iron poisoning. A therapeutic response to physostigmine is suggestive but not diagnostic of anticholinergic poisoning, because this agent can cause nonspecific arousal in patients with CNS depression of any cause. Details of antidotal therapy are described in chapters that pertain to the corresponding poison.

EMERGENCY DEPARTMENT MANAGEMENT

The management of the poisoned or potentially poisoned patient depends on the actual or predicted toxicity and the time of presentation relative to the time of exposure.[12,18] The time of presentation is important, because it reflects the phase of chemical disposition and allows a more refined prediction of toxicity based on knowledge of kinetic data.

During the *preclinical phase*—the time between exposure and the onset of clinical or laboratory evidence of poisoning—management is based solely on the history (the details of exposure). Because histories may be unreliable, the greatest possible exposure should be assumed. The assumption also should be made that all missing pills or contents of commercial products have been ingested by the child who is found with an open container. Every ingestion in suicidal adults and those with unclear histories is potentially serious. When a history is available and reliable, the maximum possible severity should be estimated from either previously reported exposures or predicted blood levels. Unless toxicity is expected to be negligible or the predicted time of peak effects has passed without incident (Table 309.6), all patients should be decontaminated and undergo a period of observation.

Early and effective decontamination (discussion follows) may prevent absorption and subsequent toxicity, or at least reduce its severity and duration. Regardless of the method used, the sooner decontamination is performed, the more effective it is. Hence, the history and physical examination should initially be brief or done concurrently with decontamination. Because the onset of toxicity may be precipitous, it is also advisable to establish intravenous access and initiate cardiac monitoring in all patients with potentially toxic exposures.

TABLE 309.6. Criteria for Nontoxic Ingestion

1. Time of ingestion and the amount and identity of each and every substance ingested is known with reasonable certainty.
2. Amount ingested relative to patient weight is less than the smallest dose known or predicted to cause toxicity.
3. Time elapsed since ingestion is greater than the longest known or predicted interval between ingestion and peak toxicity.
4. Detailed history and physical examination reveal that the patient is without symptoms and signs of toxicity.

During the *toxic phase*—from the time clinical or laboratory evidence of poisoning begins until the peak—management is based on the findings of the physical examination; the history and laboratory evaluation are of secondary importance. Resuscitation and stabilization of vital signs are the priorities. If vital signs are abnormal, the history and physical examination should initially be brief, concurrent, or even deferred. Unless toxicity is minimal and expected to remain so, all symptomatic patients should have an intravenous line, cardiac monitoring, supplemental oxygen, continuous observation, and baseline laboratory, ECG, and radiographic evaluation. Those with altered mental status, particularly coma or seizures, should be given an intravenous bolus of glucose and naloxone. Although it will not produce immediate effects, thiamine should be given whenever glucose is given. The empiric use of other antidotes may also be indicated. Unless it is predicted that complete absorption has already occurred, efforts should subsequently be directed toward decontamination and enhancement of poison elimination.

During the *resolution phase*—from the time of peak toxicity to the time of full recovery—management is based primarily on the patient's clinical status. Supportive care should continue until the patient is awake and alert and laboratory and ECG abnormalities have resolved. Clinical relapse may also develop when previously depressed GI function returns and poison still present in the gut is absorbed. A prolonged or cyclic clinical course may indicate a gastric bezoar or drug concretion, necessitating further decontamination. As in the preclinical phase, patients who become asymptomatic may require continued therapy because of a potentially toxic dose or blood level of a chemical, the metabolite of which is more harmful than the parent compound.

Decontamination

Topical Exposures

Immediate flushing with water, saline solution, or any other readily available, clear, drinkable liquid is the initial treatment for topical exposures, particularly those that involve local irritants and corrosives. If possible, particulate material should be manually removed before irrigation. A hand-held vacuum is useful for removing dry or powdered chemicals from the skin. Caregivers should use gloves to avoid contamination. A triple wash (flushing, followed by a soap scrub, and repeat flushing) is suggested for dermal decontamination.

Saline solution is the preferred fluid for eye irrigation. Buffered solutions are better tolerated than unbuffered ones. One or 2 L is usually sufficient. If ophthalmic exposure involves an acidic or alkaline chemical, the tear pH should be determined, although searching for pH paper should never delay treatment. The goal of treatment is a neutral pH (7.0). Tears, not the irrigation fluid, must be tested; the pH of unbuffered normal saline solution averages 5.5.

Patients with inhalational exposures should be rapidly removed from the exposure scene and treated with fresh air or supplemental oxygen. A rescuer should never enter a hazardous gas, vapor, fume, or dust environment without adequate eye, skin, and respiratory protection. Liquid chemicals can be removed from body cavities (e.g., vagina or rectum) by irrigation. Accessible solids (e.g., drug packets and pills) should be removed manually under visual guidance.

Ingestions

The goal of GI decontamination is to prevent the absorption of ingested poisons.[12] Decontamination is accomplished by inducing the evacuation of GI contents either orally or rectally. Syrup of ipecac (SOI), gastric lavage (GL), and activated charcoal (AC), singly or in combination, are the methods most commonly used. Charcoal, in repetitive doses, is also used to enhance the elimination of absorbed poisons. Whole-bowel irrigation (WBI) and endoscopic or surgical removal of the ingested poison are reserved for special situations. Cathartics and dilution are used in conjunction with other modalities but are not, by themselves, effective methods of GI decontamination.

Experimentally, ipecac, lavage, and charcoal are all effective in decreasing poison absorption if used within an hour of the ingestion. The greater the delay between poison intake and initiation of decontamination, the less effective treatment becomes. Unfortunately, the mean time from ingestion of an overdose to presentation to the emergency department is 1 to 2 hours for children and 3 to 4 hours for adults. Not surprisingly, the benefit of performing GI decontamination in most overdose patients has not been clearly established.[2–7] Although it is often argued that recovery of pills or pill fragments after ipecac or lavage equates with efficacy of treatment, estimation of drug removal by visual inspection of lavage effluent has not been found to correlate with the measured amount of drug removed. The explanation for this apparent discrepancy is that most pills consist mainly of insoluble excipients. Except for sustained-release formulations, pills are designed so that the drug fraction dissolves and is absorbed rapidly.

Despite these limitations, most overdose histories are uncertain, and it is often difficult to predict which patients will benefit from GI decontamination. Hence, such treatment is recommended for many overdose patients unless the ingestion is clearly nontoxic (see Table 309.6). Because absorption may be delayed or prolonged after an overdose, it is reasonable to perform decontamination unless more than 2 to 4 hours have elapsed since the time of ingestion. Decontamination may be effective at later times in patients with coma and in those who have ingested agents that have slow dissolution and absorption characteristics (e.g., carbamazepine, enteric-coated tablets, lithium, phenytoin, salicylates, sustained-release preparations, large amounts of solids), form bezoars or concretions (e.g., barbiturates, enteric-coated tablets, glutethimide, iron and other heavy metals, meprobamate, salicylates), or slow gastric emptying and intestinal motility (e.g., anticholinergics, narcotics, sedative–hypnotic agents, salicylates).

The need for decontamination in a particular patient also depends on the predicted severity of poisoning. The method selected should be based on the relative efficacy and contraindications of the different choices or procedures and the nature, severity, and risk of treatment complications as they relate to the substance(s) ingested and clinical toxicity. There is no role for decontamination as an aversive, preventive, or punitive measure in patients who have attempted suicide.

As a guideline, because AC has comparable or greater experimental efficacy and fewer complications and contraindications than ipecac or lavage, it is the preferred method of decontamination for most patients. Awake patients who are easily arousable, coherent, and verbally responsive and who can sit up and drink without assistance can be given charcoal by mouth. The gag reflex alone is not a reliable indicator of the ability to protect the airway. In patients who are uncooperative, awake but confused, or unresponsive, charcoal can be given by a standard-sized nasogastric tube with a negligible risk of complications. In unresponsive patients, an initial dose of charcoal can be given while evaluation, monitoring, and supportive measures are being performed.

Alternative methods of decontamination may be necessary when charcoal is unavailable or the ingested agent is not well absorbed by AC. The safety of ipecac for the home management of asymptomatic patients with accidental ingestions, reliable histories, and mild predicted toxicity is well established. However, there should be compelling reasons (e.g., witnessed ingestion of a potentially severe or lethal overdose) to justify the use of a large-bore lavage tube in a patient with minimal or no symptoms. Much too often, a serious iatrogenic complication (e.g., esophageal perforation) results from the forcible insertion of a large-bore orogastric tube in an uncooperative patient with a trivial ingestion.

Syrup of Ipecac. SOI contains the alkaloids cephaeline and emetine, which produce emesis by irritating gastric mucosa and by stimulating the chemoreceptor trigger zone in the medulla. Emesis can remove ingested material from the stomach and proximal small intestine.[3]

SOI causes emesis in more than 90% of overdose patients, including those who have ingested antiemetic drugs. The administration of a second dose of SOI results in vomiting in virtually all remaining patients. The mean time from administration of SOI to the onset of emesis is about 20 minutes. Most patients experience three or four episodes of vomiting in the first few hours after administration.

The efficacy of SOI in preventing poison absorption under controlled conditions (i.e., human volunteers taking nontoxic doses of drugs and animals given overdoses of drugs and other chemicals) averages 57% (range, 28% to 73%) if it is given within 5 minutes of poison ingestion, and 30% (range, 2% to 45%) if administration is delayed 30 to 60 minutes. In comparative studies, SOI is less effective than charcoal. It is probably equal in efficacy to lavage. In overdose patients, SOI offers no advantage over charcoal alone (when both treatments are potentially effective), and its use is associated with more complications.

SOI is given orally in a dose of 30 mL for adults, 15 mL for children aged 1 to 12 years, and 10 mL for infants aged 6 to 12 months. The coadministration of water, another clear drinkable liquid, or milk in an amount of 5 to 10 mL/kg is recommended. The incidence, time of onset, and number of episodes of emesis are independent of the amount of fluid given. The effect of fluid volume on the efficacy of drug removal has not been studied.

Advantages of SOI include ease of administration, widespread availability, and a relatively low incidence of complications. Disadvantages are that vomiting is noxious and delayed in onset, and prevents the administration of charcoal and other oral treatments. Vomiting lasts for more than 1 hour (sometimes as long as 8 hours) in 8% to 17% of patients, and may result in electrolyte and fluid imbalances. Giving nothing by mouth for 1 to 2 hours after the onset of vomiting may decrease the incidence of protracted vomiting. Rare but sometimes fatal complications of emesis include tears and perforations of the esophagus and stomach, pneumomediastinum, diaphragmatic rupture, and cerebral hemorrhage in the elderly. Delayed onset of action allows time for pill dissolution, gastric emptying, and drug absorption. Hence, SOI given before charcoal negates the therapeutic advantage of the latter. Aspiration can occur if the patient becomes comatose or has a seizure while vomiting. This complication has been reported in up to 5% of emergency department patients given SOI. Atypical lethargy is a side effect noted in 12% of children given SOI.

SOI is contraindicated in patients with an increased risk of GI perforation (e.g., recent GI surgery, corrosive ingestions) or aspiration (e.g., coma, seizures, ingestion of low-viscosity hydrocarbons and rapidly acting CNS poisons). It should be used with extreme caution, if at all, in patients with altered mental status, pronounced hypertension, or significant cardiovascular or cerebrovascular disease, and in women who are in the third trimester of pregnancy. Because of its prolonged effects, it is not recommended in those with acetaminophen overdoses who are likely to require antidotal therapy.[16]

Ipecac poisoning may occur in patients with bulimia or anorexia nervosa who chronically abuse SOI. In addition to complications of vomiting, cardiac dysrhythmias and conduction disturbances, myocardial infarction, myocarditis, and generalized myopathy may occur.

Other methods of inducing emesis include apomorphine, copper sulfate, liquid dishwashing detergent, mechanical stimulation of the pharynx, mustard powder, and salt water, but these are either ineffective or associated with significant toxicity and are not recommended.

Gastric Lavage. GL is a process that removes ingested poisons from the stomach.[4] Fluid is repeatedly instilled by a nasogastric or orogastric tube, then aspirated or siphoned off. Experimentally, GL decreases the absorption of potential poisons an average of 69% (range, 54% to 84%) if performed within 5 minutes of ingestion, 31% (range, 26% to 38%) if performed at 30 minutes, and 11% (range, 8% to 13%) at 60 minutes. In comparative studies, its efficacy is similar to that of SOI but less than that of charcoal.

GL is performed with the patient in both a left lateral decubitus and a Trendelenburg position. It can be safely performed in nonobtunded patients without an endotracheal tube. Conversely, the presence of a cuffed endotracheal tube does not preclude aspiration if correct patient positioning is neglected. Although it is recommended that the lavage tube be as large as possible (40F for adults, 28F for children) to increase the efficacy of particulate matter removal, no studies support this practice. On the contrary, lavage with a 16F tube was found to be just as effective in removing dissolved drugs as lavage with a 32F tube. Even with the largest tubes, simply comparing the size of the pill with that of the tube's openings and internal diameter will show that removal of intact pills is physically impossible for many drugs. Mercury-weighted, thumb-sized (46F) tubes may overcome this obstacle but are not generally available.

If a large-bore tube is used, it should be inserted orally to avoid nasal trauma. Because of potentially serious complications, only a physician should insert the tube, and struggling patients must be carefully restrained during the procedure. If restraints are necessary, the use of a short-acting sedative such as midazolam is preferable to physical measures. After the tube is inserted, gastric contents should be aspirated before fluid is instilled.

Aliquots of 50 to 250 mL of fluid are recommended. Saline solution should be used in infants to avoid iatrogenic fluid and electrolyte disturbances; for others, tap water is safe. A reusable plastic funnel can be inserted into the lavage tube for fluid instillation and removed during drainage. Gravity (raising and lowering the lavage tube) is preferable to the use of pressure and suction for fluid administration and recovery. Gastric lavage should be continued until the effluent is clear. The use of more than 5 L of fluid is usually not helpful.

Suggestions for increasing the efficacy of GL include epigastric massage (to enhance the mixing and suspension of gastric contents), the use of warmed fluids (to increase pill dissolution), and the instillation of air (to prevent stomach collapse and obstruction of lavage tube openings by gastric mucosa). Experimentally, the administration of a dose of charcoal before, as well as after, GL is more effective than the usual practice of giving charcoal only after lavage is completed. Charcoal is also a readily visible marker that can be used to assess the completeness of GL.

The main advantage of GL is that it can be used in obtunded patients. The disadvantages are that it is an invasive, noxious, and skilled procedure, with the risk of significant complications if incorrectly performed. Although significant fluid and electrolyte derangements are uncommon, aspiration occurs in up to 10% of patients. The incidence of serious complications, such as esophageal and gastric perforation and inadvertent tracheal insertion and pulmonary lavage, may be as high as 1%. In one series, complications of GL were thought to have contributed to death in over one-third of lavaged patients who subsequently died.[20] Due to an increased risk of complications, GL is generally contraindicated in patients with low-viscosity hydrocarbon and corrosive ingestions. The use of alternative decontamination measures should strongly be considered before resorting to gastric lavage, particularly in patients who are not seriously ill or who present more than 1 to 2 hours after ingestion.

Activated Charcoal. AC is an odorless, tasteless, insoluble, fine, black carbon powder that is produced (activated) by the pyrolysis and oxidation of carbon-containing materials such as petroleum and wood. Each particle of AC has an extensive internal network of branching, irregular, interconnecting channels (pores) ranging from 10 to 105 nm in diameter. Pores account for the large surface area—950 to 2,000 m^2/g for commonly used preparations.

The adsorption (adherence) of substances to the external and internal surfaces of AC occurs within 1 to 2 minutes of contact and is reversible. Increasing the ratio of AC to poison decreases the amount of free (unadsorbed) poison. At an AC–poison ratio of 10:1 or greater, *in vitro* studies indicate that 90% or more of most drugs is adsorbed to AC. The maximum amount of a chemical that can be adsorbed by AC (the binding capacity) varies from a few milligrams to more than 1,000 mg/g of AC.

The greater the surface area of AC and the greater the molecular size, dissolution rate (only molecules in solution are adsorbable), lipid solubility, and electrical neutrality of the poison, the greater the binding capacity. Hence, small, highly charged (ionized), readily dissociable inorganic molecules, such as those of mineral acids, alkalis, and salts of cyanide, fluoride, iron, and lithium, are poorly adsorbed by AC.

AC prevents the absorption of ingested poisons by binding them within the gut lumen, allowing the AC–poison complex to be evacuated per rectum.[5] Cathartics are often used concurrently to enhance the rectal evacuation of the complex and to prevent constipation. Experimentally, AC decreases the absorption of potential poisons an average of 68% (range, 14% to 99%) when given within 5 minutes of poison administration, 50% (range, 17% to 75%) when given at 30 minutes, and 50% (range, 9% to 78%) at 60 minutes. Analogous to the results of *in vitro* studies, an AC–poison ratio of 10:1 or greater decreases the absorption of most agents by more than 90%. Diluting charcoal in large volumes of lavage fluid is less effective than giving the same dose in a concentrated bolus, probably due to mass action effects on the binding equilibrium.

The ability of AC to prevent poison absorption usually correlates directly with its ability to adsorb drugs *in vitro*. However, cyanide, malathion, and tolbutamide are poorly adsorbed to charcoal *in vitro*, yet their absorption or activity is significantly reduced by AC *in vivo*. Conversely, ethanol (and probably other low-molecular-weight hydrocarbons), ipecac, and *N*-acetylcysteine are relatively well adsorbed by AC *in vitro*, yet AC has minimal effects on their *in vivo* absorption and activity. Hence, antidotal efficacy should ultimately be determined by *in vivo* testing and clinical studies.

Experimentally, AC is equal or superior to SOI and GL in preventing poison absorption. Analogous results are noted in clinical studies. In awake overdose patients, AC is equal or superior to SOI when improvement or deterioration in clinical status, length of stay in the emergency department, and complications of treatment are used to measure efficacy. In obtunded patients, AC alone is as effective as GL followed by AC in patients who present more than 1 hour after overdose. It is unclear whether it is equally or less effective than combined treatment in those who present within 1 hour of ingestion.

AC is given as a suspension in water, using 8 mL of diluent per gram of AC powder if a premixed formulation is unavailable. Commercial preparations may contain propylene glycol and carboxymethylcellulose as lubricants and sorbitol as a cathartic. The recommended dose is at least ten times the weight of the ingested poison, or as much as possible if the amount ingested is unknown. Because of volume constraints, the maximum amount of AC that can be given as a single dose is limited to 1 to 2 g/kg. Hence, large-surface-area charcoals are theoretically preferable, particularly for large ingestions (5 to 10 g or more).

AC can be given by a drinking glass, nippled bottle (for infants), or gastric tube. Acceptability and palatability may be increased by giving it through a straw from a covered opaque container. Adding a sweetener or flavoring agent may improve palatability but decreases the absorptive capacity.

The advantages of AC are its safety, ease of administration, rapidity of action, and lack of contraindications. The main disadvantages are limited patient and staff acceptability because of its color, gritty taste, and ability to stain clothing and its low binding capacity for some poisons. Side effects include nausea, vomiting, abdominal cramps, diarrhea, and constipation. It is unclear whether these effects are due to charcoal itself, excessive fluid volume, the ingested poison, or coadministered cathartics. Because charcoal is inert and nonabsorbable, complications are mechanical in nature and include aspiration pneumonitis and mechanical obstruction of the airway and bowel due to inspissated charcoal. Because of pH changes, acidic agents such as aspirin may become ionized and desorb from AC and be absorbed from the small intestine; the use of large or multiple doses of AC may prevent such occurrences. AC may also prevent the enteral absorption (or enhance the elimination) of therapeutically administered agents, necessitating the use of larger-than-usual doses.

Although AC may not be beneficial in patients who have ingested agents that it adsorbs poorly, it should be given to those who have an equivocal history or who have ingested multiple agents. It is not recommended for pure ingestions of nonabsorbable corrosives (e.g., most acids and alkalis) because it may obscure endoscopic assessment of damage to the GI tract.

Whole-Bowel Irrigation. WBI prevents poison absorption by enhancing its rectal evacuation.[7] Although experimental data are limited, WBI is more effective than either SOI or GL and more or less effective than AC in preventing poison absorption. It may be advantageous in patients who have ingested potentially toxic foreign bodies, drug packets, iron, and enteric-coated or sustained-release medications. Continuous WBI may also be effective in enhancing the elimination of drugs that are already absorbed by dialyzing the GI tract.

WBI is performed by giving a bowel-cleansing solution that contains electrolytes and polyethylene glycol (e.g., Colyte, GoLYTELY), orally or by a gastric tube, until the rectal effluent is clear. The patient must be in a sitting position. The recommended rate of fluid administration is 0.5 L/h in children and 2 L/h in adults. Fluid and electrolyte derangements are potential complications.

Endoscopy and Surgery. The absorption of poisons may also be prevented by removing them from the stomach by endoscopic snares and baskets or from anywhere along the GI tract by surgery. Endoscopy may be indicated when a potentially toxic foreign body fails to pass beyond the pylorus, when pill bezoars or concretions are present in the stomach, or when a potentially lethal dose of a heavy metal such as arsenic, iron, mercury, or thallium is radiographically visible in the stomach. Endoscopy should not be used for the removal of ingested drug packets, because the endoscope may rupture them.

Immediate surgical intervention is indicated in patients who ingest large numbers of cocaine packets and become toxic due to leakage or rupture of the packaging. Surgery should also be considered for the same situations as endoscopy when the latter is unsuccessful.[16]

Cathartics. Cathartics include osmotically active salts such as magnesium citrate, magnesium sulfate (Epsom salt), and sodium sulfate (Glauber's salt) and saccharides such as mannitol and sorbitol, which promote the rectal evacuation of GI contents by causing fluid retention, and hence increased bowel motility.[6] They are primarily used as an adjunct to AC to enhance its evacuation. When used alone or with SOI or GL, they have little, if any, benefit.

Sorbitol, the preferred agent, is the most effective cathartic in terms of shortening the GI transit time of bowel contents. Sorbitol is available as a 70% solution and with AC in premixed suspensions. The recommended dose is 1 to 2 g/kg. Saline cathartics are available in various concentrations and are given in a dose of about 250 mg/kg. Castor, mineral, and vegetable oil; phenolphthalein; and disodium phosphate (Fleets salt) are not recommended.

Side effects include nausea, abdominal cramps, vomiting, and excessive diarrhea. Dehydration and electrolyte abnormalities may result from repeated dosing and are sometimes fatal. Hypermagnesemia with lethargy, weakness, loss of reflexes, and even coma may occur with multiple doses of magnesium-containing salts. Hypocalcemia and hypernatremia may also occur. Cathartics are contraindicated in patients with corrosive ingestions or spontaneous diarrhea, and should be used with extreme caution in patients with congestive heart failure or renal failure.

Dilution. Dilution is used to decrease the local effects of ingested corrosives by lowering their concentration. It is accomplished by having the patient drink up to 5 mL/kg of water or another clear, drinkable liquid. Greater amounts of fluid may precipitate emesis due to gastric distention and should be avoided. To be effective, dilution must be accomplished immediately (within minutes) but is generally given "as soon as possible." As with cathartics, dilution alone is ineffective in preventing poison absorption; in fact, dilution may facilitate the dissolution of pills and drugs, thus enhancing absorption.

Supportive Care

The goal of supportive therapy is to maintain physiologic homeostasis until detoxification is accomplished. It is also necessary to prevent or treat secondary complications, such as aspiration, bedsores, cerebral and pulmonary edema, rhabdomyolysis, sepsis, and generalized organ dysfunction. Although supportive care is not specific to the management of poisoned patients, aspects of special relevance are discussed subsequently. The reader is referred to poison-specific chapters for further details.

The need for oxygenation and mechanical ventilation is best determined by arterial blood gas analysis. Although this need may be obvious in patients with severe CNS depression or excitation, clinical assessment of these parameters is not always reliable. In addition, because aspiration is a preventable complication of treatment (e.g., GI decontamination), as well as of poisoning, prophylactic endotracheal intubation is often required for airway protection. The gag reflex alone is not a reliable indicator of the need for intubation: Many healthy people have an absent gag reflex, and many comatose patients will gag with sufficient stimulation. Similarly, patients may be able to maintain a patent airway while being stimulated but not if left unattended. Hence, those who cannot respond to and by voice, or who cannot sit up and drink fluids without assistance, are best managed by intubation. A short-acting sedative or muscle relaxant is useful in facilitating intubation in patients with low-grade coma. Patients with high-grade physiologic excitation may require intubation for airway protection and to allow the pharmacologic control of seizures or behavioral agitation, to prevent or limit the extent of complications (e.g., hyperthermia, acidosis, rhabdomyolysis).

The initial treatment of pulmonary edema in poisoned patients should also include early endotracheal intubation. Because many cases are noncardiac in etiology (e.g., acute respiratory distress syndrome due to inhalational injury, prolonged apnea, or shock), the use of positive end-expiratory pressure is often beneficial. Iatrogenic fluid overload and myocardial depression often contribute to pulmonary edema in hypotensive patients. In such cases, an inotropic vasopressor (e.g., dopamine) is the treatment of choice. Only when the blood pressure has been normalized should a diuretic be given.

Supraventricular tachycardia associated with generalized physiologic stimulation is usually not hemodynamically compromising and requires only observation or nonspecific sedation (e.g., a benzodiazepine). However, if extreme hypertension, chest pain, or ECG evidence of ischemia is present, specific therapy is indicated. The use of a nonselective adrenergic blocker (e.g., labetalol) or both a beta blocker and a vasodilator (e.g., esmolol or propranolol and nitroprusside) is preferred for patients with sympathetic hyperactivity. Physostigmine is the treatment of choice for those with a purely anticholinergic cause.

Lidocaine is generally safe to use for ventricular tachyarrhythmias of any etiology. Procainamide and other class IA antiarrhythmics should be avoided in patients with poisoning by membrane-active agents because of their similar (and hence additive) electrophysiologic effects. Sodium bicarbonate may be therapeutic for dysrhythmias caused by cyclic antidepressants and other membrane-active agents. Patients with torsades de pointes and digitalis poisoning may respond to magnesium. Overdrive pacing (by isoproterenol or electricity) may be necessary in those with prolonged Q-T intervals. Antibody therapy as well as pacing should be considered for dysrhythmias caused by digitalis.

Bradyarrhythmias associated with hypotension should initially be treated with atropine, isoproterenol, and intravenous fluids. In patients with beta-blocker and calcium-channel blocker poisoning, the administration of calcium and glucagon may obviate the need for cardiac pacing. The treatment of bradycardia secondary to hypertension or increased intracranial pressure should be directed at the primary cause. In patients with a dysrhythmia, underlying metabolic abnormalities and extremes of temperature must be corrected.

Hypotension in poisoned patients is more often due to loss of vascular tone than to cardiac depression. It should initially be treated with crystalloids. If vasopressors are subsequently required, direct-acting agents (e.g., norepinephrine, high-dose dopamine) are preferred, because some chemicals (e.g., cyclic antidepressants) deplete endogenous catecholamines. Advanced cardiovascular and pulmonary supportive measures, such as extracorporeal membrane oxygenation, intraaortic balloon pump counterpulsation, and partial cardiopulmonary bypass pump assistance, should also be considered in severe but reversible poisoning.

Seizures caused by central excitatory neuroreceptor stimulation (e.g., those caused by sympathomimetics, hallucinogens, or drug withdrawal) or inhibitory neuroreceptor depression (e.g., the antagonism of gamma-aminobutyric acid [GABA] and glycine receptor activity by isoniazid and strychnine, respectively) are best treated with a GABA "agonist," such as a benzodiazepine or a barbiturate. Pyridoxine, which is converted to a cofactor required for GABA synthesis, is usually necessary to stop seizures caused by isoniazid, because this agent inhibits GABA synthesis and because GABA agonists act, at least partially, by causing GABA release from presynaptic nerve endings.

In contrast, seizures caused by agents that stabilize neuronal membranes (e.g., beta blockers, cyclic antidepressants) are best treated with phenytoin, a membrane-active agent. For neurobehavioral hyperactivity resulting from central dopaminergic stimulation (e.g., phencyclidine poisoning), the dopamine antagonist haloperidol is preferred. Specific antidotes may be necessary in certain cases, such as anticholinergic, cyanide, or opioid poisoning.

Regardless of the cause, it is always prudent to give dextrose. Because prolonged convulsions can lead to rhabdomyolysis and severe acidosis (each resulting in additional complications), the use of paralyzing neuromuscular blocking agents is indicated in refractory cases. Continued seizure treatment, as indicated by electroencephalographic monitoring, is necessary to prevent permanent neurologic damage. In all patients, contributing metabolic and physiologic abnormalities (e.g., cerebral edema or ischemia) should be corrected.

Antidotal Therapy

Antidotes are chemicals that counteract the effects of poisons. They act by a variety of mechanisms: neutralization by antibody–antigen reactions, chelation, or chemical binding; physiologic antagonism by blocking or reversing the interaction of a chemical and its target site; activation or inhibition of an opposing division of the nervous system; and altered disposition by enhancing or inhibiting metabolism, excretion, or secretion. Although antidotes can reduce morbidity and mortality, relatively few poisons and toxic syndromes have antidotes (Table 309.7). Antidotes can themselves be toxic, so their indiscriminate use should be avoided. Details regarding the use of antidotes are provided in the appropriate poisoning chapters.

Enhancement of Elimination

Although the elimination of many chemicals can be accelerated by various therapeutic interventions (Table 309.8), the clinical efficacy of such interventions is often insignificant. Pharmacokinetic efficacy requires that a significant fraction of a chemical dose be eliminated at a rate significantly greater than that accomplished by intrinsic mechanisms. Clinical efficacy implies a shortened duration of toxicity and improved patient outcome. In most instances, if vital signs can be adequately supported, the poison will be intrinsically detoxified and full recovery will follow. Hence, the decision to use an active removal procedure should be based on the actual or predicted maximal severity of the poisoning and the risk (i.e., invasiveness, complications) of the procedure. In addition, invasive procedures are expensive and require technical expertise and specialized equipment. Diagnostic certainty, usually by way of laboratory confirmation, is therefore a prerequisite.

The use of extracorporeal procedures should be limited to patients who would not otherwise have a favorable outcome: those with severe clinical or laboratory toxicity who do not respond to supportive care and noninvasive elimination therapy; those with blood levels predictive of a significant risk of severe, irreversible, or prolonged toxicity, particularly if an invasive procedure is the only or most effective method of enhancing elimination; those who lack the capacity for self-detoxification because of liver or kidney failure; and those who have serious underlying illnesses or complications of poisoning that would adversely affect recovery.

Chelation therapy is covered in the chapters on heavy-metal poisoning. Hyperbaric oxygenation is discussed in the chapters on carbon monoxide, hydrogen sulfide, and cyanide poisoning and methemoglobinemia. Intestinal dialysis has been discussed in this chapter.

Multiple-Dose Activated Charcoal

When given in repeated doses, AC can enhance the elimination of absorbed poisons by adsorbing them in the gut lumen as they undergo biliary excretion, intestinal secretion, or passive diffusion from higher concentrations in blood perfusing intestinal surfaces to low concentrations in luminal fluids (i.e., enterocapillary exsorption).[8] The efficacy of multiple-dose AC (MDAC) therapy depends on the adsorbability of the poison to AC and its pharmacokinetic properties but is independent of the initial route of poison absorption (e.g., orally versus intravenously). As with other dialysis techniques, efficacy is probably greatest with agents that have relatively low molecular weights, small volumes of distribution, low protein binding, and high lipid and water solubility. Experimentally, MDAC therapy is effective in enhancing the elimination of most substances tested, but its clinical efficacy (i.e., shortened duration of toxicity) remains to be

TABLE 309.7. Chemicals and Related Syndromes with Specific Antidotes

Acetaminophen	Cholinergics	Hypoglycemics
Anticholinergics	Cyanide	Isoniazid
Anticoagulants	Digitalis	Methanol
Benzodiazepines	Ethylene glycol	Methemoglobinemia
Beta blockers	Envenomations	Opioids
Calcium channel blockers	Fluoride	Sympathomimetics
	Heavy metals	Vacor (PNU)
Carbon monoxide	Hydrogen sulfide	

TABLE 309.8. Methods of Enhancing Chemical Elimination

Chelation therapy	Forced diuresis
Extracorporeal techniques	Gastrointestinal dialysis
Peritoneal dialysis	Hyperbaric oxygenation
Hemodialysis	Multiple-dose activated charcoal
Hemoperfusion	Urine pH manipulation
Hemofiltration	
Plasmapheresis	
Exchange transfusion	

proven. For some agents (e.g., phenobarbital, theophylline), its efficacy approaches that of hemodialysis.

In patients with normal bowel activity, MDAC in a dose of 0.5 g/kg of AC every 4 hours is usually well tolerated. Increasing the cumulative dose of AC by giving it in larger individual doses or at more frequent intervals increases efficacy. In patients with decreased GI motility or vomiting, MDAC may be better tolerated if given in smaller doses at more frequent intervals or by slow, continuous nasogastric infusion. The dosage of AC should be reduced or eliminated in the event of regurgitation or gastrostasis. Although the coadministration of cathartics is recommended, magnesium-containing agents should not be used, and the dose must be carefully titrated to bowel activity to avoid excessive diarrhea with fluid and electrolyte losses.

Enhanced Urinary Excretion

Diuresis and ion trapping by altering the urinary pH may prevent the passive renal tubular reabsorption of chemicals that enter the urine by glomerular filtration and active tubular secretion, and thus increase their excretion.[11] Because biologic membranes are more permeable to un-ionized molecules than to their ionized counterparts, acidic (low pK_a) chemicals are ionized and trapped in an alkaline urine, and basic chemicals are ionized and trapped in an acid urine. Saline diuresis can enhance the excretion of bromide, calcium, lithium, potassium, and isoniazid. Alkaline diuresis is effective for acidic herbicides (i.e., 2,4-D and 2,4,5-T), chlorpropamide, phenobarbital (and probably other long-acting barbiturates), and salicylates. Acid diuresis, although it enhances the excretion of amphetamines, cocaine, phencyclidine, quinine, quinidine, and strychnine, is not recommended, because the risks are significant and clinical efficacy has not been established.

The goal of diuresis is a urine flow of at least 3 mL/kg/h; that of alkalinization is a urine pH of 7.5 or greater. An intravenous alkaline diuresis solution can be prepared by adding one to three ampules (44 to 132 mEq) of sodium bicarbonate to 1 L of appropriately hypotonic fluid so that the final solution is roughly isotonic. The carbonic anhydrase inhibitor acetazolamide should not be used to alkalinize the urine, because it may produce a concomitant acidemia and enhance the tissue distribution of acidic chemicals. Acid–base, fluid, and electrolyte parameters as well as clinical response must be carefully monitored during therapy. Contraindications include congestive heart failure, kidney failure, and cerebral or pulmonary edema.

Extracorporeal Elimination

Extracorporeal techniques (see Table 309.7) theoretically can remove any diffusible chemical from the bloodstream.[17] Dialysis is most effective in enhancing the elimination of agents with a low molecular weight (less than 500 daltons), high water solubility, low protein binding, small volume of distribution (less than 1 L/kg), slow intrinsic elimination (i.e., long half-life), and high dialysis clearance relative to total body clearance. The efficacy of other extracorporeal procedures is not limited by molecular weight, water solubility, or protein binding.

Chemicals considered dialyzable with respect to both kinetic and clinical efficacy include bromide, chloral hydrate, ethanol, ethylene glycol, isopropyl alcohol, lithium, heavy metals, methanol, and salicylate. Although hemoperfusion may be more effective in removing some of these poisons, it does not readily correct associated acid–base and electrolyte abnormalities. Hemoperfusion is the preferred technique for enhancing the elimination of chloramphenicol, disopyramide, sedative–hypnotics (e.g., barbiturates, ethchlorvynol, glutethimide, meprobamate, methaqualone), phenytoin, and theophylline. Both techniques require central venous access and systemic anticoagulation, and may cause hypotension and bleeding complications. Hemoperfusion may also result in hemolysis, hypocalcemia, and thrombocytopenia.

Peritoneal dialysis is less effective, but it may be used when other extracorporeal procedures are unavailable, contraindicated, or technically difficult (e.g., in infants). Exchange transfusion is also less effective, but it may be used in the same situations, as well as for poisons that cause severe hemolysis or methemoglobinemia. The role of other extracorporeal techniques has not been defined. After the termination of any invasive elimination procedure, clinical relapse or a rebound increase in the blood level of a chemical may occur as it undergoes tissue redistribution.

DISPOSITION

After evaluation, treatment, and an appropriate observation period, asymptomatic patients may be discharged from the emergency department. The disposition of symptomatic patients depends on the actual or predicted severity and the need or potential need for therapeutic interventions. Most patients develop only mild toxicity and can be observed in the emergency department or comparable facility until asymptomatic. Those with significant (grade 3 or 4) physiologic stimulation or depression, hypoxia, hypercarbia, acid–base disturbances, metabolic abnormalities, extremes of temperature, and cardiac conduction or rhythm abnormalities should be admitted to an intensive care unit.[10,14] Patients who require close monitoring of antidotal therapy or high-risk elimination procedures, those showing progressive clinical deterioration, and those with significant underlying medical problems are also candidates for the intensive care unit.

Patients with moderate toxicity can be admitted to a general medical floor, intermediate care unit, or emergency department observation area, depending on the anticipated duration of toxicity and the level of monitoring needed (e.g., intermittent clinical observation versus continuous clinical, cardiac, and respiratory monitoring). Lack of resources for the constant behavioral observation of suicidal patients may require a higher level of care than is medically necessary.

Consultation with a poison control center or toxicologist is recommended whenever the treating physician is not completely familiar with the specific chemical(s) involved in a given exposure or poisoning. Consultation with other specialists is dictated by the nature of the injury and its actual or potential severity.

The possibility of reexposure and its prevention must be addressed before discharge. Suicidal patients require psychiatric assessment, disposition, and follow-up. Prescriptions given to depressed or psychotic patients should be written for a limited amount of the drug and a limited number of refills. Such patients also require close monitoring for compliance with and response to therapy. Drug abusers should be referred for counseling and given the opportunity for rehabilitation.

The environment of all children must be poison-proofed. Parents and other caretakers should be instructed to store alcoholic beverages; medications; all automotive, cleaning, cosmetic, fuel, painting, and pet care products; nonedible plants; vitamins; and toiletries above or out of the child's reach or in cabinets with locks or childproof latches. Safety caps are always advisable, but are not necessarily sufficient to prevent access by children.

Adults with accidental home exposures should be instructed regarding the safe use of drugs and other chemicals. They should be advised to read the instructions on the label carefully and to avoid circumstances that caused the current problem. In environmental or workplace exposures, the appropriate governmental agency (e.g., EPA, OSHA, NIOSH, local health department) should be notified. Unsafe working conditions should also be brought to the attention of the employer. Assistance with the administration of medications should be arranged for confused patients with accidental exposures due to dosing errors. Preventive education is particularly important in cases of dosing errors committed by health-care providers.

COMMON PITFALLS

- Failure to consider the diagnosis of poisoning in patients with unexplained signs and symptoms of any nature
- Failure to appreciate the limitations of toxicology screening
- Failure to initiate routine and advanced supportive care when clinically indicated
- Failure to treat the patient, not the poison (or, with few exceptions, its blood level)
- Using ipecac syrup in patients who have ingested hydrocarbons, corrosives, or rapidly acting CNS and cardiovascular poisons
- Failure to appreciate that activated charcoal is the most effective and least hazardous method of GI decontamination
- Failure to address preventive measures before discharge

References

1. Aabakken L, Johansen KS, Rydningen EB, et al. Osmolal and anion gaps in patients admitted to an emergency medical department. *Hum Exp Toxicol* 1994;13:131.
2. American Academy of Clinical Toxicology/European Association of Poisons Centres and Clinical Toxicologists position statements on gastrointestinal decontamination: introduction. *Clin Toxicol* 1997;24:695.
3. American Academy of Clinical Toxicology/European Association of Poisons Centres and Clinical Toxicologists position statements on gastrointestinal decontamination: syrup of ipecac. *Clin Toxicol* 1997;24:699.
4. American Academy of Clinical Toxicology/European Association of Poisons Centres and Clinical Toxicologists position statements on gastrointestinal decontamination: gastric lavage. *Clin Toxicol* 1997;24:711.
5. American Academy of Clinical Toxicology/European Association of Poisons Centres and Clinical Toxicologists position statements on gastrointestinal decontamination: single-dose activated charcoal. *Clin Toxicol* 1997;24:721.
6. American Academy of Clinical Toxicology/European Association of Poisons Centres and Clinical Toxicologists position statements on gastrointestinal decontamination: cathartics. *Clin Toxicol* 1997;24:743.
7. American Academy of Clinical Toxicology/European Association of Poisons Centres and Clinical Toxicologists position statements on gastrointestinal decontamination: whole-bowel irrigation. *Clin Toxicol* 1997;24:753.
8. American Academy of Clinical Toxicology/European Association of Poisons Centres and Clinical Toxicologists position statements on gastrointestinal decontamination: multi-dose activated charcoal. *Clin Toxicol* 1997;24:731.
9. Brett AS. Implication of discordance between clinical impression and toxicology analysis in drug overdose. *Arch Intern Med* 1988;148:437.
10. Brett AS, Rothschild N, Gray R, et al. Predicting the clinical course of intentional drug overdose: implications for utilization of the intensive care unit. *Arch Intern Med* 1987;147:133.
11. Garrettson LK, Geller RJ. Acid and alkaline diuresis: when are they of value in the treatment of poisoning? *Drug Saf* 1990;5:220.
12. Goldberg MJ, Spector R, Park GD, et al. An approach to the management of the poisoned patient. *Arch Intern Med* 1986;146:1381.
13. Hepler BR, Sutheimer CA, Sunshine I. Role of the toxicology laboratory in the treatment of acute poisoning. *Med Toxicol* 1986;1:61.
14. Kulling P, Persson H. Role of the intensive care unit in the management of the poisoned patient. *Med Toxicol* 1986;1:375.
15. Olson KR, Pentel PR, Kelley MT. Physical assessment and differential diagnosis of the poisoned patient. *Med Toxicol* 1987;2:52.
16. Perrone J, Hoffman RS, Goldfrank LR. Special considerations in gastrointestinal decontamination. *Emerg Med Clin North Am* 1994;12:285.
17. Pond SM. Diuresis, dialysis and hemoperfusion: indications and benefits. *Emerg Med Clin North Am* 1984;2:29.
18. Spyker DA, Minocha A. Toxicodynamic approach to the management of the poisoned patient. *J Emerg Med* 1988;6:117.
19. Sue YJ, Shannon M. Pharmacokinetics of drugs in overdose. *Clin Pharmacokinet* 1992;23:93.
20. Wright N. Common errors in the management of poisoning. *J Royal Coll Phys* 1980;14:114.

CHAPTER 310
Acetaminophen Poisoning

Jeffrey Brent

Acetaminophen (*N*-acetyl-*p*-aminophenol, or APAP) is one of the most common over-the-counter medications used in the United States. Given its widespread use and availability, it is an extremely common overdose. Because many laypeople underestimate its toxicity, suicide gestures may result in actual suicides. In 1998, over 100,000 potential APAP poisonings were reported in the American Association of Poison Control Centers' annual report. These are undoubtedly only a fraction of the total number of cases.

Acetaminophen itself is a nontoxic molecule. It is almost entirely metabolized in the liver by the pathways shown in Fig. 310.1. About 94% of an ingested dose of APAP is metabolized to glucuronide (42%) or sulfate (52%) conjugates and excreted as such in the urine.[7] Of the remaining APAP, about half is excreted unchanged in the urine and a similar amount is metabolized by the hepatic P-450 mixed-function oxidase (MFO) system to form a highly reactive intermediate.[7] With therapeutic doses, this intermediate is conjugated to glutathione and excreted as the inactive mercapturate conjugate plus other minor metabolites.[7,17] Toxicity occurs when stores of glutathione are depleted by about 70%, thus rendering the cell vulnerable to the effects of the MFO product.[7,10] Histologically, necrosis occurs at centrilobular (or perivenular) portions of the hepatic lobule.[5]

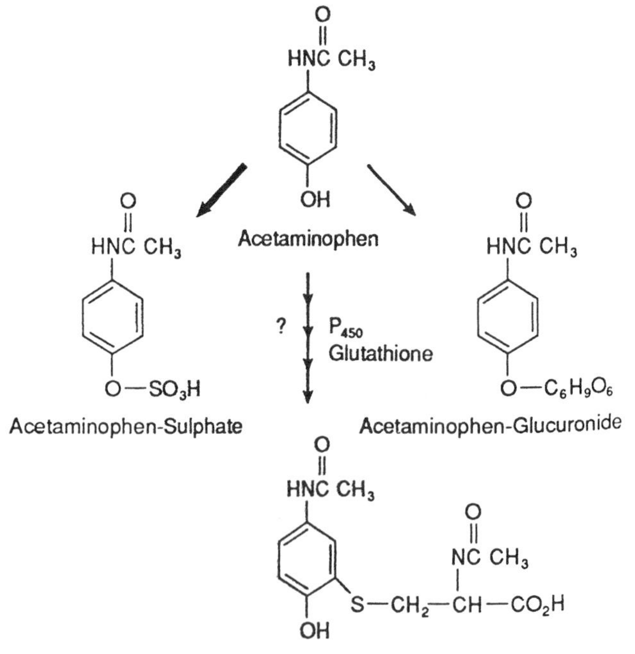

Figure 310.1. Proposed metabolic pathways for acetaminophen metabolism in children. (From Peterson RG, Rumack BH. Hgc as a variable in acetaminophen overdose. *Arch Intern Med* 1981;141:391, with permission.)

Although the clinical picture of APAP overdose is predominantly one of hepatotoxicity, some patients also have nephrotoxicity.[20] This is probably most commonly due to renal APAP metabolism by kidney MFOs. In addition, renal failure is an occasional concomitant complication of severe APAP-induced hepatotoxicity due to the hepatorenal syndrome.

The first stage of APAP poisoning is a relatively subtle period in which APAP is being absorbed and metabolized, glutathione stores are being consumed, and hepatotoxicity is beginning. This phase typically lasts less than 24 hours. Interventions to blunt the evolving hepatotoxicity are most effective during this early phase.

The second phase is entirely different. During this period, which usually begins late on the day of the ingestion, there is little APAP in the plasma. The hepatotoxic effects of MFO metabolites that have not been inactivated by glutathione become manifest during this time. The predominant clinical picture becomes one of hepatotoxicity.

There is a clear relation between the plasma level of APAP and the potential for toxicity, as demonstrated by the nomogram developed by Rumack and Matthew (Fig. 310.2).[14] The nomogram stratifies patients into risk categories of "probable" or "possible" hepatotoxicity. The validity of this nomogram was confirmed in a national multicenter study.[18] The "possible risk" category actually is a region in which toxicity would not be expected to occur, but it represents a 25% margin of error to account for possible errors in establishing the time of ingestion. The value of treating low-risk patients in the "possible toxicity" region of the nomogram has been questioned.[1] The nomogram begins at 4 hours after ingestion. Plasma APAP levels obtained before this time—during the absorption and distribution phases—are difficult to interpret. However, early APAP levels of less than 100 μg/mL predict a lack of risk for toxicity.[3]

The APAP nomogram is based on presenting levels. Repeat levels offer no further useful information and should not be routinely obtained. Based on the known volume of distribution of APAP of 0.9 to 1.0 L/kg, an ingestion of 10.5 g APAP in a 70-kg adult, or 150 mg/kg in a child, may cause toxic levels. The current nomogram is derived from adults. Although children with toxic plasma levels appear to be less susceptible to APAP toxicity than are adults,[13] the same nomogram should be used.

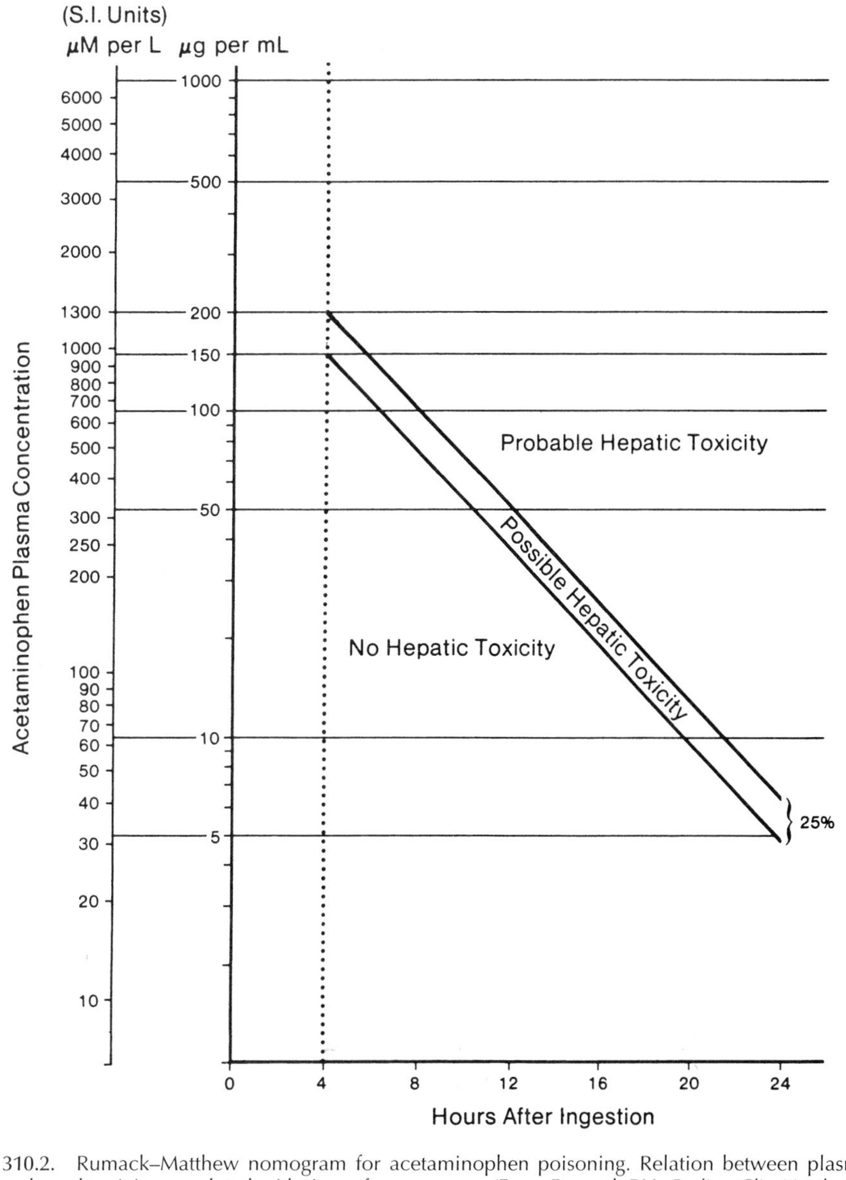

Figure 310.2. Rumack–Matthew nomogram for acetaminophen poisoning. Relation between plasma APAP levels and toxicity correlated with time after exposure. (From Rumack BH. *Pediatr Clin North Am* 1986;33:691, with permission.)

Patients who have ingested a potentially toxic amount of APAP and have a history of alcoholism, chronic liver disease, or malnutrition may be more susceptible to APAP hepatotoxicity because of decreased glutathione stores. Conversely, patients with liver disease, and, consequently, poorly functioning MFOs, may be relatively protected because of inability to generate the toxic metabolite. These patients should also be evaluated using the standard nomogram. Alcoholics without liver disease, who have both induced MFO systems (which generate the toxic metabolite) and depressed hepatic glutathione stores, and patients with acute illnesses associated with poor oral food intake (i.e., acute starvation) appear to be more susceptible to the hepatotoxic effects of APAP. However, given the large therapeutic index for APAP, this population would not be expected to be at enhanced risk when normal therapeutic doses are used.

CLINICAL PRESENTATION

The evolution of APAP toxicity can be divided into four sequential stages (Table 310.1). In the first 24 hours, patients may experience only nausea, vomiting, and malaise. Patients who present in stage II or III may have right upper quadrant pain, nausea, vomiting, jaundice, bleeding, encephalopathy, and symptoms of fulminant hepatic failure. Associated with this is a progressive increase in bilirubin, alanine aminotransferase (ALT), and aspartate aminotransferase (AST) levels, and prothrombin time. These liver function abnormalities can be dramatic in their magnitude, with ALT and AST levels of 10,000 to 20,000 not uncommon. In most cases, these abnormalities peak in 48 to 96 hours (stage III) and gradually resolve. Liver function test results usually return to normal within days after they peak (stage IV).

The occasional patient with severe, untreated APAP toxicity exhibits a pattern of rising prothrombin time and bilirubin and ammonia levels as the AST and ALT decline. This pattern signifies severe hepatic failure. However, most patients, even those with severe hepatotoxicity, eventually recover, with normal livers.

DIFFERENTIAL DIAGNOSIS

In the earliest stage of APAP poisoning, the diagnosis is made by a history suggestive of overdose. No consistently reliable or pathognomonic signs or symptoms can be expected. Hence, the physician must consider the possibility of occult APAP poisoning when confronted with any overdose patient. The finding of any APAP in the plasma must alert the clinician to the possibility of a toxic APAP ingestion.

The patient who presents in stage II, III, or IV of APAP toxicity is another kind of diagnostic challenge. By this time, there may be little detectable APAP in the serum, so the diagnosis depends on the history and clinical suspicion.

The differential diagnosis of hepatic injury includes, most commonly, viral or chemical etiologies. Virtually any drug can cause hepatotoxicity as an idiosyncratic reaction. The correct diagnosis requires an astute history supplemented by laboratory studies. One particularly difficult diagnostic quandary is distinguishing between Reye syndrome and APAP toxicity in the child given acetaminophen for an antecedent viral syndrome. The chemistry profiles typically seen with the different types of hepatitis are shown in Table 310.2. As shown in Fig. 310.3, liver function test results may not rise dramatically until a day after the ingestion.

EMERGENCY DEPARTMENT EVALUATION

In all overdose patients, excessive APAP ingestion should be ruled out by a nontoxic APAP level. For patients who have detectable plasma APAP levels, the time of ingestion must be determined as accurately as possible. If this cannot be done, the possibility of a toxic ingestion at an unknown time must be considered. Therefore, if there is detectable APAP and an unknown time of ingestion, or if the patient has abnormal liver function tests, possibly resulting from an APAP overdose, *N*-acetylcysteine (NAC) therapy should be instituted (Table 310.3). If the patient needs treatment, baseline liver function tests (AST, ALT, and total bilirubin levels and prothrombin time) and renal func-

TABLE 310.1. Stages in the Clinical Course of Acetaminophen Toxicity

Stage	Time after Ingestion	Characteristics
I	1/2–24 h	Anorexia, nausea, vomiting, malaise, pallor, diaphoresis
II	24–48 h	Resolution of above; right upper quadrant abdominal pain and tenderness; elevated bilirubin, prothrombin time, hepatic enzymes; oliguria
III	72–96 h	Peak liver function abnormalities; anorexia, nausea, vomiting, malaise may reappear
IV	4 d–2 wk	Resolution of hepatic dysfunction or fulminant hepatic failure

Modified from Linden CH, Rumack BH. Acetaminophen Overdose *Emerg Med Clin North Am* 1984;2:103.

TABLE 310.2. Laboratory Values in the Common Acute Hepatitides: Viral, Alcoholic, Acetaminophen

Hepatotoxin	Acute Viral Studies	AST (IU/L)	ALT (IU/L)
Viral	Usually positive	Hundreds to low thousands	Variable but less than AST
Alcohol	Negative	Usually <300 or 10 × normal	Usually 100 and ALT/AST >2
APAP	Negative	May be very high	Much less than AST

AST, aspartate aminotransferase; ALT, alanine aminotransferase.

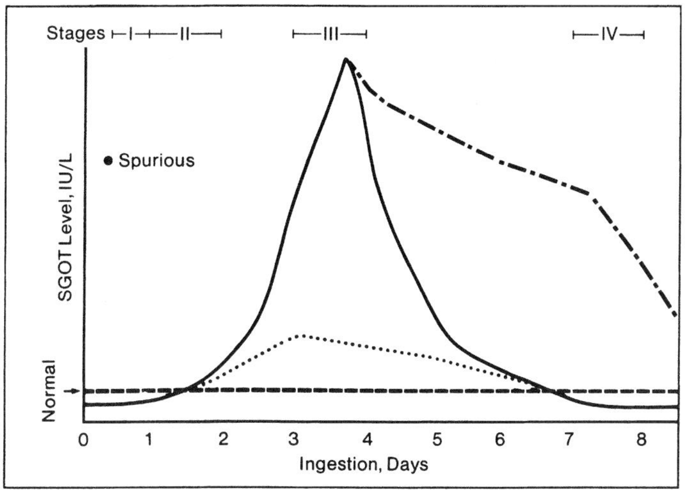

Figure 310.3. *Dotted line:* the course of those who received acetylcysteine. *Solid line:* those with natural a course. *Dotted–dashed line:* those with a severe course. (From Rumack BH, et al. Acetaminophen overdose. *Arch Intern Med* 1981;141:380, with permission.)

tion tests (blood urea nitrogen and creatinine levels and urinalysis) should be obtained.

EMERGENCY DEPARTMENT MANAGEMENT

After advanced life-support measures are performed, if necessary (e.g., for coingested agents), treatment of the patient with an acute APAP overdose includes stopping absorption and administering NAC when indicated.

Patients who have overdosed on APAP should receive activated charcoal if they present within 4 hours of ingestion. Because charcoal therapy does not have a clinically significant effect on NAC levels, it is unnecessary to increase the NAC dose when the patient is receiving both of these therapies.[2] However, charcoal and NAC should not be mixed together before administration. The routine use of gastric emptying, by syrup of ipecac or lavage, appears to have little role and should be avoided.

If an APAP level is unavailable by 8 hours after ingestion, a history (or suspicion of APAP overdose) is sufficient to warrant the initiation of NAC therapy until the plasma APAP levels are known.

The most efficacious treatment for APAP overdose is the administration of NAC.[12,15,18,19] NAC is metabolized by hepatocytes to cysteine, a precursor of glutathione. NAC also enhances APAP sulfation, potentially leaving less APAP available to the MFO system (see Fig. 310.1). NAC therapy is almost 100% effective in preventing APAP toxicity if it is started within 8 hours of the ingestion, independent of the plasma APAP level.[18] Delay in starting therapy beyond this time results in a progressive diminution of the effectiveness.[15,18]

Three protocols are in use for the treatment of APAP overdose (see Table 310.3). The only one approved by the Food and Drug Administration (FDA) is the 72-hour oral protocol. Preliminary evidence shows that the 48-hour intravenous protocol is at least as efficacious, and it is hoped that FDA approval for this will be forthcoming.[19]

The use of intravenous NAC has other advantages. Giving oral NAC can be challenging. Because it tastes and smells like rotten eggs, it is poorly tolerated. Emesis after NAC ingestion is common; if it occurs within an hour of the dose, the dose should be repeated in full. NAC is available as the mucolytic agent Mucomyst in a 10% or 20% solution. Before administration, it should be diluted to 5% in a soft drink to increase its palatability. It is also helpful to have the patient drink it through a straw from a closed container to prevent the unpleasant vapors from causing emesis. If emesis occurs during NAC administration, droperidol (Inapsine; 1.25 to 2.5 mg [0.5 to 1.0 mL] in adults, 0.1 to 0.15 mg/kg [0.04 to 0.06 mL] in children), metoclopramide (Reglan; 0.1 to 1.0 mg/kg), or ondansetron (Zofran, 0.15 mg/kg intravenously) may be given and repeated as necessary. There are no known adverse effects of giving these agents in association with an APAP overdose. If these measures fail, NAC may be given as a drip through a nasogastric tube over about 1 hour for each dose. Standard Mucomyst preparations are not approved for intravenous use. However, the practice of giving the

TABLE 310.3. Protocols for *N*-Acetylcysteine Administration

	Length	Administration	Loading Dose	Subsequent Doses	FDA Approval	Reference
I	72 h	Oral	140 mg/kg	70 mg/kg q4h for 17 doses	Yes	15
II	20 h	IV	150 mg/kg over 15 min	50 mg/kg over 4h, followed by 100 mg/kg over 16 h	No	12
III	48 h	IV	140 mg/kg	70 mg/kg q4h	No	19

oral preparation intravenously through an in-line filter is widespread and generally considered to be acceptable practice by most medical toxicologists and poison control centers.[4,11]

APAP crosses the placenta, so when a pregnant patient overdoses on APAP, fetal hepatotoxicity is possible. NAC may not cross the placenta.[6] The advantage, if any, of immediate delivery of a preterm infant, so that NAC therapy can be given, is questionable.[9] If spontaneous delivery occurs while the mother is receiving NAC, a full course of NAC should be given to the newborn.

A particularly perplexing group of patients are those who have taken a potentially toxic cumulative amount of APAP but have done so by ingesting multiple nontoxic doses over a period of time.[16] One approach would be to treat for potential APAP toxicity any patient who has ingested more than 10.5 g or 150 mg/kg during the preceding 24 hours. However, this strategy would result in many patients being treated who would not require this therapy. All patients with a toxic plasma level according to the nomogram, based on the time since the last dose of APAP, should be treated with NAC.

The management of patients with APAP-induced hepatic or renal failure consists of NAC and supportive care.[8] Patients who appear to have fulminant hepatic failure are candidates for transplantation. However, transplantation should not be done simply on the basis of an elevated transaminase level, because this does not portend a poor prognosis. Transplant teams should be considered necessary for patients with prothrombin times greater than 100 seconds, renal failure, and coma. Persistent metabolic acidosis should also be considered grounds for transplantations.

DISPOSITION

Any patient who is potentially APAP toxic by the nomogram requires admission and treatment. All intentional overdose patients should have a psychiatric evaluation before discharge. Patients who present more than 24 hours after ingestion, with abnormal liver function test results, should receive NAC therapy until the hepatotoxicity resolves.[8]

COMMON PITFALLS

- Failure to consider an occult APAP overdose in all patients with intentional overdose or unexplained hepatitis
- Withholding activated charcoal because of concern about its effect on NAC therapy
- Delaying NAC treatment beyond 8 to 10 hours while waiting for APAP levels

References

1. Brandwene E, Williams SR, Tunget-Johnson C, et al. Refining the level of anticipated hepatotoxicity in acetaminophen poisoning. *J Emerg Med* 1996;14:691–695.
2. Brent J. Are activated charcoal/N-acetylcysteine interactions of clinical significance? *Ann Emerg Med* 1993;22:1860.
3. Douglas DR, Smilkstein MJ, Rumack BH. APAP levels within 4 hours: are they useful? *Vet Hum Toxicol* 1994;36:350.
4. Falk JL. Oral N-acetylcysteine given intravenously for acetaminophen overdose: we shouldn't have to, but we must. *Crit Care Med* 1998;26:7.
5. James O, Roberts SH, Douglas AP, et al. Liver damage after paracetamol overdose: comparison of liver function tests, testing serum bile acids, and liver histology. *Lancet* 1975;2:579.
6. Johnson D, Simone C, Koren G. Transfer of N-acetylcysteine by the human placenta. *Vet Hum Toxicol* 1993;35:365.
7. Jollow DG, Thorgelrsson SS, Potter WZ, et al. Acetaminophen-induced hepatic necrosis. IV. Metabolic disposition of toxic and nontoxic doses of acetaminophen. *Pharmacology* 1974;12:251.
8. Keays R, Harrison PM, Wendon JA, et al. Intravenous acetylcysteine in paracetamol-induced fulminant hepatic failure: a prospective controlled trial. *BMJ* 1991;303:1026.
9. McElhatton PR, Sullivan FM, Volans GN, et al. Paracetamol poisoning in pregnancy: an analysis of the outcomes of cases referred to the Teratology Information Service of the National Poisons Information Service. *Hum Exp Toxicol* 1990;9:147–153.
10. Mitchell JR, Jollow DJ, Potter WZ, et al. Acetaminophen-induced hepatic necrosis. I. Role of drug metabolism. *J Pharmacol Exp Ther* 1973;187:185.
11. Perry HE, Shannon MW. Efficacy of oral versus intravenous N-acetylcysteine in acetaminophen overdose: results of an open-label, clinical trial. *J Pediatr* 1998;132:149–152.
12. Prescott LF, Illingworth RN, Critchley JAJH, et al. Intravenous N-acetylcysteine: the treatment of choice for paracetamol poisoning. *BMJ* 1979;2:1097.
13. Rumack BH. Acetaminophen overdose in young children; treatment and effects of alcohol and other additional ingestants in 417 cases. *Am J Dis Child* 1984;138:428.
14. Rumack BH, Matthew H. Acetaminophen poisoning and toxicity. *Pediatrics* 1975;55:871.
15. Rumack BH, Peterson RG, Koch GC, et al. Acetaminophen overdose: 662 cases with evaluation of oral acetylcysteine treatment. *Arch Intern Med* 1981;141:380.
16. Schiodt FV, Rochling FA, Casey DL, et al. Acetaminophen toxicity in an urban county hospital. *N Engl J Med* 1997;337:1112–1127.
17. Slattery JT, Knapp JR, Levy G. Acetaminophen pharmacokinetics after overdose. *J Toxicol Clin Toxicol* 1981;18:111.
18. Smilkstein MJ, Knapp GL, Kulig KW, et al. Efficacy of oral N-acetylcysteine in the treatment of acetaminophen overdose. Analysis of the national multicenter study (1976–1985). *N Engl J Med* 1988;319:1557.
19. Smilkstein MJ, Bronstein AC, Linden C, et al. Acetaminophen overdose: a 48-hour intravenous N-acetylcysteine treatment protocol. *Ann Emerg Med* 1991;20:1058.
20. Wilkinson SP, Moodle H, Arrogo VA, et al. Frequency of renal impairment in paracetamol overdose compared with other causes of acute liver damage. *J Clin Pathol* 1977;30:141.

CHAPTER 311
Anticholinergic Poisoning

Jeffrey Brent and Kenneth W. Kulig

The toxic effects that result from inhibition of normal cholinergic transmission are collectively known as the anticholinergic syndrome (ACS). The manifestations of this syndrome can be divided into those secondary to central or to peripheral nervous system effects. Some of the many toxins capable of causing the ACS are listed in Table 311.1.

The peripheral sites of cholinergic transmission are shown in Fig. 311.1. The major effects associated with the inhibition of cholinergic transmission are given in Table 311.2. Only at high doses do these drugs have any nicotinic blocking effects, such as sympathetic ganglionic blockage, resulting in cutaneous vasodilatation ("atropine flush"). Even at extremely high doses, the neuromuscular junction is relatively spared. Quaternary ammonium anticholinergic compounds, such as glycopyrrolate, have more pronounced antinicotinic effects but, being charged, are poorly absorbed and therefore ineffective when taken orally.[3]

Acetylcholine is a ubiquitous neurotransmitter in the central nervous system (CNS), and the central effects can be a significant or, occasionally, a predominant feature of the ACS.[6,17] Because of the altered sensorium produced, these agents are occasionally deliberately abused.[5,11] In the past, the antiparkinsonian agent trihexyphenidyl (Artane) had been among the most popular, probably because of its euphoric properties. The practice of ingestion of jimson weed (usually the seeds or flowers but sometimes a tea brewed from other plant parts), a widely available and free-for-the-picking intoxicant, is common, particularly among teenagers.[6,12]

TABLE 311.1. Agents That Cause Anticholinergic Syndrome

MEDICATIONS	
Aerosolized bronchodilators	Mydriatic eye drops
Antihistamines	Neuroleptics
Antiparkinsonian agents	Orphenadrine
Belladonna alkaloids	OTC cough and cold remedies
Cyclobenzaprine	OTC sleep aids
Drugs for motion sickness	Tricyclic antidepressants
Glutethimide	
PLANTS	
Angel's trumpet (*Datura sawolens*)	Jimson weed (*Datura stramonium*)[a]
Black henbane (*Hyoacyamus niger*)	Jerusalem cherry (*Solanum pseudocapsicum*)
Black nightshade (*Atropa belladonna*)	Matrimony vine (*Lycium halimifolium*)
Blue Bonnet (*Lupine* species)	Night-blooming jasmine (*Cestrum nocturnum*)
Bittersweet (*Solanum dulcamara*)	Nutmeg (*Myristica fragrans*)
Deadly nightshade (*Atropa belladonna*)	Potato (*Solanum tuberosum*)
Ground cherry (*Physalia heterophylla*)	Wild sage (*Lantana camara*)
	Wild tomato (*Solanum carolinensis*)

[a] Also known as Jamestown weed, stinkweed, thorn apple, and devil's apple.
OTC, over-the-counter.

TABLE 311.2. Anticholinergic Effects

Site of Blockade	Effects
Peripheral muscarinic synapses	Tachycardia
	Dilated pupils
	Loss of accommodation
	Dry skin and mucous membranes
	Flushed skin
	Decreased bowel motility
	Urinary retention
	Fever
Central nervous system	Delirium
	Seizures
	Coma
	Agitation
	Psychotic behavior
	Extrapyramidal signs
	Respiratory depression
	Cardiovascular collapse

CLINICAL PRESENTATION

The patient with the ACS may present with peripheral or central manifestations, or both. Usually the former predominates, with some component of the latter. Commonly seen as a result of cholinergic receptor blockade are mydriasis, tachycardia, dry skin and mucous membranes, fever, and altered mentation.[1,8] These features provide the basis for the mnemonic "hot as a hare, mad as a hatter, red as a beet, dry as a bone." Although this describes many of the features of the ACS, it ignores tachycardia, one of the most consistent and reliable clinical findings.[9] However, in infants, the elderly, alcoholics with autonomic neuropathy, and patients taking beta blockers or calcium channel blockers, tachycardia may be absent. Hence, the absence of tachycardia does not rule out the ACS.

Cardiac conduction delays are occasionally reported following very large overdoses.[10,15,18] It is unknown whether these are consistent features of massive anticholinergic poisonings or relate to other actions of the agents ingested. The presence of significant cardiac conduction abnormalities in the setting of anticholinergic poisoning should always prompt an evaluation for alternative causes of these effects.

Central effects vary with the ability of an agent to penetrate the CNS. Central manifestations have been colorfully described in patients who were found confused and inappropriately and scantily dressed after ingesting alcoholic beverages adulterated with scopolamine eye drops.[8]

Patients with a severe ACS can present with such extreme findings as seizures, hypotension, rhabdomyolysis, and respiratory or cardiac arrest.[20] It is unclear whether these complications are direct anticholinergic effects, are the end result of severe physiologic stimulation, or are due to other pharmacologic properties of the agents involved. Most patients have a self-limited course, the extent and duration of which are determined by the amount and nature of the agent.

Although tricyclic antidepressants can predominantly cause the ACS when taken in small overdoses, the clinical presentation of large overdoses of these agents is usually dominated by hypotension, seizures, and dysrhythmias resulting from non-anticholinergic effects.

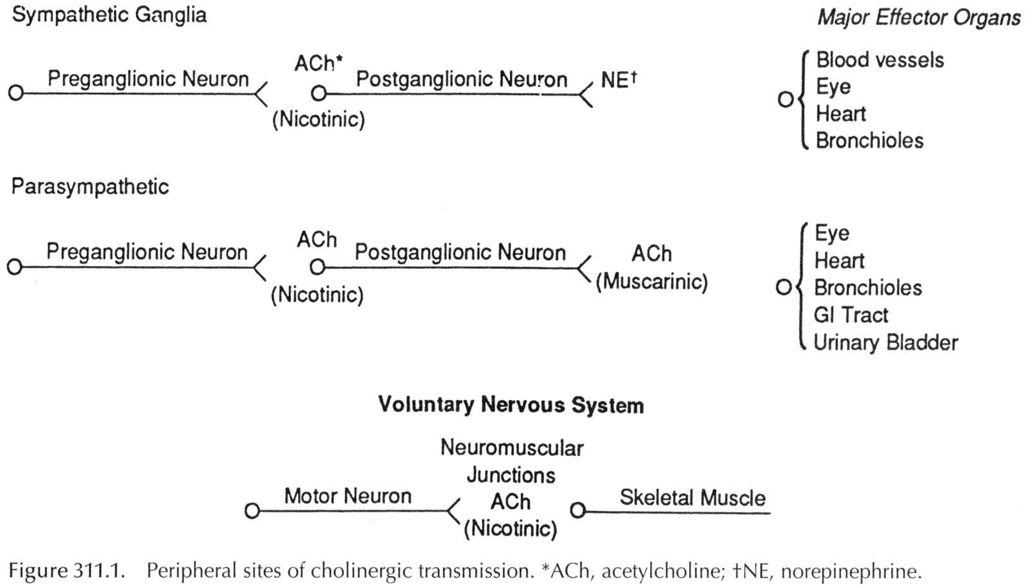

Figure 311.1. Peripheral sites of cholinergic transmission. *ACh, acetylcholine; †NE, norepinephrine.

DIFFERENTIAL DIAGNOSIS

The ACS should be included in the differential diagnosis of any patient who presents with altered mental status, fever, urinary retention, tachycardia, or seizures. The history and physical examination are often crucial in ascribing a patient's symptoms to the ACS. The history should focus not only on prescribed medications, but also on over-the-counter agents, plant or mushroom ingestions, anticholinergic eye drops, antihistamine-containing skin lotions, or circumstances in which illegitimate use of these agents may be a possibility. However, the history alone can often be misleading, and it may be left to the astute clinician to diagnose an ACS without a supporting history. For example, there have been well-documented instances of street heroin being cut with significant amounts of the anticholinergic alkaloid scopolamine. Patients using this heroin presented to emergency departments with a history of only heroin use but a clinical picture of an ACS, causing considerable initial confusion.[2] It is also important to remember that seemingly minor, and therefore historically ignored, exposure to anticholinergic agents, such as to over-the-counter medications, drops to treat infantile colic,[13] or even anticholinergic eye drops used as mydriatics for funduscopic examinations,[4] can cause life-threatening anticholinergic toxicity. The physical examination should look for features of anticholinergic poisoning, namely delirium and hallucinations, tachycardia, mydriasis, dry skin, decreased bowel sounds, and a distended bladder.

Although several *Amanita* mushrooms (*A. muscaria, A. pantherina, A. gemmata*) have been implicated in causing an ACS, the toxidrome they usually induce is clinically and physiologically distinct (see Chapter 355). Because mydriasis and altered mentation occur during this toxidrome, it is often mistaken for an ACS. This toxidrome should, however, be included in the differential diagnosis.

Often, the clinical characteristics of an intoxication are a combination of anticholinergic features and other manifestations of the additional pharmacology of the ingested agent. For example, phenothiazines can cause an ACS complicated by the sedating and alpha-adrenergic blocking properties (e.g., coma, hypotension) of these drugs.

Given the clinical features of the ACS, it may easily be misdiagnosed as a CNS infection, dehydration, psychiatric disorder, or sepsis.

EMERGENCY DEPARTMENT EVALUATION

A detailed history and complete physical examination are essential. The physical examination should specifically search for the features of an ACS. Flushing of the skin may also be present as a result of excessive ingestion of anticholinergic agents, but this occurs infrequently. Cardiac monitoring and a 12-lead electrocardiogram (ECG) should be obtained on all patients, particularly in the presence of tachycardia. If seizures or altered mentation are present, particularly with fever, a full neurologic evaluation, including a computed tomography (CT) study of the head and a lumbar puncture, is required if it cannot be proven that these effects are secondary to anticholinergic poisoning. Physostigmine (discussion follows) can be helpful in quickly distinguishing between an ACS and a CNS infection.

If there is any question of the diagnosis, a toxicology screen for common anticholinergic agents should be obtained. If a particular drug is suspected of causing the syndrome, this should be communicated to the laboratory personnel. However, because many of the medications and all of the plants that cause the ACS are not detected by many toxicology screens, the diagnosis is made predominantly by the history and physical examination.

If an ACS is suspected to be due to misuse of drugs, through either intent or misunderstanding, the possibility of an occult simultaneous acetaminophen overdose should be ruled out by a quantitative acetaminophen level. If the patient has ingested a plant, it may be helpful to have the ingestant identified by a botanist. Medical toxicologists and regional poison control centers are usually aware of local resources available for help in this regard.

EMERGENCY DEPARTMENT MANAGEMENT

After any necessary advanced life-support measures have been performed and a preliminary history and physical examination have been completed, attention should be directed to preventing further drug absorption. Activated charcoal is the preferred method of gastrointestinal decontamination and should be administered to patients with recent ingestions. Eye drop exposure is treated by irrigation of the conjunctival recesses.

Most patients with an ACS can be treated supportively. The specific antidote for the ACS is physostigmine salicylate (Antilirium), a reversible inhibitor of acetylcholinesterase derived from the West African vine *Physostigma venenosum*. Because of physostigmine's ability to penetrate the CNS, it can reverse both central and peripheral anticholinergic effects.[16] However, the cholinergic effects of physostigmine can be profound. Although such effects are rare, physostigmine may induce seizures, heart block, bradyarrhythmias, and asystole.[14,19] Most of these adverse effects occur with patients who have ingested tricyclic antidepressants.[7,14,19] Because of these effects, physostigmine should be reserved for extreme extrapyramidal movement disorders, recurrent or refractory seizures, severe agitation or hallucinations (causing patients to be dangerous to themselves or others and unresponsive to sedating medications), or ventricular or hemodynamically significant supraventricular tachyarrhythmias unresponsive to standard management, or if the diagnosis is in doubt. Both central and peripheral ACS manifestations should also be present to ensure a correct diagnosis. Because of its significant cholinergic effects, physostigmine is considered to be contraindicated in patients with bowel obstruction, significant cardiac or peripheral vascular disease, asthma, chronic obstructive pulmonary disease, cardiac conduction abnormalities on the ECG, or urinary tract obstruction. It is also contraindicated when excessive doses of tricyclic antidepressants have been ingested The latter can be ruled out by an ECG. In the absence of a large R wave in lead AVR, it is very unlikely that the patient is experiencing any significant toxic effects of a cyclic antidepressant.

Due to its potential adverse effects, physostigmine should be given with cardiac monitoring, resuscitation equipment at the bedside, and in the presence of a physician. The cholinergic effect of physostigmine is expected to cause a reduction in heart rate. Because most patients with an ACS have sinus tachycardia, the syndrome itself provides an extra margin of safety for the use of physostigmine. This agent should be used with great caution, if at all, in patients without tachycardia. The adult dose of physostigmine is 1 to 2 mg intravenously, repeated every 5 to 20 minutes until the life-threatening features of the ACS resolve. Although no pediatric dose has been formally established, children have been treated with 0.02 mg/kg intravenously (up to 1 to 2 mg per dose), repeated as needed.[16] Physostigmine has unpredictable intramuscular absorption patterns, and thus should not be given by that route. Doses of physostigmine should be given over no less than 2 minutes; however, because of its short half-life, it is ineffective if given over a period longer than a few minutes. Because it is a cholinergic agent, the treatment of physostigmine-induced complications is atropine. The dose of atropine is half of the amount of physostigmine administered.[16]

Atropine has a longer duration of action than physostigmine and must be used very cautiously in this setting. If standard doses of physostigmine are given and contraindications heeded, it is unlikely that significant complications will arise. Because the pharmacologic effects of physostigmine last from 30 minutes to 2 hours, it may be necessary to repeat treatment if life-threatening manifestations of an ACS reappear. In true anticholinergic poisoning, dramatic resolution of the syndrome is expected to occur within minutes of physostigmine administration. Thus, a lack of definitive response to physostigmine should cause the diagnosis of ACS to be questioned.

Benzodiazepines may be useful in patients with mixed signs and symptoms of the central ACS. Neuroleptic agents such as phenothiazines or butyrophenones should be avoided in the ACS because of their associated anticholinergic effects.

DISPOSITION

Any patient with a significant ACS should be observed until the clinical signs, including tachycardia, resolve and the patient has normal mentation. Often, this requires admission to a monitored unit.

In accidental poisoning, the physician must review the genesis of the ACS with patients or their caretakers so that a repetition can be avoided. Any patient who has deliberately overdosed on an anticholinergic substance needs emergency psychiatric evaluation or referral for substance-abuse treatment after their mentation has normalized.

Patients who have had a seizure caused solely by the ACS do not require chronic anticonvulsant medications.

If the physician is unfamiliar with the evaluation, management, or disposition of patients with the ACS, a medical toxicologist should be consulted.

COMMON PITFALLS

- Failure to consider the diagnosis of the ACS in patients with unexplained confusion, hallucinations, tachycardia, urinary retention, fever, or seizures
- Using physostigmine to treat minor manifestations of the ACS
- Failure to get an ECG and check for contraindications before giving physostigmine
- Using physostigmine without adequate monitoring and resuscitation capability
- Using neuroleptics to treat behavioral effects (agitation and hallucinations) of the ACS

References

1. Amitai Y, Almog S, Singer R, et al. Atropine poisoning in children during the Persian Gulf crisis. *JAMA* 1992;268:630.
2. Anonymous. Scopolamine poisoning among heroin users. *JAMA* 1996; 274: 92–93.
3. Brown JH. Atropine, scopolamine, and related antimuscarinic drugs. In: Gilman AG, Rall TW, Nies AS, et al., eds. *Goodman and Gilman's the pharmacologic basics of therapeutics,* 8th ed. New York: Pergamon Press, 1990.
4. Brunner GA, Fleck S, Pieber TR, et al. Near fatal anticholinergic intoxication after routine fundoscopy. *Intensive Care Med* 1998;24:730–731.
5. Dilsaver SC. Antimuscarinic agents as substances of abuse: a review. *J Clin Psychopharmacol* 1988;8:14.
6. Faquet RA, Rowland KF. "Spice cabinet" intoxication. *Am J Psychiatry* 1978;135:680.
7. Goldberger AL, Curtis GP. Immediate effects of physostigmine on amitriptyline-induced QRS prolongation. *Clin Toxicol* 1982;19:445.
8. Goldfrank L, Flomenbaum N, Lewin N, et al. Anticholinergic poisoning. *J Toxicol Clin Toxicol* 1982;19:17.
9. Greenblatt DJ, Shader RF. Anticholinergics. *N Engl J Med* 1973;288:1215.
10. Hestand HE, Teske DW. Diphenhydramine hydrochloride intoxication. *J Pediatr* 1977;90:1017.
11. Hidalgo HA, Mowers RM. Anticholinergic drug abuse. *Ann Pharmacother* 1990;24:40.
12. Klein-Schwartz W, Oderda GM. Jimson weed intoxication in adolescents and young adults. *Am J Dis Child* 1984;138:737.
13. Myers JH, Moro-Sutherland D, Shook JE. Anticholinergic poisoning in colicky infants treated with hyoscyamine sulfate. *Am J Emerg Med* 1997;15:532–535.
14. Newton RW. Physostigmine salicylate in the treatment of tricyclic antidepressant overdosage. *JAMA* 1975;231:941.
15. Rinder CS, D'Amato SL, Rinder HM. Survival in complicated diphenhydramine overdose. *Crit Care Med* 1988;16:1161.
16. Rumack BK. Anticholinergic poisoning: treatment with physostigmine. *Pediatrics* 1973;52:449.
17. Snoey ER, Bessen HA. Acute psychosis after amantadine overdose. *Ann Emerg Med* 1990;19:668.
18. Tobin JR, Doyle TP, Ackerman AD, et al. Astemizole-induced cardiac conduction disturbances in a child. *JAMA* 1991;266:2737.
19. Walker WE, Levy RC, Henenson IB. Physostigmine—its use and abuse. *J Am Coll Emerg Physicians* 1976;5:335.
20. Winn RE, McDonnell KP. Fatality secondary to massive overdose of dimenhydrinate. *Ann Emerg Med* 1993;22:1481.

CHAPTER 312
Antidysrhythmic Drug Poisoning

S. Rutherfoord Rose and James E. Cisek

The antidysrhythmic agents discussed here are those used exclusively for the treatment of dysrhythmias, specifically those in Vaughn-Williams classes IA, IC, and III (Table 312.1). Those from other classes have additional uses and activities and are covered in separate chapters.

Class I agents decrease the influx of sodium through fast channels in myocardial cell membranes during depolarization (phase zero of the action potential), thereby slowing the rate of rise of the action potential (V_{max}) in myocardial cells. This action results in decreased conduction velocity and increased QRS duration. Class I drugs are divided into A, B, and C subclasses based on their respective rates of dissociation from fast sodium channels. Class IC agents dissociate slowly and therefore produce the greatest degree of QRS prolongation, even at therapeutic doses. They also prolong the JT interval. Class IB drugs quickly dissociate from binding sites and produce no QRS prolongation at therapeutic concentrations. Class IA drugs have intermediate dissociation constants and cause mild QRS prolongation with therapeutic dosing.

Class IA drugs also have variable alpha-adrenergic blocking effects, and disopyramide has relatively potent negative inotropic effects. Propafenone has relatively weak beta-adrenergic activity, which may be clinically important in patients on high doses or in approximately 7% of patients who poorly metabolize propafenone to an active metabolite, which has class IC-like properties.

Class III drugs prolong repolarization (i.e., the refractory period) in all cardiac tissue. In addition, amiodarone has vasodilating and weak beta-adrenergic blocking properties; however, intravenous administration results in pharmacologic effects consistent with all four Vaughn-Williams classes. Sotalol is a nonselective beta-adrenergic blocker that also prolongs the refractory period throughout the conduction system, including bypass tracts.

TABLE 312.1. Classification of Antidysrhythmic Drugs

Class	Actions	Classic Drugs	New Drugs
I	Sodium channel inhibition		
A	Increased APD Increased ERP Slowed conduction	Quinidine Disopyramide Procainamide	Cibenzoline Pirmenol
B	Little/no decrease in APD Increased ERP in diseased tissue May increase conduction velocity	Lidocaine Tocainide Phenytoin	Ethmozine Mexiletine
C	Variable effect on APD Small increase in ERP Markedly slowed conduction	Flecainide Encainide	Lorcainide Propafenone
II	Beta-adrenergic blockade	Atenolol Metoprolol Propranolol	Acebutolol Bisoprolol Sotolol
III	Prolonged repolarization	Amiodarone Bretylium Sotalol	*N*-acetylprocainamide
IV	Calcium channel inhibition	Diltiazem Nifedipine Verapamil	Bepridil Gallopamil

APD, action potential duration; ERP, effective refractory period

Class IA drugs are used to treat a wide variety of dysrhythmias of both ventricular and supraventricular origin, including reentry tachycardias and Wolff-Parkinson-White syndrome. The efficacy of these drugs in preventing reentry dysrhythmias is probably due to a change from unidirectional to bidirectional block resulting from slowed conduction. Class IC drugs have very narrow therapeutic windows and are primarily used for maintenance of sinus rhythm in patients with atrial fibrillation. The Cardiac Arrhythmia Suppression Trial study demonstrated increased mortality in patients given encainide or flecainide after myocardial infarction. Encainide was subsequently withdrawn from the U.S. market in 1991; however, it may be obtained directly from the manufacturer for patients with life-threatening dysrhythmias who have previously responded to the drug. Flecainide is typically reserved for treatment of refractory supraventricular tachycardias. The class III drugs (amiodarone, sotalol) are assuming more prominent roles as initial therapy for both ventricular and supraventricular rhythm disturbances.

Overdose with antidysrhythmic drugs is rare, compared with other cardiovascular drugs (e.g., beta blockers or calcium channel blockers). Most overdoses occur in adults and are accidental. Adverse effects are common and occur in 20% to 50% of patients on chronic therapy.

Pertinent pharmacokinetic parameters are summarized in Table 312.2. The salt forms of these drugs are well absorbed orally. Peak plasma levels following ingestion of immediate-release dosage forms usually occur within 1 to 3 hours, except with amiodarone (4 to 6 hours, but up to 10 hours) and with disopyramide (due to its anticholinergic effects). Elimination from the body follows first-order (rate proportional to concentration) kinetics. Metabolites of quinidine, encainide, propafenone, and amiodarone have varying degrees of pharmacologic activity and probably contribute to overall effects. These metabolites are not monitored clinically. The principal metabolite of procainamide, *N*-acetylprocainamide (NAPA), is approved under orphan drug status for patients with procainamide-induced lupus, and most closely resembles class III

TABLE 312.2. Summary of Pharmacokinetic Parameters

Parameter	Quinidine	Disopyramide	Procainamide	Flecainide	Propafenone	Amiodarone	Bretylium	Sotalol
Protein binding (%)	80	5–65[a]	15–20	40	97	>95	1–6	Low
Distribution volume (L/kg)	2.5–3.0	0.8	1.8–2.4	6–10	2–3	7–21	6–10	1.5
Half-life (h)	4–8	5–6	2–4	14–20	4–8	50–60 d	7–12	7–18
Route of elimination (%)								
Hepatic metabolism	60–85	15–25	30–40 (to NAPA)	50–90	>95	>95	0	0–25
Renal excretion (unchanged)	15–40	40–60	50–60	10–50	<1	<1	100	75–100
Usual maximum adult daily dose (mg)	1,800	800	50 mg/kg	400	900	400–1,600	30 mg/kg over 3 doses	320
Therapeutic serum level (μg/mL)	2–5	2–5	4–12 (15–25 for NAPA)	0.2–1.0	0.1–1.0	1.0–2.5	1–2	0.5–4.0

[a] Binding decreases with increasing levels.

drugs because of its ability to prolong repolarization. Amiodarone is unique in that it has a very prolonged elimination half-life (50 days), and serum levels may continue to rise for a month after starting therapy.

All antidysrhythmic agents have relatively narrow therapeutic ranges, and therefore low margins of safety between efficacy and toxicity. Therapeutic ranges are estimates based on population averages and do not apply to all patients; some patients, in fact, must suffer some mild yet annoying side effects to achieve a desired therapeutic effects. Serum drug levels of quinidine and procainamide or NAPA are easily measured by most hospital laboratories and are reasonably correlated with clinical and, to some extent, toxic effects. Serum levels of the other compounds are not routinely monitored but could be obtained to document toxicity.

The toxic effects of antidysrhythmics result from exaggerated therapeutic activity. Dose-dependent delays in conduction lead to varying degrees of atrioventricular block and, eventually, asystole. High drug levels also result in myocardial depression (classes IA, IC, and III) and peripheral vasodilatation (classes IA and III), which can result in profound hypotension. Central nervous system (CNS) effects appear to be independent of cardiac effects unless shock is present.

There are insufficient data to determine the minimum toxic doses for most antidysrhythmic drugs. For class IA drugs, toxicity may be expected after acute ingestions of 1 g or more. Ingestions of more than 2.5 to 3.0 g may result in serious toxicity. Survival has been reported following acute doses of up to 20 g and peak serum levels of 21.4 μg/mL (quinidine) and 77 μg/mL (procainamide).[7,9,19,20] However, death has been reported in adults following estimated doses as low as 3.6 to 6.8 g and serum levels of 8.3 μg/mL (disopyramide), illustrating the variability in doses, plasma drug levels, and degree of toxicity. A 2-year-old boy died 28 hours after ingesting 600 mg of disopyramide, and a 16-year-old girl required 75 minutes of cardiopulmonary resuscitation after a reported ingestion of 2 g of disopyramide.[1,10]

Class IC drugs appear to be more toxic than class IA drugs. Severe toxicity has been reported in a 6-month-old child who ingested a 25-mg encainide tablet.[16] A healthy 46-year-old man ingested 3.0 to 3.5 g of encainide and suffered seizures, hypotension, bradycardia, and coma.[18] Ingestion of 1.8 g of flecainide was fatal in an 18-year-old, and 1.5 g produced seizures and polymorphous ventricular tachycardia.[11] An acute overdose of 1.8 g (133 mg/kg) of propafenone in a 2-year-old child resulted in hypotension, seizures, and a prolonged QT interval.[15] Ingestion of 8.1 g of propafenone caused seizures, coma, hypotension, and prolonged QRS in an adult with a propafenone serum level of 3.2 μg/mL.[12] An overall mortality of 22.5% was reported in a retrospective review of propafenone, flecainide, ajmaline, and prajmaline toxicity.[13] About half of the patients became nauseated within 30 minutes of ingestion, and severe cardiac toxicity (atrioventricular block, bradycardia, pulseless electrical activity, asystole) occurred within 30 to 120 minutes after ingestion.

There is considerably less information about the acute toxicity of class III drugs. Amiodarone doses of 2.6 to 8.0 g have produced mild bradycardia, prolonged QT interval, and a brief episode of nonsustained ventricular tachycardia, all with a delayed onset of 12 to 48 hours.[5] An inadvertent bolus of 30 mg/kg of bretylium resulted in significant hypertension (310/90 mm Hg) and subsequent hypotension (90/40) in a 58-year-old man being treated for recurrent ventricular tachycardia–fibrillation after a cardiac arrest.[2] A syndrome resembling clinical brain death was reported in a neonate who received a 12-fold (dosing error) increase in bretylium infusion and had a serum bretylium level (not peak) of 17 μg/mL. Sotalol poisoning is discussed in Chapter 320.

Excessive dosing or impaired excretion of these compounds frequently leads to toxic levels during chronic therapy. Clinical toxicity at a relatively lower serum concentration may be expected during chronic therapy due to prior saturation of tissue stores and the likelihood of preexisting cardiac disease.

CLINICAL PRESENTATION

The onset of symptoms following acute overdose usually occurs within 4 hours, and often within 1 to 2 hours. However, drug absorption may continue for many hours following the ingestion of massive amounts, sustained-release preparations, or agents with anticholinergic effects. Delayed onset of toxicity has been observed following amiodarone overdose.[5]

Extracardiac manifestations of acute toxicity include dizziness, visual disturbances, psychosis, anticholinergic symptoms (disopyramide), hypoglycemia (disopyramide), hyperglycemia (encainide), hypokalemia, and hypersensitivity reactions (e.g., fever, rash, urticaria).[9,19] Thrombocytopenia and a lupus-like syndrome (arthralgias, fever, myocarditis) with antinuclear antibodies have been well documented during chronic quinidine and procainamide therapy. The use of amiodarone is increasing despite the risk of numerous adverse effects, including corneal microdeposits, photosensitivity, hepatic dysfunction, myopathy, pulmonary fibrosis, hypo- or hyperthyroidism, and peripheral neuropathies.

Hypotension, bradycardia, CNS depression, seizures, metabolic acidosis, and cardiovascular collapse can occur in severe poisoning. Patients with disopyramide overdose may demonstrate early loss of consciousness, apnea, or cardiac failure. Seizures appear to be more prevalent with class IC drugs. Disopyramide has resulted in acute congestive heart failure at therapeutic doses in patients with heart disease. Clinical effects associated with quinidine include seizures, immune-mediated hemolytic anemia, syncope, and cinchonism. Syncope is due primarily to torsades de pointes (discussion follows), but may also be associated with adrenergic blockade (orthostasis) or, rarely, idiosyncratic reactions. Cinchonism (see Chapter 315) is associated with chronic therapy and does not appear to be dose-related. Procainamide and quinidine can predictably produce hypotension if given by too-rapid intravenous infusion. Death can result from refractory dysrhythmias or cardiovascular collapse.

Disturbances in cardiac conduction and rhythm are the electrocardiographic (ECG) hallmarks of poisoning. Excessive prolongation of the QT interval is almost always present in severe poisoning. With class IA agents, this results from prolongation of both the QRS and JT intervals, whereas with class IC and III agents, it is due primarily to QRS and JT prolongation, respectively. In general, an increase of the QRS or QT interval by 25% is considered therapeutic, and widening by 50% or more suggests toxicity. The PR interval may also be prolonged if there is sinus activity. Conduction disturbances and myocardial depression contribute to a host of supraventricular and ventricular dysrhythmias, including sinus bradycardia, atrioventricular dissociation, ventricular tachycardia or fibrillation, slow idioventricular rhythm, and asystole. Torsades de pointes is a triggered (early after depolarization) polymorphous ventricular tachycardia resulting from excessive JT prolongation, most commonly associated with class IA and III drugs (e.g., quinidine, amiodarone, high levels of NAPA).

All antidysrhythmic drugs can aggravate existing dysrhythmias or induce new ones (e.g., proarrhythmic effect) in patients being treated for supraventricular or ventricular dysrhythmias.

The incidence of proarrhythmia is estimated at 5% to 20% and most often is associated with initiation of therapy or a dosage increase.[14] The induction of dysrhythmias should always be suspected in patients on antidysrhythmic drugs who present with syncopal episodes.

Patients with preexisting renal, hepatic, or cardiac disease are at increased risk for toxicity. Although impairment of renal function does not appear to alter appreciably the elimination rate of quinidine, propafenone, or amiodarone, the elimination half-lives of procainamide and NAPA, flecainide, and sotalol are prolonged. Similar changes may occur when blood flow to the kidneys is reduced (i.e., congestive heart failure). Reduced biotransformation may be expected for quinidine, procainamide, propafenone, amiodarone, and, possibly, encainide and flecainide in the presence of hepatic dysfunction.

The correlation of serum levels with clinical effects depends on previous exposure to the drug, the presence of heart disease, and the degree of absorption, metabolite formation, and elimination. In general, serum levels exceeding 7, 8, and 15 μg/mL for quinidine, disopyramide, and procainamide (NAPA), respectively, should be considered toxic. Flecainide levels of 1.48 to 3.7 μg/mL have been observed in patients with prolonged QT intervals, ventricular dysrhythmias, and seizures, and levels of 13.0 to 16.3 μg/mL have been reported in fatal cases. Lower levels may result in toxicity in patients who coingest other cardiovascular agents. Patients on chronic therapy who take an acute overdose appear to be at greater risk for severe intoxication.

DIFFERENTIAL DIAGNOSIS

Similar bradyarrhythmias may be caused by beta blockers, calcium antagonists, cholinergic agents (carbamate and organophosphate insecticides), digitalis, clonidine, lithium, and cyclic antidepressants. QRS and QT interval prolongation may result from poisoning with antihistamines, phenothiazines, cyclic antidepressants, lithium, magnesium, or potassium. Ventricular tachyarrhythmias may occur in poisoning with sympathomimetics and drugs that cause QRS and QT prolongation.

EMERGENCY DEPARTMENT EVALUATION

The history should include the exact product and strength (immediate- or sustained-release), the amount ingested, the time ingested, and treatment before arrival. Any history of cardiovascular disease must be elucidated. Mechanisms for chronic toxicity, such as excessive dosing, exacerbation of congestive heart failure, or change in renal function, should be investigated.

The physical examination initially focuses on vital signs, with attention to cardiovascular stability and respiratory and neurologic status. A detailed examination should be performed after vital signs or rhythm abnormalities are stabilized.

A 12-lead ECG should be obtained as soon as possible. Laboratory work should include a blood glucose level; electrolyte analysis; blood urea nitrogen, creatinine, and magnesium measurement; liver function tests; and appropriate serum drug levels. Requests for NAPA should always accompany requests for procainamide levels. Chest radiography and arterial blood gas analysis are included for patients with depressed levels of consciousness or serious dysrhythmias.

EMERGENCY DEPARTMENT MANAGEMENT

Advanced life-support measures should be instituted, as necessary. All patients suspected of antidysrhythmic drug toxicity should have an intravenous line, continuous cardiac monitoring, and pulse oximetry. Supplemental oxygen is given to symptomatic patients. Unstable patients must have close hemodynamic monitoring. Acid–base, electrolyte, and magnesium derangements should be corrected. Potassium should be replaced cautiously, because hypokalemia may protect against cardiotoxicity due to quinidine (and possibly other agents). Seizures are treated with standard doses of intravenous diazepam or lorazepam, or phenobarbital.

Hypotension is initially treated with intravenous normal saline. Infusions of sodium bicarbonate can reverse hypotension associated with class IA and IC drugs. Patients with compromised left ventricular function must not be overly fluid resuscitated. Hypotension refractory to volume expansion may require the use of vasopressors or inotropes (epinephrine, norepinephrine, dopamine), aortic balloon counterpulsation, or cardiopulmonary bypass pump support.[9,19,20]

As in cyclic antidepressant toxicity (see Chapter 313), increasing the serum sodium level, the serum pH, or both, by administering sodium bicarbonate (1- to 2-mEq/kg bolus doses, as needed) can also reverse conduction delays and dysrhythmias due to class IA and IC drugs.[6] Symptomatic bradycardia or atrioventricular dissociation will probably require ventricular pacing if there is inadequate response to atropine or sodium bicarbonate. Successful pacemaker capture may require concomitant epinephrine therapy.[12]

After sodium bicarbonate, lidocaine is the drug of choice for ventricular ectopy. Other antidysrhythmic drugs in the same class are obviously contraindicated for treatment of dysrhythmias. Torsades de pointes usually responds to isoproterenol infusion (1 to 6 μg/min) and atrial or ventricular overdrive pacing.[8,19] A heart rate of 150 beats/min is usually required. Intravenous magnesium sulfate (1 to 4 g over several minutes to 1 hour, depending on the hemodynamic stability) may also be effective.

Activated charcoal is the preferred method of gastrointestinal decontamination. Repeat doses may be indicated when prolonged absorption is observed (increasing serum drug levels) and bowel sounds are present. Syrup of ipecac is not recommended, owing to its long duration of action and the potential for deterioration while the patient is still vomiting. Gastric lavage is of questionable benefit and should be reserved for patients with large overdoses who present soon after ingestion. Vagal effects secondary to passing a lavage tube could worsen conduction disturbances.

Patients whose vital signs can be supported during endogenous drug elimination usually recover fully. Efforts to enhance elimination of these compounds have had variable success. Patients should be adequately hydrated to maintain renal perfusion. Forced diuresis, however, is not recommended, due to potential problems of fluid overload and pulmonary edema. Urinary acidification is marginally effective in increasing quinidine excretion and is no longer recommended. Quinidine is poorly removed by hemodialysis, charcoal hemoperfusion, and peritoneal dialysis. Although disopyramide's pharmacokinetic profile would suggest success with extracorporeal removal, only small amounts of drug have been removed with charcoal hemoperfusion and resin hemoperfusion.[7,9] Hemodialysis and hemoperfusion both failed to remove a significant amount of flecainide in a patient with renal failure and chronic flecainide intoxication.

Extracorporeal elimination may have a role in the treatment of procainamide and NAPA toxicity. In the presence of renal failure, hemodialysis can increase the clearance of NAPA fourfold and procainamide twofold. Procainamide serum levels were halved, and clinical improvement was observed following a 6-hour treatment.[17] However, NAPA levels in a patient on chronic hemodialysis halved after 4 consecutive days of dialysis, perhaps due to extensive tissue stores and redistribution following each treatment.[8] Drug redistribution from tissues to serum may also have contributed to the success of continuous arteriovenous hemofiltration ($t_{1/2}$ of 3.1 days), compared with intermittent 4-hour hemodialysis ($t_{1/2}$ of 4.1 to 7.0 days) in the removal of NAPA.[4] Another case report documented a decrease of 19 μg/mL in the NAPA serum level following 4 hours of resin hemoperfusion.[3]

DISPOSITION

Patients who remain asymptomatic and have a normal ECG after 6 hours of observation can usually be safely discharged. A 12-hour observation period is recommended if a sustained-release preparation is involved. Patients with amiodarone overdose probably should be admitted for prolonged observation. Patients who are symptomatic or exhibit ECG evidence of cardiotoxicity from either acute or chronic intoxication need admission to a monitored bed. Those with cardiovascular instability should be admitted to an intensive care unit. A cardiologist should be consulted. A regional poison center or toxicologist can help with disposition and management decisions. Patients with severe toxicity should be admitted or transferred to a facility with cardiopulmonary bypass and aortic balloon counterpulsation capabilities. Patients presenting after intentional overdose should undergo psychiatric evaluation before discharge.

COMMON PITFALLS

- Failure to appreciate that severe toxicity can result from therapeutic doses of antidysrhythmic agents
- Failure to consider the possibility of drug-induced dysrhythmias as a cause of syncope and weakness in patients taking antidysrhythmic agents
- Failure to appreciate that sudden deterioration can occur without warning and to immediately initiate continuous cardiac monitoring in patients with antidysrhythmic overdose
- Failure to appreciate that drug-induced dysrhythmias may resemble the ones for which the drug was prescribed and to check drug levels before treating them with more drug
- Failure to consider sodium bicarbonate and magnesium for the treatment of dysrhythmias
- Giving syrup of ipecac to patients who may rapidly deteriorate
- Failure to consider invasive cardiovascular supportive therapies, such as pacing, aortic balloon counterpulsation, and cardiopulmonary bypass in patients with severe poisoning

References

1. Accornero F, Pellanda A, Ruffini C, et al. Prolonged CPR during acute disopyramide poisoning. *Vet Hum Toxicol* 1993;35:231.
2. Bodnar T, Nowak R, Tomlanovich MC. Massive intravenous bolus bretylium tosylate. *Ann Emerg Med* 1980;9:630.
3. Braden GL, Fitzgibbons JP, Germain MJ, et al. Hemoperfusion for treatment of *N*-acetylprocainamide intoxication. *Ann Intern Med* 1986;105:64.
4. Domoto DT, Brown WW, Bruggensmith P. Removal of toxic levels of *N*-acetylprocainamide with continuous arteriovenous hemofiltration of hemodialysis. *Ann Intern Med* 1987;106:550.
5. Goddard CJR, Whorwell PJ. Amiodarone overdose and its management. *Br J Clin Pharmacol* 1989;43:184.
6. Goldman MJ, Mowry JB, Kirk MA. Sodium bicarbonate to correct widened QRS in a case of flecainide overdose. *J Emerg Med* 1997;15:183–186.
7. Gosselin B, Mathieu D, Chopin C, et al. Acute intoxication with disopyramide: clinical and experimental study by hemoperfusion on Amberlite XAD 4 resin. *Clin Toxicol* 1980;17:439.
8. Herre JM, Thompson JA. Polymorphic ventricular tachycardia and ventricular fibrillation due to *N*-acetylprocainamide. *Am J Cardiol* 1985;55:227.
9. Holt DW, O'Keeffe B, Marshall CB, et al. Successful management of serious disopyramide poisoning. *Postgrad Med J* 1980;56:256.
10. Hutchison A, Kilham H. Fatal overdose of disopyramide in a child. *Med J Aust* 1978;2:335.
11. Kennedy A, Thomas P, Sheridan DJ. Generalized seizures as the presentation of flecainide toxicity. *Eur Heart J* 1989;10:950.
12. Kerns W, English B, Ford M. Propafenone overdose. *Ann Emerg Med* 1994;24:98–103.
13. Koppel C, Oberdisse U, Heinemeyer G. Clinical course and outcome in class IC antiarrhythmic overdose. *Clin Toxicol* 1990;28(2):433.
14. McCollam PL, Parker RB, Beckman KJ, et al. Proarrhythmia: a paradoxic response to antiarrhythmic agents. *Pharmacotherapy* 1989;9:144.
15. McHugh TP, Perina DG. Propafenone ingestion. *Ann Emerg Med* 1987;16:437.
16. Mortensen ME, Bolon CE, Kelley MT, et al. Encainide overdose in an infant. *Ann Emerg Med* 1992;21:998.
17. Nguyen KP, Thomsen G, Liem B, et al. *N*-acetylprocainamide, torsades de pointes, and hemodialysis. *Ann Intern Med* 1986;104:283.
18. Pentel PR, Goldsmith SR, Salerno DM, et al. Effect of hypertonic sodium bicarbonate on encainide overdose. *Am J Cardiol* 1986;57:878.
19. Shub C, Gau GT, Sidell PM, et al. The management of acute quinidine intoxication. *Chest* 1978;73:173.
20. Villalba-Pimentel L, Epstein LM, Sellers EM, et al. Survival after massive procainamide ingestion. *Am J Cardiol* 1973;32:727.

CHAPTER 313
Antidepressant Poisoning

Keith K. Burkhart

The availability of cyclic antidepressants (CAs) has provided a major therapeutic adjunct for the successful treatment of depression since the 1950s. Additional therapeutic indications have included chronic pain, migraine headaches, enuresis, and peptic ulcer disease. The term *cyclic antidepressants* refers to a family of drugs that have similar pharmacology and toxicity (Table 313.1).

Antidepressant overdoses continue to account for approximately 20% of the fatalities reported to the American Association of Poison Control Centers.[10] Worldwide, CAs are a leading cause of life-threatening drug poisoning. The ingestion of just one tablet may produce serious toxicity in pediatric patients.

A newer group of antidepressants, selective serotonin reuptake inhibitors (SSRIs), were introduced in the 1980s. This class of antidepressants offers a wider margin of safety, with less central nervous system (CNS) and cardiovascular toxicity, compared with the CAs.[1] Now SSRIs have taken a large share of the antidepressant-prescribing market.

The pharmacologic properties of the CAs contribute to their toxicity in overdose. CAs are highly lipophilic, with large vol-

TABLE 313.1. Antidepressant Agents

Class	Drug	Trade Name(s)
TRICYCLICS		
Tertiary Amines		
	Amitriptyline	Amitid, Amitril, Elavil, Endep, Etrafon, Triavil
	Clomipramine	Anafranil
	Doxepin	Adapin, Sinequan
	Imipramine	Janimine, Presamine, SK-Pramine, Tofranil
	Trimipramine	Surmontil
Secondary Amines		
	Desipramine	Norpramin, Pertofrane
	Nortriptyline	Aventyl, Pamelor
	Protriptyline	Vivactil
TETRACYCLICS		
	Maprotiline	Ludiomil
	Mianserin	Bolvidon, Norval
DIBENZOXAZEPINE		
	Amoxapine	Ascendin
SELECTIVE SEROTONIN REUPTAKE INHIBITORS		
	Fluoxetine	Prozac
	Sertraline	Zoloft
	Paroxetine	Paxil
INVESTIGATIONAL SSRIs		
	Fluvoxamine	
	Citalopram	

umes of distribution (VD) (10 to 50 L/kg). They are rapidly absorbed and quickly distributed to the target organs, thereby manifesting a characteristic rapid onset of toxicity. Delayed absorption, however, may result from the anticholinergic action that can prolong gastric emptying and decrease gastrointestinal motility. In addition to a large VD, CAs are more than 95% protein bound.

Most CAs are tertiary or secondary amines. Tertiary amines (e.g., amitriptyline and imipramine) are metabolized to their respective secondary amines (e.g., nortriptyline and desipramine), which are also active drugs. Tertiary amines block norepinephrine and serotonin reuptake, while secondary amines primarily block norepinephrine reuptake. Tertiary amines have more anticholinergic and antihistaminic effects than the secondary amines.

CAs have half-lives greater than 24 hours. Early reports described prolonged and delayed toxicity. Improved supportive care, including alkalinization therapy and the administration of activated charcoal (AC), is probably responsible for a better outcome today. Enterohepatic and possibly entero-entero recirculation may contribute to the long half-life, but may not have a significant effect on the duration of toxicity. Most CA-poisoned patients that are provided with good supportive care make a full recovery within 2 to 3 days.

SSRIs share some of the pharmacologic properties of CAs. Peak levels occur 4 to 8 hours after therapeutic dosing. SSRIs also have a large VD and are highly protein bound. Like CAs, SSRIs are eliminated extensively by hepatic metabolism. Fluoxetine and citalopram have active metabolites.

Therapeutic doses of CAs are typically less than 5 mg/kg. Tolerance does develop in chronically dosed patients. Toxicity is generally seen with ingestion greater than 10 mg/kg, while greater than 15 mg/kg may result in severe, potentially fatal ingestions.

The CNS and cardiovascular toxicity of CAs result from quinidine-like cardiac conduction disturbances, sympathomimetic and sympatholytic actions resulting from the blockade of the reuptake of norepinephrine, and anticholinergic effects. Antihistaminic and α-blocking properties may also contribute to toxicity. Some CAs produce predominantly CNS or cardiac toxicity. Amoxapine produces seizures, including status epilepticus, but cardiac conduction disturbances do not generally occur. The relative absence of quinidine-like effects, catecholamine reuptake blockade, and anticholinergic effects of the SSRIs is responsible for their increased margin of safety.

Serotonergic hyperstimulation may produce a symptom complex involving autonomic, motor, and CNS hyperactivity that has been termed the *serotonin syndrome* (see Chapter 370).[12] Excess stimulation of 5-HT1A receptors appears to be responsible. In most cases, the serotonin syndrome results from the addition of a second drug that further enhances serotonergic tone. Metabolic interactions involving cytochrome-P450 metabolism may also be involved in some cases.[2]

CLINICAL PRESENTATION

The presentation of CA poisoning may range from asymptomatic to cardiopulmonary arrest.[5] Most importantly, a patient who is alert on arrival may become comatose, have seizures, or develop hemodynamic and cardiac instability within minutes.

Patients may initially be tachycardic and mildly hypertensive (due to the blockade of norepinephrine reuptake and anticholinergic effects), or they may be hypotensive (from α_1 blockade). As norepinephrine is metabolized, a catecholamine depletion state may also develop and lead to hypotension, bradycardia, and, finally, cardiogenic shock.

Patients often develop absent bowel sounds, ileus, and urinary retention. Other anticholinergic effects, such as dilated pupils; flushed, hot skin; and dry mucous membranes, however, are not common. Central anticholinergic findings vary from agitation to psychosis to coma. Additional neurologic manifestations include choreoathetosis and ataxia. Despite coma unresponsive to painful stimuli, patients may develop severe myoclonus and status epilepticus.

Cardiac dysrhythmias may include supraventricular tachydysrhythmias and ventricular arrhythmias. Intraventricular conduction disturbances often make it difficult to distinguish a ventricular tachycardia from a supraventricular tachycardia with aberrant conduction. Polymorphous ventricular tachycardia (torsades de pointes) has been reported. Aspiration pneumonia is relatively common, and adult respiratory distress syndrome may occur. Coma-induced rhabdomyolysis and compartment syndromes are additional potential complications.

SSRI overdoses have proved to have a much better safety record when compared with CA overdoses. With a few exceptions, patients present asymptomatic and have benign clinical courses. Symptoms, when they occur, may include mild tachycardia, hypertension, orthostatic hypotension, tachypnea, dizziness, drowsiness or lethargy, tremor, diaphoresis, and vomiting. Fatality reports are rare and often lack a postmortem evaluation, including drug screening.[1,6,9]

Seizures have occasionally occurred following SSRI overdoses.[17] They have usually been self-limited, often not requiring specific treatment. Electrocardiographic changes and seizures, however, were common in a retrospective series of citalopram overdoses at Swedish hospitals.[16] Six patients ingesting greater than 600 mg developed widened QRS complexes. Premature ventricular complexes and ST-T wave changes were noted, but no serious arrhythmias occurred. Thirty-three percent of patients in this group developed seizures, but all patients fully recovered.[16] QTc prolongation and widened QRS intervals have rarely been reported with other SSRIs.

The serotonin syndrome usually presents with mild cognitive, neuromuscular, and autonomic symptoms (see Chapter 370).[19] Rarely have severe life-threatening presentations or fatalities been suggested to have resulted from the serotonin syndrome.[12,19]

DIFFERENTIAL DIAGNOSIS

The differential diagnosis of coma, seizures, and cardiac dysrhythmias includes hypoxia, metabolic abnormalities, intrinsic neurologic and cardiac disease, and poisoning by antidysrhythmics, antihistamines, antimalarials, beta blockers, calcium channel blockers, carbamazepine, phenothiazines, and propoxyphene. Anticholinergic, camphor, cocaine, chloral hydrate, isoniazid, lithium, and sympathomimetic poisoning and drug withdrawal should also be considered.

EMERGENCY DEPARTMENT EVALUATION

The potential for rapid deterioration requires that intravenous access and continuous cardiac and oxygenation monitoring be initiated immediately. Vital signs and neurologic status should initially be evaluated every 15 minutes, and a limb lead QRS duration (discussion follows) should be checked every 30 minutes.

The history should be obtained from the patient, family, friends, or prehospital personnel. If possible, the time, amount, and identity of all agents ingested should be determined. When known, the amount of CA ingested often helps anticipate the potential for deterioration.

Early into the evaluation, an electrocardiogram (ECG) should be performed. A QRS duration greater than 100 milliseconds is associated with seizures, while a QRS duration greater than 160 milliseconds is associated with ventricular dysrhythmias. More subtle, early ECG changes include a widening of the terminal 40 milliseconds of the QRS in the right frontal plane. This manifestation can be quickly assessed by looking for the presence of a widened S wave in leads 1 and AVL, and an R wave in lead AVR (Fig. 313.1). These terminal 40-millisecond changes are good indicators for CA poisoning, but they do not absolutely confirm or exclude the diagnosis.[20]

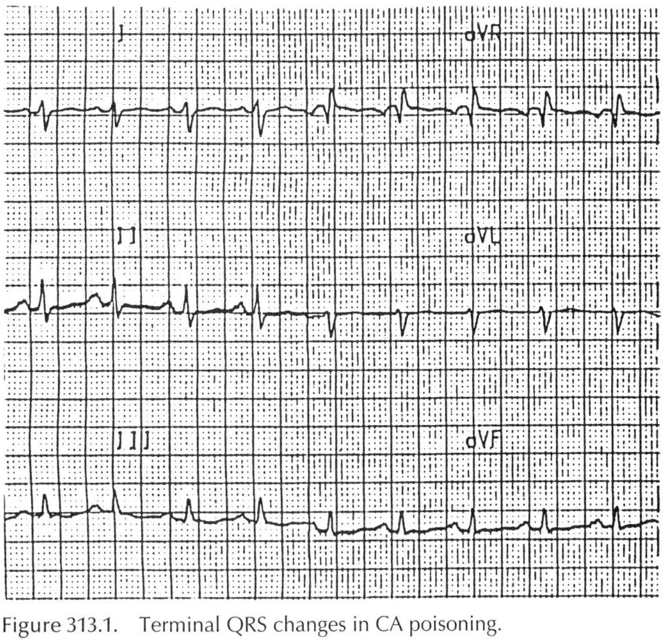

Figure 313.1. Terminal QRS changes in CA poisoning.

Other than a lactic acidosis secondary to seizures or shock, CAs are not known to produce biochemical disturbances. However, standard care of any patient with altered mental status or cardiotoxicity requires an assessment of electrolytes, blood urea nitrogen, creatinine, serum glucose, and serum osmolality. An arterial blood gas, creatine phosphokinase, calcium, magnesium, liver chemistries, and a chest x-ray should be considered in patients with abnormal vital signs, significant CNS depression, seizures, or an abnormal ECG.

Drug screening for CAs has very little impact on the management of the CA-poisoned patient. Qualitative screens may identify the presence of CAs in urine, while quantitative screens provide drug levels. Although serum levels greater than 1,000 ng/mL generally correlate with significant toxicity, levels do not assist in emergency management. Monitoring the changes on the ECG and the patient's mental status may actually be better indicators of CA toxicity. Serum levels of SSRIs are not routinely available, and no study has correlated these measurements with clinical manifestations.

EMERGENCY DEPARTMENT MANAGEMENT

The management of the CA-poisoned patient may need to begin with prehospital care directives. Field resuscitation of a patient with coma, seizures, hypotension, and arrhythmias includes endotracheal intubation; administration of anticonvulsants, crystalloids, and lidocaine; and serum alkalinization with parenteral sodium bicarbonate boluses.

While CA-induced seizures tend to be short-lived, they may deteriorate into status epilepticus.[4] A parenteral benzodiazepine such as diazepam or midazolam (5 to 10 mg), or lorazepam (2 to 4 mg), typically produces a rapid response and is the agent of choice. Higher doses may be required. Seizures will rapidly produce a lactic acidosis that may further compromise the cardiac and hemodynamic status. Hence, a bolus of sodium bicarbonate is recommended as adjunctive treatment for seizures. Neuromuscular paralysis with a short-acting agent should be considered for cases that do not respond. When intubation is required, parenteral administration of benzodiazepines may be useful for their anticonvulsant as well as sedative effects. If benzodiazepines do not completely control seizures, phenobarbital or propofol should be considered.[13] In the intubated patient, a phenobarbital loading dose of 18 mg/kg is usually sufficient. Status myoclonic activity is seen with severe poisoning. Benzodiazepines are often not effective for myoclonus.

Hypotension should be treated with crystalloid boluses up to 20 mg/kg. This treatment should overcome hypotension secondary to alpha blockade and mild dehydration. For more seriously poisoned patients, pressors may be needed. Dopamine and norepinephrine have been used successfully. However, some cases have been refractory to dopamine. Because dopamine partially acts as an indirect-acting sympathomimetic agent, by causing catecholamine release when norepinephrine stores are depleted following CA poisoning, it may lose some of its effectiveness. High infusion rates of dopamine may be tried initially, but if there is an inadequate response, norepinephrine should be given (substituted for or added to dopamine). In patients unresponsive to these measures, the insertion of a Swan-Ganz catheter and measurement of pulmonary artery pressures may be useful to guide additional management. Cardiac dysrhythmias can be terminated with the administration of sodium bicarbonate.[11,15] Many reports have described the important prophylactic and treatment role for serum alkalinization therapy in the management of CA poisoning. Sodium and bicarbonate have proven to be beneficial treatments for toxins that have quinidine-like, sodium-channel blocking actions. In experimental models of amitriptyline toxicity, sodium loading and pH elevation improved cardiac conduction, but both treatments together produced the greatest improvement.[11,18] In refractory ventricular dysrhythmias, lidocaine and bretylium should be considered, but type 1A antidysrhythmics, such as procainamide and beta blockers, should be avoided.

Dysrhythmias should be treated with at least one or two ampules of sodium bicarbonate (1 mEq/kg for pediatric patients). Sodium bicarbonate has acutely terminated ventricular tachycardia and wide complex tachycardia. The QRS duration shortens, and the terminal 40-millisecond changes become less evident. Respiratory alkalosis is advocated by many clinicians, but the pH elevation is not as instantaneous as with bolus bicarbonate administration and sustained respiratory alkalosis, which will lead to compensatory renal bicarbonate excretion, resulting in a relative deficiency state. The target pH for alkalinization is 7.45 to 7.55. Caution is also needed when sodium bicarbonate is given because of the potential to overshoot the desired pH and cause hypernatremia and ionized hypocalcemia. Additionally, the administration of large amounts of bicarbonate for a number of hours may lead to respiratory acidosis and hypoventilation.

Gastrointestinal decontamination should be accomplished following the institution of any necessary life-support measures. Syrup of ipecac is contraindicated in the setting of CA poisoning. Patients may become comatose, lose their gag reflex, and have seizures before or during emesis, resulting in airway compromise or aspiration pneumonitis. Gastric lavage probably benefits patients who present early (within an hour) after the ingestion, but its clinical utility beyond the first hour has not been proved.

AC should be administered in a dose of 1 g/kg. Because usually only a few grams of CAs are ingested, even in the most seriously poisoned patients, a single dose of AC represents a sufficiently large AC-to-drug ratio to theoretically prevent drug absorption. A clinical benefit from multiple doses of AC has not been clearly demonstrated.

The administration of Fab antibody fragments specific for CAs has resulted in hemodynamic improvement and decreased mortality in animal models.[3,8] Human clinical trials are now underway. Extracorporeal removal techniques play no role in the management of the CA-poisoned patient. Because benzodiazepines are therapeutic, flumazenil is contraindicated for patients with coma and a history or ECG suggestive of CA poisoning. Similarly, physostigmine, although it may be effective in reversing anticholinergic toxicity (see Chapter 312), has resulted in asystole when used to treat cardiac arrhythmias due to CA poisoning. It is therefore contraindicated for patients with a prolonged QRS interval or arrhythmias suggestive of CA cardiotoxicity. Anticholinergic symptoms may persist for days. Physostigmine in this recovery phase may be beneficial.

The management of the SSRI overdose is based on providing general supportive care with cardiac monitoring and intravenous access. Seizures are usually self-limited and usually terminate without therapy.

Management of the serotonin syndrome is described in detail in Chapter 370. Discontinuation of the inciting agent(s) is often all that is required.[14] Serotonin antagonists such as cyproheptadine,[7] methysergide, propranolol, chlorpromazine, and metoclopramide have been found to be of benefit in animal studies and some case reports. Benzodiazepines appear to lessen the severity without relieving the symptoms. Dopamine antagonists such as haloperidol and dantrolene have also been recommended but remain of unproven benefit. Bromocriptine increases serotonin levels and should be avoided. In severe, life-threatening syndromes, the early institution of anesthetic doses of propofol or phenobarbital may blunt neurotransmission and be protective until the clearance of the offending agent(s) can occur.

DISPOSITION

The maximal severity of a CA poisoning is usually apparent within 2 to 6 hours of an overdose. Patients who develop coma, hypotension, seizures, or arrhythmias require intensive care unit admission. A patient that remains or becomes asymptomatic after 6 hours of observation has not had a significant ingestion. These patients can be medically cleared for discharge or psychiatric evaluation (a requirement for all intentional ingestions). Patients that develop less severe symptoms, such as lethargy or tachycardia, will require prolonged monitoring and observation. Emergency department observation units or intermediate care units are appropriate.

Observation medicine is usually appropriate for serotonin overdoses and mild-to-moderate cases of the serotonin syndrome. Severe cases, however, may warrant intensive care unit admission.

A regional poison information center or toxicologist can be consulted for treatment and disposition decisions. Critically ill and complicated poisoned patients are best served at a regional poison treatment center or tertiary care facility. When indicated, transfer requires either an air ambulance or an advanced cardiac life support–equipped crew, accompanied by a nurse or physician.

COMMON PITFALLS

- Failure to appreciate that patients with recent CA overdose who are awake and appear stable may rapidly deteriorate
- Failure to administer AC
- Failure to aggressively treat seizure activity and correct the resultant metabolic acidosis
- Failure to alkalinize the serum in patients with coma, seizures, hypotension, arrhythmias, and cardiac conduction disturbances
- Failure to recognize the serotonin syndrome and to avoid prescribing multiple medications with serotonergic effects

References

1. Barbey JT, Roose SP. SSRI safety in overdose. *J Clin Psychiatry* 1998;59[Suppl 15]:42.
2. Brown TM, Skop BP, Mareth TR. Pathophysiology and management of the serotonin syndrome. *Ann Pharmacother* 1996;30:527.
3. Dart RC, Sidki A, Sullivan JB, et al. Ovine desipramine antibody fragments reverse desipramine cardiovascular toxicity in the rat. *Ann Emerg Med* 1996;27:309.
4. Ellison DW, Pentel PR. Clinical features and consequences of seizures due to cyclic antidepressant overdose. *Am J Emerg Med* 1989;7:5.
5. Frommer DA, Kulig KW, Marx JA, et al. Tricyclic antidepressant overdose: a review. *JAMA* 1987;257:521.
6. Goh KT. Fatal overdose with citalopram. *Lancet* 1996;347:1345.
7. Graudins A, Stearman A, Chan B. Treatment of the serotonin syndrome with cyproheptadine. *J Emerg Med* 1998;16:615.
8. Keyler DE, LeCouteur DG, Pond SM, et al. Effects of specific antibody fragments on desipramine pharmacokinetics in the rat in vivo and in the isolated perfused liver. *J Pharmacol Exp Ther* 1995;272:1117.
9. Kincaid RL, McMullin MM, Crookham SB, et al. Report of a fluoxetine fatality. *J Anal Toxicol* 1990;14:327.

10. Litovitz TL, Klein-Schwartz W, Caravati EM, et al. 1998 Annual report of the American Association of Poison Control Centers Toxic Exposure Surveillance System. *Am J Emerg Med* 1999;17:445.
11. Nattel S, Mittleman M. Treatment of ventricular tachyarrythmias resulting from amitriptyline toxicity in dogs. *J Pharmacol Exp Ther* 1984;231:430.
12. Martin TG. Serotonin syndrome. *Ann Emerg Med* 1996;28:520–526.
13. Merigian KS, Browning RG, Leeper KV. Successful treatment of amoxapine-induced refractory status epilepticus with propofol (Diprivan). *Acad Emerg Med* 1995;2:128.
14. Mills K. Serotonin syndrome. *Am Fam Physician* 1995;52:1475.
15. Pentel P, Benowitz NL. Tricyclic antidepressant poisoning: Management of arrhythmias. *Med Toxicol* 1986;1:101.
16. Personne M, Sjoberg G, Persson H. Citalopram overdose—review of cases treated in Swedish hospitals. *J Toxicol Clin Toxicol* 1997;35:237.
17. Riddle MA, Brown N, Dzubinski D, et al. Fluoxetine overdose in an adolescent. *J Am Acad Child Adolesc Psychiatry* 1989;28:587.
18. Sasyniuk BI, Jhamandas V. Mechanism of reversal of toxic effects of amitriptyline on cardiac Purkinje fibers by sodium bicarbonate. *J Pharmacol Exp Ther* 1984;231:387.
19. Sternbach H. The serotonin syndrome. *Am J Psychiatry* 1991;148:705.
20. Wolfe TR, Caravati EM, Rollins DE. Terminal 40-ms frontal plane QRS axis as a marker for tricyclic antidepressant overdose. *Ann Emerg Med* 1989;18:348.

CHAPTER 314
Antihistamine Poisoning

Andis Graudins

TABLE 314.1. Therapeutic Oral Adult Doses of Common Antihistamines

Agent	Dose (mg)
FIRST-GENERATION H_1 BLOCKERS	
Brompheniramine	4–8
Chlorpheniramine	4
Ciemastine	1–3
Cyclizine	50
Cyproheptadine	4
Dimenhydrinate	50–100
Diphenhydramine	25–50
Doxylamine	7.5–25
Hydroxyzine	10–50
Meclizine	25–50
Methapyriline	25
Promethazine	25
Pyrilamine	25
Trimeprazine	2.5
Tripelennamine	25–50
SECOND-GENERATION H_1 BLOCKERS	
Acrivastine	10
Astemizole	10
Cetirizine	10
Ebestine	10
Fexofenadine	60
Loratadine	10
Terfenadine	60
H_2 BLOCKERS	
Cimetidine	300
Famotidine	40
Ranitidine	150
Nizatidine	300

Histamine receptor antagonists (H_1 and H_2 blockers; Table 314.1) are a large group of drugs with wide consumer availability and multiple uses. H_1 blockers are used to relieve the symptoms of allergy and the common cold; as sedatives, antipruritics, and antiemetics; to prevent motion sickness; and to reverse dystonic reactions. These agents are available in their pure forms or combined with multiple other drugs (e.g., analgesics, sympathomimetics, caffeine, anticholinergic compounds), which can significantly alter the clinical presentation in overdose.[3] H_2 blockers are used to treat peptic ulcers and gastroesophageal reflux disease; they have also been used to treat allergic conditions.

The incidence of antihistamine overdose increased markedly following the approval of over-the-counter sale for brompheniramine, chlorpheniramine, and diphenhydramine in 1983. In 1997, antihistamines represented 4.9% of all exposures reported to poison control centers in the United States.[14] This number appears to be rising with each year and may be related to the increasing availability of these agents over the counter. Half of all exposures occurred in children under 6 years of age. Half of the ingestions were with over-the-counter medications, and half involved the use of diphenhydramine. There were 25 reported deaths with H_1-receptor antagonist ingestions but none from H_2-receptor antagonists.[14]

H_1 blockers are reversible competitive pharmacologic antagonists of histamine at H_1 receptor sites. They decrease vascular permeability, reduce pruritus, and relax smooth muscle in the respiratory and gastrointestinal (GI) tracts. The older, or first-generation, H_1 blockers are lipophilic, readily penetrate the blood–brain barrier, and cause sedation. These agents may also have anticholinergic, antiserotonergic, and alpha-sympathetic receptor blocking effects, which can become more apparent in overdose. Some of the newer second-generation agents also reduce the release of mediators of inflammation from mast cells. They are much less sedating because they are less penetrating of the central nervous system (CNS) and lack many of the unwanted side effects of the older agents.[19]

H_1 blockers can also block sodium channels in excitable tissues and have local anesthetic effects and antiarrhythmic effects similar to those of class IA antiarrhythmics (e.g., quinidine, procainamide, disopyramide; see Chapter 311). In particular, diphenhydramine and cyproheptadine are notable for prolonging the duration of cardiac muscle action potential.[4] Astemizole and terfenadine may prolong repolarization by blockade of potassium rectifier currents during myocardial repolarization, resulting in QT-interval prolongation on the electrocardiogram (ECG) and a risk of polymorphic ventricular tachycardia.[1,20] Drugs blocking terfenadine metabolism, such as ketoconazole and erythromycin, may result in accumulation of the parent compound and an increased risk of cardiac toxicity.[9,16] Fexofenadine, an active metabolite of terfenadine, is now available as an antihistamine agent. It does not possess any cardiac toxic effects in therapeutic doses or in animal studies of overdose. To date, there are no reports in the literature of human overdose.[15]

The first-generation H_1 blockers all have the basic structure of histamine. They can be divided into subgroups based on substitutions on the imidazole ring: ethanolamines (e.g., diphenhydramine, dimenhydrinate, doxylamine, clemastine); ethylenediamines (e.g., pyrilamine, methapyrilene, tripelennamine); piperazines (e.g., chlorcyclizine); alkylamines (e.g., brompheniramine, chlorpheniramine); phenothiazines (e.g., promethazine, trimeprazine); cyclizines (e.g., meclizine, hydroxyzine, cyclizine); and cyproheptadine. The second-generation H_1 blockers are less readily classifiable.

H_2 blockers primarily inhibit gastric acid secretion and have much less sedative and anticholinergic activity than the H_1 antagonists. In overdose, these agents appear to have an extremely high therapeutic index, with reported cases of ingestion of up to 15 g without clinical effect.[12] The main toxicity of these agents, particularly cimetidine, which inhibits hepatic P-450–mixed function oxidase activity, results from their interaction with the metabolism of other drugs.

Antihistamines are rapidly and extensively absorbed from the GI tract, with peak levels occurring in 2 to 4 hours. In overdose, peak levels may be delayed because of anticholinergic gastric stasis. All antihistamines are affected by extensive first-pass metabolism, with bioavailability of 40% to 60%. Some of these agents may form active metabolites; for instance, hydroxyzine is metabolized to cetirizine, a second-generation agent.[19] Protein-binding is highly variable, ranging from 20% for cimetidine to 99% for diphenhydramine. Volumes of distribution range from 1 L/kg for cimetidine to 3 to 7 L/kg for diphenhydramine. First-generation H_1 blockers are quite lipophilic and readily cross the blood–brain barrier. Most agents are metabolized in the liver, and the metabolites are excreted renally. Some of the newer agents are excreted unchanged in the urine (cetirizine, a metabolite of hydroxyzine) or fecally (astemizole).[19] Elimination half-lives are variable for the antihistamines. Most of the first-generation H_1 antagonists have half-lives of 2 to 6 hours. The half-lives of the second-generation H_1 blockers tend to be longer, allowing once-daily dosage.[19] In the elderly, those with hepatic dysfunction, and patients with overdoses, elimination may be slower.

Antihistamines have a high margin for safety, but massive overdoses of H_1 blockers have led to deaths in adults and children. Drug interactions play a role in many intentional overdoses, with potentiation of toxicity by the concurrent use of barbiturates, benzodiazepines, alcohol, or opioids. Tripelennamine may be injected in combination with pentazocine ("T's and blues") by intravenous drug users.

CLINICAL PRESENTATION

In about a third of reported exposures to H_1 blockers, there are no signs of toxicity.[14] Another third show signs of mild-to-moderate toxicity.[14] Symptoms and signs can be divided into CNS, cardiovascular, and anticholinergic effects. CNS depression (e.g., drowsiness, ataxia) is common in adults following overdosage of first-generation agents.[11] There have also been reports of patients presenting with toxic psychosis (as evidenced by hallucinations)[11] and coma (in severe overdoses). In children, CNS excitation is more common because of their sensitivity to the anticholinergic effects. Tremors, confusion, hyperpyrexia, agitation, and seizures are often seen with significant overdose and can progress to status epilepticus.[17] Children may develop anticholinergic toxicity or encephalopathy following exposure to topical antihistamines.[6,18] There have also been rare reports of anisocoria and diplopia as well as dystonias after diphenhydramine overdosage.

The most common cardiovascular effect is sinus tachycardia, which is due to anticholinergic blockade. Conduction disturbances can occur with significant overdoses. Diphenhydramine can cause QRS-interval prolongation and ventricular dysrhythmias.[4,17] Astemizole can cause QT prolongation, atrioventricular block, ventricular tachycardia, and fibrillation following overdose.[8,13] Terfenadine has also been reported to produce QT prolongation and torsades de pointes, both in overdose and in normal doses, as a drug interaction in patients concomitantly ingesting erythromycin, ketoconazole, sotalol, or cimetidine. This effect may also be apparent in patients with underlying chronic liver impairment and those with congenital QT-interval prolongation. Torsades de point has also been reported in a previously healthy individual on therapeutic doses of terfenadine.[10]

Peripheral anticholinergic effects include dry, warm skin; flushing; dry mucous membranes; mydriasis; intestinal ileus; constipation; and urinary retention. These symptoms may persist for several days. Nontraumatic rhabdomyolysis has been reported in patients following H_1-antagonist overdose.

After large ingestions, coma and seizures may occur within 30 minutes of ingestion. Patients with these findings have an increased risk of death. In children less than 2 years old, seizures have occurred with doses as little as 150 mg of diphenhydramine. Fatal doses in adults may range from 20 to 40 mg/kg; in children, as little as 500 mg may result in death.

Significant toxicity following H_2-antagonist overdose is rare.[12,14] Sinus bradycardia, atrioventricular block, and QT-segment prolongation have been reported in patients on oral or parenteral cimetidine and ranitidine.[5] Blockade of H_2 receptors and enhancement of H_1-receptor stimulation in cardiac muscle may prolong atrioventricular conduction. These drugs may also produce confusion and disorientation in therapeutic doses.[5]

DIFFERENTIAL DIAGNOSIS

A history of exposure to antihistamines is helpful in the diagnosis of poisoning but is not always available. Antihistamines are widely available as over-the-counter preparations and, as such, are often abused or used in suicide gestures. The diagnosis of H_1-antagonist poisoning should be considered in any patient presenting with signs of anticholinergic blockade, CNS depression, psychosis, or encephalopathy. Other agents capable of producing similar toxicity include antiarrhythmics, cyclic antidepressants, neuroleptics, anticholinergic medications, and plant ingestions, such as jimsonweed, henbane, and deadly nightshade. Antihistamine poisoning must be differentiated from varicella encephalitis in children with altered mental status who have chickenpox and have been treated with topical or oral antihistamines.

EMERGENCY DEPARTMENT EVALUATION

The history includes the time, amount, and identity of all agents ingested; the time of onset, nature, and progression of any symptoms; and any prehospital interventions. The physical examination begins with an assessment of vital signs and cardiovascular and autonomic function. All patients should have cardiac monitoring, and a 12-lead ECG should be obtained in symptomatic ones. In patients with intentional overdoses, routine laboratory evaluation should include electrolyte measurements; blood urea nitrogen, creatinine, and glucose levels; and toxicology screening for coingestion of acetaminophen and salicylate. In patients with abnormal vital signs, full toxicologic screening and a chest radiograph are advised. Antihistamines are not detected by standard immunoassay tests for drugs of abuse. They can be detected by thin-layer and gas chromatography, but these techniques are unavailable in most hospital laboratories.

EMERGENCY DEPARTMENT MANAGEMENT

Advanced life-support measures are instituted, as necessary. Early airway control and assisted ventilation are important to maintain oxygenation and prevent aspiration pneumonia in obtunded patients. Intravenous access is established. Hypotension is treated with intravenous crystalloid. Seizure activity and agitation may be treated with intravenous benzodiazepines (e.g., lorazepam or diazepam). In refractory cases, barbiturates and chemical paralysis may be necessary. Phenothiazines should be avoided, as they may worsen anticholinergic effects and hypotension.

Ventricular tachyarrhythmias are initially treated with lidocaine. Wide-complex tachycardia associated with massive diphenhydramine overdose may respond to hyperventilation and intravenous sodium bicarbonate infusion.[17] Torsades de pointes associated with astemizole overdose has responded to intravenous magnesium sulfate.[13] Phenytoin and bretylium might be useful in refractory cases. Class IA antiarrhythmics (e.g., procainamide) and class III agents (e.g., sotalol) should be avoided, as they may promote dysrhythmias due to prolongation of cardiac muscle cell repolarization.[7] Conduction disturbances and ventricular dysrhythmias seen with terfenadine and astemizole are often self-limiting and may require only ECG monitoring.

In patients with obvious anticholinergic toxicity, and with agitation, hallucinations, and hyperactivity refractory to benzodiazepines, the cholinesterase inhibitor physostigmine may be diagnostic and therapeutic. It may also avert unnecessary and extensive investigation of other potential causes of delirium.[2] Physostigmine should never be used in patients with ECG evidence of delayed cardiac conduction (see Chapter 312).

GI decontamination should be performed in adults who have ingested more than five therapeutic doses or in children who have ingested an adult dose. Activated charcoal orally or via a gastric tube is usually adequate in most cases. Gastric lavage should be considered only in those with massive, life-threatening ingestions, with appropriate airway protection in place. Ipecac is contraindicated in H_1-antagonist overdose because of the potential for rapid onset of coma and seizures. Antihistamines have high protein binding and large volumes of distribution, suggesting that extracorporeal methods of removal should be ineffective. A patient with cardiac toxicity resulting from diphenhydramine poisoning and refractory to serum alkalinization and bicarbonate therapy had an apparent successful response to in-series hemodialysis and hemoperfusion.[17]

DISPOSITION

Patients who become or remain asymptomatic after a 4- to 6-hour observation period may be discharged. Patients with hallucinations, agitation, coma, seizures, or cardiovascular instability should be admitted to the intensive care unit. Patients with persistent but mildly depressed levels of consciousness and stable vital signs should be admitted to a telemetry unit until symptoms have resolved. All patients with intentional overdoses should have a psychiatric evaluation before discharge.

COMMON PITFALLS

- Failing to consider antihistamines as a cause of unexplained dysrhythmias and cardiac conduction disturbances
- Failing to consider antihistamines as a cause of altered mental status in children with varicella
- Inducing emesis in patients, who may rapidly develop CNS depression, seizures, and the inability to protect the airway
- Giving physostigmine to patients with conduction disturbances on ECG
- Using physostigmine to treat CNS depression
- Giving a class IA (e.g., procainamide), IC (e.g., flecainide), or III (e.g., sotalol, amiodarone) antiarrhythmic agent to patients with ventricular tachyarrhythmias due to antihistamines
- Failing to consider the use of sodium bicarbonate and magnesium sulfate in patients with ventricular tachyarrhythmias unresponsive to lidocaine

References

1. Berul CI, Morad M. Regulation of potassium channels by non-sedating antihistamines. *Circulation* 1995;91(8):2220.
2. Burns MJ, Graudins A, Linden CH. Efficacy and safety of physostigmine for anticholinergic syndrome. *J Toxicol Clin Toxicol* 1997;35(5):564(abst).
3. Cetaruk EW, Aaron CK. Hazards of nonprescription medications. *Emerg Med Clin North Am* 1994;12:483.
4. Clark RF, Vance MV. Massive diphenhydramine poisoning resulting in wide complex tachycardia: successful treatment with sodium bicarbonate. *Ann Emerg Med* 1992;21:318.
5. Cohen N, Modai D, Golik A, et al. Cimetidine-related cardiac conduction disturbances and confusion. *J Clin Gastroenterol* 1989;11:68.
6. Danze LK, Langdorf MI. Reversal of orphenadrine-induced ventricular tachycardia with physostigmine. *J Emerg Med* 1991;9:453.
7. Feroze H, Suri R, Silverman DI. Torsade de points from terfenadine and sotalol given in combination. *Pacing Clin Electrophysiol* 1996;19(10):1519.
8. Heidemann SM, Sarnaik AP. Arrhythmias after astemizole overdose. *Pediatr Emerg Care* 1996;12(2):102.
9. Honig PK, Woosley RL, Zamani K, et al. Changes in the pharmacokinetics and ECG pharmacodynamics of terfenadine with concomitant administration of erythromycin. *Clin Pharmacol Ther* 1992;52:231.
10. June RA, Nasr I. Torsades de pointes with terfenadine ingestion. *Am J Emerg Med* 1997;15(5):542.
11. Koppel C, Ibe K, Tenczer J. Clinical symptomatology of diphenhydramine overdose: an evaluation of 136 cases in 1982 to 1985. *J Toxicol Clin Toxicol* 1987;25:53.
12. Krenzelok EP, Litovitz T, Lippold K, et al. Cimetidine toxicity: an assessment of 881 cases. *Ann Emerg Med* 1987;16:1217.
13. Leor J, Harman M, Rabinowitz B, et al. Giant U waves and associated ventricular tachycardia complicating astemizole overdose: successful treatment with intravenous magnesium [Letter]. *Am J Med* 1991;91:94.
14. Litovitz TL, Klein-Schwarz W, Dyer KS, et al. 1997 Annual reports of the American Association of Poison Control Centers Toxic Exposure Surveillance System. *Am J Emerg Med* 1998;16(5):443.
15. Markham A, Wagstaff AJ. Fexofenadine. *Drugs* 1998;55(2):269.
16. Monahan BP, Ferguson CL, Killeavy ES, et al. Torsades de pointes occurring in association with terfenadine use. *JAMA* 1990;246:2788.
17. Mullins ME, Pinnick RV, Terhes JM. Life-threatening diphenhydramine overdose treated with charcoal hemoperfusion and hemodialysis. *Ann Emerg Med* 1999;33(1):104.
18. Reilly JF, Weisse ME. Topically induced diphenhydramine toxicity. *J Emerg Med* 1990;8:59.
19. Rimmer SJ, Church MK. The pharmacology and mechanism of action of histamine H_1 antagonists. *Clin Exp Allergy* 1990;20:3.
20. Woosley RL, Chen Y, Freiman JP, et al. Mechanism of the cardiotoxic actions of terfenadine. *JAMA* 1993;269(12):1532.

CHAPTER 315
Antimalarial Poisoning

J. Ward Donovan

Agents used to treat malaria are derived from a variety of chemical compounds, and include quinolines, quinacrine, halofantrine, and dehydrofolate reductase inhibitors.[12] Of these, the quinoline derivatives quinine and chloroquine cause severe toxicity in overdoses.[4,10,12]

Quinine is the principal alkaloid derived from the bark of the cinchona tree, and has been used as an antipyretic and for the treatment of malaria, nocturnal leg cramps, and myotonia.[18] Quinine is also used as an adulterant for street cocaine and heroin, as an over-the-counter analgesic and muscle relaxant, and, in small amounts, in tonic water.[2] Quinoline derivatives have an undeserved reputation as abortifacients.[2,18] Chloroquine is also used for the treatment of rheumatoid arthritis, parasitemia, and lupus erythematosus.[17] For oral use, quinine is available as the sulfate salt, and chloroquine, as the phosphate salt. Both are available for parenteral use as the hydrochloride salt.

Most quinoline derivative poisonings are the result of attempted suicides and accidental childhood ingestions, but they may also be due to self-induced abortion attempts and to the use of street drugs. Chloroquine poisoning is associated with high fatality rates, but occurrences are infrequent in the United States.[4,12]

Quinine has local anesthetic and irritant effects, has curare-like action on skeletal muscle, is a vasodilator, has oxytocic action on the uterus, and acts centrally on the chemoreceptor trigger zone to cause emesis.[2] Chloroquine shares these properties and is also a respiratory depressant. Quinoline derivatives have type 1A antiarrhythmic cardiac effects, including negative inotropism, slowing of depolarization and conduction, increased action potential duration, and lengthened effective refractory period.[2,12]

Oral quinine and chloroquine are rapidly absorbed in the small intestine, with 80% to 90% bioavailability and peak levels occurring 1 to 3 hours after ingestion.[19] The apparent volume of distribution is 1.6 to 1.8 L/kg for quinine and 116 to 285 L/kg for chloroquine, with plasma protein binding of 89% and 55%, respectively.[19] The elimination of quinine is primarily by hepatic microsomal oxidation, but 20% is excreted unchanged in the urine.[2] Because it has a pK_a of 8.4, urinary quinine excretion increases as the pH falls, but urinary flow rate may be more important than pH in determining clearance.[1,2] The elimination half-life of quinine is 10 to 12 hours, but in malaria patients, it increases to 16 to 18 hours, owing to reduced hepatic elimination and an increase in drug distribution.[12] In overdose, the elimination half-life increases to 26 to 34 hours, probably because of decreased (saturable) metabolism.[1] Chloroquine is eliminated by slow hepatic degradation, and 55% is excreted in the urine as chloroquine and its metabolites.[12] The elimination half-life is 75 to 278 hours, with slower elimination seen with higher drug concentrations.[12]

The toxic effects of quinoline derivatives are caused by their antiarrhythmic, cytotoxic, and irritant properties. Oculotoxicity develops in 17% to 42% of patients with quinine poisoning, and appears to be caused by a direct toxic effect on the photoreceptor and ganglion cell layers of the retina.[2–4,9] Constriction of retinal arterioles occurs secondarily and has been the focus of many unsuccessful therapies.[1,10]

The toxic dose of quinine in adults ranges from 1.8 g to 4.0 g, but a lethal dose cannot be readily identified.[1,12] Chloroquine has a narrow margin of safety, with toxicity occurring at doses as low as 1.0 g to 1.5 g, or 20 mg/kg, which is only twice the therapeutic dose.[12] Doses greater than 2 g in adults almost always produce toxic effects, and doses greater than 5 g are usually lethal.[17] There is a good correlation between plasma quinine and chloroquine concentrations and the development of toxicity. Quinine levels of only 2 μg/mL can cause mild, reversible hearing loss.[6] Levels of 6 to 15 μg/mL are normally associated with the development of toxic effects, although levels of 10 μg/mL may be tolerated in malaria patients because of enhanced drug protein binding.[1,10] Levels greater than 15 μg/mL are often associated with cardiac arrhythmias, irreversible blindness, and death, but survival has occurred with levels as high as 23.5 μg/mL.[1,4,10] Concentrations higher than 13 μg/mL at 5 hours and 6 μg/mL at 20 hours postingestion predict serious toxicity.[1,4,10] Chloroquine levels greater than 3 μg/mL are usually toxic, and death is likely if the level is greater than 8 μg/mL.[12,17]

CLINICAL PRESENTATION

In quinine overdose, cinchonism is the most common early feature, and occurs in about 75% of patients.[10] Symptoms usually begin within 4 hours of ingestion but may appear as early as 2 hours after ingestion or be delayed for 8 to 12 hours.[4,10] Cinchonism is characterized by tinnitus, hearing loss, nausea, vomiting, vertigo, ataxia, diaphoresis, headache, flushing, lethargy, and hypotension.[2,11,12] It may result from acute or chronic poisoning from any quinoline derivative.

Cardiac toxicity in quinine toxicity is typically mild, with sinus tachycardia and minor electrocardiographic (ECG) changes. However, ventricular arrhythmias, including torsades de pointes, conduction disturbances, and complete atrioventricular dissociation, may occur.[2] ECG abnormalities include prolonged P-R and Q-T intervals, ST- and T-wave changes, U waves, bundle-branch blocks, and QRS widening.[4,10] Convulsions, coma, respiratory depression, adult respiratory distress syndrome, and cardiac arrest may occur in large overdoses.[4,9,10]

Visual disturbances are often delayed for 6 to 24 hours after ingestion, and may present with progressive blurring of vision or sudden blindness.[10,13] The pupils may become dilated and fixed before vision loss. Peripheral visual field defects, color misperceptions, diplopia, and poor dark adaptation can occur and either progress to total blindness or clear rapidly.[2,11,13] The fundus usually is normal at the onset of visual defects, but retinal arteriole constriction, macular edema, and a cherry-red macular spot may develop within hours.[13] Optic atrophy may be seen later in serious cases.[2] Laboratory findings may include hypoglycemia, hypokalemia, and thrombocytopenia.[12] Hypoglycemia may occur due to quinine-induced inappropriate insulin secretion by the pancreas.[2] Quinine is seldom successful in inducing abortion but frequently causes fetal abnormalities and maternal deaths.[18]

Chloroquine toxicity differs in that it produces a much more rapid onset of symptoms, severe cardiovascular effects, greater respiratory depression, marked hypokalemia, and milder and transient ocular and auditory toxicity.[12,17] Cardiovascular collapse is common within 2 hours of ingestion and is due to marked myocardial depression and ventricular arrhythmias.[12] Toxicity can be predicted by the degree of hypokalemia, which is probably caused by intracellular shifts, and a QRS greater than 0.12 second.[12,17] Toxic effects are usually short-lived, despite persistently high plasma levels of the drug.[17]

Other quinoline derivatives, such as primaquine, amodiaquine, and piperaquine, do not cause cardiovascular or other severe toxicities. They are associated with gastrointestinal distress, hemolytic anemia, and, at least in the case of primaquine, methemoglobinemia.[12] The acridine derivative, quinacrine, may cause nausea, vomiting, confusion, hallucinations, and seizures.[12] Halofantrine, a phenanthrenemethanol, causes only mild gastrointestinal distress.[12] Of the dehydrofolate reductase inhibitors, pyrimethamine is the most toxic and may cause ataxia, seizures, coma, blindness, and deafness, as well as folate deficiency with megaloblastic anemia.[12] Dapsone may cause acute methemoglobinemia and hemolytic anemia.[12]

DIFFERENTIAL DIAGNOSIS

Quinoline derivative toxicity may resemble the presentation from other agents that cause visual, auditory, or cardiac effects. Methanol, ergot derivatives, and heavy metals (e.g., lead and mercury) should be considered in the differential of visual disturbances from an unknown agent. Unlike the quinolines, methanol causes a marked anion gap acidosis and osmolal gap. Manifestations of cinchonism are similar to those of salicylate toxicity, but the latter causes an elevated anion gap, acid–base imbalances, and no visual effects.[4] Quinidine, an isomer of quinine, causes similar cardiac effects but no visual deficits.[12] Cyclic antidepressants cause similar cardiovascular and electrocardiographic effects but do not cause auditory or visual loss.

EMERGENCY DEPARTMENT EVALUATION

In the overdose patient who presents with visual, auditory, and cardiovascular symptoms of unknown cause, the history should include availability or antimalarial agents and drugs for leg cramps, lupus, and arthritis. Attempted abortion by quinine should be suspected in a pregnant patient with these complaints. Physical examination must be directed at the vital signs, cardiac rhythm, auditory and visual acuity, pupillary size and reaction, funduscopic findings, visual field testing, and cerebellar status. Studies to assist in the differential include determination of quinine, quinoline, salicylate, electrolyte, glucose, liver enzyme, blood urea nitrogen, and creatinine levels; complete blood count; platelets; serum osmolality; and ECG. If available, electroretinograms and visual evoked response testing may detect signs of retinal damage in quinine overdose.[11]

EMERGENCY DEPARTMENT MANAGEMENT

A suspected ingestion of antimalarials requires immediate attention to the vital signs, cardiac monitoring, and gastric decontamination. Prevention of absorption is probably only effective in the first 2 to 3 hours, but it must be aggressively attempted because of the direct relation of peak plasma levels to toxicity. Activated charcoal binds very effectively to chloroquine and quinine, and its immediate use is likely to be more efficacious than induced emesis or gastric lavage.[14] Gastric emptying procedures may be complicated by rapid onset of central nervous system (CNS) depression, particularly with chloroquine overdose.

Hypotension usually responds to fluids but may require a vasopressor (e.g., dopamine or norepinephrine) and powerful inotropes (e.g., epinephrine, isoproterenol, or dobutamine).[2,5,12,17] Beta agonists (e.g., isoproterenol) or combined beta and alpha agonists (e.g., epinephrine) may be more beneficial in preventing ventricular arrhythmias than alpha agonists, by increasing heart rate and shortening the effective refractory period.[5] Hypotension, ventricular arrhythmias, and cardiac conduction abnormalities are also likely to respond to serum alkalinization to a pH of 7.50.[8,12] This may be accomplished by sodium bicarbonate administration, hyperventilation, or a combination of both. Lidocaine has been used but may potentate the arrhythmias, like all class IA and IC antiarrhythmics. Torsades de pointes may require overdrive pacing.[5]

Benzodiazepines, combined with mechanical ventilation and inotropes, are of significant benefit in chloroquine toxicity.[5,12,17] Diazepam at doses of 0.5 mg to 3.0 mg/kg may counteract the hemodynamic and ECG changes, perhaps by an antiarrhythmic effect or pharmacokinetic interaction.[5,16,17] Alternatively, the benefit may derive from its anticonvulsant and sedating effects.[5] The use of other sedating and anticonvulsant agents, such as barbiturates and thiopental, risk exacerbation of hypotension and have been both discouraged and proposed in severe chloroquine toxicity.[5,7] The use of high doses of any sedating agent to induce coma and prevent seizures is probably more important than the agent selected. Because cardiac toxicity is similar to that caused by hyperkalemia, hypokalemia need not be corrected unless it is severe. In fact, potassium administration may be harmful and should initially be avoided.[12]

Repeated doses of activated charcoal have been reported to reduce the elimination half-life of quinine by passive diffusion of the drug into the gastrointestinal lumen. The half-life in healthy volunteers taking a therapeutic dose was reduced by 50%, and, in overdoses, was shortened from over 24 hours to 8 hours.[15] Doses of activated charcoal should total 200 to 400 g, given as 25 to 50 gm every 2 to 4 hours.

Acidification of the urine, despite its theoretic potential for enhanced quinine elimination, is unproved, risks increased cardiotoxicity, and should not be used. Resin and charcoal hemoperfusion, hemodialysis, peritoneal dialysis, plasmapheresis, and exchange transfusion have all been tried in attempts to enhance drug elimination. However, because of their high volumes of distribution and plasma protein binding, these techniques remove only a small portion of the total body drug load, and clinical improvements are more likely due to the natural course of recovery.[1,2,9,12]

Attempts at reversal of retinal arteriolar vasospasm by way of stellate ganglion block, anterior chamber paracentesis, retrobulbar injections, and systemic vasodilators have not been effective and can produce significant complications.[2,4,9,10,12] Hyperbaric oxygenation therapy has been promoted on the premise that retinal hypoxia secondary to arteriolar vasoconstriction contributes to visual loss.[20] However, the reported benefit may well represent natural recovery.

Recovery from quinoline overdose is usually gradual and complete, but visual deficits from quinine may resolve only partially.[2,4,10,13] Resolution of visual toxicity may occur within hours to months, but, often, the patient is left with peripheral field deficits, color impairment, and night blindness.

Specific therapies for other antimalarials are methylene blue for methemoglobinemia (see Chapter 352) and multiple-dose charcoal therapy to enhance dapsone removal.[12] Leucovorin and folic acid may be useful in patients with chronic dehydrofolate reductor poisoning.

DISPOSITION

Patients suspected of ingesting a toxic amount of a quinoline derivative should be observed for 6 to 8 hours. Symptomatic patients should be admitted to an intensive care unit. Consultation with a medical toxicologist or the regional poison center should be considered. An ophthalmologist should be consulted in patients with visual symptoms. If such services are not available, transfer to a tertiary center with complete toxicology, cardiac, and ophthalmologic services should be done rapidly and with full advanced life-support capabilities en route.

COMMON PITFALLS

- Failure to consider antimalarial poisoning in patients with auditory, visual, cardiac, and neurologic abnormalities of unknown cause

- Failure to appreciate and be prepared for very rapid neurologic and cardiac deterioration from chloroquine overdose
- Reluctance to administer the very large doses of sedatives to prevent arrhythmias and seizures in patients with chloroquine overdose
- Failure to perform prompt gastrointestinal decontamination and to administer repeated doses of activated charcoal
- Failure to recognize that invasive procedures are unlikely to be of benefit and may have significant complications

References

1. Bateman DN, Blain PG, Woodhouse KW, et al. Pharmacokinetics and clinical toxicity of quinine overdosage: lack of efficacy of techniques intended to enhance elimination. *Q J Med* 1985;54:125.
2. Bateman DN, Dyson EH. Quinine toxicity. *Adverse Drug React Acute Poisoning Rev* 1986;4:215.
3. Berglund F. Toxicity of quinine. *Toxicology* 1989;58:237.
4. Boland ME, Roper SMB, Henry JA. Complications of quinine poisoning. *Lancet* 1985;1:384.
5. Buckley NA, Smith AJ, Dosen P, et al. Effects of catecholamines and diazepam in chloroquine poisoning in barbiturate anaesthetized rats. *Hum Exp Toxicol* 1996;15:909.
6. Claessen FA, Van Boxtel CJ, Perenboom RM, et al. Quinine pharmacokinetics: ototoxic and cardiotoxic effects in healthy Caucasian subjects and in patients with falciparum malaria. *Trop Med Int Health* 1998;3:482.
7. Clemessy JL, Taboulet P, Hoffman JR, et al. Treatment of acute chloroquine poisoning. *Crit Care Med* 1996;24:1189.
8. Curry SC, Connor DA, Clark RF, et al. The effect of hypertonic sodium bicarbonate on PRS duration in rats poisoned with chloroquine. *Clin Toxicol* 1996;34:73.
9. Dyson EH, Proudfoot AT. Quinine amblyopia: is current management appropriate? *Clin Toxicol* 1985;23:571.
10. Dyson EH, Proudfoot AT, Prescott LF, et al. Death and blindness due to overdose of quinine. *BMJ* 1985;291;31.
11. Guly U, Driscoll P. The management of quinine-induced blindness. *Arch Emerg Med* 1992;9:317.
12. Jaeger A, Suder P, Kopferschmitt J, et al. Clinical features and management of poisoning due to antimalarial drugs. *Med Toxicol* 1987;2:242.
13. Mackie MA, Davidson J, Clarke J. Quinine acute self-poisoning and Acular toxicity. *Scot Med J* 1997;42:8.
14. Neuvonen PJ, Kivisto KT, Laine K, et al. Prevention of chloroquine absorption by activated charcoal. *Hum Exp Toxicol* 1992;11:117.
15. Prescott LF, Hamilton AR, Heyworth R. Treatment of quinine overdosage with repeated oral charcoal. *Br J Clin Pharmacol* 1989;27:95.
16. Rajah A. The use of diazepam in chloroquine poisoning. *Anesthesia* 1990;45:955.
17. Riou B, Barriot P, Rimailho A, et al. Treatment of severe chloroquine poisoning. *N Engl J Med* 1988;318:1.
18. Smit JA, McFadyen ML. Quinine as unofficial contraceptive—concerns about safety and efficacy [Editorial]. *S Afr Med J* 1998;88:865.
19. White NJ. Clinical pharmacokinetics of antimalarial drugs. *Clin Pharmacokinet* 1985;10:187.
20. Wolff RS, Wirtshafter D, Adkinson C. Ocular quinine toxicity treated with hyperbaric oxygen. *Undersea Hyperb Med* 1997;24:131.

CHAPTER 316
Aromatic Hydrocarbon Poisoning

Jeffrey Tucker

Aromatic hydrocarbons are a group of compounds derived from benzene, a six-membered ring compound that has alternating single and double bonds between its carbon atoms. Common aromatic hydrocarbons include naphthalene and the benzene derivatives, such as toluene (methylbenzene), xylene (dimethylbenzene), styrene, paradichlorobenzene, cresols, and phenols. Aromatic hydrocarbons are found in household and industrial products such as felt-tipped markers, glue, mothballs, shoe polish, solvents, degreasers, paints, paint removers, gasoline, preservatives, and pesticides.[14] Styrene is used in the manufacturing of polystyrene plastics. Although *p*-dichlorobenzene has replaced the more toxic naphthalene in most deodorizers and mothballs, many old-fashioned preparations may still contain naphthalene or camphor. Differences in solubility and density can help differentiate these compounds. Turpentine can dissolve a *p*-dichlorobenzene mothball in 60 minutes, whereas at least 25% of a naphthalene mothball will remain after the same period. When placed in water and saturated-salt solutions (3 tablespoons NaCl per 4 oz H_2O), camphor and *p*-dichlorobenzene float and sink, respectively, in both solutions; naphthalene sinks in water but floats in the salt solution.

Toxicity from aromatic hydrocarbons most often follows intentional inhalation, although accidental industrial and household exposures, including ingestion may occur. Volatile substance abuse (VSA) or inhalant abuse refers to the intentional inhalation of aromatic and other volatile hydrocarbons for the purpose of achieving an euphoric state.[4,7,9,14] VSA is a widespread problem among adolescents. Preteens and young teens have higher rates of abuse than do older adolescents.[16,17] Volatile hydrocarbons are abused by "sniffing," "huffing," or "bagging." Sniffing is direct inhalation of the volatile substance from an open container. Huffing involves the inhalation of the volatile substance from a piece of cloth after it has been soaked. In bagging, the volatile substance is placed in a paper or plastic bag. The user then breathes in and out of the bag. Such practices result in exposure to vapor concentrations hundred of times greater than the occupational standards for the safe use of solvents in industry.[14]

Inhalation results in the rapid distribution to the brain due to high volatility at room temperature, excellent absorption by the lungs, high lipid solubility, and bypass of first-pass hepatic metabolism. Clinical effects are seen within seconds to minutes and are related to the vapor concentration of the agent, cardiac output, and minute ventilation.

Aromatic hydrocarbons are central nervous system (CNS) depressants and neurotoxins. CNS effects are similar to those seen in ethanol intoxication, except for the presence of hallucinations, more rapid onset, and shorter duration.[7] Euphoria results from depression (disinhibition) of higher cortical function. Although pharmacologic effects were believed to be due to alterations in membrane function, recent data suggest that binding to specific GABA and glutamate receptors may represent the mechanism of action.[3,6]

Aromatic hydrocarbons are myocardial irritants and depressants. They can sensitize the heart to the dysrhythmic effects of endogenous as well as exogenous catecholamines. Sudden sniffing death results from ventricular fibrillation.[2]

They are also respiratory tract, skin, and mucous membrane irritants. Exposure to very high vapor concentrations can lead to pulmonary edema. Ingestions may be accompanied by aspiration pneumonitis. Cresols and phenols are corrosives.

CLINICAL PRESENTATION

Patients may present with altered mental status, gastrointestinal (GI) complaints, respiratory symptoms, trauma, weakness, syncope, or cardiac arrest.[2,5,7,8,10,14,15,18] Early effects include euphoria, agitation, and hallucinations. Visual hallucinations are more common than auditory hallucinations. With increasing toxicity, depressant effects predominate, with manifestations progressing from slurred speech, ataxia, and impaired manual dexterity, response, speed, and coordination to delirium and coma. Inhalational abusers may have glazed eyes and a vacant expression, and they may appear drunk. Workers exposed to styrene may develop drowsiness, dizziness, nausea, and headache ("styrene sickness"). CNS effects usually last less than an hour after a single acute exposure.

Patients with VSA will usually not seek treatment in the emergency department (ED) unless there has been a complication. They are typically brought in by friends, relatives, ambulance, or police. Findings suggestive of VSA include glue or paint on the hands and face, solvent odor on the breath, and a "glue sniffer's rash" (erythematous spots around the nose and mouth).

The typical history in a patient with sudden sniffing death is sudden collapse occurring during a period of excited behavior or exertion (e.g., running) shortly after an acute inhalation.[2] Dysrhythmias have been reported during the use of phenols for removing skin wrinkles ("facial peels"). Toluene abuse has also been associated a myocardial infarction.[11]

Acute exposure to concentrated cresols and phenols can result in corneal, skin, and GI burns. All aromatics can cause an irritant dermatitis. Children with unintentional mothball ingestions rarely become symptomatic. In contrast, the ingestion of other aromatics is often accompanied by choking, cough, dyspnea, cyanosis, and other manifestations of pulmonary aspiration, along with nausea, vomiting, abdominal cramps, and diarrhea. Systemic effects may ensue.

Chronic inhalational abuse and occupational exposure may result in neurologic, cardiac, hematologic, and renal toxicity. Neurologic effects include cognitive impairment, encephalopathy, dementia, corticospinal tract dysfunction, oculomotor abnormalities, tremor, peripheral neuropathy, parkinsonism, and deafness.[8,10,19] Subjective symptoms include fatigability, irritability, memory difficulty, changes in personality or mood, and impaired intellectual function. Dilated cardiomyopathy has been reported.

Chronic exposure to benzene is associated with a number of hematologic effects, including leukemia, aplastic anemia and multiple myeloma. Other aromatic hydrocarbons have been reported to cause similar hematologic effects, but this is probably due to contamination with benzene. The oxidative metabolites of naphthalene, alpha-naphthalene and naphthol, can cause methemoglobinemia and hemolytic anemia. Infants and patients with G6PD are at increased risk. Chronic or massive exposure to *p*-dichlorobenzene can lead to aplastic anemia, renal dysfunction, and hepatotoxicity.

Chronic exposure to toluene can cause distal renal tubular acidosis (i.e., bicarbonate wasting), Goodpasture syndrome, formation of urinary calculi, and reversible renal failure.[14,15] Patients with renal tubular acidosis may present with diffuse weakness associated with hypokalemia and hypophosphatemia, often with accompanying rhabdomyolysis. Either a high-anion-gap metabolic acidosis or a hyperchloremic non-anion-gap acidosis may be seen. Toluene is oxidized to benzoic acid and conjugated with glycine to form hippuric acid, crystals of which may be seen on urinalysis. Chronic toluene abusers may also present with abdominal pain, vomiting, and dehydration. Toluene abuse during pregnancy has been associated with an embryopathy similar to that of fetal alcohol syndrome.[1,12,20]

Laboratory evaluation may reveal evidence of rhabdomyolysis, blood dyscrasias, normal or high-anion-gap metabolic acidosis, renal failure, and profound hypokalemia. The urine may turn brown following exposure to cresols and phenols.

DIFFERENTIAL DIAGNOSIS

The diagnosis of aromatic hydrocarbon intoxication is made on the basis of history and clinical findings. Laboratory studies may be supportive if abnormal. An ethanol level should be determined because of the similarity in clinical presentations. Patients may be mistakenly triaged for psychiatric evaluation. The differential diagnosis includes other causes of altered mental status and weakness, such as drug intoxication, trauma, infection, neurologic disorders, and metabolic abnormalities of other causes. Similar metabolic abnormalities may be seen in poisoning caused by salicylates, methanol, ethylene glycol, and ethanol (ketoacidosis). Toxicologic analysis of blood and urine may be necessary to exclude these possibilities.

EMERGENCY DEPARTMENT EVALUATION

The history should include the identity of the offending agent(s) and the details surrounding the exposure (e.g., amount, time, duration, intent). The physical examination should focus on the vital signs and neurologic and cardiorespiratory functions. A detailed mental status and neurologic examination should be performed. The presence or absence of muscle tenderness should be noted. Because intoxicated patients may not perceive pain, the history and physical must also address the possibility of occult trauma.

Ancillary evaluation should include oxygen saturation measurement or arterial blood gas analysis, a complete blood count, electrolytes, blood urea nitrogen, creatinine, glucose, creatinine phosphokinase, urinalysis (for pH, crystals, and myoglobin), and electrocardiogram. Liver function tests should also be obtained in patients with chronic exposures. A chest radiograph should be obtained in patients with respiratory symptoms or abnormal breath sounds. Symptomatic patients with ingestions of cresols and phenols should be evaluated for the presence of oral, esophageal, and GI burns (see Chapter 330). A computed tomography scan or magnetic resonance imaging of the head may be useful in patients with chronic exposures and neurologic complaints.[4,13]

EMERGENCY DEPARTMENT MANAGEMENT

In industrial or environmental accidents, prehospital personnel should not enter an area of potential exposure without adequate respiratory and skin protection.

Management of aromatic hydrocarbon intoxication is supportive. Advanced life-support measures should be instituted, as necessary. Activated charcoal, with or without antecedent gastric aspiration via nasogastric tube, is recommended for patients with recent ingestions. However, if signs and symptoms of corrosive ingestion are present (e.g., with cresols and phenols), aspiration alone is preferred. Seizures, cardiac dysrhythmias, and coma are managed with standard therapy. Epinephrine and beta agonists should be used with caution, as they could precipitate or worsen dysrhythmias. Patients with metabolic acidosis should be treated with intravenous sodium bicarbonate as an infusion, not as a bolus. Volume replacement with normal saline and potassium may be necessary. Rhabdomyolysis should be treated with fluids and, possibly, bicarbonate.

Patients with acute psychiatric symptoms should be reassured and observed in a calm, protective environment. Physical or pharmacologic restraint may be required.

DISPOSITION

Patients with syncope, coma, or dysrhythmias should be admitted to a monitored bed. Those with altered mental status or metabolic abnormalities that persist after 4 to 6 hours of ED observation and treatment should also be admitted.

A neurologist should be consulted for patients with persistently abnormal mental status or peripheral neuropathy. A nephrologist should be consulted for patients with rhabdomyolysis, metabolic abnormalities, or renal dysfunction. Patients with persistent psychiatric symptoms may be referred to a psychiatrist or detoxification center if they are otherwise healthy. Those with hematologic abnormalities should be referred to a hematologist.

Long-term follow-up is usually necessary in patients with chronic aromatic hydrocarbon exposure, particularly to benzene, which may cause leukemia. All patients should be advised to avoid reexposure. VSA patients should be referred for substance-abuse treatment.

COMMON PITFALLS

- Misdiagnosing aromatic hydrocarbon poisoning as psychiatric illness, alcohol intoxication, gastroenteritis, Guillain-Barré syndrome, or dehydration
- Failing to examine blood and urine for hematologic, metabolic, electrolyte, and renal function abnormalities
- Failing to refer patients for appropriate evaluation and follow-up
- Failing to warn patients that they should avoid reexposure and that sudden death may occur during solvent inhalation
- Failing to perform GI decontamination after ingestions for fear of causing aspiration
- Failing to monitor for cardiac dysrhythmias and for hypoxia

ACKNOWLEDGMENT

The author gratefully acknowledges the contribution of Kusum Saxena, who wrote the previous version of this chapter.

References

1. Arnold GL, Kirby RS, Langendoerfer S, et al. Toluene embryopathy: clinical delineation and developmental follow-up. *Pediatrics* 1994;93:216.
2. Bass M. Sudden sniffing death. *JAMA* 1970;212:2075.
3. Balster RL. Neural basis of inhalant abuse. *Drug Alcohol Depend* 1998;51:207.
4. Caldenmeyer KS, Armstrong SW, George KK, et al. The spectrum of neuroimaging abnormalities in solvent abuse and their clinical correlation. *J Neuroimaging* 1996;6:167.
5. Committee on Substance Abuse and Committee on Native American Child Health. Inhalant abuse. *Pediatrics* 1996;97:420.
6. Cruz SL, Mirshahi T, Thomas B, et al. Effects of the abused solvent toluene on recombinant N-methyl-D-aspartate and non-methyl-D-aspartate receptors expressed in Xenopus oocytes. *J Pharmacol Exp Ther* 1998;286:334.
7. Dinwiddie SH. Abuse of inhalants: a review. *Addiction* 1994;89:925.
8. Filley CM, Heaton RK, Rosenberg NL. White matter dementia in chronic toluene abuse. *Neurology* 1990;40:532.
9. Harwood HJ. Inhalants: a policy analysis of the problem in the United States. *NIDA Res Monogr* 1995;143:274.
10. Hormes J, Filley C, Rosenberg N. Neurologic sequelae of chronic solvent vapors abuse. *Neurology* 1986;36:698.
11. Hussain TF, Heidenreich PA, Benowitz N. Recurrent non-Q wave myocardial infarction associated with toluene abuse. *Am Heart J* 1996;3:615.
12. Jones HE, Balster RL. Inhalant abuse in pregnancy. *Obstet Gynecol Clin North Am* 1998;25:153.
13. Kamaran S, Bakshi R. MRI in chronic toluene abuse: low signal in the cerebral cortex on T2-weighted images. *Neuroradiology* 1998;40:519.
14. Linden CH. Volatile substances of abuse. *Emerg Med Clin North Am* 1990;8:559.
15. Meadows R, Verghese A. Medical complications of glue sniffing. *South Med J* 1996;89:455.
16. Neumark YD, Delva J, Anthony JC. The epidemiology of adolescent inhalant drug involvement. *Arch Pediatr Adolesc Med* 1998;152:781.
17. Spiller HA, Krenzelok EP. Epidemiology of inhalant abuse reported to two regional poison centers. *J Toxicol Clin Toxicol* 1997;35:167.
18. Streichen M, Gabow P, Moss A, et al. Syndromes of solvent sniffing in adults. *Arch Intern Med* 1981;94:758.
19. Uitti RJ, Snow BJ, Shinotoh H, et al. Parkinsonism induced by solvent abuse. *Ann Neurol* 1994;35:616.
20. Wilkins-Haug L. Teratogen update: toluene. *Teratology* 1997;55:145.

CHAPTER 317
Barbiturate Poisoning

Margaret M. McCarron

Barbiturates are barbituric acid derivatives that reversibly depress excitable tissues, particularly those of the central nervous system (CNS). The term *short-acting barbiturates* (SABs) includes the pharmacologic categories of short-acting (less than 3 hours) and intermediate-acting (3 to 8 hours) barbiturates, and distinguishing between the two has no clinical relevance in overdosage.[9,10] Barbiturates are available as tablets, capsules, or elixirs for oral use and as parenteral products for intravenous or intramuscular use.

SABs are sedative–hypnotic prescription drugs (Drug Enforcement Administration [DEA] schedule II) with elimination half-lives of usually less than 40 hours (Table 317.1). SABs used to be widely prescribed as sleeping pills and were the leading cause of coma from drug overdose. Although their abuse has markedly declined in recent years, SABs are still available on the street and remain popular with drug abusers. Most SAB overdoses are suicide attempts, but some are recreational. The usual route of intoxication is oral ingestion; rarely, tablets are dissolved in water and injected intravenously.[9]

Long-acting barbiturates (LABs) are anticonvulsant prescription drugs (DEA schedule IV) with elimination half-lives of usually more than 40 hours (see Table 317.1). Although LABs have sedative effects, they are used primarily to treat tonic, clonic, and partial seizures. Some intoxications occur because of excessive therapeutic dosage, but most are suicidal ingestions of phenobarbital, taken by epileptic patients or their family members. Most LABs have active metabolites: Mephobarbital is metabolized to phenobarbital (15%); primidone is metabolized to phenobarbital (15% to 25%) and phenylethylmalonamide (PEMA; 50% to 70%).

Barbiturates act by enhancing gamma-aminobutyric acid (GABA) inhibition in excitable tissues of the CNS, skeletal muscle, smooth muscle, and heart.[11,12] GABA increases chloride flow from the chloride channel to cell membranes, thereby inhibiting depolarization. In addition, phenobarbital decreases the paroxysmal firing of nerve cells by a mechanism that is unknown but different from GABA inhibition.

Barbiturates enhance the metabolism of many drugs by interacting with cytochrome P-450, which binds substrates of the hepatic microsomal drug-metabolizing enzyme system. Although phenobarbital is a strong inducer of cytochrome P-450, it does not induce its own metabolism and appears to have a longer half-life after chronic use.[19] Barbiturates also increase the production of delta-aminolevulinic acid, a precursor of porphobilinogen, and may precipitate an attack of acute intermittent porphyria in patients with porphyria. Ethanol and barbitu-

TABLE 317.1. Barbiturate Classification and Kinetic Data

Generic Name	U.S. Trade Name	pKa	Protein-Binding (%)	Volume of Distribution (L/kg)	Therapeutic Half-Life (h)
SHORT-ACTING BARBITURATES[a]					
Amobarbital	Amytal	7.9	59	0.9–1.4	15–40
Aprobarbital	Alurate	8.1	55–70	0.6–0.7	14–34
Butabarbital	Butisol	7.9	—	—	34–42
Pentobarbital	Nembutal	7.9	65	0.5–1.0	20–30
Secobarbital	Seconal	7.9	46–70	1.6–1.9	22–29
Talbutal	Lotusate	9.4	—	—	15
LONG-ACTING BARBITURATES					
Barbital[b]		7.8	25	0.4–0.6	48
Mephobarbital	Mebaral	7.8	40–60	2.6	48–52
Metharbital	Gemonil	8.5	—	—	—
Phenobarbital[c]		7.2	50	0.5–0.6	48–144
Primidone	Mysoline	—	0–20	0.5–1.0	6–22
PEMA[d]		—	0–20	—	24–48

[a] Other short-acting barbiturates include butalbital (found in analgesic-sedative preparations such as Esgic and Fiorinal) and hexobarbital (not available in United States).
[b] Metabolite of metharbital.
[c] Metabolite of mephobarbital and primidone.
[d] Phenylethylmalonamide, metabolite of primidone.

rates are synergistic: Coingestion of ethanol and an SAB significantly decreases the LD_{50} of the barbiturate in rats.

Chronic use of barbiturates leads to tolerance, physical dependence, and withdrawal symptoms.

The therapeutic effects of SABs—decreased motor activity (sedation), followed by induction of sleep (hypnosis)—occur at doses of 0.5 to 3.0 mg/kg, begin within 30 minutes, and last for 3 to 8 hours. Therapeutic serum concentrations are 6 to 14 μg/mL.[9]

The maximum recommended anticonvulsant loading dose of phenobarbital is 20 mg/kg; the sedative dose is much lower (30 to 60 mg). Maintenance anticonvulsant doses of LABs are 200 to 600 mg/d for mephobarbital, 100 to 800 mg/d for metharbital, 60 to 200 mg/d for phenobarbital, and 750 to 1000 mg/d for primidone. The therapeutic serum concentration of phenobarbital usually ranges from 15 to 40 μg/mL, but levels up to 50 μg/mL may be necessary to control seizures in some patients. Therapeutic serum levels are 5 to 12 μg/mL for primidone; concomitant metabolite levels average 10 to 20 μg/mL for phenobarbital and 15 μg/mL for PEMA. Therapeutic serum levels for other LABs are not well defined. They are less than 5 μg/mL for mephobarbital and metharbital, with concurrent barbital and phenobarbital metabolite concentrations of 10 to 30 μg/mL. Because their lipid solubility is lower than that of SABs, LABs accumulate more slowly in tissue, and peak effects may not be seen for several hours with therapeutic dosing. Their duration of action ranges from 6 to 24 hours after a single dose.

Barbiturates are well absorbed from the intestinal tract, except for mephobarbital, which is about 71% to 75% absorbed. Food in the stomach decreases the rate of absorption but not the total amount absorbed. Barbiturates are distributed to all tissues and body fluids and concentrate in the brain, liver, and kidneys. SABs are almost entirely metabolized in the liver to inactive metabolites that are excreted in the urine as glucuronides. However, 7.5% to 17.5% of a dose of aprobarbital is excreted unchanged in the urine over 4 days.[17]

Liver metabolism of barbital, phenobarbital, primidone, and PEMA is limited because of the lower lipid–water partition coefficients. Hence, urinary excretion accounts for 95% of barbital, 25% to 33% of phenobarbital, 15% to 42% of primidone, and 95% of PEMA elimination. In addition, phenobarbital undergoes enterohepatic recirculation, which contributes to its long half-life.

Because phenobarbital is a weak acid, it is markedly enhanced by alkalinization of the urine. Increasing the urine pH increases the fraction of ionized drug in the urine, and thus decreases the amount of un-ionized drug available for passive tubular reabsorption, a process known as *ion trapping*. With alkalinization of the urine, the renal clearance of phenobarbital may be increased up to ten times and its half-life shortened by one-half to two-thirds. Although not proven, alkalinization of the urine would be expected to have similar effects on LABs that are excreted unchanged in the urine. The elimination of phenobarbital is enhanced by multiple oral doses of activated charcoal.[3]

Although not studied, a similar effect on SAB elimination would be expected. The relatively low volume of distribution, protein binding, and lipid solubility of barbiturates makes them amenable to removal by extracorporeal techniques. Elimination half-lives for phenobarbital are roughly 30 to 60 hours with alkaline diuresis, 8 to 14 hours with hemodialysis, 6 to 8 hours with hemoperfusion, and 6 to 45 hours with multiple-dose activated charcoal.

The benzodiazepine antagonist CGS 846 has shown some antidotal activity against phenobarbital in animals.[11]

Barbiturate kinetics in overdosage are largely unknown. There is some evidence that SAB elimination is constant (zero-order) at high concentrations and exponential (first-order) at lower concentrations, indicating saturable (Michaelis-Menten) metabolism.[16]

Toxic effects of barbiturates result from intensification of GABA inhibition. The cerebral cortex and reticular activating system are affected first, producing generalized CNS depression. Skeletal muscle and smooth muscle of the gastrointestinal (GI) tract, urinary bladder, and uterus may lose their tone. Depressed tissue metabolism may result in hypothermia. As the intoxication intensifies, the respiratory and vasomotor centers in the brainstem become depressed. In severe overdoses, depressive effects may extend to cardiac muscle. Cardiac dysrhythmias are unusual, but congestive heart failure may occur.[9] Hypotension may result from vasodilatation, fluid loss, or low cardiac output. In most cases, hypotension is due to hypovolemia associated with arterial constriction and normal or low central venous pressure.[14]

For nonaddicts, the acute fatal oral dose of SABs is about 3 to 6 g. Barbiturate addicts may tolerate higher doses. One adult survived a reported ingestion of 20 g.[18] Serum SAB levels correlate with the severity of intoxication (Table 317.2). For a given level of consciousness, serum SAB concentrations are higher than those listed in addicted patients and lower in those who have coingested other CNS depressants or who have medical complications such as anoxia. The highest reported serum concentration with lack of significant toxicity occurred in an SAB addict, who was drowsy when his serum SAB level was 42 μg/mL.[9]

The acute fatal oral dose of phenobarbital is about 6 to 9 g in nonaddicted patients. As with SABs, addicts may tolerate larger doses. The correlation between LAB concentrations and level of consciousness has not been precisely defined. Coma (as defined in Table 317.2) may occur with therapeutic levels in patients not previously exposed to LABs who have coingested other CNS depressants (e.g., ethanol). In contrast, patients who chronically use or abuse LABs may have levels of 100 μg/mL without manifesting coma. The highest reported serum phenobarbital level with survival was 580 μg/mL in a patient who survived after hemodialysis and alkaline diuresis, during which 11.4 g of phenobarbital was recovered in the dialysis fluid and urine.[5]

Some patients, especially the elderly, become excited, depressed, and confused after taking relatively small doses of barbiturates. Patients with hypothyroidism, myasthenia gravis, or impaired cardiac, renal, or respiratory function are sensitive to the effects of barbiturates. Except for phenobarbital and primidone, quantitative serum barbiturate measurements may not be routinely available.

CLINICAL PRESENTATION

The diagnostic signs are CNS depression, decreased motor activity, and some degree of hypothermia. About 40% of patients who present with severe toxicity have aspiration pneumonia.[9] One report described a patient who presented with shallow respirations, no obtainable pulse or blood pressure, and a rectal temperature of 69.8°F (21.0°C) after ingesting 3 g phenobarbital; his serum SAB was 27 μg/mL.[8] He recovered after peritoneal dialysis with warm fluids. Urinary retention and GI atony with acute gastric dilatation may occur. Patients with SAB intoxication may initially have a high output of almost colorless (dilute) urine. In severe cases, coma with apnea and hypotension may be present. "Barbiturate burns"—erythematous areas over pressure points that blister and heal with a black eschar—may be seen in deeply comatose patients.[1] Complications include rhabdomyolysis and renal failure. Permanent brain damage and multiple organ failure may result from anoxia. Nonocclusive intestinal infarction requiring ileostomy has been reported during phenobarbital coma.[13] Inadvertent intraarterial injection of barbiturates may result in arterial spasm and tissue necrosis.[7]

Common laboratory abnormalities include hypoglycemia and electrolyte disturbances. Alterations in acid–base and fluid balance may be present. A chest radiograph may show aspiration pneumonia or pulmonary edema. The electrocardiogram (ECG) is usually normal. The electroencephalogram (EEG) shows diffuse slowing during barbiturate-induced coma. Three patients with isoelectric EEGs had complete recovery of cerebral function.[6,15]

In SAB overdose, symptoms usually begin less than an hour after ingestion, and toxicity is usually well established by 4 to 6 hours. In LAB overdose, initial symptoms appear within an hour or two of ingestion, but toxicity may not peak for more than 10 hours.

The severity of barbiturate poisoning is judged by the degree of CNS depression and the vital signs (see Table 317.2). Expected serum SAB concentrations at the seven states of intoxication in Table 317.2 apply to patients who have taken only SABs, have no medical complications that would affect the level of consciousness, and are not addicted to barbiturates. Patients with multiple drug ingestions or medical complications such as anoxia have lower serum levels. Patients addicted to the drug have higher serum levels.

The usual clinical course for patients with drowsiness to stage 3 coma is gradual improvement within a day or two for SABs and recovery in 3 to 7 days for LABs. For patients with stage 4 coma from SAB or LAB, intractable shock and adult respiratory distress syndrome or other pulmonary complications may lead to death.

DIFFERENTIAL DIAGNOSIS

A similar clinical picture may be produced by overdosage of other sedative–hypnotics, benzodiazepines, alcohol, narcotics, clonidine, phenothiazines, or carbon monoxide, and, sometimes, phencyclidine, cyclic antidepressants, or methyl bromide.

TABLE 317.2. USC Coma Scale and Short-Acting Barbiturate Serum Concentrations

Stage	Definition	Serum Level (μg/mL)
Alert	No signs of CNS depression	6
Drowsy	All degrees of CNS depression between alert and stupor	8 ± 2
Stupor	Markedly sedated; responds but does not awaken to verbal or tactile stimuli	14 ± 3
Coma—1	Responsive to painful stimuli but not to verbal or tactile stimuli, with no disturbances in respiration or blood pressure	18 ± 2
Coma—2	Unconscious, not responsive to painful stimuli, with no disturbances in respiration or blood pressure	22 ± 2
Coma—3	Unresponsive, or abnormally responsive to painful stimuli, with spontaneous respirations that are slow, shallow, or rapid, or with low but adequate blood pressure, or both	26 ± 2
Coma—4	Unresponsive, or abnormally responsive to painful stimuli, with apnea or inadequate respirations, inadequate blood pressure, or both	34 ± 6

Drug-induced coma must be differentiated from hypoglycemia and other medical causes, head trauma, cerebrovascular insults, and CNS infections.

EMERGENCY DEPARTMENT EVALUATION

The history includes the identity of the drug, time of ingestion, treatment at the scene, known medical or psychiatric illnesses, and current drug therapy, especially use of sleeping pills or treatment for epilepsy. The physical examination focuses on the vital signs, including rectal temperature. The classification of coma includes vital signs, eye opening, best verbal response, best motor response, muscle tone, and deep tendon and central reflexes, such as gag, eyelash, corneal, and oculocephalic reaction. The skin is examined for redness or blisters over pressure points. A succussion splash elicited in the left upper quadrant is a sign of acute gastric dilatation; absent bowel sounds signify GI atony. Suprapubic percussion may reveal a distended urinary bladder.

Routine laboratory tests should include a complete blood count; determination of serum levels of electrolytes, blood urea nitrogen, creatinine, and glucose; and urinalysis. Serum alcohol and barbiturate concentrations should be quantified, if possible. If the history is unobtainable or unreliable, full toxicology screening should be done. Stuporous or comatose patients should have a chest radiograph, ECG, and arterial blood gas and serum chemistry analyses, including liver function tests and muscle enzymes. Patients in stage 3 or 4 coma and those with focal neurologic findings should have a computed tomography scan of the head to rule out cerebral edema and structural causes of coma. A lumbar puncture may be necessary to rule out meningitis.

EMERGENCY DEPARTMENT MANAGEMENT

The treatment of acute barbiturate poisoning is primarily supportive, including an intravenous line, administration of oxygen, cardiac monitoring, intubation, and mechanical ventilation, as necessary. Patients with CNS depression are given intravenous glucose and naloxone. For patients with significant hypotension, assessment of the central venous or pulmonary artery and pulmonary capillary (wedge) pressure is necessary. Those with normal or low pressures and no evidence of pulmonary edema require fluid resuscitation. Fluid administration in patients in stage 3 or 4 coma should be carefully monitored by a Swan-Ganz catheter. Patients with cardiogenic pulmonary edema, high central venous or pulmonary artery pressure, or adult respiratory distress syndrome are treated with dobutamine or dopamine. Furosemide may be given slowly intravenously in small doses (20 to 60 mg). The goal of therapy is to maintain a systolic pressure of 90 mm Hg with adequate tissue perfusion. Mild or moderate hypothermia is treated with blankets to prevent further heat loss; core rewarming is necessary for severe hypothermia.

After resuscitation and stabilization, all patients should undergo GI decontamination. Activated charcoal absorbs barbiturates quite well; repeated oral doses of activated charcoal are recommended for all stuporous and comatose patients with bowel sounds.

In LAB intoxication, the urine should be alkalinized in the absence of renal failure and cerebral or pulmonary edema. Therapy should not be started until fluid and acid–base balances have been restored. One method for alkalinizing the urine is to add 1.5 mEq/kg sodium bicarbonate to 1 L dextrose 5% in 0.45% sodium chloride solution and infuse it at a rate of 200 to 250 mL/h until a urine pH of 7.5 to 8.0 and a volume of 100 to 150 mL/h are attained. If the urine pH has not increased sufficiently after 4 hours, additional doses of bicarbonate in increments of 0.5 mEq/kg may be needed. Treatment continues until the patient regains consciousness.

In addition to vital signs and the cardiovascular measurements noted, the amount of fluid given, urine output, acid–base balance, and oxygenation status must be carefully monitored to prevent fluid overload and alkalosis. These parameters should initially be checked hourly.

Alkalinization of the urine is not indicated for SAB intoxication, because SABs are not significantly excreted in the urine as active drugs.

A major controversy in the treatment of barbiturate intoxication concerns the use of hemoperfusion or hemodialysis. Many experts advocate extracorporeal drug removal only when the patient has failed to respond to supportive measures. Because mortality in comatose patients is related to the presence of apnea, shock, hypothermia, pulmonary complications, and the duration of coma,[20] I recommend charcoal or resin hemoperfusion for patients in stage 4 coma with high serum concentrations of either SABs or LABs, and for patients with lesser degrees of coma from LAB toxicity, to shorten the duration of coma. Patients treated with hemoperfusion are usually conscious at the end of the procedure, and rebound toxicity is not expected.[4]

If the patient has pulmonary edema, renal failure, or severe electrolyte imbalance, hemodialysis may be a better choice, although it is not as effective as hemoperfusion in removing barbiturates. Peritoneal dialysis is not as effective as hemodialysis or hemoperfusion.[2]

Serial barbiturate levels should be obtained to assess the efficacy of all forms of therapy.

DISPOSITION

A regional poison control center or toxicologist should be consulted if the treating physician is not completely familiar with the management of barbiturate intoxication. Nephrology consultation should be obtained when hemodialysis or hemoperfusion is being considered. Psychiatric consultation is required for all suspected suicide attempts as soon as the patient is alert enough to be interviewed.

Awake patients who have ingested SABs may be observed for 4 to 6 hours and then discharged if symptoms are mild and the serum barbiturate level is low. For patients who have ingested LABs, the observation period should be 10 hours. Barbiturate levels should be repeated before discharge to ensure they are not increasing. All stuporous or comatose patients should be admitted to an intensive care unit.

Patients who require intensive care monitoring or hemoperfusion may need to be transferred if such facilities are unavailable. A patient should not be transferred until advanced life-support measures have been instituted and GI decontamination has been performed.

COMMON PITFALLS

- Failing to consider head trauma and barbiturate withdrawal in patients with seizures
- Misinterpreting an isoelectric EEG as evidence of brain death if the patient has very high serum levels of barbiturates
- Failing to perform GI decontamination, regardless of the time of ingestion. Pills can remain in an atonic stomach for many hours.

- Failing to use crystalloids to treat hypotension initially if the patient has normal or low central venous pressure. Vasoconstriction associated with shock may be aggravated by administering dopamine or norepinephrine.
- Failing to monitor fluid and acid–base balances and respiratory status scrupulously during therapy to avoid iatrogenic complications
- Failing to treat patients with LAB overdose with alkaline diuresis and multiple-dose activated charcoal
- Failing to consider extracorporeal drug removal in patients with severe poisoning

References

1. Beveridge GW, Lawson AAH. Occurrence of bullous lesions in acute barbiturate intoxication. *BMJ* 1965;1:835.
2. Bloomer HA. Limited usefulness of alkaline diuresis and peritoneal dialysis in pentobarbital intoxication. *N Engl J Med* 1965;272:1309.
3. Boldy DAR, Vale JA, Prescott LF. Treatment of phenobarbitone poisoning with repeated oral administration of activated charcoal. *Q J Med* 1986;235:997.
4. Jacobson D, Wiik-Lassen E, Dahl T, et al. Pharmacokinetic evaluation of haemoperfusion in phenobarbital poisoning. *Eur J Pharmacol* 1984;26:109.
5. Kennedy AC, Briggs JD, Young N, et al. Successful treatment of three cases of very severe barbiturate poisoning. *Lancet* 1969;1:995.
6. Kirshbaum RJ, Carollo VJ. Reversible isoelectric EEG in barbiturate coma. *JAMA* 1970;212:1215.
7. Klatte EC, Brooks AL, Rhamy RK. Toxicity of intra-arterial barbiturates and tranquilizing drugs. *Radiology* 1969;92:700.
8. Lash RF, Burdette JA, Ozdil T. Accidental profound hypothermia and barbiturate intoxication. *JAMA* 1967;201:123.
9. McCarron MM, Schulze BW, Walberg CB, et al. Short-acting barbiturate overdosage—correlation of intoxication score with serum barbiturate concentration. JAMA 1982;248:55.
10. Mark LC. Archaic classification of barbiturates. *Clin Pharmacol Ther* 1969;10:287.
11. Mendelson WB, Davis T, Paul SM, et al. Do benzodiazepine receptors mediate the anticonflict actions of pentobarbital? *Life Sci* 1983;32:2241.
12. Olsen RW. GABA-benzodiazepine-barbiturate receptor interactions. *J Neurochem* 1981;37:1.
13. Olson KR, Pond SM, Verrier ED, et al. Intestinal infarction complicating phenobarbital overdose. *Arch Intern Med* 1984;144:407.
14. Shubin H, Weil MH. Shock associated with barbiturate intoxication. In: Matthew H, ed. *Acute barbiturate poisoning*. Amsterdam: Excerpta Medica, 1971.
15. Silverman D. Cerebral death and the EEG; report of the Ad Hoc Committee of the American Electroencephalogram Society on EEG criteria for determination of cerebral death. *JAMA* 1969;209:1505.
16. Sumner DJ, Kalk J, Whiting B. Metabolism of barbiturate after overdosage. *BMJ* 1975;1:335.
17. Svendsen AB, Brockmann-Hanssen E. Gas chromatography of barbiturates. II. Application of the study of their metabolism and excretion in humans. *J Pharmacol Sci* 1962;51:494.
18. Terplan M, Unger AM. Survival following massive barbiturate ingestion. *JAMA* 1966;198:322.
19. Viswanathen CT, Booker HE, Welling PG. Pharmacokinetics of phenobarbital following single and repeated doses. *J Clin Pharmacol* 1979;19:282.
20. Wagner DP, Knaus WA, Draper EA. Physiologic abnormalities and outcome from acute disease—evidence for a predictable relationship. *Arch Intern Med* 1986;146:1389.

CHAPTER 318
Arsenic and Mercury Poisoning

Jay L. Schauben

Arsenic is found in rodenticides, insecticides, herbicides, paints, veterinary medicinals, and folk remedies. It is also present in drinking water and seafood and is used in the production of glass and metals (e.g., computer chips). An estimated 1.5 million exposures to arsenic occur each year. It is the most common cause of acute heavy-metal poisoning and is second only to lead as a cause of chronic intoxication. Arsine gas is formed when arsenic compounds interact with acids.

Arsenic most commonly exists in trivalent (arsenite) and pentavalent (arsenate) forms. The average dietary intake is about 2 mg/d in adults. The trivalent form exhibits rapid gastrointestinal (GI) absorption, with more than 80% of the ingested dose absorbed. The pentavalent form is even more readily absorbed. Blood arsenic levels may be as high as 60 μg/L in normal people, with urine arsenic concentrations ranging from 10 to 300 μg/L. A seafood dinner can transiently elevate arsenic urine levels to 20 to 1,700 μg/L.

Arsenic is an intracellular toxin that appears to act by combining with sulfhydryl groups of enzymes and proteins involved in the Krebs cycle, thereby interfering with oxidative phosphorylation processes. It has also been postulated that arsenic is capable of substituting itself for the phosphate moiety in many cellular reactions, resulting in the loss of high-energy bonds. The pentavalent form appears less toxic than the trivalent form but may be converted to it at the cellular level. An acute dose of 100 to 200 mg is potentially fatal, whereas larger cumulative doses can be tolerated when exposure is chronic.

In poisoned patients, blood arsenic levels usually exceed 100 μg/L, with urine concentrations ranging from several hundred to several thousand micrograms per liter. Arsenic levels tend to remain elevated with chronic exposure but decrease rapidly over a period of several days after acute exposure.

The major route of arsenic elimination is renal excretion, with small amounts excreted in bile, feces, and saliva. The elimination curve is biphasic, apparently because of protein binding and redistribution of arsenic into the extravascular compartment.

Mercury was used as a folk remedy for GI problems, an antiseptic, an antisyphilitic, an unguent, a purgative, and a cure for adynamic ileus during the latter half of the nineteenth century. It is still used medically in dental amalgam and as a germicide, bactericide, diuretic, and laxative. In industry, it is used as a chemical intermediate, in the manufacture of electrical apparatus, and as an antifouling agent, a paint pigment, an instrument fluid, a fungicide, and a catalyst in the production of plastics and paper.

Mercury is found in elemental, inorganic, and organic forms. Toxic effects vary considerably with the chemical form of the metal, as well as the duration and intensity of exposure. There is evidence that *in vivo* conversion exists between the various forms of the metal, and that these forms may accumulate in tissue by binding to proteins. Mercury crosses the placenta and can be secreted into breast milk. Normal blood mercury levels may be 20 μg/L or higher as a result of its presence in dietary fish. Urine concentrations are normally less than 50 μg/L.

Elemental mercury exposure commonly results from the accidental ingestion of the contents of a broken thermometer (0.1 mL), suicidal ingestion, rupture of mercury-containing balloons used for GI procedures, inhalation of mercury vapor, or intravenous or subcutaneous injection.[18] Although mercury is present in dental amalgam, there is little evidence that mercury-containing restorations are hazardous to health.[4,17] Elemental mercury volatilizes slowly at room temperature (more rapidly with heat), producing mercury vapor that is absorbed through the lungs. It is poorly absorbed from the GI tract but may be absorbed through the skin if applied in a suitable vehicle. The solubility of the lipophilic elemental form, and therefore its potential to cause toxicity, depends on its oxidation to the mercuric ion. This conversion is enhanced with exposure to heat, acids, and strong oxidants. As is true of arsenic, the ionic form of mercury combines with the sulfhydryl groups of various proteins, leading to the inhibition of enzyme systems. Excretion is primarily through the urine and feces, with a half-life of up to 60 days. What constitutes a toxic dose is poorly defined.

In general, bivalent inorganic mercuric salts (e.g., sulfide, chloride, and oxide) are more soluble and more toxic than monovalent ones (e.g., mercurous chloride or calomel). They are irritating, occasionally producing dermatitis with or without vesication, discoloration of the nails, and burns of mucous membranes. The potentially fatal acute oral dose is about 100 mg. Percutaneous absorption can also result in systemic toxicity.[20] Once absorbed, inorganic salts are converted to the mercuric form and are concentrated in the kidneys. They do not penetrate the blood–brain barrier to any significant extent, consistent with its limited CNS effects. Excretion is mainly through the urine and feces, with a half-life of about 40 days.

Exposure to organic mercury compounds (merbromin, Merthiolate, thimerosal, methylmercury, ethylmercury, and phenylmercuric salts) is most often due to the ingestion of contaminated fish, shellfish, or grain and to the inhalation of vaporized organomercurials. Consumption of seafood from Minamata Bay, which contained high levels of methylmercury, resulted in an outbreak of chronic organic mercury poisoning (Minamata disease). Mass poisoning has also resulted from the ingestion of grain treated with methylmercury fungicide. Organic forms of mercury are well absorbed by the GI and respiratory tracts, but the potential for dermal absorption appears low.

Alkyl mercury compounds (e.g., methyl and ethylmercury) are highly lipid-soluble, become distributed widely throughout the body, become concentrated in the blood and central nervous system (CNS), and easily pass the placental barrier. Long-chain aryl and alkyl compounds (e.g., phenyl and methoxyethyl mercury) are converted *in vivo* to the inorganic form. The shorter chain alkyl agents undergo enterohepatic recirculation, with final excretion in the feces and a half-life approaching 70 days. The potentially fatal acute oral dose of organic mercurials is about 1 g.

CLINICAL PRESENTATION

Manifestations of acute arsenic poisoning begin 30 minutes to 2 hours after ingestion and usually consist of violent gastroenteritis, with vomiting, profuse diarrhea, colicky abdominal pain, and, in severe cases, GI hemorrhage. Rapidly progressive toxicity, with hypotension, renal failure, Q-T prolongation with ventricular dysrhythmias (e.g., torsades de pointes), rhabdomyolysis, and CNS depression may occur.[2] Severe, generalized capillary damage can lead to massive third-spacing, resulting in cardiovascular collapse, adult respiratory distress syndrome, and massive proteinuria.

Delayed neurologic, dermatologic, and hematologic effects can occur after acute arsenic poisoning and are similar to the manifestations of chronic intoxication. Symmetric polyneuropathy, involving both sensory and motor nerve fibers, is common. Symptoms can resemble those of the Landry-Guillain-Barré syndrome.[7] Histologic studies demonstrate axonal degeneration of large myelinated fibers. However, recent evidence supports a demyelinating polyradiculopathy, evolving to an axonal degeneration neuropathy.[15] Recovery is slow (as long as 6 years) and often incomplete. An encephalopathy resembling Wernicke's or one characterized by prominent disinterest and anosognosia of peripheral neurologic deficits can be seen. Dermatologic manifestations may include diffuse exfoliative dermatitis, palmar hyperkeratosis, and Mees lines (transverse white bands on the nails). Normochromic, normocytic anemia, leukopenia, and thrombocytopenia may develop. Chronic exposure may also cause edema, sore throat, stomatitis, pruritus, coryza, alopecia, lacrimation, salivation, weakness, and restrictive or obstructive lung disease.[13]

Symptoms of arsine gas inhalation include abdominal pain, headache, weakness, malaise, nausea, and vomiting. Laboratory manifestations include hemolysis, renal failure, hyperkalemia, and anemia. These findings may be delayed up to 24 hours after milder exposures.

Elemental mercury is relatively nontoxic when ingested, due to poor GI absorption and slow oxidation to a more absorbable form. The oral LD_{10} for humans has been reported to be in the range of 1,429 mg/kg, or about 100 g in a 70-kg adult.[20] With ileus or leakage of mercury into the peritoneal cavity, mercuric oxide or sulfide salts may form, be absorbed, and cause systemic inorganic mercury poisoning. Without an ileus or GI perforation, systemic absorption is unlikely, and the elemental mercury usually passes uneventfully per rectum.

Aspiration of elemental mercury into the lungs can cause acute respiratory distress, pneumonitis, hemoptysis, cyanosis, tachycardia, hypotension, hematuria, and bloody diarrhea. This type of exposure may also lead to chronic respiratory and systemic problems.[11]

Intravenous injection of elemental mercury has caused abscess and granuloma formation at the injection site, hemoptysis, pulmonary embolization of mercury with consequent pulmonary dysfunction, and elevated blood and urine mercury levels.[18] Systemic manifestations include weeping dermatitis, leukopenia, anemia, diarrhea, salivation, liver damage, and kidney damage. Subcutaneous injection has also caused local inflammation, abscess and granuloma formation, and elevated mercury concentrations.[14]

Exposure to elemental mercury within a confined space may cause toxicity as a result of inhalation of fumes. Heat and oxidative processes accelerate the formation of mercury vapor (mercuric oxide). Symptoms usually begin within a few hours of exposure and include cough, dyspnea, chills, fever, weakness, salivation, nausea, vomiting, diarrhea, and a metallic taste. Respiratory symptoms may subside or progress to interstitial pneumonitis with patchy bilateral infiltrates, pulmonary edema, atelectasis, pneumothorax, necrotizing bronchiolitis, and, possibly, death. Systemic effects similar to those of inorganic mercury poisoning and CNS depression can occur. Fumes can also cause skin and mucous membrane irritation, with manifestations similar to the mucocutaneous lymph node syndrome (Kawasaki disease).[1]

Chronic exposure to mercury vapor can result in mild-to-moderate CNS dysfunction, including increased irritability, emotional instability, memory loss, and insomnia.[17] GI complaints, renal failure, chronic pneumonitis, constriction of visual fields, discoloration of the lens capsule, dermatitis, anorexia, and tremor may also be present. Hyperthyroidism and autonomic findings similar to those seen with pheochromocytoma have been described.[10,14] Findings typically associated with chronic inorganic mercury poisoning (acrodynia) have also been reported.

Acute exposure to the inorganic mercury salts may cause tachycardia, hypotension or hypertension, and sudden cardiovascular collapse. The corrosive nature of such salts often causes nausea, vomiting, abdominal pain, bloody diarrhea, edema, and necrosis of the GI tract. Symptoms may progress over 1 to 3 days to include mercurial stomatitis (glossitis and ulcerative gingivitis), loosening of teeth, jaw necrosis, proximal renal tubular necrosis resulting in transient polyuria, albuminuria, cylindruria, hematuria, anuria, and acidosis.[20] Hepatic necrosis can also occur.

Chronic exposure to inorganic mercury salts may result in acrodynia ("pink disease"). Originally reported in children exposed to elemental mercury or teething powders containing calomel, it is characterized by redness of the palms and soles, edema of the hands and feet, rashes, diaphoresis, tachycardia, hypertension, photophobia, irritability, and anorexia.

Poisoning by organic mercurials is usually much more insidious than that which results from inorganic mercury. Symptoms may not occur for as long as several weeks after exposure. Nausea, vomiting, diarrhea, and abdominal pain are common GI complaints. Phenylmercury (and other aryl compounds), however, can cause acute malaise and myalgias, and the alkylmercurials (methylmercury and ethylmercury) are irritating to skin and mucous membranes, possibly resulting in burns and dermatitis. Neurologic effects range from paresthesias, confusion, hallucinosis, irritability, sleep disturbances, ataxia, memory loss, slurred speech, auditory defects, narrowing of the visual fields, emotional instability, and inability to concentrate to stupor, coma, and death. Chronic exposure to organic mercurials can result in similar neurotoxicity.

DIFFERENTIAL DIAGNOSIS

Arsenic or mercury poisoning should be suspected in patients with acute or chronic GI and neurologic symptoms and multiple organ dysfunction of unknown etiology. Similar GI symptoms may be caused by viral or bacterial pathogens or the ingestion of other heavy metals (e.g., iron, thallium), food-borne toxins, and a variety of plants, mushrooms, and toxic agents (e.g., theophylline, ricin, abrin, cholinergics, corrosives, lithium, laxatives, alcohol, hydrocarbons, and fluoride). Solvents, hydrocarbons, other heavy metals, alcohol, and vitamins, as well as the possibility of organic disease, should be considered in the differential diagnosis of neurotoxicity. Multiple organ failure can occur after the ingestion of antimetabolites, colchicine, or other heavy metals and exposure to carbon monoxide or cyanide.

EMERGENCY DEPARTMENT EVALUATION

The history should include identification of the product and the route, dose, and duration of exposure. For ingestions, the physical examination should focus on vital signs, assessment of hydration, the abdomen, the cardiovascular system, and neurologic function. The mucosa should be checked for corrosive injury, and airway patency should be confirmed. For mercury inhalation or injection, the examination should also focus on respiratory function.

Ancillary studies include cardiac monitoring, electrocardiogram, chest radiograph, abdominal radiographs (for ingestions), and routine blood work (oxygen saturation or arterial blood gas analysis; complete blood count; serum levels of electrolytes, blood urea nitrogen, creatinine, and glucose; liver function tests; prothrombin time; partial thromboplastin time; creatine phosphokinase; and urinalysis). Blood and 24-hour urine arsenic or mercury levels (with or without chelation, depending on the presence or absence of acute symptoms) should be obtained.

EMERGENCY DEPARTMENT MANAGEMENT

Advanced life-support measures are instituted, as necessary. Patients with acute ingestions of arsenic or inorganic mercury salts and those with arsine gas inhalation commonly require aggressive intravenous fluid resuscitation. Maintenance fluids should be sufficient to sustain a brisk urine output. Central venous pressure monitoring and bladder catheterization with urine-output monitoring may be necessary. Exposure to elemental mercury fumes may necessitate endotracheal intubation.

For acute ingestions of arsenic and inorganic or organic mercurials, gastric aspiration and lavage are preferred initial methods of GI decontamination, with consideration given to the corrosive effects of the inorganic mercury salts. Activated charcoal should also be given for arsenic and inorganic mercury salt ingestions, and continued until charcoal stool is noted. Whole-bowel irrigation should also be considered for large ingestions or cases in which abdominal radiographs show the persistent presence of radiopaque material in the GI tract. In patients with progressive toxicity and persistent metal present on x-ray despite these interventions, endoscopic or surgical removal may be warranted. GI decontamination is not recommended for acute elemental mercury ingestion or chronic exposures. The patient exposed to arsine gas should have dermal decontamination.

Chelation therapy is warranted in acutely symptomatic patients and possibly in asymptomatic patients who present to the emergency department early after a significant exposure to arsenic and inorganic or aryl mercury compounds. Dimercaprol (BAL in peanut oil) should be initiated with an intramuscular loading dose of 3 to 5 mg/kg and followed by doses of 2.5 to 3.0 mg/kg every 4 to 6 hours during the first 2 days, then every 8 to 12 hours thereafter. If the integrity and function of the gut are intact, D-penicillamine (Cuprimine) or succimer (dimercaptosuccinic acid [DMSA]; Chemet), both oral chelators, may also be given. The dose of D-penicillamine is 100 mg/kg/d (maximum, 2 g/d) in four divided doses, and that of succimer is 10 mg/kg every 8 hours for 5 days, and then the same dose every 12 hours. Some investigators have advocated an optimal adult succimer dose of 30 mg/kg/d for 5 days.[3,5,9] The duration of the initial chelation course varies, depending on the severity of the exposure. A 5- to 7-day course may be adequate in mild intoxications, but it seems prudent with severe exposures to continue the initial course for 10 to 14 days. Thereafter, 24-hour urine arsenic levels should be followed, with repeat 5- to 14-day courses of chelation therapy prescribed until the 24-hour urine arsenic or mercury level falls below 50 μg/L. Courses of therapy should be interrupted by a 5- to 10-day abstinence period to allow for redistribution of arsenic from peripheral tissues into the blood and more effective subsequent chelation.

Hemolysis caused by arsine gas exposure is usually not responsive to dimercaprol therapy, but exchange transfusion or blood replacement may help. Alkalinization of the urine may benefit patients with significant rhabdomyolysis and hemoglobinuria. The use of chelation therapy in organic and elemental mercury poisoning is controversial, although succimer has shown some promise in the treatment of elemental mercury exposures.

D-penicillamine or succimer therapy is also indicated for asymptomatic patients with an elevated arsenic or mercury body burden (as indicated by blood and urine levels) or for patients exhibiting very mild symptoms who can be treated on an outpatient basis. They may be given in the same dosages described previously. The course may be repeated on the basis of the measurement of urine arsenic or mercury excretion after a 10- to 14-day abstinence period. With prolonged D-penicillamine treatment courses, some authorities have recommended decreasing the dosage to 35 mg/kg/d. Dimercaprol should be used instead of D-penicillamine if the latter cannot be taken orally, if significant renal impairment is evident, or if the patient is allergic to penicillin or succimer.

Dimercaprol can cause a dose-dependent rise in blood pressure accompanied by tachycardia. Other adverse reactions include pain at the injection site, urticaria, hyperpyrexia, CNS stimulation, headache, nausea, vomiting, conjunctivitis, a burning sensation around the mouth and throat, blepharospasm, and diaphoresis. Because dimercaprol undergoes biliary excretion, it can be used in patients with renal impairment.

D-penicillamine administration has been associated with generalized pruritus, fever, rash, leukopenia, eosinophilia, thrombocytopenia, and other symptoms consistent with penicillin allergy. Nausea, vomiting, diarrhea, nephrotoxic reactions, bone marrow suppression, and a pyridoxine-responsive optic neuritis have also been reported. Due to the possibility of cross-reactivity, D-penicillamine should be avoided in patients with a documented penicillin allergy. It should not be used in renal failure unless concurrent hemodialysis is planned. Complete blood count and renal function should be monitored during therapy.

Although succimer is approved by the Food and Drug Administration (FDA) only for the treatment of lead poisoning in children, it is now advocated for the management of mercury or arsenic toxicity in children or adults.[3,5,8,9,16] Succimer has the advantage of being relatively nontoxic. GI complaints are among the most common adverse effects. Mild and transient elevations in serum transaminase levels have been reported, so it is prudent to monitor liver function tests during therapy. Thrombocytosis, eosinophilia, and dysrhythmias occur infrequently. Pharyngitis, rhinorrhea, nasal congestion, rash, and mucocutaneous eruptions have also been reported. Because it is primarily eliminated in the urine, it should be used with caution in patients with renal impairment.

N-acetyl-D, L-penicillamine, an investigational oral chelator, appears to be more specific for chelating mercury than is D-penicillamine. It has been effective in reversing neurotoxicity due to chronic elemental and inorganic mercury exposures.[12] The dosage regimen is similar to that for D-penicillamine: Adults receive 250 to 500 mg four times a day (children, 30 mg/kg/d) for 6 to 10 days.

Dimercaptopropane sulfonate (DMPS) is an effective chelator of arsenic, elemental mercury, and inorganic mercurial salts. It is used in Europe and is also available (without FDA approval) in the United States. It can be given by a variety of parenteral routes (intravenous, intramuscular, subcutaneous) as well as orally. For chronic arsenic chelation, an oral regimen of 100 mg, administered three times a day for 3 weeks, has been used for up to 9 months. For the management of mercury exposures, 5 mg/kg of a 5% solution has been administered intramuscularly or subcutaneously three to four times within the first 24 hours, two to three times a day on day 2, and then one to two administrations daily on subsequent days.

N-acetylcysteine has also shown some promise in the treatment of arsenic and inorganic mercury salt exposures.[6,19] It could be used in the same doses as for acetaminophen poisoning. Limited experience suggests that hemodialysis (in conjunction with chelation therapy) performed within the first 24 hours of acute arsenic or mercury poisoning may remove a significant percentage of the ingested toxin before distribution into tissues, possibly averting, or at least minimizing, the toxic effects. It is ineffective later in the course, when there is relatively little metal in the blood. Hemodialysis is, however, indicated for the removal of chelated mercury or arsenic when renal dysfunction impairs its clearance.

DISPOSITION

Patients with acute poisoning after ingesting inorganic arsenic or mercury salts and long-chain aryl organic mercurials, or inhaling arsine or elemental mercury should be admitted. Patients with significant chronic toxicity should also be admitted for initial therapy. The level of care (intensive care unit or floor bed) should be dictated by the clinical presentation. The asymptomatic patient should be observed for 6 to 8 hours before discharge, with arrangements made for next-day follow-up. Patients who present with asymptomatic exposures or mild-to-moderate chronic toxicity may be treated as outpatients.

Consultation with a regional poison control center or a clinical toxicologist and a nephrologist should be part of the treatment plan. Although chelation therapy is not technically difficult, the details of treatment must be individualized, and optimal management requires the guidance of an experienced consultant. If antidotes and experts are not available locally, transfer of the patient to a tertiary care facility may be necessary. Patients with intentional exposures require psychiatric evaluation prior to discharge.

COMMON PITFALLS

- Failure to consider the possibility of acute arsenic or mercury poisoning in patients with intense abdominal pain and violent gastroenteritis of unknown cause
- Failure to appreciate that acute poisoning by inorganic arsenic or mercury salts can be rapidly progressive and that cardiovascular collapse may ensue if vigorous fluid resuscitation is not undertaken
- Failure to appreciate that the effects of mercury vary considerably with the form of the metal and the route, duration, and intensity of the exposure
- Failure to appreciate that the ingestion of liquid elemental mercury is usually benign, whereas inhalation of elemental mercury vapor may result in severe acute toxicity
- Failure to treat poisoning by long-chain aryl organomercurials the same as for inorganic salts, because the former is converted to the latter *in vivo*
- Failure to appreciate that the type of exposure, clinical severity, GI and renal function, and potential side effects of therapy influence the choice of chelating agent
- Failure to seek expert advice regarding treatment, particularly chelation

References

1. Adler R, Boxtein D, Schaft P, et al. Metallic mercury vapor poisoning simulating mucocutaneous lymph node syndrome. *J Pediatr* 1982;101:967.
2. Beckman KH, Bauman JL, Pimental PA, et al. Arsenic-induced torsades-de-pointes. *Crit Care Med* 1991;19:290.
3. Bond GR, Bloom A, Pinar A, et al. Use of succimer to enhance elimination of mercury in 6 human beings. *Vet Hum Toxicol* 1992;34:353.
4. Eley BM, Cox SW. The release, absorption and possible health effects of mercury from dental amalgam: a review of recent findings. *Br Dent J* 1993;175:355.
5. Fournier L, Thomas G, Garnier R, et al. 2,3-Dimercaptosuccinic acid treatment of heavy metal poisoning in humans. *Med Toxicol* 1988;3:499.

6. Girardi G, Elias MM. Effectiveness of N-acetylcysteine in protecting against mercuric chloride-induced nephrotoxicity. *Toxicology* 1991;67:155.
7. Goddard MJ, Tanhehco JL, Dau PC. Chronic arsenic poisoning masquerading as Landry-Guillain-Barré syndrome. *Electromyogr Clin Neurophysiol* 1992;32:419.
8. Graziano JH. Role of 2,3-dimercaptosuccinic acid in the treatment of heavy metal poisoning. *Med Toxicol* 1986;1:1051.
9. Graziano JH, Cuccia D, Friedheim E. Potential usefulness of 2,3-dimercapto-succinic acid for the treatment of arsenic poisoning. *J Pharmacol Exp Ther* 1978;207:1051.
10. Henningsson C, Hoffman S, McGonigle L, et al. Acute mercury poisoning mimicking pheochromocytoma in an adolescent. *J Pediatr* 1993;122:252.
11. Janus C, Klein B. Aspiration of metallic mercury: clinical significance. *Br J Radiol* 1982;55:675.
12. Markowitz L, Schaumburg NH. Successful treatment of inorganic mercury neurotoxicity with *N*-acetyl-penicillamine despite an adverse reaction. *Neurology* 1980;30:1000.
13. Mazumder DNG, Gupta JD, Santra A, et al. Chronic arsenic toxicity in West Bengal—the worst calamity in the world. *J Indian Med Assoc* 1998;96:4.
14. McCann M, Sheckner S. Hyperthyroidism associated with mercury poisoning. *Clin Pharm* 1991;10:742.
15. McFall TL, Richards JS, Matthews G. Rehabilitation in an individual with chronic arsenic poisoning medical, psychological, and social implications. *J Spinal Cord Med* 1998;21:142.
16. Muckter H, Liebl B, Reichl F, et al. Are we ready to replace dimercaprol (BAL) as an arsenic antidote? *Human Exp Toxicol* 1997;16:460.
17. Ratcliffe HE, Swanson GM. Human exposure to mercury: a critical assessment of the evidence of adverse health effects. *J Toxicol Environ Health* 1996;49:221.
18. Roden R, Fraser-Moodie A. Self-injection with mercury. *Injury* 1993;24:191.
19. Shum S, Skarbovig J, Habersang R. Acute lethal arsenic poisoning in mice: effect of treatment with N-acetylcysteine, d-penicillamine and dimercaprol on survival time. *Vet Hum Toxicol* 1981;23[Suppl 1]:39.
20. Von Burg R. Inorganic mercury. *J Appl Toxicol* 1995;15:483.

CHAPTER 319
Benzodiazepine Poisoning

Thomas R. Caraccio, Howard C. Mofenson, and Robin McFee

Benzodiazepines are widely used as anxiolytics, muscle relaxants, and anticonvulsants. Some of the newer benzodiazepines are primarily intended as anticonvulsants or neuroleptics (Table 319.1). Fifteen benzodiazepines are marketed in the United States.

Although the incidence of abuse and overdose is second only to that of alcohol, serious toxicity and fatalities are seldom encountered unless benzodiazepines are combined with other central nervous system (CNS) depressants.[7]

Benzodiazepines (BZDs) potentiate gamma-aminobutyric acid (GABA) neurotransmission at all levels of the neurologic axis and increase the efficacy of GABA synaptic inhibition at the postsynaptic GABA subtype A (GABA-A) receptor sites.[19] Potentiation of GABA molecules increases the rate at which chloride ion channels open, remain open, and allow chloride influx. Enhanced chloride ion permeability renders the postsynaptic sites less excitable. Several BZD receptor sites have been identified in the CNS that modulate anxiolytic, hypnotic, neuroleptic, and anticonvulsant properties. Receptor antagonists, such as the imidazodiazepine flumazenil, may be useful in the treatment of BZD poisoning.

The gastrointestinal tract rapidly and completely absorbs most of the BZDs, but absorption by the intramuscular route is sometimes erratic and delayed. The rate of absorption from the gastrointestinal tract, rather than lipophilicity, determines the onset of action. Diazepam, alprazolam, and triazolam are the most rapidly absorbed oral agents; prazepam is the slowest. Peak levels occur in 1 to 3 hours, but ethanol enhances absorption and may cause the peak level to be doubled at 1 hour.

The volume of distribution (V_D) for diazepam is 0.95 to 2.0 L/kg; for lorazepam, 1.3 L/kg; and for chlordiazepoxide, 0.3 to 6.0 L/kg. The range for other drugs in the class is 0.26 to 6 L/kg (see Table 319.1). The more lipophilic BZDs, such as diazepam and midazolam, have a shorter duration of action after a single dose than do less lipid soluble derivatives, such as lorazepam and chlordiazepoxide, because increasing lipophilicity enhances drug distribution into peripheral sites (adipose tissue). This leads to the rapid egress of the drug out of blood and brain into inactive storage sites, thus diminishing its effects on the CNS. The BZDs are highly protein bound (85% to 99%). Hepatic metabolism is their primary route of elimination. The two principal pathways involve either hepatic microsomal oxidation (*N*-dealkylation or aliphatic hydroxylation) or glucuronide conjugation (Fig. 319.1).

BZDs are substrates for CYP 2c19 and CYP 3A4 hepatic enzymes. CYP 3A4 is the predominant P-450 enzyme for xenobiotic metabolism, and is inducible by a variety of drugs, including rifampin, phenobarbital, and phenytoin. Elimination half-life can be increased by microsomal enzyme inhibitors, thus producing a potentially hazardous interaction, especially with midazolam. Examples of inhibitors include clotrimazole, erythromycin, estrogens, isoniazid, and ketoconazole. The elimination half-life is prolonged in elderly men, owing to unknown mechanisms. The elimination half-life is also prolonged in obese patients because of an increased V_D and in patients with hepatic dysfunction because of impaired metabolism. Pharmacokinetic parameters and duration of action of the various BZDs are listed in Table 319.1.

Massive overdoses of BZDs of up to 2,000 mg of chlordiazepoxide and 1,400 mg of diazepam have minimal toxic effects, and recovery is rapid and complete.[8] A lethal dose for BZDs has not been established; other CNS depressants enhance sedation and respiratory depression. Intravenous diazepam and midazolam are more toxic than the oral forms, and rapid administration may result in apnea and hypotension, because propylene glycol is used as a vehicle.[9] Concern about the ability to produce abuse, dependence, and delayed withdrawal reaction has led to restricting the range of indications for dispensing these agents.[5,13] Dependence on diazepam is produced by a dosage of 60 mg/d for 40 days; dependence on chlordiazepoxide is produced by a dosage of 200 mg/d for 60 days.

Flunitrazepam (trade name, Rohypnol; street names, "roofies," "Mexican Valium," "parachute," "roach 2") is a long-acting BZD agonist sold by prescription in over 60 countries worldwide, but it is not legally available in the United States. It has anxiolytic, anticonvulsant, and sedative effects; it also causes amnesia, muscle relaxation, and sleep induction. Flunitrazepam is sold illegally in the United States and is abused as a "date rape" drug because of the antegrade amnesia associated with its use.[1]

Flunitrazepam readily mixes with alcohol-containing beverages, although the manufacturer (Roche) has produced tablets that will break down into particles and turn the beverage blue. It is touted as a remedy for the depression that often follows a stimulant high, hence the street name "parachute." The pharmacokinetics include an onset of 1.5 to 2.0 hours, an oral peak of 2 hours and a duration of action of 8 hours or more after a 2-mg dose.

TABLE 319.1. Benzodiazepines: Dosage and Kinetics

Agent	Adult Daily Oral Dosage Range (mg) (h)	Time to Peak Plasma Concentration (h)	Half-life* (h)	Major Active Metabolites (half-life)	Protein Binding (%)	Volume of Distribution (L/kg)
ANXIOLYTICS						
Alprazolam (Xanax)	0.75–4	0.7–1.6	6–26	Yes	68–80	0.7–1
Chlorazepate+ (Tranxene)	15–60	1–2.5	48–96	Desmethyldiazepam (50–100 h) Elimination	NA	0.1–0.8
Chlordiazepoxide (Librium)	15–100	2–4	5–30	Desmethylchlordiazepoxide, demoxepam, desmethyl diazepam (50–100 h)	95	0.3
Clobazam (Frisium)++	20–80	1–3	11–77	N-desmethylclobazam	85	1
Diazepam (Valium)	6–40	1–2	14–100	Desmethyldiazepam (50–100 h) Oxazepam (active)	98	0.9–1.1
Halazepam (Paxipam)	60–160	1–3	14–16	3-Hydroxy, desmethyldiazepam (50–100 h)	NA	1–3.4
Lorazepam (Ativan)	2–6	2–5	10–20	None	85–95	NA
Oxazepam (Serax)	30–120	1–2	4–11	None Elimination	97	0.6–2
Prazepam (Centrax)	20–60	6	0.6–2	3-Hydroxy, desmethyldiazepam	NA	9–19
HYPNOTICS						
Estazolam (Pro-Som)	1–2	1–2	10–24	1-oxo-estazolam	93	NA
Flurazepam (Dalmane)	15–60	0.5–2	48–96	Desalkylflurazepam (50–100 h)	NA	1–1.3
Flunitrazepam (Rohypnol)*	1–2	<1	9–25	7-Aminoflunitrazepam (23h), *N*-desmethylfluni-	78	3.4–5.5
Midazolam (Versed)	5–30	0.3–0.8	1–4	α-hydroxymidazolam	97	0.8–1.7
Nitrazepam (Mogadon)*	5–10	2	17–48	No data Not currently available	87	2–5
Quazepam (Doral)	15	2	39–53	*N*-Dealkkylquazepam	95	NA
Temazepam (Restoril)	15–30	2–3	3–13	None	96	0.7–1.5
Triazolam (Halcion)	0.125–0.5 0.125–0.5	0.5–1.5 (2–5)	2–5	None trazepam(31h)	90	0.8–1.3
Zolpidem (Ambien)+	5–20	1–2	1.5–4.5	3 inactive	92%	0.5–0.7
ANTICONVULSANTS						
Clonazepam (Klonopin)	1.5–20(2) 0.1–0.2 mg/kg/24h	1–4 2–3 d	18–60	Desmethyldiazepam (50–100 h)	74–80	3.2
Diazepam (see above)						

NA = not available
*Half-lives include active metabolites.
+ Not a benzodiazepine chemically but an imidazopyridine, which is a selective benzodiazepine-1 receptor agonist.
++ Not yet marketed in U.S.

```
CHLORDIAZEPOXIDE (LIBRIUM)-> Desmethylchlordizepoxide -> Demoxepam

                      -> Desmethyldiazepam (Nordiazepam)->OXAZEPAM (Serax)
                                                        ->LORAZEPAM (Ativan)
                       ->TEMAZEPAM (Restoril)

DIAZEPAM (VALIUM))
CHLORAZEPATE (TRANXENE)  Desmethyldiazepam (Nordiazepam)->OXAZEPAM (Serax)
                                                       ->LORAZEPAM (Ativan)

PRAZEPAM (CENTRAX)     -> 3-Hydroxyprazepam
HALAZEPAM (PAXIPAM)    -> n-3-Hydroxyhalazepam
-
FLURAZEPAM (DALMANE)->N-Hydroxyethylflurazepam -> N-Desalkylflurazepam -> 3-Hydroxy-derivative

ALPRAZOLAM (XANAX)  -> a-Hydroxyalprazolam

TRIAZOLAM (HALCION) -> a-Hydroxytriazolam
```

Figure 319.1. Metabolism of benzodiazepines. Compounds in boldface capitals have active metabolites. Compounds in regular-face capitals are active drugs without active metabolites. Compounds in lowercase bold are active metabolites. Compounds in regular-face letters are clinically insignificant in active metabolites.

Flunitrazepam can be identified in urine from 4 to 30 days after ingestion. Although routine drug screens check for BZDs, they usually do not identify flunitrazepam. However, Hoffman-LaRoche has made available a free testing service for cases in which "date rape" drugs are suspected. For testing authorization, emergency departments, rape crisis centers, and law enforcement agencies can call 1-800-608-6540. National Medical Services, at 1-800-522-6671 or 1-215-657-4900, also has a date-rape drug-testing service. They test for flunitrazepam, ketamine, or gamma-hydroxybutyric acid (GHB). There is a fee charged for this service.

Zolpidem (Ambien) is a non-BZD, imidazopyridine sedative–hypnotic drug. Imidazopyridines are thought to interact with the same GABA receptor–chloride channel complex as the BZDs by high affinity with the "central-type" BZD receptors.[11] Zolpidem is approved only for short-term treatment of insomnia. Its metabolism is prolonged in the elderly.

Like the BZDs, zolpidem overdose usually does not produce severe respiratory depression unless other agents are coingested. However, caution should be exercised in patients with obstructive sleep apnea. Adverse effects are headache, nausea, diarrhea, miosis, and next-day drowsiness. Confusion in the elderly can occur at doses over 20 mg. Cases of withdrawal and tolerance have been reported.[8,12]

CLINICAL PRESENTATION

Manifestations of acute BZD poisoning include ataxia, lateral nystagmus, hypotonia, drowsiness, slurred speech, and coma.[36] Even when BZD is given in large doses, a resultant deep coma, causing cardiorespiratory depression and loss of deep tendon reflexes, is rare. The ultrashort-acting agents are important exceptions, however. Triazolam has been reported to produce apnea and coma within 1 hour of a dose of 2 to 5 mg.[14] Two fatal poisonings have also been associated with temazepam overdose. The toxic dose of flunitrazepam for a child is 0.1 mg/kg.[17]

Paradoxic excitement, including hallucinations, hostility, and seizures, has been reported to result from BZD overdose.[3] A sensitivity to triazolam in the healthy elderly has been reported. Triazolam has been noted to produce delirium and psychosis. Nitrazepam also has been associated with swallowing disturbances in children, which may result in aspiration.[12]

The elderly and very young children are more susceptible to the CNS depressant action of BZDs. In rare instances, the adult respiratory distress syndrome has developed after a 30-mg intravenous dose of chlordiazepoxide and a massive flurazepam ingestion.[16,18]

Long-term use of high therapeutic doses of BZDs produces manifestations of anxiety, insomnia, anorexia, headache, muscle spasm, and weakness. A spectrum of affective disorders (psychosis, agitation, confusion, hallucinations, and delirium) and motor dysfunction (tremors, restlessness, myoclonic jerks, and seizures) may develop on withdrawal when diazepam has been taken in daily doses of 60 to 300 mg.

Seizures are rare, and most commonly develop 7 to 8 days after withdrawal (range, 2 to 12 days). Withdrawal symptoms develop in an average of 3 to 4 days after discontinuation (range, 1 to 11 days), peak in 5 to 6 days, and resolve by 4 weeks, but minor symptoms may persist for months.[6,13] Earlier onset and peak and shorter duration of withdrawal may be seen with shorter acting agents.

Most patients with acute BZD poisoning recover without sequelae within 24 hours. Patients with preexisting medical conditions, such as hepatic disease, may be more susceptible to toxicity. Chronic BZD use may cause mild leukopenia and abnormal liver function tests.

Quantitative plasma BZD levels are useful only for diagnostic confirmation, not for evaluation or management. Tolerance, drug coingestion, active metabolites, and distant tissue-binding sites result in poor correlation between blood concentrations and clinical effects. Although diazepam levels of 5 to 20 mg/mL are often associated with toxicity and levels over 20 mg/mL may be seen in lethal cases, chronic daily consumption of large doses may result in blood concentrations of 5 to 6 mg/mL without signs of toxicity.

DIFFERENTIAL DIAGNOSIS

The presence of deep coma, apnea or significant respiratory depression, hypotension, multiple organ involvement, or a prolonged time for recovery should prompt a search for coingestants (i.e., sedatives, narcotics, sympatholytics, cholinergics, or alcohols) or another cause (i.e., CNS lesions, trauma, infection, or metabolic disturbances).

EMERGENCY DEPARTMENT EVALUATION

The history should include the time and intent of all agents ingested and the amount and duration of chronic daily BZD use. Concomitant medications and medical history should also be documented. The physical examination should focus on vital signs and neurologic and cardiorespiratory function and the ability to protect the airway.

Except for measurement of oxygen saturation, routine laboratory tests are not necessary in the verbally responsive patient. Hematologic and metabolic profiles, urinalysis, and arterial blood gas analysis are recommended for those who are unresponsive to voice. Qualitative or semiqualitative BZD analysis of the blood and urine by immunoassay or thin-layer chromatography may confirm the presence of the drug but does not guide clinical management. It should be noted, however, that immunoassay screening techniques will only detect BZDs that are metabolized to desmethyldiazepam or oxazepam and that most BZDs are not detected in thin-layer chromatography of the urine due to low drug concentrations. Immunoassays show cross-reactivity, such that false-positive results can occur with nonsteroidal antiinflammatory drugs (NSAIDs). Thin-layer chromatography, gas chromatography, and mass spectroscopy successfully discriminate between BZDs and NSAIDs.[28,29]

EMERGENCY DEPARTMENT MANAGEMENT

Advanced life-support measures should be instituted, as necessary. Supportive therapy is usually all that is necessary when a BZD is the sole agent involved.[20] Gastrointestinal decontamination is indicated for patients who present within 1 hour of ingestion.[1,36] Forced diuresis and hemodialysis are ineffective in enhancing BZD elimination because of high protein binding and V_D. Full recovery can be expected within 12 to 24 hours.

Flumazenil (Romazicon) is available in 5-mL and 10-mL vials containing 0.1 mg/mL. It is a specific competitive BZD receptor antagonist that blocks the effect of inhibitory neurotransmitters (GABA) and reverses BZD-induced CNS depression. It also appears to be effective in reversing the sedative effects of zolpidem and endogenous BZD receptor agonists associated with hepatic encephalopathy. It does not antagonize other portions of the GABA receptor (e.g., barbiturate, ethanol, general anesthetic-binding sites) and does not affect the bioavailability, plasma concentration, or elimination half-life of BZDs. Most importantly, it may not reverse BZD-induced hypoventilation.[10] Airway protection and mechanical ventilation are definitive treatment for respiratory distress or failure.

In intravenous doses of 0.1 to 0.2 mg, flumazenil is partially antagonistic. In doses of 0.4 to 1.0 mg, onset of action and reversal of the CNS effects are evident within 1 to 2 minutes. An 80% response occurs within 3 minutes, and the peak effect is noted within 6 to 10 minutes. Duration and degree of reversal are related to the dose and the plasma concentration of BZD. In general, flumazenil has a short duration of action. Because flumazenil has a shorter duration of action than most BZDs, the effects from the exposure may recur. A 1-mg bolus usually lasts about 60 minutes but can last as long as 6 hours.[10]

Indications for flumazenil include reversal of the sedative effect of BZDs when they have been used therapeutically (e.g., for conscious sedation, see Chapter 413) and for the management of accidental or intentional BZD overdose. In overdose situations, flumazenil is best reserved for patients with pure, acute BZD overdose who are verbally unresponsive and have no history of long-term BZD use or recent treatment of a medical condition (e.g., seizures) with BZDs. The use of flumazenil as a diagnostic and therapeutic tool in patients in coma of uncertain etiology is controversial, and generally not recommended.

Studies suggest that there is an increase in GABA-ergic tone in hepatic encephalopathy. BZD has been detected in the cerebrospinal fluid of patients with hepatic encephalopathy, and the use of flumazenil has led to the improvement of clinical as well as electrophysiologic responses in such patients. While the response rate in case studies is approximately 65%, additional research is necessary to further characterize the role of flumazenil in hepatic encephalopathy.

The suggested treatment protocol for using flumazenil in patients with known or suspected BZD overdose is shown in Fig. 319.2. An initial a dose of 0.1 mg is recommended for patients who are potentially addicted to BZDs and at risk for withdrawal. Patients who do not use BZDs chronically can be given an initial dose of 0.2 mg. For the reversal of therapeutic sedation, the initial dose in adults is 0.3 mg intravenously, followed by 0.1 mg every minute until the patient is awake or a total dose of 2 to 5 mg has been administered. It may be repeated in boluses of 0.1 mg or administered as an infusion of 0.1 to 0.5 mg/h, if necessary.

Patients who respond to flumazenil must be continuously monitored for resedation. Furthermore, because flumazenil does not reverse hypoventilation, patients who awaken must often be repeatedly "reminded" to breath (e.g., they must be prompted to "take a deep breath"), and the adequacy of ventilation must be frequently reassessed. Emergence reactions fol-

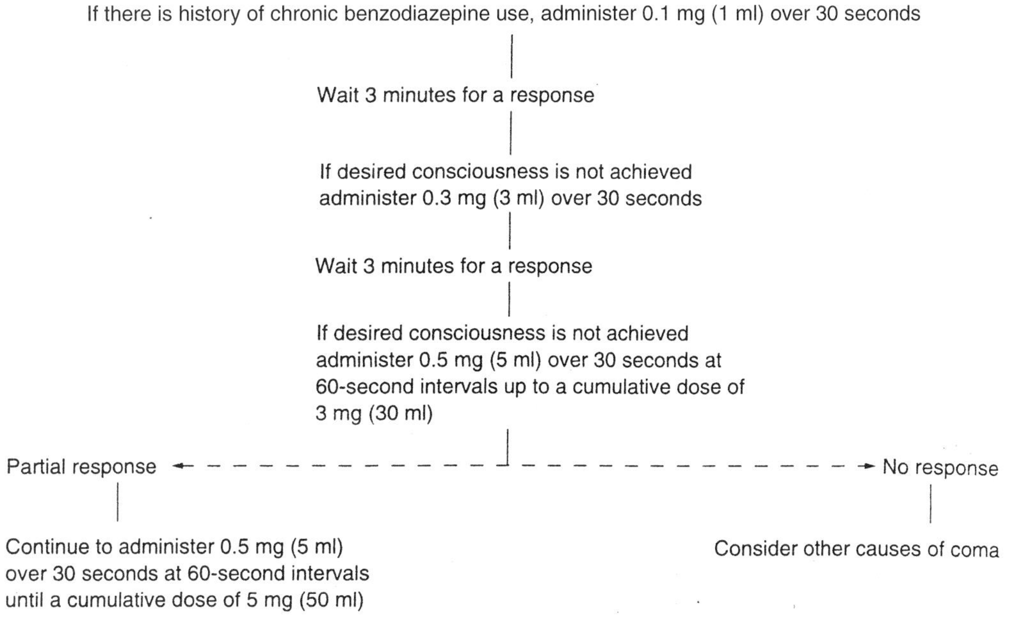

Figure 319.2. Flumazenil dosing for benzodiazepine poisoning.

lowing flumazenil administration (e.g., anxiety, agitation, confusion) are relatively common, particularly when flumazenil is given in higher doses or more rapidly than recommended.

Flumazenil has no significant intrinsic pharmacologic activity. It may cause withdrawal and seizures in BZD-dependent patients, however, and it should be used in such patients with extreme caution, if at all. Lower-than-recommended doses and slower administration should be used if the benefits outweigh the risks. Seizures have also been reported in patients with CNS trauma and cyclic antidepressant, cocaine, and isoniazid intoxication who were given flumazenil. Because BZDs have therapeutic roles (i.e., as anticonvulsants) in these conditions, flumazenil should not be given to such patients. Serious cyclic antidepressant poisoning is an absolute contraindication to the use of flumazenil. QRS-interval prolongation on an electrocardiogram is a sensitive indicator of cyclic antidepressant toxicity (see Chapter 313); this finding in a patient with an unknown or mixed overdose should be considered a contraindication to flumazenil administration. A flumazenil-related dystonic reaction has also been reported. There is no role in the treatment of BZD poisoning for stimulants such as aminophylline–theophylline, naloxone, or physostigmine.

Stopping the use of BZDs in any patient who has been maintained on these drugs longer than 6 weeks should be done gradually over a minimum of 3 weeks and up to 2 to 3 months, depending on previous dosage and duration of treatment. BZD withdrawal is managed by institution of oral diazepam (10 to 60 mg) for several days, followed by tapering the dose by 10% daily, usually over several weeks. Physician visits every 5 to 7 days are necessary to assess both physical symptoms and coping mechanisms.

DISPOSITION

Consultation with a specialist is rarely indicated, because most BZD overdoses alone do not produce significant toxicity. Psychiatric evaluation is necessary before discharge, unless the exposure is accidental.

Patients with mild clinical toxicity (i.e., they are lethargic or asleep but respond to verbal stimuli) can often be observed in the emergency department until they recover. Those who respond only to painful stimulation, regardless of whether flumazenil is given, probably require 12 or more hours of monitoring and treatment. If emergency department observation is not possible, these patients should be admitted to an intensive care unit.

Outpatient referral and follow-up are required for patients who have evidence of chronic abuse, dependence, or psychological problems, such as depression.

Transfer is indicated only if the initial facility lacks the equipment or personnel to deliver the level of support needed to maintain the patient or to provide the appropriate specialized evaluation and treatment of sequelae or complications of the overdose.

COMMON PITFALLS

- Failure to consider concomitant poisoning or other causes, especially in patients with severe CNS depression
- Failure to administer oxygen, glucose, thiamine, and naloxone to comatose patients
- Failure to appreciate that patients with poisoning from BZDs alone usually only require 6 hours of observation, not hospital admission.
- Failure to appreciate that many BZDs are not detected by immunoassay screening techniques
- Administering large initial doses of flumazenil to patients with a history of chronic BZD use, thereby precipitating withdrawal and possibly seizures
- Use of flumazenil in overdose patients with seizures or conduction delays on their electrocardiogram and in those who have coingested agents known to cause these conditions

References

1. Armstrong R. Sexual assault: clinical issues. When drugs are used for rape. *J Emerg Nurs* 1997;23:378–381.
2. Bailey DN. Blood concentrations and clinical findings following overdose of chlordiazepoxide alone and chlordiazepoxide plus ethanol. *J Toxicol Clin Toxicol* 1984;22:433.
3. Byrd JC. Alprazolam associated rage reaction. *J Clin Psychopharmacol* 1985;5:86.
4. Cavallaro R, Regazzetti HG, Covelli G, et al. Tolerance and withdrawal with zolpidem [Letter]. *Lancet* 1993;342(8867):374–375.
5. Catalon J, Gath DH. Benzodiazepines in general practice. Time for a decision. *BMJ* 1985;290:1374.
6. Ellenwood EH, Linnoilon M, Easler ME, et al. Onset of peak impairment after diazepam and after alcohol. *Clin Pharmacol Ther* 1981;30:534.
7. Greenblatt DJ, Shader RI, Abernethy DR. Current status of benzodiazepines. Part 1. *N Engl J Med* 1983;309:354.
8. Greenblatt DJ, Shader RI, Abernethy DR. Rapid recovery from massive diazepam overdose. *JAMA* 1978;240:1872.
9. Hall SC, Ovassapian A. Apnea after intravenous diazepam therapy. *JAMA* 1977;238:1052.
10. Kulka PJ, Lauven PM. Benzodiazepine antagonist: an update of their role in emergency care of overdose patients. *Drug Saf* 1992;7:381.
11. Lheureux P, Debailleul G, DeWitte O, et al. Zolpidem intoxication mimicking narcotic overdose: response to flumazenil. *Hum Exp Toxicol* 1990;9:105–107.
12. Murphy JV, Sawasky F, Marquardt MS, et al. Deaths in young children receiving nitrazepam. *J Pediatr* 1987;111:145.
13. Nutt DJ. Benzodiazepine dependence in the clinic: reason for anxiety? *Trends Pharmacol Sci* 1986;7:457.
14. Olson KR, Yin L, Osterloh J, et al. Coma caused by trivial triazolam overdose. *Am J Emerg Med* 1985;3:210.
15. Raphan H, Adams MH. False positive benzodiazepine urine test due to oxaprozin [Reply Letter]. *JAMA* 1995;273:1905–1906
16. Richman S, Harris RD. Acute pulmonary edema associated with Librium use. *Radiology* 1972;103:57.
17. Ronald OK, Dahl V. Flunitrazepam intoxication in a child treated with the benzodiazepine antagonist flumazenil. *Crit Care Med* 1989;17:1335–1356.
18. Stringer MD. Acute respiratory distress syndrome associated with flurazepam overdose. *J R Soc Med* 1985;78:74.
19. Tall JF, Paul SM, Skolnick P. Receptors for the age of anxiety: pharmacology of the benzodiazepines. *Science* 1980;207:274.
20. Trager SM, Haug MT. Reduction of diazepam serum half-life and reversal of coma by activated charcoal in a patient with severe liver disease. *Clin Toxicol* 1986;24:329.

CHAPTER 320
Beta-Blocker Poisoning

Christopher H. Linden

Beta blockers are used to treat a wide variety of conditions, including angina pectoris, pheochromocytoma, thyrotoxicosis, hypertension, aortic dissection, congestive cardiomyopathy, dysrhythmias, glaucoma, tremors, stage fright, mitral valve prolapse, migraine headache, portal hypertension, and alcohol withdrawal, and to prevent reinfarction and sudden death after myocardial infarction. These agents competitively inhibit the binding of norepinephrine and epinephrine to β-adrenergic neurohumoral receptors. This, in turn, inhibits the production of cyclic adenosine monophosphate (cAMP) by adenylate cyclase and decreases the physiologic effects resulting from the stimulation of β1 and β2 receptors (Table 320.1). Decreased levels of cAMP also inhibit sodium and calcium influx during phase zero (depolarization) of the action potential. This latter effect defines beta blockers as class II antidysrhythmics.

TABLE 320.1. Beta Receptors and Their Activity

Receptor Type	Organ	Response to Receptor Stimulation
Beta-1	Eye	Aqueous humor production
	Heart	Increased automaticity, conduction velocity, contractility, refractory period
	Kidney	Renin production
Beta-2	Blood vessels	Smooth muscle contraction
	Bronchioles	Smooth muscle contraction
	Fat	Lipolysis
	Liver	Gluconeogenesis, glycogenolysis
	Pancreas	Insulin release
	Skeletal muscle	Increased tone, potassium uptake
	Uterus	Smooth muscle relaxation

While all beta blockers block one or both subtypes of β receptors, their pharmacologic profiles differ in other respects (Table 320.2). So-called first-generation agents are nonselective and inhibit both β_1 and β_2 receptors. The second-generation, or cardioselective, beta blockers act primarily on β_1 receptors, and third-generation agents have additional alpha-adrenergic receptor blocking activity. Some beta blockers also have partial agonist (sympathomimetic) activity, and others have quinidine-like myocardial membrane-stabilizing effects. Carvedilol has antioxidant activity and sotalol has electrophysiologic properties similar to class III antidysrhythmic agents. Especially in high concentrations, sotalol prolongs the duration of the action potential in the ventricle and Purkinje fibers, which, in turn, results in a prolonged Q-T interval.[15]

Most beta-blocker preparations are racemic mixtures of the *d* and *l* isomers, with the *l* isomer responsible for most of their activity. They are available as immediate- and sustained-release pills for oral use and as solutions for intravenous and ocular use. All beta blockers are well absorbed, and peak effects occur 1 to 2 hours after a single therapeutic dose. Although most have relatively short durations of action (less than 6 hours), extended-release formulations allow for once-daily dosing. Beta blockers differ markedly in protein binding, elimination, absorption, and first-pass hepatic metabolism (Table 320.3). There is a rough correlation between volume of distribution, lipid solubility, and membrane activity.

After overdose, the cardioselectivity of second-generation agents may be lost, and membrane effects may occur with all agents.[7,9,12,20] Excessive beta-receptor blockade and membrane depression are responsible for cardiovascular, central nervous system (CNS), and metabolic toxicity. Drugs with similar activity, such as quinidine and calcium channel blockers, synergistically add to the cardiovascular toxicity when used concurrently. Patients with underlying heart, kidney, or liver disease are at increased risk for toxicity.[12]

Chronic use of beta blockers results in an increased density of adrenergic receptors and a supersensitivity to catecholamines

Table 320.2. Pharmacology of Beta Blockers

		Pharmacologic Activity			*Pharmacokinetics*					
Drug	Dose (mg)[a]	Cardio-selective	Partial Agonist	Membrane Stabilization	Absorption (%)	First-Pass Metabolism	Protein Binding (%)	Volume of Distribution (L/kg)	Route of Elimination	Half-Life (h)
Acebutolol	200–400	+	+	+	70	Yes	25	2.3	Renal	6
Atenolol	50–100	++	0	0	50	No	15	0.7	Renal	6–9
Betaxolol	10–40	++	0	+	100	Yes	50	6.1	Hepatic	14–22
Bisoprolol	5–40	+	0	0	90	No	30–36	2.7–3.1	Hepatic	11
Carteolol	2.5–10	0	++	0	80	No	23–30	4	Renal	6
Carvedilol[b,c]	3.125–25	0	0	0	>90	Yes	98	1.6	Hepatic	7–10
Esmolol	IV only	++	0	0	NA	NA	55	3.4	Serum esterase	0.15
Labetalol[c]	200–400	0	0	0	>90	Yes	50	10.0	Hepatic	3–4
Metoprolol	50–400	++	0	0	>90	Yes	12	5.5	Hepatic	3–4
Nadolol	40–320	0	0	0	30	No	30	2.1	Renal	14–24
Penbutolol	20–80	0	+	0	100	No	80–98	32–42	Hepatic	5
Pindolol	2.5–30	0	++	+	>90	No	57	2.0	Renal	5–12
Propranolol	20–120	0	0	++	>90	Yes	93	3.6	Hepatic	3–6
Sotalol[d]	80–480	0	0	0	70	No	0	0.23	Renal	5–12
Timolol	20–60	0	+	0	>90	No	10	1.5	Renal	4–5

NA, not applicable.
[a]Single oral adult dose
[b]Also has antioxidant activity
[c]Also has alpha-adrenergic blocking activity
[d]Also depresses repolarization (increases Q-T interval)

TABLE 320.3. Pharmacokinetics of Beta Blockers

Agent	Absorption (%)	First-Pass Metabolism	Protein Binding (%)	Volume of Distribution (L/kg)	Route of Elimination	Half-Life (h)
Acebutolol	70	Yes	25	2.3	Renal	6
Atenolol	50	No	15	0.7	Renal	6–9
Betaxolol	100	Yes	50	6.1	Hepatic	14–22
Bisoprolol	90	No	30–36	2.7–3.1	Hepatic	11
Carteolol	80	No	23–30	4	Renal	6
Esmolol	NA	NA	55	3.4	Serum esterase	0.15
Labetalol	>90	Yes	50	10.0	Hepatic	3–4
Metoprolol	>90	Yes	12	5.5	Hepatic	3–4
Nadolol	30	No	30	2.1	Renal	14–24
Penbutolol	100	No	80–98	32–42	Hepatic	5
Pindolol	>90	No	57	2.0	Renal	5–12
Propranolol	>90	Yes	93	3.6	Hepatic	3–6
Sotalol	70	No	0	0.23	Renal	5–12
Timolol	>90	No	10	1.5	Renal	4–5

on drug withdrawal. Hence, large doses of beta blockers are usually well tolerated when the drug dose is gradually increased, but the same dosage can result in toxicity if the patient is not accustomed to beta blockers. In addition, receptor supersensitivity may result in a sympathomimetic withdrawal syndrome after the abrupt termination of beta-blocker therapy.[13]

The minimal dose necessary to produce toxic effects varies with the particular agent. In general, toxicity may result from the ingestion of an adult dose by a child or a high therapeutic dose by a previously unexposed adult. The ingestion of more than 1 g of any beta blocker may cause serious or fatal toxicity.

CLINICAL PRESENTATION

Manifestations of toxicity usually begin within 30 minutes and peak within 2 hours of an acute oral overdose.[7,9,20] Exceptions to this are sustained-release preparations and sotalol, which may produce severe dysrhythmias up to 20 hours after ingestion.[2,14,15] Factors that influence the severity of poisoning include the type and amount of beta blockers ingested, the patient's age, the presence of underlying cardiovascular disease, tolerance to beta blockers, and the concurrent ingestion of other cardiodepressants, such as calcium channel blockers and quinidine.

The level of consciousness and the degree of hypotension reflect the severity of the intoxication.[7,9,20] In mild and moderate poisoning, symptoms include nausea, vomiting, bradycardia, and normal or slightly decreased blood pressure. The patient may be alert or slightly confused and lethargic. Hypotension can occur in the absence of bradycardia. In severe overdoses, marked bradycardia, hypotension, coma, respiratory depression, and convulsions may be present. Electromechanical dissociation, asystole, ventricular tachycardia, and ventricular fibrillation have also been reported.[5,14,16] The skin is often pale and clammy; cyanosis, both central and peripheral, has been reported. Pulmonary edema, congestive heart failure, and bronchospasm may also be seen, particularly in patients with underlying cardiac or pulmonary disease. Oliguric renal failure and mesenteric ischemia are rare complications. Beta blockers with high lipid solubility and membrane-stabilizing effects (e.g., propranolol) produce more pronounced CNS disturbances. Agents with partial sympathomimetic activity (e.g., pindolol) may cause hypertension and tachycardia.[9]

Metabolic abnormalities include hypoglycemia and hyperkalemia. Diabetics and children are at greatest risk for hypoglycemia. Metabolic (lactic) acidosis may be present in patients with shock. With increasing severity of poisoning, ECG manifestations include sinus bradycardia, progressive atrioventricular block, loss of P waves, early repolarization, increased QRS duration with either a nonspecific or bundle-branch block pattern, and asystole. Early repolarization and ST-segment elevation have also been reported.[6] Interventricular conduction delays are more common with agents that have greater membrane-stabilizing activity. Sinus tachycardia, prolongation of the Q-T interval, ventricular tachycardia (including torsades de pointes), ventricular fibrillation, and asystole may be seen with sotalol poisoning.[15] Labetalol (and probably carvedilol) may cause severe hypotension, presumably due to its concomitant alpha-blocking activity. The chest radiograph may demonstrate pulmonary edema with or without cardiomegaly. Dilated cardiomyopathy may be seen on echocardiogram.[13] Angina pectoris, myocardial infarction, and a hyperadrenergic state may result when longstanding beta-blocker therapy is abruptly discontinued.[12] Beta blockers are not detected by enzyme immunoassay toxicology screening tests, and are variably detected by thin-layer chromatography. Quantitative blood levels are not routinely available and serve only to confirm an overdose.

DIFFERENTIAL DIAGNOSIS

The differential diagnosis is that of cardiovascular collapse and includes anaphylaxis, cardiogenic shock, pulmonary emboli, hypovolemia, sepsis, and other overdoses. Beta-blocker poisoning should be suspected in patients who suddenly develop hypotension, bradycardia, or seizures that are resistant to standard therapies. Agents that may cause similar toxicity include antidysrhythmic agents, calcium channel blockers, carbamate and organophosphorus insecticides, centrally acting antihypertensive drugs, cyanide, digitalis, narcotics, sedative–hypnotics, and tricyclic antidepressants. The serum glucose level may be helpful in differentiating beta-blocker poisoning from calcium channel–blocker poisoning. Hypoglycemia may be present in the former, and hyperglycemia in the latter. Hyperkalemia is another diagnostic clue.

EMERGENCY DEPARTMENT EVALUATION

The history should include the time, type, and amount of beta blocker (and any other agents) ingested; current medications; and a medical history. The physical examination should focus on vital signs, the cardiopulmonary system, and the neurologic status. All patients should have cardiac monitoring, frequent monitoring of vital signs, and an initial rhythm strip, as well as a 12-lead ECG. In symptomatic patients, the physician should also obtain serum electrolyte measurements; glucose, blood urea nitrogen, and creatinine levels; a complete blood count; oxygen saturation or arterial blood gas analysis; and a chest radiograph. Severely poisoned patients should also have liver function tests. In unclear cases, toxicology screening tests may be useful in identifying beta blockers or coingestants.

EMERGENCY DEPARTMENT MANAGEMENT

Advanced life-support measures should be instituted as necessary. Prehospital personnel should follow advanced cardiac life-support (ACLS) guidelines for the treatment of symptomatic bradycardia, hypotension, and dysrhythmias. Endotracheal intubation and assisted ventilation may be necessary in patients with CNS or respiratory depression. Patients with altered mental status, particularly those with coma or seizures, should be given intravenous dextrose 50% in water and naloxone. Dextrose is particularly important, because beta-blocker poisoning may cause hypoglycemia. For severe cases of known etiology that are unresponsive to standard ACLS measures, prehospital personnel should also give glucagon and calcium, if available.

Patients with bradycardia and a normal blood pressure need only close monitoring. Bradycardia with hypotension should be treated initially with pharmacologic measures such as intravenous fluids, atropine, beta agonists (e.g., epinephrine, isoproterenol), glucagon, calcium, and vasopressors (e.g., dopamine, norepinephrine). Combined therapy with multiple agents may be effective when a single agent is not. Dobutamine may be useful for patients with concomitant pulmonary edema or congestive heart failure. Glucagon is the most consistently effective single agent for treating cardiovascular toxicity. Atropine usually reverses bradycardia but does not necessarily reverse hypotension.[10]

The utility of beta agonists and vasopressors is often limited: A therapeutic response often requires doses three to four times the normal levels, and toxic reactions may occur.[7,9,20] Invasive (peripheral and pulmonary artery pressure) monitoring may be necessary to optimize the treatment of persistent hemodynamic instability.

All severely poisoned patients should be given glucagon, either alone or in combination with other agents. Glucagon effectively increases the heart's contractility, as well as the heart rate and blood pressure, by activating adenylate cyclase, which, in turn, stimulates nonadrenergic membrane receptors.[17] Glucagon is more effective in reversing hypotension (86%) than either epinephrine (50%) or isoproterenol (22%), even when it occurs in the absence of concomitant bradycardia.[4] It is given as an initial bolus of 5 to 10 mg intravenously (50 to 150 μg/kg in children), diluted in 10 mL of saline, followed by an infusion of 1 to 5 mg/h (10 to 50 μg/kg/h in children).

Intravenous calcium, given in the same dose as for poisoning by calcium channel blockers (see Chapter 321), may also reverse hypotension.[8,16] Preliminary data suggest that the glucose–insulin–potassium regimen used for calcium channel blocker poisoning may also be effective for beta blockers.

Theophylline, which stimulates endogenous catecholamine release and inhibits the enzymatic inactivation of cAMP by phosphodiesterase, has a synergistic effect with glucagon in canine studies, but its clinical effectiveness is not well substantiated.[19]

Prenalterol, a cardioselective beta agonist, has been successful in reversing both bradycardia and hypotension but is not yet approved for use in the United States.

Amrinone produces an inotropic effect that is not inhibited by alpha- or beta-receptor blockade. It has been used successfully in conjunction with glucagon to treat hypotension caused by a calcium channel poisoning and is effective in canine beta-blocker poisoning. The dosage of amrinone for heart failure is a slow intravenous bolus of 0.75 mg/kg, followed by a continuous infusion of 5 to 10 μg/kg/min. If necessary, the bolus dose may be repeated 30 minutes after beginning therapy.

If pharmacologic therapy fails to restore hemodynamic stability, the physician should consider invasive measures such as cardiac pacing (transcutaneous or transvenous), intraaortic balloon pump, cardiopulmonary bypass, and extracorporeal membrane oxygenation.[10,11,14]

Patients with hypertension and sinus tachycardia due to sotalol poisoning usually require only close monitoring. If the blood pressure or heart rate is dangerously high, or if there is evidence of organ ischemia, short-acting agents (e.g., nitroprusside and esmolol) should be used. Ventricular dysrhythmias, including torsades de pointes, may result from the prolonged Q-T interval as well as the bradycardia, which lends itself to the R-on-T phenomenon. Treatment of ventricular tachyarrhythmias includes lidocaine, magnesium (2 to 4 g intravenously over several minutes to an hour, depending on patient stability), phenytoin, or overdrive pacing with either isoproterenol or electricity.[2,15,18] Prophylactic magnesium may be useful for patients with a prolonged Q-T interval. Sodium bicarbonate (see Chapter 311) should also be considered in the treatment of ventricular tachydysrhythmias and conduction disturbances caused by membrane-active agents.[5] Class IA antidysrhythmics, such as procainamide, and class III agents, such as bretylium, should be avoided.

Seizures that are not caused by hypoglycemia or responsive to glucose should be treated with diazepam, phenytoin, or a barbiturate. Bronchospasm may require the use of inhaled beta agonists, subcutaneous epinephrine, and intravenous aminophylline, alone or in combination. Exacerbation of hypotension is a potential side effect of these agents.

Gastrointestinal (GI) decontamination should be done as soon as possible. Activated charcoal is the preferred method. Whole-bowel irrigation may have some benefit in the ingestion of sustained-released tablets. Ipecac should be avoided because of the potential for vagally mediated cardiovascular collapse secondary to vomiting and the risk of aspiration if coma or seizures develop. A prophylactic dose of atropine (e.g., 0.5 mg intravenously for adults and 0.01 mg/kg for children) may inhibit the detrimental vagal effects that may result from endotracheal or gastric intubation. Repeated doses of activated charcoal are recommended for symptomatic patients.

Although charcoal hemoperfusion has been used successfully in a case of metoprolol poisoning, pharmacokinetic efficacy has not been documented.[3] Except for atenolol and sotalol, extracorporeal measures are unlikely to remove significant amounts of beta blockers because of unfavorable kinetic parameters.[4,7,18,20]

Clinical toxicity seldom lasts longer than 24 to 48 hours.[1,7,9,16] If vital signs can be supported, most patients will completely recover. The treatment of withdrawal involves treatment of ischemic complications and reinstitution of beta-blocker therapy, with a slow tapering of the dose over a 2-week period.

DISPOSITION

Patients who ingest immediate-release formulations and have mild or absent toxicity can usually be discharged, or referred for psychiatric evaluation, if they remain or become asymptomatic and have a normal ECG after 4 to 6 hours of emergency department observation. Patients who ingest sustained-released formulations should be observed for 12 hours. Patients who manifest any symptoms or signs of poisoning during the observation period should be admitted for 24 hours of cardiac monitoring. Those with abnormal vital signs, nonsinus rhythm on ECG, coma, or seizures should be admitted to an intensive care unit. Physicians unfamiliar with beta-blocker poisoning should consult a poison center or toxicologist. The services of a cardiologist or vascular surgeon may be required if electrical pacing or invasive measures are needed for hemodynamic support. If intensive care and invasive treatments are necessary but unavailable, patients should be transferred to another institution by advanced life-support units and should be accompanied by personnel familiar with potential or required therapies.

COMMON PITFALLS

- Failure to appreciate that GI decontamination may increase vagal tone and worsen or precipitate cardiovascular toxicity
- Giving ipecac to patients who may rapidly deteriorate
- Failure to determine whether the preparation ingested was an immediate- or sustained-release preparation
- Failure to appreciate that beta blockers can cause hypoglycemia, and to give dextrose to patients with altered mental status, especially those with coma and seizures
- Failure to appreciate that glucagon is the treatment of choice for bradycardia and hypotension
- Failure to appreciate that combined drug therapy may be effective for cardiovascular toxicity when a single agent is not
- Failure to consider invasive measures for hemodynamic support when drug therapy is ineffective

ACKNOWLEDGMENT

The author gratefully acknowledges Daniel A. Muse who contributed the previous version of this chapter.

References

1. Abbasi I, Sorsby S. Prolonged toxicity from atenolol overdose in adolescents. *Clin Pharm* 1986;5:836.
2. Adlerfliegel F, Leeman M, Demaeyer PH, et al. Sotalol poisoning associated with asystole. *Intensive Care Med* 1993;19:57.
3. Anthony J, Jastremski M, Elliott W, et al. Charcoal hemoperfusion for the treatment of a combined diltiazem and metoprolol overdose. *Ann Emerg Med* 1986;15:1344.
4. Critchley JA, Ungar A. The management of acute poisoning due to beta-adrenoceptor antagonists. *Med Toxicol Adverse Drug Exp* 1989;4:32.
5. Donovan KD, Gerace RV, Dreyer JF. Acebutolol-induced ventricular tachycardia reversed with sodium bicarbonate. *Clin Toxicol* 1999;37:481.
6. Gwinup GR. Propranolol toxicity presentation with early repolarization, ST segment elevation, and peaked T waves on the ECG. *Ann Emerg Med* 1988;17:171.
7. Heath A. β-Adrenoceptor blocker toxicity: clinical features and therapy. *Am J Emerg Med* 1984;2:518.
8. Henry M, Kay MM, Viccellio P. Cardiogenic shock associated with calcium-channel and beta blockers: reversal with intravenous calcium chloride. *Am J Emerg Med* 1985;3:334.
9. Jackson CD, Fishbein L. A toxicological review of beta-adrenergic blockers. *Fundam Appl Toxicol* 1986;6:395.
10. Kenyon CJ, Aldinger GE, Joshipura P, et al. Successful resuscitation using external cardiac pacing in beta-adrenergic antagonist–induced bradyasystolic arrest. *Ann Emerg Med* 1988;107:711.
11. Lane AS, Woodward AC, Goldman MR. Massive propranolol overdose poorly responsive to pharmacologic therapy: use of intra-aortic balloon pump. *Ann Emerg Med* 1987;16:1381.
12. Lewis RV, McDevitt DG. Adverse reactions and interactions with β-adrenoceptor blocking drugs. *Med Toxicol* 1986;1:343.
13. Lifshitz M, Zucker N, Zalstein E. Acute dilated cardiomyopathy and central nervous system toxicity following propranolol intoxication. *Pediatr Emerg Care* 1999;15:262.
14. Love JN, Litovitz TL, Howell JM, et al. Characterization of fatal beta blocker ingestion: a review of the American Association of Poison Control Centers data from 1985 to 1995. *Clin Toxicol* 1997;35:353.
15. Neuvonen PJ, Elonen E, Vuorenmaa T, et al. Prolonged Q-T interval and severe tachyarrhythmias, common features of sotalol intoxication. *Eur J Clin Pharmacol* 1981;20:85.
16. Pertoldi F, D'Orlando L, Mercante WP. Electromechanical dissociation 48 hours after atenolol overdose: usefulness of calcium chloride. *Ann Emerg Med* 1998;31:777.
17. Peterson CD, Leeder JS, Steiner S. Glucagon therapy for β-blocker overdose. *Drug Intell Clin Pharm* 1984;18:394.
18. Singh S, Lazin A, Cohen A, et al. Sotalol-induced torsades de pointes successfully treated with hemodialysis after failure of conventional therapy. *Am Heart J* 1991;2:601.
19. Sugg MF, Latham RD, Bruce JE, et al. Potentiation of glucagon by theophylline in the intact canine model with complete beta-adrenoreceptor blockade by propranolol. *Ann Emerg Med* 1987;16:482.
20. Weinstein RS. Recognition and management of poisoning with beta-adrenergic blocking agents. *Ann Emerg Med* 1984;13:1123.

CHAPTER 321
Calcium Channel Blocker Poisoning

G. Randall Bond

Calcium channel blockers (CCBs) are a structurally diverse group of drugs that are used for the treatment of supraventricular arrhythmias, hypertension, angina, heart failure, and subarachnoid hemorrhage, and in the prevention of migraine headaches. Ten CCBs are currently approved for use in the United States: verapamil, diltiazem, nifedipine, nicardipine, felodipine, isradipine, amlodipine, nisoldipine, nimodipine, and bepridil.

Calcium channels are found in the membranes of many cells, especially those of vascular smooth muscle, the myocardium, and the specialized pacemaker and conducting fibers of the heart. Membrane depolarization leads to the influx of calcium ions by way of the calcium channels. As intracellular calcium concentration rises in muscle cells, actin–myosin interaction inhibition ceases and muscle contraction occurs. In the pacemaker cells of the sinoatrial and atrioventricular (AV) nodes, the influx of calcium by way of slow channels during phase 4 of the action potential accounts for spontaneous depolarization. In His-Purkinje cells, calcium influx by way of slow channels contributes to phase 2 (plateau) as well as to phase 4 of the action potential. CCBs act by depressing the activation, inactivation, and recovery of slow calcium channels, and are thus classified as class IV antiarrhythmics. Cardiovascular responses to therapeutic doses vary considerably (Tables 321.1 and 321.2). Serum calcium and ionized calcium levels remain normal in therapeutic use and overdosage, and do not reflect the pharmacologic loss of calcium activity.

CCBs are well absorbed after oral administration. With verapamil, onset of action is noted within the first hour, and peak effects occur approximately 5 hours after ingestion. Nifedipine, nicardipine, and diltiazem, on the other hand, are more rapidly absorbed and show peak effects in 30 minutes to 2 hours after ingestion. Symptom onset and peak effects are usually delayed 6 to 18 hours after the ingestion of sustained-release preparations. CCBs are significantly protein-bound (80% to 98%), have a moderate volume of distribution (1.4 to 4.3 L/kg), are extensively metabolized by the liver, and are excreted in the urine and bile. Verapamil, diltiazem, and bepridil have active metabolites. The elimination half-life for most CCBs is 2 to 9 hours in therapeutic doses. Amlodipine and bepridil have longer half-lives, ranging from 24 to 60 hours. After overdose, the half-life of diltiazem remains unchanged; those of verapamil and nifedipine increase slightly.[4,9,11,15]

Most of the CCB clinical toxicology experience is based on three agents: verapamil, diltiazem, and nifedipine. Nicardipine, felodipine, nisoldipine, isradipine, amlodipine, and nimodipine are members of the same class as nifedipine (dihydropyridines) and can be expected to have similar toxicity. Bepridil is a unique agent, with actions both as a CCB and a type Ia antiarrhythmic (see Chapter 311). The toxic cardiovascular effects of CCBs are due to an exaggeration of their therapeutic effects. Peripheral vascular resistance is always decreased, but cardiac output may be normal, increased, or decreased. Central nervous system effects are secondary to hypoperfusion. Hypoperfusion may also lead to lactic acidosis. Inhibition of calcium-dependent insulin release may cause hyperglycemia. With overdosage, the drug-specific effects noted in Table 321.1 are often lost.[13,16]

Because people ingest drugs that are readily available to them, an unusually large percentage of CCB poisoning occurs in older people. Most of these are intentional, but some result from confusion or failing vision. Toxic doses are at least one to two times the usual total daily dose.[16] Significant toxicity has been reported after ingestion of a single tablet of by a child.[18] The elderly are susceptible to lower toxic doses.[16] Toxicity can also be seen when these agents are used in therapeutic doses with other

TABLE 321.1. Cardiovascular Response to Drug Therapy

	Verapamil	Diltiazem	Nifedipine and Other Dihydropyridines	Bepridil
Heart rate (sinoatrial node)	↑ or ↓	↓	↑	↓
Atrioventricular nodal conduction	↓↓	↓	↑	↓
Smooth-muscle tone	↓↓	↓	↓↓↓	↓
Blood pressure	↓	↓	↓↓	↓
Contractility (*in vivo*)	↓↓	↓	↑ or ↓	↓

TABLE 321.2. Therapeutic Doses of Calcium Channel Blockers

Drug	Trade name	Usual Dose	Therapeutic Range
Verapamil	Calan, Isoptin, Verelan		
Oral		80–160 mg t.i.d.	15–100 ng/mL
Intravenous		5–10 mg	
Diltiazem	Cardizem, Dilacor	30–90 mg q.i.d.	30–130 ng/mL
Nifedipine	Adalat, Procardia	10–40 mg t.i.d.	25–100 ng/mL
Nicardipine	Cardene	20–40 mg q.i.d.	28–50 ng/mL
Nimodipine	Nimotop	60 mg q4h	7–96 ng/mL
Felodipine	Plendil	5–20 mg qd	0.7–8.0 ng/mL
Isradipine	DynaCirc	2.5–10.0 mg b.i.d.	2–8 mg/mL
Nisoldipine	Sular	20–40 mg qd	
Amlodipine	Norvasc	2.5–10.0 mg qd	5–15 mg/mL
Bepridil	Vascor	200–400 mg qd	

myocardial depressants, such as β-adrenergic blockers and quinidine-like agents.

CLINICAL PRESENTATION

Signs and symptoms of toxicity usually develop within 30 minutes of ingestion but may be delayed as long as 16 hours after overdose of sustained-released preparations. Findings include hypotension, bradycardia, drowsiness, confusion, thready pulse, and peripheral cyanosis. Older patients may experience chest pain and myocardial ischemia and infarction. Inadequate perfusion may also result in cerebral, renal and bowel ischemia, or infarction in patients of all ages. In severe cases, coma, seizures, and respiratory distress associated with pulmonary edema are described. The electrocardiogram (ECG) often shows decreased rate and first-, second-, or even third-degree AV block, and may have changes indicative of ischemia or infarction.[16] Chest radiography may show pulmonary edema. Laboratory abnormalities include metabolic acidosis and hyperglycemia. Serum drug levels are not readily available and have not proved useful in the management of these patients.

Toxic effects typically last 24 to 36 hours. Duration may be longer after ingestion of bepridil, amlodipine, and sustained-release preparations. Complications have required longer hospitalizations in many patients.

DIFFERENTIAL DIAGNOSIS

Patients with primary myocardial infarction, as well as those with overdosage of β-adrenergic blockers, digoxin, clonidine, guanabenz, imidazolines, angiotensin converting enzyme inhibitors, cholinergic agents (nicotine, organophosphate and carbamate insecticides, and myasthenic agents), tricyclic antidepressants, α-methyldopa, and veratrum alkaloid-containing sneezing powders, may present similarly to those with CCB ingestion. β-Adrenergic blocking agents are more likely to cause hypoglycemia, and CCBs are more likely to cause hyperglycemia. With cholinergic agents salivation, nausea, vomiting, diarrhea, and weakness dominate the presentation. Tricyclic antidepressant overdosage infrequently presents with heart block and bradycardia. The QRS complex is often prolonged in tricyclic antidepressant ingestion but is usually normal with CCB overdosage.

EMERGENCY DEPARTMENT EVALUATION

The history should include time of ingestion and all other substances ingested or available to the patient. Physical examination should focus on the pulse, blood pressure, central nervous system function, heart, lungs, and peripheral perfusion. All patients should have cardiac monitoring, an ECG, and frequent monitoring of blood pressure. Those with symptoms, abnormal vital signs, or an abnormal ECG should have arterial blood gas analysis and determination of serum electrolytes, glucose, blood urea nitrogen, and creatinine. Continuous peripheral and pulmonary artery pressure monitoring may be necessary in patients with shock.

EMERGENCY DEPARTMENT MANAGEMENT

Advanced life-support measures should be initiated as necessary. Intravenous access should be established in all patients. Early management should include gastrointestinal decontamination. Activated charcoal is the preferred method.

Mild hypotension may respond to a fluid challenge with 1 to 2 L of saline solution (10 to 20 mL/kg in children). When bradycardia, with or without AV block, is also present, atropine (1.0 mg intravenously; 0.01 mg/kg in children) can be tried. Response is infrequent but may be improved following calcium administration.[8,16]

Hypotension and symptomatic bradycardia should also be treated with calcium chloride (1 g intravenous slow push; 10 to 20 mg/kg in children).[16] Calcium gluconate (3 g intravenous slow push; 30 to 60 mg/kg in children) may be given if calcium chloride is unavailable. This dose may be repeated several times in patients who show incomplete, transient, or no response.[2,6,13,14] Care must be taken to avoid extravasation, which can result in severe tissue damage. A continuous infusion at the rate of 1 g/h of calcium chloride or gluconate may be used to support heart rate and blood pressure in patients who relapse after an initial bolus. Doses as high as 30 g of calcium gluconate in 12 hours have been used with success.[2] Calcium levels should be monitored in patients receiving more than two doses, but very high serum calcium levels are not a reason to discontinue treatment. Response and survival have been associated with dosing that resulted in a peak serum calcium level of 23.8 mg/dL.[2] In another patient who responded to high-dose calcium, irreversible hypotension occurred when calcium gluconate was discontinued, solely because the serum calcium level had reached 17.7 mg/dL.[13]

Hemodynamically compromising bradycardia or heart block unresponsive to atropine and calcium may respond to an infusion of glucagon or isoproterenol, but a pacemaker is often required.[3,16] Hypotension unresponsive to fluids and calcium should be treated with pressors. Pressors may be given without regard to the coincident presence of heart disease or acute myocardial infarction, because they are titrated to reverse the adverse pharmacologic effect of the calcium blocking agent. Dopamine, dobutamine, norepinephrine, isoproterenol, and combinations of these have been used with success. Beta-agonist (inotropic) activity may be more important than alpha-agonist (peripheral vasoconstricting) activity, particularly following verapamil and diltiazem ingestions. Glucagon may also be considered in this setting. Intravenous doses of glucagon, 5 and 10 mg, have each been reported to produce a significant response.[3,19] Amrinone has produced additive effects, with isoproterenol in one case report and glucagon in another.[5,20] The use of an intraaortic balloon pump should be considered in patients who are unresponsive to pharmacologic therapies. Cardiopulmonary bypass was also used to sustain a child until hepatic metabolism of verapamil occurred.[7]

Hyperinsulinemia–euglycemia therapy, which facilitates myocardial metabolism and enhances myocardial contractility, significantly improved hemodynamics and survival over controls and epinephrine-treated, calcium-treated, and glucagon-treated dogs.[12] Human experience is limited. Five humans with severe hypotension and bradycardia, considered unresponsive to conventional therapy, were treated with regular insulin (0.1 to 0.2 U/kg as a bolus, followed by 0.1 to 1.0 U/kg/h) along with glucose (25 g as a bolus, followed by 1 g/kg/h as a 20% infusion) and potassium sufficient to maintain euglycemia and normokalemia.[10] Blood pressure normalized in all five, and all five survived. Two had transient asymptomatic hypoglycemia.

Limited information exists regarding the use of multidose charcoal to enhance CCB elimination in the overdose setting, but when used, it has not been shown to be of benefit.[17] Although enhanced elimination using charcoal hemoperfusion was described in a patient with diltiazem overdose,[1] it should not be regarded as standard therapy. If supportive measures can maintain a pulse and blood pressure sufficient to allow hemoperfusion, there is little to be gained from this procedure. Full recovery can be expected, unless prolonged shock has resulted in irreversible end-organ damage.

DISPOSITION

Asymptomatic patients should be observed for 4 to 6 hours after ingestion of standard formulations and 18 to 24 hours following ingestion of sustained-release ones. Those who remain asymptomatic may be discharged or referred for psychiatric evaluation. Symptomatic patients should be admitted to an intensive care unit. A regional poison center or a toxicologist should be consulted if the physician is unfamiliar with the management of CCB overdosage. Transfer may be necessary if an intensive care unit bed is unavailable and should be arranged as soon as the ingestion is recognized, because cardiovascular performance may rapidly deteriorate. The patient should be transferred in an advanced life-support unit with an adequate supply of cardiovascular drugs, including calcium chloride and glucagon, on hand.

COMMON PITFALLS

- Failure to consider CCB poisoning in patients with hypotension, bradycardia, or AV block, particularly when hyperglycemia is present
- Failure to observe asymptomatic patients with overdoses of sustained preparations for an extended period of time
- Failure to administer calcium, a specific antidote, for hypotension or bradycardia
- Failure to administer chronotropic agents and pressors to patients with myocardial ischemia secondary to hypoperfusion
- Failure to appreciate that refractory hypotension and bradycardia may respond to glucagon or high-dose insulin and glucose therapy
- Failure to consider invasive hemodynamic monitoring and cardiovascular support in patients with shock

ACKNOWLEDGMENT

Richard Gerkin, M.D., contributed to previous versions of this chapter.

References

1. Anthony T, Jastremski M, Elliot W, et al. Charcoal hemoperfusion for the treatment of a combined diltiazem and metoprolol overdose. *Ann Emerg Med* 1986;15:1344.
2. Buckley N, Whyte I, Dawson H. Overdose with calcium channel blockers [Correspondence]. *BMJ* 1994; 308: 1639.
3. Doyon S, Roberts JR. The use of glucagon in a case of calcium channel blocker overdose. *Ann Emerg Med* 1993;22:1229–1233.
4. Ferner RE, Monkman S, Riley S, et al. Pharmacokinetics and toxic effects of nifedipine in massive overdose. *Hum Exp Toxicol* 1990;9:309–311.
5. Goenen M, Col J, Compete A, et al. Treatment of severe verapamil poisoning with combined amrinone-isoproterenol therapy. *Am J Cardiol* 1986;58:1142.
6. Haddad LM. Resuscitation after nifedipine overdose exclusively with intravenous calcium chloride. *Am J Emerg Med* 1996;14:602–603.
7. Hendren WG, Schieber RS, Garrettson LK. Extracorporeal bypass for the treatment of verapamil poisoning. *Ann Emerg Med* 1989;18(9):984–987.
8. Howarth DM, Dawson AH, Smith AJ, et al. Calcium channel blocking drug overdose: an Australian series. *Hum Exp Toxicol* 1994;13:161–166.
9. Jablowski AT, Mizgala HF. Effect of diltiazem overdose. *Am J Cardiol* 1987;60:932.
10. Kerns R. Are we ready to utilize insulin-glucose as routine therapy for calcium channel blocker toxicity? *Int J Med Toxicol* 1998;1(5):23.
11. Kivisto K, Neuvonen PJ, Tarssanen L. Pharmacokinetics of verapamil in overdose. *Hum Exp Toxicol* 1997;16:35–37.
12. Kline JA, Leonova MS, Raymond RM. Beneficial myocardial metabolic effects of insulin during verapamil toxicity in the anesthetized canine. *Crit Care Med* 1995;23:1251–1263.
13. Koch AR, Vogelaers DP, Decruyenaere JM, et al. Fatal intoxication with amlodipine. *J Toxicol Clin Toxicol* 1995;33(3):253–256.
14. Luscher TF, Noll G, Sturmer T, et al. Calcium gluconate in severe verapamil intoxication [Correspondence]. *N Engl J Med* 1994;330:718–719.
15. Malcolm N, Callegari P, Goldberg J, et al. Massive diltiazem overdosage: clinical and pharmacokinetic observations. *Drug Intell Clin Pharm* 1986;20:888.
16. Ramoska EA, Spiller HA, Winter M, et al. A one-year evaluation of calcium channel blocker overdoses. Toxicity and treatment. *Ann Emerg Med* 1993;22(2):196–200.
17. Roberts D, Honcharik N, Sitar DS, et al. Diltiazem overdose. Pharmacokinetics of diltiazem and its metabolites and effect of multiple dose charcoal therapy. *J Toxicol Clin Toxicol* 1991;29(1):45–52.
18. Spiller HA, Ramoska EA. Isradipine ingestion in a 2 year old. *Vet Hum Toxicol* 1992;34:329(abst).
19. Walter FG, Frye G, Mullen JT, et al. Amelioration of nifedipine poisoning associated with glucagon therapy. *Ann Emerg Med* 1993;22:1234–1237.
20. Wolf LR, Spadafora MP, Otten EJ. Use of amrinone and glucagon in a case of calcium channel blocker overdose. *Ann Emerg Med* 1993;22(7):1225–1228.

CHAPTER 322

Carbamazepine Poisoning

Marco L. A. Sivilotti

Carbamazepine (CBZ) is an anticonvulsant drug widely used for the management of epilepsy, trigeminal neuralgia, chronic pain syndromes, and affective disorders. Its main actions are to reduce the permeability of neuronal membranes to sodium and potassium ions, and to block norepinephrine reuptake. CBZ is an iminostilbene derivative, structurally related to the tricyclic antidepressants. Despite the structural resemblance between CBZ and the tricyclic antidepressants, there is only partial overlapping in their toxicity after overdose. Notably, the therapeutic index of CBZ is much greater than the tricyclic antidepressants.

CBZ is available in 100- and 200-mg tablets and as a 100-mg/5 mL suspension. Although CBZ is almost completely absorbed, the rate of absorption can be erratic. Peak concentrations, usually found 4 to 8 hours after therapeutic dosing, may be delayed 24 to 72 hours after massive ingestions. At therapeutic concentrations (4 and 10 mg/L), CBZ is 75% bound to plasma proteins, with a volume of distribution of 0.8 to 1.2 L/kg and a total body clearance of about 1.3 mL/kg/min (adult). CBZ is predominantly metabolized to CBZ 10,11 epoxide (CBZE), which, in turn, is metabolized and excreted principally as glucuronides in the urine.[5] CBZE is pharmacologically active, possessing both anticonvulsant and toxic properties. Concentrations of CBZE are usually about 20% of those of CBZ, but can be as high as 50% after overdose. CBZE is less protein-bound (50%) and has a smaller volume of distribution (0.74 L/kg) and a shorter half-life than CBZ, but it has a comparable total body clearance.

Within weeks of therapeutic use, CBZ induces its own metabolism by hepatic P-450 enzymes, especially CYP 3A3 and 3A4. Consequently, patients naive to CBZ eliminate it with a half-life of 20 to 65 hours, much slower than that of the chronic user (8 to 17 hours). The half-life of CBZE is 8 to 14 hours. Other anticonvulsants, such as phenobarbital, phenytoin, valproic acid, and felbamate, may further increase the metabolism of CBZ by heteroinduction. CBZ metabolism is inhibited by erythromycin, propoxyphene, isoniazid, calcium channel blockers, cimetidine, fluvoxamine, ketoconazole, and other CYP 3A3 and 3A4 inhibitors, at times resulting in toxicity despite therapeutic CBZ dosing.

After overdose, significant toxicity can be expected after ingestion of 20 to 30 mg/kg in an adult patient not regularly taking CBZ,[14] and life-threatening effects may occur after ingestion of 140 mg/kg.[3] Ingestions of greater than 20 g have been associated with fatal outcome.[16] In a patient regularly taking CBZ, and thus with induced metabolism, survival has been reported after acute ingestion of 640 mg/kg.[15] One patient survived an ingestion of 80 g.[14] After an overdose, even in patients on chronic therapy, the half-life of CBZ is prolonged to about 19 hours.[8] This may be due to saturation of the rate-limiting epoxidation to CBZE as well as ongoing gastrointestinal (GI) absorption.

CLINICAL PRESENTATION

The clinical manifestations of CBZ toxicity involve four main areas: central nervous system (CNS), ocular, cardiac, and motor.[11,16] Although a sequential progression is classically described, individual patients may present at any stage and may, at times, progress rapidly to profound coma and cardiac instability.[13] Initial symptoms include restlessness, confusion, excitation, and aggression. Dizziness, ataxia with nystagmus and diplopia, nausea, and vomiting are often present. As toxicity progresses, drowsiness, coma, and respiratory depression may occur, often after some hours.[20] Hypotension (preceded by hypertension) and rhythm disturbances may be seen in severe poisoning.[13] Loss of P waves, premature ventricular beats, QRS prolongation, and complete atrioventricular block have been described, and tend to occur in the elderly or patients with underlying cardiac disease.[9,10] In severe poisoning, the pupils may be fixed and dilated and the gaze disconjugate.

Abnormal motor findings include tremor, choreoathetoid movements, and hemiballismus. Reflexes may initially be hyperactive with clonus. Seizures can occur, usually in patients with underlying seizure disorder.[17] The electroencephalogram may be helpful in such patients, and may show occipital delta activity (usually suggestive of a brainstem disorder), which regresses as plasma CBZ concentrations subside.[7] In the deeply comatose patient, adynamic ileus, hypothermia, and pulmonary edema may be present. Complications include aspiration and sequelae of hypoxia and seizures. Hyponatremia may result from an antidiuretic effect.[4,16] Older patients may develop bradycardia or atrioventricular block, at times progressing to Adams-Stokes syncope or ventricular standstill.[9] Chronic intoxication may result in hypokalemia as well as hyponatremia.

Confusion, lethargy, and ataxia are usually associated with peak plasma CBZ concentrations of 15 mg/L; coma may be seen with concentrations higher than 20 mg/L. Coma, cardiovascular disturbances (hypotension, dysrhythmias), seizures, and death typically occur in patients with peak plasma concentrations higher than 40 mg/L.[6,11,17,18,20] It is important to note that these concentrations represent peak concentrations, which may occur hours or days after ingestion. Initial drug levels correlate only weakly with clinical course, and they are imperfect prognosticators of outcome.[11,16] Because of the long half-life after overdose, continued absorption over many hours, and the additive effects of the active metabolite CBZE, the clinical course is typically prolonged.[8] Severely poisoned patients may require more than a week to make a full recovery. Cyclic coma, in which partial recovery is followed by a relapse into a coma, presumably due to resumption of absorption as the "gut wakes up," has been described.[6,17,19]

DIFFERENTIAL DIAGNOSIS

Mild poisoning may present in a manner similar to that of hypoglycemia, neurologic disease, serotonin syndrome, or intoxication by ethanol. In severe poisoning, the clinical picture may mimic that of overdose with tricyclic antidepressants, anticholinergic agents, or other anticonvulsants. Other physiologic depressants, coexistent trauma, and coingestions should also be considered. A prolonged postictal state in a patient with a history of seizures should raise suspicion for poisoning with CBZ or another anticonvulsant.

EMERGENCY DEPARTMENT EVALUATION

A directed history should be obtained from the patient, prehospital care providers, or available friends and family members. Attempts should be made to ascertain recent dosing changes or whether the patient has been prescribed other medications that may inhibit CBZ metabolism. The physical examination should include a full set of vital signs pupil position, size, and reactivity; bowel sounds; and a focused neurologic examination, including level and content of consciousness, responsiveness to stimuli, reflexes, motor tone, and cerebellar function. A 12-lead electrocardiogram (ECG), cardiac monitoring, and serum electrolyte and glucose determinations are indicated in symptomatic patients. Comprehensive toxicology testing and computed tomography scanning of the head should be performed when there is diagnostic uncertainty.

Frequent measurements of CBZ concentrations are mandatory to detect continued absorption in patients with acute overdose. Serial levels should be obtained until the patient is asymptomatic and levels have clearly peaked and fallen below 10 mg/L. Rebounds in levels coinciding with clinical deterioration are well described. Serum CBZ and CBZE concentrations can be separately determined by high-performance liquid chromatography. A CBZ/CBZE ratio above 2.5 suggests ongoing absorption of CBZ from the GI tract. Many centers, however, use immunologic assays, which cannot distinguish between CBZE and the parent compound.

EMERGENCY DEPARTMENT MANAGEMENT

Advanced life-support measures should be instituted, as necessary. As always, stabilization of the airway has the highest priority. Most deaths from CBZ overdose are secondary to complications such as pulmonary aspiration and respiratory depression. Level of consciousness and vital signs should be monitored. Hypotension should be managed with intravenous fluids and, if necessary, invasive pressure monitoring and pressors such as norepinephrine. Fluids, however, should be carefully monitored to avoid fluid overload, an inherent risk due to CBZ's antidiuretic effect. Arrhythmias should be treated as described for cyclic antidepressants.

Activated charcoal is the preferred method of GI decontamination and is recommended for all symptomatic patients (regardless of time to presentation) and for those with significant ingestions by history. Multiple-dose charcoal therapy enhances the elimination of CBZ and should be instituted for patients with significant symptoms or CBZ levels above 20 mg/L.[1,12,18] This treatment should be continued until levels have fallen into the therapeutic range or lower (based on whether the patient is dependent on the anticonvulsant properties of CBZ).

Forced diuresis, peritoneal dialysis, and hemodialysis are of no value in CBZ poisoning. Although CBZ is effectively cleared from the blood during charcoal hemoperfusion,[2,10,14] only a small proportion of the CBZ ingested can be removed, and hemoperfusion is difficult to obtain in a timely fashion in most centers. Hemoperfusion should be considered only for those with significant dysrhythmias, hypotension, or prolonged coma and extremely elevated CBZ levels despite multiple-dose activated charcoal.

DISPOSITION

Patients who are symptomatic or who have a CBZ level that is rising or higher than 20 mg/L should be admitted. Those with moderate or severe clinical toxicity, rising drug levels, or an abnormal ECG should be treated in an intensive care unit. A regional poison center or clinical toxicologist should be consulted if the physician is unfamiliar with CBZ poisoning. Psychiatric evaluation should be obtained for patients with intentional overdose.

COMMON PITFALLS

- Failure to appreciate that CBZ absorption is slow and erratic and that peak levels may not be seen for many hours or days after acute overdose
- Being falsely reassured by a low CBZ concentration shortly after ingestion and failure to obtain serial drug levels after acute overdose
- Failure to appreciate that although CBZ is an anticonvulsant, overdosage can cause or exacerbate seizures
- Failure to appreciate that CBZ is structurally similar to tricyclic antidepressants and can cause similar CNS and cardiovascular toxicity
- Failure to appreciate that activated charcoal may be useful, even many hours after ingestion
- Failure to consider the use of multiple-dose charcoal therapy for enhancing CBZ elimination
- Failure to appreciate that CBZ has active metabolites and that clinical toxicity may take days to resolve

ACKNOWLEDGMENT

Andrew J. W. Heath contributed to previous versions of this chapter.

References

1. Boldy DAR, Heath A, Ruddock S, et al. Activated charcoal for carbamazepine poisoning. *Lancet* 1987;1:1027.
2. De Groot G, Van Heijst ANP, Maes RAA. Charcoal hemoperfusion in the treatment of two cases as of acute carbamazepine poisoning. *Clin Toxicol* 1984;22:349.
3. Drenck NE, Risbo A. Carbamazepine poisoning, a surprisingly severe case. *Anaesth Intensive Care* 1980;8:203.
4. Edge W, Edmonds J. Serum sodium and carbamazepine overdose. *Clin Toxicol* 1992;30:479.
5. Eichelbaum M, Tomson T, Tybring G, et al. Carbamazepine metabolism in man: induction and pharmacogenetic aspects. *Clin Pharmacokinet* 1985;10:80.
6. Hojer J, Malmlund HO, Berg A. Clinical features in 28 consecutive cases of laboratory confirmed massive poisoning with carbamazepine alone. *J Toxicol Clin Toxicol* 1993;31:449.
7. Howard RS, Trend P, Townsend HRA. EEG appearances in acute carbamazepine toxicity. *Hum Exp Toxicol* 1990;9:313.
8. Hundt HKL, Aucamp AK, Muller FO. Pharmacokinetic aspects of carbamazepine and its two major metabolites in plasma during overdosage. *Hum Toxicol* 1983;2:607.
9. Kasarskis EJ, Juo C-S, Berzer R, et al. Carbamazepine-induced cardiac dysfunction: characterization of two distinct clinical syndromes. *Arch Intern Med* 1992;152;186.
10. Leslie PJ, Heyworth R, Prescott LF. Cardiac complications of carbamazepine intoxication: treatment by haemoperfusion. *BMJ* 1983;286:1018.
11. Montgomery VL, Richman BJ, Goldsmith LJ, et al. Severity and carbamazepine level at time of initial poison center contact correlated with outcome in carbamazepine poisoning. *J Toxicol Clin Toxicol* 1995;33:311.
12. Montoya-Cabrera MA, Sauceda-Garcia JM, Escalante-Galindo P, et al. Carbamazepine poisoning in adolescent suicide attempters. Effectiveness of multiple-dose activated charcoal in enhancing carbamazepine elimination. *Arch Med Res* 1996;27:485.
13. Mordel A, Sivilotti MLA, Linden CH. Fatal TCA-like cardiotoxicity following carbamazepine overdose. *Clin Toxicol* 1998;36:472.
14. Nilsson C, Sterner G, Idvall J. Charcoal hemoperfusion for treatment of serious carbamazepine poisoning. *Acta Med Scand* 1984;216:137.
15. Patsalos PN, Krishna S, Elyas AA, et al. Carbamazepine and carbamazepine 10,11 epoxide pharmacokinetics in an overdose patient. *Hum Toxicol* 1987;6:241.
16. Schmidt S, Schmitz-Buhl M. Signs and symptoms of carbamazepine overdose. *J Neurol* 1995;242:169.
17. Spiller HA, Krenzelok EP, Cookson E. Carbamazepine overdose: a prospective study of serum levels and toxicity. *J Toxicol Clin Toxicol* 190;28:445.
18. Stremski ES, Brady WB, Prasad K, et al. Pediatric carbamazepine intoxication. *Ann Emerg Med* 1995;25:624.
19. Sullivan JB Jr, Rumack BH, Peterson RG. Acute carbamazepine toxicity resulting from overdose. *Neurology* 1981;31:621.
20. Tibballs J. Acute toxic reaction to carbamazepine: clinical effects and serum concentrations. *J Pediatr* 1992;121:295.

CHAPTER 323
Carbon Monoxide Poisoning

Kent R. Olson

Carbon monoxide (CO) is a colorless, odorless gas produced by the combustion of any carbon-containing material. It is found in automobile exhaust and in gas and coal heaters, and it is an important toxin in smoke inhalation victims of fires (see Chapter 396).[5,14] CO is also produced *in vivo* by the metabolism of inhaled methylene chloride.[6] In the 10-year period from 1979 through 1988, a total of 56,133 deaths in the United States were attributed to CO poisoning. Of these, 25,889 were suicides, 15,523 were associated with severe burns or house fires, and 11,547 were classified as unintentional.[1] By most statistics, CO is one of the leading agents of fatal poisoning in the United States.

CO produces toxicity by three possible mechanisms: hypoxemia, ischemia, and cellular asphyxia.[9] It combines with hemoglobin with an affinity approximately 250 times greater than that of oxygen. Thus, at even low levels, significant saturation of hemoglobin-binding sites may occur, decreasing the oxygen-carrying capacity of the blood. In addition, CO binding to hemoglobin alters the shape of the oxygen–hemoglobin dissociation curve, effectively shifting it to the left, resulting in further lowering of intracellular oxygen concentrations. CO may also produce toxicity by decreasing cardiac output and causing hypotension, resulting in ischemic organ damage.[4] Finally, it has been proposed that CO may bind to intracellular cytochromes, interfering with oxygen utilization.[13,20]

The dose required to produce toxicity varies, depending on the rate of ventilation, the underlying health of the victim, and the presence of other toxins. Equilibrium is reached more rapidly in people who perform vigorous physical activity. As little as 0.1% CO (1,000 ppm) may produce potentially fatal 50% saturation of hemoglobin at equilibrium. The exposure limit in the workplace is 25 ppm as an 8-hour time-weighted average. The level considered immediately dangerous to life or health is 1,200 ppm. People with underlying pulmonary or cardiovascular disease may not be able to tolerate hypoxia produced by even mild or moderate CO levels. Infants and fetuses are more susceptible to CO poisoning, because fetal hemoglobin has an even higher affinity for CO.[11]

CO is rapidly absorbed from the lungs. After removal from exposure, CO slowly desaturates hemoglobin, with an apparent half-life in room air of about 4 to 5 hours.[9,13] The apparent half-life of CO produced by methylene chloride metabolism is substantially longer.

CLINICAL PRESENTATION

The signs and symptoms of CO poisoning are highly variable and nonspecific. At low levels, headache, dizziness, nausea, vomiting, and diarrhea are common. With higher levels, confusion, syncope, shortness of breath, and angina pectoris may occur. Severe poisoning may cause coma, seizures, hypotension, cardiac arrhythmias, and death (Table 323.1).[4,8,9,13] Although the severity of intoxication usually parallels the CO–hemoglobin level, there are reports of patients with severe intoxication with relatively low levels and of patients with high levels but minimal symptoms.[2] Survivors of severe poisoning are often left with permanent neurologic injury, which may be gross (blindness, deafness, seizures, parkinsonism, or vegetative state) or subtle (memory loss or personality changes).[4,8,9,13,19]

The physical examination may reveal cherry-red coloration of the skin, mucous membranes, and venous blood, owing to the bright red color of the CO–hemoglobin complex. This finding is inconsistently noted in patients with CO poisoning, and its presence or absence cannot be considered diagnostic.[9] Retinal hemorrhage may be present. Neurologic examination usually reveals altered mental status, which may rapidly improve after the patient is removed from the poisoned atmosphere and oxygen is administered. Arterial blood gas analysis and serum electrolyte levels often reveal metabolic acidosis, which is caused by tissue hypoxia–ischemia. The arterial PO_2, and hence the calculated oxygen saturation, are usually normal, because dissolved oxygen in the serum is not affected by CO. Although the oxygen saturation measured directly by co-oximetry is less than that calculated from the PO_2 (by an amount roughly equal to the percent CO–hemoglobin), the oxygen saturation measured by pulse oximetry is falsely normal.[16] Signs of myocardial ischemia are frequently present on the electrocardiogram (ECG), and, occasionally, myocardial infarction occurs.

DIFFERENTIAL DIAGNOSIS

Other causes of coma and altered mental status should be sought, such as hypoglycemia, head trauma, meningitis, and drug or alcohol intoxication. Many suicidal patients ingest medications and alcohol as they poison themselves with CO. Other toxic gases should be considered in any patient with smoke inhalation. Cyanide, hydrogen sulfide, agents that cause methemoglobinemia, and other toxins may produce symptoms and signs of systemic hypoxia that are similar to those of CO.[4,9,14]

TABLE 323.1. Signs and Symptoms of Carbon Monoxide Poisoning

Carbon Monoxide–Hemoglobin Level (%)	Signs and Symptoms
0–10	Usually none
10–20	Headache, dyspnea with minimal exertion, angina in patients with coronary disease
20–30	Moderate headache, dyspnea, nausea, dizziness
30–40	Severe headache, vomiting, fatigue, poor judgment
40–50	Confusion, syncope, tachypnea, tachycardia
50–60	Syncope, seizures, coma
60–70	Coma, hypotension, arrhythmias, death
>70	Rapidly fatal

EMERGENCY DEPARTMENT EVALUATION

Immediate evaluation in the emergency department should include rapid neurologic assessment and determination of the specific carboxyhemoglobin saturation (this may be performed on a venous or arterial sample). History that may be helpful in raising suspicion of CO poisoning includes being found in a car with the engine running, riding in the back of a pick-up truck, multiple victims found in a common room, smoke inhalation, and use of paint strippers or solvents that contain methylene chloride in a poorly ventilated area. Depending on severity, arterial blood gas analysis (using a co-oximeter), routine laboratory evaluation, ECG, and chest radiography may be indicated. Patients with suspected trauma should have a computed tomography scan of the head.

EMERGENCY DEPARTMENT MANAGEMENT

Advanced life-support measures should be instituted as needed. Oxygen (100%) should be provided through a tight-fitting mask or a nonrebreather mask with oxygen reservoir, or by way of an endotracheal tube. If the patient is hypotensive, 1 to 2 L of crystalloid solution should be administered. ECG, arterial blood gases, and the carboxyhemoglobin level should be monitored. Mild-to-moderate metabolic acidosis (i.e., serum pH 7.2 to 7.3) should not be treated, because acidosis may facilitate oxygen delivery to the tissues by moving the oxygen–hemoglobin dissociation curve to the right.

Decontamination is performed by removing the victim from the toxic environment; the rescuer should take care not to become exposed during the rescue (a self-contained breathing apparatus is recommended). Administer 100% oxygen, which shortens the half-life of CO to 40 to 80 minutes. Hyperbaric oxygen (HBO), 100% oxygen provided under pressures greater than 1 atm, may further speed removal of CO to a half-life of 20 minutes or less.[9,13,18] Some clinicians believe that HBO may also drive CO from intracellular sites, although this has not been proved. Animal studies suggest a potential protective effect of HBO against CO-induced postischemic reperfusion injury, although this benefit may be nonspecific and could have broader application for other anoxic–ischemic injuries.

Controversy remains about which patients should receive HBO treatment. Most hospitals do not have ready access to a chamber, which means that unstable patients may require transport over long distances at a time when arrhythmias and hypotension are more likely to occur. Because the half-life of CO–hemoglobin in 100% oxygen at 1 atm is less than 1 hour, in most cases, the level has already dropped to low levels by the time the HBO chamber is ready. Despite numerous case reports and uncontrolled case series supporting the use of HBO, its value has not been settled. Proponents of HBO argue that it may provide protection against late neurologic sequelae, but this claim has never been proved.[13,15,18] Up until recently, no randomized controlled studies were available to compare HBO with normobaric oxygen (NBO). In a study that failed to show a benefit of HBO compared with 100% oxygen at normal pressure, only patients without a reported loss of consciousness were randomized, a subgroup that has an expected good outcome anyway.[10] Although a greater incidence of delayed neuropsychiatric sequelae was observed in patients who received NBO compared with HBO, all patients reportedly had resolution of their symptoms within 77 days.[13] Moreover, this and other previous studies did not blind patients and health-care providers to the treatment received.

Recently, two double-blind, randomized, and placebo-controlled ("sham" HBO) studies were completed, and both found no difference in outcome between HBO and NBO.[12,17] Both studies randomized all patients regardless of severity. In one, extensive follow-up neuropsychiatric testing was performed.[17]

Pregnant women and infants pose a special problem in CO poisoning, because fetal hemoglobin has a greater affinity for CO than does normal hemoglobin.[11,13] Prolonged oxygen therapy and a lower threshold for HBO are often recommended, although, once again, studies are lacking.

The prognosis after severe CO poisoning is unpredictable but grim. As many as 40% of victims have permanent neurologic injury. Patients with an abnormal computed tomography, SPECT scan, or magnetic resonance imaging scan on admission appear to be at higher risk for permanent sequelae.[3,19]

DISPOSITION

All patients with loss of consciousness or with seizures should be admitted to the hospital, as should those with evidence of myocardial infarction or ischemia. Similarly, infants, young children, and pregnant women require intensive or prolonged treatment and should be admitted. Most authorities would also automatically admit any patient with a CO–hemoglobin level greater than 25%, regardless of symptoms. One investigator has developed a neuropsychiatric screening protocol to help determine which patients with low CO levels should be admitted for aggressive therapy.[7]

Despite the lack of conclusive scientific data, many experts recommend HBO therapy for patients with any of the following: coma (including a history of loss of consciousness), cardiovascular dysfunction (including ECG evidence of ischemia), pulmonary edema, significant acidosis, CO–hemoglobin level greater than 30% to 40%, symptoms that persist despite NBO therapy, or delayed-onset neuropsychiatric complaints. Patients with mild symptoms who become asymptomatic after several hours of oxygen therapy and who have a CO level less than 10%, a normal physical examination, and normal arterial blood gas parameters may be discharged.

A regional poison center or medical toxicologist may provide assistance with the decision to use HBO and may also know the location of nearby HBO chambers. If the patient is experiencing cardiac arrhythmias or hypotension, a critical care nurse or physician should accompany the patient during transport to an HBO facility. Once the acute episode of poisoning has resolved, patients should be referred for follow-up neuropsychiatric evaluation. Those discharged from the emergency department should be instructed to return immediately if any signs of neurologic dysfunction develop.

COMMON PITFALLS

- Failure to appreciate that signs and symptoms of CO poisoning are often nonspecific and that the diagnosis may be missed if there is no accompanying history of exposure
- Failure to consider CO the diagnosis of CO poisoning in patients presenting with a severe headache. Despite common belief, the victim's skin is seldom noted to be cherry-red.
- Failure to appreciate that the arterial blood gas Po_2, calculated oxygen saturation, and pulse oximetry oxygen saturation are usually normal despite severe CO poisoning
- Failure to consider the ingestion of alcohol or other drugs in patients with suicidal exposure to carbon monoxide

References

1. Cobb N, Etzel RA. Unintentional carbon monoxide-related deaths in the United States, 1979 through 1988. *JAMA* 1991;266(5):659.
2. Davis SM, Levy RC. High carboxyhemoglobin level without acute or chronic findings. *J Emerg Med* 1984;1:539.
3. Gale SD, Hopkins RO, Weaver LK et al. MRI, quantitative MRI, SPECT, and neuropsychological findings following carbon monoxide poisoning. *Brain Inj* 1999;13(4):229–243.
4. Ginsberg MD. Carbon monoxide intoxication: clinical features, neuropathology, and mechanisms of injury. *J Toxicol Clin Toxicol* 1985;23:281.
5. Hampson NB, Norkool DM. Carbon monoxide poisoning in children riding in the back of pickup trucks. *JAMA* 1992;267(4):22,538.
6. Horowitz BZ. Carboxyhemoglobinemia caused by inhalation of methylene chloride. *Am J Emerg Med* 1986;4:48.
7. Messier LD, Myers RA. A neuropsychological screening battery for emergency assessment of carbon-monoxide-poisoned patients. *J Clin Psychol* 1991;47(5):675.
8. Mofenson HC, Caraccio TR, Brody GM. Carbon monoxide poisoning. *Am J Emerg Med* 1984;2:254.
9. Olson KR. Carbon monoxide poisoning: mechanism, presentation, and controversies in management. *J Emerg Med* 1984;1:233.
10. Raphael JC, Elkharrat D, Jars-Guincestre MC, et al. Trial of normobaric and hyperbaric oxygen for acute carbon monoxide intoxication. *Lancet* 1989;2(8660):414.
11. Rudge FW. Carbon monoxide poisoning in infants: treatment with hyperbaric oxygen. *South Med J* 1993;86(3):334.
12. Scheinkestel CD, Bailey M, Myles PS, et al. Hyperbaric or normobaric oxygen for acute carbon monoxide poisoning: a randomised controlled clinical trial. *Med J Aust* 1999;170(5):203–210.
13. Thom SR, Keim LW. Carbon monoxide poisoning: a review. Epidemiology, pathophysiology, clinical findings, and treatment options including hyperbaric oxygen therapy. *J Toxicol Clin Toxicol* 1989;27(3):141.
14. Thom SR. Smoke inhalation. *Emerg Med Clin North Am* 1989;7(2):371.
15. Thomson LF, Mardel SN, Jack A, et al. Management of the moribund carbon monoxide victim. *Arch Emerg Med* 1992;9(2):208.
16. Vegfors M, Lennmarken C. Carboxyhaemoglobinaemia and pulse oximetry [see comments]. *Br J Anaesth* 1991;66(5):625.
17. Weaver LK, et al. Double-blind, prospective randomized clinical trial in patients with acute carbon monoxide poisoning: outcome of patients treated with normobaric oxygen or hyperbaric oxygen—an interim report. *Undersea Hyperb Med* 1995; 22[Suppl]:14(abst).
18. Weiss LD, Van Meter KW. The applications of hyperbaric oxygen therapy in emergency medicine. *Am J Emerg Med* 1992;10(6):558.
19. Zagami AS, Lethlean AK, Mellick R. Delayed neurological deterioration following carbon monoxide poisoning: MRI findings. *J Neurol* 1993;240(2):113.
20. Zhang J, Piantadosi CA. Mitochondrial oxidative stress after carbon monoxide hypoxia in the rat brain. *J Clin Invest* 1992;90(4):1193.

CHAPTER 324
Centrally Acting Antihypertensive Agent Poisoning

James R. Roberts and Sharona Bryant

Centrally acting antihypertensives include clonidine, guanabenz, guanfacine, methyldopa, and reserpine. Clonidine hydrochloride is available in tablet form (Catapres: 0.1 mg, 0.2 mg, 0.3 mg), in combination with the diuretic chlorthalidone (Combipres), or as a transdermal patch (Catapres TTS) designed to be worn for a week and slowly release 0.1 mg, 0.2 mg, or 0.3 mg per day. Significant amounts of clonidine may remain in used patches, and children have mistaken discarded patches as Band-Aids or stickers, resulting in clonidine toxicity from transdermal absorption, oral ingestion, or mouthing of patches. Although it has no known teratogenicity in humans, clonidine use in pregnancy has been associated with transitory hypertension in neonates and hyperactivity and sleep disturbances in children; therefore, this drug is not recommended for use during pregnancy. Maintenance therapy (0.2 to 0.8 mg/d) may be associated with side effects, most commonly dry mouth, fatigue, sedation, constipation, sexual dysfunction, and nonpostural dizziness. In addition to its use as an antihypertensive agent, clonidine has been used to ameliorate the symptoms associated with alcohol, narcotic, and nicotine withdrawal; as an adjunct to sedation and pain management; to reduce postmenopausal flushing; as migraine headache prophylaxis; and for acute pancreatitis.[1,5,6] Clonidine has been increasingly used to treat attention deficit disorder in children.

Clonidine, an imidazole first used as a nasal decongestant, is the prototype of a group of centrally acting agents (including guanabenz and methyldopa) that produce their antihypertensive effect by stimulation of presynaptic α_2-adrenergic receptors in the medulla oblongata, resulting in a decreased sympathetic outflow from the central nervous system (CNS).[2,14] Although clonidine is primarily a central α_2-adrenergic agonist, it also possesses some peripheral α_1-adrenergic receptor agonist properties. The therapeutic effect of clonidine is attributed primarily to a reduction in heart rate and cardiac output rather than to a significant reduction in total peripheral resistance.

Guanabenz and guanfacine are structurally and pharmacologically similar to clonidine and produce similar toxicity.[7] Proprietary preparations may also contain thiazide diuretics. Mild withdrawal symptoms have been noted after abrupt cessation of maintenance therapy. As in clonidine overdose, there are no specific laboratory studies that are helpful in the diagnosis or treatment of guanabenz overdose. Guanabenz is not detected in standard toxicologic analysis, and quantitative levels are usually unavailable. If ingestion has been recent and significant, gastrointestinal decontamination, with oral activated charcoal alone, should be accomplished. There is no known benefit of hemodialysis, charcoal hemoperfusion, or forced diuresis. There are no known antidotes. Neither naloxone nor tolazoline has been reported to be useful. Cardiovascular and respiratory derangements are treated supportively.

After efficient absorption from the gastrointestinal tract, clonidine is 20% to 40% protein bound and highly lipid soluble, with excellent CNS penetration. Forty percent to 60% of the drug is excreted unchanged in the urine, and the remainder undergoes hepatic metabolism. Onset of action is 30 to 60 minutes, peaking in 2 to 3 hours. The elimination half-life is 5 to 13 hours, with minimal accumulation in renal failure. There are no known pharmacologically active metabolites. The volume of distribution is 3.2 to 5.6 L/kg.

After abrupt cessation of long-term clonidine therapy, a well-described withdrawal syndrome may occur, producing varying degrees of rebound hypertension, tachycardia, tremulousness, insomnia, anxiety, sweating, and palpitations.[4] The syndrome is usually mild and not life-threatening; however, significant cardiac arrhythmias and hypertensive crises have been reported, as well as one case of myocardial infarction thought to have resulted from acute clonidine withdrawal.[13] The withdrawal syndrome results from an unbalancing of central adrenergic activity; as clonidine's inhibitory effect at α_2-adrenergic receptors is removed, upregulated α_1-adrenergic receptors and elevated catecholamine levels operate to increase sympathetic outflow.

Except for one poorly documented fatality attributed to a massive ingestion in a child, deaths have not been reported from clonidine poisoning alone. Clonidine overdose can result in significant respiratory and cardiovascular instability and CNS depression. Deaths have been reported when clonidine has been taken with other drugs in suicide attempts.[15] A combined overdose of clonidine and methylphenidate, drugs used to treat attention deficit disorder, has anecdotally been associated with sudden death.

Guanfacine (Tenex) and guanabenz (Wytensin) are structurally and pharmacologically similar to clonidine and produce similar toxicity.[7] The usual adult dose is 1 to 2 mg for guanfacine and 2 to 4 mg for guanabenz. Proprietary preparations may also contain thiazide diuretics. Mild withdrawal symptoms have been noted after abrupt cessation of maintenance therapy. There are no known deaths related to a pure guanabenz or guanfacine overdose.

Methyldopa (Aldomet) is metabolized α-methylnorepinephrine, which may stimulate α_2-adrenergic receptors, indirectly reduce plasma renin activity, or act as a "false" (i.e., inactive) neurotransmitter.[17] Peripheral vascular resistance is decreased, while cardiac output is maintained. The usual adult dose is 250 to 500 mg, which can be given intravenously as well as orally. Methyldopa preparations commonly include a thiazide diuretic. Sedation is a prominent side effect encountered during methyldopa therapy. A positive direct Coombs' test develops in about 25% of patients taking methyldopa, but hemolysis is seldom a clinical problem. Hepatitis occurs in 6% of patients using methyldopa. A mild rebound syndrome (mainly hypertension) has been associated with the abrupt cessation of maintenance therapy.

The pharmacologic effects of reserpine (and other rauwolfia alkaloids) are attributed to a depletion of catecholamine and serotonin in the brain and adrenal medulla. The usual adult dose of reserpine ranges from 0.1 to 0.25 mg. Most preparations also contain a thiazide diuretic. Depression and other adverse side effects, such as increased gastrointestinal motility, nasal congestion, and parkinsonian-like effects, have limited its current use. No fatalities have been reported after overdose.

CLINICAL PRESENTATION

In adults, significant clinical toxicity occurs after the ingestion of 1 to 2 mg of clonidine. A specific lethal dose has not been determined. Children seem to be particularly susceptible to even small doses of clonidine, and serious symptoms have been precipitated by ingestion of a single adult therapeutic dose (0.1 to 0.3 mg).[9,18] Toxicity has been reported in children who have sucked on a used transdermal patch containing residual clonidine.[8] Signs and symptoms of toxicity usually occur within 30 to 60 minutes after ingestion, producing a clinical scenario that resembles a narcotic overdose, consisting of bradycardia, respiratory depression, coma, and miosis. With serious toxicity, hypotension, hypothermia, and hyporeflexia are common. A peculiar intermittent apnea, responsive to physical or auditory stimuli, has been noted in children. Clonidine interacts with other CNS depressants, such as alcohol and barbiturates, and the concomitant ingestion of these substances or sedative–hypnotics can increase CNS depression. Seizures are rare after overdose and are likely related to hypoxia rather than a direct effect.

Hypertension may be seen in the initial phases of clonidine overdose and is associated with high plasma drug levels. It is due to vasoconstriction resulting from the stimulation of peripheral α_1-receptors. This phase is transient, resolves spontaneously, and is quickly and precipitously followed by prolonged or serious hypotension. Rebound hypertension and other withdrawal symptoms may subsequently develop 2 to 4 days after an overdose if the patient has been on maintenance clonidine therapy.

There are few reports of serious guanabenz or guanfacine overdose in the literature, but significant ingestion may produce lethargy, bradycardia, and hypotension. With methyldopa overdose, a benign clinical course is generally seen.[11] Drowsiness, lethargy, bradycardia, hypotension, and atrioventricular conduction abnormalities have been reported.

Significant reserpine ingestion may cause drowsiness, lethargy, hypotension, and bradycardia.[12]

DIFFERENTIAL DIAGNOSIS

Clonidine, guanabenz, and guanfacine poisoning may be clinically indistinguishable from toxicity caused by naphazoline, oxymetazoline (Afrin), tetrahydrozoline (Visine), and xylometazoline. These compounds are found in nasal decongestant and topical ophthalmic preparations. In children, the ingestion or topical application of such preparations has resulted in signs and symptoms that are identical to clonidine poisoning. Centrally acting antihypertensive agent poisoning may also resemble overdose from other substances, particularly narcotics, β-adrenergic blockers, calcium channel blockers, digitalis, and sedative–hypnotics. Hypoglycemia, sepsis, hypothermia, cerebrovascular accident, and head trauma should also be considered in the differential diagnosis.

EMERGENCY DEPARTMENT EVALUATION

Patients with known or suspected centrally acting antihypertensive agent overdose should be treated in a facility with capabilities for close clinical observation, frequent vital sign determinations, and continuous electrocardiographic (ECG) monitoring. Special attention should be directed toward the clinical assessment of airway and breathing abnormalities, cardiovascular status, and evaluation for concomitant trauma.

The diagnosis of poisoning is based on the history and clinical findings. There are no laboratory or clinical tests that are of specific diagnostic or therapeutic value. These agents are not detected on routine drug screening. Quantitative levels are unavailable in the clinical setting and are of no value in management. If the diagnosis is certain, ancillary studies will be of no additional value. Radiographic imaging, routine laboratory tests, and toxicologic analysis are useful only to rule out or confirm concomitant pathology.

EMERGENCY DEPARTMENT MANAGEMENT

Prehospital care is supportive. The routine administration of naloxone and evaluation for hypoglycemia are warranted in symptomatic patients. Because of the rapidity of onset of clonidine toxicity, prehospital use of ipecac should be avoided. Activated charcoal alone is the preferred form of gastrointestinal decontamination. Continuous ECG monitoring and intravenous access should be maintained during the prehospital care and emergency department evaluation.

Treatment is primarily supportive and symptomatic, with therapy aimed at reversing specific derangements in cardiovascular and respiratory status. Hypotension usually responds to crystalloid infusion. Occasionally, vasopressors, such as dopamine and norepinephrine, are required. Bradycardia secondary to clonidine usually responds to intravenous atropine, with repeated doses titrated against heart rate and blood pressure. Dopamine, epinephrine, and cardiac pacing are of theoretic benefit, but their use in clonidine poisoning has not been described. Respiratory depression is a serious consequence of clonidine overdose, and tracheal intubation and assisted ventilation may be required. In the unusual case in which transient hypertension is noted, antihypertensive treatment should generally be avoided because of the potential for subsequent serious and prolonged hypotension.[3] Hypertension usually requires only observation, although, occasionally, a short-acting antihypertensive such as nitroprusside may be warranted. Hypothermia and coma are treated with supportive care. Clinical recovery is usually noted within 24 to 48 hours. Hemodialysis, charcoal hemoperfusion, and forced diuresis are of no proven value. Because clonidine is excreted unchanged in the urine, adequate urine output should be assured. Antacid therapy has been recommended to counter hyperchlorhydria during reserpine overdose.

There are no proven antidotes for centrally acting antihypertensive agent overdose. Naloxone has been used to reverse clonidine toxicity, but the response is inconsistent. The improvement in mental status and hemodynamic parameters noted after naloxone has been explained on the basis of a reversal of clonidine's opiate-like activity in the CNS. Its use is acceptable as a therapeutic trial in patients with depressed mental status. The optimal dose is unknown, but doses similar to those used for narcotic poisoning have been suggested. Both hypertension and hypotension have been temporally associated with the use of naloxone to reverse clonidine overdose. Patients who are given naloxone should be closely observed for potential hemodynamic deterioration.

Tolazoline, a central and peripheral α-adrenergic blocking agent, was once touted as an antidote for clonidine toxicity.[16] Because its efficacy is based on sporadic case reports and it has potentially serious side effects (e.g., hypotension, tachycardia, and arrhythmia), its use is not recommended.

Yohimbine, a centrally acting α_2-adrenergic antagonist, may be expected to have clinical activity opposite that of clonidine. Yohimbine has been suggested as a possible antidote for clonidine overdose, but little evidence is available to support its use, and no clinical guidelines are available.

The clonidine withdrawal syndrome is best treated by the reinstitution of clonidine therapy that is tapered over 5 to 10 days. Clonidine may be used to supplement standard therapy for the inpatient or outpatient treatment of alcohol, narcotic, and nicotine withdrawal. The drug is titrated to control symptoms, particularly tremor, tachycardia, and agitation; a suggested starting dose is 5 to 8 μg/kg/d (divided into three to four doses), tapered over 5 to 10 days. Excessive sedation and orthostatic hypotension are the main side effects, limiting outpatient use.

DISPOSITION

If vital signs are normal and the patient remains or becomes asymptomatic within 4 to 6 hours of ingestion, he or she may be discharged from the emergency department with appropriate psychiatric or social service follow-up. Symptomatic patients require admission to the hospital for observation and monitoring. A toxicology consultant or the drug and poison information center may be helpful in providing advice regarding the use of particular antidotes or final disposition. There is no known cyclical nature to clonidine overdose, and improvement is not followed by relapse. Patients may be safely transferred to another facility with paramedic-level transportation.

COMMON PITFALLS

- Failure to render the correct or complete diagnosis, either by attributing the clinical scenario to other agents or diseases or by failing to recognize coexisting trauma or concomitant ingestions
- Failure to appreciate that clonidine poisoning may result in respiratory depression
- Misdiagnosis of clonidine poisoning as narcotic overdose because of clinical similarities

- Overly aggressive treatment of early but transient hypertension, especially with long-acting agents
- Reliance on unproved antidotes rather than supportive care in the treatment of toxicity
- Failure to consider the possibility of child abuse or attempted homicide in children with overdose and to address psychiatric issues in patients with suicide attempts

ACKNOWLEDGMENT

J. Frank Bonfiglio and David G. Hassard contributed to previous editions of this chapter.

References

1. Baumgartner GR, Rower RC. Clonidine vs chlordiazepoxide in the management of acute alcohol withdrawal syndrome. *Arch Intern Med* 1987;147:1223.
2. Bousquet P, Feldman J, Tibirica E, et al. New concepts on the central regulation of blood pressure: alpha-2-adrenoreceptors and imidazoline receptors. *Am J Med* 1989;87[Suppl 3C]:3C-10S.
3. Campbell BC, Reid JL. Regimen for the control of blood pressure and symptoms during clonidine withdrawal. *Int J Clin Pharmacol Res* 1985;5:215.
4. Geyskes GG, Boer P, Mees EJD. Clonidine withdrawal: mechanism and frequency of rebound hypertension. *Br J Clin Pharmacol* 1979;7:55.
5. Glassman AH, Stetner F, Walsh T. Heavy smokers, smoking cessation, and clonidine. *JAMA* 1988;259:2863.
6. Gold MS, Pottash AL, Sweeney DR, et al. Efficacy of clonidine in opiate withdrawal. *Drug Alcohol Depend* 1980;6:201.
7. Hall AH, Smolinske SC, Kulig KW, et al. Guanabenz overdose. *Ann Intern Med* 1985;102:787.
8. Harris J. Clonidine patch toxicity. *DICP (Ann Pharmacol)* 1990;24:1191.
9. Heideman S, Sarnaik A. Clonidine poisoning in children. *Crit Care Med* 1990;18:618.
10. Klein-Schwartz W, Gorman R, Oderda GM, et al. Central nervous system depression from ingestion of non-prescription eyedrops. *Am J Emerg Med* 1984;2:217.
11. Lawson DH, Glass D, Jick H. Adverse reactions to methyldopa with particular reference to hypotension. *Am Heart J* 1978;96:572.
12. Loggie JMH, Saita H, Kahn I, et al. Accidental reserpine poisoning: clinical and metabolic effects. *Clin Pharmacol Ther* 1967;8:692.
13. Nakagawa S, Yamamoto Y, Koiwaya Y. Ventricular tachycardia induced by clonidine withdrawal. *Br Heart J* 1985;53:654.
14. Oster J, Epstein M. Use of centrally acting sympatholytic agents in the management of hypertension. *Arch Intern Med* 1991;152:1638.
15. Sanklecha M, Jog A, Raghavan J. Clonidine casualty. *Indian J Pediatr* 1993;60:611.
16. Schieber RA, Kaufman ND. Use of tolazoline in massive clonidine poisoning. *Am J Dis Child* 1981;135:77.
17. Van Zwieten PA, Thoolen MJMC, Timmermans BMWM. The hypotensive activity and side effects of methyldopa, clonidine, and guanfacine. *Hypertension* 1984;5(Pt II):28.
18. Wiley J, Wiley C, Torrey S, et al. Clonidine poisoning in young children. *J Pediatr* 1990;116:654.

CHAPTER 325

Chemical and Biologic Warfare Agent Poisoning

Michael J. Burns and Christopher H. Linden

The deliberate use of chemicals, microorganisms, and toxins to impede, incapacitate, or kill the opposition has been attempted throughout history. It is only within the past decade, however, that these weapons of mass destruction have attracted global concern. Despite international treaties that ban the development, production, and stockpiling of chemical and biologic weapons, certain countries have recently weaponized and deployed these agents. Iraq is known to have used mustard gas in its war with Iran and against its own Kurdish civilians in the 1980s and, more recently, has weaponized aflatoxin, anthrax, and botulism.[4] Currently, 17 countries are suspected of having an offensive biowarfare program, and it is feared that troops may be exposed to such weapons in future military conflicts.[6]

Of more concern is the threat that chemical and biologic agents could be deployed by terrorists against unprotected civilian populations. The release of Sarin in the Tokyo subway in 1995 by the terrorist group Aum Shinrikyo resulted in over 5,000 civilian casualties, legitimizing this concern.[12] Concern is heightened further when one considers that chemical and biologic agents are easy to acquire, synthesize, and use; are fairly inexpensive; and could result in a catastrophic number of casualties if deployed under appropriate conditions.[4,16] The use of bioweapons by terrorists would be difficult to predict, detect, or prevent; the aerosolized release of an agent would be silent, invisible, odorless, and tasteless, and the first evidence of a such a covert release may not occur until patients start seeking medical treatment for symptoms several days later. Additionally, the civilian medical community has limited experience with the diagnosis and treatment of poisoning from chemical and biologic agents and is ill equipped to care for the large numbers of civilian casualties that may result from their successful deployment. The 1997 Defense Against Weapons of Mass Destruction Act directed the Department of Defense to establish a domestic preparedness program that will improve the ability of local, state, and federal agencies to respond to chemical and biologic incidents.[2,4] It is imperative that emergency physicians become involved with this program and equip themselves with the knowledge necessary to rapidly recognize and treat chemical and biologic agent casualties.

Chemical and biologic warfare agents generally fall into one of eight major categories: chemical choking agents, vesicating or blister agents, lacrimating agents, nerve agents, vomiting agents, systemic asphyxiants, biologic toxins, and infectious agents (Tables 325.1 and 325.2). Chemical agents are intended to either stun or kill, and hence can be further classified as lethal or nonlethal. The "code" refers to their U.S. military designation. Biologic agents may also be intended to either debilitate or kill. Although almost any microbial organism could theoretically be used as a biowarfare agent, only a few possess the necessary characteristics (e.g., infectivity, toxicity, ease of production, atmospheric stability, ideal size for aerosolized dissemination) to create mass casualties.[4,6,16] The likelihood that a chemical or biologic agent achieves its desired effect (e.g., lethality) ultimately

TABLE 325.1. Chemical Warfare Agents

Classification	Military Code	Chemical Name/Common Name
LETHAL AGENTS		
Blood agents	AC	Hydrogen cyanide
	CK	Cyanogen chloride
	SA	Arsenic trihydride/arsine
Choking agents	CL	Chlorine
	CG	Carbonyl chloride/phosgene
	DP	Trichloromethyl chloroformate/diphosgene
Vesicating agents		
Mustards	HD	bis(2-chloroethyl)sulfide/distilled mustard
Nitrogen mustards	HN-1	2,2-dichlorotriethylamine
	HN-2	2,2-dichloro-N-methylethylamine
	HN-3	2,2,2-trichlorotriethylamine
Arsenicals	MD	Methyldichloroarsine
	PD	Phenyldichloroarsine
	ED	Ethyldichloroarsine
	L	Dichloro(2-chlorovinyl)arsine/lewisite
Oximes	CX	Dichloroform oxime/phosgene oxime
Mixes	HL	None/ML mix (mustard-lewisite mixture)
	HT	None/HT mix (mustard-T mixture)
(Not produced)	Q	4,bis(methylchloroethyl sulfide)/Q
	T	bis(2-chloroethyl sulfide)monoxide/T
Nerve agents	GA	Ethyl *N,N*-dimethyl phosphoamicocyanidate/Tabun
	GB	Isopropyl methyl phosphonofluoridate/Sarin
	GD	Pinacolyl methyl phosphonefluoridate/Soman
	GF	Cyclohexyl-methyl phosphonofluoridate/ cyclosarin
	VX	Ethyl S-2-diisopropyl aminoethyl methylphosphonothiolate/VX
NONLETHAL AGENTS		
Vomiting agents	DA	Diphenylchloroarsine
	DC	Diphenylcyanoarsine
	DM	Diphenylaminochloroarsine/adamsite
Lacrimating agents	CA	Bromobenzeneacetonitrile/camite
	CN	2-chloro-1-phenylethanone/chloroacetophenone
	CNB	None/chloroacetophenane, carbon tetrachloride, benzene mix
	CNC	None/chloroacetophenane chloroform mix
	CNS	None/chloroacetophenane, chloroform, chloropicrin mix
	CS	*o*-chlorobenzlidene malonitrile/CS (tear gas)
	—	Capsaicin/pepper gas

depends on the dose and physicochemical properties of the agent, nature of exposure, availability and timeliness of treatment, immune status of the enemy, and atmospheric conditions.

Exposure to chemical and biologic agents may occur intentionally following terrorist or military attack or accidentally during the manufacture, transportation, storage, and deployment of these weapons. Lacrimating agents are currently used by civilians for personal protection and by law enforcement personnel for crowd dispersal and incapacitation of criminal suspects.

Chemical and biologic agents can be delivered in multiple ways. They may be aerosolized as a spray from hand-held or vehicle-mounted pressurized tanks, low-flying aircraft, crop-dusters, cruise missiles, or spray bottles. These agents may also be dispersed as liquid droplets or vapor from low-flying aircraft, artillery, missiles, detonated bombs, and hand-held devices. The geographic area affected by warfare agents typically depends on prevailing weather conditions and the method of delivery used. In the Tokyo terrorist incident, Sarin was dispersed by evaporation from punctured plastic bags that were left on subway cars.[12] If an agent is highly toxic, it may be added to the enemy's water supply or food source. In 1984, the intentional contamination of restaurant salad bars in Oregon by a religious cult resulted in 751 cases of salmonellosis.[18] Bioagent contamination of most United States water supplies is unlikely to be successful due to the excessively large amounts of bioagent required and water purification techniques currently used.[16] The aerosolized dispersal of both chemical and biologic agents is the mode most likely to result in the maximum number of casualties and is thus the method most likely to be used by terrorists and military groups.[3,4,16,20] Unexpected and uncontrollable spread of these agents by wind, water, or humans may affect unintended populations.

CHEMICAL TOXINS

Blood Agents

Incorrectly labeled "blood agents" by the military, these agents include the systemic asphyxiant gases cyanogen chloride and hydrogen cyanide (see Chapter 331), hydrogen sulfide (see Chapter 344), and the hemolytic gas arsine, derived from arsenic (see Chapter 318). Sodium monofluoroacetate (see Chapter 366)

TABLE 325.2. Biologic Warfare Agents

Classification	Examples
BIOLOGIC TOXINS	
	Abrin
	Aflatoxins
	Clostridium botulinum/ botulism
	Clostridium perfringens epsilon toxin
	Clostridium tetani toxin
	Conotoxins
	Fusarium nivale + *Fusarium tricinctum*/trichothecene mycotoxins (T-2)
	Ricin
	Saxitoxin
	Shigella species shigatoxin
	Staphylococcal enterotoxins
	Tetrodotoxin
INFECTIOUS AGENTS	
Bacteria	*Bacillus anthracis*/anthrax
	Brucella species/brucellosis
	Chlamydia psittaci/psittacosis
	Coxiella burnetii/Q fever
	Francisella tularensis/tularemia
	Rickettsia rickettsii/Rocky Mountain spotted fever
	Rickettsia prowazekii/epidemic typhus
	Salmonella typhimurium/typhoid fever
	Vibrio cholerae/cholera
	Yersinia pestis/plague
Fungi	*Coccidioides immitis*/coccidioidomycosis
Parasites	*Trypanosoma* species/trypanosomiasis
Viruses	Crimean-Congo hemorrhagic fever virus
	Dengue fever virus (flavivirus)
	Ebola viruses
	Encephalitis viruses (e.g., arboviruses, herpesviruses)
	Hantavirus
	Influenza virus (orthomyxovirus)
	Lassa fever virus
	Marburg virus
	Rift Valley fever virus (bunyavirus)
	Variola major virus (smallpox virus)
	Yellow fever virus (flavivirus)

is another cellular asphyxiant proposed for military use. As a chemical warfare agent, the efficacy of cyanide is limited due to its high volatility, resulting in nonpersistence in open air, and its relatively low toxicity compared with nerve agents.

Choking Agents

Introduced in World War I, the choking agents chlorine, phosgene, and diphosgene act principally as pulmonary irritants (see Chapter 346). Chlorine, a dense, low to moderately water soluble, yellow-green gas that smells like concentrated bleach, is toxic to all tissue surfaces it contacts—skin, eyes, and respiratory and gastrointestinal (GI) tracts. The injury is proportional to the gas concentration, duration of contact, and water content of exposed tissue. Chlorine reacts with tissue water to form hydrochloric acid and oxygen free radicals, which produce corrosive and cytotoxic effects to the lung and other tissues.

Phosgene (carbonyl chloride), which replaced chlorine, is thought to have been responsible for more than 80% of all chemical agent fatalities in World War I.[20] It is a colorless gas that is heavier than air and smells like freshly mown hay. Odor is not a reliable indicator of exposure. Phosgene's propensity to settle into low-lying areas, such as trenches, led to its tactical success. Phosgene vapor is poorly soluble in water and is only mildly irritating to the eyes and upper respiratory tract on initial contact; exposure may temporarily go unnoticed. Phosgene hydrolyzes with terminal bronchial and alveolar mucosal water to produce hydrochloric acid. This and other toxic by-products of phosgene stimulate the synthesis of leukotrienes and other inflammatory products, which leads to pulmonary edema. The rate and extent of pulmonary injury depend on the concentration and duration of exposure, but it typically occurs slowly over hours.

Diphosgene (trichloromethyl chloroformate) was created shortly after World War I and is simply phosgene with chloroform attached to it. The chloroform moiety allowed diphosgene to penetrate the crude chemical filters of the day, with the phosgene moiety being responsible for its toxicity. Diphosgene causes a more immediate irritation to the eyes, nose, and respiratory tract than does phosgene, due to its higher chlorine content.

Vesicating Agents

Vesicating agents cause blistering of exposed surfaces and include mustard gases and organic arsenicals. Sulfur mustard (2,2,-dichlorodiethyl sulfide) is the most well known and extensively used agent. It was used in World War I and in the Iran–Iraq war.[4,13,20] Sulfur mustard is not immediately lethal but has several properties that make it useful for warfare. It is simple to produce, easily disseminated, and difficult to protect against, and it effectively incapacitates its opponents. Sulfur mustard has a low volatility and persists for several days in temperate climates, thereby restricting enemy use of contaminated equipment and terrain.[4]

Sulfur mustard is an oily amber liquid that smells like burning garlic or mustard. It becomes aerosolized by spraying or volatilized by an exploding military shell or high ambient temperature and is rapidly absorbed on inhalation or contact with the skin or eye. Mustard irreversibly binds with tissue cellular components within 2 minutes of exposure.[1,13] Its cellular toxicity results from the spontaneous formation of highly reactive and unstable episulfonium compounds, which irreversibly alkylate nucleic acids and cellular proteins. This leads to DNA strand breaks and inhibition of DNA replication, protein synthesis, and enzyme function. In the process of cellular DNA repair, depletion of nicotinamide adenine dinucleotide (NAD^+) occurs, glycolysis is inhibited, cellular proteases are released, and cell death occurs. Additionally, cellular toxicity may result from mustard agent binding to cellular glutathione and resultant depletion of this free radical scavenger. Depletion of glutathione results in an inactivation of sulfhydryl-containing enzymes, loss of calcium homeostasis, lipid peroxidation, cellular membrane breakdown, and cell death. The nitrogen mustards [HN] have identical cytotoxicity. They are used medically in the intravenous form as alkylating chemotherapeutic agents and can cause severe local tissue damage if, inadvertently, intravenous extravasation occurs.

Because mustards are alkylating agents, they may be mutagenic and carcinogenic.[1,13] The mortality rate from mustard injuries during World War I was less than 2%; rates of 3% to 4% were reported in the Iran–Iraq war.[1,13,17] Death results from respiratory failure or bone marrow suppression. Most of the mustard injuries in World War I were nonfatal but disabling; nearly all of the victims suffered skin burns, 86% suffered eye burns, and 75% sustained respiratory injury.[1,20] Although the lethality of sulfur mustard is considerably less than that of other chemical agents, dermal exposure to as little as 1.0 to 1.5 teaspoons of liquid is potentially lethal to a 70-kg adult.[20]

Lewisite (2-chlorovinyldichloroarsine) is the best known of the organic arsenicals. It was developed in 1918 to complement sulfur mustard as a semipersistent blistering agent. Many countries have generated large stockpiles of lewisite, but its actual use in combat is not well documented.[17,20] It may have been used by Iraq in the Iran–Iraq war. Lewisite is an amber, oily liquid that smells like geraniums. It persists in the environment for up to 24 hours under temperate conditions due to low water solubility.[4] Under normal conditions, lewisite is moderately volatile, making inhalational toxicity a concern. Its vapor is about seven times heavier than air and will flow into lower terrain.[20]

Lewisite enters the body most rapidly through vapor inhalation or liquid absorption through breaks in the skin. It penetrates intact skin within 15 minutes, more rapidly than mustard agents, due to its moderate lipid solubility.[20] In the dermis, it hydrolyzes to hydrochloric acid and chlorovinylarsenious oxide, the vesicating agent. Its organic arsenical moiety has additional systemic toxicity (see Chapter 318). Arsenicals also increase capillary permeability and cause extensive interstitial fluid losses, resulting in hypovolemia; this phenomenon is called "lewisite shock."[20] Lung capillaries are particularly sensitive to lewisite, and inhalation may result in severe pulmonary edema.[20]

Nerve Agents

Nerve agents are similar in structure and function to commonly used organophosphorus pesticides (see Chapter 361) but are more potent and typically have a more rapid onset and shorter duration of clinical symptoms. The first three nerve agents, the "G" (short for "German") agents Tabun (GA), Sarin (GB), and Soman (GD), were developed in Germany between 1936 and 1944.[22] The fourth, VX, with the "V" standing for "viper," was synthesized in 1952 in England.

Although commonly referred to as nerve gases, these agents are colorless, odorless liquids under temperate conditions. They are dispersed as vapors or liquid aerosols by spraying or explosive blasts and are significant vapor hazards at higher ambient temperatures. Vapors are heavier than air and, thus, will concentrate closer to the ground. The G agents are moderately volatile, evaporate within several hours, and are environmentally nonpersistent.[15] Sarin is the most volatile, with a volatility similar to that of water. Vapor inhalation causes symptoms within seconds to several minutes.[5,15,20] The human lethal inhaled dose of the G agents is estimated to be 1 mg.[15,20] VX is an oily compound that is much less volatile and persists for several weeks after dispersion.[20] It is not a major inhalation hazard (unless ambient temperatures are high) and exhibits most of its toxicity by skin absorption. It is the most potent of the nerve agents on a weight basis. All the agents rapidly penetrate skin and clothing, with onset of symptoms within 30 minutes to 18 hours after skin exposure.[5,20] The time of onset is determined by the dose and the agent. VX has the most efficient percutaneous absorption, with a 10-mg dose applied to the skin expected to be lethal to 50% of unprotected individuals.[20]

Toxicity results primarily from phosphorylation and inactivation of acetylcholinesterase (AChE) at its serine active site (see Chapter 361). Acetylcholine accumulates at nerve terminals, initially stimulating, then paralyzing, cholinergic neurotransmission. Once inactivated, AChE may undergo three processes. The phosphorylated enzyme may spontaneously reactivate via endogenous hydrolysis, be reactivated by nucleophilic oximes, or become incapable of reactivation. Endogenous hydrolysis is insignificant, due to tight binding of nerve agents to AChE. Reactivation of AChE occurs if an oxime binds the phosphate moiety of the nerve agent more avidly than the serine residue of AChE. Reactivation is impossible once dealkylation ("aging") of the phosphorylated cholinesterase occurs, and *de novo* AChE synthesis is required for enzyme replenishment. The rate of aging varies among the nerve agents. It occurs within 2 minutes after Soman exposure, 5 to 8 hours after Sarin exposure, and more than 40 hours after Tabun or VX exposure.[20]

AChE inhibition is not solely responsible for nerve agent toxicity. Tabun, Sarin, and Soman are direct partial agonists at nicotinic receptor sites, and VX blocks nicotinic receptor ionic channels.[5,20] They also bind directly to cardiac muscarinic receptors, antagonize GABA neurotransmission, and stimulate glutamate *N*-methyl-*d*-aspartate receptors. These latter actions may contribute to nerve agent–induced seizures and central nervous system (CNS) neuropathology.[15] Some compounds that are protective in nerve agent toxicity do not reactivate AChE. CNS-active oximes (e.g., Pro-2-PAM) are no more efficacious in nerve agent treatment than oximes that do not reactivate brain AChE. There is poor correlation between clinical toxicity and levels of AChE activity.[5]

Vomiting Agents

The vomiting agents are typically nonlethal, arsenic-based compounds used for riot control.[20] These agents are normally solids that vaporize on heating and then condense to form aerosols. Vomiting agents were developed near the end of World War I but were not frequently used. They produce rapid irritation of the eyes, skin, and respiratory and GI tracts. Features of systemic arsenic toxicity are discussed in Chapter 318.

Lacrimating Agents

Lacrimating agents (tear gases), also known as riot-control and harassing agents, are pulmonary irritants (see Chapter 346) and mild corrosives (see Chapter 330). They were introduced in World War I and have since been used regularly for the temporary incapacitation of criminals, civilian crowds, and enemy armies. Most of the original compounds have become obsolete. Agents currently in common use include *o*-chlorobenzylidenemalonitrile (CS), *w*-chloroacetophenone (CN or Mace), and capsaicin (pepper spray). The noxious effects of lacrimating agents are typically transient, but lethal toxicity may occur.

Before CS was developed in the 1950s, CN was the agent most widely used by civilian and military authorities. CN is typically dispersed as a smoke of suspended particles or liquid aerosol. It is more toxic than CS and, at high concentrations, can result in permanent corneal epithelial damage, contact dermatitis with skin blistering, and noncardiogenic pulmonary edema.[20] At least five deaths from CN grenades have been reported when CN was used in confined spaces.[20] Persistent toxic effects are unlikely if CN is used in open spaces. CN effects usually last less than 20 minutes.

CS is now the riot-control agent of choice in the United States. It is about ten times more potent as a lacrimator than CN but is much less toxic to tissues.[20] Symptoms begin within 20 seconds of exposure; long-lasting ocular effects are uncommon. Chemical pneumonitis and fatal pulmonary edema have been reported. CS is delivered as a vapor or cloud of suspended solid particles (a smoke) produced by a thermal grenade. Newer CS formulations consist of an unheated micropulverized powder (CS1, CS2) that can remain active in the environment for several weeks. CS powders were used by the U.S. military during the Vietnam war.

Capsaicin, a chemical irritant found in many plants of the genus *Capsicum,* can produce cutaneous, GI, and respiratory irritation in humans. The oleoresin of capsicum is used frequently by civilians for personal protection and by law enforcement personnel for immobilization of assailants. "Pepper Mace" can contain CS, oleoresin of capsicum, or both. It is a lipid-soluble alkaloid that first stimulates release of substance P from nociceptive neurons and then blocks its synthesis and transport. Substance P depolarizes neurons to produce dilatation of blood vessels, stimulation of smooth muscle, and activation of sensory nerve endings that mediate pain. With repeated application, nociceptive fiber response and number are decreased (desensitization). This forms the basis for the medicinal use of capsaicin as a topical analgesic (counterirritant).

BIOLOGIC TOXINS

Biologic toxins are the poisonous by-products of microorganisms, plants, and animals. Toxins tend to be more stable than microorganisms, because they are not living. To be most effective as biowarfare agents, toxins need to be disseminated to target populations in the form of respirable aerosols. These agents are neither volatile nor dermally active.

Of all biologic toxins, the exotoxin formed by the anaerobic, spore-forming, gram-positive bacillus, *Clostridium botulinum,* poses the most credible threat as a biologic warfare agent.[4,20] Although unsuccessful in producing disease, the Aum Shinrikyo cult aerosolized botulinum toxin in Japan on several occasions before the Tokyo Sarin attack.[4] Botulinum toxin is relatively easy to manufacture and the most lethal toxin known, with an LD_{50} of 0.001 μg/kg.[20] It is 15,000 times more toxic than VX and 100,000 times more toxic than Sarin. Botulinum toxin is actually eight distinct protein by-products of *C. botulinum* metabolism.[3] Types A, B, E, and F are toxic to humans. Botulism may result from the inhalation, ingestion, or wound contamination of either the microbial spores or preformed toxin (see Chapter 205). It is characterized by progressive descending paralysis. Botulinum toxin inhibits the release of acetylcholine from presynaptic neurons at the neuromuscular end-plate and cholinergic autonomic neurons.

Other potent biotoxins include the naturally occurring trichothecene mycotoxins. Nivalenol and T2, the best known, are derived from wheat and corn contaminated by the fungi *Fusarium nivale* and *Fusarium tricinctum*, respectively. Since 1976, there have been claims that the Soviet and Vietnamese governments used trichothecenes against Indochinese refugees in Southeast Asia.[20] "Yellow rain" is allegedly due to small yellow particles of trichothecenes released from low-flying planes.

Trichothecene mycotoxins are potent inhibitors of protein synthesis and electron transport.[20] Rapidly proliferating tissues are affected most. T2 toxin is well absorbed orally, achieving peak tissue levels by 1 to 4 hours. The highest mycotoxin concentration is reached in the liver. Elimination half-life is about 22 hours, with 50% excreted as metabolites in the feces.

Other possible toxins (see Table 325.2) include those derived from plants (e.g., ricin, abrin), marine organisms (e.g., saxitoxin, tetrodotoxin), and snake venoms (e.g., bungarotoxins).

INFECTIOUS AGENTS

Of the biologic agents, anthrax, smallpox, and plague represent the greatest potential for use as weapons.[4,7,20] Anthrax is caused by *Bacillus anthracis,* an aerobic, spore-forming, gram-positive bacillus found ubiquitously in soil. Spores of *B. anthracis* are easily disseminated by military munitions and can persist in the environment for decades.[20] Anthrax is normally acquired by human skin contact with infected livestock. The spores are inoculated via skin breaks and produce cutaneous black eschars. The mortality rate for cutaneous anthrax is less than 1% with early penicillin therapy. The aerosolized delivery of anthrax spores will result in inhalational exposure and is the most likely means of military and terrorist attack.[1,20] Anthrax spores are of ideal size (1 to 5 μm) to reach alveoli. Inhalational anthrax, as contrasted to cutaneous anthrax, is a highly fatal disseminated infection. The lethal potential of aerosolized anthrax was demonstrated in 1979, when accidental release of anthrax spores from a Soviet military facility in Sverdlovsk resulted in 79 cases of inhalational anthrax, with 68 being fatal.[9] Following inhalation, spores of *B. anthracis* are phagocytized by alveolar macrophages and transported to mediastinal lymph nodes.[3] After a variable latency period (2 to 60 days), spores germinate into bacilli, which release toxins that lead to hemorrhage, edema, and necrosis.[3,9,20] Anthrax bacilli can also seed the general circulation and lead to overwhelming septicemia.

Smallpox (variola) virus is highly infectious by aerosol, environmentally stable, and associated with high mortality and secondary spread rates.[3,4,20] The virus can survive for 24 hours or more in the environment. Currently, the majority of the United States population has no immunity, and there is little available vaccine and no effective treatment for the disease. Release of the virus into any major metropolitan area would have devastating consequences. Although the virus was globally eradicated in 1980 and is currently retained in only two approved laboratories (in the United States and Russia), clandestine stockpiles may exist. Humans are infected by inhaling the virus, which enters the respiratory tract and multiplies locally. After an incubation period of 7 to 17 days, virions are hematogenously transported within macrophages (primary viremia) to regional lymph nodes, where additional multiplication occurs. Secondary viremia subsequently occurs, during which the virus localizes to small dermal blood vessels. This leads to endothelial swelling and infection of epidermal cells. Intraepidermal vesicles form in the skin and mucous membranes. Smallpox infection is usually incapacitating and frequently fatal, with mortality occurring in 30% of unvaccinated individuals.

Plague is caused by the gram-negative, bipolar-staining coccobacillus, *Yersinia pestis. Y. pestis* is usually spread to humans from infected rodents by a flea vector. Following skin inoculation by the bite of a flea, bacteria migrate to local lymph nodes, are phagocytized but not killed by mononuclear cells, replicate locally, and result in enlarged suppurative lymph nodes (buboes) after 1 to 8 days.[3,20] Bacteria subsequently spread by lymphatics and blood to distant sites. Secondary spread to the lung (secondary pneumonic plague) occurs in 10% of patients. In the United States, 85 to 90% of plague that occurs naturally is the bubonic form, with only 1% being the primary pneumonic form.[20] As a biowarfare agent, however, it would be deployed as an infectious aerosol and result in primary pneumonic plague. Pneumonic plague is readily spread person to person by respiratory droplets and, untreated, has a mortality rate approaching 100%.

Numerous other microorganisms, including bacteria, rickettsiae, viruses, and fungi, have been investigated as possible agents for use in biologic warfare. Biologic engineering makes it possible to alter current strains of these microorganisms so that they are resistant to known forms of treatment.

CLINICAL PRESENTATION

Choking Agents

Clinical symptoms begin within minutes after significant chlorine exposure and include lacrimation, conjunctival irritation, rhinorrhea, cough, sore throat, chest burning, dyspnea, sputum production, nausea, headache, and respiratory failure. Corneal abrasions and cutaneous burns may result from eye and skin exposure, respectively. Following significant chlorine exposures, pulmonary edema may develop within 2 to 4 hours and peaks at 12 to 24 hours.[20] The chest radiograph may be normal or may display noncardiogenic pulmonary edema. After a typical latency period of 4 to 6 hours (range, 1 to 24 hours), patients with significant phosgene exposure present with dyspnea, chest tightness, cyanosis, hemoptysis, hypotension, and pulmonary edema. Chest radiographic findings of pulmonary edema are rather late and nonspecific, occurring 6 to 8 hours after exposure. Diphosgene produces identical signs and symptoms. Following significant pulmonary agent exposure (e.g., chlorine gas), patients may subsequently develop reactive airways dysfunction syndrome, a chronic asthma-like condition.

Vesicating Agents

After mustard exposure, there is typically a latency period of 4 to 12 hours before the onset of symptoms. The latency period is shorter with high concentrations and long exposures, with increased ambient temperature and humidity, and in victims previously exposed to or innately susceptible to mustard.[1,13,17,20] Sites of injury principally involve the skin, eye, and respiratory tract and may follow vapor or liquid exposure. Heavy exposure may lead to systemic effects such as bone marrow depression and sloughing of intestinal mucosa.

Cutaneous injury resulting from mustard exposure ranges from erythema to vesication and skin necrosis. The moist, thinner skin of the neck, axilla, and groin is more severely affected. After an asymptomatic period of 4 to 12 hours, erythema and edema develop. Vesication typically starts within 24 hours and evolves over several days. Vesicles coalesce into blisters, and skin necrosis occurs over 24 to 72 hours.[17,20] Blister fluid does not contain active mustard and is not toxic. Skin denudation occurs over 6 to 9 days, and healing may take 4 to 10 weeks.

The eye is the organ most sensitive to sulfur mustard. Tissue injury occurs rapidly, but symptoms develop gradually over 4 to 8 hours and include eye pain, lacrimation, photophobia, and blurred vision. Physical findings include blepharospasm, eyelid edema, conjunctival injection and edema, chemosis, anterior chamber cellular infiltrates, and decreased vision. Corneal edema begins within 1 hour after exposure, and the corneal epithelium vesicates and sloughs within 4 to 36 hours.[13,17,20] Resolution of injury depends on the severity of exposure and typically takes 1 to 2 weeks. About 90% of victims are visually disabled for 10 days with conjunctivitis, photophobia, and corneal swelling. The remaining 10% are severely affected and are at risk for permanent blindness from corneal opacification, scarring, and ulceration.

Respiratory epithelial damage occurs several hours after exposure. Victims may develop rhinitis, nasal bleeding, sinus discomfort, hoarseness, sore throat, cough, sputum production, and dyspnea of increasing severity. Hemorrhagic inflammation and erosions of the upper airway mucosa are followed by fibrinous pseudomembrane formation and sloughing of necrotic, ulcerated mucosa. Bronchospasm and partial airway obstruction result. After high-dose exposures, severe bronchitis, secondary bronchopneumonia, and respiratory failure may develop within 24 to 48 hours.[1,13,20] Pulmonary edema is not a characteristic finding, as mustard does not typically affect the pulmonary parenchyma.

In the presence of high concentration or prolonged exposure, bone marrow and GI mucosal toxicity may be seen. Leukopenia develops within 5 to 7 days, with the white cell nadir occurring 10 days after exposure. Thrombocytopenia and anemia typically follow. The development of hematologic effects from mustard poisoning is a grave prognostic sign.[13,20]

The clinical manifestations of lewisite poisoning are similar to those of sulfur mustard, although lewisite causes immediate severe pain on contact with the skin, eyes, and nasal mucosa. Vapor condensing on the skin causes erythema within 30 minutes and blister formation within 2 to 3 hours.[17,20] The eyes are very sensitive to lewisite, and permanent blindness from corneal destruction may result if decontamination is not initiated within 1 minute. Inhalation of lewisite vapor can result in death within 10 minutes from rapid respiratory mucosal sloughing and bleeding, leading to asphyxiation.

Nerve Agents

Clinical manifestations of nerve agent exposure are described in detail in Chapter 361. Toxicity may occur after inhalation of vapor, skin contact with vapor or liquid, or ingestion. The rate of onset and severity of effects are determined by the route of exposure and dose.[5] At high ambient temperature, skin absorption is rapid, and increasing amounts of the agent are volatilized, leading to increased inhalation.[15] A small amount of vapor affects the eyes, nose, and lungs, causing miosis, rhinorrhea, mild dyspnea, cough, and wheezing.[5,15,20] This can occur within seconds to minutes. Symptoms of mild poisoning include eye pain, blurred and dim vision, headache, and dizziness.[12] As the dose of vapor increases, nausea and vomiting, increased respiratory difficulty, progressive muscular weakness, and agitation develop. A high vapor concentration causes rapid loss of consciousness, seizures, flaccid paralysis, and respiratory arrest within seconds to minutes. In the Tokyo Sarin gas attack (vapor exposure), the most prominent signs and symptoms for patients with moderate-to-severe poisoning included miosis (99%), headache (75%), dyspnea (63%), nausea (60%), eye pain (45%), blurred vision (40%), and vomiting (37%).[12] Tachycardia and hypertension were common, but bradycardia and bronchorrhea were not. Victims of vapor exposure are unlikely to deteriorate once removed from exposure.[5,12] In contrast, those with dermal exposure may subsequently worsen. Skin absorption of a lethal dose may occur within 1 to 2 minutes, yet symptoms are commonly delayed and develop after a latency period of 30 minutes to 18 hours.[1,5,20] Skin exposure may result in local sweating and twitching or fasciculations before systemic toxicity. In contrast to vapor exposure, miosis is absent early following skin exposure.[5]

Ingestion of food or water contaminated with a nerve agent may produce symptoms within 30 minutes.[20] Death from nerve agent exposure is primarily due to respiratory failure secondary to depression of the central respiratory drive.[5,20] Respirations cease before significant neuromuscular blockade or bronchoconstriction occurs.

Lacrimating Agents

Tear agents cause intense eye discomfort, blepharospasm, lacrimation, stinging and burning of the mouth and nose, salivation, rhinorrhea, irritation of the respiratory tract and stomach with coughing and vomiting, and skin irritation leading to burning pain and erythema within seconds to minutes of exposure.[20] Tear agents are miscible in sweat, and skin irritation is amplified in areas of increased sweat, such as the axilla, popliteal and antecubital areas, inguinal region, and buttocks. Skin effects are heightened in warm, moist environments. Prolonged exposure may produce malaise, skin blistering, chest tightness, shortness of breath, and a feeling of suffocation.

Biologic Toxins

The clinical manifestations of inhalational botulism are identical to those following ingestion of tainted food. Symptoms are likely to appear 1 to 4 days following exposure and are described in detail in Chapter 205.[3,20] Signs and symptoms begin within minutes to hours of oral, dermal, or inhalational exposure to trichothecene mycotoxins. Toxic effects include corneal, cutaneous, and mucous membrane inflammation and necrosis; GI inflammation and hemorrhage; petechiae; ecchymosis; and hematologic and immunologic suppression. Southeast Asian victims exposed to Yellow Rain experienced painful burning, irritation, rash, and blistering of the skin; vomiting; diarrhea; lightheadedness; and dyspnea. Some experienced rapid onset of asphyxiation, hemorrhage, and death.[20] Survivors developed a radiation-type illness. Trichothecene exposure may also result in alimentary toxic aleukia, a condition similar to radiation toxicity. Manifestations include fever, fatigue, weakness, headache, dizziness, nausea, vomiting, diarrhea, leukopenia, diffuse bleeding, and sepsis. Routine laboratory analysis does not aid in diagnosis. Leukopenia, thrombocytopenia, and anemia take 2 to 4 weeks to develop.

Infectious Agents

Inhalational anthrax has a typical incubation period of 1 to 6 days, but fatal human disease has occurred with a latency as long as 43 days.[3,6,9] Initial manifestations are nonspecific and "flulike" and include headache, low-grade fever, nonproductive cough, malaise, and myalgias. After 2 to 3 days, the disease progresses rapidly and is characterized by high fever, diaphoresis, dyspnea, stridor, hypoxia, hemoptysis, and cyanosis. Bacteremia, mediastinitis, meningitis, and septic shock frequently occur. Most patients die within 24 hours despite antibiotic therapy. Characteristic findings on the chest radiograph are mediastinal widening, indicative of hemorrhagic mediastinitis, and pleural effusions. Pneumonia, however, is not present.

Small pox is characterized by an incubation period of 7 to 17 days, followed by the abrupt onset of high fever (102°F to 106°F), headache, malaise, myalgias, rigors, abdominal pain, back pain, and vomiting.[3,20] Two to 3 days later, these prodromal symptoms subside and macules develop on the face, hands, forearms, and legs. At this juncture, patients are infectious to others and shed virus from oropharyngeal and respiratory secretions. Over the next 3 to 7 days, the lesions increase in number, spread centrally, and evolve to vesicles, then pustules. Greater numbers of lesions are found on the face and extremities, and lesions are in similar stages of development on each body region. In the second week of illness, skin lesions scab over and may subsequently leave depigmented scars. Bacterial pneumonia and superinfection of skin lesions may occur. Laboratory findings include leukopenia and thrombocytopenia during the prodromal illness and leukocytosis during the pustular stage.

Pneumonic plague is characterized by an incubation period of 2 to 3 days, followed by the abrupt onset of high fever, malaise, fatigue, chills, headache, myalgias, and cough productive of blood-tinged sputum.[3,20] Sputum is loaded with *Y. pestis* and is highly contagious when aerosolized by coughing. Chest radiography commonly reveals a patchy or consolidated multilobar pneumonia. Patients develop rapidly progressive respiratory failure, shock, cyanosis, and disseminated intravascular coagulation.

DIFFERENTIAL DIAGNOSIS

Chemical or biologic warfare agent poisoning should be suspected when an increased number of patients present with a disseminated disease with fulminant course and high mortality in a compressed time frame, particularly if the disease is rare, not endemic to the area, or presents in an unusual pattern (e.g., predominance of respiratory symptoms, associated with infected or dead animals).[4,16] Prompt recognition that an attack has occurred enables health-care personnel to implement measures to protect themselves and others from secondary illness and plan an appropriate medical and public health response.

It is also important to recognize the differences between chemical and biologic exposures. Following a chemical attack, clinical effects will occur within minutes to hours, and large numbers of symptomatic patients will present to medical facilities within a short period of time.[2,4] Although the nature of the exposure may not be immediately known, the release site of the weapon ("hot zone") is quickly discoverable and may be cordoned off. The distribution of affected patients is rapidly ascertained. Decontamination is an important aspect of treatment. In contrast, following a bioagent attack, clinical effects are delayed due to the incubation period of the illness.[3,6,7,16] After several days, patients will present insidiously, often with nonspecific signs and symptoms. It is often difficult to identify the release site of the weapon, and the geographic distribution of patients may be wide by the time symptomatic disease develops. Decontamination of patients is not usually necessary.[4,7]

Familiarity with the clinical syndromes associated with various chemical and biologic agents and their differentiation from other illnesses are equally important. The diagnosis is made by history, physical examination, and initial diagnostic testing.

Irritant or corrosive gas inhalation, hydrocarbon aspiration, and vesicating agent and high-dose lacrimating agent exposures may produce pulmonary signs and symptoms similar to those caused by choking agents. Exacerbations of asthma and chronic obstructive pulmonary disease and allergic or infectious pneumonitis may present similarly. The vesiculobullous skin lesions that result from vesicating agents may mimic those resulting from Stevens-Johnson syndrome, toxic epidermal necrolysis, pemphigus vulgaris, bullous pemphigoid, scalded skin syndrome, thermal and chemical burns, and hypersensitivity reactions. Nerve agent poisoning is nearly identical to organophosphate and carbamate pesticide poisoning. Other agents and conditions that can produce similar clinical effects are botulism; nicotine; cholinergic drugs such as bethanechol, carbachol, edrophonium, methacholine, neostigmine, pilocarpine, physostigmine, pyridostigmine, and succinylcholine, and muscarine-containing mushrooms. Nerve agents or cyanide should be suspected if victims of a suspected chemical weapons incident become comatose or seize within minutes of exposure.[15,20] Lacrimating agents cause effects similar to those of irritant gas and lewisite exposure.

Botulism must be differentiated from other conditions that produce generalized paralysis, such as Eaton-Lambert syndrome, neurotoxic snake envenomation, Guillain-Barré syndrome, myasthenia gravis, tick paralysis, diphtheria, familial periodic paralysis, shellfish poisoning, organophosphate or nerve agent poisoning, poliomyelitis, and transverse myelitis. Trichothecene mycotoxicosis is similar to radiation, chemotherapeutic, and vesicant toxicity and sepsis. The acute fulminant pneumonitis resulting from *Y. pestis* may be clinically indistinguishable from that caused by numerous bacterial pneumonias. Anthrax may present similarly to Legionnaire disease, Q fever, tularemia, and overwhelming bacterial or viral infections. Anthrax should be suspected if chest radiography reveals a widened mediastinum in a previously healthy patient with an overwhelming flulike illness.[6] Unlike pneumonic plague, inhalational anthrax is not characterized by pneumonia. Conditions resembling smallpox are chickenpox, herpes zoster, disseminated herpes zoster, herpes simplex virus infection, monkeypox, other disseminated viral infections, drug eruptions, Stevens-Johnson syndrome, and eczema herpeticum. Smallpox is distinguished from chickenpox by the centrifugal distribution of its rash and the presence of lesions that remain synchronous in their stage of development.[3] Fulminant hemorrhagic smallpox may closely resemble meningococcemia. Anxiety and hysterical reactions must also be considered in the differential diagnosis of patients exposed to warfare agents.

EMERGENCY DEPARTMENT EVALUATION

An attempt should be made to document the amount, time, nature, and duration of exposure. The color and odor of the toxic agent may provide clues to its identity. The time of onset, nature, progression, and severity of symptoms should be noted. If numerous patients have been affected, the epidemic should be characterized similarly. A case definition should be established, the number of cases identified, and the attack rate determined.

Physical examination should first focus on vital signs and an assessment of neuromuscular and cardiopulmonary function, and then on the eyes, skin, and GI tract. Ideally, all patients should have continuous cardiac and oxygen saturation monitoring, but priority must be given to the most severely affected patients in mass casualty situations. The initial evaluation of numerous victims from a mass casualty incident will require rapid implementation of a hospital- and community-wide disaster plan (see Chapter 399).

If signs and symptoms of choking, vesicating, or lacrimating agent toxicity are present, ancillary studies should include a chest radiograph, electrocardiogram (ECG), and arterial blood gas analysis, depending on the severity of symptoms. There are no specific diagnostic tests for choking agents. Additional laboratory evaluation after exposure to a vesicating agent should include baseline complete blood count and serum electrolyte, blood urea nitrogen, creatinine, and glucose levels. Patients with eye symptoms should have fluorescein and slit-lamp examinations.

Patients with signs and symptoms of nerve agent toxicity should have a chest radiograph, ECG, arterial blood gas analysis, routine admission laboratory studies, and measurement of peak expiratory flow rate and plasma or erythrocyte cholinesterase activity (see Chapter 361). Routine toxicology testing will not identify nerve agents in serum or urine. Treatment decisions should be clinically based, particularly because the results of cholinesterase activity will not be readily available and do not always correlate with the severity of disease.[5,20] In the Tokyo Sarin attack, 27% of patients with clinical manifestations of moderate poisoning had plasma cholinesterase levels in the normal range.[12]

Patients with suspected botulism from the ingestion of contaminated food should have blood and feces samples sent for bioassay identification of botulinum toxin. Following inhalational exposure, however, the diagnosis is made by enzyme-linked immunosorbent assay (ELISA) detection of toxin from swabs obtained from nasal and oral mucosa within 24 hours of exposure.[3,20] Spirometry and arterial blood gas analysis should also be performed. Routine laboratory studies are not helpful in the diagnosis.

With trichothecene exposure, ancillary studies should include a complete blood count and a coagulation profile. Although trichothecene mycotoxins can be identified in human tissue samples, the technology is not readily available.

Patients with suspected inhalational anthrax should have a chest radiograph, arterial blood gas analysis, routine admission laboratory studies, blood cultures, serology, and Gram-staining of unspun peripheral blood. New rapid diagnostic tests to detect *B. anthracis* and its proteins have been developed and include polymerase chain reaction, ELISA, and direct fluorescent antibody testing.[3,6,20] Currently, these tests are available only at national reference laboratories. The definitive diagnosis of anthrax is made by culturing bacteria from blood. Blood cultures from patients with systemic infection are almost always positive. Results are usually available by 24 hours. Microbiology personnel should be informed when anthrax is suspected so that *B. anthracis* is correctly identified. Antibiotic-susceptibility testing should be performed on all bacterial isolates, because strains may be deliberately modified by terrorists to enhance antibiotic resistance.

Ancillary studies in suspected smallpox depend on the clinical appearance. A chest radiograph, complete blood count, electron microscopic analysis of vesicle scrapings, and culture are recommended.[20] Acute and convalescent serologic analysis should also be performed. Polymerase chain reaction techniques have been developed and promise more rapid and accurate diagnosis. Currently, definitive diagnosis of smallpox involves viral isolation from skin lesions, the oropharynx, or urine or serology.

Patients with suspected pneumonic plague should have a chest radiograph, arterial blood gas analysis, routine admission laboratory studies, blood cultures, serology, and Gram-staining of unspun peripheral blood and sputum. Disseminated intravascular coagulation screening should be performed for patients that are critically ill. A preliminary diagnosis can be made if gram-negative coccobacilli with bipolar, safety-pin morphology are detected in the blood, sputum, or other body fluids.[3,20] The diagnosis of plague is confirmed when *Y. pestis* is detected by direct fluorescent antibody staining or culture of blood and sputum. Polymerase chain reaction techniques have been developed and can facilitate rapid diagnosis.

EMERGENCY DEPARTMENT MANAGEMENT

Advanced cardiac and trauma life-support measures are instituted, as necessary. Important facets of treatment include self-protection of health-care workers, patient decontamination, supportive care, and specific antidotal and antimicrobial therapy.

In the event of a suspected chemical weapon attack, emergency field personnel will be responsible for performing on-scene triage, decontamination, and initial treatment prior to patient transport. Emergency field personnel must be equipped with the appropriate personal protective equipment (PPE) until patients can be decontaminated and the threat of secondary exposure is no longer present. If the hazardous substance is unknown, this consists of an encapsulated, vapor-impermeable, and chemical-resistant suit; chemical-resistant gloves and boots; and a self-contained breathing apparatus (level A PPE).[2] The importance of first-responder personal protection was illustrated in the Matsumoto and Tokyo Sarin gas attacks in which 10% to 35% of rescuers developed mild toxicity.[10,12] In each incident, patients were not decontaminated, and rescuers wore standard work clothing without respiratory protection.

Initial victim management includes establishing and maintaining the airway, breathing, and circulation, and gross decontamination (brushing off chemical powder, removal of clothing and jewelry and of the patient from the contaminated environment). Clothing should be discarded in impervious plastic bags, particularly leather items (e.g., shoes and watchbands), which absorb chemicals and act as a depot. The next priorities are further medical stabilization and decontamination. If exposed, the eyes are irrigated with copious amounts of water or saline. A topical anesthetic may be used, if available. Skin should be decontaminated with a triple wash, which includes initial irrigation with tepid water, followed by 0.5% hypochlorite solution (household bleach diluted 1:10 with water) or alkaline soap, and then repeated, thorough water rinsing.[2,7,20] The waste water should be collected and isolated, if possible. For inhalation exposure, initial treatment includes administration of 100% humidified oxygen, assisted ventilation, as necessary, and removal from the vapor source. Once the patient is decontaminated, more definitive field supportive care and antidotal therapy can be delivered while the patient is taken to the hospital.

Police, fire department, emergency medical, and HAZMAT (hazardous materials) personnel should inform hospital personnel of the nature and magnitude of exposure, the number and severity of casualties, and the manifestations of illness. On recognition of a mass casualty incident, emergency physicians must implement the hospital disaster plan as well as establish a well-demarcated decontamination area outside the emergency department for patients that arrive without prior decontamination.[2] Details of disaster planning and management are discussed in Chapter 399. Emergency department personnel performing initial decontamination should wear a non-encapsulated, chemically resistant body suit, gloves, and boots, and a full-face mask with air purifier (level C PPE) until threat of secondary exposure is no longer viable.[2] Rapid dermal decontamination is critical following exposure to the liquid or aerosolized form of an agent but less important following exposure to vapor.[2,5] Patient decontamination was inadequately performed in the Tokyo Sarin gas exposure (vapor), yet secondary injury to hospital staff was minimal and did not necessitate treatment.[11]

Following a bioagent attack (exposure by aerosol), decontamination of patients is not likely necessary unless gross contamination of the skin is evident. In a publicized attack, asymptomatic victims should be instructed to remove their clothing and place it in well-sealed plastic bags, wash their hands, and shower thoroughly with soap and water.[7] This may be performed at home or in a preestablished decontamination area of the emergency department. For patients who present with symptomatic illness after a covert attack, decontamination is likely unnecessary, but health-care provider protection is critical. Standard infection control precautions (gown, mask with eyeshield, and gloves) provide adequate protection from most agents.[7] Of the potential biologic agents, only smallpox, plague, and viral hemorrhagic fevers are spread person to person and require airborne, contact, and droplet precautions.[3,7] If patients present with respiratory symptoms or a rash, they should be placed in a private negative-pressure room, and medical personnel caring for the patient should wear N95 high-efficiency particulate air filter respirators pending the results of a more complete evaluation.[7]

Choking Agents

Treatment of choking agent poisoning is primarily supportive and consists of copious saline irrigation of exposed skin and eyes, humidified oxygen, bronchodilators, ventilatory support, intravenous crystalloids for hypotension, and antibiotic administration for secondary infection.[20] Although sometimes recommended for chlorine and phosgene exposure, corticosteroids have no proven benefit. Preliminary animal studies suggest that tomelukast, a leukotriene-receptor antagonist, and *N*-acetylcysteine, an antioxidant, may limit the development of pulmonary edema following phosgene exposure. Preliminary human evidence suggests that nebulized 2% sodium bicarbonate may provide symptomatic relief following acute chlorine gas exposure.

Vesicating Agents

Treatment of sulfur mustard victims focuses on rapid decontamination, followed by symptomatic therapy. Mustard reacts irreversibly with tissue macromolecules within minutes of exposure; immediate removal of mustard from the skin is the best form of treatment.[1,13,20] Decontamination prevents further absorption and tissue damage, but only supportive care can be given once mustard is tissue-bound. Street clothing offers no protection, but military protective garments (chemical-resistant suit) can provide up to 6 hours of protection following exposure.[1]

The recommended method of decontamination is to wash with standard 5% household bleach, diluted 1:10, or copious amounts of soap and water. Water alone is ineffective, as mustard is relatively water-insoluble. Bleach produces "free" chlorine, which inactivates the mustard compound. Dry decontamination can be performed by applying absorbent powders (flour, baking soda [sodium bicarbonate], talcum powder, activated charcoal, or Fuller's earth) to the skin and wiping off with moist paper towels.[1] Skin can also be decontaminated by irrigating with 10% sodium thiosulfate. Copious water or saline irrigation is the favored method of ocular decontamination.

General supportive care focuses on the skin, eyes, and respiratory system. Skin care involves aggressive burn management of skin lesions with irrigation when appropriate, application of topical agents such as silver sulfadiazine, and surgical debridement of blisters and necrotic skin. Ocular injury requires urgent ophthalmologic consultation. Treatment may include topical anesthetics, antibiotic ointment to prevent infection, and mydriatic or cycloplegic medication to prevent adhesions between iris and cornea.[1,20] Respiratory toxicity is managed by aggressive pulmonary toilet, supplemental oxygen, inhaled bronchodilators, antibiotics for superinfection, and mechanical ventilation with positive end-expiratory pressure, when indicated.

Preliminary studies have identified several potential antidotes for sulfur mustard toxicity including mustard scavengers (glutathione, *N*-acetylcysteine, thiosulfate), antioxidants (vitamin E), NAD^+-level stabilizers (niacin and nicotinamide), anti-inflammatory drugs (corticosteroids), and nitric oxide synthase inhibitors (L-nitroarginine methyl ester).[13,20] Bone marrow suppression may respond to granulocyte colony-stimulating factor.

Treatment of lewisite exposure involves washing the skin with water, soap and water, or solutions of dilute chlorine bleach (0.5%) or baking soda (sodium bicarbonate).[20] Dry decontamination may also be efficacious. Neither scrubbing nor hot water is appropriate, because both enhance lewisite absorption and toxicity. Blisters, shown to contain arsenic, should be opened and drained of fluid. Management is otherwise identical to that of thermal burns.

The systemic manifestations of lewisite poisoning can be effectively countered by its chelator antidote, British antilewisite (BAL, 2,3-dimercaptopropanol, or dimercaprol). BAL is given intramuscularly for systemic treatment (see Chapter 318). It has also been used topically as a 5% ointment for skin lesions and as a 5% to 10% oil solution for ocular symptoms. Newer, less toxic dithiol analogs of BAL have been developed that can be given orally or intravenously. These agents include 2,3-dimercapto-1-propan-sulfonic acid (DMPS) and meso-dimercaptosuccinic acid (DMSA, marketed as Succimer or Chemet; see Chapters 318 and 348). These agents have lower mammalian toxicity than BAL and equal efficacy.

Nerve Agents

The first priority in nerve agent treatment is self-protection and decontamination. Self-protection minimally involves a well-sealed respirator with a charcoal filter and heavy-butyl rubber gloves.[5] Use of a chemical-resistant suit and self-contained breathing apparatus provides the best protection. Victims of vapor exposure manifest maximal toxicity rapidly and will not worsen after hospital arrival.[5,12] They pose little threat to hospital personnel following removal of the clothing. Patients with liquid contamination of skin and clothing, however, may develop toxicity insidiously and pose a significant vapor and skin contact risk to rescuers.[5,20] Patient clothing should be removed rapidly and the skin decontaminated. Skin can be decontaminated with a triple wash—irrigation with tepid water, followed by 0.5% hypochlorite solution or alkaline soap, and repeated, thorough water rinsing.[2,5,15,20] The U.S. military decontamination kits contain towelettes impregnated with a hypochlorite solution. The skin should not be scrubbed, because abrading the skin will increase absorption. Water alone does not hydrolyze the nerve agents but does serve to dilute the poison. Eye decontamination involves copious saline irrigation. Hypochlorite should not be used in the eye.

Intubation, mechanical ventilation, and the use of atropine and pralidoxime antidotes may be necessary. The use of succinylcholine to assist intubation is discouraged, as it may result in prolonged neuromuscular blockade due to nerve agent–induced plasma cholinesterase inhibition.[5] Antidotal therapy is discussed in Chapter 361. Cumulative atropine doses of 10 to 20 mg are usually adequate over the first 2 to 3 hours, with little or no therapy required thereafter.[5,12,15,20] This differs from organophosphate pesticide poisoning, which frequently requires significantly greater amounts and a longer duration of atropine therapy. In the Tokyo Sarin attacks, only 19% of poisoned patients required more than 2 mg of atropine.[12] Severely poisoned patients required 1.5 to 15.0 mg of atropine (mean, 6 mg).[10–12] Atropine therapy is dictated by symptoms and titrated to the desired clinical effect. Heart rate and pupil size are poor clinical indicators of adequate atropinization. U.S. soldiers carry three atropine autoinjectors, each containing 2 mg, for rapid intramuscular self-injection. Topical mydriatic–cycloplegic eye drops (e.g., tropicamide) may be used for patients with intractable eye pain due to ciliary spasm. Eye drops are not recommended for those patients with miosis as their only ocular finding. Because nerve agents age extremely rapidly, pralidoxime must be given as soon as possible after exposure to be effective. Toxicity from pralidoxime includes hypertension and tachycardia. U.S. soldiers also carry three pralidoxime autoinjectors, each containing 600 mg of the oxime to be injected intramuscularly along with each atropine injection.[20] In the Tokyo Sarin attacks, severely poisoned patients required 1 to 36 g pralidoxime (mean 11 g).[10–12]

Seizures resulting from nerve agent exposure are treated with high-dose benzodiazepines, such as diazepam 10 mg intravenously (0.2 to 0.4 mg/kg). Experimental animal data suggest that prophylactic diazepam reduces the incidence of seizures and pathologic brain injury following nerve agent exposure.[5,20] Military physicians recommend diazepam prophylaxis for all severely exposed victims.[17,22] During Operation Desert Storm, military personnel carried 10-mg diazepam autoinjectors for intramuscular use following nerve agent exposure. Recent evidence suggests that glutamate antagonists are also effective treatment for nerve agent-induced seizures. In primates poisoned with Sarin, the administration of the glutamate antagonist, GK-11 (gacyclidine), prevented seizures, mortality, and delayed neuropathology and accelerated clinical recovery.[8]

An additional approach to limit nerve agent toxicity is to pretreat at-risk personnel with a reversible (carbamate) AChE inhibitor, such as physostigmine or pyridostigmine. Nerve agents cannot bind cholinesterase that is carbamylated (bound to carbamate), which spontaneously reactivates or is regenerated with oxime therapy, leaving the victim with enough AChE to function normally. Pyridostigmine pretreatment carbamylates 20% to 40% of erythrocyte AChE. Soman exposure results in such rapid aging that standard atropine and pralidoxime therapy is unlikely to significantly increase survival. The addition of pyridostigmine pretreatment to the treatment regimen greatly reduces Soman lethality.[20] Pretreatment does not enhance protection from Sarin and VX exposures, wherein the aging phenomenon is more prolonged. Pralidoxime is useful therapy for these exposures. Pyridostigmine does not afford any protection by itself without the use of antidotes.[20] Carbamates have direct nicotinic receptor, ionic channel actions, which may contribute to their efficacy independent of AChE carbamylation.

During the Persian Gulf war, soldiers at risk for nerve agent exposure were given pyridostigmine bromide in blister packs containing twenty-one 30-mg tablets.[20] Pyridostigmine was taken orally every 8 hours without causing impaired performance. Side effects were reported to be minimal, but they can mimic those of mild nerve gas poisoning. Pyridostigmine does not cross the blood–brain barrier and offers no protection from CNS nerve agent toxicity.[15] Physostigmine, which does cross the barrier, has proved too toxic for pretreatment.

Conventional oximes (pralidoxime preparations, obidoxime, trimedoxime) are not clinically useful against Soman. Newer H-series oximes (named after their inventor, Inge Hagedorn) are superior in their ability to reactivate unaged Soman-inhibited AChE. Their greater efficacy is partly due to greater oxime group potency and enhanced reactivation of phosphorylated AChE. H-series oximes also have direct antimuscarinic and antinicotinic (ganglia-blocking and nondepolarizing neuromuscular-blocking) actions but do not protect from nerve agent–induced seizures.[14,20] Although they do not readily cross the blood–brain barrier and do not regenerate CNS AChE in animal studies, they provide some CNS protection, presumably from a direct cholinolytic action.

HI-6, the most well-studied agent, is the only oxime clinically efficacious against Soman. It also provides protection against other agents, and no significant side effects from its use have been reported in human studies.[14] HI-6 is given intramuscularly at an adult dose of 250 to 500 mg every 6 hours. Animal studies have shown that HI-6 use alone after Soman exposure protects from lethality.[14,20] Efficacy was enhanced when it was used with atropine. Animal studies suggest that the bispyridium dioxime, HLö 7, is more efficacious than HI-6.[19]

Promising treatments are being researched. Human monoclonal antibodies to the various nerve agents may provide passive protection before exposure.[20] Soman lethality is decreased when animals are preloaded with excess cholinesterase. The circulating cholinesterase presumably scavenges nerve agent and protects tissue AChE.

Lacrimating Agents

Medical treatment is frequently unnecessary after tear agent exposure, because the initial effects resolve quickly. Symptomatic patients, however, require prompt decontamination and supportive care. Health-care personnel should wear rubber gloves; if contamination is heavy, airway protection may also be necessary. The skin is washed thoroughly with soap and water or a mild alkaline solution such as 6% sodium bicarbonate or 1% benzalkonium chloride.[20] Ambulatory patients can be bathed in a shower. Contact dermatitis may respond to topical corticosteroids and antipruritics. Tearing usually irrigates the eyes adequately, but topical anesthetics and saline irrigation may be necessary. Chemical conjunctivitis may require symptomatic treatment with topical vasoconstrictors. Corneal injuries are treated with cycloplegics, topical antibiotics, and ophthalmologic referral (see Chapter 99). Some argue that patients exposed to high gas concentrations, as in enclosed spaces or near exploding tear gas canisters, should be observed for several days because of delayed pulmonary effects.[20] Treatment of pulmonary toxicity consists of humidified oxygen, bronchodilators, and assisted ventilation, as needed. Powder may linger in clothing and hair and may repoison the patient at a later time.

Biologic Toxins

Treatment of suspected botulism involves close respiratory monitoring and supportive care. Mortality is less than 5% if assisted ventilation is provided in a timely manner.[3,20] A trivalent (ABE) equine antitoxin (immunoglobulin) and investigational, heptavalent (A-G), equine, $F(ab')_2$ fragment antitoxin are available for emergent treatment of disease (see Chapter 205). After aerosol exposure, the $F(ab')_2$ fragment antitoxin is protective only if given before the onset of clinical symptoms. It will not bind toxin that has already entered nerve terminals. If there is no ileus and exposure was by ingestion, cathartics and enemas may be used to enhance elimination of unabsorbed toxin. An investigational, pentavalent (A-E) botulinum toxoid has been developed that prevents symptomatic disease following all routes of exposure. This vaccine was used to immunize Operation Desert Storm troops as a protective measure.

Treatment of trichothecene mycotoxicosis is entirely supportive. Skin decontamination with soap and water has prevented skin lesions up to 6 hours following exposure.[20] Superactivated charcoal binds T-2 toxin avidly and should be administered as soon as possible following inhalational and oral exposures. Monoclonal antibodies against T-2 toxin have been developed but are still investigational.

Infectious Agents

Treatment of inhalational anthrax includes supportive care, antibiotics, and postexposure vaccination for asymptomatic patients. Traditionally, high-dose intravenous penicillin G (2 million U every 2 hours) has been the preferred therapy.[3,6] The threat of biologic terrorism brings with it the threat of resistant strains of *B. anthracis*. Experts currently recommend intravenous ciprofloxacin (400 mg every 12 hours for adults; 20 to 30 mg/kg/d, divided in two daily doses for children) as preferred initial therapy for symptomatic patients pending the results of susceptibility testing. Doxycycline is an acceptable alternative. Recommendations for pregnant women are no different. Chemoprophylaxis and vaccination are recommended for asymptomatic patients following known or suspected exposure to *B. anthracis*. The antibiotic regimen is the same as for symptomatic patients, but drug dosages are given orally and prophylaxis is continued for 60 days.[6] Victims should be immunized with a licensed, inactivated, cell-free vaccine at 0, 2, and 4 weeks.[3,6,20] Prophylactic antibiotic administration may be discontinued at 30 to 45 days for patients that have been immunized. U.S. troops in the Persian Gulf war were immunized against anthrax as a protective measure; no serious adverse effects have been associated with the vaccine.[20]

Treatment of smallpox is mainly supportive. The antiviral, cidofovir, has demonstrated efficacy *in vitro* against variola virus and may have a therapeutic role in treatment.[3] Strict quarantine with respiratory isolation is recommended for patients (until lesions are scabbed over) and their close contacts (for 17 days).[20] Immediate vaccination with the licensed, attenuated vaccinia virus vaccine is recommended for postexposure prophylaxis. Vaccination is highly effective if accomplished within a few days of exposure. Vaccinia immune globulin should be given to patients who are pregnant, are immunocompromised, have eczema, or experience severe vaccination reactions. The United States stock of vaccinia vaccine is maintained at the Centers for Disease Control and Prevention (CDC) in Atlanta.

Streptomycin (15 mg/kg every 12 hours) by intramuscular injection has been the traditional treatment of plague pneumonia. If streptomycin is not available, intravenous gentamicin (1.75 mg/kg every 8 hours) or doxycycline (200 mg initially, followed by 100 mg every 12 hours) may be given.[3,20] For hemodynamically unstable patients and those with meningitis, intravenous chloramphenicol (50 to 75 mg/kg/d in four divided doses) is recommended. Treatment should be continued for 10 days. All patients with pneumonic plague should be isolated, with respiratory precautions. Postexposure prophylaxis is recommended for close contacts of infected patients and all asymptomatic exposure victims. Prophylaxis consists of oral tetracycline, doxycycline, or trimethoprim–sulfamethoxazole in standard doses for 6 days. A licensed, killed, whole-cell vaccine is available but will not protect against pneumonic plague.

Most U.S. military personnel are immunized against yellow fever, cholera, tetanus, typhus, typhoid fever, poliomyelitis, diphtheria, meningococcal meningitis, hepatitis A and B, and influenza. Vaccines against tularemia, Rift Valley fever, chikungunya, Q fever, Argentine hemorrhagic fever, Venezuelan equine encephalitis, Eastern equine encephalitis, and Western equine encephalitis have also been produced. Depending on the agent involved, treatment may include immune globulin and antibiotics, as described in other chapters.

DISPOSITION

Consultation with a toxicologist, regional poison control center, experienced military physician, infectious disease specialist, epidemiologist, and public health specialist is recommended for all chemical or biologic agent poisoning except civilian exposures to the lacrimating agents. The CDC (770-488-7100) and the United States Army Medical Research Institutes for Infectious Diseases (USAMRIID) (1-888-USA-RIID) have 24-hour hotline services to assist physicians with biologic agent inquiries. Any suspected or confirmed case of chemical or biologic agent poisoning should prompt an immediate call to local law enforcement authorities, the local Federal Bureau of Investigation field office, and local or state health department and laboratory. An ophthalmologist or plastic surgeon should be consulted for patients with corneal or skin burns.

Asymptomatic patients are observed and monitored for at least 6 hours after choking agent exposure. Mild to moderately symptomatic patients may be discharged safely after several hours of observation if symptoms have improved or resolved with treatment. Some argue that all patients with a history of phosgene exposure should be admitted and closely observed because of phosgene's varying latency period and high potential morbidity. Asymptomatic patients should be observed and monitored for 12 hours after vesicating agent exposure and 24 hours after skin exposure to nerve agent liquid or aerosolized droplets. Following exposure to nerve agent vapor, patients with signs and symptoms confined to the eyes may be discharged safely after a short period of observation.[5,12] Victims of lacrimating agents may be treated and released if there is no significant pulmonary toxicity. The disposition of asymptomatic patients following biologic agent exposure depends on the agent. Patients exposed to *C. botulinum* are admitted and observed, those exposed to smallpox should be quarantined for 17 days, and those exposed to trichothecene mycotoxins, *B. anthracis,* and *Y. pestis* may be discharged following appropriate chemoprophylaxis. All patients with systemic symptoms, pulmonary toxicity, and severe or extensive dermal injury should be hospitalized. Patients with moderate-to-severe poisoning from chemical or biologic agents should be admitted, with the level of care dependent on clinical severity.

COMMON PITFALLS

- Failure to adequately protect rescuers and medical personnel from secondary contamination
- Failure to decontaminate victims of chemical agent exposure in a timely fashion
- Failure to appreciate the differences between chemical and biologic warfare agent exposures
- Lack of familiarity with chemical and biologic warfare agent toxidromes
- Failure to maintain appropriate isolation of infectious patients
- Failure to observe asymptomatic victims for appropriate periods of time

References

1. Borak J, Sidell FR. Agents of chemical warfare: sulfur mustard. *Ann Emerg Med* 1992;21:303.
2. Brennan RJ, Waeckerle JF, Sharp TW, et al. Chemical warfare agents: emergency medical and emergency public health issues. *Ann Emerg Med* 1999;34:191.
3. Franz DR, Jahrling PB, Friedlander AM, et al. Clinical recognition and management of patients exposed to biological warfare agents. *JAMA* 1997;278:399.
4. Henderson DA. The looming threat of bioterrorism. *Science* 1999;283:1279.
5. Holstege CP, Kirk M, Sidell FR. Chemical warfare: nerve agent poisoning. *Med Toxicol* 1997;13:923.
6. Inglesby TV, Henderson DA, Bartlett JG, et al. Anthrax as a biological weapon: medical and public health management. *JAMA* 1999;281:1735.
7. Keim M, Kaufmann AF. Principles for emergency response to bioterrorism. *Ann Emerg Med* 1999;34:177.
8. Lallement G, Clarencon D, Masqueliez C, et al. Nerve agent poisoning in primates: antilethal, anti-epileptic and neuroprotective effects of GK-11. *Arch Toxicol* 1998;72:84.
9. Meselson M, Guillemin J, Hugh-Jones M, et al. The Sverdlovsk anthrax outbreak of 1979. *Science* 1994;266:1202.
10. Morita H, Yanagisawn, Nakajima T, et al. Sarin poisoning in Matsumoto, Japan. *Lancet* 1995;346:290.
11. Noxaki H, Aikawa N, Shinozawa Y, et al. Sarin poisoning in Tokyo subway [Letter]. *Lancet* 1995;345:980.
12. Okumura T, Takasu N, Ishimatsu S, et al. Report on 640 victims of the Tokyo subway sarin attack. *Ann Emerg Med* 1996;28:129.
13. Papirmeister B, Feister AJ, Robinson SI, et al. *Medical defense against mustard gas: toxic mechanisms and pharmacological implications.* Boca Raton, FL: CRC Press, 1991.
14. Shih T-M, Whalley C, Valdes J. A comparison of cholinergic effects of HI-6 and pralidoxime-2-chloride (2-PAM) in Soman poisoning. *Toxicol Lett* 1991;55:131.
15. Sidell FR, Borak J. Chemical warfare agents: nerve agents. *Ann Emerg Med* 1992;21:865.
16. Simon JD. Biological terrorism: preparing to meet the threat. *JAMA* 1997;278:428.
17. Smith WJ, Dunn MA. Medical defense against blistering chemical warfare agents. *Arch Dermatol* 1991;127:1207.
18. Török TJ, Tauxe TV, Wise RP, et al. A large community outbreak of salmonellosis caused by intentional contamination of restaurant salad bars. *JAMA* 1997;278:389.
19. Worek F, Widmann R, Knopff O, et al. Reactivating potency of obidoxime, pralidoxime, HI 6 and HLö 7 in human erythrocyte acetylcholinesterase inhibited by highly toxic organophosphorus compounds. *Arch Toxicol* 1998;72:237.
20. Zajtchuk R, Bellamy RD, eds. *Textbook of military medicine: medical aspects of chemical and biological warfare. Part I.* Washington, DC: Office of the Surgeon General, U.S. Dept of the Army. 1997.

CHAPTER 326
Cocaine

Richard D. Shih and Judd E. Hollander

Cocaine (benzoylmethylecgonine) has been used for social, religious, and medicinal purposes for many centuries. Over the past several decades, its illicit use as a drug of abuse has risen dramatically. An estimated 23 million Americans have used cocaine at least once, and approximately 5 million use it regularly.[15] Further, among visits to emergency departments due to drugs of abuse, cocaine is the most commonly involved drug.[12]

Cocaine is well absorbed on contact with mucous membranes or by pulmonary inhalation. It is derived from the *Erythroxylon coca* plant, which is found in abundance in Central America, South America, the West Indies, and Indonesia. In the manufacturing process, leaves are initially dissolved in hydrochloric acid to form the cocaine hydrochloride salt. This is the form most often abused via nasal insufflation or intravenous injection. Crack cocaine or cocaine free base are the alkaloid forms of cocaine that are produced by an extraction process utilizing a basic solution, a solvent (usually ether), and heat. The free-base form is close to 100% purity, while crack approximates 75%. These forms are heat stable, and thus can be smoked and absorbed by the lungs.

By the intravenous or inhalational routes, cocaine is rapidly distributed throughout the body and central nervous system (CNS), with peak effects in 3 to 5 minutes. With nasal insufflation, absorption is slower and effects are delayed, peaking at approximately 20 minutes. Although not a typical route of abuse, oral ingestion delays absorption even further, with peak effects occurring at 40 to 60 minutes.

Cocaine has a half-life of 0.5 to 1.5 hours. It is predominantly metabolized to the active metabolites ecgonine methyl ester and benzoylecgonine (BE) by hydrolysis. These two metabolites account for approximately 80% of cocaine metabolism. They have half-lives of 4 to 8 hours and many effects similar to their parent compound, cocaine. Other metabolites include cocethylene, ecgonine, and norcocaine. Urine drug tests typically test for BE, and this cocaine metabolite is typically present for 48 to 72 hours after use.[1]

Cocaine has a number of pharmacologic effects peripherally and in the CNS. It acts to augment the peripheral sympathetic system, producing such findings as tachycardia, hypertension, diaphoresis, arterial vasoconstriction, and dilated pupils. Additionally, cocaine has local anesthetic effects. In the amide group of topical anesthetic agents, it is the only one that has vasoconstrictive effects, which help control secretions and bleeding. Because of these properties, it has frequently been used for otolaryngology procedures and wound repair. The central effects of cocaine are very complex and not completely understood. It has effects on a number of neurotransmitters in the CNS. However, the net effect is the augmentation of the sympathetic nervous system.

"Body stuffers" and "body packers" are individuals who have ingested containers of an illicit drug (most commonly cocaine and heroin).[5] These containers can be plastic bags, plastic vials, elastic wraps, elastic condoms, or other packaging material. A "stuffer" is someone who hastily ingests containers just prior to being arrested by police in order to conceal the evidence.[17] A packer, or "mule," is an individual who ingests a large number of carefully wrapped containers of highly pure drug as a means of concealing and smuggling it into the United States from a foreign country or into jail.

CLINICAL PRESENTATION

Cocaine toxicity can be manifested in a number of different organ systems. The most commonly seen manifestations in the emergency department involve the cardiovascular and neurologic systems.[2] Signs and symptoms of mild cocaine intoxication include normal or minimally increased blood pressure, pulse, respiratory rate, and temperature; agitation; anxiety; euphoria; headache; hyperreflexia; nausea; vomiting; mydriasis; pallor; diaphoresis; tremors; and twitching. Moderate intoxication may result in hypertension, tachycardia, dyspnea, tachypnea, hyperthermia, confusion, hallucinations, marked hyperactivity, increased muscle tone and deep tendon reflexes, abdominal cramps, formication, and generalized but brief tonic–clonic seizures. Severe intoxication is manifested by hypotension, tachycardia (or preterminal bradycardia), ventricular dysrhythmias, Cheyne-Stokes respirations, apnea, cyanosis, malignant hyperthermia, coma, flaccid paralysis, and status epilepticus.

Chest pain is the most common chief complaint. Myocardial infarction due to cocaine is well established[7,8] and occurs in approximately 6% of patients presenting with this complaint. Cocaine causes coronary ischemia through coronary artery vasoconstriction,[10] *in situ* thrombus formation, platelet activation, and inhibition of endogenous fibrinolysis, as well as triggering an increase in the myocardial oxygen demand through generation of tachycardia and hypertension.[7] Chronic users develop premature atherosclerosis and left ventricular hypertrophy, which can further exacerbate the oxygen supply–demand mismatch that results from chronic use.[7] Other less common but equally important cardiovascular complications of cocaine use include atrial and ventricular dysrhythmias, both systolic and diastolic congestive heart failure, coronary and aortic dissection, dilated cardiomyopathy, and ischemia in other vascular beds (e.g., intestinal, renal, etc.).

Euphoria, the impetus for the recreational use of cocaine, is typically short-lived and without serious sequelae. The stimulatory effects of cocaine can lead to seizures, both bland and hemorrhagic cerebral infarction, and subarachnoid hemorrhage. Severe, persistent lethargy with an altered mental status can occur following prolonged and intense cocaine usage and has been termed the *cocaine wash-out syndrome*. This diagnosis should be made only after exclusion of the aforementioned neurologic catastrophes (i.e., after a normal computerized tomography (CT) of the head and lumbar puncture, if indicated). The syndrome is thought to be due to such excessive cocaine usage that essential neurotransmitters are depleted. Symptoms will generally abate within 12 to 24 hours.

Rhabdomyolysis is another common manifestation of cocaine toxicity. Cocaine's stimulatory effects lead to severe agitation and marked muscular agitation and rigidity. Ischemia of the skeletal muscle beds may also contribute. Profound elevations in creatinine kinase (CK) may be seen. Concurrent development of severe hyperthermia and acute renal failure can be life-threatening.[9] Hyperthermia is most commonly due to a combination of environmental exposure and heat production from excessive muscle activity. Renal failure is due to muscle breakdown and renal tubular precipitation of the released muscle myoglobin.

Cocaine has a number of direct and indirect effects on the lungs. Many of the effects of cocaine are due to the method of abuse rather than direct toxin effects. Asthma exacerbations have been frequently reported with crack cocaine usage. This is most likely due to particulate by-products of combustion. Further, crack usage is typically associated with deep Valsalva maneuvers to maximize drug delivery. This can cause pneumothorax, pneumomediastinum, and noncardiogenic pulmonary edema. Other less common effects on the lung include pulmonary infarction, bronchiolitis obliterans, pulmonary artery hypertrophy, and alveolar hemorrhage. Treatment of these conditions follows standard management protocols, whether they are related to cocaine, or not.

The intestinal vascular system is very sensitive to the effects of cocaine. Acute intestinal vascular infarction has been associated with all routes of administration.

The amount of drug released in the gastrointestinal (GI) tract in stuffers is relatively low and unlikely to cause serious toxicity.[5]

Although oral ingestion is not a common route of abuse, local intestinal and systemic effects can occur when containers of cocaine leak or rupture in body stuffers and packers. Body packers most often present asymptomatically, having been discovered by customs officers.

Habitual cocaine usage during pregnancy is associated with low birth weight, small head circumference, developmental problems, and a number of birth defects. Acute toxicity can also cause the induction of premature labor, eclampsia, and abruptio placentae. After delivery, neonates exposed to cocaine *in utero* are at risk for the development of neonatal withdrawal. This diagnosis of exclusion is manifested as irritability, jitteriness, and poor eye contact.

EMERGENCY DEPARTMENT EVALUATION

The diagnostic evaluation of patients manifesting cocaine toxicity relies on a history of cocaine use, recognition of signs and symptoms consistent with sympathomimetic toxidrome, and evaluation of specific organ system complaints. The history should include the total amount and time of cocaine use in relation to symptom onset. Friends (or witnesses) of confused patients should be questioned about a history of seizures or syncope and antecedent activities. New-onset seizures, epistaxis, hypertension, myocardial infarction, intracranial hemorrhage, or psychiatric illness, especially in young patients, should suggest the possibility of cocaine use. Many patients deny cocaine use unless approached with reassurance and compassion or confronted with a positive urine test.

The physical examination should include a complete set of vital signs and a detailed examination of the cardiac, pulmonary, and neurologic systems. All patients should initially have continuous cardiac monitoring.

When the history is clear and symptoms are mild, laboratory evaluation is unnecessary. In contrast, if the history is absent or unreliable or the patient manifests moderate or severe toxicity, routine laboratory evaluation should include a complete blood count; determination of electrolyte, glucose, blood urea nitrogen, and creatinine levels; arterial blood gas analysis; urinalysis; and CK. Qualitative toxicologic analyses of blood and urine can confirm the diagnosis and rule out other intoxicants. Toxicology testing is indicated only when confirmation of drug use would change management, counseling, or referral patterns.

A chest radiograph and electrocardiogram (ECG) should be obtained in patients with chest pain or moderate-to-severe toxicity. Those with prolonged, unexplained pain should have serial ECG and cardiac enzyme measurements to rule out myocardial infarction. Many of the clinical parameters to assess ischemia or infarction are not as reliable as when they are used for patients with traditional coronary artery disease (CAD).[4] The ECG is less sensitive and specific for identifying ischemia or infarction in this setting, the CK is often elevated due to associated rhabdomyolysis, and false elevations in the MB fraction can occur. Cardiac troponin I testing can help distinguish true-positive from false-positive CK-MB elevations.[9]

Persistent headache despite normalization of blood pressure requires evaluation by CT scan and lumbar puncture to rule out intracranial hemorrhage. Patients with abdominal or back pain must be evaluated for intestinal or renal infarction. The urine should be inspected and the CK level determined, because myoglobinuric renal failure may develop.

Occult infections must be excluded in patients with fever, even though fever can be due solely to cocaine toxicity. A brief seizure clearly related (temporally) to cocaine use in an otherwise healthy person should be evaluated with CT to exclude serious underlying pathology, but it does not require further workup, provided the patient is alert and coherent, has no headache, and has a normal neurologic examination. Patients suspected of body packing or stuffing should be evaluated by abdominal radiographs (including contrast imaging) and cavity searches (digital or visual examination of the rectum or vagina). Toxicity lasting for more than 4 hours suggests continued drug absorption and should prompt a similar workup.

The route of administration may influence the patient's chief complaint or which organ system is affected. Intravenous users may present with fever and malaise secondary to infectious complications such as cellulitis, endocarditis, hepatitis, pneumonia, and the acquired immunodeficiency syndrome. Chronic nasal use may lead to rhinitis, septal perforation, and epistaxis. Inhalational use may produce dyspnea, cough, or hemoptysis from reactive airway disease, "crack lung" pneumonitis, or pulmonary edema, or may result in pulmonary barotrauma (e.g., pneumothorax, pneumomediastinum, pneumopericardium) as a result of the Valsalva maneuver or from blowing smoke into the mouth of a partner. Patients with barotrauma may also complain of neck and chest pain and demonstrate tachypnea, subcutaneous emphysema, or Hamman's sign.

Behavioral disorders (e.g., agitation, combative behavior), headache, back pain (renal infarction or aortic dissection), abdominal pain (mesenteric ischemia), altered level of consciousness, or cardiopulmonary arrest are other common presentations that may follow the use of cocaine by any route. Patients may present as victims of trauma, because of the violent, irrational, and risk-taking behavioral associated with drug use. Delayed cardiovascular complications can sometimes occur. Myocardial ischemia can occur in the first few days after cocaine use. Intestinal and myocardial infarction have been reported 1 to 2 weeks after last use.[14]

Manifestations of chronic cocaine abuse include anorexia, insomnia, formication, depression, impotence, weight loss, paranoia, and psychosis. Halo vision (lights around objects) and "snow lights" (flashes in the peripheral fields) have also been described.

DIFFERENTIAL DIAGNOSIS

Similar toxicity can be caused by a variety of physiologic stimulants (see Table 309.4). A sympathomimetic toxidrome can also be seen with hypoglycemia, environmental and malignant hyperthermia, pheochromocytoma, psychiatric conditions, status epilepticus, and thyroid storm. Patients with persistent altered mental status need to be evaluated for possible meningitis and CNS lesions. Table 326.1 lists the differential diagnosis of chest pain related to cocaine use.

EMERGENCY DEPARTMENT MANAGEMENT

Management depends on the specific complaint and presentation (Table 326.2). Patients presenting with a sympathomimetic toxidrome are at risk for hyperthermia and rhabdomyolysis. After initial attention to the airway and cardiovascular status, management should focus on lowering core body temperature (see Chapter 209), halting further muscle agitation and heat production, and giving intravenous fluids to ensure a good urinary output. The agents of choice for muscle relaxation in this setting are benzodiazepines.[3] Supranormal cumulative doses may be necessary in severely agitated individuals.

Patients with severe hypertension or tachycardia necessitating pharmacologic measures can usually be safely treated with benzodiazepines. When large doses of benzodiazepines are not effective, intravenous nitroprusside or phentolamine should be considered. Beta antagonists or compounds with partial beta-blocking effects are contraindicated. The use of beta antagonists in the setting of cocaine intoxication can lead to unopposed alpha stimulation, with resultant marked increases in hypertension and worsening coronary vasoconstriction.[7,11,18]

Patients with suspected cocaine-induced ischemia or myocardial infarction should be treated similarly to those with traditional CAD, with some notable exceptions.[7,11] Aspirin, nitroglycerin, and heparin remain important initial therapies. Intravenous benzodiazepines should be provided as early management. They will decrease the central stimulatory effects of cocaine, thereby indirectly reducing the cardiovascular toxicity of cocaine.[3,7] Beta antagonists should not be used. They are contraindicated, as they exacerbate cocaine-induced coronary artery vasoconstriction.[5,11,18] Another management difference in the setting of cocaine use relative to patients with traditional

TABLE 326.1. The Differential Diagnosis of Cocaine-Associated Chest Pain

Aortic dissection	Bacterial endocarditis
Bronchospasm	Esophageal illnesses
Gastrointestinal illnesses	Musculoskeletal injury
Myocarditis	Myocardial infarction
Myocardial ischemia	Pericarditis
Pleurisy	Pneumonia
Pneumothorax	Pneumomediastinum
Pulmonary emboli	Pulmonary infarction

TABLE 326.2. Treatment of Specific Cocaine-Related Medical Diseases

Medical Problem	Treatment
Dysrhythmias	
Sinus tachycardia	Observation
	Oxygen
	Diazepam 5–10 mg i.v. or lorazepam 2–4 mg i.v. titrated to effect
Supraventricular tachycardia	Oxygen
	Diazepam 5 mg i.v. or lorazepam 2–4 mg i.v.
	Diltiazem 20 mg i.v. or verapamil 5 mg i.v.
	Adenosine 6 mg or 12 mg i.v. for AV node reentry
	Digoxin 0.5 mg i.v.
	Consider verapamil 5–10 mg i.v.
	Cardioversion if hemodynamically unstable
Ventricular dysrhythmias	Oxygen
	Sodium bicarbonate
	Lidocaine 1.5 mg/kg i.v. bolus, followed by 2-mg/min infusion
	Defibrillation if hemodynamically unstable
	Diazepam 5 mg i.v. or lorazepam 2–4 mg i.v.
Ischemic chest pain	Oxygen
	Diazepam 5–10 mg i.v. or lorazepam 2–4 mg i.v.
	Soluble aspirin 325 mg
	Nitroglycerin 1/150 sublingual ×3 every 5 minutes, followed by a drip titrated to a mean arterial pressure reduction of 10% or relief of chest pain
	Morphine sulfate 2 mg i.v. titrated to pain relief
	Phentolamine 1 mg i.v.; repeat in 5 minutes
	Verapamil 5–10 mg i.v.
	Heparin 5,000-U bolus, followed by 1,000 U/h
	Mechanical reperfusion (angioplasty)
	Thrombolytic therapy
Hypertension	Observation
	Diazepam 5–10 mg i.v. or lorazepam 2–4 mg i.v. titrated to effect
	Phentolamine 1 mg i.v.; repeat in 5 minutes
	Nitroglycerin or nitroprusside drip titrated to effect
Pulmonary edema	Lasix 20-40 mg i.v.
	Morphine sulfate 2 mg i.v. titrated to pain relief
	Nitroglycerin drip titrated to blood pressure or respiratory status
	Consider phentolamine or nitroprusside
Hyperthermia	Cool environment with minimal activity
	Sedation with benzodiazepines
	Tepid water with fans, cool water, or ice baths
Neurologic symptoms	
Anxiety and agitation	Diazepam 5–10 mg i.v. or lorazepam 2–4 mg i.v. titrated to effect
Seizures	Diazepam 5–10 mg i.v. or lorazepam 2–4 mg i.v. titrated to effect
	Phenobarbital 25–50 mg/min up to 10–20 mg/kg
Intracranial hemorrhage	Neurosurgery consult
Rhabdomyolysis	Cardiac monitor
	Serial potassium determination
	Intravenous hydration to maintain urine output at 3 cc/kg/h.
	Sodium bicarbonate titrated to an alkaline urine
	Hemodialysis, as necessary for renal failure
Cocaine washed-out syndrome	Supportive care
Body packers	Activated charcoal
	Whole-bowel irrigation
	Admission to monitored setting, even if asymptomatic
	Laparotomy or endoscopic retrieval for obstruction or symptoms

i.v., intravenously; AV, atrioventricular.

Adapted from Hollander JE, Hoffman RS. Cocaine. In: Goldfrank LR, Flomenbaum NE, Lewin NA, et al., eds. *Goldfrank's toxicologic emergency*, 6th ed. Stamford, CT: Appleton & Lange, 1998:1071-1089.

acute coronary syndromes is a preference for percutaneous interventions (angioplasty) over thrombolysis. Thrombolysis in the setting of cocaine-associated myocardial infarction has no proven efficacy, a possible reduced safety profile, and a high likelihood of being administered to patients who are not sustaining an acute infarction (because young patients with recent cocaine use have a high prevalence of early repolarization and "false-positive" ST-segment elevations on the ECG). Such therapy should, therefore, be used with caution. Finally, there are anecdotal reports of the safety and efficacy of phentolamine, an alpha antagonist, for treatment of cocaine-associated acute coronary syndromes.[6,7] Verapamil reverses cocaine-induced vasoconstriction,[16] but several animal experiments suggest that it exacerbates CNS toxicity. Therefore, it may have a role in patients with continued ischemia who do not have signs of central stimulation from cocaine.

Supraventricular dysrhythmias may be difficult to treat. Adenosine can be administered, but its effects may be temporary. Use of calcium channel blockers in association with benzodiazepines appear to be most beneficial. Beta blockers should be avoided.[7]

Ventricular dysrhythmias may be due to excess adrenergic tone or cocaine's sodium channel blocking effects. Management with benzodiazepines, lidocaine, and/or sodium bicarbonate appears to be most useful.[7,19] Bicarbonate is preferred when patients have dysrhythmias directly following the use of cocaine. In this setting, the dysrhythmias are presumably related to the type I effects of cocaine. Bicarbonate reverses cocaine-associated QRS widening. Lidocaine can be used when dysrhythmias appear to be related to cocaine-induced ischemia. ECG evidence for the type I effects of cocaine has often disappeared by the time symptomatic ischemia develops.

Cocaine-induced seizures are typically brief and self-limited. For refractory cases, benzodiazepines and phenobarbital are the first- and second-line agents, respectively. Phenytoin is not recommended.

Patients with suspected cerebrovascular infarctions and hemorrhage should be treated the same as other patients with these conditions. Intracranial and systemic hypertension necessitating treatment is accomplished using standard therapies, except that beta blockers should not be utilized.

The main concern in asymptomatic body stuffers and packers is eliminating the packages out of the GI system. Whole-bowel irrigation with subsequent radiologic verification of passage of all drug-filled containers may is warranted.[5]

Body stuffers who manifest clinical signs of toxicity should be treated similarly to other cocaine-exposed individuals. In addition, GI decontamination with activated charcoal should be administered liberally.[20]

Symptomatic body packers should be treated more aggressively, because rapid deterioration and severe toxicity can result from their potentially massive exposures. Immediate surgical removal of the ruptured package(s) may be lifesaving. Aggressive supportive care with activated charcoal and benzodiazepines is warranted as preparation for surgery occurs.[5,13]

DISPOSITION

Patients with severe agitation, hyperthermia, and possible rhabdomyolysis need to be admitted. Those with cocaine-associated chest pain need admission if myocardial ischemia cannot be excluded. Patients with severe hypertension, hypotension, hyperthermia, and any dysrhythmias also need to be admitted. All of these patients should have cardiac monitoring. Those with behavioral or cardiovascular instability should be admitted to an intermediate or intensive care unit. Consultation with a cardiologist, medical toxicologist, or poison control center may be warranted for patients who do not readily respond to treatment. The disposition of patients with neurologic complications is the same as for other patients with these conditions. The likelihood of compliance with outpatient follow-up should be considered when contemplating the discharge of patients who may need further evaluation. If definitive care cannot be provided at the site of presentation, transfer may be necessary. Patients requiring transfer should be accompanied by personnel with advanced life-support training. All patients should be referred for substance abuse counseling and treatment.

COMMON PITFALLS

- Failure to recognize the dangers of using beta-adrenergic antagonists to treat any manifestation of cocaine toxicity
- Failure to utilize benzodiazepines as a first-line agent in treating all cocaine-related toxicities
- Failure to consider cocaine toxicity in the differential diagnosis of patients with chest pain, seizures, agitation, altered mental status, and arrhythmias
- Failure to recognize the limitations of the ECG in the evaluation of cocaine-related chest pain
- Failure to appreciate differences between the management of cocaine-related chest pain and that of traditional CAD
- Failure to ensure adequate passage of cocaine-filled packages in treating body stuffers and body packers

References

1. Ambre J. The urinary excretion of cocaine and metabolites in humans: a kinetic analysis of published data. *J Anal Toxicol* 1985;9:241–245.
2. Brody SL, Wrenn KD, Wilber MM, et al. Predicting the severity of cocaine associated rhabdomyolysis. *Ann Emerg Med* 1990;19:1137–1143.
3. Catravas JD, Waters IW. Acute cocaine intoxication in the conscious dog: studies on the mechanism of lethality. *J Pharmacol Exp Ther* 1981;217:350–356.
4. Gitter MJ, Goldsmith ER, Dunbar DN, et al. Cocaine and chest pain: clinical features and outcome of patients hospitalized to rule out myocardial infarction. *Ann Intern Med* 1991;115:277–282.
5. Hoffman RS, Smilkstein MJ, Goldfrank LR. Whole bowel irrigation and the cocaine "bodypacker": a new approach to a common problem. *Am J Emerg Med* 1990;8:523–527.
6. Hollander JE, Carter WC, Hoffman RS. Use of phentolamine for cocaine-induced myocardial ischemia. *N Engl J Med* 1992;327:361.
7. Hollander JE. Management of cocaine-associated myocardial ischemia. *N Engl J Med* 1995;333(19):1267–1272.
8. Hollander JE, Hoffman RS, Burstein J, et al., and the Cocaine Associated Myocardial Infarction Study (CAMI) Group. Cocaine associated myocardial infarction. Mortality and complications. *Arch Intern Med* 1995;155:1081–1086.
9. Hollander JE, Levitt MA, Young GP, et al. The effect of cocaine on the specificity of cardiac markers. *Am Heart J* 1998;135(2):245–252.
10. Lange RA, Cigarroa RG, Yancy CW, et al. Cocaine-induced coronary-artery vasoconstriction. *N Engl J Med* 1989;321:1557–1561.
11. Lange RA, Cogarroa RG, Flores ED, et al. Potentiation of cocaine-induced coronary vasoconstriction by beta-adrenergic blockade. *Ann Intern Med* 1990;112:897–903.
12. MacDonald DI. Cocaine leads emergency department drug visits. *JAMA* 1987;258:2029.
13. McCarron MM, Wood JD. The cocaine body packer syndrome. *JAMA* 1983;250:1417–1420.
14. Nademanee K, Gorelick DA, Josephson MA, et al. Myocardial ischemia during cocaine withdrawal. *Ann Intern Med* 1989;111:876–880.
15. National Institute of Drug Abuse. *National household survey on drug abuse. Population estimates, 1991.* DHHS number (ADM) 92-1887, Rockville, MD: Department of Health and Human Services, 1992.
16. Negus BH, Willard JE, Hillis LD, et al. Alleviation of cocaine induced coronary vasoconstriction with intravenous verapamil. *Am J Cardiol* 1994;73:510–513.
17. Roberts J, Price D, Goldfrank L. The body stuffer syndrome: a clandestine form of drug overdose. *Am J Emerg Med* 1986;4:21–27.
18. Sand IC, Brody SL, Wrenn KD, et al. Experience with esmolol for the treatment of cocaine associated cardiovascular complications. *Am J Emerg Med* 1991;9:161–163.
19. Shih RD, Hollander JE, Hoffman RS, et al., and the Cocaine Associated Myocardial Infarction Study (CAMI) Study Group. Clinical safety of lidocaine in cocaine associated myocardial infarction. *Ann Emerg Med* 1995;26:702–706.
20. Tomaszewski C, McKinney P, Phillips S, et al. Prevention of toxicity from oral cocaine by activated charcoal in mice. *Ann Emerg Med* 1993;22:1804–1806.

CHAPTER 327
Complications of Alcohol Abuse

Cynthia K. Aaron and Thomas A. Brunell

Few diseases or conditions are as pervasive, if not unavoidable, in the emergency department as is alcoholism. Although encountered frequently, *alcoholism, alcohol use, alcohol dependence,* and *alcohol abuse* remain nebulous terms, the definitions of which lack consensus among physicians. In 1992, the Joint Commission for the Diagnosis of Alcoholism, a subgroup of the National Council on Alcoholism and Drug Dependence, and the American Society of Addiction Medicine revised the definition of *alcoholism* as,

> a primary chronic disease with genetic, psychosocial, and environmental factors influencing its development and manifestations. The disease is often progressive and fatal. It is characterized by impaired control over drinking, preoccupation with the drug alcohol, use of alcohol despite adverse consequences, and distortions in thinking, most notably, denial. Each of these symptoms may be continuous or periodic.[12]

The World Health Organization, instead, attempts to stratify a patient's drinking habits: "[H]azardous consumption" is present if the patient places himself or herself at physical or psychological risk through his or her drinking, and "harmful consumption" is present when drinking has resulted in physical or psychological complications.[16]

As of 1992, The National Longitudinal Alcohol Epidemiologic Study found that 44% of the adult population of the United States was currently drinking alcohol. The current prevalence of alcohol abuse and dependence is estimated between 7.4% to 9.7%, with a lifetime prevalence between 13.7% and 23.5%, with 43% of all adults reporting alcoholism in their families.[13,17] Among college students, 45% admit to binge drinking.[11] It is unclear how many patients proceed unknowingly from social "binging" to pathologic drinking during these years.

Alcohol is associated with between 100,000 and 200,000 deaths annually, with a total economic burden of greater than $100 billion each year in the United States alone. It is estimated to be responsible for 15% of the nation's annual health-care costs. Alcohol is involved with 64% to 70% of homicides, 75% of stabbings, 30% to 50% of all motor vehicle fatalities, 69% of beatings, and 56% of domestic violence cases. It also is a significant factor in fires, gunshot wounds, pedestrian accidents, falls, and suicides.[3,11]

Alcohol is the leading contributor to death in people between ages 15 and 45 and contributes to 85% of the 11,000 deaths per year from liver disease.[6,7,11] The disease has both a genetic and familial predisposition and is associated with immunosuppression, myocardial disease, and an increased propensity toward oral, pharyngeal, laryngeal, esophageal, and liver cancers.[2] Studies suggest that women are at an increased risk for ethanol-related morbidity at lower levels of ingestion than men, perhaps because ethanol has less presystemic metabolism and a lower volume of distribution in this population.

It can be difficult to recognize alcoholism. Despite the recent impetus to increase physician participation in recognition and treatment of the alcoholic patient, in the generalist's office, as many as 50% of patients with alcoholism go undiagnosed and untreated.[13] Despite its role in trauma, 79% of trauma centers do not screen patients for alcohol abuse.[3] Detection and treatment often are delayed for women—due perhaps to cultural and social value systems, in which it may be less acceptable for a woman to have an alcohol or substance abuse disorder.

Criteria mandating a diagnosis of alcoholism include alcoholic hepatitis, blackouts, drinking despite social contraindications, and withdrawal symptoms. A number of simple questionnaires can be used to rapidly identify high-risk patients in the emergency department (see Appendix, Tables 327.A1 through 327.A5).[8] High-risk groups include adolescents, patients involved in violent activity or trauma (one-car crashes), caretakers accused of child abuse, spouses of known alcoholics, suicidal patients, and those presenting with neuropsychiatric disturbances.[16] Other risk factors include male sex, unemployment, homelessness, polysubstance use or abuse, and tobacco use.[19] The vast preponderance of emergency department patients who present with ethanol levels of 300 mg/dL or greater score high in response to two or more CAGE questions (see Appendix). Yet even when the CAGE questionnaire is successfully utilized, it is often unclear what clinical approach to take with the patient identified at risk—beyond the chief complaint that brought him or her to the emergency department.[17]

Many of the metabolic problems caused by alcoholism result from the metabolism of ethanol. Ethanol oxidation to acetaldehyde is accomplished via three separate pathways.[5,9,10] The simplest pathway, catalase, generates H_2O from H_2O_2. Metabolism through the microsomal ethanol oxidizing system oxidizes the reduced cofactor nicotinamide adenine dinucleotide phosphate (NADPH) to $NADP^+$. This reaction generates free radicals, which then interact with glutathione, eventually leading to glutathione depletion and possibly contributing to hepatotoxicity (see Chapter 309).

The principal metabolic pathway involves alcohol dehydrogenase (ADH) and nicotinamide adenine dinucleotide (NAD^+) as a cofactor. During this reaction, NAD^+ is reduced to NADH. The conversion of NADH back to NAD^+ requires large amounts of oxygen. When excessive amounts of ethanol are metabolized, oxygen requirements in the centrilobular areas of the liver exceed those delivered. The relative hypoxia that results in these areas is believed to contribute to hepatic damage.

Increased oxygen demand also shifts the redox potential of the cell. The result is both an increased ratio of lactate to pyruvate, and a favoring of the glycolytic pathway—depleting available glycogen stores. The increase in free hydrogen radicals (H^+) tends to favor ketone formation and fatty acid generation. Excess H^+ depresses the citric acid cycle and decreases the use of free fatty acids as an energy source. This favors hypercholesterolemia and fatty liver formation.[5,14] Gamma glutamyl transferase, the most sensitive indicator of hepatic injury, rises in patients who have had more than five drinks a day for several weeks.[1] A carbohydrate-deficient transferrin test (if possible) is highly sensitive and specific for detecting alcohol abuse.[13]

Ethanol-induced metabolic derangements, especially in the setting of poor nutritional intake, increase the patient's risk of developing ketoacidosis and hypoglycemia. Renal magnesium wasting, secondary to ethanol's inhibitory effect on magnesium resorption, combined with intestinal malabsorption of magnesium, make the chronic alcoholic prone to hypomagnesemia. Thiamine, a water-soluble nutrient, has limited stores in the body. Lack of thiamine (usually secondary to poor nutrition) can lead to life-threatening lactic acidosis. Pyruvate, which is normally catalyzed to acetyl coenzyme A through thiamine cofactors, is converted instead to lactate, causing the acidosis.[15]

CLINICAL PRESENTATION

The clinical presentations suggestive of alcohol abuse are listed in Table 327.1. Certain presenting complaints and background history should prompt the physician to consider an underlying ethanol problem.

An adolescent with a drinking problem may present to the emergency department with myriad nonspecific complaints, none of which may directly point to alcohol abuse as a possible underlying etiology. Obtaining a history from family members can be invaluable. The adolescent may have recently undergone significant changes in personality, behavior, or peer contacts and peer relations. College-age alcoholics, who may use the emergency department as their only source of health care, can present with vague flulike symptoms, headache, insomnia, chest palpitations, trauma, gastrointestinal (GI) disturbances, or psychiatric complaints.

An alcoholic who is still able to function socially or occupationally may present with chief complaints of memory difficulties, GI dysfunction (including abdominal pain, diarrhea, vomiting, hematemesis, and hepatitis), respiratory complaints, frequent infections, weakness, polysubstance use, withdrawal, or recurrent trauma.[1,20] Electrolyte imbalances (hypokalemia, hypomagnesemia, and hypocalcemia) are more common in the chronic alcoholic, but may occur in the setting of acute intoxication as well.[3,14]

Young, otherwise healthy males presenting with chest palpitations, showing paroxysmal atrial fibrillation, atrial tachycardia, or frequent atrial extrasystoles, should have a thorough ethanol history investigated. "Holiday heart," resulting from binge drinking (often over a weekend or holiday), is a paroxysmal (usually atrial) dysrhythmia that represents chronic cardiac toxicity and may be an early indication of ventricular dilatation and interstitial fibrosis.[1,18] Studies have demonstrated that patients with alcohol-induced atrial fibrillation are less likely to complain of palpitations are than patients with atrial fibrillation from another cause.[18]

Chronic cardiomyopathy requires a relatively constant high intake of alcohol over an extended period. Studies have demonstrated that alcohol has direct toxic effects on skeletal and cardiac muscle. Chronic cardiomyopathy requires the ingestion of at least 70 mL a day of absolute ethanol (seven shots of hard liquor or seven bottles of beer) for several months, but, more often, the exposure time is several years.[18]

Female alcoholics may present with symptoms of anxiety, increased fatigue, insomnia, depression, or irregular menses.[16] Geriatric alcoholics may be brought to the department by their families with complaints of altered mental status, daytime sleepiness, and irrational behavior.

TABLE 327.1. Clinical Presentations of Alcohol Abuse

CNS	**HEMATOLOGIC**
Inebriation	Myelosuppression
Seizures	Coagulopathies
Dementia	Microcytic anemia
Coma	Megaloblastic anemia
Wernicke-Korsakoff psychosis	Thrombocytopenia
Polyneuropathy	**INFECTIOUS**
CV	Pneumonia
Autonomic dysfunction	Meningitis
Alcoholic congestive myopathy	Endocarditis
"Holiday heart"	Cellulitis
GI	Bacteremia
Alcoholic hepatitis	Spontaneous bacterial peritonitis
Alcoholic cirrhosis	**METABOLIC**
Peptic ulcer disease	Ketoacidosis
GI bleeding	Electrolyte abnormalities
Pancreatitis	Vitamin deficiencies
Pancreatic pseudocyst	Hypothermia
Varices and hemorrhoids	**MUSCULOSKELETAL**
Ascites	Myopathies
Malabsorption and malnutrition	Gout
Cancers of the GI tract	Rhabdomyolysis
GU	**PULMONARY**
Uric acid nephropathy	Sleep apnea
Acute tubular necrosis	Chronic respiratory insufficiency
Hepatorenal syndrome	TB
BEHAVIORAL	
Anxiety, insomnia	
Irrational behaviors	
Polysubstance abuse	
Sexual dysfunction	

DIFFERENTIAL DIAGNOSIS

Because alcoholic patients have myriad nonspecific complaints, they represent a complex diagnostic challenge. The indigent or homeless alcoholic may present as a marked contrast to the affluent alcoholic. There is the danger of the emergency physician developing negative attitudes toward the acutely intoxicated patient due to prior poor interactions. It is important not to overlook potentially lethal or devastating pathology by negatively stereotyping alcoholic patients.

Ethanol use can have serious deleterious effects on virtually all organ systems and tissues.[9,11,18] The differential diagnosis can include hypoglycemia, sepsis, drug or other toxin exposures, carbon monoxide poisoning, Wernicke-Korsakoff syndrome, tumors, blunt trauma, meningitis, epidural or subdural hematoma, subarachnoid hemorrhage, dementia, and a host of others.[1,3,9,16,20] There is always the danger that an alcoholic may use other, potentially lethal alcohols in addition to or instead of ethanol. These could include isopropol alcohol, methanol, ethylene glycol, or other solvents or toxins.

EMERGENCY DEPARTMENT EVALUATION

The initial evaluation of the alcoholic is identical to the evaluation of any other potentially ill patient. Give immediate attention to the "ABCs" of airway, breathing, and circulation. Establish intravenous access, and protect or provide a definitive airway, if necessary. Obtain a full set of vital signs, including core temperature, and continuously monitor them. Patients with abnormal vital signs and cardiorespiratory or nonspecific constitutional symptoms should have continuous electrocardiogram (ECG) monitoring and a 12-lead ECG to evaluate for ischemia and arrhythmias (especially atrial arrhythmias). Patients should also be evaluated for hematologic and metabolic abnormalities.

Patients demonstrating altered mental status require a stat fingerstick blood glucose determination. The patient should be disrobed and carefully examined for signs of trauma. Serial examinations may reveal subtle injuries that were not identified on prior examinations. Signs of trauma may become apparent as the patient becomes less intoxicated. If trauma is suspected, full spinal immobilization may be required until the patient is sober and can cooperate with a thorough examination.[9]

An alcoholic presenting with respiratory complaints or altered mental status should also be evaluated for pneumonia and tuberculosis. Chest radiography may be required even if signs of infection are absent.[20] Complaints of vomiting or GI distress warrant an evaluation for gastritis, ulcers, varices, electrolyte abnormalities, and pancreatitis. Table 327.2 summarizes some of the important aspects of the laboratory and radiologic assessment. When alcoholism is suspected, obtaining liver function tests and determining red cell mean corpuscular volume may be supportive in making the diagnosis.

Because alcohol intoxication can mimic as well as mask disease and injury, a blood or breath ethanol level should be obtained to assess the contribution of alcohol in all patients with systemic complaints. The serum ethanol level can be expected to fall by 15 to 45 mg/dL/h, depending, in part, on individual variables and the timing of the ethanol ingestion, allowing the physician to estimate if or when the patient will be functionally (or legally) sober. In chronic alcoholics, sobriety typically occurs at blood levels of 100 to 300 mg/dL. Such levels may even be accompanied by signs and symptoms of withdrawal. Once meeting sobriety criteria, the patient may be able to be safely discharged. If the patient fails to improve within a reasonable time, or if there is a disparity between the patient's clinical examination and his or her blood alcohol level, further investigation is mandatory in order to exclude occult head trauma or another severe comorbidity.[3,4,9,11]

TABLE 327.2. Laboratory and Radiographic Evaluation

LABORATORY	RADIOLOGIC
CBC	Chest radiograph
Cell counts for evaluation of	Pneumonitis
marrow function	Aspiration
Indices for folate, iron,	Tuberculosis
pyridoxine, B_{12} deficiencies	Pneumothorax
Electrolytes/BUN/creatinine/glucose	Fractured ribs/trauma
Anion gap	Cardiac size
Hypoglycemia or hyperglycemia	Abdominal radiograph
Renal failure	Pancreatic calcifications
Electrolyte imbalance	Free air
Calcium/magnesium/phosphorus	Ileus
Hypocalcemia	Limb radiograph
Hypomagnesemia	Fractures
Hypophosphatemia	Dislocations
Hyperphosphatemia	Osteomyelitis
Coagulation profile	Foreign bodies
Hepatic insufficiency reflected in	CT scan
elevated PT and aPTT and	Extraaxial hemorrhage
abnormal liver function tests	Intracerebral
Arterial blood gas with co-oximeter	hemorrhage
Hypoxemia	Intracerebral contusion
Acid-base disturbances	Intraabdominal trauma
Carbon monoxide exposure	
Therapeutic drug monitoring	
Anticonvulsant levels	
ECG	
Arrhythmia	
Evidence of electrolyte	
abnormalities	
Ischemia	
Osborn waves (hypothermia)	
Urinalysis	
Crystalluria	
Myoglobinuria	
Hemoglobinuria	
Liver function tests	
GGT elevation	
AST elevation	
ALT elevation	

EMERGENCY DEPARTMENT MANAGEMENT

In the prehospital setting, the patient with altered mental status should receive 50 to 100 mL of 50% dextrose solution intravenously (or have a fingerstick blood sugar), 100 mg parenteral thiamine, and high-flow oxygen (or pulse oximetry). If opiate use is suspected, parenteral naloxone 0.1 mg to 2.0 mg should be given. Cervical spine and full spinal immobilization should be instituted if the possibility exists that there has been trauma to the head or neck or some other part of the body.

In the department, chronic alcoholics, particularly those who are malnourished, should also receive parenteral folate (1 mg) and magnesium (2 g), and be hydrated with an electrolyte solution containing glucose. Glucose is important, as many alcoholics have inadequate glycogen stores and will become hypoglycemic with stress.[10] Oxygenation should be followed and maintained. The patient's temperature should be followed serially and treated aggressively if abnormal.

Intoxicated patients frequently are uncooperative, belligerent, or violent. Judicious use of chemical and physical restraints may be necessary to protect emergency department staff and other patients from such patients. The risks associated with chemical or physical restraint are far outweighed by the benefit of controlled, thorough, serial examinations that can assess for subtle injury or pathology. Concomitant medical or surgical problems are treated through standard measures. Treatment of withdrawal (see Chapter 375) may also be required.

DISPOSITION

The decision to admit or discharge the patient depends on the nature and severity of comorbid illness or injury as well as the patient's ability to care for himself or herself. If the patient is admitted, the potential for ethanol withdrawal needs to be considered.

Legal precedents suggest that the patient can be discharged when no longer drunk, although no specific criteria exist to determine clinical sobriety. Blood ethanol levels that define "driving under the influence" vary from state to state and range from 50 to 120 mg/dL. Even if the alcoholic patient is observed until his or her blood level is below such limits, there remains the risk of iatrogenically induced withdrawal. In general, however, if a patient is functionally sober and demonstrates no signs of injury or comorbidity, he or she can be safely discharged. It is important, as always, to accurately document all aspects of the physical and neurologic examination on the patient's chart.

The inebriated patient who wishes to leave the emergency department against medical advice (either before or after evaluation and treatment) should be considered analogous to a patient with altered mental status who requests discharge. It is the emergency department's responsibility to protect patients who do not have the capacity to make competent decisions for themselves. Documentation of a blood ethanol level greater than the state's legal limit offers support for the emergency physician's decision that the patient was not competent and left against medical advice. Psychiatric consultation may also be helpful if there is any question concerning the patient's competency. When in doubt, it is prudent to err on the side of safety by restraining the patient in the emergency department.

Prior to discharge, the patient should be offered any available social assistance, and arrangements should be made for medical follow-up. Patients should be offered medical detoxification or an appropriate referral. All such arrangements and discussions should be carefully documented on the patient's chart. If the patient consents to medical detoxification, transfer him or her directly, if possible, to the detoxification facility from the emergency department.

COMMON PITFALLS

- Failure to consider that an altered mental status may be due to something other than intoxication
- Failure to obtain a full set of vital signs, including core temperature
- Failure to fully disrobe and examine an alcoholic patient
- Failure to evaluate fully an agitated, combative, and uncooperative patient
- Failure to obtain a stat fingerstick glucose or to empirically give 50% dextrose and thiamine to the alcoholic patient with altered mental status
- Failure to consider cervical spine trauma and to appropriately immobilize the intoxicated patient with evidence of head trauma
- Failure to appreciate that intoxication in an adolescent may be a suicide attempt
- Failure to consider carbon monoxide poisoning in the obtunded and homeless alcoholic
- Failure to reevaluate the patient frequently and to document this
- Failure to evaluate the alcoholic with constitutional symptoms for metabolic abnormalities and occult infection
- Failure to detain an inebriated patient in the emergency department until functionally sober
- Failure to restrain an intoxicated but ill or injured patient who is attempting to leave against medical advice
- Failure to involve social services and to advise or arrange for detoxification services

References

1. Alcohol: a problem at any age. *Emerg Med* 1982;30:22.
2. Brown C. Alcohol. *Ann Emerg Med* 1986,15:989.
3. Gentilello LM, Donovan DM, Dunn CW, et al. Alcohol interventions in trauma centers: current practice and future directions. *JAMA* 1995;274(13):1043–1048.
4. Gibb K. Serum alcohol levels, toxicology screens, and use of the breath alcohol analyzer. *Ann Emerg Med* 1986;15:349.
5. Groover JR. Alcoholic liver disease. *Emerg Med Clin North Am* 1990;8;4:887–901.
6. Health and Public Policy Committee, American College of Physicians. Chemical dependence. *Ann Intern Med* 1985;102:405.
7. Kamerow D, Pincus H, MacDonald D. Alcohol abuse, other drug abuse, and mental disorders in medical practice. *JAMA* 1986;255:2054.
8. Kitchens JM. Does this patient have an alcohol problem? *JAMA* 1994;273:1782.
9. Lieber CS. Medical disorders of alcoholism. *N Engl J Med* 1995;333:1058–1065.
10. Lieber CS. Microsomal ethanol-oxidizing system (MEOS): the first 30 years (1968–1998)—a review. *Alcohol Clin Exp Res* 1999;23:991–1007.
11. Martinez R. Alcoholism and society. *Emerg Med Clin North Am* 1990;8:904–909.
12. Morse RM, Flavin DK. The definition of alcoholism. *JAMA* 1992;268:1012.
13. O'Connor PG, Schottenfeld RS. Patients with alcohol problems. *N Engl J Med* 1998;338:592–602.
14. Ragland G. Electrolyte abnormalities in the alcoholic patient. *Emerg Med Clin North Am* 1990;8:761–773.
15. Romanski SA, McMahon MM. Metabolic acidosis and thiamine deficiency. *Mayo Clin Proc* 1999;74:259–263.
16. Ross SM, Chappel JN. Diagnostic dilemmas. Part II: substance use disorders—difficulties in diagnoses. *Psychiatr Clin North Am* 1998;21:803–828.
17. Samet J, Rollnick S, Barnes H. Beyond CAGE: a brief clinical approach after detection of substance abuse. *Arch Intern Med* 1996;156(20):2287–2293.
18. Urbano-Marquez A, Estruch R, Navarro-Lopez F, et al. The effects of alcoholism on skeletal and cardiac muscle. *N Engl J Med* 1989;320(7):409–415.
19. Whiteman PJ, Cerinich M, Hoffman RS, et al. Alcoholism in the emergency department: an epidemiologic study. *Vet Hum Toxicol* 1994;36:350(abst).
20. Wren KD, Larson S. The febrile alcoholic in the emergency department. *Am J Emerg Med* 1991;9:57.

APPENDIX

TABLE 327.A1. CAGE Questionnaire[a]

1. Have you felt you should **C**ut down on your drinking?
2. Have people **A**nnoyed you by criticizing your drinking?
3. Have you felt bad or **G**uilty about your drinking?
4. Have you ever had a drink first thing in the morning to steady your nerves or get rid of a hangover (**E**ye-opener)?

[a]Positive answers to two or more questions indicate a high likelihood of alcoholism.

TABLE 327.A2. TACE Questionnaire[a]

T	How many drinks does it **take** to get you high? (More than two suggests tolerance)
A	Have people **annoyed** you by criticizing your drinking?
C	Have you ever felt you ought to **cut down** on your drinking?
E	Have you ever had a drink first thing in the morning to steady your nerves? (**eye-opener**)

[a]Positive test (a score ≥1) identifies at-risk drinking in pregnant women.

TABLE 327.A3. Michigan Alcoholism Screening Test (MAST)

No.	Points	Question
1	2	* Do you feel you are a normal drinker?
2	2	Have you ever awakened the morning after some drinking the night before and found that you could not remember a part of the evening before?
3	1	* Does your spouse or parents ever worry or complain about your drinking?
4	2	Can you stop drinking without a struggle after one or two drinks?
5	1	* Do you ever feel bad about your drinking?
6	2	* Do friends or relatives think you are a normal drinker?
7	2	* Are you always able to stop drinking when you want to?
8	5	* Have you ever attended a meeting of Alcoholics Anonymous?
9	1	Have you gotten into fights when drinking?
10	2	* Has drinking ever created problems with you and your spouse?
11	2	Has your spouse or other family member ever gone to anyone for help about your drinking?
12	2	Have you ever lost friends or girlfriends/boyfriends because of your drinking?
13	2	* Have you ever gotten into trouble at work because of drinking?
14	2	Have you ever lost a job because of drinking?
15	2	* Have you ever neglected your obligations, your family, or your work for 2 or more days in a row because you were drinking?
16	1	Do you ever drink before noon?
17	2	Have you ever been told you have liver trouble? Cirrhosis?
18	2	Have you ever had delirium tremens (DTs), severe shaking, heard voices, or seen things that weren't there after heavy drinking?
19	5	* Have you ever gone to anyone for help about your drinking?
20	5	* Have you ever been in a hospital because of your drinking?
21	2	Have you ever been a patient in a psychiatric hospital or on a psychiatric ward of a general hospital where drinking was part of the problem?
22	2	Have you ever been seen at a psychiatric or mental health clinic or gone to a doctor, social worker, or clergyman for help with an emotional problem in which drinking had played a part?
23	2	* Have you ever been arrested, even for a few hours, because of drunk behavior?
24	2	* Have you ever been arrested for drunk driving or driving after drinking?

*These questions are included in the short form of the MAST

0–3 points Not alcohol-dependent

4–5 points Probably alcohol-dependent

>5 points Definitely alcohol-dependent

TABLE 327.A4. SADD Questionnaire

1. Do you find difficulty in getting the thought of a drink out of your mind?
2. Is getting drunk more important than your next meal?
3. Do you plan your day around when and where you can drink?
4. Do you drink in the morning, afternoon, and evening?
5. Do you drink for the effect of alcohol without caring what the drink is?
6. Do you drink as much as you want no matter what you are doing the next day?
7. Given that many problems might be caused by alcohol, do you still drink too much?
8. Do you know that you won't be able to stop drinking once you start?
9. Do you try to control your drinking by giving it up completely for days or weeks at a time?
10. The morning after a heavy drinking session, do you need your first drink to get yourself going?
11. The morning after a heavy drinking session, do you wake up with a definite shakiness in your hands?
12. After a heavy drinking session, do you wake up and retch or vomit?
13. The morning after a heavy drinking session, do you go out of your way to avoid people?
14. After a heavy drinking session, do you see frightening things that you later realize were imaginary?
15. Do you go drinking and the next day find that you have forgotten what happened the night before?

Questions are answered with never (0 points), sometimes (1 point), often (2 points), and nearly always (3 points). The point total is utilized to guide treatment.

From Gentilello LM, Donovan DM, Dunn CW, et al. Alcohol interventions in trauma centers: current practice and future directions. *JAMA* 1995;274(13):1043–1048.

TABLE 327.A5. The Ten-Item AUDIT Questionnaire

1. How often do you have a drink containing alcohol?
2. How many drinks do you have on a typical day when you are drinking?
3. How often do you have 6 or more drinks on one occasion?
4. How often during the last year have you found that you were not able to stop drinking once you had started?
5. How often during the last year have you failed to do what was normally expected from you because of drinking?
6. How often during the last year have you needed a first drink in the morning to get yourself going after a heavy drinking session?
7. How often during the last year have you had a feeling of guilt or remorse after drinking?
8. How often during the last year have you been unable to remember what happened the night before because you had been drinking?
9. Have you or someone else been injured as a result of your drinking?
10. Has a relative or friend or a doctor or other health worker been concerned about your drinking or suggested you cut down?

Questions are answered and scored on a 0- to 4-point scale, and the total is used as a guideline for therapy.

From Saunder JB, Aasland OG, Babor TF, et al. Development of the Alcohol Use Disorders Identification Test (AUDIT): WHO Collaborative Project on Early Detection of Persons with Harmful Alcohol Consumption-II, 1194. *Addiction* 1993;88:791–804.

CHAPTER 328

Complications of Injection Drug Use

James A. Feldman and Susan S. Fish

An estimated 1.1 to 1.8 million people in the United States currently use nonprescribed drugs by intravenous, subcutaneous, and other routes of injection, and another 2.5 million have self-injected drugs at least once. The lifestyle associated with drug use increases the risk of trauma, tuberculosis, and sexually transmitted diseases. Intravenous drug use (IDU) brings with it the risk of complications directly related to the local or systemic effects of the substances injected, the use of nonsterile methods of injection, and other aspects of injection practices (Table 328.1).

A history of IDU should be routinely obtained in all patients and considered carefully in medical decision making. While patients with IDU may accurately identify complications of injection drug use, they are *unlikely* to seek medical care for these complications. Hence, such patients should be presumed to have a serious medical condition until proven otherwise.

Cutaneous and superficial soft-tissue infections, particularly abscess formation at the site of injection, are common reasons for IDU patients to seek emergency care. The bacteriology of abscesses in IDU patients is more likely to be mixed aerobic–anaerobic infections than in non-IDU patients.[16] Although *Staphylococcus aureus* is the most common organism (36% to 50%), flora of the oropharynx are often isolated. Bacteremia is infrequent, even with extensive cutaneous infections, but 19% had positive blood cultures in a recent case series.[16] Cutaneous abscesses of the neck may lead to respiratory complications such as airway obstruction, laryngeal edema, and vocal cord paralysis.[12]

Clostridial toxin-mediated diseases and tetanus have been identified in chronic injection drug users. Wound botulism has been increasingly reported since 1982, with 35 cases identified in California during a recent 26-month study period.[14] IDU-related tetanus has been increasingly reported. Of the 67 cases of tetanus reported in California from 1987 through 1997, 40% occurred in IDU patients.[17] Skin lesions or small abscesses that appear innocuous may harbor *C. botulinum* or *C. tetani*. Injection drug users are also at risk for more serious and deeper soft-tissue infections, including necrotizing fasciitis (see Chapter 181).

Broken needles at the site of intravenous injection are usually an incidental finding noted on radiograph. Such retained needle fragments rarely embolize centrally. However, pericarditis with pericardial effusion secondary to central migration has been reported.[9]

Vascular complications related to IDU include unintentional intraarterial injection, with resultant vasospasm or thrombosis and limb ischemia; venous and arterial pseudoaneurysm formation; development of infected hematoma; and venous thrombosis and septic thrombophlebitis. Mycotic aneurysms involving central arteries, such as the hepatic, mesenteric, cerebral, and pulmonary arteries, as well as large vessel occlusive emboli may occur in the context of endocarditis and should be considered in the evaluation and treatment of patients with suspected endocarditis (see Chapter 140). The bacteriology of both arterial and venous mycotic aneurysm is polymicrobial in up to 40% of cases. *S. aureus,* frequently beta-lactam–resistant, is often cultured from the wound or blood. Anaerobic organisms have been reported in up to 20% of some series.

TABLE 328.1. Medical Complications of Injection Drug Use by Organ System

CUTANEOUS
Needle foreign body
Abscess
Necrotizing fasciitis
Gas gangrene
Cellulitis
Pyomyositis
VASCULAR
Septic phlebitis
Thrombophlebitis
Pseudoaneurysm
Infected hematoma
Intraarterial injection
MUSCULOSKELETAL
Vertebral osteomyelitis
Septic arthritis
Compartment syndrome
PULMONARY
Pneumothorax
Hemothorax
Talcosis
Septic pulmonary embolus
Pneumonia
NEUROLOGIC
Peripheral nervous system
Puncture injuries
Compression injuries
Plexitis/plexopathy
Central nervous system
Infections
Meningitis
Abscesses: cerebral, epidural, spinal
Mycotic aneurysm
Transient ischemic attacks
Mucormycosis
Stroke
INTERNAL ORGANS
Heart
Endocarditis
Myocardial infarction, ischemia
Liver
Hepatitis
Spleen
Abscess
Kidney
Nephrotic syndrome
Glomerulonephritis
Abscess
Infarct
Intestine
Mesenteric ischemia, infarction
GENERAL/OTHER
Cotton fever
Septicemia
HIV infection
Tetanus
Wound botulism
Endophthalmitis
Malaria

Pulmonary complications from IDU can result from mechanical injury to the lung during injection. "Pocket shooting," or injection into the supraclavicular fossa to access the jugular, subclavian, or brachiocephalic veins, often leads to pneumothorax, hemothorax, hydropneumothorax, or pyopneumothorax. In one review of 525 cases of pneumothorax, 20% were related to IDU. Of these, 19% were complete collapse or tension pneumothorax (two were bilateral), 43% were large, 32% moderate or small, and 6% had only an apical cap.[4]

Injection of solubilized tablets and capsules can lead to pulmonary dysfunction from injected particulate matter that deposits in the lung. Tablets are usually crushed, dissolved in water or other liquid, sometimes heated. Then the solution is drawn up into a syringe either directly or filtered through cotton. The fillers in the tablet consist usually of talc, cornstarch, or cellulose. Talc is well known to induce granulomas in and around the arterioles and capillaries of the lung, and it can also deposit in retinal vessels; this condition is referred to as "talcosis."[13] Both restrictive and obstructive pulmonary dysfunction can be seen, as well as pulmonary hypertension and cor pulmonale. Although cornstarch is not associated with granuloma formation, the resultant bland pulmonary thromboses can lead to pulmonary hypertension.

Osteomyelitis and septic arthritis secondary to IDU may result from direct contamination or hematogenous spread. Vertebral osteomyelitis is the most common form of skeletal infection in IDU patients.[11] The sites of vertebral involvement reported are lumbar (54%), cervical (27%) and thoracic (4%). The increased frequency of cervical involvement noted in IDU patients is an important variation in the distribution of vertebral osteomyelitis, compared with the general population.

The sacroiliac, sternoclavicular, costochondral, and pubic symphysis synchondroses are frequent sites of septic arthritis in IDU patients. Although these axial fibrocartilaginous joints are the most common sites of septic arthritis in IDU patients,[1] other joints, including the knees, hips, and shoulders, may be involved. While *Pseudomonas aeruginosa* and *Serratia marcescens,* in the past, had been the most common cause of osteoarticular infections, *S. aureus* has more recently replaced gram-negative bacilli and *Candida* as the primary cause of these infections.[3]

Serious central and peripheral nervous system complications have been well described in the IDU population. These patients are at increased risk of central nervous system (CNS) infections, including fungal and bacterial meningitis, cerebritis, and spinal, epidural, and brain abscesses.[6] *Candida* meningitis is usually associated with *Candida* endocarditis.[10] Indolent CNS aspergillosis, cerebral mucormycosis, and anterior spinal artery syndrome with subsequent paraplegia have been reported. A syndrome of cerebral mucormycosis has been well described in IDU patients who were seronegative for the human immunodeficiency virus (HIV).[7] Fungal endophthalmitis, caused by such organisms as *Aspergillus* and *Fusarium,* has been described in patients with IDU as the only identified risk factor for these uncommon infections.[19] Peripheral nerve injuries may result from needle-induced trauma, extrinsic compression, and direct toxic or hypersensitivity reactions to injected materials.

Systemic infections may result from exposure to skin contaminants, contaminated apparatus, contaminated injection mixture, and blood-borne pathogens transmitted by the practice of needle sharing. HIV and hepatitis B, C, and delta infections are discussed in other chapters. Infection with the HTLV virus (types I and II) is associated with injection drug use.[5] Hepatitis GB virus type C (HGBV-C), an important cause of fulminant non–A-E hepatitis, is also more commonly identified in IDU patients.[18] The lifetime seroconversion rate for hepatitis B in IDU patients is 80% to 90%, and the incidence of bacterial endocarditis is 5%.[2] A number of uncommon infections have also been described. A syndrome of disseminated candidiasis, characterized by scalp, ocular, and osteoarticular involvement, was attributed to the use of lemon juice in the preparation of brown heroin for injection.[3] Malaria, both falciparum and vivax, endophthalmitis, and tick-borne relapsing fever have been reported.

In IDU patients presenting with fever, 64% had readily identifiable major illnesses such as pneumonia, cellulitis, or endocarditis; another 4% of patients had major illnesses that were not clinically apparent on initial evaluation.[15] "Cotton fever," an acute but self-limited pyrogenic reaction induced by intravenous injection of foreign material from cotton balls used to filter injected solution, may mimic sepsis. The history, physical examination, and laboratory testing were not able to reliably differentiate cotton fever or other minor conditions from more serious causes of fever.

CLINICAL PRESENTATION

Patients with superficial abscesses complain of localized pain. Fever and systemic complaints may also be present. The classic signs and symptoms of warmth, redness, tenderness, swelling, and fluctuance may be absent in IDU patients. As many as 25% of patients with cutaneous abscesses do not have fluctuance.

Patients with broken needle fragments at injection sites may be asymptomatic or have localized complaints of pain due to the needle itself or to infectious complications. Patients may present with concerns about the risks of a retained needle fragment. They may also be unaware of its presence or fail to mention it unless asked.

Inadvertent intraarterial injection causes immediate severe pain, hyperemia, numbness, weakness, distal swelling, cyanosis, and motor deficit and, often, sensory abnormalities. Distal ischemia may progress to gangrene, myonecrosis, and associated complications. The use of crushed oral medications and the lower extremity as a site of injection appears to be associated with more severe complications.

Patients with arterial mycotic aneurysms usually present with an indurated mass, local pain, and swelling. The mass is pulsatile in approximately 50%, and a bruit is often heard over the swelling.[20] Fever and leukocytosis are common, but bleeding, although occasionally massive, is usually intermittent, minor, or absent. Claudication, paresthesias, or compression neuropathy can occur. Signs and symptoms of distal embolic phenomenon, including cutaneous purpura, may be present and may precede systemic manifestations. While upper and lower extremity arteries are most commonly involved, mycotic aneurysms of the subclavian and carotid arteries have been reported following attempted central venous injections.

Venous pseudoaneurysms are most commonly noted in the groin. Pain, swelling, and purulent drainage may be noted. Some patients may appear clinically septic, with minimal localized complaints. In these patients, either pulmonary complaints or symptoms referable to sites of metastatic septic involvement may be more prominent.

Patients with pneumothorax typically present with a history of recent neck injection, dyspnea, and pleuritic chest pain.[4] Patients with particulate-induced pulmonary dysfunction frequently complain of progressive dyspnea. Chest x-ray can show a micronodular pattern; over time, the pattern changes to show large homogenous opacities, usually in the perihilar regions and upper lobes.[13] Retinoscopy can show talc depositions (small, whitish, glistening dots) and may have a higher diagnostic yield than either chest x-ray or pulmonary function tests.

Patients with skeletal infections often present with localized pain and tenderness. Almost 20% of patients with vertebral osteomyelitis related to IDU have had pain for more than 3 months at the time of diagnosis. About 15% report a history of minor blunt back trauma, such as a fall or kick, a factor that may contribute to delayed diagnosis. Fever is usually absent or of low grade. Neurologic signs and symptoms occur infrequently (less than 15%) and are usually transient. Routine laboratory studies are usually normal. The erythrocyte sedimentation rate (ESR) usually is elevated but can be normal. Plain x-rays may demonstrate disc space narrowing (82%) or paravertebral shadows, suggesting abscess (12%), but magnetic resonance imaging (MRI) is diagnostic.

Patients with septic arthritis associated with IDU are similar in presentation to other patients with septic arthritis, except for the prominence of fibrocartilaginous joint involvement. Local signs of inflammation as well as fever, leukocytosis, and elevated ESR are usually noted. Asymptomatic HIV infection has been reported in one-third of IDU patients with septic arthritis.[1]

Patients with wound botulism usually present with neurologic complaints such as cranial palsies or descending symmetrical paralysis. Atypical signs, including asymmetric or unilateral cranial nerve weakness and peripheral motor weakness, may be present.[8] Patients with atypical presentations and false-positive edrophonium tests have been misdiagnosed with Eaton-Lambert syndrome and myasthenia gravis, resulting in prolonged delays in appropriate therapy.

Patients with tetanus present with increased muscle tone, spasm or trismus. Patients with fungal endophthalmitis usually present with severe visual loss and pain, which develop rapidly in the affected eye.[19] Patients with cerebral mucormycosis usually have headache, fever, and rapidly developing cranial nerve and motor deficits. Basal ganglia lesions on computed tomography (CT) scan should suggest this diagnosis. Patients with cotton fever may complain of dyspnea, palpitations, headache, and rigors.

Patients who inject drugs are also at risk for systemic drug or drug-contaminant toxicity (see Chapters 326, 360, and 369), withdrawal syndromes (see Chapter 375), and CNS infections (see Chapter 184).

DIFFERENTIAL DIAGNOSIS

The most important requirement for developing an appropriate differential diagnosis is obtaining the history of IDU. Biases can easily enter into the physician's decision to obtain this information. It may be necessary to consider the possibility of IDU, even if denied by the patient. In such cases, a urine screening test for drugs of abuse may be helpful. Unless the history of IDU is routinely obtained or considered, conditions such as vertebral osteomyelitis and epidural abscess may not be considered in the differential diagnosis of complaints such as back pain. The IDU patient who develops a fever or flulike symptoms is much more likely to have an infection requiring hospital admission than is a non-IDU patient who presents with similar complaints. It is very important to carefully consider clinical syndromes that are well described in patients with IDU when one is evaluating such patients.

EMERGENCY DEPARTMENT EVALUATION

The possibility of IDU, recent *or* remote, should be included in the standard "screening history." A nonthreatening question such as, "Do you smoke cigarettes, or use alcohol or other drugs?" should be routinely asked of all patients. Patients with IDU should be asked about the specifics of drug type, amount, needle sharing, preparation of materials (licking the needle, for example), and whether they have a history of hepatitis, endocarditis, HIV, pain at injection sites, recent fever, and nonprescribed antibiotic self-treatment.

The physical examination of a patient with recognized IDU should include a careful review of vital signs, particularly the temperature (tympanic or rectal). Examination of the skin for signs of endocarditis, jaundice, infection at injection sites, and markers of HIV infection, such as oral thrush, should be performed in addition to a complaint-oriented examination. Evidence of opiate withdrawal, such as diaphoresis, lacrimation, yawning, pupillary dilation, and piloerection, should also be sought.

Routine laboratory tests are of limited use. Drug screens provide little information that will affect decisions, except possibly to suggest drug use when it is denied. Although the complete blood count (CBC) and ESR lack sufficient sensitivity and specificity to guide disposition decisions, if infection is suspected or present, a very high or low white blood cell count might prompt admission, even for a simple abscess. The use of ultrasonography to identify occult abscesses that require drainage is an area of active research.

Patients with significant cutaneous abscesses or associated systemic complaints should have a culture of the abscess material. A radiograph should be routinely considered in patients with cutaneous complaints of pain and tenderness at injection sites in order to exclude retained needle foreign bodies as well as to identify gas-forming infections.

In IDU patients with fever, three sets of blood cultures, chest radiograph, urinalysis, and urine culture should be obtained. Patients with respiratory complaints should have a chest radiograph and oxygen saturation. Those with joint pain and effusion should have two sets of blood cultures and aspiration, Gram stain, and culture of affected joints. Septic synchondroses may be safely aspirated in the emergency department and should be evaluated similarly. Ultrasound may identify a perivascular abscess but is not very sensitive for detecting pseudoaneurysms. While digital subtraction angiography may be a useful diagnostic modality, color-flow duplex scans may be the diagnostic study of choice.[20] Arteriography may be necessary to confirm the diagnosis.

Two sets of blood cultures and an MRI should be obtained for suspected vertebral osteomyelitis or epidural abscess. A patient with IDU and complaints that suggest a CNS process (headache, weakness, ataxia) will require a detailed neurologic examination, CT scan or MRI, and a lumbar puncture in order to identify direct vascular complications of IDU use, opportunistic CNS infections, or malignancy (related or unrelated to HIV infection). Patients with complaints of visual loss will require a complete eye examination, usually dilation with indirect funduscopy.

EMERGENCY DEPARTMENT MANAGEMENT

Localized cutaneous abscesses without vascular involvement may be managed with routine incision and drainage. If there is a possibility of vascular involvement, needle aspiration should be performed first. Patients with localized infections involving the neck, groin, or vascular structures should be evaluated by a surgeon.

While antibiotics are not routinely required, patients with HIV infection or neutropenia may require parenteral antibiotics and hospitalization. Initial antibiotic therapy should include a penicillinase-resistant synthetic penicillin such as oxacillin. An antipseudomonal aminoglycoside (APAG) such as gentamicin should also be given if enteric organisms or *Pseudomonas* has been identified as part of the "IDU" flora.

In areas with methicillin-resistant *S. aureus*, vancomycin should be used until culture results are available. Extensive extremity infections should be evaluated by a surgeon and explored in the operating room, as inadequate drainage may prolong hospitalization. The treatment of septic thrombophlebitis involves antibiotic therapy, as described previously, as well as surgical consultation. Patients with gas-forming infections require immediate operative intervention and combination antibiotic therapy with clindamycin, high-dose penicillin G (cephalothin, if penicillin allergic), and an APAG (see Chapter 181).

In general, removal of fractured needle fragments should not be attempted by emergency physicians. Even if palpable, finding them may be difficult, important neurovascular structures nearby may be injured, and migration may occur despite the use of a proximal tourniquet. All of these reasons argue for surgical consultation and removal in the operating room.[9]

When associated with infection or vascular injury, needle fragments require urgent removal. Patients with retained needle foreign bodies without these complications may be given appropriate discharge instructions and referral to a surgeon for elective removal.

Patients with signs and symptoms of intraarterial injection require aggressive management because of the potential for distal limb ischemia. Treatment should include antibiotics and anticoagulation with heparin. Consultation with a general or vascular surgeon is essential. Measurement of extremity compartment pressures should be considered. Some authors suggest the use of intravenous dextran 40 (20 mL/h) and dexamethasone (4 mg every 6 hours) or the intraarterial injection of an arterial vasodilator such as papaverine (40 to 60 mg) or phentolamine (2 mg). Favorable results have been reported from the use of Iloprost, a prostacyclin analogue, and intraarterial thrombolysis.[20]

Patients with pseudoaneurysms require blood cultures, preoperative laboratory testing, including blood typing, and consultation with a general or vascular surgeon. Hospitalization is usually indicated. Hemorrhage control with direct pressure may be required. Local drainage should not be attempted in the emergency department, as life-threatening hemorrhage may result.

The management of pneumothorax is discussed in Chapters 102 and 149. Pulmonary dysfunction from other causes is treated by supportive measures.

Vertebral osteomyelitis and septic arthritis should be treated with vancomycin and an APAG. Consultation with an orthopedic surgeon, as well as an infectious disease specialist, should be obtained for patients with or suspected of having these complications.

Patients with cotton fever require only supportive care. This illness usually resolves within 12 to 24 hours. However, given the possibility that a serious medical condition is the etiology of fever, inpatient observation is recommended until the patient is well and the results of blood cultures are known.

DISPOSITION

Patients with cutaneous abscesses who are otherwise asymptomatic and healthy may be discharged with appropriate instructions and referral for follow-up in 24 to 48 hours. The ability of a patient to comply with outpatient therapy and follow-up should be considered. Most patients with other infectious complications require admission. Many "rule-out" diagnoses, including endocarditis, sepsis, and meningitis, will also require admission for observation pending culture results. Concomitant HIV infection may also modify the decision to admit or discharge a patient with IDU and a specific complaint.

Patients should also be educated about secondary prevention and "harm reduction," practices that have been shown to reduce the morbidity and mortality from injection drug use. These should be referred for substance abuse treatment and, if available, to needle-exchange programs. Patients who continue to use injection drugs may benefit from teaching practices, such as antiseptic skin preparation prior to injection, the use of bleach for cleaning needles and syringes, and the use condoms to prevent sexually transmitted disease.

COMMON PITFALLS

- Failure to ask about IDU in all adolescent and adult patients
- Allowing a judgmental attitude toward patients who use injection drugs to interfere with a careful medical evaluation
- Labeling patients with IDU as "pain medication seekers" without performing a careful history and physical examination
- Failure to consider infectious etiologies in the differential diagnosis of musculoskeletal complaints in IDU patients
- Failure to appreciate that patients with vertebral infections may give a history of minor trauma and have a normal neurologic examination
- Attributing fever in an IDU to a trivial illness or to cotton fever
- Attempting to drain a soft-tissue mass in proximity to a major blood vessel. Incising a mycotic aneurysm or pseudoaneurysm that has been misdiagnosed as an abscess can lead to uncontrollable hemorrhage.
- Failure to consider the possibility of arterial injection, compartment syndrome, deep-space infection, or nerve injury in patients with limb complaints
- Attempting to remove an asymptomatic needle fragment in an anatomically sensitive area
- Failure to obtain a radiograph of sites of localized infection to identify the presence of foreign bodies or gas
- Failure to appreciated that extensive abscesses cannot be adequately drained in the emergency department

References

1. Brancos MA, Peris P, Miro JM, et al. Septic arthritis in heroin addicts. *Semin Arthritis Rheum* 1991;21:81–87.
2. Brettle RP. Infection and injection drug use. *J Infect* 1992;25:121–131.
3. Cherubin CE, Sapira JD. The medical complications of drug addiction and the medical assessment of the intravenous drug user: 25 years later [see comments]. *Ann Intern Med* 1993;119:1017–1028.
4. Douglass RE, Levison MA. Pneumothorax in drug abusers. An urban epidemic? *Am Surg* 1986;52:377–380.
5. Garfein RS, Vlahov D, Galai N, et al. Viral infections in short-term injection drug users: the prevalence of the hepatitis C, hepatitis B, human immunodeficiency, and human T-lymphotropic viruses. *Am J Publ Health* 1996;86:655–661.
6. Haverkos H, Lange W. Serious infections other than human immunodeficiency virus among intravenous drug abusers. *J Infect Dis* 1990;161:894.
7. Hopkins RJ, Rothman M, Fiore A, et al. Cerebral mucormycosis associated with intravenous drug use: three case reports and review [see comments]. *Clin Infect Dis* 1994;19:1133–1137.
8. Horowitz BZ, Swensen E, Marquardt K. Wound botulism associated with black tar heroin. *JAMA* 1998;280:1479–1480.
9. Kulaylat MN, Barakat N, Stephan RN, et al. Embolization of illicit needle fragments. *J Emerg Med* 1993;11:403–408.
10. Leen C, Groux N, Elliot J. Fungal infections in drug users. *J Antimicrob Chemother* 1991;28:A83.
11. Lohr KM. Rheumatic manifestations of diseases associated with substance abuse. *Semin Arthritis Rheum* 1987;17:90–111.
12. Myers EM, Kirkland LS Jr, Mickey R. The head and neck sequelae of cervical intravenous drug abuse. *Laryngoscope* 1988;98:213–218.
13. Pare JP, Cote G, Fraser RS. Long-term follow-up of drug abusers with intravenous talcosis. *Am Rev Respir Dis* 1989;139:233–241.
14. Passaro DJ, Werner SB, McGee J, et al. Wound botulism associated with black tar heroin among injecting drug users. *JAMA* 1998;279:859–863.

15. Samet JH, Shevitz A, Fowle J, et al. Hospitalization decision in febrile intravenous drug users. *Am J Med* 1990;89:53–57.
16. Summanen PH, Talan DA, Strong C, et al. Bacteriology of skin and soft-tissue infections: comparison of infections in intravenous drug users and individuals with no history of intravenous drug use. *Clin Infect Dis* 1995;20[Suppl 2]:S279–S282.
17. Talan DA, Moran GJ. Tetanus among injecting-drug users—California, 1997. *Ann Emerg Med* 1998;32:385–386.
18. Thomas DL, Nakatsuji Y, Shih JW, et al. Persistence and clinical significance of hepatitis G virus infections in injecting drug users. *J Infect Dis* 1997;176:586–592.
19. Weishaar PD, Flynn HW Jr, Murray TG, et al. Endogenous *Aspergillus* endophthalmitis. Clinical features and treatment outcomes. *Ophthalmology* 1998;105:57–65.
20. Woodburn KR, Murie JA. Vascular complications of injecting drug misuse. *Br J Surg* 1996;83:1329–1334.

CHAPTER 329

Complications of Parenteral Drug Therapy

Robert P. Ferm

Parenteral drug administration may be accomplished by subcutaneous (SC), intramuscular (IM), intravenous (IV), intradermal (ID), intraosseous (IO), intraarterial (IA), intrathecal (IT), or intracardiac (IC) injection. Parenteral routes are used when greater efficacy, more rapid effect, and the ability to more accurately titrate the dose are desired. For some agents, a parenteral route is essential for drug effect; for others, oral formulations may be unavailable. There are unique risks associated with the inherently invasive nature of parenteral routes, but with proper techniques and precautions, these risks can be minimized.

Adverse effects due to parenteral drug administration can be divided into local and systemic complications (Table 329.1). Reactions uniquely associated with parenteral drug administration include localized pain, inflammation, and infection; infiltration or extravasation; nerve injury; vascular injury; inadvertent IV or IA administration; fluid and electrolyte overload; and diluent toxicity. The annual cost associated with complications of IV drug therapy alone was estimated at greater than $112 million.[6]

TABLE 329.1. Adverse Effects of Parenteral Drug Administration

LOCAL
Pain (all routes)
Infiltration/extravasation (IV)
Phlebitis/thrombosis/thrombophlebitis (IV)
Cellulitis (all routes)
Abscess (all routes)
Granuloma (IM, SQ)
Allergic (all routes)
Nerve injury (all routes)
Vascular injury (all routes)
Ischemia (all routes)
Inadvertent IV injection (IM, SQ)
Inadvertent IA injection (all routes)
Tissue irritation/necrosis (all routes)
SYSTEMIC
Noninfectious febrile reactions (all routes)
Sepsis (all routes)
Anaphylaxis (all routes)
Fluid overload (IV)
Diluent toxicity (IV)

CLINICAL PRESENTATION

Unless the agent is given through an indwelling catheter, patients experience some pain regardless of the route of injection. Drugs notorious for causing pain on SC or IM injection include ceftriaxone, local anesthetics, benzodiazepines, glucagon, dimercaprol or British Anti-Lewisite (BAL), and calcium and magnesium salts. Those typically causing pain on IV administration include potassium, calcium, and magnesium salts, phenytoin (because of its high pH), glucagon (because of phenol diluent), chemotherapeutic agents, adenosine, hypertonic solutions, ethanol, and propofol. Local allergic reactions and histamine release may result from the injection of some drugs, particularly morphine and protamine. Manifestations include pruritus, urticarial eruptions, localized swelling (sometimes painful), and erythema over the course of veins or lymphatics.

The earliest sign of infusion phlebitis, tenderness proximal to the infusion cannula, is followed by redness, warmth, pain, edema, and induration along the course of the vein.[19] Similar localized signs accompany tissue inflammation caused by IM or SC injections and infections secondary to any route of administration. Venous thrombosis may complicate inflammation or infection. Manifestations include a tender, palpable thrombosed cord and distal edema.

Signs and symptoms of venous extravasation include immediate or delayed pain, swelling, induration, erythema or pallor, warmth or coolness, and blistering or frank necrosis. Findings are more diffuse than with phlebitis. Underlying mechanisms include hypertonic tissue injury from hyperosmolar solutions (e.g., 50% dextrose, sodium bicarbonate, and hyperalimentation preparations), ischemia from vasoconstrictors (e.g., epinephrine, dopamine, other catecholamines, and vasopressin), and direct cellular toxicity from vesicant drugs (e.g., doxorubicin, dactinomycin, and other antineoplastic agents), highly alkaline or acidic preparations (e.g., phenytoin), or irritant vehicles (e.g., propylene glycol, phenol, and ethanol).[8] Osteomyelitis may also result from IO infusions when used for protracted periods or for the administration of hypertonic fluids.

Injection injury to a nerve most typically results in sudden, immediate onset of severe pain radiating in the distribution of the affected nerve along with a neuropathy. Motor dysfunction is often more severe than sensory deficits. Less commonly, patients may experience instantaneous or delayed neuropathy without immediate pain. Inadvertent injury to peripheral nerves has been described from several different procedures involving a number of different peripheral nerves,[4,7,11,18] but most commonly involves sciatic nerve injury from intragluteal IM injections. Inadvertent intraneural (as opposed to perineural) injection with both direct physical and chemical injury is the likely mechanism of nerve damage.

The inadvertent IV administration of drugs intended for IM or SC injection may lead to systemic effects as well as vascular injury. Systemic reactions may include pulmonary, cardiovascular, or central nervous system (CNS) toxicity due to the drug (e.g., seizures or cardiovascular collapse associated with the intravascular injection of local anesthetics) or vehicle (discussion follows).

Accidental IA injection may lead to severe pain, pallor followed by patchy blue discoloration, and infarction or gangrene of tissue supplied by the involved vessel. If retrograde flow occurs, more proximal effects may be noted. Serious injuries have been reported following IA infusion of a wide variety of agents, including antibiotics (e.g., penicillin), antiinflammatory drugs, sedatives and tranquilizers (e.g., barbiturates, phenothiazines, benzodiazepines), anticonvulsants (e.g., phenytoin), and hyperalimentation solution.[3,12–14,17]

Fluid and electrolyte overload may result from infusions of drugs given in large volumes (e.g., cisplatinum, EDTA, vancomycin) or with large salt loads (e.g., sodium and potassium salts of antibiotics).

Systemic toxicity may also be due to the vehicle or solvent in which the drug is delivered. Propylene glycol has been linked to CNS depression, seizures, hypotension, cardiac dysrhythmias, hemolysis, and lactic acidosis. Toxicity has been associated with administration of phenytoin, nitroglycerin, etomidate, and other medications at excessive rates.[1] Table 329.2 lists some drugs containing propylene glycol. Alcohol intoxication has resulted from excessive coadministration of ethanol with nitroglycerin infusions.

DIFFERENTIAL DIAGNOSIS

A history of parenteral drug administration preceding the onset of symptoms suggests the diagnosis. With such a history, the diagnosis is usually straightforward. The differential diagnosis of extravasation injuries and phlebitis includes cellulitis, trauma, thermal or topical chemical burn, and catheter breakage or embolization. The differential diagnosis for injection injury to peripheral nerves may include traumatic neuropraxia, cerebrovascular accident, or mechanical nerve root impingement, such as by compartment and impingement syndromes and vertebral disc herniation. Patients with ischemic injuries usually give a history of extravasation of vasopressor agents or the accidental discharge of an autoinjection device (e.g., EpiPen). In the absence of such a history, snake and insect bites, Raynaud's phenomenon, mechanical trauma, and topical chemical injury should be considered.

TABLE 329.2. Common Parenteral Drugs Containing Propylene Glycol (Trade Name/Generic Name)

Amidate/etomidate
Apresoline/hydralazine
Bactrim/trimethoprim–sulfamethoxazole
Berocca PN/multivitamins
Brevibloc/esmolol
Dilantin/phenytoin
Dramamine/dimenhydrinate
Dramocen/dimenhydrinate
Konakion/phytonadione
Lanoxin/digoxin
Lanoxin Pediatric/digoxin
Librium/chlordiazepoxide
Loxitane/loxapine
Luminal sodium/phenobarbital
MVC9 Plus/multivitamins
MVI-12/multivitamins
Nitro-BID/nitroglycerin
Nembutal/pentobarbital
Nitrostat/nitroglycerin
Nitroglycerin
Pentobarbital sodium
Phenobarbital sodium
Phenytoin sodium
Septra/trimethoprim–sulfamethoxazole
Tridil/nitroglycerin
Valium/diazepam

EMERGENCY DEPARTMENT EVALUATION

The history should include the time of injection, the identity and amount of drug or other fluid involved, and the time of onset, nature, and progression of symptoms. For local complications, the physical examination should focus on the skin and neurovascular function of the involved extremity. A complete blood count and blood cultures may be helpful if infection is suspected. If there is significant swelling or if neurovascular impairment is noted, ultrasound and compartment pressure measurement may be necessary to evaluate for deep venous thrombosis and compartment syndrome. If catheter breakage or embolization is suspected, a radiograph should be obtained, because most catheters are radiopaque. Nerve conduction studies may be indicated to assess the extent of dysfunction following injection injuries to nerves. For systemic reactions, evaluation should focus on cardiovascular, pulmonary, and neurologic function. Patients with an abnormal pulse or blood pressure and those with altered mental status or cardiopulmonary signs and symptoms should have cardiac monitoring and oxygen saturation measurement. Depending on the agent involved and the severity of the reaction, drug, electrolyte, and diluent levels, as well as routine laboratory testing, may be indicated.

EMERGENCY DEPARTMENT MANAGEMENT

Although not strictly a management issue, one of the most important aspects of parenteral drug therapy is the prevention of complications. Attention to sterile technique is necessary regardless of the route of administration. Proper IV access can be ensured by noting blood return on aspiration by a syringe or lowering the IV set below the access site. Pulsatile blood return and the need to use high pressure for infusion indicate inadvertent artery cannulation.

Proper placement can be confirmed by infusing 10 mL of saline before giving the drug, then observing for ease of fluid administration and absence of tissue expansion. The pain caused by the IV administration of some drugs can be prevented by first giving lidocaine (1 mL of a 1% solution). Complications can be prevented by not using a certain extremity in some situations. For instance, an extremity with an arteriovenous hemodialysis fistula or a fracture should not be used; nor should an extremity on the same side as a previous radical mastectomy or inguinal or axillary node surgery.

Risk of neurovascular injury secondary to IM injection can be reduced by careful attention to anatomic landmarks. Children under age 3 years should receive injections in the vastus lateralis muscle of the thigh or the ventrogluteal areas, rather than the dorsogluteal area of the buttock. The chance of inadvertent IV or IA injection can be minimized by routinely aspirating and noting the absence of blood return before giving an IM injection. SC or IM epinephrine injections should be avoided in areas perfused by end arteries ("fingers, nose, penis, toes, and ears"). It may be impossible to prevent systemic complications without changing to an alternate therapy, but complications can be anticipated and preemptively monitored. Avoiding excessive doses or rates of administration reduces the risk. Slowing the rate of infusion alleviates propylene glycol toxicity.

Superficial venous thrombosis without evidence of infection may be treated with warm, moist packs; elevation; and aspirin or other nonsteroidal antiinflammatories. Superficial thrombophlebitis is similarly managed with analgesia and rest of the involved limb. Antibiotics are given if infection is suspected. A more aggressive approach is advised for patients with superficial thrombophlebitis that involves a large segment of the superficial saphenous vein, particularly when it extends proximal to the knee. Such patients should receive superficial venous ligation or anticoagulation, as given to patients with a deep venous thrombosis. The treatment of deep venous thrombosis is discussed in Chapter 139.

The treatment of extravasation includes immediate cessation of the infusion and elevation of the affected area, if possible. The IV catheter should be removed unless it is to be used as a port for direct administration of antidotal therapy. Various antidotes have been used for extravasation injury (Table 329.3). Proposed agents include antiinflammatory drugs (injected and topical steroids) and local infiltration or perfusion with deactivating or precipitating agents (e.g., sodium bicarbonate), agents to decrease DNA binding (e.g., sodium thiosulfate and ascorbic acid), pharmacologic antagonists (e.g., phentolamine), and agents to promote local washout and systemic absorption (e.g., hyaluronidase). The application of heat or cold is controversial; some recommend applying ice or cold compresses to limit swelling and diffusion of drug from the area affected, and others advise heat to enhance perfusion and to wash out the agent more rapidly. If the injury is limited to hematoma formation, ice packs are recommended. Patients with evidence of local tissue necrosis should be evaluated and managed by a plastic surgeon.

Local and systemic histamine reactions may be treated with oral or parenteral systemic antihistamines, such as diphenhydramine. The treatment of accidental IV injection includes immediate cessation of the injection and supportive care for systemic reactions.

Traumatic vascular injuries usually resolve with sustained direct pressure but sometimes require evaluation and management by a vascular surgeon. Early consultation with a vascular surgeon is advised for accidental IA injections. Leaving the needle in place to allow for the infusion of antidotes and immediate

TABLE 329.3. Antidotes for Drugs Causing Extravasation Injury

Extravasated Drug	Antidote	Dose	Mechanism of Antidote
Aminophylline	Hyaluronidase 15 U/mL	5 × 0.2 mL	Increased absorption
Calcium solutions	Hyaluronidase 15 U/mL	5 × 0.2 mL	Increased absorption
Carmustine	Sodium bicarbonate 8.4%	5 mL	Chemical deactivation
Dactinomycin	Sodium thiosulfate 10%	4 mL	Decreased DNA binding
	+ sterile water	6 mL	
	Ascorbic acid injection	50 mg	Decreased DNA binding
Daunorubicin	Sodium bicarbonate 8.4%	5 mL	Decreased DNA binding
	+ dexamethasone	4 mg	Decreased inflammation
Dextrose 10%	Hyaluronidase 15 U/mL	5 × 0.2 mL	Increased absorption
Dobutamine	Phentolamine	5–10 mg	α-adrenergic blockade
Dopamine	Phentolamine	5–10 mg	α-adrenergic blockade
Doxorubicin	Hydrocortisone sodium	50–200 mg	Decreased inflammation
		Apply b.i.d.	
	Succinate		
	+ hydrocortisone cream 1%	5 mL	Decreased DNA binding
	Sodium bicarbonate 8.4%		
	+ dexamethasone	4 mg	Decreased inflammation
Epinephrine	Phentolamine	5–10 mg	α-adrenergic blockade
Mechlorethamine	Sodium thiosulfate 10%	4 mL	Rapid alkylation
	+ sterile water	6 mL	
Metaraminol	Phentolamine	5–10 mg	α-adrenergic blockade
Mithramycin	Sodium edetate	150 mg	Decreased DNA binding
Mitomycin	Sodium thiosulfate 10%	4 mL	Direct inactivation
	+ sterile water	6 mL	
Nafcillin	Hyaluronidase 15 U/mL	5 × 0.2 mL	Increased absorption
Norepinephrine	Phentolamine	10–15 mg	α-adrenergic blockade
Parenteral nutrition solutions	Hyaluronidase 15 U/mL	5 × 0.2 mL	Increased absorption
Potassium solutions	Hyaluronidase 15 U/mL	5 × 0.2 mL	Increased absorption
Radiocontrast media	Hyaluronidase 15 U/mL	5 × 0.2 mL	Increased absorption
Vasopressin	Guanethidine 10 mg in sodium chloride 0.9% 10 mL		Vasodilatation
	+ heparin 1000 U		
Vinblastine	Sodium bicarbonate 8.4%	5 mL	Chemical precipitation
	Hyaluronidase	150 U	Increased absorption
	+ heat		
Vincristine	Hydrocortisone sodium succinate	25–50 mg/mL extravasate	Decreased inflammation
	Sodium bicarbonate 8.4%	5 mL	Chemical precipitation
	Hyaluronidase	150 U	Increased absorption
	+ heat		
Vindesine	Hyaluronidase	Not stated	Increased absorption
	+ heat		

Modified from MacCara ME. Extravasation: a hazard of intravenous therapy. *Drug Intell Clin Pharm* 1983;17:713.

dilution with normal saline has been proposed. The infusion or injection of vasodilators such as papaverine, lidocaine, reserpine, nitroprusside, terbutaline, or phentolamine may be successful in reversing vasospasm. Sympathetic blockade (e.g., stellate ganglion block) has also been used.

Anticoagulation with heparin, prostacyclin, and low-molecular-weight dextran infusions and oral aspirin may also be helpful. Antiinflammatory agents such as aspirin and dexamethasone have been used. Analgesics may be necessary. Both elevation (to inhibit edema formation) and lowering (to maintain arterial flow) have been recommended in the management of limb injury, so immobilization at heart level is a reasonable compromise.

The initial management of injection injuries to peripheral nerves involves the use of antiinflammatories and analgesics, as well as protection from further injury (e.g., splinting a nonfunctional extremity). Indications for and the timing of neurolysis are controversial.[5] All injection injuries to nerves should be urgently evaluated by the appropriate surgical specialist, usually an orthopedic, vascular, or neurologic surgeon.

Treatment options for digital ischemia resulting from accidental discharge of epinephrine autoinjectors include local infiltration of phentolamine at the site of injury, perivascular phentolamine infiltration as in a digital nerve block, or both.[2,9,10] Phentolamine doses of 1.0 to 3.5 mg have been used. Local infiltration of terbutaline (e.g., 0.5 to 2.0 mL of a 0.5-mg/mL dilution) also has been reported to be an effective treatment.[16] Alternative therapies, such as lidocaine digital block and local application of nitroglycerin paste, have been used but are less effective.

Ischemia induced by infiltration of vasopressors may be treated by injecting 5 to 10 mg of phentolamine in 10 mL of saline into the area of infiltration. A lower total dose of the same formulation has been used successfully in a neonate.[15] Terbutaline infiltration (1 mg in 10 mL of normal saline) has been reported to be similarly effective.[16] Success has also been reported with the application of 2% nitroglycerin ointment to treat tissue ischemia from either catheter-induced arterial vasospasm or dopamine extravasation.[20] Hypotension may complicate nitroglycerin therapy, especially in neonates and despite careful attention to dose (4 mm/kg).

Fluid and electrolyte overload, anaphylaxis, and sepsis complicating parenteral drug therapy are managed in the usual manner, which may include diuresis, fluid restriction, ion exchange resins, antibiotics, epinephrine, or cardiovascular supportive therapy. The treatment of diluent toxicity includes discontinuing or slowing the rate of infusion, as well as standard supportive care.

DISPOSITION

Reliable patients with minor extravasations of IV fluids or nonirritating medications, localized infections (cellulitis, abscess), and local allergic reactions may be discharged and treated at home, with arrangements made for appropriate follow-up. Decisions regarding continuing care and disposition of patients with more significant local injuries should be made in consultation with the appropriate specialist (see previous discussion).

COMMON PITFALLS

- Lack of knowledge of proper injection techniques
- Failure to monitor for systemic reactions after local injections
- Failure to consult the appropriate specialist in cases of neurovascular injury
- Failure to recognize the potential significance of IV infiltrations, especially those involving vesicants (e.g., antineoplastics) or vasoconstrictors (e.g., dopamine)
- Use of epinephrine-containing anesthetic mixtures where vasoconstrictors are contraindicated
- Failure to consider the use of antidotes for extravasation injuries

References

1. Bedichek I, Kirschbaum B. A case of propylene glycol toxic reaction associated with etomidate infusion. *Arch Intern Med* 1991;151:2297.
2. Burkhart KK. The reversal of the ischemic effects of epinephrine on a finger with local injections of phentolamine [Letter, comment]. *J Emerg Med* 1992;10:496.
3. Du Toit DF, Sunshine M, Knott-Craig C, et al. Gangrene of the hand and forearm after inadvertent intra-arterial injection of pyrazole. *S Afr Med J* 1985;68:491.
4. Frederick HA, Carter PR, Littler JW. Injection injuries to the median and ulnar nerves at the wrist. *J Hand Surg* 1992;17A:645.
5. Gentili F, Hudson AR, Hunter D. Clinical and experimental aspects of injection injuries of peripheral nerves. *Can J Neurol Sci* 1980;7:143.
6. Halpern MT, Yabroff KR, Sloan EP. Costs of medical resource use associated with complications of IV drug therapy. *Formulary* 1997;32:944.
7. Linskey ME, Segal R. Median nerve injury from local steroid injection in carpal tunnel syndrome. *Neurosurgery* 1990;26:512.
8. MacCara ME. Extravasation: a hazard of intravenous therapy. *Drug Intell Clin Pharm* 1983;17:713.
9. Maguire WM, Reisdorff EJ, Smith D, et al. Epinephrine-induced vasospasm reversed by phentolamine digital block. *Am J Emerg Med* 1990;8:46.
10. Markovchick V, Burkhart KK. The reversal of the ischemic effects of epinephrine on a finger with local injections of phentolamine. *J Emerg Med* 1991;9:323.
11. Preston D, Logigian E. Iatrogenic needle-induced peroneal neuropathy in the foot. *Ann Intern Med* 1988;109:921.
12. Schulenburg CE, Robbs JV, Rubin J. Intra-arterial diazepam: a report of two cases. *S Afr Med J* 1985;68:891.
13. Sherman BW, McNamara MP, Shen S-J. Inadvertent arterial administration of parenteral hyperalimentation solution resulting in generalized seizure activity. *J Parenter Enteral Nutr* 1992;16:284.
14. Sintenie JB, Tuinebreijer WE, Kreis RW, et al. Digital gangrene after accidental intra-arterial injection of phenytoin. *Eur J Surg* 1992;158:315.
15. Siwy BK, Sadove AM. Acute management of dopamine infiltration injury with Regitine. *Plast Reconstr Surg* 1987;80:610.
16. Stier PA, Bogner MP, Webster K, et al. Use of subcutaneous terbutaline to reverse peripheral ischemia. *Am J Emerg Med* 1999;17:91.
17. Stoller KP, Losey R. Inadvertent intra-arterial injection of penicillin: an unseen danger. *Pediatrics* 1985;75:785.
18. Streib EW, Sun SF. Injection injury of the sciatic nerve: unusual anatomic distribution of nerve damage. *Eur Neurol* 1981;20:481.
19. Turco SJ. Hazards associated with parenteral therapy. *Bull Parenter Drug Assoc* 1974;28(4):197.
20. Wong AF, McCulloch LM, Solo A. Treatment of peripheral tissue ischemia with topical nitroglycerin ointment in neonates. *J Pediatr* 1992;121:980.

CHAPTER 330
Corrosive Ingestions

Robert P. Dowsett and Christopher H. Linden

Corrosive poisoning can result from exposure to compounds that cause tissue injury as the result of a chemical reaction. This chapter focuses on ingestions. The evaluation and management of exposure by other routes are discussed in Chapters 309 and 346. Hydrofluoric acid exposures are discussed in Chapter 339.

Most corrosive injuries involve acids and alkalis. Acids are defined as proton donors. They dissociate into conjugate bases and hydrogen ions (H^+) in solution. Alkalis accept protons, resulting in the formation of conjugate acids and hydroxide ions (OH^-). The acidity or alkalinity of a solution is measured by its pH, the negative log of H^+ concentration. The pH of water (7) is neutral. Acidic solutions have a pH of less than 7, and alkaline solutions, greater than 7. Solutions with a pH of less than 2 or greater than 12 are highly corrosive. Table 330.1 lists the pH of some common solutions. The pH is dependent not only on the concentration of acid or alkali in solution, but also on the ease with which the acid donates H^+ or the alkali accepts H^+.

The pK_a, which is equal to the pH of a solution in which half of the acid has dissociated, is a measure of the ease with which the acid donates a proton. For an alkali, the pK_a of the conjugate acid inversely reflects the strength of the alkali as a proton acceptor. Strong (i.e., easily dissociated) acids and alkalis are those with a pK_a of less than 0 and greater than 14, respectively. Table 330.2 lists the pK_a of common chemicals.

Acid-base reactions damage biologic tissue by altering the ionized state of molecules, which, in turn, may disrupt covalent bonds, catalyze further reactions, or alter the structure of macromolecules. Acids denature protein, resulting in the formation of a firm coagulum, or eschar (coagulation necrosis). The resulting eschar may limit tissue penetration, but this does not appear to be a major variable in determining the extent of injury.[17]

In contrast, alkalis saponify fats and dissolve proteins, resulting in the softening of tissues (liquefaction necrosis). Cell death results from the emulsification and disruption of cellular membranes. Sloughing of tissue may assist the penetration of alkalis to deeper levels. Tissue injury is exacerbated by thrombosis of small vessels and the production of heat. Heat generated during the neutralization of acids is typically greater than that of alkalis. Tissue injury progresses rapidly over the first few minutes but can continue for several hours. Bacterial invasion, inflammatory response, and development of granulation tissue ensue. Because collagen deposition may not begin until the second week, tensile strength of the healing tissue is low during the first 3 weeks. Scar retraction begins in the third week, commonly continuing for months, and may result in stricture formation and shortening of the involved segment of the gastrointestinal tract. Mucosal repair can take weeks to months.

Corrosives can also cause injury by mechanisms such as reduction, oxidation, denaturation, fixation, dissolution, or thermal injury. Reactions between strong acids and strong bases are usually highly exothermic and can be explosive. Dissolving a strong acid or base in water also generates heat. Explosive reactions can occur when water is added to metallic lithium, sodium, and potassium; to aluminum and lithium salts; and to titanium tetrachloride. Chlorine, bromine, and nitrogen oxides react with water, liberating heat and forming acids, elemental ions, and free oxygen radicals. Dissolving ammonia in water results in the exothermic production of ammonium hydroxide. Ammonia and hypochlorite bleaches generate corrosive chloramine gases when mixed. When bleach is mixed with an acid (e.g., acidic toilet bowl cleaner), another corrosive gas, chlorine, is liberated. Baking soda (sodium bicarbonate) is unique in that, when it is mixed with acid (e.g., after ingestion), large amounts of carbon dioxide gas are liberated in an endothermic reaction.

Chemicals can be classified as weak irritants, strong irritants, or corrosives to indicate the likelihood of potential tissue injury, and commercial products may carry corresponding "signal words" on their labels (Table 330.3). For acids and alkalis, the likelihood of injury depends on the number of H^+ or OH^- ions available to react with tissues. The availability of H^+ or OH^- ions depends on the concentration, volume, and pH of the solution as well as the pK_a of the acid or alkali and can be measured by the titratable reserve. The titratable reserve is expressed as the amount of sodium hydroxide or hydrochloric acid required to neutralize an acidic or basic solution.[10]

Titratable acid or alkaline reserve appears to be the best indicator of corrosive potential; however, it is usually impossible to measure in the clinical setting. Hence, product classification, signal words, pH, pK_a, volume, and concentration must be used as surrogate indicators. Concentrated solutions or large volumes of any corrosive, any concentration or amount of strong acids or alkalis, and products labeled as corrosive or dangerous should be considered highly toxic to tissues.

TABLE 330.1. Approximate pH of Some Common Solutions

Solution	pH
1.0 M HCl	0
Battery acid (1% solution)	1.4
Acid toilet cleaner (1%)	2.0
Citrus juices	1.8–4
Wines	2.8–3.8
Black coffee	5.0
Rainwater	6.5
Water (25°C)	7.0
Bleach (1% solution)	9.5–10.2
Automatic dishwasher detergents	10.4–13
Laundry detergents	11.6–12.6
Ammonia cleaners (<10%)	11.9–12.4
Alkaline drain cleaners	13.3–14
1.0 M NaOH	14
Saturated ammonia solution	15

TABLE 330.2. pK_a of Acids and Alkalis

Acids	Formula	pK_a	Alkalis	Formula	pK_a
Perchloric	$HClO_4$	–8	Calcium carbonate	$CaCO_3$	5.7
Hydrochloric	HCl	– 3	Hydrazine	N_2H_4	8
Chromic	CrO_3	0.3	Ammonia	NH_3	9.3
Bromic	$HBrO_3$	<1	Ammonium hydroxide	NH_4OH	9.3
Nitric	HNO_3	<1	Ethanolamine	$NH_2C_2H_4OH$	9.5
Oxalic	$C_2H_2O_4$	1.5	Magnesium hydroxide	H_2MgO_2	10
Sulfuric	H_2SO_4	1.9	Zinc hydroxide	$Zn(OH)_2$	11
Phosphoric	$H_2P_2O_7$	2.1	Calcium hydroxide	$Ca(OH)_2$	11.6
Arsenic	H_3AsO_4	2.3	1,6-Hexane-diamine	$(NH_2)_2C_6H_{12}$	11.8
Nitrous	HNO_2	3.3	Lithium hydroxide	LiOH	>14
Hydrofluoric	HF	3.4	Potassium hydroxide	KOH	>14
Acetic	H_3C_2OOH	4.8	Sodium hydroxide	NaOH	>14
Sulfurous	HSO_3	6.9	Calcium oxide	CaO	>14
Hydrogen sulfide	H_2S	7.0	Sodium carbonate	Na_2CO_3	>14
Boric	H_3BO_3	9.2	Potassium carbonate	K_2CO_3	>14
Hydrogen peroxide	H_2O_2	11.6	Sodium hypochlorite	NaClO	>14

TABLE 330.3. U.S. Consumer Safety Committee Recommendations (1982) for the Use of Signal Words on Product Labels

Label	Classification	Description
Caution	Weak irritant	Irritating to eyes, nose, throat, and mouth.
Warning	Strong irritant	Irritating to eyes, nose, throat, and mouth. May irritate the skin.
Danger	Corrosive	May be fatal or cause permanent damage. Vapor harmful. Causes severe burns.

Additionally, the extent and severity of injury depend on the physical state of the corrosive, the duration of tissue contact, the presence of food, and the tonicity of the pyloric sphincter. Solid compounds dissolve on contact with body fluids, producing highly concentrated solutions, which may result in severe but localized damage. Solutions of a high viscosity (e.g., concentrated alkali) tend to cause deeper burns, possibly by a similar mechanism. Solids and solutions of high viscosity tend to adhere to tissues and frequently result in injury to the oropharynx. Pain, too, may limit the amount ingested but, if swallowed, severe upper esophageal burns typically occur. When taken without water or while the patient is recumbent, medications, particularly potassium chloride, iron, quinidine, antiinflammatory agents, and sustained-release formulations, can lodge in the esophagus and cause deep mucosal ulceration.

Sites commonly affected by corrosive ingestion are the oropharynx, esophagus, and stomach, although sites as distal as the proximal jejunum may be injured.[15–18] Areas at, or immediately proximal to, points of gastrointestinal tract narrowing are particularly at risk.[13] Alkali ingestion is associated with a significantly higher incidence of esophageal lesions, whereas acids tend to affect the stomach.[1,5,6,16] There are, however, many exceptions.[16,17,19] Esophageal lesions occur predominantly in the lower half, and gastric burns are usually most severe in the antrum.[17,18] Multiple sites are affected in up to 80% of patients.[18] In the presence of food, gastric injuries tend to be less severe and involve the lesser curve and pylorus.

Systemic toxicity may sometimes accompany severe gastrointestinal injuries and is usually secondary to tissue inflammation, acidosis, infection, and necrosis. Fluid and electrolyte shifts accompanying extensive burns can cause hypovolemic shock. Although corrosives are usually neutralized on contact with tissues, products of this reaction may be absorbed and cause systemic effects.

Deaths due to the ingestion of corrosive agents constituted 2.8% of all reported deaths due to poisoning in the United States in 1997.[14] Household cleaning products represented the largest group involved in all corrosive exposures. Nearly one-third of cases involved children younger than age 6 years who had commonly ingested relatively low-toxicity disinfectants and bleaches; the incidence of significant injury was only one-fourth of that in adults. Adults, either by deliberate intent or because of concomitant intoxication, often ingest a larger amount of corrosive and are more likely to suffer severe injury.[6,8,19] The elderly are at increased risk of dying from the accidental or intentional ingestion of corrosives and accounted for nearly 25% of all deaths due to corrosives ingestion.[14]

Before 1970, domestic alkali drain cleaners containing highly concentrated sodium or potassium hydroxide caused most of the serious injuries due to corrosive ingestion.[1] The less concentrated (less than 20%) alkali drain cleaners are still responsible for the largest number of severe gastrointestinal injuries and deaths. Until very recently, acid toilet bowel cleaners were responsible for as many deaths, but none were reported in 1997.[14] Domestic liquid (but not powder) automatic dishwasher detergents, ammonia (5% to 10%), bleaches (less than 10% sodium hypochlorite), and hydrogen peroxide solutions (less than 3%) rarely cause significant injury.

CLINICAL PRESENTATION

Patients usually present with oral, retrosternal, or abdominal pain. Other symptoms and signs include dysphagia, drooling, and vomiting; less commonly, symptoms and signs include stridor, hoarseness, hematemesis, and melena.[8] Young children may refuse to drink fluids, cry excessively, or be unable to swallow their secretions. The presence of vomiting is associated with severe esophageal burns; drooling and stridor appear to be predictive of severe injuries but not necessarily of a particular site.[5,7,8,16] Patients with pill-induced esophageal injury usually present with the sudden onset of retrosternal pain and odynophagia.

Visible superficial burns are often covered with a pale membrane, whereas deeper burns are black, hemorrhagic, or friable. The presence of burns in the oropharynx is not reliably predictive of more distal injuries.[5,7,8,15–19] Burns of the larynx, however, are associated with a greater incidence and severity of esophageal lesions.[16] Laryngeal burns occur in nearly one-half of patients with serious esophageal injuries and are more commonly the cause of respiratory distress than are tracheitis or pneumonitis secondary to aspiration.[16] Usually, the epiglottis and aryepiglottic folds are involved. Initial stridor and hoarseness do not reliably predict the presence or severity of laryngeal involvement.[8] Additionally, the absence of respiratory symptoms or signs on presentation does not preclude the existence of airway burns that may require later intervention.[16]

Full-thickness injuries to the esophagus or stomach are at risk of perforation and fistula formation into the mediastinum, peritoneum, or trachea.[18] Patients with mediastinitis may have chest pain, respiratory distress, fever, subcutaneous emphysema, pleural rub, and Hamman's sign (crunching sound heard during cardiac systole on auscultation of the mediastinum). Chest radiographic findings may include mediastinal widening, pleural effusion (usually left-sided), pneumomediastinum, and pneumothorax. Peritonitis may result from viscus perforation or the extension of severe gastric burns to surrounding abdominal organs.[6,19] In addition to usual findings, patients with peritonitis may have marked third-spacing of fluids, resulting in abdominal distention and hypotension. Tracheoesophageal–aortic fistula is a potential complication in patients with extensive esophageal burns and may present with hemoptysis or hematemesis.

Esophageal strictures develop in up to 70% of patients with deep esophageal ulcers and in nearly all patients with areas of necrosis.[18,19] Ulceration superficial to the muscularis mucosa layer does not lead to stricture formation.[2,6,9,17] Half of all esophageal strictures develop during initial hospitalization, and 80% are evident within 2 months. Strictures may also develop in the mouth, pharynx, and stomach.[17–19] Esophageal carcinoma, a late sequela of alkali ingestion, has been diagnosed 22 to 81 years after ingestion. This complication has not been associated with acid burns.

Systemic toxicity has been reported following skin or gastrointestinal burns caused by acetic acid, salts of arsenic and other heavy metals, cyanide, formic acid, hydrofluoric acid, hydrazine, hydrochloric acid, nitrates, phenol, sulfuric acid, and phosphoric acid. Severe acid burns may be accompanied by metabolic acidosis.

It is unclear whether metabolic acidosis results from the absorption of an acid or is secondary to hypovolemic shock. The anion gap is usually elevated, although a hyperchloremic acidosis may be seen in hydrochloric acid ingestion. Hyperphosphatemia and hypocalcemia have occurred with phosphoric acid ingestion. Methemoglobinemia (see Chapter 352) can occur following burns with phenol. Cardiovascular collapse is the most common cause of early death following hydrochloric acid ingestion. Other findings associated with severe acid injuries include hemolysis with hyperkalemia and hemoglobinuria, nephrotoxicity, pulmonary edema, and organ dysfunction resulting from hypovolemic shock.

Coma, bradycardia, hypotension, acidosis, pulmonary edema, liver dysfunction, and coagulopathy have been reported after the ingestion or inhalation of ammonia. After absorption, ammonia is rapidly taken up by the liver, where it enters the urea cycle. Systemic toxicity occurs when the rate of hepatic clearance is exceeded. Hydrazine can be absorbed through the skin and lungs as well as the gastrointestinal tract. Systemic toxicity is due to the inhibition of enzymes involved in intermediary metabolism and may be delayed up to 14 hours after initial exposure. Hypotension, ataxia, coma, hypoglycemia, hyperglycemia, hepatitis, renal tubular necrosis, hemolysis, and, possibly, methemoglobinemia may occur in severe cases of hydrazine poisoning (see Chapters 352 and 353).

DIFFERENTIAL DIAGNOSIS

The most important diagnosis to exclude is the potential coingestion of foreign bodies or systematically absorbed chemicals. If shock or altered mental status is present soon after ingestion, a search for other causes should be undertaken. Hematemesis and esophageal perforation can result from protracted vomiting of any cause. Gastroenteritis due to the corrosive effects of ingested heavy metals and hydrocarbons can cause similar symptoms. Allergic reactions may present with some of the features of corrosive ingestion if the hypopharynx or larynx is involved. Foreign-body ingestion and infections such as epiglottitis, croup, retropharyngeal abscess, and mucosal ulceration due to herpesvirus or coxsackievirus should be considered in infants, toddlers, and elderly patients who are unable to provide an adequate history.

EMERGENCY DEPARTMENT EVALUATION

The identity, concentration, and amount of chemical or product ingested and the time and circumstances of ingestion should be determined. Product labels should be examined for ingredients and signal words. If a sample is available, the pH should be measured. A pH meter is more accurate than pH paper (e.g., pHydrion paper, which is also used for testing amniotic fluid) but is not generally available.

Initial and ongoing attention should be directed to airway patency, because obstruction may develop with progressive mucosal edema. In the absence of clinical indications for immediate endotracheal intubation, patients with respiratory symptoms should have upper airway assessment, preferably by direct fiberoptic laryngoscopy. Patients suspected of having a significant injury should have an electrocardiogram, arterial blood gas analysis, complete blood count, type and cross-match, prothrombin time, and electrolyte, glucose, and liver and renal function tests. Radiologic studies should include an upright chest radiograph and an abdominal film. Methemoglobin levels should be checked in patients who have ingested hydrazine or phenol. The evaluation of cyanide, fluoride, and heavy metal poisoning is discussed in Chapters 331, 339, and 318, respectively.

Endoscopy of the upper gastrointestinal tract should be performed in all symptomatic patients. The lack of symptoms or signs usually indicates that significant injuries (i.e., those that require treatment or are likely to lead to complications) are absent and that endoscopy is not necessary.[5,8,16] Endoscopy should be considered for apparently asymptomatic young children or patients who have intentionally ingested a strong acid or alkali if the history is unreliable. Because injuries may progress over a period of several hours, endoscopy is optimally performed 6 to 24 hours after exposure. If undertaken earlier, the full extent of injury may not be apparent; if performed later, the risk of perforation may be increased. Iatrogenic esophageal perforation has only been reported with the use of rigid endoscopes.[18] Fiberoptic endoscopy is safe as long as it is performed gently, with minimal air insufflation and avoidance of retroversion or retroflexion.

Initially, the cricopharynx and larynx should be visualized to assess any laryngeal burns and the need for intubation. If laryngeal burns are noted, prophylactic endotracheal intubation should be performed before distal evaluation is begun. When a flexible, small-diameter endoscope is used, it is not necessary to terminate the procedure at the level of the first circumferential or full-thickness lesion, although the endoscope should not be forced through a narrowed area.[18]

Contrast esophagography is less sensitive than endoscopy in assessing burn injury, although it is useful for the detection of perforation. A water-soluble contrast agent should be used. Cine-esophagography can detect esophageal motility disorders, which are predictive of stricture formation. All patients with an atonic dilated or atonic rigid esophagus and some patients with abnormal uncoordinated contractions later develop esophageal strictures.[12]

EMERGENCY DEPARTMENT MANAGEMENT

Airway management is the first priority. Any patient with respiratory distress, stridor, or inability to speak should undergo immediate endotracheal intubation. Patients who are hypoxic but not in respiratory distress should be given supplemental oxygen. If laryngoscopy reveals laryngeal mucosal edema, prophylactic intubation is advised. Patients with pneumonitis and hypoxia unresponsive to oxygen should be managed with endotracheal intubation and positive-pressure ventilation. Symptomatic patients should have an intravenous line established.

Although most tissue injury occurs within minutes of ingestion, decontamination should be considered if the patient presents within 2 hours of ingestion. Emesis is contraindicated because it may reexpose the thin-walled esophagus to the corrosive agent and may increase the risk of aspiration.[16] For this reason, antiemetics should be given to patients with persistent vomiting. Unless it is likely to prevent absorption of coingestants, activated charcoal should not be given, because it does not effectively bind corrosives and obscures endoscopic evaluation. The mouth should be rinsed liberally with water, milk, or other noncarbonated beverage in patients with oral burns or symptoms. Dilution by giving oral fluids may be beneficial. The amount swallowed should be limited to 5 mL/kg to avoid inducing emesis. This may also wash any corrosive adherent in the esophagus to the stomach, which has a thicker wall and may be less susceptible to injury.

The use of a nasogastric tube to evacuate gastric contents may be useful in patients with large intentional ingestions who present within 1 to 2 hours of ingestion. Although controversial, this procedure has not been reported to cause perforation.[13] If performed, the tube should be gently inserted, gastric contents aspirated, and the tube firmly taped in place to avoid motion. Dilution or lavage with small aliquots (5 mL/kg) of water can then be undertaken. Patients should otherwise be given nothing by mouth until the need for endoscopy is determined.

Although corticosteroids reduce the incidence and severity of esophageal strictures in animal studies, their value in humans is controversial. In animal studies, steroids were given before, coincident with, or immediately after exposure. In clinical trials in which steroids were not given until up to 24 hours after exposure, there have been conflicting conclusions as well as several points of general agreement. Patients with first-degree esophageal burns do not require steroids, because strictures do not develop in this group.[2,6,9] Steroids do not appear to influence the development of esophageal strictures in patients with extensive areas of deep ulceration or necrosis and may increase complications such as hemorrhage or perforation.[2,9] For patients between these two extremes, whose injuries consist of circumferential or extensive superficial ulceration or small areas of deep ulceration or necrosis, steroids are of potential benefit.[2,9,11] Esophageal strictures are less common after acid ingestion, and the effect of steroids has not been studied; their use deserves consideration in exceptional cases.

Animal studies show that, if steroids are to be effective, they must be given as soon as possible after exposure (i.e., on presentation). Because endoscopy is usually delayed for several hours, the first dose of steroids should be administered before endoscopy is performed. The decision to continue steroids can be based on the findings at endoscopy. Recommended dosages are 1 mg/kg/d of dexamethasone or 2 mg/kg/d of prednisolone or methylprednisolone for 3 weeks, then tapering the medication. Dexamethasone has been suggested to be superior to prednisolone in improving healing and reducing the need for stricture dilatations.[3] Active bleeding or perforation are contraindications to steroid use. Animal studies indicate that antibiotics, when used in conjunction with steroids, have a synergistic effect in the prevention of stricture formation. Therefore, patients who are to continue steroids should also be given antibiotics (e.g., cefazolin). Patients with extensive transmural ulceration or necrosis, who are not candidates for steroid therapy, should also be given antibiotics to reduce the incidence and severity of perforation.

Although they are of no benefit in promoting healing or reducing complications, antacids, sucralfate, H_2-blockers, and analgesics can provide symptomatic relief. Oral medications should generally be withheld until the results of endoscopy are known, and then they should be given only to patients with injuries limited to mucosal inflammation or small areas of superficial ulceration. These patients may be given oral fluids when they are able to swallow their own secretions. Those with more severe injuries should receive intravenous fluids and nothing by mouth. Hyperalimentation, either parenteral or by jejunostomy feeding tube, is recommended for these patients.

Silastic stents, placed in the esophagus at the time of endoscopy, may also prevent stricture formation.[4] Alternatively, a nasogastric tube or string may be inserted and left in place to maintain patency of the esophageal lumen and facilitate subsequent dilation by bougienage if strictures develop. The use of lathyrogenic compounds, such as beta-aminopropionitrile and D-penicillamine, have decreased the rate of collagen deposition and stricture formation in animal studies but have not been studied in humans. Their use is not recommended. Therapy for systemic toxicity is primarily supportive. The treatment of methemoglobinemia and systemic heavy-metal, cyanide, and fluoride poisoning is discussed in Chapters 318, 331, and 339.

Surgical exploration is indicated if perforation or full-thickness necrosis is suspected. Laparotomy and early excision of necrotic tissue have been recommended for patients with extensive full-thickness esophageal necrosis, but the advantage over more conservative treatment is unproved, and surgical mortality in this group is high. In patients who develop strictures, attempts at dilatation earlier than 3 weeks after ingestion is of unclear benefit and has been associated with an increased risk of perforation. Indications for delayed esophageal replacement are (1) inability of the patient to swallow; (2) persistent symptomatic strictures despite sequential dilatation; (3) a need for frequent esophageal dilatation, requiring extended hospitalization; and (4) perforation during dilatation. Esophageal substitutes include the colon, most commonly, but also the stomach (reverse gastric tube) and jejunum.

DISPOSITION

Patients who are asymptomatic or become asymptomatic after oral rinsing and dilution may be discharged from the emergency department if they have ingested a compound classified as a mild irritant. Admission is recommended for all symptomatic patients. The choice of bed (e.g., floor, intermediate, or intensive care unit) depends on the patient's clinical status. Patients with the potential for airway compromise should be admitted to an intensive care unit. Patients with suicidal ingestions require psychiatric evaluation and one-to-one monitoring. All symptomatic patients should be evaluated by an endoscopist (gastroenterologist or surgeon). Consultation should also be considered when significant injury is suspected in a patient who is unable or unwilling to describe symptoms and who has ingested a potentially corrosive substance. If endoscopy is unavailable, patients who require hospital admission should be transferred to a facility where it can be performed. Patients with a history, symptoms, or signs suggestive of moderate or severe injury, or endoscopic evidence of such, should also have early consultation with a general, pediatric, or thoracic surgeon, depending on local referral patterns and the location of injury. Signs and symptoms of perforation require early surgical consultation. A toxicologist or regional poison control center should be consulted regarding treatment recommendations.

After endoscopy, patients with no visible injury or with injuries limited to mucosal inflammation or small areas of superficial ulceration may be discharged or referred for psychiatric care, as long as they are able to tolerate oral fluids.[2,6,9] Patients with persistent symptoms or inconclusive findings at endoscopy should remain for observation.[1] If symptoms persist, endoscopy should be repeated. Patients with deep or extensive superficial ulceration or areas of necrosis should be managed in an intensive care setting.

COMMON PITFALLS

- Failing to positively identify the substance ingested, test its pH, or seek information on its potential for corrosive injury
- Failing to evaluate the airway and intubate patients with respiratory distress or signs of laryngeal edema
- Attempting to neutralize the ingested corrosive with weak acids or alkalis
- Giving syrup of ipecac or unintentionally inducing vomiting by giving excessive amounts of oral fluid for initial decontamination
- Assuming that the absence of oropharyngeal burns precludes the presence of significant distal injuries
- Failing to consult a gastroenterologist and surgeon regarding the evaluation of all symptomatic patients

References

1. Allen RE, Thoshinsky MJ, Stallone RJ, et al. Corrosive injuries of the stomach. *Arch Surg* 1970;100:409.
2. Anderson KD, Rouse TM, Randolph JG. A controlled trial of corticosteroids in children with corrosive injury of the esophagus. *N Engl J Med* 1990;323:637.
3. Bautista A, Varela R, Villanueva A, et al. Effects of prednisolone and dexamethasone in children with alkali burns of the oesophagus. *Eur J Pediatr Surg* 1996;6:198.
4. Berkovits RN, Bos CE, Wijburg FA, et al. Caustic injury of the oesophagus. Sixteen years experience, and introduction of a new model oesophageal stent. *J Laryngol Otol* 1996;110:1041.
5. Crain EF, Gershel JC, Mezey AP. Caustic ingestions: symptoms as predictors of esophageal injury. *Am J Dis Child* 1984;138:863.
6. Estrera A, Taylor W, Mills LJ. Corrosive burns of the esophagus and stomach: a recommendation for an aggressive surgical approach. *Ann Thorac Surg* 1986;41:276.
7. Gaudreault P, Parent M, Mcguigan MA, et al. Predictability of esophageal injury from symptoms and signs: a study of caustic ingestion in 378 children. *Pediatrics* 1983;71:767.
8. Gorman RL, Khin-Maung-Gyi MT, Klein-Schwartz W, et al. Initial symptoms as predictors of esophageal injury in alkaline corrosive ingestions. *Am J Emerg Med* 1992;10:189.
9. Hawkins DB, Demeter MJ, Barness TE. Caustic ingestions: controversies in management. A review of 214 cases. *Laryngoscope* 1980;90:98.
10. Hoffman RS, Howland MA, Kamerow HN, et al. Comparison of titratable acid/alkaline reserve and pH in potentially caustic household products. *J Toxicol Clin Toxicol* 1989;27:241.
11. Howell JM, Dalsey WC, Hartsell FW, et al. Steroids for the treatment of corrosive esophageal injury: a statistical analysis of past studies. *Am J Emerg Med* 1992;10:421.
12. Kuhn JR, Tunell WP. Cine-esophagography in caustic burns of the esophagus. *Am J Surg* 1983;146:804.
13. Linden CH. Inorganic acids and bases. In: Sullivan JB, Krieger GR, eds. *Hazardous materials toxicology: clinical principles of environmental health.* Baltimore: Williams & Wilkins, 1992:762.
14. Litovitz TL, Klein-Schwartz W, Dyer KS, et al. 1997 annual report of the American Association of Poison Control Centers. Toxic Exposure Surveillance System. *Am J Emerg Med* 1998;16:443.
15. Previtera C, Giusti F, Guglielmi M. Predictive value of visible lesions (cheeks, lips, oropharynx) in suspected caustic ingestion: may endoscopy reasonably be omitted in completely negative pediatric patients? *Pediatr Emerg Care* 1990;6:176.
16. Vergauwen P, Moulin D, Buts JP, et al. Caustic burns of the upper digestive and respiratory tracts. *Eur J Pediatr* 1991;150:700.
17. Zargar SA, Kochhar R, Nagi B, et al. Ingestion of corrosive acids. Spectrum of injury to upper gastrointestinal tract and natural history. *Gastroenterology* 1989;97:702.
18. Zargar SA, Kochhar R, Mehta S, et al. The role of fiberoptic endoscopy in the management of corrosive ingestion and modified endoscopic classification of burns. *Gastrointest Endosc* 1991;37:165.
19. Zargar SA, Kochhar R, Nagi B, et al. Ingestion of strong corrosive alkalis: spectrum of injury to upper gastro-intestinal tract and natural history. *Am J Gastroenterol* 1992;87:337.

CHAPTER 331
Cyanide Poisoning

Alan H. Hall

Acute cyanide poisoning is a rare, potentially fatal but treatable condition.[20] It may be encountered in a variety of settings: smoke inhalation, chemical exposures, thermal degradation or acid contact with chemical compounds (e.g., cyanogen, cyanogen halides, calcium cyanide), and metabolic release after systemic absorption of laetrile, amygdalin, other cyanogenic glycosides of plant origin (e.g., apricot, cherry, and peach pits) and aliphatic nitrile compounds.[3,4,6,9,18] Sodium nitroprusside therapy at high doses may sometimes cause elevated blood cyanide levels.[15]

Of the 347 cases of cyanide exposure reported to poison centers in the United States during 1997, there were seven deaths.[16] While 127 patients developed some signs or symptoms, only six who had severe cyanide poisoning survived. Antidotal treatment with amyl nitrite was administered in 47 cases, sodium nitrite in 43 cases, and sodium thiosulfate in 73.[16]

Cyanide produces intracellular hypoxia by complexing with the ferric iron of mitochondrial cytochrome oxidase, inhibiting the electron transport chain and oxidative phosphorylation, and causing anaerobic metabolism with decreased adenosine triphosphate and increased lactic acid production.[3] Tissues with the greatest oxygen demand (myocardium and brain) are most profoundly and rapidly affected. Initial central nervous system and cardiovascular stimulation is followed by depression.

Human cyanide toxicokinetics are poorly understood, but the volume of distribution is probably between 0.4 and 0.5 L/kg, and the initial half-life between 30 minutes and 1 hour. Systemic absorption by the ingestion route is nearly complete, but only a small percentage of a dose is excreted unchanged in the urine.[2,8] Whole blood cyanide levels in acute ingestion poisoning decrease rapidly after specific antidote treatment, but they may remain elevated for prolonged periods when antidotes are not administered.[8] Except in rare cases, patients with whole blood cyanide levels greater than 3.0 μg/mL have not survived unless specific antidote therapy was administered.[8,9]

Although a number of specific antidotes are in clinical use worldwide, only the amyl nitrite, sodium nitrite, and sodium thiosulfate combination (the Cyanide Antidote Kit) is available in the United States. Hydroxocobalamin, commercially available in some other countries, is less toxic and generally equally efficacious.[2,3,5,7] Oxygen has an antidotal effect of its own as well as having synergistic action with certain specific cyanide antidotes, perhaps because oxidized cytochrome oxidase resists inactivation by cyanide to a greater extent than does reduced cytochrome oxidase.[17]

CLINICAL PRESENTATION

Inhalation of high concentrations of hydrogen cyanide gas may cause sudden loss of consciousness after only a few breaths.[8] With ingestion of alkaline cyanide salts (calcium cyanide, potassium cyanide, sodium cyanide), the onset of life-threatening symptomatology may occur in 30 minutes to 1 hour.[8] In fatal cases, rapid progression to coma, seizures, arrhythmias, intractable hypotension, apnea, and death is common.

Onset of symptoms may be delayed with exposure to cyanogens such as laetrile and cyanogenic glycosides from plant sources (up to 1.5 hours), or aliphatic nitrile compounds, such as acetonitrile in artificial glue-on nail removers (up to 6 to 12 hours).[4,6,9] Systemic poisoning may occur after dermal cyanide exposure,[13] although such cases are extremely rare.

Initial signs and symptoms include central nervous system stimulation (giddiness, headache, and anxiety), hyperpnea, mild hypertension, and palpitations.[8] Later manifestations include nausea, vomiting, hypotension, generalized seizures, coma, apnea, mydriasis, noncardiogenic pulmonary edema, and a variety of cardiac effects (tachycardia or bradycardia, supraventricular and ventricular arrhythmias, atrioventricular blocks, ischemic electrocardiographic changes, and, eventually, asystole).[3,8] Patients with significant cyanide poisoning have elevated serum lactate levels and an elevated anion gap metabolic acidosis.[2,8] Cyanosis is a late sign, noted only at the stage of apnea and circulatory collapse. The retinal veins and arteries may appear nearly equally red, due to the inability of tissues to extract oxygen from the blood. Development of a diabetes insipidus–like condition secondary to severe brain damage following acute cyanide poisoning is an ominous prognostic sign.[20]

During high-dose nitroprusside infusion, whole blood cyanide levels may become elevated. However, even when this occurs, clinical signs of cyanide poisoning (e.g., elevated lactate levels, metabolic acidosis) are not necessarily present.[15] Cyanide poisoning in this setting can be prevented by the concomitant administration of sodium thiosulfate.

DIFFERENTIAL DIAGNOSIS

Early symptoms may be confused with anxiety or hyperventilation, which are common after nontoxic exposures. Development of more serious clinical signs differentiates these benign conditions from true cyanide poisoning. Hydrogen sulfide and sodium azide poisoning may cause similar findings, and diabetic decompensation has been initially suspected in patients who were later found to have ingested cyanide.

Cyanide poisoning should be suspected in patients with rapid development of unexplained coma, seizures, elevated anion gap metabolic acidosis, and intractable hypotension. Severe hypoxic signs in the absence of cyanosis also suggest the diagnosis.[8]

The following laboratory values may suggest the diagnosis when no history is available:[6,8,12,20] elevated serum lactate level, elevated anion gap metabolic acidosis, relatively normal pO_2 in ventilating patients, and an elevated peripheral venous pO_2 (greater than 40 mm Hg) or decreased arteriovenous O_2 saturation difference (central venous or mixed pulmonary artery O_2 saturation greater than 70% with a relatively normal co-oximeter–measured arterial O_2 saturation), owing to decreased tissue oxygen extraction from the blood. Hydrogen sulfide and sodium azide poisoning can also cause this combination of laboratory findings.[8,11,12] Patients exposed to hydrogen sulfide may have the odor of sulfur or "rotten eggs" on the body or clothes or in a freshly drawn tube of blood.[11]

EMERGENCY DEPARTMENT EVALUATION

Whenever possible, the history should include the specific compound involved, route of exposure, any decontamination measures already undertaken, possible dose, time since ingestion or exposure, and any preexisting allergies or chronic medical conditions. Initial physical examination should focus on vital signs (monitored frequently and serially) and the respiratory, cardiovascular, and central nervous systems. The cardiac rhythm should be continuously monitored.

Determination of serum electrolytes (with calculation of the anion gap), blood glucose levels, pulse oximetry, arterial blood gas analysis, chest radiography, and 12-lead electrocardiography should be done initially and monitored frequently if clinical signs or symptoms of cyanide poisoning are present. Whole blood cyanide levels can be measured, but these determinations usually take hours or days to obtain, and thus cannot be used to guide emergent diagnosis or treatment. They are useful only to document exposure.

EMERGENCY DEPARTMENT MANAGEMENT

Rescuers must not enter areas of potential cyanide gas exposure without a self-contained positive-pressure breathing apparatus.[8] Mouth-to-mouth resuscitation should be avoided, if at all possible. If it is unavoidable, rescuers must be careful not to inhale the victim's expired air. Prehospital care consists of airway management, administration of 100% supplemental oxygen, cardiac monitoring, placement of at least one large-bore intravenous line, administration of sodium bicarbonate if hypotension (and, presumably, metabolic acidosis) is present, decontamination of exposed skin or eyes, and administration of standard anticonvulsant or antiarrhythmic medications, if indicated. If intravenous access cannot be established or in severe poisoning cases, amyl nitrite pearls may be given by inhalation (broken in gauze and held close to the nose and mouth of spontaneously breathing patients or placed into the lips of the face mask or inside the ventilation bag in apneic patients) for 30 seconds out of each minute, using a fresh pearl every 3 to 4 minutes.[2,15,19]

Exposed skin or eyes should be copiously flushed with water. Contaminated clothing should be removed and isolated. Induced emesis must be avoided, because rapid progression to coma or seizures with potential pulmonary aspiration of gastric contents may occur. Activated charcoal has decreased mortality in experimental cyanide poisoning,[14] and 1 g may bind as much as 35 mg of cyanide.[1] An activated charcoal dose of 1 g/kg should be administered to patients who have ingested cyanide.

Supportive measures alone may be satisfactory treatment for some patients, although supportive therapy and specific antidotes have resulted in survival with higher whole blood cyanide levels.[8] Standard anticonvulsant and antiarrhythmic medications should be administered when clinically indicated. Pulse oximetry or arterial blood gases should be monitored and metabolic acidosis corrected with sodium bicarbonate. Pulse oximetry may be unreliable following administration of methemoglobin-inducing nitrite antidotes. Usually, less sodium bicarbonate is required when specific antidotes are administered.

Patients with coma, seizures, apnea, acidosis, or hypotension should be administered specific antidotes. Once intravenous access has been established, amyl nitrite inhalation should be discontinued and sodium nitrite administered intravenously. The dose is one 10-mL ampule (300 mg) of a 3% solution for adults and 0.12 to 0.33 mL/kg (3.6 to 9.9 mg/kg) for children. Sodium nitrite is a potent vasodilator; rapid administration may result in severe hypotension, which can be avoided by slow infusion. Sodium nitrite is administered by slow intravenous push over no less than 5 minutes, unless the patient is in cardiac arrest. It can be diluted in 50 to 100 mL of 5% dextrose in water. The infusion is begun slowly, with frequent blood pressure monitoring, and then increased to the most rapid infusion rate not causing hypotension. Rarely, sodium nitrite may induce excessive methemoglobinemia.[8] Methemoglobin levels should be monitored, especially if multiple doses of sodium nitrite are required, and should be kept less than 30% of total hemoglobin.

Sodium nitrite should be followed by intravenous sodium thiosulfate in a dose of one 50-mL ampule (12.5 g) of a 25% solution for adults or 1.65 mL/kg for children. When used as a cyanide poisoning antidote, no significant adverse effects due to sodium thiosulfate infusion have been reported.

Second doses of sodium nitrite and thiosulfate at one-half the initial amounts may be given 30 minutes later if there is incomplete clinical response. Continued metabolic release of cyanide from cyanogenic glycosides or aliphatic nitrile compounds may cause prolonged poisoning, necessitating multiple antidote doses.[6,8] Repeated doses or a continuous infusion (1 g/h) of sodium thiosulfate (without further sodium nitrite) should be considered in such cases.[6,10]

When available, hydroxocobalamin is administered in a dose of 4 to 5 g intravenously over 20 to 30 minutes.[2,3,5,8] Sodium thiosulfate in the preceding doses may be infused after hydroxocobalamin is given.[7]

Hyperbaric oxygen therapy may be useful in patients unresponsive to supportive and antidotal therapy.[3,17] Smoke inhalation victims (see Chapter 396) may have significant cyanide as well as carbon monoxide poisoning.[2] Inducing methemoglobinemia could be dangerous in this setting. When hyperbaric oxygen therapy is available, it is suggested that sodium thiosulfate be given first, with administration of sodium nitrite only while the smoke inhalation victim is receiving hyperbaric oxygen therapy. Extracorporeal elimination procedures such as hemodialysis and hemoperfusion have no place in the treatment of acute cyanide poisoning.

DISPOSITION

Consultation with a clinical toxicologist or regional poison center can be invaluable in guiding therapy. Physicians admitting cyanide-poisoned patients should be skilled in intensive care medicine.

Asymptomatic cyanide-exposed patients should be observed in a controlled setting for a minimum of 4 to 6 hours. With aliphatic nitrile and cyanogenic glycoside exposure, the observation period should be extended to 12 hours.[6,8] Mildly symptomatic patients can be observed in the emergency department until symptoms resolve. Those requiring antidote administration should be admitted to an intensive care unit until all symptoms have resolved, or for a minimum of 24 hours.

A few survivors of acute cyanide poisoning have developed parkinsonian-like states or more subtle neuropsychiatric deficits.[8,13] Outpatient follow-up should be arranged for patients with significant acute toxicity to screen for these rare sequelae.

If transfer is necessary, the most rapid means available should be used. Accompanying personnel should be able to initiate intravenous access, perform endotracheal intubation and mechanical ventilation, and administer specific antidotes as well as sodium bicarbonate and standard anticonvulsant and antiarrhythmic medications.

ACKNOWLEDGMENT

The author gratefully acknowledges the contribution of Barry H. Rumack who wrote the previous version of this chapter.

COMMON PITFALLS

- Failure to stock an in-date cyanide antidote kit in the emergency department or other readily available location
- Failure to consider the diagnosis of cyanide poisoning in patients with sudden-onset coma, cardiovascular collapse, or metabolic acidosis of unknown etiology
- Inappropriate antidote administration to a hemodynamically stable, conscious patient
- Failure to administer antidotes to patients with more serious symptomatology
- Rapid administration of sodium nitrite, resulting in hypotension
- Administration of adult doses of cyanide antidotes to children
- Failure to monitor methemoglobin levels in patients receiving sodium nitrite, especially in children or when multiple doses are given

References

1. Anderson AH. Experimental studies on the pharmacology of activated charcoal. *Acta Pharmacol* 1946;2:69.
2. Baud FJ, Barriot P, Toffis V, et al. Elevated blood cyanide concentrations in victims of smoke inhalation. *N Engl J Med* 1991;325:1761.
3. Beasley DMG, Glass WY. Cyanide poisoning: pathophysiology and treatment recommendations. *Occup Med* 1998;48:427–431.
4. Espinoza OB, Perez M, Ramirez MS. Bitter cassava poisoning in eight children: a case report. *Vet Hum Toxicol* 1992;34:65.
5. Forsyth JG, Mueller PD, Becker CE, et al. Hydroxocobalamin as a cyanide antidote: safety, efficacy and pharmacokinetics in heavily smoking normal volunteers. *Clin Toxicol* 1993;31:277–294.
6. Geller RJ, Ekins BR, Iknoian RC. Cyanide toxicity from acetonitrile-containing false nail remover. *Am J Emerg Med* 1991;9:268.
7. Hall AH, Rumack BH. Hydroxycobalamin/sodium thiosulfate as a cyanide antidote. *J Emerg Med* 1987;5:115–121.
8. Hall AH, Rumack BH. Cyanide and related compounds. In: Haddad LM, Shannon MW, Winchester JF, eds. *Clinical management of poisoning and drug overdose*, 3rd ed. Philadelphia: WB Saunders, 1998:899–905.
9. Hall AH, Linden CH, Kulig KW, et al. Cyanide poisoning from laetrile: role of nitrite therapy. *Pediatrics* 1986;78:269.
10. Heintz B, Bock TA, Kierdorf H, et al. Cyanid-intoxikation: Behandlung mit Hiperoxigenation und Natriumthiosulfat. *Dtsch Med Wochenschr* 1990;115:1100.
11. Hoidal CR, Hall AH, Robinson MD, et al. Hydrogen sulfide poisoning from toxic inhalations of roofing asphalt fumes. *Ann Emerg Med* 1986;15:826.
12. Johnson RP, Mellors JW. Arteriolization of venous blood gases: a clue to the diagnosis of cyanide poisoning. *J Emerg Med* 1988;6:401.
13. Kales SN, Dinklage D, Dickey J, et al. Paranoid psychosis after exposure to cyanide. *Arch Environ Health* 1997;52:245–246.
14. Lambert RJ, Kindler BL, Schaeffer DJ. The efficacy of superactivated charcoal in treating rats exposed to a lethal oral dose of potassium cyanide. *Ann Emerg Med* 1988;17:595.
15. Linakis JG, Lacouture PG, Woolf A. Monitoring cyanide and thiocyanate concentrations during infusion of sodium nitroprusside in children. *Pediatr Cardiol* 1991;12:214.
16. Litovitz TL, Klein-Schwartz W, Dyer KS, et al. 1997 Annual report of the American Association of Poison Control Centers Toxic Exposure Surveillance System. *Am J Emerg Med* 1998;16:443–497.
17. Meyer GW, Hart GB, Strauss MB. Hyperbaric oxygen therapy for acute smoke inhalation injuries. *Postgrad Med* 1991;89:221.
18. Suchard JR, Wallace KL, Gerkin RD. Acute cyanide toxicity caused by apricot kernal ingestion. *Ann Emerg Med* 1998;32:742–744.
19. Wurzburg H. Treatment of cyanide poisoning in an industrial setting. *Vet Hum Toxicol* 1996;38:44–47.
20. Yen D, Tsai ZJ, Wang L-M, et al. The clinical experience of acute cyanide poisoning. *Am J Emerg Med* 1995;13:524–528.

CHAPTER 332
Digitalis Poisoning

Richard D. Gerkin, Jr. and Thomas J. Higgins, Jr.

The term *digitalis* originally referred to the dried leaf of the *Digitalis purpurea* plant (foxglove). It is now used as a generic term to designate all cardiac glycoside (CG) drugs. CGs are found in the leaves and seeds of a variety of plants and in the skin, salivary glands, and venom glands of toads of the *Bufo* species (Table 332.1). Digoxin is the only digitalis preparation in common therapeutic use in the United States. It is used in the treatment of congestive heart failure and for certain dysrhythmias, such as atrial fibrillation or flutter and supraventricular tachycardia. CGs have a narrow therapeutic window, a characteristic that leads to frequent toxicity. Digitalis toxicity is believed to occur in 5% to 20% of all patients being treated with digitalis, and 30% of those taking CGs who are admitted to the hospital exhibit some degree of toxicity.[11]

CGs inhibit the sodium–potassium adenosine triphosphatase (ATPase) membrane pump found in cardiac cells.[2] This leads to an elevation of intracellular sodium and calcium and the loss of

TABLE 332.1. Sources of Cardiac Glycosides

Genus and Species	Common Name	Part Used
Digitalis purpurea	Purple foxglove	Leaf
Digitalis lanata	Grecian foxglove	Leaf
Strophanthus kombé		Seed
Strophanthus gratis		Seed
Urginea maritima (squill)	Sea onion	Bulb
Nerium oleander	Oleander	All parts
Thevetia neriifolia	Yellow oleander	All parts
Convallaria majalis	Lily of the valley	All parts
Bufo spp.	Toad	Skin

potassium. Magnesium is an essential cofactor for the sodium-potassium ATPase pump and may also have direct effects on membrane calcium and potassium transport.[13] The electrophysiologic effects of CGs include a decrease in the refractory period of atrial and ventricular myocardial cells, leading to improved conduction. Phase 4 of the action potential in most myocardial tissue is increased, leading to an increase in automaticity. A lowering of resting membrane potential leads to more excitability. There is an augmenting of vagal tone and a prolongation of phase 3 of the action potential in the atrioventricular (AV) node and the His-Purkinje system. The other major effect is an increase in inotropic function in the myocardium due to the amount of calcium available for the myofibrils.

The therapeutic daily dose of digoxin ranges from about 0.005 mg/kg in premature infants to as much as 0.75 mg in adults. The absorption of digoxin tablets is 70% to 80%, with capsules being 95% bioavailable. An initial small volume of distribution leads to high blood levels early after ingestion. Actual volume of distribution is about 10 L/kg in adults and more in children. The elimination half-life is about 1.5 days with renal excretion. Protein binding is only 25%.

Serum digoxin levels are measured by radioimmunoassay. Normal levels are 0.5 to 2.0 ng/mL. Some patients are toxic at levels in this range, and others manifest no toxicity at levels greater than 2.0 ng/mL. Drug levels drawn less than 8 hours after a dose, during the distribution phase, do not reflect tissue levels, and hence do not correlate with effects. Following acute ingestion, the serum digoxin level merely verifies that an ingestion has occurred: A level as high 10 ng/mL 2 hours after ingestion may be seen without significant clinical toxicity.

Oleander and *Bufo* toxins can result in an apparent or false-positive digoxin level on radioimmunoassay. In both of these instances, there appears to be partial cross-reactivity in the assay, but levels have not been correlated with toxicity. There may or may not be cross reactivity between monoclonal digoxin assays and other nondigoxin cardiac glycosides. Endogenous digoxin-like steroidal substances (EDLS), which also cross-react with digoxin assays and yield false-positive results, may be present in patients with renal insufficiency, hepatic disease, hypertension, agonal states, and pregnancy, and in premature and full-term infants.[14] Levels are usually low, but have been measured above 2.0 ng/mL. Digoxin assays can lead to large errors in excess of 50% above the true level in children with EDLS.

With therapeutic doses, the QT interval may be shortened and the PR interval relatively prolonged on the electrocardiogram (ECG). The "digitalis effect," with downsloping ST segments giving a scooped appearance, may also be noted. In atrial fibrillation, there is a slowing of the ventricular response.

Toxicity results from an exaggeration of therapeutic effects. Adverse effects may also be due to coronary vasoconstriction.[16] Excessive suppression of pacemaker function may lead to bradyarrhythmia, and increased automaticity may lead to atrial, junctional, and ventricular tachyarrhythmias (Table 332.2). Adolescents appear to be more sensitive to the toxic effects of digoxin than are younger children. In one study, ventricular ectopy was often the earliest sign of digoxin toxicity in adults, whereas sinus bradycardia and AV block were the initial dysrhythmias in children.[18] In another study, there did not appear to be any age-related differences in patients with life-threatening toxicity.[19]

Digoxin toxicity may be chronic or acute. In chronic ingestion, there is a narrow therapeutic range, with toxic amounts being only two to three times therapeutic doses. Most instances of chronic toxicity occur in the elderly. It is frequently associated with hypokalemia, which tends to exacerbate tachyarrhythmias. Chronic intoxication is associated with ventricular dysrhythmias, atrial tachycardia, and junctional tachycardia. Exercise-induced ventricular tachycardia was reported in a patient with coexisting valvular heart disease, which itself can result in oversensitivity to digoxin.[8] Many other factors are known to contribute to or predispose the patient to toxicity (Tables 332.3 and 332.4).

Acute toxicity is most often associated with an accidental or intentional massive ingestion. It is more likely to be associated with hyperkalemia, because there is massive poisoning of the sodium–potassium ATPase pump, leading to accumulation of potassium in the extracellular space. In healthy adults, single acute doses of less than 5 mg of digoxin seldom cause severe

TABLE 332.2. Digitalis-Induced Dysrhythmias

Bradyarrhythmias	Tachyarrhythmias
Sinus exit block or sinus arrest	Atrial tachycardia with block
Sinus bradycardia	Junctional tachycardia
Atrioventricular nodal block: first degree; second degree, type 1; third degree	Ventricular premature beats
	Ventricular tachycardia, especially bidirectional
	Ventricular fibrillation

TABLE 332.3. Conditions Contributing to Digoxin Toxicity

- Advanced age
- Renal impairment
- Hypoxia
- Myocardial ischemia
- Hypothyroidism
- Hypokalemia
- Hypomagnesemia
- Hypercalcemia

TABLE 332.4. Drugs Enhancing Digoxin Toxicity

Causing hypokalemia	Diuretics Amphotericin B Corticosteroids
Increasing sympathetic tone	Beta agonists Theophylline
Increasing atrioventricular nodal block	Beta blockers Verapamil Diltiazem
Increasing serum digoxin level	Quinidine Verapamil Amiodarone Propafenone Erythromycin Tetracycline Itraconazole

toxicity, and fatal doses are almost always greater than 10 mg. In this setting, sinus bradycardia and varying degrees of AV block occur, with fewer ventricular dysrhythmias.

CLINICAL PRESENTATION

Nausea and vomiting are often present. In chronic toxicity, confusion, lethargy, depression, fatigue, headache, paresthesias, weakness, scotomata, and disturbances of color vision, especially xanthopsia (yellow vision), are also common.

Many dysrhythmias can occur (see Table 332.2). The most common is ventricular premature contractions. The combination of any tachyarrhythmia with any type of block (e.g., paroxysmal atrial tachycardia with AV block; regularization of the ventricular response to atrial fibrillation due to AV block with a junctional escape rhythm) is highly suggestive is of CG toxicity. In 150 patients with acute ingestions, life-threatening complications were high-grade AV block (53%), refractory ventricular tachycardia (46%), hyperkalemia (37%), and ventricular fibrillation (33%).[1] Hypotension suggests a hemodynamically significant dysrhythmia, loss of vasomotor regulation, or the presence of coingestant.

The overall mortality rate varies with different studies but is probably about 10%. In those with suicidal or accidental ingestions, mortality ranges from 13% to 25%.[11] Ventricular tachycardia is associated with a 50% mortality rate. Other risk factors include advanced age, heart disease, male sex, high-degree AV block, or hyperkalemia.[12] In acute ingestions, poor prognostic factors are old age, a digoxin level over 15 ng/mL, and hyperkalemia.[3]

Complications such as hypoxic seizures, encephalopathy, loss of vasoregulation, and acute tubular necrosis may result from inadequate tissue perfusion secondary to dysrhythmias.[20]

EMERGENCY DEPARTMENT EVALUATION

The history should include the time, amount, route, duration, and intent of exposure. The presence of conditions and agents that can influence toxicity should be noted. Physical examination should concentrate on the vital signs and assessment of hemodynamic stability. Vital signs should include measurement of the oxygen saturation. The patient should be specifically examined for signs of congestive heart failure and inadequate peripheral perfusion. Cardiac monitoring should be routine. A 12-lead ECG should be performed. Routine laboratory studies include determination of serum electrolytes, calcium, magnesium, blood urea nitrogen, and serum creatinine levels. Serum digoxin level also should be measured. Serial levels should be obtained for at least 12 hours following an acute ingestion. Patients with abnormal cardiac rhythms, hypotension, underlying cardiac disease, or hypoxia should have a chest x-ray and arterial blood gas analysis. Those with chronic intoxication should have liver function tests.

EMERGENCY DEPARTMENT MANAGEMENT

Antidotal therapy with digoxin-specific Fab fragments of sheep IgG antibodies (Digibind) is the treatment of choice for life-threatening bradydysrhythmias. Atropine (initially 0.5 mg intravenously) can be given. Refractory or recurrent bradycardia should be treated with antidotal therapy, which appears to be more effective and safer than electrical cardiac pacing.[15] Although pacing may sometimes be necessary, the pacing wire can irritate the myocardium and precipitate ventricular dysrhythmias, and this therapy should not delay definitive therapy with Fab fragments.

Antidotal therapy is also the definitive treatment for life-threatening ventricular tachyarrhythmias. Intravenous phenytoin (25 mg/min until a desired effect is reached or about 15 mg/kg has been given) and lidocaine (1 mg/kg) can be given initially. Magnesium sulfate (2 to 3 g intravenously over 1 minute) may also be effective.[7] Refractory digoxin–induced cardiac dysrhythmias have responded to magnesium infusions (2 g/h for 4 to 5 hours).[20] Because serum magnesium represents less than 1% of the total body magnesium pool, it should be assumed that hypomagnesemia exists at the cellular level, even if the serum magnesium level is normal.[14] As usual, pulseless rhythms require defibrillation or cardioversion. Cardioversion of ventricular tachycardia is risky in digitalis toxicity because it may result in ventricular fibrillation. If possible, drug therapy should be tried first. When necessary, cardioversion should initially be performed at reduced power settings, for example, at 5 or 10 watt-seconds.

Fab fragments are indicated for life-threatening or hemodynamically compromising dysrhythmias, when standard therapy fails, and when hyperkalemia (serum potassium greater than or equal to 5.5 mEq/L) occurs after acute overdose. An elevated digoxin level is useful only to confirm toxicity and should not be used as the sole criterion for use of the Fab fragments. The prophylactic use of Fab for patients with non–life-threatening dysrhythmias and risk factors for severe toxicity has been advocated but remains to be proven.[15] In one cost analysis, even patients who did not have life-threatening dysrhythmias had lower medical costs when treated with Fab fragments.[11] In addition, older patients appear to respond to Fab fragments as well as younger patients do.[9]

The Fab fragments are given intravenously over 30 minutes unless the patient is in cardiac arrest, when it can be given as a bolus. The dosage (in vials) is estimated by dividing the acutely ingested dose in milligrams (body load) by 0.6 mg per vial. Each vial contains 38 mg of Fab fragments, with each milligram binding 0.015 mg of digoxin. The usual initial dose for acute overdose is 5 to 10 vials. In chronic toxicity, the body load in milligrams can be estimated by multiplying the steady-state serum concentration of digoxin by 5.6 times the patient's weight in kilograms divided by 1,000. The usual initial dose for chronic poisoning is 1 to 2 vials. Because Fab fragments cross-react weakly with other CGs, larger doses may be needed for toxicity involving digitoxin, oleander, or *Bufo* toxins.[4–6,12] A response is usually noted within 30 minutes of Fab administration, but it may take several hours to see the maximal effect. Doses should be repeated if there is no clinical improvement in 1 hour.

Theoretically, skin testing should be performed before treatment with Fab fragments. The necessity of this practice, however, is questionable. In a study of 717 adults with digitalis intoxication who were treated with Fab, only six had adverse reactions that may have been due to components of the antibody preparation, and all reactions were benign. In addition, nearly all patients with reactions have negative skin tests; antibodies to Fab have not been detected in such patients, and the risk of delaying Fab therapy in order to perform skin testing far outweighs the risks of an adverse reaction to Fab. It may be important to perform skin testing, however, in patients repeatedly treated with Fab fragments.[10] No case of serum sickness has been reported.

After using Fab fragments, the serum digoxin level measured by most radioimmunoassays rises because the drug is pulled out of tissue to bind with the antibodies, and the assays measure both bound and unbound drug. The free digoxin level, which can be measured only by equilibrium dialysis or ultrafiltration to remove protein, is very low if the appropriate amount of antibodies are administered. The elimination half-life of the drug–antibody complex, which is excreted renally, is about 16 hours in patients with normal renal function and 4 days in those with renal failure. A rebound increase in free digoxin, presumably due to metabolic degradation of the drug–antibody complex, may occur within 24 hours of Fab administration in patients with normal renal function and up to 8 days after Fab in those with renal failure, but recurrent clinical toxicity is rare.[17]

Activated charcoal is the preferred method of gastrointestinal decontamination for patients with acute ingestions. Vagal effects associated with vomiting and gastric lavage might worsen CG toxicity in patients with bradycardia. Subsequent doses of activated charcoal are effective in shortening the elimination half-life of digoxin, digitoxin, and probably the CGs. Resin binders such as cholestyramine are no more effective than charcoal. Elimination cannot be enhanced by increasing urine flow or by peritoneal dialysis, hemodialysis, or hemoperfusion.

Patients with altered mental status (either secondary to toxicity from digoxin or coingestants) may require endotracheal intubation for airway protection or mechanical ventilation. Hypoxia, acid–base abnormalities, and fluid and electrolyte disturbances should be corrected. Caution is advised when giving potassium to hypokalemic patients with chronic intoxication and renal failure. Hyperkalemia associated with acute overdose is a consequence rather than a cause of poisoning and should be treated with Fab. Temporizing measures include intravenous sodium bicarbonate, glucose and potassium, and inhaled beta agonists. Calcium may enhance CG toxicity and should be avoided. Because hyperkalemia reflects a change in potassium distribution and not total body overload, exchange resins, which can lead to subsequent potassium depletion and consequent problems, should also be used with caution.

DISPOSITION

When the use of Fab fragments is considered, consultation with a poison center, toxicologist, or cardiologist is advised. Patients who are acutely symptomatic or who have elevated digoxin levels and those with significant dysrhythmias should be admitted to an intensive care unit. Those with chronic intoxication who are hemodynamically stable and do not require active treatment can be admitted to a telemetry unit. If Fab fragments and pacemaker therapy are not available, patients should be transferred by advanced life-support personnel (or mobile intensive care unit, if available) to the nearest center that possesses these treatment modalities.

COMMON PITFALLS

- Failure to appreciate that a serum digoxin level drawn less than 8 hours after ingestion does not reflect toxicity or need for treatment
- Failure to recognize that CG toxicity can result from exposure to nonprescription products such as herbals or teas
- Failure to recognize that digoxin immunoassays may or may not yield a measurable digoxin level with plant or *Bufo* toxin exposures
- Failure to appreciate the differences between acute and chronic toxicity
- Failure to use Fab fragments for potentially life-threatening dysrhythmias and for hyperkalemia after an acute ingestion
- Failure to correct electrolyte abnormalities, especially those that involve potassium
- Failure to initially use low-power settings for cardioversion of tachyarrhythmias

ACKNOWLEDGMENT

The author gratefully acknowledges the contribution of Frank A. Agnone who wrote the previous version of this chapter.

References

1. Bayer MJ. Recognition and management of digitalis intoxication: implications for emergency medicine. *Am J Emerg Med* 1991;9[Suppl]:29.
2. Bigger JT. Digitalis toxicity. *J Clin Pharmacol* 1985;25:514.
3. Bismuth C. Hyperkalemia in acute digitalis poisoning: prognostic implications and therapeutic implications. *Clin Toxicol* 1973;6:153.
4. Brubacher JR, Ravikumar PR., Bania T, et al. Treatment of toad venom poisoning with digoxin-specific Fab fragments. *Chest* 1996;110(5):1282–1288.
5. Brubacher JR, Lachmanen D, Ravikumar PR, et al. Efficacy of digoxin specific Fab fragments (Digibind®) in the treatment of toad venom poisoning. *Toxicon* 1999;37:931–942.
6. Clark RF, Selden BS, Curry SC. Digoxin-specific Fab fragments in the treatment of oleander toxicity in a canine model. *Am J Emerg Med* 1991;20:1073.
7. French JH. Magnesium therapy in massive digitalis intoxication. *Ann Emerg Med* 1984;13:562.
8. Gosselink ATM, Cruns HGJM, Wiesfeld ACP, et al. Exercise-induced ventricular tachycardia: a rare manifestation of digitalis toxicity. *Clin Cardiol* 1993;16:270.
9. Hickey AR, Wenger TL, Carpenter VP, et al. Antibody therapy in the management of digitalis intoxication: safety and efficacy results of an observational surveillance study. *J Am Coll Cardiol* 1991;17:590.
10. Kirkpatrick CH. The Digibind Study Advisory Panel. Allergic histories and reactions of patients treated with digoxin immune Fab (ovine) antibody. *Am J Emerg Med* 1991;9[Suppl]:7.
11. Mauskopf JA, Wenger TL. Cost-effectiveness analysis of the use of digoxin immune Fab (ovine) for treatment of digoxin toxicity. *Am J Cardiol* 1991;68:1709.
12. Shumaik GK. Oleander poisoning: treatment with digoxin-specific Fab antibody fragments. *Am Emerg Med* 1988;17:732.
13. Specter MJ, Schweizer E, Goldman RG. Studies on magnesium's mechanism of action in digitalis-induced arrhythmias. *Circulation* 1975;52:1001.
14. Stone J, Bentur Y, Zalstein E, et al. Effect of endogenous digoxin-like substances on the interpretation of high concentrations of digoxin in children. *J Pediatr* 1990;117:321.
15. Taboulet P, Baud FJ, Bismuth C. Clinical features and management of digitalis poisoning—rationale for immunotherapy. *J Toxicol Clin Toxicol* 1993;31(2):247.
16. Tanz RD. Possible contribution of digitalis-induced coronary constriction in toxicity. *Am Heart J* 1986;111:812.
17. Wenger TL. Experience with digoxin immune Fab (ovine) in patients with renal impairment. *Am J Emerg Med* 1991;9[Suppl]:21.
18. Wolff AD, Wenger T, Smith TW, et al. The use of digoxin-specific Fab fragments for severe digitalis intoxication in children. *N Engl J Med* 1992;326:1739.
19. Wofford JL, Hickey AR, Ettinger WH, et al. Lack of age-related differences in the clinical presentation of digoxin toxicity. *Arch Intern Med* 1992;152:2261.
20. Yound IS, Goh EMS, McKillop UH, et al. Magnesium status and digoxin toxicity. *Br J Clin Pharmacol* 1991;32:717.

CHAPTER 333
Disk Battery Exposures

Toby L. Litovitz

In 1998, 1,946 button battery ingestions were reported to U.S. poison centers and logged into the American Association of Poison Control Centers Toxic Exposure Surveillance System.[8] Children less than 5 years old are at greatest risk and accounted for 57% of ingestions reported nationally in 1998, with a peak incidence in 1- to 3-year-olds. Six- to 12-year-olds were implicated in 21% of the ingestions, and adults comprised 12% of cases.

Hearing aid batteries are the most commonly ingested button cells, accounting for 46% of battery ingestions (with known source) reported to the National Button Battery Ingestion Hotline and Study during the year ending in June 1999. Games and toys were the second most common source of ingested batteries (19%). Other battery sources included musical, talking, or lighted books, greeting cards, key chains, jewelry, T-shirts, shoes, doormats, teapots, and picture frames; calculators; cameras; clocks; computers; thermometers; flashlights; laser pens and pointers; pagers; phones; remote control devices; and watches.

Nearly 21% of patients ingested the battery after mistaking it for a pill. Five percent of patients ingested the battery while it was in a hearing aid (the aid was also ingested). Unintentional ingestion also occurred while replacing a battery, using the mouth as a "third" hand, and while testing the battery using the ineffective method of placing it in the mouth to determine if there is a "buzz." One percent of cases involved intentional ingestion to avoid incarceration. Suicide attempts occurred in less than 3% of cases. Eight percent of patients swallowed more than one battery.

Most button battery ingestions have a benign clinical course.[8,13] Clinical manifestations of the ingestion occurred in only 9.9% of battery ingestion cases, and most symptoms were gastrointestinal (GI).[8] Sometimes, ingestions of larger cells (greater than 20 mm in diameter, as opposed to the more common 7- to 12-mm button cells) are followed by esophageal lodgment. Disastrous injuries are possible, ranging from minor esophageal burns to permanent esophageal injury that requires colon interposition or recurrent dilatation. Significant esophageal injury may develop in just 2 to 6 hours. At least two fatalities after battery lodgment in the esophagus have occurred in young children in whom the diagnosis of foreign-body ingestion was delayed 24 hours to 4 days.[3,11] Fortunately, most ingested disk batteries rapidly pass to the stomach and then traverse the entire GI tract without complications.

The mechanism of disk battery–induced injury is multifactorial. Leakage of the potassium hydroxide electrolyte from the battery was long accepted as the major mechanism. More recent studies have identified an alternative and possibly primary cause of injury: an external current generated between the cathode and the anode across the battery crimp area. This electric current can pass through tissue, causing hydrolysis of tissue fluids and local hydroxide generation. Thus, both the external electric current mechanism and the leakage theory have a final common denominator: alkaline-type injury to the tissue. A third, less important mechanism involves pressure necrosis of an impacted battery on adjacent tissue. More severe corrosion occurs in the acid medium of the stomach than in the more alkaline intestine.

Despite much concern regarding the role of heavy-metal leakage from button cells in subsequent injury, symptomatic cases of heavy-metal poisoning after battery ingestion have not been reported. In four cases, modestly elevated mercury levels were noted after button cells broke apart or nearly split, leaving radiopaque droplets in the GI tract without clinical manifestations of mercury toxicity.[5,8–10] The theoretic mercury hazard is minimized by the reduction of toxic mercuric oxide released from a split button cell to nearly nontoxic elemental mercury in the presence of gastric acid and iron dissolved from the corroding steel battery can.[2] In addition, in 1996, environmental concerns relating to disposal of mercury-containing batteries led to federal legislation banning the sale of mercuric oxide button cells in the United States. Whereas mercuric oxide button cells were implicated in 25% of ingested batteries in the 1980s, this percentage had declined to 2% by 1998.

CLINICAL PRESENTATION

Most battery ingestions cause no symptoms and pass through the GI tract without consequence. Symptoms are present in only 9.9% of ingestion cases and are generally minor. Most batteries pass within 72 hours, but passage requires more than a week in nearly 5% of cases, and more than 2 weeks in 1% of cases. Extremely delayed passage (up to 596 days) may occur without symptoms or adverse effects when battery transit is arrested distal to the stomach. About 1% of battery ingestion cases report a diffuse, nonspecific rash that may be caused by nickel hypersensitivity, as many button cells are nickel plated. Dietary nickel is a known factor in nickel dermatitis flare-up.[1]

In contrast, a battery that lodges in the esophagus may cause vomiting, fever, dysphagia, odynophagia, tachypnea, and refusal to eat. Failure to promptly remove a battery located in the esophagus may result in tracheoesophageal fistula, tension pneumothorax or hemothorax, or perforation through the aortic arch or its branches, with massive exsanguination and cardiac arrest.

Esophageal lodgment generally follows ingestion of larger cells (20 to 23 mm in diameter), although cells as small as 11.6 mm have caused severe injury after becoming lodged. Preliminary data suggest that lithium cells may pose a greater hazard, causing earlier and more severe symptoms when lodged, due to the higher voltage of these cells. Esophageal burns, perforation, and subsequent stenosis have occurred after battery lodgment of just 2.5 hours. Unfortunately, symptom occurrence alone cannot be used as a reliable indicator of battery position in the esophagus, as patients with batteries lodged in the esophagus may be asymptomatic initially.

A battery in the ear or nose frequently causes injury to surrounding tissue, such as tympanic membrane perforation or destruction, necrosis of the dermis of the external ear canal, destruction of the ossicles, hearing impairment, nasal septal perforation or destruction, nasal turbinate destruction, and atrophic rhinitis.[4,12] Immediate removal of a battery in the ear or nose is essential to prevent severe injury.

DIFFERENTIAL DIAGNOSIS

Most battery ingestors are asymptomatic; thus, the history of ingestion provides the best diagnostic clue. Patients who are symptomatic after ingesting a miniature battery are most frequently misdiagnosed as having a nonspecific flulike illness or upper respiratory tract illness that causes pharyngitis and subsequent dysphagia. Delayed diagnosis is likely to occur in a young child, in the case of an unwitnessed ingestion. If the battery is lodged in the esophagus, presenting symptoms are limited to pain on swallowing, fever, vomiting, and tachypnea.

When a battery is lodged in the nares, the patient is likely to present with unilateral nasal discharge or pain. This presentation mandates evaluation for a nasal foreign body. Sinusitis, trauma, chemical irritants, and upper respiratory infections may produce a similar clinical picture.

A battery in the ear is likely to be discovered when otic discharge or pain is experienced. A thorough examination to exclude a foreign body is imperative. Mastoiditis, acute perforation of the tympanic membrane in otitis media, external otitis, and trauma to the ear canal may have similar presentations.

EMERGENCY DEPARTMENT EVALUATION

Prompt evaluation and definitive management are critical to successful outcomes. All patients suspected of disk battery ingestion or placement in a body cavity must be immediately evaluated to locate the battery. When ingestion is suspected, an x-ray should be obtained to exclude esophageal impaction. When a foreign body in the ear or nose is suspected based on history, pain, or discharge, thorough, direct visualization of these orifices is essential. The type of cell involved may be identified from a replacement battery or product instructions listing the battery's imprint coding. Assistance in identifying a battery, and specific management guidelines, can be obtained by contacting the National Button Battery Ingestion Hotline and Study at 202-625-3333. Please report all cases to enhance identification of emerging product problems and to support changes in clinical management guidelines.

EMERGENCY DEPARTMENT MANAGEMENT

A battery lodged in the esophagus must be removed expeditiously by endoscopy. Any delay could convert a rather benign outcome to a lifelong disability. Emetics are ineffective and should be avoided. Removal with a magnet attached to the end of a nasogastric tube or with a balloon-tipped catheter passed beyond the battery is not recommended. Neither technique allows direct visualization, which is valuable in determining the degree of injury for subsequent management; endoscopic retrieval is less likely to cause esophageal perforation, a complication of blind intubation of the injured esophagus.

If the battery has traveled beyond the esophagus and the patient is asymptomatic, a regular diet and normal activity are advised to promote GI transit. These batteries do *not* need to be retrieved endoscopically or surgically. In routine cases, cathartics, H_2 antagonists, and metoclopramide are withheld; these therapies were investigated in the dog model without significant effect.[6] Observation of the stool for battery passage is recommended. Slow passage of batteries that are clearly beyond the esophagus, in the absence of other symptoms, should not prompt intervention. Battery passage occurred within 24 hours in 23% of cases, within 48 hours in 61%, within 72 hours in 78%, and within 96 hours in 86%.[8] Battery passage required more than 1 week in 5% of cases and more than 2 weeks in 1% of cases.

A battery that appears "hung up" in the bowel (beyond the esophagus) does not require removal, despite its persistence in a single location, as long as the patient remains asymptomatic. These batteries eventually pass. Minor GI symptoms, such as transient vomiting or stool discoloration without blood, are *not* indications for battery retrieval.

A notable exception is a battery 15 mm or more in diameter, especially when ingested by a child younger than 6 years. In these cases, if the battery fails to pass beyond the stomach within 48 hours, perhaps with the added benefit of metoclopramide and an H_2 antagonist, endoscopic removal is advised. Although no longer sold, an older 15.6-mm-diameter mercuric oxide cell is occasionally ingested, and because this type of battery is more likely to split in the GI tract, a known ingestion is an indication for more frequent x-ray evaluation (once or twice weekly). In other cases, if battery passage in the stool is not documented, an x-ray may be taken 1 to 2 weeks after the ingestion; this x-ray frequently shows that passage occurred unnoticed.

Batteries lodged in nasal or ear cavities require urgent removal. Nasal and otic medications should be avoided before battery removal because they bathe the battery in an electrolyte-rich medium and enhance corrosion, leakage, generation of an external current, and local injury. A magnetized instrument can be helpful in the removal process. Sedation and direct visualization through an operating microscope may be required. In this situation, a 1-mm 90-degree pick can be inserted, rotated behind the battery, then retracted. Treatment with nasal decongestants, oral antibiotics for sinusitis, and topical antibiotics for otitis externa should be considered after removal.

DISPOSITION

Batteries lodged in the esophagus, nose, or ear require emergent removal. Subsequent inpatient or outpatient management is determined by the rapidity of intervention and the resulting local injury.

In contrast, patients with ingested batteries located beyond the esophagus who do not have signs or symptoms indicative of significant injury to the GI tract should be managed at home. A regular diet and normal activity will promote GI transit. Stools should be checked to confirm battery passage. Patients with significant symptoms should be evaluated by an endoscopist.

COMMON PITFALLS

- Failure to obtain an x-ray to identify the location of an ingested battery
- Failure to appreciate the fact that patients with esophageal battery lodgment may initially be relatively asymptomatic and symptoms may mimic upper respiratory infections
- Failure to suspect and look for batteries in the ear or nose
- Failure to appreciate that delayed identification and removal of batteries in the ear, nose, and esophagus may cause severe, permanent injuries
- Failure to appreciate that endoscopic or surgical removal is unnecessary and should be avoided in asymptomatic patients who have ingested batteries, including batteries that have split apart, located beyond the esophagus

References

1. Agency for Toxic Substances and Disease Registry. *Toxicologic profile for nickel.* Atlanta: 1988:48.
2. Barber TE, Menke RD. The relationship of ingested iron to the absorption of mercuric oxide. *Am J Emerg Med* 1984;2:500–503.
3. Blatnik BS, Toohill RJ, Lehman RH. Fatal complications from an alkaline battery foreign body in the esophagus. *Ann Otol Rhinol Laryngol* 1977;86:611.
4. Kavanagh KT, Litovitz T. Miniature battery foreign bodies in auditory and nasal cavities. *JAMA* 1986;255:1470.
5. Kulig K, Rumack CM, Rumack BH, et al. Disk battery ingestion: elevated urine mercury levels and enema removal of battery fragments. *JAMA* 1983;249:2502.
6. Litovitz T, Butterfield AB, Holloway RR, et al. Button battery ingestion: assessment of therapeutic modalities and battery discharge state. *J Pediatr* 1984;105:868.
7. Litovitz TL, Klein-Schwartz W, Caravati EM, et al. 1998 Annual report of the American Association of Poison Control Centers Toxic Exposure Surveillance System. *Am J Emerg Med* 1999;17:435.
8. Litovitz TL, Schmitz BF. Ingestion of cylindrical and button batteries: an analysis of 2382 cases. *Pediatrics* 1992;89:747.
9. Mant TGK, Lewis JL, Mattoo TK, et al. Mercury poisoning after disc-battery ingestion. *Hum Toxicol* 1987;6:179.
10. Mofenson HC, Greensher J, Caraccio T, et al. Ingestion of small flat disc batteries. *Ann Emerg Med* 1983;12:88.
11. Shabino CL, Feinberg AN. Esophageal perforation secondary to alkaline battery ingestion. *J Am Coll Emerg Physicians* 1979;8:360.
12. Skinner DW, Chui P. The hazards of button-sized batteries as foreign bodies in the nose and ear. *J Laryngol Otol* 1986;100:1315.
13. Thompson N, Lowe-Ponsford F, Mant TGK, et al. Button battery ingestion: a review. *Adverse Drug React Acute Poison Rev* 1990;9:157.

CHAPTER 334

Disulfiram Poisoning

Edward P. Krenzelok

Disulfiram (Antabuse) is used primarily to deter the use of ethanol in highly motivated alcoholics and those with recidivistic tendencies. Although the ethics of prescribing disulfiram and its efficacy have been questioned, it is still used extensively.[8] Disulfiram is also used in the rubber industry as an antioxidant.

Disulfiram inhibits aldehyde dehydrogenase, thereby inhibiting the metabolism of acetaldehyde, the product of ethanol's metabolism by alcohol dehydrogenase, and causing acetaldehyde to accumulate and produce unpleasant effects. A metabolite of disulfiram, carbon disulfide, may also produce pyridoxine depletion, which may ultimately reduce gamma-aminobutyric acid (GABA) activity and result in the development of seizures (see Chapter 347). Disulfiram also interferes with the conversion of dopamine to norepinephrine, resulting in catecholamine depletion.

Toxicity associated with the use of disulfiram is common and sometimes serious. A disulfiram–ethanol reaction (DER) can be precipitated by ingesting small amounts of ethanol—much less than one drink (one 12-oz beer, a 5-oz glass of wine, or 1 oz of 80-proof liquor). DERs have developed after the ingestion of ethanol-containing products such as liquid cold medicine and mouthwash; the topical use of ethanol-containing products, such as aftershave lotions and even beer shampoo, may produce dermal reactions.

A blood ethanol concentration as low as 5 to 10 mg/dL may precipitate a DER and a full-blown DER is likely to occur when ethanol concentrations reach approximately 50 mg/dL.[5] Alcohol-free beers may contain ethanol in concentrations of less than 0.5%.[13] In a volunteer study, the consumption of six alcohol-free beers in 60 minutes resulted in breathalyzer ethanol concentrations of up to 100 mg/dL.[13] The breathalyzer values were not correlated with blood ethanol concentrations, and it is possible that the results reflected a "mouthwash" effect. However, alcohol-free beers should be regarded as a possible explanation for a DER in a compliant patient. In addition to ethanol, many substances produce disulfiram-like reactions when used in conjunction with ethanol.

Disulfiram is administered in a dosage of 500 mg daily for 1 to 2 weeks, followed by a maintenance regimen of 125 to 500 mg daily thereafter.[5] It is absorbed rapidly and acts quickly. Within 3 to 12 hours, the ingestion of ethanol will result in a DER.[5] Giving test doses of disulfiram and ethanol is not recommended, even under controlled medical supervision, because DERs may be associated with profound morbidity.[17]

Disulfiram is eliminated slowly, and effects may persist for 2 weeks.[5] Thus, a DER may occur well after disulfiram therapy has been discontinued. Up to 20% of the drug is eliminated unchanged in the feces; the rest is eliminated renally as metabolites.[5] Disulfiram should not be prescribed by emergency physicians; the patient needs placement in an alcohol treatment program with continuous follow-up since the medicolegal considerations are too significant.

Disulfiram also produces various adverse drug reactions, but pure overdose is uncommon. American poison centers reported only 636 exposures to disulfiram in 1997.[10] Only 12.3% were adverse reactions. Adverse effects are most prominent during the first 2 to 4 weeks of therapy and include drowsiness and general lethargy, headache, dermatitis, and a sulfur or garlic breath odor. More severe and less common reactions include sensorimotor peripheral neuropathies, psychosis, and hepatitis.

Disulfiram-induced hepatitis is reported to have a very precipitous onset.[4] Orthotopic liver transplantation has been necessitated as a consequence of disulfiram-induced hepatic failure.[14] Psychosis secondary to disulfiram therapy may be more common than thought previously.[12] Irreversible neuropsychiatric impairment has been reported.[16,20] Prenatal exposure to disulfiram has been implicated in the development of fetal malformations.[15] It is difficult to associate a direct teratogenic correlation with disulfiram use, because the concurrent or prior use of ethanol or other substances of abuse is often a complicating variable.

Overdoses of disulfiram represent extensions of the drug's pharmacology and adverse effects. The primary manifestation is central nervous system (CNS) depression, but seizures may occur because of the reduction of endogenous GABA.

CLINICAL PRESENTATION

Most DERs are mild and consist of extensive vasodilation in the head and neck, resulting in notable facial and neck flushing and throbbing, and a throbbing headache. Other common findings include dyspnea, diaphoresis, hyperventilation, nausea, vomiting, diarrhea, tachycardia, hypotension, anxiety, and confusion. Electrocardiogram (ECG) findings include sinus tachycardia with occasional premature atrial contractions, flattening of the T waves, and ST depression.

Symptoms usually begin within 30 minutes of ethanol ingestion and last several hours. Onset has been delayed for up to 12 hours, but rarely. An extended period of lethargy and somnolence may follow the reaction, and recovery without sequelae usually occurs. Intermittent myoclonus was reported as the sole neurologic manifestation of a DER.[18] Severe DERs may result in secondary complications such as dehydration, myocardial infarction, and intracranial hemorrhage, as well as severe respiratory and cardiovascular collapse, profound coma, seizures, and death.

Overdose of only disulfiram results in distinctly different toxidromes in adults and children. Significant overdose in children is associated with a symptom complex similar to that of Reye syndrome, but without elevated ammonia and transaminase levels.[1] Children are extremely susceptible to disulfiram's CNS depressant properties and become ataxic, weak, and lethargic.[1] This state may progress to coma and has a poor prognosis.[1] Serious toxicity in children has been associated with ingestions of as little as 2.5 to 3.25 g.[1] Massive basal ganglia infarction, with persistent neurologic deficits, occurred in a 5-year-old who ingested an estimated 4.75 g of disulfiram.[11]

Overdose in adults may result in excessive nausea and vomiting, mental confusion, and hemodynamic compromise. Although adults may also develop severe encephalopathy after an acute disulfiram overdose, they usually recover without sequelae.[9] Toxic manifestations are most severe within the first 24 hours, but recovery may take several days.

DIFFERENTIAL DIAGNOSIS

Manifestations of the DER, adverse reactions, disulfiram overdose, and interactions between disulfiram and other agents can be difficult to distinguish from the manifestations of alcoholism itself. Specific clues to the DER include a history of alcoholism or disulfiram use, the onset of symptoms within 15 to 30 minutes of ethanol exposure, a positive blood ethanol level, flushing, a sulfur or garlic breath odor, and recovery in about 4 hours.

Disulfiram overdose and DERs should be differentiated from other substances that produce disulfiram-like reactions, from disulfiram side effects and adverse reactions, and from interactions between disulfiram and other medications.

When a DER-like reaction occurs in a person with no history of alcoholism or disulfiram use, investigation must be directed toward medication use, recent dietary habits, and occupation. Agents that can produce disulfiram-like reactions when used in conjunction with ethanol include antimicrobials (e.g., griseofulvin, metronidazole, cephalosporins), oral hypoglycemic agents, monoamine oxidase inhibitors, mushrooms (inky caps [*Coprinus atramentarius*]), and other drugs and industrial chemicals.

Concurrent use of disulfiram with other medications, such as paraldehyde,[5] cotrimoxazole,[7] and tranylcypromine,[2] can precipitate a DER. Concomitant isoniazid use can produce behavioral and neurologic aberrations. A contemporary drug interaction reference text should be used to evaluate patients who are taking disulfiram and experiencing unexplained symptoms.

Chronic disulfiram toxicity is supported by the absence of medical problems prior to the initiation of disulfiram therapy. Psychosis usually results only after high-dose, long-term use. Nonpsychotic catatonic behavior has been linked to chronic disulfiram use.[6] Sensorimotor peripheral neuropathies are more prominent distally and occur after prolonged daily doses of 500 to 3,000 mg. Although not unique to disulfiram, a sulfur or garlic breath odor may establish the suspicion of a disulfiram-related problem in patients with a decreased level of consciousness or in those who are compromised behaviorally. Hepatotoxicity usually occurs 2 weeks to 12 months after therapy begins; it normally resolves promptly after discontinuing therapy. If the medical history fails to reveal the use of disulfiram, many of the symptoms may mistakenly be attributed to chronic alcoholism.

EMERGENCY DEPARTMENT EVALUATION

The history should include alcohol and drug use, the nature of symptoms, and the time between exposure and onset of symptoms. The physician should be persistent in tracing the source of ethanol. The physical examination should focus on vital signs and the skin, chest, abdominal, and neurologic examinations to rule out other pathology or trauma. Cardiac monitoring and an ECG are recommended if the patient is tachycardic or hypotensive or experiencing chest pain, in order to detect ischemia and dysrhythmias.

If a DER is suspected, the presence of ethanol in the blood is strong presumptive evidence. Disulfiram and metabolite concentrations are not readily available on a stat basis, and there is no established correlation between ethanol and disulfiram concentrations and the severity of DERs or patient prognosis in acute and chronic overdosage. Disulfiram interferes with a variety of laboratory tests and can also worsen the electroencephalogram. If disulfiram-induced hepatotoxicity is suspected, alanine aminotransferase is the most sensitive hepatic chemistry screening indicator.[19]

EMERGENCY DEPARTMENT MANAGEMENT

Because the DER can be life-threatening, patients should be transported to the emergency department by ambulance. Basic and advanced life-support measures should be instituted as necessary. Supportive care is the cornerstone of DER management. Profuse vomiting may occur, and the Mallory-Weiss syndrome may develop. Seizures may be treated conventionally with lorazepam, diazepam, and phenytoin.

Hypotension should be managed initially by placing the patient in the Trendelenburg position and giving intravenous crystalloid. Direct-acting pressors such as levarterenol (preferred because of catecholamine depletion) may be necessary in refractory cases. Dysrhythmias, ischemic changes, and metabolic derangements are treated conventionally. There are no specific antidotes to reverse the DER, but the use of glucose, thiamine, and naloxone should be considered in alcoholics with an altered mental status.

Fomepizole effectively inhibits alcohol dehydrogenase[3] and, therefore, may have hypothetical benefit by preventing the metabolism of ethanol to acetaldehyde. Extracorporeal methods of removal have not been useful, but hemodialysis should be considered if the patient has high ethanol concentrations and the reaction is severe and prolonged. Other drug–ethanol reactions are similarly managed.

An acute overdose of disulfiram is also treated supportively. After the patient is stabilized, gastric decontamination should be considered. Activated charcoal is the preferred method. Ipecac syrup is not recommended, because vomiting may lead to aspiration and because syrup of ipecac contains ethanol (1.0% to 2.5%).

DISPOSITION

Most DERs resolve within about 2 to 4 hours and can be managed in the emergency department. Severe DERs may be life-threatening and mandate critical care management. Indications for admission to the intensive care unit include persistent or abnormal vital signs, metabolic derangements, persistent chest pain, and ECG changes (myocardial infarction must be ruled out). Moderate responses in patients with preexisting pathology also dictate admission. Alcoholics should be referred to alcohol rehabilitation or detoxification units once their DERs have resolved. Explicit instructions should be given to avoid all sources of ethanol.

Because of delayed toxicity, all patients with disulfiram overdoses should be admitted for 12 to 24 hours of observation or treatment. Depending on severity, patients suffering from adverse drug reactions may require inpatient monitoring or outpatient follow-up. Overdose patients should be referred for psychiatric evaluation before discharge.

COMMON PITFALLS

- Attributing symptoms of a DER or a disulfiram adverse effect to ethanol or underlying physical and behavioral pathology
- Failure to appreciate that foods, medicines, and "alcohol-free" beverages can be a source ethanol and provoke the DER
- Failure to appreciate that drugs and chemicals other than disulfiram can interact with ethanol and produce a DER-like reaction
- Failure to admit all patients with disulfiram overdosage
- Discharging a patient with a DER before symptoms have resolved
- Prescribing disulfiram or initiating such therapy in the emergency department
- Failure to warn patients with a DER to avoid further exposure to all sources of ethanol

References

1. Benitz WE, Tatro DS. Disulfiram intoxication in a child. *Pediatrics* 1984;105:487.
2. Blansjarr BA, Egberts TCG. Delirium in a patient treated with disulfiram and tranylcypromine. *Am J Psychiatry* 1995;152:296.

3. Brent J, McMartin K, Phillips S, et al. Fomepizole for the treatment of ethylene glycol poisoning. *N Engl J Med* 1999;340:832.
4. Dilts SL, Dilts SL. Assessing liver function before initiating disulfiram therapy. *Am J Psychiatry* 1996;153:1504.
5. Disulfiram. In: McEvoy GK, ed. *American Hospital Formulary Service drug information 1999*. Bethesda, MD: American Society of Hospital Pharmacists, 1999:3257.
6. Fisher CM. "Catatonia" due to disulfiram toxicity. *Arch Neurol* 1989;46:798.
7. Heelon MW, White M. Disulfiram-cotrimoxazole reaction. *Pharmacotherapy* 1998;18:869.
8. Hughes JC, Cook CC. The efficacy of disulfiram: a review of outcome studies. *Addiction* 1997;92:381.
9. Kirubakaran V, Liskow B, Mayfield D, et al. Case report of acute disulfiram overdose. *Am J Psychiatry* 1983;140:1513.
10. Litovitz TL, Klein-Schwartz W, Dyer KS, et al. 1997 Annual report of the American Association of Poison Control Centers Toxic Exposure Surveillance System. *Am J Emerg Med* 1998;16:443.
11. Majahan P, Lieh-Lai MW, Sarnaik A, et al. Basal ganglia infarction in a child with disulfiram poisoning. *Pediatrics* 1997;99:606.
12. Murthy KK. Psychosis during disulfiram therapy for alcoholism. *J Indian Med Assoc* 1997;95:80.
13. Nordt SP, Williams SR, Manoguerra AS, et al. Ethanol analysis following consumption of "alcohol-free" beer. *Vet Hum Toxicol* 1999;41:94.
14. Rabkin JM, Corless CL, Orloff SL, et al. Liver transplantation for disulfiram-induced hepatic failure. *Am J Gastroenterol* 1998;93:830.
15. Reitnauer PJ, Callanan NP, Farber RA, et al. Prenatal exposure to disulfiram implicated in the cause of malformations in discordant monozygotic twins. *Teratology* 1997;56:358.
16. Ryan TV, Sciara AD, Barth JT. Chronic neuropsychological impairment resulting from disulfiram overdose. *J Stud Alcohol* 1993;54:389.
17. Sevas MC. Disulfiram-ethanol test reaction: significance of supervision. *Ann Pharmacother* 1997;31:374.
18. Syed J, Moarefi G. An unusual presentation of a disulfiram-alcohol reaction. *Del Med J* 1995;67:183.
19. Wright C, Moore RD, Grodin DM, et al. Screening for disulfiram-induced liver test dysfunction in an inpatient alcoholism program. *Alcoholism* 1993;17:184.
20. Zorzon M, Mase G, Biasutti E, et al. Acute encephalopathy and polyneuropathy after disulfiram intoxication. *Alcohol Alcohol* 1995;30:629.

CHAPTER 335

Dystonic Reactions

Mary A. McCormick and
Anthony S. Manoguerra

Dystonic reactions are seldom life-threatening, but the pain and discomfort of the bodily contortions that develop often prompt the victim to seek help in the emergency department. *Acute dystonias* (acute dyskinesias), along with parkinsonism and akathisia, are considered extrapyramidal manifestations of antipsychotic and other drug administration. These effects appear early and are reversible with reduction or discontinuation of the antipsychotic medication. *Tardive dyskinesia* refers to the sometimes irreversible involuntary movements that develop later. *Primary dystonia,* abnormal movements that occur spontaneously in the absence of drug treatment, is a separate diagnosis with similar manifestations. Dystonias may begin during infancy, childhood, adolescence, or adulthood for both the primary and secondary or environmentally produced types.[13]

Dystonias of all types probably result from an abnormality of neurotransmitter function in the basal ganglia. Several specific mechanisms have been proposed for those that are drug-induced. According to one theory, they are due to direct blockade of central dopaminergic receptors. Another theory proposes that the underlying mechanism involves both dopamine and acetylcholine, with an imbalance of neurotransmitters resulting in excessive cholinergic activity. A third theory holds that acute dystonic reactions may be caused by a combination of dopamine blockade and dopamine activation in the nigrostriatal system. The delay in onset of acute dystonias after the administration of antipsychotic medication may be explained by this mechanism. Dopamine synthesis and release have been shown to increase in response to an initial blockade of dopamine receptors. A single dose of an antipsychotic drug has also produced supersensitivity of dopamine receptors 24 to 48 hours after drug administration. This occurs at a time when plasma and red-cell drug concentrations are actually falling. Therefore, enhanced dopamine release, occurring simultaneously with the unblocking of supersensitive receptors, may result in acute dystonias.[14]

The true incidence of dystonia is unknown, but it occurs in about 2% of patients treated with phenothiazines and in about 25% of patients treated with haloperidol and the depot phenothiazines. Half of these dyskinesias develop within 48 hours, and 85% are apparent within 4 days of initiation of therapy. Such reactions are more common in men than in women.[13]

The patient who presents to the emergency department with a drug-induced dystonic reaction will probably be a young male, manifesting a buccolingual or torticollar reaction. The presence of a piperazine side chain attached to the phenothiazine nucleus increases the likelihood that a compound will produce a dystonic reaction. Symptoms seem to develop earlier with haloperidol than with other neuroleptics. The development of a dystonic reaction depends more on individual susceptibility than on the chemical structure, milligram potency, dosage, or duration of treatment. The drugs currently known or suspected to produce acute dystonic reactions are listed in Table 335.1.

Patients under age 15 and those with a family history of dystonia are at greatest risk of developing drug-induced dystonias. Another factor that may predispose a patient to dystonic reactions is a history of drug abuse (especially cocaine) or alcohol use.[14]

CLINICAL PRESENTATION

Any striated muscle group may be involved in a dystonic movement. Blepharospasm, progressing to oculogyric crisis, is the most common form of dystonia in the upper face. It usually begins with increased blinking of the eyelids. The muscles of the lower jaw most commonly involved are those of the pharynx and tongue. The term *oromandibular dystonia* describes the involvement of any combination of these muscles. Specifically, mandibular dystonia is manifested as a pulling down or up of the jaw. Lingual dystonia may present as either a sustained protrusion of the tongue or an upward deflection so that the tongue curves and touches the hard palate. In the neck region, torticollis is most common, although retrocollis and anterocollis may also occur. In most cases, the shoulder is elevated on the side toward which the chin is pointing. Jerking, rhythmic movements of the head may also occur. When the trunk is involved, twisting movements and postures such as lordosis, scoliosis, kyphosis, tortipelvis, and opisthotonos develop. Dystonic movements may begin as focal but become segmental as they spread in a contiguous manner. *Generalized dystonia* refers to involvement of the leg plus other body parts, with or without the trunk. Dystonic movements are usually continual, repetitive, and twisting, varying in speed from rapid to slow and being sustained from seconds to minutes at the height of the involuntary contraction.

The prognosis is excellent for patients with drug-induced dystonias when correctly treated. Cardiorespiratory arrest and

TABLE 335.1. Drugs Reported to Have Caused Acute Dystonic Reactions

Generic Name	Brand Name	References	Generic Name	Brand Name	References
WELL DOCUMENTED			**POORLY DOCUMENTED**		
Chlorpromazine	Thorazine	14	Alfentanil	Alfenta	14
Chlorprothixene	Taractan	14	Amphetamine	Benzedrine	7
Fluphenazine	Prolixin	14	Benztropine	Cogentin	14
Haloperidol	Haldol	14	Bethanechol	Urecholine	14
Loxapine	Loxitane	14	Bromocriptine	Parlodel	14
Mesoridazine	Serentil	14	Bupropion	Wellbutrin, Zyban	14
Metoclopramide	Reglan	14	Buspirone[b]	BuSpar	14
Perphenazine	Trilafon	14	Carbamazepine[b]	Tegretol	14
Prochlorperazine	Compazine	14	Cholinesterase inhibitor insecticides	—	14
Promazine	Sparine	14	Copper	—	14
Promethazine	Phenergan	14	Cyanide	—	14
Thiethylperazine	Torecan	14	Dextromethorphan	—	6
Thioridazine	Mellaril	14	Disulfiram	Antabuse	9
Thiothixene	Navane	14	Doxorubicin	Adriamycin	1
Trifluoperazine	Stelazine	14	Ecstasy	—	18
Triflupromazine	Vesprin	14	Ergotamine	—	15
LESS WELL DOCUMENTED			Erythromycin	E.E.S.	14
Amitriptyline	Elavil	14	Etoposide	VePesid	14
Amoxapine	Asendin	14	Flecainide	Tambocor	16
Azatadine	Optimine	14	5-Fluorouracil	Adrucil	1
Cimetidine	Tagamet	14	Levodopa	Bendopa, Dopar	13
Cisapride	Propulsid	2	Meperidine	Demerol	19
Cocaine	—	14	Methylphenidate	Ritalin	5
Clozapine	Clozaril	20	Midazolam	Versed	14
Diazepam	Valium	14	Nifedipine	Adalat, Procardia	14
Diphenhydramine	Benadryl	14	Phenobarbital	Luminal	14
Doxepin	Sinequan	14	Sumatriptan	Imitrex	12
Etomidate	Amidate	14	Trazodone	Desyrel	14
Fluoxetine	Prozac	11, 14	Verapamil[b]	Calan, Isoptin	14
Fluvoxamine	Luvox	3	Antihistamines and decongestants		
Imipramine	Tofranil	14	Chlorpheniramine and phenylpropanolamine		14
Ketamine	Ketalar	14	Pheniramine and phenylephrine		14
Methohexital	Brevital	14			
Olanzapine	Zyprexa	10			
Paroxetine	Paxil	11			
Phenelzine	Nardil	14			
Phenytoin[a]	Dilantin	14			
Pimozide	Orap	4			
Ranitidine	Zantac	8			
Risperidone	Risperdal	17			
Sertraline	Zoloft	11			
Thiopental	Pentothal	10			
Tranylcypromine	Parnate	14			

[a]Symptoms develop at toxic serum concentrations.
[b]Symptoms were of latent onset (tardive dyskinesias).

death have been linked to metoclopramide in a case in which diagnosis and treatment were delayed.

DIFFERENTIAL DIAGNOSIS

Dystonic reactions have been misdiagnosed as tetanus, hysterical conversion, and even seizure disorders. Children with such abnormal movements have been thought to have encephalitis or meningitis.

EMERGENCY DEPARTMENT EVALUATION

The patient, family, or friends should be asked about the recent use of medications. Physical examination is remarkable for abnormal posturing or movements. Urinalysis may provide information about recent drug use in a patient who is unable or unwilling to provide a history.

EMERGENCY DEPARTMENT MANAGEMENT

Because dystonic reactions are not usually associated with drug overdosage, gastrointestinal (GI) decontamination is seldom necessary. Induction of emesis, administration of activated charcoal, or gastric lavage could lead to airway compromise in the patient with abnormal head or neck posturing or swallowing difficulty. In addition, charcoal may prevent the absorption of oral antidotes. If indicated, GI decontamination should be done after the dystonic reaction has been treated.

Administration of an anticholinergic medication rapidly reverses the symptoms, presumably because of restoration of the cholinergic–dopaminergic balance in nigrostriatal neurons.

Diphenhydramine (Benadryl) and benztropine mesylate (Cogentin) are used more often than biperiden (Akineton) or trihexyphenidyl (Artane). Intravenous administration is preferable to intramuscular or oral administration. Symptoms abate within 2 minutes and completely resolve within 15 minutes when the intravenous route is used; muscle relaxation begins in 30 minutes but may not be complete for 90 minutes when the antidote is given intramuscularly or orally. Benztropine has been advocated over diphenhydramine because of fewer side effects and more rapid improvement of both objective and subjective findings, regardless of route. One report describes a patient who responded minimally to multiple doses of diphenhydramine but completely to a subsequent dose of benztropine.[14] Diphenhydramine should be used in children under age 3, because benztropine is contraindicated in this age group. Drowsiness should be anticipated as a side effect of anticholinergic administration, especially with diphenhydramine.

After reversal of the reaction, treatment should continue with an oral agent for 72 hours to prevent a relapse.

The usual dose of benztropine is 1 to 2 mg for adults and 0.02 to 0.05 mg/kg for children age 3 years or older, given intravenously over 2 minutes, followed by the same dose given orally twice a day for 3 days. The dose of diphenhydramine is 50 to 100 mg for adults and 1 to 2 mg/kg for children, given intravenously over 2 minutes, followed by 12.5 to 50.0 mg orally three or four times a day for 3 days. Some patients require more than one dose of intravenous medication to control the reaction.

DISPOSITION

The patient may be discharged after the acute dystonia resolves. Consultation with the prescribing psychiatrist is advisable if the patient is to remain on neuroleptic medication. When anticholinergics are prescribed, patients should be advised not to drive or perform potentially dangerous activities for 72 hours. They should be instructed to return if symptoms recur.

COMMON PITFALLS

- Dystonic reactions may be delayed in onset 12 to 24 hours from the time of drug ingestion.
- The timely administration of an anticholinergic medication may prove to be diagnostic as well as therapeutic.
- Dystonic reactions are not usually the result of an overdose; because of their delayed onset, GI decontamination is seldom indicated and may be dangerous in patients with head or neck involvement.
- Prescribing oral anticholinergic medication for 3 days after acute treatment may prevent relapses.

References

1. Braeshear A, Siemers E. Focal dystonia after chemotherapy: a case series. *J Neurooncol* 1997;34:163–167.
2. Bucci KK, Haverstick DE, Abercrombie SA. Dystonic-like reaction following cisapride therapy. *J Fam Pract* 1995;40:86–88.
3. Chong, SA. Fluvoxamine and mandibular dystonia [Letter]. *Can J Psychiatry* 1995;40:430–431.
4. Ernst M, Gonzalez NM, Campbell M. Acute dystonic reaction with low-dose pimozide. *J Am Acad Child Adolesc Psychiatry* 1993;32:640–642.
5. Gay CT, Ryan SG. Paroxysmal kinesigenic dystonia after methylphenidate administration. *J Child Neurol* 1994;9:45–46.
6. Graudins A, Ferm RP. Acute dystonia in a child associated with therapeutic ingestion of a dextromethorphan containing cough and cold syrup [Letter]. *J Toxicol Clin Toxicol* 1996;34:351–352.
7. Humphreys A, Tanner AR. Acute dystonic reaction or tetanus? An unusual consequence of a 'Whizz' overdose. *Hum Exp Toxicol* 1994;13:311–312.
8. Kapur V, Barber KR, Peddireddy R. Ranitidine-induced acute dystonia. *Am J Emerg Med* 1999;17:258–260.
9. Krauss JK, Mohadjer M, Wakloo AK, et al. Dystonia and akinesia due to pallidoputaminal lesions after disulfiram intoxication. *Mov Disord* 1991;6:166–170.
10. Landry P, Cournoyer J. Acute dystonia with olanzapine [Letter]. *J Clin Psychiatry* 1998;59:384.
11. Lauterbach EC, Meyer JM, Simpson GM. Clinical manifestations of dystonia and dyskinesia after SSRI administration [Letter]. *J Clin Psychiatry* 1997;58:403.
12. Lopez-Alemany M, Ferrer-Tuset C, Bernacer-Alpera B. Akathisia and acute dystonia induced by sumatriptan [Letter]. 1997;244:131–133.
13. Mark MH, Sage JI. Levodopa-associated hemifacial dystonia [Letter]. *Mov Disord* 1991;6:383.
14. McCormick MA, Manoguerra AS. Dystonic reactions. In: Harwood-Nuss A, Linden CH, Luten PC, et al., eds. *The clinical practice of emergency medicine*, 2nd ed. Philadelphia: Lippincott–Raven Publishers, 1996:1319–1321.
15. Merello MJ, Nogues MA, Leiguarda RC, et al. Dystonia and reflex sympathetic dystrophy induced by ergotamine. *Mov Disord* 1991;6:263–264.
16. Miller LG, Jankokovic J. Persistent dystonia possibly induced by flecainide. *Mov Disord* 1992;7:62–63.
17. Owens DGC. Extrapyramidal side effects and tolerability of risperidone: a review. *J Clin Psychiatry* 1994;55(5)[Suppl]:29–35.
18. Priori A, Bertolasi L, Berardelli A, et al. Acute dystonic reaction to ecstasy [Letter]. *Mov Disord* 1995;10:353.
19. Saneto RP, Fitch JA, Cohen BH. Acute neurotoxicity of meperidine in an infant. *Pediatr Neurol* 1996;14:339–341.
20. Thomas P, Lalaux N, Vaiva G, et al. Dose-dependent stuttering and dystonia in a patient taking clozapine [Letter]. *Am J Psychiatry* 1994;151:1096.

CHAPTER 336
Ergot Alkaloid Poisoning

Leslie S. Carroll and Donald B. Kunkel

Ergot alkaloids are natural and semisynthetic derivatives of compounds produced by parasitic fungi of the genus *Claviceps* (most classically, *Claviceps purpurea*).[14] Various flowering grasses and grains, particularly rye, are susceptible to fungal infestation during warm, wet weather. Historically, epidemics of ergotism resulted from the ingestion of bread made from contaminated grain. Ergotism was known as holy fire (*ignis sacer*) or St. Anthony's fire in the Middle Ages; victims claimed that a pilgrimage to the Shrine of St. Anthony relieved their symptoms. The mold *Claviceps* did not infect the rye in the area of the shrine, so spontaneous cures probably did result. Today, ergot poisoning is caused almost exclusively by the ingestion or parenteral administration of medicinal preparations.

Ergot alkaloids are derivatives of the tetracyclic compound 6-methylergoline. This compound is structurally similar to the amine neurotransmitters: dopamine, norepinephrine, and serotonin. There are three classes of ergot alkaloids, including the naturally occurring amine and amino acid groups and the synthetic dihydrogenated groups. The naturally occurring ergot alkaloids consist of a lysergic acid base; the amine alkaloids contain amine side chains, and the amino acid alkaloids contain polypeptide side chains.[10] The synthetic alkaloid also contains a lysergic acid base that has been dehydrogenated. Individual agents are listed in Table 336.1. The structural similarity between the lysergic acid nucleus of ergot alkaloids and the endogenous amines dopamine, norepinephrine, and serotonin accounts for their pharmacologic activity.[2] Effects are complex and may include simultaneous stimulation and blockade of peripheral and central neuroreceptors.

Physiologic effects are variable and depend on the particular alkaloid's affinity and specificity for receptors, the dose of the drug, individual sensitivity, the route of administration, underlying disease states, and preexisting vascular tone. For instance, ergotamine produces both partial alpha-agonist and partial alpha-antagonist effects; in addition, the drug mediates vasoconstrictor action by way of a direct effect on serotonin receptors[16] and vasodilatation secondary to central vasomotor center depression. The net clinical effect may be either vasoconstriction or vasodilation, depending on the dose taken and preexisting vascular tone. Variable activities of the ergot alkaloid derivatives may produce unexpected complications, such as acute myocardial infarction.[6]

Ergotamine, the classic ergot prototype drug, is the agent most commonly involved in poisoning. It has been used for migraine and other vascular headaches because of its cranial vasoconstrictive effect, and it can be given orally, sublingually, rectally, parenterally, and by inhalation. Rectal bioavailability is 20-fold greater than an equivalent oral dose.[17] Suppository formulations of ergotamine combined with caffeine and other products are popular and are implicated in many cases of iatrogenic ergotism. The usual recommendations for rectal ergotamine use (2 mg rectally at the beginning of a headache, not to exceed 10 mg a week) may be grossly exceeded and may produce true physical dependency with withdrawal headaches, prompting more ergotamine use.[18] Although severe vasospasm has been reported with single-dose use of ergotamine, it is the setting of cyclic and increasing self-dosing with ergotamine by any route that usually precedes vasospastic toxicity.[5]

Bromocriptine is used in the treatment of hyperprolactinemia and Parkinson disease. Because of cardiovascular toxicity, bromocriptine must be used with caution when prescribed for the suppression of postpartum lactation. Usual adult doses range from 1.25 to 7.5 mg two to six times a day and vary with the condition being treated.

CLINICAL PRESENTATION

Toxicity of two major forms—gangrenous and convulsive—has been historically recorded after ingestion of contaminated grain products. The most recent natural outbreak of ergotism was of the gangrenous form and occurred in Ethiopia from 1977 to 1978 as a consequence of the ingestion of ergot-infested wild oats.[9] In the gangrenous form of natural ergotism, the clinical progression is of early paresthesias of the extremities, vomiting, diarrhea, and, finally, excruciating extremity pain, heralding the onset of gangrene. The convulsive form terminates in painful spasms of limb muscles, culminating in epileptic-like activity.[11]

Toxicity from an acute overdose of ergot alkaloids is unusual. A 13-month-old child survived a dose of 15 mg of ergotamine (plus 1 g of phenobarbital), whereas a dose of 12 mg of ergotamine (plus 1.2 g of caffeine) was fatal to a 14-month-old child.[12] Seven cases of acute neonatal toxicity resulted from inadvertent intramuscular administration of ergotamine (0.25 to 0.5 mg), which culminated in reversible encephalopathy, seizures, peripheral vasoconstriction, and occasional oliguria.[4] An obese man who ingested 120 mg of ergotamine (plus 3 g of cyclizine and 6 g of caffeine) developed myocardial ischemia and peripheral arterial spasm.[12] Symptoms of acute toxicity may include nausea, vomiting, diarrhea, severe thirst, formication (skin tingling), chest pain, bradycardia or tachycardia, hypotension, confusion, convulsions, or coma. Overdose in a gravid female may result in fetal death.[1] The use of dihydroergotamine–heparin–lidocaine as prophylaxis against postoperative venous thrombotic disease has caused severe peripheral ischemia.[7]

Chronic toxicity of ergotamine may present with a multitude of neurologic, gastrointestinal (GI), and vascular symptoms.[20] Neurologic complications include lassitude, impaired mental function, headaches, vertigo, psychoses, convulsions, and coma. Nausea, vomiting, diarrhea, and abdominal pain may occur. As in the acute overdose, abortions may occur. Vascular effects are usually prominent and may involve both the venous and arterial circulations. Angiography may reveal spasm, formation of collaterals, and intravascular thrombi. Vascular involvement may be unilateral or bilateral, and virtually any vascular distribution may be involved. The legs are most often involved; signs and symptoms include pallor, numbness, progressive pain, progressive loss of pulses, demarcation of ischemic areas, and, finally, frank gangrene. Other complications include angina, myocardial infarction, and stroke. Factors that may accelerate ergot toxicity include tobacco smoking, concomitant use of beta-blocker medications, sepsis, and hepatic or renal disease.

Bromocriptine poisoning may result in nausea, vomiting, dizziness, lethargy, confusion, hallucinations, and either hypertension or hypotension.[13]

Sumatriptan was approved for the acute treatment of migraine headache in December 1992. The compound is structurally similar to the indole serotonin but does not have the tetracyclic structure particular to the ergots. The side-effect profile, however, is similar to the ergots secondary to vasoconstrictive properties. Sumatriptan is a serotonin 1D receptor agonist that results in extracranial vasoconstriction and resultant resolution of migraine headache. Chest tightness has been reported in 3% to 5% of patients taking sumatriptan.[19] A 47-year-old woman developed an acute myocardial infarction immediately after taking sumatriptan.[15] Two cases of severe ventricular dysrhythmias have been described subsequent to sumatriptan administration.[3] Thus, sumatriptan should be given cautiously, especially in patients experiencing chest pain after administration.

TABLE 336.1. Ergot Alkaloids

Bromocriptine
Dihydroergotamine
Dihydroergocornine[a]
Dihydroergocristine[a]
Dihydroergocryptine[a]
Ergotamine
Ergonovine
Methylergonovine
Methysergide

[a] Dihydroergotoxine (ergoloid) derivatives

DIFFERENTIAL DIAGNOSIS

The diagnosis of ergotism should become readily apparent when the history reveals the use of an ergot derivative. Unfortunately, however, patients may be reluctant to admit to self-use of ergot preparations, and the entire range of causes of vasoocclusive disease may need to be considered. Included in the differential are arteriosclerosis, compartmental and entrapment syndromes, Raynaud disease, thromboangiitis obliterans, thromboembolic disease, vasculitides, and drug-induced vasospasm (e.g., ingestion of amphetamines, cocaine, and other sympathomimetics).

EMERGENCY DEPARTMENT EVALUATION

Details regarding the use, abuse, and accidental or suicidal ingestion of ergot preparations are of paramount importance in the clinical evaluation of vasospastic disease. Physical examination should include a careful evaluation of central nervous system function, cardiovascular and peripheral vascular status, and potential pregnancy, in addition to a meticulous general examination. Doppler-technique pulse measurements, digital pulse monitoring, skin temperature recordings, and other noninvasive techniques should be considered as objective markers of peripheral vasospasm. Laboratory tests that measure plasma drug levels have been developed but are unavailable for routine use and are probably not clinically helpful.[12,16] Laboratory assessment of renal and hepatic function, baseline coagulation tests, pregnancy testing, drug screens to rule out other agents, and an electrocardiogram are indicated.

EMERGENCY DEPARTMENT MANAGEMENT

Advanced life-support measures are instituted as necessary. In the acute overdose, GI decontamination is performed. In chronic presentations, all ergot preparations, as well as caffeine and nicotine, must be discontinued. No current evidence supports the efficacy of extracorporeal removal procedures (hemodialysis and hemoperfusion) or repeated oral doses of activated charcoal. Immediate attention is directed toward treating emergent catastrophes such as acute myocardial infarction, seizures, and threatened abortion.

Ischemic extremities must be protected from trauma and should be warmed but not overheated. Numerous drugs have been recommended to reverse vasospasm, including nitroprusside (the current drug of choice for severe spasm),[20] prazosin, nitroglycerin, and nifedipine.[8] Oral cyproheptadine, a serotonin receptor antagonist, has been used adjunctively. Vascular stasis and the formation of thrombi may require the use of heparin and low-molecular-weight dextran; streptokinase has been recommended to dissolve thrombi. Intraarterial balloon dilation and the use of hyperbaric oxygen have been recommended as adjuncts to therapy. The optimal management of ergot-induced vasospasm is unsettled and requires consideration of multiple modalities.

Bromocriptine overdoses require supportive care, with attention to reversal of hypotension with fluids and protection from self-injury if confusion and agitation are present.[13]

DISPOSITION

Asymptomatic patients with acute overdoses are observed for 4 to 6 hours. Those who become symptomatic and those with vasospastic sequelae are admitted to a facility that can perform vascular diagnostic procedures (e.g., arteriography) and continuous vascular monitoring and can administer anticoagulant and vasodilatory drugs. Physicians with expertise in the management of peripheral vascular diseases and in the use of vasoactive agents (e.g., vascular surgeons) should be consulted. After the toxic episode resolves, consideration must be given to continuing care of headache symptomatology.

COMMON PITFALLS

- Failure to inform patients of the toxic effects of ergot preparations, and failure to carefully monitor ergot use
- Failure to consider ergot poisoning in the differential diagnosis of vasoocclusive disease
- Failure to appreciate that almost any vascular bed may be affected by ergot, potentially giving rise to diverse clinical presentations
- Continuing ergot therapy in the presence of early vasospastic signs or symptoms
- Failure to consider the additional toxic effects of concomitantly used drugs, such as caffeine, beta blockers, and nicotine

References

1. Au KL, Woo JSK, Wong VCW. Intrauterine death from ergotamine overdose. *Eur J Obstet Gynecol Reprod Biol* 1985;19:313.
2. Berde B, Sturmer E. Introduction to the pharmacology of ergot alkaloids and related compounds as a basis of their therapeutic application. In: Berde B, Schild HO, eds. *Handbook of experimental pharmacology,* vol 49. Berlin: Springer-Verlag, 1978.
3. Curtin T, Brooks AP, Roberts JA. Cardiorespiratory distress after sumatriptan given by injection. *BMJ* 1992;305:713.
4. Dargaville PA, Campbell NT. Overdose of ergometrine in the newborn infant: acute symptomatology and long-term outcome. *J Paediatr Child Health* 1998;34:83.
5. Harrison TE. Ergotaminism after a single dose of ergotamine tartrate. *J Emerg Med* 1984;2:23.
6. Iffy L, Ten Hove W, Frisoli G. Acute myocardial infarction in the puerperium in patients receiving bromocriptine. *Am J Obstet Gynecol* 1986;155:371.
7. Jackson JE. Postsurgical ergotism: a new form of intoxication .*Vet Hum Toxicol* 1987;29:478(abst).
8. Kemerer VF, Dagher FJ, Pais SO. Successful treatment of ergotism with nifedipine. *AJR* 1984;143:333.
9. King B. Outbreak of ergotism in Wollo, Ethiopia. *Lancet* 1979;1:1411.
10. Kunkel DB, Jallo DS. Ergot. In: Haddad LM, Winchester JF, eds. *Clinical management of poisoning and drug overdose*. Philadelphia: WB Saunders, 1990.
11. Lewis WH, Elvin-Lewis MPF. *Medical botany*. New York: John Wiley and Sons, 1977.
12. McGuigan MA. Ergot alkaloids. *Clin Toxicol Rev* 1984;6:1.
13. Mack RB. Bromocriptine (Parlodel) overdose. *N C Med J* 1988;49:17.
14. Morton JF. *Major medicinal plants*. Springfield, IL: Charles C Thomas Publisher, 1977.
15. Ottervanger JP, Paalman HJA, Boxma GL, et al. Transmural myocardial infarction with sumatriptan. *Lancet* 1993;341:861.
16. Perrin VL. Clinical pharmacokinetics of ergotamine in migraine and cluster headache. *Clin Pharmacokinet* 1985;10:334.
17. Sanders SW, Haering N, Mosberg H, et al. Pharmacokinesis of ergotamine in healthy volunteers following oral and rectal dosing. *Eur J Pharmacol* 1986;30:331.
18. Saper JR, Jones JM. Ergotamine tartrate dependency: features and possible mechanisms. *Clin Neuropharmacol* 1986;9:224.
19. Stricker BHC. Coronary vasospasm and sumatriptan. *BMJ* 1992;305:118.
20. Wells KE, Stead DL, Zajko AB, et al. Recognition and treatment of arterial insufficiency from Cafergot. *J Vasc Surg* 1986;4:8.

CHAPTER 337

Ethanol, Isopropanol, and Acetone Poisoning

Susan S. Fish

Ethanol (ethyl alcohol or "alcohol") is probably the oldest and most commonly ingested poison. In addition to beverages, sources include aftershaves, antiseptics, colognes, mouthwashes, and perfumes. Beer and ale are 2% to 8% ethanol, wine is 10% to 20% ethanol, and liquor is 20% to 95% ethanol. Other sources vary in alcohol content but may be as high as 90% ethanol.

The acute effects of ethanol are seen primarily on the central nervous system (CNS), where the drug is thought to act directly on neurons, similar to the action of general anesthetics.[3] Ethanol appears to interfere with ion transport at neuronal membranes, preventing the generation of electrical impulses. The neurons of the reticular activating system are the first to become affected as blood alcohol concentrations rise.

Ethanol is rapidly absorbed from the gastrointestinal (GI) tract, primarily the small intestine, although, in an overdose, complete absorption may not occur for up to 6 hours. Food slows absorption by delaying gastric emptying time. Alcohol distributes into body tissues and fluids with an apparent volume of distribution of about 0.6 L/kg.

Metabolism is primarily by hepatic enzymatic oxidation. Ethanol exhibits zero-order elimination (constant elimination; the serum concentration decreases by a constant amount per unit of time) at concentrations between 20 and 300 mg/dL and first-order elimination (concentration-dependent; the serum concentration decreases by half during each half-life) at concentrations below 20 mg/dL or above 300 mg/dL.[16] The average nontolerant person metabolizes about 100 mg/kg/h, reducing the blood alcohol concentration by 15 to 20 mg/dL/h. Enzyme induction in tolerant patients can increase metabolism to 175 mg/kg/h, reducing the blood alcohol concentration by 30 to 40 mg/dL/h. At high concentrations, first-order elimination half-lives of 4 to 5 hours have been reported. A lethal dose is said to be 5 to 8 g/kg in adults and 3 g/kg in children, but there is substantial interpatient variability.

Isopropanol (isopropyl alcohol) is used in the home and in industry as a disinfectant and solvent. It is an ingredient in many products, including rubbing alcohol, some radiator and fuel-line antifreezes, window cleaners, animal repellents, and aftershaves.[11] Unfortunately, these products also frequently contain ethanol or the more toxic methanol or ethylene glycol. Isopropanol is the most commonly ingested nonbeverage alcohol, despite its slightly bitter taste and distinctive odor.

Isopropanol is rapidly absorbed from the intestine after ingestion. It is also well absorbed rectally. Toxicity has been reported after sponge baths with isopropanol, but the route of absorption is not agreed on; experimental evidence supports both dermal and inhalation absorption.[12] The apparent volume of distribution is about 0.6 L/kg, that of total body water. Isopropanol, like ethanol, is metabolized by alcohol dehydrogenase.[2,10,14] The metabolite acetone is eliminated by the kidney and lungs, producing a sweet ketotic odor on the breath. Isopropanol is secreted into the saliva and gastric juices, but the amounts found in these fluids are probably clinically insignificant. Isopropanol exhibits first-order elimination, with an elimination half-life of about 6 hours in nonalcoholics and 3 to 4 hours in alcoholics. A fatal dose is said to be about 8 oz in an adult, although, as with ethanol, much variability is seen.[1]

Acetone is found in household and industrial cleaners and solvents, and is a major ingredient in most fingernail polish removers. In diabetic ketoacidosis, endogenous production due to fat metabolism can produce acetone concentrations of 10 to 70 mg/dL. Acetone is rapidly absorbed after ingestion or inhalation. The apparent volume of distribution is 0.8 L/kg. Acetone is metabolized to glucose by saturable enzymes. The major route of elimination is by the lungs, producing a fruity breath odor. Acetone is also minimally eliminated unchanged by the kidney. The elimination half-life is 20 to 30 hours in adults and about 11 hours in infants.[10,17] Toxicity in children is seen after ingestion of 2 to 3 mL/kg. An ingested dose of 200 to 400 mL in an adult produces CNS depression but no serious complications.

CLINICAL PRESENTATION

Ethanol, a CNS depressant, initially produces a paradoxical CNS stimulation due to disinhibition.[3] During this phase, an intoxicated patient may appear energized and loquacious. As ethanol levels rise, the patient may become aggressive, abusive, irritable, dysarthric, confused, disoriented, ataxic, and lethargic. Severe intoxication may lead to coma and respiratory depression. Aspiration pneumonia may occur due to suppression of the gag reflex and a tendency to vomit, caused by the irritating effects of ethanol on the GI tract. Physical examination may reveal tachycardia, hypotension, hypothermia, hypoventilation, mydriasis, and nystagmus. Rarely, alcohol induces a histamine-mediated urticaria. Hypoglycemia, common in children but rare in adults,[19] may be present primarily because of an inhibition of gluconeogenesis by ethanol; this may lead to confusion, seizures, or coma. Death may result from respiratory depression.

In nontolerant people, there appears to be a good correlation between the blood alcohol concentration and the degree of neurologic impairment, with signs of intoxication beginning as blood levels reach 50 to 100 mg/dL. When the blood alcohol concentration approaches 200 mg/dL, motor skills and speech are impaired; at 300 mg/dL, equilibrium, perception, and vision are altered; and at levels above 450 to 500 mg/dL, coma, respiratory depression, and peripheral vascular collapse occur. However, people who are tolerant to ethanol have been reported not only to survive incredibly high concentrations, but also to be resistant to many of the toxic effects. A 24-year-old woman presented to an emergency department complaining of abdominal pain and appearing agitated and confused but oriented to person and place; she was discovered to have a blood alcohol level of 1,510 mg/dL.[6]

Isopropanol is considered twice as toxic as ethanol, although some disagree whether this applies to the clinical situation.[9,11,20] The signs and symptoms of isopropanol toxicity are similar to those of ethanol toxicity with only a few exceptions. The early disinhibition seen with ethanol is absent with isopropanol. CNS depression may persist for more than 24 hours, long after levels of isopropanol are undetectable. This prolonged CNS depression is due to the metabolite acetone, which has a long elimination half-life (20 to 30 hours in adults).[10] Hypoglycemia, a result of altered gluconeogenesis, is rare but may contribute to the CNS depression. Ketonemia and ketonuria commonly occur. Pupil size varies, and both miosis and mydriasis have been reported. GI irritation, a hallmark of isopropanol toxicity, may manifest as abdominal pain, vomiting, gastritis, and hematemesis, which may lead to hypotension.[7]

Hypothermia may also be seen. Tachycardia is the most common finding. Fatalities have occurred in patients who were in deep coma and were hypotensive. Coma in the absence of hypotension did not indicate a poor prognosis.

Blood levels of isopropanol do not correlate well with toxic symptoms, although toxicity is seen with levels of 50 to 100 mg/dL.[9] Most comatose patients have levels above 125 mg/dL, and death may occur with levels above 200 mg/dL. However, patients with levels above 500 mg/dL have recovered.

The signs and symptoms of acetone intoxication are also similar to those of ethanol intoxication, and the doses required to produce toxicity are also similar. However, acetone has a greater anesthetic potency than ethanol. After an acetone ingestion, nausea, vomiting, and gastric hemorrhage may occur. Inhalation of acetone can produce coughing, bronchial irritation, and eye irritation. Pharyngeal irritation and soft-palate erythema and erosions have been reported. CNS depression causes drowsiness, weakness, dysarthria, and ataxia. Lethargy can progress to coma more rapidly with acetone than with ethanol. Mild hyperglycemia and ketonemia can mimic acute diabetic coma. Acute tubular necrosis has been reported.

DIFFERENTIAL DIAGNOSIS

The differential diagnosis should include the ingestion of other CNS depressants, as well as other causes of coma, such as metabolic derangements, CNS infection, head trauma, and tumors. Other causes of increased serum osmolality include ethylene glycol and methanol ingestion. Ketosis caused by isopropanol and acetone intoxication should be differentiated from that secondary to alcoholic and diabetic ketoacidosis, starvation ketosis, and salicylate intoxication.

Acetone interferes with the measurement of creatinine by automated chemistry analyzers that utilize a colorimetric change based on the Jaffe method and can result in a falsely elevated creatinine value.[5] Hence, the finding of an elevated creatinine in an intoxicated patient with a normal blood urea nitrogen (BUN) is suggestive of acetone or isopropanol ingestion.

EMERGENCY DEPARTMENT EVALUATION

The history should document the type, amount, and alcohol or acetone concentration of the substance ingested; the route and time of ingestion; the ingestion of any other agents; chronic use of drugs or alcohol; the nature and time of onset of symptoms; and medical history. A history of trauma or disulfiram use should be specifically elicited.

The physical examination should focus on the mental status, neurologic function, and GI and cardiopulmonary systems, with frequent monitoring of vital signs for tachycardia, hypothermia, hypotension, and hypoventilation. The breath odor may provide a clue to the diagnosis (e.g., the fruity odor of acetone and isopropanol). The patient should be examined for evidence of concomitant trauma.

Laboratory tests should include a quantitative serum level of the ingested agent, routine chemistries, and a blood glucose determination.[4] Gas chromatography is the preferred testing method. A Breathalyzer may give a quick estimate of the blood alcohol concentration, but reliable readings require patient cooperation.[8] Isopropanol, methanol, and nonalcoholic beer may also result in a positive breath analysis.[15] Factors that interfere with the Breathalyzer include recent use (within 15 to 30 minutes) of ethanol-containing products (e.g., inhaled bronchodilators), methanol or isopropanol ingestion, recent belching or vomiting, and obstructive pulmonary disease. Serum ethanol concentrations are about 10% to 15% higher than whole-blood concentrations, depending on the patient's hematocrit. Enzymatic methods using alcohol dehydrogenase do not differentiate among the alcohols (ethanol, isopropanol, methanol, and ethylene glycol) and should not be used. Deaths have occurred when blood levels continue to rise while the patient is put in a corner to "sleep it off." If there is doubt, additional levels should be obtained.

Arterial blood gas analysis and serum and urine ketone measurements may be helpful. Ketonemia and ketonuria may suggest isopropanol or acetone intoxication, but their absence does not rule out these ingestions.

Measuring the serum osmolality by freezing-point depression (not the vapor-pressure method) may be helpful if quantitative serum levels are not immediately available. A measured osmolality greater than that calculated from the serum levels of sodium, BUN, and glucose ($2 \times Na + BUN/3 + glucose/18$) of more than 10 mOsmol/kg suggests the presence of a low-molecular-weight compound such as ethanol, ethylene glycol, acetone, isopropanol, and methanol. If the agent ingested is known, its concentration may be estimated from the difference between the measured and calculated osmolalities (the osmolar gap). The gap increases by about 1 mOsmol/kg for each 4.3 mg/dL of ethanol, 5.5 mg/dL of acetone, and 5.9 mg/dL of isopropanol present.[11]

EMERGENCY DEPARTMENT MANAGEMENT

The treatment of a patient who has ingested a large amount of ethanol, isopropanol, or acetone is primarily supportive. Breathing is evaluated, and the patient is endotracheally intubated, as needed. A comatose patient is given thiamine 100 mg intravenously (i.v.), dextrose 25 g i.v., and naloxone 2 mg i.v., if indicated. Although there are reports that naloxone has reversed ethanol-induced coma, no controlled studies have shown its efficacy in this situation. Studies of flumazepil's ability to reverse ethanol-induced CNS depression have shown equivocal results. Activated charcoal is of questionable benefit, although its administration with a cathartic is probably indicated for adsorption of possible coingestants.[13] The hypothermic patient should be warmed (see Chapter 386). Sodium bicarbonate may be given if there is a substantial lactic acidosis. Fluids and electrolytes are replaced as needed. In rare cases of hypotension unresponsive to crystalloid administration, vasopressors may be necessary. Although fructose may accelerate the metabolism of ethanol by as much as 25%, the adverse effects of vomiting, abdominal pain, lactic acidosis, and shock prohibit its use.

Patients with ethanol intoxication usually recover within 12 hours, but recovery from severe isopropanol or acetone poisoning may take 2 to 3 days.[9,11] Hemodialysis can be used in severe cases unresponsive to supportive therapy to increase the elimination of all of these agents.[18]

DISPOSITION

Patients with acute ethanol intoxication seldom require admission unless a complication such as aspiration is present. Even those who are comatose improve within hours with supportive care. Only if they cannot be treated and observed in the emergency department do such patients require admission. In contrast, patients with moderate-to-severe isopropanol or acetone poisoning and high blood levels of these agents usually require a day or two for toxicity to resolve; therefore, they should be admitted. Clinical severity (e.g., need for airway protection and mechanical ventilation, severe acid–base disturbances) should be used to determine the appropriate level of hospital care.

COMMON PITFALLS

- Failure to appreciate that tolerance, trauma, coingestants, hypoglycemia, and underlying disease may alter a patient's response to a particular level of alcohol, and to treat the patient, not the alcohol level
- Failure to rule out coingestions and traumatic injuries, particularly if the clinical severity is inconsistent with the alcohol level
- Failure to appreciate that nutritional deficiencies in chronic alcoholics can also cause confusion and to consider empiric therapy with thiamine for Wernicke's encephalopathy and dextrose (or a bedside glucose level) for hypoglycemia
- Failure to recognize alcohol withdrawal and to appreciate that withdrawal can occur in the presence of a positive blood alcohol concentration
- Assuming that the alcohol level has peaked by the time the patient is examined and failing to monitor and reevaluate the intoxicated patient
- Failure to protect the airway and to evaluate and support respiratory function in patients with CNS depression
- Failure to appreciate that acetone causes falsely elevated serum creatinine levels, and diagnosing renal failure when the BUN is normal
- Failure to appreciate that enzymatic methods may underestimate isopropanol concentrations
- Failure to appreciate that the serum osmolality is useful for estimating acetone and alcohol concentrations only if it is measured by the freezing-point depression method

References

1. Alexander CB, McBay AJ, Hudson RP. Isopropanol and isopropanol deaths—10 years' experience. *J Forensic Sci* 1982;27:541.
2. Daniel DR, McAnalley BH, Garriott JC. Isopropyl alcohol metabolism after acute intoxication in humans. *J Anal Toxicol* 1981;5:110.
3. David DJ, Spyker DA. The acute toxicity of ethanol: dosage and kinetic nomograms. *Vet Hum Toxicol* 1979;21:272.
4. Goldfinger TM, Shaber D. A comparison of blood alcohol concentration using nonalcohol and alcohol-containing skin antiseptics. *Ann Emerg Med* 1982;11:665.
5. Hawley PC, Falko JM. "Pseudo" renal failure after isopropyl alcohol intoxication. *South Med J* 1982;75:630.
6. Johnson RA, Noll EC, Rodney WM. Survival after a serum ethanol concentration of 1.5%. *Lancet* 1982;2:1394.
7. Juncos L, Taguchi JT. Isopropyl alcohol intoxication: report of a case associated with myopathy, renal failure, and hemolytic anemia. *JAMA* 1968;294:732.
8. Keim ME, Bartfield JM, Racco-Robak N. Blood ethanol estimation: a comparison of three methods [Letter]. *Acad Emerg Med* 1996;3:85.
9. Kelner M, Bailey DN. Isopropanol ingestion: interpretation of blood concentrations and clinical findings. *J Toxicol Clin Toxicol* 1983;20:497.
10. Lacouture PG, Heldreth DD, Shannon M, et al. The generation of acetonemia/acetonuria following ingestion of a subtoxic dose of isopropyl alcohol. *Am J Emerg Med* 1989;7:38.
11. Lacouture PG, Wason S, Abrams A, et al. Acute isopropyl alcohol intoxication: diagnosis and management. *Am J Med* 1983;75:680.
12. Martinez TT, Jaeger RW, deCastro FJ, et al. A comparison of the absorption and metabolism of isopropyl alcohol by oral, dermal, and inhalation routes. *Vet Hum Toxicol* 1986;28:233.
13. Minocha A, Herold DA, Barth JT, et al. Use of activated charcoal in ethanol overdose. *Vet Hum Toxicol* 1985;28:318(abst).
14. Natowicz M, Donahue J, Gorman L, et al. Pharmacokinetic analysis of a case of isopropanol intoxication. *Clin Chem* 1985;31:326.
15. Nordt SP, Williams SR, Manoguerra AS, et al. Ethanol analysis following consumption of "alcohol-free" beer. *Vet Hum Toxicol* 1999;41:94.
16. O'Neill S, Tipton KF, Prichard JS, et al. Survival after high blood-alcohol levels: association with first-order elimination kinetics. *Arch Intern Med* 1984;144:641.
17. Parker KM, Lera TA. Acute isopropanol ingestion: pharmacokinetic parameters in the infant. *Am J Emerg Med* 1992;10:542.
18. Rosansky SJ. Isopropyl alcohol poisoning treated with hemodialysis: kinetics of isopropyl alcohol and acetone removal. *J Toxicol Clin Toxicol* 1982;19:265.
19. Sporer KA, Ernst AA, Conte R, et al. Incidence of ethanol-induced hypoglycemia. *Am J Emerg Med* 1992;10:403.
20. Wallgren H. Relative intoxicating effects on rats of ethyl, propyl, and butyl alcohols. *Acta Pharmacol Toxicol* 1960;16:217.

CHAPTER 338

Ethylene Glycol Poisoning

Michael J. Burns and Francis P. Renzi

Ethylene glycol (EG; 1,2-ethanediol) is a colorless, odorless, sweet-tasting, water-soluble liquid that has a wide variety of household and commercial uses.[1] Because of its low freezing point (−13°C) and high boiling point (198°C), EG is commonly used as an antifreeze–coolant. Automotive antifreeze contains about 95% EG and is the source of most EG poisonings. EG may also be found in adhesives, brake and hydraulic fluids, cosmetics, de-icers, detergents, fire extinguishers, inks, lacquers, paints, pesticides, polishes, and some windshield-washer fluids. The majority of exposures occur unintentionally through misuse or by accident. Intentional ingestion of EG for purposes of inebriation or suicide accounts for a minority of exposures but the most fatalities. Widespread availability, interesting color, and pleasant, bittersweet taste likely account for its ingestion by alcoholics seeking an ethanol substitute and by children.

Unmetabolized EG produces about the same degree of central nervous system (CNS) depression and has a similar range of toxicity as ethanol. Serious toxicity (anion gap metabolic acidosis, coma, seizures, cardiopulmonary dysfunction, and acute renal failure) results largely from accumulation of the toxic metabolites, glycolic and oxalic acids.[1,4,6,9–11]

EG is rapidly absorbed from the gastrointestinal tract and distributed throughout total body water (0.6 L/kg). Peak blood concentration occurs about 2 hours after enteral administration.[10] About 20% to 50% of EG is excreted unchanged in the urine.[10] The remaining EG is metabolized in the liver to a variety of compounds with varying toxicities (Fig. 338.1).

The first step in the metabolism of EG is its oxidation to glycoaldehyde by alcohol dehydrogenase.[9,10] Because alcohol dehydrogenase has a much higher affinity for ethanol and fomepizole (synthetic inhibitor) than for EG, these substrates are preferentially bound, when present, with EG. Their presence inhibits the metabolism of EG sixfold and prevents the formation of toxic metabolites.[1–3,5,7,9,10,17]

When formed, glycoaldehyde is rapidly metabolized by aldehyde dehydrogenase to glycolic acid, which is further metabolized slowly to glyoxylic acid. Glycolic acid oxidation is rate-limiting; for this reason, it tends to accumulate.[4,11,14] Glycolic acid accumulation correlates with the increased anion gap, decreased arterial pH, development of renal injury, and mortality associated with advanced EG poisoning.[3,4,6,10,11,14]

Glycolic acid is directly nephrotoxic and causes renal tubular damage and interstitial edema.[15] Once formed, glyoxylic acid is rapidly oxidized by one of several pathways. Its principal metabolite, oxalic acid, rapidly precipitates as calcium oxalate crystals in various organs and tissues.[11] Calcium oxalate precipitation within renal tubules contributes significantly to the development of acute tubular necrosis and renal insufficiency.[10] Crystal deposition is likely responsible for much of the end-organ injury that results from serious EG poisoning (e.g., cerebral and pulmonary edema).

Significant systemic toxicity from EG occurs only after ingestion.[1,10] Skin exposure may cause minor irritation, and direct eye contact may result in conjunctivitis, chemosis, and iridocyclitis.[18] Inhalation of EG vapors is not normally hazardous. The toxic and lethal doses of EG after acute ingestion vary. Death has

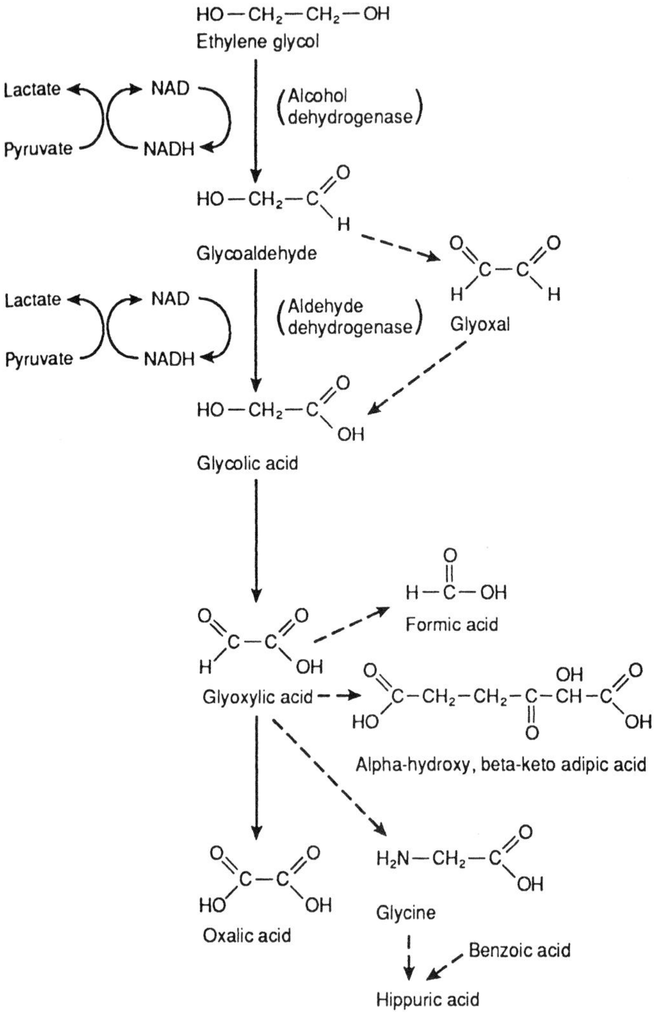

Figure 338.1. Metabolism of ethylene glycol. *Solid lines,* known pathways of metabolism; *dotted lines,* postulated pathways of metabolism.

been reported in two men who shared 60 mL of 95% EG, but one patient survived after ingesting about 2 L of EG.[17,19] Because as little as 0.1 mL/kg of pure EG may result in potentially toxic blood concentrations, the ingestion of even a mouthful of EG should be considered hazardous. Conversely, although the oral lethal dose is approximately 1.5 mL/kg, the relationship between the amount consumed and prognosis is usually poor.[5,9,10]

CLINICAL PRESENTATION

With EG poisoning, three distinct stages of organ system involvement—CNS, cardiopulmonary, and renal—have been classically described, but the onset, progression, and confluence of these stages vary widely.[1,5,10] Thirty minutes to 12 hours after ingestion, CNS signs and symptoms predominate. Initially, slurred speech, ataxia, nystagmus, and lethargy occur. The patient may appear drunk but lacks the odor of ethanol; instead, a faint, sweet, or aromatic odor may be detected on the breath. Nausea, vomiting, and abdominal pain may also be present.

At this early stage, the presence of an elevated osmolal gap may provide a clue to the diagnosis of EG poisoning.[5,9,10] The difference between the measured serum osmolality and the calculated osmolarity ([2 × sodium] + [glucose/18] + [blood urea nitrogen/2.8] + [serum ethanol concentration/4.6]) is the corrected osmolal gap. Normally, serum osmolality ranges from 280 to 300 mOsmol/kg H_2O, with an corrected osmolal gap of −2 (±6) mOsmol/kg H_2O.[8] Low-molecular-weight solutes such as EG, acetone, isopropanol, and methanol increase serum osmolality, and thus increase the osmolal gap. Osmolality measured by the freezing-point depression (not vapor pressure) method will detect these agents. A large osmolal gap (particularly if greater than 25) is suggestive of toxic alcohol poisoning.[5,10] A small osmolal gap, however, cannot be used to exclude significant EG poisoning.[8] EG poisoning should be confirmed by the presence of EG in serum or urine.

Following a latent period of 3 to 12 hours, the signs and symptoms caused by accumulated toxic metabolites develop. CNS depression progresses to stupor and coma. Hyporeflexia, tremors, tetany, and seizures (both focal and generalized) may occur. Severe CNS disturbances may reflect the development of cerebral edema and are associated with calcium oxalate deposition within the brain and leptomeninges.[10] A decreased serum bicarbonate may be seen as early as 3 hours following EG ingestion.[1,2,5,7] Hyperventilation signifies the development of an anion gap metabolic acidosis.

Cardiopulmonary signs and symptoms, such as hypertension, tachycardia, dysrhythmias, and pulmonary edema, develop 12 to 36 hours after the ingestion of EG. During this stage, tachypnea and Kussmaul respirations reflect a progressively worsening anion gap metabolic acidosis. A normal anion gap (serum sodium minus chloride and bicarbonate) is 12 (±2) mEq/L and represents unmeasured anions in the serum. The presence of nonvolatile acids, such as formic acid, keto acid, lactic acid, or, in the case of EG poisoning, glycolic acid, increases the anion gap.

If the history is not suggestive of lactic acidosis or ketoacidosis, then a high osmolal gap with anion gap metabolic acidosis strongly points toward EG or methanol poisoning.[5,10] Present in approximately 80% of patients, anion gap metabolic acidosis is the most frequently reported laboratory abnormality associated with EG poisoning.[3,13] Its absence in a patient with known EG ingestion suggests early presentation, insignificant poisoning, or the coingestion of another toxic alcohol (e.g., ethanol) that has blocked the metabolism of EG.

Urinalysis may provide additional evidence of EG poisoning. Proteinuria and microscopic hematuria may be seen in over 60% of cases.[3] Calcium oxalate crystalluria, virtually pathognomonic of EG poisoning, is present on admission in nearly 50% of patients; this percentage increases with serial urinalysis.[3,10,13] Calcium oxalate is often excreted as needle-shaped monohydrate crystals that may be misidentified as hippuric or uric acid crystals.[5,10] At higher urinary concentrations, calcium oxalate is also excreted in an evelope-shaped dihydrate form.[9,10] The formation of calcium oxalate may cause hypoglycemia with myoclonic jerks or tetanic contractions. Because fluorescein is added to many commercial antifreeze preparations, fluorescence of urine or gastric contents with a Wood lamp may support EG poisoning early after ingestion.[20] Lack of urine fluorescence, however, cannot be used to exclude EG poisoning.

Death is most common during the cardiopulmonary stage and results from cerebral edema and infarction, multiple organ failure, and irreversible shock.[10,13,15] Even with conventional treatment, mortality rates of 5% to 17% are still described.[3,13] The time elapsed between ingestion and treatment and the degree of metabolic acidosis at the initiation of treatment are the factors most closely correlated with survival.[10,13] Rapid diagnosis and treatment prevents EG bioactivation and lethality, regardless of the initial plasma EG concentration.[10,13]

Patients who survive may complain of severe flank pain and develop costovertebral angle tenderness and acute renal insufficiency 18 to 48 hours after ingestion. Renal dysfunction is seen in nearly 70% of cases and is characterized by oliguria, proteinuria, and urine with a low specific gravity and sodium content (acute tubular necrosis).[13] The high frequency of renal injury reflects the delayed presentation and diagnosis of the majority of EG-poisoned patients. The degree of metabolic acidosis or glycolic acid accumulation at the initiation of treatment is closely correlated with the subsequent development of renal injury.[3,10,13]

Conversely, patients who have normal renal function upon initiation of treatment are unlikely to develop renal insufficiency.[3,16] Although most patients treated for EG poisoning have a complete recovery, some may have protracted renal insufficiency that requires months of hemodialysis. Uncommonly, cranial neuropathies may develop 1 to 2 weeks after acute poisoning.[10]

DIFFERENTIAL DIAGNOSIS

EG intoxication can mimic a large variety of poisonings or disease states, depending on the amount of EG ingested and the degree of EG metabolism at presentation. Diagnostic clues include drunkenness without the odor of ethanol, latency between ingestion and significant illness, hyperventilation on physical examination, increased osmolal or anion gaps, metabolic acidosis, calcium oxalate crystalluria, and hypocalcemia. Similar findings may be present in methanol intoxication, but crystalluria is absent and visual complaints and an abnormal eye examination may be present. Other common diagnostic considerations that must be ruled out include alcoholic, diabetic, and starvation ketoacidosis; lactic acidosis; renal failure; and advanced, untreated acetaminophen or salicylate poisoning.

EMERGENCY DEPARTMENT EVALUATION

The history should include the time of ingestion, the volume and concentration of the ingested product, and the onset, nature, and progression of symptoms. The ingestion of any other substance, particularly ethanol, and the details of such events should be documented. Patients should be specifically asked about symptoms of ethanol-like intoxication, shortness of breath, flank pain, and urinary dysfunction.

Initially, the physical examination should focus on the neurologic status and cardiopulmonary function. A complete physical with documentation of any abdominal and back tenderness should then be performed. In symptomatic patients, routine laboratory evaluation should include a complete blood count; measurement of serum electrolytes, blood urea nitrogen, creatinine, glucose, amylase, calcium, ketones, and lactate; serum osmolality; arterial blood gas analysis; toxicologic screen; and a urinalysis.

A quantitative serum EG concentration should be obtained in all patients, preferably by gas chromatography and mass spectrometry. In all patients with intentional ingestion, a serum ethanol concentration should also be obtained. In addition, because many antifreeze products also contain methanol, a methanol concentration should be ordered if the identity of the ingested substance cannot be confirmed.

If results are not readily available, the serum EG concentration can be estimated by calculating the osmolal gap and assuming that the serum osmolality will increase the normal gap by 1 mOsmol/kg for each 6.2 mg/dL of EG (and each 4.6 mg/dL of ethanol) present.[9,10] However, the absence of an increased osmolal gap does not rule out the possibility of EG poisoning, particularly in the later stages of poisoning, when significant metabolism has already occurred.[8] Conversely, the presence of a large osmolal and anion gap is not specific to EG intoxication.[8]

Symptomatic patients should also have an electrocardiogram and a chest radiograph.

EMERGENCY DEPARTMENT MANAGEMENT

Aggressive supportive measures, including airway protection and respiratory and circulatory support with cardiac and hemodynamic monitoring, should be instituted as necessary. Initially, intravenous fluids should be liberally administered to maintain an adequate urine output; a large urine flow increases the urinary excretion of EG in those without renal failure.[9,10]

If the patient has ingested EG within 4 hours, gastric aspiration, with or without lavage, via a nasogastric tube should be performed immediately. Activated charcoal does adsorb EG but may be clinically ineffective because EG is rapidly absorbed, because of the relatively large amounts often ingested, and because the patient may delay coming to the emergency department. Regardless, the administration of activated charcoal is recommended, particularly if a coingestant is a possibility.

Specific treatment for EG poisoning consists of sodium bicarbonate to correct metabolic acidosis, calcium to correct hypocalcemia, ethanol or fomepizole to inhibit production of toxic metabolites, hemodialysis to remove EG and its toxic metabolites, and pyridoxine to theoretically enhance endogenous clearance of toxic metabolites.[1]

Correction of metabolic acidosis may require the use of large amounts of intravenous sodium bicarbonate, given slowly in 1-mEq/kg increments. The acid–base status should be frequently reevaluated to assess the response to therapy. Hypocalcemia may be worsened by sodium bicarbonate administration.[10]

Serum calcium levels should be monitored frequently. Hypocalcemia, tetany, and seizures should be treated initially with intravenous calcium chloride or gluconate (7 to 14 mEq for adults and 1 to 7 mEq for children). The 10% chloride solution contains 1.4 mEq of calcium per milliliter, while the 10% gluconate solution contains 0.46 mEq/mL. Seizures should otherwise be treated with standard drugs (diazepam, lorazepam, or a barbiturate).

Traditionally, ethanol has been used to inhibit the alcohol dehydrogenase–mediated metabolism of EG. Fomepizole (4-methylpyrazole, 4-MP; Antizol) is a potent and long-acting, competitive alcohol dehydrogenase inhibitor that appears to be a safe, easy, and effective alternative to ethanol.[1–4,6,7,10,16] It was approved by the Food and Drug Administration in 1997 for treatment of EG poisoning. Fomepizole has been shown to both attenuate and prevent metabolic acidosis and renal failure in humans and animals poisoned by EG by halting the accumulation of glycolic and oxalic acids, respectively.[1–4,6,7] Fomepizole offers several advantages over ethanol, which include a higher potency, longer duration of action, and easier dosing regimen.[1,3,9] Unlike treatment with ethanol, fomepizole treatment does not require frequent monitoring and adjustment of plasma concentrations. Additionally, fomepizole does not produce the CNS depression, hypoglycemia, gastritis, pancreatitis, and habituation that are commonly associated with ethanol therapy.[1,3,4,6,9]

Potential disadvantages of fomepizole include its high cost ($1,000 U.S. per 1.5-g vial) and incompletely established safety profile. Although likely safe, fomepizole has been associated infrequently with transient hepatic transaminase elevation, rash, eosinophilia, and seizures in humans.[1,3,7,9]

Regardless of which antidote is used, both ethanol and fomepizole preferentially bind alcohol dehydrogenase and prevent further EG metabolism. Once administered, EG can then be eliminated by urinary excretion or hemodialysis. Indications for treatment with ethanol or fomepizole include a documented history of recent EG ingestion when a serum EG concentration is not immediately available, particularly if the osmol gap is elevated; strong suspicion of EG ingestion based on abnormal clinical or laboratory findings (e.g., oxalate crystalluria, unexplained anion gap metabolic acidosis or elevated corrected osmolar gap, or a combination thereof); or a measured serum EG concentration greater than 20 mg/dL.[1,3,9,10]

For ethanol therapy, the therapeutic goal is a serum ethanol concentration of at least 100 mg/dL.[9,10] Although it can be accomplished with oral administration of ethanol,[15] intravenous administration provides a more constant serum concentration. An intravenous loading dose of 10 mL/kg of 10% ethanol (with glucose to avoid hypoglycemia), followed by a maintenance infusion of 1.5 mL/kg/h, generally produces a serum ethanol concentration of slightly greater than 100 mg/dL.[9,10] Serum ethanol and glucose concentrations should be monitored and the dose of ethanol adjusted, as necessary, to maintain a therapeutic ethanol concentration.

For fomepizole, a loading dose of 15 mg/kg should be administered, followed by doses of 10 mg/kg every 12 hours thereafter.[3] All doses are diluted in 100 cc of 5% dextrose in water or normal saline and are administered by slow intravenous infusion over 30 minutes.[3] Like ethanol, fomepizole is also effective following oral administration.[1] Antidotal therapy is continued until EG concentrations fall below 20 mg/dL.[3]

Hemodialysis rapidly removes both EG and glycolic acid.[9–11,14] Elimination half-lives are reduced to approximately 3 hours for each, as compared with 19 and 10 hours, respectively, during alcohol dehydrogenase inhibitor therapy alone.[1–3,7,11,14,16] Indications for hemodialysis include significant metabolic acidosis (arterial pH less than or equal to 7.20), renal insufficiency (serum creatinine greater than 1.2 mg/dL), as well as deterioration in these parameters or clinical status despite conventional treatment.[1,3,9,10]

Traditionally, hemodialysis has also been recommended for a serum EG concentration greater than or equal to 50 mg/dL.[5,9,10] This concentration, however, does not define toxicity, predict prolonged elimination, or correlate with patient outcome. Recent evidence suggests that patients who present before the development of metabolic acidosis and renal impairment can be effectively and safely managed with fomepizole monotherapy (no hemodialysis), regardless of initial EG concentration.[1–3,7] For these patients, EG is excreted by the kidneys, with an approximate half-life of 18 hours.[1–3,16] For patients who present with elevated serum creatinine, however, EG elimination half-life is prolonged to approximately 49 hours and hemodialysis is recommended.[3,16] These patients will also likely require hemodialysis based on the presence of a significant metabolic acidosis. When initiated, hemodialysis should be continued until acid–base and metabolic abnormalities are corrected and serum EG concentrations are below 50 mg/dL.[3,9,10]

During hemodialysis, the infusion rate of ethanol should be increased to 3 mL/kg/h to compensate for losses.[1,9,10] Because fomepizole is also dialyzable, dosing frequency should be increased to every 4 hours during hemodialysis.[3,12] If hemodialysis is unavailable or technically difficult (e.g., in infants), peritoneal dialysis can be used, although this method is considerably less effective than hemodialysis.

Pyridoxine and thiamine are cofactors in the degradation of EG to less toxic products. They theoretically shunt metabolism of glyoxylic acid away from oxalic acid. They should both be given intravenously in doses of 100 mg four times daily.[9,10]

DISPOSITION

Patients with EG poisoning almost always require admission to an intensive care unit. Early consultation with a toxicologist or local poison center is encouraged to aid in patient care and to determine the availability of EG concentrations. The need for hemodialysis should always be anticipated, and the patient should be transferred if such treatment is unavailable.

COMMON PITFALLS

- Failure to consider EG as a cause of ethanol-like intoxication and anion gap metabolic acidosis
- Failure to appreciate that a normal osmolal and/or anion gap does not exclude the presence of potentially toxic amounts of EG
- Failure to treat with ethanol or fomepizole before the results of confirmatory testing for EG when there is sufficient clinical suspicion of EG poisoning
- Failure to correct EG-induced metabolic acidosis with bicarbonate
- Failure to employ emergent hemodialysis for the EG-poisoned patient who presents with significant metabolic acidosis or renal insufficiency, regardless of the EG concentration

References

1. Barceloux DG, Krenzelok EP, Olsen K, et al. American Academy of Clinical Toxicology practice guidelines on the treatment of ethylene glycol poisoning. *Clin Toxicol* 1999;37:537–560.
2. Baud FJ, Galliot M, Astier A, et al. Treatment of ethylene glycol poisoning with intravenous 4-methylpyrazole. *N Engl J Med* 1988;319:97.
3. Brent J, McMartin K, Phillips S, et al. Fomepizole for the treatment of ethylene glycol poisoning. *N Engl J Med* 1999;340:832.
4. Clay KL, Murphy RC. On the metabolic acidosis of ethylene glycol intoxication. *Toxicol Appl Pharmacol* 1977;39:39.
5. Eder AF, McGrath CM, Dowdy YG, et al. Ethylene glycol poisoning; toxicokinetic and analytic factors affecting laboratory diagnosis. *Clin Chem* 1998;44:168.
6. Grauer GF, Thrall MA, Henre BA, et al. Comparison of the effects of ethanol and 4-methylpyrazole on the pharmacokinetics and toxicity of ethylene glycol in the dog. *Toxicol Lett* 1987;35:307.
7. Harry P, Turcant G, Bouachour G, et al. Efficacy of 4-methylpyrazole in ethylene glycol poisoning: clinical and toxicokinetic aspects. *Hum Exp Toxicol* 1994;13:61.
8. Hoffman RS, Smilkstein MJ, Howland MA, et al. *J Toxicol Clin Toxicol* 1993;31:81.
9. Jacobsen D, McMartin KE. Antidotes for methanol and ethylene glycol poisoning. *J Toxicol Clin Toxicol* 1997;35:127.
10. Jacobsen D, McMartin KE. Methanol and ethylene glycol poisonings: mechanisms of toxicity, clinical course, diagnosis and treatment. *Med Toxicol* 1986;1:309.
11. Jacobsen D, Ovrebo S, Ostborg J, et al. Glycolate causes the acidosis in ethylene glycol poisoning and is effectively removed by hemodialysis. *Acta Med Scand* 1984;216:409.
12. Jobard E, Harry P, Turcant A, et al. 4-Methylpyrazole and hemodialysis in ethylene glycol poisoning. *J Toxicol Clin Toxicol* 1996;34:373.
13. Karlson-Stiber C, Persson H. Ethylene glycol poisoning: experiences from an epidemic in Sweden. *Clin Toxicol* 1992;30:565.
14. Moreau CL, Kerns II W, Tomaszewski CA, et al. Glycolate kinetics and hemodialysis clearance in ethylene glycol poisoning. *J Toxicol Clin Toxicol* 1998;36:659.
15. Pons CA, Custer RP. Acute ethylene glycol poisoning: a clinicopathologic report of 18 fatal cases. *Am J Med Sci* 1946;211:544.
16. Sivilotti M, Burns M, McMartin K, et al. Pharmacokinetics of ethylene glycol and methanol during fomepizole therapy: results of the META trial. *J Toxicol Clin Toxicol* 1998;36:451(abst).
17. Stokes JB, Aueron F. Prevention of organ damage in massive ethylene glycol ingestion. *JAMA* 1980;243:2065. 18. Sykowski P. Ethylene glycol toxicity. *Am J Ophthalmol* 1951;34:1599.
19. Widman C. A few cases of ethylene glycol intoxication. *Acta Med Scand* 1946;126:295.
20. Winter ML, Ellis MD, Snodgrass WR. Urine fluorescence using a Wood's lamp to detect the antifreeze additive fluorescein: a qualitative adjunctive test in suspected ethylene glycol ingestions. *Ann Emerg Med* 1990;19:663.

CHAPTER 339

Fluoride and Hydrofluoric Acid Poisoning

Andis Graudins

Fluoride is found in various commercial and household products. Inorganic salts of fluoride have been extensively used as insecticides and rodenticides. Sulfuryl fluoride (Vikane) is used as a "tent" fumigant to eradicate pests in buildings. Sodium fluoride is also used in the manufacture of fertilizers and plastics. The inorganic acid of fluoride, hydrofluoric acid (HF) is an extremely corrosive substance used in the etching of glass, metal, and stone and in the electronics and semiconductor industries.

HF is also a common constituent of rust and scale removers designed for commercial and home use, often found in poorly labeled containers with little warning about the potential toxicity of HF. Fluoride is added to the municipal water supply in many communities, and to toothpaste and other dental hygiene preparations because of its role in preventing tooth decay. The recommended dose is 0.7 to 1.2 ppm in drinking water, or 0.25 to 0.5 mg/d as a dietary supplement.

Because of the variety of fluoride compounds and differences in the duration and routes of exposure, there are three primary forms of fluoride poisoning: acute systemic fluoride poisoning; acute topical exposure to HF; and chronic "fluorosis," a syndrome of osteosclerosis, brittle bones, exostoses, ectopic calcification (e.g., of ligaments and tendons), and renal calculi, which results from long-term exposure to low concentrations of fluoride.

Acute systemic fluoride poisoning may be due to the intentional or accidental ingestion of fluoride salts or to oral or dermal exposures to HF.[5,19] More than 600 deaths have been attributed to acute fluoride poisoning since the 1930s. There has been a marked increase in recent years in the number of reports of topical HF exposure, no doubt because of the rapid growth of the semiconductor industry and of other industrial applications for fluoride.[19]

Soluble fluoride salts, such as sodium fluoride and stannous fluoride, are rapidly absorbed through the gastrointestinal (GI) tract.[5] Fluoride may also be absorbed through the skin, although dermal absorption is probably limited to HF exposures. Fatal accidental and intentional fluoride poisoning has also been reported after inhalational exposure.[5,16]

Once absorbed, fluoride is distributed to virtually every tissue and organ and is slowly eliminated in the urine. Normal fluoride levels are 0.4 to 2.0 μg/dL in blood and 0.2 to 1.1 μg/mL in urine. As little as 2 g of sodium fluoride or 32 mg/kg may be lethal in an adult, and 16 mg/kg in children. A dose of more than 5 to 10 mg/kg should be considered serious and may result in hypocalcemia. GI effects may occur with lesser amounts. Severe chemical burns may result from exposures to very dilute (less than 5%) solutions of HF, and fatal systemic poisoning has resulted from relatively small (less than 5% total body surface area) burns caused by more concentrated solutions.[5,6,13,14]

Several pathologic mechanisms are involved in both local and systemic fluoride poisoning. Fluoride binds to divalent cations, especially calcium and magnesium, to form insoluble fluoride salts. The resulting hypocalcemia, hypomagnesemia, and depletion of other trace nutrients have profound effects on a number of cellular and organ functions. Fluoride is also a general protoplasmic poison, inhibiting numerous aerobic and even anaerobic metabolic enzyme systems and interfering with cellular respiration.[5] Fluoride also interferes with Na^+/K^+-ATPase and activates calcium-dependent potassium channels in cell membranes, resulting in massive leaks of potassium into the extracellular space, with subsequent hyperkalemia.[7] Precipitation of calcium also interferes with calcium-dependent clotting factors, resulting in coagulopathy. Finally, exposure to HF may produce direct corrosive injury.

The evaluation and management of HF burns and systemic fluoride toxicity are very different and require separate consideration. Systemic fluoride toxicity may accompany topical HF exposure due to absorption of fluoride, however, and HF injury may accompany systemic fluoride poisoning due to the conversion of fluoride salts to HF in an acidic medium (e.g., gastric juices).

CLINICAL PRESENTATION

Systemic fluoride poisoning is manifest by various toxic effects, including direct tissue injury at the site of absorption. Signs and symptoms usually begin within minutes of exposure. Fluoride ingestion is associated with an acute gastroenteritis, vomiting, diarrhea, and abdominal pain.[5] Fluoride inhalation is associated with pulmonary injury, including the development of noncardiogenic pulmonary edema and adult respiratory distress syndrome.[5,16] Dermal fluoride exposure produces typical HF burns.

Patients with systemic fluoride poisoning typically present with significant metabolic acidosis; it is usually ascribed to interference with intracellular metabolism. The most lethal complications are due to the severe electrolyte abnormalities produced by direct interaction with fluoride or effects on cell membranes.[5,7] Severe hypocalcemia (serum calcium level less than 5 mEq/L), frequently reported as a major finding in systemic fluoride poisoning, is presumably due to the complexing of calcium by fluoride ions. Severe hypomagnesemia and hypomagnesemia have also been reported. Most recent evidence, however, indicates that the primary cause of the lethal dysrhythmias (refractory ventricular tachycardia, ventricular fibrillation, and pulseless idioventricular rhythm) is the development of hyperkalemia. The combination of hypocalcemia and hyperkalemia is extremely harmful, but studies have shown that lethal hyperkalemia may occur despite maintenance of normal serum calcium levels.[7]

Systemic manifestations of hypocalcemia include carpopedal spasm, positive Chvostek's and Trousseau's signs, hyperreflexia, tetany, and coagulopathy. Headache, paresthesias, and visual complaints may be noted. In severe cases, coma, seizures, shock, and dysrhythmias may precede death.

A patient with an acute exposure to HF may be a difficult diagnostic problem. First, the patient may not even know that the product he or she was using contained HF, as product labels may be incomplete. Second, the patient may have been exposed to HF inadvertently, through unrecognized HF contamination of materials and work sites. Finally, the typical signs and symptoms of an acute HF injury may be delayed for many hours after an exposure, and patients may not recognize that their symptoms are related to the exposure. The onset of symptoms following acute dermal HF exposure depends on the concentration of the acid and the duration of exposure.[5] Highly concentrated (70%) HF may contain enough hydrogen ions to produce some burning sensation on the skin and may provide some degree of warning of an acute exposure with symptom onset within 1 to 2 hours. Low concentrations of HF (less than 10%), found in products such as over-the-counter rust removers, however, produce no symptoms at the time of contact, and patients may present as long as 10 to 12 hours following the initial exposure. This delay is due to the fact that the relatively small dissociation constant ($K = 3.53 \times 10^{-4}$) limits the concentration of free hydrogen ions.[19] In addition, the fact that HF tends to remain in an undissociated, neutral state enhances its ability to penetrate through the skin into deeper tissues, where its gradual dissociation into free fluoride ions leads to the characteristic local tissue injury.

The presenting complaint of acute topical HF injury is pain, often in the absence of any physical signs. HF exposure should always be considered in this situation. It is usually described as a tingling sensation that progresses to a burning pain and, ultimately, to the typical deep, throbbing, unremitting, and excruciating pain.[5,12,18,19]

Visible evidence of HF burns also follows a fairly characteristic pattern. The burn site initially becomes erythematous and may be somewhat edematous. As tissue injury progresses, the site assumes a pale, blanched appearance, which may be followed by the development of local vesiculation and frank tissue necrosis (e.g., blackened tissue). Fluoride may penetrate into underlying bone, and demineralization may ensue. This destructive process may progress over several days in inadequately treated patients, resulting in the development of deep ulceration and extensive tissue loss, including the loss of entire digits.

DIFFERENTIAL DIAGNOSIS

GI manifestations of fluoride ingestion are similar to those of infectious gastroenteritis. Although virtually any poison can cause GI symptoms, alcohols, corrosives, heavy metals, lithium, nonsteroidal antiinflammatory agents, and theophylline typically cause effects of comparable severity. The differential diagnosis of hypocalcemia includes parathyroid hormone deficiency and ethylene glycol poisoning. Hyperkalemia may be caused by alpha agonists, beta blockers, digitalis, and potassium overdose. The combination of hypocalcemia, hypomagnesemia, and hyperkalemia points to fluoride poisoning.

HF burns, when apparent, may resemble those resulting from thermal injury, frostbite, or other corrosives (e.g., acids and alkalis).

EMERGENCY DEPARTMENT EVALUATION

The history should include the dose (the amount of fluoride ingested or the concentration of HF), the time of exposure, first-aid measures taken, symptoms, and current medical problems.

Once vital signs have been obtained, the focus of the physical examination becomes the abdomen, lungs, or skin (and mucous membranes), depending on the route of exposure. Evidence of hypocalcemia (i.e., neuromuscular hyperactivity) is sought. All patients with significant ingestions, inhalations, or topical exposures (greater than 5% body surface area) should have cardiac monitoring, a 12-lead electrocardiogram (ECG), and serum calcium, magnesium, and electrolyte level measurements. A baseline complete blood count, prothrombin time, partial thromboplastin time, and kidney function studies are also recommended. A chest radiograph is ordered for patients with respiratory symptoms or severe clinical toxicity.

Serum and urine fluoride levels are not readily available or clinically useful. They can, however, be used to confirm the diagnosis retrospectively and assess the efficacy of therapy.

EMERGENCY DEPARTMENT MANAGEMENT

The treatment of systemic fluoride poisoning has two primary goals: to remove fluoride from the system and to correct electrolyte abnormalities. Patients with fluoride ingestion should receive rapid, aggressive GI decontamination, including lavage and instillation of calcium-containing substances (e.g., antacids) to complex fluoride in the gut.[3–5] Urinary fluoride excretion may be enhanced by alkalinization, and hemodialysis removes fluoride from the blood directly.

Serum calcium levels should be closely monitored, and intravenous calcium chloride should be given for replacement. Massive amounts of calcium may be required; in one case, the administration of 280 mEq of calcium increased the serum calcium level from 2.2 mEq/L to only 3.1 mEq/L.[14] Either 10% calcium chloride (14 mEq calcium/10 mL) or calcium gluconate (4.65 mEq/10 mL) may be used. The initial dose of 0.2 mL/kg is given intravenously over 5 to 10 minutes and is repeated, as needed, until serum calcium levels are normalized. Similarly, 10% magnesium sulfate, in an initial dose of 0.1 to 0.2 mL/kg, may be given for hypomagnesemia.

Hyperkalemia may first be recognized by the appearance of characteristic tall, peaked T waves on the ECG, but close monitoring of serum potassium levels is warranted, even in the absence of peaked T waves. Hyperkalemia in systemic fluoride poisoning does not respond to some traditional measures, such as insulin, glucose, and bicarbonate. Also, the ventricular dysrhythmias associated with acute fluoride poisoning are refractory to cardioversion and defibrillation, lidocaine has not been shown to be effective, and propranolol may actually exacerbate the hyperkalemia.[7] Quinidine, on the other hand, has shown promise in preventing or reversing hyperkalemia and ventricular irritability in dogs, although this method of treatment is yet to be tried in humans.[7] Hemodialysis is indicated for severe or refractory hypocalcemia, hyperkalemia, or clinical toxicity (e.g., dysrhythmias) and may also be useful for removing fluoride ions. Calcium and magnesium monitoring and replacement should continue during this procedure.

The initial step in management of an acute topical HF exposure is thorough skin decontamination with a water flush. It should be accomplished before arrival in the emergency department if prehospital personnel are involved or if the patient contacts the emergency department for advice. Unfortunately, the delayed presentation of most patients with HF burns makes it unlikely that significant amounts of HF still remain on the surface of the skin.

First-aid measures for known or suspected HF burns are the use of topical soaks, creams, and ointments. These usually contain calcium gluconate (2.5% to 10% gel), magnesium oxide (10% paste), or a quaternary ammonium salt (benzalkonium or benzethonium chloride). Topical therapies are intended to form insoluble complexes with any surface fluoride ion to prevent penetration into tissues, thereby minimizing or preventing deep cellular injury.

Animal studies have compared the efficacy of various topical therapies or infiltration techniques, with varied results.[4,8] Most of these studies involve an immediate therapeutic intervention. Many HF exposures, however, are not promptly recognized, and patients often do not present until symptoms have developed (usually many hours after exposure). Therefore, animal models do not usually reproduce the typical clinical presentation in the emergency department.

Topical treatment is probably of some benefit if applied immediately after initial decontamination of a known, recognized exposure. It may also be of benefit in patients with mild pain and minimal evidence of tissue damage (e.g., erythema only) who present late. It should be considered adjunctive, however, in patients who present with progressive pain and signs of deeper tissue injury. At worst, reliance on topical therapies delays definitive treatment and allows greater tissue injury to develop.[19]

Definitive treatment of acute HF burns involves the administration of calcium gluconate into the tissues affected by the exposure.[19] It may be achieved by a number of methods: direct tissue infiltration, regional intravenous infusion using a Bier's block technique, and intraarterial infusion. The choice of method depends on the site and concentration of HF involved.

In soft tissues with sufficient loose tissue space for injection of a volume of fluid, this is most easily accomplished by the direct injection of approximately 0.5 mL per square centimeter of 10% calcium gluconate solution at the burn site. A small needle (25- to 30-gauge) should be used to minimize discomfort and mechanical tissue damage, and care should be taken to infiltrate into, around, and beneath the burn area as completely as possible. By loading the local tissue with calcium, the mechanism of fluoride injury is terminated and even reversed by the precipitation of free fluoride and replenishment of decreased tissue calcium levels. Only calcium gluconate should be used for local infiltration; calcium chloride produces direct injury when injected into tissues.[3,5]

Digital HF burns are relatively common and deserve special consideration. Fingertip burns are particularly painful because of the rich sensory nerve supply, and are difficult to infiltrate with calcium gluconate for the same reason. In addition, only small amounts of calcium gluconate may be injected directly into the fingertips because of limited space for introduction of additional fluid volume in an end-arterial circulation region. Repeated injections are frequently necessary to neutralize all the fluoride present. HF may penetrate beneath the fingernails, and the nails must be removed before calcium gluconate is injected directly into the nail bed, to avoid the unbearable pain associated with administering even a minimal volume of fluid into the closed space between the nail plate and distal phalanx.[3,11,18,19]

Currently two techniques are available as an alternative to direct injection of calcium gluconate into digital HF burns. The first is to infuse calcium gluconate into the arterial supply of the involved digit(s). This technique involves inserting an indwelling arterial catheter into the radial or brachial artery of the involved extremity and slowly infusing a dilute solution of calcium gluconate by an infusion pump. It allows the calcium to be delivered to the affected tissues through the vascular supply and avoids the pain and tissue distention associated with direct injection.[12,19] A typical dose is 10 to 20 mL of 10% calcium gluconate in 50 to 100 mL of dextrose 5% in water given over 4 hours and repeated as necessary. Because extravasated calcium salts are themselves corrosive, the arterial waveform should be monitored during the infusion to confirm proper catheter placement. The end point for therapy should be the absence of pain at rest. In one large case series, the average number of intraarterial infusions was four, with a range of one to ten.[17]

The second technique that may be considered in the treatment of digital HF burns is regional intravenous calcium gluconate infusion using a Bier's block technique.[9,10,15,20] This technique is similar to that originally described by Bier for regional limb anesthesia and has the advantages of relative simplicity and of not requiring arterial cannulation. Success has been reported for digital, hand, and forearm exposures,[9,10,15] as well as for exposures to the leg.[15] The technique involves placing a canula in the dorsum of the hand (or foot) of the affected limb, raising the arm to exsanguinate the superficial venous system, and then inflating a surgical pneumatic tourniquet applied to the upper arm to a pressure 100 mm Hg above systolic blood pressure. Ten to 15 mL of 10% calcium gluconate is diluted to a total volume of 50 mL with normal saline and infused via the canula to the ischemic arm. The tourniquet is sequentially released after 20 to 25 minutes.[9] When successful, relief is apparent within 30 minutes of tourniquet release.

In cases in which exposure has been to high-concentration HF (greater than 20%) or multiple digits are involved, the arterial route appears to be more effective, perhaps because of the more focal provision of calcium to the site of digital exposure than is possible with the regional intravenous route. Additionally, it is possible to administer multiple infusions by intraarterial canula in patients with ongoing pain. If the intravenous route is selected as primary therapy and it is unsuccessful following one treatment, the intraarterial route should be used subsequently.

Finally, ocular HF exposures should also be mentioned; they can result in serious consequences if left untreated. The use of topical calcium gluconate drops is controversial. Animal studies suggest that they are no better than copious irrigation with normal saline and may, in fact, result in delayed corneal healing.[2] Patients should be treated as for other chemical exposures to the eye, with copious saline irrigation, local anesthetic drops for pain relief, and early ophthalmologic referral.

To date, there have been no controlled, prospective human studies comparing the techniques for the management of HF exposure. Retrospective and even prospective case series are difficult to evaluate, as the concentration, amount, and duration of HF exposure are frequently unknown. Numerous animal studies have been reported with varying results. In an *in vivo* porcine model, using high-concentration HF (49%) and comparing regional intravenous and intraarterial infusions of calcium gluconate, there was a trend toward lesser burn depth following intraarterial therapy.[1] At present, the most logical approach seems to be an initial trial of topical therapy. Invasive techniques should be used in patients who do not respond to topical therapy within 30 to 60 minutes of application of calcium gluconate gel, those who have been exposed to a known high concentration of HF, or those who have had extensive skin exposure.

DISPOSITION

Any patient who presents with persistent symptoms or signs after acute ingestion, inhalation, or topical HF exposure requires admission to a monitored bed for close observation. Many patients with severe poisoning have presented in relatively stable condition and with normal initial laboratory values, only to develop severe complications after several hours of evaluation and treatment.

Patients with HF burns require much closer follow-up than do patients with almost any other kind of corrosive injury. Repeated calcium infiltrations or infusions are frequently required, and patients with lesions that demonstrate vesiculation or necrosis before or despite adequate treatment should be referred to a plastic surgeon for wound care. Extensive HF exposures should be carefully monitored for the possibility of systemic fluoride poisoning. Unless the physician is familiar with treating this type of poisoning, initial consultation with a poison center, toxicologist, or plastic surgeon is advised. Eye exposures should be referred to an ophthalmologist as soon as possible.

COMMON PITFALLS

- Failing to appreciate that patients with fluoride or HF exposure are at risk for progressive poisoning, with life- and limb-threatening complications

- Failing to recognize and treat patients with symptomatic HF exposures despite lack of visible evidence of tissue injury
- Failing to monitor serum calcium, magnesium, and potassium and to admit patients with significant exposures
- Relying on topical therapy for HF burns when calcium gluconate infiltration or infusion is indicated
- Using calcium chloride rather than calcium gluconate for infiltration or parenteral therapy
- Failing to appreciate that large doses of parenteral calcium and magnesium may be necessary in severe cases of systemic poisoning
- Failing to arrange follow-up in 12 to 24 hours for patients who have been symptomatic after a topical exposure

ACKNOWLEDGMENT

Michael V. Vance contributed the previous editions of this chapter.

References

1. Aaron CK, Fudem GM, Hartigan CF. Treatment of extremity hydrofluoric acid burns: an in-vivo histopathological comparison of topical, locally infiltrated, intraarterial, and regional IV calcium gluconate. *Acad Emerg Med* 1996;5:419(abst).
2. Beiran I, Miller B, Bentur Y. The efficacy of calcium gluconate in ocular hydrofluoric acid burns. *Hum Exp Toxicol* 1997;16(4):223–228.
3. Bracken WM, Cuppage F, McLaury RL, et al. Comparative effectiveness of topical treatments for hydrofluoric acid burns. *J Occup Med* 1985;27(10):733–739.
4. Burkhart KK, Brent J, Kirk MA, et al. Comparison of topical magnesium and calcium treatment for dermal hydrofluoric acid burns. *Ann Emerg Med* 1994;24(1):9–13.
5. Caravati EM. Acute hydrofluoric acid exposure. *Am J Emerg Med* 1988;6(2):143–150.
6. Chan KM, Svancarek WP, Creer M. Fatality due to acute hydrofluoric acid exposure. *J Toxicol Clin Toxicol* 1987;25(4):333–339.
7. Cummings CC, McIvor ME. Fluoride-induced hyperkalemia: the role of Ca++-dependent K+ channels. *Am J Emerg Med* 1988;6:1.
8. Dunn BJ, MacKinnon MA, Knowlden NF, et al. Hydrofluoric acid dermal burns. An assessment of treatment efficacy using an experimental pig model. *J Occup Med* 1992;34(9):902–909.
9. Graudins A, Burns MJ, Aaron CK. Regional intravenous infusion of calcium gluconate for hydrofluoric acid burns of the upper extremity [see comments]. *Ann Emerg Med* 1997;30(5):604–607.
10. Henry JA, Hla KK. Intravenous regional calcium gluconate perfusion for hydrofluoric acid burns. *J Toxicol Clin Toxicol* 1992;30(2):203–207.
11. Hoffman R, Mann J, Calderone J, et al. Acute fluoride poisoning in a New Mexico elementary school. *Pediatrics* 1980;65:897.
12. Kohnlein HE, Achinger R. A new method of treatment of HF burns of the extremities. *Chir Plastica* 1982;6:298.
13. Manoguerra AS, Neuman TS. Fatal poisoning from acute HF ingestion. *Am J Emerg Med* 1988;4:362.
14. Mayer TG, Gross PL. Fatal systemic fluorosis due to hydrofluoric acid burns. *Ann Emerg Med* 1985;14(2):149–153.
15. Ryan JM, McCarthy GM, Plunkett PK. Regional intravenous calcium—an effective method of treating hydrofluoric acid burns to limb peripheries. *J Accid Emerg Med* 1997;14(6):401–404.
16. Scheuerman EH. Suicide by exposure to sulfuryl fluoride. *J Forensic Sci* 1986;31:1154.
17. Siegel DC, Heard JM. Intra-arterial calcium infusion for hydrofluoric acid burns. *Aviat Space Environ Med* 1992;63(3):206–211.
18. Trevino MA, Herrmann GH, Sprout WL. Treatment of severe hydrofluoric acid exposures. *J Occup Med* 1983;25(12):861–863.
19. Vance MV, Curry SC, Kunkel DB, et al. Digital hydrofluoric acid burns: treatment with intraarterial calcium infusion. *Ann Emerg Med* 1986;15(8):890–896.
20. Wilkes GJ. Intravenous regional calcium gluconate for hydrofluoric acid burns of the digits. *Emerg Med* 1993;5:149–244.

CHAPTER 340
Food Poisoning

Marc C. Restuccia

Despite improvements in detection and increased regulatory oversight, food-borne illness remains a serious cause of morbidity and mortality throughout the world, including the United States. With the growth in modern mass-production farms and food-handling and -processing plants, the potential for amplification of food-borne pathogens is great. Although common, the exact incidence of food-borne illness is not accurately known.[2] What is known is that each year, millions of people are affected worldwide,[1] and although the majority of persons suffer only temporary discomfort, for the very young, the old, and the immunocompromised, food-borne illnesses can be fatal.

Improper food handling, leading to fecal contamination of food, is the usual cause of most food-borne illnesses. Causative agents include bacteria, viruses, parasites, and toxins. More recently, prions, a new infectious class of agents have been implicated in causing transmissible spongiform encephalopathies.[4] This chapter focuses on the bacterial causes of food poisoning.

Alterations in normal gastrointestinal (GI) tract function are the hallmark of bacterial food poisoning. Patients with food poisoning may have some or all of the following: nausea, vomiting, diarrhea, abdominal pain, cramps, and fever.

Bacterial causes of food poisoning can be characterized as toxin induced, invasive, or inflammatory. Breaking them up like this allows easier identification of the causative agent.

Organisms such as *Staphylococcus aureus,* which produce a toxin, cause symptoms such as vomiting quickly, as little as 8 hours after ingestion. Toxins can also lead to diarrhea as the toxin disrupts intestinal sodium absorption. This, in turn, leads to massive amounts of salt and water being presented to the large intestine, with subsequent volume-overload diarrhea. Invasive bacteria, on the other hand, invade or destroy the mucosal layer, leading to bloody diarrhea with fecal leukocytes. Examples of such bacteria include *Escherichia coli, Campylobacter, Salmonella, Shigella,* and *Yersinia.*

CLINICAL PRESENTATION

Almost all types of food poisoning present with similar complaints. After a variable incubation period (Table 340.1), alterations in GI functions begin. The patient may present with all or only some of the following: fever, abdominal pain, cramps, nausea, vomiting, diarrhea (bloody or watery), myalgias, and athralgias. The pain of food poisoning is most often characterized as colicky, but can be more severe. Patients with *Salmonella* as a causative agent occasionally present with severe abdominal pain, even peritoneal signs. Bloody diarrhea is seen with the invasive organisms, such as *Campylobacter.* Watery diarrhea can be seen with any food-borne pathogen. Fever and dehydration can be seen, and the dehydration may be profound.

DIFFERENTIAL DIAGNOSIS

The actual number of cases of food-borne illness is unknown. It is a diagnosis often considered but rarely confirmed. Only in multiperson outbreaks is a diagnosis usually reached. In addition, the long incubation period of some food-borne pathogens

TABLE 340.1. Bacterial Causes of Food-Borne Illness

Agent	Incubation	Duration	Common Sources	Manifestations	Specific Treatment
Staphylococcus aureus (toxin)	4 h	20 h	Dairy products, ham, potato salad, custards, pastry	Vomit, cramp, diarrhea; – fever	None
Salmonella (invasive)	24 h	5 d	Dairy products, poultry, eggs, chocolate, coconut, dried foods	Watery, bloody diarrhea + or – fecal leukocytes, possibly bacteremia	Immunocompromised/septic: TMS, CFT, FQ, CAP
Shigella (invasive)	1–3 d	5 d	Any food contaminated with fecal material during processing; ice in developing countries	Copious bloody diarrhea, fever, cramps; rare: DIC, HUS, sepsis; children may have seizures; + fecal leukocytes	TMS or FQ
Clostridium perfringens (toxin)	12 h	24 h	Meat, meat byproducts; poultry, especially cooked and inadequate refrigeration	Nonbloody diarrhea; – fecal leukocytes	None
Campylobacter jejuni (both)	3 d	4 d	Unpasteurized milk, dairy products	Abdominal pain, diarrhea, fever, constitutional symptoms; biphasic illness; + fecal leukocytes	FQ, AG, MAC
Bacillus cereus (toxin)	3 h 10 h	12 h 36 h	Spices and grains such as fried rice, especially if inadequate refrigeration	Vomiting: Fried rice ingestion; Diarrhea; – Fecal leukocytes	None
Escherichia coli 0157:H7 (toxin)	48 h	1 wk	Raw or undercooked beef	Copious, bloody diarrhea; rare HUS, renal failure; – fecal leukocytes	None
Traveler's diarrhea					
Enterotoxigenic (toxin)	12–72 h	24–72 h	Raw vegetables, seafood, improperly cooked food from street vendors, hot-pepper sauce, tap water	Watery diarrhea, low-grade fever, – fecal leukocytes	Prophylaxis: BSS, TMS, FQ. Treatment: FQ, TMS, + antidiarrheal agent
Enteroinvasive (invasive)	12–72 h	24–72 h	Similar to above	Severe cramps, malaise; initially watery, then bloody diarrhea; + fecal leukocytes	FQ, TMS
Clostridium botulinum (toxin)	30 h	Variable	Improper home canning, unpasteurized honey	Flulike symptoms, descending weakness or paralysis, ptosis; may have no GI symptoms	Antitoxin
Yersinia enterocolitica (invasive)	15–24 h	2 wk	Foods contaminated with fecal material during processing or handling (e.g., tofu, bean sprouts, milk, milk products, contaminated water)	Diarrhea, fever, abdominal pain, vomiting, bloody stools; may be protracted; can lead to appendicitis operations; + or – fecal leukocytes	FQ, TMS, AG
Streptococcus (invasive)	1–3 d	3–5 d	Salads, meats, inadequately refrigerated, fried, boiled rice	Viral-type syndrome; pharyngitis, myalgia, fever, chills	Penicillin
Listeria monocytogenes (invasive)	1–70 d	Variable	Beef, pork, poultry, cheeses (soft "Mexican-style," Swiss); milk, contaminated after pasteurization; fruits and vegetables; other dairy products	Pregnant and immunocompromised patients more susceptible; meningitis, meningoencephalitis; + fever; may have limited GI symptoms	Amp, TMS, CAP
Cryptosporidium	6 d	6 d	Hand-pressed cider, municipal water supplies, public pools	Vomiting, diarrhea; worse in immunocompromised patients	None

TMS, trimethoprim–sulfamethoxazole; CFT, ceftriaxone; FQ, fluoroquinolones (ofloxacin or ciprofloxacin);[5] CAP, chloramphenicol; DIC, disseminated intravascular coagulation; HUS, hemolytic–uremic syndrome; AG, aminoglycoside; MAC, macrolides (azithromycin, clarithromycin, erythromycin); BSS, bismuth subsalicylate; Amp, ampicillin.

and the overlap with multiple other causes of GI disturbances can easily lead to a missed diagnosis.

Viral gastroenteritis is the most common diagnosis for patients with nausea, vomiting, and diarrhea. Common viral causes of gastroenteritis are rotavirus (in the winter), Norwalk virus, enteric adenovirus, and hepatitis A (no seasonal predilection).

Parasites are another source of gastroenteritis and often can be linked with specific habits and activities. *Giardia lamblia* is most commonly seen among hikers, campers, and travelers who are infected through drinking contaminated water. Other parasites, such as *Entamoeba histolytica, Cryptosporidium,* and *Isospora belli* are linked to either male homosexuals or the human immunodeficiency virus (HIV) infection.

Clostridium difficile can overgrow the GI tract in persons taking wide-spectrum antibiotics. The resulting pseudomembranous colitis can cause bloody diarrhea and severe abdominal pain.

Other diagnoses to consider in the differential include biliary disease, food intolerance or allergies, inflammatory bowel disease, irritable bowel disease, urinary tract infections, appendicitis, peptic ulcer disease, and gynecologic disorders.

Contamination of food with toxins, pesticides, or chemicals can lead to illness.[3]

EMERGENCY DEPARTMENT EVALUATION

In the patient with suspected food poisoning, supportive therapy should be instituted even as the diagnostic workup proceeds. Intravenous access for fluid resuscitation and to obtain blood samples for potential laboratory evaluation are usually required. Fluid resuscitation should be ongoing during the evaluation of the patient.

The history should focus on recent meals, what foods were consumed, how they were prepared, the manner in which they were kept after being prepared, and who ate with the patient and their current health. The time of onset, nature, and progression of the illness may provide diagnostic clues to uncover the etiology of the infecting agent. Any recent travel, especially to regions such as Mexico (well known for having a high incidence of food-borne infections), should be noted. Drinking water sources should be asked about, especially in campers and hikers who might have been drinking from "back country" water sources. Underlying medical conditions, such as HIV, sickle cell disease, malignancies, diabetes, cardiac or renal disorders, immunodeficiencies, and medications should be asked about.

The physical examination should be structured so as to quickly ascertain the hydration status of the patient and perform an abdominal examination. This should include a rectal examination, looking for the presence or absence of fecal blood. As is true with any patient with abdominal pain, serial examinations and vital signs are imperative to ensure that any clinical deterioration in the patient is detected quickly.

The extent of the laboratory evaluation varies from patient to patient. A white blood cell count is not usually useful; a high white blood cell count only confirms that an inflammatory process is going on. It will do little to narrow the diagnostic possibilities. On the other hand, a hematocrit and hemoglobin may be useful, especially if followed serially in patients with invasive organisms and bloody diarrhea. Anemia can occur with *Salmonella.*

Likewise, the amount of chemistries obtained varies from patient to patient. In the well-hydrated patient who appears well, routine chemistries are unlikely to add anything to the diagnosis. Patients who are dehydrated or who have the possibility of other diagnoses may require additional testing. In general, serum electrolytes, blood urea nitrogen (BUN), creatinine, blood sugar, and urinalysis are sufficient. A urine specific gravity greater than 1.025 or a BUN–creatinine ratio greater than 20:1 is consistent with severe dehydration. Likewise, a serum bicarbonate level below 20 mEq/L is consistent with significant dehydration, particularly in children.

Patients with significant abdominal tenderness or a high fever may require a more extensive evaluation. In addition to the aforementioned tests, consideration should be given to obtaining liver function tests, an amylase or lipase, a complete blood count, bilirubin, and blood cultures. Virtually any woman of childbearing age should have a human chorionic gonadotropin test performed. In patients with heme-positive stools or diarrhea, it is common to obtain stool for routine bacterial culture. As this rarely affects the acute management of the illness, it is probably not indicated. In patients who present with weeks or months of diarrhea, three separate specimens for ova and parasites may well be indicated.

In patients with clear indications of food poisoning who are otherwise healthy, do not appear seriously ill, and have little abdominal pain, radiologic evaluation is not indicated. In the elderly, infants, patients who appear very ill, and patients who have significant abdominal pain or a history of intraabdominal pain, upright views of the abdomen and chest are indicated to rule out perforation or obstruction. In the elderly, the possibility of an abdominal aortic aneurysm should be considered. If the diagnosis is uncertain, abdominal computed tomography imaging is indicated in the ill patient.

In patients with significant risk factors for coronary artery disease, or have an actual history of the same, an electrocardiogram is warranted to rule out a cardiac cause for the illness.

EMERGENCY DEPARTMENT MANAGEMENT

The first priority in treating patients with suspected food poisoning is to replace fluid and electrolyte losses. In mild or moderately ill patients who are not vomiting and can take fluids by mouth, oral rehydration is acceptable. Intravenous crystalloid, either lactated Ringer's or normal saline, with or without 5% dextrose, is indicated for moderately to severely ill patients, especially if they continue to vomit and/or are seriously dehydrated. The initial bolus should be from 5 to 20 cc/kg, depending on the patients' age, cardiovascular status, and degree of dehydration. A maintenance infusion should be initiated and further boluses tailored to the patients' clinical response to treatment. The adequacy of the resuscitation can be judged by subjective response, appearance, urinary output, vital signs, and improving laboratory parameters.

Intravenous, intramuscular, or rectal antiemetics (prochlorperazine or metoclopramide) may be helpful in patients with persistent nausea, vomiting, and abdominal cramping. Although antidiarrheal drugs (e.g., diphenoxylate [Lomotil] or loperamide [Imodium]) have traditionally been held to be contraindicated in the treatment of food poisoning, in some situations, such as traveler's diarrhea, their use may speed recovery.[5] However, they are not appropriate for use in patients with bloody diarrhea. Their use can prolong symptoms (e.g., with *Shigella*), cause perforation (with amebiasis), and increase mortality (e.g., with *Campylobacter*).

Antibiotics are usually not indicated. Patients with viral sources of diarrhea and those with many bacterial illnesses do not improve more rapidly when given antibiotics. Some organisms, such as *Salmonella,* may have prolonged colonic colonization when antibiotics are used. In patients who are septic, immunosuppressed, or HIV-positive; are elderly; or have other coexistent illnesses, antibiotics may be appropriate. Specific treatments for each causative organism are given in Table 340.1.

DISPOSITION

Most patients can be discharged once they are rehydrated and are feeling better. The ability to take fluids orally should be documented before discharge. These patients should be instructed to maintain a generous intake of clear fluids and begin frequent small feedings as soon as they can be tolerated. Patients should be advised to return to the emergency department or to contact their personal physician if symptoms have not abated within 24 hours, or to return sooner if they cannot maintain a sufficient oral intake, if they develop a high fever, or if abdominal pain persists. The parents of small children should also be warned that the hemolytic–uremic syndrome (see Chapter 211) is a potential complication.

Patients with severe dehydration, especially those with significant underlying illness or at the extremes of age, should be admitted. Those with suspected bacteremia (e.g., fever, elevated white count, or toxic appearance) and those patients who do not improve with therapy should be admitted or observed over a period of several hours. Likewise, any patient in whom the diagnosis is in doubt should be considered for admission. Patients who may not be able to seek further medical care because of social circumstances or those who cannot tolerate oral intake should be admitted. For most patients needing admission, a floor bed or observation unit will suffice. Occasionally, a patient with an underlying illness or who remains hemodynamically unstable may require an intensive care admission.

Local health authorities should be contacted if other persons in the community may be at risk. If the suspected food was bought at a store or restaurant, other members of the public may be exposed. Such actions can limit the numbers of people who become ill.[2]

COMMON PITFALLS

- Failure to consider the possibility of food poisoning in all patients with nausea, vomiting, diarrhea, and abdominal cramps
- Failure to obtain a history of antecedent antibiotic use, travel, camping, and diet in patients with nausea, vomiting, diarrhea, and abdominal cramps
- Failure to exclude life-threatening etiologies of abdominal complaints, such as appendicitis, aortic aneurysm, pyelonephritis, cholecystitis, pneumonia, and myocardial disease, and pregnancy-induced conditions
- Discharging patients who cannot take oral fluids, especially if they have been inadequately rehydrated
- Failure to consider the effects of underlying diseases in the management of patients with suspected food poisoning
- Failure to consider potential public health hazards and failing to notify public health authorities when appropriate

References

1. Bashai WR, Sears CL. Food poisoning syndromes. *Gastroenterol Clin North Am* 1993;3:579.
2. Keene WE. Lessons from investigations of foodborne disease outbreaks. *JAMA* 1999;281(19):1845–1847.
3. Poisonings associated with illegal use of Aldicarb as a rodenticide—New York City, 1994–1997. *MMWR* 1997;46(41):41.
4. Tan L, Williams MA, Khan MK, et al. Risk of transmission of bovine-spongiform encephalopathy to humans in the United States. *JAMA* 1999; 281(24):2330–2339.
5. Taylor DN, Sanchez JL, Candlor W, et al. Treatment of traveler's diarrhea; ciprofloxacin plus loperamide compared with ciprofloxacin alone. *Ann Intern Med* 1991;114;731.

CHAPTER 341
Hallucinogen Poisoning

Christopher H. Linden

Hallucinogens, also known as psychedelic or psychotomimetic agents, are chemicals whose predominant effect is the production of sensory misperceptions, disordered thought processes, and mood changes. Included in this category are lysergic acid diethylamide (LSD) and related tryptamine derivatives (Table 341.1); marijuana; mescaline and related analogues of amphetamine (Table 341.2); and phencyclidine (see Chapter 363). Hallucinogens are classified as Food and Drug Administration schedule I agents (i.e., no proven medical value) and are primarily regarded as substances of abuse. They are readily available through illicit street markets, but their use was more common during the 1960s and 1970s than it is today. Use is most prevalent in teenagers and young adults.

Marijuana and its main active ingredient THC (delta-9-tetrahydrocannabinol) are used medically to treat glaucoma, as appetite stimulants to treat cachexia (e.g., in acquired immunodeficiency syndrome patients), and as antiemetics to treat the nausea and vomiting associated with cancer chemotherapy. They are also being studied for the treatment of neuropathic pain, seizures, and spasticity. The therapeutic potential of amphetamine derivatives is being studied in patients with psychiatric disorders.

TABLE 341.1. Hallucinogenic Tryptamine Derivatives (LSD Analogues)
Tryptamine
Alpha-methyltryptamine (AMT)
4-hydroxy-AMT
5-fluoro-AMT
5-methoxy-AMT
N,N-dimethyltryptamine (DMT)
4-hydroxy-DMT (psilocyn)
4-phosphoryloxy-DMT (psilocybin)
5-hydroxy-DMT (bufotenine)
5-methoxy-DMT
N, N-diethyltryptamine (DET)
4-hydroxy-DET
N, N-diallyltryptamine (DAT)
N, N-dipropyltryptamine (DPT)

TABLE 341.2. Hallucinogenic Amphetamine Derivatives (Mescaline Analogues)
2,5-dinethaxyamphetamine (DMA)
2,4-DMA
4-bromo-DMA (DOB)
4-ethyl-DMA (DOET)
4-iodo-DMA (DOI)
4-methyl-DMA (DOM) and its *N*-alkyl analogues
4-propyl-DMA (DPO)
p-methoxyamphetamine (PMA)
3,4,5-trimethoxyamphetamine (TMA or mescaline)
Other TMAs
3,4-methylenedioxy methamphetamine (MDMA)
N-ethyl MDA (MDEA) and its *N*-alkyl analogues
3-methoxy-4,5-MDA (MMDA) and its 2-methoxy analogues
2,5-dimethoxy MDA (DMMDA) and other dimethoxy analogues
2,5-dimethoxy-4-bromo-phenylethylamine (2CB)

LSD ("acid") is a colorless, odorless, tasteless, water-soluble derivative of ergot (see Chapter 336). It is available as single doses ("hits") in tablet, capsule, or powder form and also as impregnated sugar cubes, small pieces of blotter paper ("blotter acid"), and gelatin ("windowpane"). Foods (e.g., animal crackers, gum, and fruit punch) and lickable paper materials (e.g., stamps, stickers, and decal tattoos) have also been used as vehicles.

Analogues of LSD (see Table 341.1) are most commonly synthetic and are supplied as pills or powders. Tryptamine and alphamethyltryptamine are also present in foods such as aged cheese and smoked meat. Psilocin and psilocybin are found in certain mushrooms (see Chapter 348). Bufotenin, an isomer of psilocin, is a component of the skin secretions and venoms of some frogs and toads (e.g., *Bufo, Hyla, Leptodactylus,* and *Rana* species).[13] Toad venom also contains catecholamines (e.g., dopamine, epinephrine, and norepinephrine) and digitalis-like cardiac glycosides (bufadienolides; see Chapter 337). Bufotenin, dimethyltryptamine (DMT), and 5-methoxy-DMT are found in species of *Mimosaceae,* plants that grow in South America. Analogues of LSD are also found in the seeds of plants from the morning glory (*Convolvulaceae*) family, such as the common morning glory (*Ipomoea violenceae*), Hawaiian baby woodrose (*Argyreia nervosa*), Hawaiian woodrose (*Merremia tuberosa*), and Mexican morning glory (*Rivea corymbosa*).

LSD and its analogues are usually taken orally, by chewing, licking, or swallowing. Hallucinogenic plants may also be smoked or sniffed. Dried toad skin or toxin extracts may be ingested. "Toad licking" (licking the skin of live toads), another means of exposure, is most commonly practiced by teenagers in the southeastern United States.[13]

Marijuana is a mixture of the branches, flowers, leaves, and seeds of the plant *Cannabis sativa.* Although its THC concentration usually ranges from 1% to 3%, high-potency strains such as sinsemilla, with THC concentrations of 7% to 14%, have been cultivated. Common street names include grass, Mary Jane, pot, and weed. Hashish and keefe, dried resin extracts of marijuana, usually contain 5% to 15% THC. Hash oil, the liquid resin, has a THC concentration of 30% to 50%.

Marijuana is most commonly smoked as a cigarette (known as a bone, joint, or reefer) or from a pipe. Hashish is usually smoked from a pipe. Hash oil is usually applied to marijuana or tobacco cigarettes and then smoked. Marijuana and its derivatives may also be brewed as a tea or mixed into baked goods, such as brownies, and then ingested. The intravenous injection of marijuana extracts has also been reported.

Mescaline (3,4,5-trimethoxyamphetamine) is a natural product of the peyote cactus, *Lophophora williamsii,* indigenous to the southwestern United States and northern Mexico. The San Pedro cactus of Peru, *Trichocercus pachanoi,* may also contain mescaline. The dried, brownish gray, fleshy top of the peyote cactus is cut up and sold as "buttons," reflecting their size. Peyote buttons contain 1% to 6% mescaline. The seeds of nutmeg (*Myristica fragrans*) contain psychoactive volatile oils (terpenes) as well as myristican and elemicin (MMDA and PMA, respectively; see Table 341.2).

Mescaline and its synthetic derivatives (see Table 341.2) are also available as pills and powders. These agents are almost always taken by ingestion. The most commonly abused agents of years past were DOM, also known as STP ("serenity, tranquility, and peace"), and the "love drug," MDA. Currently in vogue are MDMA ("Ecstasy," "XTC," or "Adam") and 2CB and MDEA (both known by the street name of "Eve").[7]

LSD, mescaline, and their analogues are structurally similar to the endogenous neurotransmitters serotonin (5-hydroxytryptamine), dopamine, and norepinephrine, and act by stimulating central nervous system (CNS) receptors.[10,19] The pyrrole structure of the indole ring of tryptamine derivatives and the methoxylated or methylenedioxylated catechol ring of amphetamine derivatives appear to be essential for hallucinogenic activity. Tryptamine derivatives appear to cause stimulation of type 2 serotonin receptors primarily, with lesser effects resulting from dopaminergic stimulation and monoamine oxidase inhibition. Amphetamine derivatives may act directly by stimulating catecholamine receptors or indirectly by causing the presynaptic release of endogenous transmitters, by inhibiting their presynaptic reuptake, or by preventing their synaptic degradation by monoamine oxidase. In addition, hallucinogenic amphetamines may undergo biotransformation to tryptamine analogues. Sympathetic effects also appear to be due primarily to CNS stimulation. Amphetamine derivatives may also activate the sympathetic nervous system by directly stimulating peripheral alpha- and beta-adrenergic receptors. Marijuana was originally thought to interact with membrane lipids, thereby distorting CNS neurotransmitter receptor sites.[9,15] It is now known that most of its effects result from an interaction with unique "cannabinoid receptors" in the brain.[14]

LSD is rapidly absorbed from all mucosal surfaces, with an onset of action of about 30 minutes, peak effects in 3 to 5 hours, and a duration of action of 8 to 12 hours. The hallucinogenic oral dose usually ranges from 50 to 300 μg; peak plasma levels of 1 to 4 ng/mL occur 1 to 2 hours after ingestion. LSD has a small volume of distribution (0.28 L/kg), undergoes hepatic metabolism, with a half-life of 3 to 4 hours, and can be detected in the urine for up to 5 days after an hallucinogenic dose. The potentially lethal dose is estimated to be about 100 times the hallucinogenic dose.[8,19]

Analogues of LSD are far less potent than the parent compound, with hallucinogenic doses ranging from 3 to 100 mg. A dozen Hawaiian baby woodrose, several hundred common morning glory, and one to three whole nutmeg (5 to 15 g) seeds can cause symptoms. Absorption is rapid after intravenous and inhalational use, with onset and peak effects occurring in minutes and duration of effects ranging from 2 to 24 hours. The onset of effects occurs about 30 minutes after ingestion and peaks in 1 to 6 hours. Hepatic metabolites are excreted in the urine.

Marijuana and THC are also rapidly absorbed. The onset of effects and peak plasma levels occur within 10 minutes of smoking and within 30 minutes to 3 hours of ingestion. Peak effects are noted about 30 minutes after smoking and 2 to 6 hours after ingestion. The hallucinogenic dose is 5 to 10 mg. The average marijuana cigarette contains about 30 mg of THC, but only 20% to 50% is absorbed. The amount of THC per puff increases as the cigarette is smoked, with about 25% remaining in the butt, known as a "roach" (which may also be smoked). Medical THC (dronabinol, Marinol) is given orally in daily doses of 2.5 to 20.0 mg. Peak plasma THC concentrations after smoking average 20 ng/mL after an hallucinogenic dose and are several times higher than those obtained after ingesting an equivalent dose. THC is highly lipid-soluble and has a large volume of distribution (4 to 14 L/kg). It undergoes extensive hepatic metabolism, with a half-life of 15 to 35 hours. THC metabolites can be detected in the urine for up to 1 week after a single dose in occasional users and for a month or more after the cessation of chronic intake. The estimated lethal dose of THC is several hundred times the hallucinogenic dose.[9,15]

Mescaline is readily absorbed, with the onset of effects occurring about 1 hour after ingestion. Physiologic effects usually peak within 2 hours and then abate, whereas hallucinogenic effects peak at 3 to 6 hours and last 6 to 12 hours. The hallucinogenic dose is 200 to 500 mg. Because a single peyote button contains about 45 mg of mescaline, the usual hallucinogenic dose is six to 12 buttons. Blood levels range from 2 to 4 μg/mL 2 hours after an hallucinogenic dose. Mescaline is eliminated by renal excretion as well as hepatic metabolism, with a half-life of about 6 hours. Mescaline and its metabolites can be detected in the urine for about 24 hours after intake. The potentially lethal dose is between ten and 100 times the hallucinogenic dose.[8,10,19]

Analogues of mescaline are more potent than the parent compound, with hallucinogenic doses ranging from 1 mg for DOB to 150 mg for MDMA. Effects are similar to those caused by mescaline in time of onset and time of maximal intensity, but they may last two to three times as long. As a result of their sympathetic activity, potentially lethal doses are usually only several times the usual hallucinogenic dose, but even the latter is occasionally fatal.[16,18]

Tolerance may develop after the chronic use of all hallucinogens. Cross-tolerance occurs between LSD and mescaline and their derivatives and probably between marijuana, ethanol, and barbiturates. A drug-free interval of 3 to 4 days is usually sufficient for the disappearance of pharmacokinetic tolerance, but pharmacodynamic tolerance may persist for many years. A withdrawal syndrome has been reported only with marijuana.[16,19]

CLINICAL PRESENTATION

Hallucinogen use is usually intentional, results in expected effects, and does not attract particular attention. Patients who present to the emergency department usually do so because of accidental intake; lack of experience with these agents; excessive, persistent, or unpleasant reactions; and psychotic or violent behavior. They are typically brought in by friends, family, paramedics, or police.

The hallucinogenic effects of LSD, marijuana, mescaline, and related synthetic agents are qualitatively similar.[12] Patients usually remain aware that their hallucinations are drug-induced and maintain their ability to distinguish what is real from what is not. Sensory misperceptions may take the form of auditory, gustatory, olfactory, tactile, and visual dysesthesias (i.e., exaggerated or diminished sensations) or synesthesias (i.e., one sensation interpreted as another, such as sound resulting in color perception). LSD, mescaline, and their analogues tend to cause visual hallucinations, whereas marijuana tends to provoke auditory and gustatory hallucinations. Anorexia is typical of the former, whereas an increased, sometimes ravenous appetite is often associated with the latter. Altered sense of time occurs with all agents. Disordered thought processes may result in illusions of movement, misinterpretation of the meaning or significance of an event (e.g., religious or evil connotations), impaired judgment and memory, or frankly psychotic behavior. Although the drug experience is usually considered pleasant and associated with mood elevation, it is occasionally perceived as being noxious or frightening, resulting in a panic reaction.

Catatonic, paranoid, homicidal, and suicidal behavior can also occur. The mood may swing unpredictably from one extreme to the other. Although effects usually last less than 24 hours, a few patients may develop persistent psychosis. Acute adverse reactions appear to be more common in teenagers who take single large doses, whereas persistent reactions are more common in older people who have been chronic users. Flashbacks (spontaneous, short-lived, intrusive images, such as flashes of light; halos; trails; objects appearing to be moving, enlarged, or shrunken; and double exposures; and recollections or re-creations of hallucinogenic experiences) have been described following the use of LSD, morning glory seeds, and psilocybin. Persistent and prolonged afterimages (palinopsia) can also occur after LSD use. Chronic marijuana smoking may result in adverse pulmonary effects similar to, but more pronounced than, those caused by tobacco.[19] Decreased levels of luteinizing hormone–releasing hormone, prolactin, and testosterone have been reported in experimental animals, and gynecomastia and decreased sperm count and motility have been noted in humans. Female marijuana users are more likely than nonusers to have unintended pregnancies, premature labor, abruptio placentae, low-birth-weight children, and children with features of the fetal alcohol syndrome, but these effects are more likely due to concomitant poor nutrition, low socioeconomic status, and use of alcohol, tobacco, and other drugs than to marijuana itself. Although cannabinoids are capable of suppressing immune function, evidence of a clinically significant effect is lacking. Similarly, although high doses of THC have caused fetal malformations in experimental animals, there is no evidence that marijuana is a human teratogen.

Regardless of the agent taken, CNS effects are usually associated with sympathetic hyperactivity, as evidenced by mydriasis, diaphoresis, piloerection, tremors, and mildly elevated blood pressure, pulse, respiratory rate, and temperature. Nausea, vomiting, diarrhea, blurred vision, ataxia, dizziness, and weakness may also be present. LSD, mescaline, and their analogues tend to cause pallor and salivation, whereas a dry mouth, flushing, coughing, conjunctival injection, and orthostatic hypotension are characteristic of marijuana.[4,6,8–10,15,19]

In severe intoxications, physiologic effects vary, depending on the identity of the hallucinogen. Massive LSD doses may cause hypotension, hyperthermia, coma, seizures, respiratory depression, coagulation abnormalities, and death.[4,12,19] Although seizures from usual hallucinogenic doses of LSD are poorly documented, the author has seen them in a patient who was taking a serotonin reuptake inhibitor for depression. The ingestion of marijuana, especially in children, may result in marked CNS depression.[20] Its intravenous administration has been reported to cause abdominal pain, vomiting, headache, fever, hypotension, respiratory distress, rhabdomyolysis, renal failure, and death.[5] Although mescaline itself has relatively mild sympathetic effects, more potent analogues, such as MDMA and MDEA, may cause tachyarrhythmias, marked hypertension, vasospasm with limb or organ ischemia, cardiovascular collapse, acute respiratory distress syndrome, malignant hyperthermia, coma, seizures, rhabdomyolysis, acute renal failure, disseminated intravascular coagulation, and death, probably as a result of their serotonergic effects (see also Chapter 370).[7,17] Hepatotoxicity, sometimes fatal, has also been reported as a complication of MDMA ingestion. Overall, fatalities are rare, and far more often result from physical violence caused by dangerous behavior than from direct drug effects.[16,19]

Laboratory findings include nonspecific leukocytosis and hyperglycemia in mild intoxications. Lactic acidosis, prolonged prothrombin and partial thromboplastin times, and elevated creatine phosphokinase, blood urea nitrogen, and creatinine levels may be seen with severe cases. Although ventricular ectopy is occasionally noted, the electrocardiogram (ECG) normally reveals only sinus tachycardia. The chest radiograph is usually normal. Pneumothorax, pneumomediastinum, and pneumopericardium have been reported after marijuana smoking.[3] Evidence of noncardiogenic pulmonary edema may be present in patients with severe poisoning by LSD or synthetic agents. Marked hyponatremia and consequent mental status changes, including coma and seizures, may be seen in patients who attend "rave" parties and drink large amounts of water in order to prevent dehydration and hyperthermia.

Hallucinogens are not readily detectable in the urine by routine toxicology screening (e.g., thin-layer chromatography). Their detection requires specific analysis, using techniques such as radioisotope or enzyme-linked immunoassay and gas or high-pressure liquid chromatography with fluorometry or mass spectrometry.

Abrupt withdrawal from chronic marijuana use may result in anxiety, insomnia, tremors, nausea, and, possibly, vomiting.[15]

DIFFERENTIAL DIAGNOSIS

Medical and psychiatric conditions that cause similar effects include hypoxia, hypoglycemia, hyponatremia, encephalopathy, encephalitis, meningitis, cerebral trauma, drug withdrawal, thyrotoxicosis, and major affective disorders (schizophrenia and manic–depressive illness). In patients with hyperthermia, motor hyperactivity, autonomic instability, rhabdomyolysis, the neuroleptic malignant syndrome, and the serotonin syndrome (see Chapter 370) must also be considered in the differential. Poisons that cause hallucinations with a relatively high frequency include sympathomimetics (e.g., amphetamines, cocaine, and methylxanthines), anticholinergics, local anesthetics (e.g., lidocaine), phencyclidine (PCP), ergot derivatives, aromatic and halogenated hydrocarbons, and mushrooms. PCP is distinguished by its propensity to cause amnesia, anesthesia, nystagmus, and wide fluctuations in the level of consciousness. The physiologic effects of sympathomimetics are usually much more pronounced relative to their hallucinogenic activity than is the case with LSD, marijuana, mescaline, and related agents.

Uncommon toxic causes of hallucinations include heavy metals, nutmeg (which contains an amphetamine derivative as well as volatile oils), morning glory seeds (which contain tryptamine derivatives), and toad poisons. In addition, hallucinations have been reported as idiosyncratic reactions to almost all medications.

Street-drug adulterants (e.g., cyanide, local anesthetics, quinine, quinidine, caffeine, theophylline, and strychnine) should also be considered in the differential of the cause of toxic effects of alleged hallucinogens.

EMERGENCY DEPARTMENT EVALUATION

The history includes the name or description of the hallucinogen, the time of ingestion, amount(s) taken, and the route of exposure. Slang names may provide a presumptive identity if the chemical name is not known. The time of onset and the nature of symptoms are noted. A history of previous drug use, psychiatric problems, and medical conditions, particularly cardiovascular disease, is documented. The clinician should specifically ask about the possibility of concomitant traumatic injuries.

The physical examination focuses on the mental status, neurologic evaluation, and cardiovascular system. A full set of vital signs is documented and repeated frequently. The patient is examined carefully for evidence of trauma and underlying diseases.

Ancillary testing is neither necessary nor useful in patients with mild hallucinogen intoxication, except to rule out other diagnoses. Patients with moderate or severe symptoms (e.g., excessive agitation and significantly abnormal vital signs) should have a chest radiograph; cardiac monitoring and a 12-lead ECG; complete blood count; determination of electrolyte, glucose, blood urea nitrogen, creatinine, and creatine kinase levels; and urinalysis (including myoglobin). Routine toxicology screening may be useful for detecting or excluding other agents. Specific assays of the urine are usually necessary to confirm the presence of hallucinogens. Quantitative blood (or urine) hallucinogen levels are not clinically useful or routinely available.

EMERGENCY DEPARTMENT MANAGEMENT

Although most patients with hallucinogen intoxication are physiologically stable, cognitive impairment and emotional lability place them at risk for unpredictable, self-destructive, or violent behavior. Those who are merely anxious and have normal or mildly elevated vital signs should be reassured and continuously observed in a quiet environment until symptoms abate. It is often helpful to have a friend or relative stay with the patient. Those with agitated, psychotic, or paranoid behavior require restraints to protect themselves and others from harm. Pharmacologic measures are preferable to physical ones, because the latter may predispose the patient to hyperthermia and rhabdomyolysis. Most such patients respond to treatment with a nonspecific sedative such as diazepam (5 to 10 mg) or lorazepam (2 to 4 mg), orally or intravenously, repeated as necessary. Those who are severely agitated or psychotic may require an antipsychotic agent such as chlorpromazine (0.5 to 2.0 mg/kg)[6] or haloperidol (0.05 to 0.1 mg/kg), orally, intramuscularly, or intravenously, repeated as necessary. Those with hallucinations lasting more than 12 to 24 hours should also be treated with an antipsychotic medication. Persistent LSD-induced psychosis may also respond to oral L-5-hydroxytryptophan (400 mg/d) and carbidopa (100 mg/d).[1,2]

Gastrointestinal decontamination is indicated for asymptomatic patients with recent ingestions. Activated charcoal is preferred. Except for large ingestions of marijuana, decontamination is unlikely to be of benefit in patients who present after the onset of hallucinations.

Patients with CNS depression, seizures, or significant vital sign abnormalities should have an intravenous line established and cardiac monitoring. Advanced life-support measures should be initiated as necessary. Seizures should be treated with lorazepam, diazepam, or a barbiturate. Marked tachycardia and hypertension should be treated with an adrenergic blocker such as labetalol (20 mg intravenously, with additional doses as needed) or a vasodilator–beta blocker combination (e.g., nitroprusside and esmolol or propranolol). Hypotension usually responds to fluid administration. Vasopressors (e.g., dopamine and norepinephrine) should be used for refractory hypotension. Hyperthermia should be aggressively treated with cooling measures (see Chapter 387) and pharmacologic control of behavioral hyperactivity.[11] Patients with the serotonin syndrome may respond to serotonin antagonists (see Chapter 370). Vascular spasm should be treated with nitroprusside or nifedipine and with heparin.[2] Alkaline diuresis may prevent myoglobinuric renal failure in patients with rhabdomyolysis. Symptoms of marijuana withdrawal do not require specific therapy.

DISPOSITION

Patients with hallucinations and mildly elevated vital signs can usually be observed in the emergency department and discharged (with a responsible friend or relative) once they become asymptomatic. Those with persistent hallucinations and stable vital signs should be referred for psychiatric evaluation and admission for behavioral observation and treatment. Those with coma, seizures, or abnormal vital signs requiring active treatment should be admitted to an intensive care unit. A vascular surgeon should be consulted in patients with arterial spasm. Physicians unfamiliar with the management of hallucinogen intoxication should consult a regional poison control center or a toxicologist for further advice, as needed. All patients with intentional hallucinogen use should be referred for drug-abuse counseling and rehabilitation before discharge.

COMMON PITFALLS

- Failure to closely observe the patient, to prevent physical injury to the patient and others, and to sedate and restrain the patient, if necessary

- Failure to evaluate for and treat coexisting trauma or medical problems
- Failure to obtain a complete set of vital signs, especially an accurate core temperature
- Failure to evaluate for occult rhabdomyolysis in patients with coma, seizures, hyperthermia, or behavioral or physiologic hyperactivity
- Failure to appreciate the potential severity of poisoning after the ingestion of marijuana, particularly in children
- Failure to appreciate that street drugs are frequently not what the user thinks they are and to consider adulterants or other drugs misrepresented as hallucinogens as the cause of toxicity

ACKNOWLEDGMENT

Daniel A. Muse contributed to previous versions of this chapter.

References

1. Abraham HD. L-5-hydroxytryptophan for LSD-induced psychosis. *Am J Psychiatry* 1983;140:456.
2. Altura BM, Altura BT. Pharmacologic inhibition of cerebral vasospasm in ischemia/hallucinogen ingestion, and hypomagnesemia: barbiturates, calcium antagonists, and magnesium. *Am J Emerg Med* 1983;2:180.
3. Birrer RB, Calderon J. Pneumothorax, pneumomediastinum, and pneumopericardium following Valsalva's maneuver during marijuana smoking. *N Y State J Med* 1984;12:619.
4. Blaho K, Merigian K, Winbery S, et al. Clinical pharmacology of lysergic acid diethylamide: case reports and review of the literature. *Am J Ther* 1997;4:211.
5. Brandenburg D, Wernick R. Intravenous marijuana syndrome. *West J Med* 1986;145:94.
6. Forest JAH, Tarala RA. 60 hospital admissions due to reactions to lysergide (LSD). *Lancet* 1973;2:1310.
7. Henry JA, Jeffreys KJ, Dowling S. Toxicity and deaths from 3,4-methylenedioxymethamphetamine ("ecstasy"). *Lancet* 1992;340:384.
8. Hollister LE. Clinical aspects of use of phenylalkylamine and indolealkylamine hallucinogens. *Psychopharmacol Bull* 1986;22:977.
9. Jones RT. Drug of abuse profile: cannabis. *Clin Chem* 1987;33B:72.
10. Kapadia GJ, Fayez MBE. Peyote constituents: chemistry, biogenesis, and biological effects. *J Pharm Sci* 1970;59:1699.
11. Klock JC, Boerner U, Becker CE. Coma, hyperthermia, and bleeding associated with massive LSD overdose: a report of eight cases. *West J Med* 1974;3:183.
12. Leikin JB, Krantz AJ, Zell-Kanter M, et al. Clinical features and management of intoxication due to hallucinogenic drugs. *Med Toxicol Adv Drug Exp* 1989;4:324.
13. Lyttle T. Misuse and legend in the "toad licking" phenomenon. *Int J Addict* 1993;28:521.
14. Murphy L, Bartke A, eds. *Marijuana/cannabinoids: neurobiology and neurophysiology*. Boca Raton, FL, CRC Press, 1992.
15. Nahas GG. Cannabis: toxicological properties and epidemiological aspects. *Med J Aust* 1986;145:82.
16. Reynolds PC, Jindrich EJ. A mescaline-associated fatality. *J Anal Toxicol* 1985;9:183.
17. Schmidt CJ. Neurotoxicity of the psychedelic amphetamines: methylenedioxymethamphetamine. *J Pharmacol Exp Ther* 1987;240:1.
18. Schwartz R. Mescaline: a survey. *Am Fam Pract* 1988;37:122.
19. Strassman RJ. Adverse reactions to psychedelic drugs: a review of the literature. *J Nerv Ment Dis* 1984;172:577.
20. Weinberg D, Lande A, Hilton N, et al. Intoxication from accidental marijuana ingestion. *Pediatrics* 1983;71:848.

CHAPTER 342

Halogenated Hydrocarbon Poisoning

Mohamud R. Daya

Halogenated hydrocarbons are aliphatic and aromatic organic compounds that contain one or more molecules of bromine, chlorine, fluorine, or iodine. The solvent properties of these substances make them useful for extracting, dissolving, and cleaning fats, waxes, grease, adhesives, resins, and oils that are insoluble in water. They are also used as refrigerants, aerosol propellants, fire-extinguishing agents, and fumigants (Table 342.1). They are constituents of various household cleaners, paint removers, aerosols, and office products. Due to environmental persistence and their ozone-depleting properties, some older halogenated hydrocarbons (e.g., chlorofluorocarbons [Freon], 1,1,1-trichloroethane [TCA]) are being phased out of use.

Toxicity may result from deliberate or accidental overexposure. These hydrocarbons are frequently abused by male adolescents, and as many as 20% of high-school seniors have experimented with volatile substances at least once.[1,7] These agents are readily available, conveniently packaged, easily concealed, inexpensive, and legal, and they provide a rapid state of intoxication when inhaled.[6] Abuse can be accomplished by directly inhaling vapors from an open container (sniffing), inhaling from a piece of cloth (rag or towel) soaked with the substance and placed in front of the nose and mouth (huffing), or breathing in and out of a plastic or paper bag filled with the volatile substance (bagging).[7,11]

In industry, about 10 million workers are exposed to organic solvents, a significant portion of which are chlorinated hydrocarbons. Risk of occupational inhalation exposure is determined by factors such as volatility, method of use, ventilation, and the presence of personal protective equipment. Dermal exposure is also common and may result in skin injury and systemic ab-

TABLE 342.1. Common Halogenated Hydrocarbons

SOLVENTS
Chloroform
Carbon tetrachloride
Trichloroethylene (TCE)
Tetrachloroethylene (perchloroethylene [PCE])
1,1,1-Trichloroethane (TCA)[a]
Methylene chloride (dichloromethane [DCM])[a]
Trichlorotrifluoroethane (Freon 113)
REFRIGERANTS/AEROSOLS
Ethyl chloride
Trichlorofluoromethane (Freon 11)
Dichlorofluoromethane (Freon 12)
1,2-Dichlorotetrafluoroethane (Freon 114)
Difluoroethane (Freon 152)
FUMIGANTS
Methyl bromide
Ethylene dibromide

[a] Also used as aerosol propellants.

sorption.[16] Ingestions of halogenated hydrocarbons are infrequent and usually involve accidental pediatric cases or deliberate adult suicide attempts.

These highly lipid-soluble hydrocarbons are rapidly absorbed following inhalation and ingestion. Distribution is rapid, with significant uptake in the brain and other organs of high fat content.[11] Absorption depends on the vapor concentration and minute ventilation and is increased with physical activity.[16] There is considerable variation in the extent of hepatic metabolism and route of excretion among different compounds. Freons, TCA, and tetrachloroethylene (perchloroethylene [PCE]) are primarily excreted unchanged by the lungs. Methylene chloride (dichloromethane [DCM]) is excreted after almost complete metabolism in the liver to carbon dioxide (70%) and carbon monoxide (30%).[15,16] Trichloroethylene (TCE), carbon tetrachloride, and chloroform undergo significant biotransformation in addition to excretion of the parent compound in expired air. TCE and, to a lesser extent, PCE are metabolized to trichloroacetic acid and trichloroethanol. These metabolites are excreted in the urine and may be useful for monitoring industrial exposures and compliance with abstinence from abuse.[11] Carbon tetrachloride and chloroform metabolism generates carbon dioxide along with hydrochloric acid.

Cytochrome P-450–mediated biotransformation of chloroform, carbon tetrachloride, and other halogenated hydrocarbons can produce toxic reactive intermediates (e.g., phosgene) that result in subsequent hepatic and renal damage.[9,10] Ethanol, by inducing these microsomal enzyme systems, increases the toxicity of these compounds.

CLINICAL PRESENTATION

Central nervous system (CNS) depression is the primary effect of the halogenated hydrocarbons. Changes in consciousness are similar to those of ether anesthesia. Initially, there is euphoria, in association with visual or auditory hallucinations and perceptual disturbances. An intoxicated appearance, accompanied by ataxia and disorientation, is characteristic.[20] In addition, there is often a feeling of invulnerability, which can result in impulsive and dangerous behavior. Continued exposure results in increasing CNS depression, leading to stupor and coma. Coma may be associated with respiratory depression and seizures.

The irritant effects of halogenated hydrocarbons can result in pulmonary complaints, such as cough and dyspnea, following inhalational exposures. Bronchospasm can also occur in susceptible patients, and massive exposures may result in pneumonitis or pulmonary edema. Respiratory symptoms may also be present in instances of aspiration (see Chapter 362). Nausea, vomiting, diarrhea, and abdominal pain may be prominent symptoms, especially following ingestion. Delayed or persistent gastrointestinal (GI) symptoms usually reflect direct hepatic or renal injury. Dermal exposure may result in skin rashes due to the defatting and irritating properties of these agents.

Halogenated hydrocarbons can sensitize the myocardium to the dysrhythmogenic effects of circulating catecholamines, with resultant ventricular and supraventricular dysrhythmias.[2,13,14,20] This sensitization is thought to account for the sudden deaths that occur following exposure in conjunction with agitation or strenuous physical activity.[4] Death can also result from respiratory depression, anoxia (bag-breathing), and injuries from impulsive and irrational behavior.[11] Additional cardiac effects include bradycardia, depressed contractility, decreased cardiac output, and increased autonomic reflex activity.[2,11]

Exposure to some halogenated hydrocarbons may result in distinct clinical presentations. For example, degreaser's flush is a cutaneous vascular reaction characterized by red blotches on the face, neck, and trunk that sometimes occurs following ethanol ingestion in workers recently exposed to TCE.[18] The red discoloration, due to dilatation of superficial skin vessels, peaks within 30 minutes and fades completely within 1 hour.

Intoxication with TCE has also been associated with palsies of the oculomotor, trigeminal, and abducens cranial nerves.[20] Exposure to DCM or its two-halogen analogues (methylene iodide, chlorobromomethane), which are also metabolized to carbon monoxide, may produce carboxyhemoglobin levels of 5% to 50%.[15] Although accompanying symptoms of carbon monoxide poisoning are usually mild (see Chapter 323), patients with underlying coronary artery disease can experience angina or myocardial infarction.[19] The apparent half-life of carboxyhemoglobin produced from DCM is considerably longer than that produced following carbon monoxide exposure, because of the continued metabolism of DCM that is slowly released from adipose tissue stores.[12,15]

DIFFERENTIAL DIAGNOSIS

Alternative diagnoses include intoxication from psychoactive agents such as phencyclidine, lysergic acid diethylamide, mescaline, and other hallucinogens. Anticholinergic and stimulant (cocaine, amphetamines) drug abuse should be considered in patients presenting with a toxic delirium. Drugs that produce CNS depression (e.g., opiates, ethanol, sedative–hypnotics, cyclic antidepressants, phenothiazines, gamma hydroxybutyrate) should be considered in the lethargic, obtunded, or comatose patient. Infectious, metabolic, traumatic, and other nondrug causes of altered mental status should also be considered.

EMERGENCY DEPARTMENT EVALUATION

The history should focus on the time of ingestion, the amount and identity of ingested substances, and the duration, nature, and identity of inhalational and dermal exposures. The time of onset and nature of symptoms and any prehospital interventions should be noted.

Inhalational solvent abuse should be suspected in an adolescent if bags or rags have been discovered at the scene, if he or she has a sweet, chemical breath odor, and if residual solvent stains are present around the face, hands, or clothes. The physical examination focuses on the cardiac, pulmonary, and neurologic status and the abdomen in cases of ingestion and inhalation, and on the involved area in topical exposures. An electrocardiogram and chest x-ray are obtained for symptomatic patients. Measurements of baseline liver enzymes, blood urea nitrogen, and creatinine and a urinalysis are helpful in the evaluation of renal or hepatic toxicity. Carboxyhemoglobin levels are valuable in DCM exposures.

Halogenated hydrocarbon ingestions may be confirmed by visualizing radiopaque material on abdominal radiographs.[3] A serum ethanol concentration and a urine screen for drugs of abuse may be necessary to rule out other intoxications. Qualitative and quantitative analysis of blood and other tissues, using headspace gas chromatography, may be helpful in confirming volatile substance abuse in fatal cases.

EMERGENCY DEPARTMENT MANAGEMENT

First, direct attention to advanced life-support measures, because treatment is primarily supportive. Monitor cardiac rhythm and establish intravenous access. The regional poison control center may be a useful resource for substance information and patient management issues.

Decontamination measures depend on the route of exposure.[16] The skin should be irrigated immediately with water, followed by soap-and-water washing. The eyes should be irrigated immediately with isotonic saline solution. Eye exposures should be evaluated with a slit lamp after irrigation. Antibiotic ointment may be indicated if corneal erosion is present. With significant ocular injury, consultation and follow-up with an ophthalmologist is recommended.

Patients with fumigant exposures or pulmonary symptoms after inhalation should be managed as described for irritant gas exposures (see Chapter 346). Mechanical hyperventilation may enhance the elimination of some substances and is recommended in intubated patients.[11] Adrenergic agents (beta agonists and theophylline) should be used with caution because of their potential dysrhythmogenic (cardiac sensitization) effects.[11] GI decontamination should be considered for all patients with recent ingestions, especially those with evidence of radiopaque material on abdominal radiographs. Gastric aspiration and activated charcoal are the preferred methods.

Seizures are treated with a benzodiazepine (e.g., lorazepam, diazepam), followed by phenytoin or phenobarbital. Life-threatening tachydysrhythmias following inhalational exposure are treated with beta blockers (e.g., propranolol, esmolol, metoprolol) or lidocaine. Beta blockade is also the treatment of choice for dysrhythmias encountered in chloral hydrate ingestions.[8] Hypotension is treated with volume expansion and, if necessary, pure alpha vasopressors (e.g., norepinephrine). Dopamine should be avoided, because it promotes cardiac dysrhythmias in some cases.[11] Hepatotoxicity and nephrotoxicity are managed primarily by intensive supportive care.

Several unproved but potentially beneficial treatments, including *N*-acetylcysteine (NAC), hemoperfusion, and hyperbaric oxygen (HBO), should be considered for hepatotoxic agents such as carbon tetrachloride.[5,17] These treatments must be started early if they are to be of benefit. The dosing regimen for NAC is similar to that used in acetaminophen overdose.[11] In large overdoses, treatment may have to be extended beyond the usual 18 doses, in light of continued release of solvent into the circulation from adipose tissue stores. The mechanism of action may relate to NAC's ability to bind toxic metabolites such as phosgene, or to the maintenance of intracellular glutathione concentrations. NAC and HBO may act primarily as free-radical scavengers, because their hepatoprotective effects have been related to reduced lipid peroxidation in animal models.[5]

Degreaser's flush does not generally require pharmacologic treatment but may respond to propranolol (40 to 80 mg orally).[17] The management of carbon monoxide poisoning is discussed in Chapter 323.

DISPOSITION

Patients with evidence of dysrhythmias require admission for cardiac monitoring. Those with persistent CNS and respiratory depression should also be admitted to a monitored unit. Patients with potential hepatic or renal toxicity or those with persistent GI symptoms may require admission for observation. Similarly, patients with significant DCM exposures and elevated carboxyhemoglobin levels should be admitted for oxygen therapy and serial monitoring of their carboxyhemoglobin levels. Patients who improve rapidly and become asymptomatic after a 4- to 6-hour observation period in the emergency department may be discharged. If indicated, appropriate psychiatric consultation should be obtained before discharge.

Patients must be warned to avoid circumstances that could result in future reexposure. Volatile substance abuse is a risk factor for progressive illicit drug use, and rehabilitation counseling should be offered. Employers and appropriate governmental regulatory agencies (e.g., the Occupational Safety and Health Administration) should be notified in cases of workplace exposures.

COMMON PITFALLS

- Failure to consider inhalant abuse in intoxicated patients, especially male adolescents
- Failure to use adrenergic drugs with caution in the treatment of bronchospasm and hypotension
- Failure to use beta blockers in the treatment of life-threatening tachydysrhythmias
- Failure to anticipate the need for prolonged treatment due to release of solvent from adipose tissue stores
- Failure to warn patients about the dangers of halogenated hydrocarbons and of reexposure
- Failure to notify employers and governmental agencies in cases of occupational exposures

References

1. Anderson HR, Macnair RS, Ramsey JD. Deaths from abuse of volatile substances: a national epidemiological study. *BMJ* 1985;290:304.
2. Aviado DM. Pharmacology of abused inhalants. In: Sharp CW, Carroll LT, eds. *Voluntary inhalation of industrial solvents.* Washington, DC: U.S. Government Printing Office, 1978.
3. Bagnasco FM, Stringer B, Muslim AM. Carbon tetrachloride poisoning: radiographic findings. *N Y State J Med* 1978;78:646.
4. Bass M. Sudden sniffing death. *JAMA* 1970;212:2075.
5. Burkhart KK, Hall AH, Gerace R, et al. Hyperbaric oxygen treatment for carbon tetrachloride poisoning. *Drug Saf* 1991;6:332.
6. Cohen S. Inhalant abuse: an overview of the problem. In: Sharp CW, Brehm ML, eds. *Review of inhalants: euphoria to dysfunction* (NIDA monograph 15). Washington, DC: U.S. Government Printing Office, 1977.
7. Giovacchini RP. Abusing the volatile organic chemicals. *Regul Toxicol Pharmacol* 1985;5:18.
8. Graham SR, Day RO, Lee R, et al. Overdose with chloral hydrate: a pharmacological and therapeutic review. *Med J Aust* 1988;149:686.
9. Klassen CD, Plaa GL. Relative effects of various chlorinated hydrocarbons on liver and renal function in dogs. *Toxicol Appl Pharmacol* 1967;10:119.
10. Kenna JG, Jones RM. The organ toxicity of inhaled anesthetics. *Anesth Analg* 1995;81:S51.
11. Linden CH. Volatile substances of abuse. *Emerg Med Clin North Am* 1990;8:559.
12. Ratney RS, Wegmen DH, Elkins HB. In vivo conversion of methylene chloride to carbon monoxide. *Arch Environ Health* 1974;28:223.
13. Reinhardt CF, Mullin LS, Maxfield ME. Epinephrine-induced cardiac arrhythmia potential of some common industrial solvents. *J Occup Med* 1973;15:953.
14. Reinhardt CF, Azar A, Maxfield ME, et al. Cardiac arrhythmias and aerosol sniffing. *Arch Environ Health* 1971;22:265.
15. Rioux JP, Meyers RA. Methylene chloride: a paradigmatic review. *J Emerg Med* 1988;6:227.
16. Rumack BH, ed. *PoisIndex.* Englewood, CO: Micromedex, 1999.
17. Ruprahm M, Mant TK, Flanagan RJ. Acute carbon tetrachloride poisoning in 19 patients: implications for diagnosis and treatment. *Lancet* 1985;1:1027.
18. Stewart RD, Hake CL, Peterson JE. Degreaser's flush. *Arch Environ Health* 1974;29:1.
19. Stewart RD, Hake CL. Paint-remover hazard. *JAMA* 1976;235:398.
20. Szlatenyi CS, Wang RY. Encephalopathy and cranial nerve palsies caused by intentional trichloroethylene inhalation. *Am J Emerg Med* 1996;14:464.

CHAPTER 343
Herbicide Poisoning

William J. Lewander and Christopher H. Linden

PARAQUAT

Paraquat (1,1′-dimethyl-4,4′-bipyridium) is a relatively nonselective, rain-fast, foliage-applied, contact herbicide. Although it forms an inert complex with most types of soil, becoming rapidly harmless to both plants and animals, paraquat is one of the most toxic herbicides when ingested, producing multisystem failure, pulmonary fibrosis, and death. Mortality has been estimated at 20% to 50% from accidental ingestions and is probably greater after intentional ingestions.

Paraquat is a bipyridium quaternary ammonium compound available as a dichloride or dimethyl salt. Commercial paraquat preparations contain about 20% (wt/wt) cation, and household products, 0.2% (wt/wt). Common brand names include Herbaxone, Gramoxone, Gramonol, Preglone, and Weedol. Its herbicidal activity is due to interference with electron transfer during photosynthesis. The resulting inhibition of the reduction of nicotinamide–adenine dinucleotide phosphate (NADP) to NADPH leads to the production of superoxide and peroxide radicals, reactive forms of oxygen, which destroy lipid cell membrane components.

Only 1% to 5% of paraquat is absorbed from the gastrointestinal (GI) tract. Peak concentrations are achieved within 2 hours. Although dermal absorption is minimal unless the skin is abraded, fatal cutaneous exposures have been reported after a single or chronic application of commercial concentrates.[16] Inhalation of paraquat spray is unlikely to cause systemic toxicity because its low vapor pressure and large spray droplets prevent its absorption. The smoking of paraquat-sprayed marijuana results in minimal absorption, estimated at 0.03% to 0.2%. Nevertheless, an estimated 60% to 70% of the paraquat in marijuana is converted to bipyridene when smoked, and this is a direct respiratory irritant.

Paraquat has a large volume of distribution (2 to 8 L/kg). Although it is distributed to all major organ systems, it selectively accumulates in the lungs. Its pulmonary toxicity may be accounted for by lung tissue concentrations ten to 15 times greater than plasma levels. Peak lung concentrations are achieved 4 to 5 days after ingestion. Paraquat is not metabolized. Most of an oral dose is eliminated by glomerular filtration and active tubular secretion within 48 hours, but 20% to 30% that may remain tissue-bound is excreted over 2 to 3 weeks.[3]

Although not fully understood, the mechanism of human toxicity is believed to be due to the formation of superoxides that may damage cells directly or through the generation of other active oxygen species. The lung is the site of greatest toxicity, but paraquat poisoning can cause multisystem damage involving the kidneys, liver, heart, orogastric passages, skin, eyes, and adrenal glands.

The severity of paraquat poisoning depends on the amount ingested. The ingestion of less than 20 mg/kg of paraquat results in a mild poisoning consisting of corrosive injury to the GI tract. Moderate-to-severe poisoning follows ingestions of 20 to 40 mg/kg, causing corrosive injury and the gradual (days to weeks) development of renal failure and pulmonary fibrosis. Death occurs in most patients but is usually delayed 2 to 3 weeks. An acute fulminant course with corrosive effects, multiorgan failure, and death occurs within hours to days after the ingestion of more than 40 mg/kg.[16]

The more concentrated the solution, the greater the corrosive effect. Depending on the route of exposure, burns may involve the eyes, respiratory tract, and skin, as well as the oropharynx, esophagus, and stomach. The major pathologic changes in the lung consist of alveolar epithelial destruction, with pulmonary hemorrhage and congestion progressing to intraalveolar and obliterative fibrosis. Oxygen potentiates the paraquat-induced pulmonary fibrosis.[8]

CLINICAL PRESENTATION

Exposure to dilute solutions usually results in local signs and symptoms such as dermatitis, conjunctivitis, cough, sore throat, and burning pain in the oropharynx. Exposure to more concentrated solutions can cause dermal burns, corneal abrasions, and esophageal and gastric ulcerations, causing burning of the mouth and throat, dysphagia, substernal chest pain, abdominal cramps, diarrhea, and vomiting.

Additional systemic toxicity may include acute proximal renal tubular necrosis and reversible renal failure, centrilobular hepatic necrosis, myocarditis and necrosis, and adrenal hemorrhage. In fulminant cases, severe local symptoms are accompanied by multiorgan failure, with death occurring within hours to days from pulmonary edema, seizures, and cardiogenic shock.[16] The findings of elevated serum creatinine, low serum potassium, and metabolic acidosis on presentation are associated with the development of renal failure and death within 48 hours. Stomatitis, epistaxis, and bronchial irritation have been reported after inhalation.

Renal, hepatic, and cardiac involvement may be manifested by uremia, proteinuria, and oliguria or anuria; right upper quadrant tenderness with elevated serum bilirubin and transaminase levels; and chest pain with ischemic electrocardiogram (ECG) changes or evidence of myocarditis. With adequate treatment, renal and hepatic changes may be reversible, but pulmonary fibrosis and respiratory failure usually progresses relentlessly.

Pulmonary dysfunction is manifested by dyspnea, chest pain, tachypnea, and slowly progressive cyanosis. The chest radiograph may demonstrate pulmonary infiltrates, atelectasis, and pleural effusions. Pulmonary function testing may reveal low compliance and decreased lung volumes and diffusing capacity. Blood gas analysis reflects a worsening hypoxemia, with respiratory alkalosis and metabolic acidosis. Paraquat plasma concentrations above 2.0, 0.9, 0.3, 0.16, and 0.10 g/mL at 4, 6, 10, 16, and 24 hours after ingestion, respectively, represent potentially lethal concentrations.[7]

DIFFERENTIAL DIAGNOSIS

Paraquat poisoning is either known or suspected by a history of access to paraquat-containing products at the time of presentation or is realized retrospectively based on the characteristic corrosive effects, followed by multisystem involvement, particularly progressive pulmonary failure. The initial presentation may resemble that of other corrosive exposures. Heavy-metal poisoning can cause multisystem organ toxicity as well as corrosive GI effects. Paraquat should not be confused with diquat, which, although structurally related, differs in toxicity. Diquat poisoning is associated with cerebral hemorrhagic lesions, a higher incidence of severe acute renal failure, and paralytic ileus. It has minimal corrosive effects and does not appear to cause pulmonary fibrosis.[17]

EMERGENCY DEPARTMENT EVALUATION

The history should include the concentration, amount, and route of paraquat exposure, as well as the time of onset and nature of symptoms. Vitals signs should include measurement of the oxygen saturation. The physical examination should include inspection of exposed surfaces for evidence of corrosive injury. Patients with eye exposures should have fluorescein and slit-lamp examinations. Esophagogastric endoscopy should be considered for patients with GI symptoms following ingestion.

Patients with significant ingestions should also have an ECG, chest radiograph, arterial blood gas analysis, pulmonary function tests, complete blood count (CBC), electrolytes, blood urea nitrogen (BUN), creatinine, glucose, amylase, liver function tests, cardiac enzymes, and urinalysis. Urine and serum paraquat concentrations as early as 4 hours after ingestion can confirm the exposure and may be prognostic.[7] A qualitative urine test detects paraquat concentrations greater than 1 g/mL and confirms exposure but is not prognostic. It may be performed by adding 1 mL of a 1% solution of sodium dithionite in 2N sodium hydroxide to 10 mL of urine. A blue color indicates the presence of paraquat.[7] Arrangements for quantitative paraquat assays can be made by calling ENECA (800-327-8633).

EMERGENCY DEPARTMENT MANAGEMENT

Contaminated skin should be flushed with copious amounts of water. Material splashed in the eyes should be removed by prolonged irrigation with water. Immediate and aggressive GI decontamination is critical, even when small amounts have been ingested. Unless the risk of esophageal perforation is great (i.e., the patient is unable to swallow and many hours have passed since the time of ingestion), GI decontamination should be performed. Activated charcoal is readily available and hence preferred, although Fuller's earth and 7.5% bentonite suspensions are also effective in binding paraquat in animal models.[9] Preceding activated charcoal by gastric aspiration might be helpful in those with large or intentional ingestions. Repeated doses of activated charcoal should be given until paraquat is no longer detected in the urine or blood. The patient must be monitored for development of diarrhea or an ileus, which would limit the serial use of charcoal.

Early, prolonged hemoperfusion appears to be useful in removing paraquat and limiting systemic toxicity when started within 10 hours of ingestion (15 to 20 hours in the presence of renal failure) and performed 8 hours daily or continuously for 2 to 3 weeks until paraquat can no longer be detected in the urine or blood.[14,20] Others have questioned the efficacy of hemoperfusion, particularly if initial plasma concentrations exceed 3 mg/L.[6] Further studies are needed to confirm the effectiveness of this procedure and a new technique, continuous arteriovenous hemofiltration.[14] Cyclophosphamide and methylprednisolone have been used to prevent pulmonary toxicity, but their efficacy remains to be proven.[11,12] A successful single-lung transplantation has been reported after poisoning by paraquat resulted in end-stage lung disease.[18]

Supportive care should include monitoring for and treatment of hepatic, renal, cardiac, and pulmonary dysfunction, and fluid and electrolyte abnormalities. With the exception of supplemental oxygen, standard therapies are employed. Because oxygen increases pulmonary toxicity, concentrations greater than 21% should be used only when the Po_2 falls below 50 mm Hg. Positive end-expiratory pressure may improve arterial oxygenation while obviating the need for increasing the inspired oxygen concentration.

DISPOSITION

A toxicologist or regional poison center should be consulted in all cases of paraquat poisoning. The National Pesticide Telecommunications Network also provides 24-hour-a-day consultation services (800-858-7378). Consultation with an ophthalmologist or GI endoscopist may also be required. Admission or referral to a tertiary care center capable of providing continuous hemoperfusion and supportive care is required in all but the most minor exposures.

COMMON PITFALLS

- Underestimating the potential toxicity in an asymptomatic patient who has ingested even a small quantity of paraquat
- Failure to obtain blood paraquat levels
- Failure to admit all patients with intentional ingestions or significant skin exposures
- Potentiating pulmonary toxicity with supplemental oxygen therapy when it is not absolutely required

CHLOROPHENOXY ACIDS

The chlorophenoxy acid herbicides include 2,4-dichlorophenoxyacetic acid (2,4-D), 2,4,5-trichlorophenoxyacetic acid (2,4,5-T), 4-chloro-2-methyl-phenoxypropionic acid (mecoprop), and related compounds. They act as plant hormones (auxins) to limit the growth of broadleaf and woody vegetation. Agents Orange, Green, Pink, Purple, Blue, and White (the colors of the drums that contained them) were chlorophenoxy acid herbicides used in the Vietnam War. Agent Orange was a 50:50 mixture of the *N*-butyl esters of 2,4-D and 2,4,5-T, whereas agents Green, Pink, and Purple were primarily 2,4,5-T; all contained the contaminant 2,3,7,8-tetrachlorodibenzo-*p*-dioxin (TCDD, or dioxin). TCDD is carcinogenic and teratogenic in animals, and an analogous role in humans is suspected. Agents Blue and White were related defoliants.

Only 2,4-D is currently available for general use in the United States, and its TCDD concentrations are quite low. Common brand names include Aqua-Kleen, Emulsamine, Herbidol, Weed-B-Gone, and Weedone. Serious poisoning is rare and almost always results from suicidal ingestion. Pulmonary absorption is possible but unlikely to cause systemic toxicity. Although skin absorption is low, toxicity has resulted from chronic exposure.[2]

GI absorption is slow; peak blood levels may not occur for 12 hours or longer.[1] 2,4-D has an apparent volume of distribution of 0.1 L/kg, with the highest concentrations found in the blood and heart. Elimination occurs mainly by renal excretion of unchanged 2,4-D, with a half-life of about 12 hours after low doses. With overdose, the volume of distribution and half-life appear to be much greater. Because it is a weak acid (pK_a 3.3), alkaline diuresis shortens the half-life by a factor of 10 or more.[4,15]

It is unclear how 2,4-D causes toxicity in humans, but uncoupling of oxidative phosphorylation may be involved. Rhabdomyolysis may be due to direct muscle toxicity resulting from increased activity of skeletal muscle mitochondrial enzymes. Neuronal demyelinization and rhabdomyolysis are pathologic findings. Doses of roughly 50 mg/kg produce mild toxicity, those of 100 mg/kg cause severe poisoning, and those of 250 mg/kg or more may be fatal.[15] Plasma 2,4-D levels, measured by gas chromatography, are usually in the range of 500 g/mL or more in patients with severe or fatal poisoning.

CLINICAL PRESENTATION

A burning sensation may be noted in the pharynx, chest, and abdomen after ingestion. Vomiting occurs early and may be persistent. Within a few hours, neurologic abnormalities such as agitation, confusion, headache, dizziness, lethargy, coma, and seizures may develop.[4,5,15,19] Pupils tend to be small but reactive. Deep tendon reflexes and muscle tone may be increased, decreased, or normal. Opisthotonus, myoclonus, fasciculations, and muscle tenderness have been described. Dyspnea and tachypnea are often present. In severe cases, progressive tachycardia, hypotension, and hyperthermia may ensue. Cyanosis, flushed skin, and diaphoresis have been reported. Early death may be due to ventricular fibrillation. Eye, skin, and respiratory tract irritation may follow exposure by these routes.

Laboratory abnormalities include an increased anion gap metabolic acidosis, hypoxia, hyperkalemia, hypocalcemia, leukocytosis, evidence of rhabdomyolysis (increased creatine phosphokinase level and myoglobinuria), mildly elevated hepatic enzyme levels, and renal function disturbances (elevated BUN and creatinine levels, proteinuria, and glycosuria).[11,19] The ECG may show flat or inverted T waves. Although pulmonary edema and aspiration have been reported, the chest radiograph usually is normal. Nerve conduction and electromyographic studies may show evidence of peripheral neuropathy and myopathy.[15]

In mild-to-moderate intoxications, recovery is usually complete within 2 to 3 days; in severe cases, it may take longer than 1 week. Coma and acidemia are poor prognostic signs.[4] Neuritis and myopathy with limb pain, paresthesias, twitching, tenderness, and weakness may be delayed in onset and persist for several months.[13]

DIFFERENTIAL DIAGNOSIS

The central nervous system depression seen in mild-to-moderate 2,4-D poisoning may be confused with that caused by trauma, infection, hypoglycemia, and sedative–hypnotic poisoning. In contrast to narcotic poisoning, there is no respiratory depression. Severe 2,4-D poisoning, with tachycardia, hypotension, fever, rhabdomyolysis, and metabolic acidosis, may be confused with septic shock, diabetic ketoacidosis, severe stimulant poisoning (e.g., amphetamines, cocaine, theophylline), and intoxication by methanol, ethylene glycol, and salicylates.

Other uncouplers of oxidative phosphorylation, such as the dinitrocresol and dinitrophenol herbicides and the pentachlorophenol fungicides, may produce a similar clinical picture. Cresolic and phenolic herbicides may stain the skin yellow and cause dark-colored urine. Other agents to consider when an unknown herbicide has been ingested include amide, aniline, and arsenic derivatives; carbamates and thiocarbamates; chlorates; glyphosate; paraquat; and triazines. Toxicologic analysis of the blood may be necessary for a definitive diagnosis.

EMERGENCY DEPARTMENT EVALUATION

The history should include the time, amount, and concentration of the agent(s) ingested; the onset, nature, and progression of symptoms; and the patient's health history. A similar description of circumstances should be obtained if other routes of exposure are involved.

The physical examination should focus on the vital signs, neurologic status, cardiovascular system, muscles, and skin. Laboratory evaluation in symptomatic patients should include arterial blood gas analysis; a CBC; measurement of electrolyte, calcium, magnesium, BUN, creatinine, glucose, creatine phosphokinase, and cardiac and liver enzyme levels; and urinalysis for myoglobin and routine analysis. An ECG and chest radiograph should be obtained. Nerve conduction studies and electromyography are sometimes necessary.

EMERGENCY DEPARTMENT MANAGEMENT

Advanced life-support measures should be instituted as necessary. In severe cases, endotracheal intubation and fluid resuscitation may be required. Active external cooling may be necessary in patients with hyperthermia. Because salicylates can cause uncoupling of oxidative phosphorylation, their use should be avoided. Due to slow absorption, GI decontamination may be effective long after ingestion (possibly as long as 18 hours). Activated charcoal is the preferred method. Gastric aspiration prior to activated charcoal may offer some additional benefit.

Treatment consists primarily of supportive measures. Electrolyte abnormalities should be corrected. The administration of sodium bicarbonate has three beneficial effects: correction of acidemia, enhancement of the urinary excretion of 2,4-D by ion trapping, and prevention of renal failure in patients with rhabdomyolysis. It also appears to improve survival.[4] Sodium bicarbonate should be given as a constant infusion rather than as a bolus. The urine pH must be increased to 8.0 to enhance excretion significantly.[18] A suggested initial infusion is two ampules (88 mEq) of sodium bicarbonate per liter of dextrose 5% in sodium chloride 0.45% at 150 mL/h. Adjustments in the rate and the amount of bicarbonate should be made on the basis of urine flow and pH.

The use of muscle relaxants should be considered in patients with agitation, fasciculations, myoclonus, or muscle rigidity. A benzodiazepine or nondepolarizing neuromuscular blocker may be preferable to succinylcholine because of the clinical similarity between 2,4-D muscle toxicity and early succinylcholine effects.

Plasma 2,4-D levels have been used to monitor the effect of therapy, but they are not readily available, and treatment must be based on clinical findings. The kinetic profile of 2,4-D suggests that extracorporeal removal (dialysis or hemoperfusion) may be effective, but the use of these techniques has not been reported.

DISPOSITION

Because the onset and peak of toxicity may be delayed many hours after ingestion, all patients except those with trivial ingestions (or exposure by other routes) should be admitted for observation. Symptomatic patients should be admitted to an intensive care unit. If intensive supportive care is unavailable, symptomatic patients should be transferred to a facility with such capability.

COMMON PITFALLS

- Failure to appreciate that GI decontamination may be effective many hours after ingestion
- Failure to appreciate that toxicity may be delayed in onset and to admit all patients with nontrivial ingestions for observation
- Failure to evaluate symptomatic patients for multisystem toxicity, especially rhabdomyolysis
- Failure to use alkaline diuresis to enhance 2,4-D elimination

References

1. Arnold EK, Beasley R. The pharmacokinetics of chlorinated phenoxy acid herbicides: a literature review. *Vet Hum Toxicol* 1989;31:121.
2. Feldman RJ, Maibach HI. Percutaneous penetration of some pesticides and herbicides in man. *Toxicol Appl Pharmacol* 1974;28:126.
3. Fisher HK. Paraquat poisoning—recovery from renal and pulmonary damage. *Ann Intern Med* 1971;79:731.
4. Flanagan RJ, Meredith TJ, Ruprah M, et al. Alkaline diuresis for acute poisoning with chlorphenoxy herbicides and ioxynil. *Lancet* 1990;335:454.
5. Friesen EG, Jones GR, Vaughan D. Clinical presentation and management of acute 2,4-D oral ingestion. *Drug Saf* 1990;5:155.
6. Hampson ECGM, Pond SM. Failure of haemoperfusion and haemodialysis to prevent death in paraquat poisoning: a retrospective review of 42 patients. *Med Toxicol* 1988;3:64.
7. Hart TB. A statistical approach to the prognostic significance of plasma paraquat concentrations. *Lancet* 1984;2:1222.
8. Hoet PH, Demedts M, Nemery B. Effects of oxygen pressure and medium volume on the toxicity of paraquat in rat and human type II pneumocytes. *Hum Exp Toxicol* 1997;16:305.
9. Idid SZ, Lee CY. Effects of Fuller's Earth and activated charcoal on oral absorption of paraquat in rabbits. *Clin Exp Pharmacol Physiol* 1996;23:679.
10. Kancir CB, Anderson C, Olesen AS. Marked hypocalcemia in a fatal poisoning with chlorinated phenoxy acid derivatives. *Clin Toxicol* 1988;26:257.
11. Lin JL, Leu ML, Liu YC, Chen GH. A prospective clinical trial of pulse therapy with glucocorticoid and cyclophosphamide in moderate to severe paraquat-poisoned patients. *Am J Resp & Crit Care Med* 1999;159(2):357.
12. Newstead CG. Cyclophosphamide treatment of paraquat poisoning. *Thorax* 1996;51:659.
13. O'Reilly JF. Prolonged coma and delayed peripheral neuropathy after ingestion of phenoxyacetic acid weed killers. *Postgrad Med J* 1984;60:76.
14. Pond SM. Repeated hemoperfusion and continuous arteriovenous hemofiltration in a paraquat-poisoned patient. *Clin Toxicol* 1987;25:305.
15. Prescott LF, Park J, Carrien I. Treatment of severe 2,4-D and mecoprop intoxication with alkaline diuresis. *Br J Clin Pharmacol* 1979;7:111.
16. Vale JA. Paraquat poisoning: clinical features and immediate general management. *Hum Toxicol* 1987;6:41.
17. Vanholder R, Colardyn F, DeReuck J, et al. Diquat intoxication: report of two cases and review of the literature. *Am J Med* 1981;70:1267.
18. Walder B, Brundler MA, Spilopoulos A, et al. Successful single-lung transplantation after paraquat intoxication. *Transplantation* 1997;64:789.
19. Wells WDE, Wright N, Yeoman WB. Clinical features and management of poisoning with 2,4-D and mecoprop. *Clin Toxicol* 1981;18:273.
20. Yang TS, Chang YL, Yen CK. Haemoperfusion treatment in pigs experimentally intoxicated by paraquat. *Human Exp Toxicol* 1997;16:709.

CHAPTER 344

Hydrogen Sulfide Poisoning

Daniel R. Douglas and Martin J. Smilkstein

Hydrogen sulfide (H_2S) is a colorless, irritating, heavier-than-air gas recognized at low concentrations by its characteristic rotten-eggs odor. Although less notorious than cyanide, H_2S can be just as deadly and is far more common. Natural sources include sulfur springs, crude petroleum, natural gas, volcanic gas, and bacterial decomposition of sulfur-containing proteinaceous material. Exposure may occur during digging, drilling, mining, and caisson work, or during refining (petroleum and natural gas refineries, coke ovens, and ore smelting).

Chemical reactions that involve sulfur-containing compounds may produce H_2S during rubber vulcanization, viscose rayon manufacturing, Kraft paper milling, leather and fur processing, food processing, dairy and brewery work, and production of pesticides, heavy water, felt, and glue. H_2S exposure may also occur in the setting of hot asphalt use, sewer and septic tank cleaning, and drain cleaning (reaction of acid drain cleaners with sulfur-containing sludge).[2]

Dermal absorption is negligible, but after inhalation, reversible binding of H_2S to the ferric ion of the cytochrome-aa_3 oxidase complex prevents cellular respiration and leads to cellular asphyxia and lactic acidosis.[2,13] Although H_2S is a more potent inhibitor of cytochrome oxidase than cyanide, the detoxification of H_2S and the return of cellular respiration is rapid, so that even severe symptomatology is often reversible if the toxic exposure is brief.[2,5]

Therefore, unlike toxicity from other cellular asphyxiants (cyanide and carbon monoxide), which is more persistent, removal from exposure and administration of oxygen rapidly terminate H_2S inhibition of cellular respiration. In many cases, severely poisoned victims show rapid spontaneous correction of lactic acidosis, often by the time initial resuscitation is complete.[7]

There has been speculation that sulfhemoglobin formation may contribute to cyanosis and to the pathophysiology of poisoning. Although sulfhemoglobin has been present in some cases of sulfide poisoning,[10] it has also been absent in many fatal accidental and experimental cases,[13] is difficult to assay accurately, and is probably not clinically significant.[9] Sulfhemoglobin is not readily assayable, but an "oxygen saturation gap" (calculated oxygen saturation minus measured oxygen saturation) that is not explained by the presence of other abnormal hemoglobins (carboxyhemoglobin and methemoglobin) may represent the presence of sulfhemoglobin.

Animal studies have demonstrated that the greatest central nervous system (CNS) uptake of sulfide after sodium hydrosulfide (alkali salt of H_2S) exposure is in the brainstem, which contains the medullary respiratory center.[18] Furthermore, increased levels of monoamines (epinephrine, norepinephrine, serotonin, and dopamine), as well as enhanced monoamine oxidase inhibition, have been found in the brainstem of rats acutely poisoned with sodium hydrosulfide.[19] Although the exact significance of these findings is unclear, they may play a role in the central respiratory paralysis seen after severe H_2S poisoning.[19] The metabolic fate of H_2S has not been studied in humans. Rapid oxidation of sulfide to sulfate is thought to be the primary route of detoxification,[2] and probably occurs within minutes.[3]

CLINICAL PRESENTATION

The severity of H_2S poisoning, and thus the clinical presentation, is largely determined by the intensity of the initial exposure. Low concentrations (50 to 100 ppm) may initially cause only mucous membrane irritation, whereas exposure to high concentrations (500 to 1000 ppm) may cause immediate respiratory paralysis and death, even before mucous membrane irritation develops.[2] The rotten-eggs odor of H_2S is detectable between 0.02 and 0.1 ppm and becomes intense between 20 and 30 ppm. As the sulfide concentration increases to dangerous levels (greater than 100 ppm), olfactory nerve dysfunction occurs and the sense of smell is lost.[2]

H_2S exposure may cause both local and systemic effects. The direct irritative action of H_2S on the mucous membrane results in both ocular and respiratory inflammation. Eye pain and burning, lacrimation, and blurred vision consistent with keratoconjunctivitis are typically noted first. Patients may complain of colored halos around lights ("gas eyes") due to inflammation and edema of the cornea. Rarely, corneal ulcerations may develop in more severe exposures. Mucosal irritation of the respiratory tract can result in inflammation from the nasal passages to the pulmonary parenchyma. Thus, patients may complain of nasal congestion, sore throat, hoarseness, cough, bloody sputum, and shortness of breath. Physical examination may reveal nasal and pharyngeal mucosal hyperemia or edema and auscultatory findings of wheezing, rales, and consolidation due to pneumonitis or pulmonary edema. Twenty percent of cases in one study were clinically diagnosed with pulmonary edema.[5] Both noncardiogenic and cardiogenic pulmonary edema may result from severe exposure.

CNS effects typically predominate after systemic absorption of H_2S. Severe, acute exposures typically cause rapid loss of consciousness and central respiratory paralysis. Corresponding to the possible effects of CNS anoxia, many other neurologic effects have been described, including headache, confusion, vertigo, agitation, somnolence, weakness of extremities, prolonged coma, and seizures.[5] Horizontal and vertical nystagmus has also been reported.[15] Although less common, reported cardiovascular effects include hypertension,[1,15] hypotension, tachycardia, bradycardia, conduction defects (left bundle-branch block),[15] and ischemic electrocardiogram (ECG) changes.[17] Nausea, vomiting, and abdominal cramps may occur with more subacute exposures. Vomiting combined with a depressed level of consciousness may result in aspiration.

Because of the potential for sudden loss of consciousness and collapse, the possibility of occult traumatic injuries (e.g., cervical spine injuries) must be entertained. Some form of bodily trauma was noted in 27% of 221 cases in one review.[5]

In contrast to acute H_2S poisoning, chronic toxicity (prolonged low-level exposure or intermittent moderate-level exposures) does not cause dramatic CNS effects but may result in neuropsychiatric sequelae such as fatigue, headache, dizziness, irritability, and cognitive impairment.

Laboratory and ECG findings are nonspecific but reflect the severity of the anoxic injury. In significant poisonings, arterial blood gas measurements may show a combined metabolic and respiratory acidosis. Elevated lactate levels may also be present secondary to inhibited cellular respiration; however, due to rapid correction, significant levels may not be present at the time of the emergency department evaluation if there has been adequate cardiorespiratory support. In addition, the blood gas abnormalities often described after cyanide and carbon monoxide exposure (persistent or worsening acidosis and decreased arterial–venous oxygen saturation difference) are uncommon after H_2S poisoning. There are no readily available tests to confirm the diagnosis.

Methods to assay blood sulfide at low concentrations have been developed and may be useful in determining exposure in less severe poisonings.[8] Due to the rapid detoxification and metabolism of sulfide, the sample must be taken as soon as possible after exposure, usually no later than 2 hours. Although of interest in some cases, the assay is not readily available, and the meaning of sulfide levels is unknown. Anecdotally, the H_2S odor may be detectable when the stopper is removed from blood specimens drawn from victims, but this finding is not consistently present.

DIFFERENTIAL DIAGNOSIS

The differential diagnosis includes other toxic gases capable of the same "knock-down" effect, including cyanide and simple asphyxiants (e.g., carbon dioxide and methane). Cardiovascular, CNS, and thromboembolic causes of syncope and collapse must also be considered.

EMERGENCY DEPARTMENT EVALUATION

The history is directed at documenting H_2S exposure and the severity of symptoms. The physician notes the setting and actions immediately preceding symptom onset, unusual odors, other exposures, associated trauma, the duration of exposure, and the time course (rapidity of onset and duration) of any alterations in level of consciousness.

Physical examination focuses on vital signs, mucous membrane and eye findings, and cardiac, pulmonary, and neurologic findings. An alert mental status is insufficient to rule out CNS dysfunction. A meticulous neurologic examination and mental status testing, including short-term memory, attention, and concentration, may reveal subtle abnormalities indicative of either ongoing toxicity or postasphyxiant dysfunction.

When only eye and respiratory irritation is present, without respiratory distress or alteration in mental status or vital signs, laboratory assessment is unnecessary. Arterial blood gas measurements, a chest radiograph, and an ECG should be done in patients with systemic symptoms or signs. Patients with a prolonged loss of consciousness may also warrant routine hematology, chemistry, and coagulation profiles.

EMERGENCY DEPARTMENT MANAGEMENT

Rescuers and prehospital care providers must wear self-contained breathing equipment if there is a risk of ongoing exposure. Rescue breathing by mouth-to-mouth resuscitation can be attempted if absolutely necessary, because evidence is lacking to suggest that it is potentially harmful to the rescuer. Dermal decontamination is not critical, because no significant skin absorption occurs. Ocular irrigation may provide symptomatic relief but is not an immediate treatment priority, because eye damage is usually limited to superficial irritation.

Supportive care is the mainstay of therapy. Advanced life-support measures should be initiated as needed. To maximize oxygen delivery and reduce ongoing sulfide–cytochrome binding, all patients should receive 100% oxygen. Noncardiogenic pulmonary edema may require positive-pressure ventilation. Pulmonary edema due to cardiac failure may require diuretics and other adjuncts. Routine eye care should be provided.

The use of nitrites and hyperbaric oxygen (HBO) is controversial. Nitrite-induced methemoglobin may act as a competitive inhibitor of sulfide–cytochrome binding by forming a sulfide–methemoglobin complex (sulfmethemoglobin), or it may enhance detoxification by acting as a catalyst for sulfide oxidation.[2] Despite anecdotal reports[11,15] and evidence of prophylactic (preexposure) efficacy in animal models,[14] there is no convincing evidence that nitrites are effective when given after the exposure. Laboratory studies[3] and the clinical course of patients[5] indicate that sulfide oxidation is so rapid that the amount of cytochrome-bound sulfide is probably inconsequential by the time most patients reach the emergency department. As a result, nitrite therapy should be reserved for severely poisoned patients who reach the hospital within a few minutes of exposure and fail to improve rapidly.

In such cases, the nitrite portion of the Lilly cyanide antidote kit may be given in the same dosage as for cyanide (adults, 10 mL of 3% sodium nitrite intravenously over 3 to 4 minutes; children, 0.2 to 0.33 mL/kg, up to 10 mL). If intravenous access is established, it is unnecessary to administer amyl nitrite. Nitrite therapy can cause hypotension with rapid administration and can cause significant methemoglobinemia.

HBO has mostly been studied in the treatment of acute carbon monoxide poisoning, but the exact indications for its use remain unclear. Several studies suggest that HBO therapy may decrease the incidence of neuropsychiatric sequelae after acute carbon monoxide exposure,[6,16] and most authorities recommend its use for the patient with sustained neurologic changes or depressed mental status. The indications for HBO therapy in H_2S poisoning are even less well defined. However, animal studies[4] and anecdotal reports[12,20] suggest the possible utility of HBO in treating H_2S toxicity. Although its efficacy and mechanism of action remain unproved, HBO should be considered in patients with a persistently decreased level of consciousness or neurologic changes despite treatment with the previously described measures.

DISPOSITION

Consultation with a toxicologist or poison center is advisable if the physician is unfamiliar with H_2S poisoning. Patients with only mucous membrane irritation may be treated as outpatients. Patients with mild systemic symptoms, including brief syncope (less than 1 minute), may be discharged when asymptomatic if they have no underlying cardiovascular or neurologic disease and the physical examination, arterial blood gas analysis, ECG, and chest radiograph are normal. All other patients should be admitted, and those with persistent vital sign, respiratory, or neurologic abnormalities should be admitted to an intensive care unit. Transfer of severely intoxicated patients should be considered if intensive care admission, antidotal therapy, or HBO is indicated but unavailable.

COMMON PITFALLS

- Failure to consider the possibility of H_2S poisoning in otherwise healthy patients who suddenly collapse at work
- Failure to appreciate that olfactory paralysis prevents odor detection at dangerous H_2S levels and that the absence of an odor does not imply safety
- Failure of prehospital rescuers to wear self-contained breathing gear to avoid becoming additional victims
- Failure to consider the possibility of other victims and perform a scene search when an index case is found
- Failure to evaluate patients for concomitant traumatic injuries
- Failure to appreciate that nitrite therapy has limited usefulness and entails significant risks

References

1. Audeau FM, Gnanaharan C, Davey K. H_2S poisoning associated with pelt processing. *N Z Med J* 1985;145:98.
2. Beauchamp RO Jr, Bus JS, Popp JA, et al. A critical review of the literature on H_2S toxicity. *CRC Crit Rev Toxicol* 1984;13:25.
3. Beck JF, Bradbury CM, Connors AJ, et al. Nitrite as an antidote for acute H_2S intoxication? *Am Indust Hyg Assoc J* 1981;42:805.
4. Bitterman N, Talmi Y, Lerman A, et al. The effect of hyperbaric oxygen on acute experimental sulfide poisoning in the rat. *Toxicol Appl Pharmacol* 1986;84:325.
5. Burnett WW, King EG, Grace M, et al. H_2S poisoning—review of 5 years' experience. *Can Med Assoc J* 1977;117:1277.
6. Ducasse JL, Celsis P, Marc-Vergnes JP. Non-comatose patients with acute carbon monoxide poisoning: hyperbaric or normobaric oxygenation? *Undersea Hyperb Med* 1995;22:9–15.
7. Hoidal CR, Hall AH, Robinson MD, et al. H_2S poisoning from toxic inhalations of roofing asphalt fumes. *Ann Emerg Med* 1986;15:826.
8. Lindell H, Jappinen P, Savolainen H. Determination of sulfide in blood with an ion-selective electrode by preconcentration of trapped sulfide in sodium hydroxide solution. *Analyst* 1988;113:839.
9. Park CM, Nagel RL. Sulfhemoglobinemia: clinical and molecular aspects. *N Engl J Med* 1984;310:1579.
10. Peters JW. H_2S poisoning in a hospital setting. *JAMA* 1981;246:1588.
11. Ravizza AG, Carugo D, Cerchiari EL, et al. The treatment of H_2S intoxication: oxygen vs. nitrites. *Vet Hum Toxicol* 1982;24:241.
12. Smilkstein MJ, Bronstein AC, Pickett HM, et al. Hyperbaric oxygen therapy for severe H_2S poisoning. *J Emerg Med* 1985;3:27.
13. Smith RP, Gosselin RE. H_2S poisoning. *J Occup Med* 1979;21:93.
14. Smith RP, Kruszyna R, Kruszyna H. Management of acute sulfide poisoning. *Arch Environ Health* 1976;166:166.
15. Stine RJ, Slosberg B, Beacham BE. H_2S intoxication—a case report and discussion of treatment. *Ann Intern Med* 1976;85:756.
16. Thom SR, Tabar RL, Mendiguren I, et al. Delayed neuropsychological sequelae after carbon monoxide (CO) poisoning: prevention by treatment with hyperbaric oxygen. *Ann Emerg Med* 1995;25:474–480.
17. Vanthenen AS, Emberton P, Wales JM. H_2S poisoning in a factory worker [Letter]. *Lancet* 1988;1:305.
18. Warenycia MW, Goodwin LR, Benishin CG, et al. Acute H_2S poisoning—demonstration of selective uptake of sulfide by the brain stem by measurement of brain sulfide levels. *Biochem Pharmacol* 1989;38:973.
19. Warenycia MW, Smith KA, Blashko CS, et al. Monoamine oxidase inhibition as a sequel of H_2S intoxication: increases in brain catecholamine and 5-hydroxytryptamine levels. *Arch Toxicol* 1989;63:131.
20. Whitcraft DD III, Bailey TD, Hart GB. H_2S poisoning treated with hyperbaric oxygen. *J Emerg Med* 1985;3:23.

CHAPTER 345
Iron Poisoning

Jeffrey R. Suchard and Steven C. Curry

Although iron poisoning occurs in all age groups, it is the leading cause of accidental poisoning death from pharmaceutical agents among young children. The American Association of Poison Control Centers has reported over 29,000 iron ingestions annually, with two fatal outcomes in both 1996 and 1997.[9,10] Household sources of iron are commonplace, making them readily available for impetuous ingestions. Parental iron supplements of these preparations are often found in homes with young children, and many of these preparations appear nearly identical to candy; some are even sugar-coated. Chewable multivitamins with iron are specifically designed to appeal to young children.

The amount of iron in each preparation varies, and toxicity after acute ingestion depends on the amount of elemental iron ingested (Table 345.1). Toxic doses are difficult to define, given the frequently unreliable histories surrounding accidental ingestions. In general, the ingestion of more than 20 mg of elemental iron per kilogram of body weight produces significant gastroenteritis; doses above the 40- to 60-mg/kg range are potentially fatal. Though confirmatory epidemiology studies are lacking, many physicians believe that the ingestion of children's chewable multiple vitamins with iron rarely causes severe iron poisoning, and that toxicity from such exposures is less than expected on the basis of elemental iron ingested per body weight.[8]

TABLE 345.1. Iron Compounds and Their Percent Elemental Iron Content

Compound	Percent Elemental Iron by Weight
Ferrous carbonate, anhydrous	48
Ferrous fumarate	33
Ferrous gluconate	12
Ferrous phosphate	37
Ferrous pyrophosphate	12
Ferrous sulfate	16
Ferrocholinate	12
Ferroglycine sulfate	16
Ferric pyrophosphate	12

Some poison centers choose to observe asymptomatic or only mildly symptomatic children at home after ingesting such preparations, even when the estimated ingestion exceeds 20 mg/kg of elemental iron.

About 10% of ingested iron, mainly the ferrous (Fe^{2+}) state, is absorbed each day from the small intestine. Because free, unbound iron is toxic to tissues, the body has many mechanisms to keep iron bound to proteins or other macromolecules. After absorption, iron changes to the ferric (Fe^{3+}) state and is stored in the intestinal mucosa complexed to ferritin. Transport to other tissues occurs with iron bound to transferrin. The total amount of iron that transferrin can bind is termed the *total iron-binding capacity* (TIBC). Normal serum iron concentrations vary from 50 to 150 μg/dL, while normal TIBCs can range from 300 to 450 μg/dL. Because the TIBC is far in excess of the iron concentration, there normally is no circulating unbound iron.

Excessive iron is corrosive to the gastrointestinal (GI) tract, resulting in gastroenteritis, with the potential for hemorrhage, hypovolemia, and perforation. If enough iron is absorbed, systemic and metabolic consequences of iron poisoning develop. Iron accumulates mainly in the liver after overdose but can have toxic effects in almost any organ. Iron is concentrated in mitochondria, where it disrupts oxidative phosphorylation and catalyzes the formation of oxygen free radicals, leading to lipid peroxidation and cell death. Toxic amounts of iron also produce venodilation and increase capillary permeability. The metabolic acidosis seen in iron poisoning is due to several factors, including hypovolemia, tissue hypoperfusion, a shift to anaerobic metabolism as mitochondrial function is impaired, and the hydration of the ferric ion with generation of hydrogen ions:

$$[Fe^{3+} + 3H_2O \rightarrow 3Fe(OH)_3 + 3H^+].$$

Coagulopathy may occur, even before the onset of hepatic dysfunction, from iron's ability to inhibit serine proteases as thrombin and other coagulation factors. Isolated liver damage may occur, but multiple organ system failure is possible in severe iron poisonings.[5,12,14]

CLINICAL PRESENTATION

Clinical effects of iron poisoning are usually considered in stages.[5,12,14] It is important to remember, however, that the time frame for staging is imprecise, patients present at variable times after ingestion, and distinguishing between stages can be difficult due to overlapping signs, symptoms, and laboratory manifestations, and because of rapid progression. Patients can die in any stage of iron poisoning, but for different reasons.

The first stage of iron poisoning develops within the first few hours after ingestion. It is due to the direct corrosive effects of iron on the GI tract, and is characterized by abdominal pain, vomiting, and diarrhea. Hematemesis or melena may occur if significant GI bleeding is present. Serum iron concentrations may be normal or elevated. Diarrhea may be the only manifestation in patients who ingest multiple vitamins with iron, particularly preparations intended for children. Patients with serious stage 1 iron toxicity will develop lethargy, shock, and metabolic acidosis due to hypovolemia, anemia, and tissue hypoperfusion.

Stage 2 is characterized by resolution of the clinical signs and symptoms seen in stage 1, despite continued absorption of toxic amounts of iron and increasing tissue iron burden. Sometimes unseen, this stage may last until about 24 hours after ingestion. Patients frequently lie quietly and clinically appear improved, but the resolution of gastroenteritis can be falsely reassuring. If laboratory studies are obtained, they are likely to show elevated serum iron levels and a progressive metabolic acidosis.

Stage 3 systemic iron poisoning becomes clinically evident. Stage 3 may appear early in patients with severe poisoning (bypassing stage 2) or may appear several hours after the beginning of stage 2. Toxic amounts of iron have moved from blood into tissues, disrupting cellular metabolism, causing third-spacing of fluids and producing venous pooling of blood. Shock and metabolic acidosis in this stage can result from persistent hypovolemia, anemia, hepatic dysfunction, impaired oxidative phosphorylation, heart failure, and renal failure. Fulminant hepatic failure with hypoglycemia, hyperammonemia, and coagulopathy may occur, though significant hepatic injury is unusual when peak serum iron levels remain below 500 μg/dL.

Stage 4 is characterized by gastric outlet or small-bowel obstruction. GI obstruction is an unusual occurrence but may develop several weeks after the acute toxicity has resolved, due to scarring produced by iron's corrosive effects.

Elevated serum iron levels obtained within the proper time frame are helpful in confirming the diagnosis of iron poisoning. Serum iron concentrations usually peak 2 to 6 hours after ingestion. Because it is iron in tissue that produces systemic toxicity, a patient may be seriously ill from iron poisoning and have a normal serum iron level many hours after ingestion. On the other hand, a serum iron level drawn early after ingestion may be misleadingly low if absorption is still occurring. Therefore, a normal serum iron concentration very early or many hours after ingestion does not exclude iron poisoning.

Clinical and laboratory findings can help predict the degree of toxicity. The majority of children who have vomiting or diarrhea, a white blood cell count greater than 15,000/μL, and a serum glucose level greater than 150 mg/dL after ingesting iron have a serum iron level greater than 300 μg/dL.[7] However, severely poisoned patients can still have normal white count and serum glucose levels.[6,13] The "deferoxamine challenge" test, in which the presence of *vin rosé*-colored urine after giving a dose of deferoxamine was considered an indication for chelation therapy, is no longer recommended because this color change is unreliable.[18] A kidney–ureter–bladder (KUB) radiograph may demonstrate radiopacities in the GI tract, a finding often present in patients who develop significant poisoning. However, a patient may be seriously ill from iron poisoning and have a normal KUB radiograph. About 50% of children who develop serum iron levels in excess of 300 μg/dL have a negative KUB.[7,13] Experience at our center indicates that even when iron tablets are noted initially, they are no longer visible at 24 hours in patients who receive chelation therapy and supportive care.

DIFFERENTIAL DIAGNOSIS

The initial GI signs and symptoms of iron poisoning occur in many disorders, including poisoning by acetaminophen, salicylate, hepatotoxic mushrooms, arsenic, caffeine and theophylline, caustics, copper salts, and mercurial salts. Infectious gastroenteritis, medical and surgical intraabdominal conditions, or sepsis may cause vomiting, diarrhea, acidosis, and shock. Acute iron poisoning, however, is not accompanied by fever unless produced by a sequela of iron poisoning (e.g., aspiration, bowel infarction).

EMERGENCY DEPARTMENT EVALUATION

The history should include the time and amount of ingestion, the identity of the iron preparation ingested, and the nature, severity, time of onset, and progression of symptoms. The physician should specifically ask about abdominal pain, vomiting, and diarrhea, and whether blood was noted. The amount of elemental iron ingested, in milligrams per kilogram, should be calculated. The physical examination should focus on vital signs, overall appearance, and the abdomen.

Patients who have had only one or two episodes of vomiting or diarrhea and are subsequently asymptomatic should have a complete blood count and measurement of serum electrolytes, glucose, blood urea nitrogen, creatinine, and iron levels. Those with more pronounced or persistent GI symptoms, evidence of hypovolemia, or lethargy should also have a prothrombin time, liver function studies, arterial blood gas analysis, and a KUB radiograph. A TIBC is not helpful in the evaluation of iron toxicity and should not be ordered. It does not assist in the treatment decisions, and several laboratory methods to measure the TIBC are inaccurate in the setting of iron overload.

EMERGENCY DEPARTMENT MANAGEMENT

In general, all symptomatic patients and those who ingested more than 20 mg/kg of elemental iron less than 6 hours earlier are referred by poison control centers to emergency departments for evaluation. Prehospital care of symptomatic patients includes adequate oxygenation and intravenous hydration for patients with hypotension or other evidence of hypovolemia.

Gastric decontamination measures are of questionable value in iron ingestion. Activated charcoal does not effectively bind iron, and its use should be limited to cases in which coingestion of other substances that bind to charcoal is known or suspected. If activated charcoal is administered, cathartics should be withheld, especially in patients who already have gastroenteritis, as this may exacerbate hypovolemia. Though gastric lavage is commonly employed in iron ingestions, it has never been shown to be of clinical benefit, possibly because most iron tablets are too large to evacuate by this method. Simulated overdose studies suggest that oral magnesium oxide (Milk of Magnesia)[17] or a slurry of charcoal mixed with deferoxamine[3] can reduce iron absorption, but the utility of such treatments in actual overdose patients is unknown. There are no data supporting lavage with sodium bicarbonate solutions or administration of phosphates to prevent iron absorption. Lavage with deferoxamine solutions is not recommended because of the tremendous amounts required and because only a small portion of the ingested iron is absorbed. Whole-bowel irrigation with polyethylene glycol–electrolyte lavage solutions[16] and gastrotomy to remove iron pills[2] have also been reported, but such recommendations are based on anecdotal data. Whether they are more effective than supportive care alone has not been studied in controlled trials.

Patients who remain completely asymptomatic (including no lethargy) for 6 hours after ingestion and who have a normal physical examination do not require treatment. Those who ingested more than 20 mg/kg of elemental iron but are seen within 6 hours might benefit from gastric lavage. Given the lack of data concerning the efficacy of gastric lavage in this setting, the decision to use it is made on an individual basis. Syrup of ipecac is not recommended, because the vomiting it produces cannot be distinguished from iron-induced gastroenteritis. If vomiting has already occurred, gastric lavage is of questionable benefit. Bicarbonate, phosphate, or deferoxamine solutions should not be used for lavage.[5] Activated charcoal does not prevent iron absorption and is not indicated for isolated ingestions of iron or vitamins with iron. However, a single dose of Milk of Magnesia (60 mL/g of elemental iron ingested) is recommended, as it may significantly prevent iron absorption.[5] If the serum iron concentration in an asymptomatic patient is lower than 350 μg/dL, and a repeat study documents no rise in the serum iron concentration, the patient can be released. On the other hand a KUB radiograph demonstrating numerous tablets suggests that serum iron concentrations will be rising. Patients who have suffered only a single emesis or diarrheal stool but who have remained asymptomatic for several hours and have a normal physical examination, KUB, and laboratory evaluation do not require treatment.

Patients who present with or develop more than two episodes of emesis or diarrhea, have evidence of hypovolemia, or exhibit lethargy require treatment with fluids and deferoxamine mesylate. In patients with significant symptoms of iron poisoning, treatment should not be delayed to wait for results of a serum iron determination, because the therapy is indicated regardless of the serum iron concentration. In contrast, iron ingestions are expected to raise serum iron levels above the normal range, and an "abnormal" iron level does not constitute an indication for deferoxamine or admission in the absence of clinical signs of toxicity.

With rare exceptions, all symptomatic patients are hypovolemic. Fluid challenges of 20 mL/kg of lactated Ringer's or normal saline are given to restore fluid volume and ensure a normal urine output. Patients commonly require maintenance infusions at twice normal rates to keep up with GI losses and third-spacing.

Deferoxamine mesylate is an iron-chelating agent that can remove iron from tissues and non–transferrin-bound iron from plasma. Deferoxamine binds to iron to form ferrioxamine, which is excreted in the urine over days to weeks. Ferrioxamine occasionally imparts a *vin rosé* color to the urine, but this color change is unreliable and inconsistent and should not be used to determine the need for additional treatment.[12,18] Deferoxamine mesylate can be mixed in any crystalloid and should be continuously infused at 15 mg/kg/h. Higher infusion rates are recommended in severe cases by some authorities. Rapid intravenous administration is sometimes associated with hypotension, presumably from histamine release, but this is not usually a problem with infusion rates below 45 mg/kg/h. Intramuscular deferoxamine is not recommended.

Many statements in the manufacturer's package insert for deferoxamine do not reflect the standard of care. Deferoxamine is not contraindicated for the treatment of acute iron poisoning in pregnancy. Animal data and human experience strongly suggest that toxic amounts of maternally ingested iron, deferoxamine, and ferrioxamine do not cross into the fetal circulation.[1,11] Fetal death, therefore, results from maternal demise, and a pregnant woman should be treated the same as any other person. At 15 mg/kg/h, many patients receive well over 6 g deferoxamine mesylate each day; this is safe for the short-term treatment of iron poisoning.

Deferoxamine causes falsely low serum iron concentrations.[4] Because tissue iron, not serum iron, is responsible for toxicity, a normal or low serum iron concentration by itself cannot be used to justify stopping deferoxamine. Intravenous deferoxamine should be continued until clinical toxicity has resolved, serum iron levels are normal or low, *and* any *vin rosé*-colored urine (if present) disappears.[12] A urinary iron assay, which may objectively define when to stop deferoxamine therapy, has also been described, but its clinical utility has not been proved.[18] Most patients require 12 to 24 hours of deferoxamine infusion, but occasional patients with very large overdoses require therapy for longer periods.

The use of prochlorperazine (Compazine) and deferoxamine together has produced coma in humans that has been reproduced in animals. This drug combination should therefore be avoided.

In renal failure, deferoxamine should be continued but at much lower infusion rates. Assuming that therapeutic deferoxamine levels have been obtained, anuric patients should continue to receive infusions at about 1.5 mg/kg/h, based on the known prolonged half-life in renal failure.[12]

General supportive care for attendant complications (e.g., liver failure, GI bleeding) is the same as for any other patient.

DISPOSITION

Patients who remain completely asymptomatic and those with a normal physical examination, KUB, and laboratory evaluation who have had only one or two episodes of emesis or diarrhea and then become asymptomatic 6 hours after ingestion can be discharged.

Patients with mild symptoms should have repeat labs demonstrating no rise in the serum level and no evidence of metabolic acidosis prior to discharge. Symptomatic patients should be admitted. The level of monitoring and treatment required usually necessitates intensive care. If the necessary laboratory and treatment services are not available, the patients should be transferred to a facility where such services are available. A poison center or toxicologist can be consulted for assistance with management.

COMMON PITFALLS

- Failing to administer adequate amounts of intravenous fluids to symptomatic patients
- Waiting for the result of the serum iron level before treating symptomatic patients with deferoxamine mesylate
- Using the TIBC for evaluation and treatment decisions
- Assuming that a "nontoxic" serum iron concentration excludes the diagnosis of iron poisoning or the need for treatment in a symptomatic patient
- Sending a patient home during stage 2 of poisoning because gastroenteritis has resolved
- Relying on normal serum glucose levels, white blood cell counts, and negative x-rays to exclude significant iron poisoning
- Failure to appreciate that deferoxamine may falsely lower serum iron concentration

ACKNOWLEDGMENTS

David A. Connor, MD, contributed to this chapter in a previous edition.

References

1. Curry S, Bond GR, Raschke R, et al. An ovine model of maternal iron poisoning in pregnancy. *Ann Emerg Med* 1990;19:632.
2. Foxford R, Goldfrank L. Gastronomy—a surgical approach to iron overdose. *Ann Emerg Med* 1985;14:1223.
3. Gomez HF, McClafferty HH, Flory D, et al. Prevention of gastrointestinal iron absorption by chelation from an orally administered premixed deferoxamine/charcoal slurry. *Ann Emerg Med* 1997;30:587.
4. Helfer RE, Rodgerson DO. The effect of deferoxamine on the determination of serum iron and iron-binding capacity. *J Pediatr* 1966;68:804.
5. Jacobs J, Greene H, Gendel BR. Acute iron intoxication. *N Engl J Med* 1965;273:1124.
6. Knasel AL, Collins-Barrow MD. Applicability of early indicators of iron toxicity. *J Natl Med Assoc* 1986;78:1037.
7. Lacouture PG, Wason S, Temple AR, et al. Emergency assessment of severity in iron overdose by clinical and laboratory methods. *J Pediatr* 1981;99:89.
8. Linakis JG, Lacouture PG, Woolf A. Iron absorption from chewable vitamins with iron versus iron tablets: implications for toxicity. *Pediatr Emerg Care* 1992;8:321.
9. Litovitz TL, Smilkstein M, Felberg L, et al. 1996 annual report of the American Association of Poison Control Centers Toxic Exposure Surveillance System. *Am J Emerg Med* 1997;15:447.
10. Litovitz TL, Klein-Schwartz W, Dyer KS, et al. 1997 annual report of the American Association of Poison Control Centers Toxic Exposure Surveillance System. *Am J Emerg Med* 1998;16:443.
11. McElhatton PR, Roberts JC, Sullivan FM. The consequences of iron overdose and its treatment with desferrioxamine in pregnancy. *Hum Exp Toxicol* 1991;10:251.
12. Mills KC, Curry SC. Acute iron poisoning. *Emerg Med Clin North Am* 1994;12:397.
13. Palatnick W, Tenebein M. Leukocytosis, hyperglycemia, vomiting, and positive x-rays are not indicators of severity of iron overdose in adults. *Am J Emerg Med* 1996;14:454.
14. Robotham J, Lietman P. Acute iron poisoning. *Am J Dis Child* 1980;134:875.
15. Siff JE, Meldon SW, Tomassoni AJ. Usefulness of the total iron binding capacity in the evaluation and treatment of acute iron overdose. *Ann Emerg Med* 1999;33:73.
16. Tenenbein M. Whole bowel irrigation as a gastrointestinal decontamination procedure after acute poisoning. *Med Toxicol* 1988;3:77.
17. Wallace KL, Curry SC, LoVecchio FL, et al. Effect of magnesium hydroxide on iron absorption following simulated mild iron overdose in human subjects. *Acad Emerg Med* 1998;5:961.
18. Yatscoff RW, Wayne EA, Tenenbein M. An objective criterion for the cessation of deferoxamine therapy in the acutely iron-poisoned patient. *Clin Toxicol* 1991;29:1.

CHAPTER 346

Irritant Gas Inhalation

Philip A. Edelman

The airway serves as a conduit, allowing the passage of fresh and waste gases. Extrapulmonary forces (muscles) affect inhalation, but the elastic recoil of the lung is primarily responsible for normal exhalation (bellows function). The lungs provide a large surface area for diffusion of gases between the alveolar spaces and the bloodstream. The upper airways are responsible for humidifying inspired air to prevent drying and irritation of lower airway surfaces. Lung compliance is dynamic, and contractile elements (smooth muscles), particularly those of the lower airways, respond to various stimuli by relaxing or contracting. The lung is also a metabolic and immunologically active organ. Mucous secretion (from goblet cells and mucous glands), combined with ciliary motion, is responsible for clearing particles from the airways. Any of the lung's functions may be affected by inhalation of an irritant gas.[11]

The response of the nose to inhalation of irritants may vary from rhinitis or hay fever to septal perforation (e.g., with chronic chromate exposure). The trachea and bronchi may respond by bronchoconstriction (immediate or delayed) and the development of asthma or acute tracheobronchitis. The response of lung parenchyma includes allergic alveolitis, pulmonary edema, emphysema, acute alveolitis, bronchiolitis, and interstitial fibrosis. The exact pathology depends on the nature, intensity, and duration of the exposure and the actual properties of the inhaled irritant.

Acute changes in lung function caused by irritant inhalation can be detected by several types of tests. Air flow capacity is best determined by spirometry, especially a flow-volume loop. The peak flowmeter is a simple device useful in determining the presence and severity of bronchoconstriction. In motivated and carefully trained patients, it may be a useful and readily available indicator of the need for, and response to, treatment. However, it has not been demonstrated to be an effective screening tool for patients with subtle changes in small airways resulting from early or mild exposures. The flow-volume loop provides additional information about the status of the smaller airways and probably remains better for this evaluation.

Reversibility of bronchospasm can be determined by the use of a bronchodilator and repeat testing. Changes in the alveolar–capillary permeability can be assessed by the single-breath carbon monoxide diffusing capacity (D_{LO}). A chest radiograph is also useful, particularly for visualizing inflammatory reactions of the parenchyma. Arterial blood gas analysis can assist in the assessment of blood oxygenation (PO_2) and ventilation (PCO_2). Ventilation–perfusion scanning does not usually provide significant additional information, except to rule out other processes, such as pulmonary emboli. Most important, careful physical examination may demonstrate pathology not detected by these studies, such as fine wheezes in subtle or early asthma and fine crackles in early pulmonary edema.

Toxic gases can also injure internal organs after inhalation. Absorption of gases by routes other than inhalation is usually minimal compared with the dose delivered by inhalation.

The physical characteristics of the inhalant are extremely important in determining the site and depth of lung penetration and systemic absorption, as well as local effects of the exposure. A *gas* is a material without a defined shape when unconstrained at room temperature under ambient conditions. A *fume* is a small, solid particulate dispersion formed by the coalescence of gases volatilized during an oxidative process such as combustion. Fumes are usually submicronic particles that can penetrate deeply into the lung. *Mists* are suspended liquid droplets generated by the condensation of gases or the breaking up of liquids (e.g., by splashing, atomization, or related actions). A *vapor* is the gaseous phase of a material that is normally a liquid at room temperature. Its concentration depends on the liquid's vapor pressure and temperature. Various other definitions apply to fogs, aerosols, smokes, and dusts (see Chapter 396).

The deposition and absorption of a gas or vapor in the respiratory tract are primarily governed by its water solubility. Highly soluble gases are absorbed in the upper airways, whereas less soluble materials reach the lower airways. The deposition of particulates, such as dusts, is a function of their size. Particles 5 μm or smaller reach the lower airways. Larger particles are deposited more proximally; those of submicron size may pass in and out of the airways without substantial impaction or deposition.

These concepts are important in determining the likely signs and symptoms of a person exposed to irritant gases. Highly water soluble airway irritants usually cause upper airway (eye, nose, and throat) irritation. Materials that are less water soluble may reach the lower airways and alveolar membrane, causing bronchospasm and pulmonary edema. Some common and representative irritants are discussed in this chapter.

CLINICAL PRESENTATION

Primary Pulmonary Irritants

The signs and symptoms of irritant inhalation may be immediate or delayed in onset. Primary irritants include corrosive, acid, or alkaline materials that may become airborne and inhaled. Irritant substances may also adsorb to the surfaces of otherwise inert particles, causing deeper penetration and persistence in the lungs. For example, the products of combustion in a plastics fire may include highly irritant aldehydes and organic acids that may bind to the carbonaceous particulates in smoke (see Chapter 396).

Signs and symptoms vary with the nature of the exposure. Although low-level and long-term (months to years) exposures may contribute to the development of bronchitis or related lung disease, exposures to high levels for short periods usually cause irritation of the eyes, nose, and throat, leading to lacrimation, rhinorrhea, conjunctivitis, pharyngitis, dyspnea, chest tightness, and, possibly, dysphonia. If the exposure is great enough, tracheobronchitis may occur. Chest tightness, wheezing, decreased inspiration–expiration ratio, and increased sputum production may result. Arterial blood gas analysis frequently demonstrates altered ventilatory mechanics consistent with acute airway obstruction. The chest radiograph is usually normal. Pulmonary function studies, especially a prebronchodilator and postbronchodilator flow-volume loop, usually demonstrate reversible abnormalities.

In severe exposures, pulmonary edema may occur. The diffusing capacity as evaluated by the D_{LCO} is decreased with pulmonary edema. The chest radiograph may be normal, especially at the earlier phases of injury, or it may show signs of interstitial edema. Arterial blood gas analysis may demonstrate hyperventilation with hypoxemia, or it may be normal. Bronchiolitis obliterans has been infrequently reported after these exposures.

Tear gases (see Chapter 325) can cause severe upper and lower respiratory tract irritation, and asphyxia with prolonged or high-dose exposure (e.g., in a confined space).[1]

Chloropicrin is used as an additive to fumigants such as methyl bromide (see later discussion) because it is a strong lacrimatory agent. Mercaptans and thiophene are used to odorize natural gas; they are slightly irritating in high doses, but they are generally known for their particular sulfur odors.

Oxides of sulfur react with water in the air to form sulfuric (or sulfurous) acid vapor or mists. These gases (e.g., SO_2) and vapors are responsible for urban air pollution resulting from fossil fuel combustion, smelting, and paper and rubber manufacturing. They are also used in bleaching, brewing, fumigation, tanning, preserving, and refrigeration.[4] Oxides of nitrogen and sulfur are the principal causes of acid rain.

Ozone is a by-product of bleaching, water purification, and processes that generate a spark or electric arc in the presence of oxygen (e.g., welding, mercury vapor lamps, photocopiers, and x-ray generators).[17] It is also found in the atmosphere, and higher levels are found at higher altitudes; flight at altitudes above 35,000 feet may result in transient toxicity.

Isocyanates, classically toluene diisocyanate, can cause chemically induced (occupational) asthma.[2,19] After long-term, low-level exposures, a worker may develop increasing symptoms of asthma. Alternatively, short-term, high-level exposures may produce the same problem. As there may be a delay of several hours between the exposure and the asthma (delayed hypersensitivity reaction), careful questioning for sources of exposure may be necessary. Isocyanates are used in the production of urethane foams for insulation, packaging, and the sealing and potting of electrical equipment. They are also used in many paints and finishes. Some chemicals in this class have different physiochemical and toxicologic properties—for instance, the more toxic methyl isocyanate was responsible for the deaths at Bhopal.

Oxides of nitrogen (NO, NO_2, N_2O_3, N_2O_4) are generated in many oxidative processes, including welding, fires, and industrial applications such as dye, fertilizer, celluloid, and lacquer manufacturing.[18] The accidental introduction of organic materials into nitric acid may cause combustion and release of nitrogen oxides. They may also evolve during the decomposition of plants with a high nitrate content, as in silo filler's disease. The color of the gas varies according to the exact species, but it may be clear, orange-brown, or red. Symptoms usually occur immediately after inhalation. Any portion of the respiratory tract may be involved, but frequently, only lower airway effects are noted. Pulmonary edema may be delayed for 12 hours. Asthma may develop immediately or over the first few days and may be severe, even in the nonasthmatic patient. After resolution of a moderately severe, acute reaction, relapse may occur 3 weeks later and can be more serious than the original episode.

Phosgene (carbonyl chloride, $COCl_2$) is a classic inducer of delayed pulmonary edema.[8] The main chemical warfare agent used in World War I, it is used in various chemical processes (drug, dye, insecticide, and isocyanate manufacturing). It is most frequently encountered in situations of combustion or pyrolysis when carbon, oxygen, and chlorine are available to react (e.g., burning plastics, chlorinated hydrocarbons, or carbons along with hydrochloric acid vapors). A haylike, musty odor may be noted.

Formaldehyde is a reactant or by-product in many chemical processes, such as embalming, cosmetic and resin manufacture, and sterilizing. It may evolve spontaneously from plastics, resins, insulation material, and many other occult sources.[13,15] Formaldehyde has been noted to be a carcinogen in limited rodent studies and is suspected as a human carcinogen, although no confirmatory human studies have been completed.

Inorganic acids cause immediate irritation or corrosion of tissues, depending on the concentration and the agent. Sulfuric acid is also a desiccating agent, and chromic acid is a strong oxidizer. Although most acids do not cause systemic poisoning, chromates are hepatotoxic and nephrotoxic, and hydrofluoric acid (or hydrogen fluoride) may cause systemic fluoride poisoning. Acid vapor inhalation usually causes upper airway irritation with ocular and nasopharyngeal inflammation. If the acid forms a mist, deeper pulmonary penetration may occur, resulting in pulmonary edema, bronchiolitis obliterans, or asthma.

Chlorine is a heavier-than-air, water-soluble, yellow-green gas that is irritating to the mucous membranes.[6] The warning properties of chlorine are usually adequate to alert the person to the presence of the material and afford time for escape. However, when a person is caught in a confined space or an overwhelming cloud, inhalation may cause irritation of the lower airways. Chlorine is used in many chemical industries and processes (e.g., sanitation of water) and can be generated by the action of an acid on hypochlorite, as found in bleaches. For example, the inappropriate mixing of bleach with an acid-based cleanser can generate chlorine during the cleaning of toilet bowls.[14] Mixing hypochlorite with ammonia-based cleaners can produce chloramine, another gaseous irritant.[10]

Ammonia is highly water soluble and very irritating to the upper airways.[5] In solution as ammonium hydroxide, its vapors can produce an immediate reaction. Although the odor of ammonia provides excellent warning of its presence, sudden overwhelming exposures, large clouds of the gas, or confined-space exposures can cause severe corrosive burns to the skin or eyes (with potential blindness). The oropharynx is readily burned, and hoarseness is common. Deeper injury to the lung can cause severe pulmonary dysfunction that is usually transient but can be permanent. The effects are rapid; "delayed" effects are usually the result of the progression of burns to the mucous membranes. Ammonia is used in various chemical processes, such as cleaning, fertilization, and refrigeration, and evolves during the combustion of a number of products.

Hydrocarbons comprise a wide variety of compounds. Although the irritancy of these gases or vapors cannot easily be generalized, the ketones, aldehydes, acid anhydrides, and halogenated compounds are most irritating. Aromatic compounds (e.g., benzene, xylene, and toluene) are more irritating than aliphatic ones (pentane, hexane, and butane). In addition, hydrocarbons are often systemic poisons, with central nervous system (CNS) effects predominating.

Epoxy resins, catalysts, and hardeners frequently produce vapors that can cause irritation or allergic sensitization of the airways. Styrene is used in the manufacture of boats, bathtubs, and many other products (polystyrene).

Pulmonary Irritants with Systemic Toxicity

Gases and vapors may gain entry to the body through the lungs and may inflict serious injury on a target organ remote from the portal of entry. The internal dose depends on such factors as the solubility of the gas, blood flow through the lungs (more important with materials with low blood solubility), gas distribution in the lungs, and ventilatory rate (as affected by activity). Delivery to the target organ depends on similar factors, including tissue perfusion, tissue penetration (especially lipid solubility for the liver, brain, and other organs), binding materials in the blood, and pH. Uptake into a temporary depot may occur, allowing the chemical to be redistributed to the target organ over a more protracted period (seen with highly fat soluble materials).

Arsine (AsH_3, arsenic trihydride) may be generated when arsenic-bearing materials come in contact with acids (e.g., during the processing of metals in which arsenic may be a natural contaminant, in sewer gases, and in laboratories).[9] Arsine gas is also commonly used in the manufacture of computer chips. It has a garlic odor. In addition to its irritant effects, inhalation of arsine in high doses can cause immediate death from CNS toxicity. Classically, however, arsine combines with hemoglobin, causing intravascular hemolysis. Onset is usually rapid but may be delayed. Symptoms include nausea, vomiting, abdominal pain, fatigue, and weakness. The hematocrit may drop by 50% in a matter of minutes. Examination may reveal brownish skin, hepatosplenomegaly, tachycardia, tachypnea, and dark urine. Renal failure may ensue from the effects of the free plasma hemoglobin, the sludging of red cells, and the direct effects of the arsine–hemoglobin complex on the renal cells. Anemia may result in secondary ischemic complications such as congestive heart failure. Systemic toxicity due to inorganic arsenic poisoning may ensue (see Chapter 318). The urine arsenic level may confirm exposure but is usually unavailable.

Ethylene oxide is a colorless gas with an indistinct odor or taste.[7] Manufactured by Union Carbide, it is called Oxirane. For gas sterilization, it is frequently supplied with a halogenated hydrocarbon in a nonflammable 12:88 mixture, but, at higher concentrations, it is flammable. In addition to mucosal irritation, ethylene oxide may cause CNS depression, seizures, skin and pulmonary burns, allergic reactions, and mild chemical hepatitis with transient lymphocytosis after acute exposure. It can also cause peripheral neuropathies, is a suspected human carcinogen, and is considered a reproductive hazard. It is used in many chemical industries and in hospitals (e.g., gas sterilization of products that cannot be steam-autoclaved).

Phosphine gas (PH_3, phosphorous trihydride) is used in fumigation (of grains), in silos and ship holds, in the electronics industry, and in the production of acetylene.[20] Phosphine can cause severe gastrointestinal (GI) and CNS toxicity, as well as immediate or delayed pulmonary edema. Symptoms are usually mild: headache, nausea, chest tightness, and lethargy. Coma, seizures, and shock may be seen in severe cases. Although there is no specific biologic test for exposure, a fishy or garlic odor may suggest the presence of zinc or aluminum phosphide and phosphine, respectively.

Methyl bromide is used as a fumigant.[12] When pumped into tented structures, the concentrations of gas are usually lethal. Intractable seizures, coma, and severe neurologic sequelae can result from exposure to this material. Severe acidosis may occur, presumably secondary to seizure activity. Mild exposure results in a flulike syndrome that is often delayed in onset. For fumigation, chloropicrin is usually added to methyl bromide to provide olfactory warning of its presence. Serum bromide levels above 5 mg/dL are probably consistent with exposure. If a lumbar puncture is performed to evaluate seizures or coma, determination of the bromide level in the cerebrospinal fluid may also be useful.

Sulfuryl fluoride, marketed as Vikane, is a fumigant that is primarily an irritant, although recent reports have suggested systemic toxicity.[3]

Ethylene dibromide was commonly used as a fumigant for soil, fruit, and other foods before 1984. Deaths have occurred after high-level exposure to this chemical as the result of combined dermal and inhalation absorption. Although symptoms are mainly limited to the respiratory and GI tracts, severe illness with acidosis and renal failure has been reported.[16] Because of its potential carcinogenicity, its use is now restricted.

DIFFERENTIAL DIAGNOSIS

Respiratory symptoms after irritant gas exposure are nonspecific. Similar findings may be caused by allergic and infectious etiologies. Although the onset is usually acute with toxic gas exposure, it may be delayed. In addition, a low-grade fever and leukocytosis may be present in patients with pneumonitis. Irritant-induced pulmonary edema is almost always noncardiogenic, as is that caused by severe narcotic and sedative–hypnotic poisoning. Bronchospasm may result from an exacerbation of asthma or chronic obstructive pulmonary disease due to other or unknown factors. Only a careful exposure (environmental or occupational) history will identify the correct cause.

EMERGENCY DEPARTMENT EVALUATION

The history includes medical history, previous exposures, and details of the presenting illness, such as the nature, progression, and severity of symptoms and antecedent activities. The physical examination is directed, but not limited, to the skin, eyes, nose, mouth, and chest. Depending on clinical findings, spirometry, response to bronchodilator inhalation, arterial blood gas analysis, chest radiography, D_{LCO}, and ventilation–perfusion scanning may be necessary to assess the nature and severity of signs and symptoms. Laboratory evaluation may be necessary with poisoning by systemic toxins (e.g., arsine and methyl bromide), as noted previously. Patients with respiratory distress should have an electrocardiogram.

EMERGENCY DEPARTMENT MANAGEMENT

Removal from the exposure, decontamination, and supportive care are the mainstays of prehospital treatment. A rescuer should never enter an area in which an irritant gas is potentially present without adequate skin, eye, and respiratory protection. Along with provision of supplemental oxygen, thorough flushing of irritated surfaces (skin and eyes) with water (preferably saline) may be required. Eye irrigation is especially important with acid fume, ammonia, chlorine, and tear gas exposure.

Respiratory therapy should include humidified oxygen, bronchodilators, and mechanical measures (intubation, ventilation, continuous positive airway pressure, positive end-expiratory pressure, and suctioning), as clinically indicated for bronchospasm or pulmonary edema. A course of high-dose steroids to reduce inflammation is theoretically beneficial and should be considered in patients with moderate, severe, or progressive symptoms. Data from animal experiments suggest that inhaled steroids decrease pulmonary vascular resistance and improve lung compliance and survival.

With arsine-induced hemolysis, exchange transfusion may be necessary when the resulting anemia is severe and free hemoglobin levels are high (greater than 1.5 g/dL). Chelation therapy may also be indicated if urine arsenic levels are elevated (see Chapter 318).

Other standard supportive therapies may be indicated for coexisting toxicity, such as anticonvulsant therapy for seizures and dialysis for renal failure.

DISPOSITION

The decision to admit or discharge depends primarily on the severity and progression of clinical and laboratory manifestations. Young, otherwise healthy patients who become asymptomatic or mildly symptomatic after 4 hours of emergency department observation and treatment may be discharged. Those with moderate, severe, or worsening symptoms or abnormal spirometry, arterial blood gas analysis, or chest radiograph should be admitted, especially if they are elderly or have underlying cardiac, respiratory, or other significant medical problems. If delayed toxicity is possible, patients who have persistent symptoms of any degree of severity should be admitted. Asymptomatic patients who are discharged should be instructed to return at the first sign of respiratory symptoms or systemic illness. If the physician is unfamiliar with the toxicity of a certain agent and its treatment, a poison center, toxicologist, or toxicology text should be consulted.

COMMON PITFALLS

- Failure to take an environmental or occupational exposure history
- Failure to recognize that a toxic exposure has occurred
- Failure to evaluate for systemic poisoning after irritant gas exposure
- Failure to use adequate protective equipment (in prehospital treatment) so that additional casualties are avoided
- Failure to obtain additional information and advice when unfamiliar with the toxicity of a particular gas and its management
- Failure to instruct discharged patients to return immediately if delayed symptoms develop or mild symptoms worsen; such instructions should be documented.

References

1. Beswick FW. Chemical agents used in riot control and warfare. *Hum Toxicol* 1983;2:247.
2. Brugsch HG, Elkins HB. Toluene diisocyanate (TDI) toxicity. *N Engl J Med* 1963;268:353.
3. Centers for Disease Control. Fatalities resulting from sulfuryl fluoride exposure after home fumigation. *MMWR* 1987;36:602.
4. Charan NB, Myers CG, Lakshminarayan S, et al. Pulmonary injuries associated with sulfur dioxide inhalation. *Am Rev Respir Dis* 1979;119:555.
5. Close GL, Cattin FI, Cohn AM. Acute and chronic effects of ammonia burns of the respiratory tract. *Arch Otolaryngol* 1980;106:151.
6. Das R, Blanc PD. Chlorine gas exposure and the lung: a review. *Toxicol Indust Health* 1993;9:439.
7. Deschamps D, Rosenberg N, Soler P, et al. Persistent asthma after accidental exposure to ethylene oxide. *Br J Indust Med* 1992;49:523.
8. Diller WF. Medical phosgene problems and their possible solution. *J Occup Med* 1975;20:189.
9. Fowler BA, Weissberg JB. Arsine poisoning. *N Engl J Med* 1974;291:1171.
10. Gapany-Gapanavicius M, Molko M, Tirosh M. Chloramine-induced pneumonitis from mixing household cleaning agents. *BMJ* 1982;285:1086.
11. Gordon T, Amdur MO. Responses of the respiratory system to toxic agents. In: *Casarett and Doull's toxicology: the basic science of poisons*, 4th ed. New York: Pergamon, 1991:339.
12. Greenberg JO. The neurological effects of methyl bromide poisoning. *Indust Med* 1977;27:959.
13. Harris JC, Rumack BH, Alrich FD. Toxicology of urea formaldehyde and polyurethane foam insulation. *JAMA* 1981;245:243.
14. Jones FL. Chlorine poisoning from mixing household cleaners. *JAMA* 1972;222:1312.

15. L'abbe KA, Hoey JR. Review of the health effects of urea formaldehyde foam insulation. *Environ Res* 1984;35:246.
16. Letz GA, Pond SM, Osterloh JD, et al. Two fatalities after occupational exposure to ethylene dibromide. *JAMA* 1984;252:2428.
17. Nasr ANH. Ozone poisoning in man: clinical manifestations and differential diagnosis. *Clin Toxicol* 1971;14:461.
18. Tse RL, Bockman AD. Nitrogen dioxide toxicity: report of four cases in firemen. *JAMA* 1970;212:1341.
19. Vandenplas O, Malo JL, Saetta M, et al. Occupational asthma and extrinsic alveolitis due to isocyanates: current status and perspectives. *Br J Indust Med* 1993;50:213.
20. Wilson R, Lovejoy FH, Jaeger RJ, et al. Acute phosphine poisoning aboard a grain freighter. *JAMA* 1980;244:148.

CHAPTER 347
Isoniazid Poisoning

Alan D. Woolf

Isoniazid (isonicotinic acid hydrazide, INH), a derivative of vitamin B_3 (nicotinamide), has been used for the prophylaxis and treatment of tuberculosis since 1952. With the resurgence of tuberculosis in the 1990s has come an increasing incidence also in isoniazid poisoning.[15] There were 480 isoniazid poisonings and one isoniazid-related death reported by the American Association of Poison Control Centers in 1997.[13] The incidence of self-poisoning is greatest among those adult populations with a high prevalence of both tuberculosis and depression (e.g., Native Americans, immigrant populations).[2,16]

INH is rapidly absorbed from the small intestine within 30 to 60 minutes after ingestion. Therapeutic doses are 5 to 10 mg/kg (maximum, 300 mg) daily, given orally or by intramuscular injection.[1] Peak INH serum levels (therapeutic range, 5 to 8 μg/mL) are reached within 1 to 2 hours.[19] The drug is minimally bound to plasma proteins and has a small apparent volume of distribution (0.6 L/kg).[19] INH can be detected in such diverse bodily fluids as saliva, cerebrospinal fluid (CSF), and breast milk. Up to 36% of the drug may be excreted unchanged in urine.[11] Metabolism by acetylation in the liver yields inactive metabolites that are predominantly excreted in the urine. People with normal renal function excrete 50% to 80% of a therapeutic dose of INH within 24 hours.[3]

There is great genetic variability in the metabolism of INH. Between 45% and 75% of Caucasians are "slow acetylators" and have a mean serum INH half-life of about 5 hours. By contrast, 95% of Inuit are "fast acetylators" and have an average serum half-life of 80 minutes.[12] These differences are therapeutically important: Slow acetylators can achieve sustained bactericidal drug levels on every-other-day dosage regimens, whereas fast acetylators may have inadequate levels unless they receive the drug daily.[11]

Various mechanisms are responsible for the toxic effects of INH. In acute overdoses, INH decreases the conversion of glutamic acid to gamma-aminobutyric acid (GABA) by inhibiting the pyridoxal phosphate–dependent enzyme glutamic acid decarboxylase. Because GABA is an inhibitory neurotransmitter, seizures may ensue.[20] With chronic therapy, INH hydrazone analogues, which arise spontaneously *in vivo* (especially in slow acetylators), form rapidly excreted complexes with pyridoxine and also inhibit pyridoxine kinase, thereby decreasing the conversion of pyridoxine to its active cofactor form, pyridoxal phosphate.

INH is structurally similar to nicotinic acid and may substitute for it in the synthesis of nicotinamide adenine dinucleotide (NAD), producing an inactive coenzyme. Inhibition of NAD-dependent Krebs cycle enzymes may result in hyperglycemia, and inhibition of NAD-mediated conversion of lactate to pyruvate may contribute to the profound lactic acidosis that typically accompanies seizures.

Patients who are malnourished, pregnant, alcoholic, elderly, diabetic, or uremic may be at particularly high risk for pyridoxine deficiency during chronic INH therapy.[14] In the absence of supplemental doses of pyridoxine (e.g., 10 mg/d), pyridoxine deficiency may develop and lead to peripheral neuropathies, anemia, and a lowered seizure threshold. Pyridoxine depletion can also inhibit the activity of pyridoxine-dependent decarboxylases and transaminases (leading to decreased catecholamine synthesis), cytochrome P-450 enzymes (leading to decreased drug metabolism), histaminase, and monoamine oxidase (see Chapter 354).

CLINICAL PRESENTATION

Seizures may be seen after acute overdoses of INH as low as 35 mg/kg in adults. Severe toxicity has been noted with ingestions of 5 to 7 g (80 to 150 mg/kg); death has resulted after the ingestion of as little as 3 g.[17] Although ingestions of more than 12 g in an adult have a high fatality rate, survival has been reported after the ingestion of as much as 25 g.[18] Poisoning is associated with an INH serum concentration above 30 μg/mL, although such laboratory assays for INH are not routinely available.

The initial symptoms of acute poisoning, which may occur as soon as 30 to 120 minutes after ingestion, include nausea, vomiting, slurred speech, blurred vision, and disorientation. Anticholinergic signs (e.g., mydriasis, tachycardia, and urinary retention) and hyperreflexia or areflexia may also be prominent. In severe poisonings, seizures appear abruptly and precede the development of a profound metabolic acidosis and coma, the triad of which forms the classic clinical picture. An arterial pH as low as 6.49 was recorded in an adolescent who survived INH poisoning with no sequelae.[10]

Multiple seizures over a short time period are the hallmark of INH poisoning. Other symptoms and signs of acute poisoning include confusion or hallucinations, garbled speech, hyperpyrexia, and respiratory depression. Laboratory findings include lactic acidosis, ketosis, hyperglycemia, an increased anion gap, hyperkalemia, peripheral blood leukocytosis, CSF pleocytosis, and renal defects (e.g., glycosuria, albuminuria, and oliguria). An elevated creatine phosphokinase due to rhabdomyolysis may precede myoglobinuria and renal failure. An electroencephalogram (EEG) often demonstrates diffuse slowing or paroxysmal electrical activity compatible with subclinical seizures. A chest radiograph may reveal aspiration pneumonia.

The clinical course of the untreated patient with a massive INH overdose is often unremitting seizures, resulting in death from acidosis and cardiovascular and respiratory collapse. Hepatic damage, manifested by elevated liver enzyme levels, has been documented in as many as 20.7 of 1,000 patients treated chronically with INH.[4] Although such hepatotoxicity appears transient in most cases, even with continued use of the drug, rarely do patients go on to develop acute liver necrosis, liver failure, and death.[4,8]

Toxic effects of chronic INH use also include euphoria, tinnitus, ataxia, impaired memory, encephalopathy, and optic neuritis. Allergic manifestations, such as rashes, eosinophilia, vasculitis, arthralgias, and a positive antinuclear antibody test, have also been described.[9] Progressive lethargy, garbled speech, confusion, and coma were described in a man who mistakenly treated his tuberculosis with 1,200 mg of INH daily for 6 weeks.[14]

Patients with underlying impaired renal function or hepatic disease do not metabolize INH well, have a prolonged serum half-life, and are at greater risk for intoxication. Those with a preexisting seizure disorder are at higher risk for neurotoxic effects.

DIFFERENTIAL DIAGNOSIS

Agents that can cause a clinical picture similar to that of INH overdose include salicylates, cyanide, carbon monoxide, other hydrazines, monomethylhydrazine-containing mushrooms, anticholinergics, and sympathomimetics. Neurotoxins such as pesticides, camphor, lead, narcotics, strychnine, and tricyclic antidepressants must also be ruled out.[5] Other medical conditions, such as meningitis with sepsis, diabetic ketoacidosis, uremia, meningoencephalitis, and head trauma, should also be considered in the differential of patients presenting with seizures, coma, and acidosis.[5,7]

EMERGENCY DEPARTMENT EVALUATION

INH overdose should be strongly considered in the patient who presents with seizures refractory to conventional anticonvulsants and an evolving metabolic acidosis, especially within the context of a history of a psychiatric condition (i.e., depression) and tuberculosis, with access to INH.

The physical examination focuses on vital signs and the neurologic status, including an accurate scoring of the patient's alertness. The patient is carefully evaluated for hyperreflexia, focal neurologic deficits, abnormal thought processes, and lethargy.

Laboratory tests include determination of serum electrolytes, glucose, bicarbonate levels and an arterial pH and gases. A toxicology screen of blood and urine should also be obtained. In severe or chronic cases, baseline tests of kidney and liver function are important. A chest radiograph can diagnose aspiration, and electrocardiographic monitoring is routine. An EEG may reveal diffuse slowing or seizure activity.

EMERGENCY DEPARTMENT MANAGEMENT

Advanced life-support measures should be instituted for victims of severe INH overdose, as necessary. A diagnostic clue to INH poisoning is the prompt termination of seizure activity after the administration of intravenous pyridoxine. Pyridoxine (vitamin B_6) is the specific antidote; it should be given in gram-for-gram equivalency to the estimated total amount of INH ingested.[15,18] If the total ingested dose of INH is unknown, 5 g of pyridoxine can be given empirically by slow intravenous push and repeated in 20 minutes if there is no clinical response. Typically, the seizures abate and the patient's level of consciousness slowly improves. Diazepam (5 to 10 mg intravenously) may be used as an adjunct to control seizures. Additional pyridoxine is sometimes necessary for the resolution of INH-induced coma.

Although severe metabolic acidosis should be treated with intravenous sodium bicarbonate, large doses are usually unnecessary, because the acidosis is secondary to seizures and resolves shortly after seizures have been controlled.[6,17] Diuresis is not of proven benefit in INH overdose. The use of adequate doses of diazepam and pyridoxine has essentially eliminated the need for barbiturates, paralyzing agents, anesthesia, dialysis, or exchange transfusion in the management of INH overdose. Chronic pyridoxine overdosing can cause a peripheral sensory neuropathy. Multiple large doses should be avoided because of pyridoxine's neurotoxic potential; only gram-for-gram replacement is recommended in INH poisoning.

After stabilization, instillation of activated charcoal into the gut should be done in all acute overdose patients to prevent further absorption of INH or other coingestants.

DISPOSITION

Asymptomatic or mildly symptomatic patients can be observed in the emergency department for 6 hours. A toxicologist or poison center should be consulted if the physician is unfamiliar with the management of INH poisoning. Such consultants can be helpful in assessing the patient with seizures and acidosis of unknown cause and in locating supplies of pyridoxine.

Moderately or severely symptomatic patients should be admitted to an intensive care unit. Patients with refractory seizures, severe respiratory depression, or renal failure should be transferred to a hospital with intensive care capabilities if they are not locally available.

COMMON PITFALLS

- Failure to appreciate that asymptomatic patients may rapidly deteriorate
- Using syrup of ipecac in patients who may develop seizures and coma while vomiting
- Failure to consider isoniazid poisoning in patients with metabolic acidosis and seizures refractory to conventional anticonvulsants, particularly in patients who are Native Americans or recent immigrants
- Failure to give pyridoxine at the first sign of toxicity
- Giving excessive doses of sodium bicarbonate for the treatment of metabolic acidosis, which spontaneously resolves when convulsions cease

References

1. American Tuberculosis Society. Position statement: treatment of tuberculosis and other mycobacterial diseases. *Am Rev Respir Dis* 1983;127:790.
2. Blanchard P, Yao J, McAlpine D, et al. Isoniazid overdose in the Cambodian population of Olmstead County, Minnesota. *JAMA* 1986;256:3131.
3. Bowersox DW, Winterbauer RH, Stewart GL, et al. Isoniazid dosage in patients with renal failure. *N Engl J Med* 1973;289:84.
4. Centers for Disease Control. Severe isoniazid-associated hepatitis—New York, 1991 to 1993. *MMWR* 1993;42:545.
5. Chang YD, Yang CC, Lin TJ, et al. Acute isoniazid intoxication: a case report. *Chin Med J (Taipei)* 1996;57:152.
6. Chin L, Sievers M, Herrier R, et al. Convulsions as the etiology of lactic acidosis in acute isoniazid toxicity in dogs. *Toxicol Appl Pharmacol* 1979;49:377.
7. Ehsan T, Malkoff MD. Acute isoniazid poisoning simulating meningoencephalitis. *Neurology* 1995;45:1627.
8. Gal A, Klatt E. Fatal isoniazid hepatitis in a child. *Pediatr Infect Dis* 1986;5:490.
9. Goldman A, Braman S. Isoniazid: review with emphasis on adverse effects. *Chest* 1972;62:71.
10. Hankins DG, Saxena K, Faville RJ, et al. Profound acidosis caused by isoniazid ingestion. *Am J Emerg Med* 1987;5:165.
11. Hughes H, Schmidt L, Biehl J. The metabolism of isoniazid: its implications in therapeutic use. *Transactions of the 14th Conference on the Chemotherapy of Tuberculosis*. Washington, DC: Virginia Department of Medicine and Surgery, 1976:276.
12. Jeanes C, Schaefer O, Eidus L. Inactivation of isoniazid by Canadian Eskimos and Indians. *Can Med Assoc J* 1972;106:331.
13. Litovitz TL, Klein-Schwartz W, Dyer KS, et al. 1997 annual report of the American Association of Poison Control Centers Toxic Exposure Surveillance System. *Am J Emerg Med* 1998;16:443.
14. Salkind AR, Hewitt CC. Coma from long-term overingestion of isoniazid. *Arch Intern Med* 1997;157:2518.
15. Shah BR, Santucci K, Sinert R, et al. Acute isoniazid neurotoxicity in an urban

hospital. *Pediatrics* 1995;95:700.
16. Sievers M, Cynamon M, Bittker T. Intentional isoniazid overdosage among Southwestern American Indians. *Am J Psychiatry* 1975;132:662.
17. Terman D, Teitelbaum D. Isoniazid self-poisoning. *Neurology* 1970;20:299.
18. Wason S, Lacouture P, Lovejoy F. Single high-dose pyridoxine treatment for isoniazid overdose. *JAMA* 1981;246:1102.
19. Weber W, Hein D. Clinical pharmacokinetics of isoniazid. *Clin Pharmacokinet* 1979;4:401.
20. Wood J, Peesker S. A correlation between changes in GABA metabolism and isonicotinic acid hydrazide-induced seizures. *Brain Res* 1972;45:489.

CHAPTER 348
Lead Poisoning

Steven M. Marcus

Lead is a heavy metal that exists in elemental, inorganic, and organic forms and as a contaminant of other metals. More than 900 hobbies and occupations involve contact with lead, such as metal extracting and refining, plumbing, pottery production, soldering, and painting. Children develop lead poisoning by eating chips of paint from surfaces painted with lead-based pigments or by ingesting dust, which contains lead. Data suggest that lead-contaminated house dust is, currently, the major source of lead exposure for children living in the United States. The potential for developing lead poisoning from the leaching of lead from imported lead-glazed cookware, dinnerware, and glassware and from the use of folk remedies such as azarcon, "pay-loo-ah," and maha yogran guggula by Mexican, Hmong, and Asian Indian immigrants, respectively, has received much publicity.[6,13]

Lead is principally absorbed through the gastrointestinal (GI) tract and the lungs. Although there is minimal or no absorption through the skin, absorption of lead from bullets lodged in joints (synovial fluid) or the spinal cord (cerebrospinal fluid) has been reported.[8] The degree of absorption depends on the particle size and concentration. Lead has a melting point of 327°C and a vapor pressure of 1.77 mmHg at 1,000°C. Thus, lead becomes volatilized and airborne at relatively low temperatures. Gaseous lead and particulate lead with a diameter of less than 5 μm are nearly completely absorbed through pulmonary alveoli. Inhaled lead dust particles of larger size are usually trapped by cilia or in the tracheobronchial mucus and are cleared without being absorbed.

The absorption of ingested lead depends on factors such as the concentration, coincidental or previously ingested food, the status of the metal transfer protein, and age.[7,11] In laboratory animals and humans, the younger the age, the greater the percentage of absorption of ingested lead. Iron and calcium deficiencies appear to promote absorption of lead, as does the coincidental ingestion of high-fat, low-protein, and low-phosphate meals. Unabsorbed lead is excreted in the stool.

Once absorbed, lead is principally carried on the red blood cell membrane, distributed to all parts of the body, and stored in bones. The calculated volume of distribution is quite high.[17] The average blood lead level in United States residents is currently less than 4 μg/dL.[5] Lead is not required for normal body function, nor is it metabolized. Lead is primarily eliminated by urinary excretion, with a small proportion excreted in bile and eliminated with stool. The total body elimination half-life of lead is greater than 18 months.

Lead is a protean poison that affects sulfhydryl-containing enzyme systems throughout the body—virtually all enzymes and organ systems are affected. Chief among the enzyme systems affected are those that involve heme synthesis. Inhibition of δ-aminolevulinic acid dehydratase levels has been associated with central nervous system symptoms. Interference with ferrochelatase, the enzyme that promotes the incorporation of iron into protoporphyrin to produce heme, results in elevated free protoporphyrin levels.

Acute lead poisoning occasionally occurs from exposure to high concentrations of organic lead (e.g., tetraethyl lead). Although symptoms may suggest acute intoxication, poisoning from metallic and inorganic lead is usually due to chronic or subacute exposure, and the insidious onset of symptoms before presentation can be elicited by taking a careful history.

It is extremely important to have an index of suspicion for the presence of chronic lead poisoning. Chronic lead exposure has been associated with abnormality of semen quality, sperm morphology and physiology, hearing deficits, defects in reaction time (specifically the central component [decision slowing]), decreased numbers of CD16+ cells, chronic nephropathies associated with hypertension,[10,18] gout, Fanconi syndrome (years after treatment with chelators), and a possible association with various cancers.

CLINICAL PRESENTATION

Patients with lead poisoning frequently present with headache, fatigue, malaise, abdominal pain, constipation, and vomiting. The abdominal pain is usually colicky and not responsive to standard analgesics. There may be complaints of peripheral paresthesias or hypoesthesias and occasional frank neurologic symptoms (e.g., wrist or ankle drop). Muscle weakness may also be noted. Depression and other affective disorders have been reported in lead-poisoned adults.[1] Hyperactivity, delayed development, or loss of recently acquired skills may be seen in children.[11,14] In severe cases, coma and seizures may be noted.

Physical examination is generally unrevealing, although the blood pressure may be elevated. Occasionally, in adults with poor dental care, a dark bluish-black discoloration of the gingiva at the dental border (lead lines) may be present. This finding is seldom present in children and in those with good dental hygiene. If increased intracranial pressure accompanies lead encephalopathy, examination of the optic fundi may show papilledema. Cardiac dysrhythmias such as premature ventricular contractions have been reported.

An abdominal radiograph may reveal radiopaque foreign bodies in patients with pica or accidental lead ingestion. Long-bone radiographs may show an increased density of metaphyseal lines due to disordered calcium deposition. This finding is seldom present in adults.

The laboratory evaluation usually reveals a hypochromic microcytic anemia. Lead may produce a nonautoimmune hemolytic anemia with increased red cell fragility and an elevated reticulocyte count. Basophilic stippling and eosinophilia are less often noted. Proteinuria, glycosuria, a Fanconi syndrome (with aminoaciduria and renal tubular acidosis), and increased blood urea nitrogen and creatinine levels may be seen in patients with lead nephropathy. Because lead reduces the excretion of uric acid, patients with lead toxicity are prone to develop gout.

The definitive diagnosis of lead poisoning depends on the measurement of whole-blood lead and free erythrocyte protoporphyrin (FEP). The former indicates exposure and the latter is evidence of poisoning, because it is the result of lead's effect on ferrochelatase. Lead levels as low as 5 μg/dL have been reported to produce biochemical abnormalities, and levels between 10 and 20 μg/dL may be associated with clinical pathology (e.g., decreased intelligence and neurobehavioral problems in children).[5] Lead levels above 10 μg/dL in children are currently considered to be evidence of increased lead absorption, and lead levels above 40 μg/dL in adults are considered evidence of lead poisoning serious enough to warrant intervention. FEP levels above 15 μg/dL are uncommon in healthy people. Although FEP levels over 20 μg/dL may be seen with either iron deficiency or lead poisoning, FEP levels above 35 μg/dL usually indicate lead poisoning.[16]

DIFFERENTIAL DIAGNOSIS

Lead poisoning shares symptomatology with other heavy metal poisonings. Unlike poisoning with arsenic, however, the peripheral neuropathy from lead is associated with decreased sensitivity; with arsenic, there are painful paresthesias. Unlike in thallium poisoning, there is no hair loss. Both lead and mercury poisoning are characterized by personality changes. Mercury intoxication is characterized by erythrism and rapid changes in affect, with outbursts of anger alternating with happiness. Lead poisoning is usually accompanied by depressive disorders. Urinary heavy metal analysis may be necessary for differentiation.

EMERGENCY DEPARTMENT EVALUATION

Patients who present to the emergency department with multisystem complaints, particularly chronic abdominal symptoms that have not responded to standard conservative therapy, should be suspected of having lead poisoning. The patient's occupation, hobbies, or living conditions may suggest exposure to lead. The physician should ask about subtle changes in bowel habits, behavior, mood, and cognitive function, as well as headaches, weakness, and paresthesias.

In addition to vital signs and a general examination, a detailed neurologic examination should be performed. The physician should specifically check for papilledema and gingival pigmentation. If recent lead ingestion is suspected, an abdominal radiograph may be helpful. Long-bone radiographs (knee and wrist) may suggest chronic lead exposure. The laboratory evaluation should include a complete blood count, whole-blood lead and FEP levels, serum blood urea nitrogen and creatinine levels, and a urinalysis.

Elevated blood lead levels should usually be confirmed before initiating treatment. Asymptomatic patients with mildly elevated lead levels (20 to 44 μg/dL in children, 40 to 80 μg/dL in adults) may be evaluated with the calcium disodium EDTA lead mobilization test (discussion follows).[15]

EMERGENCY DEPARTMENT MANAGEMENT

Cerebral edema should be treated by hyperventilation, elevation of the head, and restriction of fluids. Seizures should be controlled with pharmacologic agents such as diazepam, barbiturates, and phenytoin. In patients with acute encephalopathy (with or without coma or seizures), chelation therapy should be initiated before obtaining confirmatory laboratory data, because the long-term outcome is related to the length of time the vital organs are exposed to elevated lead levels. GI decontamination should be performed if there is radiopaque material in the intestine, but decontamination should *not* delay definitive chelation therapy.

Chelation therapy is usually indicated for children with lead levels above 44 μg/dL, for adults with levels above 80 μg/dL, and for patients with lower levels who have a positive lead mobilization test or evidence of lead-associated symptoms or signs (discussion follows). Dimercaprol (British antilewisite [BAL]) crosses the blood–brain barrier and forms a tight bond with lead; in patients with lead encephalopathy, it is the initial therapy of choice. An oil-based solution of dimercaprol is given intramuscularly in a usual dose of 3 to 5 mg/kg every 4 to 6 hours. Dimercaprol is painful when injected and foul-smelling, and it may produce adverse local and systemic reactions. Sterile abscesses may occur at the site of dimercaprol injection, and febrile responses are not unusual. Many patients complain of a terrible taste in their mouths and of lightheadedness.

EDTA is water soluble and can be given intramuscularly or intravenously. The lead–EDTA bond is very strong and stable at a physiologic pH. However, in acid urine, the bond is less stable, and there is the potential for release of free lead into the renal tubule and subsequent renal tubular damage. The main side effects of EDTA are phlebitis (with concentrations of greater than 0.5 mg/mL) and potential renal toxicity. Because intramuscular injections are extremely irritating and produce elevations of creatine phosphokinase, intravenous administration is preferred.[19] If the intramuscular route is used, procaine or lidocaine is usually added to produce an 0.5% concentration of the local anesthetic.

EDTA is given in a dose of 50 mg/kg/d. Intravenous EDTA is given as a continuous drip. At a concentration of 0.5 mg/mL, an enormous amount of fluid must be infused. However, if the patient can tolerate the fluid load, the incidence of side effects, particularly renal dysfunction, may be decreased. Intramuscular EDTA is given in divided doses every 4 to 24 hours. Because the use of EDTA alone may liberate carcass lead and transiently raise brain lead levels and increase symptoms,[2,3] it may be advisable to start with a dose of dimercaprol in all symptomatic patients and those with high blood lead levels (greater than 55 μg/dL in children and 100 mg/dL in adults).

The dose of EDTA for a diagnostic lead mobilization test is 1 g for adults and 25 mg/kg in children, infused over 1 to 2 hours with 250 to 1,000 mL of normal saline solution. The bladder is initially emptied, fluid intake is encouraged, and the urine is collected for 24 hours (3 days in patients with abnormal renal function) and analyzed for its lead content. If the amount of lead excreted (in micrograms) exceeds the amount of EDTA given (in milligrams), therapeutic chelation therapy may be indicated. In children, the challenge dose of EDTA can be given intramuscularly and the urine collected for 8 hours. With this regimen, chelation therapy is indicated if the urinary lead excretion (in micrograms) exceeds 60% of the dose of EDTA (in milligrams).

Two oral chelators are available. Only succimer (Chemet), or dimercaptosuccinic acid (succimer), is currently approved for use by the Food and Drug Administration. It is indicated for children with lead levels above 45 μg/dL and is as effective in clearing lead as the combination of dimercaprol and EDTA.[4] The side-effect spectrum is minimal, with a small incidence of skin rash, transaminase elevations, and GI discomfort.[12] Although not officially licensed for use in adults, its effectiveness, combined with its low order of toxicity, argues for its use in this population.[9] The published dosage in children may be used safely in adults—10 mg/kg/dose every 8 hours for 5 days, followed by 10 mg/kg per dose every 12 hours for an additional 14 days. Patients should be monitored for toxicity with weekly blood counts, chemistry profiles, and urinalysis. The presence of ketones in the urine may be used as a measure of compliance, because it is a very common accompaniment of successful treatment. A mild rash or mild transaminitis is usually not a reason to abandon therapy, but requires closer observation, with more frequent laboratory investigation.

The other oral chelator, D-penicillamine, a derivative of penicillin, is given orally at a dosage of 30 mg/kg/d, with the average adult dose of about 1.0 to 1.5 g/d.[12,20] It is usually used only for adults with mild or no symptoms but high lead levels. Side effects include diarrhea, renal toxicity, leukopenia, and, occasionally, a rash. Penicillamine is less effective than dimercaprol or EDTA.

If renal toxicity develops as a result of antidotal therapy, fluid input should be increased in an attempt to dilute the lead content of the urine. Alkalinization of the urine may also be helpful.

Therapy should be continued until the lead level drops below 20 μg/dL in children and 40 μg/dL in adults. Maximum lead excretion occurs during the first 3 days of chelation therapy and falls off rapidly. After 5 days of therapy, it is unlikely that there will be further significant plumburesis without a rest period to allow lead to redistribute from tissue compartments to the blood. Hence, chelation therapy is usually limited to a 5-day course, followed by a treatment-free interval of 2 to 7 days. Additional courses of therapy are indicated if symptoms persist or blood lead levels remain elevated. Repeat lead levels and perhaps reinstitution of therapy, depending on the rebound in lead level, should be considered. Children with lead levels below 20 μg/dL and adults with levels below 40 μg/dL should be managed by preventing further exposure by environmental and educational interventions (see discussion in next section). Follow-up evaluation and periodic monitoring are required.

The vast majority of lead-poisoned patients survive. The final neurologic outcome may not be known for many weeks or months after treatment. Patients with cerebral edema have a poor prognosis.

DISPOSITION

All patients with evidence of encephalopathy should be admitted. Although chelation with EDTA, penicillamine, and succimer can be done on an outpatient basis, it is advisable to admit all patients who are symptomatic or who have markedly elevated lead levels (requiring dimercaprol therapy). However, because blood lead levels are not immediately available at the time of initial evaluation, patients who are not acutely ill can be discharged and admitted later if blood lead analysis or an EDTA mobilization test confirms the suspected diagnosis.

Further exposure to lead must be prevented. Environmental and occupational investigations should be performed to determine the most likely source of lead so that it can be eliminated. Involvement of the public health department, primarily in dealing with a child with lead poisoning, is imperative. The Occupational Safety and Health Administration may be helpful in investigating cases of occupational lead exposure. Many states also have active divisions of occupational and environmental health that may be helpful in the long-term treatment of patients.

Although chelation therapy is not difficult, some of the nuances are appreciated only after treating many patients. Hence, the physician unfamiliar with the evaluation and therapy of lead exposure and poisoning is advised to consult an experienced pharmacologist, toxicologist, or nephrologist.

All patients should be seen within 2 weeks of chelation therapy for repeat lead and FEP levels, because lead will be mobilized from storage sites and blood levels will rebound after treatment. It is not uncommon for the lead level at 2 weeks after therapy to equal or exceed the initial level.

COMMON PITFALLS

- Failure to consider the diagnosis of lead poisoning in patients with cognitive dysfunction, neurologic symptoms, and GI complaints
- Failure to appreciate that elevated lead levels without coincidental elevations in FEP may be seen with recent exposures
- Failure to consult a lead-poisoning expert for management advice
- Failure to treat the patient with an extremely high lead level and a normal FEP level
- Failure to appreciate that, in many states, lead poisoning is a reportable illness, and both state and local health officials must be notified
- Failure to identify the source of lead and to prevent reexposure

References

1. Baker EL, Feldman RG, White RF, et al. The role of occupational lead exposure in the genesis of psychiatric and behavioral disturbances. *Acta Psychiatr Scand* 1983;67[Suppl]:38.
2. Chisolm JJ. Mobilization of lead by calcium disodium edetate—a reappraisal. *Am J Dis Child* 1987;141:1256.
3. Cory-Slechta DA, Weiss B, Cox C. Mobilization and redistribution of lead over the course of Ca-EDTA therapy. *J Pharmacol Exp Ther* 1987;243:804.
4. Graziano JH, Sins ES, LoIacono N, et al. 2,3-Dimercaptosuccinic acid as an antidote for lead intoxication. *Clin Pharmacol Ther* 1985;37:431.
5. Harvey B. Should blood lead screening recommendations be revisited? *Pediatrics* 1994;93:201.
6. Hasegawa S, Nakayama K, Iwakiri K, et al. Herbal medicine-associated lead intoxication. *Intern Med* 1997;36(1):56–58.
7. Johnson NE, Tenuta K. Diets and lead blood levels of children who practice pica. *Environ Res* 1979;18:369.
8. Kilkano GE, Strange KC. Lead poisoning in a child after a gunshot injury. *J Fam Pract* 1992;34:498.
9. Lifshitz M, Hashkanazi R, Phillip M. The effect of 2,3 dimercaptosuccinic acid in the treatment of lead poisoning in adults. *Ann Med* 1997;29(1):83–85.
10. Lin JL, Ho HH, Yu CC. Chelation therapy for patients with elevated body lead burden and progressive renal insufficiency. A randomized, controlled trial. *Ann Intern Med* 1999;130(1):7–13.
11. Mahaffey K, Michaelson A. Interactions between lead and nutrition. In: Needleman HL, ed. *Low-level lead exposure: the clinical implications of current research.* New York: Raven Press, 1980:159.
12. Marcus SM. Experience with D-penicillamine in treating lead poisoning. *Vet Hum Toxicol* 1982;24:18.
13. Natelson EA, Fred HL. Lead poisoning from cocktail glasses: observations of two patients. *JAMA* 1976;236:2527.
14. Needleman HL, Gunnoe CG, Leviton A, et al. Deficits in psychological performance and classroom behavior in children with elevated dentine lead levels. *N Engl J Med* 1979;300:689.
15. Piomelli S, Rosen JF, Chisolm JJ, et al. Management of childhood lead poisoning. *J Pediatr* 1984;105:523.
16. Piomelli S, Seaman C, Zullow D, et al. Threshold for lead damage to have synthesis in urban children. *Proc Natl Acad Sci U S A* 1982;79:3335.
17. Rabinowitz MB, Wetherill GW, Kopple JD. Kinetic analysis of lead metabolism in healthy humans. *J Clin Invest* 1976;58:260.
18. Sanchez-Fructusos AI, Torralbo A, Arroyo M, et al. Occult lead intoxication as a cause of hypertension and renal failure. *Nephrol Dial Transplant* 1996;11(9):17775–17780.
19. Santiago M, Charnock R, Whitehead B, et al. Toxicity of EDTA in treating lead poisoning: IM vs IV. Platform session, American Association of Poison Control Centers, American Academy of Clinical Toxicologists, American Board of Medical Toxicologists, Annual Meeting, Boston, 1983. *Vet Hum Toxicol* 1983;25[Suppl 1]:67.
20. Vitale LF, Rosalinas-Bailon A, Brennan JF, et al. Oral penicillamine therapy for chronic lead poisoning in children. *J Pediatr* 1973;83:1041.

CHAPTER 349
Lithium Poisoning

Kenneth W. Kulig

The primary use of lithium is in the treatment of bipolar disorders. Other uses have included the treatment of drug and alcohol abuse, episodic aggression, anorexia nervosa, Huntington's chorea, tardive dyskinesia, SIADH, neutropenia, and Felty syndrome.[1]

In the United States, lithium is available as lithium carbonate tablets in regular (300 mg; 8.12 mEq) or slow-release (450 mg; 12.18 mEq) form, and as lithium citrate syrup (8 mEq/5 mL). Common adult daily doses are 900 to 2400 mg. Numerous adverse drug reactions and drug–drug interactions have been reported, and serum levels must be monitored carefully to avoid toxicity. Therapeutic lithium levels vary slightly from one laboratory to another but are generally cited as being within the range of 0.5 to 1.5 mEq/L.

The exact mechanism of action of lithium in the treatment of bipolar disorders is unknown. Therapeutic doses have no psychotropic effect in humans who do not have a bipolar disorder. Although lithium can replace sodium in supporting a single action potential in a nerve cell, it cannot maintain membrane potentials. Its ability to substitute for other cations, such as potassium, calcium, and magnesium at the cell membrane, has uncertain physiologic effects. Changes in the release or reuptake of norepinephrine and serotonin or modified hormonal responses mediated by adenyl cyclase have been postulated.

Understanding the kinetics of lithium, particularly its distribution, is important in the proper management of lithium overdose patients. Lithium ions are completely absorbed from the gastrointestinal (GI) tract. Absorption, which is rapid after therapeutic doses, may be delayed after large overdoses, in the presence of food, or if the patient has decreased intestinal motility from coingestants. Slow-release preparations result in lower peak concentrations, which occur at a later time.[3,5]

Lithium is initially distributed into the extracellular space and then more slowly into tissues, including the primary target organ of toxicity, the brain. After an acute overdose, the patient may initially appear well, with a high serum level, but deteriorate as the levels fall. The blood is not a target organ but is only an indirect measure of the total body burden of lithium. Invasive measures to remove lithium, such as hemodialysis or venovenous hemofiltration, may be more effective during the distribution phase in select patients, when the drug is still found in the intravascular compartment.[8,10] The volume of distribution is about that of body water—0.8 to 1.2 L/kg.

Lithium is entirely eliminated by renal excretion. The renal handling of lithium is similar to that of sodium; it is filtered and reabsorbed by the proximal tubule. Reabsorption is enhanced and toxicity is more likely in the setting of hyponatremia, volume depletion, renal hypoperfusion, and diuretic use.[1] Lithium, itself, may be nephrotoxic.[6,13] After a single dose, the serum half-life is 9 to 13 hours. At steady state, the half-life may be 30 to 58 hours. After an overdose, the serum half-life depends on how much lithium has been distributed into tissues; the figure is meaningful only after absorption is complete.

CLINICAL PRESENTATION

The toxicity seen depends on the dose, the time since ingestion, underlying medical conditions such as renal disease or dehydration, concomitant ingestions, and the patient's age. It is sometimes useful to classify the overdose as acute (single ingestion), acute on top of chronic therapy, or chronic. Because the latter situation is likely to result in the greatest lithium distribution into tissues, it is the most dangerous. There can be overlap among these categories. The clinical classification given in Table 349.1[7] is valuable in the initial assessment.

Patients may move from one category to another with time, depending primarily on the tissue distribution of lithium, which is not accurately measured by the serum level.[3,5,14,18] Electrocardiographic (ECG) changes are nondiagnostic and may occur in patients with therapeutic levels who are not clinically toxic.[13] Common changes include nonspecific ST-T wave changes, first-degree atrioventricular block, mild intraventricular conduction delay, and prolonged Q-T interval. These ECG changes may be responsible for the common misconception that lithium is primarily toxic to the heart, when the brain is, in reality, the primary target organ. Cardiovascular collapse generally occurs only as a result of severe central nervous system toxicity.

DIFFERENTIAL DIAGNOSIS

The classic painless rigidity, tremor, and hyperreflexia may not be present early in the clinical course. Other neurologic manifestations might mimic a cerebrovascular accident, a postictal state, metabolic disorders such as hypercalcemia or hyperthyroidism, or meningitis. The common nausea and vomiting seen after an acute overdose may be easily confused with gastroenteritis or another intraabdominal process. Particularly in the elderly, parkinsonism or tardive dyskinesia should be considered. Coingestants should be considered, especially other psychiatric medications such as antipsychotics and antidepressants. Carbamazepine and sodium valproate are also used to treat bipolar illness and may be coingestants.

EMERGENCY DEPARTMENT EVALUATION

Attention should focus on the mental status and a neurologic examination, searching particularly for tremor, myoclonus, hyperreflexia, and stiffness. Hydration status, renal function, and diuretic use should be assessed. When lithium toxicity is suspected, serum electrolytes should be measured, paying particular attention to the sodium, blood urea nitrogen, and creatinine. A lithium level should be taken when the patient has symptoms or signs consistent with lithium toxicity or if an acute overdose is suspected. Lithium levels are not included in broad toxicology screens and must be ordered separately. The screen is indicated if the patient is ill enough to require admission to the hospital. More than one lithium level should be drawn if the patient has taken an acute overdose,[15,17,18] particularly if the preparation is of the sustained-release type.[3,5]

An ECG should be performed to serve as a baseline and to help rule out coingestants such as the tricyclic antidepressants. ST-T abnormalities are common with therapeutic dosing and do

TABLE 349.1. Severity of Lithium Poisoning

Grade 1 (mild): Nausea, vomiting, tremor, hyperreflexia, agitation, muscle weakness, ataxia
Grade 2 (moderate): Confusion, dysarthria, rigidity, hypertonia, hypotension, stupor
Grade 3 (severe): Convulsions, myoclonic jerking, coma, cardiovascular collapse

not necessarily mean cardiotoxicity.[12] Obtaining the patient's pill bottles or calling the pharmacy where the patient gets the medications can also help to rule out coingestants. Medications such as acetaminophen, which do not cause early symptoms, should also be considered.

Vital signs, including temperature, should be measured often. Serial neurologic examinations, including a mental status examination, should be performed. A Foley catheter to monitor urine output should be placed if the patient exhibits moderate or severe toxicity.

EMERGENCY DEPARTMENT MANAGEMENT

Advanced life-support measures are instituted as necessary. An intravenous line of normal saline should be started, and the patient should be rehydrated aggressively. However, once euvolemia and normal urine output have been established, there may be little added advantage to aggressive saline diuresis. Fluid overload may occur from overly aggressive saline administration.

The use of ipecac should be avoided, as it is unlikely to remove significant quantities of drug; it also interferes with patient assessment, because vomiting is an early sign of lithium toxicity. Lavage is also unlikely to remove much lithium from the stomach and should probably be considered only if the patient presents very soon after an acute ingestion.

Activated charcoal does not bind lithium, but it should be given if coingestants are suspected. If only lithium was ingested, or if the patient is chronically lithium-intoxicated without other drugs involved, activated charcoal is unnecessary.

Sodium polystyrene sulfonate (Kayexalate) is an ion-exchange resin usually used to treat hyperkalemia. There is experimental evidence that Kayexalate can both prevent absorption of lithium and enhance its removal once absorbed.[4,11,19] The clinical efficacy of this therapy is unproved, and it is probably best reserved for patients who have taken a massive overdose, have high or rising levels, or are otherwise severely ill. The optimum dose and dosing intervals have not been defined; 15 to 50 g orally or by nasogastric tube every 4 to 6 hours might be a reasonable starting point. Kayexalate can cause nausea, vomiting, and constipation. The serum potassium level should be carefully monitored to prevent hypokalemia.

Whole-bowel irrigation has also been recommended as a GI decontamination measure for lithium overdose.[9,16] It is uncertain whether this technique is as effective as using Kayexalate, or whether, in fact, either approach is necessary.

Hemodialysis is the most efficient method of removing lithium from the intravascular compartment, allowing lithium to redistribute into it from the brain.[1,8,10] Because this redistribution is relatively slow, however, clinical improvement lags behind the fall in serum lithium levels. It may take days or weeks for toxicity to resolve, despite hemodialysis. For a critically ill lithium-intoxicated patient or a patient with a very high (greater than 3 mEq/L) or rising lithium level, a nephrologist should be consulted regarding hemodialysis. Permanent neurologic sequelae (e.g., encephalopathy) can result from lithium intoxication.[2,17,20] Whether late hemodialysis can prevent such complications is unclear. Peritoneal dialysis is much less effective and is not usually considered in this setting.

DISPOSITION

A patient with an acute lithium overdose cannot usually be medically cleared on the basis of a single lithium level, unless it is zero or very near zero and it has been hours since the reported ingestion. In most cases, a second level should be measured to ensure that delayed absorption is not occurring. In all cases of overdose with suicidal intent, psychiatric consultation should be obtained before discharge.

Patients should be admitted if they have any neurologic symptoms from lithium, such as altered mental status, tremor, or stiffness. If patients are dehydrated, are in renal failure, or have a high or rising lithium level, they should be admitted to an intensive care unit.

It is difficult to give a precise lithium level above which all patients need to be admitted or hemodialyzed. Patients on chronic therapy may manifest toxicity even within the therapeutic range. Other patients may be relatively asymptomatic with levels of 5 to 8 mEq/L following acute overdose.[8,15] Clinical judgment, preferably by a physician experienced in the treatment of lithium-poisoned patients, is necessary in making these important decisions. Consulting a regional poison center or toxicologist can be very helpful.

COMMON PITFALLS

- Failure to appreciate that severe lithium poisoning can lead to permanent neurologic impairment
- Failure to consider the kinetics of lithium and whether toxicity is acute, acute on chronic, or chronic when interpreting serum lithium levels
- Failure to consider the possibility of lithium poisoning and to obtain a serum lithium level in patients taking lithium who present with an illness predisposing them to dehydration
- Failure to obtain serial lithium levels in patients with acute overdose
- Failure to treat dehydration and hyponatremia aggressively
- Failure to consider dialysis in the early stages of care in patients with significant clinical toxicity or very high lithium levels

References

1. Amdisen A. Clinical features and management of lithium poisoning. *Med Toxicol Adverse Drug Exp* 1988;3:18.
2. Apte SN, Langston JW. Permanent neurological deficits due to lithium toxicity. *Ann Neurol* 1983;13:453.
3. Astruc B, Petit P, Abbar M. Overdose with sustained-release lithium preparations. *Eur Psychiatry* 1999;14:172–174.
4. Belanger DR, Tierney MG, Dickinson G. Effect of sodium polystyrene sulfonate on lithium bioavailability. *Ann Emerg Med* 1992;21:1312.
5. Bosse GM, Arnold TC. Overdose with sustained-release lithium preparations. *J Emerg Med* 1992;10:719.
6. Gitlin M. Lithium and the kidney. *Drug Saf* 1999;20:231–243.
7. Hansen HE, Amdisen A. Lithium intoxication: report of 23 cases and review of 100 cases from the literature. *Q J Med* 1978;47:123.
8. Jaeger A, Sauder P, Kopferschmitt J, et al. When should dialysis be performed in lithium poisoning? A kinetic study in 14 cases of lithium poisoning. *Clin Toxicol* 1993;31:429.
9. Kirshenbaum LA, Mathews SC, Sitar DS, et al. Whole bowel irrigation versus activated charcoal in sorbitol for the ingestion of modified-release pharmaceuticals. *Clin Pharmacol Ther* 1989;46:264.
10. Hazouard E, Ferrandiere M, Rateau H, et al. Continuous veno-venous haemofiltration versus continuous veno-venous haemodialysis in severe lithium self-poisoning: a toxicokinetics study in an intensive care unit. *Nephrol Dial Transplant* 1999;14:1605–1606.
11. Linakis JG, Eisenberg MS, Lacoutre PG, et al. Multiple-dose sodium polystyrene sulfonate in lithium intoxication: an animal model. *Pharmacol Toxicol* 1992;70:38.
12. Mateer JR, Clark MR. Lithium toxicity with rarely reported EKG manifestations. *Ann Emerg Med* 1982;11:208.
13. Rose SR, Klein-Schwartz W, Oderda GM, et al. Lithium intoxication with acute renal failure and death. *Drug Intell Clin Pharm* 1988;22:691.
14. Sadosty AT, Groleau GA, Atcherson MM. The use of lithium levels in the emergency department. *J Emerg Med* 1999;17:887–891.
15. Sawyer D, Kulig K. Lithium overdose superimposed on chronic therapy—lack of indication for dialysis. *Vet Hum Toxicol* 1983;25:273(abst).
16. Smith SW, Ling LW, Halstenson CE. Whole bowel irrigation as a treatment for acute lithium overdose. *Ann Emerg Med* 1991;20:536.

17. Strayhorn JM, Nash JL. Severe neurotoxicity despite "therapeutic" serum lithium levels. *Dis Nerv Syst* 1977;38:107.
18. Timmer RT, Sands JM. Lithium intoxication. *J Am Soc Nephrol* 1999;10:666–674.
19. Tomaszewski C, Musso C, Pearson JR, et al. Lithium absorption prevented by sodium polystyrene sulfonate in volunteers. *Ann Emerg Med* 1992;21:1308.
20. Von Hartitzch B, Hoenich NA, Leigh RJ, et al. Permanent neurological sequelae despite hemodialysis for lithium intoxication. *BMJ* 1972;4:757.

CHAPTER 350
Local Anesthetic Poisoning

Donna L. Seger and Heeten Desai

In 1940, lidocaine was introduced as a local anesthetic agent. Lidocaine causes anesthesia in peripheral nerves by decreasing conduction and membrane stability through reduced permeability to sodium ions, which prevents transmembrane polarization and subsequent propagation of the action potential. Lidocaine is a group II (amide-type) local anesthetic; it does not contain a *p*-aminophenyl group. Other members of group II include dibucaine (Nupercainal), mepivacaine (Carbocaine), prilocaine (Citanest), bupivacaine (Marcaine), and etidocaine (Duranest).

In contrast, group I anesthetics contain esters of benzoic acid, *p*-aminobenzoic acid, and meta-aminobenzoic acid and include cocaine (see Chapter 326), tetracaine (Pontocaine), procaine (Novocain), proparacaine (Opthaine), butethamine (Monocane), and ethyl aminobenzoate. Patients who are allergic to an anesthetic in group I are allergic to all group I anesthetics but may safely be given a group II anesthetic, and vice versa.

Lidocaine, also known as lignocaine, became popular as an antidysrhythmic agent in 1960. Lidocaine blocks fast sodium channels during phase zero of the action potential (depolarization). This action, as well as local anesthetic activity, is shared by all class I antidysrhythmics (see Chapter 311). Lidocaine, along with phenytoin (see Chapter 364), mexiletine, and moricizine, and tocainide, are grouped as class 1B agents because they shorten the action potential duration. In contrast, class IA agents (quinidine and procainamide) lengthen it, and class IC agents (flecainide, encainide, and propafenone) have little effect on the action potential duration (see Chapter 311). Lidocaine also diminishes the slope of phase four depolarization (suppressing automaticity and membrane responsiveness) in the His Purkinje system. Lidocaine prevents reentry impulses and increases uniformity of conduction in ischemic tissue where action potential duration is prolonged and propagation of reentry rhythms is enhanced.

Lidocaine is well absorbed through mucous membranes and the gastrointestinal (GI) tract. Peak plasma concentrations are reached within 2 minutes of intravenous administration, within 10 minutes of endotracheal administration, and within 30 to 60 minutes of ingestion. Lidocaine is 50% protein bound. Protein binding is concentration dependent, with a greater amount bound at increased serum concentration. Seventy percent is bound to alpha-1 glycoprotein, and 30% is bound to albumin. Unbound fraction (free) is increased in newborns and in patients with hepatitis or conditions with decreased alpha-1 glycoprotein. The volume of distribution is 1.7 L/kg, meaning the drug is largely tissue bound.

Following intravenous injection, lidocaine is rapidly distributed to well-perfused tissue (brain and heart), with subsequent slower distribution to less well perfused tissues (skeletal muscle and fat). The initial distribution serum half-life is approximately 10 minutes. The peak serum concentration, which depends on the rate of administration, rapidly declines. Because of this biphasic pattern of distribution, an infusion is required to maintain therapeutic serum concentrations following intravenous bolus. A standard intravenous dosing regimen is 1.0 to 1.4 mg/kg, followed in 10 minutes by an additional bolus of 0.7 mg/kg and a maintenance infusion of 1 to 4 mg/min (20 to 50 μg/kg/min for children).

Lidocaine is metabolized to two active metabolites: monoethylglycinexylidide (MEGX) and glycine xylidide (GX). These metabolites achieve peak concentrations in 1 to 2 hours after an oral dose. The plasma elimination half-life of lidocaine ranges from 1.5 to 2.0 hours. The elimination half-lives of MEGX and GX are 3 and 5 hours, respectively. All are excreted in the urine. Only 5% to 10% of the parent drug is excreted unchanged. High concentrations of MEGX may produce toxic effects even though serum lidocaine concentrations are low.[16] The risk of lidocaine toxicity is increased in patients with hepatic dysfunction, congestive heart failure, and shock due to alterations of metabolism, hepatic blood flow, and volume of distribution. The volume of distribution of lidocaine in patients with congestive heart failure can be decreased by 30%. Conversely, in patients with chronic hepatic disease, an increase of parent drug in the circulation and a decrease in alpha-1 glycoprotein may increase the volume of distribution by 30% to 40%. Both of these conditions decrease the hepatic extraction ratio. Cimetidine decreases splanchnic circulation and hepatic blood flow (decreasing metabolism), which may cause toxic concentrations of lidocaine.

Mexiletine (Mexitil) and tocainide (Tonocard) have chemical structures and electrophysiologic properties that are similar to those of lidocaine.[14,17] Moricizine (Ethmozine), a phenothiazine, depresses sodium current but does not affect phase 4 depolarization.[16] Because of the proarrhythmic activity and increased mortality associated with their use (see Chapter 311), these agents are generally reserved for patients with dysrhythmias refractory to other drugs who have shown a positive response to them on electrophysiologic testing.[7] Usual adult doses are 200 to 400 mg every 8 hours for all agents. All are well absorbed from the GI tract and are hepatically metabolized. Unlike lidocaine, they do not undergo significant first-pass metabolism and are 90% to 100% bioavailable after ingestion. Because 40% of the parent drug is excreted unchanged in the urine, tocainide clearance is decreased in patients with renal disease. The half-life is 10 to 12 hours for mexiletine, 1.5 to 3.0 hours for moricizine, and 15 hours for tocainide. Pharmacokinetics do not seem to be altered by concurrent administration of other drugs.[2,8,16,19]

CLINICAL PRESENTATION

Although intravenous, subcutaneous (infiltration), topical, or oral administration of lidocaine may cause toxicity,[1,3,15] the emergency department physician most frequently encounters symptoms of toxicity during intravenous infusion.[4,5,9] Manifestations of toxicity occur in the central nervous system (CNS) and the cardiovascular (CV) system. CNS effects have been reported in up to 47% of patients receiving intravenous lidocaine. Initial symptoms, such as lightheadedness, dizziness, drowsiness, and euphoria, may occur at therapeutic concentrations. At higher concentrations, more serious symptoms include confusion, hearing loss, dysarthria, visual disturbances, ataxia, agitation, and muscle twitching, which may lead to seizures and coma. Seizures may be prolonged.[4,5]

Cardiovascular toxicity is rare and usually occurs from rapidly administered intravenous infusions. When serum concentrations are above 11 μg/mL, the refractory period is decreased, automaticity and myocardial contractility are depressed, and hypotension and bradycardia ensue.[18] Conduction abnormalities include sinus bradycardia, atrioventricular block, complete heart block, and sinus arrest. Conduction defects may be more common in patients with preexisting bundle-branch abnormalities.[11]

Although extensive first-pass metabolism occurs following intestinal absorption, mucosal absorption bypasses hepatic metabolism, and significant drug is bioavailable. A number of case reports have documented seizures in children following mucosal application of 10 mL of 2% to 4% viscous lidocaine solution. [5,15,20] Administration of topical or oral lidocaine for the treatment of painful oral lesions in children should be recommended with caution, if at all.

Seizures have been reported following lidocaine infiltration. During laceration repair, the total dose for infiltration of lidocaine without epinephrine should not exceed 4.5 mg/kg, nor should the dose exceed 7.0 mg/kg of lidocaine with epinephrine.

The toxicity of other local anesthetics is similar to that of lidocaine, and the toxicity of other antidysrhythmics is similar to that of other class I agents (see Chapter 311). Many local anesthetics have also been reported to cause methemoglobinemia (see Chapter 352).

DIFFERENTIAL DIAGNOSIS

Physiologic stimulants and metabolic disturbances should be considered in the differential diagnosis of patients with CNS manifestations, and agents with membrane activity should be considered in those with CV system toxicity (see Table 309.4). Methemoglobinemia (see Chapter 352) should be considered in a patient who becomes cyanotic and is responding poorly to oxygen therapy after exposure to local anesthetics.

EMERGENCY DEPARTMENT EVALUATION

The history and physical examination should focus on the concomitant use of prescription and nonprescription drugs, as well as CNS and CV signs and symptoms. Symptomatic patients should have continuous cardiac and oxygen saturation monitoring, as well as a 12-lead electrocardiogram. As always, hypoglycemia should be excluded in those with altered mental status. Those with unexplained toxicity should have serum electrolyte determinations and liver and kidney function tests. Serum levels of lidocaine and tocainide may confirm clinical toxicity but are often unavailable in an emergency situation. Remember that toxicity can occur at therapeutic serum concentrations.

EMERGENCY DEPARTMENT MANAGEMENT

Treatment is primarily supportive. Advanced life-support measures should be instituted as necessary. If the patient becomes symptomatic while receiving intravenous lidocaine, the infusion should either be decreased or discontinued.

Seizures and other manifestations of CNS excitation may be controlled with intravenous lorazepam (adult, 2 to 4 mg intravenously as needed; child, 0.05 to 0.1 mg/kg initially) or diazepam; pay close attention to potential respiratory depression. Severe CV toxicity from lidocaine may require support of blood pressure and pulse by crystalloid, pressor agents, atropine, or a temporary pacemaker.[4–6] Sodium bicarbonate should be considered in patients with tachydysrhythmias due to related antidysrhythmic agents (see Chapter 311). The use of other class IB agents, however, should be avoided.

Although exchange transfusion has been reported for severe lidocaine toxicity, its efficacy has not been substantiated.[11] There is no evidence that hemodialysis or forced diuresis effectively increases lidocaine elimination.[13] Even in severe cases, patients usually recover if vital signs can be supported (e.g., by aortic balloon counterpulsation or extracorporeal bypass pump) while the drug is eliminated.[11]

DISPOSITION

Patients with mucosal exposure or ingestion should be observed for 4 hours. Patients who remain asymptomatic may be discharged. Those who are or become symptomatic should be observed and have cardiac monitoring until signs and symptoms of toxicity have resolved. The appropriate level of care should be determined by the severity of clinical toxicity. If such care is not available, the patient should be transferred by advanced life-support personnel to a facility capable of providing it. Depending on the nature and severity of toxicity, consultation with a regional poison control center, toxicologist, or cardiologist may be appropriate.

COMMON PITFALLS

- Failure to adhere to recommended dosing guidelines and to check the dose and concentration of parenteral local anesthetic solutions, resulting in iatrogenic poisoning
- Failure to perform cardiac monitoring on patients receiving systemic infusions of lidocaine, intravenous regional blocks with local anesthetics, and large doses of local anesthetics by infiltration
- Failure to appreciate that local anesthetics can cause CNS excitation as well as depression
- Failure to appreciate that class IB antidysrhythmics can cause dysrhythmias and that they can do so at therapeutic as well as toxic doses
- Failure to appreciate that multiple doses of oral viscous lidocaine can be toxic and to warn patients and parents of children that it should not be swallowed

ACKNOWLEDGMENT

Theodore B. Tong contributed to previous versions of this chapter.

References

1. Alfaro SN, Leicht MJ, Skiendzielewski JJ. Lidocaine toxicity following subcutaneous administration. *Ann Emerg Med* 1984;13:465.
2. Alpert JS, Haffajee CI, Young MD. Chemistry, pharmacology, antiarrhythmic efficacy and adverse effects of tocainide hydrochloride, an orally active structural analog of lidocaine. *Pharmacotherapy* 1983;3:316.
3. Amitai Y, Whitesell L, Lovejoy FH. Death following accidental lidocaine overdosage in a child. *N Engl J Med* 1986;314:181.
4. Brown DL, Skiendzielewski JJ. Lidocaine toxicity. *Ann Emerg Med* 1980;9:627.
5. Bryant CA, Hoffman JR, Nichtes LS. Pitfalls and perils of intravenous lidocaine. *West J Med* 1983;139:528.

6. Burlington B, Freed C. Massive overdose and death from prophylactic lidocaine. *JAMA* 1980;243:1036.
7. Campbell TJ. Proarrhythmic actions of antiarrhythmic drugs: a review. *Aust N Z J Med* 1990;20:275–282.
8. Clarke CWF, El-Malde EO. Fatal oral tocainide overdosage. *BMJ* 1984;228:760.
9. Finkelstein F, Kreeft J. Massive lidocaine poisoning. *N Engl J Med* 1979;301:50.
10. Follath F, Canzinger U, Schultz E. Reliability of antiarrhythmic drug plasma concentration monitoring. *Clin Pharmacokinet* 1983;8:63.
11. Freedman MD, Gal J, Freed CR. Extracorporeal pump assistance: novel treatment for acute lidocaine poisoning. *Eur J Clin Pharmacol* 1982;22:129.
12. Gupta P, Lichstein E, Claade K. Lidocaine-induced heart block in patients with bundle-branch block. *Am J Cardiol* 1976;33:487.
13. Jacobi J, McGory RW, McCoy H, et al. Hemodialysis clearance of total unbound lidocaine. *Clin Pharm* 1983;2:54.
14. Kutatek SP, Morgan Roth J, Horowitz W. Tocainide: a new oral antiarrhythmic agent. *Ann Intern Med* 1985;103:387.
15. Mofenson HC, Caraccio TR, Miller H, et al. Lidocaine toxicity from topical mucosal application. *Clin Pediatr* 1983;22:190.
16. Pieper JA, Slaughter RL, Anderson GD, et al. Lidocaine: clinical pharmacokinetics. *Drug Intell Clin Pharm* 1982;16:291.
17. Pottage A. Clinical profiles of newer class I antiarrhythmic agents—tocainide, mexiletine, encainide, flecainide and lorcainide. *Am J Cardiol* 1983; 52[Suppl]:24C.
18. Promisloff RA, Dupont DC. Death from ARDS and cardiovascular collapse following lidocaine administration. *Chest* 1983;3:585.
19. Roden DM, Woosley RL. Tocainide. *N Engl J Med* 1986;315:41.
20. Rothstein P, Dornbusch J, Shaywitz BA. Prolonged seizures associated with the use of viscous lidocaine. *J Pediatr* 1982;134:323.

CHAPTER 351
Methanol Poisoning

Dag Jacobsen

Poisoning may occur after the accidental or intentional ingestion of methanol. Although most cases are isolated, epidemics of methanol poisoning may occur when methanol is mistakenly substituted for ethanol by, for instance, alcoholics, or when methanol contaminants are used to ferment (e.g., wine) or illicitly distill (e.g., moonshine whisky) alcoholic beverages.

Methanol (methyl alcohol, "colonial spirit," "wood alcohol," "solvent alcohol") is a colorless, volatile, highly flammable liquid with a density of 0.81 g/mL and a weak smell that resembles that of ethanol. Methanol is widely used industrially as a solvent and in the production of formaldehyde and methylated compounds. It is found in commercial products such as gasoline, antifreeze, gasohol, windshield washer fluid, copy machine fluid, canned heat (Sterno), paint, shellac, and solvents for removing wood finishes. The lethal dose of methanol is variably given as 30 to 240 mL, with 1 g/kg as the best estimate.[11,19] The minimum dose that can cause permanent visual defects is unknown. Because a potentially toxic methanol level (20 mg/dL) may result from the ingestion of 0.14 mL/kg of pure methanol, one swallow should be considered potentially toxic.

Methanol is rapidly absorbed after ingestion and distributes in the total body water compartment (about 0.6 L/kg). It is metabolized first to formaldehyde and then to formic acid, which is responsible for the toxic effects in methanol intoxication.[11] The metabolism of formate depends on the folate pool.[11] Primates have a small folate reserve and are the only species that accumulates formate and, thus, suffers from methanol toxicity.[10] The metabolism of methanol by alcohol dehydrogenase, which accounts for 90% of its elimination, is zero order, with a rate of 8.5 mg/dL/h in one case.[8] Small amounts are excreted in expired air and urine.

In the early stage, the toxic effects are due to the increasing metabolic acidosis caused by the accumulation of formic acid.[5] In late stages, when more formate is accumulated, the toxicity is mainly caused by the histotoxic effects of formate as it inhibits the mitochondrial respiration within the cell. This leads to lactate production, which increases the acidosis and the toxicity of formate as more formate is protonated and thereby able to penetrate the blood–brain barrier.[6] Thus, a vicious *circulus hypoxicus* is initiated (Fig. 351.1).[9] Why the eye is the primary target organ for methanol's toxic effects is unknown.[11,15,16]

Ethanol and fomepizole bind to alcohol dehydrogenase with a higher affinity than does ethylene glycol, and hence block the production of toxic metabolites. Ethanol is metabolized by alcohol dehydrogenase, but fomepizole is not. When these antidotes are present, the elimination half-life of methanol increases to 30 to 60 hours.

CLINICAL PRESENTATION

Usually 6 to 24 hours elapse from the time of ingestion to the occurrence of symptoms. It takes this much time for sufficient amounts of formic acid to be produced by methanol metabolism. This latent period may be longer, especially if ethanol is coingested, because ethanol competitively inhibits methanol metabolism by alcohol dehydrogenase. A latent period up to 90 hours has been reported when ethanol is coingested.[10]

Methanol itself has few direct effects. Mild central nervous system (CNS) depression (ethanol-like intoxication) has been reported.[11] With concentrated methanol solutions, nausea, vomiting, and abdominal pain may develop shortly after ingestion. The diagnosis is confirmed by detection of methanol in the serum. Because of its low molecular weight (32), at high concentrations methanol increases the serum osmolality, as do other alcohols and low-molecular-weight solutes (see Table 309.5). This effect can be detected easily by calculating the difference be-

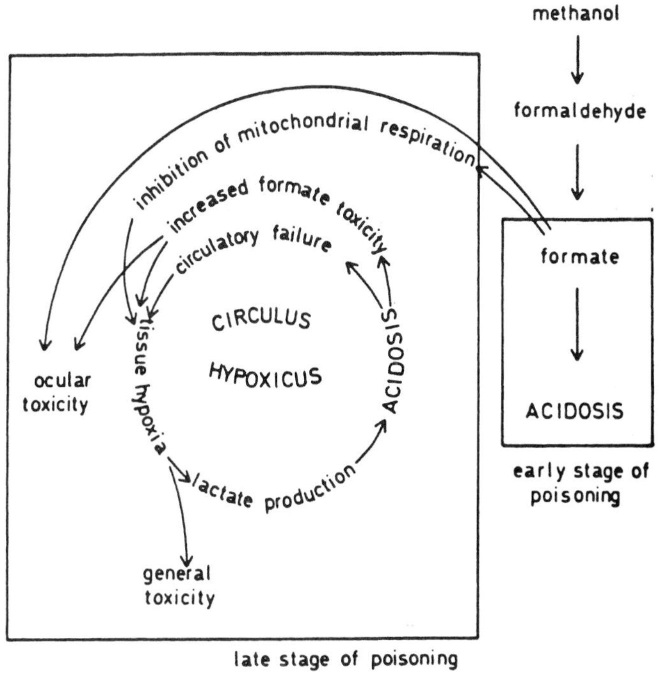

Figure 351.1. The "circulus hypoxicus" resulting from methanol ingestion.

tween the measured osmolality (om) and the calculated osmolality (oc) (oc = 2 × sodium + blood urea nitrogen/3 + glucose/18). The "normal" range for the osmolal gap in unselected patients is 5 ± 7 mOsmol/kg H_2O (mean ± SD).[1] An osmolal gap above 19, therefore, strongly indicates exogenous osmoles of some kind.[5,11] If a serum methanol level is not immediately available, it can be estimated by multiplying the excess osmolal gap by 2.6 mg/dL, the amount of methanol that increases to osmolality by 1 milliosmol per kilogram of water. In this early stage, metabolic acidosis is absent as the metabolism of methanol to formate is just beginning.

The first clinical features of systemic toxicity are usually a feeling of weakness, anorexia, headache, nausea, and vomiting, accompanied or followed by increasing hyperventilation as a result of progressive increased anion gap metabolic acidosis.[11,18,19] The "normal" range for the anion gap ([Na + K] – [Cl + HCO_3]) in unselected, acutely hospitalized patients is 13 ± 4 mmol/L (mean ± SD).[1] Visual symptoms (blurred vision, decreased acuity, halo vision, tunnel vision, photophobia, and "snowfields") may appear first or with the aforementioned symptoms. Usually, ocular symptoms precede objective signs such as dilated pupils that are partially reactive or nonreactive to light and funduscopy showing optic disk hyperemia with blurring of the margins. At this stage, the diagnosis is confirmed by detecting methanol or formate in the serum; the osmolal gap may or may not be elevated. A few cases may also present as acute abdomen, probably because of acute pancreatitis.[11,12]

Without treatment, coma and respiratory and circulatory failure may ensue. A few patients may also develop methemoglobinemia with cyanosis, probably because of an interaction between formate and the ferric part of hemoglobin. In the late stages of methanol poisoning, when most or all of the methanol is metabolized to formate, the anion gap is elevated but the osmolal gap is normal, methanol may be undetectable, and formate detection is the only way to confirm the diagnosis.

The toxic effect on the putamen does not lead to detectable signs and symptoms in the acute stage because it is concealed by pronounced CNS depression. Survivors may later manifest a Parkinson-like syndrome.[2,13]

DIFFERENTIAL DIAGNOSIS

If quantitative methanol and formate levels are unavailable, all other causes of metabolic acidosis and increased serum osmolality should be considered in the differential diagnosis (Fig. 351.2; see also Figure 309.1). Increased anion and osmolal gaps occur in ethylene glycol intoxication as well as in methanol poisoning. Differentiating the two may be difficult, but the treatments are essentially the same. Visual complaints suggest methanol poisoning, whereas hypocalcemia, seizures, and urine oxalate crystals indicate ethylene glycol poisoning.[11]

EMERGENCY DEPARTMENT EVALUATION

The history should include the amount, concentration, and time of methanol ingestion; the nature and onset of symptoms; and whether ethanol was coingested. Patients should be questioned carefully about the presence or absence of visual complaints, GI symptoms, and a feeling of intoxication.

The physical examination should focus on vital signs (especially respiratory rate) and the neurologic, visual, and cardiopulmonary status. Visual acuity and funduscopic examinations should be documented.

Laboratory evaluation should include arterial blood gas analysis; complete blood count; measurement of electrolytes,

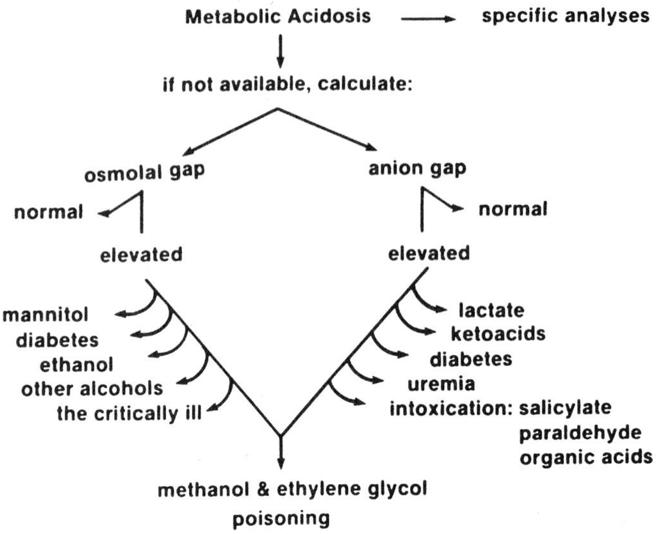

Figure 351.2. Causes of an increased anion and osmolal gap.

blood urea nitrogen, creatinine, glucose, and amylase; urinalysis; and quantitative serum methanol or formic acid level. A chest radiograph and an electrocardiogram are obtained if clinical toxicity is pronounced.

If the diagnosis is based on the osmolal and anion gaps, osmometry must be performed by the freezing-point depression technique and not by the vapor pressure technique, as the latter does not detect the increased osmolality caused by volatile alcohols. A computed tomography scan or MRI of the brain may show necrosis of the putaminal areas, a finding seen late in the course of methanol poisoning.[2,13]

EMERGENCY DEPARTMENT MANAGEMENT

General treatment measures include intensive supportive care and GI decontamination. If the patient is seen soon after ingestion (within 2 hours) immediate gastric aspiration, preferably with a nasogastric tube, is recommended. Emesis induction and activated charcoal alone are probably of limited value because of slow onset and limited binding, respectively.

Specific treatment of methanol poisoning includes bicarbonate to combat the metabolic acidosis, antidotal therapy with ethanol or fomepizale to inhibit methanol metabolism to formate, and hemodialysis to remove methanol and formate. Folinic acid (leucovorin), 1 mg/kg up to 50 mg intravenously every 4 hours, may be of value in increasing the metabolism of formate.[17] If folinic acid is unavailable, folic acid, in the same dose, can be used.

Metabolic acidosis is aggressively treated by infusing sodium bicarbonate. As much as 400 to 600 mEq may be required during the first few hours. The goal should be full correction of the acidosis. Bicarbonate treatment also decreases the amount of undissociated formic acid, resulting in less access of formate to the CNS.[6,19] Hence, metabolic acidosis resulting from methanol poisoning, in contrast to other types of metabolic acidosis, should always be treated with bicarbonate.

Alkali treatment must be accompanied by administration of ethanol or fomepizole; otherwise, the acidosis becomes bicarbonate-resistant, as more formic acid will be produced from the metabolism of methanol. If a methanol level cannot readily be obtained, ethanol therapy should be started in any patient with acidosis, symptoms, or a history of a potentially toxic ingestion. Antidotal treatment can be discontinued when the methanol level drops below 20 mg/dL, provided that the acid–base status is normal and there are no complications.

Most authors recommend a therapeutic blood ethanol level of at least 100 mg/dL. However, the amount of ethanol necessary to block methanol metabolism depends on the concomitant methanol level, because there is a dynamic competition for the enzyme alcohol dehydrogenase in the liver. If the blood methanol level is known, the molar–ethanol concentrations should be at least one-fourth of the molar–methanol concentration.[11,14]

A blood ethanol level of 100 mg/dL may be achieved by giving a bolus dose of 0.6 mg/kg, followed by 66 to 154 mg/kg/h intravenously or orally, with the higher maintenance dose for heavy drinkers. Mixing 50 mL of absolute ethanol with 500 mL isotonic glucose yields a 10% solution if a 10% ethanol solution for intravenous use is unavailable. With this solution, a bolus of 8 mL/kg (over 0.5 h), followed by 1.5 mL/kg/h, will produce the desired ethanol concentration. The maintenance infusion should be increased or decreased according to measured ethanol levels.

Monitoring the blood ethanol level is important, especially during hemodialysis, as this procedure also removes ethanol. As a rule of thumb, the maintenance dose of ethanol should be doubled during hemodialysis. If not, methanol metabolism can resume when the ethanol level drops, resulting in worsening toxicity despite hemodialysis.

Fomepizole (4-methylpryazole; Antizol) is commercially available, but it has been approved only for the treatment of ethylene glycol poisoning.[3,8] So far, only a few methanol-poisoned patients treated with fomepizole have been reported.[4,7] The results from these studies are so favorable, however, that fomepizole should be considered an alternative to ethanol for methanol as well as ethylene glycol poisoning. The dosing of fomepizole and therapeutic considerations are the same as for ethylene glycol (see Chapter 338).

Hemodialysis effectively removes methanol and formate and also counteracts metabolic acidosis.[11] The only absolute indication for hemodialysis is visual impairment of any degree in a patient with metabolic acidosis or a detectable methanol level. Other indications include severe metabolic acidosis (particularly if unresponsive to bicarbonate and ethanol therapy), a blood methanol level above 50 mg/dL (because of the very slow elimination of methanol during antidotal therapy), and ingestion of more than 1 g/kg of methanol.

Hemodialysis is continued until the blood methanol level is below 20 mg/dL and the acidosis is corrected. If methanol analyses are unavailable, hemodialysis should be continued for at least 8 hours. Peritoneal dialysis may also remove methanol but not as effectively as hemodialysis. Hemoperfusion is ineffective.

DISPOSITION

Consultation with a poison center or toxicologist is strongly recommended if the physician is unfamiliar with the management of methanol poisoning. In addition, information on where to obtain methanol or formate levels may be provided. When the diagnosis of methanol poisoning is made or suspected, a nephrologist should be consulted, as many patients ultimately require hemodialysis, especially when admitted in a late stage.

If a methanol level is unavailable, all patients with suspected methanol poisoning should be admitted to the hospital for continued clinical and laboratory evaluation. Every patient with a definite diagnosis of methanol intoxication should be admitted and have an initial and follow-up examination by an ophthalmologist.

If hemodialysis is unavailable, the patient who needs it, or will probably need it, should be transferred to a facility with this capability. Alkali administration and antidotal therapy (if available) should be given prior to and during transport.

COMMON PITFALLS

- Failure to appreciate that even small amounts of concentrated methanol may be toxic
- Failure to consider methanol poisoning in the differential diagnosis of metabolic acidosis of unknown origin
- Failure to consider the possibility of multiple victims when the source of methanol is unknown or is known to be contaminated ethanol
- Failure to appreciate that the absence of early symptoms and the presence of normal anion and osmolal gaps do not exclude a potentially toxic methanol ingestion
- Failure to observe all patients with known or suspected methanol ingestion until a methanol level can be obtained
- Failure to appreciate that ethanol and fomepizole are removed by hemodialysis and to adjust their dosing during this procedure accordingly
- Failure to have visual function formally assessed by an ophthalmologist in patients with methanol poisoning

References

1. Aabakken L, Johansen KS, Rydningen EB, et al. Osmolal and anion gaps in patients admitted to an emergency medical department. *Hum Exp Toxicol* 1994;13:131.
2. Aquilonius SM, Bergstrom K, Enoksson P, et al. Cerebral computed tomography in methanol intoxication. *J Comput Assist Tomogr* 1980;4:425.
3. Baud FJ, Galliot M, Astier A, et al. Treatment of ethylene glycol poisoning with intravenous 4-methylpyrazole. *Ann Emerg Med* 1997;30:829.
4. Burns MJ, Graudins A, Aaron CK, et al. Treatment of methanol poisoning with intravenous 4-methylpyrazole. *Ann Emerg Med* 1997;30:829.
5. Enger E. Acidosis, gaps and poisonings. *Acta Med Scand* 1982;212:1.
6. Herken W, Rietbrock N, Henschler D. Zum mechanismus der Methanol-Vergiftung. Toxisches Agens und Einfluss der Sure-Basenstatus auf die Giftwirkung. *Arch Toxicol* 1969;24:214.
7. Hantson P, Wallemacq P, Brau M, et al. Two cases of acute methanol poisoning partially treated by oral 4-methylpyrazole. *Intensive Care Med* 1999;340:879.
8. Jacobsen D. New treatment for ethylene glycol poisoning. *N Engl J Med* 1999;340:879.
9. Jacobsen D. *Studies in methanol and ethylene glycol poisonings: acidosis—kinetics—management*. Thesis, University of Oslo, 1985.
10. Jacobsen D, Jansen H, Wiik-Larsen E, et al. Studies on methanol poisoning. *Acta Med Scand* 1982;212:5.
11. Jacobsen D, McMartin KE. Methanol and ethylene glycol poisonings: mechanism of toxicity, clinical course, diagnosis and treatment. *Med Toxicol* 1986;1:309.
12. Jacobsen D, Webb R, Collins TD, et al. Methanol and formate kinetics in late diagnosed methanol intoxication. *Med Toxicol* 1988;3:418.
13. Kuteifan K, Oesterele H, Tajahmady T, et al. Necrosis and haemorrhage of the putamen in methanol poisoning shown on MRI. *Neuroradiology* 1998;40:158.
14. Makar AB, Tephly TR, Mannering GJ. Methanol metabolism in the monkey. *Mol Pharmacol* 1968;4:471.
15. Martinasevic MK, Green MD, Baron J, et al. Folate and 10-formyltetrahydrofolate dehydrogenase in human and rat retina: relation to methanol toxicity. *Toxicol Appl Pharmacol* 1996;141:373.
16. McKellar MJ, Hidajat RR, Elder MJ. Acute ocular methanol toxicity: clinical and electrophysiological features. *Aust N Z J Ophthalmol* 1997;25:225.
17. Osterloh JD, Pond SM, Grady S, et al. Serum formate concentrations in methanol intoxication as criterion for hemodialysis. *Ann Intern Med* 1986;104:200.
18. Roe O. The metabolism and toxicity of methanol. *Pharmacol Rev* 1955;7:399.
19. Roe O. Species differences in methanol poisonings. *CRC Crit Rev Toxicol* 1982;10:275.

CHAPTER 352
Methemoglobinemia

Steven C. Curry and David A. Tanen

Reduced hemoglobin (deoxyhemoglobin) normally contains four heme groups, each with a ferrous (Fe^{2+}) ion capable of binding oxygen. Oxidative stress within the red cell produces methemoglobinemia, Heinz body hemolysis, or both. When the iron in reduced hemoglobin is oxidized to the ferric state (Fe^{3+}), methemoglobin is formed. The oxidation of protein in hemoglobin results in denaturation of protein, splenic sequestration of damaged erythrocytes, and hemolysis. Denatured erythrocytic protein can easily be visualized as Heinz bodies by using specialized staining.

Under normal conditions, methemoglobin levels are less than 1% to 2% of total heme pigments.[12] Higher fractions are termed *methemoglobinemia*.

Oxyhemoglobin is red, but methemoglobin is dark brown and cannot transport oxygen, resulting in a functional anemia. Also, the presence of ferric heme groups impairs the unloading of oxygen by oxygenated (ferrous) heme, producing a leftward shift in the oxyhemoglobin dissociation curve.[3,12] The physiologic consequences of methemoglobinemia are thus due to decreased tissue oxygenation.

The production of cyanosis requires 5 g/dL blood of reduced hemoglobin, but only 1.5 g/dL of methemoglobin produces noticeable discoloration. In the nonanemic patient, 10% to 20% methemoglobinemia produces asymptomatic cyanosis. Headache, dyspnea on exertion, tachypnea, tachycardia, and mild hypertension can be noted with methemoglobin levels of 15% to 35%. Higher fractions can result in confusion, coma, seizures, apnea, ventricular dysrhythmias, bradyarrhythmias, hypotension, and lactic acidosis. Death is frequently seen with methemoglobin fractions above 70%.

What can be confusing is an arterial blood gas report of a normal Po_2 *and* a normal percentage of oxyhemoglobin (percentage saturation) despite cyanosis. This is because most blood gas instruments do not measure oxyhemoglobin fractions, but only calculate and report what the percentage hemoglobin saturation should be, assuming the absence of methemoglobin, carboxyhemoglobin, and sulfhemoglobin, and assuming no shift in the dissociation curve from changes in erythrocytic 2,3-diphosphoglycerate concentrations.

A co-oximeter is needed to measure true percentage saturation and other hemoglobin pigments. Co-oximeters most commonly used in hospitals can measure and report the total hemoglobin concentration as well as percentages of oxyhemoglobin, methemoglobin, and carboxyhemoglobin in less than 2 minutes. Sulfhemoglobin is usually recognized as methemoglobin by these instruments. The difference between the percentage of hemoglobin saturation calculated by the blood gas analyzer and the saturation measured by the co-oximeter is called the *saturation gap*. A large saturation gap in arterial blood is almost always due to carboxyhemoglobin or methemoglobin. To interpret blood gas reports accurately, the emergency physician must know whether reported percentage saturations on arterial blood gas samples are determined by co-oximetry.

Hyperlipemia, such as that seen after infusions of lipid emulsions (e.g., Intralipid, Liposyn) or in patients with diabetes mellitus, interferes with the measurement of hemoglobin pigments by co-oximeters, resulting in falsely elevated methemoglobin concentrations.[13] Total blood and plasma free hemoglobin concentrations also can be falsely elevated in patients with lipemic plasma or serum. In these instances, the patient with a normal hemoglobin concentration and without cyanosis does not have serious methemoglobinemia.

Methemoglobinemia does not affect the measurement of hemoglobin concentration, such as in a complete blood count or hemogram. Pulse oximeters (e.g., ear or finger oximeters) usually measure only oxyhemoglobin and deoxyhemoglobin. They do not predictably or accurately recognize the presence of methemoglobin or carboxyhemoglobin. Therefore, a pulse oximeter can report a falsely normal percentage hemoglobin oxygen saturation in the presence of methemoglobinemia or carboxyhemoglobinemia.[8]

If accurate determination of methemoglobin concentration by co-oximetry is unavailable, a drop of the patient's blood can be placed on filter paper and allowed to dry. If the blood appears obviously brown, as compared with a drop of blood from a healthy person, then a level of at least 15% methemoglobin is present, assuming a normal total hemoglobin concentration.[3] Furthermore, venous blood from a healthy person becomes bright red when shaken in the air as oxyhemoglobin is formed. Venous blood that contains elevated methemoglobin concentrations remains dark brown after shaking.

Besides determining the methemoglobin fraction, the physician should also seek evidence of hemolysis.[2,14] Heinz bodies usually are not visible on a normal Wright stain of blood and can be seen only with special staining. Therefore, a hemoglobin–hematocrit, Heinz body stain, and plasma free hemoglobin concentration should be ordered.

Because hemoglobin is slowly oxidized to methemoglobin under normal conditions, the erythrocyte contains enzymes that can catalyze the reduction of methemoglobin back to reduced hemoglobin (Fig. 352.1). More than 95% of methemoglobin reduction is accomplished by the transfer of electrons from NADH (the reduced form of nicotinamide-adenine dinucleotide, which is generated in glycolysis) to cytochrome-b_5 and then to methemoglobin by way of the enzyme variously known as NADH-dependent methemoglobin reductase, diaphorase I, and, most recently, NADH cytochrome-b_5 reductase (EC 1.6.2.2).[6,12]

In normal persons, enzymatic reduction of methemoglobin occurs at a rate 200- to 300-fold greater than its spontaneous formation. However, congenital deficiencies in NADH cytochrome-b_5 reductase[12] or in cytochrome-b_5 itself[6] can cause methemoglobinemia, or can greatly predispose a person to developing methemoglobinemia after exposure to methemoglobin-producing agents. Neonates, especially those with a metabolic acidosis,[15] are at increased risk for developing methemoglobinemia after oxidant stress (e.g., drugs, toxins, sepsis)

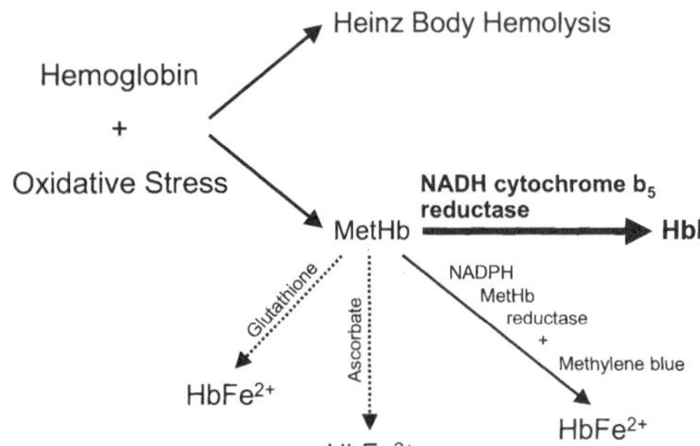

Figure 352.1. Pathways of hemoglobin oxidations and methemoglobin reduction.

because they have lower levels of NADH cytochrome-b_5 reductase and cytochrome-b_5.[3,6,12]

A second enzyme, NADPH (the reduced form of nicotinamide-adenine dinucleotide phosphate) methemoglobin reductase, can facilitate the reduction of methemoglobin by transferring electrons from NADPH (produced in the hexose monophosphate shunt) to an intermediate compound and then to methemoglobin.[3,12] There is apparently no endogenous cofactor for this enzyme; consequently, it has little or no physiologic role in maintaining methemoglobin levels at low concentrations. However, exogenously administered methylene blue can act as an intermediate for electron transfer and greatly increase the activity of this enzyme. People with depressed levels of erythrocytic NADPH (e.g., glucose-6-phosphate dehydrogenase [G6PD] deficiency) or a congenital lack of the NADPH-dependent reducing enzyme do not normally suffer from and are not predisposed to developing methemoglobinemia. If they do develop methemoglobinemia, however, treatment with methylene blue is ineffective and can even trigger massive hemolysis in those with G6PD deficiency.[11]

Exposure to a variety of agents may result in acquired methemoglobinemia (Table 352.1). Not all of the compounds are direct oxidants, implying that their metabolites or oxidizing intermediates (e.g., free radicals) are responsible for producing methemoglobin in some cases. The most commonly reported therapeutic agents that cause methemoglobinemia are local anesthetics, nitroglycerin, phenazopyridine (Pyridium), and diaminodiphenylsulfone (dapsone).[3,4] Local anesthetics injected or applied topically (e.g., infant teething ointments) are well-documented causes of methemoglobinemia. Aniline and related aromatic amines are potent inducers of methemoglobinemia. The conversion of nitrates to nitrites by bacteria in the gastrointestinal (GI) tract has resulted in fatal methemoglobinemia in infants who ingested well water high in nitrates. Bacteria colonizing burn wounds treated with silver nitrate have been reported to oxidize nitrate to nitrite and produce methemoglobinemia.[3] The recreational use of inhalable nitrites such as isobutyl nitrite has resulted in large numbers of casualties.[7] With toxins such as chlorates and arsine, massive hemolysis can be as detrimental as the methemoglobinemia, or more so.[2,14]

TABLE 352.1. Some Methemoglobin-Producing Agents

Acetanalid	Aminophenols	Amyl nitrite
Aniline dyes	Arsine	Aniline
Chlorates	Chlorobenzene	Benzocaine
Dapsone	Dinitrophenol	Bismuth sulfate
Food additives	Hydrazines	Chromates
Inks	Isobutyl nitrite	Commercial marking crayons[a]
Local anesthetics	Methylene blue	Dinitrotoluene
Mushrooms	Metoclopramide	Flutamide
Nitrites	Naphthylamines	Hydroxylamine
Pamaquine	Nitrobenzene	Lidocaine
Phenylazopyridine	Phenacetin	Naphthalene
Prilocaine	Phenylenediamine	Nitrates
Quinones	Primaquine	Nitric oxide
Sulfonamides	Silver nitrate	Nitroglycerin
Trinitrotoluene	Sulfones	Phenols
		Plasmoquine
		Pyridine
		Shoe dye or polish
		Toluidine

[a] Children's crayons no longer contain methemoglobin-producing dyes. Commercial marking crayons may still contain ingredients that produce methemoglobinemia.

CLINICAL PRESENTATION

Nonanemic patients with 10% to 20% methemoglobinemia usually present with unexplained cyanosis and no other symptoms. Headache, dyspnea on exertion, tachypnea, tachycardia, and mild hypertension can be noted with methemoglobin levels of 15% to 35%. Higher fractions can result in confusion, coma, seizures, apnea, ventricular dysrhythmias, bradyarrhythmias, hypotension, and lactic acidosis. Death is frequently seen with methemoglobin fractions above 70%.

Patients with underlying cardiovascular or cerebrovascular disease are more susceptible to the effects of hypoxia. Those with preexisting anemia or with concomitant Heinz body hemolytic anemia suffer greater toxicity at a given methemoglobin level, because the remaining functional hemoglobin concentration is lower. Also, cyanosis is not apparent until a greater percentage of methemoglobin is present, as compared with the nonanemic patient. Hence, anemic patients can suffer from significant methemoglobinemia without exhibiting cyanosis.

The cyanosis of methemoglobinemia is refractory to the administration of oxygen and is present despite a normal or elevated arterial Po_2. A metabolic acidosis develops with severely compromised oxygen delivery to tissues. Pink plasma from hemoglobinemia may be noted in severe cases of hemolysis. The electrocardiogram (ECG) may reveal tachycardia, bradycardia, ventricular dysrhythmias, and changes suggestive of myocardial ischemia.

DIFFERENTIAL DIAGNOSIS

Cyanosis due to methemoglobinemia may be differentiated from that due to hypoxia by the presence of a normal Po_2 and by the fact that it is unresponsive to oxygen. A peculiar and poorly characterized cyanosis may also be seen in some cases of hydrogen sulfide or tellurium poisoning. Both carbon monoxide and sulfhemoglobinemia produce a noticeable saturation gap with a normal arterial Po_2. Sulfhemoglobinemia, a rare cause of cyanosis, causes noticeable discoloration at only 0.5 g/dL blood. Most co-oximeters measure sulfhemoglobin as methemoglobin. Fortunately, sulfhemoglobin is rarely (if ever) severe enough to cause life-threatening symptoms. Topical contact with blue dyes (e.g., new towels or clothing) may cause blue skin. Generalized discoloration from excessive administration of methylene blue may also be confused with cyanosis.[5]

EMERGENCY DEPARTMENT EVALUATION

A careful history should be taken from the patient and family regarding medications, occupational exposures to chemicals, family history of methemoglobinemia, recreational drug use, and, in the case of children, any substances in the house that could have been ingested. The physical examination should focus on vital signs, skin color, and any evidence of dysfunction of the central nervous system or cardiovascular system. Laboratory studies should include a complete blood count, arterial blood gas analysis, urinalysis, ECG, a blood methemoglobin concentration or oxygen saturation measured by co-oximetry, Heinz body stain of peripheral blood, plasma free hemoglobin, and serum haptoglobin, electrolytes, blood urea nitrogen, and serum creatinine, and glucose. A bedside screening test for methemoglobin may also be helpful.

EMERGENCY DEPARTMENT MANAGEMENT

Patients with methemoglobinemia should be placed on oxygen to maximize the oxygen-carrying capacity of normal hemoglobin. Intravenous access should be established, and the patient should be placed on a cardiac monitor.

Most patients are blue but asymptomatic and do not require treatment.[3] Once exposure to the offending agent is terminated, methemoglobin levels usually return to normal within 12 to 36 hours. Patients with symptoms unrelieved by oxygen, those with methemoglobin fractions above 30%, those with ECG changes, or those with a metabolic acidosis should receive antidotal therapy with methylene blue, provided there is no history of G6PD deficiency. Methylene blue is usually available as a 1% solution (10 mg/mL) and should be given intravenously over 3 to 5 minutes at an initial dose of 2 mg/kg (0.2 mL/kg of a 1% solution).[3] A dramatic response with resolution of cyanosis is usually noted within 15 minutes, although more time is sometimes required. If the patient is seriously symptomatic and no response is noted within 15 minutes, or if the patient remains moderately symptomatic after 15 to 30 minutes, repeat doses of 1 mg/kg (0.1 mL/kg of 1% solution) can be given. If methemoglobin levels are readily available, repeat determinations of methemoglobin concentration should be performed before repeat doses of methylene blue are given, because large doses of methylene blue themselves can cause discoloration of skin.[3,5] The total dose of methylene blue during the first 2 to 3 hours should not exceed 5 to 7 mg/kg.[3]

Adverse effects of methylene blue include dysuria, substernal chest pain, and anxiety.[10] Urine frequently turns blue and then green as the drug is excreted. Single doses of methylene blue as low as 5 mg/kg can cause methemoglobinemia in animals.[9]

Methylene blue should never be given to patients with G6PD deficiency. Such patients have low erythrocytic NADPH concentrations, making augmentation of the NADPH-dependent, methemoglobin-reducing enzyme by methylene blue impossible. More important, methylene blue can trigger massive hemolysis in such patients, further compromising oxygen delivery to tissues.[11] About 15% of African American males are thought to be deficient in G6PD; men and women of Mediterranean ancestry also have an increased incidence of this enzyme deficiency.

As soon as time allows, GI and skin decontamination should be performed to limit continued absorption of the offending agent. Decontamination is particularly important after acute dermal exposures to chemicals or after intentional ingestions of toxic agents. Dermal decontamination can be performed with a triple wash (water rinse, soap scrub, water rinse). GI decontamination is discussed in Chapter 309.

If the drug or chemical causing methemoglobinemia cannot be readily eliminated from the body (e.g., dapsone), methemoglobinemia may continually recur for hours or days after successful treatment with methylene blue. In this instance, serial measurements of methemoglobin levels are required, and a constant intravenous infusion of methylene blue at a rate of 0.1 mg/kg/h has been used successfully to maintain methemoglobin concentrations at a safe level.[1] Repeated oral doses of activated charcoal also enhance the elimination of dapsone. High-dose intravenous cimetidine has been shown to lessen dapsone-induced methemoglobin production. Renal failure is a relative contraindication to using a constant infusion or frequently repeated doses of methylene blue, because the drug is mainly excreted by the kidneys.

Treatment with hyperbaric oxygen or exchange transfusions should be considered for patients with G6PD deficiency or for those who do not respond satisfactorily to methylene blue. Hyperbaric oxygenation can provide enough dissolved oxygen to support life in the presence of 100% methemoglobinemia.

Symptomatic hemolytic anemia may require treatment with blood transfusions. Because massive hemolysis may cause hyperkalemia and acute renal failure, efforts should be made to maintain a good rate of urine flow.

Ascorbic acid also reduces methemoglobin to hemoglobin (nonenzymatically). A dose of 0.5 to 1.0 g ascorbic acid every 6 hours may be given intravenously or orally in conjunction with methylene blue. However, ascorbic acid works too slowly to be useful in the treatment of acute, acquired methemoglobinemia.[3]

DISPOSITION

Patients with methemoglobinemia should be admitted after emergency department evaluation and management. Patients are best managed at a facility where methemoglobin concentrations can be measured easily and quickly. Physicians unfamiliar with the management of methemoglobinemia should consult a toxicologist or hematologist or the regional poison center. If transfer is necessary, advanced life-support services should be provided and should include a supply of methylene blue, if available. In the case of an accidental or intentional poisoning, the physician must evaluate and treat other toxic effects of methemoglobin-producing agents. All patients who receive methylene blue should be observed for recurrence of symptomatic methemoglobinemia and for adverse effects such as hemolysis.

An asymptomatic and otherwise healthy patient who has been cyanotic for several days while taking therapeutic doses of an offending drug does not necessarily require admission if the total hemoglobin concentration is normal (e.g., no significant hemolysis), the methemoglobin level is below 20%, exposure to the offending agent is terminated, and reliable follow-up is available. Methemoglobin concentrations will return to normal in these patients as the offending drug is cleared from the body. A wise and conservative approach would be to admit all young children and elderly patients for observation, serial methemoglobin concentrations, and, when indicated, serial ECGs.

Any patient who unexpectedly develops methemoglobinemia after ingestion of therapeutic doses of drugs should be referred to a hematologist for evaluation of possible heterozygous NADH cytochrome-b_5 reductase deficiency. Any patient with methemoglobinemia that is unresponsive to treatment with methylene blue should be evaluated, after full recovery, for G6PD deficiency or, much less commonly, NADPH methemoglobin reductase deficiency.

COMMON PITFALLS

- Failing to consider the diagnosis of methemoglobinemia in patients with cyanosis unresponsive to oxygen
- Failing to appreciate that a normal arterial Po_2 and normal oxygen saturation (as measured by pulse oximetry or calculated from arterial blood gases) do not rule out methemoglobinemia
- Failing to appreciate that symptomatic methemoglobinemia may be present in the anemic patient despite lack of cyanosis
- Failing to evaluate for Heinz body hemolytic anemia in patients with methemoglobinemia
- Giving methylene blue to asymptomatic patients who are suffering from mild methemoglobinemia or to patients with G6PD deficiency
- Failing to evaluate and treat other toxic effects produced by agents that cause methemoglobinemia

- Failing to recognize that resolution of cyanosis in a patient with methemoglobinemia may be due to accompanying hemolysis, with actual worsening of oxygen delivery to tissues

References

1. Berlin G, Brodin B, Hilden J-O. Acute dapsone intoxication: a case treated with continuous infusion of methylene blue, forced diuresis, and plasma exchange. *J Toxicol Clin Toxicol* 1985;22:537.
2. Chan TK, Mak LW, Ng RP. Methemoglobinemia Heinz bodies and acute massive intravascular hemolysis in Lysol poisoning. *Blood* 1971;38:739.
3. Curry S. Methemoglobinemia. *Ann Emerg Med* 1982;11:214.
4. Gibson GR, Hunter JB, Raabe DS, et al. Methemoglobinemia produced by high-dose intravenous nitroglycerin. *Ann Intern Med* 1982;96:615.
5. Goluboff N, Wheaton R. Methylene blue-induced cyanosis and acute hemolytic anemia complicating the treatment of methemoglobinemia. *J Pediatr* 1961;58:86.
6. Hegesh E, Hegesh J, Kaftory A. Congenital methemoglobinemia with a deficiency of cytochrome b_5. *N Engl J Med* 1986;314:757.
7. Horne MK III, Waterman MR, Garriott JC, et al. Methemoglobinemia from sniffing butyl nitrite. *Ann Intern Med* 1982;91:417.
8. Kulick RM. Pulse oximetry. *Pediatr Emerg Care* 1987;3:127.
9. Lovejoy FH. Methemoglobinemia. *Clin Toxicol Rev* 1984;6:1.
10. Nadler JE, Green H, Rosenbaum A. Intravenous injection of methylene blue in man with reference to its toxic symptoms and effect on the ECG. *Am J Med Sci* 1934;188:15.
11. Rosen PJ, Johnson C, McGehee WG, et al. Failure of methylene blue treatment in toxic methemoglobinemia; association with glucose-6-phosphate dehydrogenase deficiency. *Ann Intern Med* 1971;75:83.
12. Schwartz JM, Reiss AL, Jaffe ER. Hereditary methemoglobinemia with deficiency of NADH cytochrome b_5 reductase. In: Stanbury JB, Wyngaarden JB, Fredrickson DS, et al., eds. *The metabolic basis of inherited disease,* 5th ed. New York: McGraw-Hill, 1983.
13. Spurzem JR, Bonekat HW, Shigeoka JW. Factitious methemoglobinemia caused by hyperlipemia. *Chest* 1984;86:84.
14. Teunis BS, Leftwich El, Pierce LA. Acute methemoglobinemia and hemolytic anemia due to toluidine blue. *Arch Surg* 1971;101:527.
15. Yano SS, Danish EH, Hsia YE. Transient methemoglobinemia with acidosis in infants. *J Pediatr* 1982;100:415.

CHAPTER 353
Methylxanthine Poisoning

Pierre Gaudreault

Methylxanthines, methylated derivatives of xanthine, include theophylline, caffeine, diphylline, pentoxifylline, and theobromine. Theophylline (1,3-dimethylxanthine) is used to treat asthma, apnea of premature infants, and chronic obstructive pulmonary disease (COPD), and as an analgesic adjunct. It is available as anhydrous theophylline or as a variety of salts (Table 353.1). Aminophylline is theophylline ethylenediamine, and oxtriphylline is 7-choline theophyllinate. Available formulations include intravenous solutions of aminophylline and suspensions, capsules, tablets, and sustained-release formulations for oral use. Therapeutic oral doses range from 13 to 24 mg/kg/d, usually administered in divided doses.

Caffeine (1,3,7-trimethylxanthine) is a naturally occurring alkaloid contained in beverages such as coffee (60 to 180 mg/5 oz), tea (20 to 60 mg/5 oz), chocolate milk (2 to 7 mg/8 oz), and cola soft drinks (45 mg/12 oz) and in chocolate candy bars (7 mg per bar). It is also contained in analgesic preparations and over-the-counter diet and stimulant ("wake-up" or "stay awake" pills) formulations in doses of 15 to 100 mg. Street-drug capsules that contain caffeine, phenylpropanolamine, and ephedrine are sold as stimulants. These products are called "look-alikes" because they are usually prepared to resemble prescription amphetamines.[9] Since 1983, it has been illegal in the United States to market products that contain combinations of caffeine and ephedrine, pseudoephedrine, or phenylpropanolamine.

TABLE 353.1. Theophylline Salts

Drug	Anhydrous Theophylline (%)
Aminophylline, anhydrous	84–86
Aminophylline, dihydrate	78–82
Oxtriphylline	62–66
Theophylline calcium salicylate	48–50
Theophylline monohydrate	91
Theophylline olamine	73–75
Theophylline sodium acetate	55–65
Theophylline sodium glycinate	49

Methylxanthines are rapidly absorbed after ingestion, with peak blood levels occurring in 1 to 2 hours. With sustained-release preparations, peak levels are maintained for 6 to 24 hours. Absorption is prolonged, and peak blood levels are delayed after overdosage, particularly with sustained-release preparations. Theophylline is 60% protein-bound, and caffeine is 35% protein-bound, mainly to albumin. Protein binding decreases with acidemia (resulting in increased free drug) and increases with alkalemia. The volume of distribution averages 0.5 L/kg (range, 0.3 to 0.7 L/kg) for theophylline and 0.4 L/kg for caffeine. Therapeutic serum levels are 10 to 20 μg/mL. Caffeine levels ranging from 12 to 36 μg/mL are effective in preventing neonatal apnea, but levels are only 3 to 10 μg/mL following usual adult doses.

Theophylline is eliminated by hepatic metabolism (90%) and urinary excretion of unchanged drug (10%). The half-life is age-dependent and influenced by concomitant drug therapy and illnesses. It averages 20 hours in newborns, 6 to 7 hours in infants, 3 to 5 hours in ages 6 months to 18 years, and 4 to 6 hours for adults. Hepatic elimination is increased by beta agonists, smoking, rifampin, and antiepileptic drugs (carbamazepine, phenobarbital, and phenytoin) and is decreased by allopurinol, beta blockers (nonselective), calcium channel blockers, cimetidine, congestive heart failure, fever, influenza virus vaccine, interferon, liver disease, macrolide antibiotics, mexiletine, oral contraceptives, and quinolones. Active metabolites include 3-methylxanthine, caffeine, and theobromine. Metabolism is saturable at serum theophylline levels near or above 20 μg/mL, resulting in a prolonged half-life after overdose. Metabolites may also contribute to overdose toxicity. The kinetics of caffeine are similar, with half-lives ranging from 2 to 12 hours in infants, children, and adults. In newborns, the half-life of caffeine is about 4 days, because up to 85% is excreted unchanged in the urine.

Therapeutic, adverse, and toxic effects of methylxanthines are due to the inhibition of adenosine synthesis, resulting in central nervous system (CNS) stimulation, reduction of the ventricular fibrillation threshold, smooth muscle relaxation, and gastric acid and pepsin secretion. Cardiovascular effects also result from epinephrine and norepinephrine release (low theophylline concentrations) and inhibition of phosphodiesterase, leading to increased cyclic adenosine and guanosine monophosphate (high theophylline concentrations).[10] Tachydysrhythmias may result from a decrease of the ventricular fibrillation threshold, a nonuniform increase in the cardiac conduction velocity that favors reentry phenomena, and the liberation of catecholamine. Hypokalemia and a reduced oxygen delivery in the face of increased demand by the myocardium seen with theophylline overdoses might also be contributory. Caffeine, the most potent CNS stimulant of the methylxanthines, stimulates the cortex (increases alertness and enhances performance), increases the spontaneous activity of the reticular formation and directly stimulates the respiratory center located in the medulla, and increases its sensitivity to the stimulatory effects of carbon dioxide. Theophylline and caffeine cause peripheral vasodilation, yet cerebral vasoconstriction. The latter effect may be involved in the pathogenesis of CNS toxicity.

Poisoning may result from chronic (therapeutic) oral overdose, acute ingestion of more than 10 mg/kg, or excessive intravenous dosing. The chronic use of caffeine can lead to a dependence syndrome. Abrupt withdrawal in dependent persons is characterized by headache, lethargy, and depression.

CLINICAL PRESENTATION

Initial symptoms of poisoning include nausea, vomiting, and abdominal pain. Diarrhea and gastrointestinal (GI) bleeding may develop later. Spontaneous vomiting may limit drug absorption, especially with caffeine ingestions. However, serum drug levels may continue to rise despite vomiting, particularly when sustained-release preparations have been ingested. Additional signs and symptoms may include headache, insomnia, agitation, delirium, tinnitus, tremors, motor hyperactivity and hypertonicity, jitteriness, hyperventilation, polyuria, seizures, coma, GI bleeding, hyperthermia, and ventricular and supraventricular tachyarrhythmias.[1,10,16,19] At low doses, theophylline induces a mild and transitory hypertension. At high doses, the direct effect of theophylline on the beta-2 adrenoreceptors reduces the total peripheral resistance, inducing hypotension. This may partly explain why hypotension is seen with acute, but not chronic, overdose. Laboratory evaluation may reveal leukocytosis, hyperglycemia, hypokalemia, hypophosphatemia, ketosis, metabolic acidosis, and respiratory alkalosis.[10,16,17] Decreased serum calcium and magnesium levels, elevated serum amylase and uric acid levels, and evidence of dehydration (elevated blood urea nitrogen and creatinine levels) or rhabdomyolysis (elevated creatine phosphokinase level and myoglobinuria) may be noted.[20]

The risk of tachydysrhythmias depends on the duration of exposure, drug concentration, and age. After an acute overdose (single ingestion), patients aged 6 months to 60 years may develop life-threatening dysrhythmias or seizures when serum concentrations exceed 80 μg/mL.[10] For the same age group, serious toxic manifestations can occur with serum concentrations above 60 μg/mL with chronic intoxication. Patients younger than age 6 months or older than age 60 years may experience serious toxic manifestations with serum concentrations above 30 μg/mL, regardless of the type of intoxication. Patients over age 40 are at risk of developing serious cardiac dysrhythmias when serum concentrations are above 35 μg/mL. In contrast, serum concentrations higher than 50 μg/mL are necessary to induce serious arrhythmias in younger patients (age 40 or less).[12]

Seizures are usually generalized but can be focal. The neurotoxicity of theophylline seems to be dose-dependent, but other factors also influence the development of neurotoxicity. Indeed, patients younger than age 6 months or older than age 60 years who are chronically intoxicated or have a history of neurologic problems (e.g., seizures, cerebrovascular insufficiency) are at greater risk of seizing.[8,16] Permanent neurologic damage (e.g., encephalopathy) is not uncommon in patients with prolonged coma or intractable seizures and appears to correlate with their duration.

DIFFERENTIAL DIAGNOSIS

Because the clinical effects of methylxanthine poisoning can be characterized as a "beta-adrenergic storm," poisoning by direct-acting beta agonists (e.g., albuterol and related bronchodilators, terbutaline) can cause an indistinguishable clinical picture. Poisoning by amphetamines, sympathomimetics, anticholinergics, hallucinogens, monoamine oxidase inhibitors, and epinephrine should also be considered in the differential diagnosis. Agitated psychiatric states, drug withdrawal, and medical conditions such as CNS infection, electrolyte disturbance, hypoglycemia, hypocalcemia, pheochromocytoma, and thyroid storm may cause similar signs and symptoms.

EMERGENCY DEPARTMENT EVALUATION

The history should include the time, amount, and formulation of theophylline or caffeine ingested; past or recent therapeutic use of these agents; and routine medical history. Symptoms before arrival should be noted. The maximum possible serum drug level (micrograms per milliliter) can be estimated by doubling the acutely ingested dose (milligrams per kilogram).

The physical examination should focus on vital signs, mental status and neurologic evaluation, cardiorespiratory status, and GI function. Vomitus and stool should be checked for overt or occult blood. Laboratory evaluation should include a quantitative theophylline or caffeine level; complete blood count; determination of electrolyte, glucose, blood urea nitrogen, and creatinine levels; and urinalysis. Drug levels should be repeated every 2 to 4 hours following acute ingestions, until the level is no longer rising. Patients with elevated theophylline levels and moderate or severe clinical toxicity should also have measurements of serum amylase, calcium, creatine phosphokinase, ketones, magnesium, and phosphorus levels, urine myoglobin, and arterial blood gas analysis.

Cardiac monitoring and an electrocardiogram (ECG) should be obtained on all patients. Patients with respiratory symptoms, an abnormal pulmonary examination or ECG, or coma or seizures should have a chest radiograph.

EMERGENCY DEPARTMENT MANAGEMENT

Advanced life-support measures are instituted, as necessary. Activated charcoal significantly reduces the absorption of theophylline and is the preferred method of GI decontamination. The repetitive administration of activated charcoal also enhances the total body clearance of theophylline.[3] The effects of charcoal on the absorption and elimination of other methylxanthines are predicted to be similar. Because serum concentrations may not peak for many hours after ingestion (up to 24 hours with slow-release preparations), every patient with an oral theophylline overdose should receive activated charcoal, regardless of the alleged time of ingestion. A dose of 0.5 to 1.0 g/kg of body weight should be given every 2 to 4 hours until drug levels are in the therapeutic range. If the patient cannot tolerate charcoal because of persistent vomiting, the administration of smaller but more frequent doses (by continuous infusion by way of nasogastric tube, if necessary), metoclopramide (up to 10 mg), ranitidine (50 mg intravenously), droperidol (2.5 mg intravenously), or odensatron (8 to 32 mg intravenously) may be used.[2,11]

Gastric drug bezoar has been reported after sustained-release theophylline overdose.[4] Endoscopic evaluation and drug mass removal, if necessary, should be considered in patients with rising drug levels and severe poisoning. Although often recommended, whole-bowel irrigation did not add to the benefit of multiple-dose activated charcoal in an experimental sustained-release theophylline overdose.[7]

Seizures should be treated aggressively. A benzodiazepine (e.g., diazepam, lorazepam, midazolam) should be given first. If the seizures do not stop rapidly or if they recur, phenobarbital (15 to 20 mg/kg) should be administered intravenously. If seizures do not stop within 20 to 30 minutes, thiopental should be given; a loading dose of 3 to 5 mg/kg, followed by an infusion of 2 to 4 mg/kg/h is usually efficacious, but these doses can be increased, if necessary. Phenytoin unlikely to be effective.[6] Neuromuscular paralysis (e.g., pancuronium) may be necessary to stop muscle contractions, facilitate ventilation, and prevent hyperthermia and rhabdomyolysis. Electroencephalographic monitoring and continued treatment of seizures are necessary during paralysis. Treatment should also include correction of accompanying acidemia, as this may promote dysrhythmias.

Propranolol is the drug of choice to treat supraventricular and ventricular arrhythmias after acute overdose. Intravenous doses of 1 mg in adults or 0.02 mg/kg in children should be given slowly and repeated every 5 to 10 minutes until dysrhythmias stop, or to a maximal dose of 0.1 mg/kg.[5] Lidocaine may also be used for ventricular dysrhythmias. Although propranolol is normally contraindicated in patients with asthma or COPD, it has been used without adverse effects in asthmatics with acute theophylline poisoning. In such patients, the short-acting beta antagonist esmolol has been used.[15] However, because esmolol is selective for beta-1 receptors, it could theoretically worsen hypotension resulting from beta-2 stimulation. Propranolol may also be effective in treating theophylline-induced seizures.[14] Clinical evidence of bronchospasm is an absolute contraindication to the use of beta blockers. In patients with atrial tachyarrhythmias exacerbated by theophylline intoxication, verapamil has been effective.[11] Correction of hypoxemia, acidemia, hypokalemia, and other metabolic abnormalities is also important. Because hypokalemia is due to an intracellular shift of potassium rather than a total body deficit, overly aggressive therapy for this condition may result in hyperkalemia as toxicity resolves and should be avoided. Hyperglycemia is transitory and well tolerated and usually does not necessitate insulin therapy.

Hypotension is initially treated with fluid administration. Persistent hypotension may be treated with pressors (e.g., dopamine and norepinephrine) or propranolol (because of its beta-2 blocking effect).[5] Hyperthermia and rhabdomyolysis should be treated with standard measures.

Charcoal hemoperfusion can enhance the elimination of theophylline and should be considered for patients with the following criteria: persistently unstable hemodynamic parameters; seizures; or theophylline serum concentrations above 80 to 100 μg/mL after an acute ingestion, above 60 μg/mL after chronic ingestion, and above 40 μg/mL after an acute or chronic intoxication if age is less than 6 months or above 60 years or there is severe underlying cardiovascular disease.[10–12,18] Similar parameters should be used in patients with caffeine poisoning.

Hemodialysis also enhances the elimination of theophylline and should be used if hemoperfusion is not immediately available. A tandem set-up (in-line hemodialysis and hemoperfusion) can be used for patients with severe metabolic abnormalities as well as high drug levels. Exchange transfusion has also been used in neonates with caffeine intoxication when hemoperfusion is technically difficult.[13]

DISPOSITION

Patients with a serum theophylline concentration above 35 μg/mL should be admitted to a monitored bed. Those with severe neurologic or cardiotoxic manifestations or serum concentrations above 50 μg/mL should be admitted to an intensive care unit. Those with levels under 35 μg/mL and mild symptoms can usually be treated in the emergency department and discharged when they become asymptomatic. A nephrologist should be consulted for patients who meet or are approaching criteria for extracorporeal elimination therapy. If intensive care unit and extracorporeal treatment are not available, the patient should be transferred to a facility with these capabilities.

COMMON PITFALLS

- Failure to consider the effects of age, underlying disease, and potential drug interactions on drug kinetics and dosing when prescribing theophylline
- Failure to appreciate that patients with chronic exposures develop toxicity at lower drug levels than those with acute or acute-on-chronic overdose
- Failure to consider the patient's age, the type of intoxication (acute vs. chronic), and underlying diseases (previous neurologic or cardiac problems) when interpreting theophylline serum concentrations
- Failure to appreciate that hypotension (not hypertension) is characteristic of severe, acute (but not chronic) caffeine or theophylline poisoning
- Failure to obtain serial theophylline levels to assess for delayed and prolonged absorption and to assess the results of treatment
- Failure to administer activated charcoal in single and multiple doses and to give antiemetics, if necessary
- Failure to treat seizures aggressively to prevent acidemia, hyperthermia, rhabdomyolysis, and permanent neurologic damage
- Failure to appreciate that beta blockers can reverse much of the toxicity caused by theophylline overdose but that the risks must be weighed against the benefits in patients with asthma or COPD
- Failure to consider enhanced elimination therapy with hemoperfusion or hemodialysis and to consult a nephrologist in patients with severe poisoning

References

1. Albert S. Aminophylline toxicity. *Pediatr Clin North Am* 1987;34:61.
2. Amitai Y, Yeung AC, Moye J, et al. Repetitive oral activated charcoal and control of emesis in severe theophylline toxicity. *Ann Intern Med* 1986;105:386.
3. Berlinger WG, Spector R, Goldberg MJ, et al. Enhancement of theophylline clearance by oral activated charcoal. *Clin Pharmacol Ther* 1983;33:351.
4. Bernstein G, Jehle D, Bernaski E, et al. Failure of gastric emptying and charcoal administration in fatal sustained-release theophylline overdose: pharmacobezoar formation. *Ann Emerg Med* 1992;21:1388.
5. Biberstein MP, Fiegler MG, Ward DM. Use of B-blockade and hemoperfusion for acute theophylline poisoning. *West J Med* 1984;141:485.
6. Blake KU, Massey KL, Hendeles L, et al. Relative efficacy of phenytoin and phenobarbital for the prevention of theophylline-induced seizures in mice. *Ann Emerg Med* 1988;17:1024.
7. Burkhart KK, Wuerz RC, Donovan JW. Whole bowel irrigation as adjunctive treatment for sustained-release theophylline overdose. *Ann Emerg Med* 1992;21:1316.
8. Covelli HD, Knodel AR, Heppner BT. Predisposing factors to apparent theophylline induced seizures. *Ann Allergy* 1985;54:411.
9. Garriott JC, Simmons LM, Poklis A, et al. Five cases of fatal overdose from caffeine-containing "look-alike" drugs. *J Anal Toxicol* 1985;9:141.
10. Gaudreault P, Guay J. Theophylline poisoning: pharmacological considerations and clinical management. *Med Toxicol* 1986;1:169.
11. Minton NA, Henry JA. Treatment of theophylline overdose. *Am J Emerg Med* 1996;14:606.
12. Olson KR, Benowitz NL, Woo OF, et al. Theophylline overdose: acute single ingestion versus chronic repeated overmedication. *Am J Emerg Med* 1985;3:386.
13. Perrin C, Debruyne D, Lacotte J, et al. Treatment of caffeine intoxication by exchange transfusion in a newborn. *Acta Paediatr Scand* 1987;76:679.
14. Schneider SM, Borok A, Michelson EA. Beta-blockade for acute theophylline-induced seizures. *Vet Hum Toxicol* 1987;29:451.

15. Seneff M, Scott J, Friedman B, et al. Acute theophylline toxicity and the use of esmolol to reverse cardiovascular instability. *Ann Emerg Med* 1990;19:671.
16. Sessler CN. Theophylline toxicity: clinical features of 116 consecutive cases. *Am J Med* 1990;88:567.
17. Shannon M. Hypokalemia, hyperglycemia, and plasma catecholamine activity after severe theophylline intoxication. *Clin Toxicol* 1994;32:41.
18. Shannon MW. Comparative efficacy of hemodialysis and hemoperfusion in severe theophylline intoxication. *Acad Emerg Med* 1997;4:674.
19. Shum S, Seale C, Hathaway D, et al. Acute caffeine ingestion fatalities: management issues. *Vet Hum Toxicol* 1997;39:228.
20. Wren K, Oschner I. Rhabdomyolysis induced by a caffeine overdose. *Ann Emerg Med* 1989;18:94.

CHAPTER 354
Monoamine Oxidase Inhibitor Poisoning

Michael J. Burns

The monoamine oxidase (MAO) inhibitors have been available for the treatment of major depression since the 1950s.[15] They were largely replaced by the less toxic tricyclic antidepressants in the 1970s.

Although effective, MAO inhibitors are infrequently prescribed because of their risk for producing dangerous food and drug interactions and serious toxicity following overdose. These agents are generally reserved for the management of atypical, drug-resistant, neurotic, and reactive depression. MAO inhibitors are also occasionally used to treat anxiety states, bulimia, hypertension, migraine headaches, narcolepsy, obsessive-compulsive disorder, Parkinson disease, and phobias. Newer selective, reversible inhibitors of MAO have a lower propensity for adverse effects and may lead to a resurgence of MAO inhibitor use.[1,4–7]

These agents block the oxidative deamination of endogenous and exogenous monoamines by means of MAO, a flavin-containing enzyme located in the outer mitochondrial membranes of most tissues.[15] Two subtypes of MAO exist (MAO-A and MAO-B), which differ in their substrate and inhibitor specificities and tissue distribution.[4,6,8,9,12,15,18] MAO-A is found in the brain (monoaminergic neurons), peripheral sympathetic postganglionic neurons, intestinal mucosa, and liver. MAO-B is located in the brain (glial cells and some serotonergic neurons), platelets, and liver, with smaller amounts in the intestinal mucosa.

Noradrenergic neurons contain predominantly MAO-A; serotonergic neurons contain both. Substrates primarily deaminated by MAO-A include epinephrine, metanephrine, norepinephrine (NE), and 5-hydroxytryptamine (5-HT, or serotonin). Substrates metabolized primarily by MAO-B include beta-phenylethylamine, methylhistamine, phenylethanolamine, and benzylamine. Many substrates are metabolized by both enzymes, including tyramine, dopamine (DA), octopamine, and tryptamine. Substrate specificity is not absolute and is primarily dependent on the relative concentrations of substrate and MAO subtype in a particular anatomic location. Inhibition of MAO-A is necessary for therapeutic efficacy in the treatment of depression.[15]

MAO enzymes function to maintain low body concentrations of monoamines.[4,6,15,18] Hepatic and intestinal MAOs prevent the absorption of and systemic effects from dietary monoamines (e.g., tyramine). Intraneuronal MAO maintains a low cytoplasmic concentration of monoamine neurotransmitters that allows for net reuptake and termination of effect of extracellular monoamines.[4,6,15] Glial cell MAO scavenges monoamines and prevents their accumulation within the central nervous system (CNS).[4,6]

All MAO inhibitors are false substrates for the MAO enzyme; they bind to the active site of MAO and prevent it from further activity.[1,15] MAO inhibitors may be classified by their differential selectivity for MAO subtypes, reversibility of MAO binding (inhibition), or by chemical structure (Table 354.1). The oldest MAO inhibitors in use are nonselective irreversible ("suicide") inactivators of MAO. Initially, they bind reversibly to the flavin active site of MAO but are subsequently oxidized to a reactive intermediate, which forms an irreversible covalent bond with the enzyme. New enzyme must be synthesized before the function of MAO returns to normal.

Currently, only irreversible inhibitors of MAO are available for clinical use in the United States. The nonselective inhibitors include isocarboxazid, phenelzine sulfate, and tranylcypromine sulfate. Procarbazine, an antitumor agent used primarily for patients with Hodgkin disease, also has weak MAO inhibitor activity. Selegiline, an inhibitor of MAO-B used to treat Parkinson disease, is the only selective inhibitor currently available in the United States.[8] It is not associated with dangerous food and drug interactions at doses used clinically. Its specificity for MAO-B, however, is dose-dependent and lost at supratherapeutic doses.[8]

More recently, reversible selective inhibitors of MAO-A (brofaromine, cimoxatone, moclobemide, and toloxatone), often termed *RIMAs,* have been developed and are used clinically

TABLE 354.1. Classification of Monoamine Oxidase Inhibitors

Agent (Trade Name)	Inhibition	Selectivity	Structure
Brofaromine	Reversible	MAO-A	Piperidine
Clorgyline	Irreversible	MAO-A	Amine
Iproniazid (Marsilid)	Irreversible	Nonselective	Hydrazine (Hydrazide)
Isocarboxazid (Marplan)	Irreversible	Nonselective	Hydrazine (Hydrazide)
Moclobemide (Aurorix)	Reversible	MAO-A	Benzamide
Nialamide	Irreversible	Nonselective	Hydrazine
Pargyline (Eutonyl)	Irreversible	MAO-B	Amine
Phenelzine (Nardil)	Irreversible	Nonselective	Hydrazine
Procarbazine (Matulane)	Irreversible	Nonselective	Hydrazine
Selegiline, deprenyl (Eldepryl)	Irreversible	MAO-B	Amine
Toloxatone (Humoryl)	Reversible	MAO-A	Benzamide
Tranylcypromine (Parnate)	Irreversible	Nonselective	Amine

outside the United States.[1,4–7] These agents bind competitively (with respect to natural amine substrate) and reversibly at the active site of MAO-A. MAO inhibition is short-lived (enzyme activity commonly restored within 24 hours) and may be overcome by increasing levels of amine substrate. Initial experience with these agents has demonstrated greater safety following overdose and a significant reduction of adverse effects when combined with other pharmaceutical agents or dietary amines.

MAO inhibitors have traditionally been classified by chemical structure into hydrazines (iproniazid, isocarboxazid, and phenelzine) and nonhydrazines (clorgyline, pargyline, selegiline, and tranylcypromine).[9,10,15] The hydrazine moiety imparts distinct pharmacologic and toxic effects to these agents (discussion follows). Structurally, most MAO inhibitors are similar to amphetamines and other sympathomimetic agents.[15] In fact, both selegiline and tranylcypromine are partly metabolized to amphetamine and methamphetamine.[8,10,13,15] This characteristic also accounts for additional pharmacologic activity.

MAO inhibitors exert their pharmacologic and toxic effects by increasing neuronal and synaptic concentrations of biogenic amines (see Figure 354.1).[6,14,15] By decreasing the degradation of MAO substrates, MAO inhibitors result in expansion of cytosolic and vesicular storage pools of NE, DA, and 5-HT in presynaptic nerve terminals. Increased presynaptic neurotransmitter

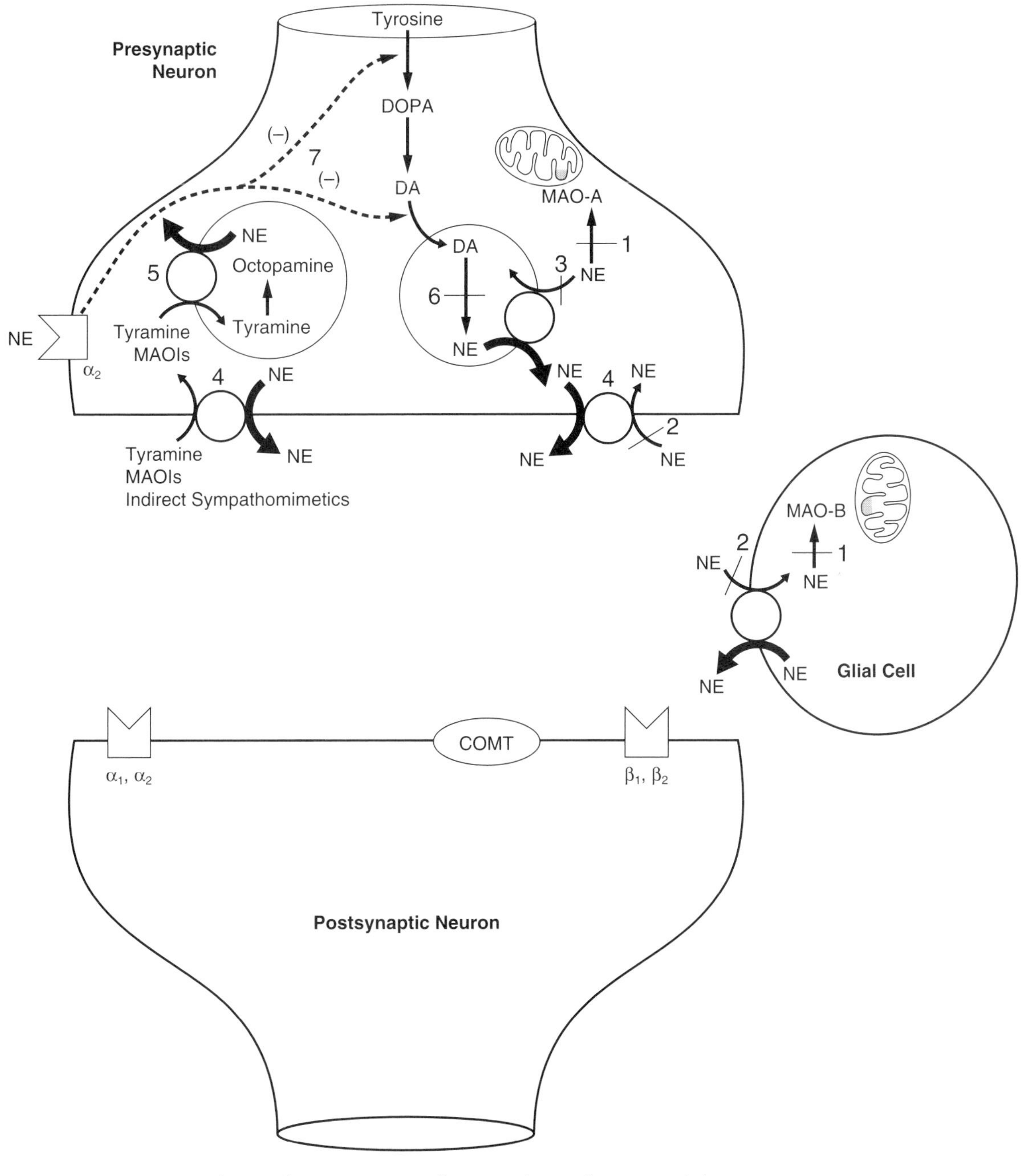

Figure 354.1. Diagram of a noradrenergic synapse illustrating the mechanisms underlying monoamine oxidase inhibitor (MAOI) toxicity: *(1)* Inhibit MAO to prevent nonephedrine (NE) degradation; *(2)* inhibit NE reuptake by monoamine transporter; *(3)* inhibit NE reuptake by vesicles; *(4)* promote reverse transport of NE from nerve ending; *(5)* promote reverse transport of NE from vesicles; *(6)* block dopamine (DA) beta-hydroxylase; *(7)* indirectly inhibit enzymes necessary for production of NE. Similar mechanisms operate at dopaminergic and serotonergic nerve endings. α and β refer to adrenergic receptors; COMT= catechol-O-methyltransferase, another enzyme that degrades catecholamines.

concentrations increase their quantal release from vesicles during normal neurotransmission, cause spontaneous spill-over into the synaptic cleft independent of nerve activity, and decrease concentration-dependent reuptake by nerve-ending amine transporters.[4,6,15,18] Spontaneous hypertensive episodes that occur in patients taking therapeutic doses of MAO inhibitors (in the absence of dietary indiscretions or drug interactions) likely result from the spontaneous release of NE from nerve terminals.[10,12,15,18]

As amphetamine congeners and indirect-acting sympathomimetics themselves, MAO inhibitors further enhance the release of cytoplasmic amines from the nerve ending in the absence of vesicle exocytosis.[6,10,15] They bind competitively to the amine uptake transporter and prevent reuptake of natural amine neurotransmitters. When the MAO inhibitor is transported into the neuron, reverse transport of cytosolic biogenic amines occurs that further increases their synaptic concentrations. MAO inhibitors similarly prevent uptake from glial cell transporters that scavenge extracellular (synaptic) monoamines.[4,6]

Overdose of MAO inhibitors produces an exaggeration of these neuronal effects and may result in profound hyperadrenergic, hyperdopaminergic, and hyperserotonergic states. The delayed appearance of signs and symptoms following overdose is attributed to initial reversible binding with MAO and the time required for significant enzyme inhibition and cumulative effects to occur (e.g., neuronal accumulation of NE, DA, 5-HT).[10,12] Although effects from NE and DA contribute significantly, the neuromuscular abnormalities (e.g., rigidity, myoclonus), hyperthermia, and unusual ocular movements associated with MAO overdose appear to be mediated primarily by enhanced serotonergic neurotransmission in the brainstem and spinal cord.[9,14]

Stimulation of 5-HT_{1A} receptors from raphe bulbospinal neurons results in myoclonus and rigidity. These neuromuscular effects combined with stimulation of 5-HT_2 receptors in the diencephalon result in hyperthermia. Enhanced raphe serotonergic neurotransmission, which controls saccadic eye movements, may produce an unusual "ping-pong" gaze in patients with severe MAO inhibitor toxicity.[3,9] These effects are also seen in the serotonin syndrome (Chapter 370).

The most serious adverse reactions associated with MAO inhibitor therapy result from drug and food interactions and are also the result of exaggerated neuronal effects. The administration or ingestion of any agent that increases CNS serotonin levels may result in potentially life-threatening toxicity known as the serotonin syndrome (see Chapter 370).[9,14,18] The use of indirectly acting sympathomimetic agents (e.g., amphetamine, cocaine, ephedrine, phenylpropanolamine, methylphenidate), which act primarily by causing the release of NE from the presynaptic nerve terminal, may result in the release of the expanded pool of NE and signs and symptoms of catecholamine poisoning (e.g., hypertensive crisis).[10–12,18]

A similar adverse sympathomimetic effect, called the "cheese reaction," may occur when foods containing large amounts of tyramine (e.g., aged cheeses; aged, pickled, or smoked meats; yeast extracts; certain beers; and red wines) and other indirectly acting monoamines (e.g., phenylethylamine, phenylethanolamine, tryptamine, octopamine) are ingested.[11] Inhibition of MAO in the liver and intestinal mucosa allows for systemic absorption of these amines. Like other indirect-acting amines, they may precipitate a rapid, massive release of NE when taken up into noradrenergic nerve endings.

Chronic MAO inhibition increases intraneuronal concentrations of false monoamine neurotransmitters (e.g., tyramine, phenylethylamine, octopamine), which are normally present in very small amounts. With the scavenging function of hepatic and intestinal MAO blocked, dietary monoamines gradually accumulate within noradrenergic nerve endings and displace NE from synaptic vesicles (see Fig. 354.1).[11,15,18] Stimulation of sympathetic neurons results in release of these false neurotransmitters, which have minimal postsynaptic effect. Functional blockade of sympathetic neurotransmission is manifested clinically by hypotension. This hypotensive effect is potentiated by other adaptive responses that result from chronic MAO inhibition and include upregulation of inhibitory presynaptic receptors and downregulation of postsynaptic receptors.[11,15,17]

In addition, MAO inhibitors, through feedback inhibition and via direct effects, inhibit tyrosine hydroxylase, L-amino acid decarboxylase, and DA decarboxylase, enzymes necessary for the production of catecholamine neurotransmitters.[11,15,18] These pharmacologic effects likely contribute to the profound sympatholytic phase that follows an initial sympathomimetic phase in severe MAO inhibitor poisoning.[10] After the initial massive catecholamine release, neuronal stores of these neurotransmitters are depleted, and there is the inability to rapidly regenerate new neurotransmitter. Hypotension and cardiovascular collapse result.

The acute and chronic toxic effects of MAO inhibitors are mediated by several additional mechanisms. MAO inhibitors interfere with the production, activation, supply, and function of pyridoxine and gamma-amino butyric acid (GABA) by binding to and inhibiting pyridoxine, pyridoxine phosphokinase, L-amino acid decarboxylase, and the GABA-A receptor.[15,16] These effects may mediate seizures that are occasionally associated with acute overdose and chronic use of MAO inhibitors. Hydrazine MAO inhibitors inhibit diamine oxidase, an enzyme that, in addition to MAO, metabolizes histamine.[10,16] Flushing and hypotension may result from these effects.

Hydrazine MAO inhibitors also inhibit hepatic cytochrome P-450 enzymes, and thus may potentiate the effects of alcohol, antihistamines, barbiturates, opioids, neuroleptics, anticonvulsants, benzodiazepines, and warfarin.[12,15,16] Additionally, the hypoglycemic effects of insulin and oral antidiabetic drugs may be potentiated by MAO inhibitors.[12] Hydrazine MAO inhibitors are also occasionally associated with the development of severe hepatotoxicity. Hepatic injury is likely mediated by a toxic metabolite that binds irreversibly to hepatocellular macromolecules. The hydrazine MAO inhibitor, iproniazid, was withdrawn from the market because of severe hepatotoxicity associated with its use.[15,16]

MAO inhibitors are rapidly and completely absorbed from the GI tract, with peak plasma concentrations ranging from 1 to 4 hours after ingestion.[1,5,8,10,13] Plasma elimination for these agents is also rapid, with half-lives ranging from 1 to 3 hours. For the irreversible MAO inhibitors, plasma drug concentrations do not correlate with level of MAO inhibition, and toxic plasma concentrations have not been defined.[10,12,18] Maximal inhibition of MAO occurs after 5 to 10 days of therapy with these agents.[16]

For reversible inhibitors, however, maximal MAO inhibition is achieved within a few hours after the first dose.[1,4–6] MAO inhibitors are extensively metabolized in the liver, often by many different enzymes.[1,5,8,13] With irreversible MAO inhibitors, the potential for drug or dietary interactions may last for 2 to 3 weeks after discontinuation of treatment.[11,12,15,16] For reversible agents, MAO activity is restored within 24 hours after the last dose, and the potential for drug and dietary interactions is much less.[1,5]

The ingestion of 2 to 3 mg/kg or more of an irreversible MAO inhibitor should be considered potentially life-threatening.[10,12] Fatal amounts have been reported to be 4 to 6 mg/kg.[10,19] Death has been reported after the ingestion of 170 to 650 mg of tranylcypromine and 375 to 1,500 mg of phenelzine.[10,19] Survival after larger ingestions has also been reported.[10,16,19]

CLINICAL PRESENTATION

Drug or food interactions with MAO inhibitors are a common problem. The incidence of hypertensive crisis for MAO inhibitor–treated patients is 1% to 8%.[12] The clinical presentation may include headache, hypertension, tachycardia (or reflex bradycardia), diaphoresis, agitation, hypertonicity, hyperreflexia with myoclonus, rigidity, seizures, and coma.[11,12] Hyperpyrexia, intracranial hemorrhage, and death may occur.[11] Toxicity begins within 30 to 90 minutes of the ingestion or administration of sympathomimetic amines. The duration of effect is variable but often resolves within a few hours.

Nonselective irreversible MAO inhibitor overdose follows a distinctly different time course.[2,3,10,19,20] The absence of early symptomatology is typical. The onset of toxicity is usually delayed from 6 to 12 hours after the overdose, peaks from 24 to 48 hours for severe cases, and may last for 72 to 96 hours.[10,17,19] A latent period as long as 29 hours has been described following tranylcypromine overdose.[20]

During the latent phase, the patient usually appears well or mildly sedated.[10,19,20] Poisoning is characterized by alterations in behavior, cognition, autonomic nervous system function, and neuromuscular activity and may be classified as mild, moderate, or severe (Table 354.2).[10] Signs and symptoms vary greatly in their onset, severity, and duration. Patients with early or mild toxicity may demonstrate mild lethargy or restlessness, dysarthria, nausea, headache, ataxia, palpitations, flushing, shivering, sweating, tremor, nystagmus, incoordination, or hyperreflexia. Signs and symptoms of moderate toxicity may include confusion, hallucinations, disorientation, agitated delirium, mutism, salivation, diarrhea, marked diaphoresis, myoclonus, fasciculations, trismus, writhing movements, and mild-to-moderate elevations of temperature, pulse, respiratory rate, and blood pressure. Severe toxicity may be characterized by unresponsive coma; fixed, dilated pupils; "ping-pong" gaze; pathologic reflexes; generalized rigidity; seizures; hyperpyrexia (temperature greater than 104°F); marked tachypnea or respiratory depression; extreme sinus tachycardia or bradycardia; malignant cardiac arrhythmias; hypotension; and death.[2,3,10,19] Death from cardiovascular collapse is most likely to occur in patients with severe hyperpyrexia.[19]

Although seizures may occur following MAO overdose, they are uncommon and can be confused with neuromuscular hyperactivity produced by these agents.[9,19] Secondary complications may occur in patients with moderate-to-severe toxicity and include aspiration pneumonitis, adult respiratory distress syndrome, rhabdomyolysis, acute renal failure, metabolic acidosis, and disseminated intravascular coagulation (DIC).[10] The likelihood of secondary complications (e.g., rhabdomyolysis, DIC) and death is related to the degree and duration of hyper-

TABLE 354.2. Clinical Course of Monoamine Oxidase Inhibitor Poisoning

Phase-Severity[a]	Time after Ingestion[a]	Cognitive-Behavioral Dysfunction	Autonomic Dysfunction	Neuromuscular Dysfunction
0-Latent	0–24 h	Mild lethargy	Absent	Absent
I-Mild	6–12 h	Mild lethargy	Nausea	Mild tremor
		Dysarthria	Flushing	Hyperreflexia
		Ataxia	Diaphoresis	Incoordination
		Headache	Shivering	Nystagmus
		Irritability	Mydriasis	
		Anxiety		
		Insomnia		
II-Moderate	10–24 h	Confusion	Mild hyperthermia(temperature <104°(F)	Myoclonus
		Disorientation	Marked diaphoresis	Fasciculations
		Agitated delirium	Salivation	Trismus
		Mumbling/rambling speech	Piloerection	Facial grimacing
		Mutism	Hypertension	Writhing extremities
		Hyperactivity	Sinus tachycardia (P <150 beats/min)	
			Hyperventilation	
III-Severe	16–72 h	Incomprehensible speech	Hyperventilation to respiratory arrest	Generalized rigidity
		Coma	Extreme sinus tachycardia to sinus bradycardia	Opisthotonus
		Seizures	Malignant dysrhythmias (VT, VF, bradyasystole)	Fixed, dilated pupils
			Hypotension	"Ping-pong" gaze
			Pale, clammy, mottled skin	Pathologic reflexes (decorticate, decerebrate, Babinski)
			Severe hyperthermia (temperature <104°F)	
IV-Complications	24–96 h	Aspiration pneumonitis	Anion gap metabolic acidosis	Rhabdomyolysis
		Adult respiratory distress syndrome		Hemolysis Acute renal
failure				
				Disseminated intravascular coagulation
				Hepatic failure

[a] Signs and symptoms vary greatly in their onset, severity, and duration.

thermia. Patients with severe toxicity can manifest fixed, dilated pupils; posturing; and extensor plantar response yet make a complete neurologic recovery.[2,3,17,19]

When taken alone, reversible inhibitors of MAO-A appear to have a benign course following acute overdose. At doses as high as 20.5 g, no fatalities have been reported following overdose with moclobemide alone.[5] Large overdoses are characterized by mild CNS depression, agitation, tachycardia, hypertension, and mydriasis.[5] Mixed-drug overdoses are more serious. Patient deaths have been reported from serotonin syndrome when moclobemide has been combined with other serotonin-potentiating drugs (e.g., citalopram, clomipramine).[5]

Patients with chronic toxicity from irreversible nonselective inhibitors may manifest tremors, insomnia, hyperhidrosis, agitation, hypomanic behavior, hallucinations, confusion, and seizures.

DIFFERENTIAL DIAGNOSIS

Toxicity from amphetamines, cocaine, and other sympathomimetic agents (including over-the-counter appetite suppressants) may produce a clinical picture similar to the hypertensive reactions associated with MAO inhibitors and dietary and drug monoamines. The clinical presentation of MAO inhibitor overdose may be similar to anticholinergic, hallucinogen (e.g., lysergic acid diethylamide, phencyclidine), lithium, salicylate, sympathomimetic (e.g., amphetamines, cocaine), and strychnine poisoning. MAO inhibitor toxicity may be confused with the neuroleptic malignant syndrome and withdrawal from alcohol or sedative–hypnotic agents. The serotonin syndrome has clinical features nearly identical to those following overdoses with MAO inhibitors. Medical emergencies such as hypoglycemia, malignant hyperthermia, intracranial hemorrhage, meningitis, encephalitis, pheochromocytoma, septicemia, tetanus, and thyrotoxicosis may present in a similar manner.

EMERGENCY DEPARTMENT EVALUATION

There are no pathognomonic physical findings or laboratory abnormalities. Accurate and complete historical data are essential in differentiating the toxic syndromes related to MAO inhibitors. Initial testing for patients with suspected intentional overdose should include an electrocardiogram and measurements of serum electrolytes, glucose, renal function, and acetaminophen and salicylate levels. Patients who present with signs and symptoms of toxicity should also have a complete blood count; prothrombin and partial thromboplastin times; creatine phosphokinase, calcium, magnesium, and liver function tests; and a urinalysis. Patients with altered mental status should have a bedside fingerstick glucose determination and appropriate intervention, as necessary. A lumbar puncture and computed tomography scanning may be necessary to differentiate drug intoxication from intracranial hemorrhage, meningitis, and encephalitis.

Toxicology screening may be useful to exclude other intoxications, but it rarely detects MAO inhibitors because of their low concentrations in blood and urine samples.[10] Overdose of selegiline or tranylcypromine, however, may produce a positive qualitative screen for amphetamines.[8,10,13,15] Quantitative MAO inhibitor levels are not generally available and have not been shown to correlate with the severity of poisoning.[10,12,19] Similarly, the degree of MAO enzyme activity inhibition does not correlate with clinical toxicity.

EMERGENCY DEPARTMENT MANAGEMENT

Supportive care is the primary treatment for MAO inhibitor overdose. Advanced life-support measures should be instituted, as necessary. The administration of glucose, oxygen, naloxone, and thiamine should be considered for patients with altered mental status. Activated charcoal is the preferred method of GI decontamination for recent acute MAO inhibitor overdose. Before any drug or food is given, the potential for an adverse interaction with MAO inhibitors must be considered.

Agitation, neuromuscular hyperactivity, and seizures should be treated promptly with liberal doses of benzodiazepines (e.g., diazepam, lorazepam) or barbiturates (e.g., phenobarbital).[10] Phenytoin is unlikely to be as effective for seizures associated with MAO inhibitors. Pyridoxine administration is recommended for seizures that occur following overdose with a hydrazine MAO inhibitor.

Rapid cooling is essential to minimize patient morbidity and mortality from hyperthermia. Because it is almost invariably associated with CNS agitation and neuromuscular hyperactivity, initial treatment with benzodiazepines or barbiturates is recommended. In conjunction with these initial pharmacologic measures, evaporative and convective cooling methods, using wet sheets or cool mist sprays and fans, are recommended.[10,19] Antipyretics and cooling blankets are generally ineffective. If these initial maneuvers do not provide rapid patient cooling, neuromuscular blockade with nondepolarizing paralyzing agents is strongly recommended.

Evidence from animal studies and human case reports suggests that neuromuscular paralysis is effective for the treatment of severe hyperthermia.[2] Cooling times of less than 1 hour have been achieved with this method of treatment. Although dantrolene (2.5 mg/kg orally or intravenously every 6 hours) has also been reported to be effective,[17] it is itself toxic and does not terminate muscular rigidity and hyperthermia as rapidly as paralyzing agents. Because the pathophysiology of serotonin syndrome overlaps considerably with MAO inhibitor overdose, nonspecific serotonin receptor antagonists (e.g., cyproheptadine, methysergide; see Chapter 370) could be of benefit. Because of the lack of any clinical data, however, their use cannot yet be recommended for MAO inhibitor overdose.

Severe hypertension may be treated with the intravenous administration of rapid-onset, short-acting agents such as sodium nitroprusside or phentolamine.[10,12,16,19] Phentolamine (5 to 10 mg intravenously) is pharmacologically attractive because it can block alpha-adrenergic receptors and antagonize the effects of NE. It has proven effective for the treatment of hypertension associated with the "cheese reaction."[11] Long-acting agents (tolazoline, clonidine) also have been used but are not recommended, as hypertension is often followed by severe hypotension.[10]

Hypotension should initially be treated with fluid resuscitation. When pressors are required, direct-acting agents (e.g., epinephrine, NE) are recommended.[10,12] The use of indirect-acting agents (e.g., DA), which require the release of intracellular amines for their pressor effect, may either precipitate a hypertensive crisis or be ineffective on account of depleted stores of catecholamines. Additionally, MAO inhibition is less likely to potentiate the effects of exogenously administered, direct-acting pressors, which circulate extracellularly and are primarily metabolized by catechol-*o*-methyltransferase. Regardless, low doses of direct-acting pressors should be used initially to minimize the risk of an exaggerated pressor response. Phenylephrine, a direct-acting agent, has been associated with an exaggerated pressor response and is not recommended for the treatment of hypotension in MAO inhibitor poisoning.[11]

Ventricular dysrhythmias and severe bradycardias, usually premorbid signs, should be treated according to current advanced cardiac life-support protocols. Bretylium, however, is not recommended for the treatment of refractory ventricular dysrhythmias; it has initial catecholamine-releasing effects that may potentiate the cardiotoxic effects of MAO inhibitors.[10,12]

Diuresis, urinary acidification, hemodialysis, and hemoperfusion play no role in the management of MAO inhibitor poisoning.[10,12,19]

DISPOSITION

Because of the delayed onset of toxicity, all patients with suspected MAO inhibitor overdose should be admitted for extended observation (24 hours) in a monitored setting. Symptomatic patients and those with abnormal vital signs should be admitted to an intensive care unit. If intensive care is unavailable, patients should be transferred to an institution with this capacity.

Patients who present with drug or dietary interactions may not require hospital admission if the clinical response has been mild. Patients with severe reactions, those with persistent symptoms after a 4- to 6-hour observation period, and those with symptoms that necessitate active intervention should be admitted. The level of in-hospital care required (intensive care or floor) depends on the severity of symptoms. For patients well enough to eat, an MAO inhibitor diet (e.g., low tyramine) should be ordered.

COMMON PITFALLS

- Failure to check for MAO inhibitor use before prescribing sympathomimetics or giving pain medications, particularly meperidine
- Failure to appreciate that the onset of toxicity may be delayed and gradual in onset after MAO inhibitor overdose and to admit all patients with MAO inhibitor overdose for observation
- Failure to appreciate that the history is key to differentiating acute overdose from drug and food interactions, including the serotonin syndrome
- Failure to rapidly and aggressively cool the patient with hyperthermia
- Failure to appreciate that early sympathetic stimulation may be followed by catecholamine depletion and cardiovascular collapse in patients with acute MAO inhibitor overdose
- Failure to exclude other CNS pathology in patients who present with fever, altered mental status, hypertension, or neuromuscular hyperactivity

References

1. Amrein R, Allen SR, Guentert TW, et al. The pharmacology of reversible monoamine oxidase inhibitors. *Br J Psychiatry* 1989;155[Suppl 6]:66.
2. Ciocatto E, Gagiano G, Bava GL. Clinical features and treatment of overdosage of monoamine oxidase inhibitors and their interaction with other psychotropic drugs. *Resuscitation* 1972;1:69.
3. Erich JL, Shih RD, O'Connor RE. "Ping-pong" gaze in severe monoamine oxidase inhibitor toxicity. *J Emerg Med* 1995;13:653.
4. Finberg JPM. Pharmacology of reversible and selective inhibitors of monoamine oxidase type A. *Acta Psychiatr Scand* 1995;91[Suppl 386]:8.
5. Fulton B, Benfield P. Moclobemide: an update of its pharmacological properties and therapeutic use. *Drugs* 1996;52:450.
6. Haefely W, Burkard WP, Cesura AM, et al. Biochemistry and pharmacology of moclobemide, a prototype RIMA. *Psychopharmacology* 1992;106:S6.
7. Hartmann D, Cesura AM, Schmid-Burgk W, et al. Relevance of reversible inhibitors of monoamine oxidase type A and reuptake inhibition for noradrenaline turnover. *Acta Psychiatr Scand* 1995;91[Suppl 386]:14.
8. Heinonen EH, Lammintausta R. A review of the pharmacology of selegiline. *Acta Neurol Scand* 1991;84[Suppl 136]:44.
9. Lieberman JA, Kane JM, Reife R. Neuromuscular effects of monoamine oxidase inhibitors. *Adv Neurol* 1986;43:231.
10. Linden CH, Rumack BH. MAO inhibitor overdose. *Ann Emerg Med* 1984;13:1137.
11. Lippman SB, Nash K. MAO inhibitor update: potential adverse food and drug interactions. *Drug Saf* 1990;5:195.
12. Lipson RE, Stern TA. Management of monoamine oxidase inhibitor-treated patients in the emergency and critical care setting. *J Intensive Care Med* 1991;6:117.
13. Mallinger AG, Smith E. Pharmacokinetics of MAO inhibitors. *Psychopharmacol Bull* 1991;27:493.
14. Marley E, Wozniak KM. Interactions of non-selective monoamine oxidase inhibitors, tranylcypromine and nialamide, with inhibitors of 5-hydroxytryptamine, dopamine, or noradrenaline uptake. *J Psychiatr Res* 1984;18:191.
15. McDaniel KD. Clinical pharmacology of monoamine oxidase inhibitors. *Clin Neuropharmacol* 1986;9:207.
16. Tollefson GD. Monoamine oxidase inhibitors: a review. *J Clin Psychiatry* 1983;44:280.
17. Verrilli MR, Salanga VD, Kozachuk WE, et al. Phenelzine toxicity responsive to dantrolene. *Neurology* 1987;37:865.
18. Wells DG, Bjorksten AR. Monoamine oxidase inhibitors revisited. *Can J Anaesth* 1989;36:64.
19. White K, Simpson GM. Management of MAOI overdoses and hyperthermic crises. In: Shader RI, ed. *MAOI therapy*. New York: Audio Visual Medical Marketing, Inc., 1988:53.
20. Young S, Walpole BG. Tranylcypromine and chlordiazepoxide intoxication. *Med J Aust* 1986;144:166.

CHAPTER 355
Mushroom Poisoning

Christopher H. Linden and Robert P. Dowsett

Mushrooms (or toadstools) is a common name for the fruit of certain kinds of fungi. Although foraging for wild mushrooms has long been commonplace in other parts of the world, it has only recently become popular in the United States. Even though the incidence of mushroom poisoning, also known as mycetism, appears to be rising, it remains uncommon. Of the thousands of ingestions reported each year, only a few hundred result in serious toxicity; however, mycetism is sometimes fatal.

Mushroom poisoning is most common during the late summer and early fall, when wild mushrooms are most abundant. Victims include young children who accidentally ingest mushrooms, recreational drug users who intentionally ingest hallucinogenic species, and foragers (and their families and friends) who confuse poisonous mushrooms with edible ones.[6,8,10,20] Serious poisoning in children is rare and is usually due to the ingestion of mushrooms served to them by adults. Poisoning may also occur after the inhalation of toxic vapors during the cooking (i.e., the attempted detoxification by boiling) of gyromitrin-containing mushrooms.[10] Sometimes, hallucinogenic mushrooms are prepared to be brewed in tea, snorted, smoked, or injected intravenously.[11–13]

Edible mushrooms may also cause poisoning. Allergic reactions such as mushroom worker's alveolitis, food allergy, and hemolytic anemia can occur, and they are subject to bacterial, insecticidal, and chemical contamination. Adulteration with phencyclidine has been reported. Idiosyncratic reactions, most likely of genetic origin, such as gastrointestinal (GI) intolerance to *Agaricus bisporus,* the most prevalent grocery store species, are relatively common. Mushrooms containing coprine are edible, but toxic reactions can occur if they are coingested with alcohol.

Only about 100 of the many thousands of species of mushrooms are considered poisonous. They can be divided into eight groups, based on their toxins (Table 355.1).[2,7–10,12,17] Amatoxins are found in species of the *Amanita, Conocybe, Galerina,* and *Lepiota* genera, such as *Amanita phalloides* (death cap) and *Amanita virosa* (destroying angel). These cyclic octapeptides can cause delayed and potentially fatal liver and kidney necrosis. Additional cyclic heptapeptides (phallotoxins) may contribute to GI cytotoxicity. Orellanine and cortinarins are present in some species of the *Cortinarius* genus. These toxins can cause a renal tubulointerstitial nephritis, which does not become apparent until many days after ingestion. Although toxic *Cortinarius* species are found primarily in Europe, *Amanita smithiana,* which is indigenous to North America and sometimes mistaken for the edible pine mushroom or matsutake (*Tricholoma magnivelare*), contains toxins (allenic norleucine and pentynoic acid) that cause similar toxicity.[19] Gyromitrins are contained in mushrooms of the *Gyromitra, Paxina,* and *Sarcosphaera* genera. An example is the "false morel," or *Gyromitra esculenta.* The active metabolites of gyromitrins are hydrazines that can oxidize hemoglobin and cause delayed hepatic, neurologic, and renal cytotoxicity. Muscarine is found in species of the *Boletus, Clitocybe,* and *Inocybe* genera, such as *Clitocybe dealbata* (the sweater). An aminofuran alkaloid, muscarine, stimulates peripheral parasympathetic nerves soon after ingestion. Ibotenic acid and its active metabolite muscimol are present in some species of *Amanita,* such as *Amanita muscaria* (fly agaric) and *Amanita pantherina* (panther cap). These isoxazole derivatives have a structural skeleton similar to that of γ-aminobutyric acid, but they have complex interactions with multiple types of central and peripheral neurotransmitters and their receptors. Small amounts of muscarine may also be present. The net effect is the early onset of hallucinations and either cholinergic or anticholinergic symptoms. Psilocin is the active metabolite of psilocybin. These dimethyltryptamines are serotonin analogues that cause the rapid onset of hallucinations and sympathetic stimulation. They are present in species of *Conocybe, Gymnopilus, Panaeolus,* and *Psilocybe.* Coprine is found in *Clitocybe calvipes* and species of *Coprinus,* such as *Coprinus atramentarius* (inky cap). This compound inhibits aldehyde dehydrogenase and results in a disulfiram-ethanol–like reaction if consumed with ethanol. A wide variety of mostly identified (miscellaneous) toxins are present in mushrooms from many genera (e.g., *Boletus, Chlorophyllum, Entoloma, Gomphus, Hebeloma, Lactarius, Omphalotus, Paxillus, Pholiota, Ramaria, Russula, Tricholoma,* and *Verpa*); toxicity is limited to the GI tract and occurs within a short time of ingestion.

The nature and severity of poisoning depends on the dose, maturity, growing conditions (e.g., geographic location, food source, amount of rainfall, and temperature), method of storage and preparation, route of administration, and species of mushroom, and age and underlying health status of the victim. Mushrooms that contain amatoxins are responsible for most fatalities in the United States. The ingestion of one to three phalloides or 15 to 20 of the smaller *Galerina* species is potentially lethal. The overall mortality rate from amatoxin poisoning is estimated to be less than 5%, but it has been as high as 50% in some series. Children appear to be more susceptible than do adults, probably because of the ingestion of a proportionately greater dose when they partake of a mushroom meal. In some areas of Europe, mushrooms that contain gyromitrin (and sometimes orellanine) account for a significant number of deaths. Serious or fatal poisoning from other mushroom toxins is rare.

CLINICAL PRESENTATION

Except with mushrooms containing hallucinogens, symptoms typically begin with some combination of nausea, vomiting, abdominal cramps, and diarrhea. Associated or subsequent systemic toxicity depends on the type of toxin in the mushroom ingested. For a particular toxin, the higher the dose, the earlier the onset and the greater the severity of poisoning.

GI symptoms after amatoxin mushroom ingestion are characteristically delayed 6 to 24 hours after ingestion but are abrupt in onset, severe, and prolonged.[4,7–11,14,17,20] Diarrhea may be profuse, occasionally bloody, and may result in severe dehydration and metabolic acidosis. Leukocytosis and hyperamylasemia may be present. There may be a period of apparent im-

TABLE 355.1. Mushroom Toxins

Onset of Toxicity	Mechanism of Action	Principal Effects[c]
DELAYED[a]		
Amatoxins	Inhibition of RNA polymerase II	Hepatic and renal cytotoxicity
Orellanine/orelline	Inhibition of alkaline phosphatase	Renal cytotoxicity
Gyromitrins	Inhibition of pyridoxal phosphate-dependent and cytochrome P-450 enzymes	CNS, hepatic, and renal cytotoxicity
EARLY[b]		
Muscarine	Stimulation of postganglionic parasympathetic receptors	Cholinergic syndrome
Ibotenic acid/muscimol	Interaction with CNS neuroreceptors	Hallucinations, anticholinergic or cholinergic syndrome
Psilocin/psilocybin	Stimulation of serotonin receptors	Hallucinations, sympathetic syndrome
Miscellaneous GI toxins	Irritation and stimulation of mucosa	Gastorenteritis
VARIABLE		
Coprine	Inhibition of acetaldehyde dehydrogenase	Disulfiram-ethanol–like reaction

[a] Onset more than 6 h after ingestion.
[b] Onset less than 3 h after ingestion.
[c] Usually includes GI symptoms regardless of toxin involved.
CNS, central nervous system; GI, gastrointestinal.

provement occurring 24 to 48 hours after ingestion in less severe cases. Biochemical evidence of hepatotoxicity may occur as early as 24 hours after ingestion, but it typically begins at 48 hours and becomes maximal in 4 to 5 days. Hypoglycemia, elevated serum bilirubin, transaminase, and ammonia levels (ten to 30 times normal), and increased prothrombin and partial thromboplastin times are common. Physical findings include mild but tender hepatomegaly, jaundice, lethargy, and confusion. There may be concomitant or subsequent acute renal failure with elevated blood urea nitrogen and creatinine levels, and oliguria, hematuria, and proteinuria. With good supportive care, most patients slowly recover, but, in severe cases, progressive hepatic failure may end in death within 1 week. Delayed polyneuropathy and chronic active hepatitis have also been reported.

GI symptoms caused by *Cortinarius* species are typically mild, transient, and delayed (2 to 3 days after ingestion).[2,15–17] They can occur within 20 minutes after ingesting *A. smithiana.* Constipation, rather than diarrhea, may occur. Associated symptoms include headache, chills, polyuria, thirst (intense, burning), and nightsweats. Renal failure may become apparent between 3 days and 3 weeks after ingestion and is associated with flank pain and tenderness. Hematuria, marked albuminuria, and red cell casts may be seen on urinalysis. In 50% to 70% of cases, renal function gradually returns to baseline over a period of several weeks to several months.

The gastroenteritis that follows the ingestion of mushrooms that contain gyromitrins is usually delayed 6 to 24 hours and is moderate in severity and duration.[8–10,17] The onset may be earlier after inhalation exposure to vapors during cooking. Agitation, ataxia, headache (often severe), hyperreflexia, muscle cramps, vertigo, and weakness may ensue. Methemoglobinemia with cyanosis and associated Heinz body hemolytic anemia, hepatitis with encephalopathy, hyperthermia, and renal failure may develop in severe cases. Hepatic failure may be fatal.

In muscarine poisoning, GI symptoms occur within 15 minutes to 2 hours of mushroom ingestion and are relatively mild and of short duration (2 to 10 hours).[8–11,17] Associated findings include diaphoresis, headache, lacrimation, miosis, blurred vision, urinary frequency, and salivation. In severe cases, bronchorrhea, bronchospasm, bradycardia, hypotension, and, rarely, seizures and liver function abnormalities may occur.

GI symptoms after the ingestion of mushrooms that contain ibotenic acid and muscimol are typically absent, although short-lived vomiting may be noted.[1,8–11,17] Drowsiness, dizziness, and lethargy may occur within 20 minutes to 2 hours of ingestion and be followed by agitation, euphoria, confusion, delirium, hallucinations (visual misperceptions of color and shape, often with religious associations), and psychosis. Cholinergic (e.g., bradycardia, miosis, salivation) or anticholinergic (e.g., dry skin, fever, hypertension, mydriasis) may be noted. Symptoms in children include crying, screaming, and incoherent babbling. Muscle fasciculation, twitching, hyperreflexia, and myoclonus may also be seen. A fluctuating level of consciousness is common with severe poisoning. Coma and seizures may occur, but symptoms seldom last for more than 6 to 8 hours.

Nausea and vomiting occur in a minority of patients with psilocin and psilocybin intoxication and, if present, they are mild and transient.[8–13,17] Symptoms begin within 30 to 60 minutes of mushroom ingestion and typically include dysphoria followed by disorientation, incoordination, and hallucinations (usually visual but sometimes auditory and tactile as well). Associated signs and symptoms include mydriasis, blurred vision, mild tachycardia, hypertension, hyperreflexia, and irrational, antisocial, and sometimes suicidal behavior. Symptoms typically last for 4 to 6 hours, but flashbacks may occur for several months. Cyanosis with both hypoxia and methemoglobinemia, arthralgias, myalgias, fever, chills, and mild kidney and liver function abnormalities have been noted after intravenous injection.[3] Seizures, coma, hyperthermia, and death have occurred in children.

Mushrooms that contain coprine, although they are edible, may result in a disulfiram-ethanol–like reaction within 15 to 30 minutes of ethanol ingestion.[8–11,17] The reaction may occur 2 hours to 5 days after mushroom ingestion and typically lasts for 3 to 6 hours. In addition to GI symptoms, which may be severe, manifestations include diaphoresis, flushing, headache, dyspnea, chest tightness, palpitations, tachycardia, paresthesias, vertigo, and weakness. Hypotension (orthostatic or supine), confusion, coma, arrhythmias (atrial fibrillation and premature beats), and ischemic electrocardiographic changes may occur in severe cases.

Gastroenteritis is usually the only manifestation of poisoning by the miscellaneous mushrooms.[8–10,17] Symptoms begin within 30 minutes to 6 hours, are of variable severity, and last for 4 to 48 hours. In severe cases, diarrhea may become bloody, and dehydration may ensue. Other symptoms include chills, headache, diaphoresis, light-headedness, myalgias, paresthesias, carpopedal spasm, and weakness.

DIFFERENTIAL DIAGNOSIS

Without a history of mushroom ingestion, GI symptoms may be mistaken for food poisoning or viral gastroenteritis. Acetaminophen, chlorinated hydrocarbon, and heavy-metal poisoning may cause toxicity similar to that of amatoxin mycetism. Poisoning by isoniazid and other hydrazines or hydrazones is similar to that caused by the ingestion of mushrooms that contain gyromitrins. Carbamate and organophosphate insecticide poisoning may mimic that caused by ingestion of muscarine-containing mushrooms. Intoxication caused by ibutenic acid and muscimol is similar to the anticholinergic syndrome caused by a number of drugs. Lysergic acid diethylamide and amphetamine and tryptamine analogues cause effects that are similar to those that result from psilocin and psilocybin poisoning.

EMERGENCY DEPARTMENT EVALUATION

All patients with gastroenteritis, hallucinations, or an unexpected reaction to ethanol should be asked if they have ingested wild mushrooms. If such a history is elicited, the number, types, description, and method of preparation of the mushrooms should be noted, and an attempt should be made to obtain a fresh sample of the mushroom. Ideally, the mushroom or its parts should be identified by an experienced mycologist. Experts may be located at botany departments of colleges and universities, botanical gardens, poison centers, and local, state, or regional mycologic societies. If necessary, the suspect mushroom can be dried by hot air, light, or oven (not a microwave) and sent in a paper container to a mycologist. Alternatively, a field guide for mushroom identification can be consulted. Attempting to identify a mushroom from spores obtained from leftovers, vomitus, or stool is seldom fruitful. When mushroom samples are not available, those described as puffballs or as having a white cap, a ring on the stalk, or a sack at the base should be suspected to be one of the deadly *Amanita,* and those described as brainlike should be assumed to be a lethal *Gyromitra*. Any wild mushroom that is not available for positive identification should be assumed to be one that can cause serious or lethal poisoning.

The interval between the time of ingestion and the onset of symptoms, and the nature of symptoms should be determined. The onset of GI symptoms 6 hours or more after ingestion suggests potentially fatal poisoning by a mushroom containing an amatoxin, orellanine, or gyromitrin cytotoxin.[8–10,17] In these patients, laboratory evaluation should include a complete blood count; determination of electrolyte, blood urea nitrogen, creatinine, glucose, and methemoglobin levels; prothrombin time; partial thromboplastin time; liver function tests; and urinalysis. Severe GI symptoms suggest amatoxin poisoning. Thirst, polyuria, and renal abnormalities 3 or more days after ingestion are consistent with orellanine poisoning, and severe headaches, neurologic dysfunction (in the absence of severe dehydration), methemoglobinemia, and hemolysis suggest mycetism caused by gyromitrins. The subsequent development of hepatic and renal failure is consistent with either amatoxin or gyromitrin mushroom intoxication, whereas renal failure alone suggests orellanine poisoning.

The onset of symptoms within 3 hours of mushroom ingestion indicates poisoning by a noncytotoxic mushroom containing muscarine, ibotenic acid–muscimol, psilocin–psilocybin, coprine, or a GI irritant.[8–10,19] It does not, however, rule out poisoning by a cytotoxic species if more than one kind of mushroom has been ingested, nor does it exclude poisoning by *A. smithiana*. Hallucinations with mild or absent GI symptoms indicate ibotenic acid–muscimol or psilocin–psilocybin mushroom poisoning. A fluctuating level of consciousness, central nervous system depression, and either cholinergic or anticholinergic findings suggest the former, whereas signs of sympathetic stimulation occur with the latter. Manifestations of cholinergic hyperactivity imply intoxication by a muscarine-containing mushroom. Flushing, headache, and "beta sympathomimetic" findings after ethanol ingestion suggest an interaction with a mushroom that contains coprine, and symptoms limited to the GI tract suggest ingestion of a mushroom that contains one of the miscellaneous GI irritants.

All patients with prolonged GI symptoms or abnormal supine or orthostatic vital signs should have baseline determinations of electrolyte, blood urea nitrogen, creatinine, and glucose levels and urinalysis. Stool and vomitus should be tested for occult blood. Patients with hypotension, dyspnea, or chest pain should have cardiac rhythm monitoring and an electrocardiogram. Except for muscarine, which can be identified by thin-layer chromatography, mushroom toxins are not detected by routine toxicology screening.

EMERGENCY DEPARTMENT MANAGEMENT

Activated charcoal should be given to all patients, even if spontaneous vomiting and diarrhea are present. Ipecac is not recommended, because it may add to the emetic effects of mushrooms themselves and delay or prevent the administration of charcoal. If a cytotoxic species has been ingested within 6 hours, gastric lavage, preceded and followed by administration of charcoal, may be optimal. Whole-bowel irrigation should also be considered. Repeated dosing of charcoal should be continued for 2 to 4 days or until symptoms resolve. Metoclopramide may facilitate the administration of charcoal in patients with protracted vomiting.

Many patients also need large amounts of intravenous crystalloids to compensate for significant GI fluid losses. Glucose and electrolytes should be included in the replacement solution. A bolus of glucose should be given immediately to patients with altered mental status, particularly those with evidence of liver dysfunction.

Specific therapy primarily depends on the clinical (presumptive) diagnosis of the type of mushroom poisoning, based on the time of onset and nature of symptoms. Positive identification of the species of mushroom ingested is secondary. Patients with delayed symptoms or early symptoms after the ingestion of multiple unidentified species should be assumed to have ingested a cytotoxic mushroom.

If amatoxin ingestion is possible or confirmed, charcoal hemoperfusion may enhance toxin elimination if performed in the first 24 hours.[4,17,18] Repeated administration of activated charcoal is recommended, even for late presentation, to interrupt enterohepatic circulation of amatoxins.[17,20] Forced diuresis is no longer recommended, but maintenance of a normal urine output is essential. Possible antidotal treatments include the use of silibinin or penicillin to reduce the hepatocyte uptake of amatoxins.[4,6,17,18,20] When high-dose intravenous penicillin is used, the total dose and rate of administration should take into account the potassium content (up to 1.5 mEq per million units) and the risk of penicillin toxicity (e.g., resulting in encephalopathy and seizures), especially if renal impairment is present. A suggested dosing regimen is 1 million units per kilogram per day for the first day, followed by 0.5 million units per kilogram per day for 2 more days. Penicillin should be given in multiple, small, divided doses. Silibinin, an extract of milk thistle, has been used successfully when given within 48 hours of amatoxin ingestion, but it is not available in the United States.[6] The recommended dosage is 5 mg/kg intravenously over 1 hour, followed by a constant infusion of 20 to 50 mg/kg/d until hepatic recovery. Silimaryn, a dietary supplement available in capsules from health food stores, contains silibinin. Oral doses of 1.4 to 4.2 g/d have been suggested as an alternative to intravenous silibinin, but the efficacy of this formulation is unknown.[6] *Amanita*-induced hepatotoxicity is similar to that caused by toxins that undergo mixed-function oxidase P-450 activation, and cimetidine, an inhibitor of these enzymes, has shown efficacy in experimental animals. Doses of cimetidine of up to 2 g every 4 hours have been used in humans.

Hyperbaric oxygen has been used and should be considered if readily available, but its efficacy is unproved. The use of *N*-acetylcysteine and the iridoid glycosides aucubin and kutkin is also being investigated. Corticosteroids and thioctic acid are no longer recommended.[17,20] Hepatic and renal failure should be treated by standard measures. Patients with severe liver dysfunction should be tissue-typed and have arrangements made for transfer to a liver transplantation center.[20] Liver transplantation should not be performed prematurely (sooner than 1 week), because some patients with significant hepatic failure recover with medical therapy. Patients who develop chronic active hepatitis, a common sequela, may also be candidates for liver transplantation.

Patients with orellanine and orelline exposure may benefit from hemoperfusion if it is performed within 1 week of mushroom ingestion.[15,16] Hemodialysis should be used supportively. Patients with permanent renal failure may be candidates for kidney transplantation.

Neurologic dysfunction or severe systemic toxicity owing to gyromitrin poisoning should be treated with pyridoxine (vitamin B_6).[5] A dose of 25 mg/kg should be given intravenously every 15 to 30 minutes (up to four doses) for coma or seizures. A similar dose every 6 hours may be used for recurrent or less severe symptoms. Larger doses have been used, but they are unlikely to be of additional benefit and increase the risk of pyridoxine toxicity. Theoretically, methemoglobinemia could require treatment with methylene blue (see Chapter 352). Hemolysis usually requires only fluid therapy to prevent renal complications.

Poisoning by other mushroom toxins is treated symptomatically. Agitated behavior and hallucinations may be treated with a benzodiazepine or haloperidol, but phenothiazines should be avoided.[13] Seizures may be treated with diazepam, a barbiturate, or phenytoin. Coprine–ethanol reactions are treated the same as those caused by disulfiram and ethanol (see Chapter 334).[11,17] Severe anticholinergic symptoms may require the use of physostigmine (see Chapter 312).[11,17] Patients with excessive secretions, bronchospasm, or bradycardia with hypotension should be given small doses (less than or equal to 0.01 mg/kg) of intravenous atropine.[5,11,17] Because atropine may increase toxin absorption by slowing its rectal evacuation, however, it should not be given solely for GI symptoms unless they are markedly prolonged or severe.

DISPOSITION

Patients with confirmed or possible cytotoxic mushroom ingestion or those with severe or persistent symptoms from other mushrooms should be admitted to the hospital. Patients with noncytotoxic mushroom ingestions who become asymptomatic after emergency department treatment and observation may be discharged. Those with intentional hallucinogenic mushroom ingestion should be referred for drug abuse counseling.

It is advisable to consult a poison center or toxicologist in all cases of mushroom ingestion. Depending on clinical evaluation and the type of mushroom involved, consultation with or referral to a gastroenterologist, nephrologist, psychiatrist, or transplant surgeon may be necessary. Patients may need to be transferred if intensive or specialized care is necessary but not available.

COMMON PITFALLS

- Failure to appreciate that, contrary to common folklore, there is no easy way to differentiate poisonous mushrooms from edible mushrooms
- Failure to include wild mushroom ingestion in the differential diagnosis of gastroenteritis, altered mental status, and liver or kidney dysfunction of unknown cause
- Assuming that a potentially lethal mushroom has not been ingested along with noncytotoxic species simply because symptoms began soon after ingestion
- Failure to admit patients with possible cytotoxic mushroom ingestion
- Failure to appreciate that therapy is based primarily on clinical symptoms and should not be delayed or withheld because the mushroom itself has not been identified

References

1. Benjamin DR. Mushroom poisoning in infants and children: the *Amanita pantherina/muscaria* group. *J Toxicol Clin Toxicol* 1992;30:13.
2. Bouget J, Bousser J, Pats B, et al. Acute renal failure following collective intoxication by *Cortinarius orellanus*. *Intensive Care Med* 1990;16:506.
3. Curry SC, Rose MC. Intravenous mushroom poisoning. *Ann Emerg Med* 1985;14:900.
4. Floersheim GL. Treatment of human amatoxin mushroom poisoning: myths and advances in therapy. *Med Toxicol* 1987;2:1.
5. Hanrahan JP, Gordon MA. Mushroom poisoning: case reports and review of therapy. *JAMA* 1984;251:1057.
6. Hruby K, Csomos G, Fuhrmann M, et al. Chemotherapy of a *Amanita phalloides* poisoning with intravenous silibinin. *Hum Toxicol* 1983;2:183.
7. Koppel C. Clinical symptomatology and management of mushroom poisoning. *Toxicon* 1993;31:1513.
8. Lampe KF. Toxic fungi. *Annu Rev Pharmacol Toxicol* 1979;19:85.
9. Lampe KF. Differential diagnosis of poisoning by North American mushrooms, with particular emphasis on *Amanita phalloides*-like intoxication. *Ann Emerg Med* 1987;16:956.
10. Lincoff G, Mitchell DH. *Toxic and hallucinogenic mushroom poisoning: a handbook for physicians and mushroom hunters*. Reinhold, NY: Van Nostrand, 1977.
11. McCormick DJ, Avbel AJ, Gibbons MC. Nonlethal mushroom poisoning. *Ann Intern Med* 1979;90:332.
12. McDonald A. Mushrooms and madness: hallucinogenic mushrooms and some psychopharmacological implications. *Can J Psychiatry* 1980;25:586.
13. Peden NR, Bisset AF, Macauly KEC, et al. Clinical toxicology of magic mushroom ingestion. *Postgrad Med J* 1981;57:543.
14. Ramirez P, Parrilla P, Bueno FS, et al. Fulminant hepatic failure after *Lepiota* mushroom poisoning. *J Hepatol* 1993;19:51.
15. Schumacher T, Hoiland K. Mushroom poisoning caused by species of the genus *Cortinarius fries*. *Arch Toxicol* 1983;53:87.
16. Short ALK, Watling R, MacDonald MK, et al. Poisoning by *Cortinarius speciosissimus*. Lancet 1980;2:942.
17. Spoerke DG, Rumack BH. *Handbook of mushroom poisoning: diagnosis and treatment*, 2nd ed. Boca Raton, FL: CRC Press, 1994.
18. Vesconi S, Langer M, Iapichino G, et al. Therapy of cytotoxic mushroom intoxication. *Crit Care Med* 1985;13:402.
19. Warden CR, Benjamin DR. Acute renal failure associated with suspected *Amanita smithiana* mushroom ingestions: a case series. *Acad Emerg Med* 1998;5:808.
20. Yamada EG, Mohle-Boetani J, Olson KR, et al. Mushroom poisoning due to amatoxin. *West J Med* 1998;169:380.

CHAPTER 356
Neuroleptic Poisoning

Christopher H. Linden

Neuroleptics, also known as antipsychotic agents and major tranquilizers, are used to treat schizophrenia, the manic phase of bipolar disorders, and agitated behavior. They are also used for nausea, vomiting, sedation, hiccoughs, and tics. The older or classic agents are mainly effective for treating the positive symptoms of schizophrenia (e.g., agitation, hallucinations), whereas the newer or atypical antipsychotic agents are also effective for treating negative and cognitive symptoms (e.g., alogia, avolition, flattened affect, social withdrawal).[3,12,16] These agents are a structurally diverse group of compounds containing two to five aliphatic, aromatic, or heterocyclic rings (Table 356.1). Formulations include tablets, capsules, liquids, sustained-release preparations, suppositories, and injectable solutions.

Poisoning may be due to adverse reactions following therapeutic doses or may result from accidental or intentional overdosage. Poisoning in two infants has been reported after treatment with topical promethazine cream.[18] Side effects include the anticholinergic syndrome (see Chapter 312), dystonic reactions (see Chapter 335) and other extrapyramidal syndromes (e.g., akathisia, parkinsonism, perioral tremor, tardive dyskinesia), the neuroleptic malignant syndrome (NMS; see Chapter 209), hypotension, and sedation.[3,4] Phenothiazines have also been associated with sleep apnea, sudden infant death syndrome, and sudden death in adults.[8] Most deaths result from either suicidal overdose by psychotic or depressed adults or the NMS. Clozapine can cause agranulocytosis during therapeutic use.

The mechanism of action of neuroleptic agents is complex and incompletely understood. These drugs block alpha-adrenergic (α_1 and α_2), dopamine (primarily D_2, but also D_1 and D_4), histamine (H_1), muscarinic (primarily M_1), and serotoninergic (primarily 5-HT_{1A}, 5-HT_{2A}, and 5-HT_{1C}) receptors.[3,12,16]

TABLE 356.1. Neuroleptic Agents

Structural Class	Generic Name	Trade Name	Oral Dose (Adult, mg)
TRADITIONAL AGENTS			
Butyrophenone	Droperidol	Inapsine	2.5–10.0[c]
	Haloperidol	Haldol	0.5–2.0
Dibenzoxazepine	Loxapine	Loxitane	10–50
Diphenylbutylpiperidine	Pimozide	Orap	0.5–1
Indole	Molindone	Moban	5–25
Phenothiazine	Chlorpromazine	Thorazine	25–50
	Fluphenazine	Prolixin	2.5–10
	Mesoridazine	Serentil	25–100
	Perphenazine	Trilafon	4–16
	Prochlorperazine	Compazine	5–10
	Promazine	Sparine	25–100
	Promethazine[a]	Phenergan	25–50
	Thiethylperazine[a]	Torecan	10–30
	Thioridazine	Mellaril	25–100
	Trifluoperazine	Stelazine	2–5
	Triflupromazine	Vesprin	5–15[c]
	Trimeprazine[b]	Temaril	2.5
Thioxanthene	Chlorprothixene	Taractan	25–50
	Thiothixene	Navane	2–15
ATYPICAL ANTIPSYCHOTICS[d]			
Benzisoxazole	Risperidone	Risperdal	1–3
Dibenzodiazepine	Clozapine	Clozaril	200–600
Dibenzothiazepine	Quetiapine	Seroquel	50–250
Thienobenzodiazepine	Olanzapine	Zyprexa	10–15

[a] Used only as antiemetic.
[b] Used only as antipruritic.
[c] Parenteral dose.
[d] Atypical agents available outside the United States include raclopride, remoxipride, sertindole, sulpiride, and ziprasidone.

Antipsychotic activity, extrapyramidal effects, and the NMS appear to be due to interference with central nervous system (CNS) (cortical, limbic, basal ganglia) D_2 neurotransmission. Antiemetic activity and the ability to increase prolactin secretion also appear to result from inhibition of dopaminergic receptors (in the chemoreceptor trigger zone of the medulla and in the hypothalamus, respectively). Hypothalamic dysfunction may also be responsible for disordered temperature regulation. The atypical antipsychotic agents have lower and more selective (mesolimbic) D_2 potency and higher M_1 and/or 5-HT_{2A} antagonist activity than the traditional agents. Although higher doses are required for antipsychotic effect, they are less likely to cause acute dystonia and tardive dyskinesia. They also have minimal or no effect on prolactin secretion. Anticholinergic (M_1) potency correlates directly with sedative activity and inversely with the incidence of extrapyramidal reactions. Chlorpromazine, chlorprothixene, and thioridazine have potent sedative effects, whereas fluphenazine, haloperidol, trifluoperazine, and triflupromazine are commonly associated with extrapyramidal side effects. Of the atypical agents, only clozapine, olanzapine, and quetiapine have significant M_1 activity. Risperidone can cause extrapyramidal effects. Most antipsychotic agents are much more potent H_1 blockers than diphenhydramine.

Extrapyramidal side effects may occur early (within days) or late (after 3 months) in the course of therapy, particularly in patients treated with high-potency agents. Early effects include dyskinesia, akathisia, and parkinsonism; late effects include tardive dyskinesia, tardive dystonia, and the "rabbit syndrome" (focal perioral tremor).

Hypotension and miosis (common with chlorpromazine) appear to be due to peripheral alpha-adrenergic blockade as well as central effects. Hypotensive effects are primarily orthostatic and systolic in nature and tend to correlate in incidence and severity with sedative potency. Concomitant therapy with beta agonists (e.g., epinephrine) or beta blockers (e.g., propranolol) may result in severe hypotension.

Phenothiazines also have local anesthetic and quinidine-like (class 1a) antidysrhythmic and myocardial depressant effects. They frequently produce electrocardiogram (ECG) changes with therapeutic doses (most commonly with thioridazine and its metabolite mesoridazine).[5] Sertindole blocks cardiac potassium channels and can delay repolarization.[15] Many antipsychotic agents lower the seizure threshold and can induce epileptiform encephalogram (EEG) discharge patterns.[19] Ventricular dysrhythmias or asphyxia due to seizures, aspiration, or respiratory depression have been postulated as etiologies of sudden death in patients taking therapeutic doses of phenothiazines.

Because neuroleptic agents have a relatively flat dose–response curve, therapeutic doses vary widely (see Table 356.1) and are adjusted on the basis of clinical response and side effects, not by monitoring drug levels. Pharmacologic effects generally last 24 hours or more, allowing once-a-day dosing.

Most antipsychotic agents have an unpredictable pattern of gastrointestinal (GI) absorption, with peak levels 2 to 4 hours after ingestion. Their bioavailability with parenteral administration is two to ten times greater than with oral dosing, due to presystemic (GI and hepatic) metabolism following ingestion. Hence, therapeutic intravenous or intramuscular doses are substantially less than oral ones. After absorption, neuroleptic agents are highly bound to plasma proteins (90% to 99%). Because they are highly lipophilic, volumes of distribution are large (10 to 40 L/kg) and therapeutic drug levels are low (1 to several hundred ng/mL). Neuroleptics tend to accumulate in the brain and easily cross the placenta.

Elimination of these drugs occurs slowly by hepatic metabolism, with serum concentration half-lives averaging 20 to 40 hours. Small amounts (1% to 3%) are excreted unchanged by the kidney. As a rule, hepatic metabolism yields multiple metabolites, some of which are pharmacologically active (e.g., mesoridazine is an active metabolite of thioridazine). Metabolites are eliminated by urinary and, to some extent, by biliary excretion and can be detected in the urine for a month or more after cessation of chronic therapy.[3] Concomitant use of agents that inhibit or stimulate hepatic cytochrome oxidases can increase or decrease, respectively, the blood level and effect of these agents.[3,4]

Toxic effects following overdosage result from exaggerated pharmacologic activity. Central effects include CNS and respiratory depression and occasional delirium.[20] Central and peripheral anticholinergic effects can occur (see Chapter 312). Hypothermia may be due both to hypothalamic depression and peripheral vasodilatation. Seizures are rare and occur mainly in patients with underlying epilepsy and in those with loxapine overdoses.[14] Rhabdomyolysis may occur with prolonged convulsions. Cardiovascular effects include hypotension (often with reflex tachycardia), cardiac conduction disturbances, dysrhythmias, and, rarely, pulmonary edema.[6,11] Conduction delays (prolonged QRS and Q-T intervals) and associated ventricular tachyarrhythmias are most common with thioridazine overdoses.[5] They can also occur during high-dose intravenous haloperidol therapy.[19]

Antipsychotic agents have a high therapeutic index. Of the thousands of overdoses reported each year, only 1% to 2% of patients develop serious toxicity; only about one in 50 overdoses proves fatal. Thioridazine (because of its tricyclic antidepressant–like cardiotoxicity) or mixed overdoses are involved in most successful suicides.

Toxic doses are not well established. In general, acute ingestion of the maximal therapeutic dose results in significant side effects, and ingestion of five to ten times this amount can result in serious toxicity. Death of an infant has been reported after the ingestion of only 350 mg of chlorpromazine. Adult fatalities have been reported with ingestions of 600 mg of olanzapine, 2 g of chlorpromazine and clozapine, 2.5 g of loxapine and mesoridazine, and 1.5 g of thioridazine. Many patients, however, have survived much higher ingestions.

CLINICAL PRESENTATION

Although nausea and vomiting may develop soon after overdose, CNS and cardiovascular effects dominate the clinical picture of acute poisoning.[1,5–7,10,13] Findings in mild cases include ataxia, confusion, lethargy, slurred speech, tachycardia, and diastolic or orthostatic hypotension. Anticholinergic signs (Chapter 312) and hyperreflexia may also be present. ECG changes such as prolonged P-R and Q-T intervals, ST-segment depression, T-wave abnormalities (biphasic, blunting, inversion, notching, widening), and increased U waves may be seen with both therapeutic and excessive doses, particularly with thioridazine and mesoridazine.[5] A prolonged Q-T interval is also common with sertindole use and overdose.[4]

Signs and symptoms of moderate poisoning include mild coma with respiratory depression and systolic hypotension. Miosis is common, but mydriasis may also be seen. Hypothermia (occasional) and hyperthermia (rare) may be present. Paradoxical agitation, delirium, and tachypnea have been reported. Sialorrhea may be seen following clozapine overdose.

In severe cases, coma, with loss of brainstem and deep tendon reflexes, apnea, hypotension, and cardiac dysrhythmias (especially with thioridazine and mesoridazine), may develop. Bradyarrhythmias include all degrees of atrioventricular block, bundle-branch block, QRS widening, and asystole.[5,6] Tachyarrhythmias include ventricular premature beats, ventricular tachycardia and fibrillation, and polymorphic ventricular tachycardia in the setting of Q-T interval prolongation (torsades de pointes). Pulmonary edema has been reported.[11] Loxapine poisoning is unique in that quinidine-like effects are not seen, but it causes severe, prolonged convulsions, leading to rhabdomyolysis and subsequent renal failure.[14]

The onset of poisoning occurs within 1 to 2 hours, with maximal severity usually apparent within 2 to 6 hours of ingestion. The presentation is the same regardless of age and whether the overdose is acute or chronic. Children appear more sensitive than adults to the effects of neuroleptic agents.

Extrapyramidal symptoms are usually related to a change in medication or dosing rather than to acute overdose (Chapter 335). Akathisia, a subjective sensation of motor restlessness, occurs in about 20% of patients treated with traditional neuroleptics and is sometimes associated with severe parkinsonism (see Chapter 208). It occurs in up to 50% of those treated with intravenous prochlorperazine for headache, nausea, and vomiting. Women are affected more often than men. Patients complain of feeling restless, jittery, and tense; they cannot sit or stand still, and when standing may shift their weight from foot to foot as if walking in place. Vital signs remain normal. Semipurposeful or purposeless limb movements (especially of the lower extremities), frequent shifting of body position, and tremors and myoclonic jerking may be noted.

The NMS (Chapter 209) usually occurs on initiation or increased intensity of neuroleptic therapy. A similar presentation has been reported following acute overdose.[2]

DIFFERENTIAL DIAGNOSIS

Poisoning by antidysrhythmic, anticholinergic, antiepileptic, narcotic, and sedative–hypnotic agents and the veterinary tranquilizer xylazine may cause similar CNS or cardiovascular effects. It may be impossible to distinguish tricyclic antidepressant from thioridazine or mesoridazine poisoning without laboratory assistance. CNS infection, infarction, and trauma should also be considered in the differential diagnosis. Akathisia is commonly misdiagnosed as anxiety or agitation related to an underlying psychiatric disorder.

EMERGENCY DEPARTMENT EVALUATION

A complete history should be obtained from the patient and, to corroborate the patient's history, from the person who either found or brought the patient to the emergency department. The name, quantity, and time of ingestion should be determined. In patients taking chronic neuroleptic medication, the physician should determine whether there was a recent medication or dosage change or a recent illness.

The physical examination should focus on the vital signs, cardiovascular system, neurologic function, and evidence of coexisting trauma. An initial rhythm strip and subsequent 12-lead ECG should be evaluated. Arterial blood gas analysis and a chest x-ray should be ordered in patients with severe poisoning. Because phenothiazines can be radiopaque, abdominal radiographs may be useful if the identity of the overdose agent is unknown. However, the lack of x-ray visualization does not rule out an ingestion and does not necessarily imply successful gastric decontamination. Routine laboratory evaluation should include a complete blood count and measurements of electrolytes, blood urea nitrogen, creatinine, and glucose to rule out concomitant abnormalities. In patients with seizures or hyperthermia, the laboratory evaluation should also include urinalysis (routine and for myoglobin); measurement of serum muscle enzymes (creatine phosphokinase, aldolase, alkaline phosphatase), calcium, magnesium, and phosphate; and a coagulation profile. Toxicologic analysis of the urine and serum by chromatography or immunoassay may be useful to confirm the identity of the agent and rule out other ingestants. Quantitative drug levels are not helpful in predicting clinical toxicity or in guiding treatment. Although neither sensitive nor specific, the Forest, Mason, and Phenistix colorimetric tests are rapid urine screens that may be positive with phenothiazine ingestions.

EMERGENCY DEPARTMENT MANAGEMENT

Supportive care is the priority for patients with neuroleptic overdose. The tempo and sequence of interventions depend on clinical severity. Advanced life-support measures should be instituted as necessary. All patients require cardiac and respiratory monitoring and intravenous access. Those with hyper- or hypothermia should have continuous (rectal or axillary probe) temperature monitoring. Patients with altered mental status or seizures should receive supplemental oxygen and empiric therapy with naloxone, dextrose, and thiamine.

Hypotension is initially treated with intravenous crystalloids. Norepinephrine and high-dose dopamine are the drugs of choice for refractory hypotension. Seizures are treated with incremental doses of lorazepam (initial dose 0.05 mg/kg intravenously) or diazepam (initial dose 0.1 mg/kg intravenously), followed by a loading dose of phenytoin (18 mg/kg intravenously; maximal rate, 50 mg/min) and then a barbiturate (e.g., amobarbital 10 to 15 mg/kg intravenously, maximal rate 100 mg/min; or phenobarbital 20 mg/kg intravenously, maximal rate 30 mg/min), if necessary. Refractory convulsions may require a paralyzing agent to prevent complications such as hyperthermia and rhabdomyolysis. Because succinylcholine itself may cause malignant hyperthermia, a nondepolarizing neuromuscular blocker such as pancuronium (0.06 to 0.1 mg/kg intravenously) or vecuronium (0.08 to 0.1 mg/kg intravenously) should be used. Treatment of seizures, as indicated by continuous or serial EEG monitoring, should be continued during the period of paralysis. Diuresis and alkalinization of the urine may prevent myoglobinuric renal failure in patients with rhabdomyolysis. Physostigmine can be given to control delirium in those with other anticholinergic findings who have normal cardiac conduction intervals (see Chapter 312).[17]

Stable ventricular tachyarrhythmias should be treated with lidocaine. Underlying metabolic abnormalities should be corrected. Sodium bicarbonate (1 mEq/kg intravenously) may be given if the QRS complex is wide (see Chapters 311 and 313). Type Ia (disopyramide, quinidine, procainamide) and II (beta blockers) antidysrhythmic drugs should be avoided. Unstable rhythms should be treated with electrical cardioversion. Torsades de pointes ventricular tachycardia may respond to magnesium (50 to 100 mg/kg intravenously over 1 hour) or overdrive pacing using isoproterenol or electricity.[9] Increasing the heart rate may shorten a prolonged Q-T interval, and thus facilitate conversion of this dysrhythmia. Hypotension may complicate isoproterenol therapy. Bradyarrhythmias are treated according to current Advanced Cardiac Life Support (ACLS) protocols. Complete heart block may require temporary cardiac pacing.

After stabilization, treatment should focus on GI decontamination in cases of acute oral overdosage. Activated charcoal and gastric lavage are preferred. Because of the risk of aspiration in patients who may develop CNS depression, seizures, and dystonic reactions, syrup of ipecac should be reserved for asymptomatic patients who can be treated within 30 minutes of ingestion. Drug-induced decreased GI motility may allow for effective decontamination many hours after the overdose. Measures to enhance the elimination of neuroleptic agents, such as diuresis, dialysis, and hemoperfusion, have not been shown to be effective. Repeated oral doses of activated charcoal are of potential but unproven benefit.

Recovery from acute poisoning can be expected within several hours to several days, depending on the severity. Mortality, due to early dysrhythmias or to late cerebral edema, pulmonary edema, disseminated intravascular coagulation, renal failure, or infectious complications, is estimated at 5% to 10%.

Patients who develop akathisia after a single therapeutic dose of a neuroleptic (e.g., prochlorperazine for migraine or vomiting) should be reassured that symptoms will resolve within 24 hours. Diphenhydramine or lorazepam can be given if necessary. Pretreatment with diphenhydramine may prevent this complication. Those with akathisia who require continued neuroleptic therapy can be managed by reducing the dose, switching to an agent of lower potency, or giving additional agents. Benzodiazepines, benztropine, clonidine, propranolol, and short-acting barbiturates have been used with moderate success.

DISPOSITION

Role of the Consultant

Physicians unfamiliar with the details of the evaluation and management of neuroleptic poisoning should consult a poison center or toxicologist for advice.

Indications for Admission

Asymptomatic patients with an acute overdose should be observed for 6 hours. Symptomatic patients should be observed until alert. Those with hypotension, significant CNS depression, seizures, or dysrhythmias should be admitted to an intensive care unit or a similarly equipped observation area. Alert patients with a history of overdose and quinidine-like ECG findings present a difficult disposition problem, because such ECG changes can be seen with therapeutic doses, yet they have been implicated in sudden death. It seems safest to admit these patients for 24 hours of cardiac monitoring.

Extrapyramidal symptoms, although worrisome to the patient, are not life-threatening. The patient's medications may need to be adjusted; this should be done in consultation with the patient's psychiatrist.

Transfer Considerations

Patients requiring transfer to a facility capable of providing intensive care should be accompanied by advanced life-support personnel and should have cardiac monitoring en route. Because treatment may require the use of agents not included in standard ACLS protocols, if possible, a physician should accompany the patient. Air as well as ground transportation is appropriate for this type of transfer.

COMMON PITFALLS

- Failing to obtain an accurate temperature
- Failing to institute cardiac monitoring and obtain an ECG, especially in patients with thioridazine, mesoridazine, and sertindole overdose

- Failing to appreciate that loxapine can cause intractable seizures, leading to rhabdomyolysis in the absence of cardiotoxicity
- Indiscriminate use of syrup of ipecac in patients with acute neuroleptic overdose
- Failing to institute aggressive treatment of hyperthermia, seizures, and muscle hyperactivity
- Failing to consider magnesium, isoproterenol, and overdrive pacing in the treatment of the torsades de pointes variety of ventricular tachycardia

ACKNOWLEDGMENT

The author gratefully acknowledges the contribution of Ross S. Carol who wrote the previous version of this chapter.

References

1. Acri AA, Henretig FM. Effects of risperidone in overdose. *Am J Emerg Med* 1998;16:498.
2. Baker PB, Merfian KS, Roberts JR, et al. Hyperthermia, hypertension, hypertonia, and coma in a massive thioridazine overdose. *Am J Emerg Med* 1988;6:346.
3. Baldessarini RJ. Drugs and the treatment of psychiatric disorders. Psychosis and anxiety. In: Hardman JG, Limbird LE, Molinoff PB, et al., eds. *Gilman & Goodman's the pharmacological basis of therapeutics,* 9th ed. New York: McGraw-Hill, 1996:399.
4. Brown CS, Markowitz JS, Moore TR, et al. Atypical antipsychotics. Part II: adverse effects, drug interactions, and costs. *Ann Pharmacother* 1999;33:210.
5. Buckley NA, White IM, Dawson AH. Cardiotoxicity more common in thioridazine overdose than with other neuroleptics. *Clin Toxicol* 1995;33:199.
6. Elkayan U, Frishman W. Cardiovascular effects of phenothiazines. *Am Heart J* 1980;100:397.
7. Harmon TJ, Benitez JG, Krenzelok EP, et al. Loss of consciousness from acute quetiapine overdose. *Clin Toxicol* 1998;36:599.
8. Kahn A, Blum D. Phenothiazines and sudden infant death syndrome. *Pediatrics* 1982;70:75.
9. Kemper A, Dunlop R, Pietro D. Thioridazine-induced torsades de pointes: successful therapy with isoproterenol. *JAMA* 1983;249:2931.
10. LeBlaye I, Donatoni B, Hall M, et al. Acute overdosage with clozapine: a review of the available clinical experience. *Pharm Med* 1992;6:169.
11. Li C, Gefter WB. Acute pulmonary edema induced by overdose of phenothiazines. *Chest* 1992;101:102.
12. Markowitz JS, Brown CS, Moore TR, et al. Atypical antipsychotics. Part I: pharmacology, pharmacokinetics, and efficacy. *Ann Pharmacother* 1999;33:73.
13. O'Malley GF, Seifert S, Heard K, et al. Olanzepine overdose mimicking opioid intoxication. *Ann Emerg Med* 1999;34:279.
14. Peterson C. Seizures induced by acute loxapine overdose. *Am J Psychiatry* 1981;138:1089.
15. Rampe D, Marawsky K, Grau J, et al. The antipsychotic sertindole is a high affinity antagonist of the human cardiac potassium channel. *J Pharmacol Exp Ther* 1998;286:788.
16. Richelson E. Receptor pharmacology of neuroleptics: relation to clinical effects. *J Clin Psychiatry* 1999;60[Suppl 10]:5.
17. Schuster P, Gabriel E, Kufferle B, et al. Reversal by physostigmine of clozapine-induced delirium. *Clin Toxicol* 1977;10:437.
18. Shawn DH, McGuigan MA. Poisoning from dermal absorption of promethazine. *Can Med Assoc J* 1984;130:1460.
19. Wilt JL, Minnema AM, Johnson RF, et al. Torsade de pointes associated with the use of intravenous haloperidol. *Ann Intern Med* 1993;119:391.
20. Zaratzian VL. Psychotropic drugs—neurotoxicity. *Clin Toxicol* 1980;17:231.

CHAPTER 357
Nicotine, Pyrethrin, and Chlorinated Hydrocarbon Insecticide Poisoning

William K. Chiang, Richard Y. Wang, and Ronald B. Mack

NICOTINE

Nicotine, the primary alkaloid of tobacco, is a naturally occurring pesticide obtained from *Nicotiana tabacum, Nicotiana rustica,* and other plants. It is also used in gum, nasal inhalers, and transdermal patches to aid in the cessation of smoking. Nicotine binds to nicotinic cholinergic (acetylcholine) receptors in the sympathetic and parasympathetic ganglion cells, neuromuscular junction, adrenal medulla, and the central nervous system (CNS).[17] An initial transitory stimulation of nicotinic receptors is followed by a more persistent depression and paralysis as a result of desensitization. Clinical symptoms may reflect receptor stimulation, depression, or both.

Absorption occurs through intact skin, the gastrointestinal tract, and the respiratory tree. Nicotine has a pK_a of 8.5 and is not well absorbed in the acid milieu of the stomach; alkalinization markedly increases absorption.[7] The apparent volume of distribution is approximately 1 L/kg. Protein binding is 20%. Once absorbed, 80% to 90% of the chemical is detoxified into cotinine in the liver and 20% is excreted unchanged by the kidneys. The elimination half-life in smokers is 0.8 hours and in nonsmokers, 1.3 hours. Elimination is complete in about 16 hours.

Tobacco leaves contain 1% to 6% nicotine; a cigarette contains 15 to 20 mg of nicotine, with one-fourth remaining in the butt; snuff contains 4.6 to 15.0 mg of nicotine per gram of moist material; chewing tobacco contains 2.5 mg of nicotine per gram of dry material; a cigar contains 15 to 20 mg of nicotine. Nicotine gum (e.g., Nicorette) contains 2 mg of nicotine buffered to a pH of 8.5 to enhance absorption. Transdermal nicotine patches (Habitrol, Nicoderm, Nicotrol, Prostep) release 7 to 21 mg of nicotine per day. However, the total nicotine content may range from 8.3 mg to 114.0 mg per patch.

Poisoning from nicotine can occur from any of the following: exposure to nicotine sulfate insecticides (Table 357.1); percutaneous absorption of nicotine in tobacco harvesters who pick and brush up against wet tobacco leaves[5]; ingestion of tobacco products, such as cigarettes, snuff, chewing tobacco, and cigars; chewing or ingestion of nicotine chewing gum; and improper

TABLE 357.1. Common Nicotine Insecticide Preparations

Black-Leaf 40	Nic-Dust
Destruxol Orchid Spray	Nicocide
Emo-Nik	Nico-Fume
Fumetobac	Nic-Sal
Mach-NIC	Ortho N-4 and N-5 dusts
Niagra PA Dust	Tendust

use or ingestion of nicotine patches.[20] Infants and young children are most susceptible to nicotine poisoning because of their small body size and the lack of tolerance to nicotine. Nicotine-related fatalities are rare because of its decreasing usage as a pesticide.

The toxic dose of nicotine varies. As little as 4 mg can cause symptoms; 40 to 60 mg is potentially fatal in an adult. In a small child, 1 mg of nicotine may cause symptoms.[9] Ingestion of one cigarette, three cigarette butts, one cigar butt, or any amount of nicotine chewing gum or patch should be considered potentially toxic in a child.

CLINICAL PRESENTATION

Onset of toxicity is rapid and can be seen within 15 minutes of exposure. Initial signs and symptoms include nausea, vomiting, salivation, bronchorrhea, abdominal pain, and diarrhea from parasympathetic stimulation and tachycardia; hypertension; and diaphoresis as result of sympathetic and adrenal stimulation. Early CNS effects include dizziness, headache, confusion, agitation, incoordination, and seizures. Muscular fasciculations may result from neuromuscular junction stimulation.

As the symptoms progress, hypotonia, muscle paralysis, respiratory failure, coma, bradycardia, and hypotension may ensue.[1,12] Because of both stimulatory and inhibitory effects on multiple systems, the signs and symptoms vary by the time, dose, and route of exposure. In severe cases, such as nicotine pesticide poisoning, the progression from stimulation to inhibition of the various systems may be rapid.[9]

In mild exposures, the symptoms can last for several hours. In severe cases, clinical toxicity can endure for 18 to 24 hours or more. Severe cases involve seizures and coma within 30 minutes, with respiratory arrest and death within 1 hour or less, especially with concentrated nicotine products. Patients who survive the first 4 hours usually recover fully.

Radiographic and electrocardiographic (ECG) findings are nonspecific. Nicotine can be detected in the urine by chromatographic drug assays. Leukocytosis and glycosuria may be noted.

DIFFERENTIAL DIAGNOSIS

Without a history of exposure, there are no pathognomonic signs of nicotine poisoning. It could be confused with acetylcholinesterase inhibitor poisoning, such organophosphate or carbamate insecticides, and carbamate drugs (edrophonium, physostigmine, and pilocarpine). In nicotine poisoning, however, there is no depression of the red blood cell cholinesterase.

Direct-acting cholinomimetic agents such as bethanechol, carbachol, and methacholine can also produce cholinergic effects similar to those of nicotine. However, because these agents have minimal effects on nicotinic receptors (except for carbachol), they produce minimal or no sympathetic or muscular symptoms.[17] Central and peripheral sympatholytics (alpha-adrenergic and beta-adrenergic receptor blockers, clonidine, guanabenz, topical decongestant imidazoline derivatives, and calcium blockers) can mimic the later stages of nicotine poisoning. These agents will not produce any muscarinic symptoms or neuromuscular weakness. Tree tobacco (*Nicotiana glauca*) contains the alkaloid anabasine, an isomer of nicotine that can cause similar symptoms.[11] Other substances to consider are the insect repellent diethyltoluamide; *Veratrum* and sabadilla plants; *Clitocybe* and *Inocybe* mushroom species; and poison hemlock (*Conium maculatum*).

EMERGENCY DEPARTMENT EVALUATION

The history should document the time, agent, dose, route, intent, and duration of exposure and the nature and course of symptoms. A complete physical examination should be performed, with particular attention to assessing cardiovascular, respiratory, and neurologic function. Patients with vital sign abnormalities should have an ECG. Symptomatic patients should have cardiac and oxygen saturation monitoring. No specific laboratory tests are diagnostic. The presence of nicotine in the urine of a nonsmoker is supportive. Plasma nicotine levels are not useful. Arterial blood gas analysis, blood chemistries, and hematologic analysis should be obtained based on clinical severity.

EMERGENCY DEPARTMENT MANAGEMENT

Activated charcoal is the preferred method of gastrointestinal decontamination. Except for recent ingestion (less than an hour) of large quantities of a nicotine pesticide, gastric aspiration or lavage would not likely provide additional benefit. Because emesis is usually rapid and spontaneous, ipecac is not advised. In addition, seizures and coma can occur rapidly, and emesis increases the risk of aspiration. If present, the transdermal patch should be removed. Exposed skin areas should be washed with soap and water. Exposed eyes should be irrigated with copious amounts of water for 15 minutes.

The patient should be closely monitored for the first few hours after exposure. Supportive care should be instituted as necessary. Seizures should be treated with intravenous benzodiazepines such as diazepam (for adults, 5 to 10 mg initially, repeated every 5 to 10 minutes as necessary, up to 30 mg; for children, 0.25 to 0.4 mg/kg per dose) or lorazepam (0.05 to 0.1 mg/kg; may be repeated twice every 15 minutes as necessary). If seizures cannot be controlled with diazepam or lorazepam, a barbiturate such as phenobarbital may be given.

Excess parasympathetic stimulation (e.g., marked bronchial secretions) can be controlled by atropine (for adults, 0.5 mg intravenously, repeated every 5 minutes as necessary, to a maximum of 2 mg). For children, the dose is 0.01 to 0.02 mg/kg intravenously, not to exceed 0.4 mg. Hypotension should be treated initially with administration of intravenous fluids; if it fails, dopamine or norepinephrine may be added. Artificial ventilation and oxygen therapy may be necessary. Mecamylamine (Inversine) is a specific nicotine antagonist; it is available only in tablets, however, and is not a practical form of therapy in a patient who is vomiting, convulsing, or hypotensive. Multiple-dose charcoal has not been evaluated, nor have hemodialysis and hemoperfusion.

DISPOSITION

Patients with mild symptoms can be observed for several hours and discharged once they become asymptomatic. All others should be admitted to the hospital, observed, and treated supportively. Because the cardiorespiratory system requires monitoring, intensive care unit (ICU) admission is advised. If such facilities are unavailable, the patient should be transferred. Advanced life-support measures and anticonvulsants should be available during transport. If necessary, consultation can be obtained by calling a regional poison control center or the National Pesticide Telecommunications Network (800-858-7378).

COMMON PITFALLS

- Failure to discover a nicotine patch unintentionally stuck to the skin of an infant or toddler with altered mental status because they were not completely undressed
- Inducing emesis with syrup of ipecac
- Being unprepared to manage seizure activity
- Failure to diagnose and treat respiratory failure, the primary cause of death in nicotine poisoning
- Failure to appreciate that administering antacids for gastrointestinal symptoms may increase the absorption of ingested nicotine

PYRETHRINS

Pyrethrins and pyrethroids are widely used as bug sprays because of their rapid incapacitating ("knock-down") effects on insects. Most are formulated in petroleum distillates for spray applications; many are marketed in pressurized cases. Synergists such as piperonyl butoxide, *N*-octyl-bicycloheptene dicarbonimide, and sesame oil derivatives are commonly added to inhibit the metabolism of pyrethrins and thus increase their efficiency. Pyrethrins and pyrethroids are also used for the treatment of head lice and scabies and as insect repellents (Table 357.2).

Pyrethrins are naturally occurring insecticides extracted from chrysanthemum flowers; they are esters of pyrethric and chrysanthemic acid.[15] Pyrethroids (e.g., permethrin, deltamethrin) are synthetic pyrethrins that are more stable (resist photolysis) in the natural environment and have greater insecticide potency than do pyrethrins. They can be separated into two classes based on their chemical structures: Type II agents contain a cyano group at the alpha carbon, and type I agents do not.[4]

In insects, pyrethrins and pyrethroids rapidly cause death by paralyzing the nervous system. They inactivate sodium channels in nerve axons by binding and prolonging the opened state. Other potential mechanisms of toxicity include the inhibition of adenosine triphosphatases and direct effects on membrane integrity. Type II pyrethroids also antagonize inhibitory chloride channels at the GABA binding site.[4] In general, type I agents are less toxic than the type II agents.

These compounds are rapidly degraded and leave almost no residuum in the environment. They are considered less toxic to mammals than any other major class of insecticides. Human toxicity is limited by factors such as a large first-pass effect by the liver, poor bioavailability, and rapid metabolic breakdown by ester hydrolysis, followed by hepatic oxidation.[13] Ingestion of amounts up to 5 mg/kg is unlikely to cause significant toxicity. The toxic oral dose is estimated to be more than 100 to 1,000 mg/kg, with a lethal dose estimated to be 10 to 100 g.[2] Synergists also have low human toxicity.[6]

TABLE 357.2. Common Pyrethrin/Pyrethroid Preparations

SHAMPOOS FOR HEAD LICE	
Elimite	
Nix-Creme Rinse	
Rid	
ENVIRONMENTAL SPRAYS	
Ambush	Pydrin
Atroban	Pynamin
Cesso 7c	Rondo
Dragon	Time Mist
Insectiban	Torpedo
Pounce	

CLINICAL PRESENTATION

Direct toxicity is uncommon. Adverse effects are usually due to hypersensitivity and include bronchospasm, vasomotor rhinitis, contact dermatitis, and, rarely, anaphylaxis.[19] Following inhalation, the most common presentation is a stuffy nose with clear discharge and a "scratchy" throat. In rare cases, sudden bronchospasm, swelling of the laryngeal mucosa, and shock (anaphylaxis) can occur. Patients allergic to ragweed have a higher risk of developing allergic reactions to pyrethrins. Synthetic pyrethroid is less likely to cause these reactions than natural pyrethrins.

Direct dermal exposure to pyrethrins can produce a contact dermatitis consisting of redness, blisters, burning, stinging, and numbness. Ocular exposure to hydrocarbon propellants can cause eye irritation and corneal abrasions. Massive exposure to type II pyrethroids can cause tremors, salivation, paresthesia, ataxia, choreoathetosis, and seizures. Similar exposure to type I agents can result in tremors, agitation, and hyperthermia.[4]

DIFFERENTIAL DIAGNOSIS

Pyrethrins and pyrethroids should be included in the differential diagnosis of patients who present with an apparent hypersensitivity reaction of the skin or respiratory system when exposed to flora, insecticides, or insect bites. Because almost all of the insecticides containing these compounds are in a hydrocarbon base, the risk of hydrocarbon pneumonitis must be considered in humans ingesting these products.

EMERGENCY DEPARTMENT EVALUATION

The history should include details of exposure as described for nicotine, and the physical examination should focus on the respiratory tract, neurologic status, and skin. Chest radiographs, oxygen saturation measurement or arterial blood gas analysis, and pulmonary function tests can help to assess respiratory function and possible aspiration in patients with wheezing, dyspnea, cough, and fever.

EMERGENCY DEPARTMENT MANAGEMENT

Gastrointestinal, skin, and eye decontamination should be performed. Pyrethrins and pyrethroids are lipophilic, so milk, cream, or substances that contain animal or vegetable fats should not be administered. Supportive care should be instituted as necessary. Anaphylaxis should be treated as described in Chapter 217. Hydrocarbon aspiration should be treated supportively (see Chapter 316). If seizures occur, diazepam or lorazepam should be administered. Refractory seizures may be treated with phenobarbital or other barbiturates. Atropine may be required for the control of secretions from type II agents. Contact dermatitis should be treated with topical corticosteroids.

DISPOSITION

Assistance in management can be provided by the sources described in the Nicotine section. Asymptomatic patients with oral ingestions should be observed for 6 hours; if they become symptomatic, admission to an ICU is advised. Patients with allergic reactions can usually be discharged after treatment. Depending on severity, those with persistent symptoms may require admission to a floor or ICU.

COMMON PITFALLS

- Failure to appreciate that most cases of pyrethrin poisoning are allergic reactions and not direct toxicity
- Failure to recognize and treat anaphylactic reactions
- Failure to consider the possibility of aspiration (hydrocarbon) pneumonitis in patients with respiratory symptoms

CHLORINATED HYDROCARBONS

Chlorinated hydrocarbon (organochlorine) insecticides are low-molecular-weight, fat-soluble aliphatic, aromatic, and complex hydrocarbons that contain chlorine (Table 357.3).[6,14,16] The Environmental Protection Agency has banned the use of many of these pesticides in the United States because they are stored indefinitely in human tissue.[16] Chlordane and toxaphene are still available, but their use is restricted. Other available agents include methoxychlor, dicofol, and the miticide and scabicide lindane (gamma benzene hexachloride).

Organochlorines can be absorbed from the skin, lungs, and gastrointestinal tract. Enteral absorption is efficient and increased in the presence of animal or vegetable fat. To a lesser extent, they are absorbed across pulmonary membranes, but only 10% or less of a dermally applied dose (e.g., lindane) is absorbed. Different compounds exhibit different tissue-storage and hepatic elimination rates. Many (e.g., chlordane, dieldrin, and heptachlor) can induce hepatic enzymes.

As the body stores decrease, their half-lives markedly increase, due to either altered lipoprotein binding or lessened chemical concentration gradient across body compartments. It may require months to years to eliminate mirex, kepone, DDT, and the beta isomer of benzene hydrochloride; weeks to months for aldrin, dieldrin, heptachlor, and hexachlorobenzene; and hours to several days for endrin, chlordane, toxaphene, endosulfan, methoxychlor, and chlorobenzilate. Most residents of the United States have detectable organochlorine residues in their bodies, especially in fat. These compounds are excreted in the feces and can be found in breast milk.

TABLE 357.3. Chlorinated Hydrocarbon Insecticides

Insecticide	Brand/Trade Name
Aldrin	Aldrex, Aldrite, Drinox
Chlorobenzilate	Acaraben, Folbex, Kop-Mite
Chlordane	1068, Belt, Chlor Kill, Niran
Chlordecone	Depone, Tat Ant Trap
DDT	Anofex, Dinocide, Pentech
Dieldrin	Albit, Dorytox, Octalox
Endrin	Agrine, Endrex, Hexadrin
Heptachlor	Velaicol, 53-CS-17
Lindane	Agrocide, Isotox, Kwell
Methoxychlor	DMDT, Marlate, Moxie
Mirex	Dechlorane, Ferriamide
Toxaphene	Alltox, Camphoclor, Motox

Toxicity is due primarily to interference with the axonal transmission of nerve impulses. Organochlorines interfere with the normal flow of sodium and potassium ions across the axon membrane as nerve impulses pass.[16] Unlike organophosphate insecticides, they do not depress cholinesterase enzymes.

The acute toxic potential of organochlorines varies with the different compounds and their rates and routes of absorption. The highest risk occurs from endrin, dieldrin, aldrin, chlordane, and toxaphene.[14] Intermediate-risk products include kepone, endosulfan, heptachlor, mirex, and DDT. The lowest risk products are methoxychlor, perthan, kelthane, chlorobenzilate, and hexachlorobenzene. Lindane is potentially toxic if applications to the skin are multiple.[10] Dermal and inhalational exposures most commonly occur in workers who spray organochlorine insecticides. Oral exposure may result from the ingestion of contaminated food or drinking water.[3] The estimated oral lethal dose in adults is 3 to 7 g for aldrin, 6 g for chlordane (less than 2 g can cause stupor and seizures), 1 to 5 g for dieldrin, and 10 to 30 g for lindane (as little as 1.6 g can cause seizures in children).[14]

CLINICAL PRESENTATION

The onset of symptoms following exposure may vary from minutes to hours, depending on the route and method of exposure and the physicochemical properties of the agent.[3] Nausea, vomiting, and diarrhea can occur as soon as 45 minutes after acute ingestion. Initial CNS effects include apprehension, headache, dizziness, tremors, ataxia, and disorientation. Stupor, coma, and seizures with respiratory depression may be seen in severe cases. Arrhythmias may result from increased myocardial sensitivity to catecholamines. Aspiration of formulations containing a petroleum distillate can result in a chemical pneumonitis. CNS toxicity, including seizures, can also occur in children following prolonged or excessive topical lindane exposures during the treatment of lice or scabies.[10] In severe cases, potential complications include lactic acidosis, rhabdomyolysis, and disseminated intravascular coagulation.

Chronic exposure to organochlorines can cause hepatomegaly. Extensive or prolonged dermal contact can result in skin irritation. Chronic ingestion of hexachlorobenzene has been associated with cutaneous porphyria. Cases of leukemia have been associated with the use of chlordane or heptachlor to control termites in homes.

DIFFERENTIAL DIAGNOSIS

Acute organochlorine insecticide poisoning must be distinguished from any condition that produces "gastroenteritis" with an altered mental status, especially ataxia, tremors, and seizures. CNS disease, drug withdrawal, stimulant intoxication (e.g., from sympathomimetics, xanthines, anticholinergics, hallucinogens, and isoniazid), and infectious etiologies should be considered.

EMERGENCY DEPARTMENT EVALUATION

Details of exposure should be elicited as described for nicotine. The physical examination should focus on the neurologic and cardiovascular systems. Symptomatic patients should have chest radiography, ECG, arterial blood gas analysis, and routine blood tests. Chlorinated hydrocarbons can be measured in the serum by using gas chromatography, but levels are not useful for clinical management.[8]

EMERGENCY DEPARTMENT MANAGEMENT

Activated charcoal is the preferred method of gastrointestinal decontamination. Because organochlorine compounds have an extensive enterohepatic recirculation, repeat doses of activated charcoal are recommended to enhance their elimination. Multiple doses of cholestyramine resin are also effective, but cholestyramine is less well tolerated than charcoal. Powder contaminating the skin should first be vacuumed off. Contaminated clothing should be removed, and the skin, hair, and nails scrubbed. Extracorporeal procedures are not effective in enhancing organochlorine elimination.

Supportive care, including oxygen, endotracheal intubation, and assisted ventilation, should be instituted as necessary. Benzodiazepines and barbiturates should be given for seizure control (see Nicotine section). Phenytoin may be less effective than barbiturates and may actually increase the incidence of seizures.[18] Intravenous fluids and cardiac monitoring are indicated for all but mild intoxications. Respiratory distress due to bronchospasm is managed with inhaled bronchodilators and humidified oxygen. Parenteral administration of adrenergic amines (e.g., epinephrine) is not recommended, because myocardial irritability may be enhanced.

DISPOSITION

Assistance may be obtained by consulting the sources noted in the Nicotine section. All patients who are symptomatic after an acute exposure should be admitted for observation and treatment. Patients with significant CNS depression or seizures should be admitted to an ICU. If such facilities are not available, the patient should be transferred. Advanced life-support measures should be available during transport. Patients remaining asymptomatic after a 6-hour period of observation following an acute exposure may be discharged with appropriate follow-up. Those with chronic exposures can generally be treated as outpatients.

COMMON PITFALLS

- Mistaking organochlorine insecticides for organophosphate insecticides (and vice versa), resulting in incorrect treatment
- Failure to consider the possibility of pulmonary aspiration after ingestion
- Failure to administer multiple doses of activated charcoal for oral exposures
- Failure to properly decontaminate patients with dermal exposures
- Inducing emesis with syrup of ipecac
- Being unprepared to manage seizure activity

References

1. Borys DJ, Setzer DJ, Ling LJ. CNS depression after ingestion of tobacco. *Vet Hum Toxicol* 1988;30(1):21.
2. Casida JE, Kimmel EC, Elliott M, et al. Oxidative metabolism of pyrethrins in mammals. *Nature* 1971;230:326.
3. Chugh SN, Dhawan R, Agrawal N, et al. Endosulfan poisoning in Northern India: a report of 18 cases. *Int J Clin Pharmacol Ther* 1998;36:474.
4. Dorman DC, Beasley R. Neurotoxicology of pyrethrin and pyrethroid insecticides. *Vet Human Toxicol* 1991;33:238.
5. Gehlbach SH, Williams WA, Perry LD, et al. Green tobacco sickness. *JAMA* 1974;229:14.
6. Hayes WJ Jr. *Pesticides studied in man*. Baltimore: Williams & Wilkins, 1982.
7. Ivey KJ, Trigg EJ. Absorption of nicotine in the human stomach and its effect on gastric ion fluxes and potential difference. *Am J Dig Dis* 1978;23:809.
8. Kutz FW, Strassman SC, Sperling JF, et al. A fatal chlordane poisoning. *J Toxicol Clin Toxicol* 1983;20:167.
9. Lavoie FW, Harris TM. Fatal nicotine ingestion. *J Emerg Med* 1991;9:133.
10. Lee B, Groth P. Scabies: transcutaneous poisoning during treatment. *Pediatrics* 1977;59:643.
11. Mellick LB, Makowski T, Mellick GA, et al. Neuromuscular blockade after ingestion of tree tobacco (*Nicotiana glauca*). *Ann Emerg Med* 1999;34:101.
12. Mensch AR, Holden M. Nicotine overdose after a single piece of nicotine gum. *Chest* 1984; 86:801.
13. Miyamoto J. Degradation, metabolism and toxicity of synthetic pyrethroids. *Environ Health Perspect* 1976;14:15.
14. Morgan DP. Solid organochlorine pesticides. In: *Recognition and management of pesticide poisoning*. Publication EPA-540/9-80-005. Washington, DC: US Environmental Protection Agency, 1982:14.
15. Ray DE. Pesticides derived from plants and other organisms. In: Hayes WJ Jr, Law ER, eds. *Handbook of pesticide toxicology*. San Diego: Academic Press, 1991:585.
16. Sharp DS, Eskenazi B, Harrison R, et al. Delayed health hazards of pesticide exposure. *Annu Rev Publ Health* 1986;8:441.
17. Taylor P. Agents acting at the neuromuscular junction and autonomic ganglia. In: Hardman JG, Limbird LE, Molinoff PB, et al., eds. *Goodman & Gilman's the pharmacological basis of therapeutics*, 9th ed. New York: McGraw-Hill, 1996:192.
18. Tilson HA, Hong JS, Mactutus CF. Effects of 5,5 diphenylhydantoin on neurobehavioral toxicity of organochlorine pesticides and permethrin. *J Pharmacol Exp Ther* 1985;233:285.
19. Wax PM, Hoffman RS. Fatality associated with inhalation of a pyrethrin shampoo. *Clin Toxicol* 1994;32:457.
20. Woolf A, Burkhart K, Caraccio T, et al. Self-poisoning among adults using multiple transdermal nicotine patches. *Clin Toxicol* 1996;34:691.

CHAPTER 358

Nonsteroidal Antiinflammatory Agent Poisoning

Marco L. A. Sivilotti

Nonsteroidal antiinflammatory drugs (NSAIDs) are a heterogeneous group of agents that have antiinflammatory, analgesic, and antipyretic activity. Excluding salicylates (discussed in Chap. 367), there are a variety of NSAIDs, which can be classified by target specificity and structure (Table 358.1). With widespread use and over-the-counter availability of some NSAIDs, it is not surprising that NSAIDs constitute one of the most common medications encountered in intentional overdose.

Three-fourths of these ingestions involve ibuprofen, the first nonsalicylate NSAID to be approved for over-the-counter use in the United States. Despite this frequency, most NSAID overdose patients develop minimal symptoms, and death is rare. In contrast, major sequelae due to side effects of therapeutic use of (e.g., gastrointestinal [GI] bleeding) are a much greater health concern.

The primary pharmacologic effects of NSAIDs result from the inhibition of cyclooxygenase (COX), the enzyme involved in the initial step of prostaglandin (PG) synthesis. Two isoforms of COX have been identified: COX-1, constitutionally present in platelets, endothelium, gastric mucosa, and the kidney; and COX-2, induced by inflammatory mediators and suppressed by glucocorticoids. Because the antiinflammatory properties of

TABLE 358.1. Pharmacokinetics of NSAIDS after Therapeutic Doses

Drug	Brand Name	Time to Peak Level (h)	Half-life (h)	Maximum Recommended Daily Adult Dose (mg)
NONSELECTIVE COX INHIBITORS				
Acetic acids				
Diclofenac sodium[a]	Voltaren	2–3	1.2–1.8	225
Diclofenac potassium	Cataflam	0.3–2.0	1.2–1.8	150
Etodolac[a]	Lodine	1–2	7.3	1,200
Indomethacin[a,b,c]	Indocin	1–2	4.5–6.0	200
Ketorolac[c]	Toradol	0.5–1.0	2.4–8.6	IM 120 PO 40
Nabumetone[d]	Relafen	2.5–4.0	22–30	2,000
Sulindac[e]	Clinoril	1–2	7.8	400
Tolmetin	Tolectin	0.5–1.0	1.1–1.5	2,000
Fenamic acids				
Mefenamic acid	Ponstel	1–3	2–4	1,000
Meclofenamate	Meclomen	0.5–2.0	2	400
Oxicams				
Meloxicam[f]	Mobic	5–6	20	22.5
Piroxicam	Feldene	3–5	30–60	20
Propionic acids				
Fenoprofen	Nalfon	1–2	2–3	3,200
Flurbiprofen	Ansaid, etc.	1–2	3–4	200
Ibuprofen[b]	Motrin, Advil, Nuprin	0.5–2.0	1.8–2.5	3,200
Ketoprofen[a]	Orudis, etc.	0.5–2.0	1.5–4.0	300
Naproxen[a,b]	Naprosyn, Aleve	2–4	12–15	1,500
Naproxen sodium[a]	Anaprox	1–2	12–15	1,375
Oxaprozin	Daypro	3–5	42–50	1,800
Carprofen	Rimadyl			1,200
Pyrazolones				
Oxyphenbutazone	Oxalid		27–72	600
Phenylbutazone	Azolid, Butazolidin	1–4	50–100	600
Salicylates				
Acetylsalicylic acid	Aspirin, etc.	1–2	2–30	4,000
Diflunisal	Dolobid	1–2	5–20	1,500
SELECTIVE COX-2 INHIBITORS				
Celecoxib	Celebrex	3–5	11	400
Rofecoxib[g]	Vioxx			

[a] Available as a sustained-release product.
[b] Available as a liquid formulation.
[c] Also available as parenteral formulation.
[d] Prodrug metabolized to 6-methoxy-2-naphthylacetic acid (6 MNA).
[e] Prodrug metabolized to sulindac sulphide (half-life 16.4 h).
[f] Preferential COX-2 inhibitor, but selectivity lost at therapeutic doses.
[g] Pharmacokinetic data not available.

NSAIDs appear to result from COX-2 inhibition, NSAIDs with selective COX-2 inhibition have recently been developed, with the promise of reduced side effects (see Table 358.1).[8] The significance and conservation of COX-2 selectivity in overdose are unknown.

Inhibition of COX may result in increased shunting of arachidonic acid to leukotrienes, at times precipitating severe allergic reactions. Inhibition of PGD_2, PGE_2 and $PGF_{2\alpha}$, which maintain the gastric mucosal barrier, local irritant effects, and inhibition of platelet thromboxane A_2 production, and hence platelet aggregation, are responsible for adverse GI effects such as gastritis and ulceration. Similarly, inhibition of PGI_2 and PGE_2, which have vasodilatory and natriuretic activity in the kidney, has been linked to the salt and water retention and acute renal failure that can occur with NSAID ingestion.[5]

NSAIDs are rapidly and almost completely absorbed.[3,17] They are weak acids with pK_as ranging from 3.5 to 5.6, have small volumes of distribution (0.08 to 0.4 L/kg; celecoxib, at 6 L/kg, is an exception), and are highly protein bound (more than 90%).[3,17] Metabolic acidosis after ibuprofen overdose is probably related to high levels of acidic drug and metabolites.[9,10] Elimination depends on hepatic metabolism primarily via the CYP2C subfamily of cytochrome P-450 enzymes, with subsequent renal excretion of metabolites conjugated with glucuronide. As much as 50% of ketorolac and 30% of indomethacin are excreted in the urine unchanged.[3] Only small quantities (less than 10%) of other NSAIDs are excreted unchanged in the urine, limiting the utility of urinary alkalinization in promoting elimination. Indomethacin, sulindac, etodolac, phenylbutazone, miloxicam, and piroxicam undergo enterohepatic recirculation.[17] The renal clearance of naproxen and oxaprozin is increased at high plasma concentrations as a result of saturable protein binding.[17] Only phenylbutazone exhibits dose-dependent (Michaelis-Menten) elimination.[17] Pharmacokinetic data are summarized in Table 358.1.

Except for pyrazolones and fenamic acids, NSAIDs seldom cause serious toxicity, even in large doses.[4,16] There is inadequate information to determine the minimum toxic or lethal dose for most NSAIDs. In a series of ibuprofen overdoses, all children who ingested less than 100 mg/kg remained asymptomatic, whereas those who ingested more than 400 mg/kg were at risk of developing significant toxicity.[7] In adults, the correlation between the amount ingested and subsequent development of symptoms was poor, with those ingesting between 6 and 54 g of ibuprofen at risk for potentially serious toxicity. In contrast, seizures have been reported with mefenamic acid ingestions of as little as 2.5 g in a 12-year-old child.[4] Phenylbutazone has caused death with as little as 2 g in a 1-year-old child and 2.5 g in an alcoholic adult.[4,15]

CLINICAL PRESENTATION

Most patients remain asymptomatic or develop only mild GI or neurologic symptoms following acute overdose. Specific signs and symptoms are summarized in Table 358.2. Death is rare and usually results from secondary complications such as aspiration or sepsis. In the absence of acute renal failure or secondary complications, full recovery can be expected within 6 to 24 hours. The elderly have an increased propensity to develop adverse effects with therapeutic doses and may be at increased risk of toxicity with overdoses because of preexisting disease. There is very little known about the new selective COX-2 inhibitors in overdose.

In contrast, the pyrazolones and fenamates can cause severe toxicity. Phenylbutazone and its active metabolite oxyphenbutazone can cause coma, seizures, arrhythmias, cardiogenic shock, respiratory alkalosis, and metabolic acidosis.[4,16] Tinnitus, deafness, and a rash may be present. Hepatic necrosis, without other symptoms, may develop 24 hours after overdosage. A red discoloration of the urine caused by the metabolite rubazonic acid may be observed. Mefenamic acid has a propensity to cause muscle twitching and tonic–clonic seizures. In one series, 15 of 54 patients had muscle twitching, and 11 of these progressed to grand mal seizures.[1] One 12-year-old patient seized after taking 2.5 g of mefenamic acid, and four adult patients seized after ingesting less than 5 g.[4] The time between ingestion and onset of seizures varies between 0.5 and 12.0 hours. Both cardiac and respiratory arrest may follow seizures.

Propionic and acetic acid derivatives are associated with relatively low toxicity. Of these agents, fenoprofen appears to be the most toxic.[4] Indomethacin, an indole structurally similar to serotonin, frequently causes headaches, even in therapeutic doses. It is also more often associated with tinnitus than are other NSAIDs. Zomepirac was withdrawn from markets because of a high incidence of severe allergic reactions, benoxaprofen because of fatal liver toxicity, and suprofen because of acute renal failure.

TABLE 358.2. Signs and Symptoms of NSAID Overdose

Gastrointestinal: nausea, vomiting, anorexia, abdominal pain, diarrhea, gastritis, gastrointestinal bleeding, occasional hepatocellular injury, rare cholestasis
Neurologic: dizziness, nystagmus, diplopia, blurred vision, headache, tinnitus, restlessness, lethargy, ataxia, confusion, coma, muscle fasciculations, seizures
Respiratory: hyperventilation, respiratory depression with cyanosis, apnea, diaphoresis
Cardiovascular: hypotension, bradycardia, occasional tachycardia, rare cardiac arrest
Renal: sodium retention and edema, proteinuria, hematuria, acute oliguric or nonoliguric renal failure
Hematologic: decreased platelet aggregation, prolongation of prothrombin time and partial thromboplastin time
Other: occasional metabolic acidosis, rare electrolyte imbalance

After piroxicam overdose, two patients who ingested 300 to 400 mg developed dizziness with blurred vision, and one who ingested 600 mg presented with coma but responded to pain and regained consciousness within 1 hour.[4] Because of the long elimination half-life of piroxicam, overdose symptoms can be prolonged.[11,13] Multisystem toxicity was noted in a 2-year-old who ingested 100 mg of piroxicam.[12] Initial effects included severe GI symptoms with fluid and electrolyte imbalance, mental confusion, and a generalized seizure. Liver and kidney dysfunction was evident by day 3, and pancytopenia with bone marrow aplasia and coagulopathy developed later. The white blood cell count nadir and liver enzyme peak were seen on day 9. Although the hospital course was complicated by sepsis, the child recovered by day 46. Experience in the overdose of other NSAIDs with long half-lives (oxaprozin and nabumetone) is limited, but prolonged toxicity should be anticipated. NSAID plasma levels are not routinely available and are not necessary for the treatment of acute ingestion. A rough correlation between ibuprofen plasma levels and clinical toxicity has been noted.[7]

DIFFERENTIAL DIAGNOSIS

Because GI symptoms, neurologic symptoms, and respiratory depression are common to many drug ingestions and medical illnesses, NSAID overdose cannot be diagnosed by clinical findings alone. The diagnosis is made primarily on the basis of history and the exclusion of other etiologies.

The central nervous system (CNS) depression that occurs with NSAID overdose is usually mild; coma unresponsive to stimulation is uncommon. Benzodiazepines, which may cause a similar degree of CNS and respiratory depression, should be considered in the differential diagnosis. Deep coma, marked hypotension, and severe respiratory depression suggest the presence of other drugs. The metabolic acidosis caused by ibuprofen is relatively mild and short-lived compared with that caused by the ingestion of salicylates, isoniazid, ethylene glycol, and methanol.[10]

EMERGENCY DEPARTMENT EVALUATION

A detailed history, including all medications available in the household, should be obtained; it may provide the only clue to NSAID overdose. The amount and time of ingestion and the onset, nature, and progression of symptoms should be noted. The physical examination should include complete vital signs and assessment of mental status and cardiorespiratory function, including oxygen saturation measurement. Evaluation for occult GI bleeding should be considered for patients with abdominal pain.

A complete blood count, electrolytes, blood urea nitrogen, creatinine, glucose, and urinalysis should be obtained in all symptomatic patients, those with underlying kidney dysfunction, and the elderly. Etodolac may cause a false-positive urine bilirubin and a false-positive urine ketone test when dipstick methods are used. Because the time of onset of renal failure varies and is poorly defined, it has been recommended that these tests be performed in all adults with ibuprofen overdoses of more than 6 g.[6] Arterial blood gases should be monitored in patients with significant mental status changes or respiratory depression. In patients with pyrazolone overdose, liver function tests should also be obtained.

Urine and blood samples should be sent for a toxicology screen in cases of altered sensorium of unknown cause. NSAIDs are difficult to detect and correctly identify using common screening procedures. Hence, a negative screen does not necessarily rule out overdose of these agents. Toxicology analysis may also help to rule out other drugs that cause similar symptoms.

EMERGENCY DEPARTMENT MANAGEMENT

Initial management consists of standard supportive care and GI decontamination. Mechanical ventilation may be necessary in severe poisonings. Hypotension can be managed with intravascular volume expansion using crystalloids. Vasopressors are seldom necessary. Atropine may be used for symptomatic bradycardia, and benzodiazepines are indicated for seizures. Sodium bicarbonate should be given to patients with significant metabolic acidosis. GI bleeding should be treated by standard measures. Coagulopathy can be corrected by administering fresh-frozen plasma and vitamin K1.

Activated charcoal is the preferred method of GI decontamination. It should be considered in all patients with intentional overdoses, adults with accidental ingestions of more than ten therapeutic doses, and children with accidental ingestions of more than five adult doses who present within 4 hours of ingestion.[16] Fenamic acids or pyrazolones may cause serious toxicity with even a couple of doses, and decontamination may be appropriate for all patients with these ingestions. Multiple-dose activated charcoal therapy has not been studied with most NSAIDs. Although the elimination half-life of phenylbutazone was decreased by 30% after therapeutic doses,[14] the clinical efficacy of this treatment is likely to be minimal, even for NSAIDs that undergo enterohepatic recirculation. Because most NSAIDs are highly protein bound and rapidly metabolized, diuresis or dialysis is not expected to remove a significant amount of active drug. Charcoal hemoperfusion may benefit patients with severe phenylbutazone poisoning.[2]

DISPOSITION

Patients should be observed for 4 to 6 hours after ingestion.[6,16] Those with minor symptoms should be observed until they become asymptomatic. Those with minor symptoms following the ingestion of fenamic acids or pyrazolones should be monitored for at least 12 hours. Patients with significant toxicity (coma, respiratory depression, seizures, or renal failure) should be admitted to a medical intensive care unit.

Patients with an abnormal urinalysis or underlying renal dysfunction should have follow-up kidney function tests. A complete blood count and kidney and liver function tests should be repeated 24 to 48 hours after pyrazolone overdose. Follow-up liver function tests should be obtained in symptomatic piroxicam overdose patients.

Transfer should not ordinarily be necessary. If acute renal failure develops, a nephrologist should be consulted. Psychiatric evaluation is necessary for all intentional ingestions.

COMMON PITFALLS

- Failure to appreciate that, in contrast to other NSAIDs, pyrazolones and fenamates can cause severe toxicity following overdose
- Failure to consider the possibility of other ingestions in patients with significant CNS depression, metabolic acidosis, or vital sign abnormalities
- Inducing emesis in a patient likely to develop seizures or coma
- Failure to observe the patient for 4 to 6 hours after overdose
- Failure to recognize that a negative toxicology screen does not necessarily exclude NSAID poisoning

ACKNOWLEDGMENT

The author gratefully acknowledges the contribution of Paula L. Townsend who wrote the previous edition of this chapter.

References

1. Balali-Mood M, Proudfoot AT, Critchley JAJH, et al. Mefenamic acid overdosage. *Lancet* 1981;1:1354.
2. Berlinger WG, Spector R, Flanigan MJ, et al. Hemoperfusion for phenylbutazone poisoning. *Ann Intern Med* 1982;96:334.
3. Brater DC. Clinical pharmacology of NSAIDs. *J Clin Pharmacol* 1988;28:518.
4. Court H, Volans GN. Poisoning after overdose with non-steroidal anti-inflammatory drugs. *Adverse Drug React Acute Poisoning Rev* 1984;3:1.
5. Dunn MJ. Nonsteroidal antiinflammatory drugs and renal function. *Annu Rev Med* 1984;35:411.
6. Hall AH, Rumack BH. Treatment of patients with ibuprofen overdose [Letter]. *Ann Emerg Med* 1988;17:184.
7. Hall AH, Smolinske SC, Conrad FL, et al. Ibuprofen overdose. 126 cases. *Ann Emerg Med* 1986;15:1308.
8. Hawkey CJ. COX-2 inhibitors. *Lancet* 1999;353:307.
9. Lee CY, Finkler A. Acute intoxication due to ibuprofen overdose. *Arch Pathol Lab Med* 1986;110:747.
10. Linden CH, Townsend PL. Metabolic acidosis after acute ibuprofen overdosage. *J Pediatr* 1987;111:922.
11. Lo GCC, Chan JYW. Piroxicam poisoning. *BMJ* 1983;287:798.
12. Macdougall LG, Taylor-Smith A, Rothberg AD, et al. Piroxicam poisoning in a 2-year-old child. *S Afr Med J* 1984;66:31.
13. Mosvold J, Mellem H, Stave R, et al. Overdosage of piroxicam. *Acta Med Scand* 1984;216:335.
14. Neuvonen P, Elonen E. Effect of activated charcoal on absorption and elimination of phenobarbitone, carbamazepine and phenylbutazone in man. *Eur J Clin Pharmacol* 1980;17:51.
15. Okonek S, Reinecke H. Acute toxicity of pyrazolones. *Am J Med* 1983;75(5A):94.
16. Vale JA, Meredith TJ. Acute poisoning due to non-steroidal anti-inflammatory drugs: clinical features and management. *Med Toxicol* 1986;1:12.
17. Verbeeck RK, Blackburn JL, Loewen GR. Clinical pharmacokinetics of nonsteroidal anti-inflammatory drugs. *Clin Pharmacokinet* 1983;8:297.

CHAPTER 359
Nutritional Supplements and Vitamins

Andrew R. Topliff

Vitamins are organic substances that are provided in small amounts in the normal diet to sustain the normal metabolic functions of life. These substances differ in chemical structure, biologic action, and, in most cases, dietary sources. The physiologic functions of each vitamin are complex and may depend on several related compounds. The use of vitamins includes treatment of vitamin deficiencies, treatment of inborn errors of metabolism, and self-prescribed dietary supplements to treat or prevent various medical conditions. Clinical disease may result from vitamin deficiency or vitamin excess.

Vitamin preparations may be solid or liquid oral dosage forms, parenteral solutions, and, in some cases, topical preparations. Most vitamins are available as a single entity or combined with other vitamins in multivitamin preparations.

In the United States, an estimated 23% of adults regularly use vitamin supplements, with higher proportions among females, Caucasians, and people living on the West Coast.[3] Several million of these take vitamins in excess of the recommended daily allowance (RDA; Table 359.1).[10,15] While such self-therapy may be costly (some have stated that Americans have the most expensive urine in the world), there is little doubt that some of the substances have potent antioxidant-free radical quenching activity, with potential to possibly prevent genetic mutation and carcinogenic activity and other forms of disease secondary to free radical mechanisms.[4]

The ubiquitous distribution of vitamins results in a relatively large number of acute poisonings, either accidental or intentional, many of which are treated in emergency departments. In 1997, there were 48,633 vitamin exposures reported.[9] About 78% involved children under age 6, 91% were accidental, and 11% were treated in a health-care facility. Less than 1% had moderate adverse effects, only 0.04% had major adverse effects, and there were no deaths. The majority of adverse reactions were seen in multivitamins that contained significant amounts of iron (see Chapter 345).

Data regarding chronic vitamin toxicity consists primarily of isolated case reports of severe toxicity, some resulting from self-prescribed "megadosing." Megadosing has been defined as the daily intake of more than five to ten times the RDA for longer than 4 weeks. However, even at large doses, chronic vitamin toxicity rarely occurs and, when present, is typically secondary to fat-soluble vitamins and to a few water-soluble vitamins.

Fat-soluble vitamins typically regulate specific metabolic activities, and water-soluble vitamins function as coenzymes. Fat-soluble vitamins include vitamins A, D, E, and K. Water-soluble vitamins include thiamine (B_1), riboflavin (B_2), nicotinic acid (B_3), pantothenic acid (B_5), pyridoxine (B_6), cyanocobalamin (B_{12}), biotin, folic acid, and ascorbic acid. While there are many nutritional substances that are taken for a variety of reasons, other commonly used substances include androstenedione and dihydroepiandrostenedione (DHEA), tryptophan, and melatonin. Herbal agents are discussed in Chapter 365.

FAT-SOLUBLE VITAMINS

Vitamin A is comprised of several closely related compounds (e.g., retinol, retinal, retinyl esters, and retinoic acid), all of which are biologically active but have different functions. Retinol functions in reproductive processes, retinal in vision, and retinoic acid in epithelial cell growth and differentiation. Interconversion between these isomers occurs readily in the body. Retinol is preferentially stored in the liver and transported to tissue sites by retinol-binding protein (RBP). Aqueous emulsions of synthetic retinol result in higher blood levels and lower fecal elimination than the older, oily preparation, thus producing toxicity at lower dosage levels.[12] Carotenoids (i.e., beta carotene) are precursors of retinol, but they are rarely associated with toxicity because biotransformation is relatively inefficient.

Vitamin A toxicity appears to result from exaggeration of retinol's normal physiologic action.[7,12] Retinol acts similarly to a hormone, stimulating mitosis and epithelial cell turnover rates. Thus, excess retinol results in eczema, excessive desquamation, alopecia, bony exostoses, metaphyseal flare, decreased bone remodeling, rarefaction of long bones, and congenital defects. It also appears that unbound retinol and retinyl esters may have membranolytic properties; this may occur when RBP becomes saturated. Diseases that alter RBP levels may increase the risk of toxicity. Preexisting liver disease, protein–calorie malnutrition, cystic fibrosis, febrile infection, proteinuria, and pregnancy have been associated with low RBP levels. When RBP levels are low, less retinol is required to saturate binding sites and increase circulating unbound retinol.[12] Patients with preexisting renal disease have impaired renal catabolism of RBP and elevated RBP levels and are also at increased risk of toxicity. Elevated plasma retinol and plasma retinyl ester levels have also been noted in patients with type V hyperlipoproteinemia.[6] Vitamin A has teratogenic activity, and doses significantly greater than the RDA should be avoided by women of childbearing age unless there is evidence of a deficit.

Pseudotumor cerebri occasionally occurs and may be related to altered cellular membrane function in the choroid plexus. Hepatic Ito cells also accumulate excess retinol and lipids, leading to fatty hepatic changes, enhanced hepatic collagen production, and, eventually, obstruction of sinusoidal blood flow and cirrhosis.

Vitamin D, a steroid-like substance, is formed by ultraviolet light acting to convert 7-dehydroxycholesterol to cholecalciferol. Cholecalciferol is then hydroxylated by the liver to 25-hydroxycholecalciferol (25-OHD), which is then metabolized by the kidneys to a more potent metabolite, 1,25-hydroxycholecalciferol (1,25-OHD). The latter metabolite regulates calcium and phosphorus absorption from the gut and resorption from bone. The mechanisms of vitamin D toxicity are related to exaggerated physiologic effects (i.e., increased calcium absorption and in-

TABLE 359.1. Recommended Dietary Allowances for Vitamins

	Fat-Soluble Vitamins			*Water-Soluble Vitamins*			
Age Group	Vitamin A (μg RE)*	Vitamin D (μg)†	Vitamin E (mg TE)‡	Vitamin C (mg)	Thiamine (mg)	Niacin (mg NE)§	Pyridoxine (mg)
Infant (< 1 yr)	375	7.5–10	3–4	30–35	0.3–0.4	5–6	0.3–0.6
Child (1–10 yrs)	400–700	10	6–7	40–45	0.7–1.0	9–13	1.0–1.4
Male > 10 yrs	1,000	5–10	10	50–60	1.2–1.5	15–20	1.7–2.0
Female > 10 yrs‖	800	5–10	8	50–60	1.0–1.1	13–15	1.4–1.6

* Retinol equivalents, 1 retinol equivalent = 1 μg retinol = 6 μg beta-carotene = 3.3 IU.
† As cholecalciferol, 10 μg cholecalciferol = 400 IU of vitamin D.
‡ Alpha-tocopherol equivalents. 1 mg d-alpha-tocopherol = 1 alpha-tocopherol equivalent (1 TE) = 1.49 IU.
§ Niacin equivalents. 1 niacin equivalent = 1 mg niacin = 60 mg of dietary tryptophar.
‖ Pregnant or lactating women require larger amounts of all vitamins.
From *Recommended dietary allowances*, 10th ed. Committee on Dietary Allowances, Food and Nutrition Board, National Research Council, 1989.

creased levels of the metabolite 25-OHD). 25-OHD may saturate normal protein-binding sites and become bound to albumin, allowing increased cellular membrane damage. 1,25-OHD, the metabolite with more potent physiologic activity, does not appear to be responsible for toxicity, and serum levels may be normal or even depressed.

Vitamin E comprises at least eight naturally occurring tocopherols. Alpha-tocopherol is the most important because it is the most abundant in animal tissue sources and has the greatest biologic activity. The d optical isomer is more active than the l isomer; most synthetic alpha-tocopherol preparations are mixed dl isomers. Tocopherols function as antioxidants by protecting lipids from oxidation by cellular components. Vitamin E toxicity is minimal, and its mechanism has not been elucidated.

Two naturally occurring substances have vitamin K activity: phytonadione (K_1) and a series of closely related compounds called menaquinones (K_2). The former is found in plants; the latter are synthesized by gram-positive bacteria in the intestinal tract. Menadione (K_3) is a synthetic derivative with vitamin K activity that is available as a water-soluble salt. Vitamin K promotes biosynthesis of clotting factors II, VII, IX, and X.

Vitamin K_3 toxicity is caused by the action of menadione as an oxidizing hemolysin.[12]

WATER-SOLUBLE VITAMINS

Most water-soluble vitamins are relatively nontoxic and their mechanisms of toxicity are unknown.[12,16] Severe toxicity and death from water-soluble vitamins is exceedingly rare, except for hypersensitivity reactions.

Thiamine (B_1) is converted by adenosine triphosphate to its active form, thiamine pyrophosphate, which functions as a coenzyme in the decarboxylation of alpha-keto acids and in the use of pentose in the hexose monophosphate shunt.

Nicotinic acid (niacin, B_3) is the functional component of nicotinamide adenine dinucleotide (NAD) and nicotinamide adenine dinucleotide phosphate (NADP). These coenzymes activate several dehydrogenases important to cellular respiration. Nutritional requirements can also be satisfied by nicotinamide (niacinamide) and tryptophan. The vasodilatory effects of nicotinic acid are thought to result from direct action on small blood vessels and histamine release.

Several naturally occurring substances have pyridoxine-related biologic activity, including pyridoxine, pyridoxal, and pyridoxamine. All three forms are converted to pyridoxal phosphate, which acts as a coenzyme for biotransformations of amino acids. The specific biochemical cause of their neurotoxicity has not been identified.

Several substances also have activities similar to ascorbic acid, but ascorbic acid itself is the most potent and the most commonly available. Ascorbic acid is reversibly oxidized to dehydroascorbic acid. Both function in oxidative biochemical reactions.

NUTRITIONAL SUPPLEMENTS

Androstenedione and DHEA are precursors for steroid synthesis and may have some steroidal activity of their own. DHEA levels, in particular, have been shown to be elevated in younger animals and tend to fall off with age, poor health, obesity, certain infections, and other disorders. In some animal models, DHEA appears to be partially protective against infection with certain viruses and may inhibit certain types of cancer.[13,19] Individuals often take this substance as an "antiaging" supplement, to promote health, in an attempt to build muscle mass, and for its purported aphrodisiac effect (a commonly held belief, given that it is a precursor to testosterone synthesis).

Melatonin is a substance released by the pineal gland during times of decreased light. It serves to promote a resting state, alters other neuroendocrine function, and, in animals, appears to affect the ovulatory cycle, gonadal maturity, thyroid function, and the release of other pituitary hormones. It is often taken as a soporific in supraphysiologic amounts of 1 to 3 mg or more. It has also been prescribed in very large amounts, for its immunomodulatory effects, during certain kinds of chemotherapy.

Tryptophan, an essential amino acid, was taken by many individuals in the 1980s in large amounts (up to 8 g or more for extended lengths of time) as a soporific and antidepressant (thought to increase serotonin levels). At that time, approximately 1,500 individuals taking an L-tryptophan agent developed eosinophilia–myalgia syndrome.[17] Its sale was then restricted, but it was later found that a contaminant was likely the responsible etiology, as virtually all of the cases were from tryptophan that was produced by manufacturers using a new production process.

5-Hydroxytryptophan, a direct precursor of serotonin, is currently sold as an antidepressant. The eosinophilia–myalgia syndrome has not been reported with its use, and the valvulopathy seen with high serotonin states and the appetite suppressants fenfluramine and dexfenfluramine has also not been seen.

CLINICAL PRESENTATION

Patients with a single acute exposure to vitamins often present to the emergency department with either no symptoms or mild gastrointestinal (GI) distress, unless other, toxic agents were coingested. Vitamin formulations that contain significant iron are most likely to cause GI symptoms and other adverse sequelae (see Chapter 345). Notable exceptions include hypersensitivity reactions and nicotinic acid–induced flushing. Patients with toxicity from chronic megavitamin therapy may present to the emergency department with vague, nonspecific clinical findings (see specific vitamins). The key to diagnosis is to ask about vitamins and other supplements. Some patients may deny exposure to vitamins, either because they do not recognize them as drugs or because they perceive megavitamin therapy as unacceptable to physicians.

Fat-Soluble Vitamins

Acute vitamin A toxicity has been reported in Arctic explorers who have eaten polar bear or husky liver, which contains large amounts of vitamin A secondary to a marine diet. Acute toxicity from a single large overdose of vitamin A generally requires more than 25,000 IU/kg (4 million U in an adult and 300,000 U in children have caused toxicity). In adults, manifestations include severe headaches, dizziness, vomiting, diarrhea, and erythematous skin, which can develop within 8 hours. Later, skin typically cracks and peels.[12] In infants and children, anorexia, hyperirritability, vomiting, and bulging fontanelles (secondary to increased intracranial pressure) have been occasionally noted. Within a few days, these infants' skin also cracked and peeled. Symptoms resolved in all age categories, with no apparent long-term sequelae.

Other effects include increased intracranial pressure (pseudotumor cerebri). This condition is most common in women in their 30s to 40s, who often present with headaches, blurred vision, and diplopia. Elevated intake of vitamin A can also lead to hepatic disease.

Chronic vitamin A toxicity is usually associated with 4,000 IU/kg for months, although, occasionally, toxicity can develop with lower dosages (30 to 50,000 IU in adults and dosages of ten times the RDA in children).[12] The minimum toxic dose varies between patients, depending on age, health status, and dosage preparation. Skin and mucous membrane effects (e.g., erythema; eczema; pruritus; dry, cracked skin; epistaxis; conjunctivitis; palmar and plantar peeling; and alopecia) are the most common and first signs of toxicity. Musculoskeletal pain and tenderness over the long bones of the upper and lower extremities is common. Epiphyseal cupping and premature epiphyseal fusion may occur in children. Hypercalcemia has been reported but is not consistently present. Retinal crystals have been noted in patients ingesting carotene for tanning purposes.[18]

Neurologic symptoms include frontal headaches, blurred vision and diplopia. Hepatotoxicity, usually a later stage of toxicity, is manifested by hepatomegaly, splenomegaly, abnormal liver function tests (primarily aminotransferases, bilirubin, and alkaline phosphatase), and, eventually, portal hypertension, cirrhosis, and ascites. Liver biopsies reveal perisinusoidal, central vein sclerosis and hypertrophy of Ito cells. Normal retinol levels are 30 to 70 μg/dL, and a level greater than 80 μg/dL would be suggestive of toxicity; however, normal levels do not rule out toxicity, as the majority of vitamin A is hepatically stored.

Acute vitamin D toxicity is exceedingly rare, even with the consumption of rodenticides containing cholecalciferol. In a huge overdose, hypercalcemia would be expected. Chronic vitamin D toxicity, although more common, is also rare. This may occur in ingestion of the parent compound or the cholecalciferol metabolite. Chronic daily doses above 1250 μg of cholecalciferol in adults may cause toxicity. Patients with diseases such as hypoparathyroidism, vitamin D–resistant rickets, and osteomalacia who are taking physician-prescribed calciferol are at risk. Those with sarcoidosis, mycobacterial infections, and idiopathic hypercalcemia and hypercalciuria may develop toxicity with doses of 25 μg of cholecalciferol daily.

Chronic vitamin D toxicity has been associated with nausea, vomiting, constipation, anorexia, polydipsia, polyuria, hyperlipemia, hypercalcemia, and hyperphosphatemia. Hypercalcemia may be present without any symptoms, or it may cause pruritus, calcium deposits in soft tissue, and renal calculi.[12] Children and infants appear to be more susceptible to toxic effects and can develop cardiovascular, renal, and central nervous system injury.

Acute toxicity from vitamin E is virtually nonexistent, with only mild GI complaints expected. Chronic vitamin E toxicity is quite rare, even at dosages of ten times the RDA,[2] and many individuals have taken 800 IU or more daily for several years without apparent toxicity. Minor symptoms, such as nausea, fatigue, headaches, diplopia, muscle weakness, creatinuria, and elevated serum creatine kinase levels, can occur with extremely high doses. It appears that large amounts of vitamin E can hinder the absorption of other fat-soluble vitamins and can cause the inactivation of vitamin K, possibly explaining the minor elevation in prothrombin time in individuals on coumadin.[2]

E-Ferol, a discontinued parenteral dosage of vitamin E used in neonates, was associated with ascites, hepatomegaly, hyperbilirubinemia, azotemia, and thrombocytopenia, possibly caused by the emulsificants (polysorbate 20 and 80), which were used in the formulation.[11]

No adverse effects have been seen after the ingestion of oral vitamin K. Premature infants given menadione (the synthetic analogue) in parenteral doses of 5 to 25 μg daily have developed hemolytic anemia, hyperbilirubinemia, or kernicterus, and fatalities have rarely been reported. Patients with glucose-6-phosphate dehydrogenase deficiency and premature infants with hypoglycemia are at increased risk for these hemolytic effects. Intravenous phytonadione injections have occasionally resulted in chest pain, hypotension and dyspnea, asystole, and seizures. Chronic toxicity is not usually a concern, as phytonadione is rarely used long term and is not readily stored

Water-Soluble Vitamins

Single, acute thiamine ingestions have not resulted in toxicity. With older preparations and multiple dosing, parenteral administration was associated with tachycardia, hypotension, cardiac dysrhythmias, anaphylaxis, vasodilatation, headache, weakness, paralysis, and convulsions. Toxicity would not be expected in doses of 100 mg (or even much larger dosages) given intramuscularly or intravenously over 1 to 2 minutes as part of the "coma cocktail." It is unlikely that any chronic toxicity exists.

Most patients who use niacin experience flushing. These effects have been noted with oral doses of 100 mg and intravenous doses of 20 mg and are sometimes accompanied by pruritus, headache, and increased intracranial blood flow. These effects are more common in individuals just starting nicotinic acid therapy. High doses may be associated with nausea, diarrhea, and heartburn. Rarely, near syncopal spells are seen. These symptoms subside rapidly and do not usually require treatment. Nicotinamide has not been associated with these effects.

Chronic nicotinic acid therapy has been implicated as the cause of hepatotoxicity with centrilobular cholestasis and necrosis. This typically occurs at large dosages (3 g) used to treat hyperlipidemia (up to 100 times the RDA).[5,14] The hepatotoxicity, although rare, also appears to be correlated with using a sustained-release product and, possibly, the dose and frequency. Nicotinamide appears to be more hepatotoxic than nicotinic acid. Acute gouty arthritis has been precipitated secondary to elevated serum uric acid levels. Coagulopathies and hyperglycemia have rarely been reported.

Acute toxicity from pyridoxine is extremely rare but has occurred at extremely large doses (greater than 100 g in adults), resulting in dorsal root and sensory ganglia deficits.[1,16] Chronic toxicity often results in a nonspecific (primarily sensory) polyneuropathy, which is often, at least partially, reversible with discontinuance. Some studies have suggested that dosages greater than 200 mg/d could be neurotoxic, but toxicity is probably more common at dosages of a gram per day or more in adults.[16]

Ascorbic acid may cause diarrhea, nausea, and abdominal cramps with single doses as low as 1 to 2 g in adults. Ascorbic acid may cause a false-negative test for occult blood in the stool, spurious blood and urine glucose determinations, and inaccurate liver function (enzyme) tests. Massive intravenous dosages (greater than 40 g) of vitamin C can result in oxalate crystal precipitation and subsequent renal failure.[8]

With chronic ascorbic acid megavitamin therapy, excessive excretion of oxalate (an ascorbic acid metabolite) may increase the risk for kidney stones. The risk of nephrolithiasis formation (secondary to oxalate) is rare but occurs. This is exacerbated with increased fractional urinary excretion of uric acid and urine acidification, both resulting from chronic high-dose ascorbic acid therapy.

Nutritional Supplements

Acute androstenedione and DHEA overdose would not be expected to cause toxicity. In chronic use, there is a slight potential for all of the effects that are seen with anabolic steroids (which generally are reversible on discontinuation). It is possible that masculinization may occur, as well as possible hepatotoxicity, acne, gonadal suppression, and alterations of lipoproteins. It is also possible that individuals with hormone-sensitive cancers (i.e., prostate) could possibly have acceleration of their carcinoma. Although charcoal would likely bind these substances, it is unclear whether such therapy would be needed. Chronic overdose could be expected to cause these effects.

In acute melatonin overdose, symptoms include mild sedation, headache, and lethargy. Chronically, it has the potential to effect the neuroendocrine axis and possibly ovulation, and may worsen seasonal affective disorder in predisposed individuals (who probably have high endogenous levels of melatonin).

The eosinophilia–myalgia syndrome associated with L-tryptophan consists of the sudden onset of severe myalgias, pulmonary complaints, sclerodermal-like cutaneous involvement, eosinophilia and, rarely, a polyneuropathy.[17] It is possible that tryptophan and 5-hydroxytryptophan could cause serotonin syndrome when taken in large amounts or, more likely, when taken with antidepressants or certain other drugs. In acute overdose, sedation, fatigue, and, occasionally, emesis are the most common symptoms.

DIFFERENTIAL DIAGNOSIS

Given that the symptoms of vitamin toxicity, both acute and chronic, can be quite vague and nonspecific, it is important to consider this etiology in any patient with unexplained complaints. Vitamin A toxicity should be included in the differential diagnosis of dry eczematous skin, hepatic disease, or symptoms consistent with increased intracranial pressure. Pseudotumor cerebri can be caused by or associated with a variety of medications (e.g., corticosteroids, oral contraceptives, tetracyclines, thyroxin) and medical conditions (e.g., hypertension, hyperthyroidism, lupus, obesity, pheochromocytoma, pregnancy, sarcoidosis, ulcerative colitis), and it is also frequently idiopathic. Some cases have been misdiagnosed as acute encephalitis and subsequently treated with surgery. Signs and symptoms have also been attributed to optic neuritis and psychiatric illness. The differential of hypercalcemia should include vitamin A and D toxicity, malignancy (osteolytic metastases and malignancies associated with excess production of parathyroid hormone), sarcoidosis, multiple myeloma, milk–alkali syndrome, thyrotoxicosis, adrenal insufficiency, idiopathic hypercalcemia of infancy, and secondary complications in patients undergoing chronic hemodialysis. For neuropathy, causes in addition to pyridoxine include alcohol, heavy metals, solvents, other toxins, various drugs (e.g., isoniazid, nitrofurantoin, phenytoin), diabetes, collagen vascular diseases, and malignancy.

EMERGENCY DEPARTMENT EVALUATION

The history should routinely include asking about over-the-counter medications, vitamins, and herbals. A careful history directed toward medications and all over-the-counter products is necessary to ensure that important details are not missed. It is important to exclude the possibility that the supplements contain large amounts of iron.

Physical examination is frequently nonspecific. Papilledema and a desquamating rash suggest vitamin A toxicity. Serum calcium and, possibly, liver enzyme studies may be important tests for vitamin A and D toxicity. Radiographic changes may be present in vitamin D toxicity. The diagnosis is dependent on the history and the demonstration of persistently elevated blood levels of the vitamin in question.

EMERGENCY DEPARTMENT MANAGEMENT

Therapy is primarily supportive. Most of the signs and symptoms of vitamin intoxication are usually reversible. GI symptoms and niacin-induced flushing usually resolve in a few hours, but resolution of hepatic, metabolic, and neurologic toxicity may takes days to weeks. For acute exposures, GI decontamination may be indicated. Charcoal can be administered, depending on clinical likelihood of toxicity and the presence of coingestants. Patients with symptoms secondary to chronic exposure require discontinuation of vitamin therapy. Occasionally, it may be appropriate to begin intravenous fluids to maintain good urine output and promote excretion of calcium or water-soluble vitamins. Hypercalcemia can be treated with intravenous fluids and diuretics. Prednisone, calcitonin, chelators, and dialysis can be used if necessary. Low-grade pseudotumor cerebri typically resolves spontaneously. Diuretics, mannitol, steroids, and daily lumbar punctures may be required for more severe cases. Red cell transfusion and exchange transfusion or dialysis may be needed for neonates with significant hemolysis secondary to parenteral menadione.

DISPOSITION

Most patients can be referred for appropriate outpatient follow-up. Patients with hypercalcemia and evidence of increased intracranial pressure should be admitted. Women exposed to vitamin A during the first trimester of pregnancy should be referred to an obstetrician. Those with sensory neuropathies should be referred to a neurologist. Patients taking megadose vitamins should be warned about the dangers of chronic toxicity. Those with intentional overdose should be referred for psychiatric evaluation.

COMMON PITFALLS

- Failure to appreciate that vitamins, particularly fat-soluble vitamins, can cause poisoning
- Failure to ask about vitamin use and to include vitamin intoxication in the differential diagnosis of unexplained constitutional symptoms, hypercalcemia, and increased intracranial pressure
- Failure to determine whether iron was present in the vitamin preparation in cases of acute overdose
- Failure to warn patients about the dangers of megadose vitamin self-treatment

ACKNOWLEDGMENT

William Banner, Jr., and Newell E. McElwee contributed to previous versions of this chapter.

References

1. Albin RL, et al. Acute sensory neuropathy-neuronopathy from pyridoxine overdose. *Neurology* 1987;37:1729–1732.
2. Bendich A, et al. Safety of oral intake of vitamin E. *Am J Clin Nutr* 1988;48:612–619.
3. Block G, Cox C, Madans J, et al. Vitamin supplement use by demographic characteristics. *Am J Epidemiol* 1988;127:297.
4. Block G, et al. Fruit, vegetables, and cancer prevention: a review of the epidemiological evidence. *Nutr Cancer* 1992;18:1–29.
5. Dalton TA, et al. Hepatotoxicity associated with sustained release niacin. *Am J Med* 1992;93:102–104.
6. Ellis JK, Russell RM, Makrauer FL, et al. Increased risk of vitamin A toxicity in severe hypertriglyceridemia. *N Engl J Med* 1986;105:877.
7. Goodman DS. Vitamin A and retinoids in health and disease. *N Engl J Med* 1984;310:1023.
8. Lawton JM, et al. Acute oxalate nephropathy after massive ascorbic acid administration. *Arch Intern Med* 1985;145:950–951.
9. Litovitz TL, et al. 1997 Annual report of the American Association of Poison Control Centers National Data Collection System. *Am J Emerg Med* 1994;12:546.
10. Marcus R, Coulson AM. The vitamins. In: *Goodman & Gilman's the pharmacological basis of therapeutics,* 8th ed. New York: Macmillan, 1990:1523.

11. Martone WJ, Williams WW, Mortensen ML, et al. Illness with fatalities in premature infants: association with an intravenous vitamin E preparation, E-Ferol. *Pediatrics* 1986;78:591.
12. Miller DR, Hayes KC. Vitamin excess and toxicity. In: Hathcock JN, ed. *Nutritional toxicology,* vol 1. New York: Academic Press, 1982:81.
13. Pashko LL, et al. Topical DHEA inhibits tumors. *Carcinogenesis* 1984;5(4): 463–466.
14. Rader JI, et al. Hepatic toxicity of unmodified and time release preparations of niacin. *Am J Med* 1992;92:77–81.
15. *Recommended dietary allowances,* 10th ed. Committee on Dietary Allowances, Food and Nutrition Board, National Research Council, National Academy of Sciences, Washington, D.C. 1989.
16. Schaumburg H, Kaplan J, Windebank A, et al. Sensory neuropathy from pyridoxine abuse: a new megavitamin syndrome. *N Engl J Med* 1983;309:445.
17. Vargas J, et al. The cause and pathogenesis of the eosinophilia-myalgia syndrome. *Ann Intern Med* 1992;116:140–147.
18. White GL, Beesley R, Thiese SM, et al. Retinal crystals and oral tanning agents. *Am Fam Pract* 1988;37:125.
19. Yen SS, et al. Replacement of DHEA in aging men and women—potential remedial effects. *Ann N Y Acad Sci* 1995;774:128–142.

CHAPTER 360
Opioid Poisoning

William H. Dribben and Brent Furbee

Opioid poisoning is relatively common. The 1997 annual report of the American Association of Poison Control Centers noted 37,300 opioid exposures from pharmaceuticals, with 750 resulting in major toxicity and 113 in death. Heroin has recently made a resurgence in the United States, particularly among adolescents. There are an estimated 325,000 current past-month users (compared with 41,000 in 1990) and 810,000 chronic heroin users. The 1997 National Household Survey on Drug Abuse found that the mean age of initiation declined from 27.3 years in 1988 to 18.1 in 1996, the lowest since 1972. Increased availability of high-purity heroin has made snorting and smoking more common and has profoundly altered the pattern of heroin use. The Drug Abuse Warning Network (DAWN) estimated 72,010 heroin-related emergency department visits in 1997. DAWN received 9,484 reports of drug-abuse deaths in 1996, and 68.5% of those deaths had narcotic analgesics reported by the medical examiners' office as a contributory cause.

Regional fentanyl epidemics have been associated with hundreds of fatal overdoses, particularly among heroin users who have purchased it as "synthetic heroin" or "China White."[20] In 1982, cases of severe, acute parkinsonism occurred after illicit use of a meperidine analogue synthesized in a clandestine laboratory.[8] Affected individuals were known as "frozen addicts." A metabolite of the contaminant MPTP (1-methyl-4-phenyl-1,2,3,6-tetrahydropyridine), which selectively destroys dopamine-containing substantia nigra cells through inhibition of oxidative phosphorylation, was found to be responsible.

The term *opioid* applies to all agonists and antagonists with morphine-like activity, including both naturally occurring and synthetic compounds (Table 360.1). Additional agonists include levomethadyl, levorphanol, and sufentanil. Buprenorphine is another agonist–antagonist. Dextromethorphan is an agonist used only as an antitussive. It is low in potency, but doses of 100 times the therapeutic one can cause moderate toxicity. The distinction between different opioids is important from the standpoint of therapeutic effectiveness (potency), side effects, duration of action, and detectabilty by drug screens.

TABLE 360.1. Comparison of Common Opioids

Drug	Dose and Route	$T_{1/2}$	Duration of Action	Equiv. Dose (10 mg of MSO_4)
NATURAL				
Codeine	60 mg PO	2.9 h	4–6 h	120 mg
Morphine sulfate	2–10 mg IM/IV 60 mg PO	1.5–2.0 h	4–5 h	10 mg
SEMISYNTHETIC				
Heroin	3 mg IM/IV	as MSO_4	3-4 h	3 mg
Hydrocodone	5–10 mg IM/IV 25–30 mg PO	3.8 h	4-8 h	—
Hydromorphone	1–2 mg IM/IV 2 mg PO 3 mg per rectum	2.6 h	4-5 h	1.5 mg
Oxycodone	5 mg PO	—	3–4 h	10 mg
Oxymorphone HCl	0.5–1.0 IM/IV	—	3–6 h	1.1 mg
SYNTHETIC				
Diphenoxylate	5 mg PO	12–14 h	6–8 h	—
Fentanyl	0.05 mg IM/IV	2–4 h	30–60 min IV	0.125 mg
Meperidine	50–100 mg IM/IV	3.5 h	2–4 h	80–100 mg
Methadone	5–15 IM/IV	15 h	36–48 h	—
Propoxyphene	65–100 mg PO	3.5 h	2–4 h	240 mg
Tramadol	50–100 mg PO	6.3 h	4–6 h	—
AGONIST–ANTAGONIST				
Butorphanol	1 mg IV 2 mg IM 1 mg intranasally	3–4 h	3–4 h	—
Nalbuphine	10 mg IM/IV	5 h	3–6 h	—
Pentazocine	30 mg IM/IV 50 mg PO	2 h 3.6 h	2–3 h	—

Opioids are rapidly absorbed by all routes. Those with high lipid solubility can even be absorbed transdermally. Most opioids are metabolized by hepatic conjugation, with 90% excreted in the urine as inactive compounds. Significant first-pass metabolism results in lesser effects after oral administration than after parenteral administration of the same dose. Opioids have a large volume of distribution (1 to 4 L/kg) and variable penetration of the blood–brain barrier. The rate of metabolism of opiates does not accelerate with ongoing usage.[3]

Opioids act by binding to and activating specific receptors in the central and peripheral nervous system. At least three opioid receptor classes, some of which have been divided into subtypes, have been identified: the mu, kappa, and delta sites (Table 360.2). The sigma receptor, originally described as an opioid receptor, has since been reclassified because of its affinity for dextrorotatory isomers (opioid receptors prefer levorotatory isomers).

Central nervous system (CNS) opioid receptors modulate the transmission or perception of painful stimuli.[3] They are coupled to G-proteins and, when stimulated, inhibit adenylate cyclase. This results in blockage of voltage-gated calcium channels, activation of potassium efflux channels, hyperpolarization of the nerve terminal, and suppression of neurotransmitter release.[15] Opioid receptors also have inhibitory effects at postsynaptic sites, interrupting pain sensations at afferent nerves (Fig. 360.1).[9] Endogenous CNS peptide neurotransmitters (met- and leu-enkephalins, beta endorphins, and dynorphins) are opioid receptor agonists.[12] These substances may play an important role in drug tolerance and withdrawal.[3]

Therapeutic effects of pure opioid agonists are predominately mu-receptor–mediated, whereas the newer agonist–antagonist agents have antagonist activity at mu receptors and agonist activity at kappa receptors. Although tramadol has only weak affinity for mu receptors, it enhances serotonin release and inhibits serotonin and norepinephrine uptake, effects that may contribute to its analgesic activity.

Mechanisms implicated in opioid-induced seizures include hypoxia, decreased release of the inhibitory neurotransmitter gamma-aminobutyric acid (GABA), inhibition of inhibitory interneuron transmission, and membrane destabilization. Miosis stems from increased activity of the parasympathetic input to the pupil (Edinger-Westphal nucleus). The cause of pulmonary edema remains obscure, but several theories exist. Currently, the most accepted theory is that it involves a neurogenic process initiated by CNS hypoxia. Many opioids have a nonspecific ability to activate mast cell G-proteins, inducing degranulation of histamine-releasing vesicles. Opioids cause an initial stimulation and subsequent depression of the chemoreceptor zone of the medulla. Decreased gastrointestinal motility and increased sphincter tone (e.g., anal, ampulla of Vater) are secondary to mu-receptor stimulation. Cardiotoxicity (and seizures) due to propoxyphene and its metabolite norpropoxyphene is thought to be secondary to sodium channel blockade (also known as quinidine-like or membrane effect).[17] On a molar basis, propoxyphene and its metabolite have greater sodium channel blocking properties than quinidine or procainamide.

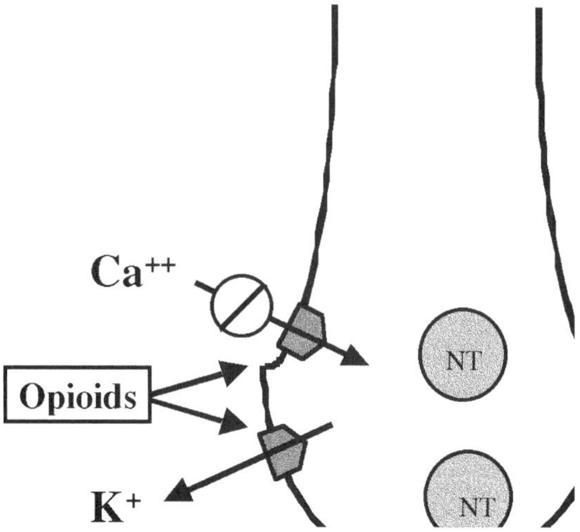

Figure 360.1. Mechanism of action: Opioids work at the presynaptic nerve ending by inhibiting calcium influx and promoting potassium efflux, preventing release of neurotransmitter *(NT)*; at the postsynaptic nerve terminal, opioids have similar effects, hyperpolarizing the cellular membrane, preventing effective propagation of nerve impulses.

TABLE 360.2. CNS Opioid Receptors

Receptor	Effects
Mu$_1$ (μ_1)	Supraspinal analgesia Peripheral analgesia Euphoria Prolactin release
Mu$_2$ (μ_2)	Spinal analgesia Respiratory depression Physical dependence Gastrointestinal dysmotility Miosis Pruritus Bradycardia
Kappa$_1$ (κ_1)	Spinal analgesia Miosis
Kappa$_2$ (κ_2)	Psychotomimesis Dysphoria
Kappa$_3$ (κ_3)	Supraspinal analgesia
Delta (δ)	Spinal analgesia Modulation of mu-receptor function Modulation of dopaminergic neurons

Opioid antagonists competitively bind to opioid receptors, reversing the effects of agonists and permitting increased transmission of painful stimuli. Additionally, antagonists are thought to alter the configuration of the receptor, thereby decreasing the availability of agonist-binding sites. Pure antagonists (naloxone, nalmefene, and naltrexone) avidly bind to all opioid receptor subtypes, but their activity at sigma receptors is variable.[7]

Tolerance, a well-known phenomenon whereby steadily increasing dosages are required to produce the same physiologic response, is most pronounced in the euphoric, analgesic, and sedative effects of opioids, whereas constipating and miotic effects show little or no tolerance.[3] Some tolerance to the respiratory depressant effects occurs, but the therapeutic index rapidly diminishes as the dose is increased to maintain the same euphoric or analgesic effects. The recurrent administration of exogenous opioids decreases endogenous production and secretion. If exogenous opioid administration is suddenly stopped, inadequate amounts of endogenous opioids are present to preclude neuronal firing; this hyperexcitability state may add to withdrawal symptoms.[3] Unlike benzodiazepine, barbiturate, or alcohol withdrawal, opioid withdrawal is generally not life-threatening. It can, however, cause seizures in neonates.[1,4]

CLINICAL PRESENTATION

Poisoning may occur after intravenous, intramuscular, intranasal, inhalational, oral, subcutaneous, intradermal, or transdermal exposure. Unintentional poisoning in addicts or persons seeking to get "high" and intentional use in suicide attempts are relatively common. In injection, inhalational, and intranasal drug users, poisoning typically occurs in novice users, during binging, or when an experienced user obtains a new supply of heroin (from a different source or dealer) and accidentally miscalculates the dose due to differences in purity. The possibility of an intentional self-overdose or attempted homicide must also be considered. Unintentional exposure is most common in children, although iatrogenic poisonings (therapeutic misadventures) do occur. Children may ingest pills or apply or ingest transdermal patches (that sometimes become stuck on the roof of the mouth). Elderly patients, particularly those on chronic opioid therapy for pain control of systemic illness, also constitute a high-risk group for unintentional poisoning.

The onset of symptoms is nearly immediate after injection, inhalation, and nasal insufflation. Although effects are usually noted within 30 minutes of ingestion, absorption can be erratic and delayed, particularly in children and with sustained-release formulations. Lomotil (diphenoxylate and atropine) is particularly notorious for causing delayed toxicity, perhaps because both constituents can inhibit gastrointestinal motility.[14] The effects of transdermal medications also begin about 30 minutes after application. They can, however, develop or progress after the patch is removed.

CNS depression, miosis, and respiratory depression are the three hallmark signs of opioid poisoning. CNS effects range from drowsiness to deep coma. In some cases, however, paradoxic excitation may be seen. Mixed agonist–antagonists such as pentazocine and butorphanol can cause dysphoric reactions or even psychosis because of their sigma-agonist activity. Seizures can occur in a pure opioid overdosage, particularly in children, but are most common in propoxyphene, tramadol, and meperidine poisoning.[17] They have also been reported with therapeutic doses of tramadol.[11] Increased muscle tone, tremors, or twitches may be seen with meperidine, and muscle rigidity has been associated with fentanyl.

Miosis is present in most cases.[6] Mydriasis or midrange pupils do not rule out opioid poisoning; in these instances, diphenoxylate, meperidine, hypoxic injury, hypoglycemia, a postictal state, or a cointoxicant should be considered. Atypical presentations are listed in Table 360.3.

Initially, the rate (but not the depth) of respirations is decreased. With increasing severity, cyanosis and extreme bradypnea are noted. Rapid, shallow respirations may be noted in patients with noncardiogenic pulmonary edema (NCPE). In such patients, an arterial blood gas analysis reveals hypoxemia, hypercarbia, and a respiratory acidosis.[2] NCPE can occur with any route of exposure. It is observed in a large percentage of heroin overdose fatalities[5] and often occurs after opioid antagonist administration. Respiratory decompensation develops within minutes to several hours, but radiographic evidence may be delayed up to 24 hours.[16] Patients who have not been comatose and apneic do not appear to be at risk for this complication. Manifestations include copious pink, frothy sputum and rhonchi, rales, or wheezes. Central venous pressure is normal or low. Hence, jugular venous distention and an S_3 gallop are absent. Chest radiograph findings include a normal-size heart and a variable pattern of pulmonary edema ranging from unilateral localized infiltrates to classic hilar-based bilateral infiltrates. Due to the CNS depressant effects of opioids, aspiration pneumonitis must also be considered as the cause of abnormal pulmonary findings on examination and radiograph.[2] These entities may be difficult to differentiate in the emergency department. Aspiration is more likely the cause when the chest radiograph abnormalities do not resolve within 48 hours.

Opioids have limited effects on the cardiovascular system. They increase venous capacitance (a therapeutic benefit when using morphine to treat cardiogenic pulmonary edema), which may cause a slight decrease in both systolic and diastolic pressures. In the supine patient, this effect often goes unnoticed. Except for propoxyphene, meperidine, or pentazocine, opioids have no direct inotropic or chronotropic effects.[17] Although significant hypotension can occur in propoxyphene poisoning and as a consequence of nonspecific histamine release, it is usually secondary to hypoxia, a cointoxicant, or shock from other etiologies. Likewise, although rhythm disturbances can occur in propoxyphene poisoning,[17] they otherwise suggest hypoxia or a coingestant. Propoxyphene can cause QRS widening, ventricular ectopy, decreased contractility, and hypotension.[17] Other electrocardiographic (ECG) abnormalities include right bundle-branch block, left bundle-branch block, first-degree atrioventricular block, ventricular bigeminy, and ventricular fibrillation. A murmur in an intravenous abuser should raise the possibility of endocarditis. Pulmonary hypertension with cor pulmonale may result from the injection of adulterants or contaminants.

Gastrointestinal effects include nausea and vomiting, decreased bowel sounds, and abdominal distention. Other complications of opioid overdose include urinary retention due to the increased sphincter tone, rhabdomyolysis, hypoglycemia, and hypothermia. Acute parkinsonism in a young person suggests the use of illicitly synthesized meperidine.

TABLE 360.3. Atypical Presentations of Opioid Poisoning

Agent	Prominent/Atypical Features
Propoxyphene (Darvon)	Rapid, sudden onset of opioid effects Seizures, psychosis (unresponsive to naloxone) Hypotension Prolongation of PR, QRS, and ventricular tachycardia Delayed onset of membrane depressant effects Low dose is life-threatening (11 mg/kg) Higher doses of naloxone needed to antagonize narcotic effects
Diphenoxylate (Lomotil)	Initial anticholinergic features Delayed onset of opioid effects Children at high risk for toxicity
Meperidine (Demerol)	Mydriasis Prolonged half-life of metabolite Seizures Increased muscle tone; serotonin syndrome
Pentazocine (Talwin)	Higher doses of naloxone needed to antagonize effects
Tramadol (Ultram)	Seizures unresponsive to naloxone Serotonin syndrome

DIFFERENTIAL DIAGNOSIS

Opioid poisoning should be considered in any patient with altered mental status (including seizures), miosis, and respiratory depression. Anticonvulsant, antidepressant, antihistamine, ethanol, muscle relaxant, neuroleptic, and sedative–hypnotic intoxication should be included in the differential diagnosis. Pontine hemorrhage, cholinergic agents, clonidine and other imidazolines, phencyclidine, and phenothiazines may cause also cause miosis. In pontine hemorrhage, the patient exhibits tachypnea (central neurogenic hyperventilation) and hypertension. Cholinergic agents (e.g., organophosphate insecticides) may cause a diagnostic dilemma initially, because the patient may appear to have pulmonary edema (profuse oral secretions, wheezing, and rales). The gastrointestinal tract is stimulated rather than depressed, however, resulting in hyperactive bowel sounds, recurrent vomiting, and diarrhea. Similarly, clonidine and other imidazolines (e.g., tetrahydrozoline, guanabenz) overdosage may result in bradycardia, hypotonia, and bradypnea. Phencyclidine intoxication is usually accompanied by tachycardia, hypertension, and muscle rigidity or tremor. In phenothiazine poisoning, hypotension and tachycardia occur in conjunction with coma. Hypothermia, encephalopathy, postictal state, CNS trauma or infection, cerebral vascular accident, and metabolic or electrolyte abnormalities, including hypoglycemia, hypercalcemia, hyponatremia, and hypernatremia, should also be considered in the differential diagnosis.

EMERGENCY DEPARTMENT EVALUATION

The history should include the identity of the opioid and any cointoxicants and the amount, time, intent, and route of exposure. The physical examination should initially focus on assessing the patency of the airway and the adequacy of ventilation. Patients should be placed on a cardiac monitor and have an oxygen saturation measured or an arterial blood gas analysis. Intravenous access should be established and blood obtained for determination of glucose (at the bedside for patients with altered mental status), electrolytes, blood urea nitrogen, and creatinine. Extra blood should be obtained for potential additional studies. A chest x-ray and ECG should be obtained in patients with unstable vital signs, hypoxia, or abnormal findings on cardiopulmonary examination (after antagonist therapy). An ECG should also be performed in patients with propoxyphene ingestions or abnormal rhythm or conduction intervals on cardiac monitoring. Creatine kinase and urine for myoglobin should be checked in patients with coma. Toxicology testing is appropriate to exclude cointoxicants such as acetaminophen (found in combination with opioids in many prescription medications) in cases of oral overdose. It is unnecessary in nonsuicidal patients with a history of injection drug use or recreational misadventures. Urine screening and comprehensive toxicology testing for drugs of abuse can detect some, but not all, opioids. Hence, a negative toxicology screen does not rule out opioid poisoning. In contrast, a lack of response to opioid antagonists virtually excludes this diagnosis. A positive response to opioid antagonists, although usually diagnostic, must be interpreted with caution, as poisoning with clonidine and valproate (and rarely benzodiazepines, ethanol, and chlorpromazine) sometimes responds to naloxone.

EMERGENCY DEPARTMENT MANAGEMENT

Supplemental oxygen and assisted ventilation should be provided, as necessary. With the expeditious use of opioid antagonists and ventilation temporarily provided by bag-valve-mask, endotracheal intubation can often be avoided. The application of four-point restraints should be considered before antagonist administration, because the patient may become uncooperative and combative. Suction equipment should be set up in advance, because vomiting may occur after naloxone administration.[19]

Opioid antagonists are indicated primarily for the treatment of respiratory depression. They may also be effective for opioid-induced seizures and can be used for diagnostic purposes in patients with altered mental status of unknown etiology.[6] In suspected addicts, a low initial dose of naloxone (0.1 to 0.4 mg intravenously) should be administered to avoid precipitating a severe withdrawal reaction. This dose may be repeated every minute until a total of 2 mg has been given or respiratory depression is reversed and the patient awakens. If the patient is not a suspected addict, 0.4 to 2.0 mg of naloxone can be given as the initial bolus. Because some opioid overdoses (e.g., propoxyphene and methadone) are relatively resistant to naloxone, increments of 2 mg every 2 to 5 minutes, up to a total of 10 mg, should be given if there is little or no response to the initial 2-mg bolus.[6] The dose of nalmefene is essentially the same as for naloxone.[7] Although longer acting than naloxone (4 to 8 hours vs. 30 to 100 minutes), this antagonist is more expensive. Naltrexone, an oral opioid antagonist, is only used for abstinence maintenance.

If intravenous access cannot be obtained, naloxone may be administered intramuscularly, subcutaneously, or endotracheally. The time to response after intramuscular administration is about the same as that required to start an intravenous line and give the drug intravenously. Indeed, because intramuscular administration has less risk of needlestick injury (and attendant potential for infections such as hepatitis and the human immunodeficiency virus) to health-care workers than attempting to start an intravenous line in an uncooperative patient or in one with sclerosed veins from injection drug use, this route is preferred by many, particularly prehospital care providers.

Because naloxone has a shorter duration of action—shorter than almost all of the opioid agents it antagonizes—opioid toxicity can recur (primarily after oral overdose and particularly with diphenoxylate and methadone), and repeat doses of naloxone may be necessary. A continuous naloxone drip may be appropriate in such situations. An infusion of two-thirds of the initial dose of naloxone required to reverse respiratory depression, given every hour, should maintain arousal. It may be necessary to give one-half of the original dose as an additional bolus 15 to 20 minutes after initiation of the drip.[10] Health-care providers must be diligent in monitoring patients placed on a naloxone drip.

A partial response to naloxone requires a careful search for other accompanying illness, injury, or intoxicants. Endotracheal intubation is necessary in patients with hypercarbia, hypoxia, or an inability to protect their airway. A neuromuscular blocking agent (e.g., succinylcholine) may be needed to perform an atraumatic intubation in some patients. Fluid restriction and positive end-expiratory pressure are also useful in the treatment of noncardiac pulmonary edema, but morphine and diuresis are inappropriate. Seizures unresponsive to naloxone should be treated with intravenous benzodiazepines (diazepam or lorazepam) or phenobarbital. Ongoing seizures suggest a cause other than pure opiate poisoning.

Hypotension is usually not a prominent feature of pure opioid overdose, and its presence should be managed initially with a crystalloid fluid bolus and an aggressive search for another cause.[3] Propoxyphene, however, can cause hypotension, necessitating aggressive use of vasopressors such as dopamine.[17] Likewise, cardiac rhythm disturbances or cardiogenic shock should suggest that pure opioid poisoning (except with propoxyphene) is unlikely.[6,17] Arrhythmias due to propoxyphene are similar to those of the tricyclic antidepressants and may respond to sodium bicarbonate therapy in a similar fashion (see Chapter 313). Naloxone will not reverse propoxyphene cardiotoxicity. Although naloxone only partially inhibits tramadol-mediated analgesia, it reverses respiratory depression and coma due to this agent. Patients with oral overdoses should receive activated charcoal. Delayed gastric emptying may slow drug absorption and make gastric decontamination efforts effective many hours after ingestion.

DISPOSITION

Careful observation is required for any patient who has demonstrated clinical evidence of opioid poisoning requiring naloxone administration. Although it is often recommended that patients with intravenous overdose be observed for a minimum of 6 hours for evidence of relapse or the development of noncardiac pulmonary edema, this may not be necessary. Such patients usually have taken only slightly more heroin than necessary to achieve the desired effect. In addition, complications, if they develop, are usually evident soon after presentation. In contrast, all patients who require naloxone after an oral overdose should be admitted to an intensive care unit with cardiac and respiratory monitoring (and suicide precautions, as needed). They should not be discharged until they are symptom-free for 12 hours. Adults who are or become asymptomatic during a 6-hour observation period after oral overdose may be discharged, whereas all children with an oral overdose should be admitted to the hospital for observation and monitoring for 12 to 24 hours. Psychiatric or social work follow-up must be arranged for all intentional or pediatric poisonings. Asymptomatic patients who have been treated with narcotic antagonists should be monitored.

COMMON PITFALLS

- Failure to consider opioid overdose in patients who present with altered mental status, including seizures or combativeness, as well as CNS depression
- Failure to apply restraints, thereby risking injury to staff, before giving naloxone to suspected addicts
- Failure to admit all patients who require naloxone after oral overdose and all symptomatic children
- Failure to evaluate for pulmonary complications, aspiration, and concomitant traumatic and medical illness
- Failure to examine thoroughly for medication patches (i.e., Fentanyl)

References

1. Doberczak TM, Kandall SR, Wilets I. Neonatal opiate abstinence syndrome in term and preterm infants. *J Pediatr* 1991;118:933.
2. Duberstein JL, Kaufman DM. A clinical study of an epidemic of heroin intoxication and heroin-induced pulmonary edema. *Am J Med* 1971;51:704.
3. Goldfrank L, Bresnitz E, Weisman R. Clinical aspects of drug intoxication: opioids and opiates. *Heart Lung* 1983;12:114.
4. Herzlinger RA, Kandall SR, Vaughan HG. Neonatal seizures associated with narcotic withdrawal. *J Pediatr* 1971;91:638.
5. Hine CH, Wright JA, Alison DJ, et al. Analysis of fatalities from acute narcotism in a major urban area. *J Forensic Sci* 1982;27:372.
6. Hoffman JR, Schriger DL, Luo JS. The empiric use of naloxone in patients with altered mental status: a reappraisal. *Ann Emerg Med* 1991;20:246.
7. Kaplan JL, Marx JA. Effectiveness and safety of intravenous nalmefene for emergency department patients with suspected narcotic overdose: a pilot study. *Ann Emerg Med* 1993;22:187.
8. Langston JW, Irwin I. MPTP: Current concepts and controversies. *Clin Neuropharmacol* 1986;9:485.
9. Lewis J, Mansour A, Khachaturian H, et al. *Opioids and pain regulation*, vol 9. Basel: Karger, 1987.
10. Lewis JM, Klein-Schwartz W, Benson BE, et al. Continuous naloxone infusion in pediatric narcotic overdose. *Am J Dis Child* 1984;138:944.
11. Lewis KS, Han NH. Tramadol: a new centrally acting analgesic. *Am J Health Syst Pharm* 1997;54:643.
12. Lutz RA, Pfister HP. Opioid receptors and their pharmacological profiles. *J Recept Res* 1992;12:267.
13. Martin M, Hecker J, Clark R, et al. China White epidemic: an eastern United States emergency department experience. *Ann Emerg Med* 1991;20:158.
14. Rumack BH, Temple AR. Lomotil poisoning. *Pediatrics* 1974;53:495.
15. Sarne Y, Fields A, Keren O, et al. Stimulatory effects of opioids on transmitter release and possible cellular mechanisms: overview and original results. *Neurochem Res* 1996;21:1353.
16. Sey MJ, Rubenstein D, Smith DS. Accidental methadone intoxication in a child. *Pediatrics* 1971;48:294.
17. Strom J. Acute propoxyphene self-poisoning. *Dan Med Bull* 1989;36:316.
18. Way EL. Sites and mechanisms of basic narcotic receptor function based on current research. *Ann Emerg Med* 1986;15:1021.
19. Yealy DM, Paris PM, Kaplan RM, et al. The safety of prehospital naloxone administration by paramedics. *Ann Emerg Med* 1990;19:902.
20. Ziporyn T. A growing industry and menace: makeshift laboratory's designer drugs. *JAMA* 1986;256:3061.

CHAPTER 361
Organophosphate and Carbamate Insecticides

Jeanmarie Perrone and Stephanie B. Abbuhl

Organophosphates were first synthesized in the early 1800s. During World War II, German scientists developed the highly toxic "nerve gas" agents Sarin, Soman, and Tabun and highlighted their toxic potential for chemical warfare (see Chapter 325). Although large-scale production of these nerve gas agents followed, it was not until March 20, 1995, when a container of Sarin gas was released in a crowded Tokyo subway car, that mass exposure resulting in human poisoning occurred. Over 5000 people were injured, and many required emergency treatment.[20] This terrorist act stimulated efforts in the United States and other countries to be prepared for a potential nerve gas exposure in any large city. Emergency physicians must be familiar with the manifestations and treatment of organophosphate poisoning, because they will be integral in the medical management of exposure victims.

Organophosphates and carbamates are more commonly encountered during their use as pesticides (Tables 361.1 and 361.2). Human exposures most often occur inadvertently in the agricultural setting or from intentional ingestion of products used to control pests around the home. Organophosphates are a very common cause of completed suicide attempts in developing countries such as India.[10] World health statistics estimate that 3 million serious pesticide poisonings occur worldwide annually.[7] Rarely, pesticide residues on crops have led to multiperson outbreaks of cholinergic poisoning.[6] Unintentional pediatric and some adult exposures occur when these toxic products are left in open or unmarked containers and are inadvertently ingested. Poison center data revealed 4,400 patients evaluated in health-care facilities and five deaths secondary to organophosphate or carbamate exposures in 1997.[8]

Organophosphates and carbamates are also used as pharmaceuticals. Malathion (Ovide) is used topically for the treatment of head lice. Echothiophate, a long-acting topical miotic utilized

TABLE 361.1. Toxicity of Selected Organophosphate Insecticides[a]

HIGHLY TOXIC
Tetraethyl pyrophosphate, TEPP (Bladan, Kilmite 40, Tetron, Vapatone)
Mevinphos (Phosdrin)
Sulfotepp (Bladafum, Dithione)
Methyl parathion (Dalf, Penncap-M)
Ethyl parathion (Parathion)
Methamidophos (Monitor)
Bonnyl (Swat)
MODERATELY TOXIC
Leptophos (Phosvel, Abar)
Dichlorvos, DDVP (Vapona, No Pest Strip)
Chlorpyridos (Lorsban, Dursban)
Fenthion (Baytex, Entex, Tiguvon, Spotton, Lysoff)
Dichlofenthion (Mobilawn, Bromex, Nemacide)
Diazinon (Spectracide, Diazide, Gardentox)
Trichlorfon (Dylox, Dipterex, Neguvon)
Acephate (Orthene)
Merphos (Folex)
Malathion (Cythion, Karbofos, Malamar)
Temephos (Abate, Abathion)
Ronnel (Korlan, Trolene, Viozene)

[a] The common name is followed by some examples of trade names in parentheses. Agents are listed in approximate order of decreasing toxicity within each toxicity grouping. Highly toxic organophosphates have oral LD_{50} values less than 50 mg/kg in rats and are usually restricted to agricultural use. Moderately toxic organophosphates have oral LD_{50} values greater than 50 mg/kg in rats and may be sold in formulations for household use.

Adapted from Morgan DP, *Recognition and management of pesticide poisonings*, 3rd ed. Washington, D.C.: US Environmental Protection Agency, 1982, and Mortensen ML. *Pediatr Clin North Am* 1986; 33:431, with permission.

TABLE 361.2. Toxicity of Selected Carbamate Insecticides[a]

HIGHLY TOXIC	MODERATELY TOXIC
Aldicarb (Temik)	Promecarb (Carbamult)
Methomyl (Lannate, Nudrin)	Methiocarb (Mesurol, Draza)
Carbofuran (Furadan)	Propoxur (Baygon)
Aminocarb (Matacil)	Primicarb (Pirimor, Aphox, Rapid)
Dimetilan (Snip Fly Bands)	Bufencarb (Bux)
	Carbaryl (Sevin)

[a] The common name is followed by some examples of trade names in parentheses. Agents are listed in approximate order of decreasing toxicity within each category. Highly toxic carbomates have oral LD_{50} values less than 50 mg/kg in rats and are usually restricted to agricultural use. Moderately toxic carbamates have oral LD_{50} values greater than 50 mg/kg in rats and may be sold in formulations for household use.

From Morgan DP. *Recognition and management of pesticide poisonings*, 3rd ed. Washington, D.C: US Environmental Protection Agency, 1982; and Mortensen ML. *Pediatr Clin North Am* 1986;33:431, with permission.

in the treatment of glaucoma, is also an organophosphate. Pyridostigmine, neostigmine, physostigmine and donepezil (Aricept), a new agent for treatment of Alzheimer disease, are carbamates.

Organophosphates and carbamates are rapidly absorbed from the skin and respiratory and gastrointestinal (GI) tracts. They are acetylcholinesterase inhibitors and potentiate acetylcholine at sites of cholinergic neurotransmission in the parasympathetic, sympathetic, and central nervous systems and at the neuromuscular junction (Figs. 361.1 and 361.2). Organophosphates inactivate the enzyme by phosphorylation; the resulting enzyme complex is stable, and thus binding is irreversible. Carbamates bind to the acetylcholinesterase enzyme but form an unstable complex, which spontaneously hydrolyzes within 24 to 48 hours, regenerating acetylcholinesterase and limiting toxicity. Acetylcholine released into the synapse in the presence of either type of acetylcholinesterase inhibitor is prevented from degradation, and excess acetylcholine activates postsynaptic receptors.

CLINICAL PRESENTATION

Acute Toxicity

Patients with organophosphate poisoning are often critically ill.[2,11,14,17] Cholinergic findings (see Fig. 361.2) may be subtle or obvious, depending on the exposure. Vital signs may be unstable, including depressed respirations and heart rate. Respiratory failure may result from excess pulmonary and oropharyngeal secretions, central nervous system (CNS) depression and neuromuscular weakness. CNS toxicity may include altered mental status, confusion, lethargy, seizures, and coma. Overstimulation of postsynaptic receptors at the neuromuscular junction results initially in fasciculations and then muscle fatigue and weakness. In the autonomic nervous system, parasympathetic effects predominate as muscarinic cholinergic nerve fibers are stimulated. The mnemonic DUMBBELS (see Fig. 361.2) is helpful in describing the cholinergic muscarinic findings due to parasympathetic stimulation of hollow viscous organs and glands. Sympathetic ganglia effects may result in hypertension and tachycardia. Diaphoresis occurs commonly due to direct cholinergic stimulation of sympathetic sweat glands. Pancreatitis and rhabdomyolysis are relatively common complications.

The severity and extent of cholinergic toxicity is dependent on dose, route, and agent of exposure. The onset of symptoms is generally most rapid after inhalation and most prolonged after skin exposure. Symptoms have been reported as early as 5 minutes after ingestion but usually occur by 12 to 24 hours. Highly fat soluble agents such as fenthion may cause delayed or prolonged toxicity.[4,13] Generally, toxicity is less with carbamate exposures. The organophosphates are a widely variable class, and some may produce protean cholinergic effects, while others may produce selected toxicity. The nerve gas agents (Sarin, Soman) characteristically produce more CNS effects and fewer peripheral signs of cholinergic toxicity. Therefore, characteristic muscarinic findings (DUMBBELS) may be absent despite significant exposures. The elderly are at especially high risk for complications, including aspiration and pneumonia, severe neurologic toxicity, and prolonged weakness. Patients with myasthenia gravis who intentionally or inadvertently develop toxicity from their own medications, such as pyridostigmine, may develop more severe cholinergic findings due to their compromised acetylcholine neurotransmission at baseline.

Intermediate Syndrome

In 1987, a syndrome of recrudescent organophosphate neurotoxicity was described in a series of patients 1 to 4 days following acute organophosphate poisoning.[19] Although all had initially improved following therapy with atropine and pralidoxime, cranial nerve palsies and a progressive truncal and proximal limb weakness became evident; 40% of the affected patients required intubation. Symptoms lasted 5 to 15 days, and one patient died. Subsequent prospective studies have demonstrated that this syndrome occurs frequently following exposure to highly fat soluble organophosphates and is related to prolonged cholinesterase inhibition.[5] It is proposed that redistribution of organophosphates from tissue reservoirs causes recrudescent toxicity at a time when atropine and oxime therapy have been completed.[3]

Delayed Peripheral Neuropathy

A distinct polyneuropathy may occur 1 to 3 weeks following organophosphate exposure. This syndrome was first described in 1930, when an estimated 40,000 persons became symptomatic due to contamination of an alcoholic beverage by tri-ortho-cresyl phosphate (TOCP), an organophosphate.[16] The debilitating distal flaccid paresis resulting from the neuropathy was termed the *Jamaican ginger paralysis* after the contaminated beverage, a ginger extract imported from Jamaica. The neuropathy resulting from organophosphate-induced inhibition of the enzyme, *neuropathy target esterase*, is characterized by axonal degeneration followed by myelin degeneration, with the large distal neurons affected first.[1] Patients with underlying medical problems such as alcoholism or nutritional deprivation may be at higher risk for developing delayed peripheral neuropathy. Recovery is incomplete in many cases, and motor symptoms are often persistent.

DIFFERENTIAL DIAGNOSIS

Identical manifestations can be seen in patients poisoned with direct-acting cholinergic agonists such as bethanechol, pilocarpine, and Urecholine. Digitalis, clonidine, calcium- or beta-receptor antagonist poisoning, myocardial ischemia, or conduction disease should be considered in patients who present with altered mental status and bradycardia, without other obvious signs of cholinergic toxicity. Miosis, bradycardia, lethargy, and respiratory depression would lead to a consideration of opioid toxicity. Lethargy and prominent sialorrhea or salivation may be seen with certain neuroleptic agents, such as clozapine and risperidone. Organophosphate-induced bronchorrhea and pulmonary edema may be difficult to distinguish from any other etiology of pulmonary edema. Patients with nicotine poisoning due to ingestion of tobacco products or harvesting wet tobacco may have similar findings, including vomiting, diarrhea, fascic-

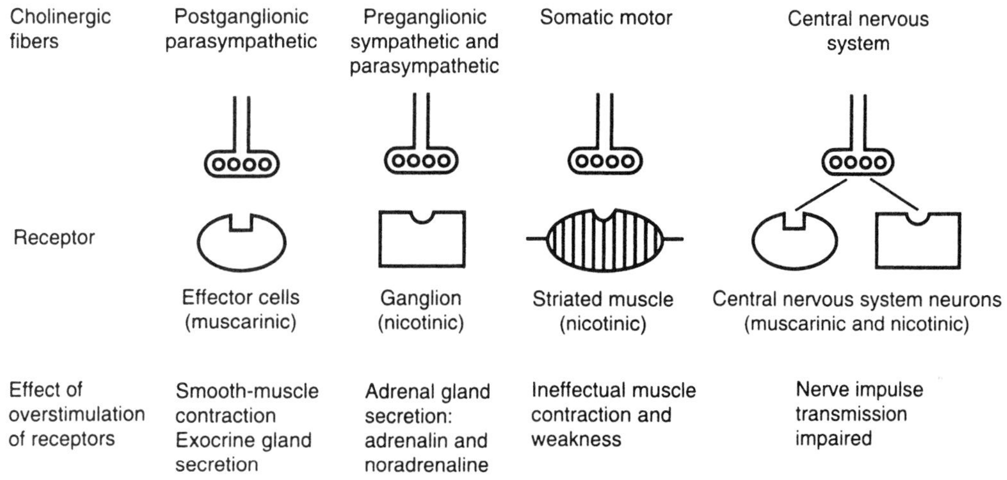

Figure 361.1. Acetylcholine (depicted as *open circles*) released by cholinergic nerve endings combines with four different groups of receptors to produce characteristic effects in different organs. Organophosphate poisoning leads to decreased destruction of acetylcholine and overstimulation of the receptors (cholinergic crisis). (From Bardin PG, van Eeden SF, Moolman JA, et al. Organophosphate and carbamate poisoning. *Arch Intern Med* 1994;154:1435.)

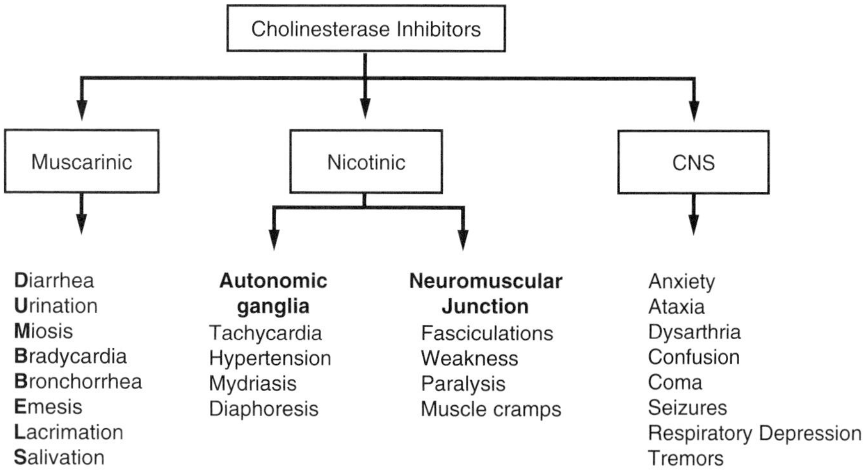

Figure 361.2. Cholinergic toxidrome.

ulations, weakness, altered mental status, and autonomic instability.

EMERGENCY DEPARTMENT EVALUATION

The history should document the amount, time, and route of exposure and the identity of the agent involved. Cardiac monitoring and pulse oximetry are crucial, because bradycardia may be marked and bronchial secretions and pulmonary edema may limit oxygenation. The physical examination should focus on the vital signs and assessment of cardiopulmonary and neuromuscular function, especially motor strength and respiratory effort. Cholinergic signs, particularly respiratory tract secretions, should be noted. Arterial blood gas analysis, forced vital capacity, and bedside spirometry should be performed to quantify respiratory dysfunction. An electrocardiogram, chest radiograph, and routine blood work, including complete blood count, electrolytes, blood urea nitrogen, creatinine, glucose, creatine phosphokinase, amylase, and liver function tests, should be obtained on symptomatic patients.

The diagnosis is confirmed by documenting decreased red blood cell (RBC) cholinesterase and plasma pseudocholinesterase activity. RBC cholinesterase activity is more specific, but plasma pseudocholinesterase activity tests are less expensive and more widely available. Although results are usually unavailable in a clinically relevant time frame, they can be helpful in cases in which the diagnosis is uncertain and in the evaluation of occupationally exposed patients. Specimens should be obtained prior to the administration of pralidoxime, because this antidote can increase measured enzyme activity.

Enzyme depression usually occurs rapidly. Following acute exposure, a 50% decrease in enzyme activity is associated with mild symptoms, and a 90% decrease with severe poisoning. Pseudocholinesterase activity may remain depressed for days to weeks, and RBC cholinesterase activity for 1 to 3 months following organophosphate exposure. In carbamate poisoning, activity may return to normal within minutes to hours. Interpretation of results may be difficult due to the variability in baseline values, which are subject to variety of factors. Pseudocholinesterase activity can be reduced in advanced liver disease, chronic alcoholism, dermatomyositis, malnutrition, and pregnancy, and following exposure to birth control pills, carbon disulfide, ciguatoxin, organic mercury compounds, benzalkonium salts, and solanins. Activity is genetically low than the norm in about 3% of the population. RBC cholinesterase activity is reduced in those with decreased red cell lifespan, such as in patients with hemolytic anemia and sickle cell disease. In some cases (e.g., chronic or occupational exposures), serial activity levels, showing a return to baseline with time, may be necessary. Specific pesticides can also be identified by detecting alkyl phosphates, phenols, and other metabolites in the urine.

EMERGENCY DEPARTMENT MANAGEMENT

Health-care providers should gown and glove appropriately in advance of treating the patient with potential organophosphate poisoning. Many of these patients carry significant dermal contamination, which can be dispersed unknowingly onto health-care providers. Organophosphates are absorbed via any body surface, and, therefore, nitrile or neoprene gloves, impervious gowns, masks, and head and shoe covers are recommended for the treatment team.

Advanced life-support measures should be instituted, as necessary. This may require endotracheal intubation by emergency medical services in the field. Atropine may be initiated prehospital in patients with bronchorrhea and/or bradycardia, because this may be effective in decreasing respiratory compromise. GI and skin decontamination should be undertaken as soon as the patient is stabilized. Activated charcoal is the preferred method for GI decontamination. Gastric aspiration or lavage should precede administration of activated charcoal in any patient requiring endotracheal intubation.

Patients with muscarinic findings, particularly excessive pulmonary secretions, should be given a trial of atropine immediately: 2 to 4 mg intravenously (0.02 to 0.05 mg/kg intravenously in children). Atropine acts by competitively blocking acetylcholine at muscarinic receptors, thereby reversing the excessive parasympathetic stimulation. It is only partially effective in treating CNS symptoms and has a variable effect on seizures and altered mental status. It has no effect on nicotinic receptors and, therefore, will not reverse muscle weakness or sympathetic ganglionic effects.

Patients who require intubation in the emergency department should undergo a rapid-sequence protocol. Because the duration of effect of succinylcholine may be much longer than usual due to the concomitant inhibition of cholinesterases that degrade succinylcholine,[18] an alternative, short-acting, nondepolarizing neuromuscular blocking agent such as mivacurium may be preferable.

Repeated doses of atropine may be needed to decrease bronchorrhea and oropharyngeal secretions. Atropine should be titrated to the clearing of these secretions, and not to irrelevant end points such as mydriasis or tachycardia. Very often, tachycardia is a result of dyspnea and inadequate atropine dosing. Atropine may be repeated every 5 to 15 minutes, with consideration of an atropine infusion (0.02 to 0.08 mg/kg/h) if frequent doses are needed. Atropine requirements are highly variable; patients with significant poisoning may require as much as 40 mg/d; one reported case describes a patient requiring 1,000 mg of atropine in a 24-hour period.[17]

Any patient who requires treatment with atropine should also receive pralidoxime (2-PAM). This should be initiated in the emergency department or as soon as the drug becomes available. Pralidoxime may be infused as a bolus therapy: 1 to 2 g in saline and administered over 30 minutes (20 to 40 mg/kg; maximum, 1 g per dose in children). The dose may be repeated in 1 to 2 hours if fasciculations are still present, and then at 6- to 12-hour intervals for 24 to 48 hours. Alternatively, it may be administered as a continuous infusion of 500 mg/h. Pralidoxime initially binds to cholinesterase enzymes and then to the inhibitor. The inhibitor–pralidoxime complex detaches from the acetylcholinesterase enzyme, returning it to a functional state. Pralidoxime is most effective in reversing the nicotinic effects, and it is synergistic with atropine at muscarinic receptors. Pralidoxime effects are rapid; improvement in muscle strength is noted within 10 to 40 minutes. Although it is not thought to cross the blood–brain barrier, pralidoxime may reverse some CNS effects.[9,17] Benzodiazepines may be needed for neurotoxic effects such as agitation and seizures.

Certain organophosphates have "aging" properties, which refer to their ability to bind permanently to acetylcholinesterase and not respond to pralidoxime. While many organophosphates share this capability, aging occurs at different rates. The hallmark of the "nerve gas" agents is their ability to age quickly, thereby becoming resistant to any antidotal intervention (see Chapter 325). Because carbamates undergo spontaneous hydrolysis from the acetylcholinesterase enzyme, early studies raised concerns about the need and safety of treating patients with carbaryl (a carbamate) poisoning with 2-PAM. Recent data support treating any poisoned patient requiring atropine with 2-PAM, regardless of the anticholinesterase agent.[12]

Therapy for the intermediate syndrome includes additional pralidoxime and, possibly, atropine, as well as supportive care. No specific therapy exists for peripheral neuropathy.

DISPOSITION

Patients with an unintentional exposure who remain asymptomatic following at least 6 hours of observation may be discharged home with a family member. Those requiring treatment with atropine or pralidoxime and those with evolving toxicity should be admitted to an intensive care unit (ICU) for close observation and monitoring. If the patient needs to be transferred to an ICU for admission, advance cardiac life-support (ACLS) personnel should accompany the patient. Prophylactic intubation prior to initiating transport may be advisable in patients with respiratory compromise. Consultation with a regional poison control center or medical toxicologist is advised for all exposures. Even asymptomatic patients need follow-up with their family doctor, because peripheral neuropathy can occur even in the absence of initial cholinergic manifestations.[15]

COMMON PITFALLS

- Failure to decontaminate the skin of patients with dermal exposures and to take appropriate precautions to prevent secondary exposure to health-care workers
- Failure to appreciate that death is usually due to respiratory failure and to administer oxygen, perform timely endotracheal intubation, and assist ventilation
- Failure to treat based on the presence of characteristic signs and symptoms rather than on the results of laboratory testing for cholinesterase inhibition
- Failure to appreciate that atropine therapy should be titrated to drying of secretions rather than to heart rate or pupil size and that doses far exceeding standard ACLS recommendations may be necessary
- Failure to treat all patients requiring atropine with pralidoxime
- Failure to appreciate that pralidoxime therapy must be initiated early in order to prevent "aging" of the cholinesterase inhibitor to the acetylcholinesterase enzyme and to decrease atropine requirements
- Failure to appreciate that highly fat soluble organophosphates may caused delayed, prolonged, or recurrent toxicity

References

1. Abou-Donia MB, Lapadula DM. Mechanisms of organophosphorus ester induced delayed neurotoxicity: type 1 and type II. *Ann Rev Pharmacol Toxicol* 1990;30:405.
2. Bardin PG, van Eeden SF, Moolman JA, et al. Organophosphate and carbamate poisoning. *Arch Intern Med* 1994;154:1433.
3. Benson B, Tolo D, McIntire M. Is the intermediate syndrome in organophosphate poisoning the result of insufficient oxime therapy? [Editorial] *J Toxicol Clin Toxicol* 1992;30:347.
4. Borowitz SM. Prolonged organophosphate toxicity in a 26-month-old child. *J Pediatr* 1988;112:302–304.
5. De Bleecker J, Van Den Neucker K, Colardyn F. Intermediate syndrome in organophosphorus poisoning: a prospective study. *Crit Care Med* 1993;21:1706–1711.
6. Green MA, Heumann MA, Wehr M, et al. An outbreak of watermelon-borne pesticide toxicity. *Am J Publ Health* 1987;77:1431–1434.
7. Jayaratnam J. Acute pesticide poisoning: a major global health problem. *World Health Stat Q* 1990;43:139–144.
8. Litovitz TL, Klein-Schwartz W, Dyer KS, et al. 1997 Annual report of the American Association of Poison Control Centers Toxic Exposure Surveillance System. *Am J Emerg Med* 1998;16:443–497.
9. Lotti M, Becker C. Treatment of acute organophosphate poisoning: evidence of a direct effect on central nervous system by 2-PAM (pyridine-2-aldoxime methyl chloride). *J Toxicol Clin Toxicol* 1982;19:121–127.
10. Malik GM, Mubarik M, Romshoo GJ. Organophosphorous poisoning in the Kashmir Valley, 1994–1997. *N Engl J Med* 1998;338:1078.
11. Marrs TC. Organophosphate poisoning. *Pharmacol Ther* 1993;58:51.
12. Mercurio-Zappala M, Hack J, Salvador A, et al. Carbaryl poisoning: 2-PAM or not 2-PAM. *J Toxicol Clin Toxicol* 1998;36:428(abst).
13. Merril D, Milton F. Prolonged toxicity of organophosphate poisoning. *Crit Care Med* 1982;10:550–551.
14. Minton NA, Murray VSG. A review of organophosphate poisoning. *Med Toxicol* 1988;3:350.
15. Moretto A, Lottei M. Poisoning by organophosphorus insecticides and sensory neuropathy. *J Neurol Neurosurg Psychiatry* 1998;64:463–468.
16. Morgan JP. The Jamaica ginger paralysis. *JAMA* 1982;248:1864–1867.
17. Namba T, Nolte C, Jackrel J, et al. Poisoning due to organophosphate insecticide. *Am J Med* 1971;50:475.
18. Selden BS, Curry SC. Prolonged succinylcholine-induced paralysis in organophosphate insecticide poisoning. *Ann Emerg Med* 1987;16:215–217.
19. Senanayake N, Karalliedde L. Neurotoxic effects of organophosphorus insecticides. An intermediate syndrome. *N Engl J Med* 1987;316:761–763.
20. Suzuke T, Morita H, Ono K, et al. Sarin poisoning in Tokyo subway. *Lancet* 1995;345:980.

CHAPTER 362

Petroleum Distillate Poisoning

Sophia Dyer and Michael W. Shannon

Products of the fractional distillation of natural petroleum include kerosene, mineral seal oil, gasoline, mineral spirits, naphtha, diesel fuel, motor oil, xylene, toluene, and benzene. Petroleum distillates begin as crude oil, which is heated in columns and separated on the basis of volatility. Petroleum distillates are typically classified as either aliphatic (straight-chain) or aromatic (benzene derivatives). Many are mixtures of both. Aromatic compounds are discussed in Chapter 316. Petroleum distillates are found in many household products, and improper storage of these products can result in inadvertent exposure.

Petroleum distillates are also referred to as hydrocarbons. The term *hydrocarbon*, however, describes structure rather than origin and includes compounds derived from plants (e.g., turpentine, pine oil, vegetable oil), animal fats, and coal. Therefore, whereas all petroleum distillates are hydrocarbons, not all hydrocarbons are petroleum distillates.

For clinical purposes, petroleum distillates are either toxic or nontoxic. Nontoxic petroleum distillates are those that have minimal gastrointestinal absorption and systemic toxicity, such as mineral oil. In contrast, halogenated and aromatic hydrocarbons and halogenated derivatives (Chapter 342) can be absorbed and produce substantial systemic effects. Petroleum distillates are also utilized as components of products such as pesticides.

Until recently, petroleum distillates were a leading cause of poisoning and death in children.[19] There are over 50,000 hydrocarbon exposures reported to U.S. poison centers each year. Over 20,000 occur in children under 6 years of age, with gasoline, kerosene, and lighter fluid most often involved. The majority of these exposures have minor effects. In adults, petroleum distillate poisoning is less common, usually occurring after occupational exposure, intentional ingestion, or accidental ingestion during the siphoning of fuels.[19] Data suggest a marked decrease in the overall frequency of petroleum distillate exposure in the United States. In developing countries, however, exposure remains common and results in significant morbidity and mortality.[10,14]

The greatest toxicity of petroleum distillates is to the respiratory tract. If they are aspirated, they lead to severe, diffuse chemical pneumonitis. The ratio of the LD_{50} of petroleum distillates when instilled intratracheally versus intragastrically is 1: 140 in animals. Petroleum distillate pneumonitis is characterized by the development of hemorrhagic bronchitis or alveolitis, loss of surfactant, alveolar collapse, respiratory failure, and death.[6,19] These complications are not seen after ingestion without aspiration, supporting the belief that petroleum distillates are poorly absorbed from the gastrointestinal tract and that pulmonary toxicity occurs only after direct contact with the respiratory epithelium.[4,8,20] Destruction of surfactant is a major contributor to pulmonary injury from petroleum distillates.

Many petroleum distillates have a central nervous system (CNS) narcotic effect that is the basis of sniffing or huffing, an increasingly common method of substance abuse in adolescents. Whether inhaled, injected, or ingested, such petroleum distillates can cause light-headedness, euphoria, incoordination, and impaired judgment. Inhalational injury and burns secondary to ignition of gasoline, while abusing it for CNS intoxication effects, have been reported. CNS effects may impair judgment and place the user at risk for thermal burns.[17]

Two independent physical characteristics govern the pulmonary and CNS effects of the petroleum distillates: viscosity and volatility (Table 362.1).[19] Viscosity (fluidity) is measured in units of Saybolt seconds universal (SSU) and correlates with aspiration risk. The lower the viscosity, the more likely a petroleum distillate will be aspirated. Substances of less than 60 SSU, such as kerosene and mineral seal oil, pose a significant aspiration risk, whereas those greater than 60 SSU do not. Volatility, measured by vapor pressure, determines the potential for CNS effects. The more volatile a substance, the greater the likelihood of pulmonary absorption and subsequent narcosis.

CLINICAL PRESENTATION

Following inhalation, pulmonary toxicity is usually negligible, but systemic effects are common. As many as 28% of intentional abusers have lethargy and coma.[19] Seizures, cardiac arrhythmias, including ventricular fibrillation, and permanent encephalopathy can occur. Lipoid pneumonia has been reported from chronic inhalation of aerosolized aliphatic petroleum distillates as well as the chronic ingestion or acute aspiration of mineral oil.[5] Inhalation of leaded gasoline has also been associated with the development of organic lead poisoning.[19]

Although the intravenous injection of petroleum distillates is a relatively uncommon event, several reports describe altered mental status, pneumonitis, thrombophlebitis, local cellulitis, venous thrombosis, abscess formation, and necrotizing myositis with an associated compartment syndrome.[11,15]

The ingestion of petroleum distillates is almost always followed by nausea and abdominal cramping. Spontaneous vomiting is also common, occurring in up to 40% of cases, and is associated with an increase in the likelihood of aspiration.[14] Oral pain, dysphagia, drooling, or hematemesis may also result from mucosal irritation. Additional signs of petroleum distillate ingestion include altered mental status or loss of consciousness (in up to 60% of children), fever (17%), and leukocytosis.[18,19] In children, intravascular hemolysis, hemoglobinuria, and disruptions of the omentum have also been reported.[1,19]

Aspiration of petroleum distillates leads to immediate coughing and gagging. Depending on the distillate and the amount aspirated, these symptoms may rapidly progress to tachypnea, nasal flaring, and respiratory distress.[12] Physical examination may reveal use of accessory respiratory muscles and cyanosis, and chest auscultation may reveal diffuse wheezes and rales. In severe cases, arterial blood gas analysis shows marked hypoxia, hypercapnia, and acidosis. Radiographic findings include atelectasis, patchy perihilar and midlung densities, pneumothorax, and pneumomediastinum.[16] Abnormalities on chest radiograph may lag behind clinical manifestations by several hours, but most will be evident within 12 hours.

Symptoms of pneumonitis usually worsen over 1 to 5 days and then resolve. Even after clinical illness has resolved, radiographic abnormalities may persist for days to weeks. Pneumatoceles have been reported presenting up to 15 days after exposure.[3] Although there are usually no overt long-term sequelae, some children have shown evidence of subclinical disturbances in pulmonary function 8 to 14 years after pneumonitis.[6]

TABLE 362.1. Influence of Volatility and Viscosity on the Clinical Effects of Petroleum Distillate Exposure

Volatility	Viscosity	Examples	Clinical Effect
High	Low	Kerosene, gasoline	CNS, respiratory
High	High	Toluene, xylene, benzene	CNS
	Low	Mineral seal oil	Respiratory
	High	Mineral oil, motor oil	No toxicity

DIFFERENTIAL DIAGNOSIS

Gastrointestinal symptoms resulting from petroleum distillate ingestion are similar to those of corrosive ingestion, infectious gastroenteritis, and food poisoning. A hydrocarbon odor on the breath or vomitus may suggest the correct diagnosis. Similarly, although symptoms of aspiration may resemble those caused by asthma, allergic reactions, pulmonary infections, and the inhalation of irritant gases (see Chapter 346), the history and physical examination usually disclose the correct cause.

EMERGENCY DEPARTMENT EVALUATION

The history should include the identity, amount, and concentration of the petroleum distillate ingested, the time of ingestion, and any symptoms present before arrival at the emergency department, particularly respiratory symptoms and vomiting at the time of ingestion. Because a number of different petroleum distillates may be found in a given product, all ingredients should be determined.

The physical examination should focus on the vital signs, respiratory system, mental status, and gastrointestinal system. Oxygen saturation should be obtained on all patients. Serial or continuous oximetry should be performed to identify the appearance of pulmonary decompensation. A chest radiograph should be obtained on any patient with respiratory symptoms. Arterial blood gases should be obtained in those who have an oxygen saturation of less than 90%. They should also be considered in patients with oxygen saturations less than 95% if significant tachypnea is present.

Routine laboratory studies (e.g., complete blood count, determination of electrolyte levels, blood urea nitrogen, creatinine, and glucose, and urinalysis) should also be obtained in patients with toxic petroleum distillate ingestion or evidence of aspiration. Depending on the specific agent ingested and the suspicion of coingestants, a toxic screen or other laboratory studies may also be indicated.

EMERGENCY DEPARTMENT MANAGEMENT

Management of ingestions depends on whether the compound has the potential to cause systemic toxicity. If a potentially toxic aromatic or halogenated agent has been ingested, gastrointestinal decontamination may be indicated. The risk of aspiration is equally increased by both gastric lavage and ipecac-induced emesis.[12,13] Because petroleum distillates are liquids, gastric aspiration (without lavage) may be effective and less risky and is the preferred method of gastric emptying. A small-bore nasogastric tube should be sufficient. In the patient with altered mental status, gastric evacuation should be preceded by endotracheal intubation.

Vomiting should be prevented and activated charcoal, which may produce emesis, should not be administered.[7] The efficacy of activated charcoal for petroleum distillate adsorption is unknown but is thought to be minimal. Similarly, sorbitol, a commonly used cathartic, has significant emetic potential and should not be administered. Because the greatest toxicity of the petroleum distillates results from aspiration and not gastrointestinal absorption, nontoxic petroleum distillates that are ingested do not require removal, regardless of the amount ingested.

All patients with respiratory symptoms should be given supplemental oxygen. The management of severe petroleum distillate aspiration includes early intubation and positive end-expiratory pressure to prevent alveolar collapse. Recent attention has been focused on the respiratory support of the patient with hydrocarbon- or petroleum distillate–induced lung injury. Alternative methods of ventilation are extracorporeal membrane oxygenation, high-frequency jet ventilation, and partial liquid fluorocarbon ventilation.

The clinician caring for a patient with a severe petroleum-induced lung injury should discuss the role of alternative methods of ventilation with a toxicologist or critical care specialist. Bronchodilators should be administered for bronchospasm. Artificial surfactant has been found to improve lung compliance and capillary stability and to increase pO_2. Cardiac monitoring is essential, because these agents may aggravate myocardial irritability due to hypoxia and precipitate dysrhythmias.

Data have consistently shown that corticosteroids are ineffective in the treatment of aspiration pneumonitis and may promote bacterial overgrowth.[18,19] Similarly, the prophylactic use of broad-spectrum antibiotics may lead to the overgrowth of resistant pathogens and should be avoided.[18,19] Antibiotics should be given on the basis of a positive sputum culture or Gram stain. However, because petroleum distillate aspiration may cause fever and leukocytosis, antibiotics (e.g., penicillin and clindamycin) are often given empirically.[9,18]

DISPOSITION

The disposition of patients with suspected aspiration depends on clinical, laboratory, and chest radiograph findings.[3] If patients are symptomatic and their chest radiographs and oxygen saturation or arterial blood gas analyses are abnormal, they should be admitted to the hospital for further observation. If their chest radiographs are normal, patients should be reevaluated in 2 to 6 hours. If they remain symptomatic or hypoxemic, or their chest radiographs become abnormal, they should be admitted.

If patients become asymptomatic and have normal oxygenation and normal repeat chest radiographs, they may be discharged. Patients who initially have symptoms suggesting aspiration, but who are asymptomatic on presentation, should also be observed and have a delayed chest radiograph after 2 to 6 hours. If their radiographs are normal and they remain asymptomatic, with normal oxygenation, they may be discharged.

COMMON PITFALLS

- Failure to appreciate that only those petroleum distillates with low viscosity and high volatility represent aspiration hazards
- Failure to differentiate between petroleum distillates that cause systemic toxicity and those that do not when assessing the need for gastrointestinal decontamination
- Failure to appreciate that gastric evacuation procedures may increase the risk of aspiration and are not routinely indicated
- Failure to appreciate that radiographic evidence of aspiration may lag behind clinical findings
- Failure to admit symptomatic patients to the hospital, even if the chest radiograph and pulmonary examination are normal

References

1. Algren JT, Rodgers GC. Intravascular hemolysis associated with hydrocarbon poisoning. *Pediatr Emerg Care* 1992;8:34.
2. Anas N, Namosonthi V, Ginsburg CM. Criteria for hospitalizing children who have ingested products containing hydrocarbons. *JAMA* 1981;246:840.
3. Bergeson PS, Hales SW, Lustgarten MD, et al. Pneumatoceles following hydrocarbon ingestion. *Am J Dis Child* 1975;129:49.
4. Dice WH, Ward G, Kelley J, et al. Pulmonary toxicity following gastrointestinal ingestion of kerosene. *Ann Emerg Med* 1982;11:138.
5. Glynn KP, Gale NA. Exogenous lipoid pneumonia due to inhalation of spray lubricant (WD-40 Lung). *Chest* 1990;97:1265.
6. Gurwitz D, Kattan M, Levinson B, et al. Pulmonary function abnormalities in asymptomatic children after hydrocarbon pneumonitis. *Pediatrics* 1978;62:789.
7. Litovitz T. Hydrocarbon ingestions. *Ear Nose Throat J* 1983;62:142.
8. Mann MD, Piro DJ, Wolfdorf J. Kerosene absorption in primates. *J Pediatr* 1977;91:495.
9. Marks MI, Chicoine I, Legere G, et al. Adrenocorticosteroid treatment of hydrocarbon pneumonia in children. A cooperative study. *J Pediatr* 1972;81:366.
10. Nagi NA, Abdulallah ZA. Kerosene poisoning in children in Iraq. *Postgrad Med J* 1995;71:419.
11. Neeld EM, Limacher MC. Chemical pneumonitis after the intravenous injection of hydrocarbons. *Radiology* 1978;129:36.
12. Ng RC, Darwish H, Steward DA. Emergency treatment of petroleum distillate and turpentine ingestion. *Can Med Assoc J* 1974;111:537.
13. Press E, Adams WC, Chittenden RF, et al. Cooperative kerosene poisoning study. Evaluation of gastric lavage and other factors in the treatment of accidental ingestion of petroleum distillate products. *Pediatrics* 1962;29:648.
14. Reed RP, Conradie FM. The epidemiology and clinical features of paraffin (kerosene) poisoning in rural African children. *Ann Trop Paediatr* 1997;17:49.
15. Rush MD, Schoenfeld CN, Watson WA. Skin necrosis and venous thrombosis from subcutaneous injection of charcoal lighter fluid (Naptha). *Am J Emerg Med* 1998;16:508.
16. Sharma A, Nain K, Nanda S. Pneumomediastinum, pneumothorax and subcutaneous emphysema with kerosene oil. *Indian J Chest Dis Allied Sci* 1996;38:211.
17. Sheridan RL. Burns with inhalation injury and petrol aspiration in adolescents seeking euphoria through hydrocarbon inhalation. *Burns* 1997;22:566.
18. Steele RW, Conklin RH, Mark HM. Corticosteroids and antibiotics for the treatment of fulminant hydrocarbon aspiration. *JAMA* 1972;219:1434.
19. Truemper E, DeLaRocha SR, Atkinson SD. Clinical characteristics, pathophysiology, and management of hydrocarbon ingestion: case report and review of the literature. *Pediatr Emerg Care* 1987;3:187.
20. Wason S, Greiner PT. Intravenous hydrocarbon abuse. *Am J Emerg Med* 1986;4:543.

CHAPTER 363

Phencyclidine Poisoning

Andis Graudins

Phencyclidine (PCP) is an arylcyclohexylamine related to the "dissociative" anesthetic ketamine. PCP was used briefly in the 1950s as an intravenous anesthetic agent and was used as a veterinary anesthetic agent until 1979, when legal production was stopped. Illicit use of PCP began in the late 1960s, peaked in the early 1980s, and has seen a steady decline since then. PCP use is currently sporadic and relatively infrequent. Ketamine ("K," "Special K"), a dissociative anesthetic agent with a similar pharmacodynamic action, is also sporadically abused for its hallucinogenic properties. Use of both agents seems to be more common in inner-city areas. PCP, also commonly known on the street as "angel dust," is sometimes misrepresented as tetrahydrocannabinol (THC) or crystal. It is frequently taken by mouth, by inhalation from tobacco or marijuana cigarettes, and occasionally by intravenous injection.

The powdered form, angel dust, is usually relatively pure, consisting of 50% to 100% PCP; other forms usually contain 10% to 30% PCP. PCP is easy to synthesize, although the process often yields other 1-phenylcycloalkylamines, such as phenylcyclohexamine (PCE), phenylcyclohexylpiperidine (PCPP), phenylcyclohexylpyrrolidine (PHP), and thienylcyclohexylpiperidine (TCP), which have similar pharmacologic activity. In addition, the street drug may be contaminated with piperidinocyclohexane carbonitrile (PCC), which can cause cyanide poisoning (see Chapter 331).

PCP shows saturable, high-affinity binding to specific receptor sites in brain tissue, such as opioid sigma receptors.[11] PCP is an *N*-methyl-D-aspartate (NMDA) receptor antagonist similar to ketamine. These receptors, usually stimulated by glutamate, are the main excitatory neurotransmitters in the central nervous system (CNS). PCP antagonism at the NMDA receptor may be responsible for the cataleptic state seen with use of this drug. Adrenergic, cholinergic, and serotoninergic agonist or antagonist effects occur at concentrations 100- to 1,000-fold higher than are necessary to produce maximal neurologic or behavioral toxicity. Phencyclidine-induced psychosis is thought to resemble schizophrenia: Decreased glutaminergic neurotransmission by PCP results in a decrease of gamma-aminobutyric acid release from the nucleus accumbens, striatum, and hippocampus, which, in turn, may result in inhibition of tonic release of dopamine from the nucleus accumbens and striatum.[19]

PCP is well absorbed after oral or mucosal administration and inhalation. The onset of effects is rapid (minutes). Termination initially results from redistribution (half-life, about 10 to 15 minutes) and later from elimination (half-life, 8 to 12 hours). The main route of drug elimination is hepatic metabolism, with almost no active drug being excreted in the urine. With chronic use, PCP probably equilibrates with a "deep" compartment, which includes the fatty tissue of the CNS, leading to detectable levels in many tissues days after the last dose.[3] PCP has also been experimentally detected in hair root clippings as early as 6 hours following its administration.[7]

The most profound changes observed with PCP are psychological. Doses of about 0.1 mg/kg (5 to 10 mg total dose) consistently cause disorganized thinking, drowsiness, apathy, psychomotor retardation, perceptual distortions, disorientation, and dreamlike experiences.[1] Hostility, paranoia, and stereotyped behavior are common. True hallucinations have not been reported. Other effects include diplopia, nystagmus, nausea, vomiting, increased muscle tone, hyperreflexia, and ataxia. Larger doses cause progressively more obtundation until seizures begin in the 50-mg range. An intravenous dose of 0.25 mg/kg produces optimal surgical anesthesia. Although delirium usually resolves over hours to days, psychotic behavior may occur over the next few weeks, most commonly manifested by intermittent paranoid delusions and anxiety.[2,9,16] Chronic PCP use may lead to long-term behavioral changes.[1,18]

Death from PCP alone is unusual, with fewer than 30 deaths reported. With vigorous supportive care, patients have survived ingestions of gram quantities, but tissue levels from coroners' cases suggest that such massive ingestions are usually rapidly fatal. Most PCP deaths are due to behavioral effects leading to automobile accidents, lethal self-injury, and drowning. Death may also be due to complications of the intoxication. Status epilepticus, aspiration pneumonia, rhabdomyolysis and renal failure, hyperthermia with massive hepatic necrosis, primary respiratory arrest, or hypertensive intracerebral hemorrhage have all resulted in the demise of patients following poisoning.

Naloxone does not bind to either the PCP receptor site or the sigma receptor site, and no specific receptor antagonists for PCP have been identified.[8,11] Experimental monoclonal Fab antibodies have been developed against PCP. These have been used *in vivo* in animal models with good success but have not been used in humans to date.[7] Although no withdrawal syndrome is apparent, PCP is avidly self-administered by rhesus monkeys, and a two- to fourfold tolerance appears to develop in both monkeys and rats.[1]

CLINICAL PRESENTATION

The most striking manifestations of PCP intoxication are behavioral, ranging from agitation and belligerence to coma and seizures. Intoxication may occur in three stages. Mild intoxication, the first and most common stage of presentation, is manifested primarily by lethargy, bizarre or violent behavior, agitation, and euphoria. The second stage is characterized by stupor and coma with intact deep pain responses. Finally, patients do not respond to deep pain stimuli.[12] Other major symptom patterns may include a catatonic syndrome, toxic psychosis, or an acute brain syndrome.[9] Nystagmus (including rotatory and vertical forms), ataxia, hypertension, increased muscle tone (including twitching, tremors, facial grimacing, localized dystonias, and hyperreflexia), diaphoresis, sialorrhea, and hyperthermia may be noted on physical examination.

Variability is the most striking characteristic of PCP intoxication. The inhaled dose is usually small and limits the drug's effects. Signs and symptoms resolve over 4 to 6 hours. Ingestion often results in a larger exposure and produces more severe and prolonged symptoms. A patient may present with a minor syndrome, such as bizarre behavior, fairly early after an ingestion, and progress to coma rapidly in the emergency department.

Medical complications and traumatic injuries are responsible for most of the morbidity and mortality in hospitalized patients. Rhabdomyolysis is common, particularly in restrained patients.[10] In most cases of myoglobinuric renal failure, if urine flow is maintained, complete recovery can be expected.[4,14] Aspiration pneumonia is the next most common complication. Lactic acidosis and profound hyperthermia may result from muscular hyperactivity. Fatal intracerebral hemorrhage has been reported.[5] Prolonged psychosis for 3 weeks, with persistently elevated serum PCP levels, has been observed in a patient who swallowed a plastic bag containing PCP. Symptoms resolved when the bag was passed.[20] PCP-intoxicated patients may sustain severe injuries without awareness of pain.[2,10]

The diagnosis of PCP intoxication is supported by the detection of PCP in the urine. Toxicologic screening for drugs of abuse will not detect PCP unless it is specifically included in the drug panel. Thin-layer and gas chromatography or mass spectroscopy do not reliably detect PCP. A specific assay, such as gas–liquid chromatography, high-performance liquid chromatography, EMIT (*e*nzyme-*m*ultiplied *i*mmunoassay *t*echnique), or radioimmunoassay, must be requested.

DIFFERENTIAL DIAGNOSIS

PCP intoxication should be considered in any patient who presents with an altered mental state, particularly the young patient with acute onset of bizarre behavior or psychosis, or apparent intoxication without evidence of alcohol. Diagnostic clues include irritability and hostility, nystagmus, hypertension, sweating, hypersalivation, fever, stiffness, and dystonias. The constellation of fluctuating mental status, dystonias, nystagmus, and diaphoresis is quite suspicious, as is the combination of coma and rigidity without profound respiratory depression. PCP intoxication should also be considered in trauma patients with prolonged coma, unusual rigidity, hypertension, hyperthermia, or seizures. In patients with coma or seizures, structural neurologic causes must be considered, particularly because hypertension from PCP can lead to intracranial hemorrhage. Localized dystonias may be seen with PCP intoxication.

Patients with the neuroleptic malignant syndrome have autonomic instability rather than sustained hypertension, and the limbs show "lead pipe" rigidity rather than diffuse hypertonia. Poisoning by sedative–hypnotics (which cause nystagmus but also hypotonia and hypotension), tricyclics (which can cause anticholinergic effects and electrocardiographic abnormalities), and narcotics (characterized by pinpoint pupils and respiratory depression) should be considered in the differential diagnosis. The agitated, paranoid state of amphetamine intoxication can mimic PCP intoxication, but muscle rigidity, nystagmus, and sialorrhea are seen only with PCP. Encephalitis, meningitis, and cranial trauma should also be considered. Occasionally, alcohol or sedative–hypnotic withdrawal may be mistaken for PCP intoxication. A history of recent abstinence, continuous resting tremors, visual hallucinations, and lack of dystonias points to a withdrawal syndrome.

EMERGENCY DEPARTMENT EVALUATION

The history should be obtained from sources other than the patient, when necessary. A general physical examination and mental status examination should be performed, with a search for focal neurologic findings as well as evidence of trauma, aspiration pneumonia, and other complications.

Urinalysis (including myoglobin); measurement of electrolyte, glucose, and creatine phosphokinase levels; and renal function studies should be done. If coma, hyperthermia, or rhabdomyolysis is present, additional workup should include arterial blood gas analysis, complete blood count, coagulation profile, liver function studies, and measurement of calcium, magnesium, and phosphorus levels. Urine drug screening is unlikely to influence acute medical management of patients with PCP intoxication but may help with the subsequent psychiatric management.

EMERGENCY DEPARTMENT MANAGEMENT

Treatment of PCP intoxication consists of behavior control and standard measures for medical complications and supportive care for traumatic injuries. Activated charcoal should be considered for gut decontamination if patients present within 4 to 6 hours of ingestion and are symptomatic. Care should be taken when attempting to administer charcoal with undue force to aggressive or combative patients. Complications such as charcoal aspiration and esophageal perforation may result from forceful attempts at gastric tube placement. Obtunded and combative patients should have activated charcoal instilled by a gastric tube once the airway is secured and appropriate sedation and neuromuscular paralysis have been achieved.

Behavioral control is best achieved with parenteral haloperidol (5 to 10 mg intramuscularly or intravenously every 20 to 60 minutes; up to 30 mg in the first hour).[6] Chlorpromazine (25 to 50 mg intramuscularly every 30 to 60 minutes, up to 300 mg) is also effective; it is less likely to cause dystonias and more likely to result in hypotension. Oral diazepam has been used successfully for agitation associated with mild intoxications. Intravenous diazepam or midazolam may be effective in calming obtunded patients who are struggling against their restraints.[2,10]

Neuromuscular paralysis may be needed to control neuromuscular hyperactivity in severe cases. Minimizing stimulation is likely to be more effective than attempting to "talk down" an agitated or psychotic patient. Although physical restraints may be needed to control violent behavior until pharmacologic therapy takes effect, they clearly increase the risk of rhabdomyolysis and should be removed at the earliest possible instance.

Rhabdomyolysis should be treated with adequate intravenous volume replacement, careful attention to electrolyte balance, and monitoring of urine output. Severe hyperthermia should be treated with physical cooling measures, sedation, and neuromuscular paralysis, if necessary.

Hypertension usually responds to sedation with antipsychotic agents or benzodiazepines. If diastolic pressure stays above 115 mm Hg or if the patient is symptomatic or has known coronary or cerebrovascular disease, specific treatment is indicated. Chlorpromazine may be useful because of its alpha-blocking effects.[9] Persistent hypertension may rarely require treatment with vasodilators (e.g., nitroprusside or hydralazine).

Urinary acidification has not been shown to be of clinical value. It is potentially harmful and is *not* recommended. Although PCP is a weak base, and urinary clearance increases dramatically when the urine pH is lowered from 7.5 to 5.0, urinary acidification has only a minimal effect on overall drug elimination, because PCP is metabolized primarily by the liver, with little active drug excreted in the urine.[13,15] Further, urinary acidification may increase the renal toxicity of myoglobin (from rhabdomyolysis) and complicate fluid and electrolyte management. Hemodialysis and hemoperfusion are ineffective in removing significant amounts of PCP because of its high volume of distribution, protein binding, and hepatic clearance.

DISPOSITION

Patients with coma, delirium, catatonia, violent behavior, major trauma, hyperthermia (temperature greater than 38.5°C), aspiration pneumonia, sustained hypertension (greater than 200/115 mm Hg), or significant rhabdomyolysis should be hospitalized. Most will require admission to an intensive care unit. Other patients should be observed for at least 1 hour after all symptoms (except nystagmus) have resolved.

Patients with persistent behavior problems who do not require restraints and have no medical complications should be referred to a psychiatrist. All discharged patients should have observation by friends or family, with clear instructions to seek medical assistance if behavior problems recur.

COMMON PITFALLS

- Failure to consider the diagnosis of PCP intoxication, particularly in young patients with agitation, psychosis, or trauma
- Failure to evaluate and treat patients for medical complications (rhabdomyolysis, aspiration pneumonia, hyperthermia)
- Failure to appreciate that PCP-intoxicated patients may have major trauma without apparent pain
- Failure to appreciate that PCP is not detected by commonly used toxicology screening tests and that a specific assay must be requested
- Premature discharge from the emergency department after a brief but transient period of mental clarity
- Acidifying the urine in an attempt to enhance PCP elimination

References

1. Aniline O, Pitts FN Jr. Phencyclidine (PCP): a review and perspectives. *Crit Rev Toxicol* 1982;10(2):145–177.
2. Aronow R, Done AK. PCP overdose: an emerging concept of management. *J Am Coll Emerg Physicians* 1978;7:56.
3. Bailey DN, Shaw RF, Robinson PT, et al. PCP: studies of tissue concentrations in the rat, monkey, and man. *J Anal Toxicol* 1979;3:235.
4. Barton CH, Sterling ML, Vaziri ND. Phencyclidine intoxication: clinical experience in 27 cases confirmed by urine assay. *Ann Emerg Med* 1981;10:243.
5. Bessen HA. Intracranial hemorrhage associated with phencyclidine abuse. *JAMA* 1982;248:585.
6. Giannini AJ, Eighen MS, Loiselle RH, et al. Comparison of haloperidol and chlorpromazine in the treatment of phencyclidine psychosis. *J Clin Pharmacol* 1984;24(4):202–204.
7. Hardin JS, Wessinger WD, Proksch JW, et al. Pharmacodynamics of a monoclonal antiphencyclidine Fab with broad selectivity for phencyclidine-like drugs. *J Pharmacol Exp Ther* 1998;285:1113.
8. Kemp JA, Foster EC, Wong HF. Noncompetitive antagonists of excitatory amino acid receptors. *Trends Neurosci* 1987;10:294.
9. McCarron MM, Schulze BW, Thompson GA, et al. Acute PCP intoxication: clinical patterns, complications, and treatment. *Ann Emerg Med* 1981;10:290.
10. McCarron MM, Schulze BW, Thompson GA, et al. Acute PCP intoxication: incidence of clinical findings in 1000 cases. *Ann Emerg Med* 1981;10:237.
11. Mendelson LG, Kerchner GA, Kalra V, et al. PCP receptors in rat brain cortex. *Biochem Pharmacol* 1984;33:3529.
12. Milhorn HT Jr. Diagnosis and management of phencyclidine intoxication. *Am Fam Physician* 1991;43:1293.
13. Owens SM, Harwick WC, Blackall D. Phencyclidine pharmacokinetic scaling among species. *J Pharmacol Exp Ther* 1987;242:96.
14. Patel R, Das M, Palazzolo M, et al. Myoglobinuric acute renal failure in PCP overdose—report of observations in eight cases. *Ann Emerg Med* 1980;9:549.
15. Perez-Reyes M, DiGuisseppi S, Brine DR, et al. Urine pH and phencyclidine excretion. *Clin Pharmacol Ther* 1982;32:635.
16. Rainey JM, Crowder MK. Prolonged psychosis attributed to PCP: a report of three cases. *Am J Psychiatry* 1975;132:1076.
17. Sakamoto T, Endo M, Nagasake A, et al. Evaluation of hair root analysis for acute phencyclidine poisoning and behavior of phencyclidine metabolites in rat hair root. *Pharmazie* 1998;53(5):310–314.
18. Stillman R, Petersen RC. The paradox of PCP abuse. *Ann Intern Med* 1979;90:428.
19. Thornberg SA, Saklad SR. A review of NMDA receptors and the phencyclidine model of schizophrenia. *Pharmacotherapy* 1996;16:82.
20. Young JD, Crapo LM. Protracted phencyclidine coma from an intestinal deposit. *Arch Intern Med* 1992;152:859.

CHAPTER 364
Phenytoin Poisoning

Thomas E. Kearney

Phenytoin, formerly called diphenylhydantoin, is an anticonvulsant belonging to the chemical class known as hydantoins, which also includes mephenytoin and ethotoin. It is effective for a variety of seizure disorders, including generalized tonic–clonic, partial-complex, and other focal seizures. It has also been used in the management of trigeminal neuralgia and toxin-induced seizures. It is used as well as a type IB antiarrhythmic, especially for digitalis- and tricyclic antidepressant–induced conduction defects and ventricular dysrhythmias.

Phenytoin, a weak acid with a pK_a of 8.5, is readily soluble only in a highly alkaline medium, and therefore requires formulation in a special diluent (propylene glycol) and adjustment of pH with alkali (sodium hydroxide) for parenteral administration. Although this preparation may precipitate if added to other acidic parenteral solutions, it may be added to normal saline solution if properly diluted and used immediately. Intramuscular injection may result in erratic absorption, muscle pain, and necrosis.

A new preparation and prodrug of phenytoin, fosphenytoin (Cerebyx), has a more neutral pH (8.6 to 9.0) and greater water solubility. It is compatible with common intravenous preparations and lacks the cardiotoxic diluent propylene glycol and the high alkalinity responsible for local soft-tissue injuries; additionally, it may be administered intramuscularly.[5] Because of its higher cost, however, fosphenytoin has not replaced parenteral phenytoin.

Oral preparations categorized according to their dissolution rates include extended-release and prompt-release capsule formulations of sodium salt, chewable tablets, and suspension of the free acid. Phenytoin poisoning commonly results from acute accidental ingestion by children or from suicidal ingestion and even illicit use by adolescents and adults.[6,10,14,16,18] In addition, therapeutic misadventures and iatrogenic poisonings frequently result from drug–drug or drug–disease interactions that affect its distribution, protein binding, and clearance; excessive dosing, with administration of a daily amount of phenytoin greater than the patient's metabolic capacity for elimination; or improper parenteral administration.[8,16]

Toxicity may also result from improper mixing of phenytoin suspensions before use and switching between products with different absorption characteristics. Non–dose-related, idiosyncratic, or hypersensitivity-type toxic effects may be associated with its therapeutic use, particularly in patients with neurologic deficits or occult neurologic lesions.[18]

As an anticonvulsant, phenytoin is essentially devoid of hypnotic effects at therapeutic levels. It prevents the spread of abnormal neuronal discharges by stabilizing neuronal membranes. This effect is achieved by altering fluxes of sodium, calcium, and potassium ions in neuronal conducting membranes and by reducing the posttetanic potential of synaptic transmission. It may also deplete folate in the central nervous system (CNS), red blood cells, and bone marrow. In addition, phenytoin may have an excitatory effect on Purkinje cell discharge in the cerebellum that, in turn, activates GABA-nergic inhibitory pathways in the cerebral cortex. Phenytoin may, however, produce or unmask focal neurologic deficits in patients with GABA receptor supersensitivity resulting from hypoxic or ischemic insults. Serotonergic and dopaminergic activity may also be enhanced by phenytoin, as evidenced by its precipitation of movement disorders.

Phenytoin's effects on the myocardium parallel those of lidocaine. It inhibits sodium channels, decreases the effective refractory period and automaticity in Purkinje fibers, and has little or no effect on the QRS and action potential duration.

Phenytoin's anticonvulsant and antiarrhythmic effects are usually achieved at plasma levels in the range of 10 to 20 μg/mL. This level can be quickly attained with an intravenous loading dose of 15 to 20 mg/kg of phenytoin or PE (phenytoin equivalent) units of fosphenytoin. Because of potential toxicity from the propylene glycol diluent (cardiac arrhythmias and hypotension), phenytoin should be given no faster than 50 mg/min.[12]

Fosphenytoin, despite its lack of propylene glycol, may be associated with similar cardiovascular toxicity if administered at high infusion rates and doses. Hence, the rate of fosphenytoin administration should not exceed 150 PE units/min in adults (3 mg/kg/min in children). Phenytoin concentrations should not be monitored until conversion of fosphenytoin to phenytoin is complete, 2 hours and 4 hours after intravenous infusion and intramuscular administration, respectively. The maintenance dose of phenytoin is usually 4 to 6 mg/kg/d as single or divided doses. Neonates may require higher loading doses (15 to 20 mg/kg) and maintenance doses (5 to 8 mg/kg/d).[4]

Phenytoin is poorly soluble, and hence sparingly absorbed, in the acid milieu of the stomach. Absorption from the duodenum and lower gastrointestinal (GI) tract is extremely variable and depends on the oral dosage form, gastric emptying time, and bowel motility. Peak serum levels are observed at 2.6 to 8.9 hours after a single dose of extended-release capsule (i.e., Dilantin). After overdosage with this formulation, absorption has continued for up to 12 days.[6] This lengthy absorption period may be due to the formation of a slowly disintegrating mass of capsules (pharmacobezoar) or decreased GI motility.

Phenytoin is metabolized predominantly in the liver. Up to 70% of a given daily dose is converted by parahydroxylation to 5-(*p*-hydroxyphenyl)-5-phenylhydantoin (HPPH), which is then conjugated with glucuronide into a more water-soluble metabolite and excreted renally.[16] About 1% to 5% of phenytoin is excreted unchanged in the urine. Phenytoin is actively secreted into the gut and undergoes enterohepatic recirculation.

The enzyme system responsible for parahydroxylation of phenytoin is "saturable" at plasma levels around 10 μg/mL. Below this level, phenytoin follows first-order elimination kinetics, with an average half-life of 22 hours (range, 7 to 55 hours) in adults. Above this level, it follows zero-order kinetics, resulting in a much longer half-life. Metabolic enzymes are subject to inhibition or induction by other drugs or may be deficient because of inherited genetic traits or liver disease (Table 364.1).

Phenytoin has a relatively low volume of distribution (0.6 L/kg in adults) and preferentially distributes to the cerebellum and brainstem.[7] It is 90% bound to plasma protein, mostly albumin. Decreased protein binding, resulting from competition with protein receptors by endogenous or exogenous substrates or reduced albumin levels, increases free (pharmacologically active) drug levels as well as the volume of distribution. Because only total serum phenytoin levels are routinely monitored, decreased protein binding results in therapeutic and toxic effects at lower-than-usual serum concentrations (see Table 364.1).

Toxic effects result from exaggerated pharmacologic activity, folate depletion, altered collagen metabolism, idiosyncratic reactions, and propylene glycol toxicity with parenteral administration. Numerous teratogenic effects (fetal hydantoin syndrome) have also been reported.[3]

Acute poisoning may result from single ingestions of 20 mg/kg or more. Death is rare but has been reported in children aged 3 to 7 years with ingestions of 100 to 220 mg/kg.[10,17] The cause of death is CNS depression with respiratory insufficiency and hypoxia-related sequelae. Survival has been noted after acute ingestion of 249 mg/kg in a 2.5-year-old child, who had a level of 112 μg/mL at 70 hours.[19] Reported cases of adult phenytoin poisoning have demonstrated moderate CNS toxicity with recovery after ingestion of 12 to 25 g, with the highest recorded level of 130 μg/mL at 96 hours after ingestion.[2]

CLINICAL PRESENTATION

Because tolerance to phenytoin has not been described, dose- and level-related toxic effects are similar for both acute and chronic overdosage.[4] Phenytoin initially affects cerebellar and vestibular function, with cerebral depression occurring later. At serum levels of 20 to 40 μg/mL, signs and symptoms of mild intoxication include dizziness, ataxia, tremors, lethargy, nausea, vomiting, slurred speech, diplopia, blurred vision, normal-to-dilated pupils, and nystagmus (coarse, horizontal, or vertical).[9] An initial excitatory phase has also been reported. At levels of 40 to 90 μg/mL, confusion, psychosis, hallucinations, and progressively deeper CNS depression with suppression of nystagmus

TABLE 364.1. Factors That Influence Phenytoin Kinetics

Pharmacokinetic Effects	Condition or Concomitant Drug Use	Pharmacologic Effect
Decreased protein binding	Acidosis, age (neonates) Uremia Hepatitis Hypoalbuminemia Valproic acid Nonsteroidal antiinflammatory agents	Increased (higher free fraction of circulating phenytoin)
Decreased clearance	Amiodarone, chloramphenicol Isoniazid, disulfiram (metabolic inhibitors) Genetic deficiency of liver enzyme system	Increased (accumulation of phenytoin during chronic dosing due to prolonged half-life)
Increased clearance	Phenobarbital Carbamazepine Ethanol (hepatic enzyme inducers) Pregnancy	Decreased (shortened half-life results in less accumulation during chronic dosing)

and sluggish ocular and deep tendon reflexes may be noted.[16] Levels above 90 μg/mL are associated with severe toxicity and manifest by coma with respiratory depression.[19] "Paradoxical intoxication" with increased seizure frequency, dystonias, dyskinesias, choreoathetoid movements, and decerebrate rigidity may be noted in patients with underlying seizure disorders.[14,16] In addition, those with focal neurologic lesions may develop contralateral deficits (e.g., hemianopia, hemianesthesia, and hemiparesis). Other etiologies should be considered for seizures that occur in phenytoin-intoxicated patients without preexisting seizure or neurologic disorders. Laboratory abnormalities are limited to hyperglycemia and decreased thyroxine levels.[20] The electroencephalogram characteristically shows slowing of alpha-wave activity. With severe intoxication, brainstem evoked potentials may be absent.

Unless complications due to anoxia or sepsis ensue, recovery is usually complete once the drug is eliminated. Depending on the phenytoin level, elimination may take longer than a week. In rare cases, chronic poisoning has resulted in encephalopathy and cerebellar degeneration with persistent ataxia.[7]

With chronic use, folate depletion may occur and result in megaloblastic anemia and peripheral neuropathy. In addition, altered collagen metabolism may lead to gingival hyperplasia, hirsutism, and hypertrichosis.

Idiosyncratic or hypersensitivity reactions include fever, rash, eosinophilia, hepatitis, lupus-like syndrome, lymphadenopathy ("pseudolymphoma"), myositis, rhabdomyolysis, nephritis, vasculitis, and hemolytic anemia.[18]

The rapid infusion of propylene glycol (at phenytoin rates above 50 mg/min) may result in bradycardia, hypotension, ventricular fibrillation and asystole, conduction defects, congestive heart failure, and respiratory arrest.[12] These effects are usually transient and seldom persist for more than 1 hour after the infusion is stopped. The rapid infusion of high doses of fosphenytoin has also resulted in severe cardiovascular toxicity in infants.[11]

Phenytoin may induce the "purple glove syndrome" (limb edema, discoloration, and pain) after peripheral intravenous administration.[15] It can occur hours after infusion, in the absence of clinical signs of extravasation, and can lead to limb ischemia and necrosis from a compartment syndrome.

DIFFERENTIAL DIAGNOSIS

The differential diagnosis of phenytoin intoxication includes intoxication with other anticonvulsants, sedative–hypnotics, and CNS depressants; seizure disorders; postictal states; CNS trauma and tumors; and extrapyramidal disorders. Phenytoin poisoning may also mimic ketotic and nonketotic hyperglycemic coma.[18] Although it has been stated that nystagmus is pathognomonic of phenytoin toxicity, this finding is neither sensitive nor specific. It can be present with therapeutic levels and absent with toxic levels, and may be present in a variety of other conditions and intoxications.

EMERGENCY DEPARTMENT EVALUATION

The history should include the time, amount, and preparation of phenytoin taken; the onset and nature of symptoms; chronic medications; and past and current medical problems. The clinician should also note previous use of phenytoin and preexisting seizure disorders.

The physical examination should focus on vital signs, cardiopulmonary findings, and a detailed neurologic assessment. Serum phenytoin and glucose levels and an electrocardiogram (ECG) should be included in the initial evaluation. Other routine laboratory studies, toxicology screening, and a chest radiograph should be obtained as clinically indicated. Because phenytoin absorption and elimination may be greatly prolonged after overdosage, two (or more) serum levels taken several hours apart, along with serial clinical evaluations, are necessary to assess the degree and progression of toxicity.

Patients with the purple glove syndrome should be evaluated for limb ischemia; intracompartmental pressure measurement may be useful in guiding therapy in those with manifestations of arterial insufficiency.

EMERGENCY DEPARTMENT MANAGEMENT

Advanced life-support measures should be instituted as necessary. Patients with a preexisting seizure disorder should be placed on seizure preventives because of the possibility of paradoxical seizures during the acute intoxication phase and breakthrough seizures if serum levels drop too low. Although cardiovascular toxicity has not been reported after oral overdose, cardiac monitoring is advisable for patients with severe CNS toxicity as well as during intravenous administration.

In addition to stopping the infusion, it may be necessary to administer crystalloids to patients who develop hypotension during intravenous administration. Dysrhythmias usually resolve spontaneously upon stopping the infusion but can be treated according to advanced cardiac life-support guidelines, if necessary.

Seizures caused by phenytoin toxicity require discontinuation of the drug and treatment instead with another agent, such as diazepam or a barbiturate. Hyperglycemia usually resolves with discontinuation of phenytoin and seldom requires insulin unless the patient has diabetes.

Administration of activated charcoal is the preferred method of GI decontamination. Multiple oral doses of activated charcoal can enhance the elimination of phenytoin after systemic absorption.[13] Controlled evidence is lacking, however, that multiple-dose therapy shortens the duration of toxicity or improves outcome. For patients taking phenytoin for therapeutic purposes, an extended observation period may be necessary to ensure that phenytoin levels do not become subtherapeutic.

Because of phenytoin's high degree of protein-binding and hepatic elimination, procedures such as forced diuresis with ion trapping, hemodialysis, and peritoneal dialysis have not been beneficial.[19] Although hemoperfusion has resulted in a minimal increase in clearance in one reported case,[1] patients with phenytoin poisoning usually have a favorable outcome with good supportive care alone. Hence, the risk of hemoperfusion usually outweighs its possible benefit.

Idiosyncratic or hypersensitivity reactions and complications of chronic therapy are treated by drug withdrawal and supportive measures. A vascular surgeon should be consulted for the management of patients with purple glove syndrome who have signs of vascular compromise.

DISPOSITION

Asymptomatic patients who accidentally ingest less than 20 mg/kg of phenytoin, do not have a preexisting neurologic disorder, and are not taking phenytoin chronically can be observed at home and followed by telephone contact. All other patients should be evaluated at a health-care facility.

Nonsuicidal patients with mild-to-moderate toxicity (those who can sit up, feed themselves, and walk with assistance) can be discharged with home observation after documentation of declining drug levels. Suicidal patients, those with severe toxicity or rising drug levels after several measurements, and those without responsible friends or relatives to assist and observe them at home should be admitted. Inpatient level of care (floor vs. intensive care unit) should be determined by the degree and progression of toxicity and underlying medical problems. Any facility that can provide intensive respiratory therapy should be able to manage uncomplicated cases of phenytoin poisoning. Patients who are transferred should be accompanied by personnel trained in advanced life support.

COMMON PITFALLS

- Failure to recognize that nystagmus is of limited value in the diagnosis of phenytoin poisoning
- Failure to consider alterations in protein binding when interpreting phenytoin levels
- Failure to appreciate that phenytoin can exacerbate preexisting neurologic problems
- Failure to consider the risks of using ipecac, flumazenil, and multiple-dose activated charcoal therapy in patients with seizure disorders and phenytoin toxicity
- Failure to appreciate that phenytoin absorption and elimination may be prolonged after overdosage and that serial drug levels should be obtained
- Failure to appreciate that cardiovascular toxicity can occur with high infusion rates and doses of fosphenytoin as well as phenytoin
- Failure to appreciate that patients with uncomplicated phenytoin poisoning do well with supportive care and that extracorporeal drug removal measures are ineffective or unnecessary
- Failure to appreciate that purple glove syndrome may occur hours after peripheral intravenous administration of phenytoin.

References

1. Baechler RW, Work J, Smith W, et al. Charcoal hemoperfusion in the therapy for methsuximide and phenytoin overdose. *Arch Intern Med* 1980;40:1466.
2. Blair AAD, Hallpike JF, Lascelles PT. Acute diphenylhydantoin and primidone poisoning treated by peritoneal dialysis. *J Neurol Neurosurg Psychiatry* 1968;31:520.
3. Bodendorfer TW. Fetal effects of anticonvulsant drugs and seizure disorders. *Drug Intell Clin Pharm* 1978;12:14.
4. Borofsky LG, Louis S, Kutt H, et al. Diphenylhydantoin efficacy, toxicity and dose-serum relationships in children. *J Pediatr* 1972;81:995.
5. Browne TR. Fosphenytoin (Cerebyx) review. *Clin Neuropharmacol* 1997;20(1):1–12.
6. Chaikin P, Adir J. Unusual absorption profile of phenytoin in a massive overdose case. *J Clin Pharmacol* 1987;27:70.
7. Luef G, Burtscher J, Kremser C, et al. Magnetic resonance volumetry of the cerebellum in epileptic patients after phenytoin overdosages. *Eur Neurol* 1996;36:273–277.
8. Kutt H. Interactions of antiepileptic drugs. *Epilepsia* 1975;16:393.
9. Kutt H, Winters W, Kokenge R. Metabolism of diphenylhydantoin, blood levels and toxicity. *Arch Neurol* 1964;11:642.
10. Laubscher FA. Fatal diphenylhydantoin poisoning. *JAMA* 1966;198:1120.
11. Lieber BL, Snodgrass WR. Cardiac arrest following large intravenous fosphenytoin overdose in an infant. *J Toxicol Clin Toxicol* 1998;36:473(abst).
12. Louis S, Kutt H, McDowell F. The cardiocirculatory changes caused by intravenous Dilantin and its solvent. *Am Heart J* 1967;74:523.
13. Mauro LS, Maruo VF, Brown DL. Enhancement of phenytoin elimination by multiple-dose activated charcoal. *Am J Emerg Med* 1987;16:1132.
14. Murphy JM, Motiwala R, Devinsky O. Phenytoin intoxication. *South Med J* 1991;84:1199.
15. O'Brien TJ, Cascino GD, So EL, et al. Incidence and clinical consequence of the purple glove syndrome in patients receiving intravenous phenytoin. *Neurology* 1998;51:1034–1039.
16. Patel H, Crichton JU. The neurologic hazards of diphenylhydantoin in childhood. *J Pediatr* 1968;73:676.
17. Petty CS, Muelling RJ, Sindell HW. Accidental poisoning with diphenylhydantoin (Dilantin). *J Forensic Sci* 1957;2:279.
18. Powers NG, Carson SH. Idiosyncratic reactions to phenytoin. *Clin Pediatr* 1987;26:120.
19. Tenckhoff H, Sherrard DJ, Hickman O, et al. Acute diphenylhydantoin intoxication. *Am J Dis Child* 1968;116:422.
20. Wagner KJ, Zeil M, Leiken JB. Metabolic effects of phenytoin toxicity. *Ann Emerg Med* 1986;15:509.

CHAPTER 365
Plant Poisoning

David G. Spoerke

Exposures to potentially poisonous plants account for about 10% of calls made to poison centers in the United States. Of the over 100,000 exposures that occur annually, most involve accidental ingestions by children, and only a small number are truly life-threatening.[10] Most adult exposures are intentional, but the intent is usually self-treatment rather than self-harm.

There is no single characteristic that differentiates a poisonous plant (Appendix 365.A) from a nonpoisonous one (Appendix 365.B). Plants contain a large number of different toxins, which can affect any organ system. Almost any sign or symptom may be seen. There are rarely specific antidotes or treatments; most commonly, symptomatic and supportive care is the only treatment available or necessary.

Increasingly, herbal medications, commercially available without prescription, are promoted and used for a wide variety of illnesses. While most are relatively innocuous when taken in small quantities and for short duration, serious poisoning can occur with excessive dosing and chronic exposure. Severe idiosyncratic reactions have also been reported.

CLINICAL PRESENTATION

The most common symptoms and signs of plant exposure are referable to the skin, gastrointestinal (GI) tract, and the central nervous system (CNS). Dermal exposure can cause skin irritation as a result of mechanical, chemical, or allergic reactions, or a combination of these (Appendix 365.C).

Cacti are prime examples of plants that cause mechanical damage to the skin. Once the offending thorn, hair, spine, or glochid has been removed, pain resolves. Secondary infection is also possible.

Nettles and *Mucuna* spp. have hairs that penetrate, causing mechanical skin damage, and then release a chemical irritant into the wound to produce a secondary inflammatory reaction. Some *Euphorbia* spp. have spines as well as chemical irritants or allergens (diterpenes).

Euphorbia myrsinites also contains diterpenes (e.g., euphorbin, phorbol), but they are released on the skin rather than into a wound, causing an irritation that resembles branding.[9] Other plants in the *Euphorbia* genus, such as the pencil tree, snow-on-the-mountain, and crown of thorns, also have similar effects.

Euphorbia spp. also contain toxins that may produce both a chemical and allergic reaction. Poison ivy, poison oak, and other toxicodendrol-containing plants are additional examples. Exposure typically causes an erythematous papulovesicular eruption, often in streaks.

Plants in the parsley family contain psoralens that cause photodermatitis. An erythematous papular rash, sometimes with blisters, may not occur immediately but only after exposure to the sun. This produces unusual distributions (e.g., rash only on the face, hands, or back of forearms). Psoralens are also found in limes, lemons, and celery.

Many types of phytochemicals cause nausea, vomiting, and diarrhea; only the most common are covered here. Examples of GI toxins are colchicine, emetine, and lycorine. Many other unidentified plants and their toxins cause GI irritation. Abdominal cramping is also common. The toxic principles of daphne (daphnetoxin and mezereon) may cause abdominal symptoms that resemble those of acute appendicitis.

Alkaloids are a diverse group of plant toxins that may cause GI irritation, among other symptoms. Examples include amaryllis, hyacinth, and spider lily, all of which contain lycorine.

A variety of glycosides cause gastroenteritis. The mechanism of action and toxic concentration differ by genus. Sample species are aloe and golden shower (*Cassia fistula*), which contain emodin, and Japanese aucuba, which contains aucubin.

Many plants that initially cause GI symptoms have additional systemic effects. Saponins are glycosides of terpenoid aglycones that also have surfactant properties and may lyse red blood cells. They are widely distributed in the plant kingdom, often occur along with other toxins, and are found in blue cohosh (*Caulophyllum thalictroides*), buckeye (*Aesculus glabra*), horse chestnut (*Aesculus hippocastanum*), and ivies (*Hedera* sp.).

Several cardiac glycoside–containing plants are found in the United States (Table 365.1).[19] Signs and symptoms are similar to those of digitalis overdose (see Chapter 332) and include CNS dysfunction and cardiotoxicity as well as GI effects.[6,7] Digoxin radioimmunoassays can be used to detect digitalis glycoside (from *Digitalis purpurea*) and may be able to detect other cardiac glycosides as well. Interpretation of quantitative results for these other glycosides is impossible.

Oxalates are found in many common house and garden plants. Representatives are anthurium (*Anthurium andreanum*), dumbcane (*Dieffenbachia* sp.), elephant's ear (*Alocasia* sp.), jack in the pulpit (*Arisaema triphyllum*), philodendron (*Philodendron* sp.), and Virginia creeper (*Parthenocissus tricuspidata*). In addition to gastroenteritis, they may cause a burning sensation in the mouth, throat, lips, and tongue if chewed prior to ingestion. Erythema and edema may be noted on examination. The severity of symptoms varies considerably, depending on both the species involved and the plant part ingested. Upper airway obstruction may occur in severe cases.

Baneberry, clematis, and pasqueflower contain protoanemonin, which is a skin irritant and vesicant as well as a GI irritant.

Lectins (toxalbumins) are found in black locust (*Abrus precatorius*), castor bean (*Ricinus communis*), European mistletoe (*Viscum* sp.), North American mistletoe (*Phoradendron* sp.), and monkey pistol (*Hura crepitans*). These proteins can cause severe gastroenteritis, with hematemesis, tenesmus, and bloody diarrhea. Cyanosis, convulsions, and circulatory collapse can also occur.[11] Onset may be delayed for 2 to 24 hours.

The chronic ingestion of grain contaminated with weed seeds or certain herbal teas and medications (e.g., comfrey, seneca) containing pyrrolizidine alkaloids can cause venoocclusive hepatic disease. Other plants containing these alkaloids include seaside heliotrope (*Heliotropium curassavicum*), *Senecio* species, rattlebox (*Crotalaria* sp.), and viper's vulgare (*Echium* sp.).

Although the toxin is normally excreted within 24 hours, symptoms may not occur for days or weeks, making the diagnosis difficult. It is often made when other causes of hepatitis are ruled out and a history of herbal use is obtained.[10]

In addition to causing GI symptoms, plants containing essential or volatile oils, such as camphor (see Chapter 372), catnip, citrus oils, eucalyptus oil, eugenol, laurel oil, menthol, and pine oil, may produce CNS depression, followed by CNS stimulation and seizures.

Some plants cause CNS depression, and others cause CNS stimulation. CNS depression may be light to severe, depending on the dose, but most accidental ingestions produce mild-to-moderate effects. A wide variety of chemicals are involved, some known and some not yet identified (e.g., holly).

Plants containing solanine cause delayed-onset CNS depression. Representative species include apple of Sodom (*Solanum sodomeum*), bittersweet (*Solanum dulcamara*), Carolina horse nettle (*Solanum carolinense*), deadly nightshade (*Solanum nigra*), eggplant (*Solanum melongena*), false Jerusalem cherry (*Solanum capsicastrum*), Jerusalem cherry (*Solanum pseudocapsicum*), nipplefruit (*Solanum mammosum*), potato (*Solanum tuberosum*), and star potato vine (*Solanum seaforthianum*).

The isoquinolone alkaloids are well known for their sedative effect.[19] The extent of the depression depends on the type of toxin, the part of the plant, and the amount ingested. Examples are celandine poppy (*Chelidonium majus*), opium poppy (*Papaver somniferum*), and yellow pea (*Thermopsis montana*).

CNS stimulation can include seizures, which may be sudden in onset. It may be caused by a variety of plants whose mechanisms of action are quite different (Table 365.2). Camphor is discussed in Chapter 372 and strychnine in Chapter 366.

Well-known hallucinogenic or perception-altering plants are marijuana and the peyote cactus; less familiar are the morning glory, four o'clock, and nutmeg (see Chapter 341). Anticholinergic plants, such as jimsonweed and belladonna, also produce hallucinations (see Chapter 312). The vomiting associated with nutmeg and morning glory prevents common abuse.

The ingestion of cyanogenic glycosides, contained in the seeds or pits of apple (*Malus* sp.), cherry (*Prunus* sp.), cotoneaster (*Cotoneaster* sp.), loquat (*Eriobotrya japonica*), and peach (*Prunus* sp.), can cause cyanide poisoning (see Chapter 331).

These compounds, when mixed with water and plant enzymes such as emulsin or prunasin, are hydrolyzed and release

TABLE 365.1. Cardiac Glycoside–Containing Plants

Common (Botanical) Name	Toxin
European spindle tree (*Euonymus europaea*)	Evomonoside
Foxglove (*Digitalis purpurea*)	Digitalis
Lily-of-the-valley (*Convallaria majalis*)	Convallatoxin
Oleander (*Nerium oleander*)	Oleandrin
Poison bulb (*Acokanthera* spp.)	Quabain-like
Yellow oleander (*Thevetia peruviana*)	Thevetin

TABLE 365.2. Plants Containing CNS Stimulants

Common (Botanical) Name	Toxin
Camphor	Volatile oils
Fool's parsley (*Aethusa cynapium*)	Aethusanol
Poison hemlock (*Cornum maculatum*)	Coniine
Strychnine (*Strychnos nux vomica*)	Strychnine
Water hemlock (*Cicuta* spp.)	Cicutoxin

cyanide. The amount of glycoside is usually small, and the liberation of cyanide is a slow, incomplete process. Although boiling or roasting may detoxify these toxins, it should not be done in a confined area because of the potential release of hydrogen cyanide gas.

Herbal exposure can cause a wide variety of toxic effects, including allergic reactions, cardiovascular and CNS disturbances, skin and GI irritation, hematologic abnormalities, liver damage, renal dysfunction, and offensive odor and taste (Table 365.3).[1–4,14–16] The administration of herbal teas to young children has resulted in water intoxication, with hyponatremia and seizures.[12] Some herbals are contaminated with drugs or heavy metals (e.g., arsenic, lead).[13,18] Neonatal jaundice has occurred after *Artemisia scoparia* administration.[20] Another means by which a plant herbal can cause toxicity is by drug–plant interaction (Table 365.4).

EMERGENCY DEPARTMENT EVALUATION

A history of exposure is critical in alerting the clinician to the possibility of plant or herbal intoxication. Plant and herbal intoxication can cause any number of signs or symptoms, so questions concerning the use of or contact with plants and herbals should be asked when a patient presents with an illness of uncertain cause. Adults should be asked whether they have taken any homeopathic or folk remedies over the past few weeks. In children, even if an ingestion were not observed, questions should be asked about plant availability. Evidence of plant exposure may include plant material on a child, missing parts on a plant in or around the home, or plant material in the stool or vomitus. Any suspect plant (or a sample) should be brought with the patient, if possible, for identification.

Plants and herbals may have multiple common and scientific names. If the patient provides a common name of a plant, the correct identity should be confirmed by a botanic description. This description should include leaf structure, flower shape and color, fruits, and general size and shape. Because few emergency physicians have the expertise to identify plants, groups such as garden clubs, botanic gardens, floral or garden shops, and university agricultural departments may be of value. Poison centers and other sources, such as a toxicology laboratory, may help with plant identification and possible treatment.[3,4,8,10]

Depending on the nature of complaints, a complete or focused physical examination may be appropriate. All patients should have a complete set of vital signs. Depending on the history and physical findings, rhythm or electrocardiogram interpretation may be indicated to evaluate for cardiovascular toxicity, and laboratory testing may be necessary for the assessment of fluid and electrolyte, hematologic, and liver or renal function abnormalities. With few exceptions (e.g., digitalis and heavy-metal poisoning), toxicology testing is unlikely to be helpful.

EMERGENCY DEPARTMENT MANAGEMENT

Supportive care and decontamination are the primary treatment modalities. Although rarely necessary, advanced life-support measures should be instituted when appropriate. Supportive

TABLE 365.3. Examples of Herbal Toxicity

Allergic reactions: alfalfa, chamomile (*Chamomilla* species), dandelion (*Taraxacum officinale*), echinacea (*Echinacea pallida*), garlic (*Allium sativum*), ginger (*Zingiber officinale*), propolis.

Anticholinergic poisoning (see also Chapter 312): burdock root (*Arctium lappa*), jimson weed (*Datura stromonium*), lobelia (*Lobelia inflata*), mandrake (*Mandragon officinarum*)

Coagulopathy: melilot (*Melilotus officinalis*), tonka beans (*Coumarouna oppisitifolia*), woodruff (*Galium odoratum*)

Cardiovascular depression: astragalus, codopsis, cardiac glycosides (see Table 365.1), goldenseal (*Hydratis canadesis*), prunella, sage (*Salvia* species), hellebore (*Veratrum* species), juniper (*Juniper communis*), monkshood or wolfsbane (*Aconitum napellus*; also found in many Chinese medicines), passion flower (*Passiflora caerulea*), snakeroot (*Rauwolfia serpentina*),

Cardiovascular stimulation: figwort or xuan shen (*Scrophularia* species), khat (*Catha edulis*), monkshood or wolfsbane (*Aconitum napellus;* also found in many Chinese medicines), ma-juang (*Ephedra sinica*), mormon tea (*Ephedra nevadensis*), yohimbine (*Coryanthe yohimbe*)

CNS depression: kavakava (*Piper methysticum*), peony, peppermint (*Mentha pulegium*), snakeroot (*Rauwolfia serpentina*), St. John's wort (*Hypericum perforatum*), tang-kuei, valerian root (*Valeriana* species)

CNS stimulation (see also Table 365.2): absinthe (wormwood, mugwort; *Artemisia* species), eucalyptus, ginseng (*Panax quinquefolium*), hyssop (*Hyssopus officinalis*), juniper (*Juniper communis*), khat (*Catha edulis*), majuang (*Ephedra sinica*), mormon tea (*Ephedra nevadensis*), passion flower (*Passiflora caerulea*), periwinkle (*Vinca* species), sage (*Salvia* species), yohimbine (*Coryanthe yohimbe*)

Gastroenteritis: common; can be severe with buckthorn (*Hipthothae rhamnoides*), poke root (*Phytolacca americana*), and senna (*Cassia angustifola*).

Hematologic suppression: goldenseal (*Hydratis canadensis*), podophyllin (*Dysosma pleianthum, Podophyhyllum* species)

Hepatitis: chaparral (*Covillea tridentata, Larrea tridenta, L. divaricata*), germander (*Teucrium chamaedrys*), jin bu huan (traditional Chinese medicine), kombucha, ma-juang (*Ephedra* species), pennyroyal (*Hedeoma pugelioides* or mentha pulegium), periwinkle (Vinca species)

Hepatic venoocclusive disease: coltsfoot (*Tussilago farfara*), comfrey (*Symphytum officinale*), *Crotalaria* species, gordolobo (*Senecio longilobus*), groundsel (*Senecio vulgaris*), *Heliatropim* species, maté (*Ilex paraguayensis*), tansy ragwort (*Senecio jacobea*), t'u-san-chi (*Gynura segetum*)

Nephrotoxicity: aloe, astralgalus, burdock, dandelion, juniper (*Juniper communis*), licorice (*Glycyrrhiza* species), peony

Obstructive airway disease: betel nut (*Areca catechu*), sabah (*Sauropus androgynus*), wild or squirting cucumber (*Ecbalium elaterium*)

TABLE 365.4. Potential Herbal–Drug Interactions

Herb	Drug	Mechanism/Result
Acacia	Oral drugs	Reduces absorpt. rate
	Ferric iron salts	Acacia gelatinized
Alfalfa	Decr. warfarin activity	High vitamin K content
Aloes (chr.)	Pot. cardiac glyc.	Possible K+ loss
	Incr. thiazide diuretic toxicity	Possible K+ loss
	Licorice root	Possible K+ loss
	Glibenclamide incr. activity	Hypoglycemic agent
Ashwagandha	Barbiturates	Potentiation
Belladonna	Amantadine	Incr. A/C activity
	Quinidine	Incr. A/C activity
	Tricyclic antidepressants	Incr. A/C activity
Betel nut	Phenothiazine (antiparkinsonian)	Decr. eff.
	Flupenthixol (antiparkinsonian)	Decr. eff.
	Fluphenazine (antiparkinsonian)	Decr. eff.
	Procyclidine (A/C eff.)	Reduced
Bitter melon	Antihyperglycemics	Reduces blood sugar
Black pepper (piperidine)	Phenytoin	Incr. absorpt., decr. elim.
	Propranolol	Incr. absorpt.
	Theophylline	Incr. absorpt.
Bromelain	Tetracyclines	Incr. plasma/urine levels
Buckthorn (chr.)	Pot. cardiac glyc.	Possible K+ loss
	Incr. thiazide diuretic toxicity	Possible K+ loss
	Licorice root	Possible K+ loss
Bugleweed	Radioisotope interference	Unknown
	Thyroid hormones	Blocks thyroxin to T3
Burdock	Antidiabetic agents	Incr. hypoglycemic eff.
Cascara sagrada (chr.)	Pot. cardiac glyc.	Possible K+ loss
	Incr. thiazide diuretic toxicity	Possible K+ loss
	Licorice root	Possible K+ loss
Cassia cinnamon	Tetracyclines (absorption)	Decr.
Cinchona bark	Anticoagulant activity incr.	Unknown
Clover (sweet)	Aspirin	Incr. anticoagulant eff.
	Bromelain	Incr. anticoagulant eff.
Coffee	Iron absorption	Decr.
	Adenosine	Inhibits eff.
	CNS stimulants	Enhances eff.
	Lithium	Reduced levels
Cola nut	CNS stimulants	Pot. activity
Dan shen	Warfarin	Incr. activity
Ephedra	Cardiac glyc.	Heart rhythm abnor.
	Halothane	Heart rhythm abnor.
	Guanethidine	Incr. sympathomimetic eff.
	Oxytocin	Hypertension
Fenugreek	Antidiabetic agents	Potentiation of eff.
Flaxseed	All drugs: mucilage	May alter absorpt.
Ginkgo	Aspirin	Incr. bleeding
Ginseng	Warfarin	Potentiation of eff.
	Caffeine (13 wk, 3 g/d ginseng dose)	
	Hypoglycemic agents	Incr. hypoglycemic eff.
Henbane	Amantadine	Incr. A/C activity
	Antihistamines	Incr. A/C activity
	Phenothiazines	Incr. A/C activity
	Procainamide	Incr. A/C activity
	Tricyclic antidepressants	Incr. A/C activity
Indian snakeroot	Digitalis	Bradycardia
	Barbiturates	Potentiation
	L-dopa	Decr. effectiveness
	Sympathomimetics	Incr. blood pressure
Kava-kava	Alcohol	Potentiation
	CNS depressant drugs	Potentiation
Licorice root	Thiazide diuretics	Incr. K+ loss
Lily-of-the-valley	Cardiac glyc.	Incr. effectiveness
	Quinidine	Incr. effectiveness
Maté	CNS stimulant drugs	Incr. stimulation
Oak bark	Alkaloids	Reduced absorpt.
	Alkaline drugs	Reduced absorpt.
Pheasant's eye	Cardiac glyc.	Contains cardiac glyc.
	Quinidine	Pot. eff.
Scopolia root	Amantadine	Incr. A/C activity
	Quinidine	Incr. A/C activity
	Tricyclic antidepressants	Incr. A/C activity
Scotch broom	MAOIs (tyramine content)	Hypertension

TABLE 365.4. *(Continued)*

Herb	Drug	Mechanism/Result
Senna (chr.)	Pot. cardiac glyc.	Possible K+ loss
	Incr. thiazide diuretic toxicity	Possible K+ loss
	Licorice root	Possible K+ loss
Siberian ginseng	Monomycin antibiotic activity	Incr.
	Kanamycin antibiotic activity	Incr.
Squill	Quinidine	Incr. effectiveness
	Corticosteroids (prolonged therapy)	Incr. effectiveness
St. John's wort	Antidepressants	Incr. effectiveness
Stinging nettle	Diclofenac	Incr. effectiveness
Uva ursi	Drugs that cause an acid urine	Decr. effectiveness
Yohimbine	Clomipramine	Hypertension
	Imipramine	Hypertension
	Clonidine (antihypertensive eff.)	Reversed
	Guanabenz (antihypertensive eff.)	Reversed
	Naloxone (oral)	Incr. side eff.

abnor., abnormalities; absorpt., absorption; A/C, anticholinergic; chr., chronic; decr., decreased; eff., effect; elim., elimination; glyc., glycosides; incr., increased; pot., potentiates.

therapy includes replacement of volume deficits with intravenous crystalloids and correction of electrolyte abnormalities. Patients with CNS depression may require airway protection and ventilatory support. Seizures and CNS stimulation usually respond to treatment with benzodiazepines. Phenytoin and phenobarbital can be given for refractory seizures. Allergic reactions and hematologic, liver, and renal toxicity are treated with standard measures.

Decontamination varies with the route and nature of the exposure. Dilution with small amounts of clear liquids or milk is usually sufficient for the ingestion of plants that only cause gastroenteritis. Because many plant toxins are large molecules, activated charcoal should be effective and is the preferred method of GI decontamination for recent ingestions of agents with potential systemic toxicity.

Skin and eye exposures are treated with thorough irrigation. Some cactus spines can be removed with tweezers or forceps. Fine spines (glochids) have been removed with tape, facial masks, glue mixtures, and wood pastes applied to the skin and then peeled off. Oily materials, such as the toxicodendrol oils, should be washed thoroughly with soap and water to prevent spread to other parts of the body or to emergency room staff.

Antihistamines for itching and antiinflammatory agents or analgesics for pain may be required for some dermal exposures. Topical antiseptics and tetanus prophylaxis may be useful if there are puncture wounds.

There are few antidotes for plant poisonings, and when an antidote is considered useful, it is generally similar in effectiveness and dosage to a nonplant exposure to the same toxic substance. For example, cardiac glycoside poisoning due to *Digitalis* species may be treated with digoxin-specific Fab fragment antibodies (see Chapter 332). Anticholinergic plant poisoning may be treated with physostigmine (see Chapter 312). Patients with cyanogenic glycoside poisoning should be treated with cyanide antidotes (see Chapter 331).

DISPOSITION

Patients with acute ingestions of a potentially toxic plant should be observed for 4 hours or until symptoms have resolved. Those with irritant and oxalate ingestions may be discharged as soon as their discomfort is under control, they can take fluids orally, and there is no evidence of airway edema. Patients who are symptomatic after ingesting plants containing cardiac glycoside and CNS toxins should be admitted for observation, monitoring, and, if necessary, treatment. The level of care should be dictated by clinical severity. If severe, patients with allergic reactions and hematologic, liver, or renal toxicity may also require admission. Patients with a history of pyrrolizidine alkaloid plant ingestion and those with abnormal laboratory findings require outpatient referral and follow-up.

COMMON PITFALLS

- Failure to appreciate that plant and herbal poisoning can affect virtually any organ system.
- Failure to ask about self-treatment with plants, herbals, and folk and homeopathic remedies, especially when the clinical picture does not suggest a specific diagnosis
- Failure to recognize potential drug–plant interactions
- Failure to obtain information on plant toxicity from textbooks, poison control centers, or a toxicologist
- Failure to appreciate that, as the use of herbals increases, previously unreported toxicity may be encountered
- Failure to appreciate that the data on plant and herbal poisoning found in textbooks is sometimes conflicting, antiquated, or nonexistent and to consult an expert or perform a literature search for additional information

References

1. Abebe W. Adverse effects of traditional drug preparations. *J Ethnopharmacol* 1992;36:93.
2. Blumenthal M, Busse WR, Goldberg A, et al. *The Complete German Commission E Monographs. Therapeutic guide to herbal medicines.* Boston: Integrative Medicine Communications, 1998.
3. Brinker F. *Herb contraindications and drug interactions.* Sandy, OR: Eclectic Medical Publications, 1998.
4. Corrigan D. Educating the pharmacist about herbal medicines. *Pharm Int J* 1985;1:22.
5. Frohne D, Pfander HJ. *A colour atlas of poisonous plants.* London: Wolfe, 1984.
6. Hardin JW, Arena J. *Human poisoning from native and cultivated plants,* 2d ed. Durham, NC: Duke University Press, 1974.
7. Hayes BE, Bessen HA, Wightman WD. Oleander tea: herbal draught of death. *Ann Emerg Med* 1985;14:350.
8. Huxtable RJ. Novel aspects of pyrrolizidine poisoning in the United States. *Perspect Biol Med* 1980;24:1.
9. Kinghorn AD, ed. *Toxic plants.* New York: Columbia University Press, 1979.
10. Kunkel DB. Plant poisonings in children. *Pediatr Ann* 1987;16:927.
11. Lampe KF, McCann MA. *AMA handbook of poisonous and injurious plants.* Chicago: American Medical Association, 1985.

12. Lewis WH, Smith PR. Poke-root herbal tea poisoning. *JAMA* 1975;242:2759.
13. Lipsitz DJ. Herbal teas and water intoxication in a young child. *J Fam Pract* 1984;18:933.
14. Ridker PM. Toxic effects of herbal teas. *Arch Environ Health* 1987;42:133.
15. Rumack BH, Spoerke DG, Smolinske SC, eds. *PoisIndex system—plants: cardiac glycosides.* Denver: Micromedex, 1994.
16. Spoerke DG. Herbal medications: use and misuse. *Hosp Formul* 1980;15:941.
17. Spoerke DG, Evans B, Linaburg B. *The hidden hazards in house and garden plants.* Missoula, MT: Pictorial Histories Publishing, 1991.
18. Trotter RT. Folk medicine in the Southwest—myths and medical facts. *Postgrad Med* 1985;78:167.
19. Tyler VE, Brady LR, Robbers JE. *Pharmacognosy*, 8th ed. Philadelphia: Lea & Febiger, 1981.
20. Yeung CY, Leung CS, Chen YZ. An old traditional herbal remedy for neonatal jaundice with a newly identified risk. *J Paediatr Child Health* 1993;29:292.

APPENDICES

The following series of tables gives information about the potential toxicity of various plants. Toxicity is often difficult to assess in an exposure because it depends on the part ingested, the amount, the person's susceptibility, and other "environmental" aspects.

Toxic Part Key: A/P, all parts; B, berry; Bk, bark; Bu, bulb; F, fruit; Fl, flowers; Fol, foliage; L, leaves; N, nut; R, rhizomes; Rt, root; S, seed; Sa, sap or latex; T, thorns, spines, glochids; U/F, unripe fruit; W, wood.

References for the tables in the appendices are 5, 6, 10, 11, 15, 17, and 19.

APPENDIX 365.A. Potential Ingestion Hazards

Scientific Name	Common Name	Toxin Type	Toxic Part
Abrus precatorius	Rosary pea	Toxalbumin	S
Aconitum napellus	Monkshood	Aconitine	A/P
Actaea rubra	Baneberry	Protoanemonin	S,Rt,B
Aesculus hippocastanum	Horse chestnut	Saponins	L,N,F
Aesculus glabra	Buckeye	Saponins	L,N,F
Aethusa cynapium	Fool's parsley	CNS stimulant	A/P
Allamanda cathartica	Yellow allamanda	Cathartic	A/P
Amaryllis belladonna	Belladonna lily	Lycorine	Bu
Anemone hupehensis	Japanese anemone	Protoanemonin	A/P
Areca cathecu	Betel nut	Alkaloids	N,S
Arnica montana	Wolf's bane	Sesquiterpenes	A/P
Atropa belladonna	Deadly nightshade	Atropine	A/P
Aucuba japonica	Japanese laurel	Aucubin	A/P
Brugmansia species	Angel's trumpet	Atropine	A/P
Caesalpinia gilliesii	Bird of paradise	Tannins	S
Caltha palustris	Marsh marigold	Protoanemonin	Fol
Celastrus scandans	Viny bittersweel	Unknown	Fol
Cestrum nocturnum	Night Jessamine	Saponins	S,F
Cicuta maculata	Water hemlock	Cicutoxin	A/P
Clematis species	Virgin's bower	Protoanemonin	A/P
Clivia miniata	Kaffir lily	Lycorine	Bu
Consolida ambigua	Larkspur	Alkaloids	S,Fol
Colchicum autumnale	Autumn crocus	Colchicine	A/P
Conium maculatum	Poison hemlock	Coniine	A/P
Convallaria majalis	Lily-of-the-valley	Glycoside	L,F,S
Crinum asiaticum	Spider lily	Lycorine	Bu
Cystisus scoparius	Scotch broom	Cytisine	Fol
Daphne mezereum	Daphne	Diterpene	A/P
Datura stramonium	Jimson weed	Atropine	A/P
Delphinium elatum	Delphinium	Alkaloids	F,Fol
Digitalis purpurea	Foxglove	Glycosides	A/P
Duranta repens	Pigeon berry	Saponins	B
Euonymus europaea	Spindle tree	Glycoside	L,Bk,F
Gelsemium sempervirens	Carolina jessamine	Alkaloids	A/P
Gloriosa superba	Glory lily	Colchicine	A/P
Hyacinthus orientalis	Hyacinth	Lycorine	Bu
Hymenocallis species	Spider lily	Lycorine	Bu
Hyoscyamus niger	Henbane	Atropine	A/P
Ilex aquifolium	English holly	Saponins	B
Ipomoea violacea	Morning glory	Clavine alkal	S
Jatropha curcas	Physic nut	Toxalbumin	S
Kalmia latifolia	Mountain laurel	Grayanotoxin	A/P
Laburnum anagyroides	Golden chain tree	Cytisine	S
Lantane camara	Lantana	Unknown	U/B
Ligustrum species	Privet	Syringin	S
Melia azedarach	Chinaberry tree	Neurotoxins	F
Myristica fragrans	Nutmeg	Myristicin	S
Narcissus species	Narcissus	Lycorine	Bu
Nerium oleander	Oleander	Glycosides	A/P
Nicotiana glauca	Tree tobacco	Nicotine	A/P
Phoradendron species	American mistletoe	Toxalbumin	B
Phytolaeca americana	Pokeweed	Phytolacatoxin	A/P

APPENDIX 365.A. Potential Ingestion Hazards (continued)

Scientific Name	Common Name	Toxin Type	Toxic Part
Ranunculus species	Buttercups	Protoanemonin	Fol
Rhododendron species	Azalea	Grayanotoxins	A/P
Ricinus communis	Castor bean	Toxalbumin	S
Robinia pseudoacacia	Black locust	Toxalbumin	S
Solanum dulcamara	Bittersweet	Solanine	A/P
Solanum tuberosum	Potato	Solanine	L,Sprouts
Taxus species	Yew	Taxine	L/S
Thevetia peruviana	Yellow oleander	Glycosides	A/P
Veratrum virde	Indian poke	Veratrum alk	R
Wisteria sinensis	Wisteria	Lectin	S
Zigadenus species	Death camas	Zygadenine	Bu

APPENDIX 365.B. Nontoxic Houseplants

These houseplants are generally considered nontoxic or very minimally toxic, or have no evidence of toxicity.

Scientific Name	Common Name	Scientific Name	Common Name
Achimenes erecta	Cupid's bower	*Calathea crocata*	Flowering calathea
Acorus gramineus veriagatus	Sweet flag	*Calathea makoyana*	Peacock plant
Adiantum hispidulum	Australian maidenhair	*Calathea zabrina*	Zebra plant
Adiantum raddianum	Maidenhair fern	*Calceolaria herbeohybrida*	Slipper flower
Aeonium arboreum		*Calliandra inaequilatera*	Powderpuff plant
Aeonium tabulaeforme	Saucer plant	*Callisia elegans*	Striped inch plant
Aeschynanthus lobbianus	Lipstick vine	*Callistemon citri*	Bottlebrush plant
Ageratum houstonianum	Ageratum	*Calthea argyraea*	Calthea
Aglaomorpha meyeniana	Bear's paw fern	*Camellia japonica*	Camellia
Aglaonema species	Chinese evergreen	*Campanula isophylla*	Italian bellflower
Akchmea fasciata	Urn plant	*Celosia cristata*	Cockscomb
Albutilon hybridum	Flowering maple	*Celosia plumosa*	Plume flower
Albutilon megapotamicum	Trailing albutilon	*Centaurea cyanus*	Cornflower
Albutilon striatum thompsonii	Spotted flowering maple	*Cephalocerus senilis*	Old man cactus
Aloe vera	Burn plant	*Cereus peruvianus monstrosus*	Rock cactus
Ampelopsis brevipedunculata		*Ceropegia woodii*	Rosary vine
Andromischus cooperi		*Chamaecereus silvestrii*	Peanut cactus
Antirrhinum majus	Snapdragon	*Chamaedorea elegans*	Parlour palm
Aphelandra squarrosa	Zebra plant	*Chamaedorea erumpens*	Bamboo palm
Aponogenion senetralis	Madagascar lace plant	*Chamaedorea seifrizii*	Reed palm
Aporocactus flagelliformis	Rat's tail cactus	*Chamaerops humilis*	European fan palm
Aralia elegantissima	False aralia	*Chinodoxa luciliae*	Glory of the snow
Aralia sieboldii	Japanese aralia	*Chlorophytum comosum*	Spider plant
Araucaria heterophylla	Norfolk Island pine	*Chrysalidocarpus lutescens*	Butterfly palm
Ardisia crenata	Coral berry	*Cibotium schiedei*	Mexican fern tree
Areca lutescens	Areca palm	*Cissus antartica*	Kangaroo vine
Argyroderma testiculare	Living stone	*Cocos weddeliana*	Dwarf coconut palm
Asparagus densiflorus sprengeri	Emerald fern	*Coilinia elegans*	Parlor palm
Asparagus falcatus	Sicklethorn	*Clarkia elegans*	Clarkia
Aspelenium bulbiferum	Mother fern	*Cleistocactus staussii*	Silver torch
Aspelenium nidus	Bird's nest fern	*Cleyera japonica tricolor*	
Aspidistra elatior	Cast iron plant	*Clianthus formosus*	Glory pea
Astrophytum capricorne	Goat's horn cactus	*Coleus blumei*	Coleus
Babiana stricta	Baboon root	*Columnea banksi*	Goldfish plant
Beaucarnea recurvata	Pony tail	*Cordyline indivisa*	Dracena
Begonia semperflorens-cultorum	Wax begonia	*Cordyline terminalis*	Ti plant
Begonia tuberhybrida	Tuberous begonia	*Cotyledone tomentosa*	Bear feet
Belechnum braziliense	Brazilian tree fern	*Crassula argentea*	Jade plant
Belechnum gibbum		*Crassula falcata*	Propeller plant
Beloperone gutta	Shrimp plant	*Crassula lycopodioides*	Rat tail plant
Billbergia nutans	Queen's tears	*Creopegia woodii*	String of hearts
Bougainvillea glabra	Paper flower	*Cyanotis kewensis*	Teddy bear vine
Bouvardia domestica	Bouvardia	*Cyclamen persicum*	Persian violet
Brassaia actinophylla	Schefflera	*Davallia canariensis*	Hare's foot fern
Breynia nivosa roseopicta	Leaf flower	*Dicentra spectabilis*	Bleeding hearts
Brodiaea laxa	Brodiaea	*Dichorisandra reginae*	Queen's spiderwort
Browallia speciosa	Bush violet	*Didymochlaena truncatula*	Cloak fern
Brunfelsia calycina	Yesterday, today & tomorrow	*Dizygotheca elegantissima*	False aralia
Bryophyllum tubiforum	Chandelier plant	*Draceana fragrans massangeana*	Corn plant

APPENDIX 365.B. Nontoxic Houseplants (continued)

Scientific Name	Common Name	Scientific Name	Common Name
Dracearia dereminensis	Janet Craig	*Pelargonium domesticum*	Geranium
Draceana marginata	Madagascar dragon	*Pellaea rotundifolia*	Button fern
Echium vulgare	Blue devil	*Pellionia daveauana*	Satin pellionia
Euphorbia pulcherrima	Poinsettia	*Peperomia* species	Peperomias
Fatshedera lizei	Ivy tree	*Pilea* species	Creeping Charlie
Fatsia japonica	Japanese aralia	*Plectranthus oertendahlii*	Swedish ivy
Ficus lyrata	Fiddleleaf fig	*Polypodium vulgare*	Wall fern
Fittonia argyroneura	Silver net leaf	*Rechsleineria cardinalis*	Cardinal flower
Fittonia verschaffeltii	Painted net leaf	*Rhapis excelsia*	Little lady palm
Gardenia radicans	Gardenia	*Rhochea coccinea*	Crassula
Gibasis geniculata	Tahitian bridal veil	*Rhoicissus rhomboidea*	Grape ivy
Glechoma hederaceae	Creeping Charlie	*Rhoicissus capensis*	Cape ivy
Gynura sarmentosa	Velvet plant	*Rochea falcata*	Propeller plant
Helxine soleirolii	Baby tears	*Ruellia makoyana*	Monkey plant
Hemigraphis alternata	Red ivy	*Senecio mikanioides*	German ivy
Heptapleurum arboricola	Parasol plant	*Senecio rowleyanus*	String of beads
Hoya exotica	Wax plant	*Setcreasea purpurea*	Purple heart
Hydrangea species	Hydrangea	*Smithiantha hybrida*	Temple bells
Impatiens species	Impatiens	*Sparaxis tricolor*	Harlequin flower
Kalanchoe tubiforum	Chandelier plant	*Strelitzia reginae*	Bird of paradise
Livisona chinensis	Chinese fan palm	*Strobilanthes dyeranus*	Persian shield
Lysimachia ucnummularifolia	Creeping Jenny	*Tetrastigma voinieranum*	Chestnut ivy
Maranta makoyana	Peacock plant	*Tillandsia ionantha*	Air plant
Maranta tricolor	Herringbone plant	*Tolmiea menziesii*	Piggyback plant
Mikania ternata	Plush vine	*Tradescantia blossfeldiana*	Wandering Jew
Mimosa pudica	Sensitive plant	*Viriesea splendens*	Flaming sword
Neanthe bella	Parlor palm	*Zinnia elegans*	Zinnia
Nephrolepsis exaltata	Sword fern	*Zebrina pendula purpusii*	Wandering Jew
Nephrolepsis exaltata bostoniensis	Boston fern	*Zygocactus truncatus*	Christmas cactus
Nolia tuberculata	Elephant foot		

APPENDIX 365.C. Plants That May Cause a Dermal Reaction (*May be irritant, mechanical, or allergic*)

Scientlfic Name	Common Name	Scientlfic Name	Common Name
Abutilon hybridum	Chinese lantern	*Dicatamnus albus*	Gas plant
Acalypha hispida	Chenille plant	*Dirca palustris*	Leatherwood
Acalypha milkesiana	Copper leaf	*Euphorbia corollata*	Flowering spurge
Achillea millefolium	Yarrow	*Euphorbia cotinifolia*	Poison spurge
Ackanthera oblongifolia	Wintersweet	*Euphorbia esula*	Leafy spurge
Agapanthus orientalis	African blue lily	*Euphorbia helioscopia*	Sun spurge
Agave picta	Maguey	*Euphorbia lactea*	Candelabra cactus
Ailanthus altissima	Tree of heaven	*Euphorbia lathyris*	Caper spurge
Ambrosia artemisiifolia	Ragweed	*Euphorbia maculata*	Eyebane
Ammi majus	Bishop's weed	*Euphorbia marginata*	Snow on the mountain
Anacardium occidentale	Cashew nut	*Euphorbia milii*	Crown of thorns
Ananas comosus	Pineapple	*Euphorbia myrsinites*	Donkeytail
Anemone patens	Pasqueflower	*Euphorbia tirucalli*	Pencil tree
Anthemis cotula	Dog fennel	*Excoecaria agallocha*	Blinding tree
Aralia spinosa	Devil's club	*Ficus benjamina*	Weeping fig
Arnica montana	Mountain tobacco	*Ficus carica*	Common fig
Artemesia species	Mugwort	*Ficus pumila*	Creeping fig
Asarum caradense	Wild ginger	*Heracleum lantanum*	Cow parsnip
Asimina triloba	Papaw	*Heracleum mantegazaianum*	Giant hogweed
Asparagus cetaceus	Asparagus fern	*Hesperocnide* species	Western stinging nettles
Cactus	Cactus	*Hippomane mancinella*	Manchineel
Calendula officinalis	Pot marigold	*Hypericum perforatum*	St. John's wort
Calotropis gigantea	Crown flower	*Laportea canadensis*	Wood nettle
Caltha palustris	Marsh marigold	*Mangifera indica*	Mango
Campsis radicans	Trumpet creeper	*Metopium toxiferum*	Poison wood
Carex mitis	Tufted fishtail palm	*Opuntia* species	Beaver tail cactus
Carex urens	Wine fishtail palm	*Pastinacea sativa*	Parsnip
Catalpa species	Catalpa	*Plumeria* species	Frangipani
Caulophyllum thalicroides	Blue cohosh	*Rheo spathacea*	Moses in a boat
Chelidonium majus	Celandine	*Ruta graveolens*	Rue
Chimaphila umbellata	Prince's plume	*Schinus terebinthifolius*	Brazilian pepper
Chrysanthemum species	Chrysanthemum	*Stillingia sylvatica*	Queen's delight
Citrus aurantiifolia	Lime	*Synadenium grantii*	African milk bush
Clematis virginiana	Virgin's bower	*Toxicodendron diversilobum*	Western poison oak
Cnidoscolus species	Spurge nettle	*Toxicodendron quercifolium*	Eastern poison oak
Codiaeum variegatum	Croton	*Toxicodendron radicans*	Poison ivy
Cotinus coggygria	Smoke tree	*Toxicodendron vernix*	Poison sumac
Dahlia variabilis	Pot dahlia	*Tulipa* species	Tulips
Daucus carota	Queen Anne's lace	*Urtica dioica*	Stinging nettles

CHAPTER 366
Rodenticide Poisoning

Richard D. Shih and Robert S. Hoffman

A large number of chemically distinct compounds with varied toxicities are utilized as rodenticides. One system for classifying rodenticides was developed as part of the federal Insecticide, Fungicide, and Rodenticide Act.[7] This system categorizes rodenticides as high, moderate, or low toxicity based on their 50% lethal dose (LD_{50}) in rats (Table 366.1). Although useful for comparing the potential human toxicity of the different agents, animals may be more or less sensitive to specific agents than are humans.

A more clinically useful classification of rodenticides is based on the time of onset of symptoms (Table 366.2). The time of symptom onset, with respect to the time of exposure along with the nature of the symptoms, allows for a presumptive diagnosis in patients with exposure to an unknown rodenticide, a not uncommon clinical scenario.

Medically significant, unintentional rodenticide exposures are uncommon. Most occur in children, especially those under 6 years old, and result in minimal or no toxicity.[14,18] Adults with intentional ingestions, however, often develop significant morbidity and mortality.

TABLE 366.1. Rodenticide Toxicity

HIGHLY TOXIC
(LD_{50} <50 mg/kg in rats)
Arsenic
Oral anticoagulants ("superwarfarin" types)
Sodium monofluoracetate
Strychnine
Thallium
Vacor
Yellow phosphorus
Zinc phosphide
MODERATELY TOXIC
(LD_{50} 50–500 mg/kg in rats)
Alpha-naphthylthiourea
Cholecalciferol
LOW TOXICITY
(LD_{50} 500–5000 mg/kg in rats)
Norbormide
Red squill
Oral anticoagulants ("non-superwarfarin" types)

Adapted from Goldfrank L, Flomembaum N, Weisman RS. Rodenticides. *Hosp Physician* 1981;17:87.

TABLE 366.2. Onset of Symptoms in Rodenticide Poisoning

EARLY ONSET
Alpha-naphthylthiourea
Arsenic
Norbormide
Organophosphates
Red squill
Sodium monofluoroacetate
Strychnine
Thallium
Vacor
Yellow phosphorus
Zinc phosphide
LATE ONSET
Oral anticoagulants
Cholecalciferol

CLINICAL PRESENTATION

Patients exposed to rodenticides with a rapid onset of action can be expected to manifest symptoms within 6 hours of ingestion. Those with exposure to rodenticides that have a delayed onset typically manifest symptoms beginning 12 hours or more after ingestion. Because signs and symptoms differ and depend on the particular toxin involved, agents are discussed individually.

Alpha-Naphthylthiourea

Alpha-naphthylthiourea (ANTU) is relatively nontoxic in humans. Its mechanism of action is unknown, but the lung is the principal target organ. Dyspnea, cough, and pleuritic chest pain can occur but are not typically life-threatening. However, patients with large, acute exposures can rapidly develop noncardiogenic pulmonary edema by an unknown mechanism.

Anticoagulants (Oral)

Oral anticoagulants are the most commonly used rodenticides.[3,6,12] They are either hydroxycoumarin or indandione derivatives. Toxicity results from inhibition of the cyclic regeneration of vitamin K, a cofactor required for the activation of coagulation factors II, VII, IX, and X.[19] Although vitamin K depletion occurs almost immediately, no anticoagulant effect is seen until the activity of at least one clotting factor is diminished to below 25% of normal.[6] Because factor VII has the shortest half-life among the clotting factors affected ($t_{1/2} = 5$ hours), at least three half-lives (15 hours) are usually required before any toxicity is manifested.

Conventional anticoagulant rodenticides contain low concentrations of active ingredients. For example, a typical warfarin rodenticide may contain 0.025% to 0.05% of the toxin (100 to 200 mg in a pound of bait). These products were designed to kill rodents who ingest this bait daily over a period of several weeks. Because of this low concentration, acute, single, unintentional exposures in humans are unlikely to cause toxicity.

The widespread use of warfarin-containing rodenticides resulted in many rodent populations becoming resistant to their effects. As a result, higher-potency agents—"superwarfarins"—were developed. These agents can produce toxicity for prolonged periods after ingestions of smaller doses. Although children who unintentionally ingest superwarfarins are unlikely to develop toxicity, adults with intentional ingestions or children with repeated ingestions often develop a coagulopathy within 24 or, at the latest, 48 hours.[18] If this goes untreated, bleeding complications may develop. The most common sites of bleeding are the GI and genitourinary tracts.[3,8,12]

Arsenic

This heavy-metal rodenticide, used more commonly in the past, was a leading cause of rodenticide-related deaths in the 1950s and 1960s. Professional exterminators still have access to this compound. Arsenic causes rapid onset of toxicity by combining and inhibiting sulfhydryl enzymes. Patients with acute ingestions may be distinguished by a garlic odor on their breath and severe vomiting and diarrhea, dehydration, dysrhythmias, and central nervous system (CNS) and cardiovascular depression (see Chapter 318).

Cholecalciferol

Cholecalciferol is relatively nontoxic in acute exposures, but with large doses, symptoms consistent with hypervitaminosis D (see Chapter 359) and hypercalcemia might occur. These symptoms include gastrointestinal (GI) complaints such as nausea, vomiting, constipation, and abdominal pains; mental status depression; and rare cardiac dysrhythmias.

Norbormide

Norbormide is relatively nontoxic in humans, but, in rodents, it causes diffuse vasoconstriction and ischemia. Although the mechanism is not entirely understood, rodent smooth muscle has a specific norbormide receptor that, when stimulated, leads to these effects. No human fatalities have been reported from this agent.

Organophosphates and Carbamates

Organophosphate compounds are not sanctioned for use as rodenticides in the United States. However, they can be used as an active ingredient for this purpose by foreign manufacturers. These products have reached the United States and been sold as rodenticides.[13] Exposure can occur by the oral, dermal, or inhalational routes. Signs and symptoms include salivation, lacrimation, urination, defecation, nausea, vomiting, GI cramping and/or pain, diarrhea, mental status change, seizures, muscle fasciculations, or weakness[9,13] (see Chapter 361).

Red Squill

Red squill is a cardiac glycoside derived from the plant *Urginea maritima*. Its toxicity relates to its ability to block sodium–potassium ATPase similar to digoxin. This toxin is poorly absorbed in humans because of its potent emetic effects. In rodents, however, whose vomiting mechanism is less well developed, the toxin is fairly effective. If large amounts are ingested, a presentation similar to digoxin poisoning may occur; patients may have GI symptoms, cardiac dysrhythmias, and hyperkalemia (see Chapter 332).

Sodium Monofluoroacetate

Sodium monofluoroacetate (SMFA) is a white, odorless, tasteless, water-soluble salt typically available as a powder. Although toxicity can occur by inhalation, ingestion is the most common route of severe poisoning. Once absorbed, SMFA (and the closely related compound fluoroacetamide) rapidly enters the Krebs cycle, where it is converted to fluorocitric acid, which inhibits the Krebs cycle, blocking aerobic glycolysis. Initial symptoms include nausea and apprehension, followed shortly by severe lactic acidosis, pulmonary edema, coma, hypokalemia, hypocalcemia, seizures, and dysrhythmias. Poor prognosis is associated with hypotension, early onset of acidosis, and increased creatinine levels.[2]

Strychnine

Strychnine, a natural alkaloid derived from the native Indian tree *Strychnos nux-vomica*, has been used as a rodenticide since the 1600s. It is a potent neurotoxin that acts by competitively inhibiting glycine postsynaptically. Because glycine is the predominant inhibitory neurotransmitter in the spinal cord, its inhibition results in muscular hyperexcitability. The increased motor activity seen in severe cases results from maximal firing of peripheral muscle groups and can cause opisthotonos, facial spasm (risus sardonicus), and decorticate posturing. Patients are often mistakenly described as having generalized "seizures," but the mental status is normal. Prolonged muscle activity can lead to hyperthermia, rhabdomyolysis, lactic acidosis, and death, often from respiratory dysfunction.

Thallium

Thallium is an odorless, tasteless, highly toxic heavy metal. Although it can penetrate intact skin, it is more readily absorbed when ingested. Thallium, like arsenic, binds to and inhibits sulfhydryl-containing enzymes. Unlike arsenic, however, it preferentially affects mitochondria, and many of its clinical effects may be delayed 12 to 24 hours after ingestion. Initially, GI symptoms such as nausea, vomiting, diarrhea, constipation, and abdominal pain predominate. Characteristically, extremely painful paresthesias then develop in the extremities and are unique in their intensity. In severe cases, dysrhythmias occur and can cause death. Respiratory failure has also been described. Survival is characterized by a period of alopecia and neurologic findings such as neuropathies, paresis, ataxia, choreiform movements, and optic nerve atrophy.[16]

Vacor

When first introduced, Vacor was thought to have no human toxicity. After numerous cases of severe poisoning occurred, it was withdrawn from the market in 1979. Vacor is selectively toxic to pancreatic beta islet cells, producing a chemically induced form of insulin-dependent diabetes mellitus. The exact mechanism for the islet cell destruction is unclear, but it may be due to Vacor's ability to deplete beta islet cells of nicotinamide adenine dinucleotide.[5,15] Exposed patients develop rapid loss of glucose control and the onset of severe diabetic ketoacidosis (DKA). Along with DKA, patients often present with abdominal pain from acute pancreatitis, autonomic instability, and peripheral paresthesias.[15] Survivors of Vacor exposure are characterized by brittle insulin-dependent diabetes as well as accelerated microvascular diabetic disease.[5]

Yellow Phosphorus

Yellow phosphorus has a garlic odor, is soluble in oils, and is usually sold as a paste. It is often mixed with molasses or peanut butter and spread on bread for rodents to eat. Because it resembles food, the risk of unintentional childhood exposure is high. When yellow phosphorus comes into contact with moisture, it often ignites, and dermal exposures can result in second- and third-degree burns. In addition, this toxin is a protoplasmic poison that uncouples oxidative phosphorylation in the GI tract, liver, kidneys, and bone.

The clinical manifestations of acute ingestions occur in three stages.[20] Initially, there is a rapid onset of severe GI symptoms, including nausea, vomiting, hematemesis, diarrhea, and abdominal pain. The stool and vomitus often have a garlic odor and a luminescent appearance ("smoking stools").[17] If death occurs at this stage, it is typically from cardiovascular collapse. The second stage constitutes a relatively asymptomatic phase lasting 2 to 3 days. In the third stage, hepatorenal syndrome develops, as well as CNS symptoms such as altered mental status and coma.

Zinc Phosphide

A dark gray powder with a "rotten fish" odor, zinc phosphide is highly toxic. Although inhalational toxicity has been reported, it is most toxic after ingestion. In the presence of water and stomach acid, zinc phosphide is degraded to zinc and phosphine gas and is accompanied by the rapid development of profuse, black vomitus and abdominal pain. Phosphine gas is then inhaled and absorbed by the lungs, causing noncardiogenic pulmonary edema, liver and renal damage, dysrhythmias, and circulatory collapse.[4]

DIFFERENTIAL DIAGNOSIS

When a patient presents with an unknown rodenticide exposure, the differential diagnosis includes all of the aforementioned entities. The most useful piece of information is the name of the ingested product. A family member should be asked to return home and try to get this information. The actual container or list of active ingredients is preferred over the commercial name, because many commercial names have been used for several products with different active ingredients.

If this information is unavailable, the time of symptom onset (see Table 366.2) and clinical manifestations may suggest the identity of the offending agent. When symptoms are rapid in onset, cholinergic findings suggest organophosphate poisoning; muscular hyperactivity suggests strychnine; seizures, coma, and metabolic acidosis suggest SMFA; severe GI symptoms suggest arsenic or yellow phosphorus; respiratory manifestations suggest ANTU or zinc phosphide; hyperglycemia suggests Vacor; and GI symptoms with cardiac dysrhythmias suggest red squill.

The odor may also serve as a clue to the diagnosis. Arsenic and yellow phosphorus smell like garlic. Zinc phosphide smells like rotten fish. Patients with Vacor-induced DKA have a ketone odor on their breath.

Lack of symptoms during the first 6 hours after exposure to an unknown rodenticide suggests a nontoxic exposure to a rapidly acting agent or a potentially toxic exposure to a rodenticide with a delayed onset of toxicity (i.e., an oral anticoagulant or thallium). The most common cause of delayed rodenticide poisoning is superwarfarin anticoagulants.

EMERGENCY DEPARTMENT EVALUATION

The approach to the patient with an unknown rodenticide poisoning is detailed in the differential diagnosis section. The same principles hold true for a known rodenticide exposure, but the evaluation is more focused with the knowledge of the pathophysiology of a specific toxin. While the diagnostic evaluation is proceeding, consideration and institution of therapy (discussion follows) must occur simultaneously, as many of these poisons cause rapid and potentially fatal toxicity.

The initial assessment should always address the airway, breathing, and circulation. Although uncommon, respiratory distress may be a problem with the toxins that have pulmonary effects, such as zinc phosphide and ANTU. Strychnine may cause respiratory failure secondary to tonic muscle contractions and inability to ventilate. Toxicity from several of the other rodenticides can evolve rapidly to produce cardiovascular collapse.

Vital signs should be obtained immediately. Hyperthermia may occur with strychnine poisoning, due to increased muscle activity, or from yellow phosphorus, secondary to the uncoupling of oxidative phosphorylation.

Clinical clues from the physical examination include specific odors associated with the different toxins and the quality and amount of emesis or diarrhea. "Smoking," luminescent stools have been reported with yellow phosphorus poisoning.[17] Signs of bleeding in the GI or genitourinary tract may indicate oral anticoagulant exposure, although these findings would be delayed in onset.

Blood chemistries and a complete blood count are rarely useful in the absence of clinical findings. A low serum bicarbonate concentration might be found in symptomatic patients with SMFA, yellow phosphorus, strychnine, or Vacor exposures. An elevated serum glucose level, especially in association with a metabolic acidosis, would indicate Vacor-induced DKA. A prothrombin time should be considered in patients with anticoagulant ingestions, although shortly after ingestion, it would most likely be normal. In chronic anticoagulant exposures or in patients who present several days after exposure with active bleeding, this test may be diagnostic.

The need for radiographic assessment should be guided by the toxin involved. Exposure to agents that produce pulmonary toxicity (i.e., ANTU, zinc phosphide) mandate a chest x-ray. Abdominal radiography may help detect opacities in the gut in recent ingestions of the heavy-metal toxins (arsenic, thallium, zinc phosphide). If a sample of an unidentified rodenticide is obtained, a radiograph of it may help to determine its heavy-metal content.[11]

EMERGENCY DEPARTMENT MANAGEMENT

Treatment begins with stabilization of vital signs; advanced life-support measures are instituted, as appropriate. Once the patient is stable, gastric decontamination should be considered to prevent absorption or to increase elimination of the toxin. For the asymptomatic patient who has ingested an unknown rodenticide, activated charcoal is the preferred method. Although not useful for arsenic poisoning, activated charcoal has minimal toxicity and may reduce the severity of most other exposures, as well as potential coingestants. Syrup of ipecac–induced emesis is contraindicated because numerous toxins can cause rapid decompensation. Orogastric lavage may be used in any patient giving a history of recent ingestion (within 2 to 4 hours) of a highly toxic rodenticide. Although little data exist on the efficacy of orogastric lavage, this intervention seems justified given the severe toxicity and lack of effective antidotes for most of the compounds in the highly toxic group. Activated charcoal should also be given.

Management of asymptomatic patients with unknown ingestions involves checking coagulation studies daily for 48 hours to see if anticoagulant toxicity has manifested. Prophylactic treatment of these cases with vitamin K is not recommended in the absence of documented toxicity.

The treatment of symptomatic patients depends on the specific toxin involved.

Anticoagulants (Oral)

Fresh-frozen plasma is given to patients with life-threatening bleeding. Vitamin K should also be given. If coagulopathy exists but the patient does not have significant bleeding, vitamin K alone should be used. Not all vitamin K preparations are effective; phytonadione (AquaMEPHYTON, vitamin K_1) is recommended for this purpose. The dose needed, as well as the duration of treatment, varies with the type and amount of anticoagulant ingested and the patient's rate of toxin metabolism. Doses of up to 100 mg/d of vitamin K_1 for as long as 10 months have been necessary for superwarfarin poisoning.[10]

Alpha-Naphthylthiourea

There is no specific antidotal therapy for this toxin. Treatment involves supportive care.

Arsenic

Management includes supportive care and chelation therapy (see Chapter 318).

Norbormide

Minimal toxicity is expected; treatment is supportive if any problems develop.

Organophosphates and Carbamates

Treatment includes atropine and pralidoxime along with supportive measure (see Chapter 361).

Red Squill

Human toxicity is rare. Treatment of cardiac glycoside toxicity is similar to the management of cardiac glycoside toxicity from other causes (see Chapter 332).

Sodium Monofluoroacetate

Suggested antidotal treatments for SMFA toxicity include the use of glycerol monoacetate and ethanol, although neither approach has been well studied. Glycerol monoacetate is theorized to work by bypassing the site of blockage in the Krebs cycle; ethanol may inhibit the conversion of SMFA to fluorocitrate and allow for excretion of the nontoxic parent compound.[1] Given the availability and relative safety of ethanol administration and the severe toxicity of SMFA, ethanol administration appears warranted.

Strychnine

Treatment of muscle overactivity, the main problem that leads to the life-threatening complications of this toxin, includes high doses of benzodiazepines and, if necessary, neuromuscular paralysis. If the patient is hyperthermic, aggressive rapid cooling (see Chapter 387) is the most important intervention.

Thallium

The management of this toxin is controversial. There are limited data on the efficacy of proposed treatments. Prussian blue (ferric ferrocyanide) has been advocated by some investigators and is used routinely in Europe, but it is not approved for use in the United States.[15] Other investigators advocate using potassium diuresis to increase thallium excretion; still others propose using hemodialysis or hemoperfusion. Although it is unclear which form of treatment is beneficial, we recommend repeated doses of activated charcoal and Prussian blue (250 mg/kg/d with a cathartic in divided doses), both of which bind thallium and may enhance its elimination as well as prevent its absorption, as the main therapeutic measures.

Vacor

Patients presenting with DKA are managed like other diabetic patients with this presentation. Niacinamide (nicotinamide) has been shown to be an effective antidote in experimental animals. In these animals, the earlier the antidote was given after exposure, the better the outcome. Niacin is not an effective substitute. The dose of niacinamide is 500 mg initially, followed by 100 to 200 mg every 4 hours for 2 days. If an intravenous formulation is not available, it should be given orally.

Yellow Phosphorus

No specific antidote exists for this toxin. Treatment involves aggressive supportive care.

Zinc Phosphide

Because the toxicity of this compound depends on the conversion to zinc and phosphine gas in an acid and aqueous environment (the stomach), treatment involves measures to prevent this conversion, along with supportive care. Alkalinization of the stomach with oral bicarbonate, antacid, and H_2 antagonists is recommended, although the efficacy of these modalities is unclear.

DISPOSITION

The disposition depends on the toxin involved. For symptomatic patients exposed to any rodenticide in the highly toxic group (see Table 366.1), hospital admission to a monitored setting is warranted. Because of the relative rarity of these exposures, toxicology and poison center consultations are recommended early in the presentation.

Patients with unintentional exposures who remain asymptomatic after a period of observation (6 hours) can be discharged. For patients exposed to superwarfarin or long-acting oral anticoagulants, follow-up coagulation studies are needed at 24 and 48 hours after ingestion. These studies may be performed in the outpatient setting for patients with unintentional ingestions, if adequate family and social supports are in place. All other patients, including those with intentional ingestions, are best managed as inpatients.

COMMON PITFALLS

- Failure to send relatives, paramedics, or friends to the site of exposure to obtain a sample or container for identifying the ingested agent
- Misidentification of the rodenticide because an identical or similar brand or market name is used for more than one agent
- Failure to consider oral anticoagulant and thallium poisoning in a patient with an unknown rodenticide exposure who remains asymptomatic after a period of observation
- Using the wrong type of vitamin K to treat oral anticoagulant toxicity
- Failure to make a laboratory diagnosis of superwarfarin toxicity before beginning vitamin K treatment
- Failure to consider agents that are no longer marketed but still available in homes in the differential diagnosis

References

1. Chenoweth MB, Kandel A, Johnson LB, et al. Factors influencing fluoroacetate poisoning—practical treatment with glycerol monoacetate. *J Pharmacol Exp Ther* 1951;102:31.
2. Chi CH, Chen KW, Chan SH, et al. Clinical presentation and prognostic factors in sodium monofluoroacetate intoxication. *J Toxicol Clin Toxicol* 1996;34:707.
3. Chua JD, Friedenberg WR. Superwarfarin poisoning. *Arch Intern Med* 1998;158:1929.
4. Chugh SN, Aggarwal, Mahajan SK. Zinc phosphide intoxication symptoms: analysis of 20 cases. *Int J Clin Pharmacol Ther* 1998;36:406.
5. Feingold KR, Lee TH, Chung MY, et al. Muscle capillary basement membrane width in patients with Vacor-induced diabetes mellitus. *J Clin Invest* 1986;78:102.

6. Freedman MD. Oral anticoagulants: pharmacodynamics, clinical indications, and adverse effects. *J Clin Pharmacol* 1992;32:196.
7. Goldfrank L, Flomembaum N, Weisman RS. Rodenticides. *Hosp Physician* 1981;17:87.
8. Hoffman RS, Smilkstein MJ, Goldfrank LR. Evaluation of coagulation factor abnormalities in long-acting anticoagulant overdose. *J Toxicol Clin Toxicol* 1988;26:233.
9. Lima JS, Reis CA. Poisoning due to illegal use of carbamates as a rodenticide in Rio De Janeiro. *J Toxicol Clin Toxicol* 195;33:687.
10. Lipton RA, Klass EM. Human ingestion of a "superwarfarin" rodenticide resulting in a prolonged anticoagulant effect. *JAMA* 1988;252:3004.
11. Meggs WJ, Hoffman RS, Shih RD, et al. Malicious thallium poisoning: rapid diagnosis by x-ray, laboratory and clinical evaluation. *Vet Hum Toxicol* 1993;35:317.
12. Morgan BW, Tomaszewski C, Rotker I. Spontaneous hemoperitoneum from brodifacoum overdose. *Am J Emerg Med* 1996;14:656.
13. Nelson LS, Hoffman RS, Rao R, et al. Poisonings associated with illegal use of aldicarb as a rodenticide—New York City, 1994–1997. *MMWR* 1997;46:961.
14. Parsons BJ, Day LM, Ozanne-Smith J, et al. Rodenticide poisoning among children. *Aust N Z J Publ Health* 1996;20:488.
15. Pont A, Rubino JM, Bishop D, et al. Diabetes mellitus and neuropathy following Vacor ingestion in man. *Arch Intern Med* 1979;139:185.
16. Saddique A, Peterson CD. Thallium poisoning: a review. *Vet Hum Toxicol* 1983;25:16.
17. Simon FA, Pickering LK. Acute yellow phosphorus poisoning: "smoking stool syndrome." *JAMA* 1980;244:148.
18. Smolinske SC, Scherger DL, Kearns PC, et al. Superwarfarin poisoning in children: a prospective study. *Pediatrics* 1989;84:490.
19. Sutie JW. Warfarin and vitamin K. *Clin Cardiol* 1990;13:16.
20. Winek CL, Collom WD, Fusia EP. Yellow phosphorus ingestion—three fatal poisonings. *Clin Toxicol* 1973;6:541.

CHAPTER 367
Salicylate Poisoning

Christopher H. Linden

The incidence of pediatric salicylate poisoning has declined steadily since 1965 due to safety packaging, legislation limiting the number of tablets in bottles of children's aspirin, and decreased use because of the association between aspirin use and Reye syndrome. Similarly, the increased use of nonsalicylate aspirin substitutes has resulted in a reciprocal decrease in the incidence of adult salicylate poisoning. Despite these trends, salicylate intoxication continues to be a major cause of poisoning morbidity and mortality. In addition, patients with salicylate poisoning are still mistreated and misdiagnosed with alarming frequency.[1,15]

Aspirin (acetylsalicylic acid) is available in tablet, capsule, and suppository formulations, often in combination with anticholinergic, antihistamine, muscle-relaxing, narcotic, and neuroleptic agents. The recommended dosage of aspirin is 10 to 15 mg/kg every 4 to 6 hours, not to exceed 80 mg/kg/d. Aspirin, a weak acid (pK_a 3.5), is mostly nonionized (absorbable) but poorly soluble at gastric pH. Hence, most absorption occurs in the small intestine.

Aspirin is rapidly hydrolyzed by plasma esterases, with a half-life of about 15 minutes, to its active metabolite salicylic acid.[11,14] Salicylic acid (salicylate) is also available from other sources (Table 367.1). Benorylate and diflunisal are conjugates of salicylic acid. Only benorylate is metabolized to free salicylate, but diflunisal may cause a false-positive salicylate reaction on blood or urine testing.

TABLE 367.1. Nonaspirin Sources of Salicylate

Formulation (Brand Name)	Percentage of Salicylate
Aspirin 75	
Bismuth subsalicylate (Pepto-Bismol)	37
Choline and magnesium salicylate (Trilisate)	76
Choline salicylate (Arthropan)	56
Homomenthyl salicylate (sunscreen)	51
Magnesium salicylate (Doan's; Magan)	90
Methyl salicylate (oil of wintergreen)	89
Salicylic acid (topical keratolytic)	100
Salicylsalicylic acid (Disalcid; Salsalate)	96
Sodium salicylate (Pabalate)	84

The therapeutic effects of salicylates (analgesic, antiinflammatory, and antipyretic) are due to the inhibition of central and peripheral prostaglandin synthesis.[11] In contrast to aspirin, other salicylates do not inhibit platelet aggregation and are less likely to cause gastrointestinal (GI) bleeding. After a single oral dose, pharmacologic effects begin within 30 minutes, peak in 1 to 2 hours, and last for about 4 hours. Peak blood levels of 10 to 20 mg/dL occur 1 to 2 hours after ingestion. Therapeutic concentrations range from 10 to 30 mg/dL. High therapeutic levels, required for maximal antiinflammatory effects, are seen only with chronic dosing. Salicylic acid is extensively (up to 90%) bound to serum proteins, predominantly albumin. The apparent volume of distribution is small (0.15 L/kg), not only because of high protein binding, but also because, at physiologic pH, salicylic acid (pK_a 3.0) is greater than 99% ionized, and hence poorly diffusible across cell membranes. Salicylate is primarily eliminated by hepatic metabolism to inactive metabolites with a half-life of 2 to 3 hours (Table 367.2). Metabolites are excreted unchanged or after further metabolism, in the urine.

Salicylate kinetics differ markedly after the ingestion of multiple therapeutic doses or a single large overdose.[11,14,17] After an overdose, gastric emptying is slowed and salicylate tablets may form concretions, resulting in delayed and prolonged absorption. This is particularly true of enteric-coated and sustained-release formulations. As serum levels increase, protein binding decreases (to 50% or less) and both free salicylate concentrations and the volume of distribution increase to more than 0.35 L/kg. In the presence of acidemia, as occurs in poisoning, the fraction of nonionized (diffusible) salicylate also increases, leading to further tissue distribution. Because of increased distribution, tissue salicylate levels increase proportionately more than serum drug levels.

TABLE 367.2. Elimination of a Single Dose of Salicylic Acid

Pathway	Product(s)	Percentage
Conjugation with glycine	Salicyluric acid	75*
Conjugation with glucuronic acid	Salicyl phenolic glucuronide	10*
	Salicyl acyl glucuronide	5
Hydroxylation	Gentisic acid	<1
Urinary excretion	Salicylic acid	10

*Saturable pathways

From Flower RJ, et al. Analgesic–antipyretics and anti-inflammatory agents. In: *Goodman and Gilman's the pharmacological basis of therapeutics*. 7th ed. New York: Macmillan, 1985:674.

The two main pathways of hepatic metabolism (see Table 367.2) become saturated when salicylate levels reach or exceed the high therapeutic range and elimination changes from first order (i.e., proportional to the level) to zero order (i.e., constant), as described by the Michaelis-Menton equation. Hence, with chronic dosing, the salicylate "half-life" increases to 6 to 12 hours, and a small increase in dose results in a much (proportionately) greater increase in serum and tissue salicylate levels, with the potential for chronic intoxication. For the same reason, the salicylate "half-life" may increase to 20 to 40 hours after a large acute overdose.

When hepatic metabolism becomes saturated, urinary excretion becomes the major route of salicylate elimination.[11,14,17] The amount of salicylate excreted depends on the balance among glomerular filtration of nonionized salicylate, active proximal tubular secretion of ionized salicylate (by the organic anion active membrane transport system), and passive distal tubular reabsorption of nonionized drug. Increasing urine flow increases glomerular filtration and tubular secretion and decreases reabsorption. Raising the urine pH decreases reabsorption by way of ion trapping (conversion of urinary salicylate to the ionized, nondiffusible form). These mechanisms are the rationale for alkaline diuresis in the treatment of salicylate poisoning. Raising the serum pH also increases the ionized fraction and limits tissue distribution. With such therapy, the renal elimination of salicylate can be increased by a factor of 20 or more. Conversely, low urine output and pH, as may occur with illnesses associated with fever, dehydration, and aciduria, decrease salicylate excretion and predispose the patient using salicylates to toxicity. Similar conditions, which develop as a result of salicylate poisoning itself (discussion follows), may lead to increased severity and duration of toxicity.

The mechanisms underlying salicylate poisoning are complex.[3,8,17,18] When salicylate concentrations exceed therapeutic levels, direct stimulation of the medullary chemoreceptor trigger zone and respiratory center causes nausea and vomiting, and hyperventilation, respectively. Increased carbon dioxide production may also contribute to respiratory stimulation. These effects result in dehydration, not only from GI and insensible fluid losses, but also from diuresis caused by the excretion of bicarbonate in response to alkalemia. Because sodium and potassium are excreted with bicarbonate (in exchange for hydrogen ion reabsorption), there is concomitant depletion of these electrolytes. Alkalosis may also cause functional hypocalcemia (decreased ionized calcium) with cardiac irritability, tetany, and seizures.

As toxicity progresses, the accumulation of intracellular salicylate causes uncoupling of mitochondrial oxidative phosphorylation, inhibition of Krebs cycle enzymes (aminotransferases and dehydrogenases) and amino acid metabolism, and stimulation of gluconeogenesis, glycolysis, and lipid metabolism. These derangements result in increased but ineffective metabolism, with increased glucose, lipid, and oxygen consumption and increased amino acid, carbon dioxide, glucose, ketoacid (acetoacetic and beta-hydroxybutyric), and lactic and pyruvic acid production. The accumulation of these organic acids, with a small additional contribution from salicylic acid and its metabolites, leads to an increased anion gap metabolic acidosis.[2,18] The associated diaphoresis, fever, and osmotic diuresis (due to the renal excretion of organic acids) cause further electrolyte and fluid losses and aciduria.

When high salicylate levels are sustained, progressive metabolic derangements and increasing levels of organic acids may cause increased pulmonary capillary permeability, central nervous system (CNS) and respiratory depression, cerebral and pulmonary edema, cardiovascular collapse, and acute renal failure (acute tubular necrosis).

Acute salicylate poisoning may result from a single ingestion of more than 150 mg/kg of aspirin. Ingestions of 150 to 300 mg/kg may cause mild toxicity, those of 300 to 500 mg/kg may cause moderate toxicity, and those of more than 500 mg/kg may result in severe or fatal poisoning.[3,18] Salicylate levels may be quite high during the first 6 to 18 hours after an acute overdose without significant clinical or laboratory evidence of toxicity. Conversely, minimally elevated or even "therapeutic" salicylate levels may be seen with severe poisoning after chronic overdose or late in the course of an acute overdose. Hence, the severity of poisoning is defined by clinical and metabolic abnormalities, not by the salicylate level. Decisions regarding management should be based on direct assessments of severity rather than the widely publicized salicylate (Done) nomogram. This nomogram, which attempted to define severity with a timed salicylate level following acute overdose, was never useful for chronic poisoning and sustained-release aspirin overdose, and it has subsequently been shown to have poor predictive value in acute overdoses.[7]

Salicylate poisoning may also result from the topical (skin or gum) application of methyl salicylate or salicylic acid.[3,17] It may occur in breast-fed infants whose mothers chronically take salicylates and in the fetuses or neonates of mothers who ingested salicylates. The ingestion of salicylic acid preparations (e.g., Compound W) may cause corrosive injury to the GI tract in addition to salicylate poisoning.

CLINICAL PRESENTATION

Vomiting may occur shortly after ingestion as a consequence of direct gastric irritation. The early (postabsorption) phase of salicylate poisoning, which develops 3 to 8 hours after acute overdose (at any time after chronic overdose), is characterized by mild dehydration, respiratory alkalosis, and alkaline urine (Table 367.3). Signs and symptoms are mild and include nausea, vomiting, abdominal pain, headache, tinnitus (may occur at therapeutic levels), obvious tachypnea or hyperpnea (may be subtle), ataxia, dizziness, agitation, and lethargy. Mild increases or decreases in serum glucose, potassium, and sodium levels may be noted. Blood urea nitrogen (BUN), creatinine, sodium, and potassium levels may remain normal, however, despite total body fluid and electrolyte deficits.[3,8,17–20]

Moderate poisoning, which usually occurs 12 to 24 hours after an acute overdose, is characterized by an increased anion gap metabolic acidosis with respiratory alkalosis, alkalemia, moderate-to-severe dehydration, and "paradoxical" aciduria (see Table 367.3). GI and neurologic symptoms worsen. Fever, asterixis, diaphoresis, deafness, pallor, confusion, slurred speech, disorientation, hallucinations, tachycardia, tachypnea, and mild or orthostatic hypotension may be present. Leukocytosis, thrombocytopenia, increased or decreased glucose and sodium levels, hypokalemia, and increased BUN, creatinine, ketone, and lactate levels may be seen on laboratory evaluation.

Severe or late salicylate poisoning usually develops 24 or more hours after an acute overdose and is characterized by severe dehydration, metabolic acidosis, acidemia, and aciduria (see Table 367.3).[5,19] Respiratory acidosis and hypoxia also may be present in a few patients. Findings include coma, seizures, papilledema, respiratory depression, hypothermia or hyperthermia, hypotension, pulmonary edema, congestive heart failure, tachycardia, dysrhythmias, and oliguria. The laboratory abnormalities seen with moderate intoxication become more pronounced. The chest radiograph may show pulmonary edema with a normal-size heart, and a computed tomography (CT) scan of the head may reveal cerebral edema and hemor-

TABLE 367.3. Stages and Treatment of Salicylate Poisoning

Stage/Severity	Plasma pH	Urine pH	Intravenous Solution	$NaHCO_3$* (mEq/L)	Potassium* (mEq/L)
Early/mild	>7.4	>6	D_5 NS	50	20
Intermediate/moderate	≥7.4	<6	D_5 1/2 NS	100	40
Late/severe	<7.4	<6	D_5 W	150	60–80

* Added to intravenous solution.
Adapted from Linden CH, Rumack BH. The legitimate analgesics: aspirin and acetaminophen. In: Hanson W Jr, ed. *Toxic emergencies*. New York: Churchill Livingstone, 1984:118.

rhage. Electrocardiographic (ECG) abnormalities, other than sinus tachycardia, reflect metabolic abnormalities or the effects of coingested drugs.

GI bleeding, hepatic toxicity, pancreatitis, proteinuria, abnormal urinary sediment, an increased prothrombin time, and a low serum uric acid level (due to salicylate's uricosuric effect) may be seen with therapeutic as well as toxic salicylate levels. Clinically significant bleeding, GI perforation, blindness, and inappropriate antidiuretic hormone secretion are rare complications of acute poisoning. Chronic salicylate intoxication, especially in elderly patients, tends to be more severe than acute poisoning, and children tend to progress to moderate toxicity faster than adults.[1,8,9] Adults appear to be more prone to pulmonary complications. Although the overall mortality rate is much less than 1%, it may be as high as 15% in patients with severe poisoning.[17,18]

DIFFERENTIAL DIAGNOSIS

Occult salicylate poisoning should be considered in any patient with an unexplained acid–base disturbance.[1,8,15] Although an increased anion gap metabolic acidosis is said to be a characteristic feature, it occurs as the sole acid–base abnormality in only about 20% of patients with salicylate poisoning.[8] Metabolic acidosis with respiratory alkalosis is actually the most common finding (in more than 50% of patients), and respiratory alkalosis alone is seen in another 20% to 25%. Other poisons that cause an anion gap metabolic acidosis include methanol and ethylene glycol, but lactic acidosis may occur in any poisoning that is complicated by hypoxia, hypertension, or seizures. A persistently normal metabolic workup (arterial blood gas analysis and determination of serum levels of electrolytes) in a patient who remains symptomatic many hours after an unknown overdose rules out salicylate poisoning.

Up to 60% of patients with chronic salicylate poisoning are initially (sometimes fatally) undiagnosed.[1,8,15] These patients are often elderly, are chronically taking nonaspirin salicylates, and have serious underlying medical problems. Unless specifically questioned, the use of salicylates may not be discovered, and signs and symptoms of salicylate poisoning may be attributed to other illnesses (e.g., anxiety, cardiopulmonary disease, cerebrovascular disease, chronic obstructive pulmonary disease, dementia, encephalopathy, alcohol ketoacidosis and withdrawal, viral meningitis, pancreatitis, Reye syndrome, psychiatric disorders, and sepsis).[1,2,13,15]

Not infrequently patients give a history of aspirin ingestion or overdose when they actually (unknowingly) have taken acetaminophen, or vice versa. Unless the agent or product ingested (or its container) is available for positive identification or the history can be confirmed by a witness, a serum level of both drugs should be obtained.

In children, chronic salicylate poisoning may be indistinguishable from Reye syndrome on the basis of signs, symptoms, and routine laboratory evaluation. Low (subtherapeutic) cerebrospinal fluid salicylate levels and a liver biopsy showing fatty infiltration rule out salicylate intoxication and confirm Reye syndrome.

EMERGENCY DEPARTMENT EVALUATION

The history should include the time of ingestion, the amount ingested, and the specific product ingested in cases of acute overdose. In all cases of intentional ingestion and in those with an unclear history, a serum salicylate level should be obtained. If the patient is symptomatic or the salicylate level is elevated, arterial blood gas analysis; serum levels of electrolytes, glucose, BUN, and creatinine; and a urinalysis should be obtained. If acid–base abnormalities are present, further evaluation should include serum calcium, magnesium, and ketone levels; liver function tests; complete blood count; prothrombin time; partial thromboplastin time; ECG; and a chest radiograph. A toxicology screen may be useful to rule out the coingestion of other detectable poisons.

The physical examination should focus on vital signs, neurologic function, and cardiorespiratory findings. Accurate measurement of the respiratory rate and temperature is important but is often done in cursory fashion. The fundi should be examined for papilledema, and any vomitus and stool should be tested for occult blood. The presence of peritoneal signs necessitates evaluation for surgical complications. Salicylates, especially magnesium and bismuth (Pepto-Bismol) salts and enteric-coated or sustained-release formulations, may be evident on abdominal radiographs.

Because of delayed absorption, serial salicylate levels should be obtained until levels are noted to be declining. A single nontoxic salicylate level soon after ingestion does not rule out a significant overdose, particularly with ingestions of enteric-coated or sustained-release formulations.

If levels continue to rise, repeated metabolic evaluation is necessary.

EMERGENCY DEPARTMENT MANAGEMENT

Advanced life-support measures are instituted as necessary. Patients with altered mental states should receive intravenous dextrose (or have an immediate fingerstick blood sugar check), naloxone, and thiamine in standard doses. Glucose administration is essential in salicylate poisoning because CNS hypoglycemia may occur with a normal serum glucose concentration.[3,19] Because nearly all patients with salicylate poisoning are volume-depleted, treatment should begin with intravenous crystalloid administration (e.g., 20 mL/kg of dextrose 5% in 0.45%, or 0.9% sodium chloride with or without sodium bicarbonate, 25 mEq/L; and potassium, 10 to 20 mEq/L, over the first hour or two), provided there is no evidence of cerebral or pulmonary edema. In patients with hypernatremia, a hypotonic solution is used.

Because the immediate goal is to reverse dehydration and establish a good flow of urine, bladder catheterization is usually necessary for monitoring purposes. If hypotension or oliguria is present or persists, central venous or pulmonary artery catheterization is recommended. Patients with elevated right-sided pressures should be treated with dopamine. Furosemide may also be used in an attempt to reverse oliguric renal failure unresponsive to volume replacement.

Seizures should be treated initially with standard agents (glucose, diazepam, phenobarbital, or phenytoin). If there is papilledema or CT scan evidence of cerebral edema, elevation of the head, hyperventilation, and administration of mannitol or furosemide, and dexamethasone should be considered. Diuretics are used cautiously, if at all, in patients with hypovolemia. Pulmonary edema is treated with intubation and positive end-expiratory pressure ventilation. Vitamin K is given to patients with coagulation abnormalities. Those with overt bleeding should also receive fresh-frozen plasma. Underlying metabolic derangements are corrected. Insulin is unnecessary for nondiabetics with hyperglycemia and may be dangerous, particularly if there is coexisting hypokalemia. Similarly, hyperkalemia does not usually require specific therapy and usually resolves with fluid administration and correction of acidosis. Because acetaminophen is unlikely to be effective, physical measures (e.g., cooling blankets and sponging) are preferred for the treatment of fever. Although tetany resulting from respiratory alkalosis may respond to paper-bag breathing, the slow intravenous administration of 10% calcium chloride or gluconate (0.1 to 0.2 mL/kg) is effective, lasts longer, and can safely be given to patients with normal serum calcium levels.

GI decontamination should be done in patients with accidental ingestions of more than 150 mg/kg and in all patients with intentional overdoses. Charcoal alone is superior to ipecac followed by charcoal in simulated overdose patients[6] and is the preferred method in those with mild-to-moderate overdoses. Because charcoal binds neutral agents better than ionized ones, salicylate may desorb from charcoal in the alkaline milieu of the small intestine.[5] Therefore, at least two doses of charcoal should be given. Even in patients with spontaneous vomiting, large amounts of salicylate have been recovered as long as 18 hours after ingestion, hence the adage, "It's never too late to aspirate [the stomach] with salicylate." Optimal decontamination in patients with large overdoses may be to give a dose of charcoal before and after gastric lavage.[4] Whole-bowel irrigation should be considered in patients with large ingestions of enteric-coated or sustained-release preparations.[20] Serial salicylate levels should be obtained to assess the efficacy of GI decontamination. Levels that continue to rise despite such therapy suggest a gastric drug concretion or bezoar formation. Evaluation and treatment by gastric endoscopy should be considered if drug levels become markedly elevated or clinical toxicity is severe or progressive.

Salicylate elimination can be enhanced by giving repeated oral doses of activated charcoal,[10] alkaline diuresis,[3,11,16–20] and extracorporeal removal.[12] Although data from experimental studies are conflicting, multiple-dose charcoal shortened the salicylate half-life to 2 to 4 hours in patients with salicylate levels as high as 66 mg/dL after acute overdosage. However, in this study, the brand of charcoal used (Medicoal) was an effervescent preparation containing bicarbonate. Oral bicarbonate may have trapped salicylate in the gut (decreased its absorption) or been absorbed and caused concomitant urinary alkalinization (enhanced elimination). Until further data become available, multiple-dose charcoal therapy is nevertheless recommended.[10] It can be given to almost all patients but may be less effective in those with chronic poisoning or higher levels. Recent evidence suggest that glycine (or *N*-glycylglycine) administration may prevent glycine depletion and saturation of the salicylic acid pathway (see Table 367.2) and also enhance the elimination of salicylate. Clinical experience is limited, and this therapy should be considered experimental.

Alkaline diuresis can shorten the salicylate half-life to 6 to 12 hours in acute overdose patients with salicylate levels less than 70 mg/dL.[16] Although urinary alkalinization alone was reported to be more effective than either diuresis alone or alkaline diuresis, patients treated by "alkalinization alone" actually received 375 to 500 mL/h over the treatment period.[16] Animal studies have shown that alkalinization and diuresis are both important. Alkaline diuresis is likely to be less efficacious in patients with chronic salicylism or very high salicylate levels.

Indications for alkaline diuresis include acid–base abnormalities, the presence of symptoms, and elevated salicylate levels (greater than 30 mg/dL) within 18 hours of an acute overdose. Patients who present more than 18 hours after an acute ingestion or have chronic poisoning may require treatment despite "therapeutic" salicylate levels. Contraindications to alkaline diuresis include cerebral and pulmonary edema, oliguric renal failure, and a serum pH above 7.55. It should be performed with caution in patients with a history of congestive heart failure. Adequate hydration and urine output should be established before initiating alkaline diuresis. The rate of fluid administration and amount of sodium bicarbonate administered should be based on the severity of poisoning (see Table 367.3). Therapy should be individualized according to laboratory findings. Isotonic solutions of sodium bicarbonate at rates of 2 L/h for at least 3 hours have been recommended.

The goal of alkaline diuresis is a urine pH of 7.5 or more and a brisk (3 to 6 mL/kg/h) urine output. However, even during early (mild) intoxication, when the urine pH is alkaline, low doses of bicarbonate should be given to replace ongoing renal losses. Carbonic anhydrase inhibitors (e.g., acetazolamide) should not be used to alkalinize the urine, because they also may cause acidemia, increased ionized drug, and enhanced tissue distribution of salicylate. This may result in increased CNS salicylate levels and clinical deterioration, and increased mortality.[20] Because potassium reabsorption occurs at the expense of bicarbonate reabsorption and hydrogen ion excretion, it is often stated that alkalinization of the urine is impossible until potassium deficits are corrected. Whether this is true or not is controversial.[20] In one study, no correlation was found between serum potassium levels and urinary pH.[16] While correction of hypokalemia is clearly indicated, such therapy should not delay the administration of bicarbonate. Complications of alkaline diuresis include excessive alkalemia, hypokalemia, hypocalcemia, hypernatremia, and fluid overload with cerebral and pulmonary edema, particularly in the elderly and those with severe poisoning. Hence, all patients treated with alkaline diuresis should have cardiac monitoring, frequent vital signs, mental status and cardiorespiratory examinations, laboratory evaluation (arterial blood gas analysis and serum electrolytes), and hourly monitoring of fluid intake, urinary output, and urine pH. If intake should persistently exceed output, diuresis may be enhanced by giving furosemide.

Hemodialysis is the treatment of choice for patients with severe salicylate poisoning.[12] A reduction in the salicylate half-life to 2 to 3 hours can be achieved. Although hemoperfusion is slightly more effective in removing salicylate, it is technically more difficult and does not correct associated acid–base, fluid, and electrolyte abnormalities. Peritoneal dialysis (with 5% albumin added to compete with serum proteins for salicylate binding) and exchange transfusion are less effective and should be used only if hemodialysis is unavailable, contraindicated, or technically impossible (e.g., in infants or in patients with active or recent bleeding complications).

Indications for hemodialysis include coma, seizures, cerebral or pulmonary edema, renal failure, and clinical deterioration or failure to improve despite intensive noninvasive therapy.[2,12,15] Although, in acute poisoning, severe toxicity is usually associated with very high salicylate levels (greater than 100 mg/dL), patients with high levels without complications do not necessarily need hemodialysis. Conversely, acute or chronic overdose patients with severe toxicity or underlying cardiopulmonary disease should be treated with hemodialysis even if salicylate levels are not markedly elevated.

DISPOSITION

Patients with mild or absent clinical and laboratory toxicity after acute overdose can often be treated in the emergency department if the peak salicylate level is less than 60 mg/dL. Patients with chronic poisoning, higher levels, underlying medical problems, and moderate or severe toxicity should be admitted to an intensive care unit. A nephrologist should be consulted if poisoning is severe. If hemodialysis is unavailable, patients with severe poisoning or moderate poisoning with very high (or rising) salicylate levels should be transferred to a facility where such treatment is available.

COMMON PITFALLS

- Failure to ask specifically about salicylate ingestion and to obtain a serum salicylate level on patients with unexplained acid–base disturbances, particularly in those patients with altered mental status
- Failure to obtain quantitative levels of both aspirin and acetaminophen in patients whose history cannot be verified by a third party or by examination of the drug or its container
- Failure to obtain serial salicylate levels to rule out delayed absorption and to assess the efficacy of decontamination and elimination therapies
- Failure to appreciate the differences between acute and chronic salicylate poisoning
- Failure to monitor for complications of salicylate poisoning and its treatment
- Failure to recognize the limitations of salicylate levels and the salicylate nomogram and to base treatment on clinical and laboratory findings, not drug levels

References

1. Bailey RB, Jones SR. Chronic salicylate intoxication: a common cause of morbidity in the elderly. *J Am Geriatr Soc* 1989;37:556.
2. Bartels PD, Lund-Jacobsen H. Blood lactate and ketone body concentrations in salicylate intoxication. *Hum Toxicol* 1986;5:363.
3. Brenner BE, Simon RR. Management of salicylate intoxication. *Drugs* 1987;24:335.
4. Burton BT, Bayer MJ, Barron L, et al. Comparison of activated charcoal and gastric lavage in the prevention of aspirin absorption. *J Emerg Med* 1984;1:411.
5. Chapman BJ, Proudfoot AT. Adult salicylate poisoning: deaths and outcome in patients with high plasma salicylate concentrations. *Q J Med* 1989;72:699.
6. Curtis RA, Barone J, Giacon N. Efficacy of ipecac and activated charcoal/cathartic: prevention of salicylate absorption in a simulated overdose. *Arch Intern Med* 1984;144:48.
7. Dugandzic RM, Tierney ME, Dickinson GE, et al. Evaluation of the validity of the Done nomogram in the management of acute salicylate poisoning. *Ann Emerg Med* 1989;18:1186.
8. Gabow PA, Anderson RJ, Potts DE, et al. Acid–base disturbances in the salicylate-intoxicated adult. *Arch Intern Med* 1978;138:1481.
9. Gaudrealt P, Temple AR, Lovejoy FH. The relative severity of acute vs. chronic salicylate poisonings in children: a clinical comparison. *Pediatrics* 1982;70:566.
10. Hillman RJ, Prescott LF. Treatment of salicylate poisoning with repeated activated charcoal. *BMJ* 1985;291:1472.
11. Insel PA. Analgesics, antipyretics and anti-inflammatory agents; drugs employed in the treatment of rheumatoid arthritis and gout. In: Hardman JG, Limbird LE, Molinoff PB, et al., eds. *Goodman and Gilman's the pharmacological basis of therapeutics,* 9th ed. New York: McGraw-Hill, 1996:617.
12. Jacobsen D, Wiik-Larsen E, Bredesen JH. Haemodialysis or haemoperfusion in severe salicylate poisoning? *Hum Toxicol* 1988;7:161.
13. Leatherman JW, Schmitz PG. Fever, hyperdynamic shock, and multiple system organ failure: a pseudo-sepsis syndrome associated with chronic salicylate poisoning. *Chest* 1991;100:1391.
14. Levy G. Comparative pharmacokinetics of aspirin and acetaminophen. *Arch Intern Med* 1981;141:279.
15. McGuigan MA. A 2-year review of salicylate deaths in Ontario. *Arch Intern Med* 1987;147:510.
16. Prescott LF, Balali-Mood M, Critchley JAJH, et al. Diuresis or urinary alkalinization for salicylate poisoning? *BMJ* 1982;285:1383.
17. Proudfoot AT. Toxicity of salicylates. *Am J Med* 1983;75:99.
18. Temple AR. Acute and chronic effects of aspirin toxicity and their treatment. *Arch Intern Med* 1981;141:364.
19. Thisted B, Krantz T, Strom J, et al. Acute salicylate poisoning in 177 consecutive patients treated in ICU. *Acta Anaesthesiol Scand* 1987;31:312.
20. Yip L, Dart RC, Gabow PA. Concepts and controversies in salicylate toxicity. *Emerg Med Clin North Am* 1994;12:351.

CHAPTER 368
Seafood Toxin Poisoning

Robert P. Dowsett

Seafood poisoning can result from the ingestion of fish, shellfish, or other marine life that contains toxic substances. Often, these toxins originate from dinoflagellates and are closely related. Other toxins are endogenously produced or result from bacterial action. Dinoflagellates, which form the major component of phytoplankton, are unicellular eukaryotic marine algae of the division Pyrrophyta.

Some dinoflagellates proliferate extensively under certain weather conditions, resulting in the surface discoloration of seawater known as a "red tide" or algae bloom. Other species live below the water, attached to macroalgae, and their growth is not as obviously affected by environmental disturbances. They lie at the bottom of a food chain of which humans may be the ultimate consumers. Dinoflagellate toxins are concentrated in the viscera of filter feeders such as shellfish, herbivorous fish, and crustaceans, often causing them no harm. They are among the most potent natural toxins known.

Ciguatera, paralytic shellfish, tetrodotoxin, and scombroid poisoning are relatively well known. Neurotoxic shellfish, diarrheic shellfish, hallucinatory fish, clupeotoxic fish, fish roe, palytoxin, domoic acid (mussel) and red whelk poisoning, and Haff disease are less commonly recognized and reported. However, expanding international tourism, the importation of exotic seafood, and the harvesting of seafood from more remote waters, as coastal fishing grounds are exhausted, are likely to increase the frequency of seafood poisoning seen in domestic health facilities.

CIGUATERA

Ciguatera poisoning results from eating tropical or subtropical fish contaminated with toxins produced by dinoflagellates living in coral reef waters. *Gambierdiscus toxicus* and several other species produce toxins that accumulate in fish feeding on algae. The toxins, which appear to be harmless to fish, are passed up the food chain from herbivores to their predators and eventually to humans. Ciguatoxin is a heat-stable, lipid-soluble, highly oxygenated polyether. Several other toxins, including maitotoxin and scaritoxin, have been identified. They are concentrated in the visceral organs of fish, particularly the liver and gonads, and can remain for several years.

Environmental factors such as water temperature, salinity, and light affect the growth of *G. toxicus*. Large-scale environmental disruptions such as storms, earthquakes, underwater dredging, pollution, and global climatic changes are also thought to influence toxic dinoflagellate populations. *G. toxicus* and related species are found in coral reef waters between 35° south and 35° north latitude.

Ciguatera is endemic in Australia and the Caribbean and South Pacific islands; French Polynesia has the highest prevalence.[9] Outbreaks have been reported worldwide, and over 400 species of fish, mostly reef fish, have been implicated. Barracuda, grouper, red snapper, amberjack, eel, sea bass, and Spanish mackerel are most commonly involved. Fish larger than 2 kg are more likely to be contaminated with significant quantities of toxin.

Ciguatoxin is colorless and tasteless and is not destroyed by cooking or gastric acid. It is detectable in affected fish by mouse biologic assay or immunoassay. Ciguatoxin can be transferred across the placenta and by semen or breast milk. It acts by increasing sodium permeability through neuronal voltage-gated sodium channels, resulting in prolonged refractoriness and decreased conduction velocity.[5] A similar mechanism is suggested to occur in cardiac tissue. Ciguatoxin also may increase central and peripheral cholinergic activity, but this is probably not clinically significant.

PALYTOXIN

Palytoxin is a thermostable terpenoid toxin produced by zoanthid coral of the genus *Palythoa*. The conditions under which corals become toxic are unknown. Poisoning is most common in the South Pacific after ingestion of fish (mackerels, triggerfish, filefish, butterfly fish) and xanthrid crabs that feed on coral.[11] Palytoxin may also be found in dinoflagellates. The livers of fish have a high palytoxin content. Palytoxin binds to the ouabain receptor site on Na^+/K^+-ATPase, allowing the influx of sodium and resulting in depolarization of nerves and muscles. Although clinical effects are similar to those seen in ciguatera poisoning, additional toxicity results from vasoconstriction, norepinephrine release, and sustained contraction of skeletal and smooth muscle.[11]

NEUROTOXIC SHELLFISH POISONING

Neurotoxic shellfish poisoning also results in a ciguatera-like syndrome but is generally less severe. It is caused by brevetoxins from *Ptychodiscus brevis*, a dinoflagellate found off the coast of southeastern North America and western Europe during algae blooms. The toxins are accumulated by bivalve mollusks, predominantly clams and oysters. Brevetoxins A, B, and C are polycyclic ethers that bind to the Na^+ channel near the binding site for ciguatoxin. They are toxic to some marine life and birds and cause extensive losses in susceptible species. Brevetoxins can be aerosolized by wave action and carried several kilometers inland, resulting in respiratory irritation.

PARALYTIC SHELLFISH POISONING

Paralytic shellfish poisoning results from the ingestion of bivalve and gastropod mollusks (mussels, clams, oysters, scallops, and cockles) and occasionally some univalve mollusks, starfish, crustaceans, and fish. These creatures become toxic when dinoflagellates, especially *Gonyaulax* spp., multiply explosively, causing red tides. Toxic shellfish are commonly found in the cold, temperate waters of North America, the western coast of Europe, and the coastal waters of Japan, but are increasingly reported in warmer climates. Saxitoxin, gonyautoxins (I to IV), and neosaxitoxin have been identified.

The relative proportion of toxins varies by geographic region and the dinoflagellate species and life stage. The toxins do not affect shellfish but are concentrated in viscera and can take several weeks to be eliminated. Seabirds, several fish species, and mammals are susceptible to poisoning. Saxitoxin, a potent, heat-stable, water-soluble neurotoxin, acts by blockading fast sodium channels in nerve and muscle during depolarization, resulting in a conduction block that principally affects motor neurons and muscle. There is no reliable taste, smell, or color to identify contaminated shellfish. Saxitoxin can be detected in shellfish meat by a mouse bioassay. A level above 80 μg of purified saxitoxin per 100 g of raw shellfish meat is considered toxic.

TETRODOTOXIN

Tetrodotoxin, a heat-stable, water-soluble neurotoxin chemically similar to saxitoxin, is found in the skin and viscera of puffer fish (saltwater and fresh-water varieties), porcupine fish, sunfish, toadfish, the blue-ringed octopus, some species of salamanders, and *Atelopid* frogs. A dinoflagellate or bacterial origin has been suggested, but, at least in some species, tetrodotoxin is endogenously produced. It has been identified in a dinoflagellate (*Alexandrium tamarense*), which also contain saxitoxin. Tetrodotoxin has been isolated from scallops, during a bloom of *A. tamarense*, that were associated with paralytic shellfish poisoning.

Puffer fish, the most common source of tetrodotoxin, is eaten as a delicacy in some Southeast Asian countries. Although tetrodotoxin is concentrated in the fish's skin and internal organs, all parts of the fish may contain it. Like saxitoxin, tetrodotoxin inhibits fast sodium channels during depolarization, but at a separate site. The major effect of tetrodotoxin is to reduce conduction of peripheral motor, sensory, and autonomic nerves. Tetrodotoxin also acts on the medulla, stimulating the chemoreceptor trigger zone and possibly depressing the respiratory and vasomotor centers. In high doses, it may have direct effects on cardiac conduction, vascular smooth muscle, and skeletal muscle. Tetrodotoxin can be detected in fish by a bioassay and in serum or urine by gas chromatography or mass spectrometry.

CLUPEOTOXIN POISONING

Clupeotoxinism is a poorly documented but severe poisoning that is more lethal than other forms of seafood poisoning. It is caused by fish of the order Clupeiformes (herrings, anchovies, and sardines), particularly those caught in summer, offshore of tropical islands after heavy rains or floods. The identity of the toxin, which primarily affects the central nervous system, is unknown. A phytoplankton origin has been postulated. It appears to be thermostable and concentrated in the viscera of fish. Toxicity does not depend on the size of the fish or its freshness.[10]

SCOMBROID POISONING

Scombroid poisoning is associated with ingestion of fish of the family Scombroidea (mackerel, skipjack, and tuna) and other fish with dark flesh, such as dolphin fish (mahi mahi), bluefish, and amberjack (yellowtail). The muscles of these fish contain large amounts of free histidine. Fish become toxic when left unrefrigerated (above 20°C), allowing bacteria, particularly *Proteus morganii,* to decarboxylate histidine to histamine. This effect can occur during harvesting, transportation, storage, processing, or preparation for consumption.

Ingested histamine is normally metabolized by the intestinal mucosa and has little systemic effect. Other toxins isolated from contaminated fish, putrescine and cadaverine, both short-chain aliphatic diamines, may facilitate the absorption of ingested histamine or compete for its metabolism by diamine oxidase. Patients taking isoniazid, an inhibitor of diamine oxidase, are more sensitive to scombroid. Nonspecific monoamine oxidase inhibitors also inhibit diamine oxidase. The histamine content of spoiled flesh can vary considerably throughout a fish, being highest near the gut cavity. Individual sensitivity to scombroid also varies considerably; females are suggested to be more susceptible.

Scombroid toxins are heat-stable. Affected fish can appear spoiled and have a peppery or sharp taste, but these findings are not always present.[6] Symptoms are consistent with the known systemic effects of histamine and resemble IgE-mediated food allergies. The histamine content of dark fish flesh is normally less than 5 mg/100 g of flesh. Toxicity can occur at levels above 20 mg/100 g, although the Food and Drug Administration has set a hazard action level of 50 mg/100 g.

OTHER SEAFOOD TOXINS

Diarrheic shellfish poisoning is caused by consumption of shellfish, particularly mussels, that have eaten dinoflagellates of *Dinophysis* and *Prorocentrum.* These dinoflagellates are widely distributed but do not usually form noticeable algae blooms. Toxins have been identified as dinophysistoxins (okadaic acid and derivatives), pectenotoxins, and yessotoxins and have predominantly gastrointestinal (GI) effects.

Hallucinatory fish poisoning has been described following the ingestion of reef fish from the South Pacific and the Indian Ocean. Toxins similar to indole compounds from the algae *Microcoleus lyngbyaceus* have been implicated as a source of the poisoning.[18]

Several other outbreaks of GI and neurologic poisoning have resulted from the ingestion of various kinds of seafood. The causative toxins have not been clearly identified, but clinical toxicity has features of ciguatera or paralytic shellfish poisoning, or a combination of both.

Outbreaks of GI and neurologic toxicity have occurred on the eastern coast of Canada following the consumption of mussels contaminated by domoic acid produced by *Nitzschia pungens,* a phytoplankton associated with algae blooms.[16] Domoic acid is a heat-stable neuroexcitatory amino acid that is structurally related to glutamic acid but is 40 to 100 times more potent. Neuronal loss in the hippocampus and amygdaloid nucleus is seen in severe poisoning. Domoic acid–producing dinoflagellates have been isolated in other parts of the world but have not yet been related to human poisoning.

Raw carp bile is eaten in rural Asia in the belief that it improves visual acuity and treats hypertension and rheumatism. Five species of carp are known to be poisonous. Fish longer than 1 m or heavier than 3 kg are considered more likely to be toxic. Bile salts are thought to be responsible for toxicity.[15] Fish roe poisoning may result from eating the eggs of numerous species of fresh-water and saltwater fish during the reproductive cycle (spring and early summer). The nature of the toxin is unclear, but it does not appear to be destroyed by cooking.[12] Red whelk (*Neptunea antiqua*) and related species, except the common whelk (*Buccinum undatum*), contain tetramine, a heat-stable neurotoxin found in their salivary glands.[8] Hypervitaminosis A (see Chapter 359) may occur following the ingestion of the liver of marine mammals and several species of shark.[10]

Haff disease is a neuromyodystrophic disease that occurs after ingestion of carp from the Baltic Sea and lakes in Scandinavia and Russia. The causative toxin is heat-stable and is thought to originate from a species of blue-green algae.[19]

Several coelenterates (sea anemones) contain proteinaceous toxins that are poisonous only when eaten raw. Species from Samoa contain heat-stable toxins that produce GI toxicity, cardiovascular collapse, and muscle paralysis. Some echinoderms (sea cucumbers) contain saponins, which can cause GI symptoms. Abalone poisoning results from contamination with pyrophenophorbide A, a derivative of algal chlorophyll A, which causes a photosensitization reaction. Outbreaks of poisoning with GI and neurologic toxicity due to unknown toxins have resulted from the ingestion of squid and octopus.

CLINICAL PRESENTATION

Ciguatera

Symptoms and signs of ciguatera poisoning typically occur 6 to 12 hours after ingestion, with a range of 30 minutes to 30 hours. GI and neurologic symptoms predominate, typically beginning with vomiting, diarrhea, and myalgias. These are followed by circumoral and peripheral paresthesias, vertigo, and ataxia.[9] Patients may present initially with only neurologic symptoms; these may be delayed up to 72 hours after ingestion or may occur without GI symptoms. Hypotension is common and may be due to fluid loss, bradycardia, peripheral vasodilatation, or myocardial depression.[1] Symptoms vary between patients and depend on where the fish was caught and what parts of it were eaten.[1] More severe toxicity, especially hypotension and bradycardia, occurs in patients previously poisoned by ciguatera.

A classic feature of ciguatera poisoning is erroneously described as a paradoxical or reversed temperature perception: Cold objects feel hot, and hot objects feel cold. This feature is probably due to hyperstimulation of pain receptors at temperatures below 25°C, manifest by an intense burning sensation on exposure to cold. Warmth relieves these dysesthesias, and patients can accurately sense temperature changes.[4]

Other common neurologic symptoms include asthenia, paresis, tremors, and pain affecting the joints, head, and abdomen.[1] Paresthesias are often poorly defined and do not conform to dermatomal or peripheral nerve distribution. A sensation of looseness of the teeth is another unusual symptom. Insomnia, neurosis, depression, and hallucinations may occur. Other features include dyspnea, diaphoresis, salivation, tearing, chills, neck stiffness, pruritus, rashes, and tachycardia.[1] In pregnant patients, violent fetal movements have been described. Less commonly, transient blindness, convulsions, rhabdomyolysis, or paralysis may occur. Death, although uncommon, may result from severe dehydration or cardiac or respiratory failure.

Symptoms are often exacerbated by the ingestion of nontoxic seafood, nuts, grains, or alcohol and by exercise. Medications containing cyclic ethers, such as opiates, barbiturates, and paraldehyde, may exacerbate symptoms.[18] No specific laboratory abnormalities are characteristic. Electrolyte disturbances may occur secondary to dehydration and rhabdomyolysis. Ventricular extrasystoles and T-wave changes may be seen on the electrocardiogram.

Acute GI symptoms usually resolve by 24 to 48 hours, and neurologic symptoms by 3 weeks, but the latter may persist for up to 2 months.

Palytoxin

Features of palytoxin poisoning are similar to those of ciguatera and include weakness, sweating, GI distress, paresthesias, muscle spasms, and tremors. Severe poisoning may result in generalized, painful tonic contraction of muscles, mimicking seizures, and in rhabdomyolysis, myoglobinuria, hemolysis, hyperkalemia, respiratory failure, bradycardia, and renal failure.[11]

Neurotoxic Shellfish Poisoning

Neurotoxic shellfish poisoning also produces a similar clinical picture but is less severe. Symptoms often begin with circumoral paresthesias, which become more generalized and can be associated with headaches, dilated pupils, tachycardia, and muscle cramps. In severe cases, seizures have occurred, but no cases of paralysis or death have been reported. Symptoms of brevetoxin inhalation include a nonproductive cough, shortness of breath, lacrimation, and irritation of the eyes, nose, and throat. Patients with asthma may develop bronchospasm.

Paralytic Shellfish Poisoning

Symptoms begin 30 minutes to 2 hours after ingestion and typically include numbness of the fingertips, tongue, and lips, often accompanied by nausea and abdominal pain.[17] These symptoms are followed by paresthesias of the face and extremities and progressive muscle paralysis. Bulbar muscles are often affected, causing dysarthria, dysphagia, diplopia, and loss of the gag reflex. Other features include vertigo, ataxia, transient blindness, altered temperature perception, hypotension, headache, and low back pain. Vomiting is not a consistent feature but may result from concomitant bacterial or viral contamination.[17] Ingestion of large doses of saxitoxin can lead rapidly to coma, diaphragmatic paralysis, and respiratory failure. Children appear to be more susceptible.[17] Patients who survive the first 12 hours generally have a complete recovery after 1 to 3 days. Nonspecific T-wave changes and a rise in creatine kinase and its MB fraction have occurred in the absence of myocardial infarction or other signs of cardiac toxicity.

Tetrodotoxin

Patients usually present 10 to 45 minutes after ingesting a tetrodotoxic fish. Very early or mild poisoning reportedly results in a feeling of exhilaration—the reason such fish is eaten in countries such as Japan. Because inadvertent overdose may be fatal, chefs must be licensed in the preparation of this "delicacy."

Four stages of poisoning have been described. Initially, circumoral paresthesias, salivation, nausea, and vomiting occur, followed by peripheral paresthesias and numbness. Sensory symptoms then become more generalized, with ascending paralysis of the extremities, although deep tendon reflexes remain intact. In the third stage, ataxia and paralysis of peripheral and bulbar muscles occur. Finally, respiratory muscles are affected, although patients may still be conscious. In the most severe cases, patients may become unconscious and completely paralyzed, with dilated nonreactive pupils and loss of all brainstem reflexes. Uncommon complications include neurogenic diabetes insipidus and hypertensive cardiac failure. Patients who survive beyond 24 hours have a good prognosis. Recovery occurs over a period of days and, unless complicated by anoxia, is complete. Death is usually due to paralysis of the respiratory muscles.

Clupeotoxin Poisoning

Symptoms begin with a sharp, metallic taste, followed by severe GI upset and cardiovascular collapse. Violent headaches, paresthesias, muscle cramps, and progressive muscular paralysis may occur. Seizures and coma may intervene rapidly, resulting in death within 15 minutes of ingestion.

Scombroid

The clinical presentation of scombroid poisoning is similar to that of IgE-mediated food allergies. Symptoms typically begin within 1 hour of ingestion and are usually mild.[2] Common features are flushing of the face and upper trunk, nausea, abdominal cramps, diarrhea, and headache. Pruritus and urticaria, burning sensations of the mouth and throat, fever, and palpitations can occur. Severe reactions, such as bronchospasm, hypotension, and supraventricular tachyarrhythmias, are more likely to occur in patients with preexisting cardiac or respiratory disease. Symptoms usually resolve in 6 to 12 hours (range, 3 to 36 hours).

Other Seafood Toxins

Diarrheic shellfish poisoning results primarily in GI symptoms. Symptoms of hallucinatory fish poisoning occur within 2 hours of ingestion and typically include ataxia, hallucinations, chest tightness, and a sense of impending doom.[10] GI distress and facial and pharyngeal paresthesias are also common.

Domoic acid mussel contamination results in vomiting, diarrhea, abdominal pain, and headache, occurring about 6 hours after ingestion (range, 15 minutes to 38 hours). Toxic encephalopathy resulting in confusion, disorientation, and memory deficits occurs in one-fourth of patients. Severe poisoning can result in profuse airway secretions, hemiplegia, hypotension, cardiac dysrhythmias, myoclonus, seizures, and coma. Resolution of cognitive deficits can take up to 12 weeks, but memory deficits and peripheral neuropathy appear to be permanent.

Patients poisoned by carp bile present 10 minutes to 12 hours after ingestion, with GI upset and diarrhea, followed by fever, chills, bradycardia, hypotension, hematuria, headache, and oliguria.[15] Acute tubular necrosis and toxic hepatitis may occur; both resolve after 2 to 3 weeks. Symptoms of fish roe poisoning develop within several hours of ingestion, with GI symptoms, hypotension and tachycardia, tinnitus, and weakness.[12] Ingestion of red whelk may result in progressive weakness that may include the respiratory muscles. Also seen are GI symptoms and hypotension due to vagal-induced bradycardia and peripheral vasodilatation.[8]

Haff disease affects motor neurons of the brain, anterior horn cells of the spinal cord, and myocardial muscle cells. Clinical manifestations also include hypertension, tachycardia, diaphoresis, rhabdomyolysis, myoglobinuria, and renal failure.[19]

DIFFERENTIAL DIAGNOSIS

The clinical presentation of ciguatera, neurotoxic shellfish, palytoxin, tetrodotoxin, and paralytic shellfish poisoning may be difficult to distinguish, as all may involve symptoms of paresthesias, weakness, and ataxia.[13] Predominant symptoms and the nature of the fish eaten are used to determine the specific etiology. A common shellfish origin has been found for toxins associated with tetrodotoxin and paralytic shellfish poisoning

The differential diagnosis of toxic seafood poisoning includes infectious gastroenteritis. Common seafood pathogens are hepatitis A, Norwalk virus, *Vibrio* spp. (*V. cholerae, V. parahaemolyticus,* and *V. vulnificus*), *Clostridium botulinum, Escherichia coli, Giardia lamblia,* and species of *Campylobacter, Shigella,* and *Salmonella*.[7]

Scombroid poisoning can usually be differentiated from true allergic or anaphylactic reactions by the history of fish ingestion. Rarely, histamine poisoning indistinguishable from that caused by scombroid may result from the ingestion of aged cheese. Symptoms similar to scombroid fish poisoning can result from the ingestion of Japanese Callista clams, the ovaries of which have a high content of choline during the summer spawning season. Additional symptoms include paralysis or numbness of the throat, mouth, and tongue, and recovery takes up to 2 days.

The differential diagnosis of skin flushing also includes poisoning by niacin, vancomycin, rifampin, monosodium glutamate, and ethanol or disulfiram reactions.

EMERGENCY DEPARTMENT EVALUATION

The diagnosis of seafood poisoning is based on exposure history, clinical manifestations, and epidemiologic information. A history of seafood ingestion in the past 48 hours should be sought from patients presenting with GI, allergic, or unusual neurologic symptoms. If possible, the origin of the seafood should be identified; this information may help differentiate poisonings specific to certain regions. Public health officials may be able to assist in this process and provide information about similar cases or known quarantined fishing areas.

The physical examination focuses on vital signs, a neurologic evaluation, and assessment of respiratory function. In patients with significant GI symptoms, orthostatic vital signs are taken. The skin is examined for rashes. Peritoneal signs on abdominal examination suggest alternative pathology. Laboratory evaluation includes a complete blood count; measurements of electrolytes, blood urea nitrogen, creatinine, glucose, and creatine kinase; and urinalysis. Unless other diagnoses or complications are considered, additional laboratory tests are of no help. Assays for detecting seafood toxins are not readily available for clinical use but may be used by government agencies for epidemiologic investigations.

EMERGENCY DEPARTMENT MANAGEMENT

General Measures

Patients with bulbar paralysis, respiratory muscle weakness, or depressed consciousness require close observation of airway patency and respiratory function. Intubation and mechanical ventilation are performed, if necessary. The treatment of bradycardia and other cardiac problems should follow standard advanced cardiac life-support guidelines. Volume losses are replaced with intravenous normal saline. Hypotension unresponsive to fluids is treated with dopamine. Dobutamine may be required to treat hypotension in paralytic shellfish poisoning. Calcium gluconate (1 g intravenously over 30 minutes, followed by 2 to 4 g/d as a constant infusion) has also been used to treat hypotension secondary to ciguatera.

Most seafood toxins are readily absorbed by activated charcoal, and this therapy should be used in patients who present within 4 hours of ingestion. Control of emesis may be necessary first. Cathartic agents should be avoided, as they exacerbate diarrhea. Ipecac or gastric lavage is unnecessary.

There are no specific antidotes for any form of seafood poisoning. In most cases, supportive care, with fluid replacement and symptomatic relief, is the mainstay of treatment.

Specific Therapy

Several specific therapies have been tried for ciguatera poisoning. Mannitol appears to be the most effective treatment for control of acute toxicity. Neurologic symptoms often respond within minutes and resolve completely within 48 hours.[14] GI symptoms do not appear to respond as well. Mannitol is given intravenously as a 20% solution in a dose of 1 g/kg, up to 50 g, at 250 to 500 mL/h. Fluid and electrolyte abnormalities must be corrected before it is given. Mannitol is most effective if given within 48 hours of poisoning but may have some effect even when given late or if symptoms return.[20]

Pralidoxime was originally used because it was erroneously thought that ciguatoxin had anticholinesterase activity. Although pralidoxime can be used to control excessive secretions, it may worsen other symptoms, and its efficacy remains unproved. Amitriptyline, which may act by blocking sodium channels, in doses of 25 to 75 mg/d, usually provides some relief from the chronic neurologic symptoms of ciguatera poisoning. Other agents used with varying degrees of success include fluoxetine, nifedipine, vitamins B_{12} and C, calcium gluconate (1 to 3 g intravenously over 24 hours), lidocaine, and tocainide. Indomethacin and cyproheptadine are commonly used to relieve arthralgias and pruritus. Opiates and barbiturates should be avoided. Steroids are ineffective. Seafood, nuts, grains, alcohol, and exercise should be avoided for 3 to 6 months after exposure.

Patients with systemic anaphylactoid reactions secondary to scombroid poisoning should be treated with intravenous epinephrine, inhaled albuterol, and steroids. Less severe reactions can be treated with antihistamines. Type 2 histamine receptor blockers such as cimetidine appear more effective than type 1 blockers such as diphenhydramine.[3] Nausea and vomiting may respond to prochlorperazine. Once stabilized, patients with scombroid poisoning can be discharged on oral antihistamines for 48 hours.

Edrophonium and neostigmine have been used to reverse motor paralysis due to tetrodotoxin poisoning but have not been studied in controlled trials. Diuresis and transfusion of red cells may be necessary in patients with palytoxin poisoning who have rhabdomyolysis and hemolysis, respectively.

For all toxic seafood poisonings, prevention is the best treatment. In areas where ciguatera poisoning is endemic, people should avoid eating fish larger than 2 kg or those known to be frequently affected; for instance, the sale of barracuda is banned in Miami. Eating any viscera, especially the liver and gonads, should always be avoided. Outbreaks of paralytic shellfish poisoning are prevented by periodic testing of susceptible mollusks. When toxin levels are high, affected areas are quarantined. In some areas, harvesting of susceptible shellfish is banned during the summer. Quarantines also may be introduced during algae blooms. Failure to heed quarantines invites disaster.

Puffer fish should be eaten only if prepared by a licensed chef. Scombroid poisoning can be prevented by proper refrigeration of fish. Obviously, any fish that appears spoiled or has an unusual taste should be avoided.

DISPOSITION

Most patients can be treated in the emergency department and then discharged with outpatient follow-up. Those with abnormal vital signs, persistent or severe dehydration, systemic anaphylactoid reactions, and neurologic symptoms should be hospitalized. The level of care required depends on clinical severity. A toxicologist, regional poison control center, or public health agency can be consulted for current trends and treatment advice. Local or state departments of health should be notified of all cases of suspected seafood poisoning, because timely intervention may prevent additional exposures.

COMMON PITFALLS

- Failing to obtain a history of seafood ingestion, including the identity and source, in patients presenting with gastroenteritis or allergic symptoms
- Failing to consider seafood poisoning in patients presenting with unexplained or atypical neurologic symptoms
- Failing to assess airway control and respiratory function in patients with bulbar paresis, muscle weakness, or altered mental status
- Failing to replace fluid losses
- Failing to report cases of possible seafood poisoning to public health agencies

References

1. Bagnis R, Kuberski T, Laugier S. Clinical observations on 3009 cases of ciguatera fish poisoning in the South Pacific. *Am J Trop Med Hyg* 1967;28:1067.
2. Bartholomew BA, Berry PR, Rodhouse JC, et al. Scombrotoxic fish poisoning in Britain: features of over 250 suspected incidents from 1976 to 1986. *Epidemiol Infect* 1987;99:775.
3. Blakesley ML. Scombroid poisoning: prompt resolution of symptoms with cimetidine. *Ann Emerg Med* 1983;12:104.
4. Cameron J, Capra MF. The basis of the paradoxical disturbance of temperature perception in ciguatera poisoning. *J Toxicol Clin Toxicol* 1993;31:571.
5. Cameron J, Flowers AE, Capra MF. Electrophysiological studies on ciguatera in man (part II). *J Neurol Sci* 1991;101:93.
6. Dickinson G. Scombroid fish poisoning syndrome. *Ann Emerg Med* 1982; 11:487.
7. Eastaugh J, Shepherd S. Infectious and toxic syndromes from fish and shellfish consumption. *Arch Intern Med* 1989;149:1735.
8. Fleming C. Case of poisoning from red whelk. *BMJ* 1971;3:520.
9. Gillespie NC, Lewis JL, Pearn JH, et al. Ciguatera in Australia. *Med J Aust* 1986;145:584.
10. Halstead BW. Miscellaneous seafood toxicants. In: Ragelis EP, ed. *Seafood toxins*. Washington, DC: American Chemical Society, 1984.
11. Kodama Y, Hokama Y, Yasumoto T, et al. Clinical and laboratory findings implicating palytoxin as cause of ciguatera poisoning due to *Decapterus macrosoma* (mackerel). *Toxicon* 1989;27:1051.
12. Listernick R. Fish roe poisoning in childhood. *J Pediatr* 1987;111:729.
13. Mills AR, Passmore R. Pelagic paralysis. *Lancet* 1988;1(8578):161.
14. Palafax NA, Jain LG, Pinano AZ, et al. Successful treatment of ciguatera poisoning with intravenous mannitol. *JAMA* 1988;259:2740.
15. Park SK, Kim DG, Kang SK, et al. Toxic renal failure and hepatitis after ingestion of raw carp bile. *Nephron* 1990;56:188.
16. Perl TM, Bédard L, Kosatsky T, et al. An outbreak of toxic encephalopathy caused by eating mussels contaminated with domoic acid. *N Engl J Med* 1990;322:1775.
17. Rodrigue DC, Etzel RA, Hall S, et al. Lethal paralytic shellfish poisoning in Guatemala. *Am J Trop Med* 1990;42:267.
18. Sims JK. A theoretical discourse on the pharmacology of toxic marine ingestions. *Ann Emerg Med* 1987;16:1006.
19. Solomon M. Haff disease. *Arch Intern Med* 1990;150:683.
20. Swift AEB, Swift TR. Ciguatera. *J Toxicol Clin Toxicol* 1993;31:1.

CHAPTER 369
Sedative–Hypnotic Poisoning

Barbara Insley Crouch and Fred M. Henretig

Nonbarbiturate, nonbenzodiazepine "sedative–hypnotic" agents are used for the relief of anxiety and as sleeping aids. They include buspirone, chloral hydrate, ethchlorvynol, glutethimide, meprobamate, methaqualone, zolpidem, and gamma-hydroxybutyrate (GHB) and its congeners, gamma-butyrolactone (GBL) and 1,4 butanediol (BD). GHB and related agents were originally marketed as sleep aids and body-building nutritional supplements but are currently widely abused as recreational substances.

Overdoses of ten- to 20-fold the recommended dose may cause life-threatening central nervous system (CNS) depression and coma for many of these agents. All may be toxic at a relatively low dose in combination with alcohol or other CNS depressants. Most have a lower margin of safety than the benzodiazepines, although buspirone and zolpidem, the newest members of this class, appear to have a more favorable safety profile. As a class, sedative–hypnotics are notorious for their abuse potential, given their propensity to cause tolerance and dependence. Abstinence may cause severe effects, including a delirium tremens–like syndrome and convulsions. Methaqualone in particular had such a high abuse potential that it was made a class I agent and withdrawn from the market in the United States in 1983. GHB has no current medical indications, and its sale in the United States was banned in 1991.

All sedative–hypnotics are metabolized in the liver, and several induce hepatic enzymes, so that drug interactions with other liver-dependent agents must be borne in mind (i.e., decreased response to warfarin in patients taking ethchlorvynol), and they should not be used in patients with porphyria (particularly ethchlorvynol and meprobamate). Pharmacokinetic data for these agents are summarized in Table 369.1.

Buspirone, an azaspirodecanedione derivative, does not seem to interact with the benzodiazepine–gamma-aminobutyrate (GABA) receptor complex. Rather, it is thought to act primarily as a partial serotonin 1A agonist.[2] The drug is completely absorbed in the gastrointestinal (GI) tract, with peak concentrations reached in 40 to 90 minutes. It is 95% protein-bound, with a volume of distribution in excess of 400 L, and it is metabolized in the liver to pyrimidinyl piperazine (active), with a plasma half-life of 2 hours. A typical adult daily dose is 20 to 30 mg.

Chloral hydrate is one of the oldest known hypnotics. It was first synthesized in 1832 and used as a hypnotic as early as 1869.[17] The first cases of poisoning were reported in 1890. Chloral hydrate use in adults has declined considerably in recent years, but it is still popular for procedural sedation in children at doses ranging from 50 to 100 mg/kg. The toxic dose in adults is 5 to 10 g. As little as 1.5 g has resulted in significant toxicity in a toddler. It is rapidly absorbed, has a volume of distribution of 0.6L/kg, and is rapidly metabolized to trichloroethanol (TCE), which is believed responsible for its hypnotic effects. The half-life of TCE is 8 hours at therapeutic doses, but may be prolonged to 12 to 35 hours after overdose. The combination of alcohol and chloral hydrate ("Mickey Finn") is particularly potent, as these agents not only have additive

TABLE 369.1. Summary of Pharmacokinetic Data for Nonbarbiturate, Nonbenzodiazepine Sedative–Hypnotic Agents

						Blood Levels		
	$t_{1/2}$ (h)	PB (%)	VD (L/kg)	Renal (%)	Active Metabolite	Th	T (μg/mL)	L
Buspirone	2	95	6–7	1	Pyrimidinyl piperazine	NA	NA	NA
Chloral hydrate	8–35[a]	40[a]	0.6	0	TCE	10	100	250
Ethchlorvynol	1–3/10-25[b]	35–50	3–4	10	None	5	20	150
Gamma hydroxybutyrate	1–2	NA	0.4–0.58	<2-5	None	NA	>52	NA
Glutethimide	10–12	35–59	>TBW	<1	4-HEPG	0.2	19	30–100
Meprobamate	6–16	20	0.75	10–12	None	10	80–120	200
Methaqualone	10–40	70–90	2.4–6.4	<1	None	5	10–30	30
Methyprylon	3–6	60	0.97	3	6-Ohmethyprylon 5-Methylpyrithylin	10	30–60	100
Zolpidem	2	92	0.54	<1	None	0.2	>0.5	NA

PB, protein binding; V_D, volume of distribution; renal, percentage eliminated unchanged; TBW, total body water; 4-HEPG, 4-hydroxy-2-ethyl-2-phenylglutarimide; TCE, trichloroethanol; Th, therapeutic; T, toxic; L, lethal; NA, data not available.

[a] Data for TCE

[b] Distribution of $t_{1/2}$ of 1-3 h, with elimination $t_{1/2}$ of 10-25 h.

CNS depressant effects, but also inhibit each other's metabolism. In 1997, 461 cases of chloral hydrate exposure were reported to the American Association of Poison Control Centers' Toxic Exposure Surveillance System (TESS); three were fatal.[12]

Ethchlorvynol, an agent with a rapid onset and relatively short duration of action, has been used for more than 30 years. It is available in capsule sizes of 100, 200, 500, and 700 mg. The usual adult hypnotic dose is 500 to 700 mg. In 1997, 100 ethchlorvynol overdoses were reported to TESS; none was fatal.[12] GI absorption is rapid after therapeutic doses, with onset of effect in 15 to 30 minutes and peak concentrations in 60 to 90 minutes. The drug is initially distributed to fatty tissue, with a redistribution phase occurring at 7 to 10 hours. Protein binds 50% to 60% of free drug in plasma. The elimination half-life is about 10 to 25 hours after therapeutic dosage, but as much as 100 hours after overdose. Generally, 4 to 5 g will lead to toxic effects in an adult. A 5-g overdose has been fatal, but a patient who ingested 50 g has survived after a prolonged coma. As little as one capsule has caused toxic symptoms in toddlers, and 2.5 g coingested with alcohol has caused death in an adult. Symptomatic patients usually have concentrations above 19 to 20 mg/L, and concentrations above 38 mg/L are associated with coma. Ethchlorvynol can cross the placenta, and a neonatal withdrawal syndrome has been described.

Illicit use of GHB was reported in 1990.[4] Prior to 1991, it was available in health-food stores and by mail order as a supplement for body-building (presumably due to its growth hormone–stimulating properties), as well as a diet and sleep aid. Until very recently, it was widely available by mail order or over the Internet as kits for home production. Such kits provided GBL, sodium hydroxide, and instructions for converting GBL to GHB. Abuse of GBL itself, which is rapidly converted to GHB *in vivo,* and BD, which are still legal for sale in many states and produce effects nearly identical to those of GHB, has obviated the need for purchasing these kits.

GHB is structurally related to the inhibitory neurotransmitter GABA, and GHB receptors (probably $GABA_b$ receptors) have been identified in animal models. GHB may also have neurotransmitter and neuromodulator effects. GHB appears to increase brain dopamine levels and to effect endogenous opioids. GHB may also induce a normal sequence of rapid eye movement (REM) and non-REM sleep and has been investigated in the treatment of narcolepsy. It has also been evaluated as an anesthetic agent, but its value was limited by its lack of analgesic effects and its tendency to induce both petit mal and grand mal seizures. It is typically available as the sodium salt in a white powder or tablet form. One teaspoon of the powder provides 2.8 g of GHB. Doses range from one-fourth teaspoon to several tablespoons. GBL and BD are typically sold as liquids. Amnesia occurs after GHB doses of up to 10 mg/kg, somnolence and euphoria after 20 to 30 mg/kg, and anesthetic coma after 50 mg/kg. Doses above 50 mg/kg may be associated with seizures and cardiorespiratory depression. GHB is well absorbed orally. Onset of effects is typically within 15 minutes.[10] Peak concentrations occur in 1.5 to 2.0 hours. The volume of distribution is 0.4 to 0.58 L/kg, the elimination half-life is 1 to 2 hours, and the duration of action ranges from 2 to 8 hours.

Glutethimide, introduced in 1954, was popular as a substance of abuse prior to its being withdrawn from U.S. markets. It was often taken orally with codeine (with cough syrup, called "pancakes and syrup," or with Tylenol Compound 3 or 4, known as "loads," "packs," or "4s and Dors," from the Doriden brand of glutethimide), a combination that purportedly simulates the high of heroin. In 1997, only ten glutethimide overdoses were reported to TESS, with no deaths.[12] GI absorption is relatively erratic for this poorly water-soluble drug. Plasma protein binding is about 50%. The elimination half-life varies from 5 to 22 hours in therapeutic doses but may be 40 to 100 hours or more after overdose. There are two active metabolites. One (4-hydroxy-2-ethyl-2-phenylglutarimide) was thought to correlate with clinical effects and to be responsible for the characteristic fluctuation in level of coma seen with this agent. However, a subsequent case report has documented a lack of correlation between the 4-hydroxy metabolite concentrations and depth of coma.[5] The fluctuating level of consciousness is now felt to be due to erratic absorption, perhaps related to anticholinergic effects on GI motility. Thus, as the drug concentration falls, coma lightens, and gut activity increases, absorption of residual intraluminal drug occurs and results in deepening coma. Glutethimide induces hepatic microsomal enzymes. The toxic effects of glutethimide are due primarily to global CNS depression. It also has significant anticholinergic activity. Death is usually due to cardiovascular collapse. An acute dose of 500 mg in a young child or 5 g in an adult will produce severe poisoning. The lethal dose is reportedly 10 to 20 g, although survival after prolonged comas has occurred after ingestion of 45 g. Fatal overdoses have been associated with concentrations of 2 to 80 mg/L. Tolerance and physical dependence are characteristic of chronic abuse. Glutethimide can cross the placenta, and neonatal withdrawal has been reported.

Meprobamate, originally synthesized and used as a muscle relaxant in the late 1940s, was introduced in the United States for use as an anxiolytic agent in 1955. Although still used today for this purpose, there is little evidence that it is effective. It is available in 200-, 400-, and 600-mg tablets, and in 200- and 400-mg sustained-release capsules. In 1997, there were 229 poison exposures to meprobamate reported to TESS; four had fatal outcomes.[12] A carbamate ester, meprobamate is structurally related to the skeletal muscle relaxants carisoprodol, methocarbamol, and chlorphenesin, and to the anticonvulsant felbamate. Meprobamate itself has anticonvulsant and skeletal muscle relaxant properties. Its mechanism of action is similar to that of barbiturates, although it is thought to be more selective in its depression of areas in the cerebral cortex. It also suppresses polysynaptic reflexes in the spinal cord, which probably contributes to its skeletal muscle relaxation properties. The therapeutic dose of meprobamate for adults is usually 1.2 to 1.6 g daily, in three or four doses; the maximal daily dose is 2.4 g. Therapeutic blood concentrations are said to be between 5 and 30 μg/mL, although therapeutic drug monitoring is usually not performed. Meprobamate is well absorbed from the GI tract, with peak plasma concentrations within 1 to 3 hours after ingestion. It binds very little to plasma proteins and has volume of distribution of 0.7 L/kg. Meprobamate induces hepatic microsomal enzymes to some degree. The half-life is reported to be about 12 hours, although this may be markedly prolonged after an overdose. Toxic effects may occur after ingestions of as little as 2 to 4 g. Death has been reported with as little as 12 g, but survival has been reported after ingestions of up to 40 g.[1] Drug concentrations do not correlate well with clinical effects, although concentrations above 100 μg/mL are associated with severe toxicity. Fatal concentrations in 12 cases ranged from 142 to 346 μg/mL, with a mean concentration of 226 μg/mL.[6]

Methaqualone, a quinazoline derivative, was introduced in 1965 as a nonaddicting substitute for the barbiturates. It rapidly became popular as a drug of abuse, however. Abused for its euphoric and aphrodisiac effects, methaqualone was nicknamed the "love drug." In 1997, only 19 poison exposures were reported to TESS.[12] The therapeutic dose is 150 to 300 mg of the methaqualone base or 200 to 400 mg of the hydrochloride salt. Methaqualone is rapidly absorbed from the GI tract. Effects are noted within 30 minutes and peak at 1 to 2 hours. Methaqualone is widely distributed, especially adipose tissue, and is slowly eliminated. The distribution half-life is about 2 to 4 hours, and the elimination half-life is more than 24 hours. Protein binding is 70% to 80%. Toxic effects usually occur with ingestions of more than 2 g. Ingestion of 8 g has resulted in death, but survival was noted after ingestion of 22 g.[18] Patients with reported overdoses of 2.5 to 7.5 g of methaqualone in the form of Mandrax (methaqualone and diphenhydramine) were minimally responsive or unresponsive to deep painful stimuli and had plasma concentrations of 9 to 47 μg/mL.[9] Serum concentrations appeared to correlate with clinical findings in this study but not in another.[14]

Zolpidem, an imidazopyridine derivative that is structurally unrelated to the benzodiazepines, selectively bind to the central benzodiazepine receptor subtype BZ_1 located in the $GABA_A$ receptor complex. Unlike benzodiazepines, it does not appear to possess significant anticonvulsant or muscle relaxant properties. Oral bioavailability is 70%, due to significant first-pass metabolism. It is rapidly absorbed, and peak concentrations are reached within 30 to 120 minutes following an oral dose. It is highly protein bound (92%) and has a volume of distribution of 0.54 L/kg and a half-life of approximately 2 hours following 5- to 200-mg therapeutic doses. Ingestions of up to 300 mg without the development of symptoms have been reported.[16] An ingestion of 1,000 mg resulted in tachycardia and agitation only.[7] No deaths attributable to zolpidem alone have been reported.

CLINICAL PRESENTATION

Experience with buspirone overdose is limited. Amounts up to 300 mg have been reported to cause dysphoria, transient CNS depression, miosis, vomiting and diarrhea, and mild decreases in heart rate and blood pressure. Paresthesias and dystonic reactions have also been described. CNS depression usually resolves within 6 hours. One recent report, however, describes generalized seizures 36 hours after the ingestion of 420 mg.[2]

Chloral hydrate overdose resembles that due to barbiturates, with coma, miosis and hypotension.[17] It is also a GI irritant and commonly causes nausea and vomiting. Hemorrhagic gastritis and gastric necrosis or perforation occur rarely. As a halogenated hydrocarbon, chloral hydrate can also cause hepatic injury, renal failure, and cardiotoxicity. It reduces myocardial contractility, shortens the refractory period, sensitizes the myocardium to circulating catecholamines, and can precipitate cardiac dysrhythmias.

With an acute ethchlorvynol overdose, symptoms range from lethargy, ataxia, and nystagmus to deep coma with respiratory and cardiovascular depression. A hallmark of massive ethchlorvynol overdose is prolonged coma.[19] Pulmonary edema can occur, especially after intravenous overdose, but also 24 to 48 hours after an oral overdose. Hypothermia, bradycardia, hypotension, and excess salivation are seen in severe cases. Gastric fluid is pink, with a minty odor. Skin bullae similar to those seen with barbiturate poisoning may also be noted.[3] Complications include those of prolonged coma, especially pneumonia and pressure necrosis of the extremities.

Ingestion of GHB, GBL, or BD results in vomiting, drowsiness, hypotonia, and dizziness within 15 to 60 minutes.[4,10] These effects may soon be followed by coma, mydriasis (miosis has been noted infrequently), irregular and slowed respirations, tremor, agitation, hallucinations, myoclonus, and, possibly, seizures. Bradycardia and hypotension have also been described. Effects typically resolve within 8 hours, although dizziness may last for several days. Pulmonary aspiration is very uncommon.[4] Death has been reported, but coingestants and underlying medical conditions have complicated the interpretation of many of these cases.

Prolonged, fluctuating coma is the predominant effect of severe glutethimide overdose.[13] Anticholinergic manifestations may include mydriasis, ileus, urinary bladder retention, and hot, flushed, dry skin. Cerebral and pulmonary edema is regularly reported in severe overdoses. Ocular and neurologic signs can be dramatic: papilledema; nystagmus; unilateral or bilateral pupillary dilation; ataxia; tonic spasms and seizures; coma progressing to loss of deep tendon, corneal, gag, and pupillary light reflexes; and an isoelectric electroencephalogram. Both hypothermia and fever may be encountered. Bullous skin lesions analogous to those seen in barbiturate overdose may be noted. Hypotension can occur, and apnea may develop suddenly. The effects of coingestants (e.g., codeine with or without acetaminophen) may also be present. Complications include those of severe coma, particularly pneumonia and pulmonary edema.

Meprobamate overdose may produce lethargy, ataxia, slurred speech, and coma. Depending on the level of consciousness, respirations may or may not be depressed. Meprobamate is unique among sedative–hypnotic agents in that it often causes hypotension.[1] The observation that hypotension may occur without respiratory depression suggests a direct myocardial depressant effect. Tachycardia is also common. Miosis, mydriasis, nystagmus, respiratory depression, disconjugate gaze, seizure activity, hallucinations, and hypothermia have been reported. Meprobamate has a tendency to clump in the stomach, resulting gastric pharmacobezoar formation. Methaqualone commonly causes muscle hyperactivity, including hyperreflexia, twitching, and clonus, in addition to CNS depression.[9,14] Hypotension and respiratory depression occur infrequently. Dysrhythmias and myocardial infarctions have been noted in a few patients. Fixed drug eruptions have been noted in methaqualone abusers; lesions resolved once the drug was withdrawn. Bleeding tendencies, believed to be caused by coagulopathy and abnormal platelet count or aggregation, have been reported, with retinal hemorrhage being described in one case.

Zolpidem overdose appears to be relatively benign. In a series of 35 patients, 51% developed no symptoms.[15] The remainder had mild CNS effects, including dizziness, slurred speech, and lethargy. Four patients complained of nausea, vomiting, and abdominal discomfort. Only two patients in this series had deep sedation. Of cases reported to a poison center, 28% did not have symptoms, and over half of those that did had concomitant ingestions.[7] Of patients who ingested zolpidem alone, the majority experienced only drowsiness. Vomiting occurred in seven; coma without respiratory depression in four; mydriasis, agitation and tachycardia in three each; and confusion and hypotonia in two. Effects noted in only a single patient included hyporeflexia, gait disturbances, incoherent speech, memory impairment, tachypnea, visual hallucinations, blurred vision, bradycardia, dizziness and hypotension.

DIFFERENTIAL DIAGNOSIS

Poisoning by alcohols, anticonvulsants, barbiturates, benzodiazepines, beta blockers, calcium channel blockers, centrally acting antihypertensives, cyclic antidepressants, opioids, and skeletal muscle relaxants can cause similar signs and symptoms. Hypotension out of proportion to the degree of CNS depression suggests meprobamate, a cardiovascular agent, or a cyclic antidepressant. Cyclic coma suggests glutethimide or a gastric drug bezoar. CNS infection and trauma, hypoglycemia, hypernatremia, hypercalcemia, and hypermagnesemia should also be considered.

EMERGENCY DEPARTMENT EVALUATION

The history should include the time and amount of drug(s) ingested, the time of onset and the nature of symptoms, and medical history, including the pattern and extent of sedative–hypnotic drug use. The physical examination focuses on vital signs and the neurologic and cardiopulmonary status.

Symptomatic patients should have baseline blood work (oxygen saturation or arterial blood gas analysis, complete blood count, and determination of electrolyte, blood urea nitrogen, creatinine, and glucose concentrations), urinalysis, an electrocardiogram (ECG), a chest radiograph, and liver function tests, as indicated by clinical severity. Patients with deeper comas should also be evaluated for possible rhabdomyolysis by serum creatine phosphokinase and urine myoglobin tests. Comprehensive urine toxicology screening tests can confirm the presence of all sedative–hypnotics except GBH and its derivatives. Drugs of abuse immunoassays will not detect these agents. In general, quantitative serum drug levels are neither readily available nor clinically useful.

EMERGENCY DEPARTMENT MANAGEMENT

Generally, therapy involves stabilization and support of vital signs and gut decontamination, with the administration of activated charcoal being the preferred modality. Patients normally respond well to good supportive measures. If a patient starts to deteriorate after apparent recovery, or is deteriorating despite good supportive care, a drug mass in the stomach should be suspected. Endoscopy can be both diagnostic and therapeutic in such cases. Gastrotomy has been used for meprobamate pharmacobezoar removal.[16] If hypotension fails to respond to fluids, or if the patient is already fluid-overloaded, a trial of agents with positive inotropic activity, such as dopamine and epinephrine, is indicated. Unless hypoxic injury is present, full recovery can be expected once these drugs have been eliminated. Hence, invasive cardiovascular support (e.g., partial or full bypass and intraaortic balloon pump therapy) should be included in the supportive care of hemodynamically unstable patients.

Ventricular dysrhythmias due to chloral hydrate are often refractory to treatment.[17] Lidocaine, magnesium (especially for torsades de pointes), beta blockers, and overdrive pacing have been used with success. Pressor agents should be avoided, if possible, to decrease the risk of precipitating refractory dysrhythmias. Hemodialysis may be considered in extremely severe cases with profound hypotension and unstable arrhythmias.

The use of extracorporeal methods for enhancing the elimination of ethchlorvynol is controversial. Plasma half-life can be decreased with hemodialysis. Resin hemoperfusion, although not widely available, is even more efficacious.[19] Such therapy should be considered only in patients with high drug levels and life-threatening toxicity unresponsive to intensive supportive care.

Patients with GHB poisoning may require endotracheal intubation for airway protection or for respiratory support while obtunded and vomiting. Because the duration is short, many can be managed effectively with noninvasive airway support (recovery position with suction, oxygen, close monitoring, and stimulation) and careful observation for up to 6 hours in the emergency department. [10] Benzodiazepines may be required for seizures, and atropine for bradycardia.

Glutethimide's anticholinergic effects may cause delayed gastric emptying and absorption, so decontamination may be useful many hours after ingestion. Repeated doses of activated charcoal may also be helpful, given the prolonged and fluctuating degree of intestinal absorption. Efforts to enhance elimination with hemodialysis and hemoperfusion have shown limited benefit, probably due to the agent's extensive tissue distribution. In patients who have coingested codeine, the administration of naloxone (see Chapter 360) may be partially effective. Those who have coingested a codeine product containing acetaminophen should have an acetaminophen concentration measured and be treated accordingly.

Fluids should be given with caution in treating the hypotensive effects of meprobamate, because its myocardial depressant properties increase the risk of pulmonary edema. Hemodialysis, resin and charcoal hemoperfusion, and continuous arteriovenous hemoperfusion (CAVHP) have been used successfully in the treatment of life-threatening meprobamate overdoses.[8,11] These methods should be reserved for patients who are unresponsive to supportive measures. Proponents of CAVHP note its efficacy in hypotensive patients, as well as its potential availability in smaller community hospitals.

Patients with methaqualone poisoning may require pharmacologic paralysis for control of neuromuscular hyperactivity.

The benzodiazepine antagonist, flumazenil (see Chapter 319), can reverse CNS depression due to zolpidem.

DISPOSITION

Patients with mild symptoms may be observed in the emergency department until asymptomatic. Except with GHB and related compounds, those with moderate or severe symptoms require admission, because prolonged close monitoring and supportive care are necessary. Intensive care unit admission is advisable. Patients with unstable vital signs or very deep coma may be candidates for extracorporeal elimination procedures and should be transferred to a facility that is capable of such treatment. Advanced life-support equipment and staff should accompany the patient during transfer.

COMMON PITFALLS

- Failure to consider the possibility of gastric drug bezoar and continuing drug absorption in patients with progressive, prolonged or cyclic coma, particularly that due to glutethimide and meprobamate, and to consider interventions such as endoscopy and multiple-dose charcoal
- Failure to appreciate that meprobamate can cause hypotension in the absence of severe CNS depression
- Failure to appreciate that buspirone, GHB and its congeners, and methaqualone can cause agitated coma (i.e., neuromuscular hyperactivity or seizures in addition to CNS depression)
- Failure to appreciate that the effects of GHB, GBL, and BD are short-lived and that endotracheal intubation and intensive care unit admission may not be necessary
- Failure to monitor for pulmonary edema, especially in patients who require fluid resuscitation for hypotension
- Failure to perform toxicology testing to rule out occult coingestants (e.g., acetaminophen), especially in comatose patients
- Failure to consider invasive hemodynamic support and elimination therapies in patients with severe poisoning unresponsive to noninvasive treatment
- Failure to anticipate and treat withdrawal syndromes in patients chronically taking these drugs

References

1. Bailey DN. The present status of meprobamate ingestion: a 5-year review of cases with serum concentrations and clinical findings. *Am J Clin Pathol* 1981;75:102.
2. Catalano G, Catalano MC, Hanley PF. Seizures associated with buspirone overdose: case report and literature review. *Clin Neuropharmacol* 1998;21:347–350.
3. Chamberlain JM, Klein-Schwartz W, Gorman R. Pressure necrosis following ethchlorvynol overdose. *Am J Emerg Med* 1990;8:467.
4. Chin RL, Sporer KA, Cullison B, et al. Clinical course of gamma-hydroxybutyrate overdose. *Ann Emerg Med* 1998;31:716–722.
5. Curry SC, Hubbard JM, Gerkin R, et al. Lack of correlation between plasma 4-hydroxyglutethimide and severity of coma in acute glutethimide poisoning. *Med Toxicol* 1987;2:309.
6. Felby S. Concentrations of meprobamate in the blood and liver following fatal meprobamate poisoning. *Acta Pharmacol Toxicol* 1970;28:334.
7. Garnier R, Guerait E, Muzard D, et al. Acute zolpidem poisoning—analysis of 344 cases. J Toxicol Clin Toxicol 1994;32:391–404.
8. Hoy WE, Rivero A, Marin MG, et al. Resin hemoperfusion for treatment of a massive meprobamate overdose. *Ann Intern Med* 1980;93:455.
9. Lawson AAH, Brown SS. Acute methaqualone (Mandrax) poisoning. *Scot Med J* 1967;12:63.
10. Li J, Stokes SA, Woeckner A. A tale of novel intoxication: a review of the effects of gamma-hydroxybutyric acid with recommendations for management. *Ann Emerg Med* 1998;31:729–736.
11. Lin JL, Lim PS, Lai BC, et al. Continuous arteriovenous hemoperfusion in meprobamate poisoning. *J Toxicol Clin Toxicol* 1993;32:645.
12. Litovitz TL, Klein-Schwartz W, Dyer KS, et al. 1997 Annual report of the American Association of Poison Control Centers Toxic Exposure Surveillance System. *Am J Emerg Med* 1998;16:443–497.
13. Maher JF, Schreiner GE, Nestervelt FB. Acute glutethimide intoxication. I. Clinical experience (22 patients) compared to acute barbiturate intoxication (63 patients). *Am J Med* 1962;33:70.
14. Matthew H, Proudfoot AT, Brown SS, et al. Mandrax poisoning: conservative management of 116 patients. *BMJ* 1968;2:202.
15. Mercurio M, DeRoos F, Hoffman RS. Zolpidem (Ambien): exposure assessment of a new nonbenzodiazepine GABA agonist. *Vet Human Toxicol* 1994;36:371.
16. Schwartz HS. Acute meprobamate poisoning with gastrotomy and removal of a drug-containing mass. *N Engl J Med* 1976;295:1177.
17. Sing K, Erickson T, Amitai Y, et al. Chloral hydrate toxicity from oral and intravenous administration. *J Toxicol Clin Toxicol* 1996;34:101–106.
18. Skoutakis VA, Acchiardo SR. Methaqualone poisoning: diagnosis and treatment. *Clin Toxicol Consult* 1983;5:23.
19. Yell RP. Ethchlorvynol overdose. *Am J Emerg Med* 1990;8:246–250.

CHAPTER 370
The Serotonin Syndrome

Andis Graudins

The serotonin syndrome is due to pharmacologic overstimulation of central nervous system (CNS) 5-hydroxytryptamine (5-HT) or serotonin receptors. It may result from drug interactions during therapeutic dosing or from overdose with one or multiple serotonin-specific antidepressant agents. These antidepressants include the selective serotonin reuptake inhibitors (SSRIs) fluoxetine, sertraline, paroxetine, citalopram, and fluvoxamine; the nonselective serotonin (and norepinephrine) reuptake inhibitors (NSRIs) venlafaxine and nefazodone; and the reversible inhibitor of monoamine oxidase A (MAO-A), moclobemide.[1,5,6,12,13,17]

Most reports of the syndrome are either single case reports or small case series. There is no obvious gender or age preference.

In a study of 204 patients exposed to serotonergic antidepressants, there was a 10% incidence of serotonin syndrome. Seventy percent of the cases were the result of overdose; the remainder were due to therapeutic drug interactions. A single agent was involved in 50%, and two were involved in 45%.[4] Drug interactions often result from substituting a new antidepressant for one with a long elimination half-life (e.g., fluoxetine) or duration of action (e.g., a monoamine oxidase inhibitor [MAOI]; see Chapter 354) without an adequate wash-out period (i.e., allowing the previously used agent to be completely eliminated).

Drug interactions also may be precipitated by the addition of a second serotonergic antidepressant when a patient is already taking one. Finally, patients may be taking an antidepressant and unknowingly be given another medication with serotonergic activity (e.g., the use of meperidine or dextromethorphan in a patient taking an MAOI or serotonergic antidepressant).[3,7,20] The severe hyperthermic response sometimes seen following methylenedioxymethamphetamine (MDMA, "ecstasy") abuse may also be due to the serotonin syndrome.[9]

Serotonin is a neurotransmitter found widely throughout the body. Large amounts are stored in the enterochromaffin cells of the gastrointestinal tract (greater than 90% of body stores), where it produces stimulation of vascular and gastrointestinal smooth muscle contraction. Lesser amounts (8% of body stores) are found in platelets, where it causes their aggregation. In the CNS, which contains a relatively small amount of serotonin (2% of body stores), its main action is the inhibition of excitatory neurotransmission. Animal models of serotonin syndrome suggest that excessive stimulation of brainstem 5-HT-1a and cortical 5-HT-2 receptors is responsible for the serotonin syndrome.[10,19] Various drugs and mechanisms of action may be involved[15,16] (Table 370.1).

The high and increasing frequency of serotonergic drug use requires that caution be exercised in prescribing other serotonergic agents, particularly meperidine, for patients seen in the emergency department. Meperidine is absolutely contraindicated in patients taking MAOIs.[15,20] Morphine does not have any serotonin reuptake inhibition properties and should be used as the analgesic of choice in this population.

CLINICAL PRESENTATION

Original criteria proposed for the diagnosis of the serotonin syndrome included a recent increase or addition of a serotonergic agent to a medication regimen and at least three of the following clinical features: mental status change, agitation, myoclonus, hyperreflexia, diaphoresis, shivering, tremor, diarrhea, incoordination, and fever. In addition, they required that other etiologies be excluded; additionally, the patient must not have been exposed to neuroleptic agents.[19] These criteria may exclude a number of patients who have the serotonin syndrome, particularly those exhibiting severe toxicity.[16]

It is now recognized that signs and symptoms fall into three major categories: altered mental status, autonomic nervous system instability, and neuromuscular hyperactivity (Table 370.2). Milder forms of the syndrome may present with abnormalities in only one or two of these categories. A review of 127 cases of the serotonin syndrome found that the most common clinical findings were myoclonus, hyperreflexia, confusion, hyperthermia, diaphoresis, and sinus tachycardia.[16] The diagnosis remains one of exclusion and should be considered in patients with a history of recent exposure to serotonergic agents and findings in any of the major categories.

The time of onset of symptoms following exposure to serotonergic agents is variable. Symptoms are often reported to develop within 1 to 2 hours of ingestion.[6,12] The syndrome has also been reported to occur after several days following gradual increases in dosing of antidepressant medications.[2] There appears to be no relationship between the amount of drug ingested and the risk of serotonin syndrome, as it can occur both with therapeutic dosing and in overdosage. Reported serum levels of drugs measured in patients with the serotonin syndrome have been either at therapeutic or below therapeutic levels in up to 90% of cases.[16]

The clinical course of the serotonin syndrome is usually self-limiting. Symptoms and signs tend to subside with withdrawal of the offending drugs. Milder forms of the syndrome may resolve after a period of 6 to 12 hours. More severe cases may be symptomatic for 24 to 48 hours. Death has been reported but is rare.[17,19]

TABLE 370.1. Drugs Affecting Central Nervous System Serotonin Concentrations with the Potential to Produce Serotonin Syndrome

Increased serotonin production	L-tryptophan
Increased presynaptic serotonin release	Amphetamines MDMA Cocaine
Decrease serotonin breakdown by monoamine oxidase	Irreversible inhibitors of MAO-A and MAO-B Phenelzine, tranylcypromine, isocarboxazid Reversible inhibitors of MAO-A Moclobemide Reversible inhibitors of MAO-B Selegeline
Inhibition of serotonin reuptake	Serotonin-specific reuptake inhibitors Fluoxetine, citalopram, paroxetine, sertraline, fluvoxamine, cyclic antidepressants, meperidine, dextromethorphan Serotonin-noradrenaline reuptake inhibitors Venlafaxine, nefazodone
Direct agonists of postsynaptic receptors	Bromocriptine, lithium, levo-DOPA, electroconvulsive therapy

Data from refs. 9, 16, and 18.

TABLE 370.2. Summary of Potential Clinical Findings Associated with Serotonin Syndrome

Autonomic Instability	Altered Mental Status	Neuromuscular Hyperactivity
Tachycardia	Anxiety	Myoclonus
Fluctuating blood pressure	Confusion	Hyperreflexia
Diaphoresis	Drowsiness	Muscle rigidity
Flushed skin	Hallucinations	Tremor
Hyperthermia	Coma	Agitation
Tachypnea	Insomnia	Restlessness
Mydriasis	Dizziness	Ataxia
Unreactive pupils		Nystagmus
Diarrhea		Trismus
Abdominal pain		Opisthotonus
Excessive salivation		

DIFFERENTIAL DIAGNOSIS

Meningitis, encephalitis, septicemia, hypoglycemia, and neurotrauma should be considered in the differential diagnosis of patients presenting with mental status changes, autonomic instability, or hyperthermia. Intoxication with amphetamine, cocaine, or hallucinogens and withdrawal from alcohol and benzodiazepine should be considered when agitation, hallucinations, and sympathetic excess are present. In these conditions, the characteristic neuromuscular features of serotonin syndrome are usually absent.

Neuromuscular hyperactivity may be seen in dystonic reactions, tetanus, strychnine poisoning, and lithium intoxication. Lithium toxicity and tetanus may have additional features suggestive of the serotonin syndrome. The most similar condition, however, is the neuroleptic malignant syndrome (NMS; see Chapter 356). In contrast to patients with the serotonin syndrome, those with NMS have a history of recent commencement of, or increase in, dosage of neuroleptic medications. Symptoms tend to develop (and later resolve) over days rather than hours; muscular hyperactivity is characterized by sustained "lead pipe" rigidity rather than by myoclonus; and hyperreflexia is rarely, if ever, seen.[16]

EMERGENCY DEPARTMENT EVALUATION

The history should focus on drug use. Specifically, any evidence of drug overdose and use of multiple serotonergic medications, drugs of abuse, and over-the-counter medications containing dextromethorphan should be sought. The time course of onset and progression of symptoms is important in discriminating between NMS and serotonin syndrome.

Both the history and physical examination should focus on excluding other causes of the clinical picture. Vital signs should include an accurate temperature. A thorough search for evidence of trauma should be made. Features of serotonin syndrome that are present should be documented. The vital signs should be repeated frequently, as autonomic instability can result in fluctuating blood pressure and pulse. Patients should be questioned about the presence of visual or auditory hallucinations and examined for neuromuscular features of serotonin syndrome. A finger-stick blood sugar should be performed on patients with altered mental state.

Laboratory investigation should focus on excluding other causes of the clinical picture as well as evaluating for potential complications of the serotonin syndrome. A complete blood count, electrolytes, glucose, blood urea nitrogen, creatinine, and urinalysis and creatine kinase (to rule out rhabdomyolysis) are suggested. A coagulation profile, liver function tests, cultures, chest x-ray, head computed tomography scan, and lumbar puncture may be necessary in severely ill or hyperthermic patients to exclude sepsis, cranial trauma, meningitis, and complications such as multiorgan failure and coagulopathy (disseminated intravascular coagulation). Although toxicology testing is unlikely to be of any benefit in the acute management, detecting a serotonergic agent can support the diagnosis when a history of drug ingestion cannot be obtained.

EMERGENCY DEPARTMENT MANAGEMENT

First and foremost, management consists of supportive care. Advanced life-support measures should be instituted, as necessary. Airway control and assisted ventilation may be required in obtunded patients with severe forms of serotonin syndrome to maintain oxygenation and prevent aspiration pneumonia. Patients presenting with agitation, myoclonus, hypertonia, or hyperpyrexia should initially be treated with intravenous benzodiazepines, crystalloids, and external cooling measures. If no response is observed, chemical neuromuscular paralysis with sedation should be used to reduce muscle tone and decrease hyperthermia.[6,7]

Seizures should be treated with intravenous benzodiazepines and barbiturates. Continuous electroencephalographic monitoring should be considered in paralyzed patients with suspected seizures. In milder forms of the syndrome, benzodiazepines can be used in an attempt to reduce anxiety, restlessness, and tremor, but they may be ineffective on their own.[16] Serotonergic medications must be discontinued and avoided. Gastrointestinal decontamination, using activated charcoal, should be considered for patients with acute overdoses.

Serotonin-receptor antagonists can be considered as adjunctive therapy. Cyproheptadine (Periactin), a first-generation antihistamine with 5-HT-1a and 5-HT2 receptor-blocking effects, has been used in a number of cases of serotonin syndrome with apparent success.[12–14,19] It appears to be relatively free of potential major adverse effects. The initial adult dose is 4 to 8 mg, orally or by gastric tube, with repeat doses every 2 to 4 hours until a response is noted. It is then continued at a dose of 4 mg every 6 to 8 hours for a period of 24 hours. The maximum recommended dose is 32 mg in 24 hours. In patients with signs and symptoms of mild-to-moderate severity, a response is typically noted in 1 to 2 hours.[12] Cyproheptadine may not produce an obvious response in severe cases.

Chlorpromazine, a nonspecific serotonin receptor antagonist, has been used successfully in doses of 50 to 100 mg intravenously and intramuscularly.[8,11,19] Administration should be preceded by adequate intravenous fluid hydration to prevent hypotension. Other side effects include anticholinergic effects and dystonic reactions. The use of chlorpromazine in patients with NMS wrongly diagnosed as serotonin syndrome has the potential to worsen this condition. Conversely, the use of bromocriptine, a dopaminergic agonist with indirect serotonergic effects, in the treatment of serotonin syndrome misdiagnosed as NMS may result in worsening of serotonergic symptoms.[9] Other medications used with varying success in the treatment of serotonin syndrome include propranolol, methysergide, and dantrolene.[9,19]

DISPOSITION

Most patients with serotonin syndrome require admission and 12 to 24 hours of close observation and cardiac monitoring in a telemetry or intensive care unit until symptoms and signs resolve. Severe cases or those with evidence of complications require intensive care. In mild forms of the syndrome, symptoms may resolve spontaneously, or following use of a specific serotonin antagonist such as cyproheptadine, in a shorter time. All patients with a history of intentional overdose require psychiatric assessment prior to discharge. The risk of recurrent serotonin syndrome must be weighed against the benefits of therapy and alternative treatments when considering reinstitution of serotonergic medications.

COMMON PITFALLS

- Failure to appreciate the variety of drugs with serotonergic activity and to take a detailed history of recent drug exposure
- Failure to recognize the serotonin syndrome and to exclude other conditions causing similar signs and symptoms
- Failure to provide aggressive supportive care; overreliance on antidotal therapies

- Prescribing meperidine for pain relief or dextromethorphan as a cough suppressant to patients taking serotonergic medications, particularly MAOIs

References

1. Baetz M, Malcolm D. Serotonin syndrome from fluvoxamine and buspirone [Letter]. *Can J Psychiatry* 1995;40:428–429.
2. Brodribb TR, Downey M, Gilbar PJ. Efficacy and adverse effects of moclobemide [Letter]. *Lancet* 1994;343:475.
3. Chan BS, Graudins A, Whyte IM, et al. Serotonin syndrome resulting from drug interactions. *Med J Aust* 1998;169:523–525.
4. Chan BS, Graudins A, Braitberg G, et al. A survey of serotonin syndrome by the New South Wales Poison Information Centre. *Proc Aust Soc Exp Clin Pharmacol* 1997;4:63.
5. Daniels RJ. Serotonin syndrome due to venlafaxine overdose. *J Accid Emerg Med* 1998;15:333–334.
6. Francois B, Marquet P, Desachy A, et al. Serotonin syndrome due to an overdose of moclobemide and clomipramine. A potentially life-threatening association. *Intensive Care Med* 1997;23:122–124.
7. Gillman PK. Possible serotonin syndrome with moclobemide and pethidine [Letter]. *Med J Aust* 1995;162:554.
8. Gillman PK. Successful treatment of serotonin syndrome with chlorpromazine [Letter]. *Med J Aust* 1996;165:345.
9. Gillman PK. Ecstasy, serotonin syndrome and the treatment of hyperpyrexia. *Med J Aust* 1997;197:109–110.
10. Goodwin GM, DeSouza RJ, Green AR. The pharmacology of the behavioural and hypothermic responses of rats to 8-hydroxy2-(di–propylamino)tetralin (8-OH-DPAT). *Psychopharmacology* 1987;91:506–511.
11. Graham PM. Successful treatment of the toxic serotonin syndrome with chlorpromazine [Letter]. *Med J Aust* 1997;166:166–167.
12. Graudins A, Stearman A, Chan B. Treatment of the serotonin syndrome with cyproheptadine. *J Emerg Med* 1998;16:615–619.
13. Kolecki P. Venlafaxine induced serotonin syndrome occurring after abstinence from phenelzine for more than two weeks [Letter]. *J Toxicol Clin Toxicol* 1997;35:211–212.
14. Lappin RI, Auchinschloss EL. Treatment of serotonin syndrome with cyproheptadine [Letter]. *N Engl J Med* 1994;331:1021–1022.
15. Meyer D, Halfin V. Toxicity secondary to meperidine in patients on monoamine oxidase inhibitors: a case report and critical review. *J Clin Psychopharmacol* 1981;1:319–321.
16. Mills KC. Serotonin syndrome. *Crit Care Clin* 1997;13:763–783.
17. Neuvonen PJ, Pohjola-Sintonen S, Tacke U, et al. Five fatal cases of serotonin syndrome after moclobemide-citalopram or moclobemide-clomipramine overdoses. *Lancet* 1993;342:1419.
18. Saunders-Bush E, Mayer SE. 5-Hydroxytryptamine (serotonin) receptors agonists and antagonists. In: Hardman JG, Limbird LE, eds. *Goodman and Gillman's the pharmacological basis of therapeutics,* 9th ed. New York: McGraw-Hill, 1996:249–263.
19. Sternbach H. The serotonin syndrome. *Am J Psychiatry* 1991;148:705–713.
20. Weiner AL. Meperidine as a potential cause of serotonin syndrome in the emergency department. *Acad Emerg Med* 1999;6(2):156–158.

CHAPTER 371
Sympathomimetic Poisoning

Christine Haller and Paul R. Pentel

The sympathomimetic drugs discussed in this chapter are structural analogues of catecholamines that share their ability to stimulate adrenergic receptors. These drugs are less rapidly metabolized than catecholamines and have half-lives long enough to make oral administration feasible. The activity of sympathomimetics at various adrenergic receptors varies and, in part, explains their clinical uses (Table 371.1). Alpha-mediated vasoconstriction of the nasal mucosa is responsible for decongestion.

TABLE 371.1. Sympathomimetics

Drug	Common Uses
PRESCRIPTION	
Amphetamine, dextroamphetamine, benzphetamine, methamphetamine	Narcolepsy, anorectic agents
Methylphenidate, pemoline	Narcolepsy, attention deficit disorder
Diethylpropion, phenmetrazine, phentermine, phendimetrazine, fenfluramine	Anorectic agents
Terbutaline, albuterol	Bronchodilators
NONPRESCRIPTION	
Ephedrine	Decongestant, bronchodilator
Pseudoephedrine	Decongestant
Phenylpropanolamine	Decongestant, anorectic agent
Propylhexedrine, desoxyephedrine	Inhaled bronchodilator

$Beta_2$ stimulation causes bronchodilation. Anorectic effects are centrally mediated, but the mechanisms involved are unclear. The dopaminergic action of amphetamines may be an important determinant of amphetamine abuse. The cardiovascular toxicity of sympathomimetics is largely due to alpha- and $beta_1$-agonist activity.

Several sympathomimetics occur as optical isomers. Dextroamphetamine is a more potent central nervous system (CNS) stimulant than racemic or *l*-amphetamine. Ephedrine is a more effective bronchodilator than its isomer, pseudoephedrine. Phenylpropanolamine (PPA) is a racemic mixture sometimes referred to as *d,l*-norephedrine. *l*-PPA is more active than *d*-PPA in animals, but the relative activities of the isomers in humans are unknown. Some Australian compounds called PPA (and reported as such in the literature) may have been single isomers of PPA or another compound with the same chemical formula, norpseudoephedrine. Literature regarding these compounds must, therefore, be interpreted cautiously.

When used as decongestants, sympathomimetics are usually formulated in combination with antihistamines, anticholinergics, analgesics, or caffeine. Each of these additional drugs may add to the toxicity of sympathomimetic overdose by increasing heart rate or contributing to cardiac dysrhythmias or seizures.

Prescription sympathomimetics, particularly amphetamines, may be abused for their stimulant properties. Toxicity results from excessive doses or prolonged periods of use. Nonprescription (over-the-counter [OTC]) stimulants are often sold illicitly to buyers who think they are getting amphetamine or cocaine. Because their CNS actions are weak compared with amphetamine or cocaine, unpleasant peripheral effects (tremors and tachycardia) or toxicity is common when these drugs are abused for their weak stimulant properties. Sympathomimetic overdose may also result from excessive use of diet pills, inadvertent use of several different OTC products that all contain sympathomimetics, or suicidal ingestion.

Ephedrine and related isomers are the active constituents extracted from botanical *Ephedra* species and sold commercially as *ma huang*. Combinations of ma huang and plant-derived caffeine (e.g., kola nut and guarana), as well as other herbs, such as ginseng and willow bark, are currently marketed as herbal weight loss aids and sold as dietary supplements. Also known as "fat burners," "herbal fen-phen," and "herbal ecstasy," these products are widely promoted and used to stimulate weight loss, increase energy, build strength, and enhance athletic performance. There is no scientific basis to the claim that ephedrine alkaloids derived from a botanical source would have different biologic activity than synthetic compounds. In fact, the toxicity of ephedrine may be greater in combination with caffeine and multiple other ingredients found in herbal supplements because of synergistic effects and alterations in clearance and metabolism. Since 1993, the Food and Drug Administration (FDA) has received more than 800 reports of adverse events associated with the use of ephedrine-containing dietary supplements. Adverse events ranged in severity from insomnia and nervousness to seizures, strokes, cardiac arrhythmias, and death. The FDA has issued a number of public health warnings and proposed requirements for warning statements and dose limits of 8 mg of ephedrine per serving.[16] Approximately 21 states have limited or banned sales of ephedrine-containing products.

Various other forms of, or derivatives of, sympathomimetics are also subject to abuse. "Ice," relatively pure crystalline methamphetamine hydrochloride, is volatile enough that it can be smoked.[13] A naturally occurring amphetamine-like compound, cathinone, is the active substance in khat.[8] The leaves of the khat shrub are commonly chewed in East Africa for their stimulant properties. A derivative, methcathinone (CAT) is a drug of abuse that is growing in use and popularity in the United States and has been classified as a schedule I substance.[7] Many other "designer drug" derivatives of amphetamine have been synthesized; they are psychoactive at lower doses but may produce sympathomimetic effects with overdose (see Chapter 341).

OTC sympathomimetics are usually safe when taken by healthy people in recommended doses, but their therapeutic index is low. Although dose-response relations for toxicity are not well documented, available data suggest that ingestion of as little as four or five times the usual dose may produce toxicity.[5,11] Patients with orthostatic hypotension due to autonomic neuropathy exhibit marked sensitivity to the pressor effect of both prescription and OTC sympathomimetics, even in subtherapeutic doses, and should avoid these drugs. Concurrent use of monoamine oxidase inhibitors may also exaggerate the effects of sympathomimetics.

With chronic use of prescription sympathomimetics such as amphetamine or methylphenidate, considerable tolerance may develop. A toxic dose is therefore difficult to establish. When chronic use is discontinued, users may demonstrate fatigue, hunger, and dysphoria. Unlike withdrawal from sedative–hypnotics, this syndrome poses no medical risk except for the possibility of suicidal depression.

Sympathomimetic toxicity is typically greatest 1 to 4 hours after oral drug ingestion and lasts for 4 to 8 hours, but sustained-release formulations may alter this time course. Onset of toxicity with intravenous use is within minutes. Ephedrine, pseudoephedrine, and PPA are eliminated almost entirely by renal excretion.[20] Because these drugs are weak bases, excretion is quickest when the urine pH is low. At the usual urine pH (5.0 to 6.5), half-lives are about 3 to 6 hours.[10] Renal failure or a very alkaline urine could prolong the duration of toxicity. Amphetamine undergoes both hepatic and renal elimination, and metabolites may contribute to toxicity. The elimination half-life of amphetamine and methamphetamine is 4 to 5 hours when the urine is acidic but considerably longer (up to 20 hours for amphetamine) when it is alkaline.[6]

Sympathomimetic toxicity is primarily mediated by excessive adrenergic stimulation. Hypertension is the most common and most important feature. Hypertension is due primarily to alpha-mediated vasoconstriction and may be aggravated by concomitant $beta_1$-mediated increases in heart rate or cardiac contractility. Hypertension caused by PPA alone is usually accompanied by reflex bradycardia or atrioventricular block; however, coingestion of drugs such as anticholinergic agents that increase heart rate may aggravate hypertension by preventing the reflex slowing of heart rate.[17] Most other sympathomimetics have more $beta_1$ activity than does PPA, and hypertension is usually accompanied by sinus tachycardia. Atrial tachyarrhythmias, premature ventricular beats, and ventricular tachycardia are presumably due to excessive $beta_1$ stimulation.

The mechanisms by which sympathomimetics produce CNS toxicity are less clear. Symptoms of CNS stimulation, including insomnia, agitation, mania, psychosis, and seizures, may result from sympathomimetic triggered release of dopamine and other neurotransmitters in the brain. Hyperthermia is associated with increased heat production caused by agitation or seizures, and impaired heat loss is caused by cutaneous vasoconstriction. Toxicity may rarely result from contaminants of illicitly synthesized drugs, as in one episode of lead poisoning from methamphetamine.[1]

CLINICAL PRESENTATION

The most common life-threatening toxic effect of sympathomimetics is hypertension. If severe, hypertension may result in headache, hypertensive encephalopathy, or intracerebral hemorrhage.[4,9] However, hypertension may be asymptomatic, even at blood pressures that require urgent treatment. Most deaths from sympathomimetic overdose are due to hypertensive intracerebral hemorrhage. Dysrhythmias include sinus or supraventricular tachycardia, premature ventricular beats, and ventricular tachycardia.[19] Patients may present with palpitations or with hypotension due to hemodynamic compromise. Sympathomimetic overdose may rarely produce transient chest pain, ischemic electrocardiographic (ECG) changes, and elevation of the creatine kinase MB isoenzyme, simulating myocardial infarction.[18] This lesion may be due to diffuse myocardial necrosis rather than to focal coronary artery disease. Chronic intravenous use of propylhexedrine has been associated with cardiomyopathy and biventricular congestive heart failure.[3]

CNS toxicity of amphetamine overdose includes anxiety, agitation, confusion, psychosis, and seizures.[14,] Psychotic behavior usually occurs during drug use but has been noted to persist during abstinence in chronic amphetamine abusers. Seizures have been reported when overdoses of OTC sympathomimetics are taken in combination with antihistamines or caffeine.[15] Patients may present with focal neurologic signs or symptoms, most commonly caused by intracerebral hemorrhage. Several cases of ischemic stroke with angiographic changes suggestive of cerebral vasculitis have been reported in patients taking amphetamine or PPA.[12] Chronic amphetamine abuse has also been associated with renal or systemic vasculitis, mimicking polyarteritis nodosa.[2] The mechanisms of these toxic effects are unknown.

Pupils may be dilated or normal. Hyperthermia is most common in patients who are agitated, active, or seizing. Rhabdomyolysis and myoglobinuric renal failure may occur due to these same factors.

DIFFERENTIAL DIAGNOSIS

The dominant feature of sympathomimetic overdose is hypertension. Differentiation from essential hypertension is important, because patients with sympathomimetic overdose are at risk for intracerebral hemorrhage at blood pressures much lower than those of patients with accelerated or malignant hypertension of other causes (see Emergency Department Management section). Essential hypertension can be distinguished by history or the finding of funduscopic changes indicative of long-standing hypertension. Patients with acute cerebrovascular accidents may have secondary hypertension. These patients may be recognized by the finding of focal neurologic deficits, or focal lesions on a head computed tomography (CT) scan. Diagnosis of a cerebrovascular accident is important, because treatment of hypertension in patients with ischemic stroke may worsen the neurologic deficit, and may be contraindicated. Other causes of drug-induced hypertension include cocaine poisoning, phencyclidine poisoning, monoamine oxidase inhibitor interactions with drugs or food, tricyclic antidepressant or anticholinergic overdoses, clonidine withdrawal (or, rarely, overdose), and alcohol or sedative–hypnotic withdrawal syndromes.

Headache is a common, nonspecific finding in patients with sympathomimetic-induced hypertension, but it may also be due to intracerebral hemorrhage. Seizures may also occur as a direct toxic effect or due to secondary complications such as intracerebral hemorrhage.

EMERGENCY DEPARTMENT EVALUATION

Sympathomimetic toxicity should be considered in patients with unexplained hypertension, dysrhythmias, or CNS stimulation. Blood pressure monitoring is essential. Core temperature should be measured immediately. A 12-lead ECG should be obtained and continuous cardiac monitoring instituted. The physical examination is directed toward evaluating the optic fundi and performing a neurologic examination. Laboratory evaluation should include electrolytes, blood urea nitrogen, creatinine, glucose, creatine kinase, and urinalysis. If intracerebral hemorrhage is suspected because of focal neurologic findings, seizures, a depressed level of consciousness, severe headache, or headache that persists after hypertension resolves, a head CT scan is indicated. Most sympathomimetics can be detected in urine by thin-layer chromatography or enzyme-multiplied immunoassay technique (EMIT). Methods for measuring serum concentrations are not usually available.

EMERGENCY DEPARTMENT MANAGEMENT

Initial management is directed at treating severe hypertension, life-threatening dysrhythmias, seizures, and hyperthermia. This should take precedence over gastric decontamination or a head CT scan. Patients with sympathomimetic overdose usually do not have chronic hypertension, nor do they have the shift in cerebral blood flow autoregulation that allows patients with chronic hypertension to tolerate very high blood pressures. Encephalopathy or intracerebral hemorrhage may therefore develop with blood pressures as low as 170 mm Hg systolic or 110 mm Hg diastolic. A blood pressure exceeding these values should be treated as an emergency, with a goal of lowering the blood pressure to less than 170/110 mm Hg within 15 minutes. This can be done with intravenous nitroprusside (0.5 to 5.0 μg/kg/min) or phentolamine (1- to 5-mg bolus initially, repeated at 5- to 10-minute intervals as needed). If intravenous access cannot be established rapidly, "sublingual" or chewed nifedipine is an alternative. Propranolol is not recommended as a single agent for treatment of hypertension caused by sympathomimetics, because paradoxical worsening of the hypertension may result from blockade of $beta_2$-mediated vasodilatation. Supraventricular tachycardias seldom require therapy. Premature ventricular beats or ventricular tachycardia may be treated with the short-acting $beta_1$-selective blocker esmolol (loading dose 500 μg/kg; maintenance dose 50 to 100 μg/kg/min intravenously). Reflex bradycardia or atrioventricular block in patients with PPA overdose is a normal response that serves to limit hypertension; reversal of the bradycardia (e.g., with atropine) can worsen hypertension and is not indicated. Hyperthermia may be managed by sedation or paralysis to decrease heat production, and active external cooling with sponge bathing and evaporative cooling.

Agitation or psychotic behavior does not usually necessitate drug therapy but may be managed with intravenous benzodiazepines (diazepam 0.1 to 0.2 mg/kg, lorazepam 0.05 to 0.1 mg/kg, midazolam 0.02 to 0.05 mg/kg, or haloperidol 2 to 5 mg in adults), if needed, with a goal of calming the patient but not obscuring the neurologic examination. Seizures may be treated with a benzodiazepine, although data regarding efficacy are lacking.

Gastric decontamination is best accomplished with oral activated charcoal. Gastric lavage may be indicated for patients with massive, recent ingestions, but it should be performed only after initial treatment to lower the blood pressure. Urine acidification is not usually needed, because the normal urine pH is normally already low and because toxicity is normally brief and can be managed with the previously mentioned measures.[4] Moreover, if rhabdomyolysis occurs, acidification of the urine may aggravate renal injury. For similar reasons, there is little benefit from hemodialysis or hemoperfusion for sympathomimetic toxicity.

DISPOSITION

When toxicity resolves, monitoring is no longer needed, and admission is indicated only for evaluation or management of concurrent psychiatric diagnoses. Patients with mild signs or symptoms may be monitored in the emergency department, because the duration of toxicity is often brief. Patients with persistent or severe hypertension, dysrhythmias, or CNS stimulation should be monitored in a medical intensive care unit. Patients with headache or neurologic signs that persist when hypertension resolves may need an urgent CT scan of the head and neurologic consultation.

COMMON PITFALLS

- Failure to measure the temperature in seizing or agitated patients and to diagnose and treat hyperthermia
- Failure to evaluate symptomatic patients, especially those with agitation, hyperactivity, seizures, hyperthermia, and vital signs abnormalities, for the presence of rhabdomyolysis
- Failure to appreciate that persistent headache, even without focal signs or symptoms, may be due to intracerebral hemorrhage and should be evaluated with a CT scan of the head
- Failure to appreciate that a blood pressure above 170/110 mm Hg in a previously normotensive person should be treated as an emergency
- Failure to appreciate that bradycardia or atrioventricular block in patients with hypertension due to PPA is a normal (reflex) response that serves to limit hypertension and that treatment with atropine will probably aggravate hypertension and is not indicated
- Failure to inquire about the use of herbal remedies or dietary supplements as part of the medication history

References

1. Anonymous. Lead poisoning associated with intravenous methamphetamine use—Oregon, 1988. *MMWR* 1989;38:830.
2. Citron BP, Halpern M, McCarron M, et al. Necrotizing angiitis associated with drug abuse. *N Engl J Med* 1970;283:1003.
3. Croft CH, Firth BG, Hillis LD. Propylhexedrine-induced left ventricular dysfunction. *Ann Intern Med* 1982;97:560.
4. Delaney P, Estes M. Intracranial hemorrhage with amphetamine abuse. *Neurology* 1980;30:1125.
5. Drew CDM, Knight GT, Hughes DTD, et al. Comparison of the effects of D-(−) ephedrine and L-(pl)-pseudoephedrine on the cardiovascular and respiratory systems in man. *Br J Clin Pharmacol* 1978;6:221.
6. Gunne LM, Anggard E. Pharmacokinetic studies with amphetamines—relationship to neuropsychiatric disorders. *J Pharmacokinet Biopharm* 1973;1:481.
7. Gygi MP, Gibb JW, Hanson GR. Methcathinone: an initial study of its effects on monoaminergic systems. *J Pharmacol Exp Ther* 1996;276(3):1066–1072.
8. Kalix P. Catha edulis, a plant that has amphetamine effects. *Pharm World Sci* 1996;18(2):69–73.
9. Kizer KW. Intracranial hemorrhage associated with overdose of decongestant containing phenylpropanolamine. *Am J Emerg Med* 1986;2:180.
10. Lonnerholm G, Grahnen A, Lindstrom B. Steady-state kinetics of sustained-release phenylpropanolamine. *Int J Clin Pharmacol Ther Toxicol* 1984;22:39.
11. MacNab MW, Seaman JJ, Schumann PR, et al. Phenylpropanolamine HCl and blood pressure. *Clin Pharmacol Ther* 1988;43:163(abst).
12. Matick H, Anderson D, Brumlik J. Cerebral vasculitis associated with oral amphetamine overdose. *Arch Neurol* 1983;40:253.
13. Meng Y, Dukat M, Bridgen DT, et al. Pharmacological effects of methamphetamine and other stimulants via inhalation exposure. *Drug Alcohol Depend* 1999;53(2):111–120.
14. Mueller SM. Neurologic complications of phenylpropanolamine use. *Neurology* 1983;33:650.
15. Mueller SM, Solow EB. Seizures associated with a new combination "pick-me-up" pill. *Ann Neurol* 1982;11:322.
16. Nightingale SL. New safety measures are proposed for dietary supplements containing ephedrine alkaloids. *JAMA* 1997;278(1):15.
17. Pentel PR, Mikell F. Reaction to phenylpropanolamine-chlorpheniramine-belladonna compound in a woman with unrecognized autonomic dysfunction. *Lancet* 1982;1:274.
18. Pentel PR, Mikell FL, Zavoral JH. Myocardial injury after phenylpropanolamine ingestion. *Br Heart J* 1982;47:51.
19. Peterson RB, Vasquez LA. Phenylpropanolamine-induced arrhythmias. *JAMA* 1973;233:324.
20. Wilkinson GR, Beckett AH. Absorption, metabolism and excretion of the ephedrines in man. I. The influence of urinary pH and urine volume output. *J Pharmacol Exp Ther* 1968;162:139.

CHAPTER 372
Terpene Poisoning

Louis J. Ling

Terpenes are a class of unsaturated, aliphatic cyclic hydrocarbons. These volatile substances are found naturally in oils and oleoresins of plants and flowers. Camphor, pine oils, and turpentine are the most common terpenes involved in poisoning. Terpenes also are present in volatile oils of plants (see Chapter 365).

Camphor, a naturally occurring cyclic ketone obtained from the camphor tree or synthesized from turpentine oil, has minimal medicinal value[1] but is still widely available in up to a 10% concentration in over-the-counter products. It is used as a rubefacient in external analgesic rubs, causing vasodilatation and a sensation of warmth. When inhaled, it causes a cooling sensation, and the odor gives a strong, reassuring effect. Turpentine is a pine tree distillate consisting of pinene, diterpenes, and other terpenes. It is commonly used as a thinner for paints and varnishes. Pine oils contain a variety of terpene alcohols and are found in household cleaners (e.g., Pine Sol) in concentrations of up to 20% to 35%. The toxicity of naphthalene, a terpene found in mothballs, is discussed in Chapter 316.

Camphor is well absorbed orally. Absorption also may occur through the skin.[18] It is classified as very toxic (class 4); lethal doses in humans range from 50 to 500 mg/kg.[11] The smallest lethal dose was reported in a 19-month-old child, who died after a 1-g ingestion,[3] but an adult has survived after ingesting 42 g.[12] Typically, ingestions of 10 to 30 mg/kg—equivalent to one swallow of camphorated oil—may result in minor symptoms. Major symptoms are uncommon with ingestions below 50 mg/kg.[8] The acute toxic dose of turpentine has never been well defined, and case reports have given a wide range of effects; vomiting makes dose estimates unreliable. Gastrointestinal (GI) symptoms have occurred in children after ingestions of 15 to 60 mL, and 120 to 180 mL is a potentially lethal dose in adults.[6] Turpentine ingestions of more than 2 mL/kg should be considered potentially toxic.[6] Pine oils have about one-fifth the toxicity of turpentine in animals,[2] and a suggested lethal dose for adults is 60 to 120 g,[15] although survival after a 400-mL ingestion has been reported.[6]

Camphorated oil, with 20% camphor, was removed from the market in 1982, and camphor products are now limited to 11%. Turpentine is highly volatile. Vapors are easily inhaled, and aspiration of the liquid may occur during ingestion. It is well absorbed from the GI tract.[10] Most ingestions are accidental and involve small amounts. It is rare to see toxicity from GI absorption of pine oil, but aspiration is a common problem.

CLINICAL PRESENTATION

Patients with terpene ingestion frequently have a strong odor of camphor, turpentine, or pine oil on the breath, in vomitus, or in the urine. Mild camphor poisoning results in GI symptoms such as nausea, vomiting, and a burning sensation in the mouth, esophagus, and stomach. In some cases, central nervous system (CNS) toxicity initially presents as stimulation and restlessness. CNS depression with delirium, hallucinations, confusion, muscle irritability, and seizures may follow.[1] Symptoms can occur as soon as 5 to 30 minutes after ingestion,[19] and seizures have occurred as soon as 4 minutes after ingestion.[18]

Turpentine causes similar GI irritation and CNS symptoms; however, seizures appear to be less common than with camphor. Direct skin contact with turpentine can be irritating. A single case of acute renal failure and hemorrhagic cystitis several days after ingestion has been reported.[13] Turpentine has been implicated in the pathogenesis of thrombocytopenic purpura.[20]

The breath odor of a patient with pine oil ingestion is characteristically violet-like, from the metabolites that are excreted in exhaled air.[15] Patients usually present with gastroenteral symptoms and respiratory symptoms from aspiration. CNS toxicity (e.g., somnolence, ataxia) is usually mild and develops within 90 minutes. Ataxia is much more common in children, but lethargy and coma may be present in children or adults.[3] Facial erythema has been reported.[15] Renal failure is rare.

Patients with camphor poisoning may show a transient leukocytosis and modest abnormalities on liver function tests.[19] Hepatotoxicity has also been reported after massive pine oil ingestions.[19] Patients who ingest turpentine or pine oil may have concomitant aspiration and resultant respiratory symptoms (see Chapter 362).

DIFFERENTIAL DIAGNOSIS

If the history is vague or unavailable, the odor of the patient's breath, vomitus, or urine may be a valuable diagnostic clue.

Naphthalene, paradichlorobenzene, and other volatile oils have a vaguely similar aroma.

EMERGENCY DEPARTMENT EVALUATION

As in all toxic exposures, the product name and contents, the amount ingested, the time since exposure, and symptoms must be sought. Physical examination should focus on CNS and GI symptoms. Patients should be assessed for signs and symptoms of aspiration (see Chapter 362).[17] Any emesis should be tested for blood. Routine laboratory studies for symptomatic patients include a baseline complete blood count with platelets; determination of electrolyte, blood urea nitrogen, creatinine, and glucose levels; and urinalysis. Arterial blood gas analysis or oxygen saturation measurement and chest radiography should be performed if aspiration is suspected (see Chapter 362).

EMERGENCY DEPARTMENT MANAGEMENT

Because the onset of seizures and pulmonary toxicity may be rapid with camphor, an ambulance should be used to transport these patients.[19] Advanced life-support measures are instituted, as necessary. Patients who are symptomatic and have ingested more than 2 g[18] or 30 mg/kg of camphor[6] or 2 mL/kg of turpentine[6] should have gastric emptying. Because of the risk of aspiration with CNS depression and seizures, syrup of ipecac should not be used after camphor ingestion. Gastric lavage very early after ingestion may be considered.[19] A small tube may be adequate for a liquid preparation. Activated charcoal has not absorbed camphor well in animals.[4] Terpenes have hydrocarbon characteristics, which make them unlikely to be absorbed by activated charcoal.[4,19] Mineral oil and vegetable oil were formerly recommended as solvents or cathartics for camphor, but because their use may increase the risk of aspiration and enhance the absorption of camphor, they are no longer recommended.[15]

Renal, hepatic, and bone marrow complications are treated supportively. Lipid hemodialysis against soybean oil[9] and Amberlite resin hemoperfusion[14] have been used in patients with severe camphor poisoning. These measures are not of benefit in patients who have ingested pine oil because of its large volume of distribution.[15] Patients with pine oil aspiration recover faster; these aspirations are not as serious as other hydrocarbon aspirations.[3]

DISPOSITION

Patients who remain asymptomatic or have only mild GI symptoms during the 6 hours after ingestion are at low risk for serious complications and may be discharged.[8,15] Patients with systemic symptoms, those with aspiration with persistent or progressive symptoms,[16] and those who have clearly ingested more than 3 g of camphor should be admitted for observation.[15] Patients with seizures or CNS depression should be admitted to an intensive care unit. Symptomatic patients should also be monitored for hematologic, renal, and hepatic complications. Patients with persistent seizures or coma after camphor ingestion should be considered for hemodialysis or hemoperfusion. Although rare deaths have been reported, patients with pine oil ingestion should be expected to recover readily with minimal supportive care.[3,7]

COMMON PITFALLS

- Failure to appreciate that small amounts of camphor may be toxic (e.g., a swallow of 10% camphor)
- Failure to establish intravenous access and to be prepared to treat seizures, which can occur early and without warning
- Failure to recognize the risk of aspiration with syrup of ipecac or gastric lavage
- Failure to check hematologic, renal, and hepatic function parameters in symptomatic patients
- Failure to advise patients who are discharged to return if any respiratory symptoms develop

References

1. Aronow R. Camphor poisoning [Editorial]. *JAMA* 1976;235:1260.
2. Beamon RF, Siegel CJ, Landers G, et al. Hydrocarbon ingestion in children: a 6-year retrospective study. *J Am Coll Emerg Physicians* 1976;5:771.
3. Brook MP, McCarron MM, Mueller JA. Pine oil cleaner ingestion. *Ann Emerg Med* 1985;18:391.
4. Cooney DO. *Activated charcoal in medical applications*. New York: Marcel Dekker Inc, 1995:28.
5. Dean BS, Burdick JD, Beotz CM, et al. In vivo evaluation of the adsorptive capacity of activated charcoal for camphor. *Vet Hum Toxicol* 1992;34:297.
6. Ellenhorn MJ. Household poisonings. In: Ellenhorn MJ, Schonwald S, Ordog B, et al., eds. *Ellenhorn's medical toxicology*. Baltimore: Williams & Wilkins, 1997:1081.
7. Erickson T, Popiel R, Hyrhorczuk DO, et al. Pine oil cleaners in prison. *Ann Emerg Med* 1990;19:445.
8. Geller RJ, Spyker DA, Garrettson LK, et al. Camphor toxicity: development of a triage strategy. *Vet Hum Toxicol* 1984;2[Suppl 2]:8.
9. Ginn HE, Anderson KE, Mercier RK, et al. Camphor intoxication treated by lipid dialysis. *JAMA* 1968;203:164.
10. Goldfrank LR. Camphor and moth repellants. In: Goldfrank LR, Lewin NA, et al., eds. *Goldfrank's toxicologic emergencies*, 6th ed. Stamford, CT: Appleton & Lange, 1998:1377–1381.
11. Gosselin RE, Smith RP, Hodge HC. *Clinical toxicology of commercial products*, 5th ed. Baltimore: Williams & Wilkins, 1984.
12. Haft HH. Camphor liniment poisoning. *JAMA* 1925;84:1571.
13. Klein FA, Hackler RH. Hemorrhagic cystitis associated with turpentine ingestion. *Urology* 1980;16:187.
14. Kopelman R, Miller S, Kelly, et al. Camphor intoxication treated by resin hemoperfusion. *JAMA* 1972;241:727.
15. Koppel C, Tenczer J, Tonnesmann U, et al. Acute poisoning with pine oil—metabolism of monoterpenes. *Arch Toxicol* 1981;49:73.
16. Machado B, Cross K, Snodgrass WR. Accidental hydrocarbon ingestion cases telephoned to a regional poison center. *Ann Emerg Med* 1988;17:804.
17. Ng RC, Darwish H, Stewart DA. Emergency treatment of petroleum distillate and turpentine ingestion. *Can Med Assoc J* 1974;111:537.
18. Siegel E, Wason S. Camphor toxicity. *Pediatr Clin North Am* 1986;33:375.
19. Sue YJ, Pinkert H. Baby powder, borates and camphor. In: Haddad LR, Shannon MW, Winchester JF, eds. *Poisoning and drug overdose*, 3rd ed. Philadelphia: WB Saunders, 1998:1161–1168.
20. Wahlberg P, Nyman D. Turpentine and thrombocytopenic purpura [Letter]. *Lancet* 1969;2:215.

CHAPTER 373

Thyroid Hormone Poisoning

Milton Tennenbein

Thyroid hormones are used as replacement therapy for hypothyroid states and as pituitary suppressants in the treatment or prevention of euthyroid goiters. The two available types are tetraiodothyronine (thyroxine, or T_4) and triiodothyronine (T_3). A given preparation may be of natural (beef or pork thyroid extract) or synthetic origin and contain one or both of these hormones (Table 373.1).

TABLE 373.1. Thyroid Hormone Preparations

Thyroid Preparation	Thyroid Hormone Content
NATURAL PREPARATIONS	
Thyroid extract	T_4, T_3
Armour thyroid (USV)	
S-P-T (Fleming)	
Thyroglobulin	T_4, T_3
Proloid (Parke-Davis)	
SYNTHETIC PREPARATIONS	
Levothyroxine sodium	T_4
Synthroid (Flint)	
Levothyroid (USV)	
Liothyronine sodium	T_3
Cytomel (SKF)	
Liotrix	T_4, T_3 (4:1)
Euthroid (Parke-Davis)	
Thyrolar (USV)	

In addition to being important in the regulation of growth and development, thyroid hormones increase heat production and oxygen consumption by body tissues and stimulate the cardiovascular system. The usual daily adult replacement dose is 100 to 300 μg of T_4, 25 to 75 μg of T_3, and 60 to 180 mg of thyroid extract or its liotrix equivalent. The normal serum concentration is 4 to 12 μg/dL for T_4 and 110 to 250 ng/dL for T_3. T_3 is well absorbed from the stomach (greater than 90%), but the absorption of T_4 is less efficient (50% to 90%). Peripheral tissues convert T_4 to T_3, the metabolically active thyroid hormone. More than 99% of circulating thyroid hormones are metabolized by deiodination; most of the remainder are conjugated before excretion, with some being excreted intact. The half-life of a therapeutic dose of T_4 is 4 to 7 days; it is about 1 day for T_3.

Acute oral overdose of thyroid hormones seldom produces serious toxicity, and no deaths have been reported. Thus, the minimal toxic and lethal doses are unknown, and there is no correlation between serum T_4 concentration and clinical severity. Children are resistant to the effects of large overdoses.[20] Elderly patients with compromised cardiovascular function may be more sensitive, but there are no data to support this speculation.

To assess toxic risk, it is important to differentiate between the different types of thyroid hormone supplements. Because T_3 is the active thyroid hormone, acute toxicity would be predicted. Only one case of its ingestion has been reported,[4] and although the onset of toxicity was within a few hours, it was minor and of brief duration (12 hours) despite a documented serum concentration 50 times normal. Eighty tablets were ingested (or 80 therapeutic doses); this patient coingested significant amounts of an antidepressant and an antihistamine, which may have contributed to the observed toxicity.

In contrast, T_4 overdose is relatively common.[6,8,10,11,13,14,17,20] There has been no evidence of toxicity in children who have ingested up to 1.5 mg of T_4.[14] Ingestions of up to 30 mg have produced negligible toxicity,[20] as have serum T_4 concentrations of 84.7[20] and 90 μg/dL.[17] Thus, there is a large tolerance for acute massive ingestion of levothyroxine. Several factors contribute to this inherent low toxicity. Conversion of T_4 to T_3 takes several days, and is regulated by a negative-feedback loop. The presence of excess T_4 inhibits endogenous secretion of this hormone, inhibits the peripheral conversion of T_4 to T_3,[2] increases the disposal rates of both T_4 and T_3,[2] and downregulates the T_3 nuclear receptors.[19] Also, elevation of serum concentrations of reverse T_3 (an inhibitor of thyroid hormones) has been observed in two T_4 overdose patients.[11,16] Therefore, it is expected that the occurrence of toxicity would be less likely and its onset later (several days).

The only reported case of serious toxicity occurred in a 2-year-old boy who took 18 mg of levothyroxine.[10] At about 6 hours after ingestion, his serum thyroxine concentration was 117.4 μg/dL, and he had two seizures 7 days later. There have been reports of minor toxicities such as asymptomatic tachycardia, low-grade fever, diarrhea, and hyperactivity.[6,8,13,14]

The ingestion of products that contain both T_3 and T_4 may theoretically result in biphasic toxicity with early (within hours) and late (after several days) phases. In fact, only one of the six reported patients with acute combined overdose developed significant toxicity.[5,9,12] This 15-month-old boy was seriously ill within 6 hours, but asymptomatic by 24 hours.[12]

The repeated ingestion of excessive amounts of thyroid hormones on a daily basis (chronic overdose or abuse) will probably produce toxicity. Overt hyperthyroidism and even death may occur.[1,7,15,18] Such patients may be abusing thyroid hormones to lose weight or because of emotional instability or frank psychiatric illness. They often deny thyroid ingestion.

CLINICAL PRESENTATION

Most patients with acute thyroid overdoses are asymptomatic on presentation, and it is uncommon for signs and symptoms to develop. The few patients who manifest toxicity have the features of hyperthyroidism (fever; tachycardia; warm, moist skin; diarrhea; restlessness; and anxiety). For T_4, the onset is between many hours and several days; for T_3, the onset is within a few hours. However, chronic rather than acute overdose is more likely to produce this picture. Such patients may have virtually all the signs of hyperthyroidism except for exophthalmos.

DIFFERENTIAL DIAGNOSIS

The differential diagnosis of chronic thyroid hormone abuse includes metabolic conditions (e.g., pheochromocytoma and hypoglycemia), central nervous system infection, organic brain syndrome, overdose with psychoactive drugs (e.g., amphetamine, cocaine, anticholinergics, and hallucinogens), acute withdrawal states, and acute psychotic illness. For patients with elevated serum T_4 concentrations, the chief differentiation is from endogenous hyperthyroidism, in which the serum thyroglobulin concentration is elevated. It is depressed in patients with exogenous hyperthyroidism.[15]

EMERGENCY DEPARTMENT EVALUATION

The history includes the identity of the ingestant, the dose, the time of ingestion, symptoms of hyperthyroidism, the reason for ingestion, and prior medical conditions. The identity of the hormones involved is important because of their differing clinical courses after overdose. The physical examination is directed toward eliciting the findings of hyperthyroidism. In the case of acute ingestions, the T_4 concentration is measured 4 to 6 hours after ingestion if the patient has ingested more than 2 mg of levothyroxine or its equivalent. This amount identifies patients who require follow-up; this measurement should be done in all patients with chronic thyroid overdose.

EMERGENCY DEPARTMENT MANAGEMENT

Supportive measures are instituted as necessary. Gastrointestinal decontamination should be considered for patients who have ingested more than 2 mg of thyroxine or its equivalent. For the uncommon patient who develops symptoms after acute ingestion, acetaminophen for fever and propranolol for sympathetic hyperactivity can be considered.[6,8,13] The oral administration of iopanoic acid (Telepaque, 125 mg per day in a 2.5-year-old), an iodine-containing radiocontrast agent that inhibits the conversion of T_4 to T_3, has also been used with apparent success.[3] The use of prophylactic antithyroid therapy (cholestyramine, prednisone, propylthiouracil, and propranolol) in asymptomatic patients is controversial, but experience has demonstrated that it is unnecessary.[6,11,14,20] For the symptomatic patient with chronic thyroid ingestion, thyroid supplements should be discontinued, and the patient should be treated as for endogenous hyperthyroidism and thyroid storm. Enhanced elimination by extracorporeal removal has not been shown to be of benefit.[20]

DISPOSITION

Patients with significant T_3 overdoses (20 therapeutic doses or more) should be admitted to an observation or inpatient unit. Vital signs, cardiac rhythm, and clinical status should be monitored for 12 to 24 hours. Because patients with acute T_4 overdose are at risk only for delayed toxicity, immediate inpatient observation is unnecessary. Toxicity after acute T_4 overdose has not been reported with serum concentrations under 25 μg/dL; daily assessment for the next 10 days is required if this value is exceeded. Symptomatic patients should be treated, as necessary. Patients who present with hyperthyroidism due to chronic abuse usually require admission. Consultation with an endocrinologist is advisable.

COMMON PITFALLS

- Failing to differentiate between T_3 and T_4 overdose
- Failing to differentiate between acute and chronic overdose
- Failing to appreciate that acute overdoses of levothyroxine or thyroid extract may result in delayed toxicity. Arrangements should be made for close follow-up.
- Using overzealous therapy (prophylactic antithyroid drugs, extracorporeal removal) in asymptomatic patients

References

1. Bhasin S, Wallace W, Lawrence JB, et al. Sudden death associated with thyroid hormone abuse. *Am J Med* 1981;71:887.
2. Braverman LE, Vagenakis A, Downs P, et al. Effects of replacement doses of sodium l-thyroxine on the peripheral metabolism of thyroxine and triiodothyronine in man. *J Clin Invest* 1973;52:1010.
3. Brown RS, Cohen JH, Braverman LE. Successful treatment of massive thyroid hormone poisoning with iopanoic acid. *J Pediatr* 1998;132:903.
4. Dahlberg PA, Karlsson FA, Wide L. Triiodothyronine intoxication. *Lancet* 1979;2:700.
5. Gerard P, Malvaux P, de Visscher M. Accidental poisoning with thyroid extract treated by exchange transfusion. *Arch Dis Child* 1972;47:980.
6. Golightly LK, Smolinske SC, Kulig KW, et al. Clinical effects of accidental levothyroxine ingestion in children. *Am J Dis Child* 1987;141:1025.
7. Gorman CA, Wahner HW, Tauxe WN. Metabolic malingerers: patients who deliberately induce or perpetuate a hypermetabolic or hypometabolic state. *Am J Med* 1970;48:708.
8. Gorman RL, Chamberlain JM, Rose SR, et al. Massive levothyroxine overdose: high anxiety—low toxicity. *Pediatrics* 1988;82:666.
9. Jahr HM. Thyroid "poisoning" in children. *Nebr State Med J* 1936;21:388.
10. Kulig K, Golightly LK, Rumack BH. Levothyroxine overdose associated with seizures in a young child. *JAMA* 1985;254:2109.
11. Lehrner LM, Weir MR. Acute ingestions of thyroid hormones. *Pediatrics* 1984;73:313.
12. Levy RP, Gilger WG. Acute thyroid poisoning. *N Engl J Med* 1957;256:459.
13. Lewander WJ, Lacouture PG, Silva JE, et al. Acute thyroid ingestion in pediatric patients. *Pediatrics* 1989;84:262.
14. Litovitz TL, White JD. Levothyroxine ingestions in children: an analysis of 78 cases. *Am J Emerg Med* 1985;3:297.
15. Mariotti S, Martino E, Cupini C, et al. Low serum thyroglobulin as a clue to the diagnosis of thyrotoxicosis factitia. *N Engl J Med* 1982;307:410.
16. Nystrom E, Lindstedt G, Lindbert PA. Minor signs and symptoms of toxicity in a young woman in spite of massive thyroxine ingestion. *Acta Med Scand* 1980;207:135.
17. Roesch C, Becker PG, Sklar S. Management of a child with acute thyroxine ingestion. *Ann Emerg Med* 1985;14:1114.
18. Rose E, Sanders TP, Webb WL Jr, et al. Occult factitial thyrotoxicosis—thyroxine kinetics and psychological evaluation in three cases. *Ann Intern Med* 1969;71:309.
19. Samuels HH, Stanley F, Shapiro LE. Dose-dependent depletion of nuclear receptors by l-triiodothyronine: evidence for a role in induction of growth hormone synthesis in cultured GH_1 cells. *Proc Natl Acad Sci U S A* 1976;73:3877.
20. Tenenbein M, Dean HJ. Benign course after massive levothyroxine ingestion. *Pediatr Emerg Care* 1986;2:15.

CHAPTER 374
Valproate Poisoning

Gregory G. Gaar

Valproic acid, valproate sodium, and divalproex sodium are used either alone or in combination with other anticonvulsants primarily in the treatment of absence seizures, both simple and complex. Although not currently included in the labeling approved by the Food and Drug Administration, they are also used to treat temporal lobe seizures, myoclonic seizures, and generalized tonic–clonic seizures. They are now approved for use in the treatment of migraine headaches and the manic phase of bipolar illness.

The compounds are carboxylic acid derivatives that differ structurally from any of the other commercially available anticonvulsants.[14] Although valproic acid's mechanism of action has not been fully elucidated, it is believed to exert some effects through modulation of levels of gamma-aminobutyric acid (GABA), an inhibitory central nervous system (CNS) neurotransmitter.

In the United States, forms for oral use include capsules of valproic acid (250 mg), a solution of valproate sodium (250 mg valproic acid per 5 mL), a "sprinkle capsule" containing coated granules of divalproex sodium (equivalent to 125 mg of valproic acid), and enteric-coated tablets of divalproex sodium (equivalent to 125, 250, and 500 mg of valproic acid).[14] Depakene and Depakote are the most widely used brands of valproate sodium and divalproex sodium, respectively. The initial starting dosage is 15 mg/kg/d (maximum, 600 mg/d). Once weekly, the dosage may be increased by 5 to 10 mg/kg/d until adequate seizure control is established or adverse effects necessitate smaller dosages. The manufacturer does not recommend a dosage of more than 60 mg/kg/d. Although definite therapeutic or toxic serum levels have not been established, it is generally accepted that therapeutic concentrations are in the range of 50 to 100 μg/mL.[14]

Absorption of valproic acid is rapid and complete from either capsule or solution formulation. Although valproate sodium must be converted to valproic acid to be absorbed, this reaction occurs rapidly in the stomach. Peak plasma concentrations occur within 1 to 4 hours of a single oral dose of valproic acid. Food in the gastrointestinal (GI) tract decreases the rate of absorption but not the total amount.[14,] When enteric-coated tablet or granule preparations are used, the compound must dissociate into valproate in the jejunum before absorption can occur.

The enteric coating slows this process, so the peak plasma level occurs later, usually within 3 to 5 hours of a single oral dose.[7,14]

The volume of distribution ranges from 0.1 to 0.4 L/kg.[14] Therefore, distribution is mostly into plasma and extracellular water. Protein-binding is significant in the therapeutic range; at concentrations of 80 μg/mL, almost 90% is bound to proteins.[7,14] At concentrations above 100 μg/mL, saturation of these proteins occurs and the percentage of drug bound to plasma protein decreases.[14] Accordingly, after the acute ingestion of toxic amounts, the percentage of circulating "free" drug increases markedly.[8]

The elimination half-life ranges from 7 to 15 hours.[7,14] Valproic acid is metabolized by the liver; the metabolites are usually conjugated with glucuronide and then eliminated in the urine. Small amounts of drug are excreted unchanged in the urine and feces.[14] Other antiepileptic drugs used concomitantly can alter the half-life of valproic acid, usually reducing it.[7] In contrast, concomitant use of valproate may inhibit the metabolism of phenobarbital and increase phenobarbital levels.[11]

Valproic acid can be toxic both after acute overdoses and during chronic therapy. In acute ingestion, there are no absolute guidelines for predicting toxicity based on the amount ingested. A 19-month-old infant survived an ingestion of 204 mg/kg, with a serum drug level of 185 μg/mL, and adults have recovered from ingesting as much as 75 g.[9,13,16] In one large series, patients were likely to be unconscious only after ingesting more than 200 mg/kg.[9] Death from complications of pneumonia has been reported after an ingestion of 15 g (705 mg/kg) in a 20-month-old boy.[17]

Toxic manifestations have occurred during chronic use at therapeutic dosages. Blood levels above 100 μg/mL may cause unusual neurologic effects or potentiate seizures. Dosages of 2.2 to 2.5 g/d have caused CNS effects.[6] Hepatotoxicity can occur with chronic therapy and may be fatal.[5] Hyperammonemia and hyperglycinemia have occurred secondary to inhibition of enzymes involved in intermediate cell metabolism, independent of hepatotoxicity. Acute pancreatitis is rare.[3]

CLINICAL PRESENTATION

The predominant symptoms and signs of toxicity after acute overdosage with valproate relate to the CNS. Drowsiness, confusion, and change in mental status are the most common.[6,13] Coma may ensue, with subsequent respiratory failure.[9,13,17] Seizures and myoclonic movements have been reported.[9] Pupils may be pinpoint and sluggishly reactive to light.[1] GI toxicity includes nausea, vomiting, and diarrhea. Hypotension and cardiorespiratory arrest are rare.[17]

Toxicity during chronic valproate usage includes mental status changes such as drowsiness, confusion, and social withdrawal.[6] Nausea, emesis, and abdominal pain have been observed. Elevated liver enzyme levels, hepatocellular necrosis, and fatal cholestatic hepatitis are rare. Hyperammonemia has been noted.[12] Hematologically, thrombocytopenia and impaired platelet aggregation have been seen.

DIFFERENTIAL DIAGNOSIS

The differential diagnosis of a patient with impaired mental status due to the acute ingestion of a toxic amount of valproate includes trauma, hypoglycemia, hypoxia, other toxins (barbiturates, opiates, tricyclic antidepressants), infections, metabolic disorders (diabetic ketoacidosis and Reye syndrome), intracranial tumors, and the postictal state. An elevated serum valproate level and the exclusion of other causes confirm the diagnosis.

EMERGENCY DEPARTMENT EVALUATION

The history includes questions about the amount of valproate presumed to be ingested, other substances available for ingestion in the patient's environment, and the time of the ingestion (or the last time the patient was in his or her usual state of health). The patient's preexisting health status is noted. The events that occurred between the time of the ingestion and presentation to the emergency department are documented.

The physical examination initially focuses on the CNS and cardiorespiratory function. Cardiorespiratory monitoring and pulse oximetry are instituted in patients with a known ingestion of toxic amounts or in patients demonstrating toxic effects. A quantitative valproate level is ordered to confirm the diagnosis. Serial levels are obtained after an acute overdose. As most patients with seizure disorders have access to multiple medications, an "anticonvulsant screen" is often useful. Full toxicology testing should be considered in patients with intentional overdoses. In symptomatic patients, routine laboratory evaluation includes a complete blood count; measurement of serum electrolytes, blood urea nitrogen, creatinine, and glucose; and hepatic function tests. A chest x-ray and arterial blood gas analysis should be obtained in patients with severe poisoning.

For patients on chronic valproate therapy, monitoring should include a complete blood count with differential, a platelet count, liver function tests (including serum ammonia), and serum electrolyte measurements.

EMERGENCY DEPARTMENT MANAGEMENT

Initial management of the patient suspected of having ingested an overdose of valproate is immediate support of vital functions. In patients with coma of unknown cause, appropriate doses of naloxone, glucose, and thiamine are given. Naloxone reportedly reverses CNS depression secondary to valproate poisoning,[1] but no study of a series of patients has replicated this finding, and responses have been inconsistent.

Prevention of absorption is the next consideration. Activated charcoal is the preferred method of preventing absorption of valproic acid. Charcoal adsorbs valproate.[16] Emesis with syrup of ipecac is not recommended, as the patient could develop an altered mental status from drug effects during emesis. Gastric lavage should be reserved for patients who are comatose and present within 30 minutes to 1 hour after the ingestion. In patients who have ingested large amounts of enteric-coated tablets, whole-bowel irrigation might, theoretically, be advantageous.[2]

Hemodialysis and hemoperfusion were used in an adult who ingested 75 g[15] of valproate and in another who had a valproic acid level of 1,262 μg/mL.[18] Although both recovered, pharmacokinetic data were not available to prove the efficacy of extracorporeal removal. Given the complications of these procedures and the fact that toxicity is usually responsive to good supportive care, extracorporeal removal is not routinely recommended.[10] Forced diuresis is ineffective.

There is evidence supporting the use of repeated doses of activated charcoal. In one case, continuous nasogastric infusion of charcoal appeared to increase the elimination of valproic acid.[8] However, the effect of this therapy on other drugs must be considered in the management of patients who may be on multiple anticonvulsants.

Most patients recover fully. Sequelae are rare, although a report of visual disturbances has been published.[4]

DISPOSITION

All patients with changes in mental status or respiratory function after an acute overdose of valproic acid should be hospitalized in a facility capable of providing continuous cardiorespiratory monitoring. Appropriate consultation from physicians trained in clinical toxicology, intensive care, and pulmonary medicine may be indicated, depending on the clinical course. If intensive care necessitates transfer to another facility, stabilization—including appropriate airway management, intravenous access, and maintenance of circulatory status—should precede advanced cardiac life-support–capable transport to the appropriate institution.

Patients who have ingested rapidly absorbed products should have valproate levels monitored for at least 6 hours after the overdose; those who have ingested enteric-coated preparations should be monitored for 8 to 10 hours. If drug levels are decreasing and there are no clinical signs of toxicity, they can be discharged. Psychiatric consultation should be obtained before discharge on all patients with intentional overdose.

COMMON PITFALLS

- Failure to appreciate that the onset of toxicity may be delayed, particularly after overdose of enteric-coated or granule formulations of divalproex sodium
- Failure to obtain serial drug levels after an acute overdose, in order to determine whether further observation is necessary
- Failure to appreciate that therapy is primarily supportive and depends on the clinical condition, not the drug level
- Failure to appreciate that the benefit–risk ratio does not justify the routine use of extracorporeal elimination procedures, even with markedly elevated drug levels

References

1. Alberto G, Erickson T, Popiel R, et al. CNS manifestations of a valproic acid overdose responsive to naloxone. *Ann Emerg Med* 1989;18:889.
2. American Academy of Clinical Toxicology and European Association of Poison Centres and Clinical Toxicologists. Position statements on gastrointestinal decontamination. *J Toxicol Clin Toxicol* 1997;7:695.
3. Anderson GO, Ritland S. Life threatening intoxication with sodium valproate. *J Toxicol Clin Toxicol* 1995;33:279.
4. Bigler D. Neurological sequelae after intoxication with sodium valproate. *Acta Neurol Scand* 1985;72:351.
5. Bryant AE, Dreifuss FE. Valproic acid hepatic fatalities. III. U.S. experience since 1986. *Neurology* 1996;46:465.
6. Chadwick DW, Cumming WJK, Livingston I, et al. Acute intoxication with sodium valproate. *Ann Neurol* 1979;6:552.
7. Davis R, Peters DH, McTavish D. Valproic acid: a reappraisal of its pharmacological properties and clinical efficacy in epilepsy. *Drugs* 1994;47:332.
8. Farrar HC, Herold DA, Reed MD. Acute valproic acid intoxication: enhanced drug clearance with oral activated charcoal. *Crit Care Med* 1993;21:299.
9. Garnier R, Boudignat O, Fournier PE. Valproate poisoning. *Lancet* 1982;2:97.
10. Graeme K, Higgins T, Curry S, et al. Markedly elevated valproate levels do not serve as an indication for hemodialysis or hemoperfusion. *J Toxicol Clin Toxicol* 1999;37:636.
11. Keys PA. Valproic acid: interactions with phenytoin and phenobarbital. *Drug Intell Clin Pharm* 1982;16:737.
12. Kulick SK, Kramer DA. Hyperammonemia secondary to valproic acid as a cause of lethargy in a postictal patient. *Ann Emerg Med* 1993;22:610.
13. Lakhani M, McMurdo MET. Survival after severe self-poisoning with sodium valproate. *Postgrad Med J* 1986;62:409.
14. McEvoy GK, ed. *Drug information 1999*. Baltimore: American Society of Health-System Pharmacists, 1999:1888.
15. Mortensen PB, Hansen HE, Pedersen B, et al. Acute valproate intoxication: biochemical investigations and hemodialysis treatment. *Int J Clin Pharmacol Ther Toxicol* 1983;21:64.
16. Neuvonen PJ, Kannisto H, Hirvisalo EL. Effect of activated charcoal on absorption of tolbutamide and valproate in man. *Eur J Clin Pharmacol* 1983;24:243.
17. Schnabel R, Rambeck B, Janssen F. Fatal intoxication with sodium valproate. *Lancet* 1984;1:221.
18. Tank JE, Palmer BF. Simultaneous "in series" hemodialysis and hemoperfusion in the management of valproic acid overdose. *Am J Kidney Dis* 1993;22:341.

CHAPTER 375
Withdrawal Syndromes

Paul M. Wax

The clinical presentation of the withdrawal syndrome varies significantly among patients. Patients who present with symptoms and signs of withdrawal and admit to a history of substance abuse are easily identified; those who present with withdrawal symptoms (e.g., seizures) but initially deny ethanol and drug use are not. In patients who present with medical and surgical complications of ethanol and drug abuse, such as pneumonia, pancreatitis, skin abscess, or subdural hematoma, the physician must carefully look beyond the primary process to recognize manifestations of a withdrawal process. Finally, patients may present with an unrelated problem, such as a myocardial infarction or motor vehicle accident, and develop withdrawal symptoms while waiting for admission. To recognize and manage these diverse groups of patients expeditiously, emergency physicians must be familiar with the clinical manifestations and treatment strategies of ethanol and drug withdrawal.

Ethanol withdrawal is the most common withdrawal syndrome seen in the emergency department (Table 375.1). Ethanol withdrawal, as well as the less commonly seen withdrawal from sedative–hypnotics such as benzodiazepines, barbiturates, chloral hydrate, glutethimide, ethchlorvynol, and meprobamate, may result in life-threatening manifestations. Anticipating and recognizing the early signs of ethanol and sedative–hypnotic withdrawal allow for timely treatment and prevent the development of serious withdrawal manifestations. Opioid withdrawal tends to follow a much more benign course. Withdrawal from cocaine may result in lethargy, dysphoria, and depression; withdrawal from tricyclic antidepressants may result in anxiety, insomnia, malaise, and gastrointestinal (GI) symptoms, but the importance of emergent recognition and treatment of these conditions is less well defined.

Physical tolerance and dependency to a drug are a prerequisite for the development of a withdrawal syndrome from that drug. The dose of the drug, duration of effect, frequency of administration, and duration of abuse all contribute to the development of dependency. More severe withdrawal phenomena may be associated with a longer period of abuse or a history of previous withdrawal episodes. Sporadic use of a drug does not generally cause the altered pharmacodynamic and pharmacokinetic responses required for the development of withdrawal symptoms.

Withdrawal from ethanol and other sedative–hypnotics is characterized by intense sympathetic stimulation. The exact

TABLE 375.1. Withdrawal Syndromes Seen in the Emergency Department

Type of Withdrawal	Onset of Symptoms
Ethanol	6–8 h
Sedative–hypnotic (e.g., benzodiazepines, barbiturates)	3–7 d (long-acting drugs)
Opioids	4–8 h (heroin); 36–72 h (methadone)
Cocaine	Within hours after binge
Tricyclic antidepressants	Few days

mechanism has not been fully elucidated, but it has been theorized that this hyperadrenergic state may result, in part, from unopposed compensatory central nervous system (CNS) mechanisms that counteract the depressant effects of ethanol intoxication. Elevated levels of plasma and urinary catecholamines and a decrease in the inhibitory activity of presynaptic $alpha_2$ receptors have been demonstrated in patients withdrawing from ethanol.

Other contributory mechanisms to ethanol withdrawal may involve changes in gamma-aminobutyric acid (GABA; an inhibitory neurotransmitter), glutamate (an excitatory neurotransmitter), and dopamine-receptor activity.[1] Chronic ethanol abusers have been shown to have a decrease in GABA activity. Ethanol withdrawal results in reduced sensitivity to GABA inhibition. The "excitotoxicity" associated with ethanol withdrawal may also be partially due to upregulation in *N*-methyl-D-aspartate (NMDA) glutamate receptors, thereby increasing calcium flux through these receptors.[5] Increased dopaminergic transmission may contribute to ethanol withdrawal hallucinations.[10]

Withdrawal from opioids may also involve an increase in sympathetic discharge, but to a lesser extent than ethanol withdrawal and by a different mechanism. Unlike ethanol, opioids have a specific, well-defined receptor. A decrease in exogenous opioid binding to opioid receptors increases catecholamine release in the locus ceruleus of the CNS. Severe catecholamine storm, however, is not observed during opioid withdrawal.

In all withdrawal scenarios, the precipitant is a decrease or elimination of the dependent drug. An absolute serum drug level of zero is not required to make the diagnosis of ethanol or drug withdrawal. In chronic alcoholics who routinely maintain high ethanol blood levels, withdrawal symptoms may occur at serum levels of 100 mg/dL or more.

CLINICAL PRESENTATION

The clinical presentation of ethanol withdrawal varies in intensity and duration. There are four different symptom stages: tremulousness, seizures, hallucinations, and delirium.[19] Because these stages may coexist and overlap, the physician should categorize ethanol withdrawal as mild, moderate, or severe.

Tremulousness and anxiety characterize mild ethanol withdrawal. Because ethanol is a short-acting agent, withdrawal may begin relatively quickly, within 6 to 8 hours after the patient stops or reduces ethanol intake. Other symptoms may include insomnia, anorexia, nausea, and vomiting. The physical examination may be remarkable for mild autonomic and CNS hyperactivity characterized by tachycardia, hypertension, irritability, and hyperreflexia. Unlike patients with delirium tremens, patients with mild ethanol withdrawal have a clear mental status. Most patients with mild withdrawal recover uneventfully after a few days, but 20% to 25% develop more serious withdrawal manifestations.

Seizures and hallucinations are evidence of moderately severe withdrawal. About 25% of patients with ethanol withdrawal demonstrate seizure activity. Seizures usually occur within 48 hours of decreased ethanol intake. These patients may or may not have tremulousness and other sympathetic hyperactivity before seizure activity begins. Seizures tend to be of the generalized tonic–clonic type. They may occur singly or as a brief flurry with normal sensorium between seizures. Status epilepticus is uncommon. As many as a third of patients with seizures progress to delirium tremens.

About 25% of patients with ethanol withdrawal experience some form of false perceptions, including hallucinations and illusory experiences. Most of the hallucinations appear to be visual (e.g., insects crawling on the wall). Some patients complain of auditory hallucinations, often of a persecutory nature. This distinctive presentation, known as acute alcoholic hallucinosis, may not be accompanied by sympathetic hyperactivity. Acute alcoholic hallucinosis usually lasts for at least several days but may persist for months; it may resemble paranoid schizophrenia.[18]

Delirium tremens, characterized by an altered sensorium and dramatic sympathetic hyperactivity, is the most severe form of ethanol withdrawal. Although only 5% of patients with ethanol withdrawal progress to delirium tremens, a study of inpatients admitted for ethanol detoxification or withdrawal showed that 24% developed delirium tremens.[6] It appears to be more common in patients with a long history of ethanol use, a prior history of significant withdrawal, more days since last ethanol use, and concurrent acute medical illness.

Delirium tremens usually begins 48 to 72 hours after cessation or reduction of ethanol. These patients are truly delirious, demonstrating global confusion, agitation, hallucinations, and delusions. Picking at the bedclothes is common. Tachycardia, hypertension, tachypnea, hyperthermia, diaphoresis, and mydriasis may occur, as may tachyarrhythmias. In the untreated patient, mortality usually results from severe dehydration, coexisting medical conditions, or hyperthermia. Although, in the past, mortality rates have been as high as 35% in untreated patients, early recognition of the problem and aggressive treatment should eliminate mortality in patients without significant underlying disease.

Other sedative–hypnotic withdrawal syndromes may be indistinguishable from ethanol withdrawal except for differences in the time course. Because most benzodiazepines have a much longer elimination half-life than ethanol and have active metabolites, withdrawal manifestations may be delayed up to 1 week or more after cessation of drug use. Mild withdrawal symptoms include anxiety, apprehension, irritability, dysphoria, and insomnia.[14] These symptoms may be difficult to distinguish from an underlying anxiety disorder. Hallucinations, delusions, myoclonus, seizures, and agitation may appear with more severe withdrawal. Symptoms from long-acting benzodiazepine withdrawal may persist for weeks. Severe withdrawal symptoms, including seizures, may occur after the administration of flumazenil to patients chronically taking benzodiazepines.

The clinical manifestations of opioid withdrawal are usually different. Symptoms of mild opioid withdrawal include lacrimation, rhinorrhea, yawning, diaphoresis, anxiety, restlessness, and dysphoria. Piloerection is particularly characteristic. The patient may exhibit mild elevations in pulse, blood pressure, and respiratory rate, but these changes are usually not very significant. More severe opioid withdrawal is characterized by vomiting, diarrhea, abdominal pain, and dehydration. Severe agitation, seizures (except in neonatal withdrawal), mental status changes, and hyperthermia are not seen with opioid withdrawal, as they are in ethanol and sedative–hypnotic withdrawal.

The severity and time course of the opioid withdrawal syndrome depends on the pharmacokinetics of the opioid. Shorter-acting agents (e.g., heroin) tend to have a more intense course than longer-acting agents (e.g., methadone). Heroin withdrawal usually begins within 4 to 8 hours after the last dose, peaking by 36 to 72 hours. In contrast, the onset of methadone withdrawal may be delayed 36 to 72 hours after the last dose, and symptoms may persist for up to 2 weeks.[7]

In the emergency department, the sudden onset of opioid withdrawal may occur after an opioid antagonist such as naloxone is given to an unsuspected opioid-dependent patient. Due to naloxone's short half-life, withdrawal symptoms do not usually persist beyond 20 to 60 minutes. Treatment with additional opioid to reverse these effects is not indicated. Giving opioids with agonist–antagonist properties, such as pentazocine (Talwin), nalbuphine (Nubain), and butorphanol (Stadol), to the opioid-dependent patient may also precipitate withdrawal symptoms. Opioid withdrawal from the long-acting opioid antagonists naltrexone and nalmefene may result in a markedly prolonged withdrawal period lasting upwards of 1 to 2 days.

DIFFERENTIAL DIAGNOSIS

The differential diagnosis of the withdrawal state is broad and includes many other serious conditions that may require different therapy (Table 375.2). Because drug-dependent patients are particularly prone to develop many of these conditions, careful exclusion of other etiologies is critically important. Ethanol-induced hypoglycemia must be differentiated from ethanol withdrawal. Clinically, both conditions may feature diaphoresis, tachycardia, confusion, agitation, and an odor of ethanol on the breath. However, only the patient with hypoglycemia will have rapid improvement with the intravenous administration of 50 g of glucose.

Differentiating ethanol withdrawal seizures from other types of seizures may be particularly difficult. Not all seizures in the alcoholic patient are due to ethanol withdrawal: Other common causes include preexisting idiopathic epilepsy, posttraumatic epilepsy, and other complications of ethanol abuse (e.g., hypoglycemia, hypomagnesemia, hyponatremia, head trauma). Poor anticonvulsant compliance in chronic alcoholics with underlying seizure disorders may add to the diagnostic confusion.

Opioid withdrawal must be distinguished from ethanol and other sedative–hypnotic withdrawal because of the significant differences in therapy. Symptoms of significant ethanol withdrawal, such as confusion, agitation, and seizures, are not generally seen with opioid withdrawal; opioid withdrawal symptoms such as piloerection, yawning, lacrimation, and rhinorrhea are not seen with ethanol and sedative–hypnotic withdrawal. Some patients, however, may be withdrawing from both substances. GI manifestations of opioid withdrawal must be differentiated from other causes of gastroenteritis.

EMERGENCY DEPARTMENT EVALUATION

Patients presenting with possible ethanol or drug withdrawal require a comprehensive assessment. All patients initially should be connected to a cardiac monitor. A fingerstick glucose and oxygen saturation analysis should also be performed. The physician must obtain a complete history of substance abuse, previous withdrawal episodes, and all current and former medications. If possible, family, friends, and prehospital personnel are interviewed to gain additional information. Alcoholics tend to underreport their substance use; drug abusers may overreport it.

All vital signs, including rectal temperature, are recorded and closely monitored. Examination of the skin, abdomen, eyes, and pulse rate may help to distinguish an anticholinergic toxidrome (dry skin, decreased bowel sounds, urinary retention, mydriasis, tachycardia) from a sympathomimetic toxidrome (moist skin, normal bowel sounds, no urinary retention, mydri-

TABLE 375.2. Differential Diagnosis of Major Withdrawal Symptoms

Tremor	Seizures	Hallucinations	Delirium
Withdrawal	Withdrawal	Withdrawal	Withdrawal
Ethanol	Ethanol	Ethanol	Ethanol
Sedative–hypnotics	Sedative–hypnotics	Sedative–hypnotics	Sedative–hypnotics
Intoxications	Intoxications	Intoxications	Intoxications
Theophylline	Cocaine	LSD	Cocaine
Caffeine	Anticholinergics	Mescaline	Amphetamine
Beta agonists	Phenothiazines	Mushrooms	Phencyclidine
Mercury	TCAs	Peyote	Anticholinergics
Lithium	Theophylline	Phencyclidine	LSD
TCAs	Camphor	Anticholinergics	Infectious
Phenytoin	Isoniazid	Ergot	Meningitis
Metabolic	Phencyclidine	Nutmeg	Encephalitis
Hypoglycemia	Lidocaine	Infectious	Sepsis
Thyrotoxicosis	Organophosphates	Meningitis	Metabolic
Structural	Infectious	Encephalitis	Thyrotoxicosis
Cerebellar disease	Meningitis	Sepsis	Hypoglycemia
Other	Encephalitis	Metabolic	Hyperglycemia
Parkinsonism	Metabolic	Hypoglycemia	Hypocalcemia
	Hypoglycemia	Hypoxia	Hypoxia
	Hypoxia	Structural	Thiamine deficiency
	Hypothyroidism	CNS hemorrhage	Structural
	Thyrotoxicosis	Tumor	Head trauma
	Hypocalcemia	Psychiatric	CNS hemorrhage
	Hyperosmolar state	Schizophrenia	Tumor
	Hepatic failure	Bipolar disorder	Psychiatric
	Uremia	Other	Other
	Structural	Seizures	Seizures
	Head trauma	Heat-related illness	Heat-related illness
	CNS hemorrhage		
	Tumor		
	CVA		
	Other		
	Idiopathic epilepsy		
	Posttraumatic epilepsy		
	Degenerative disease		

TCAs, tricyclic antidepressants; CVA, cerebrovascular accident.

asis, tachycardia). Close attention should be directed to any stigmata of chronic liver disease or evidence of intravenous drug use.

Because these patients are at high risk for concomitant trauma, a full assessment for obvious and occult traumatic injury should be done. These patients should also be evaluated for other complications of ethanol and drug abuse, such as pneumonia, skin abscesses, bacterial endocarditis, acquired immunodeficiency syndrome, pancreatitis, liver disease, and GI bleeding.

Laboratory studies should include a complete blood count; measurement of electrolytes, glucose, blood urea nitrogen, and creatinine levels; liver function tests; coagulation profile; and ethanol level. Ethanol levels in patients with ethanol withdrawal may be 100 mg/dL or more; likewise, a urine drug screen may be positive or negative for the offending agent. In patients with significant agitation, a creatine phosphokinase determination may help detect rhabdomyolysis.

An elevated temperature requires a full sepsis workup, including urine and blood cultures, chest radiograph, and, often, a lumbar puncture. Obtaining a head computed tomography scan before lumbar puncture is critical in patients presenting with either focal neurologic deficits or high risk for intracranial hemorrhage. Patients with a first-time seizure in the setting of withdrawal should be evaluated the same as any other patient with a new seizure (see Chapter 206). Subsequent withdrawal seizures do not require reevaluation unless there are extenuating circumstances.

EMERGENCY DEPARTMENT MANAGEMENT

Withdrawal syndromes, particularly in the case of ethanol and sedative–hypnotic withdrawal, must be recognized and treated in a timely fashion. Because treatment may prevent withdrawal from progressing to a more serious stage, early treatment may significantly affect the subsequent clinical course. A successful strategy of treating withdrawal in the emergency department must address several basic goals: alleviating symptoms, preventing progression, avoiding complications, and recognizing and treating coexisting medical problems. Planning for long-term rehabilitation and drug independence is usually better done as part of inpatient management.

Initial treatment should be directed at readily correctable causes of altered mental status. Oxygen should be given if the oxygen saturation is low, and an intravenous line should be established. Fifty grams of glucose should be immediately given intravenously if hypoglycemia is present. In a patient with a borderline normal glucose level and altered mental status, glucose should also be given, in case the glucose determination is inaccurate.

To treat possible Wernicke's encephalopathy, 100 mg of thiamine should be given intravenously. If the mental status is clear, thiamine may still be given as a nutritional supplement. A "vitamin cocktail" of 100 mg of thiamine, one ampule of multivitamins, 1 mg of folate, and 2 g of magnesium sulfate is often added to the initial liter of intravenous fluid given to chronic alcoholics, due to their increased risk for malnutrition. Volume resuscitation is often necessary, particularly in patients with severe withdrawal manifestations and dehydration.

Significantly agitated patients may initially need to be physically restrained to prevent injury, establish intravenous access, and facilitate sedation. Soft restraints should be used. Prolonged use of restraints is discouraged, because continued struggling against them may lead to rhabdomyolysis, hyperthermia, and metabolic acidosis. Once intravenous access is obtained and chemical sedation has achieved behavioral control, physical restraints should be discontinued.

Achieving adequate sedation is the cornerstone of successful treatment of ethanol and other sedative–hypnotic withdrawal (Table 375.3). Sedation alleviates the excitatory manifestations of the hyperadrenergic state and may prevent progression to delirium tremens with its attendant complications.

Substitution with a cross-tolerant drug is required to achieve proper sedation and replace the dependent agent. Many agents have been used over the years, but benzodiazepines have proven to be the most effective.[11,13] Compared with other sedative–hypnotic agents, benzodiazepines are safer and produce less respiratory depression. Their dosage is easier to titrate and the effects are more predictable. Diazepam (Valium), chlordiazepoxide (Librium), and lorazepam (Ativan) are the most commonly used agents for ethanol withdrawal and can also be used for sedative–hypnotic withdrawal. These agents are preferred over benzodiazepines with shorter half-lives, which require frequent dosing, because they allow gradual drug elimination over several days.

Compared with short-acting agents, long-acting agents may be more effective in preventing withdrawal seizures and contribute to smoother withdrawal with fewer rebound symptoms.[13] Active metabolites of diazepam and chlordiazepoxide prolong their therapeutic effect. In elderly patients and those with hepatic dysfunction, lorazepam, which has no active metabolites, may be preferred. In other cases, lorazepam does not appear to offer any distinct advantage over diazepam or chlordiazepoxide.[2]

Intravenous dosing is preferred in all but the mildest cases of ethanol withdrawal: Agitation may preclude oral administration, and gastritis may impair drug absorption. Intravenous therapy can be readily titrated. Lorazepam (but not diazepam or chlordiazepoxide) is predictably absorbed intramuscularly. This route may be useful in the wildly agitated patient before intravenous access is established.

The dose of benzodiazepines required to achieve proper sedation must be individualized and varies considerably, de-

TABLE 375.3. Pharmaceutical Management of Ethanol and Drug Withdrawal

ETHANOL OR SEDATIVE–HYPNOTIC WITHDRAWAL
1st Choice: Dlazepam
5 mg i.v. bolus q5–15min until sedated
May increase dose to 20 mg q5–15min in refractory cases
Total over 24-h period may >1,000 mg
Do not exceed 5 mg/min
2nd Choice: Lorazepam
1–2 mg i.v. bolus q5–15min until sedated
Not as long-acting as diazepam
Preferable in cases of hepatic failure or recurrent seizures
3rd Choice: Pentobarbital
100 mg i.v. bolus
Continued titration to sedation or 600 mg total
Potential for more respiratory depression than benzodiazepines
Do not exceed 50 mg/min
Alternatives:
Chlordiazepoxide, secobarbital, phenobarbital
OPIOID WITHDRAWAL
1st Choice: Clonidine
0.1–0.2 mg PO test dose in emergency department
If tolerated well this dose may be continued q4–6h for several days
2nd Choice: Methadone
5–25 mg i.m. or PO
Give if needed to patients who require admission; do not use for patients sent home

pending on the patient's tolerance to the drug. Symptom-triggered therapy is as efficacious as fixed-schedule therapy and decreases both the amount of benzodiazepine used and treatment duration.[16] Frequent intravenous boluses should be given until the patient has achieved a restful state. When using diazepam, 5 to 20 mg can be given every 5 to 15 minutes until the patient is sleepy but arousable. Sometimes, very large doses of diazepam (1,000 mg or more over 24 hours) are necessary to achieve adequate sedation. Usually, sedation is obtained before respiratory depression develops, but close airway observation is always required.

Failure to obtain immediate sedation need not prompt switching to an alternative agent. Mixing different drugs or different routes of administration may increase the risk of adverse effects, particularly respiratory depression. However, if a patient does not respond completely to the chosen benzodiazepine, the use of another cross-tolerant agent may be valuable. Intermediate-acting or long-acting barbiturates such as pentobarbital, secobarbital, or phenobarbital are recommended in these situations. Doses of 100 mg of pentobarbital may be given intravenously every 5 to 10 minutes until sufficient sedation is achieved or a total dose of 600 mg is given.

Phenobarbital may also be used, although its onset of action may be delayed. Phenobarbital's long duration of effect, however, requires less frequent dosing and allows gradual self-tapering. Phenobarbital may be particularly helpful in withdrawal patients with idiopathic or posttraumatic epilepsy who require maintenance anticonvulsant levels. The barbiturates are more likely to cause excessive sedation and respiratory depression.[20]

The use of midazolam (a short-acting benzodiazepine) by continuous intravenous infusion has been suggested to treat for ethanol withdrawal.[12] This approach, however, requires more vigilant monitoring, especially in the patient who is not intubated, and does not provide the advantages of a long-acting agent. More recently, propofol has been suggested as an effective alternative to benzodiazepines for refractory delirium tremens.[3] Such an approach, however, has not been subject to controlled trials. Paraldehyde and ethanol itself, both used in the past, are considerably more toxic and difficult to titrate than the benzodiazepines and are no longer recommended.[13]

Withdrawal seizures should also be treated with benzodiazepines. Lorazepam, which has a longer anticonvulsant effect than does diazepam, has been shown to decrease the risk of recurrent seizures related to ethanol and is the agent of choice in this situation.[4] Phenobarbital is a useful alternative. Phenytoin is ineffective in treating or preventing withdrawal seizures.[15] It should be reserved for patients with a history of an underlying chronic seizure disorder who require maintenance phenytoin therapy.

Neuroleptics such as the phenothiazines and butyrophenones (e.g., haloperidol) should never be used as monotherapy in the treatment of ethanol and sedative–hypnotic withdrawal. Although sometimes used for severe agitation, these neuroleptics are not cross-tolerant with ethanol or sedative–hypnotics and do not prevent or suppress withdrawal. Hypotension, impaired thermoregulation, a lowered seizure threshold, and dystonic reactions may result from their use. Uncontrolled clinical experience suggests that neuroleptics may be considered as adjunctive therapy for patients with refractory agitation and hallucinations.[17] They may also be useful in treating concomitant nausea, vomiting, and GI cramps.

Sympatholytic therapy with beta blockers (e.g., propranolol) and central adrenergic agonists (e.g., clonidine) has been used for ethanol or sedative–hypnotic withdrawal, but these agents offer little benefit in the emergency department setting. Sympatholytics are not cross-tolerant with ethanol or sedative–hypnotics and do not prevent agitation, confusion, or seizures. Their ability to normalize vital signs may mask a deteriorating clinical situation.

For opioid withdrawal, clonidine may offer symptomatic relief because it decreases sympathetic activity in the locus ceruleus. An initial oral dose of 0.1 to 0.2 mg is recommended. Because hypotension may be particularly problematic after the first dose, the blood pressure should be monitored for 2 hours while the patient remains in the emergency department. A dose of 0.1 to 0.2 mg every 4 to 6 hours may help prevent recurrence of opioid withdrawal symptoms.[7] Nonspecific sedation with benzodiazepines is also an option.

For patients who will be hospitalized with other medical problems, methadone may be given to relieve the symptoms of significant opioid withdrawal.[8] A dose of 5 to 25 mg intramuscularly or orally blocks most manifestations of physiologic withdrawal. Parenteral administration guarantees absorption in the vomiting patient. Symptomatic improvement usually occurs within 30 to 60 minutes. Daily maintenance doses average 50 mg and range from 25 to 150 mg. Shorter-acting preparations such as morphine or meperidine are not indicated.

Federal regulations restrict the use of methadone to Food and Drug Administration–designated programs.[7] While this legislation does not prohibit the use of methadone in opioid addicts who are admitted for other reasons, unless the facility has an approved program, methadone should not be given to those admitted solely for the treatment of opioid withdrawal. Similarly, legislation prohibits prescribing methadone for the outpatient treatment of withdrawal without a specific license.

DISPOSITION

Patients with moderate-to-severe ethanol and sedative–hypnotic withdrawal should be admitted. Because withdrawal usually persists for several days, admitted patients should be closely monitored for signs of progression and treated as necessary. The level of care necessary depends on clinical severity. Because of potential complications, patients requiring intravenous sedation are best managed in an intensive or intermediate care unit. Patients with less severe withdrawal may be managed and observed on a medical floor, psychiatric floor, hospital-based detoxification unit, or detoxification unit outside of the hospital. Patients with mild withdrawal may also need to be admitted for the evaluation and treatment of concomitant medical problems that have not been adequately addressed in the past due to poor use of outpatient services. The inpatient setting also provides a protected environment away from the temptations of ethanol and street drugs.

Prescriptions for benzodiazepines should not usually be given to patients with ethanol withdrawal who are being discharged home from the emergency department. The ingestion of ethanol by a patient taking benzodiazepines may result in fatal respiratory depression, or the benzodiazepines may simply be sold on the street. Outpatient management should be attempted only if the patient can be discharged home with a supportive family member or friend and appropriate outpatient follow-up can be arranged. Supervised withdrawal in the home setting, under the direction of a visiting nurse, may be appropriate in some of these circumstances.[9]

Patients who present to the emergency department with opiate withdrawal may be discharged home if they do not have other concomitant medical problems that require hospital admission and they can tolerate oral fluids. Offering the patient a limited supply of clonidine (if tolerated in the emergency department) may help prevent further withdrawal symptoms. Prescriptions for opioids should not be given.

Social service, detoxification, or substance-abuse counseling and psychiatric referrals should be offered to all patients with a history of substance abuse.

COMMON PITFALLS

- Failure to consider the possibility of ethanol and drug withdrawal in all patients with altered mental status and elevated vital signs
- Failure to appreciate that ethanol and sedative–hypnotic withdrawal are potentially life-threatening, whereas opioid withdrawal, although bothersome, does not usually cause significant morbidity
- Failure to appreciate that ethanol withdrawal is not synonymous with delirium tremens but that those with other withdrawal symptoms are at risk of progressing to delirium tremens if not treated
- Failure to exclude other etiologies of fever and altered mental status (e.g., hypoglycemia, head trauma, infection) in patients with suspected withdrawal
- Failure to appreciate that long-acting intravenous benzodiazepines such as diazepam or lorazepam are the treatment of choice for ethanol and sedative–hypnotic withdrawal
- Failure to appreciate that neuroleptics do not cross-react with ethanol and are generally not indicated in the treatment of ethanol withdrawal
- Failure to evaluate for and treat the dehydration that often accompanies withdrawal
- Failure to admit patients with signs and symptoms of moderate or severe ethanol and sedative–hypnotic withdrawal, particularly those with underlying medical problems

References

1. Adinoff B. The alcohol withdrawal syndrome: neurobiology of treatment and toxicity. *Am J Addict* 1994;3:277–288.
2. Bird R, Makela E. Alcohol withdrawal: what is the benzodiazepine of choice? *Ann Pharmacother* 1994;28:67–71.
3. Coomes TR, Smith SW. Successful use of propofol in refractory delirium tremens. *Ann Emerg Med* 1997;30:825–828.
4. D'Onofrio G, Rathlev N, Ulrich S, et al. Lorazepam for the prevention of recurrent seizures related to alcohol. *N Engl J Med* 1999;340:915–919.
5. Dodd P. Neural mechanisms of adaptation in chronic ethanol exposure and alcoholism. *Alcohol Clin Exp Res* 1996;20:151A–156A.
6. Ferguson JA, Suelzer CJ, Eckert GJ. Risk factors for delirium tremens development. *J Gen Intern Med* 1996;11:410–414.
7. Freitas PM. Narcotic withdrawal in the emergency department. *Am J Emerg Med* 1985;3:456.
8. Fultz JM, Senay ED. Guidelines for the management of hospitalized narcotic addicts. *Ann Intern Med* 1975;82:815.
9. Hall W, Zador D. The alcohol withdrawal syndrome. *Lancet* 1997;349: 1897–1900.
10. Heinz A, Schmidt K, Baum SS, et al. Influence of dopaminergic transmission on severity of withdrawal syndrome in alcoholism. *J Stud Alcohol* 1996; 57:471–474.
11. Holbrook AM, Crowther R, Lotter A, et al. Meta-analysis of benzodiazepine use in the treatment of acute alcohol withdrawal. *Can Med Assoc J* 1999; 160:649–655.
12. Lineaweaver WC, Anderson K, Hing DN. Massive doses of midazolam infusion for delirium tremens without respiratory depression. *Crit Care Med* 1988;16:294.
13. Mayo-Smith M. Pharmacological management of alcohol withdrawal: a meta-analysis and evidence-based practice guideline. *JAMA* 1997;278:144–151.
14. Petursson H. The benzodiazepine withdrawal syndrome. *Addiction* 1994;89:1455–1459.
15. Rathlev NK, D'Onofrio GD, Fish SS, et al. The lack of efficacy of phenytoin in the prevention of recurrent alcohol-related seizures. *Ann Emerg Med* 1994;23:513–518.
16. Saitz R, Mayo-Smith M, Roberts M et al. Individualize treatment for alcohol withdrawal: a randomized double-blind controlled study. *JAMA* 1994;272: 519–523.
17. Sellers EM, Kalant H. Management of the alcohol withdrawal syndrome. *Annu Rev Med* 1991;42:323–340.
18. Tsuang JW, Irwin MR, Smith TL, et al. Characteristics of men with alcoholic hallucinosis. *Addiction* 1994;89:73–78.
19. Victor M, Adams RD. The effects of alcohol on the nervous system. *Proc Assoc Res Nerv Ment Dis* 1953;32:526.
20. Young GP, Rores C, Murphy C, et al. Intravenous phenobarbital for alcohol withdrawal and convulsions. *Ann Emerg Med* 1987;16:847.

SECTION VII

Section Editor: Christopher H. Linden

Environmental Emergencies

PART I
Bites and Stings

CHAPTER 376
Black Widow Spider Envenomations

Steven C. Curry and Thomas J. Higgins, Jr.

The common name "black widow spider" was initially limited to *Latrodectus mactans,* but several other species of the genus *Latrodectus* are now referred to as black widow spiders.[7] Although the males are too small to produce significant envenomation, both immature and adult female spiders can produce significant envenomation after a bite.

Mature females have globular abdomens and leg spans ranging up to 40 mm. *L. mactans* of southern North America and *Latrodectus hesperus* of the western United States are shiny black, with a red hourglass on the ventral surface of the abdomen. In *Latrodectus variolus,* found in the eastern United States and Canada, the triangles of the hourglass do not quite meet. The red widow, *Latrodectus bishopi,* found in central Florida, has an orange carapace, sternum, and legs, with a black abdomen. The abdomen may have red spots surrounded by a yellow border. The brown widow, *Latrodectus geometricus,* is found in southern Florida. There may be regional variations in appearance of all black widow spiders.[7] Furthermore, immature yet venomous spiders may be brown or cream-colored with spots, and sometimes exhibit broad red markings on the dorsal surface of the abdomen.

Most bites occur in the warmer months and result from accidental encounters between humans and spiders. In Arizona, the spiders can be found in almost every crawl space, fence corner, storage shed, or other partially concealed location. They commonly nest in porch furniture or in the metal tubing of lawn chairs and baby strollers kept outside or in the garage.

Latrodectus venom from all species appears to have identical action, although structural differences can be demonstrated on electrophoresis.[5,7] The most important action of the venom is to cause the release of neurotransmitters from both noradrenergic and cholinergic nerve endings.[2,6,7] Ca^{++} may be mobilized from intracellular stores to cause neurotransmitter release.[7] Early studies suggested that neurotransmitter release was accompanied by Ca^{++} influx into nerve endings, but other studies have failed to document this. *Ex vivo* studies document greater neurotransmitter release when extracellular Ca^{++} concentrations are increased, suggesting that it is irrational to give calcium to patients suffering from black widow spider bites.[8] Excessive release of acetylcholine from cholinergic nerve endings results in diaphoresis and muscle cramping. Although frequently not recognized as such by the patient, it is the cramping that is thought to cause the severe pain that characterizes serious envenomations. Excessive release of catecholamines from adrenergic nerve endings and the adrenal medulla can result in hypertension and tachycardia.

Older literature alludes to deaths after black widow spider bites, but mortality is extremely rare with modern supportive care. From 1983 through 1997, there were 30,782 black widow spider bites reported without a single death.[1] However, stress from severe pain and catecholamine release may compromise the very young, the elderly, and those with cardiopulmonary disease.

CLINICAL PRESENTATION

Bites by black widow spiders are usually felt, although not necessarily recognized as such. A brief, sharp pain resembling a needle stick is often noted. Over the next 30 minutes to several hours, pain described as deep, burning, aching, or numbing may begin near the bite, such as in an arm or a leg. Children may present with unexplained persistent crying. A history of onset of crying shortly after the child was placed in a stroller or other item kept in the garage or outside should raise the possibility of a black widow spider bite in areas where these spiders are common.

Examination of the bite site may reveal two minute puncture wounds but no necrosis or significant swelling. A close examination also frequently reveals a halo lesion consisting of a circular area of pallor surrounded by a ring of erythema.[10] Multiple bites are fairly common, and halo lesions may be noted at each site.[10] Halo lesions are especially helpful in making the diagnosis in the absence of a history of a spider bite (e.g., in young children).

Most patients who seek medical care do so to obtain relief from pain. In those suffering significant envenomations, symptoms may not peak for 12 to 18 hours and can last up to several days. Mild-to-moderate symptoms may then persist for 2 to 3 weeks. Muscle cramping and pain typically occur in major muscle groups such as the back, neck, thighs, flanks, abdomen, and chest. Patients frequently move about intermittently in attempts to find comfortable positions. On occasion, abdominal muscles may become rigid and tender, sometimes mimicking an acute abdomen. Diaphoresis is frequently noted over the site of the bite. Sometimes, diaphoresis is localized to areas distant to the bite. For example, a bite to the arm could result in diaphoresis limited to the nose or to the lower legs and feet without other evidence of sweating. An occasional patient suffers severe diaphoresis over the entire body, drenching sheets and covers.

Mild-to-moderate hypertension is common but usually not severe enough to require treatment. Less frequent findings include vomiting, headache, chest tightness, hyperesthesias, weakness, priapism, lacrimation, salivation, and, especially in children, bilateral periorbital ecchymosis. Rare reports describe paresthesias, weakness, and atrial fibrillation. Herpes zoster has been reported after envenomation, although a causal relation has not been established.

Pregnant women who suffer black widow spider bites may develop uterine muscle contractions and abort the fetus.[8] We have seen one woman in her first trimester of pregnancy develop vaginal bleeding while suffering severe pain and muscle cramping after a bite. Antivenin completely relieved symptoms and halted further bleeding, resulting in successful delivery at 40 weeks.

DIFFERENTIAL DIAGNOSIS

The differential diagnosis includes almost any illness that can produce severe pain. Pain localized to the back or flanks may suggest renal colic or infection, but the urinalysis is normal. Severe muscle pain from envenomation may be confused with rhabdomyolysis; a normal or minimally elevated total serum creatine kinase level rules out the latter. Severe abdominal pain has resulted in unnecessary exploratory surgery. In older patients with prolonged chest pain, myocardial ischemia may need to be ruled out, even if a black widow envenomation is known to have occurred. The presence of fever should suggest an alternative or accompanying diagnosis.

Patients who suffer black widow spider envenomations often stay in one position for a few seconds or minutes before moving to a new position. In contrast, severe scorpion envenomation results in constant writhing and abnormal eye movements. In addition, scorpion stings do not produce halo lesions.

EMERGENCY DEPARTMENT EVALUATION

The physician should ask about the circumstances surrounding the suspected bite (e.g., witnessed bite, unexplained crying after the child was placed in a stroller), the description of the spider, and the progression of symptoms.

The physical examination should include a search for minute puncture wounds or halo lesions suggestive of black widow envenomation. The skin should be examined for unexplained diaphoresis, even in areas remote from the bite site. Vital signs should be examined for the presence of hypertension and tachycardia. No laboratory studies specific for black widow spider envenomations are available. Evaluation for other causes of pain may be necessary, even in patients with known black widow spider bites.

EMERGENCY DEPARTMENT MANAGEMENT

Advanced life-support measures should be instituted, as necessary. As with any puncture wound, a primary tetanus immunization or booster should be given, if indicated. Efforts should then be directed at relieving pain. Patients with mild pain can usually be treated with oral analgesics. Those with moderate pain may require agents such as hydrocodone or hydromorphone. Those with severe pain or moderate pain refractory to oral analgesics require parenteral agents. We prefer morphine for analgesia and lorazepam for sedation and amnesia. Doses of these drugs vary tremendously, depending on the patient's age and weight, other central nervous system (CNS) depressants the patient may be taking, preexisting diseases, and individual responses to these agents. An initial intravenous dose of 6 mg of morphine sulfate and 1 mg of lorazepam may be given to an otherwise healthy adult in severe pain. Further doses of morphine sulfate may be given every 2 to 5 minutes until the pain is controlled or until excessive CNS depression limits further doses.

L. mactans antivenin, a horse serum product, is effective in reversing all signs and symptoms caused by envenomations by any species of *Latrodectus*. The main indications are severe pain or dangerous hypertension. It is also reasonable to give antivenin to pregnant women who suffer moderate-to-severe envenomations and to those with mild symptoms and threatened abortion. Antivenin is contraindicated in patients allergic to horse serum, and it is ill-advised in patients taking beta-adrenergic blocking agents, as these drugs may predispose to anaphylactic reactions that can be refractory to treatment.

The manufacturer recommends skin testing before administration, although information obtained from skin testing may not be reliable in predicting who will or will not suffer an anaphylactic response to the antivenin (unless the skin test itself produces anaphylaxis). Therefore, it is prudent to administer the antivenin in a controlled critical care setting such as the emergency department or intensive care unit and to be prepared to immediately treat life-threatening anaphylaxis. We mix one vial of antivenin in 50 mL of crystalloid solution and give it intravenously over 20 to 30 minutes, regardless of the patient's age or weight. Symptoms usually begin to resolve in about 40 minutes, and the patient is usually completely asymptomatic within 60 to 90 minutes. Rarely, if ever, is a second vial of antivenin required. There have been case reports of antivenin being effective in the treatment of latrodectism as long as 12 days after envenomation in patients who remain symptomatic.[11]

Because of the minimal volume of horse serum in a single vial of *Latrodectus* antivenin, serum sickness is an uncommon late occurrence.[9] If it does occur, symptoms are easily controlled with oral corticosteroids and hydroxyzine.

Patients not treated with antivenin may require therapy to control hypertension or excessive diaphoresis. Hypertension may be treated with a vasodilator (e.g., nitroprusside, nifedipine, hydralazine). Severe diaphoresis may be treated with low doses of subcutaneous atropine sulfate.

Patients suffering from *L. hesperus* envenomation benefit little, if at all, from intravenous calcium salts.[3] There are anecdotal reports of dramatic pain relief from intravenous calcium after envenomations by other species, but there are no meaningful studies documenting calcium's efficacy. The same is true for centrally acting muscle relaxants (e.g., methocarbamol), which have little or no muscle-relaxing activity independent of their CNS depressant activity. In fact, methocarbamol has been reported to be even less effective than calcium.[4]

DISPOSITION

Patients with mild-to-moderate symptoms who respond to oral analgesics may be discharged from the emergency department with prescriptions for analgesics. They should be warned that symptoms may continue to worsen for 12 to 18 hours after envenomation and should be told to return if symptoms are not relieved with medication. Patients who receive antivenin without complications may also be discharged when asymptomatic. They should be told that they are likely to be allergic to horse serum in the future, should be warned of the signs and symptoms of serum sickness, and should be instructed to see a physician if this complication develops.

Patients who require parenteral narcotics and do not receive antivenin should be admitted to the hospital. They can be discharged when the pain has lessened enough that it can be controlled with oral analgesics, usually in 2 to 4 days.

COMMON PITFALLS

- Sending patients with moderate-to-severe pain home with a prescription for oral analgesics without ensuring that they respond to such agents in the emergency department
- Risking anaphylaxis and serum sickness by giving antivenin to patients with only mild symptoms
- Giving antivenin to a patient taking a beta-adrenergic blocking agent, which can make anaphylaxis, if it occurs, difficult to treat
- Mistaking severe abdominal, back, or chest pain for other disease processes
- Failure to appreciate that chest pain in a patient at risk for heart disease may be due to myocardial ischemia, even if a black widow spider bite is known to have occurred

References

1. American Association of Poison Control Centers. Toxic Exposure Surveillance System: Published in September issues of *Am J Emerg Med* 1983–1997 annual reports.
2. Baba A, Cooper JR. The action of black widow spider venom on cholinergic mechanisms in synaptosomes. *J Neurochem* 1980;34:1369.
3. Clark RF, Wethern-Kestner S, Vance MV, et al. Clinical presentation and treatment of black widow spider envenomation: a review of 163 cases. *Ann Emerg Med* 1992;21:782.
4. Key GF. A comparison of calcium gluconate and methocarbamol (Robaxin) in the treatment of latrodectism (black widow spider envenomation). *Am J Trop Med Hyg* 1981;30:273.
5. McCrone JD. Comparative lethality of several *Latrodectus* venoms. *Toxicon* 1964;2:201.
6. Picotti GB, Bondiolotti GP, Meldolesi J. Peripheral catecholamine release by alpha-latrotoxin in the rat. *Arch Pharmacol* 1982;320:224.
7. Rauber A. Black widow spider bites. *J Toxicol Clin Toxicol* 1984;21:473.
8. Russell FE, Marcus P, Streng JA. Black widow spider envenomation during pregnancy—report of a case. *Toxicon* 1979;17:188.
9. Timms RK, Gibbons RB. Latrodectism—effects of the black widow spider bite. *West J Med* 1986;144:315.
10. Vance M, Curry S, Gerkin R, et al. The "target lesion": a pathognomonic sign of black widow spider (*Latrodectus* spp.) envenomation. *Vet Hum Toxicol* 1986;28:485.
11. Wells CL, Spring WJ. Delayed but effective treatment of red-back spider envenomation. *Med J Aust* 1996;164(7):447.

CHAPTER 377

Brown Recluse Spider Envenomations

Gary S. Wasserman

Spiders of the genus *Loxosceles* from the family Loxoscelidae are distributed throughout the world. *Loxosceles reclusa,* the most important species in the United States, can be found coast to coast but is most common in the southern Midwestern states. Depending on the temperature, it prefers living outdoors (under rocks, woodpiles, and debris) or in structures (basements, attics, and storage areas). The name "reclusa" describes its behavior: It is nocturnal, avoids areas of activity, hides its web, and is seldom seen. Bites are most common from April to October, usually involve an extremity, and seldom occur unless the spider is disturbed or threatened. Most victims are bitten while asleep, dressing, or working in the yard or house, and they may not initially be aware that envenomation has occurred.

L. reclusa measures 1 to 5 cm leg to leg, is fawn to dark brown, and has on its dorsal cephalothorax a violin-shaped, dark brown to yellow marking with the larger end toward the head. The body of a large spider will measure 1 cm in length by 0.5 cm in width. The short-haired body is oval, and the legs are long and slender. Three pairs of eyes, rather than four, is a distinctive but not unique feature of the genus. Although all *Loxosceles* species are often called "brown," "violin," or "fiddleback" spiders, the name "brown recluse" should be used only for *L. reclusa.*

Loxosceles venom contains proteins, mostly enzymes (e.g., protease, phospholipase, hyaluronidase, collagenase, esterase, sphingomyelinase), which cause both local and systemic toxicity.[7–9,11,13] Dermonecrosis (ulceration) is mainly due to ischemia secondary to inflammation caused by leukocyte infiltration, hemolysis, complement activation, and intravascular coagulation.[5,16]

CLINICAL PRESENTATION

Cutaneous and systemic toxicity (arachnidism) may occur, and the systemic reaction is not necessarily proportional to the local reaction. Systemic symptoms may develop before a necrotic lesion. Severity relates to the amount of venom injected, the bite location, and the victim's immune status. Many bites have a relatively benign course.[4] Children and debilitated victims are at greater risk for severe reaction, but the elderly are often asymptomatic, possibly because of immunity that developed following earlier bites.

Typically, the bite itself feels like a pinprick that, in a few hours, may itch, tingle, swell, and become tender and red or blanch. Often, a blister or purpura forms, or both. Necrosis with induration and eschar formation may occur within hours or as late as 2 weeks after the bite; the eschar falls off, leaving an ulceration that may take months to heal. The most severe necrotic lesions occur in fatty areas such as the abdomen, thighs, and buttocks.[18] Occasionally, an erythematous or violaceous reaction at the bite site, surrounded by a ring of pallor ("halo," "target," or "bull's eye" lesion), may be seen soon after envenomation. Vast edema may occur to the general bite site, especially on the neck and face.

Systemic effects develop within 96 hours after the bite and include fever, chills, malaise, weakness, nausea, vomiting, arthralgia, myalgia, and rash. Laboratory findings may include anemia, thrombocytopenia, leukocytosis, and evidence of hemolysis and disseminated intravascular coagulation. Hemolysis may directly result in hemoglobinuria, renal failure, and shock, or indirectly cause congestive heart failure, coma, convulsions, liver injury, and death due to anemic hypoxia.[17,18,20] The seldom-seen rash, a transient, early, diffuse, faint, macular, or speckled erythematous eruption over the trunk and flexural areas, may be a favorable prognostic sign, because it is often observed when a skin lesion suddenly involutes and resolves. A scarlatiniform rash may appear within days and is thought to often represent a toxigenic erythroderma reaction to the venom rather than a *Streptococcus* or *Staphylococcus* infection.

DIFFERENTIAL DIAGNOSIS

At least five other genera of spiders in the United States can cause necrotic lesions.[2,14,18] The differential diagnosis also in-

TABLE 377.1. Differential Diagnoses of Necrotic Lesion(s)

SPIDER BITES (COMMON NAME)	OTHER BITES AND STINGS
Acanthoscurria	Assassin bugs
Argiope (orbweaver)[a]	Bed bug
Atrax	Fly bite
Avicularia	Grasshoppers
Chiracanthium (running or sac spider)[a]	Hymenoptera
Loxosceles[a]	Infected flea bites
Lycosa (wolf spider)[a]	Jerusalem crickets
Megaphobema	Kissing bug (*Triatoma protracta*)
Pamphobeteus	Mites
Phidippus (jumping spider)[a]	Other orthopterans (biting insects)
Phormictopus	Scorpaenidae (scorpionfish, stonefish, lionfish)
Tegenaria agrestis (northwestern brown spider)[a]	Scorplons
Teraphosa	Snakes
Xenesthis	Solenopsis (fire ant)
	Solpugids (kind of venomous ant or spider)
	Ticks
	Vesicating beetle
MEDICAL CONDITIONS	
Artifactual ulcers	Infections
Diabetic ulcer	Injections
Drugs—heparin, coumadin, warfarin, ergot, bromoderma (bromine)	Keratin-mediated response to a fungus
Emboli	Lyell syndrome (toxic epidermal necrolysis)
Erythema chronicum migrans	Lymphoid papulosis
Erythema multiforme	Malignancy causing arterial obstruction
Erythema nodosum	Periarteritis nodosa
Fat herniation with infarction	Poison ivy
Focal vasculitis	Poison oak
Foreign bodies	Pyoderma gangrenosum
Frostbite	Purpura fulminans
Gonococcal hemorrhagic lesion	Scleroderma
Herpes simplex	Sporotrichosis
Hypersensitivity angiitis	Stevens-Johnson syndrome
	Thrombi

[a] Genera found in United States.
Data from Ellenhorn M, Barceloux D. Medical toxicology, New York: Elsevier, 1988:1149; Russell F. *Emerg Med* 1986;18(8):13; Russell F, et al. *Toxicon* 1983;21:337; Wasserman G, et al. *Toxicol Clin Toxicol* 1983;21:451.

cludes other bites and stings as well as many medical conditions (Table 377.1).[6,14,15,18] Erythema that evolves into a violaceous macule distinguishes a necrotic envenomation from a nonnecrotic bite. In addition, as the macule widens, the edge becomes uneven and the center sinks below skin level; nonnecrotic lesions remain edematous, raised, and red.[1] Unless an offending spider is positively identified, a generic diagnosis such as "cutaneous necrosis," "necrotic arachnidism," or "necrotic arthropod bite or sting" should be used rather than a definitive one such as "brown recluse envenomation" or "loxoscelism." Other natural toxins causing hemolysis are Coelenterata (Portuguese man-of-war jellyfish), Hymenoptera (bees, wasps, hornets), snakes, *Clostridium* infections, and streptococcal and staphylococcal infections.

EMERGENCY DEPARTMENT EVALUATION

The history should include the time and circumstances of a bite and a description of the spider (although this information is seldom known), as well as the nature and progression of symptoms. The skin should be examined closely for typical lesions in patients with acute hemolysis and coagulopathy of unknown cause. The general examination should focus on vital signs, heart, lungs, and neurologic function.

All patients with possible envenomation should have a baseline complete blood count and Dipstix or urinalysis. Those with evidence of hemolysis or systemic reactions may also require plasma and urine free hemoglobin levels, a reticulocyte count, coagulation studies (prothrombin time, partial thromboplastin time, fibrinogen, and D-dimers), and antiglobulin tests (i.e., Coombs' test). Other tests that should be performed include type, crossmatch, and screen; liver function studies (alkaline phosphatase, alanine aminotransferase, aspartate aminotransferase, creatine phosphokinase, and bilirubin); renal function studies (electrolytes, blood urea nitrogen, creatinine); and serum amylase. Rarely necessary are a serum haptoglobin level, haptoglobin binding capacity, biopsy, culture, or Gram stain. A passive hemagglutination inhibition test performed from skin lesion exudate is sensitive, specific, and reproducible but, at present, is only a research tool because it is cumbersome to prepare.[3]

EMERGENCY DEPARTMENT MANAGEMENT

Treatment of necrotic or cutaneous arachnidism should be the same, regardless of the culprit. A "benign neglect" approach nearly always results in an excellent outcome. It is impossible to make an early prediction about which bite will result in a disfiguring lesion. General wound care usually suffices. Corticosteroids injected locally or systemically, as well as vasodilators, have not proved helpful.[1] Antibiotics are not needed routinely, but they may be needed for secondary bacterial infection. An antipruritic or antianxiety drug is often comforting, as well as cool compresses (avoid heat, because it may stimulate a cascade of inflammatory reactants).

Analgesics can be given for pain, but nonsteroidal antiinflammatory drugs are contraindicated because of possible bleeding problems. Although still performed by some surgeons, early wide excision is ineffective, unnecessary, and expensive; produces complications (such as allowing venom to penetrate deeper into tissues); and may cause disability or worsen scarring. Corrective surgery should be delayed for 6 to 8 weeks, when the necrosis is clearly demarcated.[18,19] Necrotizing fasciitis or abscess would warrant emergency surgery.

Some authorities suggest that a polymorphonuclear leukocyte inhibitor such as dapsone (25 to 100 mg orally twice a day for 1 to 2 weeks) may prevent ulceration if started early.[12] Dapsone should be reserved for nonpregnant, healthy adults with rapidly progressive blistering and hemorrhage or impending ulceration in a cosmetic area such as the face or digits, and a strongly suggestive or confirmed history of spider envenomation. Glucose-6-phosphate dehydrogenase deficiency is a contraindication for dapsone therapy, and patients treated with this agent must be carefully monitored for drug toxicity (hemolysis, methemoglobinemia, superinfection, leukopenia, rash). There is no controlled study proving the effectiveness of hyperbaric oxygen, although it may be beneficial in a subgroup of patients with a history of poor wound healing.

The treatment of systemic arachnidism is mainly aggressive, symptomatic, and supportive care. Corticosteroids (methylprednisolone, 10 to 40 mg intravenously every 6 hours) ameliorate hemolysis and are needed for only 3 to 7 days. Alkalinization of the urine can protect against renal failure secondary to hemoglobinuria. Anemia and thrombocytopenia should be treated with component therapy (e.g., platelets, packed red cells), as needed. As complement or unknown factors in whole blood may react with venom components and contribute to red blood cell destruction, this product is not recommended.[10]

DISPOSITION

Physicians unfamiliar with arachnidism should consult a regional poison control center or toxicologist for advice. A telephone call to an envenomation expert may be necessary. Patients who present immediately after a bite should be followed as outpatients with 24- to 48-hour rechecks for 3 to 5 days. Patients who present with or develop large ulcers should be referred to a plastic surgeon for follow-up. Patients with significant systemic symptoms, clinical toxicity, or hematologic abnormalities should be admitted with an appropriate level of monitoring. Those with a benign course and stable physical and laboratory evaluations can be discharged with follow-up in 24 to 48 hours. Liberal admission for observation may be prudent in very young or debilitated patients and in those judged to be unreliable regarding follow-up.

COMMON PITFALLS

- Diagnosing "brown recluse spider bite" rather than "necrotic arthropod bite or sting" or "necrotic or cutaneous arachnidism" when positive identification of the offending species has not been made
- Failure to appreciate that hemolysis secondary to *L. reclusa* envenomation may occur rapidly or be insidious
- Failure to perform laboratory evaluations on patients with skin lesions highly suspicious of loxoscelism
- Failure to warn patients about potential but unpredictable complications, such as hemolysis, coagulopathies, and secondary infections
- Failure to provide adequate follow-up
- Failure to discuss therapeutic options, controversies, and complications

References

1. Anderson P. Necrotizing spider bites. *Am Fam Physician* 1982;26:198.
2. Atkin J, Wingo C, Sodeman W. Probable cause of necrotic spider bite in the Midwest. *Science* 1957;126:73.
3. Barrett SM, Romine-Jenkins M, Blick KE. Passive hemagglutination inhibition test for diagnosis of brown recluse spider bite envenomation. *Clin Chem* 1993;39:2104.
4. Berger R. The unremarkable brown recluse spider bite. *JAMA* 1973;225:1109.
5. Berger R, Adelstein E, Anderson P. Intravascular coagulation—the cause of necrotic arachnidism. *J Invest Dermatol* 1978;61:142.
6. Ellenhorn M, Barceloux D. *Medical toxicology, diagnosis and treatment of human poisoning*. New York: Elsevier Science, 1988:1149.
7. Forrester L, Barrett J, Campbell B. Red blood cell lysis induced by the venom of the brown recluse spider: the role of sphingomyelinase D. *Arch Biochem Biophys* 1978;187:355.
8. Geren C, Chan T, Hewell D, et al. Partial characterization of the low-molecular-weight fractions of the extract of the venom apparatus of the brown recluse spider and its hemolymph. *Toxicon* 1975;13:233.
9. Geren C, Chan T, Hewell D, et al. Isolation and characterization of toxins from brown recluse spider venom (*Loxosceles reclusa*). *Arch Biochem Biophys* 1976;174:90.
10. Hardman J, Beck M, Hardman P, et al. Incompatibility associated with the bite of a brown recluse spider (*Loxosceles reclusa*). *Transfusion* 1983;23:233.
11. Hufford D, Morgan P. C-reactive protein as a mediator in the lysis of human erythrocytes sensitized by brown recluse spider venom. *Proc Soc Exp Biol Med* 1981;167:493.
12. Rees R, Altenbern P, Lynch J, et al. A comparison of surgical excision versus dapsone and delayed surgical excision. *Ann Surg* 1985;202:659.
13. Rees R, Nanney L, Yates R, et al. Interaction of brown recluse spider venom on cell membranes: the inciting mechanism? *J Invest Dermatol* 1984;83:270.
14. Russell F. A confusion of spiders. *Emerg Med* 1986;(June 15):8.
15. Russell F, Gertsch W. Letter to the editor. *Toxicon* 1983;21:337.
16. Smith C, Micks D. The role of polymorphonuclear leukocytes in the lesion caused by the venom of the brown spider, *Loxosceles reclusa*. *Lab Invest* 1970;22:90.
17. Taylor E, Denny W. Hemolysis, renal failure and death, presumed secondary to the bite of brown recluse spider. *South Med J* 1966;59:1209.
18. Wasserman G, Anderson P. Loxoscelism and necrotic arachnidism. *J Toxicol Clin Toxicol* 1983;21:451.
19. Wasserman G. Wound care of spider and snake envenomations. *Ann Emerg Med* 1988;17:1331.
20. Wasserman G, Mydler TT, Sharma V. Brown recluse spider envenomation as a cause of hemolysis and hemoglobinuria. *Vet Hum Toxicol* 1991;33:359.

CHAPTER 378

Crotalid Snake Envenomations

Richard C. Dart and John B. Sullivan, Jr.

There are several thousand poisonous snakebites in the United States each year, resulting in approximately five deaths.[10] Most of these bites involve members of the Crotalidae family and include the genera *Crotalus* (rattlesnakes), *Agkistrodon* (copperheads and water moccasins or cottonmouths), and *Sistrurus* (pygmy rattler and massasauga). Although all states except Alaska, Hawaii, and Maine have poisonous snakes, most bites occur in the southeast, southwest, and western regions. The incidence is greatest between March and October, when snakes and victims are the most active.

Crotalidae have a temperature (prey)-sensing pit below and in front of the eye (the pupil of which is elliptical)—hence the common name "pit viper." Venom is injected through a pair of fangs attached to the maxilla. Venom is mainly a mixture of digestive enzymes that cause local tissue necrosis and systemic vascular damage, hemolysis, fibrinolysis, and neuromuscular dysfunction. Venom shock and pulmonary injury result from increased vascular permeability and coagulopathy, leading to edema and hemorrhage. Direct cardiac depressant effects may also contribute to shock.[12] Venom composition varies with the species.

Up to 25% of bites do not result in envenomation (dry bites).[12] Most envenomations result in a combination of local and systemic effects. However, some populations of Mojave rattlesnakes have a venom (type a) that may cause presynaptic neuromuscular blockade with delayed respiratory failure and mild or absent local effects.[2,6,8] Envenomations by *Agkistrodon* and *Sistrurus* species tend to be less severe than those of *Crotalus* species.

The size and species of snake, the location and depth of the bite, the victim's size and health, first-aid measures performed, the time to definitive therapy, and the type of therapy influence the severity and outcome. The worst scenario is a small, unhealthy victim deeply bitten by a large snake in the central body. Improper first-aid measures, delay in arriving at medical care, delayed diagnosis, and inadequate or unnecessary treatment adversely affects the outcome.

Bites by exotic snakes may occur in zoo and pet snake handlers and require specific antivenoms. A regional poison center or zoo can provide information on snake identification, expected toxicity, and antivenom location. A 24-hour Antivenom Index Service can be reached by calling your certified regional poison center. Physicians unfamiliar with the management of snake envenomation should consult a toxicologist or regional poison center.

CLINICAL PRESENTATION

Dry bites produce no signs or symptoms other than those of a puncture wound. If envenomation has occurred, the victim (often an intoxicated male) typically notes sudden, severe pain at the bite site, soon followed by progressive swelling and, sometimes, paresthesias.

Examination may show two puncture wounds exuding bloody fluid. However, there are many reports of serious envenomation associated with scratches and single or multiple puncture wounds. Other local findings include erythema, ecchymosis, bullae, and, eventually, necrosis and ulceration. Severity is graded using several factors (Table 378.1). Bites about the face may lead to airway obstruction; those of the extremities may lead to compartmental syndromes. Wound infection is a potential complication.[7]

Systemic symptoms include nausea, vomiting, diarrhea, perioral paresthesias, salivation, lethargy, and weakness. Severe envenomations may lead to cardiovascular collapse, coma, seizures, dyspnea, respiratory depression, and gastrointestinal and pulmonary hemorrhage. Initial vital signs often show tachycardia and mild hypertension. Laboratory evaluation may reveal hemolysis, anemia, thrombocytopenia, coagulopathy (including severe fibrinolysis), and blood, protein, and glucose in the urine in severe cases. In severe cases, the chest radiograph may reveal pulmonary edema, and the electrocardiogram (ECG) may show dysrhythmias or ischemic changes. Systemic findings are also used to assess the severity of envenomation (see Table 378.1). An initially mild envenomation may progress over a period of hours to become moderate, severe, or even life-threatening. Coagulation abnormalities may peak as late as 3 days after envenomation.

DIFFERENTIAL DIAGNOSIS

Victims at the extremes of age, those with altered mental states, and those who are bitten while reaching into concealed areas may not realize they have been bitten. Snakebite may be misdiagnosed as a nonvenomous bite or sting or as puncture wounds and scratches from thorns and brush. The possible diagnosis of snake venom poisoning can be excluded only by prolonged observation, documenting a lack of progressive local and systemic manifestations.

EMERGENCY DEPARTMENT EVALUATION

On the patient's arrival in the emergency department, vital signs and a rapid patient survey should be performed to determine the patient's clinical stability. The time and circumstances of the bite, the nature and severity of symptoms, the first-aid measures taken before arrival, and any history of allergies, medical problems, previous bites, and antivenom therapy are noted. The bite site should be examined, noting the nature and extent of local findings. Distal neurovascular status should be noted in extremity bites. In the early course, the local evaluation should be repeated every 15 minutes. The general examination should focus on the cardiovascular, pulmonary, and neurologic systems. Laboratory tests in questionable or initially minimal bites should include complete blood count; determination of electrolytes, blood urea nitrogen, and creatinine levels; prothrombin time; platelet count; and urinalysis. In severe cases or in patients who worsen, creatine kinase, fibrinogen, fibrin split products, arterial blood gas analysis, and blood typing should be included. A chest radiograph and an ECG should be obtained in patients with systemic signs or symptoms.

EMERGENCY DEPARTMENT MANAGEMENT

Advanced life-support measures should be instituted, as necessary. Prehospital personnel should be directed to establish in-

TABLE 378.1 Grading of Envenomation by Signs and Symptoms

Dry Bite	Minimal	Moderate	Severe
Puncture wound, pain, little or no swelling. No systemic symptoms or progression. Normal laboratory studies.	Localized pain, edema, ecchymosis. No systemic symptoms or progression. Normal laboratory studies.	Progressive pain, edema, ecchymosis. Variable systemic symptoms. Stable vital signs. Mild laboratory abnormalities.	Massive edema, ecchymosis. Unstable vital signs. Coma, seizure, respiratory depression or distress, clinical coagulopathy. Markedly abnormal laboratory

travenous access, to give oxygen, and to transport victims of venomous snakebites to a medical facility that possesses antivenom. If a tourniquet has been placed, it should not be removed until intravenous access has been established. The limb should be maintained in a neutral position. Loose (lymphatic) tourniquets, incision and suction, and cooling an extremity may be effective if used within 30 minutes of envenomations, but they are not substitutes for definitive care. Local wound care and tetanus prophylaxis should be provided. Worsening of local or systemic manifestations provides a guide for appropriate administration of Wyeth equine polyvalent Crotalidae antivenom. Immunoglobulins in the antivenom neutralize venom proteins by antigen–antibody complex formation. If, after several hours, pain and edema remain localized to the bite site and coagulopathy is not progressing, antivenom is unnecessary. Continued observation for signs of local progression and laboratory abnormalities cannot be overemphasized. The extent of swelling should be outlined with a marking pen, and the limb circumference should be measured at several sites above and below the bite. If any of these parameters worsen, antivenom therapy is usually warranted.

The skin test should not be performed unless a definite decision to give antivenom has been made. Unstable patients and those with obvious systemic involvement should be tested immediately. A negative skin test suggests, but does not guarantee, that an antivenom reaction will not develop. Although a positive test (erythema or induration) is an important warning, it does not absolutely preclude administration of antivenom.[13] Patients with moderate or severe envenomation who require antivenom can be pretreated with diphenhydramine, cimetidine, and, if necessary, epinephrine.[11,12]

Each vial of antivenom should be diluted to 10 mL, using the diluent supplied with the vial. This requires 20 to 30 minutes of gentle mixing, so preparation should begin at the same time as skin testing. Each vial is further diluted twofold to fivefold in intravenous fluid before infusion, and tenfold in patients with an allergic response.

Initially, the antivenom should be given slowly, while observing for allergic or hypotensive reactions. If none occurs, the infusion rate should be rapidly increased so that the antivenom dose is completed in 1 hour. Antivenom should be given only in a critical care setting with epinephrine and antihistamines readily available. It can reverse coagulopathy up to 72 hours after envenomation.

Patients with minimal envenomations with progression and those with moderate envenomations should receive five to ten vials of antivenom initially. Patients with severe envenomations require ten to 20 vials initially. Life-threatening envenomations require higher dosages. Management decisions are outlined in Fig. 378.1. Subsequent antivenom doses are guided by clinical response.

Concomitant supportive care (e.g., fluids and pressors for hypotension, blood component replacement for severe hematologic abnormalities, and respiratory support) is extremely important but often neglected.[9] Blood products should be used only if the patient is actively bleeding or cannot receive antivenom.[1]

The effectiveness of antivenom in the treatment of snake venom poisoning has been extensively documented. However, fasciotomy and supportive care without antivenom have been proposed in some areas as definitive treatment of snakebite. Experimental evidence in animals shows no beneficial effect.[4,5] Only in patients with documented increased intracompartmental pressure unresponsive to limb elevation, mannitol (1 to 2 g/kg intravenously), and antivenom (five to ten vials) should fasciotomy be considered. Cultures and antibiotic therapy should be initiated if clinical signs of infection develop.

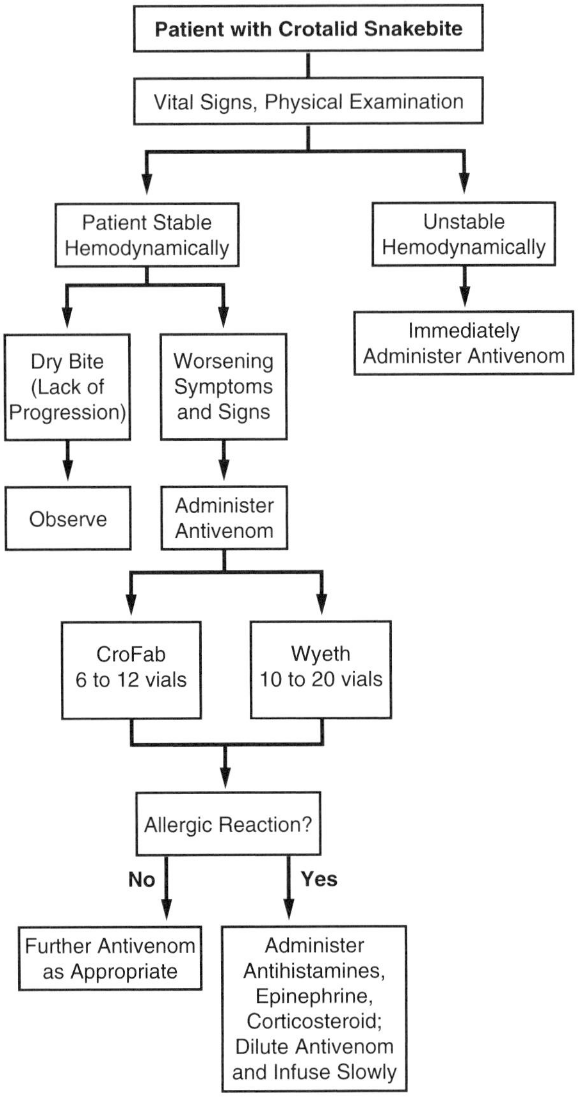

Figure 378.1. Algorithm for the management of crotalid snakebite.

DISPOSITION

Patients with dry bites may be discharged after an 8- to 12-hour observation period. Those with severe or life-threatening bites and those receiving antivenom should be admitted to an intensive care unit. Admission to a floor bed is appropriate for the observation of patients with mild or moderate envenomations. Mobilization of the affected extremity can begin when the progression of swelling has ceased. Discharge is appropriate when swelling is decreasing, any coagulopathy has completely reversed, and the patient is ambulatory. Outpatient follow-up may be necessary for several days to monitor for infection and serum sickness. Serum sickness may range from a mild viral-like illness to severe urticarial rash, arthralgias, and other complications. Most patients who receive more than five vials will develop serum sickness.[3] Most cases can be treated as outpatients, with antiinflammatory analgesics, antihistamines, and corticosteroids.

COMMON PITFALLS

- Failure to diagnose envenomation because of a lack of history or inadequate observation of patients with suspicious wounds of unclear cause

- Performing inappropriate skin testing in patients who do not need antivenom
- Failure to monitor closely for allergic reactions in patients receiving antivenom, even though they may have had a negative skin test. Epinephrine and diphenhydramine must be available at the bedside.
- Using antivenom unnecessarily, or giving inadequate doses
- Failure to provide supportive care as well as antivenom to patients with severe reactions
- Failure to recognize that horse serum allergy is not an absolute contraindication to antivenom administration

References

1. Burgess JL, Dart RC. Snake venom coagulopathy: use and abuse of blood products in the treatment of pit viper envenomation. *Ann Emerg Med* 1991;20:795.
2. Castilonia R, Pattabhiramin T, Russell FE. Neuromuscular blocking effects of the Mojave rattlesnake (*Crotalus scutulatus scutulatus*) venom. *Proc West Pharmacol Soc* 1980;23:103.
3. Corrigan P, Russell FE, Wainschel J. Clinical reactions to antivenom. *Toxicon* 1978;[Suppl]:457.
4. Garfin SR, Castilonia RR, Mubarak SJ, et al. Rattlesnake bites and surgical decompression: results using a laboratory model. *Toxicon* 1984;22:177.
5. Garfin SR, Castilonia RR, Mubarak SJ, et al. The effect of antivenom on intramuscular pressure elevation induced by rattlesnake venom. *Toxicon* 1985;23:677.
6. Glenn J, Straight R, Wolfe M. Geographical variation in *Crotalus scutulatus scutulatus* (Mohave rattlesnake) venom properties. *Toxicon* 1983;21:119.
7. Goldstein E, Citron D, Gonzales H, et al. Bacteriology of rattlesnake venom and implications for therapy. *J Infect Dis* 1979;140:818.
8. Hardy D. Envenomation by the Mohave rattlesnake (*Crotalus scutulatus scutulatus*) in Southern Arizona, USA. *Toxicon* 1983;21:111.
9. Hardy D. Fatal rattlesnake envenomation in Arizona: 1969–1984. *Clin Toxicol* 1986;24:1.
10. Langley RL, Morow WE. Deaths resulting from animal attacks in the United States. *Wild Environ Med* 1997;8:8.
11. Otten EJ, McKimm D. Venomous snakebite in a patient allergic to horse serum. *Ann Emerg Med* 1983;12:624.
12. Russell FE. *Snake venom poisoning*. Great Neck, NY: Scholium International, 1983.
13. Spaite D, Dart RC, Sullivan JB. Skin testing in cases of possible crotalid envenomation. *Ann Emerg Med* 1988;17:105.

CHAPTER 379
Elapid Snake Envenomations

Richard C. Dart and John B. Sullivan, Jr.

North American representatives of the elapid family are the coral snakes. These brightly colored snakes are known for the potency of their venom. Fortunately, few bites occur, because these snakes are usually small, nocturnal, and reticent.

Coral snakes found in the United States include the Eastern coral snake (*Micrurus fulvius fulvius*), the Texas coral snake (*Micrurus fulvius tenere*), and the Arizona (Sonoran) coral snake (*Micruroides euryxanthus*). The Eastern coral snake is found in the deep southeast United States; the Texas and Arizona subspecies are found primarily in the states whose name they bear.[3] All these snakes are brightly colored, with black, red, and yellow rings that encircle their bodies. The red and yellow rings touch in coral snakes but are separated by black rings in nonpoisonous snakes, hence the rhyme, "Red on yellow, kill a fellow; red on black, venom lack." Unfortunately, victims may confuse the rhyme, especially when intoxicated (e.g., "Red on yellow, good fellow."). Elapids lack facial pits and have nearly round pupils.

Coral snakes are docile. When biting, they hold on or chew, allowing them to envenomate. Their venom is discharged through grooves on two small, fixed anterior fangs. Their small size makes it difficult, but not impossible, to envenomate humans seriously. The Eastern and Texas subspecies are larger and have seriously envenomated many patients, but the Sonoran coral snake has not caused severe envenomation.[3]

CLINICAL PRESENTATION

Coral snake envenomation can be difficult to diagnose and easy to underestimate. The typical bite shows little local damage and few initial systemic symptoms. Minor pain without swelling may be present. This may be followed by numbness and weakness of the affected part as the envenomation syndrome advances. Systemic symptoms, which may take hours to develop, include drowsiness, apprehension, weakness, fasciculation, tremors, difficulty swallowing, dyspnea, salivation, nausea, and vomiting.[1]

Physical examination may show fang marks and associated scratches. It is often possible to express a drop of blood. However, the history is particularly important, because significant envenomation without any apparent marks, despite close examination, has occurred. In such cases, injecting lidocaine under the suspected area may show minute beads of serosanguineous fluid exuding from fang punctures. Signs of systemic toxicity may be delayed in onset and include weakness of extraocular muscles, miotic pupils, bulbar paralysis, respiratory depression, and convulsions. In severe cases, arterial blood gas analysis may show hypoventilation and an elevated creatine kinase level.

DIFFERENTIAL DIAGNOSIS

The diagnosis of coral snake envenomation is usually clear, because the snake frequently hangs on to the victim and has bright, identifiable coloring. When the patient cannot clearly communicate, the rapidity of onset and usually short duration of venom poisoning distinguish it from other motor neuron diseases. Laboratory testing may be necessary to rule out poisoning by agents such as botulism, heavy metals, and central nervous system depressant medications.

EMERGENCY DEPARTMENT EVALUATION

The time and circumstances of the bite, a description of the snake, first-aid treatment before arrival, allergies, previous bites and antivenom therapy, medical history prior to presentation, and the onset, progression, and nature of symptoms should be established. The physical examination focuses on neurologic assessment, particularly the cranial motor nerve, and respiratory muscle function. Tidal volume, arterial blood gas analysis, and other routine studies (laboratory, chest radiograph, electrocardiogram) are obtained, if clinically indicated. Although positive identification of the offending snake is helpful, it should not delay treatment.

EMERGENCY DEPARTMENT MANAGEMENT

Prehospital care should consist of intravenous line insertion, maintenance of airway, and timely transport to a health-care facility capable of full life-support and antivenom therapy. Constriction bands or pressure bandages to retard venom spread may be useful.

Wound cleansing and tetanus prophylaxis are provided. Patients who have clearly been bitten or who have developed symptoms or signs of envenomation are given at least five vials of *M. fulvius* antivenom (equine) by intravenous infusion. Waiting until systemic manifestations develop before giving antivenom may not always reverse them or prevent further deterioration. If symptoms progress, the dose of antivenom is repeated. Although *M. fulvius* antivenom is neither effective nor necessary in Sonoran coral snake envenomation, the aforementioned protocol should be followed unless a positive identification of this species has been made. The elective intubation of patients with bulbar signs or symptoms may prevent aspiration pneumonia.[1]

The prognosis is excellent. There is normally no tissue loss or permanent neurologic dysfunction. Even without antivenom treatment, recovery can be expected if appropriate supportive care is provided.[2] Hence, patients with allergic reactions to horse serum or antivenom can be managed successfully without antivenom.

DISPOSITION

All patients in whom the diagnosis of coral snake envenomation is entertained should be admitted to an intensive care area for at least 12 hours of close monitoring of vital signs and neurologic function. This disposition applies to patients with a definite bite, either by history or examination, regardless of whether they are symptomatic. Patients with no evidence of envenomation after 12 hours of observation may be discharged. Those with severe envenomations may require several days of hospitalization.

COMMON PITFALLS

- Delaying antivenom administration until systemic signs and symptoms are present
- Failure to admit and monitor all patients with possible coral snake envenomation
- Failure to monitor for progression of toxicity after antivenom administration, and failure to provide concurrent, aggressive supportive care
- Using antivenom inappropriately in patients with documented Arizona (Sonoran) coral snake envenomation and in those with allergic reactions to horse serum or antivenom
- Failure to take the same precautions as described for crotalid antivenom when giving coral snake antivenom

References

1. Kitchens CS, Van Mierop LHS. Envenomation by the Eastern coral snake (*Micrurus fulvius fulvius*). *JAMA* 1987;258:1615.
2. Mosely T. Coral snake bite: recovery following symptoms of respiratory paralysis. *Ann Surg* 1966;163:943.
3. Russell FE. *Snake venom poisoning*. Great Neck, NY: Scholium International, 1983.

CHAPTER 380
Mammal Bites and Associated Infections

Stephen J. Playe and Richard V. Aghababian

Thousands of people throughout the world are killed each year by sharks, crocodiles, pachyderms, big cats, and other large carnivores.[4] Ten to 20 fatal dog attacks occur in the United States each year, almost always involving children. Morbidity is extensive. More than a million Americans seek care for animal bites each year, accounting for about 1% of emergency department visits. One percent to 2% of these patients require hospital admission. Dogs and cats inflict 95% of the bites, and tend to bite the extremities of adults and older children and the face and scalp of younger children and infants. Infectious complications are often responsible for serious morbidity and mortality.

Bite wounds are unique in several respects. Dog bites are usually crush-type lacerations with devitalized adjacent tissue. About 10% of full-thickness dog bites become infected.[1,2] Cat bites tend to be puncture wounds, with an infection rate of up to 50%.[1] Human bites are thought to be third most frequent after dog and cat bites. Although occlusional human bites of the extremities or trunk are mechanically similar to dog bites, the epidemiology and microbiology of human bites are different. Occupational exposure can occur in dental professionals, caretakers of the mentally impaired, daycare workers, and medical personnel involved in airway management or the care of seizing or combative patients. "Love bites" can be incurred, often involving the neck, breasts, or genitalia, during passionate sexual encounters. Biting off the tip of the nose as punishment for adultery is reported in some cultures. Teeth marks (wound imprints) have been used by forensic dental pathologists to help identify assailants. Clinched-fist injuries ("fight bites"), which occur when a fist strikes teeth during altercations, are the most serious of human bites. The microbes contained in plaque and deposits around teeth may be carried to deep structures and relatively avascular tissue planes. The patient may present with an innocuous-appearing laceration, initially offer an alternative explanation of the mechanism of injury, and subsequently develop tenosynovitis, septic arthritis, or osteomyelitis. Persistent infections can necessitate amputation. Animal bites may inoculate the site with a host of potentially pathologic microorganisms, including tetanus and rabies viruses, *Staphylococcus* spp., *Streptococcus* spp., *Corynebacterium* spp., and anaerobes.[14] The human oral flora frequently includes *Eikenella corrodens*. Transmission of hepatitis B, hepatitis C, and human immunodeficiency virus (HIV) must also be considered.

Pasteurella species, small gram-negative rods that are part of the normal mouth flora of many animals, have been implicated in up to 50% of infected dog bites (most often *P. canis*) and in up to 75% of infected cat bites (most often *P. multocida* subspecies *multocida* and *septica*).[5,12,14] These organisms typically produce a rapidly developing inflammatory response in the wound, often with purulent drainage, within 24 hours. *Pasteurella* species may also cause cellulitis, abscess, osteomyelitis, septic arthritis, meningitis, and septicemia.

Capnocytophaga canimorsus (DF-2), a fastidious gram-negative bacillus, can infect dog and cat bites and can lead to often rapidly fatal bacteremia, disseminated intravascular coagulation, or meningitis. Although most common in immunocompromised patients,[15] these infections have been reported in normal hosts.[13,16]

The organism thought responsible for cat-scratch disease, *Bartonella henselae,* is a small pleomorphic bacillus identified by Warthin-Starry stain of lymph node or skin biopsies.[7] The gram-negative organisms *Streptobacillus* moniliformis and *Spirillum minus* cause rat-bite fever. *Francisella tularensis* is a gram-negative coccobacillus that causes tularemia.

Herpesvirus simiae (B virus) is carried by rhesus and other macaque monkeys. It is spread to humans by bites or scratches and can lead to fatal encephalitis.[9]

CLINICAL PRESENTATION

Animal bites can lead to trauma of the skin, tendons, joints, bones, major vessels, viscera, brain, and other organs. Death in immediately fatal cases is usually due to hemorrhagic shock. Crush lacerations over the dorsum of the proximal phalanges or metacarpophalangeal joints should be presumed to be due to clenched-fist bites, even when patients are reluctant to offer this history. Patients who present more than 24 hours after injury usually have signs of established local or systemic infection. This is often the case with clenched-fist injuries.

Patients with cat-scratch disease present with headache, fever, malaise, and tender regional lymphadenopathy about a week (range, 3 days to 6 weeks) after a cat scratch or bite.[7] A tender papule that develops at the inoculum site and subsequently blisters and heals with eschar formation or a transient macular or vesicular rash may be noted. A significant number of patients give a history of cat exposure without a wound or primary lesion. Lymph nodes may suppurate and drain spontaneously or become nontender but remain palpable over a period of weeks to months. Complications and associated conditions include encephalitis, Parinaud syndrome (granulomatous conjunctivitis), mesenteric adenitis without splenomegaly, osteolytic bone lesions, purpura with both normal and low platelet counts, and erythema nodosum.

Patients with rat-bite fever caused by *S. moniliformis* typically develop sudden fever, chills, headache, and myalgias several days (range, 1 to 22 days) after a bite by a wild, laboratory, or pet rodent or carnivore, or the ingestion of food contaminated by rat excreta.[4] A rash (macular, petechial, purpuric, or pustular; centripetal or generalized) and asymmetric polyarthralgia or arthritis may also be present. Complications include soft-tissue and brain abscesses and endocarditis. Patients with *S. minus* infection usually develop relapsing fever, headache (with nausea, vomiting, and photophobia), and signs of nonpurulent local infection with regional lymphangitis and adenopathy several weeks (range, 1 to 36 days) after the initial healing of the bite wound. A rash (macular, brown or purple) may be noted on the extremities. Endocarditis has been reported.

Patients with tularemia usually present with fever, chills, headache, malaise, myalgias, tender hepatosplenomegaly, wound ulcer, and regional adenopathy 2 to 5 days after a bite or direct or indirect skin contact with virtually any animal (e.g., amphibians, birds, fish, or mammals).[4] Skin inoculation most frequently results from exposure to wild rabbits (usually cottontails) during skinning and preparation for eating and from bites from insect vectors (e.g., ticks, deer flies, mosquitoes). Other animals that commonly harbor *F. tularensis* include beavers, cats, cattle, muskrats, sheep, and squirrels. The initial skin lesion (a bite or puncture wound or contaminated scratch) develops into a well-defined ulcer with a black base and yellow exudate. A macular rash may be present, and lymph nodes may suppurate and drain spontaneously. Contamination of the eye, throat and intestines (ingestion), or lung (inhalation) may also lead to conjunctivitis, pharyngitis, gastroenteritis, or pneumonia, all of which are associated with regional lymphadenopathy. Complications include endocarditis, meningitis, osteomyelitis, pericarditis, and peritonitis.

The presentation of human rabies varies with the time elapsed after exposure. An asymptomatic incubation period (generally 20 to 60 days) is followed by a prodrome of 2 to 10 days characterized by symptoms that may include pain, paresthesias, or pruritus at the site of the bite and nonspecific symptoms such as fever, headache, nausea, vomiting, and malaise. The ensuing acute neurologic phase lasts 2 to 10 days. In about 80% of cases, the "furious" signs of hyperactivity predominate; these include agitation, hallucinations, thrashing, biting, and the classic hydrophobia caused by an exaggerated respiratory tract protective reflex. In about 20% of cases, paralytic signs predominate; this is termed *dumb rabies* and is characterized by progressive paralysis with intact sensorium. If patients do not succumb during the acute neurologic phase, they then become comatose and die within 2 weeks.[8]

Routine laboratory findings in cat-scratch disease, rat-bite fever, and tularemia are nonspecific (e.g., elevated leukocyte count and erythrocyte sedimentation rate). Cat-scratch disease is confirmed by antigen skin testing or microscopic examination of the primary skin lesion or lymph node. Rat-bite fever is confirmed by culture or antibody response to *S. moniliformis* or examination (Wright's stain or dark-field microscopy) of blood, skin lesion, or lymph node drainage in *S. minus* infections. These infections may result in false-positive syphilis tests. Tularemia is confirmed by serologic response.

DIFFERENTIAL DIAGNOSIS

Concomitant envenomations should be considered in bites by lizards (i.e., Gila monster), snakes, marine animals, and the short-tailed shrew. The differential diagnosis of cat-scratch disease, rat-bite fever, and tularemia is extensive and includes infections such as plague, syphilis, lymphogranuloma venereum, sporotrichosis, anthrax, histoplasmosis, coccidioidomycosis, infectious mononucleosis, toxoplasmosis, brucellosis, bacterial adenitis, and infections with *Mycobacterium, Rickettsia, Staphylococcus,* and *Streptococcus.* Sarcoid, lymphoma, and cysts and tumors of the neck should also be considered.

Rabies must be differentiated from other infectious causes of encephalitis, including herpes, arbovirus, tetanus, malaria, rickettsia, typhoid, poliomyelitis, and botulism. Noninfectious diseases that must be considered include Guillain-Barré syndrome, poisoning, alcohol withdrawal, acute porphyria, and behavioral disorders.[8]

EMERGENCY DEPARTMENT EVALUATION

Initial evaluation of acute injuries should include a primary survey, with attention to the basics of trauma care, particularly when a small victim is attacked by a large animal. The history should include details of the biting event: the time, the offending animal and its identity (wild or domestic, immunization and health status, captured or not), and the nature of the attack (provoked or unprovoked). The patient's underlying health status should also be determined.

The patient should be assessed not only for skin wounds, but also for deep-structure injury, particularly of the brain, vessels, viscera, nerves, tendons, joints, bones, and spinal cord. Puncture wounds are particularly prone to cause deep and often undiagnosed injuries. Location of the wound on the hand, wrist, foot, or joint or on the face and scalp of an infant increases the likelihood of deep-structure injury. Because clenched-fist injuries occur in flexion, they must be carefully explored throughout flexion in addition to extension to identify retained tooth fragments or tendon, joint, or bone injury. Radiographs should be obtained.

Local infectious complications include wound infection, cellulitis, abscess, osteomyelitis, prosthesis infection, and septic arthritis (even when the joint is not penetrated). Local wound infections that develop less than 24 hours after the bite are probably caused by either *P. multocida* or streptococci. Local infections that develop more than 48 hours after the bite are most frequently caused by *S. aureus*. Systemic complications include bacterial sepsis, meningitis, disseminated intravascular coagulation, cat-scratch disease, rat-bite fever, tetanus, tularemia, and rabies. The risk of infection is high in patients who are very young, very old, or immunocompromised (alcoholism, splenectomy, diabetes mellitus, liver dysfunction, acquired immunodeficiency syndrome, or immunosuppressive medication); those who have prosthetic joints or valves; and those who have peripheral vascular or lymphatic compromise. Other risk factors include cat bites; puncture wounds; location on a hand, wrist, foot, or joint; and treatment delay beyond 8 hours.

Although Gram stain and culture of fresh bites do not predict infection, a Gram stain and culture (aerobic and anaerobic) should be obtained in clinically infected wounds. If sepsis is suspected, the Gram stain of the peripheral blood should be examined for evidence of C. *canimorsus*, and blood cultures (anaerobic and aerobic) should be obtained. Complete blood count; determination of blood urea nitrogen, glucose, electrolyte, and creatinine levels; prothrombin time; partial thromboplastin time; fibrin split products; and lumbar puncture with cerebrospinal fluid (CSF) analysis and culture should be obtained, if clinically indicated.

Extremity radiographs are useful to evaluate the possibility of joint penetration, fracture, foreign body, and osteomyelitis. Skull radiographs and computed tomography scanning of the head are indicated for infants with face and scalp bites.

The patient who presents with fever, constitutional symptoms, and regional adenopathy should be questioned about animal bites, scratches, or exposures and a history of rash or skin lesions. The extent of adenopathy and tenderness and the size of the lymph nodes, liver, and spleen should be noted. The patient should also be examined for evidence of endocarditis, meningitis, and other complications. Further assessment should include complete blood count, serum electrolyte levels, liver and kidney function studies, blood cultures, and a chest radiograph. Lumbar puncture, peripheral blood smear, lymph node and skin biopsy examination, skin testing, and antibody titers (acute and convalescent) may be necessary.

EMERGENCY DEPARTMENT MANAGEMENT

For acute injuries, prehospital care should initially focus on life-support measures. Wound care should include copious irrigation with sterile saline solution or clean tap water. Wounded extremities should be immobilized and elevated.

In the emergency department, extremity wounds should be assessed for distal function and neurovascular status before local or regional anesthesia. Extremity tourniquets may facilitate exploration and repair. The most important aspect of wound care is copious irrigation with sterile saline solution, 1% povidone–iodine solution (1:10 dilution of the commercial 10% solution), or Pluronic-68. Devitalized tissue should be debrided with a scalpel or fine dissection scissors. Excision of puncture wounds has been recommended but never proved to be effective. Abrasions should be cleansed and treated with topical antibiotics.

Primary closure of animal bite wounds is controversial. When successful, the benefits are early return of function and optimal cosmetic results. As a rule, normal hosts with relatively clean lacerations, especially of the face, can safely be sutured, primarily if seen within a few hours of injury. Alternatively, sterile skin tapes may result in a lower incidence of infection. Delayed primary closure, often a prudent alternative, and healing by secondary intention are less apt to result in infection. Buried sutures should be avoided whenever possible. All wounded extremities should be immobilized, and strict elevation should be advised.

Clenched-fist bite wounds are best treated by delayed primary closure or secondary intention. In gaping wounds, the edges can be loosely approximated with a minimum of sutures, provided that sufficient space is allowed for drainage. All wounds should be carefully explored, copiously irrigated, splinted, and elevated. Admission to the hand, orthopedic, or plastic surgery service should be considered if there is any injury to the tendon, joint, or bone or if signs of infection are present. Intravenous antibiotics should be administered in all cases. Abscesses and infections that involve deep structures such as tendon sheaths and joints should also be referred to a surgeon, because they may require concomitant operative management. Antibiotics should again be administered intravenously. Patients may be discharged only after consultation and only when reliable, early follow-up can be assured.

Although "prophylactic" antibiotics are often prescribed, there are no prospective controlled studies with sufficient numbers of patients to demonstrate their effectiveness definitively or the superiority of a particular regimen. It seems, however, that antibiotics significantly decrease the incidence of infection in high-risk situations.[3,6]

Antibiotics, whether "prophylactic" or as empirical treatment of established infections, should cover *Pasteurella* spp. streptococci, staphylococci, *C. canimorsus*, and anaerobes. Amoxicillin–clavulanic acid (Augmentin 875 twice a day), a second-generation cephalosporin with anaerobic activity (e.g., cefuroxime 500 mg twice a day), or penicillin combined with a first-generation cephalosporin or with a semisynthetic penicillin, all offer an appropriately broad spectrum of activity.[14] Many authors have suggested semisynthetic penicillins or first-generation cephalosporins alone. These agents are not sufficiently effective against *P. multocida*. Penicillin-allergic patients can be given the combination of clindamycin (300 mg three times a day) with a fluoroquinolone (e.g., levofloxacin 500 mg daily) or doxycycline alone (100 mg twice a day for 7 days). Azithromycin (10 mg/kg, up to 500 mg on day 1; then 5 mg/kg, up to 250 mg daily for up to 4 more days) can be used in penicillin-allergic patients who are pregnant, nursing, or under 9 years old. Intravenous antibiotic administration (e.g., ampicillin–sulbactam 2 g; penicillin G 1 million units, plus nafcillin 1 g; or doxycycline 100 mg; or azithromycin 500 mg) before wound closure, although never formally studied in bites, can produce adequate penetration of the wound coagulum and is advisable in high-risk situations.

If used prophylactically, the course of therapy should be limited to 3 to 5 days, with a follow-up wound check scheduled during this period. Seven to 10 days of oral therapy is usually sufficient for the treatment of superficial wound infections. Close follow-up should be arranged. Deeper infections should be treated initially with intravenous antibiotics. In reliable patients, this can be accomplished on an outpatient basis by scheduling them to return to the emergency department or outpatient clinic. Daily reassessment should be performed until there is improvement, at which time, therapy can be continued with an oral agent and follow-up can be done less frequently.

Septic patients with a history of recent animal bites should be given broad-spectrum intravenous antibiotics initiated in the emergency department as soon as the Gram stain and culture are obtained from wounds, blood, and CSF, if indicated. Meropenem (1 g intravenously) is a reasonable choice for initial therapy pending culture results.[3]

Cat-scratch disease resolves spontaneously in 1 to 2 months or can be treated with ciprofloxacin, gentamicin, erythromycin, or trimethoprim–sulfamethoxazole.[10] Needle aspiration of fluctuant lymph nodes can alleviate constitutional symptoms as well as local pain.

Uncomplicated rat-bite fever should be treated with a 10-day course of penicillin, tetracycline, or erythromycin (500 mg orally four times a day).

Treatments of choice for tularemia are streptomycin (10 to 15 mg/kg intramuscularly twice a day) or gentamicin (2 mg/kg intravenously for loading dose) for 7 to 10 days.

Treatment of patients exposed to B-virus (*H. simiae*) should include prophylactic acyclovir (15 mg/kg intravenously every 8 hours).[9]

Bites are tetanus-prone, and immunoprophylaxis should be provided.

Rabies is fatal, and only supportive care can be offered once symptoms develop. Prevention depends on control of exposure, aggressive local wound care, and knowledge of transmission, which is usually by means of saliva contacting a laceration, scratch, abrasion, or mucous membrane. Postexposure prophylaxis is indicated if the offending animal is known or clinically suspected to be rabid or if it is a bat or wild carnivore (e.g., a bobcat, coyote, fox, raccoon, skunk, or wolf).[4,7] The silver-haired bat variant of rabies virus is able to replicate in the superficial dermis and has been associated with several recent cases of human rabies without known history of conventional exposure. For this reason, postexposure prophylaxis is now recommended for persons who may have come in contact with a bat (e.g., an infant or a sleeping adult in a room with a bat, even if a bite or scratch wound is not apparent).[11] Livestock and unprovoked dog and cat bites should be considered individually in consultation with public health officials.

Patients bitten by healthy dogs and cats do not require immunization, provided the animal can be observed for 10 days for signs of illness. Rabbit and rodent (e.g., hamster, mouse, rat, squirrel) bites do not require treatment unless the animal is wild and rabies is endemic in the offending species. Patients who have not been previously immunized should receive both human rabies immune globulin (20 IU/kg), up to half the dose infiltrated at the bite site, if anatomically feasible, and the remainder given intramuscularly (e.g., deltoid), and human diploid cell rabies vaccine (1 mL intramuscularly on days 0, 3, 7, 14, and 28).

Because hepatitis B can be transmitted by saliva, all bites must be considered for hepatitis B prophylaxis according to the risk evaluation of the source. While saliva contains only low concentrations of HIV, there is often admixture of blood in bite situations. This is the case in occlusional bites by persons with friable gingiva or seizing patients who have bitten their tongue. Clenched-fist injuries have significant risk for HIV transmission, especially when a lip laceration was sustained at the time of the altercation. In these situations, postexposure HIV treatment should be offered.

DISPOSITION

Role of the Consultant

Consultation with an infectious disease specialist and a microbiologist (for a careful search for organisms unique to animal bites) is advisable in cases of septicemia. Infectious disease consultation should be considered in cases of possible HIV, hepatitis B, or B-virus transmission. A surgeon (general, hand, plastic, or orthopedic, depending on local practices) should be consulted when there is violation of a deep structure (such as a joint, bone, tendon, or internal organ), extensive facial damage, tissue loss, or a clenched-fist bite. Bites by potentially rabid animals should be reported to state public health officials. All bite wounds should be reported to local agencies.

Indications for Admission

Patients who sustain major trauma, significant blood loss, or injuries that require operative intervention usually need to be admitted. Those who require intravenous antibiotics (i.e., systemic, central nervous system, hand, joint, or other deep-structure infection or any infection in a high-risk patient) or who cannot receive proper care as outpatients should also be admitted. Clenched-fist bites with involvement of tendon, joint, or bone should be considered for admission. All patients who do not require admission should be rechecked in 24 to 72 hours for signs of infection. If signs of infection develop, sutures must be removed and the wound left opened for drainage.

Transfer Considerations

Transfer to another institution should be arranged whenever appropriate inpatient facilities or consultants are unavailable.

COMMON PITFALLS

- Failure to diagnose deep-structure or vital organ injury
- Failure to diagnose, fully explore, and refrain from primary closure in clenched-fist bites
- Failure to identify and admit infected immunocompromised patients
- Failure to close low-risk wounds
- Failure to immobilize and elevate injured extremities
- Failure to recheck all wounds in 24 to 72 hours
- Failure to provide rabies immunization after possible bat exposure

References

1. Aghababian RV, Conte JE. Mammalian bite wounds. *Ann Emerg Med* 1980;9:79.
2. Callaham M. Dog bite wounds. *JAMA* 1980;244:2327.
3. Callaham M. Prophylactic antibiotics in common dog bite wounds: a controlled study. *Ann Emerg Med* 1980;9:410.
4. Callaham ML. Domestic and feral mammalian bites. In: Auerbach PS, Geehr EC, eds. *Management of wilderness and environmental emergencies,* 3rd ed. St. Louis: Mosby, 1995.
5. Chapple CR, Fraser AN. *Pasteurella multocida* wound infections—a commonly unrecognized problem in the casualty department. *Injury* 1986;17:410.
6. Cummings PC. Antibiotics to prevent infection in patients with dog bite wounds: a meta-analysis of randomized trials. *Ann Emerg Med* 1994;23:535.
7. Elliot DL, Tolle SW, Goldberg L, et al. Pet-associated illness. *N Engl J Med* 1985;313:985.
8. Fishbein DB. Rabies in humans. In: Baer GM, ed. *The natural history of rabies.* Boca Raton, FL: CRC Press, 1991.
9. Holmes GP, Chapman LE, Stewart JA, et al. Guidelines for the prevention and treatment of B-virus infections in exposed persons. *Clin Infect Dis* 1995;20:421.
10. Margileth AM. Antibiotic therapy for cat-scratch disease: clinical study of therapeutic outcome in 268 patients and a review of the literature. *Pediatr Infect Dis J* 1992;11:6.
11. Morimoto K, Patel M, Corisdeo S, et al. Characterization of a unique variant of bat rabies virus responsible for newly emerging human cases in North America. *Proc Natl Acad Sci U S A* 1996;93:5653.
12. Ordog GJ. The bacteriology of dog bite wounds on initial presentation. *Ann Emerg Med* 1986;15:1324.
13. Pers C, Kristiansen JE, Scheibel JH, et al. Fatal septicemia caused by DF-2 in a previously healthy man. *Scand J Infect Dis* 1986;18:265.
14. Talan DA, Citron DM, Abrahamian EM, et al. Bacteriologic analysis of infected dog and cat bites. *N Engl J Med* 1999;340:85.
15. Underman A. Bite wounds inflicted by dogs and cats. *Vet Clin North Am Small Anim Pract* 1987;17:195.
16. Weber DJ, Hansen AR. Infections resulting from animal bites. *Infect Dis Clin North Am* 1991;5:3.

CHAPTER 381
Hymenoptera Envenomation

Paul A. Janson and Richard J. Iseke

Hymenoptera envenomations are commonly referred to as bee stings, although the order Hymenoptera also includes wasps, hornets, yellow jackets, and ants. Honeybees and bumblebees belong to the family Aphididae; yellow jackets, hornets, and wasps are of the Vespidae family; and ants, of which only a small number are venomous, belong to the Formicidae family.

There is a strong cross-reactivity between the venoms within each family, but less so between families. Stinging or "fire ants" are found predominantly in the southern United States, but winged species are ubiquitous. Yellow jackets build nests in the ground. Hornets' nests are large and are found in trees and under branches. Wasps build honeycombed nests, often under roofs. Only the honeybee leaves its stinger, often with the venom gland attached, in the skin of victims of envenomation.

The venoms of winged species contain mixtures of biogenic amines (e.g., acetylcholine, dopamine, histamine, norepinephrine, serotonin), polypeptides or protein toxins (e.g., apamin, melittin, kinins), and enzymes (e.g., hyaluronidase, phospholipases). That of bees and wasps may be more potent during the cooler autumn months. The venom of fire ants consists mostly of piperidine alkaloids, with small amounts of low-molecular-weight protein.[3,5]

Hymenoptera envenomation may result in local inflammatory reactions, immediate and delayed hypersensitivity reactions, atypical reactions, and direct systemic toxicity. Nonallergic local reactions result from alkaloid-, polypeptide-, and protein-induced histamine release from mast cells, as well as the direct action of injected amines. Immediate (type I) hypersensitivity reactions may be either local or systemic. They occur when basophils or mast cells react with antigenic venom polypeptides, proteins, and enzymes (or alkaloid haptens) and cause the release or production of intracellular histamine, serotonin, leukotrienes, and other chemicals.

Physiologic effects include bronchiolar constriction, vasodilatation, myocardial depression, increased capillary permeability, and production of mucus. Sensitized people usually have elevated levels of venom-specific serum IgE. However, different winged species have similar venom constituents, and people sensitized to one species may also react to a sting by another species, particularly one of the same family, even though those people have not been previously stung by the latter. Anaphylaxis to insect stings affects up to 0.5% of the U.S. population and accounts for about 40 deaths annually.[13]

Delayed (type III) hypersensitivity reactions are caused by IgG and IgM antibody–antigen complex–mediated local (Arthus) and systemic (serum sickness) toxicity.[11] Delayed atypical reactions, suspected to be allergic in etiology, include hematologic and neurologic disorders such as hemolytic anemia, thrombocytopenic purpura, Guillain-Barré syndrome, multiple sclerosis, optic neuritis, parkinsonism, and transverse myelitis.[11,15,19]

Direct systemic toxicity results from the absorption of large amounts of venom after multiple stings. Although most multiple stings occur when a nest has been disturbed, African honeybees ("Brazilian killer bees"), now indigenous to Central America and the southwestern United States, are notorious for large, aggressive swarms, with encounters and often resulting in multiple stings.[9,13,19] Their venom, however, is no more potent than that of other honeybees.

Hymenoptera envenomation usually causes only a transient reaction at the site of the sting. A few victims develop an excessive local inflammatory response or a generalized systemic reaction.[7,12,13,16,19] A sting in someone with no history of previous systemic reaction (including those with pronounced local reactions) results in an anaphylactic reaction less than 1% of the time.[11] However, because most victims of fatal stings have no history of a prior systemic reaction, a negative history does not rule out the possibility of a severe reaction in the future.

Adults with a history of a previous systemic reaction have up to a 60% chance of a similar reaction after subsequent envenomation. Those with a severe local reaction have about a 5% chance of a future anaphylactic reaction. Children with a systemic reaction limited to non–life-threatening urticaria or angioedema have a subsequent systemic reaction rate of less than 10%. Venom immunotherapy is 98% effective in preventing subsequent systemic reactions.[10]

Most anaphylactic fatalities are due to laryngeal edema and bronchospasm and occur within an hour of the sting.[1] Vascular collapse, coma, and seizures can also occur. Direct venom toxicity (Braphylactoid reaction) may result in vascular collapse with renal or cardiac failure. Death may occur hours to weeks after multiple stings. Depending on the size of the victim and the offending species, 20 to 300 simultaneous stings may be serious or fatal.[19] Both children and adults have survived single episodes that involved more than 1,000 honeybee stings.

CLINICAL PRESENTATION

Nonallergic local reactions are characterized by pain, wheal and flare formation, warmth, and pruritus at the sting site. Reactions to stings by winged species begin immediately and last for several hours. Fire ant stings, often in clusters, frequently develop into painful vesicles and pustules during the first 24 hours and require up to 10 days for resolution.[6] Puncture marks may be invisible without the aid of a magnifying lens.

Local allergic reactions are manifested by persistent swelling, pain, and erythema at the site of the sting. These reactions may progress to involve a large area (e.g., an entire extremity) over the first 2 to 3 days and may last for more than a week. Stings after insect inhalation or ingestion may result in swelling and obstruction of the pharynx, larynx, or esophagus.

Most anaphylactic reactions develop within minutes of envenomation and peak within an hour.[2,6,15] Rarely, they may be delayed as long as 6 hours after the sting. Recurrent reactions may occur for up to 2 days. Mild reactions are characterized by generalized flushing and urticaria. Weakness, chest or throat tightness, nausea, vomiting, diarrhea, and generalized angioedema indicate a moderate reaction. Cyanosis, dyspnea, stridor, hoarseness, confusion, coma, and collapse are seen in severe cases. Physical findings may include hypotension, tachycardia, laryngeal and pulmonary edema, and wheezing, as well as skin manifestations. Secondary complications include cerebral and myocardial infarction and coagulopathy.[9,15,18]

Delayed atypical and hypersensitivity reactions are rare.[8] Symptoms normally occur within 1 week of envenomation. Serum sickness is characterized by fever, arthralgia, myalgias, rash, adenopathy, headache, glomerulonephritis, nephrotic syndrome, and necrotizing vasculitis. Cutaneous vasculitis ("palpable purpura") may indicate an Arthus reaction. Hematologic and neurologic abnormalities may suggest one of the previously mentioned disorders or syndromes.

Signs and symptoms of direct systemic toxicity usually begin within minutes and include vomiting, diarrhea, generalized edema, collapse, loss of consciousness, confusion, headache, muscle spasms, and seizures. Hepatotoxicity and encephalopathy mimicking Reye syndrome has been described. Vital signs may reveal hypotension, tachycardia, and fever. Severe cases may be complicated by hemolysis, rhabdomyolysis and acute renal failure.[13,16,19]

DIFFERENTIAL DIAGNOSIS

Because Hymenoptera envenomation can cause a variety of reactions, the differential diagnosis is extensive. Fortunately, there is usually a history of a sting to indicate the correct diagnosis. The challenge is making the diagnosis when the history is unclear.

Limited local reactions of similar appearance may be produced by virtually any stinging or biting insect (see Chapter 382). Extensive local reactions must be differentiated from infection: Hymenoptera envenomations seldom become infected. Progressive extension of the initial reaction beginning shortly after the sting indicates an allergic reaction, whereas inflammation with fever, leukocytosis, and lymphangitis beginning more than 24 hours after envenomation suggests infection.

Anaphylactic reactions may be caused by a wide variety of proteins (e.g., pollen, food), drugs, dyes, and diagnostic and therapeutic agents. This diagnosis should be considered in any unconscious patient with hypotension and signs of airway obstruction during warm months, particularly if the patient is discovered outdoors. A careful skin examination may suggest the correct diagnosis.

Patients who present with symptoms and signs of delayed or atypical reactions should be asked about recent insect bites or stings, illnesses, and medication use (particularly passive immunization therapy) within the previous month, as it is unlikely they will volunteer such a history.

Direct systemic toxicity must be differentiated from anaphylaxis. Toxic reactions progress more slowly, require many stings, and may produce fever. Urticaria, pruritus, and wheezing suggest anaphylaxis.

EMERGENCY DEPARTMENT EVALUATION

The history should include the time and number of stings, the offending species (if known), previous Hymenoptera reactions, preexisting medical conditions, and the time of onset, progression, and nature of symptoms. The physical examination should focus on the vital signs, upper airway patency, the lungs, the cardiovascular system, and the skin. With honeybee envenomation, the stinger and venom sac may be apparent at the sting site. Patients with hypotension, chest pain, or loss of consciousness should have an electrocardiogram to rule out myocardial injury.

If the physical examination is equivocal, upper airway patency may be assessed by soft-tissue neck radiographs. Patients with persistent respiratory signs and symptoms should have arterial blood gas analysis and a chest radiograph. Patients with hypotension, loss of consciousness, or more than ten stings should have measurements of serum creatine phosphokinase, blood urea nitrogen, and creatinine levels; prothrombin time; partial thromboplastin time; and urinalysis. A complete blood count may help to differentiate local allergic reactions (eosinophilia) from infection (leukocytosis with left shift) as well as to detect hemolysis and thrombocytopenia.

EMERGENCY DEPARTMENT MANAGEMENT

The treatment for anaphylaxis due to Hymenoptera stings is the same as that for anaphylaxis of other etiologies (see Chapter 217). Advanced life-support measures should be instituted, as necessary. Epinephrine should be given at the first sign of an anaphylactic reaction, preferably by prehospital personnel.[4,6,15] The dose and route depend on the severity and nature of symptoms, as well as on the victim's underlying medical problems (see Chapter 217).

Aggressive volume replacement with crystalloid should be part of the management of patients with anaphylaxis, particularly those with hypotension. Adjunctive therapy should include oral or intravenous diphenhydramine (0.5 to 1.0 mg/kg) and oral prednisone (0.5 to 1.0 mg/kg) or intravenous methylprednisolone (1 to 4 mg/kg), depending on the severity and response to epinephrine.[14,17] Whether an H_2 blocker such as cimetidine would also be helpful is unknown.

Severe anaphylactic reactions or marked local reactions that involve the nose, mouth, and throat may require immediate airway control. Because most deaths are due to airway obstruction, early endotracheal intubation may be lifesaving in patients with respiratory distress from either upper or lower airway obstruction. Intubation should also be considered in patients with significant central nervous system depression or severe shock.

Measures to consider in recurrent or refractory anaphylaxis include continuous infusions of epinephrine or isoproterenol, and norepinephrine for hypotension. Higher-than-usual doses of adrenergic agents may be required in patients taking beta-adrenergic blocking agents and those on chronic beta-agonist medications. Isoproterenol may be preferred in patients taking beta blockers.[7]

The treatment of local reactions includes wound care and symptomatic therapy for pain, swelling, and pruritus (with analgesics; cool soaks, ice packs, and elevation; and antihistamines). Cleansing of the puncture site and tetanus prophylaxis are routine measures. Stingers with attached venom sacs should be removed, to avoid further envenomation, by brushing or scraping with the sharp edge of a needle or scalpel. Stingers without sacs may also be removed with forceps.[20] The use of topical papain (meat tenderizer), aluminum-containing antiperspirants, and parenteral heparin is controversial and of uncertain benefit.

The treatment of toxic reactions after multiple envenomations is entirely supportive. Delayed hypersensitivity reactions can usually be treated with analgesics and antihistamines. Corticosteroids may be necessary in severe cases. Complications and atypical reactions should be treated with standard measures.

DISPOSITION

Patients who present immediately after envenomation should be observed for 1 to 2 hours for signs and symptoms of anaphylaxis. Asymptomatic patients may then be discharged. Because milder anaphylactic reactions may be delayed, patients should be instructed to return immediately if systemic symptoms ensue. In asymptomatic patients with a history of previous anaphylactic reactions or severe local ones, it may be prudent to prescribe a prophylactic 3-day course of antihistamines and corticosteroids, beginning with a dose before discharge.

Patients with anaphylaxis should be treated and observed for 4 hours. Those who become asymptomatic may be discharged. Patients with persistent or recurrent symptoms (excluding isolated urticaria) and those with life-threatening reactions should be hospitalized. Similarly, those with ischemic complications, those with toxic reactions and multiple envenomations, and those without reliable home observation should be admitted. All patients with anaphylactic reactions should be treated with a 3-day course of antihistamines and corticosteroids to prevent a relapse.

Those with anaphylactic or severe local reactions should be given a prescription for epinephrine (e.g., EpiPen or Ana-kit) and referred to an allergist (directly or through the primary care physician) so that they can receive instruction regarding the self-use of epinephrine and evaluation for desensitization immunotherapy. Victims of anaphylaxis should be cautioned about outdoor work and recreation (particularly gardening, fruit picking, and eating) and advised to avoid wearing bright colors and perfumes. The use of insect repellents may be helpful. An allergy identification bracelet is also recommended.

Patients with local or delayed hypersensitivity reactions can be treated as outpatients, with emergency department or primary care follow-up. Atypical reactions may require admission and referral to an appropriate specialist. Although the role of desensitization therapy in patients with severe local reactions is controversial, such patients should be referred to an allergist.

COMMON PITFALLS

- Failure to suspect anaphylaxis caused by Hymenoptera envenomation in an unconscious patient with cardiovascular collapse during an outdoor activity in warm seasons
- Failure to recognize delayed and atypical reactions and secondary complications of anaphylaxis and massive envenomation
- Failure to intubate patients with severe upper or lower airway reactions
- Failure to give epinephrine to patients with life-threatening anaphylaxis
- Failure to prescribe antihistamines and corticosteroids for 3 days after anaphylaxis, to prevent its recurrence
- Failure to prescribe an emergency epinephrine kit for victims of severe local and anaphylactic reactions
- Failure to refer patients with severe local and anaphylactic reactions to an allergist

References

1. Barnard JH. Studies of 400 Hymenoptera sting deaths in the United States. *J Allergy Clin Immunol* 1973;52:259.
2. Barr SE. Allergy to Hymenoptera stings—review of the world literature, 1953–1970. *Ann Allergy* 1971;29:49.
3. DeShazo RD, Butcher BT, Banks WA. Reactions to the stings of the imported fire ant. *N Engl J Med* 1990;323:462.
4. Fortenberry JE, Laine J, Shalit M, et al. Use of epinephrine for anaphylaxis by emergency medical technicians in a wilderness setting. *Ann Emerg Med* 1995;25:785.
5. Ginsburg CN. Fire ant envenomation in children. *Pediatrics* 1984;73:689.
6. Golden DBK, Valentine M. Insect sting allergy. *Ann Allergy* 1984;53:444.
7. Graft DF, Schuberth KC, Kagey-Sobotka A, et al. A prospective study of the natural history of large local reactions after Hymenoptera stings in children. *J Pediatr* 1984;104:664.
8. Ingall M, Goldman G, Page LB. Beta-blockage in stinging insect anaphylaxis [Letter]. *JAMA* 1984;251:2118.
9. Levine HD. Acute myocardial infarction following wasp sting. *Am Heart J* 1976;91:365.
10. Li JT, Yunginger JW. Management of insect sting hypersensitivity. *Mayo Clin Proc* 1992;67(2):180.
11. Light WC, Reisman RE, Shimizu M, et al. Unusual reactions following insect stings. *J Allergy Clin Immunol* 1977;59:391.
12. Mauriello PM, Barde SH, Georgitis JW, et al. Natural history of large local reactions from stinging insects. *J Allergy Clin Immunol* 1984;74:494.
13. Mejia G, Arbelaez M, Henao JE, et al. Acute renal failure due to multiple stings by Africanized bees. *Ann Intern Med* 1986;104:210.
14. Muller U, Mosbech H, Henao JE, et al. Emergency treatment of allergic reactions to Hymenoptera stings. *Clin Exp Allergy* 1991;21:281.
15. Ratnoff OD, Nossel HL. Wasp sting anaphylaxis. *Blood* 1983;61:132.
16. Reisman RE. Stinging insect allergy. *Med Clin North Am* 1992;76:883.
17. Shumacher MJ, Egen NB. Significance of Africanized bees for public health; a review. *Arch Intern Med* 1995;155:2038.
18. Stan JC, Brasher GW. Wasp sting anaphylaxis with cerebral infarction. *Ann Allergy* 1977;39:431.
19. Vetter RS, Visscher PK, Camazine S. Mass envenomations by honey bees and wasps. *West J Med* 1999;170:223.
20. Visscher PK, Vetter RS, Camazine S. Removing bee stings. *Lancet* 1996;348:301.

CHAPTER 382
Insect Bites and Infestations

Constance G. Nichols

Insects are members of the phylum Arthropoda. Those commonly causing bites or infestations in the United States include fleas, flies, lice, mites, and ticks. Insect bites are frequently not recognized as such. Those frequently affected are the young, the elderly, or the mentally or physically impaired who are unable to give a history, cannot care for themselves, and live under crowded conditions (e.g., nursing homes, chronic care institutions or daycare centers).

Fleas (order Siphonaptera) are small wingless insects that carry diseases such as typhus or plague. Fleas have specially adapted legs that allow them to jump several feet at a time. They feed on the blood of animals but can survive (e.g., on carpets) for several months without a meal. Flea-bite dermatitis is an inflammatory reaction to flea saliva.[3,5]

Lice (Anoplura) are crablike, crawling parasites that require a human blood meal every 12 to 24 hours. The female lice deposit eggs ("nits") at the base of hair shafts and "cement" them to the shaft. The scalp and body are infested by the *Pediculus humanis,* while the pubic area is infested by *Phthirus pubis.* Transmission of lice occurs through such fomites as clothing, caps, hairbrushes, and linens or through direct contact. In the case of pubic lice, the patient is usually sexually active and may have other coexisting venereal diseases. Body lice are usually found in those with poor personal hygiene. The bites and saliva of the lice are responsible for symptoms. These insects are also vectors of epidemic typhus, trench fever, and relapsing fever.[8–10]

Flies and mosquitoes (Diptera) are ubiquitous winged insects that require a moist environment for larval and pupal development and feed on warm-blooded animals, including humans. The blood-sucking apparatus is a syringe-like proboscis through which the insect injects salivary material that has allergenic, vasodilatory, and anticoagulant activity. These insects range in size from 2.5-mm midges, sandflies, and "no-seeums" to 2.5-cm horseflies and deerflies. Some are vectors for diseases such as dengue fever, encephalitis, filariasis, leishmaniasis, malaria, trypanosomiasis, and tularemia.

Assassin bugs, bedbugs, and wheel bugs (Hemiptera) are large (2 to 4 cm) and winged. The assassin bug (*Triatoma protracta*), also known as the kissing, reduviid, or western cone-nosed bug, has a long proboscis with which it sucks blood painlessly from the victim. It usually lives in conjunction with mammals in the wild but can adapt to human environs.

Bedbugs (*Cimex* species) have nonfunctional wings, feed on blood, and inflict painless bites. The larvae are found in clothing, bedding, and furniture; they attack at night. A wheel bug (*Arilus cristatus*) inflicts injury by rubbing its snout on the skin, inflicting a transient abrasion and local reaction.[8,10]

Blister beetles (Coleoptera) are winged insects that live on vegetation and are in contact with humans only when disturbed. These insects do not bite or sting. Exposure to them occurs when handling plants on which the insects live. When the beetle is crushed, it releases hemolymph, a vesicant.[8]

Centipedes (Chilopeda) are long, crawling insects with one pair of legs on each body segment and fangs for injecting venom on the first segment. Millipedes (Myriapoda) excrete defensive fluid that contains a number of toxic chemicals. They have two pairs of legs per body segment. Centipedes and millipedes are most common in the tropics.[10]

Insects of the Arachnid order include mites, such as scabies and chiggers, and ticks. Scabies is caused by the barely visible female of the species, *Sarcoptes scabiei* var. *hominis,* which, after fertilization, burrows into the epidermis and lays eggs at the rate of two to three per day. The mite dies after laying a total of ten to 25 eggs, resulting in an inflammatory reaction. Scabies is spread through close contact, as the mite cannot survive more than 24 to 48 hours without human contact. Normally, only a small number of mites are present on the skin. In patients with compromised immune systems, thousands of mites may be present.[10,15]

Chiggers, the larvae of harvest mites, are prevalent in the South and Midwest. The adults live on plants and deposit their eggs there. After the larvae hatch they migrate to the ends of leaves, waiting for a vertebrate host so they may attach, feed, molt, and continue the life cycle as vegetarian adults. When the chigger attaches to the skin, it bites and feeds, releasing digestant substances that cause an allergic reaction.[2,8,15]

Ticks are divided into two morphologic types: hard (Ixodidae) and soft (Argasidae). This classification is based on the presence or absence of the scutum, a protective covering of chitin on the dorsal surface of the tick. They are found worldwide and feed on the blood of warm-blooded animals and some reptiles. Bites occur when the tick attaches itself painlessly to the skin surface. The tick is attached by its teeth and by a cement-like substance that it excretes onto the host. Soft ticks tend to feed for several hours and drop off, whereas hard ticks may remain attached for days. After the tick attaches, its saliva contaminates the host.

Ticks may transmit a variety of diseases caused by viruses or bacteria (Table 382.1). Tick paralysis occurs when a tick has been attached for 4 to 5 days; it is due to neurotoxins present in the saliva of some species. Prevention of tick-borne diseases is possible by careful examination of people who have been exposed to the outdoors, especially children.[8,13,14]

Swimmer's itch (cercarial dermatitis) is caused by the invasion of the dermis by avian blood flukes or schistosomes. Released by intermediate hosts (snails and other mollusks) and unable to find natural hosts (e.g., ducks, geese), cercariae burrow into the skin; however, unable to penetrate the dermis, they die.[6,11] Seabather's eruption is caused by the bite of planula larvae of the phylum Cnidaria, with different species responsible in varying locales.[4]

CLINICAL PRESENTATION

Flea bites are grouped welts, papules, and vesicles surrounded by urticarial areas, usually on the exposed parts of extremities. In children, the vesicles can become generalized and confused with varicella. Although the lesions usually resolve after several days, they may be intensely pruritic, with scratching leading to secondary infections. Repeated exposure to bites in sensitive people, especially children, results in more severe reactions.[5,8,10]

Lice bites are often pruritic and can cause urticaria. They can become secondarily infected from excoriation. Head lice are commonly found in schoolchildren, usually in the temporal and occipital regions. Often, the children present with lymphadenopathy and a secondarily infected area of the scalp with matted hair. They may complain of something "crawling" on their scalp. Body lice do not live on the skin but in the clothes or bedding of the affected individual. Nits can often be found in the seams of clothing. The lice are present on the person during feeding but leave after a blood meal. Lesions are often found on the back, waist, and buttocks.[8–10]

Pubic lice live at the base of hairs in the perineum, abdomen, and thighs. They can also be found in the eyelashes, axillae, and beards. Occasionally, maculae cerulae, blue-pigmented lesions up to 1 cm in diameter, thought to be due to alteration in blood pigment, can be seen at sites of louse feeding.[1,8–10]

Fly and mosquito bites initially cause intensely pruritic, painful papules. By age 5, almost all children react to such bites. Erythema, edema, and urticaria may develop later as a result of delayed hypersensitivity. Bites may become secondarily infected.[8,10]

The bites of assassin bugs are usually discovered the morning after they have occurred. They are clustered, erythematous, pruritic nodules found in areas not covered by clothing. The lesions can be large (2 to 6 cm) and often last for more than a week. Some people have more severe reactions, such as light-headedness, gastrointestinal upset, and frank anaphylaxis.

TABLE 382.1. Tick-borne Diseases

Disease	Tick Vector	Agent	U.S. Distribution
Babesiosis	Ixodes	*Babesia* spp.	Northeast
Lyme disease	Ixodes	*Borrelia burgdorferi*	Northeast, Wisconsin, Minnesota, California
Ehrlichiosis	Dermacentor	*Ehrlichia chaffeensis*	South Central, South Atlantic
Rocky Mountain spotted fever	Dermacentor	*Rickettsia rickettsii*	Southeast, West, South Central
Tularemia	Dermacentor, amblyomma	*Francisella tularensis*	Arkansas, Missouri, Oklahoma
Tick paralysis	Dermacentor, amblyomma	Toxin	Northwest, South
Relapsing fever	Ornithodoros	*Borrelia* spp.	West
Colorado tick fever	Dermacentor	*Coltivirus* spp.	West

Bedbug bites, also first noted in the morning, generally appear as reddened and sometimes hemorrhagic lesions in a linear distribution. Anaphylaxis has been reported but is extremely rare. Wheel bugs cause minute, painful lacerations with transient swelling.[8,10] Patients with blister beetle bites present 2 to 5 hours after gardening, with the development of large (5- to 50-mm) vesicles or bullae on the exposed skin.[10]

Centipede envenomation results in pain, itching, and, sometimes, local necrosis with lymphadenitis and myonecrosis. Millipede secretions initially cause a brown-stained area with some burning, which can progress to blistering with subsequent exfoliation. If the toxin gets in the eyes, there is immediate irritation, usually accompanied by pain, lacrimation, chemosis, periorbital edema, and corneal ulceration.[10]

Patients with scabies present with severe pruritus. Examination of the skin reveals excoriated, dry, scaly patches. The diagnostic lesion is a serpentine burrow usually found on the hands, especially in the finger webs. Erythematous papules occur on the skin, and nodules can appear on the penis and scrotum. A severe form of scabies found frequently in the immunocompromised patient is called "Norwegian scabies"; it presents with severe, crusting lesions. Secondary bacterial infection is common.[1,10,15]

Chigger bites cause intense, pruritic, papular, or vesicular erythematous lesions with a central punctum. The reaction begins within 3 to 24 hours of exposure. After a few days, the lesions become red, flat, and conical.[2,8,10,15] Chigger bites to the penis can result in local swelling, pruritus, dysuria, and decreased urine stream (the "summer penile syndrome"). Half of patients with this syndrome have a papule or bite puncture mark on the penis.[12]

Tick bites result in a pruritic papule that resolves in 2 to 3 days. Patients commonly present with the tick still attached to the skin. If mouthparts are left in the bite site after removal of the tick, a nodular granuloma can form. With tick paralysis, there is a 24-hour prodrome of malaise, followed by an ascending symmetric paralysis similar to that of the Guillain-Barré syndrome, often with respiratory compromise. Other neurologic findings include difficulty swallowing and involuntary eye movements. The patient is afebrile and reflexes are absent, but sensation is intact. Laboratory tests, including cerebrospinal fluid analysis, are usually normal.[8,10,14]

Patients with swimmer's itch have only a slight pruritus immediately after exposure to fresh water. Twelve hours to 2 weeks later, an intense pruritus develops along with a maculopapular or papulovesicular erythematous rash.[6,11] Seabather's eruption, often confused with insect bites, occurs after exposure to salt water and is characterized by a papular rash that is typically more intense on areas covered by a bathing suit.

DIFFERENTIAL DIAGNOSIS

Insect bites are commonly confused with contact dermatitis (allergic or chemical) and viral exanthems. Generalized vesiculation from flea bites may resemble varicella, but fever and systemic symptoms are absent. Bullous impetigo and burns may have the same appearance as reactions to blister beetles. Potential exposure by history is frequently the only diagnostic clue. Tick bite nodules may resemble tumor visually and histologically. The Guillain-Barré syndrome, myasthenia gravis, and other causes of weakness or peripheral neuropathy may be confused with tick bite paralysis if the tick is not discovered. The rash of swimmer's itch may resemble chigger bites, mosquito bites, and poison ivy or oak, scabies, or sea bather's eruption.[6,11]

EMERGENCY DEPARTMENT EVALUATION

The history should include inquiries regarding activities that occurred prior to or at the time of onset of skin lesions, exposure to animals and others with similar skin lesions, the description of any insects observed, similar reactions in the past, and what treatments have been tried prior to presentation. Evaluation should include a complete examination of the entire skin surface, as well as a general examination, to exclude systemic diseases, particular anaphylactic reactions, and infectious diseases with insect vectors. Self-medication with steroids and topical diphenhydramine (itself a cause of allergic reactions), excoriations from scratching, and secondary bacterial infection can result in atypical lesions.

EMERGENCY DEPARTMENT MANAGEMENT

General measures include cool soaks, showers, baths, and antihistamines for itching; topical steroids for inflammatory reactions; and topical or systemic antibiotics for secondary infections. Treatment should also include eradication of the insect source and prevention of reexposure, when possible. Insecticides, insect repellents, and protective clothing may be helpful for environmental control.

Flea control requires vacuuming, washing of rugs and pet beds, and, often, the use of insecticides (foggers, sprays, flea collars).[7]

Lice and scabies control often requires the treatment of institutional contacts and sexual partners, as well as the laundering of bedding and clothing. Treatment of lice and scabies infestation has historically been topical 1% lindane (gamma benzene hexachloride; Kwell, Scabene) lotion or shampoo. Toxic reactions to lindane, such as nausea, vomiting, irritability, convulsions, respiratory failure, and blood dyscrasias, have been reported when it is used improperly, especially in young children.

Permethrin cream (5%), a newer scabicide with little potential for neurotoxicity, may be preferred for children. In infants less than 2 months old, pregnant women, nursing mothers, and patients with underlying skin diseases and neurologic disorders, the recommended treatment is 10% crotamiton. This cream or lotion is rubbed into the skin on two consecutive nights and can itself cause dermatitis.[8] Alternatives for scabies include 5% to 10% sulfur in petrolatum (very messy), benzyl benzoate emulsion, and NBIN (benzyl benzoate, DDT, benzocaine, and polysorbate 80, used by the World Health Organization in underdeveloped countries). Other pediculosis treatments include malathion, benzyl benzoate, and NBIN. Hospitalized patients with scabies need to be placed on skin precautions, and hospital personnel must be gowned and gloved. Lice infestation of the eyelashes is treated by application of thick layers of petrolatum twice daily for 8 days, with mechanical removal of the nits.[1,8–10]

Tick paralysis is treated supportively. Following removal of the tick, there is rapid recovery (within 24 to 48 hours). One method of removal is to grasp the tick with forceps close to the mouthparts, flip (not twist) the tick over so that its backside is closest to the skin and pull. Other methods include suffocation of the tick with mineral oil, nail polish, petrolatum, or chloroform. Hot objects may be applied, but care must be taken to avoid causing thermal burns. During the agonal struggle from suffocation, the tick's gastric contents may be forced into the bite wound. The site should be explored for retained mouthparts. Retained mouthparts and tick-bite nodules should be removed by excision.[8,10]

Treatment of swimmer's and seabather's itch is symptomatic. Antipruritic agents are useful, along with antihistamines, and, in severe cases, corticosteroids will relieve the intense pruritus.[6,11]

COMMON PITFALLS

- Failure to elicit a history of activities with the potential for insect exposure
- Failure to consider insect bites and infestations in the differential diagnosis of rashes
- Failure to consider the possibility of concomitant insect-transmitted infections or disease in patients with insect bites
- Failure to institute infection control measures for lice and scabies and to offer treatment to those who have had close but unprotected contact with such patients

References

1. Billstein SA, Mattaliano VJ Jr. The "nuisance" sexually transmitted diseases: *Molluscum contagiosum*, scabies, and crab lice. *Med Clin North Am* 1990;74:487.
2. Blankenship ML. Mite dermatitis other than scabies. *Dermatol Clin* 1990;8:265–275.
3. Elston DM. What's eating you? Ctenocephalides fleas (dog and cat fleas). *Cutis* 1998;62:15.
4. Freudenthal AR, Joseph PR. Seabather's eruption. *N Engl J Med* 1993;329:542–544.
5. Hutchins ME, Burnett JW. Fleas. *Cutis* 1993;51:241–243.
6. Kizer KW. Aquatic infections: from the benign to the life threatening. *Emerg Med* 1991;23:77–90.
7. Levinsohn DR. Treatment of scabies and similar infestations. *West J Med* 1992;56:193.
8. Maguire JH, Speilman A. Ectoparasite infestations and arthropod bites and stings. In: Fauci AS, Braunwald E, Isselbacher KJ, et al., eds. *Harrison's principles of internal medicine*. New York: McGraw-Hill, 1998:2548–2554.
9. Meinking TL, Taplin D. Infestations: pediculosis. *Curr Probl Dermatol* 1996;24:157–163.
10. Minton, SA. Arthropod envenomation and parasitism. In: Auerbach PS, ed. *Management of wilderness and environmental emergencies*. New York: Macmillan, 1995:750–768.
11. Mulvihill CA, Burnett JW. Swimmer's itch: a cercarial dermatitis. *Cutis* 1990;46:211–213.
12. Smith GA, Sharma V, Knapp JF, et al. The summer penile syndrome: seasonal acute hypersensitivity reaction caused by chigger bites on the penis. *Pediatr Emerg Care* 1998;14(2):116–118.
13. Spach DH, Liles WC, Campbell GL, et al. Tick-borne diseases in the United States. *N Engl J Med* 1993;329:936–947.
14. Walker DH. Tick transmitted infectious diseases in the United States. *Annu Rev Publ Health* 1998;19:237–269.
15. Zabawski EJ, Costner M, Granklin G, et al. A potpourri of parasitic infestations. *Cutis* 1999;63:81–85.

CHAPTER 383
Marine Envenomations

Kenneth W. Kizer

About 1,200 species of venomous or poisonous marine animals are found throughout the oceans and seas of the world. These animals usually do not cause major medical, public health, or socioeconomic problems, but untoward encounters with these animals present unique and challenging clinical situations. Such encounters have increased in frequency in recent years because of greater use of the marine environment for recreational, commercial, and scientific activities. Unfortunately, these situations are not always medically managed most effectively.

This chapter reviews the most common marine animal envenomations, focusing briefly on the biology of the animals, their venom apparatus and mechanism of envenomation, and the clinical presentation and management of the injury. Infection is always a potential complication, and tetanus prophylaxis should be given as needed.

INVERTEBRATES

Coelenterates

The phylum Coelenterata is a diverse group of more than 9,000 species, all of which possess the basic coelenteron structure: a gastrovascular cavity that functions in both digestion and circulation and has a single opening. Coelenterates also have tentacles and a highly developed venom apparatus, used primarily to capture prey and secondarily for defense.

About 100 coelenterate species are dangerous to humans, and they collectively account for more marine envenomations than any other phylum.[1,6,9,13] These species, generally known as Cnidaria, have venom-containing stinging cells (cnidocytes) near their mouths or on the outer surface of their tentacles. Cnidaria that cause the most human envenomations are the hydrozoans (fire coral and Portuguese man-of-war), scyphozoans (true jellyfish), and anthozoans (sea anemones).

Cnidocytes contain organelles known as nematocysts, composed of a venom-filled capsule (the cnidoblast) that contains a spiral-coiled, harpoon-like eversible tube. On the cnidoblast, there is a trigger (the cnidocil) and a trapdoor-like operculum over the opening, through which the nematocyst is discharged. The cnidocil is sensitive to pressure and changes in osmolarity, so both mechanical and chemical stimulation will trigger its discharge. On penetrating the upper dermis, the viscous venom coating the harpoon is released and picked up by the victim's circulation. The amount of venom contained in a single nematocyst is extremely small, but envenomation by jellyfish or Portuguese man-of-war typically involves the discharge of hundreds of thousands or even millions of nematocysts. Venoms are complex mixtures of heat-labile peptides and proteins, including deoxyribonuclease, ribonuclease I, adenosine triphosphatase, phospholipases, catecholamines, histamine, hyaluronidase, fibrolysins, kinins, and various hemolytic, cardiotoxic, and dermatonecrotic fractions.[5,6,9,16]

Mollusks

Mollusks comprise the single largest group (45,000 species) of potentially toxic marine invertebrates. Most mollusk poisonings result from ingestion (see Chapter 340). The main molluscan envenomations of concern are cone shell stings and blue-ringed octopus bites (see subsequent discussion).

Conidae

Conidae, beautiful cone-shaped, univalve gastropods, are found primarily in the shallow tropical waters of the Indian and Pacific oceans; they are prized by shell collectors. Cones are nocturnal predatory carnivores that kill their prey by the injection of paralyzing conotoxins, delivered by a venomous radular tooth that inflicts a puncture wound.[13]

The venom consists of conotoxins, which attack neural and muscular impulse transmission at several points.[14,16] One conotoxin acts by preventing entry of calcium into presynaptic nerve terminals, thus inhibiting the release of acetylcholine. Another conotoxin inhibits acetylcholine receptors, and others block sodium channels in cell membranes, thereby abolishing action potentials.

Eighteen species of the genus *Conus* have been implicated in human envenomations, which usually result from careless handling of live specimens or from accidental encounters with burrowed animals while rummaging through sand or debris in the area of coral reefs.

Octopuses

Although octopuses are usually reclusive creatures that pose no threat to humans, severe and even fatal reactions may result from bites of the Australian blue-ringed octopus (*Hapalochlaena maculosa*). The blue-ringed octopus seldom exceeds 20 cm in length and is yellow-brown with barely visible blue rings. The rings become a brilliant iridescent blue when the animal is provoked. The principal active venom component is tetrodotoxin, which blocks sodium conduction in both central and peripheral nerves.[13,19]

Echinoderms

About 80 species of echinoderms, which include sea cucumbers, urchins, and starfish, are known to be venomous or poisonous to humans.[2,13] Only sea urchins are discussed here.

Sea urchins are globular or flattened creatures whose vital organs are encased in a calcareous shell covered with regularly arranged spines. The spines are sharp, movable, and brittle, easily breaking off after puncturing a victim's skin; they may exceed a foot in length (e.g., *Diadema* spp.). Some sea urchin spines are venomous (e.g., *Asthenosoma* and *Areosoma* spp.). In addition, some species have small, triple-jawed, pincer-like seizing organs known as pedicellariae, which also may be venomous (e.g., *Tripneustes* and *Toxoneustes* spp.). Most sea urchins that are hazardous to humans are found in the Indian and Pacific oceans and the Red Sea.

The venom consists primarily of steroid glycosides, serotonin, and acetylcholine-like substances.[16] Envenomation causes reactions that are painful but rarely life-threatening.

VERTEBRATES

There are about 200 species of fish that envenomate by spines located on their gill covers or dorsal, pelvic, or anal fins. The spine-puncture wound may be quite serious in itself. Although venomous species include sting rays, scorpionfish, catfish, weeverfish, and sea snakes, this discussion is limited to sting rays and scorpionfish.

Sting Rays

Sting rays, commonly found in tropical and subtropical waters, are peaceful, reclusive bottom feeders that usually lie buried in the sand or mud, with only their eyes, spiracles, and tail exposed. Envenomations usually occur when an unsuspecting swimmer, fisherman, wader, or scuba diver steps on the animal, causing the animal to reflexively thrust its barbed tail upward and forward, impaling the victim's leg or foot.[1,10,12,15] When the tail penetrates the skin, the integumentary sheath over the spine ruptures and venom passes along the spine's ventrolateral grooves into the wound. Wounds are usually deep, jagged, and contaminated with debris. The barb is typically retroserrate and causes further injury as it is withdrawn. Sting ray venom is a complex mixture of heat-labile peptides and proteins.

Scorpionfish

Envenomations by bony fish of the family Scorpaenidae are relatively common, extremely painful, and, depending on the species, potentially deadly. This large, diverse family consists of about 30 genera and 350 species, at least 80 of which have caused venomous injuries in humans.[10,11] They are widely distributed throughout the world but are especially prevalent in the Red Sea and the Indian and Pacific oceans, where they are usually found around coral reefs. They are masterfully camouflaged, and envenomation usually occurs when an unsuspecting scuba diver, swimmer, or fisherman naively handles or unknowingly grasps or steps on the fish. A finger or the palm is most often envenomated. In addition, thousands of lionfish are imported into the United States every year for private or commercial fish collections, resulting in envenomations of aquarists and tropical fish enthusiasts.[11]

Scorpaenids envenomate victims by erectile spines on their dorsal, anal, and pelvic fins; these pierce the victim's skin and release venom from glands located in grooves on either side of the spine. The Scorpaenidae are typified by three genera: *Pterois* (e.g., lionfish, zebrafish, and turkeyfish), *Scorpaena* (e.g., scorpionfish and bullrouts), and *Synaceja* (the stonefish). *Pterois* spp. have long, slender spines and small venom glands; *Scorpaena* spp. have long, heavy spines and moderate-sized venom glands; *Synaceja* spp. have short, thick spines and very large, well-developed venom glands. Stonefish are the most dangerous of the Scorpaenids, accounting for a number of fatalities, but they are indigenous only to the Indo-Pacific region.

Scorpaenid venom is a complex mixture of peptides and proteins that are not well characterized. The principal toxic fraction of stonefish venom (stonustoxin) is a nondialyzable, heat-labile protein that causes an inflammatory reaction and potentially lethal hypotension.[10]

CLINICAL PRESENTATION

Coelenterates

The clinical manifestations of coelenterate envenomation are both toxic and antigenic in etiology.[1,4,5,9] The most common presentation is localized dermatitis at the points of tentacle contact. For hydroids and fire coral, burning pain occurs immediately on contact with the animal; this is typically followed by development of an erythematous, papular, or urticarial eruption, which may become quite pruritic and last for several days.

In cases of jellyfish or Portuguese man-of-war stings, intense burning or stinging pain is usually followed by the appearance of linear red papules, beaded streaks, or urticaria in the areas of tentacle contact. These lesions are of variable duration, usually lasting for minutes to hours, and they may become vesicular, hemorrhagic, necrotizing, or ulcerative. The initial cutaneous eruption may be followed by localized or regional hyperhidrosis, angioedema, or lymphadenopathy.

Systemic symptoms include malaise, generalized weakness, pallor, myalgias and muscle spasms, diaphoresis, nausea, vomiting, headache, dizziness, low-grade fever, hyperpnea and respiratory distress, paresthesias and other sensory disturbances, ataxia, emotional lability, tachycardia, hypotension, and, rarely, cardiovascular collapse and death.[3] Conjunctivitis, chemosis, corneal ulcerations, visual disturbances, and lid edema have been reported in cases of eye contact. Ingestion may produce abdominal pain and cramps and a generalized cutaneous eruption.

In addition to the acute reactions, persistent, recurrent, and delayed reactions may occur. These may take the form of papular urticaria, granuloma annulare, granulomatous nodules, fat atrophy, keloid formation, hyperpigmentation, contractions, gangrene, scarring, vasospasm, mononeuritis, autonomic nerve paralysis, and renal failure.[4] Recurrent eruptions involve both type I and type IV hypersensitivity.

Fatal coelenterate envenomation may result from anaphylaxis or venom-induced cardiac or respiratory arrest or from hyperkalemia secondary to acute renal failure. Deaths from envenomation by the Pacific box jellyfish (*Chironex fleckeri*) or sea wasp (*Chiropsalmus quadrigatus*) may occur within minutes and are believed to be due to direct cardiotoxicity.[5]

Conidae

Envenomation initially causes a stinging or burning sensation, numbness, localized ischemia, and cyanosis about the wound.[1,13,15] Depending on the severity of the envenomation, swelling, numbness, and paresthesias may rapidly extend from the wound. Local paralysis may progress to generalized weakness, paralysis, and respiratory failure. Severely envenomed victims may develop dysphagia, dysphonia, diplopia, blurry vision, generalized pruritus, and nausea. Rarely, disseminated intravascular coagulation, coma, or cardiovascular collapse follows. Death may occur within 2 hours of envenomation, although symptoms more often resolve in 6 to 8 hours.

Octopuses

Most envenomations occur when the victim is handling the animal—something that should not be done. Venom is injected painlessly but under sufficient pressure that it spreads rapidly through the dermis and into the muscle fascia.[1,13,15,19] Victims are often unaware that they have been bitten. Within 10 minutes, local burning or throbbing pain is noted. Marked erythema, edema, pruritus, and pain may soon develop and spread to involve part or all of the extremity. Severe envenomations may result in systemic symptoms such as oral and lingual paresthesias, nausea, vomiting, blurred vision, dysphonia, dysphagia, generalized paresthesias, and ataxia. Neurologic symptoms may progress to generalized paralysis and respiratory failure.

Echinoderms

An immediate reaction consists of intense, localized burning pain, accompanied by erythema, swelling, and bleeding. Subcutaneous staining (e.g., purple or black) may result from dye in the spines. Without treatment, the affected area typically aches, is numb, and bleeds for several minutes to several hours. Infrequent systemic symptoms include nausea, generalized paresthesias or weakness, myalgias, ataxia, syncope, and bronchospasm.[1,2,13,15] Local swelling and discomfort may occasionally recur periodically for a year or more after the initial envenomation.

A delayed reaction sometimes occurs 1 to 2 months after the injury, consisting of either localized granuloma formation or a diffuse inflammatory process. Embedded spines can also lead to wound infection and damage to nerves or joints.

Sting Rays

Victims of sting ray envenomation usually experience immediate, sharp, excruciating pain and bleeding. Without treatment, the pain rapidly spreads to involve the entire extremity, peaking 1 to 2 hours after inoculation. Pain is usually more severe than with similar nonvenomous injuries. Marked erythema or cyanosis and swelling may also develop. Systemic manifestations include nausea, vomiting, fever, chills, tremors, myalgias and muscle cramps, weakness, paresthesias, lymphadenopathy, and syncope. Rarely, dyspnea, hypotension, cardiac dysrhythmias, convulsions, and even death may occur.[1,10,12,15]

Scorpionfish

The clinical manifestations of envenomation are relatively mild for lionfish and related species, moderate for scorpionfish, and potentially life-threatening for stonefish.[1,10–12] Intense, sharp, throbbing pain occurs immediately and rapidly radiates centrally. The wound and surrounding area typically become erythematous, ecchymotic or cyanotic, and swollen. Paresthesias or anesthesia about the wound and in the affected extremity and regional lymphadenopathy are relatively common. Localized tissue necrosis and sloughing may occur over several days. Systemic symptoms include nausea, vomiting, abdominal cramps, headache, dizziness, tremors, cardiac dysrhythmias, hypotension, myalgias, weakness or paralysis, dyspnea, pulmonary edema, syncope, and convulsions.[11] Delayed complications include neuropathies, cutaneous granulomata, and indolent ulcers. Without treatment, the pain and other local manifestations typically peak in 60 to 90 minutes and last for 8 to 12 hours, but sometimes they persist for days or weeks.

DIFFERENTIAL DIAGNOSIS

Allergic reactions, traumatic injuries, wound botulism and infections (Table 383.1), and bites and envenomations by other marine animals are the main considerations in the differential diagnosis.

Seabather's eruption ("sea lice") is an intensely pruritic maculopapular or vesicular eruption caused by contact with larvae of the jellyfish (*Linuche unguiculata*).[17] It begins within 24 hours of swimming, affects skin surfaces covered by bathing suits, and lasts 3 to 5 days. Treatment consists of antipruritics and topical or systemic steroids. Other measures used for coelenterate en-

TABLE 383.1. Marine Pathogens

FRESH-WATER ORGANISMS	
Acinetobacter calcoaceticus	*Aeromonas hydrophila*
Aeromonas sobria	*Agrobacterium sanguineum*
Alcaligenes dentrificans	*Bacillus cereus*
Bacillus sphericus	*Campylobacter jejuni*
Chromobacterium violaceum	*Coryneform group*
Enterobacter agglomerans	*Enterobacter cloacae*
Escherichia coli	*Flavobacterium breve*
Legionella pneumophila	*Listeria monocytogenes*
Mycobacterium amrinum	*Plesiomonas shigelloides*
Pseudomonas acidovorans	*Pseudomonas aeruginosa*
Pseudomonas indigofera	*Pseudomonas putida*
Salmonella typhi	*Serratia liquefaciens*
Serratia marcescens	*Shigella sonnei*
Staphylococcus aureus	*Vibrio parahaemolyticus*
Yersinia enterocolitica	
SALTWATER ORGANISMS	
Acinetobacter lwoffi	*Aerobacter aerogenes*
Aeromonas hydrophila	*Aeromonas sobria*
Bacillus cereus	*Bacillus subtilis*
Bacteroides fragilis	*Clostridium perfringens*
Clostridium tetani	*Enterobacter aerogenes*
Enterobacter cloacae	*Escherichia coli*
Klebsiella pneumoniae	*Mycobacterium marinum*
Neisseria catarrhalis	*Proteus mirabilis*
Proteus vulgaris	*Pseudomonas aeruginosa*
Pseudomonas putrefaciens	*Salmonella typhi*
Staphylococcus aureus	*Staphylococcus epidermidis*
Streptococcus iniae	*Streptococcus faecalis*
Vibrio alginolyticus	*Vibrio cholerae*
Vibrio damsela	*Vibrio damsela*
Vibrio fulnificus	*Vibrio parahaemolyticus*

venomation may be tried but are unlikely to be helpful, due to the typically late presentation. Contact with bristleworms, which have numerous silky, spine-like setae, can cause a similar eruption on exposed surfaces.[1]

Catfish envenomation can occur when these fish are handled when caught or stepped on while wading in both salt and fresh water.[20] The dorsal and pectoral fins have barbed spines with venom glands. Pain, erythema followed by cyanosis and edema, and muscle fasciculations are typical manifestations. The spines are radiopaque. Secondary infection may occur. Treatment consists of immersion in hot water, spine removal, and antibiotics for infection (discussion follows). Some shark species also have venomous dorsal fin spines.[10]

Corals, although not venomous, can produce painful cuts when the victim brushes against the reef.[1,13,15] Pruritus, erythema, urticaria, and cellulitis with ulceration and necrosis occur. Foreign-body granuloma can occur. Irrigation with hydrogen peroxide has been used to remove coral particles from the wound. Additional treatment includes routine wound care and antibiotic therapy covering *Vibrio* and *Aeromonas* species (see previous discussion).[1]

Sea snakes are found primarily in coastal waters of the Indian and Pacific oceans. All sea snakes are venomous.[18] Their venoms contain protein mixtures similar to those found in land snakes (see Chapters 378 and 379). The principal component is a neurotoxin that binds to acetylcholine and the neuromuscular junction and causes muscle weakness, pain, stiffness, spasm, and, finally, paralysis. The bite itself is usually painless and may go unnoticed unless a careful search is made for fang marks. Fangs can break off and may be visible on x-ray. Symptoms may be delayed in onset up to 2 days. Rhabdomyolysis is a common complication. Treatment consists of supportive care and antivenom administration. Australian sea snake antivenom is available from the Commonwealth Serum Laboratory in Melbourne, Australia.

Sponges can cause irritant and contact dermatitis.[1,13,15] Erythema multiforme and anaphylaxis can also occur. Spicules can be removed with adhesive tape. Soaking with vinegar may provide some relief. Treatment with topical or systemic steroids also may be necessary.

EMERGENCY DEPARTMENT EVALUATION

The history includes the identity or a description of the offending animal, the geographic location and circumstances surrounding the envenomation, and the time of onset, nature, and progression of symptoms. The physical examination focuses on vital signs and cardiovascular, respiratory, and neurologic functions. The skin is examined for puncture wounds, teeth marks, rashes, and signs of infection. All wounds are explored and x-rayed for foreign bodies. Infected wounds are cultured. Patients with abnormal vital signs or altered mental status should have routine laboratory evaluation, including a complete blood count; measurement of electrolytes, blood urea nitrogen, creatinine, glucose, and creatine phosphokinase; and an arterial blood gas or oxygen saturation measurement.

EMERGENCY DEPARTMENT MANAGEMENT

Coelenterates

Management requires recognition of envenomation, identification of the offending species, general supportive care, and specific detoxification measures.[1,4,5,9,15] Initial management includes reassurance, rinsing the involved area with sea water or isotonic saline solution (not fresh water), and species-specific measures to suppress additional nematocyst firing. Cold packs or ice is an effective first-aid measure for the treatment of pain.[8] Spraying or immersing the affected area in vinegar or other dilute acetic acid solution is effective if the offending animal is the jellyfish *C. fleckeri* or the Atlantic Portuguese man-of-war, *Physalia physalis;* a slurry of baking soda should be used for *Chrysaora quinquecirrha.* The application of a slurry of isopropyl alcohol and powdered papain (e.g., Adolph's unseasoned meat tenderizer or papaya latex) appears to be clinically effective for the Pacific Portuguese man-of-war, *Physalia utriculus,* and some jellyfish species, although alcohol has been observed to prompt nematocyst firing *in vitro.*

After the nematocysts have been inactivated, adherent tentacles are manually removed with forceps or by shaving the area. Surgical gloves should be worn for protection. The envenomed area should be immobilized for at least 30 to 60 minutes, because muscle activity tends to mobilize the venom from the inoculation site. Although some venom components are heat-labile, the application of local heat or cold is not helpful.

Systemic reactions are treated according to the severity of the reaction and the species involved. Anaphylaxis is treated in the standard manner. Severe *C. fleckeri* envenomations usually require respiratory and cardiac support. Intravenous verapamil may be useful in these cases, although this therapy is controversial.[7] Hyperimmune serum and antivenom specific for *Chironex* is available from the Commonwealth Serum Laboratory in Melbourne, Australia. Systemic corticosteroids are ineffective for toxin-mediated effects. Analgesics may be necessary for prolonged or persistent local reactions.

Conidae

Treatment is empiric, relying on nonspecific symptomatic and supportive measures.[1,13,15] Immersing the affected area in hot water (110°F to 115°F) for 30 to 60 minutes sometimes provides pain relief. Careful observation for at least 12 hours after injury is essential.

Octopuses

Treatment is symptomatic; respiratory support is crucial.[1,19] Recovery is usually rapid, with complete resolution within 24 hours.

Echinoderms

Treatment of spine-puncture injuries is primarily symptomatic.[1,2,13,15] Immersing the affected area in hot water (110°F to 115°F) for 30 to 90 minutes usually produces substantial pain relief. Systemic analgesics can also be given. Spines are carefully removed: They easily fracture. Spines are removed after they have been clearly localized by appropriate radiologic procedures and with the aid of a bloodless field and operating microscope. Retained spines may produce a local foreign-body, sarcoid-like granulomatous reaction. There is no justification for blindly probing these wounds or pounding the affected area to break up the spines. Topical agents are ineffective in relieving pain. Antibiotics are not indicated unless infection has developed, which, at times, may be difficult to differentiate from the toxic inflammatory reaction. Systemic corticosteroids are of no proven value.

Sting Rays

Treatment should begin immediately and focuses on inactivating the venom, providing symptomatic relief and necessary vital function support, and preventing infection.[1,10,12,15] Initial therapy includes immersing the affected area in hot water (110°F to 115°F) for 30 to 90 minutes, followed by thorough wound irrigation. After maximal pain relief has been achieved by hot water, systemic analgesics can be given for residual pain. Many of these wounds become secondarily infected and require treatment with a broad-spectrum antibiotic.[1] Systemic manifestations are treated symptomatically.

Scorpionfish

Initial management consists of immediate immersion of the affected area in hot water (110°F to 115°F) for 30 to 90 minutes.[1,10–12] Systemic analgesics can be given for residual pain. Other symptomatic and supportive measures are used as necessary. An antivenom is available in Australia and at a few public aquariums in the United States for stonefish stings; it is almost never needed for other types of Scorpaenid envenomations.

Secondary Infection

Given the variety of gram-positive and gram-negative organisms present in both fresh and salt water (see Table 383.1), broad-spectrum antibiotics should be given for infection that develops in wounds acquired in aquatic environments. For oral therapy, ciprofloxacin, levofloxacin, or trimethoprim–sulfamethoxazole can be used. Ceftazidime, a second-generation fluoroquinolone, or imipenem can be given for infections requiring intravenous therapy.

DISPOSITION

Patients with systemic signs and symptoms should be admitted. The level of care is dictated by the clinical severity. Patients with wound infections also may require admission. Those with skin eruptions can be managed as outpatients. Antivenoms can often be located through regional poison centers or aquariums. A poison center or toxicologist can be consulted for treatment advice.

COMMON PITFALLS

- Failure to appreciate that the pain from most spine-induced envenomations can be effectively treated with hot-water immersion
- Failure to appreciate that the pain from most coelenterate envenomations can be effectively treated by 5% acetic acid (vinegar) soaks
- Failure to appreciate that irrigation of jellyfish or coelenterate envenomations with fresh water may cause worsening of pain
- Failure to diagnose and treat associated traumatic injuries
- Failure to consider bacterial infection in the differential diagnosis and to reorganize that broad-spectrum antibiotics may be necessary
- Failure to observe for systemic toxicity
- Failure to appreciate that antivenoms are available for *Chironex* jellyfish, sea snake, and stonefish envenomations
- Failure to appreciate that envenomation may lead to anaphylactic as well as toxic reactions

ACKNOWLEDGMENT

The author gratefully acknowledges the contribution of Kenneth W. Kizer who wrote the previous versions of this chapter.

References

1. Auerbach PS. Marine envenomations. *N Engl J Med* 1991;325:486.
2. Baden HP. Injuries from sea urchins. *Clin Dermatol* 1987;5:113.
3. Bengston K, Nichols MM, Schnading V, et al. Sudden death in a child following jellyfish envenomation by *Chiropsalmus quadrumanus*. JAMA 1991;266:1401.
4. Burnett JW, Calton CJ. Jellyfish envenomation syndromes updated. *Ann Emerg Med* 1987;16:1000.
5. Burnett JW, Calton GJ. Venomous pelagic coelenterates: chemistry, toxicology, immunology, and treatment of their stings. *Toxicon* 1987;25:581.
6. Burnett JW, Calton GJ, Burnett HW, et al. Local and systemic reactions from jellyfish stings. *Clin Dermatol* 1987;5:14.
7. Burnett JW, Gean CJ, Warnick JE, et al. The effect of verapamil on the cardiotoxin of the Portuguese man-o'-war (*Physalia physalis*) and sea nettle (*Chrysaora quinquecirrha*). *Toxicon* 1985;23:681.
8. Exton RE, Fenner PJ, Williamson JA. Cold packs—effective topical analgesia in the treatment of painful stings by physalia. *Med J Aust* 1989;151:625.
9. Halstead BW. Coelenterate (Cnidarian) stings and wounds. *Clin Dermatol* 1987;5:8.
10. Halstead BW, Vinci JM. Venomous fish stings (ichthyoacanthotoxicoses). *Clin Dermatol* 1987;5:29.
11. Kizer KW, McKinney HE, Auerbach PS. Scorpaenidae envenomation: a 5-year poison center experience. *JAMA* 1985;253:807.
12. McGoldrick J, Marx JA. Marine envenomations, part 1: vertebrates. *J Emerg Med* 1991;9:497.
13. McGoldrick J, Marx JA. Marine envenomations, part 2: invertebrates. *J Emerg Med* 1992;10:71.
14. Olivera BM, Gray WR, Zeikus R, et al. Peptide neurotoxins from fish-hunting cone snails. *Science* 1985;230:1338.
15. Rosson CL, Tolle SW. Management of marine stings and scrapes. *West J Med* 1989;150:97.
16. Russell FE. Marine toxins and venomous and poisonous marine plants and animals (invertebrates). *Adv Marine Biol* 1984;21:59.
17. Tomchik RS, Russell MT, Szmant AM, et al. Clinical perspectives in seabather's eruption, also known as "sea lice." *JAMA* 1993;269:1669.
18. Tu AT, Fulde G. Sea snake bites. *Clin Dermatol* 1987;5:119.
19. Williamson JA. The blue-ringed octopus bite and envenomation syndrome. *Clin Dermatol* 1987;5:127.
20. Zemen MG. Catfish stings: a report of three cases. *Ann Emerg Med* 1988;18:211.

CHAPTER 384
Scorpion Envenomation

Jeffrey R. Suchard and Steven C. Curry

Although nearly 40 scorpion species are found in the United States, *Centruroides sculpturatus* is the only scorpion reported to produce potentially life-threatening illness after a sting. This species, also known as *Centruroides exilicauda*, or the bark scorpion, is found throughout Arizona and in parts of Texas, New Mexico, small areas of California, the northern shore of Lake Mead in Nevada, and northern Mexico.[3] *C. sculpturatus* stings may occur elsewhere, as scorpions have been known to stow away in a person's belongings (e.g., shoes, duffel bags) and be transported long distances before stinging their victims. Most other American scorpion stings produce only local pain and inflammation, which respond well to minimal supportive therapy and wound care, though the common striped scorpion, *Centruroides vittatus*, causes mild-to-moderate systemic effects in 20% of cases.[11]

C. sculpturatus specimens generally measure about 5 cm (range, 1.3 to 7.6 cm) long; have a streamlined appearance, with a thin tail and claws; and are a uniform tan, yellow, or light brown. The last (sixth) tail segment, termed a *telson*, contains a venom apparatus and stinger (Fig. 384.1). *C. sculpturatus* prefers

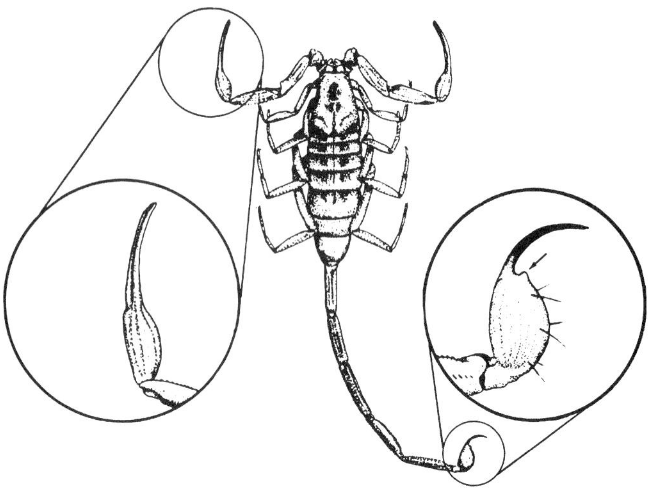

Figure 384.1. The sixth tail segment of *C. sculpturatus* (bark scorpion) contains venom apparatus and stinger.

to reside in or near trees, especially sycamore, mesquite, cottonwood, and palm. They may also hide in ground debris, camping equipment, or clothing left unattended in natural desert areas, or even in areas long-inhabited by humans. Scorpions spend the daylight hours undercover and are active at night in warm weather, lying quietly while waiting to ambush prey. In defending themselves, they grasp the victim's flesh with pincers and repeatedly sting by thrusting their tails over their bodies.

Although a sting from any scorpion can produce local pain, *C. sculpturatus* venom contains protein neurotoxins that cause repetitive firing of neurons by binding to sodium channels and preventing channel inactivation during depolarization or after repolarization.[3] No destructive enzymes are present in the venom, accounting for lack of inflammation or necrosis. Prolonged and excessive firing of parasympathetic, sympathetic, and somatic motor neurons produces various autonomic effects and uncoordinated and spontaneous activity in voluntary muscle.

Scorpion stings are fairly common in endemic areas. About 10% of all calls to the Samaritan Regional Poison Center in Phoenix, Arizona, are regarding scorpions, with several thousand stings reported annually. Fortunately, the majority of envenomations are not serious enough to warrant medical attention. Children tend to be more seriously affected by *C. sculpturatus* stings, however, and may require aggressive intervention to avoid morbidity and mortality. Death has not been reported in Arizona for many years. The lack of recent fatalities probably reflects advances in supportive medical care.

Severe envenomations by *C. sculpturatus* are seen almost entirely in children under age 10 and occur in 15% to 20% of this group. In contrast, 95% of envenomations in those older than age 10 result in only mild-to-moderate effects. The life-threatening effects (myocarditis, pulmonary edema, shock) associated with adrenergic storm and caused by the venom from scorpion species found in other parts of the world are not noted after envenomations by *C. sculpturatus*.

CLINICAL PRESENTATION

Scorpion envenomation results in the immediate onset of a painful tingling or burning sensation at the sting site. Tapping the site of the sting may produce severe pain, although no lesion is usually visible. Over minutes to several hours, pain and paresthesias may become generalized. Victims may complain of "thick tongue" and "trouble swallowing," yet lack objective abnormalities on examination. Young children frequently rub their noses, eyes, and ears, and may present with unexplained crying.

TABLE 384.1. Scorpion Envenomations: Signs and Symptoms

Grade	Description
I	Local pain and/or paresthesias at site of envenomation
II	Pain and/or paresthesias remote from the site of sting
III	Either cranial nerve or somatic skeletal neuromuscular dysfunction *Cranial nerve dysfunction:* Blurred vision, wandering eye movements, hypersalivation, trouble swallowing, tongue fasciculations, stridor, slurred speech *Somatic skeletal neuromuscular dysfunction:* Jerking of extremity(ies), restlessness, severe involuntary shaking and jerking which may be mistaken for seizures
IV	Both cranial nerve and somatic skeletal neuromuscular dysfunction

Autonomic dysfunction is characterized by tachycardia, excessive secretions, and, occasionally, vomiting and wheezing. Somatic motor abnormalities include roving eye movements, blurred vision, fasciculations (especially of the tongue), and poor control of pharyngeal muscles. Continuous jerking of extremities may be noted and misinterpreted as restlessness, seizures, or hysteria. The combination of uncoordinated pharyngeal musculature and muscles of respiration, increased secretions, and occasional wheezing may produce stridor, hypoxia, aspiration, and respiratory arrest in severe cases.

Severe envenomations may also be accompanied by metabolic acidosis, respiratory failure, sterile cerebrospinal fluid pleocytosis (9 to 20 white blood cells per microliter), coagulopathy, pancreatitis, and rhabdomyolysis.[1–3]

Envenomations can be graded on the basis of signs and symptoms (Table 384.1). In serious envenomations, abnormal motor activity may last 10 to 20 hours.[3,8] Paresthesias may last up to 3 weeks.

DIFFERENTIAL DIAGNOSIS

Bites or stings from other arthropods should be considered in the differential diagnosis of scorpion envenomation. The pain at the site of envenomation may be similar to that seen after a black widow spider bite. However, severely ill patients who suffer from scorpion stings appear unable to lie still, whereas those bitten by black widow spiders can maintain a position for short periods of time before moving in an attempt to become comfortable. Black widow envenomations do not produce abnormal eye movements, fasciculations, and paresthesias. Tapping over the site of envenomation produces severe pain in the patient stung by a scorpion, but not in someone bitten by a spider. Black widow spider bites frequently produce a characteristic halo lesion at the site of the bite; no lesion is usually visible after a *C. sculpturatus* sting.

Tachycardia, excessive secretions, wheezing, and respiratory distress accompanying serious scorpion stings may be mistaken for asthma, airway obstruction from a foreign body, or poisoning with cholinergic agents such as organophosphate insecticides. In the absence of a witnessed scorpion sting, other entities to be considered include central nervous system infections, tetanus, dystonic reactions, seizures, and intoxication with sympathomimetics, phencyclidine, and nicotine. Methamphetamine toxicity, for instance, is sometimes mistaken for *C. sculpturatus* envenomation when young children from scorpion-endemic areas present with unusual neurologic findings such as agitation or choreiform movements; this has occasionally led to the inappropriate use of antivenin.[6,8]

EMERGENCY DEPARTMENT EVALUATION

If a sting was not witnessed, it should be determined whether there are scorpions near where the patient became ill. The physical examination should focus on vital signs, the airway, and neuromuscular function. Although no specific diagnostic tests are available, patients with suspected aspiration should have an arterial blood gas analysis and a chest radiograph. Patients with severe envenomation should also have serum amylase and creatine kinase determinations and coagulation studies.

EMERGENCY DEPARTMENT MANAGEMENT

Advanced life-support measures, with particular attention to airway management, should be instituted as necessary. As with any puncture wound, a primary tetanus immunization or booster should be given, if indicated.

Patients with grade I or II envenomations are treated symptomatically. Application of ice to the sting often provides relief in lower grade envenomations. Oral analgesics are effective in most cases, but parenteral analgesia may be needed in rare cases. There are no rational or therapeutic benefits in giving barbiturates, benzodiazepines, steroids, epinephrine, calcium, or antihistamines to patients with scorpion envenomations. Barbiturates have not been found effective in lessening motor activity or in shortening the course of the illness, and they often produce serious or life-threatening respiratory depression.[10] Propranolol has anecdotally been reported to lessen the tachycardia in a severely envenomated child without affecting other neuromuscular abnormalities.[9] Beta-adrenergic blockers are not recommended, because tachyarrhythmias do not cause morbidity, bronchospasm can be seen in severe scorpion envenomations, and such therapy does not correct neurologic abnormalities.

C. sculpturatus goat serum antivenin is available for the treatment of severe envenomations. The only current source of this antivenin in the United States is the Antivenom Production Laboratory at Arizona State University, which distributes the product free of charge to hospitals within the state. This antivenin is very effective in alleviating symptoms of grade III or IV envenomations, reversing severe neurotoxicity usually within 30 to 60 minutes. Abnormal motor activity usually resolves within 60 to 90 minutes.[3,4] Patients who do not receive antivenin will continue to have symptoms for 4 to 20 hours. Antivenin has no role in the treatment of grade I or II envenomations.

Patients with grade III or IV envenomations can be successfully treated with antivenin after the institution of supportive care. Supportive measures include continuous monitoring of the airway, with respiratory assistance as needed; intravenous hydration; and loose restraints to prevent self-harm. One or two vials of antivenin mixed in 50 mL of a crystalloid solution is given intravenously over 20 to 30 minutes. Although skin testing with antivenin is suggested, it is not completely reliable in predicting which patients will suffer allergic reactions.[4] Those with a history of prolonged exposure to goats or goat's milk and those who have previously received goat serum antivenin are at increased risk for allergic reactions and should not be given antivenin. The use of beta blockers is a relative contraindication to the administration of *C. sculpturatus* antivenin, because beta-adrenergic blockade complicates the treatment of anaphylaxis, a potential complication of antivenin administration. The Samaritan Regional Poison Center in Phoenix (602-253-3334) may be contacted before giving antivenin if the physician is not completely familiar with the technique and potential risks of antivenin therapy.

Some physicians in scorpion-endemic areas do not use antivenin, but prefer to treat severely envenomated patients with supportive and symptomatic care in the intensive care unit (ICU). Such treatment requires close respiratory monitoring, as the patients are often given benzodiazepines to control neuromuscular hyperactivity and to induce sedation and amnesia.[5] We believe that routine admission unnecessarily increases cost, and that administering sedatives to patients who already have tenuous airway control unduly increases the risk of respiratory depression and aspiration in those who could potentially be safely discharged home from the emergency department if treated with antivenin.[2] The main argument against antivenin is that using animal-derived serum products places the patient at risk for potentially serious immunologic reactions. Anaphylactic reactions to antivenin can occur, but they are usually mild and can be reversed with appropriate treatment.[2,3,7] Serum sickness occurs in about 60% of patients treated with scorpion antivenin, though the symptoms typically resolve within 3 days when treated with antihistamines and corticosteroids.[2,7]

DISPOSITION

Patients with grade I or II envenomations should be observed for 3 to 4 hours after a sting for evidence of progression of symptoms. Those who do not manifest increased envenomation severity can be discharged home with oral analgesics and follow-up with their personal physician, if needed.

Patients with grade III or IV envenomations can be discharged after receiving antivenin if they are asymptomatic and aspiration pneumonia or other complications from envenomation are ruled out. Children with grade III or IV envenomations who have not received antivenin, or who have evidence of a complication after receiving antivenin, should be admitted to an ICU. Adults without respiratory difficulties who require admission for pain control may be admitted to an unmonitored bed. Those with more severe envenomations generally require intensive care.

All patients who receive antivenin should be advised of the signs and symptoms of serum sickness, which could appear 3 to 14 days after the administration of antivenin. In addition, they should consider themselves allergic to goat serum in the future. Serum sickness is easily controlled with nonsteroidal antiinflammatory agents, hydroxyzine, and tapering doses of oral corticosteroid.

COMMON PITFALLS

- Mistaking symptoms of severe envenomation for hysterical or uncooperative behavior or for seizures, especially in children
- Relying on the absence of a visible lesion at the site of the sting to rule out scorpion envenomation
- Routinely giving barbiturates, steroids, epinephrine, antihistamines, benzodiazepines, or calcium
- Using antivenin as a substitute for good supportive care
- Failure inform patients about potential allergic reactions to antivenom and to monitor for such reactions

References

1. Berg RA, Tarantino MD. Envenomation by the scorpion *Centruroides exilicauda* (*C. sculpturatus*): severe and unusual manifestations. *Pediatrics* 1991;87:930.
2. Bond GR. Antivenin administration for *Centruroides* scorpion sting: risks and benefits. *Ann Emerg Med* 1992;21:788.
3. Curry SC, Vance MV, Ryan PJ, et al. Envenomation by the scorpion *Centruroides sculpturatus*. *J Toxicol Clin Toxicol* 1984;21:417.
4. Gateau T, Bloom M, Clark R. Response to specific *Centruroides sculpturatus* antivenom in 151 cases of scorpion stings. *J Toxicol Clin Toxicol* 1994;32:165.
5. Gibly R, Williams M, Walter F. Continuous intravenous midazolam infusions for *Centruroides exilicauda* envenomations. *J Toxicol Clin Toxicol* 1998;36:460.
6. Kolecki P. Inadvertent methamphetamine poisoning in pediatric patients. *Pediatr Emerg Care* 1998;14:385.
7. LoVecchio F, Klemens J, Welch S, et al. Prospective study of immediate and delayed hypersensitivity to *Centruroides* antivenin. *J Toxicol Clin Toxicol* 1998;36:462.
8. Nagorka AR, Bergeson PS. Infant methamphetamine toxicity posing as scorpion envenomation. *Pediatr Emerg Care* 1998;14:350.
9. Rachesky IJ, Banner W, Dansky J, et al. Treatment for *Centruroides exilicauda* envenomation. *Am J Dis Child* 1984;138:1136.
10. Rimsza ME, Zimmerman DR, Bergeson PS. Scorpion envenomation. *Pediatrics* 1980;66:298.
11. Stipetic ME, Lugo A, Brown B, et al. A prospective analysis of 558 common striped scorpion (*Centruroides vittatus*) envenomations in Texas during 1997. *J Toxicol Clin Toxicol* 1998;36:461.

PART II

Cold-, Heat-, and Pressure-Related Illness and Injury

CHAPTER 385

Cold-Induced Tissue Injuries

Federico Gonzalez and Kenneth Leong

Historically, cold-induced tissue injuries have been most prevalent in military personnel. In the civilian population, those involved in outdoor sporting activities, industrial workers in cold environments, and the homeless compose the majority of individuals who suffer injury due to cold exposure. Altered mental status due to either medical illness or drugs, advanced age, malnutrition, and peripheral vascular disease are added risk factors for cold injury.[2,3,9,20]

Frostnip, the mildest form of cold-induced tissue injury, results from cold-induced vasoconstriction and resolves without epidermal or dermal damage with rewarming. *Chilblain,* or *perniosis,* a more severe form of cold injury, results from exposure to cold temperatures above freezing. This injury is characterized by a chronic vasculitis of the dermis and often results from repeated exposures to cold, usually humid air. Tissue changes are felt to reflect vascular inflammation from hypoxia secondary to cold-induced vasoconstriction. *Trenchfoot,* or *immersion foot,* is tissue injury at temperatures between 0°C and 20°C, resulting from prolonged exposure to a cold, wet environment. Tissue injury is due to skin edema and microvascular damage secondary to water absorption and cold temperatures. The role of secondary infection is controversial.

Frostbite is the destruction of tissue due to freezing and commonly occurs at temperatures below 2°C. Tissue injury can be divided into two phases: cooling or initial freeze injury, and reperfusion injury with thawing and rewarming. The first physiologic response to peripheral cooling is vasoconstriction resulting from the release of tissue factors and the generalized sympathetic response.[4,11] When tissue temperature falls to 10°C, the "hunting response" occurs. This phenomenon is characterized by 5- to 10-minute cycles of vasoconstriction and vasodilation in an attempt to preserve tissue viability while conserving core temperature. When core temperature is threatened, the hunting response is superseded by vasoconstriction alone. Once tissue temperatures reach −2°C to −4°C, extracellular ice crystals form. This usually requires an ambient temperature of −6°C. Ice crystal formation increases extracellular colloid osmotic pressure and draws fluid from the intracellular space, resulting in cellular dehydration. If tissue freezing is rapid (greater than 10°C per minute), intracellular ice formation results in cell death.[12,13] Intravascular ice crystal formation concurrent with interstitial ice formation results in hemoconcentration, leading to red blood cell sludging and cessation of blood flow. In addition to ice crystal formation, freezing temperatures also have direct effects on endothelial cell integrity, with sloughing of the endothelium from the internal elastic membrane.[11] Tissue injury due to freezing may be partially reversible with rapid warming.[12,15,18,19]

Reperfusion following rewarming results in endothelial cell damage that causes leakage of protein and fluid from endothelium damaged by freezing. Vascular intimal damage leads to increased platelet affinity, with resultant erythrostasis and vessel thrombosis. Histologic studies have revealed thrombus clogging venules within 10 minutes of thawing. By 1 hour, capillaries are thrombosed and most blood flow is through arteriovenous anastomoses. Elevated numbers of neutrophils have also been demonstrated in skin following thawing. Neutrophil aggregation and adhesion to endothelium has been hypothesized to play a critical role in tissue injury. Experimental data and clinical observation indicate that the major mechanism for tissue loss in frostbite is likely due to microvascular disruption. This hypothesis is supported by the observation that frozen and then thawed skin grafted onto normal tissue usually results in graft survival, whereas normal skin grafted onto previously frozen tissue results in graft loss.[19]

Vasoactive substances released from damaged tissue may also cause microvascular injury. Analysis of blister fluid from frostbite reveals high levels of thromboxane metabolites, which may mediate tissue ischemia through vasoconstriction. Animal and clinical studies have demonstrated a decrease in tissue ischemia after treatment with cyclooxygenase inhibitors such as ibuprofen and aspirin as well as with the thromboxane inhibitor aloe vera.[14,17]

As with other reperfusion injuries, frostbite-induced tissue damage may also be mediated by the release of oxygen free radicals. Animal models using the free radical scavengers, superoxide dismutase and deferoxamine, have shown improved tissue survival. However, clinical studies have not been as promising.[11] Studies with the use of hyperbaric oxygen, effective in reducing oxygen free radical formation, have been promising in both clinical and animal studies.[8,16]

CLINICAL PRESENTATION

Manifestations of *frostnip* include numbness, pain, paresthesias, and pallor. The fingers, toes, ears, and nose are the most common sites affected. Symptoms usually resolve within 30 minutes of rewarming.

Symptoms associated with *chilblain* include erythema, pruritus, and burning, usually of appendages, including the ears and nose. Blistering and ulceration is uncommon but may occur. Recurrence is common, particularly in patients with underlying peripheral vascular disease. Symptoms usually resolve in 1 to 3 weeks.

Patients at risk for *immersion foot* include soldiers, sailors, fishermen, and, increasingly, the homeless. Complaints may include itchiness, numbness, pain, and paresthesia, along with leg muscle cramping. Early findings include coolness, pallor, insensitivity, and wrinkling of the soles. With dorsal involvement, papules, purpura, vesicles, and edema may be present. Cyanosis, mottling, and erythema present later. Maceration with secondary infection, fever, and femoral adenopathy is common. In severe cases, blisters, ulcers, and gangrene may be present. Tissue loss is unusual, although healing with return of normal skin color, temperature, and sensation may take months.

The history given by victims of *frostbite* is usually sufficient to make a diagnosis and estimate the extent of tissue damage. The patient may present with totally or partially frozen parts. In general, the tissue is white and waxy when frozen. The subcutaneous tissue is soft and pliable prior to thawing in superficial frostbite. In more deeply injured tissues, there is little resilience in the subcutaneous tissues. The frozen part is cold and lacks sensibility. Some victims demonstrate a superimposed burn injury from attempts to rewarm the frozen, insensate part. Classification of the depth of injury is done after thawing, when frostbitten tissue takes on an appearance that is characteristic of the depth of injury (Table 385.1).

DIFFERENTIAL DIAGNOSIS

The appearance of frostbite or cold immersion may be confused with a devascularizing injury, envenomation, or a thermal or chemical burn. The history usually reveals the correct cause of tissue injury. In patients who are not communicative, the temperature of the body or the extremity will assist in making the diagnosis.

EMERGENCY DEPARTMENT EVALUATION

The early evaluation of cold-injured tissue is difficult and can be deceiving. Often, the full extent of injury may not be apparent for days after the injury. Because only 10% to 15% of patients arrive in the emergency department with the involved part still frozen, the physician must recognize the injury at various stages in its presentation. A careful history, including exposure temperature, duration of exposure, the extent of wetting involved, and the wind conditions at the time of exposure, is critical. Risk factors such as trauma, peripheral vascular disease, smoking, alcohol use, and other systemic illnesses should be investigated.

Physical examination should include the patient's core temperature and a full description of the injured part. Color, blister formation, the color of the blister fluid, temperature, consistency, capillary refill, movement, two-point discrimination, and vibratory sensibility should be observed serially, because these signs may change rapidly. The presence of peripheral pulses should be ascertained by palpation or by Doppler examination. Rarely, cold injury to the cornea may occur, necessitating visual acuity and fluorescein examination. Laboratory studies are of minimal assistance in diagnosing the frostbite injury. The frostbite patient should, however, be evaluated for hypothermia, trauma, and concomitant illness. Angiography is contraindicated due to potential injury to the vasculature. Technetium three-phase bone scanning may be helpful in determining the extent of injury and in planning surgical debridement, but does not change early therapy.

EMERGENCY DEPARTMENT MANAGEMENT

Prior to arrival, there should be no rubbing or manipulation of the frozen part, as this can exacerbate tissue injury. Refreezing of thawed parts can cause greater damage than the initial injury, so rewarming should be delayed until there is no risk of refreezing.[2,7]

Nonadherent wet or cold apparel should be removed and the patient placed under warm blankets. Clothing frozen to the skin

TABLE 385.1. Classification of Frostbite Severity

Severity	Symptoms
First degree: partial thickness	
Erythema, edema, hyperemia	Stinging, burning
No blisters or necrosis	Possible throbbing and aching
Occasional skin desquamation (5-10 d later)	Possible hyperhidrosis
Second degree: full thickness	
Erythema, significant edema	Numbness
Clear vesicles	
Blisters may desquamate and form blackened eschar	
Third degree: involves subcutaneous tissue	Initially insensate; later, shooting pains, burning, throbbing, aching
Violaceous/hemorrhagic blisters due to injury to the reticular dermis and subdermal plexus	
Skin necrosis	
Blue-gray skin	
Fourth degree: involves muscle, tendon, and bone	Possible joint discomfort
Little edema	
Initially mottled, deep red, or cyanotic	
Later dry, black, mummified	

Adapted from Britt L, Dascombe W, Rodriguez A. New horizons in management of hypothermia and frostbite injury. *Surg Clin North Am* 1991;71:345–370.

should be trimmed and removed only after it is loosened with rewarming. Systemic hypothermia should be treated prior to thawing of frozen extremities. Tetanus toxoid should be administered, if indicated. Intravenous hydration may be beneficial for hemodilution in the dehydrated patient and for redistribution of blood flow to underperfused areas to minimize tissue loss secondary to ischemia.[1]

Rewarming with dry heat is sufficient for the treatment of *frostnip, chilblain,* and *immersion foot*. Elevation and avoidance of manipulation and pressure, cleansing, topical antimicrobials (e.g., Neosporin ointment and silver sulfadiazine cream), and dressings for denuded areas are also recommended for immersion foot. Prophylactic systemic antibiotics are not indicated. Treatment of infections should be based on clinical examination as well as microscopic examination and culture results for both fungi and bacteria.

The initial care of *frostbite* is rapid thawing of the involved part in a water bath at 40°C to 42°C.[10] The water temperature should be kept constant, as cooling of the bath could allow refreezing and further tissue damage. Thawing usually takes 15 to 20 minutes; during this period, rubbing or manipulation should again be avoided. Thawing with dry heat should be avoided, because it has been associated with larger areas of tissue loss. Ultrasound therapy is contraindicated as an adjunct to thawing, because it has been associated with earlier development of wet gangrene.

With rewarming, symptoms of pain with gradual evolution to numbness may present. Throbbing pain may develop 48 to 72 hours postthaw and may persist for several weeks. With nerve regeneration, a tingling sensation may be present. Return of normal sensibility depends on the depth and extent of injury. Postthaw pain may be managed with narcotic analgesia as well as elevation and avoidance of abrasion or pressure.

Bullae containing clear fluid should be opened to remove the fluid, as prostanoid derivatives contained within may cause further tissue damage. Hemorrhagic bullae indicate injury to the subdermal vascular plexus and should be left intact to minimize further injury to the remaining viable tissue.

Additional therapies for frostbite include aloe vera (applied topically to the injured tissue every 6 hours) and ibuprofen (400 to 800 mg orally every 6 to 8 hours). Ascorbic acid (1 g orally every 12 hours), a free radical scavenger, is also recommended.[5,7] Small-vessel vasodilation and blood flow can be maximized with nifedipine (10 mg orally every 8 hours).[6] Smoking is prohibited for both patient and visitors. The patient should be restricted to bed and the injured part elevated, with no external garments or bedclothes touching it. Although clinical experience with the use of hyperbaric oxygen is limited, this therapy warrants consideration when it is available.

Other frostbite therapies should be considered experimental or of unproved benefit. Dextran has been shown to reduce tissue loss after frostbite in animal studies. There is experimental support for use of the thrombolytic agents (streptokinase and urokinase, but not tissue plasminogen activator) in frostbite injuries. The calmodulin antagonists, thioridazine and trifluoperazine, have been found to reverse frostbite tissue damage. Studies of sympathectomy, both medical and surgical, have not been conclusive. Reserpine and guanethidine have yielded long-term benefits in frostbite patients.

The amount of tissue loss following cold injury depends on the depth and extent of injury. Appropriately treated, second-degree or less frostbite or immersion foot seldom results in tissue loss. However, hypesthesia or dysesthesia may be present for a long time postinjury. Surgical intervention and debridement of tissues should be reserved for wet gangrene or late gangrene. Early surgery may injure marginally viable tissue and result in an extension of tissue necrosis.

DISPOSITION

All but the most superficially injured frostbite patient should be admitted. Surgical consultation (plastic, vascular, or general, depending on local practices) should be obtained. Corneal injuries warrant an ophthalmology consult. Discharged patients should be reevaluated within 24 to 48 hours, as tissue necrosis may be progressive and infectious complications may develop. Protective clothing and footwear, as well avoidance of future cold exposure, should be advised due to the increased sensitivity and susceptibility to subsequent exposures. Smoking should be prohibited.

COMMON PITFALLS

- Failure to evaluate and treat for concurrent systemic hypothermia
- Rubbing or manipulating frozen tissue
- Failure to rapidly warm affected parts
- Failure to monitor the temperature of the rewarming bath, which can result in refreezing or burn injury
- Failure to obtain surgical consultation
- Failure to admit patients with significant frostbite injuries for observation
- Failure to consider adjunctive therapy (e.g., thromboxane inhibitors and vasodilators)
- Failure to appreciate that the extent of irreversible tissue damage may not be evident until many days after exposure
- Failure to warn patients about the hazards of reexposure

References

1. Beitner R, Chen-Zion M, Sofer-Bassukevita Y, et al. Treatment of frostbite with the calmodulin antagonists thioridazine and trifluoperazine. *Gen Pharmacol* 1989;20:641.
2. Boswick J, Thompson J, Jonas R. The epidemiology of cold injuries. *Surg Gynecol Obstet* 1979;149:326.
3. Britt L, Dascombe W, Rodriguez A. New horizons in management of hypothermia and frostbite injury. *Surg Clin North Am* 1991;71:345–370.
4. Carpenter H, Hurley L, Hardenbergh E, et al. Vascular injury due to cold. *Arch Pathol* 1971;92:153.
5. Cummings R, Lykke A. The effects of anti-inflammatory drugs in vascular exudation evoked by cold injury. *Pathology* 1973;5:117.
6. Dowd P, Rustin M, Lanigan S. Nifedipine in the treatment of chillblains. *BMJ* 1986;293:923.
7. Foray J. Mountain frostbite; current trends in prognosis and treatment. *Int J Sports Med* 1992;13:S193.
8. Hardenbergh E. Hyperbaric oxygen treatment of experimental frostbite in the mouse. *J Surg Res* 1972;12:34-40.
9. Knize D, Weatherley-White R, Paton B, et al. Prognostic factors in the management of frostbite. *J Trauma* 1969;9:749.
10. Malhotra M, Mathew L. Effect of rewarming at various water bath temperatures in experimental frostbite. *Aviat Space Environ Med* 1978;49:874–876.
11. Marzella L, Jesudass R, Manson P. Morphologic characterization of acute injury to vascular endothelium of skin after frostbite. *Plast Reconstr Surg* 1989;83:67.
12. Meryman H. Mechanism of freezing in living cells and tissues. *Science* 1956;124:815.
13. Meryman H. Osmotic stress as a mechanism of freezing injury. *Cryobiology* 1956;8:489.
14. Miller M, Koltai P. Treatment of experimental frostbite with pentoxyfylline and aloe vera cream. *Arch Otolaryngol Head Neck Surg* 1995;121:678–680.
15. Mills W. Frostbite. Northwest Med 1966;65:119.
16. Okuboye J, Ferguson C. The use of hyperbaric oxygen in the treatment of experimental frostbite. *Can J Surg* 1968;11:78–84.
17. Raine T, London M, Goluch L, et al. Antiprostaglandins and antithromboxanes for treatment of frostbite. *Surg Forum Plast Surg* 1980;31:557.
18. Weatherley-White R, Paton B, Sjostrom B. Experimental studies in cold injury. III. Observations on the treatment of frostbite. *Plast Reconstr Surg* 1965;36:10.

19. Weatherley-White R, Sjostrom B, Paton B. Experimental studies in cold injury. II. The pathogenesis of frostbite. *J Surg Res* 1964;4:17.
20. Wrenn K. Immersion foot; a problem of the homeless in the 1990's. *Arch Intern Med* 1991;151:785.

CHAPTER 386
Hypothermia

Joseph J. Currier

Hypothermia is defined as a core temperature less than 35°C (95°F).[3,8,11,12,20] It may be acute (less than 6 hours' duration) or chronic (greater than 6 hours' duration); mild (32°C to 35°C), moderate (28°C to 32°C), or severe (less than 28°C); and primary or secondary. Primary, or "exposure," hypothermia is usually acute and occurs in healthy persons following immersion in cold water or exposure to low environmental temperatures.

In contrast, secondary, or "urban," hypothermia is generally chronic and occurs in those with predisposing illness, infirmity, intoxication, or extremes of age.[3,4] Secondary hypothermia is much more common than primary hypothermia and has a very high mortality rate (approaching 100% in severe cases). In contrast, recovery is the rule for young, healthy adults with primary hypothermia. Survival has been reported with a core temperature as low as 16°C (61°F).[17]

Body temperature is a function of the production and loss of heat.[3,10–12,20] Heat is produced by metabolism, muscular activity, and shivering. Newborns can also produce heat by nonshivering thermogenesis, in which specialized adipose tissue (brown fat) can directly transform substrate into heat due to the unusually high density of mitochondria.[18] Heat is conserved by peripheral vasoconstriction and the insulation provided by clothing.

Heat is lost by conduction (direct contact with colder objects, such as ground, snow, and water), convection (air motion across body surfaces), evaporation (from skin, lungs, or wet clothing), and radiation (from exposed surfaces). Normal heat dissipation occurs predominantly by radiation. The rate of heat loss is proportional to the difference between body and environmental temperature. Convection losses are also a function of ambient air velocity (the wind-chill factor) and humidity.

Humans, like other warm-blooded animals, normally maintain core body temperature within a very narrow range (37°C ± 0.2°C). Thermosensors in the skin, spinal cord, and gastrointestinal tract detect changes in body temperature. Efferent impulses are integrated within the spinal cord and transmitted to the hypothalamus, the central thermoregulatory center. Both neural (vasomotor) and hormonal (e.g., catecholamines, thyroxine) hypothalamic efferents control heat production and heat loss.

Any condition that results in decreased heat production, increased heat loss, or impaired temperature regulation may result in hypothermia (Table 386.1).[3,8,11,12,20] Very low ambient temperatures are not required. Without adequate insulation and intact thermoregulatory mechanisms, exposure to any temperature below 35°C can result in hypothermia. Neonates are at risk because of a relatively large body surface relative to total mass and ineffective shivering and heat production. Low fat stores, medication effects, lower metabolic rate, relative inability to detect temperature changes, and deteriorating adaptive responses place the elderly at risk.

TABLE 386.1. Predisposing Factors in Hypothermia

DECREASED HEAT PRODUCTION	INCREASED HEAT LOSS
CNS depression (metabolic or traumatic) Immobility (age, neuromuscular disorders) Endocrine failure (adrenal/pituitary/thyroid) Hypoglycemia/malnutrition	Environmental exposure: inadequate clothing/shelter, wind chill, low humidity, perspiration, wet clothing Exfoliative skin disease Vasodilatation Drugs Neuropathy Sepsis Shock Burns
HYPOTHALAMIC DYSFUNCTION	**IATROGENIC COOLING**
Acidosis/anoxia CNS hemorrhage/infarction Drugs (e.g., phenothiazines) Encephalopathy	Use of large volumes of cool (<35°C [95°F]) fluids for lavage or i.v. administration; overly aggressive treatment of hyperthermia

Ethanol and drug use may increase heat loss due to cutaneous vasodilatation and impaired shivering. Hypothalamic dysfunction and decreased ability to seek shelter from the cold also may contribute. Sepsis, endocrine dysfunction (diabetic ketoacidosis, hypoglycemia, hypothyroidism, hypopituitarism, hypoadrenalism), central nervous system (CNS) disorders (stroke, brain tumors, spinal cord injury), and skin conditions (burns, erythroderma, psoriasis, ichthyosis) are additional predisposing factors. Lengthy exposure times, cool intravenous fluid infusions, and general anesthesia contribute to the hypothermia often seen in trauma victims.[4,13,18]

The initial response to cooling includes cutaneous vasoconstriction, shivering, and increased metabolic activity.[3,4,8,10–12,20] Heart rate and respirations are usually increased, but facial immersion in cold water can cause vagally mediated bradycardia (the diving reflex) and apnea. Generalized organ dysfunction with CNS, cardiac, and respiratory depression occurs with core temperatures below 35°C. Acid–base status may vary. Mild hypothermia is accompanied by respiratory alkalosis, while more severe hypothermia is associated with respiratory acidosis.

Decreased tissue oxygenation results from hypoventilation, vasoconstriction, increased blood viscosity, ventilation–perfusion mismatch, shifting of the oxyhemoglobin dissociation curve to the left, and volume depletion due to cold-induced diuresis and ileus. Furthermore, shivering increases lactate production, which, along with poor perfusion of tissues, decreased acid excretion, and impaired hepatic metabolism, causes a metabolic acidosis. The threshold for ventricular fibrillation is decreased at temperatures below 28°C.

CLINICAL PRESENTATION

The physiologic changes that occur during hypothermia are summarized in Table 386.2.[3,4,8,10–12,20] Manifestations of mild hypothermia include apathy, confusion, lethargy, fatigue, forgetfulness, incoordination, shivering, slurred speech, withdrawal, and increased pulse and respirations. A fine, at times unilateral, muscle tremor may also be present. With progressive hypothermia, shivering stops and pulse, blood pressure, and respirations are decreased. Disorientation, stupor, inappropriate behavior, ileus, polyuria, rhonchi, and wheezing may be noted.

TABLE 386.2. Physiologic Changes during Hypothermia

Stage of Hypothermia	Organ System: Central Nervous System	Cardiovascular	Respiratory	Dermatologic/ Neuromuscular	Renal/Gastrointestinal (GI)
Mild (32.2°C–35.0°C) (Excitation Phase)	Apathy Hyperreflexia Disorientation	Tachycardia Hypertension Increased CO	Tachypnea Bronchorrhea Bronchospasm	Shivering Vasoconstriction Increased tone	Cold-induced diuresis Decreased GI motility Constipation
Moderate (28.0°C–32.3°C) (Slowing Phase)	EEG abnormal Hyporeflexia Paradoxical undressing	Bradycardia Hypotension Increased atrial arrhythmias	Bradypnea Diminished gag Decreased O_2 consumption	Decreased shivering Spasm	Ileus GI erosions Hepatic necrosis/pancreatitis
Severe (<28°C)	Coma Areflexia Flattening EEG	Asystole Ventricular arrhythmias	Pulmonary edema Apnea	Rigidity Compartment syndrome	Oliguria Decreased renal blood flow

CO, cardiac output; EEG, electroencephalogram.

The electrocardiogram (ECG) commonly shows atrial fibrillation. Paroxysmal atrial tachycardia, interval prolongation (P-R, QRS, Q-T), decreased P-wave amplitude, T-wave changes, premature ventricular contractions, or a humped ST segment adjacent to the QRS complex (Osborn wave) may also be seen.[15] Findings in severe hypothermia include coma, dilated unreactive pupils, absent reflexes, a flat electroencephalogram, muscle rigidity, hypotension, weak or absent pulse, and slow, barely detectable respirations. Rarely, transient focal neurologic findings can be seen.[17] The ECG may show marked bradycardia, asystole, or ventricular fibrillation.

Laboratory findings include respiratory alkalosis in mild hypothermia, and hypoxia, metabolic and respiratory acidosis, increased amylase and hematocrit, and leukopenia, thrombocytopenia, coagulopathy, and variable electrolyte abnormalities in moderate and severe hypothermia. Hyperglycemia and, less commonly, hypoglycemia can be seen. The chest x-ray may disclose pulmonary infiltrates characteristic of aspiration or pneumonia. Other abnormalities may be present in patients with coexisting illness or injury.

DIFFERENTIAL DIAGNOSIS

Unless an accurate core (rectal or esophageal) temperature is obtained, hypothermia may be confused with virtually any endocrine, metabolic, toxic, traumatic, or vascular condition causing CNS depression. Even after the diagnosis has been made, it is necessary to distinguish between primary and secondary hypothermia by ruling out predisposing pathology.

ECG J waves may be misidentified as early repolarization or the T-on-R phenomenon seen in cyanide poisoning. The J wave is a distinct deflection during the downstroke of the QRS complex, not an early T wave. The lack of detectable vital signs on physical examination in severe hypothermia may lead to a misdiagnosis of death; careful and prolonged observation, an ECG, intraarterial blood pressure monitoring, core temperature measurement, and reassessment after warming can prevent this error.

EMERGENCY DEPARTMENT EVALUATION

The diagnosis of hypothermia may be suggested by the setting in which the patient was found (e.g., cool or cold, indoor or outdoor environment). The length and conditions of exposure, underlying medical problems, recent illnesses, and medications are documented. Any patient with altered mental status should have a core temperature measured; the same is true for initially normothermic or hyperthermic patients treated with cooling measures or large volumes of intravenous or lavage solutions.

The physical examination initially focuses on vital signs and the neurologic, cardiovascular, and pulmonary systems. In severe cases, observation for 2 minutes or longer may be required to detect a pulse or respirations. An esophageal or rectal probe (thermocouple) or a thermometer capable of measuring low temperatures (below the usual 34°C) is required for an accurate diagnosis. A detailed examination should then be performed, searching for coexisting pathology. An ECG and chest x-ray are usually indicated.

In moderate and severe hypothermia, routine laboratory tests should include arterial blood gas measurement; a complete blood count; measurement of amylase, electrolytes, glucose, blood urea nitrogen, and creatinine; a coagulation profile; and urinalysis. Additional tests, such as a bacteriologic culture; measurement of calcium, magnesium, phosphate, lactate, ketones, cortisol, and cardiac enzymes; liver and thyroid function tests; and toxicology screening, may also be necessary to elucidate concomitant medical problems.[20]

The interpretation of arterial blood gas results in hypothermia is controversial. Because the pH increases (0.015 U/°C) and the P_{CO_2} (4.4%/°C) and P_{O_2} (7.2%/°C) decrease at temperatures below 37°C as the result of changes in gas solubility, measurement of these parameters in samples warmed to 37°C will result in a falsely decreased pH and increased P_{CO_2} and P_{O_2} levels if not corrected for temperature. However, the pH of neutrality increases as temperature decreases. Therefore, the normal pH at room temperature (7.40) is relatively acidic in a hypothermic state, and the uncorrected results of an arterial blood gas analysis may better guide therapy for acid–base disturbances.[8,9]

EMERGENCY DEPARTMENT MANAGEMENT

All patients should receive oxygen and have cardiac and temperature monitoring. An intravenous line should be established. In the prehospital setting, the patient should be protected from further cooling. Wet clothes should be removed, the ambulance should be heated, and the patient should be covered with blankets.

If a pulse is detected, cardiopulmonary resuscitation (CPR) and endotracheal intubation should not be performed, because these procedures may precipitate ventricular tachycardia, fibrillation, or asystole. Ventilations should be assisted by a bag-mask device, and the patient should be moved as little as possible. Hyperventilation should be avoided, as it may induce alkalosis and result in ventricular fibrillation.

Emergency department management depends on severity.[3,4,8,10–12,20] Nearly all patients require volume expansion. Normal saline with dextrose is preferable to lactated Ringer's, because lactate may not be metabolized during hypothermia. The volume of fluid should be determined by tissue perfusion and vital signs. Intravascular monitoring (e.g., arterial central venous, pulmonary artery) may be required in severe cases. Room-temperature intravenous fluids are acceptable for mild hypothermia, unless the rapid infusion of large volumes is necessary (e.g., patients with bleeding or severe dehydration). Otherwise, intravenous fluids should be warmed to 45°C, because room-temperature intravenous fluids are relatively hypothermic compared with most patients suffering from hypothermia. If a blood warmer is unavailable, 1 L of room-temperature intravenous fluid may be warmed in a standard microwave oven (high setting for 1 to 2 minutes, depending on wattage).[5]

Patients who require intubation for airway protection, hypoxia, or respiratory depression (CO_2 retention) should first receive 100% oxygen, topical anesthesia, and sedation. Acid–base abnormalities should be corrected. Prophylactic administration of lidocaine or bretylium may be helpful. Intubation should be done with as little airway manipulation as possible to avoid inducing dysrhythmias. Nasal intubation may be preferable to the oral route if spontaneous respirations are present.

Chemical or electrical treatment of dysrhythmias is usually ineffective at temperatures below 30°C, so warming should take precedence. Supraventricular dysrhythmias will generally convert spontaneously during or within 24 hours of rewarming. Pulseless rhythms should be treated according to advanced cardiac life-support guidelines. Because bretylium (but not lidocaine) has been shown to increase the threshold for ventricular fibrillation and to increase the success of defibrillation during experimental hypothermia, it should be considered a first-line agent for this rhythm.[14] Although open cardiac massage in conjunction with mediastinal lavage using warm saline has been advocated for pulseless rhythms, its efficacy remains to be determined.

Passive (spontaneous) rewarming is appropriate for adults with mild, primary hypothermia. Warm blankets and shivering will generally increase body temperature by an average of 0.4°C per hour. Neonates and adults with secondary hypothermia should be treated by active rewarming, as should victims of moderate and severe hypothermia. Active rewarming may be accomplished by providing warm intravenous fluids; humidified air or oxygen (by mask or ventilator) heated to 42°C to 45°C (mouth temperature); immersion in a 40°C water bath; peritoneal, gastric, bladder, or colonic lavage with 45°C fluid; covering the patient with a plastic circulating hot-air blanket (e.g., Bair Hugger); blood warming by hemodialysis (with an in-line heat exchanger) or femoral–femoral (partial) cardiopulmonary bypass pump; and pleuromediastinal lavage via thoracostomy or thoracotomy.[1–4,7,8,10–12,19,20]

Inhalational warming, using a cascade humidifier, is safe, easy, and readily available and can increase the temperature by about 1°C per hour. Gastric, bladder, colonic, and pleuromediastinal lavages are less efficacious. Bath rewarming is more effective than inhalation rewarming but makes monitoring difficult. Peritoneal lavage can increase the temperature by 2°C to 4°C per hour, whereas extracorporeal techniques can achieve rates of up to 10°C per hour. Cardiopulmonary bypass can support the circulation in lieu of prolonged CPR. Although not as rapid as cardiopulmonary bypass, hemodialysis may be advantageous in the hypothermic patient who also has a coincident drug overdose responsive to dialysis.[6] Resuscitation should not be considered unsuccessful until the core temperature has been raised to at least 32°C.[19]

The optimal rate of rewarming depends on the cardiopulmonary status and the degree of hypothermia. Animal studies suggest that slow rewarming (maintaining an intramyocardial temperature gradient of less than 2°C) minimizes the risk of ventricular fibrillation. Hence, invasive procedures should generally be reserved for hemodynamically unstable patients with severe hypothermia. When used in such instances, the most effective techniques available should be employed in order to minimize the rewarming time.

Decreases in core temperature (afterdrop) and, possibly, acidosis and hypotension due to peripheral vasodilatation and the exchange of cool peripheral blood for warm core blood have been noted during spontaneous, inhalation, or immersion rewarming.[16] Because there are both central and peripheral thermosensors, afterdrop is theoretically possible with any rewarming technique.

The magnitude and duration of afterdrop appears to be lower with bath rewarming than with spontaneous or inhalation techniques.[16] In addition, metabolic rates are increased with surface rewarming but not by inhalation.[6] It thus appears that active surface rewarming is not contraindicated, as previously speculated. Uneven surface warming (e.g., warm packs to axilla and groin), however, is not recommended. The concurrent use of multiple rewarming techniques is probably most effective and safest.

Additional measures should include correction of underlying metabolic derangements and the treatment of coexisting or secondary medical or surgical problems.

DISPOSITION

Patients with mild hypothermia should be observed until they are asymptomatic and normothermic. Those with extremes of age or coexisting underlying pathology should be admitted for further evaluation and treatment. Patients with moderate or severe hypothermia should be admitted to an intensive care unit. Those with unstable vital signs or a core temperature below 28°C should be transferred by an advanced life-support unit to a facility capable of performing extracorporeal rewarming, if such services are not available at the current facility.

COMMON PITFALLS

- Failure to consider the diagnosis of hypothermia in patients with altered mental status
- Failure to obtain an accurate (core or rectal) temperature
- Failure to search diligently for underlying causes of secondary hypothermia
- Failure to recognize that chemical and electrical treatment of dysrhythmias is generally ineffective at temperatures below 28°C
- Failure to appreciate that rough handling, airway manipulation, and invasive procedures may precipitate dysrhythmias
- Failing to continue resuscitation attempts until the core temperature is at least 32°C
- Failure to include volume replacement in resuscitative efforts
- Failing to monitor for core temperature afterdrop

ACKNOWLEDGMENT

The author gratefully acknowledges the contribution of Paul H. Klainer and Brian Mongillo who wrote the previous version of this chapter.

References

1. Baumgartner FJ, Janusz MT, Jamieson WR, et al. Cardiopulmonary bypass for resuscitation of patients with accidental hypothermia and cardiac arrest. *Can J Surg* 1992;35:184.

2. Bolgiano E, Sykes L, Barish RA, et al. Accidental hypothermia with cardiac arrest: recovery following rewarming by cardiopulmonary bypass. *J Emerg Med* 1992;10:427.
3. Curley FJ, Irwin RS. Disorders of temperature control, part III. *J Intensive Care Med* 1986;1:5.
4. Danzl DF, Pozos RS. Accidental hypothermia. *N Engl J Med* 1994;331:26.
5. Gong V. Microwave rewarming of IV fluids in management of hypothermia. *Ann Emerg Med* 1984;13:116.
6. Hernandez E, Praga M, Alcazar JM, et al. Hemodialysis for treatment of accidental hypothermia. *Nephron* 1993;63:214.
7. Ireland KW, Follette DM, Iquidbashian J, et al. Use of a heat exchanger to prevent hypothermia during thoracic and thoracoabdominal aneurysm repairs. *Ann Thorac Surg* 1993;55:534.
8. Jolly B, Ghezzi K. Accidental hypothermia. *Emerg Clin North Am* 1992;10:311.
9. Kofstad J. Blood gases and hypothermia: some theoretical and practical considerations. *Scand J Clin Lab Invest* 1996;56:224.
10. Lazar HL. The treatment of hypothermia. *N Engl J Med* 1997;337:21.
11. Lee-Chiong TL Jr, Stitt JT. Accidental hypothermia. *Postgrad Med* 1996;99:1.
12. Leikin JB, Aks SE, Andrews S, et al. Environmental injuries. *Dis Mon* 1997;43:12.
13. Marion DW, Leonov Y, et al. Resuscitative hypothermia. *Crit Care Med* 1996;24:2.
14. Orts A, Alcaraz C, Delaney KA, et al. Bretylium tosylate and electrically induced cardiac arrhythmias during hypothermia in dogs. *Am J Emerg Med* 1992;10:4.
15. Osborne L, Kamal A, El-Din AS, et al. Survival after prolonged cardiac arrest in accidental hypothermia. *BMJ* 1984;289:881.
16. Romet TT, Hoskin RW. Temperature and metabolic response to inhalation and bath rewarming protocols. *Aviat Space Environ Med* 1988;59:630.
17. Sekar T, MacDonnell K, Namsirikul P, et al. Survival after prolonged submersion in cold water without neurologic sequelae. *Arch Intern Med* 1980;140:775.
18. Sessler DI. Mild perioperative hypothermia. *N Engl J Med* 1997;336:24.
19. Steele MT, Nelson MJ, et al. Forced air speeds rewarming in accidental hypothermia. *Ann Emerg Med* 1996;27:4.
20. Weinberg A. Hypothermia. *Ann Emerg Med* 1993;22:370.

TABLE 387.1. Factors Predisposing to Heat Illness

Endogenous Factors	Exogenous Factors
INCREASED HEAT GAIN	
Infection	High ambient temperature
Drugs	Malignant hyperthermia
Stimulants	Sunlight
Hallucinogens	
Increased activity	
Exercise	
Seizures	
Drug withdrawal	
Psychosis	
Neuroleptic malignant syndrome	
Thyrotoxicosis	
DECREASED HEAT LOSS	
Lack of acclimation	High temperature
Dehydration	High humidity
Hypokalemia	Restrictive clothing
Drugs	
Anticholinergics	
Neuroleptics	
Barbiturates	
Antiparkinson agents	
Diuretics	
Beta blockers	
Alcohol	
Extremes of age	
Skin disorders	
Cystic fibrosis	
Obesity	
Debilitated/chronic disease	
Impaired voluntary responses	

CHAPTER 387
Heat- and Sun-Related Illnesses

Eric W. Schmidt and Constance G. Nichols

Heat illness can be defined as the inability of normal regulatory mechanisms to cope with a heat stress. Minor heat-related problems, such as muscle cramps, edema, rash, syncope, and tetany, account for significant morbidity. Heat exhaustion and heatstroke are major heat syndromes in that, if left untreated, they may cause organ damage or death. Among athletes, heatstroke is second only to head and cervical spine injuries as a cause of death. In elderly patients, mortality has been directly correlated with increased ambient temperature.[8] Sunburn and other photodermal ultraviolet (UV) injuries may exacerbate all other heat syndromes or may present separately.

Heat cramps are due to muscle fatigue combined with water and salt depletion. Heat syncope results from vasodilatation, usually compounded by volume depletion or the use of drugs that interfere with cardiovascular reflexes. Heat tetany apparatus to be due to hyperventilation-induced respiratory alkalosis, resulting in decreased ionized serum calcium. It may be an attempt to compensate for exercise-induced lactic acidosis. Heat rash is caused by the plugging, dilation, and rupture of sweat glands following skin maceration resulting from sweating. The etiology of heat edema is unknown.

Exposed to a variety of temperatures, humans maintain a relatively constant body temperature by balancing heat loss with heat gain. Any condition that increases heat gain or decreases heat loss may result in a major heat illness (Table 387.1). Heat gain may be due to increased endogenous heat production resulting from basal metabolism and muscle activity or may result from an environmental heat load. For example, basal metabolism generates 65 to 85 kcal/h, which may increase five- to sixfold with exertion. Underlying illness or drug ingestion may also increase endogenous heat production. Hot environments decrease heat loss as well as increase the heat load. The average sunbather may gain 150 kcal/h. Without heat dissipation, at rest, the average human temperature would increase 1.1°C /h.

In cool environments, heat is lost mainly through passive convection and radiation. As the ambient and body temperatures increase, centrally mediated mechanisms for active heat removal—cutaneous vasodilatation and sweating—begin. Radiational heat loss is first increased as the cardiovascular system adjusts blood flow to the periphery by decreasing the splanchnic and mesenteric flow and increasing heart rate and cardiac output. The second phase of active heat dissipation, sweating, is then brought into play. Sympathetic stimulation releases acetylcholine, which stimulates the sweat glands, resulting in evaporative heat loss. Acetylcholine also facilitates the secretion of kallikreins, which facilitate the formation of bradykinin from globin. Bradykinin and other peptides may contribute to superficial vasodilatation. The unacclimatized person can sweat up to 1.5 L/h, losing 1.7 kcal/mL of sweat.[1,13]

Heat exhaustion results from dehydration with inadequate fluid and electrolyte replacement. Water or salt depletion, or both, may be present. Without treatment, heat exhaustion progresses to heatstroke. Heatstroke is due to severe dehydration, with thermoregulatory failure resulting in body temperatures above 40°C (105°F to 106°F) and a mortality rate of up to 70%.

Acclimatization is a process of physiologic adaptation to repeated heat stress that occurs over 10 to 60 days. It results in decreased heat production and increased heat loss for a given amount of work. Metabolic function improves by increasing skeletal muscle mitochondria and glycogen stores, thereby enhancing the aerobic work capacity, which produces less heat. Fluid and electrolyte balance is altered by aldosterone secretion, which helps to conserve sodium stores by both sweat and renal mechanisms and by increasing extracellular volume. Cardiac efficiency is improved, with an increase in maximum cardiac output, a decreased peak heart rate, and increased stroke volume. Changes in sweating occur so that the threshold core temperature for sweating is decreased and the volume of sweat is increased. Sweat volumes may decrease with further acclimatization due to increased efficiency of the metabolic components. Potassium loss during acclimatization peaks at 8 to 10 days and often increases susceptibility to heat illness.[1,13] Although acclimatization protects against heat illness, as the wet-bulb temperature approaches 30°C (86°F), even young, well-acclimated persons are susceptible during vigorous or prolonged physical activity.[4,5]

UV exposure varies 40- to 80-fold over the course of the year for a given location. Intensity peaks between 10 a.m. and 2 p.m. daily. The degree and extent of UV injury is a direct function of the total energy absorbed. UV tissue injury occurs at multiple cellular levels. Initially, there is an inflammatory reaction similar to other tissue insults, with a cellular and humoral response involving Langerhans cells, macrophages, lymphocytes, prostaglandins, interleukins, and multiple cytokines. Individual response ranges from mild transient erythema to urticaria with exacerbation of underlying medical conditions, depending on exposure, skin type, photoallergy, or photodrug reaction (Table 387.2).[4] The maximal response may be delayed up to 30 hours and last for several days.

Phytophotodermatitis is due to skin exposure to furanocoumarins (psoralens) from fruits and vegetables, followed by sun exposure. It is an occupational hazard of harvesters and grocery workers.[11]

UVB frequencies (290 to 320 nm) are up to 1600 times more injurious than UVA (320 to 400 nm), but there is a preponderance of UVA in the environment.[4,10]

TABLE 387.2. Common Causes of Photosensitivity Reactions

DIRECT PHOTOTOXICITY
Amiodarone
Doxycycline
Furosemide
Naproxen sodium
Phenothiazines
Sulfonamides
PHOTOALLERGY
Phenothiazines
Sulfonamides
Sunscreens
PHYTOPHOTODERMATITIS
Celery
Chrysanthemums
Dill
Limes
Parsnip

CLINICAL PRESENTATION

Heat cramps are painful spasms of heavily used muscle groups. They often occur in acclimatized persons, during or up to several hours after exertion. The victim often has been sweating heavily, with insufficient or hypotonic fluid replacement for several days. Serum sodium levels are normal.[3,13]

Heat edema is manifest by ankle and wrist swelling. It occurs in the first few days of heat exposure and sometimes results in pitting.[3,13]

Heat rash (prickly heat) is most common early in acclimatization, in tropical areas, and in those wearing tight clothes. It is an intensely pruritic, red, papular, occasionally vesicular dermatitis. Complications include infection and the formation of large nonpruritic plugs, which take several weeks to desquamate. Persons with advanced heat rash are at risk for heat exhaustion or heatstroke due to loss of sweat gland function.[4]

Heat syncope is a transient loss of postural tone, with or without brief loss of consciousness, occurring early in exposure to a new heat stress. It is often preceded by dehydration or the presence of drugs that affect the body's normal compensatory mechanisms.[2] By the time victims are examined, vital signs are usually normal.

Heat tetany presents as carpopedal spasm and is frequently seen in conjunction with other heat syndromes or other causes of hyperventilation. In contrast to heat cramps, it does not involve the heavily used proximal muscles. Arterial blood gas analysis may reveal a respiratory alkalosis.[3,9]

Victims of *heat exhaustion* are usually nonacclimatized persons who have been working in the heat for several days. Symptoms caused by water depletion include thirst, weakness, dizziness, anxiety, muscular incoordination, agitation, confusion, palpitations, oliguria, and elevated temperature. Those caused by salt depletion include fatigue, weakness, headache, anorexia, vomiting, diarrhea, and skeletal muscle cramps; thirst is absent. Body temperature is usually normal or subnormal in both types of heat exhaustion; the skin is cool and clammy. Tachycardia and hypotension are common. Most victims present with a combined picture of water and salt depletion. Laboratory findings may include hyponatremia, high urinary specific gravity, and mildly elevated serum creatine phosphokinase and liver enzyme levels. Without termination of the heat stressor and immediate treatment, heat exhaustion may progress to frank heatstroke.[3,9]

Classic heatstroke usually affects the very young or the debilitated elderly and develops over several days, mostly during heat waves.[3,9] The gradual onset may result in severe dehydration and hot, dry skin. Exertional heatstroke usually occurs in an unacclimatized younger person after a few hours of severe heat stress. Victims usually can still sweat.

Vital signs show hyperthermia(usually greater than 40°C), tachycardia, tachypnea, and hypotension. Family or witnesses may describe a malaise or flulike prodrome.[2,4,13]

Because a high core temperature for a short period of time can produce the same injury as a relatively lower temperature for a longer period, the presenting temperature may not predict severity or outcome.[14] Widespread damage to almost every organ system, especially the cerebellum, has been described. The central nervous system (CNS) is one of the first systems involved and the last to recover. Mental confusion begins with a core temperature of 38°C, with cessation of function at temperatures above 42°C. Any CNS change from confusion and coma to seizure activity and posturing has been described.[13] The liver is particularly susceptible to heat injury. Serum transaminase levels may initially be in the thousands and peak up to 2 weeks later at more than 10,000. Coagulopathies and hypoglycemia are common. The kidneys are at high risk for acute tubular necrosis.

Rhabdomyolysis may contribute to renal injury in victims of exertional heatstroke.[3,9,13] Arterial blood gas measurements usually reveal a respiratory alkalosis. Lactic acidosis may also be seen following heavy exertion. Death is usually secondary to disseminated intravascular coagulation, acute renal failure, liver failure, or adult respiratory distress syndrome.[3,17]

DIFFERENTIAL DIAGNOSIS

The key to diagnosing any heat illness is a history of a heat stress. During a heat wave, the diagnosis is easily considered. Vigorous exercise in moderate temperatures, or working in a closed, hot environment, may also result in significant heat stress. The clinician should remember the predisposing factors in Table 387.1. Rhabdomyolysis should be excluded in patients with heat cramps. Electrolyte abnormalities should be ruled out in victims of heat cramps and tetany. An extensive evaluation may be necessary to exclude other causes of edema and syncope. The differential diagnosis of heatstroke includes infection, particularly meningitis, thyroid storm, drug intoxication, and the neuroleptic malignant syndrome (malignant hyperthermia). In contrast to heatstroke, patients with the neuroleptic malignant syndrome have muscular rigidity that responds to dantrolene.[13,15]

EMERGENCY DEPARTMENT EVALUATION

The history includes the duration, magnitude, and conditions of heat exposure; recent activity; the nature, progression, and duration of symptoms; medications; drug use; and underlying medical problems. In young, healthy victims, a typical history and physical examination that reveal no other pathology are all that is necessary for a diagnosis of minor heat-related problems. Normal laboratory findings will confirm the diagnosis in questionable cases and in those with advanced age or coexisting medical problems.

In victims of heat exhaustion and heatstroke, vital signs include orthostatic pulse and blood pressure measurements and a rectal temperature. Depending on the severity, laboratory evaluation should include arterial blood gas analysis; a complete blood count; measurements of electrolytes, blood urea nitrogen, creatinine, glucose, creatine phosphokinase and liver enzymes; and urinalysis. Those with elevated levels of creatine phosphokinase, abnormal electrolyte or liver enzyme levels, or high temperatures should also have coagulation studies; calcium, magnesium, phosphorus, and uric acid measurements; an electrocardiogram and a chest x-ray.[3]

EMERGENCY DEPARTMENT MANAGEMENT

Heat cramps are treated with oral or intravenous fluid and salt replacement. Fruit juices or Gatorade by mouth is sufficient for mild cases. Intravenous normal saline is recommended for severe symptoms. Heat edema is self-limited and will resolve with time if the limb is elevated and support hose are worn. Patients with heat rash should keep their skin cool and dry and avoid tight clothing. Antihistamines may be given for pruritus, but, to prevent further plugging, powders should be avoided. Desquamating agents (e.g., salicylic acid) and antibiotics effective against staphylococci may be prescribed for secondary infection. Heat syncope is treated with rest, fluids, salt, and gradual return to activity. Heat tetany should resolve with the reversal of hyperventilation (e.g., bag breathing).

The treatment of heat exhaustion centers around replacement of fluid and electrolyte losses with isotonic saline. Orthostatic patients may require 4 L or more of intravenous fluids. Oral fluids can substitute for or supplement intravenous fluid in mild cases. Rare cases will present with severe hyponatremia requiring hypertonic saline infusion.[3,9,13]

The cornerstone of heatstroke therapy is rapid cooling. Immersing or covering the patient in ice is not recommended, because skin cooling causes both vasoconstriction and shivering and could increase the core temperature.[3] Cooling rates similar to ice immersion can be achieved by using immersion in 15°C water.[7] Applying ice packs in the areas of large vessels, such as the groin and axillae, and infusing large volumes of cool intravenous fluids are useful for field management but insufficient for definitive cooling.[3,5]

Although the fastest cooling rates (0.5°C/min) have been reported with peritoneal and even thoracic lavage using iced dialysate, using evaporation (0.3°C/min) and iced gastric lavage (0.2°C/min) with water or saline is a more practical combination.[6,13,16] Evaporation is maximized without inducing shivering by keeping the patient wet with lukewarm water or wet towels and blowing air over him or her with a fan. Helicopter blade fanning has also been used.[12] The rectal temperature should be monitored with a probe capable of measuring high temperatures (up to 44°C).

Cooling is continued only until the temperature drops to 38.5°C to 39.0°C, to avoid overshoot hypothermia. Rectal temperature monitoring should be continued, as the patient may rebound hours later and be thermally unstable for days. Along with cooling, these patients frequently need sedation and intubation and large volumes of intravenous normal saline. A central venous pressure line and Foley catheter are recommended to monitor fluid therapy. Acid–base, electrolyte, and coagulation abnormalities should be corrected. Alkaline diuresis may be helpful if rhabdomyolysis is present.[3]

Shivering may be treated with chlorpromazine (25 mg intravenously), benzodiazepines, or thiopental. Seizure activity is best treated with diazepam or phenobarbital. Phenytoin is ineffective. Dantrolene sodium has not been proved efficacious in canine studies, although anecdotal reports of success do exist.[15] Poor prognostic indicators are a serum glutamic–oxaloacetic transaminase level above 1,000 after 24 hours, a coma that lasts more than 8 hours, or a presenting temperature of 42.2°C or higher.[3,5]

Prevention of sunburn is the best therapy and can be done by avoiding unnecessary sun exposure (especially between 10 a.m. and 3 p.m.); wearing protective clothing, hats, and sunglasses; using broad-spectrum sunscreens with a sun protection factor of 15 or higher on exposed areas; and avoiding artificial tanning lights.[10] Treatment is otherwise supportive. Antiinflammatory drugs and topical aloe vera and steroid spray may be useful for mild cases. More severe cases may require therapy similar to that for thermal burns (see Chapter 125).

DISPOSITION

Patients with minor heat-related problems may be discharged. Patients with heat exhaustion should be admitted to a floor bed if they have abnormal vital signs or laboratory findings or remain symptomatic after fluid therapy. Patients with heatstroke should be admitted to an intensive care unit. Discharged patients should be advised to avoid the conditions that precipitated their illness. Acclimatization with frequent water breaks and rest periods during hot-weather activity should prevent future problems. Consultation with a dermatologist may be helpful in patients with photosensitivity reactions.

COMMON PITFALLS

- Failure to recognize heat-related illness and to appreciate its nonenvironmental causes
- Failure to assess carefully for mental status changes in potential heatstroke victims
- Failure to obtain an accurate temperature (by rectal thermoresistor probe, if necessary) in patients with suspected heat illness
- Failure to cool heatstroke patients aggressively
- Overaggressive rehydration of heatstroke victims
- Failure to warn victims to avoid reexposure until acclimatization has occurred
- Prescribing medications that predispose patients to or exacerbate heat or UV reactions

References

1. Armstrong L, Maresh C. The induction and decay of heat acclimatization in trained athletes. *Sports Med* 1991;12(5):302.
2. Barrow MW, Clark KA. Heat-related illnesses. *Am Fam Physician* 1998;58(3):749–756, 759.
3. Eichner ER. Treatment of suspected heat illness. *Int J Sports Med* 1998;19(Suppl 2):S150–S153.
4. Harber LC. Abnormal responses to ultraviolet radiation: drug induced sensitivity. In: Fitzpatrick T, Eisen A, Wolff K, et al., eds. *Dermatology in general medicine,* 4th ed. New York: McGraw-Hill, 1993.
5. Khosla R, Guntupalli KK. Heat-related illnesses. *Crit Care Clin* 1999;15(2):251–263.
6. Kielblock AJ, Van Rensburg JP, Franz RM. Body cooling as a method for reducing hyperthermia. *S Afr Med J* 1986;69:378–380.
7. Magazanik A, et al. Tap water: an efficient method for cooling heat stroke victims—a model in dogs. *Aviat Space Environ Med* 1980;51:864.
8. MMWR. Heat-related illnesses and deaths—Missouri, 1998, and United States, 1979–1996. *MMWR* 1999;48(22):469–473.
9. Noakes TD. Fluid and electrolyte disturbances in heat illness. *Int J Sports Med* 1998;19[Suppl 2]:S146–S211.
10. Parhak M. Advances in photomedicine: photoprotection and sunscreens. *Photochem Photobiol* 1991;53(5):66.
11. Parish JA. Photodermatology. In: Fitzpatrick T, Eisen A, Wolff K, et al., eds. *Dermatology in general medicine,* 4th ed. New York: McGraw-Hill, 1993.
12. Poulton TJ, Walker RA. Helicopter cooling of heatstroke victims. *Aviat Space Environ Med* 1987;58:358–561.
13. Simon H. Hyperthermia. *N Engl J Med* 1993;329:483.
14. Vicarion SJ, Okabajue RMS, Haltom T. Rapid cooling in classic heatstroke: effect on mortality rates. *Am J Emerg Med* 1986;4(5):394–398.
15. Watson J, et al. Exertional heat stroke induced by amphetamine analogues. Does dantrolene have a place? *Anaesthesia* 1993;49(12):1057.
16. White JD, et al. Evaporation versus iced gastric lavage treatment of heatstroke: comparative efficacy in a canine model. *Crit Care Med* 1987;15(8):748–750.
17. Yaqub BA, et al. Heat stroke at the Mekkah pilgrimage: clinical characteristics and course of 30 Patients. *Q J Med* 1986;59(229):523–530.

PART III
Dysbaric Emergencies

CHAPTER 388
Arterial Gas Embolism

Christopher H. Linden

Arterial gas embolism (AGE) is the most feared complication of compressed-gas diving. Second only to drowning as a cause of dive-related deaths, it accounts for 12% to 55% of patients treated at centers that specialize in the treatment of diving emergencies.[8]

AGE occurs for the same reasons as all barotrauma of ascent. Scuba equipment is designed to deliver compressed gas at ambient pressure. As a diver ascends, he or she moves to an environment of progressively lower pressure. According to Boyle's law, at a constant temperature, the volume of a gas varies inversely with ambient pressure ($PV = k$, where k is a constant). Thus, all gas breathed at depth will attempt to expand as the diver approaches the surface. If compressed gas is not allowed to vent from an enclosed space, pressures may eventually rise enough to rupture that space.

Whenever transpulmonic pressure exceeds a critical value, gas may dissect into surrounding tissue and produce a "pulmonary overpressurization syndrome" (POPS). In dogs, the critical pressure is as low as 60 mm Hg.[14] Human cadaver studies and anecdotal reports suggest that a depth change of as little as 4 to 6 ft of seawater may be enough to produce significant overpressurization.[2,4] People with poor lung compliance (due to structural abnormalities or pulmonary disease) are at higher risk for such a problem.[3] Most cases of POPS are of minor clinical importance. Local extravasation of gas commonly results in interstitial, mediastinal, and subcutaneous emphysema. Pneumothorax is rare, and tension pneumothorax even more so.

Penetration of gas into the pulmonary venous circulation is more serious. If gas bubbles survive passage through the left side of the heart, they may travel via the arterial circulation to distant organs. AGE may also develop as systemic venous gas bubbles that paradoxically embolize into the arterial system via right-to-left shunts (e.g., patent foramen ovale).[13] When such emboli are large enough, catastrophic complications may ensue.

The distribution of gas emboli seems to be determined by the same gravitational and hemodynamic forces that affect the movement of other types of emboli. Clinical manifestations are determined by a target organ's tolerance of arterial occlusion and its overall importance to homeostasis. Although coronary artery embolism has been reported, cerebral air embolism (CAE) is the most common and devastating manifestation of AGE. Thus, despite the fact that AGE to many different organs has been described, from a practical standpoint, AGE is synonymous with CAE.

CLINICAL PRESENTATION

The classic presentation of AGE was long thought to be hemoptysis and unilateral neurologic findings that occurred soon after a rapid ascent. Although studies are complicated by the frequent coincidence of embolic and decompression syndromes,[7] it is now clear that AGE may present in several ways. By definition, AGE can occur only in the setting of a compressed-gas dive. Most cases are associated with some violation of standard dive protocols (e.g., rapid ascent and failure to exhale during ascent), but failure to identify such risk factors should not rule out the diagnosis. Virtually all significant cases of AGE become clinically apparent within 10 minutes of ascent, but most within 5 minutes.[4,5,8,9]

Pulmonary symptoms play a surprisingly small role in the presentation of AGE. Only 25% to 50% of patients report dyspnea, 5% to 15% note hemoptysis, and pneumothorax is rare.[8,9] Neurologic symptoms are the hallmark of AGE, which is essentially a dive-related stroke. Clinical presentation is determined by the arterial distribution(s) occluded and by whatever secondary inflammatory response may develop in surrounding brain tissue. Symptoms range from subtle mental status changes to headache, cranial nerve abnormalities, focal paralysis or paresis, altered consciousness, seizures, and total vasomotor collapse.[4,5,8–10] Some authorities have found loss of consciousness to be the most common presentation of AGE (up to 40%).[4] Others find focal limb paralysis or paresis to be far more frequent (up to 65%).[8]

Neuroimaging may or may not reveal abnormalities in patients with neurologic deficits.[12,18] Magnetic resonance imaging is more sensitive than computed tomography scanning in detecting ischemic cerebrovascular lesions, but it is often normal. Transcranial Doppler sonography can sometimes detect arterial bubbles and may sometimes be diagnostic of CAE if performed early.[13]

In addition to neurologic findings, crepitus heard on auscultation of the heart (Hamman's sign), or signs of pneumothorax, hemoptysis, or subcutaneous air should suggest pulmonary barotrauma and thereby raise suspicion of AGE. Rarely, air bubbles seen in the retinal arteries or sharply circumscribed areas of glossal pallor (Liebermeister's sign) provide direct evidence of embolization.

An elevated serum creatinine kinase level (predominantly MM isoenzyme) is common in dive-related AGE. Levels above 900 U/L may be diagnostic in an appropriate clinical setting.[12] Other laboratory abnormalities include hemoconcentration with subsequent decline in the hematocrit and elevated serum transaminases and lactate dehydrogenase.[16,17] Chest radiographs may demonstrate pulmonary infiltrates (hemorrhage), pneumothorax, pneumomediastinum, or subcutaneous emphysema.[6] Gas embolization to a coronary artery or to cerebral autonomic centers may produce electrocardiographic (ECG) abnormalities such as dysrhythmias, ischemia, and infarction.

Some divers who suffer symptomatic AGE experience spontaneous recovery within minutes to hours of onset (the so-called lucid period). Without treatment, as many as 20% to 35% of these patients relapse.[11] Therefore, even in the absence of physical, radiographic, or ECG abnormalities, any diver with a history suggestive of AGE must be assumed to have suffered it and must be managed accordingly.

DIFFERENTIAL DIAGNOSIS

When AGE presents as altered mental status, it may be difficult to distinguish from trauma, near-drowning, or hypothermia. Victims of trauma or near-drowning often ascend or are taken to the surface rapidly and may develop AGE as a secondary complication. Thus, it is best to assume that anyone with a history of altered mental status immediately after a compressed-gas dive has suffered CAE.

Neurologic decompression sickness (DCS) usually becomes manifest later than CAE and classically presents as a spinal cord rather than a cerebral syndrome. However, the two may be difficult to distinguish, and up to half of all divers who present with AGE do so in the setting of a more generalized "dysbarism syndrome."[8] Clinically, the point is moot: CAE and neurologic DCS are managed identically.

Thrombotic or vasospastic arterial occlusion and paradoxical arterial embolization of venous air, amniotic fluid, fat, foreign bodies, or thrombi cause similar clinical findings but occur in different settings.

EMERGENCY DEPARTMENT EVALUATION

Even in the presence of other likely causes, a history of altered neurologic status within 10 minutes of ascent from a compressed-gas dive must be interpreted as presumptive CAE. A history of improper or rapid ascent or evidence of pulmonary barotrauma may be supportive, but their absence does not rule out the diagnosis.

Because patients may deny symptoms, the testimony of diving partners or witnesses is often useful. Complaints of headache or weakness should raise suspicion of AGE. A history of diminished consciousness, seizures, paralysis, paresis, dizziness, vertigo, nausea, ataxia, visual problems, or difficulty speaking is virtually diagnostic. In patients with chest discomfort, dyspnea, or hemoptysis, the presence or absence of neurologic symptoms must be specifically investigated.

Although all patients should receive a complete physical examination, special attention must be given to the neurologic evaluation. Mental status, cranial nerves, motor pathways, sensation, and cerebellar function are critically important. The patient is also evaluated for evidence of pulmonary barotrauma, hypothermia, and signs of head or spinal trauma.

All patients require a complete blood count, biochemical profile (including electrolytes, blood urea nitrogen, creatinine, glucose, creatine kinase, and liver function tests), chest radiograph, and ECG. If a patient demonstrates respiratory symptoms or altered mental status, arterial blood gas analysis is indicated. History or evidence of trauma may dictate additional radiographic studies.

EMERGENCY DEPARTMENT MANAGEMENT

Advanced life-support measures are instituted as necessary. All victims of AGE must be treated in a recompression chamber as soon as possible. Any diagnostic or therapeutic interventions that unnecessarily delay such therapy are unjustifiable. *In vitro* and animal studies suggest that a high inspired FiO_2 level increases tissue oxygen levels and also increases the nitrogen pressure gradient between air bubbles and blood, thereby speeding reabsorption.[1] Patients should, therefore, be given the highest available oxygen concentration. Beyond this, in the absence of acute cardiopulmonary decompensation, most patients require only supportive care (e.g., airway, cardiac monitoring, intravenous fluids, and rewarming) while awaiting transfer to a hyperbaric facility.

Dysrhythmias are treated according to advanced cardiac life-support protocols. Seizures that do not respond to oxygenation are treated with intravenous diazepam. An empiric trial of thiamine, dextrose, and naloxone is indicated if the patient demonstrates altered mental status.

In anticipation of recompression, all AGE patients with a simple pneumothorax should have a prophylactic chest tube placed to prevent progression to a tension pneumothorax. Endotracheal tube and Foley catheter cuffs should be filled with water or saline solution, not air.

All other interventions are controversial. Many authorities believe that AGE victims should be maintained in the Trendelenburg or Durant (left lateral decubitus) position to decrease risk of further embolization. Others believe that this maneuver is more likely to harm the patient by increasing intracranial pressure.

Anecdotal reports of efficacy have led to widespread use of high-dose corticosteroids in the management of CAE and DCS.[7,9] As yet, there have been no prospective, controlled trials to document their therapeutic value in diving accidents. Enthusiasm for such agents should be tempered by their failure to prove beneficial in the management of most types of cerebral insult (e.g., trauma, infarction, hemorrhage, and infection).

When AGE is managed appropriately, the prognosis is surprisingly good. Although overall mortality is as high as 5% to 15%, only 1% to 5% mortality should be anticipated among patients who reach medical attention.[5,8,9,15] Complete recovery is seen in 60% to 65% of survivors; persistent neurologic deficits of varying severity may be seen in the rest. Eventual neurologic outcome seems to correlate well with the magnitude of hemoconcentration serum creatinine kinase elevation.[15,16] Victims who present with loss of consciousness and those who require resuscitation represent a subset at high risk for a poor outcome.[4]

DISPOSITION

All patients suspected of suffering AGE must be referred for recompression. Transfer to the closest hyperbaric facility should be done as soon as possible. If transfer is by air, further decompression should be minimized. Aircraft capable of full pressurization (1 atm absolute) or of flight below 1,000 feet are best suited for such transfers. Consultations regarding the management of diving-accident victims or the location of recompression facilities are available 24 hours a day from the Diver's Alert Network, (919)684-8111.

COMMON PITFALLS

- Failure to consider the diagnosis of AGE in a patient with a history or clinical evidence of central nervous system injury

occurring within 10 minutes of ascent from a compressed-gas dive
- Failure to consider concomitant trauma, near-drowning, and hypothermia in the differential diagnosis of AGE
- Failure to recompress all AGE victims, regardless of their condition at the time of presentation. Those who experience spontaneous recovery may later relapse.
- Failure to treat AGE victims with 100% oxygen, supportive measures, and rapid transfer to the nearest hyperbaric facility
- Failure to appreciate that the Divers Alert Network is available day and night to assist in questions of management or transfer

ACKNOWLEDGMENT

Brant L. Viner contributed to previous versions of this chapter.

References

1. Annane D, Troché G, Delisle F, et al. Effects of mechanical ventilation with normobaric oxygen therapy on the rate of air removal from cerebral arteries. *Crit Care Med* 1994;22:851.
2. Arthur DC, Margulies RA. A short course in diving medicine. *Ann Emerg Med* 1987;16:689.
3. Colebatch HJH, Smith MM, Ng CKY. Increased elastic recoil as a determinant of pulmonary barotrauma in divers. *Respir Physiol* 1976;26:55.
4. Dick APK, Massey EW. Neurologic presentation of decompression sickness and air embolism in sport divers. *Neurology* 1985;35:667.
5. Gillen HW. Symptomatology of cerebral gas embolism. *Neurology* 1968;18:507.
6. Harker CP, Newman TS, Olson LK, et al. The roentgenographic findings associated with air embolism in sport scuba divers. *J Emerg Med* 1993;11:443.
7. Kizer KW. Corticosteroids in treatment of serious decompression sickness. *Ann Emerg Med* 1981;10:485.
8. Kizer KW. Dysbaric cerebral air embolism in Hawaii. *Ann Emerg Med* 1987;16:535.
9. Leitch DR, Green RD. Pulmonary barotrauma in divers and the treatment of cerebral AGE. *Aviat Space Environ Med* 1986;57:931.
10. Neuman TS, Hallenbeck JM. Barotraumatic cerebral air embolism and the mental status examination. *Ann Emerg Med* 1987;16:220.
11. Pearson RR, Goad RF. Delayed cerebral edema complicating cerebral AGE: case histories. *Undersea Biomed Res* 1982;9:283.
12. Reuter M, Tetzlaff K, Huttzelmann A, et al. MR imaging of the central nervous system in diving-related decompression illness. *Acta Radiol* 1997;38:940.
13. Ries S, Knath M, Kern R, et al. Arterial gas embolism after decompression: correlation to right-to-left shunting. *Neurology* 1999;52:401.
14. Schaeffer KE, McNulty WP Jr, Carey C, et al. Mechanisms in development of interstitial emphysema and air embolism on decompression from depth. *J Appl Physiol* 1958;13:15.
15. Smith RM, Neumann TS. Elevation of serum creatinine kinase in divers with AGE. *N Engl J Med* 1994;330:19.
16. Smith RM, VanHoesen KB, Neuman TS. Arterial gas embolism and hemoconcentration. *J Emerg Med* 1994;12:147.
17. Smith RM, Neuman TS. Abnormal serum biochemistries in association with arterial gas embolism. *J Emerg Med* 1997;15:285.
18. Warren LP Jr, Djang WT, Moon RE, et al. Neuroimaging of scuba diving injuries to the CNS. *AJR* 1988;151:1003.

CHAPTER 389
Barotrauma

Christopher J. Degnen

Injuries due to changes in ambient pressure result primarily from two basic mechanisms: changes in volume of free gas and changes in solubility of dissolved gas. Injuries resulting from changes in volume of free gas are classified as barotrauma. Expansion (or relative contraction) of gas within a closed anatomic space results in mechanical injury. Injuries resulting from changes in solubility of dissolved gases are classified as decompression sickness (DCS). Gas coming out of solution in body fluids causes pain (in joints, bones, soft tissues) or neurologic changes (in brain, spinal cord, blood vessels).

Often, these mechanisms and their presentations overlap. For example, expansion of free gas in the pulmonary cavity (pulmonary barotrauma) can force free gas into ruptured pulmonary vessels (air embolism), which may cause neurologic symptoms (mimicking DCS). Although the etiology and pathophysiology of neurologic injuries are diverse, the therapy for all such injuries is similar.

A third category of injury occurs when pressurized air or gas mixtures are inhaled, as with scuba (self-contained underwater breathing apparatus) diving or hyperbaric chambers. Under such conditions, the partial pressure of oxygen and nitrogen in plasma can reach toxic levels (see Chapter 390).

Scuba diving accidents occur in all regions of the United States. Although sport diving is most common along both coasts, lake diving and swimming pool training sessions are universal. Cerebral air embolism from a 12-ft pool dive has been reported.[15] Scuba divers sometimes travel by air soon after a dive, and aircraft cabin pressures less than the pressure at sea level may precipitate injury in those travelers.

The weight of the gases in the earth's atmosphere at sea level, 760 mm Hg of pressure, is arbitrarily defined as 1 atmosphere (1 atm). For every 33 ft of seawater that a diver descends, the ambient pressure increases by an additional 1 atm. Boyle's law (the volume of a gas is inversely proportional to the absolute pressure) describes how the volume of a free gas varies in response to ambient pressure. The rate of change of volume proportional to change of depth is most rapid near the surface.[1] Major volume changes are possible on a shallow dive; hence, significant barotrauma can be seen even in a swimming pool dive.[2,3]

Barotrauma during descent can cause injury even on a breath-holding dive, or free dive, in which no scuba or other breathing apparatus is used. This condition is commonly called a "squeeze" and generally causes only pain unless the diver continues deeper without correcting the problem. The areas of the body most commonly affected in this situation are the ears and facial sinuses. Because external pressure on the tympanic membrane (TM) increases with increasing depth and middle ear and sinus cavity pressures remain at about 1 atm, TM rupture can result. Cerebrospinal fluid and inner ear fluid pressures also increase. Small vessels may rupture into the middle ear or sinuses, and the round or oval windows may rupture into the middle ear if adequate equalization of pressures is not accomplished.

Divers who breathe pressurized air can correct these imbalances with a modified Valsalva maneuver, in which the glottis is open and the nares and lips are held closed. A safer technique is the Frenzel maneuver, in which the glottis is closed and nasopharynx pressure is increased by facial muscle manipulation.[11] Both of these techniques are also useful during airplane descent.

Barotrauma of ascent is seen only when divers inhale air (or other gaseous mixtures) under pressure. With such equipment, divers can fully inflate their lungs (including sinuses, middle ears, and so on) at depth; these compartments can then overexpand if they remain closed during ascent. Ruptures of the TM, round or oval windows, sinus bones, and alveoli or visceral pleura are all possible. This typically occurs during a panic ascent, in which the diver forgets to exhale.

Swallowing air at depth creates the potential for abdominal viscus rupture as well. Pockets of infection with gas-producing organisms have the potential for painful squeezes on descent or ascent. Periodontal abscess is the usual source of such pain.[13] Wearing a face mask creates a potential closed space on descent only and may result in facial petechiae.

Every person who wishes to participate in compressed-air diving should first have a thorough physical examination. Medical conditions such as asthma, sinusitis, or chronic otitis media might predispose the diver to air trapping.[5,10,16] Active allergic rhinitis or upper or lower respiratory infections are also contraindications to diving.

CLINICAL PRESENTATION

Pain is typically the first and most common symptom of barotrauma. Bleeding from the nares, ears, mouth, or lungs may accompany the pain. Hearing loss, tinnitus, and potentially disabling vertigo can occur with rupture of any of the ear membranes. A transient spinning sensation, called alternobaric vertigo, may result from a disequilibrium in middle ear pressures, even when all ear membranes are intact. Pneumothorax, pneumomediastinum, and perforated viscus may also occur.

Because barotrauma is a mechanical phenomenon, symptoms are likely to be maximal as soon as, or shortly after, a diver surfaces. Unusual exceptions occur when slow leaks of air trapped in the lungs or bowel produce a progressive tension pneumothorax or pneumoperitoneum.[4]

The physical examination is consistent with the injuries. Hearing loss may be either conductive (TM rupture) or sensorineural (oval or round window rupture or fistula). Subcutaneous emphysema may be palpated about the sinuses or chest. Radiography of the affected area (e.g., chest, abdomen, sinus, skull) is the most helpful diagnostic study.

DIFFERENTIAL DIAGNOSIS

Alternate diagnoses include almost any pathologic condition that can affect a given body compartment. For this reason, divers should never descend when they have an acute illness.[8] The history of acute onset of symptoms in a previously well individual exposed to atmospheric pressure changes suggests barotrauma. The inability to establish a nondysbaric diagnosis may commit the patient to an expensive, time-consuming, and potentially dangerous recompression.

EMERGENCY DEPARTMENT EVALUATION

In divers, the history should indicate a rapid descent or ascent. Although the dive profile (see Chapter 390) should be obtained, on any single dive, a patient is equally at risk for a *de novo* barotraumatic event. The patient should describe the following: any problems in clearing the ears or sinuses on descent, swallowing air at depth, failing to exhale on ascent, when the symptoms began, and whether the dive was a breath-holding or compressed-air dive.

In addition to receiving a complaint-oriented physical examination, any victim of a dysbaric event should receive thorough ear, nose, and throat (ENT); cardiopulmonary; abdominal; and neurologic evaluations. Severe pain from a benign sinus squeeze may cause a patient to overlook minor sensory changes with a more ominous prognosis (i.e., DCS).

Plain radiographs of the affected area provide a good initial screen. Even skull films may be useful in a patient with significant headache following ear or sinus squeeze; pneumocephalus has been detected in such patients.[7] A computed tomography scan may be indicated in patients with severe unexplained headache. If plain films reveal pneumothorax or pneumoperitoneum, further laboratory tests for arterial blood gases and preoperative blood work, for example, are indicated.

If the physical examination and plain films are normal, significant barotrauma can be ruled out.

EMERGENCY DEPARTMENT MANAGEMENT

Unlike air embolism or DCS, barotrauma can often be managed definitively in the emergency department. Advanced life-support measures should be instituted, as necessary. In cases of true barotrauma, the only probable life-threatening process is tension pneumothorax, in which case, needle decompression followed by tube thoracostomy is indicated. Because barotrauma is not a spontaneous injury and other complications may develop, patients with pneumothorax or pneumomediastinum should be admitted to the hospital. Similarly, patients with free intraperitoneal air require gastric decompression via nasogastric tube and surgical evaluation and treatment. Patients with pneumocephalus require assessment and management by a neurosurgeon. Patients with severe headaches require frequent neurologic checks, and patients with severe headaches of unexplained cause should be referred for hyperbaric chamber treatment when DCS is a possible cause.

Minor ENT problems, including small TM ruptures, are best treated with decongestants and prophylactic antibiotics. Severe vertigo or unexplained hearing loss require emergent ENT referral for round or oval window evaluation. Ruptures of these membranes are generally observed and require surgery only if symptoms do not resolve.[6,12]

DISPOSITION

Patients with pulmonary, gastrointestinal, and central nervous system barotrauma should be admitted to the hospital, and patients with associated air embolism or DCS should be transferred to a hyperbaric treatment center for management. Patients with ENT problems can be discharged with referral to an ENT surgeon.

The prognosis for purely barotraumatic injuries is very good. Previous ENT barotrauma is a relative contraindication to further diving. The diver generally has warning symptoms when descending and can take corrective action or resurface. Pulmonary barotrauma is an absolute contraindication, however, because recurrences tend to be more severe.[9,14]

A local hyperbarics expert or the Diver's Alert Network ([919]684-8111) may be consulted. The Diver's Alert Network is a resource for statistics and for locations and telephone numbers of hyperbaric treatment centers.

COMMON PITFALLS

- Failure to elicit a history of rapid ascent or descent and to diagnose barotrauma as the cause of a sudden illness in patients with recent diving or air travel

- Failure to appreciate that significant barotrauma can occur even in shallow depths and even on breath-holding dives
- Failure to rule out associated decompression sickness or air embolism in patients who have been scuba diving
- Failure to advise patients with significant barotrauma of the risks of further diving and to discourage them from such activity in the future

References

1. Arthur DC, Margulies RA. A short course in diving medicine. *Ann Emerg Med* 1987;16(6):689.
2. Bennett PB, Elliott DH. *The physiology and medicine of diving and compressed air work,* 3rd ed. Baltimore: Williams & Wilkins, 1982.
3. Calder IM. Dysbarism. A review. *Forensic Sci Int* 1986;30:237.
4. Cramer FS, Heimbach RD. Stomach rupture as a result of gastrointestinal barotrauma in a scuba diver. *J Trauma* 1982;22:238.
5. Dembert ML, Keith JF. Evaluating the pediatric scuba diver. *Am J Dis Child* 1986;140:1135.
6. Garges LM. Maxillary sinus barotrauma—case report and review. *Aviat Space Environ Med* 1985;56:796.
7. Goldman RW. Pneumocephalus as a consequence of barotrauma. *JAMA* 1986;255:3154.
8. Haake R, Schlictig R, Ulstad DR, et al. Barotrauma. Pathophysiology, risk factors and prevention. *Chest* 1987;91(4):608.
9. Leitch DR, Green RD. Recurrent pulmonary barotrauma. *Aviat Space Environ Med* 1986;57:1039.
10. Martin L. Letter to the editor. *N Engl J Med* 1992;326:1497.
11. Neblett LM. Otolaryngology and sport scuba diving. Update and guidelines. *Ann Otol Rhinol Laryngol Suppl* 1985;115:1.
12. Parell BJ, Becker GD. Conservative management of inner ear barotrauma resulting from scuba diving. *Otolaryngol Head Neck Surg* 1985;93:393.
13. Rauch JW. Barodontalgia—dental pain related to ambient pressure change. *Gen Dent* 1985;33:313.
14. Strauss RH. Diving medicine. *Am Rev Respir Dis* 1979;119:1001.
15. Strauss RH, Prockop LD. Decompression sickness among scuba divers. *JAMA* 1973;223:637.
16. Szasz MS, Cooper MA. Evaluating the sport scuba diver. *Am Fam Physician* 1982;25:131.

CHAPTER 390
Decompression Sickness

Christopher J. Degnen

Records suggest that divers have used air bells (which compress air by being open to seawater) since 330 B.C.[1,3] Diving helmets became practical in 1819, and compressed air technology for caissons and tunnels was developed in 1839. In the late 1800s, decompression sickness was first recognized and was termed *caisson disease,* the *bends* (for the doubled-over gait), or the *staggers* (presumably reflecting inner-ear involvement).

The development of the self-contained underwater breathing apparatus (scuba) allowed commercial divers increased freedom and gave birth to the sport of recreational diving. About 5 million divers are certified in the United States,[10] and easy air travel allows them quick access to remote dive sites. Emergency physicians practicing anywhere in the United States may encounter patients with complications of scuba diving.

There are two types of decompression sickness (DCS). Type I, called "pain only" or musculoskeletal DCS, primarily affects the joints, bones, and soft tissues. Type II, called central or neurologic DCS, affects the brain, the spinal cord, and the cardiopulmonary process. Diving complications also include barotrauma (see Chapter 389) and nitrogen toxicity (discussion follows).

The pathophysiology of DCS is not clearly established. Evidence suggests that bubble formation on a microscopic, even subcellular, level is the initial insult.[3] Bubbles form in tissue when the ambient pressure is decreased too rapidly to allow supersaturated gases to be released from plasma into the pulmonary alveoli.

The pressure of the atmosphere at sea level (760 mm Hg) is defined as one atmosphere (1 atm). The ambient pressure on a diver increases by 1 atm for each 33 ft of seawater (FSW) descended. The scuba regulator is designed to deliver compressed air at increased (ambient) pressure as the diver descends. Hence, the alveolar gas pressure in a scuba diver is the same as ambient pressure. High external pressures would otherwise prevent normal chest expansion.

Most sport divers breathe compressed air (21% oxygen, 78% nitrogen, 0.03% carbon dioxide). Because the amount of gas dissolved in a liquid is proportional to the pressure of that gas in contact with the liquid, increasing amounts of each component of air are dissolved in plasma with increasing depth. Excess oxygen can be metabolized, but excess nitrogen cannot and is released from solution on decompression. Because helium is less toxic than nitrogen, mixtures of oxygen and helium are generally used in commercial (deep) diving.

Increased partial pressures of nitrogen are intoxicating and cause confusion and euphoria ("rapture of the deep"). This short-lived effect resolves with resurfacing but may precipitate poor judgment and slow reflexes while the diver is at depth.

In a controlled ascent, supersaturated gases are slowly released from plasma at the alveoli. If the diver ascends too rapidly, the gas can "boil out" of the liquid phase anywhere in the body, both intravascularly and extravascularly. A similar phenomenon can occur if a person at sea level ascends too rapidly in an airplane or altitude chamber.

Dissolved nitrogen can accumulate in plasma and tissues over several dives. Divers are trained to keep exact records (dive profiles) that specify the maximum depth achieved, time spent at that depth, decompression stops made during ascent, and time spent on the surface before the next dive.

Tables can tell divers how long they may stay at different depths before decompression stops (rest periods on ascent to allow off-loading of nitrogen) are required. At depths of 0 to 33 FSW, a diver can spend unlimited time without the need for a decompression stop. Descending more than 33 FSW requires stops after variable periods of time; the deeper the dive, the shorter the maximum allowable time until a decompression stop is required.

Constructing these tables is not an exact science, however: They were empirically prepared on the experience of British and U.S. Navy divers. Consequently, rare divers suffer DCS even though they adhered to the tables. DCS has also been reported in a diver who stayed within the allowable 33 FSW.[12] Also, fatal barotrauma, a different mechanism of injury, is possible at much shallower depths (see Chapter 389).

CLINICAL PRESENTATION

Decompression sickness may manifest initially as profound but nonspecific fatigue. In type I DCS, pain is most common in the large joints. Pain may be deep, mild to severe, and radiate to surrounding areas. In some cases, tenderness, edema, and paresthesias may also occur. Type I DCS can also involve the skin (itching, erysipelas-like rash or mottling) and the lymph nodes (peau d'orange edema). Avascular necrosis of bone can be seen on radiographs after a single episode of DCS. These lesions are usually asymptomatic, but crippling osteonecrosis of the large joints can occur.

Type II DCS may present with a variety of neurologic manifestations, such as back pain (radiating around to the abdomen), confusion, deafness, dysphasia, headache, fecal incontinence, paresthesias, weakness, scotoma, vertigo, and urinary retention.[4] These symptoms reflect involvement of the brain or the spinal cord. Objective neurologic deficits (e.g., motor or sensory loss) may be evident. Patients with pulmonary involvement (the "chokes") may present with dyspnea, cyanosis, cough, frothy or bloody sputum, and central chest pain with a pleuritic component. Findings include tachypnea, tachycardia, and turbulent cardiac flow murmurs. Rarely, patients may present with cardiovascular collapse or may develop evidence of kidney or liver injury or disseminated intravascular coagulation.

Patients may present with combinations of types I and II DCS, and the extent and severity of signs and symptoms may progress over time. The onset is usually gradual and may even be delayed for many hours.[2,9]

DIFFERENTIAL DIAGNOSIS

Diagnosing DCS, especially type I, can be difficult. Diving is a strenuous sport, and strains and sprains are as common as with other sports. It would be impractical to recompress every scuba diver who complains of headache; however, not doing so demands that the physician be precise in evaluating the patient.

The patient's dive profile should be reviewed. Decompression occurs when the dive tables are violated. In contrast, barotrauma does not relate to these tables but occurs when a patient descended deeper or ascended despite the onset of painful symptoms, or made an uncontrolled ascent without exhaling. If symptoms occurred immediately or within minutes of surfacing, barotrauma and air embolism are the most likely causes. Decompression symptoms generally develop over minutes to hours after surfacing, occasionally longer.

If the patient complains of pain in an extremity only, and the examination reveals no other involvement, a blood pressure cuff should be applied to the affected area. If symptoms are relieved when the cuff is inflated, type I DCS probably exists.

Should the physician need assistance in evaluating or referring a patient, a national reference center, the Diver's Alert Network, is available at Duke University on an around-the-clock basis at (919)684-8111.[6]

EMERGENCY DEPARTMENT EVALUATION

The history emphasizes the dive profile and any predisposing illnesses. If the patient has been diving on previous days, profiles should be obtained for the past 1 or 2 weeks. The time of onset, nature, and progression of symptoms are documented.

Regardless of the nature of the complaint, the patient requires a full physical examination. The neurologic examination includes mental status, memory, cranial nerves, sensation to pain, light touch and position, motor strength of individual muscles, deep tendon reflexes, Babinski reflex, cerebellar function, pronator drift, and tandem gait, if possible. The skin is examined for rash and edema. Any adventitious heart or lung sounds are documented, as well as the status of bowel sounds. Involved joints are examined for active and passive range of motion, effusion, and warmth or erythema. If the patient presents with altered mental status, coexistent intoxication or trauma is possible.

Applying a blood pressure cuff may be useful in confirming type I DCS (see earlier discussion). Laboratory tests are of little value in DCS, other than ruling out other causes. However, obtunded patients or those with unstable vital signs require blood gas analysis; a complete blood count; measurement of electrolytes, glucose, blood urea nitrogen, and creatinine; prothrombin time; an electrocardiogram; and a chest radiograph, at a minimum. If recompression cannot be performed promptly, a computed tomography or magnetic resonance imaging scan may identify lesions.[8] However, because recovery is best with rapid recompression, these studies should not delay treatment.

EMERGENCY DEPARTMENT MANAGEMENT

Victims of a significant diving accident are quite ill and often require prehospital care. Such patients should have 100% oxygen by face mask and intravenous normal saline. Endotracheal intubation with cervical precautions may be required. Debate continues over the best position for transport. The Trendelenburg position may prevent potential cerebral air embolization in pulmonary barotrauma, but may worsen cerebral edema in DCS. The supine position or a few degrees of Trendelenburg are reasonable approaches. Administration of thiamine, $D_{50}W$, and naloxone is appropriate if the patient is obtunded. Seizures are treated with benzodiazepines.

The treatment of nitrogen toxicity is decompression to 1 atm (i.e., returning to the surface for divers) until symptoms resolve. Midazolam is preferred for the treatment of seizures, because recompression will probably be necessary to treat associated DCS, and long-acting agents may obscure the detection of oxygen toxicity secondary to recompression therapy, where 100% oxygen at increased pressure is provided for limited intervals to enhance the off-gassing of nitrogen.

Treatment of DCS is designed to reduce bubble size and to force free gas back into solution. This may be achieved by returning a diver to depth at the scene, but this approach is fraught with problems. Often, these patients are uncooperative and may vomit or have seizures. Recompression is best accomplished in a hyperbaric chamber (see Chapter 389), preferably one that allows a physician or nurse to be with the patient. Typically, the patient is recompressed to 3 to 6 atm, depending on the history and symptoms.[7] While at these pressures, the patient breathes 100% oxygen in brief intervals. Recovery is often rapid and dramatic.

Emergency department management should be aimed at correcting treatable problems while simultaneously arranging for recompression therapy. The vital signs and neurologic status are monitored. DCS can cause third-spacing of fluid, and hydration should be aggressive, with 200 to 500 mL/h normal saline if the neurologic and cardiopulmonary status permit. In anticipation of recompression, plastic intravenous bags should be used. The cuffs of any endotracheal tube or Foley catheter used should be filled with saline, not air.

Various anticlotting agents (e.g., aspirin, heparin, dipyridamole, and dextran polymers) have been tried without success and are not generally recommended. Intramuscular diclofenac has been used with success to relieve pain after recompression.[5] Steroid response is variable. Because the early use of these agents has not shown any decided benefit, drug therapy can be deferred to the hyperbaric center receiving the case.

DISPOSITION

If symptoms are very mild (e.g., headache) and the history and physical examination do not immediately suggest a decompression event, the patient is observed in the emergency department or discharged home with reliable family members or friends.

Delayed recompression therapy has been successful in treating minor symptoms that develop gradually if the initial examination is normal.[9,11] Patients with significant symptoms are referred for recompression therapy. If there is doubt as to the etiology of suspicious symptoms, consultation with a hyperbaric treatment specialist is indicated. Transport to a recompression chamber may be accomplished by ambulance, low-flying helicopter, or aircraft with a fully pressurized (1 atm) cabin.

COMMON PITFALLS

- Failure to appreciate that symptoms and signs of DCS may worsen with time
- Failure to use recompression early, when it is most effective
- Failure to consider recompression as a diagnostic trial when the etiology of symptoms is in doubt
- Failure to admit patients with mild symptoms for observation
- Failure to consult a hyperbaric treatment specialist or the Diver's Alert Network

References

1. Bachrach AJ. A short history of man in the sea. In: Bennett PB, Elliott DH, eds. *The physiology of medicine of diving and compressed air work*, 3rd ed. Baltimore: Williams & Wilkins, 1982.
2. Butler FK, Pinto CV. Progressive ulnar palsy as a late complication of decompression sickness. *Ann Emerg Med* 1986;15:738.
3. Calder IM. Dysbarism: a review. *Forensic Sci Int* 1986;30:237.
4. Dick AP, Massey EW. Neurologic presentation of decompression sickness and air embolism in sport divers. *Neurology* 1985;35:667.
5. Douglas JD. Intramuscular diclofenac sodium as adjuvant therapy for type I decompression sickness: a case report. *Undersea Biomed Res* 1986;13:457.
6. Dunford R. Diver's Alert Network [Letter]. *Ann Emerg Med* 1985;14:278.
7. Green RD, Leitch DR. 20 years of treating decompression sickness. *Aviat Space Environ Med* 1987;58:322.
8. Kizer KW. The role of computed tomography in the management of dysbaric diving accidents. *Radiology* 1981;140:705.
9. Kizer KW. Delayed treatment of dysbarism: a retrospective of 50 cases. *JAMA* 1982;247:2555.
10. Melamed Y, Shupak A, Bitterman H. Medical problems associated with underwater diving. *N Engl J Med* 1992;326:30.
11. Myers RA, Bray P. Delayed treatment of serious decompression sickness. *Ann Emerg Med* 1985;14:254.
12. Rugman F, Meecham J. Spinal decompression sickness at unusually shallow depth. *J Soc Occup Med* 1985;35:103.

CHAPTER 391
High-Altitude Illness

David M. Richardson

Increasing mobility and leisure time have allowed many more people to explore wilderness worlds previously experienced only by the privileged few.[15] Interest in hiking, camping, rock climbing, mountain biking, alpine and cross-country skiing, and other high-altitude sports has grown dramatically over the past few decades. In the United States alone, tens of millions of athletes and tourists now seek mountainous destinations in every season of the year.[14] High-speed transportation now permits travel from low to high altitudes within hours.

High-altitude medical illness, better known as *acute mountain sickness* (AMS), is a spectrum of disease ranging from subclinical effects to potentially lethal high-altitude pulmonary edema (HAPE) or high-altitude cerebral edema (HACE).[18] Because barometric pressure decreases with increasing altitude, yet the fraction of inspired oxygen in air remains constant at 21%, the PaO_2 is reduced. Even a young, healthy, physically fit nonsmoker may experience PaO_2 under 60 mm Hg at 2,500 m (8,100 ft) and under 50 mm Hg at 4,500 m (14,600 ft). Symptomatic AMS is uncommon under 2,500 m but occurs in up to 25% of the population at 2,500 m, and in 75% at 4,500 m.[8,9] Repeated attacks are common (about 20%), potentially limiting high-altitude activity and requiring prophylactic medications and a slow, controlled ascent.[10]

The incidence, severity, and duration of AMS are proportional to the rate and height of ascent and are modified by individual susceptibility, physical exertion, and sleeping altitude.[6,11] Symptoms vary widely but remain consistent on repeated episodes in the same person.[11] AMS demonstrates no sexual preference,[10] but HAPE is more common in males.[11] Spontaneous diuresis occurs in response to complicated fluid shifts.[6,10] Well-being at altitude is proportional to individual diuretic response.[13] In mild cases, symptoms abate in 3 to 7 days as acclimatization occurs.

Chronic mountain sickness, or Monge disease, may develop in some patients who do not acclimatize despite prolonged altitude exposure. It is characterized by persistent hypoxia, polycythemia (hematocrit greater than 60), and development of congestive heart failure.[9]

HAPE is a form of noncardiac pulmonary edema associated with pulmonary artery hypertension. A defect in nitric oxide synthesis may be contributory.[17] It develops in 0.5% to 15.0% of persons who ascend rapidly to high altitudes and has an overall mortality of 11%. HAPE recurs in susceptible persons, thus requiring cautious reexposure.[1]

HACE affects an estimated 1% of travelers to high altitude. Symptoms are due to increased intracranial pressure. While cerebral vessels dilate in response to hypoxia, the exact pathophysiology of this condition is not known.[7,9,10,18] Recent findings indicate that the predominant underlying mechanism is vasogenic (extracellular, due to leakage of fluid and protein through the blood–brain barrier) rather than cytotoxic (intracellular, due to cellular swelling).

Hypobaric hypoxia can exacerbate preexisting cardiac or pulmonary disease.[6] Relative contraindications to high-altitude travel include advanced age, chronic diseases, coronary artery disease, chronic obstructive pulmonary disease, pulmonary hypertension, sickle cell disease, and other diseases that compromise cardiopulmonary function.[6,9]

Measures to prevent or reduce AMS in a person who is about to undergo rapid ascent to high altitude (particularly those with previous episodes) include cautious acclimatization and medication. A staged, gradual ascent is most effective to achieve acclimatization. Either remaining at 2,000 to 3,000 m (6,600 to 9,800 ft) for 2 to 5 days before going higher, or ascending less than 300 m (1,000 ft) per day above 2,500 m (8,200 ft) can significantly reduce symptomatology.[11,16] Climbing high but sleeping low can also be effective in reducing the results of hypobaric hypoxia exacerbated by nighttime hypoventilation.[6,7,13] Drinking plenty of fluids, eliminating salt intake, and limiting physical activity may restrict symptom development.[6,10,11,13]

The carbonic anhydrase inhibitor acetazolamide causes a bicarbonate diuresis, resulting in a hyperchloremic metabolic acidosis and a compensatory respiratory alkalosis.[7,11] Pretreatment with 250 mg every 6 to 12 hours or with 500 mg of the sustained-release formula each day, beginning 1 or 2 days before ascent and continuing at least 48 hours after ascent, mimics the acclimated state of acid–base balance.[6,7,10,11,13,17] Some patients may not be helped, but symptoms are lessened in 30% to 50% of patients.[11] Side effects include paresthesias, gastrointestinal distress, somnolence, and dehydration if fluid intake is insufficient.[11,13]

Dexamethasone, which stabilizes membranes, reduces vasogenic cerebral edema and AMS symptoms to a greater extent than acetazolamide, with fewer side effects.[3,4,11] The dosage is 4 mg every 6 hours, starting 48 hours before ascent and continuing 48 hours after ascent.[6,11] Combining it with acetazolamide improves efficacy over either drug alone.[20]

CLINICAL PRESENTATION

Early symptoms of AMS are nonspecific and generally develop within 8 to 24 hours of arriving at altitude (range, 6 to 48 hours).[11] Headache, anorexia, nausea, vomiting, malaise, insomnia, lassitude, shortness of breath, and dyspnea on exertion make up the most common symptom complex.[6,10,11,19] The headache is usually throbbing, bilateral, and frontal. It is worst in the morning and when supine, increases with exercise, and may be minimally responsive to aspirin or acetaminophen.[11] Sleep is generally poor and often exacerbates symptoms as a result of hypoventilatory hypoxia, so the patient feels worse on waking.[6]

Physical examination may reveal a dyspneic, tachypneic, tachycardic patient with peripheral or periorbital edema, and rales. Tachypnea and tachycardia serve to maximize oxygenation and oxygen delivery to tissues. Despite having edema, the patient is often dehydrated and hypovolemic, with oliguria, increased hematocrit, and hypercoagulable state.[6] Petechiae may indicate disturbed vascular integrity, and papilledema may be present without raised intracranial pressure.[10] High-altitude retinal hemorrhage is detectable as flame hemorrhages in up to 40% of AMS patients.[6,10,11] It is usually asymptomatic and resolves without residua. Macular involvement (less than 5%) is manifest by central scotoma.[6,10] Laboratory studies may reveal mild leukocytosis and hemoconcentration.[6,9]

Manifestations of HAPE include worsening dyspnea, cough, hemoptysis, and cyanosis.[6] Complications such as adult respiratory distress syndrome or infection may develop. The chest radiograph reveals a normal-sized heart and diffuse bilateral patchy infiltrates, in contrast to the typical butterfly distribution of alveolar edema.[6,10] Arterial blood gas analysis may show hypoxia, hypocapnia, and alkalosis. Pulmonary function tests indicate decreased vital capacity and peak expiratory flow rates.[16] Pulmonary hypertension with normal left atrial pressure and normal pulmonary artery wedge pressure would be expected if pulmonary artery catheterization becomes necessary.[17] The electrocardiogram (ECG) most often shows only sinus tachycardia, but it may show evidence of right-sided heart strain.[6,10]

Manifestations of HACE include increasing headache, nausea, and vomiting, accompanied by CNS deficits such as confusion, poor judgment, and ataxia.[6–10,18] HACE can progress to coma and death if untreated and may leave neuropsychological residual even if promptly recognized and treated.[10] White matter edema may be seen on computed tomography (CT) or magnetic resonance imaging of the brain.

DIFFERENTIAL DIAGNOSIS

The multiple nonspecific symptoms of early AMS may mimic viral upper respiratory infection or gastroenteritis. Poor central nervous system (CNS) function upon environmental exposure adds hypothermia, hypovolemia, and exhaustion to the differential diagnosis.[6] Worsening pulmonary symptoms may also be due to acute exacerbations of chronic respiratory diseases such as asthma or chronic obstructive pulmonary disease.[10] Other etiologies of noncardiogenic pulmonary edema should be considered (e.g., medications, neurologic disorders). Low-grade fever and leukocytosis expand the differential to more serious infections, including pneumonia and meningitis.[10] The differential of CNS dysfunction also includes metabolic, psychiatric, toxic, and traumatic disorders.[9]

EMERGENCY DEPARTMENT EVALUATION

A history of recent, rapid transit to high altitude should alert the physician to the potential diagnosis of AMS. A previous history of similar episodes at altitude should immediately raise suspicion. The rapidity of ascent, altitude, activities and length of stay at altitude, the time of onset, nature and duration of symptoms, and preexisting medical conditions should be noted.

The physical examination should focus on vital signs and evaluation of CNS, cardiac, and respiratory function. A funduscopic examination should also be performed. All patients should have an oxygen saturation measured. Laboratory evaluation of patients with constitutional symptoms of AMS should include a complete blood count, electrolytes, blood urea nitrogen, creatinine, and glucose. Those with tachypnea, hypoxia, altered mental status, or abnormal findings on cardiopulmonary examination should have arterial blood gas analysis, cardiac monitoring, an ECG, and a chest radiograph. A CT scan of the head should be performed in those with persistently abnormal mental status or severe headache.

EMERGENCY DEPARTMENT MANAGEMENT

Acetazolamide and dexamethasone are effective for treating mild-to-moderate AMS as well as preventing it.[5] Acetazolamide relieves symptoms, improves arterial oxygenation, and prevents further impairment of pulmonary gas exchange.[7] Multiple acetazolamide regimens are effective.[2] Administration of 250 mg orally every 8 hours until symptoms of AMS resolve is recommended.[7]

Dexamethasone is given in the same dose as that for prevention. Patients with dehydration should be given oral fluids. Those with severe symptoms require descent to a lower altitude. Patients with vomiting should be given antiemetics and hydrated with intravenous saline. Acetaminophen or a nonsteroidal antiinflammatory agent can be given for headache.

Lightweight, portable hyperbaric chambers (Gamow, Certec, PAC [or portable altitude chamber]) have become part of the field regimen to treat AMS. These pressurized, cylindrical, zipper body bags simulate descent to a lower altitude, the most effective treatment for altitude sickness. The patient is placed in the bag and air is pumped in. Bag pressure is maintained at a pressure of 100 mm Hg by means of a pop-off valve vent (usually 2 psi). The patient may also be placed on oxygen while in the chamber. Hyperbaric therapy with the Gamow bag is as effective as oxygen therapy for the immediate treatment of AMS.[12]

HAPE should be treated initially with oxygen and evacuation to a lower altitude.[1,11] Sublingual and oral nifedipine (10 mg every 4 hours until improved, then 30 mg of long-acting preparation every 12 to 24 hours) given to patients with clinical and radiologic evidence of HAPE has been shown to decrease pulmonary artery pressure, improve oxygenation, and decrease subjective symptoms of AMS.[1,11]

Nifedipine treatment offers a potential emergency measure for patients when descent or evacuation is impossible.[11]

Nifedipine should not be used prophylactically in HAPE-susceptible subjects, however, because of potential harmful side effects, such as hypotension and consequent myocardial and cerebral ischemia and infarction.[11]

Depending on severity, continuous positive airway pressure (CPAP or BiPAP) by mask or endotracheal intubation and mechanical ventilation with positive end-expiratory pressure may be necessary for patients with respiratory failure.[8,14] Inhaled nitric oxide can also improve arterial oxygenation.[16] Diuretics are not helpful and may be harmful in patients with underlying dehydration. If recognized early and treated aggressively, nearly all young, physically fit, otherwise healthy patients with all forms of AMS will improve quickly, often with full resolution of symptoms within 24 hours.

DISPOSITION

Young, healthy patients with mild-to-moderate AMS may be discharged with instructions not to resume ascent until after symptoms have subsided and only if preventative measures are taken. Medications should never be used to allow further ascent in light of persistent symptoms. Patients with HAPE, HACE, severe AMS, or moderate AMS and underlying cardiopulmonary or cerebrovascular disease, complications (e.g., ECG changes), or other significant medical problems should be admitted. Most such patients will require observation and treatment in an intensive care unit.

COMMON PITFALLS

- Failure to ask about altitude in patients who become ill when traveling
- Minimizing the signs and symptoms of AMS and attempting to remain at high altitude
- Treating AMS with medications to allow for further ascent or continued exposure
- Failure to descend immediately if HACE or HAPE is suspected
- Failure to use adjunctive medications and hyperbaric therapy (if available) when descent is not immediately possible
- Failure to treat severe HAPE with positive airway pressure by mask or positive end-expiratory pressure with endotracheal intubation and mechanical ventilation
- Giving medications used for the treatment of congestive heart failure or cardiogenic pulmonary edema to patients with HAPE

References

1. Bartsch P, Maggiorini M, Ritter M, et al. Prevention of high-altitude pulmonary edema by nifedipine. *N Engl J Med* 1991;325:1284.
2. Dickinson JG. Acetazolamide in acute mountain sickness. *BMJ* 1987;295:1161.
3. Ellsworth AE, Larson EB, Strickland D. A randomized trial of dexamethasone and acetazolamide for acute mountain sickness prophylaxis. *Am J Med* 1987;83:1024.
4. Ellsworth AE, Meyer AF, Larson EB. Dexamethasone in the prevention of acute mountain sickness during rapid, active ascent of Mount Rainier. *Clin Res* 1988;36:172a.
5. Ferrazzini G, Maggiorini M, Kriemler S, et al. Successful treatment of acute mountain sickness with dexamethasone. *BMJ* 1987;294:1380.
6. Foulke GE. Altitude-related illness. *Am J Emerg Med* 1985;3:217.
7. Grissom CK, Roach RC, Sarnquist FH, et al. Acetazolamide in the treatment of acute mountain sickness: clinical efficacy and effect on gas exchange. *Ann Intern Med* 1992;116:461.
8. Honigman B, Theis MK, Koziol-McLain J, et al. Acute mountain sickness in a general tourist population at moderate altitudes. *Ann Intern Med* 1993;118:587.
9. Houston CS. Altitude illness. *Postgrad Med* 1983;74(1):231.
10. Houston CS. Altitude illness. *Emerg Med Clin North Am* 1984;2:503.
11. Johnson TS, Rock PB. Current concepts, acute mountain sickness. *N Engl J Med* 1982;73:395.
12. Kasic J, Yaron M, Nicholas R, et al. Treatment of acute mountain sickness: hyperbaric versus oxygen therapy. *Ann Emerg Med* 1991;20:1109.
13. Milledge JS. Acute mountain sickness. *Thorax* 1983;38:641.
14. Oelz O, Maggiorini M, Ritter M, et al. Prevention and treatment of high-altitude pulmonary edema by a calcium-channel blocker. *Int J Sports Med* 1992;13:S65.
15. Rennie D. The great breathless mountains. *JAMA* 1986;256:81.
16. Scherrer U, Vollenweider L, Delabays A, et al. Inhaled nitric acid for high altitude pulmonary edema. *N Engl J Med* 1996;334:624.
17. Schoene RB. High-altitude pulmonary edema: pathophysiology and clinical review. *Ann Emerg Med* 1987;16:987.
18. Shlim DR. Treatment of acute mountain sickness. *N Engl J Med* 1985;313:891.
19. Tso E. High-altitude illness. *Emerg Med Clin North Am* 1992;10:231.
20. Zell SC, Goodman PH. Acetazolamide and dexamethasone in the prevention of acute mountain sickness. *West J Med* 1988;148:541.

CHAPTER 392
Venous Air Embolism

Christopher H. Linden

Venous air embolism may occur whenever the integrity of a vein is violated and its lumen is exposed to air or any other gas. The presence of a pressure gradient (i.e., ambient air pressure greater than venous blood pressure) is also required. Air may be forced into an open vein by positive external pressure, or it may be drawn into the venous system by negative intravascular pressure. Inspiration, which augments venous return and increases the pressure differential, facilitates aspiration of air into exposed central veins. However, air can passively enter any open vein above the level of the heart.

Venous air emboli of small volume (a few milliliters) are common during intravenous infusion but are clinically insignificant. Hence, they are frequently unrecognized or ignored and are rarely reported. In contrast, large air emboli are rare but quickly fatal, and they generally remain undiagnosed until autopsy.[14,16] Estimates of the fatal volume range from 100 to 500 mL, depending on the speed of infusion and underlying disease. Slow infusions are tolerated better than rapid ones. Emboli of intermediate size result in significant respiratory, cardiovascular, and neurologic dysfunction. Because signs and symptoms are nonspecific, knowledge of the clinical settings in which venous air embolism may occur will aid in the proper diagnosis.

Physiologically significant venous air emboli are most commonly reported after surgical procedures such as craniotomy (particularly posterior fossa surgery), sinus and neck surgery, central venous or pulmonary artery catheterization, cervical laminectomy, hemodialysis, lung and open-heart surgery, hip arthroplasty, thoracentesis, thyroidectomy, and tracheostomy.[4,5,14,16] The sitting (Fowler's) position and the noncollapsibility of intracranial veins account for the relatively high incidence during craniotomy. Preventing air emboli during central venous cannulation requires proper technique: using the Trendelenburg position and Valsalva maneuver, covering the catheter hub with a finger during placement, and securing the catheter and its connections with sutures or tape.[4]

Blunt or penetrating chest trauma with concomitant airway and venous disruption may result in either insidious or acute air embolism.[9] The same is true for blunt and penetrating head trauma and penetrating neck trauma.[1] With head trauma, air can enter the venous circulation via open skull fractures, basilar fractures crossing the cavernous sinus, and those involving dural venous (petrosal, sigmoid, sphenoparietal, transverse) sinuses and paranasal air (usually ethmoid) sinuses.

Serious emboli may also occur as a complication of any diagnostic or therapeutic procedure that uses air or another gas under pressure. Examples include arthrography, nasal sinus irrigation, positive-pressure ventilation, laparoscopy, presacral or retroperitoneal pneumography, pneumoencephalography, Rubin's test (vaginal insufflation), pressurized intravenous infusions, pneumourethrocystography, gas-cooled laser surgery of the uterus, and vacuum abortion with accidental reversal (i.e., pressurization) of the suction catheter.[3,5,14,16,17] Significant amounts of air may sometimes enter a vein during gravity infusion as a result of tubing defects, an obstructed filter, or the presence of air in a collapsible infusion bag.[5] Air may be rapidly aspirated into cervical or thoracic veins via central venous catheters that become disconnected, particularly when the patient assumes an upright position or inspires.[4] Improper ventilation of a phlebotomy collection bottle has also caused air to be forced into a vein.[5] Pressure-induced air embolism may occur in nonmedical settings, such as attempted criminal abortion, vaginal douching, insufflation of the vagina during cunnilingus (in pregnant women), recreational inhalation of helium or nitrous oxide from pressurized tanks, and the self-injection of air into the scrotum, urethra, or a peripheral vein (usually suicidal).[6,8,14,16,17]

The primary physiologic mechanism underlying clinical findings appears to be gas-bubble obstruction of the pulmonary outflow tract of the right ventricle, resulting in pulmonary vasoconstriction, pulmonary hypertension, hypoxemia, systemic hypotension, and arterial ischemia.[7,16,17] As usual, the heart and brain are the most susceptible organs. The whipping or churning of blood and air by ventricular contractions also results in platelet and red cell aggregation and fibrin and fat globule formation, with deposition in, and obstruction of, pulmonary arterioles.[11] Secondary effects include decreased lung compliance, increased airway resistance, ventilation–perfusion mismatching, and pulmonary edema leading to additional hypoxia and hemodynamic compromise.[16,17] In patients with atrial or ventricular septal defects, paradoxical embolization of venous air to the left side of the heart may sometimes result in subsequent gas-bubble occlusion of the arterial circulation, with symptoms identical to those of direct arterial gas embolism (see Chapter 388).[6,20] Paradoxical embolization may also occur through arteriovenous anastomoses in the lung.[16]

CLINICAL PRESENTATION

The severity of symptoms depends on the size of the embolus and its rate of formation. Patients with large venous air emboli that develop over a short period of time often experience sudden dyspnea or gasping, chest pain, loss of consciousness, and cardiovascular collapse. In severe cases, there may be an immediate cardiac arrest. Cyanosis, wheezing, rales, hypotension, coma, tachycardia, hemoptysis, and tachypnea are typical physical findings. Auscultation of the heart may reveal a characteristic loud churning sound or "millwheel" murmur. This coarse, continuous (systolic and diastolic), metallic or machine-like murmur is transient and heard only with large right ventricular emboli. It may be preceded or followed by tympanic, resonant, or drumlike valvular sounds, gallop rhythms, and a softer systolic murmur. Jugular venous distention may be present.

Patients with smaller emboli may complain of faintness, dizziness, shortness of breath, weakness, palpitations, and chest pain. Lesser degrees of hypotension, tachycardia, tachypnea, and central nervous system dysfunction (e.g., anxiety, confusion) may be noted on physical examination. Abnormal cardiopulmonary findings may be present. In paradoxical embolization, the patient may present with an acute stroke, myocardial infarction, or manifestations of limb or intraabdominal organ arterial insufficiency.

Hypoxia, metabolic acidosis, and an increased or decreased P_{CO_2} may be noted on arterial blood gas analysis. Thrombocytopenia is sometimes present. If continuously monitored, the end-expiratory CO_2 concentration (a reflection of the alveolar P_{CO_2}) will show an abrupt decrease. The electrocardiogram (ECG) may reveal evidence of ischemia (e.g., right ventricular ST-T wave changes), dysrhythmias, or acute cor pulmonale (e.g., right axis deviation, P pulmonale, and right bundle-branch block). Right ventricular Doppler ultrasound (usually heard best over the right third to fifth intercostal spaces) may reveal an abrupt change in heart sounds when air enters the heart. The chest radiograph may show pulmonary edema without cardiomegaly.[10,12] Rarely, intracardiac or pulmonary arterial air may be radiographically visualized; this confirms the diagnosis.[12] The central venous pressure may be normal or elevated. Aspiration of air from a central venous, right atrial, right ventricular, or pulmonary artery catheter also confirms the diagnosis.[13,19]

DIFFERENTIAL DIAGNOSIS

Venous air embolism is most often confused with pulmonary thromboembolism and acute myocardial infarction. Without prior monitoring, the clinical setting and characteristic murmur are the primary clues to the correct etiology. In pregnant patients, amniotic fluid embolism should also be considered in the differential diagnosis.[8] Signs and symptoms are similar, but amniotic fluid embolism occurs almost exclusively at or about the time of delivery and is usually associated with a coagulopathy.[18]

In patients with multiple trauma, conditions such as hemothorax, pneumothorax, hypovolemia, cardiac tamponade, tracheobronchial disruption, and aortic transection are more common causes of cardiovascular collapse. Fat embolism should also be considered. Hemoptysis and unexpected deterioration or arrest, especially if occurring immediately after intubation and positive-pressure ventilation in a patient with lung trauma, are clinical clues to the presence of venous air embolism. With paradoxical embolization, manifestations are usually those of arterial insufficiency, but signs and symptoms of venous air embolism may also be present.

EMERGENCY DEPARTMENT EVALUATION

Venous air embolism should be suspected in any patient who develops acute respiratory, neurologic, or cardiovascular decompensation following a diagnostic, therapeutic, or traumatic event involving air insufflation or potential venous disruption and a communication with an external or internal gaseous atmosphere. Details of the precipitant circumstances are documented, and the site of air entry is identified, if possible.

The physical examination focuses on the vital signs and the cardiovascular, neurologic, and respiratory status. Careful auscultation for abnormal heart sounds is essential.

The ancillary evaluation should include arterial blood gas measurements, cardiac monitoring, a 12-lead ECG, and a chest radiograph. In unstable patients with suspected venous air embolism, insertion of a central venous or, preferably, a right-sided heart (Swan-Ganz) catheter and aspiration of air may be diagnostic as well as therapeutic. Although not reported, findings on echocardiogram are also likely to be diagnostic. Measurement of the end-expiratory CO_2 concentration and evaluation of heart sounds by Doppler flowmeter are useful only if baseline parameters are known.

EMERGENCY DEPARTMENT MANAGEMENT

Advanced life-support measures are instituted as necessary. Initial treatment should include prevention of further air embolization by manually sealing, if possible, the venous portal of entry and discontinuing any insufflation procedures. The patient is placed in a head-down (Trendelenburg) or head-down, left lateral (Durant) position so that the air present in the heart can be displaced from the pulmonary outflow tracts and rise toward the apex.[2,4,14,16,17] Closed-chest cardiac massage may also be effective in forcing air out of pulmonary arteries and into smaller vessels. If vital signs remain or become stable, supportive care is all that is necessary. Small amounts of air will eventually dissolve in the blood.

All patients are given 100% oxygen to hasten the absorption of embolized air. Because air is 80% nitrogen, decreasing the partial pressure of nitrogen in the blood by giving oxygen will result in the diffusion of nitrogen from the embolus into the blood, thus decreasing the size of the air bubble.[5,17]

In patients with profound shock or cardiac arrest, direct transthoracic aspiration of air from the heart may be lifesaving, especially in the case of a massive air embolism.[5,14,16,17] To accomplish a right ventricular puncture, an 18-gauge, 3.5-in. or larger needle is inserted, with or without a catheter, into the fourth or fifth intercostal space at the left sternal border. It is directed perpendicularly to the chest wall. Alternatively, the needle can be inserted just to the left of the xiphoid process and directed toward the inferior tip of the left scapula. Because transthoracic aspiration may result in coronary artery or myocardial laceration and pericardial tamponade, the preferred treatment for patients with less severe hemodynamic compromise is to insert a central venous or Swan-Ganz catheter, with the tip placed at the junction of the superior vena cava and right atrium,[2,13,19] and to aspirate the embolus. Pulmonary edema is treated with oxygen, intubation, and mechanical ventilation, as necessary.

The management of air embolism in patients with blunt or penetrating chest trauma and profound shock or cardiac arrest requires immediate thoracotomy for diagnosis, resuscitation, and treatment. Although not generally indicated for victims of cardiac arrest due to blunt trauma, thoracotomy may be lifesaving when air embolism is the underlying pathologic event. Definitive treatment usually requires hilar cross-clamping for initial control of bronchovenous communications. Selective intubation of the right or left mainstem bronchus and ventilation of the uninvolved lung can reduce the flow of air into the venous circulation, facilitate resuscitation, and obviate the need for thoracotomy in some cases.[9] Nitrous oxide should not be used: It may diffuse into the air embolus and increase its size.[15,17]

The management of patients with paradoxical air embolization (i.e., arterial gas embolism) is described in Chapter 388. Hyperbaric oxygen therapy should be considered for patients with persistent neurologic manifestations.[19]

DISPOSITION

Symptomatic patients with documented or suspected venous air embolism are admitted. The level of care is based on the degree of hemodynamic and respiratory dysfunction. Depending on the circumstances, consultation with a cardiothoracic or trauma surgeon or a hyperbaric medicine specialist may be indicated. In patients who survive the acute event, the long-term outcome depends on the degree of anoxic injury and associated illnesses or trauma.

ACKNOWLEDGMENT

Francis P. Renzi contributed to previous versions of this chapter.

COMMON PITFALLS

- Failure to consider venous air embolism as a cause of acute hemodynamic decompensation
- Failure to recognize venous air embolism as a complication of head, neck, and chest trauma and of many diagnostic and therapeutic procedures
- Failure to recognize and follow measures designed to avoid iatrogenic air embolism
- Failure to place the patient in a head-down, left lateral position, and failing to give 100% oxygen
- Failure to consider concomitant arterial embolization (paradoxical embolization)

References

1. Adams VI, Hirsch CS. Venous air embolism from head and neck wounds. *Arch Pathol Lab Med* 1989;113:498.
2. Alvaran SB, Toung JK, Graff TE, et al. Venous air embolism: comparative merits of external massage, intracardiac aspiration and left lateral decubitus position. *Anesth Analg* 1978;57:166.
3. Banagale RC. Massive intracranial air embolism: a complication of mechanical ventilation. *Am J Dis Child* 1980;134:799.
4. Feliciano DV, Mattox KL, Graham JM, et al. Major complications of percutaneous subclavian vein catheters. *Am J Surg* 1974;138:869.
5. Gottlieb JD, Ericsson JA, Sweet RS. Venous air embolism: a review. *Anesth Analg* 1965;44:773.
6. Gronert GA, Messick JM, Cucchiara RF, et al. Paradoxical air embolism from a patent foramen ovale. *Anesthesiology* 1979;50:548.
7. Hartveit F, Lystad H, Minken A. The pathology of venous air embolism. *Br J Exp Pathol* 1968;49:81.
8. Hill BF, Jones JS. Venous air embolism following orogenital sex during pregnancy. *Am J Emerg Med* 1993;11:155.
9. Ho AM-H, Ling E. Systemic air embolism after lung trauma. *Anesthesiology* 1999;90:564.
10. Ishak BA, Seleny FL, Noah ZL. Venous air embolism: a possible cause of acute pulmonary edema. *Anesthesiology* 1976;45:453.
11. Khan MA, Alkalay I, Suetsugu S, et al. Acute changes in lung mechanics following pulmonary emboli of various gases in dogs. *J Appl Physiol* 1972;33:774.
12. Kizer KW, Goodman PC. Radiographic manifestations of venous air embolism. *Radiology* 1982;144:35.
13. Marshall WK, Bedford RF. Use of a pulmonary artery catheter for detection and treatment of venous air embolism. *Anesthesiology* 1980;52:131.
14. Michenfelder JD. Air embolism. In: Orkin FK, Cooperman LH, eds. *Complications in anesthesiology*. Philadelphia: JB Lippincott Co, 1982:268.
15. Munson ES. Effect of nitrous oxide on the pulmonary circulation during venous air embolism. *Anesth Analg* 1971;50:785.
16. O'Quin RJ, Lakshminarayan S. Venous air embolism. *Arch Intern Med* 1982;142:2173.
17. Orebaugh SL. Venous air embolism: clinical and experimental considerations. *Crit Care Med* 1992;20:1169.
18. Price TM, Baker VV, Cefalo RC. Amniotic fluid embolism: three case reports with a review of the literature. *Obstet Gynecol Surv* 1985;40:462.
19. Sink JD, Corner PB, James PM, et al. Evaluation of catheter placement in the treatment of venous air embolism. *Ann Surg* 1976;183:58.
20. Wilmhurst PT, Ellis BG, Jenkins BS. Paradoxical gas embolism in a scuba diver with an atrial septal defect. *BMJ* 1986;293:1277.

PART IV

Other Environmental Injuries

CHAPTER 393
Electrical Injuries

Peter L. Sosnow

There are approximately 1,000 deaths from electrocution each year in the United States. High-voltage electrical injuries occur in electrical, construction, and industrial workers, accounting for more than two-thirds of all electrocutions and serious electrical injuries. Accidental electrocution remains the second leading cause of death for these workers.[15] Nonfatal, high-voltage electrical injuries that require hospitalization account for 5% of all burn unit admissions.[9]

About 30% of all electrical injuries occur in children and adolescents. Inquisitive toddlers are exposed to household current in wall sockets, electrical cords, or extension cord outlets. A child who puts the receptacle block from an ordinary extension cord into his or her mouth may create an electrical arc through saliva with a temperature approaching 3,000°C, causing a burn with enormously disfiguring potential.[20] This devastating injury is still not well known or appreciated by most parents.

Another group at risk is adolescent boys, who are prone to risk-taking behavior. Climbing utility poles, trespassing through transformer substations, or playing near electrical railway lines are common scenarios in which they are exposed to high-tension electrical power.[17]

Common electrical safety practices and appliance design have greatly reduced the risks of electrical injury in the home. Less than 1% of accidental deaths in the home are caused by electrical injury. However, dangerous practices, such as failing to ground electrical appliances properly and using electrical appliances near water, are still seen.

The severity of electrical injury is determined by the voltage, current pathway, and duration of exposure. The type of current—direct (DC), alternating (AC), or radio frequency (RF)—also determines mechanism and severity of injury.[6]

Voltage is a measure of electromotive force and is usually the only variable known when obtaining the medical history. Voltages above 1,000 V are considered high tension. Ohm's law defines *current* as voltage divided by the resistance in the path of current flow. Resistance, which is usually unknown, is the most important determinant of current and magnitude of injury.

Resistance to current flow varies for different tissues and can be ranked in order of increasing resistance as nerve, blood, muscle, viscera, skin, tendon, fat, and bone. Nerve, blood, and muscle are rich in electrolytes and have the lowest tissue resistance. Current flows easily and in higher volume through these tissues, producing the greatest damage.

The skin is the most important resistor to current flow. Typical skin resistance is about 40,000 ohms, but dry, thick, heavily calloused skin will present resistance as high as 1 million ohms. Moisture, sweat, and surface contaminants can decrease skin resistance to as low as 300 ohms. Skin resistance while immersed in water (e.g., a bathtub) is as little as 150 ohms.[3]

When exposed to high voltage, skin breaks down (chars and burns), which physically removes the external barrier and allows the current to have direct access to internal tissue. Likewise, the exit point of a current path undergoes skin breakdown, usually described as an "explosive" wound.

The surface area of contact, the duration of contact, and the pathway of current flow are critical in assessing the potential and magnitude for hidden internal injury. Sudden death from ventricular fibrillation is three times more likely when current flows from arm to arm than from arm to leg.

The destructive heat generated by electrical energy is inversely related to the cross-sectional area of the current path: The smaller the cross-sectional area, the greater the current density. This explains why tissue injury is much greater in fingers compared with arms, or in arms compared with the trunk, even though the same current may have traversed them for the same length of time.

AC is much more dangerous than DC. Tetanic muscle contractions are induced by the repeated stimulation of muscle fibers. Although all muscles will be affected, flexors tend to be stronger and predominate. This causes the "freezing" or "lock-on" phenomenon, which can prolong exposure and the severity of injury. AC is also much more likely to induce ventricular fibrillation and at lower energy levels than DC.[4] The frequency of repetitive stimuli (60 cycles per second) greatly increases the likelihood of hitting the vulnerable ventricular recovery period, analogous to the well-known R-on-T phenomenon.

"Stun guns" are specialized electrical devices used by law-enforcement officials. The weapons shoot two to four electrode darts at a victim as far as 15 ft away. The darts are connected to the device by wires that deliver high-voltage (50,000 V), low-current (3 mA) pulse trains (about ten per second). These impulses induce tetanic muscular contractions and involuntary paralysis, effectively immobilizing the victim. Similar hand-held devices that utilize electrode prongs pressed directly against the skin and deliver lower voltage are also available. The overall morbidity and mortality from these devices is extremely low, especially when compared with the conventional ballistic handgun.[8,12]

CLINICAL PRESENTATION

Victims of electrical injury may present with sudden death, cardiac dysrhythmias, external and internal tissue injuries, neurologic dysfunction, associated mechanical trauma, and various secondary complications.[7,19] Sudden death is usually the result of ventricular fibrillation, asystole, or other fatal cardiac dysrhythmias. Sudden death may also result from direct insult to the brainstem, causing respiratory arrest.

Cardiac dysrhythmias and conduction disturbances are seen in as many as 25% of victims with electrical injury, especially patients who have had a transthoracic current pathway. These abnormalities include ventricular fibrillation, asystole, ventricular tachycardia, sinus tachycardia, atrial fibrillation, atrioventricular block, bundle-branch block, and various atrial and ventricular ectopic beats.[1,4] Although nonspecific ST-T changes are common, true myocardial infarction is uncommon.[2,4,5,13] This diagnosis is often confused by the fact that electrically injured skeletal muscle will produce significant elevation of CK-MB that is not of cardiac origin.[14]

The unpredictable course of electrical current through the body makes accurate, initial clinical assessment of internal injury extremely difficult. External signs are usually limited and deceptively minor. Entrance wounds are commonly found on the hands or upper extremities and demonstrate charring, depression, edema, and inflammatory changes. Exit wounds may be multiple and varied and may have an explosive appearance. They are commonly found at the point where the body is closest to the electrical ground (i.e., the feet) or where the loop of current flow is completed. In bathtub exposures, there may be no external burns or signs of electric current entry or exit.

Neurologic injuries are seen in some form in virtually all victims of electrical injury. Acute central nervous system manifestations include amnesia, altered mental status, irritability, depression, emotional lability, motor deficits, seizures, respiratory center depression, and coma.[16,18] These acute changes are often transient, and excellent recovery may be seen. Peripheral nerve injuries are common and usually result from direct electrothermal injury along the path of current. Vascular injury and compartment syndrome may also contribute to peripheral nerve deficits.

Vascular and muscle damage can be extensive and severe. Coagulation necrosis and vascular thrombosis are responsible for the immediate and delayed devastation to these tissues. The net effect is an injury pattern more closely resembling a severe crush injury than a burn. Delayed rupture of injured blood vessels may be responsible for significant and catastrophic hemorrhage. Rhabdomyolysis and acute renal failure are potential complications. The mechanisms of renal insult include decreased renal perfusion from hypovolemia, along with the deposition of myoglobin and hemoglobin pigments released from massive muscle breakdown and hemolysis.[10]

A wide variety of skeletal fractures and dislocations may be seen from the effects of tetanic muscular contractions or from the fall often associated with an electrical injury. Long-bone fractures, shoulder dislocations, and spinal compression fractures are common.

Gastrointestinal (GI) manifestations include nausea, vomiting, abdominal pain, and ileus. Stress ulcerations (Curling ulcers) of the stomach and duodenum are common. Dysfunction of the liver, gallbladder, and pancreas is also possible. Direct electrothermal damage to viscera may produce organ necrosis or bowel perforation.

Local and systemic infections associated with burned and necrotic tissues are caused by various aerobic and anaerobic organisms, including *Staphylococcus, Pseudomonas,* and *Clostridium.* Overwhelming infections and sepsis are responsible for many deaths seen after initial successful resuscitation.

Electrical injury in pregnant women has been associated with fetal death and abortion. The amniotic fluid provides a rich electrolyte medium that will efficiently transmit electrical current to the fetus, creating a high risk of cardiac arrest and death.[11]

DIFFERENTIAL DIAGNOSIS

It is important to understand and distinguish true conductive electrical injuries from burns associated with other electrothermal phenomena. Electrical flash burns result from the radiant heat produced by electrical arcs, with temperatures ranging from 3,000° to 20,000°C. These burns are usually localized to exposed surfaces and are treated in a manner similar to that for conventional thermal burns. True flame burns may also be seen as a result of ignition of clothing or other combustibles adjacent to the victim.

High-frequency electrical energy, such as that used for RF or microwave transmission, has relatively limited injury potential. RF current demonstrates the so-called skin effect, so that current flow is limited to the outermost surfaces of conductors. Accidental contact usually results in localized surface burns. True internal conductive injuries are seldom seen.

EMERGENCY DEPARTMENT EVALUATION

Victims of high-tension electrical injury should be evaluated like victims of multiple trauma. Initial assessment and stabilization of airway, breathing, circulation (the ABCs), and the cervical spine are immediate priorities. As soon as possible, supplemental oxygen, large-bore intravenous lines to initiate fluid resuscitation, and electrocardiographic (ECG) monitoring are established. A careful history is taken to determine the nature and potential severity of the electrical injury. This should include a determination of voltage, the type of current (AC or DC), the current pathway, and the duration of exposure.

Associated trauma (especially falls) must be considered as potential concurrent mechanisms of injury. A thorough, complete physical examination is mandatory to uncover potential multisystem injury. However, many important internal injuries may be missed in the emergency department evaluation. A paucity of external physical signs may belie the severity of hidden internal tissue damage.

Indications for radiographic studies are established by the history and physical examination. A 12-lead ECG should be obtained on all patients with a possible thoracic current pathway. Arterial blood gas, urinalysis, complete blood count, electrolytes, calcium, blood urea nitrogen, creatinine, cardiac enzymes, coagulation studies, and type and cross-match studies are appropriate for patients with high-voltage injuries (greater than 1,000 V). Patients with limb dysfunction or evidence of ischemia should have compartment pressure measurements, vascular assessment, and nerve function studies.

Clinical assessment of patients stunned by electrical weapons should focus on local wounding effects of the electrode darts and coexisting injuries or problems, including drug toxicity. Phencyclidine intoxication appears to be a common scenario in which this weapon may be used.[12]

EMERGENCY DEPARTMENT MANAGEMENT

Many deaths and injuries have occurred when first responders try to aid a victim of an electrical injury before the electrical hazard is safely controlled. Definitive measures to ensure safety must be taken before assistance is attempted.

Appropriate attention and priority should be given to the ABCs, including attention to and stabilization of the cervical spine. Standard advanced cardiac life-support and advanced trauma life-support protocols are used, as indicated. For victims with cardiopulmonary arrest, resuscitative measures should be maintained for extended periods, because ultimate recovery may be achieved in cases that initially appear refractory.

In patients with high-tension injuries, aggressive fluid resuscitation may be needed to treat hypovolemia and to prevent renal failure. Extensive internal tissue damage causes large intravascular fluid losses that greatly exceed the fluid replacement values usually calculated by formulas based on the percent of body surface area burned.[10] Fluid requirements should instead be established to maintain brisk urine output and to prevent myoglobinuric renal failure. A urinary catheter is mandatory to monitor urine volume continuously and to detect myoglobin. Central venous or pulmonary artery pressure monitoring may be needed in patients with hemodynamic instability or those at risk for congestive heart failure. Intravenous mannitol and diuretics are appropriate adjuncts to enhance and maintain urine output. Sodium bicarbonate should be added to intravenous infusions to alkalinize the urine and prevent further myoglobin precipitation in the renal tubules. Serial monitoring of electrolytes, calcium, and arterial blood gases is necessary to detect and treat hyperkalemia, hypocalcemia, and acidosis caused by massive tissue necrosis or renal failure.

Nasogastric suction may be needed to decompress the GI tract and treat ileus. Tetanus prophylaxis must be ensured. The management of electrical surface burns is similar to that for thermal burns.

DISPOSITION

All patients with high-voltage (greater than 1,000 V) conductive injury require admission for observation and monitoring. Consultation regarding transfer to a burn center is advisable. Patients with dysrhythmias or ECG or cardiac enzyme evidence of myocardial injury should have 24 hours of continuous ECG monitoring and serial cardiac enzyme analysis.[1,4] Admission to a telemetry unit may also be appropriate for patients with transthoracic electrical current exposure, loss of consciousness, significant burns, or other tissue damage. Myoglobinuria is another indication for hospitalization. An orthopedic or vascular surgeon should be consulted when compartment syndrome or neurovascular compromise of extremities is suspected. Children with burns to the lips or the oral cavity should have a plastic surgery consultation, no matter how benign the initial injuries appear.

Patients with low-voltage surface injuries may be discharged after appropriate evaluation, observation, and management in the emergency department. When in doubt, admission is advisable.

COMMON PITFALLS

- Failure to consider and control ongoing electrical hazards in the field, resulting in rescuer injury
- Failure to appreciate that there may be a paucity of external physical signs in patients with severe internal tissue damage
- Failure to perform cardiac monitoring and to obtain an ECG to detect dysrhythmias in patients with suspected transthoracic current pathway exposures
- Failure to provide aggressive fluid resuscitation to maintain circulatory volume and to evaluate for and treat myoglobinuria in patients with high-voltage injuries
- Failure to evaluate for compartment syndrome and neurovascular compromise in injured extremities
- Failure to appreciate that children with burns to lips from electrical appliance cords must have plastic surgical consultation to minimize scarring

References

1. Arrowsmith J, Usagaocar R, Dickson WA. Electrical injury and the frequency of cardiac complications. *Burns* 1997;23:576.
2. Browne BJ, Gaash WR. Electrical injuries and lightning. *Emerg Med Clin North Am* 1992;10:211.
3. Budnick L. Bathtub-related electrocutions in the United States, 1979–1982. *JAMA* 1984;52:918.
4. Carleton SC. Cardiac problems associated with electrical injury. *Cardiol Clin* 1995;13:263.
5. Chandra N, Siu C, Munster M. Clinical predictors of myocardial damage after high-voltage electrical injury. *Crit Care Med* 1990;18:3.
6. Fish R. Electric shock, part I: physics and pathophysiology. *J Emerg Med* 1993;11:309.
7. Fish R. Electric shock, part II: nature and mechanisms of injury. *J Emerg Med* 1993;11:457.
8. Fish R. Electric shock, part III: deliberately applied electric shocks and the treatment of electrical injuries. *J Emerg Med* 1993;11:599.
9. Fontanarosa PB. Electrical shock and lightning strike. *Ann Emerg Med* 1993;22:378.
10. Hussmann J, Kucan JO, Russel RC, et al. Electrical injuries: morbidity, outcome and treatment rationale. *Burns* 1995;21:530.
11. Jaffe R, Fejgin M, Ben Aderet N, et al. Fetal death in early pregnancy due to electric current. *Acta Obstet Gynecol Scand* 1986;65:283.
12. Koscove E. The Taser weapon: a new emergency medicine problem. *Ann Emerg Med* 1985;14:1205.
13. Leibovici D, Shemer J, Shapira SC. Electrical injuries: current concepts. *Injury* 1995;26:623.
14. McBride J, Labrosse KR, McCoy HG, et al. Is serum creatine kinase-MB in electrically injured patients predictive of myocardial injury? *JAMA* 1986;255:764.
15. Ore T, Casini V. Electrical fatalities among U.S. construction workers. *J Occup Environ Med* 1996;38:587.
16. Pliskin NH, Capelli-Schellpfeffer M, Law RT, et al. Neuropsychological symptom presentation after electrical injury. *J Trauma* 1998;44:709.
17. Rabban J, Adler J, Rosen C, et al. Electrical injury from subway third rails: serious injury associated with intermediate voltage contact. *Burns* 1997;23:515.
18. Ratnayake B, Emmanueal ER, Walker CC. Neurological sequelae following a high voltage electrical burn. *Burns* 1996;22:574.
19. VanDenburg S, McCormick GM II, Young DB. Investigation of deaths related to electrical injury. *South Med J* 1996;89:869.
20. Zubair M, Besner GE. Pediatric electrical burns: management strategies. *Burns* 1997;23:413.

CHAPTER 394
Lightning Injuries

David F. M. Brown

Lightning injuries are the leading cause of deaths due to environmental phenomena in the United States.[5] Although there is no central agency to collect data, estimates suggest that lightning is responsible for 75 to 300 deaths per year and up to 1,500 nonfatal injuries.[2,4,6,8,11,12] The most common victims are people who work or perform recreational activities outside, particularly campers, joggers, farm and construction workers, golfers, and hunters.[4] Indoor victims are likely to be using the telephone or other household appliances.[4] The incidence of lightning injuries parallels the frequency of lightning storms; hence, most injuries occur during the summer months.[4,5] Geographically, common areas include the Atlantic seaboard, the Southeast and Southwest, major mountain ranges, and river tidal basins.[1,4,9,19] The case fatality rate is between 25% and 32%, and about 74% of survivors suffer permanent sequelae.[7]

Lightning is produced after warm, moist air rises within a cold high-pressure front, allowing condensation into a cloud.

Air currents, ice particles, and water droplets within the cloud create a layering of ionic charges: The uppermost regions have a net positive charge, the lower regions a net negative charge.[7] The ground beneath the cloud becomes relatively positively charged, creating a potential difference. Electrical breakdown between positively and negatively charged areas of the atmosphere causes advancement of ionic charges in a downward-branching "stepped leader" or "leader stroke" pattern propagated at one-two thousandth the speed of light. This causes a path of air to become ionized to a plasma of positive and negative ions that is a better conductor than nonionized air. As the stepped leader pattern of ion propagation nears the ground, a "pilot stroke" or "return stroke" ascends from the ground at about one-tenth the speed of light, completing a channel of ionic movement between the cloud and the ground.[7]

Because the stepped leader, which is luminous secondary to the large quantity of ionic movement, is relatively slower than the return stroke, lightning is perceived as traveling from cloud to earth. However, the main electrical discharge is usually from earth to cloud, and it appears as an instantaneous brightening of the ionized pathway (the visible lightning flash) lasting about 0.2 seconds. In rapid succession, multiple secondary leader and return strokes (between three and 40) then typically occur until the ionic potential between cloud and ground is eliminated.[7]

Thunder results from the rapid expansion of warmed air and its subsequent contraction and implosion. Practically, although not technically, lightning behaves as direct current, with an energy level of 2,000 to 2 billion V and 2,000 to 300,000 A.[3,11] This energy is much higher than conventional electricity; however, the distinctly short duration of lightning contact (0.1 to 1.0 milliseconds) usually prohibits cutaneous penetration and commensurate deep-tissue injury.[5] Except for direct strikes, most of the lightning current "flashes over" the outside of the victim; only occasionally does enough current leak internally to interfere with cardiac automaticity, respiratory center function, and autonomic stability.[10]

There are several major mechanisms of lightning injury. A direct strike occurs when the major pathway of current runs directly through the victim; this results in the highest morbidity and mortality.[10] When the lightning current strikes an object in contact with the victim, the injury mechanism approximates a direct strike. With side flash, current splashes or sprays from an object through the air to the victim. Ground current, also known as step voltage or ground potential, occurs when lightning strikes the ground and spreads to involve the victim. The severity of injury due to ground current is inversely proportional to the distance from the ground strike.[7] If ground resistance is greater than the victim's resistance, current may enter one leg and exit through the other, perhaps accounting for the higher mortality in victims exhibiting leg burns.[7] Ground current and side-flash mechanisms often produce multiple casualties.

Associated trauma may result from myotonic extremity or neck contractions, acceleration–deceleration injuries as the victim is thrown, penetrating and blunt injuries from debris, and thermal burns exacerbated by metal jewelry or clothing fasteners or caused by ignition of clothing.

CLINICAL PRESENTATION

Because of the short duration of lightning exposure, current usually passes over the outside of the body ("flashover" phenomenon), commonly producing superficial or partial-thickness burns in a characteristic linear or arborescent pattern.[1,2,11,18,19] Entry and exit burns and deep internal burns with resultant rhabdomyolysis and myoglobinuria are rare.[3,8,16,19,20]

The most common cause of death in the lightning victim is cardiopulmonary arrest.[7–9,13] Internal propagation of the lightning electrical potential acts as a massive direct current countershock, which depolarizes the entire myocardium and causes cardiac asystole.[7,8,11–13] Due to cardiac automaticity, an organized electrical rhythm may occur, restoring spontaneous circulation.[8] However, primary respiratory arrest due to lightning-induced paralysis of the medullary center may occur concomitantly and can outlast cardiac arrest.[3,4,8,10,11] The critical factor in determining mortality appears to be the duration of apnea (which may also occur independently) rather than the duration of asystole.[19] Without prompt and prolonged ventilatory support, any return of cardiac rhythm and circulation will rapidly deteriorate to hypoxia-induced ventricular fibrillation.[3,7,8,19] Survivors of lightning exposure can exhibit a variety of cardiac abnormalities, with dysrhythmias and ST-T wave changes frequently reported.[8,13,15] Acute life-threatening (and often reversible) left ventricular dysfunction or pericardial tamponade, as demonstrated by echocardiography, appears to be limited to victims of direct strikes.[15]

Myriad neurologic effects of lightning injury are frequently encountered. Usually, the victim falls unconscious immediately.[17] In the absence of cardiopulmonary arrest, consciousness eventually returns, occasionally after a prolonged period. The next most common finding is paraplegia, occurring in up to two-thirds of seriously injured patients.[8,17] Hemiparesis, hemiplegia, localizing sensory deficits, and autonomic dysfunction may also be found.[17]

Virtually all lightning-struck patients have altered mental status and anterograde amnesia; retrograde amnesia is common as well.[7,17] When current passes through the brain, intraventricular hemorrhage, epidural and subdural hematomas, coagulation of brain parenchyma, and thrombosis of vessels can occur.[7,17] Associated trauma may cause cervical spine fracture with resultant spinal cord injury.

The extremities may initially appear cold, mottled, pulseless, and insensitive secondary to vascular spasm and autonomic instability.[5,7,8,11,18,19] Normal function usually returns.

Half the patients with lightning injuries have structural eye lesions.[4] Cataracts are common and may develop in a few days or up to several years after the injury.[3,19] Corneal lesions are also common; hyphema, iritis, vitreous hemorrhage, retinal detachment, and optic nerve injury are occasionally seen.[5] Unreactive, dilated pupil(s) due to transient autonomic instability may occur and should not be mistaken for a sign of brain death.[5,7,17]

Tympanic membrane rupture, the most common otologic injury, occurs in 50% of victims of lightning injury and is thought to be due to the shock wave of expanding hot air (thunder) during the strike.[7,17] Less common findings are hemotympanum, basilar skull fracture, and various acoustic and vestibular sensorineural deficits.[17]

DIFFERENTIAL DIAGNOSIS

Lightning injuries have been mistakenly diagnosed as a variety of disorders. Neurologic disease processes that can mimic lightning injury include cerebrovascular accidents, seizure disorders, and craniocerebral, spinal cord, or other neurologic trauma.[8] Cardiovascular disorders in the differential diagnosis of lightning injury include myocardial infarction, Stokes-Adams attacks, and cardiac dysrhythmias.[8] Also in the differential are toxic ingestions, envenomations, and physical assault. Cutaneous injuries may be misdiagnosed as electrical burns.

As in most clinical situations, the history is crucial to making the correct diagnosis. Obtaining information from bystanders is essential when the victim is incapacitated. Important points include a history of thunderstorm and outdoor occurrence of the accident. Physical findings that favor a diagnosis of lightning injury include partial or complete clothing disintegration and superficial linear, punctate, or arborescent burns. Tympanic membrane rupture is also highly suggestive.

EMERGENCY DEPARTMENT EVALUATION

The history should include the time, circumstances, and a description of events at the scene of injury. Any prehospital interventions, and their times, should be documented. Present complaints and medical history prior to presentation should also be noted.

The physical examination should focus initially on vital signs; assessment of the airway, breathing, and circulation; and evaluation for trauma and neurologic dysfunction. Serial neurovascular examinations should be performed in patients with signs of peripheral vascular insufficiency. All patients should have cardiac monitoring, an electrocardiogram (ECG), and oxygen saturation measurement. Laboratory evaluation should include a complete blood count and measurements of serum electrolytes, blood urea nitrogen, creatinine, glucose, and creatine phosphokinase. Urine should be tested for myoglobin. Patients with cardiac dysrhythmias or ischemia, respiratory arrest, or loss of consciousness should have a chest radiograph and cardiac enzyme analysis. Patients with altered mental status or neurologic deficits should also have cervical spine radiographs and a cranial computed tomography scan. Other radiographs and tests should be obtained as indicated by complaints or physical findings.

EMERGENCY DEPARTMENT MANAGEMENT

Lightning injuries may place prehospital paramedics in precarious environmental settings. Although acute medical intervention is paramount to reduce mortality,[3,7,11] care should be taken to prevent further injury to the patient and harm to rescuers. Treatment begins with assessment and stabilization of the airway, ventilation, and circulation. Victims should be treated as trauma patients, with special attention given to cervical spine immobilization.[5] Triage priorities, in a reversal of the usual dictum, should focus initially on victims in cardiopulmonary arrest.[1,3,5,7,9,11,13,14] This is because virtually all victims of lightning strike who do not suffer cardiac or respiratory arrest survive.[7] Standard advanced life-support (ACLS and ATLS) protocols should be followed. Aggressive, persistent resuscitative efforts are indicated for all victims, especially those with spontaneous cardiac rhythms and prolonged apnea or coma.[1,5,11] Ventilatory support may be required for several hours, but even in these cases, there is potential for full recovery.[3,11] Full support should be continued until cerebral function can be assessed.[1]

All patients should initially be given supplemental oxygen, have intravenous access established, and be placed on a cardiac monitor. Intravenous fluids should be minimized to reduce any risk of cerebral edema unless hemorrhage, hypotension, or dehydration is evident or rhabdomyolysis is a concern (e.g., with deep or extensive burns or associated crush injury). Rhabdomyolysis, as indicated by myoglobinuria and elevated serum muscle enzyme levels, may necessitate fluid loading, osmotic diuresis, and urine alkalinization.[20] Standard burn and wound care, as well as tetanus prophylaxis, should be given, if appropriate. Patients with cardiac or neurologic abnormalities should have serial ECGs and cardiac enzyme analyses as well as routine supportive care. All patients require comprehensive and repeated physical and neurologic examinations.

DISPOSITION

Patients with cardiac or neurologic abnormalities require admission for at least 24 to 36 hours of observation and continuous cardiac monitoring. Those with associated trauma, burns, or rhabdomyolysis also may require admission for their injuries.[1,3,13] Patients who have sustained cardiac or respiratory arrest should be admitted to an intensive care unit.

The decision to transfer a patient to another facility depends on the severity of injury and the ability of local resources to provide adequate care. If the necessary services are unavailable, the decision and the timing of transfer should be coordinated with the receiving physician at the nearest appropriate hospital. Emergency personnel with advanced life-support capability should accompany the patient.

COMMON PITFALLS

- Failure to appreciate the difference between lightning and high-voltage injuries
- Failure to give the highest priority to patients in cardiac or respiratory arrest when making triage decisions in mass casualty incidents involving lightning injury
- Misdiagnosing lightning injury as an isolated cutaneous burn or a primary neurologic or cardiovascular event
- Failure to evaluate lightning-stricken patients for associated traumatic injuries
- Misinterpreting unreactive, dilated pupils as a sign of death in patients struck by lightning
- Failure to make a prolonged effort to resuscitate patients found pulseless or apneic after a lightning strike
- Failure to appreciate the high incidence of permanent neurologic sequelae from lightning injury and to admit patients with neurologic complaints or deficits for observation

References

1. Amy BW, McManus WF, Goodwin CW, et al. Lightning injury with survival of 5 patients. *JAMA* 1985;253:243.
2. Anonymous. Lightning-associated deaths—United States, 1980–1995. *MMWR* 1998;47:391.
3. Apfelberg DB, Masters F, Robinson D. Pathophysiology and treatment of lightning injuries. *J Trauma* 1974;14:453.
4. Blount BW. Lightning injuries. *Am Fam Physician* 1990;42:405.
5. Browne BJ, Gaasch WR. Electrical injuries and lightning. *Emerg Med Clin North Am* 1992;10:211.
6. Cherington M. Lightning injuries. *Ann Emerg Med* 1995;25:516.
7. Cooper MA. Lightning injuries: prognostic signs for death. *Ann Emerg Med* 1980;9:134.
8. Cooper MA. Emergent care of lightning and electrical injuries. *Semin Neurol* 1995;15:268.
9. Cwinn AA, Cantril SV. Lightning injuries. *J Emerg Med* 1985;2:379.
10. Epperly TD, Stewart JR. The physical effects of lightning injury. *J Fam Pract* 1989;29:267.
11. Fontanarosa PB. Electrical shock and lightning strike. *Ann Emerg Med* 1993;22:378.
12. Graber J, Ummenhofer W, Herion H. Lightning accident with eight victims: case report and brief review of the literature. *J Trauma* 1996;40:288.
13. Kleiner JP, Wilkin JH. Cardiac effects of lightning strike. *JAMA* 1978;240:2757.
14. Kobernick M. Electrical injuries: pathophysiology and emergency management. *Ann Emerg Med* 1982;11:633.
15. Lichtenberg R, Dries D, Ward K, et al. Cardiovascular effects of lightning strikes. *J Am Coll Cardiol* 1993;21:531.
16. Ohashi M, Kitagawa N, Ishikawa T. Lightning injury caused by discharges accompanying flashovers: a clinical and experimental study of death and survival. *Burns* 1986;12:496.
17. Patten BM. Lightning and electrical injuries. *Neurol Clin* 1992;10:1047.
18. Robinson M, Seward P. Electrical and lightning injuries in children. *Pediatr Emerg Care* 1986;2:186.
19. Straser EJ, Davis RM, Menchey JJ. Lightning injuries. *J Trauma* 1977;17:315.
20. Wang X, Jin R, Bartle E, et al. Creatine phosphokinase values in electrical and thermal burns. *Burns* 1987;13:309.

CHAPTER 395
Radiation Accidents

Irvin N. Heifetz

Accidental exposures to radioactive substances may occur in various settings, such as medical diagnosis and treatment, scientific research, electricity generation, military programs, and transportation of materials. Facilities using radioactive material usually have in-house experts knowledgeable about their particular products. Truckers, who yearly transport several hundred thousand shipments of radioisotopes, must carry papers specifying the exact nature of their cargo, and freight containers must be plainly labeled. Industries use the radionuclides ^{60}Co, ^{137}Cs, ^{192}Ir, and uranium isotopes. Hospitals use ^{131}I, ^{99m}Tc, ^{67}Ga, ^{32}P, ^{133}Xe, ^{201}Tl, and ^{60}Co in various diagnostic and therapeutic modalities. Certain laboratories use ^{3}H, ^{14}C, ^{125}I, ^{60}Co, and ^{238}U. Many radionuclides can be found at nuclear power plants, including ^{3}H, ^{131}I, ^{137}Cs, ^{60}Co, ^{90}Sr, ^{144}Ce, and ^{238}Pu.

Radiation accidents are relatively rare. Since the start of the nuclear age (1944), 403 events have been reported worldwide.[16] Of the 133,617 exposed individuals, nearly 90% were victims of the accident at the Chernobyl nuclear reactor in the Ukraine in 1986. The worldwide number of persons known to have been exposed to significant levels of radiation is 2,965, nearly 75% of whom were outside of the United States. A *significant* exposure is defined by the Radiation Emergency Assistance Center/Training Site Registry as either a whole-body dose of 25 rem, a skin dose of 600 rem, or an absorbed dose of 75 rem to other tissues. Acute fatalities from such exposures have numbered 120. Twenty-nine of these occurred at Chernobyl when an incredible succession of five violations of proper operating procedure during a scheduled test at that plant resulted in two steam explosions. Radiation injuries and illness necessitated prompt hospitalization of 115 people. In addition to those who died (20 of whom had received exposures between 600 and 1,600 rem), 56 persons suffered severe skin burns.

Most accidents occur in the industrial setting, where radioactive materials are used for making precise measurements, such as the thickness of rolled products and coatings, density and concentration in liquids, moisture content, flow patterns, and degree of wear. In industrial radiography, a sealed radioactive source is used to detect metallurgic defects. Accidental exposures occur when the seal ruptures or, more commonly, when operators carelessly direct the source toward themselves or their coworkers. Most injuries are burns, usually of the hands. Although nuclear medicine laboratories (diagnostic and assay) constitute the largest number of facilities using radioactive materials, the low levels of activity and the short half-lives of the isotopes used make serious accidents unlikely. Inappropriate fear of the effects of radiation could be alleviated by improving public education on the subject. This would have a salutary influence on rational responses to these rare accidents.[10]

Radiation consists of the transfer of energy from a generating source to an absorbing body via space or another medium. Nonionizing radiation, which makes up most of the electromagnetic spectrum (e.g., radio waves, microwaves, visible light), is of low frequency, long wavelength, and low linear energy transfer. Although relatively harmless, it can cause thermal damage in exposed tissues, and skin cancer may result from excessive exposure to ultraviolet waves.

Two types of widely encountered nonionizing radiation, lasers and microwaves, warrant brief discussion. Despite common use of lasers in industry (especially manufacturing and telecommunications) and medicine (diagnostic instrumentation and surgical procedures), injuries are rare. Similarly, although millions of people use microwave ovens daily, few cases of harmful effects from these sources have been documented. Prolonged direct contact of the skin with a leaking oven seal can cause a thermal burn, and ovens have occasionally been implicated in cardiac pacemaker malfunctions. The damage to human tissue from lasers is similar to that caused by an electrical burn. High-output microwave sources (industrial or medical, not domestic) may cause asymptomatic testicular damage, which could result in effects on sperm several weeks after exposure. Injuries from microwaves and lasers can be prevented by carefully adhering to manufacturers' safety guidelines.

Ionizing radiation—subsequently referred to simply as *radiation*—is emitted during the decay of unstable isotopes or radionuclides (naturally occurring or manufactured). A more stable atomic configuration results from the discharge of accelerated subatomic particles and electromagnetic waves. When the particles or waves strike another atom, displacement of an electron may cause the absorbing atom to become ionized. Tissue damage occurs when DNA and other macromolecules become ionized directly or by highly reactive free radicals of water. The amount of subcellular damage may be small enough to be readily repaired (as are most spontaneous chromosomal defects) or may lead to the death or dysfunction of the cells. Clinically observable effects will not appear for hours to years, except in the rarest case of a supralethal exposure. Destruction of dividing cells will produce signs and symptoms at a time proportional to the usual cell turnover rate in the particular tissue. Thus, effects on bone marrow, gut, and skin are seen early, but carcinogenesis appears much later.

The rate at which radionuclide disintegrations (i.e., formation of ion pairs by displacement of an orbital electron) occur is called its *activity*. One disintegration per second is called a *becquerel* (Bq). Activity was formerly measured in curies (Ci), the amount of energy emanating from 1 g of radium-226 (one Ci = 3.7×10^{10} Bq). A radionuclide with a short half-life contains more curies per unit mass than does one with a long half-life. The *roentgen* (R), which measures ionizations in air, was originally defined as the quantity of radiation producing one electrostatic unit of electrical charge in air (1.6×10^{12} ionizations). The roentgen does not readily measure all types of ionizing radiation and does not accurately reflect the radiation dose in tissue. In contrast, the *rad* (radiation absorbed dose) refers to the quantity of energy imparted to a mass of matter: one rad equals 100 ergs/g. The rad has been replaced by the *gray* (Gy) in the new Système Internationale (SI) nomenclature. One rad equals 0.01 Gy or one centigray (cGy), and one Gy equals 1 J/kg.

The number of ionizations per distance traveled by an ionizing particle or wave is directly proportional to the mass and charge of a particle and inversely proportional to the speed of the particle or wave. This linear energy transfer determines the relative biologic effectiveness of the source. The quality factor (QF) times the number of rad is the number of *rems* (radiation equivalents in humans or mammals). The SI unit is a *sievert* (Sv): 1 rem equals 0.01 Sv (cSv). The effective dose equivalent is derived by factoring in the relative sensitivities of various tissue and organs (0.25 for the gonads, 0.12 for bone marrow, and 0.03 for the thyroid).

Alpha and beta particles, gamma and x-rays, and neutrons all cause ionization in exposed tissue. Most commonly involved in radiation accidents are gamma rays and beta particles. Alpha particles, which may be thought of as helium nuclei (two protons bound to two neutrons), are relatively heavy (four atomic mass units) and highly charged (2^+). They have very poor penetration (about 50 μ) and are blocked by the keratin layer of skin. They do, however, produce very dense ionizations (30,000 to 100,000 ion pairs/cm^3 of air).[7] Their high linear energy transfer and relative biologic effectiveness are reflected in a QF of 20, and they are hazardous in wounds or if ingested or inhaled.[14] Common sources are ^{239}Pu, ^{226}Ra, ^{212}Po, and radon and isotopes of uranium.

Beta particles are fast-moving electrons with small mass (about one-two hundredth atomic mass unit) and a negative charge. They produce no more than 200 ion pairs/cm^3 of air and have a QF of 1. They can penetrate several millimeters through the skin, causing serious burns, and also create significant damage when emitted internally. ^{90}Sr, ^{137}Cs, ^{131}I, ^{3}H, and ^{32}P emit beta particles.

Gamma rays and x-rays are essentially the same. The former come from reactions within the nucleus, and the latter from orbital interactions. Neither has any mass or charge. They both are deeply penetrating and have QFs of 1. Because x-rays are produced when a heavy-metal target (such as tungsten) is bombarded with accelerated electrons, their energy is determined by the amount of voltage applied to the accelerator vacuum tube. Diagnostic x-ray machines use up to 150 kilovolts (kV), and x-ray therapy devices up to 300 kV at peak (kVp). ^{192}Ir, ^{99m}Tc, ^{137}Cs, ^{131}I, ^{226}Ra, and uranium isotopes are the usual sources of gamma radiation. If these radionuclides are internalized, any alpha or beta activity will predominate over the gamma effects.

Neutrons have an atomic mass weight of 1 but are electrically neutral. They have a wide range of energies, but most are extremely penetrating, and their QFs have been estimated from less than 2 for acute effects to 20 for late effects.[7] Free neutrons are found at nuclear power plants, particle accelerators, and weapons assembly sites.

Appreciation of the magnitude of any acute exposure to ionizing radiation is possible only by comparing it with background radiation. The estimated average annual dose of whole-body radiation to people in the United States is 200 to 250 millirems (mrem), 50% to 80% of which is from natural sources. The dose from cosmic sources (average, 28 mrem; maximum, 130 mrem) varies with elevation above sea level. The terrestrial dose (average, 26 mrem; maximum, 115 mrem) varies with the amounts of radium, thorium, and uranium in the earth's crust at any given site.[20] Most of the manufactured dose is from medical diagnostic sources (78 mrem) and radiopharmaceuticals (14 mrem). Radioactive fallout and nuclear power plants contribute 4.0 mrem and 0.2 mrem, respectively.

In comparison, the radiation dose to the skin is 21 mrem for a posteroanterior chest radiograph and 682 mrem for an anteroposterior thoracic spine film. The bone marrow dose from a chest radiograph is 5 mrem; an abdominal computed tomography scan yields a dose of 500 mrem to marrow.[1] People closest to the Three Mile Island plant got an average dose of 73 mrem following the accident there. At Chernobyl, emergency personnel at the site received less than a few hundred rem, and people living within 30 km got no more than 1.5 to 20.0 rem.[6]

CLINICAL PRESENTATION

Most accidents involve local exposure of a small part of the body of one person or a few people. The skin is the organ commonly affected.[12] At doses of 300 to 600 rem, epilation and erythema are noted. Dry desquamation occurs at about 1,000 rem, and wet desquamation at about 2,000 rem. Burns from ionizing radiation often take longer (up to 2 weeks) to become clinically apparent than do thermal burns. The time to onset varies inversely with the amount of exposure. Local exposure to 1,200 rad may cause erythema, which peaks in 24 hours and fades in a few days. Above 2,000 rad, denudation, ulceration, and depletion of hair follicles and sweat glands may occur. Total body exposure to gamma rays at a dose approaching 600 rad may cause erythema in less than 24 hours. Although the initial erythema caused by ionizing radiation is painless, third-degree radiation burns are very painful, because nerve receptors generally are not damaged as they are in thermal injuries.

Whole-body exposure to more than 100 to 200 rad in a single dose may produce acute radiation syndrome (ARS).[5] There is a very rough correlation between the nature and severity of signs and symptoms and the dose received. With optimal treatment, the LD_{50} (dose causing death in 50% of exposed persons) at 60 days is about 450 rad; the LD_{90} is about 700 rad.[3] Classically, ARS begins with a prodromal stage characterized by nausea, vomiting, and, sometimes, diarrhea. The acuity of symptoms suggests the size of the dose: less than 2 hours, more than 400 rad; more than 2 hours, less than 200 rad; more than 6 hours, less than 50 rad. These symptoms last from a few hours to 2 days. At doses of 100 to 600 rad, a latent period of 2 to 3 weeks ensues, followed by a hematopoietic syndrome in which the rapidly dividing cells in the bone marrow are injured. The panmyelosuppressive effects seen are indistinguishable from those caused by other marrow-toxic agents. Bleeding occurs in the skin and gastrointestinal (GI) and genitourinary tracts as a result of thrombocytopenia. Destruction of granulocyte precursors renders the patient susceptible to infection. If death does not occur within 3 to 6 weeks after exposure, this syndrome resolves slowly.

In addition to the problems described, patients exposed to doses of 600 to 2,000 rad also experience a GI syndrome. Denudation of the proliferating cells of the bowel mucosal epithelium causes symptoms of greatly increased nausea, vomiting, and diarrhea. Enormous loses of fluid and plasma proteins, extreme disturbances of electrolyte balance, and enteric organism sepsis also supervene. Death of 80% to 100% of these patients can be expected within a week or so but may be delayed beyond a month.

When whole-body doses exceed 2,000 rad, minutes or hours after exposure, patients uniformly are subject to unparalleled nausea, vomiting, and diarrhea, and then tremor, ataxia, seizures, prostration, and shock. Death from this neurovascular syndrome usually occurs within 2 days; it may be immediate with 3,000 to 5,000 rad of exposure. To assist in teaching about the rare affliction that is ARS, an Internet-accessible database of case histories has been established using the framework of the World Health Organization Radiation Medical Emergency Preparedness and Assistance Network Centers.[9]

The late effects of radiation relate primarily to carcinogenesis (especially leukemia) and mutagenesis, although instances of genetic abnormalities have never been clearly documented in human studies.[1] The degree of risk is uncertain; the data are discrepant.

DIFFERENTIAL DIAGNOSIS

It is almost always clear from the history that exposure to an ionizing source has occurred. Infrequently, a patient may present with nausea and vomiting, swollen parotid glands, conjunctivitis, skin ulcerations or burns, or bone marrow depression without a readily elucidated etiology. In these instances, inquiring about possible radiation exposure would be prudent.

EMERGENCY DEPARTMENT EVALUATION AND MANAGEMENT

Because of the extreme rarity and potential calamity of an unexpected exposure, a formal plan to deal with such an event must be in place and must be well known and rehearsed.[11,15,17] The JCAHO requires every hospital to include such a plan in its policy and procedure manual. Prudence also dictates that every regional emergency management system include radiation accidents in its disaster management protocol.[18,19]

When notified that a radiation accident may have occurred in which many people were exposed to high levels of radiation, the physician should invoke the hospital and regional plans, following them as closely as the circumstances of the particular incident allow. The hospital's radiation safety officer, as well as the one employed at the site of the accident (or at the company whose truck has crashed, for instance), must be contacted immediately. Police and fire authorities and a public relations official should be called. The physician should communicate with the scene while the area designated in the hospital to receive patients is prepared.

It must be determined exactly what sort of accident has happened: an exposure to external radiation, contamination by radioactive matter, or possible incorporation of ionizing substances via open wounds or the GI or respiratory tracts. A history of trauma or other toxic exposures and the nature, severity, and time of onset of any symptoms should be elicited. The duration of exposure (partial or whole-body), the nature of and distance from the source, and shielding and dosimeters used, if any, all constitute important data.[13]

At the scene, rescuers should remove the patient's clothes unless he or she is in extremis; this will eliminate 80% to 90% of surface contamination and will avoid further exposure of the patient, rescuers, other caregivers, and the environment.[4] The clothes should be quickly and carefully packaged, prominently labeled, and left at the site. Before removing the clothes, any open wounds should be covered to avoid exposing mucosal surfaces and capillary beds, which would promote absorption and incorporation. Caregivers should protect themselves against contamination by wearing gowns, gloves, masks, and shoe coverings. Patients who have been irradiated only do not become contaminated, radioactive, or dangerous to others. If the patient is stable and facilities are readily available, a very quick rinsing of obviously contaminated exposed skin may be done at this time. Any clothes and water used should be appropriately sequestered. The patient then should be totally wrapped in blankets and transported to the nearest designated hospital.

At the hospital, the victim and rescuer should remain in the ambulance until directed to the special treatment area. Ideally, this should be adjacent to the emergency department but should have a separate entrance. In hospitals without such an area, the autopsy room may suffice because it is usually distant from other patient-care areas, has drainage tables for easy collection of effluent, and often has a separate ventilation system. If the emergency department itself must be used, any noncritical patients and nonessential personnel should be directed away before radiation victims enter. The room to be used, as well as the route from the ambulance dock, should be cordoned off and labeled "Danger: Radiation." The radiation safety officer or designee should monitor with a Geiger-Müller counter all patients and personnel entering or exiting the isolated room. If possible, a buffer zone also should be established, to provide both an extra margin of separation and an area through which necessary equipment and supplies may be transferred to the treatment room.

Before any patients arrive, all pathways and floors should be smoothly covered with paper, sheets, or, optimally, ribbed plastic (waterproof and nonslippery) to help minimize environmental contamination. All switches and handles should be covered with tape. Unless the room has a separate ventilation system, the system should be shut off. The area should contain all equipment and supplies common in a room used to treat acutely ill patients, as well as extra scrub suits, gowns, gloves, plastic aprons, and shoe coverings. Large plastic bags for clothes, containers for specimens, and steel barrels for contaminated water and other items also are needed.

Also required are survey meters capable of detecting both high-range (up to 500 rem/h) and low-range (up to 20 rem/h) exposures and also common (gamma and beta) or uncommon (alpha and neutron) sources. To ensure that they are in good working condition, and to obtain instruction in their proper use, these are best acquired from the radiology department or laboratories where they are frequently used. Personnel dosimeters should also be gathered from throughout the hospital for emergency use. The best are those that provide a constant readout. They should be attached to the collars of all personnel treating the accident victims. Team members should be relieved when their badges read 5 rem, although doses up to 25 rem may be permitted under unusual circumstances, and even 75 rem in a lifesaving effort.

If the patient's clothes were not removed at the accident scene, this should be done in the ambulance. Critical patients should be brought into the treatment room immediately. Advanced life-support measures are provided as needed. All patients are surveyed with a Geiger-Müller counter for contamination; findings should be recorded on anatomic charts. Cotton swabs should be used to sample and save contamination from the nose, ears, and mouth. Contaminated open wounds must be copiously irrigated with saline, resurveyed, irrigated with 3% hydrogen peroxide if contamination remains, and then debrided, if necessary, to prevent incorporation of radionuclides.

Once wounds have been cared for and covered with plastic, external decontamination should proceed from the area with the most debris to the area with least. Uncontaminated areas should be covered and taped. Using tepid water and mild soap or nonionic detergent, very gentle scrubbing should be done for 3 minutes with the patient lying either on a special decontamination table (similar to an autopsy table) or on a makeshift plastic trough placed on a stretcher in slight reverse Trendelenburg. Scanning for radioactivity and repeating this procedure as long as counts are decreasing should be done. Half-strength household bleach (5% sodium hypochlorite) may be used in later washes. Gentle brushing under nails and clipping of hair (not shaving, which might leave small open wounds) may be required. All fluids should be collected.

Less than 2 hours is available for possibly effective prevention of incorporation after ingestion or inhalation. Treatment of ingestions should begin with gastric lavage; whole-bowel irrigation, using a prep solution (e.g., GoLYTELY, Colyte) at 0.5 to 2.0 L/h until the rectal effluent is clear, may be beneficial. Activated charcoal is also recommended. Washings should be saved, surveyed, and disposed of by the radiation safety officer. Bronchoalveolar lavage may be helpful if radioactive dust has been inhaled, as confirmed by stained or radioactive sputum. Other methods to reduce absorption include administering Prussian blue for thallium, cesium, or rubidium, and barium sulfate or aluminum-based antacids for radium or strontium.

Isotopic dilution (competition) may be used to prevent incorporation of radionuclides that have already been absorbed. Potassium iodide (approximately 2 mg/kg) should be given orally if the thyroid dose from ^{131}I or other radioiodine exceeds 50 rad.[2,8] If given within 1 hour of exposure, potassium iodide blocks 90% of ^{131}I uptake but only 50% at 5 hours, and little at 12 hours. To prevent recycling of radioiodine, this treatment must continue for up to 2 weeks.

Stable strontium, calcium, phosphate, zinc, and iron can be used to compete with their radioactive counterparts. Water diuresis can increase the turnover of tritium, and diuresis can also hasten the removal of radioactive sodium and potassium. Chelating agents, in standard doses, may be helpful—deferoxamine for plutonium and iron, penicillamine for cobalt and copper, and dimercaprol for mercury, arsenic, bismuth, chromium, nickel, and lead. Available only from the Department of Energy, calcium or zinc DTPA may help remove plutonium and americium as well as other transuranic and rare-earth elements. Experts should be consulted for advice (discussion follows).

All patients should have a baseline complete blood count, absolute lymphocyte count, and platelet count. These should be repeated serially for 3 days. Additional blood should be drawn and saved for chromosomal analysis of peripheral lymphocytes. Some authorities recommend taking cultures of the throat, sputum, wounds, blood, and urine so that appropriate antibiotics can be started early in a patient who may become immunosuppressed.

The prognosis of radiation injury victims is directly related to the dose received. In addition to early clinical signs, the best indicator is the total lymphocyte count after 48 hours. Counts above 1,200/μL indicate a good prognosis; below 300, poor. The degree of chromosomal abnormalities (e.g., dicentrics and glycophorin A locus analysis) also correlates well with prognosis.[3]

The Radiation Emergency Assistance Center/Training Site at Oak Ridge, Tennessee, also should be contacted for anything more than very-low-dose external irradiation to a few persons. The people there are expert in all aspects of radiation injury and treatment and are available for emergencies 24 hours a day at (423)481-1000.

DISPOSITION

Any patient judged to have been exposed to more than 100 rad should be hospitalized. Depending on the severity of illness, consultation with specialists in infectious disease, gastroenterology, hematology, pulmonary medicine, and marrow transplantation may be appropriate. Reverse isolation also may be required. If these services are unavailable in the hospital where initial treatment is given, the patient should be transferred to the closest facility so equipped.

COMMON PITFALLS

- Failure to have a plan in place for the management of radiation victims
- Failure to review and rehearse the plan with key personnel at least annually
- Failure to appreciate that there are different types of radiation and to determine which one was involved in an exposure
- Failure to have decontamination and protective equipment available
- Failure to attend to associated injuries (e.g., burns, blasts) or exposures (e.g., nonradioactive toxins)
- Letting unrealistic fear prevent the care of patients or colleagues

References

1. Adelstein SJ. Uncertainty and relative risk of radiation exposure. *JAMA* 1987;258:655.
2. Becker D. Reactor accidents: public health strategies and their medical implications. *JAMA* 1987;258:649.
3. Champlin RE. Radiation accidents and nuclear energy: medical consequences and therapy. *Ann Intern Med* 1988;109:730.
4. Cox RA. Nuclear emergencies: medical preparedness. *Br J Radiol* 1987;60:1180.
5. Finch SC. Acute radiation syndrome. *JAMA* 1987;258:664.
6. Gale RP, Butturni A. Radiation accidents: primum non nocere. *Bone Marrow Transplant* 1993;11:421.
7. Hubner KF, Fry SA, eds. *The medical basis for radiation accident preparedness.* New York: Elsevier Science, 1980.
8. Kastengerg WE. Principal issues and future projects of nuclear energy. *Ann Intern Med* 1988;109:739.
9. Kindler H, Fliedner TM, Desnow D. Internet access to a medical case repository for teaching and analysis. *Proc AMIA Annu Fall Symp* 1997;543–547.
10. Lakey J. Informing the public about radiation—the messenger and the message: 1997 G. William Morgan lecture. *Health Phys* 1998;75(4):367–374.
11. Leonard RB, Ricks RC. Emergency department radiation accident protocol. *Ann Emerg Med* 1980;9:462.
12. Lushbaugh CC, Fry SA, Ricks RC. Medical and radiobiological basis of radiation accident management. *Br J Radiol* 1987;60:1159.
13. Mettler FA Jr, Kelsey CA, Ricks RC. *Medical management of radiation accidents.* Boca Raton, FL: CRC Press, 1990.
14. Milroy WC. Management of irradiated and contaminated casualty victims. *Med Clin North Am* 1984;2:667.
15. National Council on Radiation Protection and Measurements. *Management of persons accidentally contaminated with radionuclides.* NCRP Report No. 65. Washington DC: NCRP, 1980.
16. Nenot JC. Radiation accidents: lessons learnt for future radiological protection. *Int J Radiat Biol* 1998;73(4):435–442.
17. Ricks R. *Hospital emergency department management of radiation accidents.* Oak Ridge, TN: Oak Ridge Associated Universities, 1984.
18. Richter LL, Berk HW, Teates CD, et al. A systems approach to the management of radiation accidents. *Ann Emerg Med* 1980;9:303.
19. Saenger EL. Radiation accidents. *Ann Emerg Med* 1986;15:1061.
20. Upton A. Prevention of work-related injuries and diseases: lessons from experience with ionizing radiation. *Am J Indust Med* 1987;12:291.

CHAPTER 396
Smoke Inhalation

Christopher H. Linden

Smoke inhalation is airway or pulmonary parenchymal injury resulting from inhalation of toxic combustion products. Although the mortality from smoke inhalation in fire victims without surface burns is only 10%, this injury accounts for up to 84% of all fire-associated deaths.[3,5,9,18] Due to advances in the treatment of shock, sepsis, and skin wounds, smoke inhalation is now the major cause of death in patients with surface burns. Most smoke inhalation fatalities are associated with residential fires.[14] Many victims are clearly dead at the scene and do not enter the health-care system. Those who lack the ability to take independent escape action, such as the very young, the elderly, those with disabilities, and those impaired by alcohol or other drugs, are at greatest risk. A functioning smoke detector lowers the risk of death from smoke inhalation.

Smoke is a visible mixture of gases, vapors, fumes, liquid droplets, and solid carbon particles (dust) evolved during the combustion (the thermal degradation under conditions of high oxygen concentration) or pyrolysis (thermal degradation in an oxygen-poor environment) of organic material. Fire (a luminous gas) is not necessary for the production of smoke. In addition to fire and smoke, toxic combustion or pyrolysis products (TCPs) may include heat, invisible gases, and oxygen deprivation. Hence, pulmonary and systemic toxicity due to the smoke inhalation may occur in the absence of visible warning.

The composition of TCPs depends on the oxygen supply, rate of heating, absolute temperate, and material burned.[6,7,12] Although fire toxicology research has identified TCPs for some materials under some conditions (Table 396.1), in actual fires, many different and often unknown materials are burned under a variety of coexisting conditions, resulting in the evolution of hundreds or thousands of different TCPs. Hence, the exact nature of TCPs in a given situation is impossible to predict, but a few generalizations can be made. Heat, carbon monoxide, car-

TABLE 396.1. Common Toxic Products of Combustion and Their Sources

Product of Combustion	Common Sources
Acids/aldehydes	Cellulose acetate (film), cotton, paper, polystyrene, polyvinyl acetate, wood
Acrolein	Acrilan (carpet), acrylic, celluloid, cellulosics, polyolefins
Ammonia	Nylon, resins (melamine, phenolic), silk, wood
Carbon monoxide/dioxide	All organic material
Chlorine/hydrochloric acid/phosgene	Chlorinated acrylics and hydrocarbons (fire extinguishers and retardants)
Cyanide/hydrogen cyanide	Acrylonitriles, nylon, paper, polyurethane, nitrocellulose (film), resins, silk, wool
Halogen acids and gases (Br, F)	Halogenated hydrocarbons, films, resins, flame retardants and extinguishers
Isocyanates	Polyurethane
Nitrogen oxides	Celluloid, cellulose nitrate fabrics, paper, petroleum products, wood
Styrene	Polystyrene
Sulfur oxides/ hydrogen sulfide	Hair, hides, meat, petroleum products, rubber, wool

bon dioxide, dust, and oxygen deprivation are almost universally present. Fires involving plastics (e.g., acrylics, celluloids, polystyrene, polyurethane, polyvinyl chloride) burn faster and produce far more heat and smoke than those involving wood, paper, and most natural materials. Smoldering, enclosed-space fires have higher concentrations of TCPs than open, flaming ones.

The nature and severity of smoke inhalation depend on the identity, concentration, and temperature of the TCPs; the particle size of soot; the length of exposure; and the victim's respiratory rate and health status.[4–7] Carbon monoxide (see Chapter 323) is thought to be responsible for most deaths, especially those that occur early.[5–7,18] If measured immediately after exposure, elevated carboxyhemoglobin (COHb) fractions are likely to be seen in virtually all victims of smoke inhalation. However, as many as 40% of victims found dead at the scene have COHb fractions less than 50%, the fraction generally considered to be evidence of death from carbon monoxide in the forensic literature, 20% to 25% have fractions less than 30%, and up to 10% have fractions less than 10%.[7] Cyanide poisoning (see Chapter 331) also appears to contribute to early mortality. Blood cyanide (CN) levels are elevated in up to 90% of fire victims and correlate with the COHb fraction.[1,2,7,11,17] Potentially toxic CN levels have been noted in as many as 30% of smoke inhalation survivors and 100% of fatalities, and potentially lethal levels have been found in up to 10% of survivors and 70% of fatalities. Acrolein and hydrogen chloride reach potentially toxic levels in about 10% of fires. Methemoglobinemia has also been reported in victims of dwelling fires.[10] Although the concentrations and individual toxicity of other gases are usually low, their additive or synergistic toxicity is potentially significant.[7]

TCP gases can be divided into two groups, based on their mechanism of action and site of toxicity. *Cellular asphyxiants,* such as carbon monoxide and cyanide, cause systemic toxicity without direct pulmonary effects as the consequence of hypoxia secondary to impaired oxygen delivery and use at the cellular level. *Respiratory irritants* (see Chapter 346) cause upper and lower airway and pulmonary parenchymal injury without direct systemic toxicity. Highly water-soluble gases, such as acids, ammonia, and chlorine, tend to dissolve in the moisture of upper airway surfaces, producing laryngeal and tracheal edema, ulceration, and hemorrhage. Irritant gases with lower water solubility, such as acrolein, aldehydes, isocyanates, phosphine, and oxides of nitrogen and sulfur, tend to penetrate deeper, producing tracheobronchitis or variants of the respiratory distress syndrome (e.g., pneumonitis, pulmonary edema). The location of injury also depends on the nature of the soot (see subsequent discussion). In addition, severe systemic toxicity (e.g., shock) may result in pulmonary injury, and severe respiratory tract injury may lead to systemic effects due to hypoxia.

Carbon dioxide and oxygen concentrations at a fire scene are not often sufficiently high or low, respectively, to cause direct systemic effects. However, they increase exposure to TCPs by stimulating respiration. High atmospheric temperatures contribute to inhalation injury, especially if the humidity is also high. Thermal injury is generally more immediate than that due to respiratory irritants. Inhaling air greater than 200°C can be lethal in less than 5 minutes. Inhaling hot, dry air results primarily in upper airway edema, whereas steam inhalation may cause parenchymal damage as well as upper and lower airway injury. At a given temperature, injury and mortality increase with increasing humidity because of the greater thermal capacity of water vapor.

The soot fraction of smoke consists of carbon particles and dust of varying size. The particles themselves cause little acute irritation but they adsorb various toxic gases and liquids and act as vehicles to deliver these agents to various locations in the respiratory tract. Large quantities of soot may mechanically obstruct the airways, usually at the bronchiole level. In extremely sooty situations, however, death may result from upper airway obstruction (e.g., victims of the Mount St. Helen's volcanic eruption). Particles larger than 5 μm are filtered by the nasopharynx; those 1 to 5 μm settle on tracheobronchial surfaces; those smaller than 1 μm reach the alveoli.

The dose of TCPs delivered to the airways is proportional to the minute ventilation and the duration of exposure. In addition to high ambient carbon dioxide and low oxygen levels, anxiety, confusion, physical activity, and early respiratory tract irritation stimulate respirations and thus increase TCP exposure. Impaired mobility secondary to TCP toxicity (e.g., cognitive dysfunction, respiratory distress, incoordination, weakness), visual impairment (e.g., smoke, darkness, lacrimation), and physical obstacles (e.g., slippery surfaces, structural collapse) may increase the duration of exposure. Similarly, concurrent drug or alcohol intoxication, extremes of age, and physical handicaps may impair awareness, judgment, or mobility and increase exposure time. If the cycle continues, increasing respiratory tract injury and systemic toxicity may result in complete incapacitation, culminating in death.

CLINICAL PRESENTATION

Victims of smoke inhalation may present with manifestations of respiratory tract injury, or systemic toxicity from anoxia, carbon monoxide, CN, and methemoglobinemia, or both.[4,5,9,15,16,18,19] Respiratory tract injury may involve the upper airway, lower airway, pulmonary parenchyma, or a combination thereof. Nonspecific manifestations include cough, dyspnea, tachypnea, tachycardia, and cyanosis.

Signs of upper airway injury (eye, nose, and throat irritation) include conjunctivitis, tearing, rhinitis, pharyngitis, neck pain, dysphagia, drooling, hoarseness, and stridor. Fluorescein and slit-lamp examination of the eyes may reveal corneal burns. Examination of nasopharyngeal mucosa may reveal erythema, edema, hemorrhage, ulceration, or soot stains. Increased secretions and laryngospasm may be present. Facial burns and singed hair (head, eyebrows, or nose) are associated with a high incidence of thermal burns of the larynx and severe inhalation injury.[20] Direct or indirect laryngoscopy may reveal laryngeal burns or soot. A lateral soft-tissue radiograph of the neck may show laryngeal or periglottic edema. A swollen epiglottis may be seen (irritant or chemical epiglottitis). Signs and symptoms of upper airway injury are usually immediate in onset and peak within several hours of exposure.

Manifestations of lower airway injury include carbonaceous sputum production, bronchospasm (wheezing), rhonchi, chest pain (burning or tightness), and rales (due to atelectasis). Bronchoscopy may disclose tracheobronchial findings similar to those described in upper airway mucosal injury.[5] A pseudomembranous tracheobronchitis (mucosal sloughing) has been described. Bedside pulmonary function tests (e.g., PEFR, FEV_1) may reveal decreased airflow. An increased expiratory–inspiratory ratio on flow-volume loop measurement is more sensitive than simple spirometry in detecting small changes in airway resistance. Radioisotope (xenon-133) ventilation–perfusion lung scans may show delayed washout of gas in areas of small airway destruction. A chest radiograph may be normal, particularly if obtained soon after exposure, or it may reveal bronchial wall thickening (peribronchial cuffing), subglottic tracheal edema, or atelectasis.[13] Arterial blood gas analysis may reveal hypoxia and hypercapnia. Severe symptoms may occur immediately, particularly in those with underlying pulmonary disease. More often, symptoms are initially mild but worsen during the first 8 to 48 hours.

Pulmonary parenchymal injury causes nonspecific signs and symptoms. In contrast to localized rales from atelectasis, diffuse crackles may be heard in patients with pneumonitis or pulmonary edema. The chest radiograph may reveal patchy or diffuse infiltrates.[13] Arterial blood gas analysis may show hypoxia and hypocapnia or hypercapnia. Hypoxia may result in secondary complications (e.g., myocardial ischemia or infarction), particularly in patients with underlying cardiovascular disease. Unventilated areas on xenon lung scanning and decreased diffusing capacity are sensitive but nonspecific findings of parenchymal injury.[19] Spirometry may reveal restrictive disease due to decreased lung compliance as well as obstructive airway disease. Although pulmonary edema may sometimes develop immediately after irritant inhalation, it is usually gradual in onset and peaks 1 to 2 days (or longer) after exposure.

Bacterial pneumonia and tracheobronchitis are common complications. However, fever and leukocytosis secondary to chemically induced airway or lung inflammation may be seen in the absence of infection during the first 2 days after inhalation. Early postinhalation respiratory infections are usually due to *Staphylococcus aureus;* late infections are often caused by *Pseudomonas* and other gram-negative organisms.

Cellular asphyxia results in central nervous system (CNS) and cardiovascular depression (see Chapters 323 and 331). Manifestations include agitation, confusion, coma, seizures, hypotension, and dysrhythmias. An elevated carboxyhemoglobin fraction confirms the diagnosis of smoke inhalation, but a normal carboxyhemoglobin concentration does not exclude it.

DIFFERENTIAL DIAGNOSIS

Patients with smoke inhalation may have concomitant dermal burns, traumatic injuries, and drug or alcohol intoxication and may be victims of arson, attempted murder, or attempted suicide. In patients with coma and shock, head computed tomography scanning, whole-blood CN levels, toxicology screening tests, and invasive hemodynamic measurements (e.g., central venous and pulmonary artery pressures) may be necessary to define the etiology.

EMERGENCY DEPARTMENT EVALUATION

The history includes details of exposure; symptoms, signs, and treatment before arrival; current symptoms; allergies; and previous illnesses (especially cardiac and respiratory problems). Important points in the exposure history include the nature of the burning material (natural or synthetic), length of exposure, open- versus closed-space exposure, the presence or absence of explosion, falls, jumps, other victims (injured or dead), physical injury, steam, suicide note, mask use, and the amount, color, and odor of smoke. The likelihood of inhalation injury is greater with synthetic (plastics) fires, with closed-space and steam exposures, and with exposures longer than a few minutes. Any history of altered mental status, collapse, or loss of consciousness also suggests a high risk of inhalation injury. Patients should be specifically questioned about respiratory symptoms, chest pain, alcohol and drug use, and suicidal ideation.

In firefighters, the type of oxygen mask used is important. With minimum safety apparatus, oxygen is supplied by a demand valve requiring negative (inspiratory) pressure, and smoke inhalation can occur if the mask is not perfectly tight. With continuous positive-pressure oxygen devices (e.g., the Scott airpack), smoke inhalation is impossible unless the oxygen supply, which lasts 20 to 30 minutes, depending on activity, runs out. In addition, invisible toxic gas inhalation may occur if either type of mask is removed during the clean-up or cool-down period immediately after the fire is extinguished.

After a trauma survey, the physical examination focuses on the mental status, vital signs (especially respiration), skin, eyes, nose, pharynx, and chest. Extensive burns (greater than 15% of body surface area), facial burns, singed facial hair, and soot in the airways are associated with a higher incidence of inhalation injury.[20] As with historical risk factors, however, their absence does not rule out significant inhalation injury.

Arterial blood gas or oxygen saturation and carboxyhemoglobin level measurement, ECG, chest radiograph, and bedside spirometry are recommended for patients symptomatic on presentation, particularly those with historical risk factors, abnormal findings on physical examination, and underlying cardiopulmonary disease. Although hypoxemia, elevated carboxyhemoglobin levels (greater than 10%), abnormal breath sounds, and atelectasis or infiltrates on the chest radiograph are diagnostic of inhalation injury, these findings are absent in most patients who later develop respiratory complications.[3,5,18] Because carboxyhemoglobin levels decrease with increasing time since exposure (particularly if oxygen has been given), they must be measured early to detect small but significant exposures. Patients who remain symptomatic should be reevaluated after 3 or 4 hours, and sooner if symptoms worsen.

In patients with altered mental status of unclear etiology, toxicology screening tests and a quantitative ethanol level should be obtained. A whole-blood CN level is recommended in patients with coma, acidosis, shock, and high carboxyhemoglobin levels. Although not immediately useful, it may later confirm the diagnosis of CN poisoning in patients who may require empiric treatment for this condition. The methemoglobin level should also be measured in patients with refractory cyanosis.

Laryngoscopy (indirect or direct) may help identify mucosal damage in patients with mild-to-moderate upper respiratory tract symptoms, but it should not delay immediate intubation in those with severe symptoms and respiratory distress. Additional evaluation for inhalation injury (e.g., bronchoscopy, ventilation–perfusion lung scanning, flow-volume spirometry) is impractical and unnecessary for emergency department management and disposition.

EMERGENCY DEPARTMENT MANAGEMENT

Prehospital directives include prompt but safe removal of the victim from the scene of exposure; institution of basic and advanced life-support measures, as needed; and surface decontamination (e.g., clothing removal, irrigation of eyes and skin). All patients should be given supplemental oxygen. A rescuer should never enter a potentially toxic environment without adequate respiratory, eye, and skin protection.

Endotracheal intubation should be done in patients with any of the following: CNS depression (i.e., no spontaneous or coherent verbalization); respiratory distress with stridor or drooling; cyanosis or hypoxia (PO_2 less than 60) that does not quickly improve with maximal oxygen delivery and continuous positive airway pressure (CPAP) by mask; full-thickness burns of the face (nasolabial) or neck (circumferential); pharyngeal, laryngeal, or pulmonary edema; inability to clear secretions; or respiratory insufficiency (PO_2 greater than 50).[5,6,9,16] More liberal indications for early (prophylactic) intubation include less pronounced findings that worsen despite treatment. In patients whose full-thickness face or neck burns restrict mandible or neck mobility and in those with upper airway edema, blind nasal intubation may be successful when the larynx cannot be directly visualized. In rare cases, fiberoptic endoscopic guidance, cervical escharotomy, or cricothyroidotomy may be necessary for airway control. As always, if coexisting head or neck trauma or cervical spine injury is suspected, precautions are necessary until radiographs rule out this possibility.

Aggressive suctioning of the airway to remove mucus and inhaled debris should follow intubation. Oxygen should be humidified to prevent drying of secretions. Hypoxemia despite intubation and 100% oxygen should be treated initially with positive end-expiratory pressure (PEEP) ventilation. CPAP and PEEP may also be helpful in the prophylactic treatment of pulmonary edema. High-frequency ventilation may decrease the incidence of pneumonia and improve survival in those with severe inhalation injury. Extracorporeal membrane oxygenation procedures should be considered in patients with refractory hypoxemia. Because hyperbaric oxygen therapy requires relatively intact pulmonary function to be effective, it is unlikely to be of benefit in such patients.[8] The efficacy of partial liquid fluorocarbon ventilation remains to be determined.

In patients without respiratory distress, stridor, or drooling, racemic epinephrine by aerosol inhalation may relieve upper airway symptoms. Bronchospasm should be treated with standard asthma medications (i.e., inhaled beta agonists). Chest physical therapy, incentive spirometry, postural drainage, and encouragement of coughing may help clear secretions and inhaled particles from the lower airway. Although corticosteroids may be useful for refractory bronchospasm, they are not recommended for pneumonitis or pulmonary edema.[9,19] Despite theoretical benefits, corticosteroid treatment (or attempted prophylaxis) of parenchymal injury results in increased mortality from infectious complications. The administration of a single large dose of corticosteroids on initial presentation, however, may be beneficial and is unlikely to be harmful. Ibuprofen and other nonsteroidal antiinflammatory agents are of theoretical benefit in the prevention and treatment of pulmonary edema. The use of prophylactic antibiotics has not been shown to be beneficial.[5,9]

Fever and leukocytosis persisting or developing more than 2 days after inhalation suggest infection. Although the results of sputum Gram stain and culture should ultimately guide antibiotic use, empiric coverage for both *S. aureus* and gram-negative bacteria can be started when sputum or laboratory results are not immediately available. All patients, particularly those requiring fluid resuscitation, should be reassessed frequently for deteriorating respiratory function.

Management of carbon monoxide and CN poisoning and methemoglobinemia are discussed in Chapters 323, 331, and 352. Carbon monoxide poisoning should be treated according to the usual guidelines. It should again be noted, however, that hyperbaric oxygen therapy is unlikely to be effective in enhancing carbon monoxide elimination in patients who cannot be adequately oxygenated despite intubation and the administration of 100% oxygen. The use of the CN antidote kit in smoke inhalation victims is controversial because the induction of methemoglobinemia, which decreases the oxygen-carrying capacity of hemoglobin, could be harmful in patients with hypoxemia and elevated carbon monoxide levels.[7] Because coma, seizures, hypotension, and acidosis suggest CN poisoning, patients with these findings (in the absence of alcohol, drugs, hypovolemia, hypoxemia, carbon monoxide poisoning, and methemoglobinemia) may be candidates for CN antidote therapy if they fail to improve with supportive care. Although giving just the thiosulfate (the portion of the antidote kit that does not induce methemoglobinemia) may be safe in patients with hypoxemia and high carboxyhemoglobin levels, the use of nitrites should be reserved for those receiving concomitant hyperbaric oxygen therapy and those in extremis.

DISPOSITION

Patients with continuing respiratory symptoms (including cough and chest tightness); altered mental status; a history of loss of consciousness; abnormal lung sounds; concurrent drug or alcohol intoxication; elevated carboxyhemoglobin levels (greater than 10%); abnormal arterial blood gas measurements, chest radiograph, or ECG; facial or nasal burns; or a history of chronic cardiopulmonary disease should be admitted (simply for observation, if active treatment is not required). Depending on the severity of clinical findings and laboratory abnormalities and the coexistence of surface burns or traumatic injuries, intensive care unit, telemetry, or floor bed admission may be appropriate. Patients with carbon monoxide poisoning may require transfer for hyperbaric oxygen therapy (see Chapter 323), and those with significant surface burns or physical injuries may require transfer to a burn or trauma center. Advanced life-support capability should be available during transfer.

Patients in good general health who are asymptomatic (on arrival or after a short period of oxygen therapy) and have a normal physical examination, arterial blood gas or oxygen saturation results (while breathing room air), ECG, chest radiograph, and carboxyhemoglobin level may be discharged, but it is generally advisable to observe these patients for at least 3 or 4 hours before making a discharge disposition. Discharged patients should be instructed to return immediately if any respiratory symptoms develop. A scheduled recheck at 24 hours may be prudent.

COMMON PITFALLS

- Failure to admit symptomatic patients, despite the absence of abnormalities on the initial physical examination, laboratory evaluation, and chest radiograph
- Failure to evaluate and treat for coexisting carbon monoxide poisoning, drug or alcohol intoxication, traumatic injuries, and psychiatric problems

- Failure to give oxygen to all patients (including those with chronic obstructive pulmonary disease)
- Failure to perform endotracheal intubation when indicated
- Failure to fluid-resuscitate patients with trauma or surface burns for fear of exacerbating inhalation injury
- Failure to recognize the potential hazards of inappropriate corticosteroid, antibiotic, and CN antidote administration

References

1. Barillo DJ, Goode R, Esch V. Cyanide poisoning in victims of fire: analysis of 364 cases and review of the literature. *J Burn Care Rehabil* 1994;15:46.
2. Baud FJ, Barriot P, Toffis V, et al. Elevated blood cyanide concentrations in victims of smoke inhalation. *N Engl J Med* 1991;325:1761.
3. Blinn DL, Slater H, Goldfarb W. Inhalation injury with burns: a lethal combination. *J Emerg Med* 1988;6:471.
4. Calahane M, Demling RH. Early respiratory abnormalities from smoke inhalation. *JAMA* 1984;251:771.
5. Clark WR. Smoke inhalation: diagnosis and treatment. *World J Surg* 1992;16:24.
6. Fein A, Leff A, Hopewell PC. Pathophysiology and management of the complications resulting from fire and the inhaled products of combustion: review of the literature. *Crit Care Med* 1980;8:94.
7. Gad SC, Anderson RC. *Combustion toxicology*. Boca Raton, FL: CRC Press, 1990.
8. Hart GB, Strauss MB, Lennon PA, et al. Treatment of smoke inhalation by hyperbaric oxygen. *J Emerg Med* 1987;5:317.
9. Herndon DN, Thompson PB, Traber DL. Pulmonary injury in burned patients. *Crit Care Clin* 1985;1:79.
10. Hoffman RS, Santer D. Methemoglobinemia resulting from smoke inhalation. *Vet Hum Toxicol* 1989;31:168.
11. Kirk MA, Gerace R, Kulig KW. Cyanide and methemoglobin kinetics in smoke inhalation victims treated with the cyanide antidote kit. *Ann Emerg Med* 1993;22:1413.
12. Landrock AH. *Handbook of plastic flammability and combustion toxicology*. Park Ridge, NJ: Noyes, 1983.
13. Lee MJ, O'Connell DJ. The plain chest radiograph after acute smoke inhalation. *Clin Radiol* 1988;39:33.
14. Marshall SW, Runyan CW, Bangdiwala SI, et al. Fatal residential fires: who dies and who survives. *JAMA* 1998;279:1633.
15. Moylan JA. Smoke inhalation and burn injury. *Surg Clin North Am* 1980;60:1533.
16. Pruitt BA, Cioff WG, Shimazu T, et al. Evaluation and management of patients with inhalation injury. *J Trauma* 1990;30:563.
17. Shusterman D, Alexeeff G, Hargis C, et al. Predictors of carbon monoxide and hydrogen cyanide exposure in smoke inhalation patients. *Clin Toxicol* 1996;34:61.
18. Thorn SR. Smoke inhalation. *Emerg Med Clin North Am* 1989;7:371.
19. Wald PH, Balmes JR. Respiratory effects of short-term high-intensity toxic inhalation: smoke, gases and fumes. *J Intensive Care Med* 1987;2:260.
20. Wroblewski DA, Bower GC. Significance of facial burns in acute smoke inhalation. *Crit Care Med* 1979;7:335.

CHAPTER 397
Submersion Injuries

Gregory A. Volturo

Drowning, responsible for over 8,000 deaths per year in the United States, is the fourth most common cause of death in adults and the third most common in children.[5] Death rates from drowning are more than five times greater for males than for females, and nearly three times greater for Blacks than for Whites.

The highest incidence occurs between ages 10 and 19. Forty percent of victims are less than 4 years old. More than half of those who drown in swimming pools are under age 10. Swimming pools, however, account only for 10% of all reported drownings. Drownings are more likely in lakes, rivers, or oceans. Quarries, pits, ornamental pools, spas, and bathtubs also contribute to the toll.[6] Toddlers may even become trapped in a bucket when they lean over to play with the water inside. Nonlethal incidents occur an estimated 600 times more often than their fatal counterparts.[13] Factors that increase the likelihood of a submersion accident include alcohol and drug use, the inability to swim, seizures, hyperventilation, hypothermia, injury during diving or other water sports, and exhaustion.

Drowning is death from suffocation due to submersion in a fluid; *near-drowning* implies survival, at least temporarily, after such suffocation. Wet drowning (when fluid is aspirated) occurs in 85% to 90% of cases, and dry drowning (when fluid is not aspirated) occurs in the remainder. Dry drowning is thought to be due to laryngospasm. *Secondary drowning* is death is due to respiratory failure from the respiratory distress syndrome (RDS) that occurs within 72 hours of initial resuscitation.

RDS results from an influx of proteins and fluid into the alveoli due to loss of surfactant and leaky capillary membranes and is secondary to hypoxia and acidosis. Patients with secondary drowning have subtle respiratory compromise immediately after submersion. About 15% of near-drowning victims who are conscious when admitted to the hospital die of RDS.[5] The *immersion syndrome* is sudden death immediately following immersion in very cold water. It is appears to be due to vagally mediated bradysystolic cardiac arrest, or ventricular fibrillation.[2]

Drowning may begin with an initial period of panic, followed by a struggle, with breath-holding. Subsequently, apnea occurs, followed by swallowing of large amounts of water, which may be vomited and aspirated. The victim ultimately loses consciousness; shortly thereafter, cardiac arrest ensues.[19] More commonly, however, witnesses report that the victim was just floating on the water and became motionless or disappeared.[7]

Theoretically, in fresh-water drowning, aspirated water is hypotonic and should be rapidly absorbed across the alveolar membrane and into the intravascular space, resulting in hemodilution and hypervolemia, with lowering of serum electrolyte and protein levels. In contrast, with hyperosmolar saltwater aspiration, fluid would be expected to diffuse in the opposite direction, resulting in pulmonary edema, hypovolemia, hemoconcentration, and electrolyte abnormalities.

Although such changes may occur in those who are dead at the scene, they are of minor clinical importance in resuscitated patients, who generally have been submerged for a short period and have aspirated a relatively small volume of water (rarely greater than 3 to 4 mL/kg).[3,5] Although pulmonary injury may occur with aspiration of as little as 2 mL/kg of water, significant changes in intravascular volume are generally not seen with less than 10 mg/kg. More than 22 mL/kg is required before electrolyte changes occur, except for incidents in water with very high solute concentrations, such as the Dead Sea.[8]

Noncardiogenic pulmonary edema may occur in both freshwater and saltwater drowning but is less likely with aspiration of fresh water. Hypoxia and the direct effect of aspirated water combine to produce this abnormality in about 5% of near-drowning cases.[14] The causes of hypoxia include diffusion abnormalities and decreased lung compliance (due to the inactivation and dilution of surfactant) and increased intrapulmonary shunting (resulting from atelectasis, bronchospasm, and obstruction of alveoli by water and debris such as vomitus or sand).[5] Chlorine in swimming pools may have an additional deleterious effect on pulmonary tissues. Aspiration of bacteria may also result in pneumonia.

Acidosis is common and is due to both metabolic and respiratory causes (inadequate ventilation results in anaerobic metabolism with lactic acid production). The acidosis may be worse in warm-water drownings than in cold water.[5] Generally, all patients who are acidotic on admission (pH less than 7.3) do poorly. However, profound acidosis is still compatible with full recovery.

Cardiovascular complications may develop as a result of hypoxia and acidosis. Hypothermia may also be a contributory factor. The most common findings are arterial hypotension and cardiac arrest. Ventricular fibrillation is rare, particularly in normothermic patients. The diving reflex, a vagally mediated response to cold-water immersion, consisting of apnea, bradycardia, peripheral vasoconstriction, decreased cardiac output, and increased mean arterial blood pressure, may also be responsible for some of the cardiovascular changes seen in drowning victims.[20] While the diving reflex has been thought to have a neuroprotective role in children, it has not been shown to be active in human adults. Hypoxic stimulation of chemoreceptors in the carotid body may result in vagally mediated bradycardia, even to the point of asystole.[16]

Renal failure, although uncommon, may be due to anoxia or to hemoglobin or myoglobin deposition in the renal tubules secondary to hemolysis or rhabdomyolysis.[17] Hemolysis can occur in fresh-water drownings but is rare. Disseminated intravascular coagulation, also uncommon, may be caused by hypoxia, acidosis, or extensive pulmonary endothelial damage.

Severe neurologic damage occurs in 15% to 25% of near-drowning patients.[17] A favorable neurologic outcome is more likely in patients receiving cardiopulmonary resuscitation (CPR) and those with hypothermia (due to its protective effect on cerebral metabolism).[1,2,12] Neurologic injury is due to hypoxia, which is further complicated by metabolic acidosis and secondary cerebral hypoperfusion. As a result, cerebral edema develops and may lead to brainstem herniation and death. The degree of anoxic injury depends on the duration of hypoxia, the water temperature, and the patient's underlying physical condition.[2] From 10% to 20% of patients presenting with coma recover completely, despite initially fixed and dilated pupils.[10]

CLINICAL PRESENTATION

Victims of near-drowning may be awake, lethargic but arousable, combative, comatose, or in cardiac arrest on presentation. A history of coughing, choking, or vomiting may be given. In mild cases, the pulse, blood pressure, and respiratory rate may be elevated, but in patients with severe hypoxia, vital signs may be decreased or absent. Hypothermia may be present. Examination may reveal cool, clammy, pale, or cyanotic skin. Aspirated or regurgitated food, water, or other foreign material may be present in the mouth and airway. Rhonchi, rales, or wheezing may be audible on pulmonary examination. Gastric distention is common. In severe cases, decorticate or decerebrate posturing or flaccid paralysis with unreactive pupils and absent cranial nerve, brainstem, and deep tendon reflexes may be observed. Associated traumatic injuries may also be present. Victims of scuba-diving accidents may have signs and symptoms of concomitant barotrauma and decompression sickness (see Chapters 389 and 390).

The electrocardiogram (ECG) may reveal evidence of ischemia, sinus tachycardia or bradycardia, or ventricular ectopy, fibrillation, or asystole. Atrial fibrillation may also occur, primarily in patients with hypothermia. Arterial blood gas analysis may reveal acidosis, hypoxia, and hypercapnia. Although leukocytosis may be present, the hematocrit is usually normal. Except for a decrease in bicarbonate, serum chemistries are usually normal on presentation. Evidence of hemolysis, infection, rhabdomyolysis, and anoxic organ damage (e.g., liver and renal failure, disseminated intravascular coagulation) may appear hours or days after the initial insult.

The chest radiograph may reveal isolated or diffuse patchy infiltrates or frank pulmonary edema. An initially normal radiograph may reveal these findings if repeated several hours later. Pulmonary edema has been reported to develop as long as 12 hours after the submersion incident.[12]

DIFFERENTIAL DIAGNOSIS

In patients found unresponsive in water or other fluid, the possibility of trauma (especially head and neck), drug or chemical intoxication, cardiac arrest or stroke while swimming, cerebral air embolus (in scuba divers), and attempted suicide, murder, or child abuse or neglect should be considered.

EMERGENCY DEPARTMENT EVALUATION

The history includes details such as submersion time, medium, and temperature; events surrounding the accident; level of consciousness and vital signs at the scene; and signs, symptoms, and treatment before arrival. For children who fall into pails of liquid (e.g., detergent, insecticide), or industrial workers who may be submerged in a medium other than water, the type of liquid and its potential toxicity should be ascertained. An accident near rocks, in heavy surf, or while diving, or an unwitnessed event, may suggest traumatic injury.

The physical examination is initially brief and focuses on vital signs, cardiopulmonary status, and neurologic findings. To rule out hypothermia, a rectal temperature should be taken using a low-reading thermometer or probe. Serial coma grading (using, for instance, the Glasgow Coma Scale) is helpful in monitoring progress. In all patients, an initial cardiac rhythm and chest radiograph and, subsequently, an ECG, should be obtained. Baseline laboratory evaluation should include an arterial blood gas analysis, complete blood count, platelet count, serum chemistries (electrolytes, glucose, blood urea nitrogen, creatinine), coagulation profile, and urinalysis. Seriously ill patients should also have liver function tests and calcium, magnesium, and creatine phosphokinase measurements. Cardiac enzymes should be obtained in victims who require CPR or who have dysrhythmias or ECG evidence of ischemia. A computed tomography scan of the head should be performed to evaluate for cerebral edema, trauma, and other pathology in those who are comatose.

EMERGENCY DEPARTMENT MANAGEMENT

Rapid prehospital response and early initiation of resuscitation are the most important factors influencing morbidity and mortality. Although artificial ventilation can and should be started immediately in unconscious patients, cardiac compression is impractical and ineffective while the victim is still in the water. Hence, rapid extrication is essential. It is best performed by those trained in, and equipped for, water rescue to prevent additional casualties (e.g., accidental hypothermia or submersion injury in rescuers). As soon as possible, victims should have cervical and backboard immobilization if the history or setting suggests spinal injury.

After extrication, CPR and advanced cardiac and trauma life-support measures are instituted, as necessary. The airway should be cleared of fluid and vomitus before assisted breathing is started. Except for placing the victim in a head-down position, postural drainage procedures are not recommended, because the risks (loss of airway control, aggravation of spinal and other injuries, aspiration, and interruption of CPR) outweigh the possible but unproven benefits.[9,14] The Heimlich maneuver may be used to clear the airway if it is obstructed with particulate matter, but it is of unproven value in removing aspirated fluid. Indiscriminate use in victims with submersion injury may result in vomiting and aspiration of gastric contents.

All victims of submersion injury should receive high-flow oxygen and endotracheal intubation if clinically indicated. Wet clothing should be removed to prevent cooling and to allow inspection of traumatic injuries. In patients who remain obtunded, cyanotic, or hypotensive despite intubation and fluid resuscitation, and in those who present with cardiac dysrhythmias, acidosis is often present, and $NaHCO_3$ (1 to 2 mEq/kg) should be given empirically.[17] Naloxone and 50% dextrose (or a bedside glucose determination) should also be considered in the unconscious patient.

In the emergency department, treatment of hypoxia is of utmost importance. If not intubated on the basis of clinical indications, patients with an arterial PO_2 below 60 mm Hg and a PCO_2 above 50 mm Hg, with an oxygen saturation less than 90% while receiving high-flow O_2 by mask, should be intubated. If only hypoxia is present, continuous positive airway pressure by mask (CPAP) may be useful. In intubated patients with persistent hypoxia, mechanical ventilation with positive end-expiratory pressure (PEEP) will decrease the amount of intrapulmonary shunting, reduce ventilation–perfusion mismatch, and increase the functional residual capacity, resulting in an increased PaO_2. Its principal disadvantage is that by diminishing venous return from the head, it may result in worsening cerebral edema.[17] The use of extracorporeal membrane oxygenation or partial liquid fluorocarbon ventilation should be considered in patients unresponsive to 100% oxygen and PEEP. Because persistent hypoxia may be due to aspirated foreign material, aggressive suctioning and bronchoscopy may be necessary.

Bronchospasm can be treated with aerosolized bronchodilators and intravenous aminophylline. The administration of corticosteroids has not been shown to improve outcome and is not indicated in near-drowning.[7] Prophylactic antibiotics have not been proven useful in preventing infection after aspiration and are unnecessary, except when aspirated water is known to have been grossly contaminated (aspiration of sewage).[7]

The initial therapy for hypotension is intravenous fluid replacement with an isotonic crystalloid solution. Monitoring of central venous or pulmonary artery pressures, as well as urinary output by Foley catheter, may be necessary to guide fluid resuscitation. Adequate fluid resuscitation should be achieved before vasopressors are used. Volume status must be carefully monitored so that the patient is not overloaded with fluid, which may worsen cerebral or pulmonary edema.[4,11,17] Severe or persistent metabolic acidosis is treated with intravenous sodium bicarbonate.[9]

Gastric decompression by a nasogastric tube is recommended in any symptomatic near-drowning victim to prevent vomiting, aspiration, and further respiratory compromise.

Cerebral resuscitation depends primarily on rapid stabilization and correction of metabolic abnormalities. Moderate hyperventilation, elevation of the head, osmotic and loop diuretics, and muscle relaxation may be beneficial in patients with increased intracranial pressure. Pharmacologic treatment of agitation and seizures may also be necessary.[11] Treatments such as therapeutic dehydration, induced hypothermia (e.g., to 300°C), barbiturate coma, and paralysis are unproved.[14]

DISPOSITION

Patients who have been apneic or unconscious; those with extremes of age; those with hypoxia, dysrhythmias, ECG evidence of ischemia, or an abnormal chest radiograph; and those whose symptoms persist after emergency department evaluation and treatment should be admitted. The level of care (floor or intensive care) depends on the severity and progression of clinical and laboratory findings. Patients who are asymptomatic, or become so after 4 to 6 hours of observation, and have a normal physical examination, room-air arterial blood gas analysis, and chest radiograph may be discharged home with a responsible relative or friend.[15] They should be instructed to return immediately if any symptoms develop (e.g., cough, sneezing, dyspnea, fever).

Indications for transfer include lack of intensive care facilities and lack of a pulmonary specialist capable of performing bronchoscopy.

COMMON PITFALLS

- Failure to consider the possibility of accidental and nonaccidental trauma, cerebral air embolism, drug intoxication, hypothermia, and medical or psychiatric illness in all near-drowning victims
- Indiscriminate use of the Heimlich maneuver, which may be useful for clearing the upper airway of particulate matter but is of unproven efficacy in removing aspirated fluid
- Failure to appreciate that patients who initially appear moribund may recover completely and that, conversely, those who present with mild symptoms may later deteriorate
- Failure to observe patients with a history of near-drowning and normal findings on emergency department evaluation for at least 4 to 6 hours
- Failure to perform early evaluation and treatment of hypoxia and cerebral edema in order to prevent or minimize neurologic damage
- Failure to recognize and treat hypothermia

References

1. Chochinov AH. Recovery of a 62 year old man from prolonged cold water submersion. *Ann Emerg Med* 1998;31:127.
2. DeNicola LK. Submersion injuries in children and adults. *Crit Care Clin* 1997;13:477.
3. Harris MG. Drowning in man. *Crit Care Med* 1981;9:407.
4. Levin DL. Drowning and near drowning. *Pediatr Clin North Am* 1993;40:321.
5. Martin TG. Near-drowning and cold-water immersion. *Ann Emerg Med* 1984;13:263.
6. MMWR. Aquatic deaths and injuries—United States. August 13, 1982.
7. Modell JH. Drowning. *N Engl J Med* 1993;328:253.
8. Modell JH, Moya F. Effects of toxicity of saline solution on pulmonary injury in drowning. *Anesthesia* 1966;27:662.
9. Neal JM. Near-drowning. *J Emerg Med* 1985;3:41.
10. Oakes DA, Sherck JP, Maloney JR, et al. Prognosis and management of victims of near-drowning. *J Trauma* 1982;22:554.
11. Olshaker JS. Near drowning. *Emerg Med Clin North Am* 1992;10:339.
12. Orlowski JP. Drowning, near-drowning, and ice-water submersions. *Pediatr Clin North Am* 1987;43:75.
13. Orlowski JP, Abulleil MM, Phillips JM. Effects of toxicities of saline solutions on pulmonary injury in drowning. *Crit Care Med* 1987;15:126.
14. Oronato JP. Resuscitation of near-drowning victims. *JAMA* 1986;256:75.
15. Pratt FD, Haynes BE. Incidence of secondary drowning after saltwater submersion. *Ann Emerg Med* 1986;15:1084.
16. Redmond AD, Mallikarijun TS. Resuscitation from drowning. *Arch Emerg Med* 1984;2:113.
17. Robinson MD, Seward PN. Submersion injury in children. *Crit Care Med* 1987;3(1):44.
18. Smyrnios NA. Current concepts in the pathophysiology and management of near drowning. *J Intensive Care Med* 1991;6:26.
19. Weinstein MD. Near drowning: epidemiology, pathophysiology, and initial treatment. *J Emerg Med* 1996;14:461.
20. Wittmers LE Jr, Pozos RS, Fall G, et al. Cardiovascular responses to face immersion (the diving reflex) in human beings after alcohol consumption. *Ann Emerg Med* 1987;16:1031.

SECTION VIII

Section Editor: Christopher H. Linden

Essentials of Administrative and Clinical Issues in the Emergency Department

PART I

Administrative and Operational Aspects of Emergency Medicine

CHAPTER 398

Airmedical Services

Kenneth A. Williams

Airmedical care refers to the care of patients during aircraft transport. *Airmedicine* is occasionally confused with *aeromedicine*, the study of flight and altitude physiology. Although it is important to understand aeromedicine when practicing airmedicine, the two are distinct fields. The vehicle itself is only part of airmedical care; air ambulances represent sophisticated systems of care that alter previously held notions about patient referral and transport.

HISTORY

Although there is debate about when the first airmedical transport occurred, and whether the aircraft was a balloon or a fixed-wing airplane,[7] the history of airmedicine is linked to military conflict. The helicopter was first widely and successfully used during the wars in Korea and Vietnam, where it offered advantages of access in hostile jungle terrain and rapid transport speed for short-range patient rescue.[9] The helicopter developed significantly from an aviation perspective during the time between those two conflicts. The aircraft typically used during the Korean conflict carried the patient on externally mounted stretchers, precluding medical care in flight. During the Vietnam War, patients were usually transported inside the aircraft and received medical attention during transport. Over 100 air ambulances, performing more than 7,000 evacuations monthly by 1968, and about 900,000 total missions, were used during 11 years of operation in Vietnam.[8,13]

Civilian application of helicopter medical care within the continental United States began as personnel experienced with military airmedical helicopter operations returned from Vietnam during the 1960s and 1970s and proposed that similar technology would be beneficial in the civilian environment, particularly for trauma victims.[11] Fixed-wing airmedical care systems already existed on a small scale and were used primarily to transport medical personnel to patients. During the 1970s, other countries also developed air ambulance services, some focusing on emergent patient transport, some on delivery of medical resources to remote areas, and others on rescue.

Common sense argues that patients with a survivable illness or injury will benefit from early, high-quality medical care. Early scientific analysis of clinical helicopter medical care focused on trauma, with some consideration for cardiac, pediatric, and obstetric patients. Additional focuses included appropriateness of use, estimation of need, and clinical techniques during flight.

Although a wealth of helicopter medical literature exists, rigorous appraisal has been limited by sample size, confounding variables, and lack of concurrent control groups.[19] Education of referral facilities, coordination, and consultation with tertiary care hospitals before and during transport; increasing regionalization and specialization; and advances in emergency medical services (EMS) and emergency medicine have confounded efforts to separate the effects of airmedical care from other changes in medicine. There is relatively little literature evaluating fixed-wing airmedical care and even less on long-distance ("repatriation") care during commercial airline flights.

SYSTEM DESIGN

Multiple factors influence the design of airmedical systems, the most important of which are safety and the system mission. The type of aircraft used, the medical team composition and resources, and availability are additional considerations. Search-and-rescue operations,[15] for example, focus on finding and removing the victim from an endangering environment and require a design significantly different from that of interhospital patient transport programs, which focus on care in transport between relatively safe sites. Many (about 175 in the United States) full-time dedicated helicopter airmedical programs are based at or supported by hospitals and are staffed with medical professionals. Physicians, nurses, paramedics, and respiratory therapists are the most common members of the airmedical crew, with physician assistants, nurse practitioners, and other providers found in some systems.

Part-time fixed-wing airmedical programs utilize aircraft reconfigured from other uses and perform elective long-distance transfer of stable patients as their mission, using on-call nurse or paramedic crews. Some systems offer both fixed-wing and helicopter services, and an increasing number coordinate with or directly provide ground ambulance transfers as well. Few civilian airmedical systems in the United States focus on search-and-rescue operations, leaving that mission to the Coast Guard and other agencies. Many, however, perform limited search operations, and some train in regionally specific rescue, such as hover operations over water, snow, or wilderness terrain. In other countries, the rescue mission is often a component of airmedical systems, with winch lift and other rescue functions not unusual.

GENERAL AEROMEDICINE

The patient being transported by aircraft is subject to several forces not commonly encountered during hospital care: changes in altitude, noise, vibration, acceleration, and motion. With increasing altitude, oxygen tension is decreased and gas expands. The atmospheric pressure at 18,000 ft is half that at sea level. Hence, attention to oxygenation and any enclosed gas (e.g., pneumothorax, intestinal gas, middle ear, glass intravenous bottles, tube cuffs, splints) is required with any change in altitude of more than several thousand feet. The noise and vibration encountered in flight may increase stress for the patient and limit the effectiveness of routine medical procedures, such as auscultation of the chest and abdomen and palpation of the pulse.

Severe vibration may disturb fractures, trigger pacemakers and automatic internal defibrillators, reduce the accuracy of oscillographic blood pressure monitors, and limit the ability to perform manual procedures such as intravenous cannulation. Motions encountered in flight include yaw, roll, and pitch, with acceleration and deceleration in any direction also possible. Nausea, disorientation, and anxiety are not uncommon sequelae. Unfamiliar stimuli from being in atypical positions (lying backward, sitting sideways) and the strobe effect from helicopter rotors may also result in nausea and spatial disorientation. A patient who is afraid of flying may produce additional challenges for the crew.

AVIATION ISSUES

Aircraft

Factors influencing the choice of aircraft include the space and configuration of the patient care area, loading door size and arrangement, useful load, balance flexibility, speed and climb performance, range, altitude and pressurization limits, landing zone or runway needs, and capability for Instrument Flight Rules (IFRs) in addition to Visual Flight Rules (VFRs) flight. The Federal Aviation Administration sets rules for aircraft equipment and operation in the United States, including pilot qualifications and installation of any supplemental equipment, such as patient stretchers or medical equipment. Although electronic medical equipment is often certified for hospital use, it is rarely tested in the aviation environment for interaction with navigation instruments or other aircraft electronics. Concerns regarding possible interference with medical equipment from communications devices such as cell phones are magnified in the aircraft environment, where several radio transceivers are commonly installed with antennas in close proximity to medical equipment.

Fixed-wing aircraft typically used for airmedical care are mid-sized, twin-engine propeller or jet aircraft. Most are capable of flight in poor visibility (IFR), cruise at 200 to 400 mi/h for ranges of 1,000 to 2,000 mi with useful loads of 2,000 to 7,000 lb, and can climb to altitudes of 25,000 to 30,000 ft with pressurized cabins. These characteristics make fixed-wing aircraft most useful for missions over 150 to 200 miles, in which the delay for airport transportation at either end becomes less significant. In addition, the useful load and altitude characteristics increase the margin of safety for operating these aircraft in hot or mountainous areas.

Airmedical helicopters are generally light turbine-powered, mid-sized helicopters, with the proportion of twin-engine aircraft relative to single-engine aircraft increasing steadily. Cruising speeds of 100 to 160 mi/h, with ranges of 325 to 550 miles, a useful load of 1,500 to 3,000 lb, and service ceilings of 13,000 to 20,000 ft are typical. IFR flight is possible, but the need to avoid icing conditions and to fly between or near airports capable of instrument approaches limits the usefulness of IFR for airmedical care. The Global Positioning Satellite [GPS] system has expanded airmedical IFR capabilities in some areas, but concerns regarding decreased safety with poor visibility operations continue to be validated by aircraft accidents in such weather conditions.

Landing Zones

Helicopters are generally capable of vertical takeoff and landing, but there are some limits. From the pilot's point of view, a large, level area without wires, trees, or other overhead obstructions is ideal for landings, and a tall tower with a short runway surrounded by clear airspace is best for takeoffs. Most landing and takeoff sites are compromises, with clear approach and departure from a level, 100 × 100-ft area proving adequate for most helicopter operations. Helicopter weight, wind and temperature conditions, and nearby obstructions also influence helipad locations.

Hospital helipads should be designated sites with rapid access (within minutes) to the emergency department. Some programs inspect and catalogue potential landing sites near intersections, highways, and areas of high call volume. All sites should exceed program minimum standards and should be secured by educated personnel before landing. Laws regulating helipad designation and use may vary and should also be considered.

Programs that operate in inclement weather (Instrument Meteorologic Conditions [IMC]), using IFR, require additional capabilities at landing sites, including the means to perform an instrument approach. Fixed-wing aircraft need runway or landing strip access at both the sending and receiving ends of the transport, and at least one alternative destination if flying in inclement weather. Such services and facilities are generally available only at airports and are regulated by the Federal Aviation Administration.

Weather Limits

Airmedical programs operate within weather constraints, primarily visibility (distance) and ceiling (height above ground before cloud cover). Winds aloft, temperature, dew point, and presence of icing conditions, fog, storms, and other specific conditions may also determine their ability to respond and the type of response (VFR vs. IFR, helicopter vs. fixed-wing). High temperatures reduce engine power and blade lift due to decreased air density. Because weather forecasting is not an exact science, local conditions may vary markedly from the regional forecast.

Programs must make a decision about weather conditions and their ability to respond on a call-by-call basis. Occasionally, one program may be asked to perform a mission when another has already turned down the request. The second program should be informed that the request has previously been refused and why. This allows the second airmedical program to judge whether local or regional weather conditions allow the mission to be accomplished safely. For example, there may be inclement weather between the first program and the referring facility, but the second program may have an acceptable route. This precaution is particularly true for VFR programs, as many airmedical helicopter accidents involve inadvertent entry into IMC weather and subsequent pilot disorientation.

Speed and Range

Aircraft speed, fuel capacity, and fuel consumption rate define the useful range. The ability to pick up a patient and return to base without refueling is desirable but not essential. In many cases, refueling can occur while the patient is being prepared for transport. Refueling with the patient and crew onboard is discouraged but is possible with adequate precautions. Typically, airmedical helicopters can cover a service area radius of 120 to 140 miles without refueling. Fixed-wing aircraft generally have a useful range of several hundred to a thousand miles.

MEDICAL ISSUES

Airmedical Care

Patient care during airmedical transport must take into account environmental and temporal factors. Also, the airmedical team is typically a scarce resource, and system needs must also be considered. Because the referring facility or ambulance service often requests a transfer because they are overwhelmed by patient volume or severity, the airmedical team is usually entering a stressful environment. In addition, unless the team makes frequent visits to the same referring facility, they are also entering an unfamiliar one.

The airmedical team generally begins care by placing the patient on their stretcher and attaching various monitoring devices. Intravenous lines, endotracheal and other tubes, and other equipment may be disconnected accidentally during patient movement to the stretcher and transfer to the aircraft and must be secured. Monitoring equipment must often substitute for physical assessment of the patient, given the noisy environment and limited access to the patient. Limited access also means that performing procedures such as gastric emptying, splinting, pneumothorax decompression, and patient restraint are best done before takeoff. Delays in transport resulting from flight preparation of the patient may cause conflict with the referring staff, who desire prompt evacuation, unless the unique aircraft environment is appreciated.

Once in flight, the airmedical care team must consider aeromedical influences on their medical care, as previously discussed. Treatment may be initiated or continued, radio reports given to the receiving facility, documentation begun, and triage of upcoming requests performed. These tasks are typically performed by a two-person medical crew, while the pilot attends to the aircraft. Some programs use two pilots, particularly for IFR missions, and some use one medical crew for most missions with others used for specialized care, such as neonatal or intraaortic balloon pump transports.

Choosing a Service

Choosing an airmedical service provider to transport a patient involves the same concerns as with ground ambulances: availability, location, level of care, reliability, and past performance. Receiving hospitals usually prefer to use their own program. Some third-party payors have specific transport arrangements. Referring facilities should be aware of the capabilities and limits of area airmedical programs to facilitate arrangements when the need arises.

Patient Preparation

When preparing a patient for transfer, the referring clinician should also consider likely treatments and potential complications during flight. Preparing the patient before the aircraft arrives will save the flight crew time and facilitate evacuation. Records, test results, and other documentation should also be provided.

Patient Acceptance

The referring physician must ensure that the patient is accepted by a physician who can provide care and has adequate facilities available for that care. This is both good medical practice and a requirement of the Emergency Medical Treatment and Labor Act provisions of COBRA (see Chapter 408). Some airmedical programs have systems to arrange rapid acceptance of patients, particularly trauma and other critically ill patients referred to their own or member institutions. In other cases, acceptance by a specific physician or service may be necessary before takeoff.

Transfer of Care

After acceptance, there is a gradual transfer of responsibility from the referring to the receiving physician and facility. This responsibility transfer parallels the physical transfer of the patient and is essentially complete when the patient arrives at the receiving facility. Traditionally, the referring facility has been held legally responsible for the patient until arrival at the receiving hospital. However, this opinion was formed before the development of advanced and critical care transfer services, and airmedical staff will probably be held responsible for care provided during the transfer. Until better defined, the transition of responsibility should be mutually understood as a gradual and cooperative process. Written transfer agreements can be developed to clarify issues such as staff privileges and licensing requirements for the nurses and physicians from the airmedical program while at the referring facility or on out-of-state missions, and for the transfer of responsibility and the loan and return of patient-care equipment.

Crew Mix

The level and type of training for staff in most hospitals and ground EMS systems is well accepted, but the optimal mix of an airmedical crew remains controversial. There are supporters for physicians, nurses, paramedics, and others as airmedical crew, depending on the mission.[16] The literature, although limited by sample size and confounded by program variability, suggests that physician skill and judgment are important,[14] that airmedical experience is well accepted and considered a valuable educational experience by emergency medicine residents,[3] and that nurses and others can perform advanced skills in programs with off-line, protocol-based medical direction.[18]

Physician presence arguably makes more sense as the acuity and severity of illness or injury increases and as the transport time increases. Technical ability is important, but more relevant arguments include judgment, greater medical knowledge, and ability to operate without rigid protocols and on-line medical direction. Compliance with good medical practice during transfer, as well as with federal law (see Chapter 408), also demands that the level of care must not diminish during transfer, if possible. Thus, a patient who needs the constant presence of a physician and nurse before transfer should ideally have similar care during transfer, whereas a patient whose condition is more stable and whose likely complications could be managed by protocol could be transferred by crew with a lower level of training.

Each program should consider the issue of crew mix individually after examining patient and staff data.[17] Facilities requesting airmedical care should know the crew mix and capabilities of area programs, and choose the best option for their patient.

SAFETY

Patient safety includes access to medical therapy as well as vehicular transfer risks. A common misconception is that the patient must be stabilized before transfer. Patients who can be stabilized should be, but patients who need specialized definitive care may die without timely transfer, and stabilization may be impossible if such care is unavailable at the current location. Thus, it may be best not to delay the transfer because the patient is "too unstable to transfer," but instead provide *earlier* transfer because the patient is "too unstable to stay." Patient safety during transfer is a balance between the need for the transfer and the risks of that transfer.

In 1991, about 128,000 helicopter airmedical transfers occurred in the United States, with an accident rate of 3.10 per 100,000 transports, or 2.98 per 100,000 flight-hours, because each transport takes about 1 flight-hour.[12] The accident rate has decreased since the 1980s, but airmedical helicopters still crash at about three times the rate of non-EMS helicopters, and the fatality rate in those crashes is also higher. The rate of ground ambulance accidents is about ten times higher than the airmedical helicopter rate,[2] but the severity of injuries is lower.

Air travel, mile for mile, is safer than highway driving, but many more people are afraid to fly than to drive. Air travel generally involves less personal control, an unfamiliar environment, and greater risk of death should an accident occur. Airmedical program administrators and clinical staff should understand these perceptions and misperceptions when they educate others about their program, particularly those who resist requesting airmedical care because of unrealistic perceptions of risk.

About 90% of aircraft accidents are attributed to judgment error, usually continued flight into deteriorating weather. Airmedical helicopter accidents occur about equally during day or night; about a third occur en route, and two-thirds occur during takeoff or landing. Although a review of airmedical helicopter accidents failed to identify any other personnel causes, such as fatigue, lack of training, or drug abuse,[10] pilot fatigue tends to be cited as a factor despite the findings that accidents were not clustered at the end of shifts, late at night, or in any other way likely to be associated with fatigue.

Twin-engine helicopters are often recommended, because the redundancy of systems reduces the risk of accident from engine failure. However, because few accidents overall are caused by engine failure, it is difficult to prove with statistical significance that twin-engine helicopters are safer than single-engine aircraft. Further, it is unproved that the additional cost of twin-engine aircraft is money better spent for safety than money spent on pilot training, program design and education, and other measures to improve judgment and maintenance ability.

Helicopters, perhaps more than fixed-wing aircraft, are delicate aircraft requiring frequent preventive maintenance and inspection. However, few hospital-based helicopter airmedical programs have a hanger adjacent to their helipad. Daily inspections and most routine maintenance must then be performed outdoors, often from a ladder or while balancing on small steps built into the side of the aircraft, regardless of weather or time of day, thus forcing mechanics to work in an environment unacceptable to those who service the hospital's ground vehicles. This lack of basic aviation facilities is a significant issue for the safe operation of helicopter programs at hospitals. Support for airmedical programs may be provided directly by the hospital that buys or leases aircraft and hires personnel, by a government agency that operates the program, or by a contracted aviation vendor. Regardless of the type of support, the sponsoring institution should provide adequate resources for needed maintenance, aviation facilities, pilot and mechanic training, and other aviation services necessary to operate the program safely. An understanding of aviation operations is necessary to avoid making unsafe decisions, such as skipping maintenance, hiring unqualified personnel, or taking other measures that reduce immediate costs but risk long-term problems.

A review of factors associated with occupant survival showed that interior modifications to create patient-care capability probably increase the risk of injury, due to lack of restraint systems and load-absorbing seats and addition of loose equipment and intrusions into the head-strike area.[4] Hence, focusing on judgment training and safety-oriented interior modifications appears most likely to address the real cause of airmedical accidents and associated injuries.

COST AND CHARGES

Some argue that the true cost of operating an airmedical program should be reflected in charges for that service. However, many programs are heavily subsidized, operating under the assumption that losses will be recovered through inpatient revenue. This dichotomy creates a situation in which emergency medical services are potentially undervalued and in which the billed charges for airmedical care may vary by a factor of 10 or more for similar service. Third-party payors are understandably confused by this situation and naturally wish to pay the lowest common charge. Whether airmedical services should be subsidized or offered as a public service through taxation or other government support, and whether this undervaluing of care is damaging to emergency medicine as a specialty, remain controversial. As a system, airmedical care is less costly than similar care provided by a network of ground vehicles when critical care interfacility transport is the system's primary function.[2]

MEDICAL DIRECTION

Many airmedical programs use standing orders and protocols. All should have a medical director trained and knowledgeable in prehospital and airmedical care issues. The Air Medical Physician Association provides a handbook and other resources for interested physicians.[1] If written protocols vary from the treatment plan of the referring physician, the airmedical crew should be able to justify their suggested therapy, and should contact their medical director, if necessary, to discuss issues further with the referring physician. The medical director should develop and provide referring facilities with educational programs regarding the needs and capabilities of airmedical care.

FEEDBACK AND FOLLOW-UP

Because referring staff are concerned with the eventual outcome of their patients, airmedical programs should provide timely follow-up after each mission. A telephone call immediately after the mission, even if it provides little additional information, is more likely to find the referring staff still on duty and serves to answer immediate concerns. Written follow-up letters are important and can address the patient's interval status, indicate a contact person who can provide further information, or give the final diagnosis and disposition. If possible, these should go to all parties involved in the transfer, including EMS staff, emergency department or hospital physicians and nurses, and the patient's personal physician. However, because these letters are often posted in EMS headquarters or on emergency department walls, care should be taken to protect patient confidentiality. One way to do this is to draft the letter, using only the patient's age and gender and the time and circumstances of the transfer.

EQUIPMENT RETRIEVAL

Airmedical programs and referring facilities should develop a system for identifying, decontaminating, and returning equipment. Patient care may be compromised by a demand to remove splints, spinal immobilizers, intravenous pumps, pacemakers, or other equipment before flight because of a fear that it will be lost. A system that provides the referring staff with a written receipt for their equipment and a means to return it rapidly in safe and usable condition improves the relationship between care providers.

UTILIZATION REVIEW

Utilization review of airmedical care is important to establish guidelines for appropriate use and compliance with those guidelines. A statewide review process that uses objective criteria has been found to be both functional and useful in defending the utility of airmedical care, particularly to third-party payors.[20] Program design should include consideration of these issues when aircraft type, crew mix, equipment choice, operating area, and other choices are made that may affect use.[5]

Committee opinion based on accepted criteria may establish proper utilization but does not prove effectiveness. Studies of morbidity, mortality, specific clinical situations, effectiveness and techniques, complication rates, economics and cost per year of life saved, and other issues have been published,[6] but the effectiveness of airmedical care remains difficult to establish without a large, well-controlled study population, due to the multitude of confounding factors involved in studying care systems.

References

1. Air Medical Physician Association. 383 F Street, Salt Lake City, UT 84103. Telephone: (801)321-3699; Internet site: www.ampa.org
2. Bruhn J, Williams K, Aghababian R. True costs of air medical vs. ground ambulance systems. *Air Med J* 1993;12:262.
3. Carter G, O'Brien DJ. The impact of aeromedical helicopter programs on emergency medicine resident training: resident attitude, perceived risks, and benefits. *J Emerg Med* 1986;4:471.
4. Dodd RS. *Factors related to occupant crash survival in emergency medical service helicopters*. Doctor of Science Dissertation, School of Hygiene and Public Health, Johns Hopkins University, Baltimore, 1992.
5. Eroe ER, Eljaiek L, Mayer TA, et al. The development of a hospital-based helicopter program. *J Air Med Transport* 1992;11(7):14.
6. Gabram SGA, Jacobs LM. The impact of emergency medical helicopters on prehospital care. *Emerg Med Clin North Am* 1990;8:85.
7. Macnab AJ. Air medical transport: "hot air" and a French lesson. *J Air Med Transport* 1992;11(8):15.
8. Meier DR, Samper ER. Evolution of civil aeromedical helicopter aviation. *South Med J* 1989;82:885.
9. Moylan JA. Impact of helicopters on trauma care and clinical results. *Ann Surg* 1988;208:673.
10. National Transportation Safety Board. *Safety study: emergency medical service helicopter operations*. Report no. NTSB/SS-88/01. Washington, DC: National Transportation Safety Board, 1988.
11. Neel SH. Army aeromedical evacuation procedures in Vietnam: implications for rural America. *JAMA* 1968;204:99.
12. Preston N. 1991 Air medical helicopter accident rates. *J Air Med Transport* 1992;11(2):14.
13. Reddick EJ. Evaluation of the helicopter in aeromedical transfers. *Aviat Space Environ Med* 1979;50:168.
14. Rhee KJ, Strozeski M, Burney RE, et al. Is the flight physician needed for helicopter emergency medical services? *Ann Emerg Med* 1986;15:174.
15. Saunders CE. Aeromedical transport. In: Auerbach PS, Geehr EC, eds. *Management of wilderness and environmental emergencies,* 2nd ed. St. Louis: Mosby, 1989.
16. Snow N, Hull C, Severns J. Physician presence on a helicopter emergency medical service: necessary or desirable? *Aviat Space Environ Med* 1986;57:1176.
17. Stone CK. The air medical crew: is a flight physician necessary? *J Air Med Transport* 1991;10(11):7.
18. Thomas F, Clemmer TP, Orme JF. A survey of advanced trauma life-support procedures being performed by physicians and nurses used on hospital aeromedical evacuation services. *Aviat Space Environ Med* 1985;56:1213.
19. Vido DA. *The impact of rotorcraft aeromedical emergency care services on trauma mortality: a critical analysis of the literature*. Master of Science Thesis, University of Maryland, 1986.
20. Williams K, Aghababian R, Shaughnessy M. Statewide EMS helicopter utilization review: the Massachusetts experience. *J Air Med Transport* 1990;9(9):14.

CHAPTER 399
Disaster Planning and Management

Lucille Gans

Although disasters have occurred for centuries, their frequency appears to be increasing. Rising world population numbers and increasing areas of dense population, especially in potentially dangerous environments (e.g., flood plains), suggest that greater numbers of people will be affected by disasters. Despite the fact that public attention focuses on medical casualties, it is essential to consider numerous other factors when developing effective disaster plans and responses.[20]

Disaster may be defined as a destructive event that disrupts the normal functioning of a community. *Medical disaster* refers to a catastrophic event that results in casualties that overwhelm the health-care resources of the community involved.[2] However, in addition to health and medical requirements, the basic needs of water, food, and shelter must be addressed, as well as power supplies, transportation, and communications. Refugees and displaced populations can be both the result and the cause of disasters.[6]

Disasters may be classified as natural or human-generated. Natural disasters include earthquakes, floods, volcanic eruptions, hurricanes, tornadoes, winter storms, and other geologic and meteorologic phenomena. Human-generated or technologic disasters include explosions, chemical spills, radiation leaks, biochemical terrorism, transportation accidents, civil disturbances, and armed conflicts. Complex humanitarian emergencies generally include features of both natural and technologic disasters, such as population displacement that results from a combination of drought, famine, and political upheaval.

Disasters also may be categorized by onset and impact. For example, earthquakes and tornadoes are events that have a rapid onset, with a sudden impact on the community. In contrast, droughts and famines have a more gradual onset and generally have a prolonged impact. Numerous factors may modify the impact of a disaster on a community, including the nature of the event, time of day or year, health and age characteristics of the population affected, and the availability of resources.

Defining an event as a disaster also depends on the location in which it occurs. For example, an earthquake occurring in a sparsely populated area would not be considered a disaster if no people were injured or affected by loss of housing or essential services. In contrast, a similar quake, even one of lesser magnitude, could produce extensive losses of life and property if it occurred in a densely populated region with poor construction or limited medical resources. Similarly, a small community hospital could be overwhelmed by numbers and types of casualties that might be handled routinely by a large university hospital or metropolitan medical center.

Hospitals may further classify disasters as either internal or external. External disasters are those that do not affect the hospital infrastructure but do tax hospital resources, due to numbers of patients or types of injuries. For example, a tornado that produced numerous injuries and deaths in a community would be considered an external disaster. Internal disasters cause disruption of normal hospital function, due to injuries or deaths of hospital personnel or damage to the physical plant, as with a hospital fire, power failure, or chemical spill.[1] Features of both internal and external disasters may be present if a natural phenomenon affects both the community and the hospital, as in the case of an earthquake causing significant destruction in both the hospital and the surrounding community.

DISASTER PLANNING

Disaster planning must address the problems posed by a variety of events, ranging in scale from mass casualty incidents (MCIs), such as motor vehicle collisions with multiple victims, to extensive flooding or earthquake damage, to civil wars. The disaster planning continuum includes advance preparations, as well as event management and recovery efforts. Those people and organizations responsible for disaster plans should consider all eventualities, from the sanitation needs of crowds at mass gatherings to evacuation procedures for buildings and geographic areas.[11,15]

Effective disaster planning requires identification of potential problems for the institution or community involved. Risk analysis is an essential feature of disaster planning, in which a comprehensive inventory is created for all existing and potential hazards, including location and quantity, if applicable. Hazards may include such items as chemicals used by local industry, transportation elements such as airports and railroad stations, or collections of large groups of people in areas with limited access, such as high-rise office buildings, nursing homes, or sports stadiums. Environmental and meteorologic hazards must also be considered, such as the presence of fault lines and seismic zones and the seasonal risks posed by tornadoes, hurricanes, and snowstorms.

Risk analysis should attempt to identify any groups of people at particular risk of injury or death or loss of property from each hazard. The estimated risk may be constant over time, or it may vary by time of day, season, or location relative to the community. Risk analysis necessitates the cooperation of corporate, governmental, and community groups to produce a comprehensive listing of all potential hazards.[12,13] It may be possible to reduce the relative risk posed by some hazards. Relocating a chemical depot further away from a school would reduce the risk that children would be exposed to hazardous materials, for example. Hazards must be identified before effective disaster responses can be planned.

Another essential feature of disaster planning is resource identification. Resources include both human and physical elements, such as organizations with specialized personnel and equipment.[7,18] Disaster preparedness should include assembling lists of medical and paramedical groups, public works and other civic departments, and volunteer agencies, along with phone numbers and key contact personnel for each. Hospital departments should have readily available a complete record of all personnel, including home addresses and telephone numbers, accessible 24 hours a day. Resource availability may vary with factors such as time of day and season.

Effective disaster planning must occur at all levels, from local institutions to municipal, state and federal governments, including private, volunteer, and international agencies.[3] All groups should understand their own capabilities and limitations, as well as those of the organizations with which interactions are anticipated or intended. Disaster plans should be both structured and flexible, with provisions made for plan activation and decision making by field-level managers, if indicated.[8]

Once a plan has been devised or a strategy outlined, it should be evaluated for its effectiveness and completeness. The comprehension of people expected to implement the plan and their ability to perform duties must be assessed. In addition, more concrete concepts should be evaluated, such as availability and functioning of any equipment called for by the disaster plan. A recurring problem in disaster response is failure of communications, which may result from several conditions, including loss of infrastructure damaged by the disaster itself, as well as lack of operator familiarity, excessive demands, inadequate supplies, and lack of integration with other communications providers and technologies. Back-up communications systems, such as wireless, hardwire, and cellular telephones, may reduce the impact of disrupted standard communications, but, frequently, even advanced technology has been ineffectual during disasters.[9]

An essential step in disaster planning and preparedness is the evaluation of the disaster response. Several methods may be used to exercise the disaster plan, the most comprehensive of which would be its full implementation in an actual disaster. However, disaster drills may also provide an excellent means of testing plans for their completeness and effectiveness. Drills may take the form of full-scale multijurisdictional exercises, using moulaged victims and requiring vast resources of supplies and personnel, or they may be limited to a small segment of the disaster response, such as drills that assess the effectiveness of communications protocols or notification procedures. The disaster plan also may be assessed by using table-top exercises, paper or mock patients, computer simulations, or seminar sessions focusing on key personnel or limited aspects of the disaster response.

Improved performance during the drill, with enhanced understanding of disaster planning and response, is more likely when drills are preceded by some notification that a drill is scheduled. The specific goal of any drill should be clearly understood in advance. If drills are to be used as training sessions as well as evaluations of preparations and response plans, personnel are more likely to make the correct or most appropriate response choices during the drill if they are prepared. Consequently, they will be more likely to take appropriate actions when faced with an unexpected disaster situation in the future. The more realistic the exercise, the more likely it is that useful information about the strengths and weaknesses of both the disaster plan and the responders will be acquired. The factor common to all disasters is a shortage of available resources; without experiencing at least some of the stress which accompanies that situation, it is unlikely that the disaster plan and response will be taxed at a level that realistically simulates the circumstances of an actual disaster.

Essential features of all effective disaster drills are the inclusion of all parties likely to be involved in the disaster response and a critique, with debriefing, of all participants following the exercise. Regardless of the format used, the critique should consider comments from all individuals, groups, or agencies involved in the drill. Disaster planners should review all observations and comments and respond with modifications of the disaster plan, if necessary.[17] Any alterations in disaster plans or response procedures must be communicated to all groups involved or affected. Periodic evaluations of disaster plans are essential to ensure that personnel have adequate familiarity with their roles in disaster situations, as well as to provide for changes in regional emergency response operations, hospital renovations and closings, and other variables.

DISASTER MANAGEMENT

The philosophy of disaster management may be summed up in the phrase, "The needs of the many outweigh the needs of the few." In other words, in a disaster situation, resources may be so limited that stringent rationing is vital to the survival of the maximum number of people. Austere conditions may be alien to responders accustomed to ample quantities of medical supplies, equipment, personnel, and time, but they are commonly encountered with any large-scale disaster. In this setting, difficult triage decisions must be made in order to ensure that all assets are used in the most efficient and pragmatic manner.[19]

The goal of disaster management is to provide the most appropriate intervention and assistance based on the most accurate information available in a timely manner. Disaster response includes several phases (Table 399.1) but must begin with recognition that disaster conditions exist. (Some disasters, such as hurricanes, may be preceded by a period of time, called the preimpact phase, during which advance information may be gathered about the potential effects of the disaster. The data acquired during the preimpact phase may allow prepositioning of personnel and resources in a strategic location.) Due to a lack of verifiable facts, it may be necessary, at times, to proceed on assumptions and limited data, with efforts made to tailor and modify the response as updated information becomes available. It may be helpful to consult people and organizations with experience in such varied fields as engineering, toxicology, epidemiology, geophysics, and meteorology, to name only a few, depending on the disaster or the area affected.[14]

Inevitably, in the event of a disaster that produces significant or extensive morbidity and mortality, the physician on duty in the emergency department will be one of the first people called on to assume a leadership role. The existence of a hospital disaster plan provides a valuable resource, but, ideally, the emergency physician should be prepared to do more than refer to the plan when informed of the incident. The disaster response will evolve in a much more coordinated fashion if the physician understands both the hospital plan and the resources, capabilities, and disaster plans of the first responders and emergency medical services (EMS) system in the region. The physician may be required to coordinate or facilitate the hospital response and to provide direction for numerous aspects of the regional response. For example, the task of assigning personnel and resources may be delegated to the emergency physician at the regional trauma center if no adequate disaster plan exists for the local EMS system. The physician may also be consulted regarding the need for the deployment of agencies and resources from outside the affected region. Lack of familiarity with local resources and response plans may result in unnecessary and costly delays in implementing the most efficient response. In addition, emergency department staff should expect to be bombarded with requests for information on all aspects of the disaster and response, from family members, media, and government representatives and from the public at large, and be

TABLE 399.1. Components of a Disaster Response

ACTIVATION
Notification and initial response Scene assessment
IMPLEMENTATION
Organization of command Search and rescue Victim triage, stabilization, and transport
MITIGATION
Definitive management of scene hazards and victims
RECOVERY
Scene withdrawal Return to normal operations Debriefing

prepared to refer or respond to such questions. Early in a disaster, the emergency physician and staff will likely be expected to disseminate information about the disaster event, demonstrate expertise and leadership in the response and management efforts, and even make the initial determination that disaster conditions exist. Hospital administrators, social services, and public relations personnel can provide valuable assistance and should be notified as soon as a disaster is recognized.

In the case of damaged or destroyed health-care facilities or after a large-scale disaster, the physician may also be called on to provide medical care in unconventional settings. In the situation in which field medical care stations must be established, coordinating responses with other agencies is essential. The use of a hierarchical management system, such as the Incident Command System (ICS), to coordinate the information and resource management is essential for any large-scale disaster. It is important to remember, during the early stage of the disaster, that information available from those at the disaster area (data regarding death, injury, or damage) may not be accurate. Problems with communications are frequently the source of delays and misapplications of disaster resources. The ability of those in a region devastated by a disaster to survey the population and infrastructure may be severely curtailed by damage, such that even initial calls for help may be impossible. It is essential, therefore, that external resources of personnel and equipment be available and accessible if anticipation of potential need for them arises.[16] Conversely, due to disruption of communications and transportation, it is possible for the effects of the disaster to be overestimated. In order to minimize damage and disruption, expedient decisions must be made, with future consequences of such actions considered as well. Short-term benefits and costs must be weighed against their long-term counterparts. Disasters are costly events, but judicious initial expenditures may result in substantial savings, in both monetary and humanitarian terms, over the long haul. On the other hand, excessive spending by individuals, agencies, or organizations may result in prolonged or delayed recovery from the disaster and may restrict the capability to prepare or respond when the next disaster strikes.

In the case of a disaster that causes substantial destruction of infrastructure, the response may be prolonged, requiring that long-term health-care and support services be established. Issues such as nutrition evaluation and on-going disease surveillance may require the expertise of numerous other health-care providers and agencies.[10] In addition, mental health issues must also be considered for the victims and the responders, during both the emergency phase and the recovery. Posttraumatic stress disorder, major depression, generalized anxiety disorder, and substance abuse are frequently reported among disaster survivors who have experienced traumatic bereavement or severe disruption of their lives. Early access to mental health workers for evaluation and intervention reduces the incidence and severity of such reactions. In addition, Critical Incident Stress Debriefing (CISD) or a similar program is a standard component of many disaster-response agencies to reduce the mental health toll on rescuers and relief workers.[4,5]

COMMON PITFALLS

- Failure to prepare for a disaster by identifying potential hazards in the local environment, developing contingency plans, and reviewing and correcting errors and omissions in such plans
- Failure to appreciate that disrupted communication and transportation systems frequently cause problems in assessing and responding to disasters, and that redundancy of equipment and flexibility of use of communication and transportation resources are desirable

- Failure to consider the needs of the elderly, children, and technologically dependent people, and to include such things as diapers, formula, medications, interpreters, and special transportation requirements in disaster planning and response
- Failure to appreciate that disaster responders may become casualties themselves, that they may suffer psychological effects during and after the event, and that debriefing is crucial to identify or prevent mental illness or disruptions in the personal or professional lives of disaster responders

References

1. Aghababian RV, Lewis CP, Gans L, et al. Disasters within hospitals. *Ann Em Med* 1994;23:771.
2. Al-Madhari AF, Keller AZ. Review of disaster definitions. *Prehosp Disaster Med* 1997;12:17.
3. Auf der Heide E. Disaster planning, part II: disaster problems, issues, and challenges identified in the research literature. *Emerg Med Clin North Am* 1996;14:453.
4. Austin LS, Godelski LS. Therapeutic approaches for survivors of disaster. *Psychiatr Clin North Am* 1999;22:897.
5. Burkle FM. Acute-phase mental health consequences of disasters: implications for triage and emergency medical services. *Ann Emerg Med* 1996;28:119.
6. Centers for Disease Control. Famine-affected, refugee, and displaced populations: recommendations for public health issues. *MMWR* 1992;41(RR-13):1.
7. Cuny FC. Principles of disaster management. Lesson 2: program planning. *Prehosp Disaster Med* 1998;13:63.
8. De Lorenzo RA. Mass gathering medicine: a review. *Prehosp Disaster Med* 1997;12:68.
9. Garshnek V, Burkle FM. Telecommunications systems in support of disaster medicine: applications of basic information pathways. *Ann Emerg Med* 1999;34:213.
10. Koscheyev VS, Leon GR, Greaves IA. Lessons learned and unsolved public health problems after large-scale disasters. *Prehosp Disaster Med* 1997;12:120.
11. Leonard RB. Emergency evacuations in disasters. *Prehosp Disaster Med* 1991;6:463.
12. Leonard RB, Calabro JJ, Noji EK, et al. SARA (Superfund Amendments and Reauthorization Act), Title III: implications for emergency physicians. *Ann Emerg Med* 1989;18:1212.
13. Levitin HW, Siegelson HJ. Hazardous materials: disaster medical planning and response. *Emerg Med Clin North Am* 1996;14:327.
14. Noji EK. Disaster epidemiology. *Emerg Med Clin North Am* 1996;14:289.
15. Parillo SJ. Medical care at mass gatherings: considerations for physician involvement. *Prehosp Disaster Med* 1995;10:273.
16. Piper PS, Burkle FM, Murray RJ. Constructing a world wide web site for disaster management and humanitarian assistance. *Prehosp Disaster Med* 1997;12:92.
17. Quarantelli EL. Ten criteria for evaluating the management of community disasters. *Disasters* 1997;21:39.
18. Roth PB, Gaffney JK. The federal response plan and disaster medical assistance teams in domestic disasters. *Emerg Med Clin North Am* 1996;14:371.
19. SAEM Disaster Medicine White Paper Subcommittee. Disaster medicine: current assessment and blueprint for the future. *Acad Emerg Med* 1995;2:1068.
20. Waeckerle JF. Disaster planning and response. *N Engl J Med* 1991;324:815.

CHAPTER 400
Informatics

Kenneth A. Williams

Informatics is the study of information and its management.[10] Data become information only when presented in context; information becomes knowledge only if it is understood. For example, out of context, "5.4" means little, but when associated with "potassium level," it becomes information. When considered in light of additional information, such as a previous level of 4.3 in a patient who ran out of furosemide 2 weeks previously but continued to take potassium, knowledge has been acquired.

Problem solving involves a description of the problem, contextual analysis of objective data, the development of potential solutions, and feedback to optimize those solutions. This general plan for problem solving can be seen in traditional architectural design plans (program, site, design, evaluation), in the systems analysis approach to technology assessment (objectives and performance measures, system environment and constraints, resources, goals, management),[5] and in many management guides (goals, objective evaluation with consequences through praise and reprimand, adjustment through review and clarification).[2] In medicine, examples include the problem-oriented medical record, the subjective–objective assessment plan (SOAP) progress note, and continuous quality-improvement techniques (see Chapter 402).

Perhaps the most important element of problem solving is adequate definition of the goal or problem. Careful framing of a question facilitates finding its answer; to proceed otherwise risks the collection of data without information or knowledge. Stepping back or to the side, looking at the issue from another viewpoint, waiting for the emotion of a crisis to dissipate, and searching for opportunity mingled within a crisis are techniques useful for problem definition. This sentiment is well expressed in discussions about clinical research,[6] negotiation,[9] and the philosophy of creative lateral thought.[7]

In emergency medicine, challenges include time constraints, reliance on the patient for information, lack of previously established rapport, and the acuity and severity of patient problems. Improved information access and management can address some of the challenges.

COMPUTERS AND OTHER TOOLS

Currently available computers use application-level software to store, manipulate, and present data with a speed and capability that easily match the needs of a typical emergency department. Personal computers with the power of some mainframes are available in many formats, with features limited only by budget. Software typically falls into categories such as utilities, spreadsheets, data bases, word processing, communications packages, programming languages, and games.

Subdivisions by complexity, approach, supplier, and other factors are possible within these categories. For example, data bases may be grouped according to how they represent data, and products then categorized as flat file (data stored as textlike files), hierarchical (data stored in indexed lists), or relational (data stored in tables of related fields) data base applications. Further, hardware and software requirements vary, and products may be classified as needing a Mac (Macintosh, by Apple Computer, Inc.), Windows (a graphical user interface environment for DOS-based personal computers, by Microsoft, Inc.), and a certain amount of hard-drive space, RAM (random access memory, the type used for rapid access while the computer is on), or other machine capabilities. Some new software focuses on linkage and integration, resulting in "groupware" packages that facilitate enterprise-wide communications, information sharing, and planning. This approach emphasizes the flow of information, giving the user a tool to analyze group interaction and process as well as the product. Additional software applications of interest to medicine include search tools to gain access to medical literature;[15] encoding systems to represent medical knowledge;[3,13] large customized data base systems that manage patient statistics, hospital utilization, budget, and other operational data for a hospital or clinic; practice management systems that perform similar functions for private or group practices; networks that link data and personnel worldwide; computer-based patient record systems; image–graphics systems; diagnostic–decision support aids;[4,11,14] and educational tools.[12] Many examples of each of these computer applications are available and are often advertised in hospital and practice administration journals. There is little standardization of communication between these various medical software applications, despite efforts in that direction, and most emergency physicians probably do not use any of these applications on a daily basis. An excellent review of computer hardware and software applications relevant to the future of emergency medicine is available.[1]

As the diversity and complexity of personal computers and their environment increase, it is important to remember that they are tools first, and the computer neophyte should only need to frame an intelligent question. Computer scientists and hobbyists can then recommend the necessary software and hardware system for answering that question. Thus, to a large extent, the desired output should drive the input and processing system.

Data collection and input techniques lag behind processing and output, and are the major obstacle to widespread clinical computing. Innovations in voice recognition, links between computer networks, digital scanning, and character recognition should overcome some of these obstacles. Meanwhile, other information management technology may be used clinically to solve many problems. Flowcharts, posters, department status boards, protocol manuals, and clinical guideline manuals are commonly used information management techniques that can serve to clarify, simplify, and standardize quality care. A medium used primarily in other areas of medicine but with great promise in emergency medicine is video, including both still and motion pictures. Documentation of general patient status; the appearance of rashes, wounds, and other lesions; and patient education are some obvious applications for video in emergency medicine.

PRACTICAL INFORMATICS

The American College of Emergency Physicians Section on Emergency Medicine Informatics has compiled a directory of computer software for emergency medicine that can generally be used on personal computers and has reviewed software applications for use in emergency medicine.[8] The directory divides software into administrative, clinical, educational, combined, and reference categories. The advantages and challenges of applying this technology are briefly discussed next.

Administrative Uses

Billing

Billing programs range from utilities that assist with ICD coding to full-function electronic billing and accounting systems that track collection rates by physician. All are easier to use if they are electronically linked to other department systems, such as registration; otherwise, they require separate data entry.

Scheduling

Staff scheduling programs typically automate some aspects of scheduling. The more "intelligent" systems allow entry of individual preferences and account for factors such as grouping night shifts and avoiding the "third Thursday staff meeting" for those required to attend. All of the programs facilitate tracking and reporting of schedules, and most can now accommodate multiple facilities and providers. Some argue that the automated schedulers lack the intellectual finesse of a human scheduler, but many users of these programs find them quite acceptable, and all allow editing of the recommended schedule.

Tracking

Tracking programs include dispatch systems for ambulance and helicopter services, patient tracking during an emergency department visit, trauma registers, occupational injury database systems, and similar software. In addition, some tracking programs can index computer-stored patient records, allowing online quality assurance, risk management, and documentation of procedural skills for credentialing purposes. Data storage and manipulation are facilitated if a relational data base format is used with standardized query language (SQL) available for data queries. Standardization and upgradability become issues if one depends on such software and there is a need to share data with others.

Clinical Uses

Calculations

Arterial blood gas interpretation, intravenous drip mix calculators, and similar utilities are available, offering both "just in time" learning for some clinical situations and standardization of care. Challenges include avoiding intellectual dependence on the program and ensuring that the program is updated as new doses or medications are added.

Communications

Electronic mail (e-mail), electronic bulletin board systems (BBS), Internet browsers, and other computer-based communications techniques have long been standard in the academic, computer, and business worlds but are just becoming common in clinical medicine. These systems typically allow grouped distribution of messages (e.g., to all residents, all staff at a certain facility, all nurses on a certain floor), easing announcements and automating their receipt confirmation. Collaborative projects, including research and committee work, can proceed rapidly and without physical travel in many cases, as all involved can share drafts, comments, and other documents electronically.

Several commercial providers offer programs that support links to other e-mail systems and also provide formatted and edited special interest groups (SIGs) similar to Internet e-mail lists. Most health-care facilities have access to the Internet, where a variety of software provide similar capabilities. Several SIGs and Internet lists focusing on EMS and emergency medicine are active, allowing prompt and broad-based discussion on a multitude of issues.

Telephones and beepers require patience; electronic communications require diligence. Because e-mail reaches the recipient only when the computer is attended to, using e-mail for essential communications requires responsible attention to the system.

Order Entry

Several software vendors produce systems that computerize the entry and reporting of orders within the hospital, including laboratory tests, imaging studies, and medications. These systems may include checking rules that prompt for more efficient and correct entry, such as prompting the user that an ordered medication appears on the patient's list of allergies, or that an ordered study was recently performed. In addition to order entry, these systems typically include a data-reporting mechanism and results reporting. These features allow the hospital to automate tracking of ordered items and correlate use with providers, services, diagnoses, or location.

Charting

Programs that produce emergency physician records have sought, fairly successfully, to avoid significant use of the keyboard on the assumption that clinicians prefer other data entry means. Voice recognition, pen-screen, touch-screen, and similar systems to speed entry of standardized information have been well developed and accepted in many departments. Integrating these systems with other computer tools has lagged somewhat, but most providers can now link their computer charting system to other department and hospital systems to allow selection of patient demographics from menus, downloading of patient charts to the billing office, and so forth. The ability to produce graphics (e.g., sketches of anatomy) and store images (e.g., digitized photos of lacerations or rashes) is also possible.

Diagnostic Support

Several commercial programs provide diagnostic support in the form of decision-making assistance. Typically, these systems require input of signs, symptoms, physical and laboratory findings, and patient demographics and then use both rule- and case-based logic to rank differential diagnoses from among an encyclopedic knowledge base. Some can suggest cost-effective next steps in evaluation or provide case simulations for educational purposes. So far, emergency medicine is a domain not well covered; the knowledge bases tend to encompass internal medicine primarily.

Drugs

Pharmaceutic references are available that provide information to guide the choice of medication and dosing. More sophisticated packages assess all medications prescribed for a specific patient for possible interactions and contraindications.

Patient Instructions

Basic packages print previously prepared sheets for common problems. The next level of sophistication includes the ability to customize the instructions for a specific patient, and the most sophisticated packages are integrated with registration and charting systems, coordinating the instructions based on demographics, diagnoses, equipment dispensed, and follow-up arranged. Patient education in the emergency department is an area ripe for improvement. Several programs can print customized discharge instructions; although lengthy, they offer some education. Formats used less often include pictorial handouts, videotapes, interactive computer programs, and simulations. Topics that are taught often, such as crutch walking, wound care, inhaler use, and oral rehydration, lend themselves to presentation by one of these formats, with staff time used to confirm understanding of key points. The ability to show patients actual crutch use on stairs, the appearance of cellulitis, or recommended foods should be more effective than oral descriptions. Challenges include developing programs, making technology available at the bedside, and achieving consensus on standard educational points.

Quality Assurance/Continuous Quality Improvement

Charting, tracking, and patient instruction systems can usually provide administrative reports summarizing use for purposes of quality assurance review. Some charting programs include prompts to remind the clinician about elements of the history or examination that may be important but are often forgotten. Some programs display the computerized chart for quality assurance review on screen, and will sort all charts on a computer disk by provider and diagnostic category. Most data base and spreadsheet programs can serve as tools for those wishing to design a personal application.

Referral

Many hospitals now offer services that match physicians seeking additional office patients with patients seeking a physician. These services typically use a data base system to match patient requirements with physician availability. Computers can also be used to provide information for follow-up by electronic transfer (typically by fax) of patient data to the referral hospital.

Registration/Triage

After billing, ADT (admission, discharge, transfer) computer systems are the most common hospital computer application. Problems include the delay often involved in finding a patient in the system, the lack of a way to identify patients positively (the sharing of insurance cards can cause problems with multiple blood types and medication allergies), and the lengthy registration process. Some facilities are promoting preregistration as an efficiency and marketing tool, with registration drives at health fairs and shopping malls. Preregistered patients have given a certain amount of medical information before their visit, with the hope that positive identification and ready access to former diagnoses, medications, and allergies, for example, will make the overall system less costly and more efficient.

Triage, originally designed as a system to avoid patient deterioration while awaiting care, has become a lengthy initial data collection process in some institutions, often creating significant waits for the triage process itself. Flexible computer-based protocols that allow the triage staff to expand or contract their time with the patient to maximize utility are available. They include standardized lists of questions, recommended laboratory studies, and other data that streamline care for the next provider.

Records

Some health-care systems or facilities are placing patient summaries on their main computer networks, allowing rapid access to a summary of pertinent information on each patient. Accurate patient identification, accuracy of data, and confidentiality are challenges.

Educational Uses

Clinical Education

Clinician education is a continual challenge, with a staggering amount of information from diverse sources facing the clinician. Printed materials frequently are not current or are difficult to search for topic-specific information. Many abstracting services exist, with computerized data base interfaces available from the better ones. These can assist the busy clinician with generalized updates and topic reviews. Specific questions may be answered with primary searches of the medical literature. Several commercially available software packages are available that use direct modem or CD-ROM access to the National Library of Medicine's indexed MEDLINE database, and a variety of Internet resources allow access to the medical literature. As these packages become more sophisticated, they permit a shift in use from research and educational tools to clinical resources that can be used during patient visits as needed.

Several currently available CD-ROM systems have reached this level of utility and are used to access toxicology, product contents, hazardous materials, and other essential information during patient care. Challenges include learning the interface necessary to search for data adequately and the cost of searches or subscriptions. Promising technologies include natural language–processing interfaces that parse questions into search terminology and connection to the data base by the Internet, resulting in easier use and more rapid, less costly searches.

Physician education through simulations, quizzes, and other automated means is a growing area of computer use. The most sophisticated simulations use artificial intelligence programming to create an "artificial patient" whose responses do not follow a definite script but make sense to an expert in the field.

Cardiac emergencies, neonatal resuscitation, and trauma care are areas where this technique holds promise, because correct physician actions are critical, but education from real cases is limited by patient volume and clinician experience.

References

1. Barthell E, Kulick S, Termanini R. Preparing for the emergency department of the future: strategic information systems planning for emergency medicine. American College of Emergency Physicians Section of Computers in Emergency Medicine, American College of Emergency Physicians, Dallas. 1993.
2. Blanchard K, Johnson S. *The one-minute manager*. New York: William Morrow, 1981.
3. Board of Directors of the American Medical Informatics Association. Standards for medical identifiers, codes, and messages needed to create an efficient computer-stored medical record. *J Am Med Inform Assoc* 1994;1:1.
4. Chowdhury S, Bodemar G, Haug P, et al. Methods for knowledge extraction from a clinical database on liver diseases. *Comput Biomed Res* 1991;24:530.
5. Churchman CW. *The systems approach*. New York: Dell, 1968.
6. Cummings SR, Browner WS, Hulley SB. Conceiving the research question. In: Hulley SB, Cummings SR, eds. *Designing clinical research*. Baltimore: Williams & Wilkins, 1988:12.
7. De Bono E. *New think*. New York: Avon Books, 1967.
8. 1998 Directory of software for emergency medicine. Available from ACEP (telephone: (214)550-0911; Internet site: www.acep.org).
9. Fisher R, Ury W. *Getting to yes; negotiating agreement without giving in*. Boston: Houghton Mifflin, 1981.
10. Greenes RA, Shortliffe EH. Medical informatics: an emerging academic discipline and institutional priority. *JAMA* 1990;263:1114.
11. Miller RA. Medical diagnostic decision support systems—past, present, and future: a threaded bibliography and brief commentary. *J Am Med Inform Assoc* 1994;1:8.
12. Orthner HF. Ten years of medical informatics. *Comput Methods Programs Biomed* 1987;25:73.
13. Rada R, Blum B, Calhoun E, et al. A vocabulary for medical informatics. *Comput Biomed Res* 1987;20:244.
14. Reggia JA. Neural computation in medicine. *Artif Intell Med* 1993;5:143.
15. Schoolman HM, Lindberg DA. The information age in concept and practice at the National Library of Medicine. *Ann Am Acad Pol Soc Sci* 1988;(January):117.

CHAPTER 401
Prehospital Emergency Medical Services

Alexander P. Isakov, Lawrence Mottley, and Marc C. Restuccia

HISTORIC PERSPECTIVE

Prior to the rapid evolution of emergency medical services (EMS) in the 1960s and 1970s, only rudimentary systems of prehospital care and patient transport existed. Although hospital-based ambulance services had been functioning in Cincinnati, Ohio, since 1865, and city services were initiated in New York in 1869, private ventures that combined transport services with another trade, such as funeral services, had the greatest market share. Such enterprises delivered prehospital care with little training, regulation, or benchmark for quality.[9] The military advanced EMS in its care of wounded soldiers in Vietnam.[14] Corpsmen and medics were trained in prehospital intervention and evacuation of the critically wounded to appropriate facilities for prompt surgical attention. The mortality of trauma patients surviving to a medical treatment facility sharply decreased.[10]

In 1966, the National Academy of Sciences–National Research Council, which acts as a consulting body to the government, published what has been dubbed the "white paper" of prehospital systems, "Accidental Death and Disability: The Neglected Disease of Modern Society."[10] This document summarized the inadequate delivery of emergency care, the lack of an emergency services infrastructure, and the lack of leadership in this area. It also made specific recommendations for a funded, organized, proactive, prehospital medical delivery system, launching the modern era of civilian EMS in the United States.

The "white paper," along with others showing a rise in accidental deaths, especially on America's highways, prompted Congress to enact the National Highway Safety Act of 1966. This act authorized spending by the newly created Department of Transportation (DOT)/National Highway Traffic Safety Administration (NHTSA) for the improvement of essential prehospital infrastructure, training of personnel, and establishment of practice guidelines. Through this legislation, states developed regional EMS systems with funding for ambulances, personnel, and communication equipment. A nationally recognized curriculum for the training of ambulance attendants (emergency medical technician or EMT-A) was established in 1971.

The success of prehospital cardiac care units in Dublin[17] and of new methods of cardiopulmonary resuscitation (CPR) led EMS programs to expand their focus beyond trauma. Regional EMS demonstration projects showing favorable results led to the EMS Systems Act of 1973, which legislated further federal funding of comprehensive regional EMS systems to include money for operations, training, and research. Full-time medical directors and professional prehospital medical providers emerged.

National standards for EMT-A, EMT-I (intermediate level), and EMP-P (paramedic level) training evolved. Because some nonmedical public safety personnel were often the first to arrive at a scene with medical casualties, a first-responder curriculum was developed as well. NHTSA established such curricula, which came to be recognized as national standards.

Communications infrastructure, including 911 access, two-way radio communications, and centralized dispatch were developed, and criteria for optimal ambulance design and equipment were established. Regional EMS systems were intended to become financially independent as federal funding was phased out in favor of state discretionary funding of EMS through Preventive Health Block Grants, a product of the Omnibus Budget Reconciliation Act of 1981.[9] The result, however, was deterioration of the movement toward national standards as regional systems yielded to state and local concerns. A multitude of systems developed independently, providing a varied range of skill levels, training, and quality of care, from one community to another. Organizations like the National Association of EMS Physicians emerged to serve as a professional body for consensus in the continuing development of EMS systems. The NHTSA has maintained its leadership role in EMS oversight at the federal level.[5]

Today, EMS systems operate in an environment of increased fiscal restraint, with an increased demand for objective proof of the efficacy of prehospital interventions. While these forces may produce more efficient systems, delivering a high quality of care, they could also erode a prehospital infrastructure that took 30 years to develop.[13]

EDUCATION

The U.S. DOT first-responder curriculum trains providers to perform basic patient assessment, manage airway obstruction, control external hemorrhage, administer cardiopulmonary resuscitation (CPR), and apply automatic external defibrillation devices. Length of training is 20 hours. The EMT-A curriculum, historically the minimum level of training required by an ambulance attendant, was revised in 1994, is now known as the basic (EMT-B) curriculum, and currently requires approximately 110 hours of training. The trainee is educated in ambulance operation, communications, documentation, scene assessment, initial patient assessment, triage, patient immobilization, basic airway maneuvers, CPR, and so on. The revised training strategy departed from the traditional diagnosis-based model to an assessment-based model and generated much national debate. Less emphasis was placed on pathophysiology and more emphasis on basic recognition of illness and execution of skills. Automatic external defibrillation was added to the curriculum. Advanced airway training was offered as well.

EMT-I and EMT-P curricula, revised in 1998, are approximately 300 hours and 1100 hours, respectively, and retain a diagnosis-based strategy for patient evaluation. The EMT-I level requires successful completion of the EMT-B curriculum as a prerequisite and includes additional training in pathophysiology, assessment skills, venous cannulation, and establishment of a patent airway. The EMT-P level includes an anatomy and physiology course, as well as the EMT-B course as prerequisites, and advanced training in pathophysiology, intravenous access, definitive airway control, and the pharmacology and administration of a variety of medications.

Despite national standards for curricula at first-responder, EMT-B, EMT-I, and EMT-P levels, states have variably adopted them in the training and certification of EMS providers in their jurisdictions. As a result, approximately forty levels of EMS providers exist nationwide.[4] Each state adopts the curricula, in whole or in part, requires varying hours of formal education, and establishes scopes of practice presumably suited to its own needs. Although this diversity allows for the greatest flexibility to respond to local needs with local resources, it does not foster uniform standards of care and creates confusion regarding interstate reciprocity of privileges. NHTSA is currently sponsoring an EMS Education Task Force to author an EMS Education Agenda for the Future that will more explicitly define core educational content, scope of practice, and national standards for the education and certification of providers.

Specialized training programs have been established for EMTs and paramedics who function in settings where additional education is desirable. Critical care transport specialists may receive training in ventilator, invasive monitoring, and intraaortic balloon pump management. The wilderness curriculum prepares the EMT in search and rescue, environmental injuries, complications of prolonged evacuation and prehospital transport, and basic primary care in remote locations. The EMT-Tactical program prepares providers in comprehensive medical support for law enforcement teams and includes training in medical contingency planning, and in preventive medicine for the tactical team. It also includes medical support of extended operations, including primary care and recognition of performance decrement, hazardous materials (HAZMAT) safety, clinical forensics, and safe management of casualties in an austere, hostile environment. These specialized training programs allow medical directors to fulfill their responsibility while ensuring that providers are trained to function safely and effectively in unique settings.

The training of physicians for leadership roles in EMS is also developing. Historically, any physician who had an interest and the fortitude would serve as EMS medical director. No formal training existed. Today, emergency medicine residents are provided some training in EMS systems as part of their core curriculum in postgraduate training.[19] EMS experience, however, varies greatly from one training program to another. Postgraduate EMS fellowship training is now available through 1- and 2-year training programs. The 2-year programs concurrently offer a master's degree in public health, hospital administration, business, or other disciplines. Guidelines for a standard curriculum have been endorsed by the Society for Academic Emergency Medicine and the National Association of EMS Physicians.[7] The American Board of Emergency Medicine has yet to accept EMS as a certifiable subspecialty.

STRUCTURE

Regardless of the type of EMS system, the necessity for field personnel to obtain adequate clinical exposure cannot be overemphasized. Patient outcomes improve when each medical provider achieves a threshold of patient encounters. Regionalization of EMS systems, as has occurred in the South and West, provides not only economies of scale, but also the ability to rotate personnel to ensure adequate experience, uniform patient treatment protocols, and placement of units based on patient need rather than political boundaries. In the Northeast, where each city and town often independently maintain their own EMS service, staffing requirements and overall costs are higher, and more personnel almost certainly means diluted experience and loss of skills.

Fire-Based Systems

Many fire departments (FDs), especially in the western United States, adopted EMS as part of their mission immediately after the federal legislation was enacted. Fire-based systems allowed dispatch and deployment of EMS units within a currently existing system. In most combined EMS/fire systems, EMS accounts for about three-fourths of the call load. In small cities and towns, existing personnel and facilities may be able to perform EMS duties without adding staff or infrastructure. But because firefighters are usually among the highest-paid employees, larger systems which need additional staff will incur much higher costs compared with the other EMS models.

In addition, because the FD's first priority is fire suppression, conflicts of interest may arise and lead to underresourced patient care. As the annual number of fire-suppression calls decreases and cities look more closely at the most efficient use of available resources, more FDs are becoming interested in EMS. Integration of established EMS systems with and under the direction of FDs is a politically charged topic that currently is the subject of heated debate in many cities.

In a full-service EMS system, the FD provides both treatment and transport for all patients. Advance life-support (ALS) and basic life-support (BLS) ambulances or only ALS ambulances may transport all patients. In a paramedic service–only system, the fire department provides ALS response to all, or a subset, of calls. BLS calls are referred to a private ambulance provider on the basis of either telephone triage or on-scene assessment by paramedics. ALS patients may be transported in an FD ambulance or in a private ambulance accompanied by an FD paramedic. Many FDs now provide first-responder services regardless of the source of ambulance transport, using firefighter personnel trained to respond to immediately life-threatening conditions such as cardiac arrest, respiratory distress, chest pain, and loss of consciousness.

Private Ambulance Services

Private ambulance services often bid for an exclusive contract with a governmental entity to provide EMS services, usually to a city, town, or county. The contract often stipulates that certain indirect measures of quality and performance be met, such as that all units be equipped with defibrillators, that paramedics perform a minimum number of intubations, or that certain response-time parameters be met. The community establishes regulatory control over the private service, with oversight being provided by an EMS agency or a medical director.

Private ambulance services usually provide both ALS and BLS services. To a greater extent than any of the other EMS models, private ambulances depend on efficient management of resources, such as peak-load staffing and system status management, to meet their dual demands: adequate EMS response and being a successful business. Personnel costs for the private sector are usually significantly below those for both the FD and third-service industries. The risk, however, is that the vendor could withdraw from nonlucrative markets, leaving the region or municipality searching for a means to provide uninterrupted service.

Third-Service Systems

Third service, simply defined, is an EMS system housed in a municipal department, using municipality-owned and -operated ambulances, and kept separate from police and fire services. Many medium and large cities continue to use municipal hospital–based ambulances as all or part of their EMS systems. Some third services are part of the city's Health Department, and a few are separate city agencies. This model allows for concentration on one mission—patient care—without the distraction of managing, funding, and providing other services. EMT skill maintenance is rarely a problem in these mostly urban systems. A drawback is that the third-service agency must compete with other traditionally well-supported public service agencies for budgetary funding.

Volunteer Systems

Almost three-fourths of all rural EMS providers are volunteers. The tax base cannot support a full-time professional EMS system, and the revenue to attract a private contractor does not exist. The dedication of volunteers is remarkable, as are the challenges they face in finding medical oversight, time for training, the means to maintain their skills, and the financial resources to develop and maintain their systems' infrastructure. Depending on state regulation, some volunteer services may operate without medical direction. Turnover among these providers is high. Rural systems face the same challenge of quality care as urban ones but with drastically different resources.

AMBULANCES

Type 1 ambulances have a truck frame with a box compartment for patient care. This configuration offers the greatest amount of patient care area, the highest vehicle weight, and the greatest amount of storage area. Type 1 ambulances are ideal for busy ALS systems, systems with long transport times, as well as critical care ground transport systems. The down side of such vehicles is higher acquisition costs, higher ongoing maintenance costs, and their size, which can be problematic in tight urban systems.

Type 2 ambulances are trucks with a van body. They are less expensive to acquire and operate and are the most numerous class of ambulance. They are somewhat limited in available treatment space and are small for the management of critically ill or injured patients. They are commonly held to have lesser durability than type 1 ambulances and afford the crew less protection in front-end collisions.

Type 3 ambulances have van frames and front ends, with a box patient care area. They are intermediate in acquisition and maintenance cost. They have large patient care areas and work well for the vast majority of patients. They tend to be limited in their weight restrictions. Many municipal services, particularly the smaller ones, have chosen this type of ambulance.

Type 4 ambulances are "specialty" ambulances and include air ambulances, such as helicopters. Because of their unique role and mission profile, they cannot be directly compared with other ambulance types.

Type 5 ambulances are vehicles designed to bring EMS personnel to the patient, but, in general, will not transport the patient. ALS personnel may respond with their equipment in such ambulances, meet up with a BLS team, and accompany the patient during transport in a BLS vehicle.

State laws, which can be extremely detailed, govern the configuration of each vehicle, as well as its markings. In addition, although some latitude is afforded to type 4 vehicles, each state mandates the minimum and allowable equipment and medications carried on any ambulance. Despite these regulations, there is wide variation in the equipment and medications carried on individual ambulances. This variation reflects not only the medical director's equipment (manufacturer) preferences, judgment, and vision for the service, but also those of other personnel as well as the type and geographic location of the system.

A busy urban EMS system may stock large amounts of consumable equipment to minimize "down time" to restock. Conversely, if all runs end at the base facility, lesser amounts of such items may be required. In contrast, rural EMS agencies may stock every item they may conceivably need during a prolonged transport. Variation in equipment and supplies also reflects the level of service provided. The amount of medical equipment on a BLS ambulance is much less than on an ALS vehicle.

MEDICAL OVERSIGHT

Medical oversight of out-of-hospital providers is essential to providing the best in medical care. It may take the form of direct or indirect medical control. Direct or on-line medical control refers to the immediate direction and feedback, usually by radio or telephone, that a physician provides to an EMS provider "at the point of service." Although there is some controversy over whether such communication significantly improves the care provided,[6] it gives EMS providers direct access to someone with a greater level of training and knowledge.

In some systems, medical control is provided by a specified physician or institution at a single base hospital. In other systems, it is decentralized, with each receiving institution acting as a base station. Medical control physicians must have an in-depth knowledge of the skills and capabilities of the EMS provider on scene and the capabilities and availability of receiving institutions in the area. They must also know applicable state and/or regional or local protocols and the medicolegal implications of situations such as refusal of treatment or transport and the care of minors, do-not-resuscitate status, and deceased patients.

Indirect or off-line medical control consists of protocol development and implementation, equipment selection, assuring adherence to clinical standards, education of EMS providers, and on-going quality improvement within the system. Such functions are generally the responsibility of the EMS medical director. Although time consuming, they are necessary to ensure that high-quality care is being delivered.

Compliance with protocols and standards of care is usually accomplished by reviewing a percentage of all EMS patient care records (charts, or "run sheets"), by reviewing individual cases that were difficult or problematic, or by reviewing the charts of selected conditions (e.g., cardiac arrests, pediatric cases, intubations, deaths, refusals of care) or individuals (e.g., new hires, those with whom there may be quality-of-care concerns, those who have just returned from a leave of absence). The initial training and continuing education of EMS providers is a key element in medical direction. The implementation of new medications, interventions, and protocols is an ongoing process. Quality improvement includes not only identifying and correcting deficiencies in current practice, but also identifying areas that, although not necessarily deficient, can be improved (response time, scene time, timely completion of charts, documentation of procedures).

COMMUNICATION

EMS communications is best viewed as a chain of events that can be described using queuing theory. The call-taker queue consists of those who dial 911. In the past, most cities and towns had their own emergency call-receiving center. Many have now been consolidated into Public Safety Answering Points (PSAPs) serving one large local jurisdiction, or multiple smaller ones. Enhanced 911 (or 911E) provides the PSAP call-taker with the physical address of the phone (street address and, in apartment buildings, the apartment number) as well as the telephone number of the caller. This information is obtained by the PSAP when the caller dials the last digit of 911, even if the caller hangs up before the call is answered. Thus, patients unable to speak, whether because of stroke, asthma, or other condition, can still receive assistance. Protocols may also allow the call-taker to ask a series of yes or no questions that mute callers can answer by pushing the appropriate button (1 or 2). In this way, the correct agency(ies) can respond. Technology is also available to approximate the location of cell phones.

EMS callers are then placed in the triage queue. Modern EMS systems use written telephone medical triage guidelines to ensure consistent and appropriate triage. More important, by asking only for information that will assist in correctly prioritizing the call, they reduce the amount of time spent questioning the patient prior to dispatch. For example, if the caller is male, over 50 years of age, and has nontraumatic chest pain, no further information is necessary for triaging the call as high priority (potential cardiac etiology). Gathering additional information and attempting to make a presumptive diagnosis is not appropriate and possibly detrimental, because it wastes time and is not relevant to the dispatch decision.

Triage protocols can reduce both type 1 and type 2 errors (overtriage and undertriage). They also protect the call-taker from the abusive retrospective review that can occur after a high-profile adverse event. Because the medical director bears responsibility for the appropriateness of these medical triage guidelines, it is strongly suggested that a nationally recognized EMS Telephone Triage product be used. Many of these products are customizable (within limits) to meet local preferences.

EMS calls are usually triaged into one of three priorities: Priority One: life-threatening; Priority Two: emergent or unknown; and Priority Three: nonemergent. These categories are designed to reflect the instability of an illness or injury and its likelihood of deteriorating in a short period of time. They are not intended to characterize whether the condition justifies the use of an ambulance or how serious it is. For instance, although a fractured hip is serious and appropriate for the use of an ambulance, it is not likely to deteriorate and therefore does not have top priority.

Once the call is prioritized, it enters the dispatch queue. The dispatcher then assigns an ambulance to respond. Assigning the closest ambulance to the call is preferred, but this process is not always straightforward. As the number of ambulances in a system increases, so does the complexity of dispatch. In larger cities, the dispatcher would have to know each street and the location of each ambulance at any given time. Most ambulances are "in service" only 15% to 40% of the time, and they may be located outside their assigned districts, making it difficult to ascertain their position without polling multiple units over the radio.

Automatic Vehicle Locator (AVL) systems can help and are increasingly being used, particularly within the private sector. Using the federal government Global Positioning Satellite (GPS) system, AVLs can locate an ambulance within a few feet, calculate the travel time to a given call, and recommend the nearest units of each appropriate type—first-responder, BLS, and ALS.

EMS demand is remarkably predictable, especially in systems with a large call volume. System Status Management (SSM) is the process of managing resources based on known patterns of calls in time and place as well as current demand. Additional ambulances are placed in service during known periods of higher demand. Available units do not remain static, but are dynamically and proactively redeployed by EMS supervisors when call volume is high in certain areas. The practice of flat staffing, in which the same number of ambulances are on duty 24 hours a day, is less efficient; patients will have to wait longer than necessary during the busier times, and resources will be wasted during slack time.

EMS radio communications primarily utilize four frequency bands: VHF-Low (40 to 60 MHz), VHF-High (140 to 170 MHz), UHF (470 to 490 MHz), and the 800 band (800 to 900+ MHz). Each has performance characteristics with strengths and weaknesses. The height of the radio antenna is usually one-fourth the wavelength. VHF, especially VHF-Low, has a wavelength a few meters long and travels a great distance, but it is unable to penetrate manufactured obstacles such as buildings. This band is commonly used by agencies similar to the Highway Patrol, covering wide distances with few artificial obstructions. It is not suitable for use in urban or suburban systems.

UHF has good penetration into manufactured objects, and its antenna is of reasonable height for portable use. The 800 band is often used because there are no available channels to be licensed on the UHF frequencies. It has excellent penetration into buildings, but the wavelength is so short that communications are essentially limited to line of sight (i.e., no over-the-horizon reception). This band is ideal for the urban environment, where one well-placed transmitter can often cover an entire city. It can also be used for a newer technique, called "trunking."

A trunking 800 system usually consists of six to eight frequencies but has ten times that number in "virtual frequencies." For instance, each radio may have channels 1 through 6, and each of these channels may have ten subchannels (e.g., A through J), allowing for 60 discrete channels. Each of these channels and subchannels may have restrictions on it; that is, channel 1A may be for dispatch, and all users would have the ability to listen, while channel 4B might be for medical quality assurance, and only the personnel assigned to that group would have radios with the "privileges" for channel 4B. The central computer controlling the mobile and portable radios senses which radios are tuned to which channels. When a user broadcasts on a given channel, the computer assigns an actual frequency (e.g., 800.435 MHz) and programs only the other radios tuned to this channel to go to the frequency. A similar process is used for cell phones.

Frequencies assigned by the Federal Communications Commission (FCC) for medical control, the "Med Channels," are in the UHF band, thus allowing one radio to serve for both dispatch and hospital communication. There are ten channels in this group, eight for medical control (channels 1 through 8) and two for EMS dispatch (channels 9 and 10). Receiving hospitals may have permanently assigned med channels that allow medics to call directly, or hospitals may be part of a central medical dispatch (C-MED) system, in which medics call C-MED and are patched into the requested hospital.

Virtually all of the radio frequencies in use for EMS are duplexed: They operate on a pair of frequencies, one to send and another to receive. This set-up allows both parties to talk at the same time, so that either the physician or the paramedic can interrupt the other if necessary. Transmissions by field personnel are weak and can only be heard directly within a few blocks. If desired, the central radio can retransmit these messages with a more powerful transmitter, using the second channel, called a "repeater."

DISASTER PLANNING

Mass casualty incidents (MCIs; see Chapter 399) require the response of multiple different public safety and EMS agencies. They threaten to overwhelm the capacity of the out-of-hospital system as well as the medical facilities supporting them.[8] Each EMS agency and hospital must have a plan for dealing with MCIs in their service area. The importance of having a well-understood, rehearsed, and commonly recognized plan for responding to an MCI cannot be emphasized enough. Practicing implementation of the plan provides training for all participants, prevents needless delays, and identifies areas for improvement. Agencies should have complementary plans and train together to ensure cooperation.

Risk assessment of potential MCI scenarios in a service area should be part of the plan. It involves recognizing and characterizing likely sites of an MCI, such as industrial complexes, airports, residential stock (e.g., high-rise apartments, special-needs facilities), highways and railways, and unique facilities, such as nuclear power plants.

A communications plan is essential. Often, however, it is the part of the response that fails most rapidly in an MCI. Overloaded radio channels, cell channels, and phone lines can be expected. Loss of radio towers and telephone wires may occur. The plan should identify ways to minimize the effect of these occurrences.

Mutual aid agreements with EMS, police, and fire services, as well as medical treatment facilities in contiguous service areas should be in place. The ability to assemble out-of-hospital and hospital assets beyond the affected area is often essential for a timely response to an MCI. The plan should identify the resources, personnel, transport, equipment, and facilities that can be called on.

A clearly defined incident command structure should also be in place. In some states, the highest ranking fire officer serves as overall "incident commander," with police, EMS and other agencies functioning as subcommands under Incident Command Rules. All involved must use common nomenclature, practice, and communications protocols. There should be clear direction as to what freedom of operation prehospital providers might have without resorting to frequent on-line medical direction. Freedom of operation can be accomplished by having the medical director or designee assume EMS Command–Medical Command at the scene or via radio.

Special planning is required for HAZMAT situations, terrorist activities, weapons of mass destruction, and mass gatherings. Finally, a debriefing plan is necessary to allow for psychological recovery of involved personnel and for the planning to manage future MCIs.

FINANCING EMERGENCY MEDICAL SERVICES SYSTEMS

The expense of an EMS system is a function of personnel, administration, maintenance, training, equipment, and facilities. Other variables include the level of service provided; response-time requirements; how the cost will be apportioned among patient revenues, tax revenues, and other subsidies; the insurance coverage of the population served; and the cost of medical oversight.[15]

Funding of EMS systems varies greatly from system to system but can be divided into four major categories: taxes, fee-for-service billing, subscription program revenues, and special service contracts.[15] Local and state tax subsidies can entirely fund an EMS system, in which care is provided as a public service. Most often, this funding comes from general tax revenues and must compete with other public programs for scarce tax dollars.

In some states, the law allows citizens to approve a dedicated tax levy for specific purposes, and voters direct funding for EMS services. Because EMS has a very positive public image, EMS systems tend to enjoy a greater degree of financial support under such a system. In other systems, tax subsidies may simply offset costs that cannot be covered by revenues from EMS billing. Subsidies are often required in small communities that lack economies of scale yet operate a full-service EMS system and in urban and rural settings. It may flow through the budget of a government agency, in the case of third service or FD, or it may be a contractual agreement between a private ambulance provider and a local government. With private contracts, most cities and towns have enjoyed almost a decade of subsidy-free EMS services, as providers have received sufficient revenue from Medicare and Medicaid reimbursement. Recent changes in reimbursement from these sources have significantly reduced the ability of private ambulances to continue subsidy-free 911 contracts.

In a service that generates its revenue from a fee-for-service plan, income is derived from emergency and nonemergency patient transports, interfacility transfers, and special-event coverage. To balance the budget, these systems must have adequate economies of scale, a population base that has the means to pay, efficient management, and effective billing. Among the billed entities are Medicare, Medicaid, private insurance companies, and individual patients.

Subscription programs are marketed to the populace by a vendor who essentially enrolls people as an "insurance policy" in case they need ambulance services. This type of system also provides service to unenrolled members but at a charge significantly greater than the enrollment fee. Some arrangements also allow the company to bill third-party payors. Special-events coverage, interfacility transport, air transport, and other contracts can provide added revenue.

RESEARCH AND INITIATIVES FOR THE FUTURE

Rising costs of health care, the increasing prevalence of managed-care organizations, demands for cost analysis and demonstrated utility of services, and the changing structure of health-care delivery will all influence EMS system development.[11,12] EMS will undoubtedly continue to exist, as access to emergency services has come to be expected by our society. The permissive environment of EMS development and implementation of prehospital interventions without supporting data has ended.

The "chain of survival," as described by the American Heart Association, is a good example of the success and failure of EMS research. Efforts to study the effect of interventions for cardiac arrest demonstrated the need for comparable data between systems and fostered the development of a standard for the uniform reporting of data for out-of-hospital cardiac arrest: the Utstein Style.[2] They also documented the effectiveness of early defibrillation in witnessed cardiac arrest. However, many interventions that are now considered standard of care (e.g., endotracheal intubation and the administration of intravenous medication) were accepted without data showing that they improved patient outcome.

Of the 5,842 scientific studies on EMS in MEDLINE since 1985, only 54 were randomized controlled trials, only one examined a major outcome, such as survival, and only one other compared the studied intervention with a placebo.[1] There is little doubt that the value of EMS systems and the services they provide will come into question in a health-care system under significant financial pressure. Emerging systems may still have a window of opportunity to study these interventions and may, in fact, be obligated to demonstrate improved patient outcome to justify the cost of implementing advanced prehospital services in their areas.

Many attempts have been made in the last 30 years to provide some standard of reporting. Most recently, a Uniform Prehospital EMS Data Conference (1993) was held, again with the hope of establishing an accepted national EMS data set.[18] Uniform reporting would benefit not only research in EMS, but also system evaluation, medicolegal issues, and billing. Still left unaddressed is the linking of prehospital data with in-hospital and follow-up data, a necessary step in demonstrating the effectiveness of EMS care.

A recent assessment of state EMS systems found a lack of (1) comprehensive EMS legislation and statewide EMS plans, (2) enhanced communication systems, (3) consistent quality-assurance programs for training courses and instructors, (4) enabling legislation for trauma system development, (5) consistent and adequate funding sources, (6) priority for public information and education programs, and (7) effective data collection and evaluation systems.[13,16] Recommendations for future development include (1) integration of health services, (2) EMS research, (3) legislation and regulation, (4) system finance, (5) human resources, (6) medical direction, (7) education systems, (8) public education, (9) prevention, (10) public access, (11) communications, (12) clinical care, (13) information systems, and (14) evaluation.[3,4]

It is envisioned that

> Emergency medical services (EMS) of the future will be community-based health management that is fully integrated with the overall health care system. It will have the ability to identify and modify illness and injury risks, provide acute illness and injury care and follow-up, and contribute to treatment of chronic conditions and community health monitoring. This new entity will be developed from redistribution of existing health care resources and will be integrated with other health care providers and public health and public safety agencies. It will improve community health and result in more appropriate use of acute health care resources. EMS will remain the public's emergency medical safety net.[3,4]

Through its unique position in the community as a link to health-care access, the "scope of service" of EMS systems may expand to encompass injury prevention and preventive medicine initiatives, complementing and enhancing roles currently served separately and independently by other agencies.

References

1. Callaham M. Quantifying the scanty science of prehospital emergency care. *Ann Emerg Med* 1997;30:785–790.
2. Cummins RO, et al. Recommended guidelines for uniform reporting of data from out-of-hospital cardiac arrest: the Utstein style. *Ann Emerg Med* 1991;20:861–874.
3. Delbridge TD, Bailey B, Chew JL, et al. EMS agenda for the future: where we are . . . where we want to be. *Ann Emerg Med* 1998;31:251–263.
4. *Emergency medical services agenda for the future.* Washington, DC: NHTSA and the Health Resources and Services Administration, 1996.
5. *Emergency medical services: NHTSA leading the way.* Washington, DC: National Highway Traffic Safety Administration, 1995.
6. Klein KR, et al. Effects of on-line medical control in the prehospital treatment of atraumatic illness. *Prehosp Emerg Care* 1997;1:80–84.
7. Krohmer JR, et al. Prototype core content for a fellowship in emergency medical services. *Ann Emerg Med* 1994;23:109–114.
8. Lilja GP, et al. Multiple casualty incidents. In: Kuehl AE, ed. *Prehospital systems & medical oversight/National Association of EMS Physicians,* 2nd ed. St. Louis: Mosby, 1994.
9. Mustalish AC, Post C. History. In: Kuehl AE, ed. *Prehospital systems & medical oversight/National Association of EMS Physicians,* 2nd ed. St. Louis: Mosby, 1994.
10. National Academy of Sciences–National Research Council. *Accidental death and disability: the neglected disease of modern society.* Washington DC, 1966.
11. Neely KW, Drake MER, Moorhead JC, et al. Multiple options and unique pathways: a new direction for EMS? *Ann Emerg Med* 1997;30:797–799.
12. O'Connor RE, Cone DC, DeLorenzo RA. EMS systems: foundations for the future. *Acad Emerg Med* 1999;6:46–53.
13. Page J. Historical perspective in EMS systems. In: Roush WR, ed. *Principles of EMS systems,* 2nd ed. Dallas: American College of Emergency Physicians, 1994.
14. Rice MM, Brown JF. Military systems. In: Kuehl AE, ed. *Prehospital systems & medical oversight/National Association of EMS Physicians,* 2nd ed. St. Louis: Mosby, 1994.
15. Smith JE. Financial considerations in emergency medical services systems. *Emerg Med Clin North Am* 1990;8:155–161.
16. Snyder JA, Baren JM, Ryan SD, et al. Emergency medical service system development: results of the statewide emergency medical service technical assessment program. *Ann Emerg Med* 1995;25:768–775.
17. Spaite DW, et al. Emergency medical service systems research: problems of the past, challenges of the future. *Ann Emerg Med* 1995;26:146–152.
18. Spaite DW, et al. Uniform prehospital data elements and definitions: a report from the uniform prehospital emergency medical services data conference. *Ann Emerg Med* 1995;25:525–534.
19. Verdile VP, et al. Model curriculum in emergency medical services for emergency medicine residency programs. *Acad Emerg Med* 1996;3:716–722.

CHAPTER 402
Performance Improvement

Mary C. Burke

An essential feature of providing high-quality medical care and good risk management in the emergency department is a well-designed and thorough performance improvement plan that scrutinizes all facets of delivering patient care. From a medicolegal perspective, the high volume, high acuity, fast pace, and lack of an established patient–physician relationship make the emergency department a high-risk area of the hospital. This, along with the complexity and diversity of the providers, patients, and ancillary services encountered in the emergency department, makes a well-designed plan an absolute necessity. In addition, the highly competitive climate of delivering health care with the highest quality and highest cost efficiency requires effective measurement of the care delivered.

HISTORY

The Joint Commission on Accreditation of Healthcare Organizations (JCAHO) has required some form of quality assurance in the emergency department in order for a hospital to maintain accreditation since the 1950s. The first standards involved implicit review, such as morbidity and mortality data collection and analysis. The next generation of standards involved time-limited studies or retrospective audits. These included retrospective reviews of medical records, laboratory results, radiographs, electrocardiograms, emergency department deaths, antibiotic usage, and blood transfusions. Next came ongoing monitoring and evaluation, or "quality assurance."[1] Its purpose was to somehow measure quality, but, more often than not, the process was nothing more than a checklist approach toward the certification process. Consequently, the task of "doing" quality assurance was viewed rather skeptically by providers of care.

The JCAHO recognized this problem and subsequently endorsed an agenda for change in 1987, which refocused standards to facilitate the implementation of an integrated program of continual quality improvement. The audit process was replaced with the new paradigm of looking at improving the entire process related to the delivery of care.[3] This concept is grounded on philosophical work by numerous quality-control experts, such as Deming, Juran, Ishikawa, Crosby, and Stewhart, who introduced the concept to business with the specific goal of reducing variance, continually improving the work process, and improving the final product.[6] The JCAHO's new approach to improving performance includes designing processes, monitoring performance through data collection, analyzing current performance, and improving sustained performance.[4]

PERFORMANCE IMPROVEMENT: THE TEN-STEP APPROACH

The JCAHO supports the use of a ten-step approach for monitoring and evaluating performance improvement (Table 402.1). This methodology serves as a guideline for providers to design and implement an effective quality-improvement plan. Virtually all aspects of care can be integrated into this ten-step process. The specifics should be adapted to the size, volume, and financial capability of the department. The ten-step process is described in detail:

Step 1. Assign responsibility. The department chair is responsible for designating the individuals who will oversee the development and implementation of the department performance-improvement plan. The most successful approach is to have a team of physicians and nurses working together on a combined plan.[7] Communication, cooperation, and mutual respect are essential for success. This sets the tone for sharing responsibility, enhancing empowerment, and continually improving care.

Individuals responsible for collecting data must also be identified. They should be taught the reasoning behind the selection of data being collected; this knowledge leads to more accurate data collection. These individuals can be the department secretaries, administrative assistants, physicians, or nurses.

A clear hierarchy in the hospital performance improvement plan should also be defined, with specific reference to where the emergency department's plan fits into the overall scheme.

Step 2. Delineate scope of care. This section essentially outlines the types of clinical care that will be monitored and evaluated. The scope of care is defined by what types of services are available and provided in the department. The accreditation manual for hospitals requires that all hospitals be designated according to the scope of care provided.[2] Census data, such as the volume and disposition of medical, surgical, obstetric, gynecologic, pediatric, orthopedic, geriatric, and trauma patients seen in the emergency department, should be collected and reported. Hospital-specific services, such as a trauma center, burn unit, or organ transplant service, that affect emergency department care should also be mentioned.

Step 3. Identify important aspects of care. Each department should identify those aspects of care that are considered important. Generally, these are high-risk procedures, high-volume conditions, and problem-prone cases. It is virtually impossible to study all areas at all times. Consequently, each department should select aspects of care that are known or suspected to have problems. Table 402.2 lists a sample of important aspects of care.

Step 4. Identify indicators. After the important aspects of care are identified, it is then necessary to determine what variables can objectively measure that specific aspect of care. Indicators should be developed from the current literature, with specific reference to the practice of emergency medicine. A selection of examples are listed in Table 402.3.[6]

It is also suggested that department indicators coincide with hospital-wide indicators that may be used for interhospital comparisons. For example, the Maryland Hospital Quality Indicator Project[5] uses the following data points:

Unplanned returns to the emergency department within 72 hours of a previous visit

The number of patients admitted to the emergency department out of the total number of returns

Patients who remain in the emergency department more than 6 hours

X-ray report discrepancies between an emergency department reading and a radiology reading that require a change in follow-up or treatment

TABLE 402.1. 10-Step Process

1. Assign responsibility.
2. Delineate scope of care.
3. Identify important aspects of care.
4. Identify indicators.
5. Establish a means to trigger evaluation.
6. Collect and organize data.
7. Evaluate care.
8. Take actions to improve care and services.
9. Assess effectiveness of actions and ensure improvement is maintained.
10. Communicate relevant information to organization-wide quality improvement program.

TABLE 402.2. Some Important Aspects of Care

HIGH-RISK PROCEDURES
Conscious sedation
Thrombolytic therapy
Transfers
HIGH VOLUME
Tetanus status
Admissions
Completeness of medical record
PROBLEM-PRONE
Psychiatric cases (i.e., suicidal/violent patients)
Restraint use
"Left without being seen" patients

TABLE 402.3. Selected Indicators

VOLUME INDICATORS
Total ED patients
Acute
Urgent
Fast-track
Pediatric
Emergency department patients admitted
Emergency department patients seen by emergency department physicians
Poison control calls
Transfers in and out
Ambulance runs
Cardiopulmonary resuscitations
Trauma alerts
QUALITY INDICATORS
Percentage of patients for whom consult needed, but not requested
Percentage of inappropriate consultations
Patients left without being evaluated
Percentage with untimely treatment
Percentage with inappropriate x-rays or laboratory tests
Percentage delayed response team by attending MD
Percentage of time in triage
Number of visits longer than 2 hours
Number of visits longer than 4 hours
Delays in obtaining ICU beds
PERFORMANCE INDICATORS
Number (%) of patient complaints—clinical and nonclinical
Number (%) of complaints from the medical staff
Number (%) of discrepancies between final and ED x-ray interpretation
Number (%) of discrepancies between final and ED ECG interpretation
Percentage of ED records sampled:
Incomplete
Inadequate documentation
Unsigned
Number (%) of wound infections
RISK/COMPLICATION INDICATORS
Number of ED deaths
DOA
In ED
Within 24 h after admission
Number of unscheduled visits within 48–72 h for same complaint
Number of visits for missed diagnoses
Number of visits for complications related to ED visit
Number of patients denied ED care from the managed care plan

Patients who leave the emergency department before completion of treatment

State and regional variations influence the type of interhospital comparisons used. Familiarity with the indicators already being used will avoid the inefficiency of duplicate data collection.

Step 5. Establish a means to trigger evaluation. Triggers for evaluating care are occurrences or measurement thresholds that determine when a more detailed investigation of an important aspect of care must be done. Triggers can be singular or rate based. A sentinel event trigger requires evaluation every time the event occurs. One example of this type of trigger is a death in the emergency department. Complaints can also be sentinel event triggers and often indicate the need to study and improve both medical care and other areas related to patient satisfaction, such as communication, interpersonal skills, waiting times, and physical surroundings.[8]

Rate-based triggers should be determined by expert and departmental consensus as to what constitutes an acceptable and achievable goal. Such a determination will ensure better cooperation and compliance in improving an area if a single, specific problem arises. An example of this type of trigger is the average time that it takes to administer thrombolytics after a diagnostic electrocardiogram is obtained.

Step 6. Collect and organize data. For each indicator, it is essential to have a carefully designed data collection plan that identifies the following parameters:

Data sources/data collector
Collection methods (i.e., sampling, sampling size)
Data to be collected
Method of data analysis to be used to determine whether a threshold for action is reached

Step 7. Initiate evaluation. The results of all ongoing data collection and analysis should be reported back to the emergency department performance-improvement team and to the department director. This information is used to identify problems and determine whether further evaluation is necessary. This also triggers the cycle for continually improving care.

Step 8. Take actions to improve care and services. This step involves intensive work to address any problem that may have been identified. Specific actions should be initiated to improve the overall level of care provided. A specific time frame should be identified as to when a change should occur.

Step 9. Assess effectiveness of actions and ensure improvement is maintained. It is necessary to determine whether care has actually improved as a result of actions taken, and, if not, to determine what further actions need to occur. This step essentially closes the feedback loop in the performance-improvement process. It is also important to periodically monitor the same indicator to assure that quality is maintained.

Step 10. Communicate relevant information to organization-wide performance-improvement program. The results of the performance improvement effort should be forwarded to the hospital performance-improvement committee, hospital leaders, and the governing body.

Emergency departments also need to incorporate outcome monitors in the overall plan. Some of the indicators may be timeliness of surgical intervention for adult head injury, timeliness of patient transfers, and airway management for comatose trauma patients.

The final component of the complete performance-improvement plan involves thorough documentation of both patient satisfaction and patient complaints. These data should be maintained for both the clinical and nonclinical members of the department. The information can be used with the remaining quality-assessment findings to identify potential medicolegal problems.

References

1. *Accreditation manual for hospitals.* Chicago: Joint Commission on Accreditation of Hospitals, 1983.
2. *Accreditation manual for hospitals.* Chicago: Joint Commission on Accreditation of Healthcare Organizations, 1992:19.
3. *An introduction to quality improvement in health care; the transition from QA to CQI.* Chicago: Joint Commission on Accreditation of Healthcare Organizations, 1991.
4. Comprehensive accreditation manual for hospitals. In: *The official handbook,* update 3. Chicago: Joint Commission on Accreditation of Healthcare Organizations, August 1998:PI:1–28.
5. Maryland Hospital Association Quality Indicator Project, 1992.
6. Mayer TA. Quality improvement in emergency medicine. In: Schwartz G, Mayer TA, Cayten G, et al., eds. *Principles in practice of emergency medicine,* 3rd ed. Philadelphia: Lea & Febiger, 1992:3269.
7. Risser DT, Rice MM, Salisbury ML, et al. The potential for improved teamwork to reduce medical errors in the emergency department. *Ann Emerg Med* 1999;34:373.
8. Tucker JR, Kornberg AE. Effective management of complaints in the emergency department. *Pediatr Emerg Care* 1994;10:94.

CHAPTER 403
Triage

Anthony R. Berner

Triage, a word derived from the French verb *trier,* meaning "to choose or sort," was originally associated with battlefield or disaster situations. In such situations, in which casualties overwhelm the capabilities and resources of health-care systems, the triage officer must decide which patients need immediate treatment, which patients can wait for treatment, and which patients are so severely injured as to render treatment futile. Triage, in this context, is a major issue for prehospital providers of care and transport. In emergency department (ED) triage, patients are evaluated immediately on arrival, and a determination is made regarding how long they can wait for care and where they should receive this care.

The goals of ED triage are to define and classify the urgency of patients based on their complaint and presentation, to ensure their safety, to facilitate their care and flow through the ED, and to satisfy relevant legal requirements mandating "screening" examinations for all persons presenting for care. In some cases, this may include triaging patients away from the ED to other health-care sources and giving telephone advice.

TRIAGE WITHIN THE EMERGENCY DEPARTMENT

Most hospitals in the United States use registered nurses to perform triage in the ED. Despite evidence that specialized training improves performance,[4] many report that triage nurses are not required to have special training for this role. Licensed practical nurses (LPNs), nurse practitioners, technicians, and physician assistants are also frequently employed in triage roles. Specially trained nonmedical personnel using physician-written algorithms have been shown to be highly effective, with high levels of agreement with subsequent physician review.[19] Computerized algorithms have also been shown to be safe and effective adjuncts to triage.[3]

Triage documentation should include the chief complaint, a limited history and physical examination, vital signs, significant or relevant past medical history (e.g., immunization status), current medications, and allergies. If applicable and practical, visual acuity testing can also be performed. While excessive evaluation at the triage desk may actually prolong waiting time for sicker patients,[7] initiating some diagnostic tests (e.g., x-rays, blood tests, urinalysis) has been shown to decrease waiting times,[10] with good correlation to tests subsequently ordered by physicians.[16] In some instances, initiating treatment in the triage area (e.g., administering antipyretics, oral rehydration, and topical ophthalmic anesthetics) may also facilitate ED care.

Triage classification schemes typically utilize either three or five levels of priority. (Tables 403.1 and 403.2).

Generally, emergent problems include immediately life-threatening conditions, urgent problems require treatment within a fairly short time, and nonemergent problems are conditions in which delays in treatment are not expected to be detrimental. Five-level systems use additional levels primarily to further discriminate among patients with the most acute presentations (i.e., "emergent" in a three-level system). Such patients would be divided into immediate (i.e., resuscitation), very urgent, and urgent categories, with target times to evaluation and treatment of 0, 10, and 30 to 60 minutes, respectively. Such systems are used in Canada, Great Britain, Australia, and New Zealand, and include specific recommendations for acceptable waiting times in each category.[6] Based on the triage classification, the patient can be moved immediately to the appropriate treatment area, or can be processed for patient registration.

TABLE 403.1. Triage Classification Categories: Three Levels of Priority

EMERGENT
Complaints, vital signs, illness, or injury consistent with an acute, potentially life- or limb-threatening condition that requires immediate evaluation or treatment to prevent mortality or increased morbidity
Examples: airway obstruction, coma, uncontrolled hemorrhage, chest pain, respiratory distress, shock, multiple trauma, toxic ingestion, severely painful conditions, active labor, febrile infant, amputations, dental avulsions
URGENT
Complaints, vital signs, illness, or injury consistent with an acute, potentially life- or limb-threatening condition requiring evaluation or treatment within a few hours to prevent mortality or increased morbidity
Examples: open fracture, abdominal pain, lacerations, severe headache (afebrile), moderate difficulty breathing, sore throat with dysphagia, hip or long-bone fractures
NONEMERGENT
Complaints, vital signs, illness, or injury consistent with a subacute or chronic not life- or limb-threatening condition that does not require evaluation or management within 24 hours to prevent increased morbidity
Examples: wound check, suture removal, chronic rash, chronic joint pain, insect bites (without anaphylaxis), minor earache, minor isolated extremity trauma

TABLE 403.2. Triage Classification Categories: Five Levels of Priority

IMMEDIATE
Complaint or condition requiring immediate assessment and treatment; any delay represents an unacceptable risk to the life or limb of the patient.
Examples: cardiac arrest, obstructed airway, shock
VERY URGENT (EMERGENCY)
Complaint or condition requiring assessment and treatment within 10 minutes
Examples: chest pain, significant hemorrhage, significant difficulty breathing, major trauma
URGENT
Complaint or condition requiring assessment and treatment within 30–60 minutes
Examples: toxic ingestion, severely painful conditions
SEMIURGENT (STANDARD)
Complaint or condition requiring assessment and treatment within 1–2 hours
Examples: lacerations, abdominal pain, hip or long-bone fracture
NONURGENT
Complaint or condition requiring assessment and treatment within 2–4 hours or longer
Examples: wound check, minor rash, suture removal, isolated minor extremity trauma

TRIAGING FROM THE EMERGENCY DEPARTMENT TO OTHER SITES

Due to ED overcrowding and the high cost of ED care, many hospitals triage selected nonemergent patients out of the ED. In fact, in many discussions, the very term *triage* has come to mean refusal of ED services rather than prioritizing patients for care within the ED. If patients are to be refused care in the ED, they must receive an adequate screening examination as required by federal law, and there must be a practical alternative source of care. The prevailing consensus is that a screening examination constitutes a physician-directed evaluation, and treatment, if necessary, using all of the necessary resources routinely available in the hospital (see Chapter 408).

A study of more than 31,000 patients triaged from a university ED to alternative sites over a 5-year period showed no significant adverse outcomes. Patients who were refused care met strict inclusion and exclusion criteria. Follow-up data were available on only 34% of cases, but, of those, 26% had decided not to seek alternative care of any kind. Only 1% sought care at another ED.[5] Another study, using the same guidelines, at a different hospital concluded that the guidelines may not be sensitive enough to identify all patients who need emergency care.[14] Other studies have shown that high percentages of pediatric patients who were refused care failed to keep appointments made for them by the ED.[12] All studies of patient outcome after being refused care are limited by incomplete follow-up information. It is also clear that there is significant variability among individual practitioner's assessments regarding the urgency of patients' complaints[8] and that triage methods have not been widely standardized and statistically validated.[20]

The Society for Academic Emergency Medicine has published an ethics statement defining refusal of ED services as ethical only if an examination has determined the lack of an emergency and assured medical stability, that alternative care is available without financial or other barriers, that the patient will be seen in a timely fashion, that the alternative site is either on campus or transportation is assured, that the patient understands and agrees to transfer, that all patients are treated equitably, and that triage criteria are based on research showing them to be safe and effective.[18]

Many hospitals are developing "fast-track" or "urgent care" systems in which patients with minor illness and injuries are triaged to a separate area, which may or may not be in physical proximity to the ED, for prompt service. This type of system may be particularly suitable for patients who are unlikely to require x-rays, laboratory studies, or hospital admission, all of which prolong ED waiting time.[15] It is unclear whether fast-track centers within EDs actually realize the savings (either for the hospital or for society in general) for which they are intended.[17]

Nurse practitioners have been used to staff fast-tracks with good results, including decreased overall patient waiting times and high levels of patient satisfaction. Advanced training and physician backup are essential to a smoothly running system. Teaching hospitals have also reported good results with house officer–staffed fast-track systems, but problems can ensue when overall ED acuity is high, requiring fast-track staff to be used in other areas.

TELEPHONE ADVICE

More than 1 million telephone calls per month are made to various health information services nationwide. Studies of the types of calls made to EDs show a variety of complaints, ranging from common gastrointestinal and respiratory problems to hemorrhage and cardiopulmonary arrest. These calls are usually handled by a nurse, with or without physician backup. Because a patient cannot be examined over the telephone, the physician or nurse is limited in diagnosing or managing problems. Protocols (algorithms) for handling medical advice telephone calls have been developed and tested. Explicit training for telephone management is part of some residency programs.[11]

Telephone advice should also be considered another form of triage. Patients who would be triaged as emergent should be advise to call an ambulance for transport to the nearest appropriate facility. Those judged to have urgent complaints or conditions should be advised to come to the ED as soon as possible, by private vehicle or public transportation, if appropriate. Alternatively, they can be advised to check with their primary care provider. If patients cannot be seen by their primary care provider in a timely manner, ED evaluation should be recommended. Patients with nonemergent conditions may be referred to their personal physician, a staff physician, or an outpatient clinic. If there is any doubt about the urgency of the complaint, patients should be advised to come to the ED immediately. Because telephone triage is based solely on reported symptoms, it is important to triage to the highest possible level based on a worst-case scenario.

Simulated calls have been used to assess the quality of advice given in response to potentially serious complaints.[1] Essential information is often not sought, and inappropriate treatment is often recommended. In general, telephone advice is often inadequate and may expose the patient to medical risk and the advice-giver to legal risk. The experience and level of training of those who give advice over the telephone do not seem to guarantee the quality of the advice. In one study, nurse practitioners managed pediatric problems over the telephone better than pediatric house officers or practicing pediatricians. Among practicing pediatricians, less experienced physicians asked more questions and spent more time on each call than their more experienced colleagues. A large British study showed that nurses managed primary care phone consults as safely as physicians.[13]

Malpractice judgments have resulted from inadequate or erroneous medical advice given over the telephone.[9] If any medical advice is given, an assumption of duty may be presumed and the advice-giver can be held responsible for that advice, even though the advice-giver may neither have met the patient nor received any payment for services.

The American College of Emergency Physicians (ACEP) "recommends against any substantial diagnosis or treatment recommendation by telephone." Patients who have been recently discharged from the ED and have questions about their instructions are exceptions to this rule. Also, patients who need first aid information or information about accessing medical care should be obliged.[2] ACEP further recommends that telephone advice be given only by qualified personnel, and that the quality of advice should be maintained with explicit policies, protocols, and quality-assurance programs. Hence, secretaries should refer all calls to a nurse, preferably one trained in triage, with physician advice obtained in all but the most straightforward cases. It is also prudent to document all telephone conversations by using a logbook or patient encounter forms.

COMMON PITFALLS

- Failure to attribute presenting symptoms and signs to the most serious possible etiology, and then triage accordingly
- Failure to periodically reassess the condition of patients in the waiting room and retriage, if necessary
- Giving substantive telephone advice, especially advice to delay or avoid seeking care
- Triaging to other sites without using strict guidelines, and only after an appropriate screening examination

References

1. Aitken ME, et al. Telephone advice about an infant given by after-hours clinics and emergency departments. *N Z Med J* 1995;108(1005):315.
2. American College of Emergency Physicians. Providing telephone advice from the emergency department. *Ann Emerg Med* 1990;19:5.
3. Bermen DA, Coleridge ST, McMurry TA. Computerized algorithm-directed triage in the emergency department. *Ann Emerg Med* 1989;18:2.
4. Cook S, Sinclair D. Emergency department triage: a program assessment using the tools of continuous quality improvement. *J Emerg Med* 1997;15:6.
5. Derlet RW, Kinse D, Ray L, et al. Prospective identification and triage on nonemergency patients out of an emergency department: a 5-year study. *Ann Emerg Med* 1995;25:2.
6. *Emergency triage.* Manchester Triage Group, Mackway-Jones K, ed. London: BMJ Publishing Group, 1997.
7. George S, Read S, Williams B. Nurse triage increases emergency department waiting times. *BMJ* 1995;311:7015.
8. Gill JM, Reese CL, Diamond JJ. Disagreement among health-care professionals about the urgent care needs of emergency department patients. *Ann Emerg Med* 1996;28:5.
9. Katz HP, Wick W. Malpractice, meningitis, and the telephone. *Pediatr Ann* 1991;20:2.
10. Klassen TP, Ropp LF, Sutcliffe T, et al. A randomized, controlled trial of radiograph ordering for extremity trauma in a pediatric emergency department. *Ann Emerg Med* 1993;22:10.
11. Kosowe E, Inkelis SH, Seidel JS. Telephone T.A.L.K: a telephone communication program. *Pediatr Emerg Care* 1991;7:2.
12. Kuensting LL. "Triaging out" children with minor illnesses from an emergency department by a triage nurse: where do they go? *J Emerg Nurs* 1995;21:2.
13. Lattimer V, et al. Safety and effectiveness of nurse telephone consultation in out-of-hours primary care: randomized controlled trial. *BMJ* 1998; 17(317):1054–1059.
14. Lowe RA, Bindman AB, Ulrich SK, et al. Refusing care to emergency department patients: evaluation of published triage guidelines. *Ann Emerg Med* 1994;23:2.
15. Meislin HW, Coates SA, Cyr J, et al. Fast track: urgent care within a teaching hospital emergency department: can it work? *Ann Emerg Med* 1988;17:5.
16. Seaberg DC, MacLeod BA. Correlation between triage nurse and physician ordering of ED tests. *Am J Emerg Med* 1998;16:1.
17. Simon K, Ledbetter DA, Wright J. Societal savings by "fast tracking" lower acuity patients in an urban pediatric emergency department. *Am J Emerg Med* 1997;15:6.
18. Society for Academic Emergency Medicine. Ethics of emergency department triage: SAEM position statement. *Acad Emerg Med* 1995;2:11.
19. Wilson RP, Wilson LO, Butler AB, et al. Algorithm-directed triage of pediatric patients. *JAMA* 1980;243:15.
20. Wuerz R, Fernandes CM, Alarcon J. Inconsistency of emergency department triage. Emergency Department Operations Research Working Group. *Ann Emerg Med* 1998;32:4.

PART II

Medicolegal and Special Clinical Considerations

CHAPTER 404

General Legal Principles

Abigail R. Williams

FUNCTION OF THE LAW

The law provides behavioral rules that organize society, a way to enforce these rules, and a means to resolve disputes between parties. The legal system performs these functions with three mechanisms that differ in point of view and operation: adjudication, advocacy, and arbitration. The law has a major impact not only on the delivery of health care, but also on the management and daily operation of health-care institutions. The emergency physician should be familiar with the fact that various sources of law exist and with the general areas of law that apply to clinical practice. However, law is more often the interpretation of several potentially applicable sets of facts to a slightly unclear set of rules and cases. Rules have exceptions and special circumstances under which the law is applied differently. It is the exceptions, not the laws, that create the need for lawyers.

Sources of Law

The American legal system recognizes several sources of law, including statutory law and case law. Statutes are laws developed and codified by the elected legislative branches of federal, state, or local governments.* Case law is the accumulated body of decisions of state and federal courts.† Existing case law precedent must be followed in resolving current disputes, but variations between cases make case law more obscure and fluid than statutory law. A binding precedent in one jurisdiction may be, but does not have to be, followed by other jurisdictions. Regulations are like statutes but are promulgated by administrative agencies, generally to amplify or supplement statutes. Hence, although they are not legislated, regulations are considered administrative law. They tend to be even more fluid than case law and prone to variation with political climate. If challenged, regulations are reviewed by the courts to determine whether the regulation is within the scope and authority of the administrative body and whether it avoids abridging Constitutional rights.

*An act of the legislature declaring, commanding, or prohibiting something.[3]

†The aggregate of reported cases as forming a body of jurisprudence.[2]

CIVIL AND CRIMINAL LAW

There are two categories of legal actions—civil and criminal. Criminal proceedings arise from a charge of public offense in which a law has allegedly been broken and the aggrieved party is the government. The goal of criminal law is to punish the wrongdoer, and the punishment is usually some loss of liberty, most often incarceration or a significant monetary fine, or both. Civil disputes are actions between private parties. The goal of civil litigation is to compensate the injured or aggrieved party. Medical malpractice falls within the category of civil suits and is a tort, or a civil wrong. Torts can be either intentional, such as punching another person, or unintentional, such as hitting another person while hurrying around a corner. Within the broad category of negligence falls professional negligence, including medical malpractice. Negligence occurs when, without harmful intent or wrongdoing, one acts in a manner, either by commission of an act or omission of an act, that injures another.[9]

Most civil disputes are resolved without court trial, often with attorneys acting in an arbitration role. When it is not possible to resolve disputes privately, the courts assume that role and establish case law. Variability in case law occurs because of subtle differences in facts or laws and because there is room for human subjective interpretation in an otherwise well-defined process.

A lawyer's role is not just to interpret and argue the law, but also to understand and apply the exceptions, the special circumstances or conditions in which the general intent of the law does not apply or may be applied differently. For example, speed limits on highways may not apply to emergency vehicles during emergency operations. In many cases, the wealth of exceptions developed through case law complicates and exceeds the scope of the original law as stated, and compliance requires significant analysis and understanding of these conditions.

Malpractice

Medical malpractice is professional negligence, or medical practice falling below what is generally held to be the standard of practice for a physician with similar training in the same or similar circumstances as the physician who rendered the care in question.[10] It is generally assumed that a practicing physician is required to possess the same or similar skill level as others with similar training practicing in similar circumstances, regardless of his or her specialty. It is further assumed that the physician will exercise reasonable care in the treatment of his or her patients.

The application of these assumptions to physicians practicing in emergency departments creates some confusion. In many cases, the physician providing care in an emergency department may not be trained or board certified in emergency medicine. The standard, however, remains "same or similar training in same or similar circumstances." Therefore, physicians without emergency medicine training are not currently held to the standard of those who are trained or certified in emergency medicine when practicing in the emergency department setting. This is not to say that the standard for those certified in emergency medicine is always higher; a cardiologist moonlighting in the emergency department will probably be held to a higher standard when caring for a patient with cardiac disease than a board-certified emergency physician caring for the same patient. This situation, presumably existing because hospital credentialing criteria allow physicians without emergency medical training or certification to practice in that setting, is changing. It may reasonably be expected, based on the legal concept of detrimental reliance, that physicians practicing in emergency departments soon will be held to the standard of physicians trained and certified in that specialty. In other words, the public has a right to expect a facility offering emergency care to include access to physicians trained and competent in that specialty.

The standard-of-care definition will likely shift to require that physicians be held to the standard of a physician choosing to practice in the same setting, not to the standard of those with equal training regardless of setting. It is more logical from the patient's point of view, and as emergency physicians argue for more specialty-specific qualifications in hospital credentialing criteria, they will accelerate this shift. However, until this shift occurs, physicians practicing emergency medicine should be aware of the credentialing requirements at their facilities and comply with them meticulously. Failure to meet the credentialing requirements, or, worse, intentional misrepresentation that certain certification or training is an adequate substitute for a specified training program, may place the noncompliant physician in significant jeopardy if legal action occurs and the credentialing process is examined. In particular, self-insured hospitals may have no obligation to cover physicians who misrepresent themselves on credentialing forms. Physicians unhappy with credentialing requirements, for any of the reasons just mentioned, should work to change them rather than ignore or circumvent them.

To prevail in a malpractice, or negligence, action against a physician (defendant), the allegedly injured patient (plaintiff) must begin legal proceedings within the time period defined by the applicable statute of limitations, and prove four elements:

1. That the physician owed a duty of care to the patient
2. That the duty was not performed to the level of the generally accepted standard of care. This is known as a breach of duty.
3. That some injury occurred
4. That the breach of duty was the cause of the claimed injury

Not all bad outcomes are caused by negligent practice, just as every instance of substandard practice does not result in patient injury or legal action. Unfortunately, many patients are not informed or do not understand that a perfect outcome cannot be expected in all cases. Educating patients and their families about reasonably expected outcomes from a certain condition may help correct this misperception.

DUTY

The legal concept of a duty was created in an attempt to delineate the relationship and responsibilities between two or more parties. If one owes a duty to another, then a special relationship has been entered into—to treat another with "due care." *Due care* is defined as ordinary reasonable care, not the best care available and not the worst. Failure to act with due care results in a breach of duty.

In general, one does not have a duty to act on behalf of another unless some special relationship exists. There is no mandate that a physician must undertake to render care to a particular patient. The relationship between physician and patient is based on contract theory in which the physician has the right to choose which patients he or she will treat.‡ This means that, with a few exceptions, physicians are under no affirmative duty to render aid to a patient, even if the patient is likely to die without such aid. Should a physician not wish to enter into a treatment relationship with a patient, such limitations should be set out clearly so that they are understood and accepted by the patient. If the physician chooses to treat, payment or discussion of fees is not necessary to hold the physician liable for failing to exercise ordinary care. Even if a physician renders care gratuitously, he or she is not absolved of the duty of due care.[5]

Although at common law there is generally no right of a person to hospital admission, the freedom to choose whether to treat no longer extends to hospitals, and modifications of this general rule have been made with regard to patients who present to emergency departments.[4] Courts have found that an emergency department physician owes a duty to all persons who present for care, and that a hospital operating an emergency department owes a duty to offer care to all persons presenting for care, including admission, if warranted. This exception to the general principle requiring a special relationship before establishment of duty has developed from the theory of detrimental reliance; patients who presented to emergency departments in the past and were denied care were found to have relied, to their significant detriment, on their belief that the hospital was offering emergency care to all who presented for such care. Thus, the duty owed by emergency physicians arises out of an exception to the general principles of duty.

STANDARD OF CARE

Where a duty exists, that duty is to treat at least to the standard of care. The plaintiff in a malpractice action must show that the treatment provided by the defendant physician did not meet the standard of care, as defined by expert testimony. An expert is a physician with the same or similar training as the defendant who testifies to what care would have been reasonably appropriate in similar circumstances.[12,13] General practitioners are usually held to a local standard (county or state), and specialists, such as trained or certified emergency physicians, are held to a national standard.[1] As discussed, current common practice is that the standard for emergency physicians is often defined by specialists in other fields (e.g., cardiologists, orthopedists), either because that is the training of the defendant physician working in the emergency department or because the patient's problem clearly falls into that specialty in the mind of the plaintiff's attorney and the attorney is able to find a specialist willing to testify to their understanding of the standard of care. Therefore, some physicians, untrained in emergency medicine but working in emergency departments, are held to the standard of their own training rather than to emergency physician standards, and some physicians, trained in emergency medicine, are held to the standard of a specialist in whatever area encompasses the patient's problem. Both of these situations are changing. Many more trained and certified emergency

‡The terms of the relationship between the physician and the patient may be general or limited.[8]

physicians are making themselves available to the plaintiff's and/or defendant's bar for case analysis, expert opinions, and testimony related to the standard of emergency care. Guidelines for emergency physicians wishing to make themselves available for expert opinion work exist. Simultaneously, pressure to change hospital credentialing requirements for physicians practicing in the emergency department, increasing numbers of residency-trained emergency physicians, and other forces will probably reduce the number of physicians without emergency training or certification practicing in emergency departments. These trends, along with the development and publication of practice guidelines, should clarify the standard of care for emergency physicians.

In some circumstances, however, a higher standard of care is established by hospital policies and procedures, and these can vary significantly from facility to facility. Hospital employees must follow the policies and procedures established by the hospital.[6] Because emergency physicians are often employed by the hospital, or are considered hospital employees, they should familiarize themselves with, and adhere to, hospital policies and procedures.

A dilemma occurs when the individual physician feels that patient care, at or perhaps above the standard, is required that would conflict with a hospital policy or procedure. Ideally, relevant policies and procedures should be developed with the input and approval of the emergency physicians involved, but if not, any legal issues should be referred to an attorney skilled in emergency medical law for opinion. Continued physician disagreement, if any, with hospital policy should be clearly documented and a course of action developed. One option is for the hospital to agree, in writing, to accept liability for any claims arising out of the disputed policy. This is referred to as an indemnity agreement, whereby the hospital agrees to indemnify the physician for the particular matter. This is clearly more confrontational than a mutually agreeable policy, but it may be a useful concept in situations in which there are impassable issues related to a particular policy.

Implicit in due care is the expectation that the physician is acting in the best interest of the patient at all times. Adhering to accepted medical practice, but in a manner that is against the best interest of a given patient, may trigger a claim of negligence. If you know or believe the standards set in your institution pose unnecessary dangers to your patients, whatever precautionary measures as are appropriate should be taken to protect the patient from harm, even if that means violating hospital policy or procedure.

INJURY

The plaintiff must also prove that an injury has been suffered to prevail in a negligence action. Regardless of how bad the care, there is no case for malpractice if there is no injury. Although, traditionally, the injury suffered had to be physical, increasingly, states are allowing recovery for infliction of emotional injuries such as emotional distress,§ even in the absence of physical injury. The injury may also be to a third party if it was caused by negligent treatment of the patient. For example, a patient who is discharged in an impaired state (e.g., eye patch on, narcotics given, or intoxicated) without being warned against driving and who subsequently runs over a pedestrian (third party) has a reasonable claim that the accident was foreseeable, and both the patient and pedestrian could file claims against the emergency physician.

§Evidence that hospital employees mistakenly informed parents that a dead child was alive supports a claim for emotional distress.[11]

CAUSATION

The final element of a negligence claim is causal connection between the actions of the physician and the injury. The physician's action must be the *substantial* factor in the patient's injury. No matter how bad or unexpected the patient's outcome, or how far the care rendered to the patient was below the standard, if the negligence did not cause the outcome, there is no liability for malpractice. On the other hand, the outcome from the negligent act may be separate from the overall outcome, and no matter how good the overall outcome, the negligent act may still substantially cause an injury. For example, tissue necrosis that requires skin grafting and is caused by an extravasation of dextrose intended for intravenous injection may result in disfigurement and loss of function, despite the fact that the patient recovered from the hypoglycemic episode. If the same injury occurs during futile resuscitation attempts performed on a patient who arrives in asystole, there is no causal link between the extravasation and the patient's death, assuming that the death was not caused by untreated hypoglycemia.

APPLICATION OF GENERAL PRINCIPLES

Duty

The duty of an emergency physician to care for persons is complex and may vary depending on the person's circumstances, location, and problem. It is generally accepted that the emergency physician owes a duty to persons who come to the emergency department requesting care. Patients of private physicians who come to the emergency department to be seen only by their own private physician can create a great deal of confusion for the emergency department.[14] Determining who is responsible for evaluating the patient and rendering care is not easy in these situations without clear and complete policies and procedures. If not formally seen by the emergency physician, these patients are frequently not triaged, no record of their care exists, and the emergency physician on duty may not be aware of their presence in the emergency department. However, if these patients suffer a clinical deterioration while waiting, the emergency department may be liable for the patient's outcome. This is based on the theory that the emergency physician is responsible for all of the patients in the department, not just those who present for care by the emergency physician. Hence, all persons who physically present to the emergency department must be seen by the staff, and should have a nursing evaluation if it is standard in the facility, a medical record initiated, and evaluation by the emergency physician for any potentially emergent conditions that may exist before being allowed to wait for their private physician (see Chapter 408).

This duty may also extend to those patients who initiate contact with the department by telephone or through the emergency medical system (EMS) and may include others in the hospital or on hospital grounds (e.g., patients, visitors, employees), depending on the hospital's policies regarding the scope of responsibility for the emergency physician. A record should be made of all telephone and radio patient contacts, including the subject of the call and advice given. Records should also be kept for any physician–patient encounters that occur outside the emergency department, particularly if a formal emergency department evaluation is not subsequently performed.

There are situations in which the duty owed is expanded to include other foreseeable parties. If parents, for example, are *asked* to participate in the care of their child, the emergency department may owe a duty of care to the parents, including a duty to protect them from injury (e.g., fainting and needlesticks) while participating in that care.[7] If, however, the parent is not asked to participate in the patient's care but wishes to accompany the patient during the treatment, the emergency department does not owe the parent the duty of protection from fainting. Other foreseeable third parties to whom a duty is owed include bystanders who may be injured by an impaired patient within the department.

Immunity

In an attempt to encourage volunteerism in an emergency situation, many states have enacted Good Samaritan statutes, a form of immunity, to protect physicians as well as lay people from claims of malpractice if they undertake to render aid to another in an emergency. An immunity, defined as a benefit that is granted contrary to general rule, may be invoked by the emergency physician as a defense to a charge of malpractice if the circumstances of the encounter meet jurisdictional requirements. There are some typical elements of Good Samaritan statues. The first is a class requirement that delineates the group of people to which you must belong for the immunity to apply. Many statutes provide protection for the person who arrives at the scene of an emergency, is present when the emergency occurs, or is called to the scene of the emergency and refer specifically to nurses, physicians, and EMS providers. The second element is a compensation requirement. Most immunity statutes require that the care rendered must be uncompensated. Therefore, these statutes generally do not apply to physicians whose compensated or routine job it is to provide emergency care in emergency departments, but they may apply when the emergency physician is acting outside of normal employment, such as by providing care at the scene of an automobile accident while driving home from work. There is a good faith requirement in most statutes, which means that the care rendered is done so in good faith, with the victim's best interests in mind. There is also generally a conduct requirement, stating that there be no "grossly negligent conduct." This immunity may be invoked by the emergency physician charged with malpractice if the circumstances of the event meet local requirements. Generally, compensated practice in an emergency department does not apply. An immunity does not mean that one cannot be sued (although a reasonable plaintiff would not pursue action in such circumstances), and it only offers one defense to a suit, albeit a powerful one.

Therefore, the duty of an emergency physician to care for persons is complex and may vary depending on the person's circumstances, location, and problem. It generally extends to all persons presenting physically, and probably by other means of communication, to the emergency department, and may also include others in the hospital, such as patients or visitors, employees, and persons on or near the hospital grounds, depending on hospital policy regarding the responsibilities of the emergency physician and the department. In some cases, particularly when the care given may be "volunteer" and outside the scope of typical or normal duties, there may be no duty to care, and any care given may be immune from legal action if certain tests are met.

SUMMARY

Law may be statutory, regulatory, or arise from cases. Exceptions and jurisdictional location may significantly alter findings. Medical malpractice claims arise from civil tort law, and, therefore, are not criminal in nature. The elements required to prove malpractice are duty, breach, causation, and damages. Practical application of these principles can be complex, as illustrated with the concept of duty as it applies to emergency physicians. Additional legal issues are explored in detail in subsequent chapters.

COMMON PITFALLS

- Failure to appreciate the governing laws for your jurisdiction and their exceptions
- Failure to educate patients about potential adverse outcomes as well as expected outcomes
- Failure to understand the concept of the duty to treat
- Failure to apprise oneself of hospital policies and procedures and abide by same
- Failure to consider the duty owed to third parties and society

References

1. *Beach v. Cholle,* 166 N.E. 145 (1928).
2. Black HC. *Black's Law Dictionary,* rev. 4th ed., p. 272.
3. Black HC. *Black's Law Dictionary,* rev. 4th ed., p. 1581.
4. *Guerro v. Cooper Queen Hospital,* 112 Ariz. 104, 537 P.2d 1329 (1975).
5. *McNevins v. Lowe,* 40 Ill. 209 (1866).
6. *Niles v. The City of San Rafael,* 42 Cal. App 3d 230, 116 Cal. Rptr. 733 (1974).
7. *O'Hara v. Holy Cross Hospital,* 561 N.E. 2d 18 (1990).
8. *Osborne v. Frazor,* 425 S.W. 2d 768 (Tenn. 1968).
9. *Osborne v. Montgomery,* 302 Wis. 223, 234 N.W. 372 (1930).
10. *Prosser and Keeton on torts* (Keeton WP, 5th ed., 1984).
11. *Rivera v. Wyckoff Heights Hospital,* 184 A.2d 558 (1992).
12. *Shilkret v. Annapolis Emergency Hospital Association,* 276, Md., 187, 349 A.2d 245 (1975).
13. *Thomas v. Corso,* 265 Md. 84, 288 A.2d 379 (1972).
14. *University Hospital Bldg., Inc., d/b/a Memorial Hospital of Jacksonville v. Gooding,* 419 So. 2d 1111 (1982).

CHAPTER 405
Advance Directives

Abigail R. Williams

Medical technology is capable of sustaining patients unable to convey their wishes about further care. Physicians may discuss such matters with patients and write orders limiting therapy, and patients may create a variety of documents, known generally as advance directives, expressing their wishes or authorizing others to make medical decisions for them in the event they become unable or not competent to voice such wishes themselves. In most cases, the patient has a serious chronic medical problem and the orders or documents are intended to limit resuscitative measures that would otherwise be initiated. These orders are often referred to as "Do Not Resuscitate" or "DNR" orders, but the term *resuscitation* is so overly vague and broad in scope as to make it meaningless without further definition. Therefore, this chapter avoids use of the word *resuscitation* as defining a specific set of medical therapies, and uses it instead to refer to the concept of efforts to restore or stabilize vital functions.

Hospitalized patients cared for by physicians who know the patients' wishes often benefit from such orders or documents limiting therapy. Problems arise when patients present to emergency departments, move from one health-care facility to another, are cared for by emergency medical services (EMS) providers, or otherwise are in a setting where their primary physician does not directly control their care and their wishes are not clearly represented in an unambiguous and verifiable fashion. It is rare that patients have a copy of the order written by their physician or their advance directive when they present to the emergency department, and even more rare that such an order or document is acceptable to the emergency physician treating the patients. For example, these documents may be vague, illegible, outdated, not legally accepted in certain states, or impossible to verify. Medical records, if present, are not likely to be current and easily verifiable as accurate or reflecting the latest wishes of patients. Further complicating the situation is the need for speed if patients are to be treated. Another difficult question is whether emergency personnel should honor a third-party (the patients' families or primary care physicians) communication (orally or through documents) regarding the patients' wishes when the directive itself is unavailable. The result is that treatment may be initiated in an effort to resuscitate the patients, even though these efforts may not be in accord with their wishes. This chapter reviews the various types of advance directives and orders limiting therapy currently in use, examines some of the issues surrounding them, and makes suggestions for emergency department care.

"DO NOT RESUSCITATE" ORDERS

One of the most pressing problems facing emergency physicians in the area of limiting patient therapy is the definition of terms. The words *do not resuscitate* (DNR) mean different things to different people. American Heart Association (AHA) standards suggest that DNR orders are appropriate for a patient who is "irreversibly, irreparably ill, whose death is imminent; . . . ."[16] By *irreversible,* it is meant that there are no known therapeutic measures that would be effective in reversing the course of the illness. *Irreparable* means the time has been reached when the course of the illness has progressed beyond the capacity of existing knowledge and technique to stem it. *Imminent death* is defined as death occurring with reasonable probability within 2 weeks of the time that the DNR order is written. Even with these definitions, problems exist. There is confusion about what is ordinarily meant by *resuscitation,* even among physicians. In one study, 90% of physicians surveyed thought that DNR meant that there be no chest compression or use of defibrillators on a patient whose heart had stopped beating; about 85% thought that DNR prohibited intubation of the airway for artificial ventilation if the patient stopped breathing; and 60% thought that DNR meant that no drugs should be used to raise the patient's blood pressure.[13] If physicians are confused, then patients most likely are as well. What patients perceive as extraordinary measures will depend, in large part, on the orientation of their own physician.

Emergency physicians routinely perform procedures that are perceived by most patients, and some of the medical profession, as heroic and extraordinary. Therefore, the term *DNR* is too vague and broad for meaningful use. More specific instructions, such as "No CPR" or "No intubation" may be an improvement, but even more useful would be a clearer definition of *when* efforts should be made to treat the patient and the goal of those efforts, leaving the exact nature of the therapy to the treating physician. For example, documentation that a patient with chronic lung disease wants no therapy to reverse respiratory failure if respiratory arrest caused by the chronic disease is imminent, but instead prefers comfort as a goal, is clearer documentation than a vague "I do not wish any heroic or extraordinary measures" statement.

INFORMED CONSENT

Informed consent means that competent adults have the right to make decisions, after being informed about reasonable options, as to what medical care they will or will not receive, and the consequences of receiving or not receiving care.[4,8] The right to consent to care logically leads to the right of an individual not to consent to care or to refuse care, even if this decision results in the patient's loss of life.[2,3] Difficulties can arise, however, in emergency situations in which individuals are critically ill, incapable of receiving and processing the relevant information, or unable to convey their wishes due to a communication impairment resulting either from a chronic or acute disease process or a language barrier. In such cases, someone else (a "surrogate") will probably be called on to make health-care decisions for the incompetent or impaired individual, and those decisions will be based either on the prior expressed wishes of the patient or on the surrogate's own judgment about what is "best" for the patient.

The evolution of health-care proxies and other means for expressing personal wishes has been prompted by advances in resuscitative and supportive medical technology, increased expression of personal beliefs, and changes in the physician–patient relationship. Hospitals are required to have mechanisms in place for patients to reach therapy-limiting decisions and to ensure that this information is available to health-care providers.[9] The Patient Self-Determination Act of 1990 (PSDA) requires hospitals, nursing homes, home health agencies, hospices, and health maintenance organizations (HMOs) participating in the Medicare and Medicaid programs to address the subject of advance written directives with their patients. Its goal, presuming that the PSDA and other initiatives have led to an increased awareness on the part of health-care consumers about their right to guide their medical care, is to encourage people to plan ahead for their health care, although they may remain confused about the tools by which to document their wishes. It is unclear how these initiatives will impact treatment under emergency conditions.

The tools available to the patient (and to the physician) depend, in part, on the jurisdiction of the patient and the physician. Different types of directives are recognized in different states. Hence, the mobility of today's society creates a problem of legal recognition of documentation. For example, a patient who resides in Florida and has a valid living will may be vacationing in Massachusetts, where living wills are not recognized. Another problem is the issue of portability of the advance directive to unforeseen circumstances. For example, a cancer patient who made a decision in conjunction with her treating physician to forgo CPR and intubation should her heart stop beating, but who presents to the emergency room unconscious after a motor vehicle accident, presents a dilemma when a relative relates the wish for "no heroics."

Dealing with these complex issues requires an understanding of the different ways in which patients may express their wishes and the potential impact of those wishes on patient care.

DURABLE POWER OF ATTORNEY

One form of advance directive is the Durable Power of Attorney for Healthcare. The Uniform Durable Power of Attorney Act permits a competent individual to appoint an "attorney-in-fact" (that is, a legally authorized surrogate) for health-care decisions.[6] The surrogate may then authorize medical treatment if and when the patient becomes incompetent. The Act does not specify whether the surrogate may demand that treatment be withheld or withdrawn, especially if the treatment is arguably beneficial or lifesaving. More than half of the states have laws that permit surrogates to make medical decisions, specifically including decisions to withdraw or withhold life support.[15] Additional states have court decisions, attorney general opinions, or other statutes that interpret general power of attorney statutes to permit health-care decision making, including withdrawal or withholding of life support. Particular technical requirements for such documents may vary, making familiarity with state law crucial.

Statutes authorizing powers of attorney for health care may sometimes be interpreted as limiting the decision-making authority of the surrogate. In a Pennsylvania case, it was held that an attorney-in-fact who had been appointed pursuant to a broad but general durable power of attorney did not have the power to make critical care decisions for the patient.[14] In another example, an appeals court ruled that the court-appointed guardian of a 29-year-old man in a persistent vegetative state could discontinue the man's tube feedings, but not if discontinuation of the nutrition or hydration would be likely to result in death by malnutrition or dehydration. The court also read the new statute as limiting the authority of court-appointed guardians, because guardians act with even less guidance on their wards' wishes than do surrogates appointed by the patients themselves.[5]

HEALTH-CARE PROXY INSTRUMENTS

A health-care proxy is an instrument naming another individual to make medical decisions when the patient is incompetent, often in cooperation with the patient's physician. These documents often require witnesses or legal assistance in preparation. Physician orders limiting therapy then involve the patient's attending or primary care physician in the process, with either the patient or a named surrogate collaborating with the physician to express their mutual decision through signed medical orders. Whether the emergency physician can reasonably act as an "attending physician" for the patient in this case is unclear. Problems also arise when the need to make a proxy decision arises and the proxy named some time ago has since become incompetent or died.

LIVING WILLS

Living wills are legal instruments in which patients specify their wishes without the involvement of anyone other than the person(s) who assist in drafting the instrument. In some jurisdictions, an individual may actually make certain kinds of health-care decisions that take effect at a later date, when the drafter is unable to make or communicate treatment of his or her wishes. This advance directive stands on its own, *without the involvement of a surrogate decision maker*. Nearly all states have enacted some version of a living will statute. Some also include provisions authorizing the appointment of a health-care "proxy" or surrogate. Only Massachusetts, Pennsylvania, Michigan, and Nebraska have not yet provided for living wills.

Except for a few fairly standard provisions, living will laws vary greatly from jurisdiction to jurisdiction, and familiarity with local requirements is recommended. Almost all living will statutes include three basic provisions: directive language, immunity clauses, and pregnancy clauses. In some jurisdictions, a living will is a mandatory directive, and health-care providers who fail either to follow a legally authorized living will or to transfer the patient to the care of another provider can be subject to disciplinary action by the applicable professional licensing board and other penalties. Immunity clauses are included generally to provide immunity from legal liability for health-care providers who withhold or withdraw "life-sustaining" or "life-prolonging" treatment from a "terminal" or otherwise qualified patient. Pregnancy clauses limit a female patient's right to refuse treatment statutorily if she is pregnant at the time her living will is to take effect. Typically, such provisions invalidate a living will for the entire course of a woman's pregnancy. It has been convincingly argued that pregnancy clauses may be unconstitutional, but it remains to be seen how such a statute would be interpreted by a court.

PROBLEMS WITH ADVANCE DIRECTIVES

There are a number of problems with the interpretation and implementation of advance directives. States differ on what medical conditions are covered, and the scope of a proxy's authority varies widely and is often unclear. Statutory definitions are clinically ambiguous, leaving room for the definitional problems noted earlier. The instrument may have limited applicability if state law provides that the directive only becomes operative when death is imminent, again leaving room for definitional interpretation. The types of treatment that may be foregone vary from state to state, as they do from institution to institution and from physician to physician, and this raises the question of whether advance directives are truly informed (i.e., does the patient fully understand exactly what treatment will be withheld or withdrawn under what circumstances, and with what result?).

LEGAL CONSIDERATIONS

Legal liability for wrongful death when a physician has followed a DNR order in the inpatient setting is not likely. Courts have upheld the right of the patient to make these types of decisions and the obligation of the physician to honor the patient's decision, provided that the usual principles of informed consent were followed.[10–12] In fact, no surrogate decision maker can overcome the well-documented wishes of the patient, expressed when the patient had appropriate decisional capacity. The importance of such documentation was clearly illustrated in one case in which a patient, who was not terminally ill but had irreversible brain damage, was made DNR by her physician in consultation with her parents, who were her guardians. When the DNR order was challenged, the court found, after reasonable inquiry, that the patient's parents did not have sufficient knowledge of what the patient would have wanted, given the current set of circumstances, and, further, that the parents did not have a full appreciation of the nature of the treatment that would be denied. The court ordered that the patient not be considered DNR until there was a knowledgeable decision made by the guardians.[7]

To fit within the negligence framework, a patient claiming "wrongful life" would have to show breach of a duty owed by medical care providers to be aware of and honor the patient's previously expressed desire to forego potentially lifesaving or life-sustaining treatment, including resuscitation, and would have to demonstrate damages caused by that breach of duty. The duty, then, is owed by all medical personnel who are or should be constructively aware of the patient's wishes. A typical situation in which this duty would arise is one in which a DNR order is on the patient's chart, but resuscitation is performed by someone who is unaware of the order. While life is difficult to claim as a damage, as has been shown in failure to diagnose pregnancy cases, injury or suffering resulting from the resuscitation may be claimed as damage. One patient, who had a valid DNR order in his chart, suffered a stroke some time after being successfully resuscitated from a cardiac arrest caused by the ventricular arrhythmia for which he was being treated, and is currently suing a hospital in Ohio. The allegation is that the treatment provided for him by the hospital prevented his natural death with dignity and saddled him with thousands of dollars in unwanted expenses, and that these damages were caused by actions against his expressed wishes. Although the case was dismissed by the trial court, it was appealed by his estate and remains undecided.[1]

In an attempt to avoid some of the problems that are associated with DNR orders and similar directives, some states have enacted legislation that the patient's own physician must obtain the informed consent of the patient before the patient can execute a living will, that the patient must be diagnosed as suffering from a terminal illness, and that the diagnosis must be reduced to writing and certified by an independent physician as well.[19] In practice, however, the problem that the emergency physician faces in rapidly determining the validity of a variety of legal documents will not be resolved unless and until there is a readily recognizable and standard format adopted.

For civil liability to attach for following a DNR order, there would have to be evidence that the withholding or withdrawing of treatment was based on a negligent or deliberate failure to act in accordance with a duty that is owed to the patient. Note that the explicit refusal of a patient relieves the physician of any obligation to initiate the refused therapy.[18] The greatest potential for liability exists where there was a misdiagnosis of a terminal condition or an unjustifiable failure to secure an informed decision regarding care from the patient or family. The likelihood for liability would seem somewhat greater for the emergency physician than for the patient's primary treating physician, because the emergency physician usually makes treatment decisions involving an unfamiliar patient in conjunction with an unfamiliar family at a highly stressful time. In cases in which criminal liability has attached surrounding resuscitation decisions, it has been for medical interventions that hastened the death of a patient, such as assisted suicide in cases of active euthanasia.

ETHICAL CONSIDERATIONS

One must, therefore, question whether patients suffering from a sudden and severe illness or injury, who are conscious and capable of understanding that their situation is grave, are competent to make immediate decisions regarding their resuscitation. It could be argued that such patients are too overwhelmed to make a well-reasoned decision about whether to forego lifesaving treatment and that it is a better policy to initiate treatment and then have the patients or surrogate decision makers make a decision about continuation of life-sustaining treatment. (As an example of this point, patients often state that, in the stress of the moment, they did not understand the details of informed consent for routine operative procedures, such as breast surgery.*) Even if there were careful prior consideration of the expected course and potential treatment by patients with terminal illnesses, and if no resuscitation were desired, intent when such patients present for emergency care at the time of decompensation is open to some amount of interpretation. Many argue that such patients, or their families, would not activate the emergency system if they did not wish aggressive intervention.

There are ethical issues involved in transferring the responsibility for making a DNR decision from the private physician to a medical director or emergency physician who does not know the patient and who may be acting through agents such as emergency medical teams or paramedics when the private physician is unavailable. Application of these principles in the prehospital setting may lead to the announcement of the death of a patient, with the EMS providers then leaving a scene where the family members are unprepared for subsequent events. Some have suggested that this issue alone is reason for "moving death into the emergency department,"[17] and that this approach may be best to muster the support and logistics needed in a society in which almost no one dies at home.

Although risk tends to be ascribed to the medical care provider whose decision to resuscitate or not to resuscitate may be challenged by families or the legal community, the risk of error is really to the patients whose lives may be terminated or prolonged in a manner that is not in accordance with their wishes. The goal of any resolution to the problem is to minimize this risk to the patients. Because any decision to withdraw life-support measures is a decision that is irreversible, the practitioner, when faced with a dilemma, must err on the side of preservation of life until all procedural safeguards can be confirmed and a well-reasoned and informed decision can be reached.

COMMON PITFALLS

- Failure to appreciate the governing laws for your jurisdiction regarding advanced directives and their implementation
- Failure to educate patients and families about treatment decisions
- Failure to understand the concept of the right to refuse care and surrogate decision making
- Failure to apprise oneself of hospital policies and procedures regarding DNR orders and advanced directives, and abide by the same

*Some states, including Pennsylvania, have passed legislation requiring that patients facing breast surgery sign a complex consent form listing alternative therapies and documenting understanding of the therapeutic options. This procedure, allegedly in response to "surprise" mastectomies performed as part of a diagnose-and-treat operation, may have improved the flow of information to some patients but has scared and confused others.

References

1. *Anderson v. St. Francis-St. George Hospital*, 614 N.E. 2d 814.
2. *Bartling v. Superior Court*, 163 Cal. App. 3d 186, 209 Cal. Rptr. 200.
3. *Bouvia v. Superior Court*, 179 Cal. App. 1127, 225 Cal. Rptr. 297.
4. *Canterbury v. Spence*, 464 F.2d 772 (D.C. Cir. 1972).
5. *Couture v. Couture*, 48 Ohio App. 3d 208 (1989).
6. 8A U.L.A. 275 (1987).
7. *Hoyt v. St. Mary's Rehabilitation Center*, 711 F.2d 864 (1983).
8. *In the Matter of Farrell*, 108 N.J. 335, 529 A.2d 404 (1987).
9. *Joint Commission manual for hospitals, management and administrative services*, standard MA 1.3.7 and patient rights standard RI 2.1, 2.2, 2.4 (1992).
10. *Matter of Dinnerstein*, 380 N.E. 2d 134 (1978).
11. *Matter of J.N.*, 406 A.2d 1275 (1979).
12. *Matter of Spring*, 405 N.E. 2d 115 (1980).
13. Nelson S. Liability issues increasing ethics consultations. *Hospitals* 1987;61(9):80.
14. *Pocono Medical Center v. Harley*, 11 Fiduc. Rep. 2d 128 (1990).
15. Refusal of treatment legislation, published by Choice in Dying, 1991 update.
16. Standards and guidelines for cardiopulmonary resuscitation care. *JAMA* 1986;255(21):2841.
17. Stratton SJ. Withholding CPR in the prehospital setting. *Prehosp Disaster Med* 1996;5(1):45.
18. *Superintendent of Belchertown v. Saikewicz*, 373 Mass. 728 (1977).
19. The Texas Natural Death Act, Art. 4590(h), *Vernon's Texas civil statutes, annotated*.

CHAPTER 406

Confidentiality

Abigail R. Williams

A patient's right to privacy through the confidential relationship between a physician and patient has its roots in fourth and fourteenth amendments of the U.S. Constitution. Central to all physician–patient relationships is the notion of confidentiality grounded in the words of the Hippocratic Oath. Information that is relayed to a physician in the course of patient treatment should be kept confidential to the greatest degree possible. This reliance encourages patients to freely disclose information that may be sensitive but is necessary for their care. Courts recognize that there are few matters that are as personal and of such an intimate nature as health.[12] If confidential information is going to be shared with others, it is generally held that it should be with the express consent of the patient or required by law. Unfortunately, the design and patient volume of most emergency departments makes patient confidentiality exceedingly difficult. In departments where patient beds are separated only by curtains, where histories are obtained and examinations are conducted in hallways, and where many people have access to the patient's medical information as it is written on wall boards, announced on intercoms, and displayed on computer screens, patient confidentiality is at risk. The challenge for emergency medicine is to adequately protect patient confidentiality while providing care. To do so, an understanding of the concepts behind confidentiality and their application in emergency medicine is essential.

CONFIDENTIALITY CONCEPTS

The courts take the position that one of the duties a physician owes to a patient is that of confidentiality, and a breach of this duty may give rise to a claim of negligence.[10] Further, courts have found that part of the implied contract that exists between physician and patient includes the maintenance of a confidential relationship.[8,16] The Joint Commission on the Accreditation of Healthcare Organizations (JCAHO) has standards that relate to the maintenance of physician–patient confidential relationships, one of which is that the patient has the right to personal and informational privacy.

The concept of privacy, strictly speaking, refers to the "sanctity of the body" and protects one from exposure of one's body, but it is used synonymously with *confidentiality*. The terms *confidential* and *privileged communications* are often used interchangeably and refer to the sanctity of patient information. The terms actually refer to two different concepts related to privacy rights. Confidential communications refer to those communications between physician and patient that the patient has a right to expect will be kept private. In contrast, privilege is a specific application of the right of privacy. A privileged communication is one protected by this right, as defined by rules of evidence created by statute. These rules enable the holder of the privilege (the patient) to prohibit the person to whom the confidential information was disclosed (the physician) from testifying to that information in court. Note that that this testimonial privilege applies only to judicial proceedings. In order to invoke the testimonial privilege, there are specific conditions that must be met:

- The person to whom the statement is made must be a physician. (The exception is information provided to the physician while other health-care providers, such as nurses, are present for the purpose of continuing to provide necessary care for the patient.)
- The second element is that a physician–patient relationship must exist at the time that the information is provided. This creates the expectation that the communication is to be held in confidence and that violation of confidences would interfere with the nature of the professional doctor–patient relationship. The information must be reasonably necessary for the treatment of the patient.

There are, however, a number of circumstances in which patient information can be disclosed, such as when the patient consents to have information shared, where the law requires disclosure of patient information, and when the patient waives the right to keep some or all of their medical information private (e.g., disclosure to insurance companies for the purposes of billing). Patient consent to disclosure, providing the patient is competent to consent, allows release of the information. As with all other types of patient consent, the physician must make some reasonable determination about the patient's understanding of the scope of the disclosure. A consent to release information must be informed and made by a competent patient and should fit within all applicable state requirements intended to be patient-protective (see Chapter 407).

In a civil commitment proceeding, the contest of a will, child custody disputes, or other actions in which the patient's physical or mental state is at issue, the physician may testify without the patient's consent. The physician may also testify about the patient without his or her consent in defending against an action brought by the patient or in actions to collect payment for services provided to the patient by the physician. In all states, there are legal requirements for reporting some communicable diseases. Most states require reporting medical conditions and incidents such as venereal disease, contagious diseases, wounds inflicted by violence or animals, poisonings, abortions, industrial accidents, child and elder abuse, and rape.

A CHRONOLOGIC APPROACH TO CONFIDENTIALITY

Prior to Arrival

Patient information not infrequently reaches the emergency department before the patient does. Emergency medical services (EMS) and prehospital care providers are required, in most areas, to provide the emergency department with a notification that usually includes medical information such as the patient's age, medical history, allergies, circumstances surrounding the current need for medical care, and current medical condition. It is easy to forget that all of the information broadcast over the EMS radio may be overheard by persons casually listening to a scanner, and some link between the patient description (address and location of the dispatched call, age and gender of the patient) and the medical event may be made. Arguably, this is a breach of patient confidentiality if it is known that radio transmissions are routinely overheard. More private means of communication, including cellular phones (still fairly easy to hear by scanner) and various scrambled or otherwise encrypted radio systems, are available. The larger issue, however, has to do not with advances in technology but with intent. There are means to intercept almost any radio transmission, given time and technology. Patient confidentiality can be better preserved by behaviors that do not unreasonably identify the patient or disclose sensitive information.

Prearrival patient information, whether it comes from EMS providers or private physicians, is often verbally transmitted or posted in a conspicuous area. Although this may make it easier for staff to communicate about expected patients, it also exposes the patient's information publicly.

During Care

Challenges to confidentiality during care in the emergency department can be grouped into either those inherent in the design of the department or those inherent in its function, including staff behavior. Several special situations require different interpretations of confidentiality.

Department Design

Typical emergency department design often dictates that patients are interviewed in rooms or areas that are occupied by more than one patient or another person who is not a care provider. Curtains have poor soundproofing qualities, and it is not unusual for two adjacent patients to overhear the details of each other's histories and then be facing one another when the curtain is pulled back to allow better observation by the department staff. Staff in emergency departments often use large display boards, intercoms, and loud voices to communicate. These techniques make confidentiality challenging. Attention to department design and staff behavior can reduce these risks without compromising patient care.

Evidentiary Testing

Blood alcohol levels, toxicology screens, tests performed as part of sexual assault examinations or in alleged abuse cases, or care of patients involved in a criminal event may involve presentation of medical fact as evidence in court, and the evidentiary nature of diagnostic testing and other findings creates a need for heightened protection of patient information. Physicians are frequently asked by law enforcement agencies to release blood and blood levels for determination of ethanol intoxication or other chemical ingestion, which may impact on the liability of the patient in a motor vehicle accident. Employers are interested in impairment by drugs, and want results of similar tests. Prosecuting attorneys need properly obtained and protected evidence to prevail in sexual assault and other criminal matters involving medical care. When patient evidence is not handled appropriately, not only is the physician–patient relationship violated, but the admissibility of the evidence in a court proceeding is threatened as well. In an Indiana case, a physician released a blood specimen taken from a patient involved in a motor vehicle accident to the police. The physician was asked to testify at the patient's trial for involuntary manslaughter regarding the drawing of the blood sample and the test results. The patient successfully appealed his conviction because of his claim that the emergency department physician's testimony was privileged and should not have been admitted into evidence. The case was sent back to the trial court for a new trial that would not include the blood alcohol evidence.[1,18]

Disclosure to Family Members

The general rule that information about patients should not be released without their consent also applies to family members, with several exceptions. Taking a few extra minutes to ask patients if they want family members present or informed about their care, test results, or condition affords patients a proper measure of respect and privacy. Not all patients want their families to know the details of their medical care, and most expect the opportunity to make this decision. Exceptions to this practice include situations in which patients are incompetent or minors (not emancipated). In these cases, their family should be contacted and may be an essential part of the care process. Care should be taken to confirm the identity of a "family member" with a patient before releasing details; many persons are aware that hospitals are more forthcoming with family members and may impersonate a family member in order to obtain information about a patient. If a patient is competent, this process should be rapid. Otherwise, a reasonable effort to protect the patient's confidentiality is expected.

Triage

The triage process, originally intended to prevent patient decompensation while awaiting care, has expanded in many institutions to include significant data gathering that may include confidential information. Care should be taken to avoid unnecessary breaches of confidentiality. For example, a list for patients to sign in while awaiting triage need not list the complaint; the next patient then will not be able to read about their neighbors' woes. Interviews should be as confidential as possible, without lines of people overhearing details of history. Any examination performed should be given the same measure of respect and privacy expected in other settings; patients should not be asked to significantly disrobe or otherwise expose themselves in public.

Gossip

While discussion about patients serves an educational purpose, and the occasional joke serves to relieve tension, there is no excuse for gossip that breaches patient confidentiality. Patients and others in the department may overhear discussion about other patients, which may be unavoidable within architectural and functional limits. However, they should not hear unprofessional comments or derogatory discussions about current or former patients. These events are not infrequent, and they form the basis of many patient and family complaints. The best way to prevent this from occurring is to avoid such events through common courtesy and proper manners. Reminding staff that the charting desk, break room, back hallway, elevators, and cafeteria do not provide a forum for this type of conversation may be helpful. Awareness of the frequency with which these events occur can often be heightened by patient simulation. The healthcare provider should sit in a wheelchair or lie on a stretcher in typical patient care or transport areas and listen. He or she should not overhear confidential patient information.

After Care

A study reported by the Privacy Protection Commission, Personal Privacy in an Information Society, in 1977 noted that 51% of physicians and 70% of medical students discuss confidential patient information at social gatherings. Obviously, these disclosures can lead to significant patient embarrassment and may cause damage to the patient in the forms of loss of employment, loss of insurance, and credit denial.

In some cases, emergency access to patient medical information may be necessary by telephone or fax machine. In general, it is a good idea to limit any information provided about a patient to that required for immediate care. Hospitals must develop and implement systems for obtaining medical information by phone or by fax that provide for confirmation of the information received and for concrete identification of the information seeker's identity and reason for request. For example, such a system might include the following:

- Confirming caller identity from a list of area hospital emergency department telephone and fax numbers; even more preferable is when the caller is known to the staff receiving the request.

- Arranging for a fax machine location within a secure emergency department staff area, to prevent patient information from arriving at a public machine location, such as at the hospital switchboard or office desk
- Asking, whenever possible, for the requesting facility to send a signed patient record release form before sending a return facsimile with patient information
- Including on the facsimile cover sheet sent with patient records a reminder that the transmission includes confidential patient information and should be directed immediately to those caring for the patient

The Medical Record

The medical record is a complete record of a patient's history, condition, and treatment and may contain very personal information. It has been estimated that up to 75 persons may access any given medical record.[3] Access to the medical record is obtained for a variety of medical and nonmedical purposes, and consent of the patient is often presumed. Some of the reasons for medical record access include third-party payor information; quality-assurance purposes; JCAHO or other accreditation or investigatory review; documentation and evidence in a legal proceeding; and medical research. The medical record may be written and stored on paper or composed on a computer and stored either on paper or in an information system. The medical record is used to chronologically document the patient's interactions with the medical system, treatment rendered, response to treatment, and plans for further care. It also serves as an important legal document. The medical record is of paramount importance when a claim of negligence, against either a physician or hospital, has been raised, or when there is some dispute surrounding the origin of the injury or illness. It may be several years from the time of the illness, injury, or treatment before a claim is litigated. The medical record is frequently the only detailed documentation of what transpired before, during, and after the patient's interaction with the provider. It is not infrequent that persons who were involved in the patient's initial illness, injury, care, or treatment may no longer be available to testify in court, but the medical record provides documentation of circumstances surrounding the event in question. A well-documented medical record will enable the physician to recall the history, treatment provided, response to the treatment, and patient outcome. Failure to keep a well-organized and confidential record may destroy the utility of the record for both medical and legal purposes; in fact, it can cause both medical and legal problems.

Entries that are made in the medical record should be made clearly, concisely, and objectively. Only information that is relevant to the care and treatment of the patient should be contained in the medical record. Subjective comments, opinions about the care given by other providers, and extraneous commentary about the patient or circumstances of the encounter are not only not needed in the record, they can form the basis of legal action. Once information is documented, the original entry should never be altered, although additional information may be added if needed, providing it is identified as an addendum and dated as such. Corrections should be made in a standard way, with a single line through the incorrect entry, insertion of the correction, the reason for the correction, the time and date of the correction, and the identity of the documenter clearly noted. Patients may be upset by incorrect information in their records (e.g., gender, age, left and right errors), but they are generally more upset by improper corrections. The legal system is more than upset by alterations in a medical record that are made in an effort to reduce liability in a negligence action. As more emergency department records are produced on typewriters and computer printers, and are therefore more legible, they are being read by patients more often. The patient may request a copy of his or her record for many reasons, and they may be sent a copy as part of an insurance process. A concise, professional, legible, and thorough record that documents excellent emergency care should please the patient. A record that contains errors, information obtained without patient consent (e.g., "patient's co-workers contacted about his drug use and state. . . ."), or documentation that patient information that was shared with others without consent (e.g., "patient's boss called and informed about patient's . . .") may anger the patient and be the source of complaints or legal action.

Computers and Confidentiality

Computerized medical records present a special evidentiary problem for attorneys. Many state laws require that medical records be handwritten or typed and signed by a physician or other health-care provider. Some state laws require that medical records be documented in ink. Although computer-generated medical records may be printed out and may therefore satisfy the requirement of medical records, they may still need to be placed in a folder and located in a central place. Duplicative efforts like this raise additional confidentiality concerns. It is hoped that, as computerized medical record systems become more commonplace, statutes will be broadened to more readily accept computer documentation without the need for extensive paper archives. Access to computerized information can be significantly easier than access to paper records. While some argue that anyone in a white coat can stroll into most medical records departments and ask to see a particular record, computer terminals scattered throughout the institution, without attention to security, can offer much easier access to a broad range of data. Coordination with information systems staff to afford both ease of use and proper security (limiting who can access data and what data can be accessed) can improve the clinical utility of computerized records while protecting patient confidentiality.

MANDATORY DISCLOSURE

Reporting Laws

There are times when confidential patient information must be released. Most states have mandatory reporting laws for certain communicable diseases and certain suspected criminal activities. Certain agencies have the right to inspect or review records as part of their function. Accreditation bodies, third-party payors, and others may, depending on circumstances, have the right to access patient information. The emergency physician should understand the bounds of such mandatory disclosure situations as they apply locally and be prepared to both cooperate and limit that cooperation, as indicated.

Duty to Third Parties

As has been noted, obligations of the physician do not normally extend to persons other than the patient. The physician may have a duty, however, to warn third parties of significant dangers created by patients if the physician has a special relationship with either of the parties. The duty of a physician to warn some person or persons of potential dangers presented by a patient under his or her care has been interpreted by different courts to different degrees. Some courts have held that a patient confidence can be breached only when the intended victim is identifiable. Others recognize that the scope should be broadened to protection of the general public in the interest of public health. In a recent Michigan case, a physician was sued for failing to warn a family member about exposure to a highly contagious, potentially fatal disease. The question before the court was whether the physician owed a duty of care to the son (who died of meningitis) or to the mother, who was treated and released from the emergency department on antibiotics for an upper respiratory infection. Although a legitimate concern was raised regarding the confidential relationship between the patient and the physician, the court felt that the concerns were not sufficiently compelling to nullify the duty imposed on the physician.[15] Courts have also upheld the requirement of the physician to warn the daughter of a patient with scarlet fever, the wife of the potential danger of infection from her husband's infected wounds, and the neighbor of a patient who had smallpox. In essence, family members are foreseeable third parties, as are neighbors and classmates. Courts have also upheld physician liability for failing to warn of psychiatric dangerousness, of potential for sudden impairment due to disease process, and of potential drug side effects.[5,6,14,17,19,20]

Acquired Immunodeficiency Syndrome and Confidentiality

The unique characteristics of the acquired immunodeficiency syndrome (AIDS) present many ethical dilemmas for physicians. Patients who are human immunodeficiency virus (HIV)–positive, who have AIDS, or who seek counseling or testing for AIDS present special confidentiality problems for the emergency physician. Superimposed on the public health approach to confidential medical relationships is a flurry of regulatory and statutory activity regarding HIV-positive patients. Because of the way society reacts to persons with AIDS, there is heightened concern about the transmission of information relating to that condition, and some jurisdictions have legislated specific confidentiality laws related to AIDS. Regardless of the accuracy of the information released regarding patients who have AIDS, potential for liability arises. If the information provided to another is inaccurate, there is the potential for a defamation action. If information regarding patients is accurate, issues of invasion of privacy are raised. There are also issues raised by not releasing information about the HIV status of patients. If physicians know with reasonable certainty that patients are infected with HIV and are not planning to inform their sexual partners or those with whom they share needles, and the physicians fail to warn those identified third parties, liability may exist for failure to warn as well. Some states absolutely protect patients' right to confidentiality by requiring that an informed consent process be carried out before information about their HIV status can be revealed. Other states grant physicians immunity from liability if they decide to disclose due to fear of danger to identified parties. Many states have no special laws regarding patients who are HIV-positive. It is not clear where the courts will ultimately draw the line with HIV-positive patients, but it is possible that they will find that physicians have a duty to warn identified parties of real, significant, and proximate danger.

Legal Liability for Disclosure of Confidential Information

A majority of courts have upheld the right of patients to recover for unauthorized disclosure of confidential information. One theory noted by the courts is that physicians' disclosure of confidential information to third parties, without patients' consent, results in a violation of the patients' right to privacy. Physicians who violate patient confidence may also find that they are liable for damages based in tort or contract theory. Some courts have recognized a fiduciary duty on the part of physicians to maintain patient confidences.[7,9,11] The form of the communication about patients, even to medical colleagues, is also of concern to the courts. The communications must be made in a clear and objective manner, such that patients will not be subjected to humiliation, and must be made upon appropriate request, not just in the passage of casual information. A physician who sent information about a patient and their interactions to a medical peer, which contained disparaging information about the patient, was held to have violated his duty of "loyalty" and confidentiality to his patient. The patient prevailed in an action against the physician for libel and defamation of character.[2,4,11,13]

References

1. *Alder v. State of Indiana,* 154 N.E. 2d 716.
2. *Alexander v. Knight,* 177 A.2d 142.
3. American College of Hospital Administrators. Medical confidentiality: can it be protected? 1983;2–3.
4. *Berry v. Moench,* 331 P.2d 814.
5. *Edwards v. Lamb,* 45 A. 480.
6. *Freese v. Lemmon,* 210 N.W. 2d 576.
7. *Hammonds v. Aetna Casualty and Surety Co.,* 243 F. Supp. 793.
8. *Hammonds v. Aetna Casualty and Surety Co.,* 243 F. Supp 793 (ND Ohio, 1965).
9. *Horne v. Patton,* 287 So. 2d 824.
10. *Horne v. Patton,* 291 Ala. 71, 387 So. 2d 834 (1974).
11. *Humphers v. First Interstate Bank of Oregon,* 696 P.2d 527.
12. *John Doe v. The City of New York,* 15 F.3d 264;1994 U.S. App. LEXIS 1459.
13. *MacDonald v. Clinger,* 84 App. Div. 2d 482.
14. *Meyes v. Quesenberry,* 193 Cal. Rptr. 733.
15. *Shephard v. Redford Community Hospital,* 390 N.W. 2d 239.
16. *Simonsen v. Swenson,* 177 N.W. 831.
17. *Skellings v. Allen,* 173 N.W. 663.
18. *State of New Jersey v. Amaniera,* 334 A.2d 398.
19. *Tarasoff v. Regents of the Univ. of Cal.,* 551 P.2d 334.
20. *Welke v. Kuzilla,* 375 N.W. 2d 403.

CHAPTER 407
Informed Consent and Refusal of Care

Abigail R. Williams

A common and problematic medicolegal issue facing emergency physicians is patient consent to, or refusal of, treatment. The theory of informed consent has developed as the result of a strong judicial deference toward the constitutionally based right of a person to individual autonomy, resulting in the fostering of rational patient decisions. The environment of the emergency department challenges the traditional rules of consent and refusal, creating a necessity for the emergency physician to be familiar with the nuances of the consent and refusal process.

TYPES OF CONSENT

It has been well established in both the legal and medical arenas that competent adults have the right to make decisions about what diagnostic or therapeutic medical treatment or medication they will or will not accept.[11] Treating informed patients who competently refuse care renders the physician liable for battery.* However, allowing a patient to refuse care when that refusal is not informed and is detrimental to their health also creates liability for the physician. Three types of consent are recognized at law: express consent, consent that is implied in fact, and consent that is implied in law. Express consent may be either oral or written: It is basically the granting of authority to render treatment. Standard hospital consent forms signed during the registration process and those for surgery or other invasive treatment are examples of express consent. Consent that is implied in fact is consent derived from the conduct of the involved parties. If, for example, patients are told that their blood pressure should be checked, and they hold out their arm, there is implied consent. The legal test is behavior such that the reasonable individual witnessing the exchange would conclude from the behavior of the parties that consent had been given. Consent that is implied in law is consent that is assumed during an emergency for emergency treatment or extension of treatment necessary to save a life or preserve health. For implied-in-law consent to be recognized, two things *must* occur simultaneously. The patient must be in actual life-threatening danger *and* the patient must be unable to give consent. One without the other will not withstand the legal test. In this situation, the law assumes that the reasonable rational patient would consent to care if able. Consent is not waived in this situation; if the physician knows that the patient would not have consented to the proposed lifesaving treatment, it should not be undertaken.

VALID CONSENT

For any type of consent to be valid, it must be informed. *Informed* means that consent is made by the patient or responsible party after the treating physician (the one performing the procedure) submits a fair and reasonable explanation of the particular procedure or treatment, including reasonably likely risks and benefits. The duty to obtain informed consent rests with the physician who is going to perform the procedure.[3,5] There are certain elements that must be disclosed to the patient, including the nature of the patient's condition, an explanation of the proposed treatment or procedure, risks and benefits of the procedure, and alternatives to the planned procedure, including the risks of the alternative treatments.† In essence, the physician has a duty to disclose any substantial or material facts about a proposed procedure or treatment.‡

The legal standard is that the patient must receive all information about a proposed treatment or procedure§ that a reasonable and prudent physician knows would be regarded as material‖ by a reasonable and prudent patient. In the case of a relatively risk-free event, such as phlebotomy or physical examination, consent implied in fact is often sufficient. As the risk of the event increases, however, this form of consent is less appropriate. However, the physician, within reasonable professional judgment, is permitted to withhold certain information that would result in refusal of necessary treatment. For example, if a physician knows after discussion with family members that the patient is unreasonably terrified about a certain unlikely potential complication of therapy (e.g., diarrhea from antibiotic therapy for meningitis), this information may be withheld from the patient. This is a very difficult standard to meet when both time and treatment options may be limited and when the patient is not well known to the physician. It is imperative that the treating physician have good communication skills so that the patient is able to understand the information that the physician is trying to convey. Of equal import is the necessity of the physician to be able to understand the patient.[19]

COMPETENCE TO GIVE CONSENT

To make an informed decision regarding treatment options, the patient must be competent to consent. Competence for this purpose is judged more by a medical "reasonableness" standard than a legal one. Not all patients who present to the emergency department for care who are considered to be incompetent by a medical standard would be adjudicated incompetent by the courts and therefore have surrogate decision makers appointed for them. Competence in this medical sense is a very dynamic state and depends on a very complex set of factors and circumstances. Basically, the patient must be able to render a choice and understand information relevant to making this decision. This means that the patient must have the ability to appreciate the situation that he or she is in and its consequences. Further, the patient must have the ability for rational processing of the information provided. There are many factors that impact a patient's competence. Patients who are intoxicated or who are in some other way chemically impaired may not be competent. Patients who may have head injury, hypoxia, some metabolic derangement such as hypo- or hyperglycemia, or who are under severe emotional stress may not be competent. In such situations, if a true emergency exists and the patient is judged to be unable to consent, the implied-in-law consent doctrine applies.

MINORS AND CONSENT

Parents or legal guardians must, in general, consent for the care of the minor. Often, however, a minor patient seeks care in the emergency department in the absence of a parent. The emergency physician may be placed in a difficult position, caught between the risk of not evaluating and treating the patient and the risk of evaluating and treating the patient without consent. In such cases, it is advisable to evaluate and treat if delaying such could result in potential harm, to clearly document the reasoning for this, to attempt to contact the parents or guardian, and to document such attempts.

Emancipated Minors

Emancipated minors have a different legal status than that of other minors. They are able to consent for their own health care and are considered emancipated because of one or more of the following factors:

- Marital status. The minor is married, divorced, separated, or widowed.
- The nature of his or her physical condition. The patient believes that she is pregnant or he or she believes him- or herself to be suffering from or to have come into contact with any disease defined as a danger to public health, such as a sexually transmitted disease.
- Legal or financial status. The patient is either living on her or his own or is in some way financially independent.

*A person commits the tort of battery if he or she acts with intent to cause harmful or offensive contact, and the contact occurs.[15,17] Even the mere touching of one person by another without consent or legal justification was a battery at common law.[12]

†In failure-to-warn cases, the failure to disclose the alternative treatment must be the proximate cause of the patient's injury.[6,8]

‡The physician owes the patient a fiduciary duty of good faith and fair dealing, which gives rise to certain specific professional obligations. These obligations include not only the duty to exercise due care and skill, but also to fully inform the patient of his or her condition and to obtain the patient's informed consent to the medical treatment.[14]

§The physician is not liable for not disclosing diagnostic alternatives for illness or injury as of yet undiagnosed.[1]

‖*Material* is defined as the significance that a reasonable person, in what the physician knows to be the patient's position, would attach to the disclosed risk.[20]

- Is a member of the armed forces
- Is a parent

Many difficult issues are raised by this rule. For instance, if a minor believes herself to be pregnant and presents with abdominal pain, she can consent for care. If a pregnancy test is performed and is negative, what is the emergency physician to do? Are minors reliable? How can the physician be sure that the minor is in fact emancipated?

In general, physicians who rely, in good faith, on the representations of the patient will be protected. If a patient who reasonably met the standards of emancipation on presentation is found *not* to meet the standards after some evaluation (e.g., negative pregnancy test), the physician may proceed with reasonable evaluation and treatment indicated by the patient's condition while attempts are made to better define the patient's competency.

Mature Minors

Another category of minor who may be able to consent for their own care is the mature minor. The mature minor is emotionally and intellectually mature enough to be capable of appreciating the nature of his or her illness or injury as well as the risks and benefits of proposed treatment. In some cases, a minor originally and incorrectly felt to be emancipated may meet the standards for mature minor status. Although not frequently an issue, it is important to note that no unmarried minor can give consent for abortion or sterilization, even if otherwise mature or emancipated.

Age-related competence issues do not relate solely to minors. Geriatric patients may not be able to rationally manipulate information provided to them. Emancipated minors may not be able to understand complex information regarding their own children when those children are patients.

INCOMPETENCE

There are two types of patients who are considered "mentally incompetent" for reasons other than age: those who are adjudicated and those who are unadjudicated. Patients who have been determined by the courts to be not legally competent, and therefore not capable of making sound medical treatment decisions, are adjudicated incompetent. In this case, the court will assign someone else (a "surrogate") to make health-care decisions for the individual. Usually, the court will appoint a family member, such as a parent, spouse, or offspring. Sometimes, the court appoints someone not related to the patient to make these decisions. Treatment decisions will be based either on prior express wishes of the patient (see Chapter 405) or on the surrogate's own judgment about what is "best" for the incompetent party.

Patients who, for one reason or another, are temporarily or suddenly unable to make reasonable treatment decisions for themselves are unadjudicated incompetent. Competence may be affected by medication, fatigue, stress, disease processes, and other conditions. This situation is faced frequently in the emergency department. Input from the patient's significant others is important in this situation, and efforts to speak with family, those persons with whom the patient lives, or those with whom he or she is most closely associated may be necessary to determine the patient's wishes. The theory is that these people are most likely to know what the patient would want and will be acting in the patient's best interest. Surrogates do not have constitutional standing to substitute their own judgment for that of the incompetent patient, however.[4]

Determining under what circumstances the physician can treat against the patient's will poses a medical–legal challenge. Indications that a patient may not be competent to refuse care include, but are not limited to, the following:

- Patients with mental status changes
- Patients who appear to be intoxicated or suffering from hypoxia, acidosis, or other metabolic derangement
- Patients suffering from dementia
- Patients who have suicidal or homicidal ideation or intent
- Patients who are suffering from acute organic brain syndrome

RELIGIOUS BELIEFS AND CONSENT

Religious objectors, such as Jehovah's Witnesses, pose yet another dilemma for the emergency physician. Jehovah's Witnesses may believe that acceptance of blood products will result in an irreversible denial of eternal life, and therefore render the rest of life purposeless. The refusal of blood products should not be misconstrued to mean that they are refusing other care. Competent adults have the right to refuse medical care, and the competent Jehovah's Witness who is refusing a necessary transfusion of blood products is no exception, even if that refusal leads to his or her death.[9,10] Appointment of a temporary medical guardian for a Jehovah's Witness is an option when there is a question about the patient's wishes. In some cases, the court has found that the interests of children may override the interests of a parent, but this is not a common finding.[16]

Competent adults do not have the right to impose their religious beliefs on others, including their children. States are able to intervene on behalf of children when an emergency exists and lifesaving care is being refused by parents. This is because the state has an overriding interest in protecting the welfare of its citizens, especially those who are unable to care for themselves. Courts have also reasoned that although they are unable to interfere in the religious beliefs of parents, they may interfere with actions, given just cause.[18]

DOCUMENTING INFORMED CONSENT

Informed consent, as outlined earlier, must be obtained by the physician who proposes to treat the patient. The way in which this consent is reasonably documented varies with the nature of the emergency and the risk of the proposed treatment. In many cases, a specific written consent form, listing the reasonable risks of the specific treatment and signed by the patient, physician, and a witness, is best, but in some cases, there is inadequate time for this process. In all cases, the consent process should be documented in the patient's record whenever a procedure or treatment is performed that would typically require informed consent if performed in the hospital.

REFUSAL OF TREATMENT AND DISCHARGE

Just as a patient must give informed consent to treatment, refusal of treatment must also be informed. In fact, the criteria for refusal are more strict than those for consent. Refusal cannot be implied either in fact or in law, because the special knowledge in the situation is held by the physician and not the patient. When a physician "suggests" a medical event (e.g., taking a blood pressure), the patient may give implied consent in fact or in law, because the physician is presumed to be the expert and is therefore in possession of special knowledge that the suggested event is proper and appropriate in the situation. The converse is not true. If a physician "suggests" an event and the patient attempts to refuse in any way, that refusal cannot be assumed to be informed. If, for example, the physician asks to take a blood pressure and the patient withdraws his or her arm instead of extending it, a reasonable observer may feel that consent had been refused, but the observer would not likely understand *why* the event was refused. Therefore, only a fully informed patient can refuse suggested treatment. This includes understanding the consequences of the refusal and failing to follow the recommended course of treatment.

Informed refusal may apply to a specific test or treatment (e.g., a rectal examination or lumbar puncture), to any further care (e.g., a patient asking to leave during care or refusing admission to the hospital), or to a portion of the physician's plan of therapy (e.g., follow-up appointments, prescribed medications, or use of seat belts). The discharge of patients from the emergency department, even if amicable and mutually acceptable, includes an informed refusal process in that the patient must understand the reasonable consequences of refusing to follow the discharge instructions.

PATIENTS WHO LEAVE THE EMERGENCY DEPARTMENT

Despite the best intentions of the emergency department staff, some patients do not follow the informed refusal process outlined for discharge from the emergency department. Traditionally, these patients fall into one of three categories, with a fourth (item 2 on the following list) added recently:

1. Those who leave before significant medical evaluation or care has occurred. This is often labeled "leaving without being seen," although this label is viewed by some as internally contradictory. A more accurate label would be "leaving before evaluation." These patients may have registered and are not found when called for bed or room assignment; some do not even register. They may be considered a group that has voluntarily withdrawn their presentation for care. Although long waiting times are a commonly cited reason for leaving, these patients often have psychiatric issues, such as difficulty with being in public places, that make care in the emergency department particularly challenging. Every effort should be made to identify patients who appear uncomfortable with the emergency department process and to offer to accommodate their care and encourage them to stay.
2. Those who leave after their insurance plan has refused to pay for care. Changes in third-party payor practices have created this new category of patients, who leave before evaluation. While many feel that this situation will be corrected by federal legislation (see Chapter 408), it is a common occurrence and is distinct from patients who anonymously leave before evaluation. Handled properly under current guidelines, these patients are informed of the availability of care (including availability of a "screening examination" as defined under COBRA) and the consequences of refusing that care. They are then giving informed refusal prior to medical evaluation and are, in effect, withdrawing their request for care. The challenge with this category of patients is to clearly distinguish between a willingness to provide care and refusal of a payor to reimburse for that care. In many facilities, that distinction is seen as too complex to explain, and efforts are focused instead on contracting with payors to provide appropriate reimbursement for different levels of service for all persons who present for care.
3. Those who leave during care without informing the staff of their intent to leave. This is often called "eloping." These patients fall into two subgroups—competent and incompetent. The most concerning are those who are incompetent, and every effort should be made to return these patients for care. The competent patient who elopes may have not been given enough information to make an informed refusal of treatment, and if there is concern regarding further diagnosis and treatment, efforts should be made to locate the patient, relate any information necessary to ensure an informed decision, and document this exchange on the medical record. In many cases, patients elope after a particular phase of their care, such as x-rays or laboratory testing. Sometimes, this is because of a misunderstanding ("The technician said my x-rays were OK, so I thought I was supposed to go."), and efforts should be made to ensure that patients receive clear and basic instructions to return to the emergency department after testing. In other cases, patients may be using the system for testing purposes (e.g., pregnancy testing or x-rays), and leave after a desired result is available, even if the care process is incomplete. Again, effort should be made to identify this type of patient and emphasize the importance of educated and informed discharge. Some patients elope because of anger or frustration, often due to waiting time or staff attitude. An alert staff can help identify this type of patient and offer alternatives before they elope.
4. Those who leave after announcing their intent to leave, contrary to the best advice of the staff, are commonly described as leaving AMA (against medical advice). This does not have to be an adversarial process. The informed patient is declining one recommended course of therapy; the uninformed patient needs education. The physician should then attempt to discover the reason for such refusal (often a social need, such as lack of childcare or an apartment left unlocked) and negotiate a solution or suggest (recursively, if necessary) the next best course of therapy until one is acceptable to the patient.

RESTRAINTS

There are situations in the emergency department in which patients are unable to give informed consent to treatment or refuse to do so and there is a necessity to restrain them for their own safety or the safety of the staff and other patients. Use of patient restraints, regardless of the form of the restraint, is a significant patient care intervention, and the appropriateness of such intervention must be considered carefully. Before restraints are initiated and maintained for any period of time, a physician assessment must be performed. Documentation of the intervention must contain information about the reason that the restraints are being used; some indication that the patient was not competent to refuse treatment, if that is the reason for the restraint; and the plan for reassessment of the patient. It is assumed that the patient requires restraint due to a combination of incompetence and medical necessity, but the justification for both should be clearly documented. The least restrictive safe restraint method should be employed, given the circumstances.

False imprisonment is an intentional tort whereby there is an unlawful (unjustified) restriction of a person's movement. This restriction may be either actual (e.g., the patient is physically unable to move due to wrist and ankle restraints, spinal immobilization, or administered medications) or apparent (e.g., the patient believes that he or she is unable to move because of verbal warnings, the presence of guards, or a locked room). Because this is an intentional tort, the patient need only show that there was unjustified intent to confine and does not need to show that a damage occurred, as would be required if the suit were based in negligence. Therefore, use of restraints (even those typically thought of as splints or precautions) should be accompanied by documentation justifying their use.

Restraint of a patient must also include providing adequate protection for both patient and staff. In a New York case, a patient, while restrained, was injured when another patient attempted to rape her. The degree of care owed to the patient is related to the patient's own ability to provide for his or her own safety.¶ Staff working with patients requiring restraint should be properly trained and equipped to afford them reasonable protection from physical and other harm that may accompany the situation.

PHYSICIAN LIABILITY RELATED TO CONSENT

Expert testimony is needed to support claims of lack of informed consent and battery arising out of a medical procedure.[13] If the patient should claim that consent was not obtained, he or she would not need to show that the procedure was the cause of any injury, nor that the procedure was performed in a substandard manner, but only that it was performed at all and had not been consented to. In order to prevail, the physician must be able to show that the patient was informed of and understood known risks as well as those risks material to the particular patient.**

There are exceptions to the informed consent rule, however. A physician does not need to disclose to the patient those risks that are generally known to the public or those risks that are too remote to be considered actual risks and would cause the patient to refuse necessary treatment.[2] In an emergency, as noted previously, the physician may render lifesaving care without obtaining consent, and the physician may not disclose some material facts if he or she believes that the disclosure poses a threat to the patient's well-being.

References

1. *Bays v. St. Luke's Hospital,* 825 P.2d 319 (1992).
2. *Boyd v. Louisiana Medical Mut. Ins. Co.,* 593 So. 2d 427 (1991).
3. *Canterbury v. Spence,* 464 F.2d 772 (D.C. Cir. 1972).
4. *Cruzan v. Director, Missouri Department of Health,* 110 S. Ct. 2841 (1990).
5. *Davis v. Charles Gen. Hosp.,* 598 So. 2d 1244 (1992).
6. *Elzell v. Moore,* 587 N.E. 2d 1131 (1992).
7. *Freeman v. St. Clare's Health Center,* 548 N.Y.S. 2D 686 (New York Superior Court, Appellate Division).
8. *Harnish v. Children's Hospital Medical Center,* 387 Mass. 152 (1982).
9. *In re Brooks Estate,* 205 N.E. 2d 435 (1965).
10. *In re Osborne,* 294 A.2d 372 (1972).
11. *In the Matter of Farrell,* 108 N.J. 335, 529 A.2d 404 (1987).
12. Keeton W, et al. *Prosser and Keeton on the law of torts,* s9, at 39-42 (5th ed. 1984).
13. *LaCaze v. Collier,* 434 So. 2d 1039 (1983).
14. *Leach v. Shapiro,* 469 N.E. 2d 1047, 1052 (Ohio Ct. App. 1984).
15. *Precourt v. Frederick,* 395 Mass. 689.
16. *Public Health Trust of Dade County v. Wons,* 541 So. 2d 96 (1989).
17. Restatement (Second) of Torts ss 13, 18 (1965).
18. *Reynolds v. United States,* 98 US 166 (1978).
19. *Ruff v. Bossier Medical Center,* CA 5, no. 90-4800, 1/31/92.
20. *Wilkinson v. Vesey,* 110 R.I. 606 (1972).

¶The patient was awarded $125,000 for injuries sustained as a result of the attack.[7]

**The determination, therefore, of what is to be disclosed is a two-tiered test. First, one must decide what the risk is based on the scientific facts (i.e., the nature of the harm and the scientific likelihood that the harm will occur). Then it must be decided whether that probability of harm is a risk that the reasonable patient would consider in deciding on a treatment.

CHAPTER 408

Patient Transfers: Legal Issues

Abigail R. Williams

Patient transfers are often economically motivated. In many cases, the financial motivation is remote, and is a reflection of the economic and manpower impossibility of having the best medical technology available in every community. In other cases, concern over the patient's ability to pay for services provided is the major reason for the transfer. The practice of transferring patients for the direct economic benefit of the transferring hospital has been dubbed "patient dumping," and is driven by the continuing problem of assigning financial responsibility and attendant reimbursement for the care of some patients, particularly the medically indigent and those functionally indigent due to peculiarities of health insurance coverage.

When medical care was provided as a charity by hospitals and physicians, or, more recently, when medical insurance reimbursements were adjusted to compensate for free care and bad debt, there was less of a problem. As the cost of health care rose, the burden of the medically indigent became a great strain on some hospitals, physicians, and medical insurers. Medical indigency has reached the scale at which some 15 million Americans either do not seek or do not receive health care because they cannot afford it. Medically indigent people are defined as those who lack any or adequate health-care insurance. This group includes not only those people who are uninsured because of such causes as unemployment and self-employment, but also those who are in a high-risk medical group and are therefore uninsurable.[14]

Currently, it is estimated that economic dumping exceeds 250,000 patient transfers annually and that approximately 15% of patients transferred in 1986 were "dumped." *Dumping,* for purposes of this chapter, refers to the transfer of unstabilized patients, the transfer of stabilized patients, or the transfer of in-house patients whose insurance has run out.[11] The enormous economic burden of dumping rests mainly on public hospitals, which receive the majority of the patients. The American College of Emergency Physicians (ACEP) has published guidelines for appropriate patient transfers, and continues to address the issues raised by this process.[1,2]

The process of transfer is potentially dangerous for both patient and practitioner; the addition of economic and legal factors makes it even more risky. Hospital policy and transfer agreements, state and federal regulations and laws, professional practice standards, and other rules all have an impact on the transfer process. This chapter reviews the practice of emergency department patient transfer and proposes guidelines for improving the coordination and safety of the process.

MEDICAL AND ECONOMIC HISTORY

The increasing mobility of society, combined with an increased number of uninsured or underinsured patients, has resulted in an increased number who do not have a personal physician or an affiliation with a particular health-care institution or system and an increase in patient volumes at both emergency departments and urgent care clinics. In addition, the public has come to expect both high-quality and timely medical care, as well as complete subspecialty diagnostic and therapeutic capabilities when they present for emergency care. While basic prehospital care is all that is available in many areas, advanced life-support ambulance service is also an expectation. People want a low-cost, economically efficient health-care system, yet when faced with a personal emergency, they want the best of everything immediately.

The favored means of offering high-level care to a great number of patients—the regionalization of specialty care—currently necessitates patient transfer. Sending teams to the patient is currently common only as part of the transfer process. "Telemedicine," in which physicians receive diagnostic and therapeutic advice and even robotic surgical assistance from distant expert consultants via electronic networking, may become more common in the future, but may also result in potential liability from inaccuracies or confidentiality issues involving information transfer. The emergency physician now frequently controls prehospital care, emergency treatment, access to the hospital and advanced technologies, and patient transfer to facilities offering unique or subspecialty care, and therefore is in an important yet vulnerable position.

As individual providers, emergency physicians are often paid by either salary or fee-for-service arrangements, often with a minimum guaranteed income. Thus, there exists some direct, and certainly indirect, economic incentive to provide care for the well-insured or paying patient. Professional ethics dictate that care should be provided equally. However, at a certain point in treatment, economics may become important. Less costly alternatives are often arranged for patients who cannot afford prescribed medication, have no access to free care, or refuse admission for economic reasons.

Patients who require admission but are uninsured or have a facility-specific insurance plan may request transfer. The underinsured or uninsured patient may benefit financially from such a transfer; the truly indigent patient, who has no means of paying any medical bill, does not. The referring hospital does, however, and it may pressure the emergency physician directly or indirectly to perform such transfers. Admitting physicians may, for example, inquire about insurance coverage for legitimate reasons such as managed care contract coverage, and then encourage transfer based on economic factors. The emergency physician must always balance the risks and benefits of transfers, keeping the best interest of the patient as his or her guide.

In many areas of the country, additional economic issues are raised by managed health-care plans (MHCPs), such as health maintenance organizations (HMOs), preferred provider organizations (PPOs), and government-run health-care systems. For example, MHCPs that own or operate hospitals may enforce strict screening criteria during the triage process to prevent emergency visits by those not covered by their plan, or to prevent "unnecessary" visits by plan members. Other hospitals may have contracts with MHCPs that similarly attempt to regulate patient flow. Some institutions have capitation contracts with MHCPs, in which a fixed amount is paid on a regular basis for care of the plan's patients, giving them significant incentive to avoid unnecessary costs, sometimes by the transfer of patients, and perhaps giving significant incentive for the private physician to refer more patients to the emergency department because "the bill is already paid."

Many of the transfer issues currently faced in the emergency department are the result of other changes. The rising cost of health care has resulted in the disappearance of services that formerly were available: The intensive care unit (ICU) is full due to a nursing shortage, the only orthopedist in town moves to another state because of lower malpractice premiums, or the community hospital closes. On the other hand, advanced and expensive services that formerly were widely unavailable are now within reach via transfer and have come to be expected by the general public for problems such as cardiac disease, trauma, specialized neonatal and pediatric care, reimplantation of amputated limbs, and advanced diagnostic imaging. Emergency physicians need to be aware of the social and economic forces as well as the legal forces involved in their duty to provide care, and patients, if able, must be offered enough information to make an informed choice, and to give informed consent to a transfer if that option is proposed and is in their best interest.

DUTY TO CARE

The United States has not traditionally defined the access to health care in an emergency as a fundamental right, nor has the common law required that government provide access to health care for those people who are uninsured or underinsured.[10] Until recently, it was a relatively common hospital policy that the emergency department had no duty to care for patients who presented for care. Many hospitals did not offer emergency care for the uninsured, for those who had a personal physician in the community, or for those with particular types of insurance coverage. A two-tier health-care system, in which the rich and properly insured received better care than the poor, was developing. In parallel, specialty care hospitals became commonplace and attempted to limit access to their emergency departments to specific populations. As a result, "undesirable" patients were often denied care arbitrarily and had to seek help elsewhere or go without care.[4]

In 1946, the Hill Burton Act required that hospitals make their services available to all persons residing in the territorial area of the hospital, among other provisions, in return for federal funds for the construction and modernization of hospitals.[8] Compliance was poor, as there was little enforcement of the Act's requirements and the common law no-duty rule provided no relief at law for those who were turned away. As emergency departments expanded and visits increased during the 1960s, the consequences of denying care to patients resulted in a series of legal actions that eventually compelled hospitals with emergency departments to offer care for all patients who presented, regardless of their economic, medical, insurance, or other status. Since then, courts have developed theories under which hospitals can be held liable for refusing care.[9,15,20]

One theory is that a duty to treat may arise when a hospital undertakes to render aid, a position that is taken in the Restatement 2nd of Torts.[18] Under this section, there is a liability for harm that attaches if the actor fails to act with reasonable care, even when the undertaking is purely gratuitous. The basis for harm to the plaintiff is that the plaintiff relied on the actor's conduct and, in doing so, either did not take the precautionary measures that he or she would have otherwise taken and/or had foregone aid from another source. In other words, if a hospital holds itself out as one that will provide care in an emergency, that fact becomes generally known to the public.[19] Patients who present for care at such an emergency department and subsequently deteriorate because therapy, once initiated, is denied or delayed on the basis of an inability to pay for it, have a legitimate claim against the hospital.[9,12]

Another theory successfully used by the courts to impose a duty on emergency departments to see and treat emergency patients is that of negligence.[17] Negligence is the failure to act as the prudent emergency physician would under the same or similar circumstances, resulting in some harm to the patient. Considering the presence and maintenance of an emergency department as an undertaking, negligence may be found in an emergency department's failure to properly perform that undertaking (i.e., providing aid for those who present in search of emergent medical care).

The third theory used by the courts in finding hospitals liable when they turned away emergency patients was based on reliance. Under this theory, when a hospital establishes the custom of holding itself out as being a place where one can receive emergency care, that hospital then owes a duty to those patients who rely on that custom in seeking care.[5] Patients who relied on this promise of care, but were harmed by that reliance because the care was denied or delayed for some reason, then had a cause of action (detrimental reliance) against the hospital.

Fourth, the issue of financial motivation in limiting, delaying, or denying care has resulted in public policy intended to coerce hospitals into providing care for all persons who present for emergency care. This argument, briefly, holds that hospitals receiving public monies (and most do, through Medicare and Medicaid reimbursement and other programs) must serve the public equally.

By the late 1970s, it became well established that hospitals with emergency departments had a duty to render, in a reasonable manner, emergency care for all patients who presented for such care, regardless of insurance, ability to pay, or other factors, unless there was good cause not to do so. The duty was not limited to public hospitals, but included private facilities and those run for profit, particularly if they accepted some public money for expenses or capital improvements. It is still unclear at exactly what point an individual becomes a patient, but that threshold is certainly crossed once any care is rendered, and it may be crossed once the patient enters the facility and requests care. One opinion that "it would shock the public conscience if a person in need of medical emergency aid would be turned down at the door of a hospital having emergency service because that person could not at that moment assure payment for the service" summarizes the situation by the 1980s.[3] Unfortunately, some hospitals were meeting the minimum requirement of seeing all patients, but then unsafely transferring those unable to pay for continued care.

On April 7, 1986, Congress passed federal antidumping legislation as a part of the Consolidated Omnibus Budget Reconciliation Act (COBRA).[17] The purpose of this legislation was to prevent a hospital from transferring unstabilized emergency patients for economic reasons.[4] The COBRA law applies to all emergency departments at all hospitals that receive any form of federal funding, and to all of the persons who present there for care, regardless of their age or insurance status. Although the impact of COBRA was felt throughout the country, the problem of patient dumping remained one of significant proportions. In response to this situation, amendments to COBRA, known as the Omnibus Budget Reconciliation Act (OBRA) or the Emergency Medical Treatment and Labor Act (EMTALA), went into effect on July 1, 1990. The publicity of this event served to heighten awareness of patient dumping and has resulted in significant educational efforts on behalf of hospitals and their administrations to train their nurses and physicians in the requirements of this law. Regulations went into effect late in the summer of 1994 that fully implemented the intent of the COBRA law as amended. In September 1995, regulations requiring receiving hospitals went into effect, with an immediate increase in administrative EMTALA enforcement actions as a result. In June 1998, site review guidelines for surveyors were issued, further detailing government interpretations of the law and regulations.

THE COBRA LAW IN DETAIL

Scope of Coverage

COBRA, as implemented in Regulations, applies to all persons (and to persons on whose behalf care is sought) presenting to an emergency department for care, regardless of their indigency or insurance status, and to any hospital that operates an emergency department or equivalent (e.g., labor room or mental health screening area) and receives Medicare funding. The term *transfer* is broadly defined to include any patient who does not go to the morgue or competently leave the emergency department following an informed refusal of care process. Even patients admitted to the hospital may be covered if discharged from the hospital before being stabilized. A hospital that does not have a Medicare provider agreement may be influenced by COBRA, because it is possible that this law may be used to determine the "standard of care" for patient management. A hospital is not guilty of a violation, however, if it can show that it did not depart from its normal treatment procedure for any patient with similar complaints in the emergency department.[7]

Under the provisions of the law, patients must be offered a medical screening examination to determine whether an emergent condition (including active labor) exists. If the patient is stable (no emergent condition), then COBRA does not apply. One of the most problematic aspects of COBRA, from the perspective of the emergency department physician, is the legal definition of what are generally considered to be medical terms, such as *stability* and *medical emergency*.

Medical Screening Requirement Definitions

Presenting to the Emergency Department

Physically arriving in the department and asking for care obviously constitutes presentation, but HCFA guidelines state that any person who arrives on the premises of the hospital, seeking emergency care, should be screened. The 1994 Regulations add any presentation to the hospital's own ambulance service, if any, to the group of patients who become the responsibility of the emergency physician.[6] Patients who pass through the emergency department, including patients presenting for routine outpatient testing or patients presenting for direct admission after hours, must all be logged into the emergency department log. They have to be recorded, but not necessarily screened, according to HCFA enforcement patterns. These patients would not typically receive a medical screening examination unless they complained of acute problems or were observed to be in distress that was inconsistent with their scheduled presentation. Any patient who presents on the premises of the hospital must be logged and screened, if seeking care.

Obstetric patients presenting to the obstetrics department or psychiatric patients presenting to a psychiatric assessment unit, rather than the emergency department, are required to be logged and screened. HCFA interprets the term *emergency department* to cover all areas where a patient might present for primary assessment of a presenting condition on an unscheduled basis, and not just the specific area designated as an emergency department.

All patients presenting to a hospital-owned and -operated ambulance are likewise deemed to have presented to the hospital. Patients transported by non–hospital-owned ambulances are not deemed to have presented to the hospital until the ambulance has entered onto hospital-owned property. Hospital property includes all off-site locations operated under the same Medicare provider number as the hospital, under HCFA enforcement. Telephone or radio contact from outside the hospital's boundaries and not involving a hospital-owned ambulance is not deemed to be a presentation for HCFA enforcement purposes. Whether courts will follow the HCFA interpretations in civil litigation has yet to be determined, in part because few trial cases have been argued and individual cases focus on broader issues. Several cases, however, have dealt with the issue of having "come to the hospital," and have been consistent with the HCFA definition in their limited-fact situations.

Screening Examination

There are no specific instructions for how to do a "screening examination"; therefore, the COBRA requirement for such a screening examination creates an artificial entity. However, screening, in the epidemiologic sense, is one of the major functions of the emergency department; therefore, this type of examination is inherent in the emergency care process. According to this argument, the essence of emergency medicine is, in large measure, the recognition of signs and symptoms that may pose a risk (not recognized by the patient) of death, serious disease, or potential disability. It is this intellectual effort that distinguishes emergency medicine from other specialties.

The remainder of the practice of emergency medicine is simply treatment of the presenting or potential problem in an attempt to prevent these complications. The legal system adds credence to this argument by most often taking emergency physicians to court for failure to diagnose, rather than for errors in treatment. Therefore, according to this argument, the "screening examination" is no different from the problem-focused history and physical examination, with all indicated studies and tests, that would be performed to rule out, to a reasonable degree of medical certainty, impending death, serious disease, or potential for disability. It then follows that the screening examination should not differ from the regular evaluation performed for any patient with a similar problem.

Who Can Perform the Screening Examination

The qualifications of the person performing the screening are not specifically addressed, but the wording of COBRA amendments suggests that a physician evaluation, which is certainly a "service routinely available to the emergency department," is required. ACEP has interpreted the medical screening requirement to mean that a qualified emergency physician will determine whether a patient is presenting with a true or potential emergency and whether the patient is likely to benefit from a transfer to another facility. This position is supported by both the Joint Commission on Accreditation of Healthcare Organizations (JCAHO) in their accreditation manuals and most, if not all, state Boards of Registration for Nursing. The JCAHO takes the position that it is the physician who is responsible for the degree of medical treatment and evaluation of emergency department patients. Further supporting ACEP's position is the understanding that there are laws in all states that govern the practice of registered nurses and prohibit registered nurses from making medical diagnoses and discharging patients from the hospital without some higher level of certification. Others add the argument that the COBRA law specifically lists the responsible physician as one of the liable parties, and not the nurse, and that, therefore, the intent of the law was direct physician involvement in the screening examination.

It is important to note, however, that some hospitals (and MHCPs) have taken the alternative view that a nurse or other health-care provider is capable of performing a "medical screening" examination within the meaning of the law. This view is based on the theory that HCFA guidelines state that the physician has to be responsible for the screening examinations performed by nonphysicians but does not necessarily need to perform the examinations personally. In hospitals where a nurse may triage patients to other facilities and locations, some ambiguity remains. In facilities where all patients are seen by a physician, there should be little question that a physician screening examination is required. In either case, because the responsibility for the care of all of the patients who enter the department lies with the attending physician, and because it is the physician and the hospital who bear the ultimate responsibility for the patient and who are held financially liable by this Act (see later discussion), it can be argued that, at a minimum, a physician should make the decision about any patient stability for transfer or discharge, even if someone else performs the screening examination.

Where nonphysicians are utilized for medial screening functions, HCFA has been quick to cite violations in which the nonphysician was not specifically authorized as a qualified medical screening person by hospital board action, in which the services exceeded the scope of the state licensure, in which the services were not pursuant to a written protocol, and in which there were no clearly defined points at which a physician was required to be involved.

Final responsibility for the medical screening examination under HCFA Conditions of Participation in Medicare must rest with a physician, which leaves delegation of this function to nurses in the emergency department setting problematic. A 1996 Massachusetts case based on a rapid primary assessment by a registered nurse and subsequent discharge to a physician's office resulted in HCFA citations as well as an EMTALA lawsuit that produced a 1999 settlement of $1 million.

Actions by private physicians who see their own patients in the emergency department have been cited by HCFA as violations, and the hospital and physician held responsible for the violation. The definition of what persons the hospital may be accountable for refers to employees of the hospital or any person affiliated or associated directly or indirectly with the hospital.

ADEQUACY OF MEDICAL SCREENING

The original iteration of COBRA required that the screening examination be performed within the capabilities of the emergency department. Amendments to the original act now require that all ancillaries (e.g., laboratory testing, imaging, and diagnostic services) that are available to the emergency department be considered in the patient screening process. It also includes the use of all routinely available "on-call" subspecialty physicians for consultation.

Although the Act itself does not dictate the standard for emergency medical practice, the adequacy of the medical examination is likely to be judged in two ways. One is by the normal medical malpractice and negligence standards as to what care is standard for that hospital and physician when faced with a patient presenting with the same complaint. Another is by the patient's outcome (i.e., retrospective stability), judged against the Act's definition of an emergency medical condition: a medical condition manifesting acute symptoms of sufficient severity (including severe pain) such that the absence of immediate medical attention could reasonably be expected to result in placing the health of the individual (or the unborn child of a pregnant woman) in serious jeopardy, serious impairment to bodily functions, or serious dysfunction of any bodily organ or part (or, with respect to a pregnant woman who is having contractions, there is inadequate time to effect a safe transfer to another hospital before delivery or the transfer may pose a threat to the health or safety of the woman or the unborn child). This retrospective approach, particularly when applied using the broad and subjective definition of an emergency medical condition, implies that a thorough evaluation must be performed in order to accurately assess stability, provide the most responsible patient care, and avoid potential litigation.

OBRA changed the COBRA language in two additional areas that are pertinent to the medical screening requirement. First, the definition of *active labor* was broadened to include any pregnant woman having contractions, regardless of gestational age. Second, wording was added that prohibits delaying the screening examination or subsequent treatment to "inquire about the individual's method of payment or insurance status."

Thus, hospital contracts with MHCPs that require special approval procedures, telephone calls, or other measures that may delay care for such patients should be examined closely by legal counsel to be certain that they do not conflict with the spirit of this additional requirement. HCFA site review guidelines indicate that it is not appropriate for a hospital to request, or a managed care plan to require, prior authorization before the patient has received the medical screening examination to determine the presence or absence of an emergency medical condition or until an existing emergency medical condition has been stabilized. A hospital may request routine registration information, such as name of insurance, but may not pursue validating of that information or obtaining authorization for treatment prior to completion of the screening examination. Physicians may not alter the screening examination based on the type of insurance plan the patient has and may not refuse to screen a patient because his or her plan refused to authorize treatment or pay for screening and treatment.

Triage protocols that avoid any difference in patient care procedures for such patients would appear to be both legally prudent and medically sound. For example, contracts between the hospital and MHCP providing payment of a "screening fee" for patients retrospectively found to have nonemergent conditions and payment of mutually agreeable charges for other patients might be arranged between the hospital and MHCP, thus transferring the economic considerations to the billing office and moving money instead of patients. If any difference in procedure exists for MHCP patients, it must be clear to all that the MHCP is authorizing payment, not medical care, that the patient is being offered a screening examination, and that there is no significant economic disincentive to the patient in choosing to be examined and treated if the MHCP refuses payment authorization. If, for example, a patient is transferred or refuses care after being told that he or she will be billed for that care, the hospital and physician may be liable for damages if the patient is later found to have been unstable and can show that the reason for transfer or refusal of care was the threat of a bill for emergency services.

It is also important to note that the medical screening examination is an ongoing process rather than an isolated event. This means that there must be an ongoing monitoring of the patient's condition and that, where further diagnostic evaluation is necessary to rule out a condition that might constitute an emergency medical condition under the law, the medical screening is not yet completed and HCFA enforcement standards will deem that patient to have an emergency medical condition and unstable for EMTALA transfer purposes. The courts, however, tend to accept a physician determination of stability and not look beyond that, unless the medical record contains clear indications to the contrary or the scope of the examination was seriously deficient in light of the presenting conditions.

Stabilizing Treatment

The necessary stabilizing treatment for emergency medical conditions and labor means that once a patient is found to be suffering from an emergency medical condition (per COBRA definition) or is in active labor, the hospital must give the patient that treatment necessary to stabilize the patient's condition, unless the patient can be transferred without danger of deterioration of his or her medical condition or unless the benefits involved with the transfer and subsequent treatment at the receiving hospital outweigh the risks. This stabilizing treatment includes delivery of the fetus and placenta in the case of active labor, and includes the provision of ancillary services, including the skills of on-call specialists. OBRA eliminates emergency physician liability if an on-call consultant refuses to see and treat a patient in a timely manner. The wording requires that, should such a situation arise, where "the on-call physician fails or refuses to appear within a reasonable period of time, and the [emergency] physician orders the transfer of the individual because the [emergency] physician determines that without the services of the on-call physician the benefits of transfer outweigh the risks of transfer, the physician authorizing the transfer shall not be subject to a penalty." In addition, the "name and address of any on-call physician . . . who has refused or failed to appear within a reasonable time to provide necessary stabilizing treatment" must be included in the medical records provided to the receiving facility.

If transfer to another facility is offered and refused by the patient, this refusal should be informed and documented. This situation may arise when transfer is indicated to access stabilizing treatment. If transfer is not offered, but the patient refuses to consent to further examination and treatment for an emergent condition determined by the screening examination, this refusal should also be informed and documented. Note that this refusal provision follows the screening examination; refusal to consent to the screening examination itself may then constitute a withdrawal of the request for examination and treatment, because no determination has been made on which to base a reasonable discussion of the risks inherent in refusing the initial screening examination. Many facilities have adopted a "screening form," on which the process of such consents and refusals is documented. However, as discussed, the insertion of an additional process for a specific group of patients that delays care while determining reimbursement information may violate the law. Some have argued that the standard consent for treatment form used for other persons presenting to the emergency department covers consent for screening examinations and typically informs the patient that costs will be incurred and charges billed. It is then, according to this point of view, the responsibility of the patient and his or her third-party payor to discuss responsibility for payment. The test that is likely to be applied by the courts is whether the process used is different for any particular group of patients, whether that difference poses a potential for delayed care, and whether the care then given is standard for the presenting situation up to the point of determining whether an emergency condition exists and providing stabilizing treatment.

HCFA offices in many areas of the United States have required hospitals to remove financial consents for the initial consent documents signed prior to screening. This suggests a high risk associated with these forms and any other sign, procedure, or document that draws payment status issues to the attention of the patient prior to completion of the screening examination and stabilization.

Appropriate Transfer

The "restricting transfers until the individual is stabilized" provision means that a patient with an unstabilized emergent condition may not be transferred unless informed written request for transfer is made by the patient or responsible party, or all of the following conditions are met:

- A physician [or if not present, a qualified medical person] signs a certification that the medical benefits outweigh the risks and summarizes this argument as discussed with and consented to by the patient or responsible party.
- Treatment to minimize transfer risk is provided.
- The receiving facility has adequate capability and has accepted the patient.
- The receiving facility is provided with all pertinent records.
- The transfer is effected through qualified personnel, vehicle, and equipment.

The adequacy of the transfer arrangements will probably be judged using a standard of care test. Therefore, all the usual steps taken to arrange acceptance, send medical information, and physically transfer the patient should be met or exceeded. Reductions in level of care during transfer are problematic and should be avoided, if possible. As always, personnel accompanying the patient during transfer should also have the vehicle, equipment, training, and skill to treat all reasonably likely complications of the patient's emergency condition during the transfer. The use of hospital staff unfamiliar with emergency medicine, including the skills needed to provide care in ambulances and helicopters, should be avoided. An unstable patient, who requires the close attention of a physician and nurse while in the emergency department, probably warrants that level of care during transfer as well.

One of the primary areas in which hospitals encounter problems with the transfer regulations is in the use of private vehicles. Interhospital transfer or movement among different health system buildings generally triggers the "appropriate transfer" rules, and under these rules, a private vehicle cannot qualify as an appropriate vehicle, with appropriate medical personnel, and with life-support equipment. Hence it is a violation, unless the patient has refused ambulance transfer in writing, with the appropriate risks and benefits specifically itemized on the refusal form.

For the practitioner for whom relatively minor conditions still must be transferred for a narrow focus of care, the issue comes up as to what a patient needs to be told to justify an ambulance transfer that might not be paid for by the insurance or Medicare benefits. The answer from one regulator was to tell the patient, "This may sound stupid, but I am required by law to send you by ambulance unless you sign this refusal."

Closely associated with this situation is the use of police vehicles for transport of mental health patients, as is general practice throughout the United States. HCFA citations have been issued for use of police or private vehicles in transferring patients deemed to be a danger to themselves or others, as they are "unstable" under EMTALA standards. Although the site review guidelines indicate that stability may be achieved through the use of medications and restraint, these are not the sole criteria for stability. In addition, once there are medications administered or medical restraint orders issued, the patient is a medical patient as well and requires ambulance transfer. This definition places many hospitals in the position of following state procedures or complying with EMTALA. EMTALA specifically preempts state rules that directly conflict with its standards.

Receiving Facilities

The "nondiscrimination" requirement mandates acceptance by regional referral facilities capable of treating the patient. Although it is not specifically defined in the law, it appears that specialty referral centers are those that are able to handle medical emergencies that the sending hospital is not. Such facilities cannot refuse transfers if they have the capability to treat the patient.

Hospital-Wide Implications

Hospitals are required to have a compliance policy meeting requirements set forth by the COBRA law. Medical records, including transfer forms, are required to be maintained by the hospital for 5 years from the date of the transfer. In an effort to increase public awareness of patient rights to emergency care, hospitals are required to post signs with specific language identifying the rights of persons who present seeking care, the obligation of the hospital to provide that care, and the hospital's participation or lack thereof in the Medicaid program.

A 1999 Supreme Court decision (*Roberts v. Galin*) has specifically ruled that a case involving an inpatient who was transferred to a nursing home after 60 days of hospital care and in an allegedly unstable condition could have her EMTALA lawsuit tried, regardless of a failure to allege an intentional violation. Immediately following that decision, the United States Court of Appeals for the First Circuit (*Lopez-Soto v. Hawayek,* 1999 WL 188283) ruled that EMTALA stabilization and transfer rules apply any time a patient (or visitor or employee) on the premises of the hospital is known to have an unstable emergency medical condition as defined by EMTALA. This decision supports a prior Virginia Supreme Court ruling that EMTALA is not limited to patients presenting via the emergency department (*Smith v. Richmond Memorial,* 1992).

Enforcement Provisions

The mechanisms for enforcement under COBRA are specifically delineated within the Act itself. It is important for both physicians and hospitals to remember that that fines or termination of Medicare provider agreements can occur *even in the absence of patient injury*. The consequences of being the subject of a complaint, even if unsubstantiated, are potentially devastating. The hospital will be subject to investigations and probably to negative publicity. It will have to spend considerable time and money preparing a defense and correcting any potential deficiencies. A negative initial determination will be difficult and costly to overturn, even if the hospital is able to do so.

A hospital that knowingly, willfully, or negligently violates COBRA can be subject to suspension or termination of its Medicare provider agreement. A physician may be terminated from Medicare for gross, flagrant, or repeated violations. The Act also provides for penalties against institutions that receive inappropriate transfers if they do not report the violations within 72 hours. Patient dumping cases are initially investigated by state agencies under contract with HFCA to determine whether there is a material concern about compliance. Once that determination is made, the information is turned over to the federal government for further action. Once a physician is found to be out of compliance with the provisions of COBRA, the state medical board will become involved. If the state medical board does not take action within 30 days, the Office of the Inspector General (OIG) will step in to make a determination of whether a penalty of up to $50,000 is warranted. Civil monetary penalties for a violation are severe and are intended to provide a significant deterrent for those hospitals and physicians inclined to dump patients.

COBRA was not meant to supplant the medical malpractice process; it is a cause of action unto itself, and is not typically covered by physician's malpractice insurance, although most hospital insurers have defended and paid COBRA claims. Monetary compensations of up to $5 million for personal injury resulting from patient dumping have been awarded under this law. Sanctions may come in the form of termination of the Medicare provider agreement, civil monetary penalties of up to $50,000 per violation for both the hospital and physician, private cause of actions by the patient against the hospital for personal injury, private cause of action by the receiving facility against a transferring hospital to recover financial losses suffered as a result of an inappropriate transfer, or injunctive relief.

Prosecution of a Claim

The elements of a cause of action under COBRA[13] that must be alleged by the plaintiff are (1) that the plaintiff presented to the defendant's emergency room or covered adjuncts such as a hospital-run ambulance service (2) with an emergency medical condition, and that the hospital either (3) did not adequately screen to determine whether an emergency condition existed, (4) discharged the patient or transferred the patient before that emergency condition was stabilized, or (5) failed to follow the statutory standards for transfer.

The standard of care in the individual emergency department to which the plaintiff presented is also important. A COBRA claim can also involve being denied care or an allegation that care provided was materially different from what other patients who present under similar circumstances would receive. It may also be established by showing that the hospital did not adhere to its own policies and procedures for evaluation of patients who present with a similar complaint. Because this cause of action was not created to supplant a medical malpractice claim, one can have both a COBRA claim as well as a medical malpractice claim arising out of the same emergency department visit.

In defending actions based on COBRA, it is important to remember that the Act is reasonably specific as to what is considered to be a violation. It requires that a medical emergency or labor be present based on a screening examination, and that the patient be transferred either without adequate stabilizing treatment or improperly. The first defense is that the patient was stable. Under this Act, a stable patient may be transferred to another institution for any reason at all (although other causes of action may be problematic if the transfer results in injury). If there is documentation that the patient received an adequate screening evaluation, and that evaluation did not reveal an emergency medical condition, then the claim may be one of medical malpractice if there is a claim of negligence, but is not an action under COBRA. The key is to determine whether the patient received a medical screening examination that was the same as would be given to anyone else who presented with the same complaint, regardless of their insurance status, and the result of that screening examination is that the patient was found to be stable. It is important to differentiate between the patient's eventual diagnosis or outcome and the result of the screening examination. It is tempting for the plaintiff to claim that the screening was inadequate if the outcome was poor, but the defense must only show that the screening met the standard examination criteria. In other words, a patient who presents with a minor ankle fracture, is felt to be stable after adequate screening and is appropriately transferred, but dies the next day from a pulmonary embolus has an unfortunate outcome, but not a COBRA claim. More problematic is the same patient who develops chronic pain in the ankle after delayed care in a receiving facility, or who has an auto accident while driving to the receiving facility because of inability to use the injured ankle.

The next ground on which to base a defense is that the patient requested the transfer or voluntarily withdrew a request for care. This has become increasingly important following the increase in the managed care population. The burden of proof is on the hospital to show that the request was withdrawn by the patient and that there was no coercion on the hospital's part involved in the patient's decision to withdraw. Documentation of offers to provide care regardless of ability to pay at the time of care, particularly efforts that may mitigate any claim that the cost of offered care was an issue, such as documented effort to assist in application for free care or the offering of reduced cost care plans where applicable, is helpful in defending a claim of economic coercion. A final defense may be that the statute of limitations for the Act has run out.

Exceptions to COBRA

1. *The patient dies before transfer or discharge.* While this outcome may raise concerns about negligence, COBRA does not apply unless the death occurred *from or during* transfer or as a result of a failure to adequately screen or stabilize. A causal relationship between the violation and the adverse outcome must still be proven for litigation purposes, although regulatory enforcement does not link violations to negative outcomes. A citation may be based on a failure of EMTALA compliance without a negative outcome. Negative outcomes, however, are considered "red flags" that stimulate more detailed review.
2. *The patient leaves against medical advice.* A patient who is offered or receives a medical screening examination and competently leaves the hospital against medical advice (AMA) has no cause of action under COBRA. However, "making" all patients who leave the department after offer of a screening examination sign an AMA form dilutes the concept of "against medical advice." The AMA process should be reserved for situations in which the physician feels there is significant medical risk if the patient leaves, not for all situations in which the physician feels at legal risk. Use of a specific form for refusal of EMTALA rights would be more appropriate in most instances. In serious cases, use of both forms would emphasize the efforts taken by the hospital or physician to attempt to provide appropriate care. Use of the AMA form routinely may have the unintended effect of shutting off insurance coverage for subsequent treatment of the same or related condition.
3. *The patient is stable.* A patient is stabilized if, after a standard medical screening examination, there is no reasonable likelihood that the patient's condition will materially deteriorate from or during the transfer. However, as discussed, stability may be open to retrospective reinterpretation in some situations.
4. *The patient requests the transfer or refuses it.* An informed patient may request or refuse transfer. While any transfer performed under these circumstances should follow good medical practice, COBRA cannot then be invoked if the patient rather than the clinician initiated the transfer. Likewise, if a patient refuses transfer when recommended, the clinician should provide the next best alternative, but cannot be held liable under COBRA for the patient's informed decision. As in informed consent, a determination of patient competency must be made. Physicians must understand, however, that getting a patient's consent to a technically incorrect action under EMTALA does not waive the violation or validate the action. Similarly, pressure to get a patient to request transfer invalidates that patient's request and can expose the hospital and physicians to EMTALA citations and fines. The patient-initiated transfer or refusal must be documented in writing and signed by the patient, if possible. If not, extensive documentation of efforts made to obtain the written request or refusal must be present in the record.

COMMON PITFALLS

- Failure to appreciate the COBRA laws and their impact on the practice of emergency medicine for both patient treatment and transfer
- Failure to educate patients and families about COBRA
- Failure to understand the relationship between the MHCPs and the emergency physician's responsibility to provide a screening examination to all patients who present for care
- Failure to apprise oneself of hospital policies and procedures regarding the COBRA laws and implementation of compliance strategy

References

1. American College of Emergency Physicians. Access to emergency medical care: emergency physicians and uncompensated care. *Ann Emerg Med* 1987;16:1302.
2. American College of Emergency Physicians. Principles of appropriate patient transfer. *Ann Emerg Med* 1990;19:337.
3. *Chandler v. The Hospital Authority of the City of Huntsville,* 548 So. 2d. 1384 (1989).
4. Enfield LM, Sklar DP. Patient dumping in the hospital emergency department: renewed interest in an old problem. *Am J Law Med* 1988;13:561.
5. *Fabian v. Matzuko,* 236 Pa. Super. 267 (1975).
6. Federal Register, June 22, 1994.
7. *Gatewood v. Washington Healthcare Corp.,* 923 F.2d 1037 (1991).
8. Hill Burton, 42 U.S.C.A. sec. 291-2910 (1988 & Supp. II 1990).
9. *LeJuen Road Hospital Inc. v. Watson,* 171 So. 2d 202 (1960).
10. *Maher v. Roe,* 432 US 464.
11. McCormick B. Fifteen percent of transfers seen as dumping. *Hospitals* 1986;60(19):146.
12. *New Biloxi Hospital v. Frazier,* 245 Miss. 185 (1962).
13. 1990 U.S. Dist. LEXIS 7360.
14. Nutter DO. Medical indigency and the public health care crisis: the need for a definitive solution. *N Engl J Med* 1987;316:1156.
15. *O'Neill v. Montefiore Hospital,* 11 A.D. 2d. 132 (1960).
16. Pub. Law No. 99-272, @ 9121, 1986 U.S. Code Cong & Admin. News (100 Stat.) 82, 164-167 (Codified and amended as 42 U.S.C.A. @1395dd 1988 and sup II 1990).
17. *Reeves v. North Broward Hospital,* 191 So. 2nd. 307 (1966).
18. Restatement (2nd) of Torts @ 323 (1934).
19. *Williams v. Hospital Authority of Hall County,* 119 Ga. App. 262 (1969).
20. *Wilmington General v. Manlove,* 54 Del 15 (1961).

CHAPTER 409

Bereavement and Grief Reactions

Christopher H. Linden

Death in the emergency department is especially dramatic because of the suddenness of the loss, and because it is often traumatic and sometimes involves the young. Unexpected and untimely deaths are conspicuous because the person not only was active and visible at the time of death, but also was a significant force in the life of the survivors.[18] Intervention strategies to facilitate the grieving process may help survivors avoid developing major psychiatric illness as a sequela.

Bereavement is the total normal response to loss. *Grief* denotes the intense emotions and physical symptoms associated with the loss.[7] *Mourning* is a social expression of grief. Grief is a normal process that is usually set in motion by significant loss, such as the loss of a spouse, parent, child, or significant other. Grieving is characterized by an intensive, in-depth review of the survivor's relationship with the deceased. A grieving person reviews memories of the deceased and only gradually confronts each one with the realization that it no longer corresponds to something real. This sequence is repeated over and over. The grief response may also include physical ailments and guilt feelings, such as feeling responsible for the loss or failing to resolve personal conflicts. The grieving person gradually is reconciled to the loss and attenuates the attachment to the lost object. The psychological purposes of grieving are to break the emotional tie with the deceased person and to reinvest the attachment in living persons.

Expression of grief is determined by cultural mores.[18] Some people express grief histrionically, with loud crying and sobbing, but others remain still, with little visible expression of emotion. A person displaying no overt symptoms of grief may still be deeply affected or grieving. Several responses can be perplexing and may be misinterpreted by staff.[7] A frequent initial reaction is denial, a psychological defense that closes off perceptions of painful immediate reality. The survivor may question the physician closely for proof of the identity of the deceased or may continue to refer to the deceased as if he or she were alive.[11] At other times, survivors display antagonistic and angry feelings toward staff members, accusing them of being negligent or of not doing all they could have done. This anger often represents the survivors' own unconscious anger toward the deceased for abandoning them, or it may stem from guilt about unresolved conflicts with the deceased.

Medical education is deficient in the training of physicians in death notification.[10,13] Although death in the emergency department is relatively common, physicians find this process emotionally difficult and draining. There is often no preexisting relationship between the physician and patient, and physicians may fear being blamed. They must deal with their own emotions (e.g., feelings of defeat, guilt, impotence, and incompetence) and fears of death as well as the reactions of survivors. Physicians may attempt to reduce their own stress by delaying the news, thus increasing the family's anxiety, or by rushing in unprepared and presenting the news in an awkward manner.[1,15]

Conveying bad news compassionately and effectively requires communication skills and advanced preparation. A staff that is aware of the dynamics of grieving and the needs of survivors can facilitate the grief process, cushion the trauma of loss, and establish a basis for a healthy grief response.[5] Issues related to death notification and the processes involved are outlined in this chapter. Similar considerations apply when delivering other types of bad news to patients, their family, and their loved ones.[6,14] Explicit criteria should be met when declaring a person brain dead.[8]

CONTACTING SURVIVORS

The first intervention after sudden and unexpected death is contacting the survivors.[10] Because there is no ongoing relationship between the emergency department staff and the survivors, the person designated to call the survivors should identify himself or herself and should establish the identity of the survivor. Talk to an adult, and try to determine whether someone is present to provide emotional or physical support.

If the family is far away, it may be necessary to inform the family over the telephone. As a rule, however, do not tell relatives of deaths over the telephone; rather, tell them that their relative is in serious condition and ask them to come to the hospital immediately.[1,16] Information regarding the time, location, and nature of the event (illness or injury), and when and how they arrived can also be provided. Encourage the survivor to come to the hospital with a family member or close friend, allowing another person to drive. Ask them if they need directions and be prepared to provide them if needed. Having preprinted directions available is helpful in this regard. Be sure they write down this information, and have them read it back to you. Provide them with the name of the person to contact when they arrive at the hospital. If asked how the patient is doing, tell them that he or she is in critical condition, has just arrived, or is being attended by the doctor.

If the person you are trying to reach is not there, ask how to reach the person.[10] If a child answers, only give information regarding the contact person. If you reach an answering machine or service, state only your name, the name of your health-care facility, the date and time of the call, the name of the person you are trying to reach, and a return telephone number that will be answered by someone who can reach you or who knows what to tell them.

MEETING SURVIVORS ON ARRIVAL

When the family arrives, a staff member, chaplain, or social worker should be available to meet them immediately. Verify the identity of the survivors, and escort them to a quiet area where they can have privacy. All emergency departments should have a dedicated family room for this purpose. This room should have comfortable seating. Tissues and a telephone with long-distance access should also be available.

If the family arrives at the same time as the patient, have someone escort them to the family room, where registrars can obtain demographic information. Contrary to tradition, however, if they wish, it is also acceptable for them to be present during the resuscitation.

INFORMING SURVIVORS OF THE LOSS

Because the physician has the most authority, he or she should never delegate the task of informing the family of the death.[5,10,13] Further, the physician can answer the pertinent medical questions. He or she should obtain as much information as possible about the decedent and rehearse what will be said to the survivors prior to meeting them. If possible, wait for all family members to arrive before speaking to them. Have one or more staff members, such as a nurse, social worker, or chaplain, accompany you, for both your own and the family's support and to convey the message that a team was, and is, involved. This should preferably be someone who has already interacted with the family and who will be available after you leave. Make sure to clean yourself up if your clothes have been soiled. Introduce yourself and support personnel and identify by name and relationship those who are present. Sit down. Take your time and talk softly.

Nonverbal (body language) messages are important.[10] The family may not remember much of what is said, but they will likely remember your demeanor. Sitting down is comforting, symbolizes that you are part of the group, and avoids the misperception of an imbalance of power. Sitting forward is engaging and connotes empathy, whereas sitting back or in a relaxed posture connotes disinterest. Sitting next to the closest relative or key survivor, or crouching down before or beside them, also connotes empathy. Address the closest relative face to face and by name. Facing them squarely shows interest. Touching the key survivor's shoulder, arm, or hand is generally welcomed as a sign of closeness, regardless of their age, gender, or ethnic background. Nodding reinforces survivors' statements and encourages them to continue speaking. In most, but not all, cultures, direct eye contact shows interest and is a sign of respect and honesty. Persistent eye contact, however, may be interpreted as controlling or threatening.

With the exception of the immediate family, ask other relatives and close friends to wait outside until the news is revealed. However, family relationships are varied, so use judgment about whether additional family members or friends should be present when the news is revealed. If friends appear to be offering important emotional support, then, obviously, they should also be allowed to hear the news. If children are present, ask the key adult if they would prefer to have them wait outside initially. If they do, have a staff person take the children to an area with a television or toys.

Ask what family and friends already know about the incident. If they were present at the time of the decedent's demise, ask them to describe what happened. If not known, also ask them about the decedent's medical history and their health, physical condition, and level of function during the hours and days prior to death.

Briefly (in about 30 seconds) describe prehospital and emergency department events in chronologic order so that family members understand clearly what happened. Describe the course of events in simple, understandable language, avoiding medical jargon and graphic images. Be sure to validate the emergency medical services effort. To avoid confusion and be certain that the family understands that the patient is dead, use a "D" (dead, death, died) word rather than a euphemism such as "didn't make it," "gone," "passed away," or "expired." Refer to the decedent by last name and title (e.g., "Mr.") rather than "he," "she," or "your [relationship]." Do not be afraid to express your emotions and show sympathy. Tell them that you are sorry for their loss or that you are sorry to give them bad news, but do not apologize for the death itself or the care given, as this may make survivors think that the outcome could have been different if something more or different had been done.

Allow periods of silence so that the family can react to the news. Be prepared for reactions such as anger, disbelief, absolute or pathologic denial, guilt, fainting, and exacerbation of conditions such as angina. Anger may be directed toward the patient, those responsible for the death, or the medical staff. Do not argue with survivors and respond to anger without considering it a personal attack. If violence is possible (e.g., survivors are intoxicated or the decedent was a victim of an altercation and the adversarial party or parties are also in the emergency department), have security or police immediately available.

If resuscitation is in progress and survival seems unlikely, it is helpful to prepare the family for the expected outcome. Break away from the resuscitation and inform them that the patient's condition is grave and that you are doing everything possible to revive him or her.

Conveying the loss to a child is perplexing, not only for trained hospital staff, but also for family members. Encourage survivors to discuss the death with children. When adults avoid discussing death with children, they create an atmosphere of apprehension and anxiety for children, who are sensitive to evasion and family stress levels.[1] An honest discussion can be a corrective emotional experience and may help to decrease the fantasy and distortions that children have about death.[16] Adult family members should not lie or distort the truth. Children carry mistaken notions about specific family deaths into adulthood, with lingering anguish and, in some cases, severe bouts of recurring depression and potential suicide.[7] Encouraging religious interpretations is fine. Further, family members should openly discuss their own feelings with the child and should not attempt to alter the child's feelings about the loss. When the deceased is a parent, young children often require constant reassurance that the surviving parent will not disappear and will be able to maintain food, shelter, and family integrity.[1]

RESPONDING TO SURVIVORS' GRIEF

Physicians can facilitate grieving by being good listeners while the survivors cry or let out their emotions.[10–13] When survivors begin to display emotional reactions, encourage them to express their feelings and to review their last moments with the deceased. Be patient as survivors begin an obsessive review of the events leading up to the death, by repeating anecdotes from the life of the deceased and repeatedly raising the same questions regarding the circumstances of the death.[1] Again, touching or holding the survivor when appropriate will be appreciated.

When confronted with a patient expressing denial, guilt, or anger, be patient and understanding, and not defensive. Ultimately, survivors' defenses will give way to feelings of sadness and loss. Tell the family they did the right thing, even if they did not. Reassure them that everything that could have been done was done. If possibly true, tell them that the patient did not suffer. Answer questions but give only enough information to assure the family that everything reasonable was tried to resuscitate the decedent. Ask survivors if they need to use the telephone to call friends, relatives, or clergy. Offer them privacy. Tell them that you will attempt to contact the patient's physician. Have a list of clergy available for out-of-town residents. In complicated situations, enlist the aid of social services. Unless the family broaches the subjects of autopsy and organ donation, wait until later to address these issues.

PROVIDING FOR VIEWING THE BODY

Offer survivors the opportunity to view the body.[10] Viewing the body facilitates the grief reaction, but if they are reluctant or unwilling to do so, do not make them feel that their decision is wrong.[3] Never refer to the deceased as "the body" or "it." Instead, use the person's proper name or a personal pronoun. Warn them about the visible effects of trauma, resuscitation, and postmortem skin changes, such as cyanosis and livedo or livor mortis. Remove blood and emesis before family members see the body. Often, medical equipment must be left in place until the coroner or medical examiner completes the necessary postmortem examination, but remove unnecessary medical equipment. Describe any equipment that remains on the body and explain why it is there. Cover the body with a sheet or blanket, but leave the head and hands exposed for the family to touch, and encourage them to do this. Move the body to a private room, if possible. Let them cut off a lock of hair, if requested. Allow family to be alone with the body, unless there are legal reasons (e.g., ongoing police investigation) for not doing so. Staff should remain nearby outside of the room and should be available for support while the family is viewing the body. Most family members will leave within 15 minutes.

MAKING FINAL ARRANGEMENTS

After the family has viewed the body, it is then appropriate to have necessary documents signed.[1,10,11] Tell them the cause of death that you will put on the death certificate and offer them the use of a telephone so that they can call a funeral home. Ask again if there are any questions. Generally, no question should remain unanswered, unless the information is unavailable. Tell them how to reach you if they have questions at a later time.

Explain the role of medical examiners and police in cases of sudden, unexpected, or violent deaths and how the decedent's belongings will be handled. If an autopsy is mandatory, explain that fact to the family. If the cause of death is unclear and the physician feels the results will be helpful, inform the family of this and ask them for permission for an elective autopsy. Tell them that an autopsy will not interfere with funeral arrangements, that no pain or suffering will result, and that no major religion absolutely prohibits autopsy. At most institutions, there is no cost to the family, but this should be confirmed.

The issue of organ and tissue donation should be broached before family members leave the hospital; in fact, most states require that this option be addressed. One might ask, "Has your family ever discussed organ or tissue donation?" or "Our hospital offers organ and tissue donation. Would you like to discuss this further with someone from the transplant program?" If the family expresses an interest, contact the appropriate agency immediately.

Performing or practicing resuscitation skills and other procedures on the newly deceased for the purposes of medical education or research should be done only after obtaining consent from the family. Surveys indicate that the public is generally accepting of such practices.[2]

As mentioned, have a list of clergy available for out-of-town residents, as well a list of accommodations. Also have available a preprinted list with telephone numbers and addresses of local and national support groups that you can give to survivors. Educate them about the symptoms of grief and reassure them that these symptoms are normal.[12] Depressed mood, sleep disturbance, crying, difficulty with concentration, loss of interest, anxiety, and weight loss are the most common symptoms.[4] Provide antianxiety or hypnotic medications to survivors only if requested and only after a formal evaluation of the individual involved. Limit the supply to a few days. Arrangements should always be made for family members or friends to stay with the survivor for the next 24 to 48 hours, because suicide is a possibility, especially for a spouse who has been married for many years.[9,16] If a survivor appears to be suicidal or homicidal, ask them about this directly, and obtain a formal psychiatric consult if they are.

Unless necessary for the medical examiner or police investigation, give survivors the decedent's personal effects and any clothing removed from the body. Advise them of the condition of clothing and place it in a paper or plastic belongings bag, not a trash bag. Inform them when everything they need to do is done and that they may leave whenever they like. The physician or a designated staff member should accompany the survivors to the door.

COMMON PITFALLS

- Making remarks such as, "Everything will be okay" or "It was God's will," which may prematurely seal off the grief response
- Failure to appreciate the importance of body language
- Failure to clearly indicate that the patient has died, by using a "D" word
- Failure to allow and encourage survivors to express their feelings
- Impeding or impairing survivors' ability to grieve, by routinely prescribing medication
- Failure to address survivors' support systems
- Failure to offer family members the option of organ and tissue donation

ACKNOWLEDGMENT

The author gratefully acknowledges the contribution of William R. Dubin who wrote the previous version of this chapter.

References

1. Albrizio M. The client who is bereaved. In: Gorton JC, Partridge R, eds. *Practice and management of psychiatric care*. St. Louis: Mosby, 1982:256.
2. Alden AW, Ward KL, Moore GP. Should post-mortem procedures be practiced on recently deceased patients? A survey of relatives' attitudes. *Acad Emerg Med* 1999;6:749.
3. Cassem NH. Treating the person confronting death. In: Nicholi AM, ed. *The Harvard guide to modern psychiatry*. Cambridge, MA: Belknap Press of Harvard University Press, 1978:579.
4. Clayton P, Desmaris L, Winokur GA. A study of normal bereavement. *Am J Psychiatry* 1968;125:168.
5. Dubin WR, Sarnoff JR. Sudden unexpected death: intervention with the survivors. *Ann Emerg Med* 1986;15:54.
6. Girgis A, Sanson-Fisher RW. Breaking bad news: consensus guidelines for medical practitioners. *J Clin Oncol* 1995;13:2449.
7. Goodstein RK. Situational emergencies. In: Dubin WR, Hanke N, Nickens HW, eds. *Clinics in emergency medicine: psychiatric emergencies*. New York, Churchill Livingstone, 1984:167.
8. Halevy A, Brody B. Brain death: reconciling definitions, criteria, and tests. *Ann Intern Med* 1993;119:519.
9. Hanke N. Stress disorders. In: Hanke N, ed. *Handbook of emergency psychiatry*. Lexington, MA: Collamore Press, 1984:200.
10. Iserson KV. *Grave words: notifying survivors about sudden, unexpected deaths*. Tuscon, AZ: Galen Press, 1999.
11. Jones WH. Emergency room death: what can be done for the survivors? *Death Educ* 1978;2:231.
12. Lindeman E. Symptomatology and management of acute grief. *Am J Psychiatry* 1944;101:141.
13. Olsen JC, Buenefe ML, Falco WD. Death in the emergency department. *Ann Emerg Med* 1998;31:758.
14. Ptacek JT, Eberhardt TL. Breaking bad news: a review of the literature. *JAMA* 1996;267:496.
15. Robinson MA. Informing the family of sudden death. *Am Fam Physician* 1981;23:115.
16. Rund DA, Hutzler JC. Psychiatric emergencies associated with death. In: Rund DA, Hutzler JC, eds. *Emergency psychiatry*. St. Louis: Mosby, 1983:213.
17. Simos BG. Grief therapy to facilitate healthy restitution. *Soc Casework* 1977;58:337.
18. Weissman AD. Coping with untimely death. *Psychiatry* 1973;36:366.

CHAPTER 410

Domestic and Sociocultural Violence

Taryn Kennedy

Before the 1970s, violence in the family was considered to be infrequent and was thought to result from psychopathology of the persons involved rather than being seen as a societal problem. Only in the past 15 years have data on the prevalence and outcomes of domestic violence been gathered, and it is now recognized as an endemic problem. Responses have been wide-ranging, involving advocacy, medical care, and the mental health, criminal justice, and academic communities.[1] In 1985, the Surgeon General declared domestic violence a public health problem.

The statistics on battering are alarming. On the average, ten women per day are killed by their batterers; just over half of all women murdered in the United States are killed by their male partners, and 12% of murdered males are killed by their female partners. Every 12 seconds, a woman is beaten, and 95% of the victims are women. Fifty percent of women are battered at some stage in their lives,[6] and one-third are battered repeatedly. Battering is the most common cause of traumatic injury to females in the United States.[19] Fifty percent of homeless women and children in this country are fleeing domestic violence, and about 37% of obstetric patients across class, race, and educational lines are physically abused while pregnant.[13] In addition, the nation's police spend about one-third of their time responding to domestic violence calls. Domestic violence costs the nation $5 billion to $10 billion per year (estimates include health-care costs, investigative and protective services, criminal justice proceedings, and loss of productivity from work). Surprisingly, however, there are three times as many shelters for animals as for battered women.

Early studies indicated that 22% to 35% of females presenting to the emergency department (ED) with any complaint did so because of symptoms relating to partner abuse. Although it is likely that the true number is less, it is still a significant problem. Women are ten times more likely to present to the ED than to the police after they have been victimized. The emergency physician is often the first health-care provider to see the results of domestic violence and, as such, must be able to recognize and intervene on behalf of the victims.[12] In 1992, the Joint Commission on Accreditation of Healthcare Organizations (JCAHO) determined that hospitals need to develop policies and procedures to address the identification, evaluation, and treatment of victims of domestic violence and need to have evidence of a written plan to provide education for all health-care providers. However, even when such policies are in place, fewer than one in 25 cases are recognized by health-care providers.

Domestic violence, spouse abuse, partner violence, and battering all refer to the victimization of a person with whom the abuser has had an intimate or romantic relationship. The term *domestic violence* implies that all members of the household are equally likely to be perpetrators or victims. It is estimated that 10% of the elder population may be victims. Elders are also often unaware of the existence of programs that can offer aid. Many health-care providers fail to recognize elder patients at risk[9] and may are unaware of their states' regulations concerning reporting of suspected elder abuse.[4]

All EDs should have policies and procedures addressing the care of victims of violence. Emergency physicians must be able to recognize occult cases of domestic violence and correctly interpret associated behavior. About one in five battered women presenting to physicians have sought previous medical attention for injuries. When a diagnosis of abuse is missed, treatment is likely to be inappropriate and potentially harmful. Also, failing to diagnose abuse may further the victim's sense of entrapment and thereby contribute to victimization. Clinicians must consider battering in the differential diagnosis of a number of medical complaints, particularly when treating females.[5] Universal screening should exist for all patients.[11,14]

GANG VIOLENCE

The increase in the number and level of violence of street gangs is partly responsible for the fact that homicide is the second leading cause of death in males aged 15 to 34 years.[16] Ninety-four percent of all cities with a population greater than 100,000 have active violent street gangs. Gang membership offers a sense of belonging, protection, and status; adventure; and access to illegal monetary gains. The average age for a gang member is 15 to 21 years old.

As gang members are frequently injured, EDs need to be aware of the problems that may ensue as they treat an injured member, and also look for ways to promote violence prevention in their community.[18] Prehospital providers need to be aware of gang activity in their area and work closely with local law enforcement agencies in suspected gang-related injuries.[7]

VIOLENCE IN THE EMERGENCY DEPARTMENT

Violence within the ED is a growing problem that is probably underreported. Fifty-three percent of all hospital assaults occur within the ED, and, in 1991, nine department staff members died.[17] The ED lends itself to promotion of a violent environment due to the volume of sick patients, waiting times, availability of drugs, 24-hour accessibility, and potentially violent psychiatric patients awaiting medical clearance. In one study, 77% of the perpetrators were patients, and 23% were visitors, and 80% of the incidents occurred in the general treatment area or psychiatric treatment area.[15]

A 1993 American College of Emergency Physicians policy statement called for action by hospitals to ensure a safe environment for staff and patients alike. It addressed the provision of adequate security, coordination of hospital security with local law enforcement, the development of written protocols for violent situations in the ED, and education of staff to prevent, recognize, and deal with potentially violent situations.

CLINICAL PRESENTATION

Domestic Violence

Domestic violence cuts across all racial, ethnic, religious, educational, and socioeconomic strata. Women who are single, separated, or divorced; those between the ages of 17 and 28; those who are pregnant; those who abuse alcohol or drugs; and those whose partners abuse alcohol[3] and drugs are all at increased risk. Other populations at risk include children, disabled adults, and the elderly. Persons with disabilities, both male and female, are at increased risk of abuse. Their reliance on the caregiver and their forced dependency on others for life supports heighten their risk. Abuse can occur in the home or in institutional dwellings such as group homes, state schools, nursing homes, and hospitals.

Domestic violence may take many forms (Table 410.1).[14] These behaviors can occur alone or in combination, and sporadically or chronically. In addition to physical trauma, battered women may present with a variety of other medical problems, including chronic pain syndromes, posttraumatic stress disorder, anxiety, depression, alcoholism, and other forms of substance abuse. Common presentations of battered women are listed in Table 410.2. The risk of domestic violence escalates during pregnancy, with 13% reporting abuse for the first time and 21% to 29% reporting an escalation of abuse. This may result in a variety of injuries, such as placental separation, antepartum hemorrhage, preterm labor, miscarriage, or ruptured uterus, spleen, or liver.

TABLE 410.1. Examples of Domestic Violence

Physical abuse (any mechanism of injury may be used)
Verbal and emotional forms of assault, including intimidation, coercion, threats, or degradation
Withholding or denying access to money or other basic resources
Sabotaging employment, housing, or educational opportunities
Sexual assault or coercion (i.e., any type of sexual contact that is forced or coerced, including rape, incest, sexual harassment, indecent exposure, or unwanted touching)
Social isolation by denying communication with friends or relatives or making communication so difficult that the victim chooses to avoid it
Prohibiting access to needed health care
Forcing the partner to live beyond his or her means or misusing credit cards

TABLE 410.2. Common Presentations of Battered Women

Injuries to the face, neck, or throat
Injuries to the chest, breast, abdomen, or genitals
Bilateral injuries
Evidence of sexual assault
Chronic pain, especially when evidence of tissue damage cannot be found
Acute pain when no external injuries are visible
Injuries during pregnancy, commonly but not exclusively to the breast and abdomen
Substantial delay between time of injury and presentation to the emergency department
Multiple injuries in various stages of healing
Extent or type of injury inconsistent with patient's explanation
Repeated use of the emergency department or primary care services
Sexually transmitted diseases, especially recurrent episodes
Psychological or emotional complaints
Evidence of alcohol or drug abuse
Suicidal ideation or suicide attempts
An accompanying partner (male or female) who answers or who seems overly aggressive or agitated
Homelessness
Pregnant patient who reports getting no prenatal care

Elder abuse can include physical abuse, caretaker neglect, and financial exploitation. Frequently, the caregiver of an elderly family member may be the least socially integrated adult who is unable to cope with the responsibility. Isolation is often a factor, and impairments due to age may diminish the ability of elders to defend themselves or to escape the situation. Elders may be unable to drive or use public transportation, and they may have no social network or family contact other than the batterers.

Elders often do not report abuse or neglect, either because they deny the abuse is occurring or because they fear retaliation or abandonment. Feelings of helplessness may lead an elder to believe that reporting will not improve the situation.

Gang Violence

Victims of gang violence may present with blunt or penetrating trauma.[7] Common scenarios include walk-up or drive-by shootings, stabbings, and beatings. They may also be victims of arson and vehicular assault.

Violence in the Emergency Department

Patients may be physically violent, verbally abusive, angry, suicidal, depressed, restless, deluded, or act in a bizarre manner. They may boast of prior acts of violence, a desire to commit violence, and feelings of inability to control impulse among others. Many will manifest characteristic changes in mental attitude, posture, speech, and motor activity before displaying violent behavior. They may pace the room or hallways, clench their fists, stand against the wall, grip bed rails, and appear anxious. The tone, volume, and character of the patients' voices may indicate the potential for violence. Health-care providers may precipitate violent responses by argumentative, abrupt, or condescending attitudes or failure to provide requested services.

EMERGENCY DEPARTMENT EVALUATION AND MANAGEMENT

Domestic Violence

A history of abuse should be considered and questioned of all females presenting for emergency care.[11] Questioning should be carried out in confidence and with a nonjudgmental manner. A screening assessment should take place at triage if safety and privacy can be ensured. Physicians have four main areas of responsibility: to communicate their concern and validate the patient; to provide medical treatment; to review options and facilitate appropriate referrals and follow-up; and to assist in creating a safety plan.

Women who are known or suspected to be victims of domestic violence should be interviewed in private in a secure area of the ED without their partner or children present. If necessary for safety reasons, hospital security or police should be recruited. It is important to be aware of the legal requirements of reporting partner abuse in your state. If reporting is mandatory, it is important to inform the patient to prevent a perceived breach of confidentiality. Disabled patients have the legal right to be accompanied by their personal-care attendant or other supportive persons if they desire. Patients should be asked in private if they want their companion to accompany them into the treatment area, to minimize the chances that they will feel coerced into silence by an abusive companion. Lesbian partner abuse is a unique problem. The victim may not yet have come out publicly and may be reluctant to discuss the subject. It is important not to assume that it is safe for a female partner to accompany a patient to the treatment area. A history of previous trauma, chronic pain complaints, or psychological distress, which may be clues to diagnosis, should be sought from direct history or from the medical record. An interpreter should be provided, if necessary. For women, a woman trained in medical interpretation, who will honor confidentiality, is preferable to a family member. It is inappropriate to use a child as an interpreter when domestic violence is suspected.

Rather than directly asking questions about abuse relative to the presenting complaint, it may be better to focus on questions identified by the acronym SAFE:[2] What *Stress* do you experience in your relationships? Should I be concerned about your *Safety*? Are there situations in your relationships in which you have felt *Afraid*? Has your partner ever *Abused* you or your children? Have you ever been physically hurt or threatened by your partner? Are your *Friends* and *Family* aware that you have been hurt? Do you think you could tell them, and do you think they would be able to give you support? Assess the degree of social isolation. Do you have a safe place to go and the resources you (and your children) need in an *Emergency*? Do you have a plan of *Escape*? Would you like to talk to a social worker/counselor/me to develop an emergency plan?

Simply by asking the SAFE questions, the emergency physician alleviates the victim's alienation and offers her an opportunity to validate her worth, assess her safety, and become aware of community issues. Regardless of the severity of the presenting complaint or injury, the best indicator of danger is the patient's own assessment. The frequency and severity of previous attacks are good guides to current danger. Threats are as important as the actual injury, however, and the presence of weapons in the home is an additional risk factor.[1] Battered women are most likely to be killed when they are in the act of leaving or after they have left their abuser.

State law requires health-care providers to report all rapes and sexual assaults. Cases involving the abuse or neglect of elders, minors, and certain persons with disabilities must also be reported to the appropriate government agencies. A victim may seek a temporary protective order. Patients should be encouraged to consent to specific interventions and should be given assurances of safety and confidentiality. However, no intervention should be forced on an unwilling patient. Overriding a patient's refusal violates the ethical principle of respect of patient autonomy, and, in the case of domestic violence, further disempowers the patient.

Enlisting the services of a social worker can be valuable in helping to bring victims into contact with resources such as shelters, social services, legal assistance, and support groups. If the police are not already involved, the physician can offer to call them or help the victim to do so. The patient should be told that battering is a crime and that help is available.

If the patient chooses not to seek help at the time of the ED presentation, it is important that the physician be empathic and not lay blame. Offer constructive ways to help, such as preparing an escape route should the situation at home escalate. Offer the patient information and contact numbers, which she may use later. It is important to allow the patient to remain in control. Complete medical records are important to ensure quality care for the patient and may be vital in any subsequent legal proceedings.

Gang Violence

The ED reflects the community in which it resides. If appropriate, health-care providers should be offered training in recognition of gang members, such as specific tattoos, hand shakes and mannerisms, type of clothing worn, and evidence of previous trauma. On arrival at the scene, prehospital personnel must ensure their own safety and, where necessary, await help from police before entering a hostile area. Bulletproof vests may be necessary in some communities. Where possible, the hospital should be notified that a suspected gang member is being transported and, where possible, injured members from rival gangs should be taken to different facilities.[8]

Hospital security personnel and local law enforcement need to be involved to provide security for the injured gang member, for other patients (who may be members of rival gangs), and for the health-care providers. Limiting access to the ED, body searches, and the use of metal detectors to screen patients and visitors for weapons may be necessary. The victim's injuries are cared for in the appropriate manner. Patients should be disrobed to search for concealed weapons and treated with due respect. Avoid challenging victims or other members or showing disrespect, which could result in physical confrontation.

Access to the patient should be kept to immediate family members. Other parties may be informed of the patient's condition by updates. The patient should be admitted under a "John Doe" status to prevent further injury by rival gang members during hospitalization and to help ensure the safety of health-care providers.

Violence in the Emergency Department

Many violent encounters can be prevented. The goal is to recognize, deescalate, and control the potentially violent patient before violence occurs. Patients often act out of a sense of fear and danger of their surroundings. It is important to take steps to avoid confrontation. Health-care providers should never respond to patients' threats with threats of their own. However, assaults against medical personnel should be reported to law enforcement agencies. Not doing so allows patients to think such behavior is acceptable and makes the staff feel they are not adequately protected.

The patient should be approached from the side, while observing the surroundings for possible missiles. A nonoffensive posture, with hands out front but not raised, should be employed. The care provider should be cognizant of the patient's personal space and stay two arm lengths away. It is important to acknowledge the patient's needs and ask him or her to verbalize the problems. The patient should be informed, in a low voice, that help is available and that support will be provided but that the patient must take control of his or her own behavior. Expectations should be defined, and the consequences of aggressive behavior need to be clear. Frequently, talking to the patient and making offers of food and drinks may be calming and defuse the situation.

When possible, the patient should be interviewed alone and in private, but the care provider may keep the door ajar and sit between the patient and the door. Some patients may not respond to these measures, and here a "show of force" may be needed. Prior to interviewing the patient, assemble a group of security personnel who will remain within calling distance. Frequently, this show of force may be sufficient to help disorganized patients gain control of their thoughts and behavior.

If a patient is or becomes combative or assaultive and poses a danger to self or others, physical restraints may be needed. Explain clearly to the patient what is about to happen and why. Assemble a team, preferably with five members, four to restrain the limbs and one to act as team leader. Soft restraints (e.g., leather) are used to secure each limb to the stretcher. For the particularly violent patient, the team may employ mattresses, which are used to sandwich the patient. Once the patient is on the floor, each limb is then restrained. After the patient is restrained, he or she should be searched for weapons or objects that could inflict harm, and then moved to a quiet area. The history may be difficult to obtain, and other sources, such as family members, friends, and the patient's records, should be used. A physical examination should be performed to exclude an organic cause of the patient's behavior (Table 410.3). Blood tests, including toxicology screen and a blood sugar, should be obtained. Vital signs should be checked every 15 minutes while the patient is in restraints.

Pharmacologic intervention may be required when the patient remains disorganized and uncooperative. Haloperidol (2 to 10 mg intramuscularly or intravenously in the young and healthy and 0.5 to 2.0 mg in the elderly) is often used because of its relatively mild side effects in comparison with phenothiazines. If the patient will cooperate and take the medication orally, 10 mg every 30 minutes, to a maximum of 30 mg, may be used in healthy patients. Benzodiazepines (e.g., diazepam 5 to 10 mg, or lorazepam 2 to 4 mg, intramuscularly, intravenously, or orally) can also be used. Certain drug intoxications may require specific therapy (e.g., anticholinergic syndrome; see Chapter 312). The reason for physical or chemical restraint and measures taken to ensure the patient's comfort while in restraints should be clearly documented in the medical record.[10,20]

TABLE 410.3. Organic Causes of Violent Behavior

Drug intoxication: PCP, LSD, cocaine, barbiturates, amphetamines, and alcohol
Trauma
Infection: AIDS, herpes encephalitis, meningitis
Metabolic: Hypoglycemia, thyroid storm, renal or liver failure, adrenal crisis, ketoacidosis, hypoxia, hypothermia, and vitamin deficiency
Neurologic: tumors, epilepsy, cerebrovascular accidents, infections

DISPOSITION

Domestic Violence

The patient should be asked where she will go if she leaves the facility, and who is waiting for her outside. If necessary, she can leave through a less visible exit. She should be given a list of emergency numbers. The physician should be especially cautious if security had to be called to restrain an assailant. The option of overnight hospitalization should be discussed with the victim if she does not have an alternative safe place to go; the physician should clarify that she would be hospitalized only for her safety, not because the physician thinks she is mentally ill.

The discharge plan should include arrangements for a safe place to stay as well as other resources for daily living, such as money, personal papers, car keys, and a change of clothing for herself and her children. Victims should be informed that local programs for battered women provide free, confidential services, and that trained advocates from these programs can provide information regarding legal rights, police and court procedures for protective orders, shelter availability, support groups, and other essential resources. There are similar services for disabled and elderly victims of domestic violence. Physicians should discuss protection against sexually transmitted diseases and pregnancy, especially for those patients who have been raped or who have experienced coercive sexual activity as part of the violence. The physician should avoid prescribing tranquilizers or other sedating psychoactive medications, which could impair the victim's ability to respond appropriately should she need to flee.

Gang Violence

Whether the patient is admitted or discharged depends on the nature and severity of injury.

Violence in the Emergency Department

Some patients may be discharged after a period of observation in the ED (e.g., those with alcohol- or drug-induced violent behavior). Some may require admission because of an underlying medical condition. Other patients may require further evaluation by mental health services and admission to psychiatric facilities. Patients without medical or psychiatric problems requiring admission who are under arrest may be discharged to the custody of law enforcement authorities.

COMMON PITFALLS

Domestic Violence

- Failure to recognize victims of domestic violence and to consider battering in the differential diagnosis of medical as well as traumatic complaints, particularly when treating females
- Asking questions in a manner that might increase the patient's perceived level of danger or sense of humiliation and blame
- Asking about domestic violence in the presence of a partner or family members
- Using a child as an interpreter
- Failure to provide appropriate safety measures for the patient while in the ED
- Failure to devise an emergency or escape plan
- Failure to provide appropriate referrals and follow-up
- Prescribing tranquilizers or other sedating psychoactive drugs

Gang Violence

- Failure to be aware of gang activity in the community and to ensure the safety of both prehospital and ED personnel
- Not searching victims adequately for concealed weapons, resulting in the potential of serious injury to health-care providers
- Failure to protect the patient by admitting them under a pseudonym
- Treating gang members with disrespect or in a confrontational manner

Violence in the Emergency Department

- Failure to assess your ED for vulnerability to attack by violent patients
- Failure to recognize the patient who is starting to escalate and who could have been calmed before the situation was out of control
- Attributing violent behavior to drug or alcohol intoxication without looking for an organic cause
- Failure to report assaults on staff to the appropriate authorities

References

1. AMA Council on Scientific Affairs. Violence against women: relevance for medical practitioners. *JAMA* 1992;267:3184.
2. Ashur MS. Asking about domestic violence: SAFE questions. JAMA 1993;269:2367.
3. Cherpitil CJ. Alcohol and injuries resulting from violence: a review of emergency room studies. *Addiction* 1994;89:157–165.
4. Clark-Daniels CL, Daniels RS, Baumhover LA. Abuse and neglect of the elderly: are emergency department personnel aware of mandatory reporting laws? *Ann Emerg Med* 1990;19:970.
5. Fanslow JL, Norton RN, Spinola CG. Indication of assault related injuries among women presenting to the emergency department. *Ann Emerg Med* 1998;32(3):341–348.
6. Furbee PM, Sikara R, Williams JM, et al. Comparison of domestic violence screening methods: a pilot study. *Ann Emerg Med* 1998;31:495–501.
7. Hutson HR, Anglin D, Mallon W. Injuries and death from gang violence; they are preventable. *Ann Emerg Med* 1992;21:1234–1237.
8. Hutson HR, Anglin D, Mallon W. Minimizing gang violence in the emergency department. *Ann Emerg Med* 1992;21:1291–1293.
9. Jones JS, Veenstra TR, Seamon JP, et al. Elder mistreatment: national survey of emergency physicians. *Ann Emerg Med* 1997;30:473.
10. Kuhn W. Violence in the emergency department. Managing aggressive patients in a high stress environment. *Postgrad Med* 1999;105(1):143–154.
11. Larkin GL, Hyman KB, Mathias SR, et al. Universal screening for intimate partner violence in the emergency department: importance of patient and provider factors. *Ann Emerg Med* 1999;3(6):669–675.
12. McCoy M. Domestic violence: clues to victimization. *Ann Emerg Med* 1996;27:764–765.
13. McFarlane J, Parker B, Soeken K, et al. Assessing for abuse during pregnancy. Severity and frequency of injuries and associated entry into prenatal care. *JAMA* 1992;267:3176–3178.
14. Olson L, Anctil C, Fullerton L, et al. Increasing emergency physician recognition of domestic violence. *Ann Emerg Med* 1996;27:741–746.
15. Pane GA, Winiarski AM, Salness KA. Aggression directed toward emergency department staff at a university teaching hospital. *Ann Emerg Med* 1991;20(3):283–286.
16. Rankins RC, Hendey GW. Effect of a security system on violent incidents and hidden weapons in the emergency department. *Ann Emerg Med* 1999;33(6):676–679.
17. Rieger W. Escalating risk: violence in the ED. *QRC Advisor* 1993;9(8):1–4.
18. Rosenberg ML, Mercy JA. Assaultive violence. In: Rosenberg ML, Fenley MA, eds. *Violence in America: a public health approach*. New York: Oxford University Press, 1991:14–50.
19. Schittzer PG, Runyan CW. Injuries to women in the United States: an overview. *Womens Health* 1995;23:9–27
20. Walsh-Kelly CM, Strait R. Impact of violence and the emergency department response to victims and perpetrator. Issues and protocols. *Pediatr Clin North Am* 1998;45(2):449–455.

CHAPTER 411
Acute Pain Management

Steven Rosenzweig and Daniel Mines

Acute pain is the most common reason that patients seek emergency care. Patient survey studies consistently document that pain is often inadequately treated by physicians and that this problem is not limited to the emergency department.[1] Providing expert and compassionate pain relief remains one of the greatest challenges in the practice of emergency medicine.

Drugs used to treat pain act by reversing the underlying cause of pain (e.g., nitrates for angina and sumatriptan for migraine) or by suppressing the symptom (i.e., the perception of pain). This chapter focuses on drugs used to treat the symptom of acute pain. Related discussions elsewhere in this text include the chapters on conscious sedation (Chapter 413), chronic pain syndromes (Chapter 412), and poisoning with acetaminophen (Chapter 310), nonsteroidal antiinflammatory agents (NSAIDs) (Chapter 358), opioids (Chapter 360), and salicylates (Chapter 367).

PAIN ASSESSMENT

Pain is an experience that has both physical and nonphysical dimensions. Physiologically, pain is mediated by a set of neurochemical events. At the level of consciousness, it is an event of personal anguish or suffering. *The severity and quality of this suffering are highly individual; each person experiences and responds to pain in his or her own way.*

One of the most important aspects of the pain experience is the *meaning* it holds for the sufferer. Pain is often greater when its cause is perceived to be life-threatening or when it is associated with emotional trauma. Conversely, pain that is perceived to offer some secondary gain can be easier to bear.

The subjective nature of pain presents a challenge to today's medical practice, which emphasizes objective findings. It is imperative for all emergency care providers to understand that the patient need not *appear* in pain to actually *be* in pain.[5] There exist no objective signs for accurately gauging the magnitude of a patient's pain. Indicators such as heart rate, blood pressure, respiratory pattern, facial expression, and body posture are not reliable. The presentation of pain may be obscured by the effects of medication, a cultural bias toward stoicism, or complex coping mechanisms such as joking or maintaining a facade of calm.[1] Language and cultural barriers further confound pain assessment.

Equally unreliable is an estimate of pain severity based on its etiology. Can a toothache be more painful than salpingitis? Should an ankle sprain hurt less than pleurisy? These questions cannot be answered, because suffering depends on each individual's pain threshold and sensitivity to a particular condition.

The most reliable and valid means of assessing pain severity is the patient's self-report. Clinical judgment must always be guided by the patient's own assessment.

It can be very difficult for anyone to find words to convey either the quality of pain or its severity. Descriptions lack the preferred exactness of clinical language. People resort to imagination and simile: "My back feels as if it is caught in a vise"; "my hand feels like it is on fire." Another problem is that patients and physicians use words differently. For example, a patient may use the word *sharp* to mean *severe,* whereas the physician may assume it to mean *knifelike*.

Assessing pain in children, especially infants, is even more difficult than in adults.[17] The experience and expression of pain are affected by the developmental age of the child, the child's previous pain experiences, the response of the child to the medical environment, and the quality of relationship with parents or other care providers. Older children are able to describe their pain or point to pictures on a pain analogue scale. In infants and younger children, the quality of cry, facial expression, changes in vital signs, and impressions of the caretaker should all be taken into account.

Children are much less likely than adults to be given adequate analgesia for the same painful condition.[20] This observation has been attributed not only to the difficulties inherent to pain assessment, but also to the persistent myth that children do not experience or remember pain. As in any adult, pain in a child should be anticipated and aggressively treated.

Taking an accurate pain history, therefore, requires careful listening and clarifying. Patients can also be assisted in conveying pain intensity through descriptive scales (none—little—medium—severe—worst possible), numeric scales (rating 1 to 10), and visual analogue scales (placing a mark on a 10-cm line).

Compassion implies awareness of another's suffering, and gaining this awareness may be difficult. Physician attitudes may even interfere with pain recognition. One impediment is resistance to accepting the authority of the patient or the insight of a family member. The physician cannot be "in charge" of the assessment of pain. This situation in which the patient knows more than the doctor creates a reversal of roles that may be uncomfortable and even unacceptable for the treating physician.

Fear of creating an addiction by introducing a patient to a narcotic is generally unwarranted. Studies have shown that the short-term prescription of narcotic analgesics for acute pain syndromes is *not* associated with future dependence.[16]

Another impediment is fear of being manipulated into giving narcotics to patients who are feigning illness. Bear in mind that *pain* is the most common reason for drug-seeking behavior. Even a legitimate patient may feel the need to dramatize distress in order to convince the doctor of his or her need. It may indeed be impossible to know for certain whether the patient's complaint is a sham. The physician must always weigh the gain of thwarting the possible abuser against the risk of withholding relief from the person who is truly suffering.

The diagnosis of drug abuse is based on a pattern of behavior that is unlikely to be established during a single emergency department encounter. Nevertheless, a few precautions can be taken:

1. Perform a detailed history and physical, being alert to inconsistencies.
2. Attempt to confirm the patient's history by contacting the personal physician or checking medical records.
3. Communicate with colleagues about problem patients in order to corroborate impressions and develop specific treatment strategies.
4. Substitute nonnarcotic agents when indicated.
5. Write prescriptions for only small amounts of medication, or dispense one or two doses rather than actually writing a prescription.[7]

Emotional desensitization can also lead to suboptimal pain management. Emergency physicians habituate to crises and may become less attuned to the urgency of others' pain. Recurrent encounters with hostile patients, as well as physical and emotional fatigue, wear down the ability to respond compassionately. Facing our own vulnerability in the suffering of others may also lead physicians to withdraw from patients unintentionally. Compassion requires the physician to maintain an awareness of his or her own inner state in order to rise above these desensitizing factors.

Personal prejudices also interfere with empathy. Negative stereotyping and moral judgment lead to blaming the patient and undertreatment. The extreme case of withholding analgesia as a punitive measure can only be considered inhumane.

PAIN MANAGEMENT

Expediting Relief

Pain relief should be timely. Unnecessary delays can often be averted.

Treat before a definitive diagnosis is established. Pain can and should be treated *before* its underlying cause is known. Initial interventions can be nonpharmacologic (discussion follows). When the diagnosis depends solely on a laboratory or radiographic finding, there is no excuse for not offering pain medication while the evaluation is proceeding.

The belief that analgesics, particularly opioids, will obscure the underlying diagnosis is unfounded. Although it is common to withhold such medication from a patient with abdominal pain who may need surgical evaluation, this practice is not supported by clinical studies.[2,14] On the contrary, the judicious use of short-acting agents can serve the needs of both the patient and the consulting surgeon. Providing pain relief may actually enhance the patient's cooperation and improve the accuracy of the examination. Ironically, analgesics are often withheld in the emergency department, even after a decision has been made to take a patient to surgery. As the patient's most important advocate, the emergency physician must coordinate a rational and humane approach that takes into account the distress of the patient and the availability of the consultant.

Treat even if informed consent may subsequently be required. The practice of withholding opioids from a patient who might later need to sign a consent for surgery or other procedure should be reconsidered. Concern that these medications will compromise the competency of the patient are generally unfounded. First, pain can certainly be as mind-altering as medications. Second, it is possible to provide analgesia without clouding consciousness. Third, the implicit message that pain medication will be administered only after the consent is signed is itself coercive. And, finally, an opioid antagonist can be administered, if necessary.

Anticipate and treat pain before it develops. Good pain management involves anticipating pain prior to its onset or recurrence. Medications should be given before painful procedures (see Chapter 413). Similarly, patients should be given instructions and medication to help them cope with pain that may continue or recur following discharge.

Nonpharmacologic Therapy

A variety of simple and effective interventions can reduce pain.

Provide physical comfort measures. Attending to the overall physical comfort of the patient can alleviate factors that aggravate pain. This includes such actions as helping the patient find a more comfortable position, adjusting the lighting in the room, warming a patient who feels chilled, immobilizing injured extremities, and applying ice to closed bony and soft-tissue injuries.

Provide psychological support. Physical suffering is amplified by fear and anxiety. Fear often relates to the possibility that the cause of pain is life-threatening or permanently disabling. New pain in a cancer patient raises the specter of disease progression. Patients with chest pain often present with a fear of myocardial infarction. A laborer may associate an acute shoulder injury with the alarming possibility of permanent loss of income.

Information and reassurance, given whenever possible, reduce the need for analgesics. Family members of adult and pediatric patients should be included in this reassurance and support system. If a parent or spouse is more anxious, angry, or sleep deprived than the patient, they, too, must be helped to overcome their fear and anxiety in order for them to become calm supporters of the patient.

Anxiety may arise in response not only to sudden illness, but also to the emergency department experience itself. Unable to control their own pain, patients find themselves in a harsh and unfamiliar milieu, feeling exposed, vulnerable, and dependent on strangers. Building rapport, dignifying interactions, and restoring some sense of control to our patients are all essential in emergency pain management.

Muscular and mental tension arise out of pain, increasing distress even more. Both may respond to verbal and imagery techniques that relax the body and distract the mind. Music, videos, story telling, and imagining favorite places or activities are techniques that are frequently used for pediatric patients.

It is also important to address the patient's expectations regarding pain medications. Let the patient know from the outset how much time it will take for the medication to work, and whether to anticipate partial or complete relief. This can allay a premature concern that the drug "isn't working."

Pharmacologic Therapy

Hundreds of drugs are available to treat pain. To select the best regimen for an individual patient, several issues need to be explored. How intense is the pain? How quickly is pain relief required? Can the patient take oral medications? Are there contraindications to particular agents? The answers to these questions help direct the choice of drug, dose, and route of administration.

Nonopioid Analgesics

Aspirin and Acetaminophen. Aspirin and acetaminophen are equally effective for the relief of mild-to-moderate pain. Aspirin, the prototype NSAID, is believed to work by blocking cyclooxygenase (COX) enzymes, thereby inhibiting the synthesis of prostaglandins, which mediate both pain and inflammation. Unlike aspirin, acetaminophen lacks antiinflammatory properties, and its mechanism of action is poorly understood.

Aspirin also inhibits platelet function and commonly leads to gastrointestinal (GI) distress. It very rarely causes a hypersensitivity reaction (more common among asthmatics with nasal polyps), characterized by bronchospasm, urticaria, rhinitis, and even shock. Because acetaminophen is free of these side effects and hypersensitivity risk, it is often the preferable drug. Table 411.1 lists dosing recommendations for these drugs.

Nonsteroidal Antiinflammatory Drugs. At usual doses, NSAIDs are not as safe as acetaminophen but are generally better tolerated than aspirin. In addition to blocking COX enzymes, they may directly modulate neutrophil responses. More than a dozen are approved by the Food and Drug Administration (FDA) for analgesia, and still others are commonly used for pain relief (see Chapter 358). When given as a single full dose in the acute setting, most NSAIDs are more effective than aspirin or acetaminophen. In some settings, they provide analgesia equal or superior to certain oral opioids. Although no oral NSAID has emerged as a consistently superior analgesic, it is widely

TABLE 411.1. Dosing Information for Nonopioids

Drug	Dosage	Comments	Cost ($)[a]
Acetaminophen (Tylenol)	650 mg q4h 1,000 mg q6h	No antiinflammatory activity	Retail: 0.48/0.72
Aspirin	650–975 mg q4h		Retail: 0.12/0.60
Choline magnesium trisalicylate (Trilisate)	1,000–1,500 mg b.i.d.	Available as liquid Minimal antiplatelet activity	1.01/1.40
Diflunisal (Dolobid)	1,000-mg load; then 500 mg b.i.d.		2.88/3.24
Etodolac (Lodine)	200–400 mg q6–8h		NA/2.87
Fenoprofen (Nalfon)	200 mg q4–6h		1.07/1.94
Ibuprofen (Motrin and others)	400 mg q4–6h, or 600 mg q6–8h or 800 mg q8h	Available as liquid	Retail OTC: 0.60/1.08 By Rx: 0.53/1.12
Indomethacin (Indocin)	25–50 mg t.i.d.	FDA approved only as an antiinflammatory Frequency of adverse effects higher than other NSAIDs Available as a suppository	0.26/1.16
Ketoprofen (Orudis)	25–75 mg q6–8h		1.38/2.42
Ketorolac, oral (Toradol)	10 mg q6–8h	Not recommended for more than 5 days' use	NA/3.20
Ketorolac, parenteral	30–60 mg i.m. initially or 15–30 mg i.v. initially; . then 15–30 mg q6h i.m. or i.v	Use the lower dose in patients <50 kg or older than 65, or with renal impairment	NA/28.97
Naproxen (Naprosyn, Aleve)	500 mg; then 250 mg q6–8h, or 375 mg b.i.d. to t.i.d.	Oral liquid available	NA/2.83
Naproxen sodium (Anaprox)	550 mg; then 275 mg q6–8h		NA/2.85
Rofecoxib (Vioxx)	12.5–50 mg qd or divided b.i.d.	Selective COX-2 inhibition affords a higher safety profile. Available as a liquid.	Retail: 2.50–6.00

NA, not available; OTC, over the counter.

[a]Cost for 24 hours of therapy. Average wholesale price is quoted unless otherwise noted. For many drugs the generic price is given first, followed by the brand-name price. When a range of doses is available, the cost of the smallest one is recorded.

Adapted from Acute Pain Management Guideline Panel. *Acute pain management: operative or medical procedures and trauma. Clinical practice guideline.* AHCPR Pub. No. 92-0032. Rockville, MD: Agency for Health Care Policy and Research, Public Health Service, U.S. Dept. of Health and Human Services, 1992.

TABLE 411.2. Pediatric Dosing Guidelines for Drugs for Pain Management

Drug	Route	Dosage (mg/kg/dose)
Morphine	i.v.	0.1–0.2
Meperidine	i.v./i.m.	1.0–1.5
Fentanyl	i.v.	0.001–0.003
	Oral/transmucosal	0.005–0.015
Codeine	Oral	0.5–1.0 q4–6h
Acetaminophen	Oral/rectal	10–15 q4–6 h
Ibuprofen	Oral	5–10 q6–8 h

For further pediatric dosing guidelines, see Appendix D.

acknowledged that an individual patient may respond to one agent and not another.[4]

The onset of analgesia is within 1 hour for the majority of NSAIDs. For drugs with a relatively long half-life, such as diflunisal and naproxen, onset of analgesia is considerably longer but can be hastened by administration of a loading dose. Note that doses in the higher range are generally required to achieve antiinflammatory effects, which may not be seen for a few days.

For patients who cannot swallow pills, several agents are available in a liquid form (see Table 411.1). For patients who are vomiting or must remain NPO, rectal suppositories of aspirin, acetaminophen, naproxen, and indomethacin are available.

Costs of the NSAIDs vary considerably (see Table 411.1), ranging from pennies per dose of aspirin to more than a dollar per dose of newer, brand-name NSAIDs.

Ketorolac. Ketorolac tromethamine (Toradol) is the only NSAID also available for parenteral administration, either intramuscularly (i.m.) or intravenously (i.v.). It carries all the advantages and disadvantages of the other NSAIDs. Because of the drug's popularity in emergency medicine, practitioners need to be aware of its limitations. When studied in the emergency department setting, parenteral ketorolac does not provide superior analgesia to oral ibuprofen.[13,19] Given parenterally, ketorolac does not act any faster than many oral NSAIDs, because the drug effect is limited by time to prostaglandin inhibition, not absorption. Ketorolac is relatively expensive—a parenteral dose costs more than about ten times as much as morphine 10 mg, and 100 times as much as a full dose of ibuprofen. Repetitive dosing of ketorolac carries a higher risk of upper GI bleeding when compared with other NSAIDs. Acute renal failure has also been described. It seems reasonable to reserve parenteral ketorolac only for patients in whom the oral administration of NSAIDs should be avoided.

Selective COX-2 Inhibitors. These drugs selectively block COX-2, the form of cyclooxygenase that mediates inflammation, without affecting COX-1, the inhibition of which can produce gastric injury. In comparison, older "nonspecific" NSAIDs block both COX isoenzymes.[11]

Rofecoxib (Vioxx), the first COX-2 inhibitor approved by the FDA, is indicated for acute pain. Acute analgesia trials are underway with celecoxib (Celebrex), which is already approved for the treatment of rheumatoid arthritis and osteoarthritis. Both drugs appear to have an improved gastric safety profile compared with the older NSAIDs, but until more research is done, we should not assume that these drugs are without any GI toxicity. It is also not yet clear whether COX-2 inhibitors effectively treat crystal-induced arthritis, such as gout, or how quickly they produce analgesia compared with older agents. These agents are not likely to be any more effective than the older, less costly NSAIDs. Because their major advantage is their safety profile, they should be reserved for patients at high risk of NSAID side effects (discussion follows).

Advantages. The NSAIDs hold several advantages over the opioids. They do not cause respiratory depression and rarely cause mental clouding. Given their antiinflammatory properties, they treat the cause as well as the symptom of pain in conditions such as tendinitis, arthritis, or radiculitis. NSAIDs do not have abuse potential.

Adverse Effects. All NSAIDs can cause dyspepsia, the most common side effect. This can be minimized by administering the drug with food or an antacid. Less commonly, NSAIDs lead to ulcers and upper GI bleeding and perforation, complications that are seen more with chronic rather than short-term use and that may occur without warning.[4] NSAIDs are thus strongly contraindicated in patients with active ulcer disease, and should be given with caution to those with a history of upper GI bleeding. Other risk factors for GI complications include patient age greater than 60 years, high doses, and concurrent steroid or anticoagulant use.[10] In such high-risk patients, the chance of GI bleeding can be reduced by coadministration with a proton pump inhibitor or misoprostol, at least with long-term NSAID use. The benefit these agents offer with short courses of NSAID is less well established. Other agents that were often used for prophylaxis of NSAID-related GI complications are either ineffective (antacids, sucralfate) or marginally effective (H_2 blockers).[10] COX-2 inhibitors—without gastroprotective drugs—represent another therapeutic option in patients with risk factors for GI bleeding.

NSAIDs may also affect the kidneys, causing fluid retention and renal insufficiency, which is usually reversible. Patients at greater risk for renal complications include those with chronic renal insufficiency, congestive heart failure, and cirrhosis, as well as patients taking diuretics or angiotensin converting enzyme inhibitors. NSAIDs should generally be prescribed for no more than a few days in this patient population.

Because they interfere with platelet function, the nonselective NSAIDs predispose toward bleeding and should not be given to patients with thrombocytopenia or intrinsic clotting abnormalities. They should generally not be used in patients receiving anticoagulant therapy and in those suspected of internal bleeding, as in the case of severe headache with possible subarachnoid hemorrhage. In contrast, because the COX-2 selective NSAIDs do not inhibit platelet function, they may be used in patients with low platelet counts or in those on warfarin.

Very rarely, NSAIDs cause hypersensitivity reactions; patients who are sensitive to aspirin are at greater risk. NSAIDs are generally contraindicated during pregnancy, particularly in the third trimester.

Opioid Analgesics

Opioids are usually the first-choice drugs for the prompt relief of severe, acute pain. Unlike the NSAIDs, they have no ceiling on analgesic effect. Given intravenously, they work within minutes, and their effect can be titrated and reversed. Many patients treated with these agents, however, do not receive adequate pain relief because of physicians' misconceptions about correct dosing, route of administration, and adverse effects.[15]

Dosing Considerations. In real life, the effective analgesic dose varies considerably among patients; the *correct* dose of narcotic is the dose that works. The "optimal initial dose" published in various references is only a general guideline; the "standard" 10-mg dose of parenteral morphine is inadequate analgesia for one-third of patients in severe pain.[9] In the initial treatment of severe pain, then, it makes sense to titrate small frequent doses to effect (Tables 411.2 and 411.3).

Once satisfactory analgesia is achieved, another common pitfall is to withhold a subsequent dose until a "standard" dosing

TABLE 411.3. Dosing Guidelines for Parenteral Opioids

Drug	Route[a,b]	Dosage	Comments
Morphine	i.v.	Titrate 2–5-mg increments q5–10 min Peak analgesia in 10–20 min Average = 10 mg q3–4h	Preferred first-line agent in most situations
	i.m./s.c.	Average = 10 mg q3–4h	
Fentanyl	i.v.	Titrate 25–50-μg increments q2–3min Peak analgesia in 3–5 min Duration 30–60 min	Ideal for short procedures No histamine release
	i.m./s.c.	Not suitable for the emergency department	
Meperidine (Demerol)	i.v.	Titrate 12.5–50.0-mg increments Peak analgesia in 5–10 min Average = 100 mg q2–3h	Risk of unique CNS toxicity with repeated dosing i.m./s.c. injection is very irritating to tissue
	i.m./s.c.	Average = 100 mg q3h	
Hydromorphone (Dilaudid)	i.v.	Titrate 0.5–1.0 mg increments Peak analgesia in 5–15 min Average = 1.5 mg q3–4h	High solubility benefits s.c. injection
	i.m./s.c.	Average = 1.5 mg q3–4h	
Butorphanol (Stadol)	i.v.	Titrate 0.5–2.0-mg increments Peak analgesia in 4–5 min Average = 2 mg q3–4h	Mixed agonist-antagonist May be preferred in biliary colic
	i.m./s.c.	Average = 2 mg q3–4h	

Note: Intervals are approximate. Individual patients may require dosing either more or less frequently.
Caution: Dosing may need to be adjusted in the elderly, patients weighing less than 50 kg, and those with renal or hepatic insufficiency.
[a] Intravenous route is preferred for faster onset and ability to titrate to effect.
[b] Rapid i.v. administration increases incidence of respiratory depression, hypotension, nausea, and itching; IV administration should be slow (over 4–5 minutes), with the patient recumbent.

interval has elapsed. Statements about "average duration of action" provide only a rough estimate.[1]

Route of Administration. Intravenous administration of opioids is preferable to the more commonly used intramuscular route for several reasons. Absorption is more reliable, and repeated dosing is painless. It also leads to more rapid onset of analgesia; intravenous morphine begins to work within 5 minutes (peaks in 10 to 20 minutes), whereas intramuscular morphine requires 10 to 30 minutes until an effect is seen (peaks in 30 to 60 minutes).[12,15] It is obviously easier to titrate the opioid dose using the intravenous route (Fig. 411.1). It is also important to keep in mind that the frequency and severity of several side effects, such as respiratory depression, hypotension, histamine release, and nausea and vomiting, are related to the speed of intravenous injection. They can be minimized if drugs are injected over several minutes, rather than by rapid push.

It is not clear which is the second best parenteral route for opioid administration. While one authority[15] recommends subcutaneous (s.c.) injection as less painful than intramuscular, this benefit may be offset by an even more delayed onset of action.[12]

1. Initiate infusion of normal saline before administering opioids.
2. Keep the patient in a recumbent position.
3. Have naloxone and airway management equipment at the bedside.
4. Avoid or adjust dose downward in patients with hypotension, COPD, or potential for airway compromise.
5. Give **SLOWLY**, over 3–5 minutes.
6. Titrate to pain relief.
7. Supplement careful observation with pulse oxymetry and/or apnea monitoring.

Major risks:
- CNS depression leading to hypoventilation or aspiration
- Hypotension

Figure 411.1. How to give intravenous opioids safely.

Opioid analgesics can be given through a number of other routes as well. The oral route is most convenient and least expensive. When both intravenous and oral routes are unavailable, alternatives include rectal suppository (morphine, hydromorphone, and oxymorphone), sublingual tablet (buprenorphine), and even a nasal spray (butorphanol) and lollipops (fentanyl).

Adverse Effects. All opioid analgesics share certain side effects, although some occur more with one drug than another. A patient who has had a problem with one agent may be able to tolerate a second opioid without difficulty.

Of all the potential adverse effects, respiratory depression is the most dangerous. Using sophisticated testing, it is possible to show that therapeutic doses of most opiates cause some degree of respiratory depression in nearly all patients. Most of the time, this is not clinically important. However, patients with diminished respiratory reserve, such as those with severe chronic obstructive pulmonary disease or massive obesity, are liable to stop breathing after receiving these drugs. Even in those with normal reserve, removal of a painful stimulus, as occurs with the reduction of a dislocated joint, can precipitate respiratory depression; patients should be monitored closely after painful procedures. Except in the case of massive overdose, respiratory arrest does not occur suddenly but is heralded by a decreased respiratory rate and level of arousal.

Hypotension is the second major hazard of opioid use. Through a variety of mechanisms, opioids, particularly those given parenterally, may cause peripheral vasodilation. This seldom affects blood pressure in the supine patient, but the ambulatory patient may experience significant orthostatic hypotension. Volume-depleted individuals are at increased risk for hypotension regardless of body position. Hypotension from opioids generally resolves spontaneously within a few minutes; if necessary, intravenous fluids and possibly naloxone are effective.

Opiates occasionally trigger the release of histamine from mast cells. Because this occurs through a nonimmunologic mechanism, it is technically not an allergy. Clinical consequences include itching, urticaria, bronchospasm, and hypotension, which are not responsive to naloxone. The agents most frequently implicated in these reactions are morphine, followed by codeine and meperidine. Fentanyl has practically no potential for this complication.

Opiates commonly cause sedation and occasionally produce confusion. Therefore, patients should be warned not to drive vehicles or operate power tools when they take narcotics. Opioids present a special set of problems for head-injured patients. They may interfere with evaluation of central nervous system (CNS) function. The respiratory depressant effect of opioids is exaggerated in this group of patients, and the resultant hypoventilation may actually increase intracranial pressure, mediated by cerebral vasodilation in response to an elevated pCO_2.[12]

Opiates may cause spasm at the sphincter of Oddi and, in turn, precipitate biliary colic. Whether meperidine is less likely than morphine to do this remains unresolved. Among all opioids, the agonists–antagonists appear to have the least potential for this complication.[15] Paradoxically, even though it sometimes raises biliary tract pressures, morphine is usually successful in treating pain of biliary origin.[15] Nitroglycerin and glucagon, drugs that relax smooth muscle, as well as naloxone, have been used to treat opioid-induced biliary colic.[9,15]

Opioids have other effects on the genitourinary and GI systems. They may cause urinary retention, particularly in older men with underlying prostatism. They are constipating and can sometimes cause abdominal pain or dyspepsia. Nausea and vomiting can be minimized by administering the drug to the patient in the supine position and, if necessary, with an antiemetic.[9] GI side effects, if severe, can be reversed with naloxone.

Opioids have the potential to mask the diagnosis of serious abdominal disease. While they can be given safely to patients with abdominal pain who are under close observation, prescribing them for patients who are sent home with undiagnosed abdominal pain is potentially dangerous.

Choosing an Injectable Agent. A typical error in the use of opioids is to switch agents before the first one has been pushed to its limit, which is determined by unwanted side effects rather than an arbitrary "maximal" dose. Correct dosing is more important than the actual choice of agent.

Morphine is the traditional first-line parenteral narcotic. No other opioid is superior in relieving pain. It is also relatively inexpensive and has a relatively long duration of action.

Despite its widespread use, meperidine (Demerol) offers few, if any, advantages over morphine. Although it is less constipating, meperidine in equianalgesic doses produces the same degree of sedation, respiratory depression, and euphoria as does morphine.[9] With repeated dosing, meperidine has its own peculiar CNS toxicity, caused by normeperidine, an active metabolite. Findings include irritable mood, agitation, myoclonus, and seizures. CNS toxicity is more common in patients with renal insufficiency. Meperidine should not be given to patients receiving monoamine oxidase (MAO) inhibitors because of the potential for a poorly understood interaction, characterized by delirium and hyperthermia, which may be fatal.

Meperidine is recommended as a second-line analgesic for brief courses in otherwise healthy patients who have had a problem with morphine. Intramuscular or s.c. injection causes local irritation. A common mistake in the use of meperidine is to use too small a dose and too long a dosing interval.[1] Tables 411.2 and 411.3 list dosing guidelines.

Fentanyl is an ideal agent for performing short, painful procedures because of its very rapid onset and limited duration of action.

Partial agonist and agonist–antagonist opioids were developed to provide analgesia with less sedation, respiratory depression, nausea, and addiction potential.[8] Practical benefits, however, have been limited.[10] Pentazocine, the only drug of this class available in an oral form, produces psychotomimetic symptoms, including disorientation, paranoia, and hallucinations, in as many as 7% of treated patients. All drugs in this class can precipitate withdrawal when they are given to patients addicted to pure opioid agonist. These drugs really offer no advantages over the strong opioid agonists, except perhaps in the management of biliary pain.

Adjuvant Agents. A number of drugs have been administered along with parenteral opioids to minimize adverse effects by reducing the amount of opioid needed to treat pain. Phenothiazines can reduce GI side effects. When they are given along with an opioid, sedative effects are increased, but analgesia is not.[9]

The antihistamine hydroxyzine (50 to 100 mg i.m. or 1 mg/kg i.m.) is often combined with opioids to potentiate analgesia. Although hydroxyzine does have additive analgesic properties, this practice poses two problems. First, it requires an intramuscular injection. Second, it may not, in fact, decrease adverse effects: Hydroxyzine itself is a mild respiratory depressant.[6] No study has examined whether the combination of an opioid plus hydroxyzine produces respiratory depression less frequently than an equianalgesic dose of opioid alone.

Choosing an Oral Agent. Table 411.4 lists dosing guidelines for a number of commonly used oral opioids. Because opioids experience a significant first-pass hepatic metabolism, a higher oral than parenteral dose is necessary to achieve the same level of analgesia.

Codeine, which has gained widespread use, perhaps because of its low abuse potential, is a relatively weak analgesic with a relatively high incidence of GI side effects. The standard 60-mg dose alone is no more effective than 650 mg of aspirin or acetaminophen.[3] At higher doses, the analgesic effect does not increase significantly, but side effects do.

Oxycodone and hydrocodone are excellent oral analgesics. They can produce euphoria, and, in certain patients, this is a liability.

Meperidine and propoxyphene (Darvon) are less satisfactory oral agents. Meperidine has a short analgesic duration, produces significant euphoria, and has a unique CNS toxicity. Propoxyphene's efficacy is arguable. In some studies, it has been no more effective than placebo, but combined with aspirin or acetaminophen, it produces additional analgesia.[12] Overdose can result in seizures that are difficult to treat.

The main applications for oral morphine and hydromorphone (Dilaudid) are in cancer and sickle cell pain. Oral morphine is available as an immediate- and a sustained-release preparation.

Tramadol is an unscheduled, weak opioid agonist that also inhibits reuptake of serotonin and norepinephrine. It does not appear to produce respiratory depression or hypotension, probably because of selective opioid receptor binding. It is as effective, or less effective, than codeine or hydrocodone in combination with acetaminophen.[18] Tramadol is contraindicated in patients taking an MAO inhibitor.

Combination Therapy. Rational pain management often involves combining analgesics of different classes.[1] Adding acetaminophen (or an NSAID) to an opioid often produces better analgesia than a double dose of either agent alone.[3] One possible explanation for this is that the drugs work by different mechanisms. Combination therapy may permit a reduction in the

TABLE 411.4. Oral Opioid Dosing Information

Drug	Analgesic Equivalence[a]	Usual Starting Dose[b]	Usual Interval
Morphine (MSIR, Roxanol, others)	30 mg	15–30 mg[c]	3–4 h
Morphine: sustained release (MS Contin, Oramorph-SR)	30 mg	30 mg[c]	8–12 h
Meperidine (Demerol)[d]	300 mg	50–100 mg	2–3 h
Codeine (in Tylenol #3, others)[e]	200 mg	30–60 mg	3–4 h
Oxycodone (Roxicodone, also in Percocet, Percodan, Tylox, others)	20–30 mg	5–10 mg	3–6 h
Hydrocodone (in Lorcet, Lortab, Vicodin, others)	30 mg[f]	5–10 mg	3–6 h
Hydromorphone (Dilaudid)	7.5 mg	4–8 mg[c]	2–3 h

Note: Addition of a nonopioid may allow lower dosing of an opioid. In using combination products, be careful not to exceed the allowable dose of the nonopioid constituent.
Note: Intervals are approximate. Individual patients may require dosing either more or less frequently.
Caution: Dosing may need to be adjusted in the elderly, patients weighing less than 50 kg, and those with renal or hepatic insufficiency.
[a]Doses equianalgesic to intravenous morphine 10 mg and intravenous meperidine 100 mg.
[b]Doses in this column are not equianalgesic.
[c]Usually reserved for chronic, severe pain.
[d]Meperidine has a unique CNS toxicity with repeated dosing and is not recommended as a first-line agent. See text.
[e]Doses greater than 60 mg are not recommended. See text.
[f]Limited data available.

opioid dose and a corresponding reduction in opioid-associated side effects.

Many formulations are commercially available that combine aspirin or acetaminophen with codeine, hydrocodone, or oxycodone. Although combination products containing codeine and hydrocodone are controlled substances, they are classified as schedule III (rather than II) and do not require duplicate or triplicate prescription paper. Therapy does not need to be restricted to these fixed-ratio products; prescribing the constituents separately may permit greater therapeutic flexibility. For very severe pain, the opioid dose can be increased without risking toxic doses of acetaminophen or aspirin. Conversely, as the pain improves, the patient can easily taper off the opioid but continue the nonnarcotic. For the outpatient treatment of severe pain, we commonly prescribe ibuprofen 2,400 mg/d in divided doses along with oxycodone 5 to 10 mg every 4 to 6 hours. An acetaminophen (120 mg) and codeine (12 mg/5 mL) elixir is available for use in children.

COMMON PITFALLS

- Relying too much on "objective" signs of pain severity and not enough on the patient's self-report
- Confusing pain avoidance behavior with drug-seeking behavior
- Withholding analgesia until a definitive diagnosis is made
- Withholding analgesia because consent for surgery or other procedure may later be necessary
- Failing to use an opioid for fear of creating addiction
- Administering opioids i.m. or s.c. when the intravenous route is superior
- Choosing a dose based on standard guidelines instead of individual patient response

References

1. Acute Pain Management Guideline Panel. *Acute pain management: operative or medical procedures and trauma. Clinical practice guideline.* AHCPR Pub. No. 92-0032. Rockville MD: Agency for Health Care Policy and Research, Public Health Service, U.S. Dept. of Health and Human Services, 1992.
2. Attard AR, Corlett MJ, Kidner NJ, et al. Safety of early pain relief for acute abdominal pain. *BMJ* 1992;305:554.
3. Beaver WT. Combination analgesics. *Am J Med* 1984;77[Suppl A]:38.
4. Brooks PM, Day RO. Nonsteroidal antiinflammatory drugs—differences and similarities. *N Engl J Med* 1991;324:1716.
5. Cleeland CS. Measurement of pain by subjective report. In: Chapman CR, Loeser JD, eds. *Issues in pain management: advances in pain research and therapy,* vol 12. New York: Raven Press 1989:399.
6. Glazier HS. Potentiation of pain relief with hydroxyzine: a therapeutic myth? *Ann Pharmacother* 1990;24:484.
7. Goldman B. Desperately seeking drugs: a clinical and risk management approach. *Emerg Physician Legal Bull* 1993;4:1.
8. Hoskin PJ, Hanks GW. Opioid agonist-antagonist drugs in acute and chronic pain states. *Drugs* 1991;41:326.
9. Jaffee JH, Martin WR. Opioid analgesics and antagonists. In: Goodman-Gilman A, Ball TW, Nies AS, et al., eds. *Goodman and Gilman's the pharmacologic basis of therapeutics,* 8th ed. New York: Pergamon, 1990:485.
10. Lanza FL. A guideline for the treatment and prevention of NSAID-induced ulcers. *J Gastroenterol* 1998;93:2037–2046.
11. Mandell BF. COX-2 selective NSAIDs. Biology, promises and concerns. *Cleve Clin J Med* 1999;66:285–291.
12. McEvoy GK, ed. *American hospital formulary service drug information.* Bethesda, MD: American Society of Hospital Pharmacists, 1993.
13. Neighbor ML, Puntillo KA. Intramuscular ketorolac vs. oral ibuprofen in emergency department patients with acute pain. *Acad Emerg Med* 1998;5:118–122.
14. Pace S, Burke TF. Intravenous morphine for early pain relief in patients with acute abdominal pain. *Acad Emerg Med* 1996;3:1086–1092.
15. Paris PM, Weiss LD. Narcotic analgesics: the pure agonists. In: Paris PM, Stewart RD, eds. *Pain management in emergency medicine.* Norwalk, CT: Appleton & Lange, 1988:125.
16. Porter J, Jick H. Addiction rare in patients treated with narcotics [Letter]. *N Engl J Med* 1980;302:123.
17. Sacchetti A, Schafermeyer R, Gerardi M, et al. Pediatric analgesia and sedation. *Ann Emerg Med* 1994;23:237.
18. Turturro MA, Paris PM, Larkin GL. Tramadol versus hydrocodone-acetaminophen in acute musculoskeletal pain: a randomized, double-blind clinical trial. *Ann Emerg Med* 1998;32:139–143.
19. Turturro MA, Paris PM, Seaberg DC. Intramuscular ketorolac versus oral ibuprofen in acute musculoskeletal pain. *Ann Emerg Med* 1995;26:117–120.
20. Weisman SJ, Schechter NL. The management of pain in children. *Pediatr Rev* 1991;12:237.

CHAPTER 412
Chronic Pain Syndromes

Michael A. Turturro and Paul M. Paris

Chronic pain syndromes often challenge the emergency physician in both diagnosis and management. Some present with vague signs and symptoms and often are not definitively diagnosed on the first encounter. Treatment is often complex, requiring several regimens of varying effectiveness. Many patients have a protracted course of exacerbations and remissions, and frequently present because of inadequate pain control.

Most of the concepts that apply to acute pain management (see Chapter 411) also apply to patients with chronic pain. For example, with any type of pain, it is the patient's expectation and the emergency physician's responsibility to provide relief, and this should usually begin before a diagnosis is established. However, exacerbations of chronic pain are often due to a combination of both physical and psychological factors. Also, certain pain syndromes (e.g., neurogenic pain) may not be effectively treated by typical analgesic agents. Therefore, an understanding of both the physical and psychological pathophysiology associated with these disorders will ensure optimal treatment.

Acute pain and chronic pain differ in several ways (Table 412.1). Acute pain is generally due to actual or potential tissue damage. It typically has a rapid onset, coinciding with tissue damage, and resolves as tissue heals. Although distressing and anxiety provoking, it often can be treated effectively with proper selection and use of analgesic drugs. With chronic pain, the symptom of pain itself often becomes more of a problem than its underlying cause, altering the patient's life and frequently causing depression. Its treatment is complex and difficult. Success in treating chronic pain typically requires a multidisciplinary team approach, using various regimens of pharmacotherapy, physical therapy, and behavioral therapy.

Chronic pain may be due to prolonged tissue destruction (e.g., cancer pain) but may also occur due to dysfunction of the central nervous system (CNS) or peripheral nervous system, and it can be exacerbated by psychological factors. The pathophysiology of chronic pain without obvious tissue pathology is unclear. Prolonged noxious sensory input from the periphery may result in self-sustaining central neural activity, possibly by reducing inhibitory input into the CNS. This may produce a "memory" effect for pain perception in the CNS.

Pain due to malignancy, although chronic in nature, may be considered sustained acute pain because it is typically associated with progressive tissue damage. Although nonnarcotic analgesics and physical therapy are often used to treat malignant pain, progressively increasing doses of opioid analgesics remain the mainstay of therapy. Despite the risk of opioid dependence, opioid analgesics should never be withheld from patients with terminal malignant pain, as pain control is the most important factor contributing to overall quality of life. Acute exacerbations of malignant pain must be treated as an emergency, with aggressive opioid analgesia. Higher doses of opioids titrated more rapidly than in opioid-naive patients are typically needed, and this approach has been demonstrated to be safe and effective.[4]

TABLE 412.1. Differences between Acute and Chronic Pain

Acute Pain	Chronic Pain
Usually due to tissue damage	Often no identifiable pathology
Is related to underlying illness	Is the problem itself
Responds to typical analgesics	May not respond to typical analgesics
Straightforward treatment	Complex treatment
Causes anxiety	Causes depression

Behavioral and physical therapies are often used in managing chronic pain. Chronic pain commonly causes the patient to lose a sense of control over his or her environment. Allowing patients to become passively dependent on health-care practitioners and medical therapy only feeds this vicious cycle of illness and the helpless victim.

GENERAL EVALUATION

Each patient with chronic pain must also be evaluated for the development of worsening or new pathology. The physician should not assume that a patient's chronic pain exacerbation is nothing more than a worsening of an already existing disease process. For example, a patient with worsening chronic low back pain must be evaluated for new spinal cord dysfunction. Simply providing analgesics without an appropriate evaluation may result in missing serious disease.

Chronic pain patients should be considered valuable resources, because they often know the most effective therapies to treat their pain. The chronic pain patient with a true exacerbation should be treated with analgesics in the emergency department. Many of these patients require pain service referral, and communication between the emergency and pain service physicians fosters a team approach to the management of chronic pain exacerbations. For example, a contract may be developed between the patient, the pain service, and the emergency department as to when the patient will be expected to present for a pain exacerbation, the analgesic that will be used after appropriate evaluation, and the quantity of analgesics prescribed.

Typical doses of analgesics are sometimes ineffective for chronic pain syndromes, and many patients fail various modes of therapy. As a result, malingering or drug-seeking behavior may inappropriately be suspected. Patients may appear to be demanding or psychologically distressed, and may feel uncomfortable with a physician who has not been their regular caretaker. Establishing a rapport with the patient is essential, and the physician must not feel threatened by patient demands.

Drug abuse and addiction are unfortunate problems in our society, and drug abusers (whether or not they suffer from chronic pain) tend to patronize emergency departments on a frequent basis to obtain opioid analgesics. Because of this, emergency department staff members may develop a bias against all chronic pain patients. Because it may be difficult to differentiate patients with exacerbations of chronic pain from patients who are seeking drugs for abuse, many patients with real exacerbations of chronic pain are consequently labeled as drug abusers.

Drug abusers often have a history of multiple substance abuse, multiple visits for treatment of various nonspecific painful conditions, an unusual reluctance to try new therapies, or a report that their primary physician is unreachable. Because it is inappropriate and unethical to withhold analgesics from patients experiencing pain, unless the emergency physician is convinced that the patient is a drug abuser, the patient should be given the benefit of the doubt and a short course of analgesics should be prescribed. Sometimes, a known substance abuser may present with a truly painful condition. In these cases, pain should be adequately relieved in the emergency department, and judicious amounts of analgesics should be given on discharge. The use of opioid agonist–antagonists may be useful in these patients, as they are less likely to cause euphoria. However, they should not be given to a patient physically dependent on opioids, as they may precipitate withdrawal.

True addiction, compulsive use of opioids despite signs of toxicity and inability to function due to addiction, is unusual in patients with chronic pain. However, when pain medication is withheld, such patients may learn pain avoidance or maladaptive behaviors to obtain opioids. Giving pain medication on an as-needed basis, rather than around-the-clock dosing, contributes to this phenomenon, as the patient learns to express both symptoms and maladaptive behavior to obtain the reward of receiving pain medication.

The association between depression and chronic pain is clear, but, in some patients, the painful process produces depression, and, in others, chronic pain is a manifestation of a depressive disorder. In patients with chronic pain in whom no etiologic basis can be established, the treatment is focused on the underlying depression. Depression is also known to increase opioid analgesic requirements.

GENERAL TREATMENT

The treatment of chronic pain includes the use of many modalities (Tables 412.2 and 412.3). Opioid analgesics are the most useful drugs in treating exacerbations of chronic pain. The agents used are discussed in the chapter on acute pain (see Chapter 411), but longer acting preparations, such as sustained-release morphine, oxycodone, and hydromorphone, and methadone are more appropriate for the treatment of chronic pain. These agents also avoid the risk of aspirin or acetaminophen toxicity from the nonnarcotic component of combination products, which may occur when doses sufficient to provide adequate amounts of the opioid component are taken.

Tramadol is an oral opioid analgesic that also has a mechanism similar to the tricyclic antidepressants (TCAs) (i.e., the inhibition of monoamine neurotransmitter reuptake). Tolerance and withdrawal symptoms appear to be absent with tramadol. However, it has been demonstrated to be less effective in the management of acute pain than other opioids[14] and is associated with a high incidence of side effects. It appears to be most appropriate for adjunctive treatment of mild-to-moderate chronic pain.

TABLE 412.2. Therapies for Chronic Pain

Therapy	Indications
Opioid analgesics	Most causes of chronic pain; often ineffective in neurogenic pain
Antidepressants	Most causes of chronic pain
Anticonvulsants	Neurogenic pain
Transelectrical nerve stimulation (TENS)	Low back pain, reflex sympathetic dystrophy
Local anesthetics	Phantom limb pain, neurogenic pain
Capsaicin	Neurogenic pain, arthritic pain
Behavioral therapy	Most causes of chronic pain
Physical therapy	Reflex sympathetic dystrophy, TMJ dysfunction, tension myalgia
Surgery	Refractory trigeminal neuralgia, reflex sympathetic dystrophy, phantom limb pain

TABLE 412.3. Nonopioid Pharmacotherapy for Chronic Pain

Drug Class/ Agent	Brand Name	Dosing
TRICYCLIC ANTIDEPRESSANTS		
Amitriptyline	Elavil	50 mg PO qhs; up to 150 mg/d
Imipramine	Tofranil	50 mg PO qhs
Nortriptyline	Pamelor	25–50 mg PO qhs
Doxepin	Sinequan	25–50 mg PO qhs
ANTICONVULSANTS		
Carbamazepine	Tegretol	100 mg PO qhs;[a] increase to 100 mg PO b.i.d.; max. 1,200 mg/d
Clonazepam	Klonopin	1 mg PO qhs; up to 1 mg PO t.i.d.
Gabapentin	Neurontin	300 mg PO t.i.d.; increase as necessary to maximum of 3,600 mg/d
SKELETAL MUSCLE RELAXANTS		
Cyclobenzaprine	Flexeril	10 mg PO t.i.d.
Orphenadrine	Norflex	100 mg PO b.i.d.
Carisoprodol	Soma	200–400 mg q.i.d.
Chlorzoxazone	Paraflex, Parafon-Forte	250–750 mg PO t.i.d. or q.i.d.
Methocarbamol	Robaxin	1.5 g q.i.d.
Baclofen	Lioresal	5 mg PO t.i.d.; increase to 20 mg PO t.i.d.
SUBSTANCE P INHIBITOR		
Capsaicin	Zostrix	Apply to affected area q.i.d.

[a]Obtain baseline complete blood count.

TCAs are useful in treating chronic pain, both by controlling depression and by altering nociceptive responses to painful stimuli, thereby altering the cerebral process in pain perception. They are effective in pain control even if no evidence of depression exists. TCAs are effective in various chronic pain syndromes, particularly neurogenic pain, face pain syndromes, fibromyalgia, and arthritis. TCAs act synergistically with opioids in controlling chronic pain. It is likely that all TCAs are effective in treating chronic pain, but amitriptyline has been the most extensively studied. However, there is little evidence that the newer antidepressant drugs, such as the selective serotonin reuptake inhibitors (SSRIs), are useful. The recommended starting dose for all TCAs in managing chronic pain is half the antidepressant dose, which may be titrated up if necessary. Analgesic effects may not be evident for several days. Referral for follow-up is essential in patients started on TCAs in the emergency department.

Transcutaneous electrical nerve stimulation (TENS) may be effective in certain acute and chronic pain syndromes. It is used most often in chronic low back pain and reflex sympathetic dystrophy. Unfortunately, most patients note a decrease in analgesic effect over time. The "gate control" theory of pain postulates that, in the periphery, small unmyelinated C fibers transmit nociceptive information, and large myelinated A fibers transmit light touch and pressure sensations. Both of these fibers synapse at the substantia gelatinosa in the dorsal horn of the spinal cord. Stimulation of the A fibers inhibits the transmission of nociceptive C fiber stimuli into the CNS, thereby "closing the gate." By using electricity to stimulate the A fibers preferentially, the pain stimulus entering the CNS can be controlled.

In neurogenic pain syndromes, pain originates from peripheral nerve dysfunction. Therefore, anticonvulsants play a primary role in treating most of these disorders. In addition, because substance P may be the principal mediator of neurogenic pain, an effort to inhibit substance P may be beneficial. When applied topically, capsaicin, a substance derived from red chili peppers, releases substance P from primary afferent nerve fibers; with repeated application, capsaicin depletes substance P from these nerve fibers. Consequently, capsaicin may be useful in treating the neurogenic pain of postherpetic neuralgia, reflex sympathetic dystrophy, and metabolic neuropathy, as well as other chronic pain syndromes such as psoriatic and rheumatoid arthritis. Capsaicin causes skin redness and burning. This may also contribute to its analgesic effect, as peripheral counterirritation causes pain relief by a "gate-closing" effect, as described for TENS. However, skin irritation limits the concentration that may be used, thus reducing its potential efficacy.[9]

Behavioral and physical therapy helps patients cope with chronic pain and regain a sense of self-control, thus improving overall day-to-day function. The focus with these therapies is rehabilitation, not total pain relief. However, patients must be motivated to be successful.

The most effective ways to treat these chronic pain syndromes are the multidisciplinary approaches used by pain clinics, in which combinations of the various therapies are coordinated. Thus, the emergency physician should confer with the patient's primary care or referring physician and make arrangements for follow-up before initiating or changing therapy.

DIAGNOSIS AND MANAGEMENT OF SPECIFIC SYNDROMES

Myofascial Pain Syndromes

Myofascial Pain and Fibromyalgia

Myofascial pain syndrome and fibromyalgia are conditions in which acute or chronic muscle pain, stiffness, and tenderness occur at specific anatomic sites ("trigger points"). A trigger point is an area within a taut band of skeletal muscle that, when palpated, produces referred pain in the area where the patient complains of pain (a "reference zone"). It may be activated by physical trauma, other trigger points, or psychological stress.

Fibromyalgia and myofascial pain syndrome may be considered opposites in the spectrum of a single disorder (Table 412.4). Myofascial pain tends to be localized, and the involved muscle group may twitch involuntarily. Fibromyalgia pain tends to be diffuse and is associated with systemic symptoms such as chronic fatigue, headaches, vertigo, visual disturbances, and irritable bowel syndrome. Symptoms may begin after an acute viral illness, trauma, or psychological stress.

TABLE 412.4. Myofascial Pain Syndrome Versus Fibromyalgia

	Myofascial Pain	Fibromyalgia
Location	Regional	Generalized
Muscular twitch	Yes	No
Systemic symptoms	No	Possible
Sleep disturbances	No	Yes
Trigger-point injection useful	Yes	Sometimes
Physical therapy useful	Yes	No
Skeletal muscle relaxants useful	No	Yes

Physical findings may be nonspecific, and the patient may be told that the symptoms are unexplained or psychogenic. The differential diagnosis for fibromyalgia includes other painful systemic illnesses, such as systemic lupus erythematosus, polymyalgia rheumatica, polymyositis, metabolic myopathy, hypothyroidism, chronic fatigue syndrome, and irritable bowel syndrome. Because symptoms often overlap, the diagnosis is frequently one of exclusion.

Although it has been postulated that psychological causes may underlie the pathophysiology of fibromyalgia (e.g., patients may not respond in a normal fashion to physical or psychological stress or may have a heightened perception of bodily discomfort), elevated levels of plasma substance P and decreased levels of serotonin have been demonstrated.[12,13] Consequently, fibromyalgia patients may experience pain from stimuli that are below the painful threshold in normal patients due to neurochemical alteration of pain pathways. Complicating matters is that depression is a frequent result of fibromyalgia, and somatization disorders are more frequent in fibromyalgia patients than the general population.

The treatments of myofascial pain and fibromyalgia have certain similarities. Trigger-point injection of local anesthetics is a technique easily performed for both fibromyalgia and myofascial pain, often with rewarding results. Relief of local and referred pain and a decrease in muscle tension may be seen after injection.

Other physical techniques, such as muscle stretching, biofeedback, and exercise, are useful in myofascial pain syndrome but are of limited value in fibromyalgia. In fibromyalgia patients, analgesics usually provide only partial relief, and additional therapy with antidepressants or muscle relaxants is often needed. Cyclobenzaprine, a skeletal muscle relaxant related to the TCAs, may be particularly useful in treating fibromyalgia.[2] After initiating this therapy in the emergency department, follow-up care should be ensured.

Temporomandibular Dysfunction Syndrome

Temporomandibular joint (TMJ) dysfunction syndrome is increasingly common. Patients typically report facial pain and nonspecific headache, in addition to joint noise and difficulty in joint motion. Muscular and joint tenderness as well as limited TMJ range of motion may be found. The disorder is similar in many respects to both myofascial pain syndrome and fibromyalgia, and TMJ dysfunction syndrome is often referred to as a form of myofascial pain. Many patients with TMJ dysfunction also have fibromyalgia or other myofascial pain.

The etiology is unclear. Some patients may exhibit signs of TMJ dysfunction but may not have troubling symptoms. Many patients have coexistent psychiatric diagnoses, which often leads to the assumption that emotional stress plays a role in this syndrome. Many patients show a greater sensitivity to certain noxious stimuli than do pain-free controls.[7] Patients who clench or grind their teeth secondary to stress may develop masticatory muscle hyperactivity and fatigue, which can lead to pain and altered joint mechanics.

Patients may present before definitive diagnosis with a complaint of nonspecific facial pain, or may present during a symptom exacerbation. As in other chronic pain syndromes, treatment frequently requires analgesics, antidepressants, and nonpharmacologic therapy. Physical therapy, biofeedback, and intraoral splinting help relax the afflicted muscles and reduce discomfort. Pain control with analgesics is usually necessary. Patients should be discharged on TCAs if the diagnosis is certain and should be referred to a maxillofacial specialist so that an intraoral splint can be fitted and physical therapy started.

Neurogenic Pain Syndromes

Patients with neurogenic pain syndromes (Table 412.5) commonly present when symptoms first develop. The pain in these syndromes develops from nerve malfunction, sometimes due to physical damage to the involved nerve. In certain neurogenic pain syndromes, the pain is exacerbated by other stimuli that also stimulate the same nerve, such as light touch, temperature changes, or emotional stress. This phenomenon is known as allodynia. The pain is typically described as burning in nature, and treatment is often frustrating, because both opioid and nonopioid analgesics are typically ineffective in relieving it.

Facial Neuralgias

Trigeminal neuralgia is a relatively common, often debilitating disorder. Typically older patients (over age 50) are affected, and women develop this disorder more often than do men. The right side is more frequently involved, and bilaterality is rare. The second division of the fifth cranial nerve (V2) is most frequently affected. Attacks at the third division (V3) may also occur, but attacks at the first division (V1) are rare. The initial attacks are brief but severe and lancinating, often described as an "electric shock" sensation. Allodynia is prominent, and attacks may be triggered by touching the face, cold air blowing against the face, eating, shaving, or talking. Unlike other neuralgias, a sensory deficit is atypical and, if found, should alert the clinician to the possibility of nerve compression due to malignancy. As the condition progresses, the attacks become more frequent and a background ache may develop.

Glossopharyngeal neuralgia is less common and usually less severe than trigeminal neuralgia. It affects equal numbers of men and women. About 25% of cases are bilateral. Typically, a single episode of lancinating pain along the ninth cranial nerve sensory distribution (neck, throat, and ear) occurs. Atypical facial pain may occur, which is poorly localized but frequently involves the mandible. Unlike other facial pain syndromes, it is not clearly neurogenic and consequently does not respond as well as trigeminal neuralgia to anticonvulsants.[3]

The differential diagnosis of facial neuralgias includes cluster headaches, maxillary sinusitis, postherpetic neuralgia (especially with V1 distribution), dental pain, and TMJ dysfunction syndrome. Swallowing and chewing may trigger the pain from both facial neuralgias and TMJ dysfunction. Allodynia and the absence of TMJ tenderness suggest the former diagnosis.

The mainstay of treatment for the facial neuralgias is the administration of anticonvulsants, particularly carbamazepine.[8] Unfortunately, patients typically present in extreme pain, and anticonvulsants usually require several days before a demonstrable effect is noticed. The recommended starting dose for carbamazepine is 100 mg qhs for 3 days, then an increase to 100 mg twice a day. The dose may need to be titrated up to 1,200 mg/d. Other drugs, such as baclofen and clonazepam, may then need to be added. Because carbamazepine may cause neutropenia, a baseline complete blood count should be obtained. Carbamazepine may cause nausea, dizziness, or somnolence, which may limit patient compliance. Follow-up with the patient's primary care physician or a neurologist should be arranged. Patients who fail medical therapy for trigeminal neuralgia often need surgical destruction of the sensory distribution of the trigeminal nerve, either by percutaneous thermocoagulation, cryosurgery, microvascular decompression, or glycerol injection.

TABLE 412.5. Neurogenic Pain Syndromes

Facial neuralgias	Nerve compression pain
Trigeminal	Radiculopathy
Glossopharyngeal	Entrapment neuropathy
Metabolic neuropathy	Postherpetic neuralgia
Diabetic	Reflex sympathetic dystrophy
B_{12}	Phantom limb pain

Postherpetic Neuralgia

Postherpetic neuralgia is the most common neuropathic pain. It occurs in 10% of cases of herpes zoster, and it is more common in the elderly. It may begin during or after an attack of zoster, it typically persists for several weeks after the rash resolves, and it has no relation to the severity of the zoster attack. Burning pain occurs in the involved dermatome, which is most commonly thoracic (about 50%), V1 (about 20%), and cervical (about 20%).

Many treatments used in other neurogenic pain syndromes (e.g., diabetic neuropathy) have been recommended for the treatment of postherpetic neuralgia. However, it is difficult to determine what is truly effective because few well-designed, controlled clinical trials exist, and some cases may resolve with no treatment. The longer the condition is allowed to persist, the less likely that any one treatment will be effective.

Opioid analgesics may provide modest temporary improvement in pain, but they are typically are not useful alone in the treatment of postherpetic neuralgia. Local anesthetics have been used in intravenous forms, in topical preparations such as lidocaine ointment and EMLA (prilocaine/lidocaine) cream, and in nerve blocks: All appear to provide additional short-term relief of pain due to this condition.[10] Capsaicin appears to provide temporary but effective relief if used four times a day for 3 to 4 weeks. Anticonvulsants reportedly useful in treating postherpetic neuralgia include carbamazepine, phenytoin, valproic acid, and the antispastic drug baclofen. Gabapentin is a newer anticonvulsant that shows promise in treating the pain of postherpetic neuralgia in a dose titrated up to 3600 mg/d.[11] Antidepressants may also help relieve postherpetic neuralgia pain, but there is no clear superiority of one over another.[15] In addition, there is some evidence to suggest that preemptive treatment with antidepressants during an attack of herpes zoster may reduce the prevalence of postherpetic neuralgia.[1]

Acyclovir, valacyclovir, and famciclovir are useful in the treatment of an acute attack of herpes zoster, particularly in the immunosuppressed host, in decreasing viral shedding and the duration of lesions. Most evidence suggests that they also appear to have a modest effect on decreasing the incidence of postherpetic neuralgia.[5] Although occasionally prescribed, there is also no definite evidence that steroids are useful in preventing or treating postherpetic neuralgia.[16]

Reflex Sympathetic Dystrophy and Causalgia

Reflex sympathetic dystrophy (RSD), also known as complex regional pain syndrome, Sudeck atrophy, shoulder–hand syndrome, and algodystrophy, is characterized by a vicious cycle of pain, disuse atrophy, and peripheral autonomic dysfunction. Patients are usually 40 to 60 years old, although children are occasionally affected. It typically occurs after major extremity trauma, but it has also been related to minor trauma, cerebrovascular accident, myocardial infarction, arthritis, infection, and local tumor infiltration. Drugs such as isoniazid, ethanol, and phenobarbital have also been implicated as causative factors. It often occurs after prolonged extremity immobilization, presumably as a result of irritation of the sympathetic ganglia.

The term *causalgia* is reserved for RSD related to a major peripheral nerve injury. After nerve damage due to an extremity injury, a positive feedback loop develops in which sympathetic efferent neurons stimulate afferent pain fibers and vice versa. Stimuli that cause sympathetic efferent outflow, such as temperature changes, often trigger this vicious cycle. Peripheral nociceptors are sensitized, and, when stimulated, they, in turn, stimulate sympathetic fibers. Thus, the cycle of pain and sympathetic overflow occurs.

The median, ulnar, and femoral nerves are most commonly affected. In patients with minor trauma, the degree of initial pain is often much greater than suggested by objective findings. The first (acute) stage occurs during the first several weeks of the disease process. Symptoms include pain, swelling, sympathetic underactivity, joint stiffness, warm skin, hypertrichosis, and edema. As the disease progresses, joint stiffness, hair loss, allodynia, sympathetic overreactivity, and muscular dystrophy occur, along with paroxysms of pain. After several months, decreased joint motion and muscle and skin atrophy occur. At this stage, the extremity appears cool, pale, shiny, and hairless. Radiographs are usually normal early in the disease and later show patchy osteopenia and erosions. The differential diagnosis includes collagen vascular disease, phlebitis, degenerative arthritis, and conversion hysteria.

Treatment is difficult, and most therapies provide only temporary relief. Medications that may be helpful include beta blockers, alpha blockers, calcium channel blockers, serotonin antagonists, capsaicin, corticosteroids, antidepressants, and anticonvulsants.[6] As with other forms of neurogenic pain, opioids and nonsteroidal antiinflammatory agents are often ineffective. Regional blocks using guanethidine may be effective but can exacerbate the pain before it improves. Sympathetic blockade is often used but usually provides only temporary relief. Physical therapy is essential, and other nonpharmacologic therapies, such as TENS, may be used.

RSD can be prevented by avoiding prolonged immobilization in patients with extremity trauma. Recognizing the early stages and intervening before the disease progresses is important. Patients should be referred for early physical therapy.

Sympathetic blocks may provide temporary analgesia and allow for aggressive activity.

Phantom Limb Pain

Phantom limb pain is a poorly understood syndrome that occurs after extremity amputation. It, too, is difficult to treat. After amputation, phantom sensation is nearly universal, and usually resolves in less than a year. Persistent pain is thought to be related to neural damage postamputation. It has been postulated that the last impulses received by the limb before amputation may be stored in "memory," and if these impulses are painful, the sensation may persist. Consequently, the incidence of phantom limb pain is decreased in patients given preoperative regional anesthesia. As with other chronic pain syndromes, psychological stress exacerbates the degree of pain experienced.

There are few well-designed studies that evaluate the various treatment regimens for phantom limb pain. Anticonvulsants, analgesics, and beta-blocking agents all seem to provide temporary relief. Surgical techniques such as cordotomy, stump revision, and neuroma removal have been reported, with variable degrees of success. A combination of long-term behavioral therapy and antidepressants appears to be the most useful mode of therapy.

COMMON PITFALLS

- Missing acute disease by assuming an exacerbation of chronic pain is due to preexisting disease
- Labeling chronic pain patients who have true pain as drug seekers
- Overreliance on analgesic drugs to treat neurogenic pain
- Failure to appreciate the risk of aspirin or acetaminophen toxicity when using escalating doses of combination opioid products to treat chronic pain
- Assuming the pain from fibromyalgia or TMJ dysfunction is psychogenic
- Failure to consider nonpharmacologic modalities for the treatment of chronic pain
- Failure to confer and to arrange follow-up with the patient's primary care physician or pain clinic before initiating or changing therapy

References

1. Bowsher D. The effects or pre-emptive treatment of postherpetic neuralgia with amitriptyline: a randomized, double-blind placebo-controlled trial. *J Pain Symptom Manage* 1997;13:327–331.
2. Carette S, Bell MJ, Reynolds WJ, et al. Comparison of amitriptyline, cyclobenzaprine, and placebo in the treatment of fibromyalgia. a randomized, double-blind clinical trial. *Arthritis Rheum* 1994;37:32–40.
3. Ceylan S, Karakus A, Duru S, et al. Glossopharyngeal neuralgia: a study of 6 cases. *Neurosurg Rev* 1997;20:196–200.
4. Hagen NA, Elwood T, Ernst S. Cancer pain emergencies: a protocol for management. *J Pain Symptom Manage* 1997;14:45–50.
5. Jackson JL, Gibbons R, Meyer G, et al. The effect of treating herpes zoster with oral acyclovir in preventing postherpetic neuralgia: a meta-analysis. *Arch Intern Med* 1997;157:909–912.
6. Kasdan ML, Johnson AL. Reflex sympathetic dystrophy. *Occup Med* 1998;13:521–531.
7. Maixner W, Fillingim R, Booker D, et al. Sensitivity of patients with painful temporomandibular disorders to experimentally evoked pain. *Pain* 1995;63:341–351.
8. McQuay H, Carroll D, Jadad A, et al. Anticonvulsant drugs for management of pain: a systematic review. *BMJ* 1995;311:1047–1052.
9. Robbins WR, Staats PS, Levine J, et al. Treatment of intractable pain with topical large-dose capsaicin: preliminary report. *Anesth Analg* 1999;86:579–583.
10. Rowbotham MC, Davies PS, Fields HL. Topical lidocaine gel relieves postherpetic neuralgia. *Ann Neurol* 1995;37:246–253.
11. Rowbotham M, Harden N, Stacey B, et al. Gabapentin for the treatment of postherpetic neuralgia: a randomized controlled trial. *JAMA* 1998;280:1837–1842.
12. Russell IJ, Orr MD, Littman B, et al. Elevated cerebrospinal fluid levels of substance P in patients with fibromyalgia syndrome. *Arthritis Rheum* 1994;37:1593–1601.
13. Russell OJ. Neurochemical pathogenesis of fibromyalgia syndrome. *J Musculoskel Pain* 1996;4:61–92.
14. Stubhaug A, Grimstad J, Breivik H. Lack of analgesic effect of 50 and 100 mg oral tramadol after orthopedic surgery: a randomized, double-blind, placebo and active standard drug comparison. *Pain* 1995;62:111–118.
15. Watson CPN, Vernich L, Chipman M, et al. Nortriptyline versus amitriptyline in postherpetic neuralgia: a randomized trial. *Neurology* 1998;51:1166–1171.
16. Whitley RJ, Weiss H, Gnann JW, et al. Acyclovir with and without prednisone for the treatment of herpes zoster: a randomized, placebo-controlled trial. *Ann Intern Med* 1996;125:376–383.

CHAPTER 413
Conscious and Deep Sedation

Daniel A. Muse

Properly performed, conscious sedation of patients is an effective modality to alleviate pain and anxiety and to control unintentional and potentially harmful movement during therapeutic or diagnostic procedures such as cardioversion, incision and drainage of abscesses, chest tube thoracostomy, lumbar punc-

TABLE 413.1. Drugs Used for Conscious and Deep Sedation

Agent	Trade Name	Routes	Dosage	Duration of Action	Side Effects[a]
Etomidate	Amidate	i.v.	0.1–0.3 mg/kg	3–5 min	Hypotension, myoclonic jerking
Fentanyl	Sublimaze	i.v.	2–3 μg/kg	20–30 min	Truncal rigidity, glottic spasm, vomiting, bradycardia, pruritus, seizures
		i.m.	3–5 μg/kg		
Ketamine	Ketalar	i.v.	1–2 mg/kg	Biphasic: 15 min to 2–3 h	Emergence phenomenon, laryngospasm, emesis
		i.m.	2–6 mg/kg		
		PO	6–10 mg/kg		
		Rectal	5–15 mg/kg		
		Nasal	6 mg/kg		
Methoxital	Brevital	i.v.	1–2 mg/kg	10 min to 1 h	Hypotension: possible seizures
		i.m.	10 mg/kg		
		Rectal	20–30 mg/kg		
Midazolam	Versed	i.v.	0.03–0.07 mg/kg	1–2 h	Hypotension, laryngospasm
		i.m.	0.03–0.07 mg/kg		
		PO	0.2–0.75 mg/kg		
		Nasal	0.2–0.4 mg/kg		
Nitrous oxide	—	Inhalation	50%/50% N_2O to O_2; 70%/30% N_2O to O_2 at high altitudes	Seconds to minutes	Distention of gas-filled pockets, ear pain
Propofol	Diprivan	i.v.	1–2 mg/kg bolus, then 3–6 mg/kg/h (50–100 μg/kg/min) or 25–50 mg intermittent bolus	10–20 min	Hypotension, bradycardia, phlebitis

[a]All agents can cause respiratory depression.

TABLE 413.2. American Society of Anesthesia Physical Status Classification

Class I	A healthy patient
Class II	A patient with mild systemic disease
Class III	A patient with severe systemic disease
Class IV	A patient with severe systemic disease that is a constant threat to life
Class V	An ill patient not expected to survive without an operation

tures, fracture reductions, complex suturing, and imaging studies.[3,7,8] The advent of shorter-acting, more effective drugs (Table 413.1), the development of noninvasive monitoring devices, and well-publicized standards of care for performing conscious sedation have made it an extremely safe, practical procedure. Psychological gains for the patient, family, and staff, as well as the facilitation of testing and treatment, far outweigh the antiquated belief that sedating the patient will slow down the flow in the emergency department.

Conscious sedation is a pharmacologically induced state of sedation that allows the patient to continue to breathe spontaneously and to maintain a patent airway and protective airway reflexes. The patient should also respond appropriately to simple commands and physical stimulation.[1] *Deep sedation* is a pharmacologically induced state in which the patient is not easily aroused but continues to breathe spontaneously, has a patent airway, and has at least partial control of the protective reflexes. The patient does not easily respond to painful or verbal stimuli.[1] Due to the nature of procedures performed in the emergency department, deep sedation is often needed to ensure an appropriate level of analgesia and immobility.

Providing sedation in the emergency department requires a team approach. The staff must be trained in monitoring techniques and educated about the dosages, routes of administration, and side effects of the drugs. Protocols delineating staffing responsibilities, monitoring guidelines, approved medications, observation periods, and discharge criteria and instructions must be addressed before implementing conscious and deep sedation in the emergency department. It is helpful to enlist the expertise and assistance of the anesthesiology department.

A patient consent form outlining the risks and benefits of the procedure should be obtained whenever time and the patient's condition allow. Patients should also have a brief general history and physical examination to ensure that they are appropriate candidates for sedation in the emergency department. In general, sedation should be reserved for patients in American Society of Anesthesia classes I to III (Table 413.2).

MONITORING PROCEDURES

If possible, there should be a properly equipped room designated for conscious and deep sedation. All aspects of the procedure are documented, including consent, history, and physical examination, as well as condition at discharge. It is best to use a standardized departmental form that can be part of the patient's record. Oxygen, suction, intubation equipment, and the antidotes for narcotics and benzodiazepines (naloxone and flumazenil) should always be available. The room should have available a cart containing advanced life-support medications in the event of respiratory or cardiac arrest.

Most patients, especially adults, need intravenous access. This allows optimal dosing of medications and rapid access in the event of an untoward effect. The patient should have cardiac monitoring and vital signs should be monitored frequently until discharge. Continuous pulse oximetry is of paramount importance. Due to the nature of the medications used, hypoventilation, and the ensuing hypoxia, is the major cause of morbidity and mortality from conscious and deep sedation. Capnography, which monitors end-tidal carbon dioxide ($PETCO_2$), allows ensuing hypoxemia to be recognized by registering the rise in carbon dioxide or by triggering the apnea alarm even before the hypoxemia is clinically evident or noted by the desaturation on the pulse oximeter (see Chapter 414).

During the procedure, ventilation should be monitored by continually assessing airway patency, the depth and number of respirations, oxygen saturation, and, if available, the $PETCO_2$. Vital signs are obtained before sedation, then repeated and recorded every 3 to 5 minutes during the procedure. Times and dosages of all medications given are recorded. After the procedure, vital signs are recorded every 15 minutes until the patient has returned to a presedation level of consciousness. At discharge, the physician should reevaluate the patient and document the pulmonary, cardiac, and neurologic status, as well as any pertinent findings related to the procedure.

Naloxone and flumazenil should be given only to treat hypoventilation. They are not a substitute for monitoring and should not be given simply to reverse sedation. They have shorter half-lives than the sedative agents, and the patient could revert back to a sedated state and, if left unmonitored, develop respiratory compromise.

DRUG THERAPY

The optimal drug in conscious and deep sedation would have a rapid onset and a short duration of action. It would have minimal cardiovascular and respiratory effects, predictable dosing, and a large therapeutic window. It would have both amnesic and analgesic properties. Because no single agent can do this, agents such as an amnesic drug and a local anesthetic, or an amnesic and an analgesic agent, are often used together.

The type of procedure and the patient's age, medical history prior to presentation, and acute medical condition influence the choice of agents and the route of administration. Inhalation, rectal, and oral routes have all proved to be safe and effective for sedation in procedures such as imaging studies and repairs of lacerations in children. Painful procedures, such as reductions and cardioversion, need intravenous access so that medications can be titrated to the appropriate level of sedation and analgesia; as mentioned, obtaining intravenous access also allows the use of an antagonist or resuscitative agents if untoward effects occur.

Etomidate

Etomidate is an ultrashort-acting, nonbarbiturate sedative–hypnotic with no analgesic properties. Like methohexital, it causes deep sedation, has a very rapid onset (1 minute), and has a duration of action of 3 to 5 minutes. Etomidate has minimal cardiorespiratory effects; although respiratory depression can occur, it is usually transient and associated with the use of other respiratory depressants.

The drug is given intravenously at 0.1 to 0.3 mg/kg and is currently not approved for children under age 10. Lower doses should be used when the drug is combined with analgesics.

Side effects are uncommon. Transient respiratory depression can occur. Myoclonic jerking can occur and has been mistaken for seizures; using another agent, such as fentanyl, in conjunction with etomidate may prevent or minimize the jerking. Published experience with the use and safety of etomidate in the emergency department is lacking. This agent is more expensive than alternatives.

Fentanyl

Fentanyl, a synthetic opioid, is about 1,000 times as potent as meperidine. It is short acting, with a duration of action of 30 to 45 minutes. It does not cause histamine release and has minimal cardiovascular effects. It is highly lipophilic and rapidly crosses the blood–brain barrier. Redistribution then occurs into the peripheral tissues, where it is metabolized by the liver. Like all opioids, fentanyl is reversed by naloxone. It produces respiratory depression at higher doses or when combined with other central nervous system (CNS) depressants, such as midazolam or alcohol.

Fentanyl is best given in titrated intravenous doses until the desired level of sedation and analgesia is obtained. Dosing should begin at 0.5 to 1.0 mg/kg and is slowly titrated upward every 1 to 2 minutes until the desired effect is obtained. Adequate sedation and analgesia are usually obtained with doses of 2 to 3 mg/kg when fentanyl is used alone and 1 to 2 mg/kg when other medications, such as midazolam or etomidate, are used in combination. Lower doses should be used in elderly patients and when other CNS depressants may have been previously ingested. When mild sedation is needed and venous access may be difficult, such as in small children, intramuscular injections of 2 to 3 mg/kg may suffice. Having children suck on a fentanyl lollipop until the desired effect is obtained has also proved effective in sedating small children.[13] Due to its lack of amnesic effects, fentanyl is often combined with midazolam. Midazolam potentiates the effects of fentanyl as well as the potential for hypoxemia but does not appear to have any untoward cardiovascular effects.

Side effects of fentanyl include hypoxemia, apnea, vomiting, and pruritus. Hypotension is rare. Bradycardia may occur with high doses. Truncal rigidity and glottic spasm, which make ventilation difficult, are unique complications seen with doses above 10 mg/kg, or at lower doses if the drug is given rapidly. They can be reversed with naloxone or succinylcholine.[6]

Ketamine

Ketamine is an anesthetic that causes a dissociation between the thalamoneocortical and limbic systems. This, in turn, hinders the perception of visual, auditory, and painful stimuli, leaving the patient in a trancelike state.[10–12] After absorption, ketamine is rapidly distributed and taken up by the cerebral tissue. Effects are maintained until the drug redistributes into the peripheral tissues and is metabolized by the liver.

Ketamine can be given by multiple routes. An intravenous dose of 1 to 2 mg/kg, an intramuscular dose of 2 to 6 mg/kg, a rectal dose of 5 to 15 mg/kg, an oral dose of 6 to 10 mg/kg, or an intranasal dose of 6 mg/kg provides adequate sedation and analgesia.[10–12] Sedation is achieved within 1 minute when the drug is given intravenously, 5 minutes when given intramuscularly, and 5 to 20 minutes by other routes.

Ketamine's most common side effect is the emergence phenomenon, in which the patient wakes up hallucinating. This is more common in patients over age 10, females, and those with an underlying psychiatric disorder. It is less common with intramuscular injection and can be attenuated with benzodiazepines.

Laryngospasm and emesis are infrequent complications. Patients given ketamine may develop nystagmus, as well as muscular hypertonicity. The pharyngeal–laryngeal reflexes remain intact, although laryngospasm sometimes occurs.[12] Ketamine has minimal effects on oxygen delivery. Respiratory depression may occur with high doses or rapid intravenous infusion.[10] The drug stimulates tracheobronchial and salivary secretions; this effect can be minimized by the concomitant use of an anticholinergic such as atropine. Mild-to-moderate elevations in pulse rate and blood pressure may result from ketamine's ability to block the reuptake of catecholamines, especially with intravenous infusion.[12] Elevations in intracranial and cerebrospinal fluid pressure may result from the increase in blood pressure as well as cerebral vasodilatation, resulting in increased cerebral blood flow.[12] Twitching, hypertonus, and myoclonic jerking can occur and have been mistaken for seizures. Electroencephalographic studies, however, have shown that ketamine does not cause convulsions. In fact, it has anticonvulsant properties and has successfully been used to treat refractory seizures.[12]

Ketamine is contraindicated in patients with cardiovascular disease, chronic obstructive pulmonary disease, intracranial and intraocular injuries, and increased intracranial or intraocular pressures. It is not recommended for use in patients with a history of psychiatric illness and children under 3 months of age.

Methohexital

Methohexital is an ultrashort-acting barbiturate with sedative and hypnotic effects. It produces deep sedation but provides no analgesia; at lower doses, it may actually potentiate pain perception.[4] Methohexital produces a true unconscious state, which may be preferred for such procedures as cardioversion, chest tube insertion, or complicated reductions. It has a rapid onset of action of 30 to 60 seconds, a duration of action of 7 to 10 minutes, and a short recovery phase. Deep sedation is achieved with bolus doses of 1 to 2 mg/kg.[2,20] Intramuscular doses of 10 mg/kg produce effects that begin in 2 to 3 minutes and last almost 1 hour. Rectal methohexital is especially efficacious in children when a motionless state is needed. A dose of 20 to 30 mg/kg induces sleep within 10 minutes and lasts for about 45 minutes. Cardiorespiratory complications rarely occur with rectal administration.[4] Adverse reactions associated with the use of methohexital include dose-dependent respiratory depression and apnea. Oxygen desaturation is especially common when concomitant respiratory depressants are used. Hypotension is uncommon but can occur, especially in patients with hypovolemia and sepsis. It is easily corrected by giving intravenous fluids.[20] Hiccups can occur, and protective reflexes may be impaired. Methohexital induces epileptiform activity by electroencephalogram in seizure patients and should be avoided in patients with epilepsy.[14,20]

Midazolam

Midazolam is a benzodiazepine with amnesic and anxiolytic properties. At physiologic pH, the drug's open-ring structure closes, making it lipophilic and able to cross the blood–brain barrier rapidly; there it interacts with the gamma-aminobutyric acid receptors. Midazolam has a more rapid onset and shorter duration of action than diazepam and rarely causes phlebitis. Its amnesic properties also appear to be superior to those of diazepam. It is eliminated by hepatic metabolism. Like all benzodiazepines, midazolam has no analgesic properties and must be combined with analgesics such as fentanyl or morphine, or with regional or local anesthetics, when painful procedures are performed.

The intravenous dose is 0.03 to 1.0 mg/kg, with a maximum starting dose of 4 mg. Onset of sedation is within 3 to 5 minutes, and the duration of action is about 30 to 60 minutes. With intramuscular administration, the same dose is typically used, but the onset of sedation is delayed by 15 minutes.[19]

In children, oral, rectal, and intranasal routes are effective alternatives to intravenous sedation. Oral doses are 0.2 to 0.75 mg/kg, and sedation is achieved within 1 hour. Rectal administration is effective at doses of 0.3 to 0.5 mg/kg. The response by this route is variable due to the unpredictable effect of first-pass hepatic metabolism. It is not well tolerated or accepted by older children.[8] Intranasal administration can be used when an intravenous line is not needed or when sedation is necessary to establish one. Doses of 0.2 to 0.4 mg/kg result in sedation in about 10 to 15 minutes.[18]

Lower doses should be used when analgesic agents are given concomitantly, and in elderly patients. Prolonged effects may occur in elderly patients as a result of decreased metabolic clearance and decreased first-pass metabolism.

Side effects include dose-dependent hypoventilation and hypoxemia. At high doses, midazolam blunts the central respiratory center's sensitivity to hypercapnia.[19] Apnea is rare, except when other CNS depressants, such as narcotics, are used. Hypotension can also occur with high doses.

Nitrous Oxide

Nitrous oxide is a colorless gas that, when used in combination with oxygen, provides one of the most effective and safest forms of analgesia and sedation available. It has a long history of use in dentistry, with virtually no complications.[15] The gas diffuses rapidly across membranes, providing a rapid onset and elimination. An added safety feature is that the gas is self-administered, ensuring adequate but not excessive sedation. If excessive drowsiness occurs, the patient cannot hold onto the breathing apparatus, and treatment is thus discontinued. Patients continue to maintain their protective reflexes and remain awake, but their anxiety and pain perception diminish.[15] In patients having heart attacks, nitrous oxide provides excellent pain relief and has minimal effects on the cardiovascular system. The use of analgesics and anxiolytics in combination with nitrous oxide appears to synergistically enhance the level of sedation and pain control. Potential side effects also are compounded, however, and hypoxia may become a problem, especially when narcotics are used.

Nitrous oxide is given as a 50%/50% mixture with oxygen by a demand valve mask or a mouthpiece held by the patient. In mile-high altitudes such as Denver, a 70%/30% nitrous oxide–oxygen mixture is needed to obtain adequate analgesia and to compensate for the lower partial pressure of nitrous oxide at the higher altitude.[16] Patients should be allowed to breathe the gas for several minutes before the procedure, but they should be advised not to hyperventilate or take deep breaths, as this may cause light-headedness. Providing a passive environment and using suggestions appear to enhance the effects of the drug.[9,16] Scavenger devices and adequate room ventilation are used to minimize the escape of the gas into the air, preventing potential acute and chronic adverse effects on the staff.

Diffusion hypoxia is a potential complication after cessation of nitrous oxide use. It may occur when nitrous oxide is used with other analgesics, but is unlikely when nitrous oxide is the only agent used. Negative pressure may result in ear pain, and even tympanic perforation may occur in children. No long-term adverse effects have been noted from this complication.

Nitrous oxide is contraindicated in patients with altered levels of consciousness, such as in head injuries and drug or alcohol intoxication. Because the gas rapidly diffuses into gas-filled pockets, it potentially can worsen conditions such as pneumothoraces, small-bowel obstructions, decompression sickness, chronic obstructive pulmonary disease, and ear effusions.[9,16] Finally, the gas has the potential for abuse, and every effort should be made to safeguard against its abuse.

Propofol

Propofol is a very short acting sedative–hypnotic agent, with a rapid onset of action. It is currently approved for use in adults only, but its use in children is well described in the medical literature. Propofol is given intravenously as an initial bolus, followed by a continuous infusion or by intermittent bolus injections. It is metabolized by the liver and excreted by the kidneys. It is thought to have a secondary form of metabolism, because it can be used safely in patients with liver cirrhosis and renal failure. When propofol is used as the sole agent, patients fully recover from sedation 10 to 20 minutes after the infusion is discontinued.

Propofol is often used in combination with analgesics such as fentanyl and nitrous oxide. Studies comparing propofol with midazolam found them to have equivalent amnesic properties.

However, patients receiving propofol did not demonstrate the residual grogginess associated with midazolam and were discharged sooner.[5,15,17]

Sedation is usually achieved with a bolus of 1 to 2 mg/kg. This should be titrated with a slow push at a rate of 10 to 40 mg every 10 seconds until the sedative effects are achieved. A continuous infusion of 3 to 6 mg/kg/h (50 to 100 mg/kg/min) is then titrated to the desired level of sedation.[15,17] Alternatively, intermittent boluses of 25 to 50 mg can be used to maintain sedation in adults. Healthy adults may require higher doses; lower doses should be used when sedating elderly patients or when coadministering intravenous analgesics.

The major side effect noted with propofol has been transient apnea, which occurs when the bolus is infused rapidly, or when propofol is given in conjunction with opioids. Hypotension and bradycardia may also occur but are easily reversed with fluids or by terminating the infusion. Propofol may cause transient pain on injection, but this can be prevented by giving lidocaine (1 mL of a 1% solution) first.

References

1. American Academy of Pediatrics. Guidelines for monitoring and management of pediatric patients during and after sedation for diagnostic and therapeutic procedures. *Pediatrics* 1992;89:1110.
2. Bauman LA, Kish I, Baumann RC, et al. Pediatric sedation with analgesia. *Am J Emerg Med* 1999;17(1):1.
3. Bergen JM, Smith DC. A review of etomidate for rapid sequence intubation in the emergency department. *J Emerg Med* 1997;15(2):221.
4. Berman D, Graber D. Sedation and analgesia. *Emerg Med Clin North Am* 1992;10:691.
5. Chin NM, Tai HY, Chin MK. Intravenous sedation for upper gastrointestinal endoscopy: midazolam versus propofol. *Singapore Med J* 1992;33:478.
6. Chudnofsky CR, Wright SW, Dronen SC, et al. The safety of fentanyl use in the emergency department. *Ann Emerg Med* 1989;18:635.
7. Cote CJ. Sedation for the pediatric patient. *Pediatr Clin North Am* 1994;41:31.
8. Cote CJ, Strafford MA. *The principles of pediatric sedation.* Boston: Tufts University School of Medicine, 1998.
9. Gamis A, Knapp J, Glenski J, et al. Nitrous oxide analgesia in a pediatric emergency department. *Ann Emerg Med* 1989;18:177.
10. Green SM, Rothrock SG, Harris T, et al. Intravenous ketamine for pediatric sedation in the emergency department: safety profile with 156 cases. *Acad Emerg Med* 1998;5(10):971.
11. Green SM, Nakamura R, Johnson NE. Ketamine sedation for pediatric procedures: part 1, a prospective series. *Ann Emerg Med* 1990;19:1024.
12. Green SM, Nakamura R, Johnson NE. Ketamine sedation for pediatric procedures: part 2, review and implications. *Ann Emerg Med* 1990;19:1033.
13. Krauss B, Shannon M, Damian F, et al. *Guidelines for pediatric sedation*. Dallas: American College of Emergency Physicians, 1995.
14. Lerman B, et al. A prospective evaluation of the safety and efficacy of methohexital in the emergency department. *Am J Emerg Med* 1996;14(4):351.
15. Stephens AJ, Sapsford DJ, Curzon ME. Intravenous sedation for handicapped dental patients: a clinical trial of midazolam and propofol. *Br Dent J* 1993;175:20.
16. Stewart R. Nitrous oxide sedation/analgesia in emergency medicine. *Ann Emerg Med* 1985;14:139.
17. Swanson ER, Seaberg DC, Mathias S. The use of propofol for sedation in the emergency department. *Acad Emerg Med* 1996;3(3):234.
18. Theroux MC, West DW, Corddry DH, et al. Efficacy of intranasal midazolam in facilitating suturing of lacerations in preschool children in the emergency department. *Pediatrics* 1993;91:624.
19. Wright SW, Chudnofsky CR, Dronen SC, et al. Comparison of midazolam and diazepam for conscious sedation in the emergency department. *Ann Emerg Med* 1993;22:201.
20. Zink B, Darfler K, Salluzzo R, et al. The efficacy and safety of methohexital in the emergency department. *Ann Emerg Med* 1991;20:1293.

CHAPTER 414
Monitoring Techniques

Alan Jon Smally and C. J. Biddle

Monitoring in the emergency department and prehospital arena is part of the initial and ongoing assessment of each patient. The goals are to recognize and quantify the degree of illness and of any change in condition. The data provided become part of the overall clinical picture, which guides initiation, titration, and changes in all aspects of care.

ELECTROCARDIOGRAPH

Although initially developed in coronary care units, bedside electrocardiograph (ECG) monitoring has become the standard of care in the emergency department for many types of patients. Obviously, any patient suspected of having acute cardiac disease or whose general illness could affect an underlying cardiac condition should be monitored. In addition, any patient whose rate, rhythm, or ECG complex could serve as an indicator of change in disease process or therapy should be monitored.

The standard lead positions from the 12-lead ECG are distal on the extremities, whereas ECG monitor leads are placed on the outer chest or shoulders and the upper abdomen. Hence, monitor leads correspond inexactly to the standard limb leads (I, II, III) and the augmented limb leads (aVR, aVL, aVF).

ECG monitoring was designed initially to determine rhythm and rate, and this continues to be its most secure use. Conduction abnormalities such as first-degree, second-degree, and third-degree blocks can be determined in many cases, as can the abnormalities of the intervals (PR, QT, QRS). ECG monitoring alone can indicate conditions such as dysrhythmias, hyperkalemia, and drug overdoses and their effects that require urgent therapy. A single-lead ECG monitor is less useful for determining the etiology of wide-complex tachycardia. ECG monitoring is not a substitute for bedside attendance by the physician or nurse, and it does not replace the 12-lead ECG. Even with multilead machines, a monitor strip should not be used to diagnose myocardial infarction, although change in a given ST segment may be an indication of ongoing ischemia.

ECG monitoring equipment is expensive. Although equipment comparison is beyond the scope of this discussion, any purchase decision should be made only after detailed equipment analysis and careful comparison shopping.

To be effective, ECG monitors require continuing upkeep and proper usage. Monitors should not have their alarms turned off. In most cases, the monitors should be hard-wired from patient rooms to a central location. Current central station computerized monitoring systems have algorithms that detect arrhythmias more accurately than do human observers. When computerized arrhythmia detection is not available, the use of additional "slave" telemetry monitors near the charting areas can be helpful.

Emergency department patients are often diaphoretic and combative, and are continuously moved around for studies, examinations, and x-rays. Artifact and wandering baseline can be minimized by proper lead attachment. Bony prominences should be avoided. The skin should be properly prepared and shaved when necessary. Poor electrical contact produces poor-quality tracings and should be minimized. The skin can be cleansed with alcohol after shaving, and a dry towel or gauze used to further prepare the site. In difficult cases, it may be necessary to use tincture of benzoin or to further tape down a lead.

A common problem is that ignored alarms trigger reams of paper printouts containing artifacts until no paper remains in the monitor. New technologies have been developed to allow cancellation of 60-cycle interference, baseline wander, and muscle and movement artifact, and computerized storage of rhythm recordings.

Once the leads are in place, a lead that adequately shows the P wave, the QRS, and the T wave should be chosen for monitoring. The gain control should be adjusted so that there is adequate QRS volume to allow sensing of the rate without undercounting or overtriggering.

To detect intermittent ischemia, the use of automated serial ECGs and continuous ST-segment monitoring is becoming more widespread. This is used both to diagnose a cardiac etiology for chest pain and to monitor patients with known coronary disease. Systems are available that monitor and save, or print, up to 12-lead ECGs. The emergency physician should not completely rely on computer detection of ST-segment changes, but should periodically review ECGs. Depending on the software, changes of less than 1 mm, for instance, may not trigger as an event, yet may be apparent to the physician.[5]

When continuous 12-lead cardiac monitoring is not being done, repetition of 12-lead ECGs is appropriate. For consistency, the stick-on patch type of chest lead sensor is best, because repeat ECGs are done with the knowledge that there is no lead placement change. Also, a review can determine that the leads are indeed in the correct interspace.

Two other techniques not in general use are signal averaging and heart rate variability monitoring. The averaging method of ECG determination uses filtering and the averaging of multiple samples to eliminate random background noise. Ventricular late potentials (signals at the end of the QRS complex or in the ST segment) are determined that identify regions of delayed conduction. These late potentials are rarely found in normal people and, when found in patients with myocardial infarction, correlate highly with the risk of ventricular dysrhythmias and ventricular tachycardia. Heart rate variability monitoring is a computer-generated measure of autonomic balance. In patients that have had a myocardial infarction, abnormal variability has correlated with a risk of sudden death. The use of late potentials and heart rate variability testing in patients with syncope of unknown etiology may be useful in determining fitness for discharge.[6]

BLOOD PRESSURE

The physicist defines *pressure* as force per unit area. Blood is a liquid (i.e., it is noncompressible), and to achieve pressure determination, a system that converts energy from one type to another must be interposed between patient and provider. Such couplings provide for *indirect* measurement (even though we frequently use the term *direct* when using intraarterial catheters), which inevitably results in imperfect representations.

Auscultation

The sphygmomanometer is the most common tool used to measure blood pressure. It uses the traditional Riva-Rocci (auscultatory) method, which consists of determining the onset (systolic pressure) and disappearance (diastolic pressure) of the Korotkoff sounds (dating back to before 1905). To maintain its sensitivity, the pressure release should occur at a rate of about 3 mm Hg per second, and the stethoscope should be placed on the skin with enough pressure to create a seal just under or slightly beyond the cuff.

Five phases of Korotkoff sounds result from turbulent flow of blood traversing the externally compressed vessel (Table 414.1). Classically, the phase 5 disappearance of tones has been used to define diastole. However, muffling values are repeatedly more consistent among different recorders, particularly in mild hypertension. Auscultatory techniques are unreliable in low-flow states, do not determine mean arterial pressure, are intermittent, and are associated with subjective variation. In aortic regurgitation or thyrotoxicosis, phase 4 persists to almost 0 mm Hg, so the transition to phase 4 is used. Many other variables impact on blood pressure measurement accuracy.[9]

The historic standard for blood pressure measurement, the mercury sphygmomanometer, is being phased out of most hospitals because of potential toxicity associated with mercury exposure should it break or leak. The standard measuring device is now the aneroid manometer. This device is portable but is far more susceptible to calibration problems, particularly when bumped, dropped, or mishandled. It must be inspected and calibrated periodically (every 1 to 6 months) against a standard.[1] The interval of inspection should be lowered until the point at which most devices are within 3 to 5 mm of standard.

In determining the appropriate cuff size, a good rule of thumb is that the bladder length is of minor clinical significance as long as at least half the arm circumference is covered by the bladder. Because most of the pressure generated by cuff inflation is concentrated on a short portion of the underlying artery, a too-narrow cuff must be blown up to a falsely high pressure, and a too-wide cuff gives a falsely low reading. The cuff width should be about 20% greater than the diameter of the arm. Standard bladder sizes relative to width and length are shown in Table 414.2. If the cuff's markings indicate a correct fit, it is usually satisfactory.

Oscillation

The modern oscillometric technique (e.g., Critikon's Dinamap) is based on the detection of vascular diameter changes over the course of the cardiac cycle. Energy transmitted from the artery to the wall of a pneumatic cuff displaces and changes cuff volume. This intracuff pressure swing is electronically amplified and processed as the cuff is deflated. These oscillations peak near the mean arterial pressure.

Automated devices are convenient, but erroneous readings can occur during dysrhythmias and in low-output states, when accurate readings are critical. Complications such as vascular and nerve injury and bleeding can occur if cycled too frequently, particularly in patients with coagulopathy or those undergoing thrombolytic therapy. Users are advised to check the function of

TABLE 414.1. Korotkoff Sounds

Phase 1	Initial loud, clear, snapping tones
Phase 2	Continuous sequence of murmurs
Phase 3	Murmurs disappear; a less-marked tone develops
Phase 4	Muffling of the tones occurs
Phase 5	Tones disappear

TABLE 414.2. Standard Bladder Sizes Relative to Width and Length

Newborn arm	2.5 × 5.0 cm
Infant arm	5.0 × 11.9 cm
Child arm	9.4 × 21.0 cm
Adult arm	12.5 × 23.0 cm
Adult thigh	18 × 35 cm

the devices frequently by ensuring that the cuff bladder completely deflates between cycles.

Doppler Ultrasound

These devices detect sound waves that reflect off moving arterial walls. They are noninvasive, highly reliable, and accurate. The detection device must be placed directly over the artery; even slight movement or malpositioning leads to erroneous results. Restless, combative, or uncooperative patients are not good candidates for this approach.

Arterial Unloading or Volume Clamping/Counterpulsation

In arterial unloading, the volume of the arterial segment beneath the cuff is held constant—its outflow is mechanically obstructed by the cuff. The pressure required to "unload" the artery during the cardiac cycle is determined. The cuff is inflated and then gradually deflated, and a small infrared light directed across a digital artery determines oscillations photoplethysmographically. Maximal oscillations occur at the mean arterial pressure, at which time the cuff pressure is automatically adjusted as it senses further oscillations. A waveform is displayed as the device adjusts upward (sensing systolic pressure) and downward (sensing diastolic pressure). The device is susceptible to hydrostatic pressure as the hand and arm are moved above or below heart level. Erroneous readings may result if the arm is moved or if the extremity is not positioned at heart level.

Arterial Tonometry

A small sensor is applied over the radial artery with sufficient pressure to cause partial flattening of the artery. Several tiny transducers are built into the device so that at least one will be optimally positioned. With careful positioning, wall tension forces are not transmitted to the sensor and only intraluminal pressure is transferred to the transducer, producing a continuous pressure curve. The device is automatically recalibrated every few minutes and requires a palpable pulse. Use is likely to be widespread in the near future.

Intraarterial Catheterization

The advantages of this technique are that it is continuous, errors are generally easily detected, it provides access to blood sampling, and reliable pressures are obtained in hypotensive states. Also, various secondary information can be inferred (sometimes only crudely) by inspecting the waveform (Table 414.3).

Intraarterial approaches use saline-filled tubing that transmits the energy of the pulse wave to a transducer, which converts it to a voltage change. This change is subsequently amplified, filtered, and displayed as an arterial pressure tracing. The radial artery at the wrist is the most common site of cannulation, although, in hypotensive patients, larger arteries (e.g., femoral) may prove more accessible.

Although it is common to test for collateral circulation when cannulating the radial artery, most vascular complications related to radial artery manipulations result from embolic phenomena; therefore, the utility of such tests has been questioned.

TABLE 414.3. Data That Can Be Derived from Arterial Waveform

Heart rate
Stroke volume and cardiac output
Myocardial contractility
Resistance and compliance
Cardiac dysrhythmias

Adding an automatic recorder to blood pressure–measuring instruments can be invaluable. A formal, exact record of such data can be placed in the patient's permanent record.

Noninvasive Measurement of Cardiac Output

The noninvasive determination of cardiac output by either or both of two new methods—impedance cardiac output[13] and stroke distance[12]—may move to the emergency department. Impedance cardiac output determines cardiac output, with the use of electrodes placed on the neck and lower thorax, by passing a current through the patient, which is analyzed in conjunction with the patient's heart rate. Stroke distance monitoring determines blood flow by placing a Doppler ultrasound in the suprasternal notch and measuring stroke distance per cardiac contraction. Preliminary use of both of these methodologies is promising.

Central Venous Pressure Measurement

Although central venous access is often used for drug and fluid therapy, the benefit of central venous pressure (CVP) monitoring in the emergency department continues to be controversial. The CVP depends on many factors, including cardiac rhythm, intrathoracic pressure changes, tricuspid valve function, alteration in right ventricular compliance, and even the function of the lung and the left side of the heart.

A true CVP is determined by placing a catheter in the superior vena cava and measuring the height of a column of water above the presumed level of the right atrium. The right atrium is situated at the midaxillary line in a supine patient and is about 5 cm below the sternal angle in any semirecumbent position.

A noninvasive CVP determination is optimally made by measuring the height of pulsation above the sternal angle (plus 5 cm to approximate the right atrial pressure) of the column of blood in the internal jugular vein as the patient's torso is elevated. Unfortunately, this true CVP determination is often difficult to perform, and visualization of the external jugular veins or veins of the hand is substituted. These noncentral veins, however, collapse on entering the thorax and may provide a falsely high CVP determination.

Until relatively recently, invasive CVP monitoring was a standard of care in states of shock. A catheter threaded from an internal jugular vein, subclavian vein, or antecubital veins into the central circulation was used to measure pressure in the superior vena cava. It served as a measure of right atrial pressure and was thought to correlate with left ventricular end-diastolic pressure or preload. Except in young, otherwise healthy patients without acute cardiac or pulmonary dysfunction who are being evaluated for hypovolemic shock, however, the CVP is potentially misleading as an indicator of left-sided preload. Increased CVP can indicate dysfunction of the right side of the heart itself or by pericardial or pulmonary artery pressure elevation. Thus, in patients with cardiac tamponade, constrictive pericarditis, or massive pulmonary emboli, CVP is almost always elevated above 20 cm of water. Elevated pressure may also be seen in tricuspid stenosis or right atrial myxoma and superior vena cava syndrome.

In acute situations in which the physician needs to know only whether the CVP is significantly elevated, the neck veins and hand veins can be used to determine an increased CVP. In the patient with hypotension, significant elevation of the CVP can be confirmed by the presence of distended external jugular veins or the failure of the veins on the dorsum of the hand to collapse when the hand is raised 15 cm above the sternal angle (the

Jacobs test). In an appropriate clinical setting, this simple method of monitoring allows the physician to determine appropriate testing and therapy.

CVP also can be measured in the inferior vena cava, or the common iliac vein, with a standard 15- to 20-cm-length femoral line. It may not give accurate measurements when abdominal conditions such as tense ascites, peritonitis, or bowel obstruction are present.

CVP trends can be more helpful than a single reading. Measurements should be repeated in the same position, using a zero-point skin mark at the level of the right atrium.

OXYGENATION

Pulse Oximetry

Measurement of oxygen saturation by the pulse oximeter (PO) has become the "fifth vital sign." Although clinical estimation of oxygenation can be inaccurate, pulse oximetry, with some exceptions, is a valid and reliable measurement. When the oximeter is properly sensing vascular pulsation, the reading is generally accurate, even in states of low flow, hypothermia, and anemia. In profound hypoxemia, the reading is inexact but is low, not falsely near normal; when the saturation is less than 90%, the correlation with $Pa{O_2}$ may be inaccurate due to shifts in the oxyhemoglobin disassociation curve.[2] Although the PO can be used for both oximetric (oxygen saturation) and plethysmographic (pulse or circulation) monitoring, it monitors pulse, not electrical rhythm, and is not a substitute for cardiac monitoring.

Using 660-nm (red) and 940-nm (infrared) wavelength light, the PO analyzes the pulse-added component of absorbance at the two wavelengths and produces a ratio that is empirically related to hemoglobin saturation with oxygen ($Sa{O_2}$ or $Sp{O_2}$). Interpretation of displayed values, using the standard oxyhemoglobin dissociation curve, allows for estimation of $Pa{O_2}$ (e.g., $Sp{O_2}$ of 75 = $Pa{O_2}$ 40 mm Hg; $Sp{O_2}$ of 90 = $Pa{O_2}$ of 60 mm Hg). Large changes in $Pa{O_2}$ may occur before any change is noted by the PO on the long, flat portion of the oxyhemoglobin dissociation curve.

Table 414.4 lists factors that may cause the PO to provide specious information; if not taken into account, these may lead to an incorrect diagnosis or management. The major complications related to the use of the PO are a rare incidence of burns, pressure necrosis, and the potential for overly aggressive interventions in the presence of a false alarm or misleadingly low reading.

Cerebral Oximetry

In critical patients with peripheral circulatory failure, conventional PO often does not produce valid readings. A new technique, called cerebral oximetry, is being studied.[7] The device includes a light source placed lateral to a frontal sinus on the forehead and sensors that detect light emissions that measure frontal cortex oxygen saturation. The value correlates best with mixed venous oxygen saturation and gives a measure of circulatory and oxygenating adequacy.

VENTILATION

Respiratory Rate

The respiratory system works in concert with the cardiovascular system to change the $P{O_2}$ and the $P{CO_2}$. In the normal person at rest, diaphragmatic motion is all that is required. With obstruction or increasing respiratory needs, the abdominal muscles and the chest wall muscles are used. The anteroposterior diameter of the chest can be increased by 20% with the use of the intercostal, the sternocleidomastoid, and the anterior serrati and scaleni muscles. The use of these accessory muscles can be monitored as a measure of respiratory distress. In the respiratory center of the medulla, chemoreceptors monitor pH, an indirect measure of $P{CO_2}$, because hydrogen ions do not cross the blood–brain barrier, but carbon dioxide is freely permeable. Although the overwhelming respiratory drive is an increased $P{CO_2}$, peripheral O_2 oxygen receptors in the carotid and aortic bodies also signal the medulla to increase the respiratory rate in the presence of hypoxemia.

Classically, respiratory rate has been determined by counting chest wall expansions for 15 seconds and multiplying by 4, or, in more diligent observers, for 30 seconds or a minute. This is difficult to do, particularly when the patient is talking, and studies have repeatedly shown the inaccuracy of this measurement. There are mechanical methods of determining respiratory rate and pattern; there are even methods of continuous monitoring of tidal volume by electronic devices. Devices such as the impedance pneumograph, mercury-in-Silastic strain gauges, magnetometers, and respiratory inductive plethysmography may be used.

Capnometry

Carbon dioxide concentrations can be measured by a capnometer, graphically displayed as a capnogram, and recorded by a capnograph. The closer to the alveolus that one samples, the more accurately the capnogram indicates what is in the pulmonary venous blood (and thus the arterial blood). Intratracheal sampling is rare for technical reasons, but sampling from a point as close to the patient's mouth as possible, at the end of exhalation, will yield clinically useful information. In the intubated patient, sampling is best performed at the proximal end of the endotracheal tube with a T-piece.

Sampling by nasal cannula in nonintubated patients is also generally reliable. Although there are different approaches, most capnometers use infrared light, where asymmetric, polyatomic molecules such as carbon dioxide absorb specific wavelengths. The discussion here assumes that capnographic analysis is occurring close to, but not within, the trachea.

Emergency departments should generally use capnometers that can generate a waveform; otherwise, important clinical information will be lost. Those that report only the highest (end-tidal level) and lowest (inspired minimal level) carbon dioxide values are much less useful. Transcutaneous capnography may become useful in the emergency department in the future, but it currently is not recommended in adults, although it is more promising in younger children.

TABLE 414.4. Limitations of Pulse Oximetry

Low signal-to-noise ratio (too weak a signal or too much electrical interference)		
Probe position ("central" sites—ear, lip, tongue—may be more accurate than peripheral ones)		
Carboxy- and methemoglobin yield falsely high oxygen saturations		
Probe motion	Low perfusion states	MRI
Vasoconstrictors	Electrocautery	Nail polish
Dysrhythmias (abnormal pulsations may not be detected)		Strong or flickering ambient light

The capnogram can be divided into several distinct components, each of which provides valuable information (Fig. 414.1). Phase I (A to B) reflects initial expiration: The dead-space gas, virtually devoid of carbon dioxide, gives way to the sharply upstroking portion of the capnogram (phase II, B to C), which contains carbon dioxide–laden gas mixing with dead-space air. The morphology of this portion of the curve reflects the expiratory time and the evenness of ventilation. When this phase has a gradual rise, obstruction is suggested. Phase III (C to D) is the plateau of the curve: Alveolar gas is being sampled, with point D representing the end-tidal or alveolar concentration of carbon dioxide ($ETco_2$). The phase from points D to E represents inspiration of carbon dioxide–free gas. Unless rebreathing of exhaled carbon dioxide occurs, this should be a precipitous fall to baseline.

If ventilation and perfusion in the lungs are well matched, carbon dioxide readily diffuses across the capillary–alveolar membrane, and if no sampling errors are present, the $ETco_2$ is an excellent approximation of $Paco_2$. In the perfectly healthy person, there is a very small gradient; as ventilation–perfusion mismatch develops, this gradient increases.

Many conditions influence $ETco_2$ and must be carefully considered to optimize the utility of $ETco_2$ monitoring (Table 414.5). The $ETco_2$ may be so suspect in many emergency department patients as to be virtually worthless. In these instances, it is better to monitor the arterial blood gas analysis.

Capnography is valuable in assessing the proper placement of an endotracheal tube (differentiating esophageal from tracheal intubation), the adequacy of ventilation, alterations in dead space and perfusion, the rebreathing of carbon dioxide, and the effectiveness of chest compressions during cardiopulmonary resuscitation.[14] However, the best overall monitor of gas exchange is auscultation of the depth, rate, and clarity of gaseous exchange and observation of the level of consciousness.

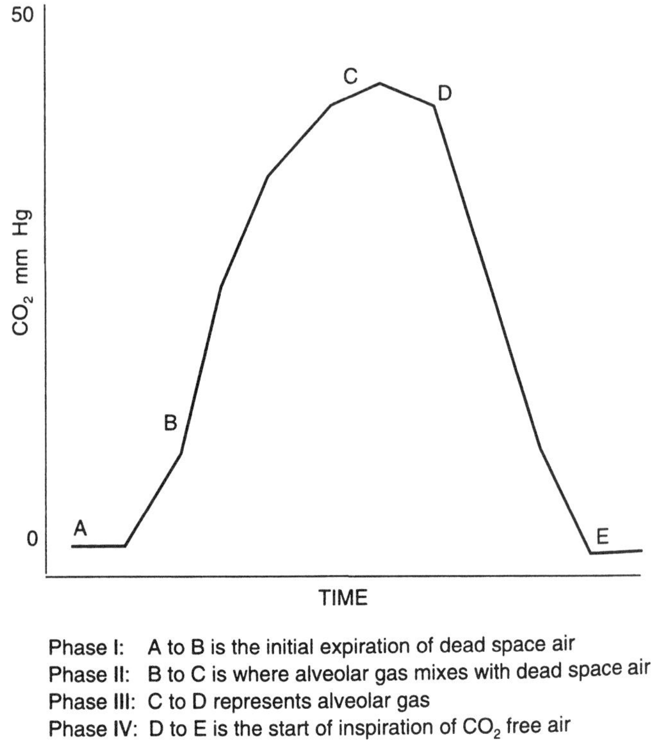
50
0
CO_2 mm Hg
TIME
A
B
C
D
E
Phase I: A to B is the initial expiration of dead space air
Phase II: B to C is where alveolar gas mixes with dead space air
Phase III: C to D represents alveolar gas
Phase IV: D to E is the start of inspiration of CO_2 free air

Figure 414.1. The component of the capnogram.

TABLE 414.5. Clinical Scenarios Influencing $ETco_2$

FACTORS THAT DECREASE $ETco_2$	FACTORS THAT INCREASE $ETco_2$
Embolic phenomena (e.g., air, thrombus, fat)	Fever or increased metabolism
Cardiac arrest	Hypoventilation–CNS depression
Shock or other low perfusion states	Hypoventilation–inadequate mechanical ventilation
Chronic obstructive pulmonary disease	Hypoventilation–CNS disease
Ventilator support disconnection	Hypoventilation–neuromuscular disease
Hypothermia or decreased metabolism	
Hyperventilation	
Mechanical factors where room air is entrained	

Pulmonary Function Tests

Monitoring of pulmonary airflow is becoming a standard of care. In asthmatic patients, the forced expiratory volume in 1 second (FEV_1), forced vital capacity (FVC), and peak expiratory flow rate (PEFR) have been shown to predict need for admission after treatment in the emergency department.[4] There are many ways of determining air flow, including spirometers, pneumotachygraphs, peak flowmeters, and minipeak flowmeters, but no one device is markedly superior to the others.

Measurements should be taken with the patient in the standing position, with three or more attempts made to obtain the best value. Current recommendations include measurement of peak flow or FEV_1 on presentation, periodically during treatment, and before decision to admit or discharge. If the patient is adequately oxygenated (pulse oximeter reading greater than 90%), has a normal mental status, is receiving maximal (steroid and beta-agonist) therapy, and is improving subjectively and on pulmonary examination, arbitrary pulmonary flow assessment is not mandated. Conversely, if there is any question of admission versus discharge or response to therapy, it may be useful (Table 414.6).

TABLE 414.6. Pulmonary Airflow Assessment Guidelines for Asthma Management

Patient Status	PEFR or FEV_1 (% of Known.Best Value or of Predicted Value)
INITIAL ASSESSMENT	
Mild asthma	80%–90% predicted
Moderate asthma	50%–80% predicted
Severe asthma	<25%–50% predicted (adults) <50% predicted (children)
Life-threatening asthma	<25% predicted
RESPONSE TO THERAPY	
Good	≥70% predicted
Incomplete	>50% but <70% predicted
Poor	≤50% but >25% predicted
Respiratory failure	≤25% predicted

Data from National Asthma Education Program. *Guidelines for the diagnosis and management of asthma.* Bethesda, MD: US Dept. of Health and Human Services, 1997 NIH Publication No. 97-4051.

GASTRIC INTRAMUCOSAL pH

An innovation in the monitoring of oxygen delivery and use in critically ill patients is the measurement of gastric intramucosal pH, or gastric tonometry.[7] A small catheter is placed into the stomach by the nasal route. Saline is used to distend a silicone balloon, which is left in contact with the gastric mucosal surface until equilibration of P_{CO_2} occurs. The P_{CO_2} value is measured and the Henderson-Hasselbach equation is used to compute the gastric intramucosal pH. This value is an indirect measure of splanchnic perfusion and oxygen extraction. A value below 7.35 suggests inadequate blood flow and oxygen delivery to the gut, serving as an indirect measure of systemic hypoperfusion.

Multiple organ system failure can be viewed as a cascade of events augmented by hypoperfusion of the gut, allowing transudation of both toxins and organisms. Thus, low values indicate the need for intensive therapy and, perhaps, for invasive hemodynamic monitoring.

Although gastric tonometry is not yet used in emergency departments, its prognostic and therapeutic implications and its minimal invasiveness may lead to its future use.

TEMPERATURE

Fever is part of an adaptive response provoked by both endogenous and exogenous mediators. The entire system is designed to defeat microbial invasion. Studies in nonhuman mammals and invertebrates have shown that artificially elevated temperature, in and of itself, reduces the morbidity and mortality of infectious diseases.

In most situations, knowing the exact temperature is unnecessary. Exceptions include hypothermia (therapy varies with the degree of hypothermia) and extreme hyperthermia (temperatures of greater than 107°F can be injurious). Generally, we need to know only whether the patient is euthermic, hypothermic, or febrile. A rectal temperature above 100.4°F (38°C) is arbitrarily defined as "fever."

To determine the accuracy of any method of temperature measurement, values obtained should be compared with true "core" temperature. By convention, this is measured in the pulmonary artery. The esophageal temperature is a close proxy. Rectal temperatures have long been the clinical standard of measurement. They tend to be 0.51°C higher than core values. With rapid temperature changes, the temperature of stool in the rectum lags behind core temperature. Thus, in moderately to severely hypothermic patients, measurement is best accomplished with an esophageal probe.

Although, traditionally, temperatures were taken with glass, mercury-filled thermometers, current electronic devices achieve suitable accuracy and have essentially replaced them. Axillary and oral sites have been used but are much less precise. Patient and environmental factors (smoking, mouth breathing, cool or hot liquid ingestion, inability to hold the thermometer in place) may alter the oral temperature. Except in newborns, the axillary temperature has been largely discarded.

Tympanic thermometry has revolutionized temperature measurement.[11] The ear canal and tympanic membrane receive blood supply from the external carotid; the hypothalamus (the brain's thermostat) receives its blood supply from the internal carotid. Thus, the common carotid artery provides both blood supplies, and, by inference, tympanic membrane temperature is another measure of core temperature. The measurement is taken by infrared sensors contained in a device that is aimed into the ear canal at the tympanic membrane. A posterior–superior tug on the pinna gives a more accurate "view" of the tympanic membrane. Most current instruments measure the core temperature and, either automatically or by a switch, add an "offset" to produce a rectal equivalent temperature. As more clinicians become familiar with the method, published studies and algorithms will use the direct reading of tympanic core temperature, and "offsets" will be discarded.

Although the evidence is conflicting, many studies have documented the accuracy of these devices in large groups of patients. Temperatures in newborns and infants less than 3 to 6 months old should probably not be measured with ear thermometry, because the correlation with rectal temperatures in published reports is not convincing, and implications of small temperature differences in defining *fever* are more significant clinically. Extremes of ambient temperature may produce false readings. In most other groups of patients, including those with otitis media and cerumen impaction, results are acceptable.

Many clinicians have the impression, through anecdotal experience, that tympanic thermometry is not accurate. This conflict with the literature is probably based on the fact that, in many emergency departments, the initial tympanic temperature is now taken at triage, and it may be an hour or more before the clinician examines the patient. During examination, the patient may "feel warm," or the total impression, based on presumed diagnosis, laboratory studies, and so forth, is that the patient should be febrile. If a rectal temperature is then obtained, whether normal or elevated, it is assumed to be the gold standard and correct. Remember that neither method is perfect.

We recommend, in patients over 6 months old, tympanic thermometry as the preferred method of screening. Specific clinical situations may dictate repeating the tympanic temperature or obtaining the temperature by rectum or other core site.

A new method of temperature assessment being used in operating rooms—deep-body thermometry—may become useful in the emergency department.[10] This method uses a 2.5-cm disk (placed on the forehead, chest, or other location) that "nulls thermal flux" and measures "deep-body" temperatures. Preliminary work shows it to closely approximate core temperature as measured in the esophagus. Disadvantages apparent at this time include a 15-minute equilibration time and the lack of confirmatory studies.

NEUROMUSCULAR PARALYSIS

Muscle relaxants facilitate endotracheal intubation, assist in the application of controlled ventilation, and allow performance of diagnostic and therapeutic interventions. Nondepolarizing muscle relaxants (e.g., pancuronium, vecuronium, atracurium) lend themselves well to titration on the basis of both clinical observation and neuromuscular function monitoring. Various strategies are available, but train-of-four (TOF) monitoring may be the most useful technique because it is simple to perform and easy to interpret. Mechanomyography (palpation of the number and strength of evoked responses) has been the standard method, although its crudeness has led to great interest in alternative methods. Electromyography (the evoked compound action potential) reflects electrical changes in the excitable membranes of one or more muscles.

Inexpensive, portable, pocket-sized neuromuscular function monitors are available. TOF stimulation involves four electrical impulses delivered over a 2-second period; the degree of blockade can be gauged by relating the height of the fourth twitch to that of the first, or by counting the number of evoked responses present in any single train (Fig. 414.2). Generally, most proce-

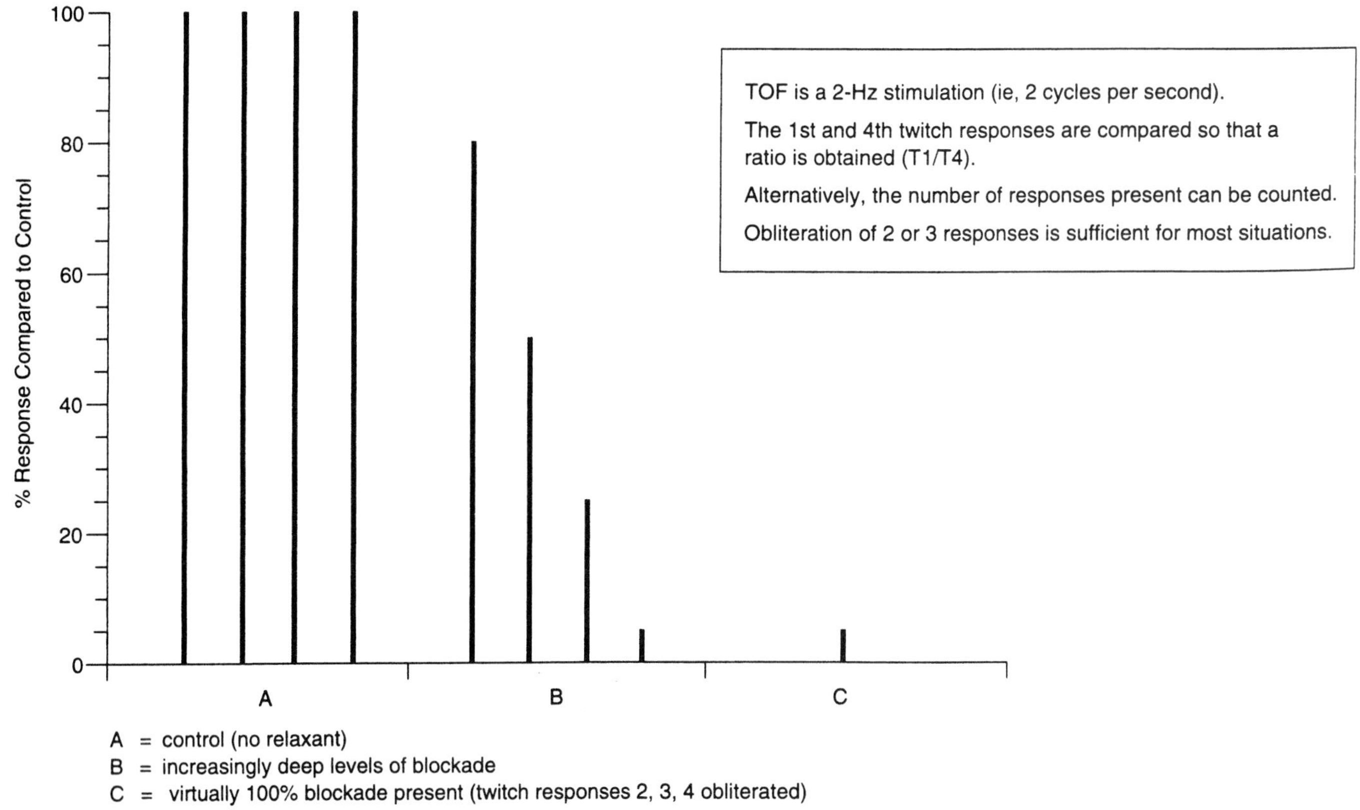
% Response Compared to Control
100
80
60
40
20
0
A
B
C
TOF is a 2-Hz stimulation (ie, 2 cycles per second).
The 1st and 4th twitch responses are compared so that a ratio is obtained (T1/T4).
Alternatively, the number of responses present can be counted.
Obliteration of 2 or 3 responses is sufficient for most situations.
A = control (no relaxant)
B = increasingly deep levels of blockade
C = virtually 100% blockade present (twitch responses 2, 3, 4 obliterated)

Figure 414.2. Train-of-four monitoring.

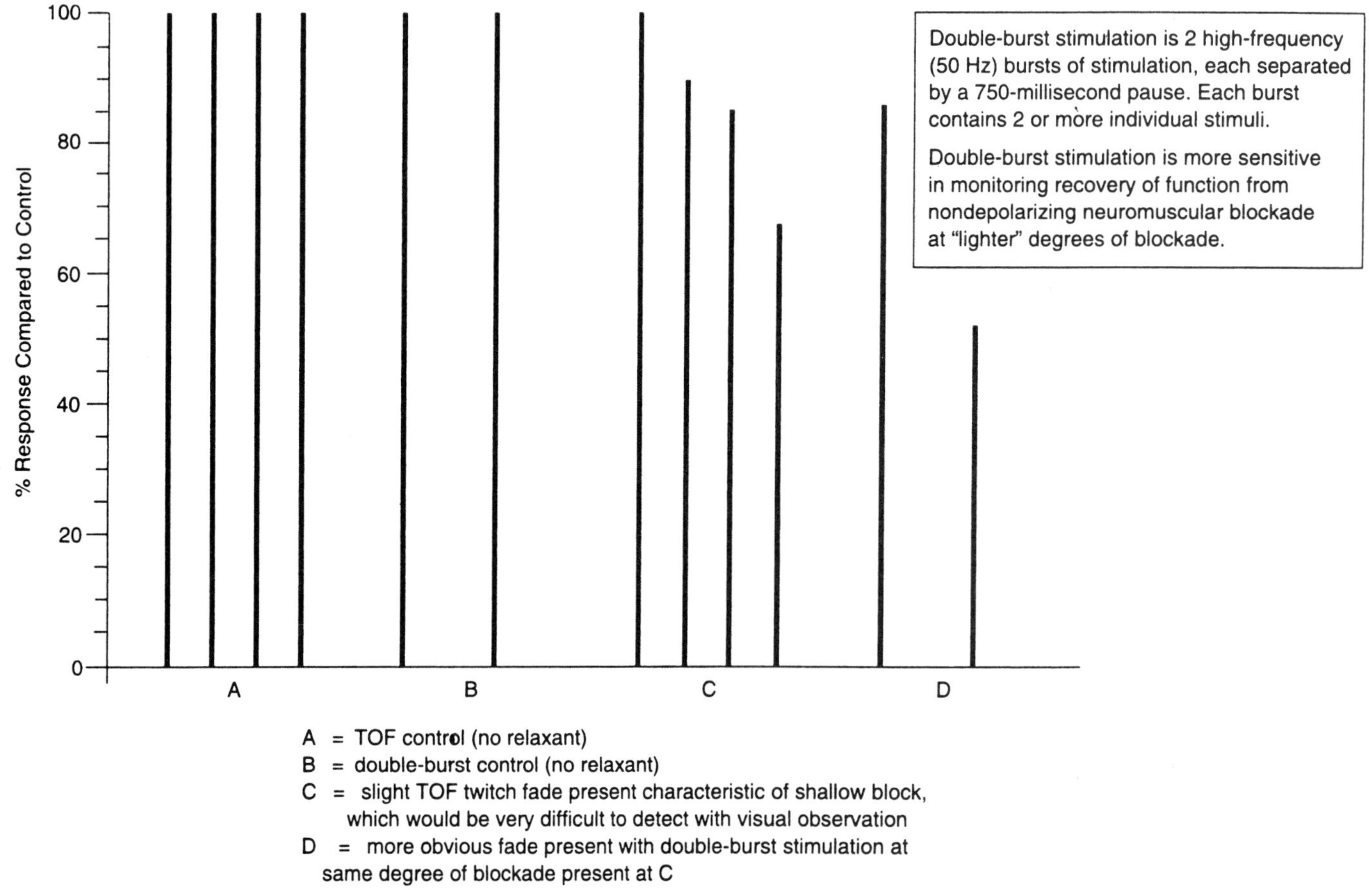
% Response Compared to Control
100
80
60
40
20
0
A
B
C
D
Double-burst stimulation is 2 high-frequency (50 Hz) bursts of stimulation, each separated by a 750-millisecond pause. Each burst contains 2 or more individual stimuli.
Double-burst stimulation is more sensitive in monitoring recovery of function from nondepolarizing neuromuscular blockade at "lighter" degrees of blockade.
A = TOF control (no relaxant)
B = double-burst control (no relaxant)
C = slight TOF twitch fade present characteristic of shallow block, which would be very difficult to detect with visual observation
D = more obvious fade present with double-burst stimulation at same degree of blockade present at C

Figure 414.3. Double-burst stimulation.

dures can be accomplished by titrating to the point at which the last two or three evoked responses are obliterated; this allows reasonable prospects for reversibility (with a combination of anticholinesterase and an anticholinergic), should the need arise. Overdosing and underdosing are thus minimized.

Double-burst stimulation has been developed to overcome some of the manual and visual difficulties associated with TOF interpretation (Fig. 414.3). In this technique, a pattern of stimulation resulting in only two evoked responses stresses the neuromuscular junction in a manner similar to that of TOF; however, double-burst stimulation appears easier to interpret. The two evoked responses are compared, rather than the first and fourth.[3] Double-burst stimulation seems best suited to evaluating the degree of residual blockade rather than as a guide to drug administration.

Patients should never be extubated after having received a muscle relaxant unless recovery is documented (as described previously) and adequate clinical signs of recovery are present (e.g., 5-second sustained head lift and adequate minute ventilation).

LEVEL OF CONSCIOUSNESS

Although not in widespread use, and just now beginning to find a foothold in operating rooms worldwide, the bispectral index (BIS) monitor is a signal-processing technique that allows information to be obtained on a patient's level of consciousness. An electroencephalograph-like, waveform, physiologic signal is used by a new signal-processing technique, bispectral analysis. A mathematic algorithm produces an objective measure of hypnosis. Clinical studies have shown correlation between the BIS and level of hypnosis (drug- or trauma-induced changes in level of consciousness).[8] The device itself is approximately the size of an end-tidal carbon dioxide monitor and is applied to the patient's forehead by using special adhesive electrodes. This tool may have important applications in emergency medicine and may offer exciting opportunities for clinical intervention, monitoring, and research.

References

1. Bailey RH, Knaus VL, Bauer JH. Aneroid sphygmomanometers. An assessment of accuracy at a university hospital and clinics. *Arch Intern Med* 1991;151(7):1409.
2. Bourdelles GL, Estagnasie P, Lenoir F, et al. Use of a pulse oximeter in an adult emergency department. *Chest* 1998;113:1042.
3. Drenick NE, Ucda N, Olsen NV, et al. Manual evaluation of residual curarization using double-burst stimulation: a comparison with train-of-four. *Anesthesiology* 1989;70:578.
4. Emond SD, Camargo CA, Nowak RM. 1997 National Asthma Education and Prevention Program guidelines: a practical summary for emergency physicians. *Ann Emerg Med* 1998;31(5):579.
5. Fesmire FM, Percy RF, Bardoner JB, et al. Usefulness of automated serial 12-lead ECG monitoring during the initial emergency department evaluation of patients with chest pain. *Ann Emerg Med* 1998;31(1):3.
6. Gomes JA, Winters SL, Ip J, et al. Identification of patients with high risk for arrhythmic mortality. *Cardiol Clin* 1993;11(1):55.
7. Gutierrez G, Bismar H, Dantzker DR, et al. Comparison of gastric intramucosal pH with measures of oxygen transport and consumption in critically ill patients. *Crit Care Med* 1992;20:451.
8. Iselin-Chaves IA, Flaishon R, Sebel PS, et al. The effect of the interaction of propofol and alfentanil on recall, loss of consciousness, and the Bispectral Index. *Anesth Analg* 1998;87(4):949.
9. Kay LE. Accuracy of blood pressure measurement in the family practice center. *J Am Board Fam Pract* 1998;11(4):252.
10. Matsukawa T, Sessler DI, Ozaki M, et al. Comparison of distal oesophageal temperature with "deep" and tracheal temperatures. *Can J Anaesth* 1997;44(4):433.
11. Rotello LC, Crawford L, Terndrup TE. Comparison of infrared ear thermometer derived and equilibrated rectal temperatures in estimating pulmonary artery temperatures. *Crit Care Med* 1996;24(9):1501.
12. Sammy I, Hanson J, James MR. Cerebral oximetry and stroke distance: the future of emergency department monitoring? *J Accid Emerg Med* 1996;13:313.
13. Shoemaker WC, Wo CJ, Bishop MH, et al. Noninvasive hemodynamic monitoring of critical patients in the emergency department. *Acad Emerg Med* 1996;3:675.
14. Ward KR, Yealy DM. End-tidal carbon dioxide monitoring in emergency medicine, part 2: clinical applications. *Acad Emerg Med* 1998;5(6):637.

CHAPTER 415
Geriatric Considerations

Robert H. Woolard, Bruce Becker, and Thomas J. Haronian

In 1985, 28.6 million U.S. citizens (12% of the population) were age 65 or over, and the elderly population is predicted to grow to 34.9 million people (22% of the U.S. population) by 2030. Elderly patients can be divided into the "young old," a group that is best considered to be enjoying healthy retirement, and the "true old," a group that includes the "frail elderly," who have significant disability. Although functional capacity, not age, creates the distinction between these groups, age 65 to 80 is usually considered "young old," and the "true old" are 80 and above. Life expectancy at age 65 is 15 years for a man and 20 years for a woman. The fastest-growing segment of the population is the 80 and above group, and, in this group, Whites and women are overrepresented. At age 65, predictors of increased longevity for men are low blood pressure, low serum glucose, not smoking, and not being obese. Continued exercise into older age is also a predictor of longevity. Emergency physicians can expect to encounter a more active and an older population in the years ahead.

Forty percent of the U.S. health-care budget is spent on the elderly. Twenty-five percent to 40% of hospital days are taken by those age 80 and above. Of all emergency department (ED) adult visits, 19.6% are by elderly patients, with 41% of these visits leading to hospitalization. The elderly also represent an ever-increasing proportion of the patients who visit EDs, and emergency physicians must understand and address the unique needs of older patients.[11]

Emergency physicians must change their conception of aging from a disease process to a gradual diminution of physiologic functions. The time course of functional loss is highly variable between individuals and is determined by both intrinsic and largely modifiable extrinsic factors such as smoking, diet, and exercise. The effects of diseases, environmental exposures, and stresses accumulate with age to limit the individual's functional capacity and his or her ability to maintain homeostasis. At age 30, the functional capacity of most organs exceeds by four to ten times that necessary to maintain homeostasis during life stresses. With each year over 30, there is a linear decline in the function of each organ system which is independent of other organ systems. Because of impaired functional reserve, diseases present after a lesser stress and at an earlier time. The manifestation of the disease often reflects the loss of homeostasis in the organ system with the least functional reserve rather than the effect of the disease on the organ system primarily attacked. Thus, common presentation of disease states in older patients, such as confusion, withdrawal from usual activities, falling, syncope, and weakness, results from myriad causes—from hyperthyroidism to CHF to appendicitis. The classic signs and symptoms of a disease may be absent, delayed, or altered in the elderly.

Vital signs change with age. The systolic blood pressure increases with age, and the maximal heart rate decreases (maximum expected heart rate = 230 − age). Orthostasis is common, with 50% of nursing home patients demonstrating a 20-mm Hg decline in systolic or a 10-mm Hg decline in diastolic pressure at 1 or 3 minutes after standing from a supine position. Elderly patients have difficulty maintaining thermoregulation and can have a lower baseline temperature or fail to mount a fever in response to infection. Twenty percent of elderly ED patients have an abnormal pulse oximetry reading (less than 95% oxygen saturation). An abnormal pulse oximetry reading prompted admission in 11% of patients and a change in treatment for 55% of patients in one study.[5]

As a group, elders have tremendous physiologic heterogeneity—more than any other age group, from elder athletes to bedridden, terminally ill patients. Expected age-related changes may cause undue concern in the patient, families, and caregivers. Bacteriuria, premature ventricular contractions, low bone mineral density, impaired glucose tolerance, and involuntary bladder contractions are common findings in older patients. Other abnormal findings may be inappropriately accepted as part of the aging process: anemia, impotence, depression, confusion, or falling.

Changes in body mass (more fat, less water) and gradual weakening of the renal, hepatic, pulmonary, cardiac, and central nervous system (CNS) functions are expected, such that some laboratory value norms must be adjusted. Others remain the same with age (Table 415.1). The changes in medical treatment necessitated by this altered physiology are only partially understood. Because elderly patients have often been excluded from clinical trials, treating them often means extrapolating from the results of trials involving younger patients.

Access to medical care and social support impacts care delivery for elders. Elderly patients often require additional time and physical space for evaluation. Access to care may be limited by factors that are not barriers for a younger population, such as narrow parking spaces and steps at an entrance. While the vast majority of elders are living independently, two-thirds of 90-year-olds need help walking. Elderly ED patients are more often acutely ill, require more diagnostic tests, and are less able to be accurately diagnosed than are younger patients. They may be misdiagnosed if a hurried, narrowly focused approach to evaluation is used. After identifying one problem and addressing it, emergency physicians may fail to recognize another problem that may be the underlying cause. In contrast to the younger patient, a single diagnosis usually does not explain all the abnormalities found in an older patient. To understand the presenting problem, deliver optimum care, and prevent future problems, the emergency evaluation must have a more comprehensive approach that includes a caregiver interview, assessment of cognitive and functional status, careful review of current and past medical problems and medications, construction of a broadened differential diagnosis, and, finally, appreciation of the resources available in the hospital and community to carry out the care plan and assure patient safety.

A systematic approach to cognitive and functional assessment should become part of routine evaluation of older patients. Using the confusion assessment method or a standard cognitive function examination, and reviewing the activities of daily living, bathing, dressing, toileting, transferring, maintaining continence, and feeding aid the physician in quantifying subtle changes in patient status. The development of delirium, or a rapid cognitive or functional decline is better appreciated by using these standard evaluation formats. The emergency physician must learn to recognize these changes as signs of potentially life-threatening illness that require investigation and hospitalization. Functional or cognitive impairment may bring the patient to the ED with failure to thrive, weakness, frequent falls, anorexia, incontinence, confusion, agitation, depression, fatigue, injury, abuse, or insomnia. A narrowly defined approach to making a rapid diagnosis may fail to identify the magnitude of the functional or cognitive impairment. Admission to the hospital or an observation area may be required to fully assess the need for treatment of an underlying illness when patients present with acute cognitive or functional decline.

Most elderly persons live alone on low incomes and find the challenge of preparing meals a burden. Loneliness, poor dentition, and decreased ability to taste, see, and move often lead to poor nutrition. Many elderly persons do not meet minimum daily nutritional requirements. Even in nursing homes, malnutrition occurs. Any elderly patient with an unintentional weight loss of 10 or more pounds in the preceding 6 months may be suffering from malnutrition. Overweight patients may suffer from protein or vitamin deficiency. One marker of malnutrition is diminished albumin. Dizziness, syncope, depression, and mental status changes, as well as chronic joint pains, may relate to subtle nutritional deficiencies.

Patients over age 65 use an average of two to six prescribed medications and one to three nonprescribed medications. An estimated 3% to 8% of all hospital admissions for elderly patients are associated with adverse drug reactions (ADRs). Most are related to aspirin, nonsteroidal antiinflammatory agents, and cardiovascular drugs. Some medications, such as propoxyphene, long-acting benzodiazepines, and long-acting oral hypoglycemics, are contraindicated in older patients. The emergency physician must have a high index of suspicion for medication-related problems. Drug effects are often more pronounced in the elderly, and ADRs particularly related to dosing are common. ADRs and adverse drug interactions (ADIs) can also result from the emergency physician's prescriptions. A review of current medications, including nonprescribed and herbal medications, must be part of every emergency evaluation of the elderly pa-

TABLE 415.1. Laboratory Values Affected by Age

VALUES THAT INCREASE WITH AGE
BUN
Creatinine
Calcium (women only)
Erythrocyte sedimentation rate
Thyroxine (T_4)
VALUES THAT DECREASE WITH AGE
Creatinine phosphokinase
Leukocyte count
VALUES UNAFFECTED BY AGE
Bicarbonate
Bilirubin
Chloride
Coagulation tests
Hemoglobin
Magnesium
Red cell indices
Sodium

Adapted from Hodkinson JM. Alterations of laboratory findings. In: Hazzard WR, Andres R, Bierman EL, et al., (eds). *Principles of geriatric medicine and gerontology*. New York: McGraw-Hill, 1990.

tient before formulating a differential diagnosis, and also prior to prescribing medications. Routine application of computerized drug-interaction programs in the ED may lead to detection of drug interactions and reduce hazardous prescribing practices among elderly patients.

The elderly patient may be a poor historian due to deafness, depression, mental deterioration, or stroke. This patient may be unable to cooperate fully with the examination. The emergency physician must overcome these barriers to obtain an adequate history and examination. It is often useful to include a family member or caregiver in the evaluation. A caregiver, present in the examination room, can provide comfort to the patient, additional history, and assistance with the physical examination.

Care after discharge is critical to satisfactory emergency treatment of elderly patients. Twenty-four percent of elderly ED patients return within 3 months of the initial visit to the ED. Patients with functional problems are more likely to return. Addressing functional problems by creating more comprehensive care plans at discharge may decrease these ED returns. Home health-care services can be integral to the treatment plan. Discussion of the patient's needs with the caregiver is an essential part of emergency care, as important as a discussion with the parent of a child treated in the ED. The patient's home-care needs and resources must be assessed before discharge. Identification of elders with needs for additional outpatient care may be accomplished by asking a few simple screening questions. In many EDs, social workers, case managers, or members of a geriatric evaluation team can carry out these assessments.

Emergency physicians may be concerned about whether it is appropriate to provide care for the elderly patient who is close to death. Many elderly persons have advanced directives concerning limitations to care. Some emergency medical service systems have taken steps that allow prehospital providers to respond in accordance with these advanced directives. Concerns about providing unwanted care may lead to suboptimal investigation and treatment. The physician must not let ageism masquerade as ethics or cost effectiveness. The patient's expressed desire to forego extraordinary measures to sustain life should not limit the clinician's diligence in seeking and treating remediable illness. When thrombolytic therapy was studied in the elderly, significant reductions in mortality were realized, with less cost per life saved, in the older patients. The emergency physician should seek to determine and follow the wishes of the elderly patient who has a desire to limit care, especially when a durable power of attorney, a living will, or orders restricting resuscitation are available. However, such desires to limit care should not be misinterpreted as desires for comfort measures only. Routine emergency care includes thorough evaluation and treatment of most medical problems.

Common emergency problems relevant to the care of elderly patients and problems unique to the elderly are reviewed in the following sections.

ABUSE AND NEGLECT

Abuse and neglect of the elderly include actions or omission of actions that result in harm or threatened harm to health or welfare.[12] Although 4% of the elderly population is subject to some type of abuse or neglect each year, this entity is often unrecognized or ignored because physicians are unfamiliar with elder abuse, unsure of how to report possible abuse, or fearful of making false accusations toward caregivers. The consequences of elder abuse include not only acute injuries, but also significant long-term morbidity, functional decline, depression, and increased mortality rates.

Physical abuse is the most commonly reported form of elder abuse, yet its actual prevalence is estimated to be lower than that of other categories. This includes acts of physical violence, sexual assault, burns, and excessive physical restraint. As with child abuse, elder abuse should be considered in patients who present with single or multiple fractures, lacerations, or contusions with inconsistent mechanisms of injury.

Psychological abuse is difficult to assess in the emergency setting, as it can be subtle. Examples include verbal harassment, insults, and threats of physical harm, institutionalization, withholding care, or even homicide. Behavioral clues of severe anxiety, passivity, fear, and shame may be observed, particularly in the presence of the caregiver. Long-term abuse of this nature can lead to, and must be considered in the differential of, depression in the elderly.

Neglect may be intentional but occasionally results when a caregiver simply cannot provide adequate care. This type of abuse most commonly affects the most debilitated elderly who cannot perform basic activities of daily living. It may include withholding medications, food, clothing, glasses, dentures, hearing aids, or walkers. Deliberate misuse of medication is also categorized as neglect. Prehospital workers often discover evidence of neglectful abuse and can provide valuable information regarding living conditions.

Financial abuse includes theft and inappropriate use or withholding of money and material goods by a caregiver. This is similar to neglect, but is associated with some sort of financial or material gain on the caregiver's part at the expense of the victim.

Most elderly patients who are subject to abuse have a physical or mental impairment that renders them dependent on others for assistance. Female gender and social isolation are risk factors. Abusers are typically family members, with daughters and sons being identified most often. Forty-five percent of abusers have a history of drug or alcohol abuse, and 64% are financially dependent on the victim. Other risk factors include a family or personal history of abuse or violence, severe external stressors, forced responsibility placed on the caregiver, and severe or increasing care needs.

Physicians must report elder abuse in all states. In the majority of states with mandatory reporting laws, failure to report suspected elder abuse is a criminal offense. Elder abuse protocols similar to those for child abuse and rape should be developed and followed. They should include appropriate forms for recording information from the patient as well as the caregiver, and objective data pertaining to the physical examination and laboratory studies. Social workers and local agencies, such as the department of elderly affairs or adult protective services should be notified, and can assist in the reporting process. However, the elderly patient, if mentally competent, has the right to refuse any intervention.

ABDOMINAL CONDITIONS

Elderly patients who present with abdominal pain are a diagnostic challenge. Chronic disease and normal physiologic changes of aging contribute to the atypical and delayed presentations of abdominal disorders. Routine laboratory tests cannot be used to reliably predict which elderly patients have an acute surgical disease or which patients which should be admitted or discharged.

Nearly half of those over age 65 have gallstones,[13] so it is not surprising that gallbladder disease is the most common cause of acute abdominal pain in the elderly. Presenting symptoms and the physical examination are often very nonspecific; less than half of geriatric patients with acute cholecystitis present with vomiting, and 25% relate no history of biliary colic. Only 30% to

55% are febrile to greater than 101°F, leukocytosis is absent in 50%, and 25% have no tenderness. Elderly patients are more likely to present with complications of cholecystitis, such as perforation, gangrenous cholecystitis, and ascending cholangitis.

Less than half of elderly patients who present with an acute complication of ulcer disease have a history of ulcers.[16] Patients with underlying coronary artery disease or cerebrovascular disease who have acute upper gastrointestinal bleeding may present only with symptoms of coronary ischemia or change in mental status. Thirty percent of elderly patients with perforated ulcers have no pain.

Five percent to 10% of all cases of appendicitis occur in patients over age 60, and these patients account for half of all appendicitis deaths.[18] In most cases of appendicitis in the elderly, the appendix is perforated at surgery. Anorexia and vomiting are less common, migration of pain to the right lower quadrant is absent in up to 60%, and half of elderly patients with appendicitis have a normal white-cell count on initial presentation.

Mesenteric ischemia is truly a disease of the elderly. In its early stages, it often goes unrecognized due to the usual presentation of vague, intermittent abdominal pain and an unremarkable physical examination. The mortality rate is up to 85%. This possibility should be considered in any elderly patient with a history of vascular disease or atrial fibrillation who presents with abdominal pain.

The incidence of abdominal aortic aneurysm (AAA) increases with age and may be as high as 11% in men over the age of 65. Symptoms of abdominal, flank, back, or groin pain should raise the suspicion of an expanding or ruptured AAA. Age alone is not a contraindication to surgery; any patient with a symptomatic AAA must be evaluated for urgent surgical intervention.

CARDIAC DISEASE

More than 25% to 33% of myocardial infarctions (MIs) in all age groups are discovered only from the appearance of new changes on routine cardiograms Thirty percent of elderly patients with cardiogram evidence of MI are asymptomatic. In studies of ambulatory monitoring of ST-segment depression, 75% of all ischemic episodes are found to be asymptomatic. Clearly, much of coronary disease is silent in elderly and other patients.

The presentation of ACSs, when not silent, become more atypical with age. In patients over age 85, atypical presentations of MI are the rule: Shortness of breath, not chest pain, is the most common presentation. The classic presentation, substernal chest pain described as a dull squeezing, is present in only 20% of patients. Abdominal or epigastric distress and fatigue or weakness are frequent complaints.[3] MIs may also present as syncope, a strokelike syndrome, or acute confusion, particularly in patients over age 75. Prodromal symptoms or anginal equivalents such as tiredness or breathlessness associated with exertion may be more helpful than acute symptoms in pointing to a cardiac origin in older patients. Elderly patients experiencing MI have a greater delay in calling 911, arriving at the ED, being examined, receiving thrombolytic therapy, and arriving at the coronary care unit (CCU). Mortality from MI is higher in the elderly. Hence, any elderly person presenting with pulmonary, cardiac, or neurologic symptoms should be quickly evaluated for myocardial ischemia with an electrocardiogram (ECG).

In elderly patients, the cardiogram is frequently abnormal, but not diagnostic.[5] The maximal heart-rate response to stress or exercise decreases with age. Modest left ventricular hypertrophy occurs with a stiffening of the ventricular wall, reduced early diastolic ventricular filling, prolonged ventricular relaxation, and reduced endocardial perfusion. Gradual loss of the elastic characteristics of the arteries increases afterload. Baseline ECG abnormalities increase with age.[2] The major changes seen with age relate to degenerative changes in the heart's conduction system. The finding of a left axis deviation with left anterior hemiblock or longer PR and QRS intervals may be due to aging. First-degree atrioventricular block is present in 10% of all elderly patients and 35% of 90-year-olds. Bundle-branch block is seen in 42% of elderly patients. Hence, an elderly patient's cardiogram may be difficult to interpret without a baseline cardiogram for comparison. In the setting of recent onset of symptoms and left bundle-branch block, early comparison with a prior ECG is necessary to determine the need for thrombolytic therapy or invasive procedures.

Aggressive treatment of acute coronary syndromes (ACSs) in elderly patients is gaining acceptance in the United States. However, procedural interventions have not proved to be as effective as thrombolytic therapy. In multiple trials, thrombolytic therapy has been shown to be effective in reducing the mortality associated with MI. In trials that have included elderly patients, the benefits of thrombolytic therapy have been demonstrated in the older group. Because the elderly have a greater mortality from MI, they stand to gain significantly from treatment. Unfortunately, the elderly have been less likely to receive treatment with thrombolytic therapy. Elders benefit from CCU admission, beta blockers, angiotensin converting enzyme inhibitors, aspirin, and aggressive treatment of complications. With improved survivorship of acute MI, a growing challenge for physicians is control and treatment of congestive heart failure (CHF). Emergency visits and admissions for CHF are growing, and 80% of patients with CHF are over age 65.

When the ECG is abnormal but not diagnostic and the history suggests a possible cardiac event, it is prudent to admit the elderly patient for observation, monitoring, and further evaluation. Rapid evaluation with serial enzymatic assays and/or imaging of the heart at rest to identify myocardial damage or an ACS can be followed by provocative testing to identify underlying coronary disease. In many EDs, elderly patients at low and moderate risk for ACSs can safely complete this evaluation during an 8- to 12-hour stay for rapid evaluation and observation.

DELIRIUM AND DEMENTIA

Fifteen percent of elderly patients admitted to medical services manifest delirium, and 25% to 35% of those who are initially lucid subsequently develop delirium. Forty-one percent of demented patients are found to be delirious, and 25% of delirious patients have underlying dementia.[14]

Delirium is an acute, reversible global disorder of cognition affecting memory, thinking, and perception. Thoughts are incoherent and chaotic, marked by delusions, paranoia, and confabulation. Disorientation is common. Memory is poor; recent memory is more affected than is remote memory. The patient may recount hallucinations and illusions. The disorder fluctuates, and periods of clarity are often interposed. Diurnal variations and unfamiliar environmental stimuli (typified by the prehospital and ED experience) often provoke delirium. Attention is decreased, as is consciousness or responsiveness. The patient may be hypoactive, with coarse tremors and asterixis, or hyperactive, with agitation and hallucinations. Many studies have suggested that the clinical diagnosis is best made by the application of the Confusion Assessment Method (CAM) coupled with multiple observation points.

Underlying disorders such as CHF, urosepsis, pneumonia, cancer, uremia, hypokalemia, dehydration, sodium depletion, right hemispheric stroke, drug intoxication (especially anticholinergics), and myriad other pathologies must be considered in elderly patients. The diagnostic workup and treatment must be directed at the underlying disease process. Patients with acute onset or decompensation should generally be admitted. Delirium can be temporarily managed by the careful use of neuroleptics (small doses of haloperidol work well) and fluids while the emergency physician performs a thorough workup, searching for the underlying cause of this reversible condition.

Dementia is a chronic, slowly progressive loss of higher mental function. There is a gradual decrease in mental capability with normal aging. Synthesis of new information, visual motor coordination, and some nonverbal processes begin declining in the third decade. However, other cortical indices actually improve with age, such as vocabulary. Most changes in learning capabilities relate more to the presence of distinct CNS disease than to age itself. Knowing the characteristics of dementia aids in separating acute nondementia illness from dementia. Alzheimer disease is, by far, the most likely etiology of dementia.

Patients typically present with memory loss, disorientation, anomia, visual spatial deficits, apraxia, and intellectual decline. Often, the patient is brought to the ED by a concerned spouse or relative because of behavioral changes, including getting lost in familiar neighborhoods; difficulties in dressing and following simple directions; loss of interest in personal habits, family, and community affairs; and forgetfulness. The patient often denies any problems. A careful neurologic examination, focusing on cognition, and a search for underlying disease should be performed. It is important to remember that elderly patients with dementia who are being treated with psychotropic agents are three to five times more likely than younger patients to develop tardive dyskinesia.

DEPRESSION

Depressive symptoms are present in up to 27% of community-dwelling elderly; full-blown clinical depression is present in up to 15%, compared with 3% in the general population.[4] The prevalence is higher in hospital inpatients and nursing home residents. Risk factors include female gender, widowhood or single life, stressful life events, and poor social support. While elders tend to report less depressed mood, they demonstrate a higher rate of anxiety than do younger patients, suggesting a depression–anxiety syndrome. Somatization is common and may represent the disorder itself or accentuation of symptoms of comorbidities. White men over age 60 have the highest rate of successful suicide.

There is a strong association between depression and dementia. Twenty percent of the demented are depressed, and up to 30% of spouses of demented patients suffer from depression. However, depression rarely presents as or masks an underlying dementia. The elderly tend not to offer symptoms of depression or dysphoria spontaneously, but will discuss them if asked directly. Often, the depression is associated with chronic illness, retirement, change in social status, new residence (to a nursing home, retirement village, or apartment), marital difficulties, or the death of a spouse. Symptoms may include insomnia or hypersomnia, fatigue, anhedonia, psychomotor agitation or retardation, difficulty concentrating, and violent outbursts. Some illnesses that mimic depression include hypothyroidism with myxedema, left-sided stroke (presenting with crying, feelings of hopelessness, anger, despair, and self-deprecation), and cancer of the pancreas.

Antidepressant medication often has adverse effects in elders. Hip fractures have been associated with antidepressant and anxiolytic medication. A study of fitness to drive reported that 88.6% of elders taking antidepressants failed to pass all the tests in a psychomotor battery.[12]

Pharmacologic agents implicated in causing depression include propranolol and methyldopa. Alcohol abuse and dependence on anxiolytics, sedatives, or hypnotics can also mimic depression. Two-thirds of elderly alcoholics are female. One-third of elderly alcoholics have an underlying illness or traumatic injury due to their alcohol problem.[1] Families often avoid discussing alcohol problems unless asked directly. Emergency medicine physicians should probably not initiate antidepressive medication; however, the newer agents, such as serotonin reuptake inhibitors, are preferred over tricyclic antidepressants because of fewer side effects.

DRUG TOXICITY

ADRs are unexpected, symptom-producing events that occur with appropriate therapeutic doses of medication. In younger patients, ADRs are generally due to idiosyncrasy (an excessive response to a therapeutic dose) or hypersensitivity. In elderly patients, however, ADRs are generally an expression of the expected actions that occur within an altered biophysiologic milieu, or they result from predictable ADIs.[6] Elderly patients are more prone to ADRs and ADIs because they often take many medications, a situation referred to as "polypharmacy." While the definition of *polypharmacy* remains controversial in the literature, it is increasingly clear that overprescription of medications to the elderly is common and results in considerable morbidity and iatrogenic complications from interactions among regularly prescribed medication. The emergency medicine physician must always try to obtain a precise list of medications and carefully consider indications, interactions, and adverse effects of any new drug added to an elder patient's regimen.

Both the pharmacokinetics (drug absorption, distribution, metabolism, and excretion) and pharmacodynamics (physiologic response to the drug) are altered in the elderly patient. While drug absorption can be impaired by achlorhydria, bacterial overgrowth, and surgical resection of digestive organs, this impairment is rarely clinically significant. Drug distribution, however, may be significantly altered due to decreased lean body mass, decreased total body water, and increased adipose tissue. Drugs that are soluble in water or hydrophilic (e.g., coumadin, digoxin, propranolol, procainamide, theophylline) have higher plasma concentrations at a given dose in the elderly. These patients demonstrate a decline in hepatic clearance of certain drugs because of a decline in liver volume and blood flow. CHF, chronic renal disease, rheumatoid arthritis, cirrhosis, protein–calorie malnutrition, and malignancy may result in hypoalbuminemia and increase the free fraction of drugs that are highly protein-bound (e.g., coumadin, phenytoin, tolbutamide, indomethacin, furosemide). Because laboratory assays generally report only the total drug concentration, the increase in pharmacologically active free drug will be occult.

Drug metabolism is impaired in the elderly. There is decreased capacity for oxidation, reduction, hydrolysis, and enzyme induction. These deficiencies are accentuated by the presence of intrinsic hepatic disease. Drug excretion decreases proportionately with impairment of the glomerular filtration rate (GFR). By age 90, the GFR falls by 50%. Serum creatinine alone is not a valid indication of GFR in the elderly person with reduced muscle mass; the creatinine clearance can be reduced to 50% of baseline with a serum creatinine in the normal range.

ADRs and ADIs must be considered in the differential diagnosis of the presenting complaint and as contributing factors to signs and symptoms in elderly patients. All currently prescribed medications should be reviewed and drug interactions considered before prescribing new medications. Unnecessary medications should be eliminated. Medications with a high potential for ADRs should generally be avoided altogether, particularly in patients who live in the community (Table 415.2).

Common ADIs in the elderly include phenytoin (metabolism inhibited by benzodiazepines, phenothiazines, and isoniazid), cimetidine (inhibits the metabolism of coumadin, phenytoin, and theophylline), digoxin (excretion decreased by quinidine, verapamil, and amiodarone), and coumadin (metabolism inhibited by allopurinol, cimetidine, metronidazole, trimethoprim–sulfamethoxazole, and quinolones).

TABLE 415.2. Drugs Considered Inappropriate for the Elderly

Agent	Reason
ANALGESICS	
Pentazocine	Seizures and cardiotoxicity from overdose
Propoxyphene	Relatively ineffective; CNS and cardiotoxicity
ANTIDEPRESSANTS	
Amitriptyline Doxepin	Anticholinergic effects and orthostatic hypotension higher than with other tricyclic antidepressants
ANTIEMETIC	
Trimethobenzamide	Less effective than other agents; may cause drowsiness, diarrhea, rash, and dystonia
ANTIHYPERTENSIVES	
Methyldopa Reserpine Propranolol	CNS side effects (all)
MUSCLE RELAXANTS	
Carisoprodol Cyclobenzaprine Methocarbamol Orphenadrine	CNS toxicity outweighs potential benefit (all)
NSAIDS	
Indomethacin	CNS toxicity greater than other NSAIDs
Phenylbutazone	Bone-marrow toxicity
ORAL HYPOGLYCEMIC	
Chlorpropamide	Long half-life; risk of SIADH
PLATELET INHIBITOR	
Dipyridamole	CNS side effects; doubtful efficacy
SEDATIVE–HYPNOTICS	
Chlordiazepoxide	Long duration of action; daytime sedation
Diazepam	Long duration of action; daytime sedation
Flurazepam	Long duration of action; daytime sedation
Meprobamate	Less safe than short-acting benzodiazepines for anxiety and insomnia
Pentobarbital	Short-acting benzodiazepines safer for sedation
Secobarbital	Short-acting benzodiazepines safer for sedation

Adapted from Wilcox SM, Himmelstein DU, Woolhandler S. Inappropriate prescribing for the community-dwelling elderly, *JAMA* 1994;272:292.

FALLS

Falls are the most common mechanism of accidental injury and death in the elderly, followed by motor vehicle accidents, burns, and assaults.[19] Over 500,000 elderly patients are admitted annually due to fall-related injuries. An estimated 30% of the geriatric population and 40% of those over age 80 living in the community fall each year. These estimates exclude falls resulting from catastrophic events such as acute cerebrovascular accidents, as well as those that occur even more frequently in constant-care facilities. Fifteen percent to 25% of falls are significant enough to require medical attention, and 5% result in fractures or acute hospitalization. Half of those who fall do so repeatedly, and falls are a contributing factor in 40% of nursing home admissions.

Intrinsic risk factors that predispose the elderly to falling include the physiologic changes of aging, acute and chronic illness, and medications. Any of these can affect physical stability and gait, which are complex functions relying on cognitive, neurologic, vestibular, sensory, and musculoskeletal interaction. Chronic impairments associated with falls include sequelae of cerebrovascular accidents, parkinsonism, normal-pressure hydrocephalus, and senile dementia. Acute infections or CNS and cardiac events may present as a fall.

Age-related visual changes associated with an increased rate of falling include decreases in acuity, contrast sensitivity, dark adaptation, and peripheral vision. Cataracts, glaucoma, and diabetic retinopathy are also common in this age group and contribute to visual impairment. Persons with poor vision rely more heavily on other sensory input, such as proprioception, vestibular reflexes, and hearing, to maintain a sense of equilibrium. Unfortunately, many elderly persons also have impaired proprioception. Peripheral neuropathy resulting from vitamin B_{12} deficiency or diabetes is a common cause. Degenerative disease of the cervical spine has also been implicated in diminished proprioception.

Age-dependent degeneration of the vestibular labyrinth and its sensory components subjects the elderly to sensations of disequilibrium, unsteadiness, and vertigo. Chronic, insidious positional vertigo is common and can lead to a gait disturbance known as vestibular ataxia.[19] Patients with this disorder develop a broad-based wandering gait and are prone to fall, particularly as a result of unexpected positional change. The elderly demonstrate a generalized slowing of reflexes, which contributes to slower preventive and protective motor responses. Muscle weakness, decreased muscle mass, degenerative joint disease, and foot disorders are some of the musculoskeletal disorders associated with an increased risk of falling. Several studies have indicated that medications with CNS side effects (see Table 415.2) are a major risk factor for falls in the elderly. The propensity to fall correlates with the degree of displacement of a person's center of gravity during activity. Daily activities such as standing, walking, and changing position are considered mildly to moderately displacing and are identified in most falls. About 12% of falls occur during markedly displacing activities (e.g., climbing on objects, participating in sports), and 5% result from clearly hazardous endeavors. Stairs are involved in 10% of falls; descending is more hazardous than ascending.

Environmental obstacles are often implicated in falls that occur in the community; however, the correlation between fall injuries and the number of obstacles in the home is unclear. Raised thresholds, uneven surfaces, scatter rugs, and small pets pose a significant risk to persons with a shuffling gait or weak ankle dorsiflexion. Other hazards include poorly fitting shoes or clothes, foot disorders, and inadequate lighting. Of the subjects who have fallen, 25% report significant limitation of daily activities due to fear of future falls. This fear of falling, coupled with poor social support, not only leads to activity curtailment, but also contributes to nursing home placement in a significant number of elderly patients. Preventive strategies, addressing medications, physical conditioning, behavioral modification, and social support, have proved to significantly reduce the incidence of falls, and should be implemented whenever an elderly patient is discharged after a fall.

INFECTIONS AND SEPSIS

The "true old" or "frail elderly," those with some degree of functional impairment, immobility, incompetence, or incontinence, are at high risk for infections and sepsis.[21] Defense against bacterial invasion is compromised by age-related decreases in skin thickness, ciliary activity, cough reflex, gastric acid, and gut motility. Pressure sores, soft-tissue edema, and indwelling catheters provide open portals for bacterial invasion. Immune response may be improved by adequate nutrition and vitamin supplementation. Vaccination for influenza and pneumococcus is cost effective and can be undertaken in the ED.

The cardinal sign of systemic infection—fever—may be absent in up to 25% of infected elderly patients. In fact, due to loss of thermoregulation, hypothermia may occur. A rectal temperature is mandatory in any elderly emergency patient with a suspected infection. Confusion, malaise, nausea, and vomiting are common presentations of infection in the elderly.

The underlying sources of sepsis are most often respiratory (13% to 58%), urinary (15% to 34%), and intraabdominal (20%). Cellulitis, endocarditis, and meningitis are less likely but must also be considered. The bacterial causes of pneumonia, skin infection, and urinary tract infection are largely the same as in younger patients, with two exceptions: Gram-negative colonization of the oropharynx and skin is much more common, and indwelling bladder catheters are associated with urinary tract infection by antimicrobial-resistant, gram-negative bacilli such as *Klebsiella, Enterobacter,* and *Proteus* spp. There is growing concern with the colonization of elderly in nursing homes and hospitals with resistant bacteria. In nursing home patients sent to the ED, methicillin-resistant *Staphylococcus aureus* was present in 15% and vancomycin-resistant enterococcus in 5%. Decubiti are a predictor of colonization with multiply resistant organisms in nursing home residents presenting to the ED.

Most elderly patients with serious infections require intravenous antibiotics. There is a growing ability to provide outpatient intravenous antibiotics. New, highly effective, broad-spectrum oral antibiotics have also been developed. These developments and earlier treatment of infection in the elderly are decreasing the need for inpatient admissions for treatment of infections. Specific guidelines have been developed to determine the need for hospital admission in patients with pneumonia.

Confusion and a raised respiratory rate or upper abdominal pain are often the only prominent findings in an elderly patient with pneumonia. Fever, chest pain, and cough may be absent, and sputum production is often minimal. Confusion or rapid functional decline may be the only sign of urosepsis in the elderly. Urinary symptoms, fever, and back pain may be absent.

Asymptomatic bacteriuria is common in elderly patients and does not require treatment. Pyuria (greater than 10 white cells per milliliter of unspun urine) is sensitive but nonspecific for bacteriuria in the elderly. However, a third of patients with pyuria do not have bacteriuria. Obstruction from prostatic enlargement or uterine prolapse is a contributing factor in many elderly patients with recurrent urinary tract infections and should be discovered on physical examination during the evaluation of a patient with recurrent infections.

Pressure sores may be missed unless the patient is fully disrobed and the areas under all dressings are inspected. Decubitus ulcers require systemic antibiotics only when cellulitis, osteomyelitis, or sepsis develops. Pressure ulcers are a marker of neglect and should alert the physician to the need for improved care or the potential of abuse.

MAJOR TRAUMA

Trauma is the fifth leading cause of death in the elderly.[15] Although persons age 65 and older make up 12% of the population, they account for up to 20% of trauma visits and 25.9% of fatal trauma injuries. In addition, trauma victims over age 80 suffer four times the mortality of those between ages 65 and 80. Elderly trauma victims require extended stays in the hospital, intensive care unit, and the rehabilitation facility. Individuals who survive the initial hospitalization continue to demonstrate higher mortality rates for at least 5 years when compared with uninjured cohorts. Although injury-severity scales are unreliable in predicting outcome in elderly patients, they demonstrate that mortality is increased in aged patients, compared with younger patients with similar injuries. Major causes of death among elderly trauma patients are multiple organ system failure and sepsis; mortality in younger trauma patients is determined predominantly by the extent of acute brain injury.

Diminished physiologic reserve renders elderly trauma patients susceptible to rapid demise. Hypothermia is more common in elderly trauma patients. Acute myocardial ischemia and cardiac dysfunction must be considered in hypotensive elderly trauma patients. The frailty of the heart and major vessels dictates a more aggressive search for occult injury and a more conservative policy on admitting these patients for observation and monitoring.

Two-dimensional echocardiography yields the most information in the shortest amount of time and should be used whenever cardiac injury is suspected. Structural evidence of contusion and abnormalities of wall motion can be identified, as can complications such as tamponade, rupture, and valvular defects. Atherosclerotic disease, decreased elasticity, and calcification of the aorta predispose to traumatic dissection as well as transection.

Diminished pulmonary reserve in the elderly is evidenced by reduced vital capacity and compliance, increased residual volume, and a higher prevalence of obstructive and restrictive disease. Kyphosis is present in two-thirds of geriatric patients, and chest-wall elasticity is reduced, resulting in less compliance and a propensity for multiple rib fractures. Elderly patients with suspected pulmonary contusion or multiple rib fractures should be admitted for close observation, pain control, and meticulous fluid management. Age over 65 is an indication for early ventilatory support in patients with flail chest, as mortality is significantly higher in elderly patients who have delayed intubation after manifestation of clinical signs of respiratory failure.

Elderly patients are particularly likely to develop subdural hematomas (SDHs).[9] Brain atrophy predisposes the cerebral cortices to move within the cranium with abrupt acceleration or deceleration forces. The parasagittal bridging veins running between the brain and dura mater are short, straight veins with no tortuosity and may tear under the added stress of brain movement. These veins also become more fragile with age and tend to rupture with less acceleration or rotational force. Leakage from one or more bridging vein results in the accumulation of venous blood between the dura and arachnoid membranes. SDHs may also result from the rupture of small cortical arteries after traumatic brain injury.

With brain atrophy, more intracranial volume can be occupied by hematoma before signs of elevated intracranial pressure develop. Headache and changes in mentation are most often present, with lateralizing motor weakness evident in about 50% of cases. New-onset paresthesias, gait disturbance, aphasia, or seizures should also raise suspicion of an acute SDH. A subacute or chronic presentation of SDH is more common than acute onset in the elderly.

Age is the most significant predictor of both acute and long-term mortality among head trauma victims. Elderly patients with acute SDH and a Glasgow score below 8 have an 82% mortality rate and only a 3.6% functional recovery, compared with a 60% mortality rate and a 24% functional recovery in adults less than age 65. Minor head trauma (defined as an admission Glasgow score of 13 to 15 and only brief loss of consciousness) can also be devastating in geriatric patients. Mortality rates are higher than in younger adults (5.0% vs. 0.35%), and prolonged neuropsychiatric deficits can occur. In patients older than age 80, a 12% mortality due to minor head injury has been reported. Elderly patients are also significantly more likely to harbor an acute intracerebral lesion and to require craniotomy.

SYNCOPE, NEAR-SYNCOPE, WEAKNESS, AND DIZZINESS

Patients over age 60 who present with syncope have a 21% incidence of major morbidity or death during the 6 months after presentation, compared with a 6% incidence in patients less than age 60.[8] An elderly patient presenting with syncope is thus at high risk and usually requires hospital admission. One study[6] found that elderly patients with near-syncope had a 30% incidence of life-threatening etiology. Thus, near-syncope should be regarded as a high-risk event.

Cardiac causes account for 30% to 35% of syncope in elderly patients. Dysrhythmias increase in prevalence and complexity with age. Atrial fibrillation occurs in up to 8% of elderly persons. Supraventricular tachycardias are the most common cause of cardiac-induced syncope in the elderly. Although less common, bradycardic syncope occurs in elderly patients and may be part of a "brady-tachy" or "sick sinus" syndrome caused, in part, by the effects of aging and ischemia on the sinus node. With cardiac disease resulting in ventricular dilation, the risk of ventricular dysrhythmia increases.

Other common causes of syncope and related symptoms in the elderly include vasovagal (40%), orthostatic (10% to 20%), postprandial (8%), autonomic, and cerebrovascular events. Conditions that cause syncope may be responsible for near-syncope, a feeling of weakness or dizziness. Other conditions that may present in a similar fashion are seizures, transient ischemic attacks (TIAs), depression, weakness, and vertigo. Witnessed seizures should be easily distinguished from syncope by motor activity. However, caution must be exercised before rejecting a cardiac cause of a brief seizure, because deprivation of oxygen to the brain from a cardiac cause can lead to a brief seizure. Transient focal neurologic symptoms are a hallmark of TIA. However, in the setting of a patchy cerebral circulation, focal symptoms may appear transiently from deprivation of oxygen to the brain from a cardiac cause. Vertigo should be distinguishable as a unique symptom that relates to neurologic disturbance and not confused with light-headedness that is cardiac in origin. A global symptom such as weakness requires an extensive history and evaluation to discover social, psychiatric, cardiac, hematologic, endocrine, or metabolic disorders.

Several age-related physiologic changes predispose the elderly to syncope.[21] Baroreflexes regulating heart rate, and blood pressure may not respond to the degree that they do in the younger patient. Medications, conduction disorders, prolonged inactivity, diabetes, and mild dehydration can impair the elderly patient's ability to mount a compensatory increase in blood flow in response to upright posture or hypovolemia. As many as 50% of elderly nursing home patients will have orthostasis on standing. Baseline hypoxia develops as the alveolar–arterial oxygen difference widens with age (to 24 mm Hg at 80 years). Exposure to cigarette smoke or inhaled toxins can further widen this gradient. Hypertension and fixed atherosclerotic plaques reset the minimal blood pressure required to maintain cerebral perfusion. Anemia and cerebrovascular disease decrease cerebral blood flow, reduce oxygen content, and can bring baseline cerebral oxygen and glucose delivery close to the threshold necessary to maintain consciousness. For these reasons, elderly patients are particularly prone to syncope.

THYROID DISEASE

Thyroid disease of the elderly primarily affects women. Symptoms of hyperthyroidism, such as weight loss, fatigue, and dyspnea, can be confused with "normal aging" and be ignored. Other symptoms, including weakness, anxiety, nervousness, and palpitations, are also common complaints in elderly patients.

The presentation can be limited to one system and may reflect an enhanced sensitivity to thyroid hormone rather than markedly increased levels.[7] Some examples of this include atrial fibrillation, often with a slow ventricular response or CHF; anorexia; and weight loss. Other presentations include bulbar myopathy (ptosis and dysphasia), with normal deep tendon reflexes (no hyperreflexia with rapid relaxation phase); agitated depression or so-called apathetic depression; and an attention deficit or emotional lability.

Patients with hypothyroidism often complain of lassitude, cold intolerance, and psychomotor slowing. Constipation affects as many as 26% of elderly men and 34% of elderly women, and may be the only clinical manifestation of early hypothyroidism. Any of these signs may be attributed to normal aging. There may be a history of thyroiditis or treated hyperthyroidism, radiation treatment to the neck for cancer, long-term lithium ingestion, or interleukin chemotherapy. The hypothyroid elderly patient may be hypothermic (less than 96°F), with hypoventilation and hypercapnia. Supraventricular or ventricular tachycardia may develop with severe hypothyroidism. Myxedema (subcutaneous glycosaminoglycans and water) of the skin, pleural, peritoneal, and pericardial cavities may be present.

Many older patients have abnormal thyroid-stimulating hormone (TSH) levels without other alterations in serum thyroid hormone levels: Subclinical hypothyroidism is present in 5% to 10%, and subclinical hyperthyroidism is present in 1% to 2%. The risks of subclinical hypothyroidism include progression to overt hypothyroidism, cardiac failure, hyperlipidemia, and neurologic neuropsychiatric symptoms. The risks of subclinical hyperthyroidism include progression to overt hyperthyroidism, dysrhythmia (especially atrial fibrillation), and osteoporosis. Elderly patients presenting to the ED with nonspecific symptoms suggestive of hyper- or hypothyroidism should be screened with a TSH level.

COMMON PITFALLS

- Failure to consider a wide differential when addressing an elderly patient's presenting problem, especially before dismissing vague and generalized complaints

- Failure to involve a family member or caregiver in all stages of the evaluation of an elderly patient, particularly in planning any treatment after discharge
- Failure to identify risk factors (such as environmental hazards and medications) that can lead to future morbidity from falls
- Failure to obtain a complete list of medications taken, including over-the-counter drugs and herbal medicines
- Failure to consider ADRs in all elderly patients and to take steps to avoid drug interactions when prescribing new medications
- Failure to appreciate that syncope in the elderly is more frequently cardiac in origin, usually requires admission, and is seldom benign
- Failure to consider infections in the elderly patient with confusing or vague complaints, even in the absence of fever or localizing signs
- Failure to provide elderly trauma patients with early ventilatory support whenever pulmonary contusion is suspected and when hypoxia is present, even if the initial chest x-ray is normal
- Failure to consider cardiac dysfunction in hypotensive elderly trauma patients
- Failure to consider bowel ischemia early in the evaluation of nonspecific abdominal pain
- Failure to consider abuse as a cause of injury in elderly patients
- Failure to consider depression and substance abuse when evaluating general symptoms such as weakness and weight loss
- Failure to recognize and treat rapid functional or cognitive decline as a sign of serious medical illness
- Failure to appreciate that suicide attempts in the elderly are always serious
- Failure to appreciate that ischemic cardiac disease in the elderly presents more often as shortness of breath or syncope than as chest pain
- Failure to respect the right of the elderly patient to participate in decision making and choose a course of therapy

References

1. Adams W, Magruder-Habib K, Trued S, et al. Alcohol abuse in elderly emergency department patients. *J Am Geriatr Soc* 1992;40:1236.
2. Bachman S, Sparrow D, Smith K. Effect of aging on the cardiogram. *Am J Cardiol* 1981;48:513.
3. Bayer AJ, Chadha JS, Farag RR, et al. Changing presentation of myocardial infarction with increasing old age. *Am Geriatric Soc J* 1981;34:263.
4. Blazer D. Depression. In: Hazzard WR, Andres R, Bierman EL, et al., eds. *Principles of geriatric medicine and gerontology*. New York: McGraw-Hill, 1990.
5. Bosker G, Jones JS, Romisher S, et al. Assessment and detection of acute coronary ischemia. In: Bosker G, Schwartz GR, Jones JS, et al., eds. *Geriatric emergency medicine*. St. Louis: Mosby–Year Book, 1990.
6. Bressler R. Adverse drug reactions. In: Bressler R, Katz MD, eds. *Geriatric pharmacology*. New York: McGraw-Hill, 1993.
7. Davis PJ, Katz PR. Disorders of the thyroid gland. In: Evans JG, Williams TF, eds. *Oxford textbook of geriatric medicine*. Oxford: Oxford University Press, 1992.
8. Day SC, Cook E, Funkenstein H, et al. Evaluation and outcome of emergency patients with transient loss of consciousness. *Am J Med* 1982;73:15.
9. Ellis GL. Subdural hematoma in the elderly. *Emerg Med Clin North Am* 1990;8:281.
10. Grabe HJ, Wolf T, Gratz S. Lawx G. The influence of polypharmacological antidepressive treatment on central nervous information processing of depressed patients. *Neuropsychobiology* 1998;37(4):200.
11. Jones J, Dougherty J, Cannon L, et al. A geriatrics curriculum for emergency medicine training programs. *Ann Emerg Med* 1986;15:1275.
12. Jones JS. Geriatric abuse and neglect. In: Bosker G, Schwartz GR, Jones JS, et al., eds. *Geriatric emergency medicine*. St. Louis: Mosby–Year Book, 1990.
13. Krasman ML, Gracie WA, Strasius SR. Biliary tract disease in the aged. *Clin Geriatr Med* 1991;7:347.
14. Lewkoff SE, Besdine R, Wetle T. Acute confusional states in the hospitalized elderly. *Annu Rev Gerontol Geriatr* 1986;6:1.
15. Martin RE, Teberian G. Multiple trauma in the elderly patient. *Emerg Med Clin North Am* 1990;8:411.
16. McCarthy D. Acid peptic disease in the elderly. *Clin Geriatr Med* 1991;7:231.
17. Mower WR, Myers G, Nicklin EL, et al. Pulse oximetry as a fifth vital sign in emergency geriatric assessment. *Ann Emerg Med* 1998;5:858.
18. Munson RJ, Fontanarosa PB, Gerson L. Acute appendicitis in the elderly: clinical features of early and delayed diagnoses. *Ann Emerg Med* 1992;21:636.
19. Nelson RC, Murlidhar AA. Falls in the elderly. *Emerg Med Clin North Am* 1990;8:309.
20. Scharenbrock C, Buggs A, Furgerson J, Manthey D. A prospective evaluation of near syncope and syncope in the elderly. *Ann Emerg Med* 1999;6(5):532.
21. Sequeira M. Syncope and dizziness. In: Bosker G, Schwartz GR, Jones JS, et al., eds. *Geriatric emergency medicine*. St. Louis: Mosby–Year Book, 1990.
22. Smith IM. Prevalence, diagnosis and treatment of infectious diseases. In: Calkins E, Davis PJ, Ford AB, eds. *The practice of geriatrics*. Philadelphia: WB Saunders, 1986.

SECTION IX

Christopher H. Linden

Appendixes

APPENDIX A
Normal Reference Laboratory Values of Commonly Ordered Tests

Chemistry

Analyte	Specimen	MGH Unit	SI Unit	Method or Instrument	Factor for Conversion to SI Unit
Adrenocorticotropin (ACTH)	P	6.0–76.0 pg/mL	1.3–16.7 pmol/L	Immunoassay	0.2202
Alanine aminotransferase (ALT, SGPT)	S			Kinetic method	0.1667
Female		7–30 U/L	0.12–0.50 μkat/L		
Male		10–55 U/L	0.17–0.92 μkat/L		
Albumin	S	3.1–4.3 g/dL	31–43 g/L	Colorimetry (bromocresol purple)	10
Aldolase	S	0–7 U/L	0.7 U/L	Kinetic method	1
Aldosterone (adult)				Immunoassay	
Supine, normal-sodium diet	S, P	2–9 ng/dL	55–250 pmol/L		27.74
Upright, normal-sodium diet	S, P	2–5 times supine value with normal-sodium diet			
Supine, low-sodium diet	S, P	2–5 times supine value with normal-sodium diet			
Urine, normal-sodium diet	U	2.3–21.0 μg/24 h	6.38–58.25 nmol/24 h		2.774
Alkaline phosphatase (adult)	S			Kinetic method	0.01667
Female		30–100 U/L	0.5–1.67 μkat/L		
Male		45–115 U/L	0.75–1.92 μkat/L		
Alkaline phosphatase, heat fractionated	S	20–35%	0.20–0.35	Kinetic method	0.01
Alpha-fetoprotein (nonmaternal)	S	<12.8 IU/mL	<9.92 μg/L	Immunoassay	0.775
Ammonia	P	12–48 μmol/L	12–48 μmol/L	Enzymatic analysis	1
Amylase	S	53–123 U/L	0.88–2.05 nkat/L	Kinetic method	0.01667
	P	43–115 U/L	0.72–1.92 nkat/L		
	U	4–400 U/L	0.07–6.67 nkat/L		
Androstenedione (adult)	S	50–250 ng/dL	1.75–8.73 nmol/L	Immunoassay	0.0349
Angiotensin converting enzyme	S			Kinetic method	1
Male		19–95 U/L	19–95 U/L		
Female		19–79 U/L	19–79 U/L		
Apolipoprotein	S			Nephelometry	
Apolipoprotein A-1		119–240 mg/dL	1.19–24 g/L		0.01
Apolipoprotein B		52–163 mg/dL	0.52–1.63 g/L		0.01
Apolipoprotein B–apolipoprotein A-1 ratio		0.35–0.98	0.35–0.98		1
Aspartate aminotransferase (AST, SGOT)	S			Kinetic method	0.01667
Female		9–25 U/L	0.15–0.42 μkat/L		
Male		10–40 U/L	0.17–0.67 μkat/L		
Beta$_2$-microglobulin	S, P	1.2–2.8 mg/L	1.2–2.8 mg/L	Immunoassay	1
	U	<200 μg/L	<200 μg/L		
Bicarbonate (HCO_3^-)	WB, S	22–26 mEq/L	22–26 mmol/L	Calculation	1
Bilirubin, direct	S	0.0–0.4 mg/dL	0–7 μmol/L	Colorimetry	17.1
Bilirubin, total	S	0.0–1.0 mg/dL	0–17 μmol/L	Colorimetry	17.1
C peptide (adult)	S, P	0.5–2.0 ng/mL	0.17–0.66 nmol/L	Immunoassay	0.33
C-reactive protein	S	0.0–12.0 mg/L	0–12 mg/L	Nephelometry	1
CA 15-3	S	0–30 U/mL	0–30 kU/L	Immunoassay	1
CA 19-9	S	0–37 U/mL	0–37 kU/L	Immunoassay	1
CA 27,29	S	0–32 U/mL	0–32 kU/L	Immunoassay	1
CA-125	S	0–35 U/mL	0–35 kU/L	Immunoassay	1
Calcitonin	S			Immunoassay	1
Male		3–26 pg/mL	3–26 ng/L		
Female		2–17 pg/mL	2–17 ng/L		
Calcium	S	8.5–10.5 mg/dL	2.1–2.6 mmol/L	Colorimetry	0.25
	U	0–300 mg/24 h	0.0–7.5 mmol/24 h	Colorimetry	0.025
Calcium, ionized	WB	1.14–1.30 mmol/L	1.14–1.30 mmol/L	Ion-selective electrode	1
Carbon dioxide content, total	P	24–30 mmol/L	24–30 mmol/L	Carbon dioxide electrode	1
Carbon dioxide, partial pressure, arterial ($PaCO_2$)	WB	35–45 mm Hg	4.7–6.0 kPa	Carbon dioxide electrode	0.1333
Carboxyhemoglobin	WB	<5% of total hemoglobin	<0.05 fraction of total hemoglobin saturation	Co-oximetry	0.01
Carcinoembryonic antigen (CEA)	P, S	0.0–3.4 ng/mL	0.0–3.4 μg/L	Immunoassay	1
Catecholamines (adult)	U			High-pressure liquid chromatography	
Epinephrine		2–24 μg/24 h	11–131 nmol/24 h		5.458
Norepinephrine		15–100 μg/24 h	89–591 nmol/24 h		5.911
Dopamine		52–480 μg/24 h	340–3134 nmol/24 h		6.53

Chemistry (Continued)

Analyte	Specimen	MGH Unit	SI Unit	Method or Instrument	Factor for Conversion to SI Unit
Total (epinephrine + norepinephrine)		26–121 μg/24 h	142–660 nmol/24 h		5.458 (as normetanephrine)
Cerebrospinal fluid (adult)	CSF				
Albumin		11–48 mg/dL	0.11–0.48 g/L	Nephelometry	0.01
Cell count		0–5 mononuclear cells/μL	0–5×10^6 cells/L	Manual count	1×10^6
Chloride		120–130 mmol/L	120–130 mmol/L	Coulometry	1
Glucose		50–75 mg/dL	2.8–4.2 mmol/L	Enzymatic analysis	0.05551
IgG		8.0–8.6 mg/dL	0.08–0.086 g/L	Nephelometry	0.01
Pressure		70–180 mm of water	70–180 arbitrary units	Manual measurement	1
Protein					
Lumbar		15–45 mg/dL	0.15–0.45 g/L	Turbidometry	0.01
Cisternal		15–25 mg/dL	0.15–0.25 g/L		
Ventricular		5–15 mg/dL	0.05–0.15 g/L		
Ceruloplasmin	S	27–50 mg/dL	270–500 mg/L	Nephelometry	10
Chloride	P	100–108 mmol/L	100–108 mmol/L	Coulometry	1
	U	Depends on diet	Depends on diet		
Cholesterol	S			Colorimetry	0.02586
Desirable		<200 mg/dL	<5.17 mmol/L		
Borderline high		200–239 mg/dL	5.17–6.18 mmol/L		
High		>239 mg/dL	>6.18 mmol/L		
Cortisol	S			Immunoassay	27.59
Fasting, 8 a.m.–noon		5–25 μg/dL	138–690 nmol/L		
Noon–8 p.m.		5–15 μg/dL	138–414 nmol/L		
8 p.m.–8 a.m.		0–10 μg/dL	0–276 nmol/L		
Cortisol, free	U	20–70 μg/24 h	55–193 nmol/24 h	Immunoassay	2.759
Creatine kinase (CK)	S			Kinetic method	0.01667
Male		60–400 U/L	1.00–6.67 μkat/L		
Female		40–150 U/L	0.67–2.50 μkat/L		
Creatine kinase isoenzyme index	S	0%–2.5% relative index	None	ng/mL / Total CK(U/L) ×100	None
Creatine kinase isoenzymes, MB fraction	S	0–5 ng/mL	0–5 μg/L	Immunoassay	1
Creatinine	P	0.6–1.5 mg/dL	53–133 μmol/L	Colorimetry	88.4
	U	15–25 mg/kg/d	0.13–0.22 mmol/kg/d		0.0884
Dehydroepiandrosterone (DHEA) (adult)	S			Immunoassay	0.03467
Male		180–1,250 ng/dL	6.24–43.3 nmol/L		
Female		130–980 ng/dL	4.5–34.0 nmol/L		
Dehydroepiandrosterone (DHEA) sulfate (adult)	S			Immunoassay	10
Male		10–619 μg/dL	100–619 μg/L		
Female					
Premenopausal		12–535 μg/dL	120–5,350 μg/L		
Postmenopausal		30–260 μg/dL	300–2,600 μg/L		
Deoxycorticosterone (DOC) (adult)	S	2–19 ng/dL	61–576 nmol/L	Immunoassay	30.3
11-Deoxycortisol (adult) (8 a.m. sample)	S	12–158 ng/dL	0.35–4.56 nmol/L	Immunoassay	0.02886
1,25-Dihydroxyvitamin D	S	18–62 pg/mL	43.2–148.8 pmol/L	Immunoassay	2.4
Estradiol	S, P			Immunoassay	3.671
Female					
Menstruating					
Follicular phase		50–145 pg/mL	184–532 pmol/L		
Midcycle peak		112–443 pg/mL	411–1,626 pmol/L		
Luteal phase		50–241 pg/mL	184–885 pmol/L		
Postmenopausal		<59 pg/mL	<217 pmol/L		
Male		<50 pg/mL	<184 pmol/L		
Fatty acids, free (adult)	S	0.17–0.95 mmol/L	0.17–0.95 mmol/L	Spectrophotometry	1
Follicle-stimulating hormone (FSH)	S, P			Immunoassay	1
Female					
Menstruating					
Follicular phase		3.0–20.0 U/L	3.0–20.0 U/L		
Ovulatory phase		9.0–26.0 U/L	9.0–26.0 U/L		
Luteal phase		1.0–12.0 U/L	1.0–12.0 U/L		
Postmenopausal		18.0–153.0 U/L	18.0–153.0 U/L		
Male		1.0–12.0 U/L	1.0–12.0 U/L		
Gastrin	S	<100 ng/L	<100 ng/L	Immunoassay	1
Globulin	S	2.6–4.1 g/dL	26–41 g/L	Calculation: total protein–albumin	10
Glucagon	P	20–100 pg/mL	20–100 mg/L	Immunoassay	1
Glucose	U	<0.05 g/dL	<0.003 mmol/L	Enzymatic analysis	0.05551
Glucose, fasting	P	70–110 mg/dL	3.9–6.1 mmol/L	Enzymatic analysis	0.05551
γ-Glutamyltransferase (GGT)	S			Spectrophotometry	1
Male		1–94 U/L	1–94 U/L		
Female		1–70 U/L	1–70 U/L		
Growth hormone (resting)	S	2–5 ng/mL	2–5 μg/L	Immunoassay	1
Hemoglobin A_{1C}	WB	3.8%–6.4%	0.038–0.064	Liquid chromatography	0.01

Chemistry (Continued)

Analyte	Specimen	MGH Unit	SI Unit	Method or Instrument	Factor for Conversion to SI Unit
High-density lipoprotein cholesterol, as major risk factor	S	<35 mg/dL	<0.91 mmol/L	Colorimetry	0.02586
Human chorionic gonadotropin (hCG) (nonpregnant women)	S	<5 mIU/mL	<5 IU/L	Immunoassay	1
5-Hydroxyindoleacetic acid (5-HIAA)	U	≤6 mg/24 h	≤31.4 μmol/d	High-pressure liquid chromatography	5.23
17-Hydroxyprogesterone (adult)	S			Immunoassay	0.03
Male		5–250 ng/dL	0.15–7.5 nmol/L		
Female					
Follicular phase		20–100 ng/dL	0.6–3.0 nmol/L		
Midcycle peak		100–250 ng/dL	3.0–7.5 nmol/L		
Luteal phase		100–500 ng/dL	3–15 nmol/L		
Postmenopausal		≤70 ng/dL	≤2.1 nmol/L		
25-Hydroxyvitamin D	S	8–42 ng/mL	20–105 nmol/L	Immunoassay	2.496
Insulin	S, P	2–20 μU/mL	14.35–143.5 pmol/L	Immunoassay	7.175
Ketone (acetone)	S, U	Negative	Negative	Colorimetry (nitroprusside)	
17-Ketosteroids	U			Modified Zimmerman reaction	3.467
Male		7–20 mg/24 h	24.3–69.3 μmol/24 h		
Female		5–15 mg/24 h	17.3–52.0 μmol/24 h		
Lactic acid	P	0.5–2.2 mmol/L	0.5–2.2 mmol/L	Enzymatic analysis	1
Lactate dehydrogenase (LDH)	S	110–210 U/L	1.83–3.50 μkat/L	Kinetic method	0.01667
Lactate dehydrogenase isoenzymes	S				
LD_1		16%–29%	0.16–0.29	Electrophoresis	0.01
LD_2		30%–41%	0.30–0.41	Electrophoresis	0.01
LD_3		15%–24%	0.15–0.24	Electrophoresis	0.01
LD_4		6%–13%	0.06–0.13	Electrophoresis	0.01
LD_5		5%–29%	0.05–0.29	Electrophoresis	0.01
Total LDH (when isoenzymes determined)		90–250 U/L	1.5–4.17 μkat/L	Kinetic method	0.01667
Lipase	S	3–19 U/dL	0.5–3.17 μkat/L	Kinetic method	0.1667
Lipoprotein(a)	S	0–30 mg/dL	0–300 mg/L	Nephelometry	10
Low-density lipoprotein cholesterol	S			Calculation	0.02586
Desirable		<130 mg/dL	<3.36 mmol/L		
Borderline high risk		130–159 mg/dL	3.36–4.11 mmol/L		
High risk		≥160 mg/dL	≥4.13 mmol/L		
Luteinizing hormone (LH)	S, P			Immunoassay	1
Female					
Menstruating					
Follicular phase		2.0–15.0 U/L	2.0–15.0 U/L		
Ovulatory phase		22.0–105.0 U/L	22.0–105.0 U/L		
Luteal phase		0.6–19.0 U/L	0.6–19.0 U/L		
Postmenopausal		16.0–64.0 U/L	16.0–64.0 U/L		
Male		2.0–12.0 U/L	2.0–12.0 U/L		
Magnesium	S	1.4–2.0 mEq/L	0.7–1.0 mmol/L	Colorimetry	0.5
Metanephrines	U			Chromatography	
Metanephrine		45–290 μg/24 h	245–1,583 nmol/24 h		5.458
Normetanephrine		82–500 μg/24 h	448–2,730 nmol/24 h		5.46
Total		120–700 μg/24 h	655–3,821 nmol/24 h		5.458
Methemoglobin	P	0.4%–1.5% of total hemoglobin	0.004–0.015	Co-oximetry	0.01
Microalbumin, random urine	U	<20 μg/mL	<20 mg/L	Nephelometry	1
5′-Nucleotidase	S	0–11 U/L	0.02–0.18 μkat/L	Kinetic method	0.01667
Osmolality	S, P	280–296 mOsmol/kg of water	280–296 mmol/kg of water	Freezing-point depression	1
Oxygen, partial pressure, arterial (PaO_2) (room air, age dependent)	WB	80–100 mm Hg	10.7–13.3 kPa	Oxygen electrode	0.1333
Parathyroid hormone	S	10–60 pg/mL	10–60 ng/L	Immunoassay	1
Parathyroid hormone–related protein	P	<1.3 pmol/L	<1.3 pmol/L	Immunoassay	1
pH, arterial	WB	7.35–7.45 pH units	7.35–7.45 pH units	pH electrode	1
Phosphorus, inorganic (adult)	S	2.6–4.5 mg/dL	0.84–1.45 mmol/L	Spectrophotometry	0.3229
	U	average, 1 g/d	average, 32 mmol/d		32.29
Potassium	P	3.4–4.8 mmol/L	3.4–4.8 mmol/L	Ion-selective electrode	1
	S	3.5–5.0 mmol/L	3.5–5.0 mmol/L		
	U	Depends on diet	Depends on diet		
Prealbumin (adult)	S	19.5–35.8 mg/dL	195–358 mg/L	Nephelometry	10
Progesterone	S, P			Immunoassay	3.18
Female					
Follicular phase		<1.0 ng/mL	<3.18 nmol/L		
Midluteal phase		3–20 ng/mL	9.54–63.6 nmol/L		
Male		<1.0 ng/mL	<3.18 nmol/L		
Prolactin	S			Immunoassay	1
Female					
Premenopausal		0–20 ng/mL	0–20 μg/L		
Postmenopausal		0–15 ng/mL	0–15 μg/L		
Male		0–15 ng/mL	0–15 μg/L		

Chemistry (Continued)

Analyte	Specimen	MGH Unit	SI Unit	Method or Instrument	Factor for Conversion to SI Unit
Prostate-specific antigen (PSA)	S			Immunoassay	1
Female		<0.5 ng/mL	<0.5 μg/L		
Male					
<40 yr old		0.0–2.0 ng/mL	0.0–2.0 μg/L		
≥40 yr old		0.04–4.0 ng/mL	0.0–4.0 μg/L		
Prostate-specific antigen (PSA), free, in males 45–75 yr old, with PSA values between 4 and 20 ng/mL	S	>25% associated with benign prostatic hyperplasia	>0.25 associated with benign prostatic hyperplasia	Immunoassay, calculation	0.01
Protein, total	S	6.0–8.0 g/dL	60–80 g/dL	Colorimetry	10
	U	<165 mg/d	<0.165 g/d	Turbidometry	0.001
Renin (adult, normal-sodium diet)	P			Immunoassay	0.2778
Supine		0.3–3.0 ng/mL/h	0.08–0.83 ng/(L-sec)		
Upright		1.0–9.0 mg/mL/h	0.28–2.5 ng/(L-sec)		
Serotonin	WB	55–260 ng/mL	0.31–1.48 μmol/L	High-pressure liquid chromatography	0.00568
Sex hormone–binding globulin (adult)	S			Immunoassay	1
Male		6–44 mmol/L	6–44 mmol/L		
Female		8–85 mmol/L	8–85 mmol/L		
Sodium	P	135–145 mmol/L	135–145 mmol/L	Ion-selective electrode	1
	U	Depends on diet	Depends on diet		
Somatomedin C (insulin-like growth factor I)	S			Immunoassay	1
16–24 yr		182–780 ng/mL	182–780 μg/L		
25–39 yr		114–492 ng/mL	114–492 μg/L		
40–54 yr		90–360 ng/mL	90–360 μg/L		
>54 yr		71–290 ng/mL	71–290 μg/L		
Testosterone, total (morning sample)	S			Immunoassay	0.03467
Female		6–86 ng/dL	0.21–2.98 nmol/L		
Male		270–1,070 ng/dL	9.36–37.10 nmol/L		
Testosterone, unbound (morning sample)	S			Immunoassay	34.67
Female					
20–40 yr		0.6–3.1 pg/mL	20.8–107.5 pmol/L		
41–60 yr		0.4–2.5 pg/mL	13.9–86.7 pmol/L		
61–80 yr		0.2–2.0 pg/mL	6.9–69.3 pmol/L		
Male					
20–40 yr		15.0–40.0 pg/mL	520–1,387 pmol/L		
41–60 yr		13.0–35.0 pg/mL	451–1,213 pmol/L		
61–80 yr		12.0–28.0 pg/mL	416–971 pmol/L		
Thyroglobulin	S	0–60 ng/mL	0–60 μg/L	Immunoassay	1
Thyroid hormone–binding index (THBI; T_3RU)	S	0.77–1.23	0.77–1.23	Immunoassay	1
Thyroid-stimulating hormone	S	0.5–5.0 μU/mL	0.5–5.0 μU/mL	Immunoassay	1
Thyroxine, total (T_4)	S	4.5–10.9 μg/dL	58–140 nmol/L	Immunoassay	12.87
Transferrin	S	191–365 mg/dL	1.91–3.65 g/L	Nephelometry	0.01
Triglycerides (fasting)	S	40–150 mg/dL	0.45–1.69 mmol/L	Spectrophotometry	0.01129
Triiodothyronine, total (T_3)	S	60–181 ng/dL	0.92–2.78 nmol/L	Immunoassay	0.01536
Troponin I	S	<0.6 ng/mL >1.5 ng/mL consistent with acute myocardial infarct	<0.6 μg/L >1.5 μg/L	Immunoassay	1
Urea nitrogen (BUN) (adult)	P	8–25 mg/dL	2.9–8.9 mmol/L	Conductivity	0.357
Urea nitrogen, urine	U	6–17 g/d	6–17 g/d	Conductivity	1
Uric acid	S			Colorimetry	59.48
Male		3.6–8.5 mg/dL	214–506 μmol/L		
Female		2.3–6.6 mg/dL	137–393 μmol/L		
Urinalysis	U			Reflectance	
pH		5.0–9.0	5.0–9.0	Spectrophotometry	1
Specific gravity		1.001	1.035		1
Chemical screens		Negative	Negative		
Urine sediment	U			Manual method	
White cells		0–2/HPF	0–2/HPF		1
Red cells		0–2/HPF	0–2/HPF		1
Vasoactive intestinal polypeptide (VIP)	P	<75 pg/mL	<75 ng/L	Immunoassay	1
Xylose				Colorimetric	
	U	4–9 g/5 h	4–9 g/5 h		1
	S (fasting)	None detected	None detected		

Toxicology and Therapeutic Drug Monitoring

Analyte	Specimen	MGH Unit	SI Unit	Method or Instrument	Factor for Conversion to SI Unit
Acetaminophen, toxicity	S	>120 μg/mL at 2–4 h	>794 μmol/L at 2–4 h	Liquid chromatography	6.62
Amikacin	S			Immunoassay	1.71
Trough		1–7 μg/mL	1.7–12 μmol/L		
Peak		15–25 μg/mL	26–43 μmol/L		
Amitriptyline	S			Liquid chromatography	3.61
Amitriptyline		120–250 μg/L	433–903 nmol/L		
Nortriptyline		50–150 μg/L	181–542 nmol/L		
Barbiturate screen	S	Negative	Negative	Liquid chromatography	
Basic drug screen	S	Negative	Negative	Liquid chromatography	
Benzodiazepine screen	S	Negative	Negative	Liquid chromatography	
Carbamazepine (adult)	S	4–12 μg/mL	17–51 μmol/L	Immunoassay	4.23
Chlordiazepoxide	S	1.0–3.0 mg/L	3.3–10 μmol/L	Liquid chromatography	3.336
Clomipramine	S	150–450 μg/L	476–1,427 nmol/L	Liquid chromatography	3.17
Clonazepam	S	10–70 μg/L	32–222 nmol/L	Liquid chromatography	3.17
Clozapine	S			Liquid chromatography	
Clozapine		150–500 μg/L	459–1,530 nmol/L		3.06
Norclozapine		100–450 μg/L	320–1,440 nmol/L		3.20
Desipramine	S	150–300 μg/L	563–1,125 nmol/L	Liquid chromatography	3.75
Diazepam	S	100–1,000 μg/L	0.35–3.50 μmol/L	Liquid chromatography	0.0035
Digoxin	S	0.9–2.0 ng/mL	1.2–2.6 nmol/L	Immunoassay	1.28
Doxepin	S	150–250 μg/L	537–895 nmol/L	Liquid chromatography	3.58
Ethanol	S	Clinical intoxication: >1,000 mg/L	Clinical intoxication: >1 g/L	Gas chromatography	0.001
Fluoxetine	S			Liquid chromatography	
Fluoxetine		50–450 μg/L	162–1,454 nmol/L		3.23
Norfluoxetine		50–450 μg/L	169–1,521 nmol/L		3.38
Fluvoxamine	S	12–240 μg/L	38–756 nmol/L	Liquid chromatography	3.15
Gentamicin	S			Immunoassay	
Trough		<2.1 μg/mL	<4.4 μmol/L		2.09
Peak		4–8 μg/mL	8.4–16.7 μmol/L		2.09
Imipramine	S			Liquid chromatography	
Imipramine		150–250 μg/L	536–893 nmol/L		3.57
Desipramine		150–300 μg/L	563–1,125 nmol/L		3.75
Lithium	S, P	0.5–1.5 mmol/L	0.5–1.5 mmol/L	Ion-selective electrode	1
Methadone	S	50–800 μg/L	0.16–2.58 μmol/L	Liquid chromatography	0.00323
Methotrexate	S			Immunoassay	1
24 h after high-dose infusion		<10 μmol/L	<10 μmol/L		
48 h after high-dose infusion		<1 μmol/L	<1 μmol/L		
72 h after high-dose infusion		<0.4 μmol/L	<0.4 μmol/L		
Nordiazepam	S	100–800 μg/L	0.37–2.95 μmol/L	Liquid chromatography	0.00369
Paroxetine	S	20–190 μg/L	61–576 nmol/L	Liquid chromatography	3.03
Phenobarbital	S	15–50 μg/mL	65–216 μmol/L	Immunoassay	4.31
Phenytoin	S	5–20 μg/mL	20–79 μmol/L	Immunoassay	3.96
Quinidine	S	1.2–4.0 μg/mL	3.7–12.3 μmol/L	Liquid chromatography	3.08
Salicylate intoxication		>500 mg/L	>3.62 mmol/L		0.00724
Sertraline	S	40–160 μg/L	130–522 nmol/L	Liquid chromatography	3.26
Sulfamethoxazole	S	5–15 mg/dL	19.8–59.2 nmol/L	Liquid chromatography	3.95
Theophylline	S	10–20 μg/mL	56–111 μmol/L	Immunoassay	5.55
For apnea control		5–15 μg/mL	28–83 μmol/L		
Thiocyanate, toxic range	S	>100 mg/L	>1,720 μmol/L	Spectrophotometry	17.2
Tobramycin	S			Immunoassay	2.14
Trough		<2.0 μg/mL	<4.3 μmol/L		
Peak		4.0–8.0 μg/mL	8.6–17.1 μmol/L		
Trazodone	S	800–1,600 μg/L	2,152–4,304 nmol/L	Liquid chromatography	2.69
Valproic acid	S	50–100 μg/mL	347–693 μmol/L	Immunoassay	6.93
Vancomycin	S			Immunoassay	0.690
Trough		<10.1 μg/mL	<7.0 μmol/L		
Peak (2 h after infusion)		18–26 μg/mL	12–18 μmol/L		

Immmunology

Analyte	Specimen	MGH Unit	SI Unit	Method or Instrument	Factor for Conversion to SI Unit
$Alpha_1$-antitrypsin (adult)	S	76–189 mg/dL	0.76–1.89 g/L	Nephelometry	0.01
Anti–glomerular basement membrane antibodies	S				
Qualitative		Negative	Negative	Western blot assay	
Quantitative		<5 U/mL	<5 kU/L	ELISA	1
Antineutrophil cytoplasmic autoantibodies, cytoplasmic (C-ANCA)	S				
Qualitative		Negative	Negative	Indirect immunofluorescence	
Quantitative (antibodies to proteinase 3)		<2.8 U/mL	<2.8 kU/L	ELISA	1
Antineutrophil cytoplasmic autoantibodies, perinuclear (P-ANCA)	S				
Qualitative		Negative	Negative	Indirect immunofluorescence	1
Quantitative (Antibodies to myeloperoxidase)		<1.4 U/mL	<1.4 kU/L	ELISA	
Autoantibodies					
Antiadrenal antibody	S	Negative at 1:10 dilution	Not applicable	Indirect immunofluorescence	
Anti–double-stranded (native) DNA	S	Negative at 1:10 dilution	Not applicable	Indirect immunofluorescence	
Antigranulocyte antibody	S	Negative	Not applicable	ELISA	
Anti–Jo-I antibody	S	Negative	Not applicable	ELISA	
Anti-La antibody	S	Negative	Not applicable	ELISA	
Antimitochondrial antibody	S	Negative	Not applicable	Indirect immunofluorescence	
Antinuclear antibody	S	Negative at 1:40 dilution	Not applicable	Indirect immunofluorescence	
Anti–parietal-cell antibody	S	Negative at 1:20 dilution	Not applicable	Indirect immunofluorescence	
Anti-Ro antibody	S	Negative	Not applicable	ELISA	
Anti-RNP antibody	S	Negative	Not applicable	ELISA	
Anti–Scl-70 antibody	S	Negative	Not applicable	ELISA	
Anti-Smith antibody	S	Negative	Not applicable	ELISA	
Anti–smooth-muscle antibody	S	Negative at 1:20 dilution	Not applicable	Indirect immunofluorescence	
Antithyroglobulin antibody	S	Negative	Not applicable	Immunoassay	
Antithyroid antibody	S	<0.3 IU/mL	<0.3 kIU/L	Immunoassay	1
Bence Jones protein	S	None detected	Not applicable	Immunoelectrophoresis	
Qualitative	U	None detected in a 50-fold concentration	Not applicable	Immunoelectrophoresis	
Quantitative	U			Nephelometry	
Kappa		<2.5 mg/dL	<0.03 g/L		0.01
Lambda		<5.0 mg/dL	<0.05 g/L		0.01
C1-esterase–inhibitor protein	S				
Antigenic		12.4–24.5 mg/dL	0.12–0.25 g/L	Nephelometry	0.01
Functional		Present	Present	Immunodiffusion	
Complement					
C3 (adult)	S	86–184 mg/dL	0.86–1.84 g/L	Nephelometry	0.01
C4 (adult)	S	20–58 mg/dL	0.20–0.58 g/L	Nephelometry	0.01
Total complement (adult)	S	63–145 U/mL	63–145 kU/L	Immunoassay	1
Factor B	S	17–42 mg/dL	0.17–0.42 g/L	Nephelometry	0.01
Cryocrit	S	None detected	Not applicable	Manual method	
Cryoproteins	S	None detected	Not applicable	Manual method	
Cryoprotein identification	S	None detected	Not applicable	Immunodiffusion	
CSF	CSF				
Agarose electrophoresis		No banding seen in an 80-fold concentration	Not applicable	Agarose electrophoresis	
Quantitation of albumin (adult)		11.0–50.9 mg/dL	0.11–0.51 g/L	Nephelometry	0.01
Quantitation of IgG (adult)		0.0–8.0 mg/dL	0.0–0.08 g/L	Nephelometry	0.01
Haptoglobin	S	16–199 mg/dL	0.16–1.99 g/L	Nephelometry	0.01
Immunofixation	S	None detected	Not applicable	Agarose electrophoresis	
Immunoglobulin (adult)					
IgA	S	60–309 mg/dL	0.60–3.09 g/L	Nephelometry	0.01
IgE	S	10–179 IU/mL	24–430 μg/L	Immunoassay	2.4
IgG	S	614–1,295 mg/dL	6.14–12.95 g/L	Nephelometry	0.01
IgM	S	53–334 mg/dL	0.53–3.34 g/L	Nephelometry	0.01
Joint fluid crystal	JF	No crystals seen	Not applicable	Microscopy	
Joint fluid mucin	JF	Only type I mucin present	Not applicable	Manual method	
Rheumatoid factor	S, JF	<30 IU/mL	<30 kIU/L	Nephelometry	1
Serum protein electrophoresis	S	Normal pattern	Not applicable	Agarose electrophoresis	
Viscosity	S	1.4–1.8 relative viscosity units, as compared	1.4–1.8 relative viscosity units, as compared with water	Ostwald viscosimetry with water	1

Hematology and Coagulation

Analyte	Specimen	MGH Unit	SI Unit	Method or Instrument	Factor for Conversion to SI Unit
Activated protein C resistance (factor V Leiden)	P	Ratio >2.0	Not applicable	Automated clotting assay	
Alpha$_2$-antiplasmin	P	80%–130%	0.80–1.30	Chromogenic assay	0.01
Antiphospholipid-antibody panel					
Partial-thromboplastin time–lupus anticoagulant screen	P	Negative	Negative	Dilute phospholipid clotting assay	
Platelet-neutralization procedure	P	Negative	Negative	Clotting assay	
Anticardiolipin antibody	S				
IgG		0–15 GPL units	0–15 arbitrary units	ELISA	1
IgM		0–15 MPL units	0–15 arbitrary units	ELISA	1
Antithrombin III	P				
Immunologic		22–39 mg/dL	220–390 mg/L	Immunoassay	10
Functional		80%–130%	0.8–1.30 U/L	Chromogenic assay	0.01
Anti-Xa assay (heparin assay)	P			Chromogenic assay	
Unfractionated heparin		0.3–0.7 IU/mL	0.3–0.7 kIU/L		1
Low-molecular-weight heparin		0.5–1.0 IU/mL	0.5–1.0 kIU/L		1
Danaparoid		0.5–0.8 IU/mL	0.5–0.8 kIU/L		1
Bleeding time (adult)		2.0–9.5 min	2.0–9.5 min	Surgicutt	1
Clot retraction	WB	50%–100%/2 h	0.50–1.00/2 h	Manual method	0.01
D-Dimer	P	<0.5 μg/mL	<0.5 mg/L	Latex agglutination	1
Differential blood count	WB			Automated cell counter or manual method	
Neutrophils		45%–75%	0.45–0.75		0.01
Bands		0%–5%	0.0–0.05		0.01
Lymphocytes		16%–46%	0.16–0.46		0.01
Monocytes		4%–11%	0.04–0.11		0.01
Eosinophils		0%–8%	0.0–0.8		0.01
Basophils		0%–3%	0.0–0.03		0.01
Erythrocyte count (adult)	WB			Automated cell counter	
Male		$4.50–5.30 \times 10^6/\mu L$	$4.50–5.30 \times 10^{12}/L$		1×10^6
Female		$4.10–5.10 \times 10^6/\mu L$	$4.10–5.10 \times 10^{12}/L$		1×10^6
Erythrocyte sedimentation rate	WB			Automated erythrocyte sedimentation rate instrument	
Female		1–25 mm/h	1–25 mm/h		
Male		0–17 mm/h	0.17 mm/h		
Factor II, prothrombin	P	60%–140%	0.60–1.40	Automated clotting assay	0.01
Factor V	P	60%–140%	0.60–1.40	Automated clotting assay	0.01
Factor VII	P	60%–140%	0.60–1.40	Automated clotting assay	0.01
Factor VIII	P	50%–200%	0.50–2.00	Automated clotting assay	0.01
Factor IX	P	60%–140%	0.60–1.40	Automated clotting assay	0.01
Factor X	P	60%–140%	0.60–1.40	Automated clotting assay	0.01
Factor XI	P	60%–140%	0.60–1.40	Automated clotting assay	0.01
Factor XII	P	60%–140%	0.60–1.40	Automated clotting assay	0.01
Factor XIII screen	P	No deficiency detected	Not applicable	Urea clot dissolution	
Factor-inhibitor assay	P	<0.5 Bethesda unit	<0.5 Bethesda unit	Automated clotting assay	1
Ferritin	S			Immunoassay	1
Male		30–300 ng/mL	30–300 μg/L		
Female		10–200 ng/mL	10–200 μg/L		
Fibrin(ogen)-degradation products	P	<2.5 μg/mL	<2.5 mg/L	Latex agglutination	1
Fibrinogen	P	175–400 mg/dL	1.75–4.00 μmol/L	Automated clotting assay	0.01
Folate (folic acid)	S, P			Immunoassay	1
Normal		3.1–17.5 ng/mL	7.0–39.7 mmol/L		
Borderline deficient		2.2–3.0 ng/mL	5.0–6.8 nmol/L		
Deficient		<2.2 ng/mL	<5.0 nmol/L		
Excessive		>17.5 ng/mL	>39.7 nmol/L		
Glucose-6-phosphate dehydrogenase (erythrocyte)	WB	No gross deficiency	Not applicable	Visual fluorescence screening	
Hematocrit (adult)	WB			Automated cell counter	
Male		37.0–49.0	0.37–0.49		0.01
Female		36.0–46.0	0.36–0.46		0.01
Hemoglobin (adult)	WB			Automated cell counter	0.6206
Male		13.0–18.0 g/dL	8.1–11.2 mmol/L		
Female		12.0–16.0 g/dL	7.4–9.9 mmol/L		
Hemoglobin A$_2$	WB	<3.5%	<0.04	Spectrophotometry	0.01
Hemoglobin F	WB	<0.02%	<0.0002	Spectrophotometry	0.01
Heparin-induced thrombocytopenia antibody	P	Negative	Negative	ELISA	
Iron	S	30–160 μg/dL	5.4–28.7 μmol/L	Colorimetry	0.1791
Iron-binding capacity	S	228–428 μg/dL	40.8–76.7 μmol/L	Colorimetry	0.1791
Leukocyte count (WBC)	WB	$4.5–11.0 \times 10^3/\mu L$	$4.5–11.0 \times 10^9/L$	Automated cell counter	1×10^6
Mean corpuscular hemoglobin (MCH)	WB	25.0–35.0 pg/cell	25.0–35.0 pg/cell	Automated cell counter	1
Mean corpuscular hemoglobin concentration (MCHC)	WB	31.0–37.0 g/dL	310–370 g/L	Automated cell counter	10
Mean corpuscular volume (MCV) (adult)	WB			Automated cell counter	1
Male		78–100 μm^3	78–100 fl		
Female		78–102 μm^3	78–102 fl		
Osmotic fragility of erythrocytes	WB	Increased hemolysis as compared with normal control	Not applicable	Spectrophotometry	
Partial thromboplastin time, activated	P	22.1–34.1 s	22.1–34.1 s	Automated clotting assay	1

Hematology and Coagulation (Continued)

Analyte	Specimen	MGH Unit	SI Unit	Method or Instrument	Factor for Conversion to SI Unit
Plasminogen	P				
Antigen		8.4–14.0 mg/dL	84–140 mg/L	Immunoassay	10
Functional		80%–130%	0.80–1.30	Chromogenic assay	0.01
Platelet aggregation	PRP	>65% aggregation response to adenosine diphosphate, epinephrine, collagen, ristocetin, and arachidonic acid	Not applicable	Platelet aggregometry	
Platelet count	WB	150–350×10^3/μL	150–350×10^9/L	Automated cell counter	1×10^4
Platelet, mean volume	WB	6.4–11.0 μm^3	6.4–11.0 fl	Automated cell counter	1
Prekallikrein assay	P	60%–140%	0.60–1.40	Chromogenic assay	0.01
Prekallikrein screen	P	No deficiency detected		Automated clotting assay	
Protein C	P				
Total antigen		70%–140%	0.70–1.40	Immunoassay	0.01
Functional		70%–140%	0.70–1.40	Chromogenic assay	0.01
Protein S	P				
Total antigen		70%–140%	0.70–1.40	Immunoassay	0.01
Functional		70%–140%	0.70–1.40	Automated clotting assay	0.01
Free antigen		70%–140%	0.70–1.40	Immunoassay	0.01
Prothrombin time	P	11.2–13.2 s	11.2–13.2 s	Automated clotting assay	1
Red-cell distribution width	WB	11.5%–14.5%	0.115–0.145	Automated cell counter	0.01
Reptilase time	P	16–24 s	16–24 s	Automated clotting assay	1
Reticulocyte count	WB	0.5%–2.5% red cells	0.005–0.025 red cells	Flow cytometry	0.01
Ristocetin cofactor (functional von Willebrand factor)	P				
Blood group O		75% mean of normal	0.75 mean of normal		
Blood group A		105% mean of normal	1.05 mean of normal		
Blood group B		115% mean of normal	1.15 mean of normal		
Blood group AB		125% mean of normal	1.25 mean of normal		
Sucrose hemolysis	WB	<10%	<0.1	Spectrophotometry	0.01
Thrombin time	P	16–24 s	16–24 s	Automated clotting assay	1
Total eosinophils	WB	70–440/μL	70–440×10^6/L	Automated cell counter	1×10^3
Vitamin B_{12}	S, P			Immunoassay	0.7378
Normal		>250 pg/mL	>184 pmol/L		
Borderline		125–250 pg/mL	92–184 pmol/L		
Deficient		<125 pg/mL	<92 pmol/L		
von Willebrand factor (vWF) antigen (factor VII:R antigen)	P			Immunoassay	
Blood group O	75% mean of normal	0.75 mean of normal			0.01
Blood group A	105% mean of normal	1.05 mean of normal			0.01
Blood group B	115% mean of normal	1.15 mean of normal			0.01
Blood group AB	125% mean of normal	1.25 mean of normal			0.01
von Willebrand factor multimers	P	Normal distribution	Normal distribution	Western blot assay	

Microbiology

Culture Specimen	Routinely Cultured for	Also Reported	Normal Flora
Throat	Group A beta-hemolytic streptococci, pyogenic groups C and G beta-hemolytic streptococci, *Arcanobacterium haemolyticum*	If a complete throat culture is requested, it will be examined for *Haemophilus influenzae, Staphylococcus aureus, Streptococcus pneumoniae, Neisseria meningitidis,* and yeast	Alpha-hemolytic streptococci, nonhemolytic streptococci, diphtheroids, coagulase-negative staphylococci, saprophytic neisseria
Sputum	Pneumococci, *H. influenzae*, beta-hemolytic streptococci, *S. aureus, Moraxella (Branhamella) catarrhalis,* pseudomonas, Enterobacteriaceae, yeast	Presence or absence of normal throat flora	Carefully collected specimens should contain few or no normal throat flora
Urine	Aerobic bacteria and yeast: abundant, $>10^5$ colony-forming units/mL; moderate, 10^4–10^5 colony-forming units/mL	Few, 10^3–10^4 colony-forming units/mL; rare, 10^2–10^3 colony-forming units/mL; no growth, $<10^2$ colony-forming units/mL; these amounts may indicate clinically significant bacteriuria if accompanied by pyuria, clinical symptoms, or both	Carefully collected specimens should not contain mixed bacterial species (i.e., two or more of the following: lactobacilli, non–beta-hemolytic streptococci, diphtheroids, coagulase-negative staphylococci, *Gardnerella vaginalis*)
Blood	Aerobic and anaerobic bacteria, yeasts	Growth in both bottles is usually more clinically significant than growth in a single bottle	None; aerobic and anaerobic diphtheroids and coagulase-negative staphylococci are common contaminants
Cerebrospinal and other fluids	Aerobic and anaerobic bacteria; yeasts, including cryptococcus	Any organism isolated	None
Feces	Enteric pathogens: salmonella, shigella, campylobacter, plesiomonas, and acromonas when predominant	Moderate or abundant yeast or *S. aureus;* presence or absence of normal gram-negative enteric flora; special cultures can be specifically requested for yersinia, *Vibrio cholerae, V. parahaemolyticus,* or hemorrhagic (O157) strains of *Escherichia coli*	Enterobacteriaceae, streptococci, pseudomonas, small numbers of staphylococci, and yeast (and anaerobes that are not cultured routinely)
Wounds	Aerobic and anaerobic bacteria, yeast		
Cervical or vaginal	Gonococci, beta-hemolytic streptococci, *S. aureus,* and *G. vaginalis* when predominant	Enteric gram-negative rods and candida, if present in large numbers	

P, plasma; S, serum; U, urine; WB, whole blood; CSF, cerebrospinal fluid; JF, joint fluid; PRP, platelet-rich plasma; ELISA, enzyme-linked immunosorbent assay; GPL, IgG phospholipid; MPL, IgM phospholipid.

From Kratz A, Lewandrowski KB. Normal reference laboratory values. *N Engl J Med* 1998;339:1063, with permission.

APPENDIX B

Dermatomes

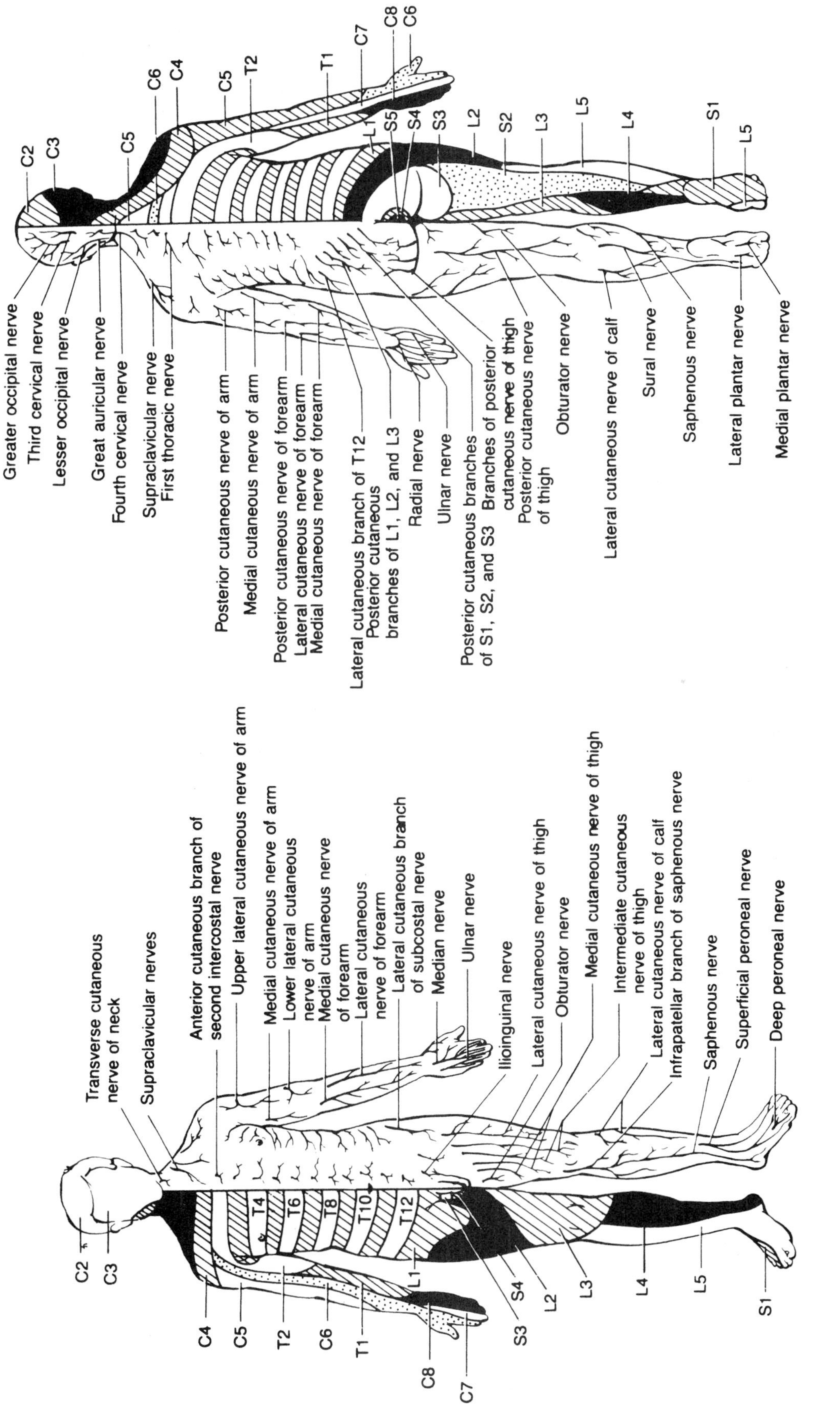

Sensory dermatomal segments.

APPENDIX C
Length-Based Equipment Chart

Item	Length (cm)						
	54–70 (4–7 kg)	70–85 (8–11 kg)	85–95 (12–14 kg)	95–107 (14–17 kg)	107–124 (18–23 kg)	124–138 (24–30 kg)	138–155 (>30 kg)
ET tube size (mm)	3.5	4.0	4.5	5.0	5.5	6.0	6.5
Lip–tip length (mm)	10.5	12.0	13.5	15.0	16.5	18.0	19.5
Laryngoscope	1 straight	1 straight	2 straight	2 straight or curved	2 straight or curved	2–3 straight or curved	3 straight or curved
Suction catheter	8F	8F–10F	10F	10F	10F	10F	12F
Stylet	6F	6F	6F	6F	14F	14F	14F
Oral airway	Infant/small child	Small child	Child	Child	Child/small adult	Child/adult	Medium adult
Bag-valve-mask	Infant	Child	Child	Child	Child	Child/adult	Adult
Oxygen mask	Newborn	Pediatric	Pediatric	Pediatric	Pediatric	Adult	Adult
Vascular access catheter/butterfly	22–24/23–25, intraosseous	20–22/23–25, intraosseous	18–22/21–23, intraosseous	18–22/21–23, intraosseous	18–20/21–23	18–20/21–22	16–20/18–21
Nasogastric tube	5F–8F	8F–10F	10F	10F–12F	12F–14F	14F–18F	18F
Urinary catheter	5F–8F	8F–10F	10F	10F–12F	10F–12F	12F	12F
Chest tube	12F–12F	16F–20F	20F–24F	20F–24F	24F–32F	28F–32F	32F–40F
Blood pressure cuff	Newborn/infant	Infant/child	Child	Child	Child	Child/adult	Adult

Directions
1. Measure patient length with centimeter tape.
2. Using measured length in centimeters, access appropriate equipment column.

Alternatively, this same information can be accessed from a single measurement directly from a Broselow tape.

Modified from Luten RC, Wears RL, Broselwo J, et al. Length-based endotracheal tube sizing for pediatric resuscitation. *Ann Emerg Med* 1995;21:900–904.

Index

Note: f after page number denotes figures/illustrations. t after page number denotes tabular material. Boldface page numbers equal major chapter discussion.